Hospital Epidemiology and Infection Control

THIRD EDITION

Editor

C. Glen Mayhall, M.D.
Professor
Division of Infectious Diseases
Department of Internal Medicine
School of Medicine
The University of Texas Medical Branch
at Galveston, and
Hospital Epidemiologist
Department of Healthcare Epidemiology
The University of Texas Medical Branch Hospitals and Clinics
Galveston, Texas

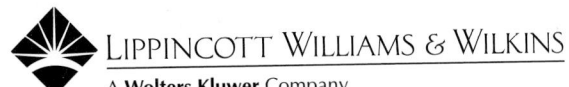

LIPPINCOTT WILLIAMS & WILKINS
A Wolters Kluwer Company
Philadelphia • Baltimore • New York • London
Buenos Aires • Hong Kong • Sydney • Tokyo

Acquisitions Editor: Ruth W. Weinberg
Developmental Editor: Joyce Murphy
Production Manager: Toni Ann Scaramuzzo
Production Editor: Michael Mallard
Manufacturing Manager: Benjamin Rivera
Cover Designer: David Levy
Compositor: Maryland Composition
Printer: Quebecor World-Kingsport

530 Walnut Street
Philadelphia, PA 19106 USA
LWW.com

Printed in the USA

Library of Congress Cataloging-in-Publication Data

Hospital epidemiology and infection control / editor, C. Glen Mayhall.—3rd ed.
p. cm.
Includes bibliographical references and index.
ISBN 0-7817-4258-7
1. Nosocomial infection—Prevention. 2. Nosocomial infections––Epidemiology. 3. Cross infection—Prevention. I. Mayhall, C. Glen.
[DNLM: 1. Cross Infection—epidemiology. 2. Cross Infection––prevention & control. 3. Bioterrorism 4. Infection Control—methods. WX 167H8292 2004]
RA969.H635 2004
614.4′4—dc22

2003065937

---

10 9 8 7 6 5 4 3 2 1

To my wife, Kathryn Ann, and my children,
Lisa Lynn, Michelle Rene, and Mark Christopher
for their abiding love and understanding through the years.

Table of Contents

III. Informatics in Healthcare Epidemiology

IV. Epidemiology and Prevention of Nosocomial Infections of Organ Systems

V. Epidemiology and Prevention of Nosocomial Infections Caused by Specific Pathogens

Part A. Bacterial Infections

VI. Epidemiology and Prevention of Nosocomial Infections in Pediatric Patients

VII. Epidemiology and Prevention of Nosocomial Infections in Special Patient Populations

VIII. Epidemiology and Prevention of Nosocomial Infections Associated with Diagnostic and Therapeutic Procedures

IX. Epidemiology and Prevention of Nosocomial Infections Related to Hospital Support Services

X. Epidemiology and Prevention of Nosocomial Infections in Healthcare Workers

XI. Disinfection and Sterilization

XII. Prevention of Infections Acquired by Patients in Healthcare Facilities Related to Construction, Renovation, Demolition and Ventilation Systems

XIII. Antimicrobial Agents in Hospital Epidemiology and Infection Control

XIV. The Literature in Hospital Epidemiology and Infection Control

XV. Organization and Implementation of Infection Control Programs

XVI. Hospital Epidemiology and Infection Control in Special Settings for Healthcare Delivery

XVII. Bioterrorism

Contributors

Joel Ackelsberg, M.D., M.P.H.
Bureau of Communicable Disease
New York City Department of Health and Mental Hygiene
New York, New York

Stuart P. Adler, M.D.
Professor and Division Chairman
Division of Infectious Diseases
Department of Pediatrics
Medical College of Virginia
Virginia Commonwealth University
Richmond, Virginia

Michael R. Albert, M.D.
Instructor, Department of Dermatology
Brown University Medical School
Providence, Rhode Island

Miriam J. Alter, Ph.D.
Associate Director for Epidemiologic Science
Division of Viral Hepatitis
Centers for Disease Control and Prevention
Atlanta, Georgia

Lennox K. Archibald, M.D.
Medical Director
Regeneration Technologies, Inc.
Alachua, Florida;
Associate Professor
University of Florida,
Gainesville, Florida

Matthew J. Arduino, Dr.P.H.
Chief, Dialysis and Medical Devices Section
Division of Healthcare Quality Promotion
Centers for Disease Control and Prevention
Atlanta, Georgia

Jeffrey D. Band, M.D.
Clinical Professor of Medicine
Wayne State University School of Medicine
Detroit, Michigan;
Director, Divisions of Infectious Diseases and Hospital
Epidemiology
William Beaumont Hospital
Royal Oak, Michigan

Neil L. Barg, M.D.
Internal Medicine Associates
Yakima, Washington

Judene Bartley, M.S., M.P.H., C.I.C.
Vice President
Epidemiology Consulting Services, Inc
Beverly Hills, Michigan

Susan E. Beekmann, R.N., M.P.H.
Nurse Epidemiologist
Department of Pathology
University of Iowa College of Medicine
Iowa City, Iowa

Debra Berg, M.D.
Bureau of Communicable Disease
New York City Department of Health and Mental Hygiene
New York, New York

Ronald G. Berglund, M.P.H.
Associate Director
Healthcare and Education
Management Resources International
Saline, Michigan

Dennis C. J. J. Bergmans, M.D., Ph.D.
Resident
Department of Internal Medicine
University Hospital Maastricht
Maastricht, The Netherlands

David Birnbaum, PhD., MPH
Adjunct Professor
Associate Member
Department of Health Care and Epidemiology
University of British Columbia
Vancouver, BC, Canada

Stephanie R. Black, M.D.
Assistant Professor
Section of Infectious Diseases
Rush Medical College
Chicago, Illinois

Mary Anne Bobinski, J.D., L.L.M.
Dean, Faculty of Law
University of British Columbia
Vancouver, British Columbia, Canada

Marc J. M. Bonten, M.D.
Infectious Disease Specialist
Department of Internal Medicine and Infectious Diseases
University Medical Center
Utrecht, The Netherlands

Janet O. Bower, M.H.A., B.S.N.
CQI Anesthesia Research Coordinator
University of Washington Medical Center
Seattle, Washington

John M. Boyce, M.D.
Clinical Professor of Medicine
Yale University School of Medicine
Chief, Section of Infectious Diseases
Hospital of Saint Raphael
New Haven, Connecticut

Joel G. Breman, M.D., D.T.P.H.
Senior Scientific Advisor
Fogarty International Center
National Institutes of Health
Bethesda, Maryland

John P. Burke, M.D.
Professor of Medicine
Chief, Department of Clinical Epidemiology and Infectious Diseases
LDS Hospital
University of Utah
Salt Lake City, Utah

Robert G. Burney, M.D.
Director
Department of Quality Improvement
US Department of State
Washington, DC

Jay C. Butler, MD, FAAP, FACP
Director, Arctic Investigations Program
Centers for Disease Control and Prevention
Anchorage, Alaska

Denise M. Cardo, M.D.
Division of Healthcare Quality Promotion
National Center for Infectious Diseases
Centers for Disease Control and Prevention
Public Health Service
U.S. Department of Health and Human Services
Atlanta, Georgia

Carol E. Chenoweth, M.D.
Clinical Associate Professor
Division of Infectious Diseases
University of Michigan Health System
Ann Arbor, Michigan;
Medical Director, Department of Infection Control and Epidemiology
University of Michigan Medical Center
Ann Arbor, Michigan

David C. Classen, M.D., M.S.
Associate Professor
Department of Medicine
University of Utah School of Medicine
Salt Lake City, Utah

Eva P. Clontz, M.Ed.
Program Coordinator
Department of Medicine
University of North Carolina at Chapel Hill
Chapel Hill, North Carolina

Stacey A. Coffin, M.D.
Staff Anesthesiologist
Department of Anesthesia
St. Luke's Hospital of Duluth
Duluth, Minnesota

Ralph L. Cordell, Ph.D.
Director, Office of Science Education
National Center for Infectious Diseases
Centers for Disease Control and Prevention
Atlanta, Georgia

Sara E. Cosgrove, M.D.
Instructor
Department of Medicine
Johns Hopkins University
Baltimore, Maryland

Donald E. Craven, M.D.
Professor of Medicine
Tufts University School of Medicine
Boston, Massachusetts;
Lahey Clinic
Section of Infectious Diseases
Burlington, Massachusetts

Kent B. Crossley, M.D.
Professor
Department of Medicine
University of Minnesota Medical School
Minneapolis, Minnesota;
Director of Education Service
Minneapolis VA Medical Center
Minneapolis, Minnesota

Burke A. Cunha, M.D., F.A.C.P.
Professor of Medicine
State University of New York School of Medicine
Stony Brook, New York;
Chief, Infectious Disease Division
Winthrop-University Hospital
Mineola, New York

Rahib O. Darouiche, M.D.
Professor and Director
Center for Prostheses Infection
Baylor College of Medicine
Houston, Texas

Franz D. Daschner, M.D.
Professor and Chief
Institute for Environmental Medicine and
Hospital Epidemiology
Freiburg University
Freiburg, Germany

Michael D. Decker, M.D., M.P.H.
Adjunct Professor
Department of Preventive Medicine and Medicine (Infectious Diseases)
Vanderbilt University School of Medicine
Nashville, Tennessee;
Vice President
Scientific and Medical Affairs
Aventis Pasteur
Swiftwater, Pennsylvania

Gerald A. Denys, Ph.D., A.B.M.M.
Clinical Associate Professor
Department of Pathology and Laboratory Medicine
Indiana University School of Medicine;
Clinical Director, Microbiology Clinical Laboratory Services, Microbiology
Clarian Health Partners, Inc, Methodist Hospital
Indianapolis, Indiana

Francesco G. DeRosa, M.D.
Assistant Clinical Professor
Department of Infectious Diseases
University of Turin
Turin, Italy

Markus Dettenkoffer, M.D.
Institute of Environmental Medicine and Hospital Epidemiology
Freiburg University
Freiburg, Germany

Samuel W. Dooley, M.D.
National Center for HIV, STD, and TB Prevention
Centers for Disease Control and Prevention
Atlanta, Georgia

Marlene Durand, M.D.
Instructor in Medicine
Department of Medicine
Infectious Disease Unit
Massachusetts General Hospital
Boston, Massachusetts

Martin E. Evans, M.D.
Professor
Division of Infectious Diseases
Department of Medicine
University of Kentucky School of Medicine
Lexington, Kentucky

Pamela S. Falk, M.P.H.
Director
Department of Healthcare Epidemiology
University of Texas Medical Branch Hospitals and Clinics
Galveston, Texas

Barry M. Farr, M.D., M.Sc.
William S. Jordan, Jr Professor of Medicine and Epidemiology
Department of Internal Medicine
University of Virginia School of Medicine
Charlottesville, Virginia

Martin S. Favero, Ph.D.
Director of Scientific and Clinical Affairs
Advanced Sterilization Products
Johnson and Johnson Medical, Inc.
Irvine, California

Jay A. Fishman, M.D.
Associate Professor
Department of Medicine
Harvard Medical School
Boston, Massachusetts;
Director, Transplant Infectious Disease and Compromised Host Program
Massachusetts General Hospital
Boston, Massachusetts

John P. Flaherty, M.D.
Associate Professor of Clinical Medicine
Department of Medicine
Northwestern University
Chicago, Illinois

Patricia M. Flynn, M.D.
Professor
Department of Pediatrics
University of Tennessee Health Science Center
Memphis, Tennessee
St. Jude Children's Research Hospital, and
Member
Department of Infectious Diseases
St. Jude Children's Research Hospital
Memphis, Tennessee

Victoria Fraser, M.D.
Professor
Division of Infectious Disease
Department of Medicine
Washington University School of Medicine
St. Louis, Missouri

Jonathan Freeman, M.D., D.Sc.
(Deceased)
Department of Epidemiology
Harvard School of Public Health
Boston, Massachusetts

G. L. French, M.D., B.Sc.
Professor, Department of Microbiology
Grey's, King's, and St. Thomas's School of Medicine;
Head of Service
Department of Clinical Microbiology
St. Thomas's Hospital
London, United Kingdom

Nelson M. Gantz, M.D.
Clinical Professor of Medicine
Penn State School of Medicine
Hershey, Pennsylvania;
Chief of Infectious Diseases
Boulder Community Hospital
Boulder, Colorado

Aditya H. Gaur, M.D.
Fellow, Department of Infectious Diseases
St. Jude Children's Research Hospital
Department of Pediatrics
University of Tennessee Health Science Center
Memphis, Tennessee

Robert P. Gaynes, M.D.
Deputy Chief, Healthcare Outcomes Branch
Division of Healthcare Quality Promotion
Centers for Disease Control and Prevention
Atlanta, Georgia

Michael S. Gelfand, M.D.
Clinical Professor of Medicine
Department of Internal Medicine
University of Tennessee, and
Chief, Division of Infectious Diseases
Methodist University Hospital
Memphis, Tennessee

Dale N. Gerding, M.D.
Professor, Department of Medicine
Northwestern University, and
Chief, Medical Service
VA Chicago Health Care System, Lakeside Division
Chicago, Illinois

Robyn R. M. Gershon, M.H.S., Dr.P.H.
Department of Sociomedical Sciences
Mailman School of Public Health
Columbia University
New York, New York

Donald A. Goldmann, M.D.
Professor, Department of Pediatrics
Harvard Medical School, and
Division of Infectious Diseases
Children's Hospital
Boston, Massachusetts

Judith G. Gordon, M.A.
President
Gordon Resources Consultants
Reston, Virginia

John N. Greene, M.D.
Professor
Department of Medicine
University of South Florida;
Chief, Department of Infectious Diseases
H. Lee Moffitt Cancer Center
Tampa, Florida

Velvl W. Greene, Ph.D., M.P.H.
Emeritus Professor
Department of Epidemiology and Public Health
Ben Gurion University Medical School
Beer Sheva, Israel

Martha J. Grimes, R.N.
Nurse Epidemiologist, Educator, Consultant
Laurel, Maryland

Peter A. Gross, M.D.
Professor and Vice-Chair
Department of Internal Medicine
New Jersey Medical School
Newark, New Jersey, and
Chair, Department Internal Medicine
Hackensack University Medical Center
Hackensack, New Jersey

Margaret A Hamburg, M.D.
Vice President
Biological Programs
NTI
Washington, DC

Bruce H. Hamory, M.D.
Executive Vice President
Chief Medical Officer
Geisinger Health System
Danville, Pennsylvania

Hend A. Hanna, M.D., M.P.H.
Assistant Professor
Department of Infectious Diseases, Infection Control and Employee Health
The University of Texas
M.D. Anderson Cancer Center
Houston, Texas

Stephen J. Harbarth, M.D., M.S.
Chef de Clinique Scientifique
Department of Internal Medicine
Geneva University Medical School
Geneva, Switzerland

Alan I. Hartstein, M.D.
Professor, Department of Medicine
University of Miami
Healthcare Epidemiologist
Jackson Memorial Hospital
Miami, Florida

R. Brian Haynes, M.D., Ph.D.
Professor and Chair
Department of Clinical Epidemiology and Biostatistics
McMaster University Faculty of Health Sciences;
Attending Staff
Department of Medicine
Hamilton Health Sciences
Hamilton, Ontario, Canada

David K. Henderson, M.D.
Deputy Director for Clinical Care
Office of the Director
Warren G. Magnuson Clinical Center
National Institutes of Health
Bethesda, Maryland

Loreen A. Herwaldt, M.D.
Professor
Department of Internal Medicine
University of Iowa College of Medicine, and
Hospital Epidemiologist
Department of Clinical Outcomes and Resource Management
University of Iowa Hospitals and Clinics
Iowa City, Iowa

Walter J. Hierholzer, Jr., M.D.
Professor Emeritus
Department of Epidemiology and Public Health
Yale University School of Medicine
New Haven, Connecticut

Karen K. Hoffmann, R.N., M.S.
Clinical Instructor
Department of Medicine
University of North Carolina at Chapel Hill
Chapel Hill, North Carolina

John Holton, M.D.
Department of Bacteriology
Windeyer Institute of Medical Sciences
Royal Free and University College London Medical School
London, United Kingdom

Cyrus C. Hopkins, M.D.
Associate Professor of Medicine
Harvard Medical School, and
Associate Director, Infection Control Unit
Massachusetts General Hospital
Boston, Massachusetts

Teresa C. Horan M.P.H.
Chief, Performance Measurement Section
Division of Healthcare Quality Promotion
Centers for Disease Control and Prevention
Atlanta, Georgia

W. Charles Huskins, M.D.
Assistant Professor Department of Pediatrics
Mayo Medical School
Senior Associate Consultant
Division of Pediatric Infectious Diseases
Department of Pediatric and Adolescent Medicine
Rochester, Minnesota

William R. Jarvis, M.D.
Director, Office of Extramural Research
National Center for Infectious Diseases
Centers for Disease Control and Prevention
Atlanta, Georgia

John A. Jernigan, M.D.
Division of Healthcare Quality Promotion
National Center for Infectious Diseases
Centers for Disease Control and Prevention
Atlanta, Georgia

Joseph F. John, Jr., M.D.
Chief, Medical Specialty Services
Ralph H. Johnson-Veterans Medical Center
Charleston, South Carolina

Stuart Johnson, M.D.
Department of Medicine
Northwestern University, and
Medical Service
VA Chicago Health Care System, Lakeside Division
Chicago, Illinois

Carol L. Joseph, M.D.
Associate Professor
Department of Medicine
Oregon Health and Science University
Portland, Oregan

Aisha O. Jumaan, Ph.D., M.P.H.
Acting Varicella Chief
National Immunization Program
Centers for Disease Control and Prevention
Atlanta, Georgia

Keith S. Kaye, M.D., M.P.H.
Assistant Professor
Department of Medicine
Duke University Medical Center
Durham, North Carolina

John H. Keene, Dr.PH.
Associate Clinical Professor
Department of Preventive Medicine and Community Health
Medical College of Virginia
Virginia Commonwealth University
Richmond, Virginia, and
President
Biohaztec Associates Inc.
Midlothian, Virginia

Venkatarama R. Koppaka, M.D., Ph.D.
Division of Global Migration and Quarantine
National Center for Infectious Diseases
Centers for Disease Control and Prevention
Atlanta, Georgia

Stephen M. Kralovic, M.D.
Assistant Professor
Division of Infectious Diseases
University of Cincinnati
Cincinnati, Ohio

Amy Beth Kressel, M.D.
Associate Professor of Clinical Medicine
University of Cincinnati
Medical Director of Infection Control
University Hospital
Cincinnati, Ohio

Stephen B. Kritchevsky, Ph.D.
Professor
Division of Geriatrics
Department of Medicine
Wake Forest University Health Sciences
Winston-Salem, North Carolina

Marcelle Layton, M.D.
Assistant Commissioner
Bureau of Communicable Disease
New York City Department of Health and Mental Hygiene
New York, New York

Elsie Lee, M.D.
Bureau of Communicable Disease
New York City Department of Health and Mental Hygiene
New York, New York

Daniel P. Lew
Professor
Infectious Diseases Division
Department of Medicine
University of Geneva Hospitals
Geneva, Switzerland

Jairam Lingappa, M.D., Ph.D.
Medical Epidemiologist
Respiratory and Enteric Viruses Branch
Centers for Diseases Control and Prevention
Atlanta, Georgia

Calvin C. Linnemann, Jr., M.D.
Professor Emeritus
Department of Medicine
Infectious Diseases Division
University of Cincinnati College of Medicine
Cincinnati, Ohio

Daniel R. Lucey, M.D., M.P.H.
Professor of Medicine
Uniformed Services University of the Health Sciences
Bethesda, Maryland;
Director, Center for Biologic Counterterrorism and Emerging Diseases
Department of Emergency Medicine
Washington Hospital Center
Washington, DC

Jon T. Mader, M.D.
(Deceased)
Departments of Internal Medicine, Pathology, Orthopedic Surgery
Division of Hyperbaric Medicine and Wound Care
University of Texas Medical Branch
Galveston, Texas

C. Glen Mayhall, M.D.
Professor, Division of Infectious Diseases
Department of Internal Medicine
School of Medicine
The University of Texas Medical Branch at Galveston;
Hospital Epidemiologist
Department of Healthcare Epidemiology
The University of Texas Medical Branch Hospitals and Clinics
Galveston, Texas

Elizabeth Linner McClure, M.D.
Center for Infectious Disease Research and Policy
University of Minnesota
Minneapolis, Minnesota

Judith Green-McKenzie, M.P.H.
Assistant Professor
Director of Clinical Practice
Associate Residency Director
Division of Occupational Medicine
Hospital of the University of Pennsylvania
Philadelphia, Pennsylvania

K. Ann McKibbon, B.Sc., M.L.S.
Research Librarian
Department of Clinical Epidemiology and Biostatistics
McMaster University
Hamilton, Ontario, Canada

Michael M. McNeil, M.D.
Epidemiology and Surveillance Division
Centers for Disease Control and Prevention
Atlanta, Georgia

James M. Melius, M.D., Dr.P.H.
Director
New York State Laborers' Health and Safety Trust Fund
Albany, New York

Kathy B. Miller, M.S., R.N.
Nursing Consultant
Richmond, Virginia

Douglas K. Mitchell, M.D.
Associate Professor
Division of Infectious Diseases
Eastern Virginia Medical School/Center for Pediatric Research
Associate Professor of Pediatrics
Children's Hospital of the King's Daughters
Norfolk, Virginia

Kelly L. Moore, M.D.
CDC Preventive Medicine Resident
Tennessee Department of Health
Nashville, Tennessee

Dorothy L. Moore, M.D.
Associate Professor
Department of Pediatrics
McGill University;
Attending Physician
Division of Infectious Diseases
Montreal Children's Hospital
Montreal, Quebec, Canada

Linda M. Mundy, M.D.
Assistant Professor of Medicine
Division of Infectious Diseases
Washington University School of Medicine
St. Louis, Missouri

Mary D. Nettleman, M.D., M.S.
Professor and Chairperson
Department of Medicine
Michigan State University
East Lansing, Michigan

Edward J. O'Rourke, M.D.
Clinical Professor of Pediatrics
Harvard Medical School;
Director, Harvard Medical International
Children's Hospital
Boston, Massachusetts

Michael Osterholm, Ph.D., M.P.H.
Director, Center for Infectious Disease Research and Policy
University of Minnesota
Minneapolis, Minnesota

Luis Ostrosky-Zeichner, M.D.
Instructor of Medicine
Division of Infectious Diseases
University of Texas Medical School
Houston, Texas

Adelisa L. Panlilio, M.D., M.P.H.
Division of Viral Hepatitis
National Center for Infectious Diseases
Centers for Disease Control and Prevention
Public Health Service
U.S. Department of Health and Human Services
Atlanta, Georgia

Mark Papania, M.D., M.P.H., F.A.A.P
Chief, Measles Elimination Activity
National Immunization Program
Centers for Disease Control and Prevention
Atlanta, Georgia

Jan Evans Patterson, M.D.
Division of Infectious Diseases
Department of Medicine
University of Texas Health Science Center
San Antonio, Texas

Trish M. Perl, M.D., M.Sc.
Associate Professor
Department of Medicine
The Johns Hopkins University, and
Hospital Epidemiologist
Department of Hospital Epidemiology and Infection Control
The Johns Hopkins Hospital
Baltimore, Maryland

Stanley L. Pestotnik, M.S. R.Ph.
President and CEO
TheraDoc, Inc.
Salt Lake City, Utah

Clarence J. Peters, M.D.
Director, John Sealy Distinguished University Chair in Tropical and Emerging Virology
Center for Biodefense
The University of Texas Medical Branch
Galveston, Texas

Didier Pittet, M.D, M.S.
Professor of Medicine
Director, Infection Control Unit
University of Geneva Hospitals
Geneva, Switzerland

Jean M. Pottinger, M.A., R.N., C.I.C.
Nurse Epidemiologist
Program of Hospital Epidemiology
University of Iowa Hospitals and Clinics
Iowa City, Iowa

Kristine A. Qureshi, R.N., D.N.Sc.
Project Director and Co-Investigator
Center for Public Health Preparedness
Columbia University
New York, New York

Issam Raad, M.D.
Professor of Medicine
Department of Infectious Diseases, Infection Control and Employee Health
The University of Texas
M.D. Anderson Cancer Center
Houston, Texas

Susan Reef, M.D.
Chief, Rubella/Mumps Activity
Child Vaccine Preventable Diseases Branch
Centers for Disease Control and Prevention
Atlanta, Georgia

Peter A. Reinhardt, M.A.
Director
Department of Environmental Health and Safety
University of North Carolina
Chapel Hill, North Carolina

John H. Rex, M.D., F.A.C.P.
Vice President
Clinical Advisor Infection Therapy Area and Global Clinical Expert
AstraZeneca
Cheshire, United Kingdom

Emily Rhinehart, R.N., M.P.H., C.I.C., C.P.H.Q.
Vice President
AIG Healthcare Management Services
Atlanta, Georgia

Bruce S. Ribner, M.D.
Professor
Division of Infectious Diseases
Department of Medicine
Emory University
Atlanta, Georgia

Louis B. Rice, M.D.
Associate Professor of Medicine
Division of Infectious Diseases
Case Western Reserve University School of Medicine
Chief, Department of Infectious Diseases
VA Medical Center
Cleveland, Ohio

Jane S. Roccaforte, M.D.
Clinical Assistant Professor
Department of Internal Medicine
University of Nebraska Medical Center;
Epidemiologist
Department Infection Control
Algent Imanual Medical Center
Omaha, Nebraska

Manfred L. Rotter, M.D., Dip.bact. (London)
Director and Professor of Hygiene and Microbiology
Institute of Hygiene and Medical Microbiology
University of Vienna
Vienna, Austria

Ulises Ruiz, M.D., Ph.D., F.A.C.S.
Associate Professor
University Institute for Health Services Assessment
Facultad de Medicina
Universidad Complutense de Madrid
Madrid, Spain

Mark E. Rupp, M.D.
Professor
Department of Internal Medicine
University of Nebraska Medical Center
Omaha, Nebraska

William A. Rutala, Ph.D., M.P.H.
Professor, Division of Infectious Diseases
University of North Carolina School of Medicine;
Director, Hospital Epidemiology, Occupational Health, and Safety Program
University of North Carolina Hospitals
Chapel Hill, North Carolina

Matthew Samore, M.D.
Chief, Division of Clinical Epidemiology
Associate Professor of Medicine
University of Utah
Salt Lake City, Utah

Susie J. Sargent, M.D., F.A.C.P.
Clinical Associate Professor
Division of Infectious Diseases
Department of Medicine
University of Tennessee
Regional Medical Center of Memphis
Memphis, Tennessee

William Schaffner, M.D.
Professor and Chairman
Department of Preventive Medicine
Vanderbilt University School of Medicine
Vanderbilt University Medical Center
Nashville, Tennessee

William E. Scheckler, M.D.
Professor
Department of Family Medicine
University of Wisconsin Medical School, and
Hospital Epidemiologist
St. Mary's Hospital Medical Center
Madison, Wisconsin

Charles J. Schleupner, M.S., M.D.
Professor of Medicine
University of North Carolina School of Medicine
Coastal Area Health Education Center
New Hanover Regional Medical Center
Wilmington, North Carolina

Jan K. Schultz
Product Manager-Liew Workshops
Healthstream, Inc
Denver, Colorado

Sebastian Schulz-Stübner, M.D., Ph.D.
Assistant Professor
Department of Anesthesia
University of Iowa Hospitals and Clinics
Iowa City, Iowa

Gordon E. Schutze, M.D.
Associate Professor
Departments of Pediatrics and Pathology
University of Arkansas for Medical Sciences;
Department of Infectious Diseases
Arkansas Children's Hospital
Little Rock, Arkansas

Thomas J. Sebastian, M.D.
Fellow
Department of Infectious Disease
University of Miami
Jackson Memorial Hospital
Miami, Florida

Marisel Segarra-Newnham, Pharm.D., BCPS
Adjunct Clinical Assistant Professor
Department of Pharmacy Practice
University of Florida College of Pharmacy
Gainesville, Florida

Lynne Sehulster, Ph.D.
Microbiologist
Division of Healthcare Quality Promotion
Centers for Disease Control and Prevention
Atlanta, Georgia

John A. Sellick, Jr., D.O., M.S.
Associate Professor of Clinical Medicine
Division of Infectious Diseases
Department of Medicine
State University of New York at Buffalo;
Hospital Epidemiologist
Veterans Affairs Western New York Healthcare System
Buffalo, New York

David L. Sewell, Ph.D.
Professor
Department of Pathology
Oregon Health and Science University
Director, Microbiology Section
Veterans Affairs Medical Center
Portland, Oregon

Ronald I. Shorr, M.D., M.S.
Associate Professor
Department of Preventive Medicine
The University of Tennessee Health Science Center
Memphis, Tennessee

José Simón, M.D.
Professor and Chairman of Physiology
University Institute Health Care Assessment
Universidad Complutense de Madrid
Madrid, Spain

Bryan P. Simmons, M.D.
Clinical Associate Professor
Department of Medicine
University of Tennessee
Medical Director, Infection Control
Methodist Hospital Systems
Memphis, Tennessee

Nina Singh, M.D.
Associate Professor of Medicine
Chief, Transplant Infectious Diseases
Veterans Affairs Medical Center
Pittsburgh, Pennsylvania

Fiona M. Smaill, M.B., Ch.B., M.Sc.
Professor
Department of Pathology and Molecular Medicine
McMaster University
Director of Microbiology
Department of Laboratory Medicine
Hamilton Health Sciences
Hamilton, Ontario, Canada

Philip W. Smith, M.D.
Professor and Chief
Section of Infectious Diseases
University of Nebraska Medical Center
Chairman of the Board
Nebraska Infection Control Network, and
Omaha, Nebraska

Steven L. Solomon, M.D.
Division of Healthcare Quality Promotion
National Center for Infectious Diseases
Centers for Disease Control and Prevention
Atlanta, Georgia

Kathleen A. Steger Craven, R.N., M.P.H.
Assistant Professor
Department of Public Health
Boston University School of Medicine;
Associate Director
Clinical AIDS Program
Boston Medical Center
Boston, Massachusetts

Valentina Stoser, M.D.
Assistant Professor
Department of Medicine
Northwestern University
Feinberg School of Medicine
Chicago, Illinois

Janet E. Stout, Ph.D.
Research Associate Professor
Department of Medicine-Infectious Disease
University of Pittsburgh
Director, Special Pathogen Laboratory
Veterans Affairs Healthcare System
Pittsburgh, Pennsylvania

Charles W. Stratton IV, M.D.
Associate Professor of Medicine and Pathology
Department of Pathology
Vanderbilt University School of Medicine
Nashville, Tennessee

Larry J. Strausbaugh, M.D.
Professor
Department of Medicine
Oregon Health Sciences University and
Hospital Epidemiologist
Veterans Affairs Medical Center
Portland, Oregon

Andrew J. Streifel M.P.H.
Department of Environmental Health and Safety
University of Minnesota
Minneapolis, Minnesota

William H. Tettelbach, M.D.
Department of Infectious Diseases
Methodist University Hospital
Memphis, Tennessee

Alan Tice, M.D.
Associate Professor
Department of Internal Medicine
John A. Burns School of Medicine
University of Hawaii
Honolulu, Hawaii

Jerome I. Tokars, M.D.
Medical Epidemiologist
Division of Healthcare Quality Promotion
Centers for Disease Control and Prevention
Atlanta, Georgia

Elizabeth A. Tolley, Ph.D.
Professor
Department of Preventive Medicine
Division of Pulmonary and Critical Care
University of Tennessee Health Science Center
Memphis, Tennessee

Ronald B. Turner, M.D.
Professor
Department of Pediatrics
University of Virginia
Charlottesville, Virginia

William M. Valenti, M.D.
Clinical Associate Professor
Department of Medicine
University of Rochester, and
Founding Medical Director
Community Health Network
Rochester, New York

Donald Vesley, Ph.D.
Professor
Department of Environmental Health
School of Public Health
University of Minnesota
Minneapolis, Minnesota

Francis A. Waldvogel
Professor, Department of Medicine
Clinique Medicale 2
University of Geneva Hospitals
Geneva, Switzerland

Cynthia J. Walker, M.L.S.
Research Associate
Department of Clinical Epidemiology and
Biostatistics
McMaster University
Hamilton, Ontario, Canada

Richard J. Wallace, Jr., M.D.
Chairman and Professor of Medicine
Department of Microbiology
University of Texas Health Center
Tyler, Texas

Jue Wang, M.D.
Hyperbaric Medicine and Surgical Infectious Diseases Fellow
Department of Orthopaedic Surgery and Rehabilitation
Division of Hyperbaric Medicine and Wound Care
University of Texas Medical Branch
Galveston, Texas

David J. Weber, M.D., M.P.H.
Professor
Division of Infectious Diseases
University of North Carolina School of Medicine
Chapel Hill, North Carolina

Robert A. Weinstein, M.D.
Professor
Department of Medicine
Rush Medical College, and
Chairman and Chief Operating Officer
Departments of Infectious Diseases and Medicine
Cook County Hospital; Core Center
Chicago, Illinois

Don Weiss, M.D., M.P.H.
Bureau of Communicable Disease
New York City Department of Health and Mental Hygiene
New York, New York

Richard P. Wenzel, M.D., M.Sc.
Professor and Chairman
Department of Internal Medicine
Medical College of Virginia
Virginia Commonwealth University
Richmond, Virginia

Cynthia J. Whitener, M.D.
Assistant Professor Division of Infectious Diseases
Department of Medicine
The Pennsylvania State University College of Medicine
Hershey, Pennsylvania

Ian T. Williams, Ph.D., M.S.
Division of Viral Hepatitis
National Center for Infectious Diseases
Centers for Disease Control and Prevention
Public Health Service
U.S. Department of Health and Human Services
Atlanta, Georgia

Walter W. Williams, M.D.
Associate Director for Minority Health
Office of the Director
Centers for Disease Control and Prevention
Atlanta, Georgia

Keith F. Woeltje, M.D., Ph.D.
Assistant Professor
Department of Internal Medicine/Infectious Diseases
Medical College of Georgia
Augusta, Georgia

Edward S. Wong, M.D.
Associate Professor
Department of Medicine
Medical College of Virginia
Virginia Commonwealth University, and
Chief, Infectious Diseases Section
Department of Medicine
McGuire Veterans Affairs Hospital
Richmond, Virginia

Rebecca Wurtz, M.D., M.P.H.
Associate Professor
Department of Preventive Medicine
Northwestern University
Chicago, Illinois

Terry Yamauchi, M.D.
Professor Department of Pediatrics
University of Arkansas for Medical Sciences, and
Vice-Chairman
Department of Pediatrics
Arkansas Children's Hospital
Little Rock, Arkansas

Tsin Wen Yeo, M.D.
Infectious Diseases Fellow
University of Utah School of Medicine
Salt Lake City, Utah

Victor L. Yu, M.D.
Professor, Department of Medicine
University of Pittsburgh, and
Chief, Infectious Diseases Section
Veterans Affairs Pittsburgh Healthcare System
Pittsburgh, Pennsylvania

John A. Zaia, M.D.
Director, Virology and Infectious Diseases
Division of Pediatrics
City of Hope National Medical Center
Duarte, California

Preface for the 3rd Edition

Again, I have been privileged to edit the Third Edition of *Hospital Epidemiology and Infection Control.* My friends and colleagues who make up the 182 authors of this edition have once again entrusted their manuscripts to me as editor to edit and integrate their works into another edition of this comprehensive reference text. I greatly appreciate the tremendous effort and sacrifice made by these authors to either create manuscripts for new chapters or to revise chapters from the previous edition that provide up-to-date and ''cutting edge'' information for the readers of the Third Edition.

Since the Second Edition of this book was published, the challenges and problems for hospital epidemiologists and infection control professionals have continued to mount. The severity of illness of hospitalized patients continues to increase, resources continue to decrease and regulatory agencies continue to promulgate more regulations for accreditation, and many of these fall to infection control programs for implementation. Added to these increasing pressures are new responsibilities for responding to bioterrorism threats and the impact of emerging infectious diseases such as SARS on our healthcare institutions. Another emerging concern in healthcare is that of medical errors. In many healthcare institutions, infection control programs will often be involved in investigating the occurrence of medical errors and in creating prevention programs.

In the Third Edition, as always, we are trying to provide the reader with up-to-date information on all subjects in healthcare epidemiology. Three new sections have been added to this edition. To provide resources for the hospital epidemiologist and infection control professional on developing programs for the control and prevention of medical errors, Section II. Healthcare Quality Improvement has been added. I am greatly indebted to Dr. David Birnbaum who helped create this section by both choosing the topics and authors and then assisting with the editing process through to the final drafts. He also wrote the introductory chapter for the section. We attempted to prepare a series of chapters that would make it possible for hospital epidemiologists and infection control professionals to apply the principles of Quality Management for solving problems of medical errors and other noninfectious nosocomial adverse outcomes.

Between the Second and Third Editions, the events of September 11, 2001 led to an emphasis on the development of programs to protect the United States against terrorism. It is clear that protecting healthcare institutions from bioterrorism and making preparations for a response to such an attack will fall to the infection control programs in our hospitals. To provide information and guidance for developing institutional programs against bioterrorism, Section XVII Bioterrorism was added to this Edition. All of the authors in this section have been and are involved at the national level in working to help provide defenses against the bioterrorism threat. I deeply appreciate the contributions of these authors who have made great sacrifices to prepare these chapters while being extremely busy in the discharge of their duties as they work diligently to help protect all of us.

Another new challenge for healthcare epidemiology is that of emerging infectious diseases which now impact significantly on our healthcare institutions. Our unfamiliarity with these diseases including lack of information on the clinical manifestations, pathogenesis, etiology, epidemiology, treatment and prevention places a heavy burden on infection control programs to provide appropriate infection control measures to prevent transmission from infected patients to other patients and hospital personnel. Section XVIII Emerging Infectious Diseases and Healthcare Epidemiology was added to address the needs of hospital epidemiologists and infection control professionals in developing infection control measures for control of these infectious diseases in hospitalized patients. The first chapter in this section is on the Severe Acute Respiratory Syndrome (SARS).

To provide additional resources for management and analysis of data in the Third Edition, Section II Computers in Hospital Epidemiology in the Second Edition has been revised and another chapter added for the Third Edition. This is now Section III Informatics in Healthcare Epidemiology. I greatly appreciate the assistance of Dr. Keith Woeltje in revising this section and the willingness of the other authors in this section, Drs. John Sellick and David Classen to make changes in their chapters to permit the reorganization of the section and accommodate a new chapter by Dr. Woeltje and Dr. Rebecca Wurtz.

Finally, in an attempt to further make the Third Edition more comprehensive other new chapters added include Chapter 19 Bacteremia, Chapter 40 Filamentous Fungi, Chapter 73 Infection in Xenotransplantation—A Model for Detection of Unknown Pathogens, Chapter 80 Vaccination of Healthcare Workers, Chapter 88. Prevention of Infections Related to Construction, Renovation and Demolition, and Chapter 93 Methodologic Review of Epidemiologic Studies in Infection Control.

Once again, it has been my pleasure to try to provide all of my colleagues in hospital epidemiology and infection control with a very comprehensive and up-to-date reference text for their use in the daily practice of Healthcare Epidemiology.

ACKNOWLEDGMENTS

I greatly appreciate the contributions made by my assistant Lydia Careaga and Joyce Murphy, Managing Editor, at Lippincott Williams & Wilkins.

C. Glen Mayhall

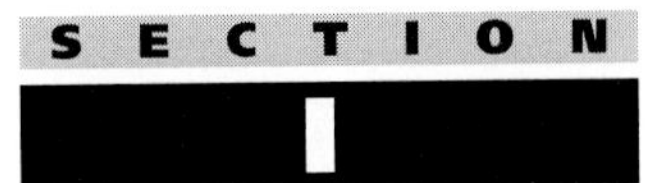

APPLIED EPIDEMIOLOGY AND BIOSTATISTICS IN HEALTHCARE EPIDEMIOLOGY AND INFECTION CONTROL

1

PRINCIPLES OF INFECTIOUS DISEASES EPIDEMIOLOGY

LENNOX K. ARCHIBALD
WALTER J. HIERHOLZER, JR.

The use of epidemiology and the accompanying statistical methods grew out of attempts to understand, predict, and control the great epidemics of our past. The study and interventions of infection control practices grew out of the need to understand and control the institutional epidemics complicating the care of the ill (1–3). The diseases of these early epidemics were infectious, and discussions of the principles of epidemiology begin with examples of methods that were first formalized in the study of transmissible microorganisms, many of which continue to cause problems today. The term *hospital epidemiology* was a modern addition by workers in the United States (4), as was the recognition of the potential use of these methods in hospitals for the study and control of noninfectious diseases (5).

The terms *hospital epidemiology* and *infection control* remain synonymous in the minds of many. However, both the terms and their associated programs have grown in definition and function in the past five decades (6,7). Interest in infection control has broadened from focused concerns with puerperal sepsis and surgical site infection to full, scientifically tested programs of surveillance, prevention, and control of all healthcare-associated infections. Using the epidemiology of the outcome of infection and infectious diseases, hospital epidemiology programs were among the earliest demonstration projects for the use of scientific methodology in analysis and improvements in patient care. In this special environment of the acute care hospital, a natural repetition of earlier studies of population-based infectious diseases provided the basic concepts for epidemiologic investigations. As happened in population epidemiology, hospital epidemiology programs are expanding their population base and applying increasingly sophisticated methodologies to the study of both infectious and noninfectious diseases outcomes in various healthcare settings (8,9).

In the current era of managed care, hospital epidemiology has expanded and become relevant beyond the acute care hospital to all settings where healthcare is delivered. The term *nosocomial infections* had been widely adopted for these adverse outcome events, reflecting their original association with hospitalized patients and the concern to separate the terminology of the events from fear of liability that might have interfered with identification and control efforts. The term *nosocomial infections* has now largely been replaced by *healthcare-associated infections.*

Traditionally, the clinical microbiology laboratory has played a key role in the control of healthcare-associated infections through accurate identification of pathogens and appropriate antimicrobial susceptibility testing of isolates. These services have grown to support the investigation and characterization of healthcare-associated infections through provision of consultation and expertise on the appropriate clinical and environmental collection of specimens and the optimum application of culture methods. Moreover, the current level of sophistication of microbiologic tests allows precise identification of clonal types for epidemiologic investigations (10–12). In conjunction with these modern methods, application of epidemiologic principles to microbiologic sampling, specimen collection, and testing is critical to the investigation and characterization of, and solution to, most healthcare-associated infection outbreaks (12). For example, using standardized methods for obtaining and processing hand cultures that are epidemiologically directed may yield far more useful data at lower costs (13) (see Chapter 102).

DEFINITIONS

Epidemiology is defined as the study of the determinants and distribution of health and disease in populations. In discussions of epidemiology, certain standard definitions have been accepted (14–16):

Attack rate A ratio of the number of new infections divided by the number of exposed, susceptible individuals in a given period, usually expressed as a percentage. Other terms are the *incidence rate* and the *case rate.*

Bias The difference between a true value of an epidemiologic measure and that which is estimated in a study. Bias may be random or systematic. There are three types of bias: selection bias, information bias, and confounding. Selection bias is a distortion in the estimate of effect resulting from the manner in which parameters are selected for the study population. Information bias depends on the accuracy of the information collected. Confounding arises from unrecognized factors that may affect interpretation of epidemiologic data. Unrecognized, systematic bias presents the greatest danger in studies by suggesting relationships that are not valid.

Carrier An individual (host) who harbors a microorganism (agent) without evidence of disease and, in some cases, without evidence of host immune response. This carriage may take place during the latent phase of the incubation period as a part of asymptomatic disease or may be chronic following recovery from illness. Carriers may shed microorganisms into the environment intermittently or continuously, and this shedding may lead to transmission. Shedding and potential transmission may be increased by other factors affecting the host, including infection by another agent.

Case An individual in a population or group recognized as having a particular disease or condition under investigation or study. This definition may not be the same as the clinical definition of a case.

Case-fatality rate A ratio of the number of deaths from a specific disease divided by the number of cases of disease, expressed as a percentage.

Cluster An aggregation of relatively uncommon events or diseases in time and/or space in numbers that are believed to be greater than are expected by chance alone.

Colonization The multiplication of a microorganism at a body site or sites without any overt clinical expression or detected immune reaction in the host at the time that the microorganism is isolated. Colonization may or may not be a precursor of infection. Colonization may be a form of carriage and is a potential source of transmission.

Communicability The characteristic of a human pathogen that enables it to be transmitted from one person to another under natural conditions. Infections may be communicable or noncommunicable. Communicable infections may be endemic, epidemic, or pandemic.

Communicable period The time in the natural history of an infection during which transmission to susceptible hosts may take place.

Confounding An illusory association between two factors when in fact there is no causal relationship between the two. The apparent association is caused by a third variable that is both a risk factor for the outcome or disease and is associated with but not a result of the exposure in question.

Contact An exposed individual who might have been infected through transmission from another host or the environment.

Contagious Having the potential for transmission.

Contamination The presence of an agent (e.g., microorganism) on a surface or in a fluid or material—therefore, a potential source for transmission.

Endemic The usual level or presence of an agent or disease in a defined population during a given period.

Epidemic An unusual, higher-than-expected level of infection or disease by an agent in a defined population in a given period. This definition assumes previous knowledge of the usual, or endemic, levels.

Epidemic curve A graphic representation of the distribution of defined cases by the time of onset of their disease.

Epidemic period The time period over which the excess cases occur.

Hyperendemic The level of an agent or disease that is consistently present at a high incidence and/or prevalence rate.

Immunity The resistance of a host to a specific agent, characterized by measurable and protective surface or humoral antibody and by cell-mediated immune responses. Immunity may be the result of specific previous experience with the agent (wild infection), from transplacental transmission to the fetus, or from active or passive immunization to the agent. Immunity is relative and governed through genetic control. Immunity to some agents remains throughout life, whereas for others it is short-lived, allowing repeat infections by the same agent. Immunity may be reduced in extremes of age, through disease, or through immunosuppressive therapy.

Immunity: cell-mediated vs. humoral Cell-mediated immune protection, largely related to specific T-lymphocytic activity, as opposed to humoral immunity, which is measured by the presence of specific immunoglobulins (antibodies) in surface body fluids or circulating in noncellular components of blood. Antibodies are produced by B lymphocytes, also now recognized to be under the influence of T-lymphocytic functions.

Immunogenicity An agent's (microorganism's) intrinsic ability to trigger specific immunity in a host. Certain agents escape host defense mechanisms by intrinsic characteristics that fail to elicit a host immune response. Other agents evoke an immune response that initiates a disease process in the host that increases cellular damage and morbidity beyond the direct actions of the microorganism itself. These disease processes may continue beyond the presence of living microorganisms in the host.

Incidence rate The ratio of the number of new infections or disease in a defined population in a given period to the number of individuals at risk in the population. "At risk" is frequently defined as the number of potentially exposed susceptibles. The rate is usually expressed as numbers of new cases per thousands (1,000, 10,000, or 100,000) per year.

Incubation period The period between exposure to an agent and the first appearance of evidence of disease in a susceptible host. Incubation periods are typical for specific agents and may be helpful in the diagnosis of unknown illness. Incubation periods may be modified by extremes of dose or by variations in host immune function. The first portion of the incubation period following colonization and infection is frequently a silent period, called the *latent period.* During this time, there is no evidence of host response(s) and evidence of the presence of the infecting agent may not be measurable. However, transmission of the microorganism to other hosts, though reduced during this period, is a recognized risk [e.g., chicken pox, hepatitis B virus, human immunodeficiency virus (HIV)]. Measurable early immune responses in the host may appear shortly before the first signs and symptoms of disease, marking the end of the latent period. Signs and symptoms of disease commonly appear shortly thereafter, marking the end of the incubation period.

Index case The first case to be recognized in a series of transmissions of an agent in a host population. In semiclosed populations, as typified by chronic disease hospitals, the index case may first introduce an agent not previously active in the population.

Infection The successful transmission of a microorganism to the host with subsequent multiplication, colonization, and invasion. Infection may be clinical or subclinical and may not produce identifiable disease. However, it is usually accompanied by measurable host response(s), either through the appearance of specific antibodies or through cell-mediated reaction(s) (e.g., positive tuberculin test results). An infectious disease may be caused by the intrinsic properties of the agent (invasion and cell destruction, release of toxins) or by associated immune response in the host (cell-mediated destruction of infected cells, immune responses to host antigens similar to antigens in the agent).

Infectivity The characteristic of the microorganism that indicates its ability to invade and multiply in the host. It is frequently expressed as the proportion of exposed patients who become infected.

Isolation The physical separation of an infected or colonized host, including the individual's contaminated body fluids and environmental materials, from the remainder of the at-risk population in an attempt to prevent transmission of the specific agent to the latter group. This is usually accomplished through individual environmentally controlled rooms or quarters, hand washing following contact with the infected host and environment, and the use of barrier protective devices, including gowns, gloves, and, in the case of airborne agents, an appropriate mask.

Morbidity rate The ratio of the number of persons infected with a new clinical disease to the number of persons at risk in the population during a defined period; an *incidence rate* of disease.

Mortality rate The ratio of those infected who have died in a given period to the number of individuals in the defined population. The rate may be *crude,* related to all causes, or *disease-specific,* related or *attributable* to a specific disease in a population at risk for the disease.

Pandemic An epidemic that spreads over several countries or continents and affects many people.

Pathogenicity The ability of an agent to cause disease in a susceptible host. The pathogenicity of a specific agent may be increased in a host with reduced defense mechanisms. For some agent–host interactions the resultant disease is due to the effects of exaggerated or prolonged action of defense mechanisms of the host.

Prevalence rate The ratio of the number of individuals measurably affected or diseased by an agent in a defined population at a particular point in time, or over a specified time period, without regard to when the process or disease began.

Pseudo-outbreak Real clustering of false infections or artifactual clustering of real infections. Often it is identified when there is increased recovery of unusual microorganisms.

Rate An expression of the frequency with which an event occurs in a defined population. All rates are ratios. Some rates are proportions, i.e., the numerator is a part of the denominator. A comparable rate is a rate that controls for variations in the distribution of major risk factors associated with an event.

Ratio An expression of the relationship between a numerator and a denominator where the two are usually distinct and separate quantities, neither being a part of the other.

Relative risk The ratio of the incidence rate of infection in the exposed group to the incidence rate in the unexposed group. Used to measure the strength of an association between exposures or risk factors and disease.

Reservoir Any animate or inanimate niche in the environment in which an infectious agent may survive and multiply to become a source of transmission to a susceptible host. Medical care workers and patients constitute the main animate reservoir for microorganisms associated with healthcare-associated infections; water-related sources are important inanimate reservoirs that have been implicated in outbreaks related to dialysis units and to air conditioning systems.

Secular trend Profile of the changes in measurable events or in the incidence rate of infection or disease over an extended period of time; also called a *temporal trend.*

Sensitivity For surveillance systems, the ratio of the number of patients reported to have an infection divided by the number of patients who actually had an infection.

Specificity For surveillance systems, the ratio of the number of patients who were reported not to have an infection divided by the number of patients who actually did not have an infection.

Sporadic Occurring irregularly and usually infrequently over a period of time.

Surveillance The ongoing systematic collection, analysis, and interpretation of healthcare data essential to the planning, implementation, and evaluation of public health practice, closely integrated with the timely dissemination of these data to those contributing data or to other interested groups who need to know. Surveillance was popularized by Langmuir and others at the Centers for Disease Control and Prevention (CDC) and has been the basic method in infection control programs in the United States since the 1960s.

Susceptibility A condition of the host that indicates absence of protection against infection by an agent. This is usually marked by the absence of specific antibodies or specific measures of cell-mediated immunity against the infecting microorganism.

Transmission The method by which any potentially infecting agent is spread to another host. Transmission may be direct or indirect. *Direct transmission* may take place by touching between hosts, by the projection of large droplets in coughing and sneezing onto another host, or by direct contact by a susceptible host with an environmental reservoir of the agent. *Indirect transmission* may be vehicle-borne, airborne, or vector-borne. In *vehicle-borne transmission,* contaminated environmental sources, including water, food, blood, and laundry, may act as an intermediate source of an infectious agent for introduction into a susceptible host. The agent may have multiplied or undergone biologic development in the vehicle.

In *airborne transmission,* aerosols containing small (1–5 μm) particles may be suspended in air for long periods and inspired into the lower respiratory tree to become a site of infection in a host. These infectious particles may be generated by evaporation of larger particles produced in coughing and sneezing *(Mycobacterium tuberculosis),* by mechanical respiratory aerosolizers *(Legionella),* or by wind or air currents (fungal spores). In *vector-borne transmission,* arthropods or other invertebrates may carry or transmit microorganisms, usually through inoculation by biting or by contamination of food or other materials. The vector may be infected itself or act only as a mechanical carrier of the agent. If the vector is infected, the agent may have multiplied or undergone biologic development in the vector. This type of transmission has been of little importance for healthcare-associated infections in the United States.

Virulence The intrinsic capabilities of an agent to infect a host and produce disease and a measure of the severity of the disease produced. In the extreme this is represented by the number of patients with clinical disease who develop severe illness or die—the case fatality rate.

CLASSIC EPIDEMIOLOGIC METHODS APPLIED TO INFECTIOUS DISEASES

The classic methods in epidemiology are used to study and characterize the various infections that occur in communities, regions, or healthcare settings; to determine the exposure-disease relationship in humans and the modes of acquisition, transmission, and spread that are essential to understand for the prevention and control of infections; and to guide rational application and practice of laboratory methods. These epidemiologic methods have been developed in an attempt to control common errors in observations that occur when one studies the association of one event (a risk or causal factor) with another later event (the outcome or disease).

Classic epidemiologic study methods are grouped as either observational or experimental. *Observational studies* are conducted in natural, everyday community or clinical settings, where the investigators observe the appearance of an outcome, but have no control over the environment or the exposure of people to a risk or an intervention. Observational epidemiologic methods are further classified as either *descriptive* or *analytic.* Analytic epidemiology primarily uses three methods of study: cohort studies, case-control studies, and cross-sectional studies.

In *experimental studies,* investigators study the effect of some factor or exposure that they control. In all studies of associations between a suspected risk factor and a disease, it is important to identify confounding factors that might be related both to the exposure of interest and causally to the disease under investigation. Confounding factors may suggest a false causal relationship between a risk factor and the disease of interest. More extensive descriptions of the use of these methods and their statistical support in hospital epidemiology and infection control programs appear in Chapters 2, 3, and 4. For more detailed discussions of the application of these methods in other population studies, see standard reference texts in epidemiology and statistics (17–20).

Descriptive Epidemiology

Observational descriptive studies establish the case definition of an infectious disease event by obtaining data for analysis from available primary (e.g., medical records) or secondary (e.g., infection control surveillance) sources. These data enable the characteristics of the population that has acquired the infection to be delineated according to (a) "person" (age, sex, race, marital status, personal habits, occupation, socioeconomic status, medical or surgical procedure or therapy, device use, underlying disease, or other exposures or events); (b) "place" (geographic occurrence of the health event or outbreak, medical or surgical service, place of acquisition of infection, travel); and (c) "time" (pre- and postepidemic periods, seasonal variation, secular trends, or duration of stay in hospital). The information from descriptive studies might provide important clues regarding the risk factors associated with infection, and in each case it is hoped that an analysis of the collected data might be used to generate hypotheses regarding the occurrence and distribution of disease or infection in the population(s) being studied.

Analytic Epidemiology

Observational analytic studies are designed to test hypotheses raised by the findings in descriptive investigations. The purposes of these studies are to establish (a) the cause and effects of infection in a population, and (b) why a population acquired a particular infection in the first place. The three most common types of observational analytic studies are cohort studies, case-control studies, and prevalence or cross-sectional studies.

Cohort Studies

In cohort studies, hypotheses that have been generated from previous (descriptive) studies are tested in a new population. A population of individuals (a cohort) that is free of the infection or disease of interest is recruited for study. The presence or absence of the suspected (hypothesized) risk factors for the disease is recorded at the beginning of the study and throughout the observation period. All members of the cohort population (e.g., all premature infants admitted to a neonatal intensive care unit during a defined time period) are followed over time for evidence or appearance of the infection or disease and classified accordingly as exposed or unexposed to specific risk factors. If the observation period begins at the present time and continues into the future or until the appearance of disease, the study is called a *prospective cohort study.* If the population studied is one that in the past was apparently free of the markers of disease on examination of records or banked laboratory specimens, it may be chosen for study if data on exposure to the suspected risk factors for disease also are available. The population may be followed to the present or until the appearance of disease. This type of study, common in occupational epidemiology, is called a *historical* or *retrospective cohort study.*

A key requirement of a cohort study is that participants be reliably categorized into exposed and unexposed groups. *Relative risk,* i.e., the ratio of the incidence rate of the outcome in the exposed group to the incidence rate in the unexposed group, is used to measure the strength of an association between exposures or risk factors and disease. Cohort studies have the advantage of allowing direct measurement of risk factors associated with disease, the incidence of infection and disease, and ascertainment of the temporal relationship between exposure and disease. Also, observational bias may be less, since the information on the presence of risk factors is recorded before the outcome of disease is known. To ensure sufficient numbers for analysis, cohort studies require continual follow-up of large populations for long periods unless the disease under investigation is one of high incidence. Thus, cohort studies are, in general, more expensive and time-consuming and are not suitable for the investigation of uncommon infections or conditions. However, they present the most convincing nonexperimental approach to information on causation.

Case-Control Studies

In a case-control study, the case-patient is an individual who is already infected or ill and meets a given case definition. A group of these case individuals is compared for the presence or history of exposure to potential risk factors with a control group of individuals who do not have the infection or illness of interest. Thus subjects are first enrolled according to whether they have acquired disease or not. The presence of significant differences in the exposure to risk factors in the case-patients versus the control subjects suggests an etiologic (causal) association between those factors and the infection or disease. In case-control studies, the search for exposure is retrospective. In an attempt to decrease bias, control subjects are frequently selected from individuals matched for certain characteristics, including age, gender, socioeconomic status, or other factors not suspected and under investigation. Case-control methods are efficient for studies of disease with low incidence rates, infections that are associated with several risk factors, for situations in which there is a long time lag between exposure and disease (outcome), or for establishing etiologic associations when there is no existing information about the cause or source of a disease or infection. Compared with cohort studies, case-control studies may be conducted in relatively shorter time, are relatively inexpensive, and may require a smaller sample size. Among the drawbacks, selection of appropriate controls may be difficult, and significant bias can appear in the selection of both case-patients and control subjects; there may be incomplete information on exposures; or risk factor data may be difficult to find (or remember). Case-control studies are not used to measure incidence rates and might not be able to establish temporal relationships between exposure and outcome.

Prevalence or Cross-Sectional Studies

In prevalence studies, both the presence of suspected risk factors and of the disease under investigation are recorded in a survey of a study population at a specific point in time or within a (short) time period. The rates of disease of those with and without the suspected risk factors are compared. Thus, cross-sectional studies can establish association but not causation for suspected risk factors. Although prevalence studies are inexpensive and rapidly accomplished, they do not allow the ascertainment of risk factors at the beginning of disease and do not allow one to establish a temporal sequence of the risk factor preceding the outcome of disease. Point prevalence, period prevalence, and seroprevalence surveys are examples of cross-sectional studies.

Experimental Epidemiology

In experimental studies, the investigator controls an exposure of individuals in a population to a suspected causal factor, a prevention measure, or therapeutic regimen. These exposure modalities are randomly allocated to comparable groups, thereby minimizing confounding factors. Both the exposed and unexposed groups are monitored thereafter for an outcome, for the appearance of infection or of disease, or for evidence of the prevention or control of the disease. Often, experimental studies are used to evaluate antimicrobial and vaccine treatment regimens for infectious diseases, or other preventive or interventional measures. Generally, experimental studies are expensive to conduct. For ethical reasons, it is rarely possible to expose human populations to potential pathogens or to withhold a preventive measure that could potentially be beneficial to the patient. Hence, the use of human volunteers in today's research environments is widely restricted, and reasonably so. Therefore, animals are frequently used as alternative populations for study. Unfortunately, many animal hosts are not naturally susceptible to the agents of human disease or react differently to these agents. Thus, one has to be careful when extrapolating epidemiologic findings in animal experimental studies to the control of infections in human subjects. Within the hospital setting, studies that investigate restriction of certain antimicrobials and promotion of use of alternative antimicrobials for the control of antimicrobial resistance could be considered under the category of experimental.

EPIDEMIOLOGY OF INFECTIOUS DISEASE: FACTORS LEADING TO INFECTION AND DISEASE

The epidemiology of infectious disease presents two processes for discussion: (a) the epidemiology of the determinants leading to infections in hosts, and (b) the epidemiology of the appearance and extent of disease related to the infection in those hosts. It is common to discuss health and disease as the result of a series of complex interactions between an agent of change, the host that is the target of the agent actions, and the mutual environment in which the host and agent are found. In studies of healthcare-associated infections, the agents are the microorganisms associated with the infections, the hosts are the patients under care or their healthcare workers, and the common environment is the acute care hospital, intensive care unit, outpatient, home, or other healthcare venues.

The interactions determining the probability of a microbiologic agent causing infection in a host may be simply presented by an equation of infection:

$$I_p = \frac{D \times S \times T \times V}{H_d}$$

where I_p is the probability of infection, D is the dose (number of microorganisms) transmitted to the host, S is the receptive host site of contact with the agent, T is the time of contact (sufficient for attachment and multiplication or not), and V represents virulence, the intrinsic characteristics of the microorganism that allow it to infect. The denominator in the equation (H_d) represents the force of the combined host defenses attempting to prevent this infection.

Any reduction in host defenses (represented by the denominator) in such an equation allows infection to take place with a similar reduction in one or more of the agent factors in the numerator. Infection may take place with a smaller dose of microorganisms. Infection may take place at an unusual site. The contact time for a microorganism to fix to an appropriate surface may be briefer, or infection may take place with an agent of lesser virulence, one that does not cause infection in the normal host. These reductions in the host defense characteristics, represented by the denominator, and the reduction of requirements to infect for the agent are typical of the interactions that allow opportunistic infections in compromised hosts, represented by many patients under care in modern hospitals. In this model, equation of infection, the environment might be considered the background or playing field on which the agent–host interaction takes place. A number of additional models of the interaction of agent, host, and environment have been suggested to help understand these processes. The three models in Fig. 1.1—the seesaw model, the triangle model, and the wheel model—have been frequently cited (18,21). Each attempts to simply visualize the interplay between the three components.

INTERACTIONS OF AGENT, DISEASE, AND ENVIRONMENT

All outcome events (diseases) have multifactorial causes. For some infectious diseases, a single unique factor or agent is *necessary* and *sufficient* for the disease to appear. This is exemplified by measles or by rabies. It is only *necessary* for the host to be exposed to and infected by an agent (the measles virus or the rabies virus) for that disease to develop. For other infectious diseases, the single factor of infectivity of the agent is *necessary* but not *sufficient* to cause disease in the host. *M. tuberculosis,* polio virus, hepatitis A, and many other agents *necessary* for specific disease in a human host infect without causing disease in a majority of cases. Within the hospital setting, exposure to a specific microorganism or colonization of an inpatient with an agent, such as vancomycin-resistant enterococcus (VRE) or *Staphylococcus aureus*, may be *necessary* but not *sufficient* to generate disease, which only develops through complex interactions between other contributory factors, such as age, state of debilitation, immune or nutritional status, device use, invasive procedures, antimicrobial usage, or susceptibility of the microorganism to available antimicrobials. The fact of the infection in these cases is not *sufficient* to produce disease in the host without

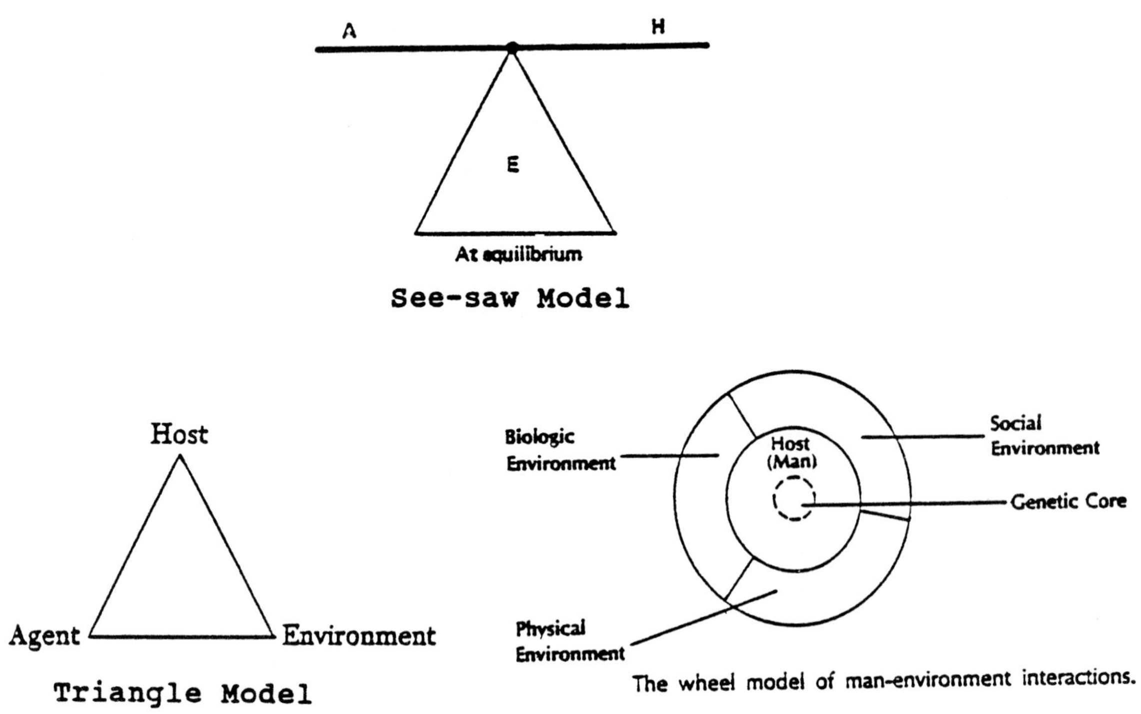

Figure 1.1. Models of interactions of agent, disease, and environment. (Seesaw model from Fox JP, Elveback L, Gatewood L, et al. Herd immunity. *Am J Epidemiol* 1971;94:171–189. Triangle model and wheel model from Mausner JS, Kramer S, eds. *Mausner & Bahn epidemiology—an introductory text.* Philadelphia: WB Saunders, 1985.)

the contribution of these latter elements in the host and the environment.

Agent

The agents causing healthcare-associated infectious diseases are microorganisms ranging in size and complexity from viruses and bacteria to protozoa and helminths. Bacteria, fungi, and certain viruses have been the agents most recognized and studied as causes of healthcare-associated infections (22). For transmission to take place, the microorganism must remain viable in the environment until contact with the host has been sufficient to allow infection. Reservoirs that allow the agent to survive or multiply may be animate, as exemplified by healthcare worker carriage of staphylococci in the anterior nares (23), or inanimate in the environment, as demonstrated by *Pseudomonas* species or *Legionella* in air-conditioning humidification systems (24,25), *Clostridium difficile* spores on inpatient work surfaces, or *Serratia marcescens* growing in contaminated soap or hand lotion preparations (26,27).

Certain intrinsic and genetically determined properties of a microorganism are important for it to survive in the environment. These include the ability to resist the effects of heat, drying, ultraviolet (UV) light, and chemical agents, including antimicrobials; the ability to compete with other microorganisms; and the ability to independently multiply in the environment or to develop and multiply within another (vector) host. Intrinsic agent factors important to the production of disease include infectivity, pathogenicity, virulence, the infecting dose, the agent's ability to produce toxins, its immunogenicity and ability to resist or overcome the human immune defense system, its ability to replicate only in certain types of cells, tissues, or hosts (vectors), its ability to persist or cause chronic infection, and its interaction with other host mechanisms, including the ability to cause immunosuppression (e.g., HIV).

Once transferred to a host surface, the agent may multiply and colonize without invading or evoking a measurable host immune response (28). Therefore, the presence of an agent at surface sites in the host does not define the presence of an infection. Nonetheless, patients so colonized may act as the reservoir source of transmission to other patients (29).

If infection takes place, a measurable immune response will develop in most hosts even if the infection is subclinical. The success of this process for the agent is increased in the nonimmune host and is most successful in the nonimmune, immunocompromised host. A microorganism's ability to infect another host vector (e.g., yellow fever virus in mosquitoes) or another nonhuman reservoir (e.g., yellow fever virus in the monkey) is important in the epidemiology of certain infectious diseases in world populations at large but plays little role in healthcare infection epidemiology.

Host

Infection depends on exposure of a susceptible host to an infecting agent. Exposure of the susceptible host to such agents is influenced by age, behavior, family associations, occupation, socioeconomic level, travel, avocation, access to preventive care, vaccination status, or hospitalization. Whether or not disease takes place in the infected host and the severity of disease when it appears depend not only on the intrinsic virulence factors of the agent, but more importantly on the pathogenicity of the interactions between the agent and the host. The host immune defenses attempt to prevent infection. Thus, any reduction in host defenses may allow infection to take place with a smaller dose of microorganisms and/or at a body site that is not usually susceptible to infection. A combination of reductions in host defense characteristics and the requirements for an agent to cause infection are typical of the interactions that allow acquisition of opportunistic infections in immunocompromised patients. A commonly cited model indicating the potential interactions between agent and host and the relationships among colonization, infection, and clinical and subclinical disease is shown in Fig. 1.2 (30).

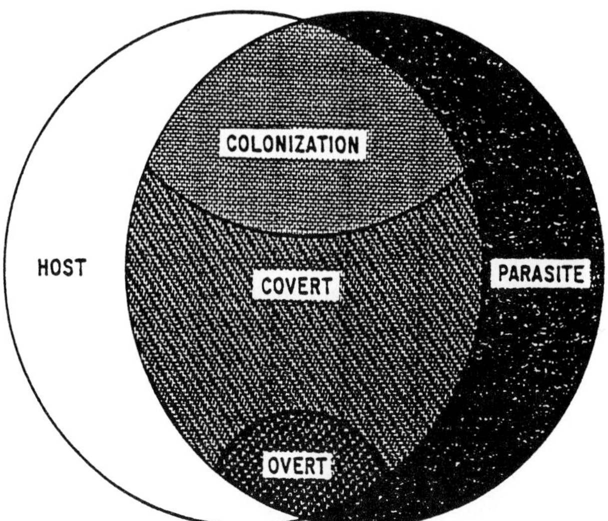

Figure 1.2. Venn diagram of agent–host interactions. An interaction between host and parasite may result in infection. Infection consists of colonization and an infectious disease. An infectious disease may be either covert (subclinical) or overt (symptomatic). (From Hoeprich PD, ed. *Infectious diseases.* Hagerstown: Harper & Row, 1972:40.)

Host factors important to the development and severity of infection or disease may be categorized as intrinsic or extrinsic. Intrinsic factors include the age at infection; birth weight; sex; race; nutritional status (31); comorbid conditions (including anatomic anomalies) and diseases; genetically determined immune status; immunosuppression associated with other infections, diseases, or therapy; vaccination or immunization status; previous experience with this or similar agents; and the psychologic state of the host (32). Extrinsic factors include invasive medical or surgical procedures; medical devices, such as intravenous catheters or mechanical ventilators; sexual practices and contraception; duration of antimicrobial therapy and hospitalization; and exposure to hospital personnel.

Environment

The environment provides the mutual background on which agent–host interactions take place and contains the factors that influence the spread of infection. The environmental factors include (a) physical factors such as climatic conditions of heat, cold, humidity, seasons, and surroundings (e.g., intensive care units, outpatient clinics, long-term care facilities, or water reservoirs); (b) biologic factors (e.g., intermediary hosts such as insect or snail vectors); and (c) social factors (socioeconomic status, sexual behavior, types of food and methods of preparation, and availability of adequate housing, potable water, adequate waste disposal and healthcare amenities). These environmental factors influence both the survival and the multiplication of infectious disease agents in their reservoirs and the behavior of the host in housing, occupation, and recreation that relate to exposure to pathogens. Food- and waterborne diseases flourish in warmer months because of better incubation temperatures for the multiplication of the agent and recreational exposures of the host, whereas respiratory agents appear to benefit from increased opportunities for airborne and droplet transmission in the closed and closer living environments of the winter. In United States hospitals, the frequency of hospital-acquired *Acinetobacter* spp. infections is increasing in critical care units and has been shown to be seasonal in nature (33). The seasonal variation in the incidence of this pathogen is thought to be due to changes in climate—summer weather increases the number of *Acinetobacter* species in the natural environment and transmission of this microorganism in the hospital environment during this season (33).

Within healthcare settings, the components of the agent, host, and environment triad interact in a variety of ways to produce healthcare-associated infections. For example, the intensive care unit is now considered the area of highest risk in the transmission of healthcare-associated infections in United States hospitals (34). Moreover, methicillin-resistant *S. aureus* (MRSA), VRE, and ceftazidime-resistant *Pseudomonas aeruginosa* are endemic in many intensive care units in these hospitals (34). More recently, the emergence of vancomycin-resistant *S. aureus* in United States institutions has highlighted the unwelcome but inevitable reality that this pathogen may become endemic in acute care settings (35). A complex interaction of factors, such as inadequate hand washing and infection control practices among healthcare workers, fluctuating staffing levels, an unexpected increase in patient census relative to staffing levels in the intensive care unit, or an unexpected increase in the number of severely ill patients with multiple invasive devices could contribute to the acquisition of hospital infections caused by one of these endemic microorganisms (36,37). Adding to the complexity of the process would be the transmission of the agent from host to healthcare worker, healthcare worker to healthcare worker, and host to environment. Thus, acceptable measures for the prevention and control of healthcare-associated infection dictate that the hospital epidemiologist look at and analyze the interrelationships among all components of the triad of agent, host, and environment.

It is well known that the social environment is extremely significant in determining personal behavior that affects the direct transmission of agents, such as HIV via breast milk in regions of high HIV endemicity, gram-negative microorganisms via artificial nails worn by healthcare workers in United States intensive care units (38), and pathogens that cause sexually transmitted diseases. What must be understood to be equally relevant is the impact of other factors in the social environment, such as the distribution of and access to medical resources; the use of preventive services (39,40); the enforcement of codes in food preparation, infection control practices, or occupational health practices; the extent of acceptance of breast-feeding for children (41,42); and the acceptance of advice on the appropriate use of antimicrobials (43–45). Also, there must be an appreciation by patients, relatives, and healthcare workers alike that extreme at-risk patients (e.g., those born very prematurely, or who have severe congenital abnormalities, or the very elderly, or those with premorbid end-stage disease), who have numerous indwelling medical devices, or who undergo multiple invasive procedures or surgeries, would be particularly susceptible to unpreventable healthcare-associated infections. There must be an informed and ethically sound willingness to reject the extraordinary application of medical technology, including the inappropriate or repeated use of resistance-inducing antimicrobials when clinical evidence and experience suggest that the condition of the sick patient is untreatable.

Special Environments

Microenvironments, including military barracks, dormitories, chronic disease institutions, ambulatory surgery centers and dialysis units, and acute care hospitals, provide special venues for agent–host interactions. Historically, these institutional environments provided the epidemic experience that drove the development and acceptance of infection control programs. Acute care hospitals, especially those offering regional secondary and tertiary care, remain the dominant examples of these environments. Changing patterns of outpatient practice and technical advances in medical care have combined to focus increasingly severely diseased and injured populations in these centers. Data from the National Nosocomial Infections Surveillance (NNIS) system, and Project Intensive Care Antimicrobial Resistance Epidemiology (ICARE) demonstrate that the changing healthcare environment is resulting in larger intensive care unit populations (34). Special units for intensive medical or surgical care for extensive burns, trauma, transplantation, and cancer chemotherapy frequently house patients with little resistance to infection and infectious diseases (46). In these patients, reduced inocula of pathogens are required to cause infection, infection may take place at unusual sites, and usually nonpathogenic agents may cause serious disease and death. Frequent opportunistic infections in these patients require repeated, broad, and extended therapy with multiple antimicrobials, leading to increasingly resistant resident microbial populations (34,45).

The emergence or reemergence in this setting of pathogens resistant to all available antimicrobials is taking place, a situation that has not been present since the 1950s (47). For example, over 80% of VRE isolates in some institutions are resistant to all available antimicrobials (48). Similarly, spiraling healthcare costs have been the major factor leading to the current shift toward managed care in the United States. The process has resulted in the downsizing of hospital work forces to cut costs and reduce patient charges. As a result, more severely ill patients are being managed or treated as outpatients or at home. For example, central venous catheters may be placed in the hospital, and kept *in situ* for long-term home infusion therapy. The trade-off is minimum exposure to the hospital environment with decreased costs to the patient. On the other hand, a patient with a central venous catheter in the home environment may be potentially at risk of bloodstream infections due to contamination of lines, dressing, and infusates in a care environment where infection control practices are not as well understood, practiced, or regulated.

SPECTRUM OF DISEASE

Once colonization or infection is established in a susceptible host, the agent may enter a silent or latent period during which there is no clinical or usual laboratory evidence of its presence. Thereafter, the host may manifest signs and symptoms of mild disease without disability, may have a rapid or slow progression of disease, or may progress to either temporary or chronic disability, or, ultimately, death. Alternatively, the patient may have a complete recovery and return to health without sequelae. In other instances, the entire process may be inapparent or subclinical without evidence of disability or disease. Subclinical cases may be recognized through laboratory testing of blood or other body fluids of the host. These tests may indicate evidence of abnormal cellular function (abnormal liver function tests), the presence of an immune response to infection (antibody to hepatitis B virus), the presence of antigens characteristic of the microorganism (positive test for hepatitis B virus antigen), or the presence of the microorganism itself.

The ability to diagnose an infection or disease is obviously easier in clinical cases and much easier in severe clinical cases wherein the typical signs and symptoms of the disease are apparent and routine tests are diagnostic of the agent. The ratio of clinical to subclinical infections varies widely by agent and is influenced by certain host factors, such as age and immune status. Certain agents may be associated with a variety of different syndromes that depend on age and vaccination status of the host, previous infection with the agent, and agent-related mechanisms that remain unclear. Polio virus is less likely to appear as a paralytic syndrome in children, and Coxsackie virus B infections may appear as myocarditis one year and more prominently as meningoencephalitis the next. Respiratory syncytial virus infections may appear as bronchiolitis in infants and as a common cold syndrome in their older caregivers. Since the ability to diagnose an infection or disease caused by a specific pathogen depends partly on the degree to which typical symptoms and physical signs develop in patients, variation in the clinical manifestation of disease underscores the difficulty in establishing causation, the importance of clinical awareness of syndromic variations of certain infections, and the importance of confirmatory laboratory evidence to precisely identify the causal agent associated with syndromes of disease outbreaks. Evans (49) provides a detailed and excellent review of the principles and issues in establishing causation in infection and disease.

MECHANISMS OF TRANSMISSION

For infection to take place, microorganisms must be transferred from a reservoir to an acceptable entry site on a susceptible host in sufficient numbers (the infecting dose) for multiplication of the agent to take place. The infecting dose of a microorganism may depend in varying degrees on the infectivity, pathogenicity, and virulence of the microorganism itself. The entire transmission process constitutes the chain of infection. Within the healthcare setting, the reservoir of an agent may include patients themselves, healthcare workers, tap water, soap dispensers, mechanical ventilators, intravenous devices and infusates, multidose vials, and other factors in the environment.

Direct transmission from another host (healthy or ill) or from an environmental reservoir or surface by direct contact or direct large-droplet spread of infectious secretions is the simplest route of agent spread. Examples of direct-contact transmission routes include kissing (infectious mononucleosis), shaking hands [common cold (rhinovirus)], or other skin contact (e.g., contamination of a wound with staphylococci or *Enterococcus* spp. during trauma, surgical procedures, or dressing changes). Transmission of *Neisseria meningitidis*, group A streptococcus, or the respiratory syncytial virus (an important cause of respiratory infection in young children worldwide) by large respiratory droplets that travel only a few feet is regarded as a special case of direct-contact transmission.

Vertical transmission of infection from mother to fetus is another form of direct-contact transmission that may occur through the placenta during pregnancy (e.g., HIV, rubella virus, hepatitis B virus, or parvovirus), by direct contact of the infant with the birth canal during childbirth (group B streptococci), or via breast milk (HIV).

Indirect transmission is the most common mechanism of transfer of the agents that cause healthcare-associated infections, and frequently takes place by the mechanical transfer of the agent on the hands of one or more healthcare workers. Indirect contact transmission may also be vehicle borne via contaminated inanimate objects (fomites), such as toys and work surfaces, contaminated food, biologic fluids (e.g., respiratory, salivary, gastrointestinal, or genital secretions, blood, urine, stool), or on shared medical devices. Rapid dissemination of agents, such as respiratory syncytial virus or the influenza virus, may occur in day-care centers through salivary contamination of shared toys and games. *C. difficile* is an important diarrheal agent transmitted from patient to patient in acute care hospitals. Its transmission is abetted by its spore-forming ability to survive in the environment, and its selection and promotion in patients by the repeated and prolonged use of certain antimicrobials (50,51). The continuing presence of *Pseudomonas* species and other gram-negative rods in potable water supplies acts as an important reservoir for these agents and a readily available source for hand transmission to patients, especially the severely ill (52,53). Medical devices contaminated with blood-borne pathogens, including hepatitis B and C viruses, cytomegalovirus, and HIV, are sources of infection for both patients and medical care personnel in healthcare institutions (54).

Airborne transmission is another indirect method of transfer. Entities transmitted by this method include droplet nuclei (1–5 μm) that remain suspended in air for long periods, spores, and shed microorganisms. The airborne transfer of droplet nuclei is the principal route of transmission of *Mycobacterium tuberculosis*, varicella (chicken pox), and measles (55,56). Treatment and control of contaminated air is a complex and expensive process, and when it became widely (and falsely) assumed that tuberculosis was a disease about to be eliminated, many institutions discontinued or did not replace their air-controlled facilities for dealing with the transmission of this type of agent. The reemergence of tuberculosis in immunocompromised individuals and the occurrence of epidemics that affected both patients and personnel were partly a result of these unwise decisions (57,58). Spores of certain fungi, such as *Aspergillus* spp., can be carried over enormous distances in hospitals from environmental reservoirs in soil and certain building sites to the lungs of highly immunocompromised patients, especially those with hematologic malignancies (59). The transmission of *Legionella* spp. through the air in droplet nuclei from cooling tower emissions, and from environmental water sites, such as air-conditioning systems, central humidifiers, and respiratory humidification devices, is another recent important example of this type of spread (60,61). Vector-borne transmission by arthropods or other insects is the final type of indirect transmission, and may be mechanical or biologic. In mechanical vector-borne transmission, the agent does not multiply or undergo physiologic changes in the vector; in biologic vector-borne transmission, the agent is modified within the host before being transmitted. Although the potential for microorganism carriage by arthropods or other insect vectors has been described (62), this type of transmission has been of little importance in the United States. In tropical countries with endemic vector-borne disease, including dengue, yellow fever, and malaria, this type of transmission is more important, requiring screening and other controls not required of medical structures in colder climates.

EPIDEMICS AND EPIDEMIC INVESTIGATION

Epidemics of infection and disease occur when an agent and an adequate number of susceptible individuals have sufficient contact for continuing transmission. An epidemic proceeds until the number of susceptible hosts in the population falls below the number at which the probability of contact, transmission, and infection becomes too low for the process to continue. This process has been studied and modeled, and the results have been compared to historical events (63,64). The modeling process has been most successful in reproducing epidemic conditions for infectious diseases of short incubation period in closed institutions such as boarding schools and chronic disease facilities. The variation in behavior, travel, and interactions in the more usual open populations has made modeling less successful in predicting onset, size, and duration of epidemics in these more complex environments. Factors that decrease transmission, such as distance (reducing contact), immunization, increasing levels of natural immunity following infection, and depression of agent reservoirs and viability by control programs or seasonal climatic change, will prevent further epidemic spread (21,65).

Epidemics may be common source or propagated. *Common source epidemics* occur when susceptible individuals have mutual exposure to the same agent in the same time period. If the exposure is continuous, as in a potable water supply contaminated with enteric microorganisms, infections and associated cases of diarrheal disease may appear sequentially, in a manner difficult to differentiate from the propagated epidemic described below. If the exposure to an infectious agent happens at a single event at a single time and place, as at an organization's picnic, it is called a *point source epidemic*. When this happens, the exposed have a similar incubation period, and the time from the common exposure event (a meal, in the case of the picnic) to the average onset of first symptoms is the natural incubation period of the agent. If the agent is known, its identified incubation period helps to define the time of the common event. For example, onset of symptoms of food poisoning cause by *S. aureus* usually occurs within 1 to 6 hours; symptoms due to *Shigella* spp. usually occur within 24 to 48 hours. The rash following infection with measles, one of the most highly communicable infectious diseases, usually appears about 14 days after infection.

Propagated epidemics occur when serial direct or indirect transmission takes place from susceptible host to susceptible host. This may occur in the form of person-to-person spread with a rapid sequence, or it may occur at a more leisurely pace in transmission of an agent with a longer incubation period from a carrier to a susceptible individual (e.g., transmission of hepatitis B from the hands of a colonized healthcare worker to a surgical wound) (66). In population epidemiology, the transmission may include serial nonhuman vectors and alternative hosts, as exemplified by the sylvan transmission of yellow fever virus from monkey to mosquito to human to mosquito to monkey or human and so on.

Steps in Investigating an Epidemic

The first and most critical step in the investigation is the ascertainment that an epidemic exists. This step assumes some previous information on the usual or endemic (baseline) rate of occurrence of the infection or disease in the population under study. When there is a perceived increase in the occurrence of an infection without reference to a baseline level, the aggregation of case-patients is known as a cluster. For this determination to take place, one must understand the etiology of the infection or disease. If the syndrome is unrecognized, a consensus definition or criteria for the condition must be established. This *case definition* must be established and fulfilled for each event that is counted as associated with the epidemic and should reflect the person, place, and time. The case definition may include a medical sign or symptom, a syndrome, an abnormal laboratory test (e.g., raised leukocyte count), the isolation of an etiologic agent (e.g., positive blood cultures for bacteremia), or the results of one of the serologic tests, such as those for serum immunoglobulin levels (e.g., immunoglobulin M group), which suggest recent infection. It is common in epidemics of unknown etiology to include combinations of clinical and laboratory findings as parts of a case definition. Depending on the data available at the onset of an investigation, a case definition may include classification of the ill as (a) definite cases, (b) probable cases, or (c) possible cases. Once the case definition is established, the number of cases of the condition in the population must be identified or ascertained. Case ascertainment is accomplished through careful examination of medical or surgical records, laboratory reports, patient census listings, administrative staffing records, death certificates, or existing surveillance data, such as frequency of medical device or antimicrobial use. Case ascertainment may require information from sources other than the hospital records: clinics, health departments, public health laboratories, physicians' offices, schools, day-care centers, or workplaces. After case ascertainment, the next steps are to prepare a line listing of the patients who meet the case definition, construct an *epidemic curve* by plotting the cases (y-axis) over time (x-axis), and identify on a geographic map the location of the cases. The line listing should contain the basic demographic data and characteristics that are relevant to the outbreak, and should include the features of the outbreak in terms of person, place, and time that were established by the case definition. The epidemic curve can graphically suggest the temporal relationship between acquisition of infection or disease and index case, the existence of a common source, the incubation period of an infectious agent, or the mode of transmission. With an initial count of the cases completed, one can determine the rates of infection and illness in the population by age group, birth weight, gender, ethnic origin, religious affiliation, socioeconomic status, water supply, food ingestion, device use, treatment regimens, or other factors that appear to be historically associated with the individuals infected.

Based on this preliminary analysis of the available information, a hypothesis is generated. Using this hypothesis, one attempts to identify the high-risk population and to characterize the specific exposures associated with the infection or disease. To test the hypothesis, a case-control or cohort study can be performed. Early in the investigation, it is important to collect appropriate microbiologic specimens from both the ill and the well study-patients to attempt laboratory isolation of an etiologic agent or to serologically define new specific host immune function. Not all cases can be expected to fit the hypothesis because, for many agents, a background rate of endemic disease must be assumed. Using the hypothesis, one then searches for additional cases, both to increase the numbers for statistical study and to include individuals with mild or subclinical disease who otherwise might have escaped evaluation.

During the course of an outbreak investigation, additional studies might be necessary. These supplementary studies include the following: (a) epidemiologically directed culture surveys of patients or healthcare personnel implicated in the epidemiologic studies (e.g., nares, hand, or stool cultures) or of the environment (e.g., agar settle plates placed in locations that are epidemiologically linked to transmission) (67); (b) observational studies of infection control practices, invasive procedures, or hand-washing techniques among healthcare personnel in the outbreak setting; or (c) engineering studies, such as measurement of airflow rates, differential pressures across operating rooms, relative humidity of the environment, or water content of sheet-rock walls (68).

With all data collected and recorded, the next step is to prepare an interpretation of the events through simple univariate analytic procedures, controlling for confounding variables or effect modification using stratification or multivariate analysis, where appropriate. If the results of the data analyses support the hypothesis, plausible areas for immediate intervention are sought; if not, the data are reviewed and reevaluated for alternative hypotheses, and another round of testing and analyses is begun. Based on the analysis and supported hypothesis, intervention and follow-up programs are outlined, including both short-term and long-term control measures. At the conclusion of the investigation, a preliminary report of the findings, immediate control measures, and other recommendations are presented to the relevant personnel.

Finally the investigation is presented in a formal report to local and regional authorities, to public health agencies, and to medical and public groups, indicating the methods, findings, nature of the outbreak, risk factors, and recommendations for future prevention and control. [For additional details on epidemic (outbreak) investigation, see Chapter 7.]

Thus, investigation of an epidemic requires a prioritized and systematic approach to the gathering and analysis of data, with careful attention to clinical and epidemiologic detail and correct interpretation of microbiologic information during each step of the investigation. The classic steps in the recommended investigation of an epidemic are outlined in Table 1.1. Published data from the Division of Healthcare Quality Promotion (DHQP), formerly the Hospital Infections Program of the CDC, suggest that the conduct of an epidemiologic investigation with subsequent epidemiology-directed laboratory investigations, such as environmental or personnel cultures, is generally a more accurate and less costly way for identifying the source and mode of transmission (12). In many DHQP outbreak investigations, subsequent laboratory studies have confirmed the epidemiologic findings, although on occasion epidemiologic findings alone without laboratory confirmation have delineated the mode of transmission in a hospital outbreak (69). Given the complexity and skill involved in obtaining and processing appropriate environmental or clinical specimens, routine culture surveys of patients, personnel, medications and other products, or the environment without a prior epidemiologic investigation may be misdirected or expensive, wasting laboratory resources without yielding results that are pertinent to the resolution of the outbreak, and are therefore not recommended.

TABLE 1.1. STEPS IN INVESTIGATING AN EPIDEMIC

Confirm the existence of an epidemic
Establish a case definition that reflects time, place, and person
Ascertain cases and create a line listing
Create an epidemic curve
Determine the extent and characteristics of cases by rapid survey
Formulate a working hypothesis
Test the hypothesis through epidemiologic studies
Initiate appropriate microbiology or other laboratory studies that are directed by the epidemiologic data
Analyze all cases for interpretation
Reassess hypothesis if not proven and initiate additional studies where warranted
Draw conclusions and inferences from investigation
Communicate with relevant personnel and recommend appropriate control and preventive measures (exit interviews and preliminary report)
Continue post-outbreak surveillance for new cases
Reevaluate control measures
Prepare a formal written report and disseminate findngs in a published manuscript

PREVENTION AND CONTROL

Measures for the prevention and control of healthcare-associated infections are directed at various links in the chain of infection. These include measures to (a) eliminate or contain the reservoirs of agents or to curtail the persistence (endemicity) of a microorganism in a specific setting, (b) interrupt the transmission of infection, or (c) protect the host against infection and disease. This approach mandates detailed knowledge of the epidemiology of infectious diseases in various healthcare settings.

Modifying Environmental Reservoirs

Measures aimed at modifying the reservoir depend on the nature of the reservoir: animate or inanimate. *Quarantine*, the restriction of movement of exposed individuals who have been exposed for the entire incubation period of the disease, is rarely used to control human disease in healthcare settings. Instead, active surveillance of exposed individuals through local health officers or (within the hospital) infection control professionals has replaced this method. However, in institutions, such as acute care hospitals or long-term care facilities, human reservoirs may be isolated from other susceptible individuals for the duration of their stay at the institution or their carriage of an agent (58, 70). Such human reservoirs include healthcare workers who are colonized with potential pathogens in their nares or hands, relatives who visit patients in intensive care units, and patients known to be colonized or infected with a particular healthcare pathogen and are transferred from one hospital to another or from one unit to another within a given institution. Since much disease is subclinical, it may be difficult to recognize and separate silent carriers from susceptible persons. Treatment of humans to eradicate their carriage of pathogens (e.g., VRE or MRSA) typically found in healthcare settings frequently fails (71,72). Commonly, removal of an individual healthcare worker, known to be a reservoir for a sentinel pathogen, from a healthcare setting with susceptible patients (e.g., bone marrow unit or surgical intensive care unit) is the only control option. Finally, ethical issues exist in exposing asymptomatic carriers or colonized but well persons to medical interventions that might have serious side effects, or render them susceptible to healthcare-associated infections or other adverse events.

In the medical care setting, reservoirs of an agent may be limited to the inanimate environment. Thus, control measures may include removing contaminated foodstuffs, intravenous infusates, or devices; handling sewage and waste appropriately; maintaining scrupulous aseptic techniques; or destroying the agent in the environmental niche (e.g., work surfaces in an intensive care unit or moisture reservoirs in mechanical ventilators) by chemical or physical means. In some healthcare settings, such as intensive care units, pathogens (e.g., VRE) may remain endemic or persistent despite identification and appropriate control of reservoirs. Such persistence may require periodic enhanced environmental cleaning (73) of the concerned intensive care unit to curtail the endemicity of the pathogen. It should be recalled that purification of potable water by filtration and chlorination; careful processing, inspection, and cooking of food; and improvements in housing, nutrition, and sanitary disposal of human waste have largely been responsible for the reduction in disease and death from infectious diseases in the industrialized world (74).

Interrupting Transmission

Many of the necessary features in the interruption of transmission are contained in the interventions for the inanimate environmental reservoirs listed above. The most important addition to these has been in the behavioral changes necessary to support improvements in the area of personal hygiene, specifically in the washing of hands between tasks in the preparation of food, caring for children, and caring for the sick (75,76). In the control of healthcare-associated infections, the use of appropriate barriers, including the use of gloves, gowns, and eye protection, has been emphasized to prevent the transmission of blood-borne pathogens (e.g., HIV and hepatitis B) between patients and healthcare workers, as has the use of high-filtration masks for protection from respiratory transmission, especially for tuberculosis (58,70,77). Nonetheless, the most important and valuable intervention for the prevention and control of healthcare-associated infections remains the routine washing of hands before, between, and after patient contacts in healthcare settings (76). One method commonly used to interrupt transmission of pathogens in healthcare settings is the isolation of patients known to be colonized or infected with a particular pathogen in a separate area so as to reduce the probability of transmission of infection to other patients. This method may include allocation of these cohorted patients to specific healthcare workers to avoid transmission of the pathogen by the healthcare workers themselves.

Protecting the Host

The risk of acquisition and transmission of infectious diseases among patient populations in healthcare settings are better characterized if the patients' immune status or immune response is known. Immunization is the most effective method of individual and community protection against epidemic diseases, and can be active or passive. Through active immunization, smallpox, one of the plagues of the world, has been eradicated (78,79), polio has been eliminated from large areas, including all of the Americas (80), and the other childhood diseases have been substantially reduced, including diphtheria, pertussis, tetanus, measles, mumps, rubella, and infections of *Haemophilus influenzae* type B (81–83). Since one of the main goals of epidemiology is to identify subgroups in the patient population that are at high risk for infection and disease, a knowledge of the vaccination status of patients is essential for the prevention of infection or disease. Institutional immunization programs have been recommended as part of the occupational health services of healthcare facilities for some time, but compliance for all healthcare workers has only recently come under mandate. Evaluation of patients for immunization during hospital admission is another program widely recommended but incompletely implemented. The residual endemic problems and periodic outbreaks of these vaccine-preventable diseases in both populations at large and in healthcare institutions have been largely the result of failure of the delivery programs for the vaccines. These have been due to poor funding, poor prioritization of the programs, the lack of political will, and the lack of organization of the vaccine effort—not to failure of the vaccine to immunize (40).

Passive immunization with hyperimmune or standard immunoglobulins is another intervention valuable in a small group of diseases, including certain genetic and acquired immunodeficiency diseases, primary antibody-deficiency disorders, hypogammaglobulinemia in chronic lymphocytic leukemia, measles, hepatitis A, varicella-zoster, hepatitis B, and immunodeficiency virus infections in children (83). Hyperimmune globulin preparations are obtained from blood plasma donor pools preselected for high antibody content against a specific antigen (e.g., hepatitis B immune globulin, varicella-zoster immune globulin, cytomegalovirus immune globulin, and respiratory syncytial virus immune globulin). Although an active search has been carried out for other immunomodulating drugs and biologics that heighten host immune function and protect the host from infection or disease (84,85), such treatment modalities have not played any significant role in the prevention and control of healthcare-associated infections.

Administering antimicrobials to ensure the presence of an antiinfective agent at the site of a potential infection is a more recent addition to the control programs protecting the host. The use of a single dose or short course of preoperative antimicrobials to reduce the probability of infection with agents commonly seen following certain procedures has become a standard part of surgical practice (86). During the nadir of immune and defense cell function following some cancer chemotherapy and certain therapeutic immunosuppression for transplantation, the use of local and systemic antiinfectives has reduced the duration of infection, reducing morbidity and death (87). The use of preprocedure antimicrobials in individuals with rheumatic heart disease is also a standard recommendation to prevent the most common types of bacterial endocarditis (88,89). Unfortunately, one of the side effects of repeated short courses of antimicrobials has been the appearance of significant resistance to these agents among pathogens in the medical care environment (34,90,91). This problem is aggravated by the misuse of antimicrobials for nonbacterial diseases by some practitioners, the over-the-counter sale of antimicrobials in many parts of the world, and the use of subtherapeutic doses of growth promoters in animal husbandry in the United States and other countries (92,93).

HEALTHCARE-ASSOCIATED INFECTIONS AND INFECTIOUS DISEASES

Inherent in all of the above measures for the prevention and control of healthcare-associated infections is the education of healthcare workers in infection control practices and procedures, and the implementation of surveillance measures to detect changes in the incidence and prevalence rates of infections caused by sentinel microorganisms commonly associated with healthcare-associated infections. The acute care hospital (inpatient, outpatient, and intensive care unit) settings and long-term care and home healthcare facilities provide special settings for the interaction of the agents of infection and patients and healthcare workers. The ongoing study of the basic epidemiologic features of agent–host interactions in these environments has led to recommendations for wide application of, and extensive testing of, surveillance, prevention, and control programs, which have proven highly successful. Descriptions of the special features of the investigations and interventions of these programs are the topics of the chapters to follow.

REFERENCES

1. Eyler JM. The conceptual origins of William Farr's epidemiology. In: Lilienfeld AM, ed. *Times, places, and persons. Aspects of the history of epidemiology.* Baltimore: Johns Hopkins University Press, 1980:1–21.
2. Lilienfeld DE, Lilienfeld AM. The French influence in the development of epidemiology. In: Lilienfeld AM, ed. *Times, places, and persons. Aspects of the history of epidemiology.* Baltimore: Johns Hopkins University Press, 1980:28–38.
3. LaForce FM. The control of infections in hospitals: 1750 to 1950. In: Wenzel RP, ed. *Prevention and control of nosocomial infections,* 2nd ed. Baltimore: Williams & Wilkins, 1993:1–12.
4. Felson JT, Wolarsky W. The hospital epidemiologist. *Hospitals* 1940; 14:41.
5. Fuerst JT, Lightman HS, James G. Hospital epidemiology. *JAMA* 1965;194:329.
6. Wenzel RP. Expanding role of hospital epidemiology: quality assurance. *Infect Control Hosp Epidemiol* 1989;10:255–256.
7. Hierholzer WJ Jr. The practice of hospital epidemiology. *Yale J Biol Med* 1982;55:225–230.
8. Wenzel RP, Pfaller MA. Infection control: the premiere quality assessment program in United States hospitals. *Am J Med* 1991;91(suppl 3b):275–315.
9. Donabedian A. Contribution of epidemiology to quality assessment and monitoring. *Infect Control Hosp Epidemiol* 1990;11:117–121.
10. McGowan JE, Weinstein RA. The role of the laboratory in control of nosocomial infection. In: Bennett JV, Brachman PS, eds. *Hospital infections,* 4th ed. Philadelphia: Lippincott-Raven, 1998:143–164.
11. Tompkins LS. The use of molecular methods in infectious diseases. *N Engl J Med* 1992;327:1290–1297.
12. Archibald LK, Jarvis WR. The role of the laboratory in outbreak investigations. *Semin Infect Dis* 2001;1:91–101.
13. Petersen NJ, Collins DE, Marshall JH. A microbiological assay technique for hands. *Health Lab Sci* 1973;10:18–22.
14. Chin J, ed. *Control of communicable diseases in man,* 17th ed. Washington, DC: American Public Health Association, 2000:567–579.
15. Evans AS. Epidemiological concepts. In: Evans AS, Brachman PS, eds. *Bacterial infections of humans,* 3rd ed. New York: Klewer Academic/ Plenum, 1998.
16. Last JM, Abramson JH. *A dictionary of epidemiology,* 4th ed. New York: Oxford Medical, 2000.
17. Hill AB, Mausner JS. *Principles of medical statistics.* New York: Oxford University Press, 1971.
18. Mausner JS, Kramer S, eds. *Mausner & Bahn epidemiology—an introductory text.* Philadelphia: WB Saunders, 1985.
19. Anderson RM. Transmission dynamics and control of infectious disease agents. In: Anderson RM, May RM, eds. *Population biology of infectious disease.* New York: Springer-Verlag, 1982:149–177.
20. Gordis L. *Epidemiology,* 2nd ed. Philadelphia: WB Saunders, 2000.
21. Fox JP, Elveback L, Gatewood L, et al. Herd immunity. *Am J Epidemiol* 1971;94:171–189.
22. Emori TG, Gaynes R. An overview of nosocomial infections, including the role of the microbiology laboratory. *Clin Microbiol Rev* 1993;6: 428–442.
23. Anderson KF, Coulter JR, Keynes DR. Staphylococcal nasal carriage in mothers, babies, and staff in a maternity hospital. *J Hyg* 1961;59: 15–27.
24. Griffith SJ, Nathan C, Selander RK, et al. The epidemiology of Pseudomonas aeruginosa in oncology patients in a general hospital. *J Infect Dis* 1989;160:1030–1036.

25. Alary M, Joly TR. Factors contributing to the contamination of hospital water distribution systems by legionellae. *J Infect Dis* 1992;165: 565–569.
26. Archibald LK, Corl A, Shah B, et al. *Serratia marcescens* outbreak associated with extrinsic contamination of 1% chlorxylenol soap. *Infect Control Hosp Epidemiol* 1997;18:704–709.
27. Morse LJ, Schonbeck LF. Hand lotions a potential nosocomial hazard. *N Engl J Med* 1968:278:376–378.
28. Niederman MS. Bacterial adherence as a mechanism of airway colonization. *Eur J Clin Microbiol Infect Dis* 1989;8:15–20.
29. Heard SR, O'Farrell S, Holland D, et al. The epidemiology of *Clostridium difficile* with use of a typing scheme: nosocomial acquisition and cross-infection among immunocompromised patients. *J Infect Dis* 1986;153:159–162.
30. Hoeprich PD, ed. *Infectious diseases.* Hagerstown: Harper & Row, 1972:40.
31. Scrimshaw NS. Malnutrition and nosocomial infection. *Infect Control Hosp Epidemiol* 1989;10:191–193.
32. Cohen S, Tyrell AJ, Smith AP. Psychological stress and susceptibility to the common cold. *N Engl J Med* 1991;325:606–612.
33. McDonald LC, Banerjee SN, Jarvis WR. Seasonal variation of Acinetobacter infections: 1987–1996. Nosocomial Infections Surveillance System. *Clin Infect Dis* 1999;29:1133–1137.
34. Archibald LK, Phillips L, Monnet D, et al. Antimicrobial resistance in inpatients and outpatients in the United States: the increasing importance of the intensive care unit. *Clin Infect Dis* 1997;24:211–215.
35. Centers for Disease Control and Prevention. *Staphylococcus aureus* resistant to vancomycin—United States, 2002. *MMWR* 2002;51: 565–567.
36. Archibald LK, Manning ML, Bell LM et. al. Patient density, nurse-to-patient ratio, and nosocomial infection risk in a pediatric intensive care unit. *Pediatr Infect Dis J* 1997;16:1045–1048.
37. Manning ML, Archibald LK, Bell LM, et al. Serratia marcescens transmission in a pediatric intensive care unit: a multifactorial occurrence. *Am J Infect Control* 2001;29:115–119.
38. Molenaar RL, Crutcher JM, San Joaquin VH, et al. A prolonged outbreak of *Pseudomonas aeruginosa* in a neonatal intensive care unit: did staff fingernails play a role in disease transmission? *Infect Control Hosp Epidemiol* 2000;21:77–79.
39. Centers for Disease Control and Prevention. Recommendations of the Advisory Committee on Immunization Practices (ACIP): use of vaccines and immune globulins in persons with altered immunocompetence. *MMWR* 1993;42(RR-4):1–18.
40. Hinman AP, Orenstein WA, Mortimer EA. When, where, and how do immunizations fail? *Ann Epidemiol* 1992;2:805–812.
41. Zembo CT. Breastfeeding. *Obstet Gynecol Clin North Am* 2002;29: 51–76.
42. Dolan SA, Boesman-Finkelstein M, Finkelstein RA. Antimicrobial activity of human milk against pediatric pathogens. *J Infect Dis* 1986; 154:722–725.
43. Javaloyas M, Garcia-Somoza D, Gudiol F. Epidemiology and prognosis of bacteremia: a 10-year study in a community hospital. *Scand J Infect Dis* 2002;34:436–441.
44. Hughes WT, Armstrong D, Bodey GP, et al. 1997 guidelines for the use of antimicrobial agents in neutropenic patients with unexplained fever. *Clin Infect Dis* 1997;25:551–573.
45. Goldmann DA, Weinstein RA, Wenzel RP, et al. Strategies to prevent and control the emergence and spread of antimicrobial-resistant microorganisms in hospitals: a challenge to hospital leadership. *JAMA* 1996; 275:234–240.
46. Pittet D, Harbarth SJ. The intensive care unit. In: Bennett JV, Brachman PS, eds. *Hospital infections,* 4th ed. Philadelphia: Lippincott-Raven, 1998:381–402.
47. Institute of Medicine, National Academy of Sciences. Committee on emerging threats to health. In: Lederberg J, Shope RE, Oaks SC, eds. *Emerging infections: microbial threats to health in the United States.* Washington, DC: National Academy Press, 1992:1–65.
48. Frieden TR, Munsiff SS, Low DE, et al. Emergence of vancomycin-resistant enterococci in New York City. *Lancet* 1993;10(342):76–79.
49. Evans AS. *Causation and disease: a chronological journey.* New York: Plenum, 1993.
50. Heard SR, O'Farrell S, Holland D, et al. The epidemiology of *Clostridium difficile* with use of a typing scheme: nosocomial acquisition and cross-infection among immunocompromised patients. *J Infect Dis* 1986;153:159–162.
51. Johnson S, Gerding DN. *Clostridium difficile*-associated diarrhea. *Clin Infect Dis* 1998;26:1027–1034.
52. Griffith SJ, Nathan C, Selander RK, et al. The epidemiology of *Pseudomonas aeruginosa* in oncology patients in a general hospital. *J Infect Dis* 1989;160:1030–1036.
53. Weinstein RA, Nathan C, Gruensfelder R. Epidemic aminoglycoside resistance in gram-negative bacilli: epidemiology and mechanisms. *J Infect Dis* 1980;141:338–345.
54. Centers for Disease Control and Prevention. Updated U.S. Public Health Service guidelines for the management of occupational exposures to HBV, HCV, and HIV and recommendations for postexposure prophylaxis. *MMWR* 2001:50(RR-11):1–43.
55. Riley RL, Mills CC, O'Grady F, et al. Infectiousness of air from a tuberculosis ward. *Am Rev Respir Dis* 1962;85:511–525.
56. Sepkowitz KA. Occupationally acquired infections in healthcare workers. Part I. *Ann Intern Med* 1996;125:826–834.
57. Centers for Disease Control and Prevention. Nosocomial transmission of multidrug-resistant tuberculosis to healthcare workers and HIV-infected patients in an urban hospital in Florida. *MMWR* 1990;39: 718–722.
58. Centers for Disease Control and Prevention. Guidelines for preventing the transmission of *Mycobacterium tuberculosis* in health-care facilities, 1994. *MMWR* 1994;43(RR-13):1–132.
59. Hahn T, Cummings KM, Michalek AM, et al. Efficacy of high-efficiency particulate air filtration in preventing aspergillosis in immunocompromised patients with hematologic malignancies. *Infect Control Hosp Epidemiol* 2002;23:525–531.
60. Centers for Disease Control and Prevention. Sustained transmission of nosocomial Legionnaires disease. *MMWR* 1997;46:416–421.
61. Alary M, Joly TR. Factors contributing to the contamination of hospital water distribution systems by legionellae. *J Infect Dis* 1992;165: 565–569.
62. Daniel M, Sramova V, Absolonova D, et al. Arthropods in a hospital and their potential significance in the epidemiology of hospital infections. *Folia Parasitol* 1992;39:159–170.
63. Anderson RM. Transmission dynamics and control of infectious agents. In: Anderson RM, May RM, eds. *Population biology of infectious disease.* New York: Springer-Verlag, 1982:149–176.
64. Cvjetanovic B, Grab B, Dixon H. Epidemiological models of poliomyelitis and measles and their application in the planning of immunization programmes. *Bull WHO* 1982;60:405–422.
65. Anderson RM, May RM. Directly transmitted infectious diseases: control by vaccination. *Science* 1982;215:1053–1060.
66. Harpaz R, Von Seidlein L, Averhoff FM, et al. Transmission of hepatitis B virus to multiple patients from a surgeon without evidence of inadequate infection control. *N Engl J Med* 1996;334:549–554.
67. Sinkowitz-Cochran R, Jarvis WR. Epidemiologic approach to outbreak investigations. *Semin Infect Control* 2001;1:85–90.
68. Kainer M, Keshavarz H, Jensen B, et al. Surgery, air, water damage, and curvularia—is being curvaceous worth the price? Oral presentation (abstract 234) at the 12th annual scientific meeting of the Society for Healthcare Epidemiology of America, Salt Lake City, Utah, April 6–9, 2002.
69. Archibald LK, Ramos M, Arduino MJ, et al. *Enterobacter cloacae* and *Pseudomonas aeruginosa* polymicrobial bloodstream infections traced to extrinsic contamination of a dextrose multidose vial. *J Pediatr* 1998; 133:640–644.
70. Garner JS, Simmons BP. CDC guideline for isolation precautions in hospitals. *Am J Infect Control* 1984;12:103–163.
71. Hachem R, Raad I. Failure of oral antimicrobial agents in eradicating gastrointestinal colonization with vancomycin-resistant enterococci. *Infect Control Hosp Epidemiol* 2002;23:43–44.
72. Hayakawa t, Hayashidera T, Katsura S, et al. Nasal mupirocin treat-

ment of pharynx-colonized methicillin-resistant *Staphylococcus aureus*: preliminary study with 10 carrier infants. *Pediatr Int* 2000;42:67–70.
73. Byers KE, Durbin LJ, Simonton BM, et al. Disinfection of hospital rooms contaminated with vancomycin-resistant *Enterococcus faecium. Infect Control Hosp Epidemiol* 1998;19:261–264.
74. McKeown T. *The role of medicine. Dream, mirage, or nemesis?,* 2nd ed. Princeton: Princeton University Press, 1979:91–113.
75. Jenner EA, Watson PWB, Miller L, et al. Explaining hand hygiene practice: an extended application of the theory of planned behaviour. *Psychol Health Med* 2002;7:311–326.
76. Boyce JM, Pittet D. Guideline for hand hygiene in health-care settings: recommendations of the healthcare infection control practices advisory committee and the HICPAC/SHEA/APIC/IDSA Hand Hygiene Task Force. *MMWR* 2002;51(RR-16):1–44.
77. Centers for Disease Control and Prevention. Leads from the MMWR. Update: universal precautions for prevention of transmission of human immunodeficiency virus, hepatitis B virus and other bloodborne pathogens in health-care settings. *JAMA* 1988;37:377–388.
78. Henderson DA. The history of smallpox eradication. In: Lilienfeld AM, ed. *Times, places, and persons. Aspects of the history of epidemiology.* Baltimore: Johns Hopkins University Press, 1980:99–108.
79. Centers for Disease Control and Prevention. Notice to readers: 25th anniversary of the last case of naturally acquired smallpox. *MMWR* 2002;51:952.
80. Centers for Disease Control and Prevention. Progress toward global eradication of poliomyelitis, *MMWR* 2002;51:253–256.
81. Centers for Disease Control and Prevention. Public health burden of vaccine-preventable diseases among adults: standards for adult immunization practice. *MMWR* 1990;39:725–729.
82. Centers for Disease Control and Prevention. Recommended childhood and adolescent immunization schedule. *MMWR* 2003;52:Q1–Q4.
83. Centers for Disease Control and Prevention. General recommendations on immunization. *MMWR* 2002;51(RR-02):1–36.
84. Lieschke GJ, Burgess AW. Colony stimulating factor and granulocyte macrophage colony-stimulating factor. *N Engl J Med* 1992;327:28–35.
85. Peters WP. Use of cytokines during prolonged neutropenia associated with autologous bone marrow transplantation. *Rev Infect Dis* 1991;13: 992–996.
86. Mangram A, Horan T, Pearson ML, et al. Guideline for prevention of surgical site infection, 1999. Hospital Infection Control Practices Advisory Committee. *Infect Control Hosp Epidemiol* 1999;20:250–278.
87. Clasener HAL, Vollaard EJ, van Saene HKF. Long-term prophylaxis of infection by selective decontamination in leukopenia and in mechanical ventilation. *Rev Infect Dis* 1987;9:295–328.
88. Dajani AS, Taubert KA, Wilson W, et al. Prevention of bacterial endocarditis: recommendation by the American Heart Association. *JAMA* 1997;277:1794–1801.
89. Durack DT. Prevention of bacterial endocarditis. *N Engl J Med* 1995; 332:38–44.
90. McGowan JE Jr. Antimicrobial resistance in hospital organisms and its relation to antibiotic use. *Rev Infect Dis* 1983;5:1033–1048.
91. Gaynes R. The impact of antimicrobial use on the emergence of antimicrobial-resistant bacteria in hospitals. *Infect Dis Clin North Am* 1997; 11:757–765.
92. Spika JS, Waterman SH, Soo Hoo GW, et al. Chloramphenicol-resistant Salmonella Newport traced through hamburger to dairy farms. *N Engl J Med* 1987;316:565–569.
93. McDonald LC, Rossiter S, Mackinson C, et al. Quinupristin-dalfopristin-resistant *Enterococcus faecium* on chicken and in human stool specimens. *N Engl J Med* 2001;345:1155–1160.

2

MODERN QUANTITATIVE EPIDEMIOLOGY IN THE HOSPITAL

JONATHAN FREEMAN
JEROME I. TOKARS

I often say that when you can measure what you are speaking about, and express it in numbers, you know something about it; but when you cannot express it in numbers, your knowledge is of a meager and unsatisfactory kind; it may be the beginning of knowledge, but you have scarcely, in your thoughts, advanced to the stage of Science, whatever the matter may be.—Lord Kelvin

The job of the hospital epidemiologist is an intensely political one, into which we can occasionally interject some science.—Jonathan Freeman

Epidemiology is the study of the occurrence of illness in human populations, and epidemiologic understanding advances through making comparisons. The study of epidemiology is essential, as there is currently extreme political pressure to measure and compare anything possibly related to the quality of healthcare. Hospital epidemiology is still in its infancy compared with chronic disease epidemiology, and the epidemiology of the measurement of quality is younger still. Two of the first attempts of the Center for Medicare and Medicaid Services (CMS, formerly the Health Care Financing Administration), a governmental agency, to measure quality were comparisons of crude death rates among hospitals and comparisons of crude self-reported hospital infection rates. As is discussed later, both attempts failed embarrassingly and had to be withdrawn. In each case, the leap to comparison occurred without sufficient understanding of the principles of epidemiology, particularly misclassification and confounding. The study of epidemiology is essential to avoid the propagation of further nonsense in the name of hospital epidemiology and quality assurance, and this chapter defines and addresses the important epidemiologic issues. After all, epidemiology is just quantified common sense.

HISTORY OF EPIDEMIOLOGY

A famous early example of applied epidemiology is the work of Dr. John Snow, a physician in London during the cholera epidemic of 1855 (1). At that time, the germ theory of disease had not been accepted and the pathogen causing cholera, *Vibrio cholera*, was unknown. Whereas the prevailing view during this period was that disease was caused by a miasm or cloud, Snow inferred from epidemiologic evidence that cholera was a waterborne illness. He constructed a spot map of cholera cases and noted a cluster of cases near a water pump on London's Broad Street, the so-called Broad Street pump. This early use of a spot map to find the putative cause of an outbreak is an example of descriptive epidemiology. He also performed several analytic studies, noting that the rate of cholera was higher for people who obtained water from more polluted areas of the Thames. His well-known intervention was to remove the handle from the Broad Street pump, thereby preventing use of this contaminated water, after which cases of cholera in the vicinity were said to have decreased. This example illustrates that epidemiologists can define the mechanism of disease spread and institute control measures before the agent causing disease is discovered. More recent examples of this power of epidemiology include Legionnaire's disease and human immunodeficiency virus (HIV) disease; for both diseases the mechanism of spread and means of prevention were inferred by epidemiologists before the microbe was discovered in the laboratory.

DESCRIPTIVE VERSUS ANALYTIC EPIDEMIOLOGY

In descriptive epidemiology, we describe characteristics of the cases and generate hypotheses. The line list of cases, case series, epidemic curves, and spot maps are examples. In analytic epidemiology, we use comparison groups, calculate statistics, and test hypotheses. Many outbreaks and other problems in healthcare epidemiology can be solved by thoughtful examination of descriptive data without the use of analytic epidemiology. However, the increasingly complex nature of healthcare and associated illness demands that we have a firm grounding in analytic or quantitative epidemiology, which is the main focus of this chapter.

MEASURES OF FREQUENCY

Proportions (synonyms are *probability, risk,* and *percentage*) are the simplest way to represent how often something occurs. A proportion is the ratio of a part to the whole, i.e., the numerator of the ratio is included in the denominator. The proportion with disease is the number of people who get the disease divided by the total number at risk for the disease, i.e., proportion ill = number ill/(number ill + number well). The probability of pulling an ace from a deck of cards is 4/52 = 7.7%. Proportions can be represented by a fraction (e.g., 0.077) or a percentage (e.g., 7.7%) and can range from 0 to 1.0 or from 0% to 100%. Proportions cannot be greater than 1.0 or 100% since, using proportions, each entry in the denominator can have at most one entry in the numerator. A proportion is unitless, because the numerator and denominator have the same units. The proportion is the measure of frequency used in cohort studies and to calculate the relative risk.

Odds represent the ratio of a part to the remainder, or the probability that an event will occur divided by the probability that it will not occur. Unlike in proportions, the numerator of the ratio is not included in the denominator. The odds of a disease occurring equal the number of people with the disease divided by the number without the disease, i.e., odds of illness = number ill/number well. The odds of pulling an ace from a deck of cards are 4/48 = 8.3%. Note that the odds of illness are always higher than a corresponding proportion ill, because the denominator is smaller for odds. Odds are unitless and have bounds of zero to infinity. Odds are used in case-control studies and to calculate the odds ratio.

A rate, in contrast to proportions and odds, has different units of measure in the numerator and denominator, as in 55 miles/hour or 20 nosocomial infections/1,000 observed patient-days. A rate can have any value from zero to infinity. Rates are used in incidence density analyses.

Common Usage

The proportion ill, especially in outbreaks, is often called an "attack rate," although strictly speaking it is a misnomer to refer to a proportion as a rate. This chapter follows common usage in using the following terms interchangeably with proportion ill: percent ill, attack rate, and rate of illness.

Cumulative Incidence versus Incidence Density

In a cumulative incidence study, time at risk is not taken into account; the denominator is the total number of persons at risk, and the proportion with disease (or proportion with potential risk factors for disease) is calculated. The cohort and case-control studies presented in the following section are examples of cumulative incidence. In an incidence density study, time at risk is accounted for; the denominator is person-time at risk and a rate of illness (e.g., infections per 1,000 patient-days) is calculated. This type of study is considered later in this chapter.

BASIC STUDY DESIGN

There are three types of analytic study: cohort, case-control, and cross-sectional. The goal of analytic epidemiologic studies is to discover a statistical association between cases of disease and possible causes of disease, called *exposures.* A first step in any such study is the careful definition of terms used, especially defining what clinical and laboratory characteristics are required to indicate a case of disease.

The Cohort Study and Relative Risk

Prospective Cohort Study

There are several subtypes of cohort study, but all have certain common features and are analyzed the same way. In the prospective cohort study, we identify a group of subjects (e.g., persons or patients) who do not have the disease of interest. Then we determine which subjects have some potential risk factor (exposure) for disease. We follow the subjects forward in time to see which develop disease. The purpose is to determine whether disease is more common in those with the exposure ("exposed") than without the exposure ("nonexposed"). Those who develop disease are called "cases," and those who do not develop disease are "noncases" or "controls."

A classic example of a prospective cohort study is the Framingham study of cardiovascular disease, begun in 1948 (1). Framingham is a city about 20 miles from Boston with a population of about 300,000, which was considered to be representative of the United States population. A random sample of 5,127 men and women, age 30 to 60 years and without evidence of cardiovascular disease, was enrolled in 1948. At each subject's enrollment, researchers recorded gender and the presence or absence of many exposures, including smoking, obesity, high blood pressure, high cholesterol, low level of physical activity, and family history of cardiovascular disease. This cohort was then followed forward in time by examining the subjects every 2 years and daily checking of the only local hospital for admissions for cardiovascular disease.

Note several features of this study. The study was truly prospective in that it was started before the subjects developed disease. Subjects were followed over many years and monitored to determine if disease occurred, i.e., if they became "cases." This is an incidence study, in which only new cases of disease were counted (because persons with cardiovascular disease in 1948 were not eligible for enrollment). In an incidence study, it is necessary to specify the study period, i.e., how long the subjects were allowed to be at risk before we looked to see whether they had developed disease.

The Framingham study allowed investigators to determine risk factors for a number of cardiovascular disease outcomes, such as anginal chest pain, myocardial infarction (heart attack), death due to myocardial infarction, and stroke. One finding of this study was that smokers had a higher rate of myocardial infarction than nonsmokers. An advantage of this study design is that it is very flexible, in that the effect of many different exposures on many different outcome variables can be determined. The disadvantages are the time, effort, and cost required.

Relative Risk

Performing hospital surveillance for surgical site infections (SSIs) is an example of a prospective cohort study. Assume that

TABLE 2.1. THE 2 × 2 TABLE AND ASSOCIATED FORMULAS

Exposure		Disease: Yes	Disease: No	
	Yes	a	b	$a + b = h_1$
	No	c	d	$c + d = h_2$
		$a + c = v_1$	$b + d = v_2$	

Exposed cases = a
Exposed noncases = b
Nonexposed cases = c
Nonexposed noncases = d
Total cases = $a + c = v_1$
Total noncases = $b + d = v_2$
Total exposed = $a + b = h_1$
Total nonexposed = $c + d = h_2$
Total subjects = $a + b + c + d = n$

Relative risk = % ill exposed/% ill nonexposed = $a/(a + b)/c/(c + d)$
Odds ratio = ad/bc

Expected values (where "ea" denotes "the expected value of cell a")
$ea = h_1v_1/n$
$eb = h_1v_2/n$
$ec = h_2v_1/n$
$ed = h_2v_2/n$

chi-square = $(a - ea)^2/ea + (b - eb)^2/eb + (c - ec)^2/ec + (d - ed)^2/ed$
Alternate "calculator" formula:
chi-square = $(ad - bc)^2(n - 1)/ (a + b)(c + d) (a + c)(b + d)$

during one year at hospital X, 100 patients had a certain operative procedure. Of these, 40 were wound class 2 to 3 and 60 were class 0 to 1. Note that wound class was determined before it was known which patients were going to develop SSI; this makes it a prospective cohort study. A subgroup or sample of patients was not selected; i.e., the entire group was studied. When the patients were followed forward in time, the following was found: of 40 patients with class 2 to 3 procedures, ten developed SSI; of 60 patients with class 0 to 1 procedures, three developed SSI.

Cohort study data are commonly presented in a 2 × 2 table format. The general form of the 2 × 2 table is shown in Table 2.1, and the 2 × 2 table for this SSI example is shown below. Notice that the columns denote whether disease (SSI) was present and the rows whether exposure (wound class 2 to 3) was present. In this example, exposed means being class 2 to 3 and nonexposed means being class 0 to 1. In the 2 × 2 table below, the total number of cases is 13, total noncases is 87, total exposed is 40, total nonexposed is 60, and total patients is 100.

Disease: Surgica Site Infection

Exposure		Yes	No	
	Class 2–3	10	30	40
	Class 0–1	3	57	60
		13	87	100

In the exposed group the proportion ill = 10/40 = 0.25 or 25%. In the nonexposed group the proportion ill = 3/60 = 0.05 or 5%. We compare the frequency of disease in the exposed versus nonexposed groups by calculating the relative risk (often called risk ratio). The relative risk of 5.0 means that patients in wound class 2 to 3 were five times more likely to develop SSI than were patients in wound class 0 to 1.

$$\text{Relative risk} = \frac{\%\,\text{ill exposed}}{\%\,\text{ill nonexposed}} = \frac{\%\,\text{ill class } 2-3}{\%\,\text{ill class } 0-1}$$

$$= \frac{a/(a+b)}{c/(c+d)} = \frac{25}{5} = 5.0$$

Retrospective Cohort Study

A retrospective cohort study is started after disease has developed. A study period (start date and stop date) is decided upon. Using patient records, we look back in time to identify a group (cohort) of subjects that did not have the disease at the start time. We then use patient records to determine whether each cohort member had a certain exposure. Again using patient records, we determine which cohort members developed disease during the study period. Finally, we calculate the percent with disease in those with the exposure and those without the exposure, and compare the two.

The following is an example of a retrospective cohort study based on the SSI example above. Hospital X noted that the overall SSI rate of 13% was higher than in previous years. We want to determine whether a new surgeon (surgeon A) was responsible for the increase. The prospective surveillance system did not routinely record the surgeon performing each procedure, so we pull the records from each procedure and record whether or not surgeon A was involved. We find that surgeon A operated on 20 patients, three of whom later developed SSI. Among the 80 other patients, ten developed SSI. The percent ill in the exposed group (surgeon A) = 3/20 = 15%. The percent ill for other surgeons (nonexposed) = 10/80 = 12.5%. The relative risk = 15%/12.5% = 1.2.

The interpretation is that patients operated on by surgeon A were 1.2 times (or 20%) more likely to develop disease than patients operated on by other surgeons. Factors to consider in deciding whether surgeon A is truly a cause of the problem are presented below (see Interpretation of Data, Including Statistical Significance and Causal Inference).

To review, this was a retrospective cohort study, since data on the exposure were collected from patient records after we knew which patients had developed SSI.

Observational versus Experimental Studies

Epidemiologic studies are generally observational, i.e., the investigator collects data but does not intervene in patient care. Patients, physicians, nurses, and random processes all play a part in assigning exposures in the hospital—only the hospital epidemiologist is left out. The goal of observational studies is to simulate the results of an experiment, had one been possible, as in an experiment of nature.

In an experimental study, a group (cohort) of subjects is identified, the investigator assigns some of them to receive treatment A (exposed) and the remainder to receive an alternate treatment B (nonexposed). The patients are followed forward in time, the cases of disease are recorded, and the rates of illness and relative risk are calculated as usual. The experimental study is a special type of a prospective cohort study where the two exposure groups are assigned by the investigator.

Epidemiology is a different sort of science from bench biology, and the closest we come to the type of standard experiment done in bench biology is in the conduct of experimental studies. In bench biology, the experimenter has control of the process and can create controls for the experiment, which usually lack one ingredient or another. Similarly, in an experimental study, the investigator can also assign the exposure (or nonexposure) according to some scheme, such as randomization.

There are three types of experimental studies. Clinical trials use patients who already have a disease as subjects, for example, in drug trials. Field trials use individuals without disease as subjects, as in a vaccine trial. Community intervention trials are field trials on a community-wide basis; an example would be fluoridation of the water supply. In all of these interventions, the experimenter can deal out the exposures in much the same way that a bench biologist allocates contrasting parts of an experiment to different vessels. The word *control* is appropriately used for a nonexposed vessel or subject in experimental studies. Experimental studies are nice to talk about, but they are relevant to only occasional situations in the hospital. They are mentioned here for contrast to the more usual observational studies in which the investigator is allowed only a relatively passive role.

Cohort Studies with Subjects Selected Based on Exposure

In this type of cohort study, subjects are selected based on exposure. We select two subgroups: one that is exposed and one that is nonexposed. Both groups are followed forward in time to see how many develop disease. Consider the SSI example and surgeon A above. We study all 20 patients operated on by surgeon A (exposed); of the 80 patients operated on by other surgeons, we randomly select 40 (nonexposed). Thus, only 60 patients of the original group of 100 are included in this study.

Note that this is a type of cohort study, not a case-control study. In a case-control study, the subjects are chosen based on whether or not they have disease. In this study, subjects were chosen based on whether or not they had exposure.

The disadvantage of this type of cohort study, where the subjects are selected based on exposure, is that only one exposure (i.e., the exposure that you selected subjects on) can be studied. However, this type of study is very useful for studying an uncommon exposure. In the SSI surveillance example used above, consider the situation if there had been 500 surgical procedures, and surgeon A had performed only 20 of them. If you performed a cohort study of the entire group, you would have to review 500 charts, which would waste time and effort. Instead, you could perform a cohort study of the 20 procedures performed by surgeon A (exposed), and 40 randomly selected procedures performed by other surgeons (nonexposed). The second alternative would be much more efficient.

Cohort Studies—Summary

Cohort studies can be prospective or retrospective, observational or experimental. They usually include a whole group of subjects, but studying two subgroups selected based on exposure is also possible. The 2 × 2 table layout and calculations are the same for all types of cohort studies. All have in common that subjects are chosen without regard to whether they develop disease.

The Case-Control Study and Odds Ratio

In a case-control study, we choose subjects for study based on whether they have disease. Since we have to know which subjects developed disease before we select them, case-control studies are always retrospective. We usually study those with disease (cases) and choose a sample of those without disease (controls). We usually study one to four controls per case. The more controls, the greater the chance of finding statistically significant results. However, there is little additional benefit from studying more than four controls per case. Controls are usually randomly selected from subjects present during the study period who did not have disease.

Example: Case-Control Study of Surgical Site Infections

This is the same example presented in the section on cohort study and relative risk. At hospital X, 100 patients had a certain operative procedure, 40 class 2 to 3 (exposed) and 60 class 0 to 1 (nonexposed), and 13 developed SSI. To perform a case-control study, we select the 13 patients with SSI (cases) and also study 26 patients who had surgical procedures but did not have SSI (controls). We studied two controls per case, but could have studied fewer or more controls. The controls were randomly chosen from all patients who had the surgical procedure under study but did not develop SSI. From their medical records, we find which of the subjects had class 2 to 3 procedures and which had class 0 to 1 procedures. Our data showed that, of 13 cases, ten had class 2 to 3 procedures. Of 26 noncases, nine had class 2 to 3 procedures. The 2 × 2 table for this example is as follows:

Disease: Surgical Site Infection

		Yes	No	
Exposure	Class 2–3	10	9	
	Class 0–1	3	15	
		13	26	39

In a case-control study, we cannot determine the percent ill in the exposed or nonexposed groups, or the relative risk. In this example, note that the percent ill among class 2 to 3 is NOT $= 10/(10+9) = 52.6\%$. However, we can validly calculate the percent of cases that were exposed, $10/13 = 76.9\%$, and the percent of noncases that were exposed, $9/26 = 34.6\%$. Note that the cases were much more likely to have the exposure than were the controls. Most importantly, we can calculate the odds ratio (also called the relative odds; Table 2.1) as follows:

$$\text{Odds ratio} = \frac{ad}{bc} = \frac{10\times15}{9\times3} = \frac{150}{27} = 5.6$$

We can interpret the odds ratio as an estimate of the relative risk. Using the case-control method, we estimated that patients in class 2 to 3 were 5.6 times more likely to develop SSI than were patients in class 0 to 1. Note that the odds ratio is similar to, but slightly higher than, the relative risk (5.0) we calculated previously. If the frequency of disease is not too high, i.e., is less than approximately 10%, the odds ratio is a good approximation of the relative risk.

The meanings of the letters (i.e., *a, b, c,* and *d*) used to represent the 2 × 2 table cells are different in cohort versus case-control studies (Table 2.1). For example, in a cohort study, *a* denotes the number of cases of disease among exposed persons; in a case-control study, *a* denotes the number exposed among a group of cases. Although this distinction may not be clear to the novice, it will suffice to keep in mind that, in a case-control study, it is not valid to calculate percent ill or relative risk, but it is valid to calculate an odds ratio.

A more in-depth explanation of the odds ratio is as follows. In a case-control study, we actually measure the odds of exposure among those with disease and the odds of exposure among those without disease. The ratio of these two odds is the exposure odds ratio; if equal to 2.0, this would be interpreted as "the odds of exposure are twice as high in those with disease versus those without disease." However, the exposure odds ratio is not a very useful quantity. Fortunately, it can be proven mathematically that the exposure odds ratio equals the disease odds ratio. Therefore, using our example of 2.0, we can say that the odds of disease are twice as high in those exposed versus those not exposed, which is closer to being useful. Finally, we use the odds ratio as an approximation of the relative risk (where the frequency of disease is not too high) and say simply that those with exposure are twice as likely to get disease.

Selection of Controls

Selection of controls is the critical design issue for a case-control study. Controls should represent the source population from which the cases came; represent persons who, if they had developed disease, would have been a case in the study; and be selected independently of exposure (2). It is always appropriate to seek advice when selecting controls, and may be worthwhile to select two control groups to compare the results obtained with each.

An example of incorrect selection of controls is provided by a case-control study of coffee and pancreatic cancer (1,3). The cases were patients with pancreatic cancer, and controls were selected from other inpatients admitted by the cases' physicians but without pancreatic cancer. The finding was that cases were more likely to have had the exposure (coffee drinking) than the controls, which translated into a significant association between coffee drinking and pancreatic cancer. The problem was that the controls were not selected from the source population of the cases (cases did not arise from hospital inpatients) and thus were not representative of noncases. The physicians admitting patients with cancer of the pancreas were likely to admit other patients with gastrointestinal illness; these control patients were less likely to be coffee drinkers than the general population, possibly because they had diseases that prompted them to avoid coffee. A better control group might have been healthy persons of similar age group to the cases.

More contemporary examples of problematic control selection are studies of the association between vancomycin receipt and vancomycin resistance (4). Cases are often hospitalized patients who are culture positive for vancomycin-resistant enterococci. Controls have often been selected from patients who were culture positive for vancomycin-sensitive enterococci. Using this control group, case-patients will be more likely to have received vancomycin than the controls, resulting in a significant association and elevated odds ratio. The problem is that controls were not representative of the source population and were less likely to have received vancomycin than other patients, since vancomycin would have suppressed or eliminated vancomycin-sensitive microorganisms. Better control groups would be hospital patients similar in age and severity of illness to the cases.

Comparison of Cohort versus Case-Control Studies

A major advantage of cohort studies is that we can calculate the percent ill and the relative risk. Cohort studies are less subject to bias than case-control studies. The potential disadvantages of cohort studies are that they are more time-consuming and expensive and may require study of a large group to collect information on a small number of cases.

Prospective cohort studies are the premier type of observational study. They provide the strongest evidence; are less subject to bias in collecting exposure data, since exposure is recorded before the subjects develop disease; and are flexible in that it is possible to study many exposures and diseases. The disadvantage is that it may be necessary to follow subjects over a long period of time to determine whether they develop disease.

The advantages of the case-control study are that we can determine risk factors while studying a relatively small group of patients; we can study as many risk factors as desired; and case-control studies are usually quicker, easier, and cheaper than cohort studies. The disadvantages are that the percent ill and relative risk are not determined; only one disease can be studied at a time; and the selection of controls can be subtle and introduces the chance of error. Deciding which is the most appropriate control group for a particular study is a matter of opinion about which even well-trained epidemiologists may disagree.

Retrospective Studies

Cohort studies may be prospective or retrospective, but case-control studies are always retrospective. The word *retrospective* has often been used pejoratively in epidemiology, which is only sometimes justified. The crucial question in hospital epidemiology is, When does this distinction matter? If one wants data on length of stay or death in the hospital, this information is usually available from the hospital administration with similar accuracy whether patients are followed prospectively or researched years later. In contrast, if one wants data on the occurrence of nosocomial infection, medical records are notoriously incomplete in this regard, and a retrospective record review might miss the majority of nosocomial infections. However, continuous prospective surveillance at the bedside presumably would identify most nosocomial infections.

Cross-Sectional or Prevalence Study

A third type of study (besides cohort and case-control) includes only subjects who are present in a locality at one point in time. Exposure and disease are ascertained at the same time. Depending on the way the subjects were selected, a cross-sectional study may be analyzed as a cohort study or a case-control study.

A cross-sectional study is clearly not an incidence study, which would include as cases only those free of disease at the start of the study and who develop disease during the study period. However, if an entire group present at one point in time is studied, the results can be analyzed in a 2 × 2 table similar to that used for cohort studies. The formula used to calculate a relative risk in a cohort study would yield a prevalence ratio in a cross-sectional study.

If the group present at one point in time is sampled as in a case-control study (i.e., the cases and a random selection of noncases are studied), then the odds ratio formula could be used to calculate a prevalence odds ratio.

Incidence versus Prevalence

Incidence includes only new cases of disease with onset during a study period; the denominator is the number of subjects without disease at the beginning of the study period. Incidence measures the rate at which people without the disease develop the disease during a specified period of time; it is used to study disease etiology (risk).

Prevalence includes both new and old cases that are present at one time and place. Prevalence measures the proportion of people who have the disease at a given point in time and is used to measure disease burden and plan for needed resources. For example, if we wanted to know how many isolation rooms would be needed for patients with resistant microorganisms, we would want to know prevalence, i.e., the total number of patients with recognized drug-resistant microorganisms of either new or old onset in the hospital at any given time.

The commonest measure of prevalence is point prevalence, which is the proportion of individuals in a certain group with a disease or condition at one point in time. Point prevalence is a unitless proportion. A different measure of prevalence, period prevalence, is the proportion of persons present during a time period with disease. Period prevalence has been criticized as an undefined mixture of both prevalent and incident cases without quantitative use, but is occasionally seen.

It is often said that prevalence equals incidence *times* duration. That is, prevalence is higher if either incidence is higher or if the duration of the illness is longer. In hospital studies, prevalence is greatly influenced by length of stay and mortality. For example, assuming that ascertainment of vancomycin-resistant enterococci is stable, the prevalence of vancomycin-resistant enterococci in a hospital may decrease because of an effective prevention program, or because patients with this microorganism are being discharged sooner or dying more commonly than had been the case previously. Nevertheless, prevalence studies may be a quick and easy way to get a general idea of disease frequency and of course are useful to assess resource needs.

Point prevalence and incidence density are mathematically linked; in a steady-state or dynamic population, one can be derived from the other. Prevalence can be derived from incidence density and distributions of durations of disease, and incidence density may be derived from prevalence and distributions of durations to date of disease (5–8).

INTERPRETATION OF DATA, INCLUDING STATISTICAL SIGNIFICANCE AND CAUSAL INFERENCE

Measures of Size of Effect and Their Interpretation

The relative risk and the odds ratio measure the size of effect, i.e., the magnitude of the association between an exposure and a disease. A relative risk of 1.3 shows a modest association, whereas a value of 20 shows a large association. In general, odds ratios are interpreted in the same manner as relative risks.

Because the relative risk = percent ill exposed/percent ill nonexposed, the relative risk can fall into three categories. First, if the two percents are approximately equal, the relative risk is approximately 1.0; this is a null result showing no association between exposure and disease. Second, if the percent ill is higher in the exposed group, the relative risk is >1.0; exposure is apparently associated with disease, is a risk factor for disease, and may be a cause of disease. Third, if the percent ill is higher in those without exposure, the relative risk is <1.0; exposure is again apparently associated with disease, but in this instance the exposure prevents disease. An example of a preventive exposure is vaccine use; persons who are "exposed" to the vaccine have a lower rate of disease than those not exposed, leading to a relative risk <1.0. Interpretation of odds ratios as equal to, greater than, or less than 1.0 is similar. To intelligently interpret relative risks and odds ratios, we must in addition understand statistical significance and the distinction between association and causation (presented below).

Relative risks can be interpreted as a percent increase or decrease. For example, a relative risk of 1.5 could be interpreted in two ways: disease is 1.5 times more likely in exposed than nonexposed, or disease is 50% more likely in exposed than nonexposed. Similarly, a protective relative risk of 0.6 could be interpreted in two ways: illness was 0.6 times as likely in exposed than nonexposed, or illness was 40% less likely in the exposed group.

Statistical Significance and *p* Values

For a given group and time period, an association between exposure and disease might occur due to chance alone. For example, suppose that over many years the rate of SSI at hospital A is the same as that of other hospitals. However, during a given quarter, the rate at hospital A may be higher or lower than average by chance alone. To tell us the probability that the SSI rate at hospital A differed from the rate at other hospitals due to chance alone, we commonly use two measures of statistical significance, the *p* value and the confidence interval.

The *p* value measures the probability that a given result, or one more extreme, could have happened by chance alone. Because computer packages calculate *p* values automatically, it is more important to know how to interpret than to calculate them. *P* values range from >0 to 1.0. By convention, a *p* value <.05

indicates statistical significance. This means that there is a <5% or <1/20 chance that the result we found (or one more extreme) could have occurred by chance alone; exposure is associated with disease. Another way of stating this is that we are 95% certain that this observed difference could not have arisen by chance alone. If the *p* value is >.05, the result is not considered statistically significant and could well have happened by chance alone; we do not have evidence that exposure is associated with disease.

The .05 cutoff was not chosen for any particular reason but now is very commonly used. There is not a meaningful difference between *p* values of .04 and .06; although the latter would not usually be considered statistically significant, in fact there is only a 6% chance that such a result could have occurred by chance alone. The adoption of the arbitrary .05 standard has its unfortunate aspects and is subject to interpretation after considering all of the sources of bias described below. Some published manuscripts describe interesting or important studies where the *p* value did not reach .05, thus allowing readers to make their own determinations of biologic importance and statistical significance not linked to the arbitrary .05 level.

Small epidemics, or epidemics that are stopped before there are sufficient cases to demonstrate statistical significance at the .05 level, may be biologically very important, so epidemiologists who work with observational data in hospitals should not consider statistical *p* values to be of primary interest. Biologic importance and size of effect are much more compelling than *p* values in the face of an ongoing problem in a hospital. One would never allow a preventable epidemic to continue unchecked simply to collect more cases for a *p* value.

In biostatistical terms, significance testing can be viewed as follows. We assume the null hypothesis that there is no true difference in rate of illness between the exposed and nonexposed groups. We then compute the *p* value, i.e., probability of the results (or results more extreme) under the null hypothesis. If the *p* value is low, then apparently the null hypothesis was wrong, and we reject the null hypothesis and embrace the alternative hypothesis, namely that there is a true difference between exposed and nonexposed (see Chapter 3).

Type I versus Type II Error

The *p* value required for statistical significance is commonly called the chance of type I error. This means that if we conclude that hospital A has a high rate of illness based on a *p* value of .05, there is a 5% chance that we are drawing this conclusion in error. The type I error then indicates the chance of concluding that a difference in rates exists when in fact there is no true difference. Type II error measures the opposite problem—that there really is a difference between the two rates but we erroneously conclude that they are the same. The power of a study (discussed below) = 1 − the probability of type II error.

Methods of Calculating p Values

P values for 2 × 2 tables may be calculated by the chi-square or Fisher exact methods. The chi-square *p* value is valid when an expected value (Table 2.1) is not <5; if an expected value is <5, the Fisher exact results should be used. Computer packages commonly calculate expected values and print out a suggestion to use the Fisher exact *p* value if appropriate. In addition to a simple or uncorrected chi-square, computer packages may compute a continuity corrected (or Yates corrected) value. The formula for continuity correction involves subtracting 0.5 from each cell in the 2 × 2 table. There are usually not great differences among these chi-square values, and many authorities suggest using the simple or uncorrected value.

The calculation of chi-square does not differ depending on whether data are from a cohort, case-control, or cross-sectional study. However, the computation of chi-square is different for incidence density data. Calculation of chi-square is shown in Table 2.1 and Question 3 in Appendix 1 at the end of this chapter. Later we suggest some simple shareware programs that do these calculations for you, both for count data and incidence density data. When one has the value for chi-square, one can determine the *p* value by looking it up in a table or by using a statistical program. In the popular spreadsheet Excel, the CHIDIST function calculates the *p* value for a given chi-square value.

P values may be one-tailed or two-tailed. Two-tailed *p* values are usually twice as great as one-tailed values. A two-tailed *p* value assumes that the rate in the exposed group could have been either higher or lower than the unexposed group due to chance alone. A one-tailed value recognizes only one of these two possibilities. Although there is not uniform agreement as to whether one- or two-tailed results should be used, the majority of authors use two-tailed *p* values. This suggests that, for uniformity and ease of comparison among studies, two-tailed *p* values should be the standard.

Confidence Intervals

The second way to judge statistical significance is the confidence interval for a relative risk or odds ratio. The confidence interval combines the concepts of size of effect (relative risk) and strength of association (*p* value). A 95% confidence interval means that, roughly speaking, we are 95% sure that the true relative risk lies between the upper and lower confidence interval limits. For example, assume that a study showed a relative risk of 5.0 with a 95% confidence interval of 1.47 to 17.05. Our best guess is that the relative risk is 5.0, which seems quite high, but we are 95% sure that it lies between 1.47 and 17.05. This is much more informative than simply reporting the probability of our results under the null hypothesis (*p* value). An additional benefit of the confidence interval is humility; a wide interval points out the uncertainty in our results.

If a 95% confidence interval does not cross 1.0, the result is statistically significant at the .05 level. Remembering the formula for the relative risk, a relative risk >1.0 with a 95% confidence interval excluding 1.0 means that we are 95% sure that the rate of illness in the exposed group is greater than the rate of illness in the nonexposed group.

Causal Inference: Association versus Causation

A statistical association between an exposure and a disease does not necessarily mean that the exposure caused the disease.

Sir Bradford Hill first described a set of logical criteria by which associations could be judged for potential causality. Fulfillment of Hill's criteria does not guarantee that an association is causal, but failure to meet these criteria generally excludes the possibility of causality. These criteria have changed somewhat over time, but here is a version appropriate for hospital epidemiology:

1. Size of effect can be estimated by the relative risk. Large effects are more likely to be causal than small effects. The magnitude of a credible relative risk must depend on the magnitude of the potential sources of bias. Generally, a relative risk >2.0 or <0.5 in a well-done study is difficult to ignore.
2. Strength of association can be measured by the *p* value. A relatively weak association can more easily be the result of random or systematic error. A *p* value near .05 would be considered a weak association. The same information is better presented by the statement that a relative risk 95% confidence bound near 1.0 would be evidence of a weak association.
3. Consistency: a particular effect should be reproducible in different populations and settings.
4. Temporality: the cause must precede the effect.
5. Biologic gradient: there should be a dose-response effect. More exposure should lead to more outcome.
6. Plausibility of the biologic model: there should be a reasonable biologic model to explain the apparent association. This includes Hill's criteria of coherence, experimental evidence, and analogy. Mathematical models of the transmission of infectious diseases would be relevant for defining and quantifying plausibility.

ERRORS IN EPIDEMIOLOGIC STUDIES

The overall goal of an epidemiologic study is accuracy in measurement with little error. However, the real definition of practical epidemiology is how to get a good-enough answer to an important biologic question at an affordable price. Epidemiologic studies, even observational studies, involve people and are usually expensive; the practical goal is to design a study that requires the least resources that will still provide a good-enough answer to a question. What is good enough? It depends on the situation, because you have to learn enough to make whatever decision has to be made, and to move on.

The perfect epidemiologic study will never be done. Thus, every epidemiologist has to be an expert on sources of error in measurement. For every question or every study, one must review the potential sources of error, estimate their likely direction and magnitude, and then decide what overall effect these distortions might have on the result of the study.

It is worthwhile to distinguish random variation, random error, and systematic error. Random variation is the statistical phenomenon of variability due to chance alone, and is sometimes called background or noise. If we were measuring SSIs, the true underlying SSI rate would vary each month according to many factors, including the mix of surgeons and patients involved; assuming hypothetically that these factors could be held stable, the SSI rate would still vary each month because of chance alone (i.e., random variation). On the other hand, random and systematic *errors* are produced by inaccuracies in finding or recording data. Random error would occur if we incorrectly measure the SSI rate to be higher than it actually is during some months and lower than it actually is in other months; over many months these random errors in measurement balance each other and the average value would be correct. Systematic error would occur if we consistently measured the SSI rate as higher or lower than the true rate, and an average over many months would be wrong; systematic error is also called *bias.* We define validity as getting the right answer, or alternately as a lack of bias.

A related concept is *precision,* which may be functionally defined as the width of the confidence interval. A narrow confidence interval indicates high precision, i.e., we are confident that the true value is within a narrow range. A confidence interval is narrower when both random variation and random error are low and vice versa. A larger sample size leads to a narrower confidence interval and greater precision. Precision may also be improved by modifying the study design to increase the statistical efficiency by which information is obtained from a given number of study subjects.

Selection Bias or Berkson's Bias

Selection bias occurs when subjects are inadvertently but systematically selected for enrollment in a study according to the exposures by which they are later compared. Thus, selection bias may be present when study subjects were selected in a manner different from the method presumed, so that the individuals in the study are not representative of the target populations. Selection bias can artifactually make an effect appear to be smaller or larger, so that relative risks estimated from a particular study may be either closer to or further from the null than the true value.

An example of selection bias is a study of mortality rates in patients with versus without nosocomial bacteremia. The problem is that blood cultures are selectively obtained from patients who appear septic, and thus mildly ill patients who may have unrecognized bacteremia are not included as cases. Therefore, cases are not representative of all patients with bacteremia. Including only the sicker cases leads to an overestimate of the mortality associated with bacteremia. In this example, one has selected patients according to a correlate of the characteristic by which they are compared (death in the hospital). Selection bias results in a permanent distortion, because it cannot be corrected later. There is no way to go back and obtain blood from the bacteremic patients who were never cultured.

Selection bias may introduce serious distortion in studies where subjects are selected for a study, such as the study of mortality with nosocomial bacteremia described above. In traditional surveillance, however, where no selection of subjects occurs, selection bias is not usually a problem.

Misclassification or Information Bias

After subjects are enrolled in a study, errors in classification of exposure and outcome are called *misclassification.* Misclassification may be nondifferential and differential. Differential misclassification means that exposure is incorrectly determined to a differing extent among those with versus without disease, or that disease is incorrectly determined to a differing extent among those with versus without exposure. Differential misclassification may bias the calculated relative risk away from the null value of 1.0, making the relative risk either falsely high (for risk factors with relative risk >1.0) or falsely low (for protective factors with relative risk <1.0).

Conversely, nondifferential misclassification would mean that exposure was recorded incorrectly to a similar extent for those both with and without disease, or disease was recorded incorrectly to a similar extent in those with and without exposure. This type of misclassification biases the relative risk toward the null value of 1.0. With nondifferential misclassification, some or all of the cells of the 2 × 2 table are not pure, as some study subjects are placed in the wrong groups, and the effect of the comparison therefore is diluted by the mixing.

Suppose that one is comparing nosocomial infections between thoracic and general surgeons. In this hypothetical hospital, the thoracic surgeons do routine urine cultures for all patients with urinary catheters, sputum cultures for all intubated patients, and vascular catheter tip cultures when catheters are removed. However, the general surgeons obtain cultures only when they feel it is necessary. A comparison of infection rates shows higher infection rates for the thoracic surgeons when all that has really happened is that infection status has been differentially misclassified according to service.

Note that mere low sensitivity does not mean that data are not useful. The reliability of data primarily depends on how consistent the sensitivity remains in the data collection. National data on sexually transmitted diseases and food-borne illnesses such as salmonella gastroenteritis have a consistent sensitivity of around 0.01 or 1%, but these data remain useful because the sensitivity has been relatively constant at that level over time, so that secular increases or decreases are evident. Data with higher levels of sensitivity but greater variability are actually less reliable in making valid comparisons. Benchmarking comparisons among facilities should be attempted only when a practitioner has some measure of the comparative sensitivities of data from different populations.

A Broader View of Bias

Bias can be more generally defined as a systematic deviation from the truth: any trend in the collection, analysis, interpretation, publication, or review of data that can lead to conclusions that are systematically different from the truth (9). In the analysis phase of a study, if one has a strong preconceived idea of what the answer should be, then a biased analysis and interpretation of the data may result. If one keeps analyzing and reanalyzing data with a view to finding something statistically significant to publish, eventually a satisfactory result will be found. This has been expressed as "If you torture data enough, it will confess to anything." Publication bias results when studies that show a statistically significant difference between study groups are published, whereas other studies of the same topic that did not show such a difference remain unpublished.

Inaccuracy of Hospital Surveillance

Errors in routine hospital surveillance for nosocomial infections could result in either reporting of spurious episodes of infection or lack of reporting of true infections. In practice, the latter problem is much more common. Patients with true nosocomial infections escape detection because (a) not all relevant data are present in the medical record or laboratory reports; (b) the data collector may overlook relevant data; and (c) the physician did not order appropriate tests to detect the infection. Estimates of the loss of sensitivity due to (a) and (b) above are shown in Table 2.2. In this table, all sensitivities are related to a composite standard, including data from multiple independent surveys of the medical record, bedside examination, and microbiology laboratory records.

The effect point (c) above was measured in the Study of the Efficacy of Nosocomial Infection Control (SENIC) (10,11). The overall culturing rate, which was the proportion of patients with signs or symptoms of any infection that had at least one appropriate culture done, was 32% in 1970 and 40% in 1975 to 1976 (10). The proportion of febrile patients from whom at least one appropriate culture was obtained was 28% in 1970 and 45% in 1975 (10). These measures varied substantially from 5% to 95% by hospital type and region of the country. Patients in academic hospitals in the northeast United States had the highest likelihood of being appropriately cultured. It follows that patients in

TABLE 2.2. SENSITIVITIES OF METHODS OF CASE-FINDING FOR NOSOCOMIAL INFECTIONS QUANTIFYING ONLY OMISSIONS FROM LIMITED DATA SOURCES AND ERRORS BY SURVEYORS

Method	Study (Reference)	Sensitivity
Reference standard: Duplicate surveys + Record review + Bedside examination + Laboratory tests		
	UVA, BCH, CDC(10)[a]	1.00
Single Survey: Record review + Bedside examination + Laboratory tests		
	BCH	0.98
Physician self-reports	CHIP (10)[a]	0.14–0.34
Micro laboratory reports	CHIP (10)[a]	0.33–0.65
Micro laboratory reports	UK (21)	0.71
Kardex clues (50% sample)	UVA (10)[a]	0.69–0.85
Record review (100% sample)	UVA (10)[a]	0.90
Kardex clues	UK (21)	0.49
Ward Ilaison	UK (21)	0.58
ICDA coded dx	BCH (9)	0.02–0.35
ICDA coded dx	Yale (22)	0.57
SENIC pliot record review	CDC (23)	0.66–0.80
SENIC project record review	CDC (24)	0.05–0.95
NNIS	CDC (25)	0.30–0.85

Note: The effects of failure of physicians to evaluate patients with suspicious clinical episodes were not included in these measures. These data do not include losses from unresolved clinical episodes.
[a] Some of these results have previously been summarized in Freeman and McGowan (17).
UVA. University of Virginia; BCH, Boston City Hospital; CDC, Centers for Disease Control and Prevention; CHIP, Community Hospital Infection Protocol; UK, United Kingdom; Yale, Yale University.
Adapted from Freeman J, McGowan JE Jr. Methodologic issues in hospital epidemiology.
I. Rates, case finding, and interpretation.
Ref infect Dis 1981; 3:658–667.

such hospitals were more likely to have a nosocomial infection documented. For urinary tract infections, pneumonias, and bacteremias, the lack of availability of objective data was a major determinant of observed rates of infection (11). The implications of these findings for benchmarking rates among hospitals are obvious.

There is a disincentive for physicians and hospitals to self-report nosocomial infections, and this leads to the paradox that hospitals that do the worst job of collecting data and documenting infections report the lowest rates. This was one of the two problems with CMS's failed infection control indicator that would have compared crude self-reported nosocomial infection rates among hospitals. Any practitioner who makes benchmarking comparisons among hospital populations without knowing the sensitivity of case reporting in all data sets is risking substantial distortion from nondifferential misclassification. In such flawed comparisons the group represented by the data set with the lowest and poorest sensitivity appears to have the lowest infection rate.

After two decades of reporting results, the National Nosocomial Infections Surveillance (NNIS) system finally conducted a study of the accuracy of reporting nosocomial infection rates in intensive care unit patients (12). The sensitivity in this study was greatly improved over that found in the SENIC project, as the NNIS hospitals correctly reported the majority of infections that occurred. Still of concern, however, was the continuing wide range in the sensitivity that varied from 30% to 85%, depending on the site of infection. In this study substantial numbers of nosocomial infections were missed by prospective monitoring and a different large group was missed by retrospective chart review.

External Validity (Generalizability)

The sections above on bias and errors concern internal validity, i.e., Are we measuring correctly within the population we selected? External validity or generalizability asks the question, Are our results applicable in other settings? Generalizability is always a matter of opinion. Selection bias and lack of generalizability of a study are often confused. The presence of selection bias implies that a study result is biased for the limited target population on which it was alleged to have been performed. A lack of bias does not guarantee generalizability. A perfectly done epidemiologic study may or may not be generalizable to a larger population.

Epidemiologists frequently choose to study unrepresentative samples of subjects in order to answer a scientific question cleanly, cheaply, practically, or safely. Although not widely generalizable, a study result may be scientifically sound for the population on which the study was performed.

In a randomized trial, for example, potential study subjects and their physicians must determine that it is safe for the study subjects to accept any of the study treatments before they can be randomized. Patients who have a contraindication to one of the treatments cannot be included in the study on the chance that they might be randomized to the contraindicated treatment. Thus, many treatable patients must ordinarily be excluded from randomized trials, rendering the sample of patients on whom the trial is actually performed highly unrepresentative of the population as a whole. This lack of representativeness does not indicate that the study is epidemiologically biased in any way, but it may limit the generalizability of the study result to a larger population.

An example was the Collaborative Antibiotic Prophylaxis Efficacy Research Study (CAPERS) trial of antibiotic prophylaxis for clean (herniorrhaphy and breast) surgery (13,14). A total of 1,218 patients were randomized into a double-blind clinical trial, and concurrently an observational study of the 3,202 patients who were not randomized was undertaken. In the clinical trial, prophylactic antibiotic administration was determined by randomization, whereas in the observational study patients received prophylaxis at the discretion of the surgeon. Patients were not included in the randomized trial for various reasons, e.g., surgeon or patient declined, or there was insufficient time to discuss randomization. The subgroup included in the randomized trial might not have been representative of all patients with these procedures, and the results of the randomized trial might not be generalizable to the larger population. The authors produced appropriate separate analyses on the randomized trial and the observational study, and in both studies about half of the SSIs were prevented by antibiotic prophylaxis. In this particular instance, the result of the randomized trial turned out to be generalizable to the larger group, but this need not have been so.

ACCOUNTING FOR TIME AT RISK

Because many nosocomial infections are related to time at risk, and because average lengths of hospital stay are decreasing, state-of-the-art studies must use methods that account for time at risk. Studies of mortality present a similar challenge: we all have one death per lifetime, and that is unavoidable, but it matters very much just when that death occurs. Methods used to account for time at risk include incidence density methods and survival analysis.

Incidence Density

Incidence density studies are a type of cohort study where the denominator is the total person-time at risk for all subjects, rather than the number of subjects. Commonly used denominators in healthcare-related incidence density studies are patient-days, (vascular or urinary) catheter-days, and ventilator-days. Of the four most commonly studied healthcare-associated infections, three are device-related and are best studied using incidence density methods: catheter-associated bloodstream infections, ventilator-associated pneumonias, and catheter-associated urinary tract infection. Only one of the four (SSI) is best studied using cumulative incidence methods, i.e., the denominator is the number of surgical procedures.

If the event being studied is a nosocomial infection, then incidence density is the number of nosocomial infections in a specified quantity of person-time in the population at risk. The population at risk is composed of all those who have not yet suffered a nosocomial infection. After a patient acquires an infection, that patient would be withdrawn from the population at risk. All hospital days for each patient who never acquired an infection would be included in the pool of days at risk, but for a patient who became infected only those hospital-days before the onset of the infection would be included.

Incidence density is the instantaneous rate of change or what used to be called the force of morbidity. For convenience in hospital epidemiology, nosocomial infection rates are usually expressed as the number of events in 1,000 hospital-days, because this usually produces a small single- or double-digit number, but we could have used seconds or years.

The basic value of this measure can be seen when comparing nosocomial infection rates in two groups with large differences in time at risk, e.g., in short-stay patients versus long-stay patients, or infection rates with peripheral venous catheters versus implanted ports. By contrast, if one looks at events that come from a point source, such as eating vanilla ice cream at a church supper, or events that are not time related, like acquiring tuberculosis during bronchoscopy with a contaminated bronchoscope, the attack rate or cumulative incidence is an excellent measure of incidence. SSIs are usually thought of as having a point source—the operation.

An incidence density rate = total events/total time at risk for an event. If we have an exposed and nonexposed group, then we define the rate ratio = rate ill in exposed/rate ill nonexposed. The rate ratio is a measure of the size of effect analogous to the relative risk used in cumulative incidence studies. Rate ratios are sometimes called incidence density ratios, relative risks, or risk ratios. Rate ratios are interpreted in a similar manner to relative risks; a rate ratio of 2 means that disease incidence was twice as great in the exposed group than in the nonexposed group. Note that the units for the denominators of incidence density divide out, so that you will find the same incidence density ratio no matter whether you use time units of seconds or millennia. *P* values for the rate ratio may be calculated by a chi-square or binomial exact method.

Multiple Events in a Single Patient

Standard statistical tests assume that each observation in a data set is independent, having no linkage with other observations. A corollary is that each subject in a study should contribute at most one event to a data set, i.e., we should study first events in an individual only. If this rule is not followed, the calculated confidence intervals and *p* values may not be valid. However, it is well known that a subset of patients will have multiple episodes of nosocomial infection and other adverse outcomes. Also, it is well established that patients with a first event are more likely to suffer a second, indicating that multiple infections in the same patients are not uncommon (15–19). For quantitative analyses, these nonindependent events cannot simply be summed and placed over a denominator. The biologic and statistical import of five infections per 100 discharges would be entirely different depending on whether it represented five sequential infections in a single moribund patient or five first infections in five different but healthy patients such as women with normal deliveries.

Furthermore, a first nosocomial infection becomes a risk factor for a second, and risk factors for multiple infections are different from the risk factors for a first infection. The simplest way to cope with multiple incident events in the same individual is to restrict quantitative analyses to first events. A second method is to stratify by number of previous infections, e.g., study the effect of exposures on risk of first infection, then on risk of second infection, and so on. These individual strata would then be combined into a summary relative risk. However, this method also violates the independence rule for conventional data analyses. A third alternative is to use statistical methods designed for longitudinal or correlated data. This type of analysis is technically complex (see Longitudinal Analysis and Repeated Measures, below).

Survival Analysis

Survival analysis is a second method for accounting for time at risk in epidemiologic studies (1). Survival analysis usually consists of the familiar Kaplan-Meier plot, where at time zero survival begins at 1.0 or 100% and gradually falls off as subjects are followed forward in time. Survival can literally mean not dying, or it can mean remaining free of infection or whatever outcome variable is being studied. The opposite of survival is termed "failure," which again may either mean death or onset of another adverse event. An extremely useful feature of survival analysis is that it can make use of subjects that are lost to follow-up or die of a disease other than that of interest; these subjects are called "censored" since we don't know if they would have failed if we had been able to follow them for a longer period of time.

Statistical packages automatically plot survival curves for two or more groups and calculate a *p* value for the difference between the two groups. Median survival (the follow-up time when the probability of survival is 0.5 or 50%) is often reported. The Kaplan-Meier plot represents a univariable analysis. Multivariable survival analysis is accomplished via regression models, the most common of which is the Cox model (discussed below).

CONFOUNDING AND EFFECT MODIFICATION

Confounding

We like to think of epidemiology in simple terms, like the occurrence of cholera in Snow's London depending on the source of drinking water or measles in a school classroom. In these stark examples, only two things really mattered: who was susceptible and who was exposed. Most diseases in epidemiology, including hospital epidemiology, are diseases of multiple causation. That is, many factors acting jointly produce the outcome, and the factors that produced the outcome in one subject may not be the factors that produced the same outcome in another. For the sake of understanding, we like to estimate the separate effects of the various causes of disease. The bench biologist has control over the situation and can accomplish this by setting up experiments to change one variable at a time. To accomplish this same end in observational epidemiology, we must somehow nullify or correct for the effects of multiple other determinants or exposures that are actually acting jointly with the exposure of primary interest.

Example of Confounding by Severity of Illness

Let's hypothetically assume that we were studying nosocomial infections at two hospitals, A and B. In our simplified example, there are two types of patients: high-risk patients who have a 10% risk of disease per hospitalization, and low-risk patients who have a 1% risk. During a time period, hospitals A and B both admit 1,000 patients, but hospital A admits 900 high-risk and 100 low-risk patients, whereas hospital B admits 100 high-risk and 900 low-risk patients. Using hospital A as the exposed group, the relative risk is 9.1/1.9 = 4.8, i.e., the risk of infection after admission to hospital A was 4.8 times higher than after admission to hospital B (Table 2.3).

This is an example of confounding. We are primarily interested in the relationship between one exposure (hospital A, which we shall denote as $exposure_1$) and disease. However, the effect of a second exposure (high- vs. low-risk patient, denoted by $exposure_2$) confuses or confounds our ability to measure the effect of $exposure_1$. This occurs because of an unequal mix of $exposure_2$ among the $exposure_1$ groups (high-risk patients comprise 90% of hospital A admissions but only 10% of hospital B admissions).

Stratified Analysis

Stratification is an important method to detect and control for confounding. First we compute a simple or crude relative risk by our usual 2 × 2 table methods (Table 2.3b). Second, we perform a stratified analysis: we calculate two relative risks (RRs), designated RR_1 and RR_2. In the above example of hospitals A and B, RR_1 measures the effect of hospital A among high risk patients and RR_2 the effect of hospital A among low-risk patients (Table 2.3c). In this example, both RR_1 and RR_2 are equal to 1.0. Third, with the help of a statistical program, we compute a Mantel-Haenszel summary relative risk (RR_{MH}), which is a weighted average of RR_1 and RR_2. In this example, the RR_{MH} was also 1.0 (i.e., null result), indicating that there was no association between hospital and infection after adjusting for patient risk.

There was an obvious case-mix difference between hospitals A and B. The RR_{MH} is our prediction of what the crude relative risk would have been if there had not been a case-mix difference between the hospitals. Calculating an RR_{MH} is a way of adjusting for a potential confounding exposure, and thus the RR_{MH} is a type of adjusted relative risk. Other methods of calculating an adjusted relative risk include indirect standardization and regression modeling (these methods are presented later in this chapter).

Calculation of Mantel-Haenszel Relative Risk and Odds Ratio

If there are i strata, the four cells of the 2 × 2 table are designated a_i, b_i, c_i, and d_i; the total number of subjects in each stratum is $n_i = a_i + b_i + c_i + d_i$; and E indicates the sum over all i strata:

$$\text{Mantel-Haenszel summary relative risk} = \frac{\Sigma a_i (c_i + d_i)/n_i}{\Sigma c_i (a_i + b_i)/n_i}$$

$$\text{Mantel-Haenszel summary odds ratio} = \frac{\Sigma (a_i d_i)/n_i}{\Sigma (b_i c_i)/n_i}$$

TABLE 2.3. SAMPLE DATA: SIMPLE AND STRATIFIED ANALYSES

a. Numbers of Patients Total and Infected, Hospitals A vs B

Hospital	High-Risk Patients		Low-Risk Patients		Overall Infection Rate
	Total	Number Infected	Total	Number Infected	
A	900	90	100	1	91/1,000 = 9.1%
B	100	10	900	9	19/1,000 = 1.9%

b. Simple (Crude) Analysis: Effect of Hospital

Hospital ($Exposure_1$)	Total Patients	No. (%) Infections	Relative Risk
A	1,000	91 (9.1)	4.8
B	1,000	19 (1.9)	—

c. Stratified Analysis: Effect of Hospital Stratified by Patient Risk

Patient Risk ($Exposure_2$)	Hospital ($Exposure_1$)	Total Patients	No. (%) Infections	Relative Risk (RR)
High	A	900	90 (10)	RR_1 = 1.0
High	B	100	10 (10)	—
Low	A	100	1 (1)	RR_2 = 1.0
Low	B	900	9 (1)	—

Mantel-Haenszel summary relative risk (RR_{MH}) = 1.0.

Recognizing Confounding

The following is a simple functional definition of confounding: if the adjusted relative risk differs to a meaningful extent from the crude relative risk, then confounding is present. There is no statistical test or firm guide for how great the difference must be. In the hospital A versus B example above, the RR_{MH} of 1.0 differed substantially from the crude relative risk of 4.9, so confounding was obviously present. We say that the effect of $exposure_1$ (hospital A vs. B) was confounded by the effect of $exposure_2$ (high- vs. low-risk patients). In order for confounding to occur, both of the following are required: $exposure_2$ must be associated with disease and $exposure_1$ must be associated with $exposure_2$.

Additional Examples of Confounding

We know that advanced age, female gender, and instrumentation of the urinary tract are all determinants or causes of nosocomial urinary tract infections. In a hospital population, patients with nosocomial urinary tract infections tend to be older and are more likely to be female than the patients without urinary tract infections. If we want to measure the effect of instrumentation alone, then we must somehow nullify the effect of age and gender. A simple 2 × 2 table analysis and relative risk will be distorted or confounded by the effects of these extraneous variables. However, confounding in this case (and in most other cases as well) is correctable if one has good enough data on the confounder (age and gender in the above example) and goes about adjusting for these extraneous influences appropriately.

Investigators in the SENIC project reported a relative risk of 0.94 for nosocomial infections in hospitals with infection surveillance and control programs compared with those lacking such programs, or a preventive effect of 6%. This relative risk of 0.94, implying prevention, could be reversed by a 7% confounding effect. These small tolerances put extreme pressure on the ability to adjust for confounding.

Methods to Deal with Confounding

We can prevent confounding in the design phase of a study by doing a randomized trial or by doing a matched case-control study. We can adjust for the effects of confounding in the analysis phase by stratification, by standardization, or by performing regression analyses.

Randomization

Randomized trials are rarely used because of their expense and difficulty, but are an effective way to avoid confounding. The process of randomization ensures that, on average, two or more similar groups will be produced. The magic of randomization is that it produces groups that are similar with respect to both known and unknown confounders. The previously mentioned CAPERS study contained both a randomized trial and an observational study of prophylactic antibiotics for clean surgery. In the trial, assignment of patients to either prophylactic antibiotics or no antibiotics was determined by randomization, and the two groups being compared were very similar. Because of randomization, there was essentially no confounding in the randomized trial (13). By contrast, in the observational study, antibiotic prophylaxis was at the discretion of the surgeon, and the group that received antibiotic prophylaxis was substantially different from the group that did not. Because of the large confounding effect of these differences in the observational study (14), logistic regression (discussed later) was ultimately employed in the analysis to adjust for these differences.

Matched Case-Control Studies

In a simple case-control study, the controls are usually a random sample of all noncases. In a matched case-control study, controls are selected by matching one or more noncases with each case according to some potentially confounding variable. For example, if we wanted to study the effects of an exposure on risk of vancomycin-resistant enterococcus, we would want to control for some well-known risk factors for vancomycin-resistant enterococcus. Therefore, for each case we could select some controls that were closest to the case in a measure of severity of illness such as Apache II score and antimicrobial receipt. To analyze the matched data, we do not do a simple 2 × 2 table analysis. Instead, we would perform a stratified analysis, where each case and its associated controls form one stratum. The Mantel-Haenszel summary odds ratio is then used rather than the simple odds ratio.

A matched design makes sense only if the potential confounders are well known and one has no need to study them further. In the matched study, one cannot calculate an odds ratio or p value for the variables that were used to match the controls (Apache II score and antimicrobial receipt, in the example above). To produce an unbiased odds ratio, we must analyze the data using the stratified method outlined above, thus reducing flexibility in the analysis phase. Also, the p value calculated in a matched study will be higher than that from a conventional 2 × 2 table, reducing the chance of finding a statistically significant result. Rather than matching, well-trained epidemiologists usually prefer to select a random sample of noncases and adjust the data using a multivariable method. However, matching clearly makes sense if an important confounding variable is common in cases and rare in noncases; under such conditions, if random sampling is done, only a few of the controls will have the confounding variable, and much effort will be expended to collect data on controls that have little relevance.

Standardization

There are two methods of standardization, direct and indirect. Direct standardization is rarely used in healthcare epidemiology and is not presented here. However, indirect standardization is a valuable method that is commonly used in healthcare surveillance. This method is typically used when stratum-specific event rates are available from a large reference population (e.g., a large number of facilities) and we want to compare a smaller group (e.g., a single facility) to this reference population. Any outcome event can be studied by indirect standardization. When applied to infections, indirect standardization produces a stan-

TABLE 2.4. EXAMPLE OF INDIRECT STANDARDIZATION TO CALCULATE A STANDARDIZED INFECTION RATIO (SIR)

Vascular Access Type	BSI Rate,[a] All Centers	Patient-Months, Center X	Expected BSI, Center X
Fistula	0.25	1709	4.27
Graft	0.53	528	2.80
Tunneled catheter	4.84	958	46.37
Nontunneled catheter	8.73	200	17.46
Total	—	3395	70.9

[a]Rate per 100 patient-months. BSI rate for all centers from ref. 52.
BSI, bloodstream infection.
Crude rate ratio = rate at Center X/rate at all centers = 2.97/1.78 = 1.67.
Standardized infection ratio = actual BSI/expected BSI = 101/70.9 = 1.42.

dardized infection ratio (SIR) and when applied to deaths a standardized mortality ratio is produced.

The following example of indirect standardization (Table 2.4) uses the incidence density approach to calculate rates and rate ratios. We want to compare the bloodstream infection (BSI) rate at a single dialysis center, center X, with the average rate of a large reference group. At center X, we observed 101 BSIs during 3,395 patient-months of follow-up, for a BSI rate of 2.97 per 100 patient-months. The crude rate ratio comparing center X to all centers was 1.67, indicating that the risk of BSI was 1.67 times higher (or 67% higher) at center X.

Vascular access type is a potential confounding variable. Rates of BSI from the reference group vary widely from 0.25 to 8.73 BSI per 100 patient-months among four vascular access types (Table 2.4). If center X treats more patients with high-risk vascular access (e.g., tunneled or nontunneled catheters) than other centers, we would expect more BSI at center X. We want to determine the intrinsic risk of BSI at center X if the mix of vascular access types at center X were the same as that at all centers.

To calculate an SIR, we first determine the expected numbers of BSI at center X for each access type by multiplying the all-center rates by the center X denominators (e.g., for nontunneled catheters, $0.0873 \times 200 = 17.46$). Second, we sum the expected values for the four access types to get total expected BSIs $= 70.9$. If the BSI rates at center X were the same as the all-centers rates, we would have expected 70.9 BSIs at center X. Finally, the SIR is calculated as the ratio of the actual to expected BSIs. The SIR is interpreted as an adjusted rate ratio, i.e., after adjusting for vascular access type the rate of BSI at center X is 1.42 times higher than that at other centers. Notice that the SIR or adjusted rate ratio (1.42) was lower than the crude value (1.67), indicating a minimal degree of confounding by vascular access type.

Confounding by Variation in the Severity of Underlying Disease—Implications for National Policy

After differential misclassification (Table 2.2), the next problem in the analysis of data from observational studies in hospital epidemiology is confounding by severity of underlying disease. In many institutions, hospital epidemiology has been broadened to include the relatively new area of quality assurance (20–22), and difficulties with confounding have been best illustrated by the initial efforts of the CMS to judge quality of hospital care through monitoring and reporting hospital death rates and rates of nosocomial infections. Both death and infection have many causes, and to measure the effect of one of these—the effect of quality (or lack of quality) of hospital care—in the analysis, one must adjust successfully for the effects of all of the other determinants of death or infection. Further research has indicated that after adjustment for severity of illness, using objective comparisons, it remains extremely difficult to detect differences in hospital care that led to excess mortality (23).

The degree to which the unalterable characteristics of the individual patient determine the inherent susceptibility to infection and probability of death are not yet well defined, but they are clearly of major importance in modern hospital epidemiology. Benchmarking comparisons should be attempted only when a practitioner has data on confounding variables and can adjust for confounding when appropriate.

Effect Modification (Interaction)

Using the terminology of exposure_1, exposure_2, and outcome, we say that effect modification is present when the effect of exposure_1 and exposure_2 together is different from what would have been predicted by their independent effects. Cigarette smoking and asbestos exposure as joint causes of lung cancer are a familiar example. Each of these is a risk factor for lung cancer individually, but when both are present the risk of cancer is particularly high, i.e., the relative risk when both are present is even higher than would be predicted from the sum or product of the two individual relative risks. The carcinogenic potential of asbestos fibers is thought to result from their unusual size, which allows them to migrate easily through the lung tissue. In smokers, these fibers become coated with the carcinogenic materials in cigarette smoke, and thus asbestos fibers become a uniquely efficient system for the delivery of powerful carcinogens from cigarettes into lung tissue. Thus, there is biologic plausibility to the epidemiologic finding of effect modification.

Recall that in the example of confounding involving hospitals A and B presented earlier (see Example of Confounding by Severity of Illness, above), the stratum-specific relative risks were equal (i.e., $RR_1 = RR_2$, Table 2.3). In contrast, effect modification would have been present if RR_1 and RR_2 were found to differ. Unlike the situation with confounding, statistical tests may be used to determine whether effect modification is present (see Chapter 3, Breslow-Day test). An example of effect modification is presented below (see Example of Confounding and Effect Modification, and Example of Logistic Regression Model: Nosocomial Infection and Neonatal Mortality, and Tables 2.7 and 2.11).

Although a single RR_{MH} can be calculated when effect modification is present, this is not recommended; instead, report RR_1 and RR_2 separately. The value of identifying effect modification and reporting separate relative risks is to identify subgroups where a certain exposure is a greater or lesser problem, or in which certain treatments may be more or less effective.

TABLE 2.5. CRUDE ASSOCIATION BETWEEN NOSOCOMIAL INFECTIONS AND DEATH

Death	Exposed	Unexposed	Totals
Outcome (+)	46	104	150
Outcome (−)	92	662	754
Totals	138	766	904

Relative risk =

$$\frac{\text{Probability of outcome (+) among exposed}}{\text{Probability of outcome (+) among unexposed}} = \frac{\frac{a}{a+c}}{\frac{b}{b+d}}$$

Crude relative risk of mortality with infection: risk ratio = 2.46.
95% Confidence intervals for crude risk ratio: (1.83–3.30).
Chi = 5.7; $p < 10^{-8}$.

Examples of Stratified Analyses

Stratification is a powerful tool to investigate confounding and effect modification. Stratification is simple, intuitive, and accessible, because the data remain visible in tables, and the origin and validity of surprising results can be investigated immediately by reference to the tables containing the data.

Example of Confounding Without Effect Modification

In the following example, the effect of nosocomial infections (exposure) on mortality (disease) was studied in the neonatal intensive care unit at the Utah Medical Center (24). Note that in this instance nosocomial infection, which we usually consider to be the disease or outcome, was instead considered the exposure. The crude relative risk was 2.46, indicating an association between infection and death (Table 2.5). However, if low birth weight is also a cause of death acting jointly with nosocomial infection, and nosocomial infection occurs preferentially in low-birth-weight infants, then the crude relative risk is incorrect, having been confounded by birth weight. To investigate this possibility, we can stratify by birth weight and see how the answers change (Table 2.6). Note that, for simplicity, we have left out several lines from each table.

TABLE 2.6. ASSOCIATION OF NOSOCOMIAL INFECTION WITH DEATH STRATIFIED BY BIRTH WEIGHT

		Nosocomial Infection		
Birth weight (g)		Exposed	Unexposed	Relative Risk
<1,000	Died	12	10	
	Total	25	30	1.44
1,000–1,499	Died	12	24	
	Total	42	107	1.27
1,500–1,999	Died	7	18	
	Total	18	142	3.07
2,000+	Died	15	52	
	Total	53	487	2.65

Mantel-Haenszel adjusted relative risk of mortality with infection: risk ratio = 1.89; 95% Confidence intervals for adjusted risk ratio (1.41–2.55).
Chi = 4.1; $p < 10^{-4}$.
Adapted from Freeman J, Goldmann DA, McGowan JE Jr. Methodologic issues in hospital epidemiology. IV. Risk ratios, confounding, effect modification, and the analysis of multiple variables. *Rev Infect Dis* 1988;10:1118–1141.

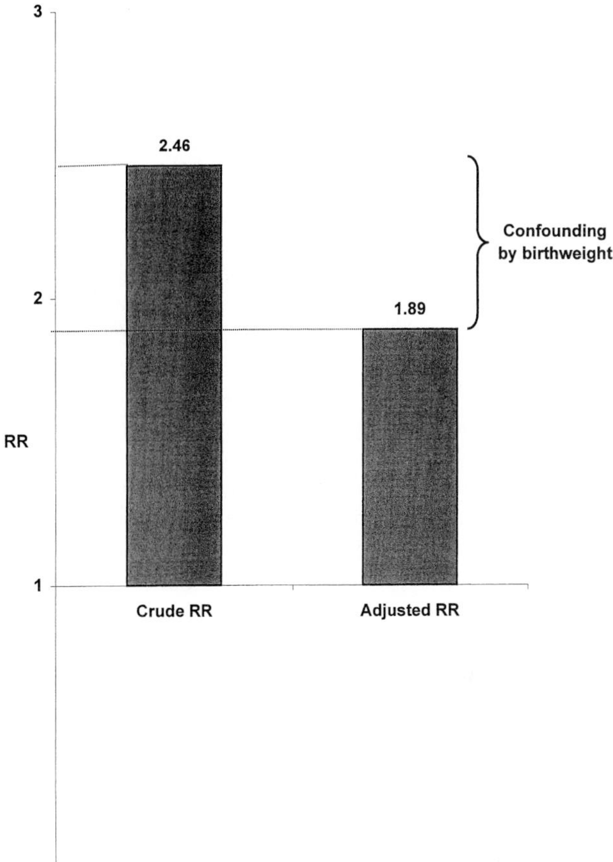

Figure 2.1. Crude and adjusted risk ratios for the association of nosocomial infection with death in neonates in Utah for Table 2.6, showing the effect of confounding by birth weight.

Adjusting for birth weight produced an adjusted relative risk of 1.89, which represents a substantial change from the crude value of 2.46 (Table 2.5 vs. Table 2.6 and Fig. 2.1). Thus, low birth weight was a substantial cause of mortality in this data set and confounded the original relative risk. The crude estimate of the relative risk of mortality with nosocomial infection of 2.46 was 30% too high—it represented the added effect of low birth weight that was mixed in with the effect of nosocomial infection in causing death (Fig. 2.1). After adjustment to remove the confounding effect of low birth weight, the relative risk was lower, chi was smaller, the associated p value was larger, and the lower bound for the relative risk was closer to the null. Note that having all the statistical trappings did not make the crude answer correct. Every aspect of the crude result was wrong. Usually we would have omitted p values and confidence intervals for relative risks that we know to be wrong, but here we included them for educational purposes.

In this example, it appears that there might have been a slight trend of increasing relative risks (from 1.44 to 2.65) as birth weight category increased. If the relative risk were significantly different in the different strata, this would represent effect modification. However, statistical testing did not show that the relative risk differed significantly among the strata, and instead the relative risks from the various strata appear to represent random variation from a true underlying relative risk. Therefore, effect modification was not present and the reporting of the RR_{MH} was appropriate. Besides the Mantel-Haenszel estimator, there are several other commonly used estimates of a uniform adjusted relative risk, but these usually do not differ very much.

Example of Confounding and Effect Modification

In another study of mortality with nosocomial infections from a different neonatal intensive care unit, data were available on underlying disease as well as birth weight (24). Infants in neonatal intensive care units have only a few different diagnoses, and of these underlying diseases, only the persistence of a patent ductus arteriosus (PDA) appeared to have any influence on the outcome (survived vs. died). The data, stratified on birth weight and PDA, are presented in Table 2.7. Again, the interest is in the effect of nosocomial infection (exposure) as a cause of mortality (outcome), but here we can also consider effect modification and confounding by the two extraneous variables birth weight and the presence of a PDA.

If we combine all of the data from this study into a single table (Table 2.7) and look at the crude effect of nosocomial infection on mortality, without stratifying by birth weight or PDA, this crude relative risk is 3.20. If we adjust for birth weight, the relative risk is 2.16, indicating confounding.

We can now investigate whether PDA modified the effect of nosocomial infection as a cause of death among these neonates. The relative risk of nosocomial infection on mortality was 0.88 for infants with PDA versus 5.01 for those without PDA (Table 2.7). This heterogeneity of the effect of infection on mortality according to PDA status was highly significant (chi-square = 7.3, p = .007), indicating that effect modification was present. Because the effect of nosocomial infection is so obviously different for neonates with and without PDA, it makes no biologic or statistical sense to combine these two groups. Thus, the crude and adjusted relative risks of mortality with nosocomial infection are presented separately for those with and without PDA. The crude and adjusted relative risks and the effect modification by PDA are presented visually in Fig. 2.2. Investigation of effect modification provides more biologic information concerning which patients (those without PDA) will be affected, and also shows how much greater the effect will be for that group.

Finally, we both stratify by PDA and adjust for birth weight. Birth weight was not a confounder among those with PDA (crude relative risk = 0.88, RH_{MH} = 0.90; Table 2.7), but was a strong confounder among those without PDA (crude relative risk = 5.01, RH_{MH} = 3.42).

Similar results are obtained when these data are analyzed by logistic regression later in this chapter (see Example of Logistic Regression Model: Nosocomial Infection and Neonatal Mortality, below, and Table 2.12).

Example of Confounding When Incidence Density Is the Outcome Measure

In hospital epidemiology, one frequently needs to correct for differing durations of exposure while investigating the effect of a specific exposure on an outcome. Incidence density data taken from an investigation of an apparent outbreak of nosocomial bacteremia with coagulase-negative staphylococci in a neonatal

TABLE 2.7. ASSOCIATION OF NOSOCOMIAL INFECTION WITH DEATH, STRATIFIED BY BIRTH WEIGHT AND PDA STATUS

		Nosocomial Infection			
		PDA Absent		PDA Present	
Birth Weight (g)		Exposed	Unexposed	Exposed	Unexposed
<1,000	Died	2	7	2	3
	Total	4	38	4	17
1,000–1,499	Died	2	12	0	6
	Total	6	107	11	27
1,500–1,999	Died	2	10	1	0
	Total	6	136	3	12
2,000+	Died	1	27	0	3
	Total	4	520	2	14
Grand total	Died	7	56	3	12
	Total	20	801	20	70

PDA, patent ductus arteriosus.
Crude relative risk[a] = 3.20.
Relative risk adjusted for birth weight[b] = 2.16.
Stratified by PDA:
With PDA, relative risk = 0.88.
Without PDA, relative risk = 5.01.
Breslow-Day test for effect modification, chi-square = 7.3, p = .007.
Stratified by PDA and adjusted for birth weight:
With PDA, relative risk[b] = 0.90.
Without PDA, relative risk[b] = 3.42.
[a] All relative risks are the relative risk of death (outcome) for infants with nosocomial infection (exposure).
[b] Mantel-Haenszel relative risk.

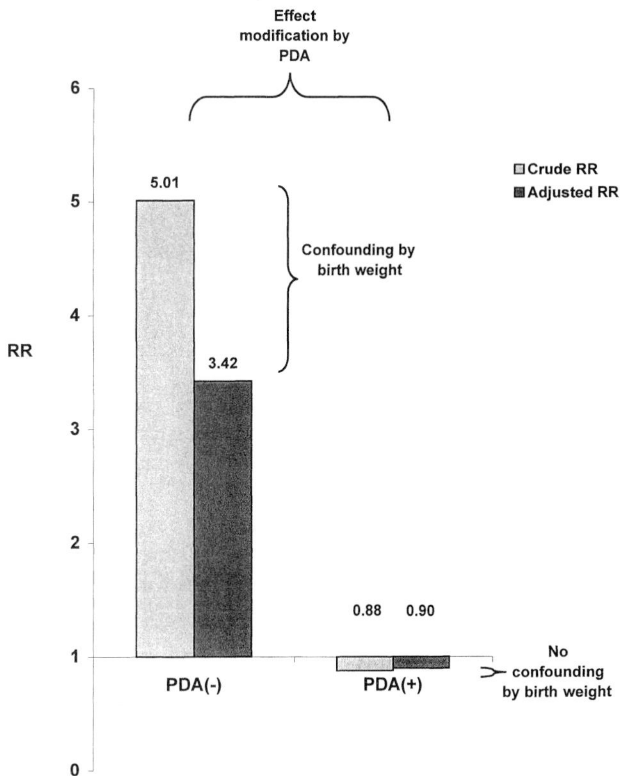

Figure 2.2. Crude and adjusted risk ratios for the association of nosocomial infection with death in neonates for Table 2.7, showing the effects of confounding by birth weight and effect modification by patent ductus arteriosus (PDA) status.

intensive care unit are presented in Table 2.8 (24). Neonatologists were convinced that an epidemic of bacteremia had occurred in 1982, so the number of individuals with first positive blood cultures for coagulase-negative staphylococci were enumerated for that year and for 1975, which was the first year such data were routinely kept. The numbers of patient-days at risk for a first positive blood culture were also accumulated for these neonates. On a simple level, the neonatologists were correct, because they had seen only eight first bacteremias in 1975, whereas they had seen twice that many, 16, in 1982, as demonstrated in the last line of Table 2.8. Thus, comparing simply the absolute numbers of bacteremias they had experienced a doubling, or a 100% increase. Using absolute numbers, the relative risk comparing the two years appeared to be 2.0. The neonatologists were, in fact, working harder.

At the next level, however, we can present these same data not as absolute numbers, but as incidence density rates, and in Table 2.8 we show how the same numbers look with denominators of time at risk for bacteremia. Here the crude rate ratio is a comparison of rates, not numbers, but these rates are still crude for birth weight. Here the crude incidence density ratio is 1.54, an apparent increase of 54%. In this incidence density ratio we have corrected for the much longer exposures to hospital experienced by the smallest neonates in 1982, and this has reduced the apparent relative risk from 2.0 to 1.54.

Finally, we can also adjust for birth weight in this analysis, and the adjusted incidence density ratio is 1.1, indicating no real change in the bacteremia rate (Fig. 2.3). Note that different programs may produce results that vary slightly depending on how they handle numerator cells with zeros. To obtain the above results, we combined the two strata containing infants with birth weights from 1,500 to 1,999 g to avoid a table with a zero marginal total (25). The shareware program dEPID (described later) yields an adjusted relative risk of 1.01, and the shareware program IDR yields an adjusted relative risk of 1.14.

TABLE 2.8. LONGITUDINAL COMPARISON OF INCIDENCE DENSITIES OF BLOOD CULTURES POSITIVE FOR COAGULASE-NEGATIVE STAPHYLOCOCCI IN A NEONATAL INTENSIVE CARE UNIT

	Positive Cultures/Days at Risk		
Birth Weight (g)	1982	1975	Incidence Density Ratio
500–749	3/535	0/10	Unbounded
750–999	8/1,034	2/358	1.4
1,000–1,249	1/424	2/821	1.0
1,250–1,499	1/213	1/567	2.7
1,500–1,749	0/179	1/233	0.0
1,750–1,999	0/455	0/351	Undetermined
2,000+	3/1,880	2/1,289	1.0
Totals	16/4,720	8/3,629	

Ratio of numbers of cases 2.0.
Risk ratio crude for birth weight = 1.54, indicating an apparent 54% increase in 1982.
Mantel-Haenszel adjusted risk ratio = 1.13 (95% confidence interval 0.44–2.86).
There was no significant heterogeneity by birth weight, $p > .05$. Adapted from. Freeman J, Goldmann DA, McGowan JE Jr. Methodologic issues in hospital epidemiology. IV. Risk ratios, confounding, effect modification, and the analysis of multiple variables. *Rev Infect Dis* 1988;10:1118–1141.

Inspection of the strata of the lowest birth weight infants

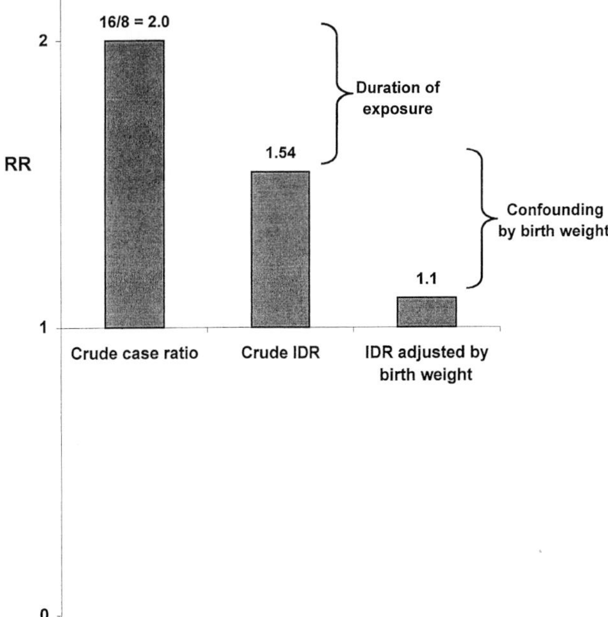

Figure 2.3. Crude, partially adjusted, and completely adjusted incidence density ratios for the longitudinal comparison of bacteremias in neonates in Table 2.8, showing the confounding effects of time at risk and of birth weight.

(those under 1,000 g) indicates that there had been a radical shift in the birth weights of infants who spent time in the neonatal intensive care unit. What we had was not an epidemic of bacteremia but *an epidemic of survival among the smallest neonates who had the majority of positive blood cultures.* More than three fourths of the apparent increase, either a perceived 100% increase or a perceived 54% increase in positive blood cultures, was the result of the increase in survival and longer occupancy of intensive care beds by the smallest infants. After adjustment for birth weight and time at risk, the true change was not substantive. These data are presented to demonstrate how stratification may be used with density data as well as count data (cumulative incidence data) in cohort studies and, additionally, how inspection of visible data explains apparently mysterious results.

Summary: Confounding and Effect Modification

To reiterate, several factors or determinants, acting jointly, are almost invariably responsible for a single outcome in hospital epidemiology. Confounding is the case-mix–induced distortion of the relative risk for one exposure by the effects of other exposures. Effect modification is the biologic interaction of two exposures to produce an unexpectedly high or low relative risk. Confounding and effect modification are compared in Table 2.9.

To detect confounding and effect modification, first calculate a crude relative risk; then perform a stratified analysis, calculating RR_1 and RR_2 separately and an RR_{MH}. If the crude relative risk and the RR_{MH} differ to a meaningful extent, then confounding is present; report the RR_{MH}. If RR_1 and RR_2 are statistically significantly different, effect modification is present; report RR_1 and RR_2 separately and do not report the RR_{MH}.

The collection of data on other prominent potential determinants of the study outcome, along with data on the exposure and outcome variables, is cheap insurance that a study will ultimately be interpretable. If a variable turns out not to confound a comparison, or not to be an effect modifier, little is lost, for data analysis is the least expensive part of an epidemiologic study. Even if all of the potentially confounding variables turn out not to influence a comparison and all potential effect modifiers do not modify, their inclusion as variables that were investigated strengthens a study. In contrast, if a relative risk is strongly distorted by confounding and no data on the confounding variable are available, the whole study is lost or, worse, misinterpreted.

A general scheme for collection and analysis of data for epidemiologic comparisons is presented in Table 2.10.

CONTINUOUS VARIABLES

Epidemiologists most commonly deal with dichotomous (e.g., exposed yes or no, infected yes or no) categorical variables. However, continuous variables that can take on an infinite number of values, such as age, height, and weight, are also seen. Continuous variables can be plotted to form a frequency distribution. These data may be approached differently depending on whether they form a normal (bell-shaped) distribution. If the data are not normally distributed, transforming the data, as by taking the logarithm, may result in a normal distribution.

If data are normally distributed, the central tendency is described by the mean and the spread (how closely the values cluster around the mean) by the standard deviation; parametric methods [i.e., t-test, analysis of variance (ANOVA)] are used to calculate *p* values that test whether the mean values in two or more groups are significantly different. If data are not normally distributed, the central tendency is best described by the median and spread by the interquartile range (the 25th to 75th percentile); nonparametric methods (i.e., Mann-Wittney U test, Wilcoxon test) are used to calculate *p* values for differences among groups.

In the following example, we determine whether maternal age was significantly related to disease in a neonatal intensive care unit (NICU) outbreak. There were nine cases and 173

TABLE 2.9 COMPARISON OF CONFOUNDING AND EFFECT MODIFICATION BY A THIRD, EXTRANEOUS VARIABLE, WHICH IS NEITHER THE EXPOSURE NOR THE OUTCOME UNDER STUDY, IN A SPECIFIC EPIDEMIOLOGIC COMPARISON[a]

	Confounding	Effect Modification
Comparison of attributes		
Effect on comparison	Always distorting: distorting effect may be positive or negative; not itself informative (see Tables 2.5–2.8)	Not distorting (unless also a confounder); provides additional Information (see Table 2.7)
Source and generalizability	One specific data set; not a feature of biology; will differ among data sets containing same comparison	Biology/the real world; likely to be similar in most data sets containing same comparison; probably a real attribute of the biology of a disease
Analytic strategies:		
Observe effect in analysis by	Comparison of crude and adjusted measures	Comparison of effect across strata
Determine quantitative importance in analysis by	Subjective observation of magnitude of distorting effect in context of a specific study (see Tables 2.5–2.8)	Objective tests for heterogeneity of effect across strata of effect modifier: subjective inspection for effects in opposite directions

Note: In an epidemiologic comparison, a single extraneous variable may be a confounder, an effect modifier, neither, or both.

[a] Suggested methods refer to epidemiologic comparisons with discrete outcomes and utilize stratification as the primary analytic strategy. Reference is made to one or more of the studies reanalyzed in this chapter by table number.

Adapted from Freeman J, Goldmann DA, McGowan JE Jr. Methodologic issues in hospital epidemiology. IV. Risk ratios, confounding, effect modification, and the analysis of multiple variables. *Rev Infect Dis* 1988;10:1118–1141.

TABLE 2.10. GENERAL APPROACH TO THE COLLECTION AND ANALYSIS OF DATA FOR EPIDEMIOLOGIC COMPARISONS WITH DISCRETE OUTCOMES[a]

Action	Details of Method
Collection and preliminary Inspection of data	
Anticipate confounding and effect modification	Collect data on multiple variables associated with exposure or outcome; include data on severity of underlying illness and indications for therapy (if therapy was used)
Preliminary stratification for inspection of data	Stratify data repeatedly over a number of extraneous variables that might confound comparisons or modify the effect of an exposure on an outcome; experiment with alternative categorizations; determine workable sizes for strata
Preliminary inspection for presence of confounding variables	Compare crude risk ratios with risk ratios adjusted for various extraneous variables; identify and retain variables for which adjustment alters the risk ratio in an epidemiologically meaningful way
Preliminary inspection for presence of effect modification	Compute stratum-specific risk ratios for different categories of various extraneous variables; Identify and retain variables for which the risk ratio appears to vary across strata: if different categories produce risk ratios in opposite directions, then any summary estimate will be misleading (see Table 2.7): plan to report stratum-specific values
Test for effect modification	If different categories produce risk ratios of varying magnitude in same direction, formally test for heterogeneity of effect over strata: if no significant heterogeneity is present, plan to use Mantel-Haenszel summary risk ratio (see Tables 2.6, 2.7, 2.8); if significant heterogeneity is present, look for pattern to heterogeneity; also, plan to use standardized summary risk ratio
Final analysis and presentation of data	
Select variables for inclusion in final analysis	Retain confounding variables and variables that modified the effect of the exposure on the outcome as stratification variables in the final analysis
Select categories for stratification of confounders and effect modifiers	Choose most efficient and Informative categories for stratification; use multiway stratification if necessary to include multiple variables simultaneously (see Table 2.7)
Present data in stratified format so readers can observe confounding and effect modification	Give summary risk ratios with confidence intervals if appropriate; compute Mantel-Haenszel estimates if there is no significant effect modification; compute standardized estimates if effect modification is present and stratum-specific risk ratios in same direction; give standard and reason for choice

[a] Suggested methods utilize stratification over levels of variables that may confound a comparison and/or modify the effect of the exposure on the outcome under study.
Adapted from Freeman J, Goldmann DA, McGowan JE Jr. Methodologic issues in hospital epidemiology. IV. Risk ratios, confounding, effect modification, and the analysis of multiple variables. *Rev Infect Dis* 1988;10:1118–1141.

noncases. The simplest approach is to dichotomize age at its median (26.5 years) and analyze the data in the familiar 2 × 2 table. This yields a relative risk = 3.5 and *p* value = .17.

		Disease: Yes	Disease: No	
Exposure	Age ≤26.5	7	84	91
	Age >26.5	2	89	91
		9	173	182

To analyze age as a continuous variable we used the statistical program EpiInfo. The mean ± standard deviation maternal age was 21.9 ± 5.3 years for cases versus 26.95 ± 6.2 for noncases. EpiInfo produces two *p* values, one parametric *p* value = .018 and a nonparametric *p* value = .0226. In this package, parametric *p* values are calculated assuming the variances are equal in the two groups; other statistical packages compute an additional parametric *p* value that assumes the variances are different in the two groups. Parametric *p* values are based on calculating the variances and are valid only if the data are normally distributed, whereas nonparametric *p* values are valid regardless of the distribution. For simplicity, nonparametric *p* values are often used in epidemiology. As in this instance, the nonparametric *p* value is usually marginally higher, i.e., less likely to be statistically significant, than the parametric value. Note that the *p* values obtained by treating maternal age as a continuous variable (*p* = .02) are lower than the value obtained in the 2 × 2 table above after converting to a dichotomous variable (*p* = .17).

The above example was for analysis of unpaired continuous variable data. Alternate methods are used for analyzing paired values, e.g., scores on a test before versus after an educational program. Rather than just averaging the mean of all scores before and comparing it with the mean of all scores after, we can take advantage of some additional available information, i.e., that we know each score before corresponds to a score after. In brief, the method is to compute the difference between the before versus after scores for each subject, so that one value per subject is obtained, and then to statistically test the null hypothesis that the difference equals zero. This provides a more precise answer and can be done by either parametric or nonparametric methods.

ADDITIONAL TOPICS IN HEALTHCARE EPIDEMIOLOGY

Hypothesis Generating versus Hypothesis Testing Studies

The classic hypothesis testing approach is to state a hypothesis, e.g., postulate an association between one or a few exposure(s) and disease(s), and then deliberately collect data to verify or refute the hypothesis. Most explanations of how to conduct and analyze epidemiologic studies refer to this approach, i.e., focusing on an exposure of primary interest and checking for confounding or effect modification from secondary exposure variables. However, in practice many modern epidemiologic studies take an alternate approach, namely to evaluate a number of exposure variables and report whether any are significantly associated with disease. Using this approach, which is one type of hypothesis generating study, there is no exposure of primary interest—all are created equal.

Repetition of data analyses with varying assumptions or methods until a statistically significant result is obtained have been called "data dredging" or "data torturing." Any complex data set will contain many apparent associations. Some of these are real and causal, whereas others are the result of random processes and represent no true association. Therefore, associations are less likely to be valid and reproducible if found in a hypothesis generating study and should be interpreted with the caveats regarding performance of multiple testing and attention to the Hill criteria for causality.

A valid approach is to use one data set for hypothesis generation and a second independent data set for hypothesis testing. If only one data set is available, this can be divided into two, with the first for hypothesis generation and the second for hypothesis testing.

Multiple Comparisons

Strictly speaking, our use of the *p* value assumes that only one potential exposure is being evaluated. If the variable is statistically significant at the .05 level, there is a 5% chance that this association occurred due to chance alone. We are willing to accept this chance of error. However, if a large number of potential exposure variables are evaluated, the probability that one or more will be significant by chance alone rises. To compensate, it has been proposed that the required level of significance be set to approximately .05 divided by the number of variables tested (Bonferroni correction). For example, if ten variables were tested, then we would require a *p* value of approximately .005 for statistical significance. This approach is occasionally seen in the literature. However, most epidemiologists prefer not to use a rigid formula such as this, but to interpret findings by considering the Hill criteria for causation as well as the *p* value and the number of variables sifted through.

Stratifying Continuous Variables and Analyzing Multilevel Tables

In data analysis, it is often necessary to construct appropriate groups from a continuous variable. An example is the grouping of neonates by birth weight. The cutoff values used to divide the groups can be chosen by allocating the same number of subjects in each group (e.g., quartiles with ¼ of the subjects in each group), dividing the group at even numbers (e.g., 750 to 1,000 g), or using cut points that are widely used and accepted. The method used should be nonbiased (i.e., the cutoff values should not be manipulated to produce a predetermined result), include an adequate number of subjects in each stratum, and include subjects with a similar risk of the outcome in individual strata. Multilevel categorical variables result from this grouping.

To analyze multilevel categorical variables, we use a variation of the 2 × 2 table methods previously presented for dichotomous or binary exposure variables. In an example of the effect of birth weight on neonatal mortality, the continuous exposure variable birth weight has been divided into four groups to form a categorical multilevel variable (Table 2.11). Note that as the birth weight increases, the percent of neonates who died decreases from 22.2% to 5.7%; this is an example of a dose-response relationship as mentioned in the Hill criteria for causality. These data are analyzed by forming multiple 2 × 2 tables with the lowest rate stratum (≥2,000 g) acting as the nonexposed group in each (Tables 2.11a–c). The number of 2 × 2 tables will be one less than the number of strata of the multilevel variable. Compared with the reference category, birth weight ≥2,000 g, which is assigned relative risk = 1.0, the risk of death was 1.44 times higher for 1,500 to 1,999 g, 2.31 times higher for 1,000 to 1,499 g, and 3.87 times higher for <1,000 g. Individual *p* values for each 2 × 2 table may be reported along with the individual relative risks. However, it is well to also calculate a test for heterogeneity among the four categories; this tests the null hypothesis that the rates are the same in the four birth weights. In this example, the chi-square value of 24.8 with three degrees of freedom indicates a highly significant difference in mortality among the birth weight groups.

Epidemic versus Endemic Disease

In every hospital, there are truly serious events with costly or even life-threatening consequences, and some of these are preventable. Epidemiologists usually have to act under great uncertainty. What to do and when to do it must be determined at least partially on a subjective basis using the best information available at the moment.

An epidemic is simply an increase in the frequency of occurrence of events above the usual level. When events with serious adverse consequences occur in epidemic form, it is in one sense convenient for an epidemiologist, because an epidemic implies that the events are noticeable. Unfortunately, about 90% of bad things that happen in hospitals are endemic and do not occur in epidemic form, which renders them even more difficult to detect (26). Strength of association is also important in epidemiology, but a hospital epidemiologist often has to act before a sample size large enough for a contrast to reach statistical significance can be collected. It would be unthinkable to allow an epidemic to continue to rage out of control in order to collect ten more deaths for the *p* value.

Statistical significance is least important in dealing with epidemics. When facing a potential epidemic, we still think back to the old saw: Two is a coincidence and three is an epidemic. This, of course, must be tempered by the seriousness of the events. A single unexpected fatality should trigger the same investigation as do multiple, less serious events (27). However, it is unlikely that three events are going to produce a contrast in which statistical significance will be reached. What is the *p* value of the one dead house officer whose potentially preventable death initiated an important study (27)? Thus an epidemiologist has to be more concerned with the biologic import of observed events, the size of the effect, and potential future events than with any statistical *p* value.

Meta-Analysis

Strictly defined, meta-analysis is the statistical analysis of a collection of analytic results from intervention studies for the

TABLE 2.11. ANALYSIS OF A MULTILEVEL VARIABLE CREATED BY CATEGORIZATION OF A CONTINUOUS VARIABLE

				Indicator Variables[b]		
Birth Weight (g)	**Died, *n* (%)**	**Survived (*n*)**	**Relative Risk[a]**	**BW1**	**BW2**	**BW3**
<1,000	14 (22.2)	49	3.87	1	0	0
1,000–1,499	20 (13.2)	131	2.31	0	1	0
1,500–1,999	13 (8.3)	144	1.44	0	0	1
≥2,000	31 (5.7)	509	1.0	0	0	0

Data collated from Table 2.7.
Test for heterogeneity, chi-square = 24.8, 3 degrees of freedom, $p < .001$.
[a] See Tables 2.11a, b, and c, below, for calculation of the relative risks.
[b] For use in logistic regression model (Table 2.12).

TABLE 2.11a.

	Died: Yes	Died: No	
Exposure			
<1000	14	49	63
≥2,000	31	509	540

Relative risk = (14/63)/(31/540) = 3.87, $p < .0001$.

TABLE 2.11b.

	Died: Yes	Died: No	
Exposure			
1,000–1,499	20	131	151
≥2,000	31	509	540

Relative risk = (20/151)/(31/540) = 2.31, $p < .004$.

TABLE 2.11c.

	Died: Yes	Died: No	
Exposure			
1,500–1,999	13	144	157
≥2,000	31	509	540

Relative risk = (13/157)/(31/540) = 1.44, $p = .3$.

purpose of integrating the findings (2,28). The results (estimates of the relative risk) of multiple trials may be pooled to produce a single estimate of the relative risk, which may be more informative and precise than any of the estimates from the individual studies. Meta-analyses may resolve uncertainty when reports disagree and produce more objective summaries of a literature than might be possible with unaided intellectual interpretation. In addition, meta-analyses may answer new questions not posed at the start of individual trials.

In the original publications the term *meta-analysis* had meaning only in terms of randomized trials, but its use has slowly been extended to observational studies. There is risk of the method becoming distorted by using it to combine the results of observational studies. The results of randomized trials are, on average, unconfounded because of the randomization process. A summary of unconfounded study results will itself be unconfounded. On the other hand, meta-analysis of confounded observational studies will produce a confounded summary result. There is the danger that meta-analysis will be used for mere technologic pooling rather than critical evaluation.

The simplest statistical method to perform meta-analysis is to perform a stratified analysis where each separate study forms one strata and an RR_{MH} is calculated. As in conventional stratified analyses, we would not want to calculate and report an RR_{MH} if the relative risks differed significantly among the strata, i.e., if there was heterogeneity of the relative risks. This amounts to a form of effect modification where the variable causing the effect modification is the study itself. Probably the most important epidemiologic issue confronted in a meta-analysis is the determination of whether there is heterogeneity among studies, and this is often more important than computing some fictional common or average effect (2,29–33). This is the same heterogeneity issue described in Table 2.7. Heterogeneity among results must be tested for rigorously. The basic question is, If heterogeneity of results is present, does it make sense to conduct a meta-analysis and present a single estimate of the relative risk? Arguments can be made on both sides.

There are two additional threats to the validity of a meta-analysis. First, publication bias, which in this instance acts as a form of selection bias, may mean that studies with a statistically significant effect were much more likely to be published and therefore to be included in the meta-analysis. Second, variations in the quality (generally forms of misclassification or confounding) of studies included may bias the result. Criteria for the quality of studies included should be set, and a detailed list of studies included in and excluded from meta-analyses (with reasons) must accompany each presentation.

An example of the use of meta-analysis was in consideration of the widely varying reports of the effectiveness of Bacille Calmette-Guérin (BCG) vaccine in preventing tuberculosis. The meta-analysis suggested that the degree of protection was partially explained by distance from the equator, which is thought to be a proxy for prevalence of prior infection with atypical mycobacteria (32). Individuals who have already been "vaccinated" by infection with naturally occurring atypicals will receive less benefit from a second vaccination with BCG. This is an example of how heterogeneity among results was explored in a meta-analysis of clinical trials and how the process resulted in a better understanding of the basic biology involved.

Sensitivity, Specificity, and Predictive Values

Suppose that we have a recognized laboratory method that we consider the "gold standard" (referred to as the "standard") and a proposed newer method (referred to as the "test") that may be cheaper, faster, or have some other advantage. We want to see how the test compares with the recognized standard. We run many specimens by both methods and arrange the data in the same format as the 2 × 2 table ("Yes" indicates a positive test and "No" indicates a negative test). This same format can be used to compare two case definitions, two methods of collecting data, etc, as long as one can be considered the accepted standard.

		Standard		
		Yes	No	
Test	Yes	a	b	a+b
	No	c	d	c+d
		a+c	b+d	

We can then define four performance characteristics of the new test:

- Sensitivity = $a/(a + c)$: Of all true positives, what proportion was identified by the test?
- Specificity = $d/(b + d)$: Of all true negatives, what proportion were identified by the test?
- Positive predictive value = $a/(a + b)$: Of those positive by the test, what proportion are true positive?
- Negative predictive value = $d/(c + d)$: Of those negative by the test, what proportion are true negative?

Sensitivity and specificity are biologic characteristics and are not influenced by the frequency of disease in the population. On the other hand, the predictive values are influenced by the frequency of disease in the population. Thus, if the disease is rare in a population, the positive predictive value will tend to be low even if specificity is high. Stated another way, if the test is applied in a population where there are few true positives, then a large number of false positives (cell *b* in the 2 × 2 table) will be found, and most of those found to be positive will in fact be false positives (cell *b* will be higher than cell *a*).

There is a trade-off between sensitivity and specificity. A change that makes the test more sensitive (more able to detect true disease) will usually make it less specific (less able to exclude nondisease). This relationship can be depicted graphically as a receiver operating curve plotting sensitivity versus 1 − specificity (34).

Sample Size and Power

Assume that there is a true difference in rates of disease in the exposed versus nonexposed populations that would be found if a very large number of subjects were studied. However, by chance alone, a study of a limited sample of these subjects might or might not find a statistically significant difference. Power is the probability of finding a significant difference between the exposed and nonexposed in your *sample* of study subjects if there really is a difference in the rates in the *populations* from which the samples were taken. Power = 1 − the probability of type II error, where type II error is the probability of not finding a significant difference when there really is a difference between the rates in the two populations.

Calculations of sample size and power involve specifying the following (1):

- The rate of illness in the nonexposed group
- The rate of illness in the exposed group (or the relative risk)
- The p value required for statistical significance (usually .05) and whether a one- or two-tailed test will be performed
- The ratio of the number of exposed to nonexposed subjects

If the above four are specified, then one can additionally specify the power desired and calculate the sample size required. Alternately one can specify the sample size and calculate the power that will be achieved. These calculations can be made easily by shareware programs such as EpiInfo (Statcalc or Epitables modules). For example, assume that the rate of SSI last year (nonexposed) was 4%, and one wanted to have 80% power to detect an SSI rate of 8% this year (exposed; relative risk = 2.0) with $p < .05$; entering these assumptions into the computer program we would find that we would need 1,202 subjects, 601 exposed and 601 nonexposed. These types of calculations should probably be used more frequently in planning hospital surveillance, so that surveillance efforts can be continued for a sufficient period of time to detect a predetermined rate of nosocomial illness.

In a prospectively planned study, it is desirable to have ≥80% power to detect a difference between exposure groups. A hypothesis testing study with marginal power to detect a true difference generally will not be worth conducting. On the other hand, power calculations may not be crucial in pilot studies or hypothesis-generating studies. Power calculations are at best only a crude estimate that cannot anticipate all the intricacies of the final data set; for example, the need to control for confounders may increase the sample size needed. Additionally, planning for sufficient power may not be possible during an outbreak investigation, where, in the interests of protecting patients, one should usually proceed even though the number of subjects involved may be too small to yield a desirable degree of power.

Simple Shareware Programs for Epidemiologic Analyses

Since the publication of the original programs for stratified analyses with the programmable calculator (25), a number of useful programs for personal computers running on the disk operating system (DOS) have been written that may be obtained at minimal expense (35). More good shareware programs appear continually so the periodic column in ref. 35 should be perused from time to time.

EpiInfo is a freeware program available from the Centers for Disease Control and Prevention (CDC) that has been updated to run in the Windows environment. This program allows one to create data entry screens, enter and manage data, sort and print data, calculate sample sizes, and perform an array of useful analyses. The data output for 2 × 2 table analysis is particularly useful (see Chapter 15).

MULTIVARIABLE REGRESSION ANALYSIS

One cannot read a scientific journal these days without being exposed to regression modeling. For most epidemiologists, it is more important to understand how to interpret results of regression models than to actually fit them. However, some insight into the regression "black box" will benefit everyone who either collects or interprets data.

Regression models are used to identify confounding and effect modification, calculate adjusted relative risks and p values that are free of confounding and reflect the independent effects of variables, find which of several potential variables are independently associated with disease, and make predictions. Regression analysis makes it much easier to sift through a large number of variables to find the few that are significant predictors. Additionally, regression models produce a more precise result (narrower confidence interval) than other multivariable methods such as stratification. However, with these advantages come the potential for abuse: fitting models has become easy enough that well-meaning but inadequately trained individuals may easily and efficiently produce incorrect results.

Problems with Multivariate Models: Survey of Published Results of Fitting Multivariate Models

Most physicians, nurses, and other medical professionals have received no instruction in the fitting of multivariate models in complex data sets, yet these methods now commonly appear in the medical literature (36). A study of articles in two medical journals in which multivariate models were frequently used showed the result of this lack of technical background. Simple identification, coding, and selection of potential confounders and effect modifiers were not described in the majority of published papers, and nonlinearity of response was not investigated in one third (36). What is visible and automatic in stratified analyses has generally been omitted from multivariate models fit by naive users. Although both stratification and the fitting of multivariate models can achieve the goals of analyzing the effects of multiple variables in complex data sets, clinician-epidemiologists without extensive training in biostatistics are more likely to obtain understandable and valid results with stratification.

Multivariate models can be validly produced only by those well trained and experienced. This section is merely an introduction and overview. Essential reading is a paper by Sander Greenland (37), which is a literate description of the use of multivariate models in epidemiologic research.

Automated Algorithms for Modeling

Statistical packages provide the capability for automated model building. This may occur by forward selection, starting with the single most highly statistically significant variable and adding one variable at time to the model; or by backward elimination, starting with all variables in the model and removing nonsignificant variables one by one. The backward elimination method may produce poor results if too many variables are under consideration. Except for some newly developed algorithms, called "change in effect algorithms" and described by Greenland (37), all common automatic algorithms in canned statistical packages use p values for selecting variables, and investigator intervention is required to select variables for reasons other than statistical significance.

These automatic algorithms for model building were written by biostatisticians for the specific purpose of selecting the best set of variables to predict a specific outcome without reference to biologic causation, confounding, effect modification, or linearity. Automatic algorithms do, in fact, produce useful prediction models, but this is not usually the purpose of an epidemiologic analysis. If causation and biologic interpretability are the reasons for fitting a multivariate model, then automatic stepwise algorithms will not provide interpretable answers, may produce substantial errors, and should not be employed. These automated methods may sometimes be used by experienced personnel as a first step in producing a model. However, they should never be relied on by inexperienced personnel to produce a final model.

Practical Aspects of Model Building

Model building requires skill and experience and cannot be reduced to a cookbook approach. It is not too difficult to fit a model involving cumulative incidence data and only a few dichotomous (e.g., yes or no) exposure variables. For this simple case a model that controls for potential confounding can be produced. Complexity is introduced by the presence of a large number of potential exposure variables, a small number of cases, multilevel exposure variables (i.e., ≥ 3 levels), continuous (e.g., age, weight) exposure variables, colinearity among exposure variables, and effect modification. Additional complications include the need to account for time at risk (as in incidence density or survival analyses) and study designs with nonindependent records (see below).

Two variables are collinear if they measure nearly the same biologic property. An example would be two severity of illness scores that include many of the same components. It is advisable to identify colinearity by exploration before multivariable analysis. If collinear variables are introduced into a model, large changes in the regression coefficients and p values may occur. It may be obvious that only one of these variables can be in the model, but there is no statistical test to indicate which to choose.

All variables should be examined by univariable (e.g., 2×2 tables) methods first, and some should be further explored in stratified analyses. Continuous variables should be explored by plotting; for the model, they should be divided into categories (e.g., quartiles) and represented by indicator variables (Table 2.11).

Criteria for inclusion of a variable in a model include:

- The variable is statistically significant (usually $p < .05$) when in the model.
- The variable is an exposure of primary interest.
- The variable is a confounder of an exposure of primary interest. An informal rule of thumb would be that the variable produces a change of $\geq 10\%$ in the regression coefficient of the variable of primary interest.
- The variable is of special biologic interest, e.g., has been found in previous studies to be an important predictor.

Variables are introduced into the model one at a time and retained in the model if they meet one of the criteria for inclusion listed above. Continuous variables should be examined in several ways: as a simple continuous variable, as the continuous variable plus its square, as a transform (e.g., logarithm, reciprocal) of the continuous variable, and (most importantly) as a series of indicator variables coding (Table 2.11) for discrete categories. If the squared value of a continuous variable is statistically significant, this suggests a curvilinear relationship between the continuous variable and the outcome variable.

The pool of variables to try in the model includes those of special biologic interest and those with less than a certain p value in univariable analysis. It may be advisable to set this p value at a relatively high level, say .2, since some such variables may prove to have lower p values in the model or to be important confounders. Remember that it is necessary that a confounder be associated with the outcome, and a very weak association as indicated by $p > .20$ cannot result in much confounding effect (37,38). Thus, if the available automatic algorithms employing p values are to be used for screening for potential confounders, the selection criterion should be set at some much larger value than .05, for instance, $p < .20$.

Effect Modification

After variables have been selected for the model, effect modification should be tested for. Interaction terms can be created by multiplying the main effect variables by one another, two at a time. These terms are then introduced into the model and checked for statistical significance. A problem is that there may be many interaction terms. A model with five main effect variables will have nine potential interaction terms, one or more of which may be significant by chance alone. If an interaction term is found to be statistically significant, one must decide whether to retain it in the final model on much the same basis as other variables, e.g., by considering factors such as the p value, size of effect, biologic plausibility, and whether it substantially changes the main effects. It may be reasonable to report models with and without interaction terms.

Additional Considerations

When the results of fitting a multivariate model to estimate relative risk differ substantively from the results of stratified analysis on the same data, the results of the multivariate analysis are wrong. Remember, again, that no analytic scheme can correct selection bias or misclassification.

Recall that two conditions must be present for an exposure (i.e., exposure_1) to be confounded by a second exposure (exposure_2): exposure_1 must be associated with exposure_2 and exposure_2 must be associated with disease. Retaining exposure_2 in a model when it is not a confounder will, by definition, not change the estimated effect of exposure_1 and therefore will not produce a wrong answer. However, there will be a statistical penalty in the sense of an increased p value and wider confidence interval for exposure_1.

Biostatisticians acknowledge that selection of variables by significant p values does not directly address confounding, but they have been appropriately concerned that the criterion used by epidemiologists to determine important confounding (i.e., biologically important change in a relative risk) is subjective. Two reasonable epidemiologists viewing the same results could reach opposite conclusions about the confounding effect of a specific variable. One way around this problem would be to report both results, one with and one without adjustment for the questionable confounding variable, and allow readers of the report to draw their own conclusions (39).

Biostatisticians have created elaborate but helpful sets of tools called regression diagnostics, including analysis of residuals, for investigating the characteristics of a regression model (36–38, 41–45). These diagnostics are extremely useful when multiple variables appear to carry the same basic information (colinearity). Other diagnostics allow one to maximize the utility of a predictive model. However, none of the biostatistical procedures relates in any way to biology or causation, and if a biologist is not making the decisions indicated by regression diagnostics, they may be of little value.

Multiple Regression Models Commonly Used in Epidemiology

Many types of regression models have been developed, but the following four are most commonly used: multiple linear regression, when the outcome variable is continuous; logistic regression when the outcome variable is dichotomous; Poisson regression for incidence density data; and the Cox model for survival analysis data.

Linear Regression

Linear regression or ordinary least squares regression is used for continuous outcome variables such as length of hospital stay or cost. The regression coefficients obtained in the model may be simply interpreted as in the following example where days of hospital stay is the outcome variable: if the regression coefficient for male gender was 2.0, then males on average had a length of stay 2 days longer than females; and if the coefficient for age ≥60 was 3.0, then patients ≥60 had an average stay 3 days longer than younger patients. The effects of the regression coefficients are combined by addition.

A number of statistical assumptions underlie this model, and one of the most important is that the outcome must be approximately normally distributed. If the outcome is not normally distributed, then the p values that arise from fitting a multiple linear regression model are uninterpretable (40–42). Confidence intervals for regression coefficients are easily calculated from standard errors and the distribution of Student's t-test. Another very useful quantity that arises from multiple linear regression is the square of the multiple correlation coefficient or the multiple R^2. The multiple R^2 represents the proportion of variation of the outcome variable that is explained by the model. In contrast to other common types of regression models, the regression coefficients in a linear model can be calculated by an exact mathematical formula.

Logistic Regression

Logistic regression, the most common type of model used in healthcare epidemiology, is used when the outcome variable is dichotomous (e.g., disease yes or no). The regression coefficient obtained for a variable is the natural logarithm of the odds ratios for that variable. Therefore, to obtain the odds ratio, the regression coefficient is exponentiated. Even in a cohort study, the relative risk cannot be directly determined using logistic regression, and therefore the odds ratio is used where logistic regression modeling is required. However, if data from a cohort study are analyzed using logistic regression, a simple formula can be used to estimate the adjusted relative risk from the adjusted odds ratio obtained from logistic regression (46). The effects of the regression coefficients are combined by adding the regression coefficients or multiplying the odds ratios (see Example of Logistic Regression Model: Nosocomial Infection and Neonatal Mortality, below).

Logistic regression requires less stringent biostatistical assumptions than linear regression but does not inherently adjust for differences in duration of exposure. There is no exact analog for multiple R^2 in logistic regression, but the area under receiver operating curves yields similar information. Unlike linear regression models, logistic regression models do not have exact algebraic solutions, and computers fit them with iterative approximation procedures. Not all models converge to a solution. Iterative fits were practically impossible before the general availability of the computer and still may be difficult for large and complex data sets (see Chapter 3).

Try study questions 8 and 9 in Appendix 1 at the end of the chapter.

Poisson Regression

Poisson regression uses incidence density data, i.e., the number of cases of disease during a certain person-time of follow-up. Like the incidence density approach, Poisson regression does not account for possible differences in disease incidence during early versus late follow-up. The regression coefficients obtained are the natural logarithm of the incidence density rate ratio. Poisson regression is a valid method to determine the rate ratio for a variable while accounting for time at risk and adjusting for potential confounding from other variables. However, Poisson regression is mainly used when data on individual subjects are not available, i.e., Poisson regression is used if we know the total number of cases and the total person-time, but do not know the person-time contributed by individual subjects or whether individual subjects were cases. If data on individual patients are known, then survival analysis (Kaplan-Meier plot or the Cox model) is used preferentially. Analogous to logistic regression, the effects of two or more exposures are predicted by adding the regression coefficients or multiplying the rate ratios.

Cox Proportional Hazards Models

Cox models were created for survival analysis and are used when the outcome variable is dichotomous and when it is desirable to account for time at risk (47,48). The terminology and methods for survival analysis were presented in an earlier section of this chapter. There are other survival analysis regression methods available, but these depend on modeling the shape of the survival curve. The Cox model represented a breakthrough, because it is not necessary to model the shape of the survival curve. The regression coefficients from Cox models are the natural logarithms of what are called hazard ratios; hazard ratios may be interpreted as incidence density rate ratios or relative risks. The effects of two or more exposures are predicted in a manner similar to that used in logistic regression. As with logistic regression models, the Cox model can be fit only by iterative processes.

The Cox model assumes that the hazard ratio for a given exposure is constant over time; this is the so-called proportional hazards assumption (47,48). This means that, if the hazard ratio for male gender is 2.0, then throughout all times of follow-up males have twice the risk of disease as females. If the hazard ratio for males were 2.0 during early follow-up but 1.0 (or anything other than 2.0) during late follow-up, this data set would not fit the proportional hazard assumption and the Cox model would not be appropriate. If the hazard ratio for a variable changes over the time of follow-up, essentially time is an effect modifier for the variable. The proportional hazards assumption can be investigated graphically or by creating a time-dependent covariate with the logarithm of time and the independent variable (47). If the hazard ratio varies significantly over time, then the proportional hazards assumption is violated. In the previous investigation of the use of multivariate models in the medical literature, checking of the proportional hazards assumption was not reported in more than 80% of publications that used Cox models (36).

An excellent program for fitting Cox models is PROC PHREG in SAS (47). In addition to routine multivariate models using survival analysis data, PROC PHREG makes it possible to define strata beforehand within which the multivariate model will be fit. For example, it is possible to group hospital patients into a small number of strata by diagnosis-related group (DRG) number, which has no inherent quantitative meaning, and then use DRG relative weight as a continuous variable in the model. This will adjust comparisons for both DRG and DRG relative weight simultaneously, one by stratification and the other by modeling. Data may be stratified by more than one variable. It seems likely that stratified Cox models fit by informed epidemiologists will become a preferred method for analysis of surveillance and other observational data in hospital epidemiology.

Cox Regression with Time-Dependent Covariates

An important variant is the Cox model with time-dependent covariates. Although some exposure variables (e.g., gender) are inherent characteristics of the subject, others may vary over a time of follow-up (e.g., neutropenia, Apache II score). Most analysis methods would require some type of compromise for variables that change value, e.g., neutropenia could be coded as never, sometimes, or always present. However, the Cox model with time-dependent covariates allows us to actually use different values for exposure variables at different times of follow-up. This elegant method allows more exact estimates and opens up exciting possibilities for future studies.

Example of Logistic Regression Model: Nosocomial Infection and Neonatal Mortality

The data for this exercise are from Table 2.7. The outcome variable was dichotomous (died or survived) and so logistic regression was used. Recall that in logistic regression we always produce odds ratios, even if the data are from a cohort study. We found in stratified analysis that nosocomial infection was a risk factor for death, birth weight was a confounder of this relationship, and PDA was an effect modifier.

Our logistic regression starts with model 1 (Table 2.12), which has only nosocomial infection (odds ratio = 3.9). We next add three indicator variables for birth weight groups (model 2); Table 2.11 shows how these indicator variables were coded. These indicator variables show the expected increase in mortality as birth weight decreases, and also that the effect of nosocomial infection decreases when we control for birth weight (odds ratio decreases from 3.9 to 2.6, suggesting confounding). We can do a statistical test for heterogeneity of the birth weight categories by taking the difference in $-2 \times$ log likelihood between models 1 and 2. This difference is 15.6, which can be evaluated as a chi-square with 3 degrees of freedom, since three variables were added to model 1 to produce model 2. The resulting p value for heterogeneity of the birth weight groups = .0014. Next, we add PDA to produce model 3; we note that PDA has a minimal

TABLE 2.12. LOGISTIC REGRESSION MODEL: CONFOUNDING AND EFFECT MODIFICATION IN A STUDY OF NEONATAL MORTALITY

Model	$-2 \times$ Log Likelihood	Variable	Regression Coefficient	Odds Ratio	Wald *p* value
1	522.4	NI	1.37	3.9	.0004
2	506.8	NI	0.97	2.6	.02
		BW1	1.41	4.1	.0001
		BW2	0.79	2.2	.01
		BW3	0.33	1.4	.3
3	506.4	NI	0.91	2.5	.03
		PDA	0.20	1.2	.6
		BW1	1.36	3.9	.0003
		BW2	0.75	2.1	.02
		BW3	0.32	1.4	.4
4	501.7	NI	1.65	5.2	.001
		PDA	0.58	1.8	.12
		BW1	1.26	3.5	.001
		BW2	0.71	2.0	.03
		BW3	0.26	1.3	.5
		NI–PDA	−1.85	0.16	.03

NI, nosocomial infection; PDA, patent ductus arteriosus; BW1–BW3, indicator variables for age group (see Table 2.11); NI–PDA, interaction term between nosocomial infections and patent ductus arteriosus.

effect on mortality (odds ratio = 1.2, p = .6). Finally, we create model 4 by adding the interaction term between nosocomial infection and PDA. This interaction term is not highly significant (p = .03) but has a substantial effect (odds ratio = 0.16).

Model 3 (Table 2.12), without an interaction term, would indicate that the odds ratio was 1.0 (reference group) for infants with no PDA and no nosocomial infection, 1.2 for infants with PDA but not nosocomial infection, 2.5 for those with nosocomial infection but not PDA, and 3.0 (the latter calculated by $1.2 \times 2.5 = 3.0$) for those with both PDA and nosocomial infection. Model 4 indicates that the risks are 1.0, 1.8, 5.2, and 1.5 (the latter calculated by $5.2 \times 1.8 \times 0.16 = 1.5$) for these four possibilities, respectively. The interaction term leads to a markedly different (in this case, lower) estimate of the risk in neonates with both PDA and nosocomial infection (3.0 in model 3 vs. 1.5 in model 4) than one would have predicted based on the separate effects of these two variables.

Longitudinal Analysis and Repeated Measures

Standard statistical techniques assume that all observations in a data set are independent. This assumption may be violated in various ways. The first and simplest is that in most healthcare studies some patients have more than one episode of the illness under study. Some patients are obviously more prone to disease than others, and two records from the same patient are not independent. Examples are that individuals who are HIV positive often have repeated bouts of illness with opportunistic infections, and some hospital patients have multiple nosocomial infections during a single hospital stay. One approach to this problem is to study only the first infection for each individual, but this wastes data and does not represent the reality that patients often have multiple events.

A second problem involves longitudinal follow-up with repeated measurements on individual patients. There are clearly situations when it is possible and even necessary to study the same individuals repeatedly over time.

A third issue involves studies carried out at a limited number of medical centers. For example, consider a study done at five hospitals with 100 patients studied at each. Individual hospitals vary greatly in patient populations and style of practice. The 500 records from five hospitals are not independent as would be the case if a random sample of 500 patients from all U.S. hospitals were studied. A recent article discusses adjustment for center in multicenter studies, including the problems of nonindependence, confounding by center, and effect modification by center (49).

To use all the data available without violating statistical assumptions, we can use methods that were developed specifically for longitudinal or repeated measures studies. The most popular method is the use of generalized estimating equations (GEEs) (50). GEE models can be fit by various statistical packages including SAS; PROC GENMOD uses GEE to fit linear, Poisson, or logistic regression models (51). The initial parameter estimates, using routine methods and not accounting for clustering (e.g., by multiple observations per patient or per medical center), are first presented; then the "robust" results that have accounted for cluster effect are produced. Fitting these models is more complicated than fitting the other models discussed above. For example, it is necessary to specify the form of the correlation matrix. It is worthwhile to compare the results obtained by various methods: standard models including all repeated events, standard models including only first events in a given patient, and the robust estimates from GEE models using various correlation assumptions. If these methods produce similar results, one can feel confident in drawing conclusions, and if they produce different results, more insight into the data is obtained. Fitting models using GEE must be done iteratively for both continuous and discrete data, and the fitting process will not always converge to a solution.

APPENDIX 1: STUDY QUESTIONS

Question 1

Reliable information on patient admissions and discharges is usually available from the hospital administration. From a list of discharges during a 6-month period, a hospital epidemiologist selected all cases that suffered at least one nosocomial urinary tract infection during hospitalization and an equal number of reference patients who did not acquire such infection during hospitalization. If the hospital epidemiologist compared the cases of nosocomial urinary tract infection with the reference subjects for mortality during hospitalization, would this be a case-control study or a cohort study? (Hint: Carefully identify the exposure and the outcome.) Suppose the noncases were matched to the cases by primary underlying illness, operation, and age. Would this change your answer?

Question 2

Consider again the situation described in question 1. Using the same cases of nosocomial urinary tract infection and the same uninfected reference patients, the hospital epidemiologist then compared the cases with the comparison subjects for events that occurred in the first week of hospitalization prior to the onset of the nosocomial infections. Specifically, the epidemiologist compared placement of indwelling bladder catheters among cases and reference patients. (Again, carefully identify the exposure and the outcome.) Would this be a case-control study or a cohort study?

Question 3

Among the discharges for a 6-month period, the hospital epidemiologist in the questions above found 200 patients who suffered first nosocomial urinary tract infections. Of these infected patients, 30 died. The next sequential uninfected patient discharged after each of these infected patients was selected as a comparison subject, and the administrative records indicated that 10 of the 200 comparison patients died. Fill in the table below and calculate the relative risk of mortality with nosocomial urinary tract infection (refer to Table 2.1).

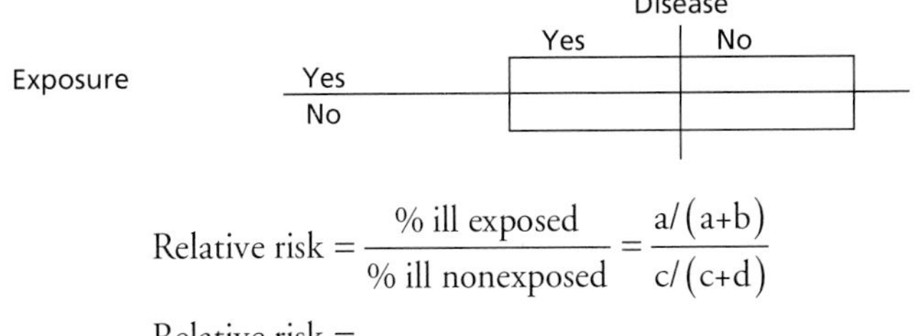

		Disease: Yes	Disease: No
Exposure	Yes		
	No		

$$\text{Relative risk} = \frac{\%\text{ ill exposed}}{\%\text{ ill nonexposed}} = \frac{a/(a+b)}{c/(c+d)}$$

Relative risk =

Optional: If you are interested, compute the value of chi-square. For a single fourfold table, the value of chi-square may be computed as:

$$\text{chi-square} = (ad-bc)^2(n-1)/(a+b)(c+d)(a+c)(b+d)$$

Question 4

If the sampling fraction were changed and ten times as many unexposed enrolled, with the same probability of infection, what would happen to the estimate of the relative risk? Optional: What would happen to the confidence intervals?

Question 5

Having decided that nosocomial urinary tract infections were a problem, the hospital epidemiologist made a first inquiry into the possible causes of these infections. The medical records of the above 400 patients were read, and the frequency of use of indwelling bladder catheters in the first week of hospitalization, prior to the onset of urinary tract infections, was determined. One hundred of the 200 infected patients had experienced prior bladder catheterization, but only ten of the noninfected patients had been catheterized. Fill in the table below and calculate the odds ratio of exposure to bladder catheterization among infected and noninfected patients (Table 2.1).

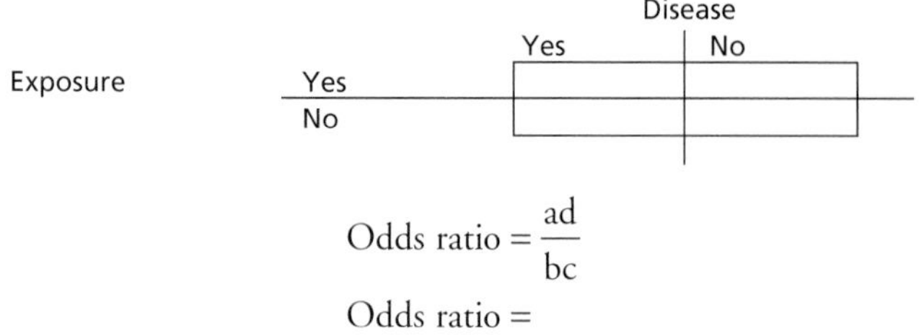

$$\text{Odds ratio} = \frac{ad}{bc}$$

Odds ratio =

Question 6

Suppose the sampling fraction among the noncases, i.e., those who were outcome-negative, was changed in question 5, and ten times as many noncases were enrolled, but the odds of having a catheter remained the same in this larger group of noncases. How would this new larger sample affect the estimate of the odds ratio in question 5? Optional: How would it affect the confidence intervals?

Question 7

Suppose you erroneously calculated the relative risk instead of the exposure odds ratio for the data in question 5. What would happen to the relative risk if the new larger sample of noncases were used in this erroneous calculation?

[Note: Questions 8 and 9 were prepared to entice you to evaluate your own assumptions. As with many things in life, these questions have no unique correct answers.]

Question 8

This is a question to help you discover how your brainstem is calibrated with respect to the additive or the multiplicative models in causal inference in epidemiology. Suppose there are two independent determinants of infection, and the first has a relative risk of 3.0, and the second has a relative risk of 5.0. If you use the conceptual framework of relative risks, this means that the relative risk of infection in the absence of either determinant of infection is defined as 1.0; the relative risk of infection with just the first determinant is 3.0; and the relative risk of infection with just the second determinant is 5.0. Now, in your view, what should be the relative risk of infection in the presence of both determinants of infection? Can you defend your choice of a relative risk of either 8.0 or 15.0 on a biologic basis? Remember that your selection of regression models makes this choice for you.

Question 9

After you have decided what the value of the relative risk should be in the presence of both determinants, consider the implications if the actual measured value of the relative risk in the presence of both determinants turns out to be less than the level you predicted (antagonism) or more than the level you predicted (synergy). Note that there are five different values for the relative risk (RR) in the presence of both determinants on which you should comment:

RR $<$ 8.0
RR = 8.0
RR $>$ 8.0 but $<$15.0
RR = 15.0
RR $>$ 15.0

APPENDIX 2: ANSWERS TO STUDY QUESTIONS

Question 1

The question is whether this is a case-control study or a cohort study. Here the outcome is survival status at discharge (lived or died), and the exposure is nosocomial urinary tract infection (or not) prior to discharge. Although individuals who acquired nosocomial urinary tract infections were called cases, infection is the exposure. Because subjects were enrolled in this study on the basis of their exposure status (infected or not) and then compared for subsequent mortality, this is an exposure-selective cohort study with count data (numbers of persons). Matching may increase statistical efficiency but has nothing to do with whether this is a case-control or cohort study.

Question 2

In this example, the situation has been reversed, and nosocomial urinary tract infection is now the outcome with prior bladder catheterization the exposure. Because subjects were enrolled in this study by their outcome status (infected or not) and then compared for prior exposure to catheters, this is a case-control study.

Question 3

		Disease: Yes	Disease: No	
Exposure	Yes	30	170	200
	No	10	190	200

$$\text{Relative risk} = \frac{30/200}{10/200} = \frac{15\%}{5\%} = 3.0$$

$$\text{RR} = 3.0; \quad \text{chi-square} = 11.08; \quad p < 10^{-3}$$

Note: The combination of the relative risk and its 95% confidence interval, 3.00 (1.57–5.73), is much more informative than just having the relative risk and the p value separately.

Question 4

If the sample of the unexposed is increased to 2,000 from 200 but the probability of the outcome remains the same, the relative risk will remain unchanged, but the value of chi-square will increase and the confidence intervals will shrink. The relative risk is 3.00 (2.06–4.37).

Question 5

		Disease: Yes	Disease: No
Exposure	Yes	100	10
	No	100	190
		200	200

$$\text{Odds ratio} = (100)(190)/(100)(10) = 19.0$$

$$\text{chi-square} = 101.3; \quad p < 10^{-8}$$

Question 6

If the sample of noncases is increased ten times from 200 to 2,000 but the odds of exposure remain the same, the odds ratio will remain unchanged, but chi-square will again increase and the confidence interval will shrink. The odds ratio is 19.0 (14.5–24.9).

Question 7

If one erroneously computes the relative risk from the above case-control study with the original sample size, relative risk = 2.64. If one then erroneously computes the relative risk with the larger sample size, relative risk = 1.82. The sampling fractions do not change the estimates of relative risks when they are calculated correctly.

Question 8

If one believes that independent effects are additive, then the relative risk in the presence of both determinants would be 3.0 + 5.0 = 8.0. If one believes that independent effects are multiplicative, then the relative risk in the presence of both determinants would be 3.0 × 5.0 = 15.0. Which is applicable depends on your point of view and the underlying biology.

Question 9

Any value less than your projected estimate would indicate antagonism between the two determinants, and any value greater than your projected estimate would indicate synergy between the two determinants. In either model, a relative risk of 7.0 in the presence of both determinants would indicate antagonism, and a relative risk of 16.0 would indicate synergy. However, if you believe in the additive model, then a relative risk of 10.0 would represent synergy, but if you believe in the multiplicative model, then the same relative risk of 10.0 would indicate antagonism. *Effect modification* is the epidemiologic term for synergy or antagonism.

REFERENCES

1. Gordis L. *Epidemiology*. Philadelphia: WB Saunders, 1996.
2. Rothman KJ, Greenland S. *Modern epidemiology,* 2nd ed. Philadelphia: Lippincott-Raven, 1998.
3. MacMahon B, Yen S, Trichopoulos D, Warren K, et al. Coffee and cancer of the pancreas. *N Engl J Med* 1981;304:630–633.
4. Harris AD, Karchmer TB, Carmeli Y, et al. Methodological principles of case-control studies that analyzed risk factors for antibiotic resistance: a systematic review. *Clin Infect Dis* 2001;32:1055–1061.
5. Freeman J, McGowan JE Jr. Methodologic issues in hospital epidemiology. III. Investigating the modifying effects of time and severity of underlying illness on estimates of the cost of nosocomial infection. *Rev Infect Dis* 1984;6:285–300.
6. Freeman J, Hutchison GB. Prevalence, incidence and duration. *Am J Epidemiol* 1980;112:707–723.
7. Freeman J, McGowan JE Jr. Day-specific incidence of nosocomial infection estimated from a prevalence survey. *Am J Epidemiol* 1981;114:888–901.
8. Freeman J, Hutchison GB. Duration of disease, duration indicators, and estimation of the risk ratio. *Am J Epidemiol* 1986;124:134–149.
9. Centers for Disease Control and Prevention. Excellence in curriculum integration through teaching epidemiology (Excite) resource library. Available at *http://www.cdc.gov/excite/library/glossary.htm.*
10. Haley RW, Culver DH, Morgan WM, et al. Increased recognition of infectious diseases in US hospitals through increased use of diagnostic tests, 1970–1976. *Am J Epidemiol* 1985;121:168–181.
11. Haley RW, Culver DH, White JW, et al. The efficacy of infection surveillance and control programs in preventing nosocomial infections in US hospitals. *Am J Epidemiol* 1985;121:182–205.
12. Emori TG, Edwards JR, Culver DH, et al. Accuracy of reporting nosocomial infections in intensive care unit patients to the National Nosocomial Infections Surveillance System: a pilot study. *Infect Control Hosp Epidemiol* 1998;19:308–316.
13. Platt R, Zaleznik DF, Hopkins CC, et al. Perioperative antibiotic prophylaxis for herniorrhaphy and breast surgery. *N Engl J Med* 1990; 322:153–160.
14. Platt R, Zucker JR, Zaleznik DF, et al. Prophylaxis against wound infection following herniorrhaphy or breast surgery. *J Infect Dis* 1992; 166:556–560.
15. Eickhoff TC, Brachman PS, Bennett JV, et al. Surveillance of nosocomial infections in community hospitals. I. Surveillance methods, effectiveness, and initial results. *J Infect Dis* 1969;120:305–317.
16. Freeman J, Rosner BA, McGowan JE Jr. Adverse effects of nosocomial infection. *J Infect Dis* 1979;140:732–740.
17. Freeman J, McGowan JE Jr. Methodologic issues in hospital epidemiology. I. Rates, case finding, and interpretation. *Rev Infect Dis* 1981;3: 658–667.
18. Freeman J, McGowan JE Jr. Methodologic issues in hospital epidemiology. II. Time and accuracy in estimation. *Rev Infect Dis* 1981;3: 668–677.
19. Brawley RL, Weber DJ, Samsa GP, et al. Multiple nosocomial infections: an incidence study. *Am J Epidemiol* 1989;130:769–780.
20. Crede W, Hierholzer WJ. Surveillance for quality assessment: I. Surveillance in infection control success reviewed. *Infect Control Hosp Epidemiol* 1989;10:470–474.
21. McGeer A, Crede W, Hierholzer WJ. Surveillance for quality assessment: II. Surveillance for noninfectious processes: back to basics. *Infect Control Hosp Epidemiol* 1990;11:36–41.
22. Crede WB, Hierholzer WJ. Surveillance for quality assessment. III. The critical assessment of quality indicators. *Infect Control Hosp Epidemiol* 1990;11:197–201.
23. Park RA, Brook RH, Kosecoff J, et al. Explaining variations in hospital death rates: randomness, severity of illness, quality of care. *JAMA* 1990; 264:484–490.
24. Freeman J, Goldmann DA, McGowan JE Jr. Methodologic issues in hospital epidemiology. IV. Risk ratios, confounding, effect modification, and the analysis of multiple variables. *Rev Infect Dis* 1988;10: 1118–1141.
25. Rothman KJ, Boice JD Jr. *Epidemiologic analysis with a programmable calculator.* Boston: Epidemiology Resources, 1982.
26. Stamm WE, Weinstein RA, Dixon RE. Comparison of endemic and epidemic nosocomial infections. *Am J Med* 1981;70:393–397.
27. Speizer FE, Regman DH, Remirez A. Palpitation rates associated with fluorocarbon exposure in a hospital setting. *N Engl J Med* 1975;296: 624–626.
28. Sacks HS, Berrier J, Reitman D, et al. Meta-analysis. In: Bailer J, Mosteller F, eds. *Medical uses of statistics.* Waltham, MA: NEJM Books, 1991.
29. Russel Sage Foundation. *Meta analysis for explanation. A casebook.* New York: Russel Sage Foundation, 1992.
30. National Research Council. *Combining information: statistical issues and opportunities for research.* Washington, DC: National Academy Press, 1992.
31. Berenson ML. Highlights meta analysis symposium. *New York Statistician* 1992;45:1–4.
32. Colditz GA, Brewer TF, Berkey CS, et al. Efficacy of BCG vaccine in

the prevention of tuberculosis: meta-analysis of the published literature. *JAMA* 1994;271:698–702.

33. DerSimonian R, Laird NM. Meta-analysis in clinical trials. *Controlled Clin Trials* 1986;7:177–188.
34. Farr BM, Shapiro DE. Diagnostic tests: distinguishing good tests from bad and even ugly ones. *Infect Control Hosp Epidemiol* 2000;21: 278–284.
35. Auerbach S, Goldman D, Oster RA, et al. Software. In: Bernier RH, Watson VM, Nowell, eds. *Episource: a guide to resources in epidemiology.* Roswell, GA: Epidemiology Monitor, 1998. (Also by the same authors: *Resources.* Roswell, GA: Epidemiology Monitor, 1998;19.)
36. Concato J, Feinstein AR, Holford TR. The risk of determining risk with multivariable models. *Ann Intern Med* 1993;118:201–210.
37. Greenland S. Modeling and variable selection in epidemiologic analysis. *Am J Public Health* 1989;79:340–349.
38. Walker AM. *Observation and inference: an introduction to the methods of epidemiology.* Chestnut Hill, MA: Epidemiology Resources, 1991.
39. Freeman J, Goldmann DA, Smith NE, et al. Association of intravenous lipid emulsion and coagulase-negative staphylococcal bacteremia in neonatal intensive care units. *N Engl J Med* 1990;323:301–308.
40. Mosteller F, Tukey JW. *Data analysis and regression: a second course in statistics.* Reading, MA: Addison-Wesley, 1977.
41. Sall J. *Technical report: A 102: SAS regression applications.* Cary, NC: SAS Institute, 1981.
42. Kleinbaum DG, Kupper LL, Muller KE, et al. *Applied regression analysis and other multivariable methods.* Pacific Grove, CA: Duxbury Press, 1998.
43. Hosmer DW, Lemeshow S. *Applied logistic regression.* New York: Wiley, 1989.
44. Breslow NE, Day NE. *Statistical methods in cancer research. I. The analysis of case-control studies.* Lyon: International Agency for Research on Cancer, 1980.
45. Breslow NE, Day NE. *Statistical methods in cancer research. II. The design and analysis of cohort studies.* Lyon: International Agency for Research on Cancer, 1987.
46. Zhang J, Yu KF. What's the relative risk? A method of correcting the odds ratio in cohort studies of common outcomes. *JAMA* 1998;280: 1690–1691.
47. SAS Institute. *SAS/STAT users guide,* version 6, 4th ed. Cary, NC: SAS Institute, 1997.
48. Harris EK, Albert A. *Survivorship analysis for clinical studies.* New York: Marcel Dekker, 1991.
49. Localio AR, Berlin JA, Ten Have TR, et al. Adjustments for center in multicenter studies: an overview. *Ann Intern Med* 2001;135:112–123.
50. Diggle PJ, Liang K-Y, Zeger SL. *Analysis of longitudinal data.* Oxford: Clarendon Press, 1994.
51. SAS Institute, Inc. *SAS/STAT software: changes and enhancements through release 6.12.* Cary, NC: SAS Institute, 1997.
52. Tokars JI, Miller ER, Stein G. A new national surveillance system for hemodialysis-associated infections: initial results. *Am J Infect Control* 2002;30:288–295.

3

BIOSTATISTICS FOR HOSPITAL EPIDEMIOLOGY AND INFECTION CONTROL

ELIZABETH A. TOLLEY

It is common knowledge that investigators face challenges during all phases of planning and implementing research protocols. Clinical and experimental researchers possess the necessary expertise for the medical and scientific aspects of their investigations. Moreover, researchers usually have some knowledge of elementary statistical methods. Some researchers find elementary statistics adequate for their purposes and need only an occasional consultation with a biostatistician. However, recent trends in clinical research, especially in hospital epidemiology and infection control, indicate increasing complexity that demands a higher level of statistical expertise. These general trends are probably going to continue for the foreseeable future—a situation that may leave a researcher feeling somewhat overwhelmed by all of the tasks to be handled in addition to mastery of subject matter. This chapter discusses the challenges and dilemmas related to statistical issues faced by the researcher during the various phases of planning and implementing a research protocol.

Statistics is the science of collecting, analyzing, interpreting, and presenting data. Descriptive statistical methods involve data reduction, summarizing many observations in a few representative numbers. Biostatistics is the application of statistical methods to biologic, biomedical, or health science problems. Data are numeric observations or measurements that result from a random phenomenon or process (1,2). A random process cannot be controlled, and the data collected can never be reproduced exactly. Data from a random process always contain some natural variation. To identify reasons for observed differences among groups of observations, the researcher must sort out the special causes that lead to systematic variation and separate these from the natural variation that is always present. Consequently, decisions will be uncertain. Before making a decision, the researcher uses statistical inference to objectively evaluate data and quantify the level of uncertainty. In addition, the researcher uses statistical models to represent data in terms of special causes and natural variation; these models aid the researcher in making inferences and decisions based on the data.

The numeric observations are in the form of variables, also called *random variables.* Certain statistical techniques apply to each type of random variable (1–9). Measurement variables may be continuous, if the number of values is very large, or discrete, if only few values (generally less than ten) are possible. Some measurement variables are actually computed variables, for example, Acute Physiology and Chronic Health Evaluation III (APACHE III) scores. A ranked variable is a measurement variable, the values of which have been placed in ascending or descending order and replaced by the ranks. Attributes must translate into numbers (e.g., frequencies of occurrence or number of infected patients). Attributes are sometimes called *categorical variables.* If an attribute can be only present or absent, the term *dichotomous variable* is frequently used.

In today's clinical studies, even the most focused research protocol can yield enormous amounts of information. The typical clinical setting contains a multitude of measuring devices that can provide exquisitely detailed measurements. Many measurements are collected because of availability rather than need. As a consequence, when a study is concluded, an investigator can be faced with the task of sorting through a huge amount of data. Certain measurements or variables are relevant to and necessary for carrying out the specific objectives of a study. An investigator determines what type of data to collect based primarily on specialized knowledge.

Two concepts have especially important implications for investigators. *Accuracy* is the closeness of the measure to the true value; lack of accuracy has to do with bias (1–3,9,10). Before recommending a study or grant for approval and/or funding, most reviewers insist that an investigator show how the results will be unbiased. Thus, the investigator's responsibility includes demonstrating the experimental validity of the study. *Precision* is the closeness of repeated measurements to each other (2,3,9). Importantly, precision has no bearing on closeness to the true value. In fact, precision without accuracy can be a problem when an investigator is trying to make statistical inferences.

Most clinical studies involve samples that are chosen from a population, instead of the entire population (2–4,8,11–13). The term *population* refers to the reference or study population. A random sample is a group chosen from a population such that each member of the sample has a nonzero probability of being chosen, independent of any other member being chosen. A simple random sample is the same as a random sample, except that each member of the population has the same nonzero probability of being chosen. Parameters of the reference population are usually unknown and unknowable. The investigator uses statistics from samples to estimate the parameters of the reference population. Because the sample is smaller than the population, information obtained from the sample is partial, and the investigator uses this information to infer something about the population. Most statistics used in hospital epidemiology and infection control require the investigator to make the assumptions that (a) the reference population is infinitely large and well defined and (b) the sample behaves like a simple random sample. In practice, the population may not be well defined or infinite. Likewise, the sample may not be random; for clinical studies, samples are often composed of those patients who have been admitted to a particular hospital over a specified period because of certain underlying diagnoses and who have undergone various medical and surgical procedures.

DESCRIPTIVE STATISTICS

In published reports, hospital epidemiologists summarize patient characteristics with descriptive statistics (1–9,11–13). Typically, a list of patient characteristics includes measures of central tendency and dispersion for continuous variables.

During the research process, the clinical investigator may start exploratory data analysis by obtaining descriptive statistics of important variables. These descriptive statistics have a variety of other practical uses. For example, a potentially important determinant of disease, such as age, may vary only slightly for those patients included in the study; consequently, the clinical investigator may decide not to consider this variable as a potential risk factor in this study. In addition, the researcher may note which variables have highly skewed distributions and, thus, might yield spurious results during data analysis. Finally, unusually high or low values can be identified and verified, if necessary. The following sections describe descriptive statistics for continuous variables.

Measures of Location or Central Tendency

Location refers to where on an axis a particular group of data is located relative to a norm or another group. Measures of central tendency or central location are used to obtain a number that represents the middle of a group of data.

Mean

Mean usually refers to the arithmetic mean or average. The mean is probably the most commonly used measure of location. However, the investigator should be aware that the mean is sensitive to extreme values—both very high and very low values. Other means exist but are used less frequently; the geometric mean is an example. An investigator computes a geometric mean by first taking the logarithm of a group of numbers, computing the mean of the transformed values, and then obtaining the antilog of the mean. Blood pH values are logarithms; however, in practice, after calculating the mean of pH values, no one takes the antilog to obtain the mean hydrogen ion concentration. The Greek letter μ is used to represent the population mean. The sample mean X is an unbiased estimator of μ regardless of the shape of the distribution. If the underlying distribution is normal, then the sample mean is the unbiased estimator with the smallest variance.

Median

The median is the 50% point or 50th percentile and, as such, is insensitive to extreme values. If an odd number of observations are ranked from smallest to largest, the median is the middle observation. If an even number of observations are similarly ranked, the median is the average of the $n/2$ and $(n/2 + 1)$ observations where n is the sample size. For example, if the sample size is 20, after ranking, the median is the average of the tenth and eleventh observations. For symmetric distributions, the mean and the median coincide. There is no standard symbol for the median of a population or a sample; however, M can be used for connoting the population parameter or the sample statistic (4).

Mode

The mode, or the value with the highest frequency, is a measure of concentration. Distributions may have more than one mode. Distributions with two modes are called bimodal. Trimodal refers to distributions with three modes. For symmetric distributions, the mean, median, and mode have the same value. No standard symbol exists for the mode of a population or a sample.

Measures of Dispersion or Spread

Range

The range is the distance between the highest (largest) and lowest (smallest) value. In hospital epidemiology, investigators often refer to the interquartile range, which is the distance between the twenty-fifth and seventy-fifth values. Researchers should report ranges with medians; in this way, information on both location and dispersion can be conveyed to others. For a sample, the range is symbolized by R.

Variance

The variance is a measure of dispersion that is often used in calculations. Another name for the variance is the mean square. For populations, the variance is called sigma squared and symbolized with the Greek letter σ^2; for samples, the variance is represented by s^2. Because of the availability of inexpensive calculators, only definitional formulas for the variance of a population and a sample are given, where n is the sample size from a population with N members, and N is much greater than n. For the population, the variance is computed as

$$\sigma^2 = \frac{\Sigma(X_i - \mu)^2}{N}$$

where X_i is the value of the random variable X, measured on each member of the population; i is a unique identifier of each member of the population; μ is the population mean for the variable X; Σ signifies summing the squared deviations of the individual values from the mean over all members; and N is the number of members in the population. For the sample, the variance is computed as

$$s^2 = \frac{\Sigma(X_i - \bar{X})^2}{n-1}$$

where X_i is the value of the random variable X, measured on each observation in the sample; i is a unique identifier of each observation in the sample; $\bar{X}$ is the sample mean for the variable X; Σ signifies summing the squared deviations over all observations; and n is the number of observations in the sample.

Standard Deviation

The standard deviation is the square root of the variance and is sometimes called the root mean square. The standard deviation is a measure of the average distance from the mean. If the standard deviation is small, the observations are crowded near the mean; if the standard deviation is large, there is substantial spread in the data. For populations, the standard deviation is symbolized with the Greek letter σ; for samples, the standard deviation is represented by s. Standard deviations correspond to means. Occasionally, an investigator must approximate the standard deviation of a future sample. The expected range (i.e., the largest value that one expects to record from a future sample minus the smallest value) divided by 4 provides an approximation when no other information is available.

Other Descriptive Measures

Measures of Skewness

Measures of skewness and kurtosis may be computed to evaluate how a distribution deviates from a normal distribution. Most clinical investigators do not routinely need these measures. In practice, the investigator may plot the distribution of the data to evaluate the presence of outliers, those observations with values much larger or smaller than the rest of the sample. A distribution that has a few to a moderate number of high values and a mean that is greater than the median is generally referred to as right or positively skewed. Conversely, a distribution that has a few to a moderate number of low values and a mean that is smaller than the median is generally referred to as left or negatively skewed. In summary, the direction in which the tail of the distribution points characterizes the direction of skew.

Kurtosis

Kurtosis refers to how flat or peaked the distribution is relative to the normal distribution. If a distribution is flatter than the normal distribution, it is called platykurtotic. On the other hand, if a distribution is more peaked than the normal distribution, it is called leptokurtotic. For kurtotic distributions, the mean and the median coincide, but the standard deviation is either larger or smaller, respectively, than it would have been if the observations were sampled from a normal distribution.

Coefficient of Variation

The coefficient of variation allows the researcher to compare two or more standard deviations, because the standard deviation has been standardized by the mean. The population coefficient of variation is $(\sigma/\mu)100\%$, and the sample coefficient of variation is $(s/\bar{X})100\%$. For most biologic data, the standard deviation increases as the mean increases. Therefore, the coefficient of variation of a particular variable tends to be rather stable over a wide range of values. For experimental studies, the coefficient of variation is an indicator of the reproducibility of the observations. The clinical investigator may use the coefficient of variation to compare variables that may be potential confounders or effect modifiers. For one group of subjects, the spread of different variables may be compared using the coefficient of variation. For two or more groups of subjects, the coefficient of variation may be used to compare the groups with respect to the spread of a particular variable.

PROBABILITY

Many patient characteristics are dichotomous attributes, which are either present or absent, such as fever. Some characteristics have the form of categorical variables with only a few possible states. For example, the investigator may categorize patients according to presence of a rapidly fatal disease, an ultimately fatal disease, or a nonfatal disease. In some statistical texts, authors apply the term *discrete variable* to a characteristic or attribute with two or more states. In published reports, hospital epidemiologists summarize these types of patient characteristics by indicating the proportion of the total group with each characteristic of interest.

During the research process, the clinical investigator often begins exploratory data analysis by considering the relationships between pairs of categorical variables. The following sections contain important rules and definitions that the clinical investigator must master before undertaking a complex study. Dichotomous variables are emphasized because many clinically important risk factors are dichotomous variables.

Definitions and Rules

Many problems in hospital epidemiology and infection control involve analysis of frequencies for various attributes (e.g., numbers of patients with and without infections). When only two outcomes are possible, the variable is called a dichotomous variable. For this example, a patient either has an infection or does not and cannot be characterized as being in both states simultaneously. Thus, having an infection is a dichotomous variable that represents mutually exclusive states. The infected state is represented by I and the noninfected state by Ī (i.e., I stricken through with a line connoting "not"). The probability that an infection is present is represented by p; the probability that an infection is not present is represented by $(1 - p)$. Some authors of statistics texts represent $(1 - p)$ as q. Mathematically, we express the probability that a patient has an infection by the expression, $Pr(I) = p$. Because the states are mutually exclusive and only these two states can occur, p and q sum to 1.0.

Probability can be expressed as a fraction with a numerator and denominator, a decimal fraction or proportion, or a percentage. In this chapter, probability is always a proportion. Probabilities can have any value between zero and 1.0, inclusive. For dichotomous variables, a probability of zero implies that an event (i.e., one of the two possible states) cannot occur; a probability of 1.0 implies that the event will always occur.

Researchers in hospital epidemiology need a basic understanding of some concepts related to probability. After mastering a few easily understood concepts (i.e., three rules and six definitions), the researcher can achieve a deeper understanding of how and when important statistics, such as risk ratio (RR), are used.

Unconditional or Total Probability

In hospital epidemiology and infection control, researchers must assess total or unconditional probabilities (1–5,8,12,13). The definition of a total probability is illustrated in the following example. The probability that a patient chosen at random has an infection may be calculated as the relative frequency of patients with infections: the numerator is the number of patients with at least one infection, the denominator is the total number of patients in the study. If 15 of 45 patients in the medical intensive care unit (ICU) have at least one infection, the empirical probability of being infected is .33. This probability may be symbolized as $Pr(I) = p = .33$. Thus, the total probability of an event occurring is the number of times the event occurs divided by the number of times that it could have occurred.

Empirical Versus Theoretical Probabilities

A clinical investigator obtains empirical probabilities from the sample of patients in the particular study. A better method for estimating the true or theoretical probability of a future patient having at least one infection would involve enumerating all infections in all the patients over a long period. The investigator could continue to expand the sample size by including other units and other hospitals and so on. Finally, after the investigator had gathered a very large group of patients from many locations, the empirical probability would approach the theoretical probability of an average hospitalized patient having an infection. Thus, the theoretical probability of infected patients is the relative frequency for cases of infection over an infinitely large sample. During an investigation of a possible outbreak of disease, infection control officers compare empirical probabilities with theoretical probabilities.

Conditional Probability

In hospital epidemiology, researchers are also interested in conditional probabilities (1,3–5,8,12,13). An example of a conditional probability is the probability of pneumonia, given that the patient has been intubated. The condition states the circumstances restricting the type of patients of interest to the researcher. A researcher obtains a conditional probability of nosocomial pneumonia given intubation by (a) enumerating the number of patients with the two characteristics (i.e., intubated patients with pneumonia) and (b) dividing by the number of patients who are intubated (i.e., those at risk for ventilator-associated pneumonia). In this example, the conditional probability of having pneumonia given that the patient is intubated may be symbolized by $Pr(P \mid V)$, where | indicates given, P symbolizes a patient with pneumonia, and V symbolizes a patient who is intubated or on a ventilator. Therefore, if 25 patients are ventilated and have nosocomial pneumonia and 100 patients are ventilated, $Pr(P \mid V) = 25/100 = 0.25$.

Joint Probability and the Product Rule

The first rule of probability consider in this chapter is the product rule (1,3–5,8,12,13). The product rule states that, for any two events A and B, the joint probability of events A and B occurring together is equal to the product of the conditional probability of A given B times the total probability of B. In this example, the probability of being intubated and having pneumonia is obtained by multiplying the conditional probability of having pneumonia given that the patient is intubated by the probability of the patient being intubated. In the ICU, the joint probability that a patient selected at random will be both intubated and have pneumonia may be symbolized mathematically by $Pr(P \text{ and } V)$, where P indicates a patient with pneumonia and V indicates a patient who is intubated or on a ventilator. In this example, if $Pr(V) = .40$ (i.e., 40% of the patients in the study are ventilated), then $Pr(P \text{ and } V) = Pr(P \mid V) \times Pr(V) = .25 \times .40 = .10$. Thus, 10% of the patients in the study have both characteristics.

Independent and Dependent Events

Often the hospital epidemiologist will want to know if there is an association between two events (1,3–5,8,12). No causal relationship can be identified without substantially more evidence than that provided by one investigation. In this example, the researcher might be looking for an association between a patient being intubated and development of nosocomial pneumonia. Therefore, the epidemiologist wishes to know if the ventilated patients in the study are more likely to develop pneumonia than expected based on the theoretical probability of nosocomial pneumonia in the particular ICU. In making this decision, the epidemiologist determines the probability of an average patient developing pneumonia and being intubated under the assumption that these two events are independent (i.e., they have no association). Under independence, $Pr(P \text{ and } V) = Pr(P) \times Pr(V)$. If 20% of the patients in the study have pneumonia, then $Pr(P) = .20$. Thus, if there is no association between being on the ventilator and developing pneumonia, $Pr(P \text{ and } V) = .20 \times .40 = .08$. This result implies that one would expect 8% of patients to be ventilated and to develop pneumonia if the assumption of independence is correct for this situation. Based on previous computations, the investigator knows that, in this study, 10% of the patients actually have both characteristics. Because the empirical probability is not the same as the theoretical probability, the conclusion is that there is evidence of an association between intubation and pneumonia. Determining whether this association is evidence of a special cause or merely a reflection of natural variability requires the researcher to use inferential statistics. Inferential methods appropriate for this example are presented in other sections.

In this example, the researcher could have reached the same conclusion by comparing total and conditional probabilities. Under independence, the probabilities are equal; therefore, $Pr(P \mid V) = Pr(P)$. For the hospital epidemiologist, this statement implies that, with respect to a patient developing pneumonia, the ventilator is neither a risk factor nor a protective factor; therefore, patients on the ventilator have the same risk of developing pneumonia as any other patient in the study. For this example, $Pr(P \mid V)$ is .25, a value that is greater than $Pr(P) = .20$. When these two probabilities are unequal, there is evidence of an association between the two variables of interest.

Addition or Total Probability Rule

The second rule is called the addition or total probability rule (1,3–5,8,13). This rule states that, for any two events A and B, the total probability of A equals the sum of the joint probability of A and B plus the joint probability of A and $\not{B}$: $Pr(A) = Pr(A \text{ and } B) + Pr(A \text{ and } \not{B})$. For convenience, these probabilities are often displayed in a 2×2 table. Accordingly, the term *marginal probability* is used interchangeably with *total probability*.

Before continuing the discussion of probability, the layout of a 2×2 table is considered. Statistically, no restriction exists that stipulates placement of exposure and disease on a particular margin or the order in which presence and absence are given on a particular margin. However, the interpretability of some measures of association, which specifically apply to epidemiology, depends on a particular arrangement. When an investigator devises a 2×2 table, the proportion of patients with the two attributes and those without the two attributes should be placed on the main diagonal (i.e., cells 1 and 4 of the following table). Epidemiologists have developed other conventions, the use of which has helped to standardize presentation of data. Furthermore, some statistical software products have specific requirements for placement of attributes.

	Exposed to ventilator	Not exposed to ventilator	Total or marginal probability of disease
Pneumonia present	P_1	P_2	$P_1 + P_2$
Pneumonia absent	P_3	P_4	$P_3 + P_4$
Total or marginal probability of exposure	$P_1 + P_3$	$P_2 + P_4$	

In the previous table, P_1, P_2, P_3, and P_4 are joint probabilities. For this example, P_1 is the joint probability of a patient having both exposure to the ventilator and pneumonia. Marginal probability of pneumonia can be calculated as the sum of the joint probabilities. In this example, $Pr(P)$ equals the sum of the joint probabilities, $Pr(P \text{ and } V)$ and $Pr(P \text{ and } \not{V})$. The other total probabilities, $Pr(\not{P})$, $Pr(V)$, and $Pr(\not{V})$, can be calculated by using the addition rule and are displayed in the following table.

	Exposed to ventilator	Not exposed to ventilator	Total or marginal probability of disease
Pneumonia present	$Pr(P \text{ and } V)$	$Pr(P \text{ and } \not{V})$	$Pr(P)$
Pneumonia absent	$Pr(\not{P} \text{ and } V)$	$Pr(\not{P} \text{ and } \not{V})$	$Pr(\not{P})$
Total or marginal probability of exposure	$Pr(V)$	$Pr(\not{V})$	1.0

Alternatively, using the definition of joint probability, the hospital epidemiologist can replace the joint probabilities P_1 and P_2 with the product of the conditional probability of disease multiplied by the respective probability of exposure. The same can be done with P_3 and P_4. Frequently, the hospital epidemiologist uses this approach when the research question involves identifying risk factors. Typically, the hospital epidemiologist asks that question before designing a prospective study.

	Exposed to ventilator	Not exposed to ventilator	Total or marginal probability of disease
Pneumonia present	$Pr(V) \times Pr(P \mid V)$	$Pr(\not{V}) \times Pr(P \mid \not{V})$	$Pr(P)$
Pneumonia absent	$Pr(V) \times Pr(\not{P} \mid V)$	$Pr(\not{V}) \times Pr(\not{P} \mid \not{V})$	$Pr(\not{P})$
Probability of exposure	$Pr(V)$	$Pr(\not{V})$	1.0

Finally, a hospital epidemiologist may wish to study a particular exposure and describe the relationship of that exposure to the presence of a particular disease. In this example, the investigator would be interested in the probability of exposure to the ventilator given that a patient has pneumonia. Usually, the hospital epidemiologist asks this question before designing a retrospective study, often a case-control study.

	Exposed to ventilator	Not exposed to ventilator	Total probability of disease
Pneumonia present	$Pr(P) \times Pr(V \mid P)$	$Pr(P) \times Pr(\not{V} \mid P)$	$Pr(P)$
Pneumonia absent	$Pr(\not{P}) \times Pr(V \mid \not{P})$	$Pr(\not{P}) \times Pr(\not{V})$	$Pr(\not{P})$
Probability of exposure	$Pr(V)$	$Pr(\not{V})$	1.0

In the hospital setting, patients are exposed simultaneously to several risk factors. By considering each exposure separately, the hospital epidemiologist can use this approach to identify the most likely route of exposure given a particular disease.

In summary, when the hospital epidemiologist investigates the relationship between two dichotomous events (e.g., exposure and disease), the 2×2 table provides a useful and flexible way of displaying the relative frequencies at which the four possible combinations of exposure and disease occur in the sample. Depending on the specific research question, the investigator chooses the most meaningful way to express P_1, P_2, P_3, and P_4.

Applications Relevant to Epidemiology

Epidemiologists measure morbidity in terms of prevalence and incidence. Several applications of probability to epidemiology require the investigator to recognize the distinction between these two measures. Prevalence is the proportion of individuals who have the disease. Stated another way, prevalence is the proportion of individuals who have the disease out of all individuals in the population (i.e., those who are at risk for the disease). Prevalence can be defined as the probability that an individual has the disease regardless of the time elapsed since diagnosis. In contrast, incidence is the rate at which new cases occur among individuals who were disease free. Incidence is the number of new cases that have occurred over a specified time divided by the number of individuals who were disease free (i.e., at risk for the disease) at the beginning of the period. Therefore, incidence can be defined as the probability that a disease-free individual will develop the disease over a specified period.

Relative Risk or Risk Ratio

RR is the ratio of the incidence of a disease among exposed persons to the incidence of a disease among unexposed persons (1,3,5,8,12–22). Often, epidemiologists use the term *risk ratio* interchangeably with *relative risk.* Values for RR are positive and range theoretically from zero to infinity; however, in practice, the denominator probability (i.e., incidence of disease in the unexposed) determines the upper limit for RR. For example, if the incidence of disease in the unexposed is 0.4, then the upper limit for RR is 2.5. This restriction limits the direct comparability of RRs across locations or studies.

If the probability of disease is equally likely for those exposed and those not exposed, the RR equals 1.0. Whenever the RR equals 1.0, exposure and disease are independent. If the probability of disease is higher for those exposed than for those not exposed, RR is greater than 1.0 and exposure is a risk factor. If the probability of disease is lower for those exposed than for those not exposed, RR is less than 1.0 and exposure is a protective factor. As the RR of disease increases or decreases from 1.0, there is evidence that the two events, exposure and disease, are associated or dependent. Using the information in a tabled display, the infection control officer can obtain two conditional probabilities: $Pr(P \mid V) = .25$ and $Pr(P \mid : Vxu) = .167$. Thus, the RR is 1.497. In this situation, the officer would conclude that, according to these data, a patient on a ventilator is about 1.5 times as likely to develop pneumonia as a patient who is not on a ventilator.

Odds Ratio

When incidence is not known, RR cannot be obtained. However, the RR can be approximated by the odds ratio (OR) (1, 5,8,12–17,19–22). If the proportion of diseased persons (i.e., prevalence) is small (i.e., less than 0.1), then the OR is usually a reasonably good approximator of the RR. Therefore, the investigator is responsible for carefully evaluating the OR as an approximator of the RR. In making this evaluation, the investigator must consider whether the disease is chronic or acute. Approximation of the RR is biased when only prevalent cases are used in the analysis. When the duration is short (because of either rapid fatality or cure), the numbers of incident and prevalent cases are very nearly the same; very little bias in approximating RR based on prevalent cases is likely. However, when duration is long, bias can be a problem. For example, when serum cholesterol is used to predict death from heart disease, the OR from prevalent cases is lower than the RR from incident cases. This downward bias occurs because the individuals with the highest cholesterol values are more likely to have a high fatality rate and thereby to escape detection as prevalent cases. In addition, the investigator should be aware that for a particular sample, the OR will have a more extreme value compared with the RR. If the estimates of the OR and RR based on the sample are greater than 1.0, the estimated OR will be larger than the estimated RR. Conversely, if the estimates of the OR and RR based on the sample are less than 1.0, the estimated OR will have a value smaller than the estimated RR.

Both RRs and ORs are very useful statistics and have many applications for observational and quasiexperimental studies. Although the clinical investigator often makes the same inferences from an OR as from a RR, these statistics are not interchangeable. Therefore, investigators should be very strict in stipulating whether an estimate is a RR or an approximation based on an OR. Furthermore, it is incumbent on the investigator to demonstrate the validity of any implicit assumption that the approximation based on an OR is a good approximation of RR. Failure to do so can have dangerous consequences involving misinterpretation of published reports and erroneous clinical decisions about patient care.

From the first table, the RR may be computed as a ratio with $P_1/(P_1 + P_3)$ in the numerator and $P_2/(P_2 + P_4)$ in the denominator. If the number of patients with pneumonia is small, P_1 will contribute very little to the quantity $(P_1 + P_3)$; likewise, P_2 will contribute very little to the quantity $(P_2 + P_4)$. The OR equals a ratio with P_1/P_3 in the numerator and P_2/P_4 in the denominator. Statistically, the OR can always be used to approximate the RR. As P_1 and P_2 become smaller, the OR may become a better approximator of the RR. Like RR, the OR ranges theoretically from zero to infinity. However, the OR has a property that can make it a more useful statistic than the RR. The OR is independent of the denominator probability (i.e., an OR of 2.0 has the same meaning regardless of the population or sample on which it was based). The OR is considered the odds of having the disease with the factor present relative to the odds of having the disease with the factor absent. The OR may be calculated from a 2 × 2 table by calculating the ratio of cross-products (multiplying diagonally): OR $= (P_1P_4)/(P_2P_3)$.

Sensitivity, Specificity, and Predictive Value

The hospital epidemiologist can use joint, conditional, and total probabilities for quantifying commonly used laboratory tests (5,8,12–26). The total or marginal probability of disease may be represented as $Pr(D^+)$; this probability is an estimate of disease state prevalence in a population. Prevalence can be thought of as the underlying probability of disease state in a particular population. Likewise, $Pr(D^-)$ can be thought of as the underlying probability of not having the disease state; it is not necessarily the probability of wellness or health.

In terms of conditional probability, the probability of a positive test result given that a patient has the disease—that is, $Pr(T^+ \mid D^+)$—refers to test sensitivity. Similarly, the probability of a negative test result given that a patient does not have the disease—that is, $Pr(T^- \mid D^-)$—refers to test specificity. The sensitivity and specificity of a test are independent of prevalence.

The hospital epidemiologist can display the various possible combinations of disease states and test results in a 2 × 2 table.

	Positive test result	Negative test result	Marginal probability
Disease present	$Pr(D^+) \times Pr(T^+ \mid D^+)$	$Pr(D^+) \times Pr(T^- \mid D^+)$	$Pr(D^+)$
Disease absent	$Pr(D^-) \times Pr(T^+ \mid D^-)$	$Pr(D^-) \times Pr(T^-) \mid D^-)$	$Pr(D^-)$
Marginal probability	$Pr(T^+)$	$Pr(T^-)$	1.0

In contrast, the predictive values of a positive test result (PV^+) and a negative test result (PV^-) depend on prevalence. In terms of conditional probability, the probability of a patient having the disease given that the test result is positive—that is, $Pr(D^+ \mid T^+)$—refers to positive predictive value of the test. Similarly, the probability of a patient not having the disease given that the test result is negative—that is, $Pr(D^- \mid T^-)$—refers to negative predictive value of the test.

	Positive test result	Negative test result	Marginal probability
Disease present	$Pr(T^+) \times Pr(D^+ \mid T^+)$	$Pr(T^-) \times Pr(D^+ \mid T^-)$	$Pr(D^+)$
Disease absent	$Pr(T^+) \times Pr(D^- \mid T^+)$	$Pr(T^-) \times Pr(D^- \mid T^-)$	$Pr(D^-)$
Marginal probability	$Pr(T^+)$	$Pr(T^-)$	1.0

Alternatively, the hospital epidemiologist may interpret this table in terms of joint probabilities. From this perspective, the epidemiologist considers the probability of an average (or random) patient having a test result that is considered true positive (TP), true negative (TN), false positive (FP), or false negative (FN). Specifically, the probability of a TP test result is a joint probability—that is, $Pr(T^+ \text{ and } D^+)$. The other three outcomes may be expressed similarly as joint probabilities. The probability of obtaining a TN result is the joint probability of testing negative and not having the disease. The probability of obtaining an FP result is the probability that a patient selected at random will test positive but not have the disease. Finally, the probability of obtaining an FN result is the probability of a patient selected at random testing negative but having the disease. In practice, these probabilities are often expressed as percentages. These probabilities may be displayed as follows.

	Test results		
Disease state	T^+	T^-	Total probability
D^+	$Pr(TP) = Pr(T^+ \text{ and } D^+)$	$Pr(FN) = Pr(T^- \text{ and } D^+)$	$Pr(D^+)$
D^-	$Pr(FP) = Pr(T^+ \text{ and } D^-)$	$Pr(TN) = Pr(T^- \text{ and } D^-)$	$Pr(D^-)$
Total probability	$Pr(T^+)$	$Pr(T^-)$	1.0

Prevalence is the sum of the probability of a TP result and the probability of an FN result. Similarly, the probability of testing positive is the sum of the probability of a TP result and the probability of an FP result. The other two marginal probabilities can be obtained in the same way.

Bayes' Theorem

In more complex situations, the hospital epidemiologist encounters more than two possible clinical signs or symptoms (symbolized as T_i, where i indicates the alternative clinical signs and symptoms) and more than two possible disease states (symbolized as D_j, *where* j indicates the alternative disease states). The 2 × 2 tables can be expanded into i columns and j rows, representing clinical findings and disease states, respectively. Bayes' theorem or rule allows the hospital epidemiologist to obtain the conditional probability of a particular disease given a particular clinical finding (1,3,5,8,12,15,16,18,25). Bayes' theorem or rule states that the conditional probability of D_1 given T_1 equals the joint probability of T_1 and D_1 divided by the sum of the joint probabilities of T_1 and each D_j:

$$Pr\left(D_1 \middle| T_1\right) = \frac{Pr\left(T_1 \text{ and } D_1\right)}{\Sigma Pr\left(T_1 \text{ and } D_j\right)} = \frac{Pr\left(T_1 \middle| D_1\right) \times Pr\left(D_1\right)}{\Sigma Pr\left(T_1 \middle| D_j\right) Pr\left(D_j\right)}$$

where (a) $Pr(D_j)$ represents the known probabilities of disease states in a specified population and the sum of all $Pr(D_j)$ values equals 1.0 and (b) the various D_j values are mutually exclusive (i.e., a patient cannot have more than one disease). When hospital epidemiologists need to choose the most likely explanation for their clinical findings, they often use Bayes' rule to assess the conditional probabilities of several disease states in light of their particular clinical findings. In published literature, epidemiologists may use conditional probabilities to discuss the merits of several alternative explanations. Clinicians may use Bayes' rule to evaluate a number of diagnostic possibilities. They realize that, although no test is absolutely accurate, positive test results do tend to increase the probability that a particular disease is present. The conditional probability of disease given certain clinical findings provides a number that quantifies the amount of confidence that can be placed in stating that a particular disease is present. Differential diagnosis, decision theory, and decision making involve applications of Bayes' rule.

HYPOTHESIS TESTING

Hypothesis testing does have a place in analysis of data related to hospital epidemiology and infection control. One-sample tests can be used to determine whether the sample is different from the reference population. Clinical investigators often use two-sample tests during exploratory data analysis to identify potentially important risk factors. The following sections address general definitions and rules for hypothesis testing for one- and two-sample tests for categorical and continuous variables using parametric and nonparametric methods.

Definitions and Rules

The hypothesis is always formulated about parameters. H_0 designates the null hypothesis and H_1 the alternative hypothesis. Based on sample statistics, the hospital epidemiologist chooses which is the true situation. For a one-sample hypothesis test, the reasons for this choice are based on how likely it is that these data could have been obtained from a specified reference population. Similarly, for a two-sample hypothesis test, the reasons are based on how likely it is that the difference between the two groups obtained from these data could have occurred given that H_0 is true. In making this decision, the epidemiologist may make errors. Naturally, minimizing the probability of making an erroneous decision is a paramount concern of the epidemiologist, even though the truth remains unknown and unknowable. The decisions that an epidemiologist can make relative to the truth (1,2,4,5,8,10,25) are displayed in the following 2 × 2 table.

	Unknown but true state of nature	
Decision in favor of:	H_0 true	H_1 true
H_0	Correct	Type II error
H_1	Type I error	Correct

Traditionally, scientific investigators have agreed on the principle of keeping the probability of a type I error as small as possible. *Pr(type I error)* is the conditional probability of rejecting H_0 when H_0 is correct. Stated another way, *Pr(type I error)* is the probability of rejecting H_0 given that H_0 is correct. Statisticians have symbolized *Pr(type I error)* as α. Another commonly used name for *Pr(type I error)* is the significance level. The interpretation of a p value is consistent with the definition of the probability of type I error; a p value gives the probability of finding a result that is at least this extreme, assuming that the H_0 is true. Stated another way, the p value qualifies the rejection of H_0 with a level of significance. An investigator rejects H_0 when the p value is less than α. The p value tells others the statistical significance of the results. Statistical significance has absolutely nothing to do with the scientific or clinical importance of findings.

Another type of error is possible—type II error. *Pr(type II error) is the conditional probability of not rejecting the* H_0 when H_1 is true. Stated differently, *Pr(type II error)* is the probability of deciding in favor of H_0 given that H_1 is correct. Statisticians have symbolized *Pr(type II error)* as β. In practice, statisticians are more concerned with power, symbolized as $1 - \beta$. Power is the probability of discriminating between H_0 and H_1, (a) given a specified sample size, a stipulated difference between the values of the parameter under H_0 and H_1, and a particular α; and (b) assuming H_1 is true. Thus, power is the probability of rejecting H_0 when H_1 is true. Power depends on α, H_0 and H_1, and sample size. As α decreases, β increases. As the difference between H_0 and H_1 decreases, power decreases. As sample size increases, power increases—power is very dependent on sample size. Investigators want power to be as large as practically possible, because power represents the probability of correctly rejecting H_0. Typical values for power are 0.80, 0.90, 0.95, and 0.99. Before recommending a clinical trial for approval and/or funding, most reviewers insist that the investigator show that the likelihood of getting conclusive results (i.e., statistical power) is high. In unplanned clinical studies, power may be as low as 0.20 or occasionally even lower. Sometimes, epidemiologists compute power after a study has been completed. Under these circumstances, power is the probability of discriminating between H_0 and H_1, given the findings of the study.

Hypothesis Tests for Categorical Data

A random variable is a numeric quantity that has different values, depending on natural variability. A discrete or categorical random variable is a variable for which there exists a discrete set of values, each having a nonzero probability. Many data from biologic and medical investigations have a common underlying structure.

Cumulative incidence and prevalence of a disease are distributed binomially (1,8,12). Variables that follow a binomial frequency distribution are characterized by the following criteria: (a) a sample is taken of n independent trials, (b) each trial may have two possible outcomes (e.g., success/failure, present/absent, alive/dead), and (c) the probabilities for the outcomes are a constant p for success and $(1 - p) = q$ for each failure for every trial. Usually a hospital epidemiologist is not concerned with the order in which the failures occurred; instead the epidemiologist is interested in the number of failures and the probability that a number as extreme or more extreme occurred given that H_0 is true.

Generally, an incidence density variable follows a binomial distribution. For variables such as incidence density, the Poisson distribution is often an accurate approximation of the binomial distribution. The Poisson distribution is a discrete frequency distribution of the number of occurrences of rare events (1,8,12). For the Poisson distribution, the theoretical number of trials is infinite and the number of possible events is also very large. Incidence density studies often involve one or more cohorts of disease-free individuals. A failure is defined as the occurrence of the disease of interest in a previously disease-free individual. The probability of k events (i.e., failures) occurring in a period T is defined for a Poisson random variable. Thus, the Poisson distribution depends on two parameters: the length of the interval, T, and the underlying λ, which represents the expected number of events per unit of time. Time may also be defined as a combination of time and level of exposure (e.g., pack-years of smoking or patient-days in the ICU). The mean and the variance of a Poisson distribution are the same. For variables that follow a binomial distribution, when n is large and p is small, the mean and variance will be similar; thus, the Poisson may be used as an approximation of the binomial.

The following two sections describe statistical methods for one- and two-sample tests on binomial proportions or rates (1, 3–8,15,18,25,27). Throughout these sections, unless otherwise stated, the significance level is .05; power is 0.80; and all tests are two-sided. In power and sample size formulas, a z-score for the 97.5th percentile is used for a two-sided test with a significance level of .05: $z_{0.975}$ is 1.96. When power of 0.80 is used to determine sample size, a z-score for the 80th percentile is used: $z_{0.80}$ is 0.842.

These sections, describing one- and two-sample tests for binomial proportions or rates, are not designed as casual reading material; instead, they provide a concise reference of commonly used statistical methods. Each section follows the same format, which is outlined in the following.

Step 1. Set up H_0 and H_1.

The investigator uses the research question to form H_0 and H_1. Generally, H_1 reflects the result that the investigator expects to find (i.e., that there is a special cause that differentiates the study group from the norm). For a one-sample hypothesis test, H_0 states that the proportion of events or rate of occurrence (p) in the study group is the same as some specified or norm value, p_0. The investigator obtains this value, p_0, from some source other than the current study. Typically, the investigator obtains p_0 from theoretically derived values or uses nationally or locally compiled values. In the one-sample situation, H_1 states that the proportion of events or rate of occurrence (p) in the group being studied differs from the specified value, p_0. The investigator estimates p from a sample. If the estimated value is sufficiently close to the specified value, p_0, the investigator decides in favor of H_0 (i.e., that the data are consistent with H_0 being true). If the data fail to support H_0, the conclusion is that the data are not consistent with H_0 being true; therefore, the investigator rejects the H_0, concluding that the rate or proportion must be some other value (i.e., higher or lower than p_0).

For a two-sample hypothesis test, H_0 states that the proportion of events or rate of occurrence (p_1) from the first group is the same as that (p_2) from the second group. For a clinical trial, the groups might reflect those receiving and not receiving the treatment. For an observational study, the groups might reflect those subjects with and without the attribute of interest. Interpretations of failing to reject and rejecting H_0 are similar to those described for the one-sample situation.

Step 2. Choose α, power, and the difference between p and p_0 (or p_1 and p_2) that is clinically meaningful. Another term for the difference between p and p_0 (or p_1 and p_2) is effect size. Frequently, investigators overlook this step. For example, the hospital epidemiologist may not have the opportunity to conduct a formal power analysis before data collection begins. However, whenever the effect size estimated from the sample is clinically meaningful but the results are consistent with H_0, the investigator should determine power retrospectively. This analysis allows the investigator to determine how much larger the sample would have to be to reject H_0, given the results of the study. Even when statistical significance is achieved, a retrospective power analysis can indicate how cautiously the results should be interpreted.

Step 3. Determine sample size, n. Sample size is extremely sensitive to the effect size chosen by the investigator.

Step 4. Obtain data.

Step 5. Compute test statistic in terms of parameters under H_0. Obtain the p value associated with the test statistic, assuming H_0 is correct. The interpretation of the p value is valid only in terms of H_0 and H_1. By choosing to make a hypothesis test, the investigator restates the research question and must decide between H_0 and H_1 based on how consistent or inconsistent the data are with H_0. The term *consistent* connotes having sufficient empirical support for the investigator to decide that the unknown true state of nature is likely to be H_0 instead of H_1. Conversely, the term *inconsistent* connotes having sufficient empirical support for the investigator to decide that the unknown true state of nature is likely not to be H_0 but rather H_1. Therefore, the p value is the probability of obtaining a result that is at least as extreme as this result, which the investigator has obtained from these data, given that H_0 is true. Stated another way, the investigator rejects H_0 when the results from the study could be called unusual if H_0 were correct. The consensus among statisticians and scientists is that, if the p value is .05 or smaller, the investigator should reject H_0 and decide that H_1 is correct. A p value of .05 indicates that this result would occur no more often than 1 in 20 times if H_0 were true.

Step 6. Decide whether to reject or fail to reject H_0. Compare the p value to α.

One-Sample Tests for a Binomial Proportion or Rate

Normal Approximation Method

The normal approximation method based on a z-test was selected because the computation of this test statistic more closely parallels the estimation of confidence limits than any of the other methods. If the normal approximation to the binomial distribution is valid (i.e., $npq > 5$), a two-sided hypothesis test is conducted as follows:

Step 1. Set up H_0 and H_1.

$$H_0{:}p = p_0 \text{ vs. } H_1{:}p \neq p_0$$

Step 2. Choose α, power, and the difference between p and p_0 that is clinically meaningful.

Step 3. Determine sample size, n. Sample size is extremely sensitive to the difference between p and p_0 and to how close these are to zero or 1.0. When no information is available, a pilot study can be conducted to get some idea of differences that can be obtained in a particular clinical situation.

$$n = \frac{\left[\left(z_{0.975} \times \sqrt{p_0 q_0}\right) + \left(z_{0.80} \times \sqrt{pq}\right)\right]^2}{\left(p - p_0\right)^2}$$

Step 4. Obtain data.

Step 5. Compute test statistic in terms of parameters under H_0, which is a z-score from the standard normal distribution, and obtain the p value as twice the probability associated with the z_s assuming that H_0 is correct. If the significance level is .05, $z_{0.975}$ is 1.96. With the wide availability of computer-based packages that contain statistical functions, many clinical investigators can obtain the p value.

$$z_s = \frac{\left|p - p_0\right|}{\sqrt{p_0 q_0 / n}}$$

where p is the estimate from the sample of the parameter p. One should note that $z^2 = \chi^2$; the squared z-score, obtained from the data (i.e., z_s), equals a chi-square test statistic with 1 degree of freedom obtained from the same data (i.e., χ_s^2). Most computer packages report a chi-square test statistic with 1 degree of freedom (i.e., χ_s^2) along with the associated p value. If the significance level is .05, $\chi^2_{0.95}$with 1 degree of freedom is 3.84, which equals 1.96^2. If the normal approximation to the binomial is not valid, p values may be obtained by the exact method.

Step 6. Decide whether to reject or fail to reject H_0. Compare the p value to α.

One-Sided Hypothesis Tests

If the hypothesis test is one-sided (i.e., $H_1{:}p > p_0$), calculate power and estimate sample size substituting $1 - \alpha$ for $1 - \alpha/2$ in the previous formulas (e.g., $z_{0.95}$ is 1.645). In addition, the p value is not multiplied by 2. It is always easier to reject a one-sided test than a similar two-sided test. In addition, an effectively larger α increases power by reducing β.

Two-Sample Tests for Binomial Proportions or Rates

When the random variable under study is classified into discrete categories, hypothesis testing and methods of inference should reflect the data structure. For the two-sample situation, there are two typical study designs: independent and paired samples. Before formulating the hypothesis, the investigator must determine whether the samples are independent or not. Two samples are independent when the data points in one sample are unrelated to the data points in the second sample. Samples that are not independent are paired. Paired samples may represent two sets of measurements on the same individuals. Alternatively, paired samples may represent measurements on different individuals chosen or matched such that each member of the pair is very similar to the other. Statistical analysis of data from clinical studies is valid only in the context of the study design; inferences are only valid in the context of research questions.

When a hospital epidemiologist investigates the relationship between two dichotomous variables, the observations are tabulated in 2 × 2 tables according to attributes. For example, suppose the epidemiologist classifies observations according to the following two attributes:

Attribute 1: *A*, :*Axu*

Attribute 2: *B*, :*Bxu*

The results will be classified into four groups that include all possible combinations of attributes 1 and 2: (*A*, *B*), ($\bar{A}$, *B*), (*A*,~~*Bxu*~~), and ($\bar{A}$, $\bar{B}$). After tabulation, data can be presented in the following format.

	B	$\bar{B}$	*Total*
A	*a*	*b*	*a* + *b*
$\bar{A}$	*c*	*d*	*c* + *d*
Total	*a* + *c*	*b* + *d*	*n*

The results of studies with either independent or paired designs may be tabulated according to the frequencies into the same four groups. Thus, this table can be obtained in different ways.

Two-Sample Test for Independent Samples

Both the table and the test statistic are the same regardless of whether the data are obtained from an observational study or a clinical trial. However, the research questions, hypotheses, and statistical tests may be different depending on the type of study. Consequently, the analyses also depend on study design.

Step 1. Set up H_0 and H_1. In many observational studies, the investigator can only control the total number of subjects; the research question involves whether the two sets of attributes are independent of each other. The statistical test is called a test of independence or association. In observational studies, the concept of independent samples stems from the notion that for a given attribute, such as pneumonia, the patients with pneumonia are unrelated to those without pneumonia. The null and alternative hypotheses may be written as follows:

$$H_0{:}p_1 = p_2 \text{ vs. } H_1{:}p_1 \neq p_2$$

where the null and alternative hypotheses are stated in terms of joint probabilities. The general approach is discussed in the earlier section on probability. For example, the investigator may record the observed joint probabilities of (a) developing pneumonia and being on the ventilator, (b) not developing pneumonia and being on the ventilator, (c) developing pneumonia and not being on the ventilator, and (d) not developing pneumonia and not being on the ventilator. The expected joint probabilities are those that would have occurred under the assumption of independence. The statistical test for association involves determining the probability of finding the observed joint probabilities if the attributes were independent.

For clinical trials, the general research question for studies with independent samples is whether the proportion of *B* (and $\bar{B}$) is the same for *A* and $\bar{A}$ [i.e., the proportion of patients who die is the same for those with the drug (treated) as for those without the drug (control subjects)]. Usually, the investigator determines not only the total number of subjects but also the number of subjects in each group. The statistical test is called a test of homogeneity of two proportions. For example, a clinical trial of a drug that may reduce the death rate associated with ventilator-associated pneumonia may be conducted. In this example, the investigator first estimates the observed conditional probabilities of death depending on whether the subject is in the treated or the control group. Next, the investigator estimates the observed marginal probabilities of death and survival using the addition rule. Using these observed marginal probabilities, the investigator then estimates the expected conditional probabilities of death independent of whether the subject is in the treated or the control group. These expected (or theoretical) conditional probabilities are based on the assumption that the death rate is the same in both groups (i.e., that H_0 is true). The statistical test involves determining the probability of finding the observed conditional probabilities if the probability of death were the same in both groups. The null and alternative hypotheses may be stated as follows:

$$H_0: P_{B|A} = p_{B|\bar{A}} \text{ vs. } H_1{:}p_{B|A} \neq P_{B|\bar{A}}$$

Step 2. Choose α, power, and the difference between p_1 and p_2 that is clinically meaningful.

Step 3. For clinical trials, determine sample size for each group, n_1 and n_2. Sample size is very sensitive to the difference between p_1 and p_2. This difference, also called the effect size, should be that difference which is biologically or clinically meaningful in the opinion of the researcher. When no information is available, a pilot study can be conducted to get some idea of differences that can be obtained in a particular clinical situation. Although the algebra is not difficult, the formula for determining sample size is quite complex; the reader is referred to the formula in Sokal and Rohlf (2), which minimizes the chances of underestimating the sample size required to detect a difference of $|p_1 - p_2|$ at given levels of significance and power. The formula in Rosner (8) yields sample size estimates that are generally about 5% smaller than those based on the Sokal and Rohlf formula:

$$n_i = \frac{\left\{\left[z_{0.975}\times\sqrt{pq\left(1+1/k\right)}\right]+\left[z_{0.80}\times\sqrt{p_1q_1+p_2q_2/k}\right]\right\}^2}{\left(p_1-p_0\right)^2}$$

$$n_2 = kn_1$$

where $p = (p_1 + kp_2)/(1 + k)$; $q = (1 - p)$; $z_{0.975} = 1.96$; $z_{0.80} = 0.842$; p_1 and p_2 are the projected true probabilities of success in the two groups; n_1 and n_2 are the numbers of observations in each group; and $k = n_1/n_2$ is the projected ratio of the two sample sizes. Unfortunately, a formula, commonly given in elementary statistical tutorials or primers, underestimates the sample size by roughly 50%. Computation of sample size can be tedious. For step 3, the investigator may wish to consult a biostatistician. Computer software is available for making some computations; however, the investigator should review documentation to determine which formulas are used and choose a software package that does not typically underestimate sample size.

Step 4. Obtain data.

Step 5. Compute test statistic in terms of parameters under H_0 and obtain the p value. If the sample size is larger than 20 and no more than 20% of the expected cell frequencies (i.e., the cell frequencies expected under the assumption of independence) are less than 5, using large sample theory and the normal approximation to the binomial distribution is valid. In this situation, the following test statistic is appropriate for both observational studies and clinical trials. The test statistic is z_s, where

$$z_s = \frac{|p_1 - p_2|}{\sqrt{pq\times(1/n_1 + 1/n_2)}}$$

where $p = (n_1p_1 + n_2p_2)/(n_1 + n_2)$; $q = (n_1q_1 + n_2q_2)/(n_1 + n_2)$; and n_1 and n_2 are the numbers of observations in each group. The p value is twice the probability associated with the test statistic, z_s, assuming that H_0 is correct.

Step 6. Decide whether to reject or fail to reject H_0. Compare the p value to α. When the two attributes are not independent of each other, there exists some form of association between the attributes. Inspecting the data will reveal what the association might be. The investigator must look closely at each of the individual cell chi-square values before making inferential statements about the nature of the association. The investigator's interpretation is based on the fact that the cells with the largest chi-square values have contributed proportionately more to the total chi-square test statistic. Note that $z^2 = \chi^2$; the squared z-score, obtained from the data (i.e., z_s), equals a chi-square test statistic with 1 degree of freedom obtained from the same data (i.e., χ_s^2). Most computer packages report a chi-square test statistic with 1 degree of freedom (i.e., χ_s^2) along with the associated p value. If the significance level is .05, $\chi^2_{0.95}$ with 1 degree of freedom is 3.84, which equals 1.96^2.

Fisher's Exact Test

If the normal approximation to the binomial is not valid, Fisher's exact test must be used to obtain the exact probability of obtaining a table with cells *a, b, c,* and *d.* This situation is described by the hypergeometric distribution. Fisher's exact test may be used to give the exact p value for any 2×2 table. Many computer packages for statistical analysis provide results based on Fisher's exact test. For a calculator-based method, the reader is referred to Rosner (8). The interpretation of the p value from Fisher's exact test is the probability of obtaining a table at least as extreme as the observed table, assuming the two attributes are independent.

Two-Sample Test for Paired Samples

Both the table and the test statistic are the same regardless of whether the data are obtained from an observational study or from a clinical trial. When matched pairs are the basic experimental unit for a clinical study, pairs are classified as to whether or not the treatment or placebo was effective for each member of the pair. Sometimes each subject is used as its own control, thereby yielding paired results. In observational studies, the pairs may be classified as to whether or not the outcome is the same for each member of the pair.

A matched pair in which the outcome is the same for both members of the pair is called a *concordant pair*—that is, (+, +) or (−, −). For example, one might consider a study in which the event of interest is death (as contrasted with survival). If both members of the pair die, this result might be symbolized as (+, +); conversely, if both members live, the result might be symbolized as (−, −). A matched pair in which the outcomes are different for the members of the pair is called a *discordant pair*—that is, (+, −) or (−, +). Rosner (8) describes a type A discordant pair as a pair in which the outcome for the member from the first group is the event and the outcome for the member from the second group is not. Using the previous example, a type A discordant pair would contain a member from the first group who died and a member from the second group who survived—that is, (+, −). According to the same logic, Rosner describes a type B discordant pair as a pair in which the outcome for the member from the first group is not the event and the outcome of the member from the second group is. Again, using the previous example, a type B discordant pair would contain a member from the first group who survived and a member from the second group who died—that is, (−, +). After tabulation, data can be presented in the following format.

Treatment or group 1	Treatment or group 2		
	+	−	
+	*a*	*b*	*a* + *b*
−	*c*	*d*	*c* + *d*
	a + *c*	*b* + *d*	*n*

Step 1. Set up H_0 and H_1. The null and alternative hypotheses may be stated as follows:

$$H_0: p_1^+ = p_2^+ \text{ versus } H_1: p_1^+ \neq p_2^+$$

where $p_1^+ = a/(a + b)$ and $p_2^+ = a/(a + c)$. The investigator tests whether the "+" proportions for the two treatments or groups are the same. Note that the only important differences between p_1^+ and p_2^+ are between b and c. Testing for differences between b and c is the same as testing that the "+" proportion for treatment or group 1 is the same as the "+" proportion for treatment or group 2. Thus, the null hypothesis could be restated as the frequency that the two types of discordant pairs are equal: $H_0: p_{+-} = p_{-+} = 0.5$ versus $H_1: p_{+-} \neq p_{-+} \neq 0.5$ where p_{+-} is $b/(b + c)$ and p_{-+} is $c/(b + c)$. This test is called McNemar's test. However, if the investigator chooses to state H_0 in terms of either p_{+-} or p_{-+}, this becomes a one-sample test with n equaling $(b + c)$. For the remainder of the procedure (i.e., steps 2 through 6), the reader is referred to the normal approximation method for one-sample tests for a binomial rate or proportion.

Two-Sample Test for Incidence-Density Variables

In many epidemiologic studies, the investigator follows subjects for varying lengths of time (e.g., length of stay in the ICU), and the outcome variable is dichotomous. For example, the variable of interest might be whether or not a nosocomial infection developed in a sample of patients. When a subject converts from a negative status to a positive status, the investigator records the time to failure. Failure connotes the event that the investigator is studying. In the simplest situation, the subjects are divided into two groups according to a single exposure (e.g., receiving or not receiving parenteral nutritional support). For this simple situation, the investigator has a choice of several methods for analyzing this type of data. Three commonly used methods are presented in this chapter. Two methods are presented in the following, and the third is discussed later (see the section on survival analysis). If the situation is more complex, the investigator must use either survival analysis or stratified analysis.

Rosner (8) presents a method that is appropriate when the investigator wishes to compare the incidence density rates of two groups. The investigator must assume that the incidence remains constant over the assessment time. Although patients are followed for varying lengths of time, the investigator knows whether a particular patient has either failed or not failed. The investigator counts the number of failures in each group. Then, the investigator computes the total number of person-time units elapsed from enrollment to the assessment time. After tabulation, data can be presented in the following format.

	Exposed	Not exposed	
Number of events	*a*	*b*	*a* + *b*
Person-time	t_1	t_2	$t_1 + t_2$

Step 1. Set up H_0 and H_1. The investigator tests whether the incidence-density (ID) is the same for the two groups of subjects. Stated another way, the investigator is interested in whether the rates of nosocomial infection per patient-day in the ICU are the same in the two exposure groups. The null and alternative hypotheses may be stated as follows:

$$H_0: \text{ID}_1 = \text{ID}_2 \text{ vs. } H_1: \text{ID}_1 \neq \text{ID}_2$$

where the estimated $\text{ID}_1 = a/t_1$ and the estimated $\text{ID}_2 = b/t_2$. The total number of events in the exposed group equals a. Similarly, the total number of events in the unexposed group equals b.

Step 2. Obtain data. Because most studies of incidence density are observational, power analyses and sample size computations are usually not completed.

Step 3. Compute test statistic in terms of parameters under H_0 and obtain the p value. If normal approximation of the binomial is valid (i.e., $V_1 \geq 5$), the test statistic is a z-score:

$$z_s = \frac{|a - E_1|}{\sqrt{V_1}}$$

where $E_1 = (a + b)t_1/(t_1 + t_2)$ and $V_1 = (a + b)t_1t_2/(t_1 + t_2)^2$. The p value is twice the probability associated with the test statistic z_s, assuming that H_0 is correct. If the normal approximation of the binomial is not valid, exact binomial probabilities must be obtained.

Step 4. Decide whether to reject or fail to reject H_0. Compare the p value to α.

The second method is probably the most commonly used test for comparing incidence rates. The Mantel-Haenszel test, also called the log rank test, does not require the assumption of a constant incidence rate over time. In this situation, the investigator may place as much importance on time to an event as on whether or not the event occurred. For example, suppose a hospital epidemiologist has a statewide surveillance program designed to detect new cases of positive tuberculin test results among nursing personnel during their first year of employment.

Step 1. H_0 and H_1 are the same as those described for the first method.

Step 2. Obtain data.

Step 3. Divide the year into shorter periods (e.g., months). Construct a 2 × 2 table for each interval. Note that subjects who have not experienced an event during a preceding interval are at risk for experiencing an event during the current interval; therefore, only the number of subjects not having the event in the preceding interval will appear in a given 2 × 2 table. Once a subject has experienced an event during a given interval, data for that subject does not appear on any table representing a subsequent interval.

Using these rules, the hospital epidemiologist constructs the table for the first time interval using the following format.

Event	Group 1	Group 2	
Yes	a_1	b_1	$a_1 + b_1$
No	c_1	d_1	$c_1 + d_1$
	$a_1 + c_1$	$b_1 + d_1$	n_1

where a_1 is the number of subjects in the first group who experienced events in the first interval; c_1 is the number of subjects in the first group who did not experience events during the first interval; $(a_1 + c_1)$ is the total number of subjects in the first group; b_1 is the number of subjects in the second group who experienced events during the first interval; d_1 is the number of subjects in the second group who did not experience events during the second interval; $(b_1 + d_1)$ is the total number of subjects in the second group; and n_1 is the total number of subjects in the study. Next, the hospital epidemiologist constructs the second table using the following format.

Event	Group 1	Group 2	
Yes	a_2	b_2	$a_2 + b_2$
No	c_2	d_2	$c_2 + d_2$
	$a_2 + c_2$	$b_2 + d_2$	n_2

where a_2 is the number of subjects in the first group who experienced events during the second interval; c_2 is the number of subjects in the first group who did not experience events during the second interval; $(a_2 + c_2)$ equals c_1 and is the total number of subjects in the first group who were at risk during the second interval; b_2 is the number of subjects in the second group who experienced events during the second interval; d_2 is the number of subjects in the second group who did not experience events during the second interval; $(b_2 + d_2)$ equals d_1 and is the total number of subjects in the second group who were at risk during the second interval; and n_2 equals $(c_1 + d_1)$ and is the total number of subjects at risk during the second interval. Continue constructing tables using the same format.

Step 4. Compute the test statistic over all the 2 × 2 tables in terms of parameters under H_0 and obtain the p value. The test statistic is the Mantel-Haenszel statistic, which may be computed with the following formula:

$$x^2_{\text{MH}} = \frac{\left\{\Sigma a_i - \left[\Sigma (a_i + b_i)(a_i + c_i)/n_i\right]\right\}^2}{\Sigma (a_i + b_i)(c_i + d_i)(a_i + c_i)(b_i + d_i)/\left[n_i^2 (n_i - 1)\right]}$$

where i indicates the individual 2 × 2 tables and the other values are defined in the discussion on construction of the various tables. Under H_0, the Mantel-Haenszel statistic, χ^2_{MH} follows a chi-square distribution with 1 degree of freedom. Therefore, for a test of significance at the .05 significance level, H_0 is rejected if χ^2_{MH} is greater than 3.84. The p value is the probability associated with χ^2_{MH} assuming that the null hypothesis is true.

Hypothesis Tests for Continuous Data

Distribution of Sample Means

The central limit theorem states that, for a large sample size regardless of the underlying distribution of the individual observations, the sample mean, $\bar{Y}$, follows a normal distribution with mean μ and variance σ^2/n (1–5,8,9,16). The mean of sample means is the same as the mean of the original population of individual values. The variance of sample means is needed to indicate dispersion or spread among $\bar{Y}$ values. The standard error is the standard deviation associated with the population of means (i.e., the standard deviation of the mean): $\sigma_{\bar{Y}} = \sigma/\sqrt{n}$. If the sample size n gets very large, the standard error approaches zero. What about the estimate from the one sample an epidemiologist actually collects? The estimated standard error (usually called simply the standard error) is $s/\sqrt{n}$, which is the standard deviation of $\bar{Y}$, regardless of whether original data follow a normal distribution.

Clinical researchers often find that hypothesis testing for continuous variables is helpful. One-sample tests can be used to determine whether the sample differs from the reference population with respect to continuous variables such as APACHE III scores. Clinical investigators often use two-sample tests during exploratory data analysis to identify potentially important continuous risk factors such as age and temperature at admission.

The following two sections describe statistical methods for one- and two-sample tests for continuous variables (1–5,7–9, 16). These sections are not designed as casual reading material; instead, they provide a concise reference of commonly used statistical methods. Each section follows the same format as has been described for hypothesis tests for categorical variables.

One-Sample Tests for a Continuous Variable

One-Sample Test for a Mean

Provided that the sample size is adequate (e.g., 20 or more) and the distribution is approximately normal, a two-sided hypothesis test is conducted as follows.

Step 1. Set up H_0 and H_1.

$$H_0 : \mu = \mu_0 \text{ vs. } H_1 : \mu \neq \mu_0$$

where μ is the mean of the population from which the sample is obtained and μ_0 is the mean of the norm group.

Step 2. Choose α, power, and the difference between μ and μ_0 that is clinically meaningful.

Step 3. Determine sample size n. Sample size is very sensitive to the difference between means, $\mu - \mu_0$, where μ is the mean of the population from which the sample is obtained and μ_0 is the mean of the norm group. This difference, also called the effect size, should be the difference that is biologically or clinically meaningful in the opinion of the researcher. When no information is available, a pilot study can be conducted to get some idea of the difference that can be obtained in a particular clinical situation.

$$n = \frac{\sigma^2 \times (z_{0.975} + z_{0.80})^2}{|\mu - \mu_0|^2}$$

where $z_{0.975} = 1.96$; $z_{0.80} = 0.842$; and σ^2 is the variance among subjects for the variable of interest.

Step 4. Obtain data.

Step 5. Compute test statistic in terms of parameters under H_0, which follows a t distribution with $(n - 1)$ degrees of freedom, and obtain the p value as twice the probability associated with the t_s, assuming that H_0 is correct. Like the standard normal distribution, the t distribution is symmetric; however, for each different degrees of freedom, there is a different distribution. If the sample size is 100 or more, the t distribution resembles the standard normal distribution.

$$t_s = \frac{\bar{X} - \mu_0}{s / \sqrt{n}}$$

where $\bar{X}$ is the estimate of the mean obtained from the sample; μ_0 is the mean if H_0 is true; and $s/\sqrt{n}$ is the standard deviation of the mean estimated from the sample. The p value is twice the probability associated with the test statistic t_s with $(n - 1)$ degrees of freedom, assuming that H_0 is correct.

Step 6. Decide whether to reject or fail to reject H_0. Compare the p value to α.

If the hypothesis test is one-sided (i.e., $H_1{:}\sigma > \sigma_0$), calculate power and estimate sample size substituting α for $\alpha/2$ in the previous formulas. In addition, the p value is not multiplied by 2. It is always easier to reject a one-sided test than a similar two-sided test. Furthermore, an effectively larger α increases power by reducing β.

One-Sample Test for a Variance or Standard Deviation

The most frequently used hypothesis test for variances or standard deviations is the two-sided test, which is conducted as follows.

Step 1. Set up H_0 and H_1 in terms of σ^2 and $\sigma_0{}^2$.

$$H_0: \sigma^2 = \sigma_0{}^2 \text{ vs. } H_1: \sigma_0{}^2 \neq \sigma^2$$

where σ^2 is the variance of the population from which the sample was chosen and $\sigma_0{}^2$ is the variance of the norm group.

Step 2. Compute test statistic in terms of parameters under H_0, which follows a χ^2 distribution with $(n - 1)$ degrees of freedom, and obtain the p value as twice the probability associated with the $\chi_s{}^2$, assuming that H_0 is correct. Unlike the standard normal distribution, the χ^2 distribution is not symmetric. For each different degrees of freedom, there is a different distribution. If the sample size is 100 or more, the χ^2 distribution resembles the standard normal distribution.

$$\chi_s{}^2 = (n - 1) \times \frac{s^2}{\sigma_0{}^2}$$

where s^2 is the sample variance for the variable of interest; n is the sample size; and $\sigma_0{}^2$ is the variance if H_0 is true. The p value is twice the probability associated with the test statistic $\chi_s{}^2$ with $(n - 1)$ degrees of freedom, assuming that H_0 is correct.

Step 3. Decide whether to reject or fail to reject H_0. Compare the p value to α.

If the hypothesis test is one-sided (i.e., $H_1{:}\sigma^2 > \sigma_0{}^2$), the p value is not multiplied by 2. Sample size and power are based on the ratio of the standard deviations that the hospital epidemiologist chooses as clinically important.

Two-Sample Tests for a Continuous Variable

When the random variable under study is a continuous variable, hypothesis testing and methods of inference should reflect the data structure. Before formulating the hypothesis, the investigator must determine whether the samples are independent or not.

Two-Sample Paired Test for Means

Paired samples are frequently encountered in biologic and health science research. For paired samples, a paired t-test is used. In follow-up or longitudinal studies, paired samples may represent two sets of measurements on the same individuals. Alternatively, paired samples may represent measurements on different individuals, matched such that each member of the pair is very similar to the other. In analyzing data from paired samples, the clinical investigator assumes that, for the variable of interest, the mean difference, Δ, between paired observations is the same for all pairs.

Step 1. Set up H_0 and H_1.

$$H_0: \Delta = 0 \text{ vs. } H_1: \Delta \neq 0$$

Step 2. Choose α, power, and the difference, Δ, that is clinically meaningful.

Step 3. Determine sample size n. Sample size is very sensitive to the mean difference. This difference, also called the effect size, should be that difference which is biologically or clinically meaningful in the opinion of the researcher. When no information is available, a pilot study can be conducted to get some idea of the mean difference that can be obtained in a particular clinical situation.

$$n = \frac{\sigma_\Delta{}^2 \times (z_{0.975} + z_{0.80})^2}{|\Delta|^2}$$

where $z_{0.975} = 1.96$; $z_{0.80} = 0.842$; and $\sigma_\Delta{}^2$ is the variance of the difference between paired observations.

Step 4. Obtain data.

Step 5. Compute test statistic in terms of parameters under H_0, which follows a t distribution with $(n - 1)$ degrees of freedom where n is the number of pairs, and obtain the p value as twice the probability associated with the t_s.

$$t_s = \frac{\bar{D}}{s_D / \sqrt{n}}$$

where $\bar{D}$ is the mean of the differences between pairs in the sample; s_D is the standard deviation of the difference between pairs in the sample; and n is the number of pairs. The p value is twice the probability associated with the test statistic t_s (assuming that H_0 is correct) with $(n - 1)$ degrees of freedom where n is the number of pairs.

Step 6. Decide whether to reject or fail to reject H_0. Compare the p value to α.

If the hypothesis test is one-sided (i.e., $H_1{:}\Delta > 0$), calculate power and estimate sample size substituting α for $\alpha/2$ in the previous formulas. In addition, the p value is not multiplied by 2. It is always easier to reject a one-sided test than a similar two-sided test. Furthermore, an effectively larger α increases power by reducing β.

Two-Sample (Independent) Test for Means

Independent samples are frequently encountered in biologic and health science research. For independent samples, a t-test for independent samples is used. Continuous variables from cross-sectional studies involving two groups are often analyzed with independent t-tests.

Step 1. Set up H_0 and H_1.

$$H_0: \mu_1 = \mu_2 \text{ vs. } H_1: \mu_1 \neq \mu_2$$

$$H'_0: \sigma_1^2 = \sigma_2^2 \text{ vs. } H'_1: \sigma_1^2 \neq \sigma_2^2$$

where μ_1 and σ_1^2 are the mean and variance of the population from which the first sample was chosen and μ_2 and σ_2^2 are the mean and variance of the population from which the second sample was chosen.

Step 2. Choose α, power, and the difference between μ_1 and μ_2 that is clinically meaningful.

Step 3. Determine sample size for each group, n_1 and n_2. Sample size is very sensitive to the difference between group means. This difference, also called the effect size, should be that difference which is biologically or clinically meaningful in the opinion of the researcher. When no information is available, a pilot study can be conducted to get some idea of differences between μ_1 and μ_2 that can be obtained in a particular clinical situation.

$$n = \frac{(\sigma_1^2 + \sigma_2^2 \times (z_{0.975} + z_{0.80})^2}{|\mu_1 - \mu_2|^2}$$

where $z_{0.975} = 1.96$ and $z_{0.80} = 0.842$. If the variances in the two groups are the same, the smallest total sample size involves equal sample sizes in each group. Sometimes it is not possible or practical to have equal sample sizes. The clinical investigator can calculate the sample sizes needed for comparing the means of two normally distributed samples for a two-sided test using the following formulas:

$$n_1 = (\sigma_1^2 + \sigma_2^2 / k)(z_{0.975} + z_{0.80})^2 / |\mu_1 - \mu_2|^2$$

$$n_2 = (k\sigma_1^2 + \sigma_2^2)(z_{0.975} + z_{0.80})^2 / |\mu_1 - \mu_2|^2$$

where $k = n_2/n_1$ is the projected ratio of the two sample sizes; $z_{0.975} = 1.96$; and $z_{0.80} = 0.842$. For one-sided tests, substitute $1 - \alpha$ for $1 - \alpha/2$ in the previous formulas.

Step 4. Obtain data.

Step 5a. Compute test statistic in terms of parameters under H'_0. If the assumption about equal variances for the two samples is doubted, the investigator can use an F-test, commonly called F', to determine the validity of this assumption. Under H'_0, $F'_s = s_1^2/s_2^2$ where s_1^2 is the variance estimated from the first sample and s_2^2 is the variance estimated from the second sample; F'_s follows an F-distribution with $\nu_1 = (n_1 - 1)$ and $\nu_2 = (n_2 - 1)$ degrees of freedom. For practical purposes, most textbooks recommend the following: label the populations (and hence the samples) such that $s_1^2 > s_2^2$ (i.e., $F'_s > 1.0$). Then reject H'_0 if $F'_s > F_{0.95}$ with ν_1 and ν_2 degrees of freedom, or $F_{0.95[\nu 1,\nu 2]}$. This is still a test at the α level of significance, but the upper tail value is used in determining the p value. If $p < .05$, the investigator rejects the assumption of equal variances and uses the Behrens-Fisher t-test, also called Satterthwaite's method. If $p > .05$, the investigator maintains the assumption of equal variances and uses Student's t-test. With general use of computers, restricting F'_s to be larger than 1.0 is no longer necessary. Therefore, the α level of significance for a comparable two-sided test is 0.10. Computer packages vary in reporting one- or two-sided p values; the investigator should check documentation to verify the nature of the p values.

Step 5b. For Student's t-test, compute test statistic in terms of parameters under H_0.

$$t_s = \frac{(\bar{X}_1 - \bar{X}_2)}{s_p \sqrt{1/n_1 + 1/n_2}}$$

where $\bar{X}_1$ is the sample mean obtained from the first sample; $\bar{X}_2$ is the sample mean obtained from the second sample; and s_p is the pooled standard deviation. The investigator obtains s_p by taking the square root of the pooled variance, s_p^2.

$$s_p^2 = \frac{\left[(n_1 - 1)s_1^2 + (n_2 - 1)s_2^2\right]}{(n_1 + n_2 - 2)}$$

The difference between two means follows a t distribution with $(n_1 + n_2 - 2)$ degrees of freedom. The p value is twice the probability associated with the test statistic t_s with $(n_1 + n_2 - 2)$ degrees of freedom, assuming that H_0 is correct.

For the Behrens-Fisher t-test

$$t_s = \frac{(\bar{X}_1 - \bar{X}_2)}{\sqrt{s_1^2/n_1 + s_2^2/n_2}}$$

where $\bar{X}_1$ is the sample mean obtained from the first sample; $\bar{X}_2$ is the sample mean obtained from the second sample; s_1^2 is the sample variance from the first sample; s_2^2 is the sample variance from the second sample; n_1 is the number of observations in the first sample; and n_2 is the number of observations in the second sample. The appropriate degrees of freedom must now be calculated based on s_1^2, s_2^2, n_1, and n_2.

$$d' = \frac{\left(s_1^2/n_1 + s_2^2/n_2\right)^2}{\left[\left(s_1^2/n_1\right)^2/(n_1 - 1) + \left(s_2^2/n_2\right)^2/(n_2 - 1)\right]}$$

The p value is twice the probability associated with the test statistic t_s (assuming that H_0 is correct) with (d') degrees of freedom.

Step 6. Decide whether to reject or fail to reject H_0. Compare the p value to α.

If the hypothesis test is one-sided (i.e., H_1:$\mu_1 > \mu_2$ or $\mu_1 < \mu_2$), calculate power and estimate sample size substituting α for $\alpha/2$ in the previous formulas. In addition, the p value is not multiplied by 2. It is always easier to reject a one-sided test than a similar two-sided test. Furthermore, an effectively larger α increases power by reducing β.

Hypothesis Tests for Ranked Data

If the central limit theorem is not applicable, the clinical investigator must use nonparametric statistical methods to analyze data and make inferences (1–5,7,8,12). A more descriptive term for these methods is *distribution-free methods.* In general, nonparametric methods are more flexible than parametric methods, because nonparametric methods require fewer or no assumptions about the shape of the underlying distribution.

Distribution-free methods are required when the data are ordinal. Ordinal data are data that can be ordered but do not have specific numeric values. Measurement data are data that lie on a scale wherein common arithmetic is meaningful. In contrast, ordinal variables cannot be given a numerical scale that makes sense biologically or clinically. Essentially, the ranks are arbitrarily assigned; these could be reversed and still retain the same meaning for the researcher. Therefore, computation of means and standard deviations is absurd, because there would be no universally accepted meaning (outside of a researcher's laboratory or clinic). Medians and ranges are used instead.

A clinical investigator can apply nonparametric tests to any measurement data. This application may be particularly appropriate when the assumption of normality appears to be grossly violated. If the actual underlying distribution is in fact normal, the clinical investigator will pay a penalty, because in this situation the nonparametric counterpart for a parametric test statistic has less power. Often, data are not normally distributed, even though a reasonable assumption has been made that the underlying (i.e., theoretical) distribution is normal. Parametric methods are often robust enough to withstand certain departures from normality. Some statisticians recommend that investigators analyze continuous data by both parametric and nonparametric methods. If the results of both analyses are consistent, the researcher is assured that the result reported from the parametric test is probably not biased. However, results from these analyses may not be consistent (i.e., the result from one analysis may be significant and the result from the other be very far from significance). In this event, the result from the parametric test is probably biased. After reviewing the data carefully, the researcher should (a) consider options for transforming the data so that the parametric test is valid or (b) report the result from the nonparametric test. Whenever it is appropriate to use nonparametric methods, these are usually more powerful than their parametric counterparts, and the results of tests are unbiased.

The following section describes nonparametric statistical methods for two-sample tests on ordinal (i.e., ranked) and continuous variables (1–5,7,8,12). These sections are not designed as casual reading material; instead, they provide a concise reference of commonly used statistical methods.

Sign Test

This test was named because it depends only on the sign of the differences in responses between matched subjects in the treatment and control groups (or, alternatively, exposed and unexposed; survivors and nonsurvivors) and not on the magnitude of the actual differences, Δ. This test can also be used for paired observations on the same individual (e.g., before and after treatment). Under some conditions, we cannot observe an actual difference, D, between two treatments but can only observe if the differences are negative or worse (i.e., $D < 0$), positive or better (i.e., $D > 0$), or not apparent or discernible (i.e., $D = 0$). The sign test is based on the number of positive (i.e., $D > 0$) differences out of the total number of nonzero differences; all differences with a zero outcome are excluded from analysis. The sign test is a two-sided test. If the number of nonzero responses is greater than or equal to 20, the normal approximation to the binomial applies and the sign test is the same as McNemar's test (see the section on two-sample test for paired samples). If the number of nonzero responses is less than 20, exact binomial probabilities must be obtained.

Wilcoxon Signed Rank Test

The Wilcoxon sign rank test may be applied to ordinal or measurement data. This test is the nonparametric counterpart for the paired t-test. This test is based on the ranks of the observations rather than on their actual values. It is more powerful than the sign test, because both sign and the magnitude of the differences, based on rank, are used in computing the test statistic. If the distribution is normal, this test has less power than the paired t-test; otherwise, it is the more powerful test. This test should be used only when the number of nonzero differences is greater than or equal to 16. For computation of the test statistic, see to Rosner (8).

Wilcoxon Rank Sum Test and the Mann-Whitney U-Test

The Wilcoxon rank sum test was developed for ranked or ordinal data; the Mann-Whitney U-Test was developed for comparisons that come from underlying distributions that are continuous. These tests are the nonparametric counterparts of the t-test for two independent samples. These tests, based on the ranks of the individual observations rather than on the actual values, should be used only when n_1 and n_2 are both greater than or equal to 10. For computation of the test statistic, see Rosner (8).

POINT AND INTERVAL ESTIMATION

In the epidemiologic literature, interval estimation is more common than hypothesis testing. Confidence intervals from a single sample can be used to determine estimated upper and lower limits for a parameter from the reference population. Often, clinical investigators divide the sample into two or more groups according to certain characteristics and estimate confidence intervals for each group. Using the previous example, the epidemiologist may be comparing the incidence of nosocomial pneumonia among patients who were ventilated to the incidence of nosocomial pneumonia among patients who were not ventilated. The following sections address general definitions and rules for estimating confidence intervals, one- and two-sided confidence intervals for categorical and continuous variables, and confidence intervals for statistics with special application to epidemiology (1–5,8,9,12,15,16,20).

Definition and Rules

First, an epidemiologist estimates parameters according to data obtained from the sample. These estimates are called point estimates. For estimating the confidence interval (CI), the epidemiologist uses the point estimate from the sample and the standard deviation of that point estimate to compute a lower confidence limit, L_L, and an upper confidence limit, L_U. The confidence limits are affected by the level of confidence that the epidemiologist wishes to place in the statement. Typically, epidemiologists report 95% CIs; 95%, called the coefficient of confidence, equals $(1 - \alpha)100\%$. Other traditional levels of confidence are 90% and 99%. It is crucial that the investigator state what level of confidence has been chosen. Often, the clinical investigator has a conflicting problem between having a high level of confidence and a CI that is not too large. For a specified level of confidence, increasing the sample size is the only option available to the epidemiologist for reducing the length of a CI. If the sample size must remain reasonably small, the epidemiologist may have to choose a lower level of confidence (e.g., 90%). The meaning of a CI is as follows: with repeated experiments, for each sample a different lower limit, L_L, and upper limit, L_U, will be computed, because both the point estimate and standard deviation of that point estimate will be different for each sample; $(1 - \alpha)100\%$ of the CIs will include the parameter and $\alpha 100\%$ will not. Thus, an investigator can state with $(1 - \alpha)100\%$ confidence that the interval based on the sample contains the parameter. How does an epidemiologist obtain confidence limits, L_L and L_U?

Point and Interval Estimation for a Continuous Variable

Point and Interval Estimation for Means

The point estimate for μ is $\bar{Y}$. A more informative way of writing this point estimate is $\bar{Y} \pm s_{\bar{Y}}$ where $s_{\bar{Y}} = s/\sqrt{n}$. The second expression tells something about the precision of the estimate of the mean—the standard error or standard deviation of $\bar{Y}$. Thus, it is not sufficient to give only $\bar{Y}$. A two-sided 95% CI for μ is calculated as follows:

$$L_L = \bar{Y} - t_{0.975/[n-1]} \times s/\sqrt{n}$$

$$L_U = \bar{Y} + t_{0.975[n-1]} \times s/\sqrt{n}$$

μ is fixed; L_L and L_U are variable so that $(1 - \alpha)100\%$ of the intervals will contain μ. $\bar{Y}$ and s both change with each new sample—thus, both location and length of the CI will change from one sample to the next. Because the t distribution is symmetric, $t_{0.025[n-1]}$ equals $-t_{0.975[n-1]}$.

Because the length of the CI depends on the sample through s, the hospital epidemiologist must know something about s before making any decisions about sample size. The length of a two-sided $(1 - \alpha)\%$ CI, L, is $2 \times t_{1-\alpha/2[n-1]} \times s/\sqrt{n}$. If the future value of σ can be estimated, sample size can be determined as follows:

$$n' = \left[(2 \times 1.96\sigma)/L\right]^2$$

This number, n', underestimates the required sample size, because $t_{0.975[n-1]}$ is always larger than $z_{0.975}$. Thus, by multiplying n' by the squared ratio of the t-score with $(n' - 1)$ degrees of freedom to the z-score, the adjusted sample, n_{adj}, can be obtained:

$$n_{adj} = n' \times \left[t_{0.975[n'-1]}/z_{0.975}\right]^2$$

For observational studies, sample size determination relies heavily on how well the actual sample reflects the assumptions used to obtain sample size. Although there are no guarantees, sample size determination gives the clinical investigator some general idea of how large a sample may be needed.

Point and Interval Estimation for Variances and Standard Deviations

The unbiased estimator of σ^2 is the sample variance, s^2. If the underlying distribution of the variable is normal, reliable estimates of CIs can be obtained. If the underlying distribution of the variable is not normal, the following methods may not be reliable. Variances do not follow a symmetric distribution. The ratio of s^2 to σ^2 follows a chi-square distribution with $(n - 1)$ degrees of freedom, $\chi^2_{[n-1]}$. Note that the χ^2 distribution is not symmetric; thus, a CI for a variance or a standard deviation is not symmetric. A CI for a variance can be estimated using the following formula:

$$L_L = (n-1)s^2/\chi^2_{0.975[n-1]}$$

$$L_U = (n-1)s^2/\chi^2_{0.025[n-1]}$$

where L_L and L_U are always positive. A CI for σ is obtained by taking the square root of L_L and L_U. As the confidence increases, the length will increase. Reducing the length requires a reduction in confidence or an increase in sample size. As the sample size increases, the CI will become less skewed. These limits are independent of the estimated mean.

Point and Interval Estimation for a Binomial Proportion or Rate

The point estimate of p is $\hat{p}$, estimated from the sample. When there is only one group with two outcome possibilities (i.e., survival and nonsurvival), the unbiased estimator of $\hat{p}$ is the proportion of the sample with the characteristic. The standard deviation of $\hat{p}$ is estimated by $\sqrt{\hat{p}\hat{q}/n}$. For a large sample, $\hat{p}$ is distributed normally with mean *acp*> and variance $\hat{p}\hat{q}/n$. Generally, the assumption of normality is valid when $n\hat{p}\hat{q}$ is greater than 5.

Under the assumption of normality, approximate CIs for p can be obtained as follows:

$$L_L = \hat{p} - z_{0.975} \times \sqrt{\hat{p}\hat{q}/n}$$

$$L_U = \hat{p} + z_{0.975} \times \sqrt{\hat{p}\hat{q}/n}$$

The length of a two-sided $(1 - \alpha)\%$ CI, L, is $2 \times z_{1-\alpha/2} \times \sqrt{pq/n}$. Sample size can be determined as follows: $n = [(2 \times 1.96pq)/L]^2$. Because the standard normal distribution is symmetric, $z_{0.025}$ equals $-z_{0.975}$.

Point and Interval Estimation for Risk Ratios and Odds Ratios

For independent samples, a clinical investigator uses data displayed in 2 × 2 tables to estimate the RR or the OR. Whether the data reflect incidence or prevalence determines which statistic is estimated. Throughout this section, it is assumed that the clinical investigator has displayed the data such that exposure to the ventilator is the first column and presence of pneumonia is the first row.

When incidence of disease for the sample is known, the epidemiologist is interested in estimating the RR of disease, which is the ratio of two conditional probabilities. In the previous example, the RR of pneumonia is $Pr(P \mid V)/Pr(P \mid \not{V})$.

Exposed to ventilator	Not exposed to ventilator	Total or marginal probability of disease	
Pneumonia present	*Pr*(*P* and *V*)	*Pr*(*P* and √*V*)	*Pr*(*P*)
Pneumonia absent	*Pr*(√*P* and *V*)	*Pr* (√*P* and √*V*)	*Pr*(√*P*)
Total or marginal probability of exposure	*Pr*(*V*)	*Pr*(√*V*)	1.0

If $Pr(P \mid V) = 0.25$ and $Pr(P \mid \not{V}) = .167$, RR equals 1.497. The interpretation of the RR is as follows: patients who are ventilated are 1.497 times as likely to have pneumonia as those who are not ventilated.

Under the assumption of normality, approximate CIs for RR can be obtained as follows:

$$L_L = \text{RR}\left(\exp\left[-z_{0.975}/s_{\text{RR}}\right]\right)$$

$$L_U = \text{RR}\left(\exp\left[z_{0.975}/s_{\text{RR}}\right]\right)$$

where RR is estimated from the sample; $z_{0.975} = 1.96$; $\exp(x) = e^x$; and

$$s_{RR} = \sqrt{\left\{\left[1 - Pr(P\,\text{B}V)\right]/n_{11} + \left[1 - Pr(P\,\text{B}\bar{V})\right]/n_{12}\right\}}$$

where n_{11} is the number of patients with pneumonia and exposure to the ventilator and n_{12} is the number of patients with pneumonia and no exposure to the ventilator.

When prevalence of disease for the sample is known, the epidemiologist estimates the odds in favor of disease based on joint probabilities. In the following table, P_1, P_2, P_3, and P_4 are joint probabilities. For example, P_1 is the joint probability of a patient having both exposure to the ventilator and presence of pneumonia. The OR equals a ratio with P_1/P_3 in the numerator and P_2/P_4 in the denominator. This expression can be simplified as follows: OR $= (P_1P_4)/(P_2P_3)$.

	Exposed to ventilator	Not exposed to ventilator	Total or marginal probability of disease
Pneumonia present	P_1	P_2	$P_1 + P_2$
Pneumonia absent	P_3	P_4	$P_3 + P_4$
Total or marginal probability of exposure			
$P_1 + P_3$			
$P_2 + P_4$			

Under the assumption of normality, approximate CIs for OR can be obtained as follows:

$$L_L = \text{OR}\left(\exp\left[-z_{0.975}/s_{\text{OR}}\right]\right)$$

$$L_U = \text{OR}\left(\exp\left[z_{0.975}/s_{\text{OR}}\right]\right)$$

where OR is the OR estimated from the sample; $z_{0.975}$ is 1.96; $\exp(x) = e^x$; and $s_{\text{OR}} = \sqrt{(1/n_{11} + 1/n_{12} + 1/n_{21} + 1/n_{22})}$ where n_{11} is the number of patients with pneumonia and with exposure to the ventilator, n_{12} is the number of patients with pneumonia and without exposure to the ventilator, n_{21} is the number of patients without pneumonia and with exposure to the ventilator, and n_{22} is the number of patients without pneumonia and without exposure to the ventilator.

For matched pairs, the clinical investigator can estimate RRs and ORs from stratified analyses. Methods for point and interval estimation are covered in that section.

Relationship Between CIs and Hypothesis Testing

CIs give a range of values within which the parameter (e.g., μ, σ, σ^2, p, RR, or OR) is likely to fall. When reporting CIs, the clinical investigator does not use a p value; however, the parameter estimate, the level of confidence, and the standard deviation of the estimate (i.e., the standard error) are reported. Conversely, when a hypothesis has been tested, the investigator should report the p value, the parameter estimate, and the standard deviation of the estimate (i.e., standard error). Sample size is as important for estimation of CIs as it is for testing hypotheses. In general, if H_0 is rejected, the corresponding CI does not contain the parameter under H_0. The one-to-one relationship between a CI and the corresponding hypothesis test is easiest to represent with the two-sided case. For completeness, it is a good practice for clinical investigators to provide enough information that both CIs and p values are obvious to anyone reading the report.

REGRESSION AND CORRELATION COEFFICIENTS

A clinical investigator uses regression or correlation analysis when the objective of the study is determining the functional relationship between two or more variables measured on the same individual. There are comparable regression and correlation methods for continuous and discrete variables.

Uses of Regression Analysis

Regression analysis has several applications that are relevant to epidemiologic studies (1,2,28). The first application is the study of causation. When looking for causal relationships, an epidemiologist must be aware that, although a cause-and-effect relationship may exist between two variables of interest, regression analysis cannot establish that the relationship is actually causal. Often, the study of causation will involve the second application of regression analysis for health science research—prediction. Nomograms, widely used in the clinical setting, have usually been developed from regression analysis. Third, the epidemiologist can use regression analysis to identify easily measured variables that can be substituted reliably for others that may be difficult, expensive, or hazardous to collect. Substituting one variable for another does require a previous experimental study to establish the relationship between the variable of interest and the surrogate variable. A fourth commonly used application is controlling for one or more extraneous or confounding variables. After controlling statistically for a variable that cannot be controlled by experimental design, the clinical investigator can make more precise inferences about the relationship between the two variables of primary interest, usually exposure and outcome (or disease). Age, sex, weight, severity of illness, and type of infection are examples of common confounding variables. In a purely experimental setting, confounding variables can often be controlled or eliminated. However, in a naturalistic setting, the investigator must rely on statistical control. Finally, inverse regression or calibration is used for obtaining many assay results.

Regression Coefficients

In the simplest situation, the clinical investigator wishes to quantify the relationship between two variables, X and Y. For regression analysis, the convention is to call X the independent variable and Y the dependent variable. Another term for X is *explanatory variable.* Clinical investigators often call Y the *response variable.* Generally, the investigator is trying to predict Y from X (i.e., $Y \mid X$, read Y given X).

In regression analysis, the clinical investigator must describe the functional relationship between X and Y in terms of an ideal mathematical relationship or model, symbolized $Y = F(X)$, which states that Y is a function (i.e., F) of X. The experienced investigator understands that the relationship between X and Y can take many forms. If the relationship is linear, the functional relationship can be symbolized as $F(X) = \alpha + \beta X$. Some relationships are curvilinear requiring the addition of a quadratic term to the mathematical model: $F(X) = \alpha + \beta X + \gamma X^2$. Some curvilinear relationships vary episodically over a day or month and can be described reasonably well with sinusoidal functions: $F(X) = \alpha + \beta \sin X$. Some relationships are not linear; two examples are $F(X) = \alpha + \beta \sqrt{X}$ and $F(X) = \alpha + \beta / X$.

For the models presented in the preceding paragraph, the investigator can make these relationships linear by using transformations of X, Y, or both. Therefore, statisticians call these relationships intrinsically linear. Intrinsically linear means that the parameters, such as α and β, are linearly related to X and Y. Some relationships are intrinsically nonlinear, meaning that the relationship of X and Y to the parameters is not linear: $F(X) = \alpha + \beta e^{-\gamma X}$. Special methods are needed for estimating regression coefficients when the relationship has a nonlinear functional form.

In nature, the observed relationship is never exact; because of natural variability, there is always some deviation from the ideal mathematical relationship or model. Thus, the clinical investigator describes the functional relationship in terms of a statistical relationship: $Y = F(X) + \epsilon$ where ϵ is distributed normally with mean 0 and variance σ_ϵ^2. Conceptually, ϵ is an error term and σ_ϵ^2 represents the variance of Y for a given X. The investigator assumes that X is measured or controlled perfectly, thereby not contributing to the natural variability of Y. Collectively, the error terms are called the residuals, which are random deviations in Y from the ideal relationship. Thus, ϵ is a random variable that measures the deviation of each individual observation, Y_i, from $\mu_{Y|X}$ (i.e., the expected value of Y_i on the regression line). Furthermore, σ_ϵ^2 is independent of X. For example, σ_ϵ^2 is the same for both small and large values of X. The clinical investigator uses the residuals to determine if there is a linear relationship based on the data.

Simple Linear Regression Coefficients

Simple linear regression is the term for linear regression with only one independent variable (1–10,12,16,28–31). For a simple linear regression, $Y = \alpha + \beta X + \epsilon$, the parameters α and β are unknown and must be estimated from the data with statistics. The line $Y = \alpha + \beta X$ is defined as the regression line, where α is the intercept (i.e., the value on the Y-axis that corresponds to $X = 0$), and β is the slope. The regression line describes the regression of Y on X. The slope may be positive, indicating that, as X increases, the expected value of Y increases. Similarly, the slope may be negative, indicating that, as X increases, the expected value of Y decreases. Finally, the slope may be zero, depicting a horizontal line and indicating that there is no relationship between X and Y. By accounting for the systematic relationship between X and Y, the investigator reduces the total variability of Y. Even if a linear relationship exists, all observations could be displayed on one axis (i.e., the Y-axis) only; however, the variation in Y would be much larger (σ_Y^2), because no attempt has been made to account or adjust for the variability in the X values that contributes to the variability of Y.

Estimating α and β

Plotting the data is an important step, because the graph is useful for suggesting whether there is a linear relationship. The difference between Y_i, the actual observation, and the corresponding expected value on the line, $\mu_{Y|X}$, reflects ϵ_i, the deviation for the particular observation. Some of these differences are positive and others are negative. The sum of the deviations (vertical deviations) is zero (i.e., $\Sigma\epsilon_i = 0$). The investigator uses the method of least squares to minimize the squared deviation between the line and the observations.

Estimate of β

The investigator estimates β from the data, using the following formula:

$$b = \frac{\Sigma(X_i - \bar{X})(Y_i - \bar{Y})}{\Sigma(X_i - \bar{X})^2} = \frac{\text{Cov}(X,Y)}{\text{Var}(X)}$$

where the numerator is the covariance between X and Y, and the denominator is the variance of X. The covariance can be either negative or positive; the variance is always positive. One should note that a small value of β does not necessarily imply that the relationship is not strong between X and Y. By itself, b (as an estimate of β) does not tell whether there is any relationship between X and Y. An experienced investigator realizes that a change of units usually makes the size of the regression coefficient change. To determine whether the relationship is strong, the investigator has to know b relative to s_ϵ^2, the estimated variance of the residuals.

Estimate of α

The estimate of α is a function of b: $\alpha = \bar{Y} - b\bar{X}$ where $\bar{Y}$ is the estimated mean of Y and $\bar{X}$ is the estimated mean of X. Estimation of α is based on the premise that two points are necessary to determine a line. Thus, every regression line goes through the point $(\bar{X}, \bar{Y})$ and the Y-intercept. If the point $(\bar{X}, \bar{Y})$ and the estimated slope b are known, then the estimate of α is based on simple algebra.

Simple Linear Regression Analysis

Interpreting Residuals

The assumptions on which linear regression is based are that the residuals are independently and identically distributed normally with mean 0 and variance σ_ϵ^2. One or more of these assumptions may be violated. In practice, a clinical investigator detects any violation of these assumptions by plotting the residuals and conducting certain hypothesis tests (1,2,28–32). The investigator applies diagnostic procedures to various plots of residuals and determines how the assumptions may be violated. Generally, lack of randomness in the residuals has some implications about possible violations. First, randomness or lack of randomness can be determined by examining a graph of the residuals plotted against the values of X. For example, plotting the residuals may reveal evidence of heteroscedasticity, which means unequal variances. In the clinical setting, heteroscedasticity is often characterized by increasing residuals as X increases. Second, systematic differences or deviations from the regression line are often revealed in a graph with actual values plotted on the X and Y axes and the predicted values superimposed on the same graph. Systematic deviations of the actual values from predicted values may indicate that a straight-line relationship is not the best fit. Third, plotting of actual values may reveal one or more points that are outliers and, as such, are influential points. Influential points often cause spurious results by drastically changing the estimated slope and intercept from what would have been expected had the influential points not been included in the analysis. Finally, the investigator chooses appropriate ways of dealing with the problem or problems. Typically, the investigator can make transformations or adjust the data in other appropriate ways so that the residuals will meet these assumptions. After the investigator has taken remedial action, the resulting graphs should reveal that the residuals meet the assumptions.

Prediction or Estimation of $\mu_{Y|X} = a + bX$

For a given value of X, $\hat{\mu}_{Y|X}$, also called $\hat{Y}$, is the corresponding point on the estimated regression line. Hence, $\hat{Y}$ is the estimate of the average response for a given X and is regarded as the predicted value of Y for a particular value of X. Interpolation within the range of the data is acceptable. Extrapolation is dangerous. Caution is needed when we are using any prediction equation outside the range covered by the X values in the study. Beyond these values, the relationship may no longer be linear.

Method of Least Squares

The numerator of the sample variance for Y is $\Sigma(Y_i - \bar{Y})^2$. Another name for this expression is the total corrected sum of squares where *corrected* refers to the deviation of each observation from the mean (i.e., corrected for the mean). In some statistics texts, the total corrected sum of squares is abbreviated as CSS. Frequently, clinical investigators use the method of least squares to partition the total corrected sum of squares for Y into two parts: (a) the sum of squares due to regression (i.e., regression SS or model SS) and (b) the residual or error sum of squares (i.e., residual SS or error SS).

As stated previously, the point $(\bar{X}\bar{Y})$ always lies on the regression line. For any sample point, the total vertical deviation of each point (X_i, Y_i) from $(\bar{X}\bar{Y})$ is the vertical distance that Y_i lies from the mean $\bar{Y}$; thus, measured on the Y-axis, the total deviation is $(Y_i - \bar{Y})$ (Fig. 3.1). The regression component of that point (X_i, Y_i) is the vertical distance from $(\bar{X}\bar{Y})$ to the predicted value on the regression line $(X_i, \hat{Y}_i)$ measured on the Y-axis; thus, on the Y-axis, the regression component is the quantity $(\hat{Y}_i - \bar{Y})$ (Fig. 3.1). Now, for any sample point, the residual component (i.e., residual) of that point about the regression line is the vertical distance from the actual observation (X_i, Y_i) to the predicted value on the regression line $(X_i, \hat{Y}_i)$; thus, on the Y-axis, the residual component is the quantity $(Y_i - \hat{Y}_i)$ (Fig. 3.1). Therefore, the total deviation $(Y_i - \bar{Y})$ of each point from the regression line can be separated into residual and regression components.

In using the least squares method, the investigator squares and sums the total deviations, the regression components, and the residuals: $\Sigma(Y_i - \bar{Y})^2 = \Sigma(\hat{Y}_i - \bar{Y})^2 + \Sigma(Y_i - \hat{Y}_i)^2$. The residual SS tells the investigator how well the regression line fits the data. However, the investigator needs a formal goodness-of-fit test to assess whether this value is large or small. Partitioning the total corrected SS allows the investigator to construct an analysis of variance (ANOVA) table. The total deviations, the regression components, and the residuals correspond to three sources of variation. These sources of variation are similarly named: regression (also called model), error (also called residual), and total. The degrees of freedom for the total variation is the denominator of the sample variance of Y: $(n - 1)$. The regression SS has 1 degree of freedom for each regression coefficient estimated; for simple linear regression, the degree of freedom is 1. The residual degrees of freedom are obtained by subtracting the regression degrees of freedom from the total degrees of freedom: for simple linear regression, $(n - 1) - 1 = (n - 2)$. The mean squares (MSs) are the values of SS divided by the respective degrees of freedom. The regression MS has a special

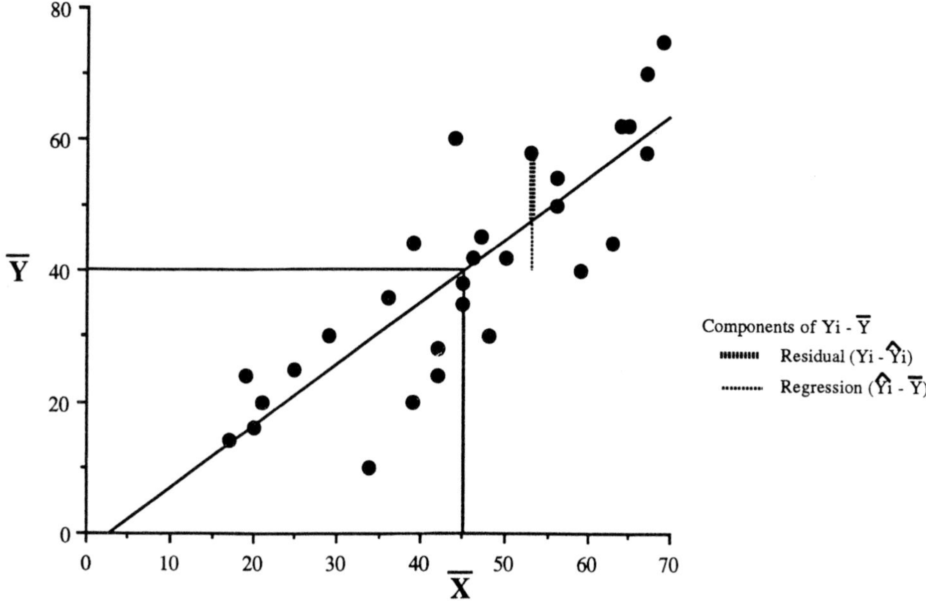

Figure 3.1. The total vertical deviation of each sample point (X_i, Y_i) from $(\bar{X}, \bar{Y})$ is divided into two components: the residual component $(Y_i - \hat{Y}_i)$ and the regression component $(\hat{Y}_i - \bar{Y})$. All three distances are measured on the Y-axis.

interpretation as the variance attributable to linear regression, $\sigma^2_{\hat{Y}}$; conceptually, the regression MS is the explained variation of Y. The residual MS also has a special interpretation as the variance attributable to Y after adjusting for X, $\sigma^2_{Y \vee \bar{X}}$; conceptually, the residual MS is the unexplained variation of Y.

The formal goodness-of-fit test is an F-test with the model MS in the numerator and the error MS in the denominator: $MS_{Model}/MS_{Error} = F_s$. F_s follows an F distribution with numerator degrees of freedom equaling 1 and denominator degrees of freedom equaling $(n - 2)$. The p value is the probability of obtaining a result this extreme, or more so, assuming that only natural or unexplained variability in Y exists. If the p value is less than .05, the investigator concludes that, according to these data, the model does account for a sufficient amount of the variation in Y to say that the model has adequate goodness of fit. Conversely, if the p value is greater than .05, the investigator concludes that, according to these data, the evidence is insufficient to say that the model has adequate goodness of fit.

ANOVA TABLE

Source of variation	Degrees of freedom	SS	MS	F_s
Regression (or model)	1	$\Sigma(\hat{Y}_i - \bar{Y})^2$	$\Sigma(\hat{Y}_i\, Y)^2$	MS_{Model}/MS_{Error}
Residual (or error)	$n - 2$	$\Sigma(Y_i - \hat{Y}_i)^2$	$\Sigma(Y_i - \hat{Y}_i)^2/(n - 2)$	
Total	$n - 1$	$\Sigma(Y_i - \bar{Y})^2$		

Tests of Hypotheses

The clinical investigator may wish to determine if there is a linear relationship between X and Y. If the slope β equals zero, there is no relationship between X and Y. Note that the magnitude of β does not tell the investigator whether the slope is different from zero. Therefore, the investigator forms the null hypothesis as $H_0{:}\beta = 0$ and the alternative hypothesis as $H_1{:}\beta \neq 0$. Single-sided alternative hypotheses (e.g., $\beta > 0$; $\beta < 0$) are allowed if there is previous knowledge that the relationship can only be either positive or negative or if a biologic phenomenon, such as growth, excludes one direction. Statistically, a one-sided test is superior to a two-sided test, because the probability of rejecting the null hypothesis is greater at the same level of significance.

Because the assumptions for regression analysis state that the residuals are normally distributed, the estimate of β (i.e., b) is also normally distributed with mean β and variance σ_b^2: $b \sim N(\beta, \sigma_b^2)$. The clinical investigator estimates the variance of b, s_b^2, from the data. The numerator of s_b^2 is the variation around the regression line (s_ϵ^2), and the denominator is the total variation of X:

$$s_b^2 = s_\varepsilon^2 / \Sigma(X_i - \bar{X})^2$$

One should note that the numerator, the variation around the regression line (s_ϵ^2), is interpreted as the amount of variation in Y remaining after taking into account or adjusting for the variation in X. Then, to test $H_0{:}\beta = 0$, the investigator computes the test statistic:

$$t_s = (b - \beta)/s_b = (b - 0)/s_b = b/s_b$$

which follows a t distribution with $(n - 2)$ degrees of freedom. Like all t statistics, the degrees of freedom for this test statistic are the degrees of freedom associated with the denominator, s_b^2. Because s_ϵ^2 is contained in s_b^2, the degrees of freedom equal the degrees of freedom for the residual SS. The p value is twice the probability associated with t_s, assuming that the null hypothesis is true. For one-sided tests, the investigator uses the same t_s but does not multiply the probability associated with t_s by 2. Rejecting H_0 implies that the data show evidence of a linear relationship between X and Y. If the investigator does not reject H_0, this conclusion implies that the data show no linear relationship between X and Y.

Confidence Intervals for β

The $(1 - \alpha)100\%$ CI for β is computed in the usual way:

$$L_L = b - t_{0.975(n-2)} s_b$$

$$L_U = b + t_{0.975(n-2)} s_b$$

Conceptually, this CI is the same as the CI for μ. Whenever the CI does not include zero, the investigator rejects H_0. If the $(1 - \alpha)100\%$ CI includes the hypothesized value, the results of the study, according to these data, are consistent with H_0. The interpretation of the CI is the following: the estimate of β is a random variable; for each sample, there will be a different estimate β and a different s_b. The slope can fluctuate within these bounds with 95% confidence that the true slope lies there.

R^2 for Simple Linear Regression

R^2 measures the proportion of the variance or variation of Y that can be explained by the variance or variation in X. Stated another way, R^2 is the proportion of the total variation in Y explained by regression. Mathematically, R^2 equals the regression SS divided by the total corrected SS: $R^2 = SS_{Reg}/CSS$. Therefore, R^2 is a summary measure of goodness of fit for simple linear regression.

For simple linear regression, the proportion of explained variance is usually expressed as r^2, instead of R^2. If the amount of explained variance is small, r^2 is small and a large proportion of the variation is unexplained by regression. Conversely, if the amount of explained variance is large, r^2 is large and a small proportion of the variation in Y is unexplained by regression. For this reason, r^2 is referred to as the coefficient of determination. Similarly, $(1 - r^2)$ is called the coefficient of nondetermination.

This concept of r^2 extends to multiple linear regression, except that r^2 is replaced by R^2, which is called the sample multiple correlation coefficient. This concept can be easily demonstrated if multiple regression is addressed from the path coefficient perspective. For an excellent explanation, see Sokal and Rohlf (2). No single quantity is the counterpart of r^2 or R^2 when the hospital epidemiologist uses logistic regression analysis or survival analysis.

Correlation Coefficients

A correlation coefficient measures the degree (in terms of both closeness and direction) of association (or relationship) between two random variables that vary together. Usually, both variables are measured on the same subject. Unlike a regression coefficient, no distinction is made between the independent and the dependent variables; generally, any distinction would be arbitrary or meaningless. Furthermore, the correlation coefficient does quantify how strong the linear relationship is between the two variables of interest. Thus, a clinical investigator reports a correlation coefficient when there is no obvious outcome or response variable. Typically, the investigator intends to describe and quantify the relationship but does not wish to use one variable to predict another.

The correlation coefficient is a dimensionless value that ranges between -1.0 and $+1.0$, inclusive. Therefore, the investigator may compare correlation coefficients obtained from different studies. Unlike the regression coefficient, the correlation coefficient is unaffected by changes in scale.

If the correlation coefficient is -1.0, there is a perfect negative correlation between the two variables; all the points lie on a straight line. If the correlation coefficient is $+1.0$, there is a perfect positive correlation between the two variables; all the points lie on a straight line. A correlation coefficient between zero and -1.0 implies that there is a negative relationship; as one variable increases, the other decreases. Similarly, a correlation coefficient between zero and $+1.0$ implies that there is a positive relationship between the two variables; as one variable increases, the other also increases. Finally, if the correlation coefficient is zero, there is no relationship between the two variables; a graph of the data reveals that the points are randomly distributed within a circle or a horizontal rectangle.

Linear Correlation Coefficient

Estimate of ρ

The linear correlation coefficient, ρ, is also called the Pearson product moment correlation coefficient (1–5,7–9,12,16). The sample Pearson correlation coefficient is used to estimate ρ when both variables are continuous variables that are both normally distributed. The investigator estimates ρ from the data using the following formula:

$$r = \mathrm{Cov}(Y_1, Y_2) / \sqrt{\mathrm{Var}(Y_1)\,\mathrm{Var}(Y_2)}$$

where the numerator is the covariance between the two random variables Y_1 and Y_2, and the denominator is the square root of the product of the variances of Y_1 and Y_2. The covariance can be either positive or negative. In the clinical setting, many more than two variables are measured on each patient. If more than one correlation coefficient is estimated, the clinical investigator should indicate which one is being discussed.

Because the assumptions for correlation analysis state that both variables are normally distributed, the estimate of ρ (i.e., r) follows a t distribution with $(n - 2)$ degrees of freedom with mean ρ and variance σ^2_ρ: $r \sim t_{(n-2)}(\rho, \sigma^2_r)$. Therefore, the clinical investigator estimates the variance of r from the data: $s^2_r = (1 - r^2)/(n - 2)$.

Hypothesis Tests

Most often, the clinical epidemiologist is interested in the question of whether or not Y_1 and Y_2 are correlated (1–5,8,9). Therefore, depending on how much information is known in advance, the epidemiologist forms the following hypotheses:

$$H_0: \rho = 0 \text{ vs. } H_1: \rho \neq 0.$$

One-sided alternative hypotheses are allowed if there is previous knowledge that the relationship can only be either positive or negative or if a biologic phenomenon, such as growth, excludes one direction. Testing these hypotheses requires the assumption that both variables are continuous and distributed normally. The epidemiologist tests H_0 according to the following test statistic:

$$t_s = (r - 0)/s_r = r/s_r$$

where s_r is $\sqrt{(1 - r^2)/(n - 2)}$. The test statistic follows a t distribution with $(n - 2)$ degrees of freedom. The p value is twice the probability associated with the test statistic, assuming that H_0 is true. For one-sided hypothesis tests, the probability is not multiplied by 2.

Confidence Intervals for ρ

The hospital epidemiologist cannot use r directly for estimating CIs (1–5,8,9). First, r is transformed with Fisher's z-transformation, as shown in the following formula:

$$z_F = 1/2\left[\ln(1+r)/(1-r)\right]$$

Then, the $(1 - \alpha)100\%$ CI for z_F is computed in the usual way:

$$L_L = z_F - z_{0.975}\left(1/\sqrt{n-3}\right)$$

$$L_U = z_F + z_{0.975}\left(1/\sqrt{n-3}\right)$$

Finally, the epidemiologist transforms L_L and L_U back to the original correlation scale. Conceptually, this CI is the same as the CI for μ. Whenever the CI does not include zero, the investigator rejects H_0. If the $(1 - \alpha)100\%$ CI includes the hypothesized value, the results of the study according to these data are consistent with H_0. The CI is interpreted as follows: the estimate of ρ is a random variable; for each sample, there will be a different estimate r and a different s_r. The linear correlation coefficient can fluctuate within these bounds with 95% confidence that the true value lies there.

Nonparametric Correlation Coefficients

The primary assumption for estimating linear correlation coefficients is that both variables are distributed normally. Sometimes the hospital epidemiologist finds that one or more of the variables of interest is not distributed normally. In this circumstance, the epidemiologist can choose to estimate a nonparametric correlation coefficient (1–5,7–9,15,16,33).

Rank Correlation

The Kendall coefficient of rank correlation, the Greek letter tau (τ), and the Spearman rank correlation coefficient, ρ_s, are nonparametric coefficients. When these are reported, the clinical investigator makes no assumptions about the distributions of the variables.

The Spearman rank correlation coefficient (also called Spearman's rho) is a sample correlation coefficient based on ranks. First, the investigator ranks the values of each variable from largest to smallest (or vice versa) and then estimates ρ_s using the Pearson product moment formula, substituting ranks for the actual values. The rationale for this estimator is that, if there were a perfect correlation between the two variables, the ranks for each subject on each variable would be the same. Thus, the change in rank (i.e., the rank of the first variable minus the rank of the second variable) would be zero for every subject. Spearman's rank correlation coefficient can also be used for estimating the correlation between ordinal (i.e., rank) variables.

Kendall's τ provides a measure of reranking. Estimation of Kendall's τ is slightly more difficult than estimation of Spearman's rank correlation coefficient. For the method, see Sokal and Rohlf (2). Usually, if both Kendall's τ and Spearman's rank correlation coefficient are estimated from the same data, the estimate of Kendall's τ is smaller than that of Spearman's rank correlation coefficient. However, the p values are usually very close to the same value. When an investigator estimates Kendall's τ, the Greek letter is used for the statistic. Kendall's τ is one of few examples of Greek letters being used for both the parameter and the statistic.

Point Biserial Correlation Coefficient

The point biserial correlation coefficient, ρ_{pb}, is used when one random variable is dichotomous and the other is continuous. Asymptotically, the point biserial correlation coefficient is the same as a Pearson product moment correlation coefficient estimated for one dichotomous variable and one continuous variable.

Biserial Correlation Coefficient

The biserial correlation coefficient, ρ_b, is used when one random variable has been forced to be dichotomous (e.g., by dividing a measurement into upper and lower halves) and the other random variable is continuous. Asymptotically, the biserial correlation coefficient is the same as a Pearson product moment correlation coefficient estimated for one dichotomous variable and one continuous variable.

Phi (ϕ) Fourfold Coefficient

The phi (ϕ) fourfold coefficient is the special name given to the measure of concordance for 2 × 2 tables (7,15). Asymptotically, the phi coefficient is the same as a Pearson product moment correlation coefficient estimated for two dichotomous variables. Thus, this statistic gives a measure of correlation or concordance for dichotomous variables. When an investigator estimates ϕ, the Greek letter is used for the statistic; ϕ is another one of few examples of Greek letters being used for both the parameter and the statistic.

Contingency Coefficient

The contingency coefficient is used to measure concordance between categorical variables depicted in r × c tables (i.e., tables in which the numbers of rows and columns are not necessarily the same) (7,33). Thus, when one or both of the categorical variables has three or more levels, the investigator would choose the contingency coefficient (C) as an estimate of the correlation coefficient.

The Kappa Statistic (κ)

The kappa statistic, κ, is used to measure concordance for 2 × 2 and square r × c tables (i.e., tables in which the numbers of rows and columns are the same) (8,33). Often, these tables reflect paired data. When an investigator estimates κ, the Greek letter is used for the statistic; κ is another one of few examples of Greek letters being used for both the parameter and the statistic.

The hospital epidemiologist may find many uses for the kappa statistic. For example, two radiologists may read radiographs of patients in a particular ICU. On a given day, which radiologist reviews radiographs often depends on a staffing schedule. In actuality, each radiograph is reviewed by only one radiologist. Therefore, one radiologist may review the radiographs for a particular patient taken on admission. The next radiograph taken on the same patient 3 days later may be read by the other radiologist. Naturally, the hospital epidemiologist would like to know whether the radiologists are likely to give the same diagnosis to the same patient based on the same radiograph. Analyzing data from patients in this ICU may require the epidemiologist to make the assumption that the diagnoses from the two radiologists are the same. Rather than making this assumption, the epidemiologist can design a study to measure the agreement (or concordance) between the two radiologists when they review the same radiographs. In a hypothetical study, one might suppose that the various diagnoses available to the radiologists are (a) definitely not interstitial disease, (b) probably not interstitial disease, (c) possibly not interstitial disease, (d) possibly interstitial disease, (e) probably interstitial disease, and (f) definitely interstitial disease. Therefore, the epidemiologist needs a measure of concordance. The epidemiologist forms the hypotheses for the kappa statistic:

$$H_0: \kappa = 0 \text{ vs. } H_1: \kappa \neq 0$$

First, the epidemiologist asks the radiologists each to review a number of radiographs. For this particular study, the epidemiologist is not as concerned about the radiologists agreeing with a gold standard as with their agreement with each other. After collecting the data, the epidemiologist tabulates the results in a 6 × 6 table with the codes *a* through *f* corresponding to the diagnoses listed previously.

		Diagnosis of the second radiologist						Marginal probability
		a	b	c	d	e	f	
Diagnosis of the first radiologist	a	**P_{11}**	P_{12}	P_{13}	P_{14}	P_{15}	P_{16}	$a_{1.}$
	b	P_{21}	**P_{22}**	P_{23}	P_{24}	P_{25}	P_{26}	$b_{2.}$
	c	P_{31}	P_{32}	**P_{33}**	P_{34}	P_{35}	P_{36}	$c_{3.}$
	d	P_{41}	P_{42}	P_{43}	**P_{44}**	P_{45}	P_{46}	$d_{4.}$
	e	P_{51}	P_{52}	P_{53}	P_{54}	**P_{55}**	P_{56}	$e_{5.}$
	f	P_{61}	P_{62}	P_{63}	P_{64}	P_{65}	**P_{66}**	$f_{6.}$
Marginal probability		$a_{.1}$	$b_{.2}$	$c_{.3}$	$d_{.4}$	$e_{.5}$	$f_{.6}$	1.0

where p_{ij} values are joint probabilities indicating the proportion of all radiographs with that particular combination of diagnoses given by the first radiologist (the rows) and the second radiologist (the columns); *i* (designating the rows) indicates the diagnosis that was given by the first radiologist; *j* (designating the columns) indicates the diagnosis that was given by the second radiologist; $a_{1.}$ through $f_{6.}$ are row marginal proportions for the first radiologist obtained by summing the proportions in each row; and $a_{.1}$ through $f_{.6}$ are column marginal proportions for the second radiologist obtained by summing the proportions in each column. Concordance is measured by the proportion of observations in the cells along the main diagonal (in bold type). The hospital epidemiologist compares the observed concordance rate (p_0) with that which would be expected (p_E) if there was no concordance among the two radiologists. In this example, the observed concordance rate is the sum of p_{11}, p_{22}, p_{33}, p_{44}, p_{55}, and p_{66}. The epidemiologist obtains the expected concordance for each of the cells along the main diagonal by multiplying the corresponding row marginal proportion by the corresponding column marginal proportion and then summing these: $p_E = a_{1.}a_{.1} + b_{2.}b_{.2} + c_{3.}c_{.3} + d_{4.}d_{.4} + e_{5.}e_{.5} + f_{6.}f_{.6}$. The epidemiologist estimates κ and the variance of κ with the following formulas:

$$\kappa = (p_0 - p_E)/(1 - p_E)$$

$$s_\kappa^2 = \left[1/n(1-p_E)^2\right]\left\{p_E + p_E^2 - \left[a_{1.}a_{.1}(a_{1.} + a_{.1})\right] \right.$$

$$\left. \cdots \left[f_6 f_6 (f_6 + f_6)\right]\right\}$$

The standard deviation of κ, s_κ, is the square root of the variance. Then, to test H_0, the epidemiologist computes the test statistic:

$$z_s = (\kappa - 0)/s_\kappa = \kappa/s_\kappa$$

which is a z-score and follows the standard normal distribution. The *p* value is the probability associated with z_s, assuming that the null hypothesis is true. Rejecting H_0 implies that the data show evidence of concordance between the two radiologists. Finally, the epidemiologist uses the following guidelines for evaluation of the estimated κ statistic: (a) a κ greater than 0.75 denotes excellent reproducibility; (b) a κ between 0.40 and 0.75, inclusive, denotes good reproducibility; and (c) a κ less than 0.40 denotes marginal reproducibility (8).

The (1 − α)100% CI for κ is computed in the usual way:

$$L_L = \kappa - z_{0.975} s_\kappa$$

$$L_U = \kappa + z_{0.975} s_\kappa$$

Conceptually, this CI is the same as the CI for μ. Whenever the CI does not include zero, the investigator rejects H_0. If the (1 − α)100% CI includes the hypothesized value, the results of the study, according to these data, are consistent with H_0. The CI is interpreted as follows: the estimate of κ is a random variable; for each sample, there will be a different estimate κ and a different s_k. The concordance can fluctuate within these bounds with 95% confidence that the true concordance lies there.

Relationship Between the Linear Regression Coefficient and the Linear Correlation Coefficient

For simple linear regression, there is a relationship among the regression coefficient, the correlation coefficient, and R^2. These relationships do not hold for multiple linear regression or other forms of regression. Conceptually, two simple linear regression coefficients exist. Usually, the investigator regresses Y on X: $Y = a + b_{Y|X}X + \epsilon$. However, the investigator could regress X on Y: $X = a' + b_{X|Y}Y + \epsilon'$. The two regression coefficients, $b_{Y|X}$ and $b_{X|Y}$, always have the same sign. The correlation coefficient, r_{XY}, is the square root of R^2; the correlation coefficient also equals the geometric mean of two regression coefficients (i.e., the square root of the product of slope from the regression of X on Y and the slope from the regression of Y on X):

$$r_{XY} = \sqrt{R^2} = \sqrt{r^2} = \sqrt{b_{X|\mathrm{B}|Y}\, b_{Y|\mathrm{B}|X}}$$

where the sign of the covariance between X and Y determines the sign of r. Thus, there is a relationship between correlation and regression. The closer the data points lie to a straight line, the stronger the relationship becomes and the larger the correlation coefficient is. The slope of the line has no bearing on the correlation. However, whenever there is a significant correlation, there will be a significant regression and vice versa. The clinical investigator can depict this relationship graphically by plotting the two regression lines (i.e., $Y = a + b_{Y|X}X + \epsilon$ and $X = a' + b_{X|Y}Y + \epsilon'$) on one set of axes; the correlation coefficient is a measure of the angle between the two regression lines. As the angle becomes larger, the correlation coefficient decreases toward zero. When the angle is 90 degrees, the lines are perpendicular, the correlation coefficient is zero, and the scatter of data is circular or rectangular. As the angle between the regression lines becomes smaller, the correlation coefficient increases toward -1.0 or $+1.0$. When the angle is 0 degrees, the lines coincide, the correlation coefficient is either -1.0 or $+1.0$, and the scatter of the data is a perfectly straight line.

The regression coefficient can also be interpreted as a rescaled version of the correlation coefficient where the scale factor is the ratio of the standard deviation of Y to that of X:

$$b_{Y|\mathrm{B}|X} = r_{XY}\left(s_Y/s_X\right)$$

and, conversely,

$$_{XY} = b_{Y|\mathrm{B}|X}\left(s_Y/s_X\right)$$

Thus, the correlation coefficient can be regarded as a standardized regression coefficient (2). The standardized regression coefficient is a dimensionless value that represents the predicted change in Y, expressed in standard deviation units, that would be expected for each change in X of one standard deviation unit. The clinical investigator can use standardized regression coefficients to compare regression coefficients obtained from several studies on a variety of patient groups.

MULTIVARIABLE ANALYSIS

Most epidemiologic investigations involve more than one or two variables of interest. Therefore, clinically based studies of disease determinants often yield data sets that require complicated analytic methods. Generally, the hospital epidemiologist identifies an outcome variable (e.g., death, infection, or time to an event). In addition, there are other selected variables, including the particular exposure, that are relevant to the investigation. The primary focus of the study is the relationship between the particular exposure and the specified outcome; complexities arise, because the epidemiologist must sort out interrelationships among other variables that affect (confound) the relationship between the outcome and exposure (see Chapter 2).

Although the epidemiologist has specialized knowledge about the disease process under investigation, usually a complete theoretical framework describing the true relationship between the exposure and the outcome variables is lacking. Furthermore, the epidemiologist cannot control or manipulate the process linking exposure to outcome in ways that may reveal the true relationship. Fortunately, statisticians have developed a variety of multivariable analytic methods that address many problems encountered in clinically based research.

What does the term *multivariable analysis* mean? Many investigators refer to the statistical analysis of one dependent variable and several descriptive or explanatory variables (i.e., several independent variables) as multivariate analysis. However, this practice reflects a misuse of a statistical term that refers to the analysis of more than one dependent variable. For this reason, I have chosen to use the term *multivariable analysis* to encompass the following statistical methods: stratified analysis, multiple linear regression, multiple logistic regression, and survival analysis.

Model Selection Process

General Problems

Dealing with more than one explanatory variable is a challenge for many clinical investigators. Kleinbaum et al. (28) suggest the following four ways in which multivariable analysis is more difficult than simple univariate analysis (i.e., one explanatory variable). First, usually more than one statistical model can be developed for the same data set to adequately describe the relationship between the exposure and outcome variable. Choice of which model is the best is generally somewhat subjective and often sample dependent. Second, on any one graph, an investigator can depict at most three dimensions. Usually, an investigator considers more than three variables. In this situation, the investigator must limit each graphic depiction to two or three variables. Third, when the model includes more than one or two explanatory variables, most clinical investigators have difficulty translating the statistical model into a clinically meaningful explanation. Finally, analysis requires the investigator to use a computer software package for statistical analysis. When the number of independent variables is large, the model selection process can be very time consuming. Many computer algorithms do not have built-in limits for the number of dependent or independent variables; the investigator has the responsibility of setting reasonable limits. The following discussion suggests some reasonable limits. Thus, in addition to specialized knowledge about the disease process, the epidemiologist must develop some expertise in multivariable analysis and acquire related computer skills.

Model Selection

Whenever the research problem involves determining which explanatory variables should be included in the analysis, a clinical investigator needs a model selection strategy. Because some relationships among variables are specific to a particular sample (i.e., they are sample dependent), many investigators find that adhering to a formal strategy is especially helpful during exploratory data analysis. In a very real sense, each data set has new information that can provide the investigator with insight into the exposure-disease relationship. If some of the intricacies of this relationship, especially those that are unique to the current study, can be dissected early in the model selection process, the investigator is more likely to understand the clinical implications of the final model.

The goal of the model selection process is to identify a statistical model that reflects important aspects of the exposure-disease relationship. Therefore, before the process begins, the investigator must perceive a theoretical framework firmly based on considerations of subject matter. The statistical methods are the mathematical tools that the investigator uses to derive empirical support for the framework and discover new aspects of the relationship that can be used to modify the framework. Both biostatisticians and epidemiologists warn against relying exclusively on any statistical package to determine the best model for a data set. Except for pharmacokinetic, pharmacodynamic, and growth models, almost all statistical models commonly used in hospital epidemiology are empirical rather than mechanistic. This distinction implies that, even though a functional relationship may exist between the exposure and disease, limited information is available on the role that other variables have in influencing how the exposure-disease process is manifested in a given patient sample. Both biostatisticians and epidemiologists also caution investigators about literally interpreting the model as an accurate reflection of the true exposure-disease process. Finally, they are adamant in stating that any type of model selection technique can be abused.

After gaining experience with multivariable analysis, a clinical investigator may develop a unique style of model selection. However, until that experience has been gained, the cautious investigator should strictly adhere to guidelines provided by a biostatistician or epidemiologist who has extensive experience in model selection. Draper and Smith (29) have summarized, in a very readable chapter, the process of planning, developing, and validating a statistical model. In their text, Rothman and Greenland (34) devoted several chapters to the modeling process. Other authors have discussed the process and provided the reader with annotated examples: Kleinbaum et al. (20,28), Myers (30), and Myers and Milton (31).

The Planning Stage

The model selection process actually begins with the statement of the problem and identification of the research question. During the planning stage, the clinical investigator selects the response variable. If there is more than one response variable of interest, the investigator should limit the number to a few—no more than five is best. For each response variable, the clinical investigator lists all variables that could possibly be related to the outcome. This list is usually very long and may include almost every variable on a patient's chart. From this extensive list, the investigator identifies those variables that can be collected and groups these collectible variables into broad categories. For example, one category might contain all demographics, another could include severity of illness indices or perhaps comorbidities, and so on. Finally, by the end of the planning stage, the investigator should have a reasonable list of variables that merit inclusion in the study.

Are there resources available that can help the investigator in selecting variables for serious consideration? Resources include (a) reports of similar investigations published in the peer-reviewed literature and (b) discussions with experts in the disease of interest. During the initial planning stages, the clinical investigator bases decisions on subject matter expertise not statistics! However, some statistical considerations become important near the end of the planning stage.

Toward the end of the planning stage, the investigator studies the feasibility of the project. Specific items that require the attention of the investigator include the number of patients required to address the problem, the number of patients available, the time needed to accrue the minimum number of patients necessary for the investigation, the costs for data collection, other budget-related issues, and the availability of skilled ancillary personnel to ensure collection of high-quality data.

Data Collection and Quality Control

Once the investigator has decided that the project is feasible, patient enrollment and data collection begins. Quality control of the data is vital to the success of the entire project. Remarkably, this is a step that some investigators overlook completely. Planning what quality control measures are needed for a clinical investigation may require advice from a biostatistician or epidemiologist. Unfortunately, despite precautions and the highest level of quality control, most data sets will contain some errors that escape detection. Reasonable goals for quality control include eliminating systematic errors, especially misclassification, and minimizing the impact of random data entry errors. Therefore, the safeguards are directed at detecting influential errors, those errors that can bias results and threaten the validity of statistical inferences. Remember that a single error, such as a 50-lb newborn human infant, can have a disastrous impact on the findings of a study.

Model Selection—Univariate Analyses

The first exploratory step in actual model selection involves obtaining descriptive statistics for the variables of interest. For continuous variables, testing for goodness of fit to the normal distribution may be important. In addition, for continuous explanatory variables, the range (or some other measure of variability) is usually an important consideration. For example, if the ages of the patients are very similar, age is not likely to influence the relationship between exposure and disease regardless of whether other studies have found that age is an important determinant of the disease of interest. Including variables with limited variability can compromise the model because of overparameterization.

The next steps in actual model selection are (a) plotting relationships between continuous variables, (b) using 2 × 2 and r × c tables to study relationships between discrete variables (i.e., attributes), and (c) estimation of Pearson and Spearman correlation coefficients for all pairs of variables. During this phase, the investigator is gaining an appreciation of which variables are associated with other variables and to what degree. The investigator should be careful about including explanatory variables in the multivariable model that are more highly correlated with each other than with the response variable. Including highly correlated independent variables in a model can lead to problems of multicollinearity. Other terms for the same phenomenon are collinearity and multiple collinearity. Multicollinearity in a statistical model occurs when two or more independent variables are strongly correlated with each other. When the explanatory variables are highly correlated with each other, the estimated coefficients are also highly correlated, thereby yielding unreasonable regression coefficients and an implausible and unusable statistical model.

At the end of the exploratory step, the investigator should have narrowed the list of potential explanatory variables to about 20 or fewer. Final models with more than five or six explanatory variables are difficult to explain. In narrowing the list, the investigator should be aware of the following rule: no fewer than five to ten observations are needed for each potentially important explanatory variable that will be included in the final model. Having at least 30 observations for each variable included in the final model is a reasonable target.

Model Selection—Multivariable Analyses

Style and philosophy influence the investigator's choice of which analytic procedures to use in developing multivariable models. Every procedure has strengths and weaknesses; all can be abused. Initially, most biostatisticians recommend using a rather liberal entrance or deletion criterion for variable selection (e.g., $p < .20$ or $p < .25$). As the final model emerges, traditional levels of significance for selected explanatory variables can be imposed. Regardless of what statistical procedure was used for model selection, most biostatisticians recommend that the investigator use appropriate diagnostic procedures to assess various aspects of the emerging statistical models and subject the results to the scrutiny of other clinical specialists with expertise in the exposure-disease process of interest. Regression diagnostics include examining the residuals and checking for systematic lack of fit.

Because more than one statistical model can provide a valid representation of the exposure-disease relationship, the investigator should select the best model and several competing models. Assessing the best model in light of competing models is a type of sensitivity analysis. The objective of this sensitivity analysis is to reveal which variables are stable in the model, reflecting the average patient, and which are seemingly sample specific (i.e., sample sensitive), reflecting small groups of patients with distinct characteristics.

Problems with Confounding

Epidemiologists apply the term *confounder variables* to variables that are partially related to both the exposure and the outcome variables (20,34). In the statistical sense, a confounder is only partially confounded (i.e., associated or correlated) with both the exposure and the outcome variables; if a confounder were completely confounded with either variable, the confounder would be completely inseparable from that variable.

Confounders create problems for the investigator. The investigator's objective is to show whether a particular exposure and the outcome are related. If the investigator ignores an important and influential confounder, the estimates of RRs, ORs, or regression coefficients are biased. Consequently, the investigator does not know whether the relationship (or lack of one) is attributable to the confounder or to the exposure (see Chapter 2).

Indications of Multicollinearity

Sometimes an explanatory variable will seem to have an important effect on a response when the variable is considered by itself with simple linear regression or correlation analysis. However, after adjusting for another explanatory variable, no significant relationship may remain. This apparent contradiction is an indication of multicollinearity. Inclusion of both variables in the statistical model may or may not be appropriate. There are rules for inclusion and exclusion, but their interpretation is subjective. Thus, the investigator must carefully assess any problems related to multicollinearity.

An investigator can learn to recognize some indications of multicollinearity. As variables are selected for inclusion or exclusion from the model, coefficients affected by multicollinearity will appear to be unstable in that their values will change dramatically. Sometimes multicollinearity can be severe enough to change the sign of an estimate. Another concomitant indication of multicollinearity is that affected coefficient estimates will often have large standard errors; sometimes the standard errors are several times larger than the estimates. Statisticians have developed several methods for detecting multicollinearity (29–32, 35,36). Condition indices, variance inflation factors, and tolerance values can be used to determine which variables in the current model are affecting the estimates of regression coefficients. Whenever multicollinearity appears to be an important problem, the clinical investigator should seek advice from a biostatistician experienced with model selection.

Indications of an Overparameterized Model

Including explanatory variables that are not statistically significant can be considered overparameterizing the model. Subjective interpretation plays a role in the distinction between overparameterization and appropriate inclusion of a variable that is not statistically significant at traditional levels. Overparameterization and multicollinearity often occur simultaneously. One serious problem with highly correlated explanatory variables is that the model becomes very difficult to interpret in terms of actual clinical applications. After all, one of the reasons for using multiple linear regression is to allow the investigator to identify which explanatory variables have a significant relationship with the response after adjusting for other significant explanatory variables. Therefore, the investigator has to carefully evaluate problems associated with overparameterizing the model.

Detection of Influential Observations

An influential observation is one that has an unusually large influence on the estimate of one or more regression coefficients. In general, influential observations are unique to a specific sample. By carefully examining the plots of each explanatory variable against the response, the investigator can identify many influential observations during exploratory analysis. However, in most large data sets, a few influential observations may emerge during model selection. In addition to examining plots of residuals, statisticians have developed several other methods for detecting influential observations (18,29–32,35,36). An investigator uses influence diagnostics for revealing which observations reflect the average patient and which are seemingly from patients with distinct characteristics. If possible, the investigator should determine why an observation has been identified as influential. Often, this process of examining influential observations reveals biologically and clinically important reasons for exclusion. After one or more influential observations have been identified, biostatisticians usually advise fitting the model after leaving out the suspect influential observations.

Stratified Analysis

As discussed previously, cumulative incidence and prevalence of a disease are distributed binomially. An important assumption is that the probabilities for the outcomes are a constant p for success and $(1 - p) = q$ for each failure for every trial. Often, in clinical studies, data from samples of patients fail to meet this assumption; other variables in addition to exposure influence the probability of the outcomes. One of the statistical methods for addressing confounders is stratified analysis (1,5,6,8,15,20, 21,34). The investigator uses stratified analysis for controlling or adjusting for the confounder and estimates an adjusted RR or OR.

Mantel-Haenszel Test

Two-way tables can be extended to multiway tables to accommodate several attributes. Typically, the Mantel-Haenszel test is used for situations in which (a) both the exposure and outcome are dichotomous variables and (b) one or more other attributes are partially confounded with the relationship between exposure and outcome. The investigator forms a number of strata based on levels of one or more confounding variables; the confounding variables must be categorical, discrete, or continuous variables that have been forced to be categorical (e.g., by dividing into quintiles). The strata are chosen so that the data within each stratum are as homogeneous as possible. Typically, strata reflect patient characteristics (e.g., age category) or institutional characteristics (e.g., medical and surgical ICUs). The investigator assumes that the strata are independent. The Mantel-Haenszel test requires a reasonably large total sample size; however, this test was developed to accommodate sparse data within strata. The Mantel-Haenszel test for 2×2 tables can be generalized to $r \times c$ tables, but that application is beyond the scope of this chapter.

Within each stratum, the investigator constructs a 2×2 table relating the exposure and outcome variables. The test statistic does not depend on a particular arrangement of the 2×2 tables as long as the arrangement is the same for all strata. Choice of which variable is designated as the rows and which is designated as the columns is arbitrary. Similarly, the order in which the data for the rows and columns are coded is arbitrary. However, certain statistical software packages may require a particular arrangement, particularly when the investigator is estimating ORs or RRs.

H_0 states that there is no association between exposure and outcome after controlling for variables that create strata; H_1 states that there is an association after controlling for the strata. Under H_0, the Mantel-Haenszel statistic, χ^2_{MH}, follows a chi-square distribution with 1 degree of freedom. Thus, for a test of significance at the .05 significance level, H_0 is rejected if χ^2_{MH} is greater than 3.84. The p value is the probability associated with χ^2_{MH}, assuming that the null hypothesis is true.

The investigator should report results based on the Mantel-Haenszel test only when there is no evidence of statistical interaction involving the strata. The Mantel-Haenszel test is still valid statistically; however, the interpretability of the results may be in question. Therefore, the investigator should not rely exclusively on the p value associated with the test statistic but should carefully study the patterns of association displayed in the various strata with a particular interest in detecting evidence of a statistical interaction involving the strata. For example, if the Mantel-Haenszel test statistic is not significant, (a) there may be no association between the exposure and the outcome (i.e., H_0 is correct) or (b) there may be opposing or inconsistent patterns among the strata. An obvious interaction is present when the pattern exhibited by some strata is in the opposite direction from the pattern of other strata. In contrast, even without the presence of opposing patterns, interaction may be present when Fisher's exact test indicates significance for some strata and lack of significance for others; in this situation, determining what constitutes an interaction is somewhat subjective. Finally, even if the Mantel-Haenszel test statistic reaches significance, there may be evidence of an interaction. In this circumstance, the issue of interpretability is addressed subjectively, according to subject matter considerations. For example, significance could be attributable to one or more dominant strata that have a strong pattern of association in one direction and overwhelm the lack of association or an opposing pattern in the remaining strata. Regardless of the significance of the test statistic, evidence of an interaction indicates that analysis of data over all strata may be inappropriate. If an investigator encounters evidence of an interaction involving the strata, he or she should seek the advice of an experienced biostatistician or epidemiologist (see also Chapter 2).

Estimates of Adjusted ORs and RRs

The Mantel-Haenszel method can be used to estimate strata-adjusted ORs and RRs along with respective 95% CIs. The reader should review the previous discussion of unadjusted ORs and RRs estimated from 2 × 2 tables. Unlike the RR, the OR is not constrained by the denominator. This property is particularly advantageous when estimated ORs are combined over strata.

Strata-adjusted estimation is based on the assumption that the parameter is the same for each stratum and that the values of estimates differ because of sampling. When estimating adjusted measures of association, the investigator should carefully study the pattern of association displayed by the various strata. The same problems of interpretability discussed for the Mantel-Haenszel test apply to estimation. However, unlike the test statistic, estimates are not valid unless the assumption of homogeneity is met. Criteria for what constitutes a violation of this assumption are somewhat subjective.

Either test-based or precision-based CIs can be estimated. For a discussion of the advantages and disadvantages of these intervals, the reader is referred to Kleinbaum et al. (20). Sometimes, extreme estimates or confidence limits are obtained because of very small observed frequencies in some cells (often as few as only one or two events).

A Special Case—Matched Pairs

For matched pairs, the clinical investigator can estimate RRs and ORs from stratified analyses with the strata representing the pairs. Methods for point and interval estimates are the same as those described previously. Usually, the investigator does not study the pattern of association for the various strata.

Breslow-Day Test

The Breslow-Day test for homogeneity tests the null hypothesis that the ORs for all strata are equal versus the alternative that the OR for at least one of the strata is different (37). The test statistic is valid only when every stratum has a large number of observations (generally more than 20). Under H_0, the test statistic follows a chi-square distribution with degrees of freedom equal to one less than the number of strata included in the test statistic. Strata with a zero column or row total are excluded from computation of the test statistic. Regardless of whether the investigator uses the Breslow-Day test, it is incumbent on the investigator to carefully study the pattern of association displayed by the various strata. When the estimates of ORs have opposing patterns, there is usually no question about the inequality of ORs over strata. However, evidence of other patterns of interaction is more subjectively determined.

Multiple Linear Regression

Multiple Linear Regression Analysis

A clinical investigator uses multiple linear regression analysis when the objective involves studying the relationship between more than two variables at the same time (1,2,4–9,18,21, 28–31). There is a single continuous dependent or response variable, but there are several independent, descriptive, or explanatory variables. The explanatory variables may be continuous or dichotomous; in addition, categorical explanatory variables can be recoded for inclusion in a multiple regression model.

The statistical model is $Y_i = \alpha + \beta_1 X_{1i} + \beta_2 X_{2i} + \ldots + \beta_p X_{pi} + \epsilon_i$ where i is the indicator for each subject and ranges from 1 to n. The data set contains n sets of $(p + 1)$ measurements where n indicates the number of subjects in the sample; a complete set of measurements is taken on every patient. Of these measurements, p values are X values, and one is a Y value. The βs values are partial regression coefficients with the intercept, α, corresponding to the intercept in simple linear regression. A partial regression coefficient quantifies the relationship between a particular explanatory variable and the response after adjusting or controlling for all other effects in the model.

The same assumptions that were necessary for simple linear regression also apply to multiple linear regression. Multiple linear regression merely reflects an expansion of the simple case to p-dimensions, each representing a different independent variable. Regardless of form, the explanatory variables are assumed to function independently. Most often, the independent variables have the form of main or direct effects (e.g., age, days on mechanical ventilation, or APACHE III score). However, some of the independent variables may represent interactions of two other independent variables, X_1X_2. As a standard practice, the investigator should include the direct effects of X_1 and X_2 in a model in which the interaction is included. An example of an interaction is the joint effect of age and APACHE III score on a particular response variable. Independent variables may represent higher powers of other independent variables, X_1^2 or X_1^3. Generally, when higher powers, such as X_1^3, are included in the model, the lower powers (X_1 and X_1^2) are also included. For example, the relationship between the response and age may not be completely linear but may increase at an increasing rate, thereby requiring the inclusion of age and age-squared.

An investigator should always be conservative in interpreting a multiple regression model. Other variables, not included in the model, may actually be the cause of differences in the response.

Polynomial or Curvilinear Regression Models

Polynomial regression is a special case of multiple linear regression for one independent variable, X, and one continuous dependent variable, Y. The highest degree polynomial that may be fit to the data is one less than the number of observations. For most biologic phenomena, biostatisticians recommend limiting the model to a cubic regression. The general rule for using polynomial regression analysis is that the investigator use as simple a model as possible but one that explains as much of the variation of Y as possible. The investigator should be aware that, as the degree of the polynomial becomes higher, the interpretation of the curve becomes more difficult. The model for a quadratic regression is $Y_i = \alpha + \beta X_i + \gamma X_i^2 + \epsilon_i$ where i is the indicator for each subject and ranges from 1 to n. Both β and γ are partial regression coefficients.

Tests of Hypotheses

Methods for regression analysis and hypothesis testing are similar to those described for simple linear regression. The same principle of least squares is used to estimate the regression coefficients by minimizing the residual sum of squares over all data points. The clinical investigator tests the overall null hypothesis that all β values equal zero versus the alternative hypothesis that at least one β value does not equal zero. Under the null hypothesis, the F_s, which is the ratio of the model or regression MS divided by the residual or error MS, follows an F distribution with p and $(n - p - 1)$ degrees of freedom. The p value is the probability associated with F_s, assuming that the null hypothesis is true.

The overall F-test will not identify which specific explanatory variables are associated with the response. The clinical investigator must perform t-tests to investigate the specific association of each independent variable with the response. For one- or two-sided t-tests on individual partial regression coefficients, the investigator uses a t statistic with $(n - p - 1)$ degrees of freedom. The p value is twice the probability associated with t_s, assuming that the null hypothesis is true.

Interval Estimation

Generally, the investigator wishes to estimate partial regression coefficients. The printed results from most computer software packages include estimates and standard deviations of the estimates. The standard deviations of the estimates may be called standard errors. The clinical investigator obtains the 95% CIs for each partial regression coefficient in the usual way:

$$L_L = b - t_{0.975(n-p-1)} s_b$$

$$L_U = b + t_{0.975(n-p-1)} s_b$$

Conceptually, this CI is the same as the CI for μ. Whenever the CI does not include zero, the investigator rejects H_0. If the $(1 - \alpha)100\%$ CI includes the hypothesized value, the results of the study according to these data are consistent with H_0. The CI is interpreted as follows: the estimate of β is a random variable; for each sample, there will be a different estimate b and a different s_b. As the variable X changes by one unit, the expected response changes by b units after controlling for all other variables in the model. Controlling for all other variables implies that the value of each of the other explanatory variables in the model has been set to the respective mean value. An investigator should always be conservative in interpreting a multiple regression coefficient. Other variables, not included in the model, may actually cause the variability of response.

Standardized Partial Regression Coefficients

The concept of standardized regression coefficients can be extended to multiple linear regression; these are called standardized partial regression coefficients. By using standardized partial regression coefficients, the clinical investigator can express relative changes that are independent of any units of measurement. In addition, the investigator can use standardized partial regression coefficients for ranking the effects of the explanatory variables in order of importance.

Partial regression coefficients are standardized by dividing the estimated partial regression coefficient by the ratio of the standard deviation of the response variable to the standard deviation of the respective explanatory variable:

$$b_{ST} = b_{Y|B|X}\left(s_X/s_Y\right)$$

Thus, the standardized regression coefficient is a dimensionless value that represents the predicted change in Y, expressed in standard deviation units, that would be expected for each change in X of one standard deviation unit after adjusting for all other variables in the model.

Partial Correlation Coefficients

The hospital epidemiologist obtains estimates of partial correlation coefficients following analyzing data by multiple regression methods. Partial correlation coefficients provide an estimate of the remaining correlation after one or more other variables are held constant (i.e., after adjusting for the other variables) (2,4,9). Partial correlation coefficients are used when there are correlations among the explanatory variables. In practice, the epidemiologist examines both the total (or unadjusted) correlation coefficients and the partial (adjusted) correlation coefficients.

Multiple Logistic Regression

A clinical investigator uses multiple logistic regression analysis when the outcome or response variable follows a binomial distribution (1,5,6,8,18,20,21,34). Generally, the objective is similar to that for multiple linear regression and involves studying the relationship between more than two variables at the same time. There is a single dichotomous dependent or response variable and several independent or explanatory variables. Typically, the investigator refers to any explanatory variables, other than the specified exposure, as confounding variables. The investigator wishes to examine the relation between the exposure and outcome after controlling for the confounding variables. These confounding variables may be continuous, dichotomous, or categorical variables. When the strata used in stratified analysis and the confounding variables used in logistic regression are defined similarly, the results from the two methods are identical. By permitting continuous variables and interactions to be included in the model as explanatory variables, logistic regression is more flexible than stratified analysis. However, logistic regression does have one potentially serious limitation—only ORs can be estimated from logistic regression. However, these ORs can be used as approximators of RRs if the study design permits.

In logistic regression, the response variable is expressed as p and is the probability that the response, Y, is an event—that is, $p = Pr(Y = 1)$. For logistic regression analysis, the presence of the event is almost always coded as one. Given that a subject has certain values for X_1 to X_k, the expected or average probability of an event is $p = Pr(Y = 1)$. The event or outcome of interest may be a particular disease or death. For this discussion, the event is disease.

The statistical model is

$$p = e^{(\alpha+\beta_1 X_1+\beta_2 X_2+\ldots+\beta_k X_k+\varepsilon)}/(1+e^{(\alpha+\beta_1 X_1+\beta_2 X_2+\ldots+\beta_k X_k+\varepsilon)})$$

Using the logit transformation, this model becomes

$$\ln\left[p/(1-p)\right] = \alpha + \beta_1 X_1 + \beta_2 X_2 + \ldots + \beta_k X_k + \varepsilon$$

The data set contains sets of $(k + 1)$ measurements on each subject. Of these measurements, k values are X values, and one is the event, Y. The β values are partial regression coefficients with the intercept, α, corresponding to the intercept in simple linear regression. In a logistic regression model, the explanatory variables are related multiplicatively to each other rather than additively as they would be in a linear model. Because of complexities that involve fitting the parameters of this model, clinical investigators rely on a computer-based iterative algorithm.

Throughout this discussion, note that the natural logarithm of the odds of disease is $\ln[p/(1 - p]$. The intercept, α, represents the natural logarithm of the baseline odds of disease (i.e., the event). The baseline odds corresponds to the odds of disease among the unexposed—that is, when all X values are set to zero. The partial regression coefficients quantify the relationships between a particular explanatory variable and the response after adjusting or controlling for all other effects in the model. When a partial regression coefficient quantifies the relationship between a dichotomous variable and the response, the β represents the natural logarithm of the additional odds of disease among those with the attribute after controlling for all other variables in the model. For a categorical or continuous variable, the multiplicative relationship between the explanatory and outcome variables becomes apparent. The β represents the change in the natural logarithm of additional odds of disease per unit change in X. Controlling for all other variables in the model implies that all other attributes occur at equal frequencies. The reader is referred to Rothman and Greenland (34) and to Kleinbaum et al. (20) for additional information on implications for epidemiologic models.

The same assumptions that were necessary for analysis of data in 2 × 2 tables and stratified analysis also apply to multiple logistic regression. In addition, logistic regression shares many similarities with multiple linear regression. Multiple logistic regression reflects k-dimensions, each representing a different independent variable. Regardless of form, the independent variables are assumed to function independently. Independent variables usually have the form of main or direct effects (e.g., presence of a nosocomial infection, age, days on mechanical ventilation, or APACHE III score). However, some independent variables may represent interactions of two other independent variables that should also be included in the model as direct effects, X_1 and X_2.

An investigator should always be conservative in interpreting a multiple logistic regression model. Other variables, not included in the model, may actually be the cause of differences in the probability of an event.

Tests of Hypotheses

Tests of hypotheses, interval estimation, and interpretation of the results are counterparts of those for multiple linear regression.

Generally, the clinical investigator does not test an overall null hypothesis that all of the explanatory variables in the model are zero. However, this test is usually available. If competing models for the same data are being compared, there are test statistics available for assessing the joint or combined significance of all explanatory variables included in the model. The Score, Akaike Information Criterion, and the Schwartz Criterion statistics are used for this purpose.

The clinical investigator can perform z-tests to investigate the specific association of each independent variable with the response. Alternatively, for two-sided hypothesis tests on individual partial regression coefficients, the investigator can use a Wald chi-square statistic, which follows a chi-square distribution with 1 degree of freedom under the null hypothesis. The p value is the probability associated with χ_s^2, assuming that the null hypothesis is true. For more information on hypothesis testing, see Lawless (36).

Interval Estimation

Generally, the investigator wishes to estimate partial regression coefficients and adjusted ORs. The printed results from most computer software packages include estimates and standard deviations of the estimates. The estimates of regression parameters are maximum likelihood estimates. Standard deviations of these estimates may be called standard errors. Sometimes the printed results also contain estimated adjusted ORs and asymptotic 95% CIs. The clinical investigator obtains the asymptotic 95% CIs for each partial regression coefficient in the usual way:

$$L_L = b - z_{0.975} s_b$$

$$L_U = b + z_{0.975} s_b$$

Whenever the CI does not include zero, the investigator rejects H_0. If the asymptotic $(1 - \alpha)100\%$ CI includes the hypothesized value, the results of the study, according to these data, are consistent with H_0. The CI is interpreted as follows: the estimate of β is a random variable; for each sample, there will be a different estimate b and a different s_b. As the variable X changes by one unit, the expected natural logarithm of additional odds of disease changes by b units after controlling for all other variables in the model.

The investigator can estimate adjusted ORs by taking the inverse of the natural logarithm of each partial regression coefficient: *exp(b)*. Approximate 95% CIs can be obtained similarly:

$$L_L = \exp(b - z_{0.975} s_b)$$

$$L_U = \exp(b + z_{0.975} s_b)$$

The interpretation of the OR is illustrated in the following example: after controlling for all other variables in the model, patients who are ventilated are 1.497 times as likely to have pneumonia as those who are not ventilated. Controlling for all other variables implies that the value of each of the continuous explanatory variables in the model has been set to the respective mean value and that each of the dichotomous variables occurs at equal frequencies. An investigator should always be conservative in interpreting an OR estimated from multiple logistic regression analysis. Other variables, not included in the model, may actually cause the variability of response.

Matched Case-Control Studies

For matched case-control studies, the investigator can use conditional logistic regression to study the effects of confounders (20). The reason for matching is that the investigator knows that certain factors are partially confounded with the relationship between exposure and outcome. However, there may be other potential confounders that the investigator wishes to consider in a multiple regression model. Because of complexities involved in fitting the parameters of this model, clinical investigators rely on a computer-based iterative algorithm.

Survival Analysis

A clinical investigator uses survival analysis when the outcome or response variable is time to an event (1,3,5,6,8,18,20,25,34, 38–40). The event is often considered a failure. Survival analysis is a form of conditional logistic regression analysis that allows for censored observations. Some survival analysis is based on parametric models that allow for left-, right-, or interval-censored observations. In clinical investigations, the most commonly used models for survival analysis are nonparametric models that allow for right-censored observations. In the clinical setting, a common feature of lifetime or survival data is the presence of right-censored observations; censoring arises from either withdrawal of subjects or termination of the study. For censored observations, the lifetime is known to have exceeded the recorded value, but the exact lifetime remains unknown. Survival data should not be analyzed by ignoring the censored observations. Among other considerations, the longer lived units are generally more likely to be censored. Therefore, the analysis must correctly use the censored observations and the uncensored observations.

The investigator regresses the survival time variable on one or more independent variables. The survival curve gives the probability of survival up to time t for each time. The hazard function is the instantaneous probability of having an event at time t given that the subject has survived up to time t. Under Cox's proportional hazards model, the hazard is modeled as $H(t) = h_0(t)e^{(\beta_1 X_1 + \ldots [SC] + \beta_k X_k)}$ where X values are independent variables and $h_0(t)$ is the baseline hazard at time t. Cox's proportional hazards model has become the method of choice for multivariable analysis of incidence density variables. By taking logarithmic transformations, the investigator can interpret the regression coefficients in a way similar to multiple logistic regression. The investigator uses similar methods for hypothesis tests and point and interval estimation of regression coefficients and conditional RR approximations of RRs. Cox's proportional hazards model can be generalized to accommodate both time-dependent and constant explanatory variables. Because of complexities involved in fitting the parameters of survival models, clinical investigators rely on statistical software.

Usually, a first step in survival analysis is the estimation of the distribution of the failure times. The survival distribution function (SDF) is used to describe the lifetimes of the population of interest. The SDF evaluated at time t is the probability that a subject sampled from the population will have a lifetime exceeding t—that is, $S(t) = Pr(T > t)$ where $S(t)$ denotes the survival function and T is the lifetime of a randomly selected subject. A likelihood ratio test may be used to test for equality of SDF between the strata. Estimates of some other functions closely related to the SDF may also be obtained. These related functions include the cumulative distribution function, the probability density function, and the hazard function. The hazard function indicates when the likelihood of failure is greatest.

Clinical investigators may select other variables for defining strata. Survival estimates within the strata can be computed and displayed using Kaplan-Meier plots for visual comparison of the results. The median survival time corresponds to that time when half the subjects have failed and half still survive. The investigator may also be interested in the times when 25% and 75% of the subjects in the sample have failed. In addition, rank tests for homogeneity can be used to indicate whether there are significant differences between strata at shorter and/or longer survival times. The Wilcoxon test places more weight on early (shorter) survival times. The log rank test places more weight on larger (longer) survival times.

Often there are additional variables, called covariates, that may be related to the failure time. These variables can be used to construct statistics that test for association between the covariate and the survival time. Two commonly used tests are the Wilcoxon and log rank tests. These tests on covariates are computed by pooling over any defined strata, thereby adjusting for the strata variables. These two tests are similar to those used to test for homogeneity.

Model Selection Techniques for Regression Analysis

Having selected a set of potential explanatory variables, the clinical investigator wishes to know which of these should be included in the final model. If there are only a few explanatory variables, the investigator can consider assessing all possible regression equations. With any more than three or four explanatory variables, the investigator should consider another technique. Statisticians have developed several techniques based on objective criteria for model selection. Before choosing one of these methods, a clinical investigator should review the section on model selection and consider consulting an experienced biostatistician or epidemiologist.

A forward inclusion procedure begins with no explanatory variables in the model. For each potential explanatory variable, the algorithm computes each variable's contribution to the model as if it alone were included in the model. Generally, for each potential explanatory variable, the p value associated with the test statistic is compared to a specified level of significance. That variable, which contributes the greatest amount of information and has a p value less than the specified value, is entered into the model. In the second step, the algorithm computes the contribution to the model (now containing one explanatory variable) for each remaining potential explanatory variable. That variable, which contributes the greatest amount of information and has a p value less than the specified value, is entered into the model. If there is none that meets the entrance criteria, the process stops. If a variable does enter the model, this process continues until there are no variables remaining that meet the criteria for entrance. Once a variable has entered the model, it stays. Models selected with a forward selection technique should be scrutinized for multicollinearity and overparameterization.

A backward elimination procedure begins with a model that includes all potential explanatory variables in the model. For each variable included in the model, the algorithm computes the amount of information contributed by that variable and the p value associated with the test statistic. The variable that contributes the least amount of information and has a p value greater than a specified value is eliminated from the model. This process continues until all variables remaining in the model yield test statistics with associated p values that are smaller than the specified value. Once a variable has been eliminated, it is gone. Although this model selection was designed to address issues of multicollinearity and overparameterization, models selected with a backward elimination technique should be scrutinized.

A stepwise algorithm combines the techniques of forward inclusion and backward elimination. As with forward inclusion, potential explanatory variables are added one by one to the model. The technique begins with no variables in the model. The algorithm computes each potentially explanatory variable's contribution to the model as if it alone were included in the model. Generally, for each potential explanatory variable, the p value associated with the test statistic is compared to a specified level of significance. The variable that contributes the greatest amount of information and has a p value less than the specified value is entered into the model. However, a stepwise algorithm differs in that variables that are already in the model do not necessarily remain there. For each variable included in the model, the algorithm computes the amount of information contributed by that variable and the p value associated with the test statistic. The variable that contributes the least amount of information and has a p value greater than a specified value is eliminated from the model. This process continues until there are no variables remaining that meet the criteria for entrance or deletion. Even though this model selection technique was developed to minimize problems related to multicollinearity and overparameterization, models selected with a stepwise algorithm should be scrutinized.

ROLE OF A CONSULTING BIOSTATISTICIAN IN CLINICAL RESEARCH

In some situations, the statistical aspects of a study become so involved that consulting with a biostatistician is essential. Throughout this chapter, I have indicated when, in my opinion, an investigator with a moderate level of both research experience and analytic skills should consider seeking the assistance of a biostatistician. Those with a lower level of either experience or skills should seek advice earlier in the research process. For some projects, a hospital epidemiologist should consider involving the biostatistician as a member of the research team. Ideally, this arrangement requires a high level of commitment on the parts of both the hospital epidemiologist and the biostatistician. Most researchers lack the time and mathematical background required to master complex statistical issues and methods (e.g., multivariable model selection). Thus, a progressively more common practice is to include a biostatistician (or a scientist with specialized training in statistics) on research teams.

The research goals and objectives of a consulting biostatistician are similar to those of researchers in other scientific disciplines: to develop and disseminate high-quality science through research. However, the biostatistician focuses on the statistical aspects of research questions. These aspects include experimental design, statistical analysis, interpretation of results, and dissemination of results through publication. As a member of a research team, a biostatistician should be capable of serving all statistical needs of the project. Occasionally, a research project presents some unique feature that has not yet been considered in the field of applied statistics. Many biostatisticians will recognize that this feature provides a research topic in biostatistics and the opportunity for developing a new statistical technique.

Qualifications, abilities, and available time will limit a biostatistician's role on a research project. Obviously, technical skills and knowledge of statistical methods are essential. Most biostatisticians have a general knowledge of many statistical methodologies. However, like most professionals, biostatisticians have special interests and, thereby, acquire practical experience in specific types of analytic methods. For example, if the study involves complex multivariable model development and selection, the investigator should attempt to seek assistance from a biostatistician who has an interest in those analytic methods and is experienced in multivariable models and model selection.

Most research questions can be addressed several ways. Constraints that are independent of the question usually make one design more desirable than another. In addition to having the necessary practical experience, possessing problem-solving abilities allows a biostatistician to appreciate practical issues and to choose efficient experimental designs and appropriate statistical methods.

Good interpersonal skills are necessary for the biostatistician to communicate effectively with the principal investigator. If the biostatistician becomes a team member, these skills are needed for communication with coinvestigators, technicians, and other ancillary staff members. Oral and written communication abilities are important team traits. Tactfulness is an interpersonal skill that is especially needed by biostatisticians who interact with individuals who may feel uncomfortable and vulnerable when they discuss statistical issues.

Typically, biostatisticians work as consultants on a large number of projects. The demand for biostatisticians exceeds the supply. Therefore, researchers will need to make compromises with biostatisticians regarding their level of involvement as members of research teams. From the biostatistician's perspective, being a member of a research team represents a long-term investment of time and effort. The biostatistician needs time to learn enough about the health science of the problem so that he or she can assist the investigator with the interpretation of results. The biostatistician needs time to complete the analyses. Because computers complete computations extremely quickly, investigators can forget that programming and exploratory data analyses can be extremely time-consuming for the biostatistician.

REFERENCES

1. Fisher LD, van Belle G. *Biostatistics: a methodology for the health sciences.* New York: Wiley, 1993.
2. Sokal RR, Rohlf RJ. *Biometry: the principles and practice of statistics in biological research,* 3rd ed. New York: WH Freeman, 1995.
3. Colton T. *Statistics in medicine.* Philadelphia: Lippincott-Raven, 1975.
4. Daniel WW. *Biostatistics: a foundation for analysis in the health sciences,* 6th ed. New York: Wiley, 1994.
5. Dawson-Saunders B, Trapp RG. *Basic and clinical biostatistics,* 2nd ed. Norwalk, CT: Appleton & Lange, 1994.
6. Matthews DE, Farewell VT. *Using and understanding medical statistics,* 2nd ed. New York: Karger, 1988.
7. Norman GR, Streiner DL. *PDQ statistics,* 2nd ed. Philadelphia: BC Decker, 1996.
8. Rosner B. *Fundamentals of biostatistics,* 4th ed. Belmont, CA: Duxbury Press, 1995.
9. Zar JH. *Biostatistical analysis,* 3rd ed. Englewood Cliffs, NJ: Prentice-Hall, 1995.
10. Bailar JC, Mosteller F, eds. *Medical uses of statistics,* 2nd ed. Waltham, MA: NEJM Books, 1992.
11. Dunn OJ. *Basic biostatistics: a primer for the biomedical sciences,* 2nd ed. New York: Wiley, 1977.
12. Elston RC, Johnson WD. *Essentials of biostatistics,* 2nd ed. Philadelphia: FA Davis, 1993.
13. Morton RF, Hebel JR. *A study guide to epidemiology and biostatistics,* 4th rev. ed. Gaithersburg, MD: Aspen, 1995.
14. Abramson JH. *Making sense of data: a self-instruction manual on the interpretation of epidemiological data,* 2nd ed. New York: Oxford University Press, 1994.
15. Fleiss JL. *Statistical methods for rates and proportions,* 2nd ed. New York: Wiley, 1981.
16. Fletcher RH, Fletcher SW, Wagner EH. *Clinical epidemiology: the essentials,* 3rd ed. Baltimore: Williams & Wilkins, 1995.
17. Greenberg RS, ed. *Medical epidemiology.* Norwalk, CT: Appleton & Lange, 1993.
18. Ingelfinger JA, Mosteller F, Thibodeau LA, Ware JH. *Biostatistics in clinical medicine,* 3rd ed. New York: McGraw-Hill HPD, 1993.
19. Kelsey JL, Thompson WD, Evans AS. *Methods in observational epidemiology,* 2nd ed. New York: Oxford University Press, 1996.
20. Kleinbaum DG, Kupper LL, Morgeenstern H. *Epidemiologic research: principles and quantitative methods.* New York: Van Nostrand Reinhold, 1982.
21. Riegelman RK, Hirsch RP. *Studying a study and testing a test: how to read the medical literature,* 2nd ed. New York: Little, Brown, 1989.
22. Sackett DL, Haynes RB, Guyatt GH, Tugwell P. *Clinical epidemiology: a basic science for clinical medicine,* 2nd ed. Philadelphia: Lippincott-Raven, 1991.
23. Bland M. *An introduction to medical statistics,* 2nd ed. New York: Oxford University Press, 1995.
24. Galan RS, Gambino SR. *Beyond normality: the predictive value and efficiency of medical diagnoses.* New York: Wiley, 1975.
25. Kramer MS. *Clinical epidemiology and biostatistics: a primer for clinical investigators and decision-makers.* New York: Springer-Verlag, 1988.
26. Lilienfeld DE, Stolley PD. *Foundations of epidemiology,* 3rd ed. New York: Oxford University Press, 1994.
27. Shuster JJ. *Practical handbook of sample size guidelines for clinical trials.* Boca Raton, FL: CRC Press, 1992.
28. Kleinbaum DG, Kupper LL, Muller KE. *Applied regression analysis and other multivariable methods,* 2nd ed. Boston: PWS-KENT, 1988.
29. Draper NR, Smith H. *Applied regression analysis,* 3rd ed. New York: Wiley, 1998.
30. Myers RH. *Classical and modern regression with applications,* 2nd ed. Boston: PWS-KENT, 1990.
31. Myers RH, Milton JS. *A first course in the theory of linear statistical models.* Boston: PWS-KENT, 1991.
32. Belsley DA, Kuh E, Welsch RE. *Regression diagnostics: identifying influential data and sources of collinearity.* New York: Wiley, 1980.
33. Agresti A. *Categorical data analysis.* New York: Wiley, 1990.
34. Rothman KJ, Greenland S. *Modern epidemiology,* 2nd ed. Philadelphia: Lippincott-Raven, 1998.
35. Hosmer DW, Lemeshow S. *Applied logistic regression.* New York: Wiley, 1989.
36. Lawless JF. *Statistical models and methods for lifetime data.* New York: Wiley, 1982.
37. Breslow NE, Day NE. *Statistical methods in cancer research, vol 1: the analysis of case-control studies,* reprinted ed. New York: Oxford University Press, 1993.
38. Cox DR, Oakes D. *Analysis of survival data.* New York: Chapman and Hall, 1984.
39. Lee ET. *Statistical methods for survival data analysis,* 2nd ed. New York: Wiley, 1992.
40. Miller RG. *Survival analysis.* New York: Wiley, 1981.

SUGGESTED READINGS

Armitage P, Berry G. *Statistical methods on medical research,* 3rd ed. Boston: Blackwell Scientific, 1994.

Conover WJ. *Practical nonparametric statistics,* 2nd ed. New York: Wiley, 1980.

Freedman D, Pisani R, Purvis R, Adhakari A. *Statistics,* 2nd ed. New York: WW Norton, 1991.

Gillings DB, Douglass CW. *Biostats: a primer for health care professionals,* 2nd ed. Chapel Hill, NC: CAVCO, 1985.

Greenland S, ed. *Evolution of epidemiologic ideas: annotated readings on concepts and methods.* Chestnut Hill, MA: Epidemiology Resources, 1987.

Hulley SB, Cummings SR, eds. *Designing clinical research: an epidemiologic approach.* Baltimore: Williams & Wilkins, 1988.

Pagano M, Gauvreau K. *Principles of biostatistics.* Belmont, CA: Duxbury Press, 1993.

Piantadosi S. *Clinical trials: a methodologic perspective.* New York: Wiley, 1997.

Schlesselman JJ. *Case-control studies: design, conduct, analysis.* New York: Oxford University Press, 1982.

4

PRINCIPLES OF HOSPITAL EPIDEMIOLOGY

MARY D. NETTLEMAN
RICHARD P. WENZEL

Epidemiology is formally defined as the study of the distribution and determinants of health and disease in populations. To many, it may be viewed simplistically as the "science of long division." That designation is meant to imply that the presentation of data involves both a numerator and a denominator. It is particularly the denominator that is missing in many case studies, and it is the denominator that helps to distinguish epidemiology from most clinical or basic science disciplines. The application of epidemiology to hospital infection control often begins with a systematic identification of major problems—surveillance. The purpose of surveillance is to calculate rates in order to prioritize the efforts of the infection control team (1). Proper analysis and interpretation of the data are essential for wise policy development and decision making.

SURVEILLANCE

Surveillance is the routine and orderly collection of data based on standard definitions of cases (2). The implication is that there will be routine analysis and thoughtful feedback of the information to important constituents. One of the fundamental goals of surveillance is to define and report various kinds of rates. In epidemiology, a rate is defined as the number of cases divided by the number of persons at risk. Prevalence and incidence rates form the foundation of epidemiologic analysis, and the distinction between the two must be understood (3).

Incidence is defined as the number of new cases divided by the number of people at risk divided by the unit of time. For example, there may be five newly diagnosed cases of nosocomial infections per 100 patients at risk per month. Prevalence is defined as the number of new and old (but still active) cases at a specific time divided by the number surveyed. For example, there may be ten nosocomial infections, both new (recently diagnosed) and old, per 100 patients surveyed on a particular day.

There is a relationship between incidence and prevalence, and it is important. In general terms, prevalence (P) equals incidence (I) times the average duration (D) of the disease: $P = I \times D$ (3). The average duration of a disease varies directly with the persistence of signs and symptoms and inversely with mortality. For example, by examining the simple formula above, one could expect an increase in the prevalence with an increase in either the incidence of the disease or the average duration of the disease. Conversely, one could expect a decrease in the prevalence resulting from either a decrease in the incidence of the disease or in the average duration of the disease. It is important to point out that the average duration of disease could decrease either as a function of improved therapy or as a function of very high and early mortality. Moreover, if one disease resolves more quickly than another, its average duration by definition is briefer than the other. As an example, one might expect that in incidence studies there would be three times as many nosocomial urinary tract infections identified through routine surveillance as nosocomial pneumonias. In prevalence studies, however, this ratio will be lower because the signs and symptoms of nosocomial urinary tract infections may last only 1 to 3 days, whereas those for nosocomial pneumonia may last 1 week or longer (Fig. 4.1).

Another important rate is the attack rate. An attack rate differs from incidence and prevalence in that there is no time unit, and it simply identifies the number of cases per number of procedures. One might examine surgical site infections as an example: the reported attack rate might be five incisional surgical site infections per 100 gallbladder operations.

Two other terms are important to define: proportion and ratio. In a proportion the numerator is part of the denominator. For example, the proportion of the total number of hospital-acquired infections due to nosocomial urinary tract infections is approximately one third. A ratio differs from a proportion in that a ratio is any numerator divided by any denominator; for example, one can talk about the ratio of lawsuits per 1,000 admissions or the ratio of deaths per 1,000 admissions. Although all proportions are ratios, not all ratios are proportions.

Monthly Report

An important function of surveillance is to develop a monthly report. For convenience, one might use monthly admissions or discharges as the denominator to represent all of those at risk, but the exposure time (days in the hospital) would not be known and the number at risk would be underestimated, since some patients admitted in the previous month and at risk would not be included in the denominator. Also, the risk of acquiring a

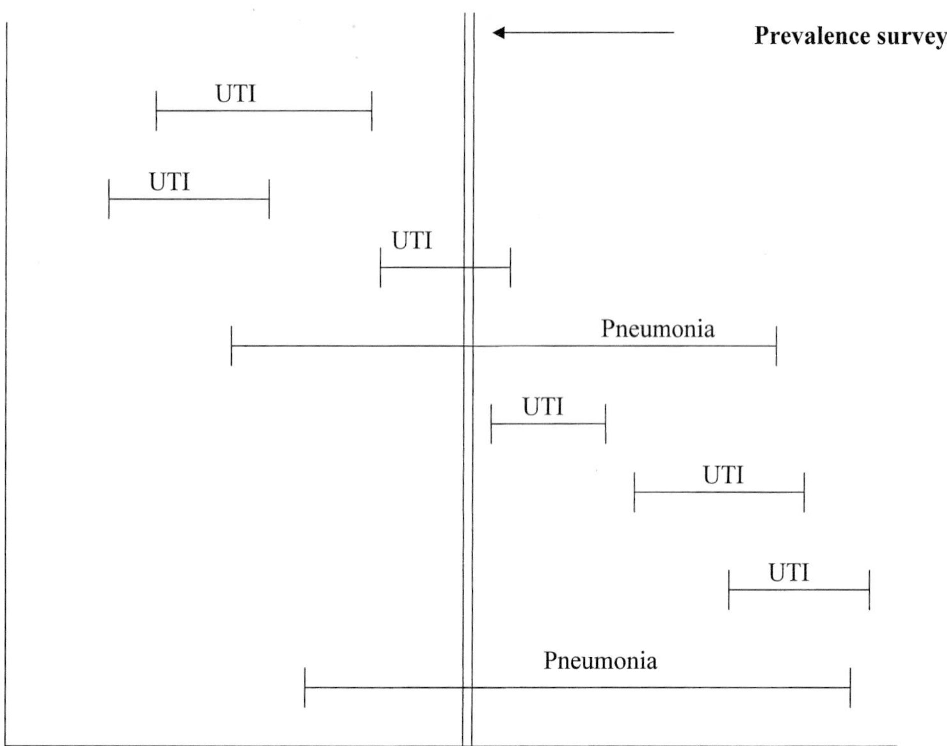

Figure 4.1. In this hypothetical data set, routine incidence surveillance identified six cases of nosocomial urinary tract infection (UTI) and two cases of nosocomial pneumonia. However, because prevalence surveys identify new and old (but active) cases, and because the symptoms and signs of pneumonia last much longer than those of urinary tract infection, the prevalence survey identified two nosocomial pneumonias and only one nosocomial urinary tract infection.

nosocomial infection would be expected to increase as the length of hospitalization, the exposure time, increases. Thus, we may talk about the number of infections per 100 admissions or per 100 discharges, but a better estimate (especially useful for comparison of different groups such as different hospitals or across different wards seeing similar kinds of patients) would be the number of infections per 1,000 patient-days. The total number of patient-days is the sum of all hospital days for all patients for the period of interest. In this case, the denominator defines the group at risk and the time at risk. This is particularly important if the average hospital stay varies from institution to institution or changes over time.

Secular trends are important, because they allow analysis of changes in rates over time. For example, one might ask: "What are the infection rates of a particular hospital over a 5-year period?" Graphically presented, such secular trends are very useful to discover if there has been a decrease or an increase in nosocomial infection rates over an extended period. However, with the changes of medical care delivery, there may be difficulties in simply comparing the crude rates from one year to another, particularly over a 5-year period. For example, the introduction of diagnosis-related groups (DRGs) in 1983 was associated with a decreased average hospital stay per patient in the United States. Length of stay may affect detection of nosocomial infections, because the patients would be discharged before some infections might become manifest. Therefore, without making some adjustments, there may be an apparent decrease in the numerator and an apparent decline in infection rate. In fact, there are a limited number of solutions for this particular problem. One is to do postdischarge surveillance for accurate case findings, and the other is to do a form of survival analysis. With respect to the latter, one might think of survival analysis as a form of analysis in which rates of infection are examined after patients are stratified by daily stay in the hospital. In survival analysis, one asks the question: What cumulative proportion of patients develop a nosocomial infection by day 3, 4, 5, etc.? With such data available, one could compare rates from one year to the next and not be concerned about average length of stay (Fig. 4.2).

There is a new argument for caution in the use of secular trends, based on the fact that one might see an increase in rates simply because the patients being admitted have more severe underlying diseases currently than previously and are at higher risk for nosocomial infections. It is obvious that rates of infection need to have additional adjustments for the severity of disease of the underlying patient population (4). One can solve that problem only if one can stratify or model the patient population; that is, stratify by various diagnoses or model the patients in general for severity of illness and then perform some type of comparison of rates of the survival curves. This discussion leads directly to the issue of statistics in hospital epidemiology (5), an issue that is important for comparing infection rates.

If we wish to compare rates from one year to another, we might, in a simple example, compare the number of infected

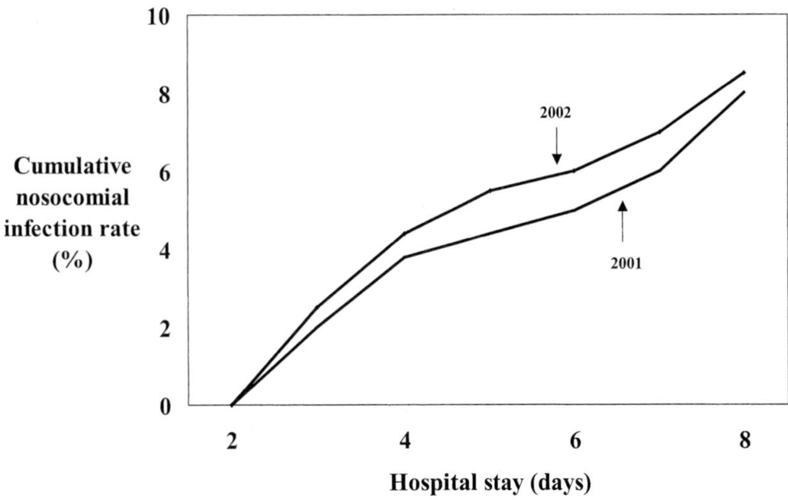

Figure 4.2. Survival curves depicting cumulative nosocomial infection rates by day in the hospital. In this hypothetical example, the 2002 rates are only slightly higher than the 2001 rates. By definition, no nosocomial infections occurred after day 28 in any month of 2001.

patients divided by the number at risk in 2001 versus that in 2002. We will come up with some statistical test showing whether or not there was a significant difference. The test result is usually given in terms of a *p* value, or probability. It is important at this point to define the *p*: the probability that the *difference observed* (or even a larger difference in annual rates) could have occurred by chance alone. For example, if the annual infection rates declined from 10% to 8%, that 20% difference in infection rates, or fall of two percentage points, may be significantly different. If the *p* was $<.05$, we conclude that it was significantly different and that there was less than a 5% probability that a difference that large—a 20% reduction—could have occurred by chance alone. It is by convention that if *p* is less than or equal to 5% or *p* is less than or equal to .05, we call that difference significant. It is also worth emphasizing that *p* has nothing to do with the success or failure of a test or test drug; instead it deals only with the probability that the difference observed occurred by chance. One might therefore view the *p* as the probability of random error.

In a study comparing two rates (e.g., 10% vs. 8%), if the *p* value reported was .01, one would conclude that the difference observed between 10% and 8% could have occurred by chance alone only one time in 100. In fact, it is possible that there was no true difference in the true rates (truth being impossible for mortals to determine), and by chance alone we saw a difference. A second possibility is that, since the probability of observing that difference by chance alone was so low, there really is a difference. Two other possibilities exist to explain a *p* less than .05: bias or confounding (Table 4.1).

TABLE 4.1. FOUR EXPLANATIONS FOR A SIGNIFICANT *p* ($p \leq .05$)

1. True difference at least as large as the one observed exists
2. The difference observed occurred by chance alone, the probability defined by the *p* value; the difference observed was in fact a random error
3. The difference observed was the result of some systematic error—bias
4. The difference observed was the result of some confounding variables

Note: With bias, there can be no adjustment for the error. With confounding, one can make adjustments and then reexamine the new *p* value.

Bias defines a systematic error (not a random error or chance) that led to the distortion of the data. For example, if in 2001 only infections detected in the first 28 days of a month were counted in the numerator, whereas in 2002 all infections for all days were counted, that systematic exclusion of days in 2001—bias—could have led to a significant *p* value. Confounding is discussed below.

CAUSE OF INFECTION

In the traditional model of epidemiology one considers the microorganism, the host, and the environment. For example, if one looks at urinary tract infections, one might look at the microorganism, for example, *Escherichia coli*; the host, for example, a patient admitted to the hospital for control of diabetes mellitus; and the environment, the management of the hospital including physicians, nurses, and various procedures, for example, a bladder catheterization performed in that particular patient (Fig. 4.3).

Each one of these—the microorganism, the host, and the environment—might be called a risk factor. It is important to know that there may be multiple risk factors as causes of infection. If one considers only the microorganism as the cause of the infection, one can conclude that to reduce or eliminate the cause or to minimize the rate, one has to affect only the microorganism. However, there are likely to be multiple additional causes, such as the influence of the integrity of the bladder mucosa, the likelihood that the mucosa has receptors for certain species of bacteria, the presence of diabetes in the host, or an environment that permits the placement of the bladder catheters

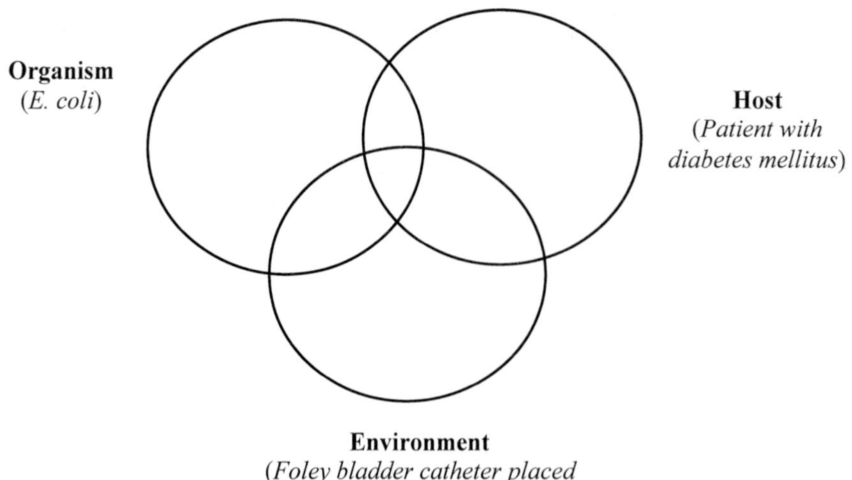

Figure 4.3. In the traditional epidemiologic model, the microorganism, the host, and the environment might all be independent risk factors for acquiring a nosocomial urinary tract infection. One might imagine the highest risk for infections being the intersection of all three risk factors.

by healthcare workers with varying degrees of skill. By modifying each one of these risk factors, one could hope to reduce the risk or rate of infection. From an infection control point of view, since outcome is multifactorial, one can modify several risk factors simultaneously. A multifactorial view of cause allows one a multifactorial approach to prevention and control. So far, true risk factors—causes—have been described in qualitative terms. One might also view them in quantitative or statistical terms—for example, in examining the cause of an epidemic.

CAUSE OF AN EPIDEMIC

A risk factor is an attribute or variable that is more likely associated with the outcome of cases than of controls. If the question is, What is the cause of a cluster of surgical site infections after thoracic cardiovascular surgery?, the cases (with pus at the sternal incision site) may be compared to controls without infection. Using standard statistical tests, certain variables from a hypothetical study may be found to be significantly associated with cases (Table 4.2).

Investigations of nosocomial infections usually involve two types of data: categorical and continuous. Categorical variables are just that: types of data that can be classified into categories. An example would be the presence or absence of a nosocomial infection. Continuous variables, such as age or temperature, are usually measured numerically and can take on any value within an interval. When comparing proportions, a test commonly used for categorical variables is the Fisher's exact test; alternatively, the chi-square test might be employed. The t-test is often used to compare continuous variables.

TABLE 4.2. VARIABLES FROM A HYPOTHETICAL STUDY

Variables	Cases	Controls	*p* Value
Average age	68	45	.01
Time of operation	180 min	130 min	.02
Exposure to surgeon no. 2	50/60	20/60	.035
Exposure to nurse no. 4	55/60	25/60	.02

If we compare each variable one by one, such as the age of cases compared to the age of controls, and do not consider other variables, we are performing a univariate analysis. Table 4.2 shows the results of a univariate analysis of a case-control study (discussed below). Recall that the p value defines the probability that the difference observed could have occurred by chance alone, given the null hypothesis that no difference is expected. For example, if one looks at age, the difference between age 68 in cases and age 45 in controls (23 years) was statistically significant. The probability that the observed difference could have occurred by chance alone is estimated at only 1%. For time of operation, the probability that the difference between 180 minutes and 130 minutes, or in other words a difference of 50 minutes, could have occurred by chance alone was only 2%. If one looks at exposure to surgeon no. 2, the probability that the difference between 50/60 in cases and 20/60 in controls could have occurred by chance alone was only 3.5%. The probability that exposure to nurse no. 4, 55/60 in cases versus 25/60 in controls, could have occurred by chance alone is defined by a p value of 2%.

The univariate analyses suggest that each one of the variables tested was a significant risk factor for sternal surgical site infections. The key question, however, is which of the variables independently predicts infection after we consider the contribution of the other variables (6). To answer this, one would have to do a multivariable analysis—that is, control for one or more variables while looking at another, or in the case of the example above, control for three variables while examining the fourth. One of the standard ways of performing multivariable analysis today is through regression analysis, particularly logistic regression. After performing a multivariable analysis, it is possible that exposure to nurse no. 4 and exposure to physician no. 2 would be the only independent risk factors. Such a mathematical analysis by itself could never prove causality but only suggest the probabilities of the important risk factors. Since we cannot prove cause-and-effect relationships in defining true risk factors, it follows that removal of the risk factor cannot guarantee a reduced rate of infection. However, one could examine this particular problem further by evaluating microbiologic data.

What would one conclude if surgeon no. 2, whose exposure is clearly a risk factor by univariate analysis, always operates with nurse no. 4? Each is therefore linked to the other and called a confounding variable for the infection. In addition, suppose that surgeon no. 2 almost always operates on patients who are over age 65, at least more so than his colleagues. Each variable (exposure to surgeon no. 2 and older age of the cases versus controls) would then be a confounding or linked variable for infection, and one would have to deal with such confounding. To go back to the independent variable question, one of the reasons to perform a multivariable analysis is to control for other variables that might be confounding the conclusion about independent risk factors.

If one knew that all of the infections in cases were caused by *Staphylococcus aureus* with a plasmid type J-1, and all the operating room team had been cultured and only one person had a nasal carriage of *S. aureus* with a plasmid type J-1, and that was nurse no. 4, exposure to nurse no. 4 would be more likely to be the true cause.

CONFOUNDING VARIABLES

A confounding variable is an extraneous variable that wholly or partially accounts for the apparent effect of the study exposure (or that masks a true underlying association). It is always a risk factor for the study disease, and it is associated with study exposure but is not the result of exposure (7). A confounding variable could be the real cause or it could be a noncausal link resulting from the confounder's association with the true causal factors. Some experts have simply thought of confounding variables as alternative causes for the outcome of interest.

As an example of confounding, one might examine penmanship skill as a function of hand size. If one imagines the data on a graph, one would see that as hand size increased (y-axis), penmanship skill increased (x-axis). That relationship defined in a simple model with two variables might be statistically significant, $p < .001$. Examining the model, a cynic might say that if one could only stretch his or her hand size, penmanship skill would increase; but a person who understood confounding would say that there is a missing link, a variable that was the true cause of penmanship skill and that was related to hand size. In this case, the confounding variable is age, because the associated skill in dexterity that is defined by age is the real cause of penmanship skill. Very young children or babies would have very poor penmanship skill, whereas those with more mature neurologic systems would have better penmanship skill.

In examining annual rates of nosocomial infections, it is important to correct for confounding variables. Examples of confounders include age of patients, severity of underlying disease, length of inpatient stay, and others. In observational studies—including surveillance—there are two ways to correct for confounding: perform a stratified analysis (stratify by age, severity of illness, stay in the hospital, etc.) or perform a multivariable analysis.

SPECIALLY DESIGNED STUDIES: HISTORICAL COHORT STUDY

One should not perform surveillance—use resources—unless the outcomes are important. There are studies specifically designed to define the importance of outcomes, particularly the excess morbidity, mortality, and costs of nosocomial infections. Cases are matched very closely to controls, and the difference in outcome between cases and controls, if properly performed, could be attributed to the infection. Such properly performed studies are called historical cohort studies, and in this case there is very tight matching of cases to controls. For example, to determine the excess or attributable outcome from a nosocomial bloodstream infection, one would want to match controls with cases by at least age, sex, service, underlying diseases, operations, and procedures. A very important additional matching variable would be length of stay in the hospital: the control must be in the hospital—exposed to the risk—for at least as long as the interval between admission and infection in the case. If one has very closely matched controls, then one can estimate the attributable outcome. For example, if 35% of cases with nosocomial bloodstream infections died (crude mortality) and 10% of closely matched controls died, the difference, 25%, is an estimate of attributable mortality—the mortality directly attributed to the bloodstream infection, apart from the underlying diseases. Historical cohort studies of nosocomial bloodstream infections have been performed (8–11), and the results have suggested that nosocomial bloodstream infections are a leading cause of death (12–14).

CASE-CONTROL STUDY

A second type of epidemiologic study, the case-control study, examines risk factors for infection. To determine risk factors, one matches cases and controls, but in this instance, instead of looking forward at outcomes, one looks backward to the admission day and asks the question: What exposures are different in cases and controls? In this situation, one would not want to match cases and controls tightly. Generally, one would match only on age, sex, and service, and again depending on which perspective one may want to examine, one could include other variables. However, it is important to point out that if one matches for a specific variable—for example, time in the hospital—then that variable can never be examined as a risk factor. One might examine, for example, intensive care unit (ICU) populations looking for the cause of *Serratia marcescens* bloodstream infections. If one matched by age, sex, underlying diseases, and the use of all transducers, one might fail to identify the true cause—the contaminated transducer—because it would be common to both cases and controls. In an epidemic situation,

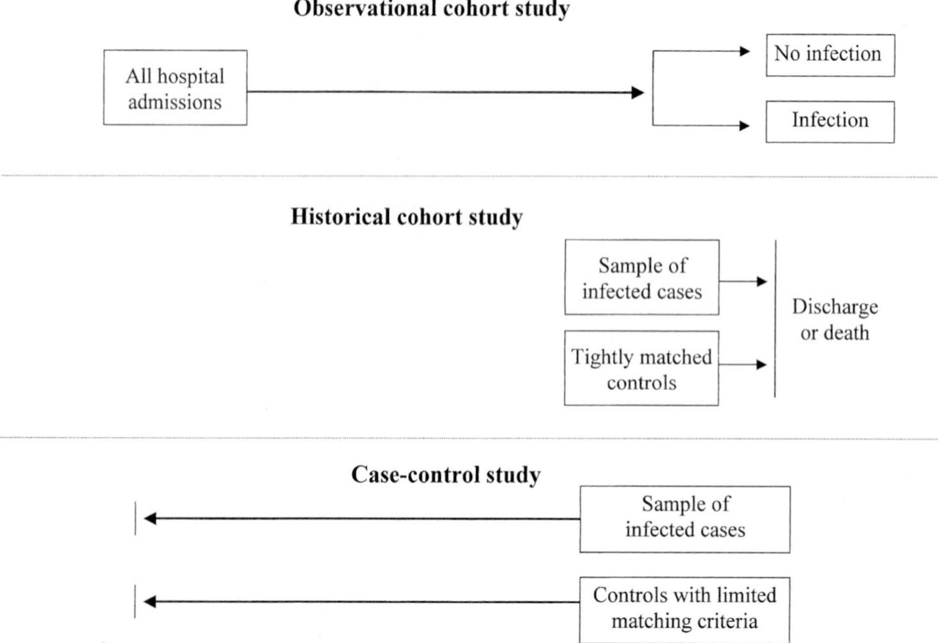

Figure 4.4. The observational cohort study is useful for determining crude rates and basic characteristics of infected and uninfected patients. Since they are prospective studies, one views the data in a forward way through time. The historical cohort study design examines tightly matched patients with uninfected controls to determine attributable (excess) morbidity, mortality, or cost due directly to the infection. In this case, even if the data are gathered retrospectively, the view of the outcome is forward in time. The case-control study design compares infected patients and controls matched on only a few variables to detect exposures (risk factors) more commonly associated with infected patients than with controls. Since one begins with infection and examines prior exposures, one views the events in a backward way through time.

one frequently is required to perform a case-control study to examine exposures more likely to have occurred in infected cases than in uninfected controls. The example of the comparison of cases with postoperative surgical site infections and controls without infections—shown above—illustrates this technique. Figure 4.4 illustrates the perspective of an observational cohort study (active, prospective surveillance), an historical cohort study to examine outcomes (patients and controls from previous admissions are examined), and a case-control study for risk factors.

In a case-control study of the risk factors for nosocomial *Candida* bloodstream infections (15), it was shown that a large number of variables in the univariate analysis predicted infection. However, when multivariable techniques were applied, only four variables predicted candidemia:

- Number of prior classes of antibiotics
- Hickman catheter
- Colonization with *Candida* species
- Hemodialysis

This study showed the importance of performing the multivariable analysis to control for the confounding variables, which appeared significant in the univariate analysis.

RISK RATIO AND ODDS RATIO

In cohort studies, all cases and controls are viewed in a time-forward fashion such as from admission to infection, or from infection to discharge or death. If cases and controls are closely matched, the differences in outcome (e.g., mortality) represent *attributable differences.* This term is important from a public health perspective. From a patient's point of view, an important question may be, "If I get infected, what is my risk of death relative to my risk without infection?" This relative risk or risk ratio is simply the mortality of cases divided by the mortality of matched controls. For example, if 39% of patients with a nosocomial bloodstream infection died and 13% of matched controls without a bloodstream infection died, the risk ratio (relative risk) would be 3.

In case-control studies, the subjects are viewed in a time-backward fashion, such as from infection to admission. The goal is to identify risk factors that are found more frequently among cases than among controls. Only estimates of risk ratios can be made in case-control studies, and the term *odds ratios* is employed.

Suppose we had the following data among cases with a nosocomial urinary tract infection and controls without a nosocomial urinary tract infection: Of 20 infected patients and 20 noninfected controls, a Foley catheter was used in 18 of the patients (and not in two of the patients) and in four of the controls (and not, of course, in 16 of the controls). The ratio 18/2 is called the odds of exposure to a Foley catheter among cases; the odds of exposure to a Foley catheter among controls is 4/16. The odds ratio refers to the odds of exposure among cases divided by the odds of exposure among controls:

$$\frac{(18/2)}{(4/16)} = \frac{(16\times18)}{(2\times4)} = 36$$

In this case, we would say that the odds of urinary tract infection among patients exposed to a Foley catheter are estimated to be 36 times that of patients not exposed to a Foley catheter. Note that the use of the term *odds* in epidemiology is different from that used in common parlance. In addition, the term *odds ratio* is used to differentiate this type of study—case-control—from a cohort study. In the case-control study, the prevalence of infection is artificial and depends on the ratio of cases to controls: 1 to 1 in the example above for a 50% prevalence. This is an important distinction between a case-control study and a cohort study, in which the normal prevalence is expected to be much lower.

DECISION ANALYSIS

Epidemiologic surveillance and the quality improvement programs that are based on surveillance require time, money, and effort—resources that are always in short supply. How does one decide where to spend limited resources? The decision is often intuitive, based on a personal assessment of the situation and a partial knowledge of the literature. For complicated problems, a more comprehensive analysis may be required. Decision analysis is a formal method for quantifying the cost and effectiveness of procedures, tests, therapies, and programs (16–18). The decision analyst views each proposed intervention as a dichotomous mixture of costs and effectiveness.

Decision analysis begins with a logical structuring of the problem at hand (19). For example, a hospital may wish to perform nasal cultures to detect patients who carry methicillin-resistant *S. aureus* (MRSA) in order to treat them. The goal would be to treat carriers and potentially prevent nosocomial spread of the microorganism. A simple decision tree would include two branches: one for the "test all patients" strategy and the other for the "do not test any patients" strategy (Fig. 4.5). To describe the problem fully, the decision tree must be expanded. More branches must be added to the tree to take into account the proportion of patients who carry MRSA but who will have falsely negative nasal cultures, the ability of medication to eradicate the carrier state, the probability of nosocomial spread from a patient who carries MRSA, etc. Creating a decision tree is more than an exercise; it requires that the problem be described completely and that its components be arranged in sequential order. Branch points, known as nodes, occur when a decision must be made—for example, whether or not to test—or when there is more than one possible outcome of a decision.

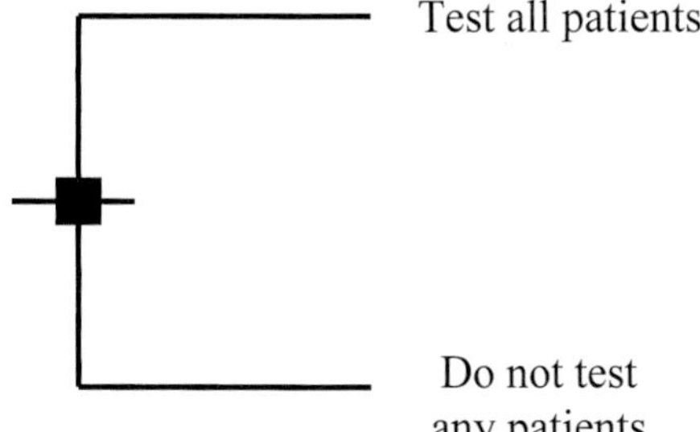

Figure 4.5. Decision tree with a single decision node.

The probability of arriving at each branch must be known or estimated. For example, what is the probability that patients with a positive test actually have disease? The answer requires an understanding of sensitivity, specificity, and predictive values. True-positive (TP) test results occur when the test is positive and the patient has the disease. False-positive (FP) results occur when the test is positive, but the patient does not have the disease. True-negative (TN) and false-negative (FN) results occur when the test is negative in patients who do not have disease and who do have disease, respectively. Sensitivity is the probability of a positive test result occurring in patients known to have disease:

$$\text{Sensitivity} = \frac{\text{TP}}{(\text{TP+FN})}$$

Positive predictive value is the probability of disease in patients with a positive test result:

$$\text{Positive Predictive Value} = \frac{\text{TP}}{(\text{TP+FP})}$$

Specificity is the probability of a negative test in patients who are free of disease:

$$\text{Specificity} = \frac{\text{TN}}{(\text{TN+FP})}$$

Negative predictive value is the probability that there is no disease in patients with a negative test:

$$\text{Negative Predictive Value} = \frac{\text{TN}}{(\text{TN+FN})}$$

After the probability of arriving at each node is determined, costs are considered. The cost of a proposed intervention need not be limited to the monetary amount required to purchase equipment and supplies or hire new workers. Although these direct costs are important, it is also useful to consider indirect costs that are not paid for immediately or that are linked tangentially to the intervention. Examples of indirect costs include time lost from work, impaired capacity to earn wages because of disability, transportation costs to and from a physician's office, maintenance costs for equipment, the cost of potential litigation, and the lost earnings due to premature mortality. If money will not be spent or earned until several years have passed, the sum must be adjusted ("discounted") to reflect the value of the dollar at the future date (20). Costs may include nonmonetary expenditures such as time lost from work or lost years of productivity.

Effectiveness, too, may be measured in many ways, and the choice depends on the desired outcome of the analysis. Effectiveness may include the number of cases of disease prevented or the number of lives or life-years saved. In the modern technologic era, prolongation of life and prolongation of enjoyable life have not always been identical. Adjustments for the quality of life are difficult to perform but may be required in some instances (21). To complete the analysis, the cost and effectiveness are expressed as a ratio (22).

The purpose of a decision analysis is to compare the cost-effectiveness ratios of different interventions. For example, one intervention might cost $5,000 per year of life saved, whereas another might cost $35 per year of life saved. Some moderately effective interventions may cost so much that one might be better to choose a series of less effective and less costly interventions. Because many assumptions about costs and probabilities must be made, it is wise to determine how sensitive the outcome of the analysis is to reasonable changes in the assumptions (sensitivity analysis). Decision analysis does not replace clinical judgment. Rather, it provides an objective perspective, allowing clinicians to examine assumptions and trade-offs inherent in healthcare decisions (23).

Resources are limited, and the ways to spend resources are countless. Decision analysis is a valuable tool for condensing problems into manageable cost-effectiveness ratios. Although intuitive judgment may suffice for simple problems, the structured approach provided by decision analysis provides a comprehensive picture of more complex problems. When combined, decision analysis and a thoughtful, intuitive approach to problem solving will maximize outcome while limiting resource expenditures.

CONCLUSION

The discipline of epidemiology includes the definition of rates; for infection control, this implies some form of active surveillance. The latter should be viewed as an observational cohort study. Once crude rates are calculated, they should be adjusted for confounding variables if one wishes to compare year-to-year or hospital-to-hospital differences. Most infections are multifactorial, and case-control studies are useful in identifying the multiple risk factors. Statistical tests can define risk factors, but even when statistically significant, no cause-effect relationship can be assigned without further confirmation (e.g., with microbiologic data). Historical cohort studies are very useful for defining the morbidity, mortality, or costs directly attributable to an infection. Decision analysis is a quantitative approach to decision making based on available data and a systematic approach to solutions.

REFERENCES

1. Edmond MB. National and international surveillance systems. In: Wenzel RP, ed. *Prevention and control of nosocomial infections,* 4th ed. Philadelphia: Lippincott Williams & Wilkins, 2003.
2. Wenzel RP, Streed SA. Surveillance and use of computers in hospital infection control. *J Hosp Infect* 1989;13:217–229.
3. Gastmeier P, Bräuer H, Sohr D, et al. Converting incidence and prevalence data of nosocomial infections: results from eight hospitals. *Infect Control Hosp Epidemiol* 2001;22:31–34.
4. Daley J, Henderson WG, Khuri SF. Risk-adjusted surgical outcomes. *Annu Rev Med* 2001;52:275–287.
5. Wenzel RP. Old wine in new bottles [editorial]. *Infect Control* 1986; 7:485–486.
6. Austin DJ. Modeling endemic and epidemic infections. In: Wenzel RP, ed. *Prevention and control of nosocomial infections,* 4th ed. Philadelphia: Lippincott Williams & Wilkins, 2003.
7. Schlesselman JJ, ed. *Case-control studies. Design, conduct, analysis.* New York: Oxford University Press, 1992.
8. Pessoa-Silva CL, Miyasaki CH, de Almeida MF, et al. Neonatal late-onset bloodstream infection: attributable mortality, excess of length of stay and risk factors. *Eur J Epidemiol* 2001;17:715–720.
9. Townsend TR, Wenzel RP. Nosocomial bloodstream infections in a newborn intensive care unit: a case-matched control study of morbidity, mortality, and risk. *Am J Epidemiol* 1981;114:73–80.
10. Landry SL, Kaiser DL, Wenzel RP. Hospital stay and mortality attributed to nosocomial enterococcal bacteremia: a controlled study. *Am J Infect Control* 1989;17:323–329.
11. Wey SB, Mori M, Pfaller MA, et al. Hospital-acquired Candidemia: the attributable mortality and excess length of stay. *Arch Intern Med* 1988;148:2642–2647.
12. Pittet D, Wenzel RP. Nosocomial bloodstream infection: secular trends in rates and mortality in a tertiary health care center. *Arch Intern Med* 1995;155:1177–1184.
13. Edmond MB, Wallace SE, McClish DK, et al. Nosocomial bloodstream infections in United States hospitals: a three-year analysis. *Clin Infect Dis* 1999;29:239–244.
14. Wenzel RP, Edmond MB. The impact of hospital-acquired bloodstream infections. *Emerg Infect Dis* 2001;7:174–177.
15. Wey SG, Mori M, Pfaller MA, et al. Risk factors for hospital-acquired candidemia: a matched case-control study. *Arch Intern Med* 1989;149: 2349–2353.
16. Detsky AS, Naglie IG. A clinician's guide to cost-effectiveness analysis. *Ann Intern Med* 1990;113:147–154.
17. Pauker SG, Kassirer JP. Decision analysis. *N Engl J Med* 1987;316: 250–258.
18. Lilford RJ, Pauker SG, Braunholtz DA, et al. Decision analysis and the implementation of research findings. *BMJ* 1998;317:405–409.
19. Detsky AS, Naglie G, Krahn MD, et al. Primer on medical decision analysis: part 1. Getting started. *Med Decis Making* 1997;17:123–125.
20. Lipscomb J. The proper role for discounting. Search in progress. *Med Care* 1996;34(suppl):DS119–123.
21. McAlearney AS, Schweikhart SB, Pathak DS. Quality-adjusted life-years and other health indices: a comparative analysis. *Clin Ther* 1999; 21:1605–1629.
22. Krahn MD, Naglie G, Naimark D, et al. Primer on medical decision analysis: part 4. Analyzing the model and interpreting the results. *Med Decis Making* 1997;17:142–151.
23. Glassman PA, Model KE, Kahan JP, et al. The role of medical necessity and cost-effectiveness in making medical decisions. *Ann Intern Med* 1997;127:165–166.

5

DATA COLLECTION IN HOSPITAL EPIDEMIOLOGY

STEPHEN B. KRITCHEVSKY
RONALD I. SHORR

Data for hospital epidemiology comes from three sources: direct ascertainment of information from subjects using questionnaires; review of medical records; and electronic sources, such as billing records, laboratory records, and medication administration records. Although we provide an overview of each of these data sources, we emphasize the development of questionnaires. After data from any of these sources is collected, it is analyzed, usually using a statistical package. We offer suggestions on the preparation and formatting of data to facilitate the transfer from data collection to data analysis.

QUESTIONNAIRES

Questionnaire Development

Questionnaires are often the most labor intensive form of data collection, but are required in situations where surveillance using electronic data sources or medical record review is inadequate.

After deciding what data need to be collected, the investigator has to decide how to collect it. This means developing the form(s) to guide data collection, identifying the data sources (e.g., individuals, proxies, medical records, direct observation), identifying data gatherers, and deciding on a mode of data collection. Decisions in each of these areas affect the others, and investigators should understand the trade-offs between them in order to make good decisions when planning an investigation.

Writing the Questions

The first step in developing a data collection form is writing the questions to elicit the information required by the study. Good questions are clear and unambiguous and match the verbal skills of prospective participants. Poorly worded questions result in answers that are unreliable or uninterpretable. Although writing good questions is something of an art, there are several common problems that can result in bad questions.

Choosing Verbiage

If respondents do not understand the words used in questions, they will not be able to answer them (or worse, they will answer them anyway). In general, the words used in the questions should be ones used by respondents in their usual conversation (e.g., use "help" rather than "assist" and "enough" rather than "sufficient"). Avoid medical jargon and abbreviations that may not be commonly understood. Be aware of regional or cultural differences in the meanings of words and the names of diseases (e.g., diabetes may be called "the sugar" by some respondents). Avoid using loaded words (i.e., those carrying excessively negative connotations).

Consider these questions:

Should smoking be banned in the hospital?
Should smoking be allowed in the hospital?

The word *banned* is loaded, and some answers to the question may be a reaction to the word itself rather than to the content of the question.

Ambiguous Questions

One of the most difficult tasks in writing a question is asking it in such a way that the respondent has the same concept in mind when answering it as the investigator did when asking it. The investigator wanting to identify current cigarette smokers might ask: "Do you smoke?" Cigar and pipe smokers will answer this affirmatively, contrary to the investigator's intention. There may also be those who have very recently quit smoking (and may soon begin the habit again). They would answer no, but the investigator might want them classified as smokers for the purposes of the study. "Have you smoked two or more packs of cigarettes in the past 2 months?" is a better version of the question. Cigarettes are specifically named, and the amount of consumption and the period are specified.

In an outbreak investigation of central line infections, hospital personnel might be asked, "Did you see patients on [a particular ward]?" This question has two ambiguous referents. Does "see" mean "care for," or is the question intended to detect less formal contact as well? Also, does the investigator mean has the respondent ever seen patients on a ward, or just during the epidemic period? A better phrasing might be, "Did you provide care for any patients on [the ward] since March of this year?"

Causes must precede effects in time. Therefore, when assessing the relationship between a behavior that may change over time and disease occurrence, it is important that the questions refer to the period prior to the onset of disease symptoms. Failure to make this clear can lead to biased results if the behavior changes in the face of symptoms. Both the failure to elicit exposure information from the appropriate period and the inclusion of irrelevant exposure information can lead to bias.

Hypotheticals

Avoid hypothetical questions. Consider a question that might be asked of nurses in an infection control project: "Is it important to wear gloves when placing an IV?" The question is problematic, because it may refer to either what is important in a hypothetical sense or what is personally important to the respondent. The responses will be a mixture of these two interpretations, with the investigator having no way of distinguishing the two.

Asking More Than One Question

Each question should try to elicit only one piece of information. Consider the question, "Have you experienced nausea, vomiting, night sweats, or loss of appetite?" This set of symptoms may be useful in arriving at a diagnosis, but in an epidemiologic investigation it may be important to document each symptom individually for later use in applying a consistent case definition. Furthermore, respondents may focus on the last symptom named. A respondent may have had night sweats but answer, "No, my appetite's fine."

Assumptions in the Questions

Answers to questions that make tacit assumptions can be difficult to interpret. Consider the example from Kelsey et al. (1): "Do you bring up phlegm when you cough?" The question assumes that a cough is present. A negative response might mean that no phlegm is produced or that the respondent does not have a cough.

Vague Questions and Answers

Avoid the use of words such as "regularly," "frequently," and "often," both in questions and as response options. Different responders will interpret these words differently. The potential for qualitative responses to introduce unwanted variability was vividly demonstrated by Bryant and Norman (2), who asked 16 physicians to assign a numerical probability to qualitative adjectives such as "probable," "normally," and "always." The numerical probability assigned to the word "probable" ranged from 30% to 95%. The probability assigned to "normally" ranged from 40% to 100%, and that to "always" ranged from 70% to 100%. Whenever possible, try to elicit a quantitative response.

Threatening Questions

Care needs to be taken when asking questions of a somewhat embarrassing nature. Embarrassing questions concern respondent behaviors that may be illegal or socially undesirable, or concern areas of life that may threaten the respondent's self-esteem. Research has indicated that the self-reported frequency of potentially embarrassing behaviors can be increased if long, open-ended questions are asked. Open-ended questions are those to which categories of set responses are not supplied by the investigator (as opposed to closed questions, in which the respondents select answers from a list of supplied alternatives). Bradburn and Sudman (3) contrasted various question styles ranging from short questions with fixed response categories to very long questions with open-ended responses. They also contrasted using the respondent's familiar term for the behavior versus a term supplied by an interviewer. Respondents were randomized in a 2 × 2 × 2 factorial design into one of eight different question formats (i.e., long vs. short response format, open vs. closed response format, and familiar vs. standard wording). One short question (with standard wording and closed response format) read: "In the past year, how often did you become intoxicated while drinking any kind of beverage?" The respondents picked a response from a list of eight alternatives. The long form (with respondent's wording and open response format) read:

> Sometimes people drink a little too much beer, wine, or whiskey so that they act different from usual. What word do you think we should use to describe people when they get that way, so that you will know what we mean and feel comfortable talking about it?
>
> Occasionally, people drink on an empty stomach or drink a little too much and become [respondent's word]. In the past year, how often have you become [respondent's word] while drinking any kind of alcoholic beverage?

The respondents were given no response categories, but asked to supply their own best estimate. The question format did not seem to affect the percentage of people reporting that they had engaged in an activity. It did, however, strongly influence the self-reported frequency of the activity. Those responding to long questions with open-ended responses using familiar terms reported significantly higher frequencies of the behavior of interest. The mean annual consumption of cans of beer calculated using responses from the long, open format with familiar wording was 320 cans; that calculated using the short, closed format with standard wording was 131 cans. Large differences in responses attributable to question format were seen for questions dealing with the frequency of sexual activity as well. Most of the difference was attributable to the use of an open-ended response format and longer questions. The effect of using familiar wording was weaker but was associated with consistently higher reported frequencies of potentially embarrassing behaviors.

Asking Questions About Events in the Past

Asking individuals about the occurrence and/or frequency of specific events in the past is a special measurement challenge. An investigator whose study depends on the validity of human recall must be particularly attuned to the shortcomings of human memory. Respondents to epidemiologic questionnaires are often asked to perform one of three memory tasks: (a) recall whether a particular event occurred to the individual, (b) recall when the event occurred, or (c) recall how frequently it occurred. Research has shown that it takes some time for people to access their memory for the occurrence of events. Longer questions seem to be useful in giving respondents more time to recall events and may increase the percentage of events recalled (4). Nevertheless, people frequently forget specific events in their past. As a rule, an event is harder to remember if (a) it occurred a long time ago, (b) it is one of a series of similar events, or (c) the respondent attaches little significance to it (4).

People also frequently misplace remembered events in time. There is a tendency to judge events that are harder to recall as less recent and, conversely, there is a tendency to date events about which a lot of detail is recalled as more recent. This problem is termed "telescoping" in survey research (4). Consider the question: "Have you been to a doctor in the past 12 months?" Respondents frequently answer affirmatively if the visit was 15 months ago. People may remember the event better than its date and import the event into the time interval of interest.

Aspects of the design and administration of questionnaires can improve both remembering and dating events. Questions starting with recent events and working backward in time can improve recall. Also, providing date cues can help. One common technique is to provide the respondent with a calendar. Before asking about events of interest, the respondent identifies personally relevant dates such as birthdays and holidays. Then, the respondent is walked back through time and assigns dates to the occurrence of the events of interest with respect to the personal landmarks. As reported by Means et al. (5), a sample of George Washington University Health Plan enrollees was asked to try to recall all health plan visits in the past year. All study participants had at least four visits in the past year. Before using the landmarking technique, participants were able to recall 41% of the health plan visits recorded in the medical record. After the landmarking, 63% of health plan visits were remembered. In a separate study group using only the landmarking technique, 57% of visits were recalled. The use of landmarking also led to an improvement in dating accuracy.

The frequency of a behavior is often of epidemiologic interest insofar as it may serve to quantify the amount and/or rate of an exposure. Humans tend to rely on two strategies for recalling the frequency of events (4). The first is simply trying to remember every instance of a behavior over a period. The second is referred to as the event decomposition method. People first estimate a rate at which a behavior is performed and then apply it over the period of interest. For example, if a respondent is asked how many times she went to a restaurant in the past 2 months, she may figure that she goes to a restaurant twice a week, and therefore, she ate at a restaurant eight times in 2 months. In general, the decomposition method seems to lead to more accurate estimates than the recall of individual events. Investigators planning studies to measure the frequency of exposure may wish to structure questionnaires to explicitly elicit these frequency estimates.

PRETESTING THE DATA COLLECTION INSTRUMENT

Prior to full-scale data collection, it is useful to pretest all study procedures. This includes pretesting any data collection documents. The pretest may include a number of steps. An expert in the field should review the data collection forms. This expert should be able to identify any content omissions. The review by nonexpert colleagues can be useful to give overall impressions, to identify troublesome questions, and to determine if the skip patterns flow logically. In the next phase of pretesting, test the data collection procedures under study conditions on a number of potential study subjects (frequently 20 to 30). In this phase of pretesting, one can identify questions that don't work and whether the needed information is indeed available from the intended data source. If the data collection form is being used to elicit information from respondents, debrief your pretest subjects to discover what they had in mind while they were answering and how some questions might be asked better. A pretest also provides the opportunity to ascertain preferences among varying question wordings and answer formats.

Schlesselman (6) describes an example indicative of the kind of problems that a pretest can identify. In a study involving analgesic use, the following series of questions were tested:

Q. HAVE YOU EVER HAD FREQUENT HEADACHES?

Yes

No

Q. HAVE YOU EVER HAD VERY SEVERE HEADACHES?

Yes

No

Q. HAVE YOU HAD HEADACHES ONCE A WEEK OR MORE DURING THE PAST MONTH?

Yes

No

The third question was used as a filter for a series of questions relating to analgesic use for headache. The purpose of the questions was to identify individuals who were likely to be frequent analgesics users for headache relief. Schlesselman states, "The third question was included under the assumption that recall is better for the most recent period, and that a person with a history of recurrent headaches in the past would retain this pattern in the present." In pretesting, however, it was found that there were many patients who had frequent headaches but for whom the past month was atypical. Thus, contrary to the intention of the investigator, a number of study participants were skipping the series of headache-analgesic questions. In light of the pretest the third question was modified to:

Q. HAVE YOU EVER HAD HEADACHES ONCE A WEEK OR MORE FOR AT LEAST ONE MONTH?

OPTIONS FOR ADMINISTRATION

The primary options for administering a questionnaire are respondent self-administered and interviewer-administered.

Self-administered questionnaires can be either given in a supervised setting or mailed to the respondent. Interviewer-administered questionnaires can be administered either in person or over the phone. Each method has its advantages and drawbacks. Self-administered questionnaires are usually less expensive to administer but need to be simpler and shorter than interviewer-administered questionnaires. Also, when a portion of the study population is of low literacy, the use of self-administered forms results in unacceptable losses of information. Interviewer-administered questionnaires can be more complicated and longer, and the literacy of the respondent is not an issue. Also, the use of an interviewer permits the probing of the respondent for clarifications and elaborations. The major drawback of using an interviewer is the cost.

Differing modes of administration have their advantages and disadvantages. Mailed questionnaires are relatively inexpensive to administer, but response rates tend to be low (typically 40–60%). Response rates can be increased by a number of techniques such as hand-addressing the envelopes, using certified mail, using postage stamps instead of metered mail, and rewarding the respondent. Data collecting over the phone is more expensive than by mail, but the response rates are higher (frequently 75–85%). Completion rates for telephone interviews can be increased by sending an introductory letter to the home introducing the study. Using the phone as the sole mode of contact may introduce subtle biases into a study. The portion of the study population that does not own a phone is systematically different from the portion that does. Also, the ability to contact certain segments of a population may differ. For example, young, single, smoking males are harder to contact by phone than some other segments of the population.

Face-to-face interviews have the highest completion rates (up to 90%), and they are also the most expensive to conduct. In face-to-face situations, visual aids and more elaborate questioning techniques can be used, providing the opportunity to improve the quality of the collected data.

MEDICAL RECORDS

Collecting data from recorded information is a part of nearly all epidemiologic studies conducted in a hospital setting. Recorded data sources include diagnostic reports, physician notes, prescription records, and culture reports. In addition to routinely collected medical data, administratively collected data are also available from billing records, insurance claim files, etc. The advantages of recorded data are clear: they provide a concurrent source of information concerning the study subject's medical experience. However, the limitations of routinely recorded data should also be borne in mind. Data are put in the medical record by a number of different individuals who are not standardized in their recording habits, and they certainly do not record information with a particular epidemiologic study in mind. Two studies illustrate the problems with the medical record as a tool for epidemiologic research.

Massanari et al. (7) compared the ability of one hospital's medical records personnel to identify and code the presence of nosocomial infections to that of an epidemiologic surveillance system. They discovered that only 43% of nosocomial infections identified through epidemiologic surveillance were reported in the discharge abstract. On inspection of a sample of incongruent cases, 44% of the cases were missed by medical records, because the physician failed to document an infection. However, medical records personnel failed to note infections clearly recorded in the chart about 16% of the time. Other studies concerning the usefulness of the medical chart in infectious diseases investigations in the hospital have documented even poorer performance (8,9).

Gerbert et al. (10) compared four methods to determine whether specific drugs had been prescribed to chronic obstructive pulmonary disease patients. The methods were a physician interview, a chart review, a patient interview, and a review of a videotape of a physician patient encounter. The four methods agreed only 36% of the time in determining whether the patient had been prescribed theophylline. According to the physician, 78% of patients were on theophylline, the medical chart indicated that 62% of patients were on the medication, and the videotape, 69%. Only 59% of the patients reported themselves to be on theophylline. The investigators determined that each method had good specificity (i.e., few respondents reported being on theophylline when they were not) and that the physician interview had the best sensitivity.

ELECTRONIC DATA

Electronic data comes from two sources: administrative data, which is used by all hospitals primarily for billing, and clinical data, such as medication administration records, laboratory, and radiology reports. The richness of clinical data available to the investigator varies among hospitals.

Administrative data from hospitals includes demographic information, admission and discharge dates, codes for principal and other diagnoses, procedure codes, disposition of the patient, and expected payment source (11). Although universally available, administrative data should be used with great caution for hospital epidemiology, primarily because of issues relating to sensitivity and specificity in diagnosis codes (12). In studies examining the reliability of discharge data forwarded to the Health Care Financing Administration, data items such as admission date, discharge date, date of birth, gender, and payment source were found to agree well with those found in the medical record (13). However, on review, the reported principal diagnosis agreed with that found in the medical record only 57% of the time. Similarly, Johnson and Appel (14) found that the diagnosis-related group reported to Medicare matched the one listed in the medical record approximately half of the time.

Even if data are reliably collected, the failure to understand how administrative databases are maintained can introduce artifactual findings. For example, Iezzoni et al. (15) found lower death rates among hospital inpatients with diabetes listed as a comorbidity in an administrative database. The reason was that the database accommodated only five comorbidities. Therefore, the relatively healthy patients (i.e., the ones with fewer acute problems) were the ones for whom the diagnosis of diabetes made it into the database.

Clinical data may be more useful for surveillance in hospital epidemiology (16–19). Classen et al. (18) described surveillance using the Health Evaluation through Logical Processing (HELP) system, of LDS Hospital in Salt Lake City, Utah. This system includes data from pharmacy, laboratory, surgery, radiology, admitting, microbiology, and pathology. Furthermore, clinical data (e.g., International Classification of Disease codes) and charge data are also a part of this system. Initial studies revealed that a computer algorithm identified more hospital-acquired infections than traditional surveillance methods, while requiring only 35% of the time (20). Several subsequent investigations of infections (21,22) and adverse drug reactions (23,24) have been conducted using this system.

PREPARING DATA FOR STATISTICAL ANALYSIS

Organization of Data Collection

Attention to the format of a data collection document can speed data collection and data entry and increase data quality. The physical appearance of the data collection document is also important. A professional-looking tool can inspire the respondent's confidence in the investigator.

A data collection form has two sections: the header and the body. The header should contain a form code, a form version number, and a unique identifier corresponding to the participant about whom data are being collected. In hospital epidemiology, a patient's medical record number is often used. The identification number allows the data collected on the form to be linked with data collected from other sources. A code for the form and its version are useful in establishing the data's provenance after computer files have been generated.

The body of the basic data collection form has three elements: the questions, the responses, and the directions. In Fig. 5.1, each element is typographically distinct. The questions are in all capital letters, the responses are in bold, and the directions to the interviewer are in italics.

The questions should flow in some sort of natural order. For instance, if the data collection form is being used to abstract a medical record, the questions should appear in the order that the information is found in the medical record. If the questionnaire is to be administered to an individual, an introduction should be included, questions on the same topic should be grouped together, and when the topic of the questions changes, a short transition statement should be included. It may be a good idea to begin questionnaires with less challenging and personal questions. This gives the respondent an opportunity to become familiar with the interview situation and to develop some rapport with the interviewer.

A different form should be developed for each data source. This allows data entry to move forward on the sections of the data collection effort that have been completed. If multiple data sources are used in a study, consider using differently colored paper for each data form. This allows quick identification of misfiled forms and incomplete sets of data forms. Do not squeeze too much type on a page. Blank space allows data collectors to make annotations as needed.

Formatting Responses to Questions

Moving information from idea to report involves three steps: (a) design of the data collection instrument, (b) data entry from data collection instrument to an electronic database, and (c) querying the database to obtain "flat files" suitable for statistical analysis. Because collected data are ultimately transferred to statistical analysis software, selecting appropriate formatting in the data collection instrument saves time and aggravation in the long term. Thus the adage "Begin with the end in mind" is particularly germane to design of the data collection instrument.

Closed- or Open-Ended Responses

An important decision is whether to have open-ended or closed-ended response formats. An open-ended response format allows the respondent to provide any answer (question 1 in Table 5.1), and is more appropriate for exploratory or hypothesis generating research. A closed-ended response format requires the respondent to select an answer from a list of possible responses supplied by the investigator (question 2 in Table 5.1). Open-ended formats allow respondents to elaborate on the answer and to provide details that may be missed by a closed-ended format. In general, however, open response formats are to be avoided. Answers can be lengthy, hard to analyze, and hard to standardize. The problem with open-ended formats can be seen in question 1 of the table. Respondents could answer "big" or "old." The responses provided in the closed-ended format cue the respondent to the frame-of-reference of the question. Because of the opportunities for misunderstandings, questionnaires using open-ended responses often need to be administered by a trained interviewer to probe incomplete answers and to lead respondents if they do not understand the intent of the question.

The answers to open-ended questions need to be assigned codes for use in data analysis. Closed-ended response formats allow data collection forms to be precoded. This means that, prior to the administration of the form, responses have already been assigned the numerical codes to be used in the data analysis. When respondents pick a response, they actually mark its code (question 3 in Table 5.1).

If there are a great number of potential responses (e.g., a respondent's occupation or place of birth), a closed-ended response may be impractical. In this case, the response is recorded for coding at a later time.

Closed-ended response categories should be exhaustive and mutually exclusive. That is to say, every possible response should be provided for, and no two responses should be logically possible at the same time. It should be recognized, however, that closed-ended responses impose the investigator's preconceptions concerning the universe of possible responses. There are certain to be unanticipated responses. A compromise between closed-ended and open-ended formats can be made.

Coding "Other" Responses

One can precode the most frequently expected responses and include an "other" category along with a space for recording what is meant by "other." These "other" responses can be logged

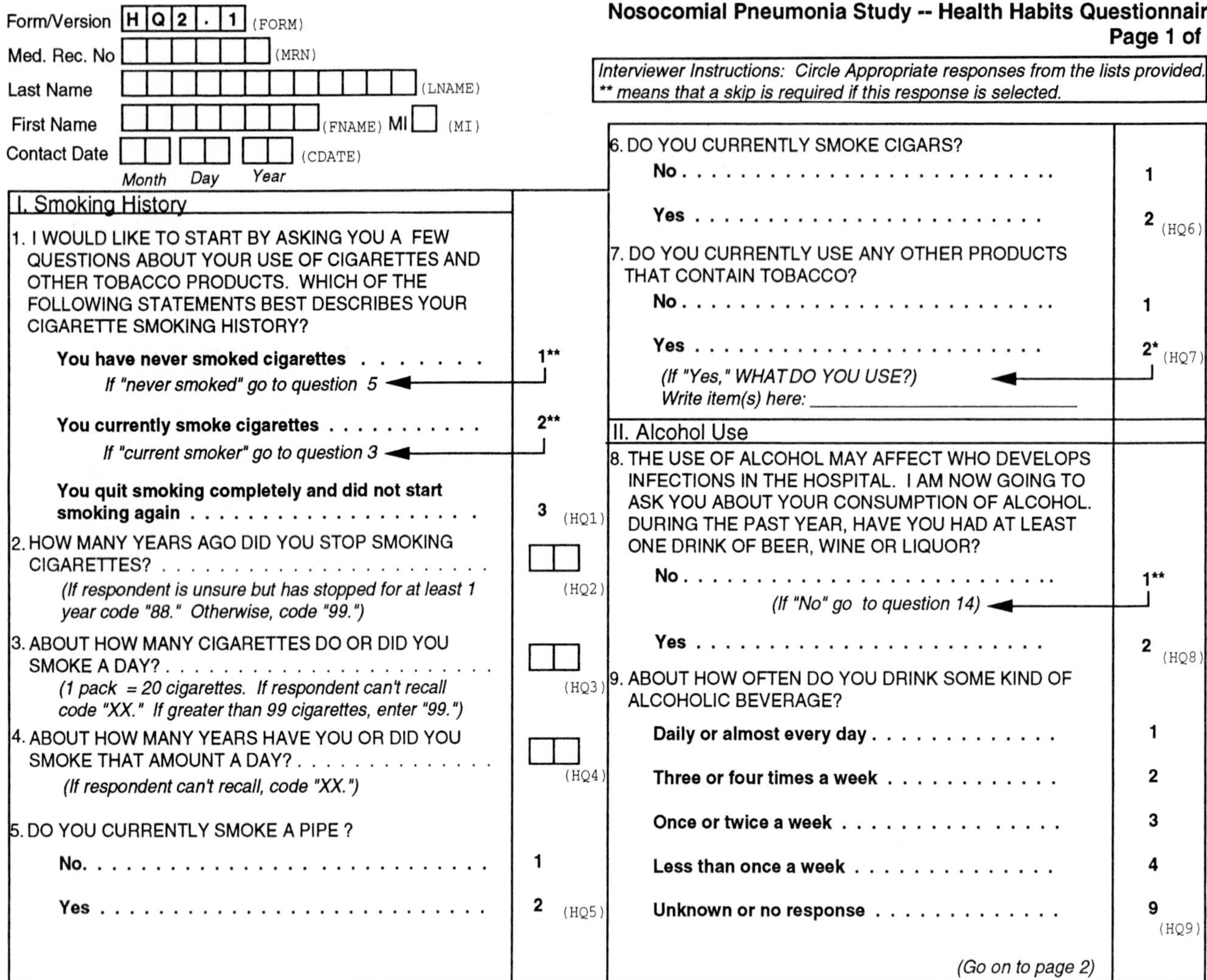

Form/Version H Q 2 . 1 (FORM)
Med. Rec. No (MRN)
Last Name (LNAME)
First Name (FNAME) MI (MI)
Contact Date (CDATE)
Month Day Year

Nosocomial Pneumonia Study -- Health Habits Questionnaire
Page 1 of 4

Interviewer Instructions: Circle Appropriate responses from the lists provided.
*** means that a skip is required if this response is selected.*

I. Smoking History

1. I WOULD LIKE TO START BY ASKING YOU A FEW QUESTIONS ABOUT YOUR USE OF CIGARETTES AND OTHER TOBACCO PRODUCTS. WHICH OF THE FOLLOWING STATEMENTS BEST DESCRIBES YOUR CIGARETTE SMOKING HISTORY?
   - **You have never smoked cigarettes** 1**
     If "never smoked" go to question 5
   - **You currently smoke cigarettes** 2**
     If "current smoker" go to question 3
   - **You quit smoking completely and did not start smoking again** 3 (HQ1)
2. HOW MANY YEARS AGO DID YOU STOP SMOKING CIGARETTES? . . . . (HQ2)
   (If respondent is unsure but has stopped for at least 1 year code "88." Otherwise, code "99.")
3. ABOUT HOW MANY CIGARETTES DO OR DID YOU SMOKE A DAY? . . . . (HQ3)
   (1 pack = 20 cigarettes. If respondent can't recall code "XX." If greater than 99 cigarettes, enter "99.")
4. ABOUT HOW MANY YEARS HAVE YOU OR DID YOU SMOKE THAT AMOUNT A DAY? . . . . (HQ4)
   (If respondent can't recall, code "XX.")
5. DO YOU CURRENTLY SMOKE A PIPE ?
   - **No.** 1
   - **Yes** 2 (HQ5)
6. DO YOU CURRENTLY SMOKE CIGARS?
   - **No** 1
   - **Yes** 2 (HQ6)
7. DO YOU CURRENTLY USE ANY OTHER PRODUCTS THAT CONTAIN TOBACCO?
   - **No** 1
   - **Yes** 2* (HQ7)
     (If "Yes," WHAT DO YOU USE?)
     Write item(s) here: ______________

II. Alcohol Use

8. THE USE OF ALCOHOL MAY AFFECT WHO DEVELOPS INFECTIONS IN THE HOSPITAL. I AM NOW GOING TO ASK YOU ABOUT YOUR CONSUMPTION OF ALCOHOL. DURING THE PAST YEAR, HAVE YOU HAD AT LEAST ONE DRINK OF BEER, WINE OR LIQUOR?
   - **No** 1**
     (If "No" go to question 14)
   - **Yes** 2 (HQ8)
9. ABOUT HOW OFTEN DO YOU DRINK SOME KIND OF ALCOHOLIC BEVERAGE?
   - **Daily or almost every day** 1
   - **Three or four times a week** 2
   - **Once or twice a week** 3
   - **Less than once a week** 4
   - **Unknown or no response** 9 (HQ9)

(Go on to page 2)

Figure 5.1. A page from a data collection form from a study of nosocomial pneumonia.

and assigned codes during the data editing process. The value of accommodating "other" responses is illustrated by the experience of Kelsey et al. (1). In a case-control study of the etiology of lumbar disc rupture, participants were asked what type of chair they sat in at work. The main difference between case-patients and control subjects was the selection of the "other" category by the case-patients. The excess of "other" responses was attributable to the omission of motor vehicle seats as a response option. This led to the finding that the vibration associated with frequent motor vehicle use was associated with disc disease, a finding that was subsequently corroborated by further epidemiologic and biomechanical studies.

A common error is to omit the categories "not applicable," "unknown," and "refused" from response lists. Their omission causes a problem when editing the data. If a "not applicable" code is omitted, then when an item is indeed not applicable, the question will be left unanswered. During editing, however, it is impossible to tell whether the question was skipped inadvertently or purposefully left blank. For record abstraction forms, a "not found" category is needed.

Do not try to force actual measurements into a closed-ended format; this may result in the unintended loss of information. Take, for example, the following question:

Q8. WHITE BLOOD CELL COUNT ON ADMISSION?
(circle the appropriate finding)

Less than 10,000	1
10,000–15,000	2
More than 15,000	3
Not ordered	8
Not found	9

Collecting data in this manner automatically constrains the investigator to analyze white blood cell count as a categorical variable. Although a categorical approach may or may not be appropriate, the investigator is further constrained, because the only categories that can be used in the analysis are those specified by the form. It is usually better to collect data in as much detail as the data source will permit, as this maintains greater flexibility in the data analysis. For example:

TABLE 5.1. EXAMPLES OF THREE DIFFERENT QUESTION RESPONSE FORMATS

A question with an open-ended response format:

1. How would you describe your residence, that is, the place where you usually live?
   __________________________ (answer here)

A question with a closed-ended response format:

2. How would you describe your residence, that is, the place where you usually live? *(Circle the correct response):*
   House
   Duplex
   Condominium
   Apartment
   Hotel
   Other

A question with a precoded closed-ended response format:

3. How would you describe your residence, that is, the place where you usually live? *(Circle the number of the correct response):*

House	1
Duplex	2
Condominium	3
Apartment	4
Hotel	5
Other	6

Q8. WHITE BLOOD CELL COUNT ON ADMISSION?
Q8. *(code 88,888 if not ordered, code 99,999 if not found)*

Again, special codes for "not found" and/or "not applicable" should be included to allow the later identification of missed items on the data form.

To ease data entry, the responses should be placed along the right margin of the form and presented as vertical lists (Fig. 5.1). Including question numbers with the responses helps data entry clerks keep their place when entering the data into a computer.

Often a number of questions do not apply to every study subject. Instructions to guide respondents past nonapplicable questions need to be clearly made. In the example (Fig. 5.1), in addition to the text instructions, visual cues are provided to guide the interviewer. Failure to skip properly can be a frequent source of error in filling out data collection forms. If the data collection form is to be self-administered by a study participant, try to keep the number of skips to a minimum.

Frequent skips are demanding even on experienced study personnel and can lead to errors in filling out study forms. Often, if there is only one question to be skipped, adding an additional response category can avoid the need for a skip instruction altogether. For example, consider the two questions:

4. DO YOU NOW SMOKE CIGARETTES?

Yes	1
No	2 *(If no, go to question 6)*

5. HOW MANY CIGARETTES DO YOU USUALLY SMOKE IN A DAY?

1 to 10	1
11 to 19	2
20 or more	3

In this situation a skip can be avoided by dropping question 4 and providing a fourth response option in question 5: "I do not currently smoke cigarettes.

Use Numeric Rather Than Text Entry

If questions are to be precoded, codings should be consistent throughout the form. Pocock (25) suggests using 1 for "No" and 2 for "Yes," because "No" is the more common response. Often an 8 is used for "not applicable" and 9 for "missing."

Questions That Require Calculation

Avoid questions that require calculation on the part of either the data collector or the respondent. If the number of days between two events is important, collect the actual dates of the events and calculate the difference later. Asking individuals to calculate simply introduces an additional opportunity for error.

CONCLUSION

Hierholzer (26) has called data the epidemiologist's sand. A lens maker takes sand, refines it, melts it, and, through a long process of grinding and smoothing, fashions a lens with which to see the world more clearly. Similarly, an epidemiologist takes data, refines it, and smooths it until a clearer picture of nature is revealed. If the sand is dirty or impure, the lens will be cloudy and distorted. If data are unreliable or invalid, the epidemiologist's understanding of nature will be clouded and distorted. By paying close attention to the data collection process, from the conception of the data collection document through the editing of the data after they are collected, the epidemiologist helps keep his sand pure so that, in the end, nature may be viewed with as much clarity as possible.

This chapter provided a practical overview of data collection in hospital settings. To find more complete discussions of issues surrounding the strengths and limitations of various data sources, and the design and administration of opinion surveys, consult several useful reviews that have served as the basis of this chapter (11,27–29).

REFERENCES

1. Kelsey JL, Thompson WD, Evans AS. *Methods in observational epidemiology.* New York: Oxford University Press, 1986.
2. Bryant GD, Norman GR. Expressions of probability: words and numbers. *N Engl J Med* 1980;302(7):411.
3. Bradburn NM, Sudman S. *Improving interview and questionnaire design.* San Francisco: Josey-Bass, 1979:26–50.
4. Bradburn NM, Rips LJ, Shevell SK. Answering autobiographical questions: the impact of memory and inference on surveys. *Science* 1987; 236(4798):157–161.
5. Means B, Nigam A, Zarrow M, et al. Autobiographical memory for health-related events. *Vital Health Stat* 1989;6(2):1–22.
6. Schlesselman JJ. *Case-control studies: design, conduct, analysis.* New York: Oxford University Press, 1982.
7. Massanari RM, Wilkerson K, Streed SA, et al. Reliability of reporting nosocomial infections in the discharge abstract and implications for receipt of revenues under prospective reimbursement. *Am J Public Health* 1987;77(5):561–564.
8. Freeman J, McGowan JE Jr. Risk factors for nosocomial infection. *J Infect Dis* 1978;138(6):811–819.
9. Marrie TJ, Durant H, Sealy E. Pneumonia—the quality of medical records data. *Med Care* 1987;25(1):20–24.

10. Gerbert B, Stone G, Stulbarg M, et al. Agreement among physician assessment methods. Searching for the truth among fallible methods. *Med Care* 1988;26(6):519–535.
11. Iezzoni LI. Assessing quality using administrative data. *Ann Intern Med* 1997;127(8 pt 2):666–674.
12. Surjan G. Questions on validity of International Classification of Diseases-coded diagnoses. *Int J Med Inf* 1999;54(2):77–95.
13. Demlo LK, Campbell PM, Brown SS. Reliability of information abstracted from patients' medical records. *Med Care* 1978;16(12): 995–1005.
14. Johnson AN, Appel GL. DRGs and hospital case records: implications for Medicare case mix accuracy. *Inquiry* 1984;21(2):128–134.
15. Iezzoni LI, Foley SM, Daley J, et al. Comorbidities, complications, and coding bias. Does the number of diagnosis codes matter in predicting in-hospital mortality? *JAMA* 1992;267(16):2197–2203.
16. Bates DW, Pappius E, Kuperman GJ, et al. Using information systems to measure and improve quality. *Int J Med Inf* 1999;53(2–3):115–124.
17. Bates DW, Evans RS, Murff H, et al. Detecting adverse events using information technology. *J Am Med Inform Assoc* 2003;10(2):115–128.
18. Classen DC, Burke JP, Pestotnik SL, et al. Surveillance for quality assessment: IV. Surveillance using a hospital information system. *Infect Control Hosp Epidemiol* 1991;12(4):239–244.
19. Classen DC, Burke JP. The computer-based patient record: the role of the hospital epidemiologist. *Infect Control Hosp Epidemiol* 1995; 16(12):729–736.
20. Evans RS, Larsen RA, Burke JP, et al. Computer surveillance of hospital-acquired infections and antibiotic use. *JAMA* 1986;256(8): 1007–1011.
21. Evans RS, Burke JP, Classen DC, et al. Computerized identification of patients at high risk for hospital-acquired infection. *Am J Infect Control* 1992;20(1):4–10.
22. Burke JP, Classen DC, Pestotnik SL, et al. The HELP system and its application to infection control. *J Hosp Infect* 1991;18(suppl A): 424–431.
23. Classen DC, Pestotnik SL, Evans RS, et al. Adverse drug events in hospitalized patients. Excess length of stay, extra costs, and attributable mortality. *JAMA* 1997;277(4):301–306.
24. Classen DC, Pestotnik SL, Evans RS, et al. Computerized surveillance of adverse drug events in hospital patients. *JAMA* 1991; 266(20): 2847–2851.
25. Pocock SJ. *Clinical trials: a practical approach.* Chichester: Wiley, 1983: 163.
26. Hierholzer WJ Jr. Health care data, the epidemiologist's sand: comments on the quantity and quality of data. *Am J Med* 1991;91(3B): 21S–26S.
27. McColl E, Jacoby A, Thomas L, et al. Design and use of questionnaires: a review of best practice applicable to surveys of health service staff and patients. *Health Technol Assess* 2001;5(31):1–256.
28. McDonald KM, Romano PS, Davies SM, et al. Measures of patient safety based on hospital administrative data: the patient safety indicators. Technical review 5. (Prepared by the University of California, San Francisco–Stanford Evidence-Based Practice Center under contract No. 290–97–013). AHRQ publication No. 02–0038. Rockville, MD: Agency for Healthcare Research and Quality, 2002.
29. Pottinger JM, Herwaldt LA, Peri TM. Basics of surveillance—an overview. *Infect Control Hosp Epidemiol* 1997;18(7):513–527.

6

DRAMATIC IMPROVEMENTS IN HEALTHCARE QUALITY: YOU CAN DO IT TOO

PETER A. GROSS

"The American health care delivery system is in need of fundamental change" (1). This opening sentence from the Institute of Medicine's (IOM's) *Crossing the Quality Chasm* report in 2000 is incontrovertible. However, evidence for a major effort to change the delivery system is hard to find. Although the change needed depends on who you are—the patient, the physician, the nurse, the hospital administrator, or the payer—and your perspective, the solution will clearly be multifactorial. So, where does one begin?

First, one must be clear on the problem and accept it. In *To Err is Human,* IOM cited two large studies that found that adverse drug events (ADEs) occurred in 2.9% and 3.7% of hospitalizations (2–4). These ADEs were fatal in 6.6% and 13.6% of patients, respectively.

In both studies, more than half of ADEs were due to preventable medical errors. Extrapolations to the entire hospital population of the United States found that 44,000 to 98,000 Americans died from medical errors in 1997. Although some have quibbled with the exact number, even if the true number is half of the quoted number it is too many. To put these numbers in perspective, one should note that 43,458 people died of motor vehicle accidents, 42,297 from breast cancer, and 16,516 from acquired immunodeficiency syndrome (AIDS) in that same year. The total national cost of preventable medical errors that resulted in injury was estimated to be between $17 billion and $29 billion. What has happened to Hippocrates' shibboleth for the medical profession—"first do no harm"?

The net result is that patients and healthcare professionals have lost faith in the system. If one defines a system as "a group of interacting, interrelated, or interdependent elements forming a complex whole" (5), one must conclude that the healthcare system is not a system at all. Inaction and even paralysis surrounds the issue of healthcare reform. The goal of the IOM reports and of this chapter is to try to break the cycle of inaction by presenting proposals to help healthcare professionals move forward and begin to correct this national disgrace.

OPERATIONAL DEFINITIONS

Before going on, a few operational definitions are needed:

- Quality is "the degree to which health services for individuals and populations increase the likelihood of desired health outcomes, and are consistent with current professional knowledge" (6).
- Safety is freedom from accidental injury.
- Error is the failure of a planned action to be completed as intended or the use of a wrong plan to achieve an aim. James Reason defines two types of errors (7):

Error of execution occurs when the correct action does not proceed as intended.

Error of planning occurs when the original intended action is not correct.

- Preventable adverse events are errors that do result in injury.
- Adverse event is an injury resulting from a medical intervention. One should note that not all errors result in an adverse event.

INTERVENTIONS TO IMPROVE HEALTHCARE QUALITY

The IOM's Quality of Health Care in America Committee, formed in 1998, made the following recommendations to address the state of disarray in healthcare. Solutions were proposed on four levels: leadership and knowledge, identification of and learning from errors, setting of performance standards and expectations for safety, and the implementation of safety systems in healthcare organizations.

Leadership and Knowledge

A Center for Patient Safety within the Agency for Healthcare Research and Quality (AHRQ) was created to set national goals for patient safety, track progress in meeting the goals, and issue an annual report. AHRQ should also develop the knowledge and understanding of errors through research and Centers of Excellence and should disseminate that information.

Identification of and Learning from Errors

A nationwide *mandatory, public reporting system* should be established through the states. They should collect standardized information on a defined list of ADEs that result in death or serious harm. The reporting should start with hospitals and then include other healthcare settings. Plans for hospital reporting are currently underway.

The core set of reporting standards should be the responsibility of the National Forum for Health Care Quality Measurement and Reporting. Funding and technical expertise should be provided to the states by the Federal government to establish or adapt their current error reporting systems. The Center for Patient Safety will analyze and aggregate reports from the states to identify patterns of failures in patient safety that must be addressed.

Separate voluntary, confidential reporting systems should be established in healthcare institutions for identifying errors and ADEs that do not result in death or serious injury but spot potential areas for improvement. Funding should be provided for reporting system pilot projects. To support this effort, Congress should pass legislation that provides protection of peer review data on patient safety and quality improvement, which is collected for internal use or shared with others for improving safety and quality.

Performance Standards and Expectations for Safety

Patient safety should be a major focus of performance standards for all healthcare organizations and should be required by regulators and accreditors. Public and private purchasers should provide incentives to healthcare organizations that meet these goals. The Joint Commission for Accreditation of Healthcare Organizations (JCAHO) has already begun this effort with its six National Patient Safety Goals.

As with healthcare organizations, healthcare professionals should also focus more on patient safety. The compliance with performance standards should be an aim of health professional licensing boards. Unsafe providers should be identified, and action should be taken by certifying and credentialing organizations. This level of professional self-discipline has not yet been instituted. Periodic reexaminations and relicensing of doctors, nurses, and other key providers should be based on competence and knowledge of safety practices.

Professional societies should establish a permanent committee dedicated to safety improvement. They should develop a curriculum on patient safety and include safety issues in training certifications processes for their members. Safety information should be disseminated at annual meetings and in periodicals from the societies. Safety issues should be included in the practice guidelines. Collaboration and coordination of their efforts with the Center for Patient Safety and other professional societies should be initiated.

The Food and Drug Administration (FDA) should focus more on safe drug use both before and after a drug is marketed. The FDA should develop and enforce standards for design of drug packing and labeling that focus on patient safety. Pharmaceutical companies should test proposed drug names to avoid sound-alike and look-alike name confusion. The FDA should work with physicians, pharmacists, consumers, drug manufacturers, distributors, pharmacy benefit managers, health plans, and other organizations to assist in identifying and preventing problems in the use of drugs.

Implementation of Safety Systems in Healthcare Organizations

Chief executive officers (CEOs) and boards of trustees should be held accountable for creating a serious commitment to a safe system of care. The organizations and their affiliated professionals should make safety a declared and serious aim by establishing patient safety programs, implementing nonpunitive systems for reporting and analyzing errors, incorporating well-understood safety principles, and establishing interdisciplinary team training programs for providers. The healthcare organization should also implement proven safe medication practices.

These four levels of intervention cannot be implemented overnight. However, concerted efforts should be made to begin the effort. After a few years of increased focus, dramatic progress should be seen.

COMPLEXITY OF BARRIERS TO HEALTHCARE IMPROVEMENT

The complexity of the problem can be seen by reviewing the litany of underuse, overuse, and misuse barriers to improvement (8).

Underuse Barriers

Underuse barriers are as follows:

- Lack of insurance (increases risk of death and disability)
- Composition of copayment and deductibles (e.g., results in decrease in hypertensive treatment)
- Benefit packages that omit preventive care
- Capitation payments
- Recent, rapid increase in medical information available

Total awareness of the medical literature expected (although an unaided human being cannot recall or act effectively on the currently available medical information)

Complexity of study analysis

Slow rate of healthcare systems to adopt sophisticated information systems

Overuse Barriers

Overuse barriers include the following:

- Fee-for-service payments (increase utilization)
- Enthusiasm to perform procedures
- Too frequent referrals to specialists by primary care providers
- Patient pressures for unnecessary treatment (e.g., antibiotics)
- National infatuation with technology [e.g., total body computed tomography (CT) scans]
- Physician fear of malpractice suits

Misuse Barriers

The following are misuse barriers:

1. Harvard Medical Practice study found the following:
   - Errors in diagnosis
   - Mishaps resulting from noninvasive, non-drug-related treatment
   - Mistakes in medication use
   - Technical complications of surgery
   - Surgical wound infections
2. Medication errors result from poor functioning of 15 different systems.
   - Errors in dissemination of knowledge about drugs to doctors and nurses
   - Mistakes in dose and identity checking
   - Mistakes stemming from lack of specific patient information
3. Faulty systems of care are responsible for error more often than individuals are.
   - "We have created systems that depend upon idealized standards of performance and that require individual physicians, nurses, and pharmacists to perform tasks at levels of perfection that cannot be achieved by human beings."

AGENDA FOR CHANGE

The IOM's effort to implement broad change was clearly iterated in *Crossing the Quality Chasm.* It was published the year after *To Err Is Human.* The title of the report comes from the concept that "between the health care we have and the care we could have lies not just a gap, but a chasm." The purpose of the report is to move beyond the patient safety issues described in *To Err Is Human* and to address the need to improve the healthcare delivery system as a whole and to effect change in all the dimensions of quality. The urgency for change is apparent, because the advances in medical knowledge have exceeded the ability to put this new information into practice for the patients' benefit. Furthermore, the lack of adequate clinical information systems to facilitate the implementation of new knowledge has been a national disgrace. Finally, as the population ages, the healthcare needs of the American public have shifted from predominantly acute, episodic care to care for chronic conditions. Chronic conditions now affect almost half of the population and are the leading cause of illness, disability, and death (9,10). The conclusion is that the current system of healthcare delivery will not get better by trying harder. The entire system has to be redesigned and the potential benefits of information technology have to be implemented.

The agenda for change is multifaceted. First, six aims for improvement must be shared goals for all groups responsible for providing care. The six aims are as follows:

1. *Safety*—avoid injury to patients from care intended to help them
2. *Effectiveness* —provide care based on the best scientific evidence when it will benefit (i.e., avoid underuse) and do not provide care when it is unlikely to benefit (i.e., avoid overuse)
3. *Patient-centered*—be respectful of, responsive to, and guided by the individuals needs, preferences, and values
4. *Timeliness*—reduce waiting time for the patient and the provider
5. *Efficiency*—avoid waste of equipment, supplies, ideas, and energy (i.e., avoid misuse)
6. *Equitable*—provide care that is the same regardless of gender, ethnicity, geographic location, and socioeconomic status

Second, a new set of principles should be adopted that will guide the redesign of the system of care. The set of ten principles are as follows:

1. *Care is based on continuous healing relationships.* This means that patients should receive care whenever they need it, 24 hours a day. Beyond face-to-face visits, care can be provided by telephone, over the Internet, and so forth.
2. *Customization is based on patient needs and values.* Although systems are designed to respond to the most common needs, it is also important that they are capable of responding to the individual patient's preferences.
3. *The patient is the source of control.* Patients should be provided with the information required to actively participate in their care. They should be given the opportunity to exercise the degree of control over their care that they choose.
4. *Knowledge is shared and information flows freely.* Patients should have access to their own medical records and to clinical information. Clinicians and patients must communicate effectively and share information.
5. *Decisions are evidence-based.* Care provided to patients is based on the best medical evidence. Care should not vary illogically from clinician to clinician or from place to place.
6. *Safety is a system property.* The care system should not harm patients. Reducing risk requires a greater focus on systems that prevent or mitigate errors.
7. *Transparency is a system property.* Information should be available that describes the system's performance on safety, evidence-based practice, and patient satisfaction. Informed patients and families can better select health plans, hospitals, or clinical practices and can choose among alternative treatments.
8. *Anticipate needs of patient.* The health system should anticipate rather than react to patient needs.
9. *Waste should be decreased continuously.* System resources or patient or provider time should not be wasted.
10. *Cooperation of clinicians is crucial.* Clinicians and institutions should commit to cooperate, collaborate, communicate, and ensure that information is exchanged in a timely fashion and that care is properly coordinated.

Third, priority health conditions that account for the majority of healthcare services delivered should be identified. Initial efforts should focus on these conditions, and innovation should be encouraged to stimulate change. The top 15 conditions are cancer, diabetes, emphysema, high cholesterol, HIV/AIDS, hypertension, ischemic heart disease, stroke, arthritis, asthma, gall bladder disease, stomach ulcers, back problems, Alzheimer's disease and other dementias, and depression and anxiety disorders.

(This list was later modified and expanded from 15 to 20 conditions, see later discussion.)

To deal more effectively with these disorders, systems should be developed that define best practices, provide prevention programs to decrease associated health risk behaviors, create the information infrastructure to support the provision of care and to measure the resultant care, and, finally, align financial incentives in the payment system.

MAJOR CHALLENGES

Organizations have at least six major challenges. They are as follows:

1. *Redesigned care processes.* One size does not fit all. Different diseases require different approaches to implement change. For chronic disorders, in particular, systems must be developed that do not forget about the patient after he or she leaves the hospital but provide for the continuum of care throughout the patient's life. Ed Wagner's chronic care model is an excellent starting point for working with a model of care that deals effectively with the care continuum (9).
2. *Investment in information technology.* Information technology enables physicians and other providers to enter orders on the computer, thereby ensuring identification of the ordering provider and permitting the provider to interact with expert rules that help reduce medical errors. In addition, the technology should eventually permit physician and other provider notes to be typed into an electronic medical record facilitating communication among providers.
3. *Better management of growth in medical knowledge.*Tools to aid the provider in accessing and applying the new knowledge should be available.
4. *Coordination of care.* Coordination of the patient's care by all providers, services, and settings will make care safer and reduce waste. Standardization of care will be facilitated with improved communication.
5. *Care provided by teams.* Team-provided care is a key to more efficient patient management. Physicians are not accustomed to functioning as part of a team. A change in mind set is necessary to accomplish all of the goals.
6. *Measurement of care processes and outcomes.* Measurement of care processes and outcomes must become widespread. As has been said, "If you are not measuring it, you are not managing it." Measurement will identify where performance is at high levels and where improvement is needed.

To accomplish the tasks described, major changes in the environment of care are needed. I have discussed the importance of dealing with new knowledge and ensuring its day-to-day application with every patient. I have also described the importance of improving the information technology infrastructure. What has not yet been considered is the alignment of payment policies and the preparation of the healthcare workforce. These are subjects for other chapters. Briefly, however, the payment of case rates to hospitals and per diem rates to physicians are counterproductive. Hospitals that try to be more efficient by shortening length of stay (although their reimbursement is on a per diem basis) are penalized because increased first-day payments are not allowed for surgical procedures. There are many other examples. Preparation of healthcare workers to orient them toward the six aims and ten principles described previously is another daunting task. Teaching this new approach to physicians, nurses, and other providers must begin in medical, nursing, and other professional schools; must be reiterated in residency and nursing training programs; and must be reinforced with attending physicians, graduate nurses, and other healthcare providers. IOM's *Crossing the Quality Chasm* is a treatise well worth reading to gain a greater understanding of what has been briefly described.

ASSESSMENT OF QUALITY

A National Health Care Quality Report has been developed (11,12). It identifies the most important questions to ask to assess the quality of care and the improvement in quality over time. It will be a barometer of health quality just as the Consumer Price Index and the Index of Leading Economic Indicators are barometers of the economic health of the nation. The quality report complements other reports on the health of the nation such as *Healthy People 2010,* but it is more oriented to personal healthcare rather than to public health.

An annual quality report will increase public awareness of the state of healthcare quality, assess progress, and monitor the effects of national policy changes. The report will point out geographic variations in care (13,14); assess care for chronic diseases such as diabetes; and monitor differences in care by ethnicity, race, gender, age, and health insurance coverage. A mosaic of data sources will be accessed because no single source will meet all the requirements.

Cognizant of the definition of quality stated earlier, two dimensions of care will be addressed. The first dimension is the components of healthcare quality. These include most of the six aims previously described—safety, effectiveness, patient-centeredness, and timeliness. The second dimension relates to the consumers' perspectives on their healthcare needs over their life cycle. These needs change during their life cycle and include the following:

- Staying healthy—preventive care
- Recovering from an illness—acute care
- Living with an illness or disability—chronic care
- Coping with the end of life—palliative care

These four consumer perspectives can be assessed with at least four of the six aims described earlier, as shown in Table 6.1.

TABLE 6.1. CLASSIFICATION MATRIX FOR MEASURES FOR THE NATIONAL HEALTH CARE QUALITY REPORT

	Components of Health Care Quality			
Consumer Perspective on Health Care Needs	Safety	Effectiveness	Patient Centeredness	Timeliness
Staying healthy				
Getting better				
Living with illness or disability				
Coping with the end of life				

Measures to Assess Achievement of High-Quality Care

Using the Table 6.1 matrix, AHRQ will apply the following ten criteria (divided into three groups) to select appropriate measures to assess the achievement of high-care quality.

1. Importance of what is being measured
   - What is the impact on health associated with this problem?
   - Are policy makers and consumers concerned about this area?
   - Can the healthcare system meaningfully address this aspect or problem?
2. Scientific soundness of the measure
   - Does the measure actually measure what it is intended to measure?
   - Does the measure provide stable results across various populations and circumstances?
   - Is there scientific evidence available to support the measure?
3. Feasibility of using the measure
   - Is the measure in use?
   - Can the information needed for the measure be collected in the scale and time frame required?
   - How much will it cost to collect the data needed for the measure?
   - Can the measure be used to compare different groups of the population (e.g., by health conditions, sociodemographic characteristics, or states)?

Structure measures will be avoided. A combination of outcome-validated process measures and condition- or procedure-specific outcome measures will be emphasized. Selection of data sources will depend on credibility and validity, national scope and potential to provide state-level detail, availability and consistency over time and across sources, timeliness, ability to support population subgroup and condition-specific analyses, public accessibility, and comprehensiveness.

The quality report will assess care at the state level. Several versions of the same information will be tailored to different audiences—policymakers, consumers, purchasers, providers, and researchers.

PRIORITY AREAS FOR IMPROVING HEALTHCARE DELIVERY

The next IOM report further defined the priority areas for improving the delivery of healthcare treatments (12). From an initially narrowed list of 60 areas, 20 priority areas were selected based on three factors:

Impact —the extent of the burden or disability, mortality, and economic costs

Improvability—the extent of the gap between current practice and best evidence-based practice

Inclusiveness—relevance to a broad range of individuals

The 20 priority areas are as follows:

- Care coordination (cross-cutting)
- Self-management and health literacy (cross-cutting)
- Asthma—appropriate treatment for persons with mild or moderate persistent asthma
- Evidence-based cancer screening—focus on colorectal and cervical cancer
- Children with special healthcare needs
- Diabetes—focus on appropriate management of early disease
- End of life with advanced organ system failure—focus on congestive heart failure and chronic obstructive pulmonary disease
- Frailty associated with old age—prevention of falls and pressure ulcers, maximization of function, and development of advanced care plans
- Hypertension—focus on appropriate management of early disease
- Immunization—children and adults
- Ischemic heart disease—prevention, reduction of recurring events, and optimization of functional capacity
- Major depression—screening and treatment
- Medication management—prevention of medication errors and overuse of antibiotics
- Nosocomial infections—prevention and surveillance
- Pain control in advanced cancer
- Pregnancy and childbirth—appropriate prenatal and intrapartum care
- Severe and persistent mental illness—focus on treatment in the public sector
- Stroke—early intervention and rehabilitation
- Tobacco dependence treatment in adults
- Obesity (emerging area)

An emerging area is one with high impact and broad inclusiveness but is one in which the evidence base for effective interventions (improvability) is still forming. The 20 areas described can also be grouped into preventive care, behavioral health, chronic conditions, end of life care, care for children and adolescents, and inpatient and surgical care with much overlap among the groups. In the future, revisions may occur in the selection criteria and priority areas as the evidence base is expanded with new knowledge. Assessment of functional status will become more important. Currently, 5 of the 20 priority areas account for 63% of the total deaths in the United States. These five conditions are heart disease, cancer, stroke, chronic obstructive pulmonary disease, and diabetes.

ROLE OF THE PROVIDER

Thus far, this chapter considered the major problems of the dysfunctional healthcare system, the laudable goals in patient care, and, finally, the priority disorders that most deserve the clinician's attention. Now, I identify how the necessary changes can be implemented so that the goal of redesigning the healthcare system can be achieved. My focus is on the new roles and responsibilities of the individual provider of care—physician, nurse, and pharmacist—not on the redesign of the economics of healthcare. The new role of physicians is emphasized.

To determine the new role of the provider, one must reconsider the rules of engagement for the provider. If one uses the currently popular phrase of "simple rules" and redefines the simple rules, then one must consider how the science of implementation can help translate recent scientific advances into practice. Finally, I explore attitudinal changes and technical innovations that will facilitate progress toward the goal of forming a more perfect health system.

In the past, the physician's rules of engagement were that he or she was the captain of the ship and was the sole provider. The physician's word was final and the physician's success or failure was self-assessed. The new simple rules are or should be that the physician is part of an interdisciplinary team of other physicians, nurses, pharmacists, and other healthcare providers. Standards of care are determined by the group, whether it is a national professional organization or a local consensus group. Lastly, physicians and other providers should get feedback on their performance from their peers. Under the new simple rules, the physician can still be captain of the ship, but the physician has to deal with more passengers.

This change in simple rules will be facilitated by the fact that "the human mind cannot possibly remember all a physician has to remember" (personal communication, David Eddy). For example, in the 1960s, approximately 100 randomized controlled trials were published. In the 1990s, the number rose to more than 10,000.

The idea of simple rules is not a new concept. The Declaration of Independence served as the simple rules for a new nation more than 200 years ago, and the Ten Commandments have helped guide the major monotheistic religions of the world.

Now that there are some simple rules to guide clinicians, I discuss some tools to help facilitate change. The implementation strategies are based on several theories for facilitating change (15,16):

- Educational theories—change is driven by the desire to learn and be competent. By interacting with peers, the group can acquire "ownership" (e.g., using local consensus groups).
- Epidemiologic theories—humans are rational beings and will reach a rational decision based on the evidence (e.g., creation of guidelines by professional organizations or performance measures by Medicare).
- Marketing theories—attractive marketing practices will change behavior (e.g., using local opinion leaders, academic detailing, or mass media).
- Behavioral theories—change results from external factors applied before, during, or after the targeted change objectives (e.g., using audit and feedback, reminders, incentives, or sanctions).
- Social influence theories—the social group is important for influencing the desired change (e.g., using local opinion leaders and audit and feedback).
- Organizational theories—altering the system of care can promote change. Hence, the emphasis on the "bad system," not the "bad provider" (e.g., CQI and PDSA cycles).
- Coercive theories—exerting pressure and control will facilitate change (e.g., Medicare laws and JCAHO regulations).

Effectiveness of Strategies

Numerous studies have been conducted to determine which of these implementation measures work all the time, some of the time, or none of the time. Generally effective strategies, variably effective strategies, and generally ineffective strategies are as follows:

1. Generally effective strategies
   - *Reminders* are effective when used sparingly.
   - *Computerized physician order entry systems* with suggestions, warnings, and reminders that pop up during the ordering process for drugs and tests are helpful.
   - *Educational outreach* when learning is *interactive* rather than didactic or when *academic detailing* is done as a one-to-one dialogue between the targeted provider and the expert is effective.
   - *Barrier-oriented interventions* in which local barriers are identified and the interventions tailored to addressing the barriers are effective.
   - *Multifaceted intervention methods* succeed when single interventions fail. Almost all interventions must be multifaceted to have a chance of success.
   - *Use of nonphysician providers* to facilitate change is gaining increasing recognition (17). Nurse practitioners, pharmacists, and other providers can supplement care to help translate research into practice. This is illustrated by the number of practitioners who have near perfect compliance with Medicare's Sixth Scope of Work performance measures sets for community-acquired pneumonia, congestive heart failure, acute myocardial infarction, atrial fibrillation, and stroke and with the Seventh Scope of Work measure sets.
2. Variably effective strategies
   - *Audit and feedback* in which performance of individual physicians is compared with peers may be effective.
   - *Local opinion leaders* are usually considered educationally influential by their peers.
   - *Local consensus groups* often facilitate adoption and can adapt the national practice guidelines or performance measures for local needs.
   - *Consumer education* in which patients are provided information on healthcare intervention that is appropriate for them has had a small effect in the past but may be more influential in the future as consumers become more sophisticated and knowledgeable about their health needs. By increasing patient involvement in healthcare decisions, physicians may be able to provide more effective evidence-based care.
3. Generally Ineffective Strategies
   - *Passive educational programs.* Ironically, this is the area that is most emphasized. Grand rounds and didactic lectures have been shown repeatedly to be ineffective in changing practices. They certainly inform, but the new knowledge usually does not result in a change in practice. Similarly, dissemination of guidelines and publication of research findings inform do not change behavior. If all of these didactic approaches were made interactive, change might follow.

SUMMARY

Awareness of the previously described tools for implementing change plus a reorientation in the attitude when approaching care will permit the redesigning of a more effective healthcare system for the twenty-first century. The ten principles outlined from *Crossing the Quality Chasm* are the starting point. I have used the previously described implementation tools in a multifaceted approach for Medicare's five diseases in the Sixth Scope of Work and have achieved at least 90% compliance for most of the measures. A nurse practitioner was the key to successful implementation (17).

Finally, one must abandon the expectation that physicians, nurses, and other clinicians will perform perfectly (8). The individual provider must function as part of a team. Evidence-based guidelines should be embraced to reduce inappropriate practice variation (13,14). Computerized systems can help to keep track of patients' past history, to increase the accuracy of medication orders, and to schedule reminders for screening tests. Clinicians' jobs must be redesigned to prevent errors and increase safety (18). Computerized systems will help clinicians to avoid reliance on memory and to keep vigilant.

Key care processes must be simplified and standardized using checklists, order sets, and other protocols. The impact of work hours, staffing ratios, and staff education in the new care systems must be evaluated. Pharmaceutical software for hospitals and offices must be designed to point out drug interactions and incorrect doses. Up-to-date evidence-based information must be readily available and incorporated into the system of care more rapidly.

Although American clinicians have come far in improving healthcare, it is still astounding to consider how infrequently best practices are implemented decades after the best practices have been described. It is even more surprising how little attention has been paid to medical error prevention. Acknowledging faults in care is the first step to eliminating those faults. With the new concepts of the importance of teamwork, especially in chronic care; greater involvement of patients in their care; communication among providers; the benefits of information technology; and the greater understanding of the science of guideline implementation the provision of nearly perfect, safe healthcare in the twenty-first century will become a reality.

ACKNOWLEDGMENT

This work was supported in part by The Robert Wood Johnson Foundation grant—Pursuing Perfection: Raising the Bar for Health Care Performance.

REFERENCES

1. Committee on Quality of Health Care in America, Institute of Medicine. *Crossing the quality chasm: a new health system for the 21st century.* Washington DC: National Academy Press, 2001.
2. Committee on Quality of Health Care in America, Institute of Medicine. *To err is human: building a safe health system.* Washington DC: National Academy Press, 2000.
3. Brennan TA, Leape LL, Laird NM, et al. Incidence of adverse events and negligence in hospitalized patients. *N Engl J Med* 1991;324: 370–376.
4. Thomas EJ, Studdert DM, Newhouse JP, et al. Costs of mechanical injuries in Utah and Colorado. *Inquiry* 1999;36:255–264.
5. *The American Heritage dictionary of the English language,* 4th ed. Boston, New York: Houghton Mifflin Company, 2000.
6. Lohr L, ed. *Medicare: a strategy for quality assurance,* vol 2. Washington DC: Institute of Medicine, National Academy Press, 1990.
7. Reason J. Understanding adverse events: the human factor. In: Vincent C, ed. *Clinical risk management: enhancing patient safety,* 2nd ed. BMJ Books, 2001:6–30.
8. Chassin M. Is health care ready for six sigma quality? *Milbank Q* 1998; 76:565–591.
9. Resources for improving chronic care. Available at *http://www.improvingchroniccare.org/resources/bibliography/ccm.html* (accessed Jan 30, 2003).
10. Bodenheimer T, Wagner EH, Grumbach K. Improving primary care for patients with chronic illness: the chronic care model, part 2. *JAMA* 2002;288:1909–1914.
11. Hurtado MP, Swift EK, Corrigan JM, eds. *Envisioning the National Health Care Quality Report.* Washington DC: Institute of Medicine, National Academy Press, 2001.
12. Adams K, Corrigan JM, eds. *Priority areas for national action: transforming health care quality.* Washington DC: Institute of Medicine, National Academy Press, 2002.
13. Fisher ES, Wennberg DE, Stukel TA, et al. The implications of regional variations in Medicare spending. Part 1: the content, quality, and accessibility of care. *Ann Intern Med* 2003;138:273–287.
14. Fisher ES, Wennberg DE, Stukel TA, et al. The implications of regional variations in Medicare spending. Part 2: health outcomes and satisfaction with care. *Ann Intern Med* 2003;138:288–298.
15. Grol R, Grimshaw J. Evidence-based implementation of evidence-based medicine. *Jt Comm Qual Improv* 1999;25:503–521.
16. Gross PA, Greenfield S, Cretin S, et al. Optimal methods for guideline implementation: conclusions from Leeds Castle meeting. *Med Care* 2001;39(8 Suppl 2):II-85–92.
17. Gross PA, Patriaco D, McGuire K, et al. A nurse practitioner intervention model to maximize efficient use of telemetry resources. *Jt Comm J Qual Improv* 2002;28:566–573.
18. Nolan TW. System changes to improve patient safety. *BMJ* 2000;320: 771–773.

7

INVESTIGATION OF OUTBREAKS

WILLIAM R. JARVIS

Although most healthcare-associated infections (HAIs) in a given healthcare facility are endemic (1), outbreaks of HAIs may occur, usually in a specific group of patients. In addition, healthcare workers (HCWs) are exposed to numerous infectious diseases and may be at risk of spreading pathogens to patients and other HCWs (2–4).

An outbreak is an increase in occurrence of a complication or disease above the background rate. This implies that surveillance for such complications exists so that a background rate is known or can be calculated from existing data or requires that a retrospective review be performed to obtain these data for comparison. An outbreak may be one episode of a rare occurrence [e.g., group A streptococcal surgical site infection (SSI), anthrax, etc.] or many episodes of a common occurrence (e.g., methicillin-resistant *Staphylococcus aureus* SSI). Outbreaks in healthcare facilities, although infrequent, can cause great concern, require extensive personnel and financial resources, and can be very time-consuming.

This chapter helps hospital epidemiologists and infection control personnel determine when a cluster of infections or other complications among patients or HCWs merits an epidemiologic investigation and how to conduct such an investigation. Although the methods described can be applied to infectious diseases, chronic diseases, occupational diseases or injuries, or other complications of healthcare delivery, this chapter focuses on outbreak investigations of HAIs.

IDENTIFICATION OF A POTENTIAL OUTBREAK

Routine surveillance for HAI provides the data to enable infection control personnel to calculate infection rates, determine secular trends in pathogens, and identify unusual pathogens or increased infection rates in patients or HCWs (see Chapter 94). The key to effective surveillance is to use common, accepted definitions and to calculate rates that permit valid interhospital or intrahospital comparisons (5–9). Rate calculations using an inappropriate denominator may be misleading and suggest an outbreak is occurring, when only a change in the population at risk has occurred. Similarly, use of variably defined numerator events may lead to an apparent increase in the rate secondary to surveillance artifact. Outbreaks of infectious diseases that are not included in routine surveillance or that occur among patients in areas where routine surveillance may not be conducted may be identified in a variety of ways. Clinical nursing or medical staff may recognize that a number of patients have the same type of infection or regular examination of microbiology or other records may reveal an increase in the isolation of a particular microorganism, thus leading to the identification of a potential outbreak.

REASONS TO INVESTIGATE A POTENTIAL OUTBREAK

Objectives

Although any cluster of patients with HAIs can be investigated, the constraints of time and resources require that each investigation have specific objectives. The most important of these is the control of further transmission (10). Other important objectives may be to advance the field of healthcare epidemiology and infection control by describing etiologic agents or describing host, virulence, or environmental factors; to assess prevention interventions; or to determine the quality of epidemiologic surveillance at the healthcare facility (11).

Evidence of Healthcare-Associated Transmission of Infectious Diseases

HAI transmission should be considered when (a) a cluster of similar infections occurs on one hospital unit or among similar patients, (b) a cluster of infections associated with invasive devices occurs, (c) HCWs and patients develop the same type of infection, or (d) a cluster of infections with microorganisms typically associated with HAIs (e.g., multidrug-resistant or opportunistic microorganisms) occurs. These clusters merit investigation to determine if HAI transmission is really occurring and to institute appropriate control measures to stop transmission. Selection bias frequently occurs in identifying outbreaks because unusual pathogens, or common microorganisms with unusual antimicrobial susceptibility patterns, are more easily recognized. For example, although *Escherichia coli* urinary tract infection outbreaks probably occur, they are either not recognized or not investigated, because the microorganism is the most common cause of urinary tract infections and typing of the strains usually is not performed. In contrast, a small cluster of unusual pathogens or common pathogens with unusual antimicrobial susceptibility patterns are easily and frequently recognized.

Determination of Risk Factors for Disease

Known host risk factors for HAI include the presence of invasive devices, severity of illness, or underlying diseases (12–14). In addition, environmental sources of infection can play a role, especially among immunocompromised patients (15–19). Investigation of outbreaks can further define both host and environmental risk factors for HAI. Infection control personnel should be constantly vigilant for complications associated with new technologies or changes in previously safe technologies (20–23).

Institution of Appropriate Control Measures

In outbreak situations, one often must introduce preventive interventions to control pathogen transmission and adverse outcomes before an investigation is initiated or completed. Control measures that have proven effective in similar HAI outbreaks in the past can be implemented immediately. This could include measures ranging from the simple (e.g., conducting hand hygiene in-service sessions for personnel) to the complex (e.g., closing a unit to new admissions or removing a product or device). The potential benefit of more drastic measures should be carefully weighed against the potential harm to patients currently residing in the facility. The epidemiologic investigation of the outbreak may help focus control measures on specific infection control or procedural techniques (10).

FIRST STEPS

Once an outbreak is suspected and an investigation is contemplated, all levels of the healthcare facility's personnel (e.g., the chief of the affected service, head nurse for the unit, director of microbiology, hospital administration, etc.) must be committed to the investigation. The cooperation of a variety of healthcare professionals is essential to efficiently conduct an investigation and to implement control measures.

A second consideration during the early stages of an outbreak investigation is the availability of microbiologic isolates for antimicrobial susceptibility testing or molecular or nonmolecular typing. Unlike community outbreaks, typing of microorganisms in HAI outbreaks may be essential to proving chains of transmission because of the ubiquitous nature of microorganisms in the hospital environment (18,24). For this reason, microbiology laboratory personnel should be informed early in the investigation, so that they can save specimens and isolates and be alert for additional isolates that may be part of the outbreak. Laboratory personnel also can suggest other specimens that should be collected from current or future patients who develop the disease being studied.

Finally, before beginning an investigation, available resources (e.g., personnel, supplies, laboratory), the lead investigator, and the person to be responsible for statistical analysis of the data should be identified. Taking these steps before initiating an investigation will allow it to proceed smoothly later.

THE INVESTIGATION

A complete investigation involves many steps; the order of steps may vary and steps may be done simultaneously. These steps, although not specific to the healthcare setting, are a useful guide in conducting an outbreak investigation (Table 7.1).

Case Definitions

One of the first tasks of the investigative team is to develop a working case definition based on the known facts of the outbreak. This definition should include time, place, person, clinical and laboratory parameters (e.g., date of onset of illness, symptoms, signs, and specific laboratory or diagnostic findings), epidemiologic parameters (e.g., a patient's presence on a specific ward or service during a specified time), and confirmed and possible cases of disease on a differential basis. The process of developing case definitions is an iterative one and should be based on balancing the need for an all-inclusive (sensitive) case definition at the beginning of the investigation and more specific case definition as the investigation proceeds and more information is acquired. Case definitions may vary from the relatively simple to the more complex (21,25) (Table 7.2). Occasionally, the case definition may need to be refined as the investigation proceeds and more information is acquired.

Case Finding

Once an initial case definition has been developed, additional case finding can be conducted. The case definition should be applied to the source population without bias as to known or potential underlying host or environmental risk factors. Sources most commonly used for finding cases are discharge diagnosis codes; microbiology, infection control, or transfusion records;

TABLE 7.1. GUIDELINES FOR EPIDEMIOLOGIC FIELD INVESTIGATIONS

1. Prepare for field work (e.g., administration, clearance, travel, contacts, designation of lead investigator, and the like)
2. Confirm the existence of an epidemic
3. Verify the diagnosis
4. Identify and count cases or exposures
   Create a case definition
   Develop a line listing
5. Tabulate and orient the data in terms of time, place, and person
6. Take immediate control measures (if indicated)
7. Formulate hypotheses
8. Test hypotheses through epidemiologic studies
9. Plan an additional systematic study (or studies)
10. Culture environment and personnel based on epidemiologic data
11. Implement and evaluate control and preventive measures
12. Initiate surveillance
13. Communicate findings
    Summarize investigation for requesting authority
    Prepare written report(s)

Modified from Goodman RA, Buehler JW, Koplan JP. The epidemiologic field investigation: Science and judgement in public health practice. *Am J Epidemiol* 1990; 132:9–16, with permission.

TABLE 7.2. EXAMPLES OF CASE DEFINITIONS FROM HOSPITAL OUTBREAKS INVESTIGATED BY THE CDC'S HOSPITAL INFECTIONS PROGRAM

1. "A case of multidrug-resistant tuberculosis was defined as any patient diagnosed with active tuberculosis from January 1989 through March 1991 whose *M. tuberculosis* isolate was resistant to at least isoniazid and rifampin."
2. "An [anaphylactic reaction] was defined as hypotension (≥30 mm Hg fall in systolic blood pressure from the pre-induction blood pressure) and at least one of the following during a general anesthesia procedure at hospital A from January 1989 through January 1991: rash, angioedema, stridor, wheezing, or bronchospasm" (21).

CDC, Centers for Disease Control and Prevention.

emergency room, outpatient clinic, or dialysis clinic logs; or patient medical records in a cohort study, if the cases are limited to a single ward or if the healthcare facility is very small (i.e., where charts can be reviewed in a short period).

Confirming an Outbreak

Confirming an outbreak begins with calculating the background rate of infection or adverse event and then comparing the outbreak period rate with the background rate. The outbreak period should include the time period from the possible incubation period for the first case of disease until the last case or time of the investigation. The background rate of the same disease should be based on existing data, which can be collected from a variety of resources, including microbiology, infection control, or patient records. Data may have to be collected for a period of months to years preceding the outbreak to determine accurate background rates. Comparison of the outbreak period attack rate to the background rate can be performed using the rate ratio:

$$\text{Rate ratio} = \frac{\text{Attack rate during epidemic period}}{\text{Attack rate during background period}}$$

Pseudo-outbreaks are increases in the incidence of infection or adverse event that are not real. This can be due to (a) clusters of positive cultures in patients without evidence of disease or (b) a perceived increase in infections because surveillance was not previously being conducted for that particular problem or because surveillance definitions, intensity, or methods have changed. Pseudo-outbreaks usually are due to either increased surveillance of an area or type of infection or laboratory errors (i.e., extrinsic or cross-contamination) (26–29). Hypotheses developed during the investigation of a presumed outbreak should include the possibility of a pseudo-outbreak, particularly if laboratory clustering of the positive cultures occurs (see Chapter 8).

Chart Review

Before beginning the lengthy process of reviewing medical records, one should determine which data are important to collect for each case-patient or case-HCW and design a questionnaire for ease of data collection (see Chapter 5 for details on questionnaire design). Some important categories of information to consider in most investigations are demographic variables (e.g., age race, ethnicity, or gender), underlying illnesses, severity of illness indicators [e.g., Acute Physiology and Chronic Health Evaluation (APACHE) or Pediatric Risk of Mortality (PRISM) scores] (30,31), ward/unit, duration of hospitalization, invasive devices or procedures, exposures to personnel or other patients; medications, and clinical aspects of the disease being studied (e.g., date of onset of illness, symptoms, and signs); for SSI outbreaks, surgical risk factors (e.g., procedure, operating room, surgeon, or surgical team members) or surgical risk index (7,32) must also be determined in addition to the other categories.

Descriptive Epidemiology

A line listing of the case-patients and pertinent demographic and clinical information serves as a useful tool to begin the process of describing the outbreak in terms of time, place, and person. Describing an outbreak in this way helps determine who is at particular risk for the disease that is being studied. In turn, knowing which population of patients or HCWs is at risk determines who should be included in further analytic studies.

Describing the outbreak over time is most easily done by graphing the case-patients or case-HCWs by onset of disease; the cases can be graphed by time (e.g., hours, days, months, or quarters), as appropriate. These graphs, often called epidemic or epi curves, can provide a great deal of information about possible sources and modes of transmission. For example, a common-source outbreak with subsequent person-to-person transmission is well illustrated by a foodborne outbreak in a retirement community (33) (Fig. 7.1). A high initial peak of onset of illness, indicating a point source of infection, followed by continued cases of illness is typical of an outbreak of gastrointestinal illness caused by a viral agent. Person-to-person transmission, on the other hand, is usually illustrated by an epidemic curve of longer duration with few, if any, peaks. A typical epidemic curve illustrating person-to-person transmission would be an outbreak of *Mycobacterium tuberculosis* HAIs (34) (Fig. 7.2).

The epidemic curve of an outbreak caused by poor infection control techniques (e.g., poor hand hygiene compliance) or contaminated patient equipment also are usually spread over a long period. For example, an *Acinetobacter baumannii* outbreak related to reusable intravascular transducers that were not adequately sterilized continued for over a year until the problem was recognized and the decontamination and disinfection technique was corrected (18) (Fig. 7.3). If HCWs and patients are both affected by the outbreak, the dates of onset of disease for patients and HCWs should be plotted together and separately to determine if transmission occurred from patient to patient, patient to HCW, HCW to patient, or HCW to HCW.

At times, the location of the outbreak is limited to a certain ward, unit, or operating room and at other times to a certain type of ward (e.g., general surgical units). The location of the outbreak may provide a clue to the mode of transmission or to certain risk factors or exposures of particular patients.

For example, an investigation in a hospital with high tuberculin skin test (TST) conversion rates among patients and HCWs revealed that many of the TST converters were patients of or

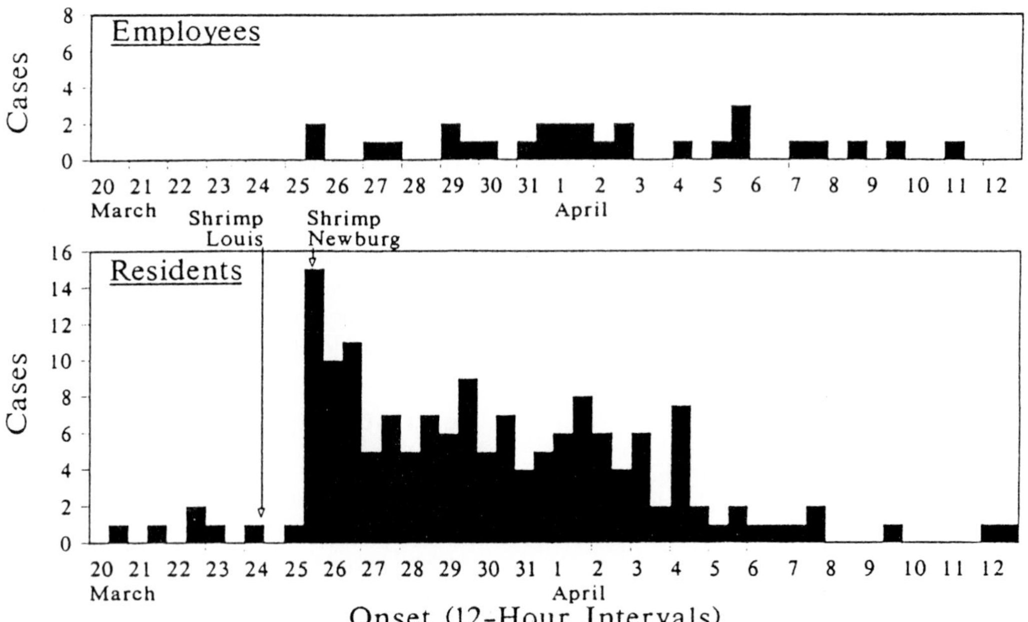

Figure 7.1. Epidemic curve from a common source outbreak with subsequent person-to-person transmission. (From Gordon SM, Oshiro LS, Jarvis WR, et al. Foodborne Snow Mountain agent gastroenteritis with secondary person-to-person spread in a retirement community. *Am J Epidemiol* 1990;131:702–710, with permission.)

workers in the outpatient human immunodeficiency virus (HIV) clinic (35). The clinic had a large room with reclining chairs for patients with acquired immunodeficiency syndrome (AIDS) to receive intravenous medications on an outpatient basis. This room was immediately adjacent to two rooms with floor-to-ceiling sliding glass doors in which aerosolized pentamidine was administered to patients with *Pneumocystis carinii* pneumonia, some of whom had active tuberculosis. Because these treatment rooms were under positive pressure relative to the intravenous medication room, patients receiving intravenous medications, and HCWs administering the medications, were exposed to patients with *M. tuberculosis* when HIV-infected patients with active tuberculosis received aerosolized pentamidine. This occurred even if the isolation room doors were closed. In addition, air in the isolation rooms and waiting area was recirculated, causing a mixture of clean and potentially contaminated air to be circulated through the room. Thus, the location of a number of the cases led to identification of risk factors for acquisition of the disease (i.e., new onset of tuberculosis or TST conversion among AIDS clinic patients or HCWs exposed to patients with active tuberculosis) and to mode of transmission (airborne spread caused by poor isolation practices and inadequate ventilation systems).

By describing the case-patients in terms of demographics and underlying disease, one can define the at-risk population and

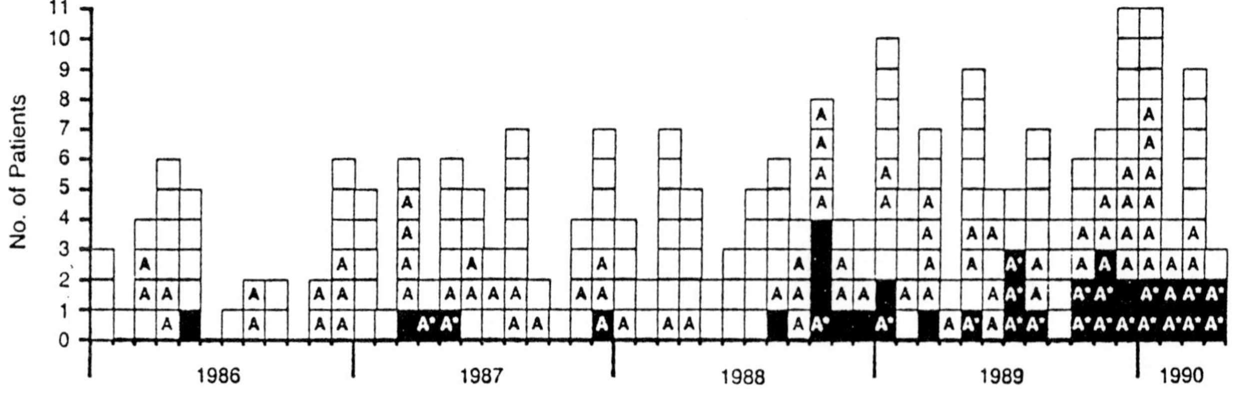

Figure 7.2. Epidemic curve illustrating person-to-person transmission. (From Edlin BR, Tokars JI, Grieco MH, et al. An outbreak of multidrug-resistant tuberculosis among hospitalized patients with the acquired immunodeficiency syndrome. *N Engl J Med* 1992;326:1514–1521, with permission.)

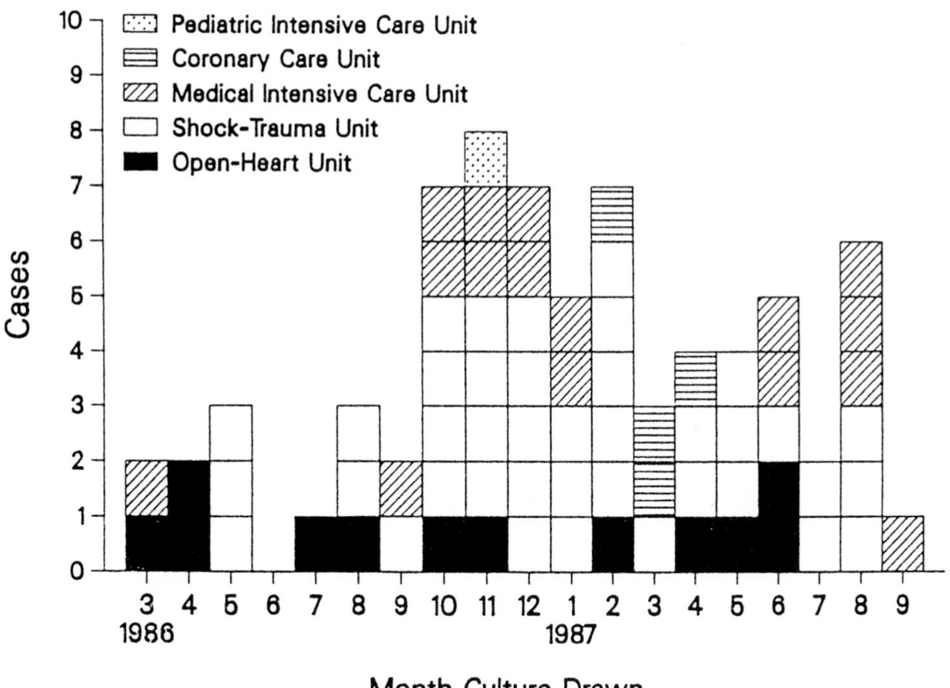

Figure 7.3. Epidemic curve of an outbreak caused by contaminated patient-care equipment. (From Beck-Sague CM, Jarvis WR, Brook JH, et al. Epidemic bacteremia due to *Acinetobacter baumannii* in five intensive care units. *Am J Epidemiol* 1990;132:723– 733, with permission.)

determine possible exposures. Certain patient populations may be at risk because of either age or underlying disease-specific exposures. The entire population that meets these identified criteria is the group of patients that would have been identified as case-patients had they developed disease (36). This is the population from which controls or the cohort to be studied should be chosen for epidemiologic studies. The comparison population (controls or noncases) should have the same opportunity for infection or disease as the case-patients.

Developing Hypotheses

Once cases are identified, and pertinent information from the medical records is abstracted, hypotheses about the cause of the outbreak can be generated. These hypotheses should be based on the available information, previously published literature, and expert opinion. Then, epidemiologic studies can be conducted to test the hypotheses.

Testing Hypotheses

Investigation of outbreaks is by nature retrospective to the development of disease. Two types of retrospective analytic studies can be performed to test hypotheses formed in an outbreak investigation: case-control or cohort studies. Each type of study has inherent advantages and disadvantages, which should be taken into account before embarking on the study. Before embarking on such an analytic study, it is important to determine whether the number of case-patients is sufficient to statistically identify or confirm the source and risk factors for infection or disease (i.e., the statistical power of the study). If the number of cases is small, an epidemiologic study may be fruitless.

Case-Control Studies

The case-patients for a case-control study have already been selected by the occurrence of the outbreak. Choosing the appropriate controls is the next step. Case-control studies require the selection of study participants on the basis of disease status. For example, if 25 affected patients or HCWs (case-patients) are enrolled, a proportional number (25, 50, 75, etc.) of unaffected members of the at-risk population should be enrolled as controls. Specific risk factors for disease then can be compared between case-patients and control subjects. Care should be taken to ensure that case-patients and control subjects have equal likelihood of the exposure.

The main advantage of case-control studies is that they require a small number of subjects [cases (n) and controls ($1n$, $2n$, or $3n$)] and can, therefore, be conducted relatively quickly. In addition, because subjects are chosen on the basis of their disease status (i.e., cases being ill and controls being well), case-control studies are well suited for rare diseases or diseases with long latency periods, and multiple exposures can be examined in the course of one study. This same feature, however, means that the design is backward (i.e., one selects subjects on the basis of disease status, then looks backward in time to look at potential exposures). This may lead to uncertainty that the exposure actually preceded the onset of disease. In addition, this backwardness may subject the study to both selection and recall bias. Another disadvantage of case-control studies is that they are unsuitable for rare exposures (disease incidence rates cannot be measured because the population at risk has not been proportionately sampled) (see also Chapter 2).

Cohort Studies

In contrast to case-control studies, cohort studies require the selection of study participants on the basis of exposure status. Such status can be determined on the basis of known facts about the case-patients or case-HCWs. Exposures that often are used to determine the cohort to be studied are underlying disease, being hospitalized on a particular ward, having a particular physician, or undergoing a particular procedure. Once the cohort of diseased (cases) and nondiseased (noncases) patients is selected, specific risk factors for development of disease can be evaluated among the cases and noncases.

Because cohort study subjects are selected on the basis of an exposure and followed forward through time (albeit historical time) for the occurrence of disease, cohort studies have the advantage of a logical temporal sequence. The selection of subjects on the basis of exposure also facilitates studying rare exposures or the many effects of one exposure. Another major advantage of the cohort study design is the ability to calculate disease incidence rates for the affected population (see also Chapter 2).

Study Design

The type of study that should be done and the population from which study subjects should be chosen depend on the particular hypotheses to be tested, the duration of the outbreak, the number of case-patients identified, and so forth. Often, it is necessary to conduct several studies, each testing hypotheses from the different levels of the outbreak. Much of the data for the case-patients or case-HCWs for either type of study has already been collected in the initial data collection and chart review procedure. The same data should be collected for the control subjects (case-control study) or noncase patients (cohort study), so that particular risk factors can be evaluated. Data should be collected similarly for cases and for controls or noncases.

Data Analysis

Descriptive Statistics

Initial data analysis should consist of descriptive statistics (e.g., frequency tables for each independent or exposure variable). For example, if information collected for cases and controls or noncases includes age, gender, hospital ward, attending physician, and surgical procedure performed, the frequency of all of the values of those variables should be examined for the study population. This type of descriptive information is very useful to direct further analyses. For example, if the study population was exposed to attending physicians A, B, and C as shown in Table 7.3, further analyses might be conducted around events associated with attending physician A.

Univariate Analysis: Categorical Variables

Categorical variables (i.e., variables with values that can be sorted into categories such as ill or well, yes or no, male or female) are compared using the 2 × 2, or cross-tabulation, table.

TABLE 7.3. FREQUENCY DISTRIBUTION OF ATTENDING PHYSICIANS FOR CASES AND CONTROLS, OUTBREAK OF UNKNOWN DISEASE, HOSPITAL X

Physician	Number of cases	Number of controls
A	14 (93%)	7 (47%)
B	0 (0%)	0 (0%)
C	1 (7%)	8 (53%)
Total	15 (100%)	15 (100%)

If a case-control study design has been used, odds ratios (ORs) should be calculated by using the following formula:

$$\text{OR} = ad/bc$$

The OR is the odds that a person with the disease was previously exposed to the risk factor of interest, compared with the odds that a person without the disease was not previously exposed to the risk factor of interest. Usually, the further away from 1.0 in either direction, the stronger the association between the variables. The OR estimates the relative risk (RR) (see later) when a case-control study design has been used. To continue with the previous example, if exposure to physicians A and C is compared with case or control status, exposure to physician A is associated with illness (Table 7.4).

When using a cohort study design, RR estimates can be calculated for the population, using the following equation:

$$\text{RR} = a(c+d)/c(a+b)$$

The RR is the risk of development of the disease if the exposure has occurred, compared with the risk of development of the disease if the exposure has not occurred. As with the OR, the further away from 1.0 the RR is, the stronger the association is between the variables. This calculation assumes that the study subjects have been selected on the basis of exposure; therefore, this calculation can only be used with a cohort study design.

Most statistical software packages also calculate 95% confidence limits around the OR or the RR. This calculation indicates that if the population were resampled a number of times, the OR or RR would fall within the calculated confidence limits 95% of the time. If the confidence limits surround 1.0, it is likely that for any given sample of the population, the real odds of disease or RR could equal 1.0, indicating no association between the variables. Thus, 95% confidence limits are one indication of the significance of the OR or RR (see also Chapter 2).

Most statistical software packages also calculate a chi square test from the 2 × 2 table to test the association between the

TABLE 7.4. TWO-BY-TWO TABLE COMPARING PHYSICIANS A AND C TO CASE CONTROL STATUS, OUTBREAK OF UNKNOWN DISEASE, HOSPITAL X[a]

	Cases	Controls	Total
Physician A	14	7	21
Physician C	1	8	9
	15	15	30

[a]Odds ratio = *ad*/*bc* = (14) (8)/(7) (1) = 16.

variables. More commonly reported in the scientific literature than the chi-square value is the *p* value, which is based on the chi-square value. If the expected value in any of the cells of the 2 × 2 table is less than 5, the Fisher's exact test (FET) is calculated instead of the chi-square value. The *p* value for the FET is calculated directly from the 2 × 2 table in this instance, rather than by using chi-square tables. For either the chi-square test or the FET, the *p* value indicates the level of certainty one has that the association between the variables is not occurring by chance alone. Both the chi-square test and the FET require that the variables be mutually exclusive and independent.

Univariate Analysis: Continuous Variables

Continuous variables, such as age or severity of illness measurement, are compared among the cases and controls or noncases by using measures of central tendency, most frequently the mean or median. If the data are normally distributed (i.e., plotting the values on a graph yields a bell-shaped, or normal, curve), the mean and its standard deviation should be calculated. If the data are not normally distributed, the median and range of the data values should be used.

Stratified and Multiple Variable Analysis

Because many HAI are multifactorial, it often is necessary to control for one or more variables while testing another. For instance, SSIs frequently are related to the surgeon's skill (usually measured as the duration of surgery), the condition of the surgical site at the time of the operation (measured by a standard surgical site classification score), and the patient's underlying health status (measured by a variety of risk factor scores).

Analytic techniques to control for all of these factors usually start with simple stratification of the data. Other techniques include logistic or linear regression models (for categorical and continuous outcome variables, respectively), which require advanced statistical software and training. In some outbreaks, the number of cases may be too small to do either stratified or regression analysis. Furthermore, two or more variables may be linearly associated so that the independent importance of each risk factor cannot be determined. Details on the use of univariate, stratified, and multivariate statistical techniques can be found in Chapter 3.

Use of Microcomputers

The analytic techniques described in this section can be accomplished with the use of microcomputers. Statistical software packages, such as Statistical Analysis System (SAS Institute Inc., Cary, NC), EpiInfo Software [Centers for Disease Control and Prevention (CDC), Atlanta, GA], and others, offer a wide variety of features. Particularly useful is the Statcalc feature of EpiInfo. It allows calculation of the necessary sample size to find significant associations; direct input of data into cross-tabulation tables for calculation of ORs or RRs and their respective chi square, FET, and *p* values; and direct input of data into a trend analysis model for continuous variables (37). Calculation of the power of the study or the sample size necessary to detect significant associations is essential before embarking on any outbreak investigation or epidemiologic study. Details on the use of microcomputers in hospital epidemiology can be found in Chapters 14 and 15.

MICROBIOLOGY LABORATORY ASPECTS OF THE INVESTIGATION

Once a potential outbreak has been identified, the microbiology laboratory should be notified, so that all appropriate specimens and positive cultures can be saved. Because of the ubiquitous nature of microorganisms in the healthcare facility environment, typing of microorganisms thought to be related to an outbreak may be essential to determine if the infected patient is indeed part of the outbreak. The first line of typing of microorganisms is species identification. This is followed by biotyping and then antimicrobial susceptibility testing. For example, during an outbreak of SSIs caused by methicillin-resistant *S. aureus,* a patient thought to be involved in the outbreak would be excluded as a case-patient if antimicrobial susceptibility testing revealed that he or she was infected with a methicillin-sensitive strain of *S. aureus.*

When antimicrobial susceptibility testing is insufficient to determine the relatedness of two microorganisms, other methods of typing can be used, including serotyping, phage typing, isoenzyme electrophoresis, and genetic fingerprinting techniques (e.g., pulsed-field gel electrophoresis, plasmid analysis, or restriction fragment polymorphism). These methods are further detailed in Chapter 102.

Although some research-oriented hospital laboratories may be capable of very sophisticated typing techniques, most infection control professionals require assistance in typing microorganisms from an outbreak. University, state health department, the CDC, or other laboratories may be able to assist with typing of isolates from an outbreak. It should be remembered that genetic typing of isolates can determine whether the isolates are the same strain (clonal) or not (nonclonal), but it cannot tell whether there is an outbreak or not; outbreaks can be caused by clonal (common source) or nonclonal (intermittent person-to-person transmission because of inadequate hand hygiene) isolates.

ENVIRONMENTAL INVESTIGATION

A thorough investigation of an infectious disease outbreak should include some inspection of the environment, particularly if an inanimate object is epidemiologically implicated as a possible means of transmission. For example, investigation of an outbreak of *Serratia marcescens* SSIs following breast reconstruction revealed that expandable breast implants were associated with a greater risk of infection than were nonexpandable implants. Furthermore, infections were more likely when the expansion procedure was performed in the surgeon's office (38). This led the investigators to sample solutions, water sources, and personnel from the surgeon's office that were involved in the expansion procedure. Positive cultures were obtained only from a specimen of saline taken from a partially used bag in the procedure room, allowing investigators to remove the contaminated solution and other bags with the same purchase date. Environmental cultures should not be taken randomly, because many surfaces are contaminated with numerous microorganisms, perhaps including the microorganism being investigated. Positive culture results from such random sampling may be misleading, difficult to interpret, and often confusing to investigators.

In addition to environmental cultures, outbreaks of diseases caused by airborne microorganisms such as *M. tuberculosis* or *Aspergillus* spp. merit a thorough inspection of airhandling systems, isolation room airflow patterns, and infection control techniques. Neither routine environmental culturing nor selected culturing of the air or room is indicated; these should only be done when epidemiologically directed. Without epidemiologic direction, such culturing usually either misses the source or leads to uninterpretable results.

INTERPRETING RESULTS

The most important part of the investigation is the interpretation of results. Meaningful associations between exposures or risk factors and the development of disease depend on numerous factors: the quality of the study design and the study population, biologic plausibility (i.e., the measured association makes biologic sense), and the exposure's preceding of the onset of the disease (39). Other qualities that lend confidence to a significant association are the statistical strength of the association, consistency with other studies, and the presence of a dose-response effect (39).

INSTITUTING CONTROL MEASURES

Control measures can be instituted as soon as a potential outbreak is discovered. For example, increased attention to hand hygiene and other infection control techniques may halt transmission. In addition, published guidelines from the CDC, Association for Professionals in Infection Control and Epidemiology (APIC), the Society for Healthcare Epidemiology of America (SHEA), Joint Commission on the Accreditation of Healthcare Organizations (JCAHO), or other organizations may lend guidance for specific situations (40–51). If the investigation implicates a particular HCW or item of patient-care equipment, specific measures should be taken to rectify the situation.

EXAMPLE OF A HOSPITAL INVESTIGATION

An excellent example of an outbreak investigation in a hospital is the investigation of SSIs caused by an unusual human pathogen, *Rhodococcus bronchialis,* after open-heart surgery (52). This outbreak provided an opportunity to assess risk factors for infection with *R. bronchialis,* mode of transmission of the microorganism, and potential sources for this unusual HAI pathogen. Logical hypotheses for the source of SSIs after open-heart surgery included preoperative (e.g., nurses, physicians, wards), intraoperative (e.g., operating room environment or personnel), or postoperative (e.g., recovery room or intensive care unit personnel) exposures. The investigators analyzed both categorical and continuous variables as measures of potential risk for infection and possible exposures as the source of infection (Table 7.5). The only factor significantly associated with infection was the presence of one operating room nurse, nurse A, during the operative procedure. Examination of nurse A's intraoperative practices revealed that she could have contaminated the sterile field after performing an activated clotting time test that involved the use of a water bath for incubation of a tube of the patient's blood. A revised hypothesis was that nurse A contaminated the sterile operative field after performing the test; this would account for all of the cases of *R. bronchialis* SSIs during the epidemic period.

To prove that nurse A was responsible for all of the cases of *R. bronchialis* SSIs at the hospital, the investigators performed numerous cultures indicated by the epidemiologic data. These included cultures of nurse A's and nurse B's hands before and after each performed the activated clotting time test; nasal swabs from all cardiac operating room personnel; swabs from nurse A's scalp, pharynx, vagina, and rectum; and swabs from environmental sites while nurse A was present in or absent from the operating room. Only cultures of nurse A's hands after performing the activated clotting test, nurse A's nasal swab, settle plates from the operating room while nurse A was present, and nurse A's scalp and vaginal cultures were positive for *R. bronchialis.* To identify the ultimate source of the microorganism, nurse A's operating room locker and her home were examined and selectively cultured. The neck-scruff skin of nurse A's dog and air vents at her home (where the dog would lay) were positive for *R. bronchialis.* Antimicrobial susceptibility testing and molecular typing showed that all of the outbreak isolates (i.e., patient, HCW, environment, and dog) were identical and distinct from nonoutbreak stock *R. bronchialis* isolates.

The role of the water bath used to incubate blood samples for the activated clotting time test was analyzed by simulating what the scrub nurses would do during surgery and by using a colorless fluorescent dye in the water bath. After simulating the beginning of an open-heart procedure (e.g., performing an activated clotting time test and opening sterile packs for the procedure), 8 of 11 circulating nurses had contaminated the sterile field with fluorescent dye from the water bath. Also contaminated with fluorescent dye were all of the nurses' hands; some of the nurses' wrists, forearms, and scrub suits; the outer surface of the water bath container; the table surface; and the floor around the water bath. This simulation showed that although the bath water was culture-negative for *R. bronchialis,* the bath water provided the mechanism for the microorganism to be spread from nurse A's hands to the sterile field. Because nurse A was epidemiologically implicated in the investigation, cultures were obtained from a variety of sources highly likely to yield positive results. Culturing of the operating room environment and other personnel earlier in the investigation would have been unfocused, increasing the work load on the laboratory without aiding the investigation. Additional selected surgical personnel and environmental sources were included in the culture survey to avoid identification of Nurse A as the source before confirming culture evidence could be obtained.

TABLE 7.5. CATEGORICAL AND CONTINUOUS VARIABLES AS MEASURES OF POTENTIAL RISK FOR INFECTION

Potential risk factor	Case patients (n = 7) no. (%)	Controls (n = 28)	Odds ratio	p value
Categorical variables				
Male sex	7 (100)	24 (86)	NC	0.6
Underlying conditions	6 (86)	22 (79)	1.6	1.0
Diabetes	1 (14)	6 (21)	0.6	1.0
Obesity	3 (43)	4 (14)	4.5	0.1
Smoking	4 (57)	9 (32)	2.8	0.4
Cancer	1 (14)	0 (0)	NC	0.2
Renal insufficiency	0 (0)	0 (0)	—	—
Treatment with steroids	1 (14)	1 (4)	4.5	0.4
Chronic lung disease	2 (29)	3 (11)	3.3	0.3
Presence of nurse A	7 (100)	6 (21)	NC	0.0003
Coronary artery bypass graft	7 (100)	28 (100)	—	—
Saphenous vein	6 (86)	26 (93)	0.5	0.5
Mammary artery	6 (86)	25 (89)	0.7	1
Transfusion	4 (57)	13 (46)	2.2	1
Continuous variables				
Preoperative stay (days)	1.8 ± 1.3[a]	1.9 ± 1.8	—	0.7
Postoperative stay (days)	6.2 ± 1.3	7.5 ± 3.7	—	0.4
Age (yr)	59.4 ± 5.4	58.5 ± 11.0	—	0.9
No. of underlying conditions	2.2 ± 1.9	1.1 ± 0.9	—	0.2
Duration of operation (min)	284 ± 64	292 ± 87	—	0.9
Duration of bypass (min)	119 ± 38	128 ± 44	—	0.7
Duration of aortic clamping (min)	67 ± 23	70 ± 27	—	0.8
Amount of blood reperfused (mL)	903 ± 236	901 ± 317	—	1.0
Cardiac index[b]	2.8 ± 0.6	3.0 ± 0.5	—	0.6
Duration of treatment (days)				
Stay in cardiac ICU	2.2 ± 0.4	2.9 ± 2.2	—	0.8
Swan-Ganz catheter	1.8 ± 0.4	2.2 ± 1.0	—	0.6
Arterial line	2 ± 0	2.3 ± 1.0	—	0.6
Mediastinal drains	2 ± 0	2.2 ± 0.8	—	0.6
Pacer wires	4.8 ± 0.4	5.0 ± 1.6	—	0.8
Ventilation	1 ± 0	1.6 ± 2.7	—	0.6
Antimicrobial prophylaxis	4.2 ± 2.2	3.7 ± 1.0	—	0.9

[a] Plus/minus values are means ± SD. ICU, intensive care unit; NC, not calculable.
[b] Cardiac index was defined as cardiac output in liters per minute per square meter of body surface area.
From Richet HM, Craven PC, Brown JM, et al. A cluster of *Rhodococcus (Gordona) bronchialis* sternal wound infections after coronary artery bypass surgery. *N Engl J Med* 1991; 324:104–109, with permission.

FINAL STEPS

After instituting control measures, assessing the efficacy of the introduced control measures is essential. Occasionally, more than one mode of transmission is present, and prevention interventions eliminate only one of the modes of transmission (53). In other situations, it is essential to ensure that previously accepted control measures really are adequate to terminate transmission (54,55).

Once an investigation is concluded, it is imperative that all of the concerned parties in the hospital and state or local health department, consultants, and other involved persons be told of the results of the investigation. In addition, if patient-care devices or products are implicated in the investigation, the appropriate divisions of the Food and Drug Administration or CDC should be alerted. Finally, during the course of the investigation, answering inquiries from the public and press may be necessary. It is good practice to have one person, usually from the public relations or legal departments of the healthcare facility, respond to these inquiries. That person should be kept informed of all developments in the investigation.

Although the investigation of outbreaks is an interesting and challenging endeavor, it may be beyond the capability of a given infection control or epidemiology department because of resource constraints or lack of expertise in analytic and epidemiologic techniques. In such cases, assistance is available from state or local health departments, the CDC, university infection control or epidemiology departments, other facility infection control personnel, or private consultants.

RESULTS USING THIS APPROACH

From July 1987 through December 1999, the previously described approach to investigation of outbreaks was consistently applied by Epidemic Intelligence Service (EIS) officers in the Investigation and Prevention Branch, Hospital Infections Pro-

TABLE 7.6. ON-SITE HAI OUTBREAK INVESTIGATIONS, HOSPITAL INFECTIONS PROGRAM, CDC, JULY 1987–DECEMBER 1999

1987 [Outbreak name-state/country (reference number)]
1. Pyrogenic reactions in hemodialysis patients–Illinois (56)
2. *Malassezia furfur* infections in neonatal intensive care unit patients—Washington D.C. (57)
3. *Acinetobacter* spp. bloodstream infections in intensive care unit patients—New Jersey (18)
4. *Yersinia enterocolitica* sepsis associated with red blood cell transfusion—Wisconsin/Texas (58)
5. *Pseudomonas cepacia* infection/colonization in attendees at a cystic fibrosis summer camp—Michigan (59)
6. Human immunodeficiency virus knowledge and compliance with CDC recommendations (NP)

1988
1. *Aspergillus flavus* pseudofungemia in bone marrow transplant patients—North Carolina (NP)
2. Methicillin-resistant *Staphylococcus aureus* surgical site Infections in cardiac surgery patients—Tennessee (NP)
3. *Mycobacterium chelonae* infections in hemodialysis patients—California (60)
4. *Aspergillus fumigatus* surgical site infections in cardiac surgery patients—Tennessee (61)
5. Epidemic hemolytic anemia in hemodialysis patients—Pennsylvania (62)
6. Gastroenteritis in a retirement facility—California (33)
7. Pyrogenic reactions and/or bloodstream infections in hemodialysis patients—Arzona (63)
8. Hemolysis in pediatric hemodialysis patients—Texas (64)
9. Invasive candidiasis in hematology-oncology patients—France (65)
10. Disseminated intravascular coagulation in open heart surgery patients—California (66)

1989
1. *Serratia marcescens* bloodstream infections in intensive care unit patients—Illinois (67)
2. Surgical site infections in patients undergoing hip replacement procedures—Maine (68)
3. Hypotension in hemodialysis patients—New York (69)
4. *Rhodococcus broncialis* surgical site infections in cardiac surgery patients—Washington (52)
5. Hepatitis A infections in neonates in a neonatal intensive care Unit—Hawaii (70)
6. *Pseudomonas cepacia* pseudobacteremia in Infants—Texas (71)
7. *Xanthamonas maltophilia* infections in intensive care unit patients—Utah (72)
8. Group A streptococcal surgical site infections—California (NP)
9. *Salmonella* spp. gastroenteritis in patients and healthcare workers—Tennessee (NP)
10. *Pseudomonas cepacia* infections in cystic fibrosis patients—Pensylvania (73)
11. Multidrug-resistant *Mycobacterium tuberculosis* infections in human immunodeficiency virus infected patients—Puerto Rico (74)
12. *Tsukamurella* spp. pseudoinfections traced to laboratory contamination—South Carolina (27)
13. *Mycobacteria gordonae* pseudoinfections traced to intrinsic product contamination—Connecticut/Georgia (26)
14. Nosocomial infections in long-term care facility residents—California (75)
15. *Serratia marcescens* surgical wound infections following augmentation mammoplasty—North Dakota (38)
16. Allergic reactions in hemodialysis patients—Virginia (76)

1990
1. Group A streptococcus bacteremia in residents of a long-term care facility (77)
2. *Clostridium difficile* enteritis in a hospital—New York (78)
3. Drug-resistant tuberculosis in hospitalized AIDS patients—New York (34)
4. *Staphylococcus aureus* infections following clean surgical procedures—Michigan (20)
5. *Candida albicans* infections following clean surgical procedures—Illinois (20)
6. *Staphylococcus aureus* infections following clean surgical procedures—Texas (20)
7. Endotoxin reactions during clean surgical procedures—Maine (20)
8. Nosocomial transmission of drug-resistant *M. tuberculosis*—Florida (35)
9. *Enterobacter agglomerans* sepsis and bacteremia in postsurgical patients—Alabama (20)
10. *Enterobacter cloacae* bacteremia in emergency room and outpatient clinic patients—New Mexico (29)
11. Carbon monoxide poisoning in surgical patients—Georgia (22,79)
12. Inadvertent injection of HIV-contaminated material during nuclear medicine procedures—California and New Mexico (80)
13. Scleritis following cataract surgery—Florida (81)
14. Gram-negative meningitis and bacteremia in neonates in a neonatal intensive care unit—Guatemala (82)

1991
1. Tuberculosis in renal transplant patients—Pennsylvania (83)
2. Anaphylactic reactions in pediatric patients—Wisconsin (21,84)
3. Pyrogenic reactions and bacteremia in hemodialysis patients—Ohio (85)
4. Multidrug-resistant *Mycobacterium tuberculosis* in New York City—New York (25)
5. *Aspergillus* spp. infections in immunocompromised patients—California (16)
6. Anaphylactic reactions in patients with spina bifida—Pennsylvania (NP)

(*continued*)

TABLE 7.6. (continued)

7. *Klebsiella* sp. sepsis in neonates in a neonatal intensive care unit—Saudi Arabia (86)
8. Bacterial sepsis associated with pooled platelet transfusions—Ohio (87)
9. Anaphylactic reactions in pediatric patients—Oklahoma (NP)
10. Fungemia in neonatal intensive care unit patients—Louisiana (88,89)
11. Invasive aspergillosis in oncology patients—Pennsylvania (90)
12. Hepatitis A in healthcare workers in a bone marrow transplant unit—Florida (91)
13. Polymicrobial bacteremia in postcardiac surgery patients—Washington (17)
14. Bacteremia in hemodialysis patients—Texas (NP)
15. Hepatitis B among nursing home residents—Ohio (NP)

1992

1. Nosocomial transmission of multidrug-resistant *Mycobacterium tuberculosis*—New York (92)
2. Pyrogenic reactions in hemodialysis patients—California (93)
3. Aluminum toxicity in chronic hemodialysis patients—Pennsylvania (94)
4. Nosocomial transmission of *Mycobacterium tuberculosis*—Georgia (4,95)
5. Gram-negative bacteremia in patients undergoing hemodialysis—Maryland (96)
6. *Aspergillus fumigatus* sternal wound infections following open heart surgery—Pennsylvania (NP)
7. Multidrug-resistant *Mycobacterium tuberculosis*—New Jersey (NP)
8. Nosocomial transmission of multidrug-resistant *Mycobacterium tuberculosis*—New York (55)
9. Nosocomial transmission of multidrug-resistant *Mycobacterium tuberculosis*—New York (97)
10. Nosocomial transmission of multidrug-resistant *Mycobacterium tuberculosis*—Florida (54)
11. *Mycobacterium fortuitum* infections/pseudoinfections associated with bronchoscopy—Kentucky (98)
12. Nosocomial transmission of multidrug-resistant *Mycobacterium tuberculosis*—New York (NP)
13. Complications of Lyme disease treatment—New Jersey (99)

1993

1. Endotoxin reactions during surgical procedures—Arizona (20)
2. *Serratia marcescens* infections in surgical patients—Arizona (20)
3. Invasive aspergillosis in cardiac transplant patients—New York (NP)
4. Nosocomial coagulase-negative staphylococcal bacteremia in neonatal intensive care unit patients—Kentucky (NP)
5. *Enterobacter hormaechei* bloodstream infections in neonatal intensive care unit patients—Pennsylvania (100)
6. *Norcardia farcinica* surgical wound infections after open heart surgery—Montana (101)
7. Adverse reactions and death during hemodialysis—Illinois (102)
8. Bloodstream and surgical site infections due to vancomycin-resistant enterococci—New York (103)
9. Surgical site infections due to methicillin-resistant *Staphylococcus aureus*—Tennessee (NP)
10. Nosocomial vancomycin-resistant enterococcal infections—Maryland (104)
11. Intravascular catheter complications in intensive care unit patients—Arizona (105)

1994

1. Bloodstream infections associated with outpatient infusion therapy—Rhode Island (106)
2. Pulmonary complications associated with total parenteral nutrition—Hawaii (107)
3. *Acremonium kiliense* endophthalmitis following cataract surgery—Pennsylvania (108)
4. Possible HIV transmission in a dialysis center—Colombia (109)
5. Acute hepatitis B infections in hemodialysis patients—Texas (110)
6. Acute hepatitis B infections in hemodialysis patients—California (110)
7. Bloodstream infections in pediatric oncology patients—California (111)
8. Methicillin-resistant *Staphylococcus aureus* (MRSA) infection colonization in wrestlers—Vermont (NP)
9. *Clostridium difficile* gastroenteritis in hospitalized patients—Canada (112)
10. Postoperative *Ochrabactrum anthropi* meningitis in pediatric patients—Utah (113)

1995

1. Nosocomial transmission of *Malassezia pachydermatis* in neonatal intensive care unit patients—New Hampshire (114)
2. Bloodstream infections in home infusion therapy patients—Texas (115)
3. *Salmonella sundsvall* infection in neonates in a neonatal intensive care unit—Oklahoma (NP)
4. *Serratia marcescens* infections in neonatal intensive care unit patients—Massachusetts (116)
5. *Enterobacter cloacae* bloodstream infections in hemodialysis patients—Canada (117)
6. Pyrogenic reactions in patients undergoing cardiac catheterization—Colorado (118)

1996

1. *Serratia marcescens* infection in cardiac intensive care unit patients—Pennsylvania (119,120)
2. Vancomycin-resistant enterococcal infections—Indiana (121,122,123)
3. Bloodstream infections associated with needleless devices—Indiana (124,125,126)
4. Fatal illness in a hemodialysis center—Brazil (127)
5. *Enterobacter cloacae* bloodstream infections in neonatal intensive care unit patients—Puerto Rico (128)
6. Hepatitis C infections possibly associated with intramuscular immune globulin—Texas (NP)

(continued)

TABLE 7.6. (continued)

7. *Staphylococcus aureus* bloodstream infections among patients undergoing electroconvulsive therapy at a psychiatric hospital—Mississippi (129)
8. Bloodstream infections in pediatric intensive care unit patients—Georgia (130)
9. Bloodstream infections in pediatric outpatients—Georgia (NP)
10. Aseptic peritonitis in peritoneal dialysis patients—Pennsylvania (131)
11. Vancomycin-resistant *Staphylococcus epidermidis* bloodstream infection in a patient—Virginia (132)
12. Invasive aspergillosis in rheumatology patients—Maryland (133)
13. *Acinetobacter* species bloodstream infection in neonatal intensive care unit patients—Bahamas (134)
14. Neurologic (loss of hearing and vision) symptoms after hemodialysis—Alabama (135)
15. Bloodstream infections associated with serum albumen—Kansas (136)
16. Overwhelming sepsis and death in newborn nursery patients—Brazil (137)

1997

1. Bloodstream infections in hemodialysis patients—Maryland (138)
2. Nosocomial vancomycin-resistant enterococcus colonization/infection—Indiana (NP)
3. Vancomycin-resistant enterococcus colonization/infection in patients in hospitals and long-term care facilities in a region—Iowa, Nebraska, South Dakota (139,140)
4. Nosocomial bloodstream infections in sickle cell anemia patients—Georgia (NP)
5. *Staphylococcus aureus* with reduced susceptibility to vancomycin—Michigan (141)
6. *Staphylococcus aureus* with reduced susceptibility to vancomycin—New Jersey (141)
7. Pyrogenic reactions in cardiac catheterization patients—Brazil (NP)
8. Dementia in solid organ transplant recipients—Maryland (NP)
9. Creutzfeldt-Jakob disease possibly associated with a dura mater transplant—Florida (142)
10. *Microbacterium* spp. bloodstream infections in oncology patients—Maine (143)
11. *Pseudomonas aeruginosa* infections in neurosurgical patients with external ventricular devices—Arizona (144)
12. Infections in pediatric oncology patients with indwelling central vascular catheters—California (145)

1998

1. Red eye syndrome associated with red blood cell transfusion—Michigan, Washington, Oregon (nationwide) (146)
2. Corneal degeneration after ophthalmologic surgery—Missouri (147)
3. *Malassezia pachydermatis* infections in neonates in a neonatal intensive care unit—Kentucky (NP)
4. Postcoronary artery bypass graft sternal wound infections—Wisconsin (148,149)
5. Hemolysis in hemodialysis patients—Nebraska, Massachusetts, Maryland (nationwide) (150)
6. Vancomycin-resistant enterococci in a long-term care facility setting—Illinois (NP)
7. Pyrogenic reactions in hospitalized patients receiving parenteral gentamicin—California (nationwide) (151)
8. Vancomycin-resistant enterococcal infection/colonization among residents of acute and long-term care facilities—Iowa, Nebraska, South Dakota (140)
9. Gram-negative bloodstream infections in bone marrow transplant patients—Washington (NP)

1999

1. *Serratia marcescens* bloodstream infections in surgical intensive care unit patients—Pennsylvania (152)
2. Cellulitis, sepsis, and death in neonates in a neonatal intensive care unit—Indonesia (NP)
3. *Klebsiella pneumoniae* bloodstream infections in neonates in a neonatal intensive care unit—Colombia (NP)
4. *Serratia marcescens* bloodstream infections in cardiac catheteritization patients—California (NP)
5. Nosocomial sepsis and meningitis in neonates in a neonatal intensive care unit—Brazil (153)
6. *Serratia liquefaciens* bloodstream infections and pyrogenic reactions in hemodialysis patients—Colorado (154)
7. Nosocomial transmission of extended spectrum beta-lactamase producing *Escherichia coli* and *Klebsiella pneumoniae* in long-term care facility patients—Illinois (NP)
8. Vancomycin-resistant enterococcal infection/colonization among residents of acute and long-term care facilities—Iowa, Nebraska, South Dakota (140)

NP, not published.

gram (currently the Division of Healthcare Quality Promotion), CDC. In nearly 150 outbreak investigations, the source was identified and the outbreak was terminated (4,16–18,20–22, 25,27,29,33–35,38,54–154) (Table 7.6). The use of this approach, has led to the identification of intrinsic product contamination [*Yersinia enterocolitica* from packed red blood cells (58), *Pseudomonas cepacia* in povidone iodine disinfectant (71), aseptic peritonitis associated with peritoneal dialysis (131), gram-negative bloodstream infections associated with serum albumin (136), sepsis and death in neonates associated with contaminated glucose infusates (137), pyrogenic reactions associated with once daily administration of gentamicin (151), and *Mycobacterium gordonae* pseudoinfections traced to culture additive contamination (26)]. Many episodes of extrinsic product contamination involving either pyrogenic reactions and/or infection were detected that were associated with reprocessing of hemodialyzers (56,60,63,85,93,94,96,102,109,110,117,127,138,154). New modes of transmission were identified, such as *R. bronchialis* SSIs or *Malazessia furfur* infections in neonates traced to the HCWs' dogs (52,114); Hepatitis A from prolonged excretion of the virus by premature neonates (70); many microorganisms from extrinsic contamination of a new anesthetic propofol (20); anaphylactic reactions in patients and HCWs traced to latex exposure (21,84), aluminum, microcystin, or fluoride toxicity in hemodialysis patients traced to an aluminum pump (94,102,127), inadequate water disinfection (127), or exhaustion of a reverse osmosis filter (102), respectively; *Mycobacterium fortuitum* infection or pseudoinfections from inadequate bronchoscopy disinfection (98); *Nocardia* SSIs traced to a colonized anesthesiologist and his contaminated home environment (101); bloodstream infections traced to needleless devices used in home infusion therapy (106,111,115,124–126); the role of the nursing shortage on increasing infection rates (105,119); and others. In addition, risk factors for transmission of *M. tuberculosis* (34, 35,74,83,92) to patients and HCWs in healthcare settings were identified, and interventions were implemented and documented to terminate such transmission (54,55,97). Similarly, risk factors for the emergence and transmission of vancomycin-resistant enterococci were identified (103,104,121–123); then interventions (including active surveillance cultures and contact isolation) were implemented and shown to be effective in reducing or eradicating transmission on a ward (103,104), in an entire hospital (123), or in an entire region of a state (all acute care and long-term care facilities) (140). In addition, new and emerging HAI pathogens were identified, such as *M. furfur* in neonates (57,114), *Y. enterocolitica* in red blood cell products (58), *P. (now Burkolderia) cepacia* in cystic fibrosis patients (59,73), multidrug-resistant *M. tuberculosis* (4,25,34,35,54,55,74,83,92,95, 97), nontuberculous mycobacteria in hemodialysis patients (60) or bronchoscopy patients (98), *R. bronchialis* or *Norcardia farcinica* in cardiac surgery patients (52,101), *Enterobacter hormaechei* in neonates (100), *Akremonium kiliense* in surgical patients (108), *Ochrabactrum anthoropi* in pediatric patients (113), vancomycin-resistant enterococci (103,104,121–123,140), and *S. aureus* with reduced susceptibility to vancomycin (141).

This approach has worked well for infectious and noninfectious diseases and in all types of healthcare settings and countries. The success of this approach illustrates the value of a combined epidemiologic and laboratory investigation; the power of using these tools together is much greater than using either one alone. When appropriately implemented, this outbreak investigative approach identifies the source and mode of transmission, assists in evaluating the efficacy of the interventions, and ultimately and effectively protects patients and HCWs by preventing further infection and disease.

REFERENCES

1. Haley RW, Tenney JH, Lindsey JO II, et al. How frequent are outbreaks of nosocomial infection in community hospitals? *Infect Control* 1985;6:233–236.
2. McNeil M, Solomon S. The epidemiology of methicillin-resistant *Staphylococcus aureus*. *Antimicrob Newslett* 1985;2:49–56.
3. Snydman DR, Hindman SH, Wineland MD, et al. Nosocomial viral hepatitis B: a cluster among staff with subsequent transmission to patients. *Ann Intern Med* 1976;85:573–577.
4. Zaza S, Blumberg H, Beck-Sague C, et al. Nosocomial transmission of *Mycobacterium tuberculosis:* role of healthcare workers in outbreak propagation. *J Infect Dis* 1995;172:1542–1549.
5. Garner JS, Jarvis WR, Emori TG, et al. CDC definitions for nosocomial infections, 1988. *Am J Infect Control* 1988;16:128–140.
6. Jarvis WR, Edwards JR, Culver DH, et al. Nosocomial infection rates in adult and pediatric intensive care units in the United States. *Am J Med* 1991;91:185s–191s.
7. Culver DH, Horan TC, Gaynes RP, et al. Surgical wound infection rates by wound class, operative procedure, and patient risk index. *Am J Med* 1991;91:152s–157s.
8. Gaynes RP, Martone WJ, Culver DH, et al. Comparison of rates of nosocomial infections in neonatal intensive care units in the United States. *Am J Med* 1991;91:192s–196s.
9. Horan TC, Gaynes RP, Martone WJ, et al. CDC definitions of nosocomial surgical site infections, 1992: a modification of CDC definitions of surgical wound infections. *Am J Infect Control* 1992;20: 271–274.
10. Goodman RA, Buehler JW, Koplan JP. The epidemiologic field investigation: science and judgement in public health practice. *Am J Epidemiol* 1990;132:9–16.
11. Jarvis WR. Nosocomial outbreaks: the Centers for Disease Control's Hospital Infections Program experience, 1980–1990. *Am J Med* 1991;91:101s–106s.
12. Beck-Sague CM, Jarvis WR. Epidemic bloodstream infections associated with pressure transducers: a persistent problem. *Infect Control Hosp Epidemiol* 1989;10:54–59.
13. Cross AS, Roup B. Role of respiratory assistance devices in endemic nosocomial pneumonia. *Am J Med* 1981;70:681–685.
14. Richet H, Escande MC, Marie JP, et al. Epidemic *Pseudomonas aeruginosa* serotype O16 bacteremia in hematology oncology patients. *J Clin Microbiol* 1989;27:1992–1996.
15. Weems JJ, Davis BJ, Tablan OC, et al. Construction activity: an independent risk factor for invasive aspergillosis and zygomycosis in patients with hematologic malignancy. *Infect Control* 1987;8:71–75.
16. Buffington J, Reporter R, Lasker BA, et al. Investigation of an outbreak of invasive aspergillosis: utility of molecular typing with the use of random amplified polymorphic DNA probes. *Pediatr Infect Dis J* 1994;13:386–393.
17. Rudnick JR, Beck-Sague CM, Anderson RL, et al. Gram-negative bacteremia in open heart surgery patients traced to probable tap water contamination of pressure monitoring equipment. *Infect Control Hosp Epidemiol* 1996;17:272–275.
18. Beck-Sague CM, Jarvis WR, Brook JH, et al. Epidemic bacteremia due to *Acinetobacter baumannii* in five intensive care units. *Am J Epidemiol* 1990;132:723– 733.
19. Lowry PW, Beck-Sague CM, Bland LA, et al. *Mycobacterium chelonae* infection among patients receiving high flux dialysis in a hemodialysis clinic in California. *J Infect Dis* 1990;161:85–91.
20. Bennett SN, McNeil MM, Bland LA, et. al. Multiple outbreaks of postoperative infections traced to extrinsic contamination of an intravenous anesthetic, propofol. *N Engl J Med* 1995;333:147–154.
21. Centers for Disease Control and Prevention. Anaphylactic reactions during general anesthesia among pediatric patients-United States, January 1990-January 1991. *MMWR* 1991;40:437, 443.
22. Centers for Disease Control and Prevention. Elevated intraoperative blood carboxyhemoglobin levels in surgical patients—Georgia, Illinois, and North Carolina. *MMWR* 1991;40:248–249.
23. Centers for Disease Control and Prevention. Nosocomial infection and pseudoinfection from contaminated endoscopes and bronchoscopes—Wisconsin and Missouri. *MMWR* 1991;40:675–678.
24. Jereb J, Burwen DR, Dooley SW, et al. Nosocomial outbreak of tuberculosis in a renal transplant unit: application of a new technique for restriction fragment length polymorphism analysis of *Mycobacterium tuberculosis* isolates. *J Infect Dis* 1993;168:1219–1224.

25. Pearson ML, Jereb JA, Frieden TR, et al. Nosocomial transmission of multidrug-resistant *Mycobacterium tuberculosis.* A risk to patients and health care workers. *Ann Intern Med* 1992;117:191–196.
26. Tokars JI, McNeil MM, Tablan OC, et al. *Mycobacterium gordonae* pseudoinfection associated with a contaminated antimicrobial solution. *J Clin Microbiol* 1990;28:2765–2769.
27. Auerbach SB, McNeil MM, Brown JM, et al. Outbreak of pseudoinfections with *Tsukamurella paurometabolum* traced to laboratory contamination: efficacy of joint epidemiological and laboratory investigation. *Clin Infect Dis* 1992;14:1015–1022.
28. Weinstein RA, Stamm WE. Pseudoepidemics in hospitals. *Lancet* 1977;2:862–864.
29. Pearson ML, Pegues DA, Carson LA, et al. Cluster of *Enterobacter cloacae* pseudobacteremias associated with use of an agar slant blood culturing system. *J Clin Microbiol* 1993;31:2599–2603.
30. Knaus WA, Draper EA, Wagner DP, et al. APACHE II: a severity of disease classification system. *Crit Care Med* 1985;13:818–829.
31. Pollack MM, Ruttimann UE, Getson PR. Pediatric risk of mortality (PRISM) score. *Crit Care Med* 1988;16:1110–1116.
32. Haley RW, Culver DH, Morgan WM, et al. Identifying patients at high risk of surgical wound infection. A simple multivariate index of patient susceptibility and wound contamination. *Am J Epidemiol* 1985;121:206–215.
33. Gordon SM, Oshiro LS, Jarvis WR, et al. Foodborne Snow Mountain agent gastroenteritis with secondary person-to-person spread in a retirement community. *Am J Epidemiol* 1990;131:702–710.
34. Edlin BR, Tokars JI, Grieco MH, et al. An outbreak of multidrug-resistant tuberculosis among hospitalized patients with the acquired immunodeficiency syndrome. *N Engl J Med* 1992;326:1514–1521.
35. Beck-Sague C, Dooley SW, Hutton MD, et al. Hospital outbreak of multidrug-resistant *Mycobacterium tuberculosis* infections; factors in transmission to staff and HIV-infected patients. *JAMA* 1992;268: 1280–1286.
36. Hennekens CH, Buring JE. Case-control studies. In: Mayrant SL, ed. *Epidemiology in medicine.* Boston/Toronto: Little, Brown, 1987: 132–142.
37. Dean AG, Dean JA, Burton AG, et al. *EpiInfo version 5: computer programs for epidemiologic investigations.* Atlanta, GA: Centers for Disease Control, 1988.
38. Pegues DA, Shireley LA, Riddle CF, et al. *Serratia marcescens* surgical wound infection following breast reconstruction. *Am J Med* 1991;91: 173s–178s.
39. Hill AB. The environment and disease: association or causation? *Proc R Soc Med (Lond)* 1965;1:295–300.
40. Boyce JM, Pittet D. Guideline for hand hygiene in health-care settings: recommendations of the healthcare infection control practices advisory committee and the HICPAC/SHEA/APIC/IDSA hand hygiene task force. *Infect Control Hosp Epidemiol* 2002;23:S3–S40.
41. O'Grady NP, Alexander M, Dellinger EP, et al. Guidelines for the prevention of intravascular catheter-related infections. *MMWR* 2002; 51:1–29.
42. Mangram AJ, Horan TC, Pearson ML, et al. and the Hospital Infection Control Advisory Committee. Guideline for the prevention of surgical site infection, 1999. *Infect Control Hosp Epidemiol* 1999;20: 247–278.
43. Updated U.S. Public Health Service guidelines for the management of occupational exposures to HBV, HCV, and HIV and recommendations for postexposure prophylaxis. *MMWR* 2001;50:1–42.
44. Tablan OC, Anderson LJ. Guideline for prevention of nosocomial pneumonia. *Respir Care* 1994;39:1191–1236.
45. Garner JS. Guideline for isolation precautions in hospitals. *Infect Control Hosp Epidemiol* 1996;17:53–80.
46. Bolyard EA, Tablan OC. Guideline for infection control in health care personnel, 1998. *Am J Infect Control* 1998;26:289–354.
47. Centers for Disease Control and Prevention. Recommendations for preventing transmission of human immunodeficiency virus and hepatitis B virus to patients during exposure-prone invasive procedures. *MMWR* 1991;40(RR8):1–9.
48. HICPAC. Recommendations for preventing the spread of vancomycin resistance. *Infect Control Hosp Epidemiol* 1995;16:105–113.
49. Centers for Disease Control and Prevention. Interim guidelines for prevention and control of staphylococcal infection associated with reduced susceptibility to vancomycin. *MMWR* 1997;46:626–628, 635.
50. Centers for Disease Control and Prevention. Guidelines for preventing the transmission of tuberculosis in health care settings, with special focus on HIV-related issues. *MMWR* 1990;39(RR17):1–29.
51. Joint Commission on Accreditation of Healthcare Organizations. Standards: infection control. In: *JCAHO, accreditation manual for hospitals.* Chicago: Joint Commission on Accreditation of Healthcare Organizations, 1990.
52. Richet HM, Craven PC, Brown JM, et al. A cluster of *Rhodococcus (Gordona) bronchialis* sternal wound infections after coronary artery bypass surgery. *N Engl J Med* 1991;324:104–109.
53. Nakashima AK, Allen JR, Martone WJ, et al. Epidemic bullous impetigo in a nursery due to a nasal carrier of *Staphylococcus aureus:* role of epidemiology and control measures. *Infect Control* 1984;5:326–331.
54. Wenger P, Otten J, Breeden A, et al. Control of nosocomial transmission of multiple drug resistant *Mycobacterium tuberculosis* among healthcare workers and HIV infected patients. *Lancet* 1995;345: 235–240.
55. Maloney S, Pearson M, Gordon M, et al. Efficacy of control measures in preventing transmission of multidrug-resistant tuberculosis to patients and healthcare workers. *Ann Intern Med* 1995;122:90–95.
56. Gordon SM, Tipple M, Bland LA, et al. Pyrogenic reactions associated with the use of processed disposable hollow fiber hemodialyzers. *JAMA* 1988;260:2077–2081.
57. Richet HM, McNeil MM, Edwards MC, et al. Cluster of *Malassezia furfur* pulmonary infections in infants in a neonatal intensive care unit. *J Clin Microbiol* 1989;27:1197–1200.
58. Tipple MA, Murphy JJ, Bland LA, et al. Sepsis associated with transfusion of red blood cells contaminated with *Yersinia enterocolitica. Transfusion* 1990;30:207–213.
59. Pegues DA, Carson LA, Tablan OC, et al. Acquisition of *Pseudomonas cepacia* at summer camps for patients with cystic fibrosis. *J Pediatrics* 1994;124:694–702.
60. Lowry PW, Beck-Sague CM, Bland LA, et al. *Mycobacterium chelonae* infections among patients receiving high-flux dialysis in a hemodialysis clinic, California. *J Infect Dis* 1990;161:85–91.
61. Richet HM, McNeil MM, Davis BJ, et al. *Aspergillus fumigatus* sternal wound infection in patients undergoing open-heart surgery. *Am J Epidemiol* 1992:135;48–58.
62. Tipple MA, Schusterman N, Bland LA, et al. Illness in hemodialysis patients after exposure to chloramine contaminated dialysate. *Trans Am Soc Artific Intern Organs* 1991;37:588–591.
63. Beck-Sague CM, Jarvis WR, Bland LA, et al. Outbreak of gram-negative bacteremia and pyrogenic reactions in a hemodialysis center. *Am J Nephrol* 1990;10:397–403.
64. Gordon SM, Bland LA, Alexander S, et al. Hemolysis associated with hydrogen peroxide at a pediatric dialysis center. *Am J Nephrol* 1990; 10:123–127.
65. Richet HM, Andremont A, Tancrede C, et al. Risk factors for candidemia in patients with acute lymphocytic leukemia. *Rev Infect Dis* 1991; 13:211–215.
66. Villarino ME, Gordon SM, Valdon C, et al. A cluster of severe postoperative bleeding following open heart surgery. *Infect Control Hosp Epidemiol* 1992;13:282–288.
67. Villarino ME, Jarvis WR, O'Hara C, et al. Epidemic of *Serratia marcescens* bacteremia in a cardiac intensive care unit. *J Clinl Microbiol* 1989;27:2433–2436.
68. Beck-Sague CM, Chong W, Roy C, et al. Outbreak of surgical wound infections associated with total hip arthroplasty procedures. *Infect Control Hosp Epidemiol* 1992;13:526–535.
69. Gordon SM, Drachman J, Bland LA, et al. Epidemic hypotension in a dialysis center caused by sodium azide. *Kidney Int* 1990;10:123–127.
70. Rosenblum LS, Villarino ME, Nainan O, et al. Prolonged virus excretion among preterm infants in a hepatitis A outbreak in a neonatal intensive care unit. *J Infect Dis* 1991;164:476–482.
71. Panlilio A, Beck-Sague CM, Siegel J, et al. Infections and pseudoinfec-

tions due to povidone-iodine solution contaminated with *Pseudomonas cepacia. Clin Infect Dis* 1992;14:1078–1083.

72. Villarino ME, Stevens L, Schable B, et al. Epidemic *Xanthamonas maltophilia* infections and colonization in an intensive care unit. *Infect Control Hosp Epidemiol* 1992;13:201–206.
73. Pegues DA, Schidlow DV, Tablan OC, et al. Possible nosocomial transmission of *Pseudomonas cepacia* in cystic fibrosis patients. *Arch Pediatr Adolesc Med* 1994;148:805–812.
74. Dooley SW, Villarino ME, Lawrence M, et al. Tuberculosis in a hospital unit for patients infected with the human immunodeficiency virus (HIV): evidence of nosocomial transmission. *JAMA* 1992;267: 2632–2634.
75. Beck-Sague CM, Villarino ME, Giuliano D, et al. Infectious diseases and death among nursing home residents: results of surveillance in 13 nursing homes. *Infect Control Hosp Epidemiol* 1994;15:494–496.
76. Pegues DA, Beck-Sague C, Woollen SW, et al. Anaphylactic reactions associated with reuse of disposable hollow-fiber dialyzers. *Kidney Int* 1992;42:1232–1237.
77. Auerbach SB, Schwartz B, Williams D, et al. Outbreak of invasive group A streptococcal infections in a nursing home. Lessons on prevention and control. *Arch Intern Med* 1992;152:1017–1022.
78. Nelson DE, Auerbach SB, Baltch AL, et al. Epidemic *C. difficile* associated diarrhea: role of second and third generation cephalosporins. *Infect Control Hosp Epidemiol* 1994;15:88–95.
79. Pearson ML, Levine WC, Finton RJ, et al. Anesthesia-associated carbon monoxide exposures among surgical patients. *Infect Control Hosp Epidemiol* 2001;22:352–356.
80. Ginsberg M, Roberto R, Trujillo E, et al. Patient exposures to HIV during nuclear medicine procedures. *MMWR* 1992;41:575–578.
81. Burwen DR, Margo CE, McNeil MM, et al. A pseudoepidemic of postoperative scleritis due to misdiagnosis. *Infect Control Hosp Epidemiol* 1999;20:539–542.
82. Pegues DA, Arathoon E, Samayoa B, et al. Epidemic gram-negative bacteremia in a neonatal intensive care unit, Guatemala. *Am J Infect Control* 1994;6:163–171.
83. Jereb J, Burwen D, Dooley S, et al. Nosocomial outbreak of tuberculosis on a renal transplant unit. *J Infect Dis* 1993;168:1219–1225.
84. Kelly JK, Pearson ML, Kurup VP, et al. Epidemiologic features, risk factors and latex hypersensitivity in patients with spina bifida who develop anaphylactic reactions during general anesthesia. *Am J Clin Allergy Immunol* 1994;94:53–61.
85. Jackson BM, Beck-Sague CM, Bland LA, et al. Pyrogenic reactions and gram-negative bacteremia in a hemodialysis center. *Am J Nephrol* 1994;14:85–89.
86. Al-Rabea AA, Burwen DR, Eldeen MA, et al. *Klebsiella pneumoniae* bloodstream infections in neonates in a hospital in the Kingdom of Saudi Arabia. *Infect Control Hosp Epidemiol* 1998;19:674–679.
87. Zaza S, Tokars JI, Jarvis WR, et al. Bloodstream infections associated with transfusion of random donor platelet pools. *Infect Control Hosp Epidemiol* 1994;15:82–88.
88. Welbel SF, McNeil M. Pramanik A, et al. Nosocomial *Malassezia pachydermetis* bloodstream infections in a neonatal intensive care unit. *Pediatr Infect Dis J* 1994;13:104–109.
89. Welbel SF, McNeil MM, Kuykendall RJ, et al. *Candida parapsilosis* bloodstream infections in neonatal intensive care unit patients: epidemiologic and laboratory confirmation of a common source outbreak. *Pediatr Infect Dis J* 1996;15:998–1002.
90. Burwen DR, Lasker BA, Rao N, et al. Invasive aspergillosis outbreak on a hematology-oncology ward. *Infect Control Hosp Epidemiol* 2000; 22:45–47.
91. Burkholder BT, Coronado VG, Brown J, et al. Nosocomial transmission of hepatitis A in a pediatric hospital traced to an anti-hepatitis A virus-negative patient with immunodeficiency. *Pediatr Infect Dis J* 1995;14:261–266.
92. Coronado VG, Beck-Sague CM, Hutton MD, et al. Transmission of multidrug-resistant *Mycobacterium tuberculosis* among persons with human immunodeficiency virus infection in an urban hospital: epidemiologic and restriction fragment length polymorphism analysis. *J Infect Dis* 1993;168:1052–1055.
93. Rudnick JR, Arduino MJ, Bland LA, et al. An outbreak of pyrogenic reactions in chronic hemodialysis patients associated with hemodialyzer reuse. *Trans Am Soc Artific Intern Organs* 1995;19:289–294.
94. Burwen DR, Olsen SM, Bland LA, et al. Epidemic aluminum intoxication in hemodialysis patients traced to use of an aluminum pump. *Kidney Int* 1995;48:469–474.
95. Zaza S, Beck-Sague CM, Jarvis WR. Tracing patients exposed to health care workerswith tuberculosis. *Public Health Rep* 1997;112: 153–157.
96. Welbel SF, Schoendorf K, Bland LA, et al. An outbreak of gram-negative bacteremia in chronic hemodialysis patients. *Am J Nephrol* 1995;15:1–4.
97. Stroud LA, Tokars JI, Grieco MH, et al. Evaluation of infection control measures inpreventing the nosocomial transmission of multidrug-resistant *Mycobacterium tuberculosis* in a New York City hospital. *Infect Control Hosp Epidemiol* 1995;16:141–147.
98. Maloney S, Welbel S, Daves B, et al. *Mycobacterium abscessus* pseudoinfection traced to an automated endoscope washer: utility of epidemiologic and laboratory investigation. *J Infect Dis* 1994;169: 1166–1169.
99. Ettestad PJ, Campbell GL, Welbel SF, et al. Biliary complications in the treatment of unsubstantiated Lyme disease. *J Infect Dis* 1995;171: 356–361.
100. Wenger PN, Tokars JI, Brennan P, et al. An outbreak of *Enterobacter hormaechei* infection and colonization in an intensive care nursery. *Clin Infect Dis* 1997;24:1243–1244.
101. Wenger PN, Brown JM, McNeil MM, et al. *Nocardia farcinica* sternotomy site infections in patients following open heart surgery. *J Infect Dis* 1998;178:1539–1543.
102. Arnow PM, Bland LA, Garcia-Houchins S, et al. An outbreak of fatal fluoride intoxication in a long-term hemodialysis unit. *Ann Intern Med* 1994;121:339–344.
103. Shay DK, Maloney SM, Montecalvo M, et al. Epidemiology and mortality of vancomycin-resistant enterococcal bloodstream infections. *J Infect Dis* 1995;172:993–1000.
104. Morris JG Jr, Shay DK, Hebden JN, et al. Enterococci resistant to multiple antimicrobial agents, including vancomycin: establishment of endemicity in a university medical center. *Ann Intern Med* 1995; 123:250–259.
105. Fridkin SK, Pear SM, Williamson TH, et al. The role of understaffing in central venous catheter-associated bloodstream infections. *Infect Control Hosp Epidemiol* 1996;17:150–158.
106. Danzig LE, Short LM, Collins K, et al. Bloodstream infections associated with a needleless intravenous infusion system in patients receiving home infusion therapy. *JAMA* 1995;273:1862–1864.
107. Shay DK, Fann LA, Jarvis WR. Respiratory distress and sudden death associated with receipt of a peripheral parenteral nutrition admixture. *Infect Control Hosp Epidemiol* 1997;18:814–817.
108. Fridkin SK, Kremer FB, Bland LA, et al. *Acremonium kiliense* endophthalmitis that occurred after cataract extraction in an ambulatory surgical center and was traced to an environment reservoir. *Clin Infect Dis* 1996;22:222–227.
109. Valendia MP, Fridkin SK, Cardenas VM, et al. Transmission of human immunodeficiency virus in a dialysis center. *Lancet* 1995;345: 1417–1422.
110. Danzig L, Hendricks K, Schulster L, et al. Outbreaks of hepatitis B virus infection among hemodialysis patients-California, Nebraska, and Texas 1994. *MMWR* 1996;45:285–289.
111. Kellerman S, Shay D, Howard J, et al. Bloodstream infections in home infusion patients: the influence of race and needleless intravascular access devices. *J Pediatr* 1996;129:711–717.
112. Do AN, Fridkin SK, Yechouron AY, et al. Risk factors for early recurrent *Clostridium difficile*-associated diarrhea. *Clin Infect Dis* 1998;26: 954–959.
113. Chang HJ, Christenson JC, Pavia AT, et al. *Ochrabactrum anthropi* meningitis in pediatric pericardial allograft transplant recipients. *J Infect Dis* 1996;173:656–660.
114. Chang HJ, Miller HL, Watkin N, et al. An epidemic of *Malassezia pachydermatis* in intensive care nursery associated with colonization of health care worker pet dogs. *N Engl J Med* 1998;338:706–711.
115. Do AN, Ray BJ, Banerjee SN, et al. Bloodstream infections associated

with needleless device use and the importance of infection control practices in home health care setting. *J Infect Dis* 1999;179:4442–448.
116. Archibald LK, Corl A, Shah B, et al. *Serratia marcescens* outbreak associated with extrinsic contamination of 1% chlorxylenol soap. *Infect Control Hosp Epidemiol* 1997;18:704–709.
117. Jochimsen EM, Frenette C, Delorme M, et al. A cluster of bloodstream infections and pyrogenic reactions among hemodialysis patients traced to dialysis machine waste-handling option units. *Am J Nephrol* 1998;18:485–489.
118. Cookson ST, Nora JJ, Kithas JA, et al. Pyrogenic reactions in patients undergoing cardiac catheterization associated with contaminated glass medicine cups. *Cathet Cardiovasc Diagn* 1997;42:12–18.
119. Archibald LK, Manning ML, Bell LM, et al. Patient density, nurse-to-patient ratio and nosocomial infection risk in a pediatric cardiac intensive care unit. *Pediatr Infect Dis J* 1997;16:1045–1048.
120. Manning ML, Archibald LK, Bell LM, et al. *Serratia marcescens* transmission in a pediatric cardiac intensive care unit: a multifactorial occurrence. *Am J Infect Control* 2001;29:115–119.
121. Singer DA, Jochimsen EM, Gielarek P, et al. Pseudo-outbreak of *Enterococcus durans* infections and colonization associated with the introduction of an automated identification system software update. *J Clin Microbiol* 1996;34:2685–2687.
122. Jochimsen EM, Singer DA, Fish L, et al. Risk factors for acquisition of vancomycin-resistant enterococci among patients on a renal ward during a community hospital outbreak. *Am J Infect Control* 2000;28: 282–285.
123. Jochimsen EM, Fish L, Manning K, et al. Control of vancomycin-resistant enterococci at a community hospital: efficacy of patient and staff cohorting. *Infect Control Hosp Epidemiol* 1999;20:106–110.
124. Cookson ST, Ihrig M, O'Mara E, Hartstein AI, et al. Use of an estimation method to derive an appropriate denominator to calculate central venous catheter-associated bloodstream infection rates. *Infect Control Hosp Epidemiol* 1998;19:28–31.
125. Cookson ST, Ihrig M, O'Mara EM, et al. Increased bloodstream infection rates in surgical patients associated with variation from recommended use and care following implementation of a needleless access device. *Infect Control Hosp Epidemiol* 1998;19:23–27.
126. Ihrig M, Cookson ST, Campbell K, et al. Evaluation of the acceptability of a needleless vascular-access system by nurses. *Am J Infect Control* 1997;25:434–438.
127. Jochimsen EM, Carmicheal WW, An J, et al. Liver failure and death after exposure to microcystins at a hemodialysis center in Brazil. *N Engl J Med* 1998;383:873–878.
128. Archibald LK, Romas M, Arduino MJ, et al. *Enterobacter cloacae* and *Pseudomonas aeruginosa* polymicrobial bloodstream infections traced to extrinsic contamination of a dextrose multidose vial. *J Pediatr* 1999; 133:640–644.
129. Kuehnert MJ, Webb RM, Jochimsen EM, et al. *Staphylococcus aureus* bloodstream infections among patients undergoing electroconvulsive therapy traced to breaks in infection control and possible extrinsic contamination of propofol. *Anesth Analg* 1997;85:420–425.
130. McDonald LC, Banerjee SN, Jarvis WR. Line-associated bloodstream infection in pediatric intensive care unit patients associated with needleless device and intermittent intravenous therapy. *Infect Control Hosp Epidemiol* 1998;19:772–777.
131. Mangram AJ, Archibald LK, Hupert M, et al. Outbreak of sterile peritonitis among continuous cycling peritoneal dialysis patients. *Kidney Int* 1998;54:1367–1371.
132. Garrett DO, Jochimsen E, Murfitt K, et al. The emergence of decreased susceptibility to vancomycin in *Staphylococcus epidermidis*. *Infect Control Hosp* 1999;17:167–170.
133. Garrett DO, Jochimsen E, Jarvis WR. Invasive *Aspergillus* spp. infection in rheumatology patients. *J Rheumatol* 1999;26:146–149.
134. McDonald LC, Walker M, Carson L, et al. Outbreak of Acinetobacter spp. Bloodstream infections in a nursery associated with contaminated aerosols and air conditioners. *Pediatr Infect Dis J* 1998;17:716–727.
135. Hutter JC, Kuehnert MJ, Wallis RR, et al. Acute onset of decreased vision and blindness traced to hemodialysis treatment with aged dialyzers. *JAMA* 2000:283;2128–2134.
136. Wang SA, Tokars JI, Bianchine PJ, et al. *Enterobacter cloacae* bloodstream infections traced to intrinsically contaminated human albumin. *Clin Infect Dis* 2000:30;35–40.
137. Garrett DO, McDonald C, Wanderly A, et al. An outbreak of neonatal deaths in Brazil associated with contaminated intravenous fluids. *J Infect Dis* 2002;186:81–85.
138. Wang SA, Levin RB, Carson LA, et al. An outbreak of gram-negative bacteremia in hemodialysis patients traced to hemodialysis machine waste drain ports. *Infect Control Hosp Epidemiol* 1999;20:746–751.
139. Trick WE, Kuehnert MJ, Quirk SB, et al. Regional dissemination of vancomycin-resistant Enterococci resulting from interfacility transfer of colonized patients. *J Infect Dis* 1999;180:391–396.
140. Ostrowsky BE, Trick WE, Sohn A, et al. Successful control of vancomycin-resistant enterococcus (VRE) colonization in acute and long-term care facility patients: working together as a community. *N Engl J Med* 2001;344:1427–1433.
141. Smith TL, Pearson ML, Wilcox KR, et al. Emergence of vancomycin resistance in *Staphylococcus aureus*. *N Engl J Med* 1999;340:493–501.
142. Dobbins JG, Belay ED, Malecki J, et al. Creutzfeldt-Jakob disease in a recipient of a dura mater graft processed in the U.S.: cause or coincidence? *Neuroepidemiology* 2000;19:62–66.
143. Alonso-Echanove J, Sha SS, Velanti AJ, et al. Nosocomial outbreak of *Microbacterium* spp. bacteremia among cancer patients. *J Infect Dis* 2001;184:754–760.
144. Trick WE, Kioski CM, Howard KM, et al. Outbreak of *Pseudomonas aeruginosa* ventriculitis among patients in a neurosurgical intensive care unit. *Infect Control Hosp Epidemiol* 2000:21;204–208.
145. Smith TL, Pullen GT, Crouse V, et al. Bloodstream infections in pediatric outpatient oncology patients—a new healthcare systems challenge. *Infect Control Hosp Epidemiol* 2002;23:381–387.
146. Alonso-Echanove J, Cairns L, Richards M, et al. Adverse ocular reactions following transfusions–United States, 1997–1998. *MMWR* 1997;47:49–50.
147. Duffy RE, Brown SE, Caldwell KL, et al. Toxic endothelial cell destruction of the cornea following intraocular surgery associated with trace element contamination of instruments sterilized by plasma gas. *Arch Ophthalmol* 2000;118:1167–1176.
148. Trick WE, Scheckler WE, Tokars JL, et al. Risk factors for radial artery harvest site infection following coronary artery bypass graft surgery. *Clin Infect Dis* 2000:30;270–275.
149. Trick WE, Scheckler WE, Tokars JI, et al. Modifiable risk factors associated with coronary artery bypass graft deep sternal site infection. *J Thorac Cardiovasc Surg* 2000;49:108–114.
150. Duffy R, Tomashek K, Spangenberg M, et al. Multistate outbreak of hemolysis in hemodialysis patients traced to faulty blood tubing sets. *Kidney Int* 2000:57;1668–1674.
151. Buchholz U, Richards C, Murthy R, et al. Pyrogenic reactions associated with single daily-dosed intravenous gentamicin. *Infect Control Hospl Epidemiol* 2000;21:771–775.
152. Ostrowsky BE, Whitener C, Brendenberg KH, et al. *Serratia marcescens* bacteremia traced to an infused narcotic. *N Engl J Med* 2002; 346:1529–1537.
153. Pessoa-Silva C, Toscano C, Moreira B, et al. Infection due to extended-spectrum beta-lactamase-producing *Salmonella enterica* subsp. *Enterica* serotype Infantis in a neonatal unit. *J Pediatr* 2002;141: 381–387.
154. Grohskopf LA, Roth VR, Feikin DR, et al. *Serratia liquefaciens* bloodstream infection and pyrogenic reactions at a hemodialysis center traced to extrinsically contaminated epoetin alfa. *N Engl J Med* 2001; 344:1491–1497.

8

PSEUDOINFECTIONS AND PSEUDO-OUTBREAKS

BURKE A. CUNHA

GENERAL CONCEPTS

Pseudoinfections and pseudo-outbreaks are an ongoing problem for infection control personnel, infectious disease physicians, and hospital epidemiologists. Pseudoinfections and pseudo-outbreaks must be differentiated from actual outbreaks. An outbreak refers to an isolate, with its usual clinical manifestations, that is over baseline incidence for the institution. With actual outbreaks, the isolate is recovered from the body site where the microorganism usually colonizes or infects, and the clinical presentation is usual for the microorganism in a particular body site. For example, an *Acinetobacter* outbreak in an intensive care unit is usually manifested by an increase in the incidence of cultures of the microorganism from respiratory secretions, which may or may not be accompanied by manifestations of infection in the form of tracheobronchitis or nosocomial pneumonia. Each institution has baseline epidemiologic data, and in such a situation there would be a dramatic increase in the numbers of *Acinetobacter* species cultured from respiratory secretions in the intensive care unit or units involved in the outbreak.

Pseudoinfection, in contrast to true infection, may involve a cluster of usual or unusual microorganism recovered from a body site. Single episodes of pseudoinfection may occur if an uncommon microorganism is isolated from a body site where it is not usually pathogenic [e.g., *Citrobacter* species isolated from the cerebrospinal fluid (CSF) in a nonneurosurgical patient]. Alternately, a common microorganism, *Hemophilus influenzae,* cultured from the urine merits attention. Because *Citrobacter* is not a usual neuropathogen and *H. influenzae* is not a usual uropathogen, the possibility of pseudoinfection should be entertained in such cases. Another presentation for isolated episodes of pseudoinfection involves the recovery of a usual or unusual microorganism from a body site, which is at variance with its usual laboratory or clinical features. For example, if *Flavobacterium meningosepticum* is recovered from the CSF in an adult with mental confusion with the CSF findings of no pleocytosis, no increase in lactic acid, no increase in protein, and no decrease in glucose, the possibility of a pseudomeningitis should be entertained because there is a discordance between the isolate and clinical findings, even though the isolate is a potential neuropathogen. The discrepancy between laboratory or clinical findings for the usual presentation of a given microorganism at a given anatomic site should lead the clinician to suspect the possibility of a pseudoinfection. If multiple patients are involved, then this situation should be termed a pseudo-outbreak. There should be no difficulty in differentiating simple contaminants from pseudoinfection. Contaminants represent normal or altered flora that are introduced into culture media during the process of specimen collection. Contaminants represent the microflora of site from which they are cultured. In contrast, pseudoinfections are usually not due to contaminants from the resident microflora at a given body site. Even when they are, there is a discordance between the patient's clinical manifestations and the usual manifestations of the isolate at the body site being cultured in pseudo-infections and pseudo-outbreaks.

PSEUDOBACTEREMIAS

The most common type of pseudoinfection is pseudobacteremia. The microorganisms associated with pseudobacteremias include a wide variety of species. The most frequently cultured microorganisms in pseudobacteremias are *Bacillus* species, *Pseudomonas* species, and streptococci. Pseudobacteremias are most often related to the introduction of normal or altered flora from the skin, to contaminated antiseptics applied to the skin before venipuncture, to contamination of the rubber gaskets and tops of culture transport media, or to contaminated culture media. Less commonly, pseudobacteremias may be related to the processing of blood culture samples. Inadequately disinfected blood culture bottle tops or inadequate needle sterilization in blood culture autoanalyzers have been associated with pseudobacteremias. Contaminated disinfectant solutions, as mentioned, may contaminate the specimen at one or more points in the blood culture collection and processing sequence of events. Rarely, actual infections have resulted from accidental reflux of contaminated blood from blood tube holders or blood tubes, contaminated disinfectants, or contaminated needles reintroduced into the patient during the process of blood culture collection. As with other types of pseudoinfections, inappropriate antimicrobial therapy is often initiated if clinicians do not recognize that a pseudobacteremia rather than a true infection is present (1–64) (Table 8.1).

TABLE 8.1. PSEUDOBACTEREMIA

Reference Year	Microorganisms	Patients affected (No.)	Patients infected (No.)	Therapy affected (No.)	Problem
[1] 1969	*Escherichia coli*	7	0	7	Contaminated penicillinase in blood culture media
[2] 1972	*Acinetobacter lwoffi*	27	3	4	Contaminated penicillinase in blood culture media
[3] 1973	*Moraxella nonliquefaciens*	8	1	1	Contaminated holders of blood culture tubes
[4] 1974	*Bacillus* species	26	0	0	Contaminated blood culture media
[5] 1976	*Pseudomonas cepacia*	79	3	4	Contaminated benzalkonium chloride used for venipuncture
[6] 1976	*Flavobacterium meningosepticum*	6	0	0	Contaminated chlorhexidine solution used for venipuncture
[7] 1976	*Serratia marcescens*	40	0	0	Cross contamination of blood cultures with bacteria form nonsterile blood collection tubes
[8] 1977	*Acinetobacter lwoffi*	11	0	2	Improper blood culture technique in a mist tent heavily contaminated with bacteria
[9] 1978	*Pseudomonas maltophila*	25	1	3	Cross contamination of blood cultures with bacteria from nonsterile blood collection tubes
[10] 1979	*Staphylococcus aureus*	11	0	5	Blood cultures contaminated by a colonized (nasopharynx) laboratory technician
[11] 1980	*Clostridium sordellii*	11	0	0	Contaminated thimerosal solution/diaphragms of blood culture media
[12] 1980	*Acinetobacter lwoffi*	22	0	0	Blood cultures contaminated
[13] 1980	*Staphylococcus aureus*	5	0	0	Blood culture media contaminated by physician
[14] 1980	*Aerococcus viridans*	7	0	0	Inadequately disinfected blood culture bottle stoppers
[15] 1981	*Pseudomonas cepacia*	30	0	0	Contaminated povidone-iodine solution used for venipuncture/disinfection of blood culture bottle stoppers
[16] 1981	*Enterobacter cloacae*	7	0	1	Contaminated thrombin in blood culture collection vials
[17] 1981	*Klebsiella pneumoniae*	13	7	6	Contaminated sampling needle in an automated blood culture analyzer
[18] 1981	Gram-negative bacilli	75	0	NA	Improper blood culture collection technique
[19] 1981	*Pseudomonas cepacia*	16	0	2	Contaminated povidone-iodine solution
[20] 1982	*Klebsiella pneumoniae*	2	0	1	Inadequate needle sterilization in automated blood culture analyzer
	Streptococcus pyogenes	1			
	Staphylococcus epidermidis	1			
[21] 1982	*Bacillus* species	36	0	0	Contaminated syringes
[22] 1982	*Serratia marcescens*	17	0	NA	Improper blood culture collection technique
[23] 1982	*Serratia marcescens*	16	0	2	Cross contamination with blood gas specimens
[24] 1982	*Pseudomonas aeruginosa*	17	0	0	Contamination of blood culture processing equipment
[25] 1983	*Bacillus* species	15	0	0	Contaminated cotton swabs used to disinfect blood culture bottles
[26] 1983	*Pseudomonas stutzeri*	24	1	21	Contaminated green soap solution
[27] 1983	*Streptococcus faecalis* (enterococcus)	8	0	2	Cross contamination in automated blood culture analyzer
[28] 1983	*Pseudomonas maltophilia*	5	0	0	Contaminated soduim citrate solution improper blood culture technique
[29] 1983	*Bacillus* species	15	0	0	Contaminated brain-heart infusion broth
[30] 1984	*Staphylococcus aureus*	11			Inadequate needle sterilization in automated blood culture analyzer
	Staphylococcus epidermidis	10			
	Streptococcus species	1	0	3	
	Escherichia coli	1			
[31] 1984	*Streptococcus bovis*	1	0	1	Inadequate cleaning of needle in automated blood culture analyzer
[32] 1984	*Bacillus* species	26	0	1	Spore contamination of needle in automated blood culture analyzer
[33] 1985	*Streptomyces* species	7	0	0	Airborne contamination of clinical specimens secondary to construction
[34] 1985	*Pseudomonas cepacia*	2	0	NA	Contaminated antiseptic handwash
[35] 1985	*Pseudomonas pickettii*	21	0	NA	Contaminated aqueous chlorhexidine solution
[36] 1985	*Pseudomonas fluorescens*	57	0	0	Cross contamination of citrated blood collection tubes

(continued)

TABLE 8.1. (continued)

Reference Year	Microorganisms	Patients affected (No.)	Patients infected (No.)	Therapy affected (No.)	Problem
[37] 1987	*Enterococcus* species	17	0	2	Contaminated radiometric blood culture device
	Staphylococcus aureus	5	0	NA	
[38] 1987	*Ewingella americana*	20	0	14	Cross contamination of blood culture bottles with bacteria from nonsterile tubes
[39] 1988	*Pseudomonas cepacia*	2	0	NA	Contaminated blood gas analyzer
[40] 1989	*Streptococcus viridans*	41	0	NA	Blood cultures contaminated by colonized laboratory technician with dermatitis
[41] 1989	Streptococci and *Staphylococcus aureus*	7	0	1	Blood cultures contaminated by a colonized laboratory technician with positive nasopharyngeal cultures
[42] 1990	*Bacillus* species	10	0	6	Blood cultures contaminated by nonsterile gloves used by phlebotomists
[43] 1991	*Candida guilliermondii*	17	0	2	Contaminated heparin vials used for blood culture collection
[44] 1991	*Aspergillus* and *Penicillium* species	13	0	0	Nonaseptic processing of culture media
[45] 1993	*Enterobacter cloacae*	27	0	0	Nonaseptic blood culture collection
[46] 1993	*Pseudomonas cepacia*	27	0	0	Contaminated EDTA in blood culture bottles
[47] 1993	*Alcaligenes xylosoxidans* (8) *Xanthomonas maltophilia* (2) *Klebsiella oxytoca* (1) *Corynebacterium aquaticum* (5)	16	0	0	Nonsterile blood culture collection/processing
[48] 1994	*Mycobacterium avium intracellulare*	30	0	1	Cross contamination of culture media
[49] 1994	*Pseudomonas fluorescens*	11	0	0	Breakdown in aseptic technique
[50] 1994	Gram-variable bacilli	1	0	1	Contaminated culture plate
[51] 1994	*Enterobacter agglomerans*	37	0	0	Nonsterile blood collection tubes
[52] 1996	*Burkholderia cepacia*	13	0	4	Contaminated blood gas analyzer
[53] 1997	*Mycobacterium abscessus*	23	0	0	Probably due to contaminated lysis centrifugation tube
[54] 1998	*Candida parapsilosis*	29	0	0	Contamination of blood culture bottles by lab technician
[55] 1999	*Pseudomonas fluorescens*	12	0	8	Contaminated lithium heparin bottles
[56] 1999	*Pseudomonas fluorescens*	53	0	0	Contaminated lithium heparin bottles
[57] 1999	*Serratia marcescens*	2	0	2	Contaminated blood glucose/lactate analyzer
[58] 1999	*Staphylococcus saccharolyticus*	6	0	NA	Inadequate venipuncture skin site preparation
[59] 1999	*Agrobacterium radiobacter*	15	0	NA	Contaminated blood culture tubes
[60] 1999	*Enterococcus faecium*	4	0	NA	Phlebotomist contaminated blood culture bottles
[61] 1999	*Pseudomonas fluorescens* *Comamonas acidovorans*	7	0	NA	Contaminated lithium heparin bottles
[62] 1999	Gram-negative microorganism	1	0	1	False-positive blood cultures
[63] 2000	*Bacillus megatherium*	1	0	0	Probably due to contaminated blood culture bottle tops
[64] 2001	*Paenibacillus macerans*	8	0	8	Contaminated blood culture bottles

NA, not available.

PSEUDOMENINGITIS

Pseudomeningitis is the next commonest type of pseudoinfection after pseudobacteremia. Pseudomeningitis is suspected when nonneuropathogens are cultured from the CSF in patients who have had a lumbar puncture for altered mental status or other neurologic findings. Gram-negative bacilli or gram-negative coccobacilli are the microorganisms most often associated with pseudomeningitis. Alternately, neuropathogens, recovered from the CSF of patients with altered mental status, may also represent pseudomeningitis. The clinical clue to the recognition of pseudomeningitis is the discrepancy between the usual clinical presentation of the neuropathogen and the discrepancy in the laboratory or clinical manifestations in the patient with pseudomeningitis. For example, if a patient has *Staphylococcus aureus* isolated from CSF and has fever and mental confusion, the clinician is faced with the possibility that either the patient has *S. aureus* meningitis or, depending on the clinical circumstances, may have a pseudoinfection. If the CSF findings are not consistent with the usual purulent CSF profile associated with *S. aureus* acute bacterial meningitis, then a pseudoinfection should be suspected. A more common situation is when a nonneuropathogen or an uncommon neuropathogen is recovered from the CSF of a patient without compatible clinical findings. For example, if *Candida albicans* is recovered from the CSF of a neonate with fever and neurologic findings, the clinician should be alert to the fact that *C. albicans* is a rare cause of fungal meningitis. Even if the CSF profile is consistent with a fungal infection, the clinician should look for extraneural manifestations of disseminated candidal infection, which is responsible for the seeding of the CSF. In the absence of clinical evidence of invasive candidiasis outside the CNS, [e.g., chorioretinitis, pustular skin lesions containing *Candida* or *Candida* recovered from a usually sterile organ (liver or spleen)], the diagnosis of pseudomeningitis should be entertained. The source of specimen contamination resulting in false-positive Gram stains or cultures may be due to extrinsic contamination in the process of CSF specimen collection or by contamination of laboratory materials (e.g., slides, tubes, culture media). Because of the mortality and morbidity associated with meningitis, many patients with pseudomeningitis receive empiric antimicrobial therapy until the diagnosis of pseudomeningitis is made (65–86) (Table 8.2).

PSEUDOPNEUMONIAS

Atypical mycobacteria, fungi, and gram-negative aerobic bacilli are the microorganisms most often associated with pseudopneumonias. Most pseudopneumonia outbreaks are associated with various microorganisms contaminating bronchoscopes. Microorganism contamination of various parts of the bronchoscope (e.g., biopsy forceps, or brush) are not uncommon. Alternately, contamination of respiratory therapy solutions or topical anesthetics has also been implicated in pseudopneumonia outbreaks. Empiric antimicrobial therapy for pseudopneumonias is less common, because many pseudopneumonias are caused by mycobacteria or fungi (87–121) (Table 8.3).

TABLE 8.2. PSEUDOMENINGITIS

[Reference] Year	Microorganisms	Positive CSF gram stain (No.)	Positive CSF culture (No.)	patients involved (No.)	patients treated (No.)	Problem
[65] 1973	Gram-negative cocci	4	0	4	0	Contaminated specimen tubes
[66] 1974	Gram-positive cocci	1	0	1	1	Contaminated slides
[67] 1976	*Flavobacterium meningosepticum*	0	1	1	1	Contaminated skin preparation soap
[68] 1978	Gram-negative bacilli	10	0	10	5	Contaminated slides
[69] 1979	Gram-negative bacilli	2	0	2	2	Contaminated transport media
[70] 1983	*Salmonella typhimurium*	0	2	2	1	Contaminated pipette
[71] 1985	Gram-negative bacilli	5	0	0	1	Contaminated specimen tubes
[72] 1985	*Acinetobacter* CDC group VE-1	1	1	1	1	Extrinsically contaminated culture media
[73] 1986	*Sporobolomyces salmonicolar*	0	3	3	0	Extrinsically contaminated culture media
[74] 1987	*Aspergillus* species	0	1	1	0	Extrinsically contaminated culture media
[75] 1988	*Bacillus* species	3	13	16	3	Contaminated culture broth
[76] 1989	*Bacillus* species	0	1	1	1	Contaminated culture media
[77] 1990	Fungal elements	1	0	1	1	Airborne contamination of staining reagent
[78] 1991	*Pseudomonas paucimobilis*	0	1	1	0	Contaminated culture media
[79] 1994	Gram-positive diplococci	1	0	0	1	Contaminated culture media
[80] 1995	*Neisseria lactamica*	1	1	1	1	Contaminated culture media
[81] 1997	*Bacillus* species	0	1	1	1	Contaminated culture media
[82] 1998	Viridans streptococci	0	1	1	0	Contaminated culture media
[83] 1999	*Acinetobacter baumannii*	1	1	1	1	Contaminated culture media
[84] 2002	*Acinetobacter lwoffi*	0	1	1	0	Contaminated culture media
[85] 2002	*Acinetobacter baumannii*	0	1	1	1	Contaminated culture media
[86] 2003	*Flavimonas oryzihabitans*	0	1	1	1	Contaminated culture media

TABLE 8.3. PSEUDOPNEUMONIA

[Reference] Year	Microorganisms	Patients affected (No.)	Patients infected (No.)	Therapy affected (No.)	Problem
[87] 1973	*Pseudomonas cepacia*	22	0	0	Contamination of topical anesthetic used during fiberoptic bronchoscopy
[88] 1976	*Mycobacterium gordonae*	7	0	0	Sputum contaminated by tap water from patients rinsing their mouths prior to specimen collection
[89] 1977	*Pseudomonas aeruginosa*	103	0	0	Contaminated fiberoptic bronchoscope
[90] 1978	*Serratia marcescens*	89	1	0	Contaminated fiberoptic bronchoscope
[91] 1979	*Mycobacterium gordonae*	52	0	1	Bronchoscopy specimens contaminated with topical anesthetic dye
[92] 1980	*Penicillium/Trichosporin* species	8	0	0	Contamination of bronchial washings with topical anesthetic (cocaine)
[93] 1982	Coccidioidomycosis	7	0	0	Spore contaminated slides
[94] 1983	*Mycobacterium gordonae*	>100	0	0	Bronchoscope contaminated by water/glutaraldehyde
[95] 1983	*Penicillium* species	21	0	0	Contaminated bronchoscope biopsy forceps
[96] 1984	*Mycobacterium marinum*	5	0	1	Specimens contaminated by laboratory personnel
[97] 1985	*Bacillus* species	17	0	0	Contaminated fiberoptic bronchoscope
[98] 1989	*Rhodotorula rubra*	30	0	0	Contaminated brushes used to clean bronchoscopes
[99] 1985	*Pseudomonas pickettii*	5	0	NA	Contaminated respiratory therapy solution
[100] 1985	*Serratia marcescens*	4	0	NA	Bronchoscopes contaminated by water
[101] 1992	*Methylobacter mesophilica*	7	0	NA	Contamination of fungal culture tubes
[102] 1994	*Mycobacterium xenopi*	21	0	0	Contaminated tap water used to process bronchoscopes
[103] 1994	*Pseudomonas aeruginosa*	8	0	0	Contaminated cleaning fluid for bronchoscopes
[104] 1994	*Mycobacterium tuberculosis*	3	0	0	Contaminated red staining solution
[105] 1995	Nontuberculous mycobacteria	9	0	8	Inadequate sterilization of culture system
[106] 1996	*Mycobacterium tuberculosis*	12	0	0	Laboratory specimen contamination
[107] 1997	*Legionella pneumophila*	3	0	0	Contaminated tap water
[108] 1997	*Mycobacterium chelonae*	28	0	0	Contaminated tap water
	M. avium-intracellulare	3			
	M. gordonae	2			
	M. fortuitum	1			
[109] 1998	*Mycobacterium tuberculosis*	9	0	0	Contaminated laboratory pipettes
[110] 1998	*Mycobacterium abscessus*	16	0	NA	Contaminated distilled water used to clean bronchoscopes
[111] 1999	*Mycobacterium tuberculosis*	12	4	NA	Contaminated bronchoscopy biopsy port
	M. avium-intracellulare				
	Pseudomonas aeruginosa				
[112] 1999	*Ralstonia pickettii*	34			Contaminated saline solution used in respiratory therapy
[113] 2000	*Mycobacterium gordonae*	5	0	4	Sputum contaminated by refrigerator water
[114] 2001	*Mycobacterium chelonae*	22	0	3	Contaminated automated endoscope washer
[115] 2001	*Mycobacterium szulgai*	31	0	NA	Contaminated water storage tank
[116] 2002	*Mycobacterium fortuitum*	19	0	1	Contaminated ice machine
[117] 2002	*Mycobacterium fortuitum*	47	0	1	Contaminated ice machine
[118] 2002	*Mycobacterium simiae*	62	0	NA	Contaminated water supply
[119] 2002	*Mycobacterium gordonae*	16	0	NA	Contaminated automated endoscope washer
[120] 2002	*Mycobacterium tuberculosis*	6	0	2	Laboratory contamination of specimens
[121] 2003	*Pseudomonas aeruginosa*	41	0	0	Inadequate bronchoscope sterilization procedure

NA, not available.

TABLE 8.4. PSEUDOBACTERIURIA

[Reference] Year	Microorganisms	Patients affected (No.)	Patients infected (No.)	Therapy affected (No.)	Problem
[122] 1982	*Pseudomonas cepacia*	44	0	0	Contaminated disinfectant solution
[123] 1987	*Mucor circinelloides*	1	0	0	Contaminated specimen by vaginal or colonic microorganisms
[124] 1988	*Serratia marcescens*	1	0	0	Contaminated ultrasound jelly
[125] 1989	*Trichosporon beigelii*	15	0	4	Contamination of urinary catheter drainage system
[126] 1997	*Klebsiella pneumoniae*	6	0	0	Contamination from transducer
[127] 1998	*Pseudomonas putida*	23	0	Some	Contaminated urine culture kits

PSEUDOBACTERIURIA

Pseudobacteriuria is the least common type of pseudoinfection. The usual mechanism of pseudoinfections for pseudobacteriuria is extrinsic contamination of the urinary drainage collecting system. Pseudoinfection is suggested if the pathogen recovered is not a usual uropathogen and pyuria is not present in the urinalysis (122–127) (Table 8.4).

MISCELLANEOUS PSEUDOINFECTIONS

A variety of other pseudoinfections have been described in the literature including pseudoendocarditis, pseudohepatitis, pseudoadenitis, and pseudowound infections. Contaminated transport media and disinfectant or soap solution are responsible for most of these pseudoinfections, and specimen contamination by laboratory technicians can also occur. Pseudoinfections may also involve contaminated specimens from multiple sites. Pseudo-outbreaks may involve multiple contaminated specimens of sputum, urine, CSF, tissue or wound, blood, bronchial washings, nasal swabs, and gastric aspirates resulting from contaminated antimicrobial solutions. Bacterial contamination of deionized water has caused false-positive smears of body fluids, contaminated transport medium, or contaminated disinfectants (e.g., povidone iodine) (6,31,43,69,128–152) (Table 8.5).

INFECTION CONTROL ASPECTS OF PSEUDOINFECTIONS AND PSEUDO-OUTBREAKS

Infection control professionals, infectious disease clinicians, and hospital epidemiologists should remain alert to the possibility of pseudoinfections or pseudo-outbreaks. The first task of the infection control staff is to differentiate true infection from pseudoinfection or pseudo-outbreak. Clusters of single isolates may occur in true outbreaks and in pseudo-outbreaks. The clue to a pseudo-outbreak is either the recovery of an unusual microorganism from a body site from which it is uncommonly isolated or the recovery of a common microorganism from an unusual body site. An abrupt increase in the incidence in colonization or infection of any body site should alert the clinician to the possibility of pseudoinfection. Individual cases of pseudoinfection are more difficult to recognize than are pseudo-outbreaks that merit attention because of their increased numbers and incidence compared with baseline. Either a common microorganism can be isolated from an unusual body site or an unusual microorganism can be isolated from a typical body site. In both situations, the clinician should be alerted that more information or investigation is necessary. The next step is to evaluate the patient and determine if there is a discrepancy between the patient's clinical manifestations and laboratory test results related to a given isolate and body site versus the usual clinical manifestations of infection caused by the microorganism as reported in the literature. The discordance or discrepancy between what the patient has and what the usual clinical expression of the microorganism is at different body sites should suggest the possibility of pseudoinfection (Table 8.6).

Pseudoinfections probably occur more commonly than they are reported and are probably, in general, underappreciated. Clinicians are most likely to encounter pseudobacteremias or pseudomeningitis as the two most common types of pseudoinfection that occur either singly or in outbreaks. Infection control personnel working in concert with the microbiology laboratory should undertake a thorough investigation that is appropriate for the potential pseudoinfection under investigation. A suggested infection control investigative approach for pseudobacteremia and pseudomeningitis is provided in tabular form (Tables 8.7 and 8.8). An organized infection control approach should try to confirm the presence of a pseudoinfection, and the epidemiologic investigation should determine the source of contamination and entry point in the sequence of specimen collection, processing, and culture. Pseudoinfections and pseudo-outbreaks should be reported to remind infection control professionals to be vigilant for the possibility of pseudoinfection. Reports of pseudoinfection also provide important information for infection control personnel in their investigative efforts to determine the source and entry point of the microorganisms involved in pseudoinfections and pseudo-outbreaks.

TABLE 8.5. MISCELLANEOUS PSEUDOINFECTIONS

[Reference] year	Microorganisms	Patients affected (No.)	Patients infected (No.)	Therapy affected (No.)	Problem
Pseudoendocarditis					
[6] 1976	*Flavobacterium meningosepticum*	1	0	0	Contaminated soap solution used for skin prep in placement of intracardiac catheter
[128] 1983	Gram-positive cocci	3	0	1	Broth contamination with nonviable gram-positive cocci
Pseudohepatitis					
[129] 1977	Acid-fast bacilli (AFB)	2	0	0	AFB specimen contaminated by laboratory personnel
[130] 1981	Hepatitis B virus	7	0	0	Contamination of automated pipette diluter
Pseudoadenitis					
[69] 1978	*Mycobacterium marinum*	2	0	0	AFB culture contaminated by laboratory technician
Pseudo-wound infection					
[6] 1976	*Flavobacterium meningosepticum*	3	0	0	Contaminated soap solution used for skin prep
[31] 1984	*Streptomyces* species	1	0	0	Contaminated Gortex graft culture
[131] 1986	Gram-negative bacilli	4	0	1	Contaminated transport medium
[43] 1991	Gram-negative bacilli	2	0	2	Contaminated transport medium
Pseudo-bone infection					
[132] 1994	*Candida parapsilosis*	1	0	1	Contaminated bone graft
[133] 1994	*Pseudomonas aeruginosa*	7	0	6	Contaminated saline diluent
[146] 1995	*Enterobacter faecium E. cloacae*	3	0	0	Contaminated CMBG tubes
[147] 1998	*Alcaligenes xylosoxidans*	2	0	0	Contaminated saline
Pseudo-diarrhea					
[150] 1995	*Salmonella hadar*	39	0	0	Contaminated selenite enrichment media
[151] 1999	*Aeromonas hydrophila*	NA	NA	NA	Inadequate disinfection of endoscopes
Pseudoinfections involving multiple sites/body fluids					
[131] 1986	*Mycobacterium gordonae*	28	0	0	Contaminated ice and water
[134] 1990	*Mycobacterium gordonae*	34	0	4	Contaminated "Panta" antimicrobial solution from improperly maintained ice machine
[135] 1990	*Pseudomonas thomasii*	28	0	0	Contaminated aqueous fluids
[136] 1990	Gram-negative rods	NA	NA	NA	Contaminated deionized water
[137] 1990	*Pseudomonas* species	13	0	NA	Contaminated transport media
[138] 1991	*Mycobacterium chelonae*	14	0	NA	Contaminated automated reprocessing machines
[139] 1992	*Tsukamurella paurometabolum*	10	0	NA	Laboratory contaminated
[140] 1992	*Pseudomonas cepacia*	6	3	3	Contaminated povidoneiodine
[141] 1992	Nonviable bacilli	2	0	1	Contaminated transport media in culture of prosthetic hip implants
[143] 1993	*Mycobacterium xenopi*	13	0	0	Contaminated potable water
[80] 1995	*Neisseria lactamica*	1	0	1	Contaminated culture media
[142] 1997	*Acinetobacter* species	14	0	0	Unrelated laboratory errors in processing of sputum, nasopharyngeal and endotracheal aspirates
[144] 1997	*Listeria monocytogenes*	3	0	0	Unknown
[145] 1997	*Mycobacterium* species	5	0	0	Faulty PPD testing materials media
[148] 1997	*Rhizopus microsporus* var. *rhizopodiformis*	17	0	0	Nonsterile specimen mixers
[149] 1997	*Cyclospora*	92	0	0	Laboratory contamination/errors
	Cryptosporidium	280	0	0	
Pseudopharyngitis					
[152] 2001	*Streptococcus pyogenes*	10	0	10	False-positive rapid Strep tests

NA, not applicable; PPD, purified protein derivative.

TABLE 8.6. AN APPROACH TO PSEUDOINFECTION OR PSEUDO-OUTBREAK INVESTIGATION

Infection control implications	Microbiology and clinical presentation		
Possible pseudoinfection	*Cluster* of *same* microorganisms	*Usual* microorganism preliminarily identified by Gram stain/culture recovered from *unusual* body site	*Unusual* microorganism preliminarily identified by Gram stain/culture recovered from *any* body site
	1. Possible outbreak 2. Investigate common denominators/epidemiologic aspects 3. Perform literature search for similar cases to determine investigative approach 4. Species isolated and body site *in agreement with the literature* and the patient's clinical presentation	1. Possible pseudoinfection/ pseudo-outbreak 2. Confirm identification of microorganism 3. Perform literature search for similar cases to determine investigative approach 4. *Discrepancy* between patient's clinical presentation and usual presentation in the literature	1. Possible pseudoinfection/ pseudo-outbreak 2. Confirm identification of microorganism 3. Perform literature search for similar cases to determine investigative approach 4. *Discrepancy* between patient's clinical presentation and usual presentation in the literature
Infection control classification	1. True outbreak	1. Pseudoinfection/pseudo-outbreak	1. Pseudoinfection/pseudo-outbreak

TABLE 8.7. EPIDEMIOLOGIC INVESTIGATION OF PSEUDOBACTEREMIA

Potential source	Focus of investigation	Items to culture
Skin disinfectants	Try to find commonality with specimens and other contaminated lots involved in the outbreak	Culture unused disinfectant fluids from same lots as involved in outbreak
Vacutainers, syringes, or needles	Look for potentially contaminated lots used in patients involved in the outbreak	Culture unused disposable syringes (inside lumen and plunger) and needles from same lots as involved in the outbreak
Intravenous fluids	Look for turbidity in the infusate (may not be present). Determine if IV infusion solutions involved in outbreak are from common lots	Culture infusate solution from bags of lots involved in the outbreak
Intravenous tubing/connectors/filters reused disposable devices	Look for cracks/breaks in equipment (may be gross/microscopic). Collect reused disposable devices	Culture filters and interior of disposable devices involved in the outbreak
Blood culture autoanalyzers	Check temperature of injecting needle, assess nearness to open windows, vents. Correlate work shifts with time of reports/culture positivity to determine relationships between potential events/personnel	Culture automated blood culture machine needle after heating Culture rubber caps/gaskets of blood culture bottles before and after applying antiseptic to rubber caps/gaskets Culture transport and culture media from lots involved in outbreak

IV, intravenous.

TABLE 8.8. INVESTIGATION APPROACH TO PSEUDOMENINGITIS

Potential source	Focus of investigation	Items to culture
Skin disinfectants	Determine if LP tray lots for patients involved in the outbreak are the same	Culture disinfectant solutions from unused LP trays from same lots involved in the outbreak
Glass slides	Examine glass slides and investigate staining procedures. Presence of water-related microorganisms in outbreak may support water source	Culture water used in slide cleaning/preparation, or staining
CSF plastic culture tubes	Determine if common LP trays are involved in the outbreak	Culture insides of CSF culture tubes and inside caps from same lots involved in the outbreak
CSF culture media	Determine if the same potentially contaminated lots are involved in the outbreak	Culture CSF liquid/solid media from lots involved in the outbreak

CSF, cerebrospinal fluid; LP, lumbar puncture.

REFERENCES

1. Norden CW. Pseudosepticemia. *Ann Intern Med* 1969;71:789–790.
2. Faris HM, Sparling FF. *Mima polymorpha* bacteremia. False-positive cultures due to contaminated penicillinase. *JAMA* 1972;219:76–77.
3. DuClos TW, Hodges GR, Killian JE. Bacterial contamination of blood-drawing equipment; a cause of false-positive blood cultures. *Am J Med Sci* 1973;266:459–463.
4. Noble RC, Reeves SA. *Bacillus* species pseudosepsis caused by contaminated commercial blood culture media. *JAMA* 1974;230: 1002–1004.
5. Kaslow RA, Machel DC, Mallison GF. Nosocomial pseudobacteremia. Positive blood cultures due to contaminated benzalkonium antiseptic. *JAMA* 1976;236:2407–2409.
6. Coyle-Gilchrist MM, Crewe P, Roberts G. *Flavobacterium meningosepticum* in the hospital environment. *J Clin Pathol* 1976;29:824–826.
7. Hoffman PC, Arnow PM, Goldmann DA, et al. False positive blood cultures—association with nonsterile blood collection tubes. *JAMA* 1976;236:2073–2075.
8. Snydman DR, Maloy MF, Brock SM, et al. Pseudobacteremia: false-positive blood cultures from mist tent contamination. *Am J Epidemiol* 1977;106:154–159.
9. Semel JD, Trenholme GM, Harris AA, et al. *Pseudomonas maltophilia* pseudosepticemia. *Am J Med* 1978;64:403–406.
10. Centers for Disease Control, Dolan J, Joachim GR. Pseudobacteremia due to *Staphylococcus aureus*—New York. *MMWR* 1979;28:82–83.
11. Lynch JM, Anderson A, Camacho FR, et al. Pseudobacteremia caused by *Clostridium sordellii. Arch Intern Med* 1980;140:65–68.
12. Jones BC, Stark FR, Reordan R, et al. Pseudo-positive blood cultures caused by contamination in a humidified incubator. *Infect Control* 1984;5:109–110.
13. Spivack ML, Shannon R, Natsios GA, et al. Two epidemics of pseudobacteremia due to *Staphylococcus aureus* and *Aerococcus viridans. Infect Control* 1980;1:321–323.
14. Centers for Disease Control, Spivack ML, Shannon R, Natsios G, et al. Nosocomial pseudobacteremia. *MMWR* 1980;29:243–249.
15. Berkelman RL, Lewin S, Allen JR, et al. Pseudobacteremia attributed to contamination of povidone-iodine with *Pseudomonas cepacia. Ann Intern Med* 1981;95:32–36.
16. Graham DR, Wu E, Highsmith AK, et al. An outbreak of pseudobacteremia caused by *Enterobacter cloacae* from a phlebotomist's vial of thrombin. *Ann Intern Med* 1981;95:585–588.
17. Greenwood GP, Highsmith AK, Allen JR, et al. *Klebsiella pneumoniae* pseudobacteremia due to cross-contamination of a radiometric blood culture analyzer. *Infect Control* 1981;2:460–465.
18. Wilson PA, Peters DW, Baker SL. An outbreak of pseudobacteraemia. *BMJ* 1981;283:866.
19. Craven DE, Moody B, Connolly MG, et al. Pseudobacteremia caused by povidone-iodine solution contaminated with *Pseudomonas cepacia. N Engl J Med* 1981;305:621–623.
20. Griffin MR, Miller AD, Davis AC. Blood culture cross-contamination associated with radiometric analyzer. *J Clin Microbiol* 1982;15: 567–570.
21. MacDonald N. Investigation of an outbreak of pseudobacteremia attributed to *Bacillus* species in a general hospital. Abstracts of the 82nd annual meeting of the American Society for Microbiology, Atlanta, March 7–12, 1982, p 83.
22. Cookson BO, Mehtar S, Sadler G. Serratia pseudobacteraemia. *Lancet* 1982;2:1276–1277.
23. Ives KN, Evans NA, Thom BT, et al. *Serratia marcescens* pseudobacteraemia on a special care baby unit. *Lancet* 1982;2:994–995.
24. Farmer JJ III, Weinstein RA, Zierdt CH, et al. Hospital outbreaks caused by *Pseudomonas aeruginosa*. Importance of serogroup 011. *J Clin Microbiol* 1982;16:266–270.
25. Berger SA. Pseudobacteremia due to contaminated alcohol swabs. *J Clin Microbiol* 1983;18:974–975.
26. Keys TF, Melton J, Maker MD, et al. A suspected hospital outbreak of pseudobacteremia due to *Pseudomonas stutzeri. J Infect Dis* 1983; 147:489–493.
27. Whiteside M, Moore J, Ratzan K. An investigation of enterococcal bacteremia. *Am J Infect Control* 1983;11:125–129.
28. Whale K. Pseudobacteremia: a bedside fault. *Lancet* 1983;2:830.
29. Crowley MM, Shannon R, Spivack M, et al. Pseudobacteremia due to intrinsic contamination of blood culture media by *Bacillus* species. *Am J Infect Control* 1983;11:150(abst).
30. Craven DE, Lichtenberg DA, Browne KF, et al. Pseudobacteremia traced to cross-contamination by an automated blood culture analyzer. *Infect Control* 1984;5:75–78.
31. Donowitz LG, Schwartzman JD. Pseudobacteremia and use of the radiometric blood culture analyzer [Letter]. *Infect Control* 1984;5: 266.
32. Gurevich I, Tafuro P, Krystofiak S, et al. Three clusters of *Bacillus* pseudobacteremia related to a radiometric blood culture analyzer. *Infect Control* 1984;5:71–74.
33. Farber BF, Rihs JD, Goetz A, et al. A pseudo-outbreak of *Streptomyces* infections linked to laboratory construction. *Am J Clin Pathol* 1984; 82:453–455.
34. Gosden PE, Norman P. Pseudobacteraemia associated with a contaminated skin cleaning agent. *Lancet* 1985;2:671–672.
35. Verschraegen G, Claeys G, Meeus G, et al. *Pseudomonas pickettii* as a cause of pseudobacteremia. *J Clin Microbiol* 1985;21:278–279.
36. Simor AE, Ricci J, Lau A, et al. Pseudobacteremia due to *Pseudomonas fluorescens. Pediatr Infect Dis* 1985;4:508–511.
37. Bradley SF, Wilson KH, Rosloniec MA, et al. Recurrent pseudobacteremias traced to a radiometric blood culture device. *Infect Control* 1987;8:281–283.
38. McNeil MM, Davis BJ, Solomon SL, et al. *Ewingella americana*: recurrent pseudobacteremia from a persistent environmental reservoir. *J Clin Microbiol* 1987;25:498–500.
39. Henderson DK, Baptiste R, Parillo J, et al. Indolent epidemic of *Pseudomonas cepacia* bacteremia and pseudobacteremia in an intensive care unit traced to a contaminated blood gas analyzer. *Am J Med* 1988;84:75–81.
40. Church DL, Bryant HE. Investigation of a *Streptococcus viridans* pseudobacteremia epidemic at a university teaching center. *Infect Control Hosp Epidemiol* 1989;10:416–421.
41. Smith GE, Cook DA. *Streptococcus pyogenes* and *Staphylococcus aureus* pseudobacteremia. *J Infect* 1989;18:194–195.
42. York MK. Bacillus species pseudobacteremia traced to contaminated gloves used incollection of blood from patients with acquired immunodeficiency syndrome. *J Clin Microbiol* 1990;28:2114–2116.
43. Yagupsky P, Dagan R, Chipman M, et al. Pseudo-outbreak of *Candida guilliermondii* fungemia in a neonatal intensive care unit. *Pediatr Infect Dis J* 1991; 12:928-32.
44. Hruszkewycz V, Ruben B, Hypes CM, et al. A cluster of pseudofungemia associated with hospital renovation adjacent to the microbiology laboratory. *Infect Control Hosp Epidemiol* 1991;13:147–150.
45. Pearson ML, Peques DA, Carson LA, et al. Cluster of *Enterobacter cloacae* pseudobacteremias associated with use of an agar slant blood culturing system. *J Clin Microbiol* 1993;31:2599–2603.
46. Dave J, Springbett R, Padmore H, et al. *Pseudomonas cepacia* pseudobacteraemia. *J Hosp Infect* 1993;23:71–75.
47. Rathbone PG, Sinickas V, Humphery V, et al. Polymicrobial pseudobacteraemias associated with non-sterile sodium citrate blood collection tubes. *J Hosp Infect* 1993;25:297–304.
48. Bignardi GE, Barrett SP, Hinkins R, et al. False-positive *Mycobacterium avium-intracellulare* cultures with the Bactec 460 TB system. *J Hosp Infect* 1994;26:203–210.
49. Anderson M, Davey R. Pseudobacteraemia with *Pseudomonas fluorescens. Med J Aust* 1994;160:233–234.
50. Jacobs JA, Hendrix MGR, Stobberingh EE. Pseudobacteremia: stowaways in commercial culture media. *J Hosp Infect* 1994;27:242–243.
51. Astagneau P, Gotto S, Gobin Y, et al. Nosocomial outbreak of *Enterobacter agglomerans* pseudobacteremia associated with non-sterile blood collection tubes. *J Hosp Infect* 1994;27:73–74.
52. Gravel-Tropper D, Sample ML, Oxley C, et al. Three-year outbreak of Pseudobacteremia with *Burkholderia cepacia* traced to a contaminated blood gas analyzer. *Infect Control Hosp Epidemiol* 1996;17: 737–740.
53. Ashford DA, Kellerman S, Yakrus M, et al. Pseudo-outbreak of septicemia due to rapidly growing Mycobacteria associated with extrinsic contamination of culture supplement. *J Clin Microbiol* 1997;35: 2040–2042.

54. Kappstein I, Krause G, Hauer T, et al. Pseudo-Outbreak of candidemia with *Candida parasilopsis. J Hosp Infect* 1998;40:164–165.
55. Collignon P, Dreimanis D, Beckingham W. Pseudobacteraemia due to *Pseudomonas fluorescens. J Hosp Infect* 1999;42:321–322.
56. Namnyak S, Hussain S, Davalle J, et al. Contaminated lithium heparin bottles as a source of pseudobacteraemia due to *Pseudomonas fluorescens. J Hosp Infect* 1999;41:23–28.
57. Neal TJ, Corkill JE, Bennett KJ, et al. *Serratia marcescens* pseudobacteraemia in neonates associated with a contaminated blood glucose/lactate analyzer confirmed by molecular typing. *J Hosp Infect* 1999; 41:219–222.
58. Reed RP, Sinickas VG, Byron KA. *Staphylococcus saccharolyticus* pseudobacteremia. *Clin Microbiol Newslett* 1999;21:38–39.
59. Rogues A-M, Sarlangue J, de Barbeyrac B, et al. *Agrobacterium radiobacter* as a cause of pseudobacteremia. *Infect Control Hosp Epidemiol* 1999;20:345–348.
60. Baddour LM, Harris E, Huycke MM, et al. Outbreak of pseudobacteremia due to multidrug-susceptible *Enterococcus faecium. Clin Infect Dis* 1999;28:1333–1334.
61. Whyte A, Lafong C, Malone J, et al. Contaminated lithium heparin bottles as a source of pseudobacteremia. *J Hosp Infect* 1999;42: 342–343.
62. Meessen NEI, van Pampus ECM, Jacobs JA. False-positive blood cultures in a patient with acute myeloid leukemia. *Clin Microbiol Infect* 1999;5:769–770.
63. Psevedos G, Minnaganti VR, Cunha BA. Pseudobacteremia due to *Bacillus megatherium. Infect Dis Pract* 2000;24:96–97.
64. Noskin GA, Suriano T, Collins S, et al. *Paenibacillus macerans* pseudobacteremia resulting from contaminated blood culture bottles in a neonatal intensive care unit. *Am J Infect Control* 2001;29:126–129.
65. Musher DM, Schell RF. False-positive gram stains of cerebrospinal fluid [Letter]. *Ann Intern Med* 1973;79:603–604.
66. Joyner RW, Idriss ZH, Wilfert CM. Misinterpretation of cerebrospinal fluid gram stain. *Pediatrics* 1974;54:360–362.
67. Ericsson CD, Carmichael M, Pickering LK, et al. Erroneous diagnosis of meningitis due to false-positive gram stains. *South Med J* 1978;71: 524–525.
68. Batt JM, Reller LB. False-positive gram stain due to nonviable organisms in sterile commercial transport medium. *MMWR Morbid Mortal Wkly Rep* 1978;27:23.
69. Hoke CH, Batt JM, Mirrett S, et al. False-positive gram-stained smears. *JAMA* 1979;241:478–480.
70. Harris A, Pottage JC, Fliegelman R, et al. A pseudoepidemic due to *Salmonella typhimurium. Diagn Microbiol Infect Dis* 1983;1:335–337.
71. Weinstein RA, Bauer FW, Hoffman RD, et al. Factitious diagnostic error due to nonviable bacteria in commercial lumbar puncture trays. *JAMA* 1985;233:878–879.
72. Ullman R, Schoch P, Cunha BA. Pseudomeningitis due to *Acinetobacter*/CDC group VE-1 organisms. *Med J Winthrop-University Hosp* 1985;7:38–41.
73. Bross JE, Manning P, Kacian D, et al. Pseudomeningitis caused by *Sporobolomyces salmonicolor. Am J Infect Control* 1986;14:220–223.
74. Strampfer MJ, Twist PF, Greensher J, et al. *Aspergillus* pseudomeningitis in a neonate. *Clin Microbiol Newslett* 1987;9:22–23.
75. Lettau LA, Benjamin D, Cantrell HF, et al. *Bacillus* species pseudomeningitis. *Infect Control Hosp Epidemiol* 1988;9:394–397.
76. Cunha BA, Cohen S. Pseudomeningitis: report of a case caused by *Bacillus* and review of the literature. *Heart Lung* 1989;18:418–420.
77. Gelfand MS, Schoch PE, Cunha BA. Fungal pseudomeningitis superimposed on *Escherichia coli* meningitis. *Heart Lung* 1990;19: 534–536.
78. Mitrani-Schwartz A, Schoch E, Cunha BA. Pseudomeningitis caused by *Pseudomonas paucimobilis. Heart Lung* 1991;20:305–307.
79. Gill VM, Shea KW, Klein NC, et al. Pseudomeningitis due to gram-positive diplococci. *Infect Dis Pract* 1994;18:91.
80. Jacobsen E, Gurevich I, Cunha BA. Pseudomeningitis due to *Neisseria lactamica. Antimicrob Infect Dis Newslett* 1995;13:67.
81. Cunha BA, Bonoan JT. *Bacillus* species pseudomeningitis. *Heart Lung* 1997;26:249–251.
82. Cunha BA, Bonoan JT. Pseudomeningitis due to viridans streptococci. *Antimicrob Infect Dis Newslett* 1998;17:76–77.
83. Cunha BA, Visvalingam B, Yannelli B. Pseudomeningitis due to *Acinetobacter* baumannii. *Am J Infect Control* 1999;27:179–181.
84. Gusten WM, Dorsainvil P, Cunha BA. *Acinetobacter lwoffi* pseudomeningitis. *Antimicrob Infect Dis Newslett* 2002:18:86–88.
85. Gusten WM, Hansen EA, Cunha BA. *Acinetobacter baumannii* pseudomeningitis. *Heart Lung* 2002;31:76–78.
86. Grinchenko T, Remé P, Cunha BA. *Flavimonas oryzihabitans* pseudomeningitis. *Am J Infect Control* 2003;31:385–386.
87. Schaffner W, Reisig G, Verrall RA. Outbreak of *Pseudomonas cepacia* infection due to contaminated anesthetics. *Lancet* 1973;1: 1050–1051.
88. Gangadarma PRJ, Lockhart JA, Awe RJ, et al. Mycobacterial contamination through tap water [Letter]. *Am Rev Respir Dis* 1976;113:894.
89. Suratt PM, Gruber B, Wellons HA, et al. Absence of clinical pneumonia following bronchoscopy with contaminated and clean bronchofiberscopes. *Chest* 1977;71:52–54.
90. Kellerhals S. A pseudo-outbreak of *Serratia marcescens* from a contaminated fiberbronchoscope. *Assoc Practitioners Infect Control J* 1978;6: 5–7.
91. Steere AC, Corrales J, von Graevenitz A. A cluster of *Mycobacterium gordonae* isolates from bronchoscopy specimens. *Am Rev Respir Dis* 1979;120:214–216.
92. Schleupner CJ, Hamilton JR. A pseudoepidemic of pulmonary fungal infections related to fiberoptic bronchoscopy. *Infect Control* 1980;1: 38–42.
93. Nuñez D, Stanley C, Robertstad GW, et al. Pseudoepidemic of coccidioidomycosis. *Am J Infect Control* 1982;10:68–71.
94. Schanbacher KJ, Stieritz DD, LeFrock JL, et al. A pseudo-epidemic of nontubercular mycobacteriosis. *Am J Infect Control* 1983;11: 150(abst).
95. Vogel R, Neu HC. A pseudoepidemic of *Penicillium* of fiberoptic bronchoscopy patients. *Am J Infect Control* 1983;11:149(abst).
96. Goodman RA, Smith JD, Kubica GP, et al. Nosocomial mycobacterial pseudoinfection in a Georgia hospital. *Infect Control* 1984;5: 573–576.
97. Goldstein B, Abrutyn E. Pseudo-outbreak of *Bacillus* species related with fiberoptic bronchoscopy. *J Hosp Infect* 1985;6:194–200.
98. Hoffman KK, Weber OJ, Rutala WA. Pseudoepidemic of *Rhodotorula rubra* in patients undergoing fiberoptic bronchoscopy. *Infect Control Hosp Epidemiol* 1989;10:511–514.
99. McNeil M, Solomon SL, Anderson RL, et al. Nosocomial *Pseudomonas pickettii* colonization associated with a contaminated respiratory therapy solution in a special care nursery. *J Clin Microbiol* 1985;22: 903–907.
100. Siegman-Igra Y, Inbar G, Campos A. An outbreak of pulmonary pseudo-infection by *Serratia marcescens. J Hosp Infect* 1985;6: 218—220.
101. Flournoy DJ, Petrone RL, Voth DW. A pseudo-outbreak of *Methylobacterium mesophilica* isolated from patients undergoing bronchoscopy. *Eur J Clin Microbiol Infect Dis* 1992;11:240–243.
102. Bennett SN, Peterson DE, Johnson DR, et al. Bronchoscopy-associated *Mycobacterium xenopi* pseudoinfections. *Am J Respir Crit Care Med* 1994;150:245–250.
103. Kolmos HJ, Lerche A, Kristoffersen K, et al. Pseudo-outbreak of *Pseudomonas aeruginosa* in HIV-infected patients undergoing fiberoptic bronchoscopy. *Scand J Infect Dis* 1994;26:663–667.
104. Shears P, Rhodes LE, Syed Q, et al. A pseudo outbreak of tuberculosis. *Commun Dis Rep CDR Rev* 1994;4:R9–10.
105. Mehta JB, Kefri M, Soike DR. Pseudoepidemic in nontuberculous Mycobacteria in a community hospital. *Infect Control Hosp Epidemiol* 1995;16:633–634.
106. Wurtz R, Demarais P, Trainor W, et al. Specimen contamination by mycobacteriology laboratory detected by pseudo-outbreak of multidrug-resistant tuberculosis: analysis by routine epidemiology and confirmation by molecular technique. *J Clin Microbiol* 1996;34: 1017–1019.
107. Mitchell DH, Hicks LJ, Chiew R, et al. Pseudoepidemic of *Legionella pneumophila* serogroup 6 associated with contaminated bronchoscopes. *J Hosp Infect* 1997;37:19–23.
108. Cox R, deBorja K, Bach MC. A pseudo-outbreak of *Mycobacterium*

chelonae infections related to bronchoscopy. *Infect Control Hosp Epidemiol* 1997;18:136–137.

109. Cronin W, Rodriguez E, Valway S, et al. Pseudo-outbreak of tuberculosis in an acute care general hospital: Epidemiology and general implications. *Infect Control Hosp Epidemiol* 1998;19:345–347.
110. Lai KK, Brown BA, Westerling JA. Long-term laboratory contamination by *Mycobacterium abscessus* resulting in two pseudo-outbreaks. Recognition with use of random amplified polymorphic DNA (RAPD) polymerase chain reaction. *Clin Infect Dis* 1998;27:169–175.
111. Centers for Disease Control and Prevention. Bronchoscopy-related infections and pseudoinfections in New York, 1996 and 1998. *MMWR* 1999;48:557–560.
112. Labarca JA, Trick WE, Peterson CL. A multistate nosocomial outbreak of *Ralstonia pickettii* colonization associated with an intrinsically contaminated respiratory care solution. *Clin Infect Dis* 1999;29: 1281–1286.
113. Lalande V, Barbut F, Varnerot A, et al. Pseudo-outbreak of *Mycobacterium gordonae* associated with water from refrigerated fountains. *J Hosp Infect* 2001;48:76–79.
114. Kressel AB, Kidd F. Pseudo-outbreak of *Mycobacterium chelonae* and *Methylobacterium mesophilicum* caused by contamination of an automated endoscopy washer. *Infect Control Hosp Epidemiol* 2001;22: 414–418.
115. Zhang Q, Kennon R, Koza MA, et al. Pseudoepidemic due to a unique strain of *Mycobacterium szulgai*: genotypic, phenotypic, and epidemiologic analysis. *J Clin Microbiol* 2002;1134–1139.
116. LaBombardi VJ, O'Brien AM, Kislak JW. Pseudo-outbreak of *Mycobacterium fortuitum* due to contaminated ice machines. *Am J Infect Control* 2002;30:184–186.
117. Gebo KA, Srinivasan A, Perl TM, et al. Pseudo-outbreak of *Mycobacterium fortuitum* on a human immunodeficiency virus ward: transient respiratory tract colonization from a contaminated ice machine. *Clin Infect Dis* 2002;35:32–38.
118. El Sahly HM, Septimus E, Soini H, et al. *Mycobacterium simiae* pseudo-outbreak resulting from a contaminated hospital water supply in Houston, Texas. *Clin Infect Dis* 2002;35:802–807.
119. Rossetti R, Lencioni P, Innocenti F, et al. Pseudoepidemic from *Mycobacterium gordonae* due to a contaminated automatic bronchoscope washing machine. *Am J Infect Control* 2002;30:196–198.
120. Bearman G, Vaamonde C, Larone D, et al. Pseudo-outbreak of multidrug-resistant *Mycobacterium tuberculosis* associated with presumed laboratory processing contamination. *Infect Control Hosp Epidemiol* 2002;23:620–622.
121. Silva CV, Magalhaes VD, Pereira CR, et al. Pseudo-outbreak of *Pseudomonas aeruginosa* and *Serratia marcescens* related to bronchoscopes. *Infect Control Hosp Epidemiol* 2003;24:195–197.
122. John JF, Twitty JA. Pseudo-bacteriuria with plasmid-containing *Pseudomonas cepacia*: contamination of rayon balls in benzalkonium chloride (abst). American Society for Microbiology Clinical Meeting, 1982, p 83.
123. Cooper BH. A case of pseudo paracoccidioidomycosis: detection of the yeast phase of *Mucor circinelloides* in a clinical specimen. *Mycopathology* 1987;97:189–193.
124. Verschraegen G, Voet D, Claeys G, et al. Pseudobacteriuria with *Serratia marcescens. J Hosp Infect* 1988;12:238–240.
125. Stone J, Manasse R. Pseudoepidemic of urinary tract infections due to *Trichosporon beigelli. Infect Control Hosp Epidemiol* 1989;10:312–315.
126. Catchpole CR, Cutter M, Layfield A. Pseudobacteriuria associated with a urine flow rate transducer. *J Hosp Infect* 1997;37:251–252.
127. Zafar AB. Pseudo-epidemic in an acute-care teaching hospital. *Infect Control Hosp Epidemiol* 1998;19:739–740.
128. Aber RC, Appelbaum RC. Pseudoepidemic of endocarditis in patients undergoing open-heart surgery. *Infect Control* 1983;1:97–99.
129. Weinstein RA, Stamm WE. Pseudoepidemics in hospitals. *Lancet* 1977;2:862–864.
130. Laxson L, Schultz A, Kane M. Pseudo outbreak of hepatitis B in a transplant unit may answer transient positive question (abst). Annual Conference, Association for Practitioners in Infection Control, 1981, pp 88–89.
131. Panwalker AP, Fuhse E. Nosocomial *Mycobacterium gordonae* pseudoinfection from contaminated ice machines. *Infect Control* 1986;7: 67–70.
132. Schiappacasse RH, Ritter S, Schleis C, et al. Contaminated collection media as a cause of pseudoinfection. *Infect Control Hosp Epidemiol* 1994;15:760–767.
133. Forman W, Axelrod P, St.John K, et al. Investigation of a pseudo-outbreak of orthopedic infections caused by *Pseudomonas aeruginosa. Infect Control Hosp Epidemiol* 1994;15:652–657.
134. Tokars JI, McNeil MM, Tablan OC, et al. *Mycobacterium gordonae* pseudoinfection associated with a contaminated antimicrobial Solution. *J Clin Microbiol* 1990;28:2765–2769.
135. Costas M, Holmes B, Sloss LL, et al. Investigation of a pseudo-outbreak of *Pseudomonas thomasii* in a special care baby unit by numerical analysis of SDS-PAGE. *Epidemiol Infect* 1990;105:127–137.
136. Medcraft JW, New CW. False-positive gram-stained smears of sterile body fluids due to contamination of laboratory deionized water. *J Hosp Infect* 1990;16:75–80.
137. Heard S, Lawrence S, Holmes B, et al. A pseudo-outbreak of *Pseudomonas* on a special care baby unit. *J Hosp Infect* 1990;16:59–65.
138. Centers for Disease Control. Nosocomial infection and pseudoinfection from contaminated endoscopes and bronchoscopes. Wisconsin and Missouri. *MMWR Morb Mortal Wkly Rep* 1991;40:675–678.
139. Auerbach SB, McNeil MM, Brown JM, et al. Outbreak of pseudoinfection with *Tsukamurella paurometabolum* traced to laboratory contamination: efficacy of joint epidemiological and laboratory investigation. *Clin Infect Dis* 1992;14:1015–1022.
140. Panlilio AL, Beck-Saque CM, Siegel JD, et al. Infections and pseudoinfections due to povidone iodine solution contaminated with *Pseudomonas cepacia. Clin Infect Dis* 1992;14:1078–1083.
141. Quale JM, Reese D. Pseudoinfection of prosthetic hip implants. *J Infect Dis* 1992;165:981.
141. Maloney S, Welbel S, Daves B, et al. *Mycobacterium abscessus* pseudoinfection traced to an automatic endoscope washer: utility of epidemiologic and laboratory investigation. *J Infect Dis* 1994;169: 166–169.
142. Sule O, Ludlam HA, Walker CW, et al. A pseudo outbreak of respiratory infection with *Acinetobacter* species. *Infect Control Hosp Epidemiol* 1997;18:510–512.
143. Sniadack DH, Ostroff SM, Karlix MA, et al. A nosocomial pseudo outbreak of *Mycobacterium xenopi* due to a contaminated potable water supply: lessons in prevention. *Infect Control Hosp Epidemiol* 1993;14:636–641.
144. La Scola B, Fournier PE, Musso D, et al. Pseudo-outbreak of listeriosis elucidated by pulsed-field gel electrophoresis. *Eur J Clin Microbiol Infect Dis* 1997;16:756–760.
145. Grabau JC, Burrows DJ, Kern ML. A pseudo outbreak of purified protein derivative skin-test conversions caused by inappropriate testing materials. *Infect Control Hosp Epidemiol* 1997;18:571–574.
146. Morris T, Brecher SM, Fitzsimmons D, et al. A pseudo-epidemic due to laboratory contamination deciphered by molecular analysis. *Infect Control Hosp Epidemiol* 1995;16:82–87.
147. Granowitz EV, Keenholtz SL. A pseudoepidemic of *Alcaligenes xylosoxidans* attributable to contaminated saline. *Am J Infect Control* 1998; 26:146–148.
148. Verweij PE, Voss A, Donnelly JP, et al. Wooden sticks as the source of a pseudoepidemic of infection with Rhizopus microsporus var. rhizopodiformis among immunocompromised patients. *J Clin Microbiol* 1997;35:2422–2423.
149. Centers for Disease Control. Outbreaks of pseudo-infection with *Cyclospora* and *Cryptosporidium*—Florida and New York City, 1995. *JAMA* 1997;277:18:1428–1429.
150. Joce RE, Murphy F, Robertson MH. A pseudo-outbreak of salmonellosis. *Epidemiol Infect* 1995;115:31–38.
151. Esteban J, Gadea I, Fernandez-Roblas R, et al. Pseudo-outbreak of *Aeromonas hydrophila* isolates related to endoscopy. *J Hosp Infect* 1999; 41:313–316.
152. Karchmer TB, Anglim AM, Drubin LJ, et al. Pseudoepidemic of streptococcal pharyngitis in a hospital pharmacy. *Am J Infect Control* 2001;29:104–108.

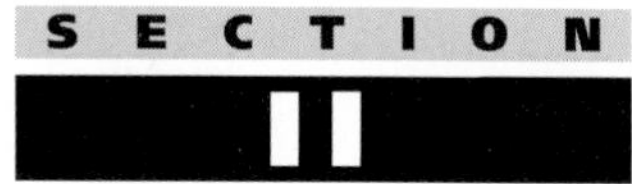

HEALTHCARE QUALITY IMPROVEMENT

9

HOW TO SELECT IMPROVEMENT PROJECTS

DAVID BIRNBAUM

Epidemiology, as a process for logical inquiry, has much in common with systems analysis or industrial engineering (also known as management engineering) (1). Similar perspectives and complementary methods shared by these disciplines make them ideal for managing healthcare quality improvement (2). However, to succeed, these disciplines must be applied in a supportive setting and on worthwhile quality improvement projects. There are underlying principles and precedents of both successes and failures; these can serve as important guides to anyone contemplating extension of epidemiologic skills from familiar areas of infection control to less familiar areas of quality improvement. Healthcare as a business sector has lagged far behind the cutting edge of other industries in advancing its methods to assure and improve service quality. Healthcare organizations have generally failed to use the full potential of epidemiology in discerning alternative strategies and informing consensus on best practices; exploring the natural course of conditions; performing cost-benefit and effectiveness analyses; surveying patient preferences; measuring organizational effectiveness; establishing indicators, criteria, and other measures; and designing and evaluating surveillance systems (3,4). Although it is noteworthy and unfortunate that epidemiology is not listed among team leadership in recent reference books and motivating reports (5,6), this reflects the simple fact that relatively few hospital epidemiologists rose to embrace challenging new opportunities.

Although some of the language in general underlying principles for selecting improvement projects might introduce foreign concepts, the principles are not complicated. Mozena and Anderson (7) list the following essential criteria to consider:

- Impact on patient care or external customer
- Impact on favorable patient outcomes
- Magnitude of potential cost savings
- Cost of implementation
- Difficulty of implementation
- Ability to measure performance of process
- Potential benefits outweigh cost of the project
- Deals with key business issue
- High error rate
- Availability of data
- Impact on profitability
- Potential for success
- Impact on ongoing quality
- Ability to quantify results
- High visibility to customers or patients
- Elimination of rework
- High risk to patients or employees

A National Demonstration Project on Quality Improvement in Health Care reported that nomination and selection of projects often is run by steering committees (a quality council) but that the best ideas come from "listening to the voice of the customer" (in which external customers are patients who receive services and internal customers are staff members who collectively provide and support service delivery) (8). Surveying customer opinion is an active way to listen; design and conduct of surveys is familiar ground in epidemiology. Relating service attributes to customer expectations may involve less familiar but still simple techniques such as Quality Function Deployment matrices (a simple two-dimensional matrix in which the strength of association between specific items and categories of customer expectations is summarized) (9,10). However, all of these criteria and methods are disjointed considerations. What is needed to bring efficiency and acceptance is an effective system for their implementation.

GUIDANCE FROM HISTORICAL PRECEDENTS

Three precedents bear consideration as effective systems to select improvement projects. Although two were successful quality improvement systems, they failed to persist and become today's North American gold standard models. Williamson's Achievable Benefits Not Achieved (ABNA) system to identify and prioritize potential projects (11) has a remarkable track record among alternatives (12). Similarly, the so-called Denver Connection of the same era is a story of successful amalgamation and reorganization of two hospitals in a way that put quality improvement supported by real-time performance data analysis as the centerpiece of medical staff departmental meetings and continuing medical education (encouraged by board-level involvement while the usual array of advisory committees was eliminated) (13). Finally, the Institute of Medicine's (IOM's) Model Process for semiquantitatively ranking alternative projects is instructive for its mathematical approach (14).

Dr. John W. Williamson developed systems for health accounting and ABNA during an impressive body of work that spans decades on the faculty of the Department of Health Services Administration at the Johns Hopkins University School of Hygiene and Public Health, Medicine and Medical Informatics at the University of Utah School of Medicine, Regional Medical Education Center of the Salt Lake Veterans Affairs Medical Center, and service on government commissions. Health accounting, conceptualized in the early 1960s, is "a management model to integrate continuing education and patient care research into an ongoing cyclic function to systematically improve the quality of medical care" (15). It is an evidence-based outcome-focused approach that selects project priorities through ABNA, a formal, efficient process refined in the 1970s. Although proven effective and cost effective in a wide range of applied research and demonstration projects at the American National Institutes of Health, Veterans Administration, and elsewhere, Williamson acknowledges that the most successful application of his system to enhance national quality is in the Netherlands (15). The fact that Williamson's name and work are unfamiliar to many members of the healthcare quality special interest group of the Society for Healthcare Epidemiology of America and the American Society for Quality's (ASQ's) Health Care Division reflects lack of recognition throughout North American hospitals. This is hauntingly reminiscent of the history of W. Edwards Deming's influence taking decades to return to North America, heeded by American manufacturers only after Japan capitalized on Deming's leadership to outperform its American counterparts (and heeded by health service organizations decades after that!). Williamson stresses the following:

1. The importance of applying principles of epidemiology, sampling, and simple statistical testing to QA-focused reviews
2. The necessity of a multidisciplinary team approach to QA, in which the consumer was the most important member of the team
3. The need to use structured group judgment methods for establishing priorities, criteria, and standards as well as QA action decisions under the usual conditions of factual uncertainty
4. The need for a unique set of statistical methods for QA that allowed comparison of measured results against consensus standards that reflected reasonably achievable projected outcomes

Consistent with concurrent surveillance methods that have become a mainstay of contemporary infection surveillance programs, Williamson recognized long ago that chart-based audits as a basis for quality assurance may be misleading and severely limit the potential impact of programs to improve quality (15). His ABNA process consists of selecting a team (ideally 7 to 11 persons, including "at least four knowledgeable and respected staff physicians" and representatives of other functional areas and the lay public), then supporting that team through two 2-hour meetings 3 to 4 weeks apart. The first meeting is a training session simulating the later priority-setting session. A master list of potential topics developed during the training session, together with team recommendations on additional "data, literature, or consultation" required, provides an indication of support materials that will be needed at the second session. Ideally, these are gathered during the 3 to 4 week hiatus. There are seven tasks in the priority-setting meeting:

1. Introductory remarks by the moderator clarify meeting purpose, tasks, and timing of the 2-hour session and review the ABNA framework (5 to 10 minutes).
2. A simple four-column form is distributed so that individual team members can each list as many topics as they wish, listing along one row for each topic:
   a. exactly who (what group) will benefit
   b. for what health problem
   c. from what action(s)
   d. by which provider(s)

   A cue sheet is provided to give examples of various patient characteristics, health problem characteristics, provider characteristics, and (inter)action types that might be considered. Time is given to work individually (10 minutes).
3. Each team member, sequentially, is then asked by the coordinator to nominate one problem from their list. The coordinator develops a summary chart; in addition to the four columns identified in step 2, when acting as coordinator I found it helpful to list in two additional columns an indication of whether the intervention is known to work (nature of evidence for efficacy or effectiveness) and whether it is feasible (information on cost, cost-effectiveness, case study, etc.). Discussion is limited to clarification at this stage, and the process repeats until all the most promising ideas from each member's list are presented (30 minutes).
4. Individuals then vote in an "initial weights" column on their form to assign a priority rank (high to low on a 5-point scale) for each project nominated (5 minutes).
5. The coordinator then collects the votes, anonymously recording both initial individual weights and their sum for each nominated project. This information, superimposed on the summary chart, is projected back to the group (10 minutes).
6. Discussion of results, one topic at a time, then examines whether priority ranking is tightly or widely dispersed, the strength of evidence, and other detailed considerations. On completion of comprehensive discussion, members are then asked to vote again on every topic, in a "revised weights" column on their form. The coordinator again collects and records votes anonymously (50 minutes).
7. The highest-ranked ABNA topics are then forwarded as recommendations from the team, along with any further recommendations for additional data or evidence required for any of the topics. The meeting is adjourned, the team thanked for completing its work, and special teams of qualified individuals then take responsibility for moving approved projects forward.

Meanwhile, also in the 1970s, radical changes under the amalgamation of the medical staffs at Denver's Swedish Medical Center and Porter Memorial Hospital occurred. Radical change was needed because as Dr. William Robinson, Director of Medical Education, noted, "In spite of the hundreds of physician hours devoted to medical staff activities, little actually was accomplished. It was almost impossible to demonstrate that quality of care was in any way influenced by the physicians' repetitive, duplicative, unrewarding medical staff activities." The usual litany of committees was reduced to just three (Executive, Professional Activities, and Credentials). A reduced number of subcommittees composed of small numbers of individuals, the bulk of whom were not physicians, served these committees, and much of the quality-related work was shifted from committees to medical staff departments supported by the work of subcommittees or research and education department employees. Medical staff members were strongly encouraged to ask questions at their departmental meetings about quality issues, then make policy decisions based on evidence delivered soon thereafter (answers supplied through real-time research capacity in their own institution) (13).

Although successful into the 1980s, by the turn of the twenty-first century the Denver Connection was so far dismantled that it no longer even existed in the institutional memory of Porter Hospital's present administration! Porter and Swedish, partners of the so-called Denver Connection formed in 1972, went their separate ways in 1992. These two hospitals serving health needs of southeast Denver had remained separate corporate entities, yet collaborated successfully for many years following formal merger of their medical staff organizations. That merger was initiated by the doctors, not the administrators, for the purpose of improving quality of care. Administrative support grew following demonstrated successes, and the hospitals cooperated in division of complementary health services instead of duplication of what the other offered solely to compete. That was before big business entered sickness. Ultimately, poor quality of management in emerging, large, managed-care corporations led to unexpected deficits in profitability of operations, and corporate vision shifted to preoccupation with that debt. A grass-roots anticompetitive way of serving the community's health needs could not sustain itself in the face of powerful market forces and growing business empires awash in corporate debt. Personal ideologies in administrative leadership compounded the difficulty of making effective alliances, and mistrust grew where open communication once thrived. Key participants later interviewed conveyed a sense of loss and regret, a realization they participated in something very unique and beneficial that was lost for illogical reasons ("nobody had any appreciation what we were doing was special or unique . . . only in retrospect we came to appreciate the specialness of what we were doing."). The influence of accreditation programs in this saga was noteworthy only for its lack of influence (16). It is tempting to speculate that this visionary effort thrived because it followed characteristic principles that seem to distinguish great companies from others (17) and that the Denver Connection ultimately fell when it strayed from core values and these fundamental principles.

The IOM Model Process to set priorities in health technology assessment addresses similar dimensions as ABNA but in a more quasinumeric than nominal group consensus manner. The IOM priority score for each technology, instead of being assigned by consensus ranking, is calculated as $\Sigma W_1 \ln S_1 + W_2 \ln S_2 + \ldots + W_7 \ln S_7$ where W_i represents the criterion weight and S_i the criterion score for ($i = 1$ to 7):

1. Prevalence (e.g., cases per 1,000 persons)
2. Burden of illness (e.g., difference in quality-adjusted life years of individuals with vs. without the condition under consideration)
3. Cost (total direct and indirect costs per person with the condition)
4. Variation in rates of use of the technology (coefficient of variation)
5. Potential to change health outcome (subjective assessment on 5-point scale)
6. Potential to change costs (subjective assessment on 5-point scale)
7. Potential of assessment result to inform ethical, legal, or social issues (subjective assessment on 5-point scale)

The first three criteria are objective measures; the remaining four are subjective and are addressed by one or more expert panels. Criterion weighting values are arbitrary choices; the process described has an expert panel select one criterion as least important, which then is assigned weight of 1. Mean weights given by panel members for each of the remaining criteria, relative to the least important one, then determine the other six weights. After discussion of results to resolve any wide disagreement, results of a second vote are final. Pilot test results with small conventional and mailed response panels are examined in the IOM report, which gives the following values: $W_1 = 1.6$, $W_2 = 2.25$, $W_3 = 1.5$, $W_4 = 1.2$, $W_5 = 2.0$, $W_6 = 1.5$, and $W_7 = 1.0$. Logarithms of criterion scores are used to make the model multiplicative rather than additive, thus responsive to relative rather than absolute differences in scores (algebraically, the formula can be restated as $\Sigma W_i \ln S_i$ which equals the product $\Pi S_i^{W_i}$ for $i = 1$ to 7). Subjective item scales, therefore, run from a value of 1 for least likely to 5 for most likely.

Health accounting provided a philosophy, the Denver Connection a forum, and ABNA a method all consistent with today's emphasis on evidence-based practice and continuous quality improvement (CQI). What lessons should one take from these all-but-forgotten precedents? Williamson reflects on lessons learned from 25 years of experience (15), naming three premises on which quality assurance or improvement is based and five principles that evolve from it:

- Because it is an inherent management function encompassing both effectiveness and efficiency of any healthcare activity, the main issue is not whether but how well it is conducted.
- As a healthcare management function, it involves the same clinical problem solving principles whether applied at an individual, institutional, regional, national, or international level.
- As a scientific endeavor, it must be built on a foundation of the health sciences integrated with other disciplines (including philosophy, quantitative disciplines like epidemiology, education, social sciences, business and management, economics, and informatics).
- It must start with clarification of individual and organization values, must be supported by management of incentives, and will be successful to the extent that it is internally motivated.
- Although it must be organized along sound management and administrative principles, it will be successful to the extent that responsibility for excellence moves closer to the bedside.
- It is inherently interdisciplinary so it will be successful to the extent that it is comprehensive in membership and vision.

- Attention should be focused on carefully targeted problems selected by consensus methods, not dispersed in shotgun approaches nor restricted to narrow problems defined by audit of single data sets.
- It must be subjected to ongoing analysis of costs and accomplishments to ensure that it maintains effectiveness and adapts to changing times.

Clearly, these premises and principles are not consistent with chart audits conducted behind closed doors, at accreditation-mandated intervals, by discipline-specific advisory committees that regarded patients or their families as recipients of care rather than members of a team. They also are not consistent with quality being viewed as a destination (viz., no evidence of negligent care) rather than as a journey nor with centralizing authority in a quality council. The Denver Connection clearly represented a journey outside the map of externally mandated routes and vaguely defined directions. It decentralized autonomy, predated by decades the Health Care Financing Administration (HCFA) (subsequently renamed the Centers for Medicare and Medicaid Services) instigated removal of infection control committees as a Joint Commission on Accreditation of Healthcare Organizations (JCAHO) requirement, inspired one other hospital to disband that committee despite accreditation standards (18), and set a coordination role for administration in an era when command and control was the norm. In short, neither of these precedents was typical of conventional programs during their era, and they documented successes in their publications. Instructively, ABNA and the Denver Connection challenged but failed to change convention and in this one is warned about the importance of establishing protective legislative, board, and administrative political perimeters around vital programs.

SURVIVAL AS A MANAGER OF CHANGE

Discussion of timing and perception is not obvious in the previous list by Mozena and Anderson but is inherent in the ABNA process. Hospital epidemiology often succeeds when implementing interventions that are motivated by frank outbreaks of disease but may not be as successful in convincing administrators to adopt new programs during normal times when competing against business cases or political agendas of line departments. One can take lessons from the social policy cycle recognized in public administration and must recognize the importance of marketing to create a sense of need before attempting to satisfy that need ("deals with key business issue" criterion). Later steps recognized in the policy cycle are familiar ground to the evidence-based nature of epidemiology; however, an initial stage of creating shared understanding of any problem (because all parties can agree on the data but disagree on the theory or meaning explaining that data and, therefore, on direction of actions required) and, second, articulating that vision to ensure sufficiently widespread acceptance or readiness to act are politically astute (19):

- Identify issues
  Problem defined
  Problem articulated
- Policy analysis
  Collect relevant data and information
  Clarify objectives and resolve key questions
  Develop options and proposals
- Undertake consultation
- Move toward decisions
- Implement
- Evaluate

Healthcare must operate in a businesslike manner but must retain at its core the values inherent in principles underlying healthcare professions, because care cannot be viewed simply as a commodity to sell. "Patients do not value health care per se, they value health; "health care" is an intermediate good that people consume (based on expert advice) in hopes of deriving a health benefit. Many patients, and especially those under duress of serious illness, do not have the time, interest, or ability to gain sufficient knowledge to be equally informed as their health care provider. So, no matter how much information patients receive, choosing your surgery is never going to be like buying a car" (20). Our primary focus should be on improving quality not on cutting cost. If experience in other industries is any guide, improving quality will lead to cost reductions. To motivate change in a business environment, program managers should consider principles of economic application to recognize the diminishing effectiveness of different arguments (excellent arguments: improving operating costs, increasing production rates, and improving product quality; good arguments: improving customer relations, improving labor relations, and increasing job pride; fair arguments: reducing injury rate, giving legislative compliance, and reducing liability potential; and poor arguments: enhancing public relations or providing personal satisfaction) (21). The experience of clinical microbiology laboratory directors who have been successful at proving cost-effectiveness as a new business skill is pertinent (22). Administrators may be more interested by projects that promise to lower variable rather than fixed costs, that work with cost rather than charge data, and that show benefit using adjusted cost estimates. Adjusting cost estimates for a diagnosis-related group (DRG) probably is not familiar to most hospital epidemiologists, but epidemiologists are aware of the "shifting base" bias potential that is inherent in an indirect adjustment (standardization) calculation (23) that hospital administrators tend to apply to compensate for differences in severity of patients within DRGs.

MANAGEMENT OF CHANGE TO ACHIEVE QUALITY MANAGEMENT

Quality management is a sustained, systematic approach to improving quality. Quality management requires an ability to chart the best courses (a task for which the technical skills of epidemiologists generically are well-suited) and to help all workers pursue specific targets along those courses. The latter task requires communication and organizational development skills and methods complementary to epidemiology. Chapters in this section are integrated and meant to be read together, unlike all but one other section (Section XVII Bioterrorism) in this book.

This chapter introduces concepts that are explained in more details elsewhere in the section. Planned data collection and effective manipulation of data are described later, but greater detail is provided in Chapters 10 and 11. Creating and maintaining a climate, a learning organization, in which such data are embraced as the basis for constructive criticism is illustrated by interdisciplinary experiences shared in Chapter 12 and illuminated by review of ideologies in Chapters 12 and 13.

STARTING ON A PATH THAT LEADS TO SUCCESS

When introducing CQI programs, it is essential to avoid early failures, because they are a dispiriting enemy of progress in promoting continuous improvement. Rather than lose momentum by failing at the start, it is better to begin with small yet meaningful projects, be successful, attract champions who sustain progressive projects, and mobilize new converts into groups that do more over the long term.

Two aspects identified in previous lists, *availability of data* and *collect relevant data and information,* are fundamental to decision criteria, policy cycles, and design of surveillance programs. Quality of healthcare data (in terms of precision, accuracy, and reliability) has been considered extensively by epidemiologists.(24–27) Therefore, this is an aspect in which the core "process" knowledge of hospital epidemiologists can guide decisions about which noninfectious diseases problems to study, whether to use available data sources, and which supplementary surveillance tools should be developed. Although other specialists probably have more "content" knowledge than the hospital epidemiologist about a given noninfectious disease, interdisciplinary collaboration between process and content experts is more likely to lead to success.

Benchmarking often is mentioned as a source of guidance. Recent volumes describe successful and cost-effective improvement projects. Although the best way to select the right improvement projects for a given organization is to understand the needs, expectations, resources, culture, and values of that organization and its own customers, there also is merit in benchmarking the success of others. The second edition of *Quality Profiles* (28), for example, profiles a selection from more than 1,100 quality improvement initiatives; these were chosen by an advisory board of experts in quality improvement from health plans, trade associations, government organizations, and individuals from National Committee for Quality Assurance (NCQA) and Pfizer (the sponsors of this volume). According to its authors, the 27 case studies selected demonstrate more sophistication and more refined use of data than initiatives in the first edition (18 months prior). Forum opportunities represent another source of research funding, benchmark information, and networking opportunities, noteworthy examples are the Breakthrough Series Collaboratives and Pursuing Perfection program (*www.ihi.org/pursuingperfection*) of the Institute for Healthcare Improvement, or The Academic Medicine and Managed Care Forum created by Aetna U.S. Healthcare (*www.aetnaushc.com*). Clinical practice guidelines provide another basis for evaluating quality of care to identify opportunities for improvement (29), an area in which the Agency for Healthcare Research and Quality (*http://www.ahrq.gov*) has a lead role, but it is important to remember that "listening to the voice of the customer" implies attempting to delight customers with unexpected extras of valued quality rather than focusing just on fixing deficient care.

CHECKPOINTS ALONG THE JOURNEY

Ensuring that project teams have sufficient time, skill, and information to make critical assessment of data from internal or external sources is an obvious but often overlooked checkpoint. Another checkpoint is influence of those teams among peers and organizational hierarchy. Availability alone is not sufficient justification for allocating resources. Credibility, willingness, and readiness form a better basis for selecting team members for each project, processes for team activities must be efficient and effective, and training needs of teams must be met.

Last, but not least, the journey must be chronicled in ways that are meaningful to all stakeholders. Deming's famed 14 Points for Management and the enumeration of "Deadly Diseases" advocate driving out fear, shifting focus from short to long term, and eliminating recognitions based on essentially random chance allocations or just doing well as an individual in the system at short-term quotas rather than attempting to improve the system. Thus, Deming advocates eliminating practices such as traditional "employee of the month" and subjective annual employee performance rating (30). In their place, CQI activities, supported by administrative models oriented toward building learning organizations and reinforced by team-building morale-boosting recognition for actual achievements, have merit. As part of your chronicle, an annotated inventory of current quality-related activities should be maintained. If quality assurance and improvement is viewed in the context of a surveillance system to detect and prevent adverse trends, then familiar methods to evaluate surveillance system performance readily apply. Forms that could be used for survey of a surveillance system are shown in Appendices A, B, and C.

Similarly, in each project, maintaining a newsworthy log of project progress and events should be an archivist's responsibility. This inventory and log can be used to promote interdisciplinary communication throughout an organization and its surrounding community and to serve as a basis to continuously monitor the value and cost-effectiveness of current measures. In addition, as a gauge of institutional culture and readiness to change, these documents can provide insight into the types of projects likely to succeed or fail at any given period in an organization's journey toward quality. Since its inception in 1987, thousands of businesses (including 44 healthcare organizations after the piloting of education and health categories in 1995 and 25 healthcare applications after formal addition in 1999) have used the more structured Malcolm Baldrige Award (*http://www.quality.nist.gov/*) application process as a way to chart progress on that journey. The comprehensive Baldrige program provides a wide-ranging audit, as do other award programs patterned after it, but a less formal annotated chronicle of an individual institution's own history also has unique worth. We may

APPENDIX A

Quality Program Survey Form

SECTION I: WHAT DOES YOUR PROGRAM ASSURE?

Quality assurance involves systems of monitoring to confirm that a specified level of quality is delivered, and systems of controls to maintain or adjust performance. As an initial step in designing an appropriate program, you need a clear understanding of current objectives and an inventory of existing activities. Section I should be completed, independently, by all participants (e.g.: the manager, director, and administrator for each quality program).

Completed by: Date (dd/mm/yy): / /

1. Please attach a copy of your statement of program philosophy, purpose or mission.

2. Please complete the following section to list your current goals and objectives; date of last review/revision; associated monitoring and/or control activities; and whether these are mandated by external requirements. Continue on the reverse side if necessary.

Goal/Objective #1:__________________________
Date Adopted (dd/mm/yy): / /
Monitoring Activities: Control Activities:

Circle as appropriate: STATUTORY, PROFESSIONAL, ACCREDITATION requirement

Goal/Objective #2:__________________________
Date Adopted (dd/mm/yy): / /
Monitoring Activities: Control Activities:

Circle as appropriate: STATUTORY, PROFESSIONAL, ACCREDITATION requirement

Goal/Objective #3:__________________________
Date Adopted (dd/mm/yy): / /
Monitoring Activities: Control Activities:

Circle as appropriate: STATUTORY, PROFESSIONAL, ACCREDITATION requirement

Goal/Objective #4:__________________________
Date Adopted (dd/mm/yy): / /
Monitoring Activities: Control Activities:

Circle as appropriate: STATUTORY, PROFESSIONAL, ACCREDITATION requirement

Adapted from MMWR 1988;37(S5) By Applied Epidemiology

have been slow to recognize the importance of sharing success stories in social and scientific exchanges (31).

External review programs that acknowledge competence and reveal organizational deficiencies or other opportunities for improvement include familiar accreditation programs, International Organization for Standardization (ISO) certification, the American Baldrige Award, the Japanese Deming award, and others. They are not identical; thus, it is important to appreciate the relative merits of the model that each establishes. It has been noted that "Baldrige and JCAHO standards are both based on the concepts of CQI but differ in so many ways that direct comparison is difficult" (32). Baldrige criteria have tended to

APPENDIX B

Quality Program Survey Form

SECTION II: HOW IS IT BEING ASSURED? PROGRAM STRUCTURE

For each of the Monitoring Activities listed in Section I, please answer the following questions. Use one page for each activity under each numbered Goal/Objective. Section II should be completed, independently, by the program manager (e.g.: Infection Control Professional), the program director (e.g.: Hospital Epidemiologist), and the administrator to whom they report.

Completed by: Date (dd/mm/yy): / /

3. This page relates to Goal/Objective #_____ Activity______________________

4. Is there written documentation (policy, procedure, instruction, etc.) covering this activity? *Yes* *No* If yes, please attach a copy or indicate location.

5. How will this activity help to assure quality? (check all that apply)
   __ Establishes baseline levels/monitors trends
   __ Detects incidents to prevent recurrence
   __ Detects incident-producing conditions before injury or damage results
   __ Other (Specify):

6. How will the information be used? By whom? Give examples

7. What information is requested or collected?

8. What sources of information are used (e.g.: medical record, lab reports, incident reports, professional activity summary reports, committee records, etc.)?

9. Who has responsibility for reporting or collecting this? Describe the flow of information.

10. What percentage of actual events is detected?
    o Have program sensitivity and specificity been measured formally?
    o How are minimum sample sizes or sampling frequencies determined?

11. After data analysis, to whom are reports sent? How frequently? Who has authority to act on this information?

12. Have objectives for this activity changed over the past 2 years; if so, why?

Adapted from MMWR 1988;37(S5) By Applied Epidemiology

be more general; accreditation agency criteria more specific and prescriptive. The Baldrige Award also differs from ISO 9000: 94 certification, but the new ISO 9000:2000 standard reportedly has the same focus as Excellence Models such as Baldrige or European Foundation for Quality Management (see Chapter 13 for more detail). As the Baldrige Web site described, "The purpose, content, and focus of the Baldrige Award and ISO 9000[:94] are very different. The Baldrige Award was created by Congress in 1987 to enhance U.S. competitiveness. The award program promotes quality awareness, recognizes quality achievements of U.S. organizations, and provides a vehicle for sharing successful strategies. The Baldrige Award criteria focus on results

APPENDIX C
Quality Program Survey Form
SECTION III: HOW WELL DOES THE SYSTEM WORK?

For each monitoring activity listed in Section II, please answer the following questions. Use one page for each numbered Goal/Objective activity. Section III should be completed by your program director; questions 19 and 20 should also be answered by your administrator.

Completed by: Date (dd/mm/yy): / /

13. This page relates to Goal/Objective #_____ Activity_______________________

14. What method(s) is (are) used to analyze the data collected?

15. What are the time delays from actual incidence to:

Detection:	__________	(unknown)
Reporting:	__________	(unknown)
Analysis:	__________	(unknown)
Dissemination:	__________	(unknown)
Action:	__________	(unknown)

16. What problems or biases can affect the activity?

17. What are the costs (in dollars or hours per week) for data collection, analysis and dissemination? Please indicate whether the figure is known (i.e.: charted to a cost center), estimated, or unknown.

18. Does this cost include everyone involved?

19. What decisions or outcomes has the activity effected? Check and provide examples:
    ___ Prompted review or corrective action:
    ___ Validated good performance:
    ___ Provided support for a (change in) policy or procedure:
    ___ Influenced allocation of resources:
    ___ Influenced educational priorities/programs:
    ___ Other:

20. Is there a mechanism for on-going evaluation of this activity's value? If yes, give details:

Adapted from MMWR 1988;37(S5) By Applied Epidemiology

and continuous improvement. They provide a framework for designing, implementing, and assessing a process for managing all business operations. ISO 9000 is a series of five international standards published in 1987 by the ISO, Geneva, Switzerland. Companies can use the standards to help determine what is needed to maintain an efficient quality conformance system. For example, the standards describe the need for an effective quality system, for ensuring that measuring and testing equipment is calibrated regularly and for maintaining an adequate record-keeping system. ISO 9000 registration determines whether a company complies with its own quality system. Overall, ISO 9000 registration covers less than 10 percent of the Baldrige

Award criteria." The Baldrige information Web pages also acknowledge that both the U.S. Baldrige Award and Japan's Deming award are based on the same purposes (to promote recognition of quality achievements and to raise awareness of the importance and techniques of quality improvement) but note that the Baldrige Award focuses more on results and service, relies on the involvement of many different professional and trade groups, provides special credits for innovative approaches to quality, includes a strong customer and human resource focus, and stresses the importance of sharing information (33). Another recent development is Industry Workshop Agreement 1, which makes ISO 9000 more specific to the healthcare industry.

LEADERSHIP

Epidemiology has long been recognized as providing the scientific foundation for public health and the evidence-based resource for health planning. Unfortunately, dissatisfied customers rather than hospital epidemiologists have been leading recent movements to initiate change and improvement in healthcare. Although the automotive industry has quality problems of its own, it recognized 20 years ago that healthcare tops its list of direct costs in the construction of automobiles (34). Now 20 years later, having not seen significant innovation and progress within healthcare, the automotive industry's division within the ASQ became the driving force for radical redirection in healthcare leadership by demanding ISO certification of its suppliers and funding consensus meetings to support initiatives of ASQ's Health Care Division that led to ISO's Industry Workshop Agreement 1 (6). There is no reason for epidemiologists to take a back seat while others drive, for as Dr. John Millar, vice-president of the Canadian Institute for Health Information, observed to a room filled with hospital epidemiologists and infection control professionals during a symposium on "Collaborations to Improve Health Care Quality," "you folks have more expertise than most people who could be in this game" (35).

REFERENCES

1. Benneyan JC, Kaminsky FC. Another view on how to measure health care quality. *Qual Prog* 1995;28(2):120–124.
2. Donabedian A. Continuity and change in the quest for quality. *Clin Perform Qual Health Care* 1993;1:9–16.
3. Donabedian A. Contributions of epidemiology to quality assessment and monitoring. *Infect Control Hosp Epidemiol* 1990;11:117–121.
4. Wenzel RP, Pfaller MA. Infection control: the premier quality assessment program in United States hospitals. *Am J Med* 1991;91(Suppl 3B):27–31.
5. Birnbaum D. Book review. *Clin Perform Qual Health Care* 1996;4: 231.
6. Birnbaum D, and the Health Care Quality Special Interest Group. A shared vision of healthcare quality improvement. *Infect Control Hosp Epidemiol* 2001;22:582–584.
7. Mozena JP, Anderson DL. *Quality improvement handbook for health care professionals.* Milwaukee, WI: Quality Press, 1993.
8. Berwick DM, Godfrey AB, Roessner J. *Curing health care, new strategies for quality improvement.* San Francisco: Jossey-Bass, 1990.
9. Glushkovsky EA, Florescu RA, Hershkovits A, et al. Avoid a flop: use QFD with questionnaires. *Qual Prog* 1995;28(6):57–62.
10. Ermer DS. Using QFD becomes an educational experience for students and faculty. *Qual Prog* 1995;28(5):131–136.
11. Williamson JW. Formulating priorities for quality assurance activity—description of a method & its application. *JAMA* 1978;239: 631–637.
12. Palmer RH, Nesson HR. Review of methods for ambulatory medical care evaluations. *Med Care* 1982;20:758–781.
13. Scher Z. *The Denver Connection.* Englewood, CO: Estes Park Institute, 1976.
14. Donaldson MS, Sox HC Jr, eds. *Setting priorities for health technology assessment, a model process.* Washington DC: National Academy Press, 1992.
15. Williamson JW. Future policy directions for quality assurance: lessons from the health accounting experience. *Inquiry*1988;25:67–77.
16. Birnbaum D, Petersen C. The Denver Connection (Porter-Swedish) experiment revisited. *Clinical Governance* 2003;8(4):337–345.
17. Collins JC, Porras JI. *Built to last: successful habits of visionary companies.* New York: HarperCollins, 1994.
18. Birnbaum D. The organization of infection surveillance and control programs: risk management vs. control committee. *Dimens Health Serv* 1981;58(12):16–19.
19. Edwards M, Howard C, Miller C. *Social policy, public policy from problem to practice.* Crows Nest NSW Australia: Allen & Unwin, 2001.
20. Birnbaum D, Berglund R, Ruiz U, and the Health Care Quality Special Interest Group of the ASQ's Health Care Division and of the Society for Healthcare Epidemiology of America. Quality and quality improvement in health care services. Available at *http://www.healthcare.org/SIG-PAPER.html* (accessed. 11/12/2003)
21. Bird FE Jr, Loftus RG. *Lo$$ control management.* Loganville GA: Institute Press, 1976:142–166.
22. Barenfanger J. Clinical microbiology laboratories can directly benefit patients. *ASM News* 2001;67(2):71–77.
23. Rothman KJ. *Modern epidemiology.* Boston: Little, Brown and Company, 1986.
24. Hierholzer WJ Jr. Health care data: the epidemiologist's sand. *Am J Med* 1991;91(Suppl 3B):21–26.
25. Sorensen HT, et al. A framework for evaluation of secondary data sources for epidemiologic research. *Int J Epidemiol* 1996;25:435–442.
26. Gross PA. Basics of stratifying for severity of illness. *Infect Control Hosp Epidemiol* 1996;17:675–686.
27. Kritchevsky SB. Data collection in hospital epidemiology. In: Mayhall CG, ed. *Hospital epidemiology and infection control,* 2nd ed. Philadelphia: Lippincott Williams & Wilkins, 1999.
28. *Quality profiles,* 2nd ed. National Committee for Quality Assurance. Washington, D.C.: NCQA, 2001.
29. *Using clinical practice guidelines to evaluate quality care,* vol 1 and 2. Washington DC: Agency for Healthcare Research and Quality, 1995.
30. Deming WE. *Out of the crisis.* Cambridge, MA: Massachusetts Institute of Technology, 1982.
31. Richards C, Emori TG, Peavy G, et al. Promoting quality through measurement of performance and response: prevention success stories. *Emerging Infect Dis* 2001;7:299–301.
32. Fisher DC, Simmons BP. *The Baldrige workbook for healthcare.* New York: Quality Resources, 1996.
33. Baldridge Award information. Available at *http://www.quality.nist.gov/* (accessed January 10, 2002).
34. Stavro B. Sick call. *Forbes* 1983;132(10):116.
35. Birnbaum D, Simmons B, Millar J, et al. Discussion. *Infect Control Hosp Epidemiol* 2001;22:593–595.

10

SELECTION OF QUALITY IMPROVEMENT TOOLS AND METHODS

ROBERT BURNEY
RONALD BERGLUND

Healthcare, like all industries, can use a process approach for improvement. In this chapter we discuss a basic process approach, which includes *design,* leading to *monitor,* leading to *repair,* leading to *improve* which of course will lead to new design and so forth. The bewildering array of tools available can make selection of the proper tools difficult, but consideration of the focus of the improvement effort will aid in the selection of appropriate tools. We list basic tools under four headings, depending on the general task at hand: design, monitor, repair, and improve. Some tools may be listed under more than one category. Each of the four headings contains several steps in which the healthcare practitioner can deploy various tools. Each tool is discussed briefly, and then a case study shows how one organization used this approach.

DESIGN

For new processes or significant modifications of existing processes, that is, breakthrough leaps, the following steps and tools may be useful.

First, one defines the requirements with tools such as customer surveys, market research, and quality function deployment (QFD). QFD is a structured process that captures the voice of the customer and translates those needs into system design. A key feature of QFD is the establishment of a traceable link between customer requirements and the product or service being produced. A product planning matrix, referred to as the house of quality, is a graphical representation of the QFD planning process. One side of the building lists customer requirements, the roof contains the technical requirements of the product, the foundation contains the values of the design (engineering characteristic), the other wall lists the customer competitive assessment (options for the customer), and within the house the relative importance of the required and desired characteristics of the product or service are calculated.

Customer surveys with double Likert scales yield excellent starting points. *Likert scales* usually contain statements with five levels of agreement from disagreement to agreement and a corresponding question that asks how important the measure is to the customer, again on a scale of one to five. Areas of importance to the customer are, thus, distinguished from those of lesser or no importance.

Second, one should establish indicators or criteria for success. How will one know if it is going well? Metrics can be displayed as control charts, which also facilitate the determination of process capability (Cp). Cp relates actual output data from the process to the customer's specification limits. Variation in the process should not exceed the customer's specified limits. A calculated Cp greater than one indicates better performance than a Cp less than one. Further refinements of Cp look at how centered the process is and account for nonsymmetrical distributions of specifications or performance.

Third, one must evaluate the design. Failure mode and effects analysis (FMEA) and mistake proofing help develop strategies to eliminate expected errors. FMEA is a systematic process to identify potential failures of a product and to assess the effects or criticality of such a failure. FMEA then identifies actions that could minimize or eliminate the potential failure. Finally, one must establish a control plan to ensure that quality control methods are deployed to minimize failure opportunities. One should install gates at various points in the process to prevent problems from continuing to the next step.

Fourth, one should verify the design through limited trials or a full design of experiments approach. *Design of experiments* activities identify the most important factors that affect the mean and the variation of a processes while minimizing the required testing and experimentation. As a final step, one must look again at user needs and reassess Cp.

Finally, one should implement the new design. The standard operating procedure (SOP) must be written, and the control plan must be finalized. One should define leading indicators that will predict future performance of the process and ensure conformity throughout the process.

MONITOR

One must keep a finger on the pulse. How does one know that it is going well? How will one know when it is not? *Control charts* indicate when a process is in control and when there is need for improvement. There are different types of control charts for continuous data and for categorical data, but the goal of any control chart is to determine the degree of process control. Is the process stable and operating within the required upper and/or lower specification limits?

A histogram compresses data for a given time period into a single snapshot. The shape of the histogram indicates whether the results of the process are centered on the customer requirements or whether the distribution is skewed. Presentation of data in a frequency bar chart (histogram) allows the display of large amounts of data that would be difficult to interpret in tabular form.

Either a control chart or a histogram will identify outliers—individual cases or results that are beyond the specification limits of the process. A *Pareto chart* helps target improvement actions for the vital few—those few causes that produce the largest number of defects. A Pareto chart is a bar chart that links the type of problem with the number of occurrences and displays the problem with the most occurrences on the left. The Pareto chart, thus, separates the most important problems from the "trivial many." Pareto charts can also track changes before and after an intervention and can compare costs to problem areas. It is one of the easiest tools to use and also one of the most powerful for prioritizing improvement efforts.

REPAIR

Tools in this category are used to analyze and fix problems that have been discovered through the monitoring process. *Root cause analysis* uses the fishbone or Ishikawa diagram to identify, select, and graphically display possible causes of a problem. This diagram looks like a fishbone with the problem statement as the head and each major category of potential contributing factors portrayed as a "bone." Typical major categories for the fishbone diagram include material, machines, measurement, environment, people, and policies. *Brainstorming* helps identify factors for consideration under each of these headings. The final outcome of a root cause analysis should be an *action plan* to correct the identified problem areas and to ensure that the problem does not recur.

The *is/is not diagram* isolates the exact location of the problem in time and place by documenting where and when it is or is not occurring. Often, the cause of the problem will become apparent when the location in time and space is identified. Again, brainstorming may provide ideas for a solution to the problem.

Mistake proofing tries to make it impossible for a mistake to happen by eliminating the human factor. For example, it is not possible to connect a nitrous oxide cylinder to the oxygen line on an anesthesia machine because the connectors do not fit.

Before implementing the solution, one must use the *plan, do, check, act* (PDCA) cycle to test the proposed solution on a small scale before wider deployment. One should look also at the cost of the repair versus the benefit to the patient before finally deploying the solution.

IMPROVE

Tweaking existing systems produces incremental improvements. Sometimes problems, new technology, or new customer requirements require leapfrog improvements. This means wiping the slate clean and redesigning the process, using the tools discussed in the section about design. Usually, the first step in any improvement is to map the existing process and to identify rework loops, redundancies, and other non-value-added steps. The *nominal group technique* is a structured process that includes all team members in the selection of the problems to work on. It is a method of selecting the problems that are most important to the problem solvers.

DIARY OF A SURGERY CENTER (A scenario to demonstrate tools and techniques)

The First Few Years

Day Zero

Valley Surgery Center (VSC) was started as a joint venture between Valley Community Hospital (VCH) and a group of local physicians. VCH had a day surgery program, but it was mixed in with the inpatient surgery area, which was scheduled for major renovation. Several of the surgeons agreed to join the hospital in this joint venture. An anesthesiologist was appointed as medical director and chairman of the planning committee. Other members of the planning committee were the business office director, an operating room (OR) nurse, and a recovery room nurse. This is the diary of that committee.

We had each read some books or gone to seminars on quality, but none of us was truly expert. We did, however, have one expert spouse who offered advice from the sidelines. Because there were two other surgery centers nearby, we knew the environment would be competitive. We determined that our response would be to know our customers better and provide better service to meet their needs. Because this was a new venture, we had the opportunity to design not only the care processes but also the building itself around stakeholder needs. Our spouse suggested QFD as a design tool. This was a quick read for us, but we decided to try. First, we identified four major stakeholder groups: patients, employees, surgeons, and payers. There were other stakeholders, but these were the ones we considered in the design process.

We surveyed each group to determine their needs regarding ambulatory surgery. We sent paper surveys by mail, held small focus groups, and conducted structured interviews by phone or in person. The results are shown in Table 10.1.

Following roughly along the QFD outline, we designed our processes to accommodate these needs as follows:

1. Patients. The anesthesia providers agreed that preoperative visits were not necessary for most patients. They developed a list of potential problems for surgeons to screen. Any patients with problems on that list will be scheduled for a phone call or visit. A "familiarization visit" will be an option for mothers with small children

   Paperwork for patients will be limited to their signature

TABLE 10.1. RESULTS OF STAKEHOLDER NEEDS ASSESSMENTS

Stakeholder group	Key needs/desires	Notes
Patients	1. No hassle. No preop visit 2. Minimal paperwork 3. No nausea/vomiting	Patients are busy too
Surgeons	1. Start on time 2. All supplies present 3. Easy scheduling	Minimal paperwork was also on their list
Employees	1. No enforced overtime 2. Fair wages and benefits 3. Opportunities for education	A "family friendly" work environment was particularly important to RNs
Payers	1. Low cost 2. Clean claims 3. Rapid billing	No one mentioned quality of care. They just want it low cost

on two forms at the time of their procedure (one for billing and one procedure permit). Patients' satisfaction with the intake process will be surveyed periodically.

Risk factors for postoperative nausea and vomiting will be included on the anesthesia preoperative evaluation form. The presence of more than one of these will prompt preventive actions, including medication. Literature on this subject will be reviewed by the anesthesia team and practices are updated at least annually. The incidence of nausea and vomiting in the recovery room will be monitored constantly and tracked by anesthesia providers. This information will presented to the board every 2 years, at the time of applications for privileging, and consistent outliers among anesthesiologists will not be granted privileges.

2. Surgeons. The actual starting time of the first case in each OR will be tracked by day of the week, by anesthesia provider, by OR nurse, and by surgeon. These data will be presented to the quality improvement (QI) committee monthly for analysis and appropriate corrective action. For this purpose, *start time* will be defined as the presence in the OR of the patient, the anesthesiologist, and the surgeon. The data will be plotted as a control chart, and any special cause variation will be investigated using a root cause analysis technique. At least quarterly, the QI committee will look for ways to minimize variation and eliminate any discrepancy between scheduled start time and actual start time.

   The circulating nurse in each OR will list every time that she or he has to leave the OR to obtain missing equipment or supplies. The OR director will submit a summary of these lists monthly to the QI committee, together with the plan for corrective action. We will use standardized kits for most procedures to minimize set up time and missing items. Any surgeon requesting special items not in the kit will be referred to the medical advisory board.

   Any surgeon scheduling more than three cases per week will be offered the opportunity to reserve block time for his or her exclusive use until 1 week ahead. We plan eventually to allow surgeons to schedule into their block time directly from their offices via an Internet connection. Surgeons' satisfaction with the scheduling process will be assessed annually. We also will meet regularly with the scheduling clerks in the surgeons' offices to resolve their problems with the process.
3. Employees. As a matter of policy, there will be no enforced overtime at VSC. The OR director will monitor the scheduling process to ensure that there is a reasonable probability of completing all scheduled cases. The medical director and the OR director will monitor progress of cases during each day. If it seems that all cases cannot be completed by the end of the schedule, patients will be invited to schedule another day for their procedure. Any cases canceled for this reason will be referred to the QI committee for analysis and corrective action.

   The business office manager will assess local and regional pay and benefits for all our categories of employees annually. Our goal will be to remain competitive and just below the comparable scale for local hospitals. Our superior work environment and profit sharing plan will provides us with a competitive edge for hiring.

   Consistent with our mission, we will encourage all employees to participate in relevant professional organizations and to obtain available certifications in their disciplines. VSC will pay the cost of any examinations that are successfully completed for certifications. In addition, there will be a tuition reimbursement plan that pays education expenses for any course, whether related to duties at VSC or not. This will offset the fact that there are no opportunities for promotion within VSC, and most employees will reach their maximum salary after 5 years.
4. Payers. VSC will remain competitive with the low-cost providers for our five most common procedures. Charges for competitors will be obtained from a state mandated reporting system and from information supplied by patients, surgeons, and our employees who have procedures done at other places.

   The number of claims rejected for missing or incorrect data will be monitored. This will be presented as a bar graph each month in the business office. Business office personnel will collect the data, and the final graph will be posted in the business office each month.

   A recovery room nurse will transfer the patient chart to the business office as soon as the patient has left the building; thus, billing should be completed on the same day for most patients and within 24 hours for all patients. The business office will monitor the number of bills submitted each month outside of this 24-hour window. These numbers will be displayed in a run chart for the current and previous months. The business office manager will be responsible for strategies to keep these numbers at or near zero.

The QFD process allowed us to design aspects of our system to accommodate the key concerns of our principal customer groups and to select monitors to ensure that we satisfy those needs on a continuous basis.

As part of our planning process, we also established a mission for VSC: "Ambulatory surgery service that is personal, professional, and profitable."

Our spouse consultant advised us to expand on the mission statement to produce a list of measurable goals to demonstrate that we are accomplishing our mission. We struggled with deter-

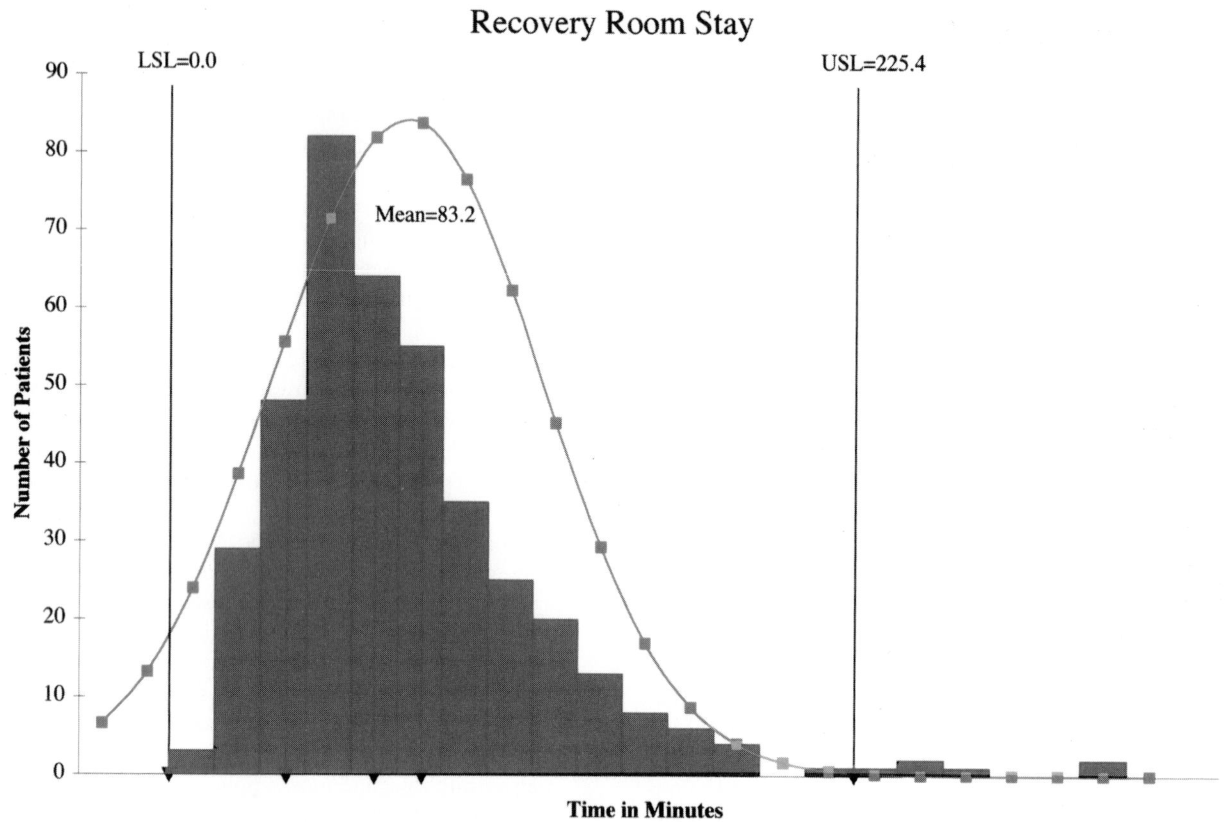

Figure 10.1. Histogram of the length of stay in recovery.

mining a measure for the first element of our mission, "personal." Finally, we asked, "What would it look like if we were successful in providing personal healthcare?" We concluded that patients would know the name of the staff taking care of them. To measure this, we included a question on our satisfaction survey, "Was any individual particularly helpful to you?" We decided to count the number of times a name was mentioned versus a position title. ("The nurse in pre op" or "the clerk at check in.") The results are presented as a bar graph that is posted in the employee lounge.

For "professional," we decided to count the number of staff in the OR and the recovery room who belonged to professional organizations, such as the Association of Operating Room Nurses (AORN) and the American Society of Post Anesthesia Nurses (ASPAN) and the number who had achieved professional certification. This too is posted in the employee lounge.

At first glance "profitable" was easier to measure, but the presentation and audience were issues. We finally decided to present "progress on the employee bonus" each month as a chart in the employee lounge. All employees receive a bonus of up to 10% of salary, depending on profits. Thus, the audience that most influences profit sees that feedback each month.

Six-Month Mark

After some "noise" in the first 30 days, our charts and graphs settled into patterns that helped us target areas for improvement. Fig. 10.1 is a histogram of the cycle times for patients. We drew a vertical line at the 3-hour mark and looked at the charts of people who stayed in the center for more than 3 hours. From the charts, we determined the reasons for the prolonged stay and plotted those as a Pareto chart (Fig. 10.2).

The Pareto chart placed the most important reason to the left, so we took action on "waiting for a ride." We held a brain-

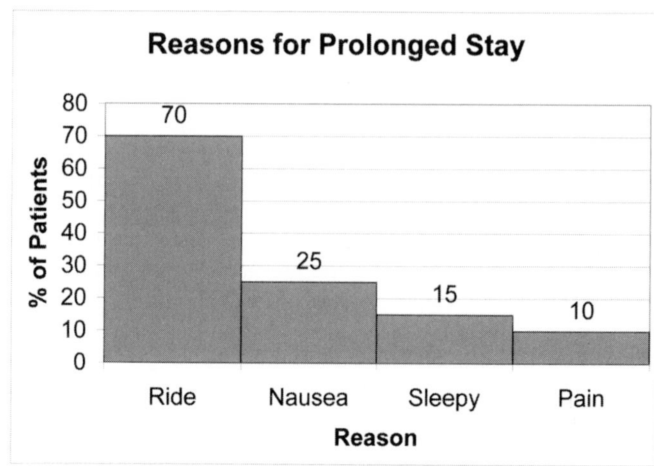

Figure 10.2. Pareto chart showing the leading causes for delayed discharge after surgery.

storming session with the discharge nurses and came up with the following strategies to decrease the time waiting for a ride after surgery:

1. Give rented beepers to spouses and page them when the patient is almost ready to leave.
2. Tell the spouse what time to come back. Because of our time data, we can give a good estimate of the time by procedure code; thus, we can tell the spouse with some degree of certainty what time to come back.
3. Produce a map of the local area, indicating restaurants and shopping areas so that spouses might remain close by.

During this period, we had one surgical site infection. A root cause analysis of this case disclosed that the patient did not receive antibiotics within the 2-hour window of beginning surgery. In this case, the surgeon did not ask for antibiotics, and no one thought to ask him if he wanted them. The medical advisory board recommended that preoperative antibiotics be provided automatically as a matter of policy for a defined list of procedures. We instituted a procedure to make this happen next time and every time.

One Year

We had two subsequent surgical site infections. However, there were predisposing factors in each, and we could discern no systematic factors. Finding cases of infection is not easy for an ambulatory facility, because patients are gone from the facility when they develop an infection. We put one of the OR nurses in charge of infection control, and she developed a process to capture information about surgical site infections in our patients. First, each month our computer generated a list of the patients who had surgery (sorted by surgeon). She sent this list with a letter to each surgeon asking if any of the patients on the list had developed an infection. Nonresponders received a personal phone call from the medical director. Because this phone call was a waste of everyone's time, we soon reached a 100% response rate without the call. In addition, the nurse took a list of all patients for the month to the hospital laboratory and cross referenced it with their list of positive cultures for the month. Because all of the surgeons used this laboratory, we could find any wound cultures this way.

Our "unexpected admissions" to the hospital ran about one per week. The medical advisory board routinely reviewed these each month, and no unreasonable pattern was noted. On closer examination of these admissions, we noted that several of these were not covered by the patient's insurance. We also discovered that many other patients would prefer to go to a supervised care area for the first night. Our medical director negotiated a contract with the hospital to lease beds in their fully staffed but underused pediatric ward. They accepted patients of any age for a fee of $100, with some limits on the care provided. (No expensive drugs.) They billed insurance when possible for their regular fees and credited our account. We paid any difference up to $100 per patient per night. On our side, we charged $100 cash to patients whose insurance did not pay for this service. The hospital makes a little money on a marginal cost basis, and we essentially break even. It is, however, a valuable service for our patients that they did not know they needed until we provided it. A common comment from patients is "What a difference a day makes!"

We had one adverse event this year: an overdose of codeine to a child by a recovery room nurse. After looking at the process for determining the dose, we felt fortunate that the overdose was so small. The patient was weighed in pounds. The dose specified in our policy was in mg per kg. The syrup was supplied in a concentration of mg per teaspoon, and the medicine cup used to measure the syrup was graduated in mL. We constructed a new dosage table that directly converts body weight in pounds to mL of syrup for patients. We also bought smaller medication cups, so that it is not possible to administer a serious overdose, even to our smallest patients. Subsequent monitoring of this process disclosed no errors, and we put this on the shelf as a solved problem.

Some of our proposed charts have not proven useful and have been dropped. For example, the infection rate was very small, and the incidence chart was not meaningful. These cases are now analyzed individually, using a root cause analysis approach. In addition, the starting time for first cases rapidly rose to almost 100%, and this chart was also dropped.

We paid our first employee bonus in December. Profits were sufficient, even in our first year of operation, to pay a full bonus to all employees. A rough calculation suggested that cost saving programs initiated by employees saved 2.5 times the cost of the employee bonus plan. This is also an important morale issue and provides us a hiring edge over other regional employers. The bonus for managers begins with the employee bonus, and the balance relates to goals in their individual areas of responsibility.

Year Two

Business is good. We paid a 32% return to our investors the first year, and this year will be at least as good. Since opening, we have had zero turnover among employees, although two new hires did not complete the 3-month probationary period.

A review of our key indicators from day zero disclosed the following:

1. Patients. We give every patient a survey and about 50% are returned. The overall results have been so favorable that we are concerned that we are asking the wrong questions. The responses have not provided us with much to work on. Some mothers did complain about having to get here 1 hour before surgery in the morning—a critical time for them at home with other children going to school and a husband leaving for work. In response, we changed our policy to 30 minutes before surgery and used more precise OR start times. There was some concern that patients might be late and thus delay the OR. The close timing is emphasized in the preoperative phone call, and our experience to date has been good.

   The incidence of nausea or vomiting (Fig. 10.3) is well below published norms and has been stable at this low level.

   There is really no paperwork for the patient to complete, other than signing the permission and billing forms. We get insurance and demographic information from the surgeon's office and merely confirm the data with the patient at check in.

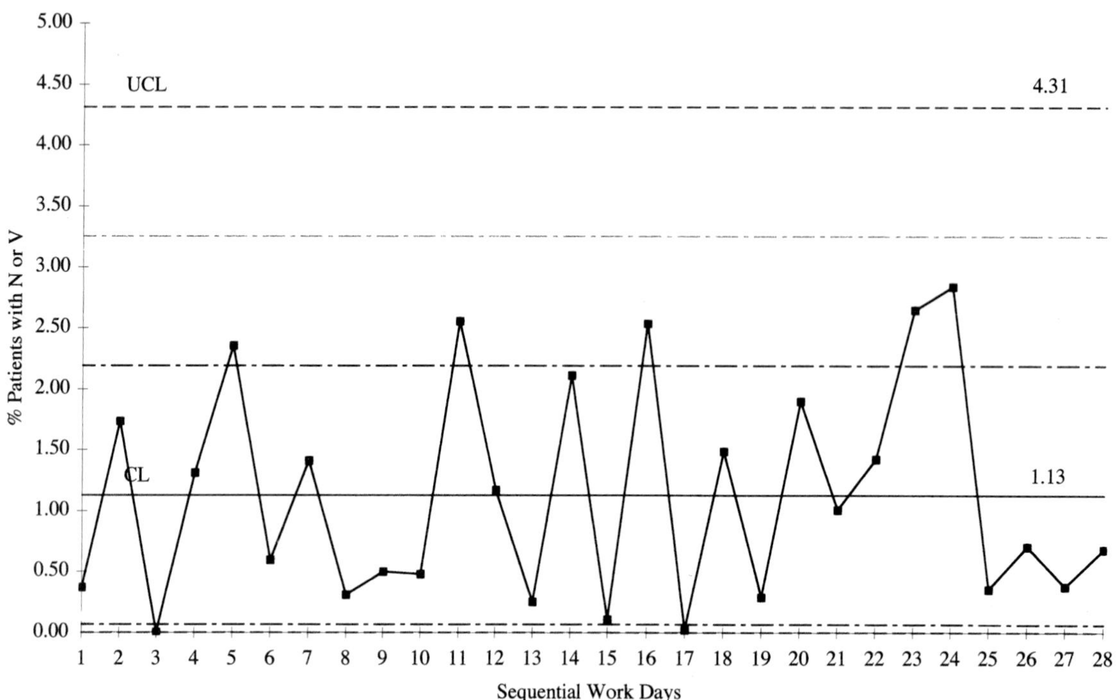

Figure 10.3. Incidence of nausea and vomiting after anesthesia.

2. Surgeons. More than 95% of our first cases now start at the appointed hour (Fig. 10.4). Initially, we had the same problem with start times as the hospital. However, once the surgeons learned that we were on time and ready to go, they began to show up on time. There was one surgeon who just could not get out of bed in the morning, so we arranged for him to start his block at 9 am and found an ear, nose, and throat (ENT) surgeon who was delighted to have a 1-hour slot to do myringotomy tubes before office hours. This was a true win-win situation.

   The supply kit concept has been extended to our 15 most common procedures, and everyone is happy with the results. Trips out of the operating room for missing items are zero for procedures that use kits and about 10% for other cases. Because our "kit cases" constitute 90% of our work, this is an acceptable number.

   We meet monthly with scheduling personnel in the surgeons' offices to facilitate scheduling. Our scheduling clerk knows every surgeon's scheduling clerk on a first name, face-to-face basis. We are now working on an Internet-based program that would allow surgeons to schedule directly into their block time from their offices without talking to anyone.
3. Employees. The few overtime hours were done on a strictly voluntary basis. We have occasionally sent patients home when the OR was running late and we would not have time to complete their surgery during normal hours.

   Every year, we survey local salary scales and share this information with all employees. We position ourselves slightly below the average for our area, because we want our employees to have compelling reasons other than money for wanting to work here. Our zero turnover record demonstrates the success of this strategy.

   We received an award from the local Association of Operating Nurses for 100% membership by our OR nurses. All of the recovery room nurses who were eligible to do so took the ASPAN certification examination. Two of our managers are enrolled in a Masters of Business Administration program at a local college, and one of our billing clerks has started nursing school. VSC contributes to all of these educational efforts. We also sent our billing clerk to a computer programming class and most of the nursing staff to a regional meeting. We believe that these opportunities for professional development compensate for the lack of upward mobility in a flat organization.
4. Payers. We remain at or close to the low-cost provider point for most of the procedures we do, as documented by the mandatory state reporting system.

   After an initial learning curve for our billing clerk, all our claims go through now without a problem. Last year, we purchased software to print claim forms, and typing errors have disappeared. Our days in accounts receivable hovers at 50 days, which is a benchmark for healthcare facilities in this area. (The hospital runs at 110 days.)

Thirty Months

We had our accreditation survey last month. The medical director left a letter to the surveyors at their hotel the night

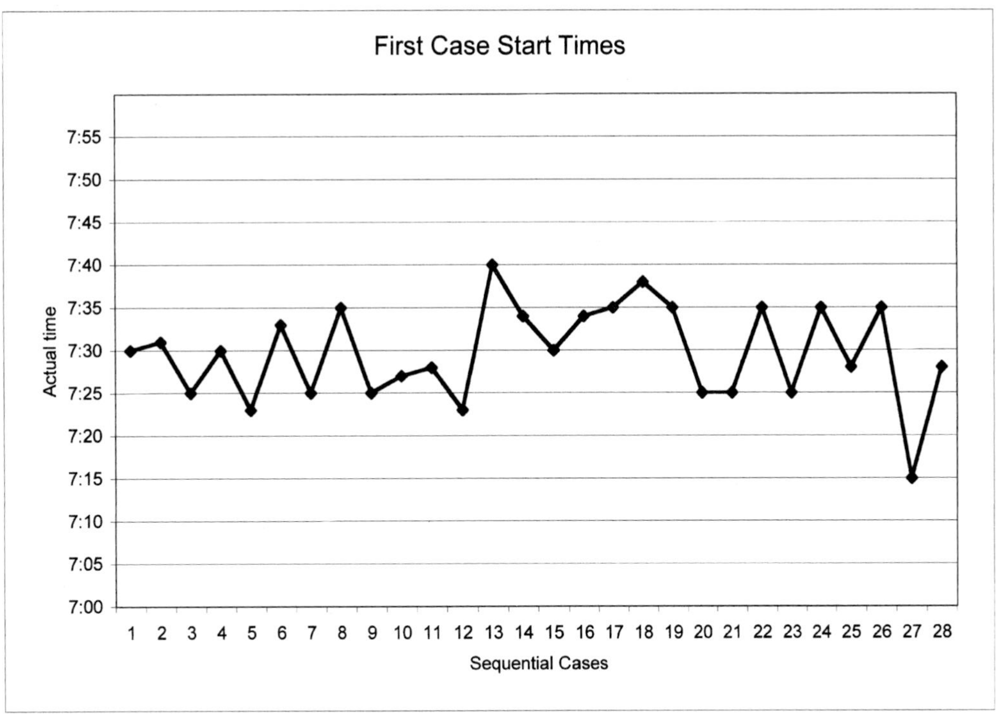

Figure 10.4. Actual start times for the first case in each operating room.

before the survey with the following points: "We know we're good. We've hired you to tell us how good, and how we can get better." They did all those things. The only recommendation in their report was that we paint the utility room floor. (We had some steam leaks there, and the floor was stained although not dirty.) There was considerable discussion about our medication error (see previous discussion), but they finally agreed that it did not meet the requirements for a sentinel event. No one had died, and the risk was not there—the medicine cup was too small for a lethal dose. Also, the area is intensely monitored. We had not done a formal root cause analysis, but many of the elements were included in our report. We discovered the root cause and fixed it by error-proofing the system.

We had our first employee resignation. Her husband was transferred out of state, and she decided to go with him after briefly considering divorce. We may face more departures in the next year, because several of our employees are married to military personnel whose tours of duty at the local base will expire in the next year. Despite a local and national shortage of nurses, we do not anticipate any difficulty replacing any employees.

We revised our patient satisfaction questionnaire and instituted a process to revise half of the questions every quarter. Some questions relate to our mission, and these will remain as a permanent core. The other questions will vary from time to time as various issues surface. Some of these come from perceptions or chance remarks by patients. For instance, a patient in the preoperative area remarked to her husband that she was cold. The nurse who overheard this provided a blanket and also reported this to the nurse in charge of the questionnaire. As a result, we included this question the following month and discovered that many patients were cold in that same location. We had a new thermostat installed, and there were no more comments about being cold. The voice of this customer was very soft, but fortunately, we were listening.

We sent our three managers to Disney World. Specifically, they went to Disney University in Orlando for a course on "The Disney Approach to Quality Management." Although Disney has nothing to do with healthcare, our managers came back with good ideas that we were able to implement in VSC. Some of the thoughts from Disney included:

- Success does not happen by accident.
- Customers have expectations that we must exceed.
- All disciplines work together to improve the overall quality.
- Give the personal touch by smiling and treating every customer as an individual.
- Courtesy is also important between employees.
- A neat appearance is important. We do not allow eating, drinking, and so forth "on stage."
- Efficiency should enhance quality and should never detract from safety or courtesy.
- It takes teamwork to run a smooth and effective show.

As a result of the previously mentioned training, we instituted several new policies. For example, no one eats or drinks at their desk or in view of the public. Some of the principles cannot be implemented by policy. Courtesy is part of our quality culture. Managers are conscious of minor disagreements and confront these before they become problems. Every employee tries to provide the extra "personal touch" for patients. One of our nurses made a preoperative visit in the parking lot so the mother would not have to awaken her sleeping child before surgery. Our maintenance man changed a flat tire so that the departing family would not have to wait for the repair truck. Things like this are done, because they are part of our culture.

The Future

The Institute of Medicine's report came out in 1999, and we plan to change our mission to consider their six aims for better healthcare quality. We sent two employees to the "Quest for Excellence" in Washington, DC to learn about the Baldrige Award (see Chapter 13). Based on their enthusiasm, we reviewed the "Criteria for Excellence in Healthcare" and plan to write an application for our state quality program.

We are also looking at the new ISO document for healthcare. Although we do not plan to become registered, this looks like a helpful tool for maintaining our accreditation, particularly for developing our quality management plan.

We purchased a book on quality tools and hope to improve the sophistication of our charts and graphs. Six Sigma has received a lot of attention recently, but at this point it seems too complex for a small organization like ours (see Chapter 13).

In general, we plan to keep getting better and to do that faster than our competition. This is a great place to work. We are easily the best healthcare facility around, and we plan to stay that way. However, as they say at Disney World, it will not happen by accident.

In Retrospect

Design

Our use of QFD as a design tool was relatively unsophisticated but effective. If we had used double Likert scales on our surveys of future customers, we could have been more objective about what was important to them. We could also have used the same technique on our customer surveys each month to determine where to focus our improvement efforts.

Monitor

The control charts, histograms, and Pareto charts were useful, and we should have done more. Specifications and control limits were arbitrary, and we did not assess Cp. However, it is not clear that these refinements would have been useful here.

Repair

Although the accreditation surveyors were happy with our disposition of the codeine overdose, it would have been a useful exercise for us to have done a formal root cause analysis. The process is not difficult and would have been useful for other issues. We did use brainstorming to good effect.

Improve

Improvement efforts were a little chaotic and responsive to problems rather than proactive. We might have appointed permanent improvement teams for each of our key processes, and the recovery room team might have used FMEA on our narcotic administration process to prevent the codeine overdose.

We also failed to segment our customers. We did respond to a complaint from mothers, but there are several other customer groups that have individual needs that we were not able to address.

SUGGESTED READINGS

Berglund RG. How close to Six Sigma are you? *Informed Outlook* 2002;(Feb):1, 28–31.

Carey RG, Lloyd RC. *Measuring quality improvement in healthcare.* Milwaukee: Quality Press, 2001.

Daniel WW. *Biostatistics: a foundation for analysis in the health sciences.* New York: John Wiley and Sons, 1998.

Tague NR. *The quality toolbox.* Milwaukee: Quality Press, 1995.

The Memory Jogger One, University of Michigan Hospitals Version, 2nd ed. Methuen, MA: AIM Goal QPC, 1998.

11

COLLECTING DATA FOR ACTIONS

STEPHEN B. KRITCHEVSKY
RONALD I. SHORR

Formalized approaches for quality improvement (QI) are known by many names, but all trace their roots to the seminal work by Shewhart on statistical process control (SPC) early in the last century (1). It is an axiom of SPC that a process must be measured to be managed, and, to be managed properly, measurements must be made properly and interpreted in the proper statistical context (2). In the past 20 years, hospitals have embraced QI methodologies to help provide better, safer, and more efficient patient care, and the collection and analysis of data have played a central role.

Data collected for quality assurance and QI provide evidence for action. If data are to be effective for this purpose, they must be of a quality that will persuade people to change behavior. Although scientists think of data as a scientific tool, in the QI context they are also a rhetorical tool: devices to convince others to act. Therefore, appropriate data collection and presentation depend not only on the problem at hand but also on the audience that is meant to react to them. Booth et al. (3) are among the few commentators who have considered data's rhetorical importance, and we use their framework here to discuss the use of data to motivate action for QI.

Table 11.1 presents key characteristics that data should have to be accepted as persuasive evidence (3). Most scientifically trained people recognize the first four criteria in other guises. Whether data are representative is often discussed in terms of selection bias and generalizability. Accuracy and precision are often discussed in science in terms of validity and reliability, and sufficiency is often discussed in terms of effect size, statistical power, and confounding. The next four criteria are discussed less frequently but are important in the QI context, because they relate to how data are received. Not all data are equally authoritative. In clinical epidemiology, for example, the randomized, placebo-controlled, double-blinded trial is considered the most authoritative research evidence, and clinicians are more likely to accept conclusions from this type of study than from observational study designs. Perspicuous data are data that are easily understood by the target audience. A sophisticated analyst can present data derived from a complex statistical model, but if the result cannot be understood by those being asked to endorse change, it will have a weaker effect. Appropriate data are data that are seen by the audience as useful for supporting a claim for action. A hospital administrator may be shown data on bleeding times of patients on anticoagulation therapy in an attempt to convince him or her to redirect resources to a project to standardize this aspect of care. The typical administrator is unprepared to interpret these data. More appropriate data would show the financial impact of the lack of control. Even if the financial data are weaker by other standards, those data might be more persuasive, because they are more appropriate to the target audience. Finally, data are presented to stimulate action. There must be a link between the data offered and the action proposed; otherwise, the data can be disregarded as irrelevant. Each of these points deserves some elaboration. We present our interpretations of these criteria based on our experience in dozens of activities in which data have been used for QI in healthcare settings.

REPRESENTATIVE DATA

Representative data can be trusted to be a fair reflection of the underlying process or outcome that they are meant to measure. In epidemiology, the failure of data to be representative can lead to misleading conclusions through selection bias. Bias

TABLE 11.1. CHARACTERISTICS OF DATA THAT SUPPORT THEIR ACCEPTANCE AS EVIDENCE FOR ACTION

- Representative
  - Do the data fairly represent the thing measured?
- Accurate
  - Do the data reflect what is intended to be measured?
- Precise
  - Is there a close correspondence between the data and the target of measurement?
- Sufficient
  - Are there enough data to act?
- Authoritative
  - Are these the best data for drawing a meaningful conclusion?
- Perspicuous
  - Can the target audience understand the data being presented?
- Appropriate
  - Are the data appropriate evidence for action?
- Relevant
  - Are the data relevant evidence for the action proposed?

Adapted from Booth WC, Columb CG, Williams JM. *The craft of research.* Chicago: University of Chicago Press, 1995: 85–148.

can also taint QI studies. Studies may focus on only certain shifts, days of the week, or floors, but it may be that most of the problems occur at other times or other places. Failure to represent these times may lead to erroneous conclusions about the process under study. Data can also fail to be representative if they do not include the full spectrum of occurrences. A study of falls that only includes falls that result in injuries includes only the most severe cases. On one hand, this might be acceptable, because it is specifically these cases that the hospital most wishes to prevent. On the other hand, these cases may have features such that they would misrepresent the true nature of the problem.

This issue was illustrated in a recently completed study to identify risk factors for falls in a hospital in Tennessee (4). During the planning phase, the only identifiable data source for identifying falls was the hospital's incident-reporting system. In this system, persons observing a fall fill out a form describing the event and then forward it to the risk management department. Despite its convenience, there were serious concerns about this system that precluded its use in a scientific study. Because incident reports take effort to complete and were intended to alert the risk management department of potential problems, it seemed likely that the falls reported by this system overrepresented the more serious falls, especially those resulting in injuries. Moreover, we were told that incident reports had been used as an index of poor nursing performance by nursing administration. Thus, nurses had a disincentive for filing incident reports, which led to an underestimate of the total number of falls. Taking these considerations together, we had little confidence that the falls reported to this system were representative of all falls occurring in the hospital. To remedy this situation, we implemented a specialized surveillance system for falls, used for the duration of the study. Each nursing unit was instructed to page a special "falls" number every time a fall was ascertained. The pager was staffed 7 days a week, 24 hours/day by residents and medical student externs who had been specially trained in the evaluation of falls. We discovered that only 77% of the falls detected by the surveillance system were also reported as incident reports to risk management.

A number of methods can be used to ensure that collected data are representative. The most straightforward method is to collect information on all occurrences. In many situations, this is impractical, and it is perfectly appropriate to use sampling strategies to obtain an unbiased sample from the process understudy. A large number of techniques have been developed for selecting representative samples, many of which require statistical advice to implement (5). Two easily implemented methods require having a list in advance of the population of interest (known as a sampling frame). The desired number of subjects n are selected from the population of size N. The proportion of subjects selected is called the sampling fraction ($f = n/N$). In the first method, a different random number is assigned to each member of the population. The list is sorted by the random number, and the first x subjects are selected. An even easier method is called systematic sampling. This method uses a number called the sampling interval *(k)* and is equal to the inverse of the sampling fraction ($1/f$). This number is rounded down to the nearest integer. One picks a random number between 1 and k. One starts with the randomly selected subject on the list and then picks every kth subject thereafter. Harrington et al. (6) used this method to select controls for a case-control study examining factors for silent aspiration among patients after coronary artery bypass graft (CABG) surgery. The investigators had a list of all CABG surgeries performed over 4.5 years (N = 5,777), from which 106 controls were required (n = 106, f= 106/5,777, k = 54). The investigators selected a random number between 1 and 54 and used this number to pick the person sampled as the first control. Every fifty-fourth patient was sampled thereafter. If a chart was missing or one of the sampled patients was found to be a case, the next patient on the list was selected. The important feature of this method is that every patient had an equal probability of being selected as a control, a criterion that ensures that the sample is representative. The QI literature also provides guidance for selecting representative samples for other uses (e.g., acceptance sampling and samples selected for the construction of control charts).

The representativeness of participants in epidemiologic studies is constantly threatened by nonresponse and loss to follow-up. Typically, a large proportion of those whom one wishes to study is not available to the investigator for one reason or another. Usually no data are available on those not included, so it is often difficult to tell how much different the observed results are from those that would have been observed given full participation. Any amount of nonresponse can introduce selection bias, but the greater the extent of the problem, the greater the threat. Cochran (7) has a more detailed discussion of assessing this problem.

ACCURATE DATA

Accurate data capture what the researcher intends. To most scientists, this is understood as the concept of validity. Whenever a new measurement instrument is developed or an old instrument is applied to a new situation, the validity of the instrument must be demonstrated. For example, in a study of hand washing in the intensive care unit (ICU), Simmons et al. (8) determined by direct observation that 22% of ICU nurses washed their hands in appropriate situations. When asked by questionnaire, nurses replied that they washed their hands appropriately between 69% and 92% of the time. Clearly, self-reported hand washing is an inaccurate representation of true behavior.

The importance of measurement validity to epidemiologic inference is demonstrated by the following equation (9, p. 61):

$$\mathrm{OR}_0 = (\mathrm{OR}_T)^z \text{ where } z = (\rho_{\mathrm{TX}})^2$$

This equation states that the observed odds ratio (OR_0) relating disease to an exposure is equal to the true odds ratio (OR_T) raised to the power of the square of the correlation between the study measurement (X) and the true measurement (ρ_{TX}). In other words, the observed odds ratio is always smaller than the true odds ratio when the measurement is imperfect. This equation holds when the correlation between the study measure and the true measure is the same for both cases and noncases. To see the effect of mismeasurement, consider the situation in which

TABLE 11.2. RELATIONSHIP BETWEEN ORDERS FOR RESTRAINTS AND OBSERVED RESTRAINT USE AT THE TIME OF FALL IN THE CASES

	Orders for restraints		
Observed restraint use	Yes	No	Total
Yes	4	11	**15**
No	18	195	**213**
Total	**22**	**206**	**228**

Kappa = 0.15 (95% CI = −0.4–0.34).
From Shorr RI, Guillen MK, Rosenblatt LC, et al. Restraint use, restraint orders, and the risk of falls in hospitalized patients. *J Am Geriatr Soc* 2002; 50: 526–529.

the correlation between the exposure measurement and the true exposure is 0.5 and the true odds ratio is 3.0; the observed odds ratio will be 1.32 ($OR_0 = 3^{(0.25)}$). Given a measure with poor validity, a nonsignificant result might indicate that no relationship exists between exposure and disease or that the relationship was too weak to overcome the attenuation resulting from inaccurate measurement.

The validity of a new study measure can be established by comparing it to a perfect measure or "gold standard." However, perfect measures are seldom available. It is possible to use a less than ideal measure to establish the validity of a new measure as long as the comparison measure's sources of error differ from the measure being evaluated (9, pp. 83–84). The validity of a measure relying on data in the medical chart, for example, could not be established by reabstracting the same medical chart, because the errors in measurement inherent in the charting process will be the same for both chart reviews. Another source of information must be found. Currently much controversy is related to the use of restraints in the prevention of falls. Studies typically rely on the medical chart to make this determination. A patient is considered restrained if an order in the chart can be found. Shorr et al. (4) used falls evaluators to look at the correspondence between the chart and the situation at the time of falls. Their data (Table 11.2) show that there is almost no correspondence between the chart and observed restraint use near the time of the fall. Inferences based on restraint orders as a measure of restraint use would, therefore, be invalid.

PRECISE DATA

A number of concepts fall under the umbrella of precision, but they all share the underlying idea of obtaining the same result time after time. In common epidemiologic use, precision can relate to either the reliability of a measure or the magnitude of the error associated with statistical inferences. The reliability of a measure is the extent to which the same result is obtained on repeated applications of the same instrument in the same situation. Reliability is a somewhat weaker test of a measurement instrument than validity is, because a highly reliable measure still may be invalid. However, a measurement instrument can be no more valid than it is reliable. Reliability studies are usually easier to conduct than validity studies are. Survey participants can be interviewed twice, or charts can be reabstracted and the results compared. If multiple data collectors are to be used, they can each collect data from a common source, and their results can be compared. Reliability studies should be a facet of a study pretest to uncover potential problems in the data collection procedures. Such studies can direct training efforts and redesign of forms and data collection instruments.

Horwitz and Yu (10) examined the reliability of medical record abstraction. Three data collectors reabstracted 102 charts from a case-control study of breast cancer. The abstractors were evaluated on ten different items found in the medical record. The intraabstractor agreement between two different reviews ranged from a low of 54% for a history of benign breast disease to around 90% for the number of children, presence of diabetes, and history of lactation. The interabstractor agreement was slightly lower and followed the intraabstractor pattern. Disagreements were ascribed either to the abstracting process or to the interpretation of the abstracted data. Errors in abstraction were categorized as conflicting data in the medical record, missed information, volumes of the medical record unavailable, and transcribing errors. These errors accounted for 31% of disagreements between abstractors. By far, the most frequent source of disagreements (60%) was the differential application of coding criteria. For example, if the chart contained no specific information indicating that a patient was hypertensive, the record might have been coded as negative for hypertension at one time and as unknown at another.

In QI applications, poor data reliability is an additional source of random error or "noise" in the data. Noise makes it more difficult to detect and interpret meaningful variation (2). Data reliability can be increased by insisting on clear, unambiguous data definitions and clear guidelines for dealing with unusual situations.

Precision can also be interpreted as statistical precision or the exactness with which the collected data characterize the process or population of interest. What if one tried to determine the length of stay for pneumonia patients by looking at six random patients? This method could be criticized because data from six patients permit only an imprecise characterization of the experience of pneumonia patients in general. The precision with which the sample reflects the underlying population is known as the standard error of the mean (SEM). If one has a sample of n measurements with mean x and standard deviation s, the SEM is given by the formula:

$$\text{SEM} = s/\sqrt{n}.$$

The smaller the SEM, the more precise the characterization of the process or population. By inspection of the formula, it can be seen that there are two strategies to reduce the SEM. First, the standard deviation can be reduced. This would typically be done by increasing the reliability of the measure or increasing the number of measures per subject (e.g., measuring in duplicate). Second, the sample size can be increased to improve the precision of the estimate. The SEM can be used to calculate the 95% confidence interval (CI) around a given sample estimate. This interval is widely used in the medical literature to provide a sense

TABLE 11.3. PRECISION INCREASES WITH SAMPLE SIZE

Sample size	Standard error	Width of 95% CI	95% CI
20	6.7%	±13.1%	0.0%, 23.1%
40	4.7%	±9.3%	0.1%, 19.3%
60	3.9%	±7.6%	2.5%, 17.6%
80	3.4%	±6.6%	3.4%, 16.6%
100	3.0%	±5.9%	4.1%, 15.9%
200	2.1%	±4.2%	5.8%, 14.1%
300	1.7%	±3.4%	6.6%, 13.4%
500	1.3%	±2.6%	7.4%, 12.6%

Event Rate is 10%

of the precision with which an estimate is known. It is given by the formula:

$$95\%\ \text{CI} = x \pm 1.96 \cdot \text{SEM}(x)$$

Technically, there is a 95% probability that the true mean of the population falls within the interval. Informally, the narrower the interval, the more precise the guess as to the value of the underlying value that one is trying to estimate.

QI projects can stall because data collection goals are too ambitious. If events are frequent, such as the processing of pharmacy orders, the volume is so daunting that worthwhile projects may never be seriously considered. In situations like this, it is rarely necessary to collect complete data. Data can be sampled as long as the sample is representative (see previous discussion). However, the question remains: how much data should be collected? The answer depends on how precise the data must be to make the decision to act. If one is interested in seeing how many lapses there are in the proper timing of a certain medication that may be given thousands of times per year in the hospital and the error rate is 10%, one can calculate what the standard errors and 95% CIs for various sample sizes would be. The standard error of a binomial variable (i.e., one that can take only two values, in this case error and no error) is given by: $\sqrt{pq/n}$ where p is the proportion of times an error is made, q is $1 - p$, and n is the sample size. Table 11.3 shows how the precision of the estimate increases with sample size. There is a substantial increase in precision as the sample size increases from 20 to 40, but a relatively modest increase as it goes from 200 to 300.

SUFFICIENT DATA

Data sufficiency implies that data are of sufficient quality and quantity to justify action. Typically, this justification is derived from the comparison of data to some standard and often entails comparisons with peers, with one's past performance, or in reference to a stated goal.

Data are insufficient when they do not differ sufficiently from the criteria of acceptability to motivate action, or they do not exclude other plausible explanations. In SPC, the statistics based on measurements from serial samples are plotted on a graph. The control chart, in its most rudimentary form, plots the historical mean of the process along with "action limits." These limits are lines placed three standard errors above and below the mean (essentially it is 99.7% CI around the historical mean level). If a point falls outside the limits, then there is sufficient evidence that the process is degrading, because it would be quite rare for a stable process to generate a measurement so distant from its historical mean. In the absence of such signals, the process is deemed to be working acceptably. The control chart uses statistics to judge when evidence is sufficient for intervention. The criterion for setting action limits in healthcare settings is an area of active controversy, with some arguing that the three standard error limit is too strict (11,12).

Statistics are used to judge sufficiency in other ways as well. If clinicians differ from each other, these differences may be ignored as evidence unless they are "statistically significantly" different from one another. This is usually taken to mean that a p value calculated for the difference under the assumption that the clinicians do not differ at all is .05 or less. There are situations in which even small amounts of data are sufficient for action. Rare or catastrophic situations (sentinel events) can be so beyond the realm of expectation that action is required regardless of any statistical consideration. Finally, just because a difference is statistically significant does not mean that it is worth acting on. There are cases when even small differences are "significant" because the sample size available for the comparison is very large.

If chance is deemed unlikely, it does not necessarily mean that action is ruled in. Selection bias and measurement errors can lead to significant differences. There may also be alternative explanations for differences. For example, if the postoperative death rate differs significantly between two hospitals, it may be due to poorer quality care at one of the institutions, but it may also be due to differences in the patient acuity or in the kinds of operations that are performed. These differences confound the comparison between the two hospitals. Administrators may be reluctant to act on such comparisons until they have sufficient data that differences in outcome are indeed attributable to actual differences in the process of care. Confounding is much less a problem with process-oriented measures than with outcome-oriented ones. A completely sufficient comparison of outcome measures would account for all alternative causes of the outcome under study.

A tension can develop around the issue of data sufficiency if there is a goal to publish the results of a QI project in the medical literature. Typically, a scientific audience will have a higher standard for data sufficiency than a hospital QI team may require. This means that data sufficient to lead to local change may not be publishable in a scientific journal. Moreover, common techniques in QI are not well known in the traditional medical literature and vice versa, leading to reduced appreciation of achievements. On the other hand, collecting sufficient data for publication may lead to lengthy delays in implementing a data collection project in the hospital and may lead to frustration with the data collection process. This tension may deter academically minded physicians from participating in QI processes, because they will not necessarily see a benefit from participation in the process. This can also mean that academically minded physicians will not accept the results of a QI study, because they think that the data are insufficient.

AUTHORITATIVE DATA

The greater the authority of the data, the more likely they are to be accepted as evidence. Authority is invested in data both by the person presenting data and by their source. Data from hospital QI projects may be rejected if such data are based solely on billing data that are often inadequate for research. Data abstracted from medical charts may be seen as more authoritative than billing data, because the abstracted data were collected for the specific purpose of the project at hand. The person presenting the data may influence how the data are perceived by the audience. Research has shown that when data are presented to physicians by peer leaders, such data have a greater effect on behavior than when data are presented by other healthcare professionals (13). If data are shown that have obvious flaws, not only will those data not be considered but also future data presented by the same spokesperson will be received with much skepticism.

In clinical science, the authority of data is often a function of the design of the study that generated the data, with results from randomized trials being held in highest esteem, and some physicians may insist on evidence from such trials before changing behaviors. Many guidelines groups explicitly consider hierarchies of evidence, investing trials evidence with the greatest authority. In reality, no one study design is appropriate for every situation, and each study must be judged on its own merits. Because small clinical trials tend to give imprecise results, some commentators believe that meta-analyses of clinical trials are the highest authority (14–16).

PERSPICUOUS DATA

If data are not understood, they will not be accepted as evidence. Audiences differ in both background and orientation. Most people understand simple graphs and charts, some understand simple statistical analyses, and a few understand the results of a statistical model. In some settings, apt anecdotes may be more effective in building the case for change than well-executed scientific studies with validated rating scales. The level of sophistication varies tremendously. In mixed audiences, presentation of data in a number of different ways will increase the chances that the data will be understood and, thus, acted on.

APPROPRIATE DATA

Because of the variety in training and professional backgrounds among those working in the hospital, it is easy to present data that are inappropriate to a given audience. In general, the data presented should be matched to the training and sphere of activities of the audience. The kind of data presented carries with it an implicit message. If an analyst shows data on antibiotic selection to hospital administrators, the implicit message is that the administrator should change the way that antibiotics are prescribed. This cannot happen because the prescription of drugs is beyond the administrators' area of professional competence. Similarly, nurses should not be presented with financial data, because the deployment of resources in most hospitals is beyond their scope of activities. Again, in mixed audiences, using many kinds of data may improve the chances that the data are acted on.

RELEVANT DATA

The idea of relevancy comes into play in the structure of the implicit argument for change. Data on the variation of medical practice may show that the average cost per patient is much higher at one hospital than at peer hospitals. The implicit argument is that this variance represents a deficiency of some kind that must be addressed. Physicians may not care about the cost of care provided, as long as they think that the care they are providing is meeting standards of good medical practice. In this case, data are seen as irrelevant, because no change in medical practice would be considered based solely on financial considerations.

Data are also considered irrelevant if they are not seen as being applicable to those reviewing the data. The financial data discussed previously would also be irrelevant if the physicians believed that the reasons for the excess charges were due to other kinds of problems, such as inefficiencies in various hospital support services or even the method that the hospital uses to calculate the cost of care.

"My patients are sicker" is a stereotypical reaction of physicians who are shown data comparing their performance to that of peers. This statement is one about the relevancy of the data to their situation. They are essentially saying that these data are irrelevant, because a physician's patients are different in some essential fashion from the comparison group. This is the idea of representativeness turned inside out. Similar appeals are used to reject data relative to hospital performance ("but our patients are of much higher acuity") and the implementation of care pathways developed at other institutions ("sure, that works in Boston, but it won't work here"). The declaration that the data are irrelevant to the local situation is difficult to address, but some techniques can be effective. There are statistical algorithms that can be used to "adjust" for differences between patients to come up with conclusions that account for how patient-related characteristics differ from one another. The problem is that these techniques tend to be poorly understood by those presented with the data and, thus, may fail as evidence on that basis. Another method is to stratify patient populations to generate comparisons that are easily understood. In this strategy, patients are selected who represent the typical patient, so that those with comorbidities and complications are purposefully deleted from the sample. This removes the "exceptions" to better see the "rule." If, after making these exclusions, the physician in question still has a higher resource use than his or her peers do, the claim of exceptionalism is much more difficult to sustain.

The relevancy of data is a major issue when trying to decide whether to collect outcome or process data. The attraction of outcomes data (e.g., patient satisfaction or mortality) is that they represent the performance of the hospital in achieving important goals (satisfied customers or good quality care). Outcome measures are integrative in the sense that they represent the net effect of all the hospital processes when applied to a specific set of patients. This integrative aspect makes their relevancy to individuals working at the hospital questionable. If a hospital had a goal of improved patient satisfaction and the datum presented as evidence of the need for change is a score on a global satisfaction question that puts the hospital at the 20th percentile of satisfaction with respect to peer institutions, it is probably useless to present this datum to the hospital's professional staff, because it is completely unclear how this fact could be translated into action. The datum certainly would not be relevant evidence to support any specific proposed action. Data would need to be proffered showing that, when "X" happens, patients are much less satisfied; therefore, the hospital would need to change to ensure that "X" happens less frequently. This demonstration would translate the outcome data of dubious relevance to a process measure of clear relevance. The science of making outcomes data relevant by understanding what processes drive the outcome is relatively underdeveloped. However, in the era of interhospital comparisons, it is essential for using outcomes data to their best advantage.

CONCLUSION

The collection of QI data should be thoughtfully planned. Much effort can be wasted collecting and analyzing data that are not meaningful. Part of the planning effort can involve some prenegotiation with stakeholders in the process under study to determine what kinds of data are going to be most persuasive in the case for change. There are many advantages to involving multidisciplinary teams in QI projects. To this list we add another. If the team represents all those who would be expected to change, then they can provide guidance on the kinds of evidence that would be required to motivate their peers to change as well. For data collection to be useful, the product must be perceived to be meaningful by those who are expected to respond to it.

REFERENCES

1. Shewhart WA. *Economic control of quality of manufactured product.* New York: Van Nostrand Reinhold, 1931.
2. Deming WE. *Out of the crisis.* Cambridge, MA: Massachusetts Institute of Technology, Center for Advanced Engineering Study, 1986.
3. Booth WC, Colomb GG, Williams JM. *The craft of research.* Chicago: University of Chicago Press, 1995:85–148.
4. Shorr RI, Guillen MK, Rosenblatt LC, et al. Restraint use, restraint orders, and the risk of falls in hospitalized patients. *J Am Geriatr Soc* 2002;50:526–529.
5. Kish L. *Survey sampling.* New York: John Wiley and Sons, 1965.
6. Harrington OB, Duckworth JK, Starnes CL, et al. Silent aspiration after coronary artery bypass grafting. *Ann Thorac Surg* 1998;65: 1599–1603.
7. Cochran WG. *Sampling techniques,* 3rd ed. New York: John Wiley and Sons, 1977:361–363.
8. Simmons B, Bryant J, Nieman K, et al. The role of hand washing in prevention of endemic intensive care unit infection. *Infect Control Hosp Epidemiol* 1990;11:589–594.
9. Armstrong BK, White E, Saracci R. *Principles of exposure measurement in epidemiology.* New York: Oxford University Press, 1992.
10. Horwitz RI, Yu EC. Assessing the reliability of epidemiologic data obtained from medical records. *J Chron Dis* 1984;37:825–831.
11. Benneyan JC. Statistical quality control methods in infection control and hospital epidemiology, part II: chart use, statistical properties, and research issues. *Infect Control Hosp Epidemiol* 1998;19:265–283.
12. Birnbaum D. Analysis of hospital infection surveillance data. *Infect Control* 1984;5:332–338.
13. Borbas C, Morris N, McLaughlin B, et al. The role of clinical opinion leaders in guideline implementation and quality improvement. *Chest* 2000;118(2 Suppl):24S–32S.
14. Sackett DL, Haynes RB, Guyatt GH, et al. *Clinical epidemiology: a basic science for clinical medicine,* 2nd ed. Boston, Little, Brown and Company, 1991:366.
15. Barton S. Which clinical studies provide the best evidence? The best RCT still trumps the best observational study. *BMJ* 2000;321: 255–256.
16. Collins R, MacMahon S. Reliable assessment of effects of treatment on mortality and major morbidity, 1: clinical trials. *Lancet* 2001;357: 373–380.

12

SELECTING CHANGE IMPLEMENTATION STRATEGIES

JAN BOWER
MARISEL SEGARRA-NEWNHAM
ALAN TICE

GENERAL DISCUSSION OF CHANGE

Change is inherent in daily life, and it is the only thing that humans can be sure of—it is a conundrum. The result of change can be unpredictable. Change can have a positive impact, a negative impact, or no impact at all. The challenge in healthcare is to create change that produces a desirable impact (change for improvement) (1).

Much has been written about change, and it is generally agreed that the concept of change is uncomfortable for most people, although in reality, everyone experiences some change each day. When a request for change is unclear or there is a perceived threat, such as to security or to comfort, human nature drives people to find creative ways to resist change. People are more apt to be open to changes if they see change as a solution to a problem, and they are involved in the whole change process, which extends from identification, through planning and implementation, and finally to evaluation and refining.

Unfortunately, change is more complicated than simply rearranging the external structure. Bridges (2) wrote that in order for external changes to be sustainable, people must go through an internal transition process. The three stages of transition are letting go of the old, the neutral zone, and the new beginning. Depending on the extent of the change, different people need different amounts of time to work through this transition process. Understanding the internal process of change, knowing that people respond differently, and being accommodating to these differences is the key to making change successful and sustainable.

Healthcare is a complicated industry and one in which change is demanded all the time at many levels. Payers want lower costs; patients want fewer bad outcomes; regulators want to eliminate fraud and abuse; and administrators want to provide safe care, be compliant with the law, maintain a financial balance sheet with a positive margin, and so on. Healthcare providers continue to feel an enormous amount of pressure to be more productive and the demands seem to be endless (3).

The challenge for healthcare leaders is to learn how to create environments where change is viewed as a natural and positive force. Savvy leaders are able to listen to care providers, those who work at the bedside, for their interpretation of the problems to identify common themes that lead to making plans for improvement. Leaders must possess the finesse to align opinions and identify core issues that can generally be agreed on so that improvement projects can move forward. Too often change projects stop, because the energy and momentum become lost from poor clarification and lack of agreement on what exactly the problem is and the result is a project that is unmanageable. When consensus is built, ideas for a solution will emerge through dialogue and brainstorming among the stakeholders. If leaders can capture this energy and provide the framework and resources needed to plan and implement the change project, the result will be positive change that is rewarding for the stakeholders involved.

Rogers (4) wrote about the natural speed of diffusion of innovation or change among a given group of people, which tends to resemble a bell curve. He demonstrated how people adopt to innovation at different rates. On the far left side of the curve the first 3% of a population are innovators, the people who invent and want to do things differently. Rogers refers to the next group (13%) as the early adopters. These are the people who move slower then the innovators, but nonetheless want to change. The next 34% are in the early majority; these are people who will watch and wait for a while and then move with the flow. The other half of the curve mirrors the first half but with the opposite drives to change. These groups are labeled late majority, laggards, and immovables.

By understanding and accepting that there will be a range of these types of personality responses to a change, most effort should be spent with the people on the left of the curve and the rest will eventually follow out of necessity. In our experience, most healthcare providers are willing to change if the change makes sense to them, if they are provided with adequate information, if their opinions are listened to, and if they are invited to be involved in the change project.

A Culture for Change

In order for a change project to be successful in healthcare, those involved in making the change must be provided with an environment that is emotionally supportive. There must be a certain level of tolerance for self-expression and even for some risk-taking behavior. A supportive culture starts with trust, which takes time to build. In healthcare this is a difficult balancing act. On one hand, patient safety is at stake and mistakes cannot be tolerated; on the other hand, if a culture is not created in which people feel safe to discuss near misses, errors, and patient harm, an opportunity for learning and making improvements will be lost.

It is becoming common knowledge that to reduce medical errors, healthcare providers must know about medical errors that have occurred, they must understand how the errors occurred, and they must have input on how to improve, or change, the system and educate others so that a similar error will not occur in the future. To do this, there must be a culture that is "blame free" so that care providers will feel safe to report medical errors or near miss events. If healthcare providers have experienced or witnessed blame and punishment for mistakes and errors (even if only subtle), human nature will drive them to be defensive or hide errors and near-miss events. They may even go so far as to cast blame on others to avoid shame, embarrassment, or punishment. To build trust and create a culture in which it is safe to report and discuss errors, healthcare providers must be made to feel valued, protected, and even emotionally rewarded for speaking up about an error they made or near-miss situation that they were involved in.

Providers must be encouraged to voice their opinion regarding what problems must be solved or what changes must be made in order for the delivery of healthcare to be safer and better. If a voice falls on "deaf ears," or if someone else uses the idea and takes the credit, a culture is created in which information is not shared and creative ideas are suppressed. In both cases there is missed opportunity for change and improvement and even worse, by remaining silent, a dangerous situation might continue to exist, which could lead to a bad outcome for a patient.

To build this culture, leaders and managers must set the tone and model the behavior that they want from their employees. Leaders who openly discuss and recount their personal stories of making mistakes and show genuine empathy toward those that are involved in situations that cause patient harm will rapidly build a culture that supports improvement changes. Additional ways to build a culture that is supportive is to make sure that healthcare providers are properly mentored. New members should be given a thorough orientation to the department, the policies, and procedures and should be provided with the information and resources that they need to do their job. Ideally, someone should be appointed to stay connected to the new employee to coach him or her through the various stages of integrating into a new system. This is just as important for the medical staff as it is for the nursing and technical staff.

Change Agent

The change agent, or person who is the leader for change is in a vulnerable position, because he or she continually is placed at risk (4). Risk of resistance, risk of making a change that turns out not to be beneficial, risk of being a threat, and so on. This is a delicate position because it is one of always gently pushing people to change, specifically to work better. To be effective, a change agent must be empathetic, listen well, and be customer focused. In healthcare, more than in other disciplines, leaders must understand that in order for care providers to provide good, safe care, they themselves must be cared for. There must be understanding of and acknowledgment of barriers to doing good work, both physical and emotional, to be able to move forward in building systems that make it easier for care providers to provide care.

Change agents can take many forms; for example, the role of the mentor is part change agent. One of the most important roles for a change agent in healthcare is to work to improve communication and to teach health workers how to better connect and help each other to prevent patient harm. The Joint Commission on Accreditation of Healthcare Organizations (JCAHO) documented that one of the most common themes in sentinel events is poor communication—both verbal and written. Lack of passing information along as the patient moves from one service to another (continuum of care), unavailable information, lack of clear effective communication with the patient and family, lack of communication among staff, and poor labeling of medications have been documented (5).

Plan-Do-Check-Act (PDCA) Cycle of Improvement

The Shewart/Deming PDCA cycle of improvement provides an excellent framework for improvement projects (6). The planning stage requires consideration and consensus, but at some point the project must move into the do stage with the knowledge that it probably will not be perfect, but by doing new issues will emerge for further consideration. It is important that the change agent work with people through these stages and reiterate that the goal is not perfection but rather learning and improvement. The check stage is used to focus on what worked well and what did not so that further changes can be made and implemented.

An example of an easy, yet powerful change project using the PDCA framework is updating the list of acceptable abbreviations for medications. Historically providers write a "U" or "u" to indicate *unit* of insulin. The U has sometimes been mistaken for a 0, which has the potential to lead to a tenfold overdose of insulin with the potential tragic outcome of death. By changing the system to disallow the use of an abbreviation for the word *unit* and require that the word be spelled out, the result will be a significant decrease of the probability of administering a tenfold overdose of insulin.

The planning stage would include looking at the evidence for change, literature review, occurrence reports, and so forth and planning the change process. The do stage would include providing education and reminders to encourage care providers to write out the abbreviations. The check stage would include a process to flag any orders that were not written properly, to educate the prescriber, and to track the incidents for trending. The act stage would be to review the incidents to determine what additional education needed to be provided, or if a few people were responsible for most errors, they may need to be reminded in a firmer manner of the change and the rationale behind the request. The cycle does not stop with one "trip" around the loop; it is continuous. The process must be monitored, because there are usually unforeseen problems, such as new employees who may not know the policies and procedures, or other unanticipated barriers to following the policies. As issues arise, improvements must be implemented and the continual nature of quality improvement will move forward.

The remainder of this chapter provides examples of how change projects were managed using the concepts and frameworks in the previous discussion. Although the PDCA cycle was used in development of the improvement projects in surgery described in the second set of examples, the PDCA cycle was applied retrospectively to the improvement projects in the first example in the pharmacy and the last example in implementing an outpatient antibiotic therapy program. In the first example, a pharmacist from the Veterans Affairs (VA) Health Care System describes how the VA system is working to decrease medication errors through three different projects that require systems and process change. A quality improvement nurse who works with surgical services wrote the second section. These examples focus on the complexity of change when many different disciplines and departments are involved. An internal medicine/infectious diseases (ID) physician who has been working with patients and care providers to move a traditional in-hospital procedure to the home environment wrote the final example. This section focuses on the benefits of the change, the challenges and how they were managed, and finally examples of data that support and exemplify the success of the project.

CREATING AND IMPLEMENTING SYSTEMS TO DECREASE MEDICATION ERRORS AT THE VETERANS ADMINISTRATION

The number of deaths from medical errors has been debated since the report *To Err is Human* was published in late 1999. Whether or not one believes the reported number of deaths, one cannot deny that errors happen, sometimes patients are harmed, and blaming a specific person for the error is not the answer. Although errors may be excusable, ignoring them is not (7). The cost of errors is estimated at $17 to $19 billion dollars per year with about half of the cost related to the management of adverse events (8). Systems of medication administration must improve to prevent medication-related errors from reaching the patient and causing harm. Medication errors have been a significant concern within the pharmacist community for many years, particularly in hospitals (9). The studies cited by the Institute of Medicine's (IOM) report *To Err is Human* are several years old, and, although improvement has been noted, there remains much to be done (7). Medication errors result in adverse events and bad outcomes that not only cause harm and distress to patients and their families but add an enormous and unnecessary cost to healthcare. Medication errors have significant implications to epidemiologists when medications are dispensed and administered improperly, resulting in prolonging disease or not curing disease.

In any system created to decrease the occurrence of errors or harm, it is important to balance the must keep some accountability while supporting a nonpunitive environment. Perfection, or decreasing to zero the number of errors, is a foolish goal (10). The true goal should be to decrease to zero the times that patients are harmed, by making these errors visible enough that they are corrected before reaching the patient (11). In many instances, decreasing errors and improving safety result from doing a lot of little things at the same time that in aggregate make a big difference. Methods for prioritizing these little things are needed. However, demanding that controlled trials be done before implementing changes, as in evidence-based medicine, is likely unrealistic and may be viewed as an excuse for inaction (12).

One of the controversies associated with medication error reporting is the temptation of comparing rates between institutions. The National Coordinating Council for Medication Error Reporting and Prevention (NCC MERP) believes that medication error rates should not be used to compare the quality of healthcare between organizations because these rates can be misleading, unless all the confounding variables such as patient's severity of illness and institutional culture regarding handling of medication error reports are taken into account (13). The goal of these reporting systems should be to continually improve the systems to prevent patient harm. The goal should not be to produce report cards for interinstitutional comparison.

Definitions

According to the IOM, an error is defined as the failure of a planned action to be completed as intended or the use of a wrong plan to achieve an aim. Errors can include problems in practice, products, procedures, and systems. One type of medical error is that related to medications. The reader is referred to Table 12.1 for the definitions of medication misadventure, adverse drug event (ADE), and adverse drug reaction (ADR) (14). Based on the definition of ADRs, allergic or idiosyncratic reactions to medications would be classified as ADRs, possibly as an ADE if injury resulted, but not necessarily as a medication error unless they were preventable (i.e., a patient with a known history of anaphylaxis to penicillin was given a cephalosporin). Some examples of medication errors are prescribing errors, omissions, wrong time, or improper dose error. The NCC MERP

TABLE 12.1. DEFINITIONS OF UNTOWARD OCCURRENCES RELATED TO THE ADMINISTRATION OF MEDICATIONS

- Medication misadventure: an iatrogenic hazard or incident
- Medication error: preventable event that may cause or lead to inappropriate medication use or patient harm
- Adverse drug event: injury from a medicine
- Adverse drug reaction: unexpected, unintended, undesired, or excessive response to a medication that requires discontinuation; requires changing of medication therapy; requires modifying dose; requires admission to a hospital; prolongs stay in a health care facility; requires supportive treatment; negatively impacts prognosis; significantly complicates diagnosis; or results in temporary or permanent harm, disability, or death

Adopted from American Society of Health-System Pharmacists. Suggested definitions and relationships among medication misadventures; medication errors, adverse drug event, and adverse drug reactions. Available at http://www.ashp.org/public/proad/mederror/draftdefin.html (cited May 22, 2002).

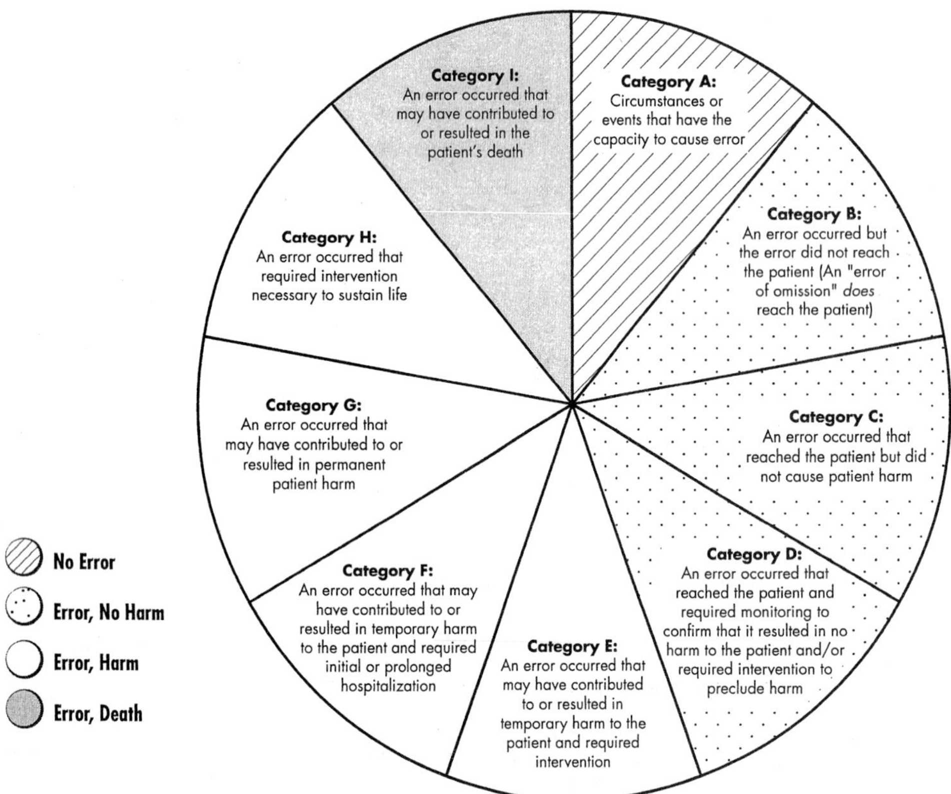
NCC MERP Index for Categorizing Medication Errors
Category I: An error occurred that may have contributed to or resulted in the patient's death
Category A: Circumstances or events that have the capacity to cause error
Category B: An error occurred but the error did not reach the patient (An "error of omission" does reach the patient)
Category C: An error occurred that reached the patient but did not cause patient harm
Category D: An error occurred that reached the patient and required monitoring to confirm that it resulted in no harm to the patient and/or required intervention to preclude harm
Category E: An error occurred that may have contributed to or resulted in temporary harm to the patient and required intervention
Category F: An error occurred that may have contributed to or resulted in temporary harm to the patient and required initial or prolonged hospitalization
Category G: An error occurred that may have contributed to or resulted in permanent patient harm
Category H: An error occurred that required intervention necessary to sustain life
No Error
Error, No Harm
Error, Harm
Error, Death
Definitions
Harm
Impairment of the physical, emotional, or psychological function or structure of the body and/or pain resulting therefrom.
Monitoring
To observe or record relevant physiological or psychological signs.
Intervention
May include change in therapy or active medical/surgical treatment.
Intervention Necessary to Sustain Life
Includes cardiovascular and respiratory support (e.g., CPR, defibrillation, intubation, etc.)
© 2001 National Coordinating Council for Medication Error Reporting and Prevention. All Rights Reserved.
* Permission is hereby granted to reproduce information contained herein provided that such reproduction shall not modify the text and shall include the copyright notice appearing on the pages from which it was copied.

Figure 12.1. Index for categorizing medication errors. (From American Society of Health-System Pharmacists. Suggested definitions and relationships among medication misadventures, medication errors, adverse drug events, and adverse drug reactions. Available at *http://www.ashp.org/public/proad/mederror/draftdefin.html* [cited May 22, 2002].) *http://www.nccmerp.org/010612_bw_index.pdf*

has created an algorithm and classification system for errors as depicted in Figs. 12.1 and 12.2 (15,16).

The United States Pharmacopoeia system receives reports from 184 hospitals (about 3% of the nation's hospitals) through its MedMARx program. In 2000 there were more than 41,000 errors reported (17). The top three types of reported medication errors continue to be omission errors, incorrect doses, and administration of the wrong drug (18). Three percent of the reported errors harmed patients, with less than 1% resulting in death. Thirty-one percent of errors did not reach the patient. Staffing issues accounted for 33% of the factors contributing to an error, and 40% reported more than one cause for error. Computer entry was fifth place in terms of the most frequently reported reason for the errors for 2000 compared with seventh place in 1999.

Medication Orders Via Computer

Historically, medicine has been practiced as a "cottage industry" in which providers have functioned independently and the improvements to the medication process have been slow and insufficient. The time has come for the medical industry, and specifically the medication process component of medicine, to be automated and brought up to a level of accuracy that is comparable to the banking industry, the freight industry, and/or the travel industry. In 1975 it was estimated that medication errors decreased by 82% with the implementation of the unit dose system (19) and by 55% when order entry was implemented in the 1980s (20). Both of these initiatives needed some level of automation. Mandates and pressure to change the way that the medical industry "does business" come from a multiple of opinion leading groups such as the IOM and Leapfrog. One common mandate from these groups has been that healthcare systems implement computerized prescriber order entry (CPOE) systems because it is estimated that 56% of errors occur during prescribing (21). One goal of the IOM is to have handwritten orders eliminated by 2010; meanwhile, one of the recommendations by the Leapfrog group is to have healthcare insurance contracts with institutions that use computer software to replace

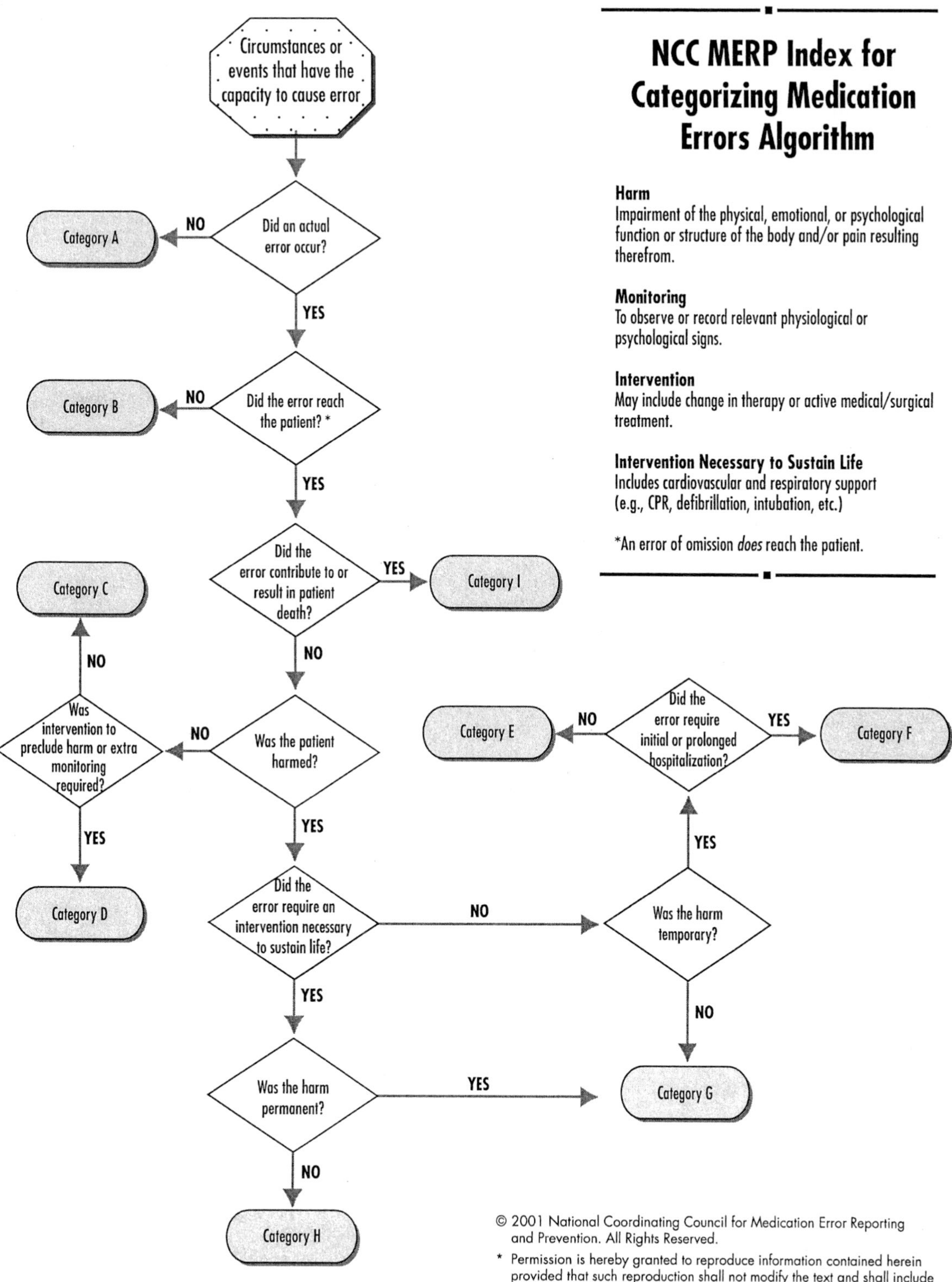

Circumstances or events that have the capacity to cause error
Did an actual error occur?
NO
Category A
YES
Did the error reach the patient? *
NO
Category B
YES
Did the error contribute to or result in patient death?
YES
Category I
NO
Was the patient harmed?
NO
Was intervention to preclude harm or extra monitoring required?
NO
Category C
YES
Category D
YES
Did the error require an intervention necessary to sustain life?
NO
Was the harm temporary?
YES
Did the error require initial or prolonged hospitalization?
NO
Category E
YES
Category F
NO
Category G
YES
Was the harm permanent?
YES
NO
Category H
NCC MERP Index for Categorizing Medication Errors Algorithm
Harm
Impairment of the physical, emotional, or psychological function or structure of the body and/or pain resulting therefrom.
Monitoring
To observe or record relevant physiological or psychological signs.
Intervention
May include change in therapy or active medical/surgical treatment.
Intervention Necessary to Sustain Life
Includes cardiovascular and respiratory support (e.g., CPR, defibrillation, intubation, etc.)
*An error of omission does reach the patient.
© 2001 National Coordinating Council for Medication Error Reporting and Prevention. All Rights Reserved.
* Permission is hereby granted to reproduce information contained herein provided that such reproduction shall not modify the text and shall include the copyright notice appearing on the pages from which it was copied.

Figure 12.2. Medication errors algorithm. (From The National Coordinating Council for Medication Error Reporting and Prevention. NCC MERP index for categorizing medication errors algorithm. Available at *http://www.nccmerp.org/010612_bw_algo.pdf* [cited Aug 30, 2002].)

paper-based ordering of drugs and medical tests. It is estimated that only 5% of hospitals have such a system (22). Although a tremendous challenge, the VA has been a leader in successfully implementing these computerized systems, by careful planning, execution, and evaluation. The reader is referred to Chapters 14, 15, and 16 for a general review of computerized systems. According to a survey by the American Society of Health-System Pharmacists (ASHP), of hospitals that have CPOE systems, only 13% have software programs in place to screen orders (23), and, in hospitals with fully implemented CPOE, more than 90% of orders continue to be handwritten (24). It appears that accepting only computer-entered orders is the only way to bring about change. The elimination of verbal or telephone orders except in emergencies will likely decrease errors resulting from misinterpretation of orders and other communication failures.

Transition to a computerized medical record is not easy. Even if it is a new facility, old habits are hard to break. Consistency is key to ensure that the providers will embrace the technology. In most cases, if providers have no other choice than to change, they will join the majority. At the West Palm Beach VA Medical Center, the Chief of Staff was very vocal about how he was able to adapt to a computerized medical record. It also helps credibility if administrators trying to convince providers to change their habits, "practice what they preach" and understand first hand the limitations and advantages of these systems. The impact of educational efforts may be weakened if what is required by the administration is not practiced by supervisors.

Systems must be well designed, but training and education of staff on the use of these systems is paramount for success with any patient safety initiative. Designing good computerized systems should be a clear goal, because using automation that has been poorly designed and tested will only make it easier and faster to achieve undesirable results. These highly automated systems must be understood by the humans who use them in order for the systems to be helpful. The computerized systems should enhance instead of restrict human performance. Automation appears to work well for repetitive tasks, and humans can spend their time with more complex tasks that require discernment, communication, cooperation, creativity, and flexibility (25). Humans are still needed to make complex decisions (11,26). These systems will avoid reliance on memory, recall, or vigilance. Similar to the aviation industry, policies must be in place about how to handle disagreements. Intimidation should not be the way unusual or problematic orders are handled. The old argument—"I am the physician and that is what I want"—should not be accepted in any setting as a reason to dispense and administer a potentially erroneous order. In the planning process it is wise to include as many users as possible so that their opinions and desires can be incorporated into the process. This nurtures the sense of "ownership" giving incentive to participate in the new process despite the unknowns and frustrations.

Recently, JCAHO decided to delete a standard that would have allowed CPOE orders to be processed and given to the patient without prospective pharmacist review (27). In some cases, as systems of CPOE are activated, some directors of pharmacy and our personal experience find that initially pharmacists may actually spend more time intervening to prevent errors. Sometimes this is due to unfamiliarity with the system and to lack of training. In some instances, pharmacists spend more time correcting orders because of provider's information and "alert" overload. For instance, if the systems are not designed and tested with the professionals who will be using them in mind, the software may be designed to alert about clinically insignificant drug interactions. Providers may become numb to the alerts and bypass ones that may be critical because of overload with insignificant alerts. Although CPOE eliminates the hassles of trying to decipher a prescriber's handwriting, it may create new problem orders resulting from typos; nonetheless, these would likely be easier to track because at least the name of the provider would be legible! One way to decrease problems with ignoring critical drug interactions is to force the prescriber to specify a reason to override the order; however, that alone should not be used by the pharmacist as a reason to dispense a medication without further review. In some cases, we have had physicians just enter several characters to bypass this alert. The technology is not advanced enough to recognize the randomly entered keys as nonsense. The availability of a clinical pharmacist specialist in care areas has been shown to decrease medication errors in the intensive care unit and other areas (28).

The implementation of a CPOE system, although daunting, can be somewhat simplified by looking at it through the PDCA framework, with an emphasis on barriers and incentives for implementing a system of such complexity. Planning for implementation of a CPOE system can be subdivided into smaller units. Some areas that must be considered are as follows:

- Breaking old habits
- Creating a culture that embraces automation
- Fear of the unknown
- Education plan
- Communication plan
- Identification and use of clinical champions
- Plan for skeptics and laggards
- Plan to include users in the planning stage
- Monitoring and evaluation plan

Implementation of the CPOE system took several years for the VA to complete. During this process different, albeit related, improvements to the medication prescribing process took place in our medical center. Three significant systems were (a) enhancing the continuity of care (specifically medication regimens) as the human immunodeficiency virus (HIV) patient population transitioned from inpatient to outpatient, (b) implementation of bar coding technology to enhance patient safety (verification), and (c) implementation of a clinical reminder system for specified patient populations. The remainder of this discussion reviews the implementation of each of these systems through the PDCA framework.

Continuity of Care for HIV Patients in Transition from Inpatient to Outpatient Status

Our planning stage consisted of reviewing our system and the literature. Theoretically it would be easier to process information if a patient is followed in the same institution for all of their healthcare needs; however, even with a computerized medical record shared between inpatient and outpatient providers, errors can still occur because of loss of information on transfer between settings (29). Although teamwork and the goal of seamless coordination of care are important, they may be difficult to achieve if the information is not shared equally within an institution. According to an ASHP survey, only 26% of health systems have integrated information systems, but integrated systems are very important. In some cases, different programs are used within the same hospital, making communication more difficult. A review of hospital discharges for patients from the HIV clinic in 1999 at the West Palm Beach VA revealed that an alarming percent were receiving incorrect doses or medications for treatment of HIV or related opportunistic infections. We learned that most of these admissions were not related to HIV and a consult to the ID service was not always done. To improve education of inpatient internal medicine providers, who are not versed in the treatment of HIV disease, the ID clinical pharmacy specialist was asked to follow patients admitted to the hospital if the ID service was not formally consulted to facilitate transfer between inpatient to outpatient and vice versa.

The do stage consisted of implementing a system whereby the pharmacist would receive an electronic-mail alert whenever an ID clinic patient is admitted to the hospital. When the pharmacist receives the e-mail, the patient is visited and their inpatient and outpatient medication regimens are reviewed and compared to previous outpatient clinic notes. Any discrepancies are reviewed with the attending physician and a "pharmacy admission progress note" is written to document any changes or recommendations. The information is then forwarded to the ID clinic staff. The check stage showed us that at least half of the recommendations provided were to avoid a potential medication error and the rest were to provide information to the inpatient provider. We were able to publish this experience (30).

The system continues at this time with a slight decrease in the number of interventions needed per patient. The act stage consists of ongoing evaluation, providing educational, and making changes as the need is presented.

The process has facilitated information sharing between the inpatient and outpatient setting. Our experience shows that even if a computer system and facilities are shared, miscommunication can still occur because of lack of familiarity with current protocols. The pharmacist serves also as a source for medication information and education for providers. For most patients, except for their primary care ID physician, the pharmacist was the professional most familiar with their history. A similar system using a summary note for the outpatient provider has also been described (31).

Implementation of Bar Coding Technology

Bar code medication administration (BCMA) systems have been suggested as a way to decrease medication errors related to the administration phase by adding another system check to the ones already performed by the pharmacist and the nurse. The BCMA system incorporates the "five rights" that the nursing profession is familiar with: right patient, right drug, right dose, right time, and right route. Nationally, the VA has reported a 75% decrease in the wrong medication being dispensed after implementation of BCMA (32). The baseline error rate was not known. At the West Palm Beach VA, beta testing of the BCMA system was started in 1999. One reason why some hospitals have been slow in incorporating the bar code technology is that manufacturers of unit dose medications are not required to print a bar code on each unit dose package. However, this may change with a proposed Food and Drug Administration rule (32). Unfortunately, the potential of this rule has resulted in manufacturers discontinuing production of unit dosage forms altogether. Smaller hospitals that do not have the equipment needed to repackage medications in bulk face problems with this change. Having to repackage medications also adds another step in the process at which errors can occur.

The planning stage for BCMA at our VA was poorly conducted and resulted in problems with the do stage. None of the most important personnel needed for the installation and training process (e.g., front-line nurses, pharmacists, and clinical informatics specialists) were included during the development phase of the system. The main emphasis was in meeting the deadline that had been set by the statewide VA network for implementation of the system by the spring of 1999.

On the first day of implementation of the BCMA system (the do stage), hundreds of e-mail messages were generated by the system every few minutes, as medications were one or two minutes "off schedule." The default was set so that an alert for a "missed dose" would be sent to all nurses and pharmacists on staff if the administration did not occur at the exact time listed in the computer. Fortunately the problem was quickly identified and fixed. However, it is very likely that if the system had been pilot tested by key personnel expected to use the system, the problem would have been corrected earlier. Because of inadequate training, it was not uncommon to initially find nurses bypassing the scanning of the patient's wristband bar code and entering the information by hand. Other VA medical centers have reported a similar problem when the BCMA system was installed at their facility (33).

After the timing of doses was adjusted and initial growing pains passed, the system was embraced by all professionals and for the most part has been used correctly. During the check stage it was discovered that some nurses were bypassing the system and so we acted (act stage) on this information by improving employee training and making it clear why it was so important not to bypass the system. We continue to improve and refine the process as problems arise.

Implementation of a Clinical Reminder System

Computerized systems can be used to improve the quality of patient care by creating reminders for preventive health initiatives such as vaccinations (34). These alerts can also be used to ensure that patients who are candidates for antibiotic prophylaxis before dental surgery receive the appropriate medication. Nationwide, the VA reports compliance of about 75% with adult vaccinations (35). We have also used the reminder systems to ensure monitoring of long-term therapy with amiodarone (i.e., thyroid function tests) and provision of antibiotic prophylaxis for HIV-positive patients according to their CD4 count. Table 12.2 has a list of the most commonly used computerized re-

TABLE 12.2. EXAMPLE OF COMPUTERIZED CLINICAL REMINDERS

- Adult vaccinations
  - Influenza during flu season
  - Pneumococcal for patients older than 65 years or with chronic conditions
  - Tetanus booster
- HIV
  - Prophylaxis against PCP for CD4 counts below 200
  - Prophylaxis against MAC for CD4 counts below 50
  - Glucose and lipid profiles before starting anti-retroviral therapy
- Diabetes
  - At least annual A1c testing
  - Annual eye examinations
  - Annual testing for microalbuminuria
- Medication-related
  - Evaluate liver enzymes every other month for first year of glitazone therapy
  - Evaluate serum creatinine for patients receiving metformin
  - Evaluate patients with CHF for use of ACE inhibitors

ACE, angiotensin-converting enzyme; CHF, congestive heart failure; HIV, human immunodeficiency virus; MAC, *Mycobacterium avium* complex; PCP, *Pneumocystis carinii* pneumonia.

minders in the VA system. Although the computer-generated alerts are useful, if the humans who receive the messages do not "process" them, improvement in quality indicators is unlikely. We have found that simplification of the processing of reminders is essential for compliance. Also, having a compliance officer who monitors the rates of addressing these reminders helps with improving the provision of preventive healthcare services.

The planning stage started with a goal of improving use of preventive health services because this process was selected as an important area to be reviewed at many VA medical centers across the country. The availability of a computerized system that allowed entry of previous vaccinations received, even if not given at the local VA, was a big asset to improve compliance with these recommendations. In addition, the system was simplified by permitting entry of the information with a single step instead of the multiple entries that were required in the past.

The program was tested and finally implemented (do stage) in 1997 at the West Palm Beach VA. The new system required entry of the patient's immunizations, whether current or past, in one step. In addition, a provider has the ability to document that the issue was addressed with the patient and that the patient declined vaccination. This allows for better tracking of providers who addressed this issue. At the West Palm Beach VA outpatient clinics, an increase in the pneumococcal vaccination rate was documented at more than 90%, well above the national average and most VA centers (35,36). To evaluate the efficacy of the project (check stage), individual feedback was provided to all the medical center staff. Almost all reports showed close to a 90% compliance rate with vaccinations for patients older than 65 years. Monitoring of these rates continues with feedback to clinicians on a quarterly basis. Information was acted on (act stage) to continue to improve the process, as needed.

As healthcare organizations move forward to automate and improve medication processes, it should become an expected norm that many different PDCA cycles will be occurring simultaneously. Every system should be continuously monitored and evaluated and the question of "how can we further improve the system?" should be asked continuously. As stated in the beginning of this discussion, change is the only certainty. The goal of the VA is to make certain that the changes enhance outcomes and not cause harm to patients.

EXPERIENCE IN THE OPERATING ROOM AND ANESTHESIA

The key elements of our anesthesia patient safety/quality improvement program at the University of Washington Medical Center are (a) a database, (b) a facilitator, (c) a weekly peer review meeting, and (d) a means for care providers to report issues. The program is driven by the care providers who report issues of concern. The facilitator (change agent) plays a key role in creating a culture for change. The facilitator collects the reports of concern and interviews the care providers with empathy. If the care provider wants to debrief or talk out a bad experience, the facilitator listens. If the facilitator senses that the care provider is embarrassed about the event, it is important to get the facts and leave the person alone. Being able to adapt to different styles and needs has the benefit of creating a supportive environment. The person who was embarrassed is well aware of his or her mistake and will most likely be more careful next time. The person who needed to talk the issue out had his or her needs met and learned from the experience. The key is to create a culture in which it is safe to discuss issues so that people can learn from each other.

Our peer review meeting provides a different format in which issues can be talked out and learning can take place. The result from all this talking about issues is that care providers learn, they are better able to teach others, and they are more willing or able to change their own practice.

Occasionally there is a care provider who has a history of poor performance and this is handled on an individual basis. For the most part, care providers inherently want to do the right thing, they want to learn, and they want support when there is patient harm, especially if they were directly involved in the care of the patient when the harm occurred.

Creating a System That Minimizes Opportunities for Error While Improving Teamwork and Communication

At one point, we discovered that our system for delivering blood to the operating rooms had many opportunities for error. In the old system, the nurse would page the hospital assistant and verbally request the blood. The hospital assistant would then pick up the blood and deliver it to the operating room. On one busy day, the wrong blood was brought into the room and hung by the anesthesiologist, who did not carefully verify that the blood paperwork matched the patient. Fortunately, the error was caught before the transfusion took place, but this was a very close near-miss and could have resulted in a sentinel event if the patient had been harmed. Rather than punishing the hospital assistant for bringing the blood to the wrong room or punishing the anesthesiologist for not checking the blood, the leadership decided to use this near-miss incident as an opportunity to change and improve the system. The event demanded that we immediately improve the process for obtaining, verifying, and administering blood products in the operating room. Our goal was to implement a change in the system that would prevent blood from being brought to the wrong patient's bedside. We then began to develop a culture that expressed "patient safety is everyone's business," which would be exemplified by better communication between care providers and improved teamwork. We chose to use the PDCA cycle as our model for the improvement process.

The planning stage started by convening a multidisciplinary team that included an operating room nurse, an anesthesiologist, a hospital assistant, the transfusion services nurse, and a quality improvement nurse who also functioned as the facilitator. Using the multidisciplinary team approach we were able to understand each member's perspective of how the work was currently being done, where the system was failing, and each member's unique insight into how the system and communications could be improved.

We learned from the nurse who was employed by the transfusion department that in other services there was a system in place that made it difficult to deliver the wrong blood to a patient. The system was simple. It consisted of the nurse handing the hospital assistant a stamped form that documented the patient's name and number and the blood products requested. This eliminated the need for the hospital assistant having to memorize the patient's name and the blood product requested. It also provided a written record of the request. Adoption of this simple process in surgical services could nearly eliminate the possibility of blood products being brought to the wrong patient's bedside. The other benefit of adopting this system would be that the process of distributing blood products to patients would be standardized throughout the entire medical center. The second part of the plan focused on building a culture of safety that would result in better teamwork and communication patterns. We choose to use education, team meetings, and individual conversations as the primary vehicles to improve and change the culture.

The do stage consisted of a presentation of the problem and proposed solution with ample time for discussion at staff meetings and e-mail reminders that described the new process. There were three separate staff meetings, one with the hospital assistants, one with the nursing staff, and one with the anesthesia staff. Ideally we should have had one large meeting, but because of schedules and tradition this was not possible. At these meetings, the members were told the story of the harm that was almost caused to a patient, which served as a compelling incentive to help the staff move through the internal transition process for adopting the new system. As a side note, the new process actually forced the change, because the laboratory technicians would not dispense blood products without the correct paper work. This made the systems change fairly easy for everyone to comply with. The challenge was a change of culture.

Through staff meetings and one-on-one conversations, we began discussing the imperative for careful communication and verification of blood products between two licensed healthcare providers. We also discussed some ways to tactfully remind each other how important it was to follow the policies and procedures when verifying and administering blood products. It is difficult to assess the level of compliance with some procedures such as ensuring that all the steps are taken to verify that blood products are correctly matched to the patient to be transfused. However, with the background knowledge of the harm that could be caused, there is more incentive for all members of the team to communicate better and to focus on complying with the policy and procedure. In conclusion, the do portion of this improvement project used a combination of forcing a change and nurturing a willingness and desire to change through knowledge of the potential serious consequences to the patient. Most people respond well to improved teamwork, because it generally makes work a more enjoyable experience.

The check stage is ongoing, because we continuously monitor the success of our improvement efforts through the anesthesia quality improvement system and transfusion support services. As issues or concerns are reported to the facilitator, education or reminders are sent out via e-mail to both the nurses and anesthesiologists. Because we are a teaching hospital and there is a significant rate of turnover, we must continually provide education and reminders to the staff about the policies and procedures and potential harms to patients that might occur if the policies and procedures are not followed. Care providers are encouraged to report any breech of the process, and it is made clear that such reporting is not for the purpose of assigning blame but rather for the purpose of discovering where there is lack of knowledge so that education can be provided.

When we identify gaps in the check phase, such as care providers failing to sign off on a transfusion record, we act (act stage) on that knowledge by sending out reminders to the care providers on how to follow the correct process. These reminders are brief, written in a friendly tone, and do not point the finger in any one direction. This process is cyclic and does not stop, because in our complex environment, there continues to be a need for education, tracking and trending, and then acting when problems are identified.

As new programs are introduced through transfusion services, such as the bloodless program for Jehovah Witness patients, we convened a multidisciplinary team to plan out a large change project but then proceed through the basic steps of the PDCA process that continues as long as the service is available. The most compelling incentives for healthcare workers to build a culture of safety are (a) leadership who responds to concerns, (b) a nonpunitive environment, and (c) a commitment to change systems and to provide information and education that promote internal and external changes in the behavior of care providers.

Understanding Roles and Creating a Supportive Culture for Change

A second example is an improvement project to decrease the incidence of surgical site infections (SSI) through appropriate preoperative antibiotic prophylaxis. Postoperative SSIs cause suffering and expense for the patients, payers, and healthcare organizations and are frequently avoidable if preventive techniques are instituted. The primary goal of this project was to improve the delivery of preoperative antibiotic prophylaxis.

As with most surgical services, we were aware that the timely delivery of preoperative antibiotics was inconsistent. We needed to implement an improvement project that provided a better system for ensuring that no patient's preoperative antibiotic was omitted. We needed to change the culture so that care providers saw this as a patient safety issue that demanded clear communication among the entire surgical team. When we began this project, it became clear that no one service had ownership of this task. However, because of the complexity of patient flow into the operating room, it became clear that everyone on the team needed to work together to ensure that all patients received appropriate preoperative antibiotic prophylaxis.

The planning stage started with identifying which processes worked, which did not, and where the gaps were. To improve delivery of preoperative antibiotics, the entire surgical team needed to be involved. The first step was to clarify everyone's roles: (a) the surgeon's job was to correctly write the order, noting any allergies that the patient might have; (b) the pharmacist's job was to verify the order, check against any allergies, and dispense the antibiotic up to an hour before surgery; (c) the presurgical nurse's or the anesthesiologist's job was to again verify the orders, check them against known allergies, and then administer the antibiotic approximately 30 minutes before incision time; and (d) the surgical nurse verified that the antibiotic was given and wrote this on the white board for the entire team to see. The white board is used to write counts, allergies, and special information about the patient that is visible to all the care providers involved in the case.

During our preliminary investigation, we discovered the considerable complexity of the process. Inpatients follow a different route into the operating room than do the outpatients and emergent patients take yet a different route. To add confusion to the variation, it was discovered that errors could include orders not written, orders not filled, resistance of anesthesiologists to give antibiotics with their induction drugs (which is valid), and resistance by some surgical nurses who did not feel it was their responsibility to "make sure the anesthesiologist gave the drug." The confusion and lack of ownership goes on and on.

It started to become clear that there was not going to be an easy systems solution and that the primary solution was to focus on the culture by making everyone in the system aware of the importance of preoperative antibiotics as a patient safety concern. It was necessary to clarify each person's role in the process and what to do when a problem was discovered.

Through education and a focus on a culture of patient safety, we were able to convince everyone that the timely delivery of preoperative antibiotics was everyone's business, because it affected patient safety. By improving communication and building in mandatory checkpoints, we were able to improve the administration of preoperative antibiotics.

The do stage involved providing education and then auditing a subset of the surgical population to verify that the antibiotics were given on time. We realized that we could force verification of preoperative antibiotic delivery if the surgical nurses had a mandatory field in their electronic operating record that required documentation of the administration of the preoperative antibiotic (or that it was not required). This would foster better communication between the anesthesiologist and nurse. We requested that surgical nurses write the time of the preoperative antibiotic administration on the white board in the operating room so that the surgeons, or any one for that matter, could quickly verify whether or not it had been administered. We also posted some fun posters such as one that has a picture of a red Ferrari and race flags and that says "Ladies and Gentlemen: start your antibiotics as you exit preoperative." This particular poster catches everyone's attention, because it is sort of a pun and so it sticks in people's minds and is effective.

The check stage involved requesting that nurses report any omissions and the reasons for the omissions, if known, so that the causes for the omissions could be discovered and addressed. This structure overlaps with the surgical peer review process. The surgeons monitor SSIs as one of their quality indicators. When a patient sustains an SSI, it is noted whether or not the preoperative antibiotic was given. This information is then brought forward to the facilitator for the project to be used to direct further improvement actions—the act stage. The PDCA process will become an ongoing process until there is evidence that most patients receive their preoperative antibiotics on time. Once this is accomplished, the system will continually be monitored for errors, the incidences of SSIs will be evaluated, and improvement action will be taken.

As better habits are formed the omission of preoperative antibiotics will become less frequent, and we will be able to move onto focusing on other factors that contribute to SSIs such as accidental placement of unsterile instruments on the sterile field, regulation of patient temperature during surgery, blood glucose levels, and proper oxygenation levels.

We plan to try continuously to identify the reasons for failure of timely delivery of antibiotics so that we can make changes to the system or provide knowledge and education to prevent future errors.

CHARTING NEW TERRITORY: IMPLEMENTATING AN OUTPATIENT INTRAVENOUS ANTIBIOTIC THERAPY PROGRAM

Outpatient parenteral antimicrobial therapy (OPAT) was a new and challenging method of treating serious infections a decade or more ago—with the potential for patient satisfaction and cost savings as well. In 1974, Rucker and Harrison (37) reported treating children with cystic fibrosis with outpatient rather than inpatient intravenous (IV) antibiotic therapy for recurrent bacterial infections. Twenty years ago in Canada and the United States, OPAT use was reported in adults, but there were concerns about its safety (38–41).

Because of this relatively novel and unexplored method of therapy, a group of ID specialists got together to form an organization called the OutPatient IntraVenous Infusion Therapy Association (OPIVITA). The objective was to share experiences, discuss mutual problems, improve patient care, and learn what the risks and benefits were for OPAT. We used the PDCA format as the framework for this complex and exciting project.

We identified several political and administrative issues among the various stakeholders that needed to be addressed before implementing an OPAT program. Some of the key concerns were (a) reimbursement for physician management would drop dramatically because charges could only be made when the patient was seen and examined in accordance with CPT coding rules. This reduced income from patient visits from seven to one or two per week; (b) some physicians were reluctant to treat patients with OPAT because they were not familiar with it; (c) payers were reluctant to pay for it because they were uncertain as to the charges and did not have established billing procedures, especially when OPAT was provided through a physician's office; (d) patients and nursing staff were not always comfortable with the idea of patients receiving IV infusion therapy at home, placing them outside the protected confines of the hospital; and (e) hospital administrators also became concerned that they might lose money through reduced bed occupancy if patients were not admitted or if they were discharged early.

The planning phase commenced with the OPIVITA members meeting to develop both clinical and business plans. We included stakeholders, who were also respected as opinion leaders, from the various groups so all interests would be represented at the table during the planning process. The clinical plan focused on the logistics of education and administration of the therapies and a monitoring plan; the business plan focused on both direct and indirect costs and cost versus benefit.

One significant concern, shared by all members, was development of a plan for monitoring patient safety and quality indicators. The group agreed that it was imperative to develop a database to track and trend information regarding patient safety and outcomes as part of the program. Because of the complexity of the project, we decided to contract with a commercial management service; thus, we interviewed several companies and found one that met our needs within budget.

We worked closely with the vendor to develop data sheets for the collection of the quality indicators that we were interested in. We wanted outcome indicators that were simple, practical, and reproducible. Examples of indicators we chose included (a) demographic data, (b) type of infection, (c) antimicrobial agent, (d) clinical outcomes, (e) bacterial cultures, (f) adverse events, (g) unplanned hospitalization, (h) death, (i) compliance issues, and (j) other.

It was imperative that we thought out the myriad of possible adverse event scenarios; to do this we used the failure mode and effects analyses process. This allowed us to identify potential adverse events and to make plans to avoid them. Through our shared experience, unique knowledge, and creative thinking, we worked diligently to ensure that no glaring safety factors were being overlooked.

As our plan developed, we were able to demonstrate to our payers, the insurance companies, who were initially very suspicious, that this method of therapy could potentially realize a cost savings of $500 per day or more compared to an inpatient method of treatment (42). The payers began to embrace our plan and even became champions of it with advertisements of this feature for their subscribers.

The focus of the project then turned to other matters such as how soon could patients be sent home on outpatient therapy, how much money could be saved, and where were the safety boundaries for offering this method of treatment. We continued to search for the limits within which we could ensure a safe environment for our patients and continued to seek and understand potential and unexpected problems.

Our do stage was met with excitement and anticipation, because we were charting new territory. We started with a small population who met strict requirements for acuity and personal history of compliance so that we would have success as we learned, trained, and developed our program. The check stage was rigorous and systematic, because we had outsourced this to a management firm. As issues were discovered, we moved swiftly into action (act stage) to address them, and, through discussion, education, change of policy, and a communication plan, we were able to take swift action to implement change. Our goal was to identify and learn from the near misses and potential failures before a critical event.

Clinical outcome was assessed by a doctor's report on the patient on the last day of OPAT therapy (43–45). The physician was simply asked whether the patient was improved, worse, or clinically the same on the last day of OPAT. The information comes from approximately 12,000 courses of OPAT entered into the registry (Fig. 12.3).

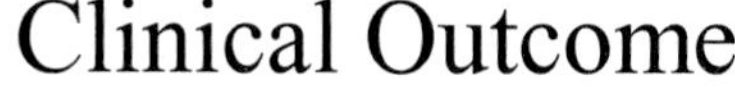

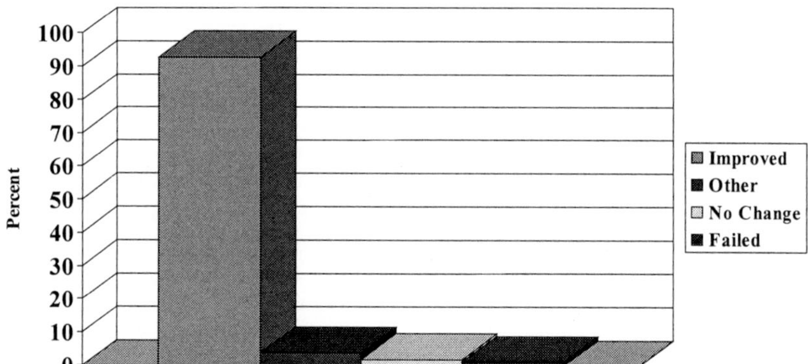

Figure 12.3. Clinical outcome for patients who received outpatient parenteral antimicrobial therapy (OPAT) for infections diseases.

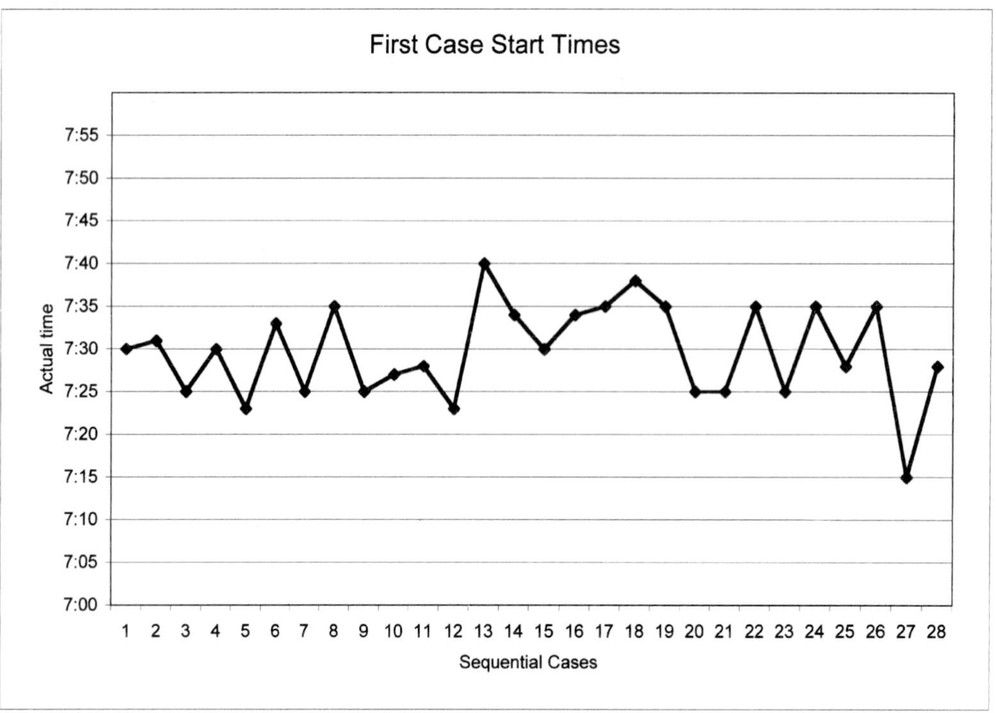

Figure 12.4. Microbial response to treatment of patients with outpatient parenteral antimicrobial therapy (OPAT).

The microbiology laboratories determined bacterial outcome. If an initial culture was done and identified a pathogen, it was possible to repeat the culture in some cases to see if the pathogen had been eradicated, had persisted, or was replaced with a new one. Repeat cultures were usually not obtained, presumably because the pathogen had been eliminated. Susceptibility panels were used in part to identify new strains of microorganisms (Fig. 12.4).

Adverse effects were also determined for each course of antibiotics administered. However, only the adverse effects that were severe enough to cause the OPAT antibiotic to be discontinued before the planned course of antimicrobial therapy ended were noted. If this occurred, the type of reaction was also indicated (Fig. 12.5).

The findings clearly demonstrate the effectiveness and safety of OPAT, and we had a pleasant serendipitous discovery. The data we collected was richer than we had anticipated, because it provided valuable information that not only documented the value of OPAT but gave us critical data to study diseases. Osteomyelitis, for example, is a frequent indication for OPAT. There are now more than 5,000 cases of bone infections entered into the registry. Of the pathogens recovered, 56% were due to *Staphylococcus aureus* with an increasing percentage of those resistant to methicillin over time. Twelve percent were due to coagulase-negative staphylococci, often with a foreign body in place. Six percent were caused by *Pseudomonas aeruginosa.* Failure rates by microorganism can be determined through the registry as well.

Data collected on 484 cases of osteomyelitis treated by our OPAT program demonstrated a higher rate of failure with the recovery of *P. aeruginosa* from cultures (15 %) than with *S. aureus* (4.5%). We were also able to demonstrate a higher rate of recurrence in 256 patients with *S. aureus* osteomyelitis treated with vancomycin (53%) compared with treatment with penicillinase-resistant penicillins (29%), cefazolin (35%), or ceftriaxone (29%) with a relative risk of failure of recurrence of 2.5 ($p < .04$).

In addition, the adverse effects can be tabulated and correlated with the antibiotic used. The analysis indicated that gentamicin and oxacillin were considerably more likely to cause an adverse event that would stop therapy (9% to 10%) than were cephalosporin antibiotics such as cefazolin (4%) and ceftriaxone (3%). The types of reactions to antibiotics also vary considerably; more than half of clindamycin reactions were due to rash, whereas the aminoglycosides were much more likely to produce nephrotoxicity and vestibular toxicity and rarely cause a rash (46).

An interactive program has been developed to help make decisions about the risks and benefits of specific antibiotic therapy in certain disease states that are commonly treated with OPAT. There is the potential to bring real-time data to the Internet, or possibly even a handheld device, so that the outcomes with different antibiotics can be assessed and displayed with automatic calculation of confidence intervals and statistical significance (47).

The OPAT Outcomes Registry has evolved out of the interest of a group of physicians who set out to document the effectiveness and safety of a new form of medical therapy. The success of OPAT is indicated by the estimate that more than 1 in 1,000 Americans receives OPAT every year. These physicians also took the information and applied it to learn more about infections

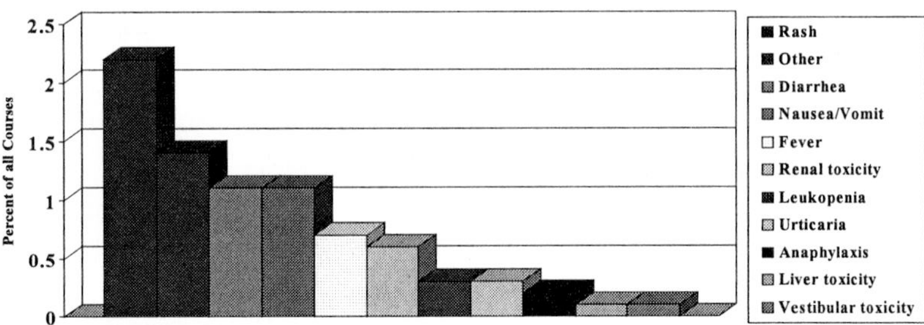

Figure 12.5. Adverse effects of antibiotics used to treat patients with outpatient parenteral antimicrobial therapy (OPAT) (10,844 courses of therapy).

and the potential adverse events with antimicrobial therapy. Whether this system can now be transformed into a means of ongoing monitoring of antimicrobials that reach market is unclear, but the need for postrelease information is growing and the need for timely assessment of outcomes is increasing, especially with the escalating problems with antimicrobial resistance.

SUMMARY AND FUTURE DIRECTION

When care providers are involved with the planning and implementation of change, there is a high probability that the attempt to bring about change will be successful. General and logical models such as the PDCA cycle of improvement provide teams with a natural framework to guide their change projects within. Healthcare is a complex and demanding field, and care providers at the "sharp end" are in the best position to identify the issues that are most apt to cause patient harm or to add unnecessary cost. By carefully listening to the voices of healthcare providers and using models, sustained changes can be made that will make a difference in our national fight against medical errors and inefficiency.

REFERENCES

1. Kohn LT, Corrigan JM, Donaldson MS, and Committee on Quality of Health Care in America (CQHCA) Institute of Medicine. *To err is human: building a safer health system.* Washington DC: National Academy Press, 2000.
2. Bridges W. *Managing transitions: making the most of change.* Reading, MA: Addison-Wesley, 1991.
3. Needleman J, Buerhaus P, Matke, S, et al. Nurse-staffing levels and the quality of care in hospitals. *N Engl J Med* 2002;346:1715–1722.
4. Rogers EM. *Diffusion of innovations,* 4th ed. New York: Free Press, 1995.
5. Sentinel event statistics. Joint Commission on Accreditation of Healthcare Organizations. Available at *http://www.jacho.org* (cited October 2002).
6. Smith DF. *Sedation, anesthesia and the JCAHO,* 2nd ed. Marblehead, MA: Opus Communications, 2001.
7. Leape LL. Institute of Medicine medical error figures are not exaggerated. *JAMA* 2000;284:95–97.
8. Valenti WM. Errors in medicine: problems and solutions for managed care. *AIDS Reader* 2000;10:647–651.
9. American Society of Hospital Pharmacists. ASHP guidelines on preventing medication errors in hospitals. *Am J Hosp Pharm* 1993;50: 305–314.
10. Pietro DA, Shyavitz LJ, Smith RA, et al. Detecting and reporting medical errors: why the dilemma? *BMJ* 2000;320:794–796.
11. Nolan TW. System changes to improve patient safety. *BMJ* 2000;320: 771–773.
12. Leape LL, Berwick DM, Bates DW. What practices will most improve safety? Evidence-based medicine meets patient safety. *JAMA* 2002;288: 501–507.
13. National Coordinating Council for Medication Error Reporting and Prevention. Statement from NCC MERP: use of medication error rates to compare health care organizations is of no value. [Cited 2002 July 16]. Available at *http://www.nccmerp.org/rec__020611.htm* (cited July 16, 2002).
14. American Society of Health-System Pharmacists. Suggested definitions and relationships among medication misadventures, medication errors, adverse drug events, and adverse drug reactions. Available at *http://www.ashp.org/public/proad/mederror/draftdefin.html* (cited May 22, 2002).
15. The National Coordinating Council for Medication Error Reporting and Prevention. NCC MERP index for categorizing medication errors [Cited 2002 August 30]. Available at *http://www.nccmerp.org/010612__bw__index.pdf* (cited Aug 30, 2002).
16. The National Coordinating Council for Medication Error Reporting and Prevention. NCC MERP index for categorizing medication errors algorithm. Available at *http://www.nccmerp.org/010612__bw__algo.pdf* (cited Aug 30, 2002).
17. United States Pharmacopeia. USP releases the MedMARx 2000 data report. Available at *http://www.onlinepressroom.net/uspharm/*(cited May 29, 2002).
18. Young D. More hospitals report medication errors, but USP finds few changes. *Am J Health Syst Pharm* 2002;59:1233.
19. Simborg DW, Derewicz HJ. A highly automated hospital medication system. *Ann Intern Med* 1975;83:342–346.
20. Bates DW, Leape LL, Cullen DH, et al. Effect of computerized physician order entry and a team intervention on prevention of serious medication errors. *JAMA* 1998;280:1311–1316.
21. Bates D, Cullen D, Laird N, et al. Incidence of adverse drug events and potential adverse drug events. *JAMA* 1995;274:29–34.
22. Brown D. The end of an error? Big business, launching a new era of reform, is pressuring hospitals to cut mistakes and costs [Cited 2002 March 28]. Available at *http://www.washingtonpost.com/wp-dyn/articles/A3955-2002Mar22.html* (cited Mar 28, 2002).
23. Cohen MR, Johns TE. Pharmacist's role expands in preventing medication errors. Mid-year clinical meeting report. 2001;30:6–7.

24. Ash JS, Gorman PN, Hersh WR. Physician order entry in US hospitals. *Proc AMIA* 1998;xx:235–239.
25. Crane VS. New perspectives on preventing medication errors and adverse drug events. *Am J Health Syst Pharm* 2000;57:690–697.
26. Bates DW. Using information technology to reduce rates of medication errors in hospitals. *BMJ* 2000;320:788–791.
27. Traynor K. JCAHO retreats on retrospective pharmacy review for CPOE system. *Am J Health Syst Pharm* 2002;59:1397–1402.
28. Leape LL, Cullen DJ, Dempsey Clapp M, et al. Pharmacist participation on physician rounds and adverse drug events in the intensive care unit. *JAMA* 1999;282:267–270.
29. Cook RI, Render M, Woods DW. Gaps in the continuity of care and progress in patient safety. *BMJ* 2000;320:791–794.
30. Segarra-Newnham M. Preventing medication errors with a "Pharmacy Admission Note" for HIV-positive patients. *Hosp Pharm* 2002;37: 34–37.
31. Geletko S, Small FJ, Piñón M. Using a pharmacist's progress-note form to manage HIV pharmacotherapy. *Am J Health Syst Pharm* 1999;56: 420–421.
32. Young D. Veterans Affairs bar-code-scanning system reduces medication errors. *Am J Health Syst Pharm* 2002;59:591–592.
33. Thompson C. FDA to develop rules for mandatory bar-code labels [Cited 2002 March 20]. Available at *http://www.ashp.org/pubnlic/news/ShowArticle.cfm?id+2745* (cited Mar 20, 2002).
34. Dexter PR, Perkins S, Overhage M, et al. A computerized reminder system to increase the use of preventive care for hospital patients. *N Engl J Med* 2001;345:965–970.
35. Butler ME. VA performance ranks high. *US Med* 2002;38(7):4.
36. Segarra-Newnham M. Utilizaton of a computerized reminder system to improve tracking of vaccination rates for HIV-positive patients. *Pharmacotherapy* 2002;22:412. Abstract
37. Rucker RW, Harrison GM. Outpatient intravenous medications in the management of cystic fibrosis. *Pediatrics* 1974;54:358–360.
38. Stiver HG, Telford GO, Mossey JM, et al. Intravenous antibiotic therapy at home. *Ann Intern Med* 1978;89:690–693.
39. Poretz DM, Eron LJ, Goldenberg RI, et al. Intravenous antibiotic therapy in an outpatient setting. *JAMA* 1982;248:336–339.
40. Rehm SJ, Weinstein AJ. Home intravenous antibiotic therapy: a team approach. *Ann Intern Med* 1983;99:388–392.
41. Tice AD. An office model of outpatient parenteral antibiotic therapy. *Rev Infect Dis* 1991;13(Suppl 2):S184–S188.
42. Tice AD. Pharmacoeconomic considerations in the ambulatory use of parenteral cephalosporins. *Drugs* 2000;59:29–35.
43. Tice AD. Documenting the value of OPAT: outcomes studies and patient registries. *Can J Infect Dis* 2000;10:45A–8A.
44. Nathwani D, Tice AD. Ambulatory antimicrobial use: the value of an outcomes registry. *J Antimicrob Chemother* 2002;49:149–154.
45. Tice AD, Hoaglund P, Shultz D. Risk factors and treatment outcomes in osteomyelitis. *J Antimicrob Chemother (in press).*
46. Tice AD, Seibold G, Martinelli LP. Adverse effects with intravenous antibiotics with OPAT. Presented at the 40th annual meeting of the IDSA, Chicago, October, 25, 2002.
47. Tice AD, Seibold GL, Martinelli LP, et al. Interactive, computer-assisted decision-making in antibiotic therapy. Presented at the 39th annual meeting of the IDSA, San Francisco, October, 2001.

13

SELECTING SUCCESSFUL HEALTH SYSTEM MANAGING APPROACHES

ULISES RUIZ
JOSÉ SIMÓN

This chapter examines the evolution of the concept of quality in healthcare, how the existing systems of healthcare fall short of what their quality should be, and what approaches are available for improving health systems operation. Integration of approaches for a comprehensive journey toward excellence is advocated.

THE QUALITY ISSUE IN HEALTHCARE

Traditionally, quality of healthcare was ensured by the technical knowledge of medical and nursing professionals who were expected to use it in the best interest of their patients. Consequently the authority to define and interpret the meaning of healthcare practice has been located solely within the healthcare professions where, for a long time, the know-how of other industrial and service sectors has been considered not applicable.

Historically, quality of care has been a major concern for leading healthcare givers. In the Hammurabi code (2000 B.C.) the physician causing the death of a wounded warrior would have the fingers of his hand amputated. The Hypocratic Oath (fourth century B.C.) established standards for medical ethics. In the Middle Ages, throughout Europe physicians and surgeons were organized into guilds and needed recognition to act as such. In the United States, authorization to practice medicine appeared in 1760, and the first medical association, the Medical College, was founded in 1787.

The American College of Surgeons and the Joint Commission on Accreditation of Healthcare Organizations

In the modern age, Nightingale's observations for normalization of care in military hospitals during the Croatian war in the 1860s led to the first attempt to improve hospital care. The Flexner report in 1910 established standards for medical education, and Codman, a surgeon at Massachusetts General Hospital, introduced the concept of "End Result Follow Up" in the early 1900s. The American College of Surgeons was founded in 1913, and translated Codman's concept into a minimum standard for surgical care and established a Hospital Standardization Program by 1917.

From the latter program, the Joint Commission on Accreditation of Hospitals came in to being in 1951. Now known as the Joint Commission on Accreditation of Healthcare Organizations (JCAHO), it revised, expanded, and updated the previously established American College of Surgeons standards of care in hospitals. These new standards related to physical structure, medical documentation, and interviews with healthcare professionals. Different levels of certification were delivered through a triennial external review, which has become a routine in most U.S. hospitals. In addition to external review, the JCAHO required a continuous internal review system through several internal committees. The so-called explicit and implicit reviewing approaches were used in the specific healthcare quality assurance (QA) approach. Explicit review meant reviewing according to written criteria, and implicit review meant following expert opinions with no reference to specific criteria.

In the 1960s, both Donabedian and Williamson introduced into healthcare, each one in their own way, approaches similar to those used in industry for product QA. Aware of these changes, the JCAHO changed its policy and its approach through the "Agenda for Change" in 1986, establishing criteria beyond the Donabedian framework and assessing the effects of healthcare on the customers.

The philosophical context of the Agenda for Change reflects the continual quality improvement approach and emphasizes (a) quality as a central priority: organization-wide devotion to quality, leadership involvement in promoting and improving quality; (b) customers: attention to customer needs, feedback from internal and external customers, customer-supplier dialog; (c) work processes: describing key clinical and managerial processes, systems approach, cross-disciplinary teams; (d) measurement: use of data, understanding variation, search for underlying causes; and (e) improvement: never-ending commitment to improvement.

The Agenda for Change had two major goals (1): (a) stimulation of healthcare organizations to create an environment focused on quality of care, whose governance, management, and clinical leaders are devoted to quality improvement and (b) development and implementation of a national performance measurement database that will help to stimulate continual improvement.

These key principles set forth by the JCAHO are similar to other sets of criteria such as the Malcolm Baldrige National Quality Award criteria and the National Committee for Quality Assurance criteria, which apply to an organization's efforts to achieve compliance with the standards and criteria of continual quality improvement.

Therefore, the JCAHO is looking for common traits in healthcare organizations that include the following: (a) strategic alignment, (b) integration of services, (c) data-based decision making, (d) current competence, and (e) continuous improvement.

In developing these traits the healthcare organizations must address the following key issues: (a) executive leadership, (b) focus on processes, (c) performance improvement, (d) patient care, (e) information management, and (f) environment.

It is noteworthy to mention that all of these key issues are a common rallying point in modern quality improvement approaches and are considered as such in the so-called excellence models [Baldrige and European Foundation for Quality Management (EFQM)] and more recently in the 2000 version of International Organization for Standardization (ISO) 9000. The JCAHO is applying the same key issues in its approach but differs in the methodology and tools applied to implement it as organizational criteria.

Thus, the reasoning behind the integration of the successful health systems managing approaches covered in this chapter is also valid for JCAHO beyond its specific healthcare criteria. These criteria are not considered in ISO or in the excellence models because the JCAHO criteria are specific for healthcare. As such, they should be the responsibility of their professional associations.

Other Approaches

In the 1960s, Donabedian (2) established a common denominator framework for both explicit and implicit inspection, defining structure, process, and outcome for care. In the early 1970s researchers started investigating the reasons for the large variation found in the process of healthcare delivery amongst the practitioners, the hospitals, and the geographical regions (3).

Also in the 1960s, Williamson introduced his health accounting approach. This approach is not well known and not recognized as a valid model for managing quality in healthcare. This approach is described in detail in Chapter 9.

More recently, using developed information systems, databases have been established in which individual professionals and healthcare organizations can search basic databases such as mortality of treated patients, resource utilization, and adherence to care protocols. Reaction of professionals to the availability of these databases has been mixed. Successful use of this kind of information system has been reported by Wennberg and Keller (4).

In the early 1980s a European Community (EC) Concerted Action Project on Health Services and "Avoidable Deaths" initiated research on a series of conditions for which mortality is considered largely avoidable given timely and appropriate medical intervention. Avoidable mortality was accepted by the European Commission and by many member countries as an important indicator of performance.

In 1988 the first edition of the *European Community Atlas of "Avoidable Death"* was published and described the avoidable mortality from 17 conditions in ten countries of the EC for the years 1974 to 1978. In its third edition published in 1997 it covers 12 EC countries; it describes avoidable death for the years 1985 to 1989 and shows time trends between this period and the previous second period from 1980 to 1984 covered by the second edition of the atlas (5).

HEALTH PROFESSIONALS, QUALITY OF CARE, AND ORGANIZATIONAL QUALITY

Responsibility for care and responsibility for running the organization should be clearly differentiated, as well as the dual role of physicians when they are both caregivers and administrators of their own clinical service as a unit of the whole organization. Thus, the traditional professional bureaucracy approach currently used by most hospitals in the developed world is shifting to focus on organizing rather than on organizational structures.

Today's healthcare centers and services are complex organizations where the work of each professional is part of a system that has to constantly be in perfect running condition, ensuring efficient, effective, and safe operation for the benefit and safety of the people who enter the system for care (6).

Healthcare professionals, both caregivers and administrators, have been confronted for a full two decades now with a most perplexing issue: the debate on how to improve the quality of the healthcare system without losing traditional roles and responsibilities (7–9), while facing an increasing recognition that healthcare providers have to respond to the preferences and values of the patients as their customers (10,11). As a result, two different perspectives for quality issues in healthcare, considered complementary, developed. First was the classical QA approach cherished by healthcare providers (12) and second the more recent approach of total quality management (TQM) imported from the industrial and service sectors (13,14). The organization's continuous quality improvement (CQI) trade off reconciles both approaches through participation and active commitment of both managers and caregivers in the search for quality (15,6).

The service perspective for healthcare systems as a nuclear concept for CQI has been the focus of extensive quality research studies for the past decade (16). Factors like customer satisfaction (17,18), return behavior (19), recommendations to others (20), choice behavior (21), and interactions with employees (22) have been considered when analyzing quality in healthcare systems.

In the health sector today, approaches like quality control (QC), QA, business process reengineering (BPR), CQI, and TQM and tools and techniques like ISO 9000:2000, Six Sigma, and Balanced Score Card (BSC) are complementary methodologies to achieve what is considered organizational excellence according to models like the Baldrige model in the United States, the EFQM model in Europe, and the Deming model in Japan.

Nowadays there is no doubt that the healthcare system's performance worldwide is unacceptably far from what it should be, and movement in that direction has been set forward by a controversial report from the Institute of Medicine (23). It has been recognized that ensuring the quality, safety, and social justice of the care provided to patient-customers is a requirement for both public and private health services, beyond the basic public health measures. Therefore, a new healthcare system has to be designed for the twenty-first century (24) recognizing criteria set forth in some of the oldest European public health services, which are also falling short of their expectations.

THE NEED TO IMPROVE THE HEALTHCARE SYSTEM

In the past, errors in medicine were considered the responsibility of caregivers rather than a design fault of the underlying system. The blame and punish approach to errors has been prevalent and still is considered valid in many healthcare systems, services, and organizations. Licenses are lost and health professionals are sued for error-induced injuries. However, only rarely are these so-called medical errors due uniquely to the carelessness or inappropriate conduct of the individual health professional.

For years, the scientific literature has shown the existence of so-called medical errors and how they can be prevented. A large study found that adverse events occurred in 3.7% of hospitalizations leading to death in 13.6%. More than half of these adverse events resulted from errors that could have been prevented (25, 26).

Basic considerations about errors in medicine, comparison of the aviation model to the medical model, and system changes to be implemented to follow the TQM approach can be found in Leape's (27) "Error in Medicine." The number of deaths associated with adverse events has been also quantified (28).

Consequently, the Institute of Medicine sponsored a National Roundtable on Healthcare Quality that stated among their conclusions that

> Serious and widespread problems exist throughout American medicine. These problems, which may be classified as underuse, overuse or misuse, occur in small and large communities alike, in all parts of the country, and with approximately equal frequency in managed care and fee-for-service systems of care. Very large numbers of Americans are harmed as a direct result. Current efforts to improve will not succeed unless we undertake a major, systematic effort to overhaul how to deliver healthcare services, educate and train clinicians, and assess and improve quality.

The findings were published in a lead article in the *Journal of the American Medical Association* (20). Other U.S. national groups published similar findings about the gaps in healthcare (29).

These findings about patient safety in U.S. medical care prompted the IOM to examine this issue through a Committee on Quality in Healthcare in America, which released its landmark report in November 1999 establishing for the first time the results of an in-depth study that names medical errors as the nation's leading cause of death and injury. The report indicates that medical errors kill more than 44,000 people in U.S. hospitals each year, which is more than from motor vehicle accidents (43,458), breast cancer (42,297), or AIDS (16,516). Total national costs of preventable adverse events are estimated between \$17 and \$29 billion (30). The report states in its conclusions that the current rates of injury from care are inherent properties of current system designs and that safer care will require new designs.

A second report of the Committee on Quality in Health Care in America, *Crossing the Quality Chasm. A New Health System for the 21st Century,* focuses on how the healthcare delivery system can be designed to innovate and improve care (24). This report endorses the purpose stated by the President Advisory Commission: "The purpose of the healthcare system is to reduce continually the burden of illness, injury and disability, and to improve the health status and function of the people of the United States."

The committee translated this statement of purpose into a set of six aims for improvement: (a) safety, (b) effectiveness, (c) patient centeredness, (d) timeliness, (e) efficiency, and (f) equity. However, in assessing the capacity of today's U.S. healthcare system to achieve these six aims the committee states that "in its current form, habits and environment, American health care is incapable of providing the public with the quality healthcare it expects and deserves."

Although no such studies are available from other countries, *The World Health Report 2000, Health Systems: Improving Performance* (31) analyzes the deficiencies of health systems around the world and when dealing with *The Potential to Improve* it states that "this report finds that many countries are falling short of their potential . . . [SC]. There are serious shortcomings in the performance of one or more functions in virtually all countries."

This may explain why all around the world the performance of healthcare systems is questioned and approaches to improve their design and performance are searched for outside the health sector. For the past two decades, the industrial and service sectors have been looking for new managing paradigms to improve their performance, and their methods and techniques are increasingly translated and used in the healthcare sector, although data are still somewhat scanty for scientifically assessing their effects.

OPTIONS FOR IMPROVING HEALTHCARE SYSTEMS

The concept of a quality management system in healthcare has emerged as a new paradigm in today's healthcare improvement arena where concepts such as quality of care, adverse events, cost of care, cost management, customer satisfaction, patient empowerment, or evidence-based practice define a new glossary for healthcare professionals to be familiar with. Thus, finding an acceptable methodology for measuring, assessing, and comparing organizational performance through valid standards and recognizing self-assessment and accreditation results is becoming a high priority in technically developed countries (32).

Although more data are still needed, the findings of a study on small and large hospitals in the United States reinforces anecdotal claims of the efficacy of quality management as a strategic orientation of the organization that affects the immediate and future performance and sustainable competitive advantage (33). Furthermore, the implementation of TQM in everyday practice requires availability of preexisting technologies, standards, procedures, and numerical representations to anchor the new customer-oriented focus culture that is counter to the traditional medicoscientific conception of the patient (34).

Therefore, it can be said that the successful implementation of this new quality management approach requires a conceptual break with the traditional interpretation of medical practice quality located solely within the medical profession. The TQM approach involves every single component and every single person of the healthcare organization. Everybody in the organization has a task, and all tasks can be considered to be a process; "process thinking" defines the new management paradigm.

Process Thinking

Regardless of what their end products or services are, the concept of *process* can be applied to each and everyone. A process is a unique combination of people, tools, methods, and materials that add value to an input to attain an output in goods and services.

Tasks (processes) link together to form systems that are aimed at achieving an end goal whose quality is prescribed in specified requirements and the goal of customer satisfaction. An individual task will have its own set of specified requirements that have to be satisfied. Every task can be broken down into the constituent elements that it needs or supplies.

The quality of task output depends as much on the quality of the inputs received at the workplace as it does on how well the task is actually performed or, as one might say, how well the process is system controlled. This basic fact has often been forgotten, and people have been blamed for results not within their control.

To function effectively and efficiently an organization has to identify and manage different linked activities, and, very often, the output from one process becomes the input to another one. The identification of processes, their interaction, and their control and the application of a system of processes within an organization is referred to as "the process approach."

Quality Management Systems

Process thinking is the nuclear concept for the so-called quality management systems. Quality management systems are the basis for a successful operation of an organization: they allow systems control and systematic management.

Once the quality management systems are operating, the organization is managed with the established requirements that are set by whatever managing approach the organization has chosen to follow. Traditionally, healthcare organizations in the United States and other English-speaking countries have used an operating model that focuses on the assessment approach. This approach was further evolved by the American College of Surgeons in 1917 and by the Joint Commission for Accreditation of Hospitals in 1954 (today's JCAHO). Similar approaches for local accreditation of healthcare organizations have evolved in Canada, Australia, and South Africa.

At present, healthcare organizations can follow several managing approaches and tools or methodologies that have been useful in industry and the service sectors and have shown their promise when applied in the healthcare sector: (a) ISO International Standard for Quality Management ISO 9000:2000, (b) Baldrige National Quality Program: Criteria for Performance Excellence, (c) EFQM Excellence Model, (d) Balanced Scorecard, and (e) Six Sigma.

Today there is a movement toward convergence of traditional approaches and managerial approaches for operating and assessing healthcare organizations. Their standardization and comparability within a country and among different countries is becoming a requirement for improving healthcare systems around the world. Political and commercial forces also favor this convergence (35). In this section, we consider ISO 9000:2000 and the North American and European Excellence Models.

ISO International Standard for Quality Management ISO 9000:2000

The ISO, established in the manufacturing and engineering industries after the World War II, is today a worldwide federation with members in 130 countries and more than 230,000 international certificates awarded. ISO has developed over 12,000 standards. The ISO 9000 series on QA released in 1987 and revised in 1994 and 2000 has been seen as the most applicable to healthcare (36). The revised ISO 9000:2000 series published in December 2000 has moved its focus from QA to quality managements systems in convergence with the excellence models (Fig.13.1).

The ISO 9000:2000 series comprises a harmonized pair of standards, 9001 and 9004, with the same approach, structure, and vocabulary. ISO 9001:2000 establishes the criteria for certifying quality management systems in organizations, and ISO 9004:2000 offers guidelines for process improvement, not for certification, once quality management systems are operative.

The ISO 9000:2000 series

> promotes the adoption of a process approach when developing, implementing and improving the effectiveness and efficiency of a quality management system to enhance interested party satisfaction by meeting interested party requirements (ISO 9001:2000, 0.2 process approach) (Fig. 13.1).

The ISO-International Workshop Agreement 1, for Healthcare

An *ISO 9004:2000 Guidelines for Process Improvement in Health Service Organizations* was published by ISO in September 2001 as the first ISO International Workshop Agreement (IWA 1) to be used in defining the fundamentals of the healthcare organization's quality system and improvement methodology not as a substitute for traditional accreditation (37). The proposal for these guidelines was made jointly to ISO by the Healthcare Division of the American Society for Quality (ASQ-HCD) and the Automotive Industry Action Group (AIAG) representing the "Big Three" automotive companies: Ford, Chrysler, and General Motors.

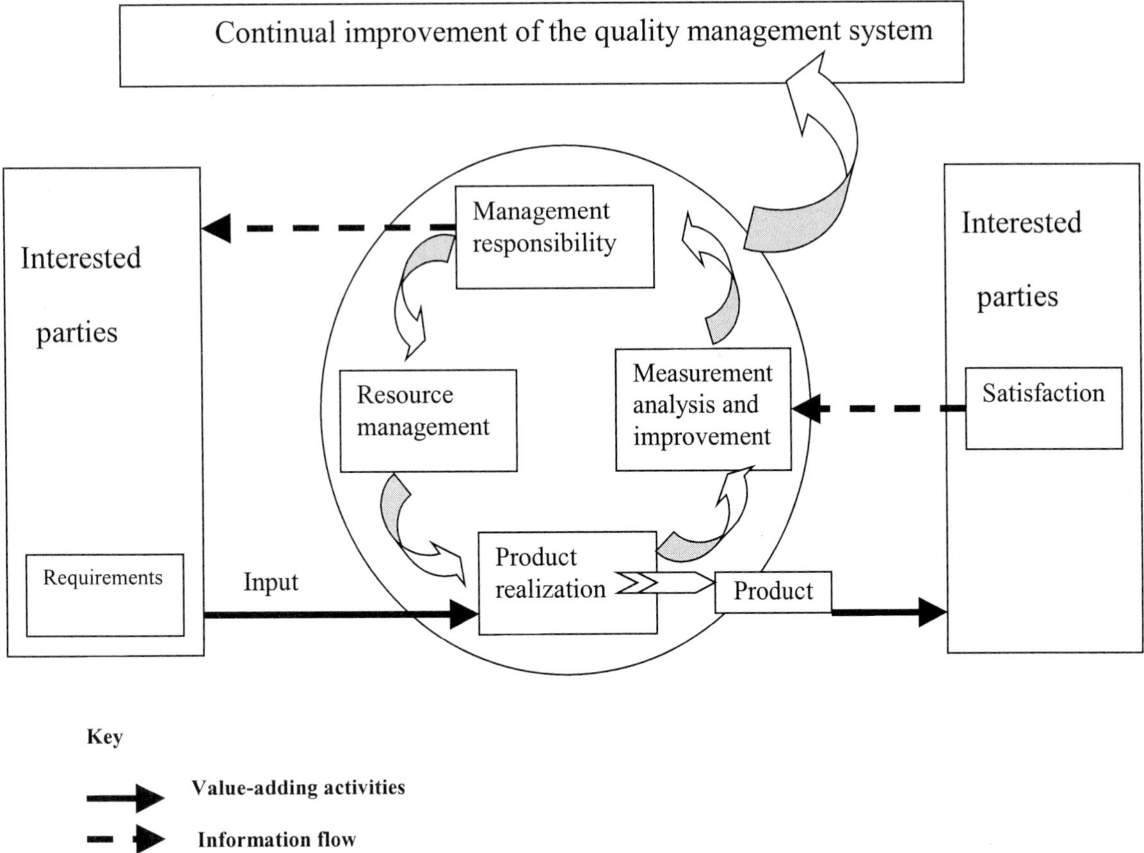

Figure 13.1. ISO 9000:2000 model.

The ASQ-HCD considered that the new series ISO 9000: 2000, published in 2000, were easily applicable to the health sector as a way to implement quality management systems in healthcare organizations and, therefore, to improve the overall quality of care. The "Big Three" deal with a large number of healthcare providers and spend large amounts of money on healthcare programs. They consider implementation of ISO by healthcare organizations a means of rationalizing the client-supplier relationship and improving the quality of care while reducing costs.

Both groups started their work independently and joined their efforts once they became aware of their common focus. An international workshop of health sector experts with 130 international attendees took place to discuss and modify the proposal that was published as an ISO document in September 2001.

IWA 1 addresses the systems deficiencies and the establishment of needed foundations for performance improvement in healthcare systems and organizations:

> The goal of this document is to aid in the development or improvement of a fundamental quality management system for health service organizations that provides for continuous improvement, emphasizing error prevention, the reduction of variation and organizational waste, e.g. non-value added activities. (IWA 1 Introduction)

These guidelines are not intended for use in third-party certification, although it could be used in the improvement of healthcare services through quality management systems in the health sector, themselves certifiable to ISO 9001:2000.

Baldrige National Quality Program: Criteria for Performance Excellence.

Created by the U.S. Congress in 1987, the Malcom Baldrige National Quality Award (MBNQA) criteria and processes are reviewed every 2 years and improved so that they remain relevant and reflect current thinking. The improvements made for the 1997 criteria are noteworthy. Improvements to the criteria's name, framework, wording, and rules have given them a new look, without changing their essence. Originally the booklet describing the criteria was called "Award Criteria"; it is now called "Criteria for Excellence."

> The Criteria are designed to help organizations use an aligned approach to organizational performance management that results in (MBNQA 2001): 1) delivery of ever improving value to customers, contributing to marketplace success; 2) improvement of overall organizational effectiveness and capabilities; and 3) organizational and personal learning.

The focus of the MBNQA is enhancing competitiveness. Its central purpose is educational—to encourage sharing of competitiveness learning and to "drive" this learning, creating and nationally evolving a body of knowledge. Its content reflects two key competitiveness thrusts: (a) delivery of ever-improving value

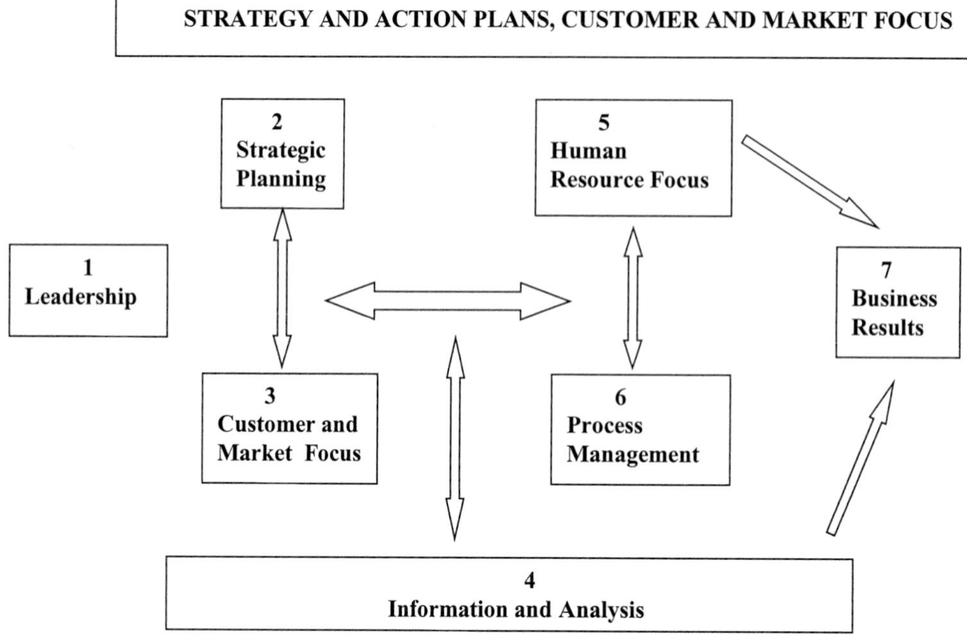

Figure 13.2. Malcom Baldrige Excellence Model.

to customers and (b) systematic improvement of company operational performance.

> The Criteria are built upon a set of interrelated Core values and Concepts. These values and concepts . . . [SC] are embedded beliefs and behaviours found in high-performing organizations. They are the foundation for integrating key business requirements within a results-oriented framework that creates a basis for action and feedback (39).

Overall, the MBNQA criteria provide an integrated, results-oriented framework for designing, implementing, and assessing a process for managing all operations (Fig. 13.2).

For almost a decade now, the healthcare community has been interested in applying the MBNQA criteria to healthcare. Its potential usefulness was advanced by Hertz et al. (39):

> A Baldrige Award program in healthcare could facilitate and accelerate the extension of the knowledge base of important concepts and results measures for quality management and improvement and could greatly enhance the sharing of successful strategies.

Since 1988, Baldrige Award Health Care Criteria have been available to healthcare organizations either for performance of a self-assessment as an internal improvement effort or as the basis for an award application. Self-assessment using all seven categories of the Health Care Criteria allows the organization to identify strengths and to target opportunities for improving its processes and results. Submitting an award application has other valuable benefits. Applicants receive a detailed feedback report based on an independent external assessment conducted by a panel of specially trained and recognized experts.

The constructs of the Baldrige Award Health Care Criteria framework have been examined to investigate whether quality management systems are related to organizational results and customer satisfaction in hospitals. Early experiences show that the Baldrige criteria can be used by healthcare organizations to conduct internal evaluations resulting in improvement of the organization's effectiveness (40,41). The Baldrige management framework was found to be useful for identification of areas of improvement and areas of achievement within a sample of VHA hospitals (42). Empirical evidence has been provided from 220 hospitals that the 19 dimensions of the Baldrige criteria lead hospitals to improvement on some dimensions of performance (43).

EFQM Excellence Model

EFQM was founded in 1988 by presidents of 14 major Europeans companies, with the endorsement of the European Union. At present, more than 600 organizations all over Europe are involved. The main aim is to promote quality management through the external assessment of an Award Scheme (the European Quality Award and national awards, inspired by the example of the Baldrige Award in the United States) and to establish a reference model that can be used for self-assessment (44).

The model conceptualizes organizations by discerning five enablers' dimensions and four results dimensions in an operative structure (Fig. 13.3). The enablers' dimensions ultimately lead organizations to excellence: excellence in customer satisfaction, employee satisfaction, impact on society, and key performance results. The European Excellence Model is used in healthcare organizations of different European countries (45–48).

Six Sigma

Six Sigma was pioneered at Motorola Corporation in the 1980s. Six Sigma is based on rigorous statistical process control.

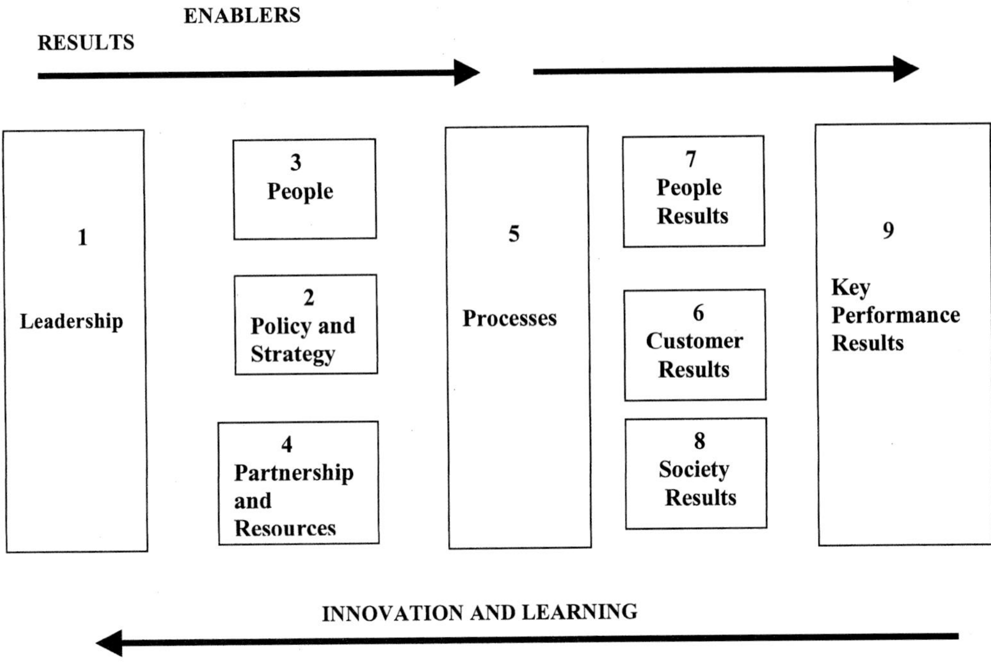

Figure 13.3. EFQM Excellence Model.

It augments the traditional quality tools with exacting statistical analysis and a systematic problem-solving approach, targeting the root causes of variations and redefining processes for long-term results. The Six Sigma methodology, is known as DMAIC:

1. Define
2. Measure
3. Analyze
4. Improve
5. Control

Six Sigma is increasingly used in healthcare as shown in the 2-day conference on "Six Sigma for Health Care Providers" in San Francisco in September 2001.

Balanced Score Card

The BSC is a framework proposed by Robert Kaplan and David Norton in 1992 to facilitate translation of strategy into action. It summarizes succinctly in a short document a set of leading and lagging performance indicators grouped into four different perspectives: financial, customer, internal processes, and learning and growth (Fig. 13.4).

The BSC and the Models of Excellence work together to bring added value to the company. The BSC is used in some healthcare institutions. A 2-day BSC conference was held on "Saving Lives, Saving Money and How Healthcare Organizations Use the Balanced Score Card to Achieve Results," in Cambridge, Massachusetts, in April 2002.

Integrated Approach

Self-assessment leading solely to certification or accreditation by an external organization should not be the only way to manage the collective knowledge gathered from this exercise. Self-assessment carried out as a regular and systematic review of organizational processes allows an organization to identify its strengths and areas that need improvement. It offers everybody in the organization an opportunity to learn from the outcomes of their improvement activities and collective wisdom ensues.

CQI through self-assessment requires defined process control within an established processes system resulting from the implementation of recognized standards and criteria. Most healthcare organizations are typical professional organizations in which the professionals establish their rules for managing the whole organization and do not allow changes that might diminish their decision power. The healthcare organizational structure requires nuclear changes so that accepted modern managerial approaches to excellence can be successfully applied.

The new International Standard ISO 9000:2000 offers an approach for establishing a system of controlled processes that offers linkage between the individual processes within the system of processes, as well as their combination and interaction. Integration of ISO 9000, traditional accreditation, and Excellence Models together with Six Sigma and BSC offer a logical journey toward excellence.

The journey starts with ISO 9000 as a foundation for the organization's quality management system, allowing traditional accreditation assessment for specific clinical standards. The Excellence Models can then be aimed at, together with tools like Six Sigma for specific improvement projects and BSC, establishing the strategic perspective of the organization. This is at present an acceptable approach toward excellence in the health sector. Integration of the different approaches at different levels and through progressive steps allows a smooth journey toward excellence of the organization (49).

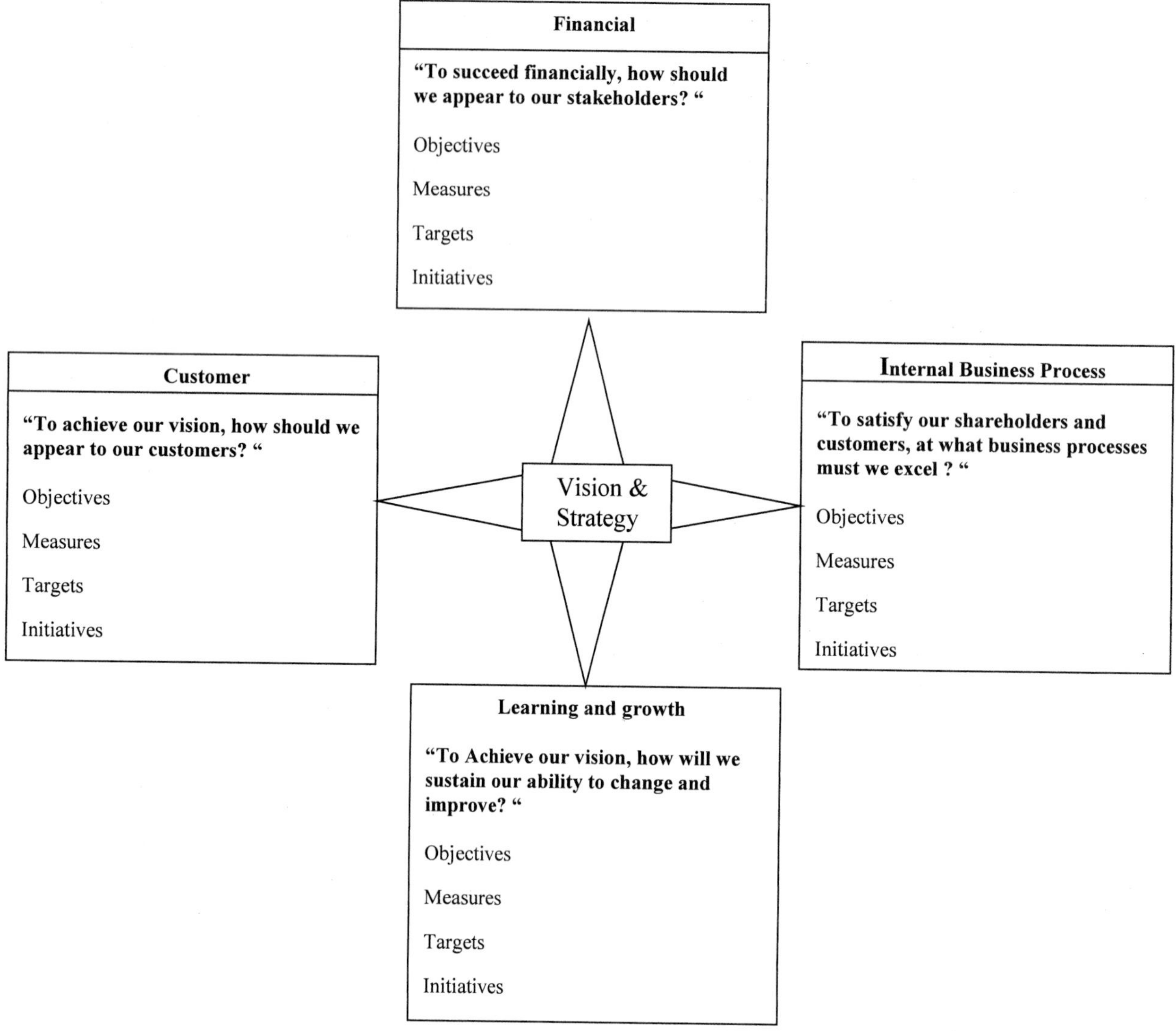

Figure 13.4. Balanced Scorecard framework.

CONCLUSIONS

1. In general, all over the world, the performance of healthcare systems falls short of acceptable standards. A WHO report in the year 2000 on the world health systems states that many countries are falling short of their potential and that there are serious shortcomings in the performance of one or more functions in virtually all countries.
2. These shortcomings are not related to the economic health of the country nor to its expenditure in healthcare. The United States is the country with the highest percentage of its Gross National Product expended in healthcare in the world. In 1999 an IOM report states that " . . . [SC]serious and widespread problems exist throughout American Medicine . . . [SC]Current efforts to improve will not succeed unless we undertake a major, systematic effort to overhaul how to deliver healthcare services, educate and train clinicians, and assess and improve quality."
3. To improve the quality, approaches used in other sectors such as the service sector and the industrial sector can be applied to the healthcare sector, where the concept of quality management systems has emerged as a new paradigm for managing healthcare systems and organizations.
4. Process thinking is the nuclear concept for quality management systems and is the focus of most of the recognized approaches to quality improvement.
5. All of those approaches are aimed at continuously improving the organization and can be integrated in a stepwise journey in pursuit of excellence.

REFERENCES

1. Joint Commission on Accreditation of Healthcare Organizations. *Overview of the Joint Commission's "Agenda for Change."* Joint Commission document. August 1987.

2. Donabedian A. Evaluating the quality of medical care. *Milbank Mem Fund Q* 1966;44:166–206.
3. Wennberg JE, Gittelson A. Small area variations in healthcare delivery. *Science* 1973;1823:1102–1108.
4. Wennberg JE, Keller R. Regional professional foundations. *Health Aff* 1994;13:257–263.
5. Holland WW et al. *European Community atlas of "avoidable death" 1985–89.* Oxford, UK: CEC Health Services Series, Oxford University Press, 1997.
6. Moss F, Garside P, Dawson S. Organisational change: the key to quality improvement. *Qual Health Care* 1998;7:S1–S2.
7. Coile RC Jr. *THE NEW MEDICINE. Reshaping medical practice and health care management.* Rockville, MD: Aspen Publishers, 1990.
8. Graham NO. Quality assurance in hospitals. Strategies for assessment and implementation, 2nd ed. Aspen Publishers, Inc., Rockville, Ma: USA, 1990.
9. Jessee WF. *Identifying health care quality problems: a practical manual for PSROs and hospitals.* HPAA Monograph, *University of North Carolina*, 1982.
10. Hughes EFX. *Perspectives on quality in American health care.* Washington DC: McGraw-Hill, 1988.
11. McLaughlin CP. *Continuous quality improvement in health care. Theory, implementation, and applications.* Rockville, MD: Aspen Publishers, 1994.
12. Vouri HV. *Quality assurance of health services,* Copenhagen, Denmark: Public Health in Europe n° 16 Regional Office for Europe, World Health Organization, 1982.
13. Arndt M, Bigelow B. The implementation of total quality management in hospitals: How good is the fit?. *Health Care Manage Rev* 1995;20: 7–14.
14. Bigelow B, Arndt M. Total quality management: field of dreams? *Health Care Manage Rev* 1995;20:15–25.
15. Blumenthal D, Epstein AM. The Role of Physicians in the Future of Quality Management-Part six of six. *N. Engl J Med* 1996;335: 1328–1332
16. Bebko CP. Consumer factors affecting the delivery of quality health services. *Health Mark Q* 1993;11:19–41.
17. Gombeski WR, et al. Patient callback program: a quality improvement, customer service, and marketing tool. *J Health Care Mark* 1993;13: 60–65.
18. Peyrot M, et al. Consumer satisfaction and perceived quality of outpatient health services. *J Health Care Mark* 1993;13:24–33.
19. John J. Patient satisfaction: the impact of past experience. *J Health Care Mark* 1992;12:56–62.
20. Reference deleted in proofs.
21. Richard MD, Allaway AW. Service quality attributes and choice behaviour. *J Serv Mark* 1993;7:59–68.
22. John J. Improving quality through patient-provider information. *J Health Care Mark* 1991;11:51–60.
23. Kohn L, Corrigan J, Donaldson M, eds. *To err is human: building a safer health system.* Washington DC: National Academy Press, 1999
24. Institute of Medicine. *Crossing the quality chasm: a new health system for the twenty-first century.* Washington DC: National Academy Press, 2001.
25. Brennan TA, Leape LL, Laird NM, et al. Incidence of adverse events and negligence in hospitalized patients: results of the Harvard Medical Practice Study, I. *N Engl J Med* 1991;324:370–376.
26. Leape LL, Brennan TA, Laird NM, et al. The nature of adverse events in hospitalized patients: results of the Harvard Medical Practice Study II. *N Engl J Med* 1991;324:377–384.
27. Leape LL. Error in medicine. *JAMA* 1994;272:1851–1857.
28. Garcia-Martin M et al: Proportion of hospital deaths associated with adverse events. *J Clin Epidemiol* 1997;50:1319–1326. 29. Advisory Commission on Consumer Protection and Quality in the Health Care Industry. *Quality first: better health care for all Americans; final report to the President of the United States.* Washington DC: US Government Printing Office, 1998.
30. Institute of Medicine. *To err is human: building a safer health system.* Washington DC: National Academy Press, 1999.
31. World Health Organization. *The world health report 2000: health systems: improving performance.* 2000. Who, Geneva, Ch.
32. Sanders NR. Health care organisations can learn from the experiences of others. *Qual Prog* 1997;(*Feb*):47–49.
33. Rapert MI, Wren BM. Service quality as a competitive opportunity. *J Serv Mark* 1998;12:223–235.
34. Hansson J. Quality in health care. Medical or managerial? *J Manage Med* 2000;14:357–361.
35. Schyve PM. The evolution of external quality evaluation: observations from the Joint Commission of Accreditation of Healthcare Organizations. *Int J Qual Health Care* 2000;12:255–258.
36. Sweeney J, Heaton C. Interpretations and variations of ISO 9000 in acute health care. *Int J Qual Health Care* 2000;12:203–209.
37. ISO. *IWA 1, quality management systems-guidelines for process improvements in health service organizations.* Available at *www.iso.ch* (accessed 12-01-03).
38. Baldrige National Quality Program. *Criteria for performance excellence.* Available at *www.quality.nist.gov* (accessed 12-01-03).
39. Hertz HS, Reimann CW, Bostwick MC. The Malcom Baldrige National Quality Award concept: could it help stimulate or accelerate health care quality improvement? *Qual Manage Health Care* 1994;2: 63–72.
40. Gaucher E, Kratochwill E. The Malcom Baldrige National Quality Award: implications and uses for healthcare organizations. *Infect Control Hosp Epidemiol* 1995;16:302–307.
41. Jensen LA. Improving health care quality. Application of the Baldrige process. J Nurs Adm 1996;26:51–54.
42. Weeks WB, Hamby L, Batalden PB. Using the Baldrige management system framework in health care: the Veterans Health Administration experience. *Jt Comm J Qual Improv* 2000;26:379–387.
43. Goldstein SM, Schweikhart SB. Empirical support for the Baldrige Award framework in U.S. hospitals. *Health Care Manage Rev* 2002; 27:62–75.
44. European Foundation for Quality Management. *The EFQM Excellence Model 1999.* Available at *www.efqm.org* (accessed 12-01-03).
45. Arcelay A, Sánchez E, Hernández L, et al. Self-assessment of all the health centres of a public health service through the European model of total quality management. *Int J Health Care Qual Assurance* 1999; 12:54–58.
46. Breinlinger-O'Reilly J, Elser J, Möller J. Quality management in German health care—the EFQM Excellence Model. *Int J Health Care Qual Assurance* 2000;6:254–258.
47. Jackson S. Exploring the suitability of the European Foundation for Quality Management (EFQM) Excellence Model as a framework for delivering clinical governance in the UK National Health Service. *Qual Assurance J* 2001;5:19–31.
48. Nabitz U, Klazinga N, Walburg J. The EFQM Excellence Model: European and Dutch experiences with the EFQM approach in health care. *Int J Qual Health Care* 2000;12:191–201.
49. Ruiz U, Simón J, Molina P, Jimenez J, et al. A two level integrated approach to self-assessment in health care organizations. *Int J of Health Care Qual Assurance* 1999;12;4:135–142.

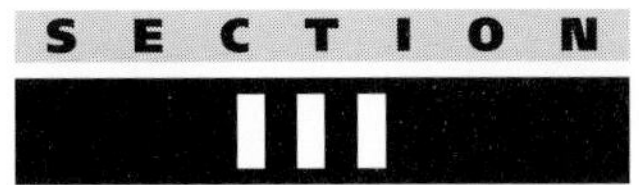

INFORMATICS IN HEALTHCARE EPIDEMIOLOGY

14

COMPUTER FUNDAMENTALS FOR HEALTHCARE EPIDEMIOLOGY

JOHN A. SELLICK, JR.

This is the information age; thus, the effective and widespread use of computers in hospital epidemiology and infection control is not only desirable but also necessary. This chapter discusses computer systems, networks, and the Internet from a high-level perspective. Because of space limitations, it is not possible to discuss each computer system, software package, network configuration, or troubleshooting program or to refer to specific products. Instead, this chapter provides a conceptual framework for discussing information services in an academic institution, hospital, or other healthcare organization. The electronic patient record, information management, and statistical analysis of data are discussed in other chapters and are not discussed here (see Chapters 3, 15, and 16).

COMPUTER SYSTEMS AND NETWORKS

Historical Perspective

The Era of the Mainframe

Historically, electronic data processing in large organizations, including hospitals, has been done on mainframe computer systems. (Minicomputers, now called midrange servers, are smaller siblings of the mainframe and are widely used in this setting as well.) These large computers were developed to support the fiscal and demographic data needs of institutions and became known as management information systems (MISs). However, they have matured to include clinical components such as laboratory information systems and order entry, which make important patient data more readily available to care providers. Data management systems for infection control and surgical demographics also are available. Data input generally is from a keyboard terminal, although optical scanning of standardized data sheets also can be used. Printing often is done at central, high-speed printers, but distributed network printers may be used as well.

Mainframe computers are monolithic not only in physical structure but also in function as well. The software operating systems (OSs) and applications software typically are cryptic and complicated, requiring extensive expertise and time for setup and maintenance. Access for end users usually is through a hardwired (directly connected) dumb terminal, essentially a cathode ray tube monitor with an attached keyboard and, sometimes, a light pen. [A personal computer (PC) with appropriate terminal emulation software as described later can function similarly.] User interaction is restricted to a set of defined keyboard commands and functions, often in the setting of predesigned menus or screens. Partially customizable infection control data management software is available in some clinical or laboratory information system software packages.

Attempts have been made to develop customized mainframe infection control software to capture relevant demographic and clinical data and then to merge them with surveillance data collected and entered for individual nosocomial events (1,2). Standard reporting templates allowed the production of a wide variety of summary reports at set intervals, and provisions were made for the retrieval of data via ad hoc queries when the standard reports were insufficient (3). These custom-developed mainframe infection control data management systems typically were developed through cooperative efforts between infection control and the information services departments of a few larger hospitals. They were usually computer OS specific and thus difficult to adapt to other institutions with different computing configurations. Their high development (1) and maintenance costs and their lack of adaptability to other computing environments have made them impractical.

The Rise of Personal Computers

In the 1970s and 1980s, desktop microcomputers, often called PCs, were developed by Apple Computer, Inc. (Cupertino, CA) and International Business Machines Corp. (Armonk, NY). They have become so ubiquitous that most people associate the term *computer* with desktop microcomputers. The terms *personal computer, desktop computer,* and *microcomputer* all describe the same machine and can be used interchangeably. These user-friendly machines sport a graphical user interface (GUI) and a control device such as a mouse or trackpad along with the ability to connect to a network and local printer. External input devices such as scanners and bar-code readers are inexpensive and easily attached, as are removable media (disk, cartridge, or tape) storage and backup devices. The standards for such connections are set by the Information Technology Working Group of the Institute of Electrical and Electronics Engineers (IEEE) and often are referred to by number.

Desktop computer hardware and software tools allow for a

large measure of autonomy in developing and maintaining data management systems independent of the hospital's information system. As a result, they have significantly altered the practice of surveillance, data management, and data analysis in healthcare epidemiology. Both specific infection control software programs and generic database management programs are available to develop customized infection control databases. Word processing, statistical analysis, charting, communications, and presentation programs fulfill the remaining needs for most healthcare epidemiology and infection control providers. Terminal emulation software, which often is included in communications software packages, may allow access to mainframe computers via telephone modem. This provides a convenient means of accessing data or electronic mail from outside of the hospital or other facility. Specific log-in procedures, often in addition to password protection, are necessary to protect the integrity of the server and its data.

Unfortunately, the learning curve for computers and software may be steep, and even software designed specifically for infection control may be difficult to use (4,5). Data often must be manually entered, which is time-consuming and leads to errors. Moreover, the distributed nature of personal computing has resulted in both duplicative and fragmented data sets throughout organizations. Similarly, the keepers of individual databases may be unwilling to share data with others and may not take the necessary steps to ensure the integrity and safety of their data.

The Advent of Client/Server Computing

The desire for both the flexibility of a microcomputer and access to the data archives and computing power of a mainframe computer system has led to the development of client/server computing. In this system, the desktop computer is a client that can connect to a host midrange server or mainframe via a network. A network is a series of hardware devices and wiring that connect any number of client or server computers, printers, storage devices, and so forth. The network also requires its own software or protocol in order for the various devices to communicate and function with one another. Ethernet is the commonest network hardware specification and communications protocol for local area networks (LANs) in use today. There are a variety of network operating system (NOS) software products available to control the services (e.g., access to files and printers) provided by the LAN.

A server may simply store files, deliver messages, or queue print jobs, or, in the true sense of client/server computing, it may be a mainframe or midrange server that provides for interaction and shared computing capability between the client and server. The potential benefits for healthcare epidemiology and infection control services of having a computer attached to an information-laden mainframe or midrange server on a LAN are readily apparent. With proper client software, the organization's demographic, clinical, laboratory, and financial databases can be searched, data analyzed, and items of interest moved to the client computer for further use or analysis. Simpler tasks such as providing backup copies of files or sharing documents and mail with other clients on the network can be accomplished with simpler file or mail servers.

The appeal and potential benefits for client/server networks is considerable but so are the potential problems of implementation. The databases on large servers generally are built using proprietary systems that require additional software and training for appropriate use. Intermediary programs, collectively called middleware, may be needed to create an interface between the client and database to extract the information desired by the healthcare epidemiology service. However, if this can be accomplished, the rewards can be great once the desired data are identified, collected, and analyzed.

Recommendations for Personal Computer Systems

It is not possible to recommend a "one size fits all" approach to computerizing a healthcare epidemiology or infection control service. As with purchasing a motor vehicle, each service must evaluate its hardware and software needs in terms of the program objectives and prerequisites of team members. Most universities and other large organizations are moving or have moved to a client/server model of computing, making it feasible for healthcare epidemiology team members to have desktop computers that may fill several roles and satisfy multiple needs. However, an appropriate mainframe-based information system software package may provide the necessary support and functions, so this option should be investigated. If a PC solution is chosen, the selection of hardware and software should take into consideration the requirements of connecting to a LAN and accessing a mainframe or other server. Consultation with the appropriate university, hospital, or other organization's information service (IS) department can provide guidance in these areas.

Hardware

If choosing a PC, the first decision to be made is whether to purchase a desktop/mini-tower or a laptop. The former traditionally have offered the potential of greater power and expandability; however, current laptop models have more than adequate power for almost all healthcare epidemiology functions. Likewise, the availability of USB (*http://www.usb.org*), IEEE 1394 (*http://www.firewire.org/firewire*), and Cardbus ports make laptops widely expandable as well. Laptops typically come with active matrix [thin film transistor (TFT)] liquid crystal diode (LCD) displays, but a display is a separate item for desktop units. High-quality cathode ray tube (CRT) monitors are available at low cost, but free-standing TFT displays also have decreased in price although they still are more expensive than CRTs for equivalent sizes. TFT displays offer superior, flicker-free viewing; take up considerably less desk space; and produce less heat than conventional CRT monitors. The ultimate decision regarding the choice of desktop versus laptop often will be a financial one, but the issues of ergonomics and security of the equipment also must be considered.

Regardless of whether a desktop or laptop unit is chosen, it is important that it have adequate random access memory (RAM) for anticipated tasks, an adequate-sized hard disk drive (at least several gigabytes), and an optical drive. The latter may be a compact disk-read only memory (CD-ROM) reader or a drive that both reads and writes CD-ROM media (CD-RW). Drives that combine CD-RW with the ability to read digital versatile disk (DVD-ROM) media also are widely available as either internal drives or external drives that can be connected via USB or IEEE 1394 interfaces. These accommodate the use of the many software titles, educational programs, and databases available on optical media. Appropriate networking connections such as Ethernet cable ports or adapters or wireless networking receivers also are necessary. If not connected to a network, a telephone modem is needed to connect to the Internet.

Information "output" is a critical part of healthcare epidemiology and infection control, and a variety of options are available. Most often a printer is used, and the two types in widespread use are the laser and inkjet varieties. The laser printer fuses microscopic plastic toner particles to a page (paper or transparency) the same way that a photocopier does, whereas inkjet printers deposit droplets of ink on the page. Laser printers generally are monochrome/grayscale, whereas almost all inkjet printers produce a full spectrum of colors, including the ability to produce photographic-quality prints. Laser printers generally cost more to purchase, but inkjet printers usually have a higher cost of "consumables," (i.e., ink cartridges and specially coated photographic paper and transparencies). It is important to compare per page costs and also individual needs (i.e., frequent presentations might argue for an inkjet printer that can produce color transparencies, whereas predominantly paper reports might favor a laser printer). It is worthwhile to investigate if a workgroup printer, available to several individuals or departments, is available because it may allow costs to be shared or even avoided.

There also are devices to print presentations to 35-mm slide film or to send them directly to electronic multimedia projectors. These devices generally are too expensive for individual or even departmental purchase, but most hospitals and universities have them available for use and/or loan. Information also can be published on an intranet or the Internet (see later) using one of the many simple software programs available.

A method to provide backup or duplicate copies of important data must be provided, whether through a local device or a network file server, so that important or unique information may be retrieved in the event of equipment failure or theft. Many organizations provide each user with "space" on a network file server for copying important files, although this usually is not large enough to copy an entire hard disk drive. A CD-RW with appropriate software is a convenient and inexpensive way to make duplicate copies of important files or even an entire hard disk drive. Larger systems or workgroups may choose to use a magnetic tape based backup system for PCs or servers.

Operating Systems

An OS is the core software that enables computers to function (i.e., communicate with the hard disk drive and other devices). Several such systems are in widespread use: Microsoft Windows (Microsoft Corporation, Redmond, WA) in one of many versions is most widely used; however, Apple MacOS and a number of UNIX variants including Solaris (Sun Microsystems, Santa Clara, CA) and freeware Linux also are popular. OS software is hardware specific: the Windows OS generally operates on x86/Pentium (Intel Corporation, Santa Clara, CA) microprocessors, whereas the MacOS operates on PowerPC (International Business Machines Corporation; Motorola Inc, Schaumberg, IL) processors. UNIX variants may operate on either of these microprocessor lines or on Sun SPARC processors. Other than applications written in Sun's Java programming language, software written for one OS does not run on computers that use a different OS. Also, application software may be specific for different versions of the same OS (e.g., Windows 98 software will not run on a computer with the Windows 3.1 OS). It is important to thoroughly understand the processor, memory, and hard disk space requirements of any OS or application software before purchasing it.

Basic Software

Aside from the OS software, application software programs (often called applications, software or programs for short) are needed to make a PC more than an expensive solitaire machine. Basic software tools include a word processor for making reports and writing correspondence; a spreadsheet for making calculations and graphing data; a database for storing information, such as surveillance data; and a presentation program for making slides, electronic slideshows, and other visual reports. These basic tools often come as part of an "office" suite of software or as part of an integrated "works" package. The former usually includes full-function ("high-end") programs, whereas the latter tend to be more compact. Price, required RAM, hard drive storage space, and expertise required for efficient use tend to follow the same pattern. Note that the works packages likely provide enough power for many hospital epidemiology-infection control activities, especially in a small facility. Before purchasing software, one should attempt to evaluate it with a demonstration version (often available from publisher Web sites) or on a colleague's PC. Universities, hospitals, and other large organizations often have site license agreements with software publishers that will provide basic software at little or no cost to employees or affiliated professionals.

Basic software also may include statistical analysis software, which no longer requires a mainframe computer to use. Many commercial packages and the freeware EpiInfo from the Centers for Disease Control and Prevention (CDC) (*http://www.cdc.gov/epiinfo*) are available for PCs.

Modern software, running on a GUI-based computer, has the ability to change typefaces (fonts); manipulate typeface styles; organize materials; and add tables, charts, or images to a document. A report of epidemiologic activity, therefore, could include text with bold headings, a table of key data, and several salient charts that result in a clear, concise, and compelling document. However, the very features that allow for this flexibility also can make the report garishly unattractive if used in excess. In general, multiple typefaces should not be used in a single document, and script or other specialty typefaces should be avoided because they are difficult to read. Likewise, underlining and ALL CAPITALS are distracting and difficult to read in a body of text; emphasis may be added with boldface or italics. Some of the most egregious violations of publishing taste occur with newsletters and information sheets that, along with excessive typeface manipulation, often contain excessive amounts of clip art and other nontext items. Many publications are available to provide guidance for creating attractive documents (6).

Personal Digital Assistants

The last several years have witnessed the explosive growth of palm or shirt-pocket size devices known as *personal digital assistants* (PDAs). These small computers originally were developed to be schedulers and a place to store names and contact information. However, they have increased in speed and memory and now can provide data retrieval, basic word processing, and statistical and database functions. Newer models also include wireless access to the Internet or to local networks using the IEEE 802.11 standard. Because these devices do not have built-in hard disk drives at this time, it is necessary to "synchronize" them with a PC to ensure data availability and safety.

As with PCs, there are competing product platforms available. The original PDAs were produced to run the Palm computing platform (Palm, Inc., Milpitas, CA), but more recently devices that run a version of Microsoft Windows also have been marketed. The software made for one platform will not run on the other. Nonetheless, there are many medical programs, textbooks, and other references available for the Palm platform, and some hospitals have begun programs to use PDAs to record and/or access patient data at the bedside using wireless technology.

THE INTERNET

The Internet has become synonymous with the information superhighway, and many of the tools and techniques of accessing and navigating the Internet have been adapted for use on intranets and LANs. Therefore, a discussion of the Internet is an appropriate prelude to a discussion of information management.

Internet Structure and Function

The Internet arose from a network of government and university computer systems that was used to exchange files and information starting in the 1970s (7–9). With the wider availability of network connections and user-friendly software tools, the number of computers attached to and accessing the Internet has grown astronomically. Much of this growth has been in commercial areas, and commercial carriers now provide most of the pipelines that connect to and constitute the Internet. However, education and healthcare resources continue to thrive as well. Interestingly, a high-speed next-generation Internet or Internet2 is in development for education and research institutions to rapidly exchange information (10) (*http://www.internet2.edu*).

Analogous to the telecommunications system that preceded it, the Internet is composed of many computers that are attached to LANs. The LANs are in turn attached to larger networks that eventually become attached to the backbone of the Internet. Most of the computers that access the Internet are on the client side, that is, seeking information, whereas the minority are servers that provide the information. Like telephones and facsimile machines, each computer on the Internet must have a unique designation to send and receive data. These are called Internet protocol (IP) addresses and have both numeric and name equivalents. IP addresses are organized by domain and particular computers or servers within the domain (e.g., wings.buffalo.edu designates the main campus information server in the University at Buffalo second-level domain, within the education top-level domain). The numerical equivalent address for this server is 128.205.200.10. Other common top-level domains are *.com* for commercial sites, *.gov* for government sponsored sites, and *.org* for noncommercial sites. Country or state designations occasionally may supersede the traditional top-level domains at the far right of the IP address (e.g., *www.health.state.ny.us* is the New York State Health Department home page). Although there is no central control agency for the Internet, IP addresses are assigned under the direction of an agency called the Internet Corporation for Assigned Names and Numbers (ICANN). This maintains order and ensures that all computers on the Internet can reliably be located.

Also analogous to the telephone system, computers on the Internet must use a common set of instructions in order for communications to move appropriately from source to destination. Most of the servers on the Internet use one of the variants of the UNIX OS, but most of the PC clients are MacOS or Windows based. To allow these diverse OSs to communicate with one another, the Internet uses a set of platform-independent protocols that are determined by an international body of experts. The most important of these standards is the networking scheme called transmission control protocol/Internet protocol (TCP/IP), which determines how the computers on the Internet connect and communicate with one another. Any computer running any OS can access the Internet if it has an appropriate network connection and is TCP/IP compliant. LANs that use proprietary networking protocols still can connect to the Internet through an appropriate router or bridge. TCP/IP also can coexist with Ethernet and the NOS on a LAN, which is important in allowing connectivity and compatibility.

Unlike the telephone system, Internet transmission uses packets of digital information rather than a continuous stream of analog data. Each file or message is converted into properly addressed packets before being sent. The address in the packet header instructs the servers on the Internet to relay the packet in a process called packet switching. This allows for many client/server connections to use the same Internet lines simultaneously, rather than keeping a line tied up as happens with telephone circuit switching. The downside of packet switching is that lost or misdirected packets, which increase with heavy Internet use, can slow the user experience to maddening levels.

Connecting to the Internet

The best connection to the Internet is from a network where a computer actually is a node or connection point on the Internet with its own IP address. Because of the nature of the wiring and routing system, this broadband connection is capable of very fast and high-capacity transmission that is compliant with Internet standards. Some networks do not permanently assign a separate

IP address to each computer but rather reserve a range of addresses that are assigned electronically to computers as needed, using the dynamic host configuration protocol (DHCP). Most universities, large hospitals, and other large organizations are able to provide direct access for staff so that they are physically connected to a LAN. Some cable television companies provide individual users with broadband connections via fiberoptic cable modems that may approach the speed of traditional Internet network connections.

Recently, the development of wireless LAN and Internet connections referred to as wireless fidelity (Wi-Fi) has given a glimpse of a future where interactive mobile computing will not be tethered to a wall outlet. A laptop computer or PDA with appropriate networking hardware based on the IEEE 802.11 standard can connect with network signals provided by an antenna connected to the Internet or a LAN. The antenna may be in the "open" or within a building or even a home. In a hospital, this would allow for real-time entry or retrieval of patient related information at the bedside. Many issues, such as signal strength (which determines effective range for service), service interruptions, and security of confidential information, remain to be resolved.

If not directly connected to a network, as might be the case in a smaller facility or private office, using a telephone modem to dial in to a host computer using the point-to-point protocol (PPP) is the next best option. The PPP server of an Internet service provider (ISP) temporarily makes a desktop computer a node on the Internet with its own dynamically assigned IP address. The bandwidth of this service is dependent on the speed of the client and server computers' modems. The development of integrated services digital network (ISDN) and asymmetric digital subscriber line (ADSL) telephone line protocols also will offer much higher bandwidth than even the fastest current telephone modem connection speeds. These, like fiberoptic cable connections, require special modems that are more expensive than standard modems, and the monthly service charge also will be significant. Bandwidth is expensive!

Some organizations, including hospitals, may provide employees with remote access to the corporate network using a *virtual private network* (VPN). VPN client and server software uses a tunneling protocol to securely transmit information over the Internet using cable or telephone modems. This could allow professionals at remote sites to access electronic mail, databases, and other network-based resources.

The least robust Internet connection is via telephone modem using the terminal emulation component of a communications software package. The user's computer becomes a dumb terminal attached to the host computer, which is a node on the Internet. The user will be faced with a keyboard command line driven, text-only interface without any of the visually rich content expected on the Internet. This form of Internet connection largely has been superseded by PPP access.

Internet Tools

As noted previously, the Internet originally was developed to allow scientists to exchange messages and files electronically. This was done with text-based software tools or clients that resided on the large Internet servers and required knowledge of the locations of files and the commands to retrieve them. Although the use of newer software tools has supplanted the older tools, descendants of the original file transfer and terminal connection tools still are valuable and are discussed further. The reader is directed to other sources for information about the other tools such as Gopher, Veronica, and Archie (8, 9,11).

Files can be moved from one computer to another using the Internet file transfer protocol (FTP), and the software program that does this is referred to as an FTP client. (Client may refer to the software application or to the computer on which it resides.) If one knows the IP address of the server that contains a file of interest, this can be entered into the FTP client and a list of the folders (directories) on the server will be returned. The appropriate folder can be opened to find the file, which then can be downloaded to the client computer. Many FTP servers allow public or anonymous access to their contents, whereas others may require user identification and passwords. As an example, the CDC server at ftp.cdc.gov contains a folder entitled "pub" that can be accessed without a password. It contains folders for CDC software and CDC publications among others, and the documents contained therein are freely downloadable.

Many files on Internet servers are compressed by special software to make the file size smaller for transfer and encoded into American Standard Code for Information Interchange (ASCHII) text format to ensure safe passage over the network. This requires that the client computer have appropriate software for decoding and decompression. Compression formats vary among computer platforms. Stuffit (.sit) for Macintosh, Zip (.zip) for DOS/Windows, and tape archive (.tar) for UNIX are common. The same is true for encoding formats; uuencoding (UNIX to UNIX; .uu) is used on all platforms and binhex (binary to hexadecimal; .hqx) is common for Macintosh. There are freeware, shareware, and commercial products available to decode and expand these files.

Telnet is the other important descendant tool. A Telnet software client application allows a client computer to connect to a server or mainframe computer. This in essence re-creates the dumb terminal situation described previously, giving the client access to the software programs and files on the host computer. This is in a text-only mode, generally with keyboard-only commands as defined by the host computer, and printing may be restricted to printers attached to the mainframe. Because Telnet gives access to the functioning parts of the host (server), password access is generally required, as it would be when logging on from a hardwired terminal. Telnet may be the only means of gaining access to mainframe computers or other servers; thus, having a Telnet client is essential for anyone who wishes to obtain information from these machines. Telnet also may be useful to access mail and other application software on a server, especially if one has slow or limited access to the Internet.

Perhaps the most significant nonhardware milestones related to the Internet have been the development of the hypertext transfer protocol (HTTP), hypertext markup language (HTML), and browsers (12). Together they have transformed the client/server interface on the Internet from a cryptic, command line, text-based system to a "point and click," visually rich environment known as the World Wide Web (WWW or Web). Hypertext and HTML make it possible to include stylized text, tables, images, and hyperlinks (links for short), which, when clicked, move the user from the current location on the Web to another. Browsers are software client applications that understand HTTP, FTP, and other IPs and make it possible to view (browse), save, or print HTML pages and to download files from HTTP or FTP sites. The user combines the desired protocol and IP address into the uniform resource locator (URL), which then instructs the browser client to attach to the desired Web server. The Web server must run appropriate software to complete the interaction and deliver the appropriate file or page. It is necessary to specify both the IP and the IP address; the URLs *http://www.cdc.gov/* and *ftp://ftp.cdc.gov* will provide the user with two very different client/server interactions. The former is the CDC's home page on the Web and is a text and graphics-rich page with links to other pages, and the latter is the CDC's FTP server as noted previously.

Graphic images such as pictures, scanned images, copies of graphs, and other nontext artwork generally appear in one of two formats on the Web: graphics interchange format (GIF; .gif), which is good for nonphotographic images because it displays only 256 colors but keeps sharp edges and joint photographic experts group (JPEG; .jpg), which can display millions of colors and is better for photographs and other complex images. Charts, scanned images of electrophoresis gels, and other items of interest to hospital epidemiologists can be saved in one of these formats and placed on a Web page. Browsers can display both image types, as can most word processor, graphic, and page layout software programs.

Java, JavaScript, and Plug-Ins

Web pages can be enhanced further with Java, JavaScript, and plug-ins (13). Java is a platform-independent computer programming language developed by Sun Microsystems. It is used to operate thin client computers and program middleware for database systems, but small Java applications known as applets provide a variety of enhancements to Web sites, such as animation, forms, and messages. Recent versions of popular browsers can run Java applets although the appearance may not be consistent on different products. Windows 3.1 cannot run Java applets.

JavaScript is a scripting language, completely unrelated to Java, developed by Netscape Communications Corp. (Mountainview, CA) to provide enhancements such as pull-down menus and scrolling messages for Web pages. It is less complex and less capable than Java but exists totally within the HTML code of a Web page rather than as a separate applet. Recent versions of browsers can interpret JavaScript, including those that run on Windows 3.1.

Plug-ins are small pieces of software that can add functions to larger software programs. They are popular for use with Web browsers as a way to add capabilities that are not part of the intrinsic browser repertoire. Plug-ins have proliferated widely but none really are necessary. Some may provide useful functions such as the Acrobat Reader plug-in, which allows the user to view a portable document format (PDF) file (see later) within the browser, or a plug-in that plays streaming (continuous) audio or video. The latter can be used for Web-based transmission of lectures or conferences.

Internet Electronic Mail

Electronic mail, or e-mail, is a way to rapidly send messages across the Internet or other networks (14,15). The sending and delivery end points of e-mail transmission are mail servers; thus, messages are delivered continuously and near instantaneously, rather than slowly and episodically as with postal or "snail" mail. Internet e-mail is governed by standards like all other Internet transmissions. An e-mail software client on a PC or other computer is linked to a mail server that uses simple mail transport protocol (SMTP) for sending mail. There are two different client/server relationships for receiving Internet e-mail: post office protocol (POP) and Internet message access protocol (IMAP). POP creates a simple relationship when the client logs into the server, whereby received messages are transferred to the client's computer e-mail program. The e-mail messages then can be sorted into folders, and address books can be maintained. IMAP maintains the e-mail and address book on the server, and the client software manipulates the mailboxes and address books. The advantage of IMAP is that stored mail messages and address books can be accessed from any computer that has IMAP-compliant mail client software. Many e-mail systems also can be set up to allow Internet access through the use of a Web browser, which allows one to remain "in contact" when traveling without a laptop computer.

Along with sending messages via e-mail, appropriately encoded documents or files can be attached to the messages. E-mail clients that are multipurpose Internet mail extension (MIME) compliant can manage messages with files and graphics embedded in them, thereby eliminating the need for encoding. When sending documents or files as attachments, one must remember that along with incompatibilities among computer OSs, there are incompatibilities among the file formats used by application software programs or even different versions of the same program. There are several approaches to this problem: (a) everyone sharing a document can use the same software, preferably in the same version. This may be possible within an organization but is highly problematic when exchanging data in an educational institution or across the Internet; (b) one of the file interchange formats that can be accessed through the open, import, save as, or export commands in most software programs can be used. Common formats are rich text format (.rtf) for word processors and dbase (.dbf) and data interchange format (.dif) or symbolic link (.slk) for spreadsheets and databases. Special formatting often is lost in these formats; (c) a document can be transmitted as an ASCII text document, which will be devoid of formatting but will contain all of the data; and (d) Acrobat Distiller or Capture software (Adobe Systems Inc., San Jose, CA) can be used to create platform- and software-independent Acrobat PDF (PDF; .pdf) files. The PDF file, when viewed or printed, provides a document that appears identical to the original. A free Acrobat Reader application is available (*http://www.adobe. com*) for most computer platforms.

Many LANs in hospitals and other organizations use proprietary e-mail software systems. These often have the advantages of having a central post office for both sending and receiving mail and a master address book for everyone who has access to the LAN. However, these systems may not be fully IP compliant, and attached files may be lost or damaged when the message is sent through a bridge to the Internet.

Network News

Network news can be thought of as a large bulletin board on the Internet where messages and responses can be posted to newsgroups, each of which is devoted to a particular topic (12). The newsgroups may be part of the established users network (Usenet) or may be restricted to a part of the Internet, such as a university. Postings to newsgroups are transmitted over the Internet by the network news transport protocol (NNTP) and posted on NNTP servers, which then make the postings available to clients who subscribe. The postings are read with a newsreader software client, which may be a stand-alone product or part of a browser or e-mail package. Like the cork bulletin board at the student center, newsgroups generally are not moderated. *Caveat lector!*

Information from the Internet

The Internet contains a wealth of information and data that may be important or useful to the healthcare epidemiologist or infection control team. Most of it is contained on the Web or may be obtained by e-mail, so these areas will be highlighted. As noted previously, along with commercial growth on the Web there is a vibrant education presence as well. This is due to the general availability of Web server space at universities and other organizations and the ease with which Web pages can be constructed.

Medical Web sites may be found in several general categories: government, bibliographic databases, professional societies and organizations, educational institutions, publications, and commercial interests. Among the government Web sites, the CDC (*http://www.cdc.gov/*) has extensive information available including the *Morbidity and Mortality Weekly Report* (MMWR), *Emerging Infectious Diseases* (EID), guidelines, course/program announcements, and surveillance reports. Many of these are available as Acrobat PDFs, which provide printed copy identical to the offset printed version available by snail-mail subscription. Included in this group are the semiannual reports of the National Nosocomial Infection Surveillance (NNIS) system; the tabular data can be printed or cut and pasted to a spreadsheet for use in internal benchmarking. The CDC WONDER site (*http://wonder.cdc.gov*) contains a search engine that can locate documents and data from several CDC and National Institute of Occupational Safety and Health (NIOSH) databases (16). Other government sites with information or data of potential use to healthcare epidemiologists include the Department of Health and Human Services Smallpox information repository (*http://www.smallpox.gov*), the Occupational Safety and Health Administration (OSHA; *http://www.osha.gov/*), and the Food and Drug Administration (FDA; *http://www.fda.gov/*). Many state health departments similarly post policies, notices, and statistics.

The key medical database of the National Library of Medicine (NLM), Medical Literature Analysis and Retrieval System (MEDLARS), has been available in electronic format for many years through MEDlars on-LINE (MEDLINE). This often has been through telephone modem access or in CD-ROM format, both of which have entailed subscription charges. NLM now provides free Web access to MEDLINE (*http://www.ncbi.nlm.nih.gov/PubMed/*) with a number of enhancements, including access to other NLM resources through PubMed Central (*http://www.pubmedcentral.nih.gov/*) and MEDLINEplus (*http://www.nlm.nih.gov/medlineplus/*). There also are commercial MEDLINE-based products that may include additional databases and search capabilities available for university or other organization servers. Some may include access to a select number of full-text journals. The latter products usually are licensed on a number-of-seats basis so access is restricted to the members of the university or organization that has purchased the product or service. Nonetheless, access to the literature of medicine, healthcare epidemiology, and infection control has never before been easier or less expensive.

The Web has provided a tremendous opportunity for many professional societies and similar organizations to interact with a global audience. These organizations can provide news, membership applications, meeting and course brochures, and links to other sources of information. Professional society Web sites of interest to healthcare epidemiologists and infection control team members include the Society for Healthcare Epidemiology of America (SHEA; *http://www.shea-online.org/*), the Association for Professionals in Infection Control and Epidemiology (APIC; *http://www.apic.org/*), the Hospital Infection Society (HIS; *http://www.his.org.uk/*), and the Joint Commission on Accreditation of Healthcare Organizations (JCAHO; *http://www.jcaho.org/*). The SHEA Web pages include an extensive set of links to other healthcare epidemiology and quality improvement resources, and the APIC site includes a searchable index of topics discussed in their Internet e-mail discussion list.

The healthcare epidemiology and infection control services of several academic institutions have Web sites that contain results of outbreak investigations or ongoing surveillance activities. Information databases, such as the Health Information Research Unit (*http://hiru.mcmaster.ca/*) of McMaster University and the National Guideline Clearinghouse (*http://www.guideline.gov/*), add to the diverse sources of critical evaluation of data. In a similar context are the sites of peer-reviewed publications that often are associated with professional societies. These sites may offer the table of contents of journal issues, article abstracts, or full text of articles. The latter usually require society membership or a subscription, and access is password controlled. Finally, it should be noted that most providers of medical products and services have Web sites for self-promotion. Some of these may include data that may be helpful in purchasing or use decisions. Many of these can be found by using an Internet search engine such as Google (*http://www.google.com/*) or Sherlock on a Macintosh.

Along with exchanging messages and files with individual colleagues, Internet e-mail can be an important source of information for the healthcare epidemiologist via mail lists. Automated e-mail list servers send a message to everyone subscribed to the list in a manner analogous to broadcast facsimile, although much more rapidly and inexpensively. Lists can be used to send notices to members of an association, announce availability of products or publications, provide breaking news, or allow list members to ask questions and read and post responses. Individuals interested in the service(s) or topic(s) covered by a mail list subscribe to it by sending an e-mail message to the list administrator or to an automatic subscription program on the list server. Subscribers then receive an e-mail message whenever that message is sent to the posting address for the list. Lists may be one way, in which a designated person is the only one who can post a message to the list, or two way, in which any message that is posted is sent automatically to all list subscribers. One-way lists may be used as a means of notification; the CDC has e-mail lists by which subscribers are notified of the availability of each edition of the *MMWR* (*http://www.cdc.gov/mmwr/mmwrsubscribe.html*) and the occurrence of important healthcare events and publications (*http://www2.cdc.gov/ncidod/hip/rns/hip__rns__subscribe.html*). Moderated discussion lists usually are one way as well; all postings must be reviewed and approved by the list moderator before being posted. Although this is not peer review, it does control the content and tone of the list. Two way-lists, along with network news groups, do not require any approval for posting messages and tend to become cluttered with redundant, unnecessary, or inappropriate postings. As a result, the volume of e-mail subscribers receive becomes large and the quality of the mail tends to suffer. Again, *caveat lector!*

Security

The widespread use of the Internet has raised many questions about the security, safety, and confidentiality of the information that is transmitted over it (9). Although the topic is too complex for detailed discussion here, some general recommendations can be made. User identification and passwords must not be shared or divulged and proper log-off procedures should be followed; this will protect users and their system by not allowing unauthorized use. E-mail is the least secure form of transmission, and sensitive data such as confidential correspondence or credit card numbers should not be sent this way unless encrypted. Web browsing, on-line purchasing, or completing surveys may be done with higher levels of security that probably make it safe to undertake these transactions at reputable sites. However, be aware that the server to which you attach may acquire information about you and your computer through bits of information, called cookies, exchanged with your browser. Other information you provide may place you on a mailing list or be shared or sold to other parties.

Downloaded software programs or some e-mail messages may be infected with small programs called viruses, macro viruses, worms, or Trojan horses. Many of these are malicious or destructive to other files on the client computer, and some may send personal information from the infected computer to another source. Others send multiple copies of themselves to all of the addresses in an e-mail account, clogging mail servers. Software programs sent by e-mail or obtained from uncertain sources never should be opened, and unsolicited messages such as these should be deleted. Many organizations require the use of an antiviral utility program by all users who download or exchange files, and incoming mail often will be scanned for malicious programs.

Analogous to junk mail, junk faxes, and recorded telemarketing calls, unsolicited e-mail has burgeoned in the past several years. Often referred to as "spam," much to the chagrin of the manufacturer of the processed meat product, such mail has ranged from nuisance to disruptive. "Spammers" use net robots to seek e-mail addresses from newsgroups, outgoing mail servers, and other sources to develop a database of target addresses. Some organizations will sell e-mail addresses obtained at the time of a Web interaction (such as opening a free mail account) to others, eventually resulting in addition to a spam list. Responding to spam messages to attempt removal of an e-mail address from a list may actually verify that an account is real and result in even more unsolicited e-mail. Some browsers have anti-spam filters, and there are a number of third-party software packages that promise to remove spam messages. None of these are perfect, but they often decrease the volume of unwanted mail. Unfortunately, the spammers often are a step ahead of the attempts to foil them. A number of Web sites, including *http://www.junkbusters.org/* have more information on avoiding and fighting spam.

Internet chain letters and hoaxes, often threatening the user or user's computer with dire consequences, also have proliferated, and these are best ignored and deleted. More information on security issues and hoaxes is available at the United States Department of Energy Computer Incident Advisory Capability (CERT) Web site (*http://www.ciac.org/ciac/*).

Recommendations for Internet Connectivity and Software

It is highly desirable for healthcare epidemiology and infection control program staff to have access to the Internet using one of the methods described previously, preferably from a desktop microcomputer directly connected to a network. An Internet e-mail account likewise is desirable, but a LAN e-mail account that can be reached from the Internet is acceptable. The basic software tools for Internet use include a browser, an e-mail client, an FTP client, a Telnet client, software for encoding and decoding files, and software for compression and expansion of files. No recommendations are made for specific products, and many freeware or low-cost shareware products are sufficiently capable to preclude the purchase of more expensive commercial products. The freeware Acrobat Reader software also is recommended. If software is available from a university or organization IS department, this should be considered for use because it is likely to be compliant with Internet or LAN standards. Training and support are likely to be available as well.

Currently, two browsers account for most WWW clients: Netscape (Netscape Communications Corp., Mountainview, CA) and Internet Explorer (Microsoft Corp., Redmond, WA). Both are freely available for most client computer OSs, and both have many features (some would say too many features) beyond basic HTTP and FTP functions. Both have an Internet e-mail client either integrated or in a closely associated stand-alone program. The choice of browser is like the choice of any computer software—very dependent on individual needs and preferences. There are several other browsers available, each with particular features and proponents. Some pages may not display properly in a particular browser but may be rendered appropriately in another. This is due to evolving standards and the willingness (or unwillingness) of a software company to follow the standards.

As noted in the beginning of this section, the same tools used for accessing data from the Internet also can be used for obtaining information on many university or hospital intranets and LANs (17).

RESOURCES

Many users enter the world of computing and the Internet with trepidation, and this is understandable. However, the potential benefits to healthcare epidemiologists and infection control team members should serve as impetus to overcome fear and ignorance so that they can take advantage of the resources that are and will become available. Introductory courses are offered at educational institutions, libraries, and in healthcare organizations and are a good starting point for the newcomer. Advanced and specific topic courses also are available.

Books about general and specific computing topics have proliferated and provide additional resources for beginners and more experienced users. Particularly useful for general audiences are the*JAVA for Dummies* (Wiley Publishing, Inc., Indianapolis, IN; *http://www.dummies.com*), *Essential Guide . . .* (Prentice Hall PTR, Upper Saddle River, NJ; *http://www.phptr.com*), and the O'Reilly book series (O'Reilly & Associates, Cambridge, MA; *http://www.oreilly.com*). These are readable, inexpensive, cover a variety of basic and advanced topics, and widely available. There are magazines for essentially every computer topic, platform, and use area, and many also have some or all of their content posted on the Web. Finally, local computer user groups and educational Web sites provide additional or more detailed information for more advanced users or on specific topics. A useful encyclopedia resource for computer technology is available (*http://www.whatis.com/*).

REFERENCES

1. Hierholzer WJ Jr, Miller SP, Streed SA, et al. On-line infection control system using PCS/IMS. In: O'Neill JT, ed. *Proceedings of the fourth annual symposium on computer applications in medical care,* November 2–5, 1980. Washington, DC: National Center for Health Service Research, 1980:540–546.
2. Evans RS, Larsen RA, Burke JP, et al. Computer surveillance of hospital infections and antibiotic use. *JAMA* 1986;256:1507–1511.
3. Hierholzer WJ Jr, Streed SA, Wood DE, et al. Extended capability of an infection data management system through routine use of an on-line report generator. Proceedings of the American Association for Medical Systems and Informatics Congress, May 2–4, 1983, San Francisco.
4. LaHaise S. A comparison of infection control software for use by hospital epidemiologists in meeting the new JCAHO standards. *Infect Control Hosp Epidemiol* 1990;11:185–190.
5. Sellick JA Jr. Infection control software. *Infect Control Hosp Epidemiol* 1990;11:408.
6. Musher DM. Visual materials for lectures. *Rev Infect Dis* 1990;12: 359–360.
7. Pallen M. Introducing the Internet. *BMJ* 1995;311:1422–1424.
8. Glowniak JV, Bushway MK. Computer networks as a medical resource. Accessing and using the Internet. *JAMA* 1994;271:1934–1939.
9. Glowniak JV. Medical resources on the Internet. *Ann Intern Med* 1995; 123:123–131.
10. Dern DP, Mace S. The Internet reinvented. *Byte* 1998;23:89–96.
11. Pallen M. Guide to the Internet. Logging in, fetching files, reading news. *BMJ* 1995;311:1626–1630.
12. Pallen M. Guide to the Internet. The world wide web. *BMJ* 1995; 311:1552–1556.
13. Walsh A. *Java for dummies,* 3rd ed. Indianapolis, IN: Wiley, 1998.
14. Pallen M. Electronic mail. *BMJ* 1995;311:1487–1490.
15. Sellick JA Jr. Electronic mail: an imperative for healthcare epidemiologists. *Infect Control Hosp Epidemiol* 1997;18:377–381.
16. Friede A, O'Carroll PW. CDC and ATSDR electronic information resources for health officers. *Am J Infect Control* 1996;24:440–454.
17. Willard KE, Connelly DP, Johnson JR. Radical improvements in the display of clinical microbiology results: a Web-based clinical information system. *Am J Med* 1996;101:541–549.

15

USING THE PERSONAL COMPUTER FOR HEALTHCARE EPIDEMIOLOGY

KEITH F. WOELTJE
REBECCA WURTZ

The basic concepts of personal computers (PCs) are covered in Chapter 14. This chapter reviews the use of these systems in healthcare epidemiology. This chapter assumes the use of standalone PCs or PCs that may happen to be on a network. These are currently the most common circumstances for healthcare epidemiologists and infection control professionals (ICPs). The use of integrated data systems and electronic medical records is discussed in the Chapter 16.

THE DECISION TO USE A COMPUTER

Given that computers are a useful tool for managing large amounts of information and that infection control requires dealing with large amounts of information, it is no surprise that PCs have been used for healthcare epidemiology since shortly after they were introduced. Schifman and Palmer (1) described an early use of the PC in infection surveillance at the Tucson Veterans Administration Medical Center (VAMC). Although PCs have been used for healthcare epidemiology for decades, their penetration has been variable. Some tasks are still done using largely manual methods. In other cases, computers have simply been turned into glorified typewriters, making little use of their capabilities. A classic example of this is a spreadsheet into which the user enters results that were obtained from a calculator; all of the necessary calculations were performed manually.

Before deciding on which program is most appropriate for a given task, one must first determine whether it is appropriate to computerize the task at all. A number of factors go into this decision. First, is there a manual system already in place? If so, is it working acceptably well? The adage "if it ain't broke don't fix it" comes to mind. Then one must consider that having data on the computer is useful in three specific areas: data backups, data sharing (networking), and data analysis.

In considering whether to develop a computer-based system, one must consider how valuable are the data. One significant advantage of a computerized system is that multiple copies of the data can be made to prevent loss of critical information. Making backups should be considered a requirement, and the time required to do so factored into the decision on whether to computerize a given process. All too often backups are not done or done so infrequently as to be almost useless. One reason for making copies of information is to protect against failures of the computer hardware. As reliable as they are, computer hard disks will fail—the only real question is when. For maximal insurance, copies of the data should be stored at a site away from the computer to protect against natural disasters. Alternatively, small fire-resistant safes provide some measure of protection for important data stored locally.

Regarding data sharing, one must consider who must have access to the data. If multiple people in a small office need access, a simple paper system may be much easier to implement than a computerized one. If the data are on one person's computer, there may be an intolerable number of work interruptions while others access the information, or the others will have to wait until the computer is free. In such a setting, a paper-based system such as a card file may work much better. However, if the data must be accessed often by persons whose offices are not in close proximity or if multiple users must access the information simultaneously, then a network-based system would be very effective.

Another data access consideration is whether there is a lot of old information already stored in an older paper system. If so, it must be determined if this old data will have to be entered into the new computerized system. All too often, trying to use a split system yields the worst of both worlds. If it is important to have access to all of the old information, the costs (in terms of time and effort) spent entering all of the old data will have to be carefully balanced against any potential gains. Often only a limited amount of the older data need to be accessed with any frequency, limiting the amount of prior information that must be entered into a new system.

Is data entry episodic? One must consider the time overhead spent launching a program, entering data, making a backup, and stopping the program each time a piece of information is obtained. Even if the decision is made to use a computer-based system, it may make sense to use paper forms as an intermediate, allowing for more data to be entered into the computer at one time. Paper intermediary forms also make sense if data are gathered away from the computer (although other options exist, as discussed in the section on data gathering).

Lastly, is there a need for complicated data analysis? This is where having information on the computer pays a large dividend. The many options for data analysis are discussed at length in this chapter.

Once a computer-based system is working, one must carefully consider whether it is worthwhile to upgrade to newer versions of software. The computer industry is notorious for promoting relatively frequent upgrades of hardware and software. In part this is because of the tremendous improvements in computing power that occurs over short periods of time. Such improvements make it feasible to include more and more software features that would have slowed older hardware to a barely perceptible crawl. Although some new software is faster, the addition of features may lead to worse performance on an older computer. The decision to upgrade to newer software should be based on actual need. Does the new software have new features that would be useful? Is it easier to use? Is the new software more stable (i.e., less prone to crash)? Even if the answers are yes, other issues still must be considered: How much effort will it take to move existing data into the new system? Does the new software use the same file formats, or will the files have to be converted? Does the new software do this conversion? Will formulas and macros (short programs written by the user in some programs) written for the old version work in the new version? Finally, will the company continue to support the older software with bug fixes and so forth? As tempting as the latest and greatest version of software may be, it may well make sense to stick with an older version of a program if it is doing everything needed. This is true even if upgrading to a new computer—the older programs should get a performance boost from the new hardware. However, it may be necessary upgrade the software to accommodate newer versions of the operating system (OS) that comes with the new hardware.

BASIC OFFICE SOFTWARE

As discussed in Chapter 14, suites of office software are included with many PCs; if not, they are usually one of the first software purchases of a PC user. Word processing and presentation software are used primarily for data dissemination, as discussed later.

Spreadsheets

Spreadsheet software (more so than word processing software) ushered in the PC era. Spreadsheet software remains one of the most versatile tools at the disposal of the healthcare epidemiologist.

Flat-File Database

The column and row design of computer spreadsheets lends itself well to use as a "flat-file" database. This is a database in which all of the information can be contained on a single page (see the discussion of databases for other types of databases). Typically the first row is used to enter headings for the information to be collected (i.e., the database "field"; e.g., Name, Age, etc.). Each subsequent row is then used to store information for one subject (i.e., a database "record").

Although database programs can also be used for such flat-file databases, using a spreadsheet for this purpose has a number of advantages. For many users, a spreadsheet is almost always included with their office suite of software, whereas a database program will probably have to be purchased separately. Some users familiar with the use of a spreadsheet for calculations can extend that familiarity more easily than learning an entirely new program. Some statistical software may be able to import data from a spreadsheet table, making the spreadsheet file format a common denominator for sharing data between programs.

One of the handiest features of spreadsheets is the "filtering" function. This allows the user to see only records that meet a certain criterion. Although the same information may be obtained from a true database program, it typically involves more work. For example, an intensive care unit (ICU) may want to keep track of the intravenous (IV) devices used on various patients. In a spreadsheet, there may be a column for patient name, and others for medical record number, date of admission to the ICU, an so forth. A column could then be made for "intravenous (IV) device used." Then "peripheral catheter" or "peripherally inserted central catheter (PICC)" or "triple-lumen catheter" could be entered into this column. By using the filter function, one could readily see all of the patients that had a PICC line. However, typically an ICU patient will have multiple types of IV catheters. One could have a column "IV catheter 1" and another column "IV catheter 2" and so on. However, one must consider what would be necessary to find all of the patients who had a triple-lumen catheter. First, one would have to filter for "triple-lumen catheter" in the "IV catheter 1" column, then in the "IV catheter 2" column, and so forth. One way to get around this is to have only one column for device, and then enter a new row for each type of catheter that the patient had. However, this would mean duplicating the patient demographic data for each row and would make a simple count of the patients or calculations, such as the mean patient age, difficult. A more effective option would be to have a column for "Triple-lumen catheter" with either "Yes" or "No" listed for each patient. A search for patients with such a catheter would only require that "Yes" be filtered for in that column. Obviously such a system would become unwieldy if there were a large number of options, but, for limited numbers of choices, looking up data can be very efficient. Many spreadsheets will filter on multiple columns, so that, for example, patients with both a PICC line and a triple-lumen would require only filtering for "Yes" in both of these columns.

Simple Calculation

Although spreadsheets can be used for simple database functions, they were designed primarily to do mathematical calculations. Spreadsheet software can easily handle the nonstatistical data needs of a healthcare epidemiologist. Users can enter very complex formulas, although for most purposes only relatively simple formulas are necessary. Rates, the fundamental calculation of the epidemiologist, are trivial calculations for these programs. Tables can be created to show rates over time such as monthly. As shown in this chapter, such time series also lend themselves to graphing the data.

A great deal of the power of spreadsheets comes from the ability to program formulas that refer to other cells, even cells that are on sheets other than the one with the formulas. This can be used to great advantage. A user can, for example, use one sheet for entering National Nosocomial Infection Surveillance (NNIS) system rates from the Centers for Disease Control and Prevention into designated cells. That way, all other pages are automatically updated for the latest rates without having to enter them into each page or formula separately.

Another powerful capability of spreadsheets is the ability to copy formulas from one cell to another. Thus, once a formula is written (e.g. for a rate calculation) it need not be reentered from scratch over and over again but can simply be copied. One must be careful to ensure that formulas are copied correctly. Each cell in a spreadsheet has a unique address, typically formed by the column letter and row number of that particular cell. Thus, the cell in column "C" on row "22" is designated "C22." Sometimes when copying formulas, the user wants the column or row number to change. Consider a column D with January SSI data. Row 8 has the number of infections and row 9 the number of procedures. Row 10 is designed to have the rates. The user can enter a formula such as (D8/D9)*100 to calculate the SSI rate per 100 surgeries in cell D10 (the exact method to designate that there is a formula within in a cell, as opposed to text alone, will vary depending on the spreadsheet software used). Column E then will represent February data. Rather than retyping the formula in cell E10, the user can copy the formula from row D10. However, the formula must read (E8/E9)*100—the February, not the January, data must be used. In other cases, for example when calculating standardized infection ratios (SIRs), the user will likely want to use the NNIS rate in multiple calculations. If the spreadsheet is set up as previously mentioned, with NNIS rates entered into designated cells, then the user must be sure that that cell reference stays the same even when formulas are copied. Spreadsheet software have different ways to designate whether the cell references can be changed when a formula is copied.

Although users can enter formulas to calculate summary data (e.g., adding up monthly numbers of VAP cases to get annual numbers of VAP cases), most spreadsheet software allows for more automated ways of doing this. These summary tables go by different names depending on the software; Microsoft Excel (Microsoft Corp., Redmond, WA) calls them "Pivot Tables," whereas OpenOffice Calc (OpenOffice.Org, *www.openoffice.org*) uses the term "DataPilot." They can be used to quickly aggregate data into a variety of formats (e.g., number of positive blood cultures by patient care unit by month) that would be tedious to program by hand.

Advanced Statistics

Spreadsheet software programs can readily handle the calculations needed for most statistics. All that one needs is the correct formula for the desired calculations. Devising and entering very complicated formulas, however, is often tedious and error prone. Fortunately, spreadsheet programs typically have a number of built-in statistical functions to facilitate statistical calculations, for example, calculating means and standard deviations.

In addition, these programs typically allow for add-ins. These add-ins are additional pieces of software that extend the functionality of the base program. Statistical add-ins may come with the spreadsheet software itself (but not installed with the basic program) or are available from commercial software houses. As an example, Microsoft Excel comes with additional tools in what is called the "Analysis ToolPak." This allows more advanced statistics, such as analysis of variance (ANOVA), to be run. These add-ins can certainly extend the capabilities of spreadsheets to do fairly advanced statistics; however, even with these functions there is still a need for a significant amount of formula entry by the user (often along with some programming using the macro language available in the software).

In addition to add-ins, spreadsheet templates may be available. These are typically spreadsheets with column or row labels that indicate where data should go. Formulas are already entered in, so that all the user must do is fill in the blanks. These are typically much easier to use than add-ins, but one must be sure that the context for which the template was designed actually fits the user's situation.

For users who are very familiar with their spreadsheet software and who are comfortable modifying formulas in templates that may have been written by others or writing complicated formulas themselves, add-ins and templates may provide a good solution for their needs. For most healthcare epidemiologists, however, a specific statistical software program may be easier to use.

Charting

The visual display of quantitative information is a critical part of communicating infection control information. In addition to performing extensive calculations, graphing data is also at the core of spreadsheet programs. Typical spreadsheet software can provide a variety of graphs. For the epidemiologist, bar graphs and line graphs will be the most often used. Bar graphs can be used to show epidemic curves. Line graphs are especially useful for showing trends over time, for example, SSI rate data. Other interesting data can be shown on the graph, such as the NNIS mean rate, the mean of the local rates, and upper control limits for process control charting (Fig. 15.1). To chart these items, typically a new row is included with the desired value. To have a line across, a value must be present in every column representing a time period. Again, the ability to copy references to other cells and copy formulas is helpful here.

Databases

Although spreadsheets are often used for data storage, there are some distinct drawbacks to doing so in many cases. Databases made in spreadsheets are often termed *flat-file* databases—with their column and row layout they are like a flat sheet of paper. Although many times data collected for epidemiology can easily be fitted to this flat-file model, all too often data are forced to fit this model in an awkward manner. This was somewhat apparent in the previous discussion on using a spreadsheet to capture ICU patient catheter data. One can imagine that if there are multiple variables to be captured, such as microorganisms cultured or which healthcare workers saw a given patient, then any

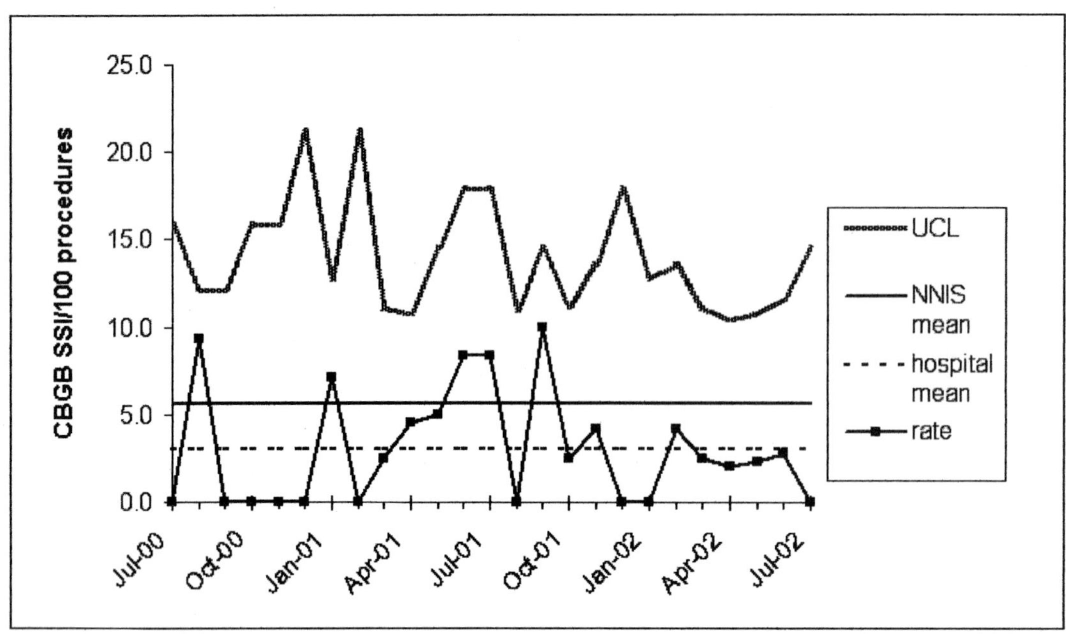

Figure 15.1. Control chart for coronary artery bypass surgery (risk category 2) produced on a personal computer (PC) with spreadsheet software. UCL, upper control limit.

of the options for using a flat-file database would be unmanageable. In such circumstances a true database program is called for.

True database programs were designed specifically for the task of organizing complicated data. There are a variety of types of databases. Some inexpensive database software provide essentially the functionality of electronic index cards. Although such software may be adequate for keeping addresses or recipes, for research purposes these are functionally flat-file databases and, thus, have all of the disadvantages of storing data in spreadsheets. A number of other database types exist, which vary in how they model or represent the data conceptually. Currently, the most popular type is the relational database model. Relational databases are popular because of their flexibility in storing data and their conceptual simplicity. They use multiple tables to store data, with a mechanism for relating the tables to one another. Thus, in the ICU line study example considered previously, one might have one table containing patient demographics, a second table containing information on IV catheters, and a third table with blood culture results. Each item would have associated with it some piece of unique information (such as a medical record number) that could be used to determine which data on one table were related to data on the other table. This relational database model is very powerful, and most large hospital systems are built around relational database systems, such as Oracle (Oracle Corp., Redwood City, CA) or DB2 (IBM, Armonk, NY), that run on mainframe computers or high-end database servers. However, very functional relational database software is available for desktop PCs. This would include programs such as FileMaker Pro (FileMaker, Inc., Santa Clara, CA), StarOffice Base (Sun Microsystem Inc, Santa Clara, CA), and Microsoft Access (Microsoft Corp., Redmond, WA). Such database software may not be included in typical software suites and must be purchased separately.

Using relational databases properly is somewhat more complicated than using spreadsheets. This is to be expected, given the more complicated structure of the information. Most PC-based database software packages have tools that dramatically simplify the use of the program. These tools also make it possible to generate attractive reports from the databases. Because their purpose is different, database programs do not have the broad range of calculating functions present in spreadsheets. Nevertheless, most of these programs can provide some simple information such as tallies or means. To design databases optimally, it is useful to have an understanding of the relational database model. There are large numbers of on-line tutorials and books available, some of which are general (2), and some of which are specific to a particular database program. Although tools and "wizards" are typically used to elicit results from the programs, advanced users can often get results not available otherwise by querying the database directly. Structured query language (SQL) is a relatively simple language designed specifically to extract information from relational databases (3). Although used more often on large-scale databases, PC-based programs typically provide an option for advanced users of querying the database directly. As with spreadsheets, PC-based databases typically allow advanced users to write programs to extend the functionality of the database.

SPECIALIZED SOFTWARE

Although a healthcare epidemiologist could manage with only a standard office suite of software, it would require extensive development work. In particular, spreadsheets and standard databases are not well suited for statistical analysis. Thus, the healthcare epidemiologist must develop familiarity with some software statistics packages. There are both general packages designed to do a broad range of statistics and specialized packages designed specifically for healthcare epidemiology and infection control purposes. These specialized packages often also have data entry, data management, charting, and reporting functions as well.

General Statistical Software

General statistical packages range from simple stand-alone programs that sometimes come bundled with introductory statistics books, to extensive multimodule programs capable of performing even esoteric statistics.

Advanced Statistical Packages

A number of commercial statistical programs are available. SAS (SAS Institute, Cary, NC), SPSS (SPSS Inc., Chicago, IL), MINITAB (Minitab Inc., State College, PA), STATISTICA (StatSoft, Tulsa, OK), and S-plus (Insightful, Seattle, WA) are among the better known. R is an open-source general-purpose statistical package (*http://www.r-project.org/*). Dozens of other general-purpose statistical software packages are available. Many of these programs have a base module with additional add-on packages. All of these programs can do basic statistics well. There are differences in their ease of use, graphics capability, ability to write macros (small programs to automate repetitive processes), and advanced statistics. Typically, the more powerful and versatile the program, the more significant is the learning curve even to do basic statistics. Also, the more advanced the software is, the more expensive the software tends to be. Most of these general-purpose statistical packages will do everything a healthcare epidemiologist needs. Once a program has been learned (perhaps in a statistics course), then there is no need to change unless a needed function is unavailable. Indeed, most of these packages are overkill for routine healthcare epidemiologic needs.

EpiInfo

EpiInfo is a program available at no charge from the CDC (4). Originally designed for Epidemiology Intelligence Service officers to perform outbreak investigations, it has grown into an extensive data management and analysis tool.

Brief History of EpiInfo

EpiInfo was released in 1985 as the Epidemiologic Analysis System. It was developed by Andrew Dean (and written in large part by his son, then a high school student). Andy Dean had been invited to the CDC in 1984 to develop software for epidemiologists. By 1986 it was renamed EpiInfo. The software provided field epidemiologists with a relatively easy to use package for obtaining, entering, analyzing, and reporting on outbreak data. It was first field tested during a syphilis outbreak in Ft. Lauderdale, FL by EIS officer Dr. Consuelo Beck-Sagué. EpiInfo was designed to run on IBM-compatible PCs running MS-DOS, which was clearly becoming the standard PC-computing environment.

Over the next 7 years more versions were released with increased capabilities. These years also saw more widespread adoption of the software. In 1992 version 6 was released, the last DOS version (4). This added even further statistical and graphical functionality. Distribution over the Internet started in 1994. Y2K corrections were added in 1997. By then the program was in use in at least 127 countries, and the manual had been translated into 13 additional languages. The most recent revisions were added in January 2001, to allow the program to run properly on faster computers (>200 MHz). This version, 6.04d, is likely to be the last DOS release of EpiInfo.

EpiInfo 2000 was released in June 2000. Rewritten from the ground up, this version of EpiInfo was a dramatic departure from the old version, providing Windows users a familiar mouse-driven interface instead of the command line driven interface of the older versions. An updated version, EpiInfo 2002, was released in the summer of 2002; this version will be referred to simply as EpiInfo in the rest of this discussion.

EpiInfo normally does not run on Macintosh computers or computers running other OSs such as Linux. Because it was written in Microsoft Visual Basic and uses Microsoft Access as the underlying file format, it is unlikely that it will ever be able to run natively on anything other than computers running MS Windows.

Survey of Tools in EpiInfo

EpiInfo consists of five main programs. One, called Nutstat, is for nutritional anthropometry. It is of limited interest to most healthcare epidemiologists. During installation of EpiInfo, it is possible to choose not to install this (or any other) component. This option may be particularly attractive for computers with limited hard disk space (such as laptop computers). The other components are MakeView, Enter, Analysis, and EpiMap. EpiInfo also has a number of utility programs for functions such as converting existing database table to EpiInfo tables and comparing data in two similar tables.

EpiInfo was designed to facilitate epidemiologic analysis from start to finish. MakeView allows the user to design data entry screens for collecting pertinent data. Data entry screens can be made more attractive and functional by allowing related data items to be gathered into a group, which may have a distinct background to aid the person entering the data. Because EpiInfo was built on a true relational database, MakeView allows for the collection of related data in separate tables. For example, a data collection tool for ventilator-associated pneumonia may have a separate table to enter the microorganism; this avoids the "entry1" and "entry2" problem noted earlier in the flat-file database discussion. Unlike most database programs, EpiInfo automatically maintains the proper relationship between the tables. To generate data collection forms, it is possible to print the data entry forms from MakeView. However, using a word processing program to design the forms will yield more control over the printed version and allow for a more aesthetic data collection tool.

The Enter program allows users to enter data into the questionnaire previously designed in MakeView. Enter also allows for searching of entered data.

EpiMap allows the user to link data contained in EpiInfo files to maps. For example, a colored scale could be used to show the number of salmonella cases by county within a state. EpiMap uses maps in the popular ESRI SHAPE file format. SHAPE files for all U.S. states and many countries are available from the EpiInfo Web site. The site also has links to other resources for understanding geographical information systems (GISs). Tools are available to create custom maps. Industrious epidemiologists could create maps of their hospitals for displaying data.

The Analysis program provides multiple options for statistical analysis of data. In addition to reading data entered using MakeView and Enter, Analysis can import data from other database and spreadsheet formats and from older versions of EpiInfo. Analysis provides a full range of data manipulation and analysis tools. Basic statistics include simple frequency tabulations; contingency tables (which can be stratified); and ANOVA, both parametric and nonparametric. Analysis also provides some basic charting functions, but the graphics are not as versatile as a spreadsheet. Advanced statistical functions include linear and logistic regression, Kaplan-Meier survival, Cox proportional hazards, and complex sample statistics (contingency tables and ANOVA). Users can also create new variables within Analysis, and can use fairly complicated rules to assign values to these new variables based on the values of existing data. Short programs for automating analyses that are done repeatedly can be written and stored in Analysis.

Overall EpiInfo 2002 provides the healthcare epidemiologist with essentially all of the statistical analysis tools that he or she will need. Like any complicated program, learning to use the entire package well takes studying and practice. However, the program is simple enough that users who are familiar with the fundamentals of statistics used in healthcare epidemiology (see Chapters 2 and 3) and who have data in a compatible format will be able to run fairly complicated analyses shortly after installing the program. The program comes with extensive on-line help. The same content can be downloaded as manuals in both Microsoft Word and Adobe Acrobat (.pdf) formats. A tutorial and exercises are included to get users up to speed with the various components of the software. A quick Internet search will turn up other tutorials and educational materials to assist new users.

Older Versions of EpiInfo and Related Software

As noted previously, EpiInfo 6.04d was the last release of the MS-DOS based versions of the program. It is still available for download from the EpiInfo Web site and continues to enjoy widespread use even for Windows-based computers. Because it is much less resource intensive, EpiInfo 6 might be able to run on older equipment even if EpiInfo 2002 cannot. Many epidemiologists have developed extensive data collection and analysis systems based on EpiInfo 6. Through years of use, they are very familiar with the commands line interface. For these users, there may be very little if any incentive to spend the time converting the system to EpiInfo 2002 (see the opening discussion of this chapter on upgrading).

For those who are comfortable doing data analysis using EpiInfo 6 but who would like a more Windows-friendly way to enter data, a program called EpiData is available (5). EpiData is a comprehensive program for data entry and data documentation. Files can be saved in EpiInfo 6 format so that data can be analyzed using EpiInfo 6. A data analysis program may be developed in the future. EpiData is currently being developed by an international team of programmers.

Other Statistical Software

In addition to full-fledged, general-purpose statistical software, there are times when all that is needed is a fairly narrow tool. There are scores (if not hundreds) of relatively limited purpose statistics programs available. A quick Internet search will usually turn these up readily. A particularly helpful program that came with EpiInfo 6 was StatCalc. This could quickly do contingency table statistics (if summary data were already available) and sample size calculations. EpiInfo 2002 includes the same StatCalc program, which is run in a DOS window. A free Windows-based program that does the same thing plus a bit more is EpiCalc 2000, written by Mark Myatt. It is available at his Web site (*http://www.myatt.demon.co.uk/*); this site also has other free utility programs available. A similar program, EpiTool, which runs on Palm OS personal digital assistants (PDAs), is available from the Johns Hopkins Healthcare Epidemiology and Infection Control Web site (*http://www.hopkins-heic.com/*). These programs are mentioned as an example of programs that we have found useful. Because Web sites can come and go rapidly and because Internet searching tools (e.g., Google; *http://www.google.com*) have become fairly dependable, one can quickly search for specialized programs.

Specialized Infection Control Programs

In addition to general purpose statistical software, software developed specifically for infection control purposes is available. AICE (ICPA, Austin, TX) and EpiQuest (EpiQuest LLC, Key Largo, FL) are two such packages. ICE Tools [Association for Professionals in Infection Control and Epidemiology (APIC), Washington DC] is actually not a stand-alone program but is an add-in program for Microsoft Excel that is designed specifically for infection control purposes. Other programs are available. Some programs popular in the past, however, such as Q-Logic II, no longer seem to be available. Some software packages are available only to participants in certain programs. One such example is IDEAS, for hospitals participating in the NNIS system, sponsored by the CDC. It allows data to be entered and sent to the CDC for aggregation. However, it also allows participant hospitals to generate reports on the surgeries they follow for NNIS.

Specialized programs guide users in selecting and analyzing data. This is especially useful for those just starting out in infection control or computers (or both). The trade off is that by nature these programs are less flexible than general-purpose tools and, thus, may be difficult to tailor to any particular circumstances or ad hoc studies. Some specialized software can be somewhat expensive. However, instead of considering the cost alone, one must consider the cost in time and effort to set up general-purpose tools to do the same thing that the specific programs can do. Unless someone locally is facile at setting up spreadsheets and databases or specific research needs are not provided by the specialized software, specialized infection control software may be a very cost effective purchase.

INFORMATION MANAGEMENT—TYING IT ALL TOGETHER

All of the capabilities reviewed previously make it clear that computers are an extremely useful tool for healthcare epidemiologists. However, they remain just that—a tool to work with. They can only work with the information they are given, and they do exactly what they are told.

Application Design

Before designing a system, several issues must be considered: What are the data going to be used for, and what information actually must be on the computer. Are the data going to be used for calculations of rates and generating graphs? Are they simply going to be used to generate text reports? Will statistical analysis be necessary? Will the data have to be queried often, and if so, how complicated will the queries be? The answers to these questions regarding the purpose will begin to suggest what program to base the system on.

Regarding what data actually must be entered, one must consider that it may not be necessary to enter every bit of information gathered into the computer, especially if data will initially be gathered on paper forms that will be retained. Some thought should be given beforehand to exactly what calculations, statistics, and queries will be needed. However, one must also consider that once information is on the computer, it will be relatively easy to manipulate this information. Uses may come to mind after the initial design is finished, and it is always easier to enter data initially than it is to go back and fill in missing data. There must be a careful balance between entering every conceivable small piece of information only because one can and being so spare with data entry that the data cannot be put to extended uses. The format of the data will also suggest what type of program to base the system on: Will the data fit easily into a flat-file format, or will a relational design be needed?

In many circumstances a single program cannot do everything desired. Fortunately, it is often quite straightforward to share data between programs. For example, a relational database might be established for data storage, but then a query could be used to generate a table that could be exported to a spreadsheet to generate a graph. Thus, there is no need to "shoe-horn" data into a bad design.

Data Types

An important consideration when using databases and many statistical programs is the notion of "data type." Spreadsheet programs also include this concept to some degree. People are typically unaware of the concept, because they are able to convert readily and intuitively between data types. Computers, however, store all information internally as a series of binary digits (zeroes and ones), as noted in Chapter 14. For example, the series "01010101" may represent the capital letter "U" or the integer 85, or it may even represent something else entirely, depending on the software that is interpreting that sequence of digits. Conversely, "1" may be represented within the computer by the sequence "00000001" (representing the actual number) or "00011111" (representing the printed character for one in a specified character set). Even numbers are represented differently depending on whether integers or real numbers (numbers with decimal points) are involved.

In order for database and other programs to manipulate the information correctly, one must tell the program what kind of data are represented in a given field. Thus, if one has a field called "Date of Birth" one could tell the program to store the entry as plain text. This may be perfectly adequate for one's purposes. On the other hand, if later one want to have the computer calculate the person's age, rather than do it manually, it would make more sense to tell the program that "Date of Birth" contained a date. Although not usually considered a number, dates are usually stored in the computer as a single number. This allows the program to easily do mathematical calculations with the date. Does it make sense to do math on dates? Certainly—one can take someone's birth date and today's date to determine how old they are in years, or one can add 7 days to today's date to get the date for next week. Thus, dates are a good candidate to store internally as a number. Another advantage of being very specific about data types is that it helps prevent data entry errors. A typist may recognize that Feb 30 is an incorrect value, but a program expecting a date to be entered will complain if someone attempts to enter that as a value.

The exact number of data types available will depend on the program involved. A few basic types are typically always available. "Text" is just that. In addition to obvious uses (e.g., names and addresses), one must consider that some entries that contain only digits are not numbers but text. (e.g., phone numbers and social security numbers). Although these are sequences of digits, are they really "numbers"? A good rule of thumb for making this decision is whether or not it makes sense to do mathematical calculations on the item under consideration. Thus, in the previous example, it made sense that computers stored dates internally as numbers, because one could do calculations on dates. However, no one would want to add a specific value to social security numbers, and taking the mean of telephone numbers makes no sense. Thus, things such as social security numbers and phone numbers are not really numbers. In the past, such items were sometimes designated as numbers to decrease the size of the resulting file (storing a social security number as text takes at least 9 bytes, whereas storing it as a single number takes as little as 4 bytes); however, in this era of inexpensive storage this approach is no longer necessary. Thus, the text data type can easily be used for these nonnumbers. Another text type may be available for long text entries (e.g., a multiline address or an extended note).

Numerical data types must be used for data that are to be manipulated mathematically. As noted previously, some non-number numbers can be stored as a numerical data type, but there is no advantage to doing so. Some programs make a distinction between integer and real numbers. Integers are numbers (positive or negative) with no fractional parts, whereas real numbers can have fractional parts. In the case of computers, it may be easiest to think of integers as numbers without decimal points. For computers, this distinction is quite important, because it affects how the numbers are stored internally. It also makes a difference in that integer arithmetic is exact, whereas mathematical calculations with real numbers may involve some rounding errors. Some programs may even distinguish between kinds of integers (e.g., integers and long integers) and kinds of real numbers (single and double). This has to do with the number of bytes used to store the information. The more bytes used, the bigger the number that can be stored (and in the case of double precision real numbers, it also allows for even smaller numbers to be stored). However, with real numbers if very small numbers are added to very large ones, the small numbers will likely be lost in rounding error. All of these distinctions are not usually significant for the healthcare epidemiologists. However, it is important to be aware of the distinctions when making choices in these programs. In some cases, integers must be used for keys in relational databases (see the database section). If given a choice, real numbers must be used for any value with a decimal point. For values that will never need a decimal point, integers are typically the better choice. However, real numbers may be used for some of these values and are a better choice if there is any chance that decimals will be used in the future. Another example is "weight"; weight may be recorded in pounds, and an integer data type may be used for the field. However, if later the decision is made to record the weight to the nearest 0.1 lb, then a real data type is required; the existing data may or may not be able to be converted, depending on the software used. If weight had been saved as real initially, then no changes would need to be made. Thus, unless the numbers involved can never occur in anything less than whole intervals, one should choose a real data type if given the option. Age should probably be saved as a real number, because, although age is usually written as an integer, an age of 40.5 years has meaning. However, the number of people present in the operating room (OR) must be an integer, and, thus, an integer data type may safely be chosen.

A variety of other data types may be available in some programs. A "Date" data type may exist. As noted previously, the date may then be stored internally as a number, allowing calculations to be performed on it. Date calculations are specialized; thus, the programs typically do not allow all mathematical operations to be done on dates (e.g., the date cannot be multiplied by 3). A "Time" data type may also be included (often associated with the date data type). A Yes/No (or True/False; also known as Boolean) data type may be available for situations in which these are the only two possible answers.

Some programs require that data types be designated explicitly. Other programs (e.g., many spreadsheets) will assign a data type based on what is entered. This "best guess" may not be immediately obvious or apparent to the user. However, if one is aware that this is going on, one may understand otherwise confusing behavior of the software. Numbers, for example, typically have leading zeros removed. Thus, if a zip code of "00258" is entered, it may show simply as "258." The column should be explicitly designated as text to ensure that all of the leading zeros are retained. Likewise, when a fragment of a date (e.g., Feb 26) is typed in, the software may assume that this is a reference to the twenty-sixth of February of the current year and assign its data type as a date, when actually a plain text type may be preferred. This can lead to confusing formatting or other issues unless the underlying data type is considered. One must be aware that the choice of data type will also affect how data are sorted. If stored as text, the following are sorted appropriately: 1, 10, 100, 2, 20, 200, whereas they would be sorted differently if stored as integers.

Aside from the actual data type, programs will also often provide a way to format the data in a particular way. This will affect how the data are displayed. For example, real numbers may only show two digits to the right of the decimal point. The program may also be able to require that the data fit a particular pattern before it is accepted. Thus, it may be possible to require that a social security number be entered as ddd-dd-dddd (where *d* is any digit), even if the data type is plain text. In some programs, commonly used data elements such as phone number may actually be incorporated as its own data type. In addition to requiring that data entered fit a certain pattern, it may also be possible to limit data entry to certain values or ranges (e.g., allowing only "M" or "F" for entry into the "Gender" field).

Data Design

Choosing a plan for organizing data and data types at the beginning of a study is sometimes difficult. For variables that may be exposure variables, the best choice may be a Yes/No (or True/False) data type—this will allow for classic 2 × 2 tables to be set up. However, if it is clear early in the study that a large number of Yes/No variables are involved, setting up (and filling out) large numbers of Yes/No questions is tedious and may lead to erroneous results because of multiple comparisons. Using related tables to capture information (e.g., a list of foods eaten for each attendee of a potluck dinner as part of a food-poisoning investigation) may be an easier solution. Fortunately, most database and statistical packages allow the creation of new variables after-the-fact. They also typically provide some means for automatically assigning the new variables a value based on the value of one or more of the existing variables. Thus, once overall data has been reviewed, a new Yes/No variable can be created for contingency table analysis. For example, after reviewing the list of foods consumed by attendees at a potluck, a few dishes may be of particular interest. A new variable "Chicken Tartare" could be created and assigned the value "Y" if it is on a person's list, and "N" otherwise. Likewise, other variables could be created for further analysis. Learning how to use the recoding functionality of any database or statistics software will pay large dividends. Data can be collected in the most efficient manner possible and yet still be subjected to any desired analysis, even if that analysis was not envisioned when the initial data collection was designed.

Data Acquisition

Manual Entry

Before computers can do anything, they need data to work on. Often, this data is entered into the computer manually. A number of things can be done to improve this process. Data entry screens should mirror paper forms to the extent possible. This will help ensure that the correct items get entered into the correct locations. If data entry locations are aligned on the screen, entry into the computer is easier (just as with a paper form, it is more visually appealing). One should try to minimize the movement of the hands—do not have one data item require the keyboard, the next the mouse, then the keyboard again, and so forth. Many programs (e.g., EpiInfo 2002) allow the user to use the "Tab" and/or "Enter" keys to advance to the next field that requires data. They may also allow the order in which the data are entered to be specified. If so, one must ensure that the data entry runs (to the degree possible) from left-to-right and top-to-bottom rather than jumping around the page (non-European languages may have different directions, but the dictum not to jump around the page holds). Similarly, spreadsheets typically allow the user to specify whether hitting the Enter key moves the cursor right or down, so that data can be entered in rows or columns easily from the keyboard.

Scanning

The availability of inexpensive scanners and form analysis software makes it possible to enter data by scanning data entry forms. Appropriate forms can be designed so that an "X" or similar mark can be interpreted by the software and entered into a database. This approach has been used successfully for infection control data entry (6).

Information from Local Computers

Even if desired information already resides on computers elsewhere in the hospital, it may be easier to enter such data manually than to try to devise and implement a way to directly transfer this data from one computer to another. Collecting this information may involve copying the data onto an intermediate paper form or reading the data from one window in the computer as it is typed into a program in another window. It may be possible to "cut-and-paste" information between two computer programs; however, issues such as formatting and data types must be considered when doing so.

Other data in the hospital may already exist in computer files that could be easily copied. This may include things such as spreadsheets of all surgeries done in the last month. An inquiry to the administrators of various departments may turn up such reports. The file may be sent via e-mail (the easiest alternative nowadays) or via direct transfer of the file using what is called file transfer protocol (FTP); software to do this is readily available but is not as convenient as e-mail. Alternatively, the file might reside on a shared directory or disk drive, from which it could be accessed. If this is the case, one must be certain not to alter data that is also used by others—making a copy to a local hard drive (if permitted to do so) will allow the data to be manipulated without interfering with other use of the files. The disadvantage to this approach is that the data may have been updated since the latest local copy was made.

For larger volumes of data, especially if it needed often, it would be worth the effort to get the information into a format that can be read directly. The software that is generating the needed data (e.g., an OR scheduling system from which surgical case denominator data is desired) may be able to readily generate a report in a format that can be used by the healthcare epidemiologist's software. This may have to be some intermediate format (i.e., it is not the format typically used by either program) but a common format that one program can write to and the other can read from. Otherwise, a file conversion program [written by the IS staff for this purpose or a commercially available program such as DBMS/Copy (Dataflux, Cary, NC)] may be needed to convert the data into a usable format.

Personal Digital Assistants and Laptops

PDAs (see Chapter 14) offer the possibility of data entry at the site of data gathering. They have the advantage of being extremely portable and relatively inexpensive. Thus, ICPs could enter data into the PDA while doing chart reviews on the wards. The information could then be "synchronized" with a desktop computer when they returned to the office. A variety of software packages are available that allow data to be collected on PDAs and then imported into desktop spreadsheet or database programs. The choice of one of these programs will largely be driven by which PDA platform is being used and which programs on the desktop computer need to import the information. Typically, these programs allow data to be exported to the PDA as well, so that all information (e.g., patient name) need not be entered directly into the PDA. The PDA software may allow the design of data entry forms with check boxes and lists of items to choose from. By minimizing text that has to be written, the speed of overall data entry is improved, and the chance for incorrect entries is minimized. However, the small screen size of the PDA may require the user to page through a number of screens to enter all of the required information.

Laptop computers are another option for data entry on-site. Unlike PDAs, laptops may be relatively heavy and certainly more expensive. Battery life limitations may require awkward set-ups with power cords, and the laptop requires desk space that may not be readily available on a nursing unit. Nevertheless, data entry is likely to be much faster than with PDAs if a lot of text entry is required. The speed of choosing from check boxes and lists is no faster than with PDAs, except for the advantage of the larger screens. Tablet computers are just being introduced. These potentially combine some of the advantages of laptops and PDAs. It is too soon to tell whether they will achieve widespread use and whether programs will be designed to take advantage of that form factor.

Data Validation and Integrity

GIGO—garbage in, garbage out. This dictum is well known to anyone who works with data. It is incumbent on the healthcare epidemiologist to ensure that the correct information is being collected. Periodic audits of data on the computer compared with primary sources will help ensure that the data being used are valid. This is especially true if the data are imported from other sources. For example, if two columns in a spreadsheet from which data are extracted are swapped for the convenience of those generating the report, this could dramatically affect any automated data input system if it were not caught immediately. For manual entry of important data, one should consider performing double entry. In this system all items are entered independently into two identical files, then the files are compared to ensure that there are no differences.

Proper data integrity requires that data be shared only with those who need the information. Healthcare epidemiologists and ICPs should have broad access to data, but this privilege is balanced by the responsibility to only copy what data are needed and to ensure that it is not released to others inappropriately. Although the Health Insurance Portability and Accountability Act of 1996 (HIPAA) is beyond the scope of this chapter, data collected by the healthcare epidemiologist or ICPs and used only for internal quality improvement purposes should not raise any patient consent or reporting issues under HIPAA. If uncertain about a particular use of data, clarification can be obtained from the hospital's HIPAA compliance office.

To ensure data integrity, frequent data backups should also be made, so that known good data can be used in the event files are lost or corrupted by computer malfunctions. The longer the time interval between backups, the more data that will have to be reentered. It may not even be possible to recreate all of the data entered if too long an interval has passed since the last backup. This would then lead to having incomplete data for subsequent use.

Data Dissemination

Just as computers can facilitate data collection, they can facilitate data dissemination. In addition to printing attractive reports, data may be sent in electronic format via e-mail. Alternatively, it may be posted to a Web site for download or even displayed on a Web site directly. For end users, it is generally better to use graphs or simple tables to convey information. For surgical site infections, use of the standardized infection ratio (SIR) may be preferable to showing extensive data for all risk categories. Unfortunately, computers can make it too easy to decorate reports and graphs with unnecessary clutter. Tufte's *The Visual Display of Quantitative Information* (7) is an excellent starting point for determining how to convey the message clearly. Other similar texts would likewise be useful.

REFERENCES

1. Schifman RB, Palmer RA. Surveillance of nosocomial infections by computer analysis of positive culture rates. *J Clin Microbiol* 1985;21: 493–495.
2. Hernandez MJ. Database Design for Mere Mortals. Reading, MA: Addison-Wesley Developers Press, 1997.
3. Hernandez MJ, Viescas JL. SQL Queries for Mere Mortals Boston: Addison-Wesley, 2000.
4. Dean AG, Dean JA, Coulombier D, et al. EpiInfo, version 6: a word-processing, database, and statistics program for public health on IBM-compatible microcomputers. Atlanta, GA: Centers for Disease Control and Prevention, Atlanta, GA, 1995.
5. Lauritsen JM, Bruus M., Myatt MA. EpiData (version 2.1). An extended tool for validated entry and documentation of data. Odense, Denmark: The EpiData Association, 2001–2002 (available at *http://www.epidata.dk*).
6. Thompson IM. Automated entry of nosocomial infection surveillance data: use of an optical scanning system. *J Hosp Infect* 1999;43(Suppl): S275–S278.
7. Tufte ER. *The visual display of quantitative information,* 2nd ed. Chesire, CT: Graphics Press, 2001.

16

THE ELECTRONIC HEALTH RECORD: AN ESSENTIAL TECHNOLOGY FOR HOSPITAL EPIDEMIOLOGY

WILLIAM H. TETTELBACH
DAVID C. CLASSEN

Healthcare is an information-intensive industry. Information management is integral to clinical practice and little occurs in the complex matrix of healthcare that does not involve information management (1–49). Clinicians, among their other unique attributes, are information managers. In the day-to-day practice of medicine they must acquire, process, store, retrieve, and apply information. This ability is paramount to the delivery of efficient and optimal healthcare. During the last 50 years, information management has risen to a pivotal role in modern healthcare (1, 2,25–28,34,42). There has been an explosion of information in healthcare. Medline now indexes approximately 360,000 new articles each year from those published in the biomedical literature. In addition to more knowledge, there has been a corollary growth in patient-specific information. The volume and complexity of patient information has increased dramatically. This increase is due to multiple factors that have occurred in healthcare, such as the greater number of patient visits, higher patient acuity, a proliferation of new data elements arising from new diagnostic techniques, and developments in the delivery system that result in many patients receiving care at multiple sites. This dramatic growth has resulted in a situation where effective clinical information management has exceeded the cognitive capabilities of the human mind. Some authors have referred to this phenomenon as "information pollution" (44). In fact, in modern healthcare we are drowning in data and starving for information.

Providing high-quality, cost-effective healthcare is an information-dependent process. Each provider and class of providers in healthcare has developed a unique set of information requirements. However, at some point in the healthcare delivery process other providers need access to those information sets. The medical record is the repository of information concerning the patient's healthcare. Virtually everyone involved in providing, receiving, and reimbursing for healthcare is affected by the medical record.

It has been estimated that as many as 22 different people need access to a hospital patient's medical record at any given time (17). An estimated 35% to 39% of total hospital operating costs has been associated with provider and patient information activities. Physicians spend an estimated 38% and nurses and estimated 50% of their time documenting in the patient's medical record. Furthermore, 70% of hospital patients' paper medical records are incomplete. This lack of detail is reflected in the fact that 40% of the time the paper medical record does not contain the patient's diagnosis and 27% of the time the patient's chief complaint is not documented. This lack of completeness also results in 11% of laboratory tests that have to be reordered, because the results are not in the patient's paper medical record.

Despite the many technologic advances in healthcare over the last 50 years and the plethora of associated problems with the typical patient record, the record has not changed much. The failure of the modern patient record to have evolved with the other technologic advances in healthcare is now creating additional stress within the already burdened U.S. healthcare system. Because of this failure, the information needs of providers, patients, administrators, third-party payers, researchers, and policy makers are often unmet.

An automated patient record, often known as the electronic health record (EHR), is a method to deal with the failures of the traditional paper record (1,14,15,17,34). The EHR could make a major contribution to improving the information management problems of healthcare. A 1991 General Accounting Office (GAO) report on automated patient records identified three major ways in which improved patient records can benefit healthcare (1). First, an automated patient record can improve healthcare delivery by providing multiple data access, faster data retrieval, and higher quality data. The EHR also provides decision-support capabilities, provides clinical reminders to assist patient care, and supports quality improvement activities. Second, computer-stored medical records have the potential to enhance outcomes research by automatically capturing clinical information for evaluation. Third, automated patient records can increase hospital efficiency by reducing costs and improving staff productivity. The GAO reported that an automated patient record system reduced hospital costs by $600 per patient in a Department of Veterans Affairs hospital because of shorter lengths of stay.

HISTORICAL PERSPECTIVE ON HEALTHCARE AUTOMATION

The current status of hospital information systems and their attendant EHRs can best be understood by recalling the retrospective cost reimbursement system in place in the United States from 1966 through the end of 1983 (2,14,17,44,50). This system created a number of inducements that suspended general economic principles and obviated most price/benefit decisions for almost two decades. The incentives created under the retrospective cost reimbursement system were mainly those to spend and fostered a hospital industry with a "blank check" mentality with little regard for expenses. These perverse incentives are most dramatically revealed by noting that inpatient hospital expenditures under Medicare have increased at a rate of about 19% per year since 1970. Retrospective cost reimbursement did little to encourage either efficient operations or the collection of data with which to systematically analyze the healthcare process. In fact, this reimbursement system fostered an environment where technologic innovations and changes in delivery of healthcare occurred with little consideration of costs or cost/benefits.

The original Medicare Act not only fostered this peculiar inducement to spend, but also helped to create a bizarre accounting system (50). The accounting system was essentially a process-costing scheme that allowed direct costs to be processed as charges. This scheme is rooted in the assumption that usual daily operations are similar enough that only direct costs need to be accounted for specifically, with the remainder absorbed as overhead. Another feature of this payment method was that retrospective reimbursement was based on the "least of costs or charges." Hospitals would simply analyze their aggregate yearly charges and compare them to their aggregate yearly costs. Based on these comparisons and analyses, a payment figure would be negotiated between the fiscal intermediary and the hospital. Since healthcare reimbursement was limited to this method, hospitals focused their information systems on capturing identifiable charges, often to the point that they were spending five dollars in processing a charge for a one-cent item (that is, the costs of capture were greater than the costs of the items) (44, 50). This flawed approach resulted in hospitals spending large sums to capture small charges that any conventional business would have included as overhead, and including the single largest component of their costs, direct labor, as overhead (a fallacious assumption that these costs were about the same for each patient). Compounding this was the willingness of the federal government and then private insurers (following the federal lead) to adopt these charge figures as their basis for reimbursement. An eventuality of this practice was "cost-sharing," since charges virtually always exceeded costs. Cost-sharing is the allocation of significant portions of reimbursements by private insurers to offset losses in other parts of the institution's operations.

Considering the importance and predominance of charges during the almost 20 years of retrospective reimbursement, most of the information systems developed in hospitals were focused on capturing charges. For all practical purposes, these information systems were financial systems and were not developed to manage or be concerned with clinical information (1,44,50). However, as these financial systems were expanded throughout the hospital to capture charges at the nursing stations and the bedside, it was realized that a "fringe benefit" of these information systems was data communication.

Another significant and interesting development in information systems during this period was stimulated with the increasing role of ancillary departments in hospitals, such as pharmacy, laboratory, and radiology. It was soon realized that even though these ancillary departments represented a low percentage of the hospital's total number of employees, peculiarities in the retrospective cost reimbursement formulas allowed each of these departments to be repaid more than their actual incurred costs. In the hospital industry these departments were referred to as "revenue centers." As a consequence of this status, ancillary departments were able to command the attention of administration as well as hospital resources out of proportion to their relative size. With this newfound influence, ancillary departments often brought pressures on administration to purchase individual ancillary information systems. A peculiar twist for this era was that the justification for these systems was usually based on service improvement and quality enhancement rather than charge recovery.

The demise of retrospective reimbursement and the concomitant rise of prospective payment or managed care, as it is now known, have changed hospitals' perspective on information and their information needs. To effectively compete in the era of healthcare reform, hospitals are now eager to have information that enhances their operations and allows them to determine their costs (as compared to charge information) and to optimize their delivery of healthcare (1,17,44). The new focus on cost/benefit relationships has forced hospitals to perform rigorous financial and administrative analysis on virtually all of the activities performed in the institution. Such analyses must be available on a patient-by-patient, provider-by-provider, resource-by-resource, and diagnosis-by-diagnosis basis. It is also impossible, in healthcare, to analyze fiscal impacts without simultaneously considering quality implications and outcomes. From an information management standpoint, these analyses and the logistical problems associated with them become seemingly insurmountable if patient information is not consolidated and integrated into a single, patient-oriented clinical record.

Hospitals discovered this harsh reality after initial attempts to gather information and perform analyses from the paper medical record failed miserably. The paper medical record is often unwieldy and the data collected inaccurate. Furthermore, the task of gathering the data for a paper medical record is often more work than performing the task that created the data. Hospitals, regulators, providers, and payers have learned that the logical solution to these problems is the EHR.

The patient is the central information unit in healthcare and patient care is the goal of the healthcare delivery system (2). The EHR provides patient-specific integrated information that is collected departmentally and is available on an institution-wide basis in an organized, comprehensive, accurate, timely, and accessible form. Uncontrolled and unorganized information (as available in the paper record) leads to "information pollution" and is a counterproductive force in an information-oriented industry (44). Information collected, presented, and available in an electronic form becomes a valuable resource.

OVERVIEW OF MEDICAL INFORMATION SYSTEMS

With any endeavor in healthcare, there are definitions and acronyms that one has to be familiar with to effectively communicate. This is particularly true in the area of healthcare information management. The glossary at the end of this chapter lists these terms. With respect to information systems, Ledley and Lusted (51) in 1960 defined an information system as consisting of three essential components: a system for organizing or documenting the information in a file; a method or a routine for accessing the information in the file; and a method to ensure that the information was current. Lindberg (52) took the definition a step further and concluded that a medical information system (MIS) contained a set of formal arrangements by which health-related facts, those concerning the individual health of the patient as well as the care of that patient, were stored and processed in computers (27–29). Based on this conception, an MIS is a complex hierarchical integration of multiple systems that include a hospital information system (HIS); an outpatient information system (OIS); and several clinical support systems (CSSs), such as pharmacy, radiology, and laboratory information systems (Fig. 16.1). When a true MIS exists, it results in a longitudinal patient record that contains the complete health status and healthcare delivery of an individual patient from birth to death. The HIS and OIS components of an MIS usually include subsystems such as an administrative information system (AIS) and a clinical information system (CIS). The AIS component of a hospital or outpatient information system is designed to meet the administrative and financial information needs of the organization. The usual or required data elements found in an AIS include the following: patient demographic, eligibility, and payer data; patient identification, registration, and appointment schedules; hospital admission, discharge, and transfer data; bed census or occupancy data; cost accounting; resource utilization; employee records; and inventory. Generally, AISs are the first computer applications in a hospital or outpatient setting.

The CIS component of a hospital or outpatient information system is designed to manage information concerning the direct care of the patient and is the foundation of the EHR. The CIS contains both objective and subjective clinical data. Because the practice of medicine and the delivery of healthcare is a dynamic process, the functional requirements of a CIS are continually changing as new treatments, procedures, and diagnostics evolve. However, certain functional requirements are always a prerequisite in a CIS. Some of these functions include an EHR that can communicate and manage patient data from multiple sources (e.g., pharmacy, radiology, surgery, laboratory, etc.) within the healthcare delivery system; provide healthcare workers with decision-support tools; provide a clinical database for epidemiologic research; support medical education; maintain patient confidentiality; and satisfy the requirement for the integrity, reliability, and security of patient data.

In the United States, the hospital has been recognized since the 1960s as the natural laboratory for automation and computerization in healthcare. This realization was partly due to the complexity of the information available in hospitals and the fact that the hospital represented the largest segment of the healthcare industry, commanding over 50% of all healthcare spending (50). Additionally, hospitals have a tradition of collecting information and developing rates for defined outcomes such as mortality, length of stay, and costs for various diagnoses and surgical procedures (53–55). Indeed, the hospital setting is probably the most sophisticated segment of the healthcare market with respect to information management. To date, no clinically functioning MIS exists. There are, however, several working examples of HISs. This chapter discusses the principles of medical computing and the EHR in the context of the HIS. These principles and lessons are applicable when discussing a functional MIS.

The basic kinds of information that hospitals require and manage have changed little since the early 1960s. What has changed is the volume of that information and the recognition that numerous providers need simultaneous access to the information. Because of these factors and healthcare's insatiable demand for information, the HIS has become a key emerging technology in U.S. hospitals. The main requirement for an HIS to meet the information management needs of a hospital is to have an integrated database (18,56–58). Friedman and Dieterle (18) have called integration the "holy grail of hospital computing." To effectively use patient-care data to improve outcomes and manage care, hospitals need access to fully integrated information. The primary function of an HIS is to communicate data (56). To perform this function, an HIS must have software and hardware components that allow the computer to acquire, process, store, retrieve, and rearrange data, and then display that data throughout the institution. The premise that underlies this design strategy is that many providers, including the medical staff, nurses, pharmacists, radiology, laboratory, respiratory therapy, physical therapy, occupational therapy, dietary, and so on, create patient-care data, and those providers need access at almost all times to a variety of patient-care data. The key is that the provider-created data must be inclusive. Within an integrated HIS, the design should allow for patient data to be entered once and then be available for all users. Ideally, data should be entered at the point of care. For example, the temperature of a patient should be entered into the HIS at the bedside, once the healthcare provider has obtained the temperature. This allows for maximum use of patient data, since clinical data are now temporally related to the course of hospitalization. This temporal relationship allows providers to analyze the patient's clinical progress and to relate outcomes to specific events during hospitalization. Point-of-care data entry goes beyond the human provider and is equally applicable to automated devices and analyzers, for example ventilators or blood chemistries. The technology to accomplish this automated point-of-care data capture is readily available.

Hospital Information System Design

The technical issues of hardware and software configuration are beyond the scope of this chapter. However, some of the more topical technical issues are briefly presented. There are currently four models for information processing in a HIS: the centralized model, the hub-and-spoke model, the network model, and the distributed model (18,21,27,28,34,58).

The centralized model, also known as a monolithic system,

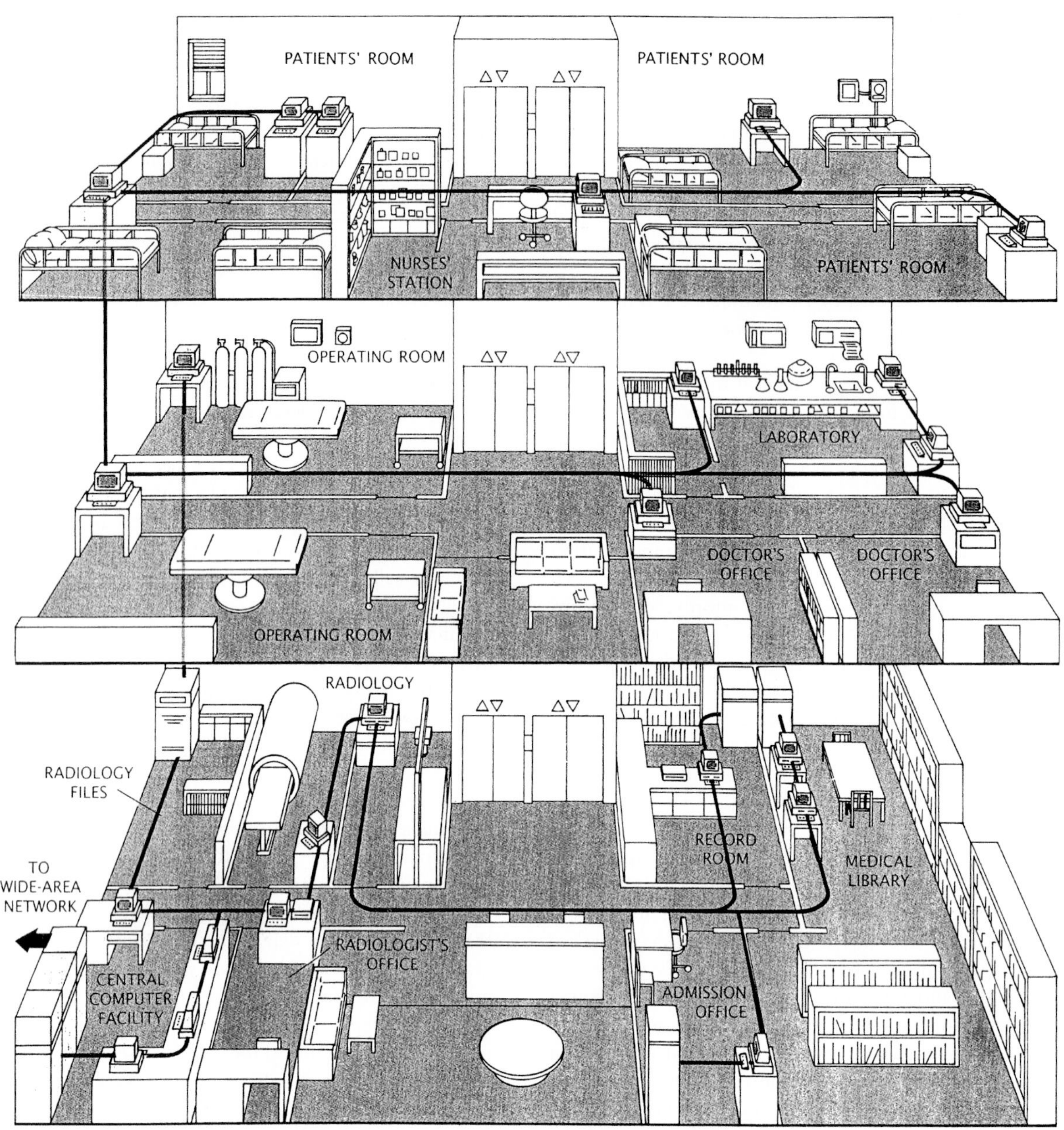

Figure 16.1. Hospital information system envisioned for the future will use a local area network to transmit not only text but also images to workstations throughout a hospital. Patient information will be entered from and transmitted to the admitting office, record room, laboratories, operating rooms, and bedside. Digitally stored results of radiographic, computer-assisted tomographic, ultrasonic, and other examinations will be transmitted by fiberoptic cables to wherever they are needed. Library material will be accessible as well, and a wide area network will bring in distant databases and medical advice systems. Unlike current systems driven from a central computer, future systems will decentralize much of the memory and processing to individual workstations. A system like this would be a more comprehensive version of the HELP system developed at the LDS Hospital in Salt Lake City.

consists of a mainframe computer with all applications existing on the mainframe. This model achieves a high degree of data integration and a common user interface. There are numerous advantages associated with this architecture. Foremost is the creation of a central patient database with all data elements going into the same file. Coincident with the creation of an EHR is the development and existence of a data dictionary (a standardized scheme for defining medical terms and patient data) (59–61). An additional benefit of a centralized database with a data dictionary is the ability to use expert system tools to provide decision support.

The centralized model removes all boundaries between departmental applications. Therefore, even if data are distributed between two or more physical computers, central processing units (CPUs) in this model, the hospital's informatics department does not need to know which computer contains a particular data element. In this system all terminals, computers, operating systems, disk drives, communications protocols, and software tools are functionally identical. Any data element that is entered in the HIS, regardless of the location in the hospital where the data were entered, is immediately available to any user on the system. The practicality of a central system is that all applications run on the same hardware, and therefore the hospital need only invest in a limited number of disk drives, terminals, CPUs, and other hardware. These surplus items can be used anywhere in the hospital without regard for the department or location of use. Furthermore, since the hardware, communication protocols, and software tools are the same throughout the hospital, the size of the informatics department and technical personnel are reduced. Likewise, the training time for users is substantially reduced since all terminals are physically connected to the mainframe, and thus the user is required to learn only one system. Centralized systems, however, have drawbacks: (a) they force the hospital to contract with one vendor; (b) in hospitals that have departmental computer systems, the interfacing of a mainframe computer with existing clinical support systems (CSS), such as a laboratory information system (LIS), is often technically difficult, laborious, and time consuming; and (c) commercially available HIS software often will not support the variety of users in a hospital. The few hospitals that have fully integrated HISs adopted the centralized model. These hospitals were forced to build their own HIS, because the marketplace was slow to develop a clinically functional and integrated HIS. Several vendors now offer centralized systems that promise an integrated EHR.

The second model of an HIS is the hub-and-spoke configuration. This HIS architecture consists of a mainframe computer, in the center, that is linked like spokes in a wheel to satellite or feeder systems. Typical satellite systems are CSSs such as a pathology laboratory or pharmacy information system. These satellite CSSs are commonly provided by multiple vendors and are interfaced to the central mainframe. A user sitting at a dumb terminal interacts primarily with the mainframe, reviewing data and placing orders. These dumb terminals are hard wired to the mainframe computer in much the same manner as in the centralized system. The mainframe computer interacts with the CSSs through interfaces. The CSSs maintain their own databases and often the mainframe only stores recent data. However, in some of the more advanced hub-and-spoke systems archived patient data (including CSS data) are available and are physically stored on the mainframe. These advanced hub-and-spoke HISs provide an EHR and are the exception in this HIS design rather than the rule. The hub-and-spoke model evolved from the centralized model to take advantage of departmental CSSs. In the past a major disadvantage of the hub-and-spoke model was that the clinical usefulness of the CSSs was constrained by the intrinsic limitations of the interfaces. To bridge these constraints, a common interface language, known as Health Level Seven (HL7), was created. HL7 is a messaging protocol specifically developed to exchange health/medical/patient information between information systems. Despite interface improvements, this model is still constrained by the intrinsic limitations of the individual CSSs. These satellite systems were developed to satisfy individual departmental needs rather than the total care of the patient. As stated above, this model of an HIS often lacks a centralized and integrated EHR and therefore ignores the information processing requirements of all healthcare providers. If this design is chosen, the system should ensure that an integrated long-term EHR will be created with an attendant data dictionary. If these two prerequisites are in a hub-and-spoke HIS, then users can take full advantage of expert system tools to provide decision support.

The third configuration used in designing an HIS is the network model (58). This model consists of a local area network (LAN) to which various host computers (CSSs and a mainframe can be host computers) are attached as nodes on the network. Computer-to-computer interfaces, like the hub-and-spoke model, are the mainstay of this system. The user sits at a terminal or a minicomputer that is attached to a backbone LAN to gain access to host computers (CSSs or the mainframe). The purpose of the backbone LAN is to provide connectivity between various host computers. The network model allows for high-speed data transfer and access. Another advantage of the network model is that the integrity and functionality of the host computers are maintained. For example, a healthcare provider could access an LIS through the LAN and have all of the flexibility that the intrinsic LIS allowed. Similar to the other models used to configure an HIS, there are disadvantages to the network model. First, the user interacts directly with the host computer and therefore does not have an integrated view of patient information. Second, a user can only access one host computer at a time. Third, the user must learn different commands to communicate with the different host computers since there is no uniform user interfaces in this model. Fourth, the burden of system interaction is shifted from standardized interface software to the healthcare provider. Current versions of this HIS architecture do not provide for an integrated EHR. To date, LAN technology in healthcare allows for only simple applications, such as results review and possibly rudimentary order entry. A bright spot in the future of this HIS design is the development and application of server technology. A server is a dedicated computer that is attached as a node on the LAN. The sole purpose of the server is to communicate with, gather, and store information from host computers. Server technology allows for merged patient data, but does not eliminate the need for interfaces.

The fourth HIS design strategy is known as the distributive model. This model is very similar to the network model in that host computers act as nodes on a LAN. What distinguishes the distributive model from the network model is that the design strives for data and system integration. This is accomplished through the use of relational database software. In the distributive model relational database software is installed on each host computer and workstation connected to the LAN. This software is not constrained by the type of hardware or operating system environments. Integration of the various heterogeneous host computers is achieved in three different ways. First, because each host computer has a relational database, Standard Query Language (SQL) (58) can be used across the entire system. The original version of SQL was developed at IBM's San Jose Research Laboratory (now the Almaden Research Center). The language was originally known as Sequel and has evolved to become known as SQL. The American National Standards Institute published an SQL standard in 1986; the last update was in 1999. Since then, SQL has become the industry-standard relational database language and is the predominate tool used to query relational databases. Second, the distributive model uses a data dictionary that standardizes medical terms and records the location of various data elements in the system. Third, the relational database software can recognize and read file structures from various host computers; the host files can be read as they exist or the software can convert them to a native relational database file format. The major advantages of the distributed model are as follows: (a) Host-to-host information exchange no longer requires interfaces. (b) An integrated EHR is created. (c) A data dictionary standardizes medical terms. (d) Users can access patient information from a workstation regardless of where it physically exists in the system. (e) Relational database software can gather all requested patient information simultaneously at the time of need, known as assembling information on the fly, and once the user has completed the task, the view disappears. This avoids the task of copying information from a CSS to a mainframe and then processing that information on the mainframe. (f) An integrated EHR provides the environment for decision-support tools (that is, expert systems).

HEALTHCARE INFORMATION MANAGEMENT IN THE MILLENNIUM: THE ELECTRONIC HEALTH RECORD

The inefficiencies of the paper medical record absorb large amounts of a hospital's budget and are directly responsible for many of the failures in the quality of care delivered, for example medication errors. Hospital information systems and their EHRs have demonstrated many benefits, but perhaps the three that will have the greatest impact on healthcare delivery and cost are (a) improved logistics and organization of the medical record to speed care, prevent duplication of data and procedures, and improve care giver's efficiency; (b) automatic computer review of the medical record to aid decision-support, limit errors, identify exceptions in care, and identify those in need of care; and (c) systematic analysis of present and past clinical experiences and outcomes to guide future practice and policies (1,14,30).

Improved Logistics and Organization of Patient Data

The EHR, with the patient as the central information unit, provides large clinical databases allowing for more comprehensive and accurate patient data collection, more complete data integration and interpretation, and greater facilitation of data analysis (1,2,17,30,34). Multiple providers can gain simultaneous access to the computer-based data, and data duplication is eliminated. Once stored in the EHR, data can be displayed in numerous different ways, providing for cost-effective utilization of services. A past investigation has demonstrated that in an emergency department with computer-displayed data, physicians ordered 15% fewer tests than when computer display of data was not available (62). Another investigation has shown that when the EHR displayed previous test results to physicians when they were ordering new tests, there was a reduction in test ordering (63). An EHR provides a cohesive, integrated, accurate, and up-to-date record that encourages and enables providers to make informed cost-conscious decisions (62–67). Computers also serve the information needs of medical, pharmacy, and nursing students (16,22,47,48,68,69) as well as the patient (70). The use of an HIS to present clinical guidelines for management of personnel with occupational exposure to body fluids was shown to improve documentation, compliance with guidelines, and percentage of charges spent on indicated activities, while decreasing overall charges (150). Wennberg and colleagues at Dartmouth's Foundation for Informed Medical Decision Making have introduced computer-aided instruction and videodisc information to patients so that they are able to make educated decisions regarding their care (70). The premise of the group at Dartmouth is that in nonemergent situations the patient should share in the decision making process with the physician so that the eventual course of action reflects the patient's preferences as well as the doctor's opinion(s).

Automatic Review of the Medical Record and Decision Support

Humans are not very good watch keepers and predictably overlook rare and uncommon events (71). A medical information system that contains an integrated EHR can continuously scan all patient data for exceptions in care and alert healthcare providers. Computer-generated reminders have been shown to dramatically affect the outcomes of many different aspects of care (62–67,71–73,151). Recent investigations into the use of hospital information systems to monitor and alter the delivery of care have resulted in remarkable cost savings and improved patient outcomes (74–95). The EHR can facilitate a healthcare system that emphasizes prevention, early diagnosis and treatment, and effective management (96).

These aspects of healthcare delivery are further facilitated by the advent of computer decision support (10,13,97–118). Six major generic uses of decision support that now exist in hospitals with integrated information systems and attendant EHRs are alerting, interpretation, assisting, critiquing, diagnostic, and management. *Alerting decision support* is defined as the automatic notification of appropriate providers of time-critical decisions. Drug–drug interactions, drug–laboratory interactions, drug–disease interactions, adverse drug reactions, and drug allergy alerts are common clinical examples of this type of decision support (79,81,82,86). These types of alerts are generated at the time of either a medication order or laboratory results reporting if alerting criteria are met. Furthermore, an HIS with this alerting function can scan patient data continuously; alerting is said to occur in the background, and if criteria are met anytime in the course of hospitalization, appropriate personnel can be notified. Notification can be escalated based on the urgency of the alert. Alerts requiring immediate attention may be sent by a pager. Less urgent alerts can be sent by e-mail or placed in an inbox to be viewed when the user logs on to the HIS.

Interpreting decision support refers to the gathering, arranging, and analyzing of patient data, resulting in a conceptual understanding of that data. One of the earliest applications of interpretive decision support in hospitals was computer analysis and interpretation of electrocardiograms (7,11,36).

Assisting decision support is used to maximize and simplify human interaction with an HIS. This model of decision support usually consists of predictive knowledge about a particular problem or task. Computer-assisted physician ordering is an example of this type of decision support (66,67,107,113–116,169,170). Assisting decision support can be as simple as fixed standing order lists or as sophisticated as computer-assisted antibiotic ordering (93,95).

Critiquing decision support is defined as computer-assisted analysis or review of human decisions for appropriateness. This type of decision support merely uses the HIS knowledge base to evaluate human decisions and to report to the user the result of the computer analysis. Critiquing decision support has been used by investigators to develop protocols for ventilator management in the intensive care unit (ICU) setting (111) and to determine the appropriateness of blood ordering (80,117).

Diagnostic decision support is defined as decision-support that provides a computer-assisted diagnosis. This type of decision support has been the most widely studied of all decision-support techniques in medical informatics (74,99,102,104,105,108, 114).

Management decision support is the automatic generation of decisions that are oriented to the total care of the patient. Management decision support differs from critiquing decision support in that in the former the computer manages patient care and suggests treatments, whereas in the latter the computer reacts to treatment plans or orders initiated by the physician. In clinical management decision support the physician critiques the computer rather than the computer critiquing the physician. Computerized clinical practice guidelines are an example of this model of decision-support. Management decision-support techniques are currently being investigated in the ICU setting to assist in the management of patients with adult respiratory distress syndrome (112,152).

Systematic Analysis of Present and Past Clinical Experiences

The third benefit of an automated patient record is the access to large amounts of archived clinical data to provide information on past clinical experience. The computer has the capability to examine large amounts of data and statistically summarize various aspects of care to answer administrative and management or clinical research questions. The ability to systematically analyze large numbers of clinical events and correlate these to different outcomes is one of the functions of CISs. Modern quality management techniques rely on these types of analysis. Investigators have realized since the late 1970s that there exists a wide variability in the patterns of clinical practice in the U.S. (119, 120). The net results of this variability in clinical practice is the inflating of the healthcare dollar and less than optimal patient care. The EHR provides the necessary tool to identify variation in all aspects of care, where it may exist (1,4,43,77,94). Once identified, corrective measures can be developed to reduce the variation.

The computer-stored medical record has become one of the "agenda items" of the federal government in its attempt to control healthcare costs and improve the quality of care. This is evidenced by the recent document of the Institute of Medicine (1) and CMS's (formerly the Health Care Financing Administration) as well as Congress's commitment of financial and political support for this initiative. Certainly, the EHR will not, in and of itself, be the sole answer to the U.S. healthcare dilemma, but it has the potential to have major impact by providing superior information to the market.

HOSPITAL INFORMATION SYSTEMS IN THE ERA OF THE INTERNET

Perhaps no technologic advance since the personal computer has had a more profound impact than the rise of the Internet and its most popular application, the World Wide Web. The Internet has revolutionized communication and provided a unique forum for the exchange of information. This forum has changed the way commerce is conducted in all businesses and has significantly altered the approach to building and using information systems in all industries. Healthcare has not been immune to this rising tide, but as always in the area of information systems, healthcare organizations have been slower to adapt this new technology (143). Because Internet development and use in healthcare is still in its infancy, it is hard to predict exactly what the final Internet-based healthcare system will look like.

We have already seen the integration of platform-independent graphical user interfaces to HISs (153,154). These types of Web-enabled interfaces have allowed clinicians to access patient data from remote locations using the Internet, thus expanding the caregiver's ability to provide continuity of care from outside of the hospital setting. An added advantage of these interfaces is that they provide a portal of access to the latest scientific information available either on the local intranet (e.g., treatment guidelines) or supplied by Internet tools such as electronic journals, Micromedex, or Up-To-Date. An Internet application has already been developed that performs global surveillance on influenza and can be used by clinicians to guide the diagnosis of influenza in their community (144).

The evolution of the Internet's potential to connect individual HISs can be witnessed in the National Nosocomial Infections Surveillance (NNIS) system's drive to automate its data reporting process. NNIS is a cooperative effort that began in 1970 between the Centers for Disease Control and Prevention (CDC) and participating hospitals to create a national nosocomial infections database. Data from participating hospitals are collected uniformly by trained infection control personnel and are reported routinely to the CDC where they are aggregated into a central database. The ultimate goal is to have all 315 participating hospitals report their data electronically via the Internet directly to the CDC's database. Exactly how this will be accomplished is still in the testing stages utilizing information management technology developed by TheraDoc, Inc., a medical informatics company that designs expert systems for health information management and clinical decision support. What is clear is that the use of Internet standards will allow enormous connectivity between existing legacy healthcare information systems, not replacing these systems but seamlessly linking them in a way that is opaque to the user who can easily access textual information, aggregated data, and video and audio images all on the same screen through the use of browser technology (145–147). Because of the pervasiveness of the Internet, the improved access to information will bring the patient directly into the healthcare organizations' computing systems. Patients will be able to access their own healthcare information as healthcare workers do now. Essentially the Internet dramatically increases the boundaries of what constitute a CIS and a computerized medical record by making this information much more broadly available. This creates an important need for electronic confidentiality, which has become a major issue especially since the U.S. Department of Health and Human Services (HHS) issued the Privacy Rule to implement the requirement of the Health Insurance Portability and Accountability Act (HIPAA) of 1996.

MOBILE COMPUTING

By any measure, the growth of mobile computing has mirrored the growth of the Internet and perhaps exceeded it. The demand for mobile devices from phones to personal digital assistants (PDAs) continues to explode. Witness:

- The number of wireless Internet users will reach 83 million by the end of 2005, or 39% of total Internet users (155).
- By the end of 2004, there will be 95 million browser-enabled cellular phones and over 13 million Web-enabled PDAs (156).
- The wireless LAN market was expected to reach $1 billion in 2001. That figure will double by 2004 (157).

Confusion often exists about the Internet and wireless; they are not synonymous. As we have seen, the Internet is a huge global network that provides access to information and applications using a browser or Web navigating application. The majority of healthcare mobile computing applications today don't interact at all with the Internet. *Mobile computing* or *wireless* refers to the underlying technology that supports the transport of data between the mobile handheld computing device and the main computer system without a wired connection between them. Mobile computing is a range of solutions that enable end-user mobility by providing access to data anytime, from any location. Mobile computing has three main components:

- Handheld computing device (a.k.a. mobile computing device, mobile device, handheld device, handheld)
- Connecting technology that allows information to pass between the site's information system and the handheld device and back
- Underlying hospital, clinic, or central information system

It is helpful to see how these work together in a clinical example. The end-user enters or accesses data—such as vital signs, charge information, clinical notes, and medication orders— using the application on the handheld computing device. Using one of several connecting technologies, the new data are transmitted from the handheld to the site's information system where system files are updated and the new data are accessible to other system users—the billing department, for example. Now both systems (the handheld and the site's computer) have the same information and are synchronized. The process works the same way starting from the other direction. For example, a physician may want to have access to all new laboratory results for today's clinic patients. This information is stored in the site's information system and now needs to be transmitted to the handheld device. Again, the connecting technology delivers the data to the handheld device, and the physician can move from room to room, accessing the appropriate information from the handheld device. The process is similar to the way a worker's desktop PC accesses the organization's applications, except that the end-user device is not physically connected to the organization's systems. The communication between the end-user device and the site's information systems uses different methods for transferring and synchronizing data, some involving the use of radiofrequency (RF) technology. This example relies on a series of data transfer approaches:

- Wireless local area network (LAN)
- Wireless Internet or wireless Web
- Hot synching or data synching uses docking cradles or docking stations that are connected to a LAN to transfer data from the device to the organization's information system.

Wireless LAN

Wireless LAN is a flexible data and communications system used in addition to, or instead of, a wired LAN. Using RF technology, wireless LANs transmit and receive data over the air, minimizing the need for wired connections and enabling user mobility. In a wireless LAN, the caregiver enters data into a handheld device such as a PDA or a laptop computer that has a special wireless LAN card. This card has an antenna that transmits the data in real time using RF technology to an access terminal, usually connected to a ceiling or wall. The access terminal is connected to the LAN and sends the data received—or requests for data—from the handheld device to the patient care information system. Conversely, data from the site's information system can be sent to the handheld device using the same technology. PDAs, the most popular approach with physicians, have a very small screen size that is best suited to only limited data viewing and data collection functions such as laboratory order entry, single results display, and clinical notes entry. Laptops and tablets provide many more processing capabilities, more data storage, and larger displays, so end users can access entire patient records and view results in a number or graphical formats. Complex applications whether inpatient or outpatient work best in a wireless LAN environment that uses these larger devices.

Wireless Internet

Wireless Internet, also known as the wireless Web, provides mobile computing access to data using the Internet and specially equipped handheld devices. For example, using a Web phone or the latest PDA phone with a micro Web browser, the end user can display data accessible from the Internet. Technically speaking, the mobile device connected to the cellular system sends the request to a computer link server. This server acts as a gateway that translates signals from the handheld device into language the Web can understand, using an access and communication protocol. One of the leading protocols is called WAP (Wireless Access Protocol). The server also forwards the request over the Internet to a Web site, such as Yahoo or AOL or the organization's site and information systems. The Web site responds to the request and sends the information back through the link server. Again the response is translated into a wireless markup language (WML) so it is viewable on a small cell phone screen. This translated response is then sent to the cellular system and finally to the Web-enabled mobile computing device. Examples of the current uses of the wireless Internet include accessing short e-mails, quick lookup capabilities (stocks, weather, flights, directions, movies, and restaurants), retailing transactions (e.g., Amazon.com) and alert messaging in healthcare.

Synchronization

Synchronization or hot synching provides many of the benefits of mobile computing without the necessity of installing wireless LAN equipment or needing access to the Internet. Information is periodically downloaded from the HIS to the handheld device and then uploaded from the device to the HIS. The major drawback of data synchronization is that it does not provide real-time access to data. Data synching is not a wireless data transfer method since data are transferred from the mobile computing device to the site's information system through a docking (or synching) cradle wired to the LAN. However, since the end-user device is only physically attached to the LAN during the batch data transfers, it is commonly grouped under the general term *wireless.*

Mobile Computing Devices

An ever-increasing number of mobile computing devices are available for use in the healthcare setting (158):

- Web phones: cellular phones with Internet access and Internet browser that allow limited e-mail, calendar, appointment scheduling, and directories. There are currently few healthcare-specific applications beyond e-mail and alert messaging.
- PDA/phone: combination of a Web phone with PDA functionality with Internet browser functions including e-mail, calendar, appointment scheduling, and directories (e.g., Trio and Blackberry). Healthcare functions include charge entry, prescription writing, and Internet access.
- PDA or pocket PC: handheld computerized information organizers (e.g., Palm Pilot, Handspring Visor, Compaq iPaq) with e-mail, calendar, appointment scheduling, and directories, including some desktop application functions (e.g., Word and Excel), pen-based system for data entry, and bar-coding functions. Healthcare applications include charge capture, prescription writing, lab results review, and multiple functions using browser technology with wireless LAN.
- Handheld PC: small hand-size personal computer with a keyboard. Much more powerful than a PDA device with some desktop application functions (e.g., Word and Excel), keyboard for data entry, voice recognition, and recording options. Healthcare functions similar to those cited above.
- Tablet/laptop: tablets are flat-paneled PCs; laptops are also known as PC notebooks with all desktop functionality. Tablets use pen or touch-screen technology and allows for multiple integrated functions, e.g., full electronic medical record (EMR) capabilities.

Mobile Computing Applications

Given the immature application market and continually advancing technology components, today's most effective applications are those focused on tasks that require data access at the point of care but do not require sophisticated infrastructures to transfer data between the device and the organization's computer system. These currently include the following:

Alert Messaging and Communication

These applications go far beyond the pagers long used by on-call physicians, often allowing them to receive test results and send messages. The biggest challenge for these products is the ability to deliver secure, uninterrupted messages. As electronic interactions between ambulatory physicians and patients become more common, devices may be able to deliver messages and alerts to physicians in that setting as well (159).

Clinical Documentation

Rapidly increasing regulatory requirements and changing payment requirements are increasing the need for clinical documentation systems. Tools with a wide range of functionality from basic notes templates on PDAs to images that can be displayed on a laptop help clinicians quickly document clinical activities, as well as organize and track patient information from one encounter to the next. Most products supporting inpatient care are focused on nursing documentation; applications for physicians in the ambulatory setting are currently supported by only a few vendors. As more physicians and other providers begin to participate in disease management, which requires increased data collection and monitoring, tools that enable providers to cope with the volume of data at the point of care will become increasingly valuable and will be accessible via mobile computing.

Charge Capture and Coding

These popular tools for both inpatient and outpatient care enable caregivers to record information at the point of care instead of after the fact. The handheld computing application replaces the antiquated index card system for recording charges. It includes coding tools for translating increasingly complex payer rules, especially in the ambulatory setting. These applications can have a positive financial impact by capturing more accurate and complete information about diagnoses, procedures, and other care-related services. In the future, charge and coding functions will likely be integrated with other clinical computing tools, thus capturing financial information as part of the automated care documentation process.

Lab Order Entry and Results Reporting

Most often found in the inpatient setting, these applications allow users to order laboratory tests and view results at the point of care. Most focus first on one aspect of the process and then move to the other. For example, one vendor decided to start with result-viewing because of the limited handheld processing and customization required, and then moved toward a total ordering and result viewing application. Lab order entry streamlines the ordering process; results reporting allows access to often-critical patient information anytime and anywhere. Because these functions require real-time interface with existing ordering and resulting systems, success so far has been limited to a few vendors who have either partnered with well-known traditional vendors or added integrating tools to their products. As the technology advances, allowing for better integration of applications, laboratory order entry and results reporting tools will likely become common.

Prescription Writing

Using a PDA or pocket PC instead of a prescription pad, physicians generate prescriptions by clicking on the patient, medication, and dose. Many e-prescribing tools can also check prescriptions for drug interactions and potential allergic reactions and transmit completed prescriptions directly to the pharmacy. Products on the market today differ in almost every step of the process, from how patient data are obtained, to where processing occurs, to how scripts are sent to the pharmacy, making this a crowded and confusing vendor field. Advancements for e-prescribing tools are likely to develop rapidly as problems of integration with patient data and data transmission are overcome (160,161).

In many ways these applications are mobile extensions of the traditional HIS. Some of the most popular inpatient applications are bedside charting, emergency room documentation, and remote access to data for physicians (162). Mobile solutions for inpatient clinical computing are likely to be offered by traditional HIS vendors; these vendors will likely partner with wireless technology providers and mobile computing vendors.

Physician use is the primary focus of mobile computing, and that is in the outpatient setting (163,164). Mobile computing devices are well suited to physician practice since physicians often spend their whole day moving between exam rooms and offices, and need continuous access to clinical data. Mobile computing also avoids the cost of hardwiring many physician offices and exam rooms. In the physician office, mobile devices that use batch synchronization of data are most common. In addition to reference tools, handheld applications are focused largely on high-stake individual processes such as charge capture or prescription management (165,166).

Mobile Computing Infectious Diseases Applications

PDAs, also known as handheld computers, pocket personal computers, and Palm Pilots, provide immediate access to vital and clinically relevant infectious diseases information at the point of care. Several infectious diseases applications are available that provide information on pathogens, diagnosis, medication, and treatment.

One study evaluated the clinical contribution of a drug database developed for the handheld computer (167). ePocrates Rx is a comprehensive drug information guide that is downloadable free from the Internet and designed for the Palm OS platform. A 7-day on-line survey of 3,000 randomly selected ePocrates Rx users was conducted observing the following parameters: user technology experience, product evaluation, usage patterns, and the effects of the drug reference database on information-seeking behavior, practice efficiency, decision making, and patient care. The survey response rate was 32%; 946 physicians who used the program reported that it saved time during information retrieval, is easily incorporated into their usual workflow, and improves drug-related decision making. They also felt that it reduced the rate of preventable adverse drug events (ADEs). The clinical and practical value of using these devices in clinical settings will clearly grow further as wireless communication becomes more ubiquitous and as more applications become available (167).

In another study, infectious diseases PDA applications were reviewed (168); these included ePocrates ID (part of ePocrates Rx Pro), the Johns Hopkins Division of Infectious Diseases Antibiotic Guide, the 2002 Sanford Guide to Antimicrobial Therapy, and Infectious Diseases and Antimicrobials Notes. Drug information, including clinical pharmacology, dosing in patients with renal insufficiency, adverse reactions, and drug interactions, were evaluated for completeness and accuracy by comparison of each application with the package insert. Treatment recommendations for six diseases using these programs were compared with current practice guidelines. Each PDA infectious diseases application reviewed was found to have unique advantages and disadvantages. This critical review will help healthcare professionals select the infectious diseases PDA application best tailored to meet their individual information needs (168).

Vendors and Communication Standards

Any chapter on the subject of computers in healthcare would be incomplete without a brief discussion of vendors and communication standards. Vendors of medical information systems have been arbitrarily divided into two types: niche vendors and total system vendors (56). Niche vendors specialize in clinical support systems, such as laboratory, administrative, or pharmacy information systems. Niche vendors are better able to support the information needs of individual healthcare departments rather than the total care system. Total system vendors are those that specialize in meeting the information management needs, both clinical and administrative, of the entire institution. However, total system vendors may enter the niche market by permitting institutions to purchase the information system in increments. They accomplish this by allowing the institution to identify which department will initially be computerized, with the goal of eventually computerizing the entire system. Total system vendors were forced into to this selling strategy because of the unwillingness of healthcare institutions to commit large budgetary allocations to an HIS or MIS purchase.

Healthcare providers with the responsibility of choosing an MIS or HIS should be aware of some the common misconceptions that vendors perpetrate (121–134). Vendors always tend to describe their systems positively and will often refer to them as "open systems." That is, they are "fully integrated" and provide universal "connectivity or interfaces." Vendors also insist that their software is reliable, secure, and provides for data integrity. Healthcare providers should be especially wary when vendors say their system is "integrated." To date, many vendors now claim to offer a total system that provides for data integration in the sense that it has been used in this chapter. But many of these claims are in marketing only and have not yet been realized in implemented systems.

Equally confusing is the issue of standards (134–137). The issue as proposed by vendors is quite simple. When they refer to standards and interfacing they are only addressing the issue of physically connecting different computers together. However, the issue of interfacing is not limited to physically connecting different computers together. To make information useful, healthcare providers not only need standards to transfer information, but standards are also needed on the content and utilization of patient information. Currently, the only standard that exists is for the transmission of data. The standard that deals with the issues involved in data transmission is HL7. However, HL7 goes far beyond data transmission issues. Currently, as proposed, HL7 consists of seven layers or protocols. Layer 1 is the physical protocol, layer 2 is the link protocol, layer 3 is the network protocol, layer 4 is the transport protocol, layer 5 is the session protocol, layer 6 is the presentation protocol, and layer 7 is the application protocol. When fully developed, HL7 has great potential. The issue of standards is even more complicated and convoluted than the above-described issues. Besides HL7, there are competing standards groups such as the American College of Radiology—National Electrical Manufacturers Association, the Institute of Electrical and Electronics Engineers, Medex, and others all developing standards. In fact, Medex with its X25 and X409 standards provide data transmission interfaces that compete with HL7 (34). The rapid rise of the Internet has forced the above groups to create standards for Internet applications in healthcare. Currently in their infancy, these Internet standards will play a major role in healthcare computing in the future. Vendors are scrambling to incorporate Web technology within their systems; purchasers of these systems should not consider any system without Web browser technology embedded within them, which will allow great connectivity between the multiple disparate legacy information systems in most healthcare organizations.

PATHWAY TO ON-LINE COMPUTERIZED SURVEILLANCE PROGRAMS

Background

Surveillance has been defined as the collection, collation, analysis, and dissemination of data (138,139). Several methods have been developed to perform this task in hospitals; the traditional method includes collection of data through extensive chart review, a time- and labor-intensive process. Computerized methods have been developed for hospital surveillance; several PC-based programs in infection control are available including Nolo 3 and NICE (121–131,140,141). In addition the CDC offers an IDEAS software program to facilitate collection of hospital data for inclusion in the NNIS system (127). These systems offer added efficiencies in the analysis of data but not in the collection of data. As surveillance in hospitals is expanded from infection control to other areas, more efficient means of data collection will be essential. The development and implementation of comprehensive HISs offers the potential for improving, enlarging, and more efficiently conducting hospital-wide surveillance. This section reviews hospital surveillance programs conducted with an HIS currently in use.

A completely computerized medical record is not necessary or even desirable before computerized surveillance can begin. Indeed, most institutions build a computerized medical record gradually over several years (29,56,57). However, certain key areas are essential before beginning hospital-wide surveillance. Virtually all hospitals have established computerized systems for admission, discharge and transfer information. These programs are driven for billing purposes, but they often collect important demographic information, including admission dates, diagnoses, length of stay, discharge status, and other information that forms the core of the inpatient medical record. Integrated clinical computer systems will have this as a foundation to which other information is added.

Laboratory Integration

Using admission/discharge/transfer information as a base, the most logical and practical approach is to first add laboratory information. Most hospitals already have computerized laboratory systems, although these systems are often targeted toward results review and billing (12,18,76,78). Unfortunately, the least computerized aspect of these laboratory systems is the microbiology laboratory. There are no published examples of infection control surveillance programs developed solely from a laboratory computer system alone. Even with demographic information integrated with the laboratory system, developing these systems to perform surveillance can be quite difficult and usually requires the creation of a more comprehensive database for management of infection control information drawn from the laboratory system. This is nicely illustrated by the work of Kahn et al. at Barnes Hospital, who have created a nosocomial infection surveillance system called *Germwatcher* (118). Not only has a specialized database been constructed, but the authors have created an artificial intelligence program with infectious disease logic that is necessary for their computerized surveillance to be clinically useful. This program uses clinical patient data and infectious disease logic to make decisions about likely nosocomial infections. There are three key components that underlie a rational computerized infection control surveillance program: first, access to computerized raw patient data; second, a special database created for the infection control application; and third, an infectious disease artificial intelligence program that can make decisions about nosocomial infections based on patient data collected in the database. This can form the nucleus for an increasingly complex group of programs that become possible as more computerized data become available from other clinical sources.

Pharmacy Integration

The next key component of a hospital-wide surveillance system is computerization of pharmacy information that allows tracking of drug use. Many hospitals have computerized pharmacy systems, but few have linked them in any meaningful way to laboratory information systems (47–49,115). Unification of the laboratory and pharmacy systems allows for the creation of numerous surveillance programs in both infection control and hospital epidemiology. This process should be an early priority in creating a computerized medical record. However, this process should not simply try to computerize drug administration records without also simultaneously creating a rational program to improve the use of drugs. An infection control application involving drug therapy will need a system that not only tracks drug use but also improves drug use. Such a system was developed at LDS Hospital beginning in 1975. All medications are ordered through the computer and the information available on each drug order includes dose, route, frequency, order time, administration time, and duration of therapy. In addition, through artificial intelligence applications, algorithms automatically identify and track potential drug interactions, including drug–drug, drug–lab, drug–food interactions, and patient drug allergies. For example, if warfarin is ordered for a patient on digoxin, an alert would be generated to the pharmacist warning of a potential drug interaction. If ampicillin was ordered for a patient with a history of penicillin allergy, an alert would be generated warning of the potential risk of an allergic reaction. Approximately 1.3 million doses of medication are given each year at LDS Hospital; with automated surveillance this leads to the generation of over 700 pharmacy alerts, 100% of which result in a therapeutic strategy change (79). The hospital epidemiology program at LDS Hospital uses this system to effect improvements in drug use and surveillance (73–95).

In addition, the drug utilization review components of the LDS Hospital system allow for weekly summaries of drug use by doses, interval, routes, service, location, physician, type of therapy, prophylaxis, and costs of use. Sophisticated algorithms involving criteria for use of drugs have been developed, and they improve drug use and the quality of patient care. For example, ongoing drug utilization review revealed that imipenem-cilastatin, an antibiotic, was being used by one physician for surgical prophylaxis, an area in which no Food and Drug Administration (FDA) indication currently exists. This system facilitated feedback to the physician and cessation of this practice.

Radiology Integration

The next step is to link a radiology information system to the above amalgam. This is practical, because many institutions have some form of computerization in the radiology department. Unfortunately, much effort has been expended in developing methods for the electronic storage of images, distracting efforts to computerize clinical information regarding interpretations of radiology studies. This information is particularly critical for infection control purposes. At the very least, free text summaries should be available for all radiology studies on the information system. However, for sophisticated surveillance systems, this information will have to be stored in a coded format, for processing by artificial intelligence programs.

Electronic Infection Control Surveillance

With the availability of admission/discharge data, laboratory data, pharmacy data, and radiology data computerized and integrated, hospital-wide surveillance is possible. In addition to these factors, a group of artificial intelligence programs are needed to process the information and to draw conclusions and make decisions. These programs are often referred to as a knowledge base. At LDS Hospital an infectious diseases knowledge base was created with input from infectious diseases physicians, which was combined with the linked system of laboratory, pharmacy, and radiology to create an automated system for the detection of all nosocomial infections. This program automatically analyzes data from the patient's electronic medical record, specifically from the microbiology and radiology modules to detect all cases of hospital-acquired infection using the rules in the infectious diseases knowledge base. Each day, the computer scans the records of all patients in the hospital and applies these data to the knowledge base and derives a list of all hospital-acquired infections, which is printed out daily for appropriate infection control follow-up. This information is then permanently stored in the patient database for future analysis and reporting (74,75).

To evaluate these computerized surveillance programs, a study was performed comparing traditional infection control surveillance methods to this automated system for the detection of nosocomial infections. Of 155 confirmed nosocomial infections (by infectious disease physician review), the computer identified 140 infections (90%) and the infection control practitioners identified 118 infections (76%). False-positive identification of infections was similar: the computer detected 42 infections (27%) and infection control practitioners detected 27 infections (17%). The adoption of this system has resulted in the savings of two full-time equivalent positions in the infection control department (74,75).

Building on this database, a computerized infectious diseases isolation program was developed and placed in operation at LDS Hospital. This program contains disease-specific isolation procedures. The system is activated by entering a patient-specific disease or category of disease in the computer, and the program then determines the appropriate specific type of isolation, generates a list of the proper isolation instructions, orders the appropriate supplies from the central services department, and sends a reminder to the infection control department for appropriate follow-up. Use of this program has resulted in significantly more patients being placed on appropriate isolation and better coordination of the infection control isolation program (74,75,84).

Using data from 150,000 individual hospital admissions, a logistic regression model for prediction of patients likely to develop a hospital-acquired infection was created. Eighteen variables known to be associated with the development of hospital-acquired infections were included in this model; ten variables were found to be associated with the development of hospital-acquired infection in this stepwise logistic regression model. Coefficients of risk for the development of hospital-acquired infection were developed, and currently all patients admitted to the hospital are assigned a risk coefficient on a daily basis. When patients' assigned coefficient exceeds an arbitrary threshold, they are identified as high risk for the development of a nosocomial infection. Preliminary data have revealed that 65% of patients predicted by this model to develop a hospital-acquired infection actually did so. In addition 50% of these patients also developed an ADE (92). This is an example of how real-time surveillance can be used to design on-line programs to prevent nosocomial infections before they occur, rather than just documenting their occurrence after the fact. Currently in progress is a randomized trial comparing usual care and aggressive infection control in this targeted high-risk group of patients.

Antibiotic Surveillance Programs

When the laboratory system, the pharmacy system, and the radiology departments are interfaced, a wide variety of hospital-wide surveillance programs are possible, many extending beyond traditional infection control surveillance. However, all of these programs fall clearly within the purview of hospital epidemiology. In 1985, a surgical knowledge base was added to LDS Hospital's HIS to study prophylactic antibiotic use in surgical patients. Computer programs were developed to track prophylactic antimicrobial timing and duration of prophylaxis in patients undergoing scheduled elective surgical procedures. Initially the exact time of the first dose of antibiotic prophylaxis was tracked with respect to the start of surgery. After studying over 12,000 surgery patients, it was found that the exact time of prophylactic antibiotic administration with respect to surgical incision correlated with the resulting rate of surgical site infections; the rate of surgical site infections was lowest when antibiotics were administered within 2 hours immediately preceding surgery, and the rate of wound infection steadily increased with each hour after surgical incision that antibiotics were begun (91). Therefore, computer-generated reminders were placed in the charts of all patients who needed antimicrobial prophylaxis based on accepted guidelines, encouraging physicians to give antibiotics in the proper time frame. During a preliminary observation period, only 40% of surgical patients received prophylactic antibiotics within 2 hours before surgical incision; with the institution of computer reminders, this increased to 58% of patients; the resulting surgical site infection rate decreased from 1.8% during the preliminary observation period to 0.9% during the study period (77).

Computer programs were also developed to follow the duration of antimicrobial prophylaxis in patients undergoing scheduled elective surgery. Using accepted guidelines for specific surgical procedures, computer-generated reminders were placed in the charts of all patients warning that the prophylactic antibiotics would be stopped after the appropriate duration unless reordered by the physician. During a 6-month preliminary observation period, surgical patients received an average of 19 doses of antimicrobial prophylaxis; after the intervention, the average duration of prophylaxis decreased to 13 doses. The average cost of antibiotics exceeding 48 hours of prophylaxis was $42 less in the study period than during the observation period. This resulted in a 6-month savings of $44,562. Currently this system is in continuous operation (81).

In 1986, the infectious diseases knowledge base was expanded to closely follow the therapeutic uses of all antibiotics on a hospital-wide basis. Computer algorithms were created to automatically determine if antimicrobial therapies were potentially inappropriate based on *in vitro* antimicrobial susceptibility data. These programs automatically searched for inconsistencies between antimicrobial therapies and corresponding microbiology susceptibility test results on individual patients. The system also screened for single- or multiple-drug therapy mismatches with microbiologic susceptibility tests. When a mismatch occurred, a therapeutic antibiotic monitor alert was generated. Three potential situations lead to an alert being generated: (a) the isolation of a microorganism in culture that was resistant to current antibiotic therapy; (b) the lack of microbial isolate susceptibility reports for current antibiotic therapy; and (c) when antibiotics were not being administered although susceptibility tests were performed for a clinically relevant microbial isolate. During a 1-year study period, a clinical pharmacist reviewed all alerts generated by the therapeutic antibiotic monitor, on a daily basis, and notified attending physicians of the alert; 620 alerts were generated from 2,157 microbiologic test results. After false-positive alerts were eliminated, 420 alerts remained. Physicians responded to these alerts by either starting or changing therapy in 125 cases (30%). Physicians were unaware of susceptibility tests in 49% of cases (82).

In 1989, the knowledge base was further expanded to aid physicians in selecting the most appropriate empiric antibiotic therapy. Five years of microbiologic test results from hospital patients were reviewed and stratified into a database of over 12,500 separate test results. This allowed for the categorization of microbiologic isolates by site of infection and by susceptibility testing. This program currently has two features. First, it allows the clinician to review in tabular form the antimicrobial susceptibility patterns for any specific microorganism. Second, it allows the clinician to review tables of site-specific types of infections by etiologic microorganism (e.g., the ten leading causes of bacteremia in hospitalized patients). In addition, susceptibility profiles and cost of therapy are included, enabling physicians to select appropriate therapy based on susceptibility and cost considerations. A randomized study was performed to evaluate the impact of this system. Physicians having access to this program empirically ordered antibiotics that covered the ultimately isolated microorganism significantly more frequently than physicians without access; in addition, the mean cost of antibiotic therapy and the duration of antibiotic therapy were significantly less in patients who had antibiotics ordered with the assistance of this program than without it. Finally, the length of stay and cost of hospitalization were less in patients whose antibiotics were selected with access to this program (93,95). Currently being implemented is an interactive computer program for direct physician ordering of antibiotics based on these algorithms.

Adverse Drug Event Surveillance Programs

An emerging area of hospital epidemiology is drug-use surveillance. Pharmacy information systems can also be adapted to target and monitor specific drugs. Such a program at LDS Hospital was used to prospectively monitor the use and safety profile of imipenem-cilastatin, a drug associated with seizures (94). Over 1,900 patients were studied and the observed seizure rate was 0.2%, which was markedly less than the 2% rate noted with the use of the drug at other centers. In addition, using creatinine clearances and other indicators of renal function that are automatically collected and stored on every patient, it was determined that all three patients experiencing seizures were receiving significant overdosage based on their renal function, thus associating the observed seizures with improper imipenem-cilastatin dosing. This system was also used for noninfectious adverse events associated with the use of midazolam, a benzodiazepine (88). In this study respiratory arrests were found to be related to drug overdosage. Both studies allowed for appropriate physician education and improved therapeutic use of both agents.

Adverse drug events from antibiotics are only the tip of the iceberg in hospital patients, and thus surveillance can be broadened to include all ADEs in hospital patients. However, the routine method for detecting and reporting ADEs at hospitals involves voluntary reporting by physicians, who are required to complete and sign an incident report and submit Form 1639 to the FDA when necessary. Computer methods have been developed to automate the detection of hospital-associated adverse drug events (87). These programs allow for both voluntary and nonvoluntary detection of ADEs. The ADE monitor allows for voluntary reporting through a menu option on all terminals in the hospital including those at every patient bedside. Physicians, nurses, and pharmacists can enter, at the computer terminals, symptoms of a potential ADE through a simple command from the main patient care menu. After entering the appropriate symptoms, algorithms are triggered that search the database for all relevant drugs administered to the patient; the reporting personnel can also enter the suspected drug. This program also allows for the nonvoluntary detection of potential ADEs. Computer programs automatically conduct surveillance on all laboratory values of all patients looking for certain arbitrary abnormalities such as eosinophilia, leukopenia, increased creatinine, and drug levels. Rule-based algorithms using medical decision logic modules of the HELP system are also used to detect ADEs. For example, pharmacy orders are automatically screened for potential antidotes, sudden stop orders, and dose reduction orders. Each day a report of all potential ADEs detected in the last 24 hours is printed out. A pharmacist reviews the records and interviews healthcare personnel relevant to all patients identified as having a potential ADE. The pharmacist then determines likely ADEs and enters his report into the patient's permanent record and the hospital ADE file. This report includes the time course of the event, pertinent subjective data, and the subsequent clinical course, all of which are stored in the ADE file. In addition, the HELP system automatically records the drug indication, administration time, duration of therapy, route of administration and the National Drug Code (NDC). ADEs are characterized as mild, moderate, or severe. Causality assessment is performed using a computer algorithm. Each patient's adverse drug event is permanently stored in the computerized medical record, and if the offending drug is reordered, an alert is generated to the pharmacist, physician, and nurse.

Over an 18-month period 36,653 hospitalized patients were monitored through the use of this system, and 731 ADEs were identified in 648 patients (86). During this period, only nine ADEs were identified using traditional means. The most common signals were diphenhydramine and naloxone use, and high serum drug levels. Physicians, pharmacists, and nurses reported only 92 of the 731 ADEs. The other 631 ADEs were detected from automated signals. The most common drug classes involved were narcotics, antibiotics, cardiovascular agents, and anticoagulants. The most common events were rash, itching, and nausea and vomiting, accounting for just over 50% of the symptoms. Of the 731 ADEs the Naranjo score averaged 9.2 (range 4–10) (86). Programs are currently implemented that have shown the capability of reducing the rate and severity of ADEs (90).

Approach to Data Analysis: Use of Personal Computers

Hospital information systems offer many advantages to the hospital epidemiologists and infection control professionals by providing comprehensive detailed and integrated clinical information in a timely and often real-time fashion that can be used to design interventional programs for the prevention and control of nosocomial events. However, the hospital epidemiologist also performs an archaeologic function by analyzing infection control data on a frequent basis to detect trends, changes, and nosocomial outbreaks. Large clinical databases have been developed that can be used for numerous epidemiologic investigations (30–33). Although HISs collect this information, analyzing it on the system is often cumbersome, expensive, and difficult if these queries compete with clinical needs of the system. For this reason, the most practical approach to data analysis is not to use the HIS for this task, but to perform those analyses on PCs using conventional database programs into which patient information is downloaded from the HIS. The PC approach allows flexibility, convenience, and efficiencies that are not often available on an HIS. In addition, there are many PC programs widely available for data analysis such as statistical packages and spreadsheet programs for report generation. Critical to this approach is deciding what information to download on each patient.

At LDS Hospital, on a periodic basis, information from the nosocomial infection monitor is downloaded to PCs for analysis and the generation of monthly and yearly infection control reports (74,75,84). Through the use of various statistical software programs, this information is analyzed in detail; when problems become apparent, further investigation can be pursued electronically. If potential outbreaks are identified, investigations are conducted with the aid of this electronic tool. Indeed, this system has been employed in the investigation of several outbreaks, including *Pseudomonas* infections in endoscopy patients, staphylococcal infections in patients undergoing coronary artery bypass grafting, streptococcal infections in bone marrow transplant patients, and in a hospital-wide outbreak of *Xanthomonas* infections. Furthermore, through the use of artificial intelligence applications, on-line prospective monitoring programs for potential outbreaks have been implemented (83). For example, a respiratory therapy program automatically tracks all ventilated patients, sputum cultures, and specific respiratory therapists looking for potential transmission of nosocomial pathogens. This illustrates a key part of the approach to surveillance, which is the creation of a separate database that can be easily manipulated for epidemiologic studies, retrospective reviews, and on-line surveillance. The most facile approach is to create the database as a distinct entity, whose use is unencumbered by the clinical demands placed on the operational mainframe of department specific systems.

Role of the Hospital Epidemiologist in Selection of Clinical Information Systems

The hospital epidemiologist has training and experience in infection control and hospital epidemiology; these fields require considerable sophistication in data collection, data analysis, statistical interpretation, and experimental study design. The hospital epidemiologist is also often involved in ongoing programs to improve antibiotic use, prevent nosocomial infections, and detect potential nosocomial outbreaks. As a practicing physician, the hospital epidemiologist is intimately involved with direct patient care and in many institutions is viewed by the medical staff as the physician's physician. The combination of medical staff credibility and a strong foundation in epidemiology offers the hospital epidemiologist a natural leadership position in directing the process of computerization of clinical information. Unfortunately, most leadership in acquisition of clinical computing systems has come from administrators who are most interested in financial systems (132). Thus, clinicians are quite frustrated with the clinical functionality of computer systems in their institutions. In some institutions physicians have taken a leading role in the procurement of computing systems often leading to the selection of systems that are clinically useful. However, the ability of these systems to perform significant epidemiologic investigations is quite limited, thus preventing their application in infection control and hospital epidemiology. Clearly an important component of a computerized medical record system is the capability for retrospective epidemiologic studies, which are an important part of infection control and hospital epidemiology. Thus, the hospital epidemiologist is in a unique position to help ask critical questions in the procurement of a computerized medical record system.

The most critical aspect of this process is defining a physician leader who can ensure that the process is brought to fruition. Often significant computer experience or a background in computer science is not necessary and can be deleterious if the physician has pet interests in computers that would narrowly focus the process to a few specific agendas. A physician leader must be able to see the broad view of clinical computerization, the institutional needs, and the goals, and not have this view poisoned by narrow interests in specific computer applications.

However, a physician leader must have experience in data collection and analysis for an understanding of the important role these issues play in a CIS. Clinical epidemiology experience is most natural, because it encompasses issues related to data collection and analysis and interpretation as well as focused investigations.

A physician leader should have clinical credibility with medical staff in order to facilitate the implementation of a CIS. Because hospital epidemiologists are viewed as the physician's physician, they thus have a significant leadership potential with the medical staff. The physician leader must use this position to establish a physician task force for selecting and implementing a CIS. Medical staff involvement at all stages of the process is critical; no other group can effectively design a CIS. The physician leader must take a strong role in setting vision and educating medical staff members about that mission.

After establishing a medical staff task force, the physician leader should form a clinical information committee that should include leaders from the institution. This committee should include the physician leader, the chief financial officer, the chief information officer, the president of the board, the medical staff president, the director of pharmacy, the chief nursing officer, and influential medical staff members. This committee should be led by the physician leader, and should not be controlled by administration or by the chief information officer.

Each institution that is considering purchasing a CIS needs not only a vision, but also, on a more practical level, a concrete set of institutional goals for information management. These goals are pivotal in setting the requirements for an information system. These goals need to consider the history and tradition as well as the mission of the institution. From this list of goals a group of needs can be generated, taking into account the existing resources at that institution. Obviously all the needs cannot be met given limited resources; thus some form of prioritization of needs is necessary. Based on this analysis, specific criteria for an information system can and must be developed. This is crucial for a rational choice among the multitude of systems available. Once these factors have been delineated, they must be presented and agreed upon by the medical staff and the administration before moving ahead to select a system.

With a clear outline of goals, needs, and priorities for information management established, and a set of criteria for selection of an information system to meet these needs, the process of selecting a system begins. It is prudent to generate a list of basic requirements from the criteria set for an information system. This facilitates the very difficult process of evaluating the multitude of different products in the area. With this list of basic requirements, one can send out a request for proposals, which can be quite laborious. A more practical solution is to send out to all the vendors a request for information. Based on a perusal of this information, the next step is to select a list of products to evaluate, initially through proposals, then through demonstrations, and finally through site visits.

Several basic questions are mandatory in evaluating a CIS: Is the system designed for direct physician use? If so, where are sites of use in the institution? Is there evidence that the system meets clinical needs? What are the speed and flexibility of the system? Have physician suggestions been incorporated into the system? What is the scope and design of the electronic medical record and the capability for a longitudinal record? Does it offer inpatient and outpatient applications? Is there a central database and a knowledge base, and who will maintain them? What are the methods for data capture? What are the interfacing capabilities and communication protocols in the system? Does it have HL7 compatibility, SNOMED (Standardized Nomenclature of Medicine) compatibility, or LOINC compatibility? Is the system Web enabled, and does it support browser applications in all of it applications. Does this system capture financial data and true cost data? What is the format for a clinical archive, and how can it be queried? What is the state of open architecture in the system, and is there any distributed computing? Can the system handle electronic mail, local and national? Does the system allow patients to directly access their own records? Does the system offer order entry, and what provisions are there for electronic signatures and security?

The next step is choosing a list of desirable systems that will be site visited. This is a vital part of the process of choosing a CIS. Quite often vendor demonstrations can lead to expectations that are not realized at institutions where their system is in operation. Vendors often boast about programs that do not exist, hence the term *vaporware* (133). This is so prevalent that the informed consumer should assume that all promised programs do not exist unless they have been personally observed in operation at a site. The site visit allows for an in-depth evaluation of each system. Site visits can become very expensive as more and more individuals are included. A priority list of personnel must be drawn up with an emphasis on interested clinicians who will actually use the system, such as nurses, pharmacists, and physicians. Given the expense of such systems, the site visit should also include an influential member of the board. A list of specific questions should be developed akin to the questions outlined above. Every effort must be made to interview clinician users of the system in a random fashion that is not staged. Observation of who is actually using the system is important, as is identifying those departments and groups that don't use the system. A critical indicator of system use is to what extent other methods are used to transmit information, such as paper transmission, telephone, fax, electronic mail, etc. Crucial issues are how often the system is being used for actual care, what is the physician adoption and use of the system, as well as physician interest in office and home use of the system. What are the capabilities for remote site access to the system? Can a computer-generated chart be used for acute care? Another critical issue is maintenance and upkeep. Thus, the cost and difficulty of these issues must be quantified. Finally, the team must draw parallels and differences between the site and its own institution.

The ultimate choice of a system will be based on an analysis of this whole process with an emphasis on the specific needs of the institution and which of the systems will best meet those needs. The overall focus should be on practical and clinically focused systems that have a track record. Selecting systems that are under development and that will be gradually installed is a very risky proposition. A critical aspect is the stability of the vendor, since system modification will clearly occur at installation and with future versions. This process requires a stable vendor who can afford to continually develop and evolve their product.

In summary, hospital epidemiologists of the future will have a much broader mission both in the inpatient and outpatient settings as the healthcare reform process moves forward and as clinical information is computerized. Not only will hospital epidemiologists be more effective in managing infection control issues in a timely and real-time basis, but their experience and background will make them invaluable in managing outcomes information in all aspect of healthcare delivery, especially as care moves to the outpatient arena. Future hospital epidemiologists must be computer literate, as they will either adapt to the electronic revolution in healthcare or become a victim of it.

MEDICAL INFORMATICS GLOSSARY

Action axiom An axiom that embodies a criterion for recommending action. Is usually in the form "IF a given condition holds, THEN the following should be done."

Admission-discharge-transfer (ADT) The core component of a hospital information system that maintains and updates the hospital census.

Aleatory Random; subject to chance.

Aleatory variable Uncertain variable. In decision analysis, aleatory variables are modeled probabilistically.

Application program A computer program designed to accomplish a user-level task.

Application research Systematic investigation or experimentation with the goal of applying knowledge to achieve practical ends.

Archie A software tool for finding files stored on anonymous file transfer protocol (FTP) site.

ARPAnet Advanced Research Projects Agency network. A computer network originally developed by the U.S. Department of Defense to link affiliated research institutions. It included the original TCP/IP protocols and developed into the Internet (see Internet and TCP/IP).

Artificial intelligence The branch of computer science concerned with endowing computers with the ability to simulate intelligent human behavior, both cognitive and perceptual.

ASCII American Standard Code for Information Interchange; the world standard code for representing characters (all the upper- and lower-case Latin letters, numbers, punctuation, etc.) as binary numbers used on computers, terminals, printers, etc. In addition to printable characters, the ASCII code includes control characters to indicate carriage return, backspace, etc. A seven-bit code for representing alphanumeric characters and other symbols.

Attention-focusing axiom An axiom that embodies a criterion for focusing attention by ranking the elements of a formal decision model in order of importance.

Axiom A proposition regarded as self-evident.

Backward reasoning Reasoning from conclusions to facts.

Baud A unit of measure that measures the speed with which information is transferred. The baud rate is the maximum number of state transitions per second; for instance, a system whose shortest pulses are $\frac{1}{300}$ second is operating at 300 baud. In practice, baud rate is equal to the number of bits per second being sent (see Bps).

BBS Bulletin board system. A computer that allows users to log in from remote terminals, exchange messages, and (usually) download files of programs, data, text, etc.

Bernoulli process A random process consisting of a series of discrete, exchangeable trials (called Bernoulli trials), each of which can either succeed or fail with a common probability of success.

Binary numbers Base-2 numbers, which are written in a positional system that uses only two digits: 0 and 1. Binary numbers are well suited for use by computers, since many electrical devices have two distinct states: on and off.

BinHex Binary hexadecimal. A file that is an encoded representation of a binary file, but consists only of printable characters arranged in lines of reasonable length. A method of converting nontext files (non-ASCII) into ASCII.

Biomedical computing The use of computers in biology or medicine.

Biomedical engineering An area of engineering concerned primarily with the research and development of medical instrumentation and medical devices.

Bit A digit that can assume the values of either 0 or 1. Shorthand for *b*inary dig*it*.

BITNET *B*ecause *i*t's *t*ime network. A wide-area network linking university computer centers all over the world. E-mail among BITNET, the Internet, and USENET is possible because of gateways.

Boolean algebra The study of operations carried out on variables that can have only two values: 1 (true) and 0 (false). Developed by George Boole in the 1850s, it was useful originally in applications of the theory logic, and has become of tremendous importance in that area since the development of the computer. A common way to represent logic in many expert systems (see Expert system).

Bps Bits per second. A measurement of the speed of data transmission. In practice bps is the same as baud. For example, a 28.8 modem can transmit data at a rate of 28,000 bps and is said to have a baud rate of 28.8 (see Baud).

Browser A client program that is used to look at various kinds of Internet resources. For example, Netscape Navigator, Microsoft Explorer, etc.

Byte A sequence of eight bits. The amount of memory space needed to store one character, which is usually eight bits.

Central computer system A single system that handles all computer applications in an institution using a common set of databases and interfaces.

Central database A database that includes common definitions of medical terms, interrelationships of medical terms, a knowledge base, and a long-term archive.

Central processing unit (CPU) The "brain" of the computer. The CPU executes a program stored in main memory by fetching and executing instructions in the program.

Client A computer that receives services from another computer (known as a server), or (on multitasking operating systems) a process that receives services from another process. The system (software running on a piece of hardware) that initiates the process or requests services in a client/server architecture (see Server).

Client/server A style of distributed computing that enables several local area network-based PCs or workstations (known as clients) to share access to a more powerful server computer. With this approach, processes are divided between two systems that work together to perform a task, such as retrieving information from a database.

Clinical decision-support system A computer-based system that assists physicians in making decisions about patient care.

Clinical prediction rule A rule, derived from statistical analysis of clinical observations, that is used to assign a patient to a clinical subgroup with a known probability of disease.

Clinical research The collection and analysis of medical data collected during patient care to improve medical science and the knowledge physicians use in caring for patients.

Clinical subgroup A subset of a population in which the members have similar characteristics and symptoms, and therefore similar likelihood of disease.

Cognitive science Area of research concerned with studying the processes by which people think and behave.

Computer-based patient monitor A patient-monitoring device that also supports other data functions, such as database maintenance, report generation, and decision making.

Consulting system A computer-based system that develops and suggests problem-specific recommendations based on user input (see Critiquing system).

Critiquing system A computer-based system that evaluates and suggests modifications for plans or data analyses already formed by a user (see Consulting system).

Data-driven reasoning Reasoning from data to conclusions.

Data mining A technique that uncovers new information from existing information by probing mammoth data sets.

Datum Any single observation or fact.

Decision support system An information-processing system designed specifically to address the information needs of decision makers. Decision support systems evolved from database and management information systems.

DECNET Digital Equipment Corporation network. A software product for networking computers made by Digital Equipment Corporation.

Deterministic Not subject to chance.

Distributed computing A collection of independent computers that share data, programs, and other resources.

Domain In decision making, the generic subject matter with respect to which the decision is being made.

Electronic medical record A patient record that resides in a system specifically designed to support users by providing accessibility to complete and accurate data, alerts, reminders, clinical decision-support systems, links to library of medical terms, and other aids.

Ethernet A type of local area network originally developed by Xerox Corporation. Communication takes place by means of radiofrequency signals carried by a coaxial cable. Different Ethernet systems use different software protocols including TCP/IP and DECNET (see TCP/IP).

Expert system A program that symbolically encodes concepts derived from experts in a field and uses that knowledge to provide the kind of problem analysis and advice that the expert might provide. Specifically, a computer system designed to capture the skills and factual knowledge of one or more individuals. A program that uses a set of rules to construct a reasoning process that can reach conclusions and generate new data. Sometimes referred to as a rule-based system.

FAQ Frequently asked question. Documents that contain and answer the most asked questions on a particular subject. A popular heading on many Internet sites.

Forward reasoning Reasoning from facts to conclusions.

FTP File Transfer Protocol. The name of a program that transfers files from one computer to another on the Internet and on other TCP/IP networks (see Internet and TCP/IP).

Fuzzy logic A formal system of reasoning developed by Lotfi Zadeh in which the values true and false are replaced by numbers on a scale from 0 to 1. The operators 0 and 1, 0 or 1, and the like are replaced by procedures for combining these numbers (see Boolean algebra). Fuzzy logic captures the fact that some questions do not have simple yes-or-no answers. Often used in expert systems (see Expert system). A rules-based system that mimics human thought, enabling the computer to think in inexact terms rather than in a definite, either/or manner.

Gateway A link between two or more computer networks.

Genetic algorithm A program based on the rule of survival of the fittest. A genetic algorithm examines data and determines by programmed stipulations what data best match a stated goal and what data do not. For example, a genetic algorithm can be used to judge which automated clinical guideline best matches a clinician's predefined objective.

Gopher A client-server program that allows for making menus of material available on the Internet.

GUI Graphical user interface. A way of communicating with the computer by manipulating icons (pictures) and windows with a mouse as opposed to a textual user interface (TUI), which requires typed commands. For example, Microsoft Windows and Apple Macintosh.

Heuristic A rule of thumb; a cognitive process used in learning or problem solving.

HTML Hypertext Markup Language. The coding language used to create hypertext documents on the World Wide Web (WWW) (see WWW).

HTTP Hypertext Transport Protocol. A formal program for moving hypertext files across the Internet (see Internet).

Hypertext A formal way of creating documents so that information can be connected in many different ways rather than in a simple sequential manner as in books. Any text that links to other documents; words or phrases in a document that can be chosen and that cause another document to be retrieved and displayed.

Inference engine A computer program that embodies one or more general-purpose problem-solving algorithms that are largely independent of any specific domain. Inference engines draw conclusions by performing simple logical operations on knowledge bases and the information supplied by users.

Information Organized data or knowledge that provide a basis for decision making.

Information science The field of study concerned with issues related to the management of both paper-based and electronically stored information.

Input The data that represents state information, to be stored and processed to produce results (output).

Integrated User works with various applications while employing the same user-interface standards, vocabulary, and functional interaction standards.

Interfaced Implies accessibility to the applications from the same desktop even though the user interface, vocabulary, and functional conventions vary greatly in different applications.

Internet An immense network of networks, connecting computers at universities, research labs, commercial settings, private homes, and military sites. Internet grew out of the original ARPAnet as well as BITNET and several other networks (see ARPAnet and BITNET).

Knowledge Relationships, facts, assumptions, heuristics, and models derived through the formal or informal analysis (interpretation) of data.

Knowledge base A collection of stored facts, heuristics, and models that can be used for problem solving.

Knowledge engineering The art of formalizing knowledge. Typically the term is used in reference to building expert systems.

Laboratory information system (LIS) A computer-based information system that supports laboratory functions for collecting, verifying, and reporting test results.

Local-area network (LAN) A network for data communication that connects multiple nodes, all typically owned by a single institution and located within a small geographic area. A system of network software and hardware components used to connect a group of end stations via wire or fiber-optic cable. A single LAN segment connects from one to several hundred end stations, usually in the same building. A large organization may have a thousand or more LAN segments and tens of thousands of end stations.

Mainframe computer A large computer designed to manage large amounts of data and complex computing tasks. A mainframe computer can be utilized by hundreds or even thousands of users. The term also describes the memory storage and computing part of a large computer system, as opposed to input or output devices, such as video monitors, keyboards, or printers.

Medical informatics A field of study concerned with the broad range of issues in the management and use of biomedical information, including medical computing and the study of the nature of medical information.

Medical information bus (MIB) A data-communication system that supports data acquisition from a variety of independent devices.

Monolithic A unified and exclusive computer system with no interfaces to other systems.

Network A set of computers that are connected together. A collection of hardware, such as printers, modems, servers, and clients, that enables users to store and retrieve information, share devices, and exchange information (see Local-area network and Wide-area network).

Neural network A highly mathematical computer learning

methodology that learns from many examples to properly categorize and characterize new examples. A computer program that models the way nerve cells (neurons) are connected together in the human brain. Neural networks enable a computer to train itself to recognize patterns in a strikingly human-like way.

Nursing information system (NIS) A computer-based information system that supports nurses' professional duties in clinical practice, nursing administration, nursing research, and education.

Open architecture An approach to computing systems that assumes heterogeneous mixture of applications and host computers, systems, and databases, which are minimally interfaced with one another by means of de facto conventions and standards.

Open scalable The flexibility to buy products from different manufacturers to meet specific needs.

Open server A network server that can accommodate multiple operating systems and myriad software products. In addition, an open server can be used in numerous hardware configurations, because it is not dependent on proprietary standards.

Output The results produced when a process is applied to input. Some forms of output are hardcopy, documents, images displayed on video display terminals, and calculated values of variables.

Patient monitor An instrument that collects and displays physiologic data, often for the purpose of watching for and warning against life-threatening changes in physiologic state.

Patient monitoring Repeated or continuous measurement of physiologic parameters for the purpose of guiding therapeutic management.

Pharmacy information system (PIS) A computer-based information system that supports pharmacy personnel.

Process In a multitasking computer system, each series of instructions that the computer is executing is called a process or task. From the user's viewpoint, processes may be programs or parts of programs.

RAID Redundant array of inexpensive disks. A method of storing data on multiple hard disk drives for faster access and/or greater reliability. Currently, there are six officially defined levels, each designed for a specific kind of application.

RAS Reliability, availability, serviceability. Key measurements of a network's life cycle.

Server A computer that provides services to another computer (called the client). On multitasking machines, a process that provides services to another process.

SHV Standard high-volume server. Readily available server that relies on open architecture.

Standards The creation of common protocols for communication between different computer systems including electronic communication and data exchange. Examples include ASTM, HL7, ISO, and MEDEX.

Stochastic Uncertain; subject to chance.

Symbolic reasoning A method of deduction that follows an explicit line of inferences.

TCP/IP Transmission Control Protocol/Internet Protocol. A standard format for transmitting data in packets from one computer to another. It is used on the Internet and various other networks (see Internet).

Telnet A command on the Internet and other TCP/IP networks that allows one to use their computer as a terminal on another computer. The command allows a user to log in from one Internet site to another (see Internet and TCP/IP).

Terminal A computer that is dependent on a single host computer for its accessibility and capability.

Three-tier architecture A client/server architecture in which the screen presentation, database, and software programs run separately on the client, host computer, and one or more application severs, respectively. This division of labor allows information to be processed more quickly and facilitates distribution of data across wide area networks.

TUI Textual User Interface. A way of communicating with a computer through typed commands. For example, DOS or Unix.

URL Uniform Resource Location. The standard method to give the address of a resource on the Internet that is part of the WWW (see Internet and WWW).

USENET A wide-area network for Unix machines exchanging files through the Unix to Unix copy (UUCP) command. A main function is to maintain a large set of newsgroups (public forums), which are transmitted mainly through the Internet (see Internet).

Vaporware Programs promised by a vendor that never materialize (an exceedingly common occurrence).

Wide-area network (WAN) A set of widely separated computers connected together. Long-distance telecommunication links and networks that connect local-area networks and end stations.

Wireless LAN A local-area network in which the computers communicate by radio signals.

Workstation A computer that is connected to a network of host and server computers and has enough local processing power to run local applications and to interface with the hosts and servers.

WWW World Wide Web. The entire available resources that can be accessed using Gopher, HTTP, Telnet, Usenet, and other tools. The universe of hypertext servers.

REFERENCES

1. Dick RS, Steen EB, eds. *The electronic health record: an essential technology for health care.* Washington, DC: National Academy Press, 1991.
2. Levinson D. Information, computers, and clinical practice. *JAMA* 1983;249:607–609.
3. Lincoln TL. Medical information science: a joint endeavor. *JAMA* 1983;249:610–612.
4. Pollak VE. The computer in medicine: its application to medical practice, quality control, and cost containment. *JAMA* 1985;253:62–68.
5. Pryor DB, Califf RM, Harrell FE, et al. Clinical databases: accomplishments and unrealized potential. *Med Care* 1985;23:623–647.
6. Miller RA, Schaffner KF, Meisel A. Ethical and legal issues related to the use of computer programs in clinical medicine. *Ann Intern Med* 1985;102:529–536.
7. Gardner RM. Computerized data management and decision making in critical care. *Surg Clin North Am* 1985;65:1041–1051.

8. Bleich HL, Beckley RF, Horowitz GL, et al. Clinical computing in a teaching hospital. *N Engl J Med* 1985;312:756–764.
9. Blum BI. Clinical information systems: a review. *West J Med* 1986; 145:791–797.
10. Shortliffe EH. Medical expert systems: knowledge tools for physicians. *West J Med* 1986;145:830–839.
11. Gardner RM. Computerized management of intensive care patients. *MD Comput* 1986;3:36–51.
12. Blum RL. Computer-assisted design of studies using routine clinical data: analyzing the association of prednisone and cholesterol. *Ann Intern Med* 1986;104:858–868.
13. Rennels GD, Shortliffe EH. Advanced computing for medicine. *Sci Am* 1987;257:154–161.
14. McDonald CJ, Tierney WM. Computer-stored medical records: their future role in medical practice. *JAMA* 1988;259:3433–3440.
15. Korpman RA, Lincoln TL. The computer-stored medical record: for whom? *JAMA* 1988;259:3454–3456.
16. DeTore AW. Medical informatics: an introduction to computer technology in medicine. *Am J Med* 1988;85:399–403.
17. Winslow R. Desktop doctors. *The Wall Street Journal* 1992 April 6: R14.
18. Friedman BA, Dieterle RC. Integrating information systems in hospitals: bringing the outside inside. *Arch Pathol Lab Med* 1990;114: 13–16.
19. Greenes RA, Shortliffe EH. Medical informatics: an emerging academic discipline and institutional priority. *JAMA* 1990;263: 1114–1120.
20. Gransden WR. Information, computers, and infection control. *J Hosp Infect* 1990;15:1–5.
21. Shortliffe EH, Perreault LE, eds. *Medical informatics: computer applications in health care.* Reading: Addison-Wesley, 1990.
22. Carter JH. Medical informatics in postgraduate training: a way to improve office-based practitioner information management. *J Gen Intern Med* 1991;6:349–354.
23. Shortliffe EH, Tang PC, Detmer DE. Patient records and computers. *Ann Intern Med* 1991;115:979–981.
24. Bloomfield BP. The role of information systems in the UK National Health Service: action at a distance and the fetish of calculation. *Soc Stud Sci* 1991;21:701–734.
25. Hannan T. Computers and clinical decision-making: overcoming data overload. *Med J Aust* 1991;155:287–288.
26. Iezzoni LI. "Black box" medical information systems: a technology needing assessment. *JAMA* 1991;265:3006–3007.
27. Ball MJ, O'Desky RI, Douglas JV. Status and progress of hospital information systems (HIS). *Int J Biomed Comput* 1991;29:161–168.
28. Collen MF. A brief historical overview of hospital information system (HIS) evolution in the United States. *Int J Biomed Comput* 1991;29: 169–189.
29. Carey TS, Thomas D, Woolsey A, et al. Half a loaf is better than waiting for the bread truck: a computerized mini-medical record for outpatient care. *Arch Intern Med* 1992;152:1845–1849.
30. Tierney WM, McDonald CJ. Practice databases and their uses in clinical research. *Stat Med* 1991;10:541–557.
31. Safran C. Using routinely collected data for clinical research. *Stat Med* 1991;10:559–564.
32. Pryor DB, Lee KL. Methods for the analysis and assessment of clinical databases: the clinician's perspective. *Stat Med* 1991;10:617–628.
33. Stead WM. Systems for the year 2000: the case for an integrated database. *MD Comput* 1991;8:103–108.
34. Ball MJ, Collen MF, eds. *Aspects of the electronic health record.* New York: Springer-Verlag, 1992.
35. Osborn JJ. Computers in critical care medicine: promises and pitfalls. *Crit Care Med* 1982;10:807–810.
36. Gardner RM, West BL, Pryor TA, et al. Computer-based ICU data acquisition as an aid to clinical decision-making. *Crit Care Med* 1982; 10:823–830.
37. Gardner RM. Computers in critical care. *Wellcomes Trends Hosp Pharm* 1992;4:6–8.
38. Gardner RM, Clemmer TP. Computers in the intensive care unit: the clinical challenge. In: Civetta JM, Taylor WT, Kirby RR, eds. *Critical care,* 2nd ed. Philadelphia: JP Lippincott, 1992:1971–1924.
39. Dasta JF. Computers in critical care: opportunities and challenges. *DICP Ann Pharmacother* 1990;24:1084–1092.
40. Friedman BA, Martin JB. Hospital information systems: the physicians role. *JAMA* 1987;257:1792.
41. McDonald CJ. Computers. *JAMA* 1989;261:2834–2836.
42. Morgan JD. The electronic health record challenges the health information management profession. *J AHIMA* 1992;63:79–85.
43. Pollack VE. Computerized medical information system enhances quality assurance: a 10-year experience in chronic maintenance hemodialysis patients. *Nephron* 1990;54:109–116.
44. Korpman RA. Using the computer to optimize human performance in health care delivery. *Arch Pathol Lab Med* 1987;111:637–645.
45. Fries JF. The chronic disease data bank model: a conceptual framework for the computer-based medical record. *Comput Biomed Res* 1992;25:586–601.
46. Gardner RM, Maack BB, Evans RS, et al. Computerized medical care: the HELP system at LDS Hospital. *J AHIMA* 1992;63:68–78.
47. Dasta JF. Enhancing the pharmacist-computer interface. *Ann Pharmacother* 1992;26:99–100.
48. Woodruff AE, Hunt CA. Involvement in medical informatics may enable pharmacists to expand their consultation potential and improve the quality of healthcare. *Ann Pharmacother* 1992;26:100–104.
49. Dasta JF, Greer ML, Speedie SM. Computers in healthcare: overview and bibliography. *Ann Pharmacother* 1992;26:109–117.
50. Mowry MM, Korpman RA. *Paying for health care: managing health care costs, quality, and technology.* Rockville, MD: Aspen Publications, 1986.
51. Ledley RS, Lusted LB. The use of electronic computers in medical data processing. *IRE Trans Med Electronics* 1960;ME-7:31–47.
52. Lindberg DAB. *The growth of medical information systems in the United States.* Lexington, MA: DC Heath, 1979.
53. Dubois RW, Rogers WH, Moxley JH III, et al. Hospital in-patient mortality: is it a predictor of quality? *N Engl J Med* 1987;317: 1674–1679.
54. Berman GD, Kottke TS, Ballard DJ. Effectiveness research and assessment of clinical outcome: a review of federal government and medical community involvement. *Mayo Clin Proc* 1990;65:657–663.
55. Crede W, Hierholzer WJ. Mortality rates as a quality indicator: a simple answer to a complex question. *Infect Control Hosp Epidemiol* 1988;9:330–332.
56. Bleich HL, Slack WV. Designing a hospital information system: a comparison of interfaced and integrated systems. *MD Comput* 1992; 9:293–296.
57. Clayton PD, Sideli RV, Sengupta S. Open architecture and integrated information at Columbia-Presbyterian Medical Center. *MD Comput* 1992;9:297–303.
58. Korth HF, Silberschatz A. *Database system concepts,* 2nd ed. New York: McGraw-Hill, 1991.
59. Pyror TA, Gardner RM, Clayton PD, et al. The HELP system. *J Med Syst* 1983;7:87–102.
60. Pryor TA. The HELP medical record system. *MD Comput* 1988;5: 22–33.
61. Kuperman GJ, Gardner RM, Pryor TA. *HELP: a dynamic hospital information system.* New York: Springer-Verlag, 1991.
62. Wilson GA, McDonald CJ, McCabe GP. The effect of immediate access to a computerized medical record on physician test ordering: a controlled clinical trial in an emergency room. *Am J Public Health* 1982;72:698–702.
63. McDonald CJ, Wilson GA, McCabe GP. Physician response to computer reminders. *JAMA* 1980;244:1579–1581.
64. Tierney WM, McDonald CJ, Martin DK, et al. Computerized display of past test results: effect on outpatient testing. *Ann Intern Med* 1987; 107:569–574.
65. McDonald CJ, Hui SL, Smith DM, et al. Reminders to physicians from an introspective computer medical record. *Ann Intern Med* 1984; 100:130–138.
66. Tierney WM, Miller ME, McDonald CJ. The effect of test ordering

of informing physicians of the charges for outpatient diagnostic tests. *N Engl J Med* 1990;322:1499–1504.

67. Tierney WM, Miller ME, Overhag JM, et al. Physician inpatient order writing on microcomputer workstations: effects on resource utilization. *JAMA* 1993;269:379–383.
68. Piemme TE. Computer-assisted learning and evaluation in medicine. *JAMA* 1988;260:367–372.
69. Rootenberg JD. Information technologies in US medical schools. *JAMA* 1992;268:3107–3107.
70. Faltermayer E. Let's really cure the health system. *Fortune* 1992;125: 46–58.
71. McDonald CJ. Protocol-based computer reminders, the quality of care and the non-perfectibility of man. *N Engl J Med* 1976:295: 1351–1355.
72. Haynes RB, Walker CJ. Computer-aided quality assurance: a critical appraisal. *Arch Intern Med* 1987;147:1297–1301.
73. Gardner RM, Evans RS. Computer-assisted quality assurance. *Group Practice J* 1992;May/June:8–11.
74. Evans RS, Gardner RM, Bush AR, et al. Development of a computerized infectious disease monitor (CIDM). *Comput Biomed Res* 1985; 18:103–113.
75. Evans RS, Larsen RA, Burke JP, et al. Computer surveillance of hospital-acquired infections and antibiotic use. *JAMA* 1986;256: 1007–1011.
76. Bradshaw KE, Gardner RM, Pryor TA. Development of a computerized laboratory information system. *Comput Biomed Res* 1989;22: 575–587.
77. Larsen RA, Evans RS, Burke JP, et al. Improved perioperative antibiotic use and reduced surgical wound infections through use of computer decision analysis. *Infect Control Hosp Epidemiol* 1989;10: 316–320.
78. Tate KE, Gardner RM, Weaver LK. A computerized laboratory alerting system. *MD Comput* 1990;7:296–301.
79. Gardner RM, Hulse RK, Larsen KG. Assessing the effectiveness of a computerized pharmacy system. *SCAMC* 1990;14:668–672.
80. Gardner RM, Golubjatnikov OK, Laub RM, et al. Computer-critiqued blood ordering using the HELP system. *Comput Biomed Res* 1990;23:514–528.
81. Evans RS, Pestotnik SL, Burke JP, et al. Reducing duration of prophylactic antibiotic use through computer monitoring of surgical patients. *DICP Ann Pharmacother* 1990;24:351–354.
82. Pestotnik SL, Evans RS, Burke JP, et al. Therapeutic antibiotic monitoring: surveillance using a hospital information system. *Am J Med* 1990;88:43–48.
83. Burke JP, Classen DC, Pestotnik SL, et al. The HELP system and its application to infection control. *J Hosp Infect* 1991;18(suppl A): 424–431.
84. Classen DC, Burke JP, Pestotnik SL, et al. Surveillance for quality assessment: IV. Surveillance using a hospital information system. *Infect Control Hosp Epidemiol* 1991;12:239–244.
85. Evans RS. The HELP system: a review of clinical applications in infectious diseases and antibiotic use. *MD Comput* 1991;5:282–315.
86. Classen DC, Pestotnik SL, Evans RS, et al. Computerized surveillance of adverse drug events in hospital patients. *JAMA* 1991;266: 2847–2851.
87. Evans RS, Pestotnik SL, Classen DC, et al. Development of a computerized adverse drug event monitor. *SCAMC* 1991;15:23–27.
88. Classen DC, Pestotnik SL, Evans RS, et al. Intensive surveillance of midazolam use in hospitalized patients and the occurrence of cardiorespiratory arrest. *Pharmacotherapy* 1992;12:213–216.
89. Classen DC, Pestotnik SL, Evans RS, et al. Description of a computerized adverse drug event monitoring using a hospital information system. *Hosp Pharm* 1992;27:774,776–779,783.
90. Evans RS, Pestotnik SL, Classen DC, et al. Prevention of adverse drug events through computerized surveillance. *SCAMC* 1992;16: 437–441.
91. Classen DC, Evans RS, Pestotnik SL, et al. The timing of prophylactic administration of antibiotics and the risk of surgical-wound infections. *N Engl J Med* 1992;326:281–286.
92. Evans RS, Burke JP, Classen DC, et al. Computerized identification of patients at high risk for hospital-acquired infections. *Am J Infect Control* 1992;20:4–10.
93. Evans RS, Pestotnik SL, Classen DC, et al. Development of an automated antibiotic consultant. *MD Comput* 1993;10:17–22.
94. Pestotnik SL, Classen DC, Evans RS, et al. Prospective surveillance of imipenem/cilastatin use and associated seizures using a hospital information system. *Ann Pharmacother* 1993;27:497–501.
95. Evans RS, Classen DC, Pestotnik SL, et al. Improving empiric antibiotic selection using computer decision support. *Arch Intern Med* 1994; 154(8):878–884.
96. Enthoven AC. A cure for health costs. *World Monitor* 1992;April: 34–39.
97. Pryor TA. Development of decision support systems. *Int J Clin Monit Comput* 1990;7:137–146.
98. Shortliffe EH. Computer programs to support clinical decision making. *JAMA* 1987;258:61–66.
99. Dasta JF. Application of artificial intelligence to pharmacy and medicine. *Hosp Pharm* 1992;27:312–315,319–322.
100. Wyatt J. Computer-based knowledge systems. *Lancet* 1991;338: 1431–1436.
101. Beyt EE. Computer monitoring—the next step in surveillance. *JAMA* 1986;256:1042.
102. Spackman KA, Connelly DP. Knowledge-based systems in laboratory medicine and pathology. *Arch Pathol Lab Med* 1987;111:116–119.
103. Kinney EL. Medical expert systems: who needs them? *Chest* 1987; 91:3–4.
104. Barnett OG, Cimino JJ, Hupp JA, et al. DXplain: an evolving diagnostic decision-support system. *JAMA* 1987;258:67–74.
105. Mabry ME, Miller RM. Distinguishing drug toxicity syndromes from medical diseases: a QMR computer-based approach. *SCAMC* 1990; 14:65–71.
106. Polaschek JX, Lenert LA, Garber AM. A computer program for statistically-based decision analysis. *SCAMC* 1990;14:795–799.
107. Lenert LA, Lurie J, Coleman R, et al. Aminoglycoside therapy manager: an advanced computer program for decision support for drug dosing and therapeutic monitoring. *SCAMC* 1990;14:982–983.
108. Mabry ME, Miller RA. Distinguishing drug toxicity syndromes from medical diseases: a QMR computer-based approach. *Comput Methods Programs Biomed* 1991;35:310.
109. Martin DK. Making the connection: the VA-Regenstrief project. *MD Comput* 1992;9:91–96.
110. Hinton GE. How neural networks learn from experience. *Sci Am* 1992;10:145–151.
111. East TD, Henderson S, Pace NL, et al. Knowledge engineering using retrospective review of data: a useful technique or merely data dredging? *Int J Clin Monit Comput* 1992;8:259–262.
112. East TD, Morris AH, Wallace CJ, et al. A strategy for development of computerized critical care decision support systems. *Int J Clin Monit Comput* 1992;8:263–269.
113. Lenert LA, Jurie J, Sheiner LB, et al. Advanced computer programs for drug dosing that combine pharmacokinetic and symbolic modeling of patients. *Comput Biomed Res* 1992;25:29–42.
114. Mabry ME. Computer-aided assessment of the adverse effects of antiepileptic drugs. *Drug Infor J* 1992;26:505–517.
115. Halpern NA, Thompson RE, Greenstein RJ. A computerized intensive care unit order-writing protocol. *Ann Pharmacother* 1992;26: 251–254.
116. Greer ML. RXPERT: a prototype expert system for formulary decision making. *Ann Pharmacother* 1992;26:244–250.
117. Lepage EF, Gardner RM, Laub RM, et al. Assessing the effectiveness of a computerized blood ordering "consultation system." *SCAMC* 1991;15:33–37.
118. Kahn MG, Steib SA, Fraser VJ, et al. An expert system for culture-based infection control surveillance. *SCAMC* 1993;17:171.
119. Berwick DM. Controlling variation in health care: a consultation with Walter Shewhart. *Med Care* 1991;29:1212–1225.
120. Chassin MR, Brook RH, Park RE, et al. Variations in the use of medical and surgical services by the Medicare population. *N Engl J Med* 1986;314:285–290.
121. Gaynes R, Friedman C, Copeland TA, et al. Methodology to evaluate

a computer-based system for surveillance of hospital-acquired infections. *Am J Infect Control* 1990;18:40–46.

122. Birnbaum D. Software for infection control data gathering. *Infect Control* 1984;5:161.
123. Ura S. Software for infection control data gathering. *Infect Control* 1984;5:161.
124. LaHaise S. A comparison of infection control software for use by hospital epidemiologists in meeting the new JCAHO standards. *Infect Control Hosp Epidemiol* 1990;11:185–190.
125. Reagan DR. The choice of microcomputer software for infection control. *Infect Control Hosp Epidemiol* 1990;11:178–179.
126. Zellner S, Polley N. Infection control software. *Infect Control Hosp Epidemiol* 1990;11:400–401.
127. Berg R. Software. *Am J Infect Control* 1986;14:139–145.
128. LaHaise S. Reply to Zellner and Polley [ref. 126 above]. *Infect Control Hosp Epidemiol* 1990;11:404.
129. Rundio A Jr. Infection control software. *Infect Control Hosp Epidemiol* 1990;11:403–404.
130. Howard B, Seymour J, Derfler FJ Jr, et al. *8th annual printer review.* New York: Ziff-Davis, 1991;110.
131. Regan DR. Product review: paradigm. *Infect Control Hosp Epidemiol* 1991;12:191–193.
132. Bria WF, Rydel RL. *The physician-computer connection.* Chicago: American Hospital Publishing, 1992.
133. Medical hardware and software buyer's guide. *MD Comput* 1992;9: 339–512.
134. Board of Directors of the American Medical Informatics Association. Standards for medical identifiers, codes, and messages needed to create an efficient computer-stored medical record. *J Am Med Inform Assoc* 1994;1:1–7.
135. Gardner RM, Tariq H, Hawley WL, et al. Editorial: medical information bus: the key to future integrated monitoring. *Int J Clin Monit Comput* 1989;6:205–209.
136. Ellis LBM, Krogh D, Werth G. Noise and validity in a practice-derived database. *SCAMC* 1990;14:271–275.
137. Thompson BD, Piland NF, Hoy WE, et al. Standard information content and procedures used in the formation of a research oriented health services database. *SCAMC* 1990;14:359–363.
138. McGeer A, Crede W, Hierholzer WJ. Surveillance for quality assessment: II surveillance for noninfectious processes: back to basics. *Infect Control Hosp Epidemiol* 1990;11:36–41.
139. Wenzel RP, Streed SA. Surveillance and use of computers in hospital infection control. *J Hosp Infect* 1989;13:217–229.
140. Schifman RB, Palmer RA. Surveillance of nosocomial infection by computer analysis of positive culture rates. *J Clin Microbiol* 1985;21: 493–495.
141. Burken MI, Zaman AF, Smith FJ. Semi-automated infection control surveillance in a Veterans' Administration Medical Center. *Infect Control Hosp Epidemiol* 1990;11:410–412.
142. Reference deleted in proofs.
143. Shortliffe EH. Healthcare and the next generation Internet [editorial]. *Ann Intern Med* 1998;129:138–140.
144. Flahault A, Dias-Ferrao V, Chaberty P, et al. FluNet as a tool for global monitoring of influenza on the web. *JAMA* 1998;280: 1330–1332.
145. Cimino JJ, Socratous SA, Clayton PD. Internet as clinical information system: application development using the World Wide Web. *J Am Med Inform Assoc* 1995;2:273–284.
146. McDonald CJ, Overhage JM, Dexter PR, et al. Canopy computing: using the web in clinical practice. *JAMA* 1998;280:1325–1329.
147. Lowe HJ, Lomax EC, Polonkey SE. The World Wide Web: a review of an emerging internet based technology for the distribution of biomedical information. *J Am Med Inform Assoc* 1996;3:1–14.
148. Reference deleted in proofs.
149. Reference deleted in proofs.
150. Schriger DL, Baraff LJ, Rogers WH, et al. Implementation of clinical guidelines using a computer charting system. Effect on the initial care of health care workers exposed to body fluids. *JAMA* 1997;278(19): 1585–1590.
151. Dexter PR, Perkins S, Overhage JM, et al. A computerized reminder system to increase the use of preventive care for hospitalized patients. *N Engl J Med* 2001;345(13):965–970.
152. Morris AH. Developing and implementing computerized protocols for standardization of clinical decisions. *Ann Intern Med* 2000;132(5): 373–383.
153. Duncan RG, Saperia D, Dulbandzhyan R, et al. Integrated web-based viewing and secure remote access to a clinical data repository and diverse clinical systems. *Proc AMIA Symp* 2001;149–153.
154. Wang DJ, Harkness KB, Allshouse C, et al. Development of a web based electronic patient record extending accessibility to clinical information and integrating ancillary applications. *Proc AMIA Symp* 1998;: 131–134.
155. Internet user will surpass 1 billion in 2005. eTForecasts, *www.etforecasts.com*, February 6, 2001.
156. WAP, not Web: 95 million browser handsets in 2004, marketers must resist imposing Web models on mobile access. Jupiter Media Metrix, *www.jup.com*, August 15, 2000.
157. Wireless LANs almost ready for widescale adoption. InformationWeek.com, *www.iweek.com*, November 14, 2000.
158. Sittig DF, Jimison HB, Hazlehurst BL, et al. Techniques for identifying the applicability of new information management technologies in the clinical setting: an example focusing on handheld computers. Proceedings of the 2000 AMIA Annual Symposium. *J Am Med Informatics Soc* 2000;symposium suppl:804–808.
159. Shabot MM, LoBue M, Chen J. Wireless clinical alerts for physiologic, laboratory and medication data. Proceedings of the 2000 AMIA Annual Symposium. *J Am Med Informatics Soc* 2000;symposium suppl: 789–793.
160. Scott L. Point of contact. *Modern Physician* 2000:38–54.
161. Physicians and the Internet: taking the pulse. *Hospitals and Health Networks.* Deloitte and Touche and Deloitte Consulting, 2001;75(2): 51–57.
162. Poussord M. Three key wireless issues to ponder. *HIS Insider Weekly* February 26, 2001:1–2.
163. Physicians and the Internet: taking the pulse. *Hospitals and Health Networks* February 2001.
164. Scott L. Point of contact. *Modern Physician* 2000:38–54.
165. Freudenheim M. Digital doctoring. *New York Times www.nytimes.-com*, January 8, 2001.
166. Wireless LANs almost ready for widescale adoption. InformationWeek.com, *www.iweek.com*, November 13, 2000.
167. Rothschild JM, Lee TH, Bae T, et al. Clinician use of a palmtop drug reference guide. *J Am Med Inform Assoc* 2002;9(3):223–229.
168. Miller SM, Beattie MM, Butt AA. Personal digital assistant infectious diseases applications for health care professionals. *Clin Infect Dis* 2003; 36(8):1018–1029.
169. Evans RS, Pestotnik SL, Classen DC, et al. A computer-assisted management program for antibiotics and other antiinfective agents. *N Engl J Med* 1998;338(4):232–238.
170. Evans RS, Pestotnik SL, Classen DC, et al. Evaluation of a computer-assisted antibiotic-dose monitor. *Ann Pharmacother* 1999;33(10): 1026–1031.

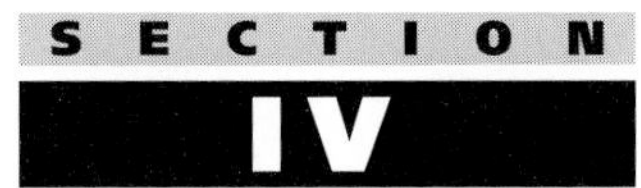

EPIDEMIOLOGY AND PREVENTION OF NOSOCOMIAL INFECTIONS OF ORGAN SYSTEMS

17

NOSOCOMIAL INFECTIONS RELATED TO USE OF INTRAVASCULAR DEVICES INSERTED FOR SHORT-TERM VASCULAR ACCESS

BARRY M. FARR

Vascular catheters have become an indispensable part of modern medicine, allowing administration of medications, fluids, electrolytes, blood products, and nutritional therapy. Specialized functions include hemodynamic monitoring, hemodialysis, and plasmapheresis. Vascular catheters are inserted into more than half of all patients admitted to hospitals in both the United States and Europe and are increasingly being used in the outpatient setting as well (1). In the United States alone, more than 150 million catheters are sold each year (2). About 3 million central venous catheters (CVCs) are inserted into patients in the United States each year (3). Although these catheters provide lifesaving therapy, they can also provide a route for microorganisms to bypass normal host defenses and cause serious infection. Infections related to short-term vascular catheters are the focus of this chapter.

DEFINITIONS

Colonization of an indwelling vascular catheter refers to significant growth of microbes on either the endoluminal surface or the external catheter surface beneath the skin. Colonization is confirmed by the results of semiquantitative culture of catheter segments growing at least 15 colony-forming units (CFUs) (4) or quantitative cultures growing at least 100 CFUs (5). For this purpose a catheter segment has usually consisted of either the distal 5 cm of the catheter (tip) or the 5-cm segment just beneath the skin (subcutaneous segment).

Local catheter-related infection is usually manifested clinically by local inflammation, which may include erythema, tenderness, warmth, and/or a purulent discharge from the catheter tract. If a culture is performed, the catheter usually is significantly colonized at the time of a local catheter-related infection.

Exit-site infection is a type of local catheter-related infection of a tunneled catheter where it exits from the skin. This has been defined clinically by the occurrence of erythema and tenderness within 2 cm of the exit site of such a catheter or by the discharge of pus at the exit site (6). A catheter segment culture would usually show colonization if performed.

Tunnel infection has been defined as the presence of erythema, tenderness, and induration extending along the tunnel of a tunneled catheter more than 2 cm from the exit site (6). Local signs of inflammation over the tunneled portion of the catheter may or may not be accompanied by signs of inflammation and/or purulent discharge at the exit site.

Catheter-related bloodstream infection has been defined as the isolation of the same microbe from blood cultures that is shown to be significantly colonizing the catheter of a patient with clinical features of bloodstream infection (most often manifested by fever alone but also possibly including hypothermia, rigors, hypotension, tachypnea, tachycardia, and confusion) in the absence of any other local infection caused by the same microbe that could have given rise to bloodstream infection (4).

Primary bloodstream infection is one that arises without apparent local infection elsewhere resulting from the same microbe. Vascular catheter-related bloodstream infection is considered to be one type of primary bloodstream infection.

PATHOGENESIS

Infection of short-term catheters has most often been due to microbes from the skin moving along the catheter surface where the catheter enters the skin (7–9). Progression of these invading microbes distally along the catheter tract can result in bloodstream infection with or without obvious local catheter-related infection. Experiments involving catheter placement in a guinea pig skin model have suggested that microbes can move rapidly along the length of a catheter placed under the skin, perhaps by capillary action (10).

By contrast, infection related to long-term catheters (i.e., those in place for more than 3 weeks) is more often due to microorganisms gaining access to the catheter through the catheter hub and then moving down the endoluminal surface of the catheter to the bloodstream (11–13). Scanning electron microscopy of the external and endoluminal surfaces of catheters after varying durations of placement has supported this hypothesis by showing more microbes on the external than endoluminal surfaces of catheters that had been in place for less than 10 days and the opposite for catheters that had been in place for more than 30 days (13) (see also Chapter 18).

CLINICAL MANIFESTATIONS

Local catheter-related infection is manifested as described previously. Clinical manifestations of bloodstream infections may include fever, rigors, hypothermia, tachypnea, hypotension, septic shock, and/or confusion. In the neonate, apnea and/or bradycardia may be prominent symptoms. The most frequent presentation for patients with catheter-related bloodstream infections is simply fever developing in a patient with a catheter in place in the absence of symptoms suggesting infection at another body site. Such a presentation has high positive predictive value for catheter-related bloodstream infections in relatively healthy outpatients with an indwelling catheter. By contrast, among patients in the intensive care unit who develop fever in the presence of an indwelling catheter, 75% to 88% of patients do not have a catheter-related infection (14–17).

In 70% of bloodstream infections related to CVCs, there are no local signs of inflammation around the catheter (18). By contrast, with bloodstream infection resulting from peripheral venous catheters, inflammation or purulent discharge is usually evident at the site of the catheter (19). Most inflammation at the site of peripheral intravenous catheters, however, is due to bland physicochemical thrombophlebitis not infection (20). This was found to remain true among patients with *Staphylococcus aureus* nasal colonization (21). Such phlebitis occurs in about 30% of patients after only 2 to 3 days of infusion therapy. Principal causes of this noninfectious phlebitis include the catheter material, inexperience of the person inserting the catheter, duration of catheter placement, the rate of infusion, and the pH and chemical composition of the infusate. A high infusion rate results in a higher risk of phlebitis, whereas a heparin lock infusing nothing is associated with a very low risk for phlebitis. Hypertonic solutions; those with low pH; and infusions containing potassium chloride or antibiotics such as vancomycin, metronidazole, or amphotericin B are more likely to cause phlebitis (20).

Catheter-related septic phlebitis is associated with local inflammation and induration over the involved vein in most but not all cases involving a peripheral intravenous catheter (22–25). In cases involving a CVC, septic phlebitis is not usually associated with signs of inflammation or of venous obstruction; these are found in only a small proportion of radiographically confirmed cases of septic thrombophlebitis. The diagnosis of septic thrombophlebitis should be suspected in patients remaining febrile and/or bacteremic despite appropriate antimicrobial therapy with drugs to which the causative microbes are susceptible.

Infective arteritis resulting from an arterial catheter is usually manifested by fever and inflammation at the site of the catheter. As the lesion develops, a pulsatile mass may become palpable. In some patients, Osler nodes, petechiae, purpura, and/or septic arthritis may occur distal to the infected aneurysm (26). Femoral neuropathy and arterial insufficiency to the leg have been reported with infection resulting from a femoral artery catheter (22–26).

Endocarditis is usually suspected clinically when a febrile patient is noted to have a new or changing murmur, splenomegaly, or embolic lesions, but such classic manifestations of endocarditis are often absent (27). Several studies suggested that nosocomial bloodstream infections and those associated with a primary focus of infection such as a vascular catheter were less likely to develop endocarditis (27–30).

New criteria for diagnosing endocarditis using echocardiography (31) were used in a recent study, which performed transthoracic and transesophageal echocardiography on all cases and found that 16 (23%) of 69 patients with catheter-related *S. aureus* bloodstream infection had developed endocarditis (32). The major criteria for diagnosing endocarditis included (a) blood culture results suggestive of endocarditis because of the species involved or the continuousness of the bacteremia and (b) evidence of endocardial involvement by echocardiography (31). The sensitivity of transthoracic echocardiography for diagnosing these cases was only 27% (32).

LABORATORY DIAGNOSIS

Sixteen different methods and 17 different variations of these methods have been proposed for the laboratory diagnosis of catheter-related bloodstream infection, but relatively few studies have examined the relative accuracy and cost-effectiveness of these different methods. A recent study found that there were sufficient publications regarding six of the different methods to allow pooling of data for a meta-analysis (33). These six methods included three methods for catheter segment culture and three methods for culture of blood drawn through the catheter. The catheter segment methods involve (a) qualitative culture of the catheter segment (i.e., dropping the segment into a tube of broth, incubating for 2 to 3 days, and identifying any microbe that grows), (b) semiquantitative culture of the segment (rolling the segment across the top of a sheep blood agar plate four times, incubating the plate for 2 to 3 days, enumerating any colonies, and identifying the microbes) (34), and (c) quantitative culture of the segment (dropping the segment into a tube containing a milliliter of culture broth and sonicating or vortexing to remove microbes from the catheter surfaces, performing serial dilutions of the resulting suspension, plating aliquots of these dilutions, incubating for 2 to 3 days, enumerating any colonies, and identifying the microbes).

The first of the three catheter blood culture methods involved qualitative culture of blood drawn through a suspect catheter (i.e., colonies were not counted). The other two methods both involved quantitative cultures of blood (i.e., serial dilutions of the original specimen were made and plated allowing precise enumeration of the concentration of microbes circulating in the blood at the time the specimen was taken). One of these two methods simply enumerates the number of CFUs per milliliter in blood drawn through the catheter and attributes the infection to an infected catheter if the concentration is higher than a certain threshold level; most of the studies used 100 CFU/mL as their threshold. The remaining method compared the result of a quantitative blood culture drawn through the catheter with one drawn percutaneously from a peripheral vein, reasoning that a higher concentration in blood from the catheter implies a catheter origin for the infection. Each of the five studies used a different threshold for diagnosing catheter involvement (one a 30-CFU absolute difference, the second a 3:1 ratio, the third a 4:1 ratio, and the fifth a 5:1 ratio). A more recent study of the paired quantitative blood culture method has advocated using a threshold of 8:1 (14).

Quantitative catheter segment culture was the only method of the six evaluated in the meta-analysis that was associated with a pooled sensitivity greater than 90% and a pooled specificity greater than 90% (94% and 92%, respectively) (33). By comparison, the test most often used by hospital laboratories in the United States, the semiquantitative catheter segment culture method, had a pooled sensitivity of 85% and a pooled specificity of 85%. Receiver operating characteristic (ROC) curve analysis found a significant increase in accuracy with increasing quantitation of the method for catheter segment culture ($p = .03$). Analysis of costs showed that the semiquantitative culture was the cheapest of the catheter segment culture methods for the laboratory to perform, at $38.63 per test. It also offered a marginally lower cost per accurate result than did the quantitative catheter segment culture ($401.38 compared with $415.62) (33).

Catheter blood culture methods showed a trend toward increasing accuracy with increasing quantitation of the method, but this did not reach statistical significance (33). This could be due to the fact that fewer and smaller studies had been performed with these methods, resulting in lower statistical power for detecting a significant difference among methods despite pooling of available data. Quantitative catheter blood culture appeared to be less sensitive albeit more specific than the catheter segment culture methods. Sensitivity of the quantitative catheter blood culture appeared to be lower in studies focusing on short-term catheters. Nevertheless, the unpaired quantitative catheter blood culture, which had a pooled sensitivity of 78%, offered the lowest cost per accurate test result ($198.18) (33). Thus, it would be preferred when evaluating for bloodstream infection in a febrile patient with a long-dwelling tunneled catheter. A new approach to diagnosing catheter-related bloodstream infection has compared time to positivity for blood drawn from a catheter with that drawn percutaneously from a peripheral vein. When blood drawn from the catheter turns culture positive more than 2 hours earlier than blood drawn from a peripheral vein, this has been shown to suggest that the catheter is the source of infection. To date, the published studies have shown this to work with long-dwelling catheters, and it remains unclear that it will work as well with short-term catheters (34,35).

INCIDENCE

Studies of the risk of catheter-related bloodstream infection with peripheral intravenous catheters have documented rates less than 1 per 1,000 catheter insertions and less than 1 per 1,000 catheter-days (36–39). Early data had found arterial catheter-related bloodstream infection after 4% of arterial catheter insertions (40), but more recent studies have found a much lower incidence. Three studies reported no episodes of arterial catheter-related bloodstream infection after 639 arterial catheter insertions (41–43). By contrast, the risk of bloodstream infection with short-term CVCs ranges from 1% to 10% of catheter insertions (2). The incidence of primary bloodstream infections during the 1980s was 0.28 per 100 discharges among patients in hospitals reporting data to the National Nosocomial Infections Surveillance (NNIS) system (44). During that decade, the rate of primary bloodstream infections increased by 70% in large teaching hospitals and by 279% in small nonteaching hospitals. Although data regarding the frequency of use of CVCs within these hospitals was not available, it is believed that increased use of such devices contributed to this large increase in catheter-related infection.

A 7-month study of the frequency of use and complications of CVC at a university hospital during 1995 documented the use of 2,806 catheters in 1,393 hospitalized adult patients (10% of all adult patients in the hospital during the study period) (45). These catheters were in place for 22,369 catheter-days, which involved 31% of all adult patient-days, including 69% of all patient days in intensive care units (ICUs) and 22% of patient-days on other adult wards. Short-term CVCs accounted for 71% of all central catheters used and 13,709 catheter-days (61% of catheter-days) (45). The overall rates of bloodstream infection during the 7-month study were 1.4 per 100 catheters inserted and 1.7 per 1,000 CVC-days. The rates were similar for patients in ICUs and hospital wards [1.7 vs. 1.6 per 1,000 CVC days, relative risk (RR) = 1.07, $p = .98$]. The rate of infection observed in this study was also similar to the rate observed during a randomized trial of catheter management in ICUs in this hospital several years before (1.5 per 100 catheter insertions) (46).

OUTCOMES

The case fatality rate associated with catheter-related bloodstream infection was found to be 14% in a meta-analysis that evaluated publications reporting 2,573 cases of catheter-related bloodstream infection and information regarding outcome (47). The authors of the original publications reported that 11.3% of patients with bloodstream infections died because of their underlying illness, accounting for 81% of the deaths in patients with catheter-related bloodstream infections. The authors of the original publications believed that 2.7% [95% confidence interval (CI): 2.0% to 3.4%] of patients with catheter-related bloodstream infection died because of the infection itself, accounting for 19% of deaths following the infections (47).

Adverse prognostic factors identified in the meta-analysis included neutropenia, bloodstream infection on a surgical service, and bloodstream infection in an ICU. Infections resulting from coagulase-negative staphylococci and enterococci were associated with lower rates of attributed mortality than for other pathogens (0.7% and 0%, respectively) (47). *Candida,* by contrast, was associated with a higher attributed mortality rate as compared with other pathogens (9%, $p = .001$) as was *S. aureus* (8.2%, $p < .001$). Another review of the outcome of catheter-related *S. aureus* bacteremias included data from 25 studies and reported 59 deaths among 177 patients for an overall case fatality rate of

33.3% (95% CI: 26.4% to 40.2%) (48). The proportion of cases in which death was attributed to the infection itself by the authors of the original publications was14.8% (95% CI: 10.8% to 18.8%), accounting for 44% of all of the deaths following catheter-related *S. aureus* bacteremia (48). A recent study found that *Candida* catheter-related bloodstream infections were associated with a sevenfold higher death rate than for coagulase-negative staphylococci (49).

Patients surviving a nosocomial bloodstream infection have remained in the hospital for an extra 7 to 24 days (50,51). This longer stay and the additional costs of antibiotics and diagnostic tests add significantly to hospital costs. The Centers for Disease Control and Prevention (CDC) estimated from data collected in the Study on the Efficacy of Nosocomial Infection Control (SENIC) conducted in the 1970s and updated in the 1980s that a nosocomial bloodstream infection added $3,517 to the cost of hospitalization (50). In 1988 Maki et al. (52) estimated that this excess cost had risen to $6,000. Pittet et al. (51) measured the costs incurred by patients suffering nosocomial bloodstream infection and control patients (matched for ICU admission, major diagnosis, number of diagnoses, and length of stay until the time of the infection in the case patient) in a surgical ICU between 1988 and 1990. Hospital costs averaged $33,268 more for case patients than for controls and $40,890 more for surviving case patients than for their matched controls.

RISK FACTORS

The most important risk factor for a catheter-related bloodstream infection in most patients has been the type of catheter used. Although peripheral intravenous catheters are used for most infusion therapy, they account for only a tiny proportion of all catheter-related bloodstream infections. CVCs account for about 2% of all catheters inserted (1,2) and 97% of all published cases of catheter-related bloodstream infections (47). Several observational studies have suggested a higher rate of infection with multilumen as compared with single-lumen CVCs (53–58), but randomized trials have produced conflicting results (59,60). One study involving multilumen catheters used in an ICU reported that only 1.5% of catheterizations resulted in bloodstream infections (46).

Total parenteral nutrition (TPN) has been considered a risk factor for catheter-related bloodstream infection, (61) but three studies found no association, suggesting that when managed properly it need not be a risk factor (7,46,62). One study found that the use of such catheters for other purposes was associated with a higher risk for infection (63). Another study found an association with infection when TPN catheters were used with a needleless infusion system (64). Infection rates associated with TPN catheters have been lower with the use of a dedicated team for the insertion and maintenance of the catheters (65–68).

A prolonged outbreak of bloodstream infections in an ICU was linked to infection of catheters being used to infuse TPN when the nurse-to-patient ratio fell below a critical level, suggesting that overworked staff may be unable to manage such high-risk devices in an optimal manner (69). A follow-up study confirmed this association between understaffing and risk for infection (70).

Hyperglycemia has been correlated with a higher rate of postoperative infections among diabetics including bloodstream infections (71), and hyperglycemia was documented more often in patients randomized to TPN than to enteral nutrition in a randomized trial (72). *Candida* and staphylococci have been the microbes most often associated with TPN catheter-related infections (17,63). Lipid infusions used with TPN have been specifically associated with risk of catheter-related bloodstream infections resulting from coagulase negative staphylococci (73,74) and *Malassezia furfur* (75). Three recent pediatric studies have also found TPN to be a risk factor for catheter-related bloodstream infection (49,76,77), and two found lipid infusions to be risk factors for fungal catheter-related bloodstream infection, one for candidemia (49) and the other for *Pichia anomola* bloodstream infection during an ICU outbreak (76). Birth weight and use of a Broviac catheter were also important predictors in one of these studies(77).

Duration of catheterization is a risk factor for infection, with the cumulative risk of infection increasing linearly as a function of catheter duration (78). The incidence density of infection does not appear to increase after the first few days of catheterization with CVCs used in the ICU (79) or for hemodialysis (80). These data were supported by studies using an experimental catheter infection model in rabbits, which showed that the highest risk of infection occurred during the first 2 days after insertion, with lower daily rates thereafter (81).

Acquired immunodeficiency syndrome (AIDS) has been a risk factor for catheter-related bloodstream infection, (82,83) but this risk appears to be somewhat lower with use of highly active antiretroviral therapy (84).

Site selection may be an important risk factor for infection because several observational studies have suggested higher infection rates for jugular than for subclavian catheters (85–89) and for femoral than subclavian catheters or internal jugular (IJ) catheters (89–91). Not all observational studies have found the same association, however (92–94). Two recent randomized controlled trials have shown higher complication rates for femoral catheters than for those in the subclavian or jugular vein (95, 96). These complications included significantly higher rates of deep venous thrombosis in both studies and of catheter-related infection in one (96).

Peripherally inserted central catheters (PICCs) have been associated with a very low incidence of bloodstream infection but have mostly been used in outpatients until recently (97,98). Limited data are available with hospitalized patients (99–101). Lower infection rates with this approach than with subclavian or internal jugular catheters could be due to lower concentrations of resident flora on the arm than the chest or neck (102,103). More randomized trials of site selection are needed.

Inexperience of the individual inserting the catheter was shown to be significantly associated with risk for infection in a study that showed an inverse correlation between the total number of catheters inserted by the physician inserting the catheter and risk for significant colonization of the catheter (104). Another observational study found a higher rate of infection when only a small sterile towel and sterile gloves were used for insertion of the catheter as compared with insertion using large sterile drapes while wearing a mask, cap, and sterile gloves and gown (85). These two studies suggest that inadvertent contamination during insertion may be an important risk factor for infection.

Several other studies suggest that management of the catheter after insertion may also significantly alter the risk for infection. In a randomized trial that preceded the onset of the use of universal or standard precautions, Klein et al. (105) documented a significantly lower overall rate of nosocomial infections and a trend toward a lower rate of primary bloodstream infections (0.3% vs. 1.3%, $p = .08$) in a pediatric ICU when gowns and gloves were routinely used for caring for patients than when they were not used. Use of a TPN catheter for other purposes than infusing TPN was found to be a risk factor for catheter-related bloodstream infection in another study referred to previously (63). The association of a higher infection rate of TPN catheters with understaffing referenced previously also suggests risk from faulty manipulation of catheters (69).

Guidewire exchanges have been found to be a risk factor in several studies of catheter infection (46,53,106–108). Failure to properly process and disinfect pressure transducers has been shown to correlate with infection in multiple outbreaks in ICUs (109).

Transparent dressings have resulted in a significantly higher rate of colonization of catheters than have cotton gauze dressings covered with tape (110,111). One randomized trial documented a significantly higher rate of bloodstream infection when catheters were covered with transparent dressings (112). Two recent outbreaks of catheter-related bloodstream infection were noted to be associated with cost-cutting measures and reliance on weekly transparent dressing changes (113,114).

Triple antibiotic ointment [polymyxin-neomycin-bacitracin (PNB)] has been associated with a halving of the rate of bacterial colonization of catheters but a fivefold increase in the rate of fungal colonization (115). One study evaluating the use of PNB ointment under a transparent dressing reported that 4 (14%) of 29 patients in a surgical ICU developed candidemia (115).

MICROBIAL ETIOLOGY

Gram-positive cocci have been the most frequent causes of primary bloodstream infection in hospitals reporting data to the NNIS system. In data collected between October 1986 and December 1990 (116), coagulase-negative staphylococci accounted for 28.2% of cases, followed by *S. aureus* (16.1%) and enterococci (12.0%) (116). These were followed by *Candida* spp. (10.2%) and *Enterobacter* spp. (5.3%). Because NNIS system data include cases diagnosed as bacteremia by physicians even if only one of many blood cultures were positive for a coagulase-negative *Staphylococcus,* these data probably overestimate the true frequency of bacteremia resulting from these microorganisms. A different approach requiring more convincing proof that coagulase-negative staphylococci actually caused catheter-related bloodstream infection provides a somewhat different relative frequency distribution. When the results of several studies were compiled using stricter definitions of catheter-related bloodstream infection, coagulase-negative staphylococci were still the most frequent cause accounting for 27 of 100 cases, but *S. aureus* was almost as frequent accounting for 26 of 100 cases (117). These were followed in order by yeast (17 of 100 cases), *Enterobacter* spp. (7 of 100 cases), *Serratia* spp. (5 of 100 cases), *Enterococcus* spp. (5 of 100 cases), *Klebsiella* spp. (4 of 100 cases), viridans species of *Streptococcus* (3 of 100 cases), *Pseudomonas* spp. (3 of 100 cases), *Proteus* spp. (2 of 100 cases), and *Yersinia* spp. (1 of 100 cases) (117).

Another study found that 32% of colonized catheters were associated with bloodstream infection resulting from the same species (118). The study found that the probability of positive blood cultures associated with a colonized catheter varied depending on the species colonizing the catheter. For example, catheters colonized by *Candida albicans* were associated with bloodstream infection resulting from the same species in 68.4% of cases, followed by *S. aureus* in 60%, *Enterobacter cloacae* in 42.9%, *Staphylococcus epidermidis* in 32.1%, *Pseudomonas aeruginosa* in 27.7%, and *Enterococcus faecalis* in 23.3%. The frequencies of bloodstream infection with *C. albicans* and with *S. aureus* significantly exceeded those for catheters colonized by the other species (118). This was confirmed by another study (119) (see also Chapter 19).

PREVENTION

Prevention of any disease involves avoidance of known risk factors for the disease. For catheter-related infection, this approach might include the following, based on the data discussed in the section on risk factors: (a) selecting a subclavian, basilic, or cephalic vein site rather than an internal jugular or femoral vein site; (b) avoiding the use of TPN catheters for purposes other than infusion of TPN; (c) using a special team for the insertion and maintenance of TPN catheters; (d) avoiding the use of triple antibiotic ointment (PNB) on CVCs (115); (e) using maximal aseptic technique for insertion of the catheter; (f) avoiding high glucose levels in diabetic patients with a CVC by careful regulation of serum glucose concentrations, especially for those receiving TPN; (g) using cotton gauze dressings; (h) avoiding understaffing in the management of patients with CVCs (69,70,120); and (i) having an experienced physician insert the catheter.

Data from randomized controlled trials provide additional support for some of these approaches. For example, a randomized trial comparing maximal aseptic technique for insertion (large sterile drapes, sterile gowns, and sterile gloves, with mask and cap being worn by the inserting physician as compared with an older approach using a mask, small drape, and sterile gloves but none of the additional barriers) confirmed the importance of using maximal sterile barrier precautions for avoiding inadvertent contamination at the time of insertion (121). Povidone-iodine ointment placed at the catheter site with dressing changes was associated with a significantly lower risk of catheter-related bloodstream infection in a randomized trial involving hemodialysis patients (122). An older study found no benefit with the ointment, however, and further studies are needed (123). Mupirocin ointment has also been found effective in preventing bacterial colonization of catheters (124) but has been associated with development of mupirocin resistance among skin flora, and recent CDC guidelines do not recommend using mupirocin at the catheter site (125).

Scheduled replacement of CVCs was used for decades for prevention of infection based on a theory that inserting a new catheter every few days should lower the patient's risk for infection. Unfortunately the strategy did not work when tested in randomized trials (46,80,107,126–128). When new site puncture was used, the infection rate was unchanged and the risk of major mechanical complications was significantly increased by scheduled replacement (46). When guidewire exchange was used for scheduled replacement, the rate of infection was paradoxically higher than if catheters were changed only as clinically necessary (46,107). The current CDC guideline for prevention of vascular device-related infections recommends against scheduled replacement of CVCs (125).

The antiseptic used for prepping the site before catheter insertion and with each dressing change was studied in multiple recent trials with all but one of them finding that chlorhexidine gluconate was associated with lower colonization and bloodstream infection rates than were povidone-iodine or alcohol (129–131). It is possible that tincture of iodine would work well for preventing catheter-related infection, but most healthcare providers have avoided using it for this purpose because of reports of increased skin rash with its use. Two recent studies suggested that it was better than povidone-iodine for antisepsis of skin before drawing percutaneous blood cultures (132,133), but one of these studies also found that tincture of iodine offered no advantage over 70% isopropyl alcohol, which was less expensive and has been associated with fewer side effects (133).

Tunneling of CVCs has been used primarily for long-dwelling catheters, but some have advocated use of tunneling even for short-term catheters in the ICU. One study with nontunneled catheters in cancer patients reported infection rates that were somewhat lower than usually reported with tunneled catheters (97), and two randomized trials found no benefit from tunneling, including one in ICU patients (134,135). Three other randomized trials showed lower infection rates with tunneled catheters (136–138). The cost-effectiveness of this approach requires further scrutiny, however.

A silver-impregnated collagen cuff placed on the catheter at the time of insertion was found to be effective in preventing bloodstream infection in two randomized trials (52,115). Catheters with an antiseptic coating have been shown to prevent catheter-related bloodstream infection (89,139–141). Antibiotic coating has been shown to work (142–146), but concern has been raised about promoting the development of antibiotic resistance from exposing the cutaneous flora of large numbers of patients to such surfaces (52,141,147).

Copper and silver-copper coatings have been shown to decrease adherence of *S. aureus* to catheters made of silicon rubber, polyvinyl chloride, and Teflon (148). A negatively charged direct current of electricity with 10 μA reduced bacterial adherence to catheters, but a positively charged current had no effect (149). Current flowing through a silver wire wrapped in a helical fashion around a catheter prevented adherence in an experimental animal model of infection (150).

Antibiotic lock therapy has been used to salvage a catheter for continued use after a catheter infection (151–159). This approach has been modified by using a periodic antimicrobial flush with vancomycin (160), taurolidine (161), or minocycline-ethylenediaminetetraacetic acid (EDTA) (162,163). Concern has been raised about the use of clinical antibiotics such as vancomycin for this purpose because of the risk of potentiating development of resistance (164).

Several recent studies evaluated novel approaches to the prevention of catheter-related infection and found no benefit from use of prophylactic intravenous immunoglobulin infusions for ICU patients in general (165), granulocyte colony stimulating factor in neutropenic ICU patients (166), or hypocaloric TPN for patients requiring TPN (167).

REFERENCES

1. Widmer AF. Central venous catheters. In: Seifert H, Jansen B, Farr BM, editors. *Catheter-related infections.* New York: Marcel Dekker, 1997:183–216.
2. Maki DG. Infections due to infusion therapy. In: Bennet JV, editor. *Hospital infections.* Boston: Little, Brown and Company, 1992:849.
3. Elliott TSJ, Faroqui MH, Tebbs SE, et al. An audit programme for central venous catheter-associated infections. *J Hosp Infect* 1995;30: 181–191.
4. Maki DG, Weise CE, Sarafini HW. A semiquantitative culture method for identifying intravenous catheter related infection. *N Engl J Med* 1977;296:1305–1309.
5. Raad I, Sabbagh MF, Rand KH, et al. Quantitative tip culture methods and the diagnosis of central venous catheter-related infections. *Diagn Microbiol Infect Dis* 1992;15:13–20.
6. Press OW, Ramsey PG, Larson EB, et al. Hickman catheter infections in patients with malignancies. *Medicine* 1984;63:189–200.
7. Maki DG, Stolz S. The epidemiology of central-venous catheter-related bloodstream infection (BSI)[abstract 67]. In: Programs and abstracts of the 34th Interscience Conference of Antimicrobial Agents and Chemotherapy, Orlando, FL, 1994.
8. Bjornson HS, Colley R, Bower RH, et al. Association between microorganism growth at the catheter insertion site and colonization of the catheter in patients receiving total parenteral nutrition. *Surgery* 1982; 92:720–727.
9. Cheesborough JS, Finch RG, Burden RP. A prospective study of the mechanisms of infection associated with hemodialysis catheters. *J Infect Dis* 1986;154:579–589.
10. Cooper CL, Schiller AL, Hopkins CC. Possible role of capillary action in pathogenesis of experimental catheter-associated dermal tunnel infections. *J Clin Micro* 1988;26:8–12.
11. Linares J, Sitges-Serra A, Garau J, et al. Pathogenesis of catheter sepsis: a prospective study with quantitative and semiquantitative cultures of catheter hub and segments. *J Clin Micro* 1985;21:357–360.
12. Moro ML, Vigano EF, Lepri AC. Risk factors for central venous catheter related infections in surgical and intensive care units. *Infect Control Hosp Epidemiol* 1994;15:253–264.
13. Raad I, Costerton W, Sabharwal U, et al. Ultrastructural analysis of indwelling vascular catheters: a quantitative relationship between luminal colonization and duration of placement. *J Infect Dis* 1993; 168:400–407.
14. Quilici N, Audibert G, Conroy MC, et al. Differential quantitative blood cultures in the diagnosis of catheter-related sepsis in intensive care units. *Clin Infect Dis* 1997;25:1066–1070.
15. Maki DG. Nosocomial bacteremia: a epidemiologic overview. *Am J Med* 1981;70:719–732.
16. Bozzetti F, Terno G, Camerini E, et al. Pathogenesis and predictability of central venous catheter sepsis. *Surgery* 1982;91:383–389.
17. Ryan JAJ, Abel RM, Abbott WM, et al. Catheter complications in total parenteral nutrition: a prospective study of 200 consecutive patients. *N Engl J Med* 1974;290:757–761.

18. Pittet D, Chuard C, Rae AC, et al. Clinical diagnosis of central venous catheter line infections: a difficult job [abstract 174]. In: Programs and abstracts of the 31st Interscience Conference of Antimicrobial Agents and Chemotherapy, Chicago, 1991.
19. Watanakunakorn C, Baird IM. Staphylococcus aureus bacteremia and endocarditis associated with a removable infected intravenous device. *Am J Med* 1977;63:523–526.
20. Maki DG, Ringer M. Risk factors for infusion-related phlebitis with small peripheral venous catheters a randomized controlled trial. *Ann Intern Med* 1991;114:845–854.
21. Lipsky BA, Peugeot RL, Boyko EJ, et al. A prospective study of *Staphylococcus aureus* nasal colonization and intravenous therapy-related phlebitis. *Arch Intern Med* 1992;152:2109–2112.
22. Farr BM. Nonendocardial vascular infections. In: Hoeprich PD, Jordanb MC, Roanld AR, eds. *Infectious diseases*. Philadelphia: JB Lippincott, 1994:1248–1258.
23. Berkowitz FE, Argent AC, Faise T. Suppurative thrombophlebitis: a serious nosocomial infection. *Pediatr Infect Dis J* 1987;6:64–67.
24. Johnson RA, Zajac RA, Evan ME. Suppurative thrombophlebitis: correlation between pathogen and underlying disease. *Infect Control* 1986;7:582–585.
25. Kaufman J, Demas C, Stark K, et al. Catheter-related septic central venous thrombosis: current therapeutic options. *West J Med* 1986; 145:200–203.
26. Cohen A, Reyes R, Kirk M, et al. Osler's nodes, pseudoaneurysm formation and sepsis complicating percutaneous radial artery cannulation. *Crit Care Med* 1984;12:1078–1079.
27. Bayer AS, Scheld WM. Endocarditis and intravascular infections. In: Mandell G, Bennet JE, Dolin R, ed. *Principles and practice of infectious diseases,* 5th ed. Philadelphia: Churchill Livingstone, 2000:857–902.
28. Nolan CM, Beaty HN. *Staphylococcus aureus* bacteremia. Current clinical patterns. *Am J Med* 1976;60:495–500.
29. Cooper R, Platt R. *Staphylococcus aureus* bacteremia in diabetic patients. *Am J Med* 1982;73:658–662.
30. Fowler VG, Olsen M, Corey GR, et al. Predictors of complications in patients with *Staphylococcus aureus* bacteremia [abstract 415]. In: Abstracts of the 41st Interscience Conference on Antimicrobial Agents and Chemotherapy, September and December, 2001.
31. Durack DT, Lukes AS, Bright DK, et al. New criteria for diagnosis of infective endocarditis: utilization of specific echocardiographic findings. *Am J Med* 1994;96:200–209.
32. Fowler VG, LI J, Corey GR, et al. Role of echocardiography in evaluation of patients with *Staphylococcus aureus* bacteremia: experience in 103 patients. *J Am Coll Cardiol* 1997;30:1072–1078.
33. Siegman-Igra Y, Anglim AM, Shapiro DE, et al. Diagnosis of vascular catheter-related bloodstream infection: a meta-analysis. *J Clin Microbiol* 1997;35:928–936.
34. Blot F, Schmidt E, Nitenberg G. Earlier positivity of central venous versus peripheral blood cultures is highly predictive of catheter related sepsis. *J Clin Microbiol* 1998;36:105–109.
35. Blot F, Nitenberg G, Chachaty E, et al. Diagnosis of catheter-related bacteraemia: a prospective comparison of the time to positivity of central vs. peripheral blood cultures. *Lancet* 1999;354:1071–1077.
36. Garland JS, Nelson DB, Cheah TE, et al. Infectious complications during peripheral intravenous therapy with Teflon catheters: a prospective study. *Pediatr Infect Dis J* 1998;6:918–921.
37. Tully JL, Griedland GH, Baldini LM, et al. Complications of intravenous therapy with steel needles and Teflon catheters a comparative study. *Am J Med* 1981;70:702–706.
38. Tager IB, Ginsberg MB, Ellis SE. An epidemiologic study of the risks associated with peripheral intravenous catheters. *Am J Epidemiol* 1983; 118:839–851.
39. Maki DG, Botticelli JT, LeRoy ML, et al. Prospective study of replacing administration sets for intravenous therapy at 48 vs 72-hour intervals: 72 hours is safe and cost effective. *JAMA* 1987;258:1777–1781.
40. Band JD, Maki DG. Infections caused by arterial catheters used for hemodynamic monitoring. *Am J Med* 1979;67:735–741.
41. Norwood SH, Cormier B, McMahon NG, et al. Prospective study of catheter-related infection during prolonged arterial catheterization. *Crit Care Med* 1988;16:836–839.
42. Leroy O, Billiau V, Beuscart C, et al. Nosocomial infections associated with long-term radial artery cannulation. *Intens Care Med* 1989;15: 241–246.
43. Furfaro S, Gauthier M, Lacroix J, et al. Arterial catheter-related infections in children. *Am J Dis Child* 1991;145:1037–1042.
44. Bannerjee SN, Emori TG, Culver DH. Secular trends in nosocomial primary bloodstream infections in the United States., 1980–1989. *Am J Med* 1991;91(Suppl 3B):87S–89S.
45. Byers KE, Anneski CJ, Anglim AM, et al. Central venous catheter utilization and complications at a university hospital [abstract]. Presented at the seventh annual meeting of the Society of Hospital Epidemiology of America, St. Louis, 1997.
46. Cobb DK, High KP, Sawyer RG, et al. A controlled trial of scheduled replacement of central venous and pulmonary-artery catheters. *N Engl J Med* 1992;327:1062–1068.
47. Byers KE, Adal KA, Anglim AM, et al. Case fatality rate for catheter-related bloodstream infections (CRBSI): a meta-analysis. *Infect Control Hosp Epidemiol* 1995;16(Part 2, Suppl):23.
48. Jernigan JA, Farr BM. Short-course therapy of catheter-related *Staphylococcus aureus* bacteremia: a meta-analysis. *Ann Intern Med* 1993; 119:304–311.
49. Saiman L, Ludington E, Pfaller M. Risk factors for candidemia in neonatal intensive care unit patients. The National Epidemiology of Mycosis Survey study group. *Pediatr Infect Dis J* 2000;19:319–324.
50. Centers for Disease Control and Prevention. Public health focus: surveillance, prevention, and control of nosocomial infections. *MMWR* 1992;41:783–787.
51. Pittet D, Tarara D, Wenzel RP. Nosocomial bloodstream infection in critically ill patients. Excess length of stay, extra costs, and attributable mortality. *JAMA* 1994;271:1598–1601.
52. Maki DG, Cobb L, Garman JK, et al. An attachable silver-impregnated cuff for prevention of infection with central venous catheters: a prospective randomized multicenter trial. *Am J Med* 1988;85: 307–314.
53. Hilton E, Haslett TM, Borenstein MT, et al. Central catheter infections: single-versus triple-lumen catheters: influence of guide wires on infection rates when used for replacement of catheters. *Am J Med* 1988;84:667–672.
54. Yeung C, May J, Hughes R. Infection rate for single lumen v triple lumen subclavian catheters. *Infect Control Hosp Epidemiol* 1988; 9: 154–158.
55. Gil RT, Kruse JA, Thill-Beharozian MC, et al. Triple-vs. single-lumen central venous catheters: a prospective study in a critically ill population. *Arch Intern Med* 1989;149:1139–1143.
56. Miller JJ, Venus B, Mathru M. Comparison of the sterility of long-term central venous catheterization using single lumen, triple lumen, and pulmonary catheters. *Crit Care Med* 1984;12:634–637.
57. Lee RB, Buckner M, Sharp KW. Do multi-lumen catheters increase central venous catheter sepsis compared to single-lumen catheters? *J Trauma* 1988;28:1472–1475.
58. Pemberton LB, Lyman B, Lander V, et al. Sepsis from triple- vs. single lumen catheters during total parenteral nutrition in surgical or critically ill patients. *Arch Surg* 1986;121:591–594.
59. Clark-Christoff N, Watters VA, Sparks W, et al. Use of triple-lumen subclavian catheters for administration of total parenteral nutrition. *J Parenteral Enteral Nutr* 1992;16:403.
60. Farkas JC, Liu N, Bleriot JP, et al. Single-versus triple-lumen central catheter related sepsis: a prospective randomized study in a critically ill population. *Am J Med* 1992;93:277.
61. Safdar N, Kluger D, Maki DG. A review of risk factors for catheter-related bloodstream infection caused by percutaneously inserted, non-cuffed central venous catheters: implications for preventive strategies. *Medicine* 2002;81:466–479.
62. Howell PB, Walters PE, Donowitz GR, et al. Risk factors for infection of adult patients with cancer who have tunnelled central venous catheters. *Cancer* 1995;75:1367–1375.
63. Snydman DR, Murray SA, Kornfeld SJ, et al. Total parenteral nutrition related infections. *Am J Med* 1982;73:695–699.
64. Danzig L, Short L, Collins K, et al. Bloodstream infections (BSIs) associated with a needleless intravenous (IV) infusion system used in

patients on home infusion therapy [abstract 195]. In: Programs and abstracts of the 34th Interscience Conference of Antimicrobial Agents and Chemotherapy, Orlando, FL, 1994.

65. Faubion WC, Wesley JR, Khalidi N, et al. Total parenteral nutrition catheter sepsis: impact of the team approach. *J Parenteral Enteral Nutr* 1986;10:642–645.
66. Freeman JB, Lemire A, Maclean LD. Intravenous alimentation and septicemia. *Surg Gynecol Obstet* 1972;135:708–712.
67. Nehme AE. Nutritional support of the hospitalized patient. The team concept. *JAMA* 1980;243:1906–1908.
68. Nelson DB, Kien CL, Mohr B, et al. Dressing changes by specialized personnel reduce infection rates in patients receiving central venous parenteral nutrition. *J Parenteral Enteral Nutr* 1986;10:220–222.
69. Fridkin SK, Pear SM, Williamson TH, et al. The role of understaffing in central venous catheter-associated bloodstream infections. *Infect Control Hosp Epidemiol* 1996;17:150–158.
70. Robert J, Fridkin SK, Blumberg HM. The influence of the composition of the nursing staff on primary bloodstream infection rates in a surgical intensive care unit. *Infect Control Hosp Epidemiol* 2000;21: 12–17.
71. Baxter JK, Babineau TJ, Apovian CM, et al. Perioperative glucose control predicts increased nosocomial infection in diabetics. *Crit Care Med* 1990;18:S207.
72. The Veterans Affairs Total Parenteral Nutrition Cooperative Study Group. Perioperative total parenteral nutrition in surgical patients. *N Engl J Med* 1991;325:525.
73. Shiro H, Muller E, Takeda S, et al. Potentiation of *Staphylococcus epidermidis* catheter-related bacteremia by lipid infusions. *J Infect Dis* 1995;171:220–224.
74. Avila-Figueroa C, Goldmann DA, Richardson DK, et al. Intravenous lipid emulsions are the major determinant of coagulase-negative staphylococcal bacteremia in very low birth weight newborns. *Pediatr Infect Dis* 1998;17:10–17.
75. Barber GR, Brown AE, Kiehn TE, et al. Catheter-related *Malassezia furfur* fungemia in immunocompromised patients. *Am J Med* 1993; 95:370.
76. Aragao PA, Oshiro IC, Manrique EI. *Pichia anomala* outbreak in a nursery: exogenous source? *Pediatr Infect Dis* 2001;20:843–848.
77. Brodie SB, Sands KE, Gray JE. Occurrence of nosocomial bloodstream infections in six neonatal intensive care units. *Pediatr Infect Dis* 2000;19:56–65.
78. Widmer AF. Intravenous-related infections. In: Wenzel RP, ed. *Prevention and control of nosocomial infections.* New York: Williams & Wilkins, 1997:771–805.
79. Stenzel JP, Green TP, Fuhrman BP, et al. Percutaneous central venous catheterization in a pediatric intensive care unit: a survival analysis of complications. *Crit Care Med* 1989;17:984–988.
80. Uldall PR, Merchant N, Woods F, et al. Changing subclavian haemodialysis cannulas to reduce infection. *Lancet* 1981;1:1373.
81. Sherertz RJ, Carruth WA, Hu Q, et al. Factors modifying the risk of *Staphylococcus aureus* infection associated with silicone catheters in a rabbit model [abstract]. Presented at the 30th Interscience Conference of Antimicrobial Agents and Chemotherapy, 1990.
82. Jacobson MA, Gellermann H, Chambers H. *Staphylococcus aureus* bacteremia and recurrent staphylococcal infection in patients with acquired immunodeficiency syndrome and AIDS related complex. *Am J Med* 1988;85:172–176.
83. Skoutelis AT, Murphy RL, MacDonell KB, et al. Indwelling central venous catheter infections in patients with acquired immunodeficiency syndrome. *J Acquir Immune Defic Syndr* 1990;3:335–342.
84. Tumbarello M, Tacconelli E, Donati KG, et al. HIV-associated bacteremia: how it has changed in the highly active antiretroviral therapy (HAART) era. *J Acquir Immune Defic Syndr* 2000;23:145–151.
85. Mermel LA, McCormick RD, Springman SR, et al. The pathogenesis and epidemiology of catheter related infection with pulmonary artery Swan-Ganz catheters: a prospective study utilizing molecular subtyping. *Am J Med* 1991;91(Suppl 3B):197S–205S.
86. Richet H, Hubert B, Nitemberg G, et al. Prospective multicenter study of vascular catheter related complications and risk factors for positive central-catheter cultures in intensive care unit patients. *J Clin Microbiol* 1990;28:2520–2525.
87. Santre CH, Georges H, Jacquier JM, et al. A comparison between semi-quantitative catheter tip cultures and non quantitative blood cultures in the diagnosis of catheter-related infections in critically ill patients [abstract 68]. In: Programs and abstracts of the 34th Interscience Conference of Antimicrobial Agents and Chemotherapy, Orlando, FL, 1994.
88. Hagley MT, Martin BM, Gast P, et al. Infectious and mechanical complications of central venous catheters placed by percutaneous venipuncture and over guidewires. *Crit Care Med* 1992;20:1426.
89. Norwood SH, Wilkins HE 3rd, Vallins VL, et al. The safety of prolonging the use of central venous catheters: a prospective analysis of the effects of using antiseptic-bonded catheters with daily site care. *Crit Care Med* 2000;28:1376–1382.
90. Goetz AM, Muder RR, Wagener MM, et al. Risk of infection due to femoral placement of central venous catheters [abstract 258]. In: Programs and abstracts of the 35th Interscience Conference of Antimicrobial Agents and Chemotherapy, San Francisco, 1995.
91. Oliver MJ, Callery SM, Thorpe KE, et al. Risk of bacteremia from temporary hemodialysis catheters by site of insertion and duration of use: a prospective study. *Kidney Int* 2000;58:2543–2545.
92. Montagnac R, Bernard C, Guillaumie J, et al. Indwelling silicone femoral catheters: experience of three haemodialysis centres. *Nephrol Dial Transplant* 1997;12:772–775.
93. Williams JF, Seneff MG, Friedman BC, et al. Use of femoral venous catheters in critically ill adults: prospective study. *Crit Care Med* 1991; 19:550–553.
94. Yurtkuran M. Catheterization of the femoral vein for chronic hemodialysis. *Angiology* 1987;38:847–850.
95. Trottier SJ, Veremakis C, O'Brien J, et al. Femoral deep vein thrombosis associated with central venous catheterization: results from a prospective, randomized trial. *Crit Care Med* 1995;23:52–59.
96. Merrer J, De Jonghe B, Bernard MD, et al. Complications of femoral and subclavian venous catheterization in critically ill patients: a randomized controlled trial. *JAMA* 2001;286:700–707.
97. Raad I, Davis S, Becker M, et.al. Low infection rate and long durability of nontunnelled silastic catheters. *Arch Intern Med* 1993;153: 1791–1796.
98. Tice AD, Bonstell RP, Marsh PK, et al. Peripherally inserted central venous catheters for outpatient intravenous antibiotic therapy. *Infect Dis Clin Pract* 1993;2:186–190.
99. Linblad B, Wolff T. Infectious complications of percutaneously inserted central venous catheters. *Acta Anaesthesiol Scand* 1985;29: 587–589.
100. Lam S, Scannell R, Roessler D, et al. Peripherally inserted central catheters in an acute-care hospital. *Arch Intern Med* 1994;154: 1833–1837.
101. Bottino J, McCredie K, Grosehel DHM, et al. Long-term intravenous therapy with peripherally inserted silicone elastomer central venous catheters in patients with malignant diseases. *Cancer* 1979;43: 1937–1943.
102. Maki DG. Marked differences in skin colonization of insertion sites for central venous, arterial and peripheral IV catheters. The major reason for differing risks of catheter-related infection? [abstract 205] In: Programs and abstracts of the 30th Interscience Conference of Antimicrobial Agents and Chemotherapy, Atlanta, GA, 1990.
103. Noble WC. Dispersal of skin microorganisms. *Br J Dermatol* 1975; 93:477–485.
104. Armstrong CW, Mayhall CG, Miller KB, et.al. Prospective study of catheter replacement and other risk factors of infection of hyperalimentation catheters. *J Infect Dis* 1986;154:808–816.
105. Klein BS, Perloff WH, Maki DG. Reduction of nosocomial infection during pediatric intensive care by protective isolation. *N Engl J Med* 1989;320:1714–1721.
106. Maki DG, Ringer M. Prospective study of arterial catheter-related infection: incidence, sources of infection, and risk factors [abstract 284]. In: Programs and abstracts of the 29th Interscience Conference of Antimicrobial Agents and Chemotherapy, Houston, TX, 1989.
107. Snyder RH, Archer FJ, Endy T, et al. Catheter infection: a comparison

of two catheter maintenance techniques. *Ann Surg* 1988;208: 651–653.

108. Cook D, Randolph A, Kernerman P, et al. Central venous catheter replacement strategies: a systematic review of the literature. *Crit Care Med* 1997;25:1417–1424.
109. Beck-Sague CM, Jarvis WR. Epidemic bloodstream infections associated with pressure transducers: a persistent problem. *Infect Control Hosp Epidemiol* 1989;10:54–59.
110. Hoffman KK, Weber DJ, Samsa GP, et al. Transparent polyurethane film as an intravenous catheter dressing: a meta-analysis of the infection risks. *JAMA* 1992;267:2072–2076.
111. Maki DG, Mermel L, Martin M, et al. A highly-semipermeable polyurethane dressing does not increase the risk of CVC-related BSI: a prospective, multicenter, investigator-blinded trial [abstract 230]. In: Programs and abstracts of the 36th Interscience Conference of Antimicrobial Agents and Chemotherapy, New Orleans, LA, 1996.
112. Conly JM, Grieves K, Peters B. A prospective, randomized study comparing transparent and dry gauze dressings for central venous catheters. *J Infect Dis* 1989;159:310–319.
113. Curchoe RM, Powers J, El-Daher N. Weekly transparent dressing change linked to increased bacteremia rates. *Infect Control Hosp Epidemiol* 2002;23:730–732.
114. Price CS, Hacek D, Noskin GA, et al. An outbreak of bloodstream infections in an outpatient hemodialysis center. *Infect Control Hosp Epidemiol* 2002;23:725–729.
115. Flowers RH, Schwenzer RJ, Kopel RJ, et al. Efficacy of an attachable subcutaneous cuff for the prevention of intravascular catheter-related infection: a randomized controlled trial. *JAMA*1989;261:878–883.
116. Jarvis WR, Martone WJ. Predominant pathogens in hospital infections. *J Antimicrob Chemo* 1992; 29(Suppl A):19–24.
117. Hampton AA, Sherertz RJ. Vascular-access infections in hospitalized patients. *Surg Clin North Am* 1988;68:57–71.
118. Sherertz RJ, Raad I, Belani A. Three year experience with sonicated vascular catheter cultures in a clinical microbiology laboratory. *J Clin Microbiol* 1990;28:76–82.
119. Peacock SJ, Eddleston M, Emptage A, et al. Positive intravenous line tip cultures as predictors of bacteremia. *J Hosp Infect* 1998;40:35–38.
120. Farr BM. Understaffing: a risk factor for infection in the era of downsizing? *Infect Control Hosp Epidemiol* 1996;17:147–149.
121. Raad I, Hohn DC, Gilbreath BJ, et al. Prevention of central venous catheter related infections by using maximal sterile barrier precautions during insertion. *Infect Control Hosp Epidemiol* 1994;15(4 Pt 1): 231–238.
122. Levin A, Mason AJ, Jindal KK, et al. Prevention of hemodialysis subclavian vein catheter infections by topical povidone iodine. *Kidney Int* 1991;40:934–938.
123. Prager RL, Silva J. Colonization of central venous catheters. *South Med J* 1984;77:458–461.
124. Hill RLR, Fisher AP, Ware RJ, et al. Mupirocin for the reduction of colonization of internal jugular cannulae-randomized controlled trial. *J Hosp Infect* 1990;15:321.
125. O'Grady N, Alexander M, Dellinger E, et al. Guidelines for the prevention of intravascular catheter-related infections. *Infect Control Hosp Epidemiol* 2002;23:759–769.
126. Bock SN, Lee RE, Fisher B, et.al. A prospective randomized trial evaluating prophylactic antibiotics to prevent triple-lumen catheter-related sepsis in patients treated with immunotherapy. *J Clin Oncol* 1990;8:161–169.
127. Powell C, Kudsk KA, Kulich PA, et al. Effect of frequent guidewire changes on triple-lumen catheter sepsis. *J Parenteral Enteral Nutr* 1988;12:462–464.
128. Eyer S, Brummitt C, Crossley K, et al. Catheter-related sepsis: a prospective, randomized study of three methods of long-term catheter maintenance. *Crit Care Med* 1990;18:1079.
129. Maki DG, Ringer M, Alvarado CJ. Prospective randomized trial of povidone-iodine, alcohol, and chlorhexidine for prevention of infection associated with central venous and arterial catheters. *Lancet* 1991; 338:339–343.
130. Mimoz O, Pieroni L, Lawrence C, et al. Prospective, randomized trial of two antiseptic solutions for prevention of central venous or arterial catheter colonization and infection in intensive care unit patients. *Crit Care Med* 1996;24:1818–1823.
131. Sheehan G, Leicht K, O, Biren M, et al. Chlorhexidine versus povidone-iodine as cutaneous antisepsis for prevention of vascular-catheter infection [abstract 414]. In: Programs and abstracts of the 33rd Interscience Conference of Antimicrobial Agents and Chemotherapy, New Orleans, LA, 1993.
132. Strand CL, Wajsbort RR, Sturmann K. Effect of iodophor vs iodine tincture skin preparation on blood culture contamination rate. *JAMA* 1993;269:1004–1006.
133. Calfee DP, Farr BM. Comparison of four antiseptic preparations for skin in the prevention of contamination of percutaneously-drawn blood cultures: a randomized trial. *J Clin Microbiol* 2002;40: 1660–1665.
134. Andrivet P, Bacquer A, Vu Ngoc C, et al. Lack of clinical benefit from subcutaneous tunnel insertion of central venous catheters in immunocompromised patients. *Clin Infect Dis* 1994;18:199–206.
135. Guichard I, Nitemberg G, Abitbol JL, et al. Tunnelled versus non-tunnelled catheters for parenteral nutrition in an intensive care unit: a controlled prospective study of catheter related sepsis. *Clin Nutr* 1986;5(Suppl 1):169.
136. Nahum E, Levy I, Katz J, et al. Efficacy of Subcutaneous tunneling for prevention of bacterial colonization of femoral central venous catheters in critically ill children. *Pediatr Infect Dis J* 2002;21:1000–1004.
137. Timsit J, Bruneel F, Cheval C, et al. Use of tunneled femoral catheters to prevent catheter-related infection: a randomized, controlled trial. *Ann Intern Med* 1999;130:729–735.
138. Timsit J, Sebille V, Farkas JC, et al. Effect of subcutaneous tunneling on internal jugular catheter-related sepsis in critically ill patients: a prospective randomized multicenter study. *JAMA* 1996;276: 1416–1420.
139. Hanley EM, Veeder A, Smith T, et al. Evaluation of an antiseptic triple-lumen catheter in an intensive care unit. *Crit Care Med* 2000; 28:366–370.
140. Veenstra DL, Saint S, Saha S, et al. Efficacy of antiseptic-impregnated catheters in preventing catheter-related bloodstream infection: a meta-analysis. *JAMA* 1999;281:261–267.
141. Maki, DG, Wheeler S, Stolz SM, et al. Prevention of central venous catheter related bloodstream infection by use of an antiseptic-impregnated catheter. A randomized, controlled trial. *Ann Intern Med* 1997; 127:257–266.
142. Kamal GD, Pfaller MA, Remple LE, et al. Reduced intravascular catheter infection by antibiotic bonding. *JAMA* 1991;265: 2364–2368.
143. Trooskin SZ, Donetz AP, Harvey RA, et al. Prevention of catheter sepsis by antibiotic bonding. *Surgery* 1985;97:547–551.
144. Sherertz RJ, Carruth WA, Hampton AA, et al. Efficacy of antibiotic-coated catheters in preventing subcutaneous *Staphylococcus aureus* infection in rabbits. *J Infect Dis* 1993;167:98–106.
145. Romano G, Berti M, Goldstein BP, et al. Efficacy of a central venous catheter (Hydrocath) loaded with teicoplanin in preventing subcutaneous staphylococcal infection in the mouse. *Int J Med Microbiol Virol Parasitol Infect Dis* 1993;279:426–433.
146. Darouiche RO, Raad I, Heard SO, et al. A comparison of two antimicrobial-impregnated central venous catheters. *N Engl J Med* 1999; 340:1–8.
147. Sampath LA, Tambe SM, Modak SM. In vitro and in vivo efficacy of catheters impregnated with antiseptics or antibiotics: evaluation of the risk of bacterial resistance to the antimicrobials in the catheters. *Infect Control Hosp Epidemiol* 2001;xx:640–646.
148. McLean RJ, Hussain AA, Sayer M, et al. Antibacterial activity of multilayer silver-copper surface films on catheter material. *Can J Microbiol* 1993;39:895–899.
149. Liu WK, Tebbs SE, Byrne PO, et al. The effects of electric current on bacteria colonizing intravenous catheters. *J Infect* 1993;27:269.
150. Raad I, Zermeno A, Dumo M, et al. In vitro antimicrobial efficacy of silver iontophoretic catheter. *Biometrics* 1996;17:1055–1059.
151. Longuet P, Douard MC, Arlet G. Venous access port-related bacteremia in patients with acquired immunodeficiency syndrome or cancer:

the reservoir as a diagnostic and therapeutic tool. *Clin Infect Dis* 2001; 32:1776–1783.

152. Krzywda EA, Andris DA, Edmiston CE. Treatment of Hickman catheter sepsis using antibiotic lock technique. *Infect Control Hosp Epidemiol* 1995;16:596–598.
153. Capdevila JA, Segarra A, Planes AM, et al. Long term follow-up of patients with catheter related sepsis (CRS) treated without catheter removal [abstract 257]. In: Programs and abstracts of the 35th Interscience Conference of Antimicrobial Agents and Chemotherapy, San Francisco, 1995.
154. Messing B, Peitra-Cohen S, Debure A, et al. Antibiotic-lock technique: a new approach to optimal therapy for catheter-related sepsis in home-parenteral nutrition patients. *J Parenteral Enteral Nutr* 1988; 12:185–189.
155. Gaillard JL, Merlino R, Pajot N, et.al. Conventional and nonconventional modes of vancomycin administration to decontaminate the internal surface of catheters colonized with coagulase-negative staphylococci. *J Parenteral Enteral Nutr* 1990;14:593–597.
156. Arnow PM, Kushner R. Malassezia furfur catheter infection cured with antibiotic lock therapy [Letter]. *Am J Med* 1982;90:128–130.
157. Douard MC, Arlet G, Leverger G, et al. Quantitative blood cultures for diagnosis and management of catheter-related sepsis in pediatric hematology and oncology patients. *Intens Care Med* 1991;17:30–35.
158. Elian JC, Frappaz D, Ros A, et.al. Study of serum kinetics of vancomycin during the "antibiotic-lock" technique. *Arch Fr Pediatr* 1992;49: 357–360.
159. Cowan CE. Antibiotic lock technique. *J Intravenous Nurs* 1992;15: 283–287.
160. Schwartz C, Henrickson KJ, Roghmann K, et al. Prevention of bacteremia attributed to luminal colonization of tunneled central venous catheters with vancomycin-susceptible organisms. *J Clin Oncol* 1990; 8:1591–1597.
161. Jurewitsch B, Lee T, Park J, et al. Taurolidine 2% as an antimicrobial lock solution for prevention of recurrent catheter-related bloodstream infections. *J Parenteral Enteral Nutr* 1998;22:242–244.
162. Raad I, Hachem R, Tcholakian RK, et al. Efficacy of minocycline and EDTA lock solution in preventing catheter-related bacteremia, septic phlebitis, and endocarditis in rabbits. *Antimicrob Agents Chemother* 2002;43:327–332.
163. Chatzinikolaou I, Zipf TF, Hanna HA, et al. Minocycline-ethylenediaminetetraacetate lock solution for the prevention of implantable port infections in children with cancer. *Clin Infect Dis* 2003;36:116–119.
164. Hospital Infection Control Practices Advisory Committee (HICPAC). Recommendations for preventing the spread of vancomycin resistance. *Infect Control Hosp Epidemiol* 1995;16:105–113.
165. Douzinas EE, Pitardis MT, Louris G. Prevention of infection in multiple trauma patients by high-dose intravenous immunoglobins. *Crit Care Med* 2000;28:8–15.
166. Gruson D, Hilbert G, Vargas F. Impact of colony-stimulating factor therapy on clinical outcome and frequency rate of nosocomial infections in intensive care unit neutropenic patients. *Crit Care Med* 2000; 28:3155–3160.
167. McCowen KC, Friel C, Stewrnberg J, et al. Hypocaloric total parenteral nutrition: effectiveness in prevention of hyperglycemia and infectious complications—a randomized clinical trial. *Crit Care Med* 2000; 28:3606–3611.

18

NOSOCOMIAL INFECTIONS RELATED TO USE OF INTRAVASCULAR DEVICES INSERTED FOR LONG-TERM VASCULAR ACCESS

HEND HANNA
ISSAM RAAD

Long-term intravascular devices have become indispensable in the modern medical care of chronically ill patients such as cancer patients, patients with renal failure requiring chronic hemodialysis, or patients requiring organ or bone marrow transplantation. In the 1960s and 1970s treatment of cancer patients through a small peripheral venous catheter used to be complicated by extravasation of vesicant chemotherapeutic agents and thrombosis of peripheral veins, which often limited anticancer chemotherapy. Long-term silicone central venous catheters (CVCs) allowed the extended, safe use of anticancer chemotherapeutic agents as well as the potential for appropriate use of total parenteral nutrition (TPN) fluids, blood products, and other intravenous therapeutic agents (1). For patients with short bowel syndrome, long-term CVCs have become the only source for nutritional support through TPN. Similarly, patients requiring hemodialysis who have had prior failure of arteriovenous fistulas or shunts become totally dependent on intravascular catheter-related access for their hemodialysis. In all of these clinical situations, the long-term CVC becomes an essential device for the maintenance of life.

There is no standard agreed-upon definition for long-term catheters in terms of the duration of catheterization. Sherertz (2) defined long-term catheters as those with a duration of placement of an average of >8 days. Rather than using an average duration, we have defined this term in a previous study to signify catheters that remain in place for >30 days (3). We also defined short-term catheterization by duration of placement of <10 days, and intermediate catheterization by duration of placement ranging between 10 and 30 days (3).

Long-term intravascular devices can be categorized into one of three groups: (a) nontunneled long-term CVCs [such as peripherally inserted central catheters (PICCs) or subclavian CVCs such as Hohn catheters]; (b) cuffed and tunneled catheters (such as Hickman/Broviac, Groshong, and tunneled Uldall catheters); and (c) implanted subcutaneous central venous ports.

NONTUNNELED CATHETERS

Traditionally it was assumed that the only method of maintaining long-term intravascular access in chronically ill patients was through surgically implantable CVCs such as the tunneled catheters and implantable ports. Over the last decades, nontunneled long-term silicone CVCs have become more accepted as a cost-effective form of intravascular access. In addition, these catheters could be maintained for a long period, up to 400 days, without complications (4). Nontunneled long-term catheters consist of two types: nontunneled subclavian silicone catheters and PICC lines. Nontunneled subclavian catheters are inserted percutaneously via the subclavian vein into the superior vena cava, in the outpatient nonsurgical setting. The advantage of these catheters is that they are associated with low cost, because their insertion does not require the use of an operating room or a special surgical technique (1). In addition, these catheters can be exchanged over a guidewire and the removed intravascular segment may be cultured if a catheter infection is suspected or if a new catheter needs to be inserted. These catheters are available as single-, double-, or triple-lumen cannulas.

The PICC lines are becoming widely used, particularly for outpatient long-term central venous therapy, such as patients requiring intravenous home antibiotics for osteomyelitis or endocarditis, cancer patients, or patients requiring TPN delivery. These catheters are usually inserted in the antecubital space, via the cephalic or basilic vein, and advanced into the central venous system. These catheters are very cost-effective, because they can be inserted in the outpatient clinic by a trained infusion therapy nurse and do not require a physician for their insertion. At our institution, these catheters can be maintained for an average of 3 months and are associated with a low infection rate and cost (4). However, their main disadvantage is a high rate of aseptic thrombophlebitis related to mechanical contact (5). Most of these catheters are made of silicone, although some are made of polyurethane.

TUNNELED CATHETERS

In 1973, Broviac et al. (6) described the first surgically implanted tunneled catheter to be used in pediatric patients requiring long-term TPN. Later, Hickman et al. (7) described another long-term tunneled catheter for cancer patients requiring bone marrow transplantation. These catheters are usually tunneled under the skin for several inches until they reach the cannulated vein. Tunneled catheters have a Dacron cuff that is located in the proximal subcutaneous segment 5 cm from the exit insertion site. After insertion, the Dacron cuff becomes enmeshed with fibrous tissue, hence anchoring the catheter and creating a tissue interface mechanical barrier against the migration of skin microorganisms along the external intracutaneous pathway. Tunneled catheters usually exit the body midway between the nipple and the sternum. Another vascular access catheter is the Groshong, which, unlike the Hickman/Broviac, is thin walled and has two slit valves adjacent to a rounded closed end that remains closed unless fluids are being infused or blood is being drawn. This decreases the risk of intraluminal blood clotting or infusion of air when the catheter is not in use. Hence, this type of catheter does not require daily heparin flushes, but rather is flushed with saline on a weekly basis.

IMPLANTABLE PORTS

To eliminate the migration of skin microorganisms from the skin insertion site in externalized catheters along the intracutaneous pathway, the surgically implanted subcutaneous central venous ports were developed where the whole catheter, including the metallic port, is placed beneath the skin (8). Hence, implantable ports consist of a metal/titanium or plastic port placed beneath the skin and connected to a catheter that enters the cannulated vein. Ports are usually placed in a subcutaneous pocket on the upper chest or, less often, in the antecubital area of the arm (peripheral port). Ports are available as single- or double-lumen catheters with or without Groshong valves and can be accessed as needed with a steel needle.

EPIDEMIOLOGY

The bloodstream infection (BSI) rates associated with long-term CVCs should be reported using catheter-days as the denominator. The Centers for Disease Control and Prevention (CDC) recommends that rates of catheter-related bloodstream infections (CR-BSI) be expressed per 1,000 device-days. This recommendation takes into consideration the varying risks of CR-BSI over time for the different types of CVCs. According to Crnich and Maki (9), although the rates of CR-BSI per 100 CVCs used are usually higher for long-term devices, the risk per 1,000 catheter-days is usually considerably lower than that for short-term CVCs. In 17 studies reviewed by Press et al. (10), 21 studies reviewed by Decker and Edwards (11), 13 studies reviewed by Clarke and Raffin (12), and 26 studies reviewed by Howell et al. (13), the average infection rate for long-term CVCs in cancer patients ranged from one to two episodes per 1,000 catheter days. Assuming this rate and the fact that half a million long-term CVCs are inserted annually in the United States, the estimated annual number of episodes of catheter-associated bacteremia that occur in the U.S. related to the use of these catheters in cancer patients is between 50,000 and 100,000.

Several studies have compared the efficacy of tunneled catheters (such as Hickman/Broviac catheters) with implantable ports. Mueller et al. (14), in a prospective, randomized study, compared the complications of the two types of long-term catheters and found no significant difference in infection rates between the two types of devices. Similarly, Keung et al. (15) conducted a retrospective study of infectious complications in 111 long-term CVCs. Multivariable analysis revealed no significant difference in infection rates between tunneled catheters and implantable ports. On the other hand, there are several studies that suggest that ports may be associated with lower infection rates. Mirro et al. (16) evaluated 266 tunneled catheters and 93 implantable ports in children with cancer, and showed that, when all causes of failure were analyzed including infectious complications, ports had a significantly longer duration of use than tunneled catheters. In a prospective observational study conducted at Memorial Sloan-Kettering on 1,630 long-term CVCs (923 tunneled catheters and 707 ports) Groeger et al. (17) found that the incidence of infection per device per day was 12 times greater with the tunneled catheter than with ports. Therefore, these data might suggest that ports are associated with a lower infection rate than tunneled catheters, even though they are not conclusive. In addition, the data should be analyzed with caution because there could be confounding variables, such as the various uses of the catheters (including the use of TPN), duration of neutropenia, and thrombotic complications that were not taken into consideration.

There are very few data in the literature comparing tunneled with nontunneled long-term CVCs in terms of infection rates. In a prospective randomized study, Andrivet et al. (18) showed that the infection rate associated with nontunneled subclavian silicone CVCs were not different from those related to tunneled silicone catheters. However, the lack of a difference could be related to the small sample size. In a prospective study evaluating nontunneled long-term CVCs at the M. D. Anderson Cancer Center, we determined that the infection rates for PICC lines and nontunneled subclavian CVCs was 1.4 per 1,000 catheter days, which was comparable to what was described for Hickman catheters in the literature (4). At the M. D. Anderson Cancer Center, the cost of insertion of nontunneled catheters, including the chest x-ray postinsertion and other related fees, is in the range of $1,190 to $1,326 as compared with more than $6,502 for the Hickman tunneled CVC. The cost of placing an implantable port at our institution is about $7,076. Given the comparable durability of all long-term catheters, the potential marginal difference in infection rates might not justify the wide difference in cost between the tunneled catheters and ports on the one hand and the nontunneled CVC (PICC lines and nontunneled subclavian catheters) on the other.

PATHOGENESIS

Microbial adherence and colonization of long-term catheters is the by-product of the interaction of several factors: (a) host-derived proteins, (b) microbial factors, (c) catheter material, and (d) iatrogenic factors.

After insertion, a thrombin sheath covers the internal and external surfaces of the catheter, which is rich in host proteins (19,20). These proteins include fibronectin, fibrinogen, laminin, thrombospondin, and collagen (1,21–25). *Staphylococcus aureus* binds strongly to fibronectin and fibrinogen, whereas coagulase-negative staphylococci bind strongly to fibronectin (21,22). In addition, *Candida albicans* has been shown to bind well to fibrin (26).

Biofilm formation represents the microbial factor involved in the enhancement of adherence of microorganisms to catheter surfaces. Microorganisms, such as coagulase-negative staphylococci, *S. aureus*, and even *C. parapsilosis*, have the potential of undergoing intrinsic phenotypic changes that result in the expression of several enzymes that lead to the production of an exopolysaccharide, thus causing the biofilm to form (27–32). Microorganisms embed themselves in this layer of biofilm (or microbial slime), and hence protect themselves from antimicrobial agents such as glycopeptides (33,34). Other microbial factors, such as hydrophobicity and the surface charges of microorganisms contribute to the adherence to catheter materials such as silicone (35,36). Hydrophobic staphylococcal microorganisms adhere better to silicone surfaces of which most long-term catheters are made, than to the polyurethane or Teflon surfaces of short-term catheters.

The material from which the catheters are made plays a role in the adherence of microorganisms to the catheter surface. The physical characteristics of the catheter surfaces, including hydrophobicity, surface charges, irregularities, and defects on the catheter surface and the thrombogenicity of the catheter surface, contribute to the process of microbial adherence (1,2). Several investigators have shown, for example, that *Staphylococcus* and *Candida* species adhere better to polyvinyl chloride catheters than to Teflon catheters (37,38). Sherertz et al. (39) have demonstrated in a rabbit model that silicone catheters are easier to infect with *S. aureus* than polyurethane, Teflon, or polyvinyl chloride catheters. This was also shown by Vaudaux et al. (40), who demonstrated that indwelling silicone catheters, after being removed from patients, were more prone to *S. aureus* adherence than were polyurethane or polyvinyl chloride catheters. This was related to the fact that silicone catheters tend to have a direct toxic effect on neutrophils, alter neutrophil chemotaxis, and cause a localized depletion of complement (41,42). (For additional information on the pathogenesis of infections associated with implantation of biomaterials, see Chapter 67).

Iatrogenic factors associated with medical interventions in high-risk patients entail a higher risk of colonization of catheter surfaces. These consist of the use of TPN fluids and lipid emulsions, interleukin-2, and long-term hemodialysis (1,2). TPN has been associated with higher rates of infection in tunneled catheters (43). The 25% dextrose and the lipid emulsions have been associated with microbial growth, particularly *Candida* species and *Malassezia furfur* (2). In addition, interleukin-2 has also been shown to predispose to catheter colonization and infection by staphylococcal microorganisms (44). It is postulated that interleukin alters neutrophil chemotaxis toward staphylococcal microorganisms, and hence leads to a higher degree of colonization of catheter surfaces with these microbial agents. Finally, chronic hemodialysis patients have a high rate of nasal carriage of *S. aureus*, ranging from 30% to 65% (45–47). *S. aureus* chronic hemodialysis carriers have a threefold higher risk of contracting catheter-related *S. aureus* BSI when compared with noncarriers (48). The majority (more than 90%) of *S. aureus* infections in carriers are caused by the same type as that carried in the nares (45).

The most common microorganisms causing catheter-associated infections in long-term CVCs are coagulase-negative staphylococci, *S. aureus*, and yeasts (1,2). This is related to the fact that staphylococci are skin microorganisms. In addition, staphylococci and *Candida* adhere well to host proteins found on catheter surfaces and tend to form a microbial biofilm (26–32). This is in contrast to gram-negative microorganisms, such as *Escherichia coli* and *Klebsiella pneumoniae*, that do not adhere well to fibronectin and fibrin and are not known to produce a biofilm. Other microorganisms that have been associated with long-term CVC infections are *Bacillus* species, *Corynebacterium* species, *Pseudomonas aeruginosa, Acinetobacter* species, *Stenotrophomonas maltophilia,* micrococcus, *Achromobacter,* rapidly growing mycobacteria, and various other fungal microorganisms such as *M. furfur* and *Fusarium oxysporum* (49).

For long-term catheters, the lumen seems to be the major site of colonization and source of CR-BSIs. This has been shown for catheters used for long-term hemodialysis and for CVCs used for total parenteral nutrition and cancer treatment (50–52). Sherertz (2) estimated that the hub/lumen contributed 66% of the microorganisms that caused infections of long-term catheters and that 26% of the microorganisms were from the skin. However, for short-term catheters with an average duration of <8 days, the skin seems to be the major source, followed by the hub/lumen (53–55). The relative contribution of contaminated infusate, hematogenous seeding from a remote infected source, or extension from a contiguous site of infection seems to be low even in long-term catheters. Using semiquantitative scanning electron microscopy studies, we have determined that the extent of biofilm formation and colonization is greater on the external surface of short-term catheters (<10 days of catheterization) than the internal surface (3). However, for catheters that remain in place for >30 days, this phenomenon is reversed with greater biofilm formation and ultrastructural colonization in the lumen of the catheter versus the external surface.

Electron microscopy studies have shown that colonization is universal (3,56). It involves all CVCs within 24 hours of insertion (56). However, although colonization is universal, only a few catheters are associated with infection. There is a quantitative relationship between the number of microorganisms (particularly free-floating microorganisms) on the catheter and the risk of BSIs. Sherertz et al. (57) studied 1,610 CVCs and found that the greater the number of microorganisms retrieved from the catheters by sonication, the greater the risk of BSI. Therefore, infection could be a function of whether the microorganisms on the catheter surface, particularly those that are free-floating, exceed a certain quantitative threshold due to various risk factors outlined above.

MANIFESTATIONS AND DEFINITIONS

The clinical manifestations of a CR-BSI for long-term catheters consist of systemic manifestations such as fever and chills, which are nonspecific, particularly in the immunocompromised patient. Clinical evidence of a local infection at an exit site, tunnel, or port pocket would be necessary to suggest the catheter as the source of the BSI. However, for PICC lines, local catheter site inflammation consisting of erythema and phlebitis could be aseptic in nature and reflect a local mechanical irritation of the vein due to the insertion of a large catheter in the relatively small basilic or cephalic veins (4). Therefore, local catheter-related infection or systemic CR-BSIs should be defined in terms of clinical manifestations associated with microbiologic data implicating the catheter as the source of the infection (Tables 18.1 and 18.2). The following definitions were proposed in a recent guideline by the CDC (58):

1. *Local catheter infection:* Local catheter infection could exist in different forms, depending on the type of catheter (nontunneled or tunneled implantable port).
   a. *Exit site infection:* either purulence or erythema, tenderness, or induration within 2 cm of the exit site of the catheter, in the absence of concomitant BSI.
   b. *Pocket infection:* purulent exudate in the subcutaneous pocket containing the reservoir of the port or erythema and necrosis of the skin over the reservoir of a totally implantable device (in the absence of concomitant BSI).
   c. *Tunnel infection:* erythema, tenderness, and induration in the tissues overlying the catheter and >2 cm from the exit site.
2. *Systemic catheter infection:* CR-BSI is defined by the CDC as the isolation of the same microorganisms (identical species and antibiogram) from a semiquantitative [>15 colony-forming units (CFU)/catheter segment] or quantitative (> 10^3 CFU/catheter segment) catheter culture and from the blood (preferably drawn from a peripheral vein) of a patient with accompanying clinical symptoms of a BSI and no other apparent source of infection (58). Most CR-BSIs are uncomplicated. However, with virulent microorganisms such as *S. aureus, C. albicans,* and *P. aeruginosa*, deep-seated infections can occur, particularly catheter-related septic thrombosis, which consists of CR-BSI with an infected thrombus (59–61). The clinical course of septic thrombosis is characterized by occasional swelling above the site of the thrombotic vein and persistent BSI on antimicrobial therapy even after the removal of the catheter. Other deep-seated infections associated with complicated catheter-related bacteremias and fungemias consist of endocarditis, osteomyelitis, and retinitis in the case of candidemia (59,60).

TABLE 18.1. DEFINITIONS OF COLONIZATION AND LOCAL CATHETER-ASSOCIATED INFECTION

Catheter colonization: The isolation of 15 colony forming units (CFUs) of any microorganism by semiquantitative culture (roll-plate method) or 10^3 CFUs by quantitative culture (e.g., sonication technique), from a catheter tip or subcutaneous segment in the absence of simultaneous clinical symptoms.

Local catheter-related infection:

- *Exit-site infection:* purulent drainage from the catheter exit site, or erythema, tenderness, and swelling within 2 cm of the catheter exit site.
- *Port-pocket infection:* erythema and necrosis of the skin over the reservoir of a totally implantable device, or purulent exudate in the subcutaneous pocket containing the reservoir.
- *Tunnel infection:* erythema, tenderness, and induration of the tissues overlying the catheter more than 2 cm from the exit site.

TABLE 18.2. DIAGNOSIS OF CATHETER-RELATED BLOODSTREAM INFECTION (CR-BSI), BEFORE OR AFTER CATHETER REMOVAL

Probable CR-BSI:

1. Common skin microorganism[a] isolated from two or more blood cultures or *Staphylococcus aureus*, enterococci, enteric gram-negative bacilli, or *Candida* isolated from one or more blood cultures
2. Clinical manifestations of infection (fever and chills)
3. No apparent source of sepsis other than the catheter

Definitive CR-BSI: All three of the criteria listed above with any one of the clinical or microbiologic findings listed below:

1. Before catheter removal:
   Clinical evidence: purulent discharge at the catheter insertion site
   Microbiologic evidence: differential quantitative blood cultures with 5 : 1 ratio of the same microorganism isolated from blood drawn simultaneously from the catheter and peripheral vein OR positive quantitative skin culture
2. After catheter removal:
   Clinical evidence: clinical sepsis that responds to antibiotic therapy upon catheter removal after being refractory to therapy in the presence of the catheter
   Microbiologic evidence: isolation of the same microorganism from the peripheral blood and from a semiquantitative or quantitative culture of a catheter segment or tip

[a]Coagulase-negative staphylococci, micrococci, and *Bacillus* and *Corynebacterium* species (except for *Corynebacterium jeikeium*).

DIAGNOSIS

Catheter-related infections are often overdiagnosed, resulting in unnecessary antimicrobial therapy and wasteful removal of the CVC. Misdiagnosis is often the result of relying on false-positive microbiologic data, such as positive blood cultures from the CVC or clinical data such as catheter-site inflammation/phlebitis associated with PICC lines in the absence of other confirmatory data. Therefore, the diagnosis of these infections is often difficult and should be the result of integrating clinical and microbiologic findings. A positive nonquantitative blood culture drawn through the CVC with a concurrent negative peripheral blood culture should be interpreted with extreme caution. Bryant and Strand (62) demonstrated that 93% of such cultures are often contaminated with microorganisms that colonize the hub or the lumen, and hence do not reflect an infection. This is particularly true for skin microorganisms such as coagulase-negative staphylococci. It has been demonstrated that the positive predictive value of a single positive blood culture for coagulase-negative staphylococci ranges from 4.1% to 26.4% (63–66). Therefore, prior to initiating antimicrobial therapy and considering whether the catheter should be removed, a single positive blood culture yielding a skin microorganism should be interpreted in light of associated clinical and microbiologic data. Because CVCs are universally colonized, a positive blood culture from the CVC could reflect intraluminal or hub colonization. Therefore, attention should be paid to other laboratory findings suggestive of BSI and which consist of (a) multiple positive blood cultures of skin microorganisms, (b) quantitative blood cultures revealing a high colony count (>35 CFU/mL of blood) (66), and (c) the same microorganisms isolated from the quantitative catheter culture and peripheral blood culture (58). All three of these factors should be considered to reflect a catheter-related infection in the setting of concurrent signs of infection such as fever and chills with no other apparent source for the infection other than the catheter.

Before or after removal of the catheter, the diagnosis should be made based on the interplay of clinical and microbiologic findings. In this chapter we use the approach of Kristinsson (67) in determining the diagnosis in these two situations. The infection is initially suspected when there is a positive blood culture in a patient with a CVC with clinical signs of infection, such as fever and chills, and no other apparent source for the BSI, such as pneumonia, urinary tract infection, intraabdominal infection, or surgical site infection (Table 18.2). This type of BSI has been termed primary BSI. In this case, the primary BSI is a probable catheter-related infection. The diagnosis becomes definitive in the presence of either confirmatory clinical or microbiologic data.

Clinical data consist of (a) local inflammation, such as catheter exit site inflammation or tunneled/port inflammatory signs (Tables 18.1 and 18.2); the presence of purulence at the insertion site, particularly in patients with *S. aureus* bacteremia, is diagnostic of catheter-related bacteremia; and (b) systemic signs of infection, such as fever and chills, that persist despite appropriate antimicrobial therapy for the BSI but resolve with catheter removal (58).

Confirmatory microbiologic data are often not available prior to catheter removal. The three best studied methods to determine the diagnosis prior to catheter removal are simultaneous quantitative blood cultures from the CVC and a peripheral vein, differential time to positivity, and, for nontunneled catheters, quantitative cultures of the skin at the exit site (68–80). In the former case, the diagnosis of CR-BSI is often suggested when the number of colonies isolated from a quantitative blood culture obtained from the catheter is severalfold (at least fivefold) more than that quantitated from a peripheral venipuncture blood culture (69–74). Differential time to positivity (DTP) is a method that was shown in cancer patients to be a simple and reliable tool for *in situ* diagnosis of catheter-related bacteremia. Blot et al. (77,78) defined DTP as the difference in time necessary for the blood cultures drawn from a peripheral vein and through the catheter to become positive. When DTP was >120 minutes, this diagnostic method was shown to be highly sensitive (100%) and specific (96.4%) for the diagnosis of CR-BSI (77). Blot et al. (78) concluded that using DTP as a diagnostic technique is mainly of value for patients requiring long-term catheterization. However, another prospective study found that DTP of >120 minutes was highly suggestive of CR-BSI associated with the use of both short-term and long-term CVCs (79). Another prospective study found that DTP does not seem to be a useful diagnostic tool for the diagnosis of CR-BSI in medical-surgical intensive care unit (ICU) patients (80). The DTP method needs to be evaluated further in different patient populations to better understand the different settings in which it can be utilized accurately. Quantitative skin cultures are most convenient in the setting of a primary BSI (75,76,81,82). Unfortunately, there is no standard method for culturing the skin around the insertion site, and criteria for positive quantitative cultures have varied in the published studies. Depending on the methodology used, a quantitative culture of >15 CFUs for a small surface area (9–10 cm^2) (81,82) or >1,000 CFUs for a large surface area (24–25 cm^2) (75,76) is suggestive of a CR-BSI in a patient with primary bacteremia/fungemia. Several other nonstandardized methods were developed to diagnose catheter-related infection in surgically implanted long-term catheters prior to removal, such as a wire brush or intraluminal brush method, Gram staining or acridine orange staining of blood drawn through the catheter, and culture of the catheter hub (83–87).

After catheter removal, semiquantitative and quantitative catheter cultures have helped in diagnosing CR-BSI. The roll-plate semiquantitative culture method is most commonly used for culturing catheters (88). However, this method is limited in that it cultures only the external surface of the catheter and may not retrieve microorganisms that are well embedded in the biofilm on the catheter surface. The fact that this method does not quantitate microorganisms from the lumen of the catheter is important for long-term indwelling catheters where colonization is mostly luminal. In a study of long-term catheters (nontunneled CVC and PICC lines) at the M. D. Anderson Cancer Center, the sensitivity of the roll-plate technique was 45% compared with 72% for the sonication technique for making the diagnosis of catheter colonization or catheter-related infection by culture of the intravascular segment of the catheter (3). Quantitative catheter cultures, particularly sonication, which retrieves microorganisms from the external and internal surfaces, have been shown to be of higher diagnostic value than the roll-plate technique, particularly for long-term CVC with predominantly luminal colonization (3,89,90). If semiquantitative or quantitative catheter cultures are not done, then a clinical response to catheter removal within 48 hours, after failure of antimicrobial therapy to resolve the infection, with the catheter *in situ*, is highly suggestive of CR-BSI.

If the bacteremia or fungemia persists after catheter removal in spite of the use of appropriate antimicrobial agents, then one has to determine whether the patient has a deep-seated catheter-related infection, such as right-sided endocarditis or septic thrombosis (59,60). In these situations, a venogram would be useful to rule out septic thrombosis, and a transesophageal echogram might be useful to detect valvular vegetations suggestive of endocarditis.

PREVENTION

Effective preventive strategies for long-term CVC-related infections should be based on an understanding of the pathogenesis

TABLE 18.3. MEASURES WITH LIMITED DATA FOR THE PREVENTION OF LONG-TERM CATHETER-RELATED INFECTIONS

Maximal sterile barriers
Skilled infusion therapy team
Tunneling of catheters
Flush solutions/antibiotic lock
New antiseptic hub
Antimicrobial coating of catheters

of these infections. Because luminal colonization is the major source of BSIs in long-term catheters, preventing colonization of the external surface of the catheter during the early phase postinsertion will not decrease the overall rate of infection. One such example is the use of the silver-impregnated cuff, which was shown to interrupt the intracutaneous migration of microorganisms and to decrease the risk of short-term catheter colonization and infection (53). However, this silver-impregnated cuff has failed to protect against infections in long-term tunneled Hickman catheters. Measures that decrease the risk of colonization of the lumen of the catheter have been shown to be of benefit in decreasing the risk of catheter-associated infection for long-term CVCs (91). However, most of the preventive measures suggested for prevention of long-term catheter-associated infections have limited data to support their use with respect to this type of catheter (Table 18.3).

Maximal Sterile Barriers

A prospective randomized study was conducted to test the efficacy of maximal sterile barriers in reducing infections associated with long-term nontunneled subclavian silicone catheters with a mean duration of placement of approximately 70 days (92). Maximal sterile barrier precautions (which involve wearing sterile gloves and gown, a cap, and using a large drape during insertion of the catheter) were compared with routine procedures (which involve wearing only sterile gloves and use of a small drape). Maximal sterile barrier precautions decreased the risk of catheter-related bacteremia from 0.5/1,000 catheter-days to 0.02/1,000 catheter-days. Long-term catheters consisted of nontunneled subclavian CVCs and PICC lines.

Skilled Infusion Therapy Team

In addition to decreasing the catheter-related infection rate by five- to eightfold, an experienced infusion therapy team has been shown to be cost-effective. Most of the studies were done with relatively short-term catheters (93–97). However, we have reported the finding that the duration of placement of nontunneled, noncuffed silicone catheters (mean duration of catheterization of 109 days) could be prolonged to approach that of the tunneled Hickman catheter with a very low infection rate of 1.4/1,000 catheter-days at the M. D. Anderson Cancer Center (4). This was attributed, at least in part, to the presence of a skilled infusion therapy team at our institution.

Tunneling

Because tunneled catheters have been associated with long durability and low infection rates, it has been assumed that tunneling decreases the risk of catheter-related infections and is the only safe option for the maintenance of long-term externalized silicone catheters. A prospective, randomized study evaluating the effect of tunneling on long-term silicone catheters was conducted by Andrivet et al. (18), wherein the catheters were used in immunocompromised patients. The risk of catheter-related bacteremia associated with tunneled as compared with nontunneled catheters was 2% and 5%, respectively. The difference was not significant, probably due to the relatively small number of patients in each group (107 and 105 patients, respectively). In another study involving short-term polyurethane catheters placed in the internal jugular vein of critically ill patients, tunneled catheters were associated with a statistically significant lower rate of catheter-related bacteremia than nontunneled catheters, suggesting that tunneling may decrease the risk of infection (98). In a prospective evaluation of more than 14,000 PICCs and 882 tunneled CVCs in cancer patients, the rate of CR-BSI associated with the use of tunneled CVCs was shown to be lower than that of PICCs (0.042 vs. 0.065 per 1,000 catheter-days, $p = .004$) (99). However, in an evaluation of more than 20,000 nontunneled subclavian CVCs, the CR-BSI rate associated with their use in cancer patients was found to be comparable to that associated with the use of tunneled CVCs (0.073 vs. 0.042 per 1,000 catheter-days, $p = .071$) (100). The main question, however, is whether tunneling is cost-effective, given the fact that surgery may incur an additional cost of about $3,600 per procedure, and long tunneled silicone catheters can be maintained for a long time with a very low infection rate (1).

Ports

The lowest rate of CR-BSI has been associated with the use of surgically implanted subcutaneous central venous ports. In a review by Crnich and Maki (9), in which they evaluated the results of 13 prospective studies of subcutaneous central venous ports, the pooled mean of CR-BSI rates associated with ports was at a low 0.2 per 1,000 catheter-days [95% confidence interval (CI) 0.1–0.2] (9). A prospective evaluation of more than 2,000 ports in cancer patients showed that they were associated with CR-BSI rates significantly lower than PICCs and than nontunneled subclavian catheters (0.0074 vs. 0.065 and 0.073/1, 000 catheter-days, respectively, $p < .0001$) (99,100). Ports are especially useful for intermittent venous access needed for short durations such as with periodic chemotherapy administrations.

Antiseptic Dressings

A novel chlorhexidine-impregnated hydrophilic polyurethane foam dressing (Biopatch, Johnson & Johnson Medical, Dallas, TX), which can be pressed firmly onto the skin at the catheter insertion site and then covered with a transparent polyurethane dressing, was shown to reduce site skin colonization as well as epidural catheter colonization (101). It also prevented infection at the site of orthopedic traction pins in an animal model (102). The chlorhexidine-impregnated sponge dressings were evaluated in a multicenter trial involving six neonatal ICU patients (103), where they were found to be similar to gauze and tape combined with periodic skin disinfection with 10% povidone-iodine, in preventing skin colonization and CR-BSI (103). However, the use of these chlorhexidine dressings was associated with 15% incidence of dermatotoxicity in low birth weight neonates (<1,000g). In another prospective randomized study, the chlorhexidine-impregnated dressings were found to decrease CR-BSI by threefold when used with PICCs or arterial catheters (104).

Intraluminal Antibiotic Locks

This prophylactic measure consists of flushing and filling the lumen of the catheter with antimicrobial agents and leaving the solution to remain in the lumen of the catheter for 6 to 12 hours. Various antimicrobial agents have been used as antimicrobial locks, often following an infection in a surgically implanted catheter in order to treat the infection without removal of the catheter (105,106). Among the antimicrobial agents used were vancomycin, gentamicin, ciprofloxacin, cefazolin, erythromycin, nafcillin, ceftriaxone, clindamycin, fluconazole, and amphotericin B. Vancomycin in combination with heparin has been used as a daily flushing solution of tunneled CVCs and has been reported to significantly decrease the frequency of catheter-related bacteremia caused by vancomycin-susceptible gram-positive microorganisms colonizing the lumen (107). In a large prospective double-blind study of 126 pediatric oncology patients, the efficacy of different flush solutions was investigated over 36,944 tunneled catheter-days (108). In that study, Henrickson et al. randomized patients to receive one of three prophylactic lock solutions: 10 U/mL heparin, heparin/25 μg/mL vancomycin, or heparin/vancomycin/2 μg/mL ciprofloxacin. The rate of total line infections including gram-positive and gram-negative line infections was significantly reduced by either heparin/vancomycin or heparin/vancomycin/ciprofloxacin compared with heparin alone. However, this study did not differentiate between local site infection and CR-BSI. In addition, Crnich and Maki (9) point out that this study also failed to evaluate the impact of using antibiotic lock solutions on nosocomial colonization with microorganisms such as vancomycin-resistant enterococci, methicillin-resistant *S. aureus*, and fluoroquinolone-resistant gram-negative bacilli. Another randomized double-blind trial in neutropenic cancer patients also found that patients who received a lock solution of 10 U/mL heparin and 25 μg/mL vancomycin had a significantly lower rate of CR-BSI than those who received a lock solution of heparin alone ($p = .05$) (109). One study revealed no difference in rates of CR-BSI between children receiving a heparin/vancomycin flush compared with those receiving heparin alone (110). However, with the emergence of resistant microorganisms, it is prudent to avoid using antibiotics that are commonly used in the therapy of BSIs (such as beta-lactam antibiotics, vancomycin, quinolones, and aminoglycosides) for prophylaxis against catheter infections. This is particularly true for vancomycin with the emergence of multidrug-resistant vancomycin-resistant enterococci.

A novel catheter flush solution consisting of low concentrations of minocycline and ethylenediaminetetraacetic acid (EDTA) has recently been developed. Minocycline is not commonly used in the treatment of systemic infections and does not have cross-resistance with vancomycin or beta-lactam antibiotics against resistant gram-positive bacteria. A flush solution of minocycline and EDTA (M-EDTA) was shown to have broad-spectrum and often synergistic activity against methicillin-resistant staphylococci, gram-negative bacilli, and *C. albicans*, and was found to prevent CR-BSIs in several complicated, high-risk patients (111). Also, in a rabbit model, M-EDTA lock solution succeeded more than heparin alone and heparin/vancomycin in preventing catheter colonization, CR-BSI, and phlebitis in all of the study animals ($p < .01$) (112). In that study, the M-EDTA lock solution also prevented tricuspid endocarditis, as did the heparin-vancomycin lock solution, more effectively than heparin alone ($p \leq .06$).

In a prospective randomized trial involving patients with long-term hemodialysis CVCs, M-EDTA flush solution significantly reduced rates of catheter colonization ($p = .005$) (113). Also, in another prospective pediatric cohort study, M-EDTA was used as a lock solution in 14 pediatric cancer patients with ports (114). There were no CR-BSIs, thrombotic events, or adverse events associated with the use of M-EDTA flush solution over a total of 2,073 catheter-days in comparison with a rate of 2.23 infections/1,000 catheter-days in a control group that received heparin flush solution.

Taurolidine, a derivative of the amino acid taurine, is an antimicrobial agent, which in high concentrations (250–2,000 μg/mL) has inhibitory as well as cidal activities against many microorganisms (115). The use of taurolidine lock solution reduced the rate of CR-BSI associated with the use of hemodialysis CVC (116) and other long-term CVCs (117). A combination of taurolidine and citrate-based catheter lock solution (Neutrollin; Biolink Corp., Norwell, MA) reduced bacterial counts in a catheter model by more than 99% (118). The microorganisms affected included *S. aureus, S. epidermidis, P. aeruginosa, E. faecalis,* and *C. albicans*. Taurolidine-citrate significantly reduced biofilm on silicone disks in modified Robbins devices more than heparin treatment (by 4.8 logs vs. 1.7 logs, $p < .01$).

The issue of resistance developing with a wide use of prophylactic antibiotic lock solutions needs to be investigated thoroughly. However, currently, the CDC guidelines for the prevention of intravascular catheter-related infections do not recommend the routine use of prophylactic antibiotic lock solutions. The guidelines recommend the use only in special circumstances, such as in treating a patient with a long-term cuffed or tunneled catheter or port who has a history of multiple CR-BSIs despite optimal maximal adherence to aseptic techniques (58).

Anticoagulant Flush Solutions

The prophylactic use of various anticoagulants, such as heparin, warfarin, and urokinase, as catheter flush solutions have shown efficacy in reducing catheter thrombosis and fibrin deposits on catheters (119–123). Since the majority of heparin solutions contain preservatives that have antimicrobial activity, it is difficult to attribute with certainty any observed efficacy to the heparin rather than to the antimicrobial activity of the preservatives (58).

Antimicrobial Coating of Catheters

Antimicrobial coating of catheters has been shown to be effective in reducing the rate of catheter-related infection in short-term polyurethane catheters. By coating the external surface of catheters with chlorhexidine plus silver sulfadiazine, Maki et al. (124) showed that this combination did decrease the risk of colonization by nearly 50% and decreased the risk of catheter-related bacteremia by at least fourfold. However, the antiinfective efficacy of catheters coated with chlorhexidine and silver sulfadiazine (CH-SS) was not confirmed in three subsequent prospective, randomized studies (125–127). In addition, these catheters were shown *in vitro* to have short-term antimicrobial activity that decreased over time, with a half-life of 3 days against *S. epidermidis* (128). A meta-analysis study analyzed the results of 12 studies investigating the efficacy of catheters impregnated with CH-SS (129). According to this analysis, the mean duration of catheterization with CH-SS catheters was between 5.1 and 11.2 days, and hence their efficacy is only proven for short-term catheterization. A second generation of catheters impregnated with CH-SS, in which the catheters are impregnated both externally and internally, significantly reduced catheter colonization more than uncoated catheters, but failed to reduce the risk of CR-BSI in two prospective randomized trials (130,131). In a prospective, randomized multicenter study when CVCs impregnated with minocycline and rifampin (M-R) on their external and internal surfaces were compared with first-generation CH-SS catheters, they were shown to be 12 times less likely to be associated with CR-BSI and three times less likely to be colonized. It was shown that the risk of catheter colonization was reduced by threefold and the risk of CR-BSIs was reduced from 5% to 0% (132). No evidence of antibiotic resistance was noted among bacteria recovered from patients with minocycline/rifampin-coated catheters. Preliminary results show that long-term nontunneled silicone catheters impregnated with minocycline/rifampin are also efficacious in reducing CR-BSI in cancer patients (133). Currently, the CDC guidelines for the prevention of intravascular catheter-related infections recommend the use of antimicrobial CVC in adults whose catheter is expected to remain in place for more than 5 days, if rates of CR-BSI remain above the goal set by the individual institution after implementing aseptic techniques, including maximal sterile barrier precautions (58).

Elimination of *S. aureus* in Nasal Carriers

S. aureus is the leading cause of long-term catheter-related infections in patients on chronic hemodialysis (134,135). BSIs in patients on chronic hemodialysis have been associated with nasal carriage of the same microorganism (45,48). In addition, it was shown that reduction of the nasal *S. aureus* carrier state resulted in a significant decrease in infection rates with *S. aureus* (136). Mupirocin ointment 2% applied to the nose two or three times daily for 5 to 7 days has resulted in eradication of the nasal carrier state in more than 80% of patients (136–138). Therefore, patients on chronic hemodialysis with at least one episode of *S. aureus* infection should be screened for possible nasal carriage and, if positive, treated with mupirocin. In addition, insertion of the catheter and maintenance care should include close adherence to aseptic technique. Topical application of povidone-iodine to exit sites of chronic hemodialysis catheters at each dressing change has been shown to be useful in decreasing the rate of infection (48).

REFERENCES

1. Raad II, Safar H. Long-term central venous catheters. Infectious complications and cost. In: Seifert H, Jansen B, Farr BM, eds. *Catheter-related infections.* New York: Marcel Dekker, 1997:307–324.
2. Sherertz RJ. Pathogenesis of vascular catheter-related infections. In: Seifert H, Jansen B, Farr BM, eds. *Catheter-related infections.* New York: Marcel Dekker, 1997:1–29.
3. Raad I, Costerton W, Sabharwal U, et al. Ultrastructural analysis of indwelling vascular catheters: a quantitative relationship between luminal colonization and duration of placement. *J Infect Dis* 1993; 168:400–407.
4. Raad I, Davis S, Becker M, et al. Low infection rate and long durability of nontunneled Silastic catheters: a safe and cost-effective alternative for long-term venous access. *Arch Intern Med* 1993;153:1791–1796.
5. Cowl, CT, Weinstock JV, Al-Jurf A, et al. Complications and cost associated with parenteral nutrition delivered to hospitalized patients through either subclavian or peripherally-inserted central catheters. *Clin Nutr* 2000;19(4):237–243.
6. Broviac JW, Cole JJ, Scribner GH. A silicone rubber atrial catheter for prolonged parenteral alimentation. *Surg Gynecol Obstet* 1973;136: 602.
7. Hickman RO, Buckner CD, Clift RA, et al. A modified right atrial catheter for access to the venous system in marrow transplant recipients. *Surg Gynecol Obstet* 1979;148:871.
8. Goodman MS, Wickman R. Venous access devices: an overview. *Oncol Nurs Forum* 1984;11:16–23.
9. Crnich CJ, Maki DG. The promise of novel technology for the prevention of intravascular device-related bloodstream infection in long-term devices. *Clin Infect Dis* 2002;34:1362–1368.
10. Press OW, Ramsey PG, Larson EB, et al. Hickman catheter infections in patients with malignancies. *Medicine* 1984;63(4):189–200.
11. Decker MD, Edwards KM. Central venous catheter infections. *Pediatr Clin North Am* 1988;35(3):579–612.
12. Clarke DE, Raffin TA. Infectious complications of indwelling long-term central venous catheters. *Chest* 1990;97(4):966–972.
13. Howell PB, Walters PE, Donowitz GR, et al. Risk factors for infection of adult patients with cancer who have tunneled central venous catheters. *Cancer* 1995;75(6):1367–1374.
14. Mueller BU, Skelton J, Callender DPE, et al. A prospective randomized trial comparing the infectious complications of the externalized catheters versus a subcutaneously implanted device in cancer patients. *J Clin Oncol* 1992;10:1943–1948.
15. Keung Y-K, Watkins K, Chen S-C, et al. Comparative study of infectious complications of different types of chronic central venous access devices. *Cancer* 1994;73:2832–2837.
16. Mirro J, Rao BN, Kumar M, et al. A comparison of placement techniques and complications of externalized catheters and implantable port use in children with cancer. *J Pediatr Surg* 1990;25(1):122–124.
17. Groeger JS, Lucas AB, Thaler HT, et al. Infectious morbidity associated with long-term use of venous access devices in patients with cancer. *Ann Intern Med* 1993;119:1168–1174.
18. Andrivet P, Bacquer A, Vu Ngoc C, et al. Lack of clinical benefit from subcutaneous tunnel insertion of central venous catheters in immunocompromised patients. *Clin Infect Dis* 1994;18:199–206.
19. Raad II, Luna M, Khalil S-A M, et al. The relationship between the thrombotic and infectious complications of central venous catheters. *JAMA* 1994;271(13):1014–1016.

20. Brismar R, Hardstedt C, Jacobson S. Diagnosis of thrombosis by catheter phlebography after prolonged central venous catheterization. *Ann Surg* 1981;194:779–783.
21. Hawiger J, Timmons S, Strong DD, et al. Identification of a region of human fibrinogen interacting with staphylococcal clumping factor. *Biochemistry* 1982;21:1407–1413.
22. Kuusela P. Fibronectin binds to *Staphylococcus aureus. Nature* 1978; 276:718–720.
23. Lopes JD, Dos Reis M, Brentani RR. Presence of laminin receptors in *Staphylococcus aureus. Science* 1985;229:275–277.
24. Hermann M, Suchard SJ, Boxer LA, et al. Thrombospondin binds to *Staphylococcus aureus* and promotes staphylococcal adherence to surfaces. *Infect Immun* 1991;59:279–288.
25. Vaudaux P, Pittet D, Haeberli A, et al. Host factors selectively increase staphylococcal adherence on inserted catheters: a role for fibronectin and fibrinogen or fibrin. *J Infect Dis* 1989;160:865–875.
26. Bouali A, Robert R, Tronchin G, et al. Characterization of binding of human fibrinogen to the surface of germ-tubes and mycelium of Candida albicans. *J Gen Microbiol* 1987;133:545–551.
27. Christensen GD, Simpson WA, Bisno AL, et al. Adherence of slime-producing strains of *Staphylococcus epidermidis* to smooth surfaces. *Infect Immun* 1982;37:318–326.
28. Christensen GD, Simpson WA, Younger JJ, et al. Adherence of coagulase-negative staphylococci to plastic tissue culture plates: a quantitative model for the adherence of staphylococci to medical devices. *J Clin Microbiol* 1985;22:996–1007.
29. Falcieri E, Vaudaux P, Huggler E, et al. Role of bacterial exopolymers and host factors on adherence and phagocytosis of *Staphylococcus aureus* in foreign body infection. *J Infect Dis* 1987;155:524–531.
30. Costerton JW, Irvin RT, Cheng KR. The bacterial glycocalyx in nature and disease. *Annu Rev Microbiol* 1981;35:299–324.
31. Pfaller MA, Messer SA, Hollis RJ. Variations in DNA subtype, antifungal susceptibility, and slim production among clinical isolates of *Candida* parapsilosis. *Diag Microbiol Infect Dis* 1995;21:9–14.
32. Sheth NK, Franson TR, Sohnle PG. Influence of bacterial adherence to intravascular catheters on in vitro antibiotic susceptibility. *Lancet* 1985;2:1266–1268.
33. Farber BF, Kaplan MH, Clogstron AG. *Staphylococcus epidermidis* extracted slime inhibits the antimicrobial action of glycopeptide antibiotics. *J Infect Dis* 1990;161:37–40.
34. Costerton JW, Lappin-Scott HM. Behavior of bacteria in biofilms. *Am Soc Microbiol News* 1989;55:650–654.
35. Hogt AH, Dankert JJ, Feijin J. Adhesion of *Staphylococcus epidermidis* and *Staphylococcus saprophyticus* onto a hydrophobic biomaterial. *J Gen Microbiol* 1985;131:2485–2491.
36. Reifsteck F, Wee S, Wilkinson BJ. Hydrophobicity-hydrophilicity of staphylococci. *J Med Microbiol* 1987;24:65–73.
37. Sheth NK, Franson TR, Rose HD, et al. Colonization of bacteria on polyvinyl chloride and Teflon intravascular catheter in hospitalized patients. *J Clin Microbiol* 1983;18:1061–1063.
38. Rotrosen D, Calderone RA, Edwards JE Jr. Adherence of *Candida* species to host tissues and plastic surfaces. *Rev Infect Dis* 1986;8: 73–85.
39. Sherertz RJ, Carruth WA, Marosok RD, et al. Contribution of vascular catheter material to the pathogenesis of infection: the enhanced risk of silicone in vivo. *J Biomed Mater Res* 1995;29:634–645.
40. Vaudaux P, Pittet D, Haeberli A, et al. Fibronectin is more active than fibrin or fibrinogen in promoting *Staphylococcus aureus* adherence to inserted intravascular devices. *J Infect Dis* 1993;167:633–641.
41. Marosok R, Washburn R, Indorf A, et al. Contribution of vascular catheter material to the pathogenesis of infection: depletion of complement by silicone elastomer in vitro. *J Biomed Mater Res* 1996;30: 245–250.
42. Lopez-Lopez G, Pascual A, Perea EJ. Effect of plastic catheters on the phagocytic activity of human polymorphonuclear leukocytes. *Eur J Clin Microbiol Infect Dis* 1990;9:324–328.
43. Fuchs PC, Gustafson ME, King JT, et al. Assessment of catheter-associated infection risk with the Hickman right atrial catheter. *Infect Control* 1984;5:226.
44. Syndman DR, Sullivan B, Gill M, et al. Nosocomial sepsis with interleukin-2. *Ann Intern Med* 1990;112:102–107.
45. Yu VL, Goetz A, Wagener M, et al. *Staphylococcus aureus* nasal carriage and infection in patients on hemodialysis. Efficacy of antibiotic prophylaxis. *N Engl J Med* 1986;315:91–96.
46. Tuazon CU. Skin and skin structure infection in the patient at risk: carrier state of *Staphylococcus aureus. Am J Med* 1984;76(suppl 51): 166–171.
47. Goldblum SE, Ulrich JA, Reed WP. Nasal and cutaneous flora among hemodialysis patients and personnel: quantitative characterization and pattern of staphylococcal carriage. *Am J Kidney Dis* 1982;2:281–286.
48. Levin A, Mason AJ, Jindal KK, et al. Prevention of hemodialysis subclavian vein catheter infections by topical povidone-iodine. *Kidney Int* 1991;40:934–938.
49. Raad I. Intravascular-catheter-related infections. *Lancet* 1998;351: 893–898.
50. Linares J, Sitges-Serra A, Garau J, et al. Pathogenesis of catheter sepsis: a prospective study with quantitative and semiquantitative cultures of catheter hub and segments. *J Clin Microbiol* 1985;21:357–360.
51. Almirall J, Gonzalez J, Rello J, et al. Infection of hemodialysis catheters: incidence and mechanisms. *Am J Nephrol* 1989;9:454–459.
52. Cheesbrough JS, Finch RG, Burden RP. A prospective study of the mechanisms of infection associated with hemodialysis catheters. *J Infect Dis* 1986;154:579–589.
53. Maki DG, Cobb L, Garman JK, et al. An attachable silver-impregnated cuff for prevention of infection with central venous catheters: a prospective randomized multicenter trial. *Am J Med* 1988;85: 307–314.
54. Flowers RH III, Schwenzer KJ, Kopel RF, et al. Efficacy of an attachable subcutaneous cuff for the prevention of intravascular catheter-related infection. *JAMA* 1989;261:878–883.
55. Mermel LA, McCormick RD, Springman SR. The pathogenesis and epidemiology of catheter-related infection with pulmonary artery Swan-Ganz catheters: a prospective study utilizing molecular subtyping. *Am J Med* 1991;91(suppl 3B):197S–205S.
56. Anaissie E, Samonis G, Kontoyiannis D, et al. Role of catheter colonization and infrequent hematogenous seeding in catheter-related infections. *Eur J Clin Microbiol Infect Dis* 1995;14:138.
57. Sherertz RJ, Raad II, Belani A, et al. Three-year experience with sonicated vascular catheter cultures in a clinical microbiology laboratory. *J Clin Microbil* 1990;28:76–82.
58. Centers for Disease Control and Prevention. Guidelines for the prevention of intravascular catheter-related infections. *MMWR* March 9, 2002;51(RR-10).
59. Raad I, Narro J, Khan A, et al. Serious complications of vascular catheter-related *Staphylococcus aureus* bacteremia in cancer patients. *Eur J Clin Microbiol Infect Dis* 1992;11:675–682.
60. Strinden WD, Helgerson RB, Maki DG. *Candida* septic thrombosis of the great central veins associated with central catheters. *Ann Surg* 1985;202:653–658.
61. Benezra D, Kiehn TE, Gold GWM, et al. Prospective study of infection in indwelling central venous catheters using quantitative blood cultures. *Am J Med* 1988;85:495–498.
62. Bryant JK, Strand CL. Reliability of blood cultures collected from intravascular catheter versus venipuncture. *Am J Clin Pathol* 1987; 88(1):113–116.
63. Fidalgo S, Vasquez F, Mondoza MC, et al. Bacteremia due to *Staphylococcus epidermidis:* microbiologic, epidemiologic, clinical and prognostic features. *Rev Infect Dis* 1990;12:520–528.
64. Ringbert H, Thoren A, Bredbert A. Evaluation of coagulase-negative staphylococci in blood cultures: a prospective clinical and microbiological study. *Scand J Infect Dis* 1991;23:321–323.
65. Kirchoff LV, Sheagren JN. Epidemiology and clinical significance of blood cultures positive for coagulase-negative staphylococci. *Infect Control* 1985;6:479–486.
66. Herwaldt LA, Geiss M, Kao C, et al. The positive predictive value of isolating coagulase-negative staphylococci from blood cultures. *Clin Infect Dis* 1996;22:14–20.
67. Kristinsson KG. Diagnosis of catheter-related infection. In: Seifert

H, Jansen B, Farr BM, eds. *Catheter-related infections*. New York: Marcel Dekker, 1997:31–57.

68. Wing EJ, Norden CW, Shadduck RK, et al. Use of quantitative bacteriologic techniques to diagnose catheter-related sepsis. *Arch Intern Med* 1979;139:482–483.
69. Raucher HS, Hyatt AC, Barzilai A, et al. Quantitative blood cultures in the evaluation of septicemia in children with Broviac catheters. *J Pediatr* 1984;104:29–33.
70. Mosca R, Curta S, Forbes B, et al. The benefits of isolator cultures in the management of suspected catheter sepsis. *Sepsis* 1987;102: 718–723.
71. Flynn PM, Shenep JL, Stokes DC, et al. In situ management of confirmed central venous catheter-related bacteremia. *Pediatr Infect Dis J* 1987;6:729–734.
72. Flynn PM, Shenep JL, Barrett FF. Differential quantitation with a commercial blood culture tube for diagnosis of catheter-related infection. *J Clin Microbiol* 1988;26:1045–1046.
73. Fan ST, Teoh-Chan CH, Lau KF. Evaluation of central venous catheter sepsis by differential quantitative blood culture. *Eur J Clin Microbiol Infect Dis* 1989;8:142–144.
74. Capdevila JA, Planes AM, Palomar M, et al. Value of differential quantitative blood cultures in the diagnosis of catheter-related sepsis. *Eur J Clin Microbiol Infect Dis* 1992;11:403–407.
75. Raad II, Baba M, Bodey GP. Diagnosis of catheter-related infections: the role of surveillance and targeted quantitative skin cultures. *Clin Infect Dis* 1995;20:593–597.
76. Bjornson HS, Colley R, Bower RH, et al. Association between microorganism growth at the catheter insertion site and colonization of the catheter in patients receiving total parenteral nutrition. *Surgery* 1982; 92:720–727.
77. Blot F, Schmidt E, Nitenberg G, et al. Earlier positivity of central venous versus peripheral blood cultures is highly predictive of catheter-related sepsis. *J Clin Microbiol* 1998;36:105–109.
78. Blot F, Nitenberg G, Chachata E, et al. Diagnosis of catheter-related bacteremia: a prospective comparison of the time to positivity of hub-blood versus peripheral-blood cultures. *Lancet* 1999;354:1071–1077.
79. Raad II, Hanna HA, Alakech B, et al. Diagnosis of catheter-related bloodstream (CRBSI): differential time to positivity (DTP) for short-term and long-term central venous catheters (CVC). In: *Program and Abstracts of the 40th Interscience Conference on Antimicrobial Agents and Chemotherapy,* Toronto, Ontario, September 17–20, 2000. Washington: American Society for Microbiology, 2000.
80. Rinjnders BJA, Verwaest C, Peeetermans E, et al. Difference in time to positivity of hub-blood versus nonhub-blood cultures is not useful for the diagnosis of catheter-related bloodstream infection in critically ill patients. *Crit Care Med* 2001;29(7):1399–1403.
81. Cercenado E, Ena J, Rodriguez-Creixems M, et al. A conservative procedure for the diagnosis of catheter-related infections. *Arch Intern Med* 1990;150:1417–1420.
82. Guidet B, Nicola I, Barakett V, et al. Skin versus hub cultures to predict colonization and infection of central venous catheter in intensive care patients. *Infection* 1994;22:43–48.
83. Kite P, Dobbins BM, Wilcox MH, et al. Evaluation of a novel endoluminal brush method for in situ diagnosis of catheter-related sepsis. *J Clin Pathol* 1997;50:278–282.
84. Tighe MJ, Kite P, Thomas D, et al. Rapid diagnosis of catheter-related sepsis using acridine orange leukocyte cytospin test and endoluminal brush. *J Parenteral Enteral Nutr* 1996;20:215–218.
85. Tighe MJ, Kite P, Fawley WN, et al. An endoluminal brush to detect the infection central venous catheter in situ: a pilot study. *BMJ* 1996; 313:1528–1529.
86. Moonens F, Alami SE, van Gossum A, et al. Usefulness of gram staining of blood collected from total parenteral nutrition catheter for rapid diagnosis of catheter-related sepsis. *J Clin Microbiol* 1994; 32:1578–1579.
87. Linares J, Sitges-Serra A, Garau J, et al. Pathogenesis of catheter sepsis: a prospective study with semiquantitative cultures of catheter hub segments. *J Clin Microbiol* 1985;21:357–360.
88. Maki DG, Weise CE, Sarafin HW. A semiquantitative culture method for identifying intravenous catheter infection. *N Engl J Med* 1977;296:1305–1309.
89. Sherertz RJ, Heard SO, Raad II. Diagnosis of triple-lumen catheter infection: comparison of roll plate, sonication, and flushing methodologies. *J Clin Microbiol* 1997;35(3):641–646.
90. Raad II, Sabbagh MF, Rand KH, et al. Quantitative tip culture methods and the diagnosis of central venous catheter-related infections. *Diagn Microbiol Infect Dis* 1991;15:13–20.
91. Groeger JS, Lucas AB, Coit D, et al. A prospective randomized evaluation of silver-impregnated subcutaneous cuffs for preventing tunneled chronic venous access catheter infections in cancer patients. *Ann Surg* 1993;218:208–210.
92. Raad II, Hohn DC, Gilbreath BJ, et al. Prevention of central venous catheter related infections using maximal sterile barrier precautions during insertion. *Infect Control Hosp Epidemiol* 1994;15:231–238.
93. Nehme AE. Nutritional support of the hospitalized patient: the team concept. *JAMA* 1980;243:1906–1908.
94. Faubion WC, Wesley JR, Khalidi N, et al. Total parenteral nutrition catheter sepsis: impact of the team approach. *J Parenter Enteral Nutr* 1986;10:642–645.
95. Freeman JB, Lemire A, MacLean LD. Intravenous alimentation and septicemia. *Surg Gynecol Obstet* 1972;135:708–712.
96. Nelson DB, Kien CL, Mohr B, et al. Dressing changes by specialized personnel reduce infection rates in patients receiving central venous parenteral nutrition. *J Parenter Enteral Nutr* 1986;10:220–222.
97. Tomford JW, Hershey CO, McLaren CE, et al. Intravenous therapy team and peripheral venous catheter-associated complications. A prospective controlled study. *Arch Intern Med* 1984;144:1191–1194.
98. Timset J-F, Sebille V, Farkas J-C, et al. Effect of subcutaneous tunneling on internal jugular catheter-related sepsis in critically ill patients. A prospective randomized multicenter study. *JAMA* 1996;276: 1416–1420.
99. Hanna HA, McFadyen S, Marts K, et al. Prospective evaluation of 1.67 million catheter-days of peripherally inserted central catheters (PICCs) in cancer patients: long durability and low infection rate. In: *Proceedings of the 41st Interscience Conference on Antimicrobial Agents and Chemotherapy* (abstract K-2045), Chicago, Illinois, September 22–25, 2001. Washington: American Society for Microbiology, 2001:439.
100. Raad II, Hanna HA, Marts K, et al. Nontunneled subclavian central venous (NTSC) vs. tunneled central venous catheters (CVCs) and ports in cancer patients. In: *Programs and abstracts of the 41st Interscience Conference on Antimicrobial Agents and Chemotherapy,* Chicago, Illinois, September 22–25, 2001. Washington: American Society for Microbiology, 2001.
101. Shapiro JM, Bond EL, Garman JK. Use of a chlorhexidine dressing to reduce microbial colonization of epidural catheters. *Anesthesiology* 1990;73:625–631.
102. DeJong ME, DeBerardino MT, Brooks DE, et al. Antimicrobial efficacy of external fixator pins coated with a lipid stabilized hydroxyapatite/chlorhexidine complex to prevent pin tract infection in a goat model. *Journal of Trauma-Injury Infection & Critical Care* 2001;50(6): 1008–1014.
103. Garland JS, Alex CP, Mueller CD, et al. A randomized trial comparing povidone-iodine to a chlorhexidine gluconate-impregnated dressing for the prevention of central venous catheter infections in neonates. *Pediatrics* 2001;107:1431–1436.
104. Maki DG, Mermel LA, Kluger D, et al. The efficacy of a chlorhexidine-impregnated sponge (Biopatch) for the prevention of intravascular catheter-related infection: a prospective, randomized, controlled, multicenter study. In: *Programs and Abstracts of the 40th Interscience Conference on Antimicrobial Agents and Chemotherapy,* Toronto, Canada, September 17–20, 2000. Washington: American Society for Microbiology, 2000.
105. Benoit J-L, Carandang G, Sitrin M, et al. Intraluminal antibiotic treatment of central venous catheter infections in patients receiving parenteral nutrition at home. *Clin Infect Dis* 1995;21:1286–1288.
106. Krzywda EA, Andris DA, Edmiston CE, et al. Treatment of Hickman catheter sepsis using antibiotic lock technique. *Infect Control Hosp Epidemiol* 1995;16:596–598.

107. Schwartz C, Henrickson KJ, Roghmann K, et al. Prevention of bacteremia attributed to luminal colonization of tunneled central venous catheters with vancomycin-susceptible microorganisms. *J Clin Oncol* 1990;8:591–597.
108. Henrickson KJ, Axtell RA, Hoover SM, et al. Prevention of central venous catheter-related infections and thrombotic events in immunocompromised children by the use of vancomycin/ciprofloxacin/heparin flush solution: a randomized, multicenter, double-blind trial. *J Clin Oncol* 2000;18(6):1269–1278.
109. Carratala J, Niubo J, Fernandez-Sevilla A, et al. Randomized, double-blind trial of an antibiotic-lock technique for prevention of gram-positive central venous catheter-related infection in neutropenic patients with cancer. *Antimicrob Agents Chemother* 1999;43(9): 2200–2204.
110. Rackoff WR, Weiman J, Jakobowski D, et al. A randomized, controlled trial of the efficacy of a heparin and vancomycin solution in preventing central venous catheter infections in children. *J Pediatr* 1995;127:147–151.
111. Raad I, Buzaid A, Rhyne, et al. Minocycline and EDTA for the prevention of recurrent vascular catheter infections. *Clin Infect Dis* 1997; 25:149–151.
112. Raad I, Hachem R, Tcholakian RK, et al. Efficacy of minocycline and EDTA lock solution in preventing catheter-related bacteremia, septic phlebitis, and endocarditis in rabbits. *Antimicrob Agents Chemother* 2002;46(2):327–332.
113. Bleyer A, Mason L, Raad I, et al. A randomized double-blind trial comparing minocycline/EDTA vs. heparin as flush solution for hemodialysis catheters. *Infect Control Hosp Epidemiol* 1999;21:100(abst).
114. Chatzinikolaou I, Zipf TF, Hanna H, et al. Minocycline-ethylenediamine-tetraacetate lock solution for the prevention of implantable port infections in children with cancer. *Clin Infect Dis* 2003;36: 116–119.
115. Torres-Viera C, Thauvin-Eliopoulos C, Souli M, et al. Activities of taurolidine *in vitro* and in experimental enterococcal endocarditis. *Antimicrob Agents Chemother* 2000;44(6):1720–1724.
116. Sodemann K, Polaschegg HD, Feldmer B. Two years' experience with Dialock and CLS (a new antimicrobial lock solution). *Blood Purif* 2001;19:251–254.
117. Jurewitsch B, Lee T, Park J, et al. Taurolidine 2% as an antimicrobial lock solution for prevention of recurrent catheter-related bloodstream infections. *JPEN J Parenter Enteral Nutr* 1998;22:242–244.
118. Shah CB, Mittleman MW, Costerton JW, et al. Antimicrobial activity of a novel catheter lock solution. *Antimicrob Agents Chemother* 2002; 46(6):1674–1679.
119. Bern MM, Lokich JJ, Wallach SR, et al. Very low doses of warfarin can prevent thrombosis in central venous catheters: a randomized prospective trial. *Ann Intern Med* 1990;112:423–428.
120. Randolph AG, Cook DJ, Gonzalez CA, et al. Benefit of heparin in central venous and pulmonary artery catheters: a meta-analysis of randomized controlled trials. *Chest* 1998;113:165–171.
121. Boraks P, Seale J, Price J, et al. Prevention of central venous catheter associated thrombosis using minidose warfarin in patients with haematological malignancies. *Br J Haematol* 1998;101:483–486.
122. Franschini G, Becker M, Bruso P, et al. Comparative trial of urokinase (uk) vs. heparin (h) as prophylaxis for central venous ports. In: *Programs and abstracts of the 27th annual meeting of the American Society of Clinical Oncology (ASCO).* Orlando, FL, ASCO: 1991:337(abst).
123. Ray CE Jr, Shenoy SS, McCarthy PL, et al. Weekly prophylactic urokinase instillation in tunneled central venous access devices. *J Vasc Interv Radiol* 1999;10:1330–1334.
124. Maki DG, Stolz SM, Wheeler SJ, et al. Prevention of central venous catheter-related bloodstream infection by use of an antiseptic-impregnated catheter. A randomized, controlled trial. *Ann Intern Med* 1997; 127:257–266.
125. Pemberton LB, Ross V, Cuddy P, et al. No difference in catheter sepsis between standard and antiseptic central venous catheters. A prospective randomized trial. *Arch Surg* 1996;131:986–989.
126. Ciresi D, Albrecht RM, Volkers PA, et al. Failure of antiseptic bonding to prevent central venous catheter-related infection and sepsis. *Am J Surg* 1996;62:641–646.
127. Heard SO, Wagle M, Vijayakumar E, et al. The influence of central venous catheters coated with chlorhexidine/silver sulfadiazine on catheter-related infections. *Crit Care Med* 1997;25(suppl):A117(abst).
128. Raad I, Darouiche R, Hachem R, et al. The broad-spectrum activity and efficacy of catheters coated with minocycline and rifampin. *J Infect Dis* 1996;173:418–424.
129. Veenstra DL, Saint S, Saha S, et al. Efficacy of antiseptic-impregnated central venous catheters in preventing catheter-related bloodstream infection: a meta-analysis. *JAMA* 1999;281:261–267.
130. Rupp ME, Lisco S, Lipsett P, et al. Efficacy of chlorhexidine/silver sulfadiazine coating on microbial colonization of central venous catheters in a multicenter trial. In: *Program and abstracts of the 41st annual meeting of the Interscience Conference on Antimicrobial Agents and Chemotherapy,* Chicago, Illinois, September 22–25, 2001.
131. Brun-Buisson C, Nitenberg G, Doyon F, et al. Randomized controlled trial of antiseptic-coated (ACC) central venous catheters (CVC). In: *Program and abstracts of the 42nd Interscience Conference on Antimicrobial Agents and Chemotherapy,* San Diego, California, September 27–30, 2002.
132. Darouiche RO, Raad II, Heard SO, et al., for the Catheter Study Group. A comparison of two antimicrobial-impregnated central venous catheters. *N Engl J Med* 1999;340(1);1–8.
133. Hanna H, Banjamin R, Chatzinikolaou I, et al. The role of long-term silicone central venous catheters impregnated with rifampin and minocycline (S-CVC-RM) in preventing catheter-related infections: a prospective randomized study. In: *Program and abstracts of the 38th Conference of the American Society of Clinical Oncology (ASCO),* Orlando, Florida, May 18–21, 2002.
134. Sherertz RJ, Falk RJJ, Huffman KA, et al. Infections associated with subclavian Uldall catheters. *Arch Intern Med* 1983;143:53–56.
135. Boelaert JR, Van Landyt HW, Godard CA, et al. Nasal mupirocin ointment decreases the incidence of *Staphylococcus aureus* bacteraemia in haemodialysis patients. *Nephrol Dial Transplant* 1993;8:235–239.
136. Holton DL, Nicolle LE, Diley D, et al. Efficacy of mupirocin nasal ointment in eradicating *Staphylococcus aureus* nasal carriage in chronic haemodialysis patients. *J Hosp Infect* 1991;17:133–137.
137. Watanakunokorn C, Brandt J, Durkin P, et al. The efficacy of mupirocin ointment and chlorhexidine body scrubs in the eradication of nasal carriage of *Staphylococcus aureus* among patients undergoing long-term hemodialysis. *Am J Infect Control* 1992;20:138–141.
138. Reagan DR, Doebbeling BD, Pfaller MA, et al. Elimination of coincident *Staphylococcus aureus* nasal and hand carriage with intranasal application of mupirocin calcium ointment. *Ann Intern Med* 1991; 114:101–106.

19

NOSOCOMIAL BLOODSTREAM INFECTIONS

MARK E. RUPP

Nosocomial bloodstream infections (BSIs) are a significant and increasing problem associated with the present-day healthcare system. A variety of factors, including central venous catheterization, predispose patients toward development of infections involving the bloodstream. Pathogens causing these infections vary according to the primary site of infection and a variety of patient factors. Preventive efforts are generally directed at the primary site of invasion. This chapter summarizes general issues related to nosocomial bacteremia. More specific information can be found in chapters covering specific primary infections and pathogens.

INCIDENCE AND IMPACT

Nosocomial BSIs are increasing in prevalence and result in significant morbidity, mortality, and economic cost. From 1975 to 1996, the proportion of nosocomial infections accounted for by BSIs increased from 5% to 14% (1,2). McGowan and Shulman (3) noted from 1975 through the early 1990s that the rate of nosocomial BSI increased dramatically from approximately 2 to 4 episodes/1,000 discharges to 15 to 20 episodes/1,000 discharges. It is estimated that each year in the United States up to 350,000 patients experience a nosocomial BSI (4).

The crude mortality associated with nosocomial BSI varies in published reports from 5% to 58% and depends on the microbial etiology and the underlying condition of the patient (3). Over a 3-year observational period from 1995 to 1998, the Surveillance and Control of Pathogens of Epidemiological Importance (SCOPE) investigators analyzed over 10,000 cases of nosocomial BSI from 49 medical centers, and noted a crude mortality rate of 27%, ranging from 21% for coagulase-negative staphylococci to 40% for *Candida* sp. (4,5). Nosocomial BSI results in dramatic increases in economic cost. The length of hospital stay is extended by 1 to 4 weeks (6--9) at a cost of up to $40,000 per survivor (7,8). There is no doubt that nosocomial BSI is a very significant problem associated with the current healthcare system and that efforts to better understand and prevent this problem are well warranted.

CLASSIFICATION AND DEFINITIONS

Although the definition of hospital-acquired BSI appears clear-cut, the application of the definition is, at times, confusing. Nosocomial BSI is typically defined as the demonstration of a recognized pathogen in the bloodstream of a patient who has been hospitalized for >48 hours. BSIs can be further categorized as primary or secondary. When a microorganism isolated from the bloodstream originated from a nosocomial infection at another site (urinary tract, surgical site, etc.), the infection is classified as a secondary BSI. Conversely, primary BSIs occur without a recognizable focus of infection elsewhere. It should be noted, that BSIs stemming from intravascular catheters are classified as primary infections.

The Centers for Disease Control and Prevention (CDC) National Nosocomial Infection Surveillance (NNIS) system defines BSI as "laboratory confirmed BSI" and "clinical sepsis" (10). Laboratory-confirmed BSI must meet at least one of the following criteria:

Criterion 1: Patient has a recognized pathogen cultured from one or more blood cultures

and

organism cultured from blood is *not* related to an infection at another site.

Criterion 2: Patient has at least *one* of the following signs or symptoms: fever (>38°C), chills, or hypotension (systolic pressure ≤90 mm Hg)

and

signs and symptoms and positive laboratory results are *not* related to an infection at another site

and

at least *one* of the following:

a. common skin contaminant (e.g., diphtheroids, *Bacillus* sp., *Propionibacterium* sp., coagulase-negative staphylococci, or micrococci) is cultured from *two* or more blood cultures drawn on *separate* occasions

b. common skin contaminant (e.g., diphtheroids, *Bacillus* sp., *Propionibacterium* sp., coagulase-negative staphylococci, or micrococci) is cultured from at least one blood culture from a patient with an intravascular line, and the physician institutes appropriate antimicrobial therapy

c. positive antigen test on blood (e.g., *Haemophilus influenzae, Streptococcus pneumoniae, Neisseria meningitidis,* or group B streptococcus).

Criterion 3: Patient ≤1 year of age has at least *one* of the following signs or symptoms: fever (>38°C rectal), hypothermia (<37°C rectal), apnea, or bradycardia

and

signs and symptoms and positive laboratory results are *not* related to an infection at another site

and

at least *one* of the following:

a. common skin contaminant (e.g., diphtheroids, *Bacillus* sp., *Propionibacterium sp., coagulase-negative staphylococci, or micrococci) is cultured from two* or more blood cultures drawn on *separate* occasions

b. common skin contaminant (e.g., diphtheroids, *Bacillus* sp., *Propionibacterium* sp., coagulase-negative staphylococci, or micrococci) is cultured from at least one blood culture from a patient with an intravascular line, and the physician institutes appropriate antimicrobial therapy

c. positive antigen test on blood or urine (e.g., *H. influenzae, S. pneumoniae, N. meningitidis,* or group B streptococcus).

The definition of clinical sepsis is intended primarily for infants and neonates, and patients with clinical sepsis must meet at least one of the following criteria:

Criterion 1: Patient has at least *one* of the following clinical signs or symptoms with no other recognized cause: fever (>38°C), hypotension (systolic pressure ≤90 mm Hg), or oliguria (<20 cc/hr)

and

blood culture *not* done or *no* organisms or antigen detected in blood

and

no apparent infection at another site

and

physician institutes treatment for sepsis.

Criterion 2: Patient ≤1 year of age has at least *one* of the following signs or symptoms with no other recognized cause: fever (>38°C rectal), hypothermia (<37°C rectal), apnea, or bradycardia

and

blood culture *not* done or *no* organisms or antigen detected in blood

and

no apparent infection at another site

and

physician institutes treatment for sepsis.

Although ambiguity is generally not encountered in evaluating patients with positive blood cultures, it is important to note that there is potentially wide practice variation with regard to procurement of blood cultures, and thus bias can be introduced when comparing rates of BSI from institution to institution or unit to unit (11). In general, it is felt that clinicians in the U.S. are very liberal in their ordering of blood cultures, and it is doubtful that many clinically significant episodes of bacteremia escape detection.

Differentiating true, clinically significant, BSI from blood culture contaminants can also, at times, offer a challenge to clinicians. This is discussed in greater detail in subsequent sections.

Another issue that has complicated the definition of nosocomial BSI is the blurring of the distinction between nosocomial and community-acquired infections. Friedman et al. (12) observed that of 504 consecutive BSIs detected at an academic medical center and two associated community hospitals, 37% were healthcare associated. Many of these patients were receiving home healthcare, including intravenous infusions and chemotherapy that, up until the recent past, would have been administered in the inpatient setting. The term "nosohusial" has been proposed to describe infections occurring in homecare subjects (13). Likewise, Siegman-Igra et al. (14) noted that 39% of 604 BSI occurring in settings traditionally classified as community acquired could be more accurately classified as healthcare associated and included patients with infections occurring shortly after discharge, infections associated with outpatient procedures (endoscopy, urethral dilatation, etc.), and infections in nursing home patients.

CLINICAL MICROBIOLOGY AND DIAGNOSTIC TECHNIQUES

The diagnosis of BSI is dependent on the capacity to recover microbes from the blood. Most large laboratories utilize various automated blood culture systems that are reasonably comparable and are often continuously monitored. These automated systems have been reviewed elsewhere (15), and an extensive discussion is beyond the scope of this chapter. In considering the reliability of recovery of nonfastidious microbes, the type of system used is probably not as important as a variety of procurement issues.

Several factors regarding blood culture reliability and contamination should be emphasized:

Skin Preparation and Culture Technique

Culture contamination is often due to poor skin preparation technique. Protocols at many centers recommend that the venipuncture site be cleansed with alcohol followed by an iodophor or tincture of iodine. Several studies have found that use of iodine tincture results in lower rates of contamination when compared to povidone iodine, which is thought to be due to the shorter drying time and rapidity of antimicrobial activity associated with iodine tincture (16–18). However, Calfee and Farr (19) observed no significant differences in contamination rates among four different skin antiseptics including povidone iodine and tincture of iodine. Mimoz et al. (20) found that skin disinfection with alcoholic chlorhexidine was more efficacious in prevention of blood culture contamination than povidone iodine. Following appropriate skin preparation, if the blood vessel must be palpated, it should be done with a sterile glove. A new needle should be utilized for each attempt at venipuncture (21). Blood should be promptly inoculated into culture bottles following disinfection of culture bottle top septums. It is not necessary to change needles between procurement of blood and inoculation of blood cultures (22,23).

Blood Volume Sampled

To maximize the diagnostic yield from blood cultures, an adequate amount of blood must be sampled. In many cases, the concentration of microorganisms in the bloodstream is ≤ 1 colony-forming unit (CFU)/mL, and therefore 10 to 20 mL of blood should be sampled to reliably detect bacteremia (24,25). Mermel and Maki (26) calculated that the yield from blood cultures in adults increased 3% per milliliter of blood obtained. Unfortunately, it is common practice to sample inadequate volumes of blood in many clinical centers (26).

Timing of Blood Cultures

The optimum time to draw blood cultures is when the number of microbes in the bloodstream is greatest, which unfortunately is 1 to 2 hours before the onset of symptoms (27). Therefore, it is recommended to obtain blood cultures as soon as symptoms occur. Although it is common to wait 30 to 60 minutes between obtaining culture sets, Li et al. (28) found no advantage associated with this practice. Issues regarding the number of blood cultures, repetitive blood cultures, the utility of anaerobic cultures, blood-to-broth ratios, and other clinical microbiology issues have been reviewed elsewhere (29–31).

Sites for Obtaining Blood Cultures

Although it is generally recommended to avoid obtaining blood for cultures via intravascular catheters because of concern for contamination, the ease of vascular access and minimization of patient discomfort has made this a common clinical practice. Studies evaluating rates of contamination of blood drawn via catheters are not conclusive, but generally indicate increased recovery of contaminants in catheter-drawn blood (32–34). In addition, due to the widespread use of automated, continuously monitored blood culture systems, many clinicians have started to use differential time to positivity to evaluate the source of fever/bacteremia in patients with central venous catheters. This technique, which is described in greater detail in Chapter 18, is based on the premise that patients with a catheter-associated infection should have a greater burden of bacteria in blood drawn from the intravascular catheter (and hence a shorter time to culture positivity) than blood drawn from the periphery. Early experience with this technique appears promising (35–37). Therefore, if clinicians are using catheter-drawn blood for culture, it should be paired with a sample drawn peripherally and the sites and times of procurement should be clearly documented.

INDICATIONS FOR BLOOD CULTURES

Indications for blood cultures are not standardized, but should be obtained as a routine study whenever there is a realistic possibility of nosocomial BSI. Fever is generally the most common clinical marker for serious nosocomial infection, and blood cultures are usually included in the evaluation of fever in hospitalized patients. However, it should be noted that fever may be absent during episodes of bacteremia in certain patient populations such as the elderly, neonates, immunocompromised hosts, and persons with end-stage renal disease. Changes in mental status or functional status may be the most prominent findings associated with bacteremia in elderly patients or patients with renal dysfunction (21,38). Likewise, bacteremia in neonates is often manifested by lethargy, feeding intolerance, apnea, cholestasis, and temperature instability rather than fever (39,40).

If a nosocomial BSI is identified by blood culture, it is generally not necessary to repeat blood cultures after appropriate treatment has been initiated. Patients who fail to improve despite appropriate antimicrobial therapy should have repeat blood cultures performed to assess for persistence of infection. Also, in the evaluation of *Staphylococcus aureus* nosocomial BSI, many authorities would recommend repeating blood cultures to help assess whether a patient has endocarditis or other deep-seated staphylococcal infection.

MICROBIAL ETIOLOGY OF NOSOCOMIAL BSI

The microbial profile of nosocomial BSI has changed markedly over the past several decades in response to changes in patient population and antibiotic use. Throughout the 1970s, Enterobacteriaceae were the most common cause of nosocomial BSI (41). During the 1980s, a relative decrease in bacteremia due to *Escherichia coli* and *Klebsiella pneumoniae* was observed, whereas the contribution due to coagulase-negative staphylococci, enterococci, and *Candida albicans* increased (42). These changes were attributed to the widespread use of antibiotics with activity against Enterobacteriaceae and the increased utilization of indwelling medical devices, particularly intravascular catheters. Banerjee et al. (43), reporting on secular trends in nosocomial primary BSIs during the 1980s, found that, depending on the type of hospital studied (small, ≤ 200 beds; large, ≥ 500

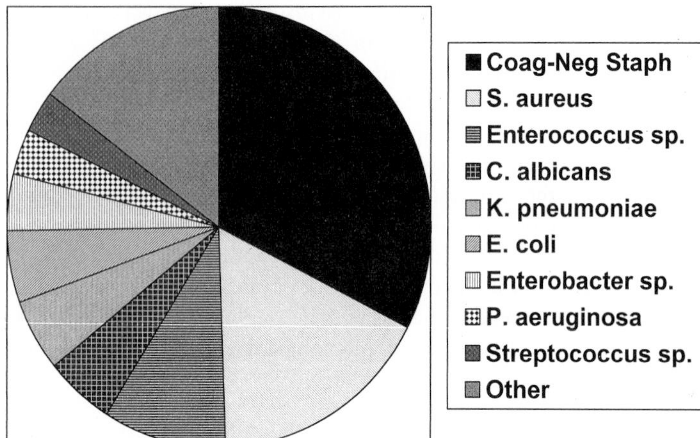

Figure 19.1. Microbial etiology of nosocomial bloodstream infection from 1990 to 1996.

beds; teaching versus nonteaching), the rate of bacteremia due to coagulase-negative staphylococci skyrocketed by 161% to 754% (43). Similarly, enterococcal bacteremia increased by 120% to 197% and *Candida* sp. fungemia increased by 75% to 487% (43). Another trend observed during the 1980s was a shift toward more antibiotic-resistant pathogens. Increased prevalence of antibiotic-resistance was observed in *Pseudomonas aeruginosa* and *Enterobacter cloacae* resistant to third-generation cephalosporins, *S. aureus* and coagulase-negative staphylococci resistant to methicillin, and enterococci resistant to high levels of aminoglycosides (42).

These trends continued in the 1990s. Figure 19.1 illustrates the distribution of over 14,000 bloodstream isolates from the CDC's NNIS hospitals from 1990 through 1996 (2). BSI accounted for approximately 14% of nosocomial infections. Gram-positive cocci predominated the profile, with coagulase-negative staphylococci, *S. aureus*, and enterococci responsible for 56% of nosocomial BSIs. Unfortunately, since the mid-1990s, due to limitations in time and personnel resources, fewer and fewer hospitals participated in the hospital-wide surveillance component of the NNIS system and it was discontinued in 1999. However, the NNIS system has continued to track nosocomial infections from targeted surveillance in intensive care units (ICUs). There was little change in the relative rank order of bloodstream isolates observed in ICU patients from 1990 to 1999 as compared to the hospital-wide data shown in Figure 19.1. Table 19.1 summarizes observations regarding nosocomial

TABLE 19.1. PATHOGENS ISOLATED FROM INTENSIVE CARE UNIT (ICU) NOSOCOMIAL BLOODSTREAM INFECTIONS, 1992–1999 (*n* = 21,943) (44)

Pathogen	Number (%)
Coagulase-negative staphylococci	8,181 (37.3)
Enterococcus sp.	2,967 (13.5)
S. aureus	2,758 (12.6)
C. albicans	1,090 (5.0)
Enterobacter sp.	1,083 (4.9)
P. aeruginosa	841 (3.8)
K. pneumoniae	735 (3.4)
E. coli	514 (2.3)
Other	3,774 (17.2)

BSI from 1992 to 1999 in ICU patients (44). Nine types of ICUs were surveyed. In burn ICUs, BSI was more frequently due to *Enterobacter* sp. or *P. aeruginosa* (11.2% and 9.5%, respectively) than other types of ICUs, whereas coronary care and cardiothoracic ICU patients experienced BSI due to *S. aureus* and coagulase-negative staphylococci with greater frequency (23.2% and 42.7%, respectively) than in other ICUs (44). These trends are supported by several recent observational studies that are summarized in Table 19.2 (5,45,46). As previously mentioned, during the 1980s a trend was observed indicating that nosocomial BSIs were increasingly being caused by antibiotic-resistant pathogens. This trend has continued in the 1990s. The most recently published data from the NNIS system, summarizing bacterial isolates from ICU and non-ICU inpatient areas from January 1998 to June 2002, indicate an alarming prevalence of antimicrobial resistance (47). These data are shown in Table 19.3.

SOURCES OF BACTEREMIA

Most episodes of primary nosocomial BSI or laboratory-confirmed nosocomial BSI without an obvious source are thought to be due to intravascular catheters. These infections are discussed in depth in Chapters 17 and 18. Prior to the widespread use of intravascular catheters, nosocomial BSIs were largely secondary to infections at other sites. During the 1960s and 1970s, approximately 75% of nosocomial BSIs were secondary to surgical site infections, intraabdominal infections, infections of the urinary tract, pneumonia, or skin and soft tissue infections (48, 49). Approximately two thirds of these infections were due to aerobic, gram-negative bacilli (48). As previously mentioned, in more recent years primary BSI has become more prevalent and staphylococci and enterococci have become more prominent pathogens. Pittet and Wenzel (50) noted that from 1981 to 1992 the proportion of nosocomial BSIs classified as primary BSIs increased from 51% to 71%. Over the same time period, the proportion of nosocomial BSIs due to coagulase-negative staphylococci increased from 12% to 30% and those due to aerobic gram-negative rods fell from 52% to 29%.

Rates of bacteremia vary due to the pathogen and site of

TABLE 19.2. PATHOGENS ISOLATED FROM NOSOCOMIAL BLOODSTREAM INFECTIONS, 1990s

	Cockerill et al. (45), 1989–1992, *n* = 9,109	Lark et al. (46), 1994–1997, *n* = 404	Edmund et al. (5), 1995–1998, *n* = 10,617
Coagulase-negative staphylococci	10.4	27.3	31.9
S. aureus	18.4	15.4	15.7
Enterococcus sp.	6.2	10.4	11.1
E. coli	11.1	5.8	5.7
Candida sp.	14	5.8	7.6
Viridans streptococci	3.2	5.2	1.4
Pseudomonas sp.	4.3	5	4.4
Klebsiella sp.	5.2	3.0	5.4
Enterobacter sp.	3.8	2.6	4.5
Other GNR	6.2	2.4	1.4
Other	17.2	6.2	10.9
Polymicrobic	NS	19.5	NS

Values represent percentage of total bloodstream isolates for pathogen in specific study.
NS, not stated; GNR, gram-negative aerobic rods.

infection. For example, although nosocomial urinary tract infections (UTIs) are common and account for 30% to 40% of nosocomial infections, they result in secondary bacteremia in only 1% to 4% of cases (51,52). The rate of bacteremia secondary to nosocomial UTI appears to be higher with pathogens such as *Serratia marcescens* (16%) and is lowest in low virulence microorganisms such as coagulase-negative staphylococci (1.8%) (53). Allen et al. (41) found that bacteremia was associated with 3.3% of nosocomial UTIs, 6.2% of surgical site infections, and 8.6% of lower respiratory tract infections. Petti et al. (54) recently noted in a community hospital setting that 9.1% of surgical site infections were associated with bacteremia. *S. aureus* surgical site infection was associated with an almost threefold increased rate of bacteremia compared to other microbes (54). Table 19.4 characterizes the relative contribution of various sites to overall rates of secondary bacteremia (45,50,55,56).

TABLE 19.3. PREVALENCE OF ANTIMICROBIAL-RESISTANT PHENOTYPES AMONG NOSOCOMIAL PATHOGENS ISOLATED IN CDC'S NATIONAL NOSOCOMIAL INFECTION SURVEILLANCE (NNIS) SYSTEM FROM JANUARY 1998 TO JUNE 2002(47)

	Mean Percentage Exhibiting Resistance Phenotype in ICU and Non-ICU Patients	
Antimicrobial-Resistant Pathogens	ICU	Non-ICU
MRSA	51.3	41.4
Methicillin-resistant coagulase-negative staphylococci	75.7	64
Vancomycin-resistant enterococci	12.8	12
Fluoroquinolone-resistant *P. aeruginosa*	36.3	27
Imipenem-resistant *P. aeruginosa*	19.6	12.7
Ceftazidime-resistant *P. aeruginosa*	13.9	8.3
Pipercillin-resistant *P. aeruginosa*	17.5	11.5
Cef3-resistant *Enterobacter* sp.	26.3	19.8
Cef3-resistant *K. pneumoniae*	6.1	5.7
Fluoroquinolone-resistant *E. coli*	5.8	5.3

MRSA, methicillin-resistant *S. aureus*; Cef3 = third-generation cephalosporine.

Two additional trends in the microbiology of nosocomial BSI should be noted. First, the proportion of infections due to a polymicrobic etiology appears to be increasing and accounts for approximately 15% to 20% of infections. Pittet and Wenzel (50) observed from 1980 to 1992 that polymicrobic nosocomial BSIs increased from eight episodes/10,000 patient-days to approximately 20 episodes/10,000 patient-days, which equated to a rise from 11% to 14%. Other investigators have observed a polymicrobic etiology for 16% to 20% of nosocomial BSIs (45, 55). Polymicrobic infections are more common in elderly patients (57), neonates (58), and patients with underlying malignancies (59). In addition, polymicrobic infections are more likely to be associated with mortality than monomicrobic infections (60). Second, a shift in the microbiology of nosocomial BSIs due to yeast has occurred. Increasingly, non-albicans *Candida* sp. are being recovered from blood cultures. Edmond et al. (5) noted that half of *Candida* BSIs were due to species other than *C. albicans*, which was mirrored in NNIS system hospitals (61). Similarly, in 34 medical centers throughout North America and Latin America, 46% of 306 episodes of candidemia were due to non-albicans species of *Candida* (62). The increasing prevalence of non-albicans species as a cause for nosocomial BSI may be related to the use of imidazole antifungal agents (63).

NOSOCOMIAL BSI IN SPECIFIC PATIENT POPULATIONS AND CIRCUMSTANCES

Nosocomial BSIs are more common in certain patient populations. Nosocomial infections in many of these specific groups of patients (elderly, neonates, ICU patients, burn patients, etc.) are discussed more thoroughly in other chapters of this text. The following is a concise summary of issues related more specifically to nosocomial BSIs.

TABLE 19.4. RELATIVE CONTRIBUTION OF ANATOMIC SITES TO OVERALL NOSOCOMIAL BLOODSTREAM INFECTION (BSI) (46,50,55,56)

	Study (Author, Reference, No. of Subjects, Years of Study)			
Site responsible for BSI	Mylotte et al. (56), n = 1,365, 1979–1987	Pittet and Wenzel (50), n = 3,464, 1980–1992	Roberts et al. (55), n = 1,244, 1984–1987	Lark et al. (46), n = 404, 1994–1997
Intraabdominal	5.5	2.0	14.5	16
Urinary tract	21.2	8.3	16.2	11
Lower respiratory tract	13.4	12	14.3	15
Skin/soft tissue	—	—	—	11
Surgical site	4.4	10	13.4	7
Bone/joint	—	—	1.8	2
Other	19.1	—	23	—
Primary	34.1	59	16.7	49

Elderly and Long-Term Care

Older age (>65 years old) has been noted as a predisposing factor for nosocomial bacteremia and an indicator for worse outcome (64–66). In addition, the rate of bacteremia in the elderly population in the U.S. appears to be increasing (67). Mylotte et al. (66) recently reviewed the literature on BSI in nursing home residents. Briefly, BSI occurred at a rate of approximately 0.3 episodes/1,000 patient-days and mortality ranged from 18% to 35%. *E. coli* (23%) was the most common cause of bacteremia followed by *Proteus* sp. (14%). *S. aureus* was responsible for 11% of cases of BSI. Over the past two decades, the urinary tract, as a site responsible for episodes of bacteremia, has been remarkably stable from study to study and caused from 51% to 56% of BSIs (66). The respiratory tract was the second most likely site to be implicated in BSI and was responsible for 7% to 11% of cases (66). Dementia and stroke were the most frequently observed underlying conditions (66) (see also Chapter 106).

Neonates and Pediatrics

General considerations regarding nosocomial infections in neonates and pediatric patients is discussed thoroughly in Section VI (Chapters 48 to 53). BSI rates in these patients are generally higher than the adult population. Neonatal BSI, during the initial period after birth, is most often a result of infection of the birth canal or maternally acquired microbes. Late-onset BSIs are usually due to hospital-acquired microorganisms. BSI was the most commonly observed nosocomial infection in neonates in the NNIS system from 1980 to 1994 and accounted for 26% to 43% of infections depending on birth weight category (68). Low birth weight is a major risk factor for nosocomial BSI. The U.S. National Institute of Child Health and Human Development (NICHD) documented that late-onset BSI was commonly due to the nosocomial pathogens coagulase-negative staphylococci (55%), *S. aureus* (9%), enterococci (5%), and *Candida* sp. (7%), and were more common in very low birth weight infants (50/100 births) than infants >2,500 g (10/100 births) (69,70). Intravascular catheter use is major risk factor for primary BSI in neonates. Data from the NNIS system from 1995 to 2002 documented BSI rates ranging from 3.6/1,000 central venous catheter (CVC) days to 10.8/1000 CVC days, depending on birth weight classification (47). Lastly, administration of certain therapies strongly increases the risk of bacteremia due to specific pathogens. For example, fungemia due to *Malassezia furfur* is seen almost exclusively in infants receiving intravenous lipids (71).

Richards et al. (72) summarized observations from the NNIS system regarding nosocomial infections in pediatric ICU patients (72). BSIs were responsible for 21% to 34% of nosocomial infections depending on the age of the patient. Similar to the experience observed in adult patients, the most frequently recovered pathogens were coagulase-negative staphylococci (37.8%), enterococci (11.2%), and *S. aureus* (9.3%) (72). *Enterobacter* sp. (6.2%) and *P. aeruginosa* (4.9%) were the most commonly observed gram-negative pathogens, and *C. albicans* was responsible for 5.5% of BSI (72).

ICU Patients

ICU patients account for a disproportional share of nosocomial infections compared to other patients. Two decades ago, Wenzel et al. (73) noted that ICU patients accounted for 45% of nosocomial BSIs, although critical care units comprised only 5% to 10% of hospital beds. More recently, in a large multicenter study in France, the risk of nosocomial BSI was noted to be 12-fold greater in ICU patients than in ward patients (74). For an extensive description of ICU-associated nosocomial BSI, see several recent reviews and studies that will be briefly discussed herein (75–78). Table 19.5 summarizes the observations from several studies concerning ICU BSI. The rate of nosocomial BSI in ICU patients has been increasing and is primarily due to intravascular catheters, lower respiratory tract infections, and intraabdominal infections. Overall mortality is approximately 40%. The microbiology of ICU bacteremia is shown in Fig. 19.2. Similar to nosocomial BSI throughout the hospital, the gram-positive cocci are the most frequent etiology. In a surgical ICU population Mainous et al. (79) noted that enterococci were the most common cause of nosocomial BSI (79). Polymicrobic infections were observed in 14.5% of bacteremic patients. The prevalence of polymicrobic infections depends on the ICU setting and is most common in surgical ICUs that care for a larger number of patients with intraabdominal infections (74).

TABLE 19.5. NOSOCOMIAL BLOODSTREAM INFECTIONS IN ICU PATIENTS

Author/Reference/ Year(s)	No. BSI	Rate of BSI (per 1,000 ICU admissions)	Sources for BSI (%)	Mortality (%)	Comment
Crowe et al. (76), 1985–1996	315	Increased from 17.7 (1985) to 80.3 (1996)	IVC 24.5, LRTI 39.7, GI 7.3, UTI 4.1, SSI 2.2, CNS 5.1, Unk 8.9	44.4	Single ICU
Valles et al. (77), 1993	590	36	IVC 37.1, LRTI 17.5, GI 6.1, UTI 5.9, SSI 2.4, Unk 28.1, Other 2.9	41.6	Multicenter study, length of ICU stay for patients with BSI 28.5 days
Edgeworth et al. (78), 1971–1995	486	Increased from 17.4 (1971–1975 to 38 (1991–1995)	IVC 62, LRTI 3, GI 6.9, UTI 2.4, SSI 3, Unk 22.5, Other 2.9	Decreased from 44% (1971–1975) to 31%(1991–1995)	Single ICU

IVC, intravenous catheter; LRTI, lower respiratory tract infection; GI, gastrointestinal/intraabdominal; UTI, urinary tract infection; SSI, surgical site/skin, soft tissue infection; CNS, central nervous system; Unk, unknown.

Blot et al. (80) recently reviewed their experience in ICU patients with nosocomial BSI due to gram-negative bacteria. In an analysis of 328 cases, older age, abdominal or respiratory tract source, and higher Acute Physiology and Chronic Health Evaluation System (APACHE) II scores correlated with mortality. *E. coli* was the most common cause of bacteremia (21.6%), but BSI due to *P. aeruginosa* or polymicrobic infections were more likely to be associated with mortality (27% and 33%, respectively). Interestingly, no increased association with mortality was observed in relation to antimicrobial resistance. Similarly, no increase in mortality was observed in patients with nosocomial BSI due to extended-spectrum beta-lactamase (ESBL)-producing Enterobacteriaceae in comparison to those with bacteremia due to non–ESBL-producing strains (81). Garcia-Garmendia et al. (82) analyzed risk factors for development of ICU nosocomial BSI due to *Acinetobacter baumannii*, a pathogen of increasing importance. *A. baumannii* accounted for 18% of 233 nosocomial BSIs observed over a 2-year period (compared to 19.7% due to *S. epidermidis*). Risk factors independently associated with *A. baumannii* BSI were immunosuppression, prior antibiotic therapy, unscheduled hospital admission, respiratory failure, prior ICU sepsis, and the invasive procedure index (82).

Neutropenia/Oncology Patients

It has long been known that patients with underlying oncologic diseases and/or neutropenia are more likely to experience nosocomial BSI (83–85). These conditions are discussed more fully in Chapters 58 and 60. Patients with hematologic malignancies are at greater risk of nosocomial BSI than patients with solid tumors (83,85). Gram-positive pathogens have replaced gram-negative pathogens as the most likely etiologic agents, which are thought to be secondary to increased use of intravascular catheters and widespread use of prophylactic agents directed at gram-negative microorganisms for patients with neutropenia (86). Risk factors for development of nosocomial BSI in this population include hematologic malignancy, cytotoxic chemotherapy resulting in neutropenia and mucositis, graft versus host disease in bone marrow transplant patients, and the presence of intravascular catheters (83,85,86).

Cirrhosis/Chronic Liver Disease

Patients with cirrhosis are predisposed to a variety of infectious complications including bacterial peritonitis and nosocomial BSI (87). Campillo et al. (88) studied 200 cirrhotic patients

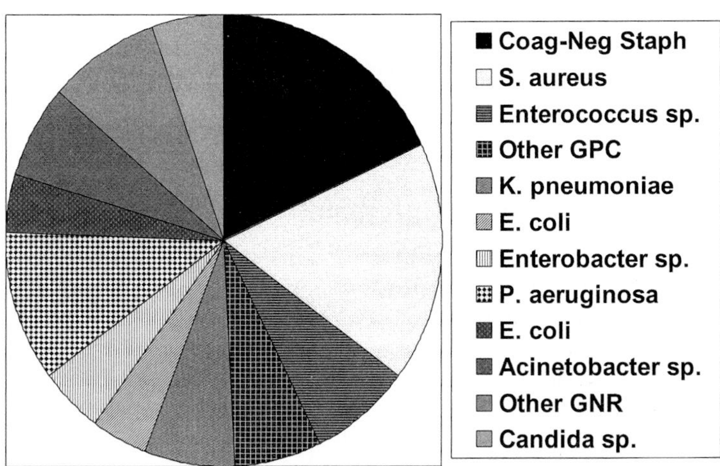

Figure 19.2. Microbial etiology of nosocomial bloodstream infections in intensive care unit patients.

in whom 194 episodes of bacterial peritonitis and 119 episodes of BSI were documented over a 5-year period; 93.3% of the BSIs were nosocomially acquired, and *S. aureus* was the most commonly observed pathogen, responsible for 39.5% of cases. The mortality rate was 49.5% for patients with nosocomial BSI versus 23.8% for patients with community-acquired BSI (88).

Burn Patients

Thermal injury destroys the barrier function of the skin and is often complicated by burn wound infection and bacteremia (89). *S. aureus* is typically the most frequent pathogen encountered in nosocomial BSI in burn patients, followed by *P. aeruginosa* and other nosocomial gram-negative bacilli (90,91). Enterococci have become more problematic in more recent years (90, 91).

Spinal Cord Injury Patients

Nosocomial BSI in spinal cord injury patients is largely secondary to UTI (25% to 47%), infected pressure sores (19%), and pneumonia (9%) (92,93). Predisposing conditions include indwelling urinary catheters, ventilator dependency in quadriplegics, and pressure sores. Prevention of BSI requires prevention of the primary infectious complications associated with spinal cord injury.

Hemodialysis

Approximately 250,000 persons are maintained on hemodialysis in the U.S. These patients experience nosocomial BSI at a rate of approximately 0.6 BSI/1,000 patient-days, which equates to approximately 50,000 BSIs per year (94). Approximately 80% of BSIs in hemodialysis patients are related to vascular access and 20% are secondary to infections at other sites, most frequently UTI and lower respiratory tract infections (11). Primary BSI is much more likely in patients whose vascular access is achieved through intravascular catheters than those with arteriovenous fistula or synthetic grafts. Tokars et al. (11) observed at 109 participating centers, from October 1999 to May 2001, that rates of bacteremia per 100 patient-months based on the type of access is as follows: fistula (0.25), graft (0.53), cuffed catheters (4.84), and noncuffed catheters (8.73). Primary nosocomial BSI in hemodialysis patients is described more fully in Chapter 64.

Solid Organ Transplant Patients

Nosocomial infections in solid organ transplant recipients are discussed in detail in Chapter 59. A few specific issues regarding nosocomial BSI are as follows:

Renal

Prior to the widespread use of posttransplant antibiotics, 50% to 70% of renal transplant patients developed UTI with a 40% incidence of bacteremia (95). Although prophylactic antibiotics have significantly reduced the incidence of UTI to 5% to 10%, UTI remains responsible for 40% to 60% of episodes of bacteremia in kidney transplant patients (96). Gram-negative bacilli are responsible for approximately 50% of bloodstream isolates, with *E. coli*, *Klebsiella* sp., and other Enterobacteriaceae most prominently represented (96).

Liver

Nosocomial BSI occurs in approximately 20% to 25% of liver transplant recipients. About half of these BSIs are due to intravascular catheters and are predominantly due to gram-positive cocci (97). Nosocomial BSIs due to gram-negative bacilli are usually secondary to intraabdominal or biliary tract infections (98,99). Antibiotic-resistant gram-positive cocci are being increasingly described as significant pathogens following liver transplantation and are associated with significant morbidity and mortality (100,101).

Small Bowel

Nosocomial bacteremia is a common complication of small bowel transplantation and is most frequently due to intravascular catheters or intraabdominal foci (102). BSI commonly occurs in patients with organ rejection due to altered permeability of the small bowel allograft (103).

Lung

Approximately 25% of lung transplant recipients experience nosocomial BSI, which most commonly arises from a pulmonary source (104). Methicillin-resistant *S. aureus* (MRSA), *P. aeruginosa*, and *Burkholderia cepacia* are commonly observed pathogens (104).

Heart

Nosocomial BSI occurs in 10% to 20% of heart transplant recipients and most commonly stems from a pulmonary, intravascular catheter, or surgical site source (105).

Pancreas

Approximately 11% of pancreatic transplant patients experience nosocomial BSI (96). UTI and surgical site infection are the most common identifiable sources for bacteremia.

Transient Bacteremia

A large variety of medical procedures can result in transient bacteremia. Although many of these episodes might not be considered "nosocomial" in a strict classification scheme, they would oftentimes qualify as "healthcare-associated" bacteremia. In many instances, transient healthcare-associated bacteremia does not result in significant infection due to efficient host defense mechanisms designed to filter and interdict circulating pathogens. However, in some groups of patients, transient bacteremia can result in infection. Roberts et al. (55) noted that 7% of almost 2,000 positive blood cultures were due to transient bacteremia; 71.6% of these episodes were due to gram-positive cocci (39% coagulase-negative staphylococci, 23% viridans streptococci). Transient bacteremia has been well documented to result from dental procedures. Although tooth brushing and tooth flossing cannot usually be considered a nosocomial source, they result in transient bacteremia in up to 86% of patients (106–108). Similarly, tooth extraction results in a very high percentage of patients experiencing transient bacteremia (109, 110), and antibiotic prophylaxis is recommended to prevent endocarditis in certain groups of patients (111). Numerous other procedures have been documented to result in transient bacteremia and occasional infection and include endotracheal intubation (112,113); lachrymal duct probing (114); burn wound manipulation (115); gastrointestinal endoscopy, including gastroscopy, scleral therapy, sigmoidoscopy, colonoscopy, esophageal dilatation, and polypectomy (116–121); chorionic villous sampling (122); nephrostomy tube manipulation (123); minor dermatologic surgery (124,125); urologic endoscopy and transurethral prostatic resection (126); replacement of intrauterine contraceptive devices (127); barium enema (128); and percutaneous liver biopsy (129). The significance of bacteremia in most of these settings is debatable and the rationale or need for antibiotic prophylaxis is often not clear (130–133).

BLOOD CULTURE CONTAMINATION OR PSEUDOBACTEREMIA

Pseudobacteremia, false-positive blood cultures, and blood culture contamination all refer to the problem in which microbes from a site outside the bloodstream are introduced into the sample of blood obtained for culture. This is a widespread phenomenon and occurs in 2% to 3% of cultures even under optimal conditions (21). Up to 50% of positive cultures may represent contamination (29,134). The implications of blood culture contamination are significant and include increased cost due to additional cultures and tests needed to investigate culture positivity, unnecessary antibiotics, side effects and toxicity due to the antibiotics, and increased length of hospital stay. The total excess cost associated with blood culture contamination was $4,385/patient in one study and $4,100/patient in another (17,135).

Means to differentiate contamination from true bacteremia include consideration of the microbe recovered from the blood, clinical presentation, number of positive cultures, and incubation time to positivity. It should be noted, however, that discounting single positive cultures with skin flora microbes (coagulase-negative staphylococci) may lead to misdiagnosis in up to 25% of clinically significant bacteremic episodes due to these microorganisms (21). Measures to prevent contamination were discussed in the section on clinical microbiology (see also Chapter 8).

PREVENTION OF NOSOCOMIAL BACTEREMIA

The prevention of nosocomial BSI requires prevention of intravascular catheter infections and other sites of infection (pneumonia, UTI, wound infection, etc.). Prevention of infection associated with intravascular catheters requires that the catheters be inserted by trained personnel using appropriate precautions (full sterile barrier precautions) and effective skin antisepsis (chlorhexidine). Additionally, great care must be exercised in accessing the catheters and routine site care. These measures are discussed in detail in Chapters 17 and 18 and in recent CDC guidelines (136). Progress in prevention of IV catheter–associated infection was documented in NNIS participating institutions during the 1990s (137).

Similarly, to prevent urinary catheter–associated infection and the potential complication of nosocomial BSI, urinary catheters should be used only when necessary, inserted with careful attention to aseptic technique, carefully maintained, and removed as soon as possible. The use of antiseptic bonded urinary catheters has shown great promise in prevention of nosocomial UTI (51,138). These preventive measures are discussed in greater detail in Chapter 20.

Prevention of nosocomial pneumonia requires a multidisciplinary approach designed for the provision of appropriate care to patients receiving mechanical ventilation and other high-risk groups. The CDC Hospital Infection Control Practices Advisory Committee (HICPAC) has recently issued a revised guideline for the prevention of nosocomial pneumonia (139) (see also Chapter 22).

Prevention of surgical site infections requires careful attention to preoperative risk factor reduction, timely administration of prophylactic antibiotics, aseptic surgical technique, and appropriate wound care. A more comprehensive discussion can be found in Chapter 21 and the 1999 CDC HICPAC guideline (140).

Specific recommendations for prevention of nosocomial infection and, hence, secondary bacteremia can be found throughout this text in sections detailing specific infections and specific patient populations and care settings.

PREDICTION MODELS FOR NOSOCOMIAL BSI AND CHALLENGES FOR THE FUTURE

Clinicians tend to make decisions regarding diagnosis and prognosis based on overall clinical judgment and anecdotal experience. Unfortunately, the inability of physicians to accurately predict the presence of bacteremia has been noted (141). Therefore, investigators have attempted to develop quantitative predictive models to assist clinicians in their recognition of bacteremic patients. Nosocomial BSIs are associated with a variety of risk factors, many of which have been previously discussed, such as age, use of intravascular catheters, underlying diseases and conditions, severity of illness, and healthcare worker understaffing. Taking many of these factors into account, a number of investigators have developed predictive models (142–145). In general, these models are not specific for nosocomial BSI, and their clinical utility remains unknown. Recently, as our understanding of the pathogenesis of sepsis has improved, a number of investigators have attempted to correlate various proinflammatory markers and other factors with bacteremia and outcome in several patient populations (146–149). These markers and models have not been specifically applied to patients with nosocomial infections, and further validation is required.

Nosocomial BSI is a significant medical problem that promises to increase in the future as the number of high-risk patients and the use of invasive devices in intensive care settings increases. In the future, the healthcare epidemiologist will be challenged to design and operate surveillance systems to monitor nosocomial BSI in the rapidly changing healthcare arena. Increased numbers of outpatient surgical procedures, shorter hospital stay, utilization of outpatient intravenous infusion services, and expanding populations of hemodialysis patients, residents of long-term care facilities, and immunocompromised hosts will influence the occurrence of BSI and must be accounted for. It is hoped that improved understanding of the pathogenesis of nosocomial BSI and the risk factors predisposing to infection will lead to better predictive models and improved preventive measures.

REFERENCES

1. Haley RW, Culver DH, White JW, et al. The efficacy of infection surveillance and control programs in preventing nosocomial infections in US hospitals. *Am J Epidemiol* 1985;121:182–205.
2. Hospital Infections Program, National Center for Infectious Diseases, Center for Disease Control and Prevention. National Nosocomial Infections Surveillance (NNIS) report, data summary from October 1986–April 1996, issued May 1996. *Am J Infect Control* 1996;24: 380–388.
3. McGowan JE Jr, Shulman JA. Blood stream invasion. In: Gorbach SL, Bartlett JG, Blacklow NR, eds. *Infectious diseases*, 2nd ed. Philadelphia: WB Saunders, 1998:645–654.
4. Wenzel RP, Edmond MB. The impact of hospital-acquired bloodstream infections. *Emerg Infect Dis* 2001;7:174–177.
5. Edmond MB, Wallace SE, McClish DK, et al. Nosocomial bloodstream infections in United States hospitals: a three-year analysis. *Clin Infect Dis* 1999;29:239–244.
6. Jarvis WR. Selected aspects of the socioeconomic impact of nosocomial infections; morbidity, mortality, cost, and prevention. *Infect Control Hosp Epidemiol* 1996;17:552–557.
7. Digiovine B, Chenoweth C, Watts C, et al. The attributable mortality and costs of primary nosocomial bloodstream infections in the intensive care unit. *Am J Respir Crit Care Med* 1999;160:976–981.
8. Pittet D, Tarara D, Wenzel RP. Nosocomial bloodstream infection in critically ill patients. *JAMA* 1994;271:1598–1601.
9. Orsi GB, DiStefano L, Noah N. Hospital-acquired laboratory-confirmed bloodstream infection: increased hospital stay and direct costs. *Infect Control Hosp Epidemiol* 2002;23:190–197.
10. U.S. Department of Health and Human Services, Centers for Disease Control and Prevention. *NNIS manual.* Washington, DC: DHHS, May, 1999.
11. Tokars JI, Miller ER, Stein G. New national surveillance system for hemodialysis-associated infections: initial results. *Am J Infect Control* 2002;30:288–295.
12. Friedman ND, Kaye KS, Stout JE, et al. Health care-associated bloodstream infections in adults: a reason to change the accepted definition of community-acquired infections. *Ann Intern Med* 2002;137: 791–792.
13. Graham DR, Kelderman MM, Klemm LW, et al. Infectious complications among patients receiving home intravenous therapy with peripheral, central, or peripherally placed central venous catheters. *Am J Med* 1991;9:95S–100S.
14. Siegman-Igra Y, Fourer B, Orni-Wasserlauf R, et al. Reappraisal of community-acquired bacteremia: a proposal of a new classification for the spectrum of acquisition of bacteremia. *Clin Infect Dis* 2002; 34:1431–1439.
15. Reimer LG, Wilson ML, Weinstein MP. Update on detection of bacteremia and fungemia. *Clin Microbiol Rev* 1997;10:447–465.
16. Strand CL, Wajsbort RR, Sturmann K. Effect of iodophor vs iodine tincture skin preparation on blood culture contamination rate. *JAMA* 1993;269:1004–1006.
17. Little JR, Murray PR, Traynor PS, et al. A randomized trial of povidone-iodine compared with iodine tincture for venipuncture site disinfection: effects on rates of blood culture contamination. *Am J Med* 1999;107:119–125.
18. Weinbaum FI, Lavie S, Danek M, et al. Doing it right the first time: quality improvement and the contaminant blood culture. *J Clin Microbiol* 1997;35:563–565.
19. Calfee DP, Farr BM. Comparison of four antiseptic preparations for skin in the prevention of contamination of percutaneously drawn blood cultures: a randomized trial. *J Clin Microbiol* 2002;40: 1660–1665.
20. Mimoz O, Karim A, Mercat A, et al. Chlorhexidine compared with povidone-iodine as skin preparation before blood culture. *Ann Intern Med* 1999;131:834–837.
21. Chandrasekar PH, Brown WJ. Clinical Issues of blood cultures. *Arch Intern Med* 1994;154:841–849.
22. Chapnick EK, Schaffer BC, Gradon JD, et al. Technique for drawing blood for cultures: is changing needles truly necessary? *So Med J* 1991; 84:1197–1198.
23. Krumholz HM, Cummings S, York M. Blood culture phlebotomy: switching needles does not prevent contamination. *Ann Intern Med* 1990;113:290–292.
24. Kellogg JA, Manzella JP, McConville JH. Clinical laboratory comparison of the 10-ml isolator blood culture system with BACTEC radiometric blood culture media. *J Clin Microbiol* 1984;20:618–623.
25. Brannon P, Kiehn TE. Large-scale clinical comparison of the lysis-centrifugation and radiometric systems for blood culture. *J Clin Microbiol* 1985;22:951–954.
26. Mermel LA, Maki DG. Detection of bacteremia in adults: consequences of culturing an inadequate volume of blood. *Ann Intern Med* 1993;119:270–272.
27. Bennett IL, Beeson PB. Bacteremia: a consideration of some experimental and clinical aspects. *Yale J Biol Med* 1954;26:241–262.
28. Li J, Plorde JJ, Carlson LG. Effects of volume and periodicity on blood cultures. *J Clin Microbiol* 1994;32:2829–2831.
29. Aronson MD, Bor DH. Blood cultures. *Ann Intern Med* 1987;106: 246–253.
30. Mylotte JM, Tayara A. Blood cultures: clinical aspects and controversies. *Eur J Clin Microbiol Infect Dis* 2000;19:157–163.
31. Bartlett JG, Dick J. The controversy regarding routine anaerobic blood cultures. *Am J Med* 2000;108:505–506.
32. Bryant JK, Stand CL. Reliability of blood cultures collected from intravascular catheter versus venipuncture. *Am J Clin Pathol* 1987; 88:113–116.
33. Tonnesen A, Peuler M, Lockwood WR. Cultures of blood drawn by catheters vs venipuncture. *JAMA* 1976;235:1877.
34. Vaisanen IT, Michelsen T, Valtonen V, et al. Comparison of arterial and venous blood samples for the diagnosis of bacteremia in critically ill patients. *Crit Care Med* 1985;13:664–667.
35. Blot F, Schmidt E, Nitenberg G, et al. Earlier positivity of central-venous-versus peripheral-blood cultures is highly predictive of catheter-related sepsis. *J Clin Microbiol* 1998;36:105–109.
36. DesJardin JA, Falagas ME, Ruthazer R, et al. Clinical utility of blood cultures drawn from indwelling central venous catheters in hospitalized patients with cancer. *Ann Intern Med* 1999;131:641–647.
37. Malgrange VB, Escande MC, Theobald S. Validity of earlier positivity of central venous blood cultures in comparison with peripheral blood cultures for diagnosing catheter-related bacteremia in cancer patients. *J Clin Microbiol* 2001;39:274–278.
38. Gleckman R, Hibert D. Afebrile bacteremia a phenomenon in geriatric patients. *JAMA* 1982;248:1478–1481.
39. Schmidt BK, Kirpalani HM, Corey M, et al. Coagulase-negative staphylococci as true pathogens in newborn infants: a cohort study. *Pediatr Infect Dis J* 1987;6:1026–1031.
40. Baumgart, Hall SE, Campos JM, et al. Sepsis with coagulase-negative staphylococci in critically ill newborns. *Am J Dis Child* 1983;137: 461–463.

41. Allen JR, Hightower AW, Martin SM, et al. Secular trends in nosocomial infections 1970–1979. *Am J Med* 1981;70:389–392.
42. Schaberg DR, Culver DH, Gaynes RP. Major trends in the microbial etiology of nosocomial infection. *Am J Med* 1991;91:72S–75S.
43. Banerjee SH, Emori TG, Culver DH, et al. Secular trends in nosocomial primary bloodstream infections in the United States, 1980–1989. *Am J Med* 1991;91:86S–89S.
44. Hospital Infections Program, National Center for Infectious Diseases, Center for Disease Control and Prevention. National Nosocomial Infections Surveillance (NNIS) report, data summary from January 1990–May 1999, issued June 1999. *Am J Infect Control* 1999;27: 520–532.
45. Cockerill FR, Hughes JG, Vetter EA, et al. Analysis of 281,797 consecutive blood cultures performed over an eight-year period: trends in microorganisms isolated and the value of anaerobic culture of blood. *Clin Infect Dis* 1997;24:403–418.
46. Lark RL, Chenoweth C, Saint S, et al. Four year prospective evaluation of nosocomial bacteremia: epidemiology, microbiology, and patient outcome. *Diag Microbiol Infect Dis* 2000;38:131–140.
47. Division of Healthcare Quality Promotion, National Center for Infectious Diseases, Center for Disease Control and Prevention. National Nosocomial Infections Surveillance (NNIS) report, data summary from January 1992–June 2002, issued August 2002. *Am J Infect Control* 2002;30:458–475.
48. Maki DG. Nosocomial bacteremia. *Am J Med* 1981;70:719–732.
49. Scheckler WE, Scheibel W, Kresge D. Temporal trends in septicemia in a community hospital. *Am J Med* 1991;91:90S–94S.
50. Pittet D, Wenzel RP. Nosocomial bloodstream infections. *Arch Intern Med* 1995;155:1177–1184.
51. Karchmer TB, Giannetta ET, Muto CA, et al. A randomized crossover study of silver-coated urinary catheters in hospitalized patients. *Arch Intern Med* 2000;160:3294–3298.
52. Bryan CS, Reynolds KL. Hospital-acquired bacteremic urinary tract infection: epidemiology and outcome. *J Urol* 1984;132:494–498.
53. Krieger JN, Kaiser DL, Wenzel RP. Urinary tract etiology of bloodstream infections in hospitalized patients. *J Infect Dis* 1983;148: 57–62.
54. Petti CA, Sanders LL, Trivette SL, et al. Postoperative bacteremia secondary to surgical site infection. *Clin Infect Dis* 2002;34:305–308.
55. Roberts FJ, Geere IW, Coldman A. A three-year study of positive blood cultures, with emphasis on prognosis. *Rev Infect Dis* 1991;13: 34–46.
56. Mylotte JM, White D, McDermott C, et al. Nosocomial bloodstream infection at a veterans hospital; 1979 to 1987. *Infect Control Hosp Epidemiol* 1989;10:455–464.
57. Muder RR, Brennen C, Wagener MM, et al. Bacteremia in a long-term-care facility: a five-year prospective study of 163 consecutive episodes. *Clin Infect Dis* 1992;14:647–654.
58. Faix RG, Kovarik SM. Polymicrobial sepsis among intensive care nursery infants. *J Perinatol* 1989;9:131–136.
59. Elting LS, Bodey GP. Septicemia due to Xanthomonas species and non-aeruginosa pseudomonas species: increasing incidence of catheter-related infections. *Medicine* 1990;69:296–306.
60. Pittet D, Li N, Wenzel RP. Association of secondary and polymicrobial nosocomial bloodstream infections with higher mortality. *Eur J Clin Microbiol Infect Dis* 1993;12:813–819.
61. Trick WE, Fridkin SK, Edwards JR, et al. Secular trend of hospital-acquired candidemia among intensive care unit patients in the United States during 1989–1999. *Clin Infect Dis* 2002;35:627–630.
62. Pfaller MA, Jones RN, Doern GV, et al. Bloodstream infections due to candida species: sentry antimicrobial surveillance program in North America and Latin America, 1997–1998. *Antimicrob Agents Chemother* 2000;44:747–751.
63. Abi-Said D, Anaissie E, Uzun O, et al. The epidemiology of hematogenous candidiasis caused by different candida species. *Clin Infect Dis* 1997;24:1122–1128.
64. Saviteer SM, Samsa GP, Rutala WA. Nosocomial infections in the elderly increased risk per hospital day. *Am J Med* 1988;84:661–666.
65. Trilla A, Gatell JM, Mensa J, et al. Risk factors for nosocomial bacteremia in a large Spanish teaching hospital: a case-control study. *Infect Control Hosp Epidemiol* 1991;12:150–156.
66. Mylotte JM, Tayara A, Goodnough S. Epidemiology of bloodstream infection in nursing home residents: evaluation in a large cohort from multiple homes. *Clin Infect Dis* 2002;35:1484–1490.
67. McBean M, Rajamani S. Increasing rates of hospitalization due to septicemia in the US elderly population, 1986–1997. *J Infect Dis* 2001;183:596–603.
68. Gaynes RP, Edwards JR, Jarvis WR, et al. Nosocomial infections among neonates in high-risk nurseries in the United States. *Pediatrics* 1996;98:357–361.
69. Stoll BJ, Gordon T, Korones SB, et al. Early-onset sepsis in very low birth weight neonates: a report from the national institute of child health and human development neonatal research network. *J Pediatr* 1996;129:72–80.
70. Stoll BJ, Gordon T, Korones SB, et al. Late onset sepsis in very low birth weight neonates: a report from the national institute of child health and human development neonatal research network. *J Pediatr* 1996;129:63–71.
71. Dankner WM, Spector SA, Fierer J, et al. Malassezia fungemia in neonates and adults: complications of hyperalimentation. *Rev Infect Dis* 1987;9:743–753.
72. Richards MJ, Edwards JR, Culver DH, et al. National infections in pediatric intensive care units in the United States. *Pediatrics* 1999; 103:1–7.
73. Wenzel RP, Thompson RL, Landry SM, et al. Hospital-acquired infection in intensive care unit patients: an overview with emphasis on epidemics. *Infect Control* 1983;4:371.
74. Brun-Buisson C, Doyon F, Carlet J, et al. Bacteremia and severe sepsis in adults: a multicenter prospective survey in ICUs and wards of 24 hospitals. *Am J Respir Crit Care Med* 1996;154:167–124.
75. Vallés J. Nosocomial bloodstream infection in the ICU. In: Rello J, Valles J, Kollef M, eds. *Critical care infectious diseases textbook.* Boston: Kluwer Academic, 2001:535–560.
76. Crowe M, Ispahani P, Humphreys H, et al. Bacteraemia in the adult intensive care unit of a teaching hospital in Nottingham, UK, 1985–1996. *Eur J Clin Microbiol Infect Dis* 1998;17:377–384.
77. Valles J, Leon C, Alvarez-Lerma F, et al. Nosocomial bacteremia in critically ill patients: a multicenter study evaluating epidemiology and prognosis. *Clin Infect Dis* 1997;24:387–395.
78. Edgeworth JD, Treacher DF, Eykyn SJ. A 25-year study of nosocomial bacteremia in an adult intensive care unit. *Crit Care Med* 1999; 27:1421–1428.
79. Mainous MR, Lipsett PA, O'Brein M. Enterococcal bacteremia in the surgical intensive care unit. *Arch Surg* 1997;132:76–81.
80. Blot S, Vandewoude K, DeBacquer D, et al. Nosocomial bacteremia caused by antibiotic-resistant gram-negative bacteria in critically ill patients: clinical outcome and length of hospitalization. *Clin Infect Dis* 2002;34:1600–1606.
81. Menashe G, Borer A, Yagupsky P, et al. Clinical significance and impact on mortality of extended-spectrum beta lactamase-producing *Enterobacteriaceae* isolates in nosocomial bacteremia. *Scand J Infect Dis* 2001;33:188–193.
82. Garcia-Garmendia JL, Ortiz-Leyba C, Garnacho-Montero J, et al. Risk factors for Acinetobacter baumannii nosocomial bacteremia in critically ill patients: a cohort study. *Clin Infect Dis* 2001;33:939–946.
83. Bodey GP. Infection in cancer patients: a continuing association. *Am J Med* 1986;81:11–26.
84. Singer C, Kaplan MH, Armstrong D. Bacteremia and fungemia complicating neoplastic disease: a study of 364 cases. *Am J Med* 1977; 62:731–742.
85. Mayo JW, Wenzel R. Rates of hospital-acquired bloodstream infection in patients with specific malignancy. *Cancer* 1982;50:187–190.
86. Bow EJ, Mandell LA, Louie TJ, et al. Quinolone-based antibacterial chemoprophylaxis in neutropenic patients: effect of augmented gram-positive activity on infectious morbidity. *Ann Intern Med* 1996;125: 183–190.
87. Caly WR, Stauss E. A prospective study of bacterial infections in patients with cirrhosis. *J Hepatol* 1993;18:353–358.
88. Campillo B, Richardet JP, Kheo T, et al. Nosocomial spontaneous

bacterial peritonitis and bacteremia in cirrhotic patients: impact of isolate type on prognosis and characteristics of infection. *Clin Infect Dis* 2002;35:1–10.
89. Luterman A, Dacso CC, Curreri PW. Infection in burn patients. *Am J Med* 1986;81:45–52.
90. Singh NP, Goyal R, Manchanda V, et al. Changing trends in bacteriology of buns in the burns unit, Delhi, India. *Burns* 2003;29: 129–132.
91. Santucci SG, Gobara S, Santos CR, et al. Infections in a burn intensive care unit: experience of seven years. *J Hosp Infect* 2003;53:6–13.
92. Waites KB, Canupp KC, Chen Y, et al. Bacteremia after spinal cord injury in initial versus subsequent hospitalizations. *J Spinal Cord Med* 2001;24:96–100.
93. Montgomerie JZ, Chan E, Gilmore DS, et al. Low mortality among patients with spinal cord injury and bacteremia. *Rev Infect Dis* 1991; 13:867–871.
94. Tokars JI. Bloodstream infections in hemodialysis patients: getting some deserved attention. *Infect Control Hosp Epidemiol* 2002;23: 713–715.
95. Rubin RH. Infectious disease complications of renal transplantation. *Kidney Int* 1993;44:221–236.
96. Wagener MM, Yu VL. Bacteremia in transplant recipients: a prospective study of demographics, etiologic agents, risk factors, and outcomes. *Am J Infect Control* 1992;20:239–247.
97. McClean K, Kneteman N, Taylor G. Comparative risk of bloodstream infection in organ transplant recipients. *Infect Control Hosp Epidemiol* 1994;15:582–584.
98. Simon DM, Levin S. Infectious complications of solid organ transplantation. *Infect Dis Clin North Am* 2001;15:521–549.
99. Winston DJ, Emmanouilides C, Busuttil RW. Infections in liver transplant recipients. *Clin Infect Dis* 1995;21:1077–1091.
100. Singh N, Gayowski T, Wagener MM, et al. Bloodstream infections in liver transplant recipients receiving tacrolimus. *Clin Transplant* 1997;11:275–281.
101. Linden PK, Pasculle AW, Manez R, et al. Differences in outcomes for patients with bacteremia due to vancomycin-resistant *Enterococcus faecium* or vancomycin-susceptible *E. faecium*. *Clin Infect Dis* 1996; 22:663–670.
102. Kusne S, Furukawa H, Abu-Elmagd K, et al. Infectious complications after small bowel transplantation in adults: an update. *Transplant Proc* 1996;28:2761–2762.
103. Sigurdsson L, Reyes J, Kocoshis SA, et al. Bacteremia after intestinal transplantation in children correlates temporarily with rejection or gastrointestinal lymphoproliferative disease. *Transplantation* 2000;70: 302–305.
104. Palmer SM, Alexander BD, Sanders LL, et al. Significance of blood stream infection after lung transplantation: analysis in 176 consecutive patients. *Transplantation* 2000;69:2360–2366.
105. Petri WA. Infections in heart transplant recipients. *Clin Infect Dis* 1994;18:141–148.
106. Bhanji S, Williams B, Sheller B, et al. Transient bacteremia induced by toothbrushing a comparison of the Sonicare toothbrush with a conventional toothbrush. *Pediatr Dent* 2002;24:295–299.
107. Schlein RA, Kudlick EM, Reindorf CA, et al. Toothbrushing and transient bacteremia in patients undergoing orthodontic treatment. *Am J Orthod Dentofacial Orthop* 1991;99:466–472.
108. Carroll GC, Sebor RJ. Dental flossing and its relationship to transient bacteremia. *J Periodontol* 1980;51:691–692.
109. Hall G, Hedström SA, Heimdahl A, et al. Prophylactic administration of penicillins for endocarditis does not reduce the incidence of postextraction bacteremia. *Clin Infect Dis* 1993;17:188–194.
110. Coulter WA, Coffey A, Saunders ID, et al. Bacteremia in children following dental extraction. *J Dent Res* 1990;69:1691–1695.
111. Dajani AS, Taubert KA, Wilson W, et al. Prevention of bacterial endocarditis. Recommendations by the American Heart Association. *JAMA* 1997;277:1794–1801.
112. Depoix JP, Malbezin S, Videcoq M, et al. Oral intubation v. nasal intubation in adult cardiac surgery. *Br J Anaesth* 1987;59:167–169.
113. Rijnders BJ, Wilmer A, Van Eldere J, et al. Frequency of transient streptococcal bacteremia following urgent orotracheal intubation in critically ill patients. *Intensive Care Med* 2001;27:434–437.
114. Eippert GA, Burnstine RA, Bates JH. Lacrimal-duct-probing-induced bacteremia: should children with congenital heart defects receive antibiotic prophylaxis? *J Pediatr Ophthalmol Strabismus* 1998;35:38–40.
115. Mozingo DW, McManus AT, Kim SH, et al. Incidence of bacteremia after burn wound manipulation in the early postburn period. *J Trauma* 1997;42:1006–1010.
116. Schlaeffer F, Riesenberg K, Mikolich D, et al. Serious bacterial infections after endoscopic procedures. *Arch Intern Med* 1996;156: 572–574.
117. Lee M, Munoz J. Septicemia occurring after colonoscopic polypectomy in a splenectomized patient taking corticosteroids. *Am J Gastroenterol* 1994;89:2245–2246.
118. Lo GH, Lai KH, Shen MT, et al. A comparison of the incidence of transient bacteremia and infectious sequelae after sclerotherapy and rubber band ligation of bleeding esophageal varices. *Gastrointest Endosc* 1994;40:675–679.
119. Low DE, Shoenut JP, Kennedy JK, et al. Prospective assessment of risk of bacteremia with colonoscopy and polypectomy. *Dig Dis Sci* 1987;32:1239–1243.
120. Camara DS, Gruber M, Barde CJ, et al. Transient bacteremia following endoscopic injection sclerotherapy of esophageal varices. *Arch Intern Med* 1983;143:1350–1352.
121. Norfleet RG, Mitchell PD, Mulholland DD, et al. Does bacteremia follow upper gastrointestinal endoscopy? *Am J Gastroenterol* 1981;76: 420–422.
122. Silverman NS, Sullivan MW, Jungkind DL, et al. Incidence of bacteremia associated with chorionic villus sampling. *Obstet Gynecol* 1994; 84:1021–1024.
123. Cronan JJ, Horn DL, Marcello A, et al. Antibiotics and nephrostomy tube care: preliminary observations. Part II. Bacteremia. *Radiology* 1989;172:1043–1045.
124. Halpern AC, Leyden JJ, Dzubow LM, et al. The incidence of bacteremia in skin surgery of the head and neck. *J Am Acad Dermatol* 1988; 19:112–116.
125. Sabetta JB, Zitelli JA. The incidence of bacteremia during skin surgery. *Arch Dermatol* 123;2:213–215.
126. Nielsen PB, Hansen RI, Madsen OG, et al. Bacteremia in connection with transurethral resection of the prostate. *Infection* 1987;15: 245–247.
127. Murray S, Hickey JB, Houang E. Significant bacteremia associated with replacement of intrauterine contraceptive device. *Am J Obstet Gynecol* 1987;156:698–700.
128. Le Frock J, Ellis CA, Klainer AS, et al. Transient bacteremia associated with barium enema. *Arch Intern Med* 1975;135:835–837.
129. Le Frock J, Ellis CA, Turchik JB, et al. Transient bacteremia associated with percutaneous liver biopsy. *J Infect Dis* 1975;131:104–107.
130. Wahl MJ. Myths of dental-induced prosthetic joint infections. *Clin Infect Dis* 1995;20:1420–1425.
131. Schembre D, Bjorkman DJ. A rational approach to giving antibiotic prophylaxis before endoscopy. Who needs it? Which procedures pose the greatest risk? *J Crit Illness* 1995;10:259–261,265–266,270–272.
132. Baker KA. Antibiotic prophylaxis for selected implants and devices. *J Calif Dent Assoc* 2000;28:620–626.
133. Strom BL, Abrutyn E, Berlin JA, et al. Dental and cardiac risk factors for infective endocarditis. *Ann Intern Med* 1998;129:761–769.
134. Weinstein MP, Towns ML, Quartey SM, et al. The clinical significance of positive blood cultures in the 1990s: a prospective comprehensive evaluation of the microbiology, epidemiology, and outcome of bacteremia and fungemia in adults. *Clin Infect Dis* 1997;24:584–602.
135. Bates DW, Goldman L, Lee TH. Contaminant blood cultures and resource utilization. The true consequences of false-positive results. *JAMA* 1991;265:365–369.
136. Centers for Disease Control and Prevention. Guideline for the prevention of intravascular catheter-related infections. *MMWR* 2002;51(RR-10):1–32.
137. Centers for Disease Control and Prevention. Monitoring hospital-acquired infections to promote patient safety—United States 1990–1991. *MMWR* 2000;49:149–153.
138. Liedberg H, Lundeburg T, Ekman P. Refinements in the coatings of

urethral catheters reduces the incidence of catheter-associated bacteriuria. *Eur Urol* 1990;17:236–240.

139. CDC. Guideline for Prevention of Healthcare-Associated Pneumonia, 2003. Recommendations of the Healthcare Infection Control Practices Advisory Committee. MMWR 2004 (*In Press*).
140. CDC HICPAC. Guideline for prevention of surgical site infection, 1999. *Infect Cont Hosp Epidemiol* 1999;20:247–278.
141. Poses RM, Anthony M. Availability, wishful thinking, and physicians' diagnostic judgments for patients with suspected bacteremia. *Med Decis Making* 1991;11:159–168.
142. Bates DW, Sands K, Miller E, et al. Predicting bacteremia in patients with sepsis syndrome. *J Infect Dis* 1997;176:1538–1551.
143. Yehezkelli Y, Subah S, Elhanan G, et al. Two rules for early prediction of bacteremia: testing in a university and community hospital. *J Gen Intern Med* 1996;11:98–103.
144. Leibovici L, Greenshtain S, Cohen O, et al. Bacteremia in febrile patients: a clinical model for diagnosis. *Arch Intern Med* 1991;151: 1801–1806.
145. Bates DW, Cook EF, Goldman L, et al. Predicting bacteremia in hospitalized patients: a prospectively validated model. *Ann Intern Med* 1990;113:495–500.
146. Kern WV, Heiss M, Steinbach G. Prediction of gram-negative bacteremia in patients with cancer and febrile neutropenia by means of interleukin-8 levels in serum: targeting empirical monotherapy versus combination therapy. *Clin Infect Dis* 2001;32:832–835.
147. Lacour AG, Gervaix A, Zamora SA, et al. Procalcitonin, IL-6, IL-8, IL-1 receptor antagonist and C-reactive protein as identificators of serious bacterial infections in children with fever without localizing signs. *Eur J Pediatr* 2001;160:95–100.
148. Aouifi A, Piriou V, Bastien O, et al. Usefulness of procalcitonin for diagnosis of infection in cardiac surgical patients. *Crit Care Med* 2000; 28:3171–3176.
149. Vales EC, Abraira V, Sanchez JCC, et al. A predictive model for mortality of bloodstream infections: bedside analysis with the Weibull function. *J Clin Epidemiol* 2002;55:563–72.

20

NOSOCOMIAL URINARY TRACT INFECTIONS

JOHN P. BURKE
TSIN WEN YEO

Urinary tract infections (UTIs) are the most common nosocomial infections in both acute care hospitals and long-term care facilities, accounting for about 40% of all hospital-acquired infections and constituting a major source for nosocomial septicemia and related mortality. The rates of nosocomial UTIs are similar in both adult and pediatric patients (1), and nearly all such infections are associated with urinary tract instrumentation. In acute care hospitals, the vast majority of UTIs occur in patients with temporary indwelling bladder catheters; the remaining ones are usually related to cystoscopy and other urologic procedures. The costs for the prevention, detection, treatment, and complications of these infections add significantly to the nation's healthcare bill.

The catheterized urinary tract is also a model of the growing problem of infections related to the placement of a foreign body in a patient's tissues. So-called device-associated infections are important both because of their high frequency and expanding number of different types of devices, and because they appear to be the most preventable of all nosocomial infections (2). Their prevention depends on the oldest and most basic tenets of infection control as well as on the promise of technologic advances to develop safer instruments (3).

Urinary catheters are characterized by site of insertion (e.g., urethral, suprapubic, or nephrostomy) and by duration of use (e.g., intermittent or indwelling). Modern catheters are typically manufactured of latex rubber, silicone- or Teflon-coated latex rubber, or solid silicone, and come in a bewildering variety of types and sizes (4). The indwelling Foley catheter with a retention balloon was first developed in 1927 by Frederick E. B. Foley to control bleeding in patients after transurethral prostatectomy (5,6) and is still essential to modern medical care. It is used today to drain the functionally or anatomically obstructed urinary tract, to control drainage in incontinent patients, and to obtain precise measurement of urinary output (7). Although the most mundane of invasive devices, it is the single most frequent cause of nosocomial infection. Major questions regarding its use and care—not to mention alternatives to its use—remain unanswered.

Infections associated with urinary catheters occur in both endemic and epidemic circumstances; common-source outbreaks are infrequent, although an estimated 15% of endemic infections occur in clusters, presumably from cross-infection (8). Most UTIs—whether endemic or epidemic—are asymptomatic, and removal of the catheter is usually curative. The usually benign nature of catheter-associated UTIs and the perception that they are easily treated by antibiotics may inhibit aggressive measures for both their prevention and their recognition.

Nevertheless, today's complacency of clinicians toward the continued high occurrence of UTIs should not diminish recognition of the remarkable achievements of the last several decades in their prevention. Indeed, this is one of the most successful chapters in the history of infection control. In the past, UTIs were generally accepted as an inevitable consequence of indwelling bladder catheterization. However, in the 1950s, the effectiveness of closed sterile urinary drainage, which had first been proposed by Cuthbert Dukes at London's St. Mark's Hospital more than 30 years earlier (9), was finally established. Its introduction proved a landmark in infection control (10–13). Commercially available systems for closed drainage into sterile plastic bags now enable the prevention of UTIs in 70% to 85% of patients with temporary indwelling catheters (14–17).

The benefits of closed drainage systems have not been fully documented because routine surveillance of nosocomial infections did not exist before the 1970s. Furthermore, current surveillance methods provide only limited data about UTIs in relation to catheter-days at risk (18). According to a recent National Nosocomial Infections Surveillance (NNIS) system report, nosocomial UTI rates ranged from 0.5 to 12.7 per 1,000 urinary catheter-days in intensive care patients (19), but similar data from other patient populations are not available.

The challenge of preventing UTIs has multiplied with changes in the character of hospitalized populations. These changes are often enumerated: the increased numbers of patients with advanced age and more severe underlying illnesses, the emergence of specialized units for the care of critically ill patients, the increased use of multiple invasive devices, the growing population of immunosuppressed patients, and the expanding use of organ transplantation. Such factors may have increased both the use of indwelling catheters and the susceptibility of catheterized patients. Even today, despite significant progress, virtually all patients with chronic indwelling bladder catheters are continuously infected. Moreover, as a result of the extensive use of broad-spectrum antimicrobial agents and the emergence of multiply resistant pathogens, patients with urinary catheter–associated UTIs also harbor an increasingly formidable reservoir of antibiotic-resistant pathogens (20–22).

All urinary catheters may induce UTIs, but indwelling catheters have additional hazards; for example, they may also obstruct the periurethral glands, producing urethritis, epididymitis, or urethral stricture. Paul Beeson (23) was one of the first, in 1958, to advise caution in the use of urinary catheters: "At times, the catheter is indispensable for therapy and there are many good indications for its use. Nevertheless, the decision to use the instrument should be made with the knowledge that it involves the risk of producing serious disease which is often difficult to treat." Many investigators, stimulated by Beeson's admonition and the controversy it aroused, have added to our knowledge of the pathogenesis, epidemiology, and prevention of these infections. Although the remaining problems should not be underestimated, the grounds for optimism have been summarized by Calvin Kunin (24): "In the current era of magnificent biotechnological advances, we should be able to solve the apparently simple but very important problem of draining the urinary bladder without producing infection."

EPIDEMIOLOGY

Catheter Use

The problem of nosocomial UTI appears to be deceptively simple: the major extrinsic risk factor is the use of a device that bypasses host defense mechanisms and allows microorganisms to grow in normally sterile body sites. Yet, the pathogenesis is far more complex than is implied by a purely mechanical model, and the epidemiology of the use and complications of urinary catheters is today understood only in its broad outlines.

The relative neglect of this problem by investigators undoubtedly reflects the low importance assigned to UTIs both by clinicians and by infection control programs. Indeed, in 2001 Jarvis (25) reported no epidemics of UTIs among 114 nosocomial outbreaks that the Centers for Disease Control and Prevention (CDC) investigated on-site in the previous decade (25). Although this could suggest that the CDC did not elect to participate for various reasons or that individual hospitals simply did not request the CDC's help, underreporting or failures of surveillance are also likely explanations.

Nosocomial UTIs present unique challenges for epidemiologists. Because endemic UTIs occur throughout the hospital and because nosocomial epidemics often involve multiple sites of infection, epidemic rates of catheter-associated UTIs may not be readily apparent unless they involve an unusual microbial species (26). Indwelling urinary catheters are used in nearly all hospital nursing units, unlike ventilators and many other devices. For this reason, nosocomial UTIs have complex behavioral, social, environmental, microbiologic, and biotechnologic determinants.

Duration of indwelling catheterization is the most important risk factor for the development of catheter-associated infection. Overall, the mean and median durations of catheterization in acute care hospitals are 2 and 4 days, respectively, and catheters are removed within 7 days in nearly 70% of patients (27). Although the prevalence of infection increases steadily with extended durations of catheterization, the daily incidence of newly acquired infection is relatively constant during closed drainage, at least for the first 10 days, with 2% to 16% of previously uninfected patients acquiring infection each day (28,29). Infection becomes nearly universal by 30 days. Nonetheless, this is a dramatic improvement over open drainage systems, for which universal infection followed just 4 days after insertion (30).

Thus, the principal benefit of closed drainage has been to delay, if not prevent, the onset of infection. True prevention begins by avoiding unnecessary catheter use. Catheters that must be used should be removed at the earliest possible time. Unfortunately, epidemiologists have not fully exploited the potential of these simple principles. Studies in many countries suggest that more restrictive policies for catheter use would be beneficial (31–43). Though patterns of use in other countries may differ from those in the United States, investigators in Denmark and Sweden determined that indwelling catheters were used in 13% of patients and 12% of hospital days, respectively, and there was great variation between hospitals for the same type of nursing service (32,33). Catheter usage is most prevalent in ICUs; in the NNIS system, urinary catheters were in place for 69% of patient days in 112 medical ICUs with a range from 44% to 88% in the lowest 10th percentile to the 90th percentile, respectively, of reporting hospitals (34). A study in Israel suggested that patients with intermediate durations of catheterization (7–30 days) and who are catheterized for the indications of obstruction or incontinence are a high-risk group that may benefit most from intervention (35). Such patients had a higher daily risk (8.6%) of acquiring infection even during the early period of catheterization. In Canada, an investigation of overutilization of indwelling urinary catheters in a large tertiary-care hospital found that 20.3% of patients admitted via the emergency room were catheterized upon admission (36). Furthermore, 50% of catheters were inserted for nonjustifiable reasons and 60% of those patients who subsequently developed UTI did not meet the study's criteria for justifiable catheterization. Another study found that 21% of catheterized medical patients did not have any initial indication for placement of the urinary catheter and that continued catheterization was unjustified in 47% of patient-days studied (37).

Other recent studies have produced similar findings. For example, 10.7% of patients on a medical service had an indwelling urinary catheter inserted within the first 24 hours, with 91% having been placed in the emergency room and 38% deemed inappropriate (38). In a point prevalence study from Spain, only 22% of patients had a correct indication with adequate drainage systems (39).

Lack of awareness of the presence of an indwelling catheter is a further problem. One group found that physicians were not aware of the catheter status in 28% of their patients and in as many as 41% of those whose catheterization was judged inappropriate (40). Thus, physicians appear to discount the importance of the urinary catheter, leading to overuse and misuse, for example, for inappropriate indications such as nursing staff convenience. In a study of patients with urinary incontinence, 37.5% were catheterized even though 55.5% of these were previously incontinent before admission to hospital and had managed this problem by other noninvasive methods. The decision to catheterize was made by physicians in 31.7% and by nursing staff in 37.3% (41).

All the above studies emphasize that catheter use is frequently inappropriate; inattention to both the proper indications for catheter use and the catheter status in patients appears to be an important factor. Potential solutions include the implementation of hospital-wide protocols for catheter insertion and continued usage, such as allowing removal of a catheter by a nurse without a physician's order, and systems for computer-based order entry of indwelling catheters (42,43).

Magnitude of the Problem

Incidence and Costs

From a broad epidemiologic perspective, the problem of catheter-associated infections acquires force from the magnitude of the population affected. Each year, 3 to 6 million of the 33 million patients admitted to acute care hospitals in the United States receive indwelling catheters. It has been estimated that about 15% to 25% of patients in general hospitals have a catheter inserted sometime during their stay (44), and that the prevalence of urinary catheters has increased over recent decades (45). The problem encompasses many different medical specialties, local practice patterns, and geographical differences. For example, in a French urology department, 52.4% of the patients received indwelling catheters and the incidence of catheter-related UTI was 13% (46). By contrast, in a pediatric population, nosocomial UTI was the fifth most common nosocomial infection and only 50% of patients with nosocomial UTIs had urethral instrumentation (47). However, there are no recent hospital-wide figures available. According to an older estimate performed by the CDC, there were 2.39 nosocomial UTIs per 100 hospital admissions in 1975–1976 (48). In 1992, the CDC estimated that more than 900,000 nosocomial UTIs occurred in the United States, and that the resulting extra charges exceeded $600 million (49). This represented nearly 14% of the total charges for nosocomial infections, estimated to be $4.5 billion.

These figures, however, may markedly understate the actual costs of UTIs, since they are based on decade-old estimates of an expected increased length of stay of only 1 day and extra charges of $680 (1992 dollars) for each UTI. Moreover, charges reflect cost shifting, and therefore are an inaccurate measure of true costs. Using attribution methods in a case-referent study of true costs at the Salt Lake City LDS Hospital from 1990 to 1992, the mean attributable difference in length of stay for patients with nosocomial UTIs was 3.8 days, and the mean increase in hospital costs was $3,803 (50). If this is representative of all U.S. hospitals, the true national cost of nosocomial UTIs is likely to be more than $3 billion.

In the managed care environment, costs are a financial loss to healthcare institutions. Thus, market forces should revive interest in preventing all nosocomial infections, including UTIs. Based on a theoretical model, the extra costs were estimated for each symptomatic nosocomial UTI to be at least $676 and for each catheter-associated bacteremia to be $2,836 (51). Another study estimated the mean costs of a nosocomial UTI to be $589, with the lowest costs associated with infections caused by *Escherichia coli* and higher costs with infections caused by other gram-negative bacilli and yeasts (52). The substantially lower estimates in this study as compared to other earlier retrospective studies were attributed to cost-containment measures implemented in the era of managed care as well as to the availability of newer oral antimicrobials with activity against gram-negative pathogens.

Mortality

The extent of mortality attributed to catheter-associated UTIs is still uncertain since these infections might be effect modifiers or simply markers of high mortality from other causes. The most generally acknowledged cause of death is related to bacteremia, which occurs in 0.3% to 3.9% of patients with nosocomial catheter-associated UTIs (53–55). Secondary bacteremia from a urinary source is generally considered unequivocal evidence of an invasive UTI. However, when a blood culture was obtained immediately after urethral catheterization from patients with sterile bladder urine, 6.5% were positive (56). Therefore, transient bacteremia secondary to urinary tract instrumentation can be a source of a remote infection, perhaps at the site of an implanted prosthetic device.

As many as 35,000 cases of bacteremia secondary to nosocomial catheter-associated UTIs occur each year in the U.S. Even though the crude case-fatality rate perhaps exceeds 30%, the mortality rate attributed specifically to bacteremic UTI in one large retrospective study was 12.7% (54). According to this estimate of the attributable mortality, as many as 4,500 deaths occur in the U.S. each year from nosocomial UTIs, but most of these deaths may occur in patients with serious underlying disease processes.

The true mortality rate from bacteremic UTIs for the U.S. in recent years is also undoubtedly lower than such extrapolations from studies in large tertiary care hospitals. In 1992, the CDC estimated that UTIs directly caused only 932 of the 19,027 deaths from nosocomial infections but contributed to an additional 6,500 of 58,092 deaths associated with nosocomial infections in U.S. hospitals (49). To appreciate recent advances, consider that, before closed drainage systems were used, Martin et al. (57) estimated that 31,000 deaths occurred in U.S. hospitals each year because of urinary catheter-related bacteremia. This study serves as the principal evidence that closed drainage markedly lowered the mortality rate and suggests that further reductions will be achieved only with great difficulty.

Additional mortality may nonetheless occur from causes unrelated to bacteremia. One study, using logistic regression analysis in a large hospital population, suggested that the actual mortality rate of nosocomial UTIs is significantly higher than estimates based on the incidence of bacteremia (58). Acquisition of catheter-related UTI predicted a nearly threefold increase in mortality that was not completely explained by clinical sepsis, documented bacteremia, or underlying disease. If this study is representative of all U.S. hospitals, the actual excess mortality associated with catheter-related infections could be as high as 56,000 deaths per year in acute care hospitals. Possible support for this conclusion also came from observations of women with long-term catheters in whom the incidence of death during fevers of suspected urinary origin was 60 times the incidence during afebrile periods (59).

Morbidity

Indwelling urinary catheters pose a risk for many infective and noninfective complications. Catheter-related infection can spread to any site in the urinary tract and can predispose patients to perinephric, vesical, and urethral abscesses as well as epididymitis, prostatitis, orchitis, and vesicoureteral reflux. The overall incidence of these complications is unknown, although 20% to 30% of patients with asymptomatic catheter-induced UTIs may develop local or systemic symptoms (51,53).

Infection may also have a role in other complications of catheterization. Bladder and renal stones, hemorrhagic pseudopolyps of the bladder (60,61), and squamous metaplasia and carcinoma of the bladder (62) have all been associated with UTIs in patients with long-term or chronic indwelling catheters. Accidental inflation of the catheter balloon in the posterior urethra has caused minor hematuria and subsequent urethral stricture as well as periurethral abscesses, sepsis, and death (63). Neglect of long-term catheters, usually in patients who are discharged from the hospital with an indwelling catheter, can lead to bladder gangrene, perforation, and peritonitis (64–66). Among noninfectious complications of indwelling urethral catheterization, some cardiovascular surgery units have reported that urethral ischemia during cardiopulmonary bypass caused urethral strictures that could be prevented by the use of silicone rather than latex catheters (67).

Nosocomial UTIs may also be a source for other nosocomial infections. In one large study, 40% of UTIs occurred in patients with multiple nosocomial infections, but the incidence of autoinfection secondary to the urinary site was not evaluated (68). In a study of patients in a university hospital in Spain, an indwelling urinary catheter used for more than 3 days more than doubled the risk of developing bacteremia (69). Nosocomial UTIs can be the source 10% to 15% of nosocomial bloodstream infections (54,55,70).

Surgical site infection secondary to a nosocomial UTI has been documented as a cause of major morbidity with an attack rate of 2.3 secondary surgical site infections per 100 surgical patients with nosocomial UTIs (71). Two reports confirm an increased rate of surgical site infections and allograft dysfunction in renal transplant recipients with nosocomial UTIs (72,73), whereas others have demonstrated associations between UTIs and infections of prosthetic heart valves (74,75), total hip replacements (76,77), and central venous catheters (78). Rare complications such as gram-negative endocarditis and septic discitis may also complicate urosepsis of nosocomial origin (79, 80).

Consequences of Antimicrobial Use

The indication for antibiotic therapy of nosocomial UTIs in acute care settings is a subject of debate and controversy. Nonetheless, treatment of symptomatic UTIs is virtually universal. In one report, among 1,233 patients with nosocomial UTIs, only a single patient was not treated (81). Yet, routine therapy increases not only drug costs but also adverse drug reactions and the emergence of antibiotic-resistant microorganisms. These adverse consequences have not been fully evaluated in epidemiologic studies, although antibiotic use during catheterization influences the patterns of microbial species causing nosocomial UTIs. The changing nature of UTIs at one medical center in the last decade was reflected by significant increases in the proportion of certain uropathogens such as yeasts, *Klebsiella pneumoniae,* and group B streptococcus (82). Antibiotic use was probably largely responsible for these changes. Other reports, such as one that tied the emergence of multidrug-resistant *K. pneumoniae* to prophylactic use of trimethoprim-sulfamethoxazole in patients with indwelling catheters (83), serve as further evidence that antibiotic use shapes the character of nosocomial UTIs.

In the report from the NNIS system with data from 1992 to 1997 for nosocomial infections in medical ICUs, fungi accounted for almost 40% of urinary isolates (34). *Candida albicans* alone accounted for 21% and was the single most frequent microorganism cultured. This was a marked change from a previous report with results from 1986 to 1989 that included all types of ICUs in which all fungi constituted 22.1% and *C. albicans* 12.8%. Extensive use of broad-spectrum antibiotics and antifungal drugs may have contributed to this increase, especially for the increasing prevalence of non-albicans *Candida.*

Epidemics of Nosocomial UTIs

Epidemics of nosocomial UTIs have garnered national attention when the causative microorganisms displayed unusually high levels of antibiotic resistance. In seven large epidemics investigated by the CDC between 1970 and 1975, asymptomatic catheter-associated UTIs were reservoirs of the epidemic microorganisms (84). The most frequently observed risk factor in these epidemics was prior exposure to broad-spectrum antibiotic therapy.

Only three microorganisms caused the seven outbreaks: *K. pneumoniae, Serratia marcescens,* and *Proteus rettgeri.* Gastrointestinal carriage was especially prominent in outbreaks caused by *K. pneumoniae,* but the epidemic microorganism was thought to be transmitted from patient to patient on the hands of healthcare workers in all seven outbreaks. Nosocomial UTIs were also sources for other nosocomial infections as the epidemic microorganism was isolated repeatedly from nonurinary sites in five of the outbreaks.

Indwelling urinary catheters and other types of urologic instrumentation have contributed to the emergence of nosocomial pathogens highly resistant to antimicrobial agents. The urinary drainage bag is a potential site for extraintestinal transfer of resistance plasmids in Enterobacteriaceae as well as an environmental reservoir for cross-infection (85). For instance, interhospital spread of multiply resistant *S. marcescens* occurred among patients with indwelling catheters in four geographically separate hospitals in one city (86). Hand carriage by personnel rotating among hospitals was the apparent mode of transmission. Indirect contact transmission of highly resistant *P. rettgeri* appeared to be important in two reported outbreaks of nosocomial UTIs (87,88).

Contaminated equipment and inadequate disinfectants have also been responsible for epidemics of UTIs. An outbreak of gentamicin-resistant *P. rettgeri* and *Providencia stuartii* UTIs in patients with chronic indwelling catheters in a rehabilitation unit was caused by contaminated urinary leg bags (89). In another hospital, a contaminated drainage pan in a cystoscopy room caused a common-source outbreak of 105 cases of multiple antibiotic-resistant *S. marcescens* UTIs following cystoscopy, and cross-infection of 29 patients on nursing units amplified the magnitude of the epidemic (90). At yet another hospital, inadequate disinfection of urologic instruments with reuse of 2% glutaraldehyde led to a 12-month-long epidemic of antibiotic-resistant *S. marcescens* UTIs after a variety of urologic procedures (91). The use of chlorhexidine for hand washing caused an outbreak due to multiply antibiotic-resistant and chlorhexidine-resistant *S. marcescens* UTIs that lasted over 19 months (92), and use of hexachlorophene solution in preparing patients and cleaning instruments for cystoscopy and transurethral resection of the prostate was associated with *Pseudomonas aeruginosa* UTIs (93). Contaminated urine measuring containers and urometers were the reservoir for *P. aeruginosa* that caused 66 catheter-associated UTIs (94). Clearly, rigorous application of existing infection control principles can prevent such epidemics.

Many of these and other reported epidemics had well-defined sources. Others occurred from previously unsuspected environmental reservoirs. For example, uninfected patients with condom catheters who had contaminated urine drainage bags served as a reservoir for infection of patients with indwelling catheters on the same hospital unit (95). Contaminated drainage bags may also mislead surveillance personnel, as false diagnoses of UTIs made from urine specimens obtained from drainage bags can skew surveillance data. Such errors at one hospital led to a pseudoepidemic of *Trichosporon beigelii* UTIs that, if not recognized, could have subjected patients to the risks of antifungal treatment (96) (see Chapter 8).

ETIOLOGIC AGENTS

The microorganisms usually responsible for catheter-associated UTIs are derived from the fecal flora native to the patient or that originate in the hospital environment. According to 1990–1992 data from the NNIS system, these include *E. coli* (25%); *Enterococcus* species (16%); *P. aeruginosa* (11%); *C. albicans* (8%); *K. pneumoniae* (7%); *Enterobacter* species and *Proteus mirabilis* (5% each); coagulase-negative staphylococci (CoNS) (4%); other fungi (3%); *Citrobacter* species, group D streptococci, other *Candida* species, and *Staphylococcus aureus* (2% each); *Acinetobacter* species, *S. marcescens*, group B streptococci, other *Klebsiella* species, other streptococcal species, and other Enterobacteriaceae (1% each) (97).

Although anaerobic bacteria have been isolated from catheter urine of patients with long-term catheters, and most secondary suppurative genitourinary infections commonly involve anaerobic bacteria, anaerobic UTIs are rarely reported (98,99). *S. aureus* is an occasional cause of catheter-associated UTI, with a high rate of secondary bacteremia, but is also frequently found in urine cultures secondary to *S. aureus* bacteremia (100–102). In addition, some microorganisms, such as CoNS, have received increased attention in recent years, although their role as uropathogens is still unsettled (103).

A single infecting species is responsible for about 80% of UTIs in patients with short-term catheters, but most patients with long-term catheters have polymicrobial infections with spontaneous turnover of individual species (104). The microbial species causing hospital-acquired UTIs have always differed from those causing community-acquired UTIs. *E. coli,* for example, causes 80% or more of the cases in outpatients (105) versus less than 50% of the nosocomial ones. As with other complicated UTIs, recognized virulence factors of *E. coli* are not prevalent among the strains causing catheter-associated UTI (106,107). The frequencies of the various pathogens also differ in chronically catheterized patients who have, for example, a particularly high risk of infection with *P. stuartii* (108).

The frequency of individual pathogens causing nosocomial UTIs has changed markedly in the last two decades. The single most important factor influencing the distribution of infecting species in the hospital is the use of antimicrobial agents. Although reduced rates of nosocomial UTIs have been associated with antibiotic use in patients who have indwelling catheters for brief periods, this possible benefit has been offset by increased acquisition of resistant species such as enterococci, *Klebsiella, Pseudomonas, Proteus, Enterobacter,* and yeast (28,34).

At Salt Lake City's LDS Hospital, antibiotic use during the period of catheterization has steadily increased: 53% of 405 catheterized patients in 1972 received antibiotics, as compared to 80% of 1,309 in 1990 (109). As a consequence, in 1990, *E. coli* accounted for only 10% to 20%, other gram-negative bacilli for 20% to 30%, enterococci for 20%, coagulase-negative staphylococci for 10%, and yeast for 20% to 30% of all isolates from urine cultures with microbial growth.

The incidence of nosocomial UTIs caused by *Candida* species and other yeasts has been increasing in recent years (34,82). The risk for candiduria has been related to duration of catheterization, duration of hospitalization, and antibiotic use (110). It is usually asymptomatic, but complications can include fungus balls in the bladder or renal pelvis, fever, renal and perirenal abscess, and disseminated candidiasis (111–114).

Viral agents have not been systematically studied in patients with indwelling catheters. Cytomegalovirus can be isolated, often intermittently, from the urine of patients infected with this agent, but the risk of transmission to healthcare workers is probably negligible (115–117). Human immunodeficiency virus type 1 (HIV-1), however, could not be detected in the urine of 48 seropositive individuals (118), and no evidence suggests that HIV can be transmitted by urine. Nevertheless, because urine can become contaminated with blood, especially after catheterization, universal precautions should apply to the handling of urine as well as blood. The proper use of gloves, particularly changing gloves between tasks, not only can protect the healthcare worker but also can theoretically prevent transmission of UTIs.

PATHOGENESIS

Role of the Catheter

Microbial colonization of bladder urine precedes most invasive UTIs. Urine is an excellent growth medium for common urinary tract pathogens (119,120). Nonetheless, the urinary tract above the distal urethra is normally free of bacteria, and micturition permits nearly complete cyclic emptying of the bladder, thereby rapidly eliminating the small numbers of microorganisms introduced through minor urethral trauma (121). The indwelling transurethral catheter breaches this normal defense mechanism, distending the urethra, and blocking the ducts of the periurethral glands. The retention balloon prevents the complete emptying of the bladder and creates a small pool of residual urine in which microorganisms can multiply. The resulting increase in susceptibility to infection is shown by observations that low-level bacteriuria progresses very rapidly to levels exceeding 100,000 colony-forming units (CFUs)/mL when any microorganisms appear in the catheterized bladder (28,122).

Since the catheter is a continuously open channel, microorganisms can migrate upstream into the bladder through the lumen of the catheter. As long ago as 1957, Dutton and Ralston (123) showed that nonmotile bacteria could ascend sterile tubing against a flow of sterile urine. In addition, the external surface of the catheter stresses the urethral surface, creating a channel for bacterial colonization and entry outside the catheter (24). It has been reemphasized in recent years that the urethra is not merely a passive conduit but has its own complex defense mechanism (124). Exfoliation of urethral cells with bound uropathogens is one example of an overlooked defense mechanism, and differences in the rates of exfoliation of cells in menstruating women or those on hormone replacement as compared with postmenopausal individuals may account for the different rates of UTIs in these populations. The effect of a foreign body on the rate of exfoliation of urethral cells and its contribution to bacteriuria has not been well defined.

The foreign material of the catheter also may promote infection by a number of other mechanisms. For instance, by blunting the local inflammatory response as shown in other types of implanted foreign bodies (125), the catheter may interfere with the removal of bacteria that gain entry to the bladder. In mouse models, Toll-like receptor 4 (TLR4) in both bladder epithelial cells and leukocytes protects against *E. coli* infection by recruiting inflammatory cells and upregulating chemokine expression needed for an innate immune response (126,127). Although the effect of the urinary catheter on the local innate immune response has not been studied, a dysfunctional TLR4 may hinder inflammation and bacterial clearance from the urinary tract (127). The possibility that the innate immune response is blunted in catheter-associated UTIs is suggested by observations that, in humans, nosocomial UTIs are seldom symptomatic (128) and the sensitivity of detecting catheter-associated UTIs by screening for pyuria is only 37% (129). Pyuria is also less frequently associated with yeast and gram-positive microorganisms than with gram-negative microorganisms colonizing the catheterized urinary tract.

Recently the function of defensins, specifically human *B*-defensin 1, which is produced by renal epithelial cells, and their role in UTI and pyelonephritis have been studied more closely. *B*-defensin 1 has activity against *E. coli*, although the concentration required is tenfold higher than is present in the urine. However, it is also possible that defensins could exist on epithelial cells to form an antimicrobial barrier, a process that may be affected by or compromised by the presence of a urinary catheter (130). Studies have shown the presence of a catheter may enhance the adherence of gram-negative bacteria to uroepithelial cells. For unknown reasons, 2 to 4 days before the onset of bacteriuria, epithelial cells harvested from the catheterized bladder show a transient increase in the adherence of gram-negative bacteria (131).

Bacteria may also adhere to and migrate along the extraluminal surface of the catheter itself. The physical and chemical properties of the catheter material, therefore, are posited as important determinants of UTI (132). In consequence, efforts have been made to develop an adhesion-resistant or colonization-resistant urinary catheter. An *in vitro* study found marked differences in the ability of various gram-positive and gram-negative bacteria to attach to red rubber catheters and those coated with either a hydrophilic substance, silicone, or tetrafluoroethylene (Teflon) (133). Most bacteria are hydrophobic, and none of the tested bacteria adhered to the hydrophilic catheter. However, studies of hydrophilic catheters in patients have demonstrated no clinical benefit (134–136). Regardless of their influence on bacterial adhesion, catheters made of Teflon-coated latex or silicone have been introduced for clinical use with the hope of improved biocompatibility, but in the absence of established infection there is little evidence of less irritation and inflammation in the urethra from these catheters than from those made of latex rubber (137, 138).

Bacteria that colonize both the external and internal surfaces of urinary catheters grow in microcolonies within a biofilm that encases the bacterial cells. When urine cultures reveal a single species, the biofilm often contains a mixed community with up to four species. In recent years there has been greater understanding of the biology of biofilms, with additional insight into the process in which planktonic or freely suspended microorganisms become surface-associated microorganisms or biofilms (139–142). A biofilm is loosely defined as a collection of microbial cells that is stably associated with a surface and enclosed in a matrix of primary polysaccharide material. The microbial cells in a biofilm are also different from their freely suspended counterparts with respect to gene transcription and growth. The initial step in the process is the formation of a conditioning film by the urine on the catheter surface followed by attachment of the microbial cell to the surface of the urinary catheter or substratum. The surface properties of the catheter appear to play a role with microorganisms more rapidly attaching to hydrophobic surfaces like Teflon and plastics than to hydrophilic substances like glass (143). It is thought that some kind of hydrophobic interaction occurs between the cell and the catheter surface and overcomes local repulsive forces, thereby enabling attachment. *In vitro* studies have also shown that the nutrient content of the aqueous medium, in this case urine, also affects the number of bacterial cells that attach to the surface. In certain bacteria, differences in bacterial surface hydrophobicity and presence of fimbriae (pili) and flagella also influence the rate and amount of attachment.

The next step in the formation of a biofilm is a change in gene expression by attached cells with both up- and downregulation of certain genes upon initial adherence (144). Most of these changes are needed for adaptation to living in a new environment and the change from a planktonic to a surface-associated form. After attachment, the bacterial cells produce extracellular polymeric substances (EPS), which will account for 50% to 90% of the total mass of the biofilm (145). The EPS is composed mainly of polysaccharides and is highly hydrated. The overall charge and composition of the polysaccharides and the amount of EPS produced can vary between different microorganisms and may contribute to antimicrobial resistance by decreasing diffusion of antibiotics through the EPS (146).

An *in vitro* study has shown that certain cell-to-cell signals are needed for biofilm formation in a process called quorum sensing (147). In a model using *P. aeruginosa*, mutants lacking two signaling genes were only able to produce a biofilm that was flat, undifferentiated, and phenotypically vastly different from the wild type and much less resistant to surfactant treatment. These signaling systems are also thought to play a role in dispersion of microorganisms from the biofilm, although the process is still not fully understood. The final architecture of the biofilm is a heterogeneous mixture of microcolonies of microbial cells surrounded by an EPS matrix with microbial colonies separated by water channels that play a role in transport of nutrients and possibly antimicrobial agents.

Several factors account for the fact that biofilm-associated infections are resistant to treatment without removal of the catheter. The rate of penetration of antimicrobial agents through the biofilm may be reduced to such an extent that they do not reach a sufficient concentration to be effective. Also, even small amounts of bacterial enzymes such as beta-lactamases might be sufficient to hydrolyze the reduced numbers of antimicrobial molecules that manage to reach the microbial cells. Another factor is the reduced metabolism and reproductive rate of the cells living within the biofilm, as some antimicrobial agents act only on rapidly dividing cells.

These mechanisms, however, do not readily explain the resistance of biofilms to the activity of fluoroquinolones that readily equilibrate across biofilms and kill non-growing planktonic cells of *P. aeruginosa*. Recently, it has been shown *in vitro* that increased concentrations of a quinolone did not result in further killing after an initial three- to four-log decrease in the bacterial population in biofilms (148,149). This small fraction of persistent cells may account for high-level resistance of biofilm-associated bacteria, although the exact mechanism accounting for this behavior has not been defined.

Bacterial Factors

Bacterial *virulence factors* (VFs) have been sought to explain each stage of UTI pathogenesis: bacterial adherence to uroepithelial cells and to the catheter surface, intraluminal migration of bacteria within the drainage tubing against the direction of urine flow, ascending infection through the ureters to the upper urinary tract, invasion of the kidney to cause pyelonephritis, invasion of the bloodstream to cause bacteremia, and persistence of bacteriuria in long-term catheterized patients. The swarming motility of *Proteus mirabilis* has been postulated as a VF for ascending infection of the ureters (150). Other virulence factors encoded by genes localized to chromosomal pathogenicity islands, including hemolysin, the siderophore aerobactin, and adhesive organelles (S pili, Dr family adhesins, P pili, and type 1 pili), have been identified in strains of uropathogenic *E. coli* (UPEC) causing urinary infection syndromes in noncatheterized patients (151). However, *E. coli* is a less common cause of infection in catheterized patients, and many strains causing urosepsis in catheterized patients typically lack these VFs (106,152). Catheterization enables otherwise avirulent microorganisms to persist and initiate infection.

The diversity of microorganisms causing catheter-associated UTIs and the relatively greater importance of host compromise make it unlikely that recognition of common virulence properties will lead to strategies capable either of blocking attachment or of predicting strains most likely to cause bacteremia. Type 1 pili that are mannose-sensitive and mediate adherence to epithelial cells and polymorphonuclear leukocytes, for example, have been found in 61% of *E. coli,* 55% of *Klebsiella* species, and 11% of *Proteus* species from catheterized patients (153). Moreover, *E. coli* flora of the urethral meatus, when present, has been shown to change frequently from isolates expressing adhesins to those without this property, perhaps resulting from on-off phase variation in phenotype (106).

In contrast, type 1 pili-mediated adherence has been correlated with persistence of *E. coli* in the long-term catheterized urinary tract (154). In an animal model of cystitis, UPEC expressing type 1 pili were able to invade and persist within bladder cells and serve as a reservoir for recurrent infection (155). So-called type 3 pili [mannose-resistant, *Klebsiella*-like (MR/K) hemagglutination] found in *Providencia, Proteus,* and *Morganella* species also may play a role in long-term catheter-associated bacteriuria through adherence to the catheter material (156), and numerous other adhesins continue to be discovered. Further evidence shows that *E. coli* strains lacking the more common virulence factors (P pili and hemolysin) often carry multiple antibiotic resistance and aerobactin plasmids and are associated with bacteremia in patients with urinary tract abnormalities (157).

Urease, a VF of *Proteus* species, is undoubtedly important, since virtually all patients with *Proteus* bacteriuria develop upper tract infection. Urea-splitting by microorganisms such as *Proteus* species and *Corynebacterium* group D2 causes alkalinization of the urine that damages the urothelium, and urease inhibitors such as acetohydroxamic acid can prevent invasion of kidney tissue (158,159).

Pathways of Infection

Clinical studies have also contributed to our understanding of the pathogenesis of catheter-related urinary infections (15, 28,29,103,160–165). Such studies have confirmed the importance of the extraluminal pathway of infection during closed drainage, and they have revealed other problems that complicate the prevention of UTIs. For example, in the hospital, indwelling catheterization may unmask community-acquired asymptomatic bacteriuria (166). The incidence of asymptomatic bacteriuria is higher in hospitalized than in nonhospitalized populations and varies from 10% to 30% in women on medical wards to 70% in men on urology wards (167).

Catheter insertion may also push microorganisms into the previously uninfected bladder, a mode of infection that has not been well studied but may account for a risk of at least 2% based on the incidence of bacteriuria after a straight in-and-out catheterization (168,169). Urethral catheterization following use of an external condom catheter system may be associated with an even higher risk of infection that is due to the introduction of a large bacterial inoculum that results from the warm moist conditions inside the condom (170). Finally, infection may be acquired, or become clinically manifest, after the catheter is removed, perhaps in association with straight catheterizations during bladder training. The relative importance of each of these patterns of infection, and, therefore, the effectiveness of prevention, depends on host factors, patient care practices, and environmental influences.

The use of sterile barriers and procedures in insertion of central venous catheters reduce the rates of nosocomial bacteremia, but the effectiveness of such maximal sterile procedures during urinary catheter insertion has not been conclusively demonstrated. Patients who had a urinary catheter inserted in an operating room had a lower incidence of early nosocomial UTIs (171), but a separate small randomized study showed no difference between sterile and nonsterile urinary catheter insertion (172). Nonetheless, catheter insertion under suboptimal conditions and with poor visualization of the urethral meatus may increase the risks of subsequent UTIs.

Closed systems are designed to block the intraluminal pathway of infection by preventing exogenous contamination from air, dust, and the environment. Modern systems for closed sterile urinary drainage consist of a plastic collection bag fused to the distal end of the collecting tube. But since the system is vented to the air and since the collection bag must be emptied frequently, the system is never truly closed. Improper emptying of the bag or nonsterile disconnection of the junction between the catheter and the collection tube may result in microbial contamination of the system. Large populations of bacteria can grow in the collection bag and travel upstream against the flow of urine to infect the bladder within a day or two (15,28,123,160,173).

After the first week of indwelling catheterization, the extraluminal pathway of infection becomes increasingly important as fecal bacteria migrate and colonize the perineal and meatal-urethral surfaces. The first direct evidence for the existence of this external pathway came many years ago from experimental application of *S. marcescens* (which was then considered a nonpathogenic microorganism) to the periurethral area; the microorganism was then recovered from catheter urine 1 to 3 days later (174). Supporting evidence came from the finding that colonization of the perineum or fossa navicularis with pathogens usually preceded the development of bladder bacteriuria by several days in catheterized urology patients (175,176). Indirect evidence indicated that more than 85% of patients had the onset of bacteriuria and colonization of the drainage bag on the same day, implying that the major pathway of infection during closed drainage is extraluminal (15,28,177).

Each pathway is accompanied, to some extent, by a characteristic pattern of infection by different species. In general, exogenous microorganisms more frequently enter through the intraluminal pathway, whereas endogenous microorganisms cause infection through the extraluminal route. Exogenous microorganisms such as *Citrobacter freundii, Pseudomonas* species, *Serratia* species, and nonfermenting gram-negative bacilli that are not part of the normal flora are commonly acquired from transient carriage on the hands of personnel or from collection containers and may be transmitted by cross-infection (178). In contrast, endogenous microorganisms that enter through the pericatheter space are generally part of the patient's normal fecal and perineal flora.

Exogenous microorganisms may become a part of the perineal flora as a consequence of hospitalization and especially of antibiotic use. Selden et al. (179) found that the gastrointestinal tract of hospitalized patients frequently became colonized with multidrug-resistant *Klebsiella,* and that the fecal reservoir then served as a source for endogenous infections, with the urinary tract being the commonest site. Systemic antibiotic use may also unmask low-level colonization with microorganisms such as *Pseudomonas* (180). Finally, many microorganisms are associated with both exogenous and endogenous infection. Bacteriuria with CoNS has been linked to disconnections of the catheter-drainage tube junction and, perhaps, exogenous sources (29), as well as to endogenous meatal colonization (103).

The effect of the duration of indwelling bladder catheterization and the relative importance of each of the possible mechanisms of bacterial entry were confirmed with 66% of nosocomial UTIs being acquired extraluminally with 18% detected within the first 24 hours (171). After this time, the extraluminal route was also more frequent. Gram-positive microorganisms and yeasts were far more likely to be extraluminally acquired, whereas gram-negative bacilli were associated with both routes equally.

Host Factors

The effective prevention of exogenous intraluminal infection by closed drainage systems has revealed differences in the risk of infection among different categories of patients (15,28). Risk factors that were identified in a study analyzed by a multivariable statistical technique include increasing duration of use, female gender, absence of systemic antibiotics, diabetes mellitus, and renal insufficiency (serum creatinine >2 mg/dL) (165). Advanced age and severe underlying illness also have been identified as risk factors by univariate analysis (28). Thus, biologic differences in the nature of patient populations account for differing rates of catheter-related UTIs. Importantly, these patient variables can distort interhospital comparisons of infection rates.

Colonization of the urethral meatus appears to be a pathogenetic link between host factors and the risk of infection. In one study of 612 patients with meatal colonization by gram-negative bacilli or enterococci, 110 (18%) developed bacteriuria as compared to 28 (5%) of 601 patients not colonized ($p < .001$) (162). Meatal colonization was more frequent for each of the high-risk groups than for their lower-risk comparison groups. For example, 72% of female patients had meatal colonization as compared with 30% of male patients ($p < .0001$). Overall, the same species was isolated from prior meatal and later urine cultures in 94 (68%) of 138 patients with catheter-induced bacteriuria—further evidence that the extraluminal spread of bacteria within the periurethral space is the major route by which bacteria enter the bladder during closed drainage.

The increased risk of bacteriuria for catheterized women has been blamed in part on the short length of the female urethra, a conclusion that is not well founded. For instance, consider the pathogenesis of bacteriuria due to CoNS. The prevalence of meatal colonization with CoNS, according to one study, was similar in both sexes, as were the rates of bacteriuria with these microorganisms; in both sexes, the rates of CoNS bacteriuria were significantly higher in those with a prior meatal culture yielding CoNS (4.5% vs. 1.5%, $p < .05$) (103). These data suggest that meatal colonization is the major risk factor and that urethral length is relatively unimportant in the catheterized patient.

Although the rates of bacteriuria due to gram-negative bacilli and enterococci are generally lower in men than in women, these differences correlated with differences in rates of meatal colonization with these microorganisms (162). For example, the rate of bacteriuria was only slightly higher in women whose meatal cultures showed negative results (12%) than in men whose meatal cultures showed positive results (8%); the extraluminal pathway predominated in both sexes. Therefore, either the intraluminal or the extraluminal pathway may predominate under given conditions, depending on the local environment, the quality of catheter care, and the nature of the catheterized population.

Unfortunately, factors influencing meatal and urethral colonization have not been studied extensively in catheterized patients. One study using serotyping of *E. coli* isolates causing urethral and rectal colonization observed that the same strains were later present in bladder urine. Systemic antibiotics were associated with a lower rate of bacteriuria while having little apparent effect on serial cultures of urethral colonization (164). In catheterized patients with spinal cord injuries or who had undergone renal transplantation, bacteria colonizing the urethral meatus were acquired after admission to the hospital (163). The density of bacterial colonization increased during catheterization, was associated with increased rates of bacteriuria, and was greater in patients on open wards than in those in reverse isolation.

By sampling the intraurethral flora using cultures of the external surface of catheters after removal, Kunin and Steele (181) documented gradually increasing colonization of the urethra with gram-negative bacilli and enterococci with extended durations of catheterization. They further found that predominantly gram-positive species could be grown from removed catheters of patients with sterile urine. Despite high concentrations of antibiotics in the urine, antibacterial activity could not be detected on the catheters, perhaps explaining the lack of effect of antibiotics on the urethral flora.

DIAGNOSIS

The differing needs of clinicians and epidemiologists are responsible for disagreements over terminology, particularly the definition of UTIs in asymptomatic catheterized patients (182). A clinician uses a diagnosis to define an illness that requires treatment and to help form a prognosis. An epidemiologist selects a pragmatic case definition for surveillance that can be proficiently applied. An investigator demands objective data regardless of cost. These considerations lead to disparate criteria for nosocomial UTIs.

The term *bacteriuria,* or, in the case of yeasts, *candiduria,* is widely used by authors when there is no clinical, histologic, or immunologic evidence of infection. Bacteriuria literally means the presence of bacteria in urine and therefore is evidence of colonization and a precursor of infection. The only generally accepted criteria for infection of the urinary tract, therefore, require the presence of symptoms or other evidence of tissue invasion in addition to recovery of a pathogen from a source within the urinary tract. However, there is no formal guideline reflecting consensus.

The CDC has developed a set of surveillance definitions, formulated as algorithms, that aim to distinguish hospital-acquired from community-acquired infections (183). These definitions exclude infections that are present or incubating at the time of hospital admission. Unavoidable incongruities occur in the use of these definitions, however. For example, unless a urine culture is performed at the time of hospital admission, preexisting asymptomatic bacteriuria may be falsely attributed to later catheterization. On the other hand, the CDC criteria do not permit classification of asymptomatic catheter-associated bacteriuria with fewer than 100,000 colonies per milliliter as an infection, even though the bacteriuria is hospital-acquired.

The common goal for diagnostic criteria is to provide a basis for predicting morbidity and mortality. Quantitative bacterial cultures of urine have proven satisfactory for this purpose. Except with very low colony counts (<100 colonies/mL), the problem of contamination and false-positive results is virtually nonexistent when urine is obtained by aseptic needle aspiration from the sampling port on the drainage tube. Evidence indicates that the diagnosis of infection associated with short-term indwelling catheterization is supported with colony counts as low as 100 microorganisms per milliliter (184). Colony counts of this magnitude are reproducibly present in the same or higher numbers, usually more than 100,000 colonies per milliliter, within 1 or 2 days except for those patients receiving antibiotics or who have infection with fastidious slow-growing microorganisms (122).

The epidemiologist must be cautious when interpreting colony counts because of their influence on comparative data. The infection rates found in clinical trials, for example, are actually rates of bacteriuria and may be markedly different from rates of clinical UTIs (29,185). Some investigators have restricted the definition of uropathogens to certain species of bacteria, which also affects the observed rate of bacteriuria. In addition, very low colony counts (100 or 1,000 colonies/mL) are commonly selected as a threshold to define bacteriuria in clinical trials, with the result that rates are higher than those from routine surveillance. This confers greater sensitivity and hence greater power to detect differences between study and control groups. Infection rates may also be higher in hospitals that use protocols for obtaining urine cultures from all patients regardless of symptoms.

From a clinical perspective, secondary bacteremia occasionally occurs in bacteriuric patients with colony counts of fewer than 100,000 microorganisms per milliliter, and some rapid tests for bacteriuria are insensitive to such low colony counts (186, 187). Colony counts may also be lower in urine aspirates from replacement catheters than in those from the original catheters, although the differences are seldom large enough to be detected by conventional urine cultures (188). One proposed method of detecting infection, the culturing of the tip of a removed Foley catheter, has proven ineffective (189).

Few studies have carefully examined the relation of bacteriuria to pyuria. Musher et al. (190) found that pyuria nearly always accompanied bacteriuria (>100,000 bacteria/mL) in catheterized male patients, but pyuria was also present in nearly 30% of urine specimens from catheterized male patients without bacteriuria. Therefore, the finding of pyuria did not help to discriminate infection from colonization. In a study of patients with spinal cord injury who underwent intermittent catheterization, bacteriuria with more than 100,000 gram-negative bacilli per milliliter, or colonization with yeast regardless of the colony count, resulted in pyuria (191). In patients with long-term indwelling catheters who had chronic pyuria and bacteriuria, neither urinalysis nor urine culture was a reliable test for symptomatic UTI (192). In contrast, in a study of patients with short-term indwelling urinary catheters, Tambyah and Maki (129) found that only 37% of patients with bacteriuria had pyuria, and similarly bacteriuria was present in 37% of patients with pyuria. The authors concluded that the differences between their results and the previous study done by Musher et al. were likely due to different patient populations.

The CDC surveillance algorithm uses symptoms to define UTI if other supporting evidence is present, but it also recognizes asymptomatic bacteriuria if the urine culture yields more than 100,000 colonies per milliliter with no more than two species of microorganisms. However, the symptoms of UTI, such as dysuria, urgency, frequency, or suprapubic tenderness, are often obscured by the presence of the catheter and, except for fever, may become evident only when the catheter is removed. Urinary catheters contribute directly to nosocomial febrile illnesses (193). However, fever may be absent in elderly, debilitated, or immunosuppressed patients who also may be unable to report other symptoms. In a companion study by Tambyah and Maki (128), more than 90% of patients with catheter-associated UTI were asymptomatic, but 52% were diagnosed by their physicians using the hospital laboratory. Interestingly, symptoms referable to the urinary tract had no predictive value for the diagnosis of infection.

Objective, reproducible, and economical methods for surveillance are obviously needed. One proposal for the surveillance of nosocomial UTIs avoids time-consuming reviews of patient records by using concurrent review of microbiology laboratory reports (194). Because evaluation of symptomatic patients usually includes a urine culture, the sensitivity of laboratory-based surveillance approaches 98% when nosocomial UTI is defined by positive urine culture on the third hospital day or later.

PREVENTION

Closed Sterile Drainage

An understanding of the major risk factors and pathways of infection should facilitate logical strategies for the prevention of nosocomial UTIs. The most successful infection control method, closed sterile drainage, reduces the risk of infection only through the exogenous pathway and requires little additional effort by healthcare workers. Nonetheless, irregularities in catheter care and resulting breaches of closed systems are pervasive problems and are therefore a target for prevention efforts (28, 29). Improper hand hygiene—with a nondisinfectant soap, for example (195)—is also an important risk factor for exogenous infection. Proper technique depends on healthcare workers and is difficult to monitor and enforce (196).

Infection Control and Surveillance Programs

The CDC's Study on the Efficacy of Nosocomial Infection Control (SENIC) remains today the major source of data regarding the preventability of nosocomial infections including UTIs (197). Complicated methodology hindered the understanding and limited the impact of the SENIC study. The multiple factors influencing UTI rates, for example, could not be independently assessed. Nonetheless, the study suggested the yet-unfulfilled potential of existing methods for prevention and the role of surveillance itself as a control measure.

The SENIC report estimated that intensive infection surveillance and control programs—those with at least one infection control practitioner (professional in current terminology) per 250 beds—might have been able to reduce the UTI rate by 33%. Unfortunately, because relatively few hospitals had effective programs in the mid-1970s, only 2% of the number of nosocomial UTIs predicted in the absence of such programs were actually prevented. A follow-up survey in 1983 found that the proportion of hospitals with effective programs had increased from 7% to 24%, with potentially 6% of the UTIs prevented (198).

Guidelines

Two decades ago, the CDC developed a guideline for the prevention of catheter-associated UTIs that has not been revised since. It emphasized principles for maintaining closed sterile drainage but overlooked the role of surveillance (199). The extent of adherence to these guidelines remains unknown, although evidence points to marked variation among institutions. Catheter care violations, such as accidental junction disconnections, improper closure of the outflow spigot, and improper positioning of the collection bag, are common and are associated with increased rates of bacteriuria. Studies at the Salt Lake City LDS Hospital reported these errors in 11% of catheter-days and overall in 29% of catheterized patients with little change over time despite intensive education of healthcare workers (29). Modifications in the design of drainage systems, such as antireflux valves and seals of the catheter-drainage tubing junction, aimed at reducing the frequency of errors in catheter care by passive means, have proved disappointing.

Adjuncts to Closed Drainage

In the past few decades, many adjuncts to closed drainage have been introduced and aggressively marketed by device manufacturers, often without adequate clinical investigation and evidence of efficacy. These efforts have focused on more effectively preventing infection by both the intraluminal and extraluminal pathways.

Randomized controlled trials (RCTs) have been useful in the evaluation of preventive measures for nosocomial UTIs. Many seemingly logical adjuncts to closed drainage have not been efficacious when evaluated in RCTs. For example, RCTs showed that a costly and once widely used procedure, daily meatal care, is not cost-effective and, in fact, that meatal care with iodophors is deleterious (200–203). However, closed sterile urinary drainage has not been evaluated in RCTs, because its efficacy has been evident from nonrandomized studies (204).

RCTs are expensive and susceptible to many limitations, including errors in design and analysis. Because of the varying importance of the different pathways for acquisition of catheter-associated UTIs in different settings and patient populations, the results of a single RCT may be valid only for the time and place a study was conducted. RCTs are also susceptible to exploitation by manufacturers. Accordingly, Kunin (205) has suggested that the efficacy of new devices for infection control should be supported with carefully controlled studies by at least three groups working independently.

RCTs relevant to nosocomial UTIs are instructive and may help identify productive areas for future investigation. The listing of 52 representative RCTs from 1962 to 2003 shown in Table 20.1 intentionally omits some studies of prophylactic antibiotic use in surgery, urology, and gynecology in which catheter-related UTI was an outcome measure. It also omits comparative trials that were not randomized, and some of those included were not randomized at the individual patient level. Furthermore, 30 of the 52 RCTs were restricted to certain types of patient populations, and the results, therefore, may not be generally applicable to all catheterized patients.

Judgments of outcomes as positive (+) or negative (−) were based on the presence or absence, respectively, of statistically significant differences ($p < .05$) between the study and control groups. Some outcomes that were otherwise negative were judged to be equivocal (+/−) if a significant difference was found in at least one subset of the population or if the authors believed a trend favored the intervention.

The majority of these RCTs (35 of 52) had either negative or equivocal outcomes. The studies ranged in size from 31 patients to 27,878 patients. Study size was correlated to outcome: 15 positive outcomes occurred in 26 studies with fewer than 200 patients, as compared to only two positive outcomes in 13 studies with more than 500 patients. Smaller studies, therefore, may have erroneous outcomes.

The types of interventions studied in these RCTs can be grouped in four categories: (a) alternative methods of bladder drainage (intermittent straight and suprapubic catheters); (b) methods to prevent extraluminal infection (urethral lubrication, meatal disinfection, and catheters coated with hydrophilic polymers or antimicrobial compounds); (c) methods to prevent intraluminal infection (antireflux valves and vents, instillation of disinfectants into the bag, irrigation of the bladder with disinfectants or antimicrobials, and junction seals); and (d) combined approaches including systemic antibiotic prophylaxis.

None of the individual interventions met criteria for efficacy in at least three RCTs. Systemic antibiotic prophylaxis, with six of seven trials having positive outcomes, and methods that included junction seals, with two positive and two equivocal outcomes among seven trials, appeared to be the most promising approaches. Yet only one of these positive outcomes—an RCT of antibiotic prophylaxis—occurred in a study of more than 500 patients. Junction seals are potentially effective, although they do not yet meet Kunin's criteria for efficacy. However, prevention of junction disconnections might reduce the incidence of bacteriuria by only about 10% (29).

An intriguing approach to antibiotic prophylaxis, evaluated in a single small trial, involved the use of ampicillin 1 hour before, at the time of, and 6 hours after catheter insertion (206). This study found significant protection for up to 1 week after use of this regimen. The use of antimicrobials during catheterization, especially fluoroquinolones—effective in two RCTs—merits further investigation but cannot yet be recommended pending large-scale clinical trials.

Methods to prevent UTIs that are effective in one patient group, such as males undergoing prostatectomy, may not be suitable for general use. All of the RCTs of antibiotic prophylaxis were restricted to certain types of patients. All three positive trials of bladder irrigation with antimicrobials involved patients undergoing urologic or gynecologic procedures, and the control group for one trial received open drainage. Ideally, preventive methods should be evaluated in general hospital use among all patient services. The only RCT of antibiotic irrigation that met this criterion showed no benefit, although the authors believed that this failure was due to an increased rate of junction disconnections in the treatment group (161).

Methods found to be efficacious in RCTs should then be evaluated for effectiveness and cost-benefit in routine clinical practice. For example, the routine use of preconnected catheters with junction seals has not been evaluated despite a strong rationale for an expected cost-benefit based on a single RCT (207). In addition, the largest RCT of the use of catheters with presealed junctions showed only a small reduction in the frequency of disconnections (208). A large RCT showed that tape seals applied after catheterization were not effective in reducing either the frequency of junction disconnections or the rate of bacteriuria (209). Thus, the protective effect of the presealed catheter junctions on the rate of bacteriuria is difficult to interpret and may be related to effects of its use other than preventing disconnections or to the fact that factory preconnection may be important.

The results from recent RCTs (210,211) and meta-analysis (212) of RCTs of silver-coated catheters were inconclusive. In a recent review of all studies of silver-coated catheters including controlled clinical trials, RCTs, systematic reviews, and meta-analyses, only seven studies satisfied the reviewers' selection criteria for adequate quality and only one had a high-quality score (213). The authors concluded that current evidence is insufficient to recommend silver-coated catheters. Moreover, several studies looking at the best possible scenarios for possible cost-benefit of reducing infection rates with the more expensive silver-coated catheters have estimated cost savings per patient of only \$4.09 (212) but annual hospital-wide savings from \$12,563 to

TABLE 20.1. RANDOMIZED CONTROLLED CLINICAL TRIALS FOR THE PREVENTION OF CATHETER-ASSOCIATED URINARY TRACT INFECTIONS, 1962–2003

First Author (Reference)	Year	No. of Patients Studied	Intervention Studied	Outcome of Trial	Comments
Martin (237)	1962	40	Constant bladder irrigation with acetic acid or neomycin-polymyxin vs. open drainage	+	Gynecology patients
Butler (238)	1968	470	Polymyxin B vs. placebo lubricant	–	
Finkelberg (239)	1969	400	Eight different closed systems	–	
Kunin (240)	1971	314	Intraurethral lubricating catheter	+/–	
Brehmer (175)	1972	40	Polymyxin B–neomycin-bacitracin spray of perineum and meatus	+	Prostatectomies
Monson (134)	1974	287	Hydrophilic, polymer-coated catheter	–	
Garibaldi (28)	1974	405	Antireflux valves in drainage bags	–	
Little (241)	1974	747	Systemic antibiotic prophylaxis	+	Prostatectomies
Monson (242)	1977	506	Top-vented vs. nonvented drainage system	+/–	
Britt (243)	1977	196	Systemic antibiotic prophylaxis	+/–	Hysterectomies
Bastable (244)	1977	223	Continuous irrigation with chlorhexidine	–	Prostatectomies
Warren (161)	1978	187	Continuous irrigation with neomycin–polymyxin B	–	
Matthew (245)	1978	87	Nitrofurantoin prophylaxis	+	Prostatectomies
Keys (246)	1979	236	Top-vented vs. bag-vented system	–	
Kirk (247)	1979	125	Chlorhexidine instillation in bladder	+	Urology service
Maizels (248)	1980	31	Hydrogen peroxide instillation in bag	+	Spinal cord injury patients
Burke (200)	1981	846	Meatal care with green soap or povidone-iodine	–	
Burke (201)	1983	428	Meatal care with polyantibiotic ointment	+/–	
Platt (208)	1983	1,494	Preconnected catheters with sealed junction	+/–	
Gillespie (249)	1983	58	Chlorhexidine instillations in bag	–	Prostatectomies
Thompson (177)	1984	668	Hydrogen peroxide instillation in bag	–	
Sweet (250)	1985	134	Hydrogen peroxide instillation in bag	–	ICU patients
Mountokalakis (206)	1985	78	Ampicillin prophylaxis before catheterization	+	Neurology patients
Klarskov (251)	1986	40	Hydrophilic catheters with junction seals; povidone-iodine applications	+	Female GU or Gyn surgery patients
Davies (252)	1987	44	Chlorhexidine vs. saline bladder instillations	–	Geriatric patients
Sethia (253)	1987	66	Suprapubic vs. urethral catheters	+/–	Surgery patients
Charton (254)	1987	95	Preoperative netilmicin prophylaxis	+	Prostatectomies
Ball (255)	1987	89	Chlorhexidine bladder irrigations	+	Prostatectomies
Hozack (256)	1988	54	Straight catheterization postop	–	Orthopedic patients
DeGroot-Kosolcharoen (257)	1988	202	Preconnected silicone vs. latex catheters	+/–	Male patients
Schaeffer (258)	1988	74	Silver-oxide/trichloroisocyanuric acid antimicrobial drainage system	+	Spinal cord injury patients
Michelson (259)	1988	96	Intermittent vs. indwelling catheters	–	Orthopedic patients
Verbrugh (260)	1988	105	Norfloxacin prophylaxis	+	Gynecology patients
Al-Juburi (261)	1989	109	Hydrophilic preconnected catheter with povidone-iodine instillations in bag	+	
Liedberg (262)	1990	120	Silver alloy–coated catheters	+	Postoperative patients
Johnson (263)	1990	482	Silver oxide–coated catheter	+/–	Selected services
Classen (202)	1991	747	Meatal care with polyantibiotic cream	+/–	
Classen (136)	1991	606	Preconnected hydrophilic catheter with povidone-iodine applied to catheter and bag	–	
Huth (209)	1992	1,740	Tape seals applied to catheter junction	–	
van der Wall (264)	1992	184	Ciprofloxacin prophylaxis	+	Surgery patients
Schneeberger (265)	1992	264	Povidone-iodine bladder irrigations	–	Urology patients
Skelly (266)	1992	67	Intermittent vs. indwelling catheters	–	Orthopedic patients
Huth (203)	1992	696	Meatal care with silver sulfadiazine cream	–	
Wille (267)	1993	181	Preconnected hydrophilic catheter with povidone-iodine instillations in bag	–	Selected units
Riley (109)	1995	1309	Silver oxide–coated catheter	–	
Maki (268)	1998	852	Silver-hydrogel impregnated catheter	+/–	
Maki (269,270)	1998, 2001	417	Nitrofurazone-coated catheter	+/–	
Darouiche (215)	1999	124	Minocycline- and rifampin-coated catheter	+	Prostatectomies
Thibon (210)	2000	199	Silver-hydrogel coated catheter	–	Selected units
Karchmer (211)	2000	27,878	Silver alloy-coated catheter	+	Selected units
Keerasuntonpong (271)	2003	153	3-day urinary bag change	–	
Srinivasan (272)	2003	3336	Silicon-based silver-impregnated catheter	–	

as much as $573,293 (211,214). In the only other recent trial of an antibiotic-impregnated urinary catheter (using minocycline and rifampin), a small number of male patients undergoing radical prostatectomy showed a statistically significant reduction in gram-positive bacteriuria but not gram-negative bacteriuria or candiduria (215).

Alternatives to Foley Catheters

Alternatives to the Foley catheter include the condom catheter for female patients, the intraurethral stent, the conformable catheter, and older approaches such as adult diapers and biofeedback training (216–218). None of these devices has been evaluated in RCTs. However, they are applicable to only certain types of patients (e.g., condoms for women with incontinence or intraurethral catheters for males with prostatic obstruction). The conformable catheter, a type of balloon catheter with a collapsible intraurethral segment that may cause less trauma to the urethra, has been tested only in women without urethral strictures and is not commercially available.

A newer method to reduce the use of indwelling catheters involves the use of a portable ultrasound device to scan the bladder before catheterization to accurately measure the volume of urine in the bladder. In a nonrandomized study, this device enabled reduced use of intermittent and indwelling urinary catheters with a reduction in the incidence of UTIs (219). Another study using this method in postoperative patients reported that the rate of urinary catheterization decreased from 31% to 16% (220).

Secondary Prevention

Secondary prevention of the complications of UTIs is desirable but has not been evaluated in RCTs. In 1968, Butler and Kunin (221) first proposed that routine monitoring of urine cultures from patients undergoing short-term catheterization could enable the use of specific antimicrobial therapy in order to reduce the number of patient-days at risk for gram-negative sepsis. Large-scale clinical trials to test this hypothesis have still not been done. The results of limited observational studies suggest that the only benefit might be the prevention of UTI symptoms in the subset of patients with chronic asymptomatic bacteriuria that precedes catheterization (53). However, treatment of asymptomatic bacteriuria in long-term catheterized patients has shown no beneficial effects (222).

Guidelines for the treatment of catheter-associated UTIs are not available despite the great frequency of this problem and the diverse approaches that have been used. There is also a dearth of well-controlled trials that could be a basis for specific recommendations. Many believe that treatment of asymptomatic bacteriuria while the catheter remains in place has little apparent benefit (184). However, even a single dose of an aminoglycoside antibiotic, if combined with a catheter change, can eradicate bacteria from the urine of catheterized patients (223). The efficacy of this approach has not been evaluated in large-scale trials, but one clinical trial found that daily treatment with a fluoroquinolone antibiotic failed more than half the time with or without a catheter change (224). The high rate of relapse and reinfection, as well as the adverse consequences of antibiotic use, has also discouraged the routine treatment of asymptomatic bacteriuria.

Wide variation by clinicians likely exists in the use of diagnostic urine cultures, in the indications for antimicrobial treatment, and in the duration of treatment. The practice of obtaining urine cultures only in symptomatic patients may prevent unnecessary treatment (225), but it also prevents an aggressive approach to the detection and management of catheter-associated bacteriuria. A common recommendation is that urine cultures should be obtained at the times of insertion and upon removal of the catheter with an appropriate follow-up culture for those who have acquired bacteriuria (226). Other clinicians recommend against routine cultures even at the time of catheter removal (227). At present, there are few studies to assist in resolving these conflicting recommendations, but evidence seems to be growing in favor of more rather than less intensive culture monitoring.

Whether to perform routine cultures to identify catheter-associated bacteriuria, especially in high-risk patients, is an important issue for hospital epidemiologists. The effective use of closed drainage requires ongoing surveillance, or periodic culture monitoring as recommended by Kunin (7), to uncover epidemic rates, evidence of cross-infection, and possible environmental sources of exogenous infection. The prevention of mortality that is not associated with bacteremia or sepsis may also challenge current approaches to asymptomatic bacteriuria (58).

The generalization that asymptomatic catheter-associated UTIs should not be treated is already outmoded for certain patient populations. Immunocompromised patients and those undergoing a urologic operation or a surgical procedure involving prosthetic material may also be at high risk for complications of untreated asymptomatic bacteriuria. One study found that asymptomatic bacteriuria in women after short-term catheterization also warranted therapy, even though the bacteriuria resolved spontaneously in 36% of patients (228). In addition, asymptomatic *S. marcescens* UTIs, known to cause a high rate of bacteremia with a prolonged lag time between the onset of bacteriuria and the development of bacteremia, may warrant treatment (55). Therefore, as hospital populations change with increasing numbers of critically ill and immunocompromised patients, many patients with asymptomatic bacteriuria should be treated.

Routine monitoring of catheter urine cultures could, in theory, promote more restrained and targeted antibiotic use in catheterized patients and could help eliminate environmental reservoirs of antibiotic-resistant microorganisms (229). More than 80% of catheterized patients receive antibiotics for treatment or prophylaxis of nonurinary infections. Selection of resistance can occur when these antibiotics remain in the drainage bag for extended periods. Virtually no studies assess the contribution of UTIs to the overall problem of antibiotic resistance or means to eliminate these reservoirs of resistant microorganisms. Furthermore, concern has been expressed that the use of antimicrobial-coated catheters may select for resistant microorganisms.

Candiduria is an emerging problem with a still unclear natural history and few controlled trials of the efficacy of treatment with antifungal agents. Catheter-associated candiduria may resolve in 35% to 40% of patients with catheter removal and in 20% with catheter change alone without antifungal therapy (230,231). On the other hand, the clearance of candiduria by treatment with fluconazole was only temporary (230). Consensus guidelines developed by the Infectious Diseases Society of America for the treatment of urinary candidiasis recommended treatment for certain types of patients, including those with symptoms, neutropenia, or renal allografts, those undergoing urologic manipulation, and low birth weight infants (232). Because use of fluconazole is a risk factor for *Candida glabrata* UTI (233) and because the benefits of treatment are still unclear, treatment of catheterized patients with this agent should be avoided if possible.

CONCLUSION

In recent years a patient safety movement has gathered momentum throughout the world, generating broad public interest in and support for efforts to prevent medical mistakes and adverse clinical outcomes. Nosocomial infections are the most common complications affecting hospitalized patients (234, 235), and catheter-associated UTIs are the most frequent and perhaps most preventable type of hospital-acquired infection. Despite several decades of investigation by clinicians and epidemiologists, advances in the prevention of such infections are disappointing. Strategies for prevention have been evaluated in randomized controlled trials more frequently for infections associated with urinary catheters than for any other type of nosocomial infection. Often, these studies were necessary because of the aggressive marketing of newer modifications of closed drainage systems by their manufacturers. Most of the well-designed large trials found no significant benefits of the new devices and saved healthcare costs through avoidance of more costly equipment. However, other trials have reduced healthcare costs by identifying widely used preventive measures that were not cost-effective or were even harmful. This frustrating history now appears to be a recurring theme with the recent marketing of antimicrobial-coated catheters accompanied by enthusiastic initial reports, followed by disappointing large-scale trials.

Despite the research efforts of a small cadre of committed investigators, hospital epidemiologists have neglected nosocomial UTIs because these infections are associated with relatively low mortality and costs. A reappraisal of the status of UTIs is overdue because of the important relation between antibiotic use in patients with urinary drainage systems and the emergence of multiply antibiotic-resistant hospital pathogens. Drug resistance is now a global problem with the threat of bacterial infections that cannot be treated with any existing antibiotic and limited prospects for the development of more effective antibiotics. Therefore, we can no longer afford to neglect a category of infection that accounts for nearly half of the hospital-acquired infections; nor can we ignore a patient population—those with indwelling urinary catheter systems—in which antibiotic use is so prevalent.

Epidemiologists must more fully examine and assure the appropriate use of urinary drainage, not simply the problem of nosocomial UTIs. Kunin (236) has emphasized that the unnecessary and prolonged use of catheters, the most obvious cause of nosocomial UTIs, must be addressed rather than waiting for the perfect technology. Epidemiologists must employ the strengths of their own discipline and not rely only on technical advances from industry.

The agenda for hospital epidemiologists is clear: to eliminate unnecessary urethral catheterization, to promote noninvasive alternatives to the Foley catheter, to reduce the duration of catheterization, and to promote aseptic care of closed drainage systems. Quality improvement programs can successfully restrict the initial use and reduce the duration of catheterization (42), and innovative methods such as the ultrasound bladder scan (219,220) can also reduce the use of indwelling urinary catheters in some clinical situations. Because marked variation is inherent in the management of urinary drainage, the techniques of quality management and continuous quality improvement may be especially suitable to identify and implement the best practices. These strategies depend on epidemiologists for the definition and measurement of important outcomes. In an era that touts outcomes research and patient safety, managing urinary drainage represents a model in which the outcomes are definable and important (see Chapters 9 to 13).

REFERENCES

1. Lohr JA, Donowitz LG, Sadler JE III. Hospital-acquired urinary tract infection. *Pediatrics* 1989;83:193–199.
2. Stamm WE. Infections related to medical devices. *Ann Intern Med* 1978:89(part 2):764–769.
3. Maki DG. Risk factors for nosocomial infection in intensive care. "Devices vs nature" and goals for the next decade. *Arch Intern Med* 1989:149;30–35.
4. Slade N, Gillespie WA. *The urinary tract and the catheter. Infection and other problems.* New York: Wiley, 1985:63.
5. Foley FEB. Cystoscopic prostatectomy. A new procedure and instrument; preliminary report. *J Urol* 1929;21:289–306.
6. Foley FEB. A hemostatic bag catheter. A one piece latex rubber structure for control of bleeding and constant drainage following prostatic resection. *J Urol* 1936;35:134–139.
7. Kunin CM. Care of the urinary catheter. In: *Urinary tract infections. Detection, prevention, and management,* 5th ed. Baltimore: Williams & Wilkins, 1997:226–278.
8. Schaberg DR, Haley RW, Highsmith AK, et al. Nosocomial bacteriuria: a prospective study of case clustering and antimicrobial resistance. *Ann Intern Med* 1980;93:420–424.
9. Dukes C. Urinary infections after excision of the rectum: their cause and prevention. *Proc R Soc Med* 1928;22:259–269.
10. Pyrah LN, Goldie W, Parsons FM, et al. Control of *Pseudomonas pyocyanea* infection in a urological ward. *Lancet* 1955;2:314–317.
11. Miller A, Gillespie WA, Linton KB, et al. Postoperative infection in urology. *Lancet* 1958;2:608–612.
12. Miller A, Linton KB, Gillespie WA, et al. Catheter drainage and infection in acute retention of urine. *Lancet* 1960;1:310–312.
13. Desautels RE. Aseptic management of catheter drainage. *N Engl J Med* 1960;263:189–191.
14. Desautels RE, Walter CW, Graves RC, et al. Technical advances in the prevention of urinary tract infection. *J Urol* 1962;87:487–490.
15. Kunin CM, McCormack RC. Prevention of catheter-induced urinary-tract infections by sterile closed drainage. *N Engl J Med* 1966;274: 1155–1161.
16. Gillespie WA, Lennon GG, Linton KB, et al. Prevention of urinary infection by means of closed drainage into a sterile plastic bag. *Br Med J* 1967;2:90–92.
17. Desautels RE. The causes of catheter-induced urinary infections and their prevention. *J Urol* 1969;101:757–760.
18. A Report from the National Nosocomial Infections Surveillance (NNIS) System. Nosocomial infection rates for interhospital compari-

son: limitations and possible solutions. *Infect Control Hosp Epidemiol* 1991;12:609–621.
19. National Nosocomial Infections Surveillance (NNIS) System Report, data summary from January 1992 to June 2002, issued August 2002. *Am J Infect Control* 2002;30:458–475.
20. Burgert SJ, Burke JP. Antibiotic resistance: will infection control meet the challenge? [editorial]. *Am J Infect Control* 1994;22:193–194.
21. Vartvarian SE, Papadakis KA, Anaissie EJ. *Stenotrophomonas (Xanthomonas) maltophilia* urinary tract infections. A disease that is usually severe and complicated. *Arch Intern Med* 1996;156:433–435.
22. Strausbaugh LJ, Crossley KB, Nurse BA, et al. Antimicrobial resistance in long-term-care facilities. *Infect Control Hosp Epidemiol* 1996; 17:129–140.
23. Beeson PB. The case against the catheter [editorial]. *Am J Med* 1958; 24:1–3.
24. Kunin CM. Can we build a better urinary catheter? [editorial]. *N Engl J Med* 1988;319:365–366.
25. Jarvis WR. Hospital Infections Program, Centers for Disease Control and Prevention on-site outbreak investigations, 1990 to 1999. *Semin Infect Control* 2001;1:74–84.
26. Villarino ME, Stevens LE, Schable B, et al. Risk factors for epidemic *Xanthomonas maltophilia* infection/colonization in intensive care unit patients. *Infect Control Hosp Epidemiol* 1992;13:201–206.
27. Scheckler WE. Nosocomial infections in a community hospital: 1972 through 1976. *Arch Intern Med* 1978;138:1792–1794.
28. Garibaldi RA, Burke JP, Dickman ML, et al. Factors predisposing to bacteriuria during indwelling urethral catheterization. *N Engl J Med* 1974;291;215–219.
29. Burke JP, Larsen RA, Stevens LE. Nosocomial bacteriuria: estimating the potential for prevention by closed sterile urinary drainage. *Infect Control* 1986;7(suppl):96–99.
30. Kass EH, Sossen HS. Prevention of infection of urinary tract in presence of indwelling catheters. Description of electromechanical valve to provide intermittent drainage of the bladder. *JAMA* 1959;169: 1181–1183.
31. Jepsen OB, Larsen SO, Dankert J, et al. Urinary-tract infection and bacteraemia in hospitalized medical patients—a European multicentre prevalence survey on nosocomial infection. *J Hosp Infect* 1982; 3:241–252.
32. Zimakoff J, Pontoppidan B, Larsen SO, et al. Management of urinary bladder function in Danish hospitals, nursing homes and home care. *J Hosp Infect* 1993;24:183–199.
33. Burman LG, Fryklund B, Nystrom B. Use of indwelling urinary tract catheters in Swedish hospitals. *Infect Control* 1987;8:507–511.
34. Richards MJ, Edwards JR, Culver DH, et al., and the National Nosocomial Infections Surveillance System. Nosocomial infections in medical intensive care units in the United States. *Crit Care Med* 1999; 27:887–892.
35. Shapiro M, Simchen E, Izraeli S, et al. A multivariate analysis of risk factors for acquiring bacteriuria in patients with indwelling urinary catheters for longer than 24 hours. *Infect Control* 1984;5:525–532.
36. Gardam MA, Amihod B, Orenstein P, et al. Overutilization of indwelling urinary catheters and the development of nosocomial urinary tract infections. *Clin Perform Quality Health Care* 1998;6:99–102.
37. Jain P, Parada JP, David A, et al. Overuse of the indwelling urinary tract catheter in hospitalized medical patients. *Arch Intern Med* 1995; 155:1425–1429.
38. Munasinghe RL, Yazdani H, Siddique M, et al. Appropriateness of use of indwelling urinary catheters in patients admitted to the medical service. *Infect Control Hosp Epidemiol* 2001; 22:647–649.
39. Bouza E, Rodríguez-Bouza H, Muñoz P, et al. Evaluation of indwelling bladder catheterization in a general hospital. *Infect Dis Clin Pract* 1994;3:358–362.
40. Saint S, Wiese J, Amory JK, et al. Are physicians aware of which of their patients have indwelling urinary catheters? *Am J Med* 2000;109: 476–480.
41. Brennan ML, Evans A. Why catheterize?: audit findings on the use of urinary catheters. *Br J Nurs* 2001;10:580–590.
42. Dumigan DG, Kohan CA, Reed CR, et al. Utilizing National Nosocomial Infection Surveillance System data to improve urinary tract infection rates in three intensive-care units. *Clin Perform Qual Health Care* 1998;6:172–178.
43. Cornia PB, Amory JK, Fraser S, et al. Computer-based order entry decreases duration of indwelling urinary catheterization in hospitalized patients. *Am J Med* 2003;114:404–407.
44. Haley RW, Hooton TM, Culver DH, et al. Nosocomial infections in U.S. hospitals, 1975–1976. Estimated frequency by selected characteristics of patients. *Am J Med* 1981;70:947– 959.
45. Huth TS, Burke JP. Infections and antibiotic use in a community hospital, 1971–1990. *Infect Control Hosp Epidemiol* 1991;12: 525–534.
46. Merle V, Germain J-M, Bugel H, et al. Nosocomial urinary tract infections in urologic patients: assessment of a prospective surveillance program including 10,000 patients. *Eur Urol* 2002;41:483–489.
47. Langley JM, Hanakowski M, LeBlanc JC. Unique epidemiology of nosocomial urinary tract infection in children. *Am J Infect Control* 2001;29:94–98.
48. Haley RW, Culver DH, White JW, et al. The nationwide nosocomial infection rate. A new need for vital statistics. *Am J Epidemiol* 1985; 121:159–167.
49. Centers for Disease Control. Public health focus: surveillance, prevention, and control of nosocomial infections. *MMWR* 1992;41: 783–787.
50. Classen DC. *Assessing the effect of adverse hospital events on the cost of hospitalization and other patient outcomes* [thesis]. Salt Lake City, Utah: University of Utah, 1993.
51. Saint S. Clinical and economic consequences of nosocomial catheter-related bacteriuria. *Am J Infect Control* 2000;28:68–75.
52. Tambyah PA, Knasinski V, Maki DG. The direct costs of nosocomial catheter-associated urinary tract infection in the era of managed care. *Infect Control Hosp Epidemiol* 2002;23:27–31.
53. Garibaldi RA, Mooney BR, Epstein BJ, et al. An evaluation of daily bacteriological monitoring to identify preventable episodes of catheter-associated urinary tract infection. *Infect Control* 1982;3:466–470.
54. Bryan CS, Reynolds KL. Hospital-acquired bacteremic urinary tract infection: epidemiology and outcome. *J Urol* 1984;132:494–498.
55. Krieger JN, Kaiser DL, Wenzel RP. Urinary tract etiology of bloodstream infections in hospitalized patients. *J Infect Dis* 1983;148: 57–62.
56. Sullivan NM, Sutter VL, Mims MM, et al. Clinical aspects of bacteremia after manipulation of the genitourinary tract. *J Infect Dis* 1973; 127:49–55.
57. Martin CM, Vaquer F, Meyers MS, et al. Prevention of Gram-negative rod bacteremia associated with indwelling urinary tract catheterization. In: Sylvester JC, ed. *Antimicrobial agents and chemotherapy—1963.* Ann Arbor, MI: Braun-Brumfield, 1964:617–623.
58. Platt R, Polk BF, Murdock B, et al. Mortality associated with nosocomial urinary-tract infection. *N Engl J Med* 1982;307:637–642.
59. Warren JW, Damron D, Tenney JH, et al. Fever, bacteremia, and death as complications of bacteriuria in women with long-term urethral catheters. *J Infect Dis* 1987;155:1151–1158.
60. Milles G. Catheter-induced hemorrhagic pseudopolyps of the urinary bladder. *JAMA* 1965;193:968–969.
61. Ekelund P, Anderström C, Johansson SL, et al. The reversibility of catheter-associated polypoid cystitis. *J Urol* 1983;130:456–459.
62. Kantor AF, Hartge P, Hoover RN, et al. Urinary tract infection and risk of bladder cancer. *Am J Epidemiol* 1984;119:510–515.
63. Sellett T. Iatrogenic urethral injury due to preinflation of a Foley catheter. *JAMA* 1971;217:1548–1549.
64. Rubinstein A, Benaroya Y, Rubinstein E. Foley catheter perforation of the urinary bladder [letter]. *JAMA* 1976;236:822.
65. Busse K, Altwein JE. Catheter-induced bladder gangrene. *J Urol* 1974; 112:461–462.
66. Merguerian PA, Erturk E, Hulbert WC Jr, et al. Peritonitis and abdominal free air due to intraperitoneal bladder perforation associated with indwelling urethral catheter drainage. *J Urol* 1985;134:747–750.
67. Elhilali MM, Hassouna M, Abdel-Hakim A, et al. Urethral stricture following cardiovascular surgery: role of urethral ischemia. *J Urol* 1986;135:275–277.

68. Brawley RL, Weber DJ, Samsa GP, et al. Multiple nosocomial infections. An incidence study. *Am J Epidemiol* 1989;130:769–780.
69. Trilla A, Gatell JM, Mensa J, et al. Risk factors for nosocomial bacteremia in a large Spanish teaching hospital: a case-control study. *Infect Control Hosp Epidemiol* 1991;12:150–156.
70. Coello R, Charlett A, Ward V, et al. Device-related sources of bacteraemia in English hospitals—opportunities for the prevention of hospital-acquired bacteraemia. *J Hosp Infect* 2003;53:46–57.
71. Krieger JN, Kaiser DL, Wenzel RP. Nosocomial urinary tract infections cause wound infections postoperatively in surgical patients. *Surg Gynecol Obstet* 1983;156:313–318.
72. Lobo PI, Rudolf LE, Krieger JN. Wound infections in renal transplant recipients—a complication of urinary tract infections during allograft malfunction. *Surgery* 1982;3:491–496.
73. Krieger JN, Tapia L, Stubenbord WR, et al. Urinary infection in kidney transplantation. *Urology* 1977;9:130–136.
74. Quenzer RW, Edwards LD, Levin S. A comparative study of 48 host valve and 24 prosthetic valve endocarditis cases. *Am Heart J* 1976; 92:15–22.
75. Dismukes WE, Karchmer AW, Buckley MJ, et al. Prosthetic valve endocarditis. Analysis of 38 cases. *Circulation* 1973;48:365–377.
76. Wroblewski BM, del Sel HJ. Urethral instrumentation and deep sepsis in total hip replacement. *Clin Orthop* 1980;146:209–212.
77. Irvine R, Johnson BL, Amstutz HC. The relationship of genitourinary tract procedures and deep sepsis after total hip replacements. *Surg Gynecol Obstet* 1974;139:701–706.
78. Kovacevich DS, Faubion WC, Bender JM, et al. Association of parenteral nutrition catheter sepsis with urinary tract infections. *J Parenteral Enteral Nutr* 1986;10:639–641.
79. Marier R, Valenti AJ, Madri JA. Gram-negative endocarditis following cystoscopy. *J Urol* 1978;119:134–137.
80. Ponte CD, McDonald M. Septic discitis resulting from *Escherichia coli* urosepsis. *J Fam Pract* 1992;34:767–771.
81. Krieger JN, Kaiser DL, Wenzel RP. Nosocomial urinary tract infections: secular trends, treatment and economics in a university hospital. *J Urol* 1983;130:102–106.
82. Bronsema DA, Adams JR, Pallares R, et al. Secular trends in rates and etiology of nosocomial urinary tract infections at a university hospital. *J Urol* 1993;150:414–416.
83. Sewell CM, Koza MA, Luchi RJ, et al. Risk factors associated with a cluster of urinary tract infections in a geriatric unit caused by *Klebsiella pneumoniae* resistant to multiple antibiotics. *Am J Infect Control* 1988; 16:66–71.
84. Schaberg DR, Weinstein RA, Stamm WE. Epidemics of nosocomial urinary tract infection caused by multiply resistant gram-negative bacilli: epidemiology and control. *J Infect Dis* 1976;133:363–366.
85. Schaberg DR, Highsmith AK, Wachsmuth IK. Resistance plasmid transfer by *Serratia marcescens* in urine. *Antimicrob Agents Chemother* 1977;11:449–450.
86. Schaberg DR, Alford RH, Anderson R, et al. An outbreak of nosocomial infection due to multiply resistant *Serratia marcescens*: evidence of interhospital spread. *J Infect Dis* 1976;134:181–188.
87. Kaslow RA, Lindsey JO, Bisno AL, et al. Nosocomial infection with highly resistant *Proteus rettgeri*. Report of an epidemic. *Am J Epidemiol* 1976;104:278–286.
88. Lindsey JO, Martin WT, Sonnenwirth AC, et al. An outbreak of nosocomial *Proteus rettgeri* urinary tract infection. *Am J Epidemiol* 1976;103:261–269.
89. Washington JA II, Senjem DH, Haldorson A, et al. Nosocomially acquired bacteriuria due to *Proteus rettgeri* and *Providencia stuartii*. *Am J Clin Pathol* 1973;60:836–838.
90. Krieger JN, Levy-Zombeck E, Scheidt A, et al. A nosocomial epidemic of antibiotic-resistant *Serratia marcescens* urinary tract infections. *J Urol* 1980;124:498–502.
91. Echols RM, Palmer DL, King RM, et al. Multidrug-resistant *Serratia marcescens* bacteriuria related to urologic instrumentation. *South Med J* 1984;77:173–177.
92. Okuda T, Endo N, Osada Y, et al. Outbreak of nosocomial urinary tract infections caused by *Serratia marcescens*. *J Clin Microbiol* 1984; 20:691–695.
93. Strand CL, Bryant JK, Morgan JW, et al. Nosocomial *Pseudomonas aeruginosa* urinary tract infections. *JAMA* 1982;248:1615–1618.
94. Marrie TJ, Major H, Gurwith M, et al. Prolonged outbreak of nosocomial urinary tract infection with a single strain of *Pseudomonas aeruginosa*. *Can Med Assoc J* 1978;119:593–598.
95. Fierer J, Ekstrom M. An outbreak of *Providencia stuartii* urinary tract infections. Patients with condom catheters are a reservoir of the bacteria. *JAMA* 1981;245:1553–1555.
96. Stone J, Manasse R. Pseudoepidemic of urinary tract infections due to *Trichosporon beigelii*. *Infect Control Hosp Epidemiol* 1989;10: 312–315.
97. Emori TG, Gaynes RP. An overview of nosocomial infections, including the role of the microbiology laboratory. *Clin Microbiol Rev* 1993; 6:428–442.
98. Alling B, Brandberg A, Seeberg S, et al. Aerobic and anaerobic microbial flora in the urinary tract of geriatric patients during long-term care. *J Infect Dis* 1973;127:34–39.
99. Brook I. Anaerobic bacteria in suppurative genitourinary infections. *J Urol* 1989;141:889–893.
100. Lee BK, Crossley K, Gerding DN. The association between *Staphylococcus aureus* bacteremia and bacteriuria. *Am J Med* 1978;65:303–306.
101. Demuth PJ, Gerding DN. *Staphylococcus aureus* bacteriuria. *Arch Intern Med* 1979;139:78–80.
102. Arpi M, Renneberg J. The clinical significance of *Staphylococcus aureus* bacteriuria. *J Urol* 1984;132:697–700.
103. Larsen RL, Burke JP. The epidemiology and risk factors for nosocomial catheter-associated bacteriuria caused by coagulase-negative staphylococci. *Infect Control* 1986;7:212–215.
104. Warren JW, Tenney JH, Hoopes JM, et al. A prospective microbiologic study of bacteriuria in patients with chronic indwelling urethral catheters. *J Infect Dis* 1982;146:719–723.
105. Hooton TM, Johnson C, Winter C, et al. Single-dose and three-day regimens of ofloxacin versus trimethoprim-sulfamethoxazole for acute cystitis in women. *Antimicrob Agents Chemother* 1991;35:1479–1483.
106. Kisielius PV, Schwan WR, Amundsen SK, et al. *In vivo* expression and variation of *Escherichia coli* type 1 and P pili in the urine of adults with acute urinary tract infections. *Infect Immun* 1989;57: 1656–1662.
107. Ikäheimo R, Siitonen A, Kärkkäinen U, et al. Virulence characteristics of *Escherichia coli* in nosocomial urinary tract infection. *Clin Infect Dis* 1993;16:785–791.
108. Hollick GE, Nolte FS, Calnan BJ, et al. Characterization of endemic *Providencia stuartii* isolates from patients with urinary devices. *Eur J Clin Microbiol* 1984;3:521–525.
109. Riley DK, Classen DC, Stevens LE, et al. A large randomized clinical trial of a silver impregnated urinary catheter: lack of efficacy and staphylococcal superinfection. *Am J Med* 1995;98:349–356.
110. Hamory BH, Wenzel RP. Hospital-associated candiduria: predisposing factors and review of the literature. *J Urol* 1978;120:444–448.
111. Ang BSP, Telenti A, King B, et al. Candidemia from a urinary tract source: microbiological aspects and clinical significance. *Clin Infect Dis* 1993;17:662–666.
112. Jacobs L, Skidmore E, Freeman K, et al. Oral fluconazole compared with bladder irrigation with amphotericin B for treatment of fungal urinary tract infections in elderly patients. *Clin Infect Dis* 1996;22: 30–35.
113. Nassoura Z, Ivtury R, Simon R, et al. Candiduria as an early marker of disseminated infection in critically ill patients: the role of fluconazole therapy. *J Trauma* 1993;35:290–295.
114. Wainstein M, Graham R, Resnick M. Predisposing factors of systemic fungal infections of the genitourinary tract. *J Urol* 1995;154: 160–163.
115. Onorato IM, Morens DM, Martone WJ, et al. Epidemiology of cytomegaloviral infections: recommendations for prevention and control. *Rev Infect Dis* 1985;7:479–497.
116. Balfour CL, Balfour HH Jr. Cytomegalovirus is not an occupational risk for nurses in renal transplant and neonatal units. Results of a prospective surveillance study. *JAMA* 1986;256:1909–1914.
117. Adler SP. Hospital transmission of cytomegalovirus. *Infect Agents Dis* 1992;1:43–49.

118. Skolnik PR, Kosloff BR, Bechtel LJ, et al. Absence of infectious HIV-1 in the urine of seropositive viremic subjects. *J Infect Dis* 1989;160: 1056–1060.
119. Stamey TA, Mihara G. Observations on the growth of urethral and vaginal bacteria in sterile urine. *J Urol* 1980;124:461–463.
120. Chambers ST, Kunin CM. Isolation of glycine betaine and proline betaine from human urine. Assessment of their role as osmoprotective agents for bacteria and the kidney. *J Clin Invest* 1987;79:731–737.
121. Bran JL, Levison ME, Kaye D. Entrance of bacteria into the female urinary bladder. *N Engl J Med* 1972;286:626–629.
122. Stark RP, Maki DG. Bacteriuria in the catheterized patient. What quantitative level of bacteriuria is relevant? *N Engl J Med* 1984;311: 560–564.
123. Dutton AAC, Ralston M. Urinary tract infection in a male urological ward with special reference to the mode of infection. *Lancet* 1957;1: 115–119.
124. Kunin CM, Evans C, Bartholomew D, et al. The antimicrobial defense mechanism of the female urethra: a reassessment. *J Urol* 2002; 168:413–419
125. Zimmerli W, Lew PD, Waldvogel FA. Pathogenesis of foreign body infection. Evidence for a local granulocyte defect. *J Clin Invest* 1984; 73:1191–1200.
126. Schilling JD, Martin SM, Hung CS, et al. Toll-like receptor 4 on stromal and hematopoietic cells mediates innate resistance to uropathogenic *Escherichia coli. Proc Natl Acad Sci USA* 2003;100: 4203–4208.
127. Anderson GG, Palermo JJ, Schilling JD, et al. Intracellular bacterial biofilm-like pods in urinary tract infections. *Science* 2003;301: 105–107.
128. Tambyah PA, Maki DG. Catheter-associated urinary tract infection is rarely symptomatic. A prospective study of 1497 catheterized patients. *Arch Intern Med* 2000;160:678–682.
129. Tambyah PA, Maki DG. The relationship between pyuria and infection in patients with indwelling urinary catheters. A prospective study of 761 patients. *Arch Intern Med* 2000;160:673–677.
130. Ganz T. Defensins in the urinary tract and other tissues. *J Infect Dis* 2001;183(suppl 1):S41–S42.
131. Daifuku R, Stamm WE. Bacterial adherence to bladder uroepithelial cells in catheter-associated urinary tract infection. *N Engl J Med* 1986; 314:1208–1213.
132. Dankert J, Hogt AH, Feijen J. Biomedical polymers: bacterial adhesion, colonization, and infection. *CRC Crit Rev Biocompat* 1986;2: 219–301.
133. Roberts JA, Kaack MB, Fussell EN. Adherence to urethral catheters by bacteria causing nosocomial infections. *Urology* 1993;41:338–342.
134. Monson T, Kunin CM. Evaluation of a polymer-coated indwelling catheter in prevention of infection. *J Urol* 1974;111:220–222.
135. Tidd MJ, Gow JG, Pennington JH, et al. Comparison of hydrophilic polymer-coated latex, uncoated latex and PVC indwelling balloon catheters in the prevention of urinary infection. *Br J Urol* 1976;48: 285–291.
136. Classen DC, Larsen RA, Burke JP, et al. Prevention of catheter-associated bacteriuria: clinical trial of methods to block three known pathways of infection. *Am J Infect Control* 1991;19:136–142.
137. Bruce AW, Plumpton KJ, Willett WS, et al. Urethral response to latex and Silastic catheters. *Can Med Assoc J* 1976;115:1099–1100.
138. Anderson RU. Response of bladder and urethral mucosa to catheterization. *JAMA* 1979;242:451–454.
139. Donlan RM. Biofilms: microbial life on surfaces. *Emerg Infect Dis* 2002;8:881–890.
140. Donlan RM. Biofilms and device-associated infections. *Emerg Infect Dis* 2001;7:277–281.
141. Donlan RM. Biofilm formation: a clinically relevant microbiological process. *Clin Infect Dis* 2001;33:1387–1392.
142. Habash M, Reid G. Microbial biofilms: their development and significance for medical device-related infections. *J Clin Pharmacol* 1999; 39:887–898.
143. Fletcher M, Loeb GI. Influence of substratum characteristics on attachment of a marine pseudomonad to solid surfaces. *Appl Environ Microbiol* 1979;37:67–72.
144. Prigent-Combaret C, Vidal O, Dorel C, et al. Abiotic surface sensing and biofilm-dependent regulation of gene expression in *Escherichia coli. J Bacteriol* 1999;181:5993–6002.
145. Flemming H-C, Wingender J, Griebe T, et al. Physico-chemical properties of biofilms. In: Evans LV, ed. *Biofilms: recent advances in their study and control.* Amsterdam: Harwood Academic, 2000:19–34.
146. Donlan RM. Role of biofilms in antimicrobial resistance. *ASAIO J* 2000;46;S47–S52.
147. Davies DG, Parsek MR, Pearson JP, et al. The involvement of cell-to-cell signals in the development of a bacterial biofilm. *Science* 1998; 280:295–297.
148. Lewis K. Riddle of biofilm resistance. *Antimicrob Agents Chemother* 2001;45:999–1007.
149. Brooun A, Liu S, Lewis K. A dose-response study of antibiotic resistance in *Pseudomonas aeruginosa* biofilms. *Antimicrob Agents Chemother* 2000;44:640–646.
150. Pazin GJ, Braude AI. Immobilizing antibodies in urine. II. Prevention of ascending spread of *Proteus mirabilis. Invest Urol* 1974;12: 129–133.
151. Johnson JR. Virulence factors in *Escherichia coli* urinary tract infection. *Clin Microbiol Rev* 1991;4:80–128.
152. Benton J, Chawla J, Parry S, et al. Virulence factors in *Escherichia coli* from urinary tract infections in patients with spinal injuries. *J Hosp Infect* 1992;22:117–127.
153. Rubinstein E, Tavdioglu B, Schwartzkopf R, et al. Screening of urinary pathogens obtained from catheterized patients for mannose-specific lectin: clinical implications. *Isr J Med Sci* 1982;18:469–473.
154. Mobley HLT, Chippendale GR, Tenney JH, et al. Expression of type 1 fimbriae may be required for persistence of *Escherichia coli* in the catheterized urinary tract. *J Clin Microbiol* 1987;25:2253–2257.
155. Mulvey MA, Schilling JD, Martinez JJ, et al. Bad bugs and beleaguered bladders: interplay between uropathogenic *Escherichia coli* and innate host defenses. *Proc Natl Acad Sci USA* 2000;97:8829–8835.
156. Mobley HLT, Chippendale GR, Tenney JH, et al. MR/K hemagglutination of *Providencia stuartii* correlates with adherence to catheters and with persistence in catheter-associated bacteriuria. *J Infect Dis* 1988;157:264–271.
157. Johnson RJ, Orskov I, Orskov F, et al. O, K, and H antigens predict virulence factors, carboxylesterase B pattern, antimicrobial resistance, and host compromise among *Escherichia coli* strains causing urosepsis. *J Infect Dis* 1994;169:119–126.
158. Soriano F, Aguado JM, Ponte C, et al. Urinary tract infection caused by Corynebacterium group D2: report of 82 cases and review. *Rev Infect Dis* 1990;12:1019–1034.
159. Musher DM, Griffith DP, Yawn D, et al. Role of urease in pyelonephritis resulting from urinary tract infection with *Proteus. J Infect Dis* 1975;131:177–181.
160. Thornton GF, Andriole VT. Bacteriuria during indwelling catheter drainage. II. Effect of a closed sterile drainage system. *JAMA* 1970; 214:339–342.
161. Warren JW, Platt R, Thomas RJ, et al. Antibiotic irrigation and catheter-associated urinary-tract infections. *N Engl J Med* 1978;299: 570–573.
162. Garibaldi RA, Burke JP, Britt MR, et al. Meatal colonization and catheter-associated bacteriuria. *N Engl J Med* 1980;303:316–318.
163. Schaeffer AJ, Chmiel J. Urethral meatal colonization in the pathogenesis of catheter-associated bacteriuria. *J Urol* 1983;130:1096–1099.
164. Daifuku R, Stamm WE. Association of rectal and urethral colonization with urinary tract infection in patients with indwelling catheters. *JAMA* 1984;252:2028–2030.
165. Platt R, Polk BF, Murdock B, et al. Risk factors for nosocomial urinary tract infection. *Am J Epidemiol* 1986;124:977–985.
166. Burke JP, Jacobson JT, Jacobson JA, et al. Origins of urinary catheter-associated bacteremia. *Clin Res* 1978;26:391A(abst).
167. Sanford JP. Hospital-acquired urinary-tract infections. *Ann Intern Med* 1964;60:903–914.
168. Guze LB, Beeson PB. Observations on the reliability and safety of bladder catheterization for bacteriologic study of the urine. *N Engl J Med* 1956;255:474–475.

169. Kass EH. Bacteriuria and diagnosis of infections of the urinary tract. *Arch Intern Med* 1957;100:709–715.
170. Hirsh DD, Fainstein V, Musher DM. Do condom catheter collecting systems cause urinary tract infection? *JAMA* 1979;242:340–341.
171. Tambyah PA, Halvorson KT, Maki DG. A prospective study of pathogenesis of catheter-associated urinary tract infections. *Mayo Clin Proc* 1999;74:131–136.
172. Carapeti EA, Andrews SM, Bentley PG. Randomised study of sterile vs non-sterile urethral catheterization. *Ann R Coll Surg Engl* 1996; 78:59–60.
173. Weyrauch HM, Bassitt JB. Ascending infection in an artificial urinary tract. *Stanford Med Bull* 1951;9:25.
174. Kass EH, Schneiderman LJ. Entry of bacteria into the urinary tracts of patients with inlying catheters. *N Engl J Med* 1957;256:556–557.
175. Brehmer B, Madsen PO. Route and prophylaxis of ascending bladder infection in male patients with indwelling catheters. *J Urol* 1972;108: 719–721.
176. Bultitude MI, Eykyn S. The relationship between the urethral flora and urinary infection in the catheterised male. *Br J Urol* 1973;45: 678–683.
177. Thompson RL, Haley CE, Searcy MA, et al. Catheter-associated bacteriuria. Failure to reduce attack rates using periodic instillations of a disinfectant into urinary drainage systems. *JAMA* 1984;251:747–751.
178. Maki DG, Hennekens CG, Phillips CW, et al. Nosocomial urinary tract infection with *Serratia marcescens*: an epidemiologic study. *J Infect Dis* 1973;128:579–587.
179. Selden R, Lee S, Wang WLL, et al. Nosocomial *Klebsiella* infections: intestinal colonization as a reservoir. *Ann Intern Med* 1971;74: 657–664.
180. Olson B, Weinstein RA, Nathan C, et al. Occult aminoglycoside resistance in *Pseudomonas aeruginosa:* epidemiology and implications for therapy and control. *J Infect Dis* 1985;152:769–774.
181. Kunin CM, Steele C. Culture of the surfaces of urinary catheters to sample urethral flora and study the effect of antimicrobial therapy. *J Clin Microbiol* 1985;21:902–908.
182. Stamm WE, Daifuku R. Bacteriuria: colonization or infection [letter]. *JAMA* 1985;253:1879.
183. Garner JS, Jarvis WR, Emori TG, et al. CDC definitions for nosocomial infections, 1988. *Am J Infect Control* 1988;16:128–140.
184. Stamm WE, Hooton TM. Management of urinary tract infections in adults. *N Engl J Med* 1993;329:1328–1334.
185. Garibaldi RA. Catheter-associated urinary tract infection. *Curr Opin Infect Dis* 1992;5:517–523.
186. Moffat CM, Britt MR, Burke JP. Evaluation of miniature test for bacteriuria using dehydrated media and nitrite pads. *Appl Microbiol* 1974;28:95–99.
187. Birch DF. Dipslide screening of hospitalized patients for bacteriuria. *Med J Aust* 1971;1:1176–1178.
188. Rubin M, Berger SA, Zodda FN Jr, et al. Effect of catheter replacement on bacterial counts in urine aspirated from indwelling catheters. *J Infect Dis* 1980;142:291.
189. Gross PA, Harkavy LM, Barden GE, et al. Positive Foley catheter tip cultures—fact or fancy? *JAMA* 1974;228:72–73.
190. Musher DM, Thorsteinsson SB, Airola VM II. Quantitative urinalysis. Diagnosing urinary tract infection in men. *JAMA* 1976;236: 2069–2072.
191. Anderson RU, Hsieh-Ma ST. Association of bacteriuria and pyuria during intermittent catheterization after spinal cord injury. *J Urol* 1983;130:299–301.
192. Steward DK, Wood GL, Cohen RL, et al. Failure of the urinalysis and quantitative urine culture in diagnosing symptomatic urinary tract infections in patients with long-term urinary catheters. *Am J Infect Control* 1985;13:154–160.
193. Filice GA, Weiler MD, Hughes RA, et al. Nosocomial febrile illnesses in patients on an internal medicine service. *Arch Intern Med* 1989; 149:319–324.
194. Costel EE, Mitchell S, Kaiser AB. Abbreviated surveillance of nosocomial urinary tract infections: a new approach. *Infect Control* 1985;6: 11–13.
195. Ehrenkranz NJ, Alfonso BC. Failure of bland soap handwash to prevent hand transfer of patient bacteria to urethral catheters. *Infect Control Hosp Epidemiol* 1991;12:654–662.
196. Simmons B, Bryant J, Neiman K, et al. The role of handwashing in prevention of endemic intensive care unit infections. *Infect Control Hosp Epidemiol* 1990;11:589–594.
197. Haley RW, Culver DH, White JW, et al. The efficacy of infection surveillance and control programs in preventing nosocomial infections in US hospitals. *Am J Epidemiol* 1985;121:182–205.
198. Haley RW, Morgan WM, Culver DH, et al. Update from the SENIC Project. Hospital infection control: recent progress and opportunities under prospective payment. *Am J Infect Control* 1985;13:97–108.
199. Dieckhaus KD, Garibaldi RA. Prevention of catheter-associated urinary tract infections. In: Abrutyn E, Goldmann DA, Scheckler WE, eds. *Saunders Infection Control Reference Service: the experts guide to the guidelines,* 2nd ed. Philadelphia: WB Saunders, 257–262.
200. Burke JP, Garibaldi RA, Britt MR, et al. Prevention of catheter-associated urinary tract infections. Efficacy of daily meatal care regimens. *Am J Med* 1981;70:655–658.
201. Burke JP, Jacobson JA, Garibaldi RA, et al. Evaluation of daily meatal care with poly-antibiotic ointment in prevention of urinary catheter-associated bacteriuria. *J Urol* 1983;129:331–334.
202. Classen DC, Larsen RA, Burke JP, et al. Daily meatal care for prevention of catheter-associated bacteriuria: results using frequent applications of polyantibiotic cream. *Infect Control Hosp Epidemiol* 1991;12: 157–162.
203. Huth TS, Burke JP, Larsen RA, et al. Randomized trial of meatal care with silver sulfadiazine cream for the prevention of catheter-associated bacteriuria. *J Infect Dis* 1992;165:14–18.
204. Burke JP. Randomized controlled trials in hospital epidemiology. Sixth annual National Foundation for Infectious Diseases lecture. *Am J Infect Control* 1983;11:165–173.
205. Kunin CM. The future of hospital epidemiology. *Infect Control Hosp Epidemiol* 1989;10:276–279.
206. Mountokalakis T, Skounakis M, Tselentis J. Short-term versus prolonged systemic antibiotic prophylaxis in patients treated with indwelling catheters. *J Urol* 1985;134:506–508.
207. Platt R, Polk BF, Murdock B, et al. Prevention of catheter-associated urinary tract infection: a cost-benefit analysis. *Infect Control Hosp Epidemiol* 1989;10:60–64.
208. Platt R, Polk BF, Murdock B, et al. Reduction of mortality associated with nosocomial urinary tract infection. *Lancet* 1983;1:893–896.
209. Huth TS, Burke JP, Larsen RA, et al. Clinical trial of junction seals for the prevention of urinary catheter-associated bacteriuria. *Arch Intern Med* 1992;152:807–812.
210. Thibon P, Le Coutour X, Leroyer R, et al. Randomized multi-centre trial of the effects of a catheter coated with hydrogel and silver salts on the incidence of hospital-acquired urinary tract infections. *J Hosp Infect* 2000;45:117–124.
211. Karchmer TB, Giannetta ET, Muto CA, et al. A randomized crossover study of silver-coated urinary catheters in hospitalized patients. *Arch Intern Med* 2000;160:3294–3298.
212. Saint S, Veenstra DL, Sullivan SD, et al. The potential clinical and economic benefits of silver alloy urinary catheters in preventing urinary tract infections. *Arch Intern Med* 2000;160:2670–2675.
213. Niël-Weise BS, Arend SM, Van den Broek PJ. Is there evidence for recommending silver-coated urinary catheters in guidelines? *J Hosp Infect* 2002;52:81–87.
214. Lai KK, Fontecchio SA. Use of silver-hydrogel urinary catheters on the incidence of catheter-associated urinary tract infections in hospitalized patients. *Am J Infect Control* 2002;30:221–225.
215. Darouiche RO, Smith JA Jr, Hanna H, et al. Efficacy of antimicrobial-impregnated bladder catheters in reducing catheter-associated bacteriuria: a prospective, randomized, multicenter clinical trial. *Urology* 1999;54:976–981.
216. Johnson DE, O'Reilly JL, Warren JW. Clinical evaluation of an external urine collection device for nonambulatory incontinent women. *J Urol* 1989;141:535–537.
217. Nissenkorn I. The intraurethral catheter—three years of experience. *Eur Urol* 1993;24:27–30.

218. Brocklehurst JC, Hickey DS, Davies I, et al. A new urethral catheter. *Br Med J* 1988;296:1691–1693.
219. Moore DA, Edwards K. Using a portable bladder scan to reduce the incidence of nosocomial urinary tract infections. *Medsurg Nursing* 1997;6:39–42.
220. Slappendel R, Weber EWG. Non-invasive measurement of bladder volume as an indication for bladder catheterization after orthopaedic surgery and its effect on urinary tract infections. *Eur J Anaesthesiol* 1999;16:503–506.
221. Butler HK, Kunin CM. Evaluation of specific systemic antimicrobial therapy in patients while on closed catheter drainage. *J Urol* 1968; 100:567–572.
222. Warren JW, Anthony WC, Hoopes JM, et al. Cephalexin for susceptible bacteriuria in afebrile, long-term catheterized patients. *JAMA* 1982;248:454–458.
223. Peloquin CA, Cumbo TJ, Schentag JJ. Kinetics and dynamics of tobramycin action in patients with bacteriuria given single doses. *Antimicrob Agents Chemother* 1991;35:1191–1195.
224. Kumazawa J, Matsumoto T. The dipstick test in the diagnosis of UTI and the effect of pretreatment catheter exchange in catheter-associated UTI. *Infection* 1992;20(suppl 3):S157–S159.
225. Hyams KC. Inappropriate urine cultures in hospitalized patients receiving antibiotic therapy. *Arch Intern Med* 1987;147:48–49.
226. Kunin CM. Surveillance cultures of the urine and catheter placement [questions and answers]. *JAMA* 1992;267:1677.
227. Davies AJ, Shroff KJ. Catheter-associated urinary-tract infection [letter]. *Lancet* 1984;1:44.
228. Harding GKM, Nicolle LE, Ronald AR, et al. How long should catheter-acquired urinary tract infection in women be treated? A randomized controlled study. *Ann Intern Med* 1991;114:713–719.
229. Jacobson JA, Burke JP, Kasworm E. Effect of bacteriologic monitoring of urinary catheters on recognition and treatment of hospital-acquired urinary tract infections. *Infect Control* 1981;2:227–232.
230. Sobel JD, Kauffman CA, McKinsey D, et al. Candiduria: a randomized, double-blind study of treatment with fluconazole and placebo. *Clin Infect Dis* 2000;30:19–24.
231. Kauffman CA, Vasquez JA, Sobel JD, et al. Prospective multicenter surveillance of funguria in hospitalized patients. *Clin Infect Dis* 2000; 30:14–18.
232. Rex JH, Walsh TJ, Sobel JD, et al. Practice guidelines for treatment of candidiasis. *Clin Infect Dis* 2000;30:662–678.
233. Harris AD, Castro J, Sheppard DC, et al. Risk factors for nosocomial candiduria due to *Candida glabrata* and *Candida albicans*. *Clin Infect Dis* 1999;29:926–928.
234. Burke JP. Infection control—a problem for patient safety. *N Engl J Med* 2003;348:651–656.
235. Gerberding JL. Hospital-onset infections: a patient safety issue. *Ann Intern Med* 2002;137:665–670.
236. Kunin CM. Nosocomial urinary tract infections and the indwelling catheter. What is new and what is true? *Chest* 2001;120:10–12.
237. Martin CM, Bookrajian EN. Bacteriuria prevention after indwelling urinary catheterization. A controlled study. *Arch Intern Med* 1962; 110:703–711.
238. Butler HK, Kunin CM. Evaluation of polymyxin catheter lubricant and impregnated catheters. *J Urol* 1968;100:560–566.
239. Finkelberg Z, Kunin CM. Clinical evaluation of closed urinary drainage systems. *JAMA* 1969;207:1657–1662.
240. Kunin CM, Finkelberg Z. Evaluation of an intraurethral lubricating catheter in prevention of catheter-induced urinary tract infections. *J Urol* 1971;106:928–930.
241. Little PJ, Pearson S, Peddie BA, et al. Amoxicillin in the prevention of catheter-induced urinary infection. *J Infect Dis* 1974;129(suppl): S241–S242.
242. Monson TP, Macalalad FV, Hamman JW, et al. Evaluation of a vented drainage system in prevention of bacteriuria. *J Urol* 1977;117: 216–219.
243. Britt MR, Garibaldi RA, Miller WA, et al. Antimicrobial prophylaxis for catheter-associated bacteriuria. *Antimicrob Agents Chemother* 1977; 11:240–243.
244. Bastable JRG, Peel RN, Birch DM, et al. Continuous irrigation of the bladder after prostatectomy: its effect on post-prostatectomy infection. *Br J Urol* 1977;49:689–693.
245. Matthew AD, Gonzalez R, Jeffords D, et al. Prevention of bacteriuria after transurethral prostatectomy with nitrofurantoin macrocrystals. *J Urol* 1978;120:442–443.
246. Keys TF, Maker MD, Segura JW. Bacteriuria during closed urinary drainage: an evaluation of top-vented versus bag-vented systems. *J Urol* 1979;122:49–51.
247. Kirk D, Dunn M, Bullock DW, et al. Hibitane bladder irrigation in the prevention of catheter-associated urinary infection. *Br J Urol* 1979; 51:528–531.
248. Maizels M, Schaeffer AJ. Decreased incidence of bacteriuria associated with periodic instillations of hydrogen peroxide into the urethral catheter drainage bag. *J Urol* 1980;123:841–845.
249. Gillespie WA, Simpson RA, Jones JE, et al. Does the addition of disinfectant to urine drainage bags prevent infection in catheterised patients? *Lancet* 1983;1:1037–1039.
250. Sweet DE, Goodpasture HC, Holl K, et al. Evaluation of H_2O_2 prophylaxis of bacteriuria in patients with long-term indwelling Foley catheters: a randomized controlled study. *Infect Control* 1985;6: 263–266.
251. Klarskov P, Bischoff N, Bremmelgaard A, et al. Catheter-associated bacteriuria. A controlled trial with the Bardex urinary drainage system. *Acta Obstet Gynaecol Scand* 1986;65:295–299.
252. Davies AJ, Desai HN, Turton S, et al. Does instillation of chlorhexidine into the bladder of catheterized geriatric patients help to reduce bacteriuria? *J Hosp Infect* 1987;9:72–75.
253. Sethia KK, Selkon JB, Berry AR, et al. Prospective randomized controlled trial of urethral versus suprapubic catheterization. *Br J Surg* 1987;74:624–625.
254. Charton M, Vallancien G, Veillon B, et al. Antibiotic prophylaxis of urinary tract infection after transurethral resection of the prostate: a randomized study. *J Urol* 1987;138:87–89.
255. Ball AJ, Carr TW, Gillespie WA, et al. Bladder irrigation with chlorhexidine for the prevention of urinary infection after transurethral operations: a prospective controlled study. *J Urol* 1987;138:491–494.
256. Hozack WJ, Carpiniello V, Booth RE Jr. The effect of early bladder catheterization on the incidence of urinary complications after total joint replacement. *Clin Orthop* 1988;231:79–82.
257. DeGroot-Kosolcharoen J, Guse R, Jones JM. Evaluation of a urinary catheter with a preconnected closed drainage bag. *Infect Control Hosp Epidemiol* 1988;9:72–76.
258. Schaeffer AJ, Story KO, Johnson SM. Effect of silver oxide/trichloroisocyanuric acid antimicrobial urinary drainage system on catheter-associated bacteriuria. *J Urol* 1988;139:69–73.
259. Michelson JD, Lotke PA, Steinberg ME. Urinary-bladder management after total joint-replacement surgery. *N Engl J Med* 1988;319: 321–326.
260. Verbrugh HA, Mintjes-de Groot AJ, Andriesse R, et al. Postoperative prophylaxis with norfloxacin in patients requiring bladder catheters. *Eur J Clin Microbiol Infect Dis* 1988;7:490–494.
261. Al-Juburi AZ, Cicmanec J. New apparatus to reduce urinary drainage associated with urinary tract infections. *Urology* 1989;33:97–101.
262. Liedberg H, Lundeberg T. Silver alloy coated catheters reduce catheter-associated bacteriuria. *Br J Urol* 1990;65:379–381.
263. Johnson JR, Roberts PL, Olsen RJ, et al. Prevention of catheter-associated urinary tract infection with a silver oxide-coated urinary catheter: clinical and microbiologic correlates. *J Infect Dis* 1990;162: 1145–1150.
264. Van der Wall E, Verkooyen RP, Mintjes-de Groot J, et al. Prophylactic ciprofloxacin for catheter-associated urinary-tract infection. *Lancet* 1992;339:946–951.
265. Schneeberger PM, Vreede RW, Bogdanowicz JFAT, et al. A randomized study on the effect of bladder irrigation with povidone-iodine before removal of an indwelling catheter. *J Hosp Infect* 1992;21: 223–229.
266. Skelly JM, Guyatt GH, Kalbfleisch R, et al. Management of urinary retention after surgical repair of hip fracture. *Can Med Assoc J* 1992; 146:1185–1189.

267. Wille JC, van Oud Alblas AB, Thewessen EAPM. Nosocomial catheter-associated bacteriuria: a clinical trial comparing two closed urinary drainage systems. *J Hosp Infect* 1993;25:191–198.
268. Maki DG, Knasinski V, Halvorson K, et al. A novel silver-hydrogel-impregnated indwelling urinary catheter reduces CAUTIs: a prospective double-blind study. *Infect Control Hosp Epidemiol* 1998;19: 682(abst).
269. Maki DG, Knasinski V, Tambyah PA, et al. A prospective investigator-blinded trial of a novel nitrofurazone-impregnated indwelling urinary catheter. Presented at the SHEA meeting, 1998.
270. Maki DG, Tambyah PA. Engineering out the risk for infection with urinary catheters. *Emerg Infect Dis* 2001;7:342–347.
271. Keerasuntopong A, Thearawiboon W, Panthawanan A, et al. Incidence of urinary tract infections in patients with short-term indwelling urethral catheters: a comparison between three-day urinary drainage bag change and no change regimens. *Am J Infect Control* 2003;31:9–12
272. Srinivasan A, Richards A, Song X, et al. A randomized evaluation of the efficacy of a silver impregnated silicon based catheter in preventing nosocomial urinary tract infections. Presented at the SHEA meeting, 2003.

21

SURGICAL SITE INFECTIONS

EDWARD S. WONG

Despite advances in operative techniques, better understanding of the pathogenesis of wound infection, and widespread use of prophylactic antibiotics, surgical site infections (SSI) continue to be a major source of morbidity and mortality for patients undergoing operative procedures. It is estimated that SSIs develop in 2% to 5% of the 27 million patients undergoing surgical procedures each year (1,2). They account for 14% to 16% of all nosocomial infections, making the surgical site the second most common site of nosocomial infections, second only to infections of the urinary tract (3). Based on the Study on the Efficacy of Nosocomial Infection Control (SENIC) by the Centers for Disease Control and Prevention (CDC), we can expect that over 500,000 SSIs will occur among adults each year in the United States (4). These infections prolong hospital stay by an average of 7.4 days at a cost of between $400 and $2,600 per wound infection, resulting in an annual cost of $130 to $845 million per year (5–7). Total cost, including indirect expenses related to SSIs, may exceed $10 billion annually.

INCIDENCE OF SURGICAL SITE INFECTIONS

The incidence of SSIs has traditionally been stratified by the type of hospital and surgical service. CDC's National Nosocomial Infections Surveillance (NNIS) system categorized participating hospitals by size and medical school affiliation. Between 1980 and 1982, nonteaching, small teaching (<500 beds), and large teaching (≥500 beds) NNIS system hospitals reported SSI rates of 4.6, 6.4, and 8.2 per 1,000 discharges, respectively (8). These were crude infection rates unadjusted for the different types of patients admitted to each category of NNIS system hospitals. The rates of SSIs also vary by service, with the highest infection rates found with cardiac surgery (2.5 infections per 100 patient discharges), followed by general surgery (1.9 per 100 discharges) and burn/trauma surgery (1.1 per 100 discharges) (8).

In contrast to SSIs among adults, the rate of SSIs among children has not been studied as extensively. SENIC specifically excluded pediatric and newborn services and children's hospitals from its study. However, medical centers with large pediatric surgical services have published their infection rates. Among these centers, the rate of pediatric SSIs varied from 3.4 per 1,000 admissions at the Children's Hospital in Buffalo (9) to 5.5 per 1,000 admissions at the University of Virginia (10) and up to 11.9 per 1,000 admissions at the Children's Hospital in Boston (11). Unlike SENIC, NNIS does include hospitals with pediatric services. From 1980 to 1982, the pediatric SSI rates for nonteaching, small teaching, and large teaching hospitals, respectively, were 0.6, 0.8, and 1.6 infections per 1,000 discharges (8). For newborns, the SSI rates for the same categories of hospitals were 0.2, 0.4, and 0.7 infections per 1,000 discharges. Compared to the overall SSI rates (adults and children) among NNIS hospitals of 4.6, 6.4, and 8.2 per 1,000 discharges for each hospital category, the SSI rates among children are approximately ten times lower.

SURGICAL SITE (WOUND) CLASSIFICATION

The risk of developing an SSI is affected by the degree of microbial contamination of the operative site. A widely accepted system of classifying operative site contamination was developed by the National Research Council for its cooperative study of the effects of ultraviolet irradiation of operating rooms on SSIs (12). This classification scheme, in a modified form, is as follows:

Clean sites (wounds): These are surgical sites in which no inflammation is encountered and the respiratory, alimentary, genital, and urinary tracts are not entered. In addition, clean wounds are primarily closed and, if necessary, drained with closed drainage. Surgical sites for operations that follow nonpenetrating (blunt) trauma should be included in this category if they meet these criteria.

Clean-contaminated sites (wounds): These are operative sites in which the respiratory, alimentary, genital, or urinary tract is entered under controlled conditions and without unusual contamination. Specifically, operations involving the biliary tract, appendix, vagina, and oropharynx are included in this category, provided no evidence of infection or major break in technique is encountered.

Contaminated sites (wounds): These include open, fresh accidental wounds or operations with major breaks in sterile technique or gross spillage from the gastrointestinal tract. Surgical sites through which there is entry into the genitourinary tract with infected urine or biliary tract with infected bile, and surgical sites in which acute, nonpurulent inflammation is encountered, fall into this category.

Dirty and infected sites (wounds): These include old traumatic wounds with retained devitalized tissue, foreign bodies, or fecal contamination. Surgical sites where a perforated viscus or pus is encountered during the operation fall into this category.

Early studies showed that this surgical site (wound) classification scheme did predict the risk of subsequent SSIs. In Cruse and

Foord's (13) study, surgery involving clean, clean-contaminated, contaminated, and dirty surgical sites had infection rates of 1.5%, 7.7%, 15.2%, and 40%, respectively. The SSI rates in the National Research Council cooperative study were 3.3% for refined clean sites, 7.4% for other clean sites, 16.4% for contaminated sites, and 28.6% for dirty sites (12). More recently, among 84,691 operations that were reported by hospitals to NNIS, the infection rates by site (wound) class were as follows: clean, 2.1%; clean-contaminated, 3.3%; contaminated, 6.4%; and dirty-infected, 7.1% (14).

The correlation of site (wound) class to the risk of SSIs would suggest that intraoperative site contamination should also be linked to the risk of subsequent infections. However, conflicting results were obtained when the microbiology of intraoperative site contamination was examined and attempts were made to correlate microorganisms isolated intraoperatively with pathogens responsible for the SSIs. Barlett et al. (15) isolated bacteria from 43 of 91 (47%) intraoperative surgical site irrigation cultures. However, they found no significant difference in the rate of subsequent SSIs between those patients with and those without positive cultures. Further, there was no relationship between the concentration of bacteria in the sites and the subsequent development of infection. In contrast, Garibaldi and Cushing (16) found that intraoperative contamination increased the risk of SSIs even after adjustments for the influences of other variables by stepwise logistic regression (odds ratio 3.0, confidence interval 2.0–4.6, $p < .001$). In spite of the association, they found the clinical usefulness of this information to be limited, as the predictive value of a positive intraoperative culture in this study was low (32%), and the rate of false-positive cultures was high (86%). They also noted that the concordance between the microorganisms isolated from the sites intraoperatively and the pathogens responsible for the SSIs was low (41%).

In retrospect, it is clear that wound classification is only a moderate predictor of infectious risk because of the existence of other variables that also influence this risk, such as host factors and operative technique (14,17). In addition, exogenous sources such as operating room personnel potentially contribute to the contamination of the operative site, and these sources are not included in the site (wound) classification scheme, which largely reflects the degree of microbial contamination from endogenous sources including microorganisms from the patient's skin or incised viscera.

DIAGNOSIS OF SURGICAL SITE INFECTION

Clinically, a surgical site can be considered infected when purulent drainage is present at the incision site. This may be associated with local swelling, erythema, tenderness, wound dehiscence, or abscess formation. However, local signs and symptoms may not always be present, nor are they necessarily due to infection when they are present. Therefore, the clinical definition of SSI that has been the most widely adopted is the simplest one—that of a surgical site draining a purulent exudate. Clinicians are encouraged to culture all purulent exudates, but neither culture nor a positive microbiologic result is required for diagnosis of an SSI.

The definition of an SSI that is to be used for surveillance and epidemiologic purposes must meet additional needs. Such a definition must be simple to use but also unambiguous so that hospitals with varying surveillance resources will be able to apply it and obtain consistent results so that comparisons between hospitals are meaningful. The CDC has previously developed and published definitions for the surveillance of surgical wound infections (now called SSIs—see below) (18), and although intended for use by hospitals participating in NNIS, they have become widely adopted for use by non-NNIS system hospitals as well. In the CDC definition, wound infection (SSI) is diagnosed on the basis of one of the following: purulent drainage from incision site or from a drain; positive results from a culture of fluid obtained from a surgical site closed primarily; the surgeon's or attending physician's diagnosis of infection; or the surgical site requires reopening. SSIs are classified as incisional (now subdivided into superficial incisional and deep incisional—see below) when they involve the skin, subcutaneous tissue, or muscle above the fascial layer; or deep (now termed organ/space SSI—see below) if they involve structures or organs beneath the area of the incision. In NNIS system hospitals, operative sites are followed for 30 days for the development of SSI, unless an implant is involved, in which case the period of surveillance is extended to a year.

MICROBIOLOGY OF SURGICAL SITE INFECTIONS

Table 21.1 depicts the most common pathogens responsible for SSIs as reported to NNIS from 1986 to 1989 and from 1990 to 1992 (19,20). Bacteria account for the majority of SSIs. *Staphylococcus aureus* and coagulase-negative staphylococci were the two most common pathogens isolated largely from clean surgical procedures. When surgery involves entry of the respiratory, gastrointestinal, or gynecologic tracts, pathogens are often polymicrobic, involving aerobic and anaerobic microorganisms endogenous to the organ resected or entered.

TABLE 21.1. PERCENTAGE OF DISTRIBUTION OF NOSOCOMIAL PATHOGENS FOR SURGICAL SITE INFECTIONS (SSIs) NATIONAL NOSOCOMIAL INFECTIONS SURVEILLANCE SYSTEM, 1986–1989 AND 1990–1992

Pathogen[a]	1986–1989 n = 16,727	1990–1992 n = 11,724
Escherichia coli	10	8
Enterococci	13	12
Pseudomonas aeruginosa	8	8
Staphylococcus aureus	17	19
Coagulase-negative staphylococci	12	14
Enterobacter spp.	8	7
Klebsiella pneumoniae	3	3
Candida albicans	2	3
Proteus mirabilis	4	3
Streptococcal spp.	3	3

[a]Pathogens with less than 2% are not shown.

In recent years, there has been noted in SSIs, as in other sites of nosocomial infections, a shift toward infections with antibiotic-resistant strains of both gram-positive and gram-negative microorganisms (19). Infections involving fungi, especially *Candida albicans* or *C. tropicalis,* are more common because of the increasing number of immunocompromised patients undergoing operative procedures. SSIs caused by unusual microorganisms are also increasingly being recognized; for example, SSIs caused by *Rhizopus rhizopodiformis* due to contaminated adhesive dressings (21–22), infections with *Mycobacterium chelonae* and *M. fortuitum* (see Chapter 38) following augmentation mammoplasty (23–24), and sternal wound infections due to rapidly growing mycobacteria and *Rhodococcus bronchialis* after coronary artery bypass surgery have been reported (25,26). Nosocomial SSIs and prosthetic valve endocarditis due to *Legionella pneumophila* after contamination by tap water have been described (27–29). Clusters of infections by such unusual microorganisms clearly warrant investigation to rule out common source exposures.

SOURCES FOR PATHOGENS CAUSING SURGICAL SITE INFECTIONS

Pathogens that cause SSIs are acquired either endogenously from the patient's own flora or exogenously from contact with operating room personnel or the environment. It is believed that, within 24 hours of an operative procedure, most surgical sites are sufficiently sealed, unless the site was closed secondarily or involved drain placement, to make them resistant to inoculation and infection. Thus, most pathogens, whether endogenously or exogenously acquired, are believed to be implanted at the time of surgery (30). Theoretically, the operative site can be seeded postoperatively by the hematogenous or lymphatic route or by direct inoculation of the closed operative site, but such mechanisms of acquisition are thought to occur infrequently (30). Ehrenkranz and Pfaff (31), however, described a cluster of sternal infections occurring postoperatively that were preceded by infections caused by the same microorganisms at remote sites (pneumonias and bacteremias). In the outbreak of *Legionella* sternal infections reported by Lowry et al. (29), patients were not exposed to contaminated tap water containing *Legionella* during bathing and dressing changes until well after cardiac surgery. Thus, there is evidence to suggest that inoculation (and infection) may occasionally occur postoperatively. Nonetheless, the period of greatest risk for infection remains the time between opening and closing the operative site.

Endogenous Sources of Pathogens

The patient's own flora at or contiguous to the site of operation accounts for the majority of SSIs (32). *S. aureus* and coagulase-negative staphylococci, the first and second most frequent causative microorganisms, are residents of skin, and presumably they are directly inoculated into the operative site during incision or subsequent manipulations. Cleansing and the use of a skin degerming agent during preparation of the operative site for surgery are currently routinely performed, and they are expected to reduce the surface population of these microorganisms. However, if the skin became heavily colonized—for example, as a result of dermatitis—resident flora may persist and be carried into the operative site. During nonclean surgery, the normal flora of the gastrointestinal, respiratory, genital, and urinary tracts can directly contaminate the operative site when these tracts are opened or when injury has occurred to one of these tracts prior to surgery.

The patient's endogenous flora at distant sites may also be a source of SSI. Wiley and Ha'eri (33) noted that human albumin microspheres (HAMs) were like human skin squames and could be used as tracer particles. When they applied HAM to the patient's skin outside the area of the incision, they demonstrated that the tracer particles could be easily recovered from the operative site (in 40 of 40 orthopedic operations), suggesting that surface microflora can migrate from distant sites and gain entrance to the operative site despite distance and the use of cloth and adhesive drapes as barriers. Finally, microorganisms causing infections at remote sites may gain access to operative sites by hematogenous or lymphogenous seeding. Untreated urinary tract, skin, and respiratory tract infections are the three most common remote infections that have been associated with an increase in the rate of SSIs (34,35).

Exogenous Sources of Pathogens

Personnel

The hands of the operative team harbor microorganisms that can contaminate the surgical site by direct inoculation during the operative procedure (36–38). This has led to the use of surgical gloves as a barrier to the transfer of microorganisms and to the surgical hand scrub to reduce the microbial population on the skin of the hands. Initially introduced as a way of protecting operating room personnel against dermatitis from Listerian antisepsis, surgical gloving has became a standard of practice as a method to prevent the passage of microorganisms from the surgeon's hands to the patient's surgical site. Whether surgical gloves are an effective barrier has been questioned, since studies have demonstrated that glove perforations occur frequently; this occurs in up to a third or more of operations (13,38). Nonetheless, with appropriate preoperative scrubbing to reduce the burden of microorganisms on the surgeon's hands, there is no evidence that such perforations of surgical gloves are of any clinical significance. Dodds et al. (39) found no difference in the rate of SSIs among 100 hernia repairs that were or were not associated with glove perforations.

In addition to the hands, other body sites in the operative team may be sources for exogenous contamination of the operative site. The hair and scalp of hospital staff (as well as of patients themselves) have been shown to harbor potentially pathogenic bacteria, including *S. aureus* and gram-negative bacteria (40). Ha'eri and Wiley (41) demonstrated that the head and neck can theoretically be sources of microorganisms that are shed into the operative site. Human albumin microspheres applied to the head and neck of operating surgeons were recovered from the operative wound in 20 of 20 experiments. Despite those observations, however, only a few outbreaks of SSIs have been traced to the hair and scalp of the operative team (40,42).

The nares and oropharynges of operating room personnel are also colonized with microorganisms that can be shed in large droplets into the surgical site. Ford et al. (43) isolated *S. aureus, S. epidermidis,* and streptococci frequently from the nasopharynges of operating room personnel and recovered the same microorganisms from the exudates of infected wounds. Although the simultaneous recovery of similar microorganisms from the nasopharynx and infected surgical site does not prove that the nasopharynx is the source, tracer particle studies have shown that this might occur. Ha'eri and Wiley (41) applied albumin microspheres to the inner surface of surgical face masks and recovered them from operative sites consistently, unless leakage around the lower edges of the mask was prevented by a hood overlapping the edges of the mask. Similarly, Letts and Doermer (44) were able to recover tracer particles that had been sprayed onto the face and nostrils of personnel from simulated surgical sites. They also noted that talking by operating room personnel increased the number of microspheres recovered, suggesting that conversation contributed to aerosolization of bacteria from the oropharynx.

Environment

The microorganisms that are isolated from the operating room environment are usually considered nonpathogens or commensals that are rarely associated with infections (45). Atypical mycobacteria are ubiquitous and can be recovered from hospital dust but are rarely incriminated in SSIs. In the clusters of infections due to *M. fortuitum* and *M. chelonae* that followed valve replacement surgery and augmentation mammoplasty (23–25), it was bone wax or gentian violet marking solution that was incriminated rather than the general operating room environment. Spores of *Clostridium perfringens* have been isolated from the ventilation system and floors of operating rooms (46), but when investigators looked for potential sources for these microorganisms that cause devastating SSIs, they concluded that *C. perfringens* was either endogenously acquired from the patient's own gastrointestinal flora (47) or acquired from contaminated surgical instruments that had been inadequately sterilized between cases (48).

In those rare instances when inanimate sources in the operating room have been incriminated, the sources have been contaminated solutions, antiseptics, or dressings. Contaminated elastic dressings have been implicated in SSIs caused by *Rhizopus* (21, 22,49) and *C. perfringens* (50). Contaminated solutions have been the source for SSIs caused by *Pseudomonas aeruginosa, P. multivorans,* and *Serratia marcescens* (51–53).

It is currently standard practice to wet-mop the floor of the operating room with a disinfectant between cases. Coupled with a more thorough wet vacuuming of the rooms and corridors at night, this routine is believed to provide a sufficiently clean environment that minimizes the risk of the operating room environmental surfaces and floors as a source of infection.

Air

The role of the operating room air as a source of infection and the need for special ventilation systems in the operating room have long been subjects of debate. The largest source of airborne microbial contamination is the staff in the operating room (44,45). It is presumed that microorganisms become airborne as a result of conversation, which creates droplet nuclei from the respiratory tract, or as a result of shedding from hair or exposed skin. Tracer particle studies using human albumin microspheres suggest that airborne microorganisms from the respiratory tract or head and neck area of operating room personnel can settle on the operative site (33,41,44). Despite this possibility, there is little evidence that the airborne route of transmission contributes significantly to SSIs. Evidence that SSI resulting from airborne contamination occurs at all is based on outbreaks of group A β-hemolytic streptococcal infections that have been reported in the literature (54–58). In these outbreaks, the evidence for airborne transmission was as follows. First, streptococci with the same serotype as the isolates from infected surgical sites were isolated from sites of colonization (anal, vaginal, or pharyngeal) in operating room personnel. Second, the sites of carriage (anal or vaginal) had no possibility of direct contact with the operative site. Moreover, some of these carriers were ancillary personnel who, while they were in the same room, did not work directly in the operative field. Finally, when settling plates were used during these investigations, the epidemic microorganism could be recovered from the air of a room during exercise by the carrier.

Additional evidence for the role of airborne transmission comes from studies on the use of laminar flow air systems and ultraviolet irradiation to provide ultraclean air. Early studies appeared to show a reduction in SSIs when special air handling systems were used to reduce airborne microbial contamination (59–62). However, many of these studies were flawed, because they were not comparative, had inadequate sample sizes, were not randomized or blinded, or included other interventions that could affect the rate of SSIs. Two well-designed studies have been published (12,63). The National Research Council study evaluated the effect of ultraviolet irradiation on microbial contamination of the operating room air and on SSIs. The results indicated that refined-clean operations were significantly less likely to be complicated by infection when they were performed in rooms illuminated with ultraviolet irradiation when compared with operations performed in rooms with standard ventilation. The second study was a multicenter European study that compared infection rates among total hip and knee replacement procedures that were performed in rooms with ultraclean air provided by special ventilation systems or body-exhaust suits with those procedures performed in conventionally ventilated rooms (63). In rooms with special ventilation systems or in which body-exhaust suits were used, the amount of airborne contamination as measured by air sampling, the microbial count of wound washing, and the frequency of SSIs in patients were all significantly less than the corresponding measurements in conventionally ventilated rooms.

In the National Research Council study, the benefits of ultraviolet irradiation did not extend to operations in the other surgical site (wound) classes (other clean, clean-contaminated, contaminated, or dirty surgery). In these other categories, it was believed that microbial contamination of the operative site from endogenous sources negated any benefit that was to be gained by a reduction in contamination from an airborne source. Thus, air as an exogenous source of pathogens is important only in clean wounds and is likely not of significance when other sources and modes of transmission result in heavier microbial contamination.

RISK FACTORS FOR THE DEVELOPMENT OF SURGICAL SITE INFECTIONS

In 1965, Altemeier and Culbertson (64) stated that the risk of an infection varies (a) directly in proportion to the dose of bacterial contamination; (b) directly in proportion to the virulence of the microorganism; and (c) inversely in proportion to the resistance of the host, that is, the patient's ability to control the microbial contamination. On the basis of animal studies, we can add a fourth key factor: the physiologic status or condition of the surgical site at the end of the operation. A surgical site in poor condition, that is, one that is poorly vascularized or that contains damaged or necrotic tissue or foreign material, is at a higher risk of infection given the same degree of microbial contamination. Surgical site condition is also determined by the underlying disease process that necessitated surgery (e.g., the severity of trauma) and by operative technique (i.e., the skill of the surgeon). These four key factors interact in a complex way to foster the development of infection.

Since the days of Altemeier and Culbertson, clinical and epidemiologic studies have identified other risk factors that are described below that also affect the rate of SSIs. These factors, however, may be viewed as secondary in that they are likely to exert their effect through interaction with the key factors—for example, by increasing the inoculum of microorganisms contaminating the surgical site or by affecting resistance of the host or the condition of the surgical site.

Prolonged Preoperative Stay

Over the years, studies have consistently demonstrated an adverse effect of prolonged preoperative stay on the rate of SSIs. The National Research Council study found that the rate of SSI rose from 6% for a preoperative stay of 1 day to 14.7% when the preoperative stay was 21 or more days (12). Cruse and Foord (13) reported that the overall infection rate was 1.1% for patients whose preoperative stay was 1 day versus 2.1% in patients who remained in the hospital for 1 week before their operation. These early studies might be criticized, because the influence of other risk factors was not specifically taken into account. Other studies, however, have used multivariate analysis methodology to adjust for potentially confounding variables (16,65–67). These studies continue to find prolonged preoperative stay to be an important independent risk factor for SSIs.

The mechanism(s) by which prolonged hospital stay brings about an increased risk of infection is unknown. A long preoperative stay may promote proliferation of endogenous microorganisms, which can then more heavily contaminate the surgical site, or such a stay may promote the acquisition of hospital-acquired multidrug-resistant pathogens. Prolonged preoperative stay also permits the performance of procedural interventions that allow microorganisms access into the body (portals of entry) or chemotherapeutic interventions that can adversely affect host resistance (e.g., steroids) or alter normal flora (e.g., through exposure to antibiotics). Researchers have found that patients who are hospitalized for cardiovascular surgery quickly become colonized with methicillin-resistant coagulase-negative staphylococci and that these microorganisms were responsible for surgical site complications including mediastinitis and prosthetic valve endocarditis (68–72). Kernodle et al. (68) believed that the methicillin-resistant staphylococci were present on admission and were selected from the patients' endogenous population by perioperative antibiotics. Archer et al. (69,71,72), in contrast, believed that these resistant staphylococci were acquired exogenously from hospital personnel and cited differences between preoperative and postoperative strains in gentamicin resistance and plasmid patterns and the similarity of isolates recovered from patients and recovery room personnel to support their contention for exogenous acquisition.

Preoperative Shave

In 1971, Seropian and Reynolds (73) compared the SSI rate among 406 surgical patients randomized to hair removal by razor or by depilatory. The rate of infection after shaving was 5.6% compared with 0.6% when hair was removed by a depilatory ($p < .02$). It was 0.6% when hair was not removed at all. In this study, the timing of hair removal also affected the infection rate. Among patients subjected to the razor, the infection rate was 3.1% when the shaving was done just before surgery versus 7.1% when the patient was shaved within 24 hours of surgery. The infection rate was greater than 20% when patients were shaved more than 24 hours before surgery. In the study by Cruse and Foord (13), similar results were obtained. Patients who were shaved with a razor had the highest rate of infection at 2.5%. Among patients who were not shaved but had their hair clipped, the infection rate was 1.7%. Patients who were shaved with an electric razor had an infection rate of 1.4%. Patients who were neither shaved nor clipped had the lowest infection rate of 0.9%.

Not all studies found that the frequency of wound infections varied by method of hair removal (74–76). The number of subjects enrolled in these studies, however, was small, limiting the studies' ability to detect small but true differences between groups. Studies by Mehta et al. (77) and Mishriki et al. (67) corroborated the earlier results of Seropian and Reynolds.

Hamilton and Lone (78) used a scanning electron microscope to examine the skin after removal of hair with a razor, electric clipper, and a depilatory. Their photographs showed that the razor caused gross skin cuts, the clipper caused less injury, and the depilatory caused no injury. Thus, the increase in SSIs may result from disruptions in the skin barrier caused by the razor, permitting an increase in colonization or actual invasion with either resident or exogenous microorganisms at the incision site.

Length of Operation

The length of surgery has long been established as an important risk factor for SSI. Cruse and Foord (13) found a direct relationship between duration of surgery and the infection rate.

Among clean wounds, the infection rates for operations lasting 1, 2, and 3 hours were 1.3%, 2.7%, and 3.6%, respectively. The SENIC study found that having an operation lasting more than 2 hours was one of four risk factors for SSI that remained significant when logistic regression techniques were applied to the SENIC database (4). In refining the SENIC risk index for NNIS, Culver et al. (14) noted that the 75th percentile of the distributions of duration of surgery for each procedure was a better predictor of infection than the common cut point of 2 hours used for all procedures in the SENIC index. Garibaldi and Cushing (16) applied stepwise logistic regression to the analysis of 1,852 procedures and found that the duration of surgery greater than 2 hours was associated with relative risk of 3 (confidence interval 1.6–3.6) for SSIs.

Exactly how lengthening duration of surgery increases the risk for SSI remains speculative. Cruse and Foord (13) listed four possible explanations: (a) an increase in the contamination of the wound with longer operations; (b) an increase in tissue damage from drying, prolonged retraction, and manipulations; (c) an increase in the amount of suture and electrocoagulation, which may reduce the local resistance of the wound; and (d) greater suppression of host defenses from blood loss and shock. Garibaldi and Cushing (16) added that the duration of surgery may be a marker for factors that are difficult to incorporate in multivariate modeling such as the skill of the surgeon and complexity of surgery. Shapiro et al. (79) suggested that increased infections after prolonged hysterectomy may be the result of decreasing effects of antibiotic prophylaxis with lengthy procedures. This is the rationale for repeat dosing of antibiotics in operations lasting for more than 2 to 3 hours.

Surgical Technique

The skill of the surgeon has a central role in SSIs. Technique directly affects the degree of contamination of the surgical site through breaks in technique or inadvertent entry into a viscus. The skill of the surgeon also affects the condition of the surgical site and therefore its resistance to infection. The risk of infection is minimized by control of bleeding, gentle traction and handling of tissue, removal of necrotic tissue, and eradication of dead space. Finally, the skilled surgeon can reduce the duration of surgery, which affects the risk of SSI (see above).

The quality of a surgeon's operative technique cannot be easily assessed without direct observation, and thus the impact of a surgeon's technical skill on SSIs has not been evaluated except indirectly. Farber et al. (80) used a statewide surveillance program to examine the relationship between surgical volume and the incidence of SSIs. They noted a highly significant relationship between a lower number of procedures performed by surgeons and a higher rate of infection for appendectomies, herniorrhaphies, cholecystectomies, colon resections, and abdominal hysterectomies. One explanation put forth was that higher volume meant more experience, and surgeons with more experience generally acquire better technique. In a follow-up study by the same group, Miller et al. (81) examined the relationship of the level of physician training and incidence of endometritis after cesarean section. Among 15 variables examined by stepwise logistic regression analysis, only the presence of a resident as the lead surgeon was associated with a higher risk for endometritis. Surgical residents presumably would have less experience and skill than attending physicians.

Presence of Remote Infections

The presence of a remote infection at the time of surgery has been shown to affect the rate of SSIs. In the National Research Council study, the presence of a remote infection increased the rate of SSI 2.7 times (18.4% vs. 6.7%) (12). Edwards (34) observed that, among 383 patients who had cultures taken from SSIs and remote sites, 55% of the wound infections were preceded by infections of the urinary tract or lower respiratory tract with the same microorganisms. In the study by Garibaldi and Cushing (16), the presence of a remote infection was significantly associated with an increased rate of infection on univariate analysis (odds ratio 2.8; confidence interval 1.5–5.3). However, when the authors used logistic regression analysis to adjust for the influence of other variables, the presence of remote infection was no longer significantly associated with SSI.

Abdominal Drains

Early observational studies suggested that surgical drains contributed to the development of SSIs (12,13,82). Experimental studies seemed to support these clinical observations. Nora et al. (83) were able to produce wound infections in dogs with drains placed before abdominal closure but not in dogs without drains. In the clinical phase of this study, the investigators observed that 17 of 50 patients with abdominal drains placed had *S. aureus* and *S. epidermidis* cultured from the interior surfaces of their drains and suggested that these microorganisms may migrate retrograde from overlying skin flora. The work of Magee et al. (84) suggested that the drains may also potentiate the risk of infection by acting as a foreign body and suppressing local tissue defenses.

Subsequent studies on the effect of drains on the risk of SSIs have produced conflicting results. Simchen et al. (85) prospectively evaluated 1,487 patients who had undergone hernia operations. Among 14 variables analyzed using multivariate analysis, the use of drains was found to significantly increase the risk of infection (odds ratio 4.1; $p < .001$). Lidwell (86) also found drains to be a risk factor when he applied regression analysis to data collected on SSIs. In contrast, neither the study by Claesson and Holmlund (87) nor the study by Mishriki et al. (67), both of which used multivariate analysis methodology, was able to incriminate drains as a risk factor for SSIs. Several prospective, randomized trials have also been published (88–91). Three studies found no difference in infection rates when drains were used (88–90). In the fourth study, Monson et al. (91) noted that patients randomized to receive high-pressure suction drainage after cholecystectomy had a significantly higher rate of SSI (15 of 239 with drains, vs. 5 of 240 without, $p < .05$). A task force of experts from the Society for Hospital Epidemiology of America (SHEA), the Association of Practitioners in Infection Control (APIC), the CDC, and the Surgical Infection Society (SIS) concluded, after review of the evidence, that the use of drains was only a possible contributor to SSIs. This was the weakest of three categories of risk factors, which included definitive and likely risk factors (92).

Host Factors

Intuitively, host susceptibility, that is, the host's intrinsic ability to defend itself against microbial invasion, should be an important determinant of the risk of infection following surgery. Over the years, studies have examined many host factors as to whether or not they affected the SSI rate, including such factors as age, obesity, nutritional status, and the presence of certain underlying diseases such as diabetes and malignancy. These factors were used, in effect, as surrogate markers for the host's intrinsic susceptibility to infection.

Of these host factors, advanced age has consistently been found to be a risk factor for SSIs (12,13,67,77,85,88). Garibaldi and Cushing (16) did not find age to be a risk factor. In their study, the lack of association might have been due to the inclusion of another marker into the regression model, the American Society of Anesthesiologists (ASA) physical status, which was a better predictor of host susceptibility than age alone.

Cruse and Foord (13) reported higher rates of SSIs in their patients with diabetes, as did Nagachinta et al. (66) in their prospective study of 1,009 cardiac surgery patients. In the latter study's regression analysis, diabetes mellitus and obesity were the two host factors that remained independently associated with sternal or mediastinal SSIs. Lidgren (93) and Mishriki et al. (67), in contrast, found no significant difference in SSI rates between diabetics and nondiabetics. The association of obesity and increased SSI rates appears to be better established. The National Research Council (12), Nagachinta et al. (66), Lilienfeld et al. (94), and Nystrom et al. (95) all demonstrated a higher infection rate among obese patients undergoing surgery. Low albumin, malnutrition, recent weight loss, cancer, and immunosuppressive therapy such as steroids are other factors that have been evaluated (12,67,82,87,96–98). Their roles as risk factors for infection, although suggested, are not well established.

PREVENTION OF SURGICAL SITE INFECTIONS

Interventional measures to prevent SSIs can be categorized as directed toward one of three strategies: (a) reducing the amount and type of microbial contamination; (b) improving wound condition at the end of the operation through better surgical technique; and (c) improving the host's defenses, that is, his or her ability to deal with microbial contamination. Because the critical event that initiates the process leading to infection occurs pre- or intraoperatively, the majority of these infection control measures are applied before or during operation, but some are applied after operation or even after the patient has been discharged.

Preoperative Measures

Preoperative Stay

A long duration of hospitalization before surgery has been established as a risk factor for SSI. As previously stated, one of the mechanisms accounting for this increased risk may be increased colonization with nosocomial pathogens. Northey (99) observed that the rate of acquisition of gram-negative colonization was 60% by the fifth day of hospitalization in the intensive care unit and virtually 100% by day 10. Similarly, Weinstein's group (100,101) documented increasing colonization and infection with antibiotic-resistant gram-negative bacteria with increasing stay in intensive care, although they noted that many were already colonized on admission to the unit.

Although a prolonged hospital stay may increase the risk for colonization, there is as yet no evidence that this leads directly to SSIs or that a reduction in stay would lead to a reduction in infections. Nonetheless, it would seem prudent to keep the preoperative hospital stay as short as possible. The ideal for elective operations would be to admit patients to the hospital on the morning of surgery or on the day prior to operation.

Host Factors

Host factors determine a patient's intrinsic susceptibility to infection. Unfortunately, the majority of host factors are not subject to modification. For example, advanced age cannot be changed. Obesity, diabetes, and malnutrition have been implicated as adding to the risk for SSI (see above). Although not all of these conditions have been proved to be risk factors, it would, nonetheless, be reasonable to attempt to control patients' blood glucose, improve their nutritional status, or have the morbidly obese individual lose weight, to the extent possible, preoperatively. Infections at other body sites should be treated prior to surgery.

Preoperative Showers

Preoperative bathing or showering with an antimicrobial product has been advocated as a preoperative measure with the goal of reducing skin colonization by bacteria that can contaminate the operative site. Cruse and Foord (13) reported that SSI rates for clean sites (wounds) were 2.3% for patients who did not shower, 2.1% for patients who showered with soap, and 1.3% for those who showered with hexachlorophene. Studies by Wihlborg (102) and Hayek et al. (103) seem to confirm the observations of Cruse and Foord. However, other trials have failed to demonstrate a significant difference in SSI rates when different methods of preoperative bathing were used. Garibaldi et al. (104) observed no significant difference in infection rates between surgical patients who showered with chlorhexidine and those who showered with povidone-iodine or bar soap. In a prospective, randomized, double-blinded trial involving 1,400 patients who bathed preoperatively with or without chlorhexidine, Rotter et al. (105) also were unable to find any significant difference in infection rates.

Hair Removal

Surgeons prefer to remove hair from the operative field so that it does not contaminate the operative site during surgery. Seropian and Reynolds (73) and other studies (13,78) showed that shaving with a razor can injure the skin and increase the risk of infection. Because lower rates of SSI have been associated with clipping or using a depilatory, these methods are preferred over shaving with a razor. If shaving is necessary, studies suggest that it should be performed immediately before the operation (73,77).

Preoperative Antibiotics

Contamination of operative sites, even clean ones, is unavoidable despite the best preparation and operative technique. Studies by Culbertson et al. (106), Howe and Marston (107), and Burke (108) have shown that potentially pathogenic bacteria, including *S. aureus*, can be recovered from up to 90% of surgical sites just before closure. The goal of prophylactic antibiotics, therefore, is to eradicate or retard the growth of contaminant microorganisms such that SSI can be avoided. The practice began with Lister and his carbolic acid wound antisepsis. The advent of antibiotics saw their use as a means of preventing SSIs. Prior to 1960, many clinical trials were conducted to evaluate the efficacy of prophylactic antibiotics. However, the results were often contradictory. The classic work of Burke (109) in 1961 provided the experimental basis for the scientific study of antibiotic prophylaxis. He showed how critically important timing was in the administration of the antibiotic. Burke administered penicillin at various times before and after intradermal inoculation of *S. aureus* into the skin of guinea pigs and found that, when the antibiotic was administered before or shortly after the inoculation, there was a marked reduction in the severity of inflammation and infection. If administration of the antibiotic was delayed for more than 3 or 4 hours after inoculation, there was no appreciable difference in the size of the dermal lesion or infection compared with animals who received no prophylaxis. The clinical importance of the timing of preoperative antibiotics was reaffirmed by Classen et al. (110). These authors prospectively monitored the effect of the timing of administration of prophylactic antibiotics on the occurrence of SSIs in 2,847 elective clean and clean-contaminated procedures. When prophylactic antibiotics were administered correctly preoperatively (during the 2 hours before incision), the SSI rate was the lowest, at 0.6%. The infection rates for early administration (2–24 hours before incision), perioperative administration (during the 3 hours after incision), and postoperative administration (3–24 hours after incision) were 3.8%, 1.4%, and 3.3%, respectively.

Many of the previously published clinical trials on antibiotic prophylaxis in surgery have been criticized because of flaws in study design. A well-designed clinical trial on prophylactic antibiotics should include the following features: (a) the study should be prospective, randomized, and double-blind; (b) standardized, written definitions of SSIs should be used; (c) host risk factors should be comparable in all arms of the study; (d) the operative procedures should be well defined and equally distributed in all arms; (e) the choice and administration of antibiotics should be appropriate; (f) the concomitant use of nonstudy antimicrobials

TABLE 21.2. ANTIBIOTIC PROPHYLAXIS FOR SURGICAL PROCEDURES TO PREVENT SURGICAL SITE INFECTION

Procedure	Expected Pathogens	Antibiotic of Choice[a]
Cardiac (coronary artery bypass, valve replacement, pacemaker insertion)	*Staphylococcus aureus*, *S. epidermidis*, GNB[b]	Cefazolin, cefuroxime, or vancomycin[c]
Vascular surgery	*S. aureus*, *S. epidermidis*, GNB	Cefazolin, or vancomycin[b]
Neurosurgery		
CSF shunt procedures	*S. aureus*, *S. epidermidis*	Cefazolin, or vancomycin[b]
Craniotomy	*S. aureus*, *S. epidermidis*	Cefazolin, or vancomycin[b]
Thoracic (lung resection)	*S. aureus*	Cefazolin
Ophthalmic (lens extraction)	*S. aureus*, *S. epidermidis*, streptococci, GNB	Topical gentamicin, or tobramycin or neomycin-gramicidin-polymyxin B or subconjunctival cefazolin
Orthopedic		
Joint replacement	*S. aureus*, *S. epidermidis*	Cefazolin, or vancomycin[b]
Amputation of lower limb	*S. aureus*, GNB	Cefoxitin
General surgery		
Gastric resection	GNB	Cefazolin
Cholecystectomy	GNB, enterococci, clostridia	Cefazolin
Colon surgery	GNB, anaerobes	Oral neomycin and erythromycin base or cefoxitin
Appendectomy	GNB, anaerobes	Cefoxitin or cefotetan
Penetrating abdominal trauma	GNB, anaerobes enterococci	Cefoxitin or cefotetan
Head and neck		
Procedures with incision through oral or pharyngeal mucosa	*S. aureus*, streptococci, anaerobes	Cefazolin or clindamycin
Gynecologic		
Hysterectomy	GNB, anaerobes, streptococci, enterococci	Cefazolin
Cesarean section	GNB, anaerobes, streptococci, enterococci	Cefazolin[c]
Abortion	GNB, anaerobes, streptococci, enterococci	Cefazolin[d]

[a]Unless indicated, route of administration is intravenous.
[b]To be used when methicillin-resistant *S. aureus* or *S. epidermidis* may be encountered or if patient is allergic to β-lactam antibiotics.
[c]Not to be used in uncomplicated elective procedures.
[d]To be used in uncomplicated abortions unless patient has history of previous pelvic inflammatory disease.
GNB, gram-negative bacilli.

should be controlled; and (g) sample size should be adequate to minimize type II (beta) error. Unfortunately, the design of many of the past studies falls short of this ideal. Chodak and Plaut (111) in 1977 reviewed 131 trials published in the English-language literature from 1960 to 1976 and found that only 24 (18%) met their criteria for adequate study design. In their review of 45 articles published from 1980 to 1981, Evans and Pollock (112) found the majority to have sufficient errors in design to make the results of doubtful clinical significance.

For many studies, the problem was of one of insufficient sample size, leading to the possibility of a type II error (not finding a difference between groups when one truly exists). This was especially a problem with trials assessing surgical prophylaxis in clean surgery where the expected rate of SSIs is low. One method of overcoming this problem is the use of meta-analysis. Baum et al. (113) used this technique to survey 26 trials of antibiotic prophylaxis in colon surgery and found a true difference of 14% ± 6% in infection rates between prophylaxis and no prophylaxis (22% vs. 36%). Similarly, Meijer et al. (114) used meta-analysis to combine the results of 42 trials of prophylaxis in biliary surgery (4,129 patients). Overall, patients who received antibiotic prophylaxis had a 9% lower SSI rate.

The consensus among experts is that antibiotic prophylaxis is appropriate when the operation is associated with a high risk of infection or when the consequences of an SSI are disastrous, even if the risk of infection may not be high—for example, in operations involving a prosthetic implant (115,116). According to this principle, surgical prophylaxis would be indicated for clean-contaminated or contaminated operative procedures. It would not be indicated for most clean surgery or dirty/infected surgical sites for which the use of antibiotics would be therapeutic and not prophylactic. The definition of "appropriate" prophylactic antibiotics also generally includes two other conditions. First, the timing of antibiotic administration should be such that there are adequate concentrations of the antibiotic in the tissue at the time contamination is likely to occur (as soon as the incision is made). Second, the antibiotic chosen should be effective against the most likely pathogen or pathogens encountered, taking into account their antibiotic susceptibilities. The surgical procedures for which antibiotic prophylaxis is currently recommended are shown in Table 21.2.

Intraoperative Measures

Preparation of the Incisional Site

The operative site is prepared first by cleaning to remove superficial bacteria and organic debris and then by application of an antimicrobial solution to reduce the deeply resident skin flora. The most commonly used preoperative skin preparation agents include iodine, chlorhexidine and iodine, or chlorhexidine-containing compounds. Both chlorhexidine and iodophors have a broad spectrum of activity and are effective in reducing the number of microorganisms on intact skin (117–119). Hexachlorophene is currently not used because of its limited activity against gram-negative bacteria (117). Chlorhexidine has a broad spectrum of activity and a substantive action after a single application; unlike the iodophors, it is not inactivated by blood and serum proteins.

Although microbiologic data exist to confirm that preoperative skin preparation agents do reduce the amount of skin colonization, there are no trials to show that this has led to a reduction in the number of surgical infections. Cruse and Foord (13) used historical controls to conclude that a povidone-iodine scrub followed by application of tincture of chlorhexidine was more effective (infection rate of 1.6%) than the routine used from 1967 to 1971, when green soap scrub and alcohol were used (infection rate of 2%). On the other hand, two studies suggest that the usual skin site preparation may be unnecessary (117,119). In these studies, mechanical scrubbing of the incisional site was omitted, and skin antisepsis was achieved through the use of an iodophor or chlorhexidine spray, with no increase in infection rates observed. Despite this, site preparation continues to be recommended and routinely performed.

Surgical Scrub

The surgical hand scrub is intended to reduce the number of microorganisms on the surgeon's hands and reduce contamination of the operative site through recognized or unrecognized breaks in surgical gloves. This is achieved through the use of an antiseptic hand scrub preparation, which the U. S. Food and Drug Administration (FDA) defines as "a nonirritating antimicrobial containing preparation that significantly reduces the number of microorganisms on intact skin" (120). Many such products are available, but according to studies using microbiologic data as an end point, solutions containing chlorhexidine gluconate appear to be the most effective in reducing microbial hand flora compared with iodophors or hexachlorophene-containing products (118,121). As with preoperative skin preparation agents, no clinical data indicate that reduction of hand flora with hand scrubs will lead to a reduction in the rate of SSIs.

The ideal duration of a surgical hand scrub is not known. Studies show 5-minute hand scrubs are as effective as 10-minute scrubs, with less risk of irritation and dermatitis (122,123). Later studies have shown that scrubs as short as 3 minutes may be just as effective as longer scrubs in reducing bacterial colony counts (124,125).

The wearing of long or artificial nails by operating room personnel may compromise the efficacy of the preoperative hand scrub. Several studies suggested that long or artifical nails enhance hand colonization with bacteria and fungi (126,127). In several investigations, such enhanced colonization were linked to outbreaks of bloodstream infections by *Pseudomonas aeruginosa* in a neonatal intensive care unit and SSIs with *Serratia marcescens* among cardiovascular surgery patients (127,128). These reports have prompted the CDC in its latest guideline to recommend that operating room team members keep their nails short and that they not wear artificial nails (category IB) (129).

Barrier Devices

Experimental studies using tracer particles suggest that microorganisms can be shed from hair, exposed skin, and mucous membranes of operating room personnel and that the patient's endogenous skin flora contiguous to or even distant from the operative site can gain access to the operative site through indirect contact (33,41). The use of masks, hoods, and gowns by operating room personnel is intended to reduce shedding of microorganisms by operative personnel. Similarly, surgical drapes are used to cover the patient except for the operative site and to act as a barrier to contamination from endogenous skin flora by indirect contact. Despite the strong theoretical rationale based on these experimental studies, no clinical studies have proved that the use of the barrier devices discussed below have led to a reduction in the rates of SSI.

Masks

Modern surgical masks are made of synthetic material and are highly effective in filtering out bacteria even when the material becomes wet or is used for a long time (130–132). Microorganisms from the nose and oropharynx probably pass around the lower edges of a mask rather than through it to contaminate the operative field, but this leakage can be minimized by positioning the edges of a mask underneath an overlapping surgical hood (41). A 1991 study found no difference in the numbers of SSIs among patients undergoing operations by surgeons who did or did not wear masks (133). Similarly, Orr (134) observed no increase in the infection rate when masks were not worn for 6 months. These studies question the importance of surgical masks as an infection control measure. The most important role of the surgical mask is to prevent contamination of the mucous membranes of the operative team.

Caps

Surgical caps are worn to prevent hair and skin squames, potentially laden with microorganisms, from falling into the operative field. As noted previously, with the exception of a few outbreaks traced to the hair as a source (40,42), there is scant evidence that hair is an important source for surgical site contamination or that caps are effective in preventing such contamination.

Gowns and Drapes

The composition and porosity of material are related to the effectiveness of gowns and drapes as barriers to bacteria and body fluids (135,136). Cotton muslin with thread counts of 140 is easily penetrated by bacteria. Beck and Collette (137) showed that when gowns and drapes became wet, microbial penetration was enhanced by a wicking effect. In areas of contact, such as the sleeve and abdominal areas of gowns, mechanical pressure from contact may also enhance microbial penetration. This has led to the practice of reinforcing these areas. Drapes and gowns made of nonwoven or more tightly woven material (280-thread-count cotton) are more resistant to penetration of bacteria, but whether or not this translates to lower SSI rates is unclear. In 1980, Moylan and Kennedy (138) found that the overall SSI rate following operations was 2.3% when gowns and drapes made from a nonwoven fabric were used compared to 6.4% when cotton muslin fabric (140- to 180-thread count) was used. In contrast, Garibaldi et al. (139) compared operations with woven and nonwoven gown and drape fabrics using two end points: the frequency of wound contamination assessed by an intraoperative wound culture just before wound closure and the SSI rate. They observed no difference in either of these outcomes. In 1987, Moylan et al. (140) compared the infection rate among operations using disposable spun-laced fabric versus 280-thread-count cotton and again noted a reduction in infections after operations in which the relatively more impermeable disposable gown and drape system were used (2.83% vs. 6.5%). Unexplained in both of Moylan's studies is why the protective effect of the more impermeable fabric system should extend to clean-contaminated surgery, where heavy endogenous surgical site contamination from a perforated viscus should outweigh the contribution of extrinsic contamination from operating room personnel. In summary, the use of gowns and drapes to prevent surgical site contamination and infection is logical, and their value is implied but not proven in clinical studies. One of the most important roles for surgical gowns is protection of the operative team from contamination by blood and body fluids.

In addition to drapes that simply cover the skin, adhesive plastic drapes are available that are applied to the skin at the operative site. The belief is that adherent coverage of skin up to the margin of the incision would more effectively prevent surgical site contamination from contiguous sites. Paradoxically, Cruse and Foord (13) noted a higher infection rate when plastic drapes were used. Other studies found no difference in infection rates when adhesive plastic drapes were compared to conventional drapes (141,142).

Shoe Covers

The use of shoe covers has been a standard practice in operating rooms. However, no studies demonstrate that their use affects SSIs. The American Hospital Association recommends shoe covers only when laundry facilities permit. The principal utility of shoe covers may be protection of the operative team's shoes from contamination by blood and other body fluids.

Reduction of Airborne Contamination in the Operating Room

Traffic and activity of operating room personnel, including talking and movement, are responsible for increasing the bacterial count in the air (41,44). These airborne microorganisms are usually attached to dust particles, squames shed by operating room personnel from uncovered skin areas, or respiratory secretions generated by conversation. Attached to particles, these microorganisms settle quickly but can contaminate operative sites located a short distance from the source of the microorganisms. Because of the relationship between the number of operating room personnel and bacterial air count, one method of reducing airborne contamination would be to control the number of people allowed in the operating room and their activity ("traffic control"). Traditionally, this included restricting the number of people allowed in the operating room, closing the doors to the operating room to prevent in and out traffic, and limiting unnecessary movement and talking once in the operating room. The use of proper operating room attire should also serve to decrease the amount of airborne contamination by decreasing the amount of shedding from exposed body areas.

Airborne contamination may be further reduced through dilution by high-volume exchanges with clean, filtered air and introduction of outside air. The standard set by the Public Health Service for the minimum number of air exchanges for the operating room is 15 air changes per hour with three exchanges of outside air (143). However, the value of such a standard requiring high air exchanges is unproven (144). Maki et al. (145) compared the results of microbiologic sampling in the operating room and SSI rates in an old and in a new hospital. The mean number of microorganisms was lower in the new hospital with 25 air exchanges per hour, compared with 16 air exchanges per hour in the old building. However, they observed no difference in the SSI rates.

Laminar flow ventilation systems and ultraviolet irradiation further decrease airborne contamination to very low levels (ultraclean air). As noted, such ultraclean air would only be expected to lower the SSI rate for clean surgery; specifically, ultraclean air might be of benefit in orthopedic surgery involving the insertion of prosthetic devices, but not for procedures in the other surgical site (wound) classes (12,63). Even then, the same benefits may be achieved through the use of prophylactic antibiotics. Indeed, a follow-up study by the British National Health Service suggested that, for total joint replacement surgery, antimicrobial prophylaxis was more cost-effective than an ultraclean air system (146). Modern rates of organ/space (deep) SSIs following total hip arthroplasty using conventional air handling systems, standard barrier techniques, and prophylactic antibiotics are comparable with rates reported with ultraclean air-handling systems (147,148).

Operative Technique

One of the important determinants of SSIs is operative technique. Good operative technique includes the use of aseptic barriers (gloves, masks, gowns); adequate hemostasis to prevent formation of hematomas and seromas; adequate debridement and removal of dead, devitalized tissue and foreign bodies; gentle traction and handling of tissue; and closure of the wound without tension (149). Good technique also includes the skill to perform surgery expeditiously without compromising any of the basic principles of good technique and sound judgment in the use of drains. Since the literature is inconclusive about whether drains increase or decrease the risk of SSIs, drains should not be used routinely as an infection control measure. Some of the accepted indications for drains include their use following mediastinal surgery to prevent tamponade, following thoracic surgery to prevent accumulation of pleural effusion or pneumothorax, and in the management of deep-seated abscesses that otherwise cannot be adequately drained (149).

SURGICAL SITE SURVEILLANCE AS AN INFECTION CONTROL MEASURE

Cruse and Foord (13) noted that the rate of SSIs among clean procedures was reduced when the information on rates were reported back to practicing surgeons. In a 5-year prospective study, Condon et al. (150) similarly observed a decline in the clean SSI rate from 3% to 1% after the institution of their surgical site surveillance program with direct reporting of the results to surgeons. Surveillance and reporting in these two studies focused on clean surgeries because of the assumption that infections in clean cases should naturally be low, and those that result from breaks in aseptic or operative techniques would be amenable to correction when surgeons were made aware of the problem. Subsequent studies by Olson et al. (151,152) and SENIC (4) suggested that the benefits of SSI surveillance and feedback extended to procedures in all wound categories. In the CDC study, Haley et al. (4) showed that establishment of a strong infection surveillance program and the feedback of SSI rates lowered the overall SSI rate by 35%, and the reduction occurred among contaminated or dirty cases as well as in clean or clean-contaminated cases. In the other study, Olson et al. (152) prospectively performed SSI surveillance with feedback to surgeons on 40,915 operations over a 10-year period. Their overall infection rate declined from 4.2% to 2.5%: the clean surgical site (wound) infection rate declined from 2.3% to 1.5%; the clean-contaminated infection rate declined from 5.4% to 2.5%; and the contaminated procedure infection rate declined from 12.8% to 7.8%.

How such feedback brings about changes in surgeons' behavior is not known. The effect may be achieved through an improved general awareness of the problem of SSIs that feedback brings about, through a learning process that surgeons undergo when they review cases of infections and identify probable errors in technique, or because of an anxiety factor as surgeons become aware that their patients' outcomes are being monitored.

These studies form the basis for the CDC's recommendation that hospitals routinely perform surveillance for SSIs and report the information back to the surgeons (129,153). These studies, however, are not without their weaknesses. In a 1988 editorial, Scheckler (154) pointed out that none of the studies that were cited to support the value of feedback of SSIs as an infection control measure included concurrent prospective controls; the studies did not control for changes in various other procedures that could affect SSIs, or the studies failed to provide for stratification of rates by an adequate index of host susceptibility toward infection (risk index) beyond surgical site contamination. In 2002, Scheckler (155) updated his review but could not find any recent studies that clearly show the independent efficacy of feedback of infection rates to surgeons in lowering SSI rates.

EVALUATION OF RISK FACTORS AND INFECTION CONTROL MEASURES IN THE PREVENTION OF SURGICAL SITE INFECTIONS

Risk Factors

Advanced age, morbid obesity, and the presence of remote infections at other body sites are well supported by clinical and epidemiologic studies as host factors that predispose to SSIs. They may be viewed as probable or possible risk factors for SSIs. Other surgically related risk factors that are well supported by studies include surgical site contamination (wound class), prolonged preoperative stay, shaving by razor (especially at prolonged intervals before surgery), prolonged duration of surgery, and the nonuse or inappropriate use of prophylactic antibiotics. The evidence for diabetes, malnutrition, cancer, and immunosuppression as host risk factors for SSIs is not as well supported. Operative technique affects surgical site contamination and the condition of the wound and, therefore, logically should be an important determinant of infection risk. However, the importance of surgical experience or technique has never been tested directly (79,80). Another surgically related factor that has not been definitively shown to contribute to SSIs is the use of drains.

Infection Control Measures

Infection control measures that are supported by sound clinical and epidemiologic studies as being effective in reducing SSIs include (a) shortening the length of preoperative stay; (b) eliminating infections at remote sites; (c) avoiding the removal of hair, but if necessary, using a depilatory or shaving with a razor just before surgery; (d) minimizing the duration of surgery; and (e) using appropriate antimicrobial prophylaxis. Interventions that may be useful but have not been shown to be definitively so include (a) preoperative scrubbing of the hands of surgeons; (b) use of barrier devices such as caps, hoods, masks, gloves, gowns, and drapes; (c) preoperative bathing; and (d) implementing a surgical site surveillance program with feedback of SSI rates to operating surgeons.

The CDC has published guidelines for prevention of SSIs (156). In 1999, the Hospital Infection Control Practices Advisory Committee (HICPAC) of the CDC published revised guidelines (129). The new guidelines contain 72 recommendations, and as in previous CDC guidelines, each recommendation is ranked by a revised scheme that takes into consideration the strength of the recommendation's scientific backing, the opinion of experts in the field, and the practicality and cost of implementation (Table 21.3). In the revised scheme, category IA and IB measures are strongly recommended for adoption by all hospitals. Category IA measures are supported by well-designed experimental or epidemiologic studies; category IB measures are not supported by definitive scientific studies, but they are backed by highly suggestive studies and are viewed as effective by experts in the field and by consensus of HICPAC. Category II recommendations are suggested for implementation by many but not necessarily all hospitals. These recommendations are backed by a strong theoretical rationale or suggestive clinical or epidemiologic studies. In the new guideline, practices for which there is insufficient supportive evidence or for which no consensus could be reached are identified as unresolved issues for which no recommendations could be made.

SURGICAL SITE INFECTIONS IN CHILDREN

As previously mentioned, SSIs among children have not been studied as extensively as those among adults. In NNIS system hospitals, the incidence of infection among pediatric patients and newborns is approximately ten times less than that reportedamong the adult surgical services from the same hospitals (8). In published studies, the pediatric SSI rate has varied from 2.9 per 1,000 admissions to a high of 150.3 per 1,000 admissions. The variation has been due, in part, to the use of different surveillance definitions, the use of different surveillance methodologies, and differences in populations among the medical centers (9–11). As in adults, the SSI rates by service are highest for cardiovascular, neurosurgery, general, and orthopedic surgery. The most common bacterial pathogens in pediatric and newborn SSIs include *S. aureus* (34.8%), *Escherichia coli* (10.6%), coagulase-negative staphylococci (10.6%), *P. aeruginosa* (10.6%), and enterococci (8). This differs only slightly from the distribution of pathogens responsible for adult SSIs.

Only a few variables have been looked at as potential risk factors for the development of SSIs among pediatric patients. Young age may be a risk factor. Doig and Wilkinson (157) showed that children younger than 5 years of age had significantly higher rates of SSI than children who were older (38.4% vs. 12.4%). Mead et al. (158) also noted that children less than 1 year of age had a greater infection rate in clean procedures (2.7%) than children who were older (0.3%). On the other hand, when Davis et al. (159) compared the age of infected and uninfected pediatric patients after clean surgical procedures, they were unable to demonstrate a significant difference. Donowitz (160) and Maguire et al. (161) both demonstrated an increased risk for SSIs among pediatric patients residing in intensive care or special care units compared to residents on pediatric wards. This is not surprising given the greater debilitation and, hence, underlying susceptibility of intensive care unit patients toward infections in general. Finally, Davis et al. (159) found that prolonged preoperative stay and prolonged length of surgery predisposed pediatric patients toward wound infections, as have been found among adult surgical patients. Although the overall SSI rates among pediatric surgical patients may be lower than those among adults, it is clear that within the population some pediatric patients are at a higher risk for infection—for example, low birth weight neonates and children housed in intensive care units. Studies are needed to identify risk factors that are unique to high-risk pediatric populations before meaningful interventional strategies can be designed and tested. Meanwhile, there is little reason not to assume that the infection control measures that have been evaluated and deemed useful in adults would be similarly useful in preventing SSIs among pediatric patients.

SURGICAL SITE INFECTIONS IN CARDIAC SURGERY

Cardiovascular operations are among the most common surgical procedures performed in large hospitals. Among 86,691 operations reported to the CDC by 44 NNIS system hospitals between 1987 and 1990, coronary artery bypass accounted for 7,553 (8.7%) of the procedures, whereas valve surgery or valve replacement accounted for another 2,074 (2.4%) (14). The incidence of serious SSIs—that is, sternal SSIs or mediastinitis (organ/space SSIs)—following these procedures ranged from a low of 0.81% as reported by Hazelrigg et al. (162) to a high of 16% reported by Conklin et al. (163). The infection rate re-

TABLE 21.3. CENTERS FOR DISEASE CONTROL AND PREVENTION (CDC) GUIDELINE FOR THE PREVENTION OF SURGICAL SITE INFECTION, 1999: PART II—RECOMMENDATIONS FOR THE PREVENTION OF SURGICAL SITE INFECTION (SSI)

1. Preoperative preparation of the patient
   a. Adequately control serum blood glucose level in all diabetic patients before elective operation and maintain blood glucose level <200 mg/dL during the operation and in the immediate postoperative period (48 hours). Category IB.
   b. Always encourage tobacco cessation. At minimum, instruct patients to abstain for at least 30 days before elective operation from smoking cigarettes, cigars, pipes, or any other form of tobacco consumption (e.g., chewing/dipping). Category IB.
   c. No recommendation to taper or discontinue steroid use (when medically permissible) before elective operation. Unresolved issue.
   d. Consider delaying an elective operation in a severely malnourished patient. A good predictor of nutritional status is serum albumin. Category II.
   e. Attempt weight reduction in obese patients before elective operation. Category II.
   f. Identify and treat all infections remote to the surgical site before elective operation. Do not perform elective operations in patients with remote site infections. Category IA.
   g. Keep preoperative hospital stay as short as possible. Category IA.
   h. Prescribe preoperative showers/baths with an antiseptic agent the night before and the morning of the operation. Category IB.
   i. Do not remove hair preoperatively unless the hair at or around the incision site will interfere with the operation. Category IA.
   j. If hair is removed, it should be removed immediately before the operation using electric clippers rather than razors or depilatories. Category IA.
   k. Thoroughly wash and clean at and around the incision site to remove gross contamination before performing antiseptic skin preparation. Category IB.
   l. Use an acceptable antiseptic agent for skin preparation, such as alcohol (usually 70–92%), chlorhexidine (4%, 2%, or 0.5% in alcohol base), or iodine/iodophors (usually 10% aqueous with 1% iodine or formulation with 7.5%). Category IB.
   m. Apply preoperative antiseptic skin preparation in concentric circles moving out toward the periphery. The prepped area must be large enough to extend the incision or create new incisions or drain sites, if necessary. Category IB.
2. Preoperative hand/forearm antisepsis
   All members of the surgical team:
   a. Keep nails short and do not wear artificial nails. Category IB.
   b. No recommendations on wearing nail polish. Unresolved issue.
   c. Do not wear hand/arm jewelry. Category II.
   d. Perform a preoperative surgical scrub that includes hands and forearms up to the elbows before the sterile field, sterile instruments, or the patient's prepped skin is touched. Category IB.
   e. Clean underneath each fingernail prior to performing the surgical scrub. Category IB.
   f. Perform the surgical scrub for a duration of 3–5 minutes with an appropriate antiseptic. Category IB.
   g. After performing the surgical scrub, keep hands up and away from the body (elbows in flexed position) so that water runs from the tips of the fingers toward the elbows. Dry hands with a sterile towel and don a sterile gown and gloves. Category IB.
3. Antimicrobial prophylaxis
   a. Select a prophylactic antimicrobial agent based on its efficacy against the most common pathogens causing SSI for a specific operation. Category IA.
   b. Administer the antimicrobial prophylactic agent by the intravenous route except for colorectal operations. In colorectal operations the antimicrobial agent is administered orally or a combination of oral and intravenous route is used. Category IA.
   c. Administer the antimicrobial agent before the operation starts to assure adequate microbial tissue levels before the skin incision is made. Ideally antimicrobial prophylaxis should be administered within 30 minutes before, but not longer than 2 hours before the initial incision. Category IA.
   d. For cesarean section, administer prophylaxis immediately after the umbilical cord is clamped. Category IA.
   e. Administer prophylactic antimicrobial agent as close as possible to the time of induction of anesthesia. Category II.
   f. Do not extend prophylaxis postoperatively. Category IB.
   g. Consider additional intraoperative doses under the following circumstances: (1) operations whose duration exceeds the estimated serum half-life of the agent, (2) operations with major intraoperative blood loss, and (3) operations on morbidly obese patients. Category IB.
   h. Do not routinely use vancomycin for prophylaxis. Category IB.
4. Intraoperative issues
   4.1. Operating room environment
   A. Ventilation
      a. Maintain positive-pressure ventilation in the operating room with respect to the corridors and adjacent areas. Category IB.
      b. Maintain a minimum of 15 air changes per hour, of which at least three should be fresh air. Category IB.
      c. Filter all air, recirculated and fresh, through the appropriate filters per the American Institute of Architects recommendations. Category IB.
      d. Introduce all air at the ceiling and exhaust near the floor. Category IB.
      e. No recommendation for the use of laminar flow ventilation or ultraviolet lights in the operating room to prevent SSI. Unresolved issue.
      f. Keep operating room doors closed except as needed for passage of equipment, personnel, and the patient. Category IB.
      g. Limit the number of personnel entering the operating room to necessary personnel. Category IB.
   B. Cleaning and disinfection of environmental surfaces
      a. No recommendation on disinfecting operating rooms between operations in the absence of visible soiling of surfaces or equipment. Unresolved issue.
      b. When visible soiling or contamination, with blood or other body fluids, of surfaces or equipment occurs during an operation, use an EPA-approved hospital disinfectant to clean the affected areas before the next operation. Category IB.[a]
      c. Wet vacuum the operating room floor after the last operation of the day or night with an EPA-approved hospital disinfectant. Category IB.
      d. Do not perform special cleaning or disinfection of operating rooms after contaminated or dirty operations. Category IA.
      e. Do not use tacky mats at the entrance to the operating room suite for infection control; this is not proven to decrease SSI risk. Category IA.
   C. Microbiologic sampling
      Do not perform routine environmental sampling of the operating room. Perform microbiologic sampling of operating room environmental surfaces or air only as part of an epidemiologic investigation. Category IB.
   D. Sterilization of surgical instruments
      a. Sterilize all surgical instruments according to published guidelines. Category IB.
      b. Perform flash sterilization only in emergency situations. Category IB.
      c. Do not use flash sterilization for routine reprocessing of surgical instruments. Category IB.

(Continued)

TABLE 21.3. CONTINUED

4.2. Surgical attire and drapes

a. No recommendations on how or where to launder scrub suits, on restricting use of scrub suits to the operating suite or for covering scrub suits when out of the operating suite. Unresolved issue.

b. Change scrub suits when visibly soiled, contaminated, and/or penetrated by blood or other potentially infectious materials. Category IB.

c. Wear a surgical mask that fully covers the mouth and nose when entering the operating room if sterile instruments are exposed, or if an operation is about to begin or already under way. Wear the mask throughout the entire operation. Category IB.[a]

d. Wear a cap or hood to fully cover hair on the head and face when entering the operating room suite. Category IB.[a]

e. Do not wear shoe covers for the prevention of SSI. Category IA.

f. Wear shoe covers when gross contamination can reasonably be anticipated. Category II.[a]

g. The surgical team must wear sterile gloves, which are put on after donning a sterile gown. Category IB.[a]

h. Use materials for surgical gowns and drapes that are effective barriers when wet. Category IB.

4.3. Practice of anesthesiology

Anesthesia team members must adhere to recommended infection control practices during operations. Category IA.

4.4. Surgical technique

a. Handle tissue gently, maintain effective hemostasis, minimize devitalized tissue and foreign bodies (e.g., sutures, charred tissues, necrotic debris), and eradicate dead space at the surgical site. Category IB.

b. Use delayed primary closure or leave incision open to close by secondary intention, if the surgical site is heavily contaminated (e.g., class III and class IV). Category IB.

c. If drainage is deemed necessary, use a closed suction drain. Place the drain through a separate incision, rather than the main surgical incision. Remove the drain as soon as possible. Category IB.

5. Postoperative surgical incision care

a. Protect an incision closed primarily with a sterile dressing for 24–48 hours postoperatively. Also ensure that the dressing remains dry and that it is not removed during bathing. Category IA.

b. No recommendation on whether or not to cover an incision closed primarily beyond 48 hours, or on the appropriate time to shower/bathe with an uncovered incision. Unresolved issue.

c. Wash hands with an antiseptic agent before and after dressing changes, or any contact with the surgical site. Category IA.

d. For incisions left open postoperatively, no recommendation for dressing changes using a sterile technique vs. clean technique. Unresolved issue.

e. Educate the patient and family using a coordinated team approach on how to perform proper incision care, identify signs and symptoms of infection, and where to report any signs and symptoms of infection. Category II.

6. Surveillance

a. Use CDC definitions of SSI without modifications for identifying SSI among surgical inpatients and outpatients. Category IB.

b. For inpatient case-finding, use direct prospective observation, indirect prospective detection, or a combination of both direct and indirect methods for the duration of the patient's hospitalization, and include a method of postdischarge surveillance that accommodates available resources and data needs. Category IB.

c. For outpatient case-finding, use a method that accommodates available resources and data needs. Category IB.

d. For each patient undergoing an operation chosen for surveillance, record those variables shown to be associated with increased SSI risk (e.g., surgical wound class, ASA class, and duration or operation). Category IB.

e. Upon completion of the operation, a surgical team member assigns the surgical wound classification. Category IB.

f. Periodically calculate operation-specific SSI rates stratified by variables shown to be predictive of SSI risk. Category IB.

g. Report appropriately stratified, operation-specific SSI rates to surgical team members. The optimum frequency and format for such rate computations will be determined by stratified case-load sizes and the objectives of local, continuous, quality improvement initiatives. Category IB.

h. No recommendations to make available to the infection control committee coded surgeon-specific data. Unresolved issue.

[a]Federal regulation of the Occupational Safety and Health Administration.
ASA, American Society of Anesthesiologists.
EPA, Environmental Protection Agency.

ported in the majority of studies, however, is approximately 2% (Table 21.4).

The type of procedure performed appears to significantly affect the risk of sternal SSI. Wells et al. (164) noted that the sternal SSI rate for intracardiac operations (valve replacement or congenital heart repair) of 2.2% was lower than the rate for coronary bypass surgery (7.5%). Similarly, in the series by Farrington et al. (165), the rate of infection was lower for intracardiac surgery than for coronary revascularization procedures (1.6% vs. 8.7%). Cullingford et al. (166), however, found the rates to be similar (1.2% vs. 1.9% for intracardiac and coronary bypass surgery, respectively). Within coronary bypass surgery, the risk of sternal SSI may be affected by the type of graft used. Three of four studies that have specifically compared coronary bypass by saphenous vein with internal mammary artery grafting suggested that the rate of infection was significantly higher when internal mammary arteries were used for bypass as opposed to saphenous veins (167–170) (Table 21.4). In the study by Hazelrigg et al. (162) the use of bilateral internal mammary arteries for bypass increased the sternal wound infection rate by five times compared to saphenous vein grafts and by three times compared with when a single internal mammary artery was used. In the study by Grossi et al. (171) the use of bilateral internal mammary artery bypass in diabetics increased the rate of SSI 13.9 times. The internal mammary arteries are the principal source of blood supply to the sternum. It is believed that mobilization of one or both internal mammary arteries for cardiac revascularization compromises the blood supply to the sternum, thereby increasing the risk for infectious complications (172).

These studies identified other risk factors that predisposed patients to sternal SSIs: prolonged preoperative stay, prolonged intensive care stay, mechanical ventilation, smoking, preexisting chronic pulmonary disease, older age, male sex, prolonged cardiopulmonary bypass, increased blood loss requiring transfusions, reoperation, diabetes mellitus, Foley catheterization, and postoperative weight gain.

The microbiology of sternal SSIs includes both gram-positive and gram-negative bacteria. *S. aureus* and coagulase-negative

TABLE 21.4. RATES OF SURGICAL SITE INFECTION IN CARDIOTHORACIC SURGERY

Reference	No. of Procedures	Overall	Intracardiac[a]	Coronary Bypass	Saphenous Vein	Single IMA	Bilateral IMA
Wells et al. (164)	454	5.5%	2.2%	7.5%			
Farrington et al. (165)	433	14.3%	1.6%	8.7%			
Cosgrove et al. (167)	500				0%	0.3%	2.4%
Hazelrigg et al. (162)	2,582			0.81%	0.43%	0.49%	1.65%[b]
Kouchoukos et al. (168)	1,566			2.4%	1.3%	1.9%	6.9%[b]
Demmy et al. (169)	1,521			2.1%			
Grossi et al. (171)	2,356			1.7%	0.8%	2.1%	3.8%[b]

[a]Intracardiac procedures include valve repairs and valve replacements.
[b]Statistically significant difference in infection rates between saphenous vein and internal mammary artery bypass procedures.
IMA, internal mammary artery.

staphylococci *(S. epidermidis)* are recovered from 40% to 50% of infected surgical sites (164–166). The most common gram-negative bacteria include *E. coli, Klebsiella* spp., *Enterobacter* spp., *Proteus* spp., and *Pseudomonas* spp. The frequency of staphylococci as causative agents suggests that direct inoculation of overlying skin microorganisms into the operative site is an important mechanism of acquisition. Both Wells et al. (164) and Farrington et al. (165) noted the similarity of the gram-negative bacteria recovered from sternal SSIs and leg SSIs at sites of saphenous vein harvest. They suggested that the leg surgical site or perineum may be the source of gram-negative bacteria that are transferred onto the sternal site when the saphenous vein is harvested. Sources exogenous to the patient may occasionally be responsible for infections. Outbreaks of sternal SSIs associated with contaminated transducers *(P. cepacia)* (171), cardioplegia solution *(Enterobacter cloacae)* (173), and suction pumps *(P. aeruginosa)* (174) have been reported. Outbreaks by unusual microorganisms have also been reported including *M. fortuitum* (25), *R. bronchialis* (26), *L. pneumophila* (29), and *C. tropicalis* (175).

CURRENT ISSUES IN POSTOPERATIVE SURGICAL SITE INFECTIONS

Risk Adjustment

In recent years, clinical outcomes have been emphasized as one way to measure and improve quality of care. An important obstacle to the use of SSIs as a quality assurance outcome indicator has been failure to adjust for differences in types of patients undergoing operations by different surgeons or admitted by different hospitals (differences in case-mix of patients). The surgical site (wound) classification scheme of the National Research Council attempted to capture the risk of subsequent infection brought on by the degree of microbial contamination of the operative site (12). However, as mentioned previously, this scheme fails to account for the patient's susceptibility to infection that is the result of underlying host conditions (the patient's intrinsic risk to infection). Until an indexing system can be developed that includes all the important determinants that affect infection risk, including different case-mix and intrinsic risks of patients and wound conditions, comparisons of individual surgeons within a hospital or comparisons between hospitals are necessarily crude and potentially misleading.

The CDC developed, as part of its SENIC project, a risk index system that was an improvement over the traditional surgical site (wound) classification system (17). By subjecting multiple variables to analysis by regression modeling, it found four risk factors that predicted 90% of SSIs among the SENIC database: (a) an operation that involved the abdomen, (b) an operation lasting longer than 2 hours, (c) an operation classified as either contaminated or dirty-infected, and (d) a patient having three or more diagnoses at discharge. The last factor, having multiple diagnoses, was, in effect, a proxy variable for a patient's intrinsic risk to infection. The presence of each risk factor added a point to the SENIC index such that each operation could be scored from 0 to 4 (low-risk to high-risk procedure). When tested, the SENIC index predicted SSI risk for all surgical patients twice as well as traditional surgical site (wound) classifications.

Despite the improved performance over the traditional surgical site (wound) classification scheme, limitations in the SENIC index were noted. First, the SENIC index stratified the length of operation in a dichotomous fashion—that is, either less than 2 hours or 2 hours or greater. Intuitively, since the technical difficulty of operative procedures vary—for example, a coronary artery bypass procedure would take more operating time than a simple hernia repair—the appropriate cut point for what would be deemed an excessive length of operation should also vary to reflect the complexity of surgery. Second, the SENIC index required the number of discharge diagnoses, information that could only be gotten retrospectively after the patient has been discharged. Its use would thus seem problematic in infection control programs conducting ongoing, prospective surgical site surveillance.

To overcome these limitations, NNIS system modified the SENIC patient risk index so that it was based on data easily obtainable at the time of surgery (14). In the NNIS risk index, each operation is scored by the presence or absence of three risk factors: (a) a patient having an ASA preoperative assessment score of 3, 4, or 5; (b) an operation classified as either contaminated or dirty-infected; and (c) an operation with duration of surgery more than *T* hours, where *T* depends on the operative procedure being performed. In the NNIS index, the ASA score becomes the proxy variable for the patient's intrinsic risk and is more easily obtainable than the discharge diagnoses used for the

SENIC index. The *T* cut point for each surgical procedure was derived from the NNIS database and was chosen to be the 75th percentile of the distribution of durations of surgery for that procedure. Unlike the SENIC risk index, where the risk factor of duration of operation is fixed at greater than 2 hours, NNIS's cutoff for excessive length of operation is variable and indexed to a specific operative procedure. The NNIS risk index ranges from 0 (low-risk procedure) to 3 (high-risk procedure).

In validation studies, the basic NNIS risk index generally has performed well in predicting the risk of SSIs (170). For the majority of operative procedures (30 of 40 procedures), a higher NNIS risk index score predicted a higher infection rate. For example, among the 35,293 cardiac surgeries reported to NNIS between 1992 and 2001, the SSI rate was 0.66% for risk index category 0, 1.63% for risk index 1, and 2.54% for risk index categories 2 and 3. Notable, however, was that in ten procedures, the NNIS risk index performed poorly, as the infection rate was the same whether patients had a risk index of 0, 1, 2, or 3.

The basic NNIS index assumes that the risk index variables of wound class, ASA score, and operative duration account for the majority of operative risk for infection from various influences and that each variable should have equal importance or weight. It is clear from the poor performance of the basic NNIS risk index among certain operative procedures that these assumptions are not necessarily valid. Analysis of SSIs among cholecystectomies, colon surgery, appendectomies, and gastric surgery suggested that the rates of infections were lower when a laparoscope was used. The finding that use of a laparoscope had a protective effect has prompted the CDC to modify its basic NNIS index by allowing subtraction by 1 to a lower risk category whenever a laparoscope is used (170). Other modifications to the basic NNIS risk index may be necessary, and indeed the optimal approach may be to develop a specific risk index for each surgical procedure based on multivariate analyses of procedure-related risk factors. Currently, CDC personnel are performing such analyses (171,172).

Surveillance for Surgical Site Infections

Before hospitals can meaningfully compare their infection rates, the surveillance systems among these hospitals must be comparable. Comparability first requires that standardized definitions be used in order to avoid "apples and oranges" comparisons. Moreover, these definitions need to be simple and unambiguous so that the same results are obtained when they are applied by different observers. Comparability also requires that the definitions be applied in a consistent manner to avoid ascertainment bias. The last condition requires that the same case-finding methods be used, or if the methods differ, that they at least have the same sensitivity so that the end result is that the same number of SSIs are identified.

STANDARDIZED DEFINITIONS: REVISED CDC DEFINITIONS OF SURGICAL WOUND INFECTION

Currently, the CDC definitions of SSIs are the most widely adopted set of definitions used by hospitals. Larson et al. (176) surveyed 297 randomly selected U.S. hospitals and found that 78.1% used the CDC definitions. They also found that many of these hospitals that had used CDC definitions for SSIs had modified them with non-CDC criteria. When study hospitals were asked to classify six cases of surgical wound infections in an exercise, 78% of the hospitals were correct, compared with 86% of 97 NNIS hospitals that also participated in this exercise (all of whom, by definition, used NNIS criteria). The results of this study affirm the importance of using standardized definitions for accurate surveillance.

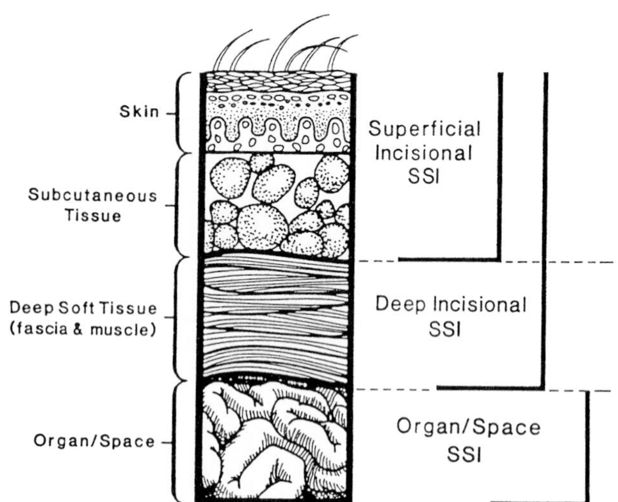

Figure 21.1. The anatomy of surgical site infections and their appropriate classifications.

In 1992, the CDC, with input from the Surgical Wound Infection Task Force, a multidisciplinary group representing SHEA, SIS, and APIC, published revised CDC definitions for nosocomial surgical wound infections (92). The two major changes in the revised definitions include (a) a change in terminology from the word *wound* to *site* because, in surgical terminology, wound only connotes the incision from the skin to deep soft tissue, and (b) a requirement for the anatomic location of a deep infection by designating the organ or space involved. The revised definitions were published with the hope that, with the backing of the task force, they would be adopted by all U.S. hospitals without modification. The new definitions are presented below, and the anatomic location of each site is depicted in Fig. 21.1

Superficial Incisional Surgical Site Infections

Superficial incisional SSIs must occur within 30 days after the operative procedure, they must involve only skin or subcutaneous tissue of the incision, and at least one of the following must be present:

1. Purulent drainage from the superficial incision
2. Microorganisms isolated from an aseptically obtained culture of fluid or tissue from the superficial incision
3. At least one of the following signs or symptoms of infection—pain or tenderness, localized swelling, redness, or

heat—and the superficial incision is deliberately opened by the surgeon, unless culture of incision is negative

4. Diagnosis of superficial incisional SSI by the surgeon or attending physician

The following should not be reported as superficial incisional SSIs: (a) stitch abscess (minimal inflammation and discharge confined to the points of suture penetration), (b) infection of an episiotomy or a neonate's circumcision site (episiotomy and circumcision are not considered NNIS operative procedures), (c) infected burn wound, and (d) incisional SSI that extends into the fascial and muscle layers (should be reported as deep incisional SSI).

Deep Incisional Surgical Site Infections

Deep incisional SSIs must occur within 30 days after the operative procedure if no implant is left in place or within 1 year if implant is in place; the infection must appear to be related to the operative procedure; the infection must involve deep soft tissues (fascial and muscle layers) of the incision; and at least one of the following must be present:

1. Purulent drainage from the deep incision but not from the organ/space component of the surgical site
2. A deep incision that spontaneously dehisces or is deliberately opened by a surgeon when the patient has at least one of the following signs or symptoms: fever (>38°C) or localized pain or tenderness, unless culture of the incision is negative
3. An abscess or other evidence of infection involving the deep incision that is found on direct examination, during reoperation, or by histopathologic or radiologic examination
4. Diagnosis of a deep incisional SSI by a surgeon or attending physician

Organ/Space Surgical Site Infections

An organ/space SSIs involve any part of the anatomy (e.g., organs or spaces), other than the incision, opened or manipulated during the operative procedure. Specific sites are assigned to organ/space SSIs to identify the location of the infection (e.g., intraabdominal site).

Organ/space SSIs must occur within 30 days after the operative procedure if no implant is left in place or within 1 year if implant is in place; the infection must appear to be related to the operative procedure; the infection must involve a part of the anatomy (e.g., organs or spaces), other than the incision, that has been opened or manipulated during the operative procedure; and at least one of the following must be present:

1. Purulent drainage from a drain that is placed through a stab wound into the organ/space
2. Microorganisms isolated from an aseptically obtained culture of fluid or tissue in the organ/space
3. An abscess or other evidence of infection involving the organ/space that is found on direct examination, during reoperation, or by histopathologic or radiologic examination
4. Diagnosis of an organ/space SSI by a surgeon or attending physician

SURVEILLANCE METHODOLOGY

For valid comparisons of rates of SSIs among hospitals, the surveillance methods for case-finding in these hospitals must be similar. Multiple case-finding methods are currently available, including (a) direct observation by infection control personnel or other surveyors and (b) indirect methods such as review of microbiology reports, Kardexes, medical records, fever charts, or antibiotic use. Often, combinations of both methods are used. For example, in the study by Olson and Lee (152), SSIs were identified by a combination of daily visits to the surgical floors (direct observation), daily review of surgical site culture reports at the microbiology laboratory, and frequent contact with ward and clinic nurses for signs and symptoms in patients that might suggest SSI (traditional infection control methods).

Direct, prospective observation of all postoperative patients for SSIs by trained personnel is generally viewed as the best method to identify SSIs (2,13,146). The sensitivity of indirect methods to detect infections has not been firmly established. The few studies that have been published suggest that indirect methods of surveillance have the following sensitivities: review of microbiology reports, 33% to 65%; presence of fever, 47%; antibiotic use, 48%; review of Kardexes, 85%; medical record review, 90% (177–179). In these studies, the outcome of interest was the detection of all nosocomial infections; thus, it is not clear whether the sensitivities would have been the same if the object of surveillance had been, specifically, SSIs. In the one published study that focused only on the sensitivity and specificity of the surveillance of SSIs using indirect methods, Cardo et al. (180) observed a sensitivity of 83.8% (95% confidence interval, 75.7–91.9%) and a specificity of 99.8% (95% confidence interval, 99–100%). In an unpublished study, Froggatt and Mayhall (181) also evaluated the ability of chart review to identify SSIs and found it to have a sensitivity of 89.7% and a specificity of 99.5% when combined with the use of outpatient clinic forms to capture late-developing infections.

NEED FOR POSTDISCHARGE SURVEILLANCE

Studies estimate that between 19% and 77% of SSIs do not become manifest until after patients are discharged from the hospital (182–187); thus, a surveillance system based solely on inpatients would greatly underestimate the rate of SSIs. With decreasing postoperative stays and the continuing shift toward same-day procedures or outpatient procedures, the likelihood of missing SSIs will only increase unless patients are followed after they are discharged from the hospital.

Although the need for postdischarge surveillance may be established, the best method to accomplish this remains unclear. Polk et al. (182) surveyed patients by letter at 6 weeks and confirmed the diagnoses of infection with their surgeons. They found that 19% of SSIs had occurred after discharge. Rosendorf et al. (184) surveyed surgeons and patients at their follow-up clinic appointments and detected an additional 44% of infections by this method. Reimer et al. (186) used a telephone survey to contact patients at 30 days after discharge and found that 77% of their SSIs occurred after discharge. However, reliance on questionnaires or telephone surveys of patients may be problematic, as one study demonstrated that patient-derived information underestimated the true number of SSIs occurring after discharge (188). The CDC recommends that surveillance for SSIs be maintained for 30 days after discharge (149). The choice of 30 days as the interval of follow-up is arbitrary, although most published studies have chosen this length of time. Weigelt et al. (187) found that 65% of SSIs occurred by the day of discharge, 82% were noted by the seventh day after discharge, 93% by the 14th day after discharge, and 97% by the 21st day after discharge. The results of this study support the choice of 30 days after discharge as the appropriate period of follow-up, since virtually 100% of the SSIs were detected within this period.

The Joint Commission on Accreditation of Healthcare Organizations (JCAHO) is considering making postdischarge surveillance mandatory to ensure that SSI rates would be accurate and a true quality of care indicator when interhospital comparisons are made. Studies are needed to establish the best method(s) for SSI surveillance, however. Until such studies become available, the recently convened Surgical Wound Task Force suggests that each institution develop and use a method that works for it based on considerations of its own resources, circumstances, and locale (92).

Alternative Method of Surveillance: Use of Automated Databases

Traditional surveillance for SSIs that rely on review of culture results, fever charts, Kardexes, medical records, or postdischarge telephone or written surveys require significant expenditure of time and effort from infection control personnel. Hence, hospitals with limited resources are often forced to choose among not performing such surveillance, limiting their surveillance to a certain time periods, e.g., 3 months out of a year (sampling), or rotating surveillance among different surgical procedural types. In the past decade, the growth and use of computers in the healthcare industry have resulted in the automated capture of heathcare data, some of which could be useful in the surveillance for SSIs. Computerized medical record systems found in today's hospitals, physicians' offices, and health maintenance organizations (HMOs) vary in their sophistication. These databases all capture administrative and demographic information, such as age, sex, underlying diagnoses, and length of hospitalization. More sophisticated databases often capture microbiology and pharmacy data, including the use of antibiotics. The most sophisticated medical record systems are usually found in tertiary referral hospitals or large HMOs. They often contain more specific operative data such as ASA score, duration of surgery, and codes for procedures like incision and drainage that more directly indicate an infection.

The availability of such automated databases provides an opportunity to use such data in novel ways to identify SSIs, with the expectation that, since data are captured automatically, such a surveillance system would require less time and personnel. Wenzel et al. (177) have shown that treatment with antibiotics during hospitalization correlates well with the presence of a nosocomial infection. For SSIs, however, antibiotic exposure by itself, although a sensitive indicator, would likely be nonspecific since antibiotics are often extended inappropriately postoperatively for prophylaxis or used to treat an infection at another site, for example, a urinary tract infection or pneumonia. Platt's group (189,190) introduced the concept of quantitative antibiotic exposure, that is, use of additional information on the timing and duration of antibiotic administration to improve the specificity of antibiotic exposure as an indicator of SSI. In their analysis of postoperative infections following cesarean section, they found that the criterion of at least 2 days of parenteral antibiotic administration following C-section had a sensitivity of 81% and a specificity of 95% compared to the performance of traditional NNIS surveillance (189). The number of antibiotic exposure days that best indicates an SSI apparently varies by procedure and is best determined by analysis of receiver-operating curves to give the optimal combination of sensitivity and specificity. For infections following coronary bypass surgery, the antibiotic threshold is at least 9 days of antibiotic administration during 30 days following the operative procedure (190). This criterion includes both oral and parenteral antibiotics, and the 30-day followup interval requirement allows the detection of patients who may be readmitted for treatment of infection. The 9-day exposure diagnostic threshold has greater sensitivity (approximately 90%) and specificity than traditional prospective surveillance.

The use of automated healthcare databases holds promise as an alternative method of performing surveillance for SSIs, one that would require less effort than traditional methods. However, quantitative antibiotic exposure thresholds have yet to be tested in a large number of hospitals with different patient casemix and automated data capture systems, although such testing is under way (191). These investigators continue to refine and improve their methodology. They have shown that the addition of certain International Classification of Diseases (ICD-9) codes and procedural codes, such as incision and drainage, to the algorithm improves on the specificity of quantitative antibiotic exposure while maintaining a high sensitivity (190,191).

EXTENDING THE USE OF PROPHYLACTIC ANTIBIOTICS TO CLEAN SURGERY

The consensus among authorities is that prophylactic antibiotics are not indicated in clean surgical procedures unless prosthetic material is implanted or the clean surgery is extensive—for example, in hip arthroplasty or cardiothoracic surgery. Studies have begun to challenge this concept. In a prospective, double-blind trial, Platt et al. (192) randomized 1,319 patients undergoing herniorrhaphy and breast surgery to either preoperative prophylactic antibiotic (cefonicid) or placebo. Study patients were followed for 4 to 6 weeks after surgery for SSIs. For breast surgery, the authors found that patients receiving antibiotics had an infection rate of 6.6% compared with 12.2% among placebo recipients. For those undergoing herniorrhaphy, infection occurred in 2.3% of cefonicid recipients compared with 4.2% of placebo recipients. Overall, the patients who received prophylactic antibiotics had a 48% reduction in the risk of SSI (Mantel-Haenszel risk ratio, 0.52; 95% confidence interval, 0.32–0.84; $p < .01$).

Studies have also established that antibiotic prophylaxis is useful in preventing superficial incisional and deep incisional SSIs in clean peripheral vascular surgery (189,194,195). Kaiser et al. (193) randomized patients to cefazolin or placebo in a prospective, double-blind trial. Among recipients of cefazolin, the infection rate was only 0.9% compared with 6.8% among recipients of placebo. Kaiser et al. calculated that the use of prophylactic antibiotics was cost-effective even for procedures with this low rate of infection. In Sweden, Hasselgren et al. (194) randomized 211 patients undergoing peripheral vascular surgery to placebo or to a 1- or 3-day regimen of cefuroxime. The two groups who received antibiotics both had a statistically significantly lower rate of SSI than did placebo recipients (3.8% and 4.3% among antibiotic recipients vs. 16.7% among placebo recipients).

Other clean surgical procedures likely will benefit from prophylactic antibiotics. However, proof may be logistically difficult to come by, since a great number of patients will have to be enrolled to yield results with reasonable statistical power, given the expected low infection rate. However, it can also be argued that, even if a reduction in infections can be realized, the margin of benefit will be small with clean surgeries that already have low rates of infection, especially when weighed against the risk of drug toxicity and the potential for the emergence of antibiotic-resistant microorganisms.

It is of interest to note that there may be other benefits to be accrued from prophylactic antibiotics. Platt et al. (192) noted that, in addition to a reduction in the rate of SSIs, patients who received cefonicid prophylaxis additionally had a lower number of urinary tract infections, nonroutine physician visits, and readmissions to the hospital and a reduction in the need for postoperative antibiotic therapy. Their findings need to be corroborated but point out that the issue of cost-benefit for antibiotic prophylaxis is complex and requires much more study. Until the studies become available, extending the use of prophylactic antibiotics in clean surgery beyond those that currently have support (herniorrhaphy, breast, and peripheral vascular surgery) must be done cautiously.

LAPAROSCOPIC SURGERY

The laparoscope had been used diagnostically since the 1930s to evaluate abdominal and pelvic organs (195). With technologic improvements and better video imaging, the laparoscope soon became an instrument of surgery. Initially, the laparoscope was used for minor ovarian, tubal, and uterine surgery. In 1987, the first laparoscopic cholecystectomy was performed by Mouret (196) and within a short period of time, the procedure has largely supplanted open cholecystectomy. In 1991, a survey of surgeons in the Southern Surgeons' Club found that only 12.1% of the cholecystectomies performed by 59 participating surgeons were open cholecystectomies (197). In 1989, the first case of laparoscopic hysterectomy was reported by Reich et al. (198). This procedure has now become commonplace (199,200). Currently, laparoscopic surgery is now being explored for multiple diseases, including the management of peptic ulcer disease and acid reflux disease, for removal of the spleen, liver, pancreas, adrenal gland, and appendix. It is being used for herniorraphies and in surgical oncology to resect tumors of the intestine (201,202).

The impetus for increasing popularity of laparoscopic surgery over traditional surgery has been reduced postoperative pain, shorter hospital stay, shorter recovery period before the patient returns to work, and better cosmetic results because smaller incisions are made. Laparoscopic surgery may also have an advantage in a lower incidence of SSIs. Early publications seem to corroborate this. In 1991, one group described only two SSIs among the first 100 laparoscopic cholecystectomies they performed (203). In a much larger study, the Southern Surgeons' Club reported only 16 SSIs (1.1%) among the 1,518 laparoscopic cholecystectomies surveyed (197). Fourteen patients had superficial infections involving the site of insertion of the umbilical trocar; two patients had a more serious intraabdominal abscess that required open or percutaneous drainage. In a review of early complications of laparoscopic hysterectomies, Harris and Danille (200) reviewed 34 publications and identified 2,412 patients who had undergone hysterectomy by traditional abdominal, vaginal, or laparoscopic procedures. The SSI rate for traditional abdominal hysterectomy was 8.4% and for vaginal hysterectomy it was 3.3%. The infection rate was lowest for laparoscopic surgery at 1.27%.

Currently, we have over a decade and a half of experience with laparoscopic surgery, and more recent publications confirm the safety of the laparoscopic surgical approach (204,205). Chang and Dellinger (205) in their recent review concluded that the use of laparoscopic surgery reduced not only the incidence of SSIs but also the severity of the infections. They reviewed 11 articles comparing infection rates between open and laparoscopic procedures in clean, noncontaminated type cases (hernia repair, Nissen procedures, and donor nephrectomies). In all but two studies, procedures done laparoscopically were associated with a reduction in the infection rate (range of reduction, 25–100%). For clean, contaminated surgeries (cholecystectomy, colectomy, gastric bypass, and band gastroplasty), again the laparoscopic approach yielded a lower infection rate when compared to the open procedure (range of reduction, 20–100%). They surmised that SSIs arising from laparoscopic surgery were less severe because of the shorter length of stay associated with laparoscopic surgery when compared to open surgery. On a national level, the CDC has gathered safety data on laparoscopic surgeries from participating NNIS system hospitals (170). Of 42,815 cholecystectomies reported to the CDC from 1992 to 1997, the rate of infection for open procedures was 1.77%, compared to 0.64% for laparoscopic procedures. For colectomies, the SSI infection rate was 4.3% for open procedures compared to 0.7% for colectomies done with the laparoscope. For these two procedures, the reduction in infection rates was consistent across NNIS system hospitals. In recognition of this protective effect, the CDC modified the SSI NNIS risk index by subtracting 1 point from the risk index when the laparoscope is used (206).

To minimize infections in laparoscopic surgery, the same considerations and recommendations on preparation of the patient for surgery, previously outlined in this chapter and by the CDC, should apply (150). For example, preoperative stay should be kept to a minimum; remote infections should be treated; the operative site should be cleaned and prepped with an approved antiseptic; and sterile barrier devices should be used by the operative team. As in other surgeries, operative technique is important. The effect of a learning curve in laparoscopic surgery has been observed by investigators who note decreasing operating room time and lower complication rates, including infections, as the experience of the operators increases (197,200,207,208). In recognition of the importance of adequate training and experience in ensuring skillful care, many surgical societies are now grappling with the issue of certification and privileging of their practitioners to perform laparoscopic surgery (208).

PREVENTION OF POSTOPERATIVE SURGICAL-SITE INFECTIONS WITH MUPIROCIN

S. aureus is the most common pathogen isolated from SSIs. This pathogen is thought to be acquired largely from the patient's own flora (endogenous acquisition). Up to 30% of healthy humans are colonized in the nares with this microorganism, and up to 50% of healthcare workers may carry this microorganism (203,209). Nasal carriage of *S. aureus* has been shown to be a risk factor for hemodialysis catheter infections and for bacteremias in patients undergoing central venous catheterizations (210–213). There is also evidence to suggest that nasal carriage with *S. aureus* is a risk factor for SSIs (209,214). Kluytmans et al. (215) demonstrated that preoperative nasal carriage with *S. aureus* was significantly associated with an increased risk of subsequent SSI (odds ratio 9.6, 95% confidence interval, 3.9–23.7). The results prompted the same group to attempt to eradicate nasal colonization as a method to prevent SSIs (216). In this trial, 752 patients about to undergo cardiothoracic surgery were treat perioperatively with intranasal mupirocin. The deep and incisional SSI rates among treated patients were 0.8% and 1.2%, respectively (total 2%) compared to 4% and 3.3% (total 7.3%) among historical controls not treated with mupirocin (relative risk, 0.44; $p = .0032$). Although not all cardiothoracic patients treated with mupirocin were colonized with *S. aureus* in this trial, a cost-effective analysis taking into account the costs of treating the whole group (752 patients) and the attributable cost of an SSI concluded that this approach was still cost-effective and saved approximately $16,000 per episode of SSI prevented (217).

An accompanying editorial by Boyce (218) noted that the study by Kluytmans et al. was not a randomized trial but instead used historical controls. In addition, significant differences were noted between the intervention group and the controls, in age ($p = .023$), frequency of valve replacement procedures ($p = .008$), and gender among the subgroup of patients undergoing valve replacement surgery. Because of these limitations and concerns about the emergence of mupirocin resistance, experts including Boyce have urged caution before proceeding with the routine use of mupirocin to prevent SSIs.

In the only randomized trial to date, Perl et al. (219) enrolled 4,030 patients about to undergo general, gynecologic, neurologic, or cardiothoracic surgery. After exclusions, 1,933 patients were randomized to receive mupirocin intranasally twice a day for up to 5 days before surgery; 1,931 patients received placebo ointment at the same schedule. At the end of the study, mupirocin treatment was found to have no effect in reducing the SSI rate caused by *S. aureus* (mupirocin treated group, 2.3% compared to placebo treatment, 2.4%). However, when the analysis was restricted to only those patients with nasal carriage of *S. aureus* before surgery, treatment with mupirocin was effective. The infection rate among 444 nasal carriers treated with mupirocin was 4%, compared to 7.7% among 447 nasal carriers treated with placebo (odds ratio 0.49; 95% confidence interval, 0.25–0.92; $p = .02$).

Given the current data, there is insufficient evidence to support the widespread use of mupirocin routinely to reduce SSIs caused by *S. aureus*, although its use in a subset of patients who are colonized in their nares with *S. aureus* may be justified. We know that the frequency of nasal colonization varies from one hospital population to another, and likely from hospital to hospital. We also know that the role of *S. aureus* as a pathogen for SSIs varies from one type of procedure to another, higher for cardiothoracic surgery as compared to gynecologic/obstetrical surgery. The effect of these variables on efficacy and cost-efficacy must be resolved before mupirocin decontamination can be considered for more than just limited use.

REFERENCES

1. Graves EJ. National hospital discharge survey: annual summary 1987. National Center for health Statistics. *Vital Stat* 1989;13:11.
2. Cruse P. Wound infection surveillance. *Rev Infect Dis* 1981;4: 734–737.
3. Hughes JM, Culver DH, White JW. Nosocomial infection surveillance, 1980–1982. *MMWR* 1983;32(suppl):1–16.
4. Haley RW, Culver DH, White JW, et al. The efficacy of infection surveillance and control programs in preventing nosocomial infections in the U.S. hospitals. *Am J Epidemiol* 1985;121:182–205.
5. Haley RW, Crossly KB, Von Allman SD, et al. Extra charges and prolongation of stay attributable to nosocomial infections: a prospective interhospital comparison. *Am J Med* 1981;70:51–58.
6. Pinner RW, Haley RW, Blumenstein BA, et al. High cost of nosocomial infections. *Infect Control* 1982;3:143–147.
7. Green JW, Wenzel RP. A controlled study of the increased duration of hospital stay and direct cost of hospitalization. *Ann Surg* 1977; 185:264–268.
8. Centers for Disease Control. Nosocomial infection surveillance, 1980–1982. *CDC Surveillance Summaries* 1983;32:1SS–16SS.
9. Welliver RC, McLaughlin S. Unique epidemiology of nosocomial infection in a children's hospital. *Am J Dis Child* 1984;138:131–135.
10. Donowitz LG. High risk of nosocomial infection in the pediatric critical care patient. *Crit Care Med* 1986;14:26–28.
11. Garner P, Carles DG. Infections acquired in a pediatric hospital. *J Pediatr* 1972;81:1205–1210.
12. National Academy of Sciences National Research Council. Postoperative wound infections: the influence of ultraviolet irradiation of the operating room and of various other factors. *Ann Surg* 1964;160(suppl 2):1–132.
13. Cruse PJE, Foord R. The epidemiology of wound infection. A 10-year prospective study of 62,939 wounds. *Surg Clin North Am* 1980; 60:27–40.
14. Culver DH, Horan TC, Gaynes RP, et al. Surgical wound infection rates by wound class, operative procedure, and patient risk index. *Am J Med* 1991;91(suppl 3B):152–157.
15. Barlett JG, Condon RE, Gorbach SL, et al. Veterans Administration cooperative study on bowel preparation for elective colorectal operations: impact of oral antibiotic regimen on colonic flora, wound irrigation cultures and bacteriology of septic complications. *Ann Surg* 1978; 188:249–254.

16. Garibaldi RA, Cushing D. Risk factors for postoperative infection. *Am J Med* 1991;91(suppl 3B):158S–163S.
17. Haley RW, Culver DH, Morgan WM, et al. Identifying patients at high risk of surgical wound infection: a simple multivariate index of patient susceptibility and wound contamination. *Am J Epidemiol* 1985;121:206–215.
18. Garner JS, Jarvis WR, Emori TH, et al. CDC definitions for nosocomial infections. *Am J Infect Control* 1988;16:128–140.
19. Schaberg DR, Culver DH, Gaynes RP. Major trends in the microbial etiology of nosocomial infections. *Am J Med* 1991;91(suppl 3B): 72–75.20. *Semiannual Report, Summary of NNIS data from 1990–1992.* Atlanta, GA: Centers for Disease Control and Prevention, May 1993.
21. Gartenberg G, Bottone EJ, Keusch GT, et al. Hospital-acquired mucormycosis *(Rhizopus rhizopodiformis)* of skin and subcutaneous tissue. Epidemiology, mycology and treatment. *N Engl J Med* 1978;299: 1115–1118.
22. Sheldon DL, Johnson WC. Cutaneous mucormycosis. Two documented cases of suspected nosocomial cause. *JAMA* 1979;241: 1032–1034.
23. Clegg HW, Foster MT, Sanders WE Jr, et al. Infection due to organisms of the *Mycobacterium fortuitum* complex after augmentation mammaplasty: clinical and epidemiologic features. *J Infect Dis* 1983; 147:427–433.
24. Safranek TJ, Jarvis WR, Carson LA, et al. *Mycobacterium chelonae* wound infections after plastic surgery employing contaminated gentian violet skin-marking solution. *N Engl J* Med 1987;317:197–201.
25. Wallace RJ Jr, Musser JM, Hull SI, et al. Diversity and sources of rapidly growing mycobacteria associated with infections following cardiac surgery. *J Infect Dis* 1989;159:708–716.
26. Richet HM, Craven PC, Brown JM, et al. A cluster of *Rhodococcus* (Gordona) bronchialis sternal-wound infections after coronary-artery bypass surgery. *N Engl J Med* 1989;324:104–109.
27. Brabender W, Hinthorn DR, Asher M, et al. *Legionella pneumophila* wound infection. *JAMA* 1983;250:3091–3092.
28. Thompkins LS, Roessler BJ, Redd SC, et al. *Legionella pneumophila* prosthetic-valve endocarditis. *N Engl J Med* 1988;318:530–535.
29. Lowry PW, Blakenship RJ, Gridley W, et al. A cluster of legionella sternal-wound infections due to postoperative topical exposure to contaminated tap water. *N Engl J Med* 1989;324:109–113.
30. Kernodle DS, Kaiser AB. Postoperative infections and antimicrobial prophylaxis. In: Mandell GL, Bennet JE, Dolin R, eds. *Principles and practice of infectious disease,* 5th ed. Philadelphia: Churchill Livingstone, 2000:3177–3191.
31. Ehrenkranz JE, Pfaff SJ. Mediastinitis complicating cardiac operations: evidence of postoperative causation. *Rev Infect Dis* 1991;13: 803–814.
32. Altemeier WA, Culbertson WR, Hummel RP. Surgical consideration of endogenous infections sources, types, and methods of control. *Surg Clin North Am* 1968;48:227–240.
33. Wiley AM, Ha'eri GB. Routes of infection. A study of using tracer particles in the orthopedic operating room. *Clin Orthop* 1979;139: 150–155.
34. Edwards LD. The epidemiology of 2056 remote site infections and 1966 surgical wound infections occurring in 1865 patients: a four-year study of 40,923 operations at Rush-Presbyterian–St. Lukes's Hospital, Chicago. *Ann Surg* 1976;184:758–766.
35. Valentine RJ, Weigelt JA, Dryer D, et al. Effect of remote infections on clean wound infection rates. *Am J Infect Control* 1986;14:64–67.
36. Devenish EA, Miles AA. Control of *Staphylococcus aureus* in an operative theatre. *Lancet* 1939;1:1088–1094.
37. Lowbury EJL, Lilly HA. Disinfection of the hands of surgeons and nurses. *Br Med J* 1960;1:1445–1450.
38. Walter CW, Kundsin RB. The bacteriologic study of surgical gloves from 250 operations. *Surg Gynecol Obstet* 1969;129:949–952.
39. Dodds RDA, Guy PJ, Peacock AM, et al. Surgical glove perforation. *Br J Surg* 1988;75:966–968.
40. Dineen P, Drusin L. Epidemics of postoperative wound infections associated with hair carriers. *Lancet* 1973;2:1157–1159.
41. Ha'eri GB, Wiley AM. The efficacy of standard surgical face masks: an investigation using tracer particles. *Clin Orthop* 1980;148:160–162.
42. Mastro TD, Farley TA, Elliott JA, et al. An outbreak of surgical-wound infections due to group A streptococcus carried on the scalp. *N Engl J Med* 1990;323:968–972.
43. Ford CR, Peterson DE, Mitchell CR. An appraisal of the role of surgical masks. *Am J Surg* 1967;113:787–790.
44. Letts RM, Doermer E. Conversation in the operating theater as a cause of airborne bacterial contamination. *J Bone Joint Surg* 1983; 65A:357–362.
45. Walter CW, Kundsin RB. The floor as a reservoir of hospital infections. *Surg Gynecol Obstet* 1960;111:1–7.
46. Fredette V. The bacteriological efficiency of air-conditioning systems in operating-rooms. *Can J Surg* 1958;1:226–229.
47. Lowbury EJL, Lilly HA. The sources of hospital infection of wounds with *Clostridium welchii. J Hyg* 1958;56:169–182.
48. Eickhoff TC. An outbreak of surgical wound infections due to *Clostridium perfringens. Surg Gynecol Obstet* 1962;114:1102–1108.
49. Everett ED, Pearson S, Rogers W. Rhizopus surgical wound infection associated with elasticized adhesive tape dressings. *Arch Surg* 1979; 114:738–739.
50. Pearson RD, Valenti WM, Steigbigel RT. *Clostridium perfringens* wound infection associated with elastic bandages. *JAMA* 1980;244: 1128–1130.
51. Basset DCJ, Stokes KJ, Thomas WRG. Wound infection with *Pseudomonas multivorans.* A water-borne contaminant of disinfectant solutions. *Lancet* 1970;1:1118–1119.
52. Thomas MEM, Piper E, Maurer IM. Contamination of an operating theatre by gram-negative bacteria. Examination of water supplies, cleaning methods, and wound infections. *J Hyg* 1972;70:63–68.
53. Ehrenkranz NJ, Bolyard E, Weiner M, et al. Antibiotic-sensitive *Serratia marcescens* infections complicating cardiopulmonary operations: contaminated disinfectant as a reservoir. *Lancet* 1980;2:1289–1292.
54. McIntyre DM. An epidemic of *Streptococcus pyogenes* puerperal and postoperative sepsis with an unusual carrier site—the anus. *Am J Obstet Gynecol* 1968;101:308–314.
55. Schaffner W, Lefkowitz LB Jr, Goodman JS, et al. Hospital outbreak of infections with group A streptococci traced to an asymptomatic anal carrier. *N Engl J Med* 1969;280:1124–1125.
56. Gyrska PF, O'Dea AE. Postoperative streptococcal wound infection. The anatomy of an epidemic. *JAMA* 1970;213:1189–1191.
57. Stamm WE, Feely JC, Facklam RR. Wound infections due to group A *Streptococcus* traced to a vaginal carrier. *J Infect Dis* 1978;138: 287–292.
58. Berkelman RL, Martin D, Graham DR, et al. Streptococcal wound infections caused by a vaginal carrier. *JAMA* 1982;247:2680–2682.
59. Bradley LP, Enneking WF, Franco JA. The effect of operating-room environment on the infection rate after Charnley low-friction total hip replacement. *J Bone Joint Surg* 1975;57A:80–83.
60. Sanderson MC, Bentley G. Assessment of wound contamination during surgery: a preliminary report comparing vertical laminar flow and conventional theatre systems. *Br J Surg* 1976;63:431–432.
61. Charnley J. Postoperative infection after total hip replacement with special reference to air contamination in the operating room. *Clin Orthop* 1972;87:167–187.
62. Salvati EA, Robinson RP, Zeno SM, et al. Infection rates after 3175 total hip and total knee replacements performed with and without a horizontal unidirectional filtered air flow system. *J Bone Joint Surg* 1982;64A:525–535.
63. Lidwell OM, Lowbury EJL, Whyte W, et al. Airborne contamination of wounds in joint replacement operations: the relationship to sepsis rates. *J Hosp Infect* 1983;4:111–131.
64. Altemeier WA, Culbertson WR. Surgical infection. In: Moyer C, et al., eds. *Surgery, principles and practice,* 3rd ed. Philadelphia: Lippincott, 1965.
65. Bruun JN. Post-operative wound infection. Predisposing factors and the effect of a reduction in the dissemination of staphylococci. *Acta Med Scand* 1970;514(suppl):1–89.
66. Nagachinta T, Stephens M, Reitz B, et al. Risk factors for surgical-

wound infection following cardiac surgery. *J Infect Dis* 1987;156: 967–973.

67. Mishriki SF, Law DJW, Jeffery PJ. Factors affecting the incidence of postoperative wound infection. *J Hosp Infect* 1990;16:223–230.
68. Kernodle DS, Barg NL, Kaiser AB. Low-level colonization of hospitalized patients with methicillin-resistant coagulase-negative staphylococci and emergence of the organisms during surgical antimicrobial prophylaxis. *Antimicrob Agents Chemother* 1988;32:202–208.
69. Archer GL, Armstrong BC. Alteration of staphylococcal flora in cardiac surgery patients receiving antibiotic prophylaxis. *J Infect Dis* 1983;147:642–649.
70. Maki DG, Stevens JA. Nosocomial colonization of cardiac surgery and cardiology patients by methicillin-resistant coagulase negative *Staphylococcus* [abstract 472]. In: *Program and abstracts of the 24th Interscience Conference on Antimicrobial Agents and Chemotherapy.* Washington, DC: American Society for Microbiology, 1984:176.
71. Archer GL. Alteration of cutaneous staphylococcal flora as a consequence of antimicrobial prophylaxis. *Rev Infect Dis* 1991;13(suppl 10):S805–S809.
72. Archer GL, Dietric DR, Johnston JL. Molecular epidemiology of transmissible gentamicin resistance among coagulase-negative staphylococci in a cardiac surgery unit. *J Infect Dis* 1985;151:243–251.
73. Seropian R, Reynolds BM. Wound infections after preoperative depilatory versus razor preparation. *Am J Surg* 1971;121:251–254.
74. Powis SJA, Waterworth TA, Arkell DG. Preoperative skin preparation: clinical evaluation of depilatory cream. *Br Med J* 1976;2: 1166–1168.
75. Balthazar ER, Colt JD, Nichols RL. Preoperative hair removal: a randomized prospective study of shaving versus clipping. *South Med J* 1982;75:799–801.
76. Alexander JW, Fischer JE, Boyajiian M, et al. The influence of hair-removal methods on wound infections. *Arch Surg* 1983;118:347–352.
77. Mehta G, Prakash B, Karmoker S. Computer assisted analysis of wound infection in neurosurgery. *J Hosp Infect* 1988;11:244–252.
78. Hamilton WH, Lone FJ. Preoperative hair removal. *Can J Surg* 1977; 20:269–275.
79. Shapiro MB, Munoz A, Tager IB, et al. Risk factors for infection at the operative site after abdominal or vaginal hysterectomy. *N Engl J Med* 1982;307:1661–1666.
80. Farber BF, Kaiser DL, Wenzel RP. Relationship between surgical volume and incidence of postoperative wound infection. *N Engl J Med* 1981;305:200–204.
81. Miller PJ, Searcy MA, Kaiser DL, et al. The relationship between surgeon experience and endometritis after cesarean section. *Surg Gynecol Obstet* 1987;165:535–539.
82. Cruse PJE, Foord R. A five-year prospective study of 23,649 surgical wounds. *Arch Surg* 1973;107:206–210.
83. Nora PF, Vanecko RM, Bransfield JJ. Prophylactic abdominal drains. *Arch Surg* 1972;105:173–176.
84. Magee C, Rodeheaver GT, Golden GT, et al. Potentiation of wound infection by surgical drains. *Am J Surg* 1976;131:547–549.
85. Simchen E, Stein H, Sacks TG, et al. Multivariate analysis of determinants of postoperative wound infection in orthopaedic patients. *J Hosp Infect* 1984;5:137–146.
86. Lidwell OM. Sepsis in surgical wounds. Multiple regression analysis applied to records of post-operative hospital sepsis. *J Hyg* 1961;59: 259–270.
87. Claesson BEB, Holmlund DEW. Predictors of intraoperative bacterial contamination and postoperative infection in elective colorectal surgery. *J Hosp Infect* 1988;11:127–135.
88. Lubowski D, Hunt DR. Abdominal wound drainage—a prospective, randomized trial. *Med J Aust* 1987;146:133–135.
89. Shaffer D, Benotti PN, Bothe A Jr, et al. A prospective, randomized trial of abdominal wound drainage in gastric bypass surgery. *Ann Surg* 1987;206:134–137.
90. Loong RLC, Rogers MS, Chang AMZ. A controlled trial of wound drainage in caesarian section. *Aust NZ J Obstet Gynecol* 1988;28: 266–269.
91. Monson JRT, Guillou PJ, Keane FBV, et al. Cholecystectomy is safer without drainage: the results of a prospective, randomized clinical trial. *Surgery* 1991;109:740–746.
92. Sheretz RJ, Garibaldi RA, Marosok RD, et al. Consensus paper on the surveillance of surgical wound infections. *Am J Infect Control* 1992;20:263–270.
93. Lidgren L. Postoperative orthopaedic infections in patients with diabetes mellitus. *Acta Orthop Scand* 1973;44:149–151.
94. Lilienfeld DE, Vlahov D, Tenny JH, et al. Obesity and diabetes as risk factors for postoperative wound infections after cardiac surgery. *Am J Infect Control* 1988;16:3–6.
95. Nystrom P, Jonstam A, Hojer H, et al. Incisional infection after colorectal surgery in obese patients. *Acta Chir Scand* 1987;153:225–227.
96. Windsor JA, Hill GL. Weight loss with physiologic impairment. A basic indicator of surgical risk. *Ann Surg* 1988;207:290–296.
97. Gil-Egea MJ, Pi-Sunyer MT, Verdaguer A, et al. Surgical wound infections: prospective study of 4,468 clean wounds. *Infect Control* 1987;8:277–280.
98. Huchcroft SA, Nicolle LE, Cruse PJE. Surgical wound infection and cancer among the elderly: a case control study. *J Surg Oncol* 1990; 45:250–256.
99. Northey D. Microbial surveillance in a surgical intensive care unit. *Surg Gynecol Obstet* 1974;139:321–326.
100. Flynn DM, Weinstein RA, Nathan C, et al. Patients' endogenous flora as the source of nosocomial enterobacter in cardiac surgery. *J Infect Dis* 1987;156:363–368.
101. Weinstein RA. Epidemiology and control of nosocomial infections in adult intensive care units. *Am J Med* 1991;91(suppl 3B):179–184.
102. Wihlborg O. The effect of washing with chlorhexidine soap on wound infection rate in general surgery. *Ann Chir Gynaecol* 1987;76: 263–265.
103. Hayek LJ, Emerson JM, Gardner AMN. A placebo-controlled trial of the effect of two preoperative baths or showers with chlorhexidine detergent on postoperative wound infection rates. *J Hosp Infect* 1987; 10:165–172.
104. Garibaldi RA, Skolnick D, Lerer T, et al. The impact of preoperative skin disinfection on preventing intraoperative wound contamination. *Infect Control Hosp Epidemiol* 1988;9:109–113.
105. Rotter ML, Larsen SO, Cooke EM, et al. A comparison of the effects of preoperative whole-body bathing with detergent alone and with detergent containing chlorhexidine gluconate on the frequency of wound infections after clean surgery. *J Hosp Infect* 1988;11:310–320.
106. Culbertson WR, Altemeier WA, Gonzalez LL, et al. Studies on the epidemiology of postoperative infection of clean operative wounds. *Ann Surg* 1961;154:599–610.
107. Howe CW, Marston AT. A study on sources of postoperative staphylococcal infection. *Surg Gynecol Obstet* 1962;158:266–275.
108. Burke JF. Identification of the sources of staphylococci contaminating the surgical wound during operation. *Ann Surg* 1963;158:898–904.
109. Burke JF. The effective period of preventive antibiotic action in experimental incisions and dermal lesions. *Surgery* 1961;50:161–168.
110. Classen DC, Evans RS, Pestotnik SL, et al. The timing of prophylactic administration of antibiotics and the risk of surgical-wound infection. *N Engl J Med* 1992;326:281–286.
111. Chodak GW, Plaut ME. Use of systemic antibiotics for prophylaxis in surgery: a critical review. *Arch Surg* 1977;112:326–334.
112. Evans M, Pollock AV. Trial on trial. A review of trials of antibiotic prophylaxis. *Arch Surg* 1984;119:109–113.
113. Baum ML, Anish DS, Chalmers TC, et al. A survey of clinical trials of antibiotic prophylaxis in colon surgery: evidence against further use of no-treatment controls. *N Engl J Med* 1981;305:795–799.
114. Meijer WS, Schmitz PIM, Jeekel J. Meta-analysis of controlled clinical trials of antibiotic prophylaxis in biliary tract surgery. *Br J Surg* 1990; 77:283–290.
115. Kaiser AB. Antimicrobial prophylaxis in surgery. *N Engl J Med* 1986; 315:1129–1138.
116. Anonymous. Antimicrobial prophylaxis in surgery. *Med Lett* 1993; 35:91–94.
117. Ritter MA, French MLV, Eitzen HE, et al. The antimicrobial effectiveness of operative-site preparative agents. *J Bone Joint Surg* 1980; 62A:826–828.

118. Peterson AF, Rosenberg A, Alatary SD. Comparative evaluation of surgical scrub preparations. *Surg Gynecol Obstet* 1978;146:63–65.
119. Brown TR, Ehrlich CE, Stehman FB, et al. A clinical evaluation of chlorhexidine gluconate spray as compared with iodophor scrub for preoperative skin preparation. *Surg Gynecol Obstet* 1984;158: 363–366.
120. The tentative final monograph for OTC topical antimicrobial products. *Fed Reg* 1978(January 6);43FR 1210:1211–1249.
121. Lowbury EJL, Lilly HA. Use of 4% chlorhexidine detergent solution (Hibiscrub) and other methods of skin disinfection. *Br Med J* 1973; 1:510–515.
122. Dineen P. An evaluation of the duration of the surgical scrub. *Surg Gynecol Obstet* 1969;129:1181–1184.
123. Galle PC, Homesley HD, Rhyne AL. Reassessment of the surgical scrub. *Surg Gynecol Obstet* 1978;147:215–218.
124. O'Shaughnessy M, O'Malley VP, Corbett G, et al. Optimum duration of surgical scrub-time. *Br J Surg* 1991;78(6):685–686.
125. Hingst V, Juditzki I, Heeg P, et al. Evaluation of the efficacy of surgical hand disinfection following a reduced application time of 3 instead of 5 min. *J Hosp Infect* 1992;20(2):79–86.
126. Pottinger J, Burns S, Manske C. Bacterial carriage by artifical versus natural nails. *Am J Infect Control* 1989;17:340–344.
127. Moolenaar RL, Crutcher JM, San Joaquin VH, et al. A prolonged outbreak of Pseudomonas aeruginosa in a neonatal intensive care unit: did staff fingernails play a role in disease transmission? *Infect Control Hosp Epidemiol* 2002:21:80–85.
128. Waring L, Armstron R, Bolding F, et al. Postoperative Serratia marcescens wound infections traced to an out-of-hospital source. *J Infect Dis* 1997;175(4):992–995.
129. Mangram AJ, Horan TC, Peason ML, et al. Hospital Infection Control Practices Advisory Committee. Guidelines for prevention of Surgical Site Infection, 1999. *Infect Control Hosp Epidemiol* 1999;20: 247–278.
130. Ford CL, Peterson DE, Mitchell CR. An appraisal of the role of surgical face masks. *Am J Surg* 1967;113:787–790.
131. Dineen P. Microbial filtration by surgical masks. *Surg Gynecol Obstet* 1971;133:812–814.
132. Quesnel LB. The efficiency of surgical masks of varying design and composition. *Br J Surg* 1975;62:936–940.
133. Tunevall TG. Postoperative wound infections and surgical face masks: a controlled study. *World J Surg* 1991;15:383–388.
134. Orr NWM. Is a mask necessary in the operating theatre? *Ann R Coll Surg Engl* 1981;63:390–394.
135. Schwartz JT, Saunders DE. Microbial penetration of surgical gown materials. *Surg Gynecol Obstet* 1980;150:508–512.
136. Lovitt SA, Nichols RL, Smith JW, et al. Isolation gowns: a false sense of security? *Am J Infect Control* 1992;20:185–191.
137. Beck WC, Collette TS. False faith in the surgeon's gown and drape. *Am J Surg* 1952;83:125–126.
138. Moylan JA, Kennedy BV. The importance of gown and drape barriers in the prevention of wound infection. *Surg Gynecol Obstet* 1980;151: 465–470.
139. Garibaldi RA, Maglio S, Lerer T, et al. Comparisons of nonwoven and woven gown and drape fabric to prevent intraoperative wound contamination and postoperative infection. *Am J Surg* 1986;152: 505–509.
140. Moylan JA, Fitzpatrick PA, Davenport KE. Reducing wound infections. Improved gown and drape barrier performance. *Arch Surg* 1987; 122:152–157.
141. Lilly HA, London PS, Lowbury EJL, et al. Effects of adhesive drapes on contamination of operation wounds. *Lancet* 1970;2:431–432.
142. Jackson DW, Pollock AV, Tindal DS. The value of a plastic adhesive drape in the prevention of wound infection. A controlled trial. *Br J Surg* 1971;58:340–342.
143. Anonymous. *Mechanical standards. Guidelines for construction and equipment of hospital and medical facilities.* Washington, DC: American Institute of Architects Press, 1987.
144. Kinmouth JB, Hare R, Tracy GD, et al. Studies of theatre ventilation and wound infection. *Br Med J* 1958;2:407–411.
145. Maki DG, Alvarado CJ, Hassemer CA, et al. Relation of the inanimate hospital environment to endemic nosocomial infection. *N Engl J Med* 1982;307:1562–1566.
146. Lidwell OM. Clean air at operation and subsequent sepsis in the joint. *Clin Orthop* 1986;91:211–218.
147. Collis DK, Steinhaus K. Total hip replacement without deep infection in a standard operating room. *J Bone Joint Surg* 1976;58A:446–450.
148. Hill C, Flamant R, Mazas F, et al. Prophylactic cefazolin versus placebo in total hip replacement. *Lancet* 1981;1:795–797.
149. American College of Surgeons Committee on Control of Surgical Infections of the Committee on Pre- and Postoperative Care. *Manual on control of infection in surgical patients,* 2nd ed. Philadelphia: Lippincott, 1984.
150. Condon RE, Schulte WJ, Malangoni MA, et al. Effectiveness of a surgical wound surveillance program. *Arch Surg* 1983;118:303–307.
151. Olson M, O'Connor M, Schwartz ML. Surgical wound infections. A 5-year prospective study of 20,193 wounds at the Minneapolis VA Medical Center. *Ann Surg* 1984;199:253–259.
152. Olson MM, Lee JT Jr. Continuous, 10-year wound infection surveillance. Results, advantages, and unanswered questions. *Arch Surg* 1990; 125:794–803.
153. Simmons BP. CDC guideline for prevention of surgical wound infections. *Infect Control* 1982;3:187–196.
154. Scheckler WE. Surgeon specific wound infection rates—a potentially dangerous and misleading strategy. *Infect Control Hosp Epidemiol* 1988;9:145–146.
155. Scheckler WE. Feedback of surgical site infection rates to surgeons: recommendations, the data and the reality. *Semin Infect Control* 2002: 2:81–85.
156. Garner JS. Guideline for prevention of surgical wound infections, 1985. *Infect Control* 1986;7:193–200.
157. Doig CM, Wilkinson AW. Wound infection in a children's hospital. *Br J Surg* 1976;63:647–650.
158. Mead PB, Pories SE, Hall P, et al. Decreasing the incidence of surgical wound infections. Validation of a surveillance notification program. *Arch Surg* 1986;121:458–461.
159. Davis SD, Sobocinski K, Hoffmann RG, et al. Postoperative wound infections in a children's hospital. *Pediatr Infect Dis* 1984;3:114–116.
160. Donowitz LG. High risk of nosocomial infection in the pediatric critical care patient. *Crit Care Med* 1986;14:26–28.
161. Maguire GC, Nordin J, Myers MG, et al. Infections acquired by young infants. *Am J Dis Child* 1981;135:693–698.
162. Hazelrigg SR, Wellons HA Jr, Schneider JA, et al. Wound complications after median sternotomy: relationship to internal mammary grafting. *J Thorac Cardiovasc Surg* 1989;98:1096–1099.
163. Conklin CM, Gray RJ, Neilson D, et al. Determinants of wound infection incidence after isolated coronary artery bypass surgery in patients randomized to receive prophylactic cefuroxime or cefazolin. *Ann Thorac Surg* 1988;46:172–177.
164. Wells FC, Newsom SWB, Rowlands C. Wound infection in cardiothoracic surgery. *Lancet* 1983;1:1209–1210.
165. Farrington M, Webster M, Fenn A, et al. Study of cardiothoracic wound infection at St. Thomas Hospital. *Br J Surg* 1985;72:759–762.
166. Cullingford AT, Cunningham JN Jr, Zeff RH, et al. Sternal and costochondral infections following open-heart surgery. A review of 2,594 cases. *J Thorac Cardiovasc Surg* 1976;72:714–726.
167. Cosgrove DM, Lytle BM, Loop FD, et al. Does bilateral internal mammary artery grafting increase surgical risk? *J Thorac Cardiovasc Surg* 1988;95:850–856.
168. Kouchoukos NT, Wareing TH, Murphy SF, et al. Risks of bilateral internal mammary artery bypass grafting. *Ann Thorac Surg* 1990;49: 210–219.
169. Demmy TL, Park SB, Liebler GA, et al. Recent experience with major sternal wound complications. *Ann Thorac Surg* 1990;49:458–462.
170. Centers for Disease Control and Prevention: National Nosocomial Infections Surveillance (NNIS) System Report. Data summary from January 1992–June 2001, August 2001. *Am J Infect Control* 2001; 404–421.
171. Grossi EA, Esposito R, Harris LJ, et al. Sternal wound infections and use of internal mammary artery grafts. *J Thorac Cardiovasc Surg* 1991; 102:342–347.

172. Arnold M. The surgical anatomy of sternal blood supply. *J Thorac Cardiovasc Surg* 1972;64:596–610.
173. Hughes CF, Grant AF, Leckie BD, et al. Cardioplegia solution: a contamination crisis. *J Thorac Cardiovasc Surg* 1986;91:296–302.
174. Stiver HG, Clark J, Kennedy J, et al. *Pseudomonas* sternotomy wound infection and sternal osteomyelitis. Complications after open heart surgery. *JAMA* 1979;241:1034–1036.
175. Isenberg HD, Tucci V, Cintron F, et al. Single-source outbreak of *Candida tropicalis* complicating coronary bypass surgery. *J Clin Microbiol* 1989;27:2426–2428.
176. Larson E, Horan T, Kotilainen H, et al. Study of the definitions of nosocomial infections. *Am J Infect Control* 1991;19:259–267.
177. Wenzel RP, Osterman CA, Hunting KJ, et al. Hospital acquired infections. I. Surveillance in a university hospital. *Am J Epidemiol* 1976;103:251–260.
178. Freeman J, McGowan JE Jr. Methodologic issues in hospital epidemiology. I. Rates, case finding and interpretation. *Rev Infect Dis* 1981; 3:658–667.
179. Thompson RL. Surveillance and reporting of nosocomial infections. In: Wenzel RP, ed. *Prevention and control of nosocomial infections.* Baltimore: Williams & Wilkins, 1987:70–82.
180. Cardo DM, Falk PS, Mayhall CG. Validation of surgical wound surveillance. *Infect Control Hosp Epidemiol* 1993;14:211–215.
181. Froggatt JW, Mayhall CG. Development and validation of a surveillance system for postoperative wound infections in a university center. Annual Meeting of the American Society for Microbiology, New Orleans, LA, May 14–18, 1989.
182. Polk BF, Tager IB, Shapiro M, et al. Randomized clinical trial of perioperative cefazolin in preventing infection in hysterectomy. *Lancet* 1980;1:437–440.
183. Burns SJ, Dippe SE. Postoperative wound infections detected during hospitalization and after discharge in a community hospital. *Am J Infect Control* 1982;10:60–65.
184. Rosendorf LL, Octabio J, Estes JP. Effect of methods of postdischarge wound infection surveillance on reported infection rates. *Am J Infect Control* 1983;11:226–229.
185. Brown RB, Bradley S, Opitz E, et al. Surgical wound infections documented after hospital discharge. *Am J Infect Control* 1987;15:54–58.
186. Reimer K, Gleed C, Nicolle LE. The impact of postdischarge infection on surgical wound infection rates. *Infect Control Hosp Epidemiol* 1987; 8:237–240.
187. Weigelt JA, Dryer D, Haley RW. The necessity and efficiency of wound surveillance after discharge. *Arch Surg* 1992;127:77–82.
188. Seaman M, Lammers R. Inability of patients to self-diagnose wound infections. *J Emerg Med* 1991;9:215–219.
189. Hirschhorn L, Currier J, Platt R. Electronic surveillance antibiotic exposure and coded discharge diagnoses as indicators of postoperative infection and other quality assurance measures. *Infect Control Hosp Epidemiol* 1993;14:21–28.
190. Yokoe DS, Shapiro MM, Simchen E, et al. Use of antibiotic exposure to detect postoperative infections. *Infect Control Hosp Epidemiol* 1998; 19:317–322.
191. Platt R, Yokoe D, Sands K, and the CDC Eastern Massachusetts Prevention Epicenter Investigators. Automated methods for surveillance of SSIs. *Emerg Infect Dis* 2001;7(2):1–11.
192. Platt R, Zaleznik DF, Hopkins CC, et al. Perioperative antibiotic prophylaxis for herniorraphy and breast surgery. *N Engl J Med* 1990; 322:153–160.
193. Kaiser AB, Roach AC, Mulherin J Jr, et al. The cost-effectiveness of antimicrobial prophylaxis in clean vascular surgery. *J Infect Dis* 1983; 147:1103.
194. Hasselgren PO, Ivarsson L, Risberg B, et al. Effects of prophylactic antibiotics in vascular surgery: a prospective, randomized, double-blind study. *Ann Surg* 1984;200:86–92.
195. Stellato TA. History of laparoscopic surgery. *Surg Clin North Am* 1992;72:997–1002.
196. Perrisat J, Vitale GC. Laparoscopic cholecystectomy: gateway to the future [editorial]. *Am J Surg* 1991;161:408.
197. A prospective analysis of 1518 laparoscopic cholecystectomies. The Southern Surgeons Club. *N Engl J Med* 1991;324:1073–1078.
198. Reich H, DeCaprio J, McGlynn F. Laparoscopic hysterectomy. *J Gynecol Surg* 1989;5:213–216.
199. Richardson RE, Bournas N, Magos AL. Is laparoscopic hysterectomy a waste of time? *Lancet* 1995;345:36–41.
200. Harris WJ, Danille JF. Early complications of laparoscopic hysterectomy. *Obstet Gynecol Surv* 1996;51:559–567.
201. Donohue JH. Laparoscopic surgical procedures. *Mayo Clin Proc* 1994; 69:758–762.
202. Scott-Conner EH, ed. *Laparoscopic surgery. Surgery clinics of North America.* Philadelphia: WB Saunders, 1996:76.
203. Kluytmans J, van Belkum A, Verbrugh H. Nasal carriage of *Staphylococcus aureus*: epidemiology, underlying mechanisms, and associated risks. *Clin Microbial Rev* 1997;10:505–520.
204. Centers for Disease Control and Prevention: National Nosocomial Infections Surveillance (NNIS) System Report. Data summary from January 1992–June 2001, issued August 2001. *Am J Infect Control* 2001;29:404–421.
205. Chang L, Dellinger EP. Impact of laparoscopy on surgical-site infections. *Semin Infect Control* 2002;102–107.
206. Horan TC. Surgical-site infection surveillance and risk adjustment: the National Nosocomial Infections Surveillance System methodology. *Semin Infect Control* 2002;2:72–80.
207. Peters JH, Ellison EC, Innes JT, et al. Safety and efficacy of laparoscopic cholecystectomy. A prospective analysis of 100 initial patients. *Ann Surg* 1991;213:3–12.
208. Dent TL. Training and privileging for new procedures. *Surg Clin North Am* 1996;76:615–621.
209. Wenzel RP Perl TM. The significance of nasal carriage of *Staphylococcus aureus* an incidence of postoperative wound infection. *J Hosp Infect* 1995;31:13–24.
210. H.W. The use of nasal mupirocin ointment to prevent *Staphylococcus aureus* bacteraemias in haemodialysis patients: an analysis of cost-effectiveness. *J Hosp Infect* 1991;19(suppl B):41–46.
211. Boelacert JR, Van Landuyt HW, Godard CA, et al. Nasal mupirocin ointment decreases the incidence of *Staphylococcus aureus* bacteraemias in haemodialysis patients. *Nephron Dial Transplant* 1993;8:235–239.
212. Yu,VL, Goetz A. Wagener M, et al. *Staphylococcus aureus* nasal carriage and infection in patients on hemodialysis. *N Engl J Med* 1986:315: 91–96.
213. von Eiff C, Beckler K, Machka K, et al. Nasal carriage as a source of *Staphylococcus aureus* bacteremia. *N Engl J Med* 2001;344:11–16.
214. Cimochowski GE, Harostock MD, Brown R, et al. Intranasal mupirocin reduces sternal wound infection after open heart surgery in diabetics and nondiabetics. *Ann Thorac Surg* 2001;71:1572–1579.
215. Kluytmans JAJW, Mouton JW, Ijzerman EPF, et al. Nasal carriage of *Staphylococcal aureus* is a major risk factor for wound infections after cardiac surgery. *J Infect Dis* 1995;171:216–219.
216. Kluytmans JAJW, Mouton JW, Vandenbergh MFG, et al. Reduction of surgical-site infections in cardiothoracic surgery by elimination of nasal carriage of *Staphylococcus aureus. Infect Control Hosp Epidemiol* 1966;17:780–785.
217. Vandenbergh MFQ, Kluytmans JAJAW, van Hont BA, et al. Cost effectiveness of perioperative mupirocin nasal ointment in cardiothoracic surgery. *Infect Control Hosp Epidemiol* 1996;17:786–792.
218. Boyce JM. Preventing staphylococcal infections by eradicating nasal carriage of *Staphylococcus aureus*. Proceeding with caution. *Infect Control hospital Epidemiol* 1996;17:775–779.
219. Perl TM, Cullen JJ, Wenzel RP, et al. Intranasal mupirocin to prevent post operative *Staphylococcus aureus* infections. *N Engl J Med* 2002; 346:1871–1877.

22

NOSOCOMIAL PNEUMONIA

DENNIS C. J. J. BERGMANS
MARC J. M. BONTEN

The substantial clinical and financial impact of nosocomial pneumonia makes this an important topic for hospital epidemiologists. According to surveillance data from the National Nosocomial Infections Surveillance (NNIS) system of the Centers for Disease Control and Prevention (CDC), pneumonia is the second most common nosocomial infection overall (1) and the most common infection in intensive care units (ICUs) (2). In addition, pneumonia is associated with significant attributable mortality (3,4) and with considerably increased costs of care (3, 5). The widespread use of tracheal intubation and mechanical ventilation to support the critically ill has defined an expanding group of patients who are at particularly high risk for developing nosocomial pneumonia. In this group of patients, the infection is usually called ventilator-associated pneumonia (VAP). Unfortunately, prevention of VAP has proved to be difficult (6).

HISTORICAL ASPECTS

During the last three decades, much has been learned about the epidemiology of nosocomial pneumonia. In the 1960s, Pierce, Sanford, and others investigated the relationship of epidemic necrotizing gram-negative pneumonia to contaminated reservoir nebulizers in respiratory therapy devices and described effective disinfection measures (7–9). During the 1970s and early 1980s, additional work described the continuing association of nosocomial pneumonia with respiratory therapy equipment (10), risk factors for postoperative pneumonia (11), and the relationship of nosocomial pneumonia with oropharyngeal (12) and gastric (13) gram-negative bacillary colonization. During the 1980s and 1990s, several preventive strategies were designed and tested with varying success, such as the use of sucralfate for stress-ulcer prophylaxis (14–17), selective decontamination of the digestive tract (SDD) (18–26), continuous subglottic aspiration (27–29), and continuous lateral rotation therapy (30–35). Moreover, controversies developed over the relevance of gastric colonization in the pathogenesis of VAP (6,36,37), the usefulness of SDD (38,39), and the necessity of bronchoscopic techniques for diagnosing VAP (40,41). In the most recent years, more general approaches for patient management, not only directed to VAP, have been applied, such as strict control of blood glucose levels, noninvasive ventilation, and sedation strategies to reduce duration of ventilation. This chapter summarizes current knowledge of diagnosis, epidemiology, and prevention of nosocomial pneumonia.

DIAGNOSIS

Pneumonia refers to inflammation of the distal lung caused by infection with microorganisms and is characterized histologically by the accumulation of neutrophils in the distal bronchioles, alveoli, and interstitium. Three types of nosocomial pneumonia can be distinguished: hospital-acquired pneumonia, early-onset VAP, and late-onset VAP. Pneumonia is defined as VAP when diagnosed in an intubated, mechanically ventilated patient after more than 48 hours of ventilation; early-onset VAP occurs within the first 4 days of mechanical ventilation, and late-onset VAP occurs thereafter (42). The relevance of a rapid and accurate diagnosis of nosocomial pneumonia is obvious. The goals are to prescribe the optimal antibiotic therapy to only those patients with infection of the lungs. Using a technique with a low sensitivity, patients will remain untreated and may suffer significant morbidity and increased risk for mortality. In contrast, a technique with high sensitivity but low specificity will lead to unnecessary use of antibiotics, resulting in unnecessary exposure of patients to toxicity, a potential delay in diagnosing the real cause of infection, increased hospital costs, and, most importantly, unnecessary selection and induction of resistant pathogenic microorganisms.

Clinical and Radiographic Findings

Traditionally, clinical and radiographic criteria have been used to identify cases of nosocomial pneumonia among patients who are not mechanically ventilated. Patients with nosocomial pneumonia are likely to have fever, purulent sputum, signs of pulmonary consolidation, and new or progressive radiographic infiltrates. Although they may complain of dyspnea, cough, and pleuritic chest pain, many patients with nosocomial pneumonia are unable to give a helpful history because of neurologic impairment or severity of illness. The CDC definitions (Table 22.1) of nosocomial pneumonia have been widely used for infection control surveillance and rely predominantly on clinical and radiographic criteria, although the results of other diagnostic tests may also be used (43).

TABLE 22.1. CDC DEFINITIONS OF PNEUMONIA

Pneumonia is defined separately from other infections of the lower respiratory tract. The criteria for pneumonia involve various combinations of clinical, radiographic, and laboratory evidence of infection. In general, expectorated sputum cultures are not useful in diagnosing pneumonia but may help identify the etiologic agent and provide useful antimicrobial susceptibility data. Findings from serial chest x-ray studies may be more helpful than those from a single x-ray film.

Pneumonia must meet one of the following criteria:

1. Rales or dullness to percussion on physical examination of chest *and* any of the following:
   a. New onset of purulent sputum or change in character of sputum
   b. Organism isolated from blood culture
   c. Isolation of pathogen from specimen obtained by transtracheal aspirate, bronchial brushing, or biopsy
2. Chest radiographic examination shows new or progressive infiltrate, consolidation, cavitation, or pleural effusion *and* any of the following:
   a. New onset of purulent sputum or change in character of sputum
   b. Organism isolated from blood culture
   c. Isolation of pathogen from specimen obtained by transtracheal aspirate, bronchial brushing, or biopsy
   d. Isolation of virus or detection of viral antigen in respiratory secretions
   e. Diagnostic single antibody titer [immunoglobulin M (IgM)] or fourfold increase in paired serum samples [immunoglobulin G (IgG)] for pathogen
   f. Histopathologic evidence of pneumonia
3. Patient ≤12 months of age has two of the following: apnea, tachypnea, bradycardia, wheezing, rhonchi, or cough *and* any of the following:
   a. Increased production of respiratory secretions
   b. New onset of purulent sputum or change in character of sputum
   c. Organism isolated from blood culture
   d. Isolation of pathogen from specimen obtained by transtracheal aspirate, bronchial brushing, or biopsy
   e. Isolation of virus or detection of viral antigen in respiratory secretions
   f. Diagnostic single antibody titer (IgM) or fourfold increase in paired serum samples (IgG) for pathogen
   g. Histopathologic evidence of pneumonia
4. Patient ≤12 months of age has chest radiologic examination that shows new or progressive infiltrate, cavitation, consolidation, or pleural effusion *and* any of the following:
   a. Increased production of respiratory secretions
   b. New onset of purulent sputum or change in character of sputum
   c. Organism isolated from blood culture
   d. Isolation of pathogen from specimen obtained by transtracheal aspirate, bronchial brushing, or biopsy
   e. Isolation of virus or detection of viral antigen in respiratory secretions
   f. Diagnostic single antibody titer (IgM) or fourfold increase in paired serum samples (IgG) for pathogen
   g. Histopathologic evidence of pneumonia

Adapted from Garner JS, Jaruis WR, Emori TG, et al. CDC definitions for nosocomial infections, 1988. *Am J Infect Control* 1988;16:128–140.

Diagnosing VAP is even more problematic than diagnosing nosocomial pneumonia in nonventilated patients (44). For scientific purposes, VAP is usually diagnosed using a modified version of the CDC's definitions (45). These criteria are a new or progressive radiographic infiltrate that has persisted for at least 48 hours plus at least two of the following: a temperature higher than 38.5°C or below 35.0°C, a leukocyte count of more than 10,000 per cubic millimeter or less than 5,000 per cubic millimeter, purulent sputum, or isolation of pathogenic bacteria from an endotracheal aspirate. An alternative for the modified CDC criteria is the Clinical Pulmonary Infection Score (CPIS) as defined by Pugin et al. (46) (Table 22.2). This scoring system, basically, uses the same criteria as in the modified CDC criteria. The range of the score is from 0 to 12, with VAP defined by a score of seven or more.

Although each of these criteria may have a reasonable sensitivity for VAP, specificity is poor. Radiographic infiltrates are sensitive indicators of VAP; however, more specific radiographic findings such as single air bronchograms, fissure abutment, or rapid progress to cavitation are infrequently present (47). Unfortunately, even the combination of clinical and radiographic criteria (as in the modified CDC criteria and the CPIS) have been unable to reliably diagnose cases of nosocomial pneumonia diagnosed by autopsy (47,48), histopathology (49), or other stringent criteria (50–52). In an autopsy study of ventilated patients, no radiographic sign predicted pneumonia more than 68% of the time, and no radiographic signs predicted pneumonia in the subgroup

TABLE 22.2. CLINICAL PULMONARY INFECTION SCORE (CPIS) USED FOR THE DIAGNOSIS OF VENTILATOR-ASSOCIATED PNEUMONIA[a]

	Number of points
1. Temperature °C	
≥36.5 and ≤38.4	0
≥38.5 and ≤38.9	1
≥39.0 and ≤36.0	2
2. Blood leukocytes, mm^3	
≥4,000 and ≤11,000	0
<4,000 or >11,000	1
<4,000 or >11,000 and band forms ≥500	2
3. Tracheal secretions[b]	
<14+ of tracheal secretions	0
≥14+ of tracheal secretions	1
≥14+ of tracheal secretions and purulent secretions	2
4. Oxygenation: PaO_2/FIO_2, mm Hg	
>240 or ARDS	0
≤240 and no evidence of ARDS	2
5. Pulmonary radiography	
No infiltrate	0
Diffuse (or patchy) infiltrate	1
Localized infiltrate	2
6. Culture of tracheal aspirate (semiquantitative: 0, 1, 2, or 3+)	
Pathogenic bacteria cultured ≤1+ or no growth	0
Pathogenic bacteria cultured >1+	1
Pathogenic bacteria cultured >1+ and same pathogenic bacteria seen on the Gram stain >1+	2

ARDS, adult respiratory distress syndrome.

[a]Total points = CPIS (varies from 0 to 12 points).

[b]Quantity of tracheal aspirates per day (for each endotracheal aspiration, the quantity of secretions was estimated from 0 to 4+; estimation of the volume of total secretions per day was calculated by adding all the + values recorded over 24 hours together).

Adapted from ref. Pugin J, Auckenthaler R, Mili N, et al. Diagnosis of ventilator-associated pneumonia by bacteriologic analysis of bronchoscopic and nonbronchoscopic "blind" bronchoalveolar lavage fluid. *Am Rev Respir Dis* 1991;143:1121–1129.

of patients with the adult respiratory distress syndrome (ARDS); when clinical and sputum culture results were added to the model, the diagnostic efficiency rose only to 72% (47). Two other reports have documented that fever and pulmonary infiltrates in mechanically ventilated patients were caused by processes other than pneumonia in 49% to 69% of cases (50,51). A variety of other conditions (e.g., drug reactions, atelectasis, chemical aspiration, congestive heart failure), alone or in combination, can mimic the clinical and radiographic presentation of nosocomial pneumonia (53); these conditions are not uncommon in patients with significant underlying medical illness. Furthermore, cultures of sputum and tracheal aspirate do not reliably identify pathogens that cause nosocomial pneumonia (53–56).

Interpretation of the usefulness of diagnostic techniques is seriously hampered because populations studied varied widely and because the use of antibiotics, which strongly influences the yield of bacteriologic procedures, was not always taken into account. The largest problem, however, is the gold standard used to verify the value of diagnostic procedures. Histologic and bacteriologic examination of lung tissue remains the optimal standard to establish the diagnosis of pneumonia. However, these techniques require an open-lung biopsy or autopsy. Although histology and bacteriology of lung tissue, usually at autopsy, have been used as the gold standard in several studies, one should realize that patients who died form a subgroup of all patients with pneumonia. In addition, in several studies, autopsy findings are compared with diagnostic procedures performed several days earlier. In such circumstances, the physiologic host response to infection, usually in combination with antibiotic therapy, may have influenced the ultimate findings. These considerations also account for the evaluation of newer diagnostic techniques.

Quantitative Bronchoscopic Techniques

Diagnostic techniques have been improved by using quantitative cultures of lower airway samples to more accurately diagnose nosocomial pneumonia and identify causative pathogens (49, 55,57–60). The rationale of bronchoscopy is to avoid contamination of culture samples with material from the upper respiratory tract. Three bronchoscopic techniques have been used to diagnose VAP: protected specimen brush (PSB), bronchoalveolar lavage (BAL), and protected bronchoalveolar lavage (PBAL) (Table 22.3).

The PSB technique uses a double-lumen bronchoscopic catheter with a telescoping cannula and distal plug (57). A bacterial burden of less than 10^4 colony-forming units (CFU) per gram in lung tissue has been associated with histologic pneumonia (61). Because the sample size with PSB is ± 0.001 mL, a quantitative culture of 10^3 CFU/mL reflects about 10^6 CFU/mL at the site of infection and is generally used as a cutoff point for VAP. Quantitative cultures of PSB specimens have been shown to accurately identify pneumonia and its causative pathogens in mechanically ventilated patients undergoing open lung biopsy (49) and in mechanically ventilated baboons with diffuse lung injury (55). Studies in normal hosts (62), patients with chronic bronchitis (63), and mechanically ventilated patients with suspected pneumonia (49,50,56) indicate that quantitative PSB cultures are considerably more specific than clinical and radiographic criteria for diagnosing nosocomial pneumonia. Based on the pooled results of published studies (49,50,55,64), one review (53) reported PSB to have a sensitivity of 83% and a specificity of 91%. False-negative results have been attributed to sampling error and to antibiotic use (56,60,64). In several studies, PSB results were compared with histologic and microbiologic evaluation of lung tissue, with sensitivities ranging from 36% to 100% and specificities ranging from 50% to 95% (Table 22.3) (49,65–68).

Some investigators have also used quantitative cultures of BAL specimens to sample a larger portion of the lung, including alveoli (58,59,69). BAL entails sampling of an area of 10^6 alveoli. The tip of the bronchoscope is wedged, under visual control, into a third- or fourth-generation midsize bronchus, according to chest radiograph appearance. Lavage is carried out using at

TABLE 22.3. SENSITIVITIES AND SPECIFICITIES OF INVASIVE DIAGNOSTIC TECHNIQUES FOR VENTILATOR-ASSOCIATED PNEUMONIA (VAP) AS COMPARED TO HISTOLOGIC AND MICROBIOLOGIC EVALUATION OF LUNG TISSUE

Reference	No. patients	No. clinical suspicion of VAP	No. histologic/ microbiologic VAP	Sensitivity	Specificity	Percent on antibiotics
Protected specimen brush (cutoff: 10^3 CFU/mL)						
Chastre et al. (49)	26	?	6 (23%)	100%	60%	54%
Torres et al. (67)	30	?	18 (60%)	50%	100%	100%
Chastre et al. (65)	20	0	11 (55%)	82%	89%	0%
Marquette et al. (66)	28	28	19 (68%)	57%	88%	47%
Papazian et al. (68)	38	?	18 (47%)	42%	95%	21%
Broncholaveolar lavage (cutoff: 10^4 CFU/mL)						
Torres et al. (67)	30	?	18 (60%)	50%	45%	100%
Chastre et al. (65)	20	0	11 (55%)	91%	78%	0%
Marquette et al. (66)	28	28	19 (68%)	47%	100%	47%
Papazian et al. (68)	38	?	18 (47%)	55%	95%	21%
Intracellular microorganisms						
Chastre et al. (65)	20	0	11 (55%)	91% (cutoff: >0%)	89%	0%
Marquette et al. (66)	28	28	19 (68%)	37% (cutoff: >5%)	100%	47%

least 120 mL of sterile isotonic saline in several aliquot portions. The dilution of alveolar secretions in the lavage fluid is 10- to 100-fold, so a colony count of 10^4 CFU/mL in lavage fluid represents 10^5 to 10^6 bacteria per milliliter of alveolar secretion (70). In mechanically ventilated baboons, this method appears to be sensitive and provides the best correlation with culture of lung tissue (69). Like PSB, quantitative culture of BAL specimens appears to be more accurate than clinical and radiographic criteria for diagnosing nosocomial pneumonia (58,59,71); however, most studies evaluating quantitative BAL have not used rigorous criteria for determining whether pneumonia was actually present. BAL samples can become contaminated with bacterial flora from the upper respiratory tract, and reduced specificity may result (58). As with PSB, antibiotic use may diminish the sensitivity of BAL (59,69). In studies using histology and microbiologic examination of lung tissue as the gold standard, sensitivities of BAL ranged from 47% to 91%, and specificities ranged from 45% to 100% (Table 22.3) (65–68).

To reduce upper airway contamination while still obtaining a representative sample of affected alveoli, Meduri et al. (60) developed a technique to obtain PBAL specimens using a balloon-tipped telescoping catheter. In a study of 46 patients, including 25 with suspected VAP, quantitative PBAL culture proved to have a sensitivity of 92% and a specificity of 97% for diagnosing bacterial pneumonia (60). Castella et al. (72) applied a similar PBAL technique and found that PBAL displayed improved sensitivity (85%) compared with PSB (62%) and improved specificity (83%) compared with BAL (44%). PBAL appears to be somewhat more demanding and time-consuming than unprotected BAL, and has been studied less often than PSB and BAL.

After several years of experience with these bronchoscopic techniques, a consensus conference proposed a new definition for diagnosing VAP, which became known as the Memphis Ventilator-Associated Pneumonia Consensus Conference criteria (Table 22.4) (61). Definite VAP is only present with radiographic evidence of abscess and a positive needle aspirate or if there is histologic proof of pneumonia at biopsy or autopsy. Probable VAP requires positive quantitative or semiquantitative cultures from PSB or BAL, blood or pleural fluid cultures of a microorganism found within 48 hours of isolation in the sputum, or abscess formation or consolidation with polymorphonuclear-cell infiltration at histologic examination.

Several technical and safety considerations pertaining to these bronchoscopic techniques warrant comment. The technique of the bronchoscopist may influence the results. The passage of the bronchoscope through the upper airway results in bacterial contamination of the suction channel, and the injection of topical anesthetic agents through the bronchoscope carries contaminants into the distal airways (57). Therefore, it is prudent to avoid suctioning or the injection of topical anesthetics before obtaining bronchoscopic samples. Other operator-dependent variables may also affect quantitative culture results. Elevated temperature, hypoxemia, increased radiographic infiltrates, bleeding, arrhythmias, and pneumothorax may be related to these bronchoscopic procedures, but serious or lasting complications appear to be rare (40,41). The use of a high FiO_2, careful monitoring of exhaled volumes and oxygen saturation, and pre-

TABLE 22.4. RECOMMENDED DEFINITIONS FOR VAP FROM THE MEMPHIS VENTILOTOR-ASSOCIATED PNEUMONIA CONSENSUS CONFERENCE

Definite pneumonia The patient meets the clinical criteria for suspicion of VAP of new (progressive) or persistent infiltrate and purulent tracheal secretions and demonstrates one of the following:

1. There is radiographic evidence, preferably computed tomography (CT) evidence, of pulmonary abscess and positive needle aspirate culture from the abscess.
2. There is pathologic evidence of pneumonia on histologic examination of lung tissue obtained by open-lung biopsy or at a postmortem examination immediately after death that demonstrates abscess formation of an area of consolidation with intense polymorphonuclear leukocyte accumulation plus a positive quantitative culture of lung parenchyma (>10^4 microorganisms per gram of lung tissue). When used to confirm the diagnosis of pneumonia made by bronchoscopy, the lung tissue for histologic examination and culture must have been obtained within 3 days of the bronchoscopic procedure.

Probable pneumonia In the absence of any of the above criteria for pneumonia, the patient meets the clinical criteria for suspicion of VAP of new (progressive) or persistent infiltrate and purulent tracheal secretions and demonstrates one of the following:

1. The presence of positive quantitative culture of a sample of secretions from the lower respiratory tract obtained by a technique that minimizes contamination with upper respiratory tract flora (PSB, BAL, PBAL).
2. The presence of positive blood culture unrelated to another source and obtained within 48 hours before or after respiratory sampling. The microorganism(s) recovered should be identical to the organism recovered from a culture of lower respiratory tract secretions.
3. The presence of a positive pleural fluid culture in the absence of previous pleural instrumentation. The microorganism(s) recovered should be identical to the organism recovered from a culture of lower respiratory tract secretions.
4. The presence of pathologic evidence of pneumonia on histologic examination of lung tissue obtained by open-lung biopsy or at a postmortem examination immediately after death that demonstrates abscess formation of an area of consolidation with intense polymorphonuclear leukocyte accumulation plus a negative quantitative culture of lung parenchyma (<10^4 microorganisms per gram of lung tissue). When used to support the diagnosis of pneumonia made by bronchoscopy, the lung tissue for histologic examination and culture must have been obtained within 3 days of the bronchoscopic procedure.

Definitive absence of pneumonia In patients not meeting the criteria for definite pneumonia, the absence of pneumonia is definitive if one of the following criteria are met:

1. Postmortem exam within 3 days of the suspicion of pneumonia showing no histologic sign of lung infection.
2. Definitive alternative etiology with no bacterial growth on a reliable respiratory specimen.
3. Cytologic identification of a process other than pneumonia (e.g., lung cancer) without significant bacterial growth on a reliable respiratory specimen.

Probable absence of pneumonia Indicated by the lack of significant growth on a reliable respiratory specimen with one of the following:

1. Resolution without antibiotic therapy of one of the following: fever, radiographic infiltrate, or radiographic infiltrate and a definitive alternative diagnosis.
2. Persistent fever and radiographic infiltrate, with a definite alternative diagnosis established.

BAL, bronchoalveolar lavage; PBAL, protected BAL; PSB, protected specimen brush; VAP, ventilator-associated pneumonia.
Adapted from Pineton SK, Fagon JY, Leeper KV Jr. Patient selection for clinical investigation of ventilator-associated pneumonia: criteria for evaluating diagnostic techniques. *Chest* 1992;102:553S–556S.

bronchoscopy assessment of risk should help prevent serious complications.

The most important question remains whether these bronchoscopic techniques influence (preferably improve) patient care in the ICU. Several studies have suggested that quantitative bronchoscopic sampling of the distal airways by PSB, BAL, or PBAL substantially improves the accuracy of diagnosing nosocomial pneumonia when compared with clinical and radiographic criteria. In this way, these techniques may help to distinguish between patients who do and patients who do not need antibiotic therapy. In one study, VAP was simultaneously diagnosed according to the modified CDC criteria, CPIS, and quantitative bronchoscopic sampling (17). Incidences of VAP were 22% using the modified CDC criteria, 20% using CPIS, 9% using the Memphis criteria for probable VAP, and 0.4% using the Memphis criteria for definite VAP. In another study, only 50% of all patients fulfilling the modified CDC criteria for VAP met the definition of probable VAP with the Memphis criteria (73).

Five studies determined the effects of withholding or withdrawing empiric antibiotic therapy if a clinical suspicion was not confirmed by a diagnostic test. In three Spanish studies, patients with a clinical suspicion of VAP were randomized to an invasive or noninvasive strategy (74–76). Because empirical therapy was not discontinued in any patient, regardless of whether the suspicion was microbiologically confirmed or not, these studies have not been included here.

Croce et al. (77) performed bronchoscopy in ten mechanically ventilated trauma patients with a clinical suspicion of VAP. The clinical suspicion was based on the presence of fever, leukocytosis, purulent sputum, and changing infiltrates on chest x-ray film. None of the patients received antibiotics before bronchoscopy. Three had $\geq 10^5$ CFU/mL in BAL fluid, and antimicrobial therapy was continued with rapid solution of signs of pneumonia. The other seven patients had less than 10^5 CFU/mL in BAL fluid, and all had their empiric therapy discontinued. Six patients survived, and one died 8 days after bronchoscopy because of head injury. All survivors had resolution of their clinical signs of infection. Only one of them developed an episode of VAP (diagnosis based on CDC criteria and quantitative culture results of BAL) 16 days after the first bronchoscopy.

Bonten et al. (73) investigated 155 mechanically ventilated patients with a clinical suspicion of VAP (CDC criteria) of whom 138 underwent bronchoscopy with BAL or PSB. In 66 patients, the clinical suspicion of infection was not confirmed by quantitative cultures. In 34 patients empiric antimicrobial therapy was started directly after bronchoscopy, and antibiotics were withdrawn in 17 patients. In the other 17 patients, the attending physicians decided to continue antimicrobial therapy because of the clinical condition, usually severe sepsis. In those patients who had not started with empiric antimicrobial therapy (n = 31), only one patient received antimicrobial therapy in the immediate period after bronchoscopy. Thus, 48 patients with a clinical suspicion of VAP that was not confirmed by quantitative culture results of BAL or PSB were not treated and did not have treatment withdrawn. The follow-up of these patients was compared with the follow-up in patients who received treatment (with and without confirmed pneumonia). There were no differences in the incidence of new episodes of VAP, ICU mortality, or hospital mortality. Withholding of antibiotic therapy or discontinuation of empiric therapy in patients with nonsignificant or no growth in quantitative bronchoscopic samples did not lead to higher rates of recurrent episodes of VAP or mortality. A simple cost analysis revealed that, under the circumstances tested, bronchoscopy would be cost effective if bronchoscopy would cost less than $191 or when the costs of antibiotics to treat VAP would be higher than $93 per day (73).

Fagon et al. (78) randomized 413 mechanically ventilated patients with a clinical suspicion of VAP to a diagnostic strategy based on semiquantitative cultures of endotracheal aspirates (n = 209) or an invasive strategy (n = 204). The invasive strategy consisted of bronchoscopy with direct microscopic examination of specimens and quantitative cultures. Quantitative cultures (PSB cutoff point $\geq 10^3$ CFU/mL, BAL cutoff point $\geq 10^4$ CFU/mL) were used to adjust or withdraw empirical treatment. In 117 of 204 patients, direct examinations yielded no bacteria. However, 20 of these patients had signs of severe sepsis and received antibiotics, although the suspicion of VAP was not confirmed. Of the remaining 97 patients, 7 had significant quantitative cultures and antibiotics were started when culture results were available. Thus, the clinical suspicion of VAP was not confirmed in 90 patients. When comparing antibiotic use between patients randomized to either of the two invasive strategies, patients undergoing bronchoscopy had more antibiotic-free days. Twenty-nine patients did not receive antibiotics up to day 28 (compared with 4 in the clinical management group), and patient survival was better among those randomized to the invasive strategy as well.

The Canadian Critical Care Group investigated the effects of an invasive diagnostic strategy in 138 patients with a clinical suspicion of VAP (79). In a nonrandomized study design, 92 patients underwent bronchoscopy and 46 did not. Although changes in antibiotic therapy occurred with equal frequency in both patient groups (66/92 vs. 37/49), in the group that underwent bronchoscopy more patients received less antibiotics (31/92 vs. 9/49). Although discontinuation of empirical antibiotics, because of negative culture results, occurred in only 9 of 34 patients, there was a trend toward reduction in overall antibiotic use following bronchoscopy. No differences were observed for duration of mechanical ventilation, length of ICU stay, and mortality.

In summary, these four studies analyzed the safety of withholding or withdrawing antibiotics when a clinical suspicion of VAP was not confirmed microbiologically. Such a diagnostic strategy was not negatively associated with patient outcome in any of these studies. Thus, based on these limited data, it seems safe to withhold or withdraw antibiotics if quantitative cultures of bronchoscopic samples fail to confirm a clinical suspicion of VAP, as long as there are no signs of severe sepsis, but more rigorously designed prospective studies are warranted.

A different approach was used by Singh et al. (80). They determined CPIS scores of patients with a clinical suspicion of VAP and randomized those with a CPIS score ≤ 6 to different therapeutic strategies—antibiotics for 10 to 21 days (n = 42) or ciprofloxacin for 3 days (n = 39)—that could be compared with withdrawing empirical therapy. Patients randomized to a short course had less antibiotic use, lower antibiotic costs, fewer superinfections with antibiotic resistant pathogens, and no increase in length of stay or mortality. Thus, it seems safe to withdraw antibiotics after 3 days in patients with CPIS scores ≤6. However, the question is whether patients with such a low CPIS score should receive antimicrobial treatment in the first place.

Investigational Methods

A number of adjunctive or alternative methods for diagnosing nosocomial pneumonia have been proposed. Several reports have evaluated nonbronchoscopic techniques for sampling distal airway secretions, including brush (56), BAL (46,68,81,82), and endotracheal aspirates (64). Although such techniques might reduce costs, they have not been adequately validated or standardized, and sampling error can occur. In one study, however, good diagnostic agreement was demonstrated between quantitative cultures from PSB and minibronchoalveolar lavage done by respiratory therapists in patients with suspected VAP (83). And in another study, using postmortem analysis as the gold standard, blind bronchial sampling had a higher sensitivity for VAP than PSB (68).

The identification of intracellular microorganisms by Giemsa stain of BAL specimens has been reported to be highly predictive of nosocomial pneumonia (46,60,84). This technique has been compared with histologic and microbiologic examination of lung tissue at autopsy in two studies, with contradictory results (Table 22.3). Specificities were high in both studies, 100% and 89% (65,66). However, sensitivity was 91% in one study when more than 5% of leukocytes containing intracellular bacteria was considered positive for VAP (65). In the other study, sensitivity was only 37%, when any leukocyte with intracellular bacteria was considered as a threshold for diagnosis of VAP (66).

Measurement of cytokines or inflammatory mediators may be adjunctive tools for diagnosing VAP in the future. Although blood levels of inflammatory mediators poorly correlated with quantitative results from bronchoscopic samples (85,86), elevated concentrations of endotoxin (>5 endotoxin units (EU)/mL) in BAL fluid had a sensitivity of 100% and specificity of 75% for diagnosing VAP (87). Other methods that cannot be recommended at present, but which may merit further investigation, include the detection of elastin fibers (46,88) and antibody-coated bacteria (89) in respiratory secretions and high-resolution computed tomography (CT) (90).

DESCRIPTIVE EPIDEMIOLOGY

Incidence

Published hospital-wide incidence rates for nosocomial pneumonia based on clinical diagnostic criteria have generally been in the range of 0.5 to 1.0 cases per 100 patients (91). The incorporation of time into the denominator may produce more reliable rates: a rate of 0.76 cases per 1,000 patient-days was estimated from a nationwide database in the Study on the Efficacy of Nosocomial Infection Control (SENIC) (92). In the United States, 275,000 cases of nosocomial pneumonia are estimated to occur annually (93).

Incidence rates of VAP among ICU patients depend on the type of ICU, the severity of illness of patients studied, and the criteria for diagnosis. The overall incidence of pneumonia decreases when the definition of pneumonia becomes more strict. Therefore, whether investigators used bronchoscopic techniques in their diagnosis of VAP or only clinical and radiographic parameters is important with regard to incidence rates of VAP. In a number of studies that aimed to ascertain incidences of VAP or to evaluate modalities to diagnose VAP or studies in which risk factors for VAP were assessed, the cumulative incidences of VAP range from 8.6% to 64.7% (Table 22.5). Moreover, in

TABLE 22.5. STUDIES ON THE CUMULATIVE INCIDENCE OF VAP IN VARIOUS PATIENT POPULATIONS USING DIFFERENT DIAGNOSTIC CRITERIA

Author and year	Population	No.	Diagnosis with bronchoscopy	No. VAP (%)
Apte (347) 1992	Medical	34	No	22 (64.7)
Kingston (348) 1991	Mixed	24	No	10 (41.7)
Craven (100) 1986	Mixed	233	No	49 (21.0)
Reusser (202) 1989	Neurologic	40	No	15 (37.5)
Rodriquez (349) 1991	Trauma	294	No	130 (44.2)
Rello (151) 1992	Trauma	161	No	38 (23.6)
de Latorre (200) 1995	Medical/surgical	80	No	12 (15.0)
Fiddian-Green (176) 1991	Mixed	62	No	8 (12.9)
Vincent (95) 1995	Mixed	2,060	No	967 (46.9)
Beck-Sague (117) 1996	Surgical	145	No	15 (10.3)
Fagon (97) 1989	Mixed	567	Yes	49 (8.6)
Rello (128) 1991	Medical/surgical	264	Yes	58 (22.0)
Papazian (136) 1996	Medical/surgical	586	Yes	97 (16.6)
Garrouste-Oregas (206) 1997	Medical/surgical	86	Yes	31 (36.0)
Fagon (350) 1996	Mixed	1,978	Yes	328 (16.6)
Torres (127) 1990	Mixed	322	Yes	78 (24.2)
Bonten (199) 1994	Mixed	64	Yes	11 (17.2)
Kollef (351) 1997	Mixed	521	Yes	77 (14.8)

VAP, ventilator-associated preumonia.

TABLE 22.6. INCIDENCE OF NOSOCOMIAL PNEUMONIA IN SELECTED PATIENT GROUPS

Group	Incidence ratio (per 100 patients)	Rate (per 1,000 patient-days)	References
Hospital-wide	0.5–1.0	0.8	(10,91,92,102,103,107,139,156,352–354)
Elderly (age ≤60–65 years)	0.7–1.7	0.9–1.7	(107,142,355,356)
Adult medical and surgical ICU, mechanically ventilated	8–54 (median 24)	5–34 (per 1,000 ventilator-days)	(13,97,101,104,116,128,357–362)
Pediatric ICU, mechanical ventilation	1.5–8	4.7–6	(99,363)
ICU, nonventilated	0.4, 6.9	0.9	(98,104)
ICU, all patients	0.5–31.5 (median 9.5)	9.8–17.6	(12,42,98,99,104,129,145,150,156,354, 364–368)
Mechanical ventilation (all patients)	3–5		(10,103,369,370)
Trauma, mechanical ventilation	5.0–44.2 (median 20.8)		(151,348,369,371)
Chest trauma	20–25		(372,373)
Head trauma and neurosurgical ICU, mechanically ventilated	23–42.2		(151,202,374,375)
Extensive burns	14	34.4	(99,376)
Postoperative, abdominal or thoracic surgery	3.8–17.5	1.72	(11,377,378)
Cancer patients, including bone marrow transplant recipients	19.5–20		(169,379,380)
Intraabdominal sepsis	22–29		(381,382)

ICU, intensive care unit.

studies on the effect of preventive measures on the occurrence of VAP, incidences of up to 78% have been reported in the control groups (94). In the European Prevalence of Infection in Intensive Care Study, 10,038 patients in 1,417 ICUs were studied on a single day; 45% of the patients were infected, and 47% of them had pneumonia. Another 18% were treated for infections of the lower respiratory tract but did not fulfill the criteria for pneumonia (95).

The cumulative risk for developing VAP during ICU stay increases until day five. In one study, the calculated rates for VAP were 3% per day in the first week, 2% per day in the second week, and 1% per day thereafter (96). Two other studies suggest that there is a relatively constant 1% to 3% risk per day for developing VAP while mechanical ventilation continues for medical and surgical ICU patients (equivalent to 10 to 30 cases per 10,000 patient-ventilator-days) (97,98). According to data from the NNIS system based primarily on clinical diagnostic criteria, median incidence rates for VAP range from 4.7 cases per 1,000 patient-ventilator-days for pediatric ICUs to 34.4 cases per 1,000 patient-ventilator-days for burn ICUs (99). Intermediate median rates were reported for combined coronary and medical ICUs (12.8 cases per 1,000 patient-ventilator-days) and combined surgical and medical-surgical ICUs (17.6 cases per 1, 000 patient-ventilator-days).

A number of studies have reported incidence rates for nosocomial pneumonia in other patient groups, such as the elderly, trauma patients, or cancer patients. These studies have relied primarily on clinical diagnostic criteria and are summarized in Table 22.6 (12,13,91,97–101).

RISK FACTORS

The strongest risk factor for nosocomial pneumonia appears to be tracheal intubation and mechanical ventilation, which results in a 3- to 21-fold increase in the risk of developing nosocomial pneumonia (10,98,101–104). Because other pathogenetic factors may be different, it is useful to consider nonventilated and ventilated patients (Table 22.7) separately when discussing risk factors.

When nonventilated or broad hospital populations are considered, factors found by multivariable analysis to significantly increase the risk of nosocomial pneumonia include chronic lung disease (101,105), severity of illness (105), upper abdominal or thoracic surgery (101,105,106), duration of surgery (105), age (101), poor nutritional state (106,107), immunosuppressive therapy (106,108), depressed level of consciousness (101,109), large volume of aspiration (101), impaired airway reflexes or difficulty handling secretions (109), nasoenteric intubation (109), neuromuscular disease (107), and male gender (105). Additional risk factors suggested by univariate analysis include duration of hospitalization (8,11), oropharyngeal colonization with gram-negative bacilli (12), obesity (11), antibiotic therapy (8), reflux esophagitis (110), and previous pneumonia (110).

The risk factors associated with the development of VAP have been determined in studies using multivariable analysis techniques, Cox regression techniques, and case-control designs or have been suggested on the basis of reviews. Determination of risk factors for VAP has several clinical implications. They offer prognostic information about the probability of developing VAP, they help to reveal the pathogenesis of VAP, and they may provide possible targets for preventive strategies. By risk stratification, one can determine which patients may benefit most from pneumonia prophylaxis (111). Risk factor analyses for ICU-acquired pneumonia (i.e., pneumonia diagnosed in ICU patients with or without mechanical ventilation) have clearly identified mechanical ventilation to be the most important risk factor (101,112–115). In general, the risk factors that have been identified can be divided into three groups: (a) risk factors that

TABLE 22.7. RISK FACTORS FOR ICU-ACQUIRED AND VENTILATOR-ASSOCIATED PNEUMONIA

ICU-acquired pneumonia	Ventilator-associated pneumonia
Identified risk factors with no or only limited possibilities for prevention	
Naso/orotracheal intubation (101,115)	Emergent intubation (349)
Duration of MV (101,112,115)	Duration of MV (118,120,127,383)
Severity of illness (112,114,384)	Severity of illness (116,349)
History of COPD (101)	History of COPD (118,119,127)
Reason for admission	Reason for admission
Trauma (101,112,113)	Trauma/head trauma/blunt trauma (96,100,349,385)
Neurologic disease (115,384)	Hypotension (349)
Thoraco/abdominal surgery (101,129)	Coma (386)
Coma (112,150)	Neurosurgery (383,385)
Age (101,113)	Acute respiratory distress syndrome (385,387,388)
	Burns (96)
	Neurologic disease (96)
	Cardiac disease (96)
	Age (116)
Identified risk factors that offer possibilities for prevention	
Antacids (384)	Antacids or H_2-antagonists (100,117,134)
Large volume aspiration (101)	Large volume aspiration (96,127,385)
Presence of nasogastric tube (129)	Enteral nutrition (383,386)
Impaired airway reflexes (112,115)	Contaminated ventilator circuits (100,389)
Depressed consciousness (101)	Reintubation (127,134,351,386,390)
	Previous antibiotic use (27,116–121,173)
	Absence of previous antibiotic use (96,173)
	Nonelevated head position (116)
	Paralytic agents (96)
Risk factors identified incidentally or needing further investigation to assess their influence on infection and possibilities for prevention	
Male gender (384)	Male gender (351)
Recent bronchoscopy (129)	Fall-winter season (100)
Thoracic drainage (384)	Failure of continuous aspiration of subglottic secretions (27)
Coagulation products (384)	Inadequate intracuff pressure (27)
	Administration of aerosols (351)
	Presence of a tracheostomy (134,351)
	Transport out of the ICU (351)
	Sinusitis (391,392)
	Multiple central venous line insertions (134)
	Positive end expiratory pressure (PEEP) (2)
	Corticosteroid therapy (383)
	Dental plaque colonization (393)
	Accidental extubation (394)

COPD, chronic obstructive pulmonary disease; ICU, intensive care unit; MV, mechanical ventilation.

are well known (intubation, duration of mechanical ventilation, etc.) but very difficult to modify and that offer no or only limited possibilities for prevention, (b) risk factors that seem to play a role in the pathogenesis of VAP and have stimulated the development of a number of preventive strategies, and (c) risk factors that have been identified only incidentally or need further investigations to assess their significance and the possibility for prevention. Several risk factor analyses identified previous antibiotic use to be significantly associated with the development of VAP (27,116,117). Rello et al. (118) reported that prior use of antibiotics was a risk factor for *Pseudomonas aeruginosa* VAP. The same conclusion was reached by Talon et al. (119) in patients who received metronidazole. Other investigators concluded that prior broad-spectrum antibiotic use was a risk factor for VAP caused by "potentially drug-resistant bacteria" (methicillin-resistant *Staphylococcus aureus, P. aeruginosa, Acinetobacter baumanii,* and *Stenotrophomonas maltophilia)* (120). In contrast, antibiotics conferred protection for VAP in a risk factor analysis (96), and the absence of prior antibiotic treatment was a risk factor for VAP caused by *Haemophilus influenzae* (121). Lately, attention has been drawn to the association between the mode of mechanical ventilation, ventilator-induced lung injury, and inflammation or infection (122,123).

Mortality

The CDC estimated that nosocomial pneumonia is a primary or contributing cause for more than 30,000 deaths annually in the United States (124). In a study of 200 consecutive hospital deaths, pneumonia was implicated in 60% of deaths for which nosocomial infection was a contributing factor (125). An attributable mortality rate of nosocomial pneumonia of 33% has been found in one matched cohort study (91). In other words, approximately one third of patients who develop nosocomial pneumonia and die would not die otherwise.

Published crude mortality rates for nosocomial pneumonia range widely from 20% to 71% for hospital-wide, ICU, and ventilated patient groups with a median of 41.5% (4,10,14,42, 91,97–101,107,116,126–128); within the wide reported range, it is not possible to distinguish between these groups. Several factors have been associated with a greater risk of mortality, most prominently *P. aeruginosa* as a pathogen, severity of underlying illness, inappropriate antibiotic therapy, and age (Table 22.8) (91,97,101,116,127,129–132).

With regard to mortality and VAP, the existing controversy is whether patients die from or die with VAP. In a number of risk factor analyses, VAP was not independently associated with mortality (100,127,133–135). Moreover, other studies also failed to demonstrate attributable mortality for VAP (85,136). In contrast, Fagon et al. (4) described an attributable mortality of 27% and a risk for death of 2.0 for patients developing VAP, and the risk ratio even increased to 2.5 when VAP was caused by *P. aeruginosa* or *Acinetobacter* species. Rello et al. (137) found an attributable mortality of 13.5% for ventilated patients developing VAP resulting from *P. aeruginosa.* The existence of attributable mortality resulting from VAP was supported by three recent prospective cohort studies (130–132). Late-onset VAP independently contributed to ICU mortality when empirical antibiotic treatment was not immediately appropriate (hazard ratio = 1.69) (130). Nosocomial pneumonia was independently associated with death in ICU in a matched risk-adjusted cohort (131). Overall odds ratio for mortality was 2.12, which increased 2.6 when VAP was caused by multiresistant microorganisms (131). VAP had a trend toward increased risk of death [relative risk (RR) = 1.32] in a matched cohort study including 173 patients with VAP, and attributable mortality was higher for medical than for surgical patients (RR = 1.65) (132).

TABLE 22.8. FACTORS ASSOCIATED WITH INCREASED MORTALITY FOR NOSOCOMIAL PNEUMONIA

Factor	References
Aerobic gram-negative bacilli as pathogen(s), particularly *Pseudomonas aeruginosa*	(98,101)
Multiresistant microorganism as pathogen(s)	(131)
Severity of underlying illness	(101,116,127, 130)
Age	(91,101,129)
Inappropriate antibiotic therapy	(101,127,130)
Shock	(127)
Bilateral infiltrates	(101)
Prior antibiotic therapy	(97)
Neoplastic disease	(91)
Duration of prior hospitalization	(91)
Supine head position in ventilated patients	(116)
Medical patients	(132)

We studied the systemic inflammatory response in patients developing and not developing VAP who were matched on variables representing the severity of underlying disease. The development of VAP was not associated with increasing circulating levels of interleukin-6 or interleukin-8 in the days just before or after diagnosis of VAP. Interleukin levels increased and were higher than in the corresponding control patients who did not develop VAP only in patients in whom VAP was associated with a clinical presentation of severe sepsis or septic shock. Overall mortality rates were similar for patients with and without VAP. However, the subgroup of patients who developed VAP with severe sepsis or septic shock (and who had higher interleukin levels) had a higher mortality than their corresponding control patients (85). These and other data (86,138) suggest that there is a dynamic equilibrium ranging from colonization without signs of infection to infection of the lungs with septic shock and elevated levels of circulating systemic inflammatory mediators. Therefore, the attributable risk of VAP appears to vary with patient population, severity of (systemic) infection, and infecting microorganism (132).

Morbidity and Cost

Nosocomial pneumonia is also associated with substantial morbidity. Reported rates of secondary bacteremia have ranged from 4% to 38% (85,91,97,100,101,127,128,134) and empyema developed in 5% to 8% of patients with nosocomial pneumonia (85,139,140).

The excess costs associated with nosocomial pneumonia are remarkable. According to estimates published by the CDC, an average of 5.9 days of increased length of stay and $5,683 in extra hospital charges (in 1992 dollars) result from each episode of nosocomial pneumonia (124). Analysis of a nationwide database suggests that no more than 5% of these excess costs would be recovered by hospitals under prospective reimbursement (141). It is not surprising that Boyce et al. (142) reported costs to exceed reimbursements for 31 of 33 Medicare patients developing nosocomial pneumonia, with a median net loss of $5,800 per patient. Published estimates of excess duration of hospitalization attributed to nosocomial pneumonia have ranged from 4 to 21 days (4,5,91,131,132,136,143–146). It is obvious that the financial constraints of prospective reimbursement and healthcare reform provide a strong incentive for preventing nosocomial pneumonia. The magnitude of this problem is highlighted by an estimate that the excess cost of nosocomial pneumonia exceeds $1 billion annually in the United States (147).

PATHOGENS

A variety of pathogens appear to be important as causes of nosocomial pneumonia. The NNIS system provides the largest database describing microorganisms isolated from both ventilated and nonventilated patients with nosocomial pneumonia. According to NNIS system data from 1992 to 1997, the most frequently isolated pathogen is *P. aeruginosa* (21%), followed by *S. aureus* (20%), *Enterobacter* species (9%), *Klebsiella pneumoniae* (8%), and *Escherichia coli* (4%) (1). Collectively, gram-negative aerobes account for 64% of pathogens cited as causes of nosocomial pneumonia in the NNIS system database. *P. aeruginosa* and *Acinetobacter* species were more commonly reported in VAP than in non-VAP. Compared with data from 1982, the proportion of Enterobacteriaceae has decreased, and the proportions of *P. aeruginosa* and *S. aureus* have increased (1).

In addition to the difference in duration of mechanical ventilation at time of diagnosis, early-onset and late-onset VAP also have a different etiologic spectrum. Early-onset VAP is mainly caused by *Streptococcus pneumoniae, S. aureus,* and *H. influenzae,* pathogens that presumably already colonize the respiratory tract at the time of intubation. Late-onset VAP is caused by nosocomial pathogens such as Enterobacteriaceae, *S. aureus,* and *P. aeruginosa.* Because these nosocomial pathogens are known to cause serious infections under certain circumstances, they are usually grouped and labeled as potentially pathogenic microorganisms (PPMO). In many studies, colonization and infection with PPMO is analyzed instead of the separate species. Although PPMO are regarded as a single group, it should be kept in mind that each species has its own characteristics with regard to preferred site of colonization, routes and vectors of transmission, and clinical spectrum.

Studies using quantitative cultures of BAL and/or PSB demonstrate that approximately 60% of all cases of VAP are associated with gram-negative bacteria, mainly *P. aeruginosa* (20%), and 35% with gram-positive bacteria (97,128,148,149). *S. aureus* is the most frequent gram-positive pathogen causing VAP (20%). In comatose multiple trauma patients, incidences of *S. aureus* VAP as high as 56% have been reported (150–153). VAP is often polymicrobial with incidences ranging from 20% to 60% of all episodes of VAP (16,148,154). The proportional distribution of the species that cause VAP within the etiologic spectrum and their antibiotic susceptibility may vary considerably between hospital settings, patient populations, and countries.

The importance of anaerobic bacteria in the pathogenesis of VAP has not been studied extensively. Isolation of anaerobic bacteria requires specific transport conditions and culture media, which usually are not systematically achieved during bacteriologic investigation of respiratory tract samples. The incidence of VAP in which anaerobic bacteria are involved, therefore, is probably underestimated. In a prospective study of 130 episodes of VAP, aerobic and anaerobic bacteria were isolated from PSB ($\geq 10^3$ CFU/mL) in 26 (20%) patients, and anaerobic bacteria only were isolated in four (3%) patients (149). In another prospective study no anaerobic microorganisms were isolated in a group of 143 patients, of whom 63 were diagnosed with VAP, despite painstaking microbiologic efforts (155). Moreover, only one nonpathogenic anaerobic microorganism was isolated in 25 patients with suspected aspiration pneumonia receiving mechanical ventilation of which 12 met the criteria of pneumonia (155).

Although less common, other pathogens may also be problematic. Additional work is needed to clarify the roles of influenza and other respiratory viruses, *Mycoplasma pneumoniae,* and *Chlamydia pneumoniae;* however, several reports suggest that these pathogens may account for a modest proportion of cases (156–163). *Legionella* can be an important cause of nosocomial pneumonia, particularly when there is colonization of the hospital hot water system (164–168). *Aspergillus* and cytomegalovirus are important pathogens in bone marrow transplant recipients (169) and other immunocompromised patients. The risk of *Aspergillus* infection may be increased by adjacent construction activity or by a faulty ventilation system (169–171). Nosocomial infections due to respiratory viruses, *Legionella, Aspergillus,* cytomegalovirus, and *Mycobacterium tuberculosis* are discussed at greater length in Chapters 35, 37, 40, and 60.

PATHOGENESIS

Colonization of the upper respiratory tract precedes the development of nosocomial pneumonia (133,172,173). For upper respiratory tract colonization and pneumonia to develop, pathogenic microorganisms must reach the distal lung and then multiply, overcoming host defenses at each step. Host defenses include filtration and humidification of air in the upper airways, epiglottic and cough reflexes, ciliary transport by respiratory epithelium, phagocytes and opsonins in the distal lung, and systemic cell-mediated and humoral immunity (174,175).

The predominant mode of inoculation is aspiration; however, inhalation (particularly *Aspergillus* and other fungal molds), seeding via the bloodstream, and reactivation of latent infection (*M. tuberculosis,* cytomegalovirus in immunocompromised patients) account for some pneumonias that develop in hospitalized patients. Translocation from the gastrointestinal tract has also been hypothesized as a mode of inoculation (176), but this has not been confirmed.

Colonization

The relation between colonization of the upper respiratory tract and the development of VAP was established by Johanson et al. (12) in 1972. Nosocomial respiratory infections developed in 23% of ICU patients with upper respiratory tract colonization but in only 3% of noncolonized patients (12). Moreover, upper respiratory tract colonization increased with severity of illness. Repeated oropharyngeal cultures obtained from 33 normal subjects revealed gram-negative bacteria in 6% of subjects, whereas these pathogens were cultured from 35% of moderately ill hospitalized patients and 73% of moribund patients (177). Since then, many variables have been determined that enhance colonization and infection of the respiratory tract in ICU patients (178). Although increased exposure to pathogens may play a role, this cannot exclusively explain increased colonization rates. Nursing and medical staff have colonization rates similar to those of normal subjects not working in a hospital setting (177). A reduced capacity to clear pathogens and/or increased adherence of microorganisms are more likely mechanisms to account for the higher colonization rates in critically ill patients. The latter mechanisms can be the result of decreased immunologic host function, destruction of epithelial surfaces (179,180), impaired mucociliary clearance, proinflammatory enzymes, and fibronectin reducing proteases (181). Furthermore, during ICU stay, approximately 60% of patients receive systemic antibiotics. Antibiotic therapy can rapidly change the commensal oropharyngeal flora, resulting in an increase in oropharyngeal and upper respiratory tract colonization with aerobic gram-negative or gram-positive bacilli and yeasts, possibly resulting from loss of the normal bacterial flora (178,182) and to selection of pathogens that are resistant to the antibiotics used (18,19,21,183,184).

Routes of Colonization

Microorganisms reach the lungs after aspiration of colonized oropharyngeal fluid. Microaspiration occurs often, both in healthy people and in critically ill patients (185,186). Pathogens colonizing the respiratory tract and causing VAP are derived from either endogenous or exogenous sources. The stomach and intestine are the most important endogenous sources. In addition, pathogens colonizing the upper respiratory tract (oropharynx, sinus cavities, the nares, and dental plaque) may be aspirated. Contaminated environment (sinks, faucets, sheets, etc.), contaminated equipment (mechanical ventilation devices, ventilator circuits, radiographic equipment, etc.), contaminated enteral feeding, and other colonized patients in ICU are potential exogenous sources.

Several routes of colonization by which pathogens are transported from their endogenous or exogenous sources to the upper respiratory tract of the patient are possible. In the gastropulmonary route of colonization (187,188), endogenous bacteria reach the upper respiratory tract via the stomach and subsequently colonize the oropharynx and trachea, after which the bacteria are aspirated into the lower respiratory tract. This route of colonization has been propagated as important in the pathogenesis of VAP for many years. The rectopulmonary route of colonization has attracted less attention. In this route, intestinal microorganisms spread from the rectal area via the patient's skin or the hands of healthcare personnel to the upper respiratory tract. Finally, transfer of pathogens from exogenous sources most probably occurs via hands of nursing and medical staff, which enables direct inoculation of microorganisms into the tracheobronchial tree during manipulation of ventilator circuits or tubes (189–191). This is called the exogenous route of colonization or cross-colonization when another patient is the exogenous source.

Essential Conditions to Study the Pathogenesis of VAP

Because colonization is not always followed by infection, infection rates with a certain pathogen form only the tip of the iceberg of the complete epidemiology (172,190). When studying the epidemiology of microorganisms in ICU, surveillance of colonization is indispensable. In clinical practice, surveillance is advised only for high-risk patients in specific clinical settings (192). However, when determining the epidemiology of ICU pathogens in detail, surveillance should include all patients within the ICU, as well as equipment and environmental surfaces for certain pathogens. Surveillance cultures from patients should be taken on admission and subsequently with a frequency high enough to study sequences of colonization from initial body sites to other body sites. Moreover, patients may be colonized or infected with multiple genotypes of the same species, both at one particular body site and at different body sites (189). Therefore, analysis of a single isolate may not accurately represent the bacterial flora. Analysis of several isolates and determination of similarity of isolates is crucial (193).

Comparison of bacterial phenotypes, such as antibiotic susceptibility patterns, serotypes, phage types, and outer membrane protein types, is relatively easy to perform but lacks specificity (193,194). Genomic DNA fingerprinting techniques, such as pulsed-field gel electrophoresis (PFGE), random amplification of polymorphic DNA, and arbitrarily primed polymerase chain reaction, have a higher specificity and discriminatory power while maintaining epidemiologic linkage. These techniques, therefore, are considered the methods of choice to determine identity of bacterial isolates in the epidemiology of nosocomial outbreaks (195–197). However, the techniques are often cumbersome and expensive and, therefore, not always feasible in routine practice.

In summary, the optimal study design to study routes of colonization that may lead to VAP includes (a) determination the incidence of VAP, preferably diagnosed by bronchoscopic techniques; (b) performance of surveillance cultures of all patients present in ICU and possibly environment and equipment; (c) culturing of several body sites on admission and with a sufficient frequency thereafter; (d) analysis of several isolates of each species, cultured from each site; and (e) determination of similarity of isolates of a certain pathogen by genotyping techniques.

Endogenous Routes

Gastric Colonization and the Gastropulmonary Route

In critically ill patients, gastric acidity may be decreased (i.e., pH value higher) because of decreased acid production, application of enteral feeding, or stress-ulcer prophylaxis [antacids, H_2-antagonists, H^+K^+–adenosine triphosphatase (ATPase) inhibitors]. If the gastric environment favors bacterial growth, bacteria may multiply; hence, colonization with gram-negative bacteria occurs often at this site (16,187,188). Because of the simultaneous occurrence of gastric colonization and the development of VAP, a causal relationship has been assumed. In the so-called gastropulmonary route of colonization, bacteria presumably reach the upper respiratory tract by retrograde movement from the colonized stomach, and bacteria are aspirated into the lower respiratory tract. Based on studies reporting correlations between development of VAP and concurrent or preceding gastric colonization with the same species, a central role in the pathogenesis of VAP was assigned to gastric colonization (13,187,198). However, in six studies, the gastropulmonary route of colonization was found to be unimportant with respect to colonization or infection of the upper respiratory tract (16,199–203), whereas another four studies did support a role for gastric colonization (13,15,204,205). In these studies the percentage of patients in whom the stomach served as a source of colonization or infection of the respiratory tract ranged from 4% to 24% for colonization and from zero to 15% for the development of VAP (6). Thus, the role of the stomach and gastropulmonary route of colonization remains a subject of debate (36). Nevertheless, based on the alleged importance of gastric colonization, modulation of colonization at this site is still used as a measure to prevent VAP.

Oropharyngeal Colonization

The results of studies performed by Johanson and co-workers (12,177) in the early 1970s pointed toward an association between colonization of the upper respiratory tract and the development of VAP. However, at that time, VAP could not be diagnosed with bronchoscopy, and the diagnosis relied on relatively nonspecific clinical, radiographic, and microbiologic criteria. Moreover, only antibiotic susceptibility patterns and serotyping were used to determine the similarity of isolates, because molecular genotyping techniques were not yet available. Remarkably, in the following years research on the pathogenesis of VAP almost exclusively focused on the role of gastric colonization and the gastropulmonary route of colonization. Approximately 20 years later, new studies on sequences of colonization in patients who developed VAP provided additional evidence in support of Johanson et al.'s earlier findings. The upper respiratory tract was the site of first colonization in 14 out of 15 cases of VAP in a study in which qualitative endotracheal aspirate cultures were used for the diagnosis of pneumonia (202). Torres et al. (187) compared pharyngeal, gastric, and respiratory tract colonization in 63 patients with and without VAP, as diagnosed by bronchoscopic techniques. They found a strong association between upper respiratory tract colonization and VAP and concluded that both pharyngeal and gastric colonization were important reservoirs for bacteria causing VAP. However, in both studies colonization was not assessed serially; thus, no conclusions could be drawn with respect to the actual sequences of colonization.

In a number of other studies, serial cultures of multiple body sites were obtained to determine sequences of colonization leading to VAP. In doing so, de Latorre et al. (200) concluded that tracheal colonization precedes VAP in most patients and that pharyngeal colonization, rather than gastric colonization, is the main source of microorganisms found in patients with VAP. Cade et al. (201) studied 100 consecutive patients, of whom 60 had positive throat cultures that were preceded by gastric colonization in 15 (25%) patients. There was no association between the presence of a positive gastric culture and the development of infection. Two studies from our group showed that 85% and 96% of the pathogens causing VAP had been isolated previously from tracheal aspirates and 50% and 75% from the oropharynx (16,199). Gastric colonization preceded VAP in only 30% and 31% of the cases (16,199). These results were confirmed later in a study by Cendrero et al. (203). Garrouste-Oregas et al. (206) analyzed oropharyngeal and gastric colonization before VAP in 86 patients. VAP was diagnosed by bronchoscopic techniques and identity of strains was based on results of PFGE. Oropharyngeal colonization (either on admission or acquired) correlated better with VAP than gastric colonization. Moreover, PFGE demonstrated that identical strains were isolated from both oropharyngeal and bronchial samples in 28 out of the 31 cases of pneumonia.

In conclusion, the evidence at hand strongly suggests an important role for the oropharynx in the pathogenesis of VAP and offers a potential target for preventive strategies.

Intestinal Colonization and the Rectopulmonary Route

The intestines are a large endogenous source of gram-negative bacteria, which may spread to the upper respiratory tract via the patients' skin or hands of healthcare personnel. This so-called rectopulmonary route of colonization, in reality, is an exogenous route for endogenous microorganisms. However, because of decreased intestinal peristalsis and gastric emptying in critically ill patients, bacteria can colonize the proximal small intestine and subsequently migrate to the stomach via duodenogastric reflux (205,207). The rectopulmonary route of colonization has attracted little attention, especially when compared with other routes of colonization. To our knowledge, only four studies have been performed with special attention to the rectopulmonary route. In one of these, the rectum was the most common primary site of colonization with *P. aeruginosa* among 153 patients admitted to a surgical ICU (208). In that study, ten (6.5%) patients acquired colonization with *P. aeruginosa* (seven from rectal swab cultures, three from nasal cultures, and three from tracheal secretions cultures), of whom one patient developed pneumonia (208). (Some patients were colonized at two sites.) In another study, the rectum was the most commonly observed colonization site for *P. aeruginosa* among 186 admissions to three hospital wards. In all, 20 patients acquired colonization with *P. aeruginosa* in the rectum or oropharynx or both; only 2 acquired oropharyngeal colonization alone. Unfortunately, data on gastric and oropharyngeal colonization were not reported in the first study (208), and data on gastric and tracheal colonization (209) are lacking in the latter study, which precludes conclusions regarding routes of colonization. Noone et al. (189) studied 27 intubated ICU patients of whom 15 were colonized with *P. aeruginosa* (rectum, pharynx, trachea, groin, toe web, or ear). Among 12 patients with rectal colonization, tracheal colonization occurred in 5 but in only 1 case with the same serotype at both sites; tracheal colonization preceded isolation from rectal swabs by two days (189). Among cardiac surgery patients receiving cefazolin prophylaxis, 58 of 87 became colonized or infected with *Enterobacter* species. At least 48% of these patients were already colonized before admission to ICU (mainly in the rectum). Moreover, the typing data strongly suggested that the *Enterobacter* strains came from endogenous sources (210).

In summary, available data suggest that rectal colonization with *Enterobacter* species and *P. aeruginosa* often occurs in critically ill patients, but secondary colonization of the upper respiratory tract seems infrequent. The relevance of rectal colonization and the rectopulmonary route of colonization in the pathogenesis of VAP remains largely undetermined.

Exogenous Routes

Data on the role of exogenous sources in colonization and infection of ICU patients are derived mainly from case reports and descriptions of outbreaks. Sinks (211–213), distilled water systems (214), faucets (215), tube-feeding formulas (216,217), and ventilator circuits (218) have been reported as exogenous sources of PPMO, causing outbreaks of nosocomial infections.

Especially *P. aeruginosa* possesses the ability to proliferate in aqueous sources throughout the hospital. In addition, patients themselves are major reservoirs of nosocomial pathogens (219). It is unlikely that airborne transmission contributes to the spread of staphylococci and gram-negative bacilli (219). Therefore, transfer of these pathogens most probably occurs via hands of nursing and medical staff or equipment (stethoscopes, blood pressure cuffs, etc.) (189–191). Direct inoculation of pathogens into the tracheobronchial tree from contaminated hands is possible during manipulation of ventilator circuits or tubes. If the tracheobronchial epithelium is able to bind pathogens, colonization and subsequent pneumonia may occur. This hypothesis is supported by studies that reported lower incidences of nosocomial infections after increasing hand-washing frequency or use of gloves or antiseptic hand-washing products (220–222).

The importance of cross-colonization in nonepidemic situations has rarely been studied. Olson et al. (190) addressed this issue in a study of 207 patients admitted to a medical-surgical ICU ward: 63 (23%) patients were colonized with *P. aeruginosa* on admission; 33 (16%) acquired colonization, and 12 (36%) of 33 acquisitions resulted from cross-colonization. In contrast, Chetchotisakd et al. (223) did not find an important role of cross-colonization in ICU. In a prospective surveillance in five ICUs during 6 months, they only found 14 (10%) of 137 isolates of bacteria (*P. aeruginosa, E. coli, K. pneumoniae, Enterobacter cloacae,* and enterococci) cultured from patients with suspected infection to be acquired by cross-colonization. Although molecular biotyping methods were used to determine identity of isolates, it is very likely that the true incidence of cross-colonization has been underestimated. Only a single isolate from a suspected site of infection was analyzed (the tip of the iceberg), without including isolates from colonized patients. Our group studied the influence of nonabsorbable antimicrobial prophylaxis of the stomach and oropharynx on respiratory colonization among patients in two identical ICUs. Prophylaxis was given to half of the patients in one of the ICUs, whereas the other half served as a control group. Patients treated in the other ICU, where no prophylaxis was given, formed the second control group. Colonization rates were lowest among patients who received prophylaxis. However, control patients who were treated in the same ward as patients receiving prophylaxis were found to be colonized less often and, if anything, later than controls in the ward where no prophylaxis was given. These findings strongly suggest that cross-colonization occurs often (224). Subsequently, we determined the importance of exogenous colonization for *P. aeruginosa* in two identical ICUs in a nonepidemic setting. In this analysis 100 patients were studied, of whom 23 were colonized with *P. aeruginosa,* 7 at the start of study or on admission to ICU and 16 of the remaining 93 patients became colonized during the study. Eight patients developed VAP due to *P. aeruginosa.* PFGE of 118 isolates yielded 11 genotypes: 8 in one patient each, 2 in three patients each, and 1 type in eight patients. Based on chronologic evaluation and genotypical identity of isolates, eight cases of cross-colonization were identified. Eight (50%) of 16 episodes of acquired colonization and two (25%) of eight cases of VAP due to *P. aeruginosa* seemed to be the result of cross-colonization. Cross-colonization occurred not only between patients in the same ICU but also between patients from different ICUs (225).

In contrast, endemicity of colonization with *P. aeruginosa* in ICU was characterized by polyclonality and seemed to be maintained by the continuous introduction of patients colonized with new strains of *P. aeruginosa* (226). Most episodes of acquired colonization resulted from endogenous selection, most likely stimulated by selective antibiotic pressure, rather than spread via cross-transmission (226). More recently, Berthelot et al. also found that for *P. aeruginosa* endogenous colonization was more important than cross-transmission (213).

In summary, multiple data have shown that cross-colonization, mainly from patient-to-patient via hands of healthcare workers or equipment, may be an important route of colonization. However, endogenous colonization, usually driven by selective pressure, may be equally or even more important, even in settings with high levels of endemic prevalence.

PREVENTION

Guidelines for the prevention of hospital-acquired or nosocomial pneumonia have been formulated by the American Thoracic Society (ATS) (227) and the CDC, with the consensus recommendations of the Hospital Infection Control Practices Advisory Committee (HICPAC) (192). Both guidelines incorporate general recommendations regarding infection control practices that undoubtedly decrease incidences of many infections, including VAP. These recommendations, however, are not specifically directed against VAP. For example, pneumococcal and influenza vaccination of at-risk populations, hand-washing protocols, and isolation of patients with multiply resistant respiratory tract pathogens are regarded as "currently available preventive strategies with probable efficacy" in the ATS guidelines (227). Similarly, the CDC guidelines strongly recommend staff education, surveillance for bacterial pneumonia in high-risk ICU patients, and vaccination as general measures. Furthermore, an extensive list of recommendations regarding interruption of transmission of microorganisms from human or inanimate sources to patients is described. These recommendations include sterilization, disinfection and maintenance instructions for ventilator systems and circuits, and hand washing and barrier precautions (192). Moreover, a number of recommendations have been added that are strongly advocated for all hospitals and that are viewed as effective on the basis of strong suggestive evidence, although comparative studies have not been done. These recommendations include discontinuation of enteral-tube feeding and removal of endotracheal and/or enteral tubes as soon as possible, routine verification of appropriate placement of the feeding tube, routine assessment of the patient's intestinal motility, and clearing of secretions above the inflated tube cuff before tube removal or moving of the tube (192).

Table 22.9 lists the recommendations from both guidelines for preventing VAP. The value categorization for each recommendation is included, as are the results of the relevant studies that evaluated the beneficial effects of these recommendations. Only studies with the occurrence of VAP as the endpoint of intervention are considered. The number of patients and epi-

TABLE 22.9. STRATEGIES TO PREVENT VENTILATOR-ASSOCIATED PNEUMONIA (VAP)

Preventive strategy	Guidelines advice		No. of studies	No. of pts with VAP/total		Relative risk reduction (95% CI)
	ATS[a]	CDC[b]		Study	Control	
Selective digestive decontamination						
Oropharyngeal, intestinal, and systemic prophylaxis vs. control (232–245, 258–260)	3	UI	17	131/1,685	377/1,542	0.68 (0.61–0.73)
Oropharyngeal, and intestinal prophylaxis vs. control (18,21,246–249,261)	3	UI	7	84/506	145/514	0.41 (0.25–0.52)
Oropharyngeal, intestinal, and systemic prophylaxis vs. systemic (19,20,250–252,262)	3	UI	6	90/438	127/446	0.28 (0.09–0.43)
Intestinal prophylaxis vs. control (253,254)	3	UI	2	3/133	14/134	0.78 (0.25–0.94)
Oropharyngeal prophylaxis vs. control (94,255,263,264)	3	UI	4	14/158	74/215	0.74 (0.56–0.85)
Oropharyngeal and systemic prophylaxis vs. control (256)	3	UI	1	13/58	23/30	0.71 (0.51–0.83)
Systemic prophylaxis vs. control (257)	3	IA	1	12/50	25/50	0.52 (0.15–0.73)
Stress-ulcer prophylaxis						
Sucralfate vs. acid neutralization (H_2-antagonists/antacids)[c]	1	II	14	231/1,318	343/1,531	0.22 (0.09–0.33)
Sucralfate vs. H_2-antagonists (15,17,281,282,288–293)	1	II	10	187/1,092	256/1,172	0.22 (0.08–0.34)
Sucralfate vs. antacids (15,16,291,294)	1	II	4	38/230	59/232	0.35 (0.06–0.55)
Sucralfate vs. antacids and/or H_2-antagonists (14,295)	1	II	2	24/109	25/117	−0.03 (−0.69–0.37)
Enteral feeding (EF)						
Total enteral nutrition vs. total parenteral nutrition (395)	2	—	1	0/29	6/30	1.00
Postpyloric feeding vs. gastric feeding (396–398)	2	UI	3	26/90	27/93	0.01 (−0.56–0.37)
Small-bore vs. large-bore tube (315)	2	UI	1	Na	Na	
Intermittent vs. continuous EF (298–300)	2	UI	3	8/65	18/61	0.58 (0.11–0.80)
Acidified vs. nonacidified EF (302)	—	UI	1	3/49	7/46	0.60 (−0.45–0.89)
Semirecumbent vs. supine body position (314)	2	IB	1	2/39	11/47	0.78 (0.07–0.95)
Subglottic secretions drainage						
Subglottic secretions drainage vs. control (28,29,308,309)	2	UI	4	45/425	81/421	0.45 (0.23–0.61)
Continuous lateral rotational therapy (CLRT)						
CLRT vs. control (30–35,316)	2	UI	7	39/247	81/250	0.51 (0.31–0.65)
Ventilator circuits						
Heat and moisture exchangers vs. heated humidifiers (340–345)	2	UI	6	42/538	65/492	0.41 (0.15–0.59)
Infrequent change vs. frequent change (332,333)	2	IA	2	34/302	33/274	0.06 (−0.47–0.40)
No change vs. change (126,334,335)	2	UI	3	82/433	94/451	0.09 (−0.19–0.30)
Closed vs. open suction catheter system (336–339)	2	UI	4	30/128	36/121	0.21 (−0.20–0.48)
Orotracheal vs. nasotracheal intubation (399)	2	UI	1	9/151	17/149	0.47 (−0.15–0.76)
Topical tracheobronchial antibiotics						
Topical tracheobronchial antibiotics vs. control (326,327,331)	3	—	3	120/764	147/663	0.29 (0.12–0.43)

Na, incidence of VAP not analyzed.
[a]Categorization of preventive strategies by the American Thoracic Society statement (227): 1, currently available and probably effective for specific populations and indications; 2, currently available, promising in efficacy, and being used by some hospitals on a regular basis; 3, currently available but of unproven value, being used in investigational studies, or on limited clinical basis; and 4, unproven regimens, still being evaluated.
[b]Categorization of Centers for Disease Control and Prevention recommendations (192): IA, strongly recommended for all hospitals and strongly supported by well-designed experimental or epidemiologic studies; IB, strongly recommended for all hospitals and viewed as effective by experts in the field and a consensus of HICPAC based on strong rationale and suggestive evidence, even though definitive scientific studies may not have been done; II, suggested for implementation in many hospitals, recommendations may be supported by suggestive clinical or epidemiologic studies, strong theoretical rationale, or definitive studies applicable to some but not all hospitals; UI (unresolved issue), no recommendation, practices for which insufficient evidence or consensus regarding efficacy exists.
[c]The results of studies comparing sucralfate to acid neutralizing prophylaxis have all been combined. Data on the comparisons with antacids and H_2-antagonists have also been analyzed separately for which the data of two studies (15,291) comparing sucralfate with antacids and with H_2-antagonists were split up. In two other studies (14,295) this was not possible, because control patients received antacids and/or H_2-antagonists, and separate analyses were not performed or reported.

sodes of VAP reported by the studies on a certain recommendation have been grouped, and from these data the relative risk reduction (RRR) with 95% confidence intervals (95% CI) were calculated. The RRR is the reduction of adverse events achieved by a treatment, expressed as a proportion of the control rate. In other words, it is the difference in event rates between the control and treatment groups, divided by the event rate in the control group. A RRR of 0 means that the incidence of VAP is equal in control and treatment group, whereas a RRR of 1.00 means that no VAP occurred in the treatment group. Thus, the closer the RRR approaches 1.00, the more effective the treatment. The use of RRR is sometimes criticized, because it does not reflect the magnitude of the risk without therapy (i.e., baseline risk) (228,229). However, because the incidences of VAP in the control groups of the analyzed studies vary considerably due to differences in the diagnostic criteria, the use of a relative risk measure is desirable. The preventive strategies most often studied and their contribution to the understanding of the pathogenesis of VAP are described in the following section.

Selective Decontamination of the Digestive Tract

In 1971 the concept of colonization resistance was proposed by van der Waaij et al. (230) who suggested a beneficial effect of the anaerobic flora in resisting colonization by aerobic gram-negative bacilli in the digestive tract. Many infections are caused by these enteric bacilli. SDD was developed to selectively eliminate the aerobic gram-negative bacilli and yeasts from the digestive tract, leaving the anaerobic flora unaffected. The first clinical studies with this technique were performed in granulocytopenic patients and showed favorable results (231). In the early 1980s, Stoutenbeek et al. (232) adapted the technique for ICU patients. The full concept of SDD aims to eradicate microorganisms from the intestine, the stomach, and the oropharynx by nonabsorbable antibiotics, which are combined with systemic antibiotic prophylaxis during the first days of ICU admission. In the SDD regimen the combination of colistin and an aminoglycoside are generally used; both are effective against gram-negative bacilli and *S. aureus.* Moreover, both agents are nonabsorbable and do not affect the anaerobic intestinal flora. Amphotericin B was added to prevent overgrowth with yeasts and systemic prophylaxis was added to prevent early infections. Since the introduction of this preventive strategy, dozens of studies in a variety of ICU populations have been performed (18–21,94,232–264). However, SDD has some potential drawbacks such as antibiotic resistance of gram-negative bacteria and the occurrence or selection of resistant gram-positive microorganisms. Although a number of studies reported no increased incidences of resistant bacteria (233,237,239,243,244,248–250,255,256), overgrowth and even infections with gram-positive bacteria, resistant to the antibiotics used for SDD, have been reported in several trials (18,19,21,183,184,238,240,241,246,251,254,258,265–267), as were increased colonization and infection rates resulting from gram-negative resistant bacteria (234,238,240,241). Moreover, the lack of cost-benefit analyses and of beneficial effects on mortality rates have further limited the widespread use of SDD (227).

Meta-Analyses

Up until now, eight meta-analyses of SDD studies have been published, with comparable results. They all conclude that SDD decreases the incidence of VAP caused by aerobic gram-negative bacteria with RRRs ranging from 0.40 to 0.78. In the latest meta-analysis the reported outcomes regarding prevention of VAP and reduction in ICU mortality were related to the methodologic quality of the individual studies (268). Of note, an inverse relationship between the quality of study design and the reported effects on VAP prevention was found: the better the study quality the less the preventive effects, although reductions remained statistically significant even for the best studies. In multivariable analysis, blinding of studies and appropriate allocation of intervention most strongly influenced treatment effect.

Beneficial effects of SDD on mortality rates are less clear, with RRR in meta-analysis ranging from 0.06 to 0.13 (22–26, 268–270). The authors of five of the eight meta-analyses, therefore, stated that the routine use of SDD cannot be recommended (24–26,268–270). In two meta-analyses, studies that combined topical and systemic therapy were associated with statistically significant reductions in ICU mortality of SDD patients as compared with control patients (23,270). No significant benefit was found for studies comparing only topical prophylaxis to control patients or when both study groups were receiving systemic prophylaxis (271). Therefore, results of these meta-analyses suggest that systemic prophylaxis was responsible for the beneficial patient outcome. Of note, study quality did not influence reported reductions in ICU mortality (268), underscoring the potential bias in studies using a study endpoint that lacks a gold standard for diagnosis, such as VAP.

Although meta-analyses are attractive in many ways, there appear to be major problems with interpretation. Because of publication bias and many other biases that may be introduced in the process of locating, selecting, and combining studies, the findings of meta-analyses may be misleading, and questions remain: Should meta-analyses include unpublished studies? Is the literature search to be restricted to the English language? Should trialists be contacted for individual patient data? Specifically with regard to SDD, one wonders whether the results of studies with different SDD regimens, different definitions of the diagnosis of VAP, and various study designs can be pooled. Therefore, the findings of the meta-analyses on SDD must be interpreted with caution.

The Full Regimen

Unfortunately, the full regimen of SDD does not help to elucidate the pathogenesis of VAP. Because SDD aims to modulate colonization at three sites—the oropharynx, stomach, and intestine in combination with systemic prophylaxis—it has remained unclear which part of SDD prevents VAP. The first study of Stoutenbeek et al. (232) addressed this topic. In a prospective open trial they consecutively compared three prophylactic antibiotic regimens (intestinal decontamination, $n = 17$; oropharyngeal and intestinal decontamination, $n = 25$; oropharyngeal and intestinal decontamination combined with systemic antibiotics, $n = 63$) with an historical control group who did not receive any prophylaxis ($n = 59$). They concluded that intestinal decontamination alone had no effect on infection rates. The addition of oropharyngeal decontamination effectively prevented secondary pneumonia. Finally, the additive effect of systemic prophylaxis [cefotaxime 50 to 100 mg/kg/day intravenous (IV), from arrival to ICU until no more pathogens were isolated from oropharynx or respiratory tract] also prevented primary pneumonia (232,272). However, this was a nonrandomized, open study with relatively few patients per group, and the diagnosis of pneumonia was not established by bronchoscopic techniques. Nevertheless, the full regimen of SDD was propagated as the method of choice for infection prevention, and since then few studies have analyzed the relevance of the various individual parts of SDD.

The full regimen of SDD (including oropharyngeal and intestinal decontamination and systemic prophylaxis) was studied in at least 17 trials (232–245,258–260) with VAP or respiratory tract infections as the endpoint (Table 22.9). Only four of these had a double-blind placebo-controlled design (236,240,258, 259). Twelve reported beneficial effects on incidences of VAP (233,235,237,240,243,258,260) or all respiratory tract infections (232,234,238,245,259), including only two of the four double-blind studies. The overall RRR of VAP in these 17 trials was 0.68 (95% CI: 0.61 to 0.73).

SDD Without Systemic Prophylaxis

The effect of selective decontamination of oropharynx, stomach, and intestines per se has been determined in 13 studies. In seven of these, no systemic prophylaxis was employed (18,21, 246–249,261), and in the other six studies all patients (study and control) received systemic prophylaxis (19,20,250–252, 262).

Four out of the seven studies on the effect of SDD without systemic prophylaxis reported beneficial effects on incidences of VAP. For instance, Korinec et al. (249) studied 123 neurosurgical patients in a randomized, double-blind, placebo-controlled design and found incidences of VAP, diagnosed by bronchoscopy, of 24% in SDD and 42% in control patients ($p <$ .04). With a similar study design, comparable results were found by Quinio et al. (246) in 148 multiple trauma patients on mechanical ventilation with incidences of VAP of 25% in SDD treated patients and 51% in controls ($p =$ .01). Furthermore, Unertl et al. (248), in a randomized study among 39 neurologic patients, reported incidences of VAP of 5% in SDD and 45% in control patients ($p < .01$). In contrast, no differences in the incidences of VAP, diagnosed by "blind" PSB, between study groups (27% in SDD group vs. 26% in control group) were found in 61 patients in a medical-surgical ICU (21). Gastinne et al. (18) also failed to find beneficial effects of SDD in 445 mechanically ventilated patients admitted to medical ICUs. Pneumonia was diagnosed in 26 (12%) of 220 SDD treated patients and in 33 (15%) of 225 control patients. Finally, in addition to these two randomized, double-blind, placebo-controlled trials, Flaherty et al. (247) studied 107 cardiac surgery patients. Randomization was performed by alternating treatment in 2-week periods to either oropharyngeal and gastrointestinal application of polymyxin, gentamicin, and nystatin or sucralfate for stress-ulcer prophylaxis. One out of 51 patients treated with SDD and 5 out of 56 patients receiving sucralfate developed pneumonia.

Among the six trials in which all patients received systemic prophylaxis, no beneficial effects were reported by the five with a double-blind and placebo-controlled design (19,20,251,252, 262). In the study by Hartenauer et al. (250), which included 200 consecutive patients in a crossover controlled trial, the incidence of VAP was 10% in study patients and 46% in controls.

In summary, the effects of oropharyngeal and gastrointestinal decontamination per se are doubtful because four out of seven studies report beneficial effects on incidences of VAP, whereas no difference in incidence rates were found in the other three. Moreover, the six studies in which all patients (study and control) received systemic prophylaxis suggested that oropharyngeal and gastrointestinal decontamination have only limited additional effect to systemic antibiotics. The RRR of VAP, as calculated from the combined results of these 13 studies, is 0.34 (95% CI: 0.22 to 0.44).

Gastrointestinal Decontamination

The effects of gastrointestinal decontamination on incidences of VAP have been evaluated in only three studies (253,254,265). Brun-Buisson et al. (254) administered neomycin, polymyxin E, and nalidixic acid in liquid form through the nasogastric tube without systemic prophylaxis or oropharyngeal paste to control a nosocomial outbreak of intestinal colonization and infection with multiresistant Enterobacteriaceae. Although the outbreak was controlled successfully, intestinal decontamination did not reduce the number of nosocomial infections: the incidence of pneumonia was 8.3% in the treated group and 14.4% in the control group. In another study, none of 97 patients receiving intestinal decontamination developed VAP (diagnosed with quantitative cultures of PSB), compared with 8 of 84 control patients ($p < .05$) (253). Finally, Cerra et al. (265) reported a decrease in the overall incidence of infections, which almost reached statistical significance ($p = .08$). Unfortunately, the incidence of VAP was not reported.

In summary, gastrointestinal decontamination alone seems to have a beneficial effect on overall infection rates, but the influence on incidences of VAP remains unclear, with one positive and one negative study. Combination of the results of the studies by Brun-Buisson and Godard yields a RRR of 0.78 (95% CI: 0.22 to 1.33). The width of the 95% CI of RRR is indicative of the need for more studies.

Oropharyngeal Decontamination

The effects of oropharyngeal decontamination alone have been assessed in four studies. In a double-blind trial Pugin et al. (94) randomized 52 patients to receive either a solution of polymyxin B, neomycin, and vancomycin or placebo in the retropharynx. Colonization with aerobic gram-negative bacteria was significantly reduced in oropharynx and stomach, resulting in a RRR of VAP of 0.79. Rodriguez-Roldán et al. (255) used an oropharyngeal paste containing tobramycin, amphotericin B, and polymyxin E. Decontamination of the oropharynx and trachea was established in 10 of 13 patients receiving active medication, none of whom developed pneumonia. In contrast, 11 (73%) of 15 patients receiving placebo medication developed pneumonia. Attention must be drawn to the high incidences of VAP in the control groups of both studies (78% and 73%, respectively), which is probably due to the use of clinical and microbiologic criteria, rather than bronchoscopic techniques, to diagnose VAP. Unfortunately, because gastric colonization was significantly decreased in the study by Pugin et al., their findings do not elucidate the relative importance of gastric and oropharyngeal colonization in the pathogenesis of VAP.

In a prospective randomized placebo-controlled double-blind study, 87 patients received topical antimicrobial prophylaxis in the oropharynx and 139 patients received placebo. The aim of the study was to prevent VAP by modulation of oropharyngeal colonization, without influencing gastric and intestinal colonization and without systemic prophylaxis. Oropharyngeal colonization present on admission was eradicated in 75% of the patients (4% among control patients) and only 10% of study patients acquired oropharyngeal colonization, as compared with 61% of control patients. There were no significant differences in gastric and intestinal colonization. This regimen resulted in a RRR for VAP of 0.62 (95% CI 0.26 to 0.98) (263).

Oropharyngeal decontamination in combination with systemic prophylaxis was studied by Abele-Horn et al. (256) in a randomized, controlled trial. The incidences of both primary (0% vs. 33%; $p < .001$) and secondary pneumonia (22% vs. 47%; $p < .001$) were reduced significantly in study patients. Pneumonia was diagnosed by quantitative cultures of tracheal aspirates ($>10^4$ CFU/mL). Again, the total incidence of pneumonia (primary and secondary) in the control group was very high (77%).

Another way to achieve oropharyngeal decontamination, when antibiotics are not used, is the use of chlorhexidine. For instance, an oral rinse of 0.12% chlorhexidine reduced the incidence of respiratory tract infections among 353 cardiosurgical patients from 9% in control patients to 3% in patients receiving oropharyngeal decontamination with chlorhexidine (273). This difference was mainly due to a reduction of infections with gram-negative pathogens. However, it is not known to what extent prolonged application of chlorhexidine will affect oral, esophageal, and gastric mucosa in critically ill ICU patients, and the risk of chlorhexidine resistance after long-term application is not known (274–276).

Systemic Prophylaxis

Prevention of pneumonia with systemic antibiotics was attempted first by Lepper et al. (277) in 1954. No reduction of tracheal colonization or infection was achieved in 72 tracheotomized poliomyelitis patients. Two other studies from that time also failed to modify the incidence of infection by antibiotic prophylaxis in unconscious patients (278) and patients with acute heart failure (279). Moreover, the latter two studies reported selection of resistant pathogens. It was not until 1989 that another attempt was made to prevent pneumonia with systemic antibiotics. Then, Mandelli et al. (280) randomized 570 ICU patients, half of whom were intubated, to receive 24 hours of either cefoxitin, penicillin G, or no prophylaxis. The incidence of early-onset pneumonia (primary outcome measure) was 6.1% in patients receiving antibiotics and 7.2% for controls (280). More recently, in a prospective, randomized, but not double-blind or placebo-controlled, trial in 100 mechanically ventilated patients with coma, systemic antibiotic prophylaxis with cefuroxime (two 1,500-mg doses) was studied. Prophylaxis resulted in a lower incidence of VAP compared with the control group [12/50 (24%) vs. 25/50 (50%); $p = .007$; RRR 0.52]. This difference was due to a reduction in the episodes of early-onset VAP in the cefuroxime group [8/50 (16%) vs. 18/50 (36%); $p = .022$; RRR 0.56], whereas the incidences of late-onset VAP were comparable (8% vs. 14%) (257). The impact of this regimen on antibiotic susceptibility of pathogens causing VAP remains to be established.

The results of all the trials with various SDD regimens and of the meta-analyses indicated that SDD reduces the incidence of VAP; may reduce ICU-mortality; and increases, in some settings, the selection of multiple resistant pathogens. Several controversies remain. A considerable portion of the studies that reported favorable results of SDD were poorly designed (nonrandomized, unblinded, historical control groups, nonbronchoscopic diagnosis of VAP, etc.). Moreover, the preventive effects of the individual parts of SDD were not fully elucidated. The systemic antibiotics within the regimen seemed to prevent early-onset, but not late-onset, VAP. The effects of gastrointestinal decontamination were scarcely investigated and remain unclear. Because the role of gastric colonization and the gastropulmonary route of colonization are regarded as less important than previously assumed, the additive effect of gastrointestinal decontamination may be minimal. In contrast, oropharyngeal decontamination may be equally effective as the full SDD regimen with regard to preventing VAP. However, more studies are needed to answer these questions and to determine the true effects of antibiotic-containing preventive measures on patient survival.

Stress-Ulcer Prophylaxis

Because critically ill patients on mechanical ventilation are prone to develop gastritis and/or gastric ulcers (281–283), stress-ulcer prophylaxis is routinely provided. In this respect, gastric acidity may be reduced by neutralization of gastric acid (antacids) or by inhibition of acid production (H_2-antagonists, H^+K^+ATPase inhibitors), both of which will decrease the natural protection against bacterial overgrowth. In contrast to these agents, sucralfate has been claimed to prevent stress ulcers without influencing gastric acidity (284). Theoretically, patients who receive sucralfate should maintain lower intragastric pH values compared with patients receiving antacids or H_2-antagonists. Moreover, *in vitro* studies demonstrated bactericidal and bacteriostatic effects of sucralfate, mainly at high pH values (285–287). As a result, sucralfate should prevent bacterial overgrowth in the stomach and, according to the alleged importance of the gastropulmonary route of colonization, also reduce the incidence of VAP. Administration of sucralfate for stress-ulcer prophylaxis has shown favorable effects on the incidence of VAP in two studies (14,15). However, 12 studies showed no significant effect on the incidence of VAP (16,17,281,282,288–295). In a prospective, randomized, double-blind study by our group in which patients were stratified on the basis of their initial gastric pH, sucralfate was compared with a fixed dosage of antacids (16). Intragastric acidity was determined by means of computerized intragastric pH monitoring. No significant differences in median pH values were observed. Colonization rates in the stomach, the oropharynx, and the trachea and the incidence of VAP were comparable in both treatment groups. However, patients colonized with PPMO in the stomach had higher median pH values compared with noncolonized patients. This underscores the relation between intragastric acidity and gastric colonization (16). The observation that sucralfate does not prevent VAP could be due to the fact that sucralfate did not decrease intragastric pH levels below 3.5 in most of the studies (6). These findings were confirmed by two other double-blind studies testing the preventive effects of sucralfate. A study by Artigas et al. (288), comparing sucralfate and ranitidine, was terminated prematurely after inclusion of 146 patients because no difference in incidence of VAP between both study groups was observed (published only in abstract form). In addition, similar data were reported in a prospective, double-blind, placebo-controlled study in which 1,200 patients had been randomized to either sucralfate or ranitidine (17).

Modulation of Enteral Feeding

In addition to stress-ulcer prophylaxis, enteral feeding, which usually has a pH of 6, may reduce intragastric acidity because of dilutional alkalization. If enteral feeding was a risk factor for the development of VAP, this would support the role of the gastropulmonary route of colonization in the pathogenesis of VAP. Several studies showed high rates of gastric colonization in patients receiving enteral feeding (296,297). Hence, modulation of enteral feeding has been used as a possible approach to interrupt the gastropulmonary route of colonization and to reduce the incidence of VAP. In this regard, intermittent enteral feeding would be expected to be superior to continuous enteral feeding, because gastric acidity increases during the periods that feeding is discontinued. Three studies have been performed with opposite results. Lee et al. (298) reported lower intragastric pH values and incidence rates of VAP in patients who received intermittent enteral feeding compared with a historical control group that received continuous enteral feeding. Skiest et al. (299) randomized 16 patients to either intermittent enteral feeding or continuous enteral feeding for a 5-day period. They concluded that intermittent enteral feeding resulted in lower postfasting gastric pH and lower rates of gastric colonization with pathogenic microorganisms. No patients developed nosocomial pneumonia during the 5-day study period. Our group (300) failed to find a beneficial effect of intermittent enteral feeding on intragastric acidity, gastric colonization, and incidence of VAP in a prospective randomized trial in which intermittent enteral feeding and continuous enteral feeding were compared in 60 patients.

The effects of acidified (pH 3.5) enteral feeding were determined in two studies (301,302). In both studies favorable results with respect to intragastric acidity and gastric colonization were found. However, the incidence of VAP was analyzed only in the latter showing no difference (6.1% in the acidified enteral feeding group vs. 15% in controls; $p = .19$) (302). Large, prospective randomized and controlled trials are needed to confirm the effects of modulation of enteral feeding as a means to decrease the incidence of VAP.

In another attempt to reduce aspiration, gastric nutrition has been compared with postpyloric feeding. Seven studies evaluated the risks for VAP in patients randomized to either gastric or postpyloric feeding (303). Although significant differences were not demonstrated in any individual study, postpyloric feeding was associated with a significant reduction in VAP in meta-analysis [RR = 0.76 (0.59 to 0.99)] (303).

Another option for infection prevention might be enteral immunonutrition. Several small studies determined the effects of enteral feeding enriched with specific immunonutrients (e.g., arginine, purine nucleotides and polyunsaturated fats) on outcome in critically ill patients (304). Several studies reported a trend toward better clinical outcome for patients receiving immunonutrition (304). In a randomized double-blind trial, immunonutrition failed to decrease hospital mortality in critically ill patients. However, in the subgroup of patients who received enteral nutrition within 72 hours after admission, reductions in the requirement for mechanical ventilation and length of hospital stay were found. Unfortunately, incidences of pneumonia were not reported (305). In another randomized and controlled study among trauma patients, enteral nutrition was enriched with glutamine, which is an important protein for lymphocytes and enterocytes. The incidence of pneumonia decreased from 43% to 17% ($p < .02$) and of bacteremia from 42% to 9% ($p < .005$). However, pneumonia was diagnosed on extremely nonspecific criteria, and colonization of the respiratory tract was not studied. Moreover, glutamine levels were only significantly elevated in study patients from day three to day five of treatment. Because almost all infections in both study groups occurred within the first week of study, the mode of action leading to prevention of pneumonia remains unclear (306). More recently a prospective, single-blind, randomized trial in a mixed ICU population ($n = 220$) comparing standard high-protein diet with high-protein diet enriched with arginine, fiber, and antioxidants showed a significant decrease in catheter-related sepsis but failed to influence the incidence of VAP and mortality (307).

Subglottic Secretions Drainage

During mechanical ventilation, subglottic secretions and oropharyngeal fluids may accumulate above the inflated endotracheal cuff. This fluid contains large amounts of microorganisms. Microaspiration of these secretions along the tracheal tube cuff results in colonization and possibly infection of the lower respiratory tract. Drainage of subglottic secretions with specifically designed devices may, therefore, prevent VAP. This preventive measure has now been evaluated in four studies, which all showed statistically significant or strong tendencies toward significant reductions in incidences of VAP (28,29,308,309). Moreover, from a theoretical decision-model analysis, it was concluded that the use of endotracheal tubes allowing subglottic suctioning may result in cost savings in mechanically ventilated ICU patients (310). Finally, Pneumatikos et al. (311) determined the effects of subglottic secretion drainage in combination with decontamination of the subglottic area with nonabsorbable antibiotics (polymyxin, tobramycin, and amphotericin B). This combined intervention reduced the incidence of VAP (RRR = 0.68). Clearly, subglottic aspiration is a promising preventive measure, and more studies, carefully addressing the diagnostic criteria for VAP, are warranted.

Body Position

Enteral feeding increases gastric volume, especially in critically ill patients who often have reduced gastric motility and delayed gastric emptying because of the underlying disease or as a result of medication (312). In these patients the risk of aspiration of gastric contents is enhanced. Torres et al. (186) analyzed gastroesophageal reflux in ventilated patients on enteral feeding, using radioactive-labeled gastric nutrition. They found that patients in the supine position had higher counts of radioactivity in endobronchial secretions compared with patients treated in a semirecumbent position. Moreover, the length of time in the supine position appeared to be a risk factor for aspiration of gastric contents. In a follow-up study in 15 patients by the same group, it was concluded that gastroesophageal reflux occurs irrespective of body position, and that the semirecumbent position does not protect completely from gastroesophageal reflux (313). These data confirmed the results reported by Ibanez et al. (185) in a similar study. Up until now, the semirecumbent patient position has been evaluated in a randomized design only once (314). In a small randomized trial a semirecumbent position was associated with a significant reduction in the incidence of VAP as compared with the supine position (5% and 23%, respectively; $p = .018$). However, the combination of a supine position while receiving enteral feeding might have been responsible for this large difference (314). Moreover, little is known about the feasibility of this intervention.

In addition to the patient's position, gastroesophageal reflux may be influenced by the presence and even the size of the nasogastric tube (185,313,315). However, the effects on incidences of VAP were not evaluated in any of these studies.

Continuous Lateral Rotational Therapy

Another potentially effective approach is continuous lateral rotational therapy. Continuous rotation is thought to stimulate mobilization of respiratory tract secretions, thereby preventing the development of atelectasis and pneumonia. Seven studies compared continuous lateral rotational therapy with turning by nursing staff every 2 hours in conventional beds. All studies reported reduced incidences of pneumonia in patients on rotation (30–35,316); the difference was statistically significant in two (32,316).

Other Preventive Strategies

Intubation and mechanical ventilation clearly are the most important risk factors for VAP. Unnecessary intubation, therefore, should be avoided at all times. Noninvasive positive-pressure ventilation (NIPPV) using a face mask could be used as an alternative ventilation mode in ICU patients. The beneficial effects of NIPPV on the development of VAP and patient survival have been determined in randomized trials for patients with acute exacerbations of chronic obstructive pulmonary disease (COPD) (317) or acute respiratory failure (318) and in immunosuppressed patients with pulmonary infiltrates, fever, and respiratory failure (319). In addition, the risk for VAP increases with duration of ventilation. As a result, strategies to reduce the duration of ventilation may decrease the risk for development of VAP. Examples of such strategies are protocols to improve methods of sedation administration (320,321) and to accelerate weaning (322). Furthermore, staffing levels may influence the length of stay of patients in ICU, with an inverse relationship between adequacy of staffing levels and duration of stay and subsequent development of VAP (323,324). Understaffing can also lead to lapses in infection control practices, facilitating transmission of antibiotic-resistant bacteria (325).

The use of topical tracheobronchial antibiotics, administered either as an aerosol (polymyxin B, gentamicin) or in a solution (gentamicin, colistin), has been attempted to reduce the incidence of pneumonia caused by gram-negative bacteria, especially *P. aeruginosa.* Four studies performed between 1973 and 1975, of which two had a controlled design (326,327), reported significantly decreased incidences of upper airway colonization and/or pneumonia caused by these microorganisms (326–329). However, the study by Klastersky et al. (327), using endotracheal administration of gentamicin, reported that bacteria isolated from treated patients were slightly more resistant to gentamicin than microorganisms recovered from the respiratory tracts of controls. Feeley et al. (329) used an aerosol with polymyxin B, which successfully prevented *P. aeruginosa* pneumonia. However, the incidence of pneumonia caused by polymyxin-resistant microorganisms (*Pseudomonas* species and *Serratia* species) and intrinsically resistant pathogens (*Proteus* species, *Flavobacterium* species, and *Streptococcus faecalis*) was high, and the overall mortality rate for patients with acquired pneumonia was 64% (329). Furthermore, a randomized study in 30 thermally injured patients with inhalation injury, using aerosolized gentamicin, reported no differences in number of patients with infiltrates on chest radiographs, necessity of mechanical ventilation, and pulmonary complications between study and control patients (330). Moreover, continued use of gentamicin in this study resulted in resistant strains of *Klebsiella* and *Pseudomonas* emerging in burn wounds and sputum (330). Because of the frequent occurrence of infection with highly resistant bacteria and the lack of (or even negative) effect on mortality, the use of topical tracheobronchial antibiotics was not recommended. Rouby et al. (331) performed a nonrandomized study in which 347 consecutive patients receiving intratracheal colistin were compared with a historical control group of 251 patients. The incidences of pneumonia caused by gram-negative bacteria and polymicrobial pneumonia were significantly reduced in the group receiving colistin. Mortality was comparable in both groups, and no increase in the number of VAP cases caused by colistin-resistant microorganisms was observed.

Bacterial contamination of the ventilator tubing circuit may predispose to the development of VAP (218). Frequent changing of these circuits (including in-line suction catheters, heat and moisture exchangers, and heated humidifiers) may be beneficial to decrease the bacterial burden. On the other hand, frequent manipulation of ventilator tubing circuits may lead to introduction of nosocomial pathogens. Five studies have addressed the effects of lengthening intervals between circuit changes on colonization of the patient and circuits and incidence of VAP (126, 332–335). They all concluded that decreasing the frequency of ventilator circuit changes did not increase incidences of VAP or patient and circuit colonization. Therefore, substantial reductions in the costs of mechanical ventilation can be obtained without apparent adverse effect. Studies using a closed-suction catheter system for endotracheal suctioning found similar incidences of pneumonia compared with the open-suction system with single-use sterile suction catheters (336–339). Finally, during mechanical ventilation, heating and humidifying of inspired gases are necessary. Heated humidifiers are used most often, but these cause accumulation of water in the circuit that may become colonized with bacteria (218). Heat and moisture exchangers are a possible alternative in which the formation of condensate in ventilation circuits is avoided due to the combination of humidification with antimicrobial filtering properties. However, heat and moisture exchangers failed to reduce the incidence of pneumonia in five studies that compared both methods (340–344). Kirton et al. (345) are the only investigators to report a significant reduction in late-onset VAP, but not early-onset VAP, with the use of heat and moisture exchangers. Recently, the effect of heat and moisture exchanger filters with different compositions of the condensation surface, either $CaCl_2$ or $AlCl_2$ based, were compared. No differences were noted in the incidences of tracheal colonization and VAP (346).

CONCLUSIONS

It remains difficult to reach firm conclusions after a critical assessment of the various studies on the prevention of VAP. Because of small numbers of patients studied, heterogeneous ICU populations, and differences in diagnostic criteria and quality of the studies, a comparison of the studies is hampered. Moreover, some strategies have scarcely been studied. Ideally, preventive strategies are studied in well-designed multicenter trials, including large numbers of comparable patients.

The use of SDD has been studied most often and seems to have the best potential to reduce the incidence of VAP. However, SDD was considered of unproven value by the ATS (category 3) and as a strategy for which insufficient evidence is available by the CDC (category UI). More studies are needed to determine whether SDD, or any other antibiotic prophylaxis, improves patient survival in a cost-effective manner. However, such strategies are probably contraindicated in ICU settings with high-levels of multiresistant microorganisms. In settings, where resistance-levels are low, the long-term effects of antibiotic prophylaxis should be carefully monitored.

The use of sucralfate for stress-ulcer prophylaxis is considered promising by the ATS (category 2) and is suggested for implementation in many hospitals (category II) by the CDC. However, most clinical trials and all randomized, double-blind, placebo-controlled trials have failed to show favorable effects of sucralfate on the incidence of VAP. Moreover, sucralfate was found to be inferior to ranitidine with regard to the prevention of clinically important gastrointestinal bleeding.

The various preventive strategies associated with enteral feeding and (prevention of) gastric aspiration are thought to be efficacious by the ATS (category 2), although very few studies on their efficacy have been performed and the results of these studies are controversial. The CDC considers these recommendations to be an unresolved issue (category UI); however, a semirecumbent body position during mechanical ventilation was strongly recommended (category IB), even though definitive scientific evidence for this recommendation is lacking. There is now one randomized trial favoring the semirecumbent position. More studies evaluating both the beneficial effects and the feasibility of this intervention are needed.

Subglottic secretions drainage and continuous lateral rotational therapy are both regarded as "promising in efficacy and being used by some hospitals on a regular basis" by the ATS (category 2), which is consistent with the scientific evidence. Continuous lateral rotational therapy has been studied only in selected patient populations, and favorable results on incidence rates of VAP have been reported. The mechanism for this beneficial effect remains to be established. Whether this technique is applicable to large numbers of patients is also unclear, especially because the associated costs of this technique are considerable. The CDC considers both these strategies to be practices for which insufficient evidence or consensus regarding efficacy exists (category UI).

Although preventive strategies aimed at ventilator circuits are categorized as promising in efficacy (category 2) by the ATS, the accessory guidelines indicate that the proposed measures (i.e., heat and moisture exchangers; frequent, infrequent, or no change of circuits; and closed-suction systems) do not seem to add to the risk of developing VAP. This is congruent with the categorization of the CDC (category UI).

REFERENCES

1. Richards MJ, Edwards JR, Culver DH, et al. Nosocomial infections in medical intensive care units in the United States. *Crit Care Med* 1999;27:887–892.
2. Centers for Disease Control (CDC). National nosocomial infections surveillance (NNIS) system report, data summary from January 1992 to June 2002, issued August 2002. *Am J Infect Control* 2002;30: 458–475.
3. Emori TG, Gaynes RP. An overview of nosocomial infections, including the role of the microbiology laboratory. *Clin Microbiol Rev* 1993; 6:428–442.
4. Fagon JY, Chastre J, Hance AJ, et al. Nosocomial pneumonia in ventilated patients: a cohort study evaluating attributable mortality and hospital stay. *Am J Med* 1993;94:281–288.
5. Kappstein I, Schulgen G, Beyer U, et al. Prolongation of hospital stay and extra costs due to ventilator-associated pneumonia in an intensive care unit. *Eur J Clin Microbiol Infect Dis* 1992;11:504–508.
6. Bonten MJM, Gaillard CA, de Leeuw PW, et al. Role of colonization of the upper intestinal tract in the pathogenesis of ventilator-associated pneumonia. *Clin Infect Dis* 1997;24:309–319.
7. Reinarz JA, Pierce AK, Mays BB. The potential role of inhalation therapy equipment in nosocomial pulmonary infection. *J Clin Invest* 1965;44:831–839.
8. Pierce AK, Edmonson EB, McGee G, et al. An analysis of factors predisposing to gram-negative bacillary necrotizing pneumonia. *Am Rev Respir Dis* 1966;94:309–315.
9. Pierce AK, Sanford JP, Thomas GD, et al. Long-term evaluation of decontamination of inhalation therapy equipment and the occurrence of necrotizing pneumonia. *N Engl J Med* 1970;282:528–531.
10. Cross AS, Roup B. Role of respiratory assistance devices in endemic nosocomial pneumonia. *Am J Med* 1981;70:681–685.
11. Garibaldi RA, Britt MR, Coleman ML, et al. Risk factors for postoperative pneumonia. *Am J Med* 1981;70:677–680.
12. Johanson WG Jr, Pierce AK, Sanford JP, et al. Nosocomial respiratory infections with gram-negative bacilli: the significance of colonization of the respiratory tract. *Ann Intern Med* 1972;77:701–706.
13. du Moulin GC, Paterson DG, Hedley-Whyte J, et al. Aspiration of gastric bacteria in antacid-treated patients: a frequent cause of postoperative colonisation of the airway. *Lancet* 1982;i:242–245.
14. Driks MR, Craven DE, Celli BR, et al. Nosocomial pneumonia in

intubated patients given sucralfate as compared with antacids or histamine type 2 blockers: the role of gastric colonisation. *N Engl J Med* 1987;317:1376–1382.
15. Prod'hom G, Leuenberger P, Koerfer J, et al. Nosocomial pneumonia in mechanically ventilated patients receiving antacid, ranitidine, or sucralfate as prophylaxis for stress ulcer: a randomised controlled trial. *Ann Intern Med* 1994;120:653–662.
16. Bonten MJM, Gaillard CA, van der Geest S, et al. The role of intragastric acidity and stress ulcer prophylaxis on colonization and infection in mechanically ventilated patients. A stratified, randomized, double blind study of sucralfate versus antacids. *Am J Respir Crit Care Med* 1995;152:1825–1834.
17. Cook D, Guyatt G, Marshall J, et al. A comparison of sucralfate and ranitidine for the prevention of upper gastrointestinal bleeding in patients requiring mechanical ventilation. *N Engl J Med* 1998;338: 791–797.
18. Gastinne H, Wolff M, Delatour F, et al. A controlled trial in intensive care units of selective decontamination of the digestive tract with nonabsorbable antibiotics. *N Engl J Med* 1992;326:594–599.
19. Hammond JMJ, Potgieter PD, Saunders GL, et al. Double-blind study of selective decontamination of the digestive tract in intensive care. *Lancet* 1992;340:5–9.
20. Ferrer M, Torres A, González J, et al. Utility of selective digestive decontamination in mechanically ventilated patients. *Ann Intern Med* 1994;120:389–395.
21. Wiener J, Itokazu G, Nathan C, et al. A randomized, double-blind, placebo-controlled trial of selective decontamination in a medical-surgical intensive care unit. *Clin Infect Dis* 1995;20:861–867.
22. Selective Decontamination of the Digestive Tract Trialists' Collaborative Group. Meta-analysis of randomised controlled trials of selective decontamination of the digestive tract. *BMJ* 1993;307:525–532.
23. D'Amico R, Pifferi S, Leonetti C, et al. Effectiveness of antibiotic prophylaxis in critically ill adult patients: systematic review of randomised controlled trials. *BMJ* 1998;316:1275–1285.
24. Heyland DK, Cook DJ, Jaeschke R, et al. Selective decontamination of the digestive tract: an overview. *Chest* 1994;105:1221–1229.
25. Vandenbroucke-Grauls CMJE, Vandenbroucke JP. Effect of selective decontamination of the digestive tract on respiratory tract infections and mortality in the intensive care unit. *Lancet* 1991;338:859–862.
26. Kollef MH. The role of selective digestive tract decontamination on mortality and respiratory tract infections: a meta-analysis. *Chest* 1994; 105:1101–1108.
27. Rello J, Sonora R, Jubert P, et al. Pneumonia in intubated patients: role of respiratory airway care. *Am J Respir Crit Care Med* 1996;154: 111–115.
28. Mahul P, Auboyer C, Jospe R, et al. Prevention of nosocomial pneumonia in intubated patients: respective role of mechanical subglottic secretions drainage and stress ulcer prophylaxis. *Intensive Care Med* 1992;18:20–25.
29. Valles J, Artigas A, Rello J, et al. Continuous aspiration of subglottic secretions in preventing ventilator-associated pneumonia. *Ann Intern Med* 1995;122:179–186.
30. Gentilello L, Thompson DA, Tonnesen AS, et al. Effect of a rotating bed on the incidence of pulmonary complications in critically ill patients. *Crit Care Med* 1988;16:783–786.
31. Kelley RE, Vibulresth S, Bell L, et al. Evaluation of kinetic therapy in the prevention of complications of prolonged bed rest secondary to stroke. *Stroke* 1987;18:638–642.
32. Fink MP, Helsmoortel CM, Stein KL, et al. The efficacy of an oscillating bed in the prevention of lower respiratory tract infection in critically ill victims of blunt trauma. *Chest* 1990;97:132–137.
33. Summer WR, Curry P, Haponik EF, et al. Continuous mechanical turning of intensive care patients shortens length of stay in some diagnostic-related groups. *J Crit Care* 1989;4:45–53.
34. de Boisblanc BP, Castro M, Everret B, et al. Effect of air-supported, continuous, postural oscillation on the risk of early ICU pneumonia in nontraumatic critical illness. *Chest* 1993;103:1543–1547.
35. Whiteman K, Nachtmann L, Kramer D, et al. Effects of continuous lateral rotation therapy on pulmonary complications in liver transplant patients. *Am J Crit Care* 1995;4:133–139.
36. Niederman MS, Craven DE. Editorial response: devising strategies for preventing nosocomial pneumonia—should we ignore the stomach? *Clin Infect Dis* 1997;24:320–323.
37. Heyland D, Mandell LA. Gastric colonization by gram-negative bacilli and nosocomial pneumonia in the intensive care unit patient: evidence for causation. *Chest* 1992;101:187–193.
38. Dever LL, Johanson WG Jr. An update on selective decontamination of the digestive tract. *Curr Opin Infect Dis* 1993;6:744–750.
39. Bonten MJM, Weinstein RA. Selective decontamination of the digestive tract: a measure whose time has passed? *Curr Opin Infect Dis* 1996;9:270–275.
40. Niederman MS, Torres A, Summer W. Invasive diagnostic testing is not needed routinely to manage suspected ventilator-associated pneumonia. *Am J Respir Crit Care Med* 1994;150:565–569.
41. Chastre J, Fagon JY. Invasive diagnostic testing should be routinely used to manage ventilated patients with suspected pneumonia. *Am J Respir Crit Care Med* 1994;150:570–574.
42. Langer M, Cigada M, Mandelli M, et al. Early-onset pneumonia: a multicenter study in intensive care units. *Intensive Care Med* 1987; 13:342–346.
43. Garner JS, Jarvis WR, Emori TG, et al. CDC definitions for nosocomial infections, 1988. *Am J Infect Control* 1988;16:128–140.
44. Bonten MJM, Gaillard CA, Wouters EFM, et al. Problems in diagnosing nosocomial pneumonia in mechanically ventilated patients: a review. *Crit Care Med* 1994;22:1683–1691.
45. Centers for Disease Control (CDC). CDC definitions for nosocomial infections, 1988. *Am Rev Respir Dis* 1989;139:1058–1059.
46. Pugin J, Auckenthaler R, Mili N, et al. Diagnosis of ventilator-associated pneumonia by bacteriologic analysis of bronchoscopic and non-bronchoscopic "blind" bronchoalveolar lavage fluid. *Am Rev Respir Dis* 1991;143:1121–1129.
47. Wunderink RG, Woldenberg LS, Zeiss J. The radiologic diagnosis of autopsy-proven ventilator-associated pneumonia. *Chest* 1992;101: 458–463.
48. Bell RC, Coalson JJ, Smith JD, et al. Multiple organ system failure and infection in adult respiratory distress syndrome. *Ann Intern Med* 1983;99:293–298.
49. Chastre J, Viau F, Brun P, et al. Prospective evaluation of the protected specimen brush for the diagnosis of pulmonary infections in ventilated patients. *Am Rev Respir Dis* 1984;130:924–929.
50. Fagon JY, Chastre J, Hance AJ, et al. Detection of nosocomial lung infection in ventilated patients: use of a protected specimen brush and quantitative culture techniques in 147 patients. *Am Rev Respir Dis* 1988;138:110–116.
51. Meduri GU, Mauldin GL, Wunderink RG, et al. Causes of fever and pulmonary densities in patients with clinical manifestations of ventilator-associated pneumonia. *Chest* 1994;106:221–235.
52. Fagon JY, Chastre J, Hance AJ, et al. Evaluation of clinical judgement in the identification and treatment of nosocomial pneumonia in ventilated patients. *Chest* 1993;103:547–553.
53. Meduri GU. Diagnosis of ventilator-associated pneumonia. *Infect Dis Clin North Am* 1993;7:295–329.
54. Andrews CP, Coalson JJ, Smith JD, et al. Diagnosis of nosocomial bacterial pneumonia in acute, diffuse lung injury. *Chest* 1981;80: 254–257.
55. Higuchi JH, Coalson JJ, Johanson WG Jr. Bacteriologic diagnosis of nosocomial pneumonia in primates: usefulness of the protected specimen brush. *Am Rev Respir Dis* 1982;125:53–57.
56. Torres A, Puig de la Bellacasa J, Xaubet A, et al. Diagnostic value of quantitative cultures of bronchoalveolar lavage and telescoping plugged catheters in mechanically ventilated patients with bacterial pneumonia. *Am Rev Respir Dis* 1989;140:306–310.
57. Wimberley N, Faling LJ, Bartlett JG. A fiberoptic bronchoscopy technique to obtain uncontaminated lower airway secretions for bacterial culture. *Am Rev Respir Dis* 1979;119:337–343.
58. Kahn FW, Jones JM. Diagnosing bacterial respiratory infection by bronchoalveolar lavage. *J Infect Dis* 1987;155:862–869.
59. Thorpe JE, Baughman RP, Frame PT, et al. Bronchoalveolar lavage for diagnosing acute bacterial pneumonia. *J Infect Dis* 1987;155: 855–861.

60. Meduri GU, Beals DH, Maijub AG, et al. Protected bronchoalveolar lavage. A new bronchoscopic technique to retrieve uncontaminated distal airway secretions. *Am Rev Respir Dis* 1991;143:855–864.
61. Pingleton SK, Fagon JY, Leeper KV Jr. Patient selection for clinical investigation of ventilator-associated pneumonia: criteria for evaluating diagnostic techniques. *Chest* 1992;102:553S–556S.
62. Kirkpatrick MB, Bass JB. Quantitative bacterial cultures of bronchoalveolar lavage fluids and protected brush catheter specimens from normal subjects. *Am Rev Respir Dis* 1989;139:546–548.
63. Swenson ER, Carlson LC, Albert RK, et al. Antibody coating and quantitative cultures of bacteria in the airways of patients with chronic bronchitis. *Chest* 1989;95:197s.
64. Pham LH, Brun-Buisson C, Legrand P, et al. Diagnosis of nosocomial pneumonia in mechanically ventilated patients: comparison of a plugged telescoping catheter with the protected specimen brush. *Am Rev Respir Dis* 1991;143:1055–1061.
65. Chastre J, Fagon JY, Bornet-Lecso M, et al. Evaluation of bronchoscopic techniques for the diagnosis of nosocomial pneumonia. *Am J Respir Crit Care Med* 1995;152:231–240.
66. Marquette CH, Copin MC, Wallet F, et al. Diagnostic tests for pneumonia in ventilated patients: prospective evaluation of diagnostic accuracy using histology as a diagnostic gold standard. *Am J Respir Crit Care Med* 1995;151:1878–1888.
67. Torres A, El-Ebiary M, Padró L, et al. Validation of different techniques for the diagnosis of ventilator-associated pneumonia: comparison with immediate postmortem pulmonary biopsy. *Am J Respir Crit Care Med* 1994;149:324–331.
68. Papazian L, Thomas P, Garbe L, et al. Bronchoscopic or blind sampling techniques for the diagnosis of ventilator-associated pneumonia. *Am J Respir Crit Care Med* 1995;152:1982–1991.
69. Johanson WG Jr, Seidenfeld JJ, Gomez P, et al. Bacteriologic diagnosis of nosocomial pneumonia following prolonged mechanical ventilation. *Am Rev Respir Dis* 1988;137:259–264.
70. Reynolds HY. Bronchoalveolar lavage. *Am Rev Respir Dis* 1987;135: 250–263.
71. Guerra LF, Baughman RP. Use of bronchoalveolar lavage to diagnose bacterial pneumonia in mechanically ventilated patients. *Crit Care Med* 1990;18:169–173.
72. Castella J, Puzo C, Ausina V. Diagnosis of pneumonia with a method of protected bronchoalveolar lavage. *Eur Respir J* 1991;4:407s.
73. Bonten MJM, Bergmans DCJJ, Stobberingh EE, et al. Implementation of bronchoscopic techniques in the diagnosis of ventilator-associated pneumonia to reduce antibiotic use. *Am J Respir Crit Care Med* 1997;156:1820–1824.
74. Ruiz M, Torres A, Ewig S. Non-invasive versus invasive microbial investigation in ventilator-associated pneumonia. Evaluation of outcome. *Am J Respir Crit Care Med* 2000;162:119–125.
75. Sanchez Nieto JM, Torres A, Garcia-Cordoba F, et al. Impact of invasive and noninvasive quantitative culture sampling on outcome of ventilator-associated pneumonia. A pilot study. *Am J Respir Crit Care Med* 1998;157:371–376.
76. Solé-Violán J, Sanchez-Ramirez C, Padron Mujica A. Impact of nosocomial pneumonia on the outcome of mechanically ventilated patients. *Crit Care Med* 1998;2:19–23.
77. Croce MA, Fabian TC, Shaw B, et al. Analysis of charges associated with diagnosis of nosocomial pneumonia: can routine bronchoscopy be justified? *J Trauma* 1994;37:721–727.
78. Fagon JY, Chastre J, Wolff M. Invasive and non-invasive strategies for management of suspected ventilator-associated pneumonia. A randomized trial. *Ann Intern Med* 2000;132:621–630.
79. Heyland DK, Cook DJ, Marshall J, et al. The clinical utility of invasive diagnostic techniques in the setting of ventilator-associated pneumonia. *Chest* 1999;115:1076–1084.
80. Singh N, Rogers P, Atwood CW, et al. Short-course empiric antibiotic therapy for patients with pulmonary infiltrates in the intensive care unit. A proposed solution for indiscriminate antibiotic prescription. *Am J Respir Crit Care Med* 2000;162:505–511.
81. Gaussorgues P, Piperno D, Bachmann P, et al. Comparison of nonbronchoscopic bronchoalveolar lavage to open lung biopsy for the bacteriologic diagnosis of pulmonary infections in mechanically ventilated patients. *Intensive Care Med* 1989;15:94–98.
82. Rouby JJ, Rossignon MD, Nicolas MH, et al. A prospective study of protected bronchoalveolar lavage in the diagnosis of nosocomial pneumonia. *Anesthesiology* 1989;71:679–685.
83. Kollef MH, Bock KR, Richards RD, et al. The safety and diagnostic accuracy of minibronchoalveolar lavage in patients with suspected ventilator-associated pneumonia. *Ann Intern Med* 1995;122: 743–748.
84. Chastre J, Fagon JY, Trouillet JL. Diagnosis and treatment of nosocomial pneumonia in patients in intensive care units. *Clin Infect Dis* 1995;21:S226–S237.
85. Bonten MJM, Froon AHM, Gaillard CA, et al. The systemic inflammatory response in the development of ventilator-associated pneumonia. *Am J Respir Crit Care Med* 1997;156:1105-1113.
86. Froon AHM, Bonten MJM, Gaillard CA. Prediction of clinical severity and outcome of ventilator-associated pneumonia. Comparison of simplified acute physiology score with systemic inflammatory mediators. *Am J Respir Crit Care Med* 1998;158:1026–1031.
87. Kollef M, Eisenberg PR, Ohlendorf MF, et al. The accuracy of elevated concentrations of endotoxin in bronchoalveolar lavage fluid for the rapid diagnosis of gram-negative pneumonia. *Am J Respir Crit Care Med* 1996;154:1020–1028.
88. Salata RA, Lederman MM, Shlaes DM, et al. Diagnosis of nosocomial pneumonia in intubated, intensive care unit patients. *Am Rev Respir Dis* 1987;135:426–432.
89. Winterbauer RH, Hutchinson JF, Reinhardt GN, et al. The use of quantitative cultures and antibody coating of bacteria to diagnose bacterial pneumonia by fiberoptic bronchoscopy. *Am Rev Respir Dis* 1983;128:98–103.
90. Winer-Muram HT, Rubin SA, Miniati M, et al. Guidelines for reading and interpreting chest radiographs in patients receiving mechanical ventilation. *Chest* 1992;102:565S–570S.
91. Leu HS, Kaiser DL, Mori M, et al. Hospital-acquired pneumonia: attributable mortality and morbidity. *Am J Epidemiol* 1989;129: 1258–1267.
92. Haley RW, Culver DH, White JW, et al. The nationwide nosocomial infection rate: a new need for vital statistics. *Am J Epidemiol* 1985; 121:159–167.
93. Dixon RE. Econimic costs of respiratory infections in the United States. *Am J Med* 1985;78(6B):45–51.
94. Pugin J, Auckenthaler R, Lew DP, et al. Oropharyngeal decontamination decreases incidence of ventilator-associated pneumonia: a randomized, placebo-controlled, double-blind clinical trial. *JAMA* 1991; 265:2704–2710.
95. Vincent JL, Bihari DJ, Suter PM, et al. The prevalence of nosocomial infection in intensive care units in Europe. Results of the European prevalence of infection in intensive care (EPIC) study. *JAMA* 1995; 274:639–644.
96. Cook DJ, Walter SD, Cook RJ. Incidence of and risk factors for ventilator-associated pneumonia in critically ill patients. *Ann Intern Med* 1998;129:433–440.
97. Fagon JY, Chastre J, Domart Y, et al. Nosocomial pneumonia in patients receiving continuous mechanical ventilation: prospective analysis of 52 episodes with use of a protected specimen brush and quantitative culture technique. *Am Rev Respir Dis* 1989;139:877–884.
98. Langer M, Mosconi P, Cigada M, et al. Long-term respiratory support and risk of pneumonia in critically ill patients. *Am Rev Respir Dis* 1989;140:302–305.
99. Jarvis WR, Edward JR, Culver DH. Nosocomial infection rates in adult and pediatric intensive care units in the United States. *Am J Med* 1991;91(3B):185s–191s.
100. Craven DE, Kunches LM, Kilinsky V, et al. Risk factors for pneumonia and fatality in patients receiving continuous mechanical ventilation. *Am Rev Respir Dis* 1986;133:792–796.
101. Celis R, Torres A, Gatell JM, et al. Nosocomial pneumonia: a multivariate analysis of risk and prognosis. *Chest* 1988;93:318–324.
102. Haley RW, Hooton RM, Culver DH. Nosocomial infections in U.S. hospitals 1975–1976. Estimated frequency by selected characteristics of patients. *Am J Med* 1981;70:947–959.

103. Wenzel RP, Osterman CA, Hunting KJ. Hospital-acquired infections; Infection rates by site, service and common procedures in a university hospital. *Am J Epidemiol* 1976;104:645–651.
104. George DL, Falk PS, Meduri GU. The epidemiology of nosocomial pneumonia in medical intensive care unit patients: a prospective study based on protected bronchoscopic sampling. 13-4-1992.
105. Hooton TM, Haley RW, Culver DH, et al. The joint association of multiple risk factors with the occurrence of nosocomial infection. *Am J Med* 1981;70:960–970.
106. Windsor JA, Hill GL. Risk factors for postoperative pneumonia: the importance of protein depletion. *Ann Surg* 1988;208:209–214.
107. Hanson LC, Weber DJ, Rutala WA, et al. Risk factors for nosocomial pneumonia in the elderly. *Am J Med* 1992;92:161–166.
108. Gorse GJ, Messner RL, Stephens ND. Association of malnutrition with nosocomial infection. *Infect Control Hosp Epidemiol* 1989;10: 194–203.
109. Gorensec MJ, Stewart RW, Keys TF, et al. A multivariate analysis of risk factors for pneumonia following cardiac transplantation. *Transplantation* 1988;46:860–865.
110. Patel PH, Thomas E. Risk factors for pneumonia after percutaneous endoscopic gastrostomy. *J Clin Gastroenterol* 1990;12:389–392.
111. Cook DJ, Kollef MH. Risk factors for ICU-acquired pneumonia. *JAMA* 1998;279:1605–1606.
112. Chevret S, Hemmer M, Carlet J, et al. and European Cooperative Group on Nosocomial Pneumonia. Incidence and risk factors of pneumonia acquired in intensive care units: results from a multicenter prospective study on 996 patients. *Intensive Care Med* 1993;19: 256–264.
113. Antonelli M, Moro ML, Capelli O, et al. Risk factors for early onset pneumonia in trauma patients. *Chest* 1994;105:224–228.
114. Cunnion KM, Weber DJ, Broadhead WE, et al. Risk factors for nosocomial pneumonia: comparing adult critical-care populations. *Am J Respir Crit Care Med* 1996;153:158–162.
115. Mosconi P, Langer M, Cigada M, et al. Epidemiology and risk factors of pneumonia in critically ill patients. *Eur J Epidemiol* 1991;7: 320–327.
116. Kollef MH. Ventilator-associated pneumonia. A multivariate analysis. *JAMA* 1993;270:1965–1970.
117. Beck-Sague CM, Sinkowitz RL, Chinn RY, et al. Risk factors for ventilator-associated pneumonia in surgical intensive-care-unit patients. *Infect Control Hosp Epidemiol* 1994;17:374–376.
118. Rello J, Ausina V, Ricart M, et al. Risk factors for infection by *Pseudomonas aeruginosa* in patients with ventilator-associated pneumonia. *Intensive Care Med* 1994;20:193–198.
119. Talon D, Mulin B, Rouget C, et al. Risks and routes for ventilator-associated pneumonia with *Pseudomonas aeruginosa. Am J Respir Crit Care Med* 1998;157:978–984.
120. Trouillet JL, Chastre J, Vuagnat A, et al. Ventilator-associated pneumonia caused by potentially drug-resistant bacteria. *Am J Respir Crit Care Med* 1998;157:531–539.
121. Rello J, Ricart M, Ausina V, et al. Pneumonia due to *Haemophilus influenzae* among mechanically ventilated patients: incidence, outcome, and risk factors. *Chest* 1992;102:1562–1565.
122. Standiford TJ. Cytokines and pulmonary host defenses. *Curr Opin Pulmon Med* 1997;3:81–88.
123. Slutsky AS, Tremblay LN. Multiple system organ failure. Is mechanical ventilation a contributing factor? *Am J Respir Crit Care Med* 1998; 157:1721–1725.
124. Public health focus: surveillance, prevention, and control of nosocomial infections. *MMWR* 1992;41:783–787.
125. Gross PA, Neu HC, Aswapokee P, et al. Deaths from nosocomial infections: experience in a university hospital and a community hospital. *Am J Med* 1980;68:219–223.
126. Dreyfuss D, Djedaini K, Weber P, et al. Prospective study of nosocomial pneumonia and of patient and circuit colonization during mechanical ventilation with circuit changes every 48 hours versus no change. *Am Rev Respir Dis* 1991;143:738–743.
127. Torres A, Aznar R, Gatell JM, et al. Incidence, risk, and prognosis factors of nosocomial pneumonia in mechanically ventilated patients. *Am Rev Respir Dis* 1990;142:523–528.
128. Rello J, Quintana E, Ausina V, et al. Incidence, etiology, and outcome of nosocomial pneumonia in mechanically ventilated patients. *Chest* 1991;100:439–444.
129. Joshi N, Localio AR, Hamory BH. A predictive risk index for nosocomial pneumonia in the intensive care unit. *Am J Med* 1992;93: 135–142.
130. Moine P, Timsit JF, de Lassence A, et al. Mortality associated with late-onset pneumonia in the intensive care unit: results of a multicenter cohort study. *Intensive Care Med* 2002;28:154–163.
131. Bercault N, Boulain T. Mortality rate attributable to ventilator-associated nosocomial pneumonia in an adult intensive care unit: a prospective case-control study. *Crit Care Med* 2001;29:2303–2309.
132. Heyland DK, Cook DJ, Griffith L, et al. The attributable morbidity and mortality of ventilator-associated pneumonia in the critically ill patient. *Am J Respir Crit Care Med* 1999;159:1249–1256.
133. Bonten MJM, Bergmans DCJJ, Ambergen AW, et al. Risk factors for pneumonia, and colonization of respiratory tract and stomach in mechanically ventilated ICU patients. *Am J Respir Crit Care Med* 1996;154:1339–1346.
134. Ibrahim EH, Tracy L, Hill C, et al. The occurrence of ventilator-associated pneumonia in a community hospital. Risk factors and clinical outcomes. *Chest* 2001;120:555–561.
135. Bregeon F, Ciais V, Carret V, et al. Is ventilator-associated pneumonia an independent risk factor for death? *Anesthesiology* 2001;94: 554–560.
136. Papazian L, Bregeon F, Thirion X, et al. Effect of ventilator-associated pneumonia on mortality and morbidity. *Am J Respir Crit Care Med* 1996;154:91–97.
137. Rello J, Jubert P, Valles J, et al. Evaluation of outcome for intubated patients with pneumonia due to *Pseudomonas aeruginosa. Clin Infect Dis* 1996;23:973–978.
138. Fox-Dewhurst R, Alberts MK, Kajikawa O. Pulmonary and systemic inflammatory responses in rabbits with gram-negative pneumonia. *Am J Respir Crit Care Med* 1997;155:2030–2040.
139. Bartlett JG, O'Keefe P, Tally FP, et al. Bacteriology of hospital-acquired pneumonia. *Arch Intern Med* 1986;146:868–871.
140. Graybill JR, Marshall LW, Charache P, et al. Nosocomial pneumonia: a continuing major problem. *Am Rev Respir Dis* 1973;108: 1130–1140.
141. Haley RW, White JW, Culver DH, et al. The financial incentive for hospitals to prevent nosocomial infections under the prospective payment system. *JAMA* 1987;257:1611–1614.
142. Boyce JM, Potter-Bynoe G, Dziobek L, et al. Nosocomial pneumonia in Medicare patients: hospital costs and reimbursement patterns under 5the prospective payment system. *Arch Intern Med* 1991;1501: 1109–1114.
143. Dixon RE. Costs of nosocomial infections and benefits of infection control programs. In: Wenzel RP, ed. *Prevention and control of nosocomial infections.* Baltimore: Williams & Wilkins, 1987:19–25.
144. Haley RW, Schaberg DR, Crossley KB, et al. Extra charges and prolongation of stay attributable to nosocomial infections: a prospective interhospital comparison. *Am J Med* 1984;70:51–58.
145. Craig CP, Connelly S. Effect of intensive care unit nosocomial pneumonia on duration of stay and mortality. *Am J Infect Control* 1984; 12:233–238.
146. Freeman J, Rosner BA, McGowan JE. Adverse effects of nosocomial infection. *J Infect Dis* 1979;140:732–740.
147. Wenzel RP. Hospital-acquired pneumonia: overview of the current state of the art for prevention and control. *Eur J Clin Microbiol Infect Dis* 1989;8:56–60.
148. Rello J, Ausina V, Ricart M, et al. Impact of previous antimicrobial therapy on the etiology and outcome of ventilator-associated pneumonia. *Chest* 1993;104:1230–1235.
149. Doré P, Robert R, Grollier G, et al. Incidence of anaerobes in ventilator-associated pneumonia with use of a protected specimen brush. *Am J Respir Crit Care Med* 1996;153:1292–1298.
150. Rello J, Quintana E, Ausina V, et al. Risk factors for *Staphylococcus aureus* nosocomial pneumonia in critically ill patients. *Am Rev Respir Dis* 1990;142:1320–1324.
151. Rello J, Ausina V, Castella J, et al. Nosocomial respiratory tract infec-

tions in multiple trauma patients: influence of level of consciousness with implications for therapy. *Chest* 1992;102:525–529.

152. Espersen F, Gabrielsen J. Pneumonia due to *Staphylococcus aureus* during mechanical ventilation. *J Infect Dis* 1981;144:19–23.
153. Rello J, Torres A, Ricart M, et al. Ventilator-associated pneumonia by *Staphylococcus aureus*: comparison of methicillin-resistant and methicillin-sensitive episodes. *Am J Respir Crit Care Med* 1994;150: 1545–1549.
154. Combes A, Figliolini C, Trouillet JL, et al. Incidence and outcome of polymicrobial ventilator-associated pneumonia. *Chest* 2002;121: 1618–1623.
155. Marik PE, Careau P. The role of anaerobes in patients with ventilator-associated pneumonia and aspiration pneumonia. A prospective study. *Chest* 1999;115:178–183.
156. Louie M, Dyck B, Parker S, et al. Nosocomial pneumonia in a Canadian tertiary care center: a prospective surveillance. *Infect Control Hosp Epidemiol* 1991;12:356–363.
157. Bates JH, Campbell GD, Barron AL. Microbial etiology of acute pneumonia in hospitalized patients. *Chest* 1992;101:1005–1012.
158. Weingarten S, Friedlander M, Rascon D, et al. Influenza surveillance in an acute-care hospital. *Arch Intern Med* 1988;148:113–116.
159. Suspected nosocomial influenza cases in an intensive care unit-Georgia. *MMWR* 1988;37:3–9.
160. Takimoto CH, Cram DL, Root RK. Respiratory syncytial virus infections on an adult medical ward. *Arch Intern Med* 1991;151:706–708.
161. Guidry GG, Black-Payne CA, Payne DK, et al. Respiratory syncytial virus infections among intubated adults in a university medical intensive care unit. *Chest* 1991;100:1377–1384.
162. Fouillard L, Mouthon L, Laporte JP. Severe respiratory syncytial virus pneumonia after autologous bone marrow transplantation: a report of three cases and review. *Bone Marrow Transplant* 1992;9:97–100.
163. Grayston JT, Diwan VK, Cooney M, et al. Community- and hospital-acquired pneumonia associated with *Chlamydia* TWAR infection demonstrated serologically. *Arch Intern Med* 1989;149:169–173.
164. Kirby BD, Snyder KM, Meyer RD, et al. Legionnaires' disease: report of sixty-five nosocomially acquired cases and review of the literature. *Medicine* 1980;59:188–205.
165. Rudin JE, Wing EJ. A comparative study of *Legionella micdadei* and other nosocomial acquired pneumonia. *Chest* 1984;86:675–680.
166. Parry MF, Stampleman L, Hutchinson JG, et al. Waterborne *Legionella bozemanii* and nosocomial pneumonia in immunosuppressed patients. *Ann Intern Med* 1985;103:205–210.
167. Doebbeling BN, Ishak MA, Wade BH. Nosocomial *Legionella micdadei* pneumonia: 10 years' experience and a case-control study. *J Hosp Infect* 1989;13:289–298.
168. Rhame FS, Streifel AJ, Kersey JH, et al. Extrinsic risk factors for pneumonia in the patient at high risk for infection. *Am J Med* 1984; 76(Suppl):42–52.
169. Pannuti C, Gingrich RD, Pfaller MA, et al. Nosocomial pneumonia in adult patients undergoing bone marrow transplantation: a 9-year study. *J Clin Oncol* 1991;9:77–84.
170. Arnow PM, Andersen RL, Mainous PD, et al. Pulmonary aspergillosis during hospital renovation. *Am Rev Respir Dis* 1978;118:49–53.
171. Arnow PM, Sadigh M, Costas C, et al. Endemic and epidemic aspergillosis associated with in-hospital replication of *Aspergillus* organisms. *J Infect Dis* 1991;164:998–1002.
172. Bonten MJM, Weinstein RA. The role of colonization in the pathogenesis of nosocomial infections. *Infect Control Hosp Epidemiol* 1996; 17:193–200.
173. Ewig S, Torres A, El-Ebiary M, et al. Bacterial colonization patterns in mechanically ventilated patients with traumatic and medical head injury. Incidence, risk factors, and association with ventilator-associated pneumonia. *Am J Respir Crit Care Med* 1999;159:188–198.
174. Pennington JE. Nosocomial pneumonias. *Curr Opin Infect Dis* 1992; 5:505–511.
175. Mason CM, Nelson S, Summer WR. Bacterial colonization. Pathogenesis and clinical significance. *Immunol Allergy Clin North Am* 1993; 13:93–108.
176. Fiddian-Green RG, Baker S. Nosocomial pneumonia in the critically ill: product of aspiration or translocation? *Crit Care Med* 1991;19: 763–769.
177. Johanson WG, Pierce AK, Sanford JP. Changing pharyngeal bacterial flora of hospitalized patients. *N Engl J Med* 1969;281:1137–1140.
178. Penn RG, Sanders WE, Sanders CC. Colonization of the oropharynx with gram-negative bacilli: a major antecedent to nosocomial pneumonia. *Am J Infect Control* 1981;9:25–34.
179. Ramphal R, Small PM, Shands JW, et al. Adherence of *Pseudomonas aeruginosa* to tracheal cells injured by influenza infection or by endotracheal intubation. *Infect Immunol* 1980;27:614–619.
180. Niederman MS, Merrill WW, Ferranti RD, et al. Nutritional status and bacterial binding in the lower respiratory tract in patients with chronic tracheostomy. *Ann Intern Med* 1984;100:795–800.
181. Woods DE. Role of fibronectin in the pathogenesis of gram-negative bacillary pneumonia. *Rev Infect Dis* 1987;9:S386–S390.
182. Estes RJ, Meduri GU. The pathogenesis of ventilator-associated pneumonia: I. mechanisms of bacterial transcolonization and airway inoculation. *Intensive Care Med* 1995;21:365–383.
183. Bonten MJM, Gaillard CA, van Tiel FH, et al. Colonization and infection with *Enterococcus faecalis* in intensive care units: the role of antimicrobial agents. *Antimicrob Agents Chemother* 1995;39: 2783–2786.
184. Sijpkens YWJ, Buurke EJ, Ulrich C, et al. *Enterococcus faecalis* colonisation and endocarditis in five intensive care patients as late sequelae of selective decontamination. *Intensive Care Med* 1995;21:231–234.
185. Ibáñez J, Peñafiel A, Raurich JM, et al. Gastroesophageal reflux in intubated patients receiving enteral nutrition: effect of supine and semirecumbent positions. *J Parent Enteral Nutr* 1992;16:419–422.
186. Torres A, Serra-Batlles J, Ros E, et al. Pulmonary aspiration of gastric contents in patients receiving mechanical ventilation: the effect of body position. *Ann Intern Med* 1992;116:540–543.
187. Torres A, El-Ebiary M, González J, et al. Gastric and pharyngeal flora in nosocomial pneumonia acquired during mechanical ventilation. *Am Rev Respir Dis* 1993;148:352–357.
188. Hillman KM, Riordan T, O'Farrell SM, et al. Colonization of the gastric contents in critically ill patients. *Crit Care Med* 1982;10: 444–447.
189. Noone MR, Pitt TL, Bedder M, et al. *Pseudomonas aeruginosa* colonisation in an intensive therapy unit: role of cross infection and host factors. *BMJ* 1983;286:341–344.
190. Olson B, Weinstein RA, Nathan C, et al. Epidemiology of endemic *Pseudomonas aeruginosa*: why infection control efforts have failed. *J Infect Dis* 1984;150:808–816.
191. Widmer AF, Wenzel RP, Trilla A, et al. Outbreak of *Pseudomonas aeruginosa* infections in a surgical intensive care unit: probable transmission via hands of a health care worker. *Clin Infect Dis* 1993;16: 372–376.
192. Tablan OC, Anderson LJ, Arden NH, et al. Guideline for prevention of nosocomial pneumonia. Part I. Issues on prevention of nosocomial pneumonia, 1994. *Infect Control Hosp Epidemiol* 1994;15:588–627.
193. Pitt TL. Epidemiological typing of *Pseudomonas aeruginosa*. *Eur J Clin Microbiol Infect Dis* 1988;7:238–247.
194. Bergmans D, Bonten M, van Tiel F, et al. Value of phenotyping methods as an initial screening of *Pseudomonas aeruginosa* in epidemiologic studies. *Infection* 1997;25:350–254.
195. Maslow JN, Mulligan ME, Arbeit RD. Molecular epidemiology: application of contemporary techniques to the typing of microorganisms. *Clin Infect Dis* 1993;17:153–64.
196. Tompkins LS. The use of molecular methods in infectious diseases. *N Engl J Med* 1992;327:1290–1297.
197. Bonten MJM, Gaillard CA, van Tiel FH, et al. A typical case of cross-acquisition? The importance of genotypic characterization of bacterial strains. *Infect Control Hosp Epidemiol* 1995;16:415–416.
198. Garvey BM, McCambley JA, Tuxen DV. Effects of gastric alkalization on bacterial colonization in critically ill patients. *Crit Care Med* 1989; 17:211–216.
199. Bonten MJM, Gaillard CA, van Tiel FH, et al. The stomach is not a source for colonization of the upper respiratory tract and pneumonia in ICU patients. *Chest* 1994;105:878–884.
200. de Latorre FJ, Pont T, Ferrer A, et al. Pattern of tracheal colonization

during mechanical ventilation. *Am J Respir Crit Care Med* 1995;152: 1028–1033.
201. Cade JF, McOwat E, Siganporia R, et al. Uncertain relevance of gastric colonization in the seriously ill. *Intensive Care Med* 1992;18: 210–217.
202. Reusser P, Zimmerli W, Scheidegger D, et al. Role of gastric colonization in nosocomial infections and endotoxemia: a prospective study in neurosurgical patients on mechanical ventilation. *J Infect Dis* 1989; 160:414–421.
203. Cendrero JAC, Solé-Violán J, Benítez AB, et al. Role of different routes of tracheal colonization in the development of pneumonia in patients receiving mechanical ventilation. *Chest* 1999;116:462–470.
204. Daschner FD, Reuschenbach K, Pfisterer J, et al. Der Einflub von Strebulcusprophylaxe auf die Häufigkeit einer Beatmungspneumonie. *Anaesthesist* 1987;36:9–18.
205. Inglis TJJ, Sherratt MJ, Sproat LJ, et al. Gastroduodenal dysfunction and bacterial colonization of the ventilated lung. *Lancet* 1993;341: 911–913.
206. Garrouste-Orgeas M, Chevret S, Arlet G, et al. Oropharyngeal or gastric colonization and nosocomial pneumonia in adult intensive care unit patients. A prospective study based on genomic DNA analysis. *Am J Respir Crit Care Med* 1997;156:1647–1655.
207. Inglis TJJ, Sproat LJ, Sherratt MJ, et al. Gastroduodenal dysfunction as a cause of gastric bacterial overgrowth in patients undergoing mechanical ventilation of the lungs. *Br J Anaesth* 1992;68:499–502.
208. Kropec A, Huebner J, Riffel M, et al. Exogenous or endogenous reservoirs of nosocomial *Pseudomonas aeruginosa* and *Staphylococcus aureus* infections in a surgical intensive care unit. *Intensive Care Med* 1993;19:161–165.
209. Murthy SK, Baltch AL, Smith RP, et al. Oropharyngeal and fecal carriage of *Pseudomonas aeruginosa* in hospital patients. *J Clin Microbiol* 1989;27:35–40.
210. Flynn DM, Weinstein RA, Nathan C, et al. Patients' endogenous flora as the source of "nosocomial" Enterobacter in cardiac surgery. *J Infect Dis* 1987;156:363–368.
211. Whitby JL, Rampling A. *Pseudomonas aeruginosa* contamination in domestic and hospital environment. *Lancet* 1972;i:15–17.
212. Griffith SJ, Nathan C, Selander RK, et al. The epidemiology of *Pseudomonas aeruginosa* in oncology patients in a general hospital. *J Infect Dis* 1989;160:1030–1036.
213. Berthelot P, Grattard F, Mahul P, et al. Prospective study of nosocomial colonization and infection due to *Pseudomonas aeruginosa* in mechanically ventilated patients. *Intensive Care Med* 2001;27: 503–512.
214. Favero MS, Carson LA, Bond WW, et al. *Pseudomonas aeruginosa*: growth in distilled water from hospitals. *Science* 1971;173:836–838.
215. Grundmann H, Kropec A, Hartung D, et al. *Pseudomonas aeruginosa* in a neonatal intensive care unit: reservoirs and ecology of the nosocomial pathogen. *J Infect Dis* 1993;168:943–947.
216. Thurn J, Crossley K, Gerdts A, et al. Enteral hyperalimentation as a source of nosocomial infection. *J Hosp Infect* 1990;15:203–217.
217. Levy J, van Laethem Y, Verhaegen G, et al. Contaminated enteral nutrition solutions as a cause of nosocomial bloodstream infection: a study using plasmid fingerprinting. *J Parent Enteral Nutr* 1989; 13:228–234.
218. Craven DE, Goularte TA, Make BJ. Contaminated condensate in mechanical ventilator circuits: a risk factor for nosocomial pneumonia? *Am Rev Respir Dis* 1984;129:625–628.
219. Maki DG. Control of colonization and transmission of pathogenic bacteria in the hospital. *Ann Intern Med* 1978;89:777–780.
220. Mayer JA, Dubbert PM, Miller M, et al. Increasing handwashing in an intensive care unit. *Infect Control* 1986;7:259–262.
221. Maki DG, Alvarado CJ, Hassemer CA, et al. Relation of the inanimate hospital environment to endemic nosocomial infection. *N Engl J Med* 1982;307:1562–1566.
222. Doebbeling BN, Stanley GL, Sheetz CT, et al. Comparative efficacy of alternative hand-washing agents in reducing nosocomial infections in intensive care units. *N Engl J Med* 1992;327:88–93.
223. Chetchotisakd P, Phelps CL, Hartstein AI. Assessment of bacterial cross-transmission as a cause of infections in patients in intensive care units. *Clin Infect Dis* 1994;18:929–937.
224. Bonten MJM, Gaillard CA, Johanson WG Jr, et al. Colonization in patients receiving and not receiving topical antimicrobial prophylaxis. *Am J Respir Crit Care Med* 1994;150:1332–1340.
225. Bergmans DCJJ, Bonten MJM, van Tiel FH, et al. Cross-colonisation with *Pseudomonas aeruginosa* of patients in an intensive care unit. *Thorax* 1998;53:x–5.
226. Bonten MJM, Bergmans DCJJ, Speijer H, et al. Characteristics of polyclonal endemicity of *Pseudomonas aeruginosa* colonization in intensive care units. Implications for infection control. *Am J Respir Crit Care Med* 1999;160:1212–1219.
227. American Thoracic Society Ad Hoc Committee of the Scientific Assembly on Microbiology TaPI. Hospital-acquired pneumonia in adults: diagnosis, assessment of severity, initial antimicrobial therapy, and preventative strategies. A consensus statement. *Am J Respir Crit Care Med* 1996;153:1711–1725.
228. Jaeschke R, Guyatt G, Shannon H, et al. Basic statistics for clinicians: 3. assessing the effects of treatment: measures of association. *Can Med Assoc J* 1995;152:351–357.
229. Laupacis A, Sackett DL, Roberts RS. An assessment of clinically useful measures of the consequences of treatment. *N Engl J Med* 1988;318: 1728–1733.
230. van der Waaij D, Berghuis-de Vries JM, Lekkerkerk-van der Wees JEC. Colonization resistance of the digestive tract in conventional and antibiotic-treated mice. *J Hyg* 1971;69:405–411.
231. Sleijfer DT, Mulder NH, de Vries-Hospers HG, et al. Infection prevention in granulocytopenic patients by selective decontamination of the digestive tract. *Eur J Cancer* 1980;16:859–869.
232. Stoutenbeek CP, van Saene HKF, Miranda DR, et al. The effect of selective decontamination of the digestive tract on colonization and infection rate in multiple trauma patients. *Intensive Care Med* 1984; 10:185–192.
233. Mackie DP, van Hertum WAJ, Schumburg T, et al. Prevention of infection in burns: preliminary experience with selectice decontamination of the digestive tract in patients with extensive injuries. *J Trauma* 1992;32:570–575.
234. Blair P, Rowlands BJ, Lowry K, et al. Selective decontamination of the digestive tract: a stratified, randomized, prospective study in a mixed intensive care unit. *Surgery* 1991;110:303–310.
235. Aerdts SJA, van Dalen R, Clasener HAL, et al. Antibiotic prophylaxis of respiratory tract infection in mechanically ventilated patients: a prospective, blinded, randomized trial of the effect of a novel regimen. *Chest* 1991;100:783–791.
236. Hammond JMJ, Potgieter PD. Is there a role for selective decontamination of the digestive tract in primarily infected patients in the ICU? *Anaesth Intensive Care* 1995;23:168–174.
237. Kerver AJH, Rommes JH, Mevissen-Verhage EAE, et al. Prevention of colonization and infection in critically ill patients: a prospective randomized study. *Crit Care Med* 1988;16:1087–1093.
238. Ulrich C, Harinck-de Weerd JE, Bakker NC, et al. Selective decontamination of the digestive tract with norfloxacin in the prevention of ICU-acquired infections: a prospective randomized study. *Intensive Care Med* 1989;15:424–431.
239. Cockerill FR III, Muller SR, Anhalt JP, et al. Prevention of infection in critically ill patients by selective decontamination of the digestive tract. *Ann Intern Med* 1992;117:545–553.
240. Rocha LA, Martin MJ, Pita S, et al. Prevention of nosocomial infection in critically ill patients by selective decontamination of the digestive tract: a randomized, double blind, placebo-controlled study. *Intensive Care Med* 1992;18:398–404.
241. Verwaest C, Verhaegen J, Ferdinande P, et al. Randomized, controlled trial of selective digestive decontamination in 600 mechanically ventilated patients in a multidisciplinary intensive care unit. *Critical Care Med* 1997;25:63–71.
242. Jacobs S, Foweraker JE, Roberts SE. Effectiveness of selective decontamination of the digestive tract in an ICU with a policy encouraging a low gastric pH. *Clin Intensive Care* 1992;3:52–58.
243. Winter R, Humphreys H, Pick A, et al. A controlled trial of selective

decontamination of the digestive tract in intensive care and its effect on nosocomial infection. *J Antimicrob Chemother* 1992;30:73–87.

244. Ledingham IMA, Eastaway AT, McKay IC, et al. Triple regimens of selective decontamination of the digestive tract, systemic cefotaxime, and microbiological surveillance for prevention of acquired infection in intensive care. *Lancet* 1988;i:785–790.
245. McClelland P, Murray AE, Williams PS, et al. Reducing sepsis in severe combined acute renal and respiratory failure by selective decontamination of the digestive tract. *Crit Care Med* 1990;18:935–939.
246. Quinio B, Albanèse J, Bues-Charbit M, et al. Selective decontamination of the digestive tract in multiple trauma patients; a prospective double-blind, randomized, placebo-controlled study. *Chest* 1996;109: 765–772.
247. Flaherty JP, Nathan C, Kabins SA, et al. Pilot trial of selective decontamination for prevention of bacterial infection in an intensive care unit. *J Infect Dis* 1990;162:1393–1397.
248. Unertl K, Ruckdeschel G, Selbmann HK, et al. Prevention of colonization and respiratory infections in long-term ventilated patients by local antimicrobial prophylaxis. *Intensive Care Med* 1987;13: 106–113.
249. Korinek AM, Laisne MJ, Nicolas MH, et al. Selective decontamination of the digestive tract in neurosurgical intensive care unit patients: a double-blind, randomized, placebo-controlled study. *Crit Care Med* 1993;21:1466–1473.
250. Hartenauer U, Thülig B, Diemer W, et al. Effect of selective flora suppression on colonization, infection, and mortality in critically ill patients: a one-year, prospective consecutive study. *Crit Care Med* 1991;19:463–473.
251. Hammond JMJ, Potgieter PD, Saunders GL. Selective decontamination of the digestive tract in multiple trauma patients—is there a role? Results of a prospective, double-blind, randomized trial. *Crit Care Med* 1994;22:33–39.
252. Hammond JMJ, Potgieter PD. Neurologic disease requiring long-term ventilation. The role of selective decontamination of the digestive tract in preventing nosocomial infection. *Chest* 1993;104:547–551.
253. Godard J, Guillaume C, Reverdy ME, et al. Intestinal decontamination in a polyvalent ICU: a double-blind study. *Intensive Care Med* 1990;16:307–311.
254. Brun-Buisson C, Legrand P, Rauss A, et al. Intestinal decontamination for control of nosocomial multiresistant gram-negative bacilli: study of an outbreak in an intensive care unit. *Ann Intern Med* 1989; 110:873–881.
255. Rodríguez-Roldán JM, Altuna-Cuesta A, López A, et al. Prevention of nosocomial lung infection in ventilated patients: use of an antimicrobial pharyngeal nonabsorbable paste. *Crit Care Med* 1990;18: 1239–1242.
256. Abele-Horn M, Dauber A, Bauernfeind A, et al. Decrease in nosocomial pneumonia in ventilated patients by selective oropharyngeal decontamination. *Intensive Care Med* 1996;23:187–195.
257. Sirvent JM, Torres A, El-Ebiary M, et al. Protective effect of intravenously administered cefuroxime against nosocomial pneumonia in patients with structural coma. *Am J Respir Crit Care Med* 1997;155: 1729–1734.
258. Sanchez Garcia M, Cambronero Galache JA, Lopez Diaz J, et al. Effectiveness and cost of selective decontamination of the digestive tract in critically ill intubated patients. A randomized, double-blind, placebo-controlled, multicenter trial. *Am J Respir Crit Care Med* 1998; 158:908–916.
259. Krueger WA, Lenhart FP, Neeser G, et al. Influence of combined intravenous and topical antibiotic prophylaxis on the incidence of infections, organ dysfunctions, and mortality in critically ill surgical patients. A prospective, stratified, randomized, double-blind, placebo-controlled clinical trial. *Am J Respir Crit Care Med* 2002;166: 1029–1037.
260. Palomar M, Alvarez-Lerma F, Jorda R, et al. and Catalan Study Group of Nosocomial Pneumonia Prevention. Prevention of nosocomial infection in mechanically ventilated patients: selective digestive decontamination *versus* sucralfate. *Clin Intensive Care* 1997;8:228–235.
261. Langlois-Karaga A, Bues-Charbit M, Davignon A, et al. Selective digestive decontamination in multiple trauma patients: cost and efficacy. *Pharm World Sci* 1995;17:12–16.
262. Lingnau W, Berger J, Javorsky F, et al. Selective intestinal decontamination in multiple trauma patients: prospective, controlled trial. *J Trauma* 1997;42:687–694.
263. Bergmans DCJJ, Bonten MJM, Gaillard CA, et al. Prevention of ventilator-associated pneumonia by oral decontamination. A prospective, randomized, double-blind, placebo-controlled study. *Am J Respir Crit Care Med* 2001;164:382–388.
264. Laggner AN, Tryba M, Georgopoulos A, et al. Oropharyngeal decontamination with gentamicin for long-term ventilated patients on stress ulcer prophylaxis with sucralfate? *Wien Klin Wochenschr* 1994;106: 15–19.
265. Cerra FB, Maddaus MA, Dunn DL, et al. Selective gut decontamination reduces nosocomial infections and length of stay but not mortality or organ failure in surgical intensive care unit patients. *Arch Surg* 1992;127:163–169.
266. Kaufhold A, Behrendt W, Kräuss T, et al. Selective decontamination of the digestive tract and methicillin-resistant *Staphylococcus aureus* [Letter]. *Lancet* 1992;339:1411–1412.
267. Lingnau W, Berger J, Javorsky F, et al. Changing bacterial ecology during a five year period of selective intestinal decontamination. *J Hosp Infect* 1998;39:195–206.
268. van Nieuwenhoven CA, Buskens E, van Tiel FH, et al. Relationship between methodological trial quality and the effects of selective digestive decontamination on pneumonia and mortality in critically ill patients. *JAMA* 2001;286:335–340.
269. Hurley JC. Prophylaxis with enteral antibiotics in ventilated patients: selective decontamination or selective cross-infection? *Antimicrob Agents Chemother* 1995;39:941–947.
270. Nathans AB, Marshall JC. Selective decontamination of the digestive tract in surgical patients. A systematic review of the evidence. *Arch Surg* 1999;134:170—176.
271. Wunderink RG. Mortality and the diagnosis of ventilator-associated pneumonia. A new direction. *Am J Respir Crit Care Med* 1998;157: 349–350.
272. Stoutenbeek CP, van Saene HKF, Miranda DR, et al. The effect of oropharyngeal decontamination using topical nonabsorbable antibiotics on the incidence of nosocomial respiratory tract infections in multiple trauma patients. *J Trauma* 1987;27:357–364.
273. DeRiso AJ II, Ladowski JS, Dillon TA, et al. Chlorhexidine gluconate 0.12% oral rinse reduces the incidence of total nosocomial respiratory infection and nonprophylactic systemic antibiotic use in patients undergoing heart surgery. *Chest* 1996;109:1556–1561.
274. Russell AD, Day MJ. Antibacterial activity of chlorhexidine. *J Hosp Infect* 1993;25:229–238.
275. Russell AD. Chlorhexidine: antibacterial action and bacterial resistance. *Infection* 1986;14:212–215.
276. Shiraishi T, Nakagawa Y. Review of disinfectant susceptibility of bacteria isolated in hospital to commonly used disinfectants. *Postgrad Med J* 1993;69:S70–S77.
277. Lepper MH, Kofman S, Blatt N. Effect of eight antibiotics used singly and in combination on the tracheal flora following tracheostomy in poliomyelitis. *Antibiotics Chemother* 1954;4:829–843.
278. Petersdorf RG, Curtin JA, Hoeprich PD. A study of antibiotic prophylaxis in unconscious patients. *N Engl J Med* 1957;257:1001–1009.
279. Petersdorf RG, Merchant RK. A study of antibiotic prophylaxis in patients with acute heart failure. *N Engl J Med* 1959;260:565–575.
280. Mandelli M, Mosconi P, Langer M, et al. Prevention of pneumonia in an intensive care unit: a randomized multicenter clinical trial. *Crit Care Med* 1989;17:501–505.
281. Fabian TC, Boucher BA, Croce MA, et al. Pneumonia and stress ulceration in severely injured patients. A prospective evaluation of the effects of stress ulcer prophylaxis. *Arch Surg* 1993;128:185–192.
282. Ben-Menachem T, Fogel R, Patel RV, et al. Prophylaxis for stress-related gastric hemorrhage in the medical intensive care unit: a randomized, controlled, single-blind study. *Ann Intern Med* 1994;121: 568–575.
283. Reusser P, Gyr K, Scheidegger D, et al. Prospective endoscopic study of stress erosions and ulcers in critically ill neurosurgical patients:

current incidence and effect of acid-reducing prophylaxis. *Crit Care Med* 1990;18:270–274.
284. McCarthy DM. Sucralfate. *N Engl J Med* 1991;325:1017–1025.
285. Kappstein I, Engels I. Antibacterial activity of sucralfate and bismuth subsalicylate in simulated gastric fluid. *Eur J Clin Microbiol Infect Dis* 1987;6:216–217.
286. Tryba M, Mantey-Stiers F. Antibacterial activity of sucralfate in human gastric juice. *Am J Med* 1987;83(Suppl 3B):125–127.
287. Bergmans D, Bonten M, Gaillard C, et al. In vitro antibacterial activity of sucralfate. *Eur J Clin Microbiol Infect Dis* 1994;13:615–620.
288. Artigas A, Campillo M, Cardona A, et al. and Collaborative LAMG Working Group. Nosocomial pneumonia and gastrointestinal bleeding in mechanically ventilated patients receiving ranitidine or sucralfate. *Am J Respir Crit Care Med* 1995;151:A721(abst).
289. Kappstein I, Schulgen G, Friedrich T, et al. Incidence of pneumonia in mechanically ventilated patients treated with sucralfate or cimetidine as prophylaxis for stress bleeding: bacterial colonization of the stomach. *Am J Med* 1991;91(Suppl 2A):125S–31S.
290. Eddleston JM, Vohra A, Scott P, et al. A comparison of the frequency of stress ulceration and secondary pneumonia in sucralfate- or ranitidine-treated intensive care unit patients. *Crit Care Med* 1991;19: 1491–1496.
291. Simms HH, DeMaria E, McDonald L, et al. Role of gastric colonization in the development of pneumonia in critically ill trauma patients: results of a prospective randomized trial. *J Trauma* 1991;31:531–536.
292. Ryan P, Dawson J, Teres D, et al. Nosocomial pneumonia during stress ulcer prophylaxis with cimetidine and sucralfate. *Arch Surg* 1993;128:1353–1357.
293. Pickworth KK, Falcone RE, Hoogeboom JE, et al. Occurrence of nosocomial pneumonia in mechanically ventilated trauma patients: a comparison of sucralfate and ranitidine. *Crit Care Med* 1993;21: 1856–1862.
294. Tryba M. Risk of acute stress bleeding and nosocomial pneumonia in ventilated intensive care unit patients: sucralfate versus antacids. *Am J Med* 1987;83(Suppl 3B):117–124.
295. Cioffi WG, McManus AT, Rue LR III, et al. Comparison of acid neutralizing and non-acid neutralizing stress ulcer prophylaxis in thermally injured patients. *J Trauma* 1994;36:541–547.
296. Pingleton SK, Hinthorn DR, Liu C. Enteral nutrition in patients receiving mechanical ventilation. *Am J Med* 1986;80:827–832.
297. Bonten MJM, Gaillard CA, van Tiel FH, et al. Continuous enteral feeding counteracts preventive measures for gastric colonization in intensive care unit patients. *Crit Care Med* 1994;22:939–944.
298. Lee B, Chang RWS, Jacobs S. Intermittent nasogastric feeding: a simple and effective method to reduce pneumonia among ventilated ICU patients. *Clin Intensive Care* 1990;1:100–102.
299. Skiest DJ, Khan N, Feld R, et al. The role of enteral feeding in gastric colonisation: a randomised controlled trial comparing continuous to intermittent enteral feeding in mechanically ventilated patients. *Clin Intensive Care* 1996;7:138–143.
300. Bonten MJM, Gaillard CA, van der Hulst R, et al. Intermittent enteral feeding: the influence on respiratory and digestive tract colonization in mechanically ventilated intensive-care-unit patients. *Am J Respir Crit Care Med* 1996;154:394–399.
301. Heyland D, Bradley C, Mandell LA. Effect of acidified enteral feedings on gastric colonization in the critically ill patients. *Crit Care Med* 1992;20:1388–1394.
302. Heyland DK, Cook DJ, Schoenfeld PS, et al. The effect of acidified enteral feeds on gastric colonization in critically ill patients: results of a multicenter randomized trial. *Crit Care Med* 1999;27:2399–406.
303. Heyland DK, Drover JW, Dhaliwal R, et al. Optimizing the benefits and minimizing the risks of enteral nutrition in the critically ill: role of small bowel feeding. *J Parent Enteral Nutr* 2002;26:S51–S57.
304. Zaloga GP. Bedside method for placing small bowel feeding tubes in critically ill patients: a prospective study. *Chest* 1991;100:1643–1646.
305. Atkinson S, Sieffert E, Bihari D. A prospective, randomized, double-blind, controlled clinical trial of enteral immunonutrition in the critically ill. *Crit Care Med* 1998;26:1164–1172.
306. Houdijk APJ, Rijnsburger ER, Jansen J. Randomised trial of glutamine-enriched enteral nutrition on infectious morbidity in patients with multiple trauma. *Lancet* 1998;352:772–776.
307. Caparros T, Lopez J, Grau T. Early enteral nutrition in critically ill patients with high-protein diet enriched with arginine, fiber, and antioxidants compared with standard high-protein diet. The effect on nosocomial infections and outcome. *J Parent Enteral Nutri* 2001; 25:299–309.
308. Kollef MH, Skubas NJ, Sundt TM. A randomized clinical trial of continuous aspiration of subglottic secretions in cardiac surgery patients. *Chest* 1999;116:1339–1346.
309. Smulders K, van der Hoeven H, Weers-Pothoff I, et al. A randomized clinical trial of intermittent subglottic secretion drainage in patients receiving mechanical ventilation. *Chest* 2002;121:858–862.
310. Shorr AF, O'Malley PG. Continuous subglottic suctioning for the prevention of ventilator-associated pneumonia. Potential economic implications. *Chest* 2001;119:228–235.
311. Pneumatikos I, Koulouras V, Nathanail C, et al. Selective decontamination of subglottic area in mechanically ventilated patients with multiple trauma. *Intensive Care Med* 2002;28:432–437.
312. Dive A, Moulart M, Jonard P, et al. Gastroduodenal motility in mechanically ventilated critically ill patients: a manometric study. *Crit Care Med* 1994;22:441–447.
313. Orozco-Levi M, Torres A, Ferrer M, et al. Semirecumbent position protects from pulmonary aspiration but not completely from gastroesophageal reflux in mechanically ventilated patients. *Am J Respir Crit Care Med* 1995;152:1387–1390.
314. Drakulovic MB, Torres A, Bauer TT, et al. Supine body position as a risk factor for nosocomial pneumonia in mechanically ventilated patients: a randomised trial. *Lancet* 1999;354:1851–1858.
315. Dotson RG, Robinson RG, Pingleton SK. Gastroesophageal reflux with nasogastric tubes. Effect of nasogastric tube size. *Am J Respir Crit Care Med* 1994;149:1659–1662.
316. Kirschenbaum L, Azzi E, Sfeir T, et al. Effect of continuous lateral rotational therapy on the prevalence of ventilator-associated pneumonia in patients requiring long-term ventilatory care. *Crit Care Med* 2002;30:1983–1986.
317. Brochard L, Mancebo J, Wysocki M, et al. Noninvasive ventilation for acute exacerbations of chronic obstructive pulmonary disease. *N Engl J Med* 1995;333:817–822.
318. Antonelli M, Conti G, Rocco M, et al. A comparison of noninvasive positive-pressure ventilation and conventional mechanical ventilation in patients with acute respiratory failure. *N Engl J Med* 1998;339: 429—435.
319. Hilbert G, Gruson D, Vargas F, et al. Noninvasive ventilation in immunosuppressed patients with pulmonary infiltrates, fever, and acute respiratory failure. *N Engl J Med* 2001;344:481–487.
320. Kress JP, Pohlman AS, O'Conner MF, et al. Daily interruption of sedative infusions in critically ill patients undergoing mechanical ventilation. *N Engl J Med* 2000;342:1471–1477.
321. Brook AD, Ahrens TS, Schaiff R, et al. Effect of a nursing-implemented sedation protocol on the duration of mechanical ventilation. *Crit Care Med* 1999;27:2609–2615.
322. Marelich GP, Murin S, Battistella F, et al. Protocol weaning of mechanical ventilation in medical and surgical patients by respiratory care practitioners and nurses. Effect on weaning time and incidence of ventilator-associated pneumonia. *Chest* 2000;118:459–467.
323. Needleman J, Buerhaus P, Mattke S, et al. Nurse-staffing levels and the quality of care in hospitals. *N Engl J Med* 2002;346:1715–1722.
324. Thorens JB, Kaelin RM, Jolliet P, et al. Influence of the quality of nursing on the duration of weaning from mechanical ventilation in patients with chronic obstructive pulmonary disease. *Crit Care Med* 1995;23:1807–1815.
325. Grundmann H, Hori S, Winter B, et al. Risk factors for the transmission of methicillin-resistant *Staphylococcus aureus* in an adult intensive care unit: fitting a model to the data. *J Infect Dis* 2002;185:481–488.
326. Klick JM, du Moulin GC, Hedley-Whyte J, et al. Prevention of gram-negative bacillary pneumonia using polymyxin aerosol as prophylaxis. II. Effect on the incidence of pneumonia in seriously ill patients. *J Clin Invest* 1975;55:514–519.
327. Klastersky J, Huysmans E, Weerts D, et al. Endotracheally adminis-

tered gentamicin for the prevention of infections of the respiratory tract in patients with tracheostomy: a double-blind study. *Chest* 1974; 65:650–654.

328. Greenfield S, Teres D, Bushnell LS, et al. Prevention of gram-negative bacillary pneumonia using aerosol polymyxin as prophylaxis. I. Effect on the colonization pattern of the upper respiratory tract of seriously ill patients. *J Clin Invest* 1973;52:2935–2940.
329. Feeley TW, du Moulin GC, Hedley-Whyte J, et al. Aerosol polymyxin and pneumonia in seriously ill patients. *N Engl J Med* 1975;293: 471–475.
330. Levine BA, Petroff PA, Slade CL, et al. Prospective trials of dexamethasone and aerosolized gentamicin in the treatment of inhalation injury in the burned patient. *J Trauma* 1978;18:188–193.
331. Rouby JJ, Martin de Lassale E, Nicolas MH, et al. Prevention of gram negative nosocomial bronchopneumonia by intratracheal colistin in critically ill patients: histologic and bacteriologic study. *Crit Care Med* 1994;20:187–192.
332. Djedaini K, Billiard M, Mier L, et al. Changing heat and moisture exchangers every 48 hours rather than 24 hours does not affect their efficacy and the incidence of nosocomial pneumonia. *Am J Respir Crit Care Med* 1995;152:1562–1569.
333. Long MN, Wickstrom G, Grimes A, et al. Prospective, randomized study of ventilator-associated pneumonia in patients with one versus three ventilator circuit changes per week. *Infect Control Hosp Epidemiol* 1996;17:14–19.
334. Kollef MH, Prentice D, Shapiro SD, et al. Mechanical ventilation with or without daily changes of in-line suction catheters. *Am J Respir Crit Care Med* 1997;156:466–472.
335. Kollef MH, Shapiro SD, Fraser VJ, et al. Mechanical ventilation with or without 7-day circuit changes; A randomized controlled trial. *Ann Intern Med* 1995;123:168–174.
336. Deppe SA, Kelly JW, Thoi LL, et al. Incidence of colonization, nosocomial pneumonia, and mortality in critically ill patients using Trach Care closed-suction system versus an open-suction system: prospective, randomized study. *Crit Care Med* 1990;18:1389–1393.
337. Johnson KL, Kearney PA, Johnson SB, et al. Closed versus open endotracheal suctioning: costs and physiologic consequences. *Crit Care Med* 1994;22:658–666.
338. Conrad SA, George RB, Romero MD, et al. Comparison of nosocomial pneumonia rates in closed and open tracheal suction system. Proceedings of the XVI World Congress on Diseases of the Chest and 55th Annual Scientific Assembly, 1989:184S–184S.
339. Combes P, Fauvage B, Oleyer C. Nosocomial pneumonia in mechanically ventilated patients, a prospective randomised evaluation of the Stericath closed suctioning system. *Intensive Care Med* 2000;26: 878–882.
340. Dreyfuss D, Djedaini K, Gros I, et al. Mechanical ventilation with heated humidifiers or heat and moisture exchangers: effects on patient colonization and incidence of nosocomial pneumonia. *Am J Respir Crit Care Med* 1995;151:986–992.
341. Branson RD, Davis K Jr, Campbell RS, et al. Humidification in the intensive care unit. Prospective study of a new protocol utilizing heated humidification and a hygroscopic condenser humidifier. *Chest* 1993;104:1800–1805.
342. Roustan JP, Kienlen J, Aubas P, et al. Comparison of hydrophobic heat and moisture exchangers with heated humidifier during prolonged mechanical ventilation. *Intensive Care Med* 1998;18:97–100.
343. Martin C, Perrin G, Gevaudan MJ, et al. Heat and moisture exchangers and vaporizing humidifiers in the intensive care unit. *Chest* 1990; 97:144–149.
344. Kollef MH, Shapiro SD, Boyd V, et al. A randomized clinical trial comparing an extended-use hygroscopic condenser humidifier with heated-water humidification in mechanically ventilated patients. *Chest* 1998;113:759–767.
345. Kirton OC, DeHaven B, Morgan J, et al. A prospective, randomized comparison of an in-line heat moisture exchanger filter and heated wire humidifiers. Rates of ventilator-associated early-onset (community-acquired) or late-onset (hospital-acquired) pneumonia and incidence of endotracheal tube occlusion. *Chest* 1997;112:1055–1059.
346. Thomachot L, Vialet R, Arnaud S, et al. Do the components of heat and moisture exchanger filters affect their humidifying efficacy and the incidence of nosocomial pneumonia? *Crit Care Med* 1999;27: 923–928.
347. Apte NM, Karnad DR, Medhekar TP, et al. Gastric colonization and pneumonia in intubated critically ill patients receiving stress ulcer prophylaxis: a randomized, controlled trial. *Crit Care Med* 1992;20: 590–593.
348. Kingston GW, Phang PT, Leathley MJ. Increased incidence of nosocomial pneumonia in mechanically ventilated patients with subclinical aspiration. *Am J Surg* 1991;161:589–592.
349. Rodriguez JL, Gibbons KJ, Bitzer LG, et al. Pneumonia: incidence, risk factors, and outcome in injured patients. *J Trauma* 1991;31: 907–914.
350. Fagon JY, Chastre J, Vuagnat A, et al. Nosocomial pneumonia and mortality among patients in intensive care units. *JAMA* 1996;275: 866–869.
351. Kollef MH, Von Harz B, Prentice D, et al. Patient transportation from intensive care increases the risk of developing ventilator-associated pneumonia. *Chest* 1997;112:765–773.
352. Horan TC, White JW, Jarvis WR. Nosocomial infection surveillance, 1984. *MMWR* 1986;35(1SS):17SS–29SS.
353. Hughes JM, Culver DH, White JW, et al. Nosocomial infection surveillance, 1980–1982. *MMWR* 1983;32(4SS):1SS–15SS.
354. Donowitz LG, Wenzel RP, Hoyt JW. High risk of hospital-acquired infection in the ICU patient. *Crit Care Med* 1982;10:355–357.
355. Saviteer SM, Samsa GP, Rutala WA. Nosocomial infections in the elderly: increased risk per hospital day. *Am J Med* 1988;84:661–666.
356. Harkness GA, Bentley DW, Roghmann KJ. Risk factors for nosocomial pneumonia in the elderly. *Am J Med* 1990;89:457–463.
357. Daschner FD, Kappstein I, Engels I, et al. Stress ulcer prophylaxis and ventilation pneumonia: prevention by antibacterial cytoprotective agents? *Infect Control Hosp Epidemiol* 1988;9:59–65.
358. Ruiz-Santana S, Jiminez AG, Esteban A. ICU-pneumonias: a multi-institutional study. *Crit Care Med* 1987;15:930–932.
359. Bryant LR, Trinkle JK, Mobin-Uddin K, et al. Bacterial colonization profile with tracheal intubation and mechanical ventilation. *Arch Surg* 1972;104:647–651.
360. Lareau SC, Ryan KL, Diener CF. The relationship between frequency of ventilator circuit changes and infectious hazard. *Am Rev Respir Dis* 1978;118:493–496.
361. Rashkin MC, Davis T. Acute complications of endotracheal intubation: relationship to intubation, route, urgency, and duration. *Chest* 1986;89:165–167.
362. Daschner F, Kappstein I, Schuster F. Influence of disposable ("Conchapak") and re-usable humidifying systems on the incidence of ventilation pneumonia. *J Hosp Infect* 1988;11:161–168.
363. Klein BS, Perloff WH, Maki DG. Reduction of nosocomial infection during pediatric intensive care by protective isolation. *N Engl J Med* 1989;320:1714–1721.
364. Potgieter PD, Linton DM, Oliver S, et al. Nosocomial infections in a respiratory intensive care unit. *Crit Care Med* 1987;15:495–498.
365. Stevens RM, Teres D, Skillman JJ, et al. Pneumonia in an intensive care unit: a 30-month experience. *Arch Intern Med* 1974;134: 106–111.
366. Nyström B, Frederici H, von Euler C. Bacterial colonization and infection in an intensive care unit. *Intensive Care Med* 1988;14:34–38.
367. Wenzel RP, Thompson RL, Landry SL. Hospital-acquired infections in intensive care unit patients: an overview with emphasis on epidemics. *Infect Control* 1983;4:371–375.
368. Nielsen SL, Roder B, Magnussen P, et al. Nosocomial pneumonia in an intensive care unit in a Danish university hospital: incidence, mortality and etiology. *Scand J Infect Dis* 1992;24:65–70.
369. Zwillich CW, Pierson DJ, Creagh CE, et al. Complications of assisted ventilation: a prospective study of 354 consecutive episodes. *Am J Med* 1974;57:161–170.
370. Schimpff SC, Miller RM, Polakavetz S, et al. Infection in the severely traumatized patient. *Ann Surg* 1974;179:352–357.
371. Allgower M, Durig M, Wolff G. Infection and trauma. *Surg Clin North Am* 1980;60:133–144.

372. Walker WE, Kapelanski DP, Weiland AP, et al. Patterns of infection and mortality in thoracic trauma. *Ann Surg* 1985;201:752–756.
373. Williams MD, Rechard PE, Knox R, et al. Steroid use is associated with pneumonia in pediatric chest trauma. *Crit Care Med* 1992;14:520–524.
374. Braun SR, Levin AB, Clark KL. Role of corticosteroids in the development of pneumonia in mechanically ventilated head-trauma patients. *Crit Care Med* 1986;14:198–201.
375. Hsieh AH, Bishop MJ, Kubilis PS, et al. Pneumonia following closed head injury. *Am Rev Respir Dis* 1992;146:290–294.
376. Pruitt BA Jr, Flemma RJ, DiVincenti FC, et al. Pulmonary complications in burn patients: a comparative study of 697 patients. *J Thorac Cardiovasc Surg* 1970;59:7–18.
377. Gaynes R, Bizek B, Mowry-Hanley J, et al. Risk factors for nosocomial pneumonia after coronary artery bypass graft operations. *Ann Thorac Surg* 1991;51:215–218.
378. Carrel T, Schmid ER, von Segesser L, et al. Preoperative assessment of the likelihood of infection of the lower respiratory tract after cardiac surgery. *Thorac Cardiovasc Surgeon* 1991;39:85–88.
379. Rotstein C, Cummings KM, Nicolaou AL, et al. Nosocomial infection rates at an oncology center. *Infect Control Hosp Epidemiol* 1988;9:13–19.
380. Jules-Elysee K, Stover DE, Yahalom J, et al. Pulmonary complications in lymphoma patients treated with high-dose therapy and autologous bone marrow transplantation. *Am Rev Respir Dis* 1992;146:485–491.
381. Richardon JD, DeCamp MM, Garrison RN, et al. Pulmonary infection complicating intra-abdominal sepsis: clinical and experimental observations. *Ann Surg* 1982;195:732–737.
382. Mustard RA, Bohnen JMA, Rosati C, et al. Pneumonia complicating abdominal sepsis: an independent risk factor for mortality. *Arch Surg* 1991;126:170–175.
383. Artigas AT, Dronda SB, Vallés EC, et al. Risk factors for nosocomial pneumonia in critically ill trauma patients. *Crit Care Med* 2001;29:304–309.
384. Kropec A, Schulgen G, Just H, et al. Scoring system for nosocomial pneumonia in ICUs. *Intensive Care Med* 1996;22:1155–1161.
385. Baraibar J, Correa H, Mariscal D, et al. Risk factors for infection by *Acinetobacter baumannii* in intubated patients with nosocomial pneumonia. *Chest* 1997;112:1050–1054.
386. Elatrous S, Boujdaria R, Merghli S. Incidence and risk factors of ventilator-associated pneumonia: a one-year prospective survey. *Clin Intensive Care* 1996;7:276–281.
387. Chastre J, Trouillet JL, Vuagnat A, et al. Nosocomial pneumonia in patients with acute respiratory distress syndrome. *Am J Respir Crit Care Med* 1998;157:1165–1172.
388. Markowicz P, Wolff M, Djedaini K, et al. Multicenter prospective study of ventilator-associated pneumonia during acute respiratory distress syndrome. Incidence, prognosis, and risk factors. *Am J Respir Crit Care Med* 2000;161:1942–1948.
389. Pingleton SK. Enteral nutrition as a risk factor for nosocomial pneumonia. *Eur J Clin Microbiol Infect Dis* 1989;8:51–55.
390. Torres A, Gatell JP, Aznar E, et al. Re-intubation increases the risk of nosocomial pneumonia in patients needing mechanical ventilation. *Am J Respir Crit Care Med* 1995;152:137–141.
391. Rouby JJ, Laurent P, Gosnach M, et al. Risk factors and clinical relevance of nosocomial maxillary sinusitis in the critically ill. *Am J Respir Crit Care Med* 1994;150:776–783.
392. Bert F, Lambert-Zechovsky N. Sinusitis in mechanically ventilated patients and its role in the pathogenesis of nosocomial pneumonia. *Eur J Clin Microbiol Infect Dis* 1996;15:533–544.
393. Fourrier F, Duvivier B, Boutigny H, et al. Colonization of dental plaque: a source of nosocomial infections in intensive care unit patients. *Crit Care Med* 1998;26:301–308.
394. de Lassence A, Alberti C, Azoulay E, et al. Impact of unplanned extubation and reintubation after weaning on nosocomial pneumonia risk in the intensive care unit. A prospective multicenter study. *Anesthesiology* 2002;97:148–156.
395. Tyler KD, Wang G, Tyler SD, et al. Factors affecting reliability and reproducibility of amplification-based DNA fingerprinting of representative bacterial pathogens. *J Clin Microbiol* 1997;35:339–346.
396. Montecalvo MA, Steger KA, Farber HW, et al. Nutritional outcome and pneumonia in critical care patients randomized to gastric versus jejunal feedings. *Crit Care Med* 1992;20:1377–1387.
397. Kearns PJ, Chin D, Mueller L, et al. The incidence of ventilator-associated pneumonia and success in nutrient delivery with gastric versus small intestinal feeding: a randomized clinical trial. *Crit Care Med* 2000;28:1742–1746.
398. Montejo JC, Grau T, Acosta J, et al. Multicenter, prospective, randomized, single-blind study comparing the efficacy and gastrointestinal complications of early jejunal feeding with early gastric feeding in critically ill patients. *Crit Care Med* 2002;30:796–800.
399. Holzapfel L, Chevret S, Madinier G, et al. Influence of long-term oro- or nasotracheal intubation on nosocomial maxillary sinusitis and pneumonia: results of a prospective, randomized, clinical trial. *Crit Care Med* 1993;21:1132–1138.

23

NOSOCOMIAL SINUSITIS

MARC J. M. BONTEN

Nosocomial sinusitis (NS) is a common, unrecognized cause of fever and even sepsis in mechanically ventilated patients. Underestimation of its incidence is at least partly due to the difficulty in diagnosing NS. The reported cumulative incidence ranges from 1% to 83% in studies specifically designed to investigate NS. Combined with pneumonia, catheter-related sepsis, and urinary tract infection, NS has been considered as one of the four "horsemen" of clinically important nosocomial infections in critically ill patients (1). NS is most often caused by enteric gram-negative bacteria or *Staphylococcus aureus.* The infection is a result of disturbances of local anatomy, colonization of the upper respiratory tract with potentially pathogenic microorganisms, and the severity of underlying illness in critically ill patients. The most important risk factors are prolonged nasotracheal intubation, mechanical ventilation, and the presence of a nasogastric tube. Basic infection control procedures and avoidance of nasotracheal intubation seem to be most important for prevention of NS.

DEFINITION

Because of the wide variation of definitions used for NS, interpretation of the whole body of literature dedicated to this topic is difficult, mainly because of the problems encountered in diagnosing NS. It is usually diagnosed using a combination of clinical suspicion of infection, with fever and leukocytosis, together with radiologic evidence of NS. The latter may be based on radiographic, ultrasonographic, or computed tomography (CT) examinations. Finally, the diagnosis is confirmed by microbiologic cultures. The value of each of these diagnostic modalities is discussed later. In what probably is the most detailed prospective study of NS, Rouby et al. (2) distinguished between radiologic maxillary sinusitis and infectious maxillary sinusitis (Fig. 23.1). Radiologic maxillary sinusitis was defined as total opacification of one or both maxillary sinuses or as the presence of an air-fluid level within one or both maxillary sinuses on CT image. Based on microbiologic cultures and Gram staining, the diagnosis of infectious maxillary sinusitis was established or refuted.

CLINICAL RELEVANCE OF NOSOCOMIAL SINUSITIS

NS was first described in 1974. Arens et al. (3) described four patients who had undergone nasotracheal intubation for coronary artery bypass surgery and who developed NS. All patients had been intubated less than 36 hours, and evidence of NS appeared in 6 to 10 days postoperatively. In later studies, NS was usually described in patients who were still intubated. The true incidence of NS and its relevance as a source of fever are unknown. Large studies determining prevalences and incidences of nosocomial infections, such as the National Nosocomial Infection Surveillance system from the Centers for Disease Control and Prevention or the European Prevalence of Infection in Intensive Care Study, did not include NS as an infectious entity (4,5). However, the cumulative incidence of NS was remarkably high in several studies carefully analyzing causes of fever in mechanically ventilated patients, with the reported cumulative incidence ranging from 1% to 83% (Table 23.1). Meduri et al. (6) subjected 50 patients with a clinical suspicion of ventilator-associated pneumonia to a systematic diagnostic protocol, which included CT scanning of the sinuses and aspiration of the maxillary sinuses for microbiologic analysis when air-fluid levels or opacifications were encountered. A definitive source of fever was identified in 45 patients and NS was diagnosed in 12 of them. NS was in all cases accompanied by another infection, which in most cases (72%) was caused by pathogens other than those isolated from maxillary aspirates. In a large prospective study in medical intensive care unit (ICU) patients with endotracheal intubation, the cumulative incidence of NS was 7.7%, with incidence rates of 12 cases per 1,000 patient-days and 19.8 cases per 1,000 nasoenteric tube days (7). Furthermore, cumulative incidences from 9% to 26% have been reported in neurosurgical ICU patients (8–10).

These studies suggest that NS may occur often in selected patient groups. However, it is unknown to what extent NS affects morbidity and patient outcome. Interestingly, NS may occur concomitantly with other infections. For instance, Borman et al. (11) described 19 patients with radiographic evidence of NS, and 10 of these patients had positive cultures of antral aspirates. Evaluation of causes of fever in these patients revealed that fever was definitely caused by NS in only one patient, possibly in two, and definitely not caused by NS in the remaining 16 patients.

CLINICAL MANIFESTATIONS AND DIAGNOSIS

Clinical Presentation

In previously healthy and ambulatory patients, acute sinusitis usually results in localized pain, nasal congestion, and purulent

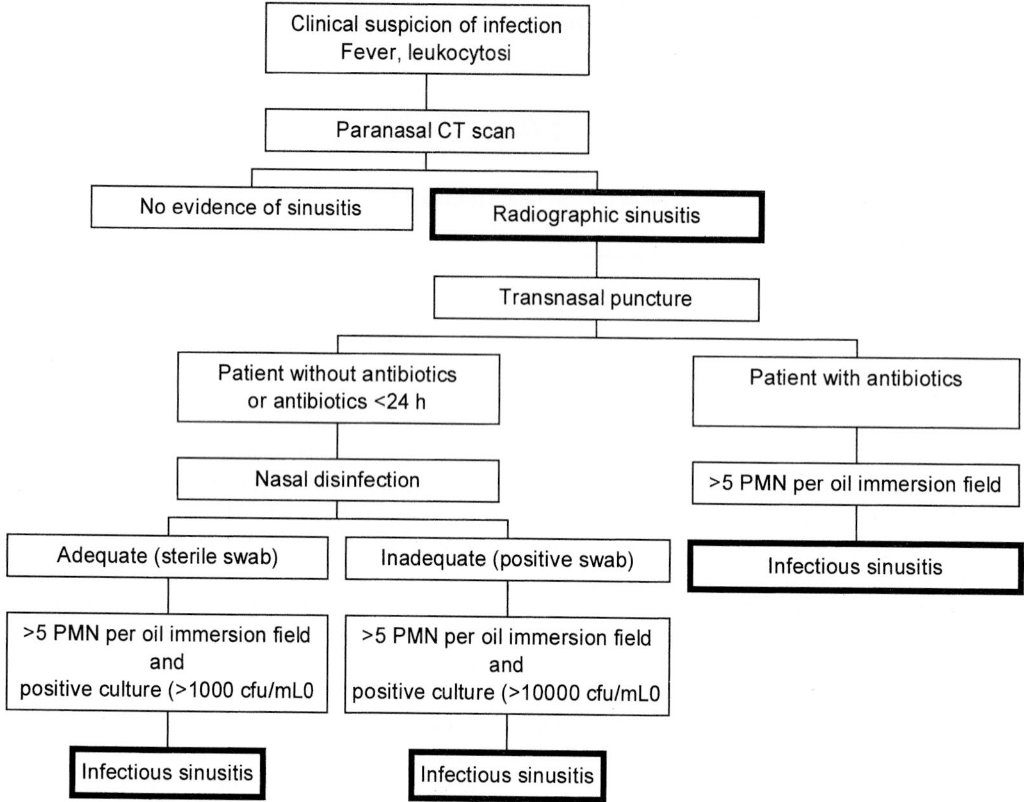

Figure 23.1. Possible diagnostic track for patients with a clinical suspicion of nosocomial sinusitis. (Modified from Rouby JJ, Laurent P, Gosnach M, et al. Risk factors and clinical relevance of nosocomial maxillary sinusitis in the critically ill. *Am J Respir Crit Care Med* 1994;150:776–783.)

nasal drainage. Sinus disease is an inherent part of the common cold syndrome, and 87% of ambulatory patients with colds have sinus cavity disease (12). In these patients, sinusitis is rarely associated with systemic symptoms or fever (13). Pain cannot be expressed by most intubated patients, and findings of physical examination, such as tenderness and purulent nasal discharge, are often absent. As a result, physical examination usually does not contribute to establishing the diagnosis of NS (14). Nonspecific symptoms such as fever or leukocytosis often are the first signs of NS. Because fever and leukocytosis, in this patient population, may have many other causes, both infectious and noninfectious, NS may not be considered as the cause of infection by clinicians. Careful radiographic and microbiologic analyses are, therefore, mandatory.

Radiologic Examination

Sinus radiography usually includes three views (15): the straight anterior-posterior view (Caldwell view) for examining the frontal and ethmoid sinuses; the Water's view to visualize the maxillary sinuses (also a straight anterior-posterior view with the patient's head tilted upward); and the lateral view to visualize the sphenoid sinus. Because of the complex labyrinthine structure of air cells separated by bony septa, the ethmoid sinus is difficult to evaluate. In addition, the sphenoid sinus is localized centrally and surrounded by bony structures and, therefore, is also difficult to evaluate. In critically ill patients, the diagnostic yields of conventional radiography are further diminished by the use of portable equipment, difficulties in placing patients in the upright position, and interference of nasogastric and nasotracheal tubes with x-ray images. Conventional multiview plain sinus radiographs, therefore, are regarded as inaccurate for diagnosing NS (16).

Computed axial tomography displays bony details and can distinguish soft tissue swelling or fluid within the sinuses. In healthy subjects, sinuses are aerated. Signs suggestive for infection include maxillary mucosal thickening, total opacification, or the presence of an air-fluid level in one or both maxillary sinuses (2). CT scanning definitely has multiple advantages over conventional radiography for diagnosing NS. However, mucosal thickening or fluid accumulation within sinus cavities are not proof of infection, and CT scan is unable to distinguish between blood and other fluids, which may be problematic in patients with facial trauma. Even total opacification of one or both maxillary sinuses or an air-fluid level within one or both maxillary sinuses had specificities for infectious maxillary sinusitis ranging from 38% to 69% (2,11,17). Furthermore, CT scan is costly and requires transport of patients, which may, in itself, be a risk factor for nosocomial infections (18).

Bedside sinus ultrasonography may be a reliable, noninvasive, and cheap alternative to CT scanning. This method, when compared with culture of antral aspirates as a gold standard, has

TABLE 23.1. CUMULATIVE INCIDENCE OF NOSOCOMIAL SINUSITIS (NS) ACCORDING TO PATIENT POPULATION AND DIAGNOSTIC TECHNIQUES USED

Study (ref)	No. of patients	No. of cases	Cumulative incidence	Population studied	Diagnostic criteria
Kaups et al. (16)	100	1	1%	Surgical ICU 54% multiple trauma 90% mechanically ventilated	Unexplained fever Bedside ultrasonography Positive antral puncture
Caplan and Hoyt (55)	2,368	32	1.3%	Trauma unit All patients admitted	Opacification or air-fluid level on bedside radiography with purulent nasal discharge or purulent aspirate from the involved sinus
Mevio et al. (56)	1,126	27	2%	ICU	Unexplained fever Imaging evidence of fluid in maxillary sinus Antral puncture
Bert and Lambert-Zechousky	4,509	103	2.3% (0.1%–8.8%)	6 ICUs All patients admitted	Clinical suspicion of NS Positive transnasal culture
Aebert et al. (58)	171	4	2.3%	Trauma ICU Nasotracheal intubation	Unexplained fever or purulent nasal discharge Opacification or air-fluid level on bedside radiography Purulent aspirate from the involved sinus
George et al. (7)	366	28	7.7%	Medical ICU Expected mechanical ventilation >3 days	Opacification or air-fluid level on bedside radiography or CT evidence of NS ≥1 microorganism in culture of aspiration fluid
Bell et al. (14)	139	11	7.8%	Trauma ICU Intubated and ventilated	Unexplained fever Opacification or air-fluid level on bedside radiography or CT evidence of NS Purulent aspirate from the involved sinus
Korinek et al. (10)	123	11	9%	Neurosurgical ICU Intubated and ventilated	Unexplained fever Opacification or air-fluid level on CT Purulent aspirate from the involved sinus
Westergren et al. (8)	15	2	13%	Neurosurgical ICU >7 days on mechanical ventilation	Unexplained fever Bedside ultrasonography Positive antral puncture after sinoscopy
Holzapfel et al. (17)	300	54	18%	Mixed ICU Expected duration of intubation >7 days	CT evidence for maxillary sinusitis Quantitative cultures from transnasal puncture
Meduri et al. (6)	50	12	24%	Medical ICU Intubated and ventilated >48 hours	CT evidence for maxillary sinusitis Cultures from transnasal puncture
Bach et al. (43)	68	17	25%	Postoperaitive patients Mechanically ventilated >4 days	Opacification or air-fluid level on bedside radiography with purulent nasal discharge or purulent aspirate from the involved sinus
Deutschman et al. (9)	43	11	26%	Neurosurgical ICU Nasotracheal intubation and ventilated>72 hours No surgery or trauma of paranasal sinuses	Clinical suspicion of NS or unexplained fever Radiography or CT evidence of NS Positive culture from transnasal puncture
Rouby et al. (2)	162	51	31%	Surgical ICU Intubated and ventilated on admission	CT evidence for maxillary sinusitis Quantitative cultures from transnasal puncture
Holzapfel et al. (26)	199	80	40%	Mixed ICU Expected duration of nasotracheal intubation >7 days	Opacification or air-fluid level on CT, purulent sinus aspiration with $\geq 10^3$ CFU/mL in quantitative culture
Guerin et al. (59)	30	25	83%	ICU Nasotracheal intubation >6 days	Evidence for sinusitis on routine CT scan Cultures from transnasal puncture

CT, computed tomography; ICU intensive care unit; VAP, ventilator-associated pneumonia.

been demonstrated to be accurate in ambulatory adults and children (19). However, clinical experience in mechanically ventilated patients is limited (8,16,20,21). In one study, 100 patients were examined with bedside sinus ultrasonography on admission and every 48 hours thereafter. CT scanning of the head was performed at the discretion of attending physicians and was performed in 61 patients. Fifteen patients had fluid within the maxillary sinus detected by ultrasonography, and in nine other patients sinus fluid was detected by a head CT scan but not by bedside sinus ultrasonography. None of these nine patients, however, had clinical sepsis without another clearly documented source. The authors concluded that the head CT scan is more sensitive but may detect abnormalities that have little clinical significance (16). In another study, left and right paranasal sinuses were examined by ultrasonography in the supine and semirecumbent position in 15 neurosurgical ICU patients in whom NS was suspected on clinical grounds. Findings of ultrasonography were compared with observations made by sinoscopy. Sensitivities of ultrasonography for the presence of fluid and edema were higher in the semirecumbent position (91% and 81%, respectively). However, specificity was only 25% for the presence of fluid. Moreover, edema and/or secretions were demonstrated in 29 of 30 sinus cavities examined, but microorganisms were cultured from only two antra (8). In a third study, A-mode ultrasonography of maxillary and frontal sinuses was performed in 50 comatose patients that needed cerebral CT for another reason than suspicion of sinusitis (21). With CT images as gold standard, ultrasonography had a specificity of 72% to 98% and sensitivity of 63% to 86% for maxillary sinuses, and of 96% to 99% and 14% to 57%, respectively, for frontal sinuses. With areas under the receiver-operating characteristic curves of 0.89 and 0.76, for maxillary and frontal sinuses, respectively, the authors concluded that ultrasonography was an accurate tool to detect secretions in maxillary sinuses (21). In addition, excellent agreement levels (with kappa statistic >0.9) between B-mode ultrasonographic examination of both maxillary sinuses and CT imaging have been reported (20). These data suggest that ultrasonography may be a useful screening test, but whether it can be used as the sole diagnostic method remains to be established.

Microbiologic Analysis

The problem of microbiologic analyses in many ICU-acquired infections is distinguishing between colonization and infection. Colonization of the upper respiratory tract (e.g., nares, oropharynx, and trachea) is universal in mechanically ventilated patients. Nasal swab cultures will grow upper respiratory tract flora and are believed to be of little value to determine pathogens causing sinusitis (22). Mucociliary clearance and drainage may keep the sinuses clean. Therefore, antral aspirate cultures are regarded as the gold standard. The frontal, ethmoid, and sphenoid sinuses can only be drained surgically and are not amenable to aspiration at the bedside. However, the maxillary sinuses can be drained, and these cavities are most often involved. CT imaging demonstrated that the maxillary sinuses are involved in almost all ICU patients who develop NS, and radiographic evidence of maxillary sinusitis was associated with radiologic abnormalities of ethmoid and sphenoid sinuses in more than 80% of ventilated patients. However, according to Rouby et al.'s (2) study, 50% of the patients with normal maxillary sinuses on CT had radiologic signs of ethmoid and/or sphenoid sinusitis, as did 92% of patients with mucosal thickening in maxillary sinuses. The contribution of infection of the ethmoid and sphenoid sinuses has never been studied.

Aspiration cultures from maxillary sinuses are representative for microorganisms causing pansinusitis, and irrigation at this site is often therapeutic. Insertion is performed with a specialized trocar, which has an inner needle obturator with an outer sleeve. Once inserted, the needle can be removed and irrigation can be performed via the hollow sleeve (15). Because of colonization of the nares, even transnasal cultures can be falsely positive because of introduction of pathogens into the sinus cavity. Adequate disinfection, therefore, has been recommended (2). Disinfection of the nares with a povidone-iodine solution proved to be totally adequate (sterile cultures) in 51%, partially effective (decrease in nasal bacterial burden) in 38%, and completely ineffective (increase in nasal bacterial burden) in 11% (2). In Rouby et al.'s study, patients underwent transnasal puncture of the affected maxillary sinus after nasal disinfection. The diagnosis was changed to infectious maxillary sinusitis when there were more than five polymorphonuclear leukocytes per oil immersion field and a positive culture from sinus aspirate. In patients who did not receive antibiotics, the diagnosis of infectious maxillary sinusitis was established by quantitative cultures depending on the effectiveness of nasal disinfection [cutoff points were $>10^3$ colony forming units (CFU)/mL with adequate nasal disinfection (sterile nasal swab) and $>10^4$ CFU/mL with inadequate nasal disinfection (positive nasal swab)] (2). Two studies reported poor correlations between endoscopically guided middle meatal cultures and cultures from antral lavage aspirates or taps in patients with clinical suspicion of NS (23,24).

A diagnostic scheme incorporating clinical, radiographic, and microbiologic evaluation is depicted in Fig. 23.1. It should be mentioned that few studies prospectively determined the incidence of NS and that the clinical relevance of this infection largely remains unknown. The scheme, therefore, should be viewed merely as a possible approach to the diagnosis of sinusitis. Whether such an extensive diagnostic approach influences patient care or will be cost-effective remains to be established.

Recent guidelines for evaluating fever in critically ill patients, developed by the Task Force of the Society of Critical Care Medicine and the Infectious Diseases Society of America, recommend that a CT scan be performed when clinical evaluation suggests that NS could be the source of fever. If CT findings are consistent with sinusitis, puncture and aspiration of the sinuses should be performed under sterile conditions, and the aspirate should be Gram stained and cultured for aerobic and anaerobic bacteria and yeasts (25). This clinical guideline has been evaluated by Holzapfel et al. (26). They randomized 399 patients to receive either standard evaluation of fever occurring during the course of ICU stay or a specific diagnostic strategy directed at the possibility of NS. The strategy included sinus CT scans on days 4 and 8 after tracheal intubation and thereafter every 7 days if fever was present. When CT scan showed an air-fluid level and/or opacification of the maxillary sinus, transnasal puncture was performed for culture, drains were placed, and antibiotics were adjusted according to culture results. Radiographic evidence of NS was observed in 55% of the patients randomized to this diagnostic strategy and 80 patients (40%) fulfilled microbiologic criteria of NS. In the control group, no patient was treated for NS. Interestingly, the incidence of nosocomial pneumonia and mortality at 2 months after randomization were lower in study patients. Although striking, the absence of a mechanism explaining this favorable outcome and the fact that all patients were nasotracheally intubated, which is not the standard of care in most ICUs, warrants a cautious interpretation of these results (27).

CAUSE

The cause of NS closely resembles the spectrum of pathogens causing other nosocomial respiratory tract infections and differs from the etiologic spectrum of acute community-acquired sinusitis in ambulatory patients. Acute sinusitis is usually caused by streptococci or *Haemophilus influenzae* (28,29), whereas gram-negative enteric bacteria (e.g., *Escherichia coli, Proteus mirabilis, Klebsiella* species, *Enterobacter* species), *Acinetobacter* species, *Pseudomonas aeruginosa* and *S. aureus,* are most often isolated from patients with NS. *Candida* species also have been identified as the cause of NS, especially in long-term intubated patients receiving broad-spectrum antibiotics (30,31). One case of NS resulting from *Legionella pneumophila* has been reported in a patient with acquired immunodeficiency syndrome (AIDS) (32). An analysis of microorganisms isolated from patients with NS as described in 33 studies yielded 723 pathogens and revealed that 60% of the pathogens were gram-negative bacteria, 31% were gram-positive bacteria, and 9% were yeasts (31). A considerable proportion (20% to 50%) of patients with NS have polymicrobial infection, usually containing a mixture of the aforementioned pathogens. When analyzed quantitatively, 60% of the microorganisms isolated from sinus aspirates from patients with infectious maxillary sinusitis grew in concentrations $\geq 10^3$ CFU/mL. Concentrations less than 10^3 CFU/mL were found exclusively in patients on antibiotic therapy, and concentrations greater than 10^4 CFU/mL were only found in patients not treated with antibiotics (2).

PATHOGENESIS AND RISK FACTORS

To humidify and clear inspired air, the nose and paranasal sinuses secrete approximately 1 L of mucus daily (15,33). Via ciliated columnar epithelial lining, the mucus flows in a specific pattern through the natural ostium of each individual sinus posteriorly toward the nasopharynx. Patency of the sinus ostia is essential for this flow to occur. Obstruction of this flow, leading to mucus stasis, may result in infection. In healthy people, obstruction may occur because of an anatomic deformity or mucosal inflammation. NS is a result of local factors such as disturbances of anatomy and colonization of the upper respiratory tract with potentially pathogenic microorganisms and systemic factors such as the severity of underlying illness in critically ill patients.

Local Factors

In ICU patients, several local factors predispose to NS. Intubation in itself impairs reflex mechanisms, such as coughing, sneezing, and nose blowing, that help to cleanse the nasal passage. Avoiding intubation, for example by using noninvasive positive-pressure ventilation, will probably reduce the incidence of NS (34). Nasotracheal intubation is considered as the most important risk factor for NS, and the risk of NS increases with the duration of intubation (2,35). Nasotracheal intubation may be preferred over orotracheal intubation, because it provides greater stability of the tube, less difficulty with removal of oral secretions, decreased vocal cord injury because of less tube motion, and less patient discomfort (15,36–39). However, nasotracheal intubation will ultimately cause irritation of the nasal mucosa, resulting in edema and possibly sinus obstruction. A large tube may directly obstruct drainage from sinus cavities. Moreover, as compared with orotracheal intubation, nasotracheal intubation took more time and was more often accompanied by nasal bleeding in cardiac surgery patients randomized to either of the intubation routes. After the procedure, bacteremia with microorganisms usually colonizing nose, mouth, and throat was demonstrated in 9% of the patients with nasotracheal and 2% of the patients with orotracheal intubation (40).

When compared with nonintubated healthy subjects, radiologic evidence of NS, such as thickening of maxillary mucosa, fluid levels in and opacification of sinuses on CT images are clearly related to any kind of intubation, whether it be naso- or orotracheal intubation (8). Sixteen patients with nasotracheal intubation were prospectively studied with CT scanning of the paranasal sinuses on the second or third day and again on the eighth day after intubation. At day 2, three patients had signs of maxillary sinusitis and three of sphenoid sinusitis, and at day 8 all patients had radiographic sinusitis of at least one sinus cavity (41). In another study, paranasal sinusitis, diagnosed by CT scan and aspiration, developed in 13 of 31 (42%) patients with nasotracheal intubation and in 3 of 65 (5%) patients with orotracheal intubation. However, these patients were not randomized to the routes of intubation (42). Associations between nasotracheal intubation and NS have been further established in a series of studies comparing the effects of both routes of intubation (Table 23.2). Strict comparison of the different studies is hampered because of differences in study populations and diagnostic criteria and modalities used. Rouby et al. (2) randomized 40 patients with no evidence of maxillary sinusitis on baseline CT scan to nasotracheal or orotracheal intubation. In addition, gastric tubes were placed accordingly. After 7 days, radiologic maxillary sinusitis was demonstrated in all but one patient with nasotracheal intubation and in only four patients with orotracheal intubation. However, the results of cultures of maxillary sinus aspirates for these patients were not reported. All patients with radiologic maxillary sinusitis also had radiologic evidence of ethmoid and/or sphenoid sinusitis.

Holzapfel et al. (17) randomized 300 ICU patients to nasotracheal (n = 149) and orotracheal (n = 151) intubation. CT scans were performed every 7 days or earlier when NS was clinically suspected. Radiographic sinusitis was observed in 45 (30%) and 33 (22%) of patients with nasotracheal and orotracheal intubation, respectively (p = .08). The radiographic suspicion of NS was microbiologically confirmed in 29 (19%) and 25 (17%) of the patients with nasotracheal and orotracheal intubation, respectively (17).

Bach et al. (43) randomized 68 postoperative patients, without infection at baseline, to nasotracheal or orotracheal intubation. Sinus radiographs were performed at regular intervals and transnasal needle punctures were performed when NS was suspected. Radiologic findings suggestive for NS were found in 47% of patients with orotracheal and in 69% of patients with nasotracheal intubation. Infectious sinusitis was confirmed by microbiologic cultures in 6% and 42% of the patients, respectively ($p < .01$).

Michelson et al. (44) randomized 20 mechanically ventilated patients to nasotracheal intubation and 24 to orotracheal intubation. With the patient in the semirecumbent position, maxillary

TABLE 23.2. RANDOMIZED STUDIES COMPARING NASOTRACHEAL AND OROTRACHEAL INTUBATION IN RELATION TO NOSOCOMIAL SINUSITIS (NS)

	No. of patients included		Cumulative incidence of radiographic NS		Outcome measures of radiographic NS (95% confidence interval)		Cumulative incidence of infectious NS		Outcome measures of infectious NS (95% confidence interval)	
Study	OT	NT	OT (%)	NT (%)	ARR	RRR	OT (%)	NT (%)	ARR	RRR
Rouby et al. (2)	18	22	4 (22)	21 (95)	0.73	0.76	—	—	—	—
Holzapfel et al. (17)	151	149	33 (22)	45 (30)	0.08	0.27	25 (17)	29 (19)	0.02	0.11
Bach et al. (43)	32	36	15 (47)	25 (69)	0.25	0.32	2 (6)	15 (42)	0.36	0.86
Michelson et al. (44)	24	20	15 (63)	19 (95)	0.32	0.34	2 (8)	7 (35)	0.27	0.77
Salord et al. (38)	53	58	1 (2)	25 (43)	0.41	0.95	—	—	—	—
Total	278	285	68 (24)	137 (47)	0.23 (0.15–0.31)	0.49 (0.33–0.65)	29 (10)	51 (18)	0.08 (0.01–0.15)	0.44 (0.07–0.81)

ARR, absolute risk reduction (incidence NT − incidence OT); NT, nasotracheal intubation; OT, orotracheal intubation; RRR, relative risk reduction [1 − (incidence OT/incidence NT)].

sinuses were sonographically examined daily for signs compatible with sinusitis. Diagnostic aspirates were performed in patients with abnormal findings on sonography. Nineteen (95%) patients with nasotracheal and 15 (63%) patients with orotracheal intubation had sonographic evidence of sinusitis after approximately 2 days in both groups. Diagnostic aspiration was performed in 22 patients (13 nasally and 9 orally intubated) and pathogenic microorganisms were cultured in 7 of 13 and 2 of 9 cultures, respectively.

Salord et al. (38) randomized 111 adult patients to orotracheal ($n = 53$) or nasotracheal ($n = 58$) intubation. All patients were ventilated for at least 2 days, and NS was diagnosed by complete opacification or an air-fluid level in the maxillary sinus on bedside radiography (reversed Waters' view). NS occurred in 2% of the patients in the orotracheal group and in 43% of the patients with nasotracheal intubation.

When the results of these studies are summarized, orotracheal intubation is, when compared with nasotracheal intubation, associated with a reduced incidence of radiologic NS, but the beneficial effects on the development of infectious NS are much smaller. Orotracheal intubation results in an absolute risk reduction for the occurrence of radiographic NS of 0.23 (95% confidence interval 0.15 to 0.31) and a relative risk reduction of 0.49 (95% confidence interval 0.33 to 0.65). For the occurrence of infectious NS, orotracheal intubation has an absolute risk reduction of 0.08 (95% confidence interval 0.01 to 0.15) and a relative risk reduction of 0.44 (95% confidence interval 0.07 to 0.81) (Table 23.2).

Nasogastric tubes are probably less harmful than nasotracheal tubes, because they are smaller and, therefore, cause less irritation. Secretions were more often found in sinuses adjacent to a nasal cavity with a nasotracheal tube than in sinuses adjacent to a nasogastric tube (8). In addition, facial and head trauma can lead to accumulation of blood and debris in the sinuses and can disrupt mucosal structures. This provides a favorable medium for proliferation of microorganisms. Furthermore, patient immobility in the supine position may further predispose to sinusitis. The role of gravity and positional changes facilitate mucus drainage in physiologic circumstances. Finally, the supine position may decrease venous blood flow from the head and neck to the heart, leading to nasal congestion and narrowing of the maxillary sinus ostia (45). This effect can be exacerbated by mechanical ventilatory support with positive inspiratory and end-expiratory pressure by virtue of increasing central venous pressure. However, patient positioning and modes of mechanical ventilation on development of NS have never been studied.

Systemic Factors

Because of the severity of their underlying illnesses, mechanically ventilated patients are prone to develop any nosocomial infection, and there is no reason to assume that this does not hold true for NS. Corticosteroids may further suppress immune function in these patients. As mentioned earlier, colonization of the upper respiratory tract (e.g., nares, oropharynx, and trachea) is universal in mechanically ventilated patients, and nasal colonization with enteric gram-negative bacteria was an independent risk factor for NS in a recent study (7). In addition, the use of sedatives and a Glasgow Coma Score ≤ 7 at admission were independent risk factors in that study.

ASSOCIATION WITH NOSOCOMIAL PNEUMONIA

Because of the resemblance of the etiologic spectrum of pathogens causing NS and nosocomial pneumonia, a causal relationship between both infections has been suggested (17,43, 46). Incidences of pneumonia were found to be higher among patients with NS as compared with unaffected patients—14/26 (54%) versus 4/85 (5%) (38)—and NS increased the risk for pneumonia by a factor of 3.8 in multivariable analysis in another study (17). In this study, pneumonia was diagnosed in 16 of 54 patients with NS, and the same microorganism was isolated from the lungs and sinus in 9 of 16 episodes (17). In a third study, incidences of pneumonia demonstrated within 7 days after evidence of maxillary sinusitis on CT scan were 67% and 43% for patients with and without pathogens isolated from sinus aspirates. However, identical pathogens were isolated from the distal airways in only 38% of the patients with previous infectious maxillary sinusitis (2). Among 271 ICU patients with bacteriologically documented NS (cultures obtained by maxillary sinus puncture) the percentage of concurrent episodes of pneumonia (cultures obtained via bronchoscopic techniques) caused by similar pathogens ranged widely. More than 25% of episodes of sinusitis caused by *S. aureus, P. aeruginosa, Acinetobacter baumannii, E. Coli,* and *Hemophilus* species were followed by episodes of pneumonia caused by the same pathogens. In contrast, NS caused by coagulase-negative staphylococci, streptococci, enterococci, *Klebsiella* species, *Proteus* species, *Enterobacter* species, and yeasts were succeeded by pneumonia caused by these pathogens in less than 10% of the cases (47). A similar pattern of concurrent recovery of pathogens from sinus cavities and lungs was reported by Rouby et al. (2). It has been hypothesized that differences between microorganisms in their capacity to adhere to mucus surrounding endotracheal tubes might influence increased colonization of the tracheobronchial tree from the sinus reservoir (48). Whether NS really leads to pneumonia or whether sinusitis just reflects extensive airway colonization and infection has not been elucidated. A recent study of patients with nasotracheal intubation suggested that early treatment of episodes of NS was associated with a reduction in incidence of nosocomial pneumonia and improved patient survival (26).

COMPLICATIONS

Failure to diagnose NS as the cause of sepsis may lead to bacteremia and even hemodynamic instability. Because of the anatomic location of the sinuses, infectious complications are prone to extend to orbital or intracranial spaces (Table 23.3). The frontal and ethmoid sinuses are separated from the orbit by a thin bony plate. Infection, therefore, may extend directly via vascular channels or neurologic foramina, resulting in periorbital cellulitis, muscle edema, and even ophthalmoplegia. When pus collects between the periorbital structures and the bony wall of the orbit, a subperiosteal abscess develops. Orbital extension of infection causes fat necrosis and may lead to orbital abscess formation.

TABLE 23.3. POTENTIAL COMPLICATIONS OF PARANASAL SINUSITIS

Orbital complications
Periorbital (preseptal) edema
Orbital cellulitis
Subperiosteal abscess
Orbital abscess
Cavernous sinus thrombosis
Intracranial complications
Meningitis
Epidural abscess
Subdural empyema
Venous sinus thrombosis
Brain abscess
Other complications
Bacteremia
Sepsis, severe sepsis, septic shock
Osteomyelitis of the skull
Pneumonia
Thoracic empyema

Modified from Seiden AM. Sinusitis in the critical care patient, New Horizons 1993; 5:261–270.

The venous system draining the nose, paranasal sinuses, and the orbital system has no valves, facilitating spread of orbital infection to the cavernous sinus. This should be suspected in case of spread of orbital cellulitis to the opposite eye, severe retinal venous engorgement, and rapid clinical deterioration. In addition to direct spread of pus, thrombosis may develop.

Secondary intracranial complications may also occur along preformed pathways resulting from retrograde thrombophlebitis or by direct hematogenous spread. Meningitis is the most common intracranial complication, most often caused by sphenoid infection. Meningitis occurs less often after ethmoidal, frontal, or maxillary sinusitis (15). Kaufman et al. (49) described 17 cases of subdural empyema induced by community-acquired sinusitis. This complication occurred most often in young men, possibly because during maturation the posterior wall of the sinus may be an incomplete barrier to intracranial spread of microorganisms. The empyemas, therefore, were usually located directly behind the sinuses.

Veins from the frontal sinus communicate directly with the dura. Spread of infection may result in epidural abscess when pus collects superficial to the dura, and a subdural empyema may result from collection of pus between the dura and pia arachnoid. Because there is little resistance to the spread of infection, cerebral abscesses may develop at multiple locations. CT scanning will establish most of the diagnoses, and surgical exploration should be considered if abscess is demonstrated.

PREVENTION

Measures to prevent the development of NS can be subdivided into general measures, device-related measures, and patient-specific measures.

General measures include the principles of conventional infection control policies (50). Colonized and infected patients and environmental contamination or common sources of microorganisms should be identified as reservoirs of pathogens. When identified, environmental contamination should be cleared by cleaning and disinfection, and common sources should be eliminated. In addition, transmission from patient to patient should be prevented by improving compliance with standard infection control practices in the ICU, such as hand washing. Barrier precautions (gloves, gowns) should be used to prevent cross-transmission of multiply resistant bacteria or when taking care of a patient with open wounds.

The most important device-specific measure to prevent NS is to avoid intubation (34) and especially nasotracheal intubation. In addition, the duration of orotracheal and nasogastric intubation should be minimized. Whether the mode of mechanical ventilation influences the development of NS is unknown; therefore, no advice on how best to ventilate patients can be provided.

With regard to patient-specific preventive measures, the relevance of adequate treatment of the underlying illness is obvious. Corticosteroids should be administered only when indicated, and antibiotic prescription policy should be restrictive and rational. The relationship between antibiotic use and subsequent colonization and superinfection with antibiotic-resistant microorganisms and/or pathogens that are difficult to treat (such as yeasts) should be known to all intensivists.

Based on the pathogenesis of NS, several preventive strategies may be hypothesized, although clinical experience is scarce or completely absent. These measures are discussed but are not (yet) recommended. Prevention of colonization of the upper respiratory tract is likely to reduce the incidence of NS. Application of topical antibiotics in the oropharynx, usually in combination with nonabsorbable antibiotics administered via the nasogastric tube and systemic antibiotics during the first days of ventilation [selective decontamination of the digestive tract (SDD)], decreases the incidence of nosocomial respiratory tract infection (51). Few studies testing the SDD concept determined its effects on NS. In one double-blind, placebo-controlled study, neurosurgical patients were randomized to receive topical antibiotics (tobramycin, polymyxin E, amphotericin B) in the oropharynx and in the stomach. Vancomycin was added to the oropharyngeal paste. NS diagnosed by CT scan and microbiologic cultures occurred in 2 of 63 (3%) study patients and 9 of 60 (15%) control patients ($p < .02$) (10). However, objections against widespread use of SDD include the lack of demonstrated benefit on patient outcome and the continuous threat of selection of antibiotic resistance (52). The same objections apply to the prophylactic use of systemic antibiotics in high-risk patients for NS, such as trauma patients with facial fractures.

Based on the physiology of mucociliary clearance from the sinus cavities, a supine position of the patient may be associated with an increased risk for development of NS. In this position, the physiologic process of mucociliary clearance may be diminished and ostia may be narrowed because of nasal congestion resulting from decreased venous blood flow to the heart. In addition, aspiration of gastric bacteria may facilitate colonization of the upper respiratory tract. Using radiolabeled enteral feeding, it has been demonstrated that, in ventilated patients, gastroesophageal aspiration occurs more often in the supine than in the semirecumbent position (53). If so, placing patients in the semirecumbent position would reduce the risk for NS. It is unknown to what extent patients are kept in the supine position when treated in ICU, and, therefore, the effects of a change in nursing care (e.g., placing patients in semirecumbent position as soon as possible) on the incidence of NS cannot be predicted.

CONCLUSION

An increasing number of studies suggest that the incidence of NS among mechanically ventilated ICU patients is underreported. However, the true incidence and clinical relevance of this infection still are unknown. NS is usually caused by those microorganisms known to colonize the upper and lower respiratory tract in ICU patients such as Enterobacteriaceae, *P. aeruginosa,* and *S. aureus.* Development of NS is a result of disturbances of local anatomy, colonization of the upper respiratory tract with potentially pathogenic microorganisms, and severe underlying illness. Nasotracheal intubation has been convincingly demonstrated to be the most important risk factor and should, therefore, be avoided. Other preventive measures include prevention of cross-colonization by standard infection control measures and avoidance of unnecessary use of antibiotics and corticosteroids. Future studies should determine the incidence of NS in large patient populations and elucidate its role as a risk for the subsequent development of pneumonia. Based on these findings, the need for specific regimens for prevention of NS can be judged. In addition, cost-benefit analyses of the different diagnostic tracks are warranted. An excellent review of the clinical entity of NS has been published by Westergren et al. (54).

REFERENCES

1. Heffner JE. Nosocomial sinusitis. Den of multiresistant thieves? *Am J Respir Crit Care Med* 1994;150:608–609.
2. Rouby JJ, Laurent P, Gosnach M, et al. Risk factors and clinical relevance of nosocomial maxillary sinusitis in the critically ill. *Am J Respir Crit Care Med* 1994;150:776–783.
3. Arens JF, LeJeune FE Jr, Webre DR. Maxillary sinusitis, a complication of nasotracheal intubation. *Anesthesiology* 1974;4:415–416.
4. Vincent JL, Bihari DJ, Suter PM, et al. The prevalence of nosocomial infection in intensive care units in Europe. Results of the European Prevalence of Infection in Intensive Care (EPIC) study. *JAMA* 1995; 274:639–644.
5. Emori TG, Gaynes RP. An overview of nosocomial infections, including the role of the microbiology laboratory. *Clin Microbiol Rev* 1993; 6:428–442.
6. Meduri GU, Mauldin GL, Wunderink RG, et al. Causes of fever and pulmonary densities in patients with clinical manifestations of ventilator-associated pneumonia. *Chest* 1994;106:221–235.
7. George DL, Falk PS, Umberto MG, et al. Nosocomial sinusitis in patients in the medical intensive care unit: a prospective epidemiological study. *Clin Infect Dis* 1998;27:463–470.
8. Westergren V, Berg S, Lundgren J. Ultrasonographic bedside evaluation of maxillary sinus disease in mechanically ventilated patients. *Intensive Care Med* 1997;23:393–398.
9. Deutschman CS, Wilton PB, Sinow J, et al. Paranasal sinusitis: a common complication of nasotracheal intubation in neurosurgical patients. *Neurosurgery* 1985;17:296–299.
10. Korinek AM, Laisne MJ, Nicolas MH, et al. Selective decontamination of the digestive tract in neurosurgical intensive care unit patients: a double-blind, randomized, placebo-controlled study. *Crit Care Med* 1993;21:1466–1473.
11. Borman KR, Brown PM, Mezera KK, et al. Occult fever in surgical intensive care unit patients is seldom caused by sinusitis. *Am J Surg* 1992;164:412–416.
12. Gwaltney JM Jr, Philips CD, Miller RD, et al. Computed tomographic study of the common cold. *N Engl J Med* 1994;330:25–30.
13. Gwaltney JM Jr. Acute community-acquired sinusitis. *Clin Infect Dis* 1996;23:1209–1225.
14. Bell RM, Page GV, Bynoe RP, et al. Post-traumatic sinusitis. *J Trauma* 1988;28:923–30.
15. Seiden AM. Sinusitis in the critical care patient. *New Horizons* 1993; 5:261–270.
16. Kaups KL, Cohn SM, Nageris B, et al. Maxillary sinusitis in the surgical intensive care unit: a study using bedside sinus ultrasound. *Am J Otolaryngol* 1995;16:24–28.
17. Holzapfel L, Chevret S, Madinier G, et al. Influence of long-term oro- or nasotracheal intubation on nosocomial maxillary sinusitis and pneumonia: results of a prospective, randomized, clinical study. *Crit Care Med* 1993;21:1132–1138.
18. Kollef MH, von Harz B, Prentice D, et al. Patient transport from intensive care increases the risk of developing ventilator-associated pneumonia. *Chest* 1997;112:765–773.
19. Rohr AS, Spector SL, Siegel SC, et al. Correlation between A-mode ultrasound and radiography in the diagnosis of maxillary sinusitis. *J Allergy Clin Immunol* 1986;78:58–61.

20. Hilbert G, Vargas F, Valentino R, et al. Comparison of B-mode ultrasound and computed tomography in the diagnosis of maxillary sinusitis in mechanically ventilated patients. *Crit Care Med* 2001;29:1337–1342.
21. Lucchin F, Minicuci N, Ravasi MA, et al. Comparison of A-mode ultrasound and computed tomography: detection of secretion in maxillary and frontal sinuses in ventilated patients. *Intensive Care Med* 1996; 22:1265–1268.
22. Westergren V, Forsum U, Lundgren J. Possible errors in diagnosis of bacterial sinusitis in tracheal intubated patients. *Acta Anaesthesiol Scand* 1994;38:699–703.
23. Kountakis SE, Skoulas IG. Middle meatal vs antral lavage cultures in intensive care unit patients. *Otolaryngol Head Neck Surg* 2002;126: 377–381.
24. Casiano RR, Cohn S, Villasuso E III, et al. Comparison of antral tap with endoscopically directed nasal culture. *Laryngoscope* 2001;111: 1333–1337.
25. O'Grady NP, Barie PS, Bartlett JG, et al. Practice guidelines for evaluating new fever in critically ill adult patients. *Clin Infect Dis* 1998;26: 1042–1059.
26. Holzapfel L, Chastang C, Demingeon G, et al. A randomized study assessing the systematic search for maxillary sinusitis in nasotracheally mechanically ventilated patients. Influence of nosocomial maxillary sinusitis on the occurrence of ventilator-associated pneumonia. *Am J Resp Crit Care Med* 1999;159:695–701.
27. Hall J. Assessment of fever in the intensive care unit. Is the answer just beyond the tip of our nose? *Am J Resp Crit Care Med* 1999;159: 693–694.
28. Evans FO Jr, Sydnor B, Moore WEC, et al. Sinusitis of the maxillary antrum. *N Engl J Med* 1975;293:735–739.
29. Hamory BH, Sande MA, Sydnor A Jr, et al. Etiology and antimicrobial therapy of acute maxillary sinusitis. *J Infect Dis* 1979;139:197–202.
30. Wolf M, Zillinsky I, Lieberman P. Acute mycotic sinusitis with bacterial sepsis in orotracheal intubation and nasogastric tubing: a case report and review of the literature. *Otolaryngol Head Neck Surg* 1988;98: 615–617.
31. Talmor M, Li P, Barie PS. Acute paranasal sinusitis in critically ill patients; guidelines for prevention, diagnosis and treatment. *Clin Infect Dis* 1997;25:1441–1446.
32. Lowry PW, Tompkins LS. Nosocomial legionellosis: a review of pulmonary and extrapulmonary syndromes. *Am J Infect Control* 1993;21: 21–27.
33. Zinreich SJ. Paranasal sinus imaging. *Otolaryngol Head Neck Surg* 1990; 103:863–869.
34. Antonelli M, Conti G, Rocco M, et al. A comparison of noninvasive positive-pressure ventilation and conventional mechanical ventilation in patients with acute respiratory failure. *N Engl J Med* 1998;339: 429–435.
35. Pedersen J, Schurizek BA, Melsen NC, et al. The effect of nasotracheal intubation on the paranasal sinuses. A prospective study of 434 intensive care patients. *Acta Anaesthesiol Scand* 1991;35:11–13.
36. Dellinger RP. Airway managment and nosocomial infection. *Crit Care Med* 1993;21:1109–1110.
37. O'Reilly MJ, Reddick EJ, Black W, et al. Sepsis from sinusitis in nasotracheally intubated patients. A diagnostic dilemma. *Am J Surgery* 1984; 147:601–604.
38. Salord F, Gaussorgues P, Marti-Flich J, et al. Nosocomial maxillary sinusitis during mechanical ventilation: a prospective comparison of orotracheal versus the nasotracheal route for intubation. *Intensive Care Med* 1990;16:390–393.
39. Heffner JE. Airway management in the critically ill patient. *Crit Care Clin* 1990;6:533–550.
40. Depoix JP, Malbezin S, Videcoq M, et al. Oral intubation v. nasal intubation in adult cardiac surgery. *Br J Anaesth* 1987;59:167–169.
41. Fassoulaki A, Pamouktsoglou P. Prolonged nasotracheal intubation and its association with inflammation of paranasal sinuses. *Anesth Analg* 1989;69:50–52.
42. Grindlinger GA, Niehoff J, Hughes SL, et al. Acute paranasal sinusitis related to nasotracheal intubation of head-injured patients. *Crit Care Med* 1987;15:214–217.
43. Bach A, Boehrer H, Schmidt H, et al. Nosocomial sinusitis in ventilated patients. Nasotracheal versus orotracheal intubation. *Anaesthesia* 1992; 47:335–339.
44. Michelson A, Kamp H-D, Schuster B. Sinusitis bei langzeitintubierten Intensivpatienten: Nasale versus orale Intubation. *Anaesthesist* 1991; 40:100–104.
45. Aust R, Drettner B. The patency of the maxillary ostium in relation to body posture. *Acta Otolaryngol* 1975;80:443–446.
46. Deutschman CS, Wilton P, Sinow J, et al. Paranasal sinusitis associated with nasotracheal intubation: a frequently unrecognized and treatable source of sepsis. *Crit Care Med* 1986;14:111–114.
47. Bert F, Lambert-Zechovsky N. Pathogens responsible for concurrent sinusitis and pneumonia in intensive care unit patients. *Infection* 1996; 24:52–53.
48. Bert F, Lambert-Zechovsky N. Pneumonia associated with nosocomial sinusitis: a different risk according to the pathogen involved. *Am J Resp Crit Care Med* 1995;152:1424–1425.
49. Kaufman DM, Litman N, Miller MH. Sinusitis: induced subdural empyema. *Neurology* 1983;33:123–132.
50. Flaherty JP, Weinstein RA. Infection control and pneumonia prophylaxis strategies in the intensive care unit. *Semin Respir Infect* 1990;5: 191–203.
51. D'Amico R, Pifferi S, Leonetti C, et al. Effectiveness of antibiotic prophylaxis in critically ill adult patients: systemic review of randomised controlled trials. *BMJ* 1998;316:1275–1285.
52. Bonten MJM, Kullberg BJ, v. Dalen R, et al. Selective digestive decontamination in patients in intensive care. *J Antimicrob Chemother* 2000; 46:351–362.
53. Torres A, Serra-Batlles J, Ros E, et al. Pulmonary aspiration of gastric contents in patients receiving mechanical ventilation: the effect of body position. *Ann Intern Med* 1992;116:540–543.
54. Westergren V, Lundblad L, Hellquist HB, et al. Ventilator-associated sinusitis: a review. *Clin Infect Dis* 1998;27:851–864.
55. Caplan ES, Hoyt NJ. Nosocomial sinusitis. *JAMA* 1982;247:639–641.
56. Mevio E, Benazzo M, Quaglieri S, et al. Sinus infection in intensive care patients. *Rhinology* 1996;34:232–236.
57. Bert F, Lambert-Zechovsky N. Microbiology of nosocomial sinusitis in intensive care unit patients. *J Infection* 1995;31:5–8.
58. Aebert H, Hunefeld G, Regel G. Paranasal sinusitis and sepsis in ICU patients with nasotracheal intubation. *Intensive Care Med* 1988;15: 27–30.
59. Guerin JM, Meyer P, Habib Y, et al. Purulent rhinosinusitis is also a cause of sepsis in critically ill patients. *Chest* 1988;93:893–894.

24

NOSOCOMIAL GASTROINTESTINAL TRACT INFECTIONS

BARRY M. FARR

Nosocomial gastrointestinal (GI) tract infections cause important morbidity, mortality, and excess costs for hospitals (1). The Centers for Disease Control and Prevention's (CDC) definition of nosocomial gastroenteritis (2) requires the acute onset of diarrhea in a hospitalized patient, characterized by liquid stool for more than 12 hours, with or without vomiting and/or fever (>38°C). A diagnosis of nosocomial gastroenteritis can also be made in a patient with two of the following symptoms with no other recognized cause: nausea, vomiting, abdominal pain, or headache—in conjunction with objective evidence of enteric infection. Such evidence can be obtained by stool culture, antigen or antibody assay of feces or blood, routine or electron microscopic examination of stool, or toxin assay.

The CDC definition also provides that there must be no evidence that the infection was present or incubating at the time of hospital admission to distinguish community-acquired from nosocomial illness. This requires that the amount of time the patient was hospitalized prior to the onset of symptoms be compared with the incubation period of the particular type of gastroenteritis. Many have used 3 days after admission as a cut point for separating nosocomial from community-acquired infections. This can sometimes be misleading, however, because some of the infectious agents have incubation periods that can be longer than 3 days. Immunosuppression can also result in reactivation of latent infection. Hospital employees and visitors sometimes import pathogens from the community, resulting in hospital spread of community pathogens. Foodborne illness may present itself in an outbreak. The evaluation of diarrhea in hospitalized patients with acquired immunodeficiency syndrome (AIDS) or those in developing countries is especially complicated. Higher background rates of diarrhea in these populations force one to consider a broad range of pathogens.

Noninfectious causes of diarrhea in hospitalized patients must also be considered. Conditions such as inflammatory bowel disease, exocrine deficiency, or fecal impaction must be excluded by history, physical examination, and laboratory tests. Pharmacologic agents such as laxatives, cathartics, and quinidine produce diarrhea. Other agents, such as cytotoxic chemotherapeutic drugs and enteral nutrition supplements, are associated with a noninfectious diarrhea but can also predispose to infectious diarrhea (Table 24.1).

INCIDENCE

Much of the information concerning nosocomial gastroenteritis has come from the data generated by the CDC's National Nosocomial Infections Surveillance (NNIS) system (3), which involves voluntary reporting of nosocomial infections by participating hospitals. Between 1985 and 1991, the rate of gastroenteritis was 10.5/10,000 discharges. This rate represented an eightfold increase as compared with that observed from 1980 through 1984, when an infection rate of 1.3/10,000 was reported (4).

In recent years, such data reflecting the entire hospital population are no longer available from NNIS. Moreover, the NNIS hospitals constitute but a small fraction of all healthcare institutions in the United States, with variable surveillance methods and voluntary reporting, so this increased infection rate could have several explanations. The incidence may have been truly increasing, but improved surveillance methods, more sensitive diagnostic technologies, or a combination of such factors could have accounted for the apparent increase in nosocomial gastroenteritis.

Changes in methods of case detection can profoundly impact data regarding nosocomial gastroenteritis. At the University of Virginia, cases of nosocomial infectious diarrhea increased from one reported episode yearly to 150 to 200 annual documented cases when surveillance criteria were modified (1). Multiple studies have demonstrated the futility of the formerly routine orders for stool ova and parasites and bacterial cultures for *Salmonella, Shigella,* and *Campylobacter* species in the evaluation of sporadic nosocomial diarrhea (5,6). By contrast, *Clostridium difficile* and rotavirus have been frequently documented as causes of nosocomial diarrhea. One study in a children's hospital found that infections of the GI tract were exceeded only by those of the respiratory tract as causes of nosocomial infection (7). These GI infections were all viral, as documented by electron microscopy of stool specimens. The study suggested that the heightened prevalence of nosocomial GI tract infections reflected meticulous diagnostic testing for viral agents not done before the 1980s.

A number of prospective surveillance studies conducted in individual hospitals have revealed rates of nosocomial gastroenteritis several hundred times higher than the rates reported by NNIS. In one study, the adult medical intensive care unit

TABLE 24.1. NONINFECTIOUS CAUSES OF DIARRHEA IN HOSPITALIZED PATIENTS

Drugs	Postgastrectomy syndrome
Laxatives	Hirschsprung's disease
Cathartics	Gastrocolic fistula
Antacids	Malabsorption
Thyroid hormone	Bile salt enteropathy
Digoxin	Pancreatic insufficiency
Quinidine	Disaccharide deficiencies
Theophylline	Sprue
Caffeine	Endocrine
Colchicine	Thyrotoxicosis
Methyldopa	Diabetes mellitus
Reserpine	Adrenal insufficiency
Guanethidine	Hypoparathyroidism
Antibiotics	Tumors
Inflammatory	Villous adenoma
Ulcerative colitis	GI lymphoma
Crohn's disease	Carcinold (serotonin)
Diverticulitis	Zollinger-Ellison syndrome (gastrin)
Mechanical	Medullary carcinoma of the hyroid
Fecal impaction	Pancreatic cholera (VIP)
Partial bowel obstruction	
Bacterial overgrowth	
Blind loop syndromes	

VIP, vasoactive intestinal peptide.

(MICU) and two pediatric wards were surveyed during 1985 and 1986, yielding an overall rate of nosocomial diarrhea of 2.6/100 admissions (8). In these selected populations, nosocomial diarrhea was the most common nosocomial infection (7.7 and 2.3 per 100 admissions in adults and children, respectively). A pathogen was identified in approximately 40% of cases.

Despite limitations imposed by analysis of voluntary reporting, NNIS hospitals demonstrate variability in infection risk among different specialty services such as medicine (15.1/10,000 discharges), surgery (11.9/10,000), pediatrics (11.3/10,000), and obstetrics (1.1/10,000) (4). Higher rates are evident on some subspecialty services, notably the burn/trauma service (23.8/10,000), general surgery (20.4/10,000), the high-risk nursery (20.3/10,000), and the oncology service (18.3/10,000).

A somewhat unexpected finding from the NNIS data is the preponderance of reported infections among the elderly: 64.4% involved patients 60 years of age or older. This may be due to a relative paucity of viral diagnostic capability in hospitals participating in the NNIS program, or to infrequent testing for viral pathogens in sporadic diarrhea, since nosocomial diarrhea in children is often viral (6,9,10).

Although gastroenteritis accounted for a negligible percentage of nosocomial infections reported from NNIS during the 1970s (11), it made up 21% of nosocomial epidemics investigated by the CDC from 1956 to 1979 primarily due to *Salmonella* species and enteropathogenic *Escherichia coli* (12). Of nosocomial epidemics investigated by the CDC between 1980 and 1991, 7.4% were gastrointestinal (4). These data may suggest that the proportion of hospital epidemics caused by gastroenteritis has declined. An increase in the ability of hospitals and local health departments to handle such outbreaks without assistance from the CDC may be another explanation.

Although data are sparse, some studies have addressed the attributable mortality of nosocomial gastroenteritis. Zaidi et al. (13), in a prospective study from a tertiary-care hospital in Mexico City, found an 18% mortality rate in patients with nosocomial diarrhea compared to a 5% mortality rate in matched controls. The study also demonstrated a 7% rate of severe complications from the diarrheal illnesses, including volume depletion, hematochezia, abdominal distention, and candidemia. An older study by Yolken et al. (14) that was conducted in bone marrow transplant recipients also found a strikingly increased mortality rate associated with nosocomial gastroenteritis. Patients infected with viral pathogens or *C. difficile* had a 55% mortality rate over the course of the study period, which spanned 9 months. Matched controls had a mortality rate of 13%. Moreover, patients with GI infections had a significantly longer average duration of hospitalization, 66 days, than the 46 days noted for control subjects.

It has been postulated that this increased mortality could be a result of an increased risk for other nosocomial infections. Lima et al. (15) found that nosocomial diarrhea was an important risk factor for other nosocomial infections, particularly urinary tract infections. In that study, nosocomial urinary tract infections were ten times more common in patients with antecedent nosocomial diarrhea than in those without diarrhea. A possible mechanism involves colonization of the urethral meatus with enteric flora from patients with diarrhea that could result in infection of the genitourinary tract (16–18). These findings were supported by the results of other studies (19,20).

Such data suggest an additional economic burden from nosocomial GI infections. A 1977 study estimated the cost of a case of nosocomial diarrhea to be $800, but this figure would now need to be adjusted for subsequent inflation (21).

RISK FACTORS: THE HOST VERSUS THE HOSPITAL ENVIRONMENT

Assessment of the risk factors in nosocomial GI tract infections necessarily involves an appreciation of the complex relationship between host defenses and the hospital environment (Table 24.2).

Physical Barriers

Certain physical aspects of the GI tract protect against invading microbial pathogens. Normal gastric acidity (pH <4.0) will kill 99.9% of ingested coliform bacteria within 30 minutes (22). In contrast, subjects with induced achlorhydria have been experimentally infected with *Vibrio cholerae* inocula 10,000 times less than those used to infect subjects with normal gastric acidity (23). Likewise, several studies have shown an increased frequency and severity of *Salmonella* infections in patients with achlorhydria or history of prior gastric surgery (24). The importance of gastric acidity in protection against nosocomial pneumonia has also been demonstrated. Patients taking antacids or H2 blockers show increased colonization of the stomach, pharynx, and trachea and a resultant increase in nosocomial pneumonia when

TABLE 24.2. RISK FACTORS FOR NOSOCOMIAL GASTROENTERITIS

Factor	Proposed Mechanism
Physical	
Achlorhydria	Diminished acidity
Antacid/H2 blockers	Diminished acidity
Antimicrobial use	Altered gut flora
Recent enema	Disrupted mucosal barrier
GI tract surgery	Achlorhydria/antibiotics
Nasogastric intubation	Exogenous contamination
Enteral feeding	Exogenous contamination
Immunologic	
Immunodeficiencies	Defective gut/systemic immunity
Immunosuppressive drugs	Defective gut/systemic immunity; mucosal barrier damage
HIV infection	Decreased gut T cells; enterolnvasive opportunistic infections
Graft-vs.-host disease	Donor lymphocytes damage host mucosa
Demographic	
Old age	Debility; age-related achlorhydria
Infancy (0–11 months)	Gut immaturity
Childhood (6 months to 6 years)	Loss of maternal antibodies; poor hygiene
Environmental	
Intensive care unit	Nasogastric intubation, antibiotic use, debllity, achlorhydria
Diapering	Poor hygiene; increased cross-infection
Number of roommates	Increased cross-infection
Length of hospital stay	Multifactorial
Low staff to patient ratio	Increased cross-infection

compared with patients taking sucralfate, an agent that preserves gastric acidity (25)(see Chapter 22).

Normal intestinal motility also contributes to protection against invading pathogens. Ingestion of drugs that attenuate gut motility, such as opiates and diphenoxylate hydrochloride with atropine, increase the incidence of bacteremia associated with *Salmonella* gastroenteritis (26) and abolish antibiotic effectiveness in *Shigella* infections (27). These intestinal paralytics have prolonged fever and shedding of pathogens and have predisposed to serious complications of antibiotic-associated colitis such as toxic megacolon or intestinal perforation (28).

The normal intestinal microflora is a vital host defense effective in preventing colonization by pathogenic bacteria (29). Loss of normal intestinal ecology is usually manifested by replacement of commensal anaerobic species with pathogenic microorganisms such as *Pseudomonas, Klebsiella, Clostridium,* and *Candida* species. In mice, antibiotic administration has been associated with a rise in intestinal pH and decreased elaboration of volatile fatty acids (30), resulting in increased susceptibility to oral challenge with pathogenic bacteria. Antecedent or concurrent use of antimicrobials most often triggers the shift in intestinal flora, although this change can be seen in hospitalized debilitated patients without the influence of antibiotics.

Alteration of the resident intestinal microflora has been shown to be a risk factor for infection (31); numerous studies of nosocomial gastroenteritis have linked prior antimicrobial use to an increased incidence of infection. Thibault et al. (32) found that the risk of *C. difficile*–associated diarrhea (CDAD) increased with the number of antibiotics administered to a patient. Risk further depended on the type of antibiotic used, with the highest odds ratio found with clindamycin use. The somewhat counterintuitive finding of an increased risk associated with metronidazole use was confounded in that study by its administration with other antibiotics.

An intact intestinal mucosa, with its overlying mucus layer, appears to be a barrier to invading pathogens. Cytotoxic chemotherapeutic drugs affect the integrity of both the mucosa and gut immunity, causing noninfectious diarrhea and also predisposing to GI infection.

Immunologic Factors

The intestinal immune system is integral to the defense against microbial antigens. The human GI tract contains as much lymphoid tissue as the spleen, and about 80% of all immunoglobulin-producing cells in the body are in the intestinal mucosa (33). The gut-associated lymphoid tissue (GALT) is composed of a complex network with three major components: the Peyer's patches, the lamina propria lymphoid cells, and the intraepithelial lymphocytes (34). These elements act in concert to identify foreign antigens, activate a systemic immune response, and initiate local cytolytic processes. Abnormalities in the immune system, either congenital or acquired, contribute to an increased risk of enteric infections due to bacterial, viral, parasitic, and fungal pathogens (35).

Profound disruption of either the GALT or the overall immune system is postulated to predispose to both invasive GI candidiasis (35–37) and *Candida*-associated diarrhea. Nosocomial esophageal candidiasis is primarily a disorder seen in patients receiving corticosteroids, radiation therapy to the thorax, or systemic chemotherapy. Considerably less common is candidiasis involving the stomach, small intestine, or colon, which has been shown to be an important precursor to candidemia (13,38,39).

Patients undergoing bone marrow transplantation experience intense and prolonged immunosuppression due to marrow-ablative therapy. They also have high rates of diarrhea, which in the past was thought to be largely due to graft-versus-host disease (GVHD) (40). A study by Yolken et al. (14) found that 40% of the bone marrow transplant patients with diarrhea had at least one pathogenic virus or *C. difficile* toxin isolated from their stool. These infections were associated with a mortality rate of 55%, compared with 13% for a control group matched for age, gender, diagnosis, and duration of neutropenia.

Patients in intensive care units constitute another risk group for nosocomial GI tract infections. Kelly et al. (41) reported diarrhea in 41% of patients admitted to an intensive care unit over a 1-year surveillance period. This high rate was due to several factors that may have increased the risk of infection, such as achlorhydria induced by H2 blockers (42), liberal use of antibiotics (32,43), the immunocompromised state, and overall illness severity (42).

Environmental Influences

Certain predisposing elements for nosocomial GI tract infections are extrinsic to the host. Nasogastric intubation (42) and enteral feeding (13) are associated with the development of nosocomial gastroenteritis. Nasogastric intubation may facilitate inoculation of the GI tract with infecting microorganisms. Enteral feeding formulas (particularly hypertonic) can cause osmotic diarrhea, but bacterial contamination of nutritional formulas has been documented as leading to GI infections in the hospital setting (44). Zaidi et al. (13) found an odds ratio of 67 for the association between nosocomial diarrhea and enteral feeding in a study analyzed by multiple logistic regression. In this study, pathogenic microorganisms were identified in 59% of cases.

Crowded hospital environments appear to increase the risk of nosocomial gastroenteritis by cross-infection. Ford-Jones et al. (9) in Toronto demonstrated a correlation between nosocomial gastroenteritis and the number of patients in a room. Infection rates were found to be 15.7 cases/1,000 patient-days for rooms with zero to one patient, 27.7 cases/1,000 patient-days for rooms with two to three patients, and 45.2 cases/1,000 patient-days for rooms with four or more patients. Risk of nosocomial gastroenteritis was also shown to be increased five times by the use of diapers, perhaps because of cross-infection from diaper changing.

MODES OF TRANSMISSION

Transmission of nosocomial GI tract infections may occur through (a) direct patient-to-patient contact, (b) dissemination among patients on the hands of hospital workers, (c) environmental contamination and subsequent direct or indirect spread, and (d) spread by a common vehicle such as contaminated medical equipment. Understanding of these various mechanisms of spread has been enhanced by newly developed techniques in molecular epidemiology (45).

Hospital-acquired gastroenteritis is known to be spread by contact, primarily by the hands of hospital personnel. Routine contact with patients colonized with *C. difficile*, especially with ungloved hands, has resulted in contamination of healthcare workers' hands in 59% of cases. Contamination was also shown to occur with physical examinations or the handling of patient charts (46). In another study, nosocomial transmission of *C. difficile* was significantly reduced by regular glove use (47). The fact that 21% of asymptomatic patients in a Veterans Administration Hospital study were found to be colonized with *C. difficile* (43) underscores the need for uniform use of barrier precautions.

Environmental contamination may also play a role in transmission (46,48,49). *C. difficile* spores have been shown to persist for as long as 5 months on surfaces in close proximity to patients with *C. difficile* infection (49). In one study, 8% of environmental cultures were positive in the rooms of uninfected patients, 29% were positive in the rooms of patients with asymptomatic carriage, and 49% were positive in the rooms of patients with *C. difficile* diarrhea (46). Surface contamination was encountered on patients' bed rails, commodes, floors, call buttons, bedpans, and windowsills.

Epidemiologic markers such as serotyping have proven useful in pinpointing transmission mechanisms of *C. difficile*. In one outbreak, a serogroup analysis detected clusters of infection on hospital wards and was used as a measure of infection control efforts (50). This method was able to discern serotypes with propensity for epidemic spread. Techniques with even greater discriminatory powers, such as restriction endonuclease analysis of chromosomal DNA, allowed detection of one particular clone as a cause of nosocomial diarrhea on several wards in a hospital (50). Thus, hospital-wide transmission was documented.

Immunoblot typing was used prospectively to study acquisition and transmission of sporadic cases of *C. difficile* infection on a medical ward (46); 22.7% of the patients acquired *C. difficile* and 37% developed diarrhea. The study demonstrated that most hospitalized patients with *C. difficile* infection acquired it in the hospital. Immunoblot typing showed person-to-person spread and geographic clusters of affected patients and caregivers. At discharge from the hospital, 82% of infected patients still had positive cultures.

Thus, a large asymptomatic reservoir of *C. difficile* exists in hospitals. McFarland et al. (46) have suggested the potential for dissemination of *C. difficile* by asymptomatic carriers of *C. difficile*. They found that 23 (25%) of 92 initially culture-negative patients acquired *C. difficile* from exposure to a roommate with a positive culture. Of these 23 patients, 14 (61%) acquired *C. difficile* from an asymptomatic roommate. In another study, 42% of asymptomatic excretors shed nontoxigenic (and nonpathogenic) microorganisms (51). Patients with diarrhea are more likely to be infected with toxigenic microorganisms and to excrete higher microbial loads disseminating fecal matter into the environment (50). (For additional details on transmission of *C. difficile*, see Chapter 36.)

Some of the principles of nosocomial transmission illustrated by *C. difficile* apply to nosocomial salmonellosis as well. A distinctive feature of nosocomial *Salmonella* gastroenteritis has been its frequent connection to foodborne institutional outbreaks (52). In the developed world, common-source epidemics due to contaminated food sources account for a majority of hospital-acquired *Salmonella* infections. Following this microorganism's introduction to the hospital environment, there often ensues a protracted period of secondary person-to-person spread (53). Hospital personnel may carry the microorganism on their hands from patient to patient (54). Insidious spread can also occur by asymptomatic excretors of the microorganism (55). These individuals (either patients or hospital workers) may possess a bacterial load sufficient to cause infection in those rendered susceptible by achlorhydria, malignancy, HIV infection, hemoglobinopathies, or prior antibiotic treatment. Thus, a foodborne epidemic may be perpetuated, in a more indolent form, by food handlers, medical personnel, or patients who carry the microorganism. In this way, nosocomial outbreaks of *Salmonella* have been documented to persist for as long as 5 years (55).

Generalizations about the transmission of nosocomial salmonellosis must take into account the large numbers of serotypes with heterogeneous virulence (56). Also to be considered are host factors that can influence the severity and risk of illness illustrated by the increased rates of bacteremia in AIDS patients (57), children, and the elderly. Nosocomial *Salmonella* gastroenteritis is most often an epidemic disease that begins with a common source. The most frequently implicated foods include eggs, poultry, meat, and protein supplements. Medications, diagnostic agents, and blood products have also been linked to epidemics (58). Before the era of recombinant technology, this mode of transmission was more common, often occurring via animal extracts of the pancreas, thyroid, pituitary, or liver (52). Finally, epidemics have been initiated with contamination of fomites such as a delivery room suction apparatus (52) and endoscopy equipment (59)(see Chapter 63).

Nosocomial salmonellosis in the developing world has provided a graphic example of how, through selective pressure of widespread antimicrobial use, hospitals can develop into important reservoirs of multiply resistant microorganisms (60). Infections with multidrug-resistant *Salmonella* species have been associated with a number of nosocomial outbreaks in such countries. These epidemics can cause substantial mortality in the immunocompromised patients who are primarily affected (54).

A Tunisian outbreak among neonates (54) of *Salmonella wien* had a 33% case-fatality rate among the infected infants with prominent secondary spread. Intensive use of cefotaxime was thought to have contributed to the evolution of a *Salmonella* species that contained plasmids coding for an extended-spectrum beta-lactamase. This particular microorganism was able to spread because of lax adherence to hospital infection control policies.

A final consideration is the importance of the reservoir of *Salmonella* among domestic food animals. These animals, which are often fed antimicrobials, are thought by many to constitute a wellspring of drug-resistant microorganisms. In fact, some researchers have been able to link approximately half of *Salmonella* outbreaks to food-producing animals (61,62). Nonetheless, despite decades of investigation, there has been no definitive evidence directly linking antimicrobials fed to livestock with development of human disease due to resistant microorganisms (63). In the United Kingdom, antibiotic use in animal feed has been tightly restricted for over 20 years because of this concern. In the United States, such controls have not been implemented, although investigation of potential health hazards continues (63).

Transmission of viral gastroenteritis within hospitals usually involves secondary spread by contact with contaminated hands or stool. Additionally, a number of reports have speculated that nosocomial viral gastroenteritis may be transmitted by aerosol (64,65). Movement of contaminated laundry was also implicated in these two reports. A recent study found that nurse understaffing was a significant risk factor for transmission of viral gastrointestinal infections (66).

A feature of nosocomial viral gastroenteritis worth highlighting is the tendency for hospital personnel to work while ill with GI symptoms (67). Such illness, usually characterized by relatively mild symptoms of brief duration in the healthy caregiver, can pose considerable risk to the hospitalized patient in whom morbidity may be much greater. Further study, using molecular epidemiologic techniques, would be useful to quantify the risk associated with this route of transmission.

No discussion of nosocomial gastroenteritis would be complete without mention of pseudoepidemics (68). False outbreaks constituted 11% of all epidemics investigated by the CDC during the years 1956 to 1975, and the GI tract was the second most common site involved, accounting for 20% of all pseudoepidemics. Errors in specimen processing, clinical misdiagnosis, and surveillance artifacts caused distortion in the spatial and temporal relationships of perceived infections. Two reports failed to distinguish community-acquired from hospital-acquired infection and, thus, incorrectly documented outbreaks of nosocomial group B *Salmonella* and enteropathogenic *E. coli* gastroenteritis. Another series of false infections was linked to a hospital laboratory's contamination with *Salmonella saint-paul* of a saline solution used to process stool specimens. A nursery outbreak allegedly due to *Staphylococcus aureus* resulted from reliance on positive stool cultures without proper clinical correlation. Such reports serve to underscore the need for careful interpretation of such epidemiologic data (see Chapter 8).

CLINICAL SYNDROMES

Antibiotic-Associated Gastrointestinal Illness

Although early reports had also implicated *S. aureus* as a cause (69), toxin-producing strains of *C. difficile* are now the most frequently identified microbial etiology of antibiotic-associated diarrhea and colitis. *C. difficile* cytotoxin has been found in 96% of patients with antibiotic-associated pseudomembranous colitis, in 20% of patients with antibiotic-associated diarrhea (AAD) without colitis, and in 2% of patients with GI disease unrelated to antimicrobial use (70). Patients with cytotoxin-negative AAD have a less severe illness, without accompanying colitis, that promptly resolves with withdrawal of the antibiotic; the antibiotics most frequently implicated have been those with profound effects on colonic flora and/or prominent enterohepatic circulation. The rate of cytotoxin-negative AAD increases proportionately with the dose and duration of treatment but is not believed to be associated with nosocomial transmission (71).

Case clusters of CDAD have been documented. CDAD can occur 6 weeks after discontinuation of antibiotic agents (72), after short courses given for perioperative prophylaxis (73), and in the setting of cancer chemotherapy (74). The illness may be severe with fever, leukocytosis, and colitis. Peritonitis, toxic megacolon, perforation, and sepsis are rare complications of CDAD. It has been suggested that *C. difficile* induces a subtle protein-losing enteropathy in patients who heretofore have been assumed to be asymptomatic carriers (75).

The presence of *C. difficile* in the colon does not indicate disease, since 5% of healthy adults (76), 21% of asymptomatic hospitalized adults (43), and 29% of neonates carry small numbers of toxigenic *C. difficile* microorganisms in their stools (77). Among hospitalized patients, acquisition of *C. difficile* was noted in 21% of patients (46,78), with asymptomatic excretors of the microorganism outnumbering those with clinical disease six to one (78). Moreover, it has been shown that asymptomatic carriers may not be at more risk of developing CDAD than those without antecedent carriage (78). The determinants of symptomatic infection appear to be host related and not contingent on virulence factors of the infecting strain. Prospective analysis of 428 patients showed that 23% of enrolled patients acquired *C. difficile* a median of 12 days after admission (46). Symptomatic and asymptomatic patients had similar strains by immunoblot as well as by analysis of cytotoxin and enterotoxin. Patients who developed overt illness were more likely to have predisposing factors such as advanced age, severe intercurrent illness, enemas, GI tract stimulants, or β-lactam antibiotics (79–84). Use of clindamycin and proximity to another patient with CDAD or AAD were significant risk factors in one study (82). Use of quinolones and/or cephalosporins has also been a significant risk factor (81,83,85). CDAD was reported to affect 15% of patients in a rehabilitation hospital (86), 5.6% of patients on a surgical ward (84), and 7% of neutropenic leukemia patients undergoing chemotherapy (87). Thus, development of CDAD can be looked upon as a phenomenon requiring not only host acquisition of *C. difficile* but also the presence of additional host risk factors to allow manifestation of clinical disease. Neonates with repeatedly toxin-positive stools were significantly more likely to have frequent and abnormal stools in one study (88).

Acquisition of *C. difficile* has been shown to occur by cross-infection between patients (46,89,90), with the source being identified as newly admitted patients who were asymptomatically colonized with *C. difficile* (91). Other studies have demonstrated that the hands of hospital personnel (46,92) and the hospital environment (93) are likely vehicles for this transmission.

The epidemiology of CDAD is complex. One study used plasmid profiling and restriction endonuclease analysis (REA) of isolates from clinical cases to study a hospital outbreak of CDAD (94). The authors showed that nosocomial transmission was evident in only one third of documented cases, but asymptomatic patients did not have cultures so transmission to and from such patients could not be detected. Nosocomial transmission within a ward was documented to occur up to 4 weeks after an index case was discovered. An identical strain was noted to infect patients on different wards over a period of 7 months. Other recent studies have found that particular strains of *C. difficile* may predominate in a hospital or even in multiple hospitals in a region (95–97) and that a strain predominating in Japan may be different from a strain predominating in the United States (96) (see also Chapter 36).

Infant Necrotizing Enterocolitis

The syndrome of infant necrotizing enterocolitis (NEC) has been recognized as a frequent cause of neonatal morbidity and mortality since the early 1960s (98) and is second only to respiratory distress syndrome (RDS) as a neonatal cause of death (99). The disorder in its classic severe form is characterized by vomiting, abdominal distention, bloody stools, and demonstration of air in the intestinal walls, portal venous system, or peritoneal cavity. It can cause intestinal perforation, peritonitis, and bacteremia. Signs and symptoms arise as a result of a diffuse necrosis of the GI tract that usually affects the terminal ileum but can occur from the ligament of Treitz to the transverse colon (100).

The pathogenesis of NEC is not clear. The necrosis of the intestinal mucosa is thought to be mediated by antecedent ischemia or hypoxia, but a single precipitant is not identifiable in all cases of NEC. Many experts, therefore, invoke three interrelated components that lead to the development of NEC: (a) intestinal mucosal injury usually resulting from gut ischemia or hypoxia; (b) abnormal or delayed bacterial colonization of the bowel; and (c) GI luminal substrate, usually enteric feeding formula (101). Some might add a fourth component, an intrinsically susceptible infant with immature intestinal mucosa (102). Other poorly defined factors, such as toxins (103), inflammatory mediators (104), oxygen free radicals (105), gut hormones (106), and bacterial fermentation products (107), may promote the intestinal mucosal injury that is the hallmark of the disorder.

Risk factors associated with the development of the disease have been identified. Premature infants, or those with very low birth weight (VLBW) of less than 1,500 g, account for about 90% of affected infants (108,109). These children are particularly apt to experience hemodynamic instability, hypoxemia, and umbilical artery/vein catheterization (110). Other risk factors associated with NEC include low Apgar scores, maternal anesthesia, premature rupture of membranes, antimicrobial therapy, cyanotic heart disease, or patent ductus arteriosus (109,111). Maternal use of cocaine also appears to increase risk of NEC (112), possibly through its intensive vasoconstrictive effects on the fetal mesenteric vasculature. Many of these risk factors have not been consistently confirmed by epidemiologic studies.

Other risk factors appear to relate to the GI tract itself. Enteral feeding, especially with hypertonic formulas, is associated with NEC. The disease develops after the initiation of enteral feeding in more than 90% of infants (101). Most strongly linked to late-occurring NEC (after 30 days of life) (113), enteral feeding is postulated to stress an immature gut mucosa, which lacks the necessary digestive enzymes (114) and secretory immunoglobulin A (IgA) (113–115) and is too permeable to macromolecules (116).

Numerous reports of epidemic NEC have prompted an exhaustive search for a causative infectious agent. NEC clinically resembles an enteroinvasive gastroenteritis: positive blood cultures [37.6% of patients in one study (117)] and peritoneal fluid cultures frequently accompany NEC. An increased risk of severe gastroenteritis and other illnesses is seen in caregivers of infants with NEC (118). The gas found in the pneumatosis has been postulated to be of microbial origin, as it contains hydrogen (119), but the number of putative etiologic agents approaches the number of reported epidemics. Implicated microorganisms include aerobic gram-negative bacilli [enterotoxigenic (120) and nonenterotoxigenic *E. coli* (121), *Klebsiella pneumoniae* (122), *Enterobacter cloacae* (123), and *Salmonella* species (124)], anaerobes [*C. difficile* (125), *C. perfringens* (126), and *C. butyricum* (127)], gram-positive cocci [*S. aureus* (128) and coagulase-negative staphylococci (129)], and viruses [rotavirus (130), coronavirus (131), echovirus type 22 (132), and coxsackievirus B2 (133)]. At this time, there is no known specific pathogen that is crucial to the development of NEC. It is possible that the bacteremia and peritonitis occur as normal enteric flora are released from bowel damaged by the noninfectious mechanisms outlined above.

The incidence of NEC has been evaluated by the hospitals participating in NNIS. The rate for the years 1985 to 1991 was 6.0/10,000 discharges for the newborn service and 60/10,000 for the high-risk nursery (4). Another study found that 17% of infants weighing less than 1,500 g developed NEC (117).

Preventive measures include judicious avoidance of risk factors when possible and meticulous attention to hygiene and infection control practices in neonatal intensive care units. New approaches are being tested, with promising results in some cases. In a randomized trial, Eibl et al. (134) found that feeding low birth weight babies an immunoglobulin mixture of 75% IgA and 25% immunoglobulin G (IgG) protected infants from NEC ($p = .014$). Another multicenter randomized trial reported a decreased incidence of NEC in infants born to women who had received prepartum corticosteroids ($p = .002$) in order to stimulate fetal lung maturity (135), perhaps related to enhanced intestinal mucosal maturity. Interestingly, postnatal steroids had no effect in decreasing the incidence of NEC but did lessen the severity of NEC in those infants who developed the disease. Other studies have demonstrated success with acidification of enteral feeding formulas (136). Manipulation of the timing, concentration, and rate of enteral feeding have had mixed results (137,138). The use of prophylactic antibiotics is controversial, having no clearly demonstrable benefit. They can also predispose to selection of antibiotic resistance (139). Prevention of prematurity would eliminate the majority of cases of this disease (see also Chapter 52).

Typhlitis

Typhlitis is also known as neutropenic enterocolitis (140) or ileocecal syndrome (141). It has been described in patients with acute leukemia (141), aplastic anemia (142), cyclic neutropenia, Felty's syndrome, bone marrow transplants (143), and AIDS (144). As it has been documented most frequently in patients who have been rendered severely immunosuppressed by aggressive cytotoxic chemotherapy for hematologic or solid malignancies, symptoms usually become apparent in the hospital.

The prevalence of typhlitis in leukemic patients at autopsy is approximately 10% to 12% (35). The actual incidence is unknown, however, as the signs and symptoms can be somewhat obscure. Classically, patients have fever, nausea, vomiting, and abdominal pain. Physical examination often reveals abdominal distention with right lower quadrant tenderness and positive fecal occult blood. Occasionally the cecum is palpable as a boggy mass. Overt lower GI bleeding may be present but is often a preterminal event (145). A distended, fluid-filled cecum with dilated small-bowel loops may be seen on plain abdominal radiograph. The diagnosis of typhlitis is best made with contrast-enhanced abdominal computed tomography (CT) by demonstrating thickened walls of the cecum (146). Blood cultures may reveal growth of enteric gram-negative bacilli or anaerobes.

The pathogenesis of typhlitis is not completely defined, but cytotoxic chemotherapy may contribute by causing mucositis, by derangement of GALT, by disruption of normal enteric flora, and by generalized immunosuppression. Some authorities have suggested that rapid dissolution of leukemic infiltrates in the intestinal wall promotes inflammation, hemorrhage, and perforation of the bowel wall (141). Certain chemotherapeutic agents, such as cytosine arabinoside, may have particular effects on intestinal mucus production and bring about denudation of the mucosa (147). Vincristine can produce an adynamic ileus, and corticosteroids can alter inflammatory processes. It is, nonetheless, important to note that typhlitis can occur in the absence of treatment with cytotoxic agents. The peculiar vulnerability of the cecum may be related to its relatively poor vascular supply or its distensibility compared with the rest of the colon. Infectious agents do not appear to play a primary role in the pathogenesis of typhlitis, but rather are opportunistic invaders that are responsible for the frequent secondary bacteremias. Typhlitis is associated with a mortality rate of greater than 50% (140).

Foodborne Gastrointestinal Diseases in Institutions

Patients in hospitals and extended-care facilities are especially vulnerable to the acquisition of foodborne GI illnesses (see Chapter 106). The food services in hospitals and other institutions are confronted with the challenge of acquiring high-quality food at low cost, properly preparing and storing such food, adequately cooking it for large numbers of patients, and promptly serving it before spoilage occurs. Moreover, the population consuming the prepared food is frequently weakened by age or debility and is poorly equipped to tolerate the effects of foodborne illness.

Of epidemics reported to the CDC from 1975 to 1987 for which the location was known, hospitals and nursing homes accounted for 3.1% of the outbreaks, 5.1% of the cases, and 24.1% of the deaths attributable to epidemic foodborne disease (148). Certain institutional case clusters have been associated with substantial morbidity and mortality. One nursing home outbreak of *E. coli* O157:H7, traced to contaminated sandwiches, resulted in a 35% mortality rate among residents affected (149). In general, most institutional epidemics, including the subset recognized, investigated, and reported to state health departments and the CDC, have far less severe effects. Salmonellosis has consistently been the major contributor to foodborne morbidity and mortality in nursing homes. For outbreaks of known etiology between 1975 and 1987, *Salmonella* was responsible for 52% of outbreaks and 81% of the deaths, with an overall case-fatality rate of 3.8% (150).

Institutional foodborne GI illness often follow a characteristic biphasic epidemic pattern with an initial point source (contaminated food) infecting a relatively large number of people. Secondary transmission of the infecting microorganism usually ensues (151), which follows a more indolent course. Secondary transmission occurs by mechanisms described previously in this chapter and can involve patients, their caregivers, family members, and visitors.

The most commonly identified microorganisms in foodborne outbreaks in hospitals and nursing homes are *Salmonella* species, *S. aureus*, and *C. perfringens* (148). Because most hospital laboratories cannot test for the Norwalk and related agents and for most pathogenic *E. coli* strains, their prevalence in foodborne nosocomial illness has not been quantified.

Specific food vehicles have been identified in many of the institutional outbreaks (Table 24.3). Epidemics involving *Salmonella* species are frequently linked to poultry, meat loaf, and egg-based foods such as eggnog and scrambled eggs. Various salads have been implicated in many of the *S. aureus* outbreaks. Dishes prepared with meat have been found to be the vehicle in cases of *C. perfringens* gastroenteritis. Contamination of enteral feeding formulas with such microorganisms as *Enterobacter sakazakii* (44,152), other *Enterobacter* species, *Yersinia* species, and

TABLE 24.3. VEHICLES IMPLICATED IN INSTITUTIONAL FOODBORNE OUTBREAKS

Pathogen	Vehicle(s)
Bacteria	
Salmonella	Eggnog, egg salad, scrambled eggs, turkey, pureed food, protein supplements, cake Icing, Brewer's yeast, dry milk, carmine dye
Staphylococcus aureus	Egg salad, chicken, chicken salad, turkey, potato salad, beef liver, pork
Clostridium perfringens	Roast beef, shepherd's pie, meat loaf, turkey, turkey salad, pea soup, stew, chicken, minced ham
Shigella	Salad
Bacillus cereus	Chicken, beef stew, rice
Campylobacter jejuni	Powdered milk
Other bacteria	Hamburger (*Escherichia coli* O157:H7) Raw vegetables (*Listeria monocytogenes*)
Parasites	Sandwiches (*Giardia lamblia*)
Chemicals	Cornmeal mush (niacin)

staphylococci has been increasingly recognized as causing nosocomial diarrhea and bacteremia.

Multiple deficiencies in food handling and preparation have been blamed for institutional outbreaks of gastroenteritis. Most often cited have been errors in storage such as a failure to refrigerate at a sufficiently low temperature. Other frequently reported problems include inadequate hygienic practices of food handlers, equipment contamination, insufficient cooking, and the use of food contaminated during manufacturing or processing (148).

If an outbreak is recognized by spatial and temporal clustering of GI illness, clues for identifying the causative pathogen can be gleaned from the patient's constellation of symptoms. Upper tract symptoms, such as vomiting, suggest *S. aureus* or a Norwalk-related agent. Complaints of fever and abdominal pain in the setting of diarrhea may be compatible with an enteroinvasive microorganism such as *Salmonella* or *Campylobacter.* Early confirmation of an enteroinvasive infection can be obtained by examining stool for fecal leukocytes.

Use of preliminary data can assist outbreak management in a number of ways. An initial differential diagnosis can guide diagnostic testing. For example, a cluster of cases of bloody diarrhea would prompt a search for verotoxin-producing *E. coli,* which may require sending stool specimens to a reference laboratory. Epidemic spread may be prevented if the propensity for secondary transmission with certain pathogens is recognized. Knowledge of the putative etiologic agent's incubation period may allow a more rapid identification of potential vehicles.

Efforts to prevent foodborne nosocomial infection focus on (a) food preparation, storage, and distribution; and (b) personal health and hygiene of the food service personnel. The crucial issues in promotion of hygienic food preparation are (a) maintenance of appropriate storage temperatures for food; (b) avoidance of contamination of cooked food by raw food, infected food handlers, or contaminated equipment; and (c) education of food-service personnel. Food handlers must know how to operate and maintain equipment, practice basic personal hygiene, and know when to seek medical attention if suffering from ailments that could result in transmission of foodborne illness. Because of fatal *E. sakazakii* infections associated with powdered infant formula, it has been recommended that this risk can be lowered by using sterile liquid formula instead (152).

Foodborne nosocomial illness is perhaps the most preventable of all hospital-acquired morbidity. As mentioned above, many of these infections, particularly *Salmonella* species and enterohemorrhagic *E. coli,* can cause substantial mortality in seriously ill hospitalized patients and particularly in the elderly nursing home population. With proper attention to routine infection surveillance, food service practices, and maintenance of employee health, foodborne nosocomial illness could become a rarity.

EVALUATION OF THE HOSPITALIZED PATIENT WITH DIARRHEA

According to the epidemiology of nosocomial gastroenteritis, it is evident that the most consistently helpful test in initial patient evaluation would be an assay for *C. difficile* toxin. Testing for rotavirus can be particularly useful in children during the winter and spring. Based on pretest probability, these tests should constitute the initial workup of nosocomial diarrhea in most patients. An examination for fecal leukocytes [or a leukocyte marker such as lactoferrin (153)] may also be done.

In other scenarios, however, there is a significantly increased likelihood that other etiologies of nosocomial diarrhea will be encountered. A cluster of cases of inflammatory diarrhea with negative tests for *C. difficile* toxin may prompt a search for pathogens that commonly cause common-source outbreaks, such as *Salmonella.* Similarly, the workup of nosocomial diarrhea in developing countries would necessarily involve attention to a broader spectrum of potential pathogens. An AIDS patient who develops diarrhea while hospitalized could have a nosocomial infection due to *C. difficile* (154) but could also have diarrhea due to a broad range of community-acquired pathogens for which diagnostic evaluation may require bacterial cultures, ova and parasite examination, acid-fast studies, and viral cultures. This more comprehensive evaluation may be indicated, at times, for any immunocompromised patient as well. In a hospitalized patient with severe diarrhea that defies diagnosis with stool studies, or in a patient with bloody diarrhea, early evaluation with sigmoidoscopy or colonoscopy is warranted (155). Biopsy material sent for both cultures and histologic examination can be invaluable in making a diagnosis in these difficult cases.

ETIOLOGIC AGENTS IN NOSOCOMIAL GASTROENTERITIS

Clostridium difficile

C. difficile is a gram-positive, spore-forming, obligate anaerobe that has been shown in multiple studies to be the most frequently identified microbial etiology in nosocomial diarrhea (Tables 24.4 and 24.5). Its role in the pathogenesis of antibiotic-

TABLE 24.4. ETIOLOGIC AGENTS IN NOSOCOMIAL GASTROENTERITIS

		Organisms									
Study (reference)	Patient population	*Clostridium difficile*	Rotavirus	Salmonellae	Adenovirus	Other viruses	Other bacteria	*Candida* species	*Entamoeba histolytica*	Frequency of isolation[a]	Comments
CDC, NNIS, 1980–1984 (11)	General	45%		12%						51%	Voluntary reporting system
Yolken, Baltimore, 1980–1981 (14)	Marrow transplant	29%	26%		29%	16%				40%	Thorough testing for viral pathogens, routine bacteria, LT-*E. coli*, and *Yersinia*: prospective study
Welliver, Buffalo, 1980–1981 (7)	Children		69%		11%	20%				56%	No bacterial GI pathogens were reported; prospective study
Larn, Hong Kong, 1982–1985 (10)	Children		78%				21%			100%	Bacterial species were not specified; identification of a pathogen was part of case definition of nosocomial gastroenteritis
Ford-Jones, Toronto, 1985 (9)	Children		43%	4%	8%	45%				95%	Bacterial testing was done only if a viral pathogen was not isolated; study was performed in winter
Zaidi, Mexico, 1987–1988 (13)	Adults	3%		1%			9%	38%	25%	59%	Study was performed in a tertiary care hospital in Mexico City
CDC, NNIS, 1985–1991 (4)	General	91%	5%							97%	Voluntary reporting system
Lima, Brazil, 1989–1993 (164)	General	33%	11%	4%			13%	42%		N/A	*Shigella flexneri*—13%; no cryptosporidia, *Giardia*, or *Entamoeba histolytica* were identified; abstract

[a]Values reflect percentages of cases with known etiology. Blank spaces indicate that data were not available from the study.
LT-*E. coli*, heat-labile *E. coli*.

TABLE 24.5. ENTERAL PATHOGENS THAT MAY CAUSE NOSOCOMIAL DISEASE

Agent	Incubation Period	Modes of Transmission	Clinical Syndrome	Symptom Duration	Pathogenesis	Diagnostic Test	Typing Method
Staphylococcus aureus	1–6 hours	F	V, ± D, A	< 24 hours	Neurotoxin	Culture, toxin assay	Phage
Bacillus cereus	1–6 hours (short); 8–16 hours (long)	F	V (short); D (long)	< 24 hours	Neurotoxin (short): (?toxin (long)	Culture	Serotype, plasmid
Clostridium perfringens	8–16 hours	F	D, A	24–72 hours	Enterotoxin	Culture	Serotype
Clostridium difficile	?	C, I	F, D, A	Until treatment	Enterotoxin/cytotoxin	Culture (CCFA), toxin assay, E	RE, immunoblot
Salmonellae	16–72 hours	C, I, F	F, ± V, D, A, + S	2–7 days	Invasion ± toxin	Culture	Plasmid, serotype, phage
Shigellae	16–72 hours	C, I, F	F, ± V, D, A	2–7 days	Invasion/cytotoxin	Culture	Serotype
Campylobacter jejuni	3–5 days	C, F	F, D, A	2–10 days	Invasion ± toxin	Culture—selective medium, filter, M	Serotype
Yersinia enterocolitica	3–7 days	C, F	F, D, A	1–3 weeks	Invasion? toxin	Culture, cold enrichment	Serotype, RE
Escherichia coli							
ETEC	16–72 hours	F	D, ± F, ± A	3–5 days	Heat-labile toxin, heat-stable toxin	Toxin assay (DNA) probe, CPE)	Serotype, plasmid
EPEC	16–48 hours	C, I, F	F, D	5–15 days	Adherence ± cytotoxin	AGG assay	Serotype, plasmid
EIEC	16–48 hours	?F	F, D, A	2–7 days	Invasion	Sereny test	Serotype, plasmid
EHEC	72–120 hours	C, I, F	D, HUS	2–12 days	Verotoxin	Toxin assay (DNA probe)	Serotype, plasmid
Clostridium botulinum	18–36 hours	F	P, ± V	Weeks to months	Neurotoxin (A, B, E)	Culture (stool), toxin assay	
Aeromonas spp.	?	F	F, D	1–7 days	Enterotoxin	Culture + oxidase test	DNA hybridization
Listeria monocytogenes	Approx. 3–70 days	F, ?C	F, S, M	Variable	Invasion/cytotoxin	Culture	MEE, serotype
Rotavirus	24–72 hours	C, I, ?As	F, V, D	4–6 days	Villi disruption	ELISA, LA, EM, PCR	RE
Norwalk agent(s)	24–48 hours	I, ?F, ?As	F, V, D	24–48 hours	Villi disruption	IEM, RIA, ELISA, PCR	IEM, ELISA
Adenovirus	8–10 days	?	F, ± V, D	8 days	?	EM, ELISA	DNA hybridization
Cryptosporidium	2–14 days	C, I, F	F, ± V, D, A	Weeks to months	Villi disruption	M, E EIA	
Entamoeba histolytica	7–14 days	C, I, F	F, D, A	Variable	Mucosal cytolysis	M, E, serology, DNA probe	PCR
Giardia lamblia	7–14 days	C, I, F	D, A	Weeks to months	Villi disruption	M, E, Enterotest, ELISA	PCR, DNA probe

ETEC, enterotoxigenic *E. coli*, EPEC, enteropathogenic *E. coli*, EIEC, enteroinvasive *E. coli*, EHEC, enterohemorrhagic *E. coli*, C, direct contact, 1, indirect contact; F, common vehicle (e.g., food, water); As, aerosol; ±, not always seen; F, tever; V, vomiting; D, diarrhea; A, abdominal pain; P, paralysis; S, sepsis; M, meningitis; HUS, hemolytic uremic syndrome; E, endoscopy with biopsy; LA, latex agglutination; M, direct microscopic examination; ELISA, enzyme-linked immunosorbent assay; RIA, radioimmunoassay; EM, electron microscopy; IEM, immune electron microscopy; CCFA, cycloserine, cefoxitin, fructose in agar; CPE, cytopathic effect, AGG, agglutination; MEE, multilocus enzyme electrophoresis; PCR, polymerase chain reaction; RE, restriction endonuclease analysis.

associated pseudomembranous colitis was first noted when it was found that hamsters treated with antibiotics were susceptible to a fatal form of colitis (156). A cytotoxin was identified in the hamster feces that was neutralized by *C. sordellii* antitoxin (157). This cytotoxin, now known as toxin B, was subsequently linked to *C. difficile* (158). The microorganism was also found to elaborate an enterotoxin (toxin A) that causes intestinal fluid secretion and hemorrhage in animal models (159). Although toxin A is thought to be primarily responsible for manifestations of clinical disease, most strains of *C. difficile* produce both toxins (71).

The test generally considered to be the gold standard for diagnosis of antibiotic-associated colitis has been the tissue culture assay to detect the cytopathic effects of toxin B. This test, when used alone, has been reported to have a sensitivity between 67% (160) and 100% (161) and a specificity of 99% (160, 162) for detecting toxigenic *C. difficile*. The test, however, is technically difficult to perform, and results are not rapidly available (71). Proper maintenance of cell lines, which may not be possible for some laboratories, is crucial for accuracy of the assay. Diagnostic accuracy also depends on appropriate selection of the dilution titer used for detection of a positive result (163).

Several studies have raised questions regarding the specificity of the cytotoxin assay. Zaidi et al. (13) found *C. difficile* toxin more frequently in asymptomatic control patients than in those with diarrhea. Another study demonstrated a 5% rate of asymptomatic toxin carriage in hospitalized adults (43).

In attempts to overcome the technical difficulties of the cytotoxin assay, a number of rapid tests for *C. difficile* toxin have been developed. Several commercial enzyme immunoassay (EIA) tests to detect toxin A, toxin B, or both, as well as latex agglutination tests, are available. They are rapid and simple to perform, but there is much variability among the different test kits, with sensitivities ranging from 71% to 92% when compared with a cytotoxin assay (163). Many kits either have insufficient sensitivity or produce too many indeterminate results to allow use as a single diagnostic test (161,164,165). Another EIA that detects both toxin A and B was shown to have sensitivity of 92% and specificity of 100% (166). Other diagnostic tests are being developed. Polymerase chain reaction (PCR), using primers from both toxin A and toxin B, has shown promise (167,168). A recent study reported the detection of 28 of 29 cytotoxin positive samples using a "real-time" PCR, which provided rapid results (169). All 27 control specimens were negative. Another study found that PCR ribotyping and arbitrarily primed PCR provided more reliable genotyping for *C. difficile* isolates than did pulsed-field gel electrophoresis (PFGE) (170).

Culture techniques to isolate *C. difficile* have used an egg-yolk agar base medium with cycloserine, cefoxitin, and fructose agar (CCFA) that is selective for *C. difficile* (171). Because the rate of asymptomatic *C. difficile* carriage in hospitalized patients has been found to be about 16% (46), culture alone cannot be used for the diagnosis of CDAD. The addition of 0.1% sodium taurocholate to CCFA can increase recovery of *C. difficile* from environmental sources by increasing spore germination (172) and may be useful for epidemiologic studies. Similarly, alcohol shock enrichment has also been shown to increase yield from cultures of suspected *C. difficile* carriers (173,174).

Because of the high rate of asymptomatic carriage of *C. difficile* in hospitalized patients, the evaluation of antibiotic-associated colitis must make use of both clinical and laboratory criteria (43,160). One study found that CDAD was associated with a significantly higher mean leukocyte count than was diarrhea of other etiologies (15.8 vs. 7.7/mm^3, p <.01) (175).

There is no role for tests of cure in patients with CDAD. After treatment, high rates of asymptomatic colonization are seen (176). Moreover, despite the uncertain role of the asymptomatic excretor in the transmission of CDAD, attempts to eradicate carriage of *C. difficile* have not been very successful and are not recommended. In one study, the use of metronidazole had no effect on excretion, and vancomycin had only a temporary influence on excretion rates (177). Therefore, the recommended measures to arrest nosocomial outbreaks of CDAD involve the use of contact precautions, glove and gown use, hand washing, and the judicious use of private rooms and cohorting if patient hygiene is poor. Some data suggest that hand washing with chlorhexidine is more effective in eradicating *C. difficile* than plain soap and water (46). For more information on *C. difficile* infections, see Chapter 36. Disinfection with a 1:10 dilution of hypochlorite solution was associated with significant reduction in CDAD in one study (178). Restriction of clindamycin usage has also been associated with significantly lower rates of CDAD (179). An experimental vaccine using inactivated toxin protected hamsters from CDAD in a dose-dependent manner from both diarrhea and death (180). Protection appeared to be due to circulating antitoxin antibodies.

Salmonella

Salmonella species continue to be important causes of nosocomial illness, although in recent years their position has been overshadowed by *C. difficile*. Up to 35% of reported cases of *Salmonella* infection in the U.S. occur in hospitals and extended care facilities (53). *Salmonella* is second only to *S. aureus* as a cause of epidemic illness in the hospital (12) and is responsible for 81% of nursing home deaths from foodborne disease (150). *Salmonella* also causes disease at the other extreme of life (about 50% of the cases of all nosocomial salmonellosis occurring in newborn nurseries and pediatric wards) (181). In contrast to adult infections, which tend to result from ingestion of a contaminated food vehicle, cross-infection plays a major role in the transmission of pediatric infection.

The nomenclature of *Salmonella* is rather confusing and perhaps has led to difficulty in interpreting older epidemiologic data. With the use of such techniques as DNA hybridization, it was appreciated that there was a fundamental homogeneity among the members of the *Salmonella* genus. This phylogenetic similarity prompted many authorities to consider *Salmonella* to be essentially one species (182). Because of variability in antigenic structure and biochemical activity among members of the *Salmonella* species, however, six serogroups were devised (183), with group 1 containing the vast majority of human pathogens. Currently, a more simplified scheme is commonly used. This method uses the serogroup as a species designation. Thus, the *Salmonella* genus is divided into three species: *S. choleraesuis* (one serotype), *S. typhi* (one serotype), and *S. enteritidis* (all of the remaining approximately 2,000 serotypes). Such discussion of taxonomy is worthwhile, as it affects the analysis of secular trends in *Salmonella* disease.

The spectrum of disease caused by *Salmonella* encompasses invasive gastroenteritis, enteric (typhoid) fever, primary bacteremia, and a variety of focal infections (including septic arthritis, osteomyelitis, meningitis, and pleuropulmonary disease). It has been widely held that a relatively large inoculum of *Salmonella* is needed to cause clinical disease. This belief is based on studies of healthy volunteers, in which the lowest inoculum causing overt illness was 10^5 microorganisms (184). In fact, when *Salmonella* outbreaks have been studied, the doses of bacteria received by patients with clinical disease were less than 10^3 microorganisms (185). Many other studies have confirmed that the manifestations of illness due to *Salmonella* result from a complex interplay of microorganism- and host-specific factors. It has been shown that age, intercurrent illnesses such as AIDS, hemoglobinopathies, and malignancies and prior/concurrent antimicrobial use may influence the infective dose of bacteria, illness severity, attack rates, and length of the incubation period. Moreover, *Salmonella* serotypes have heterogeneous virulence properties, which are reflected in varying rates of bacteremia (186).

The overwhelming majority of nosocomial outbreaks due to *Salmonella* have been related to common-source contamination (12). The vehicles identified in these epidemics have included medications, diagnostic agents, blood products, banked human milk, and yeast or raw egg supplementation of enteral feeding formulas. Also connected with outbreaks has been contaminated equipment such as endoscopes (187) and suction apparatuses (53). Food vehicles are most often eggs, poultry, and dairy products.

The role of the asymptomatic excretor of *Salmonella* in the genesis of hospital outbreaks has been controversial. Convalescent shedding of *Salmonella* is very common, occurring for a median of 5 weeks after clinical infection. This period is often extended in patients younger than 5 years and in those infected with serotypes other than *S. typhimurium* (188). Chronic carriage persists for longer than 1 year in less than 1% of patients with nontyphoidal disease and in 1% to 3% of those infected with *S. typhi.* Persistent carriage is seen most commonly in older patients and those with disease of the biliary tract (189).

Although evidence supporting dissemination of *Salmonella* by chronic carriers in the hospital environment is lacking, there is concern regarding this potential method of transmission. The spread of infection from patients who chronically excrete the microorganism can be effectively limited by strict adherence to appropriate isolation precautions (see Chapter 95). It has been shown that *Salmonella* microorganisms are present on the hands of carriers after defecation and that such contamination is eliminated by simple hand washing (190).

The hospital employee who is recovering from *Salmonella* infection is a different matter. Because of the theoretical risk of nosocomial transmission, a hospital employee with patient care and food handling responsibilities should be documented to be free of *Salmonella* before resuming duties. Documentation of clearance of infection can be problematic, as *Salmonella* excretion is often intermittent. Up to 17% of patients can have positive stool cultures after four to nine consecutive negative studies (189). It is also important to note that the use of rectal swabs, instead of stool cultures, has been shown to have greatly reduced sensitivity, with an inability to detect fewer than 10^3 microorganisms/g of feces (191).

Because of the inherent difficulty in documenting *Salmonella* clearance and the unpredictable efficacy of antimicrobial agents in eradicating carriage, the most sensible and cost-effective approach is the universal practice of hand washing by all personnel involved in patient care and food service. Employees with prolonged convalescent carriage should avoid direct contact with patients or food. For these employees, judicious consideration of ampicillin therapy to eliminate carriage can be undertaken. Studies using 4 to 5 g of ampicillin daily for 4 to 6 weeks have been successful in eliminating *Salmonella* from chronic carriers. One study demonstrated a 70% cure rate in 17 chronic carriers without cholelithiasis, but only 23% of patients with biliary stones were rendered free of *Salmonella* (192). Another study using high-dose ampicillin eradicated carriage in 13 (87%) of chronic carriers during a follow-up period of 7 to 54 months (193). Also noteworthy was the prevalence of adverse reactions in the study population, with 53% of patients developing loose stools, 40% rash, and 20% eosinophilia. To circumvent problems of drug intolerance and resistance to ampicillin, agents such as fluoroquinolones have been studied. One study reported that 10 (83%) of 12 patients completing a 4-week course of ciprofloxacin had negative cultures after 1 year (194). Cholecystectomy can be considered for an asymptomatic carrier, but it is a radical option. One study of a foodborne outbreak of salmonellosis affecting 203 nurses failed to demonstrate transmission to patients despite the fact that 77 nurses worked a total of 120 shifts while ill (195). Since none of these infected workers were exposed to neonates or immunosuppressed patients, these populations may still be vulnerable to infected workers.

It is important to recognize that antibiotic use can predispose to prolonged shedding of microorganisms (196) and promote the development of bacterial resistance. Because of the risk of disseminated disease, however, certain patients (neonates, immunosuppressed patients, or those with severe infection) should receive antibiotics. Studies of salmonellosis have found antibiotic therapy to be a significant risk factor for the acquisition of disease (197).

In the developing world, nosocomial salmonellosis is more common. The hospitals in these countries have been recognized as important reservoirs for the development and transmission of multiresistant *Salmonella* (60). *Salmonella* serotypes have developed widespread resistance to ampicillin, and many are resistant to aminoglycosides, chloramphenicol, monobactams, trimethoprim/sulfamethoxazole, and other penicillins. A children's hospital in Buenos Aires, Argentina, found that 70% of its *Salmonella* isolates were resistant to multiple antibiotics. Moreover, 59% of these multiply resistant microorganisms were nosocomially acquired. No difference in strain virulence was evident; disease caused by the resistant isolates was equal in severity to that caused by sensitive strains (198).

Shigella

In contrast to *Salmonella, Shigella* species have rarely been linked to either sporadic or epidemic nosocomial gastroenteritis.

Since *Shigella* microorganisms are among the most communicable of bacterial enteric pathogens, with an infective dose as small as 100 microorganisms (199), it is somewhat paradoxical that shigellosis was found in only 1 of the 3,363 patients reported as having nosocomial gastroenteritis as part of the NNIS system data between 1986 and 1989.

The 40 serotypes of *Shigella* are divided into four groups: group A *(S. dysenteriae)*, group B *(S. flexneri)*, group C *(S. boydii)*, and group D *(S. sonnei)*. The majority of cases of shigellosis in the U.S. are caused by *S. sonnei* followed by *S. flexneri* (200). *Shigella* microorganisms produce disease by invading the intestinal mucosa (201) but rarely penetrate beyond the mucosa. Toxin elaboration plays a secondary role in disease pathogenesis. The Shiga toxin has both enterotoxin and cytotoxin properties (202,203) contributing to mucosal ulceration and microabscess formation. *Shigella* microorganisms are confined to the colon, making prolonged carriage in such protected sites as the biliary tract unusual (204). It may be the rarity of asymptomatic carriage of microorganisms that makes nosocomial shigellosis so rare. Since patients with shigellosis tend to have obvious symptoms, they are placed on appropriate isolation precautions and are appropriately treated (see Chapter 95).

The rare instances of nosocomial *Shigella* infection arise almost exclusively from direct contact. A few small outbreaks have been documented in nurseries (205) and custodial care facilities (206), with transient contamination of the hands of personnel implicated as the primary mode of spread (207). A recent outbreak in a chronic care psychiatric hospital involved 10 patients with dysentery, of whom four died. The outbreak was controlled using isolation, cohort nursing, and an emphasis upon hand hygiene (208). A study done in Nairobi, Kenya, demonstrated the rarity of nosocomial transmission of *Shigella* despite its endemicity in the surrounding community and its concurrent presence in newly admitted patients (209).

As in the case of disease due to *Salmonella*, *Shigella* infections are diagnosed by routine stool culture. Yield is much higher if fresh stool specimens are used and if samples are taken early in the course of illness. Unlike *Salmonella, Shigella* infections should be treated with antimicrobial therapy. The use of such agents as a fluoroquinolone or trimethoprim/sulfamethoxazole will limit fecal excretion of the microorganism and shorten the duration of clinical illness. Given the rarity of nosocomial shigellosis, any case of *Shigella* infection in a hospitalized patient should be scrutinized carefully by infection control personnel.

Campylobacter jejuni

C. jejuni is increasingly recognized as an important cause of invasive gastroenteritis. It is perhaps the most common cause of bacterial diarrhea in the developed world, being more prevalent than *Salmonella* or *Shigella* (210). The microorganism is ubiquitous throughout the animal kingdom and is found among swine, sheep, goats, and cattle in addition to household pets (211). Humans usually acquire the pathogen through the consumption of contaminated meat (212) or dairy products (213,214) or by contact with household pets (e.g., dogs, cats, birds) that may asymptomatically excrete the microorganism (215). Although the majority of GI disease is caused by *C. jejuni*, other species have been reported to cause disease. A number of these microorganisms prominently cause GI symptoms in homosexual men, particularly *C. cinaedi* and *C. fennelliae* (216). *C. fetus* is more often an opportunistic species, causing bacteremia, meningitis, and vascular infections in debilitated hosts.

Infection seems to be mediated by tissue invasion with sites of mucosal injury in the colon, ileum, and jejunum (217). A cytotoxin (218) or heat-labile enterotoxin (219) may also play a role. Clinical disease most commonly takes the form of fever, abdominal cramps, and diarrhea, which can be bloody (220). As with other invasive enteritides, the constellation of symptoms may resemble appendicitis or inflammatory bowel disease. Population studies of age-specific incidence have shown a bimodal peak, with the first in children less than 1 year old and the second in patients 15 to 29 years old (221,222).

Foodborne illness from *C. jejuni* has been documented in nursing homes, with milk the reported vehicle (150). Despite the prevalence of this infection in the community, nosocomial transmission has been documented only rarely, involving a case of bacteremia from a contaminated blood transfusion (223) and vertically transmitted cases of enteritis in neonates (224). The rarity of direct nosocomial transmission between patients may relate to the observation that asymptomatic excretors of *Campylobacter* do not seem to disseminate the disease (225).

Most hospital laboratories can isolate *Campylobacter* using such selective media as Campy-BAP (220) or Skirrow's medium (226). The use of filtration techniques in conjunction with nonselective media at 37°C permits growth of *C. jejuni* as well as other enteric *Campylobacter* species that may be inhibited by the use of selective media and incubation at 42°C (227,228).

Yersinia enterocolitica

Recent decades have brought increased awareness of *Y. enterocolitica* as a potential nosocomial pathogen. Like *C. jejuni, Y. enterocolitica* is a frequent cause of community-acquired gastroenteritis in developed countries, especially in Northern Europe. Over 50 serotypes exist, but most human disease is caused by serotypes O8, O9, O27, and particularly O3 (229). As nonpathogenic serotypes are commonly isolated, it is crucial to serotype any *Y. enterocolitica* strain isolated from clinical specimens to help correlate the pathogen with the illness and to establish any potential connection between cases (230).

Clinical illness usually lasts 1 to 3 weeks and is characterized by fever, abdominal pain, and diarrhea, which can be bloody in 26% of cases (231). Because of prominent involvement of the terminal ileum, the illness may mimic appendicitis (232,233). Tissue invasion occurs, with mucosal ulceration and inflammation of the mesenteric lymph nodes being common (234). Extraintestinal symptoms, consisting of a reactive polyarthritis and/or erythema nodosum, are commonly reported in Scandinavian studies (235,236). Bacteremia occurs most often in patients compromised by such conditions as diabetes mellitus, cirrhosis, iron overload states, and immunosuppression; the mortality rate is 34% (237) to 50% (238).

Vehicles in community outbreaks have been found to be milk (239), tofu packed in spring water (240), chitterlings (241), and bean sprouts packed in well water (242). Most commonly implicated has been food derived from pigs (243). Nosocomial illness has been reported much less commonly. Transfusion of contaminated packed red cells has produced *Y. enterocolitica* sepsis in recent years. Ten cases were documented in nine states, with an overall mortality rate of 70%. When questioned, nearly half of the donors of the contaminated blood had GI symptoms within the 3 weeks prior to donation. All donors had serologic evidence of recent *Yersinia* infection and were asymptomatic at the time of donation (244,245).

Nosocomial gastroenteritis due to *Y. enterocolitica* has been reported but is less severe than the much-publicized cases of blood-borne disease. Only a few clusters of nosocomial cases have been reported since 1973 (246,247). One study by Cannon and Linnemann (248) reported surveillance data for 4 years, and they were able to document five cases acquired in the hospital. These authors confirmed that the source for these infections was most often a patient with community-acquired *Yersinia* and that in each case spread occurred to only one patient. They demonstrated that *Y. enterocolitica* can be transmitted directly only with great difficulty.

Documentation of *Yersinia* infections can be hampered when clinicians do not suspect the microorganism. It can be detected on routine enteric media; yields are increased by using cold enrichment methods (249) or a selective medium such as cefsulodin-triclosan-novobiocin agar (250). Paired serologic tests can document recent infection but are best used to supplement bacteriologic methods. Serologic response is highly variable and depends on the quality of the antigen used, the age and immune status of the patient, the site and duration of infection, and the prevalence of a given serogroup in a community. Thus, interpretation of these tests should be individualized for each case (251).

Escherichia coli

The leading cause of travel-related gastroenteritis, *E. coli*, is a very common cause of noninflammatory diarrhea in developing countries. In addition to the enterotoxigenic *E. coli* (ETEC) microorganisms, which mediate disease through a heat-labile (LT) or heat-stable (ST) enterotoxin (252), there are also enteropathogenic (EPEC) strains that are important causes of childhood diarrhea (253). Enteroinvasive (EIEC) microorganisms can invade cells and produce the clinical picture of dysentery (254). Enterohemorrhagic *E. coli* (EHEC) microorganisms elaborate a Shiga-like verotoxin, resulting in hemorrhagic colitis and an attendant hemolytic-uremic syndrome in 8% to 20% of cases (149,255,256).

The incidence of nosocomial diarrhea due to the pathogenic *E. coli* is thought to be low, although routine testing for such microorganisms is beyond the capabilities of many hospital laboratories. Furthermore, reference laboratories are not often utilized in the evaluation of a sporadic case of diarrhea. Therefore, the incidence of endemic nosocomial diarrhea caused by *E. coli* is not known. In contrast, the documentation of numerous dramatic institutional epidemics serves to illustrate the potential importance of *E. coli* as a nosocomial pathogen.

EPEC serotypes, which produce disease primarily by a plasmid-mediated adhesive process (257), were associated with epidemic infantile diarrhea several decades ago. Dozens of hospital and community outbreaks were attributed to EPEC between 1940 and 1970 (258). Nosocomial infantile diarrhea commonly occurred in newborn nurseries. In the past, outbreaks often had high attack rates and mortality rates of 50% (259). Affected children were usually afebrile, with poor feeding and irritability developing over the course of 3 to 6 days (260). The diarrhea was watery and usually devoid of mucus, pus, or blood. For reasons that some have attributed to changing virulence patterns, improved rehydration practices, or the use of antibiotics, more recent reports have noted a considerably milder illness. Formerly, some children manifested a fulminant course with severe volume depletion, shock, acidosis, and occasional peritonitis, sepsis, and death. Although less severe, modern infantile diarrhea due to EPEC still produces considerable morbidity with a prolonged course of illness and frequent hospitalizations for volume depletion (261).

The typical source of EPEC is the infant who either has acquired the microorganism at delivery or is admitted already infected with the microorganism. Special care nurseries are particularly susceptible to rapid dissemination of EPEC owing to the interaction of crowded conditions and the unique vulnerability of newborns. Neonates may have severe underlying illnesses, immature immune systems, and no protective gut flora. Asymptomatic carriers may be important in nursery transmission. For example, in one outbreak it was shown that 5% of asymptomatic pediatric patients and about one third of antepartum mothers had EPEC in their stool (262). Nosocomial diarrhea due to EPEC continues to afflict the developing countries of South America, Asia, and Africa (263) despite its conspicuous decline in the U.S. and Europe (264).

ETEC has been associated with two known nosocomial outbreaks (265,266). One outbreak lasting 9 months was caused by a heat-stable enterotoxin-producing serotype that was transmitted by contaminated enteral feedings. This particular strain did not cause colonization in adults despite a widespread presence in the special care nursery (263). The epidemic serotype was also remarkable in that genes coding for resistance to multiple antibiotics and for the enterotoxin were found in the same plasmid (267).

Heretofore viewed as a sporadic pathogen, EHEC serotype O157:H7 gained notoriety as the responsible agent in a huge four-state outbreak caused by contaminated fast-food hamburger meat. This outbreak produced illness in over 500 people, with a hemorrhagic colitis that was complicated by hemolytic-uremic syndrome in 40 cases and four deaths (257). It has served as a stark reminder of both the vulnerability of the food supply as well as the need for diligently enforced standards in food hygiene (268).

Although no hospital outbreaks have yet been documented, a number of epidemics have been reported in nursing homes (149,269). One outbreak was especially striking in its attack rate of 32.5% among residents (55 of 169)(149). Twelve of the affected residents developed hemolytic-uremic syndrome (HUS), with 11 deaths. Overall, 19 patients died (case fatality rate of 35%). The epidemic also had a prominent second phase consistent with person-to-person spread characterized by relatively high attack rates among nursing home staff. The detection of indolent outbreaks as well as sporadic cases of EHEC gastroenteritis has been shown to be improved by microscopic evaluation of the stool of all patients with HUS or thrombotic thrombocytopenic purpura (TTP) (270).

Other Gram-Negative Bacteria

In addition to EPEC, other Enterobacteriaceae are known to cause epidemic infantile diarrhea, particularly *Klebsiella* and *Citrobacter* species (271). *Pseudomonas aeruginosa* was suspected to cause an outbreak of antibiotic-associated diarrhea, with two cases responding to cessation of antibiotics and five more requiring specific antipseudomonal therapy before the diarrhea was halted (272). One diarrheal outbreak was caused by multiple species sharing an enterotoxin probably carried on a plasmid or bacteriophage (273). Such occurrences are extraordinary and are rarely uncovered using technology available in most hospital laboratories. *Helicobacter pylori* spreads by a fecal-oral route and severely ill intensive care unit patients and nurses were shown to have significantly higher *H. pylori* seropositivity than did matched controls in one study, suggesting nosocomial transmission (274).

Vibrio Species

Vibrio cholerae is a well-known cause of severe noninflammatory diarrhea, primarily in developing countries. *V. cholerae* has occasionally been linked to common-source epidemics in the developed world, involving contaminated mineral water in Portugal (275) and inadequately cooked shellfish in Italy (276). In the U.S., sporadic cases of cholera have been seen, primarily in the Gulf Coast region (277). Disease caused by the halophilic *V. parahaemolyticus* is most often a self-limited illness that follows ingestion of inadequately cooked seafood or food rinsed in seawater (278). Neither of these pathogenic *Vibrio* species has been implicated as causes of nosocomial gastroenteritis.

Aeromonas Species

These species are recognized as GI pathogens (279). They appear unlikely to cause disease in healthy adults; in volunteer studies, even large doses of microorganisms did not cause illness (280). Pathogenetic mechanisms by which *Aeromonas* species cause disease include a heat-labile cytotoxic enterotoxin (281), another enterotoxin that cross-reacts with cholera toxin (282), and mucosal invasion (283).

Geographic and seasonal variability in the microorganism's isolation rates is significant (284,285). For example, *Aeromonas* species were isolated from 52.8% of Peruvian infants hospitalized with diarrhea and from only 8.7% of control subjects (286). In contrast, another study examined Brazilian children and did not isolate *Aeromonas* in a single culture (287). In Australia, *Aeromonas* species are second only to rotavirus as a cause of sporadic childhood diarrhea (288).

Aeromonas species are ubiquitous inhabitants of water (288); the relationship between the recent ingestion of untreated water and development of infection is strong (289). The seasonal variability of *Aeromonas* infection rates has been closely correlated, with the frequency of isolation of the microorganism from community water sources peaking in the summer months (290).

Isolation of *Aeromonas* species from hospital water sources (291) suggests the potential for nosocomial epidemics. Reports of nosocomial outbreaks, however, have been sparse. One such cluster involved respiratory colonization and resultant pneumonia or extrapulmonary infections (not diarrhea) in 19 patients (292). Another apparent outbreak of *Aeromonas* occurred in a nursing home where 17 patients developed a brief illness of nonbloody diarrhea over a 3-day period (293). Of the 11 cultures submitted, four yielded *A. hydrophila*. Unfortunately, these cultures were not tested for the presence of a toxin, and in neither outbreak was a common source identified.

Laboratory screening and isolation techniques are necessary to adequately define the scope of disease caused by this pathogen. Since *Aeromonas* species usually grow well on routine enteric media, it is probably simplest to screen colonies with an oxidase test. This avoids confusing these facultatively anaerobic gram-negative rods with Enterobacteriaceae on nonselective media (294). The use of a selective media such as blood agar supplemented with cefsulodin-irgasan-novobiocin (CIN) agar can also be considered (284).

Staphylococci

Staphylococcal foodborne disease has occurred commonly in the institutional setting. Outbreaks due to *S. aureus* accounted for 8% of all hospital foodborne outbreaks and 23% of those in nursing homes reported to the CDC during the years 1975 to 1987 (148). The illness, characterized by the acute onset of nausea, vomiting, and subsequent diarrhea 2 to 6 hours after ingestion of the offending food, is mediated by a heat-stable enterotoxin (Table 24.6). Toxigenic strains of *S. aureus* may elaborate any one of five immunologically unique (A, B, C, D, E) toxins (295) that appear to act through stimulation of the area postrema in the medulla, which is likely mediated by the toxin's interaction with afferent nerve endings in the abdominal viscera (296). The very short incubation period attests to the preformed nature of the toxin, with the incubation period inversely proportional to the toxin load ingested.

The illness usually runs its course in about 8 hours. Mortality is rare, with a 0.4% case-fatality rate in the CDC nursing home survey (150). Morbidity, on the other hand, can be significant, with hospitalization rates as high as 8% (150). This morbidity results from rapid volume depletion and electrolyte derangements due to severe vomiting.

Epidemics of staphylococcal food poisoning begin with a food handler harboring *S. aureus* on the hands, usually from a skin infection. If food prepared by the carrier is stored at an improper temperature or is not served in a timely manner, foodborne staphylococcal disease can result. This sequence can be interrupted by (a) meticulous attention to employee hygiene with hand washing, the use of gloves, or the exclusion of food handlers with skin infections; (b) proper refrigeration of foods at temperatures less than 4°C, especially after partial cooking (297); and (c) rapid serving of food kept at room temperature.

In the last decade, methicillin-resistant *S. aureus* (MRSA) and coagulase-negative staphylococci have received widespread

TABLE 24.6. GASTROINTESTINAL TOXINS

Microorganism	Toxin	Thermal Stability
Preformed toxins		
Staphylococcus aureus	Neurotoxin	Stable
Bacillus cereus (short incubation)	Emetic neurotoxin	Stable
Clostridium botulinum	Neurotoxin (A, B, E)	Labile
Toxins produced in vivo		
Bacillus cereus (long incubation)	Enterotoxin	Labile
Clostridium perfringens	Enterotoxin	Labile
Clostridium difficile	Enterotoxin/cytotoxin	Labile (cytotoxin)
Salmonella	?Enterotoxin	Stable
Shigella	Enterotoxin/cytotoxin	Labile
Campylobacter jejunl	Enterotoxin/cytotoxin	Labile
Yersinia enterocolitica	Enterotoxin	Stable
ETEC	Enterotoxins; heat-labile, heat-stable	Both stable and labile toxins
EPEC	?Cytotoxin (Shiga-like toxin)	Labile
EHEC	Verotoxin	Labile
Aeromonas spp.	Enterotoxin	Labile
Listeria monocytogenes	Hemolysin	Stable—both heat and cold

ETEC, enterotoxigenic *Escherichia coli*; EPEC, enteropathogenic *E. coli*; EHEC, enterohemorrhagic *E. coli*.

attention as increasingly important nosocomial pathogens. Despite a reputation as primarily a bloodstream and wound pathogen, MRSA has been implicated as a cause of antibiotic-associated diarrhea in a few reports (298).

Listeria monocytogenes

L. monocytogenes is a motile, non–spore-forming, gram-positive rod that is found ubiquitously in the environment and among animals (299). Approximately 20% of sporadic cases (299,300) and many large outbreaks have been traced to contaminated food. Common sources of major outbreaks have been pasteurized milk (301), cheese (302), cole slaw (303), and undercooked meats (300). It also has been frequently isolated from commercially prepared foods intended for instant use, with a number of products recalled or not released as a result (304).

The spectrum of illness caused by *Listeria* is broad, ranging from transient asymptomatic carriage (299) to a sepsis syndrome and meningoencephalitis (305). Infection in pregnancy is frequent, accounting for one third of all patients affected with listeriosis in a large British survey (306). Most commonly occurring in the third trimester, listeriosis manifests as a nonspecific febrile illness. *In utero* transmission of the microorganism can have trivial effects in some cases (307). The resulting infection of the fetus, however, can have potentially devastating consequences for the infant: stillbirth, prematurity, neonatal sepsis/meningitis, and granulomatosis infantisepticum (306). *Listeria* can also present in immunocompromised patients as a focal process, such as ocular infection (308), arthritis (309), or peritonitis (310), but is usually a result of bacteremia. The reporting of GI symptoms prior to the development of invasive listeriosis has caused many to speculate that either the microorganism itself or a co-infecting pathogen may damage the intestinal mucosa, permitting the invasion of *Listeria* (311).

Although infection can be inapparent in normal hosts, those who are immunocompromised are much more likely to manifest overt illness (312). Thus, most often and most severely affected are pregnant women; neonates (306); those with diabetes mellitus, renal failure, or underlying malignancy (313); AIDS patients (314); cirrhotics (315); and those on immunosuppressive agents, particularly transplant recipients (316). The microorganism primarily affects the immunocompromised, with only 10% to 30% of patients having no identified predisposing condition (305). Despite point prevalence gut colonization rates of 0.6% to 16% in the general population and longitudinal studies showing transient carriage occurring in 70% of people (317), invasive disease is exceedingly rare, with a risk for adults of 0.5/100,000 persons (304).

Hospital-associated outbreaks of listeriosis have been described. One outbreak in 1979 involved 20 patients in eight Boston-area hospitals and was traced to raw vegetables. Ten of these patients were immunosuppressed (318). Another epidemic in a Costa Rican nursery was unique in that the index case involved an infant with neonatal listeriosis; cross-infection occurred when a bottle of mineral oil became contaminated and was used on other infants (319). Although *L. monocytogenes* is not associated with gastroenteritis, it is worthwhile to note that no other foodborne illness has a higher case-fatality rate: nonperinatal cases reported from a nationwide survey in 1986 had a case-fatality rate of 35% (304).

A feature of *L. monocytogenes* that is particularly troubling to the food industry is its thermal resistance, requiring temperatures of at least 70°C for killing of the microorganism (299). The agent can also grow at temperatures near the freezing point, which allows for cold enrichment techniques and facilitates its isolation in the microbiology laboratory (299). Utilization of appropriate isolation techniques, awareness of the importance of *L. monocytogenes* as an opportunistic pathogen, and proper interpretation of diphtheroids in cultures of normally sterile body sites all should combine to enhance detection of this potentially serious pathogen. Person-to-person transmission of infection has yet to be firmly documented, with a few reports of small outbreaks suggesting spread by fomites or hospital workers

(320). Nosocomial outbreaks should be investigated with a subtyping technique, such as multilocus enzyme electrophoresis (321), in addition to serotyping.

Clostridium perfringens

C. perfringens is another important cause of foodborne GI disease. According to CDC data, nosocomial gastroenteritis due to *C. perfringens* is common, constituting the third most frequently reported foodborne illness in hospitals and nursing homes (148). It is characterized by diarrhea and abdominal cramps, usually with minimal systemic toxicity. The clinical syndrome, which follows an incubation period of 6 to 24 hours, lasts up to 24 hours and resolves without therapy (322). Despite the self-limited nature of the illness, deaths have been reported (147).

A heat-labile enterotoxin, which is a structural component of the spore coat of type A strains of *C. perfringens* (322), produces the clinical symptoms by binding to the intestinal brush border (323). This enterotoxin has also been found in type C and type D strains (324). Diarrhea is produced by toxin induction of fluid secretion into the intestinal lumen as well as cytopathic effects on the epithelium (323). Toxin is only released during sporulation and not during vegetative growth of the microorganism (325).

Toxigenic strains of *C. perfringens* have been isolated from meats, stews, poultry, gravies, and meat pies (326) that became contaminated during prolonged cooling and storage at room temperature (327). The spores are heat stable, able to survive the cooking process, and germinate with cooling. Their optimal growth in meat is achieved at a temperature of 43° to 47°C (326). Thus, the food-handling error most likely to favor the growth of *C. perfringens* is the storage of food at inappropriate temperatures. Cooked foods must be refrigerated promptly at a temperature of no greater than 4°C, and if reheated, cooked to a temperature of at least 100°C, which will inactivate the majority of *C. perfringens* vegetative bacteria after germination of spores due to inadequate refrigeration (328).

A variety of other syndromes have been associated with *C. perfringens* beyond foodborne gastroenteritis. Sporadic diarrhea unrelated to ingestion of contaminated food has been reported. The resultant illness has a more prolonged clinical course similar to that of *Salmonella* or *Campylobacter* species (329). Cases of antibiotic-associated diarrhea have also been cited (330). *C. perfringens* (126) and *C. butyricum* (127) have been implicated in the pathogenesis of NEC. Moreover, it was the finding that *C. perfringens* type C was the etiologic agent in pigbel (331) (a syndrome of necrotizing enteritis described in highland natives of New Guinea that classically occurs after ritual consumption of a large pork meal) that prompted the notion that NEC may in fact be caused by a bacterial toxin.

Viruses

Rotavirus

In many of the countries of Latin America, Africa, and Asia, diarrheal diseases may cause half of the deaths in children under the age of 5 (332), an age group with an overall mortality rate of approximately 15% (333). Rotavirus is the major etiologic agent of childhood diarrhea and an important cause of mortality in this age group in developing nations. Mortality from diarrhea in developed countries is rare, but 35% of pediatric hospital admissions for gastroenteritis are due to rotavirus (334). The attack rate for children is highest between 6 months and 2 years of age, with 62% of children having had at least one infection by 2 years (335). Hospitalization rates for children are as high as 8.5 admissions/1,000 children (336).

The typical clinical syndrome is the sudden onset of vomiting and fever followed by diarrhea. The diarrhea is usually watery without blood or leukocytes. Associated features may include irritability and pharyngeal erythema. Upper respiratory tract symptoms, although frequently seen in some studies (335), have not been confirmed in others (337). Following an incubation period of 48 to 72 hours, symptoms last from 6 to 9 days. The fever and vomiting generally resolve within 2 days, and the diarrhea within 8 days (4). Shedding of virus in the feces is seen between the third and eighth days of illness. Any age group can have clinically inapparent infection, but children aged 6 to 24 months are most likely to have overt symptoms. Adult infection is usually asymptomatic (338).

The rotaviruses belong to the family Reoviridae and consist of double-stranded RNA enclosed in a double capsid. The intact particle is 70 nm in diameter and is recognized by its wheel (Latin: *rota*) shape. Group A rotaviruses are the archetypal rotaviruses and possess a group-specific common antigen VP6, an inner capsid protein. Group A viruses are responsible for the vast majority of human disease worldwide. Cases of gastroenteritis due to non–group A viruses have been described mostly in China (339). The mechanism whereby rotaviruses cause clinical illness has not been completely clarified. Infection of the small intestinal villous cells seems to occur, which results in a net secretion of fluid. The physical shortening of these villi and crypt hyperplasia can lead to a mild malabsorption. The colon is spared from this process (340). Infected patients may excrete high viral loads; concentrations of 1,012 microorganisms/g of feces have been described (341).

The environmental stability of the rotavirus has been demonstrated by its persistence for up to 10 days on inanimate surfaces (342). Contaminated communal toys were suspected to cause one outbreak on a pediatric ward (343). A simian rotavirus can resist acid and alkaline exposures, freeze-thawing, ether, and chloroform (344), as well as such commonly used antiseptics as chlorhexidine (345). The most effective disinfectant agent has been found to be 95% ethanol (346); glutaraldehyde and povidone-iodine also are useful (345).

Rotavirus is highly contagious. Studies in households show a 40% seroconversion rate among parents of children with rotavirus gastroenteritis (347). One survey performed in a children's hospital found rotavirus to be second only to *S. aureus* as the most common nosocomial pathogen isolated (5). The importance of rotavirus as a nosocomial pathogen was not recognized until the 1970s, when the development of electron microscopy allowed diarrheal illness to be correlated with demonstration of the virus in stool specimens. The initial series of outbreaks was reported from nurseries in England (348), Australia (349), and the U.S. (350). Many of these accounts described high attack rates, with only a fraction of infected infants having overt symptoms. Breast-fed infants were significantly less likely to acquire rotavirus infection and to have symptoms, if infected, in one study (351). Transmission has been postulated to be horizontal, as rotavirus has been demonstrated in the hand washings of asymptomatic caregivers of patients with diarrhea (352). Ungloved nasogastric feedings were found to be a significant risk factor [odds ratio (OR) = 8.8] in one recent study (353). Underscoring the importance of person-to-person spread, several studies have shown that cohorting infected patients and caregivers can terminate an outbreak (350,354). One study failed to show efficacy with the use of early screening of symptomatic patients with enzyme-linked immunosorbent assay (ELISA) testing and isolation. This study compared rates of transmission from cases of rotavirus infection identified during two separate 5-week surveillance periods. The first was in 1984, before the introduction of rapid testing, when 11 admitted children had rotavirus in their stools. The second period was in 1986 after the introduction of ELISA testing for rotavirus. During that period, 12 children with rotavirus infection were hospitalized. No difference in rates of nosocomial transmission of rotavirus was detected in this small study (355).

Prevention measures should center on patients newly admitted; diarrhea has been shown to be the most important source of nosocomial rotavirus outbreaks (356). Other efforts might include reinforcement of hygienic practices among hospital staff, who have been implicated in nosocomial spread of rotavirus (350). A recent randomized trial showed a significantly lower rate of symptomatic rotavirus diarrhea among infants and toddlers receiving lactobacillus than those receiving placebo (357).

Speculation has been raised about the potential for aerosol spread (358,359), but firm data are lacking. The frequency of simultaneous respiratory symptoms with rotavirus gastroenteritis suggests the need for further investigation of this possible mode of transmission.

Nosocomial rotavirus gastroenteritis has been documented in adults, with multiple outbreaks reported among elderly patients (354,360). One particular outbreak affected 19 of 34 patients, with six severe cases of gastroenteritis and two deaths (361). Yolken et al. (14) studied adult bone marrow transplant recipients and found that 9 of 31 patients with infectious diarrhea had disease due to rotavirus. Other studies have found this virus to be the etiologic agent in 1% to 4% of cases of nosocomial gastroenteritis in adults (262).

In some populations, rotavirus infection may be more severe than the largely uncomplicated gastroenteritis. Patients with immunodeficiencies may manifest a chronic symptomatic diarrhea with prolonged viral shedding (362). The potential for more severe illness is present for the elderly (361) and for transplant recipients (14,363), with frequent prolonged viral shedding (363).

The epidemiologic study of rotavirus has been greatly facilitated by advances in diagnostic technologies. First, case-finding has been made rapid, inexpensive, and technically simple with the use of ELISA testing. These commercially available kits are widely used to detect rotavirus inner capsid antigen in stools with a sensitivity early in the course of illness equal to that of virus isolation and visualization by electron microscopy (364). Latex agglutination tests, although less sensitive than ELISA (365), are also rapid and readily available. The use of PCR to detect rotavirus antigen has been successful at concentrations 1,000 times lower than those used for electron microscopy and immunoassay techniques (366).

Second, techniques such as polyacrylamide gel electrophoresis (PAGE) have been used to distinguish different strains of rotavirus. PAGE relies on differences in the migration patterns of the RNA segments in the virus genome to define strains and is known as electropherotyping. It is a powerful method for the analysis of outbreaks (367,368). Its ability to classify rotaviruses or analyze microorganisms over time or in widely separated outbreaks is hampered by the finding that a given electropherotype does not always correlate with DNA hybridization patterns or serotype (369,370). Despite these limitations, electropherotyping can be used to study individual outbreaks and has shown infant-to-infant transmission with involvement of multiple strains in an outbreak (371). A Japanese study characterized an outbreak with an initial predominance of one electropherotype with subsequent development of highly variable RNA segments by PAGE (372), suggesting that a rotavirus strain may evolve during an epidemic either by genetic reassortment (antigenic drift) or by introduction of other strains with multiple infections.

Control of nosocomial rotavirus infections depends on the conscientious use of good hygienic practices on the hospital wards, strict hand washing, prompt institution of appropriate isolation precautions in patients with diarrhea (see Chapter 95), and cohorting of affected patients. Vaccine development is still in progress. In 1998, a tetravalent rhesus–human reassortment vaccine was licensed in the U.S., but withdrawn within a year because of intussusception in about one of every 10,000 recipients (373). Both attenuated animal and reassortment vaccine types have shown promise but have yielded uneven results in clinical trials. Randomized trial efficacy with different vaccines has ranged from 0% to 100% (374) (see also Chapter 50), with lower efficacy generally being seen in developing countries perhaps due to genetic diversity of strains in different geographical areas (375,376).

Norwalk and Related Agents

A syndrome of acute nausea and vomiting that occurs in children and adults is common during winter months in temperate climates. This illness tends to cluster in families, most often affecting children 1 to 10 years old. Until quite recently, this illness had no known etiology; hence it was given the label "winter vomiting disease" (377).

Analysis of a very large outbreak of winter vomiting disease in Norwalk, Ohio (378), revealed the first of a family of small (20- to 35-nm), round, structured viral agents that are now known to cause gastroenteritis (379). Many of these viruses have been named for the location of their initial isolation. This expanding family of viruses has been grouped into four classes (380), with nosocomial infections known to have been caused by agents of the first three: (a) Norwalk-like viruses (including the Norwalk or Montgomery County agent, Hawaii, Snow Mountain, and Taunton agents); (b) calciviruses [although recent genomic analysis suggests that the Norwalk agent may, in fact, be a calcivirus (381)]; (c) astroviruses (including the Marin County agent); and (d) other poorly characterized small round viruses (including the Wollan, Ditchling, Cockle, Paramatta, and other agents). Of the outbreaks of acute nonbacterial gastroenteritis investigated by the CDC during the years 1976 to 1981, 42% were due to the Norwalk and related agents (382).

These viruses generally are identified by immune electron microscopy or paired serology. Other methods have been developed, such as an ELISA (383) and PCR (384) for the Norwalk agent and an ELISA for both the calciviruses (385) and astroviruses (386), but routine use is limited by availability of reagents.

The typical clinical picture is an acute onset of nausea, vomiting, and watery diarrhea that lasts about 24 hours (382). Incubation periods vary between 24 and 48 hours, with viral shedding continuing for about 24 hours after cessation of symptoms. Biopsies taken from experimentally infected volunteers have shown small-bowel villus destruction and transient depletion of mucosal enzymes (387).

Most epidemics of Norwalk-related gastroenteritis have had a common source, such as contaminated drinking water (388), shellfish (382), or salad (389). Nosocomial epidemics have been documented most frequently in nursing homes, with investigation of an outbreak in an extended care facility first identifying the Marin County agent (390). Another outbreak in an Alabama nursing home was noteworthy for its documentation of an attack rate of 64% among 120 residents and 29% among staff members (391). Substantial morbidity was also evident, with nine (12%) of the ill residents requiring hospitalization and two dying. Unfortunately, stool samples were not obtained, and a common source for the outbreak was not established. Other nosocomial outbreaks appeared to be spread by person-to-person transmission (392). In another outbreak in an emergency department, investigators found several affected patients and staff who had no history of direct contact with other ill patients and hypothesized that the moving of contaminated laundry contributed to the dissemination of viral particles (65). An aerosol route was proposed in this as well as another nursing home outbreak (64), but this mode of transmission for gastroenteritis remains unproven.

Epidemiologic study of these entities is currently very difficult. Routine testing for them is not routinely performed in clinical laboratories. Therefore, the detection of either incipient outbreaks or sporadic cases without specific prospective surveillance is nearly impossible. Furthermore, outbreaks must be investigated rapidly, since the illness is brief, and stool and blood must be obtained while symptoms are present and processed promptly for accurate evaluation using immune electron microscopy or serology (393) (see also Chapter 50).

Adenovirus

Since 1975, when they were first seen by electron microscopy in the stools of infants with diarrhea (394), adenoviruses have been firmly linked to childhood enteric disease (395). Strains linked to gastroenteritis are called enteric adenoviruses and belong to serogroups 40 and 41 (396). These strains are often called uncultivatable adenoviruses, because they are easily seen using electron microscopy but are fastidious in their growth requirements in cell cultures.

For children under 2 years old, only rotavirus is a more common cause of gastroenteritis (397,398). Serum antibodies that indicate prior infection are present in 50% of children by age 4 (399). In contrast to rotavirus, infection rates have no seasonal variation (398,400). Transmission of the virus appears to be person to person (393), with secondary spread to adults uncommonly seen (398,400). Long-term immunity is thought to be conferred by infection.

Clinical illness follows an incubation period of 8 to 10 days, with symptoms of watery diarrhea lasting about 8 days (401, 402). Vomiting and fever are seen in over half of patients but subside within 2 days of onset. In one series, respiratory symptoms were noted in 27% of patients (400). Another prospective study found that 46% of infected children were asymptomatic (397).

Nosocomial acquisition of adenovirus has been reported. A report by Flewett et al. (394) described a diarrheal illness lasting 24 to 48 hours in six of 19 children in a pediatric ward and in one nurse working on the ward. Adenovirus-like particles were evident by electron microscopy in four of the six children and in the nurse but in none of the asymptomatic children. Yolken et al. (401) found evidence of adenovirus in the stools of 14 (52%) of 27 hospitalized infants with gastroenteritis, with 13 of 14 (93%) of these affected patients having concurrent respiratory symptoms. Five of the 14 children were not excreting adenovirus at the time of admission, suggesting nosocomial acquisition. Only 1 (1.4%) of 72 asymptomatic children had adenovirus detectable on stool examination. Another prospective study of children less than 2 years old found that adenovirus caused 6.2% of cases of nosocomial diarrhea and was the third most common etiology of nosocomial diarrhea (402). A study of bone marrow transplant recipients, whose average age was 21 years, found adenovirus to be as common as *C. difficile* as a cause of gastroenteritis and associated with a 45% mortality rate (14).

The diagnosis of enteric adenovirus infection has historically been made by electron microscopy. Newer techniques include immune electron microscopy to detect serotypes 40 and 41 (403), DNA hybridization (404,405), and a commercially available EIA (406). These methods, many of which possess the necessary sensitivity, specificity, and ease of use to make wide-scale testing possible, should address a number of unanswered questions.

Other viruses have been associated with nosocomial gastroenteritis. They include coronaviruses, echoviruses, and coxsackieviruses. These agents have been primarily linked to outbreaks in infants (see also Chapter 50). Human torovirus has also been reported to cause nosocomial infections associated with less vomiting but more bloody diarrhea than were control patients with rotavirus or astrovirus infections (407).

Candida Species

Determining the role of *Candida* in GI disease has been hindered by its identity as a human commensal and its presence in approximately 65% of stool specimens from healthy persons (408). Nonetheless, awareness of its potential to cause serious nosocomial disease has heightened in the last decade. Now the syndromes of esophageal candidiasis and invasive enteritis have been recognized as consequences of the widespread use of immunosuppressive and cytotoxic therapy as well as of the spread of the AIDS epidemic. GI involvement with *Candida* assumes one of two forms: (a) invasive enteric disease in immunocompromised hosts, and (b) a noninvasive overgrowth syndrome (409).

Invasive candidiasis of the GI tract, with frequent secondary candidemia, may occur in the hospital setting in patients who are neutropenic (38) or who are receiving corticosteroids, chemotherapy, and broad-spectrum antibiotics (39). Autopsies show that the esophagus is the most commonly affected site, followed by the stomach and the small intestine (36). Esophageal involvement is usually suggested by the development of odynophagia, dysphagia, or retrosternal chest pain prompting evaluation by endoscopy or barium studies (410). Endoscopic examination usually reveals white plaques with erosions and ulcerations, often with pseudomembrane formation (36). In these immunosuppressed patients, early evaluation of these complaints is warranted, as endoscopy and biopsy are often needed to exclude other causes of erosive upper GI tract disease such as herpesvirus infection. The esophagitis commonly found in AIDS patients typically has its onset in the community setting. Invasive candidiasis of the small and large intestines more often presents in an occult manner and eludes early diagnosis, usually with only fever and positive blood cultures for *Candida*.

It has been shown in case-control studies that peripheral colonization with *Candida* is associated with the development of candidemia (38,39), with an attendant mortality rate of 38% (411). The use of restriction endonuclease digestion techniques to digest fungal DNA has demonstrated that antecedent colonizing strains are identical to those subsequently found in blood (412). This hematogenous seeding has been postulated to occur by fungal penetration through GI tract mucosa (413).

A syndrome of watery diarrhea associated with *Candida* overgrowth without invasion has been described in hospitalized patients (414). The mechanism by which *Candida* produces diarrhea is subject to speculation, with some proposing a toxin-mediated process (415) and others suggesting diminished brush border enzyme activity in the small intestine (416). Nonetheless, in neonates (417) and debilitated patients (414) in whom this condition has been described, there has been no endoscopic evidence of invasion. In addition, the diarrhea has uniformly responded to oral nystatin in two studies (414,418).

Although currently only available as a research tool, serotyping methods for *Candida* may be able to define modes of nosocomial acquisition and spread (419). Doebbling et al. (420) applied the method of contour-clamped homogeneous electric field electrophoresis to demonstrate hand carriage of *Candida* in healthcare personnel, suggesting the potential for direct spread of this microorganism. Other methods have employed combinations of DNA fingerprinting and biotyping and have shown excellent discriminatory capabilities in clinical specimens (421). Unfortunately, rapid and accurate diagnosis of invasive candidiasis is still problematic, usually requiring blood culture and biopsy. Efforts to develop rapid testing for *Candida* species, using EIA to detect either cell wall (422) or cytoplasmic (423) antigens, have shown some promise in high-risk groups. However, they have demonstrated poor specificity and positive predictive value in lower-risk patients (424) (see also Chapter 39).

Protozoa

Cryptosporidium

Cryptosporidium was first described as a human pathogen in 1976 by two separate investigators (425,426). It causes severe intractable diarrhea in AIDS patients and a less severe disease in normal hosts (427). Community acquisition has been shown to occur through contact with infected animals and humans as well as through ingestion of contaminated water (428). Nosocomial transmission has been documented to occur between patients and from infected patients to hospital personnel (429–432). In one particular outbreak, all six patients in a bone marrow transplantation unit developed cryptosporidiosis. This occurred after one of the recently admitted patients had shared a room with a patient who had diarrhea on another unit (430). Nosocomial spread of *Cryptosporidium* to roommates with AIDS was not found in a retrospective cohort study, however (433).

Cryptosporidium oocysts are extremely hardy in the environment. They resist the chlorination present in public water supplies and can withstand the effects of many commonly used disinfectants such as 3% hypochlorite, iodophors, and 5% formaldehyde. Heat (65°C for 30 minutes) and 10% formalin with either 5% ammonia or bleach appear to inactivate the microorganism (428,434).

As noted above, both the severity and duration of illness vary with immune status (435). Following an incubation period of 2 to 14 days, immunologically normal patients develop watery diarrhea and cramping abdominal pain, which are exacerbated by food intake (436). These symptoms are often fulminant at onset but usually resolve within 1 to 2 weeks. In this population, fecal shedding of oocysts can persist after resolution of the clinical syndrome but usually clears within 2 weeks of resolution of symptoms (437).

In patients with impaired immune function, cryptosporidiosis takes on a much different form. The illness may begin very subtly. Particularly with AIDS patients, the disease may accelerate with progressive deterioration of the immune system. This may culminate in a chronic voluminous diarrhea (stool outputs up to 20 L/day), anorexia, wasting, and abdominal pain. These patients often experience such complications as volume depletion, electrolyte abnormalities, and biliary tract disease (436,438). Very effective therapy is not yet available, but some patients respond to highly active antiretroviral therapy with resolution of diarrhea. Those who do not respond have been treated with paromomycin, azithromycin, or nitazoxanide with moderate effects (439–443).

Currently, the identification of cryptosporidial oocysts by clinical laboratories is most easily done by direct examination of stool using a Kinyoun acid-fast stain (444,445). Multiple studies should be performed, as it is known that oocyst shedding can be intermittent (437). Alternatively, an EIA kit is available that uses a monoclonal antibody to the oocyst wall; this kit showed a sensitivity and specificity of 100% in one study when compared with immunofluorescence (446). A concentration technique (447) may be used to evaluate a nosocomial case to detect a rare oocyst in an environmental sample or a stool specimen from a contact of a patient with cryptosporidiosis. In broad-based epidemiologic studies, serologic methods are available, such as ELISA, which has a 95% sensitivity when both IgM and IgG antibodies are used (448). Efforts to control nosocomial spread depend on identification of infected patients and appropriate isolation precautions (see Chapter 95).

Entamoeba histolytica

Despite being known as a cause of diarrhea in custodial institutions (449) and in AIDS patients (450), *Entamoeba histolytica* is not a common nosocomial pathogen. One outbreak of amebiasis, however, was traced to an inadequately disinfected colonic irrigation machine in the office of a chiropractor. Thirty-six cases of the illness were reported in a 30-month period, with six deaths (451). Nosocomial amebiasis has been reported in developing countries (13). In most cases, infection seemed to be a reactivation process, as no risk factors could be identified by logistic regression analysis. Moreover, no clustering of cases was evident. The majority of affected patients had received corticosteroids or chemotherapy, perhaps allowing reactivation of latent infection by depression of cell-mediated immunity. Horizontal transmission could not be demonstrated.

In rare instances of suspected nosocomial transmission of *E. histolytica,* the newly developed techniques of DNA hybridization (452) and PCR (453) may be of value in studying the epidemiology of this microorganism.

Giardia lamblia

Giardia lamblia is the most commonly isolated intestinal parasite in the U.S. and has been responsible for massive community outbreaks. In the years between 1965 and 1984, this pathogen contaminated inadequately maintained municipal water systems and caused 90 documented epidemics that affected over 23,000 people (454,455). *G. lamblia* has also gained notoriety for causing outbreaks of diarrhea in day-care centers (456) and custodial institutions (457), as well as one outbreak in a nursing home (458). In the community setting, giardiasis is most commonly acquired by ingestion of cysts in contaminated water. Direct person-to-person transmission is the second most common mode of spread. *Giardia* cysts can be found on inanimate surfaces (459) and are resistant to many disinfectants (460), which could lead to indirect transmission.

Infection with *Giardia* occurs after an incubation period of 7 to 14 days and may be manifested by asymptomatic cyst passage, an acute diarrheal illness, or a chronic malabsorption syndrome with attendant diarrhea, weight loss, and abdominal pain (461). The proposed mechanisms for the disease manifestations include disruption of the intestinal brush border (462) and brush border enzyme deficiencies (463).

Asymptomatic cyst passage for up to 6 months has been demonstrated in children attending day-care centers (456). In these settings, prevalence studies have shown that up to 50% of children less than 3 years old asymptomatically pass cysts. Other investigators have shown that 25% of family members of children attending day care had evidence of *Giardia* infection (464). Hand washing has been shown to effectively arrest dissemination of this parasite in the day-care environment (465).

The diagnosis of giardiasis is most easily made by direct examination of a stool for trophozoites or cysts. Either a saline wet-mount of a fresh specimen or a stained (trichrome or hematoxylin) preserved specimen can be examined microscopically. It has been reported that the use of a concentration method can increase the yield such that, after three negative stool examinations, the diagnosis of giardiasis can be excluded (466). Nonetheless, if stool examination is negative after three samples and clinical suspicion remains high, sampling of the duodenum should be considered. This can be done by either a string test (Entero-Test) (467), aspiration of duodenal fluid, or endoscopy with duodenal brushings or biopsy (468). An ELISA test has been developed that can detect *Giardia* in stool with sensitivity and specificity of over 90% (469). This rapid objective test, coupled with the use of PCR to classify subgroups of *G. lamblia* (470), should facilitate epidemiologic study.

PREVENTION OF NOSOCOMIAL GASTROENTERITIS

The avoidance of GI infections in hospitalized patients rests on the recognition that transmission occurs by the fecal-oral route. It may be spread to others by direct physical contact, indirectly on the hands of healthcare workers, or by contact with contaminated environmental surfaces. Nosocomial acquisition of GI pathogens may also occur through a common source: contaminated food, water, medication, or equipment. Prevention and control strategies require awareness of these multiple modes of transmission.

Routine hand washing between patients and use of appropriate isolation precautions must be followed by each hospital employee. Although implemented to prevent employee infection by blood-borne viral agents, universal precautions (471) have been shown to reduce nosocomial transmission of agents such as *C. difficile.* A study by Johnson et al. (47) found an 80% relative reduction in the incidence of *C. difficile*–associated diarrhea after an intensive employee educational intervention that urged the use of gloves for contact with all moist body substances. Meticulous hand washing after all patient contacts (472) and changing gloves between patients should be reinforced (473). Programs in this area need to improve hand washing compliance rates that have been measured to be 40% in intensive care units (474) and address the perception of many hospital workers that they are correctly following hand washing procedures despite actual poor compliance with hygienic practices (475).

One particularly troublesome part of employee education involves the maintenance of good personal health and hygienic practices on the part of the individual. The Study on the Efficacy of Nosocomial Infection Control (SENIC) project evaluated the perceptions of hospital employees regarding their own illnesses (476). In many hospitals, it was found that infection control professionals had very little authority to require that employees with contagious illnesses be removed from patient contact. Of note was their finding that 68% of staff nurses felt that they should come to work with diarrhea; 4% thought that they should work with a sore throat and fever. Nosocomial outbreaks of gastroenteritis due to Norwalk-like agents have been linked to employees working while symptomatic with diarrhea (67). The frequent short duration of diarrheal illnesses makes it likely that a symptomatic employee can transmit the illness at work and then experience remission of symptoms without the awareness of supervisory or infection control personnel. Thus, an active role for a hospital's employee health service can be envisioned, perhaps in conjunction with members of the infection control team (see Chapter 99). Not only does employee illness need to be recognized and evaluated, but employees must be taught that patient contact must be avoided despite perceptions that an illness (e.g., intestinal flu) is trivial. For this approach to be effective, employees must be assured that they will not be penalized for missing work because of an infectious illness (477). The rate of nosocomial GI disease outbreaks was shown to be significantly lower in long-term-care facilities with paid employee sick leave policies (478).

The employee who develops diarrhea should be evaluated by a physician and excused from direct patient or food contact for the duration of the illness. Most of these employees will have a self-limited illness. In these cases, only simple supportive measures are needed. When an inflammatory diarrhea is suspected or an outbreak in the hospital is occurring, a more extensive investigation is warranted. In such cases, stool specimens should be obtained for bacterial culture and possibly ova and parasite examination to secure a microbiologic diagnosis and assess the potential for nosocomial spread (479). The central issue, from an infection control standpoint, is to exclude microorganisms that a convalescent employee can asymptomatically excrete. For such entities as nontyphoidal *Salmonella* or *Shigella* species, an employee should be asymptomatic and have at least two negative stool cultures before returning to direct patient/food contact (480). Serial stool samples should be collected no less than 24 hours apart and at least 48 hours after discontinuation of antibiotics. Over 50% of employees recovering from salmonellosis are culture-negative within 5 weeks, and 90% are culture-negative within 9 weeks (188). A hospital worker infected with most pathogens can return to duty when symptoms remit with strong counsel to practice universal precautions and hand washing.

Environmental contamination and contamination of devices such as endoscopes (see Chapter 63) and respiratory therapy equipment have been implicated in the nosocomial spread of diarrhea and other diseases, particularly *C. difficile, Salmonella* species, and recently, *H. pylori* (48,49,59,187,481,482). Most of this equipment is semicritical as described by Spaulding (483); these objects come in contact with nonintact skin and mucous membranes and require at least high-level disinfection (see Chapter 85). A national survey revealed marked variability of procedure in the disinfection of endoscopes and similar devices (484). Moreover, the complex internal design and delicate nature of endoscopes make manual cleaning, the first and pivotal step in careful disinfection, very difficult (485). An inability to manually cleanse certain devices makes mandatory the use of prolonged contact times with high-potency germicides, such as 20 minutes in 2% glutaraldehyde or perhaps sterilization (486). Failure to completely rinse equipment after use of such solutions has been noted to produce a dermatitis in workers and a chemical colitis in patients that is often comparable in appearance to pseudomembranous colitis (487). Even the use of automated washers does not completely avoid the possibility of endoscopic contamination. Alvarado et al. (488) described an endoscope washer that was persistently colonized with *P. aeruginosa,* which resulted in nosocomial infections by the same strain. Some of the machine's internal components were heavily colonized with *Pseudomonas,* with the washer's own decontamination procedure unable to eradicate it. Rinsing of endoscope channels with 70% alcohol and drying them with forced air after being processed in the washer was successful in eliminating the colonization.

Sterilization by ethylene oxide may be considered if infections are discovered to occur due to a problem with high-level disinfection until the source of contamination is found. In fact, infections due to such problems are rare.

Clinical thermometers should be considered a semicritical item and therefore should receive high-level disinfection. This is easily accomplished with 70% to 90% isopropyl alcohol (486). Outbreaks of *C. difficile,* linked to electronic rectal thermometers, have been ended by the use of disposable thermometers (489). A prospective trial of disposable thermometers has also shown decreased rates of *C. difficile* infection (490).

Decontamination of environmental surfaces is a simpler process. Low-level disinfection of noncritical items and surfaces can be accomplished with a variety of agents such as 70% to 90% isopropyl alcohol, sodium hypochlorite, or detergents with phenol, iodophor, or ammonia (486).

Prevention efforts can also focus on the patients. Avoidance of known risk factors for nosocomial diarrhea, when possible, can reduce the potential for its development. These measures may include minimizing the number of antimicrobials administered (491), curtailing the use of enemas, and reducing the duration of nasogastric intubation. Some novel approaches have been tried with variable success. Some investigators have administered nonpathogenic bacteria and yeasts to prevent antibiotic-associated diarrhea. One group was able to show a significant reduction in the rate of antibiotic-associated diarrhea with the administration of *Saccharomyces boulardii,* a saprophytic yeast (492). Interestingly, *S. boulardii* had no effect on the carriage of *C. difficile* and its toxin.

The most certain method for preventing NEC would obviously be the elimination of prematurity, as 80% to 90% of affected infants are of low birth weight. More attainable methods have been tried. Positive results have been obtained with the administration of immunoglobulins, acidification of enteral feedings, and delayed feeding, but such data should be viewed as preliminary, because studies conflict.

Issues regarding foodborne disease must concentrate on hygienic practices of food handling and storage. Food preparation equipment as well as kitchen surfaces must be kept scrupulously clean. Food should be obtained from reliable sources, and unpasteurized products should be avoided. Perhaps most critical, food must be held at proper temperatures either above 60°C or below 7°C. Food needs to be thawed completely before cooking and preferably thawed while refrigerated. Cooked items must not be allowed to stand at room temperature for prolonged periods.

Holding temperatures in serving lines and carts should be routinely measured. The potential for cross-contamination should be removed by prohibiting practices that permit contact between raw and cooked items. Waste disposal must be a standardized process. The use of modified ultraviolet lamps has been shown to eradicate *Salmonella* species on culture plates (493), but this technique has not yet been studied in food disinfection. Finally, proper training of food service personnel cannot be overemphasized, as they, more than any others, can prevent foodborne disease transmission.

OUTBREAK DETECTION AND MANAGEMENT

Outbreaks may be initially recognized by routine surveillance. A temporal or spatial cluster of nosocomial GI infections can be discerned by regular inspection of the results of clinical specimens submitted to the microbiology laboratory. Although contingent on physician ordering and laboratory processing practices, laboratory-based surveillance can be moderately effective in the detection of hospital-acquired infections (494). Other studies have found laboratory-based surveillance to be relatively insensitive as compared with selective chart review for high-risk patients (495,496). Ideally, a hospital with sufficient resources and personnel should conduct regular ward-based surveillance of all units as well as review of all microbiology results (497).

For institutions with limited resources, an effective method for the surveillance of nosocomial gastroenteritis would involve periodic review of the results of stool cultures coupled with regular inspection of such high-risk wards as the newborn and special care nurseries, intensive care units, and oncology wards. Such an approach would combine aspects of laboratory surveillance and selective chart review.

The use of surveillance methods to detect sporadic cases of *C. difficile* diarrhea has been found to be effective in reducing further nosocomial transmission of the illness (50). With rapid reporting of positive stool assays for *C. difficile*, control measures can be initiated. Such practices should include wearing gloves, wearing gowns when soiling is likely, the use of a private room if the patient's hygiene is poor, and obligatory hand washing. Chlorhexidine has been shown to be more effective than plain soap and water in removing microorganisms such as *C. difficile* from the hands of hospital employees (46).

Once it has been ascertained that a nosocomial outbreak of gastroenteritis has occurred, epidemiologic investigation should proceed. Empiric isolation procedures should be instituted during the investigation. If the outbreak is extensive, cohorting of patients and caregivers should be considered. Epidemics should be promptly reported to local or state health authorities, as nursing homes and small hospitals may lack the required laboratory and infection control resources for an intensive investigation. Even in large hospitals, the assistance of a state health department can be invaluable in providing technology to perform serotyping and to detect certain elusive pathogens such as pathogenic *E. coli* or Norwalk and related agents.

CONSIDERATIONS FOR THE FUTURE

The importance of nosocomial GI tract infections is only just beginning to be fully understood. Although the prevalence of these infections is gradually being documented, their repercussions have yet to be fully described. For example, further study is needed to establish the morbidity, mortality, and excess cost related to these infections.

The range of pathogens causing nosocomial gastroenteritis is not entirely known. The pathogenesis of *Candida*-associated diarrhea is still unclear. Examination of the role of nosocomial gastroenteritis in the pathogenesis of other nosocomial infections is another area for further investigation.

REFERENCES

1. Farr BM. Diarrhea: a neglected nosocomial hazard? [editorial]. *Infect Control Hosp Epidemiol* 1991;12:343–344.
2. Garner JS, Jarvis WR, Emori TG. CDC definitions for nosocomial infections, 1988. *Am J Infect Control* 1988;17:128–140.
3. Emori TG, Culver DH, Horan TC. National Nosocomial Infection Surveillance System (NNIS): description of surveillance methods. *Am J Infect Control* 1991;19:19–35.
4. Hughes JM, Jarvis WR. Nosocomial gastrointestinal infections. In: Wenzel RP, ed. *Prevention and control of nosocomial infections,* 2nd ed. Baltimore: Williams & Wilkins 1993:708–745.
5. Siegal DL, Edelstein PH, Nachamakin I. Inappropriate testing for diarrheal diseases in the hospital. *JAMA* 1990;263:979–982.
6. Brady MT, Pacini DL, Budde CT, et al. Diagnostic studies of nosocomial diarrhea in children: assessing their use and value. *Am J Infect Control* 1989;17:77–82.
7. Welliver RC, McLaughlin S. Unique epidemiology of nosocomial infection in a children's hospital. *Am J Dis Child* 1984;138:131–135.
8. Guerrant RL, Hughes JM, Lima NL, et al. Diarrhea in developed and developing countries: magnitude, special settings, and etiologies. *Rev Infect Dis* 1990;12(suppl):41–50.
9. Ford-Jones EL, Mindorff CM, Gold R, et al. The incidence of viral-associated diarrhea after admission to a pediatric hospital. *Am J Epidemiol* 1990;131:711–718.
10. Lam BCC, Tam J, Nguyen MH, et al. Nosocomial gastroenteritis in pediatric patients. *J Hosp Infect* 1989;14:351–355.
11. Hughes JM, Jarvis WR. Nosocomial gastrointestinal infections. In: Wenzel RP, ed. *Prevention and control of nosocomial infections.* Baltimore: Williams & Wilkins, 1987:405–439.
12. Stamm WE, Weinstein RA, Dixon RE. Comparison of endemic and epidemic nosocomial infections. *Am J Med* 1981;70:393–397.
13. Zaidi M, Ponce de Leon S, Ortiz RM. Hospital-acquired diarrhea in adults: a prospective case-controlled study in Mexico. *Infect Control Hosp Epidemiol* 1991;12:349–355.
14. Yolken RH, Bishop CA, Townsend TR. Infectious gastroenteritis in bone marrow transplant recipients. *N Engl J Med* 1982;306: 1009–1012.
15. Lima NL, Guerrant RL, Kaiser DL, et al. A retrospective cohort study of nosocomial diarrhea as a risk factor for nosocomial infection. *J Infect Dis* 1990;161:948–952.
16. Garibaldi RA, Burke J, Britt MR, et al. Meatal colonization and catheter-associated bacteriuria. *N Engl J Med* 1980;303:316–318.
17. Schaeffer AJ, Chmiel J. Urethral meatal colonication in the pathogenesis of catheter-associated bacteriuria. *J Urol* 1983;130:1096–1099.
18. Daifuku R, Stamm WE. Association of rectal and urethral colonization with urinary tract infection in patients with indwelling catheters. *JAMA* 1984;252:2028–2030.
19. Monti S, Opal S, Palardy JE, et al. Nosocomial *C. difficile* diarrhea: risk factors, complications, and cost. Abstract of the second annual SHEA meeting, Baltimore, Maryland, April 12–14, 1992.
20. McFarland LV. Epidemiology of infections and iatrogenic diarrhea

in a cohort of general medicine patients. *Am J Infect Control* 1995; 23:295–305.
21. Ryder RW, McGowan JE, Hatch MH, et al. Reovirus-like agent as a cause of nosocomial diarrhoea in infants. *J Pediatr* 1977;90:698–702.
22. Guerrant RL. Principles and syndromes of enteric infection. In: Mandell GL, Douglas RG, Bennett JE, eds. *Principles and practices of infectious diseases.* New York: Churchill Livingstone, 1990:837–851.
23. Hornick RB, Musik SI, Wenzel R. The Broad Street pump revisited: response to volunteers to ingested *cholera vibrios. Bull NY Acad Med* 1971;47:1181–1191.
24. Giannella RA, Broitman SA, Zamcheck N. Influence of gastric acidity on bacterial and parasitic enteric infection: a perspective. *Ann Intern Med* 1973;78:271–276.
25. Driks M, Craven DE, Celli BR. Nosocomial pneumonia in intubated patients given sucralfate as compared with antacids or histamine type 2 blockers. The role of gastric colonization. *N Engl J Med* 1987;317: 1376–1382.
26. Sprinz H. Pathogenesis of intestinal infections. *Arch Pathol* 1969;87: 556–561.
27. DuPont HL, Hornick RB. Adverse effect of Lomotil therapy in shigellosis. *JAMA* 1973;226:1525–1528.
28. Novak E, Lee JG, Seckman E, et al. Unfavorable effect of atropine-diphenoxylate (Lomotil) therapy in lincomycin-caused diarrhea. *JAMA* 1976;235:1451–1454.
29. Bohnhoff M, Miller CP, Martin WR. Resistance of the mouse's intestinal tract to experimental *Salmonella* infections. *J Exp Med* 1964; 120:805–828.
30. Que JU, Casey SW, Hentges DJ. Factors responsible for increased susceptibility of mice to intestinal colonization after treatment with streptomycin. *Infect Immun* 1986;53:116–123.
31. Mentzing LO, Ringertz O. *Salmonella* infection in tourists II. Prophylaxis against salmonellosis. *Acta Pathol Microbiol Scand* 1968;74: 405–413.
32. Thibault A, Miller MA, Gaese C. Risk factors for the development of *Clostridium difficile* associated diarrhea during a hospital outbreak. *Infect Control Hosp Epidemiol* 1991;12:345–348.
33. Brandtzaeg P, Halstensen TS, Kett K. Immunobiology and immunopathology of human gut mucosa: humoral immunity and intraepithelial lymphocytes. *Gastroenterology* 1989;97:1562–1584.
34. Kagnoff MF. Immunology of the digestive system. In: Johnson LR, ed. *Physiology of the gastrointestinal tract.* New York: Raven Press, 1987:1699–1728.
35. Bodey GP, Fainstein V, Guerrant RL. Infections of the gastrointestinal tract in the immunocompromised patient. *Annu Rev Med* 1986; 37:271–281.
36. Eras P, Goldstein MJ, Sherlock P. Candida infection of the gastrointestinal tract. *Medicine* 1972;51:367–379.
37. Krick JA, Remington JS. Opportunistic invasive fungal infections in patients with leukemia and lymphoma. *Clin Haemotol* 1976;5: 249–310.
38. Karabinis A, Hill C, Leclercq B, et al. Risk factors for candidemia in cancer patients: a case-control study. *J Clin Microbiol* 1988;126: 429–432.
39. Wey SB, Mori M, Pfaller MA, et al. Risk factors for hospital-acquired candidemia. A matched case-control study. *Arch Intern Med* 1989; 149:2349–2353.
40. Slavin RE, Santos GW. The graft versus host reaction in man after bone marrow transplantation: pathology, pathogenesis, clinical features, and implication. *Clin Immunol Immunopathol* 1973;1: 472–498.
41. Kelly TW, Patrick MR, Hillman KM. Study of diarrhea in critically ill patients. *Crit Care Med* 1983;11:7–9.
42. Brown E, Talbot GH, Axelrod P, et al. Risk factors for *Clostridium difficile* toxin-associated diarrhea. *Infect Control Hosp Epidemiol* 1990; 11:283–290.
43. Gerding DN, Olson MM, Peterson LR. *Clostridium difficile* associated diarrhea and colitis in adults. A prospective case-controlled study. *Arch Intern Med* 1986;146:95–100.
44. Simmons BP, Gelfand MS, Haas M, et al. *Enterobacter sakazakii* infections in neonates associated with intrinsic contamination of a powdered infant formula. *Infect Control Hosp Epidemiol* 1989;10: 398–401.
45. Eisenstein BI. New molecular techniques for microbial epidemiology and the diagnosis of infectious diseases. *J Infect Dis* 1990;161: 595–602.
46. McFarland LV, Mulligan ME, Kwok RY, et al. Nosocomial acquisition of *Clostridium difficile* infection. *N Engl J Med* 1989;320: 204–210.
47. Johnson S, Gerding DN, Olson MM. Prospective controlled study of vinyl glove use to interrupt *Clostridium difficile* nosocomial transmission. *Am J Med* 1990;88:137–140.
48. Kaatz GW, Gitlin SD, Schaberg DR. Acquisition of *Clostridium difficile* from the hospital environment. *Am J Epidemiol* 1988;127: 1289–1294.
49. Fekety FR, Kim K-H, Brown D, et al. Epidemiology of antibiotic-associated colitis. Isolation of *Clostridium difficile* from the hospital environment. *Am J Med* 1981;70:906–908.
50. Struelens M, Maas A, Nonhoff C. Control of nosocomial transmission of *Clostridium difficile* based on sporadic case surveillance. *Am J Med* 1991;91(suppl 3B):138s–144s.
51. Gerding DN, Peterson LR, Johnson S. The silent sea of *C. difficile* [abstract A80]. Third Decennial International Conference of Nosocomial Infections, Atlanta, July 31–August 3, 1990.
52. Baine WB, Gangarosa EJ, Bennett JV, et al. Institutional salmonellosis. *J Infect Dis* 1973;128:357–360.
53. Rice P, Craven PC, Wells JG. *Salmonella heidelberg* enteritis and bacteria: an epidemic on two pediatric wards. *Am J Med* 1976;60: 509–516.
54. Hammami A, Arlet G, Ben Redjeb S. Nosocomial outbreak of acute gastroenteritis in a neonatal intensive care unit in Tunisia caused by multiply drug resistant *Salmonella wien* producing SHV-2 beta-lactamase. *Eur J Clin Micro Infect Dis* 1991;10:641–646.
55. Linnemann CC Jr, Cannon CG, Staneck JL, et al. Prolonged epidemic of salmonellosis: use of trimethoprim-sulfamethoxazole for control. *Infect Control* 1985;6:221–225.
56. Weikel CS, Guerrant RL. Nosocomial salmonellosis [editorial]. *Infect Control* 1985;6:218–220.
57. Jacobs JL, Gold JWM, Murray HW, et al. Salmonella infections in patients with acquired immunodeficiency syndrome. *Ann Intern Med* 1985;102:186–188.
58. Haley CE, Guerrant RL. Institutional salmonellosis. *Asepsis* 1982;4: 7–12.
59. Dwyer DM, Klein EG, Istre GR, et al. *Salmonella newport* infections transmitted by fiberoptic colonoscopy. *Gastrointest Endosc* 1987;33: 84–87.
60. Riley LW, Ceballos O, Tabuls LR, et al. The significance of hospitals as reservoirs for epidemic multiresistant *Salmonella typhimurium* causing infection in urban Brazilian children. *J Infect Dis* 1984;150: 236–241.
61. Holmberg SD, Wells JG, Cohen ML. Animal-to-man transmission of antimicrobial-resistant *Salmonella*: investigation of U.S. outbreaks 1971–1973. *Science* 1984;225:833–835.
62. Brunton J. Drug-resistant *Salmonella* from animals fed antimicrobials. *N Engl J Med* 1984;311:1698–1699.
63. DuPont HL, Steele JH. Use of antimicrobial agents in animal feeds: implications for human health. *Rev Infect Dis* 1987;9:447–460.
64. Gellert GA, Waterman SH, Ewart D. An outbreak of acute gastroenteritis caused by a small round structured virus in a geriatric convalescent facility. *Infect Control Hosp Epidemiol* 1990;11:459–464.
65. Sawyer LA, Murphy JJ, Kaplan JE. 25- to 30-nm particle associated with a hospital of acute gastroenteritis with evidence for airborne transmission. *Am J Epidemiol* 1998;127:1261–1271.
66. Stegenga J, Bell E, Matlow A. The role of nurse understaffing in nosocomial viral gastrointestinal infections on a general pediatrics ward. *Infect Control Hosp Epidemiol* 2002;23:133–136.
67. Butcher I, Kudesia G, Gordon J, et al. Small round structured viruses and their spread [letter]. *Lancet* 1989;1:443.
68. Weinstein RA, Stamm WE. Pseudoepidemics in hospital. *Lancet* 1977;2:862–864.

69. Altemeier WE, Hummell RP, Hill EO. *Staphylococcal enterocolitis* following antibiotic therapy. *Ann Surg* 1963;157:847–852.
70. Moskovitz M, Bartlett JG. Recurrent pseudomembranous colitis unassociated with antibiotic therapy. *Arch Intern Med* 1981;141: 663–664.
71. Bartlett JG. Antibiotic-associated diarrhea. *Clin Infect Dis* 1992;15: 573–581.
72. Fekety R. Antibiotic-associated colitis. In: Mandell GL, Douglas RG, Bennett JE, eds. *Principles and practices of infectious diseases.* New York: Churchill Livingstone, 2003:863–869.
73. Freiman JP, Graham DJ, Green L. Pseudomembranous colitis associated with single-dose cephalosporin prophylaxis [letter]. *JAMA* 1989; 262–902.
74. Cudmore M, Silva J, Fekety R, et al. *Clostridium difficile* colitis associated with cancer chemotherapy. *Arch Intern Med* 1982;142:333–335.
75. Rybolt AH, Bennett RG, Laughon BE, et al. Protein-losing enteropathy associated with *Clostridium difficile* infection. *Lancet* 1989;1: 1353–1355.
76. Fekety R, Shah AB. Diagnosis and treatment of *Clostridium difficile* colitis. *JAMA* 1993;269:71–75.
77. Viscidi R, Willey S, Bartlett JG. Isolation rates and toxigenic potential of *Clostridium difficile* isolates from various patient populations. *Gastroenterology* 1981;81:5–9.
78. Johnson S, Clabots CR, Finn FV. Nosocomial *Clostridium difficile* colonization and disease. *Lancet* 1990;336:97–100.
79. McFarland LV, Surawicz CM, Stamm WE. Risk factors for *Clostridium difficile* carriage and *C. difficile* associated diarrhea in a cohort of hospitalized patients. *J Infect Dis* 1990;162:678–684.
80. Kyne L, Sougioultzis S, McFarland LV, et al. Underlying disease severity as a major risk factor for nosocomial *Clostridium difficile* diarrhea. *Infect Control Hosp Epidemiol* 2002;23:653–659.
81. Schwaber MJ, Simhon A, Block C, et al. Factors associated with nosocomial diarrhea and *Clostridium difficile*-associated disease on the adult wards of an urban tertiary care hospital. *Eur J Clin Micro Infect Dis* 2000;19:9–15.
82. Chang VT, Nelson K. The role of physical proximity in nosocomial diarrhea. *Clin Infect Dis* 2000;31:717–722.
83. Levy DG, Stergachis A, McFarland LV, et al. Antibiotics and *Clostridium difficile* diarrhea in the ambulatory care setting. *Clin Ther* 2000; 22:91–102.
84. Kent KC, Rubin MS, Wroblewski L, et al. The impact of *Clostridium difficile* on a surgical service: a prospective study of 374 patients. *Ann Surg* 1998;227:296–301.
85. Yip C, Loeb M, Salama S, et al. Quinolone use as a risk factor for nosocomial *Clostridium difficile*-associated diarrhea. *Infect Control Hosp Epidemiol* 2001;22:572–575.
86. Mylotte JM, Graham R, Kahler L, et al. Impact of nosocomial infection on length of stay and functional improvement among patients admitted to an acute rehabilitation unit. *Infect Control Hosp Epidemiol* 2001;22:83–87.
87. Gorschluter M, Glasmacher A, Hahn C, et al. *Clostridium difficile* infection in patients with neutropenia. *Clin Infect Dis* 2001;33: 786–791.
88. Enad D, Meislich D, Brodsky NL, et al. Is *Clostridium difficile* a pathogen in the newborn intensive care unit? A prospective evaluation. *J Perinatol* 1997;17:355–359.
89. Heard SR, O'Farrell S, Holland D, et al. The epidemiology of *Clostridium difficile* with use of a typing scheme: nosocomial acquisition and cross-infection among immunocompromised patients. *J Infect Dis* 1986;153:159–162.
90. Cumming AD, Thomson BJ, Sharp J, et al. Diarrhoea due to *Clostridium difficile* associated with antibiotic treatment in patients receiving dialysis: the role of cross infection. *Br Med J* 1986;292:238–239.
91. Clabots CR, Johnson S, Olson MM, et al. Acquisition of *Clostridium difficile* by hospitalized patients: evidence for colonized new admissions as a source of infection. *J Infect Dis* 1992;166:561–567.
92. Kim KH, Fekety R, Batts DH. Isolation of *Clostridium difficile* from the environment and contacts of patients with antibiotic-associated colitis. *J Infect Dis* 1981;143:42–50.
93. Mulligan, Rolfe RD, Finegold SM, et al. Contamination of a hospital environment with *Clostridium difficile. Curr Microbiol* 1979;3: 173–175.
94. Getchell-White SI, Barrett LJ, Barton BA, et al. Nosocomial significance of *Clostridium difficile*: an epidemiologic study using molecular markers. *Med Microbiol Lett* 1992;1:49–55.
95. Samore M, Kilgore G, Johnson S, et al. Multicenter typing comparison of sporadic and outbreak *Clostridium difficile* isolates from geographically diverse hospitals. *J Infect Dis* 1997;176:1233–1238.
96. Kato H, Kato N, Watanabe K, et al. Analysis of *Clostridium difficile* isolates from nosocomial outbreaks at three hospitals in diverse areas of Japan. *J Clin Microbiol* 2001;39:1391–1395.
97. Mekonen ET, Gerding DN, Sambol S, et al. Predominance of a single restriction endonuclease analysis group with intrahospital subgroup diversity among *Clostridium difficile* isolates at two Chicago hospitals. *Infect Control Hosp Epidemiol* 2002;23:648–652.
98. Berdon WE, Grossman H, Baker DH, et al. Necrotizing enterocolitis in the premature infant. *Radiology* 1964;83:879–887.
99. McClead RE. Introduction: neonatal necrotizing enterocolitis: current concepts and controversies. *J Pediatr* 1990;117(suppl):1.
100. Kleinhaus S, Weinberg G, Gregor MB. Necrotizing enterocolitis in infancy. *Surg Clin North Am* 1992;72:261–276.
101. Kliegman RM. Models of the pathogenesis of necrotizing enterocolitis. *J Pediatr* 1990;117(suppl):2–5.
102. Kosloske AM. A unifying hypothesis for pathogenesis and prevention of necrotizing enterocolitis. *J Pediatr* 1990;117(suppl):68–74.
103. Scheifele DW, Bjornson GL, Dyer RA, et al. Delta-like toxin produced by coagulase-negative *staphylococci* is associated with neonatal necrotizing enterocolitis. *Infect Immun* 1987;55:2268–2273.
104. Caplan M, Sun XM, Hsuch W, et al. Role of platelet activating factor and tumor necrosis factor-alpha in neonatal necrotizing enterocolitis. *J Pediatr* 1990;29:1207–1212.
105. Cueva JP, Hsuch W. Role of oxygen-derived free radicals in platelet activating factor induced bowel necrosis. *Gut* 1988;29:1207–1212.
106. Aynsley-Green A, Lucas A, Lawson GR, et al. Gut hormones and regulatory peptides in relation to enteral feeding, gastroenteritis, and necrotizing enterocolitis in infancy. *J Pediatr* 1990;117(suppl):24–32.
107. Clark DA, Thompson JE, Weiner LB, et al. Necrotizing enterocolitis: intraluminal biochemistry in human neonates and a rabbit model. *Pediatr Res* 1985;19:919–921.
108. Kliegman RM, Fanaroff AA. Necrotizing enterocolitis. *N Engl J Med* 1984;310:1093–1103.
109. Wiswell TE, Robertson CF, Jones TA, et al. Necrotizing enterocolitis in full-term infants. *Am J Dis Child* 1988;142:532–535.
110. Rogers AF, Dunn PM. Intestinal perforation, exchange transfusion, and P.V.C. [letter]. *Lancet* 1969;2:1246.
111. Ryder RW, Shelton JD. Necrotizing enterocolitis: a prospective multicenter investigation. *Am J Epidemiol* 1980;112:113–123.
112. Czyrko C, Del Pin CA, O'Neill JA, et al. Maternal cocaine abuse and necrotizing enterocolitis: outcome and survival. *J Pediatr Surg* 1991;26:414–418.
113. Clark DA, Miller MJS. Intraluminal pathogenesis of necrotizing enterocolitis. *J Pediatr* 1990;117(suppl):64–67.
114. Telemo E, Westrom BR, Karlson BW. Proteolytic activity as a regulator of the transmission of orally fed proteins from the gut to the blood serum in the suckling rat. *Biol Neonate* 1982;41:85–93.
115. Burgio GR, Lanzavecchia A, Plebani A, et al. Ontogeny of secretory immunity: levels of secretory IgA and natural antibodies in saliva. *Pediatr Res* 1980;14:1111–1114.
116. Udall JN. Gastrointestinal host defense and necrotizing enterocolitis. *J Pediatr* 1990;117(suppl):33–43.
117. Uauy RD, Fanaroff AA, Korones SB. Necrotizing enterocolitis in very low birth weight infants; biodemographic and clinical correlates. *J Pediatr* 1191;119:630–638.
118. Gerber AR, Hopkins RS, Lauer BA, et al. Increased risk of illness among nursery staff caring for neonates with necrotizing enterocolitis. *Pediatr Infect Dis* 1985;4:246–249.
119. Engell RR. Studies of the gastrointestinal flora in necrotizing enterocolitis. In: *Necrotizing enterocolitis in the newborn infant. Report of the 68th Ross Conference on Pediatric Research.* Columbus, OH: Ross Laboratories, 1974:66–71.

120. Speer ME, Taber LH, Yow MD. Fulminant neonatal sepsis and necrotizing enterocolitis associated with nonenteropathogenic strain of *Escherichia coli. J Pediatr* 1976;89:91–95.
121. Cushing AH. Necrotizing enterocolitis with *Escherichia coli* heat-labile enterotoxin. *Pediatrics* 1983;71:626–630.
122. Frantz ID, L'Heureux P, Engel RR, et al. Necrotizing enterocolitis. *J Pediatr* 1975;86:259–263.
123. Powell J, Bureau MA, Pare C, et al. Necrotizing enterocolitis. Epidemic following an outbreak of *Enterobacter cloacae* type 3305573 in a neonatal intensive care unit. *Am J Dis Child* 1980;134:1152–1154.
124. Richardson RJ, Chan TK, McKenzie R, et al. Necrotizing enterocolitis and *Salmonella* group C [letter]. *Ann Trop Pediatr* 1984;4:55.
125. Han VKM, Sayed H, Chance GW, et al. Outbreak of *Clostridium difficile* necrotizing enterocolitis: a case for oral vancomycin therapy? *Pediatrics* 1983;71:935–941.
126. Kosloske AM, Ball WS, Umland E, et al. Clostridial necrotizing enterocolitis. *J Pediatr Surg* 1985;20:155–159.
127. Sturm R, Staneck JL, Stauffer LR, et al. Neonatal necrotizing enterocolitis associated with penicillin-resistant, toxigenic *Clostridium butyricum. Pediatrics* 1980;66:928–931.
128. Overturf GD, Sherman MP, Scheifele DW, et al. Neonatal necrotizing enterocolitis associated with delta-toxin producing methicillin-resistant *Staphylococcus aureus. Pediatr Infect Dis* 1990;9:88–91.
129. Mollitt BL, Tepas JJ, Talbert JL. The role of coagulase-negative Staphylococcus in neonatal necrotizing enterocolitis. *J Pediatr Surg* 1988; 23:60–63.
130. Rotbart HA, Levin MJ, Yolken RH, et al. An outbreak of rotavirus-associated neonatal necrotizing enterocolitis. *J Pediatr* 1983;103: 454–459.
131. Siegal JD, Luby JP, Laptook AR, et al. Identification of coronavirus in a premature nursery during an outbreak of necrotizing enterocolitis and diarrhea. *Pediatr Res* 1983;17:181A.
132. Birenbaum E, Handsher R, Kuint J. Echovirus type 22 outbreak associated with gastro-intestinal disease in a neonatal intensive care unit. *Am J Perinatol* 1997;14:469–473.
133. Johnson FE, Crnic DM, Simmons MA, et al. Associations of fatal coxsackie B2 viral infection and necrotizing enterocolitis. *Arch Dis Child* 1977;52:802–804.
134. Eibl MM, Wolf HM, Furnkanz H, et al. Prevention of necrotizing enterocolitis in low-birth-weight infants by IgA-IgG feeding. *N Engl J Med* 1988;319:1–7.
135. Bauer CR, Morrison JC, Poole WK. A decreased incidence of necrotizing enterocolitis after prenatal glucocorticoid therapy. *Pediatrics* 1984;73:682–688.
136. Carrion V, Egan EA. Prevention of neonatal necrotizing enterocolitis. *J Pediatr Gastroenterol Nutr* 1990;11:317–323.
137. Ostertag SG, LaGamma EF, Reisen CE, et al. Early enteral feeding does not affect the incidence of necrotizing enterocolitis. *Pediatrics* 1986;77:275–280.
138. McKeown RE, Marsh TD, Amarnath U. Role of delayed feeding and of feeding increments in necrotizing enterocolitis. *J Pediatr* 1992;121: 764–770.
139. McCracken GH, Eitzman DV. Necrotizing enterocolitis [editorial]. *Am J Dis Child* 1978;132:1167–1168.
140. Alt B, Glass NR, Sullinger H. Neutropenic enterocolitis in adults. *Am J Surg* 1985;149:405–408.
141. Sherman NJ, Woolley MM. The ileocecal syndrome in acute childhood leukemia. *Arch Surg* 1973;107:39–42.
142. Mulholland MW, Delany JP. Neutropenic colitis and aplastic anemia: a new association. *Ann Surg* 1983;197:84–90.
143. Nagler A, Pavel L, Naparstek E, et al. Typhlitis occurring in autologous bone marrow transplantation. *Marrow Transplant* 1992;9: 63–64.
144. Till M, Lee N, Soper WD, et al. Typhlitis in patients with HIV-1 infection. *Ann Intern Med* 1992;116:998–1000.
145. Meyerovitz MF, Fellows KE. Typhlitis: a cause of gastrointestinal hemorrhage in children. *Am J Radiol* 1984;143:833–835.
146. Merine DS, Fishman EK, Jones B, et al. Right lower quadrant pain in the immunocompromised patient: CT findings in 10 cases. *AJR* 1987;149:1177–1179.
147. Slavin RE, Dias MA, Saral R. Cytosine arabinoside-induced gastrointestinal toxic alterations in sequential chemotherapeutic protocols. *Cancer* 1978;42:1747–1759.
148. Villarino ME, Vugia DJ, Bean NH, et al. Foodborne disease prevention in health care facilities. In: Brachman PS, Bennett JV, eds. *Hospital infections.* Boston: Little, Brown, 1992:345–358.
149. Carter AO, Borezyk AA, Carlson JAK. A severe outbreak of *Escherichia coli* 0157:H7 associated hemorrhagic colitis in a nursing home. *N Engl J Med* 1987;327:1496–1500.
150. Levine WC, Smart JF, Archer DL, et al. Foodborne disease outbreaks in nursing homes. *JAMA* 1991;266:2105–2109.
151. Steere AC, Craven PJ, Hall WJ II. Person-to-person spread of *Salmonella typhimurium* after a hospital common-source outbreak. *Lancet* 1975;1:319–321.
152. Centers for Disease Control and Prevention. *Enterobacter sakazakii* infections associated with use of powdered infant formula—Tennessee, 2001. *MMWR* 2002;51:298–300.
153. Guerrant RL, Araujo V, Barrett LJ, et al. Measurement of fecal lactoferrin (LF) as a marker of inflammatory enteritis. *Clin Res* 1990:38; 391(abst).
154. Pulvirenti JJ, Gerding DN, Nathan C, et al. Difference in the incidence of *Clostridium difficile* among patients infected with human immunodeficiency virus admitted to a public hospital and a private hospital. *Infect Control Hosp Epidemiol* 2002;22:641–647.
155. Johnson JF, Sonnenberg A. Efficient management of diarrhea in the acquired immunodeficiency syndrome (AIDS). *Ann Intern Med* 1990; 112:942–948.
156. Lusk RH, Fekety R, Silva J, et al. Clindamycin-induced enterocolitis in hamsters. *J Infect Dis* 1978;137:464–475.
157. Rifkin GD, Fekety FR, Silva J, et al. Antibiotic-associated colitis: implications of a toxin neutralized by *Clostridium sordelli* antitoxin. *Lancet* 1977;2:1103–1106.
158. Bartlett JG. Antibiotic-associated pseudomembranous colitis. *Rev Infect Dis* 1979;1:530–539.
159. Lima AAM, Lyerly DM, Wilkins TD, et al. Effects of *Clostridium difficile* toxins A and B in rabbit small and large intestines in vivo and on cultured cells in vitro. *Infect Immun* 1988;56:582–588.
160. Peterson LR, Olson MM, Shanholtzer C, et al. Results of a prospective, 18-month clinical evaluation of culture, cytotoxin testing, and culturette brand (CDT) latex testing in the diagnosis of *Clostridium difficile* associated diarrhea. *Diagn Microbiol Infect Dis* 1988;10: 85–91.
161. Shanholtzer CJ, Willard KE, Holter JJ, et al. Comparison of VIDAS *Clostridium difficile* toxin A immunoassay (CDA) with *C. difficile* culture, cytotoxin, and latex test. *J Clin Microbiol* 1992;30: 1837–1840.
162. Barbut F, Kajzer C, Planas N, et al. Comparison of three enzyme immunoassays, a cytotoxicity assay, and toxigenic culture for the diagnosis of *Clostridium difficile* associated diarrhea. *J Clin Microbiol* 1993; 31:963–967.
163. Peterson LR, Kelly PJ. Role of the clinical microbiology laboratory in the management of *Clostridium difficile* associated diarrhea. *Infect Dis Clin North Am* 1993;7:277–293.
164. Lima NL, Farr B, Lima MEF. Etiologies of nosocomial diarrhea at a university hospital in Northeastern Brazil [abstract 1297]. Presented at the Thirty-third Interscience Conference on Antimicrobial Agents and Chemotherapy, New Orleans, October 17–20, 1993.
165. Doern GV, Coughlin RT, Wu L. Laboratory diagnosis of *Clostridium difficile* associated gastrointestinal disease: comparison of a monoclonal antibody enzyme immunoassay for toxins A and B with a monoclonal antibody immunoassay for toxin A only and two cytotoxicity assays. *J Clin Microbiol* 1992;30:2042–2046.
166. Lyerly DM, Neville LM, Evans DT, et al. Multicenter evaluation of the *Clostridium difficile* TOX A/B test. *J Clin Microbiol* 1998;36: 184–190.
167. Kato N, Ou C-Y, Kato H. Identification of toxigenic *Clostridium difficile* in stool specimens by the polymerase chain reaction. *J Infect Dis* 1993;162:455–458.
168. Gumerlock PH, Tary YJ, Weiss JB, et al. Specific detection of toxi-

genic strains of *Clostridium difficile* in stool specimens. *J Clin Microbiol* 1993;31:507–511.

169. Belanger SD, Boissinot M, Clairoux N, et al. Rapid detection of *Clostridium difficile* in feces by real-time PCR. *J Clin Microbiol* 2003; 41:730–734.
170. Bidet P, Lalande V, Salauze B, et al. Comparison of PCR-ribotyping, arbitrarily primed PCR, and pulsed-field gel electrophoresis for typing *Clostridium difficile*. *J Clin Microbiol* 2000;38:2484–2487.
171. George WL, Sutter VL, Citron D, Selective and differential medium for isolation of *Clostridium difficile*. *J Clin Microbiol* 1979;9:214–219.
172. Wilson KH, Kennedy MJ, Fekety FR. Use of sodium taurocholate to enhance spore recovery on a medium selective for *Clostridium difficile*. *J Clin Microbiol* 1982;15:443–446.
173. Clabots CR, Gerding SJ, Olson MM, et al. Detection of asymptomatic *Clostridium difficile* carriage by an alcohol shock procedure. *J Clin Microbiol* 1989;27:2386–2387.
174. Riley TV, Brazier JS, Hassan H, et al. Comparison of alcohol shock enrichment and selective enrichment for the isolation of *Clostridium difficile*. *Epidemiol Infect* 1987;99:355–359.
175. Bulusu M, Narayan S, Shetler K, et al. Leukocytosis as a harbinger and surrogate marker of *Clostridium difficile* infection in hospitalized patients with diarrhea. *Am J Gastroenterol* 2000;95:3137–3141.
176. Teasley DG, Gerding DN, Olson MM. Prospective randomized trial of metronidazole versus vancomycin for *Clostridium difficile* associated diarrhoea and colitis. *Lancet* 1983;2:1043–1046.
177. Johnson S, Homann SR, Bettin KM. Treatment of asymptomatic *Clostridium difficile* carriers (fecal excretors) with vancomycin or metronidazole. A randomized, placebo controlled trial. *Ann Intern Med* 1992;117:297–302.
178. Mayfield JL, Leet T, Miller J, et al. Environmental control to reduce transmission of *Clostridium difficile*. *Clin Infect Dis* 2000;31: 995–1000.
179. Climo MW, Israel DS, Wong ES, et al. Hospital-wide restriction of clindamycin: effect on the incidence of *Clostridium difficile*-associated diarrhea and cost. *Ann Intern Med* 1998;128:989–995.
180. Giannasca PJ, Zhang ZX, Lei WD, et al. Serum antitoxin antibodies mediate systemic and mucosal protection from Clostridium difficile disease in hamsters. *Infect Immun* 1999;67:527–538.
181. DuPont HL. Nosocomial salmonellosis and shigellosis. *Infect Control Hosp Epidemiol* 1991;12:707–709.
182. LeMinor L. Salmonella. In: Krieg NR, Holt JG, eds. *Bergey's manual of systematic bacteriology*. Baltimore: Williams & Wilkins, 1984: 427–428.
183. Farmer JJ, Davis BR, Hickman-Brenner FW. Biochemical identification of new species and biogroups of Enterobacteriaceae isolated from clinical specimens. *J Clin Microbiol* 1985;21:46–76.
184. Hornick RB, Greisman SE, Woodward TE, et al. Typhoid fever: pathogenesis and immunologic control (part I). *N Engl J Med* 1970; 283:686–691.
185. Blaser MJ, Newman LS. A review of human salmonellosis: I. infective dose. *Rev Infect Dis* 1982;4:1096–1106.
186. Taylor DN, Bied JM, Munro JS, et al. *Salmonella dublin* infection in the United States, 1979–1980. *J Infect Dis* 1982;146:322–327.
187. Chmel H, Armstrong D. *Salmonella oslo*: a focal outbreak in a hospital. *Am J Med* 1976;60:203–208.
188. Buchwald DS, Blaser MJ. A review of human salmonellosis: II. Duration of excretion following infection with nontyphi *Salmonella*. *Rev Infect Dis* 1984;6:345–356.
189. Musher DM, Rubenstein AD. Permanent carriers of nontyphoidal salmonellae. *Arch Intern Med* 1973;132:869–872.
190. Pether JVS, Scott RHD. *Salmonella* carriers: are they dangerous? A study to identify finger contamination with salmonellae by convalescent carriers. *J Infect* 1982;5:81–88.
191. McCall CE, Martin WT, Boring JR. Efficiency of cultures of rectal swabs and fecal specimens in detecting *Salmonella* carriers: correlation with numbers of Salmonellas excreted. *J Hyg (London)* 1966;64: 261–269.
192. Perkins JC, Devetski RL, Dowling HF. Ampicillin in the treatment of *Salmonella* carriers. Report of six cases and summary of the literature. *Arch Intern Med* 1966;118:528–533.
193. Simon HJ, Miller RC. Ampicillin in the treatment of chronic typhoid carriers. Report of fifteen treated cases and a review of the literature. *N Engl J Med* 1966;274:807–815.
194. Ferreccio C, Morris JG, Valdivieso C. Efficacy of ciprofloxacin in the treatment of chronic typhoid carriers. *J Infect Dis* 1988;157: 1235–1239.
195. Tauxe RV, Hassan LF, Findeisen KO, et al. *Salmonella* in nurses: lack of transmission to patients. *J Infect Dis* 1988;157:370–373.
196. Aserkoff B, Bennett JE. Effect of antibiotic therapy in acute salmonellosis in the fecal excretion of salmonellae. *N Engl J Med* 1969;281: 636–640.
197. Pavia AT, Shipman LD, Wells JG. Epidemiologic evidence that prior antimicrobial exposure decreases resistance to infection by antimicrobial-sensitive *Salmonella*. *J Infect Dis* 1990;161:255–260.
198. Maiorini E, Lopez EL, Morrow AL. Multiply resistant nontyphoidal *Salmonella* gastroenteritis in children. *Pediatric Infect Dis J* 1993;12: 139–143.
199. DuPont HL, Levine MM, Hornick RB, et al. Inoculum size in shigellosis and implications for expected mode of transmission. *J Infect Dis* 1989;159:1126–1128.
200. Blaser MJ, Pollard RA. *Shiegella* infections in the United States 1974–1980. *J Infect Dis* 1983;147:771–775.
201. LaBrec E, Schneider H, Magnani T, et al. Epithelial cell penetration as an essential step in the pathogenesis of bacillary dysentery. *J Bacteriol* 1964;88:1503–1518.
202. Keusch GT, Grady GF, Mata LJ, et al. Pathogenesis of *Shigella* diarrhea. I. Enterotoxin production by *Shigella* dysenteriae 1. *J Clin Invest* 1972;51:1212–1218.
203. Keusch GT, Grady GF, Takeuchi A, et al. Pathogenesis of *Shigella* diarrhea. II. Induced-induced acute enteritis in the rabbit ileum. *J Infect Dis* 1972;126:92–95.
204. Levine MM, DuPont HL, Khodabandelou M, et al. Long-term *Shigella* carrier state. *N Engl J Med* 1973;288:1169–1171.
205. Salzman TC, Scher CD, Moss R. Shigellae with transferable drug resistance: outbreak in a nursery for premature infants. *J Pediatr* 1967; 71:21–26.
206. DuPont HL, Gangarosa EJ, Reller LB. Shigellosis in custodial institutions. *Am J Epidemiol* 1970;92:172–179.
207. Weissman JB, Hutcherson RH. Shigellosis transmitted by nurses. *South Med J* 1976;69:1341–1346.
208. Pillay DG, Karas JA, Pillay, et al. Nosocomial transmission of *Shigella dysenteriae* type 1. *J Hosp Infect* 1997;37:199–205.
209. Paton S, Nicolle L, Mwongera M. *Salmonella* and *Shigella* gastroenteritis at a public teaching hospital in Nairobi, Kenya. *Infect Control Hosp Epidemiol* 1991;12:710–717.
210. Blaser MJ, Wells JG, Feldman RA, et al., Collaborative Diarrheal Disease Study Group. *Campylobacter* enteritis in the United States: a multicenter study. *Ann Intern Med* 1983;98:360–365.
211. Blaser MJ, Taylor DN, Feldman RA. Epidemiology of *Campylobacter jejuni* infections. *Epidemiol Rev* 1983;5:157–176.
212. Harris NV, Weiss NS, Nolan CM. The role of poultry and meats in the etiology of *Campylobacter jejuni*/coli enteritis. *Am J Public Health* 1986;76:407–411.
213. Schmid GP, Schaefer RE, Plikaytis BD. A one year study of endemic campylobacteriosis in a Midwestern city: association with consumption of raw milk. *J Infect Dis* 1987;156:218–222.
214. Warner DP, Bryner JH, Beran GW. Epidemiologic study of campylobacteriosis in Iowa cattle and the possible role of unpasteurized milk as a vehicle of infection. *Am J Vet Res* 1986;47:254–258.
215. Fang GD, Araujo V, Guerrant RL. Enteric infections associated with exposure to animals or animal products. *Infect Dis Clin North Am* 1991;5:681–701.
216. Totten PA, Fennell CL, Tenovar FC. *Campylobacter cinaedi* (sp. nov.) and *Campylobacter fennelliae* (sp. nov.): two new *Campylobacter* species associated with enteric disease in homosexual men. *J Infect Dis* 1985;151:131–139.
217. Blaser MJ. *Campylobacter* species. In: Mandell GL, Douglas RG, Bennett JE, eds. *Principles and practice of infectious diseases*. New York: Churchill, Livingstone, 1990:1649–1658.
218. Guerrant RL, Wanke CA, Pennie RA, et al. Production of a unique

cytotoxin by *Campylobacter jejuni. Infect Immun* 1987;55:2526–2530.

219. Klipstein FA, Emgert RF. Properties of crude *Campylobacter jejuni* heat-labile enterotoxin. *Infect Immun* 1977;45:314–319.
220. Blaser MJ, Berkowitz ID, LaForce FM, et al. *Campylobacter enteritis*: clinical and epidemiologic features. *Ann Intern Med* 1979;91: 179–185.
221. Riley LW, Finch MJ. Results of a first year of surveillance of *Campylobacter* infections in the United States. *J Infect Dis* 1985;151:956–959.
222. Tauxe RV, Deming MS, Blake PA. *Campylobacter jejuni* infections on college campuses: a national survey. *Am J Public Health* 1985;75: 659–660.
223. Pepersack F, Prigogyne T, Butzler JP, et al. *Campylobacter jejuni* post-transfusional septicaemia [letter]. *Lancet* 1979;2:911.
224. Karmali MA, Norrish B, Lior H, et al. *Campylobacter enteritis* in a neonatal nursery. *J Infect Dis* 1984;149:874–877.
225. Blaser MJ, Reller LB. *Campylobacter enteritis. N Engl J Med* 1981; 305:1444–1452.
226. Skirrow MB. *Campylobacter enteritis. Br Med J* 1977;2:9–11.
227. Steele TW, McDermott JN. Technical note: the use of membrane filters applied directly to the surface of agar plates for the isolation of *Campylobacter jejuni* from feces. *Pathology* 1984;16:263–265.
228. Albert MJ, Tee W, Leach A, et al. Comparison of a blood-free medium and a filtration technique for the isolation of *Campylobacter* spp. from diarrhoeal stool of hospitalized patients in central Australia. *J Med Microbiol* 1992;37:176–179.
229. Lee LA, Taylor J, Carter GP, et al. *Yersinia enterocolitica* O:3: an emerging cause of pediatric gastroenteritis in the United States. *J Infect Dis* 1991;163:660–663.
230. Jarvis WR. *Yersinia enterocolitica*: a new or unrecognized nosocomial pathogen? [editorial]. *Infect Control Hosp Epidemiol* 1992;13: 137–138.
231. Marks MI, Pai CH, Lafleur L, et al. *Yersinia enterocolitica* gastroenteritis: a prospective study of clinical, bacteriologic, and epidemiologic features. *J Pediatr* 1980;96:26–31.
232. Pai CH, Gillis F, Marks MI. Infection due to *Yersinia enterocolitica* in children with abdominal pain. *J Infect Dis* 1982;146:705.
233. Olinde AJ, Lucas JR Jr, Miller RC. Acute yersiniosis and its surgical significance. *South Med J* 1984;77:1539–1540.
234. Bradford WD, Noce PS, Gutman LT. Pathologic features of enteric infection with *Yersinia enterocolitica. Arch Pathol* 1974;98:17–22.
235. Winblad S. Arthritis associated with *Yersinia enterocolitica* infections. *Scand J Infect Dis* 1975;7:191–195.
236. Leino R, Kalliomaki JL. Yersiniosis as an internal disease. *Ann Intern Med* 1974;81:458–461.
237. Bouza E, Dominguez A, Meseguer M. *Yersinia enterocolitica* septicemia. *Am Soc Clin Pathol* 1979;74:404–409.
238. Robson AR, Hallett AE, Koonhof HJ. Generalized *Yersinia enterocolitica* infection. *J Infect Dis* 1975;131:447–451.
239. Shayegani M, Morse D, DeForge I, et al. Microbiology of a major foodborne outbreak of gastroenteritis caused by *Yersinia enterocolitica* serogroup O:8. *J Clin Microbiol* 1983;17:35–40.
240. Tacket CO, Ballard J, Harris N. An outbreak of *Yersinia enterocolitica* infections caused by contaminated tofu (soybean curd). *Am J Epidemiol* 1985;121:705–711.
241. Lee LA, Gerber AR, Lonsway DR. *Yersinia enterocolitica* O:3 infections in infants and children, associated with household preparation of chitterlings. *N Engl J Med* 1990;322:984–987.
242. Aber RC, McCarthy MA, Berman R, et al. An outbreak of *Yersinia enterocolitica* gastrointestinal illness among members of a Brownie troop in Centre County, Pennsylvania. Presented at the 22nd Interscience Conference on Antimicrobial Agents and Chemotherapy, Miami Beach, October 4–6, 1982.
243. Tauxe RV, Vandepitte J, Wauters G. *Yersinia enterocolitica* infections and pork: the missing link. *Lancet* 1987;1:1129–1132.
244. Tipple MA, Bland LA, Murphy JJ. Sepsis associated with transfusion of red cells contaminated with *Yersinia enterocolitica. Transfusion* 1990;30:207–213.
245. Centers for Disease Control. Update: *Yersinia enterocolitica* bacteremia and endotoxin shock associated with red blood cell transfusions—United States, 1991. *MMWR* 1991;40:176–178.
246. Rutnam S, Mercer E, Picco B, et al. A nosocomial outbreak of diarrheal disease due to *Yersinia enterocolitica* serotype O:5; biotype 1. *J Infect Dis* 1982;145:242–247.
247. Toivanen P, Toivanen A, Olkkonen L, et al. Hospital outbreak of *Yersinia enterocolitica* infection. *Lancet* 1973;1:801–803.
248. Cannon CG, Linnemann CC. *Yersinia enterocolitica* infections in hospitalized patients: the problem of hospital-acquired infections. *Infect Control Hosp Epidemiol* 1992;13:139–143.
249. Van Noyen R, Vandepitte J, Wauters G. *Yersinia enterocolitica*: its isolation by cold enrichment from patients and healthy subjects. *J Clin Pathol* 1981;34:1052–1056.
250. Head CB, Whitty DJ, Ratnam S. Comparative study of selective media for the recovery of *Yersinia enterocolitica. J Clin Microbiol* 1982; 16:615–621.
251. Bottone EJ, Sheehan DJ. *Yersinia enterocolitica*: guidelines for serologic diagnosis of human infections. *Rev Infect Dis* 1983;5:898–906.
252. Levine MM, Kaper JB, Black RE, et al. New knowledge on pathogenesis of bacterial enteric infections as applied to vaccine development. *Microbiol Rev* 1983;47:510–550.
253. Matthewson JJ, Johnson PC, DuPont HL, et al. Pathogenicity of enteroadherent *Escherichia coli* in adult volunteers. *J Infect Dis* 1986; 154:524–527.
254. Harris JR, Wachsmuth IK, Davis BR, et al. High-molecular-weight plasmid correlates with *Escherichia coli* enteroinvasiveness. *Infect Immun* 1982;37:1295–1298.
255. Riley LW, Remia RS, Helgerson SD, et al. Hemorrhagic colitis associated with a rare *Escherichia coli* serotype. *N Engl J Med* 1983;308: 681–685.
256. Centers for Disease Control. Update: multistate outbreak of *Escherichia coli* 0157:H7 infections from hamburgers in the Western United States. *MMWR* 1993;42:258–263.
257. Levine MM, Nataro JP, Karch H. The diarrheal response of humans to some classic serotypes of enteropathogenic *Escherichia coli* is dependent on a plasmid encoding an enteroadhesiveness factor. *J Infect Dis* 1985;152:550–559.
258. Levine MM, Edelman R. Enteropathogenic *Escherichia coli* of classic subtypes associated with infant diarrhea: epidemiology and pathogenesis. *Epidemiol Rev* 1984;6:31–51.
259. Giles C, Sangster G, Smith J. Epidemic gastroenteritis of infants in Aberdeen during 1947. *Arch Dis Child* 1949;24:45–53.
260. Levine MM, Bergquist EJ, Nalin DR. *Escherichia coli* strains that cause diarrhea but do not produce heat-labile or heat-stable enterotoxins and are non-invasive. *Lancet* 1978;1:1119–1122.
261. Bower JR, Congeni BL, Cleary TG. *Escherichia coli* O114: nonmotile as a pathogen in an outbreak of severe diarrhea associated with a day care center. *J Infect Dis* 1989;160:243–247.
262. DuPont HL, Ribner BS. Infectious gastroenteritis. In: Bennett JV, Brachman PS, eds. *Hospital infections.* Boston: Little, Brown, 1992: 641–657.
263. Western KA, St. John RK, Shearer LA. Hospital infection control—an international perspective [editorial]. *Infect Control* 1982;3: 453–455.
264. Morris KJ, Rao GG. Conventional screening for enteropathogenic *Escherichia coli* in the U.K. Is it appropriate or necessary? *J Hosp Infect* 1992;21:163–167.
265. Gross RJ, Rowe B, Henderson A, et al. A new *Escherichia coli* O-group, O159, associated with outbreaks of enteritis in infants. *Scand J Infect Dis* 1976;8:195–198.
266. Ryder RW, Wachsmuth IK, Buxton AE. Infantile diarrhea produced by heat-stable enterotoxigenic *E. coli. N Engl J Med* 1976;295: 849–853.
267. Wachsmuth IK, Falkow S, Ryder RW. Plasmid-mediated properties of heat-stable enterotoxin-producing *Escherichia coli* associated with infantile diarrhea. *Infect Immun* 1976;14:403–407.
268. MacDonald KL, Osterholm MT. The emergence of *Escherichia coli* O157:H7 infection in the United States. The changing epidemiology of foodborne disease. *JAMA* 1993;269:2264–2266.
269. Ryan CA, Tauxe RV, Hosek GW. *Escherichia coli* O157:H7 diarrhea

in a nursing home: clinical, epidemiological, and pathological findings. *J Infect Dis* 1986;154:631–638.

270. Ostroff SM, Griffin PM, Tauxe RV. A statewide outbreak of *Escherichia coli* O157:H7 infections in Washington state. *Am J Epidemiol* 1990;132:239–247.
271. Guarino A, Capano G, Malamisura B, et al. Production of *Escherichia coli* STa-like heat-stable enterotoxin by *Citrobacter freundii* isolated from humans. *J Clin Microbiol* 1987;25:110–114.
272. Kim SW, Peck KR, Jung SI, et al. *Psuedomonas aeruginosa* as a potential cause of antibiotic-associated diarrhea. *J Korean Med Sci* 2001; 16:742–744.
273. Guerrant RL, Dickens MD, Wenzel RP, et al. Toxigenic bacterial diarrhea: nursery outbreak involving multiple bacterial strains. *J Pediatr* 1976;89:885–891.
274. Robertson MS, Cade JF, Clancy RL. *Helicobacter pylori* infection in intensive care: increased prevalence and a new nosocomial infection. *Crit Care Med* 1999;27:1276–1280.
275. Blake PA, Rosenberg ML, Florencia J, et al. Cholera in Portugal, 1974. II. Transmission by bottled mineral water. *Am J Epidemiol* 1977;105:344–348.
276. Baine WB, Zampieri A, Mazzotti M, et al. Epidemiology of cholera in Italy in 1973. *Lancet* 1974;2:1370–1374.
277. Weissman JB, DeWitt WE, Thompson J. A case of cholera in Texas, 1973. *Am J Epidemiol* 1975;100:487–498.
278. Centers for Disease Control. Gastroenteritis caused by *Vibrio parahaemolyticus* aboard a cruise ship. *MMWR* 1978;27:65–66.
279. Moyer NP. Clinical significance of *Aeromonas* species isolated from patients with diarrhea. *J Clin Microbiol* 1987;25:2044–2048.
280. Morgan DR, Johnson PC, DuPont HL, et al. Lack of correlation between known virulence properties of *Aeromonas hydrophila* and enteropathogenicity for humans. *Infect Immun* 1985;50:62–65.
281. Chakraborty T, Montenegro MA, Sanyal SC, et al. Cloning of the enterotoxin gene from *Aeromonas hydrophila* provides conclusive evidence of production of a cytotonic cytotoxin. *Infect Immun* 1984;46: 435–441.
282. Shimada T, Sakazaki R, Horigome K, et al. Production of cholera-like enterotoxin by *Aeromonas hydrophila*. *Jpn J Med Sci Biol* 1984; 37:141–144.
283. Pazzaglia G, Sack RB, Bourgeois AL, et al. Diarrhea and intestinal invasiveness of *Aeromonas* strains in the removable intestinal tie rabbit model. *Infect Immun* 1990;58:1924–1931.
284. Altwegg M, Geiss HK. *Aeromonas* as a human pathogen. *Crit Rev Microbiol* 1989;16:253–286.
285. Burke V, Gracey M, Robinson J, et al. The microbiology of childhood gastroenteritis: *Aeromonas* species and other infective agents. *J Infect Dis* 1983;148:68–74.
286. Pazzaglia G, Sack RB, Salazar E, et al. High frequency of coinfecting enteropathogens in *Aeromonas*-associated diarrhea of hospitalized Peruvian infants. *J Clin Microbiol* 1991;29:1151–1156.
287. Schorling JB, Wanke CA, Schorling SK, et al. A prospective study of persistent diarrhea among children in an urban Brazilian slum. *Am J Epidemiol* 1990;132:144–156.
288. Hazen TC, Fliermans CB, Hirsch RP, et al. Prevalence and distribution of *Aeromonas hydrophila* in the United States. *Appl Environ Microbiol* 1978;36:731–738.
289. Holmberg SD, Schell WL, Fanning GR, et al. *Aeromonas* intestinal infections in the United States. *Ann Intern Med* 1986;105:683–689.
290. Burke V, Robinson J, Gracey M, et al. Isolation of *Aeromonas hydrophila* from a metropolitan water supply: seasonal correlation with clinical isolates. *Appl Environ Microbiol* 1984;48:361–366.
291. Millership SE, Stephenson JR, Tabaqchalis S. Epidemiology of *Aeromonas* species in a hospital. *J Hosp Infect* 1988;11:169–175.
292. Mellersh AR, Norman P, Smith GH. *Aeromonas hydrophila*: an outbreak of hospital infection. *J Hosp Infect* 1984;5:425–430.
293. Bloom HG, Bottone EJ. *Aeromonas hydrophila* diarrhea in a long-term care setting. *J Am Geriatr Soc* 1990;38:804–806.
294. Holmberg SD, Farmer JJ III. *Aeromonas hydrophila* and *Plesiomonas shigelloides* as causes of intestinal infections. *Rev Infect Dis* 1984;6: 633–639.
295. Bergdoll MS. The enterotoxins. In: Cohen JO, ed. The *staphylococci*. New York: Wiley, 1972:301–331.
296. Sugiyami H, Hayama T. Abdominal viscera as site of emetic action for staphylococcal enterotoxin in the monkey. *J Infect Dis* 1965;115: 330–336.
297. Bryan FL. What the sanitarian should know about staphylococci and salmonellae in non-dairy products. 1. Staphylococci. *J Milk Food Tech* 1968;31:110–116.
298. Batts DH, Silva J, Fekety R. *Staphylococcal enterocolitis*. In: Nelson JD, Grassi C, eds. *Current chemotherapy and infectious disease*, version 2. Washington, DC: American Society for Microbiology, 1980: 944–945.
299. Farber JM, Peterkin PI. *Listeria monocytogenes:* a foodborne pathogen. *Microbiol Rev* 1991;55:476–511.
300. Schwartz B, Ciesielski CA, Broome CV. Association of sporadic listeriosis with consumption of uncooked hot dogs and undercooked chicken. *Lancet* 1988;2:779–782.
301. Fleming DW, Cochi SL, MacDonald KL. Pasteurized milk as a vehicle of infection in an outbreak of listeriosis. *N Engl J Med* 1985;312: 404–407.
302. Linnan MJ, Mascola L, Lou XD. Epidemic listeriosis associated with Mexican-style cheese. *N Engl J Med* 1988;319:823–829.
303. Schlech WF, Lavigne PM, Bortolussi RA. Epidemic listeriosis—evidence for transmission by food. *N Engl J Med* 1983;308:203–206.
304. Gellin BG, Broome CV, Bibb WF, et al. The epidemiology of listeriosis in the United States—1986. *Am J Epidemiol* 1991;133:392–401.
305. Nieman RE, Lorber B. Listeriosis in adults: a changing pattern. Report of eight cases and review of the literature. *Rev Infect Dis* 1980;2: 207–227.
306. McLauchlin J. Human listeriosis in Britain 1967–1985: a summary of 722 cases. 1. Listeriosis during pregnancy and in the newborn. *Epidemiol Infect* 1990;104:181–189.
307. MacGowan AP, Gartlidge PH, MacLeod F, et al. Maternal listeriosis in pregnancy without fetal or neonatal infection. *J Infect* 1991;22: 55–57.
308. Goodner EK, Okumoto MA. Intraocular listeriosis. *Am J Ophthalmol* 1967;64:682–686.
309. Louria DB, Hensle T, Armstrong D. Listeriosis complicating malignant disease, a new association. *Ann Intern Med* 1967;67:260–281.
310. Anonymous. Clinicopathological conference. *N Engl J Med* 1974; 291:516–524.
311. Schwartz B, Hexter D, Broome CV. Investigation of an outbreak of listeriosis: a new hypothesis for the etiology of epidemic *Listeria monocytogenes* infections. *J Infect Dis* 1989;159:680–685.
312. McLauchlin J. Human listeriosis in Britain, 1967–1985: a summary of 722 cases. 2. Listeriosis in non-pregnant individuals, a changing pattern of infection and seasonal incidence. *Epidemiol Infect* 1990; 104:191.
313. Chernik NL, Armstrong D, Posner JB. Central nervous system infections in patients with cancer: changing patterns. *Cancer* 1977;40: 268–274.
314. Decker CE, Simon GL, DiGioia RA, et al. *Listeria monocytogenes* infections in patients with AIDS: report of 5 cases and review. *Rev Infect Dis* 1991;13:413–417.
315. Kendall MJ, Clarke SW, Smith WT. Spinal abscess due to *Listeria monocytogenes* in a patients with hepatic cirrhosis. *J Pathol* 1972;107: 9–11.
316. Stamm AM, Dismukes WE, Simmons BP. Listeriosis in renal transplant recipients: report of an outbreak and review of 102 cases. *Rev Infect Dis* 1982;4:665–682.
317. Lamont RJ, Postlethwaite R, MacGowan AP. *Listeria monocytogenes* and its role in human infection. *J Infect* 1988;17:7–28.
318. Ho JL, Shands KN, Friedland G, et al. An outbreak of type 4b *Listeria monocytogenes* infection involving patients from eight Boston hospitals. *Arch Intern Med* 1986;146:520–524.
319. Schuchat A, Lizano C, Broome CV, et al. Outbreak of neonatal listeriosis associated with mineral oil. *Pediatr Infect Dis* 1991;10:183–189.
320. Nelson KE, Warren D, Tomasi AM, et al. Transmission of neonatal listeriosis in a delivery room. *Am J Dis Child* 1985;139:903–905.
321. Bibb WF, Schwartz B, Gellin BG, et al. Analysis of Listeria monocyto-

genes by multilocus enzyme electrophoresis and application of the method to epidemiologic investigations. *Int J Food Microbiol* 1989; 8:233–239.

322. Shandera WX, Tacket CO, Blake PA. Food poisoning due to *Clostridium perfringens* in the United States. *J Infect Dis* 1983;147:167–170.
323. McDonel JL. Binding of *Clostridium perfringens* enterotoxin to rabbit intestinal cells. *Biochemistry* 1980;19:4801–4807.
324. Uemura T, Sskjelkvale R. An enterotoxin produced by *Clostridium perfringens* type D. *Acta Pathol Microbiol Scand* 1976;84:414–420.
325. Duncan CL. Time of enterotoxin formation and release during sporulation of *Clostridium perfringens* type A. *J Bacteriol* 1973;113: 932–936.
326. Hall HE, Angelotti R. *Clostridium perfringens* in meat and meat products. *Appl Microbiol* 1965;13:352–357.
327. Peterson LR, Musher R, Cooper GH, et al. A large *Clostridium perfringens* foodborne outbreak with an unusual attack rate pattern. *Am J Epidemiol* 1988;127:605–611.
328. Hobbs BC. *Clostridium perfringens* and *Bacillus cereus* infections. In: Riemann H, ed. *Foodborne infections and intoxications.* New York: Academic Press, 1969:131–173.
329. Larson HE, Borriello SP. Infectious diarrhea due to *Clostridium perfringens. J Infect Dis* 1988;157:390–391.
330. Borriello SP, Larson HE, Welch AR, et al. Enterotoxigenic *Clostridium perfringens*: a possible cause of antibiotic-associated diarrhea. *Lancet* 1984;1:305–306.
331. Murrell TGC, Egerton JR, Rampling A, et al. The ecology and epidemiology of the pig-bel syndrome in man in New Guinea. *J Hyg (London)* 1966;64:375–396.
332. Snyder JD, Merson MH. The magnitude of the global problem of acute diarrhoeal disease: a review of active surveillance data. *Bull WHO* 1982;60:967–974.
333. Guerrant RL, Kirchoff LV, Shields DS. Prospective study of diarrheal diseases in Northeastern Brazil: patterns of disease, nutritional impact, and risk factors. *J Infect Dis* 1983;148:986–997.
334. Ho MS, Glass RI, Pinsky PF, et al. Rotavirus as a cause of diarrheal morbidity and mortality in the United States. *J Infect Dis* 1988;158: 1112–1116.
335. Gurwith M, Wenman W, Hinde D, et al. A prospective study of rotavirus infection in infants and young children. *J Infect Dis* 1981; 144:218–224.
336. Matson DO, Estes MK. Impact of rotavirus at a large pediatric hospital. *J Infect Dis* 1990;162:598–604.
337. Koopman JS, Monto AS. The Tecumseh study XV: rotavirus infection and pathogenicity. *Am J Epidemiol* 1989;130:750–759.
338. Wenman W, Hinde D, Feltham S. Rotavirus in adults: results of a prospective family study. *N Engl J Med* 1979;301:303–306.
339. Hung T, Chen G, Wang C. Waterborne outbreak of rotavirus diarrhea in adults in China by a novel rotavirus. *Lancet* 1984;1: 1139–1142.
340. Blacklow NR, Greenberg HB. Viral gastroenteritis. *N Engl J Med* 1991;325:252–264.
341. Flewett TH. Rotavirus in the home and hospital nursery. *Br Med J* 1983;287:568–569.
342. Sattar SA, Lloyd-Evans N, Springthorpe VS. Institutional outbreaks of rotavirus diarrhoea: potential role of fomites and environmental surfaces as vehicles for virus transmission. *J Hyg (London)* 1986;96: 277–289.
343. Rogers M, Weinstock DM, Eagan J, et al. Rotavirus outbreak on a pediatric oncology floor: possible association with toys. *Am J Infect Control* 2000;28:378–380.
344. Estes MK, Palmer EL, Obijeski JF. Rotaviruses: a review. *Curr Top Microbiol Immunol* 1983;105:123–184.
345. Sattar SA, Raphael RA, Lochnan H, et al. Rotavirus inactivation by chemical disinfectants and antiseptics used in hospitals. *Can J Microbiol* 1983;29:1464–1469.
346. Tan JA, Schnagel RD. Inactivation of a rotavirus by disinfectants. *Med J Aust* 1981;1:19–23.
347. Haug KW, Orstavik I, Kuelstad G. Rotavirus infections in families. *Scand J Infect Dis* 1978;10:265–269.
348. Chrystie IL, Totterdell BM, Banatvala JE. Asymptomatic endemic rotavirus infection in the newborn. *Lancet* 1978;1:1176–1178.
349. Bishop RI, Hewstone AS, Davidson GP, et al. An epidemic of diarrhoea in human neonates involving a reovirus-like agent and enteropathogenic serotypes of *E. coli. J Clin Pathol* 1976;29:46–49.
350. Rodriguez WJ, Kim HW, Brandt CD, et al. Rotavirus: a cause of nosocomial infection in the nursery. *J Pediatr* 1982;101:274–277.
351. Gianino P, Mastretta E, Longo P, et al. Incidence of nosocomial rotavirus infections, symptomatic and asymptomatic, in breast-fed and non-breast-fed infants. *J Hosp Infect* 2002;50:13–17.
352. Samadi AR, Huq MI, Ahmed OS. Detection of rotavirus in handwashings of attendants of children with diarrhoea. *Br Med J* 1983; 286:188.
353. Widdowson MA, van Doornum GJ, van der Poel H, et al. An outbreak of diarrhea in a neonatal medium care unit caused by a novel strain of rotavirus: investigation using both epidemiologic and microbiological methods. *Infect Control Hosp Epidemiol* 2002;23:665–670.
354. Cubitt WD, Holzel H. Outbreak of rotavirus infection in a long-stay ward of a geriatric hospital. *J Clin Pathol* 1980;33:306–308.
355. Dennehy PH, Tenle WE, Fisher DJ, et al. Lack of impact of rapid identification of rotavirus-infected patients on nosocomial rotavirus infections. *Pediatr Infect Dis J* 1989;8:290–296.
356. Gaggero A, Avendano LF, Fernandez J, et al. Nosocomial transmission of rotavirus from patients admitted with diarrhea. *J Clin Microbiol* 1992;30:3294–3297.
357. Szajewska H, Kotowska M, Mrukowicz JZ, et al. Efficacy of Lactobacillus GG in prevention of nosocomial diarrhea in infants. *J Pediatr* 2001;138:361–365.
358. Stals F, Walther FJ, Bruggeman CA. Faecal and pharyngeal shedding of rotavirus and rotavirus IgA in children with diarrhea. *J Med Virol* 1984;14:333–339.
359. Santosham M, Yolken RH, Quiroz E. Detection of rotavirus in respiratory secretions of children with pneumonia. *J Pediatr* 1983;103: 583–585.
360. Holzel H, Cubitt WD, McSwiggen DA, et al. An outbreak of rotavirus infection among adults in a cardiology ward. *J Infect* 1980;2:33–37.
361. Marrie TJ, Lee SHS, Faulkner RS, et al. Rotavirus infection in a geriatric population. *Arch Intern Med* 1982;142:313–316.
362. Saulsbury FT, Winkelstein JA, Yolken RH. Chronic rotavirus infection in immunodeficiency. *J Pediatr* 1980;97:61–65.
363. Peigue-Lafeuille H, Henquell C, Chambon M, et al. Nosocomial rotavirus infections in adult renal transplant recipients. *J Hosp Infect* 1991;18:67–70.
364. Miotti PG, Eiden J, Yolken RH. Comparative efficacy of commercial immunoassays for the diagnosis of rotavirus gastroenteritis during the course of infection. *J Clin Microbiol* 1985;22:693–698.
365. Doern GV, Herrmann JE, Henderson P. Detection of rotavirus with a new polyclonal antibody enzyme immunoassay (Rotazyme II) and a commercial latex agglutination test (Rotalex): comparison with a monoclonal antibody enzyme immunoassay. *J Clin Microbiol* 1986; 23:226–229.
366. Wilde J, Yolken RH, Willoughby R, et al. Improved detection of rotavirus shedding by polymerase chain reaction. *Lancet* 1991;337: 323–326.
367. Spencer E, Avendano LF, Araya M. Characteristics and analysis of electropherotypes of human rotavirus isolated in Chile. *J Infect Dis* 1983;148:41–48.
368. Steel HM, Garnham S, Beards GM, et al. Investigation of an outbreak of rotavirus infection in geriatric patients by serotyping and polyacrilamide gel electrophoresis (PAGE). *J Med Virol* 1992;37:132–136.
369. Chanock SJ, Wenske EA, Fields BN. Human rotaviruses and genomic RNA [editorial]. *J Infect Dis* 1983;48:49–50.
370. Clark IN, McCrae MA. Structural analysis of electrophoretic variation in the genomic profiles of rotavirus field isolates. *Infect Immun* 1982; 36:492–497.
371. Rodriguez WJ, Kim HW, Brandt CD, et al. The use of electophoresis of RNA from human rotavirus to establish identity of strains involved in outbreaks in a tertiary care nursery. *J Infect Dis* 1983;148:34–40.
372. Konno T, Sato T, Suzuki K. Changing RNA patterns in rotavirus of human origin: demonstration of a single dominant pattern at the start

of an epidemic and various patterns thereafter. *J Infect Dis* 1984;149: 683–687.
373. Offit PA. The future of rotavirus vaccines. *Semin Pediatr Infect Dis* 2002;13:190–195.
374. Vesikari T. Clinical trials of live oral rotavirus vaccines: the Finnish experience. *Vaccine* 1993;11:255–261.
375. Linhares AC, Bresee JS. Rotavirus vaccines and vaccination in Latin America. *Rev Panam Salud Publica* 2000;8:305–331.
376. Palombo EA. Genetic and antigenic diversity of human rotaviruses: potential impact on the success of candidate vaccines. *FEMS Microbiol Lett* 1999;181:1–8.
377. Zahorsky J. *Hyperemesis hiemis* or the winter vomiting disease. *Arch Pediatr* 1929;46:391–395.
378. Adler JL, Zickl R. Winter vomiting disease. *J Infect Dis* 1969;119: 668–673.
379. Kapikian AZ, Wyatt RG, Dolin R, et al. Visualization by immune electron microscopy of a 27nm particle associated with acute infectious nonbacterial gastroenteritis. *J Virol* 1972;10:1075–1081.
380. Caul EO, Appleton H. The electron microscopical and physical characteristics of small round human fecal viruses. An interim scheme for classification. *J Med Virol* 1982;9:257–265.
381. Jiang X, Graham DY, Wank K, et al. Norwalk virus genome cloning and characterization. *Science* 1990;250:1580–1583.
382. Kaplan JE, Gary GW, Baron RC, et al. Epidemiology of Norwalk gastroenteritis and the role of Norwalk virus in outbreaks of acute nonbacterial gastroenteritis. *Ann Intern Med* 1982;96:756–761.
383. Herrmann JE, Nowak NA, Blacklow NR. Detection of Norwalk virus in stools by enzyme immunoassay. *J Med Virol* 1985;17:127–133.
384. DeLeon R, Matsui SM, Barrie RS. Detection of Norwalk virus in stool specimens by reverse transcriptase polymerase chain reaction and nonradioactive oligoprobes. *J Clin Microbiol* 1992;30: 3151–3157.
385. Nakata S, Estes MK, Chiba S. Detection of human calcivirus antigen and antibody by enzyme-linked immunosorbent assays. *J Clin Microbiol* 1988;26:2001–2005.
386. Herrmann JE, Nowak NA, Perron-Henry DM, et al. Diagnosis of astrovirus gastroenteritis by antigen detection with monoclonal antibodies. *J Infect Dis* 1990;161:226–229.
387. Agus SG, Dolin R, Wyatt RG, et al. Acute infectious nonbacterial gastroenteritis: intestinal histopathology, histologic and enzymatic alterations during illness produced by the Norwalk agents in man. *Ann Intern Med* 1973;79:18–25.
388. Taylor JW, Gary GW, Greenberg HB. Norwalk-related viral gastroenteritis due to contaminated drinking water. *Am J Epidemiol* 1981; 114:584–592.
389. Griffin MR, Surowiec JJ, McCloskey DI. Foodborne Norwalk virus. *Am J Epidemiol* 1982;115:178–184.
390. Oshiro LS, Haley CE, Roberto RR. A 27nm virus isolated during an outbreak of acute infectious nonbacterial gastroenteritis in a convalescent hospital: a possible new serotype. *J Infect Dis* 1981;143:791–795.
391. Pegues DA, Woernle CH. An outbreak of acute nonbacterial gastroenteritis in a nursing home. *Infect Control Hosp Epidemiol* 1993;14: 87–94.
392. Kaplan JE, Schonberger LB, Varano G, et al. An outbreak of acute nonbacterial gastroenteritis in a nursing home. Demonstration of person-to-person transmission by temporal clustering of cases. *Am J Epidemiol* 1982;116:940–948.
393. Centers for Disease Control. Viral agents of gastroenteritis: public health importance and outbreak management. *MMWR* 1990;39: 1–24.
394. Flewett TH, Bryden AS, Davies H, et al. Epidemic viral enteritis in a long-stay children's ward. *Lancet* 1975;1:4–5.
395. Uhnoo I, Wadell G, Svensson L, et al. Importance of enteric adenoviruses 40 and 41 in acute gastroenteritis in infants and young children. *J Clin Microbiol* 1984;20:365–372.
396. Horwitz MS. Adenoviruses. In: Fields BN, Knipe DM, eds. *Virology.* New York: Raven Press, 1990:1723–1740.
397. Van R, Wun C-C, O'Ryan ML, et al. Outbreak of human enteric adenovirus types 40 and 41 in Houston day care centers. *J Pediatr* 1992;120:516–521.
398. Brandt CD, Kim HW, Rodriguez WJ. Adenovirus and pediatric gastroenteritis. *J Infect Dis* 1983;151:437–443.
399. Shinozak T, Araki K, Ushijima H, et al. Antibody response to enteric adenovirus types 40 and 41 in sera of people of various age groups. *J Clin Microbiol* 1987;25:1679–1682.
400. Rodriguez WJ, Kim HW, Brandt CD. Fecal adenoviruses from a longitudinal study of families in metropolitan Washington DC: laboratory, clinical, and epidemiologic observations. *J Pediatr* 1985;107: 514–520.
401. Yolken RH, Lawrence F, Leister F, et al. Gastroenteritis with enteric type adenovirus in hospitalized infants. *J Pediatr* 1982;101:21–26.
402. Kotloff KL, Losonsky GA, Morris JG, et al. Enteric adenovirus infection and childhood diarrhea: an epidemiologic study in three clinical settings. *Pediatrics* 1989;84:219–225.
403. Wood DJ, Bailey AS. Detection of adenovirus type 40 and 41 in stool specimens by immune electron microscopy. *J Med Virol* 1987; 21:191–199.
404. Takiff HE, Seidlin M, Krause P. Detection of enteric adenoviruses by dot-blot hybridization using a molecularly cloned viral DNA probe. *J Med Virol* 1985;16:107–118.
405. Hammond G, Hannan C, Yeh T, et al. DNA hybridization for diagnosis of enteric adenovirus infection from directly spotted human fecal specimens. *J Clin Microbiol* 1987;25:1881–1885.
406. Herrmann JE, Perron-Henry DM, Blacklow NR. Antigen detection with monoclonal antibodies for the diagnosis of adenovirus gastroenteritis. *J Infect Dis* 1987;155:1167–1171.
407. Jamieson FB, Wang EE, Bain C, et al. Human torovirus: a new nosocomial gastrointestinal pathogen. *J Infect Dis* 1998;178:1263–1269.
408. Cohen R, Roth FJ, Delgado E, et al. Fungal flora of the normal human small and large intestine. *N Engl J Med* 1969;280:638–641.
409. Chretien JH, Garagusi VF. Current management of fungal enteritis. *Med Clin North Am* 1982;66:675–687.
410. Cello JP. Gastrointestinal manifestations of HIV infection. *Infect Dis Clin North Am* 1989;2:387–396.
411. Wey SB, Mori M, Pfaller M, et al. Hospital-acquired candidemia: the attributable mortality and excess length of stay. *Arch Intern Med* 1988;148:2642–2645.
412. Reagan DR, Pfaller M, Hollis RJ, et al. Characterization of the sequence of colonization and nosocomial candidemia using DNA fingerprinting and a DNA probe. *J Clin Microbiol* 1990;28:2733–2738.
413. Stone HH, Kolb LD, Currie CA, et al. *Candida* sepsis: pathogenesis and principles of treatment. *Ann Surg* 1974;179:697–711.
414. Gupta T, Ehrinpreis MN. *Candida*-associated diarrhea in hospitalized patients. *Gastroenterology* 1990;98:780–785.
415. Cutler JE, Friedman L, Milner KC. Biological and chemical characterization of toxic substances from *Candida albicans. Infect Immun* 1972; 6:616–627.
416. Barnes GL, Bishop RF, Townley RRW. Microbial flora and disaccharidase depression in infantile gastroenteritis. *Acta Pediatr Scand* 1974; 63:423–426.
417. Kozinn PJ, Taschdjian CL. Enteric candidiasis. *Pediatrics* 1962;30: 71–85.
418. Margolis BD, Tsang T-K, Kuo D. Persistent diarrhea secondary to *Candida* overgrowth [letter]. *Am J Gastroenterol* 1990;85:329–330.
419. Pfaller M. Epidemiological typing methods for mycoses. *Clin Infect Dis* 1992;149(suppl):4–10.
420. Doebbling BN, Hollis RJ, Wenzel RP, et al. Prospective evaluation of *Candida* hand carriage: molecular typing of paired isolates [abstract 261]. Interscience Conference on Antimicrobial Agents and Chemotherapy, Anaheim, CA, October 11–14, 1992.
421. Pfaller M, Cabezudo I, Hollis RJ, et al. The use of biotyping and DNA fingerprinting in typing *Candida albicans* from hospitalized patients. *Diagn Microbiol Infect Dis* 1990;13:481–489.
422. Pfaller M, Cabezudo I, Buschelman B. Value of the Hybritech ICON *Candida* assay in the diagnosis of invasive candidiasis in high-risk patients. *Diagn Microbiol Infect Dis* 1993;16:53–60.
423. Walsh TJ, Hathorn JW, Sobel JD. Detection of circulating *Candida* enolase by immunoassay in patients with cancer and invasive candidiasis. *N Engl J Med* 1991;324:1026–1031.
424. Kealey GD, Heinle JA, Lewis RW II, et al. Value of *Candida* antigen

assay in the diagnosis of systemic candidiasis in burn patients. *J Trauma* 1992;32:285–288.

425. Nime FA, Burek JD, Page DL, et al. Acute enterocolitis in a human being infected with the protozoan *Cryptosporidium. Gastroenterology* 1976;70:592–598.
426. Meisel JL, Perea DR, Meligro C, et al. Overwhelming watery diarrhea associated with a *Cryptosporidium* in an immunosuppressed patients. *Gastroenterology* 1976;70:1156–1160.
427. Current WL, Reese NC, Ernst JV, et al. Human cryptosporidiosis in immunocompetent and immunodeficient persons: studies of an outbreak and experimental transmission. *N Engl J Med* 1983;308: 1252–1257.
428. Fayer R, Ungar BLP. *Cryptosporidium* spp. and cryptosporidiosis. *Microbiol Rev* 1986;50:458–483.
429. Baxby D, Hart CA, Taylor C. Human cryptosporidiosis: a possible cause of hospital cross-infection. *Br Med J* 1983;287:1760–1761.
430. Martino P, Gentile G, Caprioli A. Hospital-acquired cryptosporidiosis in a bone marrow transplantation unit. *J Infect Dis* 1988;158: 647–649.
431. Koch KL, Phillips DJ, Aber RC, et al. Cryptosporidiosis in hospital personnel: evidence for person-to-person transmission. *Ann Intern Med* 1985;102:593–596.
432. Dryjanski J, Gold JW, Ritchie MT, et al. Cryptosporidiosis: case report in a health team worker. *Am J Med* 1986;80:751–752.
433. Bruce BB, Blass MA, Blumberg HM, et al. Risk of *Cryptosporidium parvum* transmission between hospital roommates. *Clin Infect Dis* 2000;31:947–950.
434. Tzipori S. *Cryptosporidium* in animals and humans. *Microbiol Rev* 1983;47:84–96.
435. Soave R, Armstrong D. *Cryptosporidium* and cryptosporidiosis. *Rev Infect Dis* 1986;8:1012–1023.
436. Wolfson JS, Richter JM, Waldron MA, et al. Cryptosporidiosis in immunocompetent patients. *N Engl J Med* 1985;312:1278–1282.
437. Jokipii L, Jokipii AMM. Timing of symptoms and oocyst excretion in human cryptosporidiosis. *N Engl J Med* 1986;315:1643–1647.
438. Smith PD, Quinn TC, Strober W, et al. Gastrointestinal infections in AIDS. *Ann Intern Med* 1992;116:63.
439. Fichtenbaum W, Ritchie DJ, Powderly WG. Use of paromomycin for treatment of cryptosporidiosis in patients with AIDS. *Clin Infect Dis* 1993;16:298–300.
440. White AC, Chappell CL, Hayat CS, et al. Paromomycin for cryptosporidiosis in AIDS: a prospective, double-blind trial. *J Infect Dis* 1994;170:419–424.
441. Rossignol JF, Ayoub A, Ayers MS. Treatment of diarrhea caused by *Cryptosporidium parvum*: a prospective randomized, double-blind, placebo-controlled study of nitazoxanide. *J Infect Dis* 2001;184: 103–106.
442. Hewitt RG, Yiannoutsos CT, Higgs ES. Paromomycin: no more effective than placebo for treatment of cryptosporidiosis in patients with advanced human immunodeficiency virus infection. *Clin Infect Dis* 2000;31:1084–1092.
443. White AC, Cron SG, Chappell CL. Paromomycin in cryptosporidiosis. *Clin Infect Dis* 2001;32:1516–1517.
444. Henricksen SA, Pohlenz JFL. Staining of cryptosporidia by a modified Ziehl-Neelson technique. *Acta Vet Scand* 1981;22:594–596.
445. Ma P, Soave R. Three-step stool examination for cryptosporidiosis in 10 homosexual men with protracted watery diarrhea. *J Infect Dis* 1983;147:824–828.
446. Siddons CA, Chapman PA, Rush BA. Evaluation of an enzyme immunoassay kit for detecting *Cryptosporidium* in feces and environmental samples. *J Clin Pathol* 1992;45:479–482.
447. Weber R, Bryan RT, Juranek DD. Improved stool concentration procedure for detection of cryptosporidium oocysts in fecal specimens. *J Clin Microbiol* 1992;30:2869–2873.
448. Ungar BL, Soave R, Fayer R, et al. Enzyme immunoassay detection of immunoglobulin M and G antibodies to *Cryptosporidium* in immunocompetent and immunocompromised patients. *J Infect Dis* 1986; 153:570–578.
449. Petri WA Jr, Ravdin JI. Amebiasis in institutionalized populations. In: Ravdin JI, ed. *Amebiasis.* New York: Wiley, 1988:576–581.
450. Smith PD, Lane HC, Gill VJ. Intestinal infections in patients with acquired immunodeficiency syndrome (AIDS). *Ann Intern Med* 1988; 108:328–333.
451. Istre GR, Kreiss K, Hopkins RS. An outbreak of amebiasis spread by colonic irrigation at a chiropractic clinic. *N Engl J Med* 1982;307: 339–341.
452. Samuelson J, Acuna-Soto R, Reed S, et al. DNA hybridization probe for clinical diagnosis of *Entamoeba histolytica. J Clin Microbiol* 1989; 27:671–676.
453. Acuna-Soto R, Samuelson J, De Giralami P. Application of polymerase chain reaction to the epidemiology of pathogenic and nonpathogenic *Entamoeba histolytica. Am J Trop Med Hyg* 1993;48:58–70.
454. Craun GF. Waterborne giardiasis in the United States. *Lancet* 1986; 2:513–514.
455. Kent GP, Greenspan JR, Herndon JL. Epidemic giardiasis caused by a contaminated public water supply. *Am J Public Health* 1988;78: 139–143.
456. Pickering LK, Woodward WE, DuPont HL, et al. Occurrence of *Giardia lamblia* in children in day care centers. *J Pediatr* 1984;104: 522–526.
457. Yoeli M, Most H, Hammond J, et al. Parasitic infections in a closed community: results of a 10-year survey in Willowbrook State Hospital. *Trans R Soc Trop Med Hyg* 1972;66:764–776.
458. White KE, Hedberg CW, Edmonson LM, et al. An outbreak of giardiasis in a nursing home with evidence for multiple modes of transmission. *J Infect Dis* 1989;160:298–304.
459. Flanagan PA. Giardiasis-diagnosis, clinical course and epidemiology. A review. *Epidemiol Infect* 1992;109:1–22.
460. Hoff JC. Inactivation of microbiol agents by chemical disinfectants. Water engineering research laboratory. EPA-600/2-86-067. Cincinnati: U.S. Environmental Protection Agency, 1986.
461. Meyer EA, Jarroll EL. Giardiasis. *Am J Epidemiol* 1980;111:1–12.
462. Balazs M, Szaltocky E. Electron microscope examination of the mucosa of the small intestine in infection due to *Giardia lamblia. Pathol Res Pract* 1978;163:251–260.
463. Welsh LD, Poley JR, Hensley J, et al. Intestinal disaccharidase and alkaline phosphatase activity in giardiasis. *J Pediatr Gastroenterol Nutr* 1984;3:37–40.
464. Black RE, Dykes AC, Sinclair SP, et al. Giardiasis in day-care centers: evidence of person-to-person transmission. *Pediatrics* 1977;60: 486–491.
465. Black RE, Dykes AC, Anderson KE. Handwashing to prevent diarrhea in day care centers. *Am J Epidemiol* 1982;113:445–451.
466. Paerregaard A, Kjelt K, Krasilnikoff PA. The diagnosis of childhood giardiasis. *J Pediatr Gastroenterol Nutr* 1990;10:275.
467. Bezjak B. Evaluation of a new technique for sampling duodenal contents in parasitologic diagnosis. *Am J Dig Dis* 1972;17:848–850.
468. Bendig DW. Diagnosis of giardiasis in infants and children by endoscopic brush cytology. *J Pediatr Gastroenterol Nutr* 1989;8:204–206.
469. Knisley CV, Engelkirk PG, Pickering LK, et al. Rapid detection of *Giardia* antigen in stool with the use of enzyme immunoassays. *Am J Clin Pathol* 1989;91:704–708.
470. Weiss JB, van Keulen H, Nash TE. Classification of subgroups of *Giardia lamblia* based on ribosomal DNA gene sequence using polymerase chain reaction. *Mol Biochem Parasitol* 1992;54:73–86.
471. Centers for Disease Control. Recommendations for precautions of HIV transmission in health care settings. *MMWR* 1987;36:3–18.
472. Conly JM, Hill S, Ross J, et al. Handwashing practices in an intensive care unit: the effects of an educational program and its relationship to infection rates. *Am J Infect Control* 1989;17:330–339.
473. Doebbling BN, Pfaller M, Houston AK, et al. Removal of nosocomial pathogens from the contaminated glove: implications for glove reuse and handwashing. *Ann Intern Med* 1988;109:394–398.
474. Doebbling BN, Stanley GL, Sheetz CT. Comparative efficacy of alternative hand-washing agents in reducing nosocomial infections in intensive care units. *N Engl J Med* 1992;327:88–93.
475. Simmons B, Bryant J, Neiman K, et al. The role of handwashing in prevention of endemic intensive care unit infections. *Infect Control Hosp Epidemiol* 1990;11:589–594.
476. Haley RW, Emori TG. The employee health service and infection

control in U.S. hospitals, 1976–1977. II Managing employee illness. *JAMA* 1981;246:962–966.
477. Valenti WM. Employee work restriction for infection control. *Infect Control* 1984;5:583–584.
478. Li J, Birkhead GS, Strogatz DS, et al. Impact of institution size, staffing patterns, and infection control practices on communicable disease outbreaks in New York State nursing homes. *Am J Epidemiol* 1996;143:1042–1049.
479. Williams WW. Guideline for infection control in hospital personnel. *Infect Control* 1983;4:326–349.
480. Benenson AS. *Control of communicable diseases in man,* 15th ed. Washington, DC: American Public Health Association, 1990.
481. Katoh M, Saito D, Noda T. *Helicobacter pylori* may be transmitted through gastrofiberscope even after manual Hyamine washing. *Jpn J Cancer Res* 1993;84:117–119.
482. Langenberg W, Rauws EAJ, Oudbier JH, et al. Patient-to-patient transmission of *Campylobacter pylori* infection by gastroduodenoscopy and biopsy. *J Infect Dis* 1990;161:507–511.
483. Spaulding EH. Chemical disinfection of medical and surgical materials. In: Lawrence CA, Block SS, eds. *Disinfection, sterilization, and preservation.* Philadelphia: Lea & Febiger, 1968:517–531.
484. Gorse GJ, Messner RL. Infection control practices in gastrointestinal endoscopy in the United States. *Infect Control Hosp Epidemiol* 1991; 12:289–296.
485. Favero MS. Strategies for disinfection and sterilization of endoscopes: the gap between basic principles and actual practice. *Infect Control Hosp Epidemiol* 1991;12:279–281.
486. Rutala WA. APIC guidelines for selection and use of disinfectant. *Am J Infect Control* 1990;18:99–117.
487. Jonas G, Mahoney A, Murray J, et al. Chemical colitis due to endoscope cleaning solutions: a mimic of pseudomembranous colitis. *Gastroenterology* 1988;95:1403–1408.
488. Alvarado CJ, Stolz S, Maki DG. Nosocomial infections from contaminated endoscopes: a flawed automated endoscope washer. An investigation using molecular epidemiology. *Am J Med* 1991;91(suppl 3B): 272s–280s.
489. Brooks SE, Veal RO, Kramer M, et al. Reduction in the incidence of *Clostridium difficile* associated diarrhea in an acute care hospital and a skilled nursing facility following replacement of electronic thermometers with single-use disposables. *Infect Control Hosp Epidemiol* 1992;13:98–103.
490. Jernigan JA, Giuliano K, Guerrant RL, et al. Effect of disposable thermometer use on rates of nosocomial Clostridium difficile diarrhea and total nosocomial infections: a randomized controlled study [abstract]. 33rd Interscience Conference on Antimicrobial Agents and Chemotherapy, New Orleans, October 17–20, 1993.
491. McNulty C, Logan M, Donald IP. Successful control *Clostridium difficile* infection in an elderly care unit through use of a restrictive antibiotic policy. *J Antimicrob Chemother* 1997;40:707–711.
492. Surawicz CM, Elmer GW, Speelman P, et al. Prevention of antibiotic associated diarrhea by *Saccharomyces boulardii*: a prospective study. *Gastroenterology* 1989;96:981–988.
493. Bank HL, John JF, Atkins LM, et al. Bactericidal action of modulated ultraviolet light on six groups of *Salmonella. Infect Control Hosp Epidemiol* 1991;12:486–489.
494. Glenister H, Taylor L, Bartlett C, et al. An assessment of selective surveillance methods for detecting hospital-acquired infection. *Am J Med* 1991;91(suppl 3B):121s-124s.
495. Wenzel RP, Osterman CA, Hunting KJ, et al. Hospital acquired infection I. Surveillance in a university hospital. *Am J Epidemiol* 1976; 4(suppl):245–325.
496. Lima NL, Periera CRB, Souza IC. Selective surveillance for nosocomial infections in a Brazilian hospital. *Infect Control Hosp Epidemiol* 1993;14:197–202.
497. Centers for Disease Control. *Outline for surveillance and control of nosocomial infections.* Atlanta: Centers for Disease Control, 1972.

25

NOSOCOMIAL BURN WOUND INFECTIONS

C. GLEN MAYHALL

Burn patients are among the patients at highest risk for hospital-acquired infections. These patients have lost a portion of their integument that would ordinarily be a strong barrier to invasion by microorganisms. In addition, the necrotic tissue in the burn eschar combined with the presence of serum proteins provides a rich culture medium for microorganisms. Added to the loss of integument is the adverse effect of thermal injury on both local and systemic immunity (1,2). Given these effects of burn trauma, it is easily understood why burn patients are at risk for nosocomial burn wound infections.

Data submitted from burn intensive care units to the National Nosocomial Infections Surveillance (NNIS) system at the Centers for Disease Control and Prevention (CDC) indicate that the cumulative incidence for burn wound infections is 4.5% and the incidence rate is 6.8 cases per 1,000 patient-days (R. Gaynes, personal communication, 1998). Infections are the most common cause of death in burn patients, and the most common sites of infection are the lungs and the burn wound (3). The burn wound may also initiate and perpetuate a mediator-induced septic response accompanied by multiple-organ failure in the absence of an identifiable focus of infection and with negative blood culture results (4). Thus, proliferation of microorganisms in the burn wound followed by invasion of subjacent viable tissue or the mediator-induced septic response may cause the clinical manifestations of sepsis.

Although the most important cause of death in burn patients is infection, the current overall mortality rate due to infections in the burn patient is unknown (5). However, data from the NNIS system on patients with burn wound infection who died, and for whom the relationship of infection to death was reported, indicated that 18 (12.6%) of 143 deaths were caused by burn wound infection. Burn wound infection contributed importantly to death in 104 patients (72.7%), and the burn wound infection was unrelated to death in the remaining 21 patients (14.7%) (R. Gaynes, personal communication, 1998). It has also been observed that mortality in burn patients is significantly increased by bacteremia due to gram-negative bacilli (6).

TYPES OF BURNS

Most burns are due to thermal injury. Most burn injuries in adults are due to flame burns, and accidents with flammable liquids are the most common causes of burns in teenagers and adults (7). In children, 80% of burns are caused by hot liquids and 15% by flames. The remaining 5% are made up of chemical or electrical burns, house fires, and firecracker injuries (8). Chemical and electrical burns also make up a small percentage of burns in adults (9). The discussion of burn wound infections in this chapter is limited to infections that complicate thermal injuries.

PATHOGENESIS OF BURN WOUND INFECTIONS

Loss of the integument combined with the immune defects that accompany thermal injury place the burn patient at high risk for burn wound infection. Microorganisms are present on the skin at the time of burning and are readily acquired from the patient's gastrointestinal tract after the thermal injury has been sustained. Microorganisms are rapidly acquired from the environment of the burn care facility as well as from other burn patients cared for in the same unit.

In addition to the loss of the skin barrier, the rapid colonization of the burn wound from endogenous and exogenous sources, and the excellent culture medium provided by the burn wound, thermal injury has a substantial suppressive effect on the immune system. Immunosuppression involves the nonspecific immune system (abnormal neutrophil and macrophage function) (2,5,8,10), cellular immunity (decreased ratio of helper to suppressor lymphocytes, decreased natural killer cell activity) (2, 10), and humoral immunity (activation of complement with drop in complement levels, decreased serum immunoglobulin levels) (2,8,10). There is evidence that the immunosuppression that occurs after thermal injury is due to local accumulation of cytokines in the areas of burn injury that "spill over" into the systemic circulation (11). Thus, local accumulation of multiple cytokines in the area of injury that mediate the reparative process has a marked suppressive effect on host defenses when these cytokines enter the bloodstream and are distributed throughout the body.

With the loss of the integument, immunosuppression, and availability of nutrients for microbial proliferation, microorganisms contaminating the surface of the burn wound may multiply to high concentrations. Early colonization of the wound in the first 48 hours takes place with gram-positive microorganisms from within the depths of the sweat glands and hair follicles (5, 10,12). Between 3 and 21 days, the wound becomes colonized with gram-negative bacilli from the patient's own gastrointestinal tract or from other patients in the burn care facility (5,10). If microorganisms reach a concentration of at least 10^5 colony forming units (CFUs) per gram of tissue, they may spread from the hair follicles along the dermal subcutaneous junction (12). Perivascular colonization may result in thrombosis, vascular occlusion, and necrosis of the remaining viable elements. The resultant ischemia and bacterial autolysis may convert a partial-thickness injury to a full-thickness injury. In burn wounds with unexcised eschar, invasion of the subeschar viable subcutaneous tissue results in burn wound infection or burn wound sepsis and may be complicated by bacteremia.

CLINICAL MANIFESTATIONS OF BURN WOUND INFECTIONS

In burn wounds with unexcised eschar, clinical manifestations of burn wound infection appear when microorganisms reach high concentrations in the burn eschar and invade subjacent viable tissue. Clinical signs of infection may depend, to some extent, on the type of infecting microorganism. Hyperthermia and leukocytosis tend to be more marked in patients with gram-positive infection. Infections with gram-positive microorganisms are also more often associated with irrational behavior and mental confusion. The appearance of a wound infected by gram-positive microorganisms may be characterized by maceration with a ropy tenacious exudate and surrounding cellulitis (12).

Patients with gram-negative burn wound infection are more likely to have hypothermia and leukopenia. Although they may have altered mental status with confusion, some patients with gram-negative burn wound infection may remain lucid until near death (12,13). Patients with gram-negative infection may also have glucose intolerance with hyperglycemia, ileus and abdominal distention, respiratory distress syndrome, and oliguria (13).

The wound infected by gram-negative microorganisms is characterized by (a) focal gangrene that coalesces and spreads throughout the wound; (b) conversion of a partial-thickness wound to a full-thickness wound; (c) hemorrhagic discoloration of subeschar tissue; (d) focal, multifocal, or generalized dark brown, black, or violaceous discoloration of the burn wound; and (e) changes in unburned skin at the wound margins characterized by edema and violaceous discoloration (12,13). Bacteremia is a common complication of burn wound infection, but absence of bacteremia does not rule out burn wound infection. In fact, fatal burn wound infection may occur in the absence of bacteremia, particularly when the infection is caused by gram-negative microorganisms (12).

DIAGNOSIS OF BURN WOUND INFECTION

Clinical Diagnosis

Examination of the burn wound and clinical signs and symptoms provide important clues to the diagnosis of burn wound infection. As noted above, changes in the wound characterized by dark brown, black, or violaceous discoloration; unexpectedly rapid separation of the eschar; hemorrhagic discoloration of subeschar tissue and edema; and violaceous discoloration of unburned skin at the wound margin suggest burn wound infection (13). Clinical suspicion of infection is heightened when these local wound manifestations are accompanied by hypothermia (<36°C), hyperthermia (>38°C), hypotension (systolic blood pressure ≤90 mm Hg), oliguria (<20 mL/hour), ileus with abdominal distention, glucose intolerance and hyperglycemia, or altered mental status (13,14).

Microbiologic Diagnosis of Burn Wound Infection

In a study wherein about 80% of burn wound biopsies were obtained from patients with local signs of burn wound infection, Pruitt and Foley (15) observed that 75% of patients with more than 10^5 CFU/g of burn wound tissue died. When this density of microorganisms in the burn eschar was combined with a grade 6 histologic diagnosis ("invasive infection with microbial penetration into viable tissue beyond the depth of original necrosis"), the mortality rate was 100%. Loebl et al. (16) observed that 88% of children and 63% of adults who had at least 10^4 CFU/g of burn wound tissue developed clinical signs of sepsis. In a study comparing quantitative culture of burn wound biopsies with histopathologic examination of the same specimen, 100% of patients with invasive burn wound infection by histopathologic examination had wound counts between 10^4 and 10^6 CFU/g of burn wound tissue (17). However, patients in whom no microorganisms were seen in the burn wound or only a few microorganisms were seen on the surface of the wound microscopically sometimes had wound counts between 10^3 and 10^6 CFU/g of burn wound tissue; wound counts ranged between 10^6 and 10^7 CFU/g of burn wound tissue in 100% of patients with wound involvement limited to heavy surface colonization by histopathologic examination. Thus, using a cutoff of at least 10^4 CFU/g of tissue, quantitative culture of burn wound biopsies had a sensitivity of 100% but a substantially lower specificity, which could not be determined from the data provided in the report. In another study comparing quantitative burn wound cultures and histopathologic examination of the same tissue, McManus et al. (18) observed that growth of at least 10^5 CFU/g of tissue identified burn wound infection diagnosed by histopathologic assessment of tissue 96.1% of the time. However, 64.3% of biopsies that showed negative results histopathologically also had at least 10^5 CFU/g of tissue. Thus, quantitative burn wound cultures have a high sensitivity (96.1%) but a low specificity (35.7%). Stated another way, burn wounds with less than 10^5 CFU/g of tissue are highly unlikely to be infected, whereas only about one third of burn wounds with at least 10^5 CFU/g of tissue will be infected.

Although the threshold of at least 10^5 CFU/g of burn wound tissue has a high sensitivity and low specificity for burn wound infection, a threshold of over 10^8 CFU/g of tissue is highly suggestive of burn wound sepsis and impending death in the untreated patient (19,20). Thus, even though the definitive diagnosis of burn wound infection may be made by histopathologic examination of a full-thickness biopsy of the burn wound (see below), it would appear that (a) burn wound biopsies containing less than 10^5 CFU/g of tissue suggest that burn wound infection is unlikely; (b) biopsies containing 10^5 to 10^8 CFU/g of tissue are uninterpretable; and (c) biopsies with more than 10^8 CFU/g of tissue are highly suggestive of burn wound sepsis.

One problem with the interpretation of quantitative cultures of burn wound biopsies has been the uneven distribution of microorganisms, both qualitatively and quantitatively, throughout the burn wound. In a study wherein culture results were not correlated with clinical manifestations, appearance of the burn wound, or histopathologic examination of the tissue taken for culture, Woolfrey et al. (21) concluded, "Quantitative results derived from burn wound biopsy cultures are unreliable and may be significantly misleading when used for decision-making relative to patient care." These authors divided each biopsy specimen and cultured the two portions separately. Between the two segments, an average of 4.8 microorganism types were recovered. At the 10^5 CFU/g of tissue breakpoint, the paired quantitative results agreed within the same log increment for only 38% of biopsies. Although it is clear from the data of Woolfrey et al. that there may be large qualitative and quantitative differences in burn wound microbiology between immediately adjacent areas of the wound, it is unclear how their results relate to the appearance of the burn wound (and whether biopsies were taken from areas of the wound that appeared infected on clinical examination), histopathologic examination of the tissue taken for culture, and the clinical course of the patient.

Other studies tend to support the usefulness of quantitative culture of burn wound biopsies. Volenec et al. (22) observed that bacterial counts in immediately adjacent burn wound biopsies varied little, with an estimated pooled standard deviation of 0.64 log to the base 10.

Surface swab cultures, either qualitative or quantitative, have been used in the diagnosis of burn wound infections. Steer et al. (23) compared qualitative results and quantitative bacterial counts of 141 surface swabs and 141 wound biopsies taken from 74 burn patients. They observed a significant correlation between the total bacterial counts of surface swabs and the total bacterial counts of biopsies ($p < .001$), but the predictive value of the counts obtained by one method to predict the counts obtained by the other method was poor. The qualitative correlation was also poor, and only 54% of the biopsy/swab pairs yielded the same microorganism on culture. There were two exceptions to the latter observation. When *Staphylococcus aureus* was present in the burn wound biopsy, it was present on surface culture 95% of the time, and when *Pseudomonas aeruginosa* was recovered from the burn wound biopsy, it was cultured from the surface swabs 92% of the time. Thus, although *S. aureus* and *P. aeruginosa* in the burn wound may be detected by surface swabs, qualitative and quantitative surface cultures are generally not useful for predicting the qualitative and quantitative microbiology of the burn wound.

When the diagnosis of burn wound infection is made by histopathologic examination of a full-thickness burn wound biopsy (see below), quantitative culture of a portion of the biopsy may identify the causative microorganism(s) and provide antimicrobial susceptibility data for the selection of appropriate antimicrobial therapy. McManus et al. (18) observed a 100% concordance between microorganisms seen on histopathologic examination and those recovered on culture. Thus, burn wound biopsies should be both cultured and examined histopathologically. Although quantitative cultures may not be necessary for identification of the causative microorganism(s), quantitation might be useful in separating microorganisms on and in the nonviable tissue from those invading viable tissue. It would be unlikely that microorganisms recovered at a concentration below 10^5 CFU/g of tissue would be causing burn wound infection (18).

Although some investigators have found a good correlation between the results of quantitative gram-stained preparations and quantitative cultures of biopsy tissue (24,25), others have not (26). Even with a good correlation between quantitative gram-stain and culture results, the results of microscopic examination of gram-stained tissue should not be used for diagnosis of burn wound infection, because definitive diagnosis of burn wound infection requires histopathologic examination and culture.

Histopathologic Diagnosis of Burn Wound Infection

In burn wounds with unexcised eschar, the diagnosis of burn wound infection may be made by histopathologic examination of a full-thickness burn wound biopsy. The biopsy should be taken from the area of the wound with the most pronounced local changes (see above). A lenticular tissue sample should be obtained using a scalpel. The biopsy should measure from 0.5 × 0.5 × 0.5 cm to 1 × 1 × 1 cm and should weigh between 100 and 500 mg. The biopsy must include underlying or adjacent unburned tissue in addition to the eschar. The specimen should be divided; one half should be cultured quantitatively, and the other half should be placed in 10% neutral buffered formalin solution for processing for histopathologic examination. The tissue should be stained with hematoxylin and eosin stain, Brown Hopps Gram stain, and periodic acid-Schiff stain (13,27).

Histopathologic examination may show microorganisms localized to the burn eschar surface or various degrees of penetration of the eschar. Burn wound infection or sepsis develops when microorganisms invade through the eschar and into viable tissue subjacent to the eschar. These histopathologic manifestations of burn wound infection were carefully described 35 years ago by Teplitz et al. (28) using rats as an experimental model. Their findings in the animal model appear to parallel those observed in humans with thermal injury.

Kim et al. (29) have described a frozen section technique for rapid evaluation of burn wound biopsies for burn wound infection. This technique reduces the time of processing from 4 hours (rapid technique) to 30 minutes. Application of the frozen section technique to burn wound biopsies had not been possible in the past because of the hardness of the eschar. However, advances in this technique, which made frozen sections of bone and cartilage possible, have permitted its application to burn wound biopsies as well. Frozen section diagnosis should always be confirmed by examination of permanent sections (rapid section technique).

DEFINITIONS OF BURN WOUND INFECTION

Although burn wound infection may be diagnosed by histopathologic examination of a full-thickness burn wound biopsy, and the causative agent may be established by culture of the biopsy or by histopathologic examination of the burn wound biopsy using special stains for microorganisms (e.g., periodic acid-Schiff stain for fungi), such studies may not be available in all burn care facilities. Further, when the burn wound has been excised, there may be no tissue to biopsy. Thus, case definitions are needed for surveillance and outbreak investigation that make use of other, more easily obtained data such as clinical observations, blood cultures, viral cultures, and microscopic examination of lesion scrapings for viral inclusions. Table 25.1 shows case definitions for burn wound infections used by the NNIS system.

TABLE 25.1. DEFINITIONS FOR BURN WOUND INFECTIONS

Burn infections must meet one of the following criteria:

Criterion 1:	Patient has a change in burn wound appearance or character, such as rapid eschar separation, or dark brown, black, or violaceous discoloration of the eschar, or edema at wound margin *and* histologic examination of burn biopsy shows invasion of organisms into adjacent viable tissue
Criterion 2:	Patient has a change in burn wound appearance or character, such as rapid eschar separation, or dark brown, black, or violaceous discoloration of the eschar, or edema at wound margin *and* at least *one* of the following: a. organisms cultured from blood in the absence of other identifiable infection b. isolation of herpes simplex virus, histologic identification of inclusions by light or electron microscopy, or visualization of viral particles by electron microscopy in biopsies or lesion scrapings
Criterion 3:	Patient with a burn has at least *two* of the following signs or symptoms with no other recognized cause: fever (>38°C) or hypothermia (<36°C), hypotension, oliguria (<20 mL/h), hyperglycemia at previously tolerated level of dietary carbohydrate, or mental confusion *and* at least *one* of the following: a. histologic examination of burn biopsy shows invasion of organisms into adjacent viable tissue b. organisms cultured from blood c. isolation of herpes simplex virus, histologic identification of inclusions by light or electron microscopy, or visualization of viral particles by electron microscopy in biopsies or lesion scrapings

From the National Nosocomial Infections Surveillance (NNIS) system manual, section XIII, CDC, December, 1993, unpublished.

One element missing from the NNIS definitions is that of the causative agent. Thus, if one were selecting a definition for burn wound infection in a suspected outbreak of burn wound infections caused by *S. aureus*, it would be appropriate to include culture of *S. aureus* from the burn wound in the case definition of infection. The source from which a culture must be taken to establish the cause of a burn wound infection is not described in the NNIS definitions. For bacterial infections, the culture should be taken from a full-thickness burn wound biopsy and not the surface of the burn wound. Another acceptable source is blood if no other possible site of infection can be identified. Although fungi may be cultured from a full-thickness burn wound biopsy, most fungal burn wound infections will probably be diagnosed by histopathologic examination of burn wound biopsies. Herpes simplex may be cultured from scrapings from the burn wound surface; viral inclusions may also be seen microscopically in burn wound scrapings.

The NNIS definitions are based on burn wounds containing unexcised eschar. Since burn wounds are treated in many centers now by early excision and grafting, definitions are needed for infections in surgically created wounds such as excised burns and donor sites. Further, definitions are needed for other types of infections related to the burn wound such as burn wound impetigo and burn wound cellulitis (30). For the purposes of surveillance, the NNIS system lumps all wounds related to thermal injury and its treatment together as burn infections. However, when an outbreak occurs involving sites other than burn wound containing unexcised eschar, it will be necessary to use case definitions specific to the type of infection involved in the outbreak (Table 25.2).

ETIOLOGIES OF BURN WOUND INFECTIONS

Burn wound infections may be caused by bacteria, fungi, or viruses. Although not invariably the case (31), bacteria probably cause the majority of infections in most burn care centers. Almost all burn wound infections caused by bacteria are due to aerobic microorganisms. Anaerobes cause up to 2% of all burn wound infections (32,33).

Bacteria

Bacterial etiologies of burn wound infection vary, to some extent, from country to country. The best data on bacterial causes of burn wound infection in the United States are from the NNIS system (Table 25.3). As can be seen from the table, *S. aureus* continues to be the most important cause of bacterial burn wound infections. Although data are not available from the NNIS system, many burn care facilities have encountered many strains of methicillin-resistant *S. aureus* (MRSA) over the last 15 years (34–38). Occasionally, strains of *S. aureus* that produce toxic shock syndrome toxin (TSST) and exfoliative toxin (ET) cause burn wound infection (39–42). *S. aureus* also remains the most common cause of burn wound infection in the United Kingdom (43,44). Although much less common, β-hemolytic group A streptococci may occasionally cause outbreaks of burn wound infection (45). However, groups A, B,

TABLE 25.2. PROPOSED DEFINITIONS FOR BURN WOUND INFECTIONS (INCLUDING BURN WOUND IMPETIGO, OPEN BURN-RELATED SURGICAL WOUND INFECTIONS, CELLULITIS, AND INFECTION OF UNEXCISED BURN WOUNDS)

Infection	Criterion (Must Meet the Following)
Burn wound impetigo	Infection involves loss of epithelium from a previously reepithelialized surface such as grafted burns, partial-thickness burns allowed to close by secondary intention, or healed donor sites *and* Is not related to inadequate excision of the burn, mechanical disruption of the graft, or hematoma formation *and* Requires some change of or addition to antimicrobial therapy It may or may not be associated with systemic signs of infection such as hyperthermia (temperature >38.4°C) or leukocytosis (white blood cell count >10,000/m^3)
Open burn-related surgical wound infection	Infection occurs in surgically created wounds such as excised burns and donor sites that have not yet epithelialized *and* Has a purulent exudate that is culture-positive *and* Requires change of treatment (which may include change of or addition to antimicrobial therapy, removal of wound covering, or increase in frequency of dressing changes) *and* Includes at least one of the following: 1. Loss of synthetic or biologic covering of the wound 2. Changes in wound appearance such as hyperemia 3. Erythema in the uninjured skin surrounding the wound 4. Systemic signs such as hyperthermia or leukocytosis
Burn wound cellulitis	Infection occurs in uninjured skin surrounding the burn wound or donor site *and* Is associated with erythema in the uninjured skin progressing beyond what is expected from the inflammation of the burn *and* Is not associated with other signs of infection in the wound itself *and* Requires change of or addition to antimicrobial therapy *and* Includes at least one of the following: 1. Localized pain or tenderness, swelling, or heat at the affected site 2. Systemic signs of infection such as hyperthermia, leukocytosis, or septicemia 3. Progression of erythema and swelling 4. Signs of lymphangitis and/or lymphadenitis
Invasive infection in unexcised burn wounds	Infection occurs in deep partial-thickness or full-thickness burn that has not been surgically excised *and* Is associated with change in burn wound appearance or character, such as rapid eschar separation, or dark brown, black, or violaceous discoloration of the eschar *and* Requires surgical excision of the burn and treatment with systemic antimicrobials *and* May be associated with, but not dependent on, any of the following: 1. Inflammation of the surrounding uninjured skin, such as edema, erythema, warmth, or tenderness 2. Histologic examination of the burn biopsy specimen that shows invasion of organism into adjacent viable tissue 3. Organism isolated from blood culture in absence of other identifiable infection 4. Systemic signs of infection such as hyper- or hypothermia, leukocytosis, tachypnea, hypotension, oliguria, hyperglycemia at previously tolerated level of dietary carbohydrate, or mental confusion

From Peck MD, Weber J, McManus A, et al. Surveillance of burn wound infections: a proposal for definitions. *J Burn Care Rehabil* 1998;19:386–389.

and G streptococci are the third most common cause of burn wound infections in the burn unit at the Karolinska Hospital in Stockholm (46) (see also Chapter 31).

The NNIS data indicate that *P. aeruginosa* is the second most common burn wound pathogen, but this is not true for all burn care facilities in the U.S. In 1989, McManus (47) reported that only 0.2% of patients at the U.S. Army Institute of Surgical Research admitted between 1983 and 1987 developed burn wound infections due to *P. aeruginosa*. Likewise, the percentage of burn wound infections caused by *P. aeruginosa* fell dramatically during the 1980s at three burn care facilities in the United Kingdom (43,44).

Similar to nosocomial infections in other body sites, enterococci have become one of the most important causes of burn

TABLE 25.3. BACTERIAL CAUSES OF BURN WOUND INFECTIONS

Pathogen[a]	Frequency	Percentage
Staphylococcus aureus	420	23.0
Pseudomonas aeruginosa	353	19.3
Enterococci	202	11.0
Enterobacter spp.	176	9.6
Escherichia coli	131	7.2
Coagulase-negative staphylococci	78	4.3
Candida albicans	64	3.5
Serratia marcescens	64	3.5
Klebsiella pneumoniae	48	2.6
Others	294	16.0

Data from National Nosocomial Infections Surveillance system, Centers for Disease Control and Prevention, 1980–1998.
[a] 1,830 pathogens associated with 1,234 burn wound infections.

wound infection (Table 25.3). This is likely due to the widespread use of third-generation cephalosporins over the last decade to which enterococci are resistant. In 1986, Jones et al. (48) reported on a series of cases of burn wound sepsis caused by enterococci. Enterococcal infection was diagnosed by recovery of at least 10^5 CFU/g of tissue on burn wound biopsy or by recovery of enterococci from blood cultures. They identified 38 enterococcal burn wound infections in 26 months. Twenty patients developed enterococcal bacteremia, and ten of these patients died. Enterococci appear to be not only common but also virulent burn wound pathogens. As has been noted in other patient populations in the hospital, vancomycin-resistant enterococci (VRE) have been reported to cause an outbreak of VRE colonization and infection in a burn intensive care unit (49) (see also Chapter 32).

Other important bacterial burn wound pathogens include *Enterobacter* species, *Escherichia coli, Proteus* species, *Klebsiella* species, *Serratia marcescens,* and *Acinetobacter* species (43,44,50). *Acinetobacter* continues to emerge as an important cause of infection in burn patients. Recent outbreaks of infections due to multiresistant strains of *A. baumannii* have been reported from burn treatment facilities (51–53).

Fungi

As bacterial burn wound infections have come under better control with use of topical antimicrobial agents, better isolation techniques, and, perhaps, early burn wound excision, the relative importance of fungal burn wound infections has increased. At the U.S. Army Institute of Surgical Research in San Antonio, fungal burn wound infections occur in about 7.5% of annual admissions and are the most common infectious complication involving the burn wound (54).

Candida Species

Candida species are the fungal microorganisms that most commonly colonize the burn wound but do not invade and cause infection as often as do *Aspergillus* species and other filamentous fungi (55). Thus, the surfaces of burn wounds are frequently colonized by *Candida* species, but only 0.6% to 10% of patients develop burn wound infection due to *Candida* species according to histopathologic examination of burn wound tissue (54–58). The relative proportions of the different species of *Candida* that cause burn wound infections cannot be determined from the literature.

Filamentous Fungi

The great preponderance of burn wound infections caused by fungi are due to filamentous fungi. The filamentous fungi that most often cause burn wound infections are *Aspergillus* species, Zygomycetes (*Mucor* species, *Rhizopus* species), *Geotrichum* species, and *Fusarium* species. Less commonly isolated are *Drechslera* species, *Alternaria* species, and *Microspora* species (54, 59–61). The majority of these microorganisms are identified by their morphology on histopathologic examination of burn wound biopsies, because the recovery from culture of burn wound tissue is only about 30% for all fungi that cause burn wound infections (54).

Viruses

Herpes Simplex

Herpes simplex infections may occur in burn patients. Most of these infections appear to be reactivation infections and may be symptomatic or asymptomatic. Asymptomatic infections are detected by a fourfold or greater rise in antibody titer (62). Symptomatic infections most commonly involve the burn wound and tend to occur in healing partial-thickness burn wounds that involve the face (63–65). The infection, which apparently reactivates in the healing skin after burn injury, may disseminate to involve liver, adrenal glands, lungs, spleen, gastrointestinal tract, and urinary bladder (63). No data are available on the incidence of herpes simplex infections of burn wounds. In one study, 25% of children with burns had serologic evidence of herpes simplex infection, and all were reactivation infections (62). Only one of these children had a burn wound infection due to herpes simplex.

In one study of adult burn patients, 40% had serologic evidence of herpes virus infection, but apparently there was no herpetic involvement of their burn wounds (66). About 90% of these infections were reactivation infections, and about 10% appeared to be primary infections.

Cytomegalovirus

In one published study of burn patients with a mean age of 29 years, the incidence of cytomegalovirus (CMV) infection was 33% (66). These infections were due to reactivation of latent infections in 76% of the patients. There was no evidence that transfusion of blood products increased the incidence of primary or reactivation CMV infections. These infections were apparently asymptomatic, and none involved the burn wound. In a second study, 29% of the burn patients developed CMV infection, but again, none had any clinical manifestations of infection (67).

In a series of pediatric burn patients, 33% of the patients developed CMV infections (62). Unlike the adult patients, some pediatric patients developed fever and hepatitis. In a second study from the same institution, CMV infection was found to have caused initially unexplained fevers in four patients (68). None of the patients in these two reports had involvement of the burn wound by CMV. In the former study, a few patients had adenovirus infections and reactivated Epstein-Barr virus and varicella-zoster virus (VZV) infections, but none of these infections involved the burn wound.

In pediatric burn hospitals, infections in patients due to VZV occur uncommonly but may cause serious disease such as VZV pneumonia (69). Although there has been no significant involvement of the burn wound in these cases, pneumonia may be fatal. The lower morbidity, particularly involving the burn wound, may be due to the ready availability of acyclovir and varicella-zoster immune globulin. Due to the high degree of communicability of VZV, prompt detection and isolation of cases is very important in preventing spread among burn patients. That VZV can be effectively controlled in a pediatric burn hospital was shown by Sheridan et al. (69) (see also Chapter 42).

EPIDEMIOLOGY OF BURN WOUND INFECTIONS

The epidemiology of burn wound infection involves a reservoir or source for the causative microorganisms, a means of transmission of these microorganisms to the burn wound surface, and the presence or absence of certain factors (risk factors) that may promote colonization, multiplication, and invasion of wound surfaces by newly deposited microorganisms.

Reservoirs or Sources

Burn Wounds of Patients

The collective burn wound surfaces of the patients in a burn treatment facility may make up an important reservoir of microorganisms that cause burn wound infections. The burn wound has been shown to be a reservoir for *P. aeruginosa* (70–72), *Streptococcus pyogenes* (72), and *S. aureus* (72,73). Given the shift in the etiology of burn wound infections over the last decade and the continuing trend toward early burn wound excision and closure, it is unclear how important the collective burn wounds of patients in burn care facilities are today as a reservoir for microorganisms that cause burn wound infections. Most of the data published from earlier reports involved studies of *P. aeruginosa,* which now is a less common cause of burn wound infections.

Gastrointestinal Tract

There is substantial evidence that microorganisms that colonize the burn patient's bowel may contaminate the burn wound and lead to burn wound infection (74–76). In past years when *P. aeruginosa* was a common burn wound pathogen, the areas of the burn wound most often contaminated by feces (buttocks, perineum, lower abdomen, inside of the upper thighs) were the areas most often infected by *P. aeruginosa*. The previous species name for *P. aeruginosa* was *P. pyocyanea,* and burns in the areas most often contaminated by feces were called pyocyaneus-prone burns (74). *P. aeruginosa* may reach the bowel by ingestion of these microorganisms as a result of cross-contamination from one burn patient's wound surface to the oropharynx of a patient in a nearby bed or by ingestion of food contaminated by *P. aeruginosa* (74,75). It has also been suggested that gut flora may contaminate the burn wound by translocation from the gastrointestinal tract (77).

Environment

Microorganisms that cause burn wound infections have been recovered from a number of inanimate sites in the environments of burn care facilities (53,78–86). Table 25.4 lists sites from which burn wound pathogens have been recovered in the environment of burn treatment units. Among the most important inanimate reservoirs or sources for microorganisms that cause burn wound infections is hydrotherapy equipment. Hydrotherapy treatments as a source of patient colonization and infection are covered in detail in Chapter 66.

TABLE 25.4. SITES OF ENVIRONMENTAL CONTAMINATION IN BURN CARE FACILITIES

Site	Microorganism	Reference(s)
Hydrotherapy equipment	*Pseudomonas aeruginosa*	78–81
	Acinetobacter baumannii	53
	Enterobacter cloacae	83
	Methicillin-resistant *Staphylococcus aureus*	84
Sink faucets	*P. aeruginosa*	78
Faucet handles	*P. aeruginosa*	78
Bars of soap	*P. aeruginosa*	78
Towel racks	*P. aeruginosa*	78
Paper towel dispensers	*A. baumannii*	53
Sink basins	*P. aeruginosa*	80,81
	A. baumannii	53
Blood pressure cuff	*A. baumannii*	53
Transportation equipment	*P. aeruginosa*	81
Intravenous pole	*A. baumannii*	53
Water supply	*P. aeruginosa*	81
Sink drains	*P. aeruginosa*	80
Nebulizer water	*P. aeruginosa*	80
Door handles	*A. baumannii*	53
Counter surface	*P. aeruginosa*	80
Cupboards	*A. baumannii*	53
Bed rails	*P. aeruginosa*	80
Sharps container	*A. baumannii*	53
Air	*Providencia stuartii*	82
Linen cart	*A. baumannii*	53
Chair (hydrotherapy area)	*E. cloacae*	83
Filling hose (hydrotherapy tank)	*E. cloacae*	83
Mattresses	*P. aeruginosa*	85
	Acinetobacter calcoaceticus	86
	A. baumannii	53

Endogenous Flora

Early burn wound infections caused by gram-positive cocci are due to microorganisms from the endogenous skin flora (5,8). Routine antibiotic prophylaxis to prevent these early infections, given in many burn treatment centers, has eliminated infections from this source. However, one endogenous source from which antibiotic prophylaxis would not be expected to eradicate microbial flora is the nose. Using molecular typing of strains of *S. aureus* recovered from patients' nares on admission and from sites of infection, Taylor et al. (87) observed that 42% of isolates from sites of infection were identical to admission isolates recovered from the nares. With the shift toward gram-positive coccal infections of burn wounds in the past decade (see above), the endogenous flora may become an increasingly important reservoir for microorganisms that cause burn wound infections.

Modes of Transmission

Hands of Health Care Workers

As with other nosocomial infections, there is evidence that microorganisms are transmitted between patients on the hands of their caregivers (70,75,76,78,79,82,83). Microorganisms may be transmitted directly between patients by the hands of medical personnel (patient to hands to patient) or they may be indirectly transmitted by contaminated hands (patient to hands to inanimate environmental surface to hands to patient).

Gastrointestinal Tracts of Patients

As noted above, microorganisms that gain entrance to the gastrointestinal tract of a patient may be carried to the patient's burn wound surface by feces. The gastrointestinal tract may be inoculated with a burn wound pathogen by contact of the patient's oropharynx with the contaminated hands of a healthcare worker or by ingestion of contaminated food (75). Contaminated food may carry the burn wound pathogen directly to the patient's gastrointestinal tract or may contaminate utensils used for food preparation, leading to secondary contamination of food (75).

Hydrotherapy

After hydrotherapy equipment becomes contaminated, subsequent patient contact with the equipment during hydrotherapy treatments may transfer the microorganisms to a burn patient's wounds (78–81,83,84). Transfer of microorganisms from hydrotherapy equipment to patients is covered in detail in Chapter 66.

Inanimate Environmental Surfaces

Environmental surfaces frequently become contaminated with the microorganisms that cause burn wound infections (Table 25.4). Other than hydrotherapy equipment and mattresses, it has been difficult to document transfer of microorganisms from environmental surfaces directly to the burn wound surfaces of patients.

Risk Factors

After microorganisms are transmitted to the surface of the burn wound, there are several factors that determine whether the microorganisms will survive, colonize the surface, and invade the burn wound. These factors that promote colonization and burn wound invasion may be considered risk factors for burn wound infection.

Duration of Hospitalization

Using Cox model survival analysis to analyze data from a retrospective study of bacterial wound colonization and duration of hospital stay, Manson et al. (88) observed a significant positive association between length of stay and colonization with Enterobacteriaceae or a combination of *S. aureus* and *P. aeruginosa*. Although the relationship observed by these workers was between duration of stay and wound colonization (not infection), it is likely that duration of stay is related to burn wound infection, since colonization is a necessary first step in the development of wound infection.

Burn Wound Size

Intuitively, it would seem likely that the larger the burn wound, the more likely it would be contaminated and colonized with microorganisms. In a prospective study of 53 pediatric patients with burns in which the data were analyzed by multivariable analysis, Fleming et al. (77) showed a significant relationship between colonization of burn wounds with microorganisms from patients' fecal flora and the size of their burn wounds. Again, it is likely that risk factors for colonization also place the burn wound at greater risk for infection.

In a retrospective study in which data were analyzed by multiple regression analysis, Merrell et al. (89) found a significant relationship between burn wound size and subsequent occurrence of fatal sepsis. Fifty-four percent of the fatalities were due to burn shock. Graves et al. (90) also observed a significant relationship between burn wound size and infection in a retrospective study wherein data were analyzed by logistic regression analysis. Sites of infection in the latter two studies included burn wound (89,90), lungs (89,90), multiple organs (90), and abdomen (90). In a prospective cohort study in pediatric burn patients analyzed by multivariable techniques Gastmeier et al. (91) observed a significant relationship between burn wound infections and percentage of total body surface area (TBSA) affected. The authors also noted a significant relationship between duration of ventilation and pneumonia and duration of urinary catheter use and urinary tract infections.

Transfusions

Graves et al. (90), using multivariable analysis, also found a significant relationship between number of blood transfusions and infections. Although they recognized that the relationship may be only due to the possibility that more frequent transfusion identifies patients at a higher level of severity of injury and therefore at a higher risk of infection, the authors also noted that the relationship may be due to a specific depression of resistance to infection caused by the transfusions. In an investigation of an outbreak in a burn unit caused by *A. baumannii* Simor et al. (53) identified receipt of blood products as a risk factor for acquisition of the outbreak strain. In the multivariable model the odds ratio was 10.8 with a 95% confidence interval of 3.4 to 34.4, $p < .001$. Thus, blood transfusions may further suppress host defenses already impaired by the burn injury.

Hyperglycemia

Poor plasma glucose control and the effect of hyperglycemia on the occurrence of infections and on mortality in pediatric burn patients was investigated by Gore et al. (92) in a retrospective study with analysis of data limited to univariate statistics. Quantitative cultures of burn wound were done, and poor plasma glucose control was defined as >40% of glucose values ≥7.8 mmol/L and adequate control was indicated by ≤40% of glucose values of ≥7.8 mmol/L.

There was no association between adequate glucose control and wound infections defined as $>10^5$ CFU/g of burn wound tissue. There was no association between glucose control and bacteremia. However, patients with poor glucose control had a significantly higher rate of fungemia. When controlled for length of stay, patients with poor glucose control has significantly more bacteremia and fungemia, more skin grafting procedures and a lower percentage of graft takes for each procedure. Mortality was also significantly higher in patients with poor glucose control.

Although hyperglycemia did not appear to affect the incidence of burn wound infections, wound closure was apparently more difficult in patients with hyperglycemia, and patients with hyperglycemia had significantly more bacteremias and fungemias and a higher mortality rate.

Resistance of Microorganisms to Topical Antimicrobial Agents

When microorganisms in a burn patient population become resistant to the topical antimicrobial agent used for suppression of growth of microorganisms in and on the burn wound, for any given patient the risk of uncontrolled growth of bacteria or fungi in the wound increases and invasion of viable tissue resulting in burn wound infection becomes more likely. Hendry and Stewart (93) observed that colonization of burn wounds by silver- and sulfonamide-resistant bacteria may occur within 2 weeks of admission.

Five outbreaks of burn wound infection or colonization due to gram-negative bacilli resistant (or relatively resistant) to topical antimicrobial agents have been reported (78,82,94–96). The epidemic isolates from these outbreaks have been resistant to gentamicin (78), silver sulfadiazine (82,95), or silver nitrate (94, 96). No outbreaks due to mafenide acetate–resistant microorganisms have been reported.

Resistance of Microorganisms to Systemically Administered Antimicrobial Agents

Resistance to systemically administered antibiotics may also result in a selective advantage for the resistant microorganisms and place patients at greater risk for burn wound infection. Although it has been generally assumed that antimicrobial agents do not achieve therapeutic concentrations in the avascular burn eschar, Polk et al. (97) showed that gentamicin and tobramycin frequently reached therapeutic concentrations in both the superficial and the deep layers of the burn wound. Reporting on data from the same study, Mayhall et al. (98) observed that when the concentration of antibiotic in burn wound tissue exceeded the minimum bactericidal concentration (MBC) of the microorganisms present in the tissue, the microorganisms usually were eliminated from the wound. In no case was a microorganism eliminated from tissue when its minimum inhibitory concentration (MIC) was higher than the concentration of antibiotics in tissue. Of particular importance was their observation that, during therapy, six patients developed superinfection of the burn wound with *S. marcescens* and that five of these isolates were highly resistant to the antibiotic being administered. In the five patients for whom tissue levels were available, the MICs of these strains exceeded concentrations of antibiotic present in the burn wound. Thus, when a microorganism present on the wounds of patients in a burn care unit becomes highly resistant to an antibiotic used frequently to treat burn wound infection, particularly when used empirically, use of this antibiotic may place patients at risk for burn wound infection.

PREVENTION AND CONTROL

There is good evidence that improvements in the prevention and control of infections in burn patients has led to improvements in patient survival (3,99) (Table 25.5). The approach to control of infections in burn patients may be conveniently divided into the following categories: (a) use of barrier techniques to prevent cross-contamination of patients; (b) prevention of cross-contamination of patients during hydrotherapy treatments; (c) application of topical antimicrobial agents to the burn wound to diminish the colonization and growth of microorganisms on the surface of the burn wound; (d) appropriate use of systemically administered antimicrobial agents to reduce the pressure for selection of resistant microorganisms; (e) early excision and closure of the burn wound; and (f) selective decontamination of the digestive tract.

Barrier Techniques

Barrier techniques and other related techniques for preventing cross-contamination between patients in burn care facilities have been shown to be effective in diminishing infection rates in burn patients (99,100). The most important barrier techniques are those used to prevent contact transmission of microorganisms from patient to patient by the contaminated hands and clothing of personnel who provide direct patient care. Use of gloves and an apron made of impermeable material has been shown to decrease cross-contamination of burn patients (101). Hands should be washed before donning gloves and after removing gloves. Gloves need not be sterile for routine noninvasive patient care, including dressing changes (102). In order for personnel to practice frequent hand washing, there must be enough

TABLE 25.5. PATIENT CHARACTERISTICS

	n	Burn Size (%)	Age (Years)	Predicted Mortality (%)	Observed Mortality (%)	Infection (%)
All patients						
Early group	173	28.7	29.7	26.0	26.0	28.9
Infection	50	44.4	38.4	49.4	50.0	100
No infection	123	22.3	26.1	16.5	16.3	0
Late group	213	30.4	32.6	29.6	22.5[a]	19.2[b]
Infection	41	50.4	43.8	66.0	61.0	100
No infection	172	25.7	29.9	20.9	13.4[a]	0
Patients with predicted mortality of 25–75%						
Early group	31	42.8	35.6	48.5	38.7	58.1
Infection	18	45.0	37.6	51.8	38.9	100
No infection	13	39.8	32.9	44.0	38.5	0
Late group	46	39.8	41.5	48.7	28.3[a]	30.4[c]
Infection	14	41.0	44.3	51.2	50.0	100
No infection	32	39.2	40.3	47.6	18.8[a]	0

[a] $p < .05$ vs. predicted mortality.
[b] $p < .05$.
[c] $p < .02$ vs. early group.
From Shirani KZ, McManus AT, Vaughan GM, et al. Effects of environment on infection in burn patients. *Arch Surg* 1986; 121:31–36.

hand-washing sinks appropriately located within the burn care unit to minimize the amount of time required for personnel to wash their hands (99,100). Given the evidence that gram-negative microorganisms may be difficult to remove from the hands of healthcare workers in intensive care units, hand-washing agents containing antiseptics effective against gram-negative bacilli should be provided in a suitable dispenser at each sink (103).

Prevention of Cross-Contamination from Inanimate Surfaces and Food

Given the frequent contamination of inanimate surfaces in burn care facilities (Table 25.4), attention must be paid to preventing cross-contamination via these surfaces. Each patient should be assigned his or her own stethoscope, blood pressure cuff, box of clean disposable gloves (102), and container(s) of topical antimicrobial agent. Items of equipment that must be shared between patients should be thoroughly cleaned and disinfected between patients. Particular attention should be paid to mattress covers, since two outbreaks in burn units have been related to damaged mattress covers that led to contamination of the mattress foam (85,86). Covers on mattresses should be inspected between patients, and mattresses with damaged covers should not be used for subsequent patients.

A recently discovered source of microorganisms for colonization of burn wound surfaces is that of computer keyboards (104). Neely et al. (104) noted an increase in the number of their patients being colonized with *A. baumannii* and recovered the microorganism from the plastic covers over keyboards on bedside computers. Control measures included having personnel put on gloves before using the computer and having the plastic covers over the keyboards cleaned on a daily basis.

Since raw vegetables have been shown to be a source of *P. aeruginosa* microorganisms that cause burn wound infections (75), burn patients should not be fed raw fruits and vegetables. Attention should also be paid to avoiding contamination of kitchen utensils with raw fruits and vegetables that may later contact uncontaminated foods before they are served to burn patients.

Prevention of Cross-Contamination from Convalescent Patients

McManus et al. (100) showed that convalescent burn patients may be a reservoir of microorganisms for cross-contamination and infection of burn patients in the acute phase of care. They caution that patients in nonintensive care areas of burn treatment facilities should be included in microbial surveillance and infection control programs. These patients are the least likely to become infected but may be ignored as a reservoir for patients in intensive care. Consideration might be given to assignment of nursing staff to either the intensive care unit or convalescent care area without crossover of nursing staff between these two patient care areas.

Hydrotherapy

Prevention of cross-contamination in the hydrotherapy treatment area also includes use of barrier techniques but is considered separately from barrier techniques because of the unique risks for cross-contamination encountered in this area. Hydrotherapy is provided in a common area using common equipment and involves exposure to water. Effective decontamination of complex equipment between patients in a limited period may be a major challenge to burn care personnel. Unlike the hands of personnel and inanimate surfaces, water in hydrotherapy tanks contacts the entire burn wound surface. To decrease the contamination of the burn wound surface that occurs with immersion hydrotherapy, many burn care facilities have replaced immersion hydrotherapy with showering patients on a flat surface (84). In two studies the lowest rates of burn wound colonization and infection occurred when all wound care was done at the patients' bedsides (81,84). The prevention of cross-contamination of burn patients during hydrotherapy is covered in detail in Chapter 66.

Topical Antimicrobial Agents

Topical antimicrobial agents are applied to the burn wound surface to diminish colonization and multiplication of microorganisms on the surface of the wound. Multiplication of microorganisms on the burn wound surface may lead to invasion of the wound. For burn wounds with unexcised eschar, continued multiplication of microorganisms may lead to invasion of the subeschar space and then to invasion of the subeschar viable tissue and burn wound sepsis.

The most commonly used agents are silver sulfadiazine, mafenide acetate, and silver nitrate. Silver sulfadiazine is the most commonly used agent among these (105). Cerium-nitrate-silver-sulfadiazine is used in some centers but is not commercially available in the U.S. Silver sulfadiazine has the fewest side effects of the three most commonly used agents; these side effects include rare crystalluria and methemoglobinemia and common but mild transient leukopenia (105). Microbial resistance has been reported for all of the topical agents, but resistance to mafenide acetate has been uncommon. Some centers alternate use of topical agents in an attempt to delay emergence of resistance, but there are no data to indicate that such a practice is effective in preventing the development of resistance.

It should be kept in mind that resistance to the topical antimicrobial agent(s) in use in a burn care facility may develop and may be associated with an outbreak of infections caused by the resistant microorganism(s). When confronted with an outbreak, hospital epidemiologists and infection control professionals should keep in mind the possibility that the epidemic strain may be resistant to the topical antimicrobial agent in use at the time of the outbreak. Testing the outbreak strain for resistance to the topical antimicrobial agent in use prior to onset of the outbreak should be considered (93,95,96).

Systemic Antimicrobial Agents

The extensive use of systemically administered antimicrobial agents in burn care facilities for the treatment of burn wound infections frequently leads to selection of resistant microorganisms. Continued use of the same antibiotics provides a selective advantage for these microorganisms, and they are able to proliferate and displace the susceptible microorganisms in and on the burn wounds of the patients in the unit. Continued colonization of patients with large numbers of multiply resistant microorganisms with an epidemiologic advantage may lead to an outbreak. Polk et al. (97) showed that systemically administered antimicrobial agents penetrate the avascular burn wound, and Mayhall et al. (98) observed that susceptible microorganisms in the wound may be rapidly replaced by highly resistant gram-negative bacilli.

Thus, prevention of the emergence of such resistance depends on the appropriate use of antimicrobial agents. Use of antibiotics should be limited to clearly indicated situations, and their selection should be based, when possible, on the results of cultures and antimicrobial susceptibility tests. During outbreaks, control efforts should include examination of prescribing patterns, and appropriate changes and limitations in the use of antibiotics should be implemented. Detection and treatment of superinfection of burn wounds by multiply resistant microorganisms may require culture of burn wound biopsies.

Burn Wound Excision and Closure

Theoretically, early excision and closure of burn wounds should diminish the incidence of burn wound infection. If early excision and closure does reduce the rate of burn wound infections, it could be considered an important modality for prevention of burn wound infections. However, there is no scientific evidence that such treatment of burn wounds does reduce infection rates. Several studies have shown apparent reductions in burn wound infection rates related to early burn wound excision and closure (106–109). However, these studies suffer from a number of flaws such as use of small study populations, absence of randomization, use of historical controls, and failure to define burn wound infection or nonuniformity of definitions. These are important defects, because many aspects of burn care improved while early excision and wound closure were being introduced.

There have been three randomized prospective studies of early burn wound excision and closure versus nonoperative or exposure treatment published. In a study in which patients with burns of less than 20% total body surface area were randomized to either early excision and grafting or nonoperative treatment, Engrav et al. (110) make no mention of burn wound infection in either group. Sørensen et al. (111) randomized burn patients with burns of all sizes to either acute excision or exposure treatment. They observed a significantly lower rate of burn wound infections only in patients with burn wounds of 1% to 15% of body surface area. Herndon et al. (112) randomized patients with greater than 30% total body surface area second-degree and greater than 20% total body surface area third-degree burns to early excision or conservative therapy. They noted no difference in the number of septic days between patients treated with early excision and those treated conservatively. They specifically noted that early excision did not prevent septic episodes in large burns.

McManus et al. (31) have made the point that if excision of the burn wound is to be cited as the reason for improvement in the survival of burn patients, this conclusion can be validated only by studies that include concurrent controls. They further note that the extent to which the reduction in the rate of burn wound infections can be attributed to burn wound excision is unclear. There is also some concern that the increased number of blood transfusions needed for early burn wound excision may increase patients' risk of blood-borne infections.

In spite of the fact that early burn wound excision has not been scientifically proven to be an effective modality for the prevention of burn wound infections, it is a widely held belief among burn surgeons that early burn wound excision and closure significantly reduces burn wound infection and mortality from thermal injury (113–117). In the absence of randomized clinical trials, two recent publications provide evidence that early excision does reduce the incidence of burn wound infection (118, 119).

In the first study the authors prospectively studied 20 children with burns (118). Patients admitted to the authors' hospital within 24 hours of burn injury had early burn wound excision. Patients transferred from other hospitals at 7 ± 2 days had burn wound excision at the time of admission. At the time of burn excision, specimens were taken from excised burn eschar and excised burn wound bed for quantitative cultures. The 12 patients in the early excision group had less than approximately 10^4 CFU/g of tissue in burn eschar and less than approximately 10^2 CFU/g of tissue in the excised wound bed. For the eight patients in the late excision group, burn eschar had more than approximately 10^5 CFU/g and in some cases had 10^6 CFU/g of tissue. Bacterial counts in the excised wound bed were less than approximately 10^4 CFU/g of tissue.

None of the patients in the early excision group had burn wound infections or graft loss. In the late excision group three patients had infections and graft loss and two patients had sepsis after surgical excision of the burn wound. High bacterial counts and infection rates were associated with delayed excision ($p < .01$). Although this study was not a controlled trial and differences in potentially important variables between groups of patients could not be controlled for, this study lends further support to the widely held belief that early excision significantly reduces the incidence of burn wound infections.

In the second prospective study the authors investigated the effects of early versus delayed wound excision on hypermetabolism, catabolism, and sepsis in children with burns (119). The authors measured resting energy expenditure, skeletal muscle protein catabolism, and the concentration of microorganisms in burn wound tissue. Patients were divided into three groups: an early group (arrival within 72 hours of injury), a middle group (arrival 3 to 10 days after injury), and a late group (arrival at least 10 days after injury). The authors noted increased muscle catabolism in 1 to 3 weeks in the middle and late excision groups compared to the early excision group. Sepsis appeared to increase as excision and aggressive feeding were progressively delayed among the treatment cohorts ($p = .07$). The concentration of microorganisms in quantitative cultures taken 1 week after initiation of surgical and nutritional therapy was progressively increased with treatment delay ($p < .05$). Again, although not a controlled study, the data from this investigation show the benefit of early burn wound excision for reducing burn wound infections and muscle catabolism. In the absence of controlled clinical trials, these two studies provide further evidence that early burn wound excision significantly reduces the incidence of burn wound infections. However, it remains unclear how early burn wound excision and wound closure affect the epidemiology of burn wound infections in burn care facilities.

Selective Decontamination of the Digestive Tract

Selective decontamination of the digestive tract (SDD) has been suggested as a preventive measure for burn wound infections. It is postulated that the elimination of potentially pathogenic microorganisms from the gastrointestinal tracts of burn patients by the oral administration of nonabsorbable antibiotics will diminish colonization and infection of burn wounds. To date, the efficacy of such a practice remains hypothetical.

The first of only two randomized studies included only 27 patients and found no evidence that SDD decreased or delayed the colonization of the burn wound by enteric microorganisms (120). On the contrary, *Pseudomonas* appeared earlier on the wound and in blood cultures of the treated group when compared with the control group. Enteric microorganisms appeared earlier in the blood cultures of the treatment group than in those of the control group. Thirty-three percent of the treated group had complications severe enough that prophylaxis had to be discontinued early. One study of 48 patients was uncontrolled (121), and another study of 91 patients compared two regimens for SDD but contained no placebo control group (122). In a prospective, nonrandomized study, Jarrett et al. (123) assigned 20 patients to receive SDD and compared them to ten patients assigned to receive no SDD. No placebo was used for the control group. All of these patients were also treated in a laminar airflow burn unit using strict reverse isolation techniques. These authors observed a significant delay in burn wound colonization in the SDD group, but no significant differences were found in burn wound biopsies that yielded positive results ($>10^5$ CFU/g of tissue) or in the occurrence of bacteremia, burn wound sepsis, urinary tract infections, pneumonitis, or cellulitis. Mackie et al. (124) studied 64 patients in a nonrandomized study wherein 31 patients given SDD were compared with 33 historical control subjects. They noted a marked reduction in positive fecal culture results for Enterobacteriaceae and *Pseudomonas* and a significant decrease in burn wound colonization with gram-negative microorganisms in the SDD group. In addition, they noted significant reductions in respiratory infections and in septicemia. The mortality rate was also significantly lower in the SDD group. The authors did not report any differences in burn wound sepsis. No increase in antimicrobial resistance was observed after introduction of SDD.

The best study on SDD published to date is that of Barret et al. (125), who carried out a prospective, randomized, double-blinded, placebo-controlled clinical trial. The treatment regimen was a suspension containing polymyxin E, tobramycin, and amphotericin B. The suspension was given by a nasogastric tube four times a day for the duration of the study. The placebo solution was Ringer's lactate. Oral nystatin was administered as "swish-and-swallow" to prevent oral and esophageal candidiasis. Routine cultures of sputum, urine, blood, wound, stool, and gastric aspirates were taken on admission and twice weekly during the study. Eleven patients were randomized to the treatment group and 12 to the placebo group. There were no significant differences in infections at various sites and no significant differences in results of cultures between the two groups. There was however a significant difference in the occurrence of diarrhea (82% in the SDD group versus 17% in the placebo group, $p = .003$).

From the available published data, it must be concluded that SDD is unproven as an effective modality for prevention of burn wound infection. Further the side effects of such therapy may well outweigh any benefit. Finally, data are insufficient to determine whether such prophylaxis will lead to selection of resistant microorganisms in burn care facilities.

REFERENCES

1. Deitch EA, Bridges RM, Dobke M, et al. Burn wound sepsis may be promoted by a failure of local antibacterial host defenses. *Ann Surg* 1987;206:340–348.
2. Heideman M, Bengtsson A. The immunologic response to thermal injury. *World J Surg* 1992;16:53–56.
3. Pruitt BA Jr, McManus AT. The changing epidemiology of infection in burn patients. *World J Surg* 1992;16:57–67.
4. Deitch EA. The management of burns. *N Engl J Med* 1990;323: 1249–1253.
5. Luterman A, Dacso CC, Curreri PW. Infections in burn patients. *Am J Med* 1986;81(suppl 1A):45–52.
6. Mason AD Jr, McManus AT, Pruitt BA Jr. Association of burn mortality and bacteremia. *Arch Surg* 1986;121:1027–1031.
7. Demling RH. Burns. *N Engl J Med* 1985;313:1389–1398.
8. Dodd D, Stutman HR. Current issues in burn wound infections. *Adv Pediatr Infect Dis* 1991;6:137–162.
9. Herndon DN, Curreri PW, Abston S, et al. Treatment of burns. *Curr Probl Surg* 1987;24:341–397.
10. Mooney DP, Gamelli RL. Sepsis following thermal injury. *Compr Ther* 1989;15:22–29.
11. O'Sullivan ST, O'Connor TPF. Immunosuppression following thermal injury: the pathogenesis of immunodysfunction. *Br J Plast Surg* 1997;50:615–623.
12. Robson MC. Burn sepsis. *Crit Care Clin* 1988;4:281–298.
13. Pruitt BA Jr, Goodwin CW Jr. Current treatment of the extensively burned patient. *Surg Ann* 1983;15:331–364.
14. Garner JS, Jarvis WR, Emori TG, et al. CDC definitions for nosocomial infections, 1988. *Am J Infect Control* 1988;16:128–140.
15. Pruitt BA Jr, Foley FD. The use of biopsies in burn patient care. *Surgery* 1973;73:887–897.
16. Loebl EC, Marvin JA, Heck EL, et al. The method of quantitative burn-wound biopsy cultures and its routine use in the care of the burned patient. *Am J Clin Pathol* 1974;61:20–24.
17. Mitchel V, Galizia J, Fournier L. Precise diagnosis of infection in burn wound biopsy specimens. Combination of histologic technique, acridine orange staining, and culture. *J Burn Care Rehabil* 1989;10: 195–202.
18. McManus AT, Kim SH, McManus WF, et al. Comparison of quantitative microbiology and histopathology in divided burn-wound biopsy specimens. *Arch Surg* 1987;122:74–76.
19. Bharadwaj R, Joshi BN, Phadke SA. Assessment of burn wound sepsis by swab, full thickness biopsy culture and blood culture—a comparative study. *Burns* 1983;10:124–126.
20. Tahlan RN, Keswani RK, Saini S, et al. Correlation of quantitative burn wound biopsy culture and surface swab culture to burn wound sepsis. *Burns* 1983;10:217–224.
21. Woolfrey BF, Fox JM, Quall CO. An evaluation of burn wound quantitative microbiology. I. Quantitative eschar cultures. *Am J Clin Pathol* 1981;75:532–537.
22. Volenec FJ, Clark GM, Mani MM, et al. Burn wound biopsy bacterial quantitation: a statistical analysis. *Am J Surg* 1979;138:695–697.
23. Steer JA, Papini RPG, Wilson APR, et al. Quantitative microbiology in the management of burn patients. I. Correlation between quantitative and qualitative burn wound biopsy culture and surface alginate swab culture. *Burns* 1996;22:173–176.
24. Magee C, Haury B, Rodeheaver G, et al. A rapid technique for quantitating wound bacterial count. *Am J Surg* 1977;133:760–762.
25. Taddonio TE, Thomson PD, Tait MV, et al. Rapid quantification of bacterial and fungal growth in burn wounds; biopsy homogenate gram-stain versus microbial culture results. *Burns* 1988;14:180–184.
26. Woolfrey BF, Fox JMK, Quall CO. An evaluation of burn wound microbiology: the quantitative gram stain. *J Burn Care Rehabil* 1982; 3:171–175.
27. Kim SH, Hubbard GB, Worley BL, et al. A rapid section technique for burn wound biopsy. *J Burn Care Rehabil* 1985;6:433–435.
28. Teplitz C, Davis D, Mason AD Jr, et al. Pseudomonas burn wound sepsis. I. Pathogenesis of experimental Pseudomonas burn wound sepsis. *J Surg Res* 1964;4:200–216.
29. Kim SH, Hubbard GB, McManus WF, et al. Frozen section technique to evaluate early burn wound biopsy: a comparison with the rapid section technique. *J Trauma* 1985;25:1134–1137.
30. Peck MD, Weber J, McManus A, et al. Surveillance of burn wound infections: a proposal for definitions. *J Burn Care Rehabil* 1998;19: 386–389.
31. McManus WF, Mason AD Jr, Pruitt BA Jr. Excision of the burn wound in patients with large burns. *Arch Surg* 1989;124:718–720.
32. Lawrence JC. The bacteriology of burns. *J Hosp Infect* 1985;6(suppl B):3–17.
33. Smith DJ Jr, Thomson PD. Changing flora in burn and trauma units: historical perspective—experience in the United States. *J Burn Care Rehabil* 1992;13:276–280.
34. Saroglou G, Cromer M, Bisno AL. Methicillin-resistant *Staphylococcus aureus:* interstate spread of nosocomial infections with emergence of gentamicin-methicillin resistant strains. *Infect Control* 1980;1:81–89.
35. Linnemann CC Jr, Mason M, Moore P, et al. Methicillin-resistant *Staphylococcus aureus:* experience in a general hospital over four years. *Am J Epidemiol* 1982;115:941–950.
36. Boyce JM, White RL, Causey WA, et al. Burn units as a source of methicillin-resistant *Staphylococcus aureus* infections. *JAMA* 1983; 249:2803–2807.
37. Rode H, Hanslo D, de Wet PM, et al. Efficacy of mupirocin in methicillin-resistant *Staphylococcus aureus* burn wound infection. *Antimicrob Agents Chemother* 1989;33:1358–1361.
38. Matsumura H, Yoshizawa N, Narumi A, et al. Effective control of methicillin-resistant *Staphylococcus aureus* in a burn unit. *Burns* 1996; 22:283–286.
39. Egan WC, Clark WR. The toxic shock syndrome in a burn victim. *Burns* 1988;14:135–138.
40. Blomqvist L. Toxic shock syndrome after burn injuries in children. Case report. *Scand J Plast Reconstr Hand Surg* 1997;31:77–81.
41. Johnson D, Pathirana PDR. Toxic shock syndrome following cessation of prophylactic antibiotics in a child with a 2% scald. *Burns* 2002;28:181–184.
42. Oyake S, Oh-i T, Koga M. Staphylococcal scalded skin syndrome developing during burn treatment. *J Dermatol* 2001;28:557–559.
43. Frame JD, Kangesu L, Malik WM. Changing flora in burn and trauma units: experience in the United Kingdom. *J Burn Care Rehabil* 1992; 13:281–286.
44. Lawrence JC. Burn bacteriology during the last 50 years. *Burns* 1992; 18(suppl 2):523–529.
45. Gruteke P, VanBelkum A, Schouls LM, et al. Outbreak of group A streptococci in a burn center: use of pheno- and genotypic procedures for strain tracking. *J Clin Microbiol* 1996;34:114–118.
46. Appelgren P, Björnhagen V, Bragderyd K, et al. A prospective study of infections in burn patients. *Burns* 2002;28:39–46.
47. McManus AT. *Pseudomonas aeruginosa:* a controlled burn pathogen? *Antibiot Chemother* 1989;42:103–108.
48. Jones WG, Barie PS, Yurt RW, et al. Enterococcal burn sepsis. A highly lethal complication in severely burned patients. *Arch Surg* 1986; 121:649–653.
49. Falk PS, Winnike J, Woodmansee C, et al. Outbreak of vancomycin-resistant enterococci in a burn unit. *Infect Control Hosp Epidemiol* 2000;21:575–582.
50. Green AR, Milling MAP. Infection with *Acinetobacter* in a burns unit. *Burns* 1983;9:292–294.
51. Lyytikäinen O, Köljalg S, Härmä M, et al. Outbreak caused by two multi-resistant *Acinetobacter baumannii* clones in a burns unit: emergence of resistance to imipenem. *J Hosp Infect* 1995;31:41–54.
52. Wisplinghoff H, Perbix W, Seifert H. Risk factors for nosocomial bloodstream infections due to *Acinetobacter baumannii*: a case-control study of adult burn patients. *Clin Infect Dis* 1999;28:59–66.
53. Simor AE, Lee M, Vearncombe M, et al. An outbreak due to multiresistant *Acinetobacter baumannii* in a burn unit: risk factors for acquisi-

tion and management. *Infect Control Hosp Epidemiol* 2002;23: 261–267.

54. Becker WK, Cioffi WG Jr, McManus AT, et al. Fungal burn wound infection. A 10-year experience. *Arch Surg* 1991;126:44–48.
55. Spebar MJ, Pruitt BA Jr. Candidiasis in the burned patient. *J Trauma* 1981;21:237–239.
56. Prasad JK, Feller I, Thomson PD. A ten-year review of *Candida* sepsis and mortality in burn patients. *Surgery* 1987;101:213–216.
57. Desai MH, Rutan RL, Heggers JP, et al. *Candida* infection with and without nystatin prophylaxis. *Arch Surg* 1992;127:159–162.
58. Grube BJ, Marvin JA, Heimbach DM. *Candida.* A decreasing problem for the burned patient? *Arch Surg* 1988;123:194–196.
59. Wheeler MS, McGinnis MR, Schell WA, et al. Fusarium infection in burned patients. *Am J Clin Pathol* 1981;75:304–311.
60. Chakrabarti A, Nayak N, Kumar PS, et al. Surveillance of nosocomial fungal infections in a burn care unit. *Infection* 1992;20:132–135.
61. Burdge JJ, Rea F, Ayers L. Noncandidal, fungal infections of the burn wound. *J Burn Care Rehabil* 1988;9:599–601.
62. Linnemann CC Jr, MacMillan BG. Viral infections in pediatric burn patients. *Am J Dis Child* 1981;135:750–753.
63. Foley FD, Greenawald KA, Nash G, et al. Herpesvirus infection in burned patients. *N Engl J Med* 1990;282:652–656.
64. Brandt SJ, Tribble CG, Lakeman AD, et al. Herpes simplex burn wound infections: epidemiology of a case cluster and responses to acyclovir therapy. *Surgery* 1985;98:338–343.
65. Garcia H. Edwards MS. Herpes simplex infection of burn wounds. *South Med J* 1981;74:991–992.
66. Kagan RJ, Naraqi S, Matsuda T, et al. Herpes simplex virus and cytomegalovirus infections in burn patients. *J Trauma* 1985;25: 40–45.
67. Kealey GP, Bale JF, Strauss RG, et al. Cytomegalovirus infection in burn patients. *J Burn Care Rehabil* 1987;8:543–545.
68. Deepe GS Jr, MacMillan BG, Linnemann CC Jr. Unexplained fever in burn patients due to cytomegalovirus infection. *JAMA* 1982;248: 2299–2301.
69. Sheridan RL, Weber JM, Pasternak MM, et al. A 15-year experience with varicella infections in a pediatric burn unit. *Burns* 1999;25: 353–356.
70. Lowbury EJL, Fox J. The epidemiology of infection with Pseudomonas pyocyanea in a burns unit. *J Hyg* 1954;52:403–416.
71. Kohn J. A study of *P. pyocyanea* cross infection in a burns unit. Preliminary report. In: Wallace AB, Wilkinson AW, eds. *Research in burns.* Edinburgh: E and S Livingstone, 1966:491.
72. Wormald PJ. The effect of a changed environment on bacterial colonization rates in an established burns centre. *J Hyg* 1970;68:633–645.
73. Hambraeus A. Dispersal and transfer of *Staphylococcus aureus* in an isolation ward for burned patients. *J Hyg* 1973;71:787–797.
74. Barclay TL, Dexter F. Infection and cross-infection in a new burns centre. *Br J Surg* 1968;55:197–202.
75. Kominos SD, Copeland CE, Delenko CA. *Pseudomonas aeruginosa* from vegetables, salads and other foods served to patients with burns. In: Young VM, ed. *Pseudomonas aeruginosa: ecological aspects and patient colonization.* New York: Raven Press, 1977:59–75.
76. Chitkara YK, Feierabend TC. Endogenous and exogenous infection with Pseudomonas aeruginosa in a burns unit. *Int Surg* 1981;66: 237–240.
77. Fleming RYD, Zeigler ST, Walton MA, et al. Influence of burn size on the incidence of contamination of burn wounds by fecal organisms. *J Burn Care Rehabil* 1991;12:510–515.
78. Shulman JA, Terry PM, Hough CE. Colonization with gentamicin-resistant Pseudomonas aeruginosa, pyocine type 5, in a burn unit. *J Infect Dis* 1971;124(suppl):518–523.
79. Stone HH, Kolb LD. The evolution and spread of gentamicin-resistant Pseudomonads. *J Trauma* 1971;11:586–589.
80. MacMillan BG, Edmonds P, Hummel RP, et al. Epidemiology *Pseudomonas* in a burn intensive care unit. *J Trauma* 1973;13:627–638.
81. Tredget EE, Shankowsky HA, Joffe AM, et al. Epidemiology of infections with *Pseudomonas aeruginosa* in burn patients: the role of hydrotherapy. *Clin Infect Dis* 1992;15:941–949.
82. Wenzel RP, Hunting KJ, Osterman CA, et al. *Providencia stuartii,* a hospital pathogen: potential factors for its emergence and transmission. *Am J Epidemiol* 1976;104:170–180.
83. Mayhall CG, Lamb VA, Gayle WE Jr, et al. *Enterobacter cloacae* septicemia in a burn center: epidemiology and control of an outbreak. *J Infect Dis* 1979;139:166–171.
84. Embil JM, McLeod JA, Al-Barrak AM, et al. An outbreak of methicillin resistant *Staphylococcus aureus* on a burn unit: potential role of contaminated hydrotherapy equipment. *Burns* 2001;27:681–688.
85. Fujita K, Lilly HA, Kidson A, et al. Gentamicin-resistant *Pseudomonas aeruginosa* infection from mattresses in a burns unit. *Br Med J* 1981; 283:219–220.
86. Sherertz RJ, Sullivan ML. An outbreak of infections with *Acinetobacter calcoaceticus* in burn patients: contamination of patients' mattresses. *J Infect Dis* 1985;151:252–258.
87. Taylor GD, Kibsey P, Kirkland T, et al. Predominance of staphylococcal organisms in infections occurring in a burns intensive care unit. *Burns* 1992;18:332–335.
88. Manson WL, Pernot PCJ, Fidler V, et al. Colonization of burns and the duration of hospital stay of severely burned patients. *J Hosp Infect* 1992;22:55–63.
89. Merrell SW, Saffle JR, Larson CM, et al. The declining incidence of fatal sepsis following thermal injury. *J Trauma* 1989;29:1362–1366.
90. Graves TA, Cioffi WG, Mason AD Jr, et al. Relationship of transfusion and infection in a burn population. *J Trauma* 1989;29:948–954.
91. Gastmeier P, Weigt O, Sohr D, et al. Comparison of hospital-acquired infection rates in paediatric burn patients. *J Hosp Infect* 2002;52: 161–165.
92. Gore DC, Chinkes D, Heggers J, et al. Association of hyperglycemia with increased mortality after severe burn injury. *J Trauma* 2001;51: 540–544.
93. Hendry AT, Stewart IO. Silver-resistant Enterobacteriaceae from hospital patients. *Can J Microbiol* 1979;25:915–921.
94. McHugh GL, Moellering RC, Hopkins CC, et al. *Salmonella typhimurium* resistant to silver nitrate, chloramphenicol, and ampicillin. *Lancet* 1975;1:235–240.
95. Gayle WE Jr, Mayhall CG, Lamb VA, et al. Resistant *Enterobacter cloacae* in a burn center: the ineffectiveness of silver sulfadiazine. *J Trauma* 1978;18:317–323.
96. Bridges K, Kidson A, Lowbury EJL, et al. Gentamicin- and silver-resistant *Pseudomonas* in a burns unit. *Br Med J* 1979;1:446–449.
97. Polk RE, Mayhall CG, Smith J, et al. Gentamicin and tobramycin penetration into burn eschar. Pharmacokinetics and microbiological effects. *Arch Surg* 1983;118:295–302.
98. Mayhall CG, Polk RE, Haynes BW. Infections in burned patients. *Infect Control* 1983;4:454–459.
99. Shirani KZ, McManus AT, Vaughan GM, et al. Effects of environment on infection in burn patients. *Arch Surg* 1986;121:31–36.
100. McManus AT, McManus WF, Mason AD Jr, et al. Microbial colonization in a new intensive care burn unit. A prospective cohort study. *Arch Surg* 1985;120:217–223.
101. Lee JJ, Marvin JA, Heimbach DM, et al. Infection control in a burn center. *J Burn Care Rehabil* 1990;11:575–580.
102. Sadowski DA, Pohlmans, Maley MP, et al. Use of nonsterile gloves for routine noninvasive procedures in thermally injured patients. *J Burn Care Rehabil* 1988;9:613–615.
103. Knittle MA, Eitzman DV, Baer H. Role of hand contamination of personnel in the epidemiology of gram-negative nosocomial infections. *J Pediatr* 1975;86:433–437.
104. Neely AN, Maley MP, Warden GD. Computer keyboards as reservoirs for *Acinetobacter baumannii* in a burn hospital [letter]. *Clin Infect Dis* 1999;29:1358–1359.
105. Monafo WW, Freedman B. Topical therapy for burns. *Surg Clin North Am* 1987;67:133–145.
106. Gray DT, Pine RW, Harnar TJ, et al. Early surgical excision versus conventional therapy in patients with 20 to 40 percent burns. A comparative study. *Am J Surg* 1982;144:76–80.
107. Kagan RJ, Matsuda T, Hanumadass M, et al. Serious wound infections in burned patients. *Surgery* 1985;98:640–647.
108. Chicarilli ZN, Cuono CB, Heinrich JJ, et al. Selective aggressive burn excision for high mortality subgroups. *J Trauma* 1986;26:18–25.

109. Merrell SW, Saffle JR, Larson CM, et al. The declining incidence of fatal sepsis following thermal injury. *J Trauma* 1989;29:1362–1366.
110. Engrav LH, Heimbach DM, Reus JL, et al. Early excision and grafting vs. nonoperative treatment of burns of indeterminant depth: a randomized prospective study. *J Trauma* 1983;23:1001–1004.
111. Sørensen B, Fisker NP, Steensen JP, et al. Acute excision or exposure treatment? Final results of a three-year randomized controlled clinical trial. *Scand J Plast Reconstr Surg* 1984;18:87–93.
112. Herndon DN, Barrow RE, Rutan RL, et al. A comparison of conservative versus early excision. Therapies in severely burned patients. *Ann Surg* 1989;209:547–553.
113. Tompkins RG, Remensnyder JP, Burke JF, et al. Significant reductions in mortality for children with burn injuries through the use of prompt eschar excision. *Ann Surg* 1988;208:577–585.
114. Papini RPG, Wilson APR, Steer JA, et al. Wound management in burn centres in the United Kingdom. *Br J Surg* 1995;82:505–509.
115. Nguyen TT, Gilpin DA, Meyer NA, et al. Current treatment of severely burned patients. *Ann Surg* 1996;223:14–25.
116. Wurtz R, Karajovic M, Dacumos E, et al. Nosocomial infections in a burn intensive care unit. *Burns* 1995;21:181–184.
117. Pruitt BA Jr, McManus AT, Kim SH, et al. Burn wound infections: current status. *World J Surg* 1998;22:135–145.
118. Barret JP, Herndon DN. Effects of burn wound excision on bacterial colonization and invasion. *Plast Reconstr Surg* 2003;111:744–750.
119. Hart DW, Wolf SE, Chinkes DL, et al. Effects of early excision and aggressive enteral feeding on hypermetabolism, catabolism and sepsis after severe burn. *J Trauma* 2003;54:755–764.
120. Deutsch DH, Miller SF, Finley RK Jr. The use of intestinal antibiotics to delay or prevent infections in patients with burns. *J Burn Care Rehabil* 1990;11:436–442.
121. Manson WL, Westerveld AW, Klasen HJ, et al. Selective intestinal decontamination of the digestive tract for infection prophylaxis in severely burned patients. *Scand J Plast Reconstr Surg* 1987;21: 269–272.
122. Manson WL, Klasen HJ, Saver EW, et al. Selective intestinal decontamination for prevention of wound colonization in severely burned patients; a retrospective analysis. *Burns* 1992;18:98–102.
123. Jarrett F, Balish E, Moylan JA, et al. Clinical experience with prophylactic antibiotic bowel suppression in burn patients. *Surgery* 1978;83: 523–527.
124. Mackie DP, VanHertum WAJ, Schumburg T, et al. Prevention of infection in burns: preliminary experience with selective decontamination of the digestive tract in patients with extensive injuries. *J Trauma* 1992;32:570–575.
125. Barret JP, Jeschke MG, Herndon DN. Selective decontamination of the digestive tract in severely burned pediatric patients. *Burns* 2001; 27:439–445.

26

NOSOCOMIAL OCULAR INFECTIONS

MARLENE DURAND
DAVID J. WEBER
WILLIAM A. RUTALA

The eye is an uncommon site for nosocomial infections. However, conjunctivitis of the newborn remains a significant worldwide problem, and postoperative ocular infections remain an important source of morbidity for patients undergoing procedures such as cataract extraction or corneal replacement. This chapter focuses on nosocomial ocular infections including their incidence, etiology, clinical presentation, associated risk factors, and prevention. Readers interested in a more extensive treatment of ocular infections, including their diagnosis and treatment, are referred to textbooks of infectious diseases (1–4), general textbooks of ophthalmology (5,6), textbooks focusing on ocular infections (7,8), or focused monographs (9–11).

INCIDENCE OF NOSOCOMIAL OCULAR INFECTIONS

Only limited data are available on the overall incidence of nosocomial ocular infections. Peacock (12) has reported data accumulated by the National Nosocomial Infections Surveillance (NNIS) system at the Centers for Disease Control and Prevention (CDC) for the period 1986 to 1991. Hospital-acquired infections of the eye were estimated to occur at a median rate of 0.24 infections per 10,000 discharges. Overall, they represented less than 0.5% of all nosocomial infections. The rates of ocular infection varied considerably by hospital service, being almost zero on obstetrics and gynecology wards to 1.8 infections per 10,000 discharges on pediatric wards. Common pathogens included *Staphylococcus aureus* (24%), coagulase-negative staphylococci (23%), *Pseudomonas aeruginosa* (13%), streptococcal species (8%), and *Escherichia coli* (7%). However, as Peacock noted, the lack of emphasis placed on these infections and often poor documentation of their occurrence in the patient record likely means that these numbers significantly underestimate the true incidence of disease.

APPROACH TO OCULAR INFECTIONS

Ocular infections are best classified by the anatomic part of the eye involved in the infection (12–14) (Table 26.1). An appropriate history and physical examination allows determination of the structure(s) of the eye involved in infection. Contiguous structures may be involved in infection, including the skin (cellulitis), sinuses (sinusitis), cavernous sinus (cavernous venous sinus thrombosis), orbital cavity (orbital abscess), and brain (meningitis, subdural empyema). Other disease processes, such as allergies, foreign body irritation, endocrine disorders, rheumatologic disorders, and immunologic disorders, may mimic infectious syndromes. Physicians unfamiliar with the diagnosis and treatment of ocular infections should consult specialists in infectious diseases or ophthalmology, because improperly treated ocular infections may lead to vision loss and other severe complications.

Nosocomial ocular infections are best understood by considering infections unrelated to surgery separately from infections related to surgery.

SURVEILLANCE DEFINITIONS

The CDC has delineated surveillance criteria for conjunctivitis and other ocular infections (15). However, these criteria are quite limited in scope. As noted by Peacock (12), "The clinical (ophthalmologic) manifestations of ocular infections are sufficiently distinct to provide an adequate basis for definitive diagnosis, even in the absence of supportive microbiologic data." Isolation of a pathogen remains important in determining the proper therapy for ocular infections and, occasionally, in eliminating noninfectious causes of disease.

Standard time intervals should be used to define nosocomial ocular infections. Postsurgical infections are defined as clinical infections arising in the postoperative period and related to the surgery performed. In the absence of an implanted foreign body, this period extends to 30 days; in the presence of a foreign body (e.g., intraocular lens), this period extends to 1 year. A nonsurgical nosocomial ocular infection should be diagnosed if the infection was not present or incubating at the time of hospital admission. Practically, this is generally interpreted to exclude infections that manifest themselves within 48 hours of admission. Ocular infections that develop 7 to 14 days after discharge should be considered nosocomial in the absence of epidemiologic evidence suggesting community acquisition (12).

TABLE 26.1. SYMPTOMS AND SIGNS OF OCULAR INFECTION

Symptoms and Signs	Blepharitis	Conjunctivitis	Keratitis	Retinitis	Endophthalmitis
Vision	Normal	Normal	Decreased	Decreased	Decreased
Pain	0	0	0 to +	++	0 to ++
Photophobia	0	0	0 to ++	++	++
Discharge	0	++	++	0	0 to ++
Injection	+/–	++	++	0 to +	0 to ++
Corneal haze	0	0	++	0	0 to ++
Pupil	Normal	Normal	Normal or miotic	Decreased reactivity	Decreased reactivity
Smear	WBC (occ.)	WBC	WBC	0	WBC
Community acquired pathogens	*S. aureus*	*S. aureus*	Herpes simplex	CMV	Coag-negative staphylococci
		Streptococci	Herpes zoster	*T. gondii*	*Streptococcus* species[a,b]
		S. pneumoniae	*S. aureus*	*Toxocara*	*Bacillus cereus*[a,b]
		Haemophilus species	*Streptococcus* species	*Histoplasma*	GNR[a]
		Moraxella	*Moraxella*	*M. tuberculosis*	
		Adenovirus	*P. aeruginosa*[c]		*B. burgdorferi*
		Enterovirus			
Nosocomial pathogens	*S. aureus*	*S. aureus*	S. aureus	*T. gondii*	Staphylococci
	Streptococci	*Streptococcus* species	*Streptococcus* species	CMV	Enteric GNR
	P. aeruginosa	Viruses	Viruses	*Candida* species	Fungi
		N. gonorrhoeae[d]	Enteric GNR	Herpes simplex	
		Chlamydia[d]	Herpes zoster		
		Enteric GNR			

[a] Related to posttraumatic infections.
[b] Related to metastatic infections.
[c] Most common cause of keratitis in persons wearing contact lens. CMV, cytomegalovirus; GNR, gram-negative bacilli; WBC, white blood count.
[d] Etiologic agents in conjunctivitis of the newborn. 0, absent; +, mild; ++, severe.

POSTSURGICAL OCULAR INFECTIONS

Eye surgery is commonly performed in the United States. Cataract surgery, corneal transplantation surgery, surgery to repair detached retinas, and most recently LASIK (laser *in situ* keratomileusis) procedures to correct refractive errors, are performed on millions of patients in the U.S. annually. Each procedure may result in acute postoperative infection. As noted above, eye infections are considered to be nosocomial if they develop within 30 days postoperatively, but based on the time frame for postoperative infections, 6 weeks postoperatively would be a better endpoint.

Infections After Corneal Transplant

Corneal transplant, or penetrating keratoplasty (PK), is performed in 46,000 patients in the U.S. each year. The major indications for transplantation include keratoconus, pseudophakic bullous keratopathy, Fuch's dystrophy, herpetic corneal infection, and trauma (16). In the U.S., cadaver donor corneas are stored by local eye banks in an antibiotic-containing solution by protocols established by the Eye Bank Association of America (EBAA). During the transplant procedure, the surgeon trephines a central disk from a donor cornea and uses this to replace the central disk of the patient's native cornea. The donor cornea is sutured to the residual rim of the patient's native cornea. The patient uses topical corticosteroid eyedrops for at least 6 months to prevent rejection. Sutures are left in place for months to years. Nosocomial infections include donor–host transmission of systemic infections, keratitis (infection of the cornea), and endophthalmitis (infection of the vitreous).

Systemic donor infections have rarely been transmitted through PK. Premorbid bacterial sepsis in the donor appears to have no effect on the incidence of posttransplantation endophthalmitis in the recipient (17,18). Diseases transmitted from donors to recipients via corneal transplantation that have been reported in the literature include three cases of Creutzfeldt-Jakob disease) (19,20), eight cases of rabies (21–26), and two cases of hepatitis B virus from the same donor (27). Data supporting the ability of corneal transplants to transmit certain diseases have been reviewed by Hogan and Cavanagh (28). Hepatitis B surface antigen (HBsAg) has been detected in the tears of HBsAg-positive persons (29) and in the washings of corneal donors with HBsAg-positive blood (30). HBsAg has been found in 10 of 61 corneas taken from HBsAg-seropositive donors, and hepatitis B virus core DNA in 15 of the corneas (31). Hepatitis B virus has been experimentally transmitted to chimps by inoculating their corneal surfaces with hepatitis B infected human plasma (32), and human infection occurred in a healthcare worker following mucosal exposure to HBsAg-positive blood (33).

The possibility of transmission of herpes simplex virus (HSV) from donor cornea to recipient has been long suspected, but this was only recently demonstrated (34). HSV in the donor cornea may cause primary graft failure and keratitis after transplantation (35). Cases of nosocomial herpetic graft infection are rare, however. Other viruses that potentially could be transmitted through PK include human immunodeficiency virus (HIV), cytomegalovirus (CMV), Epstein-Barr virus (EBV), adenovirus, and rubella (36). The EBAA requires review of the donor's medical history and recommends serologic screening for hepatitis B, hepatitis C, and HIV-1 and -2 (37). Patients who have died from progressive encephalopathy are also excluded as cornea donors. The recommended screening is highly effective. Eye banks affiliated with EBAA provided over 400,000 corneas during a recent 12-year period, and there were no cases of donor to recipient transmission of a systemic infectious disease during this time (37).

A more common infectious complication after PK is infectious keratitis. Many cases occur beyond the postoperative time period and would not be considered nosocomial. A retrospective review of 885 transplants performed over a 16-year period revealed a 4% overall incidence of infectious keratitis, but a 1.5% incidence over the initial 2 months postoperatively (38). A similar study of 285 patients who received transplants over a 5-year period found a 2.5% incidence of keratitis in the first 3 months, but an overall incidence of 7% (39). Bacteriology in these studies was not specified by time of onset of infection, but *Streptococcus pneumoniae, Staphylococcus aureus, Pseudomonas aeruginosa,* and *Serratia marcescens* were the most common pathogens. Risk factors for keratitis included persistent corneal epithelial defects and suture abscesses. Suture abscesses may develop months after surgery. One study of 18 suture abscesses found they developed one to 53 months postoperatively (mean 21 months), so few would be considered nosocomial (40). Bacteriology included six cases of *S. epidermidis,* four cases of *S. aureus,* two cases of viridans streptococci, and four cases of gram-negative bacilli.

Endophthalmitis is a rare but potentially devastating complication of PK that occurs in 0.2% to 0.4% of recipient eyes (41, 42). Onset of symptoms is within 2 months of surgery, but most cases occur within 2 weeks. Both bacterial and fungal endophthalmitis have resulted from PK. In a U.S. study of 1,010 corneal transplants, streptococci caused three cases and *Candida* one case of posttransplant endophthalmitis (42). In a Saudi Arabian study, there were three fungal and three bacterial endophthalmitis cases (41). Another study from Saudi Arabia reported a cluster of endophthalmitis that developed in four patients 1 week after PK (three *Enterococcus faecalis,* one *Candida glabrata*) (43). Contamination of the donor corneas during storage was the likely source of infection. Endophthalmitis due to aminoglycoside-resistant *Alcaligenes* has been described, and this is significant because aminoglycosides are the only antibiotics present in standard tissue storage media (44). Eye bank corneal storage media contain either gentamicin (McCarey-Kaufman media) or gentamicin plus streptomycin (Optisol GS). No antifungal agent is present, and candidal endophthalmitis has occurred in several patients who received *Candida*-contaminated corneal tissue (45, 46).

The source of infection in nearly all cases of post-PK endophthalmitis is thought to be microbial colonization of the donor cornea. Most corneal surgeons routinely culture the unused rim of the donor cornea at the time of surgery in an attempt to predict patients at risk for endophthalmitis. Unfortunately, there is little correlation between a positive donor rim culture and subsequent endophthalmitis, and the value of this practice is unclear. From 5% to 10% of routine donor rim cultures are positive, yet subsequent endophthalmitis is rare and may occur in recipients of culture-negative corneas. This was illustrated by a study of 774 donor corneal rim cultures in which 5% were positive, yet no patient who received these corneas developed endophthalmitis (47). The only two patients in this study who did develop endophthalmitis received culture-negative corneas.

Infections After LASIK

LASIK is rapidly becoming the most commonly performed eye surgery. Unlike other eye surgeries, LASIK is performed in patients who have normal eyes except for refractive error, i.e., the need for glasses. Over one million LASIK procedures were performed in the U.S. in 2000, up from 400,000 procedures in 1998 and 200,000 in 1997 (48,49). The LASIK uses a microkeratome to cut a thin, hinged flap across the corneal surface, exposing the corneal stroma beneath. A laser then ablates some of this central stroma and the flap is replaced, leaving a flattened cornea. The procedure is often performed using only semisterile technique (e.g., the microkeratome blade is sterile but the microkeratome handle is not). The procedure is an outpatient procedure and is often performed in free-standing LASIK centers. Many centers are owned by the ophthalmologist who performs the procedures, so underreporting of complications is likely.

A major postoperative complication of LASIK is diffuse lamellar keratitis (DLK). This syndrome, also called "sands of the Sahara" because of the granular appearance of the corneal flap/stroma interface, occurs in 1% to 5% of eyes (49). The etiology is unknown, and cultures are negative. One outbreak in 52 patients in which cultures were negative was thought to be related to endotoxins. Sterilizers used at the center were found to have reservoirs contaminated with gram-negative bacterial biofilms, and it was postulated that these biofilms produced endotoxins that contaminated the instruments during sterilization (50).

The most common infectious complication of LASIK is keratitis. The reported incidence is approximately 0.1% (49), but significant underreporting in the U.S. is likely and most case reports are from other countries (51–54). Khan et al. (49) reviewed the world literature through 2001 and found reports of 39 infections (35 patients). Most patients presented with typical signs of keratitis: pain, photophobia, eye redness, blurred vision. In the 31 eyes with positive cultures, the major pathogens were *S. aureus* 32% and rapidly growing nontuberculous mycobacteria 29%, primarily *Mycobacterium chelonae.* There were no gram-negative bacterial infections. Molds (e.g., *Aspergillus, Curvularia*) caused 16% of cases, but this high incidence may reflect the contribution of case reports from tropical regions where fungal keratitis is relatively common. Nontuberculous mycobacteria and *S. aureus* were also the major pathogens in a study of 13 patients (15 eyes) with post-LASIK keratitis referred to an eye institute in Miami from centers in Florida and South America (55). Nontuberculous mycobacteria (e.g., *M. chelonae, M. abscessus*) caused six of 15 cases, whereas *S. aureus* caused four. Two cases involved gram-negative bacilli (*Pseudomonas, Stenotrophomonas*). Excluding two patients with late (>6 months) onset of keratitis due to molds and related to trauma, patients developed keratitis symptoms an average of 16 days postoperatively (range 2–65 days).

Post-LASIK *S. aureus* keratitis likely represents contamination from normal colonizing eye flora, and the incidence may be increased in patients with chronic meibomian gland dysfunction (e.g., marginal blepharitis). These patients should be free of any signs of eyelid disease at the time of the procedure to minimize infectious complications. The nontuberculous mycobacterial infections likely represent environmental contamination at the time of the procedure. For this reason, some authors recommend that LASIK be performed with sterile technique, including sterile instruments, sterile plastic bags covering portions of the laser that can't be sterilized, sterile gloves and drapes, eyelid antisepsis with povidone iodine, and prophylactic topical antibiotics (55).

Scleral Buckle Infections

Retinal detachments occur with an incidence of 18 per 100,000 persons in the U.S. (56). One method used to reattach the retina is a scleral buckling procedure. In this procedure, either a hard silicone band is placed around the eyeball, encircling it like a cinch, or one or more soft silicone "sponges" are sutured to the episclera. In each case, the underlying sclera is pressed inward against the detached retina, allowing reattachment.

Chronic scleral buckle infections may be subacute in onset and can occur years after surgery (57). They are often associated with buckle extrusion through the conjunctiva. Nosocomial scleral buckle infections, however, are acute, often occurring within 2 weeks of surgery. Patients typically present with signs of orbital cellulitis, with eye pain, chemosis, and proptosis. Vision may be decreased due to sympathetic vitreous inflammation. The vitreous is usually sterile, although in severe cases endophthalmitis may also be present. The incidence of acute scleral buckle infections is 0.4 to 0.8%, and was 0.6% in one large retrospective study (58). In this study of 4,480 scleral buckle procedures, 15 patients developed severe infections 4 to 47 days postoperatively. The main pathogens were *S. aureus* (58% of the 12 culture-positive cases) and *S. epidermidis* (25%). Staphylococci are the major pathogens in other studies as well (59). Atopic dermatitis may increase the risk of postoperative *S. aureus* scleral buckle infections. In a study from Japan of 293 eyes with scleral buckles placed between 1995 and 1997, seven developed acute infections and all were due to methicillin-resistant *S. aureus*. Six of these seven patients had atopic dermatitis, giving an infection rate of 19% in patients with atopic dermatitis, but only 0.4% in those without this condition (60).

Prophylactic preoperative intravenous antibiotics are not routinely used in scleral buckle surgery, and there are no studies evaluating the efficacy of systemic antibiotic prophylaxis. Scleral buckles are often soaked in antibiotics just prior to placement intraoperatively, based on the results of a 1974–1981 prospective study (61). In this study, half of the patients received Silastic sponges ("soft" scleral buckles) that had been soaked for 30 minutes in penicillin plus gentamicin solution, and half received nonsoaked sponges. More patients who received nonsoaked sponges than soaked sponges developed acute infections (1/450 versus 9/471, $p = .01$). This study has not been repeated.

Postcataract Endophthalmitis

Cataract surgery is one of the most common surgical procedures performed in the U.S., with over 2 million cases annually. Surgery has been performed on an ambulatory basis since 1985, when Medicare instituted a policy that covered only outpatient cataract surgery. Surgery involves making a small incision through either the sclera or cornea, removing the native lens pulp (leaving the posterior lens capsule intact), and replacing it with a synthetic intraocular lens (IOL). The most popular technique for native lens removal is phacoemulsification, in which the lens is ultrasonically broken up and aspirated. This allows for a very small incision that may be left unsutured, as it self-seals. A recent advance is "clear cornea" surgery, where the incision is made through the cornea (rather than tunneled through the sclera) and is usually not sutured. There is some concern that clear cornea surgery carries a higher risk of postoperative endophthalmitis than does traditional scleral tunnel surgery (62).

Incidence and Outcome

The major infectious complication of cataract surgery is endophthalmitis, or infection of the vitreous. This occurs in 0.08% to 0.3% of cases (63–66), with the lower rates cited from studies that include only culture-positive cases. Endophthalmitis often results in some permanent decrease in vision in the affected eye at long-term follow-up. In one prospective multicenter study of 420 patients with postcataract endophthalmitis, half were left with less than 20/40 vision in the affected eye, and 10% were left with little (<5/200) or no vision in that eye (67). Visual outcome depends on the infecting microorganism, with the best outcomes seen in cases where vitreous cultures are either negative (30% of cases) or grow only coagulase-negative staphylococci, the major pathogen.

Etiologic Agents

Postoperative endophthalmitis may be caused by a variety of bacteria and fungi. A multicenter study of postoperative endophthalmitis was able to isolate potential pathogens from 82.1% of clinically infected eyes (67,68). Gram-positive pathogens were identified in 69.3% of patients, most commonly coagulase-negative staphylococci (70.0%), *S. aureus* (9.9%), and *Streptococcus* species (9.0%) (Table 26.2). Gram-negative pathogens were identified in 5.9% of patients. Polymicrobial growth occurred in 9.3% of patients. The worst outcomes occur in endophthalmitis due to *S. aureus*, gram-negative bacilli, and streptococci of any type. However, the presenting visual acuity was more powerful than microbiologic factors in predicting visual outcome and favorable response to vitrectomy.

Clinical Features

Endophthalmitis following cataract extraction may present in one of three ways: acute, delayed acute, and chronic (Table 26.3) (69). Hughes and Hill (69) note that delayed acute endophthalmitis is similar to acute endophthalmitis but is usually associated with some complication; examples include a broken suture, suture removal, inadvertent filtering bleb, wound dehiscence, or a vitreous wick. Chronic endophthalmitis is characterized by a more indolent course. Acute endophthalmitis typi-

TABLE 26.2. MICROBIOLOGY OF POSTOPERATIVE ENDOPHTHALMITIS

Pathogen	Frequency (%)
Gram-positive bacteria	94.2
Coagulase-negative staphylococci	70.0
Staphylococcus aureus	9.9
Streptococcus species	9.0
Enterococcus species	2.2
Corynebacterium species	1.2
Bacillus species	0.6
Diphtheroids	0.6
Propionibacterium species	0.6
Gram-negative bacteria	5.9
Proteus mirabilis	1.9
Pseudomonas aeruginosa	0.9
Other pseudomonal species	0.6
Morganella morganii	0.6
Citrobacter diversus	0.6
Enterobacter species	0.6
Serratia marcescens	0.3
Flavobacterium species	0.3

Adapted from Han DP, Wisniewski SR, Wilson LR, et al. Spectrum and susceptibilities of microbiologic isolates in the endophthalmitis vitrectomy study, *Am J Ophthalmol* 1996; 122:1–17.

cally presents 2 to 4 days after an operation (70). The onset of symptoms (eye pain, redness, decreased vision) in postcataract endophthalmitis occurs within 1 week of surgery in 75% of patients, and within 1 month in nearly all patients. A hyperacute picture is often associated with *S. aureus, S. pneumoniae,* or a gram-negative infection, whereas less virulent microorganisms such as coagulase-negative staphylococci follow a more indolent course (69,71). A review of 60 patients with coagulase-negative staphylococcal endophthalmitis found that 12% of cases presented more than 30 days after surgery (71). Fungal endophthalmitis has an even greater delay and "usually mimics chronic iridocyclitis and vitreitis with minimal pain." Late-onset endophthalmitis most frequently follows glaucoma surgery (72). Hughes and Hill (69) have summarized the characteristics of acute and chronic postoperative endophthalmitis (Table 26.3). Several reports have called attention to the fact that postoperative endophthalmitis may be painless (71,73).

TABLE 26.3. CHARACTERISTICS OF ACUTE AND CHRONIC ENDOPHTHALMITIS

	Acute	Chronic
Presentation	2–4 days	>30 days
Symptoms	Ocular pain	Reduced vision
	Reduced vision	Minimal pain
	Headache	
Signs	Lid edema	Bacterial
	Conjunctival hyperemia	Steroid-responsive iritis
	Chemosis	Capsular plaque
	Purulent discharge	Granulomatous iritis
	Corneal edema	Vitritis
	Anterior chamber reaction	Localized vitreous reaction
	Hypopyon	Fungal
	Vitritis	Not usually steroid responsive
	Poor red reflex	Stringy vitreous reaction
		Fungus ball

Adapted from Hughes DS, Hill RJ. Infections endophthalmitis after cataract surgery. *Br J Ophthalmol* 1994; 78:227–232.

Treatment of endophthalmitis is discussed in detail elsewhere (74), but the IOL does not need to be removed except in cases of endophthalmitis due to molds or in some cases of indolent infections due to *Propionibacterium acnes.*

Outbreaks

Clusters of endophthalmitis cases due to contaminated instruments or ophthalmic solutions have been described, but are rare. Three outbreaks due to *P. aeruginosa,* two in Europe and one in the U.S., have been linked to use of a contaminated phacoemulsifier (75–77). In all three outbreaks the outbreak pathogen was found contaminating the internal pathways of the phacoemulsifier. Intrinsically contaminated fluids or lens used in ocular surgery have led to outbreaks with *P. aeruginosa* or *Bacillus* species (78), *P. aeruginosa* (79), or *Paecilomyces lilacinus* (80,81). Contamination of humidifier water in a ventilation system with *Acremonium kiliense* led to four cases of endophthalmitis in an ambulatory surgical center (82). *Aspergillus* endophthalmitis occurred in five patients during a period of hospital construction, which again demonstrates the need to follow standard guidelines during renovation or new construction (83).

Pathophysiology

Nearly all cases of postcataract endophthalmitis are due to microorganisms introduced into the aqueous humor at the time of surgery from the patient's own ocular surface flora. Contamination of the aqueous humor during surgery with surface flora is common, with between 8% and 43% of aqueous cultures positive at the end of surgery in uncomplicated cases (84–87). Endophthalmitis is rare, however, presumably because of aqueous turnover rate (every 100 minutes) and the immune system's ability to clear small inocula of bacteria from the aqueous (88). The vitreous is gel-like and permanent, so it is much less resistant to infection than the aqueous. If the posterior lens capsule is broken during surgery, allowing communication with the vitreous, the risk of endophthalmitis increases 14-fold (89). Other risk factors are diabetes and wound dehiscence or leak (74).

Prevention

There has been great interest in prophylactic measures that may reduce bacterial contamination during cataract surgery (90). Speaker and Menikoff (91), in an open-label nonrandomized trial, compared 5% povidone-iodine topical solution as prophylaxis in one operating room suite with silver protein solution prophylaxis in another suite. Surgeons continued to use "their customary prophylactic antibiotics." The study found a significantly lower incidence of culture-positive endophthalmitis in the suite using the povidone-iodine (0.06% vs. 0.24%). Since this study was published, it has been generally accepted that 5%

povidone-iodine solution should be used on the conjunctiva during preoperative preparation. Whether the iodine should be then flushed with sterile saline is unknown. Other nonrandomized studies have advocated intraoperative irrigation of the anterior chamber with antibiotics, antibiotic injection into the aqueous at the end of the case, and postoperative subconjunctival antibiotic injections (90). Preoperative topical antibiotics (e.g., polymyxin/trimethoprim) are routinely used, although the optimal timing and frequency of prophylactic eye drops is unknown. Even the efficacy of prophylactic antibiotic eye drops in cataract surgery is unknown, as there have been no prospective randomized trials to assess prophylactic use of eye drops. Such a trial would require a very large study population to achieve statistical significance, since the incidence of culture-positive endophthalmitis (0.1%) is so low. Prevention strategies have been summarized in several reports (Table 26.4) (92,93).

Environmental controls include the following. First, adhere to standard operating room environmental air controls (i.e., >15 air exchanges per hour, air filtered through filters of at least 90% efficiency for particles >3 μm). Second, all operative equipment and irrigating fluids should be sterile prior to use. Third, limit the use of multiple-dose dispensers and pay careful attention to manufacturer's recommendations regarding use of ophthalmic solutions.

TABLE 26.4. RECOMMENDATIONS FOR THE PREVENTION OF POSTOPERATIVE ENDOPHTHALMITIS

Preoperative
- Careful preoperative assessment of patients for risk factors
- Treatment of eyelid and lacrimal system infections/abnormalities prior to surgery
- Treatment of systemic infections prior to surgery
- Topical antibiotic therapy up to 24 hours prior to surgery: tobramycin, polymyxin-B, trimethoprim, and quinolone antibiotics are currently recommended
- Systemic antibiotic prophylaxis is of uncertain benefit but may be considered in high-risk cases such as secondary intraocular lens implantation and intraocular procedures in immunocompromised patients (e.g., diabetes)

Intraoperative
- Sterile draping to exclude lids and lashes from the operative field
- Use of 5% povidone-iodine solution to prepare the ocular surface, and 10% povidone-iodine solution for the eyelids and surrounding skin; lid margin scrubs may be omitted
- Antibiotic use in infusion fluids is of unproven benefit
- Irrigation of intraocular lens prior to insertion to remove potentially adherent bacteria
- Minimize the duration of exposure of intraocular lens to the operating room environment prior to insertion
- Systemic antibiotic prophylaxis may be considered in prolonged cataract surgery complicated by vitreous loss
- Meticulous no-touch surgical technique
- Careful wound closure by any technique
- Subconjunctival antibiotic injections at the end of surgery are of unproven benefit and carry the risk of inadvertent injection into the eye

Postoperative
- Postoperative antibiotic drops and ointment may be beneficial
- For patients with prolonged surgery, vitreous loss, or severe diabetes, consider closer postoperative follow-up
- Careful suture removal

Adapted from Staudenmaier C. Current views on the prevention of postoperative infectious endophthalmitis. *Can J Ophthalmol* 1997; 32:297–302.

NOSOCOMIAL OCULAR INFECTIONS NOT RELATED TO SURGERY

Conjunctivitis

Conjunctivitis is one of the most common infections in the Western Hemisphere. Symptoms include injection, conjunctival edema, photophobia, a foreign-body sensation, and production of copious secretions, which may range from watery to extremely purulent. Although a thick conjunctival discharge may cloud vision (it clears with blinking), true visual impairment is not present. Conjunctivitis is frequently associated with either blepharitis or keratitis.

Nosocomial conjunctivitis falls into two major groups: conjunctivitis of the newborn; and viral conjunctivitis, most commonly due to type 8 adenovirus.

Conjunctivitis of the Newborn

Conjunctivitis of the newborn is the term used by the World Health Organization (WHO) for any conjunctivitis with discharge occurring during the first 28 days of life. This term is more inclusive than the old term, *ophthalmia neonatorum,* which was previously used to describe a hyperacute purulent conjunctivitis occurring in the first 10 days of life, usually caused by *Neisseria gonorrhoeae.* Conjunctivitis of the newborn continues to be an important problem worldwide.

Etiology and Incidence

The causes of conjunctivitis of the newborn in the U.S. include *Chlamydia trachomatis, N. gonorrhoeae,* other bacterial microbes, herpes simplex, and chemical conjunctivitis due to the instillation of silver nitrate into the newborn's eye (Table 26.5) (94). The relative importance of each of these etiologic agents around the world depends on the prevalence of *C. trachomatis* and *N. gonorrhoeae* genital infections in women giving birth and whether silver nitrate prophylaxis is used. Mild chemical conjunctivitis due to silver nitrate administration is a common cause of conjunctivitis of the newborn. In one study, about 90% of neonates receiving silver nitrate prophylaxis developed conjunctivitis in the first 6 hours of life, but the majority of cases cleared within 24 hours (95). Chemical conjunctivitis following prophylaxis with tetracycline or erythromycin is rare.

Clinical Features of Infection

N. gonorrhoeae causes hyperacute conjunctivitis with marked purulent exudate, chemosis, and injection. Severe complications include corneal ulceration and perforation, which may lead to visual loss. Inadequate prophylaxis may delay the onset of disease or minimize its severity. *C. trachomatis* conjunctivitis is characterized by mild unilateral or bilateral purulence, lid edema, conjunctival injection, and profuse exudate. Newborns lack

TABLE 26.5. MAJOR AND MINOR PATHOGENS IN OPHTHALMIA NEONATORUM

Etiology of Ophthalmia Neonatorum	Percent of Cases	Incubation Period (Days)	Severity of Conjunctivitis[a]	Associated Problems
Chlamydia trachomatis	2–40	5–14	+	Pneumonitis 3 weeks to 3 months
Neisseria gonorrhoeae	<1	2–7	+++	Disseminated infection
Other bacterial microbes[b]	30–50	5–14	+	Variable
Herpes simplex virus	<1	6–14	+	Disseminated infection; keratitis and ulceration also possible
Chemical	Varies with silver nitrate use	1	+	—

[a] +, mild; +++, severe.
[b] *Staphylococcus* species; *Streptococcus pneumoniae; Haemophilus influenzae*, nontypeable; *Streptococcus mitis*; group A and B streptococci; *Neisseria cinerea; Corynebacterium* species, *Moraxella catarrhalis; E. coli; Klebsiella pneumoniae; Pseudomonas aeruginosa.*
Adapted from American Academy of Pediatrics. *1997 red book: report of the Committee on Infections Diseases,* 25th ed. Elk Grove Village, IL: American Academy of Pediatrics, 2003: 778,781,787.

lymphoid tissue and fail to develop an acute follicular conjunctivitis, which is typical of the adult infection. Chlamydial conjunctivitis may be associated with other sites of chlamydial infection, especially pneumonia.

Prophylaxis

The American Academy of Pediatrics (94) and the CDC (96) continue to recommend topical 1% silver nitrate, 0.5% erythromycin, and 1% tetracycline as prophylaxis for conjunctivitis of the newborn, since all are considered equally effective for preventing gonococcal infection (Table 26.6). Each agent is available in single-dose tubes. Prophylaxis should be given shortly after birth, preferably within 1 hour. If prophylaxis is not provided in the delivery room, hospitals should establish a check system to ensure that all infants are treated. Povidone-iodine in a 2.5% solution may also be useful but is not currently available in the U.S. Silver nitrate causes more chemical conjunctivitis than other agents but is recommended in areas where the incidence of penicillinase-producing *N. gonorrhoeae* (PPNG) is appreciable. The efficacy of erythromycin or povidone-iodine prophylaxis against PPNG is not known, but one study has demonstrated that tetracycline is effective. Infants born by cesarean section should receive prophylaxis against neonatal gonococcal ophthalmia. Although gonococcal and chlamydial infections are usually transmitted to the infant during passage through the birth canal, infection by the ascending route also occurs (94).

TABLE 26.6. PROPHYLAXIS OF CONJUNCTIVITIS OF THE NEWBORN

Recommended agents
- Silver nitrate (1%) aqueous solution in a single application *or*
- Erythromycin (0.5%) ophthalmic ointment in a single application *or*
- Tetracycline ophthalmic ointment (1%) in a single application

Administration: Before administering local prophylaxis, each eyelid should be wiped gently with sterile cotton. Two drops of a 1% silver nitrate solution or a 1-cm ribbon of antibiotic ointment are placed in each lower conjunctival sac. The eyelids should then be massaged gently to spread the ointment. After 1 minute, excess solution or ointment can be wiped away by sterile cotton. None of the prophylactic antibiotic agents should be flushed away from the eye after instillation. Comparative studies of the efficacy of silver nitrate prophylaxis with and without flushing are lacking, but anecdotal reports suggest that flushing may reduce the efficacy of prophylaxis without reducing the incidence of chemical conjunctivitis.

Adapted from American Academy of Pediatrics. *1997 red book: report of the Committee on Infectious Diseases,* 25th ed. Elk Grove Village, IL: American Academy of Pediatrics, 2003: 778,781,787; and Centers for Disease Control are Prevention. 1998 guidelines for treatment of sexually transmitted diseases. *MMWR* 2002; 451(RR-6):1–78.

Infants who develop conjunctivitis of the newborn should receive an appropriate evaluation. Early diagnosis and adequate therapy of ophthalmia neonatorum, especially gonococcal infections, can prevent corneal ulceration and blindness. Infants born to women with untreated gonococcal infections should receive one dose of ceftriaxone sodium (25–50 mg/kg intravenously or intramuscularly, not to exceed 125 mg) or cefotaxime sodium (100 mg/kg, intravenously or intramuscularly). Infants who have gonococcal ophthalmia should be hospitalized.

Epidemic Keratoconjunctivitis

Conjunctivitis may be caused by a variety of viruses. Acute hemorrhagic conjunctivitis is caused by enterovirus type 70 and coxsackievirus type A 24. Herpes simplex is an uncommon cause of follicular conjunctivitis. Pharyngoconjunctival fever, an acute and highly infectious illness, is characterized by fever, pharyngitis, and acute follicular conjunctivitis. It is caused by adenoviruses, most commonly types 3, 4, and 7, but has also been associated with types 1, 5, 6, and 14. The most serious of the adenoviral illnesses and the one most commonly associated with nosocomial outbreaks is epidemic keratoconjunctivitis (EKC). EKC has most commonly been associated with adenovirus types

8 and 19, but also has been reported with other serotypes, including types 2 to 4, 7 to 11, 14, 16, and 29. All types produce a similar clinical picture, but types 8 and 19 are much more likely to be involved in large epidemics.

The prevalence and incidence of EKC are unknown (97). During outbreaks in medical facilities, attack rates as high as 25% have been reported (Table 26.7). More cases are reported in the fall and winter months (6). The incubation period is approximately 8 days, and disease is unilateral initially, although most cases become bilateral via self-contamination. In patients who progress to bilateral disease, the second eye becomes involved in 4 to 5 days.

Ford et al. (97) have summarized the symptoms and signs of EKC reported in the literature. Ocular symptoms included a foreign body sensation (43%), photophobia (15%), lacrimation (99%), and eye redness (98%). Extraocular symptoms included fever/malaise (1–33%), upper respiratory tract symptoms (1–63%), diarrhea (2–3%), nausea/vomiting (2–14%), and

TABLE 26.7. SELECTED OUTBREAKS OF EPIDEMIC KERATOCONJUNCTIVITIS IN MEDICAL FACILITIES, 1950–2000

Reference	Year of Outbreak	Site	Number of Infections	Attack Rate (%)	Risk Factors/Environmental Sources
Cockbum et al. (98)	1951	Glaucoma clinic	9	23.5	Tonometry
Leopold (99)	1953	Hospital	17	—	Giant ophthalmoscope
Schnieder et al. (100)	1953	Nursing home	20	—	Eyedrops
Quilligan et al. (101)	1957	Eye clinic	58	—	Tonometer probable
Davidson (102)	1961	Hospital	56	8.5	—
Dawson and Darrell (103)	1961	Medical office	27	21.4	Contact with infected physician
					Tonometry
					Slip-lamp examination
					Minor surgery
					Therapeutic eyedrops
Laibson et al. (105)	1967	Eye hospital	102	—	Contact with infected physicians
Dawson et al. (106)	1967	Hospital	16	—	Indirect ophthalmoscopy
					Minor surgery
CDC (104)	1974	Hospital ward and eye clinic	20	—	Tonometer
Vastine et al. (107)	1974–75	Eye infirmary	52	—	—
Tullo and Higgins (108)	1977–78	Eye hospital	17	—	—
Keenylside et al. (109)	1977–78	Ophthalmologist's office	83	—	—
D'Angelo et al. (110)	1977–78	Ophthalmologist's office	86	29.4	Ophthalmic procedures (e.g., tonometry)
					Ophthalmic solutions
					Physician contact
		Nursing home	16	2.5	—
		Nursing home	6	25.0	—
Darougar et al. (111)	—	Eye hospital	13	—	Minor surgical procedures
Nagington et al. (112)	1979	Eye department	14	—	—
Richmond et al. (113)	1981	Emergency room	200	—	—
Buehler et al. (114)	1981	Ophthalmologist's office	39	1.8	Contact with specific caregivers[a]
					Invasive procedures[a]
					Tonometry[a]
					Foreign-body removal[a]
Reilly et al. (115)	1984	Eye infirmary	186	—	—
Warren et al. (116)	1985–86	Eye infirmary	110	0.47	Pneumotonometry[a]
Takeughi et al. (117)	1985	Hospital	30	—	—
Insler and Kern (118)	1986	Ophthalmologist's office	24	—	—
Jernigan et al. (119)	1986	Eye clinic	126	7.3	Pneumotonometry[a]
					Multiple clinic visits[a]
					Contact with infected physician[a]
Colon (120)	1986	Hospital eye clinic	132	—	Pneumotonometer
Koo et al. (121)	1987–88	Eye clinic	102	16.7	Pneumotonometry[a]
					Contact with specific caregiver[a]
Buffington et al. (122)	1990	Nursing home	47	49.5	—
Birenbaum et al. (123)	—	Hospital	7	—	—
Ankers et al. (124)	1991	Eye hospital	23	—	Contact with infected physician
Tabery (125)	1993	Eye clinic	33	—	Contact with infected physician
					Multidose dropper bottle
Curtis et al. (126)	—	Eye department	22	—	—
Montessori et al. (127)	1994	Hospital eye clinic	39	—	Contact with specific caregiver
					Diagnostic lens applied to eye
Cheung et al. (128)	1999	Hospital eye clinic	19	—	Invasive procedures
Piednoir et al. (129)	2000	Long-term care facility	41	50.8	Person-to-person via indirect contact

[a] Risk factor statistically significant ($p < .05$).

myalgias (2–12%). Ocular signs include conjunctival hypertrophy (95–96%), chemosis (26–50%), pseudomembranes (1–38%), focal epithelial keratitis (55–65%), diffuse epithelial keratitis (42%), stromal edema (18–47%), anterior uveitis (11%), preauricular adenopathy (15–94%), and decreased visual acuity (17–78%). Keratitis often begins 3 to 4 days after the onset of corneal opacities. Usually, these opacities resolve within several months and do not result in permanent loss of vision.

Large outbreaks of EKC have occurred in medical facilities (98–129) (Table 26.7). The major modes of transmission are person-to-person via the hands of medical caregivers and ophthalmic instruments (e.g., tonometers, slit lamps) or ophthalmic solutions (e.g., wash stations, topical anesthetic solutions). Infected healthcare workers may serve as both a reservoir for infection and a means of transmission of infection to other patients. In more than half of the outbreaks summarized in Table 26.7, a healthcare worker became infected. The direct cost of a single outbreak was calculated as approximately $30,000 (129).

Adenovirus type 8 is extremely hardy when deposited on environmental surfaces, and this accounts for the fact that fomites play a significant role in nosocomial transmission. Gloves should be worn for contact with patients infected with adenovirus for two reasons. First, hand washing with soap has been shown to be ineffective in eliminating infectious virus (119). Second, adenovirus can be recovered from the hands of approximately 50% of patients with adenoviral conjunctivitis (130). Adenovirus can be recovered from plastic and metal surfaces for more than 30 days (131). The CDC (132) and the Association of Professionals in Infection Control and Epidemiology (133) recommend that the tips of tonometers be cleaned with soap and water (or an alternative agent suggested by the manufacturer) and disinfected by soaking for at least 5 to 10 minutes in a solution containing 500 ppm chlorine, 3% hydrogen peroxide, 70% ethyl alcohol, or 70% isopropyl alcohol. After disinfection the device should be thoroughly rinsed in tap water and dried before use (Table 26.8). The Public Health Committee of the American Academy of Ophthalmology has stated that physicians may wish to follow the previous recommendations of the CDC, including a 5-minute soak in diluted sodium hypochlorite or in a 3% solution of hydrogen peroxide (134). Only limited data are available on the efficacy of different methods for disinfection of tonometers. Threlkeld et al. (135) have demonstrated that a tonometer contaminated with adenovirus type 8 could be sterilized by wiping or soaking for 5 minutes with isopropyl alcohol, hydrogen peroxide, or an iodophor. However, alcohol swabs have been shown ineffective in eliminating adenovirus type 5 from experimentally contaminated eyelid speculums (136). Further, two studies have found that disinfection of pneumotonometer tips between patients with a 70% isopropyl alcohol wipe contributed to an outbreak of epidemic keratoconjunctivitis (119,121).

Because of the highly contagious nature of epidemic keratoconjunctivitis, the CDC recommends the following work restrictions for healthcare workers with conjunctivitis: "Restrict personnel with epidemic keratoconjunctivitis or purulent conjunctivitis caused by other microorganisms from patient care and the patient's environment for the duration of symptoms" (Table 26.8). "If symptoms persist longer than 5 to 7 days, refer personnel to an ophthalmologist for evaluation of continued infectiousness" (137).

TABLE 26.8. GUIDELINES FOR THE PREVENTION OF EPIDEMIC KERATOCONJUNCTIVITIS (EKC)

Evaluate all medical personnel with conjunctivitis for EKC
Furlough all medical personnel with clinically diagnosed EKC for the duration of their illness (approximately 2 weeks)
All patients with known or suspected EKC should be seen in a separate area of any outpatient facility
All hospital personnel should wear disposable gloves when examining and caring for patients with known or suspected EKC; careful hand washing with an antimicrobial agent should precede and follow all patient contacts
All equipment that comes into contact with the mucous membranes of the eye should be sterilized or undergo high-level disinfection between patient uses; appropriate disinfection methods include immersion for 5 to 10 minutes in 3% hydrogen peroxide, sodium hypochlorite (500 ppm chlorine), 70% ethyl alcohol, or 70% isopropyl alcohol; after disinfection, the device should be thoroughly rinsed in tap water and dried before use
Only single-use vials of ophthalmic solutions should be used when examining patients with EKC
All persons with EKC should be cautioned against sharing towels, face cloths, glasses, goggles, or any other item that might come into direct contact with the eyes of another individual
All hospitalized patients with EKC should be placed on contact precautions; EKC should be considered potentially contagious for 10–14 days

In an evaluation of effectiveness of an infection control program to control epidemic keratoconjunctivitis, Gottsch et al. (138) reviewed the experience of EKC in a large teaching eye institute from 1984 to 1997. Following the implementation of an infection control program, the number of annual outbreaks fell from 3.89 to 0.543 ($p < .005$) and the number of affected patients from 54.09 per 100,000 visits to 5.66 per 100,000 patient visits ($p < .0005$). The infection control program included patient screening and isolation, hand hygiene, instrument disinfection, medication distribution, and furlough of infected employees.

Conjunctivitis Due to Other Microbes

Community-acquired conjunctivitis is most commonly due to *S. aureus, S. pneumoniae, Streptococcus pyogenes,* and *Haemophilus* species. Both endemic (139) and epidemic nosocomial (140) infections may be caused by these pathogens. Intrinsic contamination of a triclosan-containing soap with *Serratia marcescens* led to an outbreak of conjunctivitis in a newborn nursery (141). Nosocomial infections with resistant pathogens such as methicillin-resistant (139) or erythromycin-resistant (140) *S. aureus* have been reported. Therefore, it is important to obtain a Gram stain and culture of conjunctival secretions.

Keratitis

Keratitis or inflammation of the cornea may be the result of infection or due to trauma, hypersensitivity, or other immune-mediated reactions (142). Symptoms include a unilateral red eye with moderate to severe pain, photophobia, tearing, and decreased vision. Etiologic agents include, most commonly, viruses (e.g., adenovirus, herpes simplex) and bacteria (e.g., *S. aureus, P. aeruginosa*). Most infectious agents require a defect in the ocular surface for invasion. Any corneal inflammation should be considered potentially sight-threatening, since perforation and loss of the eye can occur within 24 hours after invasion by a pathogenic microorganism such as *S. aureus* or *P. aeruginosa* (142).

Nosocomial keratitis most commonly occurs in elderly and/or debilitated patients (143–145). The most common pathogen reported has been *P. aeruginosa* (143–146). Intubation and tracheal suctioning have been reported as predisposing factors, presumably because the suction catheter is dragged across the patient's eye, resulting in both a corneal abrasion and contamination of the conjunctivae with respiratory flora (144, 145,147). Nosocomial *P. aeruginosa* conjunctivitis, which in some patients led to corneal scarring, has also been reported in children, in whom it was associated with tracheostomy, endotracheal intubation, administration of oxygen by hood, or suctioning (148). Unconscious patients should receive appropriate eye care, which includes regular eye examinations, application of lubricating ointment, and consideration of mechanically apposing the lids with adhesive tape (146).

Topical medications for use in the conjunctivae in the home have frequently been found to be contaminated, mainly with gram-negative bacteria (149). Further, it has been shown that conjunctival colonization with pathogenic microorganisms is more likely in patients using contaminated medications (149). The use of contaminated eye drops had led to keratitis with *P. aeruginosa* (143) and *S. marcescens* (150). For hospitalized patients, therefore, it is prudent to use only single-dose vials. If multiple-dose vials are used, care must be taken to administer the drops so as to avoid touching the eye and contaminating the dropper bottle. If a separate eye dropper is used, it should be disinfected between uses.

Contact lens care systems may become contaminated with bacteria (especially *P. aeruginosa*) or *Acanthamoeba* when nonsterile water or inappropriate disinfection methods are used (151,152). Although nosocomial outbreaks due to *Acanthamoeba* have not been described, appropriate disinfection practices must be followed if hospitalized patients are allowed to use their own lens care systems. Recommendations on lens care for healthcare workers who wear contact lens have been published (153).

Endophthalmitis

Endophthalmitis is defined as an inflammatory process that involves the vitreous body, and retinal and uveal layers of the eye. It may be classified according to the mode of entry of the microbial pathogen, location within the eye, and type of etiologic agent. Endophthalmitis most commonly occurs as a complication of ocular surgery but may also occur as a sequela to penetrating ocular trauma or systemic infection (154). Infectious agents include viruses, bacteria, fungi, protozoa, and parasites. The infecting flora depends highly on the mode of entry of the microbial pathogen(s) (see below). Although not present in all cases, pain and decreased vision are the cardinal clinical features of endophthalmitis. Other symptoms include pink eye, headache, and ocular discharge. Signs include conjunctival injection, lid and/or corneal edema, poor light reflex, and orbital cellulitis.

Infections following trauma, although not a nosocomial problem, are an important source of morbidity for patients. Etiologic agents include gram-positive microorganisms (*Bacillus cereus, S. aureus, Streptococcus* species, coagulase-negative staphylococci), gram-negative bacilli (*Enterobacter* species, *Citrobacter freundii, Klebsiella* species), anaerobes, fungi, or mixed pathogens.

Nosocomial endophthalmitis not associated with surgery is most commonly due to metastatic infection of the eye via hematogenous spread. In most cases of hematogenous bacterial endophthalmitis, a septic focus is usually apparent before intraocular inflammation occurs (155). Gamel and Allansmith (155) have summarized the septic foci in 20 cases of metastatic endophthalmitis: meningitis, six; abdominal infection, four; endocarditis, two; unknown site, two; and one each of pneumonia, otitis media, breast abscess, paronychia, pharyngitis, and lymphadenitis. Endocarditis must always be considered in hospitalized patients who develop endophthalmitis without an obvious distal focus (156). Common pathogens reported in the literature included *S. pneumoniae, Streptococcus* species, *Neisseria meningitidis, S. aureus, B. cereus, Haemophilus influenzae,* and fungi *(Candida, Aspergillus).* Uncommon pathogens include *Nocardia* and group B streptococcus (157). In a review of the literature, Greenwald et al. (158) concluded that the bacteriology of metastatic endophthalmitis has changed. Comparing cases reported from 1976 to 1985 with cases reported from 1935 to 1975, they noted that infections due to *S. pneumoniae* and *N. meningitidis* were less common and cases due to *B. cereus* and gram-negative bacilli *(Haemophilus, E. coli, Klebsiella, Serratia, Salmonella)* were more common. They attribute the increasing prevalence of microorganisms of relatively low pathogenicity to increased numbers of immunocompromised patients. Similarly, in a series by Okada et al. (11), endophthalmitis occurred in patients debilitated with chronic diseases such as diabetes mellitus or malignancy, or in association with surgical procedures or intravenous hyperalimentation. Involvement of both eyes has been noted in approximately 25% of cases (158). About two-thirds of patients have been reported to lose vision as a result of infection, and more than 10% have died as a result of sepsis (158). Preservation of vision depends on rapid diagnosis and institution of appropriate treatment (154,158,159).

Candida is increasingly reported as an etiologic agent of nosocomial infections. Contributing factors for the increased prevalence of *Candida* infections likely include widespread use of broad-spectrum antibiotics, increased use of invasive procedures and parenteral hyperalimentation, and increased numbers of immunocompromised patients (premature infants, organ transplantation, bone marrow transplantation) (160) (see Chapter 39). Candidal endophthalmitis has been reported to accompany candidal sepsis in approximately 30% of patients (154,161,162). Occasionally, candidal chorioretinal lesions may develop in the absence of positive blood cultures (163). Non-*albicans* species of *Candida* have also been reported to cause endophthalmitis in the setting of fungemia but at a lower frequency than *C. albicans* (163).

CONCLUSION

Ocular infections are infrequently hospital-acquired. However, ocular infections are a well-recognized and serious adverse event following ocular surgery. Multiple outbreaks of ocular infections, especially epidemic keratoconjunctivitis have been reported. Infection control guidelines should be followed both to minimize postoperative ocular infections and to prevent outbreaks.

REFERENCES

1. Feigin RD, Cherry JD, eds. *Textbook of pediatric infectious diseases,* 5th ed. Philadelphia: WB Saunders, 2004.
2. Mandell GI, Douglas RB, Bennett JE, eds. *Principles and practices of infectious diseases,* 5th ed. New York: Churchill Livingstone, 2000.
3. Reese RE, Betts RF, eds. *A practical approach to infectious diseases,* 4th ed. Boston: Little, Brown, 1996.
4. Gorbach SL, Bartlett JG, Blacklow NR, eds. *Infectious diseases,* 3rd ed. Philadelphia: WB Saunders, 2004.
5. Tasman W, Jaeger EA, eds. *Duane's clinical ophthalmology.* Philadelphia: JB Lippincott, 1993.
6. Albert DM, Jakobiec FA, eds. *Principles and practice of ophthalmology,* 2nd ed. Philadelphia: WB Saunders, 1999.
7. Tabbara KF, Hyndiuk RA. *Infections of the eye,* 2nd ed. Boston: Little, Brown, 1995.
8. Seal DV, Bron AJ, Hay J. *Ocular infection.* St. Louis: Mosby, 1998.
9. Barza M, Baum J. Ocular infections. *Infect Dis Clin North Am* 1992; 6(4):769–1003.
10. Hibberd PI, Schein O, Baker AS. Intraocular infections: current therapeutic approaches. In: Remington J, Swartz MN, eds. *Clinical topics in infectious diseases,* vol. 11. Boston: Blackwell Scientific, 1991: 118–169.
11. Okada AA, Johnson RP, Liles WC, et al. Endogenous bacterial endophthalmitis: report of a ten-year retrospective study. *Ophthalmology* 1994;10:832–838.
12. Peacock JE. Eye infections. In: Wenzel RP, ed. *Prevention and control of nosocomial infections,* 3rd ed. Baltimore: Williams & Wilkins, 1997: 977–993.
13. Hirst LW. Ocular and periocular infections. *Aust Fam Physician* 1991; 20:979–988.
14. Syed NA, Hyndiuk RA. Infectious conjunctivitis. *Infect Dis Clin North Am* 1992;6:789–805.
15. Garner JS, Jarvis WR, Emori TG, et al. CDC definitions for nosocomial infections, 1988. *Am J Infect Control* 1988;16:128–140.
16. Naeno A, Naor J, Lee HM, et al. Three decades of corneal transplantation: indications and patient characteristics. *Cornea* 2000;19:7–11.
17. Robert PY, Camezind P, Drouet M, et al. Internal and external contamination of donor corneas before in situ excision: bacterial risk factors in 93 donors. *Graefes Arch Clin Exp Ophthalmol* 2002;240: 265–270.
18. Spelsberg H, Reinhard T, Sengler U, et al. Organ-cultured corneal grafts from septic donors: a retrospective study. *Eye* 2002;16: 622–627.
19. Heckmann JG, Lang CJG, Petruch F, et al. Transmission of Creutzfeldt-Jacob disease via a corneal transplant. *J Neurol Neurosurg Psychiatry* 1997;63:388–390.
20. Rutala WA, Weber DJ. Creutzfeldt-Jacob disease: Recommendations for disinfection and sterilization. *Clin Infect Dis* 2001;32:1348–1356.
21. Centers for Disease Control. Human-to-human transmission of rabies by a corneal transplant, Idaho. *MMWR* 1979;28:109–111.
22. Houff SA, Burton RC, Wilson RW, et al. Human-to-human transmission of rabies by corneal transplantation. *N Engl J Med* 1979;300: 603–604.
23. Centers for Disease Control. Human-to-human transmission of rabies via a corneal transplant, France. *MMWR* 1980;29:25–26.
24. Centers for Disease Control. Human-to-human transmission of rabies via corneal transplant—Thailand. *MMWR* 1981;30:473–474.
25. Gode GR, Bhide NK. Two rabies deaths after corneal grafts from one donor. *Lancet* 1988;2:791.
26. Javadi MA, Fayaz A, Mirdehghan SA, et al. Transmission of rabies by corneal graft. *Cornea* 1996;15:431–433.
27. Hoft RH, Pfugfelder SC, Forster RK, et al. Clinical evidence for hepatitis B transmission resulting from corneal transplantation. *Cornea* 1997;16:132–137.
28. Hogan RN, Cavanagh HD. Transplantation of corneal tissue from donors with diseases of the central nervous system. *Cornea* 1995;14: 547–553.
29. Darrell RW, Jacob GB. Hepatitis B surface antigen in human tears. *Arch Ophthalmol* 1978;96:674–676.
30. Raber IM, Friedman HM. Hepatitis B surface antigen in corneal donors. *Am J Ophthalmol* 1987;104:255–258.
31. Khalil A, Ayoub M, el-Din Abdel-Wahab KS, et al. Assessment of the infectivity of corneal buttons taken from hepatitis B surface antigen seropositive donors. *Br J Ophthalmol* 1995;79:6–9.
32. Bond WW, Peterson NJ, Favero MS, et al. Transmission of type B viral hepatitis via eye inoculation of a chimpanzee. *J Clin Microbiol* 1982;15:533–534.
33. Kew MC. Possible transmission of serum (Australia-antigen-positive) hepatitis via the conjunctiva. *Infect Immun* 1973;7:823–824.
34. Remeijer L, Maertzdorf J, Doornenbal P, et al. Herpes simplex virus 1 transmission through corneal transplantation. *Lancet* 2001;357:442.
35. Biswas S, Surech P, Bonshek RE, et al. Graft failure in human donor corneas due to transmission of herpes simplex virus. *Br J Ophthalmol* 2000;84:701–705.
36. O'Day DM. Diseases potentially transmitted through corneal transplantation. *Ophthalmology* 1989;96:1133–1138.
37. Glasser DB. Serologic testing of cornea donors. *Cornea* 1998;17: 123–128.
38. Tavakkoli H, Sugar J. Microbial keratitis following penetrating keratoplasty. *Ophthalmic Surg* 1994;25:356–360.
39. Akova YA, Onat M, Koc F, et al. Microbial keratitis following penetrating keratoplasty. *Ophthalmic Surg Lasers* 1999;30:449–455.
40. Leahey AB, Avery RL, Gottsch JD, et al. Suture abscesses after penetrating keratoplasty. *Cornea* 1993;12:489–492.
41. Cameron JA, Antonios SR, Correr JB, et al. Endophthalmitis from contaminated donor corneas following penetrating keratoplasty. *Arch Ophthalmol* 1991;109:54–59.
42. Kloess PM, Stulting RD, Waring GO 3rd, et al. Bacterial and fungal endophthalmitis after penetrating keratoplasty. *Am J Ophthalmol* 1993;115:309–316.
43. Cameron JA, Badr IA, Risco J, et al. Endophthalmitis cluster from contaminated donor corneas following penetrating keratoplasty. *Can J Ophthalmol* 1998;33:8–13.
44. Khokhar DS, Sethi HS, Kumar H, et al. Postkeratoplasty endophthalmitis by *Alcaligenes faecalis*: a case report. *Cornea* 2002;21:232–233.
45. Merchant A, Zacks CM, Wilhelmus K, et al. Candidal endophthalmitis after keratoplasty. *Cornea* 2001;20:226–229.
46. Sutphin JE, Pfaller MA, Hollis RJ, et al. Donor-to-host transmission of *Candida albicans* after corneal transplantation. *Am J Ophthalmol* 2002;134:120–121.
47. Everts RJ, Fowler WC, Chang DH, et al. Corneoscleral rim cultures: lack of utility and implications for clinical decision-making and infection prevention in the care of patients undergoing corneal transplantation. *Cornea* 2001;20:586–589.
48. Glazer LC, Azar DT. Refractive errors and their treatment. In: Azar DT, Koch DD, eds. *LASIK: fundamentals, surgical techniques, and complications.* New York, Basel: Marcel Dekker, 2003:1–20.
49. Khan BF, Chang M, Jain S, et al. Management of infections, inflammation, and lamellar keratitis after LASIK. In: Azar DT, Koch DD, eds. *LASIK: fundamentals, surgical techniques, and complications.* New York, Basel: Marcel Dekker, 2003:477–490.
50. Holland SP, Mathias RG, Morck DW, et al. Diffuse lamellar keratitis related to endotoxins released from sterilizer reservoir biofilms. *Ophthalmology* 2000;107:1227–1234.
51. Pache M, Schipper I, Flammer J, et al. Unilateral fungal and mycobac-

terial keratitis after simultaneous laser in situ keratomileusis. *Cornea* 2003;22:72–75.
52. Freitas D, Alvarenga L, Sampaio J, et al. An outbreak of *Mycobacterium chelonae* infection after LASIK. *Ophthalmology* 2003;110:276–285.
53. Levartovsky S, Rosenwasser G, Goodman D. Bacterial keratitis after laser in situ keratomileusis. *Ophthalmology* 2001;108:321–325.
54. Garg P, Bansal AK, Sharma S, et al. Bilateral infectious keratitis after laser *in situ* keratomileusis: a case report and review of the literature. *Ophthalmology* 2001;108:121–125.
55. Karp CL, Tuli SS, Yoo SH, et al. Infectious keratitis after LASIK. *Ophthalmology* 2003;110:503–510.
56. Rowe JA, Erie JC, Baratz KH, et al. Retinal detachment in Olmsted County, Minnesota, 1976 through 1995. *Ophthalmology* 1999;106:154–159.
57. Smiddy WE, Miller D, Flynn H. Scleral buckle removal following retinal reattachment surgery: clinical and microbiologic aspects. *Ophthalmic Surg* 1993;24:440–445.
58. Folk JC, Cutkomp J, Koontz FP. Bacterial scleral abscesses after retinal buckling operations: pathogenesis, management, and laboratory investigations. *Ophthalmology* 1987;94:1148–1154.
59. Holland SP, Pulido JS, Miller D, et al. Biofilm and scleral buckle-associated infections: a mechanism for persistence. *Ophthalmology* 1991;98:933–938.
60. Oshima Y, Ohji M, Inoue Y, et al. Methicillin-resistant *Staphylococcus aureus* infections after scleral buckling procedures for retinal detachments associated with atopic dermatitis. *Ophthalmology* 1999;106:142–147.
61. Arribas NP, Olk J, Schertzer M, et al. Preoperative antibiotic soaking of silicone sponges: does it make a difference? *Ophthalmology* 1984;91:1684–1689.
62. Cooper BA, Holekamp NM, Bohigian G, et al. Case-control study of endophthalmitis after cataract surgery comparing scleral tunnel and clear corneal wounds. *Am J Ophthalmol* 1993;136:300–305.
63. Allen HF, Mangiaracine AB. Bacterial endophthalmitis after cataract extraction. II. Incidence in 36,000 consecutive operations with special reference to preoperative topical antibiotics. *Arch Ophthalmol* 1974;91:3–7.
64. Javitt JC, Vitale S, Canner JK, et al. National outcomes of cataract extraction: endophthalmitis following inpatient surgery. *Arch Ophthalmol* 1991;109:1085–1089.
65. Aaberg TM Jr, Flynn HW, Schiffman J, et al. Nosocomial acute-onset postoperative endophthalmitis survey: a 10-year review of incidence and outcomes. *Ophthalmology* 1998;105:1004–1010.
66. Kattan HM, Flynn HW, Pflugfelder SC, et al. Nosocomial endophthalmitis survey: current incidence of infection after intraocular surgery. *Ophthalmology* 1991;98:227–238.
67. Endophthalmitis Vitrectomy Study Group. Results of the Endophthalmitis Vitrectomy Study: a randomized trial of immediate vitrectomy and of intravenous antibiotics for the treatment of postoperative bacterial endophthalmitis. *Arch Ophthalmol* 1995;113:1479.
68. Han DP, Wisniewski SR, Wilson LA, et al. Spectrum and susceptibilities of microbiologic isolates in the endophthalmitis vitrectomy study. *Am J Ophthalmol* 1996;122:1–17.
69. Hughes DS, Hill RJ. Infectious endophthalmitis after cataract surgery. *Br J Ophthalmol* 1994;78:227–232.
70. Lam SR, Tuli R, Menezes A, et al. Bacterial endophthalmitis follow extracapsular cataract extraction: recommendations for early detection. *Can J Ophthalmol* 1997;32:311–314.
71. Ormerod LD, Becker LE, Cruise RJ, et al. Endophthalmitis caused the coagulase-negative staphylococci. *Ophthalmology* 1993;100:724–729.
72. Braun C. Late infections associated with glaucoma surgery. *Int Ophthalmol Clin* 1996;36:73–85.
73. Deutsch TA, Goldberg MF. Painless endophthalmitis after cataract surgery. *Ophthalmic Surg* 1984;15:837–840.
74. Durand ML, Heier JS. Endophthalmitis. In: Remington JS, Swartz MN, eds. *Current clinical topics in infectious diseases,* vol 20. New York: Blackwell Science, 2000:271–297.
75. Cruciani M, Malena M, Amalfitano G, et al. Molecular epidemiology in a cluster of cases of postoperative *Pseudomonas aeruginosa* endophthalmitis. *Clin Infect Dis* 1998;26:330–333.
76. Zabuski S, Clayman HM, Karsenti G, et al. *Pseudomonas aeruginosa* endophthalmitis caused by contamination of the internal fluid pathways of a phacoemulsifier. *J Cataract Refract Surg* 1999;25:540–545.
77. Hoffmann KK, Weber DJ, Gergen MF, et al. *Pseudomonas aeruginosa*-related postoperative endophthalmitis linked to a contaminated emulsifier. *Arch Ophthalmol* 2002;120:90–93.
78. Centers for Disease Control and Prevention. Outbreaks of postoperative bacterial endophthalmitis caused by intrinsically contaminated ophthalmic solutions—Thailand, 1992, and Canada, 1993. *MMWR* 1996;45:491–494.
79. Ayliffe GA, Barry DR, Lowbury EJ, et al. Postoperative infection with *Pseudomonas aeruginosa* in an eye hospital. *Lancet* 1966;1:1113–1117.
80. Miller GR, Rebell G, Magoon RC, et al. Intravitreal antimycotic therapy and cure of mycotic endophthalmitis caused by *Paecilomyces lilacinus* contaminated pseudophakos. *Ophthalmic Surg* 1978;9:54–63.
81. Pettit TH, Olson RJ, Foos RY, et al. Fundal endophthalmitis following intraocular lens implantation. *Arch Ophthalmol* 1980;98:1025–1039.
82. Fridkin SK, Kremer FB, Bland LA, et al. *Acremonium kiliense* endophthalmitis that occurred after cataract extraction in an ambulatory surgical center and was traced to an environmental reservoir. *Clin Infect Dis* 1996;22:222–227.
83. Tabbara KF, Jabarti AA. Hospital construction-associated outbreak of ocular aspergillosis after cataract surgery. *Ophthalmology* 1998;105:522–526.
84. Dickey JB, Thompson KD, Jay WM. Anterior chamber aspirate cultures after uncomplicated cataract surgery. *Am J Ophthalmol* 1991;112:278.
85. Sherwood DR, Rich WJ, Jacob JS, et al. Bacterial contamination of intraocular and extraocular fluids during extracapsular cataract extraction. *Eye* 1989;3:308–311.
86. Speaker MG, Milch FA, Shah MK, et al. Role of external bacterial flora in the pathogenesis of acute postoperative endophthalmitis. *Ophthalmology* 1991;98:639–649.
87. Tervo T, Ljungberg P, Kautianinen T, et al. Prospective evaluation of external ocular microbial growth and aqueous humor contamination during cataract surgery. *J Cataract Refract Surg* 1999;25:65–71.
88. Maxwell DP Jr, Brent BD, Orillac R, et al. A natural history study of experimental *Staphylococcus epidermidis* endophthalmitis. *Curr Eye Res* 1993;12:907–912.
89. Menikoff JA, Speaker MG, Marmor M, et al. A case-control study of risk factors for postoperative endophthalmitis. *Ophthalmology* 1991;98:1761.
90. Starr MB, Lally JM. Antimicrobial prophylaxis for ophthalmic surgery. *Surv Ophthalmol* 1995;39:485–501.
91. Speaker MG, Menikoff JA. Prophylaxis of endophthalmitis with topical povidone-iodine. *Ophthalmology* 1991;98:1769–1775.
92. Staudenmaier C. Current views on the prevention of postoperative infectious endophthalmitis. *Can J Ophthalmol* 1997;32:297–302.
93. Ng EWM, Baker AS, D'Amico DJ. Postoperative endophthalmitis: risk factors and prophylaxis. *Int Ophthalmol Clin* 1996;36:109–130.
94. American Academy of Pediatrics. *1997 Red Book: report of the Committee on Infectious Diseases,* 25th ed. Elk Grove Village, IL: American Academy of Pediatrics, 2003:778,781,787.
95. Nishida H, Risemberg HM. Silver nitrate ophthalmic solution and chemical conjunctivitis. *Pediatrics* 1975;56:368–373.
96. Centers for Disease Control and Prevention. 1998 guidelines for treatment of sexually transmitted diseases. *MMWR* 2002;451(RR-6):1–78.
97. Ford E, Nelson KE, Warren D. Epidemiology of epidemic keratoconjunctivitis. *Epidemiol Rev* 1987;9:244–261.
98. Cockburn TA, Nitowsky H, Robinson T, et al. Epidemic keratoconjunctivitis. *Am J Ophthalmol* 1953;36:1367–1372.
99. Leopold IH. Characteristics of hospital epidemics of epidemic keratoconjunctivitis. *Am J Ophthalmol* 1957;43:93–97.
100. Schnieder J, Kornzweig A, Feldstein M. Epidemic keratoconjunctivitis. *Am J Ophthalmol* 1956;42:266–269.

101. Quilligan JJ, Adrian J, Alena B. The isolation of 21 strains of type 8 adenovirus. *Am J Ophthalmol* 1959;48:238–246.
102. Davidson C. Epidemic keratoconjunctivitis. *Br J Ophthalmol* 1964; 48:573–580.
103. Dawson C, Darrell R. Infections due to adenovirus type 8 in the United States. *N Engl J Med* 1963;268:1031–1034.
104. Centers for Disease Control and Prevention. Keratoconjunctivitis due to adenovirus type 19—Canada. *MMWR* 1974;23:185–186.
105. Laibson PR, Ortolan G, Dupre-Strachan S. Community and hospital outbreak of epidemic keratoconjunctivitis. *Arch Ophthalmol* 1968;80: 467–473.
106. Dawson CR, Hanna L, Wood TR, et al. Adenovirus type 8 keratoconjunctivitis in the United States. *Am J Ophthalmol* 1970;69:473–480.
107. Vastine DW, West CE, Yamashiroya H, et al. Simultaneous nosocomial and community outbreak of epidemic keratoconjunctivitis with adenovirus types 8 and 18 adenovirus. *Trans Am Acad Ophthalmol Otolaryngol* 1976;81:826–840.
108. Tullo AB, Higgins PG. An outbreak of adenovirus keratoconjunctivitis in Bristol. *Br J Ophthalmol* 1979;63:621–626.
109. Keenlyside RA, Hierholzer JC, D'Angleo LJ. Keratoconjunctivitis associated with adenovirus type 37: an extended outbreak in an ophthalmologist's office. *J Infect Dis* 1983;147:191–198.
110. D'Angelo LJ, Hierholzer JC, Holman RC, et al. Epidemic keratoconjunctivitis caused by adenovirus type 8: epidemiologic and laboratory aspects of a large outbreak. *Am J Epidemiol* 1981;113:44–49.
111. Darougar S, Grey RHB, Thaker U, et al. Clinical and epidemiological features of adenovirus keratoconjunctivitis in London. *Br J Ophthalmol* 1983;67:1–7.
112. Nagington J, Sutehall GM, Whipp P. Tonometer disinfection and viruses. *Br J Ophthalmol* 1983;67:647–676.
113. Richmond S, Burman R, Crossdale E, et al. A large outbreak of keratoconjunctivitis due to adenovirus type 8. *J Hyg (London)* 1984;93: 285–291.
114. Buehler JW, Finton RJ, Goodman RA, et al. Epidemic keratoconjunctivitis: report of an outbreak in an ophthalmology practice and recommendations for prevention. *Infect Control* 1984;5:390–394.
115. Reilly S, Dhillon BJ, Nkanza KM, et al. Adenovirus type 8 keratoconjunctivitis—an outbreak and its treatment with human fibroblast interferon. *J Hyg (London)* 1986;96:557–575.
116. Warren D, Nelson KE, Farrar JA, et al. A large outbreak of epidemic keratoconjunctivitis: problems in controlling nosocomial spread. *J Infect Dis* 1989;160:938–943.
117. Takeuchi R, Nomura Y, Kojima M, et al. A nosocomial outbreak of epidemic keratoconjunctivitis due to adenovirus type 37. *Microbiol Immunol* 1990;34:749–754.
118. Insler MS, Kern MD. Keratoconjunctivitis due to adenovirus type 8: a local outbreak. *South Med J* 1989;82:159–160.
119. Jernigan JA, Lowry BS, Hayden FG, et al. Adenovirus type 8 epidemic keratoconjunctivitis in an eye clinic: risk factors and control. *J Infect Dis* 1993;167:1307–1313.
120. Colon LE. Keratoconjunctivitis due to adenovirus type 8: Report on a large outbreak. *Ann Ophthalmol* 1991;23:63–65.
121. Koo D, Bouvier B, Wesley M, et al. Epidemic keratoconjunctivitis in a university medical center ophthalmology clinic: need for re-evaluation of the design and disinfection of instruments. *Infect Control Hosp Epidemiol* 1989;10:547–552.
122. Buffington J, Chapman LW, Strobierski G, et al. Epidemic keratoconjunctivitis in a chronic care facility: risk factors and measures for control. *J Am Geriatr Soc* 1993;41:1177–1181.
123. Birenbaum E, Linder N, Varsano N, et al. Adenovirus type 8 conjunctivitis outbreak in a neonatal intensive care unit. *Arch Dis Child* 1993; 68:610–611.
124. Ankers HE, Klapper PE, Cleator GM, et al. The role of a rapid diagnostic test (adenovirus immune dot-blot) in the control of an outbreak of adenovirus type 8 keratoconjunctivitis. *Eye* 1993;7(suppl): 15–17.
125. Tabery HM. Two outbreaks of adenovirus type 8 keratoconjunctivitis with different outcome. *Acta Ophthalmol Scand* 1995;73:358–360.
126. Curtis S, Wilkinson GWG, Westmoreland D. An outbreak of epidemic keratoconjunctivitis caused by adenovirus type 37. *J Med Microbiol* 1998;47:91–94.
127. Montessori V, Scharf S, Holland S, et al. Epidemic keratoconjunctivitis outbreak at a tertiary referral eye care clinic. *Am J Infect Control* 1998;26:399–405.
128. Cheung D, Bremner J, Chan JTK. Epidemic keratoconjunctivitis—do outbreaks have to be epidemic? *Eye* 2003;17:356–363.
129. Piednoir E, Bureau-Chalot F, Merle C, et al. Direct costs associated with a nosocomial outbreak of adenoviral conjunctivitis infection in a long-term care institution. *Am J Infect Control* 2002;30:407–410.
130. Azar MJ, Dhaliwal DK, Bower KS, et al. Possible consequences of shaking hands with your patients with epidemic keratoconjunctivitis. *Am J Ophthalmol* 1996;121:711–712.
131. Gordon YJ, Gordon RY, Romanowski E, et al. Prolonged recovery of desiccated adenoviral serotypes 5, 8, and 19 from plastic and metal surfaces in vitro. *Ophthalmology* 1993;100:1835–1840.
132. Centers for Disease Control and Prevention. Epidemic keratoconjunctivitis in an ophthalmology clinic—California. *MMWR* 1990; 39:598–601.
133. Rutala WA. APIC Guideline for selection and use of disinfectants. *Am J Infect Control* 1996;24:313–342.
134. American Academy of Ophthalmology. *Updated recommendations for ophthalmic practice in relation to the human immunodeficiency virus and other infectious agents (information statement).* San Francisco: American Academy of Ophthalmology, 1992.
135. Threlkeld AB, Froggatt JW, Schein OD, et al. Efficacy of a disinfectant wipe method for the removal of adenovirus type 8 from tonometer tips. *Ophthalmology* 1993;100:1841–1845.
136. Woodman TJ, Coats DK, Paysse EA, et al. Disinfection of eyelid speculums for retinopathy of prematurity examination. *Arch Ophthalmol* 1998;116:1195–1198.
137. Bolyard EA, Tablan OC, Williams WW, et al. Guideline for infection control in health care personnel, 1998. *Am J Infect Control* 1998;26: 289–354.
138. Gottsch JD, Frogatt JW, Smith DM, et al. Prevention and control of epidemic keratoconjunctivitis in a teaching eye institute. *Ophthalmic Epidemiol* 1999;6:29–39.
139. Brennan C, Muder RR. Conjunctivitis associated with methicillin-resistant *Staphylococcus aureus* in a long-term-care facility. *Am J Med* 1990;88:14–17.
140. Hedberg K, Ristinen TL, Solar JT, et al. Outbreak of erythromycin-resistant staphylococcal conjunctivitis in a newborn nursery. *Pediatr Infect Dis J* 1990;9:268–273.
141. McNoughton M, Mazinke N, Thomas E. Newborn conjunctivitis associated with triclosan 0.5% antiseptic intrinsically contaminated with *Serratia marcescens. Can J Infect Control* 1995;10:7–8.
142. O'Brien TP, Green WR. Keratitis. In: Mandell GL, Douglas RB, Bennett JE, eds. *Principles and practices of infectious diseases,* 4th ed. New York: Churchill Livingstone, 1995:1110–1119.
143. Alfonso E, Kenyon KR, Ormerod D, et al. *Pseudomonas* corneoscleritis. *Am J Ophthalmol* 1987;103:90–98.
144. Hutton WL, Sexton RR. Atypical *Pseudomonas* corneal in semicomatose patients. *Am J Ophthalmol* 1972;73:37–39.
145. Van Meter WS, Conklin J. Penetrating keratopathy for corneal perforation in an obtunded patient. *Ophthalmic Surg* 1992;23:137–139.
146. Parkin B, Turner A, Moore E, et al. Bacterial keratitis in the critically ill. *Br J Ophthalmol* 1997;81:1060–1063.
147. Hilton E, Uliss A, Samuels S, et al. Nosocomial bacterial eye infections in intensive-care units. *Lancet* 1983;1:1318–1320.
148. King S, Devi SP, Mindorff C, et al. Nosocomial *Pseudomonas aeruginosa* conjunctivitis in a pediatric hospital. *Infect Control Hosp Epidemiol* 1988;9:77–80.
149. Schein OD, Hibberd PL, Starck T, et al. Microbial contamination of in-use ocular medications. *Arch Ophthalmol* 1992;110:82–85.
150. Templeton WC, Eiferman RA, Synder JW, et al. *Serratia* keratitis transmitted by contaminated eyedroppers. *Am J Ophthalmol* 1982; 93:723–726.
151. Donzis PB, Mondino BJ, Weissman FA, et al. Microbial of contact lens care systems contaminated with *Acanthamoeba. Am J Ophthalmol* 1989;108:53–56.

152. Donzis PB, Mondino BJ, Weissman FA, et al. Microbial analysis of contact lens care systems. *Am J Ophthalmol* 1987;104:325–333.
153. Hay J, Seal DV. Contact lens wear by hospital health care staff: is there cause for concern? *J Hosp Infect* 1995;30(suppl):275–281.
154. Shrader SK, Band JD, Lauter DB, et al. The clinical spectrum of endophthalmitis: incidence, predisposing factors, and features influencing outcome. *J Infect Dis* 1990;162:115–120.
155. Gamel JE, Allansmith MR. Metastatic staphylococcal endophthalmitis presenting as chronic iridocyclitis. *Am J Ophthalmol* 1974;77: 454–458.
156. Burns CL. Bilateral endophthalmitis in acute bacterial endocarditis. *Am J Ophthalmol* 1979;88:909–913.
157. Weissgold DJ, D'Amico DJ. Rare causes of endophthalmitis. *Int Ophthalmol Clin* 1996;36:163–177.
158. Greenwald MJ, Wohl LG, Sell CH. Metastatic bacterial endophthalmitis: a contemporary reappraisal. *Surv Ophthalmol* 1986;31:81–101.
159. Peyman GA, Bassili SS. A practical guideline for management of endophthalmitis. *Ophthalmic Surg* 1995;26:294–303.
160. Samiy N, D'Amico DJ. Endogenous fungal endophthalmitis. *Int Ophthalmol Clin* 1996;36:147–162.
161. Brooke RB. Prospective study of *Candida* endophthalmitis in hospitalized patients with candidemia. *Arch Intern Med* 1989;149: 2226–2228.
162. Joshi N, Hamory BH. Endophthalmitis caused by non-*albicans* species of *Candida. Rev Infect Dis* 1991;13:281–287.
163. Henderson DK, Edwards RE, Montgomerie JZ. Hematogenous *Candida* endophthalmitis in patients receiving parenteral hyperalimentation fluids. *J Infect Dis* 1981;143:655–661.

27

NOSOCOMIAL CENTRAL NERVOUS SYSTEM INFECTIONS

NELSON M. GANTZ

Nosocomial infections related to the central nervous system (CNS) are a relatively small but important category of hospital-acquired infections. These infections span a spectrum from superficial wound infections, to ventricular shunt infections, to deep-seated abscesses of the brain parenchyma. The patient populations affected are equally diverse, involving neonates, children, and adults, with occurrence on nearly all medical and surgical services.

Nosocomial infections of the CNS are usually serious, if not life threatening, and are frequently associated with a poor outcome (1–13). These nosocomial infections present many challenges in diagnosis. There are also many controversies over effective prophylaxis and proper management. In addition, the identification of a particular infection as nosocomial may not be clear-cut; thus, overlaps and ambiguities concerning acquisition are unavoidable. Fortunately, a heightened awareness has fostered declining rates of infection. In spite of improving techniques and new preventive strategies, however, the threat is constant, and the stakes remain painfully high. The first part of this chapter focuses on the clinical and epidemiologic aspects of infections related directly to neurosurgical and neuroinvasive procedures as well as infectious processes that invade the CNS secondarily from other sites. The second part of this chapter discusses prevention and control of these infections.

RISK FACTORS

General Risk Factors

Not surprisingly, the patients at greatest risk for acquiring nosocomial CNS infections are neurosurgical patients. Patients with surgical site infections (SSIs) are drawn entirely from this population. These patients are subjected to procedures that traverse the skin and scalp, violate meningeal coverings, impinge upon the paranasal sinuses, implant foreign bodies, and expose tissues to hematogenous sources of infections. Infection in this setting is often facilitated by the presence of a cerebrospinal fluid (CSF) leak that occurs when the dura is disrupted and the subarachnoid space communicates with the skin, nasal cavity, paranasal sinuses, or middle ear (14–19). This group includes adult and pediatric patients undergoing common neurosurgical and neuroinvasive procedures such as craniotomy, spinal fusion, laminectomy, insertion of halo pins, burr hole placement, and implantation of ventricular shunts and reservoirs. Less common procedures include stereotactic brain biopsy, hypophysectomy, paranasal sinus surgery, acoustic neuroma resection, temporary ventricular drainage, placement of intracranial monitoring devices, nerve stimulator placement, lumbar puncture, spinal anesthesia, myelography, and skull/spinal fixation.

Patients who have suffered accidental head trauma are another population at increased risk to develop meningitis. These individuals have sustained trauma or fractures to the basilar skull and facial bones, facilitating the formation of a CSF fistula. This posttraumatic condition substantially increases the likelihood of CSF infection, particularly bacterial meningitis (20–22). In one series, a CSF leak was a predisposing factor in approximately 9% of cases of nosocomial bacterial meningitis (5).

The majority of nosocomial CNS infections reported from the National Nosocomial Infections Surveillance (NNIS) system at the Centers for Disease Control and Prevention (CDC) occurred in newborn nurseries and on surgical services (Table 27.1). All other hospital services account for a small but still substantial number of cases. Patients from this smaller population generally have a parameningeal source of infection that is

TABLE 27.1. NOSOCOMIAL CENTRAL NERVOUS SYSTEM (CNS) INFECTIONS BY HOSPITAL SERVICE IN NNIS HOSPITALS 1986–1992

	Percentage of Total Infections		
Service	Meningitis	Intracranial	Spinal Abscess
Neurosurgery	43	60	14
High-risk nursery	23	13	0
Well-baby nursery	10	2	0
Medicine	7	6	29
Pediatrics	5	2	14
Surgery	3	6	14
Bum/trauma	3	4	0
Oncology	2	6	0
Orthopedics	1	0	0
OB/GYN	1	0	14
Cardiac surgery	<1	0	14
Total	100	100	100

NNIS, National Nosocomial Infections Surveillance system.
Source: Centers for Disease Control and Prevention/NNIS.

either contiguous (e.g., sinusitis) or occult (e.g., unsuspected CSF leak), reactivation of latent infection, or an infection that has hematogenously seeded the CNS from a distant site. Patients with malignancies (especially lymphoma and leukemia), patients with organ transplants, and other immunocompromised hosts frequently fall into this last category.

Risk factors for SSIs can be classified into host factors and surgical factors. Examples of host factors include age, sex, American Society of Anesthesiologists physical status classification, underlying diseases such as diabetes mellitus, nutritional status, presence of other remote infections, and duration of preoperative stay. Surgical factors include whether the procedure was an emergency or elected, hair removal technique, surgeon, use of perioperative antibiotics, duration of surgery, type of operation, site of surgery, and whether gloves were punctured (23). (See Chapter 21 on SSIs.) One study showed that when patients underwent a neurosurgical procedure, the presence of a postoperative CSF leak was associated with a more than 13-fold increase in the infection risk (24). Also, a remote concurrent infection increased the infection risk six times, whereas use of perioperative antibiotics was associated with a decrease in the infection rate of about 20%. Three other risk factors—paranasal sinus entry, placement of a foreign body, and use of postoperative drains—were associated with an increased risk of infection, although this association was not statistically significant. Factors that were not associated with an increased risk of infection included obesity, surgical reexploration, use of the operative microscope, steroid administration, and acute therapy for seizures. Length of surgery was also not a factor associated with an increased risk of infection. In the same study, there were insufficient data to determine if diabetes mellitus was a risk factor (24). A prospective study of postoperative neurosurgical infections demonstrated a validated five-category classification system for neurosurgical infections based on specific definitions. It was found that infection rates were highest for contaminated cases (contamination known to occur, 9.7%), followed by dirty cases (established sepsis at the time of surgery, 9.1%), clean contaminated (risk of contamination of operative site during surgery, 6.8%), clean with temporary or permanent foreign body (6.0%), and clean (no identifiable risk factors present, 2.6%). In this study, surgery lasting longer than 4 hours was associated with an infection rate of 13.4% (25).

In addition to patients undergoing neurosurgery and neonates (see Chapter 52), patients undergoing invasive diagnostic or therapeutic procedures that penetrate the CNS are at risk for developing a nosocomial CNS infection (see Chapter 70). A subgroup of neurosurgery patients at high risk for nosocomial CNS infections is those with ventricular shunts. Since most shunt infections (70%) have an onset within 2 months of surgery, it is likely that the infecting microorganism is introduced during surgery or in the postoperative period (10). Risk factors for shunt infections are discussed in Chapters 49 and 67. There appears to be no association between the shunt infection rates and type of shunt and underlying disease. The rate of infection also varies with the neurosurgeon (26). The efficacy of prophylactic antibiotics in preventing shunt infection is controversial and is discussed below (see Prevention). Patients undergoing diagnostic or therapeutic procedures that penetrate the CNS, such as the installation of dyes or drugs, are more likely to develop nosocomial meningitis (27). Although such infections occur infrequently in the present era, they should be considered in the appropriate setting.

Device-Related Risk Factors

Infection is a well-recognized complication of ventriculostomy catheters used for monitoring and drainage (28). Aucoin et al. (29) noted that the rate of infection was associated with the type of monitor used. The lowest infection rate was associated with the subarachnoid screw (7.5%), followed by a rate of 14.9% for the subdural cup catheter and a 21.9% rate for the ventriculostomy catheter. An intracranial monitoring technique, the Camino intraparenchymal fiberoptic catheter system, is associated with an infection rate of 2.5% (30). The method of ventriculostomy insertion using the tunneled technique has been associated with the lowest rates of infection (28). Other factors predisposing patients to infection included open trauma or hemorrhage, use of an irrigating solution such as bacitracin, and duration of intracranial pressure (ICP) monitor greater than 4 days (29). Use of prophylactic antibiotics did not reduce significantly the risk of infection. In a study by Mayhall et al. (9) of ventriculostomy-related infections, risk factors significantly associated with infection included an intracerebral hemorrhage with intraventricular hemorrhage, a neurosurgical operation, ICP of 20 mm Hg or higher, ventricular catheterization for longer than 5 days, and irrigation of the system. The incidence of infection was not related to where the catheter was inserted when the intensive care unit was compared with the operating room. Infection rates were also not reduced by the use of nafcillin prophylaxis. Two additional studies confirm the relationship of ventriculitis to monitoring duration and supports removal of ICP monitors as soon as possible (31,32). Risk factors associated with ventriculitis were sepsis, pneumonia, depressed skull fracture requiring surgery, craniotomy, and intraventricular hemorrhage. To reduce the risk of ICP monitor–related infections, it is recommended that the device be inserted using aseptic technique, that the device be removed as soon as possible and preferably before 5 days, and that a closed system be maintained. The use of prophylactic catheter exchange and extending the duration of catheterization to 10 days has been proposed, but more data are needed (28). The type of ICP monitor device used influences the rate of infection, with epidural tunneled monitors having the lowest rates.

SOURCES OF INFECTION

Sources of Infecting Microorganisms

Nonsurgical Infections

Nosocomial CNS infections can be classified into those infections unrelated to surgery and postsurgical infections. In patients with nonsurgical-related infections, the microorganisms can compose a patient's normal flora, such as *Streptococcus pneumoniae,* or arise from an exogenous source, such as from a contaminated solution or device (27). Gram-negative bacilli are usually responsible for infections related to contaminated solutions or devices (33). Microorganisms can gain access to the CSF by hematogenous spreading of an infectious agent, spread to the CSF from contiguous foci, such as an infected sinus, or via a communication of the CSF with the flora of the skin, sinuses, or other mucosal surfaces (34,35). CSF leakage can be obvious in a patient with rhinorrhea or otorrhea, or occult if the subarachnoid space communicates with a paranasal sinus. Rarely, neoplasms erode into the subarachnoid space and produce a fistula. Microorganisms can also gain access to the CSF by direct inoculation of the agent in a patient having a lumbar puncture, especially if a substance is injected. Microorganisms acquired in this manner are usually gram-negative rods (36,37). It is extremely unusual to develop meningitis following a lumbar puncture unless a solution is injected into the CSF.

Infection (incidence 4.3%) is a well-recognized complication of chronic epidural catheters and intracerebroventricular devices (38) used for control of pain in patients with AIDS or malignancy (39) (see Chapter 61). Other complications include meningitis and epidural abscess, but prolonged surgery during catheter placement has been found to be the only factor associated with catheter infection (40). Infection may also complicate the use of an Ommaya reservoir (41). Repeated access of these devices may permit skin flora microorganisms such as *Staphylococcus aureus, S. epidermidis,* or diphtheroids to produce ventriculitis and meningitis. The source of the infecting microorganisms may also be the hands of the hospital personnel accessing the device, although powder contamination from gloves has also been implicated (42).

Neurosurgical Infections

Although many sources of contamination of a neurosurgical operation have been described, it is usually impossible to document with certainty the source for a given SSI. Probably most infections occur at the time of surgery from either direct inoculation of residual flora of the patient's skin or from contiguous spread from infected host tissue. Direct inoculation of microorganisms can also occur occasionally from the hands of surgical team members via a tear in a glove. Rarely, the source of infection is traced to contaminated surgical material such as a solution, device, or instrument. In two neurosurgical patients with postoperative *Bacillus cereus* meningitis, the source of the microorganisms was found to be heavily contaminated linen (43). Occasionally, during the postoperative period, an SSI results from direct inoculation of microorganisms. Airborne contamination at the time of surgery, either from the patient or from operating room personnel, accounts for some neurosurgical infections (1, 44). Lastly, a postoperative infection rarely results from hematogenous seeding of a wound from an infected intravenous line or other remote infection.

Outbreaks of neurosurgical infections occur infrequently today, and when they have been described, they have occurred mainly in hospitalized neonates (45–47).

INCIDENCE AND DISTRIBUTION

Nosocomial infections of the CNS (excluding wound or SSIs) are relatively uncommon, accounting for approximately 0.4% of all nosocomial infections (R. Gaynes, personal communication). Meningitis accounts for 91% of these infections, followed by intracranial suppurations (8%) and isolated spinal abscess (1%) (R. Gaynes, personal communication). When infection rates are examined using data reported from 163 hospitals participating in the NNIS system, 0.56 CNS infections per 10,000 hospital discharges occurred from 1986 through early 1993 (R. Gaynes, personal communication). Comparable rates over the past 25 years have shown a slow decline from approximately 1 infection per 10,000 hospital discharges to the present lower rate (48). While these numbers are relatively small, it must be noted that CNS infections directly related to neurosurgical procedures (SSIs) are not reflected in these numbers. The majority of nosocomial CNS infections occurring in this setting are designated under the larger category of SSIs (16% of all nosocomial infections) by CDC/NNIS system surveillance criteria (see below). These infections accounted for 8% of hospital-acquired infections following craniotomy and 34% of infections after spinal surgery in NNIS system hospitals from 1986 to 1992 (49). In addition, certain nosocomial CNS infections may represent a greater proportion of specific types of infection. For example, a retrospective study of acute bacterial meningitis in adults over a 27-year period at the Massachusetts General Hospital found 40% of 493 total episodes to be nosocomial in origin (5).

Nosocomial surgical site and CSF infections among neurosurgical patients is a primary focus of this chapter. Among NNIS system hospitals in the period 1986 through 1992, CNS infections and SSIs were responsible for 3.3% and 12% of all nosocomial neurosurgical infections, respectively. Table 27.2 shows the distribution of SSIs complicating neurosurgical procedures and illustrates the significant proportion of deep infections that occur in relation to the surgical site. Infection rates as reported in the general neurosurgical literature are often difficult to interpret and compare for a variety of reasons, including differences in definitions, methodology, reporting techniques, and use of prophylactic antibiotics. Not uncommonly, postoperative infections unrelated to the surgical site or CNS are included in the rate calculation (2). An overview of infection rates associated with neurosurgery from some of the more rigorously performed (although nonstandardized) studies over the last 30 years is shown in Table 27.3. Taking into account some of the problems mentioned above, most hospital series report infection rates of less than 5%. When individual neurosurgical procedures are compared, differences in infection rate become more apparent. The incidence of all CNS infection following typically clean craniotomy may vary from less than 1% to nearly 9%, whereas the rates following laminectomy range from 0.6% to 5%. Postoperative meningitis after clean craniotomy has a reported incidence of 0.5% to 2% when perioperative antibiotics are given (50–54). Without antibiotic prophylaxis, other studies have found rates ranging from 2% to 7% (54–56). Infection rates for selected neuroinvasive procedures are shown in Table 27.4. Again, differences in methodology, definition, and duration of follow-up greatly affect the reported rates. Analysis of infection rates following ventricular shunt surgery is particularly complex. Depending on the use of a case rate (occurrence per patient) or operative rate (occurrence per procedure) of infection and the duration of follow-up, an extremely wide variation in incidence

TABLE 27.2. SURGICAL SITE INFECTIONS FOLLOWING NEUROSURGICAL PROCEDURES

	Surgical site									
Procedure	Men	SA	SSI	DSI	IC	IAB	Bone	Disc	Other	Total
Craniotomy (n = 191)	22%	—	60%	2%	12%	—	—	—	4%	100%
Laminectomy (n = 615)	1%	3%	75%	11%	—	—	4%	6%	—	100%
Ventricular shunt (n = 93)	76%	—	18%	—	—	4%	—	—	2%	100%
Head and neck (n = 324)	3%	—	77%	13%	—	—	2%	—	5%	100%
Miscellaneous (n = 49)	8%	2%	82%	—	—	8%	—	—	—	100%

Men, meningitis; SA, spinal abscess; SSI, superficial surgical site infection; DSI, deep surgical site/soft tissue infection; IC, intracranial infection; IAB, intraabdominal abscess; bone, osteomyelitis; disc, discitis.
Source: CDC/NNIS

TABLE 27.3. INFECTION RATES IN NEUROSURGERY

	Procedures		All Laminectomy		Craniotomy	
Series (year)	No.[a]	%	No.	%	No.	%
Odum (1962)			3,774	0.6	2,342	1.3
Cairns (1963)					1.169	4.4
Wright (1966)			2,085	4.1	2,148	5.7
Green (1974)	1,770	2.3	529	2.3	692	2.6
Savitz (1974)	495	3.6	239	3.8	214	4.2
El-Gindi (1965)			650	0.8		
Madeja (1977)	1,129	3.8				
Quadery (1977)	357	4.8	40	5.0	144	5.7
Haines (1982)	1,663	1.7				
Lindholm (1982)			3,576	0.8		
Chan (1984)					338	4.7
Jomin (1984)					500	3.0
Puranen (1984)			1,100	0.7		
Blomstedt (1985)	1,039	5.7			622	8.0
Tenney (1985)	936	5.5			494	7.3
Savitz (1986)					872	0.2
Ingham (1988)					1,167	3.3
Cartmill (1989)	423	0.7				
Winston (1992)					312	0.3

[a]Number of operations performed.
Data from refs. 50, 51, 77–80, 86, 91, 101, 109, 147, 154, 351–357.

TABLE 27.4. INFECTION RATES IN SELECTED NEUROINVASIVE PROCEDURES

Procedure	Infection Rate
Ventricular shunt	
Operative	3–13%
Case	9–41%
Cerebrospinal fluid reservoir	4–23%
Ventriculostomy[a]	0–11%
Burr hole	1–5%
Spinal anesthesia	<0.5%
Lumbar puncture	<2%
Epidural catheter	0–4%
Stereotactic biopsy	<1%
Myelography	Rare

[a]Includes external drainage and intracranial pressure monitoring devices.
Data from refs. 9, 10, 29, 39, 91, 109, 146, 155, 156, 160, 163, 206, 233, 302, 313, 319, 331, 358–375.

may be seen. Perhaps, when in 1916 Cushing (57) stated, "There has never been any infection, even of a stitch in the scalp, in something over 300 cranial operations in the writer's series," he underestimated the situation. A procedure-oriented risk factor analysis is covered in a later section, and additional details are discussed elsewhere in this text (see Chapters 49, 61, 67, and 70).

Examination of SSIs reported from NNIS system hospitals shows infection rates in uncomplicated procedures with minimum risk factors to be 0.56/100 operations for craniotomies, 0.70/100 operations for spinal fusion, and 3.85/100 operations for ventricular shunts (58). The last rate is the fifth highest among all operative procedures (58). Importantly, these surveillance rates by definition include both superficial and deep infections related to operative site (59). The addition of one or more complications (surgical risk factors) will increase most of the figures to varying degrees (58).

The incidence of both community- and hospital-acquired CNS infections in immunocompromised hosts has been estimated to range from less that 1% to over 10%, depending on the host population (60–63). Classic studies at the Memorial Sloan-Kettering Cancer Center in the early 1970s revealed an incidence of CNS infections approximating 0.02% of total hospitalizations (64). These infections occurred most commonly in lymphoma patients (33%), followed by neurosurgical patients (30%) and leukemic patients (20%). Overall, meningitis accounted for the majority of infections (71%), followed by brain abscess (27%) and encephalitis (2%). Of note, intracerebral abscess in leukemic patients was responsible for 70% of CNS infections in this group. It has been postulated that conventional incidence figures may significantly underestimate the actual magnitude of CNS infections in this population (60). Other studies have shown similar patterns in cancer patients, with perhaps a higher incidence of CNS infection in transplant recipients estimated at 5% to 12% (62,63). Brain abscess seems to be particularly common in the transplant group, accounting for 35% to 44% of CNS infections after heart and heart-lung transplantation (61,65). Bacterial meningitis in the febrile neutropenic patient is often indolent in presentation and masked by the early use of broad-spectrum antibiotics. Disseminated fungal infections are not uncommon in the compromised host and are frequently difficult to diagnose; *Candida* is reported to involve the CNS in up to 50% of cases (66,67). Although the absolute number of nosocomially acquired infections in this population cannot easily be determined, the proportion is likely to be high, as many occur after multiple or prolonged hospitalizations and are caused by typical hospital-acquired pathogens.

TYPES OF NOSOCOMIAL CENTRAL NERVOUS SYSTEM INFECTIONS

Nosocomial infections related to the CNS may be broadly divided into two major categories (Table 27.5): postsurgical infections and nonsurgical infections, including those related to neuroinvasive or neurodiagnostic procedures. The first category consists of SSIs (49). Infections of this type may occur following craniotomy, ventriculostomy, and spinal column surgery. Rarely, SSIs complicate other neurosurgical operations, such as peripheral nerve surgery and carotid endarterectomy. SSIs are further classified as superficial or deep incisional SSIs, using the fascial plane as divider. Previously termed deep surgical infections unrelated to soft tissues are now classified as organ/space SSIs by the aforementioned CDC criteria (49). These infections may present as a local and/or diffuse infectious process. Local suppurative infections complicating neurosurgical procedures include the following: parenchymal brain abscess, subdural empyema, epidural abscess, discitis, subgaleal collection, and osteomyelitis of the cranium or spine. Diffuse infection of the subarachnoid space defines meningitis or ventriculitis if the process is related to a prior ventriculostomy and essentially remains localized. This latter distinction is somewhat arbitrary. Meningoencephalitis is an infrequent diffuse nosocomial CNS infection generally due to prions or viruses transferred during neuroinvasive procedures or via organ transplantation (68–74).

Nonsurgical infections constitute a smaller, but equally important, class of nosocomial CNS infections. These infections are acquired by a variety of routes that include spread from a contiguous focus, posttraumatic/CSF leak, and neuroinvasive procedures, as well as hematogenous spread. Meningitis, brain abscess, subdural empyema, and epidural abscess all may occur in this setting.

TABLE 27.5. NOSOCOMIAL CENTRAL NERVOUS SYSTEM INFECTIONS

Postsurgical	Nonsurgical
Surgical site infections	Contiguous focus or hematogenous
Superficial	Epidural abscess
Deep	Subdural empyema
Local suppurative infections	Brain abscess
Osteomyelitis	Meningitis
Discitis	Meningoencephalitis
Subgaleal collection	
Epidural abscess	
Subdural empyema	
Brain abscess	
Diffuse infections	
Meningitis	
Ventriculitis	
Meningoencephalitis	

DEFINITIONS, DIAGNOSTIC CRITERIA, AND CLINICAL PRESENTATION

It is essential for the purposes of identification, surveillance, and management that nosocomial infections be defined and diagnosed with as much sensitivity and specificity as possible. Unfortunately, factors such as colonization and aseptic inflammation prevent the establishment of gold standards and place many conditions within a spectrum of disease. Recognition of an infection as nosocomial is often not straightforward, and CNS infections are no exception. Doubt over hospital versus community acquisition of an infection is a constant problem compounded by the ubiquity of the major pathogens. The time course that defines specific nosocomial infections is neither consistently defined, easy to determine, nor universally accepted. Although the CDC outlines strict definitions and diagnostic criteria, the length of hospitalization prior to an infection being classified as nosocomial is not specified. For SSIs related to implantable devices, nosocomial infection may be diagnosed up to 1 year after surgery, according to CDC criteria. Some experts consider 60 days a more reasonable length of time for nosocomial ventricular shunt infections, as the majority of infections occur within this period (75). In addition, the diagnosis of infection ultimately may be left to the discretion of the attending physician and is inherently subjective. A prospective study by Taylor et al. (76) demonstrated that 40% of neurosurgical wound infections were diagnosed using nonstandardized criteria by the surgeon. The potential effect on infection rates is obvious. Ventricular shunt infections illustrate several of these problems. CSF profiles may be nondiagnostic, the microorganism involved may be from the normal flora, and the infection may become evident weeks after hospital discharge. This section integrates the CDC definitions with additional clinical criteria to facilitate proper identification and diagnosis of nosocomial infections related to the CNS. The CDC surveillance definitions for nosocomial surgical site and specific CNS infections have been previously published (49,59).

Surgical Site and Related Surgical Infections

Studies dealing with SSIs in neurosurgical patients have used a variety of both strict and less stringent diagnostic criteria for identification (2,4,12,25,77–84). Commonly, these infections are classified in the surgical literature as either superficial or deep. Superficial neurosurgical infections are considered to be limited by the cranial or lumbodorsal fascia. Deep wound infections encompass soft tissue infections below the fascia, discitis, osteomyelitis, and bone flap infections. However, infections below the dura (ventriculitis, meningitis, brain abscess) have been included under this heading as well (24,51,78). To improve surveillance and clarify potential overlap in reporting, the CDC definitions include the category of organ/space SSI to cover additional sites adjacent to the operative site. Specific organ/space SSIs related to neurosurgery include the following: meningitis, ventriculitis, disc space infection, osteomyelitis, intracranial abscess, and spinal abscess (49). With the exception of infections related to implantable devices, infection occurs within 30 days of the operative procedure. Since the organ/space SSI category includes several non–soft tissue infections, the definitions are relatively liberal. Diagnosis of some of these infections are covered in subsequent sections, as they also occur unrelated to surgical procedures. More detail on SSIs in general may be found elsewhere in the text (Chapter 21).

Incisional Surgical Site Infections

From a practical point of view, the diagnosis of SSIs is usually made clinically. Neurosurgical site infections must be promptly identified because of the propensity to spread to deeper spaces (85). Superficial incisional SSIs tend to be diagnosed at an early stage, usually within the first postoperative week (86–88). Generally, the area is swollen and erythematous with local tenderness. Purulent discharge and/or microorganisms isolated from drainage or a wound aspirate complete the picture. Temperature and the white blood count (WBC) are not uniformly elevated; the erythrocyte sedimentation rate (ESR) and C-reactive protein (CRP) may be increased (2,84). Deep incisional SSIs present later postoperatively with a course that may be insidious or progressive. The average time between surgery and the diagnosis of a deep infection in spinal surgery may vary from 10 to 15 days, with the range extending several weeks (84,89). A relatively normal appearance of the overlying surgical site contributes to this delay in many cases (89). Elevations of temperature, WBC, ESR, and CRP, as well as the presence of fever/chills or hyperglycemia in diabetic patients, while clearly nonspecific signs, are not infrequently seen (84,87,89). Patients often complain of increased pain at the surgical site (90).

Infections of bone flaps following craniotomy are well described and account for up to one half of infections following this procedure (1,51,91,92). By definition, infection involves either the free (devitalized) or osteoplastic bone flap following a supratentorial craniotomy. These infections may be obviously symptomatic with high fever, scalp tenderness, and suppuration (4,93) or more indolent with a persistent fistula (2). In one series, 12 of 13 bone flap infections were diagnosed within 30 days of surgery (88). Sequential nuclear scanning with technetium 99 may have enhanced diagnostic accuracy for cranial flap osteomyelitis, especially to rule out this infection (93). Indium 111–labeled leukocyte scanning is a useful technique (94,95). Plain skull radiographs are helpful, if positive, but lack sufficient sensitivity to be useful routinely (91). The use of computed tomography (CT) or magnetic resonance imaging (MRI) is invaluable in establishing a diagnosis. In general, a cranial bone flap infection is diagnosed clinically with either radiographic or microbiologic confirmation (4). A subgaleal abscess occasionally occurs adjacent to a scalp surgical site. In this case, a localized collection forms in the space between the galea of the scalp and the pericranium. Scalp tenderness, erythema, fever, and regional adenopathy may be seen. Osteomyelitis or intracranial spread of infection can occur secondarily if the underlying skull integrity has been compromised. Diagnosis of most deep incisional SSIs may be established clinically, via culture of a deep aspirate, or, rarely, with the assistance of radiologic studies. Evaluation of a soft tissue fluid collection with sonography or CT scan can be helpful.

Organ/Space Surgical Site Infections

Discitis (infection of the intervertebral disc space) is a relatively uncommon but potentially serious postoperative complication of spinal surgery (96–99). The fact that almost 20 years of surgery passed before this infection was recognized illustrates the difficulties encountered in diagnosis (100). Patients typically present with recurrent back pain and muscle cramping 1 to 8 weeks after surgery and initial improvement of preoperative symptoms (80,101–103). In a series of 111 cases of discitis described by Iversen et al. (104), back pain appeared at an average of 16 days postoperatively. Occasionally, overt infection occurs immediately after surgery (101,105). Patient examination discloses paraspinal muscle spasm with an abnormal straight leg raising test (80,101,106). Neurologic deficits are unusual. Fever is variably present, and the superficial surgical site frequently appears normal. Most notable is the severe and persistent low back pain out of proportion to the findings on physical examination. Routine laboratory studies such as the WBC are generally unremarkable, with the exception of the ESR (101,104,106). Following spine surgery, the ESR rises rapidly (peak 90–110) and falls steadily to near-normal levels within several weeks (107, 108). A significantly elevated ESR more than 2 weeks postoperatively correlates positively with disc space infection (107–110). Others have found this test less valuable, especially with early infections (104).

Several radiographic modalities are helpful in establishing the diagnosis of discitis. Plain films are of little utility in the early weeks, as most decreases in disc height are expected postoperatively. More characteristic findings occur weeks to months later with blurring of the end plate and irregularity and lytic destruction of the subchondral surface (111). Osteomyelitis of the adjacent vertebrae may occur in advanced cases. These findings are visualized in greater detail with CT scans (112). Currently, MRI with gadolinium enhancement has become the procedure of choice for the so-called failed back syndrome following spinal surgery (113). Early changes on MRI may distinguish disc space and vertebral body infection from the normal postoperative spine with a high degree of accuracy (103,114–117). Nuclear imaging is of limited value because of the high level of background positivity (109). Sequential technetium 99 and gallium 67 scans improve sensitivity but require at least 48 hours to perform (118). Although somewhat controversial, diagnosis of infectious discitis should be confirmed by biopsy despite a consistent clinical and radiographic picture. Tissue sampling allows discrimination between septic and aseptic (chemical or avascular discitis) processes and facilitates directed antibiotic therapy. Peripheral blood cultures are rarely positive for the offending microorganism (80,119). Percutaneous needle aspiration of the affected disc space under fluoroscopic or CT guidance is the method of choice. Ideally, antibiotics should be withheld until after the procedure is complete. The results of the Gram stain and/or culture are diagnostic in up to 70% of cases, and histologic examination may indicate a septic picture in cases lacking positive microbiology (106,110).

Isolated vertebral osteomyelitis is very uncommon following laminectomy and related procedures. When present, it is usually associated with progressive infection of the contiguous disc space (spondylodiscitis) (103,119–121). Clinical presentation and diagnosis are virtually the same as outlined above for discitis.

Meningitis

The diagnosis of nosocomial meningitis requires a high index of clinical suspicion and support from CSF analysis. Excluding ventricular shunt infections, most cases of meningitis following neurosurgery are diagnosed in the early postoperative period. Several series have shown that the majority of cases develop within 10 days of surgery, and virtually all are diagnosed within 28 days (3,6,7,52,91,122). Nosocomial meningitis unrelated to surgical procedures has a more variable time course. Posttraumatic bacterial meningitis associated with a CSF leak may occur days to years after the initial injury (21,123). Although some of these infections may develop in the hospital, acquisition of the infecting microorganism likely has occurred in the community environment (21,22,124). Since the CDC definitions do not specify a period during or after hospitalization that distinguishes nosocomial from community-acquired infection, evidence for hospital acquisition must be sought (59). In a review of 197 episodes (157 patients) of nosocomial meningitis by Durand et al. (5), 97% of patients were diagnosed more than 48 hours after admission or within 1 week of discharge (5). Interestingly, 41 episodes (10 patients) in this study were recurrent during the same hospitalization. Other studies indicate a similar pattern of presentation (7,21). We consider it reasonable to view nonsurgical nosocomial meningitis as developing several days after hospitalization and unrelated to an obvious community-acquired infection. Unfortunately, these distinctions are not always easy to make.

The standard clinical signs and symptoms suggestive of meningitis are often of little help in diagnosing nosocomial infection. Fever appears to be the most ubiquitous finding in all nosocomial cases (3,6,7,52,122). Neurosurgical patients commonly demonstrate an altered level of consciousness, neck stiffness, and headache reflecting some combination of their underlying disease and the surgical procedure itself in the absence of infection. These relatively nonspecific findings may become more useful if a change over time is noted or a new fever develops. Findings indicative of meningeal irritation are more useful in nonsurgical patients, especially when combined with fever and a change in mental status. Aseptic meningeal inflammation is a common postoperative condition that may further confound the diagnosis. Clinical parameters have been consistently unable to distinguish aseptic from bacterial meningitis (125,126). The use of corticosteroids may blunt the signs and symptoms of inflammation in both surgical patients and compromised hosts (62,127). Neutropenic hosts cannot mount an inflammatory response, and the resultant symptoms are often minimal (127). Low-grade fever, lethargy, and/or headache may be the only clues in these patients (63). Concurrent medical conditions or extremes of age often modify the typical clinical presentation (6,128,129). Finally, the administration of perioperative antibiotics may alter the natural course of clinical responses and laboratory findings (see below).

The signs and symptoms of posttraumatic bacterial meningitis are often similar to those seen in acute bacterial meningitis (130). However, as with the neurosurgical patient, clinical findings may be more difficult to interpret in the patient with considerable head trauma. CSF infection should be considered when there has been any change in neurologic status, or when fever or neck stiffness is noted that was not present initially (21,131). In these patients at increased risk, it is important to establish evidence of CSF leakage when meningitis is a concern. The most common signs of a CSF leak are rhinorrhea, otorrhea, hemotympanum, Battle's sign, and cranial nerve palsies (22, 132). Detection of CSF rhinorrhea is critical and may be performed at the bedside using a glucose oxidase reagent strip (Dextrostix) to detect increased glucose in nasal secretions (21). Unfortunately, a negative result does not rule out the presence of a fistula (133). Identification of transferrin in nasal secretions using immunofixation or electrophoresis has shown promise as a useful indicator of CSF leakage (134–136). A fluorescein dye test can also be used to identify suspected cases of CSF otorrhea and localize the source (137). Radiographic studies are the procedures of choice to document and localize CSF leakage. CT scanning and MRI are superior to plain films in diagnosing basilar skull fractures and identifying fistulae (138,139). Radioisotope cisternography using ^{111}In diethylenetriamine pentaacetic acid (DTPA) is highly sensitive, but specificity is a problem and localization is poor (140). Metrizamide CT cisternography is currently the best test for diagnosing active CSF fistulas and accurately defines the site of leakage (138,141). Considering the diagnostic subtleties associated with nosocomial meningitis, examination of the CSF assumes a critical role.

Analysis of CSF obtained from hospitalized patients at risk for developing meningitis is often difficult. Neurosurgical patients commonly have abnormal CSF profiles secondary to underlying disease (tumor), procedures, intracranial bleeding, and seizure activity. Perioperative antibiotics will influence the results of cultures of CSF. Nonsurgical patients are likely to be receiving concurrent antibiotics for other infections. Compromised patients may have blunted inflammatory reactions or abnormal CSF profiles from noninfectious processes (e.g., carcinomatous or leukemic meningitis). Despite these limitations, the results are often revealing, and examination of the CSF should be performed routinely in all suspected cases.

The CDC definition for nosocomial meningitis does not specify abnormal values for routine CSF parameters. As with community-acquired bacterial meningitis, most cases of nosocomial meningitis are associated with an increased CSF white cell count, neutrophilic pleocytosis, elevated protein, and depressed glucose (2,3,5,7,20,52,85,122,130,142). Neurosurgical patients with culture-proven meningitis generally have more than 100 WBCs/mm^3 with over 50% neutrophilia (7,52,85,122). In the series by Berk and McCabe (122), all patients were noted to have over 100 WBCs/mm^3, with the majority having more than 1,000 cells/mm^3 (median 2,500). In 72 episodes of culture-negative nosocomial meningitis described by Durand et al. (5), 97% of patients had more than 300 WBCs/mm^3, and 96% had more than 50% neutrophils. Since an intracerebral bleed or subarachnoid hemorrhage allows both WBCs and RBCs to enter the CSF, a correction formula may be used to better approximate the number of abnormal white blood cells (143). A CSF protein level greater than 100 mg/dL and a glucose level less than 40 mg/dL are present in the majority of nosocomial cases (5,7,52,85,122,126). Unfortunately, several studies have found no significant difference in cell counts and other CSF parameters in (early) postoperative patients with septic versus aseptic meningitis (125,126). In these patients, a significantly lowered glucose level (less that 20 mg/dL) might be the best indicator of an infectious etiology in the absence of culture data (52). The administration of MUROMONAb-CD3 (OKT3) to organ transplant recipients during rejection has been associated with the development of aseptic meningitis (144,145).

Routinely, the CSF should be Gram-stained and set up for bacterial culture. In immunocompromised patients, fungal cultures, mycobacterial studies, and viral cultures may be indicated as well. The yield on Gram-stained CSF is lower than in community-acquired cases and approximates 50% overall (5,146). Although a positive culture remains the gold standard, it is impossible to make this requirement for nosocomial cases if the clinical data and CSF profile are otherwise supportive. In one large retrospective study, a positive culture was obtained in 83% of nosocomial cases and a comparable percentage of community-acquired cases (5). Since concurrently positive cultures are often obtained from sites outside the CNS, cultures from blood, adjacent wounds, and urine are suggestive in the appropriate setting (3,7,52,85,91,122,147).

Clearly, the diagnostic value of CSF sampling, under any circumstance, can be greatly influenced by the administration of intravenous antibiotics. The effect of antibiotics prior to lumbar puncture is most marked on the Gram stain and culture with little alteration of the other standard parameters (148,149). A negative Gram stain and culture will commonly occur after 24 hours of appropriate therapy (150). The CSF glucose and white cell count usually remain abnormal for at least several days (143). When combined with the baseline abnormal CSF of the craniotomy patient or the tempered inflammatory reaction of the neutropenic host, the effect of prior antibiotics on diagnosis is substantial, and second-line tests assume greater importance. Several tests are commercially available to detect bacterial antigens in the CSF; available antigens include those from *Neisseria meningitidis, Haemophilus influenzae,* and *S. pneumoniae.* The latter two microorganisms are common pathogens in posttraumatic meningitis (21). Latex agglutination and coagglutination are rapid tests with good sensitivity and specificity. The latex agglutination text is preferable because of speed, ease of use, and high yield. Antigen detection tests are most useful when initial microbiologic studies are unrevealing or the patient has been partially treated with antibiotics (151). Latex agglutination to detect the capsular polysaccharide of *Cryptococcus neoformans* is a highly efficacious test in immunocompromised patients (63,127).

Final mention should be made concerning the role of neuroimaging in the diagnosis of bacterial meningitis. Although contrast enhancement of meninges may be seen on CT or MRI early in the course of illness, these findings are nonspecific and contribute little to establishing the diagnosis (113). A better use of these modalities is to exclude other CNS pathology or to diagnose intracranial complications of meningitis (152).

CEREBROSPINAL FLUID SHUNT INFECTIONS

A variety of temporary and permanent prosthetic devices are used to access, drain, divert, and monitor the CSF. These devices may be internalized for chronic use or externalized for use in the acute setting. Internalized devices consist of shunts (ventriculoperitoneal, ventriculoatrial, ventriculoureteral, lumboperitoneal) and reservoirs (lumbar, ventricular). Externalized devices facilitate drainage (ventriculostomy, lumbar drain, external shunt) or measure ICP when the device (intraventricular, epidural, subdural) is connected to a transducer. Insertion of a ventriculoperitoneal shunt is the most common surgical procedure performed for the long-term control of hydrocephalus. Infections complicating these devices may occur at any site or compartment traversed by the prosthesis. Proximal infections include meningitis, ventriculitis, empyema, abscess, and infection involving the surgical site (wound infection, cellulitis, osteomyelitis). Distal infections include tunnel infections along the catheter tract, bacteremia, pleuritis, peritonitis, and related intra-abdominal infections. Infections of temporary devices are almost always nosocomial, because their insertion and use requires hospitalization. The current CDC guidelines define infection secondary to an implantable device as nosocomial if it occurs within 1 year of the operative procedure and the two appear to be related (49). Such a designation must often be based subjectively on the type of infection, clinical setting, and responsible microorganism. Because of the clustering of shunt infections within 60 days of implantation (10,153–157), shorter periods have been suggested to designate a shunt infection as nosocomial (75). Because of the considerable overlap among infections of different CNS prosthetic devices, this discussion can focus on the diagnosis of CSF shunt infections as the prototype for this group. Certain specific infections potentially related to CSF shunts have already been covered in detail earlier in this chapter (SSIs) or are covered in later sections (intracranial suppurations).

The most important risk factor for the development of CNS shunt infection is the level of training of the neurosurgeon, with neurosurgical trainees having a higher rate of infection. Variables such as year of placement of the shunt, age of the patient, length and time of the operation, and exact placement of the distal drain did not increase the risk of infection (153,158). Additionally, elevated CSF protein content does not appear to increase the risk of shunt infection (159).

The clinical manifestations of infections related to CSF shunts, reservoirs, and monitoring devices are quite variable and often nonspecific. Infections of the surgical site or subcutaneous tunnel in the early postoperative period are the most easily recognized, as purulent drainage, erythema, warmth, and tenderness are usually present (10,155,160,161). As will be discussed, infections at these sites are intimately associated with the pathogenesis of deeper and more extensive infections. It has been suggested that CSF shunts be viewed as composed of a proximal and a distal segment with specific signs and symptoms of infection referable to each section (162). Since infection of one shunt section may spread contiguously to involve the entire length of the prosthesis, a patient may present with any combination of signs and symptoms related to the proximal, distal, and intervening sections of the shunt (163–167).

In general, fever appears to be the most constant feature of shunt infection (168,169). Several studies have shown that virtually all patients have a temperature greater than 100°F with the majority febrile to 102°F or higher (10,163,170,171). Unfortunately, the absence of fever cannot be used to rule out infection, as others have demonstrated a small but significant percentage of asymptomatic patients (160). Proximal infection of shunts with a ventricular origin is usually associated with symptoms secondary to shunt obstruction or malfunction (10, 155,160,172). Typical clinical manifestations include nausea, vomiting, seizure, malaise, lethargy, irritability, headache, and other indications of increased ICP (10,13,160,168,169, 171–173). Classic signs of meningeal irritation (meningismus, photophobia) are present in only one third of patients (10,130). This is due to the inability of CSF to pass into the subarachnoid space of patients with obstructive hydrocephalus or to eventual closure of the aqueduct of Sylvius in shunted patients with communicating hydrocephalus (174). Meningeal signs are more frequently seen in patients with infected lumboperitoneal shunts (163). Manifestations of distal shunt infection depend on the site of the terminal portion. Nearly one third of patients with infected ventriculoperitoneal shunts present primarily with abdominal symptoms in the absence of ventriculitis (171,175,176). Early inflammation about the shunt catheter may result in impaired CSF absorption and loculation of fluid with formation of a peritoneal cyst (177,178). This CSF-oma may present as a palpable mass in younger patients and may represent either a sterile process or an overt infection (179). Multiloculated hydrocephalus, a complication of CNS shunt infection, is more commonly seen as a result of failure to clear a gram-negative bacillus shunt infection following external drainage (180).

Progressive inflammation results in full-blown peritonitis with fever and abdominal tenderness (168,169). An acute abdomen similar to appendicitis may be seen, and intestinal obstruction, bowel perforation, and intraabdominal abscess have all been described in small numbers (167,176,181–186). Infection complicating a ventriculopleural shunt can lead to formation of an empyema (187,188). In contrast, patients with vascular shunt (ventriculoatrial) infections tend to present subacutely with lethargy and fever (10,155). The often-indolent presentation of a chronic low-grade vascular infection may delay the correct diagnosis several weeks or longer (189). These patients are also more likely to manifest bacteremia, immune complex nephritis, hypocomplementemia, and thromboembolic complications (190–192). Septicemia, not an uncommon complication in the early years of vascular shunting, is rarely seen today (164,193). A syndrome of immune complex glomerulonephritis (shunt nephritis) is seen in a small number of patients with staphylococcal infections of vascular shunts (10,194–196). Immunoglobulin G and immunoglobulin M antigen-antibody immune complexes are deposited along the basement membrane of renal glomeruli with activation and subsequent depletion of circulating complement (197–200). The nephrotic syndrome may follow generally with mild to moderate impairment of renal function (201,202). Clinically, the patient may have fever, hepatosplenomegaly, proteinuria, hematuria, and an increased ESR (189,194,202). Resolution of the infection usually results in return of the renal function to normal (189,195). Vascular shunt infections may also be accompanied by any of the proximal manifestations mentioned above.

Definitive diagnosis of CSF shunt infections depends on recovery of the etiologic agent from cultures of CSF. However, the physician must always strongly suspect such infection in any patient with fever or evidence of shunt malfunction, as CSF cultures may be negative, particularly if the patient has received prior antibiotic therapy (203–205). As with the clinical presentation, the usefulness and yield of various diagnostic tests differ according to the type of shunt. A recommended diagnostic approach based on the clinical presentation is shown in Table 27.6. The peripheral WBC is generally elevated but may be below 10,000/mm^3 in 25% of patients (9,10,169,205). In patients with ventriculoatrial shunts and chronic bacteremia, positive blood cultures may be obtained in 90% of patients who have not recently received antibiotics (10,155,163,168,171). Conversely, ventriculoperitoneal shunts have a rate of blood culture positivity that approximates only 25% (155,163,171). Urinalysis is indicated when shunt nephritis is suspected, and urine cultures may be useful in patients with ventriculoureteral or lumboureteral shunts. In the early postoperative period, cultures of an infected surgical site or of aspirate obtained from an erythematous subcutaneous tract are always indicated, but the correlation with more definitive CSF cultures is less than perfect. Aspiration of any fluid collection adjacent to the shunt apparatus is also helpful, as a communication with the CSF pathway often exists. Lumbar punctures in patients with ventriculoperitoneal shunts may not reveal evidence of more proximal infection (162). These limitations make direct sampling of the CSF from the shunt apparatus the most reliable diagnostic test (10,162,171,203,204).

Performing a shunt aspiration enables assessment of shunt function as well as a detailed fluid analysis. Sampling of lumber CSF is of little use, as cultures are usually negative (205). Routine chemical tests are of little value, as an elevated protein or depressed glucose level is a nonspecific and inconsistent finding

TABLE 27.6. CLINICAL PRESENTATION OF SHUNT INFECTIONS AND SUGGESTED DIAGNOSTIC STEPS

Clinical Presentation	Major Diagnostic Steps
Meningitis or ventriculitis	Shunt tap and lumbar puncture
Shunt malfunction	Check shunt function by pumping reservoir, shunt tap, contrast radiographic studies of shunt, computed tomography
Wound or shunt tract inflammation	Culture aspirate from inflamed area, shunt tap
Bacteremia (acute or chronic)	Blood cultures, shunt tap, evaluate for endocarditis
Thrombophlebitis or pulmonary embolism	Blood cultures, shunt tap, ventilation-perfusion scan
Cardiac complications (valve insufficiency, atrial perforation, tamponade)	Blood cultures, shunt tap, cardiac catheterization, echocardiography
Abdominal pain or mass	Culture aspirate from inflamed area along distal ventriculoperitoneal catheter, shunt tap, evaluate surgical abdomen clinically and radiographically
Glomerulonephritis	Blood cultures, shunt tap, urine sediment examination, evaluate for endocarditis

From Gardner P, Leipzig T, Sadigh M. Infections of central nervous system shunts. *Topics Infect Dis* 1988;9:185–214.

(168,203,204). The CSF WBC averages 75 to 150 cell/mm^3; greater than 100 cell/mm^3 correlates with a subsequent positive culture in 90% of confirmed cases (11,203,206). When the cell count is under 20 cell/mm^3, a positive culture is obtained in less than 50% of cases (10,155,203). All CSF specimens should be immediately Gram stained, cultured aerobically and anaerobically, and examined for fungus, especially if the host is immunocompromised. The yield of Gram stain approaches 50% overall and markedly increases with a concurrently elevated CSF cell count or with gram-negative infection (155,170). Although cultures of the CSF appear to be positive in 80% of patients later documented to have infected shunts after removal, the false-negative rate of this test has never been firmly established (13, 163). The predictive value of a negative CSF culture may also be substantially decreased in patients whose distal catheters are blocked (207). Supplemental laboratory tests that have been used in diagnosing shunt infection include determination of antistaphylococcal antibody titers and CRP and detection of immune complexes in serum (207–211). In general, the poor sensitivity and specificity of these studies severely limits any clinical utility (13,207). Neuroradiologic studies such as CT or MRI may give indirect evidence of infection by suggesting obstruction of CSF circulation.

Infection that is essentially restricted to the distal portion of a ventriculoperitoneal shunt is more difficult to diagnose. Peritoneal signs may be present with a normal functional assessment of the shunt and laboratory assessment of the CSF, especially if obtained proximally (165,177). Diagnosis may necessitate a trial of externalization of the distal end with appropriate cultures and close observation for prompt clinical improvement (157,176,181).

Infections of ICP monitoring devices present as proximal shunt infections do. Fever is the most frequent indication of infection, as signs of meningeal irritation are usually absent, and these patients often have an altered sensorium (168,212). Infection of the surgical insertion site, ventriculitis, or meningitis is the typical clinical presentation (9,174,212).

In summary, an infection should be strongly suspected in any febrile patient with an indwelling CNS prosthesis. It is important to always consider occult infection as a potential cause of shunt dysfunction (160). All available clinical and laboratory parameters must be utilized in an effort to make an accurate diagnosis. Blood cultures are usually positive in patients with ventriculoatrial shunts, and CSF cultures are positive in the majority of patients with ventriculoperitoneal shunts. Again, it should be emphasized that the CSF may be sterile in a significant number of documented infections. Antibiotic-coated catheters have been proposed as a mechanism to decrease shunt-related infections; however, the protective effect is short lived (up to 56 days) and clinical trials have not yet been performed (213). A recent review outlines an approach to treatment of shunt infections using decision analysis (214). This report recommends use of both antibiotics plus shunt removal as the best method to cure shunt infections.

Meningoencephalitis

Meningoencephalitis implies a global CNS inflammation involving the meninges as well as the brain parenchyma. These uncommon nosocomial prion and viral infections have been reported following neurosurgical and neurodiagnostic procedures, corneal transplantation, and cadaveric dural grafting (68–73,215). More details on these uncommon infections can be found elsewhere in this text (see Chapter 47), and only a brief overview is offered here.

Generally, meningoencephalitis is characterized by fever and early mental status changes that may later progress to obtundation or coma. The altered level of consciousness and impairment of cognitive functioning may be more impressive than typical meningitis. Focal neurologic features, including sensory disturbances and seizures, are universal findings. Patients with Creutzfeldt-Jakob disease (CJD) develop sensory dysfunction (i.e., ataxia), myoclonus, and cognitive and behavioral abnormalities that progress to overt dementia and finally coma over weeks to months (216). The clinical manifestations of rabies virus have been previously reviewed (217,218). A prodrome of nonspecific symptoms and fever is usually followed by an acute neurologic syndrome manifested by either hyperactivity or progressive paralysis (218). Subsequent coma and death complete the classic picture. Incubation periods of 18 months for CJD and 5 weeks for rabies have been reported in the small number of transplant cases (71,73).

Routine analysis of the CSF is not particularly helpful and usually reveals a nonspecific pleocytosis, elevated protein content, and normal glucose level. The diagnosis of rabies is made by isolation of the virus from saliva, CSF, or brain tissue, or by measurement of neutralizing antibodies in the serum or CSF (217,219). Immunofluorescent staining for rabies antigen may be applied to corneal epithelial cells or to sensory nerves obtained from a full-thickness skin biopsy of the neck (217,220). Histopathologic examination reveals pathognomonic Negri bodies in the majority of cases (221). Patients with CJD exhibit markedly abnormal electroencephalogram results and evidence of cortical atrophy on CT scan (222). Definitive diagnosis of CJD must ultimately be made from brain tissue. Demonstration of pathologic lesions of the cerebral cortex or identification of specific polypeptides (scrapie-associated protein) by immunostaining confirms the diagnosis (223). Identification of four abnormal proteins in the CSF by gel electrophoresis allows discrimination of CJD from other neurologic diseases (224).

It should be noted that certain bacteria and fungi may cause meningoencephalitis in compromised hosts. The clinical presentation and approach to diagnosis in these patients is essentially the same as for meningitis.

Cranial Epidural Abscess

An epidural abscess or empyema represents a relatively uncommon infection that occurs between the dura mater and overlying bone of the cranium (a "potential space") or spine (a "true space"). Signs and symptoms are largely based on mass effect, and as these infections often coexist with subdural infections, a composite clinical picture is frequently seen (225,226). Conditions predisposing to the development of a cranial epidural abscess (CEA) include head trauma, craniotomy, osteomyelitis, paranasal sinusitis, mastoiditis, otitis, and the application of skull tongs (1,86,227–232). Risk factors for a spinal epidural abscess

(SEA) include hematogenous spread from multiple sources, adjacent osteomyelitis, spinal wound, decubitus ulcers, lumbar puncture, nonpenetrating back trauma, epidural catheters, spinal anesthesia/injection, and spinal surgery (233–246). Few studies have estimated the number of total cases (as opposed to the incidence per procedure or per hospital admissions) that clearly qualify as nosocomial according to the CDC guidelines. However, the reported risk of these infections related to the most common neurosurgical and neuroinvasive procedures appears to be relatively small.

Nosocomial CEA generally occurs as a complication of craniotomy or head trauma. Symptoms include fever, headache, altered mental status, local swelling, erythema, focal neurologic signs, and occasionally seizures (226,232,247). Progression of the abscess is often accompanied by subdural extension and can lead to deterioration of neurologic status, increased ICP, and cerebral herniation (248). The peripheral WBC and ESR are usually elevated, and the CSF profile (lumbar puncture may be contraindicated) reflects parameningeal infection (225,234). The diagnosis is best established by CT, as contrast scanning will reveal a hypodense epidural collection with some degree of ring enhancement (230,249). MRI is likely to be an equally useful modality, but experience remains limited.

Spinal Epidural Abscess

Although hematogenous spread is possible, most hospital-acquired cases of SEA are more likely to be related to spinal procedures (e.g., laminectomy, anesthesia, epidural catheter, injection). Approximately 10% of all SEAs occur in this setting and are located primarily in the lumbar spine (241). By definition, nosocomial infection becomes evident within 30 days of the procedure, and this is certainly the typical time frame for postoperative cases (233,235,238,241). However, infection might have been introduced at surgery weeks to months prior to presentation, blurring the distinction between hospital and community acquisition (240). Patients with an SEA secondary to spinal anesthesia develop symptoms from 72 hours to 5 months after catheter placement (244,245) (see also Chapter 61).

The clinical evolution of an epidural abscess as described by Heusner (250) occurs in four progressive phases: spinal ache, nerve root pain, radicular weakness, and paralysis. This classic presentation has been well documented in many series, although the rates of neurologic deterioration have been quite variable (233,234,240,241,251,252). Backache and spinal tenderness are the most common clinical findings occurring in over 90% of patients (225,226,233,238,252). Other typical symptoms in approximate decreasing order of prevalence include motor radiculopathy, paraparesis, bowel/bladder dysfunction, sensory deficit, meningismus, and encephalopathy (233,240,252,253). Fever, peripheral leukocytosis, and an increased ESR are present in the majority of cases (233,240,241,253). Rarely, sepsis dominates the clinical picture and the neurologic symptoms go unnoticed (238). In hospitalized patients, initial manifestations may be subtle or difficult to detect because of concurrent conditions, and fever with persistent pain may be the only clue. A small series of postoperative SEAs found a notable absence of fever and peripheral leukocytosis and a paucity of neurologic features (235). Pain and tenderness localized to the surgical site was uniformly present by the second postoperative week (235). Clinical presentations of SEA have also been classified as acute and chronic based on the presence of symptoms for less than or more than 2 weeks, respectively (233,240). Acute cases are likely to be hematogenous in origin, whereas chronic cases are usually related to a contiguous focus of infection (111). Although the possibility of an SEA might be considered earlier in nosocomial cases, most studies indicate that this is uncommonly the initial diagnosis (241).

In patients with SEA, CSF analysis usually reflects a parameningeal process with a pleocytosis and elevated protein (234,240, 253). It might be expected that this profile would overlap considerably with CSF sampling from a relatively early postoperative spinal surgery patient. The CSF white cell count seems to vary inversely with the duration of symptoms (241). Gram stain and culture of the CSF rarely are revealing; blood cultures are often positive (240,241). Intraoperative cultures are usually positive (240,253).

The diagnosis of an SEA is best confirmed by a neuroradiographic examination showing displacement of intrathecal contrast and/or direct visualization of the abscess. Myelography remains a highly sensitive tool but suffers from the inability to delineate the full extent of the abscess and can cause complications. CT scanning with intrathecal contrast is both highly sensitive and relatively specific but is accompanied by some element of risk (253–255). In selected cases of presumed SEA, CT-guided needle aspiration is useful diagnostically and perhaps therapeutically (256,257). MRI with gadolinium-DTPA contrast is currently the initial examination of choice in patients with suspected spinal infection (113,115,258). MRI is highly sensitive and essentially noninvasive and allows accurate visualization of the full length of an epidural abscess in addition to any contiguous infectious processes (253,259–261). Plain films and radionuclide scans are low-yield nonspecific studies that offer little diagnostic utility. In conclusion, any clinical suspicion should always prompt an imaging study, as rapid neurologic deterioration of the patient may ensue.

Subdural Empyema

Subdural empyema refers to a collection of pus in the space between the dura and arachnoid. Infection can progress rapidly, as there is little anatomic barrier to spread in this space (230). As with CEAs, most cranial subdural empyemas (CSEs) are related to paranasal sinusitis, otitis media, trauma, and neurosurgical procedures. CSEs may be found in conjunction with an osteomyelitis or epidural abscess in 50% of cases. Mortality, near 100% before effective antibiotic therapy, has declined to 9% in one series (262). Clinically, patients present with rapid onset of altered sensorium, meningismus, seizures, focal neurologic findings, and signs of increased ICP following a period characterized by headache and fever (230,232,262–265). A more subacute presentation of CSE has been described in postoperative infections (266). Peripheral leukocytosis and a neutrophilic pleocytosis in the CSF are usually present (263,264). Differentiation from a brain abscess may be difficult on clinical grounds alone. CT scanning or MRI is currently the procedure of choice for diagnosis of CSE, although false negatives may occur (258,267–271). A contrast study will show a crescent-shaped hypodense area with intense enhancement at the brain periphery (222,268).

Spinal subdural empyema is extremely rare; the few cases reported in the literature have been associated with distant sources of infection (230,272,273). Presentation is similar to that of SEA except that spinal tenderness on examination may be absent (273). The diagnosis is best made by CT myelogram (274).

Intracranial Septic Thrombophlebitis

Any intracranial suppuration may be associated with septic thrombophlebitis or thrombosis affecting the dura, lateral, sagittal, or cavernous sinuses. Subdural empyema may be complicated by septic venous thrombosis, which can result in brain abscess and infarction. Cortical vein thrombosis has been observed in approximately 25% to 30% of cases and is often associated with a poor outcome (263,265). Clinical presentation may resemble parenchymal brain abscess with focal neurologic signs often related to the cranial nerves (275). Similarly, the compressive effects of an SEA may result in thrombosis, thrombophlebitis, and congestion of the epidural venous system (225,233). Again, CT and MRI are the diagnostic methods of choice (113, 222).

Brain Abscess

A brain abscess is a focal suppurative process confined to the brain parenchyma. The most common conditions associated with brain abscess include contiguous sources of infection, such as sinusitis, otitis, mastoiditis, dental infection, and cranial trauma (surgical or accidental), or metastatic infection, as in endocarditis or cyanotic heart disease (154,226,231,276–279). Hospital-acquired brain abscess is an unusual complication of routine neurosurgical procedures, paranasal sinus infection, sinus surgery, and transient bacteremia, but may occur following penetrating craniocerebral trauma and in immunocompromised patients (63,91,280–282). Gunshot injuries to the head associated with retained bone fragments constitute a particularly high-risk condition (283). Brain abscesses have also rarely complicated the application of cranial tongs and halo fixation devices (284, 285). Finally, a brain abscess may follow cranial wound infections, meningitis, shunt infections, or any of the previously discussed CNS-related nosocomial infections.

The clinical presentation of a nosocomially acquired brain abscess may vary from a relatively acute postcraniotomy suppuration to a more subacute or chronic infection developing secondary to a gunshot wound or indwelling ventricular shunt. Although published data are few, most of these infections appear to present within several weeks of a neuroinvasive procedure. As expected, the nosocomial etiology of these infections is often difficult to determine, and supportive evidence is derived from the clinical setting and available microbiology. The presenting features of a brain abscess depend on the size, location, virulence of the microorganism, and condition of the host. Abscesses that evolve secondarily by direct intracranial extension are usually solitary and typically found in the frontal and temporal lobes (277,278,286–289). Infections related to cranial surgery or trauma generally occur in close proximity to the wound (or foreign body), whereas hematogenously spread infection may cause multiple lesions predominantly in a middle cerebral artery distribution (283,286,290). Fever, headache, and focal neurologic findings (the classic triad) are the most common clinical manifestations, seen in approximately 50% of all cases (287, 290,291). Nausea, vomiting, papilledema, seizures, and meningismus are seen in 25% to 50% of patients (286,290,291). Unfortunately, most of these signs and symptoms are difficult to interpret in the neurosurgical patient. The differential diagnosis includes a variety of underlying conditions (e.g., tumor, hydrocephalus, hemorrhage, infarction, thrombosis, and other CNS infections). Any unexpected alteration in mental status or change in the neurologic examination, especially if combined with fever, should prompt a more detailed evaluation (see below). In immunocompromised patients, the abscess must by strongly suspected, as the onset of symptoms may be indolent and the diagnostic clues often are subtle. In these patients, a careful physical examination might disclose purulent drainage or a black eschar on the nasopharyngeal mucosa suggestive of rhinocerebral mucormycosis (292). Proptosis, periorbital cellulitis, ophthalmoplegia, and, ultimately, coma make up the classic rhinocerebral syndrome (127). The spectrum of *Aspergillus* species infections include cellulitis, sinusitis, and pneumonia that may extend to the CNS directly or, more commonly, hematogenously (293). Because of the angiotropic nature of this pathogen, cerebral hemorrhage, thrombosis, or seizure is not uncommon with *Aspergillus* species invasion of the CNS (62).

Peripheral blood studies are rarely useful in the diagnosis of a brain abscess. The WBC may vary from normal to moderately increased, the ESR is nonspecifically elevated in most cases, and blood cultures are nearly always negative (290,294). Lumbar puncture is generally contraindicated in any patient suspected of having a CNS mass lesion because of the high risk and low yield. When obtained, CSF fluid analysis reveals a mild pleocytosis, elevated protein, and normal glucose consistent with a parameningeal focus of infection (276,290,294). Cultures are rarely positive unless there is a concurrent meningitis or ventricular rupture has occurred (295). Rapid clinical deterioration and death (presumably from tentorial or brainstem herniation) may occur when CSF is sampled in the presence of a brain abscess, further substantiating the poor risk/benefit ratio of this procedure (286,287,294).

The best approach for the early diagnosis and subsequent management of a brain abscess is provided by radiographic imaging. Previously utilized radionuclide brain scanning with technetium 99 remains a highly sensitive technique (especially in the early cerebritis phase) but has essentially been replaced by newer studies (222,296). The advent of CT scanning has provided a rapid, sensitive, and relatively specific method for diagnosing this intracranial infection. The early phases of cerebritis are characterized by a low-density region on noncontrast scans representing the necrotic center of the abscess. Ring enhancement with contrast occurs variably but may become apparent if delayed images are obtained (282). With formation of a collagen capsule, ring enhancement with contrast is seen in early images surrounding a hypodense center (282). Both edema and contrast enhancement may be attenuated by corticosteroids with minimal effect on a mature lesion (297). Although the sensitivity of CT scans exceeds 95%, the typical findings mentioned above are not pathognomonic and may be seen with neoplasm, infarction, resolving hematoma, and radiation necrosis (255,297,298). Features favoring the diagnosis of abscess include intraparenchymal gas, ependymal or leptomeningeal enhancement, corticomedullary location, multiloculation, ring thickness, and homogeneous capsular enhancement (282,298).

MRI may be the most accurate imaging technique for the diagnosis of brain abscess (113,271). Subtle edema and cerebritis may be detected at an earlier stage on gadolinium-enhanced T2-weighted MRI images than on a corresponding CT scan (299–301). Other potential advantages of MRI over CT include the use of nonionizing radiation, minimal artifact from bone, better delineation of the posterior fossa, and increased ability to differentiate edema from liquefaction necrosis (299). Although the sensitivity of MRI is impressive, the clinical superiority of MRI over CT has not been established (291).

Despite the proper clinical setting and suggestive radiology, an interventional procedure is frequently required to establish the diagnosis, define the etiology, and assist therapeutically. The initial procedure of choice is currently a CT-guided stereotactic aspiration. This highly efficacious technique has an overall diagnostic accuracy exceeding 90% with a reported complication rate (e.g., hematoma, infection, seizure) of approximately 1% (302–304). Specific indications for this procedure include (a) the presence of multiple lesions, (b) deep-seated lesions, (c) evaluation for noninfectious etiologies, and (d) the need for external drainage (303,304). Significant coagulopathy is the most common contraindication (305,306). Laboratory evaluation of aspirated material should include histologic examination, Gram stain, cultures for aerobic and anaerobic bacteria, wet mount, fungal cultures, and viral studies if appropriate. The application of stereotactic biopsy has largely circumvented the use of completely empiric antibiotics as well as the need for a craniotomy.

ETIOLOGY OF NOSOCOMIAL CENTRAL NERVOUS SYSTEM INFECTIONS

The etiologic agents involved in hospital-acquired CNS infections may be viewed from several perspectives. Because a limited number of agents are responsible for the majority of infections, examining this information as a function of all nosocomial CNS infections is most useful (Fig. 27.1). Coagulase-negative staphylococci, *S. aureus,* and gram-negative aerobic bacilli account for nearly 70% of infections collected through the NNIS system from 1986 to 1992. Breaking down infections into major site categories (Fig. 27.1) changes the distribution of pathogens somewhat, most notably for spinal abscess, with which gram-negative microorganisms are rarely involved. Unfortunately, since many nosocomial CNS infections are classified as SSIs, only part of the overall picture is reflected in these data. Table 27.7 shows the pathogens involved in specific neurosurgical site infections. As expected, gram-positive cocci are responsible for the majority of skin and soft tissue infections associated with neurosurgical procedures. *Propionibacterium acnes,* a gram-positive anaerobic rod, continues to be an increasingly recognized pathogen in craniotomy infections. Organ/space SSIs may include meningitis, discitis, and intracranial or spinal abscess. Gram-negative aerobic bacilli are major pathogens in this group, often with significant resistance to antibiotic regimens. Yeast (mostly *Candida albicans*) and filamentous fungi (mostly *Aspergillus* species) are involved in an increasing number of CSF shunt infections as the number of susceptible hosts becomes larger. Although the use of rigorous standards makes the NNIS/CDC data extremely useful, further examination of the pathogens responsible for specific nosocomial CNS infections, and in specific host populations, is worthwhile. The pathogens in certain infections can be observed to change with the host population (e.g., oncology patients), a particular device, or the duration of follow-up (e.g., CSF shunts). With a few exceptions, the experience with most nosocomial infections in the literature correlates well with NNIS/CDC surveillance data.

To a great extent, the pathogens responsible for skin and soft tissue infections following neurosurgery are similar to those found in other surgical infections (see Chapter 21). The close proximity to and often open communication with the CNS underscores the importance of these infections. As will be discussed in the next section, there is a strong association between microorganisms cultured from neurosurgical wounds and isolates obtained from the CSF. *S. aureus* is generally the most common isolate from superficial and deep wound infections following both craniotomy and laminectomy procedures (1,4,24, 51,81,84,91,306,307). Several studies have identified gram-negative bacilli among the top three isolates; Aucoin et al. (29) found these microorganisms to be the most common isolates from ventriculostomy-related wound infections. Other important microorganisms in decreasing frequency of occurrence include *S. epidermidis,* streptococci, diphtheroids (including *P. acnes*), and *Clostridium* species (1,24,29,51,78,81,91).

As discussed previously, meningitis is responsible for over 90% of all nosocomial CNS infections. The largest single institutional study of bacterial meningitis in adults was published by Durand et al. (5) at the Massachusetts General Hospital. They identified 197 episodes of nosocomial meningitis in 151 patients over a 27-year period. The majority of patients had had recent neurosurgery or a neurosurgical device (65%), evidence of immune system compromise (20%), or a CSF leak (9%). The most common pathogens included gram-negative bacilli (38%), *S. aureus* (9%), coagulase-negative staphylococci (9%), *Streptococcus* species (9%), *H. influenzae* (4%), *Listeria monocytogenes* (3%), and *Enterococcus* species (3%). The relatively lower incidence of gram-positive infections in this series may reflect changing epidemiologic trends, the increased number of procedures, and improving culture techniques inherent in a long study period. Of note, 41 episodes of recurrent meningitis occurred in this group and were caused primarily by gram-negative bacilli (46%).

Studies examining meningitis following neurosurgery have repeatedly implicated gram-negative bacilli as the predominant pathogen responsible for up to 69% of cases (3,7,52,122). In a series of 23 cases of neurosurgical meningitis reported by Buckwold et al. (3), 19 cases were due to gram-negative bacilli and

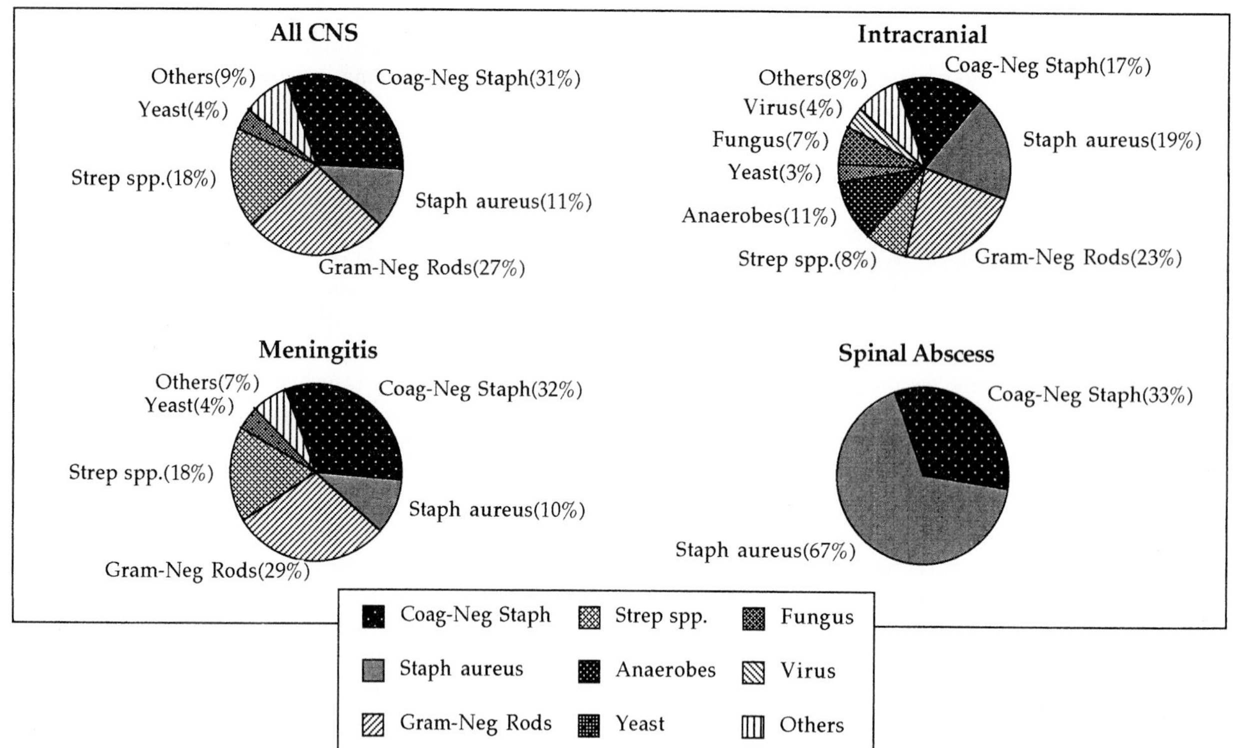

Figure 27.1. Nosocomial central nervous system infections by pathogen in National Nosocomial Infections Surveillance (NNIS) hospitals, 1986–1992.

TABLE 27.7. NOSOCOMIAL PATHOGENS IN NEUROSURGERY BY SITE: NNIS HOSPITALS 1986–1992

	Surgical Site									
	Craniolomy			Laminectomy			CNS Shunt		Other	N/S[a]
Microorganism	SI	DI	OS	SI	DI	OS	SI	OS	SI	OS
Coagulase-negative staphylococci	18%	33%	24%	17%	14%	22%	24%	44%	6%	18%
Staphylococcus aureus	41%	67%	24%	43%	41%	43%	59%	22%	47%	36%
Enterococci	6%	—	8%	7%	6%	4%	—	3%	6%	9%
Streptococcus species	4%	—	5%	5%	3%	4%	6%	5%	—	—
Gram-positive anaerobes	5%	—	1%	—	—	2%	—	1%	—	—
Pseudomonas aeruginosa	3%	—	3%	7%	5%	3%	—	5%	2%	
Acinetobacter species	3%	—	7%	1%	—	—	—	1%	—	—
Citrobacter species	1%	—	1%	1%	—	1%	—		2%	—
Enterobacter species	3%	—	8%	5%	12%	4%	—	4%	6%	9%
Klebsiella pneumoniae	4%	—	4%	1%	1%	1%	—	3%	2%	—
Escherichia coli	1%	—	4%	6%	6%	5%	—	5%	13%	9%
Gram-negative rods	7%	—	7%	6%	9%	6%	—	4%	14%	10%
Bacillus fragilis	—	—	—	—	—	—	—	—	—	9%
Yeast	2%	—	—	—	1%	—	6%	3%	2%	—
Fungi	—	—	—	—	—	—	6%	—	—	—
Viruses	—	—	1%	—	—	—	—	—	—	—
Others	—	—	—	—	—	—	—	—	—	—
Total	100%	100%	100%	100%	100%	100%	100%	100%	100%	100%

[a] Other neurosurgical procedures (i.e., burr hole placement, carolid endarterectomy).
SI, superficial incisional surgical site infection; DI, deep incisional surgical site infection; OS, organ/space infection. Data from CDC/NNIS.

four cases to *S. epidermidis* (3). *Enterobacter* species and *Klebsiella* species were the most common microorganisms. Looking at the entity of gram-negative meningitis as a whole, approximately 50% of cases are related to neurosurgery (7,52,122). *Klebsiella-Enterobacter* species, *Escherichia coli, Pseudomonas aeruginosa,* and *Acinetobacter* are the most frequent isolates. So-called diphtheroids (*Corynebacterium, Bacillus* species, and *P. acnes*) are also important pathogens in neurosurgical patients (see below). Wound infection due to *P. acnes,* with and without meningitis, has been reported after neurosurgical procedures (308–310).

In studies similar to those yielding the NNIS system data in Table 27.7, staphylococcal species are isolated from approximately 60% to 80% of CSF shunt infections in large series, whereas gram-negative bacilli are found in 5% to 27% of cases (10,13,130,155,160,163,168,169,171,205,311,312). Coagulase-negative staphylococci (mostly *S. epidermidis*) are isolated in 50% to 75% of cases followed by *S. aureus* in 10% to 25% of cases (163,311,313), although McGirt et al. (205) reported that a hospital stay of >3 days at the time of shunt insertion and prior *S. aureus* as the pathogen. There appears to be little difference in the pathogens involved in early versus late shunt infections, although one study suggested that gram-negative pathogens, especially *H. influenza,* may be more common in late infections (155,205). Similarly, the location of the distal end of the shunt catheter does not seem to significantly affect the distribution of pathogens unless intestinal perforation has occurred (171,314). Other commonly encountered pathogens include streptococcal species and diphtheroids. *P. acnes* is particularly important, as it has been reported to be the second most common pathogen in some series (315,316). Whether the incidence of this pathogen is truly increasing or underestimation occurs secondary to inadequate anaerobic culturing remains unclear (317). *Bacillus* species have also been implicated in shunt infections (318). Anaerobic bacterial and fungal shunt infections have been reported but are seen much less frequently.

The microbiology of infections complicating other CNS prosthetic devices closely parallels the profile seen with ventricular shunts. Gram-positive cocci account for the majority (70–75%) of infections complicating the placement of CSF reservoirs, with the remainder caused primarily by gram-negative microorganisms and diphtheroids (41,319). Ohrstrom et al. (320) found gram-positive cocci in almost 90% of 27 ventriculostomy-associated CSF infections. In a large prospective study of ventriculostomy-related infections, Mayhall et al. (9) described nearly equal numbers of gram-positive (47%) and gram-negative (53%) pathogens. Coagulase-negative staphylococci were the predominant species, accounting for 32% of isolates. Aucoin et al. (29) noted an increase in gram-negative ventriculomeningitis (approximately 75%) in patients with ICP monitors compared with craniotomy alone. *B. cereus* meningitis was reported in two patients with external ventricular drainage and could be traced to contaminated linen used during surgery (43).

The infectious agents responsible for deep CNS and neurosurgical infections (organ/space infections) have generally been well described in the literature. Unfortunately, although significant numbers of these cases are hospital-acquired, information relating specific pathogens to nosocomial cases is relatively limited. Most nosocomial cases of cranial epidural abscess and cranial subdural empyema occur in the setting of trauma, surgery, or paranasal sinus infection (225,262). Infections originating from the sinuses or mastoids are usually caused by anaerobes, streptococci, enterococcus, or *S. aureus* (262,263,321,322). Postsurgical and posttraumatic suppurations are usually due to *S. aureus,* streptococci, or gram-negative bacilli (263,323). Khan and Griebel (324) found that most cases of postsurgical and posttraumatic subdural empyemas were caused by *S. epidermidis* or *S. aureus.* Spinal epidural abscess is caused by *S. aureus* in 50% to 65% of cases, followed in frequency by streptococci (9–14%), gram-negative bacilli (8–16%), and *S. epidermidis* (3–9%) (228,233,240,241,252,321). Again, although varying numbers of these infections were hospital acquired, correlation to specific pathogens was not performed. However, a small series of iatrogenic cases of spinal epidural abscess reported by Ericsson et al. (238) describes a distribution of pathogens quite similar to the studies cited above. Disc space infection in adults is usually a postsurgical complication, although hematogenous spread occurs as well (111). *S. aureus* is the most common pathogen followed by *E. coli, S. epidermidis,* and other gram-negative microorganisms (80,101,106). Comparison with more recent data in Table 27.7 illustrates the increasing role of coagulase-negative staphylococci in laminectomy infections.

Nosocomial brain abscess is an uncommon infection that usually occurs in association with neurosurgical procedures or penetrating head trauma (91,226,282,283,290). A smaller number of cases may occur in the setting of sinus infection or generalized bacteremia (286). If present, the abscess is usually related to the surgical site, and staphylococci are usually isolated (131, 290,291,325). Other prevalent pathogens in this setting include streptococci, gram-negative aerobic bacilli, and *Clostridium* spp. (279,326). Anaerobes, streptococci, and, less commonly, *S. aureus* and gram-negative microorganisms are involved when a paranasal sinus or mastoid source of infection is present (287, 290,325). Hematogenous seeding of the brain may occur during the course of staphylococcal endocarditis (rarely nosocomial) and with gram-negative bacterial or fungal dissemination in immunocompromised hosts (see below) (63,127).

In the hospital setting, immunocompromised patients are at risk for a somewhat different spectrum of CNS infectious agents than their counterparts with normal immune function. In is important to recognize the close relationship between the duration and type of specific immune defect and the infections to which the host is susceptible. Table 27.8 illustrates the association between host immune status, typical CNS pathogens, and the clinical syndromes they cause. Several important pathogens (e.g., *Cryptococcus, Toxoplasma, Nocardia*) in this group are not included, as hospital acquisition would be unusual. Studies by Chernik et al. (64) identified the pathogens responsible for CNS infections among patients at a large cancer hospital. Of potential nosocomial pathogens, gram-negative bacilli (50% *P. aeruginosa*) were the most frequent cause of meningitis, followed by *L. monocytogenes,* streptococci, and, rarely, fungi. Various gram-negative bacilli were also responsible for three quarters of the brain abscesses, although *Aspergillus* was the most common isolate (60). The majority of cases developed during the course of hospitalization. In a follow-up to their initial studies, the same authors noted a high incidence of fungal CNS involvement on postmor-

TABLE 27.8. NOSOCOMIAL CNS INFECTIONS IN IMMUNOCOMPROMISED PATIENTS

Defect/Patients	Pathogens	Clinical Syndromes
Cell mediated		
Chronic steroids	*Listeria*	Meningitis, encephalitis
Lymphoma	*Aspergillus*	Brain abscess
Hodgkin's disease	Mucorales	Brain abscess
Solid organ transplant and AIDS	Mycobacterial	Brain abscess
Neutrophils		
Aplastic anemia	*Pseudomonas*	Meningitis
Acute leukemia	Enterobacteriaceae	Meningitis, brain abscess Meningoencephalitis
Chemotherapy	*Candida*	Meningitis, brain abscess
Radiation therapy	*Aspergillus*	Brain abscess
	Mucorales	Brain abscess
	Pseudallescheria boydii	Brain abscess
Mixed		
Bone marrow transplant	Enterobacteriaceae[a]	Meningitis, brain abscess Meningoencephalitis
	Candida	Meningitis, brain abscess
	Aspergillus	Brain abscess

[a] During the period of neutropenia in the early posttransplant period (0–30 days).

tem examination alone (60). Other reports have also described an increase in CNS candidiasis with systemic involvement, suggesting a higher-than-expected prevalence of this pathogen (67, 327). *Aspergillus* invasion of the CNS is often cited as the most common intracranial infection in cardiac and renal transplant patients (328). Needless to say, these patients are also at risk for the common nosocomial pathogens that may complicate neuroinvasive procedures.

OUTCOME

The considerable morbidity and mortality associated with infections involving the CNS place them among the most serious of hospital-acquired infections. Morbidity may be manifested by varying degrees of neurologic deficit, ranging from paresthesia to permanent paralysis. Intellectual impairment can be a particularly devastating consequence. Mortality due to CNS infection is frequently difficult to establish with certainty in critically ill patients with other significant medical problems. These patients may have died for reasons apart from nosocomial CNS infections, severely limiting the usefulness of most mortality data. Hospitals reporting through the NNIS system determine (subjectively) whether nosocomial infections were a contributing factor in patient death. For the period 1988–1993, nosocomial CNS infections were deemed to be related to death in 49 of 53 patients (92%) who died with a diagnosed nosocomial CNS infection (R. Gaynes, personal communication). This finding suggests that nosocomial CNS infections may contribute significantly to mortality. In addition, the economic costs of nosocomial CNS infections are often substantial and are associated with the need for extended hospitalization, intravenous antibiotics, sophisticated imaging, and multiple surgical procedures.

Superficial SSIs in neurosurgery, although often prolonging hospitalization, are rarely associated with any mortality by themselves (78). The majority of bone flap infections resolve with antibiotics and/or debridement, and a small number develop chronic persistent drainage (4,93). The real danger of these infections lies in intradural extension leading to increasing complications and deaths (1).

The reported mortality related to nosocomial meningitis (not associated with prosthetic devices) ranges from 20% to 67% (3, 5–7,52,122). Durand et al. (5) found the mortality rate to be 35% for nosocomial cases, compared with 25% for community-acquired infections. The complication rate (i.e., seizures) is also high and may be up to 50% in some series (7). As discussed above, many of these cases involve gram-negative bacilli, and some authors have demonstrated that increased mortality occurs with these microorganisms (3).

Of all infectious complications related to neurosurgery, CSF shunt infections are probably responsible for the largest volume of morbidity and mortality. Walters et al. (163) found patients with infected shunts required three times the number of surgical procedures as noninfected patients, and had greatly prolonged hospitalizations and double the case fatality rate. Schoenbaum et al. (10) found long-term mortality to approach 40% in patients with infected shunts as compared to 17% in shunted patients without infection. Yogev (329) performed an extensive review of success rates in treatment of CSF shunt infections by compiling multiple studies over a 25-year period. Cure rates were directly related to the therapeutic modality as follows: (a) 36% for antibiotics alone; (b) 65% for antibiotics and immediate shunt replacement; and (c) 96% with antibiotics, shunt removal, and external drainage or repeated ventricular aspirates. In a similar analysis by Kaufman and McLone (162), cure rates were nearly identical in each category, with mortality rates decreasing from approximately 24% with intravenous antibiotics alone to less than 10% with antibiotics plus externalization. One potential drawback of the latter method is secondary contamination of the ventriculostomy and complications related to a new infection. Retrospective studies have shown that shunt infections are associated with deterioration of intelligence quotient (IQ) scores (330). Infections related to other CNS prosthetic devices are also associated with significant mortality, especially in the setting of gram-negative involvement (9,29,58). Mayhall et al. (9) found no untreated patient survived a ventriculostomy-related infection; Smith and Alksne (331) found 100% mortality when *P. aeruginosa* was the pathogen.

Unfortunately, the precise relationship between most hospital-acquired organ/space CNS infections and outcome cannot easily be determined from reviewing the literature. Therefore, and because of the low incidence of these infections, only general trends can be examined. Spinal epidural abscess is an infection in which significant neurologic deficit is probably the most common complication. Mortality ranges from 5% to 33%, and persistent neurologic abnormalities (weakness, paraparesis, paralysis) can be seen in 10% to nearly 50% of cases (233,238,240, 241,252). Two large series found paralysis or death in 23% of patients (240,241). Cranial subdural empyema carries a mortality rate of 15% to 35% with a high incidence of seizures and disabling neurologic sequelae (223,263,265,324,332,333). Kaufman et al. (263) described four cases of postoperative subdural empyema in which two patients died and another suffered a permanent neurologic deficit. In a retrospective review of subdural empyema, Dill et al. (262) reported an overall mortality of 9%, but 55% had neurologic deficiency at time of hospital discharge. The prognosis of a nosocomial brain abscess is particularly difficult to estimate because of the low frequency of occurrence and the often-concurrent existence of another serious intracranial infection (91,282). In general, advances in diagnosis and treatment have resulted in a current overall mortality rate of approximately 10% to 32% (279,334,335). Adverse prognostic factors include delay in diagnosis, ventricular rupture, depressed mental status at the time of diagnosis, large and/or multiple lesions, extremes of age, and specific gram-negative or fungal etiology (286,287,290,294,295,336). Since most patients with nosocomially acquired brain abscess have one or more of these risk factors, morbidity and mortality can be expected to be high in this population. Even successfully treated brain abscesses can result in appreciable long-term neurologic complications. Chronic seizure disorders and persistent focal neurologic deficits can develop in up to 50% of patients (286,294,295,337,338). Neurologic outcome is most influenced by location of the abscess and the age of the patient (337). Cognitive and behavioral function may be permanently impaired, especially in younger patients (336,339). Lastly, postoperative disc space infection (usually nosocomial) is rarely associated with mortality but may cause significant morbidity. Chronic pain unrelated to the primary problem occurs in many; 39% to 88% of patients are able to return to work after treatment (80,109,340).

The consequences of infection from pathogens of even low virulence are frequently devastating in the immunocompromised patient. CNS infections are often caused by gram-negative bacteria and fungus; eradication of these microorganisms from the CNS is difficult enough in immunocompetent hosts. Chernik et al. (60,64) found mortality from CNS infections to be related primarily to the microorganism and the underlying disease of the patient. The highest overall mortality for intracranial infections was seen in leukemic patients (90%), followed by lymphoma patients (77%) and patients with head and spine tumors (59%). Survival was lowest with gram-negative bacterial infection (10–22%) and highest with infections caused by *L. monocytogenes* (63%) and *S. aureus* (76%). Notably, no patient with noncryptococcal fungal infection of the CNS survived in their series. Other series have also described overall mortality rates exceeding 50% from CNS infections in immunocompromised patients (62,341). Subsequent reports in organ transplant patients have documented rare survival with intracerebral aspergillosis (342). Rhinocerebral infection with Mucorales can be cured in over 50% of cases with aggressive medical-surgical therapy and control of acidosis in diabetic patients (292).

PREVENTION

Prevention of Craniotomy Infections

Prior to the 1980s, use of prophylactic antibiotics in neurosurgery was based mainly on data from uncontrolled trials. In the 1980s and 1990s, data from prospective randomized placebo-controlled trials demonstrated the efficacy of antibiotic prophylaxis in patients having clean neurosurgery. A meta-analysis of 2,075 patients evaluating antibiotic prophylaxis prior to neurosurgery found a fourfold reduction in wound infection rate when antibiotic prophylaxis was given (343). Table 27.9 demonstrates at least a three- to fourfold reduction in the incidence of infection after craniotomy using an antistaphylococcal antibiotic such as

TABLE 27.9. RANDOMIZED TRIALS OF ANTIBIOTIC PROPHYLAXIS IN NEUROSURGICAL PROCEDURES

			Infection Rate (%)	
Author	Year	Antibiotic(s)	Prophylaxis	No Prophylaxis
Savitz	1976	Clindamycin	1.2	10.9
Shapiro	1986	Vancomycin/gentamicin	2.8	11.7
Young	1987	Cefazolin/gentamicin	1.0	3.8
Blomstedt	1988	Vancomycin	1.8	7.3
Bullock	1988	Piperacillin	2.1	5.9
Van Ek	1988	Cloxacillin	3.3	10.3
Djindjian	1990	Oxacillin	0.6	4.9

Data from refs. 54, 344, 376–379, 381.

cefazolin or vancomycin. Some studies have also added gentamicin to the antistaphylococcal antibiotic. There are no data comparing the various antibiotics for prophylaxis. Antibiotic prophylaxis is usually administered for 24 hours. Some of the studies used, in addition to the parenteral antibiotics, a bacitracin irrigation solution. In a study of 356 patients given oxacillin or placebo for prolonged clean neurosurgery, there was an eightfold reduction in the incidence of infection in those given parenteral oxacillin compared with the placebo group (344). Use of an antibiotic irrigating solution in that study was not mentioned.

In an uncontrolled study to assess the efficacy of intravenous cloxacillin prophylaxis in patients undergoing craniotomy, the infection rate was 4% (345). Patients with a penicillin allergy received erythromycin. Antibiotics were given for 24 hours. In operations ($n = 17$) when prophylactic antibiotics were inadvertently omitted, the infection rate was 27%. The authors concluded that an antistaphylococcal penicillin such as cloxacillin was effective in reducing the incidence of craniotomy infections to less that 5% compared with the usual rates of 5% to 15% without additional prophylaxis.

The *Medical Letter on Drugs and Therapeutics* recommends the use of either cefazolin or vancomycin for a patient having craniotomy, since the most likely pathogens are either *S. aureus* or *S. epidermidis* (346).

Prevention of Cerebrospinal Fluid Shunt Infections

The majority of neurosurgical shunt infections occur within 2 months of surgery. Most infections result from the direct inoculation of bacteria during surgery and in the perioperative period. Antibiotic prophylaxis is usually directed against coagulase-negative staphylococci, the most frequent cause of shunt infections. Numerous studies have been undertaken to determine if antibiotic prophylaxis is effective in decreasing the number of infections that complicate the implantation of CSF shunts (59, 347). These studies have yielded conflicting results. In a meta-analysis of 12 controlled randomized trials (1,359 patients), antibiotic prophylaxis at the time of CSF shunt placement decreased the rate of infection by 50% (348). However, only a single trial of these 12 studies achieved statistical significance (91). Most of the studies were performed in a pediatric population and are discussed in Chapters 49 and 67. In the one study including adult patients, oxacillin reduced the infection rate from 20% in the control group to 3.3% in the treated group ($p = .1$) (344). Various antimicrobial agents were used in these trials, including cloxacillin, trimethoprim-sulfamethoxazole, cephalosporins such as cephalothin, vancomycin, and gentamicin (349). The duration of prophylaxis ranges from less than 24 hours to up to 48 hours after surgery. The ideal agent to prevent CSF shunt infections is unknown, since comparative studies are unavailable. Based on the results of susceptibility testing, vancomycin might be the preferred drug, but in one trial a histamine-like rash was noted in 35% of patients, despite the antibiotic's being infused over 1 hour (155). Despite the suggested benefit from antibiotic prophylaxis in the meta-analysis of the 12 studies, infection rates in the treated group still averaged 6.8%, with a range of 1.9% to 17% (348). Infection rates in the control groups for these studies averaged 13%, with a range of 5.5% to 24% (348). Such high rates in the groups that received prophylaxis for clean surgery suggest the need for other approaches to prevent infection such as the use of shunts with antimicrobial or antiadherence properties.

Prevention of Infections After Spinal Surgery

In a classic retrospective study, prophylactic antibiotics reduced the infection rate in patients undergoing a laminectomy for lumbar disc disease (81). However, infection rarely occurs after spinal surgery such as a lumbar discectomy, and antibiotics are usually not given. However, in spinal procedures involving fusion or for operations that are prolonged, antibiotics are often used, although randomized prospective controlled trials are lacking. In addition, spinal procedures in immunocompromised hosts or procedures involving implantation of hardware are usually given antibiotic prophylaxis, although controlled data are lacking. Use of a first- or second-generation cephalosporin is suggested, although studies supporting this approach are unavailable (84).

Prevention of Infection with a Cerebrospinal Fluid Leak

The value of antimicrobial prophylaxis in any patient with a CSF leak remains unclear. Definitive studies to resolve this issue are lacking, and at present their use cannot be recommended (350).

ACKNOWLEDGMENT

I would like to recognize Eliot Godofsky, M.D., who contributed significantly to the original edition of this chapter, and Lisa Tkatch, M.D., for her work on the second edition.

REFERENCES

1. Reichert MF, Medeiros ES, Ferraz FP. Hospital-acquired meningitis in patients undergoing craniotomy: incidence, evolution, and risk factors. *Am J Infect Control* 2002;30:158–164.
2. Blomstedt GC. Craniotomy infections. *Neurosurg Clin North Am* 1992;3:375–385.
3. Buckwold FJ, Hand R, Hansebout RR. Hospital-acquired bacterial meningitis in neurosurgical patients. *J Neurosurg* 1977;46:494–500.
4. Chou SN, Erickson DL. Craniotomy infections. *Clin Neurosurg* 1976; 23:357–362.
5. Durand ML, Calderwood SB, Weber DJ, et al. Acute bacterial meningitis in adults. A review of 493 episodes. *N Engl J Med* 1993;328: 21–28.
6. Morris A, Low DE. Nosocomial bacterial meningitis, including central nervous system shunt infections. *Infect Dis Clin North Am* 1999; 13:735–50.
7. Parodi S, Lechner A, Osih R, et al. Nosocomial enterobacter meningitis: risk factors, management, and treatment outcomes. *Clin Infect Dis* 2003;37:159–166.
8. Pople IK, Quinn MW, Bayston R. Morbidity and outcome of shunted hydrocephalus. *Z Kinderchir* 1990;1:29–31.

9. Mayhall CG, Archer N, Lamb VA, et al. Ventriculostomy-related infections—a prospective epidemiologic study. *N Engl J Med* 1984; 310:553–559.
10. Schoenbaum SC, Gardner P, Shillito J. Infections of cerebrospinal fluid shunts: epidemiology, clinical manifestations, and therapy. *J Infect Dis* 1975;131:543–552.
11. Spanu G, Karussos G, Adinolfi D, et al. An analysis of cerebrospinal fluid shunt infections in adults. A clinical experience of twelve years. *Acta Neurochir (Wien)* 1986;80:79–82.
12. Van Ek B, Bakker F, Van Dulken H, et al. Infections after craniotomy: a retrospective study. *J Infect* 1986;12:105–109.
13. Walters BC. Cerebrospinal fluid shunt infection. *Neurosurg Clin North Am* 1992;3:387–401.
14. Lyke KE, Obasanjo OO, Williams MA, et al. Ventriculitis complicating use of intraventricular catheters in adult neurosurgical patients. *Clin Infect Dis* 2001;33:2028–2033.
15. Papagelopoulos PJ, Sapkas GS, Kateros KT, et al. Halo pin intracranial penetration and epidural abscess in a patient with a previous cranioplasty. *Spine* 2001;26:E463–E467
16. Eljamel MS, Foy PM. Acute traumatic CSF fistulae: the risk of intracranial infection [see comments]. *Br J Neurosurg* 1990;4:381–385.
17. Gordon DS, Kerr AG. Cerebrospinal fluid rhinorrhea following surgery for acoustic neurinoma. Report of two cases. *J Neurosurg* 1986; 64:676–678.
18. Haddad FS, Hubballa J, Zaytoun G, et al. Intracranial complications of submucous resection of the nasal septum. *Am J Otolaryngol* 1985; 6:443–447.
19. Myers DL, Sataloff RT. Spinal fluid leakage after skull base surgical procedures. *Otolaryngol Clin North Am* 1984;17:601–612.
20. Swartz MN, Dodge PR. Bacterial meningitis—a review of selected aspects. *N Engl J Med* 1965;272:725–731,779–787,842–848, 898–902.
21. Hand WL, Sanford JP. Posttraumatic bacterial meningitis. *Ann Intern Med* 1970;72:869–874.
22. Hirschman JV. Bacterial meningitis following closed cranial trauma. In: Sande MA, Smith AL, Root RK, eds. *Bacterial meningitis.* New York: Churchill Livingstone, 1985:95–104.
23. Garibaldi R, Cushing D, Lerer R. Risk factors for postoperative infection. *Am J Med* 1991;91(suppl 3B):158S–163S.
24. Mollman HD, Haines SJ. Risk factors for postoperative neurosurgical wound infection. *J Neurosurg* 1986;64:902–906.
25. Narotam PK, vanDellen JR, duTrevou MD, et al. Operative sepsis in neurosurgery: a method of classifying surgical cases. *Neurosurgery* 1994;34:409–416.
26. McCarty M, Wenzel R. Postoperative spinal fluid infections after neurosurgical shunting procedures. *Pediatrics* 1977;59:793.
27. Sautter R, Mattman L, Legaspi R. *Serratia marcescens* meningitis associated with contaminated benzalkonium chloride solution. *Infect Control* 1984;5:223–225.
28. Lozier AP, Sciacca RR, Romagnoli MF, et al. Ventriculostomy-related infections: a critical review of the literature. *Neurosurgery* 2002;51: 170–182.
29. Aucoin P, Kotilainen H, Gantz N, et al. Intracranial pressure monitors: epidemiologic study of risk factors and infections. *Am J Med* 1988;80:369–376.
30. Bruder N, Zoghe NP, Graziani N, et al. A comparison of extradural and intraparenchymatous intracranial pressures in head injured patients. *Intensive Care Med* 1995;21:850–852.
31. Paramore CG, Turner DA. Relative risks of ventriculostomy infection and morbidity. *Acta Neurochir* 1994;127:79–84.
32. Holloway KL, Barnes T, Choi S, et al. Ventriculostomy infections: the effect of monitoring duration and catheter exchange in 584 patients. *J Neurosurg* 1996;85:419–424.
33. Seigman-Igra Y, Bar-Yosef S, Gorea A, et al. Nosocomial *Acinetobacter* meningitis secondary to invasive procedures: report of 25 cases and review. *Clin Infect Dis* 1993;17:843–849.
34. Robinson E, Woods M, McGee Z. Extrinsic factors that put patients at risk of acquiring central nervous system infections. *Am J Med* 1984; 76:203–214.
35. Jensen A, Espersen F, Skinhoj P, et al. *Staphylococcus aureus* meningitis. A review of 104 nationwide, consecutive cases. *Arch Intern Med* 1993;153:1902–1908.
36. Sarubbi FJ, Wilson M, Lee M, et al. Nosocomial meningitis and bacteremia due to contaminated amphotericin B. *JAMA* 1978;239: 416–418.
37. De Jong J. I. Lumbar myelography followed by meningitis [letter]. *Infect Control Hosp Epidemiol* 1992;13:74–75.
38. Ballantyne JC, Carr DB, Berkey CS, et al. Comparative efficacy of epidural, subarachnoid, and intracerebroventricular opioids in patients with pain due to cancer. *Reg Anaesth* 1996;21:542–556.
39. Wang LP, Hauerberg J, Schmidt JF. Incidence of spinal epidural abscess after epidural analgesia. *Anesthesiology* 1999;91:1928–1936.
40. Byers K, Axelrod P, Michael S, et al. Infections complicating tunneled intraspinal catheter systems used to treat chronic pain. *Clin Infect Dis* 1995;21:403–408.
41. Seigal T, Pfeffer R, Steiner I. Antibiotic therapy for infected Ommaya reservoir systems. *Neurosurgery* 1988;22:97–100.
42. Green M. Powder contamination of extradural catheters and implications for infection risk. *Eur J Surg* 1997;suppl 579:39–40.
43. Barrie D, Wilson JA, Hoffman PN, et al. *Bacillus cereus* meningitis in two neurosurgical patients: an investigation into the source of the organism. *J Infect* 1992;25:291–297.
44. Duhaime AC, Bonner K, McGowan KL, et al. Distribution of bacteria in the operating room environment and its relation to ventricular shunt infections: a prospective study. *Childs Nerv Syst* 1991;7: 211–214.
45. Stamm W, Colella J, Anderson R, et al. Indwelling arterial catheters as a source of nosocomial bacteremia. An outbreak caused by *Flavobacterium* species. *N Engl J Med* 1975;292:1099–1106.
46. Basset D, Thompson S, Page B. Neonatal infections with *Pseudomonas aeruginosa* associated with contaminated resuscitation equipment. *Lancet* 1965;1:781–784.
47. Berkowitz F. *Acinetobacter* meningitis—a diagnostic pitfall: a report of 3 cases. *S Afr Med J* 1982;61:448–449.
48. Bennett J. Incidence and nature of endemic and epidemic nosocomial infection. In: Bennett J, Brachman P, eds. *Hospital infections.* Boston: Little, Brown, 1979:233–238.
49. Horan T, Gaynes R, Martone W, et al. CDC definitions of nosocomial surgical site infections, 1992: a modification of CDC definitions of surgical wound infections. *Am J Infect Control* 1992;20:271–274.
50. Savitz MH, Malis LI, Meyers BR. Prophylactic antibiotics in neurosurgery. *Surg Neurol* 1974;2:95–100.
51. Tenney JH, Vlahov D, Salcman M, et al. Wide variation in risk of wound infection following clean neurosurgery. Implications for perioperative antibiotic prophylaxis. *J Neurosurg* 1985;62:243–247.
52. Mangi RJ, Quintiliani R, Anmdriole VT. Gram-negative bacillary meningitis. *Am J Med* 1975;59:829–836.
53. Haines S. Antibiotic prophylaxis in neurosurgery. The controlled trials. *Neurosurg Clin North Am* 1992;3:355–358.
54. Blomstedt GC, Kytta J. Results of a randomized trial of vancomycin prophylaxis in craniotomy. *J Neurosurg* 1988;69;216–220.
55. Young R, Lowner P. Perioperative antibiotic prophylaxis for the prevention of postoperative neurologic infections. A randomized clinical trial. *J Neurosurg* 1987;66;701–705.
56. Geraghty J, Freely M. Antibiotic prophylaxis in neurosurgery. A randomized controlled trial. *J Neurosurg* 1984;60:724–726.
57. Cushing H. Surgery of the head. In: Deen WW, ed. *Surgery, its principles and practice.* Philadelphia: WB Saunders, 1916:17–276.
58. Culver D, Horan T, Gaynes R, et al. Surgical wound infection rates by wound class, operative procedure, and patient risk index. *Am J Med* 1991;91(suppl 3B):152S–157S.
59. Garner JS, Jarvis WR, Emori TG, et al. CDC definitions for nosocomial infections, 1988. *Am J Infect Control* 1988;16:128–140.
60. Chernik N, Armstrong D, Posner J. Central nervous system infections in patients with cancer. Changing patterns. *Cancer* 1977;40:268–274.
61. Hall W, Martinez A, Dummer S, et al. Central nervous system infections in heart and heart-lung transplant recipients. *Arch Neurol* 1989; 46:173–177.
62. Hooper D, Pruitt A, Rubin R. Central nervous system infection in the chronically immunosuppressed. *Medicine* 1982;61:166–188.

63. Rubin RH, Hooper DC. Central nervous system infections in the compromised host. *Med Clin North Am* 1985;33:281–293.
64. Chernik N, Armstrong D, Posner J. Central nervous system infections in patients with cancer. *Medicine* 1973;52:563–581.
65. Britt R, Enzmann D, Remington J. Intracranial infection in cardiac transplant recipients. *Ann Neurol* 1981;9:107–119.
66. Buchs S, Pfister P. *Candida* meningitis: course, prognosis, and mortality before and after introduction of the new antimycotics. *Mykosen* 1982;26:73–81.
67. Lipton S, Hickey V, Morris J, et al. Candidal infection in the central nervous system. *Am J Med* 1984;76:101–108.
68. Will R, Matthews W. Evidence for case-to-case transmission of Creutzfeldt-Jakob disease. *J Neurol Neurosurg Psychiatry* 1982;45:235–238.
69. Masullo C, Pocchiari M, Macchi G, et al. Transmission of Creutzfeldt-Jakob disease by dural cadaveric graft. *J Neurosurg* 1989;71: 954–955.
70. CDC. Update: Creutzfeldt-Jakob disease in a second patient who received a cadaveric dura mater graft. *MMWR* 1989;38:37–38.
71. Duffy P, Collins G, Devoe A, et al. Possible person-to-person transmission of Creutzfeldt-Jakob disease. *N Engl J Med* 1974;290: 692–693.
72. Bernoulli C, Sigfried J, Baumgartner G, et al. Danger of accidental transmission of Creutzfeldt-Jakob disease by surgery. *Lancet* 1977;1: 478–479.
73. Houff S, Burtono R, Wilson R, et al. Human-to-human transmission of rabies virus by corneal transplant. *N Engl J Med* 1979;300: 603–604.
74. Valenti WM, Hruska JF, Menegus MA, et al. Nosocomial viral infections: III. Guidelines for prevention and control of exanthematous viruses, gastroenteritis viruses, picornaviruses, and uncommonly seen viruses. *Infect Control* 1981;2:38–49.
75. Scheld WM, Farr BM. Central nervous system infections. In: Bennett JV, Brachman PS, eds. *Hospital infections.* Philadelphia: Lippincott-Raven, 1998:563–569.
76. Taylor G, McKenzie M, Kirkland T, et al. Effect of surgeon's diagnosis on surgical wound infection rates. *Am J Infect Control* 1990;18: 295–299.
77. Winston KR. Hair and neurosurgery. *Neurosurgery* 1992;31: 320–329.
78. Quadery LA, Medlery AV, Miles J. Factors affecting the incidence of wound infection in neurosurgery. *Acta Neurochir (Wien)* 1977;39: 133–141.
79. Madeja C. Postoperative infections on a neurosurgical service. *J Neurosurg Nurs* 1977;9:84–86.
80. Lindholm TS, Pylkkanen P. Discitis following removal of intervertebral disc. *Spine* 1982;7:618–622.
81. Horwitz NH, Curtin JA. Prophylactic antibiotics and wound infections following laminectomy for lumbar disc herniation. *J Neurosurg* 1975;43:727–731.
82. Vlahov D, Montgomery E, Tenney JH, et al. Neurosurgical wound infections: methodological and clinical factors affecting calculation of infections rates. *J Neurosurg Nurs* 1984;16:128–133.
83. Zentner J, Gilsbach J, Daschner F. Incidence of wound infection in patients undergoing craniotomy: influence of type of shaving. *Acta Neurochir (Wien)* 1987;86:79–82.
84. Massie JB, Heller JG, Abitol JJ, et al. Postoperative posterior spinal wound infections. *Clin Orthop* 1992;284:99–107.
85. Chavenou D, Schlemmer B, Jedynak C, et al. Post-neurosurgical purulent meningitis: 31 cases. *Presse Med* 1987;16:295–298.
86. Wright RL. *Craniotomy infections.* Springfield, IL: Charles C Thomas, 1966.
87. Gepstein R, Eismont FJ. Postoperative spine infections. In: Garfin SR, ed. *Complications of spine surgery.* Baltimore: Williams & Wilkins, 1989:302–322.
88. Rasmussen S, Ohrstrom JK, Westergaard L, et al. Post-operative infections of osteoplastic compared with free bond flaps. *Br J Neurosurg* 1990;4:493–495.
89. Keller RB, Pappas AM. Infections after spinal fusion using internal fixation instrumentation. *Orthop Clin North Am* 1972;3:99–111.
90. Heller JG, Whitecloud TS III, Butler JC, et al. Complications of spinal surgery. In: Rothman RH, Simeone FA, eds. *The spine.* Philadelphia: WB Saunders, 1992:1817–1837.
91. Blomstedt GC. Infections in neurosurgery: a retrospective study of 1143 patients and 1517 operations. *Acta Neurochir (Wien)* 1985;78: 81–90.
92. Rish B, Billon J, Meirowsky A, et al. Cranioplast: a review of 1030 cases of penetrating head trauma. *Neurosurgery* 1979;4:381–385.
93. Blumenkopf B, Hartshorne MF, Bauman JM, et al. Craniotomy flap osteomyelitis: a diagnostic approach. *J Neurosurg* 1987;66:96–101.
94. Schauwecker DS, Park HM, Mock BH. Evaluation of complicating osteomyelitis with Tc-99m MDP, In-111 granulocytes, and Ga-67 citrate. *J Nucl Med* 1984;25:849–853.
95. Raptopoulos V, Doherty P, Gross T, et al. Acute osteomyelitis: advantage of white cell scans in early detection. *AJR* 1982;139:1077–1082.
96. Ducker TB. Disc space infection. *J Spinal Disord* 1988;1:236–237.
97. Dei AK, Kessel HA, Meinig G. Clinical follow-up after surgery of lumbar disc prolapses. A critical analysis. *Neurosurg Rev* 1990;13: 201–203.
98. Mayfield FH. Complications of laminectomy. *Clin Neurosurg* 1976; 23:435–439.
99. Rawlings CE, Wilkins RH, Gallis HA, et al. Postoperative intervertebral disc space infection. *Neurosurgery* 1983;13:371–376.
100. Turnbull F. Postoperative inflammatory disease of lumbar discs. *J Neurosurg* 1953;10:469–473.
101. El Gindi S, Aref S, Salama M, et al. Infections of intervertebral discs after operation. *J Bone Joint Surg* 1965;58B:114–116.
102. Thibodeau AA. Closed space infection following removal of lumbar intervertebral disc. *J Bone Joint Surg* 1968;50A:400–410.
103. Nielsen VA, Iversen E, Ahlgren P. Postoperative discitis. Radiology of progress and healing. *Acta Radiol* 1990;31:559–563.
104. Iversen E, Nielsen VA, Nansen LG. Prognosis in postoperative discitis. A retrospective study of 111 cases. *Acta Orthop Scand* 1992;63: 305–309.
105. Lang EF. Postoperative infection of the intervertebral disc space. *Surg Clin North Am* 1968;48:649–660.
106. Fernand R, Casey KL. Postlaminectomy disc space infection. *Clin Orthop* 1986;209:215–218.
107. Bircher MD, Tasker T, Crawshaw C, et al. Discitis following lumbar surgery. *Spine* 1988;13:98–102.
108. Jonsson B, Soderholm R, Stromqvist B. Erythrocyte sedimentation rate after lumbar spine surgery. *Spine* 1991;16:1049–1050.
109. Puranen J, Makela J, Lahde S. Postoperative intervertebral discitis. *Acta Orthop Scand* 1984;56:461–465.
110. Fouquet B, Goupille P, Jattiot F, et al. Discitis after lumbar disc surgery. Features of aseptic and septic forms. *Spine* 1992;17:356–358.
111. Black P, LeFrock JL. Infection of the spine. In: Long DM, ed. *Current therapy in neurological surgery.* St. Louis: CV Mosby, 1985:120–124.
112. Price A, Allen J, Eggars F, et al. Intervertebral disc space infection: CT changes. *Radiology* 1983;149:725–729.
113. Edelman RR, Warach S. Magnetic resonance imaging (first of two parts). *N Engl J Med* 1993;328:708–715.
114. Kramer J, Stiglbauer R, Wimberger D, et al. MRI of spondylitis. *Bildgebung* 1992;59:147–151.
115. Djukic S, Lang P, Morris J, et al. The postoperative spine. Magnetic resonance imaging. *Orthop Clin North Am* 1990;21:603–624.
116. Boden SD, Davis DO, Dina TS, et al. Postoperative diskitis: distinguishing early MR imaging findings from normal postoperative disk space changes. *Radiology* 1992;184:765–771.
117. Ross JS. Magnetic resonance assessment of the postoperative spine. Degenerative disc disease. *Radiol Clin North Am* 1991;29:793–808.
118. Modic M, Feiglin D, Paraino D, et al. Vertebral osteomyelitis: assessment using MR. *Radiology* 1985;157:157–166.
119. Schofferman L, Schofferman J, Zucherman J, et al. Occult infections causing persistent low-back pain. *Spine* 1989;14:417–419.
120. Blankstein A, Rubinstein E, Ezra E, et al. Disc space infection and vertebral osteomyelitis as a complication of percutaneous lateral discectomy [see comments]. *Clin Orthop* 1987;225:234–237.
121. Noble RC, Overman SB. *Propionibacterium acnes* osteomyelitis: case report and review of the literature. *J Clin Microbiol* 1987;25:251–254.

122. Berk SL, McCabe WR. Meningitis caused by gram-negative bacilli. *Ann Intern Med* 1980;93:253–260.
123. Okada J, Tsuda T, Takasugi S, et al. Unusually late onset of cerebrospinal fluid rhinorrhea after head trauma. *Surg Neurol* 1991;35: 213–217.
124. Wilson NW, Copeland B, Bastian JF. Posttraumatic meningitis in adolescents and children. *Pediatr Neurosurg* 1990;16:17–20.
125. Blomstedt GC. Post-operative aseptic meningitis. *Acta Neurochir (Wien)* 1987;89:112–116.
126. Rahal JJ. Diagnosis and management of meningitis due to gram-negative bacilli in adults. In: Remington JS, Swartz MN, eds. *Current clinical topics in infectious diseases.* New York: McGraw-Hill, 1980: 68–84.
127. Tunkel AC, Scheld WM. Central nervous system infections in the immunocompromised host. In: Rubin R, Young L, eds. *Clinical approach to infection in the compromised host.* New York: Plenum, 1994: 163–210.
128. Keroack MA. The patient with suspected meningitis. *Emerg Med Clin North Am* 1987;5:807–826.
129. Gorse G, Thrupp L, Nudleman K, et al. Bacterial meningitis in the elderly. *Arch Intern Med* 1984;144:1603–1607.
130. Kaufman BA, Tunkel AR, Pryor JC, et al. Meningitis in the neurosurgical patient. *Infect Dis Clin North Am* 1990;4:677–701.
131. Katz PM, Cooper PR. Infectious complications of neurosurgical trauma. *Infect Surg* 1985;4:22–32.
132. Clark RA, Hyslop NE Jr. Posttraumatic meningitis. In: Schlossberg D, ed. *Infections of the nervous system.* New York: Springer-Verlag, 1990:50–63.
133. Myers DL, Sataloff RT. Spinal fluid leakage after basilar skull surgical procedures. *Otolaryngol Clin North Am* 1984;17:601–611.
134. Porter MJ, Brookes GB, Zeman AZ, et al. Use of protein electrophoresis in the diagnosis of cerebrospinal fluid rhinorrhoea. *J Laryngol Otol* 1992;106:504–506.
135. Keir G, Zeman A, Brookes G, et al. Immunoblotting of transferrin in the identification of cerebrospinal fluid otorrhea and rhinorrhoea. *Ann Clin Biochem* 1992;29(pt 2):210–213.
136. Zaret DL, Morrison N, Gulbranson R, et al. Immunofixation to quantify beta 2–transferrin in cerebrospinal fluid to detect leakage of cerebrospinal fluid from skull injury. *Clin Chem* 1992;38:1908–1912.
137. Schuknecht HF, Zaytoun GM, Moon CN Jr. Adult-onset fluid in the tympanomastoid compartment. Diagnosis and management. *Arch Otolaryngol* 1982;108:759–765.
138. Wakhloo AK, Van Velthoven V, Schumacher M, et al. Evaluation of MR imaging, digital subtraction cisternography, and CT cisternography in diagnosing CSF fistula. *Acta Neurochir (Wien)* 1991;111: 119–127.
139. Zlab MK, Moore GF, Daly DT, et al. Cerebrospinal fluid rhinorrhea: a review of the literature. *Ear Nose Throat J* 1992;71:314–317.
140. Park JI, Strelzow VV, Friedman WH. Current management of cerebral spinal fluid rhinorrhea. *Laryngoscope* 1983;93:1294–1300.
141. Ahmadi J, Weiss M, Segall H, et al. Evaluation of cerebrospinal fluid rhinorrhea by metrizamide computed tomographic cisternography. *Neurosurgery* 1985;16:537–539.
142. Geisler PJ, Nelson KE, Levin S, et al. Community acquired purulent meningitis: a review of 1316 cases during the antibiotic era, 1954–1976. *Rev Infect Dis* 1980;2:725–745.
143. Conley JM, Ronald AR. Cerebrospinal fluid as a diagnostic body fluid. *Am J Med* 1983;75:102–107.
144. Martin MA, Massanari RM, Nghiem DD, et al. Nosocomial aseptic meningitis associated with the administration of OKT3. *JAMA* 1988; 259:2002–2005.
145. Figg WD. Aseptic meningitis associated with muromonab-CD3 [letter]. *DICP* 1991;25:1395.
146. Marton KI, Grean AD. The spinal tap: a new look at an old test. *Ann Intern Med* 1986;104:840–848.
147. Cairns H. Bacterial infections during intracranial surgery. *Lancet* 1963;1:1193–1198.
148. Blazer S, Berant M, Alon U. Bacterial meningitis: effect of antibiotics on cerebrospinal fluid. *Am J Clin Pathol* 1983;80:386–387.
149. Saez-Llorens X, McCracken GH Jr. Bacterial meningitis in children. *Lancet* 2003;361:2139–2148.
150. Roos KL, Tunkel AR, Scheld MR. Acute bacterial meningitis in children and adults. In: Scheld MR, Whitely RJ, Durack DT, eds. *Infections of the central nervous system.* New York: Raven Press, 1991: 335–409.
151. Dougherty JM, Roth RM. Cerebral spinal fluid. *Emerg Med Clin North Am* 1986;4:281–297.
152. Lin TY, Nelson JD, McCracken GH. Fever during treatment for bacterial meningitis. *Pediatr Infect Dis J* 1984;3:319–322.
153. Kulkarni AV, Drake JM, Lamberti-Pasculli M. Cerebrospinal fluid shunt infection: a prospective study of risk factors. *J Neurosurg* 2001; 94:195–201.
154. Green JR, Kanshepolsky J, Turkian B. Incidence and significance of central nervous system infection in neurosurgical patients. *Adv Neurol* 1974;6:223–228.
155. Odio C, McCracken GJ, Nelson JD. CSF shunt infections in pediatrics. A seven-year experience. *Am J Dis Child* 1984;138:1103–1108.
156. Renier D, Lacombe J, Pierre KA, et al. Factors causing acute shunt infection. Computer analysis of 1174 operations. *J Neurosurg* 1984; 61:1072–1078.
157. Scarff TB, Nelson PB, Reigel DH. External drainage for ventricular infection following cerebrospinal fluid shunts. *Childs Brain* 1978;4: 129–136.
158. Borgbjerg BM, Gjerris F, Albeck MJ, et al. Risk of infection after cerebrospinal fluid shunt: an analysis of 884 first-time shunts. *Acta Neurochir* 1995;136:1–7.
159. Brydon HL, Hayward R, Harkness W, et al. Does the cerebrospinal fluid protein concentration increase the risk of shunt complications? *Br J Neurosurg* 1996;10:267–273.
160. O'Brien M, Parent A, Davis B. Management of ventricular shunt infections. *Childs Brain* 1979;5:304–309.
161. Haines SJ, Taylor F. Prophylactic methicillin for shunt operations. Effects on incidence of shunt malfunction and infection. *Childs Brain* 1982;9:10–22.
162. Kaufman BA, McLone DG. Infections of cerebrospinal fluid shunts. In: Scheld WM, Whitley RJ, Durack DT, eds. *Infections of the central nervous system.* New York: Raven Press, 1991:561–585.
163. Walters BC, Hoffman HJ, Hendrick EB, et al. Cerebrospinal fluid shunt infection. Influences on initial management and subsequent outcome. *J Neurosurg* 1984;60:1014–1021.
164. Sayers MP. Shunt complications. *Clin Neurosurg* 1976;23:393–400.
165. Redman JF, Seibert JJ. Abdominal and genitourinary complications following ventriculoperitoneal shunts. *J Urol* 1978;119:295–297.
166. Loeser JD, Sells CJ, Shurtleff DB. The management of patients with cerebrospinal fluid shunts. *J Fam Pract* 1978;6:285–289.
167. Agha FP, Amendola MA, Shirazi KK, et al. Abdominal complications of ventriculoperitoneal shunts with emphasis on the role of imaging methods. *Surg Gynecol Obstet* 1983;156:473–478.
168. Bisno AL. Infections of central nervous system shunts. In: Bisno AL, Waldvogel FA, eds. *Infections associated with indwelling medical devices.* Washington, DC: American Society of Microbiology, 1989:93–109.
169. Gardner P, Leipzig T, Phillips P. Infections of central nervous system shunts. Symposium on infections of the central nervous system. *Med Clin North Am* 1985;69:297–314.
170. Yogev R, Davis AT. Neurosurgical shunt infections: a review. *Childs Brain* 1980;6:74–81.
171. Forward KR, Fewer HD, Stiver HG. Cerebrospinal fluid shunt infections: a review of 35 infections in 32 patients. *J Neurosurg* 1983;59: 389–394.
172. Mori K, Raimondi AJ. An analysis of external ventricular drainage as a treatment for infected shunts. *Childs Brain* 1975;1:243–250.
173. Quigley MR, Reigel DH, Kortyna R. Cerebrospinal fluid shunt infections. Report of 41 cases and a critical review of the literature. *Pediatr Neurosci* 1989;15:111–120.
174. James HE. Infections associated with cerebrospinal fluid prosthetic devices. In: Sugarman B, Young EJ, eds. *Infections associated with prosthetic devices.* Boca Raton, FL: CRC Press, 1984:23–41.
175. Brok I, Johnson N, Overturf G, et al. Mixed bacterial meningitis. a

comparison of ventriculo- and lumboperitoneal shunts. *J Neurosurg* 1977;47:961–964.
176. Reynolds M, Sherman JO, McLane DG. Ventriculoperitoneal shunts as an acute surgical abdomen. *J Pediatr Surg* 1983;18:951–954.
177. Parry SW, Schumacher JF, Llwellyn RC. Abdominal pseudocysts and ascites formation after ventriculoperitoneal shunt procedures. *J Neurosurg* 1975;43:476–480.
178. Latchaw JJ, Hahn JF. Intraperitoneal pseudocyst associated with peritoneal shunts. *Neurosurgery* 1981;8:469–472.
179. Dean DF, Keller IB. Cerebrospinal fluid ascites: a complication of a ventriculoperitoneal shunt. *J Neurol Neurosurg Psychiatry* 1972;35: 474–476.
180. Jamjoom AB, Mohammed AA, Al-Boukai A, et al. Multiloculated hydrocephalus related to cerebrospinal fluid shunt infection. *Acta Neurochir* 1996;138:714–719.
181. Rekate HL, Yonas H, White RJ, et al. The acute abdomen in patients with ventriculoperitoneal shunts. *Surg Neurol* 1979;11:442–445.
182. Fischer EG, Greene CJ, Winston KR. Spinal epidural abscess in children. *Neurosurgery* 1981;9:257–260.
183. Ivan LP, Choo SH, Ventureyra EC. Complications of ventriculoatrial and ventriculoperitoneal shunts in a new children's hospital. *Can J Surg* 1980;23:566–568.
184. King P. The peritoneal complications of ventriculo-peritoneal shunts. *Aust N Z J Surg* 1976;46:372–377.
185. Paone RF, Mercer LC. Hepatic abscess caused by a ventriculoperitoneal shunt. *Pediatr Infect Dis J* 1991;10:338–339.
186. Peterfy CG, Atri M. Intrahepatic abscess: a rare complication of ventriculoperitoneal shunt [letter]. *Am J Roentgenol* 1990;155:894–895.
187. Iosif G, Fleischman J, Chitkara R. Empyema due to ventriculopleural shunt. *Chest* 1991;99:1538–1539.
188. Hoffman HJ, Hendrick EB, Humphreys RP. Experience with ventriculo-pleural shunts. *Childs Brain* 1983;10:404–413.
189. Finney HL, Roberts TS. Nephritis secondary to chronic cerebrospinal fluid—vascular shunt infection: shunt nephritis. *Childs Brain* 1980; 6:189–193.
190. Eknoyan G, Dillman RO. Renal complications of infectious diseases. *Med Clin North Am* 1978;62:979–1003.
191. Drucker MH, Vanek VW, Franco AA, et al. Thromboembolic complications of ventriculoatrial shunts. *Surg Neurol* 1984;22:444–448.
192. Kim Y, Michael AF. Chronic bacteremia and nephritis. *Annu Rev Med* 1978;29:319–325.
193. Naito H, Toya S, Shizawa H, et al. High incidence of acute postoperative meningitis and septicemia in patients undergoing craniotomy with ventriculoatrial shunt. *Surg Gynecol Obstet* 1973;137:810–812.
194. Wald SL, McLaurin RL. Shunt-associated glomerulonephritis. *Neurosurgery* 1978;3:146–150.
195. Haffner D, Schindera F, Aschoff A, et al. The clinical spectrum of shunt nephritis. *Nephrol Dial Transplant* 1997;12:1143–1148.
196. Samtleben W, Bosch T, Bauriedel G, et al. Internal medicine complications of ventriculoatrial shunt. *Med Klin* 1995;90:67–71.
197. Groenveld AB, Nommensen FE, Millink H, et al. Shunt nephritis associated with *Propionibacterium acnes* with demonstration of the antigen in the glomeruli. *Nephron* 1982;32:365–369.
198. Peeters W, Mussche M, Becaus I, et al. Shunt nephritis. *Clin Nephrol* 1978;9:122–125.
199. Dobrin RS, Day NK, Quie PG, et al. The role of complement, immunoglobulin and bacterial antigen in coagulase-negative staphylococcal shunt nephritis. *Am J Med* 1975;59:660–673.
200. Stickler GB, Shin MH, Burke EC, et al. Diffuse glomerulonephritis associated with infected ventriculoatrial shunt. *Am Heart J* 1970;79: 426–427.
201. Rames L, Wise B, Goodman JR, et al. Renal disease with *Staphylococcus albus* bacteremia. A complication in ventriculoatrial shunts. *JAMA* 1970;212:1671–1677.
202. Arze RS, Rashid H, Morley R, et al. Shunt nephritis: report of 2 cases and review of the literature. *Clin Nephrol* 1983;19:48–53.
203. Myers MG, Schoenbaum SC. Shunt fluid aspiration: an adjunct in the diagnosis of cerebrospinal fluid shunt infection. *Am J Dis Child* 1975;129:220–222.
204. Pfisterer W, Muhlbauer M, Czech T, et al. Early diagnosis of external ventricular drainage infection: results of a prospective study. *J Neurol Neurosurg Psychiatry* 2003;74:929–932.
205. McGirt MJ, Zaas A, Fuchs HE, et al. Risk factors for pediatric ventriculoperitoneal shunt infection and predictors of infectious pathogens. *Clin Infect Dis* 2003;36:858–862.
206. Shurtliff DB, Christie D, Foltz EL. Ventriculoauriculostomy-associated infections. A 12-year study. *J Neurosurg* 1971;35:686–694.
207. Bayston R, Spitz L. Infective and cystic causes of malfunction of ventriculoperitoneal shunts for hydrocephalus. *Z Kinderchir* 1977;22: 419–425.
208. Bayston R. Serological investigations in children with colonized Spitz-Holter valves. *J Clin Pathol* 1972;25:718–720.
209. Holt R. The early serological detection of colonisation by *Staphylococcus epidermidis* of ventriculo-atrial shunts. *Infection* 1980;8:8–12.
210. Van Lente F. The diagnostic utility of C-reactive protein. *Hum Pathol* 1982;13:1061–1063.
211. Schena F, Petrossa G, Pastore A, et al. Circulating immune complexes in infected ventriculoatrial and ventriculoperitoneal shunts. *J Clin Immunol* 1983;3:173–177.
212. Rosner MJ, Becker DP. ICP monitoring: complications and associated factors. *Clin Neurosurg* 1976;23:494–519.
213. Bayston R, Lambert E. Duration of protective activity of cerebrospinal fluid shunt catheters impregnated with antimicrobial agents to prevent bacterial catheter-related infection. *J Neurosurg* 1997;87:247–251.
214. Schreffler RT, Schreffler AJ, Wittler RR. Treatment of cerebrospinal fluid shunt infections: a decision analysis. *Pediatr Infect Dis J* 2002; 21:632–636.
215. DuMoulin MG, Hedley WJ. Hospital associated viral infection and the anesthesiologist. *Anesthesiology* 1983;59:51–65.
216. Brown P, Cathala F, Cataigne P. Creutzfeldt-Jakob disease: clinical analysis of a consecutive series of 230 neuropathologically verified cases. *Ann Neurol* 1986:20:597–602.
217. Anderson L, Nicholson K, Tauxe R, et al. Human rabies in the United States, 1960–1979: epidemiology, diagnosis and prevention. *Ann Intern Med* 1984;100:728–735.
218. Fishbein D. Rabies. *Infect Dis Clin North Am* 1991;5:53–71.
219. Rudd RJ, Trimarchi VC, Abelseth MK. Tissue culture technique for a routine isolation of street strain rabies virus. *J Clin Microbiol* 1980; 12:590–593.
220. Blenden DC, Creech W, Torres-Anjel MJ. Use of immunofluorescence examination to detect rabies virus antigen in the skin of humans with clinical encephalitis. *J Infect Dis* 1986;154:698–701.
221. Dupont JR, Earle KM. Human rabies encephalitis—a study of forty-nine fatal cases with a review of the literature. *Neurology* 1965;15: 1023–1034.
222. Sarwar M, Ralkoff G, Naseem M. Radiologic techniques in the diagnosis of CNS infections. *Neurol Clin* 1986;4:41–68.
223. Brown P, Coker-Vann M, Pomeroy K, et al. Diagnosis of Creutzfeldt-Jakob disease by Western blot identification of marker protein in human brain tissue. *N Engl J Med* 1986;314:547–551.
224. Harrington M, Merril C, Asher D. Abnormal proteins in the cerebrospinal fluid of patients with Creutzfeldt-Jakob disease. *N Engl J Med* 1986;315:279–283.
225. Krauss WE, McCormick PC. Infections of the dural spaces. *Neurosurg Clin North Am* 1992;3:421–433.
226. Benson CA, Harris AA. Acute neurologic infections. *Med Clin North Am* 1986;70:987–1011.
227. Kaplan RJ. Neurologic complications of infections of the head and neck. *Otolaryngol Clin North Am* 1976;9:729–749.
228. Bleck TP, Greenlee JE. Subdural empyema. In: Mandell G, Douglas R, Bennett J, eds. *Principles and practices of infectious disease,* 5th ed. New York: Churchill Livingstone, 2000:1028–1031.
229. Tindal GT, Flanagean JF, Nashold BS. Brain abscess and osteomyelitis following skull traction. *Arch Surg* 1959;79:638–641.
230. Silverberg A, DiNubile M. Subdural empyema and cranial epidural abscess. *Med Clin North Am* 1985;69:361–374.
231. Samuel J, Fernandes CM, Steinberg JL. Intracranial otogenic complications: a persisting problem. *Laryngoscope* 1986;96:272–278.
232. Hlavin ML, Kaminski HJ, Fenstermaker RA, et al. Intracranial suppu-

ration: a modern decade of postoperative subdural empyema and epidural abscess. *Neurosurgery* 1994;34:974–981.
233. Baker AS, Ojemann RG, Swartz MN, et al. Spinal epidural abscess. *N Engl J Med* 1975;293:463–468.
234. Soehle M, Wallenfang T. Spinal epidural abscesses: clinical manifestations, prognostic factors, and outcomes. *Neurosurgery* 2002;51:79–87.
235. Spiegelmann R, Findler G, Faibel M, et al. Postoperative spinal epidural empyema. Clinical and computed tomography features. *Spine* 1991;16:1146–1149.
236. Nickels JG, Poulos JG, Chaouki K. Risks of infection from short-term epidural catheter use. *Reg Anaesth* 1989;14:88–89.
237. Lee HJ, Bach JR, White RE. Spinal epidural abscess complicating vertebral osteomyelitis: an insidious cause of deteriorating spinal cord function. *J Am Paraplegia Soc* 1992;15:19–21.
238. Ericsson M, Algers G, Schliamser S. Spinal epidural abscesses in adults: review and report of iatrogenic cases. *Scand J Infect Dis* 1990;22:249–257.
239. Auletta JJ, John CC. Spinal epidural abscesses in children: a 15-year experience and review of the literature. *Clin Infect Dis* 2001;32:9–16.
240. Darouiche RO, Hamil RJ, Greenberg SB, et al. Bacterial spinal epidural abscess. Review of 43 cases and literature survey. *Medicine (Baltimore)* 1992;71:369–385.
241. Danner RL, Hartman BJ. Update on spinal epidural abscess: 35 cases and review of the literature. *Rev Infect Dis* 1987;9:265–274.
242. Beaudoin MG, Klein L. Epidural abscess following multiple spinal anaesthetics. *Anaesth Intensive Care* 1984;12:163–164.
243. Abdel-Magid R, Kotb H. Epidural abscess after spinal anesthesia: a favorable outcome. *Neurosurgery* 1990;27:310–311.
244. Ferguson CC. Infection and the epidural space: a case report. *AANA J* 1992;60:393–396.
245. Kee WD, Jones MR, Thomas P, et al. Extradural abscess complicating extradural anaesthesia for caesarean section. *Br J Anaesth* 1992;69:647–652.
246. North JB, Brophy BP. Epidural abscess: a hazard of spinal epidural anaesthesia. *Aust N Z J Surg* 1979;57:351–353.
247. Hanedl SF, Klein WC, Kim YW. Intracranial epidural abscess. *Radiology* 1974;111:117–120.
248. Smith HP, Hendrick EB. Subdural empyema and epidural abscess in children. *J Neurosurg* 1983;58:392–397.
249. Sharif HS, Ibrahim A. Intracranial epidural abscess. *Br J Radiol* 1982;55:81–84.
250. Heusner AP. Nontuberulous spinal epidural infections. *N Engl J Med* 1948;239:845–854.
251. Reihsaus E, Waldbaur H, Seeling W. Spinal epidural abscess: a meta-analysis of 915 patients. *Neurosurg Rev* 2000;232:175–204.
252. Kaufman DM, Kaplan JG, Litman N. Infectious agents in spinal epidural abscesses. *Neurology* 1980;30:844–850.
253. Hlavin M, Kaminski H, Ross J, et al. Spinal epidural abscess: a ten year perspective. *Neurosurgery* 1990;27:177–184.
254. O'Sullivan R, McKenzie A, Hennessy O. Value of CT scanning in assessing location and extent of epidural and paraspinal inflammatory conditions. *Australas Radiol* 1988;32:203–206.
255. Weisberg LA. The role of CT in the evaluation of patients with intracranial CNS infectious-inflammatory disorders. *Comput Radiol* 1984;8:29–36.
256. Wheeler D, Keiser P, Rigamonti D, et al. Medical management of spinal epidural abscesses: case report and review [see comments]. *Clin Infect Dis* 1992;15:22–27.
257. Obanna WG, Rosenblum ML. Nonoperative treatment of neurosurgical infections. *Neurosurg Clin North Am* 1992;3:359–373.
258. Weingarten K, Zimmerman RD, Becker RD, et al. Subdural and epidural empyemas: MR imaging. *AJR* 1989;152:615–621.
259. Tsuchiya K, Makita K, Furui S, et al. Contrast-enhanced magnetic resonance imaging of sub- and epidural empyemas. *Neuroradiology* 1992;34:494–496.
260. Sharif HS. Role of MR imaging in the management of spinal infections. *AJR* 1992;158:1333–1345.
261. Hanigan WC, Asner NG, Elwood PW. Magnetic resonance imaging and the nonoperative treatment of spinal epidural abscess. *Surg Neurol* 1990;34:408–413.
262. Dill SR, Cobbs CG, McDonald CK. Subdural empyema: analysis of 32 cases and review. *Clin Infect Dis* 1995;20:372–386.
263. Kaufman DM, Miller MH, Steigbigel NH. Subdural empyema: analysis of 17 recent cases and review of the literature. *Medicine (Baltimore)* 1975;54:485–498.
264. Harris LF, Haws FP, Triplett JJ, et al. Subdural empyema and epidural abscess: recent experience in a community hospital. *South Med J* 1987;80:1254–1258.
265. Bhandari YS, Sakari NBS. Subdural empyema: a review of 37 cases. *J Neurosurg* 1970;32:35–39.
266. Post EM, Modesti LM. Subacute postoperative subdural empyema. *J Neurosurg* 1981;55:761–765.
267. Dunker RO, Khakoo RA. Failure of computed tomographic scanning to demonstrate subdural empyema. *JAMA* 1981;246:1116–1118.
268. Zimmerman RD, Leeds NE, Danziger A. Subdural empyema: CT findings. *Radiology* 1984;150:417–422.
269. Moseley IF, Kendal BE. Radiology of intracranial empyemas, with special reference to computed tomography. *Neuroradiology* 1984;26:333–345.
270. Baum PA, Dillon WP. Utility of magnetic resonance imaging in the detection of subdural empyema. *Ann Otol Rhinol Laryngol* 1992;101:876–878.
271. Levy RM. Brain abscess and subdural empyema. *Curr Opinion Neurol* 1994;7:223–228.
272. Lownie SP, Ferguson GG. Spinal subdural empyema complicating cervical discography. *Spine* 1989;14:1415–1417.
273. Fraser RAR, Ratzan K, Wolpert SM, et al. Spinal subdural empyema. *Arch Neurol* 1973;28:235–238.
274. Theodotou B, Woosley RE, Whaley RA. Spinal subdural empyema: diagnosis by spinal computed tomography. *Surg Neurol* 1984;21:610–612.
275. Shaw RE. Cavernous sinus thrombophlebitis: a review. *Br J Surg* 1952;40:40–48.
276. Garvey G. Current concepts of bacterial infections of the central nervous system. Bacterial meningitis and bacterial brain abscess. *J Neurosurg* 1983;59:735–744.
277. Mathews TJ, Marus G. Otogenic intradural complications (a review of 37 patients). *J Laryngol Otol* 1988;102:121–124.
278. Parker GS, Tami TA, Wilson JF, et al. Intracranial complications of sinusitis. *South Med J* 1989;82:563–569.
279. Sharma BS, Khosla VK, Kak VK, et al. Multiple pyogenic brain abscesses. *Acta Neurochir* 1995;133:36–43.
280. Tenney JH. Bacterial infections of the central nervous system in neurosurgery. *Neurol Clin* 1986;4:91–114.
281. Graus F, Rogers L, Posner J. Cerebrovascular complications in patients with cancer. *Medicine* 1985;64:16–35.
282. Osenbach RK, Loftus CM. Diagnosis and management of brain abscess. *Neurosurg Clin North Am* 1992;3:403–420.
283. Rish B, Caverness W, Dillon J, et al. Analysis of brain abscess after penetrating craniocerebral injuries in Vietnam. *Neurosurgery* 1981;9:535–541.
284. Dennis G, Clifton G. Brain abscess as a complication of halo fixation. *Neurosurgery* 1982;10:760–761.
285. Kaye AH, Briggs M. Brain abscess after insertion of skull traction. *J Bone Joint Surg* 1982;64B:500–502.
286. Mathisen GE, Johnson JP. Brain abscess. *Clin Infect Dis* 1997;25:763.
287. Yang SH. Brain abscess. A review of 400 cases. *J Neurosurg* 1981;55:794–799.
288. Small M, Dale BA. Intracranial suppuration 1968–1982—a 15 year review. *Clin Otolaryngol* 1984;9:315–321.
289. Maniglia AJ, Goodwin WJ, Arnold JE, et al. Intracranial abscesses secondary to nasal, sinus, and orbital infections in adults and children. *Arch Otolaryngol Head Neck Surg* 1989;115:1424–1429.
290. Nielsen H, Gyldensted C, Harmsen A. Cerebral abscess. Aetiology and pathogenesis, symptoms diagnosis and treatment. *Acta Neurol Scand* 1982;65:609–622.
291. Wispelwey B, Dacey R Jr, Scheld W. Brain abscess. In: Scheld W,

Whitely R, Durack D, eds. *Infections of the central nervous system.* New York: Raven Press 1991:457–486.
292. Lehner RI, Howard OH, Sypherd PS. Mucormycosis. *Ann Intern Med* 1980;93:93–108.
293. Meyer R, Young L, Armstrong D, et al. *Aspergillus* complicating neoplastic diseases. *Am J Med* 1973;54:6–15.
294. Carey ME, Chou SN, French LA. Long-term neurologic residua in patients surviving brain abscess with surgery. *J Neurosurg* 1971;34: 652–656.
295. Chun HC, Johnson JD, Hofstetter M. Brain abscess. A study of 45 consecutive cases. *Medicine (Baltimore)* 1986;65:415–431.
296. Cowan RJ, Mody DM. Radionuclide techniques for brain imaging. *Neurol Clin* 1984;2:835–851.
297. Britt RH, Enzmann DR. Clinical stages of human brain abscesses on serial CT scans after contrast infusion. Computerized tomographic, neuropathologic, and clinical correlations. *J Neurosurg* 1983;59: 972–989.
298. Whelan MA, Hilal SK. Computed tomography as a guide in the diagnosis and follow-up of brain abscesses. *Radiology* 1980;135: 663–671.
299. Haimes A, Zimmerman R, Morgello S, et al. MR imaging of brain abscess. *AJR* 1989;152:1073–1085.
300. Burke JW, Podrasky AE, Bradley WG. Benign postoperative enhancement on MR images. *Radiology* 1990;174:99–102.
301. Brant-Zawadski M, Enzmann D, Placone R, et al. NMR imaging of experimental brain abscess. Comparison with CT. *AJNR* 1983;4: 250–253.
302. Apuzzo M, Chandrasoma P, Choen D, et al. Computed imaging stereotaxy: experience and perspective related to 500 procedures applied to brain masses. *Neurosurgery* 1987;20:930–937.
303. Wild AM, Xuereb JH, Marks PV, et al. Computerized tomographic stereotaxy in the management of 200 consecutive intracranial mass lesions. Analysis of indications, benefits and outcome. *Br J Neurosurg* 1990;4:407–415.
304. Duma CM, Kondziolka D, Lunsford LD. Image-guided stereotactic management of non-AIDS related cerebral infection. *Neurosurg Clin North Am* 1992;3:291–302.
305. Anderson RE, Thomas DG, Du BG. Radiological aspects of CT-guided stereotactic neurosurgical procedures. *Neuroradiology* 1983; 24:163–166.
306. Van Ek B, Dijkmans B, Van Dulken H, et al. Effect of cloxacillin prophylaxis on the bacterial flora of craniotomy wounds. *Scand J Infect Dis* 1990;22:345–352.
307. Dernbach PD, Gomez H, Hahn J. Primary closure of infected spinal wounds. *Neurosurgery* 1990;26:707–709.
308. Skinner P, Taylor A, Coakham H. Propionibacteria as a cause of shunt and postneurosurgical infections. *J Clin Pathol* 1984;31:1085–1090.
309. Kamme C, Soltesz V, Sundbarg G. Aerobic and anaerobic bacteria in neurosurgical infections. Peri-operative culture with flexible contact agar film. *J Hosp Infect* 1984;5:147–154.
310. Maniatis A, Vassilouthis J. *Propionibacterium acnes* infection complicating craniotomy. *J Hosp Infect* 1980;1:261–264.
311. Choux M, Genitori L, Lang D, et al. Shunt implantation: reducing the incidence of shunt infection. *J Neurosurg* 1992;77:875–880.
312. Venes J. Infections of CSF shunt and intracranial pressure monitoring devices. *Infect Dis Clin North Am* 1989;3:289–299.
313. McCullough DC, Kane JG, Presper JH, et al. Antibiotic prophylaxis in ventricular shunt surgery. I. Reduction of operative infection rates with methicillin. *Childs Brain* 1980;7:182–189.
314. Sells C, Shurtleff D, Loeser J. Gram-negative cerebrospinal fluid shunt-associated infections. *Pediatrics* 1977;59:614–618.
315. Everett E, Eikhoff T, Simon R. Cerebrospinal fluid shunt infection with anaerobic diphtheroids (*Propionibacterium* species). *J Neurosurg* 1976;44:580–584.
316. Rekate H, Ruch T, Nulsen F. Diphtheroid infections of cerebrospinal fluid shunts. The changing pattern of shunt infections in Cleveland. *J Neurosurg* 1980;52:553–556.
317. Collignon PJ, Munro R, Sorrell TC. *Propionibacterium acnes* infection in neurosurgical patients. Experience with high-dose penicillin therapy. *Med J Aust* 1986;145:408–410.
318. Tuazon C, Murray H, Levy C, et al. Serious infections from *Bacillus* sp. *JAMA* 1979;241:1137–1140.
319. Lishner M, Perrin R, Feld R, et al. Complications associated with Ommaya reservoirs in patients with cancer. *Arch Intern Med* 1990; 150:173–176.
320. Ohrstrom J, Skou J, Ejlertsen T, et al. Infected ventriculostomy: bacteriology and treatment. *Acta Neurochir* 1989;100:67–70.
321. Bleck TP, Greenlee JE. Epidural abscess. In: Mandell G, Douglas R, Bennett J, eds. *Principles and practice of infectious diseases,* 5th ed. New York: Churchill Livingstone, 2000:1031–1033.
322. Bannister G, Williams B, Smith S. Treatment of subdural empyema. *J Neurosurg* 1981;55:82–88.
323. Swartz MN, O'Hanley P. Central nervous system infections. In: Rubenstein E, Federmann D, eds. *Scientific American medicine.* New York: Scientific American, 1987:24–25.
324. Khan M, Griebel R. Subdural empyema: a retrospective study of 15 patients. *Can J Surg* 1984;27:283–285.
325. De Louvois J. The bacteriology and chemotherapy of brain abscess. *J Antimicrob Chemother* 1978;4:395–413.
326. Ariza J, Casanova A, Fernandez VP, et al. Etiological agent and primary source of infection in 42 cases of focal intracranial suppuration. *J Clin Microbiol* 1986;24:899–902.
327. Bayer A, Edwards JJ, Seidel J, et al. *Candida* meningitis: report of seven cases and review of the English literature. *Medicine* 1976;55: 477–486.
328. Conti D, Rubin R. Infection of the central nervous system in organ transplant recipients. *Neurol Clin* 1988;6:241–260.
329. Yogev R. Cerebrospinal fluid shunt infections: a personal view. *Pediatr Infect Dis J* 1985;4:113–118.
330. McLone D, Czyzewski D, Raimondi A, et al. Central nervous system infections as a limiting factor in the intelligence of children with myelomeningocele. *Pediatrics* 1982;70:338–342.
331. Smith R, Alksne J. Infections complicating the use of external ventriculostomy. *J Neurosurg* 1976;44:567–570.
332. Mauser HW, Tulleken CA. Subdural empyema. A review of 48 patients. *Clin Neurol Neurosurg* 1984;86:255–263.
333. Miller ES, Dias PS, Uttley D. Management of subdural empyema: a series of 24 cases. *J Neurol Neurosurg Psychiatry* 1987;50:1415–1418.
334. Mampalam T, Rosenblum M. Trends in the management of bacterial brain abscesses: a review of 102 cases over 17 years. *Neurosurgery* 1988; 23:451–458.
335. Alderson D, Strong A, Ingham H, et al. Fifteen-year review of the mortality of brain abscess. *Neurosurgery* 1981;8:1–86.
336. Renier D, Flandin C, Hirsch E, et al. Brain abscesses in neonates. A study of 30 cases. *J Neurosurg* 1988;69:877–882.
337. Carey ME, Chou SN, French LA. Experience with brain abscesses. *J Neurosurg* 1972;36:1–9.
338. Caliauw L, de Praetere P, Verbeke L. Postoperative epilepsy in subdural suppurations. *Acta Neurochir (Wien)* 1984;71:217–223.
339. Gruszkiewicz J, Doron Y, Peyser E, et al. Brain abscess and its surgical management. *Surg Neurol* 1982;18:7–17.
340. Pilgaards. Discitis (closed space infection) following removal of lumbar intervertebral disc. *J Bone Joint Surg* 1969;51A:713–716.
341. Armstrong D, Wong B. Central nervous system infection in immunocompromised hosts. *Annu Rev Med* 1982;33:293–308.
342. Weiland D, Ferguson R, Peteron P, et al. Aspergillosis in 25 renal transplant patients. Epidemiology, clinical presentation, diagnosis, and management. *Ann Surg* 1983;198:622–629.
343. Barker FG. Efficacy of prophylactic antibiotics for craniotomy: a meta-analysis. *Neurosurgery* 1994;35:484–492.
344. Djindjian M, Febrier M, Otterbein G, et al. Oxacillin prophylaxis in cerebrospinal fluid shunt procedures: results of a randomized open study in 60 hydrocephalic patients. *Surg Neurol* 1986;25:178–180.
345. Van Ek B, Dijkmans B, Van Dulken H, et al. Efficacy of cloxacillin prophylaxis in craniotomy: a one year follow-up study. *Scand J Infect Dis* 1991;23:617–623.
346. Anonymous. Antimicrobial prophylaxis in surgery. *Med Lett* 2001; 43:92–97.
347. Rebuck JA, Murry KR, Rhoney DH, et al. Infection related to intra-

cranial pressure monitors in adults: analysis of risk factors and antibiotic prophylaxis. *J Neurol Neurosurg Psychiatry* 2000;69:381–384.

348. Langley J, LeBland J, Drake J, et al. Efficacy of antimicrobial prophylaxis in placement of cerebrospinal fluid shunts: meta-analysis. *Clin Infect Dis* 1993;17:98–103.
349. Lang J, Kerr AG. Pneumatization of the posteromedial air-cell tract. *Clin Otolaryngol* 1989;14:425–427.
350. Haines SJ. Antibiotic prophylaxis in neurosurgery. The controlled trials. *Neurosurg Clin North Am* 1992;3:355–358.
351. Odum G, Hart D, Johnson Smith W, et al. A seventeen-year survey of the use of ultraviolet radiations. Proceedings of the 24th Meeting of the American Academy of Neurologic Surgery, New Orleans, 1962.
352. Ingham H, Kalbag R, Sisson P, et al. Simple perioperative antimicrobial chemoprophylaxis in elective neurosurgical operations. *J Hosp Infect* 1988;12:125–133.
353. Haines SJ. Topical antibiotic prophylaxis in neurosurgery. *Neurosurgery* 1982;11:250–253.
354. Savitz MH, Katz SS. Prevention of primary wound infection in neurosurgical patients: a 10-year study. *Neurosurgery* 1986;18:658–688.
355. Cartmill T, Al Zahawi M, Sisson P, et al. Five days versus one day of penicillin as prophylaxis in elective neurosurgical operations. *J Hosp Infect* 1989;14:63–68.
356. Chan R, Thompson G. Morbidity, mortality, and quality of life following surgery for intracranial meningiomas. *Neurosurgery* 1984;60: 52–60.
357. Jomin M, Leosin F, Lozes G. 500 ruptured and operated intracranial arterial aneurysms. *Surg Neurol* 1984;21:13–18.
358. Lunsford L, Coffey R, Cojocaru T, et al. Image-guided stereotactic surgery. A 10-year evolutionary experience. *Stereotact Funct Neurosurg* 1990;54:375–387.
359. Eng R, Seligman S. Lumbar puncture-induced meningitis. *JAMA* 1981;245:1456–1559.
360. Weisel J, Rose D, Silver A, et al. Lumbar puncture in asymptomatic late syphilis: an analysis of the benefits and risks. *Arch Intern Med* 1985;145:465–468.
361. Fine PG, Hare BD, Zahniser JC. Epidural abscess following epidural catheterization in a chronic pain patient: a diagnostic dilemma. *Anesthesiology* 1988;69:422–424.
362. Barreto R. Bacteriology cultures of indwelling epidural catheters. *Anesthesiology* 1962;23:643–646.
363. Poppen J. Ventriculostomy as a valuable procedure in neurosurgery. Report of a satisfactory method. *Arch Neurol Psychiatry* 1943;50: 587–589.
364. Shurtleff D, Stuntz J, Hayden P. Experience with 1201 cerebrospinal fluid shunt procedures. *Pediatr Neurosci* 1985–1986;12:49–57.
365. Browne M, Dinndorf P, Perek D, et al. Infectious complications of intraventricular reservoirs in cancer patients. *Pediatr Infect Dis J* 1978; 6:182–189.
366. Joacos A, Clifford P, Kay H. The Ommaya reservoir in chemotherapy for malignant disease in the CNS. *Clin Oncol* 1981;7:123–127.
367. Obbens E, Leavens M, Beal J, et al. Ommaya reservoirs in 387 cancer patients: a 15-year experience. *Neurology* 1985;35:1274–1278.
368. Shapiro W, Posner J, Ushio Y, et al. Treatment of meningeal neoplasms. *Cancer Treat Rep* 1977;61:733–743.
369. Ratcheson R, Ommay A. Experience with the subcutaneous cerebrospinal-fluid reservoir. *N Engl J Med* 1968;279:1025–1031.
370. Constantini S, Cotev S, Rappaport H, et al. Intracranial pressure monitoring after elective intracranial surgery. *J Neurosurg* 1988;69: 540–544.
371. Strong W. Epidural abscess associated with epidural catheterization: a rare event? Report of two cases with a markedly delayed presentation. *Anesthesiology* 1991;74:943–946.
372. Schelkun S, Wagner K, Blanks J, et al. Bacterial meningitis following Pantopaque myelography. A case report and literature review. *Orthopedics* 1985;8:73–76.
373. Worthington M, Hills J, Tally F, et al. Bacterial meningitis after myelography. *Surg Neurol* 1980;14:318–320.
374. Shintani S, Tanaka H, Irifune A, et al. Iatrogenic acute spinal epidural abscess with septic meningitis: MR findings. *Clin Neurol Neurosurg* 1992;94:253–255.
375. DeJong J, Barrs A. Lumbar myelography followed by meningitis [letter]. *Infect Control Hosp Epidemiol* 1992;13:74–75.
376. Savitz M, Malis L. Prophylactic clindamycin for neurosurgical patients. *NY State J Med* 1976;76:64–67.
377. Shapiro M, Wald U, Simchen E, et al. Randomized clinical trial of intra-operative antimicrobial prophylaxis of infection after neurosurgical procedures. *J Hosp Infect* 1986;8:283–295.
378. Van Ek B, Dijkmans B, Van Dulken H, et al. Antibiotic prophylaxis in craniotomy: a prospective double-blind placebo-controlled study. *Scand J Infect Dis* 1988;20:633–639.
379. Djindjian M, Lepresle E, Homs JB. Antibiotic prophylaxis during prolonged clean neurosurgery. Results of a randomized double-blind study using oxacillin. *J Neurosurg* 1990;73:383–386.
380. Gardner P, Leipzig T, Sadigh M. Infections of central nervous system shunts. *Topics Infect Dis* 1988;9:185–214.
381. Bullock R, van Dellen JR, Ketelbey W, et al. A double-blind placebo-controlled trial of perioperative antibiotics for elective neurosurgery. *J Neurosurg* 1988;69:687–691.

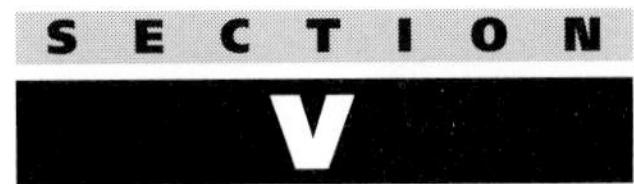

EPIDEMIOLOGY AND PREVENTION OF NOSOCOMIAL INFECTIONS CAUSED BY SPECIFIC PATHOGENS

A

Bacterial Infections

28

STAPHYLOCOCCUS AUREUS

JOSEPH F. JOHN, JR.
NEIL L. BARG

Staphylococcus aureus is the preeminent scourge of *Homo sapiens*. Though not a requirement for homeostasis, its ready incorporation into the flora of the anterior nares and other moist or hairy bodily areas in nearly 30% of healthy people suggests that *S. aureus* may function symbiotically at those sites. One constant element of pathogenesis is that nasal carriage constitutes the major risk factor for subsequent infection (1,2). After years of tedious delineation of its multiple virulence factors, publication of the whole genome and new functional studies on regulation and pathogenesis provide new insights into the mechanism for invasion of the skin, endovasculature, and solid organs by *S. aureus* (3,4). Studies of specific genes such as *mec*A, which encodes broad resistance to beta-lactam antibiotics in methicillin-resistant *S. aureus* (MRSA) (5), have revealed the complexity of gene expression in pathogenic strains of *S. aureus* (6). Since the expression of other virulence genes such as those involving surface adherence are highly regulated like *mec*, many years of additional study will likely be required to understand pathogenesis and to design strategies to reduce invasive nosocomial infections (7,8).

S. aureus as a community pathogen is best known for its ability to produce furuncles and infect soft tissue. An array of additional and emerging infections also threaten hospitalized patients who possess special risks for acquiring *S. aureus* infections (9). Historically, hospital-acquired infections were almost exclusively caused by *S. aureus* until the 1960s, when the prevalence of infections due to gram-negative bacilli increased noticeably (10). The ascent of gram-negative bacteria as the new threat in hospitals lulled hospital physicians into thinking that their old nemesis—*S. aureus*—would remain of historical interest. In the early 1990s, data from the National Nosocomial Infections Surveillance (NNIS) system at the Centers for Disease Control and Prevention (CDC) indicated that *S. aureus* was again increasing in incidence as a nosocomial pathogen (11). With broadening resistance to newer antimicrobials and disinfectants, MRSA along with methicillin-susceptible *S. aureus* (MSSA) have become the dominant nosocomial pathogens in hospitals worldwide (3,12). New strategies are needed to limit nosocomial spread and consequent morbidity due to *S. aureus* (13). This chapter reviews the role MSSA continues to play in healthcare-related infections and serves as an introduction to Chapter 29, which discusses MRSA.

HISTORICAL PERSPECTIVE

There are several early biblical descriptions of staphylococcal infection. Of the ten plagues brought by Yahweh on the Egyptian Pharaoh, the sixth cast boils or sores upon man and beast (Exodus 9:8–12) (14). The boils arose after Moses took ashes and sprinkled them aloft, filling the air over Egypt with dust that induced outbreaks of boils on man and beast, wretched in their appearance but not fatal. In another biblical passage Job is stricken by Satan with boils (or ulcers) that made his body turn black (Job 2:7). There is little information about furunculosis during the next century, though it must have remained a major problem. The so-called high Middle Ages has been described as a period that was remarkably disease free, though, ironically, it was followed by centuries of epidemics of plague with little attention to other bacterial infections (15). With the advent of Pasteur's techniques to culture bacteria, the coagulase-positive *Staphylococcus* was isolated and assigned a species name in the 1880s (16). Since that time, the number of species of the genus has grown to over 32. Using automated techniques, any clinical laboratory is able to distinguish among the 13 species indigenous to humans (17,18).

Not until the 20th century was a connection made between colonization by specific bacteria and subsequent nosocomial infection. The increasing importance of *S. aureus* as a cause of hospital sepsis resounds from the documentary writing of Dr. Wesley Spink (19). In the preantibiotic era, mortality due to staphylococcal sepsis secondary to pneumonia, osteomyelitis, and cellulitis was as high as 82% (20). Osteomyelitis due to *S. aureus*, especially of the long bones, was often disabling, although mortality due to staphylococcal sepsis was lower in patients with osteomyelitis. The use of sulfonamides from 1937 to 1942 was not much better than maggots in the treatment of local or osseous staphylococcal infection (19). Penicillin became available in 1942 and quickly reduced the mortality rate of staphylococcal infection from 80% to 35%. Penicillin resistance, however, developed rapidly in *S. aureus*, and in hospitals where penicillin was heavily used there were frequent epidemics caused by strains of penicillin-resistant *S. aureus* (19,21). Multiple advisory groups in the late 1940s assembled to make recommendations for control of staphylococcal epidemics. Pharmaceutical companies, spurred on by the early success of penicillin, mobilized to develop new antistaphylococcal agents (19).

In the 1950s, Spink and his colleagues established the connection between carriage in the nasopharynx of hospital employees and the frequent contamination of wounds (19). After penicillin resistance became widespread, Spink's Minnesota group showed again that the reservoir of *S. aureus* was hospitalized patients and hospital personnel. Spink stated that the rise in mortality due to penicillin-resistant *S. aureus* was due to cross-infection of "traumatic and surgical wounds transmitted by healthy hospital carriers or from other patients with sepsis. Patients and hospital personnel were found to be heavily parasitized by highly resistant strains of pathogenic staphylococci primarily within bacteriophage type Group III" (19). Indeed, the problem of staphylococcal sepsis in United States hospitals during the early 1950s was the major stimulus for development of infection control committees (10). Such committees under the direction of hospital epidemiologists created strict isolation units that, over the next several years, reduced the number of infections at the University of Minnesota and other centers. Despite early successes in infection control of staphylococcal infection, Spink's prescient, cautious words resound today: *"The skin and respiratory tract will remain as the major portals of entry, and staphylococcal sepsis will continue to challenge medical practice."*

Fifty years later we have forgotten the intensity of infection control measures that were required for staphylococcal sepsis in the 1950s. During the 1960s and 1970s, newer antibiotics, particularly the semisynthetic penicillins, reduced the risk of nosocomial staphylococcal infection. Extensive use of these agents over the next three decades, however, ushered in international nosocomial epidemics due to related strains of MRSA. (10). In a study comparing the rates of *S. aureus* infection in a tertiary care hospital from the periods 1971 to 1976 and 1989 to 1992, all but one of the MRSA strains from the later period were acquired in the hospital or in a nursing home, whereas about 80% of the infections due to MSSA were community-acquired (D. Musher, personal communication). Since the second edition of this text was published, the problem of nosocomial MRSA and its ensuing literature have clearly burgeoned worldwide.

MICROBIOLOGY OF *STAPHYLOCOCCUS AUREUS*

Species Characteristics

Species Identification

S. aureus has traditionally been defined by phenotypic traits that distinguish it from micrococci and other staphylococci (18). *S. aureus* is a catalase-negative, coagulase-positive, nonmotile coccus that appears as bluish-black tetrads or clusters after Gram staining. *S. aureus* grows as 6- to 8-mm colonies that are usually hemolytic on blood agar and salt tolerant; they become gold-pigmented after 24 to 48 hours of incubation. Laboratory identification can be aided by observing anaerobic acid production from glucose, production of acid from glycerol in the presence of 0.4 μg/mL erythromycin, and mannitol fermentation, as well as by susceptibility to lysostaphin (17). *S. aureus* also produces a thermonuclease that is useful in identifying the species (22). Salt tolerance is probably due to the stability of the *S. aureus* cell wall derived from the glycine pentapeptide cross-linked *N*-acetyl glycosamine residues. Ribitol teichoic acid polymers also link the peptidoglycan (3). Alterations in this structure can actually reduce the minimum inhibitory concentration (MIC) to antistaphylococcal penicillins (23). *S. aureus* has other survival genes including those to respond to low pH and some of these genes are regulated by sigma factors like σ (24).

Staphylococci can be identified by both conventional or rapid laboratory methods. Several marketed kits allow rapid species identification with 70% to 90% accuracy (17,18). Mannitol-salt agar has traditionally been the selective culture method of choice for isolation of *S. aureus*. Newer media such as CHROMagar appear superior to mannitol salt agar (25). Methods such as restriction fragment length polymorphism (RFLP) of RNA genes (ribotype) and detection of the *S. aureus nuclease* gene by polymerase chain reaction (PCR) or fluorescein tagging are available commercially to differentiate *S. aureus* from other species (26) and in the future may also become very useful for rapid surveillance of *S. aureus* nosocomial infection/colonization.

Strain Identification

The hospital epidemiologist may find it necessary to distinguish among multiple endemic versus epidemic strains of *S. aureus* for purposes of tracing the source of the infecting isolate, identifying reservoirs of antibiotic-resistant *S. aureus*, monitoring the colonization of patients or personnel, and, possibly, identifying virulent subtypes. Identification of epidemiologically related microorganisms at the subspecies level may help determine whether the observed clustering of isolates represents distinct strains or several isolates of the same strain that are causing an outbreak. A typing system is adequate if there is a high probability that two random isolates that are epidemiologically unrelated are indeed different. An ideal typing system would generate about 20 groups with even distribution of random isolates. A

TABLE 28.1. NONMOLECULAR AND MOLECULAR METHODS OF TYPING *STAPHYLOCOCCUS AUREUS*

Molecular Methods	Nonmolecular Methods
Plasmid content	Antibiotic susceptibility
Chromosomal REA	Phage typing
	Serotyping
Plasmid REA	Capsule typing
RFLP	Alloenzyme patterns
Gene polymorphism	Immunoblotting
Random PCR	
Repetitive element PCR	Multilocus enzyme focusing
PFGE	SDS-PAGE
	Multilocus sequence typing

PCR, polymerase chain reaction; PFGE, pulsed-field gel electrophoresis; REA, restriction endonuclease analysis; RFLP, restriction fragment length polymorphism; SDS-PAGE, sodium didocyl sulfate, polyacrylamide gel electrophoresis.

high proportion of isolates must be typeable, and the method must be reproducible, easy to perform, and inexpensive, and it must avoid the necessity of a second typing system to provide further discrimination. Nonmolecular and molecular methods of typing *S. aureus* are shown in Table 28.1.

Nonmolecular Methods of Typing

Typing systems have been based on differences in antigenic structure, phage susceptibility, antibiotic susceptibility, biochemical profiles, and DNA composition. One antigenic typing method uses antibodies to the 11 known capsular polysaccharides. Nosocomial isolates, however, are predominately composed of only two types, 5 and 8 (27), though 24% of strains remain untypeable by this system.

One antigenic system is based on 30 soluble protein or carbohydrate determinants (28). Antigen expression by specific strains depends on the selected growth media, which may be why the antibodies necessary for these systems are not available commercially.

Phage typing has been in use since 1952 and is a laborious method that is performed only by reference laboratories. The international set of typing phages is shown in Table 28.2 (10). The phage reactions are relatively stable; lysis is graded from weak to strong, and if no lysis develops at 100 times routine test dilution, the strain is considered untypeable. Strains are considered different if the phage pattern differs by two or more phage reactions that show strong lysis. Yet, the same lysis pattern does not necessarily equal epidemiologic relatedness. Phage typing methods are further limited, because many strains are not lysed by the available phages and are therefore untypeable. Phage-typing patterns can change when *in vitro* selected vancomycin-resistant strains are compared to their vancomycin-susceptible parents (29). Although pulsed-field gel electrophoresis (PFGE) patterns between susceptible parents and resistant selectants remained the same, phage types frequently changed or selectants became nontypeable.

TABLE 28.2. PHAGES AND PHAGE GROUPS OF *STAPHYLOCOCCUS AUREUS*

Phage Group	Standard Phages that Lyse
I	29, 52, 52a, 79, 80
II	3a, 3c, 55, 77
III	6, 42e, 47a, 53, 54, 75, 83a, 84, 85
IV	Bovine strains
V	94, 96
Miscellaneous	81, 95

An elegant antigenic typing method, termed immunoblotting, uses pooled human sera for detecting various antigens among *S. aureus* strains by Western blotting (30). Immunoblotting identified eight patterns using different batches of pooled sera that correlated with phage typing. The method was more discriminating than plasmid profiles, but between 2% and 28% of immunotypes were discrepant on repeat testing. The method was capable of identifying strains that were clinically and epidemiologically related. Immunoblotting combined with antibiograms has been used to discriminate a new outbreak strain from an endemic strain of MRSA (31). Applied in another study, immunoblotting could differentiate 43 strains into only two major groups, making it only as good as endonuclease digestion of plasmid DNA (32).

Antibiograms can be useful when a unique resistance pattern prevails. A given resistance phenotype, however, may result from different arrangements of multiply resistant genes, thus not ensuring DNA sequence identity. Furthermore, resistance (R) plasmids mediating traits such as antibiotic resistance are not always stable. The loss of R plasmids would allow otherwise identical parent strains to be typed as different using antibiograms. A clever way to circumvent this problem is through the use of multiplex PCR that will simultaneously generate multiple amplicons signifying presence or absence of specific resistance determinants like mecA, aacA, tetM, etc. (33). Multiplex PCR is the current extension of "resistotype" identification suggested by Elek et al. (34) over 30 years ago.

Biochemical typing (biotyping) is based on enzyme activities, including the commercial methods of such companies as API and Vitek. Color changes are based on acid production from carbohydrates. Although such typing is relatively inexpensive and easy to perform, the traits may vary over time and geographic areas. They are not highly discriminating and need to be combined with other typing methods. Differences in single enzymes, such as esterase, have been used in typing but are also not discriminatory when used alone (35,36).

Multilocus enzyme electrophoresis (MLEE) is based on small differences in electrophoretic mobility of chromosomally encoded metabolic enzymes. Proponents of MLEE feel that each pattern of enzymes determines a clone. MLEE has identified 11 types of *S. aureus*, though the predominance of type 15 in nosocomial outbreaks may limit its usefulness to the hospital epidemiologist (37). Because it is technically difficult to perform (38), MLEE is also not ideal for hospital outbreaks. Another method analyzes differences in the cell wall peptidoglycan. This method, termed peptidoglycan fingerprinting, separates cell wall components by thin-layer chromatography. Unfortunately, this method is difficult to perform and yields an insufficient number of bands for discriminating among endemic and epidemic strains (39).

Molecular Typing

Molecular typing takes advantage of modern molecular biologic techniques. DNA analysis can differentiate strains with similar phenotypic traits that are actually encoded by different genes (40). Plasmid analysis by visualization of individual plasmid bands in agarose gels is a classic molecular method that has been used for almost 20 years but has five major limitations. First, unlike coagulase-negative staphylococci, *S. aureus* seldom has more than three plasmids, so there is a poor chance of generating a complex fingerprint, thus limiting discrimination. Second, as with other bacteria, *S. aureus* strains may lose plasmids, thus limiting the reproducibility of the method. Third, many strains lack plasmids and are thus untypeable. Fourth, very large plasmids that migrate near the top of the gel may be difficult to differentiate; therefore, precise comparisons between strains with large plasmids would be difficult. Lastly, co-migration of plasmid bands from different strains does not ensure identity. Restriction endonuclease digestion of both large and small plasmids restriction endonuclease analysis with visualization of individual restriction fragments reduces the ambiguity of plasmid size comparison (41).

Methods for analyzing genomic DNA overcome many of the limitations of plasmid analysis. The easiest method, analysis of chromosomal restriction enzyme patterns (42), uses restriction enzymes that recognize frequently occurring unique sequences (restriction sites). Limited studies have shown the value of restriction endonuclease analysis (REA) when analyzing outbreaks due to MRSA on adult wards (43,44) and in neonatal intensive care units (NICUs) (45). Electrophoresis of such preparations, however, produces patterns with huge numbers of fragments, making interpretation very difficult. It is difficult to compare a large number of complex patterns on one gel. Small differences in patterns are difficult to resolve, and accurate comparison of bands greater than 15 megadaltons (Md) (22 kb) may be difficult.

Enzymes such as *Sma*I and *Sst*II cut the staphylococcal chromosomal DNA at rare restriction sites, producing fewer fragments (37–41) that can be easily interpreted (46). *Sma*I digests have been shown to be stable after repeated subculture. Although such enzymes generate fewer fragments than REA, *Sma*I fragments are too large to permit electrophoresis with conventional apparatus and require both an expensive, specialized apparatus to deliver a complex electrical stimulus (e.g., pulse field, orthogonal field) and preparation of genomic DNA in agarose blocks to prevent shearing. Designating MRSA strains as different when the pulse field pattern differs by more than three bands was established by Tenover et al. (47). As a general guideline, for strains to be considered related, no more than three bands (out of 20) should be different (Fig. 28.1).

A mathematical approximation of differences between strains is determined from the proportion of fragments with identical sizes. As long as the total number of fragments is not too numerous, the patterns can be subjected to a numerical analysis. A similarity coefficient can be calculated that approximates the number of nucleotides that are different (46). Such a number is based on a formula proposed by Dice (48):

$$S_d = \{2N \times 100\}/F$$

where the Dice coefficient S_d equals twice N, the number of shared restriction fragments times 100 divided by F, the total number of restriction fragments generated by enzyme digestion (48). Computer software such as GelCompar can be used to establish a DNA similarity matrix based on the Dice coefficient (49).

The utility of PFGE has made the technique the gold standard for bacterial molecular epidemiology. Early PFGE studies proved useful for typing MSSA but did not find enough differences among MRSA isolates using *Sma*I (50). New studies of MRSA such as one in the university hospital in Besancon, France, have been able to determine that of 15 clones present

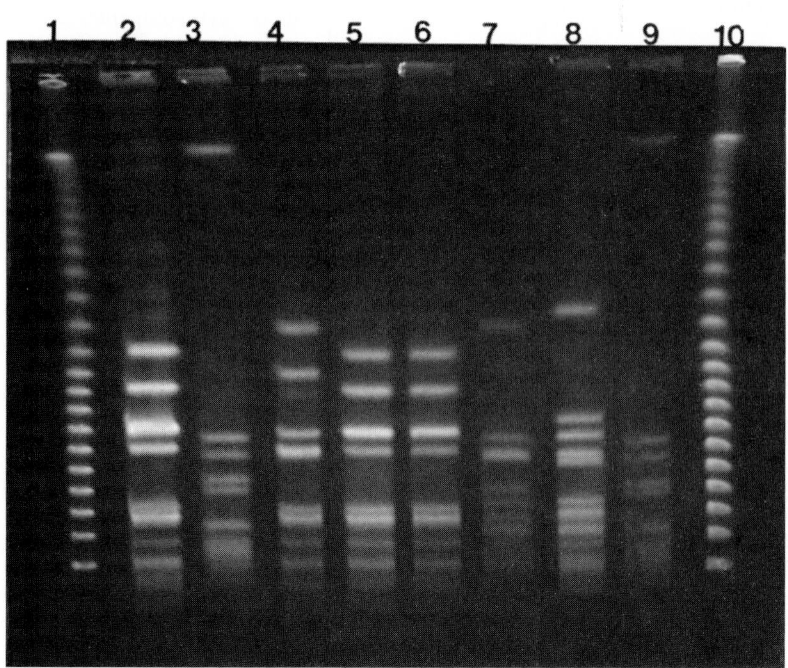

Figure 28.1. Pulsed-field gel electrophoresis (PFGE) of *Staphylococcus aureus* strains from a neonatal intensive care unit in Toronto. Genomic DNA was isolated from 0.75 mL of an overnight culture, formed into acrylic agarose plugs, digested with *Sma*I, and electrophoresed at 12°C for 24 hours on a CHEF-DR pulsed-field apparatus. Lanes 1 and 10 are molecular weight controls. Lanes 2, 5, 8, and 9 are from neonates with bacteremia. Strains in lanes 5 and 6 have the same restriction pattern, whereas the other patterns are all different. (Courtesy of Dr. Don Low.)

over a 4-year period, two epidemic clones comprised almost 90% of the strains (49). Such studies can help determine if clonal fitness is more important than antibiotic selection in determining the predominance of a clone.

Other infrequent-cutting restriction endonucleases can be used with PFGE. Another study identified 8 to 22 well-resolved *Sst*II fragments with good integral reproducibility. Using more than one band difference, 23 types of MRSA were identified. MRSA was found to be more closely related (one predominant type) than MSSA. Strains similar by PFGE were also epidemiologically related. REAP was also good, but only bands higher than 2.5 kb were analyzed. Strains were considered the same if differences of fewer than three bands existed. Using the same strains, only 50% were phage typeable. The authors concluded that clonality should be determined in the frame of reference of the ongoing study using contemporary alike and different control strains to derive the definition of same (51). PFGE has also been used successfully to discriminate between strains of *S. aureus* isolated from patients and strains isolated from personnel (52).

Although PFGE is highly discriminatory and reproducible within a laboratory, methods and technician experience differ among various laboratories and lead to differences that may arise in gel appearance and difficulties when comparing results from different laboratories. Matching of PFGE types from different sources to implicate spread from one source to another has been recently facilitated through standardization of methods and conditions for performing PFGE among ten European PFGE laboratories (53). This standardization practice was termed "harmonization."

A third method of analyzing genomic DNA is RFLP. This method compares the size of a group of restriction fragments, within which a specific gene or genes can be located. Probes constructed to detect a known sequence are labeled by isotopic or nonisotopic methods and hybridized to restriction fragments of chromosomal DNA. Probes highlight restriction site heterogeneity particularly when a gene is located in multiple or variable sites (54). For example, the use of *Tn*554, a transposon common in MRSA (not MSSA), and an insertion element, IS256, have identified epidemiologically related strains (54,55). Gentamicin-resistant *S. aureus* strains also contain IS256 as part of the gentamicin resistance transposon *Tn*4001. The distribution of this element is not uniform in the bacterial chromosome (56). At least 16 types were identified by RFLP of gentamicin-resistant strains.

Ribotyping also capitalizes on RFLP. This method employs as a probe ribosomal RNA, which hybridizes to the 23s, 16s, and 5s ribosomal protein genes that occur in 1 to 11 copies within the bacterial chromosome. Ribotyping of *S. aureus* has been compared with three other typing systems. Although 12 highly similar patterns resulted, the authors felt that epidemiologically related strains were discriminated (57). It could be argued, however, that the lack of variability of the ribotype pattern might limit the usefulness of this method in the analysis of other outbreaks. Our own experience revealed marked similarities in the ribotype pattern among epidemiologically related and unrelated strains.

Gene polymorphisms, a method based on interstrain differences in specific genes, may prove to be a useful approach to differentiate *S. aureus* strains (58). For example, the coagulase gene contains a variable region at its 3′ end based on an 81 base pair repeated section that results in numerous allelic variants. An *Alu*I restriction site occurs within some of these 81 base pair segments. PCR of the fragment at the 3′ termini of the coagulase gene followed by *Alu*I digestion discriminated among *S. aureus* strains and identified a cluster of epidemiologically related MRSA. This method identified 19 distinct groups and was more discriminating than MEE. Because some *S. aureus* strains will not hybridize to the selected PCR primer, this method is more limited than REAP or PFGE.

Newer methods like repetitive element sequence-based PCR and random amplified polymorphic DNA employ single short primers with arbitrary nucleotide sequences for amplification of genomic DNA (59,60). Not all strains hybridize with a given random primer; thus, the method may require the use of multiple primers and may not discriminate as well as PFGE. Once additional primers are needed, the expense and labor of this method approach those of PFGE. Reproducibility within and between laboratories may make these two primer based methods less useful for temporally or geographically diverse collections of strains.

Analysis of sequence similarity of ubiquitous genes such as protein A may add additional discrimination to that afforded by PFGE and RFLP due to lineage-specific polymorphisms, probably due to the number of repeats of these genes (61). Comparison of such sequences may be particularly useful in analyzing the evolution of clones of MSSA and MRSA that have become endemic in many hospitals (61). (For a general discussion of microbial typing techniques, see Chapter 102.)

A recently published method termed multilocus sequence typing (MLST) has been used for analyzing large collections of bacterial strains from several genera (Table 28.3). This method overcomes the problems with reproducibility and interpretation created by gel-based DNA typing systems. In this method for typing *S. aureus*, seven housekeeping genes have been chosen from 14 genes analyzed that exist with frequent but minute variations in DNA sequence (Fig. 28.2). Published primers are used to amplify segments from each of these housekeeping genes. The amplified fragments are then sequenced and submitted to the MLST Web site for comparison to known allelic variants. Based on the gene sequence of each of the seven alleles, a sequence type (ST) is determined. Further comparisons between STs can be performed using one of several algorithms. BURST is one such algorithm *(www.mlst.net)*. Clonal complexes consisting of related groups of strains are thus generated. This strategy has been used to show marked similarities among a highly diverse

TABLE 28.3. HOUSEKEEPING GENES AMPLIFIED BY MULTILOCUS SEQUENCE TYPING (MLST) PRIMERS

arc	Carbamate kinase
aro	Shikimate dehydrogenase
glp	Glycerol kinase
gmk	Guanylate kinase
pta	Phosphate acetyltransferase
tpi	Triosephosphate isomerase
yqi	Acetyl coenzyme A acetyltransferase

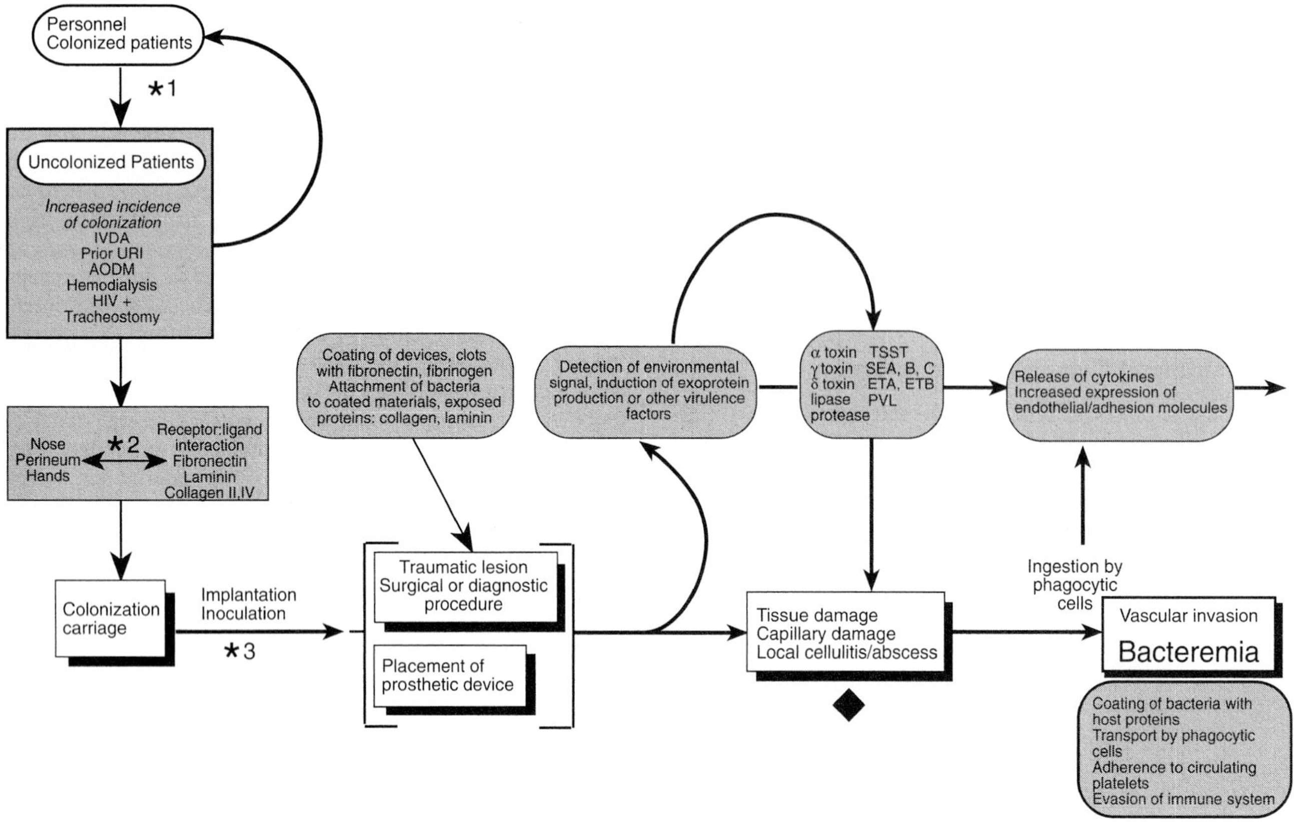

Figure 28.2. Pathogenesis of nosocomial infection caused by *Staphylococcus aureus*. *Potential strategies to interrupt the development of a nosocomial *S. aureus* infection: 1, barrier precautions, decolonization procedures; 2, bacterial receptor [microbial surface components recognizing adhesive matrix molecules (MSCRAMMs)] antagonists, competitive colonization; 3, perioperative prophylaxis, antibiotic impregnated materials, materials to which *S. aureus* adheres poorly; 4, prompt institution of effective antimicrobials, cytokine antagonists, MSCRAMM inhibitors; 5, prolonged treatment of bacteremia to cure foci of metastatic infection.

collection of MRSA and MSSA (62). This method is the most discriminatory method available currently because of the large number of possible sequence types that can potentially exist. The ability to perform PCR and rapid DNA sequencing have limited this method to research laboratories. However, it should be possible for commercial or university laboratories to adopt the methods and rapidly sequence PCR products generated from epidemiologically important isolates. Aires de Sousa and de Lencastre (63) combined the MLST technique with RFLP for tracking genomic islands that may insert into different genetic backgrounds to show elegantly the evolution of MRSA strains from ancestral MSSA strains.

PATHOGENESIS OF NOSOCOMIAL INFECTIONS

Clinical laboratories have observed an increased incidence of bacteremia caused by *S. aureus* since 1980 (64). In a study of hospital-acquired bacteremia of unknown origin, both *S. aureus* and *Pseudomonas aeruginosa* caused 15% of the cases (65). *S. aureus* also caused 50% of catheter-related bacteremias, the majority of infections associated with insertion of prosthetic materials, and the majority of cases of septic arthritis and osteomyelitis. Understanding the pathogenesis of such a diverse group of infections arising both in the community and in the hospital can be approached by examining the stages of host–pathogen interaction: colonization, attachment, adherence, tissue damage, invasion, dissemination, and metastatic infection (Fig. 28.2) (3).

Colonization

Relationship of Colonization to Infection

The major reservoir of *S. aureus* is the anterior nares. Carriage there influences carriage at other sites, including the axillae, perineum, denuded dermis, and mucous membranes (3,66–68). People may harbor *S. aureus* persistently or intermittently, with intermittent carriage occurring in as much as 90% of a sampled population (3,69). Factors that promote colonization include coincident respiratory infection, prolonged hospitalization, needle use (as in intravenous drug users), diabetics, patients requiring hemodialysis and patients receiving allergy shots, exposure to cold weather, and dermatologic conditions such as eczema (3,70). The elderly, even when they are inpatients, seem to have no higher rate of colonization (71). Antibiotic administration also promotes an ecologic, nasal niche, perhaps through

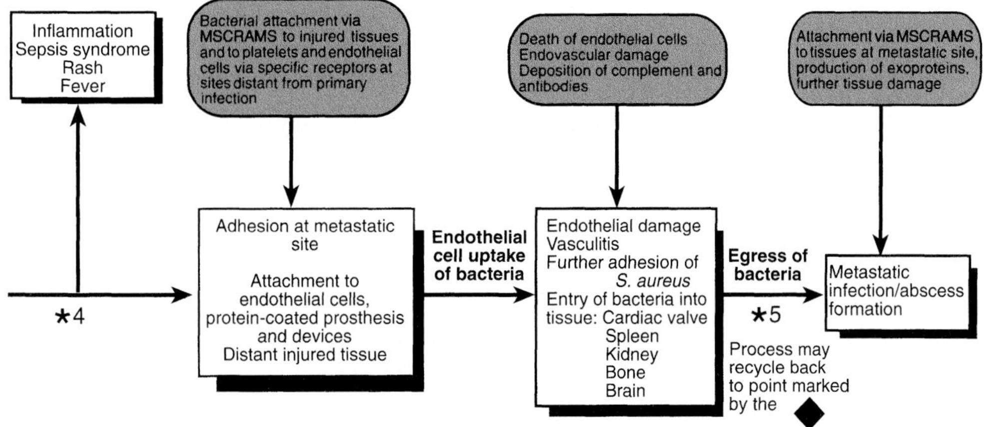

Figure 28.2. *Continued.*

alteration of normal flora that is known to provide resistance to *S. aureus* colonization (72). Once a patient is colonized with *S. aureus*, the particular strain may disseminate by person-to-person contact, particularly by spread on the hands of personnel (73), or by the dispersion of *S. aureus* carried on rafts of desquamated skin (74). In this manner, *S. aureus* strains spread among hospitalized patients. Colonization with *S. aureus* is an important risk factor, since it usually precedes infection. The importance of concomitant colonization is shown by analysis of pathogens in surgical site infections (SSIs) and device-related infections. SSI rates were higher in colonized patients than in noncolonized patients (75,76). This relationship is also quantitative: when the density of colonizing flora exceeds 10^6 colony-forming units (CFU), rates of postoperative infections are higher among carriers than among noncarriers. Patients in one surgical ICU study who were nasal carriers not only induced cross-colonization but also were significantly more likely to incur a staphylococcal infection than noncarriers (77). Treatment upon admission to the ICU with nasal antistaphylococcal ointment was associated with a lower rate of *S. aureus* colonization while in the ICU. RFLP patterns were identical for those strains colonizing the nares and causing SSI. Molecular analysis has been used in clusters of SSIs after heart operations to show identity between the nasal strain and the strains isolated from SSIs or blood (78).

The relationship between nasal carriage and subsequent SSIs is not straightforward. For example, in a study of 414 patients undergoing elective surgery in Khartoum, Sudan, only 6 of the 98 nasal carriers incurred SSIs caused by the strain inhabiting the nose (79). Besides demonstrating that nasal carriage was not a significant risk factor for development of SSI, the elegant molecular analysis further demonstrated that noncarriers were at significant risk of acquiring an independent SSI caused by strains with a high degree of genetic heterogeneity.

Further implicating *S. aureus* carriage, the same strains colonizing nonsurgical patients on admission are often the infecting strains (68). Specifically, the same strain colonizing the noses of drug addicts with endocarditis is recovered from blood cultures. Hemodialysis patients are more frequently infected if anterior nares are colonized; 93% of hemodialysis-related infections are caused by the phage type colonizing the anterior nares (80). The same relationship between colonizing and infecting strains was observed for patients on peritoneal dialysis. Nasal carriers had a fourfold higher incidence of dialysis catheter exit site infections (81). It has been estimated that there is a 4% to 16% probability of catheter loss in patients with *S. aureus* peritonitis who are nasal carriers, compared with a negligible risk for noncarriers (82). Finally, in hospitalized patients there may be preferential colonization of nonnasal sites, e.g., the oropharynx in patients undergoing long-term endotracheal intubation (83). Patients admitted to a large hospital in Meunster, Germany, who developed *S. aureus* bacteremia were found to be infected 80% of the time with their own nasal colonizing strain (2). MRSA strains were not a problem at the time of that study. A larger analysis done in Oxford, England, of the relationship of nasal colonizing strains to subsequent invasive disease was conducted by Day et al. (84) using MLST exclusively for characterizing isolates. The major implication of this landmark study was to show that hypercolonizing community strains mirror the invasive strains, thus having far-reaching implications for infection control in the community as well as in the hospital.

Adherence and Attachment

Once a *S. aureus* strain contacts a new patient, the strain must adhere to tissue or a surface; this is a crucial step in the initiation of infection. Access and adherence to host tissues or implanted materials is probably mediated by a surface receptor that involves host protein interactions. More specifically, the interaction occurs between adhesins of the bacterial cell wall surface and target structures of the eukaryotic cell. For procedures in which foreign materials are implanted or that result in a thrombus at the surgical site, plasma proteins are immediately deposited on the materials. Host proteins then act as bridging molecules in the adherence of *S. aureus* to protein-coated surfaces (85).

Adherence is mediated by a group of surface protein adhesins called microbial surface components recognizing adhesive matrix molecules (MSCRAMMs) and regulated by the *sar/agr* system (7,86). There are three major groups of MSCRAMMs depending on whether they bind fibronectin, collagen, or fibrinogen.

Early adhesion is facilitated by upregulation of *sar*-mediated MSCRAMMs. Furthermore, *Sar*S, a *sar* homologue is an activator of *S. aureus* protein A (87) (Fig. 28.3).

S. aureus binding can be blocked by antibodies specific for a particular receptor (88). An additional effect of staphylococcal-protein interaction may allow evasion of the immune system (89). Binding of host proteins to the staphylococcal cell wall effectively coats the bacteria and may prevent host recognition of the microbe. *S. aureus* may also adhere to uncoated foreign material through electrostatic forces. This interaction is mediated by surface charge and hydrophobicity of the material and bacteria. *S. aureus* has a net negative charge due to ribitol teichoic acid and protein A (90). Multiple receptors probably exist that facilitate binding to a variety of tissue substrates. Therefore, prevention of infection may require blockade of more than one receptor.

Studies that examine the binding of *S. aureus* to an extracellular matrix typically use a foreign material such as methylmethacrylate coated with a specific protein. Except for albumin, which markedly diminishes *S. aureus* binding to polymethylmethacrylate (PMMA), most host proteins augment attachment. For example, *S. aureus* binding to PMMA is markedly enhanced when fibronectin is present, and this binding is not strain dependent. Fibronectin coats implanted prosthetic material and plastic surfaces and is a major component of the fibrin matrix of clots. Staphylococcal adherence to fibrin clots is increased in the pres-

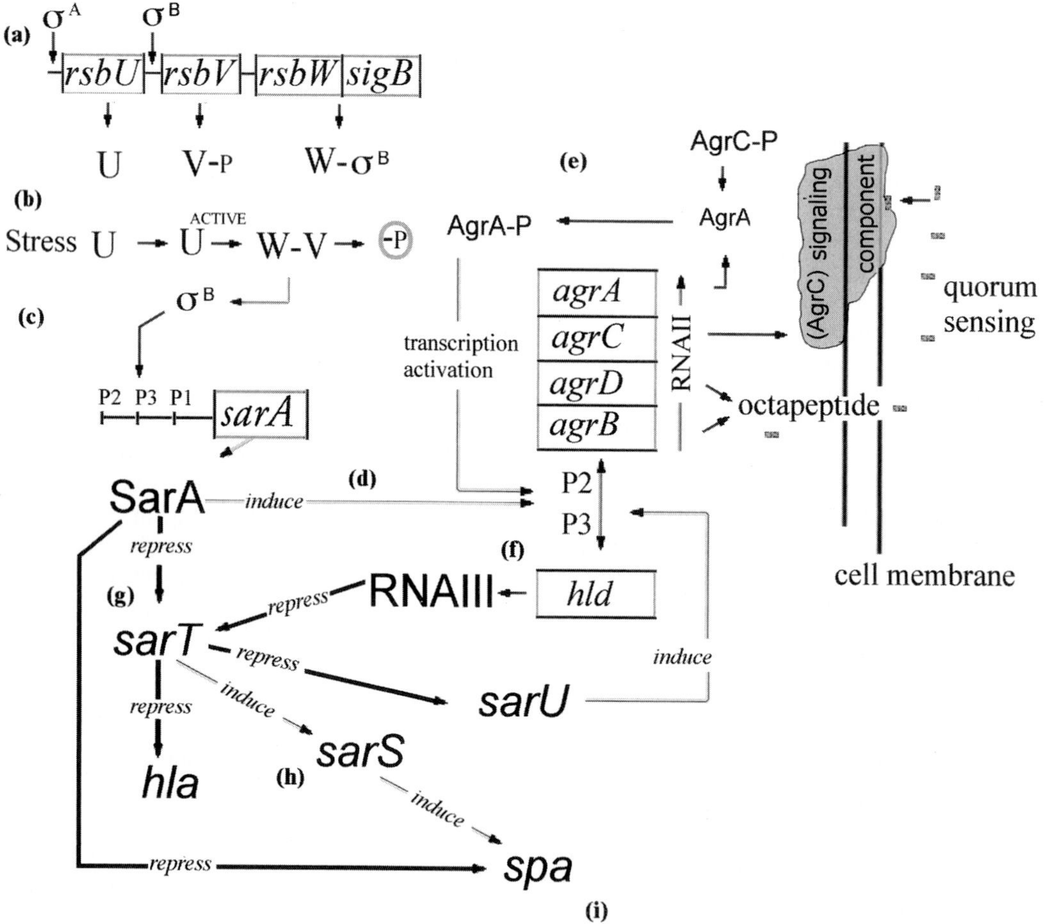

Figure 28.3. Overview of the predicted regulatory pathways involved in gene expression for *S. aureus:* (a) the *sigB* operon, transcribed under regulation of τ^A, encodes *rsbU, rsbV, rsbW,* and *sigB*. RsbW is an anti-τ^B factor that binds to τ^B, blocking its activity; (b) stress (e.g., high temperature, high osmolarity, or low pH) activates RsbU to dephosphorylate RsbV. RsbV binds to RsbW, releasing τ^B; (c) τ^B binds to a consensus sequence on the *sarA* P3 promoter, activating transcription of *sar*A (as well as other promoters); (d) *sar*A binds to the interpromoter region between P2 and P3 of the accessory gene (*agr*) locus, stimulating transcription of *agr* RNAII, which encodes *agrB, agrD, agrC,* and *agrA*, elements of a two-component quorum-sensing system. *Agr*B and *agr*D produce an octapeptide that diffuses through the membrane to bind to and activate *agr*C, a membrane-associated signaling component; (e) activated *agr*C phosphorylates *agr*A, which induces transcription of *agr* RNAIII; (f) RNAIII, a pleiotropic regulator for expression of virulence proteins, represses *sarT*; (g) increased expression of *sarT* during exponential growth causes repression of *sarU,* an inducer of RNAIII expression. *Sar*T represses expression of *hla* (encoding α-hemolysin), and induces expression of *sarS*; and (h) *sar*S induces expression of *spa* (protein A). *Sar*A represses expression of *spa*. (Courtesy of Katherine A. Schmidt and Ambrose Cheung.)

ence of fibronectin (91). Binding to fibronectin is mediated by two related fibronectin-binding proteins, FnBPA and FnBPB, that have specific ligand binding domains that recognize the N terminal and the C terminal region of fibronectin. When fibronectin coats surfaces, the N terminal end enhances binding of *S. aureus*. Fibronectin also binds well to albumin-coated substances and mediates the adherence of *S. aureus* to collagen, endothelial cells, fibroblasts, platelets, and platelet-fibrin thrombi (92). Strains of *S. aureus* that bind avidly to fibronectin are more likely to produce endocarditis in a rabbit model of catheter-induced endocarditis, probably because fibronectin first is deposited on valvular endothelial cells traumatized by the catheter (93). In another experiment, fibronectin binding was shown to be crucial in the pathogenesis of endocarditis. Fibronectin-binding deficient mutants were less likely to adhere to damaged heart valves than was the intact parent strain (94).

Similar interactions between *S. aureus* and other surfaces may also initiate infection. Fibrinogen enhances *S. aureus* binding to and may be preferentially deposited on intravenous (IV) devices (95,96). Staphylococcal clumping factor has been shown to be the staphylococcal surface protein that binds to fibrinogen (97, 98). Phase 2 clinical trials are underway to assess the therapeutic value of products that block clumping factor (99). Laminin, a major component of the basement membrane, also binds *S. aureus* by a specific receptor like fibronectin. However, only a small enhancement of *S. aureus* binding to PMMA was shown (85). Laminin binding may not be a significant factor in the production of intravascular infections, since laminin serum levels are so low. On the other hand, there may be a role for laminin in the production of primary tissue infections, since basement membrane may be exposed after traumatic injury to epithelial surfaces (100).

S. aureus binds to heparin and other glycosaminoglycans by two bacterial cell wall–associated proteins. Glycosaminoglycans are linked with proteins to form proteoglycans and are found in connective tissue, basement membranes, and eukaryotic cell surfaces. These substances bind to heparinized catheters (101); however, the binding is not specific. Other components of connective tissue bind *S. aureus* as well. Type IV collagen binds less avidly than fibronectin and laminin to *S. aureus* (102) but is exposed at the site of tissue injury. Adherence of *S. aureus* to type IV collagen is enhanced in the presence of fibronectin. In addition, *S. aureus* binds to type II collagen by a unique receptor, which has been cloned and sequenced. Strains with type II collagen receptors isolated from patients with osteomyelitis and septic arthritis were shown to bind well to cartilage (89). Cutaneous injury may promote exteriorization of cytocollagen 10, providing substrate binding not possible in normal skin (103,104).

Götz (105) has recently summarized the genetic and molecular basis of biofilm formation in staphylococci, initiated first by the adherence of cells to a surface and second by accumulation to form multilayered cell clusters. The so-called slime substance is a polysaccharide composed of beta-1,6-linked *N*-acetyl glucosamines with partly deacetylated residues. Mutations in the corresponding biosynthesis genes (*ica* operon) lead to a pleiotropic phenotype wherein staphylococcal cells are less adherent and invasive. Several biofilm-negative mutants have been isolated in which polysaccharide intercellular adhesin (106) production appears to be unaffected. Other proteins involved in biofilm formation include accumulation-associated protein (AAP), the clumping factor A (ClfA), the staphylococcal surface protein (SSP1), and the biofilm-associated protein (Bap). New antimicrobials are needed that penetrate and disrupt biofilm formation or that are combined with new polymers to resist adherence and attachment (105).

Virulence and Invasion

Several regulatory systems that control virulence have been described in *S. aureus* (Fig. 28.3). The most important of these are *sar* and *agr*, both affecting RNAIII, which is a global effector molecule capable of upregulating transcription of many staphylococcal virulence genes. Ironically, staphylococcal binding to platelets also causes release of platelet-bound peptide antibiotics that may ameliorate local infection (3). The production of specific virulence factors by staphylococci results in a complicated cascade of effects depending on the interaction of the regulatory components present. The effects that cause the most severe infections may be produced by strains that harbor a particular complement of regulatory and toxin encoding genes.

Early events in abscess formation are *sar* mediated. Subsequent exoprotein and toxin production is regulated by *agr*. There are 34 known exoproteins elaborated by *S. aureus* and their genetic determinants are grouped in pathogenicity islands throughout the chromosome. Certain proteins are highly toxic and are considered virulence factors. These enterotoxins (A, B, $X_{1,2,3}$, Δ, and E) and toxic shock syndrome toxin-1 (TSST-1) compose a related family of toxins causing staphylococcal food poisoning and toxic shock syndrome and act as superantigens once they enter the systemic circulation (107). Superantigens cause activation of certain T-cell populations, and subsequent cytokine production overwhelms the immune system, preventing a coordinated response to antigen processing. The net result of this activation, paradoxically, is similar to endotoxin-induced shock wherein excessive quantities of cytokines induce tissue damage (3,108).

More limited in activity, the epidermolytic toxins (ETAs), exfoliatins A and B specifically, attack the epidermis, causing exfoliation seen in toxic epidermal necrolysis (TEN) and staphylococcal scalded skin syndrome (SSSS). The gene for *ETA* is located on the chromosome, whereas the exfoliatin B gene *(etb)* is located on a plasmid. The major pathologic effect of these toxins occurs at a site remote from the site of infection.

Unlike enterotoxins and exfoliative toxins, membrane-damaging toxins produce damage at the site of infection. α-Toxin (heat labile), one of four known hemolysins (α, β, γ, δ), is a major pathogenic factor in that it produces tissue damage after the establishment of infection (109–111). Using allelic replacement to create isogeneic toxin-positive and toxin-negative strains, no lesions were generated by the toxin-negative strain in a murine model of mastitis (111). α-Toxin is the only staphylococcal toxin known to damage actively growing nucleated animal cells and is both dermonecrotic and lethal (30 μg/kg) in a murine model (109,111,112). When α-toxin is injected subcutaneously, vasoconstriction and subsequent tissue ischemia result

(113). β-Toxin (a heat labile sphingomyelinase) and δ-toxin (a heat stable peptide) are dermonecrotic at high doses but are less potent than α-toxin (109,114). β-Toxin is not produced in many strains because of a converting phage inserted in the *hlb* gene (112). A staphylokinase (SAK) is carried by the phage and upregulated by *agr*. SAK-deficient isolates were more than four times as likely to cause a fatal outcome (115). Nasal strains conversely were much more likely to have SAK intact.

The δ-toxin peptide is a 26-residue translation product of the *hla* gene located near the 5′ end of RNAIII encoded by the *agr* locus. Leukocidin (heat labile), which is toxic to neutrophils and macrophages, also is a potent dermonecrotic toxin (114). It is composed of two proteins, F (32 kd) and S (38 kd), and induces formation of a transmembrane potassium channel (116). Both components are necessary for toxicity. Leukocidin and γ-toxin belong to the same family of bicomponent toxins (117). The genes for all the dermotoxins *(hla, hlb, hld, hlg)* are located in the chromosome. Panton-Valentine leukocidin (PVL)-expressing strains of *S. aureus* carry an increased risk for necrotizing and fatal pneumonia among community-acquired cases of MRSA infection but the extent of the PVL determinant in MSSA strains is not as well studied (118).

Other exoproteins, such as proteases, collagenase, hyaluronidase, and lipase, probably act as virulence enhancers and are not as destructive to tissues (112). Although staphylococcal exoproteins are otherwise dissimilar, the expression of at least 12 genes (including α- and β-toxins, exfolitins, enterotoxins B, D, TSST-1, proteases, protein A, and coagulase) are upregulated by an accessory gene regulator *(agr)* (119). The *agr* locus is involved in a two-component regulatory system controlling the expression of virulence genes in other bacteria (120). Other regulatory elements, several of which are *Sar* homologs, have been recently identified. Thus, the complexity of the regulatory elements suggest that virulence factor expression is most likely responding to a variety of environmental and physiologic conditions specific to the host.

Dissemination and Metastatic Infection

After the establishment of local infection, *S. aureus* may disseminate to other sites. Spread of microorganisms from a localized cutaneous infection to the bloodstream and then to deep tissue to form abscesses or to cause endocarditis requires access to the bloodstream and rebinding to potential target sites. In part, *S. aureus* may gain access to the capillary vascular tree as a result of local inflammation and tissue damage invoked by specific highly regulated exoproteins. Phagocytic cells may also contribute to vascular entry by carrying viable microorganisms back into the capillaries. Once entry into the bloodstream occurs, binding to serum proteins would follow, and eventually bacteria might stick to a target cell bearing a receptor to either a staphylococcal cell wall component or a serum component bound to the staphylococcal cell wall.

S. aureus can also bind to platelets (121,122) and the binding may increase the capacity of platelets to bind to injured endothelium. Thus, staphylococci may be transported to a distant site and establish a metastatic focus. The ability of bacteria to bind to platelets correlates with the capacity to induce infective endocarditis. *S. aureus*, with its high capacity to bind platelets, more often caused endocarditis in an animal model than did *Escherichia coli,* with its minimal platelet-binding capacity. Binding of staphylococci to platelets is direct, rapid, and saturable, suggesting that this property is receptor mediated and dependent on the number of receptors present. Platelet binding is not dependent on protein A. The staphylococcal ligand is most likely a surface carbohydrate and, perhaps, capsular based. This ligand is resistant to proteases and susceptible to agents that modify carbohydrates and specific anticapsular antigens (123).

After dissemination, *S. aureus* must attach to distant tissues to cause a metastatic suppurative infection. Metastatic infections may develop through interactions of blood-borne staphylococci and endothelial cells. These infections may involve endovascular structures or deep tissues. This may be due, in part, to the higher degree of attachment and invasion of endovascular tissue exhibited by staphylococci (124). The interaction of endothelial cells and *S. aureus* is so efficient that these bacteria adhere to uninjured endothelial cells. Affinity for a specific site usually leads to infection at that site; *E. coli* microorganisms have been shown to attach to specific uroepithelial cell receptors, and this interaction is a prerequisite for urinary tract infection (125). *S. aureus* appears to have a specific receptor for endothelial cell surface proteins, which promotes adherence and, perhaps, the initiation of endocarditis and graft infections. As with platelet binding, bacteria that bind avidly to endothelial cells are more likely to cause endocarditis than bacteria that bind poorly and consequently rarely cause endocarditis (126). Thus, *S. aureus* more often causes endocarditis in clinical and experimental settings than does *E. coli.*

S. aureus is also a common cause of prosthetic valve endocarditis. Binding of *S. aureus* to a porcine cardiac valve is a specific receptor-mediated event. In this instance, a binding protein of 120 kd was identified as a potential receptor. This protein was not related to fibronectin. Unlike injured tissues, fibronectin may not augment *S. aureus* binding to endothelial cells. No fibronectin is expressed on the luminal surface of endothelial cells, and no fibronectin is produced by valvular endothelial cells (127). However, fibronectin may augment the binding of *S. aureus* to injured endothelial surfaces. If fibronectin binding is blocked, there is a decrease in adherence to subendothelial surfaces exposed after endothelial injury (128).

Investigators have also shown that endothelial cells ingest attached staphylococci. A 50-kd protein from umbilical vein endothelial cell membrane binds to *S. aureus* and facilitates uptake into endothelial cells (129). This protein was shown to be different from fibronectin using a fibronectin antibody assay. Binding is also specific, since albumin or fibrinogen does not inhibit this interaction. Bovine aortic endothelial cells actively phagocytosed *S. aureus*; 65% of bacteria applied to the endothelial cells were ingested. This action can be blocked by cytochalasin B and was independent of fibronectin and complement (130,131). Complement-activated endothelial cells, conversely, have increased fibronectin binding. Although *S. aureus* cells that were ingested did not multiply within endothelial cells, the endothelial cells eventually died, leading to exposed subendothelial surfaces. Adherence alone does not induce apoptosis since studies show that viable intracellular *S. aureus* is needed to induce apoptosis (132). Ingestion and endothelial cell death, however, do depend on strain and inoculum (133). The clinical impact, ultimately, is that intracellular *S. aureus* may not be affected by most antibiotics, particularly β-lactams, that fail to penetrate eukaryotic cells. Endothelial cell infection would consequently initiate invasion and infection of deeper tissues.

Subsequent interactions between the ingested *S. aureus* and the endothelial cell may lead to local vascular damage. Uptake of *S. aureus* by endothelial cells also increases expression of Fc receptors on the cell surface, hypothetically initiating vasculitis by the adherence of neutrophils and platelets to the endothelial cells. Immune complex deposition would next activate complement or initiate the coagulation cascade. These events could augment further metastatic seeding and invasion (134). Finally, host factors elicited by extravascular infection may alter endothelial cells and increase bacterial adherence. For example, staphylococcal adherence to vascular endothelium is upregulated by *sar* and enhanced in the presence of tissue necrosis factor-α (TNF-α). TNF may further increase the endothelial leukocyte adhesion molecule-1 (ELAM) and intracellular adhesion molecule-1 (ICAM) (135). Also, the exposure of endothelial cells to lipopolysaccharide increases adherence of bacteria. This effect is duplicated by incubation of cells with the cytokine interleukin-1 (136). Classic agents like aspirin downregulate many pathways associated with complications of endothelial infection and by downregulating global staphylococcal regulons, create novel therapeutic strategies (123).

Specific capsular types of *S. aureus* play a critical role in abscess induction, as well as in avoiding host phagocytic uptake. Capsules are produced by most clinical strains, and serotype 5 and 8 together account for up to 50% of clinical isolates (137).

More than 80% of nosocomial isolates from bacteremic patients produce capsule type 5 or type 8 (27). Clinical strains with a type 5 or 8 capsule are more resistant to opsonophagocytosis (138). In a mouse bacteremia model of infection a capsule type 5 strain sustained a higher level of bacteremia than two capsule-defective mutants, likely due to the antiphagocytic nature of CP5 since *in vitro* assays indicated that the parental strain was only susceptible to phagocytic killing by human polymorphonuclear leukocytes (PMNs) in the presence of capsular antibodies and complement (139,140). Although capsule types 1 and 2 confer resistance to complement-mediated opsonophagocytosis by PMNs, strains producing these capsule types do not cause clinical disease. CP5 production has also been shown to block adherence of *S. aureus* to endothelial cells in culture (141). Similarly, in a rat model of catheter-induced *S. aureus* endocarditis, both the type 5 and 8 parental strains are less pathogenic when compared with capsule-deficient mutant strains (142). These findings suggest that CP5 and CP8 may interfere with staphylococcal attachment to the damaged aortic valve *in vivo.* Data from mouse models show that a capsule-defective mutant fails to persist in the murine nares (143). Ways to exploit these observations to reduce the risk of nosocomial infection await further study.

SCOPE OF NOSOCOMIAL INFECTIONS CAUSED BY *S. AUREUS*

Bacteremia and Endocarditis

Bacteremia is a dreaded sequel of localized *S. aureus* infection that often results in production of metastatic foci in almost any organ. *S. aureus* bacteremia is hospital-acquired 20% to 60% of the time, depending on the preponderance of certain variables such as intravenous drug users in the population at large (144, 145). Up to 30% of patients with bacteremia fail to be cured when treated with parenteral antimicrobials (146). In the recently completed Surveillance and Control of Pathogens of Epidemiologic Importance (SCOPE) program, *S. aureus* was the second most common cause of nosocomial bacteremia, with its coagulase-negative counterpart ranking first. Of 2,340 strains of staphylococci reported, 787 were *S. aureus*, 602 *S. epidermidis*, 61 *S. haemolyticus*, 45 *S. hominis*, and the rest different staphylococcal species (147). One third of the cases of community-acquired *S. aureus* bacteremia are associated with endocarditis (145). In the preantibiotic era, as many as 15% of patients with nosocomial staphylococcal bacteremia developed endocarditis, whereas one modern study uncovered no cases of endocarditis associated with nosocomial staphylococcemia, perhaps because of the preponderance of hospital infections associated with IV catheters (145). Conversely, in hospitalized patients with prosthetic valves, *S. aureus* bacteremia often results in the development of new endocarditis (146).

Nosocomial *S. aureus* bacteremia has been closely studied over the last 50 years (148,149). The variable rate of all *S. aureus* bacteremias that are acquired in the hospital—40% to 60%—depends on the type of patients treated at the individual institution (144,149). In 1989 the rate of *S. aureus* bloodstream infections per 1,000 discharges was lowest in small nonteaching and large nonteaching hospitals (0.46 and 0.44, respectively) and higher in small teaching and large teaching hospitals (0.89 and 1.13, respectively) (150). The rate is also increasing in long-term-care facilities, where *S. aureus* is the most common species causing bacteremia and accounts for about 15% of all cases (151). In some countries new MRSA strains may be particularly virulent and produce epidemics alongside endemic MSSA bacteremia (152). The concern about the rising risk of bacteremic strains being MRSA led workers at Detroit Receiving Hospital to develop a prediction model. The model earmarks patients with a history of hospitalization, a longer hospitalization, comorbid conditions, and exposure to antimicrobials as at risk for MRSA bacteremia, whether hospital or community associated (153).

Patients most susceptible to *S. aureus* bacteremia have underlying conditions such as cirrhosis, diabetes, chronic obstructive pulmonary disease, congestive heart failure, and renal failure requiring dialysis. In one fourth of bacteremic patients, however, the source cannot be found (149). Patients who have the greatest change in their Acute Physiology and Chronic Health Evaluation (APACHE II) score after admission to an ICU tend to have the worst outcome (154). Interestingly, nasal MRSA carriage had a relative risk for bacteremia of 3.9 compared to MSSA carriage in 488 patients admitted to an ICU (154). The severity of illness induced by *S. aureus* bacteremia relates to the risk of dying, but poor outcome was not associated with poor opsonic activity (154). Over the last 20 years, the proportion of nosocomial bacteremias associated with vascular access devices has increased to 30% to 59% (149,155,156). At Crawford Long Hospital in Atlanta, the number of device-related bacteremias increased eightfold from 1980–1983 to 1990–1993 (157).

Some studies suggest that part of the increase may be due to the emergence of certain clonal strains sharing a common phage type. For example, in a Danish study of 15,000 strains of *S. aureus* isolated from patients with bacteremia from 1977 to 1989, phage type 95 increased from 3.8% to 18.8% during a time when no methicillin resistance was detected (158). Follow-up Danish studies indicate that MSSA is the primary cause of staphylococcal bacteremia and that death is most often associated with septic shock, age over 60, and a daily dose of a penicillinase-stable penicillin less than 4 g (159).

Adults and children with leukemia or cancer (160), particularly those with granulocytopenia, are also at high risk for *S. aureus* bacteremia associated either with the persistent nature of their *S. aureus* nasal carriage (161) or with preventive antimicrobial chemotherapy. The rate of *S. aureus* bacteremia in patients with cancer increased from 5% in 1973 to 30% by 1979 (162), though in Japan the reported rate was 6% (163). Interestingly, in a group of patients with leukemia who developed *S. aureus* bacteremia, endocarditis was an unusual outcome (164).

Patients with human immunodeficiency virus (HIV) infection are also at increased risk of acquiring *S. aureus* bacteremia; half of these cases are nosocomial (165). IV catheters were considered the likely source of nosocomial bacteremia. Both nosocomial and community-acquired cases had a higher rate of late complications (35%) than was reported in earlier studies not involving HIV-infected patients. Hospitalized hemophiliacs with acquired immunodeficiency syndrome (AIDS) compared to non-AIDS control subjects tended to have *S. aureus* bacteremia more frequently; this association was again related to increased exposure to antibiotics and central IV catheters (166). In HIV-infected patients, colonization and infection due to MRSA are related to prior hospitalization, exposure to broad-spectrum antibiotics, presence of dermatologic disease, and presence of a central venous catheter (167,168) (see Chapter 57).

Bacteremia isolates of *S. aureus* contain, as Becker et al. (169) describe, an habitual feature of classical members of the pyrogenic toxin superantigen (PTSAg) gene family comprising the staphylococcal enterotoxin (SE) genes *sea-see* and the TSST-1 gene test (169). PTSAg/ET genes *seg* and *sei* were found in combination by a multiplex PCR in 55% of strains, which were found strictly in combination in 55.0% of the *S. aureus* isolates tested. The *tst* gene was found in 20.3%. Overall, about half of *S. aureus* isolates tested harbored genes of the classical members of the PTSAg family and ETs (50.8%), and an even higher percentage if the newer toxin genes were included. Newer biologic therapies may be necessary to ameliorate the effect of groups of toxins.

Burns

S. aureus is a threat to patients with burns throughout the course of their treatment. Burns units worldwide continue to report *S. aureus* along with *P. aeruginosa* as the major pathogens affecting these patients (170). In a Brazilian burn unit from 1993 to 1999, 55% of 320 patients developed hospital infection, with primary bloodstream infection in 189 patients being the most common (171). Overall, *S. aureus* was responsible for 24% of all infections, followed by *P. aeruginosa* (18%) and *Acinetobacter* species (14%). Modern topical therapy reduces the concentration of microorganisms on the burn wound surface, and thus the potential for cross-infection (172). Nevertheless, studies from one unit that discharges burn patients only when their wounds have healed completely have shown that burn wound colonization with *S. aureus* results in prolongation of hospital stay (173). Additionally, burn units allow facile dispersion of *S. aureus* strains, since burn patients disperse *S. aureus* more readily than other hospital patients (174). Moreover, burn patients represent a threat of introducing multiresistant staphylococci to new treatment care areas (175). Bacterial isolation environments have been developed that reduce cross-infection, but they have not enjoyed widespread use. Isolation rooms in burn units have served a similar purpose, but studies are lacking to prove that such rooms actually reduce cross-infection due to *S. aureus* (176). Quantitative culture of burn wound biopsies has been reported, in some studies, to relate to the development of burn wound sepsis (177). The epidemiology of bacterial infections in burn units is discussed in Chapter 25.

Dialysis

Hemodialysis

As early as 1967, *S. aureus* had become the most frequent pathogen causing hemodialysis shunt infections (178). It has been known for many years that the skin flora in patients undergoing hemodialysis becomes dominated by *S. aureus* (179). Increased nasal carriage leads to colonization of arm shunts. Replacement of perineal normal flora by *S. aureus* also leads to colonization of shunts in the lower extremity. Colonization of any shunt site results in a shunt infection in two thirds of the sites and in bacteremia in one third (180). When studied carefully, carriage of *S. aureus* at nasal, perineal, or shunt sites was either persistent or, more often, intermittent (179). Even the throat may be a secondary site of colonization (77,180). Since the rates of colonization for dialysis outpatients were just as high as rates for dialysis inpatients, dialysis support staff members with known high rates of *S. aureus* colonization may contribute to the colonization of both groups of patients (180); other factors undoubtedly contribute to *S. aureus* colonization (181). Endocarditis may result from *S. aureus* infections in hemodialysis patients. An early study showed that 70% of access site infections and 50% of the cases of endocarditis in hemodialysis patients were due to *S. aureus* (182).

Because of the association of carriage with subsequent serious *S. aureus* infection, studies have been directed at development of prophylaxis. Intravenous vancomycin reduced the risk of shunt infections but has been impractical for widespread use. Oral rifampin, which can eradicate nasal *S. aureus* carriage, was also effective in preventing *S. aureus* infections in patients on hemodialysis (80). Nasal mupirocin clearly is effective in eliminating nasal as well as hand carriage in hemodialysis patients (183). In another study, Dutch workers evaluated 172 patients to determine the efficacy of decolonization with mupirocin; 67 (39%) were determined to be *S. aureus* carriers (184). Mupirocin given twice a day for 5 days eliminated carriage in 98.5%, of whom 94% and 91% remained negative at 3 and 6 months, respectively. Bacteremia occurred at a significantly lower rate in treated patients (0.03 per patient year) than in an untreated historical control group (0.25 per patient year, $p < .001$). Despite these early optimistic data, there has been an emergence of mupirocin resistance in nasal strains of *S. aureus,* particularly common in long-term mupirocin therapy in dialysis patients (185). The current threat of mupirocin resistance suggests the need for development of new decolonizing agents and strategies other than antimicrobial chemotherapy to alter the carrier state (186–188) (see Chapter 64).

Peritoneal Dialysis

As with hemodialysis, *S. aureus* infections in patients on continuous ambulatory peritoneal dialysis (CAPD) relate to nasal carriage. Using molecular tools, Pignatari et al. (189) showed that peritonitis was caused by the same subtype as that carried in the nose. In a 10-month study of 63 carriers and 77 noncarriers, the 11 episodes of peritonitis due to *S. aureus* occurred only in carriers, as did 22 of 24 exit-site infections. Exit-site and tunnel infections in these patients are particularly troublesome and are caused by *S. aureus* 44% of the time. Nasal carriage again seems to be the major risk factor (190). Carriage and resultant infection can be more effectively reduced by intranasal application of mupirocin than by neomycin (191). It is not known if hospitals are the origin of *S. aureus* strains colonizing these patients, although the proximity of many hemodialysis units to inpatient units implies a close connection. The morbidity of *S. aureus* infections can probably be reduced by effective decolonization of the *S. aureus* carriers who enter CAPD programs, but the evidence for efficacy in CAPD patients is less convincing than for hemodialysis patients (192) (see Chapter 65).

Gastrointestinal *S. aureus* Infections

Staphylococcal enterocolitis is a controversial disease, since the finding of *S. aureus* in the stool is not unusual and assays for cellular cytotoxicity of stool isolates are tedious to perform. Enterocolitis has been associated with indwelling feeding catheters, antimicrobial exposure, and high-risk neonates (193). In the last group, a small outbreak of necrotizing enterocolitis was due to a strain of *S. aureus* that produced δ-toxin (194). Wound strains more frequently produce staphylococcal enterotoxin C compared to diarrheal strains that more often produce staphylococcal enterotoxin B (SEB) (195). The potential for enterotoxin production by nosocomial strains may assume greater importance since SEB-producing strains have been associated with toxic shock–like illness and TSST-1 production. SEB behaves like a superantigen capable of nonspecific cytokine stimulation (196). As many as one fourth of asymptomatic *S. aureus* carriers have strains that produce at least one type of enterotoxin (197), though it is not known if the hospital environment selects out toxin-producing strains. MRSA as well as MSSA clearly have the capacity to cause enterocolitis. An interesting observation from Japan found that enterocolitis caused by the same MRSA PFGE type was preexistent in the respiratory tract (198).

Institutional outbreaks of *S. aureus* gastroenteritis are often overlooked, because the major manifestation is vomiting. In a food-borne outbreak in a Florida prison, 65% of inmates had diarrhea, vomiting, or both. *Salmonella infantis* and *S. aureus* phage type 29/52 and 52A (weak) were isolated from leftover turkey (199). *S. aureus* phage type 29/52 was isolated from two of ten food handlers. Thus, such food-borne outbreaks in institutions can involve multiple enteric pathogens including *S. aureus* (see also Chapter 24).

Meningitis—Central Nervous System Infections

Most adult cases of *S. aureus* meningitis are community-acquired and are secondary to focal staphylococcal disease and endocarditis. Modern neurosurgery with its plethora of cerebrospinal fluid access devices has created a new setting for nosocomial *S. aureus* meningitis. Prior neurosurgery, placement of ventricular shunts (200), IV catheter–induced bacteremia (201), and postpartum endometritis (202) are risk factors for the majority of nosocomial cases. Very low birth weight newborns with sepsis constitute another major group who acquire nosocomial meningitis (203). In this group, predictors of cure included central nervous system (CNS) shunt infections, age less than 1 year, and normal results with neurologic examinations. Predictors of mortality in adults included diabetes mellitus, age over 60 years, obtundation or coma on presentation, and bacteremia. With the increasing frequency of MRSA carriage in hospitalized patients, it is now more likely that neurosurgery-induced meningitis will be caused by MRSA as reflected by the experience in Taiwan over the last decade (204) (See Chapter 27).

Pneumonia

Pneumonia caused by *S. aureus* has traditionally been a community-acquired illness associated with influenza virus infection, intravenous drug use, septic thrombophlebitis, and right-sided endocarditis (205). Patients are at higher risk in contracting *S. aureus* nosocomial pneumonia if they are under 25 years of age, suffer trauma, or are infected with HIV (206) (see Chapter 22). The advent of the pandemic of MRSA nosocomial infections allows a more precise determination of the prevalence of nosocomial *S. aureus* infection, since most of these strains reside within the hospital. Epidemiologic studies of MRSA suggest that nosocomial *S. aureus* pneumonia is more frequent than generally is appreciated. In fact, the most recent NNIS system data reveal that 20% of all nosocomial pneumonia is due to *S. aureus* (11, 207).

Other countries do not necessarily reflect this high incidence of nosocomial pneumonia caused by *S. aureus.* In a Spanish study of 15,803 isolates of *S. aureus* from nosocomial infections, the highest rates were 21% from the skin and 14.7% from the blood (208). Perhaps this discrepancy is due to the high percentage of patients hospitalized in the U.S. who require mechanical ventilation, a major risk factor for *S. aureus* pneumonia. In a study of 1,000 consecutive hospitalized patients, 21.9% developed bacterial pneumonia, and in 23.2% of these the pneumonia was caused by *S. aureus;* six additional patients had polymicrobial pneumonia from which *S. aureus* was isolated (209). Ventilator-associated pneumonia due to MSSA and MRSA has increased over the last decade (210). For example, ventilator-associated pneumonia in 11 of 49 episodes was caused by MRSA, and these MRSA-infected patients were much more likely to have received antimicrobials and to have a fatal outcome (211). In German ICUs, *S. aureus* has become the most common (24%) pathogen followed by *P. aeruginosa* (17%) (210). *S. aureus* can be recovered by the protected specimen brush in 20% of ventilator patients who develop pneumonia and, although some experts advocate bronchoscopic sampling to best guide therapy, some studies suggest quantitative endotracheal aspirate cultures are equally useful (212–214).

Newborns

S. aureus infection has always been a problem in the nursery, where many factors serve to perpetuate colonization and infection. About 20% of newborns are colonized with *S. aureus* upon leaving the nursery; this figure doubles by 6 weeks after birth. These rates appear to be independent of whether neonatal care is given in a well-baby nursery or in an NICU. Other factors, such as the type of device used for circumcision, influence *S. aureus* colonization (215). In neonates, *S. aureus* infections are probably related more to colonization of the umbilicus than of the nares (216). Umbilical infection can be reduced by decolonization of the area (217).

Epidemics due to MRSA in modern NICUs suggest that such strains are hospital-acquired (218–220). Some clones are clearly transferred from adult wards, as can be shown by using a combination of PFGE and *spa* typing (221). Some outbreaks are so difficult to control that at times neonatal units have to be closed to break the cycle of cross-infection (222). Methicillin resistance is not the only resistance marker that can be linked to outbreak strains, as was demonstrated by an erythromycin-resistant strain that caused conjunctivitis in several neonates in one nursery (223). TSST-1 production in nursery strains has been another marker used to follow the spread of a strain causing the toxic shock syndrome in a nursery (224).

Another molecular study has shown that multiple strains of *S. aureus* may circulate in some nurseries. Whereas phage typing could distinguish only nine strains, molecular analysis suggested that at least 20 strains from 23 neonates were involved (45).

Crystal violet reactions of neonatal isolates of *S. aureus* may be a promising marker for detecting strains that persist after discharge from the nursery. In a study that showed a rise in the rate of colonization from 18% at discharge to 40% by 6 weeks after discharge, the purple reacting strains, usually of phage groups I and III, were more likely to persist than strains from other phage groups (225). It is becoming increasingly important to conduct surveillance of *S. aureus* clones in neonatal units. One recent study suggested that microbiologic surveillance using nasal cultures is sufficient for detection of MRSA isolates (226) (see Chapter 52).

Prosthetic Devices

There is a broadening spectrum of infection associated with insertion of prosthetic devices including intraocular lenses, cerebrospinal fluid shunts, prosthetic joints, vascular biomaterials, genital prostheses, and breast prostheses. The staphylococci predominate in these infections (227). It is well known that coagulase-negative staphylococci tend to form biofilms on biomaterials more efficiently than *S. aureus*, but almost any staphylococcal species can produce a complex infection on prosthetic material, which may include selection of small colony variants (SCVs), making treatment of prosthetic infection difficult (228). A prospective study of Spanish patients with joint prostheses showed that an etiologic diagnosis could be made in 60% and most of the 58% of gram-positive infections were staphylococcal (227). Seeding of prostheses after *S. aureus* bacteremia is surprisingly common, as was shown by a collaborative study between Duke University and an institution in Auckland, New Zealand, which reported that 15 of 44 (34%) of patients with *S. aureus* bacteremia had subsequent infection of the indwelling prosthesis (see Chapter 67).

Skin and Soft Tissue

In the preantibiotic era, pustules, carbuncles, furunculosis, cellulitis, and surgical site sepsis were common nosocomial infections in the U.S., and they continue to be major problems in large areas of the world (10,110). In modern hospitals, nosocomial staphylococcal cellulitis often occurs as a manifestation of infected indwelling intravascular devices and prosthetic implants. Pyoderma in healthy neonates and decubitus ulcers in residents of long-term-care facilities remain problems and are addressed elsewhere in this text (see Chapters 52 and 106). Specific problems may arise in NICUs. For example, a group III phage type 42E/54/75 strain of *S. aureus* caused the scalded skin syndrome, which spread through a six-room special care nursery (229).

Surgical Site Infection

Patients undergoing surgical procedures are at increased risk of developing a nosocomial infection; SSIs are the most common type of infection (230). Through 1960, *S. aureus* was by far the most common cause of SSIs (231). Studies done in the early 1960s found that SSI was associated with *S. aureus* nasal carriage and hospitalization during the month of January; this trend was consistently observed over 3 years (69). In the most recently published data from the NNIS system, *S. aureus* accounted for 19% of 11,724 SSIs (11). In developing countries, rates are even higher (i.e., *S. aureus* causes almost half of the SSIs) (232). In-hospital SSI data are always affected by delayed infections—often due to *S. aureus*—that are manifested months or even years after surgery (233). Diagnosis of other surgical infections, like mediastinitis, can also be difficult. Tammelin et al. (234) in Uppsala did an exhaustive microbiologic study over 2 years of sternotomy patients who were reexplored. Using strict criteria for tissue infection and multiple tissue samples, they found *S. aureus* in 10/32 and *S. epidermidis* in 10/32 infected patients. By PFGE they found eight different patterns among 40 *S. aureus* isolates. Interestingly, the surgeon was readily identified as the source for all cases of *S. aureus* infection but could only be suspected as the source for 30% of the infections due to coagulase-negative staphylococci.

Guidelines for prevention of SSIs have been published many times and, if followed, probably reduce the rate of SSIs to 1% to 2% (235). Adherence to these guidelines is important, because most SSIs result from exogenous strains of bacteria (236,237), some of which are carried in the nares and on the hands of hospital personnel who contact surgical patients. For example, as many as 50% of ungloved examiners may carry *S. aureus* on their hands (238). Because hair carriers have been associated with epidemics of SSI, proper head covering is mandatory during surgery (239). Body coverings and face masks, however, do not guarantee containment of *S. aureus* during surgery. Mask wiggling contributes to an increase in recovery of *S. epidermidis* and *S. aureus* from cultures taken around the operating table (240). In staff working in a cardiothoracic unit, the risk for hand carriage in nasal carriers was 7.4 [95% confidence interval (CI), 2.7 to 20.2; $p < .001$] (241). At least half of these hand carriers carried strains self-inoculated from their own nares.

The preponderance of *S. aureus* as a primary cause of SSI has spawned extensive research into the mechanism of SSIs using animal models. Progress has been slow, but several concepts are worth noting. SSis are influenced by many complex variables in the operating room. The size of the inoculum of *S. aureus* delivered to the surgical site is related to development of infection (242). In an animal model, by increasing the inoculum from 3×10^6 to 8×10^6 CFU, the infection rate rose from almost 0% to 45%. Surgeons have recognized this fact for years and have tried using quantitative bacterial cultures to predict the likelihood of subsequent infection (243). Size of the inoculum is only one element, however, in a complex process that produces SSIs. For example, the presence of remote infection, including those due to *S. aureus*, may increase the SSI rate two to five times (244). Another study has shown that personnel working overtime (because of understaffing) resulted in an increase in the number of SSIs (245).

For surgery involving exposure of tissues at the surgical site to adjacent contaminated or colonized sites, perioperative antimicrobial prophylaxis using antistaphylococcal agents is now universally advised. Even though antimicrobial prophylaxis is aimed primarily at *S. aureus*, it has been reported as the most common cause of SSI in cardiothoracic surgery (246). β-lactamase production in *S. aureus* may be one factor that has reduced the efficacy of prophylactic cephalosporins to prevent *S. aureus* mediastinal infections (247). New studies will be necessary to establish which prophylactic antimicrobial regimens are effective in this era of multiresistant staphylococci.

Infections after surgical procedures categorized as clean-contaminated, contaminated, and dirty are more likely to be due to nonstaphylococcal species. Yet, *S. aureus* infections after gastroduodenal procedures occur in up to 15% of cases (248), suggesting a need to broaden traditional antibacterial coverage before certain operations. Specific procedures like placement of percutaneous enteral gastrostomy (PEG) feeding tubes, perhaps because of the cutaneous interface, are increasingly complicated by *S. aureus* infection (249) (see Chapter 21).

Toxic Shock Syndrome

After being initially described in 1978, toxic shock syndrome (TSS) gained increased notoriety during the early 1980s. The first nosocomial cases were associated with SSIs (250), often after minor surgery. In 12 of 12 patients described, *S. aureus* was isolated from the surgical site. Four patients were men and four were menstruating women. Classic signs of TSS including fever, profound multisystem dysfunction, and desquamative erythroderma usually began within 48 hours of the operation. A gentamicin-resistant strain of *S. aureus* that produced TSST-1 caused recurrent TSS in a nurse working in a burn unit. The strain was shown to spread to patients and other workers (251). Relatively benign procedures (252), including simple mastectomy in a male (253), correction of a bat ear (254), nasal packing after septoplasty, abdominoplasty (255), and arthroscopy (256, 257), have also been associated with TSS. Another report of an erythromycin-resistant TSST-1 producing strain carried by a neurosurgeon resulted in TSS in two of his patients; the strain from the neurosurgeon and those from the patients were shown to be related by endonuclease restriction-length polymorphism seen with *Tn*554 hybridization studies (258). A moderate number of hospital strains of *S. aureus* produce TSST-1. In a study of 997 strains of *S. aureus*, 128 occurred with confirmed or probable cases of TSS. Following in frequency those strains associated with menses were those isolated from patients with septicemia, burns, and surgical sites (259). A recent discovery by Kikuchi et al. (260) at Tokyo's Women's Medical University involved TSST-1 in MRSA strains that caused a disease termed neonatal toxic shock syndrome–like exanthematous disease (NTED). Clonal TSST-1 strains of MRSA were widespread in an NICU and a general neonatal and maternal ward where 12.9% of 62 newborns carrying such strains developed NTED.

These studies collectively suggest that nosocomial strains of TSS may circulate among patients and hospital personnel. The diagnosis of nosocomial TSS should be suspected in hospitalized patients who have undergone surgical procedures and who manifest multisystem organ failure and fever and shock with or without rash and in all neonates with fever. Clustering of such cases that may involve a limited number of clones should alert the hospital epidemiologist to search diligently for a carrier of a TSST-1–producing strain of *S. aureus*.

Urinary Tract Infection

Unlike the dogma for the significance of gram-negative bacillary urinary tract infections, there are no quantitative standards for evaluating the clinical significance of staphylococci in urine. Several studies have shown that *S. aureus* is infrequently cultured from urine (261,262). The clinical significance of small numbers of *S. aureus* in the urine of hospitalized patients remains unclear (261). Bacteriuria occurs in about one fourth of patients with *S. aureus* bacteremia, but its significance is not known (263). Nevertheless, *S. aureus* can infect multiple sites in the urinary tract of hospitalized patients. Renal carbuncles, which complicate *S. aureus* bacteremia, are localized to the cortex of the kidney and may release small numbers of microorganisms into the urine (205). *S. aureus* bacteriuria in concentrations of at least 10^5

CFU/mL also occurs in the absence of renal infection. In one study using a criterion of $\geq 10^5$ CFU/mL as indicating infection, *S. aureus* was isolated from only 3.3% of the isolates from 17,437 urine cultures. Of 373 patients with *S. aureus* isolated from urine, 132 had $\geq 10^5$ CFU/mL of *S. aureus* in pure culture, and 96 had *S. aureus* in mixed culture.

Up to 50% to 81% of cases of *S. aureus* urinary tract infections are nosocomial in origin and, as such, carry a moderate risk of producing bacteremia. Of 69 patients who did not receive appropriate therapy for their *S. aureus* urinary tract infection, 11% had secondary bacteremia, compared with none of 63 who received appropriate therapy (262). Predisposing factors included an indwelling catheter, urinary obstruction, surgical manipulation, or malignancy—factors similar to those predisposing to nosocomial gram-negative bacillary urinary tract infection (see Chapter 20). Urologic patients may carry separate risks for *S. aureus* UTI. In a large 10-year study from Japan of 139 patients with *S. aureus* UTI, (45 MSSA, 94 MRSA), a febrile response was associated with certain toxin genes, and those genes were more common in MRSA than MSSA isolates (264).

Vascular Access Device Infections

S. aureus causes about half of the cases of IV catheter–related phlebitis and bacteremia (265). Over a 10-year period at a hospital in Atlanta, nosocomial device-related bacteremias increased eightfold, and 56% of these were due to *S. aureus* in the period 1990 to 1993 (157). It is important to remember that phlebitis is evident in fewer than half of the patients with IV catheter–related sepsis and that sepsis is infrequent when a catheter has been in place less than 4 days. Many studies have used semiquantitative or quantitative culture techniques to identify the catheter as a source of bacteremia, but the positive predictive value of a single catheter culture remains low.

The suggestion that an IV catheter is the source of *S. aureus* bacteremia has heretofore prompted many clinicians to use short-course antimicrobial therapy. This approach to therapy is surprising, since the frequency of late unpredictable complications of IV catheter–related bacteremia ranges from 0% to almost 70%. These complications include endocarditis, osteomyelitis, and pyelitis (266). With current technology, it is not possible to predict prospectively which patients will develop late complications. Nevertheless, short-course therapy has become popular for patients with *S. aureus* bacteremia thought to be related to an IV catheter. In those studies of short-course therapy, the combined late complication rate was 6.1%, which is probably an unacceptably high figure for most clinicians (266). Specifically, endocarditis develops in 2% of patients with catheter-related bacteremia, compared with 6% in other bacteremia patients (267). Thus, short-term therapy (10–14 days) should be reserved for only those patients carefully selected to be at minimal risk for metastatic disease (268). The quantitation of *S. aureus* adherent to a catheter or its related parts may become more meaningful when it helps identify those patients who will benefit from short-course therapy (269).

With time, the extraluminal or luminal colonization of the IV device predisposes to phlebitis and subsequent bacteremia. The mechanism of colonization involves development of a biofilm resistant to the bactericidal effects of serum or antimicrobial agents. The role of colonization by *S. aureus* at sites distant to the IV device remains unclear. In fact, one study suggests that nasal colonization with *S. aureus* may reduce the likelihood of phlebitis (270). The authors suggest that immune mechanisms that reduce nasal colonization may also protect the catheter site from inflammation. In that study, the presence or absence of *S. aureus* at the phlebitis site was not investigated, so more studies of this nature need to be performed.

Patients with catheter-related *S. aureus* bacteremia are at increased risk for developing septic thrombosis or deep-seated infections exclusive of endocarditis. The development of these sequelae is heralded by persistence of fever for more than 3 days (271). One of the most severe complications due to extension of the infected thrombosis is suppurative thrombophlebitis (see Chapters 17 and 18).

S. aureus accounts for 81% of bacteremias associated with permanent endocardial pacemakers (272). Although this infection may present like an intravascular sepsis, the portal of entry most often is the subcutaneous site where the pacing system is implanted. Similarly, permanently implantable cardioverter defibrillators (ICDs) are a newly recognized risk for development of local and systemic *S. aureus* infection (273). Cure usually requires removal of part (the generator) or all of the ICD (274) (see Chapter 62).

EPIDEMIOLOGY

Along with the work of Spink et al. already described, the careful study of the epidemiology of *S. aureus* infections in hospital patients performed by Finland and Jones (21) shortly thereafter established the basis for modern hospital infection control. The spread of infections caused by phage type 80/81 is analogous to the problem with infections caused by MRSA in hospitals today. That phage type was responsible for many serious hospital outbreaks of furuncles, carbuncles, pneumonia, and SSI (275). So pervasive was *S. aureus* infection, that, at the University of Iowa Hospital in 1957, *S. aureus* caused infections in 17% of all surgical and 12% of all medical patients; 38% of these infections in both groups were nosocomial.

Since the outbreaks of the 1950s, *S. aureus* has continued to be the preeminent nosocomial pathogen. Recent surveys by the NNIS system found that *S. aureus* was the cause of 12% of 70,411 nosocomial infections. As an individual species, it was the number-one cause of SSIs (19%), pneumonia (20%), and infections at all other sites (17%) (11). The most striking change since the last published NNIS data from 1980 to 1989 (276) was the increase in numbers of cases of nosocomial pneumonia caused by *S. aureus* (from 17% to 20%), probably due to the increase in respiratory infections caused by MRSA strains. Among NNIS hospitals, the percentage of infections due to MRSA rose from 2.4% in 1975 to 29% in 1991 (11).

The rise in the number of infections caused by MRSA has also brought attention to staphylococcal infection in long-term-care facilities (see Chapter 106). Rates of *S. aureus* infections in a nursing home care unit ranged from 0.29 to 0.47 per 1,000 resident-care days (277). Demographics for patients with MSSA and MRSA infections were similar. One study in a skilled-nursing facility found that 35% of residents were colonized with *S. aureus* at least once during a 1-year prospective surveillance study. Rectal carriage alone was present in 13% of residents who became colonized during their stay (278). Outbreaks of MRSA infections have occurred in pediatric residential care facilities as well. One such outbreak was reported in an Arkansas state facility for mentally retarded children (279). From 1978 to 1981, in one cottage, an average of ten *S. aureus* infections occurred per month, affecting 29 of 35 cottage residents. In July 1981, residents and workers in this cottage were decolonized with antibiotics, and all residents and personnel were inoculated intranasally with *S. aureus* strain 502A.

Reservoirs

The many studies of the inanimate hospital environment suggest that *S. aureus* persists on surfaces and fomites in hospitals (280). Since there is usually a human component of contagion during hospital epidemics, it is always difficult to incriminate environmental sources alone (73). Indeed, the contamination of the environment by skin scales from humans is a general index for human colonization (74). In the surgical suite, both settle plate techniques and air sampling have been used to evaluate the potential for contamination. Such studies have not proven a cause-and-effect relationship but suggest that the environment may serve as a way station for strains that preferentially colonize hospital personnel.

Modes of Transmission

Staphylococci are efficiently transmitted by contact and less efficiently by the airborne route (281). It is likely that strains from patients with *S. aureus* pneumonia or burn infections may spread by the airborne route in the hospital. It is more likely that epidemics are most efficiently maintained by human carriers, both patients and workers, who carry the microorganism in their nares and contaminate other parts of their body, particularly their hands. Modern studies have shown that contemporary MRSA strains, like earlier 80/81 phage types (282), can spread quickly and can displace susceptible nasal flora in hospital patients and personnel (220).

One group of nasal carriers who efficiently spread the microorganism are so-called shedders; 13% of male and 5% of female carriers have a heavy nasal inoculum and disperse, with normal movement, large numbers of microorganisms from their lower extremities and perineum into the air around them (283). One physician who contracted an upper respiratory infection (URI) was incriminated in a MRSA outbreak (284). The physician carried large numbers of MSSA ($2.8–4.5 \times 10^5$) in both nares and fewer MRSA in either nare. After an experimentally induced rhinovirus infection, the physician dispersed *S. aureus* up to 20 feet away, giving rise to the term *cloud adult,* in the tradition of cloud babies who similarly spread *S. aureus* in the nursery (285). In the operating room, dispersal is likely related to the wearing of permeable clothing, including scrub suits (286), and is blocked by polyethylene covering the lower extremities. Walter et al. (287) performed many studies to show that orderlies and anesthetists in the operating suite may have twice the *S. aureus* carriage rate as surgeons and nurses and that carriage may be persistent or intermittent.

There has been a historical debate between proponents of the airborne versus the contact routes of spread of *S. aureus* in hospitals. Goldmann (280) has aptly summarized the debate, emphasizing that whereas older outbreaks caused by one *S. aureus* phage type may have incriminated a point-source shedder of airborne *S. aureus,* modern outbreaks that feature multiple strains of *S. aureus* are probably initiated and perpetuated by contact transmission. That overview should not totally discount earlier work that showed that personnel who were shedders of *S. aureus* and worked in the operating room were associated with outbreaks of SSIs (287) and that removal of shedders implicated in these outbreaks from the clinical area resulted in cessation of the epidemics (287–290). Yet a causal relationship between colonization among personnel and subsequent *S. aureus* sepsis in patients remains unclear after years of study.

The nares are not the only site of *S. aureus* colonization. In women followed in a maternity unit, 33% were nasal carriers, but 25% carried *S. aureus* in their perineal region (291). Earlier, in his classic studies, Solberg (74) found that 12% of carriers harbored *S. aureus* at multiple sites.

Hospitalization is a risk for colonization with *S. aureus.* Patients become progressively colonized throughout their hospitalization, though the maximum carriage rate is about 25% in studies from hospitals in the Western Hemisphere (289). A deterministic model tested against data derived for the acquisition of tetracycline-resistant *S. aureus* demonstrated that, by about 35 days of hospital stay, the nasal carriage rate stabilizes at 25% (292).

Tracing Spread of Nosocomial Strains

The question of how many different strains of *S. aureus* circulate through a hospital at one time is not easy to answer. Historically, phage typing of strains formed the basis of epidemiologic analyses. One study of MSSA strains at Walter Reed Army Medical Center found four predominant phage types of 31 *S. aureus* bacteremic strains during a 6-month period in 1979 (182). Control measures reduced bacteremia but not carriage. In the former East Germany, the prevalence of the 94/96 phage complex increased from 9% in 1978 to 16% by 1985 (293). These strains were very similar with regard to biochemical reactions, antigenic structure, and the presence of 16-Md plasmids determining resistance to cadmium and penicillin. Yet, additional experimental phage reactions and the sites of resistance determinants on the plasmids could further differentiate the strains. Such studies raise the question of how far an investigation should proceed in an attempt to establish a relationship between strains. Newer molecular methods already discussed may simplify this process somewhat (see above). Whatever technique is chosen, it is necessary to determine discriminative indices among strains to establish a strong epidemiologic relationship and draw valid conclusions.

More advanced typing methods using staphylococcal genomics are just now being applied to MSSA strains, suggesting that relationships among nosocomial *S. aureus* strains are complex and certainly beyond the implications of phage susceptibility (see Molecular Typing, above) (84). At times, one or two molecular methods can produce incriminating DNA fingerprints, implying that a particular strain is the cause of an epidemic; such a relationship may have been undetectable by traditional epidemiologic investigations (294). Newer multicenter molecular analysis of *S. aureus* strains from nosocomial outbreaks suggest that multiple methods may be needed to establish clonal relationships among nosocomial strains (63,295).

PREVENTION AND CONTROL OF NOSOCOMIAL INFECTIONS

S. aureus has persisted as the predominant cause of nosocomial infections. This microorganism is the second most common isolate from blood (16.5%), the most common isolate from SSIs (17.1%), and the second most common respiratory isolate (16.1%) (296). Outbreaks within hospitals continue to occur and have been controlled, historically, by the institution of meticulous infection control measures. Less commonly, epidemics were controlled by the identification and treatment of carriers who were implicated in the transmission of *S. aureus* during such outbreaks (297). The close relationship between colonization and subsequent infection has most recently been reemphasized by the work of von Eiff et al. (2). In Meunster, Germany, they found that over 80% of patients with bacteremia at the time of or after admission has a bloodstream clone that matched their nasal clone present on admission. Perl et al. (298) further demonstrated that the largest impact in decolonizing nasal carriers was a reduction in SSIs. Thus, the most effective measures for the prevention of staphylococcal infections are those that diminish or eliminate colonization.

Perioperative Prophylaxis

The appropriate use of perioperative antimicrobials has been shown to reduce the rate of clean SSIs at practically any site studied. Such prophylaxis has had a major impact on lowering the incidence of *S. aureus* SSIs, although the emergence of more resistant strains threatens that success. In reviewing prophylaxis policies, one should follow several principles. First, determine whether published studies have shown that prophylaxis leads to a significant decrease in infections for the specific procedure. If so, choose an antibiotic with a spectrum that includes the microorganisms most likely to cause infection resulting from the specific procedure, realizing that no antimicrobial agent is capable of preventing infection by all pathogens. Next, determine if the chosen antibiotic achieves effective tissue levels at the site of the procedure. Also, consider the incidence of adverse reactions to the antimicrobial agent. Antimicrobials with high rates of allergic reactions would be undesirable as prophylactic agents. Finally, consider the cost of the antimicrobial agent. Less expensive, but efficacious, agents would control costs because of the large number of patients requiring prophylaxis. For all sites studied at which *S. aureus* is a predominant pathogen, cefazolin or a nearly equivalent cephalosporin (cefamandole, cefuroxime) has been the agent of choice (299–302). In practice, the best agent is often chosen on the basis of cost.

The addition of vancomycin to prophylaxis regimens could be considered if there is a significant incidence of SSIs caused by methicillin-resistant staphylococci. In a study whose findings suggested value in the use of vancomycin prophylaxis in this setting, the vancomycin prophylaxis group had fewer SSIs than the cefazolin and cefamandole prophylaxis groups, respectively (303). However, there were several SSIs in the vancomycin treatment group due to cephalosporin-resistant coagulase-negative staphylococci. It is important to remember that antimicrobial prophylaxis may cause alterations in the normal flora. When compared to control patients not receiving antibiotics, two studies have shown the emergence of bacteria, including staphylococci, resistant to the prophylactic agents in patients administered prophylactic antimicrobials (304,305) (see Chapter 21).

Thus, antimicrobial prophylaxis cannot prevent all *S. aureus* infections including those caused by susceptible strains. Many patients do not receive prophylactic antimicrobials for certain procedures such as intravascular catheter insertions or dialysis. Other patients may develop SSIs with susceptible strains of *S. aureus* despite adequate perioperative antimicrobial prophylaxis (247). As previously stressed, the initiating event in nosocomial *S. aureus* infection is colonization. Patients colonized with *S. aureus* prior to a procedure are more likely to develop a staphylococcal infection after the procedure than are those patients who are not colonized (306). Up to 80% of adults may be colonized if repeated cultures are obtained (307), and patients become infected with the strains colonizing the anterior nares (308). For these reasons, numerous strategies for reducing surface colonization have been tried.

Use of preoperative showers with a topical antiseptic scrub is a simple decolonization strategy. One study compared povidone-iodine, chlorhexidine, and soap. Only chlorhexidine significantly reduced the numbers of staphylococci inhabiting skin sites. This study did not examine the effect on infection rates (309). A variety of topical and oral agents have also been studied. Topical gentamicin eliminated carriage rapidly. However, recolonization occurred within 10 days and was usually with the same phage type noted on initial sampling. With oral trimethoprim/sulfamethoxazole, eradication was not observed in a high proportion of patients, and resistance to this agent emerged frequently among patients in the study group (310). Oral clindamycin has also been tried, but resistant strains frequently emerged (311). In a study with limited enrollment, Klempner and Styrt (312) found that clindamycin was useful; three of 11 untreated patients versus nine of 11 treated patients were free of infection after 3 months, but relapse of colonization was common.

Rifampin has been used in three studies either as a single agent or in combination with other antimicrobials. Chow and Yu (313) reported that rapid resistance to rifampin was observed if this agent was used alone. In a second study, the application of a topical antibiotic, bacitracin, to the external nares plus orally administered rifampin decreased the recovery of *S. aureus* on the forearm and from air samples and eliminated nasal carriage of *S. aureus* in hemodialysis patients. Infection rates were significantly lower in decolonized patients (80). An earlier study, however, showed that application of bacitracin alone was ineffective but that the combination of bacitracin and rifampin was better; the latter combination was not as effective as rifampin alone

(314). Widespread use of rifampin and the subsequent increase in rifampin resistance would limit the long-term use of this agent for decolonization. Oral ciprofloxacin appeared promising, as most staphylococci were susceptible to ciprofloxacin. Ciprofloxacin was successful as a single agent in eradicating colonization, but resistance emerged in 7 of 22 patients. If patients were recolonized, the new strain was more resistant to ciprofloxacin than the initial isolate. Eradication did not occur rapidly and required treatment for 2 to 3 weeks (310). Another study corroborated the frequent emergence of strains resistant to ciprofloxacin (315). Other than the bacitracin and rifampin combination, none of the decolonization strategies above could be recommended. Rifampin plus an older antimicrobial, novobiocin, seems to be a promising alternative for decolonization (41).

The topical antibacterial mupirocin (pseudomonic acid) has been shown to eradicate carriage of *S. aureus* in several studies. Reagan et al. (316), in a double-blinded study, reported that mupirocin decreased nasal carriage. Three months after therapy, 71% of treated subjects versus 18% of controls remained free of colonization ($p < .0001$). Casewell and Hill (317) reported similar success with attempts at eradication. In an analysis of six different double-blinded, independently randomized clinical trials of healthy carriers of *S. aureus*, nasal carriage was eliminated based on cultures taken 48 to 96 hours after completion of treatment in 91% of volunteers receiving mupirocin but in only 6% of placebo-treated control subjects (318). The effect lasted at least 4 weeks after therapy. In a smaller study, topical mupirocin eliminated *S. aureus* carriage in 100% of volunteers. In 60% of these subjects, carriage relapsed within 1 year (319). Decolonization of surgical ICU patients with mupirocin has been shown to be effective in preventing subsequent infections with *S. aureus* [relative risk (RR) 2.78, 95% CI 1.00–7.78] (77). In this study an added potential benefit of decolonization was evidence that bronchopulmonary strains were identical to nasal strains and bronchopulmonary colonization was decreased by nasal decolonization.

On a cautionary note, high-level resistance to mupirocin has been reported (320). A study performed at a long-term-care facility illustrates this point. A prospective study evaluated the effect of mupirocin on MRSA colonization and endemic infections. Carriage was eliminated from 94.7% when both nares and wounds were treated. Nares treatment alone did not significantly decrease overall colonization. The overall rate of recurrence was 34%. Unfortunately, the infection rate did not change with reduction in colonization. Resistance to mupirocin was detected and was mostly low level (MIC = 3.1–62.5 μg/mL); however, for one strain, an MIC greater than 5,000 μg/mL was reported. High-level mupirocin resistance was transferable and plasmid mediated. Low-level resistant strains were cleared. Because of these findings, the authors did not recommend the use of mupirocin in long-term-care patients. These investigators predicted that mupirocin resistance will increase with continued use (321). At a Canadian hospital, mupirocin resistance increased in MRSA strains from 2.5% in 1990 to 65% in 1993 (186). In Brazil, emergence of resistance was related to the extent of mupirocin use: 63% of MRSA strains were resistant in a district hospital where mupirocin was used daily compared to a rate of 6.1% in a region where the topical agent was used infrequently (322).

Resistance to topical and systemic antimicrobials remains the major limitation of antibiotic-based decolonization treatments. One must not overlook the fact that *S. aureus* colonizes other sites in addition to the nares. A prospective study has shown that hospitalized patients without nasal colonization may be colonized with *S. aureus* at other sites. The axillae were colonized in 7% of patients, the perineum in 12%, and the toe webs in 5% (323). Up to 13% of nursing home residents may harbor *S. aureus* only in the rectum (278). Therefore, it may be worthwhile to choose strategies for decolonization that are effective at multiple sites. Although nasal carriers may disseminate and spread microorganisms to other body areas, heavy shedders also disseminate from the perineum (324). Few studies have shown that widespread decolonization of hospitalized patients actually reduces the rate of infection. Moreover, in regard to carriers, less than 1% of hospital outbreaks have been caused by colonized personnel (325). Except for selected groups of high-risk patients during MRSA outbreaks or those on hemodialysis, widespread and prolonged use of antimicrobial agents for decolonization is not indicated (326). The role of decolonization in MSSA outbreaks remains to be determined. Several new agents may soon be available for topical use. Lysostaphin has been shown to be rapidly bactericidal against *S. aureus* and able to decolonize cotton rates quickly in one or two intranasal applications (327). Alkyl esters are also gaining some attention as topical antistaphylococcal agents since they select minimally for resistance in serial passage (328).

Bacterial Interference

Several other new strategies for prevention of infection besides decolonization have been tried. Competitive interference using a strain of *S. aureus* of low pathogenicity (the 502a strain) was used in nurseries by application of a bacterial suspension to the umbilical stump. The incidence of infections was reduced, but outbreaks caused by the 502a strain occurred (329). Use of this method requires previous treatment with antibiotics to establish 502a colonization. This method has also been used successfully to treat adult patients with recurrent skin infections (330). A major disadvantage of bacterial interference is the ease with which the interfering strain may be eradicated with the additional use of antibiotics. Nevertheless, several worldwide centers are proceeding with studies of recolonization using interfering *S. aureus* strains after decolonization of pathogenic strains.

Vancomycin Resistance

Over 40 resistance genes have already been identified in strains of *S. aureus* (331). Vancomycin has been utilized for staphylococcal infections for over 30 years. Even after the emergence of widespread vancomycin resistance in enterococci, resistance in *S. aureus* to vancomycin remained theoretical. The long-awaited appearance of strains of *S. aureus* with decreased (intermediate) susceptibility to vancomycin [vancomycin-intermediate *S. aureus* (VISA)] finally occurred in Japan in May 1996 (332). The first patient was a 4-month-old child who had undergone open-heart surgery and developed a chronically draining sternal SSI. The patient was treated with several courses of vancomycin and subsequently, after decreased susceptibility to vancomycin was determined, with other antimicrobial regimens. Therapy with all of the antimicrobial regimens failed, and only deep debridement ultimately eradicated the VISA.

The *S. aureus* strain responsible for this first vancomycin-resistant infection termed Mu-50 grows well in 4 μg/mL of vancomycin and displays a heteroresistance to vancomycin in concentrations up to 10 μg/mL. The whole genome sequence has been published by the group in Japan at Juntendo University (4). Another strain, Mu3, isolated from a Japanese man with pneumonia in January 1996 displayed an even greater heteroresistance, i.e., 99.99% of the population was killed by 4 μg/mL (333). These strains have a variable response to vancomycin presumably because vancomycin is sequestrated in cell walls that have altered cross-linkages of peptidoglycan (334). VISA are defined by Hiramatsu et al. (332) as *S. aureus* with an MIC of 8 μg/mL or above and heteroresistant VISA as those that give vancomycin resistance at a frequency of 10^{-6} colonies or higher, making it almost impossible to detect such a strain in standard susceptibility testing. Of particular epidemiologic interest are data from PFGE banding patterns of heteroresistant strains, suggesting Mu3 and Mu50 are highly related to a common MRSA clonotype II-A in Japanese hospitals. Early surveys conducted in Japan reveal that 1.3% of MRSA strains from nonuniversity hospitals and over 9% of strains from university hospitals display heteroresistance to vancomycin (335). When examined for expression of heteroresistance, Dutch workers found a surprisingly high (7.6%) rate of isolates with reduced susceptibility to vancomycin (336).

Several cases of VISA have originated in the U.S. Most of these patients have had extensive exposure to vancomycin (335, 337). Those patients with MRSA infections who fail vancomycin therapy, particularly after long-term therapy, should signal a need for determination of heteroresistance in the causative strain.

Initial recommendations for control of VISA emphasized extremely stringent isolation of the patient particularly by limiting the number of healthcare workers caring for the patient. Nosocomial transmission, when documented, should trigger closure of the ward to new admissions (338). Subsequent recommendations published by the CDC also emphasize similar stringent isolation and emphasize the importance of enforcing compliance with contact precautions (339) (Table 28.4). In our experience with one VISA false alarm, the most difficult aspect of implementing these recommendations is the one-on-one care for the suspected colonized/infected patient, particularly during off hours. With much alarm, in 2003 the first strains of *S. aureus* with high-level vancomycin resistance (VRSA) surfaced in two American patients (340,341). In both strains, the *vanA* gene commonplace in strains of vancomycin-resistant enterococci (VRE) was found to be located on a plasmid in both VRSA strains. If VISA and VRSA strains appear nationwide and worldwide, hospitals will have to wrestle with the issue of how many resources they can expend on the infection control and epidemiologic analysis of these multiply-resistant strains of *S. aureus.*

TABLE 28.4. RECOMMENDATIONS TO PREVENT THE SPREAD OF VANCOMYCIN-RESISTANT *STAPHYLOCOCCUS AUREUS*

The laboratory should immediately notify infection-control personnel, the clinical unit, and the attending physician

Infection-control personnel, in collaboration with appropriate authorities, including the state health department and the CDC, should initiate an epidemiologic and laboratory investigation

Medical and nursing staff tasks
- Isolate the patient in a private room and use contact precautions (gown, mask, gloves, and antibacterial soap for hand washing) as recommended for multidrug-resistant microorganisms
- Minimize the number of persons with access to colonized/infected patients
- Dedicate specific healthcare workers to provide one-on-one care for the colonized/infected patient or the cohort of colonized/infected patients

Infection-control personnel tasks
- Inform all personnel providing direct patient care of the epidemiologic implications of such strains and of the infection control precautions necessary for their containment
- Monitor and strictly enforce compliance with contact precautions and other recommended infection control practices
- Determine whether transmission has already occurred by obtaining baseline cultures (before initiation of precautions) for staphylococci with reduced susceptibility to vancomycin from the nares and hands of all healthcare workers, roommates, and others with direct patient contact

Assess efficacy of precautions by monitoring healthcare personnel for acquisition of staphylococci with reduced susceptibility to vancomycin as recommended by consultants to the state health department or CDC

Avoid transferring infected patients within or between facilities and if transfer is necessary, fully inform the receiving institution or unit of the patient's colonization/infection status and appropriate precautions

Consult with the state health department and CDC before discharge of a colonized/infected patient

CDC, Centers for Disease Control and Prevention.

Future Possibilities for Control

Future methods for control of nosocomial *S. aureus* infections may include use of genetically engineered interfering strains of *S. aureus* with inactivation of key virulence genes. Novel antimicrobial agents such as defensins or lantibiotics and other inhibiting peptides may provide additional topical or parenteral agents to aid in decolonization and therapy. Catheters impregnated with antimicrobial compounds have been shown to reduce catheter-related infections and bacteremia, but their long-term efficacy is not known (342). New materials used for wound care such as hydrophobic wound dressings would absorb bacteria and tissue proteins. Alternative strategies, such as blockade of surface protein receptors with antireceptor compounds, may decrease colonization of tissue surfaces and prosthetic materials. One study showed that fibronectin analogues blocked the binding of *S. aureus* to plastic surfaces coated with human proteins (343). The use of antibiotics at subinhibitory levels, which inhibits protein synthesis (clindamycin, erythromycin), has been shown to prevent endocarditis in an animal model by reduction in the number of fibronectin receptors (92). Aspirin has recently been shown to mitigate the effects of *S. aureus* endocarditis (123). Such measures may diminish or eliminate colonization and lower nosocomial infection rates while reducing antimicrobial selective pressure on susceptible strains. Clearly new vaccine strategies are needed to reduce the morbidity of staphylococcal bacteremia

(344,345). For example, a cellulitis model in mice was used to show that vaccination with RAP reduced cellulitis and decreased death. There are other vaccine targets in the complex regulatory pathways of *S. aureus* that await exploitation (Fig. 28.3) (8,278, 346).

ACKNOWLEDGMENTS

The authors thank Paula King for help with the manuscript, Jean Lee, Greg Bohach, and Ken Bales for help with specific sections, and Katherine Schmidt for work on the *sar/agr* graphic.

REFERENCES

1. Wenzel RP, Perl TM. The significance of nasal carriage of *Staphylococcus aureus* and the incidence of postoperative wound infection. *J Hosp Infect* 1995;31:13–24.
2. von Eiff C, Becker K, Machka K, et al. Nasal carriage as a source of *Staphylococcus aureus* bacteremia. Study Group. *N Engl J Med* 2001; 344:11–16.
3. Lowy FD. *Staphylococcus aureus* infections. *N Engl J Med* 1998;339: 520–532.
4. Kuroda M, Ohta T, Uchiyama I, et al. Whole genome sequencing of methicillin-resistant *Staphylococcus aureus. Lancet* 2001;357: 1225–1240.
5. Abramson MA, Sexton DJ. Nosocomial methicillin-resistant and methicillin-susceptible *Staphylococcus aureus* primary bacteremia: at what costs? *Infect Control Hosp Epidemiol*1999;20:408–411.
6. Abbott KC, Agodoa LY. Etiology of bacterial septicemia in chronic dialysis patients in the United States. *Clin Nephrol*2001;56:124–131.
7. Foster TJ, Hook M. Surface protein adhesins of *Staphylococcus aureus. Trends Microb* 1998;6:484–488.
8. Schmidt KA, Manna AC, Cheung AL. *Sar*T influences *sar*S expression in *Staphylococcus aureus. Infect Immun*2003;71:5139–5148.
9. John JF. Staphylococcal infection: emerging clinical syndromes and their presentations of disease. In: Ala'Aldeen D, Hiramatsu H, eds. *Staphylococcus aureus: molecular and clinical aspects.* Chichester, UK: Horwood, 2004:1–30.
10. Wise RI, Ossman EA, Littlefield DR. Personal reflections on nosocomial staphylococcal infections and the development of hospital surveillance. *Rev Infect Dis* 1989;11:1005–1019.
11. Emori TG, Gaynes RP. An overview of nosocomial infections. *Clin Microbiol Rev* 1993;6:428–442.
12. McClure AR, Gordon J. In-vitro evaluation of povidone-iodine and chlorhexidine against methicillin-resistant *Staphylococcus aureus. J Hosp Infect* 1992;21:291–299.
13. Boyce JM. Understanding and controlling methicillin-resistant staphylococcus *aureus* infections. *Infect Control Hosp Epidemiol* 2002;23: 485–487.
14. Dreamworks Productions. *The Prince of Egypt.* 1998.
15. Gottfried RS. *The Black Death, natural and human disaster in medieval Europe.* New York: Macmillan, 1983.
16. Wilson GS, Topley MA. *Topley and Wilson's principles of bacteriology, virology and immunity.* Baltimore: Williams & Wilkins, 1975.
17. Kloos W. Systematics and the natural history of staphylococci. 1. In: Jones D, Board R, Sussman M, eds. *The staphylococci.* Boston: Blackwell Scientific, 1990:25S–37S.
18. Kloos W. Taxonomy and systematics of staphylococci indigenous to humans. In: Crossley KB, Archer GL, eds. *The staphylococci.* New York: Churchill Livingstone, 1997:113–137.
19. Spink WW. *Infect diseases. Prevention and treatment in the nineteenth and twentieth centuries.* Minneapolis: University of Minnesota Press, 1978.
20. Skinner D, Keefer CS. Significance of bacteremia caused by *S. aureus*; study of 122 cases and review of literature concerned with experimental infection in animals. *Arch Intern Med* 1941;68:851–875.
21. Finland M, Jones JWF. Staphylococcal infections currently encountered in a large municipal hospital: some problems in evaluating antimicrobial therapy in such infections. *Ann N Y Acad Sci* 1957;65: 191–205.
22. Brakstad OG, Maeland JA. Detection of *Staphylococcus aureus* with biotinylated monoclonal antibodies directed against staphylococcal TNase complexed to avidin-peroxidase in a rapid sandwich enzyme-linked immunofiltration assay (sELIFA). *J Med Microbiol* 1993;39: 128–134.
23. Hurlimanndalel RL, Ryffel C, Kayser FH, et al. Survey of the methicillin resistance-associated genes mecA, mecR1-mecI, and femA-femB in clinical isolates of methicillin-resistant *Staphylococcus aureus. Antimicrob Agents Chemother* 1992;36:2617–2621.
24. Cotter PD, Hill C. Surviving the acid test: responses of gram-positive bacteria to low pH. *Microb Molecular Biology Rev*2003;67:429–453.
25. Baron EJ, D'Souza HA. (2003). CHROMagar Staph *Aureus* is superior to mannitol salt for detection of *Staphylococcus aureus* in complex mixed infections (abstract D-1681). 43rd Interscience Conference on Antimicrob Agents Chemother, Chicago, September 14–17, 2003.
26. Monzon-Moreno C, Aubert S, Morvan A, et al. Usefulness of three probes in typing isolates of methicillin-resistant *Staphylococcus aureus* (MRSA). *J Med Microbiol* 1991;35:80–88.
27. Arbeit RD, Karakawa WW, Vann WF, et al. Predominance of two newly described capsular polysaccharide types among clinical isolates of *Staphylococcus aureus. Diagn Microbiol Infect Dis* 1984;2:85–91.
28. Flandrois J, Fleurette J, Behr H. Evaluation of *S. aureus* serotyping method. *Zentralbl Bakteriol Hyg* 1978:A241:279–285.
29. Gustafson JE, O'Brien FG, Coombs GW, et al. Alterations in phage-typing patterns in vancomycin-intermediate *Staphylococcus aureus. J Med Microbiol*2003;52:711–714.
30. Mulligan M, Kwok R, Citron D, et al. Immunoblots, antimicrobial resistance, and bacteriophage typing of oxacillin-resistant *Staphylococcus aureus. J Clin Microbiol* 1988;26:2395–2401.
31. Goetz M, Mulligan M, Kwok R, et al. Management and epidemiologic analyses of an outbreak due to methicillin-resistant *Staphylococcus aureus. Am J Med* 1992;92:607–614.
32. Coia J, Thomson-Carter F, Baird D, et al. Characterization of methicillin-resistant *Staphylococcus aureus* by biotyping, immunoblotting and restriction enzyme fragmentation patterns. *J Med Microbiol* 1990; 31:125–132.
33. Strommenger B, Kettlitz C, Werner G, et al. Multiplex PCR assay for simultaneous detection of nine clinically relevant antibiotic resistance genes in *Staphylococcus aureus. J Clin Microbiol*2003;41:4089–4094.
34. Elek SD, Davies JR, Miles R. Resistotyping of Shigella sonnei. *J Med Microbiol*1973;6:329–345.
35. Bouvet A, Fournier J, Audurier A, et al. Epidemiological markers for epidemic strain and carrier isolates in an outbreak of nosocomial oxacillin-resistant *Staphylococcus aureus. J Clin Microbiol* 1990;28: 1338–1341.
36. Branger C, Goullet P. Genetic heterogeneity in methicillin-resistant strains of *Staphylococcus aureus* revealed by esterase electrophoretic polymorphism. *J Hosp Infect* 1989;14:125–134.
37. Musser J, Schlievert P, Chow A, et al. A single clone of *Staphylococcus aureus* causes the majority of cases of toxic shock syndrome. *Proc Natl Acad Sci USA* 1990;87:225–229.
38. Musser J, Kapur V. Clonal analysis of methicillin-resistant *Staphylococcus aureus* strains from intercontinental sources: association of the mec gene with divergent phylogenetic lineages implies dissemination by horizontal transfer and recombination. *J Clin Microbiol* 1992;30: 2058–2063.
39. Barzilai A, Hyatt A, Hodes D. Demonstration of differences between strains of *Staphylococcus aureus* by a peptidoglycan fingerprinting. *J Infect Dis* 1984;150:583–588.
40. Arbeit RD. Laboratory procedures for epidemiologic analysis. In: Crossley KB, Archer GL, eds. *The staphylococci in human disease.* New York: Churchill Livingstone, 1997:253–286.
41. Walsh TJ, Standiford HC, Reboli AC, et al. Randomized double-blind trial of rifampin with either novobiocin or trimethoprim-sulfa-

methoxazole against methicillin-resistant *Staphylococcus aureus* colonization: prevention of antimicrobial resistance and effect of host factors on outcome. *Antimicrob Agents Chemother* 1993;37:1334–1342.
42. Hadjiliadis D, Howell DN, Davis RD, et al. Anastomotic infections in lung transplant recipients. *Ann Transplant*2000;5:13–19.
43. Venezia R, Harris V, Miller C, et al. Investigation of an outbreak of methicillin-resistant *Staphylococcus aureus* in patients with skin disease using DNA restriction patterns. *Infect Control Hosp Epidemiol* 1992; 13:472–476.
44. Nicolle L, Bialkowska-Hobrzanska H, Romance L, et al. Colonal diversity of methicillin-resistant *Staphylococcus aureus* in an acute care institution. *Infect Control Hosp Epidemiol* 1992;13:33–37.
45. Pekkala D, Low D, Wyper P, et al. The utility of restriction endonuclease analysis and phage typing in the epidemiologic investigation of a *Staphylococcus aureus* outbreak in a neonatal nursery. *Diagn Microbiol Infect Dis* 1992;15:307–311.
46. El-Adhami W, Roberts L, Vickery A, et al. Epidemiological analysis of methicillin-resistant *Staphylococcus aureus* outbreak using restriction fragment length polymorphisms of genomic DNA. *J Gen Microbiol* 1991;137:2713–2720.
47. Tenover FC, Arbeit RD, Goering RV, et al. Interpreting chromosomal DNA restriction patterns produced by pulsed-field gel electrophoresis: criteria for bacterial strain typing. *J Clin Microbiol* 1995;33: 2233–2239.
48. Dice L. Measures of the amount of ecological association between species. *Ecology* 1945;26:297–302.
49. Thouverez M, Muller A, Hocquet D, et al. Relationship between molecular epidemiology and antibiotic susceptibility of methicillin-resistant *Staphylococcus aureus* (MRSA) in a french teaching hospital. *J Med Microbiol*2003;52:801–806.
50. Carles-Nurit M, Christophle B, Broche S, et al. DNA polymorphisms in methicillin-susceptible and methicillin-resistant strains of *Staphylococcus aureus. J Clin Microbiol* 1992;30:2092–2096.
51. Struelens M, Deplano A, Godard C, et al. Epidemiologic typing and delineation of genetic relatedness of methicillin-resistance *Staphylococcus aureus* by macrorestriction analysis of genomic DNA by using pulsed-field gel electrophoresis. *J Clin Microbiol* 1992;30:2599–2605.
52. Linhardt F, Ziebuhr W, Meyer P, et al. Pulsed-field gel electrophoresis of genomic restriction fragments as a tool for the epidemiological analysis of *Staphylococcus aureus* and coagulase-negative staphylococci. *FEMS Microbiol Lett* 1992;95:181–186.
53. Murchan S, Kaufmann ME, Delpano A, et al. Harmonization of pulsed-field gel electrophoresis protocols for epidemiological typing of strains of methicillin-resistant *Staphylococcus aureus*: a single approach developed by consensus in 10 European laboratories and its application for tracing the spread of related strains. *J Clin Microbiol*2003; 41:1574–1585.
54. Kreiswirth B, Kornblum J, Arbeit RD, et al. Evidence for a clonal origin of methicillin resistance in *Staphylococcus aureus. Science* 1993; 259:227–230.
55. Wei M-Q, Udo E, Grubb W. Typing of methicillin-resistant *Staphylococcus aureus* with IS256. *FEMS Microbiol Lett* 1992;99:175–180.
56. Dyke KG, Aubert S, el Solh N. Multiple copies of IS256 in staphylococci. *Plasmid* 1992;28:235–246.
57. Meugnier H, Fernandez M, Bes M, et al. rRNA gene restriction patterns as an epidemiological marker in nosocomial outbreaks of *Staphylococcus aureus* infections. *Res Microbiol* 1993;144:25–33.
58. Goh S-H, Byrne S, Zhang J, et al. Molecular typing of *Staphylococcus aureus* on the basis of coagulase gene polymorphisms. *J Clin Microbiol* 1992;30:1642–1645.
59. Van der Zee A, Verbakel H, Van Zon J-C, et al. Molecular genotyping of *Staphylococcus aureus* strains: Comparison of repetitive element sequence-based PCR with various typing methods and isolation of a novel epidemicity marker. *J Clin Microbiol* 1999;37:342–349.
60. Saulnier P, Bourneix C, Prevost G, et al. Random amplified polymorphic DNA assay is less discriminant than pulsed-field gel electrophoresis for typing strains of methicillin-resistant *Staphylococcus aureus. J Clin Microbiol* 1993;31:982–985.
61. Frenay HM, Theelen JP, Schouls LM, et al. Discrimination of epidemic and nonepidemic methicillin-resistant *Staphylococcus aureus* strains on the basis of protein A gene polymorphism. *J Clin Microbiol* 1994;32:846–847.
62. Enright MC, Day NP, Davies CE, et al. Multilocus sequence typing for characterization of methicillin-resistant and methicillin-susceptible clones of *Staphylococcus aureus. J Clin Microbiol*2000;38:1008–1015.
63. Aires De Sousa M, de Lencastre H. Evolution of sporadic isolates of methicillin-resistant *Staphylococcus aureus* (MRSA) in hospitals and their similarities to isolates of community-acquired MRSA. *J Clin Microbiol* 2003;41:3806–3815.
64. McGowan JJ. Changing etiology of nosocomial bacteremia and fungemia and other hospital-acquired infections. *Rev Infect Dis* 1985; 7(suppl 3):S357–S370.
65. Leibovici L, Konisberger H, Pitlik S, et al. Bacteremia and fungemia of unknown origin in adults. *Clin Infect Dis* 1992;14:436–443.
66. Casewell M, I-Ell R. The carrier state: methicillin-resistant *Staphylococcus aureus. J Antimicrob Chemother* 1986;18(suppl A):1–12.
67. Williams REO. Healthy carriage of *Staphylococcus aureus*: its prevalence and importance. *Bacterial Rev* 1963;27:56–71.
68. Sheagren J. Staphylococcal infections of the skin and skin structures. *CUTIS* 1985;36:3–6.
69. Fekety F. The epidemiology and prevention of staphylococcal infection. *Medicine* 1964;43:593–596.
70. Hoeger PH, Lenz W, Boutonnier A, et al. Staphylococcal skin colonization in children with atopic dermatitis: prevalence, persistence, and transmission of toxigenic and nontoxigenic strains. *J Infect Dis* 1992; 165:1064–1068.
71. Parnaby RM, O'Dwyer G, Monsey HG, et al. Carriage of *Staphylococcus aureus* in the elderly. *J Hosp Infect* 1996;33:201–206.
72. Tuazon C. Skin and skin structure infections in the patient at risk: carrier state of *Staphylococcus aureus. Am J Med* 1984;15:166–171.
73. Rammelkamp C, Mortimer E, Wolinsky E. Transmission of streptococcal and staphylococcal infections. *Ann Intern Med* 1964;60: 753–758.
74. Solberg CO. A study of carriers of *Staphylococcus aureus* with special regard to quantitative bacterial estimations. *Acta Med Scand* 1965; 436(suppl):1–96.
75. Kune GA, Moritz V, Carson P, et al. Postoperative wound infections: a study of bacteriology and pathogenesis. *Aust N Z J Surg* 1983;53: 245–248.
76. Calia F, Wolinsky E, Mortimer E Jr, et al. Importance of the carrier state as a source of *Staphylococcus aureus* in wound sepsis. *J Hyg (London)* 1969;67:49–57.
77. Talon D, Rouget C, Cailleau V, et al. Nasal carriage of *Staphylococcus aureus* and cross-contamination in a surgical intensive care unit: efficacy of mupirocin ointment. *J Hosp Infect* 1995;30:39–49.
78. Ruef C, Fanconi S, Nadal D. Sternal wound infection after heart operations in pediatric patients associated with nasal carriage of *Staphylococcus aureus. J Thorac Cardiovasc Surg* 1996;112:681–686.
79. Ahmed AO, van Belkum A, Fahal AH, et al. Nasal carriage of *Staphylococcus aureus* and epidemiology of surgical-site infections in a Sudanese university hospital. *J Clin Microbiol* 1998;36:3614–3618.
80. Yu VL, Goeta A, Wagener M, et al. *Staphylococcus aureus* nasal carriage and infection in patients on hemodialysis. *N Engl J Med* 1986;315: 91–96.
81. Luzar MA, Coles GA, Faller B, et al. *Staphylococcus aureus* nasal carriage and infection in patients on continuous ambulatory peritoneal dialysis. *N Engl J Med* 1990;322:505–509.
82. Churchill DN. Risk of CAPD complications in carriers of *Staph. aureus. Semin Dial* 1993;6:71.
83. Mir N, Sánchez M, Baquero F, et al. Soft salt-mannitol agar-cloxacillin test: a highly specific bedside screening test for detection of colonization with methicillin-resistant *Staphylococcus aureus. J Clin Microbiol* 1998;36:986–989.
84. Day NP, Moore CE, Enright MC, et al. A link between virulence and ecological abundance in natural populations of *Staphylococcus aureus. Science* 2001;292:114–116.
85. Herrmann M, Pierre E, Didier P, et al. Fibronectin, fibrinogen and laminin act as mediators for adherence of clinical staphylococcal isolates to foreign material. *J Infect Dis* 1988;158:693–701.

86. Foster TJ, Hook M. Surface protein adhesins of *Staphylococcus aureus. Trends Microbiol* 1998;6:484–488.
87. Cheung AL, Schmidt KA, Bateman B, et al. *SarS*, *SarA* homolog repressible by *agr*, is an activator of protein A synthesis in *Staphylococcus aureus. Infect Immun*2001;69:2448–2455.
88. Mota GFA, Carneiro CRW, Gomes L, et al. Monoclonal antibodies to *Staphylococcus aureus* laminin-binding proteins cross-react with mammalian cells. *Infect Immun* 1988;56:1580–1584.
89. Switalski L, Patti J, Butcher W, et al. A collagen receptor on *Staphylococcus aureus* strains isolated from patients with septic arthritis mediates adhesion to cartilage. *Mol Microbiol* 1993;7:99–107.
90. Wädstrom T. Molecular aspects on pathogenesis of wound and foreign body infections due to staphylococci. *Zentralbl Bakteriol Mikrobiol Hyg A* 1987;266:191–211.
91. Valentinweigand P, Timmis KN, Chhatwal GS. Role of fibronectin in staphylococcal colonisation of fibrin thrombi and plastic surfaces. *J Med Microbiol* 1993;38:90–95.
92. Hamill RJ. Role of fibronectin in infective endocarditis. *Rev Infect Dis* 1987;9:S360–S371.
93. Scheld W, Strunk R, Balian G, et al. Microbial adhesion to fibronectin in vitro correlates with production of endocarditis in rabbits (42205). *Proc Soc Exp Biol Med* 1985;180:474–482.
94. Kuypers JM, Proctor RA. Reduced adherence to traumatized rat heart valves by a low-fibronectin-binding mutant of *Staphylococcus aureus. Infect Immun* 1989;57:2306–2312.
95. Lindblad B, Johansson A. I125-Fibrinogen uptake on peripheral venous cannulas: a comparison between different cannula materials and coatings. *J Biomed Mater Res* 1987;21:99–105.
96. Hawiger J, Timmons S, Strong DD, et al. Identification of a region of human fibrinogen interacting with staphylococcal clumping factor. *Biochemistry* 1982;21:1407–1413.
97. McDevitt D, Vaudaux P, Foster T. Genetic evidence that bound coagulase of *Staphylococcus aureus* is not clumping factor. *Infect Immun* 1992;60:1514–1523.
98. Boden M, Flock J. Evidence for three different fibrinogen-binding proteins with unique properties from *Staphylococcus aureus* strain Newman. *Microb Pathog* 1992;12:289–298.
99. Josefsson E, Hartford O, O'Brien L, et al. Protection against experimental *Staphylococcus aureus* arthritis by vaccination with clumping factor A, a novel virulence determinant. *J Infect Dis* 2001;184:1572–1580.
100. Lopes JD, dosReis M, Brentani RR. Presence of laminin receptors in *Staphylococcus aureus. Science* 1985;229:275–277.
101. Liang O, Ascencio F, Fransson L, et al. Binding of heparan sulfate to *Staphylococcus aureus. Infect Immun* 1992;60:899–906.
102. Vercellotti G, McCarthy J, Lindholm P, et al. Extracellular matrix proteins (fibronectin, laminin and type IV collagen) bind and aggregate bacteria. *Am J Pathol* 1985;120:13–21.
103. Akiyama H, Huh WK, Yamasaki O, et al. Confocal laser scanning microscopic observation of glycocalyx production by *Staphylococcus aureus* in mouse skin: does *S. aureus* generally produce a biofilm on damaged skin? *Br J Dermatol* 2002;147:879–885.
104. O'Brien LM, Walsh EJ, Massey RC, et al. *Staphylococcus aureus* clumping factor B (ClfB) promotes adherence to human type I cytokeratin 10: implications for nasal colonization. *Cell Microbiol* 2002;4:759–770.
105. Gotz F. *Staphylococcus* and biofilms. *Mol Microbiol* 2002;43:1367–1378.
106. Olina M, Cametti M, Guglielmetti C, et al. [External otitis]. *Recenti Prog Med*2002;93:104–107.
107. Marrack P, Kappler J. The staphylococcal enterotoxin and their relatives. *Science* 1990;248:705–711.
108. Zumla A. Superantigens, T cells, and microbes. *Clin Infect Dis* 1992;15:313–320.
109. Rogolsky M. Nonenteric toxins of *Staphylococcus aureus. Mibrobiol Rev* 1979;43:320–360.
110. Shrayer D. *Staphylococcal disease in the Soviet Union. Epidemiology and response to a national epidemic.* Falls Church, VA: Delphic Associates, 1989.
111. O'Reilly M, de Azavedo JCS, Kennedy S, et al. Inactivation of the alpha-haemolysin gene of *Staphylococcus aureus* 8325-4 by site-directed mutagenesis and studies on the expression of its haemolysins. *Microb Pathog* 1986;1:125–138.
112. Iandolo J. Genetic analysis of extracellular toxins of *Staphylococcus aureus. Annu Rev Microbiol* 1989;43:375–402.
113. Thelestom M. Modes of membrane damaging action of staphylococcal toxins. In: Easmon CF, Adlam C, eds. *Staphylococci and staphylococcal infections.* New York: Academic Press, 1983:705–744.
114. Ward P, Turner W. Identification of staphylococcal Panton-Valentine leukocidin as a potent dermonecrotic toxin. *Infect Immun* 1980;27:393–397.
115. Jin T, Bokarewa M, McIntyre L, et al. Fatal outcome of bacteraemic patients caused by infection with staphylokinase-deficient *Staphylococcus aureus* strains. *J Med Microb*2003;52:919–923.
116. Finck-Barbancon V, Prevost G, Piemont Y. Improved purification of leukocidin from *Staphylococcus aureus* and toxin distribution among hospital strains. *Res Microbiol* 1991;142:75–85.
117. Supersac G, Prevost G, Piemont Y. Sequencing of leucocidin R from *Staphylococcus aureus* P83 suggests that staphylococcal leucocidins and gamma-hemolysin are members of a single, two-component family of toxins. *Infect Immun* 1993;61:580–587.
118. Dufour P, Gillet Y, Bes M, et al. Community-acquired methicillin-resistant *Staphylococcus aureus* infections in France: emergence of a single clone that produces Panton-Valentine leukocidin. *Clin Infect Dis* 2002;35:819–824.
119. Vandenesch F, Kornblum J, Novick R. A temporal signal, independent of *agr*, is required for *hla* but not *spa* transcription in *Staphylococcus aureus. J Bacteriol* 1991;173:6313–6320.
120. Miller J, Mekalanos J, Falkow S. Coordinate regulation and sensory transduction in the control of bacterial virulence. *Science* 1989;243:916–922.
121. Yeaman M, Sullam P, Dazin P, et al. Characterization of *Staphylococcus aureus*-platelet binding by quantitative flow cytometric analysis. *J Infect Dis* 1992;166:65–73.
122. Baker AS, Ramos MD, Menzies BE, et al. Hyperproduction of alpha-toxin by staphylococcus *aureus* results in paradoxically reduced virulence in experimental endocarditis–host defense role for platelet microbicidal protein. *Infect Immun*1997;65:4652–4660.
123. Kupferwasser LI, Yeaman MR, Nast CC, et al. Salicylic acid attenuates virulence in endovascular infections by targeting global regulatory pathways in *Staphylococcus aureus. J Clin Invest*2003;112:222–233.
124. Tompkins D, Blackwell L, Hatcher V, et al. *Staphylococcus aureus* proteins that bind to human endothelial cells. *Infect Immun* 1992;60:965–969.
125. Leffer H, Svanborg-Eden C. Glycolipid receptors for uropathogenic *Escherichia coli* on human erythrocytes and uroepithelial cells. *Infect Immun* 1981;34:920–929.
126. Ogawa SK, Yurberg ER, Hatcher VB, et al. Bacterial adherence to human endothelial cells in vitro. *Infect Immun* 1985;50:218–224.
127. Johnson C, Hancock G, Goulin G. Specific binding of *Staphylococcus aureus* to cultured porcine cardiac valvular endothelial cells. *J Lab Clin Med* 1988;112:16–22.
128. Campbell K, Johnson C. Identification of *Staphylococcus aureus* binding proteins on isolated porcine cardiac valve cells. *J Lab Clin Med* 1990;115:217–223.
129. Tompkins DC, Hatcher VB, Patel D, et al. A human endothelial cell membrane protein that binds *Staphylococcus aureus* in vitro. *J Clin Invest* 1990;85:1248–1254.
130. Hamill RL, Vann JM, Proctor RA. Phagocytosis of *Staphylococcus aureus* by cultured bovine aortic endothelial cells: model for postadherence events in endovascular infections. *Infect Immun* 1986;54:833–836.
131. Cunnion KM, Frank MM. Complement activation influences *Staphylococcus aureus* adherence to endothelial cells. *Infect Immun* 2003;71:1321–1327.
132. Menzies BE, Kourteva I. Internalization of *Staphylococcus aureus* by endothelial cells induces apoptosis. *Infect Immun* 1998;66:5994–5998.
133. Vann JM, Proctor RA. Ingestion of *Staphylococcus aureus* by bovine

endothelial cells results in time- and inoculum-dependent damage to endothelial cell monolayers. *Infect Immun* 1987;55:2155–2163.

134. Bengualid V, Hatcher V, Diamond B, et al. *Staphylococcus aureus* infection of human endothelial cells potentiates Fc receptor expression. *J Immunol* 1990;145:4279–4283.
135. Cheung AL, Fischetti VA. The role of fibrinogen in mediating staphylococcal adherence to fibers. *J Surg Res* 1991;50:150–155.
136. Thomas P, Hampson F, Hunninghake G. Bacterial adherence to human endothelial cells. *J Appl Physiol* 1988;65:1372–1376.
137. Lee JC, Liu MJ, Parsonnet J, et al. Expression of type 8 capsular polysaccharide and production of toxic shock syndrome toxin 1 are associated among vaginal isolates of *Staphylococcus aureus. J Clin Microbiol*1990;28:2612–2615.
138. Xu S, Arbeit R, Lee J. Phagocytic killing of encapsulated microencapsulated *Staphylococcus aureus* by human polymorphonuclear leukocytes. *Infect Immun* 1992;60:1358–1362.
139. Thakker M, Park JS, Carey V, et al. *Staphylococcus aureus* serotype 5 capsular polysaccharide is antiphagocytic and enhances bacterial virulence in a murine bacteremia model. *Infect Immun* 1998;66: 5183–5189.
140. Bhasin N, Albus A, Michon F, et al. Identification of a gene essential for O-acetylation of the *Staphylococcus aureus* type 5 capsular polysaccharide. *Mol Microbiol* 1998;27:9–21.
141. Pohlmann-Dietze P, Ulrich M, et al. Adherence of *Staphylococcus aureus* to endothelial cells: influence of the capsular polysaccharide, the global regulator *agr*, and the bacterial growth phase. *Infect Immun* 2000;68:4865–4871.
142. Baddour LM, Lowrance C, et al. *Staphylococcus aureus* microcapsule expression attenuates bacterial virulence in a rat model of experimental endocarditis. *J Infect Dis* 1992;165:749–753.
143. Kiser KB, Cantey-Kiser JM, Lee JC. Development and characterization of a *Staphylococcus aureus* nasal colonization model in mice. *Infect Immun*1999;67:5001–5006.
144. Gransden WR, Eykyn S, Phillips I. *Staphylococcus aureus* bacteraemia: 400 episodes in St. Thomas's Hospital. *Br Med J* 1984;288:300.
145. Mortara LA, Bayer AS. *Staphylococcus aureus* bacteremia and endocarditis. *Infect Dis Clin North Am* 1993;7:53–68.
146. Fang G, Keys TF, Gentry LO, et al. Prosthetic valve endocarditis resulting from nosocomial bacteremia. A prospective, multicenter study. *Ann Intern Med* 1993;117:560–567.
147. Marshall SA, Wilke WW, Pfaller MA, et al. *Staphylococcus aureus* and coagulase-negative staphylococci from blood stream infections: frequence of occurrence, antimicrobial susceptibility, and molecular (mecA) characterization of oxacillin resistance in the SCOPE program. *Diagn Microbiol Infect Dis* 1998;30:205–214.
148. Nolan CM, Beaty HN. *Staphylococcus aureus* bacteremia. *Am J Med* 1976;60:495–500.
149. Michel MF, Priem CC, Verbrugh HA, v*Staphylococcus aureus* bacteremia in a Dutch teaching hospital. *Med Verlag* 1985;6:267–272.
150. Banerjee SN, Emori TG, Culver DH. Secular trends in nosocomial primary bloodstream infections in the United States 1980–1989. *Am J Med* 1991;91:86–89.
151. Muder RR, Brennen C, Wagener MM, et al. Bacteremia in a long-term-care facility: a five-year prospective study of 163 consecutive episodes. *Clin Infect Dis* 1992;14:647–654.
152. de Oliveira CL, Wey SB, Castelo A. *Staphylococcus aureus* bacteremia: comparison of two periods and a predictive model of mortality. *Braz J Infect Dis* 2002;6:288–297.
153. Lodise TP, McKinnon PS, Rybak M. Prediction model to identify patients with *staphylococcus aureus* bacteremia at risk for methicillin resistance *Infect Control Hosp Epidermol* 2003;24:655–661.
154. Yzerman EP, Boelens HA, Tjhie JH, et al. Delta APACHE II for predicting course and outcome of nosocomial *Staphylococcus aureus* bacteremia and its relation to host defense. *J Infect Dis* 1996;173: 914–919.
155. Shah M, Watanakunakorn C. Changing patterns of *Staphylococcus aureus* bacteremia. *Am J Med Sci* 1979;278:115–121.
156. Libman H, Arbeit RD. Complications associated with *Staphylococcus aureus* bacteremia. *Arch Intern Med* 1984;144:541.
157. Steinberg JP, Clark CC, Hackman BO. Nosocomial and community-acquired *Staphylococcus aureus* bacteremias from 1980–1993: impact of intravascular devices and methicillin resistance. *Clin Infect Dis* 1996;23:255–259.
158. Schonheyder H, Jensen KT, Pers C, et al. Spread of *Staphylococcus aureus* strains of phage-type 95 in Denmark 1968–1989. *J Hosp Infect* 1992;20:25–34.
159. Jensen AG, Wachmann CH, Espersen F, et al. Treatment and outcome of *Staphylococcus aureus* bacteremia: a prospective study of 278 cases. *Arch Intern Med* 2002;162:25–32.
160. Ladisch S, Pizzo PA. *Staphylococcus aureus* sepsis in children with cancer. *Pediatrics* 1978;61:231–234.
161. Plaut ME, Palaszynski F, Bjornsson S, et al. Staphylococcal bacteremia in a germ-free unit. *Arch Intern Med* 1976;136:1238–1240.
162. Carney DN, Fossieck BE, Parker RH, et al. Bacteremia due to *Staphylococcus aureus* in patients with cancer: report on 45 cases in adults and review of the literature. *Rev Infect Dis* 1982;4:1–12.
163. Funada H, Yoneyama H, Machi T, et al. *Staphylococcus aureus* bacteremia in patients with hematologic disorders. *Jpn Assoc Infect Dis* 1992; 66:1436–1443.
164. Sotman SB, Schimpff SC, Young VM. *Staphylococcus aureus* bacteremia in patients with acute leukemia. *Am J Med* 1980;69:814–818.
165. Jacobson JA, Kasworm E, Daly JA. Risk of developing toxic shock syndrome associated with toxic shock syndrome toxin 1 following nongenital staphylococcal infection. *Rev Infect Dis* 1989;11:S8–S13.
166. Weber DJ, Becherer PR, Rutala WA, et al. Nosocomial infection rate as a function of human immunodeficiency virus type 1 status in hemophiliacs. *Am J Med* 1991;91(suppl 3B):206S–211S.
167. Weinke T, Schiller R, Fehrenbach FJ, et al. Association between *Staphylococcus aureus* nasopharyngeal colonization and septicemia in patients infected with the human immunodeficiency virus. *Eur J Clin Microbiol Infect Dis* 1992;11:986–989.
168. Onorato M, Borucki MJ, Baillargeon G, et al. Risk factors of colonization or infection due to methicillin-resistant *Staphylococcus aureus* in HIV-positive patients: a retrospective case-control study. *Infect Control Hosp Epidemiol* 1999;20:26–30.
169. Becker K, Friedrich AW, Lubritz G, et al. Prevalence of genes encoding pyrogenic toxin superantigens and exfoliative toxins among strains of *Staphylococcus aureus* isolated from blood and nasal specimens. *J Clin Microbiol* 2003;41:1434–1439.
170. Komolafe OO, James J, Kalongolera L, et al. Bacteriology of burns at the Queen Elizabeth Central Hospital, Blantyre, Malawi. *Burns*2003;29:235–238.
171. Santucci SG, Gobara S, Santos CR, et al. Infections in a burn intensive care unit: experience of seven years. *J Hosp Infect*2003;53:6–13.
172. Demling RH. Burns. *N Engl J Med* 1985;313:1389–1401.
173. Manson WL, Pernot PC, Fidler V, et al. Colonization of burns and the duration of hospital stay of severely burned patients. *J Hosp Infect* 1992;22:55–63.
174. Ransjo U. Isolation care of infection-prone burn patients. *Scand J Infect Dis Suppl* 1978;11:1–46.
175. Troelstra A, Kamp-Hopmans TE, Wessels FJ, et al. Epidemic of methicillin-resistant *Staphylococcus aureus* due to the transfer of 2 Dutch burn patients from a hospital outside of the Netherlands; who suffers the consequences? *Ned Tijdschr Geneeskd*2002;146:2204–2207.
176. Burke JF, Quinby WC, Bondoc CC, et al. The contribution of a bacterially isolated environment to the prevention of infection in seriously burned patients. *Ann Surg* 1977;186(3):377–385.
177. Buchanan K, Heimbach DM, Minshew BH, et al. Comparison of quantitative and semiquantitative culture techniques for burn biopsy. *J Clin Microbiol* 1986;23:258–261.
178. Martin AM, Clunie GJA, Tonkin RW, et al. The aetiology and management of shunt infections in patients on intermittent haemodialysis. *Proc Eur Dial Transplant Assoc* 1967;4:67–72.
179. Noble WC, Rebel MH, Smith I. An investigation of the skin flora of dialysis and transplant patients. *Br J Dermatol* 1974;91:201–207.
180. Kirmani N, Tuason CU, Murray HW, et al. *Staphylococcus aureus* carriage rate of patients receiving long-term hemodialysis. *Arch Intern Med* 1978;138:1657–1659.
181. Goldblum SE, Reed WP, Ulrich JA, et al. Staphylococcal carriage

and infections in hemodialysis patients. *Dialy Transplant* 1978;7: 1140–1163.

182. Cross AS, Zierdt CH, Roup B, et al. A hospital-wide outbreak of septicemia due to a few strains of *Staphylococcus aureus. Am J Clin Pathol* 1983;79:598–603.
183. Boelaert JR, van Landuyt HW, Gordts BZ, et al. Nasal and cutaneous carriage of in hemodialysis patients. *Infect Control Hosp Epidemiol* 1996;17:809–811.
184. Kluytmans JAJW, Manders M-J, van Bomel E, et al. Elimination of nasal carriage of in hemodialysis patients. *Infect Control Hosp Epidemiol* 1996;17:793–798.
185. Annigeri R, Conly J, et al. Emergence of mupirocin-resistant *Staphylococcus aureus* in chronic peritoneal dialysis patients using mupirocin prophylaxis to prevent exit-site infection. *Perit Dial Int*2001;21: 554–559.
186. Miller MA, Dascal IA, Portnoy J, et al. Development of mupirocin resistance among methicillin-resistant *Staphylococcus aureus* infections after widespread use of nasal mupirocin ointment. *Infect Control Hosp Epidemiol* 1996;17:811–813.
187. Mond LL, Kokai-Kun JF, Walsh SM, et al. Lysostapin cream eradicates nasal colonization in a cotton rat model. *Antimicrob Agents Chemther* 2003;47:1589–5977.
188. Matsuzaki S, Yasuda M, Nishikawa H, et al. Experimental protection of mice against lethal *staphylococcus aureus* infection by novel bacteriophage phi MR11. *J Infect Dis* 2003;187:613–614.
189. Pignatari A, Pfaller M, Hollis R, et al. *Staphylococcus aureus* colonization and infection in patients on continuous ambulatory peritoneal dialysis. *J Clin Microbiol* 1990;28:1898–1902.
190. Piraino B. A review of *Staphylococcus aureus* exit-site and tunnel infections in peritoneal dialysis patients. *Am J Kidney Dis* 1990;2:89–95.
191. Perez-Fontan M, Rosales M, Rodriguez-Carmona A, et al. Treatment of *Staphylococcus aureus* nasal carriers in CAPD with mupirocin. *Adv Perit Dialy* 1992;8:242–245.
192. Peacock SJ, Mandal S, Bowler IC. Preventing *Staphylococcus aureus* infection in the renal unit. *Q J Med*2002;95:405–410.
193. Christie CDC, Lynch-Ballard E. Staphylococcal enterocolitis revisited: cytotoxic properties of *Staphylococcus aureus* from a neonate with enterocolitis. *Pediatr Infect Dis J* 1988;7:791–795.
194. Overturf GD, Sherman MP, Scheifele DW, et al. Neonatal necrotizing enterocolitis associated with delta toxin-producing methicillin-resistant *Staphylococcus aureus. Pediatr Infect Dis J* 1990;9:88–91.
195. Adesiyun AA, Lenz W, Schaal KP. Phage susceptibility, enterotoxigenicity and antibiograms of *Staphylococcus aureus* strains isolated from human wounds and diarrhoea. *Int J Med Microbiol* 1992;277: 250–259.
196. Bohach GA, Fast DJ, Nelson RD, et al. Staphylococcal and streptococcal pyrogenic toxins involved in toxic shock syndrome and related illnesses. *Rev Microbiol* 1990;17:251–272.
197. de Andrade GP, Zelante F. Simultaneous occurrence of enterotoxigenic *Staphylococcus aureus* on the hands, mouth and feces of asymptomatic carriers. *Rev Saude Publica* 1989;23:277–284.
198. Watanabe H, Masaki H, Asoh N, et al. Enterocolitis caused by methicillin-resistant *Staphylococcus aureus*: molecular characterization of respiratory and digestive tract isolates. *Microbiol Immunol*2001;45: 629–634.
199. Meehan PJ, Atkeson T, Kepner DE, et al. A foodborne outbreak of gastroenteritis involving two different pathogens. *Am J Epidemiol* 1992;136:611–616.
200. Schlesinger LS, Ross SC, Schaberg DR. *Staphylococcus aureus* meningitis: a broad-based epidemiologic study. *Medicine* 1987;66:148–150.
201. Tumang-Tecson FT. Nosocomial *Staphylococcus aureus* meningitis as presumed complication of intravenous catheterization. *Infect Control* 1977;8:120–123.
202. Ali MA, Kabins SA. Subacute staphylococcal meningitis secondary to postpartum endometritis. *South Med J* 1977;70:368–369.
203. Tessin I, Trolfors BKT. Incidence and etiology of neonatal septicaemia and meningitis in western Sweden 1975–1986. *Acta Pediatr Scand* 1990;79:1023–1030.
204. Lu CH, Huang CR, Chang WN, et al. Community-acquired bacterial meningitis in adults: the epidemiology, timing of appropriate antimicrobial therapy, and prognostic factors. *Clin Neurol Neurosurg*2002; 104:352–358.
205. Musher DM, Olbricht McKenzie S. Infections due to *Staphylococcus aureus. Medicine* 1977;56:383–409.
206. Rello J, Quintana E, Ausina V, et al. Risk factors for *Staphylococcus aureus* nosocomial pneumonia in critically ill patients. *Am Rev Respir Dis* 1990;142:1320–1324.
207. Sanford BA, Thomas VL, Ramsay MA, et al. Characterization of clinical strains of *Staphylococcus aureus* associated with pneumonia. *J Clin Microbiol* 1986;24:131–136.
208. Vindel A, Trincado P, Martin de Nicolas MD, et al. Hospital infections in Spain. I. *Staphylococcus aureus* (1978–1991). *Epidemiol Infect* 1993;110:533–541.
209. Rello J, Quintana E, Ausina V, et al. Incidence, etiology, and outcome of nosocomial pneumonia in mechanically ventilated patients. *Chest* 1991;100:439–444.
210. Gastmeier P, Geffers C, Sohr D, et al. Surveillance of nosocomial infections in intensive care units. Current data and interpretations. *Wien Klin Wochenschr*2003;115:99–103.
211. Rello J, Torres A, Ricart M, et al. Ventilator-associated pneumonia by comparison of methicillin-resistant and methicillin-sensitive episodes. *Am J Respir Crit Care Med* 1994;150:1545–1549.
212. George DL, Falk PS, Wunderink RG, et al. Epidemiology of ventilator-acquired pneumonia based on protected bronchoscopic sampling. *Am J Respir Crit Care Med* 1998;158:1839–1847.
213. Chastre J, Fagon JY. Ventilator-associated pneumonia. *Am J Respir Crit Care Med*2002;165:867–903.
214. Wu CL, Yang D, Wang NY, et al. Quantitative culture of endotracheal aspirates in the diagnosis of ventilator-associated pneumonia in patients with treatment failure. *Chest*2002;122:662–668.
215. Wiswell TE, Curtis J, Dobek AS, et al. *Staphylococcus aureus* colonization after neonatal circumcision in relation to device used. *J Pediatr* 1991;119:302–304.
216. Stark V, Harrisson SP. *Staphylococcus aureus* colonization of the newborn in a Darlington hospital. *J Hosp Infect* 1992;21:201–211.
217. Watkinson M, Dyas A. *Staphylococcus aureus* still colonizes the untreated neonatal umbilicus. *J Hosp Infect* 1992;21:131–136.
218. Wanger AR, Morris SL, Ericsson C, et al. Latex agglutination-negative methicillin-resistant *Staphylococcus aureus* recovered from neonates: epidemiologic features and comparison of typing methods. *J Clin Microbiol* 1992;30:2583–2588.
219. Ish-Horowicz MR, McIntyre P, Nade S. Bone and joint infections caused by multiple-resistant *Staphylococcus aureus* in a neonatal intensive care unit. *Pediatr Infect Dis J* 1992;11:82–87.
220. Reboli AC, John JF, Platt CG, et al. Epidemic methicillin-resistant *Staphylococcus aureus* outbreak at a Veterans Affairs Medical Center: importance of carriage of the organism by hospital personnel. *Infect Control Hosp Epidemiol* 1990;11:291–300.
221. Saiman L, Cronquist A, Wu F, et al. An outbreak of methicillin-resistant *Staphylococcus aureus* in a neonatal intensive care unit. *Infect Control Hosp Epidemiol* 2003;24:317–321.
222. Nambiar S, Herwaldt LA, Singh N. Outbreak of invasive disease caused by methicillin-resistant *Staphylococcus aureus* in neonates and prevalence in the neonatal intensive care unit. *Pediatr Crit Care Med*2003;4:220–226.
223. Hedberg K, Ristinen TL, Soler JT, et al. Outbreak of erythromycin-resistant staphylococcal conjunctivitis in a newborn nursery. *Pediatr Infect Dis J* 1990;9:268–273.
224. Meguro H. MRSA infections in the neonatal unit. *Jpn J Clin Med* 1992;50:1117–1121.
225. Freeman R, Hudson SJ, Burdess D. Crystal violet reactions of fresh clinical isolates of *Staphylococcus aureus* from two British hospitals. *Epidemiol Infect* 1990;105:493–500.
226. Singh K, Gavin PJ, Vescio T, et al. Microbiologic surveillance using nasal cultures alone is sufficient for detection of methicillin-resistant *Staphylococcus aureus* isolates in neonates. *J Clin Microbiol*2003;41: 2755–2757.
227. Gomez J, Rodriguez M, Banos V, et al. [Infections in joint prostheses: epidemiology and clinical presentation. A prospective study 1992–1999]. *Enferm Infecc Microbiol Clin*2002;20:74–77.

228. Nair SP, Williams RJ, Henderson B. Advances in our understanding of the bone and joint pathology caused by *Staphylococcus aureus* infection. *Rheumatology (Oxford)*2000;39:821–834.
229. Florman AL, Holzman RS. Nosocomial scalded skin syndrome. Ritter's disease caused by phage group 3*Staphylococcus aureus. Am J Dis Child* 1980;134:1043–1045.
230. Haley RW, Hooton TM, Culver DH. Nosocomial infections in U.S. hospitals, 1975–1976: estimated frequency by selected characteristics. *Am J Med* 1981;70:947–959.
231. Artz CP, Grogan JB. Staphylococcal infections: incidence, environmental and laboratory studies. *Ann Surg* 1961;1:573–594.
232. Prabhakar P, Raje D, Castle D, et al. Nosocomial surgical infections: incidence and cost in a developing country. *Am J Infect Control* 1983; 11:51–56.
233. Davis JM, Wolff B, Cunningham TF, et al. Delayed wound infection. *Arch Surg* 1982;117:113–117.
234. Tammelin A, Hambraeus A, Stahle E. Mediastinitis after cardiac surgery: improvement of bacteriological diagnosis by use of multiple tissue samples and strain typing. *J Clin Microbiol*2002;40:2936–2941.
235. Simmons BP. CDC guidelines for the prevention and control of nosocomial infections. Guideline for prevention of surgical wound infections. *Infect Control* 1983;11:133–141.
236. Taylor G, Wiens R, Miedzinski L. Failure of preoperative cultures to predict development of *Staphylococcus aureus* wound infections after cardiac surgery. *Can J Surg* 1989;32:128–130.
237. Kropec A, Huebner J, Riffel M, et al. Exogenous or endogenous reservoirs of nosocomial *Pseudomonas aeruginosa* and *Staphylococcus aureus* infections in a surgical intensive care unit. *Intensive Care Med* 1993;19:161–165.
238. Thomas M, Hollins M. Epidemic of postoperative wound infection associated with ungloved abdominal palpation. *Lancet* 1974;2: 1215–1217.
239. Dineen P, Drusin L. Epidemics of postoperative wound infections associated with hair carriers. *Lancet* 1973;2:1157–1159.
240. Schweizer RT. Mask wiggling as a potential cause of wound contamination. *Lancet* 1976;2:1129–1130.
241. Tammelin A, Klotz F, Hambraeus A, et al. Nasal and hand carriage of *Staphylococcus aureus* in staff at a department for thoracic and cardiovascular surgery: endogenous or exogenous source? *Infect Control Hosp Epidemiol*2003;24:686–689.
242. Roettinger W, Edgerton MT, Kurtz LD, et al. Role of inoculation site as a determinant of infection in soft tissue wounds. *Am J Surg* 1973;126:354–358.
243. Marshall KA, Edgerton MT, Rodeheaver GT, et al. Quantitative microbiology: its applications to hand injuries. *Am J Surg* 1976;131: 730–733.
244. Valentine RJ, Weigelt JA, Dryer D, et al. Effect of remote infections on clean wound infection rates. *Am J Infect Control* 1986;14:64–67.
245. Russell B, Ehrenkranz NJ, Hyams PJ, et al. An outbreak of *Staphylococcus aureus* surgical wound infection associated with excess overtime employment of operating room personnel. *Am J Infect Control* 1983; 11:63–67.
246. Wells FC, Newsom SW, Rowlands C. Wound infection in cardiothoracic surgery. *Lancet* 1983;1:1209–1210.
247. Kernodle D, Classen D, Burke J, et al. Failure of cephalosporins to prevent *Staphylococcus aureus* wound infections in cardiac surgery. *JAMA* 1990;263:961–966.
248. LoCicero J, Nichols RL. Sepsis after gastroduodenal operations: relationship to gastric acid, motility and endogenous microflora. *South Med J* 1980;73:878–880.
249. Chaudhary KA, Smith OJ, Cuddy PG, et al. PEG site infections: the emergence of methicillin resistant *Staphylococcus aureus* as a major pathogen. *Am J Gastroenterol* 2002;97:1713–1716.
250. Bartlett P, Reingold AL, Graham DR, et al. Toxic shock syndrome associated with surgical wound infections. *JAMA* 1982;247: 1448–1450.
251. Arnow PM, Chou T, Weil D, et al. Spread of a toxic-shock syndrome associated strain of *Staphylococcus aureus* and measurement of antibodies to staphylococcal enterotoxin F. *J Infect Dis* 1984;149:103–107.
252. Tobin G, Shaw RC, Goodpasture HC. Toxic shock syndrome following breast and nasal surgery. *Plast Reconstr Surg* 1987;80:111–114.
253. Portnoy D, Hinchey EJ, Marcus-Jones OW, et al. Postoperative toxic shock syndrome in a man. *Can Med Assoc J* 1982;126:815–817.
254. Frame JD, Hackett M. Toxic shock syndrome after a minor surgical procedure. *Lancet* 1988;1:1330–1331.
255. Molloy M, Vukelja SJ, Yelland G, et al. Postoperative toxic shock syndrome: a case report and review of the literature. *Milit Med* 1989; 154:74–76.
256. Allen ST, Liland JB, Nichols CG, et al. Toxic shock syndrome associated with use of latex nasal packing. *Arch Intern Med* 1990;150: 2587–2588.
257. Farber BF, Broome CV, Hopkins CC. Fulminant hospital-acquired toxic shock syndrome. *Am J Med* 1984;77:331–332.
258. Kreiswirth BN, Kravitz GR, Schlievert PM, et al. Nosocomial transmission of a strain of *Staphylococcus aureus* causing toxic shock syndrome. *Ann Intern Med* 1986;105:704–707.
259. Marples RR, Richardson JF, Newton FE. Staphylococci as part of the normal flora of human skin. *J Appl Bacteriol* 1990;19:93–99.
260. Kikuchi K, Takahashi N, Piao C, et al. Molecular epidemiology of methicillin-resistant *Staphylococcus aureus* strains causing neonatal toxic shock syndrome-like exanthematous disease in neonatal and perinatal wards. *J Clin Microbiol*2003;41:3001–3006.
261. Demuth PJ, Gerding DN, Crossley K. *Staphylococcus aureus* bacteriuria. *Arch Intern Med* 1979;139:78–80.
262. Arpi M, Renneberg J. The clinical significance of *Staphylococcus aureus* bacteriuria. *J Urol* 1984;132:697–700.
263. Lee BK, Crossley K, Gerding DN. The association between *Staphylococcus aureus* bacteremia and bacteriuria. *Am J Med* 1978;65:303–306.
264. Araki M, Kariyama R, Monden K, et al. Molecular epidemiological studies of *Staphylococcus aureus* in urinary tract infection. *J Infect Chemother*2002;8:168–174.
265. Maki DG. Nosocomial bacteremia. *Am J Med* 1981;70:719–732.
266. Jernigan JA, Farr BM. Short-course therapy of catheter-related *Staphylococcus aureus* bacteremia: a meta-analysis. *Ann Intern Med* 1993; 119:304–311.
267. Knudsen AM, Rosdahl VT, Espersen F, et al. Catheter-related *Staphylococcus aureus* infections. *J Hosp Infect* 1993;23:123–131.
268. Gold HS, Karchmer AW. Catheter-associated *Staphylococcus aureus* bacteremia. *Hosp Pract* 1996;31:133–137.
269. Sherertz RJ, Heard SO, Raad II. Diagnosis of triple-lumen catheter infection: comparison of roll plate, sonication, and flushing methodologies. *J Clin Microbiol* 1997;35:641–646.
270. Lipsky BA, Peugeot RL, Boyko EJ, et al. A prospective study of *Staphylococcus aureus* nasal colonization and intravenous therapy-related phlebitis. *Arch Intern Med* 1992;152:2109–2112.
271. Raad I, Narro J, Khan A, et al. Serious complications of vascular catheter-related *Staphylococcus aureus* bacteremia in cancer patients. *Eur J Clin Microbiol* 1992;11:675–682.
272. Camus C, Leport C, Rafi F, et al. Sustained bacteremia in 26 patients with a permanent endocardial pacemaker: assessment of wire removal. *Clin Infect Dis* 1993;17:46–55.
273. Spratt KA, Blumberg EA, Wood CA, et al. Infections of implantable cardioverter defibrillators: approach to management. *Clin Infect Dis* 1993;17:679–685.
274. Karchmer AW, Longworth DL. Infections of intracardiac devices. *Cardiol Clin*2003;21:253–271.
275. Blair JE, Carr M. Bacteriophage typing of staphylococci. *J Infect Dis* 1953;91:1–73.
276. Schaberg D, Culver D, Gaynes R. Major trends in the microbial etiology of nosocomial infection. *Am J Med* 1991;91:72S–75S.
277. Spindel SJ, Strausbaugh LJ, Jacobson C. Infections caused by *Staphylococcus aureus* in a Veterans Affairs nursing home care unit: a 5-year experience. *Infect Control Hosp Epidemiol* 1995;16:217–223.
278. Lee YL, Cesaria T, Gupta G, et al. Surveillance of colonization and infection with *Staphylococcus aureus* susceptible or resistant to methicillin in a community skilled-nursing facility. *Am J Infect Control* 1997;25:312–321.
279. Steele RW, Ashcraft EW, Payton TS, et al. Recurrent staphylococcal

infection in a pediatric residential care facility. *Am J Infect Control* 1983;11:217–220.
280. Goldmann D. Epidemiology of *Staphylococcus aureus* and group A streptococci. In: Bennett J, Brachman P, eds. *Hospital infections,* 3rd ed. Boston: Little, Brown, 1992:767–787.
281. Williams R, Blowers R, Garrod L, et al. Staphylococcal infections: introduction. In: Williams REO, ed. *Hospital infection causes and prevention,* 2nd ed. London: Lloyd-Luke (Medical Books), 1966:22–41.
282. Lidwell OM, Brock B. Some aspects of the dispersal of *Staphylococcus aureus* in hospital wards. In: Laboratory CPH, ed. *Transmission in hospitals.* London: Central Public Health Laboratory, 1970:454–461.
283. Hare R, Thomas CGA. The transmission of *Staphylococcus aureus. Br Med J* 1956;2:840–844.
284. Sheretz RJ, Regan DR, Hampton KD, et al. A cloud adult: the *Staphylococcus aureus*-virus interaction revisited. *Ann Intern Med* 1996;124: 539–547.
285. Eichenwald H, Kotsevalov O, Fasso LA. The cloudy baby: an example of bacterial-viral interaction. *Am J Dis Child* 1960;100:161–173.
286. Blowers R, Hill J, Howell A. Shedding of *Staphylococcus aureus* by human carriers. In: Hers JFP, Winkler KC, eds. *Dispersal of bacteria from the human body surface.* New York: Halsted, 1972:432–434.
287. Walter CW, Kundsin RB, Brubaker MM. The incidence of airborne wound infection during operation. *JAMA* 1963;186:908–913.
288. Sompolinsky D, Samra Z, Karakawa W, et al. Encapsulation and capsular types in isolates of *Staphylococcus aureus* from different sources and relationship to phage types. *J Clin Microbiol* 1985;22:828–834.
289. Ayliffe GAJ, Collins BJ. Wound infections acquired from a disperser of an unusual strain of *Staphylococcus aureus. J Clin Pathol* 1967;20: 195–208.
290. Payne RW. Severe outbreaks of surgical sepsis due to *Staphylococcus aureus* of an unusual type and origin. *Br Med J* 1967;4:17–20.
291. Dancer SJ, Noble WC. *Staphylococcus aureus* among women: identification of strains producing epidermolytic toxin. *J Clin Pathol* 1991; 44:681–684.
292. Goonatilake PCL. Application of deterministic epidemic theory to nasal carriage of *Staphylococcus aureus. Int J Biomed Comput* 1982;14: 345–352.
293. Witte W. *Staphylococcus aureus* strains of the 94/96 complex isolated in the German Democratic Republic: incidence and discrimination of strain clones. *Zentralbl Bakteriol Mikrobiol Hyg A* 1987;265:243–252.
294. Black NA, Linnemann CC, Pfaller MA, et al. Recurrent epidemics caused by a single strain of erythromycin resistant *Staphylococcus aureus*: the importance of molecular epidemiology. *JAMA* 1993;270: 1329–1333.
295. Tenover FC, Arbeit R, Archer G, et al. Comparison of traditional and molecular methods of typing isolates of *Staphylococcus aureus. J Clin Microbiol* 1994;32:827–893.
296. Jarvis W, Martone W. Predominant pathogens in hospital infections. *J Antimicrob Chemother* 1992;29(suppl A):19–24.
297. Bartzokas C, Paton J, Gibson MF, et al. Control and eradication of methicillin-resistant *Staphylococcus aureus* on a surgical unit. *N Engl J Med* 1984;311:1422–1425.
298. Perl TM, Cullen JJ, Wenzel RP, et al. Intranasal mupirocin to prevent postoperative *Staphylococcus aureus* infections. *N Engl J Med*2002;346: 1871–1877.
299. Kaiser A. Zero infection rate: an achievable irreducible minimum in clean surgery? *Infect Control* 1986;7(suppl 2):107–109.
300. Gentry LO, Zeluff BJ, Colley DA. Antibiotic prophylaxis in open-heart surgery: a comparison of cefamandole, cefuroxime, and cefazolin. *Ann Thorac Surg* 1988;167–171.
301. Conklin CM, Gray RJ, Neilson D, et al. Determinants of wound infection incidence after isolated coronary artery bypass surgery in patients randomized to receive prophylactic cefuroxime or cefazolin. *Ann Thorac Surg* 1988;46:172–177.
302. Edwards WH Jr, Kaiser AB, Kernodle DS, et al. Cefuroxime versus cefazolin as prophylaxis in vascular surgery. *J Vasc Surg* 1992;15: 35–41.
303. Maki D, Bohn M, Stolz S, et al. Comparative study of cefazolin, cefamandole, and vancomycin for surgical prophylaxis in cardiac and vascular operations. *J Thorac Cardiovasc Surg* 1992;104:1423–1434.
304. Kernodle D, Barg N, Kaiser A. Intrinsic methicillin resistance and phage complex 94/96 of *Staphylococcus aureus. J Infect Dis* 1988;155: 396–397.
305. Flynn DM, Weinstein RA, Nathan C, et al. Patients' endogenous flora as the source of nosocomial *Enterobacter* in cardiac surgery. *J Infect Dis* 1987;156:363–368.
306. Weinstein H. The relation between the nasal-staphylococcal-carrier state and the incidence of postoperative complications. *N Engl J Med* 1959;260:1303–1307.
307. Wheat L, Kohler RB, White A. Treatment of nasal carriers of coagulase-positive staphylococci. In: Maibach HI, Aly R, eds. *Skin microbiology: relevance to clinical infection.* New York: Springer, 1981:50–58.
308. Sheagren JN. *Staphylococcus aureus*: the persistent pathogen (second of two parts). *N Engl J Med* 1984;310:1437–1442.
309. Kaiser A, Kernodle D, Barg N, et al. Influence of preoperative showers on staphylococcal skin colonization: a comparative trial of antiseptic skin cleansers. *Ann Thorac Surg* 1988;45:35–38.
310. Mulligan M, Ruane P, Johnson L, et al. Ciprofloxacin for eradication of methicillin-resistant *Staphylococcus aureus* colonization. *Am J Med* 1987;82(suppl 4A):215–219.
311. Strausbaugh U, Jacobson C, Sewell D, et al. Antimicrobial therapy for methicillin-resistant *Staphylococcus aureus* colonization in residents and staff of a Veterans Affairs nursing home care unit. *Infect Control Hosp Epidemiol* 1992;13:151–159.
312. Klempner M, Styrt B. Prevention of recurrent staphylococcal skin infections with low-dose oral clindamycin therapy. *JAMA* 1988;260: 2682–2685.
313. Chow JW, Yu VL. *Staphylococcus aureus* nasal carriage in hemodialysis patients. *Arch Intern Med* 1989;149:1258–1262.
314. McAnally TP, Lewis MR, Brown DR. Effect of rifampin and bacitracin on nasal carriers of *Staphylococcus aureus. Antimicrob Agents Chemother* 1984;25:422–426.
315. Peterson LR, Quick JN, Jensen B, et al. Emergence of ciprofloxacin resistance in nosocomial methicillin-resistant *Staphylococcus aureus* isolates. *Arch Intern Med* 1990;150:2151–2155.
316. Reagan D, Doebbeling B, Pfaller M, et al. Elimination of coincident *Staphylococcus aureus* nasal and hand carriage with intranasal application of mupirocin calcium ointment. *Ann Intern Med* 1991;114: 101–106.
317. Casewell MW, Hill RL. Minimal dose requirements for nasal mupirocin and its role in the control of epidemic MRSA. *J Hosp Infect* 1991;19:35–40.
318. Doebbeling BN, Breneman DL, Neu HC, et al. Elimination of *Staphylococcus aureus* nasal carriage in health care workers: analysis of six clinical trials with calcium mupirocin. *Clin Infect Dis* 1993;17: 466–474.
319. Bulanda M, Gruszka M, Heczko B. Effect of mupirocin on nasal carriage of *Staphylococcus aureus. J Hosp Infect* 1989;14:117–124.
320. Gilbart J, Perry C, Slocombe B. High-level mupirocin resistance in *Staphylococcus aureus*: evidence for two distinct isoleucyl-tRNA synthetases. *Antimicrob Agents Chemother* 1993;37:32–38.
321. Kauffman C, Terpenning M, He X, et al. Attempts to eradicate methicillin-resistant *Staphylococcus aureus* from a long-term-care facility with the use of mupirocin ointment. *Am J Med* 1993;94:371–378.
322. Netto Dos Santos VR, de Souza Fouseca L, Gontiju Filho PP. Emergence of high-level mupirocin resistance in methicillin-resistant *Staphylococcus aureus* isolated from Brazilian university hospitals. *Infect Control Hosp Epidemiol* 1996;17:813–816.
323. Crossley K, Ross J. Colonization of hospitalized patients by *Staphylococcus aureus, Staphylococcus epidermidis* and enterococci. *J Hosp Infect* 1985;5:179–186.
324. Hill R, Duckworth G, Casewell M. Elimination of nasal carriage of methicillin resistant *Staphylococcus aureus* with mupirocin during a hospital outbreak. *J Antimicrob Chemother* 1988;22:377–384.
325. Boyce J, Medeiros A. Role of β-lactamase in expression of resistance by methicillin-resistant *Staphylococcus aureus. Antimicrob Agents Chemother* 1987;31:1426–1428.
326. Bertino JS. Intranasal mupirocin for outbreaks of methicillin resistant *Staphylococcus aureus. Am J Health Syst Pharm* 1997;54:2185–2191.
327. Mond JJ, Kokai-Kun JF, Walsh SM, et al. Lysostaphin Cream Eradi-

cates *Staphylococcus aureus* nasal colonization in a cotton rate model. *Antimicrob Agents Chemother* 2003;47:1589–1597.

328. Rotger M, Rouse MS, Scholz M, et al. In vitro activity and emergence of resistance to mupirocin (MPC) and alkyl ester (AE) 128774-23A and 128774-23B in *Staphylococcus aureus* (SA) (abstract F-2151). 43rd Interscience Conference on Antimicrobial Agents and Chemotherapy, Chicago, September 14–17, 2003.
329. Drutz D, Van Way M, Schaffner W. Bacterial interference in the therapy of recurrent staphylococcal infections. Multiple abscesses due to the implantation of the 502A strain of *Staphylococcus. N Engl J Med* 1966;275:1161–1165.
330. Wheat L, Kohler R, White A. Prevention of infections of skin and skin structures. *Am J Med* 1984;76:187–190.
331. Paulsen IT, Firth N, Skurry RA. Resistance to antimicrobial agents other than β-lactams. In: Crossley KB, Archer GL, eds. *The staphylococci in human disease.* New York: Churchill Livingstone, 1997: 75–212.
332. Hiramatsu K, Hanaki H, Ino T, et al. Methicillin-resistant *Staphylococcus aureus* clinical strain with reduced vancomycin susceptibility. *J Antimicrob Chemother* 1997;40:135–136.
333. Hiraatsu K, Aritaka N, Hanaki H, et al. Dissemination in Japanese hospital of strains of *Staphylococcus aureus* heterogeneously resistant to vancomycin. *Lancet* 1997;350:167–173.
334. Hanaki H, Labischinski H, Inaba Y, et al. Increase of non-amidated muropeptides in the cell wall of vancomycin resistant (VISA) strain Mu50. *Jpn J Antibiot* 1998;51:272–280.
335. Tusco TF, Melko GP, Williams JR. Vancomycin intermediate-resistant *Staphylococcus aureus. Ann Pharmacother* 1998;32:758–760.
336. Van Griethuysen A, Van 't Veen A, Buiting A, et al. High percentage of methicillin-resistant *Staphylococcus aureus* isolates with reduced susceptibility to glycopeptides in the Netherlands. *J Clin Microbiol* 2003; 41:2487–2491.
337. Fores PA, Gordon SM. Vancomycin-resistant *Staphylococcus aureus*: an emerging public health threat. *Cleve Clin J Med* 1997;64:527–532.
338. Edmond MB, Wenzel RP, Pasculle AW. Vancomycin-resistant *Staphylococcus aureus*: perspectives on measures needed for control. *Ann Intern Med* 1996;124:329–334.
339. CDC. Interim guidelines for prevention and control of staphylococcal infection associated with reduced susceptibility to vancomycin. *MMWR* 1997;46:626–628,635.
340. Centers for Disease Control and Prevention. *Staphylococcus aureus* resistant to vancomycin—United States, 2002. *MMWR* 2002;51: 565–567.
341. Centers for Disease Control and Prevention. Public health dispatch: vancomycin-resistant *Staphylococcus aureus*—Pennsylvania, 2002. *MMWR* 2002;51:902–904.
342. Maki DG, Stolz SM, Wheeler S, et al. Prevention of central venous catheter-related bloodstream infection by use of an antiseptic-impregnated catheter. A randomized, controlled trial. *Ann Intern Med* 1997; 127:257–266.
343. Raja R, Raucci G, Hook M. Peptide analogs to a fibronectin receptor inhibit attachment of *Staphylococcus aureus* to fibronectin-containing substrates. *Infect Immun* 1990;58:2593–2598.
344. Lee JC. An experimental vaccine that targets staphylococcal virulence. *Trends Microbiol* 1998;6:461–463.
345. Balaban N, Goldkorn T, Nhan RT, et al. Autoinducer of virulence as a target for vaccine and therapy against *Staphylococcus aureus. Science* 1998;280:438–440.
346. Giacometti A, Cirioni O, Gov Y, et al. RNA III inhibiting peptide inhibits in vivo biofilm formation by drug-resistant *Staphylococcus aureus. Antimicrob Agents Chemother* 2003;47:1979–1983.

29

METHICILLIN-RESISTANT *STAPHYLOCOCCUS AUREUS*

ALAN I. HARTSTEIN
THOMAS J. SEBASTIAN
LARRY JAMES STRAUSBAUGH

Throughout the antibiotic era, strains of *Staphylococcus aureus* have developed resistance to the antimicrobial agents employed against them. Over the last two decades concerns about resistant strains of *S. aureus* have reached new heights as these microorganisms have become predominate in hospitals and disseminated into the community. These resistant strains have not only increased in absolute numbers but they have also acquired resistance to multiple agents, leaving few therapeutic options for some infected patients. This chapter reviews the origin, dissemination, and control of methicillin-resistant *S. aureus* (MRSA).

Soon after the introduction of penicillin, Spink and Ferris (1) reported in 1945 on a penicillin inhibitor that permitted penicillin resistance in strains of *S. aureus*. This type of resistance, resulting from penicillinase production, was initially uncommon but then spread rapidly. Attempts to understand and manage infection by penicillin-resistant *S. aureus* led to the classic investigations of the epidemiology of staphylococcal infections, the results of which form the basis for many current infection control policies. The epidemics resulting from the penicillin-resistant "golden staph" that occurred in the 1950s had many characteristics that are echoed in today's problems with methicillin resistance and vancomycin (glycopeptide) insensitivity and resistance.

Methicillin was the first semisynthetic penicillinase-resistant penicillin released. Within 2 years of its introduction, naturally occurring resistant strains of *S. aureus* were recognized (2,3). These strains were called MRSA, and they subsequently proved resistant to the isoxazolyl penicillins such as oxacillin, cloxacillin, and dicloxacillin. The acquisition of methicillin resistance provided *S. aureus* with a mechanism that made all members of the largest and most useful family of antimicrobials, the β-lactam antibiotics, ineffective as therapeutic agents against these bacteria (4). Since discovery of the first clinical isolate 4 decades ago, MRSA strains have spread rapidly throughout many parts of the world. Evolutionary changes in the microorganism in association with ineffective infection control practices and the intensified selective pressure fomented by increased antimicrobial use probably account for its phenomenal dissemination (5).

HISTORY AND GEOGRAPHICAL DISTRIBUTION OF MRSA

The international spread of MRSA following its original recognition has been and continues to be one of the most difficult challenges to the control and treatment of hospital-acquired infections (4). The first clinical MRSA isolate in Europe was in a British hospital in 1961, and the first Danish blood isolates were recovered in 1963 (4). In some European countries, such as Switzerland, Denmark, and France (6–8), MRSA became a recognized cause of nosocomial infections in the 1960s. MRSA prevalence decreased in some of these locations, and it increased in others such as Greece (9). Serious epidemics also occurred in parts of Australia in the 1960s (10). MRSA cases are now increasing in frequency in many global areas (11), but geographic variability in MRSA rates remains poorly understood. Differences in laboratory capacities for recognition of MRSA and screening practices may account for some of the apparent variation.

The possibility that we are in the midst of a widespread 30-year epidemic of MRSA, as suggested over a decade ago by Wenzel et al. (12), finds support in data from the SENTRY Antimicrobial Surveillance Program, which tracks resistance trends among nosocomial and community isolates on a global scale (11,13). During the period 1997 through 1999, the overall prevalence of MRSA from all sites of infection were as follows: Western Pacific region—46%, United States—34.2%, Latin America—34.9%, and Europe—26.3%. Hong Kong and Japan reported the highest rates (73.8% and 71.6%, respectively). During this interval, Canada had substantially lower rates—MRSA accounted for only 5.7% of all *S. aureus* isolates. However, as summarized by Simor et al. (14), the incidence of MRSA among inpatients in sentinel Canadian hospitals increased (194 vs. 4, 507 cases in 1995 and 1999, respectively). Nosocomial bloodstream MRSA infections were more frequent than community-associated bloodstream MRSA infections. However, both nosocomial and community MRSA bloodstream infections in the United States increased during the 3-year surveillance period (Fig. 29.1) (13). In Europe, 25% of all isolates were MRSA. High MRSA prevalence was also noted in southern Europe, namely in Portuguese (54%), Italian (43% to 58%), and Turkish

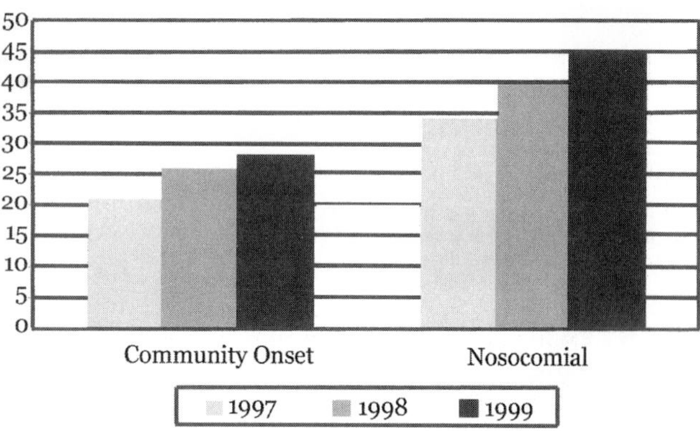

Figure 29.1. Methicillin resistance rates of *Staphylococcus aureus* causing bloodstream infections in the United States, SENTRY program, 1997–1999. (From Diekema DJ, Pfaller MA, Schmitz FJ, et al. Survey of infections due to *Staphylococcus* species: frequency of occurrence and antimicrobial susceptibility of isolates collected in the United States, Canada, Latin America, Europe, and the Western Pacific region for the SENTRY Antimicrobial Surveillance Program, 1997–1999. *Clin Infect Dis* 2001;32(Suppl 2):S114–132.)

(37.5%) hospitals. Switzerland and The Netherlands had the lowest prevalence (2%) (13).

Since the initial discovery of the first clinical isolate in the United States in 1968, MRSA has become highly endemic in many geographic areas. Initially a problem centered in tertiary care referral hospitals affiliated with medical schools (15,16), MRSA has become prevalent in American hospitals of all sizes since the late 1980s (17). Among National Nosocomial Infection Surveillance (NNIS) system hospitals, the prevalence of methicillin resistance among *S. aureus* isolates from intensive care unit (ICU) patients increased from 2.1% in 1975 to 55.3% by 2000 (18). Moreover, it can no longer be assumed that MRSA is almost always a nosocomial pathogen. Community-associated and community-acquired strains of MRSA either infecting or colonizing hosts—with or without recognized risk factors—are increasingly identified (19,20). From 1991 to 1999, a community-based survey of intravenous (IV) drug abusers in the San Francisco Bay area found that up to 35% of *S. aureus* carriers had MRSA isolates (20). A study from Chicago documented a 25-fold increase in the number of children admitted to the hospital with an MRSA infection without an identifiable risk factor for prior MRSA colonization. In two day-care centers in Dallas, Texas, 3% and 24% of the children in the respective centers were colonized with MRSA. Forty percent of the children colonized had no contact with a healthcare facility or a household member with such contact within the previous 2 years. These reports provide evidence that MRSA strains are increasingly prevalent in the community, and they have emerged as important pathogens in this setting.

MICROBIOLOGY

Mechanism and Heterogeneous Expression of Methicillin Resistance

MRSA are resistant to methicillin and other β-lactamase–resistant penicillins and cephalosporins, because they produce a unique, low-affinity penicillin-binding protein called PBP 2a (21–23). A chromosomal gene, *mec*A, contained within a region designated *mec,* encodes this abnormal protein. The *mec*A gene and PBP 2a have been detected in all strains of *S. aureus* that are fully resistant to methicillin (24,25), and this form of resistance is called intrinsic resistance. Neither *mec*A nor PBP 2a can be found in strains that are not intrinsically resistant to methicillin. This includes *S. aureus* isolates that are fully methicillin susceptible and those that have reduced susceptibility to methicillin because of other mechanisms (24–26). These latter microorganisms, sometimes called borderline-resistant *S. aureus* (BORSA) and methicillin-intermediate *S. aureus* (MODSA), are less susceptible to methicillin, because they have hyperproduction of normal staphylococcal penicillinase (BORSA) or because they have essentially normal penicillin-binding proteins with relatively low affinity for β-lactam antibiotics (MODSA) (26–29). BORSA and MODSA are genetically distinct from MRSA and are of unknown clinical and epidemiologic significance. Unlike MRSA infections, infections caused by BORSA and MODSA appear to be effectively treated with β-lactamase–resistant penicillins and cephalosporins (30–32).

The phenotypic expression of methicillin resistance among MRSA isolates varies considerably. Resistance levels are dependent on efficient PBP 2a production and are modulated by chromosomal factors (21,33–35). Most MRSA demonstrate a heterogeneous expression of resistance. This is due to the segregation of a more highly resistant subpopulation on challenge with methicillin. Only a small proportion of the bacterial population (such as one out of every 10^3 to 10^6 cells) in a given culture manifests high-level resistance under standard test conditions (36–38). Maximal expression of resistance by PBP 2a requires the efficient and correct synthesis of the peptidoglycan precursor. Genes involved in cell wall precursor formation and turnover, regulation, transport, and signal transduction may determine the level of resistance that is expressed (35). Resistance expression can be increased by physical maneuvers such as raising the pH, increasing the tonicity of the incubating media, and decreasing the temperature of incubation (20,38,39). Isolation and subculture of a highly resistant minority population on increased concentrations of methicillin produces bacterial cells that are once again heterogeneous.

Isolates of many species of coagulase-negative staphylococci are often methicillin-resistant (see Chapter 30). As with MRSA, these isolates also demonstrate the *mec* gene, PBP 2a, and heterogeneous expression of methicillin resistance (24,40). Unlike MRSA, methicillin-resistant coagulase-negative staphylococci are ubiquitous, and outbreaks caused by the spread of a single strain are not common (41) (see Chapter 30). Because of this, the isolation or confinement of patients colonized or infected with methicillin-resistant coagulase-negative staphylococci has not been advocated.

Laboratory Identification and Antimicrobial Susceptibility Testing

The ideal and most precise methods for the identification of methicillin resistance in MRSA are the direct detection of *mec, mec*A, or the product, PBP 2a (21,24,25,42–44). Also, relatively simple screening tests for PBP 2a and *mecA* are now available, and they yield results that are as or more accurate than testing for drug resistance (45–49). However, these tests are not yet performed routinely in most clinical laboratories. Hence, identification of the intrinsic methicillin-resistant phenotype remains the standard identification method. Staphylococci are considered resistant to methicillin if the minimum inhibitory concentration (MIC) is greater than or equal to 16 μg/mL, or if the oxacillin MIC is greater than or equal to 4 μg/mL (50). Oxacillin is usually chosen for testing, because it is more stable than methicillin.

Advocated testing methodologies to detect MRSA have been outlined by the National Committee for Clinical Laboratory Standards (NCCLS) (50) and are presented in Table 29.1. Accuracy depends on testing a high inoculum of cells and incubation at 35°C for 24 hours for all three tests. In addition, medium supplemented with sodium chloride is used in the oxacillin agar screen and broth microdilution tests. Decreasing the concentration of oxacillin to 2 μg/mL and the temperature of incubation to 30°C has recently been suggested to further improve the sensitivity of the oxacillin agar screen test (49). All of these test characteristics are especially important, because they increase the ability to detect heterogeneous strains of MRSA. If one of these NCCLS-supported methods is used, it is uncommon for an isolate lacking intrinsic resistance to be misidentified as MRSA or for a strain of MRSA to escape recognition.

Unfortunately, key methodologic variables are often not dealt with precisely, leading to underidentification of MRSA (51). Another problem, overreporting of MRSA, has been associated with laboratories testing fewer than 500 isolates per year (52). One additional major problem is that the accurate determination of susceptibilities to other β-lactam drugs is even more difficult despite careful observation of standard test guidelines (39,53). Awareness of the heterogeneously expressed resistance of MRSA to the other β-lactam antibiotics (including other penicillins, cephalosporins, carbapenems, and agents with β-lactamase inhibitors) is essential; clinical failures in animal models and patients are evidence of the presence of intrinsic resistance that sometimes cannot be detected in the laboratory (38,54). Although the potential role for some penicillins in combination with clavulanate is somewhat controversial (55), the NCCLS recommends that isolates determined to be MRSA should not be tested for susceptibility to other β-lactam agents and that such test results should not be reported to clinicians (50).

Automated, semiautomated, and turbidimetric methods of antimicrobial susceptibility testing are less reliable for identifying MRSA (27,38,39,53–58). The relatively small inoculum used in these tests may fail to include enough cells that express resistance. False-negative test results at the MIC cutoff points are common. Methods that have been suggested to minimize false-negative results include testing any isolate with a borderline susceptibility (with an MIC as low as two twofold dilutions below the breakpoint of a reference method) using one of the susceptibility tests presented in Table 29.1 and using these methods for any isolate that is found to be multiresistant (to antimicrobials of many classes) independent of β-lactam test results (27,57). Isolates with intrinsic resistance are more often resistant to agents such as erythromycin, clindamycin, tetracycline, trimethoprim, sulfonamides, fluoroquinolones, and aminoglycosides than are microorganisms that are fully susceptible to methicillin or are resistant because of other mechanisms (21,22,59–63). Unfortunately, the latter strategy is no longer an appropriate consideration, because many community-acquired or associated MRSA isolates are not multiresistant (see later). Finally, an algorithm involving the addition of a second test (such as the E-test) may help to improve correlation with *mecA* detection (64).

Relative Virulence of Intrinsically Resistant *Staphylococcus aureus*

The relative virulence of MRSA and fully methicillin-susceptible *S. aureus* (MSSA) has been scrutinized. Most *in vitro* studies demonstrate equivalent adherence; intraleukocytic survival; phagocytic destruction; and production of hemolysins, enzymes, and toxins (65–69). Virulence of MRSA and MSSA in animal models also appears similar (68–70). Most case-control studies or those using multivariate analysis disclose no differences in morbidity or mortality when patients with MRSA infections are compared to patients with MSSA infections (16,71–81). A few reports suggest increased virulence of MRSA. One identified

TABLE 29.1. MOST ACCURATE PHENOTYPIC TEST METHODS FOR DETECTION OF MRSA

Method	Medium	Antibiotic	Inoculum	Temperature and time of incubation	Values for defining MRSA
Disk diffusion	Mueller-Hinton agar	1 μg oxacillin or 5 μg methicillin disk	1×10^8 CFU/mL by swab inoculation of agar surface	35°C, 24 hours	Oxacillin zone <10 mm Methicillin zone <9 mm
Oxacillin agar screen	4% NaCl supplemented Mueller-Hinton agar	6 μg/mL oxacillin in test medium	1×10^8 CFU/mL by direct spot inoculation	35°C, 24 hours	Distinct spot of growth on agar surface
Broth microdilution	2% NaCl supplemented Mueller-Hinton broth	2-fold dilutions of oxacillin or methicillin	5×10^5 CFU/mL by direct suspension	35°C, 24 hours	Oxacillin MIC >16 μg/mL Methicillin MIC >4 μg/mL

MIC, minimum inhibitory concentration; MRSA, methicillin-resistant *Staphylococcus aureus*.
Adapted from NCCLS. *Performance standards for antimicrobial susceptibility testing*, 12th informational supplement, NCCLS document M100-S12. Wayne, PA: NCCLS, 2002.

lipase production by MRSA more often than in control strains (82). Another report suggested that MRSA might be more easily transmitted than MSSA among patients in a surgical ICU (83). A clinical report reviewing the natural history of persistent nasal *S. aureus* colonization among long-term care facility (LTCF) patients (84) showed that patients colonized with MRSA were more likely to develop infection than those colonized with MSSA. However, MRSA-colonized patients were in the institution longer, were followed longer, and more often required a higher intensity of care compared with MSSA-colonized patients. Other articles document a higher mortality rate among patients with MRSA bacteremia, and a higher rate of bacteremia among patients with MRSA colonization when compared to those with MSSA (85–88). Again, these studies are confounded, because MRSA-affected patients had major additional findings or factors placing them at greater risk for poor outcomes or a more complicated course. However, a recent meta-analysis did support the contention that MRSA bacteremia is associated with a significantly higher mortality rate than MSSA bacteremia (89). Most evidence, including research that involves adjustment for confounders (77,79–81,90), supports the concept that MSSA and MRSA have an equivalent potential for causing colonization and disease.

Typing of Isolates for Epidemiologic Investigations

Typing of MRSA isolates was formerly thought to be of no use, because methicillin resistance was presumed to be an obvious marker for nosocomial origin and spread. In addition, MRSA appeared to be derived from the same or closely related clones, which were expected to demonstrate little evolutionary diversity (91–94). Thus, isolates of epidemiologically unrelated MRSA were considered likely to be the same or similar. Although horizontal spread of highly genomically related strains over large geographic areas has been documented (4,13,95), MRSA strains have evolved multiple independent times. The *mec* gene has been found present in up to eight distinct *S. aureus* lineages that are highly differentiated in overall chromosomal gene content (96, 97). Also, strains of MRSA are now ubiquitous among patients in some hospitals and extended care facilities and are now often community-acquired (see the section on epidemiology). Unfortunately, in many settings, the endemic presence of MRSA is the new norm rather than the old exception (11,13,18,20). Furthermore, a newly identified colonized or infected patient who is in the hospital setting may have a community-acquired microorganism that was not cultured at or near the time of facility admission. Examination of the number and rate of newly affected patients and their epidemiologic associations may suggest the presence of cross-transmission. If good means for isolate discrimination exist, the demonstration of strain identity or difference among patients with positive cultures can be convincing evidence to support or refute epidemiologic hypotheses (98–101).

Specific typing methods for *S. aureus* are described in Chapter 28. Published comparisons of the more recently described and highly discriminatory typing tests using epidemiologically related and unrelated isolates of MRSA are still relatively few in number or examined only a limited number of isolates (102–113). Although no single method is ideal for all outbreak and large region investigations (111,114), pulsed-field gel electrophoresis of genomic DNA and polymerase chain reaction (PCR)-based typing tests are currently considered the tests that offer the best combination of ease of use and interpretation, high discriminatory power, intralaboratory and interlaboratory reproducibility, setup cost, and cost per test (102,108,115–117). These newer genotyping methods are becoming more available as epidemiologists and infection control professionals increasingly recognize the importance of typing tests for isolate discrimination, control of antimicrobial resistance, and outbreak or other epidemiologic investigations (108,115–117).

EPIDEMIOLOGY

Colonization and Infection—Rates and Risk Factors

MRSA colonization and infection contributes to the increased overall cost of healthcare (118), and the incidence of MRSA colonization and infection has risen despite implementation of infection control programs (5,119). Risk factors for MRSA colonization and infection include those for MSSA. Characteristics of endemic strains, patient populations, institutional eradication policies, and the outcome of eradication efforts contribute to variations in long-term MRSA carriage rates (5, 119,120). Patient groups that have high rates of staphylococcal colonization include those receiving hemodialysis or continuous ambulatory peritoneal dialysis; injection drug users; patients with dermatologic diseases (e.g., psoriasis, eczema, chronic skin ulcers, *S. aureus* skin infections); insulin-dependent diabetics and others requiring repeated injections; liver transplant recipients; and patients with hepatic cirrhosis, human immunodeficiency virus (HIV) or acquired immunodeficiency syndrome (AIDS), qualitative or quantitative defects in leukocyte function, malignancies, Wegener's granulomatosis, nasal abnormalities, and rhinosinusitis (120–128).

The literature describes diverse durations for MRSA carriage. One study found the prevalence of MRSA culture positivity was 67% to 70% at 2½ years or less after hospital discharge (129). Scanvic et al. (119) documented that the median time for clearance was 8.5 months. In another study, carriage rates among neonates discharged from the hospital decreased to 36% after 3 months (130). Among 32 families with mothers and babies colonized or infected during a maternity hospital MRSA outbreak, 22 had a mother or baby still colonized 4 weeks later (131). In contrast, in a study of 36 patients who were screened 2 to 3 years after becoming carriers in the hospital, only 3 (8%) were still positive (one with cystic fibrosis, one with a fistula, and one with a colostomy). None of the 44 family members of the original 36 patients were culture positive (132). MacKinnon and Allen (120) reported in their study of long-term MRSA carriers that patients with chronic skin lesions had the highest risk for having positive MRSA cultures on hospital readmission. The link between chronic skin lesions and MRSA carriage was also demonstrated in a Dutch multicenter study (133). Three fourths of chronic carriers typically have chronic medical problems as well [e.g., chronic obstructive pulmonary disease (COPD), ischemic heart disease, diabetes mellitus] (120).

Risk factors for MRSA colonization in residents of LTCFs relate, in general, to poor functional status, conditions that cause skin breakdown, presence of invasive devices, prior antimicrobial therapy, and a history of antecedent colonization (134). Specific risk factors identified in studies using multivariate analysis include male gender (135); urinary incontinence (135); fecal incontinence (136); limited mobility (137); total dependence on healthcare workers for activities of daily living (138); presence of wounds (137,139), pressure ulcers (135,136,139), nasogastric intubation (140), or urinary catheters (137); antibiotic therapy (138,140); hospitalization within the previous 3 to 6 months (136,137); and residence in a medium-sized facility (137). Studies employing only univariate analysis have delineated similar types of factors (134). Two studies conducted in Veteran's Administration (VA) facilities have examined risk factors for MRSA infection in LTCFs using multivariate analysis. Muder et al. (84) found persistent MRSA colonization and dialysis were significantly associated with infection, whereas Terpenning et al. (139) found that diabetes mellitus and peripheral vascular occlusive disease increase the risk for MRSA infections in this setting.

From a hospital perspective, patients with MRSA tend to be older, have more chronic illnesses, and have a recent history of hospitalization. Special populations in hospitals are also at increased risk such as those hospitalized in ICU and burn units (see later) (13,15–17,141,142). A French ICU study suggested that a higher severity of illness on admission and MRSA colonization were independent risk factors for the occurrence of either MRSA or MSSA infections (143). Another study reported that *S. aureus* colonization rates of medical personnel were not higher than colonization rates among nonmedical personnel (144).

Rates of MRSA colonization are also influenced by the existence and extent of surveillance programs, and ratios of infection to colonization may vary within and among institutions (5). The infection ratio is also highly dependent on the distribution of risk factors for infection among the colonized patients (119-128,145–147). As examples, Boyce (57) reported that 30% to 60% of hospitalized carriers developed infection, whereas Muder et al. (84) and Bradley et al. (148) found that only 5% to 15% of colonized residents of LTCFs became infected.

Nasal cultures are most often used in hospitals to provide an estimate of MRSA colonization rates. Nasal carriage is a major risk factor toward the development of *S. aureus* infections in various clinical settings (surgical site infections, continuous ambulatory peritoneal dialysis and hemodialysis, HIV-infected patients, etc.), but the overall rate of developing infection is low (<5%). Most MRSA infections result from autoinfection by the patient's own strain of *S. aureus* (126). A study that investigated patients receiving chronic peritoneal dialysis found that MRSA infections were eight times more common for carriers of MRSA than for noncarriers (149). Another study assessed the effect of MRSA carriage on the epidemiology of hospital-acquired infections in cirrhotic patients. Prior antibiotic use, prolonged hospitalization, and end-stage liver disease contributed to MRSA carriage, and all of these factors (including MRSA carriage) were strong predictors of subsequent infections (147).

Cross-sectional surveys of healthy adult populations have reported *S. aureus* nasal carriage rates between 20% and 55% (126). Nasal carriage rates differ between individuals. Based on longitudinal studies, 10% to 35% of persons carry *S. aureus* persistently, 20% to 75% carry intermittently, and 5% to 50% are never carriers. Children, especially males, are more prone to be persistent carriers. In addition, persistent carriers tend to be colonized with one strain, whereas intermittent carriers may carry many different strains over time. Persistent carriage may have a protective effect on the acquisition of new strains (150). However, Maslow et al. (151) suggested that long-term MRSA carriers often have different strains of MRSA that change over time in association with removal or resolution of a colonized focus and the recurrence of mucocutaneous defects.

Antibiotic exposure may also influence the frequency or rate of persistent colonization. A double-blind, placebo-controlled trial of decolonization therapy revealed that the probability of persistent MRSA colonization was almost two times greater among patients with more than one body site colonized and among those who had prior fluoroquinolone therapy (152). In two reported MRSA outbreaks in Germany and in a national surveillance study from Belgium, fluoroquinolone use was deemed an independent risk factor for MRSA carriage (153–155). The increase in fibronectin-binding proteins produced when fluoroquinolone-resistant MRSA are exposed to low levels of ciprofloxacin may promote increased adhesion and carriage, thus explaining its role as a risk factor (156,157).

Reservoirs and Sources

It is generally accepted that people serve as the major reservoir for MRSA and that other sources for the microorganisms are relatively unimportant except in special circumstances. Many investigations have focused on nasal carriage as the principal reservoir, and the presence of staphylococcal nasal colonization has been associated with infection for the individual patient (158). However, the evidence to link nasal carriage with transmission to others is far less convincing (72,159–176).

Healthcare workers are thought to be a potential reservoir, but probably they are most often only transiently colonized. Reported rates of nasal colonization of healthcare workers have varied widely. For example, a surprisingly low rate of 0.8% was detected during a burn unit outbreak (16), but approximately 50% of personnel tested were colonized in an endemic setting (177). Reasons for the disparities are not clear but probably include frequency of sampling. Hand carriage has also been well documented for personnel and, like nasal carriage, may be transient or persistent (161,178–181). It may be crucial to distinguish between transient colonization, which is likely to be inconsequential for the individual and the institution, and persistent colonization, which is more likely to precede infection and to present a risk for dissemination to others. There have been a number of outbreaks convincingly traced to colonized personnel. In most cases, these disseminators have had some factor in addition to nasal colonization, such as dermatitis or chronic recurrent staphylococcal infections or an active viral respiratory infection (161,178–184). The healthcare worker with transient nasal colonization is not likely to have the same epidemiologic impact as a patient with an extensive heavily colonized pressure sore, although the two individuals may often be treated alike by the dictates of the infection control program.

For healthcare workers, the environment of care may function as a reservoir for colonization and infection. ICUs and LTCFs may act as reservoirs. In a French study surveying 43 hospitals over a 2-month period, the risk of MRSA acquisition was greatest in ICUs, but medical and surgical wards and rehabilitation and long-term care units accounted for a larger reservoir (as much as four times greater) of the MRSA population (185). Burn units can also serve as reservoirs of MRSA affecting other patient populations within a facility (141,186). Many body sites of patients in these units can be colonized. These include the respiratory tract, any site on the skin (including surgical sites, burns, pressure sores, tracheostomy sites, sites of other foreign bodies, and normal skin), and the perineum and rectum (which may reflect intestinal colonization). It is evident that carriers are not a homogeneous group. Nasal cultures may not be adequate to detect carriers in some of these settings. Cultures of wounds, tracheostomy sites, and sputum were most helpful for detecting carriers in one study (187).

The role of environmental contamination as a reservoir for MRSA has been difficult to determine. MRSA has been recovered from many surfaces in hospitals, including stethoscopes, floors, linens, air vents, charts, tourniquets, furniture, hydrotherapy tubs, bed sheets, and dry mops (187–190), but only isolated reports have indicated that these are important in transmission. In one pediatric unit outbreak, a contaminated infant milk feed prepared by a colonized milk bank worker was considered responsible (191). A common bathtub used by patients with dermatitis or other skin lesions was implicated in another setting (192). Bures et al. (193) suggested that computer keyboards and faucet handles in ICUs contributed to an increased MRSA colonization rate. Environmental surfaces in burn units may be heavily contaminated by staphylococci and, in this setting, may constitute a very important reservoir (16,160,161,181,194, 195).

Modes of Transmission

The principal mode of transmission of MRSA within an institution is considered to be from one colonized or infected patient to another via the hands of healthcare workers (16,71,196). The healthcare worker need not be a long-term carrier of MRSA but may have only transient colonization (16,71,182,194). One study suggested that healthcare workers were almost twice as likely to become at least transiently colonized with MRSA from patients when they did not wear a mask when caring for patients with MRSA (197). Some hospital personnel who were chronic carriers or had chronic or recurrent infections have been identified as reservoirs and as vectors for direct transmission, although this appears to be uncommon (161,179,182,184,197,198). Nasal carriers are often identified in investigations of outbreaks, but in most cases a role in transmission cannot be ascribed to them with any certainty (16,71,194,199–203).

Airborne transmission is a consideration for any patient with staphylococcal pneumonia (see Chapter 22) and may be important in burn units as well (16,141,194). Farrington et al. (204) reported an inability to control spread in a burn unit using methods that were effective in a neonatal unit and attributed this to the additional problems of environmental contamination and airborne routes of dissemination.

Special Problems

Epidemic Versus Endemic MRSA

A wide variety of outbreaks of MRSA have been reported, often with rapid spread to involve many patients (16,71,72,160, 161,164,178,180,205–207). Some of these outbreaks were due to a single strain of the microorganism that could be traced readily and controlled relatively easily by prompt application of multiple infection control measures. Early identification and control of outbreaks has sometimes resulted in eradication of MRSA or at least control of the epidemic. Unfortunately, MRSA is usually not eradicated, becomes an established endemic pathogen (12,13,208) and a persistent cause of nosocomial infection (129). Prolonged survival in the hospital environment may be one of the determinants of spread and persistence of MRSA (13, 18,20,209). MRSA colonization may be acquired by up to 1% of all hospitalized patients if MRSA is highly endemic (160, 194).

Despite stringent control measures in endemic settings, MRSA eradication is very hard to achieve. Wenzel et al. (12) suggested that the spread of MRSA in an institution is an indication of the failure of simple infection control measures such as hand washing. MRSA infections have also been viewed as serious preventable infections, partly because they do not simply replace infections resulting from susceptible strains but actually add to nosocomial infection rates (210). However, epidemic infections superimposed on chronic endemic infections and colonization may often respond to special control measures (211). Even reemphasis of simple measures may be helpful (212).

Intensive Care, Liver Transplant, and Burn Units

Patients in ICUs typically have multiple risk factors for colonization and infection due to MRSA. These units have often been the site of outbreaks and continue to be an appropriate focus for special efforts to control the microorganism. Understaffing and overcrowding also contribute to the likelihood of MRSA outbreaks in ICUs (210). The type of ICU is a consideration as well (213,214). Surgical ICUs (83) and neonatal units have been the settings for frequent outbreaks, whereas coronary care units have not.

Garrouste-Orgeas et al. (143) investigated the impact of MRSA colonization on the occurrence of *S. aureus* infections among ICU patients. This study revealed that *S. aureus* infections occurred more often in patients colonized with MRSA on admission to the hospital. The crude ICU death rate was also higher in colonized versus noncolonized individuals (37.7% vs. 20.4%). The acquisition of MRSA, however, did not influence mortality in these patients, even in the presence of infection.

Liver transplant patients with prior nasal carriage of MRSA tend to develop MRSA infections sooner after transplantation than those without nasal carriage. Impaired neutrophil function as a result of corticosteroid therapy or liver disease itself may make these patients more susceptible to MRSA infections. In a study from the University of Pittsburgh, nearly one third of all MRSA infections occurred within 14 days and one half within 30 days of transplantation (215). This was in contrast to nontransplantation patients in whom MRSA infections generally occurred after very prolonged ICU stays.

Burn units constitute a special problem (204). The extensive loss of skin integrity places burned patients at high risk for staphylococcal colonization and infection and influences some of the likely modes of transmission. MRSA colonization has been associated with loss of skin grafts and delayed wound healing. Environmental reservoirs and airborne spread of MRSA also appear to be much more important in burn units than for other patient populations. Contamination of topical agents such as silver sulfadiazine cream and of environmental sites such as hydrotherapy equipment (16,141,216) are among some of the special problems that have been identified. Interestingly, a case-control study of burn unit patients did not demonstrate a difference in mortality between colonized and infected patients with MRSA (142).

Long-Term Care Facilities

During the last two decades, MRSA has become an important pathogen in LTCFs in the United States (78,84,136,148, 217–222). The number of nursing homes in the United States reporting colonization or infections with MRSA has steadily increased since the first reported outbreaks in the 1980s (223). Surveys in three states conducted over a decade ago indicated that 12%, 31%, and 81% of LTCFs in Minnesota, Oregon, and New York, respectively, had experienced MRSA cases (134). Prevalence studies conducted in 10 other locales identified MRSA colonization in 4.9% to 34% of LTCF residents (134, 138,224). Prevalence studies in France, Belgium, and Germany have reported similar rates of colonization (134,225,226). In some U.S. medical centers, the proportion of MRSA among *S. aureus* isolates in long-term care units (33%) exceeds that in the inpatient setting (14%) (223). Moreover, Muder et al. (84) found more staphylococcal infections in nursing home residents colonized with MRSA than in those colonized with MSSA.

Colonization rates vary considerably among different types of LTCFs. Rates in VA LTCFs (11% to 34%) have often exceeded those in community facilities (5% to 22%) (134,138, 224–226). A 1991 to 1992 study comparing rates in one VA and three community LTCFs found a 27% prevalence of MRSA colonization in the former and an 8% prevalence in the latter (136). The VA system may not be representative of all long-term care institutions, because VA facility residents tend to be younger, predominantly male, and sicker. Regardless, colonization rates appear to be influenced by other factors as well—geographic location, facility size, prevalence of MRSA in the referring acute-care institutions, severity of illness of the patient population, and institutional infection control practices (134, 227).

Sites of colonization in LTCF residents include the nose, throat, perineum, and urinary tract, but anterior nares and wounds are most often positive. The only body site consistently screened in all nursing home studies has been the nares (134, 228). A combination of testing the nose, throat, and wound/skin lesions may improve the yield of MRSA detection in this setting. However, 77% to 83% of MRSA-positive individuals in these settings are nasal carriers.

MRSA strains appear to enter LTCFs via infected or colonized patients transferred from hospitals or other LTCFs. Once present in a facility, these strains tend to become endemic. Few facilities have managed to eradicate them although a Finnish group recently reported this accomplishment (229). Long-term care residents remain colonized for long periods ranging from months to years (228), but only a small percentage become infected (134). Although some studies have reported higher mortality rates in MRSA-colonized nursing home residents, this appears to reflect their poor functional status and comorbidities rather than death from MRSA infection (223).

LTCFs act as reservoirs for MRSA, often introducing or reintroducing MRSA into hospitals when they transfer colonized or infected residents who need acute care (219,230). In a recent prospective study, Mylotte et al. (231) detected MRSA carriage in 13 of 92 residents transferred from LTCFs to their hospital during a 2-month period. Ironically, some LTCFs may refuse to accept MRSA culture-positive patients, thereby influencing the management of hospitalized patients, in some cases delaying their discharge (219,232,233). The Long-Term Care Committee of the Society for Healthcare Epidemiology of America has addressed this concern and the management of MRSA and other antibiotic-resistant pathogens in LTCFs (234).

Community-Acquired and Associated MRSA

Community-acquired MRSA cases in the United States were first reported in 1980, and most were identified in LTCFs and among IV drug users (127,235). Risk factors for newly identified community cases of MRSA now include recent hospitalization; admission from another hospital; prior antimicrobial use; being a child in a day-care center; and underlying illnesses such as cardiovascular and pulmonary disease, diabetes, malignancy, and chronic skin disease. Outbreaks of MRSA have also occurred in prisons, residential care facilities, and among students participating in sporting events (13,19,20). Community MRSA cases have also been described without known predisposing risk factors (19). Two university hospitals in Chicago reported increased community MRSA cases among their pediatric admissions that did not have any predisposing risk factors (19). Several studies of community MRSA cases concluded that uncomplicated skin and soft tissue infections were the most common sites of culture positivity (127).

Different reports variably defined what was a community-acquired case of MRSA. As an example, one study defined a community-acquired MRSA case as any outpatient or inpatient with culture-confirmed MRSA infection that had no history of hospitalization, surgery, renal dialysis, or residence in an LTCF within 1 year before the MRSA culture date (236). Perhaps the most useful distinctions divide new cases of MRSA bloodstream infections into three categories: (a) those occurring in hospitals (nosocomial); (b) those that were healthcare-associated; and (c) those that did not fall into either of these two categories and were, therefore, community-acquired. In this scheme, healthcare-associated cases were defined as not being a nosocomial case and (a) those who received IV therapy, wound care, or specialized nursing care at home within 30 days of a bloodstream infection; (b) those who attended a hospital or hemodialysis unit or received IV chemotherapy within 30 days of bloodstream infection; (c) those who were admitted in an acute care hospital within 90 days of bloodstream infection; or (d) those who resided in a nursing home or LTCF. Community-acquired cases were defined as those cases with a positive culture obtained at hospital admission or within 48 hours after admission and not fulfilling a healthcare-associated criteria (237). In this analysis of MRSA bloodstream infections, Friedman et al. (237) found that the incidence of MRSA in healthcare-associated and nosocomial bloodstream infections were equivalent, whereas MRSA was uncommon among patients with community-acquired bloodstream infections. Regularly using such a scheme for clinical decision-making and reporting purposes has the potential to improve patient care and clarify the literature on this subtopic.

The spread of MRSA to the community is secondary to multiple mechanisms. This includes the movement and subsequent spread of nosocomial MRSA strains into the community along with patients who are discharged earlier and/or receiving significant home-based care and the de novo appearance of community strains resulting from the transfer of genetic material from MRSA to MSSA strains (127). The emergence of MRSA as a truly community-acquired pathogen has apparently occurred at a relatively slow pace because methicillin resistance is not easily transferred to methicillin-susceptible strains of *S. aureus* (127).

The reported prevalence of MRSA in the community has been variable, and this is somewhat secondary to different applied definitions. As examples, a 1995 epidemiology study found that 28% to 41% of new MRSA cases were in adult patients from the community (238). Alternatively, community outbreaks have occurred among IV drug users; aboriginals in Canada, New Zealand, and Australia; Native Americans in North America; and even athletes participating in close contact sports (239,240). Linnemann et al. (241) reported that in their institution an initial outbreak was due to an epidemic nosocomial strain of MRSA but that a second epidemic involved multiple strains with 28% of patients judged to have had community acquisition. It is thought that children at day-care facilities may be reservoirs for MRSA. In a Japanese study, 42.9% of *S. aureus* strains among day-care attendees were MRSA (242). The overall reported MRSA rate was 7.7%. Adcock et al. (243) reported that the incidence of MRSA carriers in children attending day-care centers in the United States was 10.9%. Although most cases of community MRSA infections have been effectively managed, four fatal cases were reported in Minnesota and North Dakota (244). These cases emphasize that community infections caused by MRSA, like MSSA, can be potentially life threatening.

Isolates from community MRSA cases have shown variable antimicrobial susceptibility patterns. Some sets of isolates have resistance patterns similar to nosocomial MRSA strains, whereas others demonstrated resistance to only β-lactam antibiotics. Many of the community MRSA cases originally seen among residents of LTCFs and IV drug users were thought to be caused by nosocomial strains because both of these groups had exposures to hospitals (127). Until recently, most community MRSA cases had preceding stays in hospitals or nursing homes (223). The study by Almer et al. (238), conducted to assess the antimicrobial susceptibility profile for pretreatment MRSA isolates in cases of community-acquired respiratory infections, showed that the MRSA from the community had antimicrobial susceptibility profiles similar to those reported for nosocomial MRSA case isolates. These results agreed with those of Pfaller et al. (245) who found reduced susceptibility in 395 MRSA community isolates to erythromycin, clindamycin, and ciprofloxacin. This is in contrast to several other reports describing increased susceptibility to multiple antibiotics except penicillin. Most infections caused by MRSA with this unique susceptibility pattern (resistance limited to β-lactam antibiotics) have occurred in healthy children (235). A retrospective study conducted in Hawaii from 1992 to 1996 compared isolates from MRSA community-infected patients to isolates from MRSA community-colonized patients. The latter isolates were more likely to be susceptible to ciprofloxacin and erythromycin. In a Saudi Arabian study, most community-acquired MRSA isolates showed multidrug susceptibility (127). A study from Minnesota reported that community MRSA isolates were susceptible to all antibiotics tested except for methicillin and erythromycin (236). No community-acquired isolates studied thus far have exhibited reduced susceptibility to vancomycin. What these reports reveal is that community-acquired MRSA have more heterogeneous antibiotic susceptibility patterns than nosocomial or healthcare-associated MRSA. With susceptibility to many other antibiotics, these strains can be treated with drugs other than vancomycin.

The increasing prevalence of MRSA in the community (healthcare-associated and community-acquired) thus poses an increasing challenge for clinicians and public health officials. More surveillance data are needed to determine epidemiologic patterns and to monitor the trends in each community. Approaches such as tracking infections from sentinel hospitals or performing periodic cross-sectional surveys should be considered. The Centers for Disease Control and Prevention (CDC) advocate a national antimicrobial resistance surveillance plan as top-priority in addressing this emerging problem (246).

Vancomycin-Intermediate or Insensitive S. Aureus (VISA) and Vancomycin Resistant *S. aureus* (VRSA)

Over the last several years a new and most disturbing development has taken place—the emergence of *S. aureus* isolates with reduced susceptibility to glycopeptide antibiotics. The terms VISA and glycopeptide-intermediate *S. aureus* (GISA) have been used in the United States to describe *S. aureus* with reduced susceptibility to vancomycin. Although the term GISA is more accurate, reflecting that *S. aureus* strains were less susceptible to the glycopeptides vancomycin and teicoplanin, the term VISA is more commonly used and applied here. The NCCLS defines staphylococci as "susceptible" to vancomycin with MICs ≤ 4 μg/mL. Those requiring 8 to 16 μg/mL of vancomycin for inhibition are categorized as "intermediate," and those requiring ≥ 32 μg/mL are "resistant" (50).

The first VISA case was identified in France in 1995 from a child receiving vancomycin for an MRSA line infection (247). The following year, another clinical strain of VISA was isolated from a 4-month-old infant with a surgical-site infection in Japan

(248). In June 1997, the first clinical VISA isolate in the United States was reported in Michigan (249). As of June 2002, eight patients with VISA infections were confirmed in the United States and several more isolates were reported worldwide (250).

Several common factors exist among all of these VISA cases (250–253). All VISA strains were also MRSA and were isolated from ill patients after prolonged exposure to vancomycin (range from 6 to 18 weeks of therapy in the 3 to 6 months before VISA detection). Most of the cases reported in the United States presented with renal failure. It is unclear whether this was an independent risk factor or whether it served to increase the risk of MRSA infection, which in turn resulted in vancomycin use. Strains also had similar pulsed-field gel electrophoresis patterns to those of the patients' previous infecting MRSA strains, supporting the likelihood that they were derived from the original vancomycin-susceptible MRSA strain that was never fully eradicated.

The exact mechanism of vancomycin nonsusceptibility in *S. aureus* is not known. It was initially thought that the *van* genes that coded for *Enterococcus* species resistance to vancomycin (VRE) contributed to resistance by plasmid transfer. This was initially demonstrated *in vitro* (250). In a small study Franchi et al. (254) demonstrated that 28.6% of patients colonized with VRE were also colonized with MRSA, and the MIC of vancomycin for most (77%) of these staphylococci was 1.5 or 2 μg/mL. However, neither the *van* genes nor their altered peptidoglycan products were recovered in VISA strains. Several investigators have shown that VISA isolates have upregulated cell wall synthesis and turnover leading to thicker and more disorganized cell walls. VISA exhibits less cross-linking in the peptidoglycan component of the cell wall. It has been proposed that this thicker, disorganized cell wall can actually trap vancomycin at the periphery of the cell, therefore, blocking its action. In addition, the altered cell walls appear to have a reduced affinity for vancomycin (253).

The first case of VRSA (MIC ≥32 μg/mL) in a patient was identified in June 2002 in Michigan from a swab obtained from a catheter exit site (250). Like the VISA cases, this patient was treated intermittently with multiple antibiotic courses (including vancomycin) for chronic foot ulcerations. The MIC results for vancomycin, teicoplanin, and oxacillin were greater than 128 μg/mL, 32μg/mL, and >16μg/mL, respectively. This isolate, however, contained the *vanA* vancomycin resistance gene also present in an *Enterococcus faecalis* isolate cultured from the same ulcer. This contradicted what was described earlier among VISA strains (249). A second case of VRSA was identified in Pennsylvania in October 2002 with reconfirmation by E test (MIC = 64 μg/mL) and by broth dilution (MIC = 32 μg/mL). This isolate also grew from a chronic foot ulcer, also exhibited the *vanA* gene, and appeared to be unrelated to the Michigan strain (255).

Heteroresistant VRSA strains have also been described. These are defined as *S. aureus* subpopulations that grow on brain heart infusion (BHI) screening agar containing 4 to 6 μg/mL of vancomycin. These subpopulations have been subsequently selected, propagated, and tested for vancomycin susceptibility. These isolates typically have MICs two to eight times higher than the parent colonies from which they are derived. The MICs reported are usually those of the daughter colonies (251).

VISA can be difficult to detect in the laboratory. Tests have shown that disk diffusion using standard 30 μg vancomycin disks erroneously labeled some VISA strains as susceptible. Automated methods like Microscan and Vitek had shown limitations also. Current recommendations are to use nonautomated MIC determinations by broth microdilution, BHI agar dilution, or by an E test to determine vancomycin susceptibility (50,64). Interestingly, VISA and VRSA strains from the United States have been found susceptible to trimethoprim-sulfamethoxazole and tetracycline (252,253).

SURVEILLANCE, PREVENTION, AND CONTROL OF MRSA

Guidelines for the surveillance, prevention, and control of MRSA in healthcare facilities vary greatly. Controversies exist because of (a) an increasing endemicity of MRSA in acute and chronic care facilities in most areas within and outside of the United States (11,13,14,18,256,257); (b) the fact that MRSA eradication from a facility is extremely difficult and eradication efforts often end in failure (57); (c) an increasing prevalence of community-acquired MRSA cases in the United States and elsewhere (see previous discussion); (d) relatively poor success in eliminating MRSA from colonized and infected patients, who are the most important reservoir (258–262); (e) a paucity of controlled or randomized trials of interventions to minimize the spread of MRSA within healthcare facilities (208,263); and (f) recognition that vigorous containment strategies are or may be very expensive, disruptive of overall care, and at odds with the unique goals of different facilities (208,211,230,263–269). In addition, containment strategies are typically based on outbreak experiences rather than on prevention or minimization of endemic spread. Recommendations vary from a minimalist or very directed approach (unless there is clear evidence of an outbreak with intrainstitutional spread) (76,269,270) to highly elaborate systems involving isolation wards, extensive on-admission patient culturing, regular staff culturing, strict isolation, aggressive and special attempts to decontaminate the environment, and attempts at decolonizing patients and staff and repetitive culturing following attempted decontamination (271–274).

Table 29.2 outlines measures advocated by different groups, including academic VA physicians (275); a task force of the American Hospital Association (276); the Dutch approach (274); and the combined working party of the British Society for Antimicrobial Chemotherapy, the Hospital Infection Society, and the Infection Control Nurses Association (277). As can be seen in this table, agreement is far from complete. It is suggested that efforts be directed primarily toward pragmatic and realistic goals (i.e., recognition, containment, and control of cross-transmission of MRSA that subsequently causes infections in patients) (268,269,278). With these goals in mind, surveillance and control strategies can be adapted to the needs of a given institution or patient population. Recent large-scale surveys indicated that most acute and chronic healthcare facilities

TABLE 29.2. MEASURES ADVOCATED FOR SURVEILLANCE, PREVENTION, AND CONTROL OF MRSA IN HEALTH CARE FACILITIES

Measure	Mulligan et al. (275)	Boyce et al. (276)	Verhoef et al. (274)	Combined working party (277)
Interfacility transfer should not be discouraged or delayed because of positive MRSA cultures (but transferring facility should notify receiving facility of positive MRSA sites)	Supported	Supported	Not addressed	Transfers should be minimized
Issues specific to extended care facilities addressed	Yes	Yes	No	No
Surveillance cultures, patients	Discouraged unless outbreak	Discouraged unless outbreak	All patients from hospitals outside The Netherlands	Encouraged among some patients in general wards and strongly recommended in high-risk units (ICUs; burn, transplant, cardiothoracic, orthopedic, trauma and vascular units)
Surveillance cultures, staff	Discouraged unless outbreak	Discouraged unless outbreak	All staff caring for any patient found culture positive for MRSA (daily cultures done if care continues)	Encouraged for all those in contact with MRSA-positive patients and with any evidence of spread
Decontamination and decolonization therapy for patients and staff	Discouraged except for prevention of recurrent infections in an individual or as part of special interventions to stop an outbreak	Consider only during hospital outbreaks, when MRSA is highly endemic, or when persistently colonized and epidemiologically linked healthcare personnel are identified; should not be the major component of an overall control program and is seldom warranted in extended-care facilities	All patients and staff found colonized or infected (antiseptic detergents and oral rifampin-minocycline)	Staff and visitors to routinely use hand antiseptic detergent or alcohol; affected patients should routinely use an antiseptic detergent for washing and bathing; mupirocin in various forms should be used on colonized sites; use systemically active agents in certain exceptional circumstances
Routine isolation precautions, acute care hospital	Single room or cohort with other MRSA patient(s); contact precautions unless colonization limited to nares or rectum (then only gloves); gowns, masks, and gloves only advocated when patient has extensive and noncontained skin involvement or lower respiratory tract infection	Single room or cohort with other MRSA patient(s); hand washing and liberal use of gloves for all direct contacts with patient and environment stressed; except in burn units, gowns and masks for routine use are discouraged	All patients from hospitals outside The Netherlands quarantined until proven to be culture-negative. All MRSA-positive patients isolated in a separate room All staff caring for MRSA-positive patients to wear a mask, cap, gown, and gloves	Infected patients and carriers isolated in a single room or preferably in an isolation unit with designated staff, preferably with negative pressure ventilation; gloves and disposable plastic aprons for contact with the patient or his environment
Hand-washing agent before and after contact (even when gloves are worn)	Yes, with standard soap and water	Yes, with standard soap and water	Disinfection of hands	Yes, with antiseptic detergent or alcohol (70%)
Maintain MRSA patient list for reference in case of readmission	Supported	Supported	Not addressed	Strongly supported
Cohort affected patients together, with care by designated staff not involved with unaffected patients (when possible)	Consider for epidemic control or with high endemicity when other control measures have been unsuccessful	Should be considered only in hospitals with high levels of MRSA transmission	Entire unit closed to new admissions on first recognition of two cases on a ward or one case in an intensive care unit	Strongly supported on ongoing basis

MRSA, methicillin-resistant *Staphylococcus aureus*.

need, or will need and use, a strategy to monitor or control the spread of MRSA (11,13,14,18,20).

Strategies to Understand, Contain, and Control MRSA Transmission

Clinical Laboratory-Based Surveillance

MRSA has caused more reported nosocomial outbreaks than any other microorganism in recent times (279). In addition, MRSA is now cultured from patients in most acute and long-term care facilities in the United States (11,13,14,18,20,209, 217,223,227,256). Because of its prevalence and potential to cause outbreaks, it is considered appropriate to focus some special attention on MRSA. A review of clinical culture and susceptibility test results on a regular basis is practical for all facilities. The frequency of newly identified patients with MRSA and rates of new patients' culture positive for MRSA, using admissions, discharges, or census days as the denominator, can easily be tracked. An increase from a baseline or rates judged to warrant more concern or special attempts at control should lead to further review or study.

MRSA Case Line Listing

Developing a case line listing follows laboratory surveillance in importance. Basic case information should include name, date of admission, demographic data (e.g., age, gender), room number or nursing unit, primarily responsible clinical service or physician, sites of infection or colonization, the date and site of the first positive culture for MRSA, the name of the transferring facility (if applicable), and the antimicrobial susceptibility pattern of the isolate. Particular attention should be paid to identifying prior culture positivity by record review or patient interview and to noting patients who have positive cultures at or shortly after admission. Clusters of newly identified patients with MRSA isolates not representative of the former two groups should be evaluated. If MRSA was recovered from any patient site in the past, the new isolate is highly likely to represent ongoing or relapse of colonization or infection rather than a new microorganism acquisition (260–262,280,281). Positive cultures from patients who have not been admitted to a facility but are detected at the time of admission (or shortly thereafter) represent extrainstitutional acquisition. The number of patients who meet the latter definition of community-acquired or associated MRSA colonization or infection is an important measure of MRSA prevalence outside of the facility (19, 230,237,238,241,278, 282–291). Cases of newly identified patients with MRSA-positive cultures many days after admission do not necessarily represent nosocomial transmission or acquisition of MRSA; often they simply remained undetected until late in their hospital course. MRSA is often present in individuals within many communities and extended care facilities (19,78,84,98,99,148, 217–223,227,236–238,241–243,256,278,283–291) and, like MSSA, often causes prolonged colonization (72,84,119,120, 129–131,133,148,161,217,261,280,292).

After such cases are accounted for, clusters or increased rates of new cases that are somehow associated should be the stimulus for further evaluation and action. Examples of associations of importance include those (a) occurring over short intervals, (b) not involving patients with backgrounds of known high MRSA prevalence (e.g., patients transferred from an institution with a known high MRSA endemicity), (c) occurring in the same geographic area of the facility, (d) cared for by the same healthcare provider or clinical service (182,184,293), (e) with first isolates recovered from identical sites, and (f) demonstrating MRSA isolates with identical antimicrobial susceptibilities.

Clusters occurring in high-risk areas such as ICUs and burn units are of special importance. Microorganism transmission is accelerated and morbidity is greater when patients in these areas are affected (16,57,72,83,143,161,173,204,209,212,241,279, 294–296). Neither identity nor difference of antimicrobial susceptibility patterns among isolates from clustered cases can be assumed to definitively confirm or refute MRSA cross-transmission. However, clustered cases with isolates demonstrating an apparently new pattern of drug susceptibility should not be overlooked. Such isolates have heralded a number of nosocomial outbreaks (166,179,211,241,293,297,298).

Surveillance Cultures

Surveillance cultures can be used to address specific questions. Whether MRSA is endemic or epidemic, periodic prevalence culture surveys of patients not known to harbor MRSA in acute care hospitals can identify additional cases (typically 20–30%) that would not be identified by cultures performed for clinical indications (166,187,194,297,299). Anterior nares cultures detect most, and wound and medically placed tube site cultures in addition to nares cultures detect almost all individuals not otherwise identified (148,167,173,187,194,297,299–304). A combination of anterior nares and perineum cultures has a sensitivity to detect carriers that exceeds 90% (305). The use of enrichment broth cultures can significantly improve the sensitivity of surveillance cultures to identify colonized patients but is more time consuming and expensive (302,306,307). Selective media can be used to decrease the laboratory work associated with culture surveys (308–310). Culture surveys can thus help establish the prevalence of MRSA in a facility at a given time.

Culturing of patients on admission can be used to help define whether nosocomial acquisition is or is not the cause of newly identified cases who are first cultured after a number of days of hospitalization. Also, if special precautions are being used for all colonized and infected patients, regular surveillance culture surveys are important to identify most of the patients who need the special intervention (311). This may be particularly relevant for patients transferred from affiliated institutions with known high endemic rates of MRSA (98,178,230) and for selected patients when line-listed information suggests an out-of-facility reservoir (288). Some have also suggested doing surveillance cultures on all patients at high risk for MRSA colonization as a means to identify the reservoir, isolate cases, and therefore prevent spread; some have suggested that such programs may even be cost-effective (296,311–317). This may be practical in some acute care hospitals with a low prevalence of MRSA or as an important adjunct to contain ongoing outbreaks in specific high-risk areas or settings. Unfortunately, many factors often preclude such an approach on an institution-wide basis, such as (a) the very high prevalence of MRSA in many hospitals and high-risk units (11,13,18), (b) the high frequency of risk factors associated with MRSA colonization (e.g., recent hospitalization, recent receipt of an antibiotic, residence in an LTCF, recent medical care, etc.)(20,127,237), and (c) the ever-changing epidemiology of MRSA (19,245,304). The needs to maximize bed use and to abide by modern methods of patient management are also very real and well-known hindrances of such potential surveillance culture and patient isolation programs (318,319), particularly in institutions with high prevalence rates of MRSA.

As examples, the vigorous use of multiple site, on-admission surveillance cultures of patients coming from outside Denmark or The Netherlands has been an intervention associated with control of MRSA in these countries (273,274). However, overall control measures include (a) placing in isolation any patient transferred from a hospital outside the country; (b) discontinuing isolation of such patients only after screening cultures have revealed that they are not colonized with MRSA; (c) routinely screening all patients and personnel exposed to a patient with MRSA; (d) treating (decolonizing) all patient and staff as MRSA carriers; (e) strict control of antimicrobial prescribing for all patients; and (f) wearing a mask, a gown, and gloves whenever entering the room of a patient with MRSA.

Routine on-admission surveillance cultures for MRSA are difficult to justify. It is not likely to help overall control unless MRSA colonization is common among newly admitted patients, these otherwise unidentified colonized patients serve as a major source for subsequent transmission, and multiple other special precautions and interventions are taken and are effective in limiting spread. Routine surveillance cultures have often been and will continue to be an important component of outbreak control, particularly in high-risk clinical settings (197,311,317). The feasibility and effectiveness of routine surveillance cultures to contain and control the spread of MRSA in highly endemic regions and hospitals has not been demonstrated outside of Denmark and The Netherlands.

Isolate Typing

Newer methods for typing isolates are used more often to support or refute MRSA transmission within facilities (102-111, 320–324) and are now viewed as an essential component of a comprehensive infection control program (325–329). This is particularly true because of the rising prevalence of MRSA in outpatients, communities, LTCFs, and hospitals, all of which confounds investigations of possible cross-transmission (11,13, 18,20,78,101,105,109,113,114,217–223,227,228,232,278, 283,290,292,323). Finally, recognition that stringent and special MRSA control practices are expensive, are of variable efficacy, and often are not needed makes accurate and discriminating typing a useful tool in many situations (146,173,208,263, 266,278,291,330–333).

Many typing tests are available; most have greatly improved value for strain identification and differentiation (increased proportion of isolates typeable, as well as better reproducibility and discriminatory power) (102–117,328,329). Strain identity of MRSA isolates cultured from epidemiologically related patients by a discriminatory typing test strongly support cross-transmission or common source transmission, whereas strain differences support the concept that common source or cross-transmission has not occurred.

Staff Culturing

Culturing of staff, a low-yield activity in most circumstances (16,166,173,208,259,263,330,331,333), is another laboratory-based strategy advocated for MRSA control. Most personnel are only transiently colonized and not a likely persistent source for MRSA spread. Personnel with infected skin lesions, hand dermatitis, upper respiratory infections, or persistent nasal carriage may be more likely to transmit MRSA (161,179,182,184,196,198, 293). Screening of personnel by nasal cultures should be limited to those who are epidemiologically linked to clusters of patient cases (275,276,308,332,334). In addition, the demonstration of identity by typing of patient and personnel isolates is advised to confirm or support epidemiologic relationships (101,192,332, 334). Even if the isolates are identical, colonized personnel may be only recipients and not transmitters of the identified strain.

Rapid Identification of MRSA

Conventional laboratory testing to determine the species and presence or absence of methicillin resistance in clinical isolates of staphylococci generally takes one full day following the growth of visible colonies on an agar surface (50). Highly sensitive and specific tests are now available that can reliably confirm or refute the presence of methicillin resistance (by detecting *mecA* or PBP2A) from *S. aureus* colonies within 15 minutes to a few hours (45–49,335–340). PCR-based tests have also been described that can simultaneously and directly identify MRSA in blood cultures within 6 hours of detected growth and confirmation of the presence of gram-positive cocci by Gram-stained smears (341,342). Such tests may be helpful to more rapidly identify or institute infection control measures for those patients with MRSA. Moreover, earlier reporting of MSSA rather than MRSA to physicians may lead to a reduction in unnecessary or less effective and empirically prescribed vancomycin therapy to those patients with MSSA infections (343) and the appropriate prescription of vancomycin therapy for those with MRSA infections (344). Although promising, such testing has not yet been documented as an important or effective component of an overall MRSA control program or as substantially improving clinical outcomes of patients with *S. aureus* bacteremia (345).

Environmental Control

MRSA is usually demonstrable in the immediate environment of colonized and infected patients (184,187–190,192,193, 222,346,347), may survive on fabrics and plastic surfaces for very long periods (348), and can become airborne and disseminated within a patient room during bed making (349). One study also suggested that outbreak strains of MRSA have superior survivability in the environment compared with sporadic strains of MRSA (350).

Despite these findings, environmental contamination is rarely viewed as the proximate cause of MRSA transmission. Exceptions include outbreaks in burn units (16,141,160,161,181,198, 204,216) or unusual circumstances such as that reported from a critical care unit in which gloves used for universal precautions were not regularly changed between patients (351). In another critical care unit, damaged contaminated mattresses were identified as a possible source for MRSA spread (352). Also, enhanced hospital hygiene (increasing domestic cleaning time, emphasizing removal of dust by vacuum cleaning, and allocating responsibility for the routine cleaning of shared medical equipment), along with additional interventions, has been associated with termination of a clonal outbreak of MRSA in a surgical ward (353). Standard housekeeping practices, in general, appear to be adequate for routine MRSA control.

Hand Washing

Hand washing is a time-honored principle of routine infection prevention and control and is considered effective for eliminating transient hand contamination with MRSA (194) and other pathogens acquired from patients or the environment. A simple 10-second wash with soap and water performed by personnel in facilities with a moderate endemic rate of MRSA showed an absence of MRSA on 96% of cultured individuals' hands (354). Unfortunately, attempts to establish and sustain higher frequencies of hand washing between patient contacts have often been disappointing (355). Although hand antisepsis with agents containing povidone-iodine or alcohol have been found to more effectively remove MRSA from artificially contaminated hands of volunteers (356), the increased efficacy of antimicrobial soaps versus standard soap to contain and control MRSA has not been convincingly demonstrated. One report did suggest that the substitution of hexachlorophene for chlorhexidine as the hand-washing agent was necessary to eradicate MRSA from a neonatal ICU (195). More recently, a hospital-wide program promoting hand hygiene, with special emphasis on bedside, alcohol-based hand disinfection was associated with improved hand hygiene compliance and a reduction in attack rates of MRSA (357). Maintaining a high level of compliance with hand washing is an essential element of MRSA control. Unfortunately, improved hand hygiene is unlikely to compensate for other problems related to control of MRSA in areas of high endemicity and intensive care (358).

Isolation, Segregation, and Cohorting

Stringent isolation of affected patients has been one of many interventional components reported to contribute to containment and control of MRSA outbreaks (263,273—275,277). However, some lessening in the stringency of isolation has not been associated with subsequent increases in transmission in acute care or chronic care facilities with endemic MRSA (212, 230,263,297,308,330,359,360). There is little justification for the routine application of strict isolation (including masks, gowns, and gloves for all patient contacts) for colonized or infected patients to control endemic MRSA. The exception to this may be as a component of a series of special controls in burn units with high-level transmission (263,264,276,308). Many authors and agencies suggest only hand-washing reminders, the routine use of gloves for all patient contacts (278,361,362), universal body substance isolation, or the application of contact precautions (315,363) for general MRSA control purposes. Advocacy of one over another of these approaches for endemic MRSA control is not supported by a critical literature review (263). A stepwise approach using progressively more stringent barrier interventions can be applied when clusters or outbreaks of MRSA are recognized, with return to the usual facility routine when the problem is controlled (278,361,364).

Segregation of patients with MRSA in private rooms is generally advocated in the acute care setting. Roommate-to-roommate transmission in extended care facilities is infrequent (148,217, 264,292), and the number of private rooms may be limited. Sharing a room with an unaffected patient may be acceptable under this circumstance, particularly if the unaffected roommate seems to be at low risk for MRSA acquisition or MRSA infection (276).

Comprehensive cohorting has contributed to the control of a number of MRSA outbreaks (171,263,273,275,277,308). Cohorting should be considered when a high level of MRSA transmission is documented, transmission continues despite alternative interventions, and personnel staffing and available facilities allow for the establishment of a cohort plan. Ideally, all colonized and infected patients should be transferred to the same geographic area and cared for by a designated staff group. Unaffected patients should not be admitted or transferred to the cohort area, and the designated staff group caring for MRSA patients should not care for unaffected patients. Culturing of designated staff members before allowing them to return to normal work activities and treatment as needed if MRSA colonization is detected have also been advocated (273,274,277,365). Cohorting of patients or staff members providing care is neither practical nor warranted for endemic MRSA control.

Decolonization of Patients and Staff

Treatment of patients and staff members who are infected with MRSA is obviously indicated. Although it may decrease the numbers of microorganisms that can be cultured from a given site, antimicrobial treatment for infection usually fails to eliminate concomitant MRSA colonization. Patients with MRSA infection or colonization are considered the most important reservoir for transmission of the microorganism to unaffected patients, and patient colonization tends to be prolonged (84,119,120,129–131,148,161,217,292). In addition, colonization is a risk factor for subsequent infection for some patients (84). Staff who are epidemiologically related to clusters of patient cases are occasionally found to harbor MRSA (101,179,192, 208,264,295,308), and such staff may be disseminators of the microorganism (366). Hence, it is not surprising that microorganism eradication or decolonization therapy would be considered an adjunct for MRSA control. Recently favored regimens include systemically absorbed orally administered antimicrobials (often rifampin in combination with another agent) or the topical agent mupirocin applied to the site(s) of colonization (12, 54,178,201,260,261,364,367–377). Simultaneous baths or showers with chlorhexidine or other antistaphylococcal agents are also often advocated.

These measures may be useful as part of a comprehensive plan for MRSA outbreak control (12,178,274,275,277,308, 375–377). This is particularly true when epidemiologically implicated and culture-positive staff members are identified, removed from patient care, and given decolonization therapy (366). Personnel not necessarily responsible for dissemination of MRSA may also respond, but identification and decolonization therapy of culture-positive staff members is not advocated under these circumstances (275,276,308). Successful decolonization of patients who are debilitated and colonized at multiple sites is much less likely (259,260,261,368,378,379). Unfortunately, it is these patients who tend to get subsequent MRSA infections (84). Evidence also suggests that a large proportion of patients who achieve negative culture status after decolonization therapy subsequently become culture positive if followed for a sufficient period (54,136,259,261,262,275,308,368,379,380). Typing of sequential isolates typically supports relapse rather than new colonization or infection as the cause of the return to a culture-positive state (260,262). Treatment with orally administered antibiotics (e.g., rifampin, trimethoprim-sulfamethoxazole, ciprofloxacin, clindamycin) and topical mupirocin has been associated with the development of resistance among MRSA isolates cultured from patients who fail or relapse following decolonization therapy (54,259,260,378,381,382), and these newly resistant isolates may spread throughout a facility (211,259, 383–389). The decision to use decolonization therapy should be accompanied by a commitment to monitor for development of resistance to the agents used.

An attempt at decolonization therapy is indicated for the few patients who have relapsing infections caused by MRSA and for personnel who are colonized with MRSA and are epidemiologically associated with nosocomial clusters or outbreaks (366,376). It would be ideal to have documentation of strain identity of personnel and patient case isolates before personnel decolonization attempts. A third indication for decolonization may be minimizing the frequency of new cases in the face of an outbreak that continues despite other interventions (375,377). Decolonization therapy for most patients and most colonized personnel as a major component of endemic MRSA control is usually not efficacious and encourages the induction and spread of more resistant microorganisms.

Improvements in Antimicrobial Prescribing

Preceding antibiotic therapy for a prolonged period is well recognized as a major risk factor for subsequently documented MRSA colonization and infection (16,57,145,194,218, 390–396). Three recent studies suggest that decreasing broad-spectrum antibiotic therapy can reduce the rate of nosocomial MRSA colonization and infection. Japanese investigators showed that reducing the use of second- or third-generation cephem antibiotics in burn patients decreased nosocomial MRSA cases (397). Frank et al. (398) demonstrated that the implementation of an antimicrobial prescribing improvement program at a midwestern United States university hospital, which led to a major reduction in the use of many broad-spectrum β-lactam antibiotics, was also associated with a significant drop in the frequency and rate of nosocomial MRSA cases throughout the hospital. Landman et al. (399) described a significant reduction in the monthly number of new patients with MRSA following hospital formulary changes resulting in decreased use of cephalosporins, imipenem, clindamycin, and vancomycin. Although further confirmation of these findings is needed (400), it seems reasonable to consider antibiotic-prescribing improvement or control programs as interventions that can reduce MRSA endemicity in institutions or among specific populations of patients.

Maintenance of Reasonable Nursing Workloads

Problems with nursing staffing have recently been associated with increased nosocomial infection rates (401), and this includes difficulties in containing MRSA. Farrington et al. (402) demonstrated that MRSA outbreaks in an English hospital typically occurred when staffing gaps were most severe. Vicca (403) found that the incidence of new cases of MRSA in an ICU at a tertiary referral center over a 19-month interval correlated with peaks of nursing staff workload and times of reduced nurse-to-patient ratios. Thus, it is very reasonable to review nursing staffing as a component of MRSA surveillance and control. Any deficiencies found should be addressed as part of a comprehensive MRSA control program.

Approach to VISA and VRSA

Currently, only a limited number of patients in the United States and elsewhere have been identified as colonized or infected with VISA or VRSA, and all have also been MRSA (250–255). Thus far, transmission of VISA or VRSA from patient-to-patient or to several epidemiologically related patients has not been identified. In association with the current low prevalence of VISA and VRSA, and the limited available therapeutic armamentarium for these microorganisms, it seems very reasonable to establish special precautions to investigate, contain, and control the spread of this problem. Multifaceted interim guidelines have been recommended in the United States and include (a) rapid laboratory reporting to infection control and unit personnel, the attending physician, the state health department, and the CDC; (b) epidemiologic and laboratory investigation to identify possible spread; (c) placement in a private room and use of contact precautions (gown, mask, and gloves) and antibacterial soap for hand washing; (d) monitoring of compliance; (e) avoidance of the transfer of affected patients within or between facilities if possible; and (f) consultation with the state health department and the CDC before discharge (404).

REFERENCES

1. Spink WW, Ferris V. Quantitative action of penicillin inhibitor from penicillin-resistant strains of staphylococci. *Science* 1945;102:221.
2. Jevons MP. "Celbenin"-resistant staphylococci. *BMJ* 1961;1: 124–125.
3. Barber M. Methicillin-resistant staphylococci. *J Clin Pathol* 1961;14: 385–393.

4. Crisostomo MI, Westh H, Tomasz A, et al. The evolution of methicillin resistance in *Staphylococcus aureus*: similarity of genetic backgrounds in historically early methicillin-susceptible and resistant isolates and contemporary epidemic clones. *PNAS* 2001;98:9865–9870.
5. Boyce JM. Understanding and controlling methicillin resistant *Staphylococcus aureus* infections. *Infect Control Hosp Epidemiol* 2002;23: 485–487.
6. Kayser FM. Methicillin-resistant staphylococci, 1965–75. *Lancet* 1975;2:650–653.
7. Siboni K, Poulsen L, Digman E. The dominance of methicillin-resistant staphylococci in a country hospital. *Dan Med Bull* 1968;15: 161–165.
8. Chabbert YA, Baudens JG, Acar JF, et al. The natural resistance of staphylococci to methicillin and oxacillin. *Rev Fr Etud Clin Biol* 1965; 10:495–506.
9. Giamarellou H, Papapetropoulou M, Daikos GK. Methicillin-resistant *Staphylococcus aureus* infection during 1978–79. Clinical and bacteriological observations. *J Antimicrob Chemother* 1981;7: 649–655.
10. Rountree PM, Beard MA. Hospital strains of *Staphylococcus aureus* with particular reference to methicillin-resistant strains. *Med J Aust* 1968;2:1163–1168.
11. Fluit AC, Wielders CLC, Verhoef J, et al. Epidemiology and susceptibility of 3,051 *Staphylococcus aureus* isolates from 25 university hospitals participating in the European SENTRY study. *J Clin Microbiol* 2001;39:3727–3732.
12. Wenzel RP, Nettleman MD, Jones RN, et al. Methicillin-resistant *Staphylococcus aureus*: implications for the 1990s and effective control measures. *Am J Med* 1991;91(Suppl 3B):221–227.
13. Diekema DJ, Pfaller MA, Schmitz FJ, et al. Survey of infections due to *Staphylococcus* species: frequency of occurrence and antimicrobial susceptibility of isolates collected in the United States, Canada, Latin America, Europe, and the Western Pacific region for the SENTRY Antimicrobial Surveillance Program, 1997–1999. *Clin Infect Dis* 2001;32(Suppl 2):S114–132.
14. Simor AE, Ofner-Agostini M, Bryce E. The evolution of methicillin-resistant *Staphylococcus aureus* in Canadian hospitals: 5 years of national surveillance. *Can Med Assoc J* 2001;165:21–26.
15. Haley RW, Hightower AW, Khabbaz RF, et al. The emergence of methicillin-resistant *Staphylococcus aureus* infections in United States hospitals. Possible role of the house staff-patient transfer circuit. *Ann Intern Med* 1982;97:297–308.
16. Crossley K, Landesman B, Zaske D. An outbreak of infections caused by strains of *Staphylococcus aureus* resistant to methicillin and aminoglycosides. II. Epidemiologic studies. *J Infect Dis* 1979;139:280–287.
17. Panlilio AL, Culver DH, Gaynes RP, et al. Methicillin-resistant *Staphylococcus aureus* in U.S. hospitals, 1975–1991. *Infect Control Hosp Epidemiol* 1992;13:582–586
18. National Nosocomial Infections Surveillance (NNIS) system report, data summary from January 1992–June 2001, Issued August 2001. *Am J Infect Control* 2001;29:404–421.
19. Herold BC, Immergluck LC, Maranan MC, et al. Community-acquired methicillin-resistant *Staphylococcus aureus* in children with no identified predisposing risk. *JAMA* 1998;279:593–598.
20. Chambers HF. The changing epidemiology of *Staphylococcus aureus*? *Emerg Infect Dis* 2001;7:178–182.
21. Chambers HF. Methicillin-resistance in staphylococci: molecular and biochemical basis and clinical implications. *Clin Microbiol Rev* 1997; 10:781–791.
22. Lyon BR, Skurray R. Antimicrobial resistance of *Staphylococcus aureus*: genetic basis. *Microbiol Rev* 1987;51:88–134.
23. Hackbarth CJ, Chambers HF. Methicillin-resistant staphylococci: genetics and mechanisms of resistance. *Antmicrob Agents Chemother* 1989;33:991–994.
24. Archer GL, Pennell E. Detection of methicillin resistance in staphylococci by using a DNA probe. *Antimicrob Agents Chemother* 1990;34: 1720–1724.
25. Gerberding JL, Miick C, Liu HH, et al. Comparison of conventional susceptibility tests with direct detection of penicillin-binding protein 2a in borderline oxacillin-resistant strains of *Staphylococcus aureus. Antimicrob Agents Chemother* 1991;35:2574–2579.
26. Tomasz A, Drugeon HB, DeLencastre HM, et al. New mechanism for methicillin resistance in *Staphylococcus aureus*: clinical isolates that lack the PBP 2a gene and contain normal penicillin-binding proteins with modified penicillin-binding capacity. *Antimicrob Agents Chemother* 1989;33:1869–1874.
27. Jorgensen JH. Mechanisms of methicillin resistance in *Staphylococcus aureus* and methods for laboratory detection. *Infect Control Hosp Epidemiol* 1991;12:14–19.
28. McDougal LK, Thornsberry C. The role of B-lactamase in staphylococcal resistance to penicillinase-resistant penicillins and cephalosporins. *J Clin Microbiol* 1986;23:832–839.
29. Montanari MP, Tonin E, Biavasco F, et al. Further characterization of borderline methicillin-resistant *Staphylococcus aureus* and analysis of penicillin-binding proteins. *Antimicrob Agents Chemother* 1990;34: 911–913.
30. Chambers HF, Archer G, Matsuhashi M. Low-level methicillin-resistance in strains of *Staphylococcus aureus. Antimicrob Agents Chemother* 1989;33:424–428.
31. Kline MW, Mason EO Jr, Kaplan SL. Outcome of heteroresistant *Staphylococcus aureus* infections in children. *J Infect Dis* 1987;156: 205–208.
32. Massanari RM, Pfaller MA, Wakefield DS, et al. Implications of acquired oxacillin resistance in the management and control of *Staphylococcus aureus* infections. *J Infect Dis* 1988;158:702–709.
33. Tomasz A, Nachman S, Leaf H. Stable classes of phenotypic expression in methicillin-resistant clinical isolates of staphylococci. *Antimicrob Agents Chemother* 1991;35:124–129.
34. Hartman BJ, Tomasz A. Expression of methicillin resistance in heterogeneous strains of *Staphylococcus aureus. Antimicrob Agents Chemother* 1986;29:85–92.
35. Berger-Bachi B, Rohrer S. Factors influencing methicillin resistance in staphylococci. *Arch Microbiol* 2002;178:165–171.
36. Sabath LD. Mechanisms of resistance to beta-lactam antibiotics in strains of *Staphylococcus aureus. Ann Intern Med* 1982;97:339–344.
37. Boyce JM, Medieros AA, Papa EF, et al. Induction of beta-lactamase and methicillin resistance in unusual strains of methicillin resistant *Staphylococcus aureus. J Antimicrob Chemother* 1990;25:73–81.
38. Hackbarth CJ, Chambers HF. Methicillin-resistant staphylococci: detection methods and treatment of infections. *Antimicrob Agents Chemother* 1989;33:995–999.
39. Jorgensen JH, Redding JS, Maher LA, et al. Salt-supplemented medium for testing methicillin-resistant staphylococci with newer beta-lactams. *J Clin Microbiol* 1988;26:1675–1678.
40. Chambers HF. Coagulase-negative staphylococci resistant to beta-lactam antibiotics in vivo produce penicillin-binding protein 2a. *Antimicrob Agents Chemother* 1987;31:1919–1924.
41. Wenzel RP. Methicillin-resistant *Staphylococcus aureus* and *Staphylococcus epidermidis* strains: modern hospital pathogens. *Infect Control* 1986;7(Suppl):118–119.
42. Ligozzi M, Rossolini GM, Tonin EA, et al. Nonradioactive DNA probe for detection of gene for methicillin resistance in *Staphylococcus aureus. Antimicrob Agents Chemother* 1991;35:575–578.
43. Murakami K, Minamide W, Wada K, et al. Identification of methicillin-resistant strains of staphylococci by polymerase chain reaction. *J Clin Microbiol* 1991;29:2240–2244.
44. Salisbury SM, Sabatini LM, Spiegel CA. Identification of methicillin-resistant staphylococci by multiplex polymerase chain reaction assay. *Am J Clin Pathol* 1997;107:368–373.
45. Swenson JM, Williams PP, Killgore G, et al. Performance of eight methods, including two new rapid methods, for detection of oxacillin resistance in a challenge set of *Staphylococcus aureus* organisms. *J Clin Microbiol* 2001;39:3785–3788.
46. Sakoulas G, Gold HS, Venkataraman L, et al. Methicillin-resistant *Staphylococcus aureus*: comparison of susceptibility testing methods and analysis of *mecA*-positive susceptible strains. *J Clin Microbiol* 2001;39:3946–3951.
47. Arbique J, Forward K, Haldane D, et al. Comparison of the Velogene Rapid MRSA Identification Assay, Denka MRSA-Screen Assay, and

BBL Crystal MRSA ID System for rapid identification of methicillin-resistant *Staphylococcus aureus. J Clin Microbiol* 2002;40:3764–3770.
48. Smyth RW, Kahlmeter G, Liljequist BO, et al. Methods for identifying methicillin resistance in *Staphylococcus aureus. J Hosp Infect* 2001;48:103–107.
49. Merlino J, Watson J, Rose B, et al. Detection and expression of methicillin/oxacillin resistance in multidrug-resistant and non-multidrug-resistant *Staphylococcus aureus* in central Sydney, Australia. *J Antimicrob Chemother* 2002;49:793–801.
50. National Committee for Clinical Laboratory Standards (NCCLS). *Performance standards for antimicrobial susceptibility testing,* 12th informational supplement. NCCLS document M100-S12. Wayne, PA: NCCLS, 2002.
51. Pfaller MA, Wakefield DS, Hammons GT, et al. Variations from standards in *Staphylococcus aureus* susceptibility testing. *Am J Clin Pathol* 1987;88:231–235.
52. Fleming DW, Helgerson SD, Mallery BL, et al. Methicillin-resistant *Staphylococcus aureus*: how reliable is laboratory reporting? *Infect Control* 1986;7:164–167.
53. Aldridge KE, Janney A, Sanders CV, et al. Interlaboratory variation of antibiograms of methicillin-resistant and methicillin susceptible *Staphylococcus aureus* strains with conventional and commercial testing systems. *J Clin Microbiol* 1983;18:1226–1236.
54. Chambers HF. Treatment of infection and colonization caused by methicillin-resistant *Staphylococcus aureus. Infect Control Hosp Epidemiol* 1991;12:29–35.
55. Franciolli M, Bille J, Glauser MP, et al. B-lactam resistance mechanisms of methicillin-resistant *Staphylococcus aureus. J Infect Dis* 1991;163:514–523.
56. Coudron PE, Jones DL, Dalton HP, et al. Evaluation of laboratory tests for detection of methicillin-resistant *Staphylococcus aureus* and *Staphylococcus epidermidis. J Clin Microbiol* 1986;24:764–769.
57. Boyce JM. Methicillin-resistant *Staphylococcus aureus*: detection, epidemiology and control measures. *Infect Dis Clin North Am* 1989;3:901–913.
58. Ender PT, Durning SJ, Woelk WK, et al. Pseudo-outbreak of methicillin-resistant *Staphylococcus aureus. Mayo Clin Proc* 1999;74:885–889.
59. Lyon BR, Iuorio JL, May JW, et al. Molecular epidemiology of multiresistant *Staphylococcus aureus* in Australian hospitals. *J Med Microbiol* 1987;17:79–89.
60. Maple PAC, Hamilton-Miller JMT, Brumfitt W. World-wide antibiotic resistance in methicillin-resistant *Staphylococcus aureus. Lancet* 1989;1:537–540.
61. Turnidge J, Lawson P, Munro R, et al. A national survey of antimicrobial resistance in *Staphylococcus aureus* in Australian teaching hospitals. *Med J Aust* 1989;150:65–72.
62. Then RL, Kohl I, Burdeska A. Frequency and transferability of trimethoprim and sulfonamide resistance in methicillin-resistant *Staphylococcus aureus* and *Staphylococcus epidermidis. J Chemother* 1992;4:67–71.
63. Blumberg HM, Rimland D, Carroll DJ, et al. Rapid development of ciprofloxacin resistance in methicillin-susceptible and -resistant *Staphylococcus aureus. J Infect Dis* 1991;163:1279–1285.
64. Farrel DJ. The reliability of Microscan conventional and rapid panels to identify *Staphylococcus aureus* and detect methicillin resistance: an evaluation using tube coagulation and mecA PCR. *Pathology* 1997;29:406–410.
65. Ward TT. Comparison of in vitro adherence of methicillin-sensitive and methicillin-resistant *Staphylococcus aureus* to human nasal epithelial cells. *J Infect Dis* 1992;166:400–404.
66. Duckworth GJ, Jorden JZ. Adherence and survival properties of an epidemic methicillin-resistant strain of *Staphylococcus aureus* compared with those of methicillin-sensitive strains. *J Med Microbiol* 1990;32:195–200.
67. Vaudaux O, Waldvogel FA. Methicillin-resistant strains of *Staphylococcus aureus*: relationship between expression of resistance and phagocytosis by polymorphonuclear leukocytes. *J Infect Dis* 1979;139:547–552.
68. Peacock JE, Moorman D, Wenzel RP, et al. Methicillin-resistant *Staphylococcus aureus*: microbiologic characteristics, antimicrobial susceptibilities, and assessment of virulence of an epidemic strain. *J Infect Dis* 1981;144:575–582.
69. Cutler RR. Relationship between antibiotic resistance, the production of virulence factors, and virulence for experimental animals in *Staphylococcus aureus. J Med Microbiol* 1979;12:55–62.
70. Hewitt H, Sanderson PJ. The effect of methicillin on skin lesions in guinea pigs caused by methicillin-sensitive and methicillin-resistant *Staphylococcus aureus. J Med Microbiol* 1974;7:223–228.
71. Peacock JE Jr, Marsik FJ, Wenzel RP. Methicillin-resistant *Staphylococcus aureus*: introduction and spread within a hospital. *Ann Intern Med* 1980;93:526–532.
72. Boyce JM, Landry M, Deetz TR, et al. Epidemiologic studies of an outbreak of nosocomial methicillin-resistant *Staphylococcus aureus* infections. *Infect Control* 1981;2:110–116.
73. Sorrell TC, Packham DR, Shanker S, et al. Vancomycin therapy for methicillin-resistant *Staphylococcus aureus. Ann Intern Med* 1982;97:344–350.
74. Lewis E, Saravolatz LD. Comparison of methicillin-resistant and methicillin-sensitive *Staphylococcus aureus* bacteremia. *Am J Infect Control* 1985;13:109–114.
75. Law MR, Gill ON. Hospital-acquired infection with methicillin-resistant and methicillin-sensitive staphylococci. *Epidemiol Infect* 1988;101:623–629.
76. McManus AT, Mason AD Jr, McManus WF, et al. What's in a name? Is methicillin-resistant *Staphylococcus aureus* just another *Staphylococcus aureus* when treated with vancomycin? *Arch Surg* 1989;124:1456–1459.
77. Harbarth S, Rutschmann O, Sudre P, et al. Impact of methicillin resistance on the outcome of patients with bacteremia caused by *Staphylococcus aureus. Arch Intern Med* 1998;158:182–189.
78. Lee YL, Cesario T, Gupta G, et al. Surveillance of colonization and infection with *Staphylococcus aureus* susceptible or resistant to methicillin in a community skilled-nursing facility. *Am J Infect Control* 1997;25:312–321.
79. Soriano A, Martinez JA, Mensa J, et al. Pathogenic significance of methicillin resistance for patients with *Staphylococcus aureus* bacteremia. *Clin Infect Dis* 2000;30:368–373.
80. Selvey LA, Whitby M, Johnson B. Nosocomial methicillin-resistant *Staphylococcus aureus* bacteremia: is it any worse than nosocomial methicillin-susceptible *Staphylococcus aureus* bacteremia? *Infect Control Hosp Epidemiol* 2000;21:645–648.
81. Tumbarello M, de Gaetano Donati K, Tacconelli E, et al. Risk factors and predictors of mortality of methicillin-resistant *Staphylococcus aureus* (MRSA) bacteraemia in HIV-infected patients. *J Antimicrob Chemother* 2002;50:375–382.
82. Gedney J, Lacey RW. Properties of methicillin-resistant staphylococci now endemic in Australia. *Med J Aust* 1982;1:448–450.
83. Vriens MR, Fluit AC, Troelstra A, et al. Is methicillin resistant *Staphylococcus aureus* more contagious than methicillin-susceptible *Staphylococcus aureus* in a surgical intensive care unit. *Infect Control Hosp Epidemiol* 2002;23:491–494.
84. Muder RR, Brennen C, Wagener M, et al. Methicillin-resistant staphylococcal colonization and infection in a long-term care facility. *Ann Intern Med* 1991;114:107–112.
85. Romero-Vivas J, Rubio M, Fernandez C, et al. Mortality associated with nosocomial bacteremia due to methicillin-resistant *Staphylococcus aureus. Clin Infect Dis* 1998;21:1417–1423.
86. Pujol M, Pena C, Pallares R, et al. Nosocomial *Staphylococcus aureus* bacteremia among nasal carriers of methicillin-resistant and methicillin-susceptible strains. *Am J Med* 1996;100:509–516.
87. Whitby M, McLaws M, Berry G. Risk of death from methicillin-resistant *Staphylococcus aureus* bacteraemia: a meta-analysis. *Med J Aust* 2001;175:264–267.
88. Blot SI, Vandewoude KH, Hoste EA, et al. Outcome and attributable mortality in critically ill patients with bacteremia involving methicillin-susceptible and methicillin-resistant *Staphylococcus aureus. Arch Intern Med* 2002;162:2229–2235.
89. Hurley JC. Risk of death from methicillin-resistant *Staphylococcus au-*

reus bacteraemia: a meta-analysis [Letter]. *Med J Austr* 2002;176: 188–189.

90. Cosgrove SE, Sakoulis G, Perencevich EN, et al. Comparison of mortality associated with methicillin resistant and methicillin-susceptible *Staphylococcus aureus* bacteremia: a meta-analysis. *Clin Infect Dis* 2003; 36:53–59.
91. Lacy R, Kruczenyk S. Epidemiology of antibiotic resistance in *Staphylococcus aureus. J Antimicrob Chemother* 1986;18(Suppl C):207–214.
92. Branger C, Goullet P. Esterase electrophoretic polymorphism of methicillin-sensitive and methicillin-resistant strains of *Staphylococcus aureus. J Med Microbiol* 1987;24:275–281.
93. Skurray RA, Rouch DA, Lyon BR, et al. Multiresistant *Staphylococcus aureus*: genetics and evolution of epidemic Australian strains. *J Antimicrob Chemother* 1988;21(Suppl C):19–39.
94. Branger C, Goullet P, Boutonnier A, et al. Correlation between esterase electrophoretic types and capsular polysaccharide types 5 and 8 among methicillin-susceptible and methicillin-resistant strains of *Staphylococcus aureus. J Clin Microbiol* 1990;28:150–151.
95. Kreiswirth B, Kornblum J, Arbeit RD, et al. Evidence for a clonal origin of methicillin resistance in *Staphylococcus aureus. Science* 1993; 59:227–230.
96. Fitzgerald JR, Sturdevant DE, Mackie SM, et al. Evolutionary genomics of *Staphylococcus aureus*: insights into the origin of methicillin-resistant strains and the toxic shock syndrome epidemic. *PNAS* 2001; 98:8821–8826.
97. Wielders CLC, Fluit AC, Brisse S, et al. *mecA* gene is widely disseminated in *Staphylococcus aureus* population. *J Clin Microbiol* 2002;40: 3970–3975.
98. Trilla A, Nettleman MD, Hollis RJ, et al. Restriction endonuclease analysis of plasmid DNA from methicillin-resistant *Staphylococcus aureus*: clinical application over a three-year period. *Infect Control Hosp Epidemiol* 1993;14:29–35.
99. Lugeon C, Blanc DS, Wenger A, et al. Molecular epidemiology of methicillin-resistant *Staphylococcus aureus* at a low-incidence hospital over a 4-year period. *Infect Control Hosp Epidemiol* 1995;16:260–267.
100. Couto I, Melo-Cristino J, Fernandes ML, et al. Unusually large number of methicillin-resistant *Staphylococcus aureus* clones in a Portuguese hospital. *J Clin Microbiol* 1995;33:2032–2035.
101. Kreiswirth BN, Lutwick SM, Chapnick EK, et al. Tracing the spread of methicillin-resistant *Staphylococcus aureus* by Southern blot hybridization using gene-specific probes of mec and Tn554. *Microb Drug Resist* 1995;1:307–313.
102. Tenover FC, Arbeit R, Archer G, et al. Comparison of traditional and molecular methods of typing isolates of *Staphylococcus aureus. J Clin Microbiol* 1994;32:407–415.
103. van Belkum A, Kluytmans J, van Leeuwen W, et al. Multicenter evaluation of arbitrarily primed PCR for typing of *Staphylococcus aureus* strains. *J Clin Microbiol* 1995;33:1537–1547.
104. Yoshida T, Kondo N, Hanifah JA, et al. Combined use of ribotyping, PFGE typing and IS431 typing in the discrimination of nosocomial strains of methicillin-resistant *Staphylococcus aureus. Microbiol Immunol* 1997;41:687–695.
105. Tambic A, Power EGM, Talsania H, et al. Analysis of an outbreak of non-phage-typeable methicillin-resistant *Staphylococcus aureus* by using a randomly amplified polymorphic DNA assay. *J Clin Microbiol* 1997;35:3092–3097.
106. Nada T, Ichiyama S, Osada Y, et al. Comparison of DNA fingerprinting by PFGE and PCR-RFLP of the coagulase gene to distinguish MRSA isolates. *J Hosp Infect* 1996;32:305–317.
107. Byun DE, Kim SH, Shin JH, et al. Molecular epidemiologic analysis of *Staphylococcus aureus* isolated from clinical specimens. *J Korean Med Sci* 1997;12:190–198.
108. Olive DM, Bean P. Principles and applications of methods for DNA-based typing of microbial organisms. *J Clin Microbiol* 1999;37: 1661–1669.
109. Deplano A, Schuermans A, Van Eldere J, et al. Multicenter evaluation of epidemiological typing of methicillin-resistant *Staphylococcus aureus* strains by repetitive-element PCR analysis. *J Clin Microbiol* 2000;38: 3527–3533.
110. Grady R, Desai M, O'Neill G, et al. Genotyping of epidemic methicillin-resistant *Staphylococcus aureus* phage type 15 isolates by fluorescent amplified-fragment length polymorphism analysis. *J Clin Microbiol* 1999;37:3198–3203.
111. Weller TMA. Methicillin-resistant *Staphylococcus aureus* typing methods: which should be the international standard? *J Hosp Infect* 2000; 44:160–172.
112. Wichelhaus TA, Hunfeld K, Boddinghaus B, et al. Rapid molecular typing of methicillin-resistant *Staphylococcus aureus* by PCR-RFLP. *Infect Control Hosp Epidemiol* 2001;22:294–298.
113. Peacock SJ, de Silva GDI, Justice A, et al. Comparison of multilocus sequence typing and pulsed-field gel electrophoresis as tools for typing *Staphylococcus aureus* isolates in a microepidemiological setting. *J Clin Microbiol* 2002;40:3764–3770.
114. Shopsin B, Kreiswirth BN. Molecular epidemiology of methicillin-resistant *Staphylococcus aureus. Emerg Infect Dis* 2001;7:323–326.
115. Tenover FC, Arbeit RD, Goering RV, et al. How to select and interpret molecular strain typing methods for epidemiologic studies of bacterial infections: a review for healthcare epidemiologists. *Infect Control Hosp Epidemiol* 1997;18:426–439.
116. Pfaller MA, Herwaldt LA. The clinical microbiology laboratory and infection control: emerging pathogens, antimicrobial resistance, and new technology. *Clin Infect Dis* 1997;25:858–870.
117. Arbeit RD. Laboratory procedures for the epidemiologic analysis of microorganisms. In: Murray PR, Baron EJ, Pfaller MA, et al., eds. *Manual of clinical microbiology.* Washington DC: ASM Press, 1999: 116–137.
118. Stone PW, Larson E, Kwar LN, et al. A systematic audit of economic evidence linking nosocomial infections and infection control interventions: 1990–2000. *Am J Infect Control* 2002;30:145–152.
119. Scanvic A, Denic L, Gailon S, et al. Duration of colonization by methicillin-resistant *Staphylococcus aureus* after hospital discharge and risk factors for prolonged carriage. *Clin Infect Dis* 2001;32: 1393–1398.
120. MacKinnon M, Allen K. Long-term MRSA carriage in hospital patients. *J Hosp Infect* 2000;46:216–221.
121. Godfrey ME, Smith IM. Hospital hazards of staphylococcus sepsis. *JAMA* 1958;166:1197–2000.
122. Kirmani N, Tuazon CU, Murray HW, et al. *Staphylococcus aureus* carriage rate of patients receiving long term hemodialysis. *Arch Intern Med* 1978;138:1657–1659.
123. Tuazon CU, Sheagren JN. Increased staphylococcal carrier rate among narcotic addicts. *J Infect Dis* 1974;129:725–727.
124. Forfar JO, Gould JC, Maccabe AF. Effect of hexachlorophene on the incidence of staphylococcal and gram-negative infection in the newborn. *Lancet* 1968;2:177–179.
125. Tuazon CU, Perez A, Kishaba T, et al. *Staphylococcus aureus* among insulin-injecting diabetic patients; an increase carrier rate. *JAMA* 1975;231:1272.
126. Nouwen J, van Belkum A, Verbrugh H. Determinants of *Staphylococcus aureus* nasal carriage. *Neth J Med* 2001;59:126–133.
127. Bukharie H, Abdelhadi M, Saeed I, et al. Emergence of methicillin-resistant *Staphylococcus aureus* as a community pathogen. *Diagn Microbiol Infect Dis* 2001;40:1–4.
128. Onarato M, Borucki M, Baillargeon G, et al. Risk factors for colonization or infection due to methicillin-resistant *Staphylococcus aureus* in HIV-positive patients: a retrospective case-control study. *Infect Control Hosp Epidemiol* 1999;20:26–30.
129. Sanford M, Widmer A, Bale M, et al. Efficient detection and long-term persistence of the carriage of methicillin-resistant *Staphylococcus aureus. Clin Infect Dis* 1994;19:1123–1128.
130. Mitsuda T, Arai K, Ibe M, et al. The influence of methicillin-resistant *Staphylococcus aureus* (MRSA) carriers in a nursery and transmission of MRSA to their households. *J Hosp Infect* 1999;42:45–51.
131. Hicks NR, Moore EP, Williams EW. Carriage and community treatment of methicillin-resistant *Staphylococcus aureus*; what happens to colonized patients after discharge? *J Hosp Infect* 1991;19:17–24.
132. Frenay HM, Vanderbroucke-Grauls CM, Molkenboer MJ, et al. Long-term carriage and transmission of methicillin-resistant *Staphylococcus aureus* after discharge from hospital. *J Hosp Infect* 1992;22: 207–215.

133. Blok H, Vriens M, Weersink A, et al. Carriage of methicillin-resistant *Staphylococcus aureus* (MRSA) after discharge from hospital: follow-up for how long? A Dutch multi-centre study. *Hosp Infect Soc* 2001:325–327.
134. Strausbaugh LJ. Methicillin-resistant *Staphylococcus aureus.* In: Yoshikawa TT, Ouslander JG, eds. *Infection management for geriatrics in long-term care facilities.* New York: Marcel Dekker, 2002:383–409.
135. Murphy S, Denman S, Bennett RG, et al. Methicillin-resistant *Staphylococcus aureus* colonization in a long-term-care facility. *J Am Geriatr Soc* 1992;40:213–217.
136. Mulhausen PL, Harrell LJ, Weinberger M, et al. Contrasting methicillin-resistant *Staphylococcus aureus* colonization in Veterans Affairs and community nursing homes. *Am J Med* 1996;100:24–31.
137. von Baum H, Schmidt C, Svoboda D, et al. Risk factors for methicillin-resistant *Staphylococcus aureus* carriage in residents of German nursing homes. *Infect Control Hosp Epidemiol* 2002;23:511–515.
138. Trick WE, Weinstein RA, DeMarais PL, et al. Colonization of skilled-care facility residents with antimicrobial-resistant pathogens. *J Am Geriatr Soc* 2001;49:270–276.
139. Terpenning MS, Bradley SF, Wan JY, et al. Colonization and infection with antibiotic-resistant bacteria in a long-term care facility. *J Am Geriatr Soc* 1994;42:1062–1069.
140. Thomas JC, Bridge J, Waterman S, et al. Transmission and control of methicillin-resistant *Staphylococcus aureus* in a skilled nursing facility. *Infect Control Hosp Epidemiol* 1989;10:106–110.
141. Rutala WA, Katz EBS, Sherertz RJ, et al. Environmental study of a methicillin-resistant *Staphylococcus aureus* epidemic in a burn unit. *J Clin Microbiol* 1983;18:683–688.
142. Cook N. Methicillin-resistant *Staphylococcus aureus* versus the burn patient. *Burns* 1998;24:91–98.
143. Garrouste-Orgeas M, Timsit JF, Kallel H, et al. Colonization with methicillin-resistant *Staphylococcus aureus* in ICU patients: morbidity, morbidity, and glycopeptide use. *Infect Control Hosp Epidemiol* 2001;22:687–692.
144. Cespedes C, Miller M, Quagliarello B, et al. Differences between *Staphylococcus aureus* isolates from medical and nonmedical hospital personnel. *J Clin Microbiol* 2002;40:2594–2597.
145. Pujol M, Pena C, Pallares R, et al. Risk factors for nosocomial bacteremia due to methicillin-resistant *Staphylococcus aureus. Eur J Clin Microbiol Infect Dis* 1994;13:96–102.
146. Doebbeling BN. The epidemiology of methicillin-resistant *Staphylococcus aureus* colonization and infection. *J Chemother* 1995;7(Suppl 3):99–103.
147. Campillo B, Dupeyron C, Richardet JP. Epidemiology of hospital-acquired infections in cirrhotic patients: effect of carriage of methicillin-resistant *Staphylococcus aureus* and influence of previous antibiotic therapy and norfloxacin prophylaxis. *Epidemiol Infect* 2001;127:443–450.
148. Bradley SF, Terpenning MS, Ramsey MA, et al. Methicillin-resistant *Staphylococcus aureus*: colonization and infection in a long-term care facility. *Ann Intern Med* 1991;115:417–422.
149. Lye WC, Leong SO, Lee EJ. Methicillin-resistant *Staphylococcus aureus* nasal carriage and infections in CAPD. *Kidney Int* 1993;43:1357–1362.
150. Noble WC, Williams REO, Jevons MP, et al. Some aspects of nasal carriage of staphylococci. *J Clin Pathol* 1964;17:79–83.
151. Maslow JN, Brecher S, Gunn J, et al. Variation and persistence of methicillin-resistant *Staphylococcus aureus* strains among individual patients over extended periods of time. *Eur J Clin Microbiol Infect Dis* 1995;14:282–290.
152. Harbarth S, Liassine N, Dharan S, et al. Risk factors for persistent carriage of methicillin-resistant *Staphylococcus aureus. Clin Infect Dis* 2000;31:1380–1385.
153. Manhold C, von Rolbicki U, Brase R, et al. Outbreaks of *Staphylococcus aureus* infections during treatment of late onset pneumonia with ciprofloxacin in a prospective, randomized study. *Intensive Care Med* 1998;24:1327–1330.
154. Dziekan G, Daschner FD, Grundmann HJ. MRSA epidemic: case-control study to investigate hospital specific risk factors [abstract T2-11]. Fourth decennial conference on Nosocomial and Health Care Associated Infections (Atlanta, GA). *Infect Control Hosp Epidemiol* 2000;21;135.
155. Crowcroft NS, Ronveaux O, Monnet DL, et al. Methicillin-resistant *Staphylococcus aureus* and antimicrobial use in Belgian hospitals. *Infect Control Hosp Epidemiol* 1999;20:31–36.
156. Bisognano C, Vaudaux PE, Lew DP, et al. Increased expression of fibronectin-binding proteins by fluoroquinolone-resistant *Staphylococcus aureus* exposed to subinhibitory levels of ciprofloxacin. *Antimicrob Agents Chemother* 1997;41:906–913.
157. Bisognano C, Vaudaux PE, Rohner P, et al. Induction of fibronectin-binding proteins and increased adhesion of quinolone-resistant *Staphylococcus aureus* exposed to subinhibitory levels of ciprofloxacin. *Antimicrob Agents Chemother* 2000;44:1428–1437.
158. Yu VL, Goetz A, Wagener M, et al. *Staphylococcus aureus* infection in patients on hemodialysis: efficacy of antibiotic prophylaxis. *N Engl J Med* 1986;315:91–96.
159. Law MR, Gill ON, Turner A. Methicillin-resistant *Staphylococcus aureus*: associated morbidity and effectiveness of control measures. *Epidemiol Infect* 1988;101:301–309.
160. Boyce JM, White RL, Causey WA, et al. Burn units as a source of methicillin-resistant *Staphylococcus aureus* infections. *JAMA* 1983;249:2803–2807.
161. Locksley RM, Cohen ML, Quinn TC, et al. Multiply antibiotic-resistant *Staphylococcus aureus*: introduction, transmission, and evolution of nosocomial infection. *Ann Intern Med* 1982;97:317–324.
162. Linnemann CC Jr, Mason M, Moore P, et al. Methicillin-resistant *Staphylococcus aureus*: experience in a general hospital over four years. *Am J Epidemiol* 1982;115:941–950.
163. Bacon AE, Jorgensen KA, Wilson KH, et al. Emergence of nosocomial methicillin-resistant *Staphylococcus aureus* and therapy of colonized personnel during a hospital-wide outbreak. *Infect Control* 1987;8:145–150.
164. Bradley JM, Noone P, Townsend DE, et al. Methicillin-resistant *Staphylococcus aureus* in a London hospital. *Lancet* 1985;1:1493–1495.
165. Hill RL, Duckworth GJ, Casewell MW. Elimination of nasal carriage of methicillin-resistant *Staphylococcus aureus* with mupirocin during a hospital outbreak. *J Antimicrob Chemother* 1988;22:377–384.
166. Bitar CM, Mayhall CG, Lamb VA, et al. Outbreak due to methicillin- and rifampin-resistant *Staphylococcus aureus*: epidemiology and eradication of the resistant strain from the hospital. *Infect Control* 1987;8:15–23.
167. Dacre J, Emmerson AM, Jenner EA. Gentamicin-methicillin-resistant *Staphylococcus aureus*: epidemiology and containment of an outbreak. *J Hosp Infect* 1986;7:130–136.
168. Hill SF, Ferguson D. Multiply-resistant *Staphylococcus aureus* (bacteriophage type 90) in a special care baby unit. *J Hosp Infect* 1984;5:56–62.
169. Lejeune B, Buzit-Losquin F, Simitzis-Le Flohic AM, et al. Outbreak of gentamicin-methicillin-resistant *Staphylococcus aureus* infection in an intensive care unit for children. *J Hosp Infect* 1986;7:21–25.
170. Michel MF, Priem CC. Control at hospital level of infections by methicillin-resistant staphylococci in children. *J Hyg* 1971;69:453–460.
171. Murray-Leisure KA, Geib S, Graceley D, et al. Control of epidemic methicillin-resistant *Staphylococcus aureus. Infect Control Hosp Epidemiol* 1990;11:343–350.
172. Price EH, Brain A, Dickson JA. An outbreak of infection with a gentamicin and methicillin-resistant *Staphylococcus aureus* in a neonatal unit. *J Hosp Infect* 1980;1:221–228.
173. Rao N, Jacobs S, Joyce L. Cost-effective eradication of an outbreak of methicillin-resistant *Staphylococcus aureus* in a community teaching hospital. *Infect Control Hosp Epidemiol* 1988;9:255–260.
174. Shanson DC, Kensit JC, Duke R. Outbreak of hospital infection with a strain of *Staphylococcus aureus* resistant to gentamicin and methicillin. *Lancet* 1976;2:1347–1348.
175. Tuffnell DJ, Croton RS, Hemingway DM, et al. Methicillin-resistant *Staphylococcus aureus*; the role of antisepsis in the control of an outbreak. *J Hosp Infect* 1987;10:255–259.
176. Pearman JW, Christiansen KJ, Annear DI, et al. Control of methicil-

lin-resistant *Staphylococcus aureus* (MRSA) in an Australian metropolitan teaching hospital complex. *Med J Aust* 1985;142:103–108.
177. Opal SM, Mayer KH, Stenberg MJ, et al. Frequent acquisition of multiple strains of methicillin-resistant *Staphylococcus aureus* by health care workers in an endemic hospital setting. *Infect Control Hosp Epidemiol* 1990;11:479–485.
178. Ward TT, Winn RE, Hartstein AI, et al. Observations relating to an inter-hospital outbreak of methicillin-resistant *Staphylococcus aureus*: role of antimicrobial therapy in infection control. *Infect Control* 1981; 2:453–459.
179. Coovadia YM, Bhana RH, Johnson AP, et al. A laboratory confirmed outbreak of rifampin-methicillin resistant *Staphylococcus aureus* (RMRSA) in a newborn nursery. *J Hosp Infect* 1989;14:303–312.
180. Craven DE, Reed C, Kollisch N, et al. A large outbreak of infections caused by a strain of *Staphylococcus aureus* resistant to oxacillin and aminoglycosides. *Am J Med* 1981;71:53–58.
181. Bartzokas CA, Paton JH, Gibson MF, et al. Control and eradication of methicillin-resistant *Staphylococcus aureus* on a surgical unit. *N Engl J Med* 1984;311:1422–1425.
182. Gaynes R, Marosok R, Mowry-Hanley J, et al. Mediastinitis following coronary artery bypass surgery: a 3 year review. *J Infect Dis* 1991;163: 117–121.
183. Shanson DC, McSwiggan DA. Operating theatre acquired infection with a gentamicin-resistant strain of *Staphylococcus aureus*: outbreak in two hospitals attributable to one surgeon. *J Hosp Infect* 1980;1: 171–172.
184. Sheretz RJ, Reagan DR, Hampton KD, et al. A cloud adult: the *Staphylococcus aureus*-virus interaction revisited. *Ann Intern Med* 1996; 124:539–547.
185. The Hopital Propre II Study Group. Methicillin-resistant *Staphylococcus aureus* in French hospitals: a 2-month survey in 43 hospitals, 1995. *Infect Control Hosp Epidemiol* 1999;20:478–486.
186. Fang FC, McClelland M, Guiney DG, et al. Value of molecular epidemiologic analysis in a nosocomial methicillin-resistant *Staphylococcus aureus* outbreak. *JAMA* 1993;270:1323–1328.
187. Walsh TJ, Vlahov D, Hansen SL, et al. Prospective microbiologic surveillance in control of nosocomial methicillin-resistant *Staphylococcus aureus*. *Infect Control* 1987;8:7–14.
188. Shiomori T, Miyamoto H, Makishima K, et al. Evaluation of bedmaking-related airborne and surface methicillin-resistant *Staphylococcus aureus* contamination. *J Hosp Infect* 2002;50:30–35.
189. McNeil MM, Soloman SL. The epidemiology of MRSA. *Antimicrobial Newslett* 1985;2:49–56.
190. Oie S, Kamiya A. Survival of methicillin-resistant *Staphylococcus aureus* (MRSA) on naturally contaminated dry mops. *J Hosp Infect* 1996; 34:145–149.
191. Parks YA, Noy MF, Aukett MA, et al. Methicillin resistant *Staphylococcus aureus* in milk. *Arch Dis Child* 1987;62:82–84.
192. Venezia RA, Harris V, Miller C, et al. Investigation of an outbreak of methicillin-resistant *Staphylococcus aureus* in patients with skin disease using DNA restriction patterns. *Infect Control Hosp Epidemiol* 1992; 13:472–476.
193. Bures S, Fishbain JT, Uyehara C, et al. Computer keyboards and faucet handles as reservoirs of nosocomial pathogens in the intensive care unit. *Am J Infect Control* 2000;28:465–470.
194. Thompson RL, Cabezudo I, Wenzel RP. Epidemiology of nosocomial infections caused by methicillin-resistant *Staphylococcus aureus*. *Ann Intern Med* 1982;97:309–317.
195. Reboli AC, John JF Jr, Levkoff AH. Epidemic methicillin-gentamicin-resistant *Staphylococcus aureus* in a neonatal intensive care unit. *Am J Dis Child* 1989;143:34–39.
196. Klimek JJ, Marsik FJ, Bartlett RC, et al. Clinical, epidemiologic and bacteriologic observations of an outbreak of methicillin-resistant *Staphylococcus aureus* at a large community hospital. *Am J Med* 1976; 61:340–345.
197. Karchmer TB, Durbin LJ, Simonton BM, et al. Cost-effectiveness of active surveillance cultures and contact/droplet precautions for control of methicillin-resistant *Staphylococcus aureus*. *J Hosp Infect* 2002;51: 126–132.
198. Arnow PM, Allyn PA, Nichols EM, et al. Control of methicillin-resistant *Staphylococcus aureus* in a burn unit: role of nurse staffing. *J Trauma* 1982;22:954–959.
199. Rhinehart E, Shlaes DM, Keys TF, et al. Nosocomial clonal dissemination of methicillin-resistant *Staphylococcus aureus*. *Arch Intern Med* 1987;147:521–524.
200. Alvarez S, Shell C, Gage K, et al. An outbreak of methicillin-resistant *Staphylococcus aureus* eradicated from a large teaching hospital. *Am J Infect Control* 1985;13:115–121.
201. Davies EA, Emmerson AM, Hogg GM, et al. An outbreak of infection with a methicillin-resistant *Staphylococcus aureus* in a special care baby unit: value of topical mupirocin and of traditional methods of infection control. *J Hosp Infect* 1987;10:120–128.
202. Ellison RT, Judson FN, Peterson LC, et al. Oral rifampin and trimethoprim/sulfamethoxazole therapy in asymptomatic carriers of methicillin-resistant *Staphylococcus aureus* infections. *West J Med* 1984;140: 735–740.
203. Shanson DC, Johnstone D, Midgley J. Control of a hospital outbreak of methicillin-resistant *Staphylococcus aureus* infections: value of an isolation unit. *J Hosp Infect* 1985;6:285–292.
204. Farrington M, Ling T, French GL. Outbreaks of infection with methicillin-resistant *Staphylococcus aureus* on neonatal and burn units of a new hospital. *Epidemiol Infect* 1990;105:215–228.
205. Duckworth GJ, Lothian JL, Williams JD. Methicillin-resistant *Staphylococcus aureus*: report of an outbreak in a London teaching hospital. *J Hosp Infect* 1988;11:1–15.
206. Cafferkey MT, Hone R, Keane CT. Sources and outcome for methicillin-resistant *Staphylococcus aureus* bacteremia. *J Hosp Infect* 1988; 11:136–143.
207. Roman RS, Smith J, Walker M, et al. Rapid geographic spread of a methicillin-resistant *Staphylococcus aureus* strain. *Clin Infect Dis* 1997; 25:698–705.
208. Boyce JM. Strategies for controlling methicillin-resistant *Staphylococcus aureus* in hospitals. *J Chemother* 1995;7(Suppl 3):81–85.
209. Andersen B, Lindemann R, Bergh K, et al. Spread of methicillin-resistant *Staphylococcus aureus* in a neonatal intensive unit associated with understaffing, overcrowding and mixing of patients. *J Hosp Infect* 2002;50:18–24.
210. Boyce JM, White RL, Spruill EY. Impact of methicillin-resistant *Staphylococcus aureus* on the incidence of nosocomial staphylococcal infections. *J Infect Dis* 1983;148:763.
211. Goetz MB, Mulligan ME, Kwok R, et al. Management and epidemiologic analysis of an outbreak due to methicillin-resistant *Staphylococcus aureus*. *Am J Med* 1992;92:607–614.
212. Guiguet M, Rekacewicz C, Leclercq B, et al. Effectiveness of simple measures to control an outbreak of nosocomial methicillin-resistant *Staphylococcus aureus* infections in an intensive care unit. *Infect Control Hosp Epidemiol* 1990;11:23–26.
213. Haley RW, Cushion NB, Tenover FC, et al. Eradication of endemic methicillin-resistant *Staphylococcus aureus* infections from a neonatal intensive care unit. *J Infect Dis* 1995;171:614–624.
214. Merrer J, Santoli F, Appere-De Vecchi C, et al. "Colonization pressure" and risk of acquisition of methicillin-resistant *Staphylococcus aureus* in a medical intensive care unit. *Infect Control Hosp Epidemiol* 2000;21:718–723.
215. Singh N, Paterson D, Chang F, et al. Methicillin-resistant *Staphylococcus aureus*: the other emerging resistant gram-positive coccus among liver transplant recipients. *Clin Infect Dis* 2000;30:322–327.
216. Saroglou G, Cromer M, Bisno AL. Methicillin-resistant *Staphylococcus aureus*: interstate spread of nosocomial infections with emergence of gentamicin-methicillin resistant strains. *Infect Control* 1980;1:81–89.
217. Hsu CCS. Serial survey of methicillin-resistant *Staphylococcus aureus* nasal carriage among residents in a nursing home. *Infect Control Hosp Epidemiol* 1991;12:416–421.
218. Strausbaugh LJ, Jacobson C, Sewell DL, et al. Methicillin-resistant *Staphylococcus aureus* in extended-care facilities. *Infect Control Hosp Epidemiol* 1991;12:36–45.
219. Hsu CCS, Macaluso CP, Special L, et al. High rate of methicillin resistance of *Staphylococcus aureus* isolated from hospitalized nursing home patients. *Arch Intern Med* 1988;148:569–570.

220. Bradley SF. Methicillin-resistant *Staphylococcus aureus* infection. *Clin Geriatr Med* 1992;8:853–868.
221. Lee Y, Gupta G, Cesario T, et al. Colonization by *Staphylococcus aureus* resistant to methicillin and ciprofloxacin during 20 months surveillance in a private skilled nursing facility. *Infect Control Hosp Epidemiol* 1996;17:649–653.
222. Bradley SF. Methicillin-resistant *Staphylococcus aureus* in nursing homes. *Drugs Aging* 1997;10:185–198.
223. Bradley S. Methicillin-resistant *Staphylococcus aureus*: long-term care concerns. *Am J Med* 1999;106(5A);2S–10S.
224. Rahimi AR. Prevalence and outcome of methicillin-resistant *Staphylococcus aureus* colonization in two nursing centers in Georgia. *J Am Geriatr Soc* 1998;46:1555–1557.
225. Talon DR, Bertrand X. Methicillin-resistant *Staphylococcus aureus* in geriatric patients: usefulness of screening in a chronic-care setting. *Infect Control Hosp Epidemiol* 2001;22:505–509.
226. Hoefnagels-Schuermans A, Niclaes L, Buntinx F, et al. Molecular epidemiology of methicillin-resistant *Staphylococcus aureus* in nursing homes: a cross-sectional study. *Infect Control Hosp Epidemiol* 2002; 23:546–549.
227. McNeil S, Mody L, Bradley S. Methicillin-resistant *Staphylococcus aureus*: management of asymptomatic colonization and outbreaks of infection in long-term care. *Geriatrics* 2002;57:16–27.
228. O'Sullivan NP, Keane CT. The prevalence of methicillin-resistant *Staphylococcus aureus* among the residents of six nursing homes in the elderly. *J Hosp Infect* 2000;45:322–329.
229. Kotilainen P, Routamaa M, Peltonen R, et al. Eradication of methicillin-resistant *Staphylococcus aureus* from a health center ward and associated nursing home. *Arch Intern Med* 2001:161:859–863.
230. Strausbaugh L J, Jacobson C, Yost T. Methicillin-resistant *Staphylococcus aureus* in a nursing home and affiliated hospital: a four-year perspective. *Infect Control and Hosp Epidemiol* 1993;14:331–336.
231. Mylotte JM, Goodnough S, Tayara. Antibiotic-resistant organisms among long-term care facility residents on admission to an inpatient geriatric unit: retrospective and prospective surveillance. *Am J Infect Control* 2001;29:139–144.
232. Gradon JD, Wu EH, Lutwick LI. Aerosolized vancomycin therapy facilitating nursing home placement. *Ann Pharmacother* 1992;26: 209–210.
233. Bryce EA, Tiffin SM, Isacc-Renton JL, et al. Evidence of delays in transferring patients with methicillin-resistant *Staphylococcus aureus* or vancomycin-resistant *Enterococcus* to long-term-care facilities. *Infect Control Hosp Epidemiol* 2000;21:270–271.
234. Strausbaugh LJ, Crossley KB, Nurse BA and SHEA Long-Term Care Committee. Antimicrobial resistance in long-term care facilities—a SHEA position paper. *Infect Control Hosp Epidemiol* 1996;17: 129–140.
235. Gorak E, Yamada S, Brown J. Community-acquired methicillin-resistant *Staphylococcus aureus* in hospitalized adults and children without known risk factors. *Clin Infect Dis* 1999;29:797–800.
236. Naimi T, LeDell K, Boxrud D, et al. Epidemiology and clonality of community-acquired methicillin-resistant *Staphylococcus aureus* in Minnesota, 1996–1998. *Clin Infect Dis* 2001;33:990–996.
237. Friedman ND, Kaye KS, Stout JE, et al. Health care-associated bloodstream infections in adults: a reason to change the accepted definition of community-acquired infections. *Ann Intern Med* 2002;137: 791–797.
238. Almer L, Shortridge V, Nilius A, et al. Antimicrobial susceptibility and molecular characterization of community-acquired methicillin-resistant *Staphylococcus aureus*. *Diagn Microbiol Infect Dis* 2002;43: 225–232.
239. Culpepper R, Nolan R, Chapman R, et al. Methicillin-resistant *Staphylococcus aureus* skin or soft tissue infections in a state prison—Mississippi, 2000. *MMWR* 2001;50:919–922.
240. Shahin R, Johnson I, Jamieson F, et al. Methicillin-resistant *Staphylococcus aureus* carriage in a child care center following a case of disease. *Arch Pediatr Adolsc Med* 1999;153:864–868.
241. Linnemann CC, Moore P, Staneck J, et al. Reemergence of epidemic methicillin-resistant *Staphylococcus aureus* in a general hospital associated with changing staphylococcal strains. *Am J Med* 1991;91(Suppl 3B):238–244.
242. Masuda K, Masuda R, Nishi J, et al. Incidences of nasopharyngeal colonization of respiratory bacterial pathogens in Japanese children attending day-care centers. *Pediatr Int* 2002;44:376–380.
243. Adcock PM, Pastor P, Medlley F, et al. Methicillin-resistant *Staphylococcus aureus* in two child care centers. *J Infect Dis* 1998;178:577–580.
244. Four pediatric deaths from community-acquired methicillin-resistant *Staphylococcus aureus*—Minnesota and North Dakota, 1997–1999. *MMWR* 1999;48:707.
245. Pfaller M, Jones R, Doern, et al. Survey of blood stream infections attributable to gram-positive cocci: frequency of occurrence and antimicrobial susceptibility of isolates collected in 1997 in the United States, Canada, and Latin America from the SENTRY Antimicrobial Surveillance Program. SENTRY Participants Group. *Diagn Microbiol Infect Dis* 1999;33:283–297.
246. Interagency Task Force on Antimicrobial Resistance. A public health action plan to combat antimicrobial resistance. Part 1. Domestic issues. Available at http://www.cdc.gov/drugresistance/actionplan/index.htm [accessed January 2003].
247. Ploy M, Grelaud C, Martin C, et al. First clinical isolate of vancomycin-intermediate *Staphylococcus aureus* in a French hospital. *Lancet* 1998;351:1212.
248. Hiramatsu K, Aritaka N, Hanaki H, et al. Dissemination in Japanese hospitals of strains of *Staphylococcus aureus* heterogeneously resistant to vancomycin. *Lancet* 1997;350:1670–1673.
249. Update: *Staphylococcus aureus* with reduced susceptibility to vancomycin—United States, 1997. *MMWR* 1997;46:813–815.
250. *Staphylococcus aureus* resistant to vancomycin—United States, 2002. *MMWR* 2002;51:565–567.
251. Fridkin S. Vancomcycin-intermediate and -resistant *Staphylococcus aureus*: what the infectious disease specialist needs to know. *Clin Infect Dis* 2001;32:108–115.
252. Geisel R, Schmitz F, Fluit A, et al. Emergence, mechanism, and clinical implications of reduced glycopeptide susceptibility in *Staphylococcus aureus*. *Eur J Clin Microbiol Infect Dis* 2001;20:685–697.
253. Srinivasan A, Dick J, Perl T. Vancomycin resistance in staphylococci. *Clin Microbiol Rev* 2002;15:430–438.
254. Franchi D, Climo M, Wong A, et al. Seeking vancomycin resistant *Staphylococcus aureus* among patients with vancomycin-resistant Enterococci. *Clin Infect Dis* 1999;29:1556–1558.
255. Vancomycin-resistant *Staphylococcus aureus*—Pennsylvania, 2002. *MMWR* 2002;51:902.
256. Mylotte JM, Karuza J, Bentley DW. Methicillin-resistant *Staphylococcus aureus*: a questionnaire survey of 75 long term care facilities in western New York. *Infect Control Hosp Epidemiol* 1992;13:711–718.
257. Speller DCE, Johnson AP, James D, et al. Resistance to methicillin and other antibiotics in isolates of *Staphylococcus aureus* from blood and cerebrospinal fluid, England and Wales, 1989–95. *Lancet* 1997; 350:323–325.
258. Preheim LC, Rimland D, Bittner MJ. Methicillin-resistant *Staphylococcus aureus* in Veterans Administration Medical Centers. *Infect Control* 1987;8:191–194.
259. Strausbaugh LJ, Jacobson C, Sewell DL, et al. Antimicrobial therapy for methicillin-resistant *Staphylococcus aureus* colonization in residents and staff of a veterans affairs nursing home care unit. *Infect Control Hosp Epidemiol* 1992;13:151–159.
260. Walsh TJ, Standiford HC, Reboli AC, et al. Randomized double-blinded trial of rifampin with either novobiocin or trimethoprim-sulfamethoxazole against methicillin-resistant *Staphylococcus aureus* colonization: prevention of antimicrobial resistance and effect of host factors on outcome. *Antimicrob Agents Chemother* 1993;37: 1334–1342.
261. Kauffman CA, Terpenning MT, He X, et al. Attempts to eradicate methicillin-resistant *Staphylococcus aureus* from a long-term-care facility with the use of mupirocin ointment. *Am J Med* 1993;94:371–378.
262. Harbath S, Dharan S, Liassine N, et al. Randomized, placebo-controlled, double-blind trial to evaluate the efficacy of mupirocin for eradicating carriage of methicillin-resistant *Staphylococcus aureus*. *Antimicrob Agents Chemother* 1999;43:1412–1416.

263. Crossley, Thurn JR. Control measures for MRSA—can the cost be reduced? In: Cafferkey MT, ed. *Methicillin-resistant Staphylococcus aureus*. New York: Marcel Dekker, 1992:187–196.
264. Kauffman CA, Bradley SF, Terpenning MS. Methicillin-resistant *Staphylococcus aureus* in long-term care facilities. *Infect Control Hosp Epidemiol* 1990;11:600–603.
265. Mylotte JM. Control of methicillin-resistant *Staphylococcus aureus*: the ambivalence persists. *Infect Control Hosp Epidemiol* 1994;15:73–77.
266. Hartstein AI. Improved understanding and control of nosocomial methicillin-resistant *Staphylococcus aureus*: are we overdoing it? *Infect Control Hosp Epidemiol* 1995;16:257–259.
267. Humphreys H, Duckworth G. Methicillin-resistant *Staphylococcus aureus* (MRSA)–a reappraisal of control measures in the light of changing circumstances. *Infect Control Hosp Epidemiol* 1997;36:167–170.
268. Barrett SP, Mummery RV, Chattopadhyay B. Trying to control MRSA causes more problems than it resolves. *J Hosp Infect* 1998;39: 85–93.
269. Teare EL, Barrett SP. Stop the ritual of tracing colonized people. *BMJ* 1997;314:665–666.
270. Rahman M, Sanderson PJ, Bentley AH, et al. Revised guidelines for control of MRSA in hospitals: finding the most useful point. *J Hosp Infect* 1999;42:71–72.
271. Haley RW. Methicillin-resistant *Staphylococcus aureus*: do we just have to live with it? *Ann Intern Med* 1991;114:162–164.
272. Vandenbroucke-Grauls CM, Frenay HME, van Klingeren B, et al. Control of epidemic methicillin-resistant *Staphylococcus aureus* in a Dutch university hospital. *Eur J Clin Microbiol Infect Dis* 1991;10: 6–11.
273. Rosdahl VT, Knudsen AM. The decline of methicillin-resistance among Danish *Staphylococcus aureus* strains. *Infect Control Hosp Epidemiol* 1991;12:83–88.
274. Verhoef J, Beaujean D, Blok H, et al. A Dutch approach to methicillin-resistant *Staphylococcus aureus*. *Eur J Clin Microbiol Infect Dis* 1999;18:461–466.
275. Mulligan ME, Murray-Leisure KA, Ribner BS, et al. Methicillin-resistant *Staphylococcus aureus*: a consensus review of the microbiology, pathogenesis, and epidemiology with implications for prevention and management. *Am J Med* 1993;94:313–328.
276. Boyce JM, Jackson MM, Pugliese G, et al. Methicillin-resistant *Staphylococcus aureus* (MRSA): a briefing for acute care hospitals and nursing facilities. *Infect Control Hosp Epidemiol* 1994;15:105–113.
277. Report of a combined working party of the British Society for Antimicrobial Chemotherapy, the Hospital Infection Society and the Infection Control Nurses Association: revised guidelines for the control of methicillin-resistant *Staphylococcus aureus* infection in hospitals. *J Hosp Infect* 1998;39:253–290.
278. Hartstein AI, LeMonte AM, Iwamoto PKL. DNA typing and control of methicillin-resistant *Staphylococcus aureus* at two affiliated hospitals. *Infect Control Hosp Epidemiol* 1997;18:42–48.
279. Wendt C, Herwaldt LA. Epidemics: identification and management. In: Wenzel RP, ed. *Prevention and control of nosocomial infections*, 3rd ed. Baltimore: Williams & Wilkins, 1997:175–213.
280. Hartstein AI, Phelps CL, Kwok RYY, et al. In vivo stability and discriminatory power of methicillin-resistant *Staphylococcus aureus* typing by restriction endonuclease analysis of plasmid DNA compared to other molecular methods. *J Clin Microbiol* 1995;33:2022–2026.
281. Herwaldt LA, Pottinger JM, Coffman S, et al. Molecular epidemiology of methicillin-resistant *Staphylococcus aureus* in a Veterans Administration medical center. *Infect Control Hosp Epidemiol* 2002;23: 502–505.
282. Lugeon C, Blanc DS, Wenger A, et al. Molecular epidemiology of methicillin-resistant *Staphylococcus aureus* at a low-incidence hospital over a 4-year period. *Infect Control Hosp Epidemiol* 1995;16:260–267.
283. Moreno F, Crisp C, Jorgensen JH, et al. Methicillin-resistant *Staphylococcus aureus* as a community organism. *Clin Infect Dis* 1995;21: 1308–1312.
284. Layton MC, Hierholzer WJ Jr, Patterson JE. The evolving epidemiology of methicillin-resistant *Staphylococcus aureus* at a university hospital. *Infect Control Hosp Epidemiol* 1995;16:12–17.
285. Jernigan JA, Clemence MA, Stott GA, et al. Control of methicillin-resistant *Staphylococcus aureus* at a university hospital: one decade later. *Infect Control Hosp Epidemiol* 1995;16:686–696.
286. Steinberg JP, Clark CC, Hackman BO. Nosocomial and community-acquired *Staphylococcus aureus* bacteremias from 1980 to 1993: impact of intravascular devices and methicillin resistance. *Clin Infect Dis* 1996;23:255–259.
287. Kayaba H, Kodama K, Tamura H, et al. The spread of methicillin-resistant *Staphylococcus aureus* in a rural community: will it become a common microorganism colonizing among the general population? *Surg Today* 1997;27:217–219.
288. Hamoudi AC, Palmer RN, King TL. Nafcillin resistant *Staphylococcus aureus*: a possible community origin. *Infect Control* 1983;4:153–157.
289. Layton M, Hierholzer W, Patterson JE. The evolving epidemiology of methicillin-resistant *Staphylococcus aureus* at a university hospital. *Infect Control Hosp Epidemiol* 1993;13:763.
290. Rimland D, Killum E, Roberson B. Secular trends of infections due to methicillin-resistant *Staphylococcus aureus* at the Atlanta VA Medical Center. *Infect Control Hosp Epidemiol* 1993;13:764.
291. Dammann TA, Wiens RM, Taylor GD. Methicillin-resistant *Staphylococcus aureus*: identification of a community outbreak by monitoring of hospital isolates. *Can J Public Health* 1988;79:312–314.
292. Aeilts GD, Sapico FL, Canawati HN, et al. Methicillin-resistant *Staphylococcus aureus* colonization and infection in a rehabilitation facility. *J Clin Microbiol* 1982;16:218–223.
293. Boyce JM, Opal SM, Potter-Bynoe G, et al. Spread of methicillin-resistant *Staphylococcus aureus* in a hospital after exposure to a health care worker with chronic sinusitis. *Clin Infect Dis* 1993;17:496–504.
294. Noel GJ, Kreiswirth BN, Edelson PJ, et al. Multiple methicillin-resistant *Staphylococcus aureus* strains as a cause for a single outbreak of severe disease in hospitalized neonates. *Pediatr Infect Dis J* 1992; 11:184–188.
295. Miller MR, Keyworth N, Lincoln C, et al. Methicillin-resistant *Staphylococcus aureus* in a regional neonatology unit. *J Hosp Infect* 1987; 10:187–197.
296. Herwaldt LA. Control of methicillin-resistant *Staphylococcus aureus* in the hospital setting. *Am J Med* 1999;106(5A):11S–18S.
297. Ribner BS, Landry MN, Gholson GL. Strict versus modified isolation for prevention of nosocomial transmission of methicillin-resistant *Staphylococcus aureus*. *Infect Control* 1986;7:317–320.
298. Archer GL, Mayhall CG. Comparison of epidemiological markers used in the investigation of an outbreak of methicillin-resistant *Staphylococcus aureus* infections. *J Clin Microbiol* 1983;18:395–399.
299. Dunkle LM, Naqvi SH, McCallum R, et al. Eradication of epidemic methicillin-gentamicin-resistant *Staphylococcus aureus* in an intensive care nursery. *Am J Med* 1981;70:455–458.
300. Rimland D, Roberson B. Gastrointestinal carriage of methicillin-resistant *Staphylococcus aureus*. *J Clin Microbiol* 1986;24:137–138.
301. Sewell DL, Potter SA, Jacobson CM, et al. Sensitivity of surveillance cultures for the detection of methicillin-resistant *Staphylococcus aureus* in a nursing-home-care unit. *Diagn Microbiol Infect Dis* 1993;17: 53–56.
302. Wagenvoort JHT, Werink TJ, Gronenschild JMH, et al. Optimization of detection and yield of methicillin-resistant *Staphylococcus aureus* phage type III-29. *Infect Control Hosp Epidemiol* 1996;17: 208–209.
303. Forward KR, Arbique JC. Cumulative yield from patient surveillance cultures for methicillin-resistant *Staphylococcus aureus* during a hospital outbreak. *Infect Control Hosp Epidemiol* 1997;18:776–778.
304. Manian FA, Senkel D, Zack J, et al. Routine screening for methicillin-resistant *Staphylococcus aureus* among patients newly admitted to an acute rehabilitation unit. *Infect Control Hosp Epidemiol* 2002;23: 516–519.
305. Coello R, Jimenez J, Garcia M, et al. Prospective study of infection, colonisation and carriage of methicillin-resistant *Staphylococcus aureus* affecting 900 patients. *Eur J Clin Microbiol Infect Dis* 1994;13:74–81.
306. Gorss EB. Prospective, focused surveillance for oxacillin-resistant *Staphylococcus aureus*. In: Isenberg HD, ed. *Clinical microbiology procedures handbook*. Washington DC: American Society for Microbiology Press, 2002:11.15–11.15.2.
307. Gardam M, Brunton J, Willey B, et al. A blinded comparison of three

laboratory protocols for the identification of patients colonized with methicillin-resistant *Staphylococcus aureus. Infect Control Hosp Epidemiol* 2001;22:152–156.

308. Boyce JM. Methicillin-resistant *Staphylococcus aureus* in hospitals and long-term care facilities: microbiology, epidemiology, and preventive measures. *Infect Control Hosp Epidemiol* 1992;13:725–737.
309. Van Enk RA, Thompson KD. Use of a primary isolation medium for recovery of methicillin-resistant *Staphylococcus aureus. J Clin Microbiol* 1992;30:504– 505.
310. Kunori T, Cookson B, Roberts JA, et al. Cost-effectiveness of different MRSA screening methods. *J Hosp Infect* 2002;51:189–200.
311. Farr BM, Jarvis WR. Would active surveillance cultures help control healthcare-related methicillin-resistant *Staphylococcus aureus* infections? *Infect Control Hosp Epidemiol* 2002;23:65–68.
312. Harbath S, Martin Y, Rohner P, et al. Effect of delayed infection control measures on a hospital outbreak of methicillin-resistant *Staphylococcus aureus. J Hosp Infect* 2000;46:43–49.
313. Jernigan JA, Titus MG, Groschel DH, et al. Effectiveness of contact isolation during a hospital outbreak of methicillin-resistant *Staphylococcus aureus. Am J Epidemiol* 1996;143:496–504.
314. Papia G, Louie M, Tralla A, et al. Screening high-risk patients for methicillin-resistant *Staphylococcus aureus* on admission to the hospital: is it cost effective? *Infect Control Hosp Epidemiol* 1999;20: 473–477.
315. Girou E, Pujade G, Legrand P, et al. Selective screening of carriers for control of methicillin-resistant *Staphylococcus aureus* (MRSA) in high-risk areas with a high level of endemic MRSA. *Clin Infect Dis* 1998;27:543–550.
316. Chaix C, Durand-Zaleski I, Alberti C, et al. Control of endemic methicillin-resistant *Staphylococcus aureus*: a cost-benefit analysis in an intensive care unit. *JAMA* 1999;282:1745–1751.
317. Arnold MS, Dempsey JM, Fishman M, et al. The best hospital practices for controlling methicillin-resistant *Staphylococcus aureus*: on the cutting edge. *Infect Control Hosp Epidemiol* 2002;23:69–76.
318. Humphreys H. Control of methicillin-resistant *Staphylococcus aureus* in hospitals. An impossible dream? *J Med Microbiol* 2002;51: 283–285.
319. Cooper CL, Dyck B, Ormiston D, et al. Bed utilization of patients with methicillin-resistant *Staphylococcus aureus* in a Canadian tertiary-care center. *Infect Control Hosp Epidemiol* 2002;23:483–484.
320. Bannerman TL, Hancock GA, Tenover FC, et al. Pulsed field gel electrophoresis as a replacement for bacteriophage typing of *Staphylococcus aureus. J Clin Microbiol* 1995;33:551–555.
321. Adcock PM, Pastor P, Medley F, et al. Methicillin-resistant *Staphylococcus aureus* in two child care centers. *J Infect Dis* 1998;178:577–580.
322. Suh K, Toye B, Jessamine P, et al. Epidemiology of methicillin-resistant *Staphylococcus aureus* in three Canadian tertiary-care centers. *Infect Control Hosp Epidemiol* 1998;19:395–400.
323. Roberts RB, de Lencastre A, Eisner W, et al. Molecular epidemiology of methicillin-resistant *Staphylococcus aureus* in 12 New York hospitals. *J Infect Dis* 1998;178:164–171.
324. Macfarlane L, Walker J, Borrow R, et al. Improved recognition of MRSA case clusters by the application of molecular subtyping using pulsed-field gel electrophoresis. *J Hosp Infect* 1999;41:29–37.
325. Hacek DM, Suriano T, Noskin GA, et al. Medical and economic benefit of a comprehensive infection control program that includes routine determination of microbial clonality. *Am J Clin Pathol* 1999; 111:647–654.
326. Pfaller MA, Acar J, Jones RN, et al. Integration of molecular characterization of microorganisms in a global antimicrobial resistance surveillance program. *Clin Infect Dis* 2001;32:S156–167.
327. Peterson LR, Noskin GA. New technology for detecting multi-drug resistant pathogens in the clinical microbiology laboratory. *Emerg Infect Dis* 2001;7:306–311.
328. van Belkum A, Struelens M, de Visser A, et al. Role of genomic typing in taxonomy, evolutionary genetics and microbial epidemiology. *Clin Microbiol Rev* 2001;14:547–560.
329. Pfaller MA. Molecular approaches to diagnosing and managing infectious diseases: practicality and costs. *Emerg Infect Dis* 2001;7: 312–318.
330. Cohen SH, Morita MM, Bradford M. A seven year experience with methicillin-resistant *Staphylococcus aureus. Am J Med* 1991;31(Suppl 3B):233–237.
331. Kauffman CA, Bradley SF, Terpenning MS. Methicillin-resistant *Staphylococcus aureus* in long-term care facilities. *Infect Control Hosp Epidemiol* 1990;11:600–603.
332. Rahal JJ. Resistant staphylococcal infection. *Ann Intern Med* 1991; 114:911.
333. Wlodaver CG, McNabb SJ. MRSA in perspective. *Ann Intern Med* 1991;114:704–705.
334. Lessing MPA, Jordens JZ, Bowler ICJ. When should healthcare workers be screened for methicillin-resistant *Staphylococcus aureus*? *J Hosp Infect* 1996;34:205–210.
335. Kearns AM, Seiders PR, Wheeler J, et al. Rapid detection of methicillin-resistant staphylococci by multiplex PCR. *J Hosp Infect* 1999;43: 33–37.
336. van Leeuwen WB, van Pelt C, Luijendijk A, et al. Rapid detection of methicillin resistance in *Staphylococcus aureus* by the MRSA-screen latex agglutination test. *J Clin Microbiol* 1999;37:3029–3030.
337. Marriott DJE, Kearney P. Further evaluation of the MRSA-screen kit for rapid detection of methicillin resistance. *J Clin Microbiol* 1999; 37:3783–3784.
338. Louie L, Matsumara SO, Choi E, et al. Evaluation of three rapid methods for detection of methicillin resistance in *Staphylococcus aureus. J Clin Microbiol* 2000;38:2170–2173.
339. Yamazumi T, Marshall SA, Wilke WW, et al. Comparison of the Vitek gram-positive susceptibility 106 card and the MRSA-screen latex agglutination test for determining oxacillin resistance in clinical bloodstream isolates of *Staphylococcus aureus. J Clin Microbiol* 2001; 39:53–56.
340. Grisold AJ, Leitner E, Muhlbauer G, et al. Detection of methicillin-resistant *Staphylococcus aureus* and simultaneous confirmation by automated nucleic acid extraction and real-time PCR. *J Clin Microbiol* 2002;40:2392–2397.
341. Shrestha NK, Tuohy MJ, Hall GS, et al. Rapid identification of *Staphylococcus aureus* and the *mecA* gene from BacT/ALERT blood culture bottles by using the LightCycler system. *J Clin Microbiol* 2002;40: 2659–2661.
342. Maes N, Magdalena J, Rottier S, et al. Evaluation of a triplex PCR assay to discriminate *Staphylococcus aureus* from coagulase-negative staphylococci and determine methicillin resistance from blood cultures. *J Clin Microbiol* 2002;40:1514–1517.
343. Gonzalez C, Rubio M, Romero-Vivas J, et al. Bacteremic pneumonia due to *Staphylococcus aureus*: a comparison of disease caused by methicillin-resistant and methicillin-susceptible organisms. *Clin Infect Dis* 1999;29:1171–1177.
344. Hierholzer WJ, Garner JS, Adams AB, et al. Recommendations for preventing the spread of vancomycin resistance. Hospital Infection Control Practices Advisory Committee (HICPAC). *Infect Control Hosp Epidemiol* 1995;16:105–113.
345. Alllaouchiche B, Jaumain H, Zambardi G, et al. Clinical impact of rapid oxacillin susceptibility testing using a PCR assay in *Staphylococcus aureus* bacteremia. *J Infection* 1999;39:198–204.
346. Boyce JM, Potter-Bynoe G, Chenevert C, et al. Environmental contamination due to methicillin-resistant *Staphylococcus aureus*: possible infection control implications. *Infect Control Hosp Epidemiol* 1997; 18:622–627.
347. Oie S, Hosokawa I, Kamiya A. Contamination of room door handles by methicillin-sensitive/methicillin-resistant *Staphylococcus aureus. J Hosp Infect* 2002;51:140–143.
348. Neely AN, Maley MP. Survival of enterococci and staphylococci on hospital fabrics and plastic. *J Clin Microbiol* 2000;38:724–726.
349. Shiomori T, Miyamoto H, Makishima K, et al. Evaluation of bedmaking-related airborne and surface methicillin-resistant *Staphylococcus aureus* contamination. *J Hosp Infect* 2002;50:30–35.
350. Wagenvoort JHT, Sluijsmans, Penders RJR. Better environmental survival of outbreak vs. sporadic MRSA isolates. *J Hosp Infect* 2000; 45:231–234.
351. Maki DG, McCormack RD, Zilz MA, et al. A MRSA outbreak in an SICU during universal precautions: new epidemiology for nosocomial

MRSA: downside for universal precautions [abstract 473], 30th Interscience Conference on Antimicrobial Agents in Chemotherapy, Atlanta, 1990.

352. Ndawula EM, Brown L. Mattresses as reservoirs of epidemic methicillin-resistant *Staphylococcus aureus*. *Lancet* 1991;337:488.
353. Rampling A, Wiseman S, Davis L, et al. Evidence that hospital hygiene is important in the control of methicillin-resistant *Staphylococcus aureus*. *J Hosp Infect* 2001;49:109–116.
354. Larson E, Bobo L, Bennett R, et al. Lack of care giver hand contamination with endemic bacterial pathogens in a nursing home. *Am J Infect Control* 1991;19:11–15.
355. Simmons B, Bryant J, Neiman K, et al. The role of handwashing in prevention of endemic intensive care unit infections. *Infect Control Hosp Epidemiol* 1990;11:589–594.
356. Guilhermetti M, Hernandes SED, Fukushigue Y, et al. Effectiveness of hand-cleansing agents for removing methicillin-resistant *Staphylococcus aureus* from contaminated hands. *Infect Control Hosp Epidemiol* 2001;22:105–108.
357. Pittet D, Hugonnet S, Harbarth S, et al. Effectiveness of a hospital-wide programme to improve compliance with hand hygiene. *Lancet* 2000;358:1307–1312.
358. Grundmann H, Hori S, Winter B, et al. Risk factors for the transmission of methicillin-resistant *Staphylococcus aureus* in an adult intensive care unit: fitting a model to the data. *J Infect Dis* 2002;185:481–488.
359. Fazal BA, Telzak EE, Blum S, et al. Trends in the prevalence of methicillin-resistant *Staphylococcus aureus* associated with discontinuation of an isolation policy. *Infect Control Hosp Epidemiol* 1996;17:372–374.
360. Adeyemi-Doro FAB, Scheel O, Lyon DJ, et al. Living with methicillin-resistant *Staphylococcus aureus*: a 7-year experience with endemic MRSA in a university hospital. *Infect Control Hosp Epidemiol* 1997;18:765–767.
361. Hartstein AI, Denny MA, Morthland VH, et al. Control of methicillin-resistant *Staphylococcus aureus* in a hospital and an intensive care unit. *Infect Control Hosp Epidemiol* 1995;16:405–411.
362. Mishal J, Sherer Y, Levin Y, et al. Two-stage evaluation and intervention program for control of methicillin-resistant *Staphylococcus aureus* in the hospital setting. *Scand J Infect Dis* 2001;33:498–501.
363. Pittet D, Safran E, Harbarth S, et al. Automatic alerts for methicillin-resistant *Staphylococcus aureus* surveillance and control: role of a hospital information system. *Infect Control Hosp Epidemiol* 1996;17:496–502.
364. Wenzel RP, Reagan DR, Bertino JS Jr, et al. Methicillin-resistant *Staphylococcus aureus* outbreak: a consensus panel's definition and management guidelines. *Am J Infect Control* 1998;26:102–110.
365. Cookson B, Peters B, Webster M, et al. Staff carriage of epidemic methicillin-resistant *Staphylococcus aureus*. *J Clin Microbiol* 1989;27:1471–1476.
366. Wang JT, Chang SC, Ko WJ, et al. A hospital-acquired outbreak of methicillin-resistant *Staphylococcus aureus* infection initiated by a surgeon carrier. *J Hosp Infect* 2001;47:104–109.
367. Reagan DR, Doebbeling BN, Pfaller MA, et al. Elimination of coincident *Staphylococcus aureus* nasal and hand carriage with intranasal application of mupirocin calcium ointment. *Ann Intern Med* 1991;114:101–106.
368. Smith SM, Eng RH, Tecson-Tumang F. Ciprofloxacin therapy for methicillin-resistant *Staphylococcus aureus* infections and colonizations. *Antimicrob Agents Chemother* 1989;33:181–184.
369. Reboli AC, John JF Jr, Platt CG, et al. Methicillin-resistant *Staphylococcus aureus* outbreak at a Veterans Affairs Medical Center: importance of carriage of the organism by hospital personnel. *Infect Control Hosp Epidemiol* 1990;11:291–296.
370. Arathoon EG, Hamilton JR, Hench CE, et al. Efficacy of short courses of oral novobiocin-rifampin in eradicating carrier state of methicillin-resistant *Staphylococcus aureus* and in vitro killing studies of clinical isolates. *Antimicrob Agents Chemother* 1990;34:1655–1659.
371. Darouiche R, Wright C, Hamill R, et al. Eradication of colonization by methicillin-resistant *Staphylococcus aureus* by using oral minocycline-rifampin and topical mupirocin. *Antimicrob Agents Chemother* 1991;35:1612–1615.
372. Doebbeling BN, Breneman DL, Neu HC, et al. Elimination of *Staphylococcus aureus* nasal carriage in health care workers: analysis of six clinical trials with calcium mupirocin ointment. *Clin Infect Dis* 1993;17:466–474.
373. Rumbak MJ, Cancio MR. Significant reduction in methicillin-resistant *Staphylococcus aureus* ventilator-associated pneumonia associated with the institution of a prevention protocol. *Crit Care Med* 1995;23:1200–1203.
374. Mayall B, Martin R, Keenan AM, et al. Blanket use of intranasal mupirocin for outbreak control and long-term prophylaxis of endemic methicillin-resistant *Staphylococcus aureus* in an open ward. *J Hosp Infect* 1996;32:257–266.
375. Back NA, Linnemann CC, Staneck JL, et al. Control of methicillin-resistant *Staphylococcus aureus* in a neonatal intensive-care unit: use of intensive microbiologic surveillance and mupirocin. *Infect Control Hosp Epidemiol* 1996;17:227–231.
376. Meier PA, Carter CD, Wallace SE, et al. A prolonged outbreak of methicillin-resistant *Staphylococcus aureus* in the burn unit of a tertiary medical center. *Infect Control Hosp Epidemiol* 1996;17:798–802.
377. Nicolle LE, Dyck B, Thompson G, et al. Regional dissemination and control of epidemic methicillin-resistant *Staphylococcus aureus*. *Infect Control Hosp Epidemiol* 1999;20:202–205.
378. Hartstein AI, Ward TT, Bryant RE, et al. Decolonization therapy with rifampin and trimethoprim-sulfamethoxazole for control of methicillin-resistant *Staphylococcus aureus* infections in hospitals. Proceedings of the 13th International Congress of Chemotherapy. 1983;74:40–43.
379. Boyce JM. MRSA patients: proven methods to treat colonization and infection. *J Hosp Infect* 2001;48(Suppl A):S9–S14.
380. Bradley SF. Effectiveness of mupirocin in the control of methicillin-resistant *Staphylococcus aureus*. *Infect Med* 1993;10:23–31.
381. Irizarry L, Rupp J, Griff J. Frequency of high-level mupirocin-resistant *Staphylococcus aureus*. *Antimicrob Agents Chemother* 1996;40:1967–1968.
382. Annigeri R, Conly J, Vas SI, et al. Emergence of mupirocin-resistant *Staphylococcus aureus* in chronic peritoneal dialysis patients using mupirocin prophylaxis to prevent exit-site infection. *Peritoneal Dial Int* 2001;21:554–559.
383. Bradley SF, Ramsey MA, Morton TM, et al. Mupirocin resistance: clinical and molecular epidemiology. *Infect Control Hosp Epidemiol* 1995;16:354–358.
384. Boyce JM. Preventing staphylococcal infections by eradicating nasal carriage of *Staphylococcus aureus*: proceeding with caution. *Infect Control Hosp Epidemiol* 1996;17:775–779.
385. Miller MA, Dascal A, Portnoy J, et al. Development of mupirocin resistance among methicillin-resistant *Staphylococcus aureus* after widespread use of nasal mupirocin ointment. *Infect Control Hosp Epidemiol* 1996;17:811–813.
386. Eltringham I. Mupirocin resistance and methicillin-resistant *Staphylococcus aureus* (MRSA). *J Hosp Infect* 1997;35:1–8.
387. dos Santos KRN, Fonseca LdS, Filho PPG. Emergence of high-level mupirocin resistance in methicillin-resistant *Staphylococcus aureus* isolated from Brazilian university hospitals. *Infect Control Hosp Epidemiol* 1996;17:813–816.
388. Vasquez JE, Walker ES, Franzus BW, et al. The epidemiology of mupirocin resistance among methicillin-resistant *Staphylococcus aureus* at a Veterans' Affairs hospital. *Infect Control Hosp Epidemiol* 2000;21:459–464.
389. Leski TA, Gniadkowski M, Skoczynska A, et al. Outbreak of mupirocin resistant staphylococci in a hospital in Warsaw, Poland, due to plasmid transmission and clonal spread of several strains. *J Clin Microbiol* 1999;37:2781–2788.
390. Ayliffe GAJ. The progressive intercontinental spread of methicillin-resistant *Staphylococcus aureus*. *Clin Infect Dis* 1997;24(Suppl I):S74–S79.
391. Rello J, Torres A, Ricart M, et al. Ventilator-associated pneumonia by *Staphylococcus aureus*: comparison of methicillin-resistant and methicillin-sensitive episodes. *Am J Respir Crit Care Med* 1994;150:1545–1549.
392. Washio M, Kajioka T, Yoshimitsu T, et al. Risk factors for methicillin-

resistant *Staphylococcus aureus* (MRSA) infection in a Japanese geriatric hospital. *Public Health* 1997;111:187–190.
393. Troillet N, Carmeli Y, Samore MH, et al. Carriage of methicillin-resistant *Staphylococcus aureus* at hospital admission. *Infect Control Hosp Epidemiol* 1998;19:181–185.
394. Monnet DL. Methicillin-resistant *Staphylococcus aureus* and its relationship to antimicrobial use: possible implications for control. *Infect Control Hosp Epidemiol* 1998;19:552–559.
395. Crowcroft NS, Ronveaux O, Monnet DL, et al. Methicillin-resistant *Staphylococcus aureus* and antimicrobial use in Belgian hospitals. *Infect Control Hosp Epidemiol* 1999;20:31–36.
396. Monnet DL, Frimodt-Moller N. Antimicrobial drug use and methicillin-resistant *Staphylococcus aureus. Emerg Infect Dis* 2001;7:1–3.
397. Matsumura H, Yoshizawa N, Narumi A, et al. Effective control of methicillin-resistant *Staphylococcus aureus* in a burn unit. *Burns* 1996; 22:283–286.
398. Frank MO, Batteiger BE, Sorensen SJ, et al. Decrease in expenditures and selected nosocomial infections following implementation of an antimicrobial-prescribing improvement program. *Clin Perform Qual Health Care* 1997;5:180–188.
399. Landman D, Chockalingam M, Quale JM. Reduction in the incidence of methicillin-resistant *Staphylococcus aureus* and ceftazidime-resistant *Klebsiella pneumoniae* following changes in a hospital antibiotic formulary. *Clin Infect Dis* 1999;28:1062–1066.
400. Rice LB. Editorial response: a silver bullet for colonization and infection with methicillin-resistant *Staphylococcus aureus* still eludes us. *Clin Infect Dis* 1999;28:1067–1070.
401. Jackson M, Chiarello LA, Gaynes RP, et al. Nurse staffing and health care-associated infections: proceedings from a working group meeting. *Am J Infect Control* 2002;30:199–206.
402. Farrington M, Trundle C, Redpath C, et al. Effects on nursing workload of different methicillin-resistant *Staphylococcus aureus* (MRSA) control strategies. *J Hosp Infect* 2000;46:118–122.
403. Vicca AF. Nursing staff workload as a determinant of methicillin-resistant *Staphylococcus aureus* spread in an adult intensive therapy unit. *J Hosp Infect* 1999;43:109–113.
404. Interim guidelines for prevention and control of staphylococcal infections associated with reduced susceptibility to vancomycin. *MMWR* 1997;46:626–628, 635.

30

COAGULASE-NEGATIVE STAPHYLOCOCCI

JOHN M. BOYCE

Although *Staphylococcus aureus* has been acknowledged as an important cause of nosocomial infections for many years, recognition of coagulase-negative staphylococci as nosocomial pathogens occurred after the development of surgical techniques for repair of congenital and acquired heart diseases and other types of surgery involving implantation of prosthetic devices. In the early 1950s, cases of endocarditis due to coagulase-negative staphylococci following mitral commissurotomy were recognized to be of nosocomial origin (1,2). In 1958, Smith et al. (3) reported that 1.5% of staphylococcal bacteremias seen at University of Iowa between 1936 and 1955 were due to coagulase-negative staphylococci. Subsequently, nosocomial infections due to coagulase-negative staphylococci were described in patients undergoing surgery involving implantation of prosthetic material such as cardiac valves or patches, cerebrospinal fluid (CSF) shunts, and prosthetic hips (4). Some children with infected ventriculoatrial shunts had multiple episodes of coagulase-negative staphylococcal bacteremia over periods of several months, because the importance of removing the infected device was not appreciated initially, and the microorganism was felt to be avirulent (4). The role of these pathogens in causing bacteremia and septicemia in patients who had not undergone such procedures was not widely appreciated until the late 1970s and early 1980s (3,5–7).

Better recognition of the importance of these microorganisms was due in part to the increasing incidence of infections associated with short- and long-term indwelling intravascular catheters and an ever-expanding array of surgically implanted devices. In the 1970s, *Staphylococcus epidermidis* accounted for less than 4% of pathogens recovered from nosocomial infections diagnosed in hospitals participating in the National Nosocomial Infections Surveillance (NNIS) system at the Centers for Disease Control and Prevention (CDC), and was the eighth most common pathogen isolated (8). However, in the period 1992 to 1998, surveillance conducted in medical-surgical intensive care units revealed that coagulase-negative staphylococci were the most common cause of primary bloodstream infections, and the second most common microorganism recovered from surgical site infections (9). In 1998, coagulase-negative staphylococci accounted for 45% of central line–associated primary bloodstream infections in such patients.

MICROBIOLOGY

In the 1950s and 1960s, most coagulase-negative staphylococci recovered from hospitalized patients were referred to as *Staphylococcus albus*. Later, such strains were classified as either *S. epidermidis* or *Staphylococcus saprophyticus*. However, the genus *Staphylococcus* now includes 32 species, most of which are coagulase-negative (10). Coagulase-negative staphylococci that have been recovered from humans include *S. epidermidis, S. saprophyticus, S. haemolyticus, S. lugdunensis, S. warneri, S. hominis, S. schleiferi, S. simulans, S. cohnii, S. capitis, S. saccharolyticus, S. auricularis, S. caprae,* and *S. xylosus* (11,12). *S. epidermidis* appears to be the most virulent of the coagulase-negative staphylococci, and is without question the most common species recovered from patients with nosocomial infections (13,14). *S. lugdunensis* may cause infections that have clinical features that resemble serious *S. aureus* infections (15,16).

Identification of Coagulase-Negative Staphylococci

The most widely used, reliable test for differentiating coagulase-negative staphylococci from *S. aureus* is the tube coagulase test, which detects free coagulase produced by *S. aureus* (11). Slide coagulase tests, which detect cell-bound coagulase (clumping factor), are also used in many laboratories, and yield a negative result with most coagulase-negative staphylococci. However, 10% to 15% of *S. aureus* strains yield negative results with slide coagulase tests, but such strains are coagulase-positive if subsequently tested by the tube coagulase method (10).

Positive slide coagulase tests may occur with some staphylococcal species such as *S. schleiferi* and *S. lugdunensis* (17). Coagulase-negative staphylococci grown on media with high salt concentrations may also yield false-positive slide coagulase test results. Therefore, colonies present on selective media such as mannitol-salt agar should be restreaked onto nonselective media before testing by slide coagulase methods.

A number of commercial latex agglutination and hemagglutination assays have been licensed for rapid detection of *S. aureus*, and most of these systems reliably differentiate coagulase-negative staphylococci from *S. aureus* (18,19). However, on occasion, such systems may yield either false-positive or false-negative results. *S. saprophyticus, S. lugdunensis,* and *S. warneri* may give positive reactions when tested with commercial rapid agglutination slide tests (18–21). In contrast, capsular serotype 5 strains of methicillin-resistant *S. aureus* may yield false-negative results when some of the commercial agglutination slide tests are used (18,19,22,23). Therefore, some authorities recommend that all isolates that are coagulase negative by slide tests be subsequently tested by the tube coagulase method to confirm if they are coagulase-negative or coagulase-positive (11,18).

Identification of isolates to the species level may be helpful in differentiating clinically relevant isolates from contaminants, and when supplemented with typing systems may be, in some instances of epidemiologic significance. Conventional methods as described by Kloos et al. (11) and a variety of commercial identification kits and automated systems can be used to speciate coagulase-negative staphylococci (11,12,14,24,25). Most of the commercial kits or automated systems identify *S. epidermidis, S. haemolyticus,* and *S. hominis* (the most common species recovered from clinical specimens) with an accuracy of >80% (12).

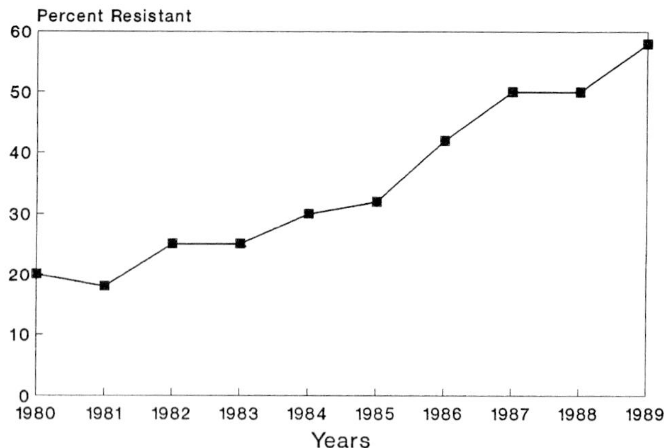

Figure 30.1. Proportion of coagulase-negative staphylococci from the National Nosocomial Infections Surveillance system reported as resistant to methicillin, oxacillin, or nafcillin, 1980–1987 (n = 27,150). (From Schaberg DR, Culver DH, Gaynes RP. Major trends in the microbial etiology of nosocomial infection. *Am J Med* 1991;91:72S–75S, with permission.)

Antimicrobial Susceptibility Tests

Antimicrobial susceptibility testing of coagulase-negative staphylococci can usually be performed using the same tests that are recommended for testing *S. aureus* (26–28). However, current interpretive criteria for oxacillin may occasionally yield inaccurate results, especially for *S. saprophyticus* and *S. lugdunensis* (28,29). The National Committee for Clinical Laboratory Standards (NCCLS) recommends that isolates with oxacillin inhibitory zones of 18 mm or greater be categorized as susceptible, and those with zone diameters of 17 mm or less be categorized as resistant. Isolates with a minimal inhibitory concentration (MIC) of 0.25 μg/mL or less are defined as susceptible, and those with an MIC of 0.5 μg/mL or more are categorized as resistant to oxacillin. Oxacillin/salt screening plates commonly used to detect oxacillin resistance among *S. aureus* isolates are no longer recommended for testing coagulase-negative staphylococci. A rapid latex agglutination test to detect PBP-2a accurately detects oxacillin resistance among coagulase-negative staphylococci (30). Laboratories need to ensure that current procedures and breakpoints are used when testing coagulase-negative staphylococci.

Antimicrobial Resistance Among Coagulase-Negative Staphylococci

Methicillin Resistance

Methicillin-resistant strains of coagulase-negative staphylococci were first reported in 1960 (31). Resistant strains were recovered from nasal cultures obtained from newborns in a nursery where methicillin was being aerosolized in an effort to reduce *S. aureus* infections. Shortly thereafter, methicillin-resistant strains of coagulase-negative staphylococci were recovered from children with ventriculocaval shunt infections and from blood cultures in other hospitals (4,32,33).

Studies conducted since the late 1970s have noted an increasing frequency of methicillin resistance among strains recovered from hospitalized patients (34–39) (Fig. 30.1). Data from the NNIS system have revealed that more than 85% of coagulase-negative staphylococci causing nosocomial infections in intensive care unit patients are resistant to methicillin (40).

All methicillin-resistant coagulase-negative staphylococci, including strains of *S. epidermidis, S. haemolyticus, S. saprophyticus, S. hominis, S. simulans, S. sciuri, S. warneri, S. capitis,* and *S. caprae* have been shown to contain a *mec*A gene or its gene product, PBP-2a (41–45). The strong similarities between the *mec*A genes and PBP-2a found in *S. aureus* and in coagulase-negative staphylococci suggest that the same *mec*A gene has spread to all methicillin-resistant staphylococci, possibly on a transposon (43–46). Although methicillin-resistant coagulase-negative staphylococci may appear susceptible to other beta-lactam antibiotics such as cephalosporins or imipenem on the basis of routine antimicrobial susceptibility tests, they are not susceptible to beta-lactams *in vivo* (42,47). Therefore, beta-lactam antibiotics should not be used for treating methicillin-resistant coagulase-negative staphylococcal infections.

Resistance to Other Antimicrobial Agents

Resistance to multiple agents such as penicillin, methicillin, erythromycin, clindamycin, trimethoprim, and gentamicin is common among *S. epidermidis* and *S. haemolyticus* isolates recovered from hospitalized patients (13,34,36,37,48–52). Erythromycin resistance in *S. epidermidis* has been shown to be due to the *erm*C gene, which resides on a plasmid (51). Trimethoprim resistance genes may reside on either conjugative or nonconjugative plasmids, or may occur on the chromosome (52). Gentamicin resistance determinants often reside on conjugative plasmids, and transfer of gentamicin resistance between species of coagulase-negative staphylococci and between *S. epidermidis* and *S. aureus* has been demonstrated (49,53–56). These findings suggest that *S. epidermidis* may serve as a reservoir of antimicrobial resistance determinants in hospitals (49,51).

Although a majority of strains are susceptible to the fluoroquinolones, resistance to ciprofloxacin has emerged in settings where the agent was used frequently for empiric treatment of neutropenic patients (57). Resistance to the glycopeptide antibiotic teicoplanin has been noted among strains of *S. haemolyticus*, and to a less extent among strains of *S. epidermidis* (58–61). In a few hospitals in Europe where teicoplanin is used, teicoplanin-resistant strains account for up to 18% of coagulase-negative staphylococcal bacteremias among patients with hematologic malignancies (62).

Most coagulase-negative staphylococci are susceptible to vancomycin, which is presently the mainstay of therapy for nosocomial infections caused by multiresistant coagulase-negative staphylococci. Therefore, it is particularly concerning that strains of *S. haemolyticus* that test intermediate or resistant to vancomycin have been described (58,63,64). Strains of *S. epidermidis* and *S. capitis* that possess heterogeneous resistance to vancomycin have also been described (65,66). Theoretically, continued widespread use of vancomycin could select for strains with greater degrees of resistance to vancomycin (65).

Epidemiologic Typing Systems

Because coagulase-negative staphylococci are normal inhabitants of human skin, growth of these microorganisms in clinical cultures may represent contamination of the specimen with skin flora, or true infection. In general, infection is more likely to be present if multiple isolates of the same strain have been recovered from the patient. Phenotypic or genotypic typing of isolates can help establish whether multiple isolates represent the same strain or different, unrelated strains. Moreover, if a cluster of coagulase-negative staphylococcal infections occurs among several patients over a short time period, determining if the isolates represent the same strain or not is necessary to establish if an outbreak is occurring. Finally, differentiating closely related strains from unrelated strains is important during epidemiologic studies designed to establish modes of transmission and sources of coagulase-negative staphylococci in healthcare settings.

Phenotypic and genotypic typing systems that have been used to study coagulase-negative staphylococci include speciation of isolates, analysis of antibiotic susceptibility patterns (antibiograms), biotyping, serotyping, phage typing, immunoblotting, cellular fatty acid profiles, analysis of plasmid DNA, restriction endonuclease digestion of total cellular DNA or chromosomal DNA using standard or pulsed-field gel electrophoresis (PFGE) and DNA hybridization methods using rRNA probes (ribotyping) or antibiotic resistance probes (24).

Phenotypic Typing Systems

Speciation of isolates, by itself, is of limited value since *S. epidermidis* accounts for a majority of clinical isolates. However, in those instances when other species are isolated, identification of the microorganism may be of clinical or epidemiologic significance.

Biotyping has been evaluated by many investigators as a potential epidemiologic marker for coagulase-negative staphylococci (48,67–74). Because many epidemiologically unrelated strains belong to the same biotype, and biotypes are not always reproducible, most authorities recommend against using biotyping alone as an epidemiologic marker for these microorganisms.

Serotyping has been used for epidemiologic studies of coagulase-negative staphylococci, but has poor discriminatory power and appropriate reagents are not readily available (71,75). Whole-cell polypeptide profiles, immunoblotting, and cellular fatty acid analysis have also been studied as markers for coagulase-negative staphylococci, but are not practical and do not appear to have advantages over other typing systems (75–77).

Phage typing was used for many years for investigating clusters of coagulase-negative staphylococci, but the proportion of isolates that are typeable varied from 20% to 90% (48,67,68, 70,73,78,79). This method also suffers from problems with reproducibility and limited discriminatory power.

In many hospitals, analysis of the antibiograms represents the major, if not the only, method for differentiating between strains of coagulase-negative staphylococci. Its advantages include availability in most hospitals, low cost, quick turnaround times, and ability of all strains to be typed using this method. In several common-source outbreaks involving *S. epidermidis* strains with unusual susceptibility patterns, antibiograms were used successfully to differentiate epidemiologically linked isolates from unrelated strains (69,80). The fact that isolates with the epidemic antibiogram represented the same strain was confirmed by using restriction endonuclease analysis of plasmid DNA in one of these outbreaks (80) (Fig. 30.2). Hartstein et al. (81) demonstrated that a carefully chosen panel of antibiotic susceptibility tests, when used in conjunction with a susceptibility coding system, was able to determine if multiple isolates from a given patient were related or unrelated. Other investigators have also reported examples of how antibiograms performed well in establishing the relatedness of multiple isolates recovered from a individual patient (73,82). However, analysis of antibiograms has several shortcomings. Some investigators have reported problems with the reproducibility of antibiograms, although others have not found this to be a problem (68,72,83). The fact that many strains responsible for nosocomial infections are multidrug resistant and demonstrate little variability in their susceptibility pattern despite differences in their genetic makeup also makes interpretation of antibiograms problematic (34,36,67,84). Finally, over a period of time, the antimicrobial susceptibility of a strain may change if the microorganism gains or loses plasmids containing antimicrobial resistance determinants (79,85).

Genotypic Typing Systems

Plasmid analysis, using either whole plasmid profiles or restriction endonuclease digestion of plasmid DNA, has been used in the past for evaluating multiple isolates from individual patients (70,71,73,74,81–83,86) and isolates from apparent outbreaks of infection caused by coagulase-negative staphylococci (79,80,84). In many instances, plasmid analysis appropriately differentiated epidemiologically related isolates from unrelated strains, and has greater discriminatory power than antibiograms and other phenotypic typing systems, especially when evaluating isolates from possible outbreaks (70,81,84,85). However, 5% to 20% of isolates were not typeable, because they contained only

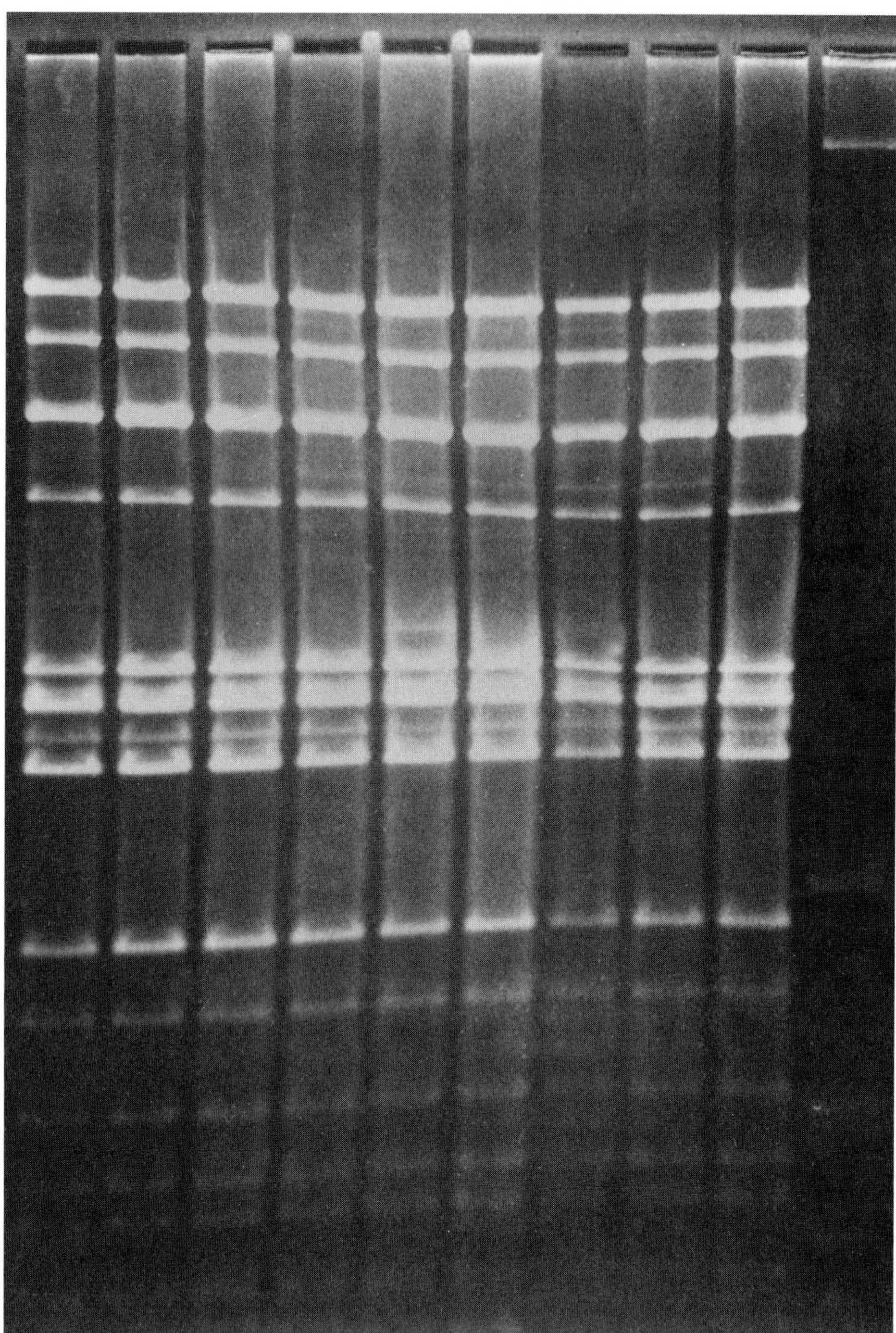

Figure 30.2. *Eco*RI restriction endonuclease digests of nine isolates of the epidemic strain of *S. epidermidis*. Lanes 1 and 8, blood cultures from patients with prosthetic valve endocarditis; lanes 2 and 3, blood cultures from cardiotomy line late during bypass; lane 4, from sternal wound of valve surgery patient; lanes 5 and 7, from sternal wounds of coronary artery bypass graft patients; lane 6, from hands of surgeon A; lane 9, from patient with septic arthritis. (From Boyce JM, Potter-Bynoe G, Opal SM, et al. A common-source outbreak of *Staphylococcus epidermidis* infections among patients undergoing cardiac surgery. *J Infect Dis* 1990;161:493–499, with permission.)

one or contained no plasmids. Also, the plasmid profile of a strain can change over time as the microorganism gains or loses plasmids (49,74,79). The latter has not been a major problem when isolates have been recovered over periods of weeks or a few months (79–83,86), but may lead to misinterpretation of results when isolates are collected over periods of one year or longer (49). Finally, dissemination of plasmids among genetically (and epidemiologically) unrelated strains may result in similar plasmid profiles among isolates that do not constitute an outbreak (74).

More recently, restriction endonuclease analysis of total cellular or chromosomal DNA has been used to study the clonality of *S. epidermidis* (71,73,74,82,87). However, standard constant-voltage gel electrophoresis of genomic DNA produces so many restriction fragments that comparison of strain patterns is difficult. To overcome this problem, DNA can subsequently be transferred to a nitrocellulose membrane and the DNA fragments can be checked for their ability to hybridize with a variety of different probes. Using an *Escherichia coli* ribosomal RNA (rRNA) gene probe (ribotyping) has made it easier to differentiate among different strains (75,82,87,88). However, the discriminatory power of ribotyping may not equal that of some other molecular typing systems. Other probes that have been used to examine restriction fragment length polymorphisms include genes encoding for aminoglycoside resistance, or resistance genes plus a portion of an insertion sequence (75).

Polymerase chain reaction (PCR)-based random amplification of polymorphic DNA (RAPD) has also been used for molecular typing of coagulase-negative staphylococci, and appears to have good discriminatory power (89–91).

Another approach to analysis of genomic DNA utilizes restriction endonucleases that cut the DNA into 10 to 20 large fragments, which are then separated by performing gel electrophoresis using pulsed current (field inversion gel electrophoresis (FIGE) or PFGE (82,88). PFGE appears to have excellent discriminatory power when used with a variety of pathogens including coagulase-negative staphylococci (88,92) and is currently one of the best methods for molecular typing of these microorganisms (89–91).

PATHOGENESIS

Host Factors

Coagulase-negative staphylococcal infections seldom occur among healthy individuals. Host factors that pose the greatest risk of infection by these microorganisms include defects in mucosal membranes or skin, immunosuppression, and most importantly the presence of a foreign body. A number of studies have shown that nosocomial infections caused by coagulase-negative staphylococci are more likely to occur among patients with malignancies, especially those who develop chemotherapy-induced damage to mucosal surfaces and neutropenia (93,94). When such patients become colonized in their gastrointestinal tracts with coagulase-negative staphylococci, the microorganisms subsequently may penetrate the damaged mucosa and cause bacteremia or other infections (64,86,93). Patients with systemic or localized defects in opsonophagocytic activity are also at increased risk of infection by these microorganisms. Decreased opsonic activity of serum may be responsible in part for the increased risk of such infections in low birth weight neonates (95), and decreased opsonic activity of peritoneal fluid may predispose patients on chronic ambulatory peritoneal dialysis to infection with *S. epidermidis* (96). In neonates, administration of intravenous lipid emulsions has also been identified as an independent risk factor for coagulase-negative staphylococcal bacteremia (97). It is not clear whether the lipid emulsions promote the growth of bacteria lodged on the catheter surface, or whether there may be effects of lipid on neutrophil and macrophage function. Although preceding antibiotic therapy is not responsible for colonization with susceptible strains of coagulase-negative staphylococci, it is clearly a risk factor for acquisition of, and subsequent infection by, multidrug resistant strains (34, 58,98).

The single most important risk factor associated with coagulase-negative staphylococcal infections is the presence of an indwelling catheter or implanted foreign body, including intravascular catheters (36,99,100), transvenous pacemaker leads (101, 102), peritoneal dialysis catheters (103,104), prosthetic heart valves or patches (37), vascular grafts (105), CSF shunts (4, 106,107), prosthetic joints (108,109), breast implants (110), intraocular lens (111–113), left ventricular assist devices (114), and genitourinary implants (115). Coagulase-negative staphylococci may enter the patient's body from the skin surface at the catheter exit site, or may be inadvertently inoculated into the operative site at the time of implantation of prosthetic devices.

Microbial Factors

S. epidermidis possesses a number of virulence factors that contribute to its ability to cause foreign-body–related infections. In 1972, Bayston and Penny (116) noted that valve surfaces of CSF shunts removed from children with coagulase-negative staphylococcal shunt infections were covered with clumps of staphylococci that were embedded in a thick layer of a mucoid substance, and that isolates from these devices produced large amounts of this substance when grown *in vitro*. Subsequent studies of intravenous catheters removed from patients or contaminated *in vitro* revealed that staphylococci were clumped together and embedded in a thick, multilayered biofilm (also called slime), especially at sites where there were physical defects on the catheter surfaces (117–120).

The pathogenesis of foreign-body–related infections caused by coagulase-negative staphylococci involves adherence of microorganisms to polymeric surfaces, followed by accumulation of cells into the biofilm. Initial adherence of coagulase-negative staphylococci to uncoated foreign bodies is affected by nonspecific physiochemical forces such as van der Waals forces, polarity, and hydrophobic interactions; by staphylococcal surface proteins (SSP-1 and -2), and the cell surface-associated autolysin AtlE; and by a capsular polysaccharide/adhesin (PS/A) (120–124). Soon after implantation of foreign bodies, surfaces of these devices become coated by host-derived proteins such as fibrinogen, vitronectin, and von Willebrand factor that can promote adherence of coagulase-negative staphylococci (120,125). Host-factor–binding proteins such as the surface-associated autolysin

AtlE produced by *S. epidermidis* also binds to the extracellular matrix protein vitronectin, and an autolysin (Aas) produced by *S. saprophyticus* binds to fibronectin (120). Other proteins produced by *S. epidermidis,* such as fibrinogen-binding protein (Fbe) and SdrG also contribute to binding of the microorganism to host proteins, and teichoic acid has been shown to facilitate adherence of *S. epidermidis* to fibronectin.

Once staphylococci have adhered to a polymeric surface, they multiply and form clusters of bacteria in the biofilm coating the surface of the device. Accumulation of bacteria in biofilms involves intercellular adhesion, which is promoted by PS/A and by the *S. epidermidis* polysaccharide intercellular adhesion (PIA) (120,126). PS/A production is also correlated to encapsulation, protection of the microorganism from complement-mediated phagocytic killing, and virulence in animal models of prosthetic valve endocarditis (121,124,127,128). It appears that PS/A and PIA are structurally related, and that production of both is mediated by the *icaADBC* gene cluster (120).

Biofilm also may protect adherent coagulase-negative staphylococci from both host defenses and antibiotics. Biofilm has been shown to inhibit neutrophil chemotaxis and phagocytosis, to inhibit the blastogenesis of T and B lymphocytes, and to inhibit immunoglobulin production by B cells (129–131). It has also been suggested that biofilm may protect adherent staphylococci from antibiotics by acting as a physical barrier, and may cause the microorganisms to be less susceptible to antibiotics (132, 133). Some of the latter effect may be due to the fact that microorganisms embedded in slime are often in a stationary phase of growth.

Although biofilm production is a major virulence factor for *S. epidermidis* and some other coagulase-negative staphylococci, some biofilm-negative strains cause clinically significant infections. Other microbial factors that may contribute to the virulence of *S. epidermidis, S. lugdunensis,* and *S. schleiferi* include their ability to produce a variety of other extracellular substances such as alpha and gamma hemolysins, lipase, esterase, and protease (120,134). *S. saprophyticus* adheres to uroepithelial cells to a greater degree than most other staphylococci. Slow-growing, hemin-dependent small colony variants of *S. epidermidis* and *S. capitis* have occasionally caused pacemaker-related infections (135).

INFECTIONS CAUSED BY COAGULASE-NEGATIVE STAPHYLOCOCCI

Intravascular Device-Associated Infections

The reported incidence of coagulase-negative staphylococcal primary bloodstream infections (most of which are intravascular catheter related) increased dramatically in the period 1980 through 1989 (136), and coagulase-negative staphylococci are now the most common cause of nosocomial bloodstream infections, accounting for about 30% of cases (137). These microorganisms are the most common cause of infections related to short-term peripheral and central venous catheters, pulmonary artery catheters and arterial catheters used for hemodynamic monitoring, total parenteral nutrition, percutaneous hemodialysis and long-term Broviac or Hickman catheters, subcutaneous ports used for vascular access, left ventricular assist devices, and long peripheral catheters used for home infusion therapy (24,114,138, 139). A majority of such infections are caused by *S. epidermidis,* but other species such as *S. warneri, S. capitis, S. haemolyticus, S. hominis, S. caprae,* and *S. simulans* may also cause vascular catheter-related infections (64,140–142). Host factors associated with catheter-related bloodstream infections include age, gender, serious underlying diseases, and neutropenia. Other frequently identified risk factors include inexperience of the operator inserting the catheter, insertion with less than maximal sterile barriers, placement of a central venous catheter in the internal jugular or femoral vein rather than subclavian vein, heavy colonization of the insertion site, placement in an old site by guidewire exchange, duration of catheterization greater than 7 days, contamination of the catheter hub, catheter composition, insertion conditions, and certain first-generation needleless device systems (143–148).

Coagulase-negative staphylococcal bacteremia causes fever in most affected patients, and one half to two thirds of patients develop leukocytosis or leukopenia (141,149). About 20% of bacteremic patients experience hypotension, and 10% to 15% develop septic shock accompanied by disseminated intravascular coagulation (139,141,149). Some patients grow coagulase-negative staphylococci [$\geq 10^5$ colony-forming units (CFU)/mL] from urine cultured at the time of their bacteremia (149). Occasionally, affected patients develop pneumonia, suppurative phlebitis, vertebral osteomyelitis, or infective endocarditis as a complication of catheter-related bacteremia (36,139,150,151). Such bacteremias prolong the patient's hospital stay by an average of 7 days, and from 10% to 15% of affected patients die as a result of their coagulase-negative staphylococcal bacteremia (141) (see also Chapters 17 and 18).

Bacteremia

Although most coagulase-negative staphylococcal bacteremias are due to intravascular catheters, and to a lesser extent other indwelling prosthetic devices, bacteremia and septicemia can also occur in the absence of such devices. Immunosuppressed patients, particularly those with severe neutropenia, are at increased risk of bacteremia caused by these microorganisms (57, 86,93,94,150). Several studies have demonstrated that colonization of the nasopharynx, rectum, or skin by coagulase-negative staphylococci often precedes the development of bacteremia in such patients (86,93,94). Chemotherapy-induced breaks in normal mucosal barriers, or skin or soft tissue infections, probably represent the portals of entry in such patients (86,93,94) (see also Chapter 19).

Surgical Site Infections

Surgical site infections (formerly termed surgical wound infections) may be divided into three categories: (a) superficial incisional and (b) deep incisional infections, which together account for about two thirds of all surgical site infections; and (c) organ/space infections, which account for the remaining one third (152–154). Coagulase-negative staphylococci are the second most common nosocomial pathogen recovered from surgical site infections, exceeded only by *S. aureus* (137). Although isolates recovered from surgical site infections are not speciated in many hospitals, the majority of isolates are probably *S. epidermidis*, with a few infections being caused by *S. caprae, S. schleiferi,* and *S. lugdunensis* (90,142,155). Coagulase-negative staphylococci are more frequently recovered from superficial incisional wound infections than from deep incisional infections (156). However, the relative frequency with which these pathogens are recovered varies to some extent by the type of surgery. For example, they are a common cause of deep surgical site infections and mediastinitis following open heart surgery, but are a less common cause of postoperative endometritis (156–158).

Risk factors for surgical site infections caused by these organisms are presumably the same as for postoperative infections caused by other microorganisms, namely severity of underlying illness (e.g., diabetes mellitus, high American Society for Anesthesiology score), duration of surgery, obesity, advanced age, malnutrition, trauma, and loss of skin integrity (39,159). The clinical signs and symptoms associated with coagulase-negative staphylococcal surgical site infections include fever, local erythema, warmth and edema, and purulent drainage, which are sometimes accompanied by an elevated peripheral white blood cell count. The interval between surgery and the onset of signs and symptoms is quite variable, but is often 3 to 7 days with superficial surgical site infections. Mediastinitis, a type of organ/space surgical site infection, often presents initially as fever without obvious changes involving the incision. Purulent drainage from the sternal incision, sternal click or instability, and wound dehiscence often occurs a matter of days or more than a week after the onset of fever.

The degree of morbidity associated with coagulase-negative staphylococcal surgical site infections is quite variable. Some incisional infections are easily cured with local wound care alone, whereas others require specific antimicrobial therapy and cause considerable morbidity. Serious surgical site infections result in prolongation of hospital stays and utilization of resources for which hospitals are not adequately reimbursed (see also Chapter 21).

Prosthetic Valve Endocarditis

Prior to the advent of open-heart surgery, coagulase-negative staphylococci were responsible for very few cases of endocarditis (160). Endocarditis due to these microorganisms began to occur more frequently when surgical procedures for treatment of congenital and acquired cardiac valvular diseases were developed in the late 1940s and early 1950s (1,2,161). Since the development of prosthetic heart valves, coagulase-negative staphylococci have become one of the most common causes of endocarditis following cardiac valve surgery (162–165). These microorganisms account for 30% to 67% of cases that present within 2 months of surgery, and for 20% to 28% of cases presenting more than 2 months following surgery (166). Most cases are due to *S. epidermidis*, but cases have also been caused by *S. haemolyticus, S. cohnii*, and *S. lugdunensis* (10,37).

The onset of symptoms and signs of nosocomial coagulase-negative staphylococcal prosthetic valve endocarditis may occur as early as a few days after surgery to as long as 12 months following surgery, with a peak incidence at about 6 weeks (69, 80,164,167). The fact that most cases with onset within the first year after surgery are due to methicillin-resistant strains, and that cases occurring later are usually methicillin-susceptible, supports the concept that cases due to hospital-acquired staphylococci may have onset up to 12 months after surgery (37). Most patients presenting soon after surgery have fever and a new regurgitant murmur or other signs of prosthetic valve dysfunction (166). Patients with late-onset endocarditis also have signs of valve dysfunction, and are somewhat more likely to have splenomegaly or peripheral stigmata of endocarditis (167). Involvement of valve ring tissue or adjacent myocardium is common, and may present as progressive congestive heart failure, valve dehiscence, worsening regurgitant murmur, or cardiac conduction disturbances (37,166). Mortality rates among patients with cases caused by coagulase-negative staphylococci have varied from 43% to 74% (37) (see also Chapter 67).

Vascular Graft-Related Infections

Early published series dealing with vascular graft infections reported that *S. aureus* was the most common pathogen (168, 169). However, in later series, coagulase-negative staphylococci have been the most common cause of prosthetic vascular graft infections (105,170,171). The major risk factor for development of prosthetic vascular graft infection is the use of a groin incision for aortic or lower extremity bypass procedures (170,172). Aortic grafts not involving the groin are much less prone to infection. Other risk factors include diabetes mellitus, surgical revision of a graft, emergency aortic aneurysm surgery, the occurrence of an inguinal surgical site infection, hematoma, or lymphocele, or preexisting infected lower extremity ulcer or gangrene (169,170, 172). Although some studies have suggested that infection rates were higher with woven Dacron graft material than with velour knitted Dacron or polytetrafluoroethylene grafts, the type of material used does not have a major impact on the infection rate (170,172).

Coagulase-negative staphylococcal infections may occur at any time following surgery, but the more common onset is months to years after surgery (105,173,174). Prosthetic vascular graft infections that occur within 30 days of surgery often present with fever, leukocytosis and cellulitis, local abscess formation, or purulent drainage from the inguinal incision (169,171). Cases presenting months to years after surgery are more likely to present with fistula formation or false aneurysm or hemorrhage at the site of the anastomosis (169–171,175). Infections of aortic grafts may present as perigraft infection, graft-enteric erosion or fistula, or aortic stump sepsis (169). Aortic perigraft infections may present with overt sepsis, persistent low-grade fever, or retroperitoneal hemorrhage.

Although infections are relatively uncommon following prosthetic vascular graft surgery, the morbidity and mortality associated with such infections are considerable. Lower extremity amputation may be required in 15% to 30% of patients with infected aortofemoral grafts, and in 36% to 53% of those with infected femoral-popliteal grafts (168,170,175). Mortality rates have ranged from 10% to 48% with aortic graft infections and

10% to 25% with infected femoral-popliteal grafts (168,170, 171,175) (see also Chapter 67).

Prosthetic Joint Infections

When total hip replacement surgery became common in the early 1960s, it became apparent that infection was a major complication, affecting 7% to 9% of patients who underwent surgery at that time (176). *S. aureus* was the most common pathogen recovered from infected hip implants during the 1960s and early 1970s, with coagulase-negative staphylococci accounting for a smaller proportion of cases (176–178). However, in later series, coagulase-negative staphylococci have emerged as a major pathogen (179). A majority of such infections are caused by *S. epidermidis,* although a few have been caused by *S. lugdunensis* (180).

The risk of prosthetic joint infections is increased with previous surgery involving the joint, prolonged duration of surgery, remote infection at the time of surgery, and rheumatoid arthritis (177,179,181). Also, the risk is higher with total replacement of the knee or elbow, if a surgical site infection not involving the prosthesis develops, or if the patient has an underlying malignancy or history of previous arthroplasty (182–184). Infections are often classified on the basis of the interval between surgery and the onset of signs or symptoms of infection (181). Stage I infections occur in the first 3 months after surgery, often represent infected hematomas, and are more likely to be due to *S. aureus.* Stage II infections occur between 3 months and 2 years after surgery, and often present as gradual reappearance of hip pain without fever or purulent drainage. It is these indolent stage II infections that are particularly likely to be due coagulase-negative staphylococci. Stage III infections often present as the acute onset of hip pain with or without fever more than 2 years after surgery, and are usually caused by hematogenous spread of microorganisms from dental, intraabdominal, or urinary tract sources to the prosthesis (181).

Aseptic loosening of hip prostheses may also be caused by coagulase-negative staphylococci (185) (see also Chapter 67).

Central Nervous System Shunt Infections

In an early series published by Schimke et al. (106), 17% of patients who underwent ventriculoatrial shunt procedures developed coagulase-negative staphylococcal bacteremia attributable to shunt infection. Later experience has revealed that shunt infections occur in 2% to 20% of patients who undergo ventriculoatrial and ventriculoperitoneal shunting procedures (107, 186–189). Coagulase-negative staphylococci are the most common pathogen, accounting for 40% to 60% of such infections (107,186,187,189).

Factors that increase the risk of infection following shunt placement include age less than 6 months old, reinsertion following shunt removal for infection, preexisting eschar or dermatitis of the scalp, postoperative wound dehiscence or scalp necrosis, duration of surgery, and the experience of the operating surgeon (186,187,189). Signs and symptoms related to shunt infection develop within 4 months of surgery in 78% of cases (107). Fever is the single most important sign associated with shunt infections. In early series of shunt infections, low-grade fever without signs of overt sepsis was documented for months in children who were treated with antibiotics without removal of the shunt (4,106). Other signs include evidence of infection at the site of the surgical incision, erythema overlying the subcutaneous catheter tract, nausea, vomiting, and signs of increased intracranial pressure or shunt malfunction. Only a third of patients have overt signs of meningitis (107). Patients with infected ventriculoatrial shunts that are not removed promptly may develop hypocomplementemic glomerulonephritis as a complication of chronic coagulase-negative staphylococcal bacteremia (107). Bone flap infections due to coagulase-negative staphylococci represent another complication of craniotomy for shunt therapy (187). Patients who undergo short-term ventriculostomy for monitoring of intracranial pressure are also at risk of developing ventriculitis or meningitis. In a prospective study performed by Mayhall et al. (190), 9% of such patients developed ventriculostomy-related infections, and coagulase-negative staphylococci were the most common microorganism recovered from the CSF of affected patients (see also Chapters 27, 49, and 67).

Infections in Continuous Ambulatory Peritoneal Dialysis Patients

Since peritoneal dialysis was first developed, peritonitis has represented an important complication. Even with the development of improved dialysis catheters, peritonitis remained a major detractor to chronic ambulatory peritoneal dialysis when bottled dialysis was used (104). However, with further technical advances and the use of fewer connections and plastic bags rather than bottles, the incidence of peritonitis associated with continuous ambulatory peritoneal dialysis (CAPD) has decreased to one episode or less per patient-year in some centers (191,192). Coagulase-negative staphylococci have for many years been the single most common cause of CAPD-related peritonitis, accounting for 25% to 50% of all cases (104,191–195). *S. epidermidis* accounts for about 80% of episodes caused by coagulase-negative staphylococci, with *S. haemolyticus, S. capitis, S. warnerii,* and *S. simulans* accounting for the remaining cases (103,195,196). Host factors that place patients at increased risk of coagulase-negative staphylococcal CAPD-related peritonitis have not been well delineated. Peritoneal dialysis catheter exit site infections precede some cases of peritonitis, but a majority of patients with peritonitis do not have concomitant exit site or tunnel infections due to the same strain of coagulase-negative staphylococcus (192,194,195). Some patients seldom experience peritonitis, whereas others have multiple episodes per year (192). The factors responsible for this phenomenon are poorly understood, but low peritoneal immunoglobulin G (IgG) concentrations may serve as a risk factor in some patients (197). About 50% of patients with CAPD-associated peritonitis have fever, and 80% complain of abdominal pain (191). One third develop nausea, and a few have diarrhea. About 70% to 80% have some degree of abdominal tenderness on physical examination, and 50% have overt rebound abdominal tenderness (191) (see also Chapter 65).

Infections in Neonates

During the early 1980s, coagulase-negative staphylococci were recognized as true pathogens, and dramatic increases in the incidence of coagulase-negative staphylococcal bacteremia among neonates were reported (7,198–202). These microorganisms now account for 31% of all nosocomial infections in neonatal intensive care units (NICUs), and are the most common cause of bacteremia and septicemia in such units (203–207). Initially, the rising number of reported cases of coagulase-negative staphylococcal bacteremia in neonates appeared to be due to increasing use of umbilical catheters and central venous catheters for monitoring of blood gases and administration of parenteral nutrition to premature infants, and partly to greater realization that *S. epidermidis* bacteremia was a complication of intravascular catheters (7,198,199,201,202,204). However, subsequent studies in some centers revealed that the incidence of blood cultures positive for coagulase-negative staphylococci had not increased, and that the dramatic increase in reported cases was due in large part to a greater probability that a positive blood culture would be interpreted by physicians as bacteremia (206, 208), and to increased utilization of NICU beds by very-low-birth-weight infants, who are much more likely to develop nosocomial bacteremia (201,209).

Newborns become colonized with coagulase-negative staphylococci within several days of admission to an NICU (208,210). Sites frequently colonized include the skin, umbilicus, nares, and pharynx. *S. epidermidis* is the most common species isolated, followed by *S. haemolyticus* (211,212). *S. warneri* and *S. capitis* have also been recovered from infants in NICUs (66,213). Infections due to these microorganisms are relatively uncommon during the first week of hospitalization. The average age of neonates who develop coagulase-negative staphylococcal bacteremia in NICUs is 3 to 4 weeks old (198,204,209,214). The major risk factors associated with *S. epidermidis* bacteremia are birth weight less than 1,500 g, central venous catheters, and total parenteral nutrition, especially intravenous lipid emulsions (97,199,201, 202,204,208,209). It is postulated that lipids, which are rich in nutrients, may facilitate the rapid growth of *S. epidermidis*, similar to their effect on *Malassezia furfur*, a lipophilic yeast that colonizes the skin of infants (97,215).

The most common signs and symptoms observed in neonates with coagulase-negative staphylococcal bacteremia include apnea, bradycardia, lethargy, feeding difficulties, abdominal distention, temperature instability, and neutropenia or thrombocytopenia (199,202,204,214,216,217). Some affected infants also develop metabolic acidosis, hyperglycemia, or signs of infection at the site of intravascular catheters. Most bacteremias occur in neonates with indwelling intravascular catheters, but serious bacteremias may also occur in the absence of vascular catheters in infants who have skin lesions or respiratory tract or gastrointestinal colonization caused by *S. epidermidis* (202,204,214).

Coagulase-negative staphylococci may also cause omphalitis, skin or wound abscesses, pneumonia, urinary tract infections, and possibly meningitis and enterocolitis in neonates (204,214, 217–220). Fortunately, coagulase-negative staphylococcal infections in neonates are seldom fatal (199,216,217). However, affected infants often suffer considerable morbidity, and those with bacteremic infection require more days of antimicrobial therapy and remain hospitalized an average of 20 days longer than comparable neonates without bacteremia (216) (see also Chapter 52).

Infections Associated with Breast Implants

Breast implants that have been used for augmentation mammoplasty are composed of a silicone rubber envelope filled with silicone gel, a silicone envelope filled with saline, or a double-lumen prosthesis with a small compartment containing silicone and a larger compartment containing saline (110). Breast implants may be placed beneath the mammary gland, but superficial to the underlying muscle, or can be implanted below the musculature. Skin flora, including *S. epidermidis*, may reside in the ducts of the glandular tissue of the breast, and may occasionally gain access to the periprosthetic space. Infections involving breast implants are relatively uncommon. When infection does occur, the most common pathogens are *S. aureus*, followed by *S. epidermidis* (110,221). When acute infection occurs in the periprosthetic space, patients often develop erythema, pain, swelling, and drainage. These signs of acute infection often occur within several weeks of implantation. Some investigators believe that chronic, low-grade infection of implants may contribute to the capsular contracture that affects some women with breast implants, but this issue is controversial (222) (see also Chapter 67).

Infections Following Intraocular Lens Implantation

Endophthalmitis related to intraocular lens implantation (pseudophakic endophthalmitis) is an uncommon, but serious complication of cataract surgery. Coagulase-negative staphylococci account for 40% to 60% of cases of pseudophakic endophthalmitis (111–113). Signs and symptoms of infection often begin within days to weeks after lens implantation. Affected patients usually present with pain or decreased vision, or both, involving the affected eye (111,223). Less common symptoms include photophobia, headache, and purulent discharge. Physical examination may reveal conjunctival injection in 66% of cases, evidence of anterior chamber inflammation such as hypopyon or flare (66%), and corneal edema and poor or absent red reflex in a majority of cases (111). Affected patients are usually afebrile, and may or may not have an elevated white blood cell count. Although these infections can cause considerable morbidity and residual visual impairment, the chances of maintaining useful vision are better following treatment of *S. epidermidis* pseudophakic endophthalmitis than with infection caused by other gram-positive cocci or by Gram-negative bacilli (112).

Infections of Genitourinary Prostheses

Coagulase-negative staphylococci are also a recognized cause of infections involving penile prostheses and artificial urinary sphincters (115). *S. epidermidis* has been reported to cause 40% to more than 50% of infections related to penile prostheses (115, 224,225). The onset of signs or symptoms of infection may begin anywhere from several weeks to a year after the device has been implanted (225). Patients with infected penile prostheses often present with local pain, and swelling and erythema of the penis, with few systemic signs of infection. Some complain of induration of the inferior aspect of the penis, fistula formation, or malfunction of the device (115,224).

Infections in Transplant Patients

Patients who undergo organ transplantation are also at increased risk of developing nosocomial infections caused by coagulase-negative staphylococci, because they often require prolonged intravascular catheterization, and are immunocompromised due to neutropenia or immunosuppressive therapy (150, 226). In addition, one study found that high-dose interleukin-2 therapy was associated with an increased risk of staphylococcal bacteremia (227).

S. epidermidis bacteremia is the most common form of infection in such patients. Less commonly, patients develop other infections such as mediastinitis or endocarditis following heart transplant surgery (228). In patients who have undergone implantation of Jarvik-7-100 total artificial hearts, *S. epidermidis* has caused infections associated with drive lines, bacteremia, and pseudopericardial sac abscesses (229,230).

DIAGNOSIS OF COAGULASE-NEGATIVE STAPHYLOCOCCAL INFECTIONS

Intravascular Catheter-Related Infections

The presence of inflammation or purulence at the catheter insertion site suggests possible catheter-related infection. However, coagulase-negative staphylococci (the most common cause of such infections) seldom cause overt signs of infection at the catheter site. As a result, examination of the catheter site has a very low sensitivity for detection of catheter colonization or infection (231). Early attempts to diagnose intravascular catheter-related infection using nonquantitative cultures of catheter tips in broth media yielded a high rate of false-positive cultures, and such methods have been abandoned. Maki et al. (232) developed a semiquantitative method for culturing intravascular catheters, and this technique has contributed considerably to our understanding of catheter-related infections. Subsequently, Gram stain or acridine orange stain of catheter tips (233,234), culture of the skin at the insertion site (235), quantitative cultures of catheter tips or central venous catheter hubs (140, 236–239), and quantitative blood cultures obtained through the catheter and from peripheral veins have been evaluated for their utility in diagnosing catheter-related infections (240,241). The semiquantitative roll plate method has been the most widely used, but recent studies suggest that this method may miss a substantial number of episodes of significant catheter colonization when only the catheter tip segment is cultured (242). Nonetheless, it is still used in many laboratories because of its simplicity and clinical utility. Sonication of both the tip and the subcutaneous segment of a catheter is slightly more time-consuming, but may detect catheter-related bloodstream infections with greater sensitivity (242). When catheter-related infection is suspected in patients with nontunneled central catheters, quantitative cultures of the skin at the catheter exit site may help establish the presence of catheter-related infection (243). However, such cultures have poor sensitivity for detecting catheter-related infections in low-risk patients. In patients with implanted catheters or ports, paired quantitative blood cultures drawn through the catheter and from a peripheral vein suggest catheter-related bloodstream infection when the colony count of the culture drawn through the catheter is five- or tenfold higher than that drawn from a peripheral vein (244). Also, if a blood culture drawn through a catheter becomes positive 2 hours or more before a culture drawn from a peripheral vein, it is likely that the catheter is the source of the bloodstream infection (244).

When *S. epidermidis* or other coagulase-negative staphylococci are recovered from multiple blood cultures and from catheter segments or hubs, isolates should be compared with respect to their species and antimicrobial susceptibility pattern. The diagnosis of *S. epidermidis* catheter-related bloodstream infection is likely if all isolates represent the same species and have similar or identical antimicrobial susceptibility patterns (81). Whenever possible, it is also desirable to compare blood and catheter isolates using genotypic typing systems such as electrophoresis of restriction endonuclease digests of plasmid DNA or pulsed-field gel electrophoresis of chromosomal DNA (81,245) (see also Chapters 17 and 18).

Bacteremia

Although most coagulase-negative staphylococcal bacteremias are associated with indwelling intravascular catheters, hospitalized patients may develop bacteremia unrelated to vascular catheters. Because coagulase-negative staphylococci are common contaminants of blood cultures and may also cause bacteremia or septicemia, establishing the clinical significance of blood cultures yielding these microorganisms is problematic. This dilemma often results in unnecessary utilization of laboratory tests and antibiotics, and may prolong hospital stays (246). Unfortunately, there are no standard criteria for diagnosing coagulase-negative staphylococcal bacteremia, and many different definitions have been used (5,36,141,149,247). The following factors need to be considered in assessing the significance of blood cultures positive for *S. epidermidis*:

1. Is there an indwelling foreign body such as a prosthetic vascular graft, ventriculoatrial shunt, or prosthetic joint that would put the patient at increased risk for a coagulase-negative staphylococcal infection?
2. Does the patient have any underlying conditions such as widespread dermatitis or a focal infection caused by coagulase-negative staphylococci that would increase the risk of the microorganism entering the bloodstream?
3. What percent of blood cultures obtained from a given patient yielded coagulase-negative staphylococci?
4. When multiple cultures yield the microorganism, are the isolates the same species and do they have the same antimicrobial susceptibility pattern, plasmid profile, or chromosomal DNA restriction endonuclease digest pattern?
5. What is the interval between the day the cultures were obtained and the day the cultures first showed detectable growth?
6. Does the patient have clinical signs or symptoms of infection?

When multiple blood cultures obtained from a patient with signs of infection yield isolates that are the same species and have identical antibiotic sensitivity patterns or genotypic characteristics, then true bloodstream infection is usually present. In contrast, if only one of several sets of blood cultures inoculated yields the microorganism after 4 or 5 days of incubation, the isolate often represents a contaminant. However, even patients with a single blood culture positive for these microorganisms must be evaluated carefully, especially if a foreign body is present (141,149) (see also Chapter 19).

Surgical Site Infections

The diagnosis of surgical site infections caused by coagulase-negative staphylococci should be based on criteria recommended by the CDC (152,153). *S. epidermidis* or other coagulase-negative staphylococci are often considered the cause of a surgical site infection if the microorganism is recovered in pure culture or as a predominant pathogen, even if accompanied by other potential pathogens, from an abscess or purulent drainage from the affected site (see also Chapter 21).

Endocarditis

Establishing the diagnosis of nosocomial coagulase-negative staphylococcal endocarditis is often difficult, and there is no consensus regarding the criteria that should be used (37,166, 248–250). Patients may develop hospital-acquired coagulase-negative staphylococcal endocarditis from a few days up to 1 year after valve replacement, or occasionally after insertion of a pacemaker or long-term intravascular catheter (166,248). It is reasonable to make the diagnosis of prosthetic valve endocarditis if the following criteria are met: (a) two or more blood cultures yield the same strain of coagulase-negative staphylococcus, and (b) there is either a clinical illness compatible with bacterial endocarditis or histopathologic evidence of endocarditis at surgery or autopsy (37,248). Most patients have fever and prosthetic valve dysfunction accompanied by a new or changing regurgitant murmur (166). Demonstration of valvular dysfunction, a vegetation, or valve ring abscess by echocardiography can help establish the diagnosis in some cases.

Pacemaker Infections

The criteria for diagnosing coagulase-negative staphylococcal infections involving an implantable pacemaker or cardioverter defibrillator include: (a) recovery of the microorganism (often moderate to heavy growth) from the generator, defibrillator, or electrodes at the time of removal or from purulent material obtained from the affected site; and (b) local inflammation, pain, or abscess formation involving the pacemaker generator or defibrillator pocket or the skin overlying the subcutaneous portions of the device leads (249,251,252). Fever may or may not be present. Bacteremia due to an infected pacemaker is usually accompanied by fever and chills, but local signs or symptoms of infection may be absent (249,251). Blood cultures usually yield the same strain of coagulase-negative *Staphylococcus* from multiple blood cultures. Differentiating uncomplicated bacteremia from endocarditis may be difficult in patients who have an infected pacemaker (see also Chapter 62).

Vascular Grafts

The diagnosis of a vascular graft infection is often suggested by the presence on physical examination of erythema or purulence involving the surgical incision, or formation of a sinus tract or pseudoaneurysm at the site of the vascular anastomosis (175). If a sinus tract develops, a sinogram can help establish if the graft is likely to be involved.

When graft material is excised from patients with suspected infection, culturing the graft with a swab that is then used to inoculate agar media alone will often result in false-negative cultures. Culturing graft material in broth media increases the likelihood of recovering *S. epidermidis* (105,253). However, if possible, a portion of the excised graft material should be disrupted using a tissue grinder and then placed in broth media, or placed in broth and ultrasonically oscillated for several minutes before incubation (173,174,253). These procedures release microorganisms that may be trapped in biofilm, and maximize the chances of recovering *S. epidermidis* from explanted vascular grafts.

Prosthetic Orthopedic Devices

Specific diagnosis of prosthetic joint infection often requires aspiration of the joint and culture of synovial fluid. Both aerobic and anaerobic cultures should be performed if sufficient fluid is obtained. In some instances, culturing tissue obtained by arthrotomy or debridement of the incision may be necessary. There are no widely accepted criteria for establishing the diagnosis of prosthetic joint infection caused by coagulase-negative staphylococci. If large numbers of colonies are obtained from synovial fluid or tissue specimens, or the same microorganism is recovered from a second joint aspiration, it is likely to be the causative agent.

Cerebrospinal Fluid Shunts and Intracranial Pressure Monitoring Devices

The diagnosis of coagulase-negative staphylococcal ventriculoperitoneal shunt infection should be suspected if the patient develops unexplained fever within 2 months of insertion, especially if there is evidence of shunt dysfunction (254). Occasionally, patients develop abdominal pain or signs of peritonitis.

The diagnosis is confirmed by isolating the microorganism from CSF obtained from cerebral ventricles or from the shunt. (187,254). If signs of meningeal irritation are present, and fluid obtained from the shunt is nondiagnostic, fluid for cultures should be obtained by lumbar puncture. In most instances, spinal fluid cultures planted on agar as well as broth cultures will yield *S. epidermidis*, and CSF neutrophilic pleocytosis will be present. A mononuclear pleocytosis accompanied by elevated CSF protein is common in infants with shunts, and should not be construed as indicating infection (254). Recovery of coagulase-negative staphylococci from the shunt itself at the time of removal can also establish the diagnosis (187). Ventriculoatrial shunt infection is usually diagnosed by finding multiple blood cultures positive for the same strain of coagulase-negative *Staphylococcus* (254).

In patients who have undergone ventriculostomy, the diagnosis of meningitis or ventriculitis is made by recovering coagulase-negative staphylococci from CSF obtained by lumbar puncture or through the ventricular catheter (190). In such patients, pleocytosis alone is not sufficient to establish the diagnosis of CSF infection.

In patients who have epidural catheters in place for up to 2 weeks, recovery of coagulase-negative staphylococci from the skin at the catheter entry site or from quantitative or semiquantitative catheter cultures is relatively common. However, isolation of these microorganisms from such cultures usually reflects colonization or superficial infection of the entry site or catheter colonization, not epidural abscess (255) (see also Chapters 27, 49, and 67).

Continuous Ambulatory Peritoneal Dialysis–Related Infections

Coagulase-negative staphylococci cause 30% to 45% of cases of CAPD-related peritonitis, and can be recovered from effluent peritoneal fluid in 90% of cases if at least 30 mL of fluid is concentrated, centrifuged, or filtered before being cultured (191, 193). Whenever possible, about 20 mL should be either filtered through a 0.45-μm filter or centrifuged at 5,000 *g* for 15 minutes, and then cultured aerobically and anaerobically (193,256). Filters can be divided into halves for plating on different media. Some authorities favor dividing an additional 10 mL of effluent fluid into two aliquots, and injecting these into aerobic and anaerobic blood culture media (193).

The diagnosis of coagulase-negative staphylococcal exit site infection is usually based on the presence of erythema or purulence at the catheter exit site, accompanied by recovery of moderate to heavy growth of the microorganism from cultures obtained from the affected area (see also Chapter 65).

Infections in Neonates

Many different criteria have been used for diagnosing coagulase-negative staphylococcal bacteremia in neonates (7,199,201, 202,204,206–208,214). Interpretation of blood cultures yielding coagulase-negative staphylococci is more difficult in neonates, because the volume of blood drawn is often small (0.1 to 1.0 mL), and only a single culture is obtained in some instances because of the small blood volume of neonates (202). As a result, determining if a positive culture represents a contaminant versus true bacteremia is sometimes based on the results of a single blood culture and other laboratory and clinical parameters.

The diagnosis of coagulase-negative staphylococcal bacteremia would appear likely if two or more blood cultures obtained at separate venipunctures yield the microorganism (same species and same antimicrobial susceptibility pattern) (201,214). However, it is also reasonable to make the diagnosis of bacteremic infection if a single blood culture is positive and the patient has laboratory evidence of infection (e.g., increased number of immature neutrophils or increased C-reactive protein level in serum) and clinical signs suggestive of infection (199,202). The diagnosis of coagulase-negative staphylococcal infection at other body sites is usually made on the basis of recovery of the microorganism from pus or normally sterile body fluids, sometimes accompanied by a positive blood culture (204) (see also Chapter 52).

Endophthalmitis Following Intraocular Lens Implantation

In cases of suspected endophthalmitis, specimens of vitreous and aqueous obtained at the time of vitrectomy should be submitted for both Gram stain and culture (111,223). The responsible microorganism is isolated from vitreous specimens in most cases; anterior chamber cultures have a lower yield. Because coagulase-negative staphylococci commonly colonize conjunctival surfaces and the eyelids, and can contaminate specimens obtained at the time of ophthalmic surgery, the diagnosis of *S. epidermidis* pseudophakic endophthalmitis is usually based on the recovery of the same microorganism on two or more media, or heavy (or repeated) growth of the same microorganism on a single medium (111,112,223).

EPIDEMIOLOGY OF NOSOCOMIAL INFECTIONS CAUSED BY COAGULASE-NEGATIVE STAPHYLOCOCCI

In the early 1990s, coagulase-negative staphylococci accounted for 11% of all pathogens recovered from nosocomial infections (38,39). Of the estimated 2.1 million nosocomial infections that occur annually in the United States, coagulase-negative staphylococci probably account for approximately 230,000 (Table 30.1) (39,257).

Data from the NNIS system indicate that coagulase-negative staphylococci are the third most common pathogen, after *E. coli* and *S. aureus*. The proportion of nosocomial urinary tract infections and lower respiratory tract infections caused by coagulase-negative staphylococci has remained low (4% and 2%, respectively) over the years (Fig. 30.3). The increasing role of these microorganisms as nosocomial pathogens is due primarily to the increased frequency with which they have been recovered from primary bloodstream infections and surgical site infections. Data from surveillance conducted in medical-surgical intensive care units revealed that these pathogens account for 39% of isolates recovered from primary bloodstream infections, 12% of those from surgical site infections, and a smaller proportion of isolates recovered from infections at other major body sites (9).

The overall incidence of nosocomial coagulase-negative staphylococcal bloodstream infections, including both primary and secondary bacteremias, has been reported to be about 4.5 episodes/1,000 discharges (141,258). The incidence of primary bloodstream infection due to these microorganisms varies considerably, depending on the type and size of institution. In institutions reporting to NNIS, the incidence is 0.31/1,000 discharges in small nonteaching hospitals, 0.67/1,000 discharges in large nonteaching hospitals, 1.10/1,000 discharges in small teaching hospitals, and 1.83/1,000 discharges in large teaching hospitals (136). A majority of these *S. epidermidis* primary bloodstream infections are related to intravascular catheters. Coagulase-negative staphylococcal bloodstream infections occur with the highest incidence in intensive care units (including high-risk

TABLE 30.1. ESTIMATED NUMBER OF NOSOCOMIAL INFECTIONS YIELDING COAGULASE-NEGATIVE STAPHYLOCOCCI ANNUALLY IN THE UNITED STATES

Site	Percent of All Infections[a]	Estimated Number of Infections Per Year[b]	Percent Positive for Coagulase-Negative Staphylococci[a]	Estimated Number of Infections Positive for Coagulase-Negative Staphylococci
UTI	33.1	695,100	4%	27,800
SSI	14.8	310,800	14%	43,500
BSI	13.1	275,100	31%	85,300
Pn	15.5	325,500	2%	6,510
Other	23.5	493,500	14%	69,100

[a] Data from Emori and Gaynes (39).
[b] Data from Haley et al. (257).
UTI, urinary tract infection; SSI, surgical site infection; BSI, bloodstream infection; Pn, pneumonia.

nurseries) and on general surgery and medical services, and are least common on obstetrics and gynecology services. In neonates who require prolonged intensive care, the incidence of coagulase-negative staphylococci bloodstream infection varies among hospitals, based in part on the percent of neonates who weigh less than 1,500 g and on the frequency with which umbilical or central line catheters are used (device utilization rates) in the respective institutions (259).

Surgical site infections are much more common than implant-related infections, and occur on general and subspecialty surgical services. Table 30.2 lists the estimated incidence of coagulase-negative staphylococcal infections related to various implanted prostheses. A majority of urinary tract infections caused by these microorganisms are probably associated with the use of indwelling bladder catheters.

Most nosocomial infections caused by coagulase-negative staphylococci represent endemic infections. However, epidemics due to these pathogens have been reported. Several clusters or outbreaks of infection following cardiac surgery have been reported, and in each instance, various phenotypic or genotypic typing systems were used to establish that the outbreaks were due to transmission of a single strain or closely related strains (48,50,69,78–80,84,167,260,261). In addition, small outbreaks of septicemia or other serious infections have been reported in intensive care units (5,36,57,71,75,207). Such outbreaks may be documented with greater frequency in the future as more hospitals adopt genotypic typing systems that can establish the degree of genetic relatedness of isolates recovered from infected patients.

Reservoirs or Sources of Infection

Nosocomial coagulase-negative staphylococcal infections may be caused by endogenous strains that are colonizing the patient at the time of admission, or by strains acquired in the hospital. Since areas of normal skin may be populated with 10 to 10^5 CFU/cm^2 of coagulase-negative staphylococci, even careful aseptic technique cannot remove these microorganisms from the skin at the time of invasive procedures (17,262,263). It is widely believed that coagulase-negative staphylococci on the skin adjacent to catheter entry sites or surgical incisions are often the source of catheter-related infections, surgical site infections, and infected implanted prostheses (107,111,115,168,171,186,254, 264,265). Genotypic typing systems have been used to confirm

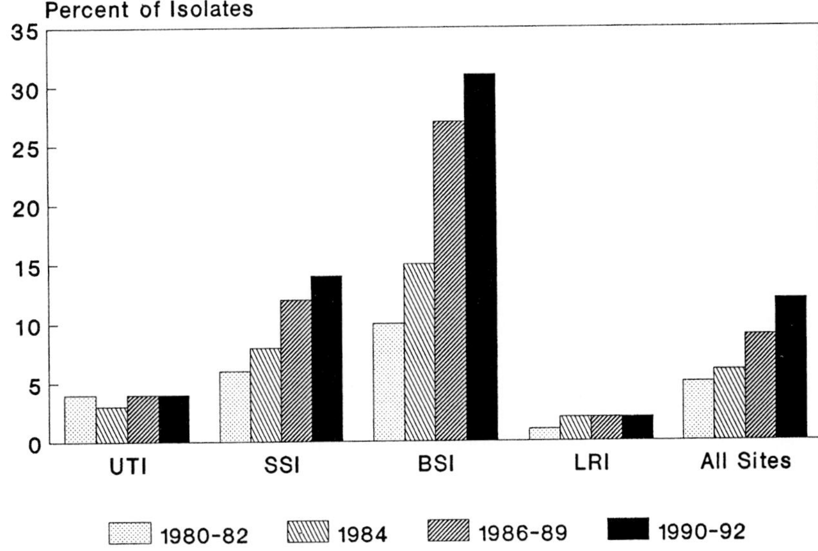

Figure 30.3. Percent of isolates from nosocomial infections in National Nosocomial Infections Surveillance system hospitals that were coagulase-negative staphylococci, for the periods 1980–1982, 1984, 1986–1989, and 1990–1992, by body site. UTI, urinary tract infection; SSI, surgical site infection; BSI, bloodstream infection; LRI, lower respiratory infection.

TABLE 30.2. OVERALL FREQUENCY OF INFECTIONS AND PERCENT OF INFECTIONS. DUE TO COAGULASE-NEGATIVE STAPHYLOCOCCI FOLLOWING SURGICAL IMPLANTATION OF PROSTHESES

Procedure	Overall Rate of Infection (%)	Percent Due to Coagulase-Negative Staphylococci	No. of Coagulase-Negative Staphylococci Infections 100 Procedures
PVE	1–4	30	0.3–1.2
Cardiac pacer	4–6	30–45	1.5–2.3
Prosthetic joints			
THR	0.5–1	30	0.15–0.3
TKR	3		
CSF shunts	4–8	40–66	1.6–5.3
CAPD peritonitis		25–50	1–2/pt/year
Lens implants	0.1	40–60	0.04–0.06
Breast implants	1		
GU implants	2–5	40–50	0.8–2.5

PVE, prosthetic valve endocarditis; THR, total hip replacement; TKR, total knee replacement; CSF, cerebrospinal fluid; CAPD, chronic ambulatory peritoneal dialysis; GU, genitourinary.

the genetic relatedness of isolates colonizing the patient's skin and those recovered from clinical infections (196,245, 266–268). Coagulase-negative staphylococci from the patient's skin may contaminate the catheter hub, which can then serve as a source of bacteremia. In patients undergoing chronic ambulatory peritoneal dialysis, many episodes of *S. epidermidis* peritonitis are not preceded by catheter exit site infection, suggesting that microorganisms from the patient's hands or other skin surfaces enter the peritoneal dialysis catheter by touch contamination or colonized skin squames that enter the system during bag changes (193,194,266). In neonates and immunocompromised patients, coagulase-negative staphylococci that are colonizing the patient's mucous membranes may also be a source of microorganisms that subsequently cause infection (86,93,204). It has also been suggested that lymph nodes or arterial aneurysms may contain coagulase-negative staphylococci that could contaminate the wound during vascular surgery (175,269). However, there is only limited evidence to support this viewpoint.

Community-acquired strains of *S. epidermidis* are most likely to cause nosocomial infections in individuals who have short preoperative stays, and have had little opportunity to become colonized with microorganisms acquired in the hospital. Most community-acquired strains responsible for colonizing or infecting patients are susceptible to methicillin (37,262). However, up to 20% of isolates that appear to be community-acquired may be methicillin-resistant (37,262). Patients who become colonized with resistant coagulase-negative staphylococci while hospitalized may also serve as a source from which further transmission may occur (98,267).

Colonized healthcare workers are an important source from which patients acquire coagulase-negative staphylococci in hospitals. In the 1950s, Koiwai and Nahas (1) obtained intraoperative cultures of fingers of surgeons who were performing digital mitral valve commissurotomy procedures without using gloves. One patient who underwent this procedure subsequently developed endocarditis due to a coagulase-negative *Staphylococcus* of the same type recovered from the surgeon intraoperatively. Later studies used genotypic typing systems to confirm that strains of *S. epidermidis* colonizing the hands of cardiac surgeons were identical to those recovered from patients with prosthetic valve endocarditis or sternal wound infections (69,80,260). Outbreaks of infection related to these surgeons stopped when the offending microorganism was eradicated from the surgeons' hands (69, 80).

Studies demonstrating that ultra-clean air systems, surgical isolator systems, and the use of body exhaust suits by surgeons reduce intraoperative contamination of wounds and infection rates related to implantation of prosthetic devices provide additional, albeit indirect, evidence that healthcare workers are a source from which coagulase-negative staphylococci may be transmitted (186,270,271). The fact that only a fraction of the coagulase-negative staphylococci that contaminate the operative field during implant surgery can be traced to the patient's skin also suggests that surgical personnel may be the source of coagulase-negative staphylococci responsible for foreign body infections (265,272,273). Finally, the same strains of multidrug resistant *S. epidermidis* responsible for colonization or infection in patients have been isolated from healthcare workers, suggesting that personnel may serve as a reservoir (5,36,48–50,78,98,205, 274). NICU personnel may well serve as a source of resistant staphylococci that colonize neonates, whose skin is usually sterile prior to birth. Acquisition of coagulase-negative staphylococci from the mother during birth is not a major source of these microorganisms (275).

Since coagulase-negative staphylococci may be shed from the skin into the environment on skin squames, it is possible that contaminated environmental surfaces could serve as a reservoir for these microorganisms (276). However, the potential role of the inanimate environment as a source of nosocomial coagulase-negative staphylococci has received very little attention. On a few occasions, contaminated parenteral fluids have been identified as the source of nosocomial coagulase-negative staphylococcal bacteremia (6,200). These microorganisms have also been recovered from medical equipment and irrigating solutions used during surgery, from the clothing of personnel and from environmental surfaces, but the epidemiologic significance of these findings is not clear (5,50,166,188,226).

Modes of Transmission

Because appropriate methods for differentiating one strain of coagulase-negative *S. epidermidis* from another have become available only recently, our understanding of how these microorganisms are transmitted is limited. Direct contact transmission occurs in some instances, as evidenced by outbreaks of infection related to cardiac surgeons whose hands were contaminated with the epidemic strain (1,69,80,260). In three outbreaks, contamination clearly occurred during the surgical procedure, suggesting that the microorganism was spread directly from the surgeon's hands to the operative field (1,69,80). In one instance, only the surgeon's hands were colonized with the epidemic strain, essentially eliminating transmission by other routes such as droplet spread or airborne transmission (80). During surgical procedures, surgeons frequently tear their gloves, which would allow microorganisms colonizing their hands to fall into the operative field (264,277). Recovery of antibiotic-resistant strains of coagulase-negative staphylococci from the hands of personnel also suggests that the microorganism may be spread from colonized personnel to patients by direct contact transmission (50,78,274). Poor handwashing practices or failure to change gloves between patients may result in transmission of the microorganism from one colonized patient to another by personnel.

Airborne transmission is another route by which coagulase-negative staphylococci may be spread from hospital personnel to patients, although convincing evidence for this is limited. Blakemore et al. (278) recovered the same strain of *S. albus* (*S. epidermidis*) from air samples and from blood samples obtained from a cardiopulmonary bypass machine during surgery. Since about 2 cubic feet of air per minute is aspirated through the coronary suction line when it is not being used to suction blood from the operative field, numerous airborne bacteria (including coagulase-negative staphylococci) can be aspirated from operating room air into the blood supply of the bypass machine (278, 279). Bacteria can also be recovered from the air adjacent to the operative field, which raises the possibility that airborne microorganisms may contaminate the wound during surgery (273,278). A majority of such bacteria are coagulase-negative staphylococci. These microorganisms are presumably shed from operating room staff, since the number of airborne bacteria is highest when many personnel are present in the room (80,278). The fact that ultra-clean air handling systems and surgical isolator systems, which reduce the number of airborne bacteria in the operative field, reduce infection rates among patients undergoing implant surgery also suggests that airborne transmission accounts for some cases of nosocomial coagulase-negative staphylococcal infection (186,270,271). *S. epidermidis* has been isolated from air samples or settle plates on wards where colonized or infected patients were located, but the extent to which airborne staphylococci contribute to transmission in these settings is not clear (50,57,205,226). Additional studies are needed to establish the relative importance of airborne transmission in the spread of these pathogens.

It is possible that indirect transmission of coagulase-negative staphylococci by fomites such as clothing of personnel or contaminated medical equipment may occur, but appropriate studies to address this issue have not been done (226).

Prevention and Control

No control measures have been evaluated specifically for their ability to reduce the incidence of nosocomial coagulase-negative staphylococcal infections. However, there is evidence that many general measures may be used either to reduce the risk of infection caused by endogenous strains of staphylococci, or to reduce the risk that nosocomial strains will colonize and infect the patient.

Since coagulase-negative staphylococci are sometimes transmitted via the hands of personnel, new CDC recommendations for healthcare worker hand hygiene should be followed (280). To reduce the incidence of intravascular catheter-related bloodstream infections caused by coagulase-negative staphylococci, hospitals should adopt general guidelines designed to prevent intravascular catheter-related infections (281). Of the many measures recommended, major emphasis should be placed on (a) educating and training healthcare workers who insert and maintain catheters; (b) using maximal sterile barrier precautions for insertion central venous catheters; (c) using a chlorhexidine preparation for cleaning the skin at the insertion site; (d) avoiding routine replacement of central venous catheters as a strategy to prevent infection; and (e) using antiseptic- or antimicrobial-coated impregnated central venous catheters if the rate of catheter-related bloodstream infections remains high despite adherence to the first three recommendations cited above (281). Although several studies have found that antimicrobial-impregnated catheters can reduce catheter-related bloodstream infections (282,283), there is presently considerable controversy over exactly when (in which clinical settings or patient subpopulations) catheters coated with intraluminal plus extraluminal minocycline/rifampin or chlorhexidine/silver sulfadiazine are cost-effective (284–287).

General recommendations for preventing surgical site infections were issued by the CDC in 1999 (288). The measures recommended can be expected to reduce the incidence of incisional and organ/space infections as well as foreign body-related infections due to *S. epidermidis.*

General guidelines for preoperative hand antisepsis and sterilization of operating room instruments should lower the risk of surgical site infections caused by *S. epidermidis* (280,288). Preoperative use of an alcohol-based hand rub with persistent activity is now considered an appropriate alternative to scrubbing hands with an antimicrobial soap (280), and one prospective clinical trial demonstrated that the incidence of surgical site infections among patients whose surgeons cleaned their hands with an alcohol-based hand rub was identical to the rate among patients whose surgeons cleaned their hands using a traditional antimicrobial soap regimen (289). Changing gloves promptly following glove tears may lower the risk of infection, particularly during cardiac or implant surgery. It has been suggested that clamping the coronary suction tubing when not in use may reduce contamination of the operative field by airborne coagulase-negative staphylococci during cardiac surgery (278). Some surgeons favor soaking synthetic vascular grafts or other prosthetic devices in an antibiotic-containing solution prior to implantation, but the efficacy and safety of this practice has not been established (115,169,254).

Since personnel are one of the sources of coagulase-negative staphylococci that may contaminate operating room air as well as the surgical field, the number and movement of personnel in the operating room should be kept to a minimum. Limited published data also suggest that use of plastic isolator systems during implantation of CSF shunts and genitourinary prostheses may reduce the incidence of foreign body–related infections (115,186,271). Operating rooms with conventional ventilation should maintain at least 15 air exchanges per hour. Hospitals that perform more than 100 total hip or knee replacement procedures per year may find it cost-effective to use an ultra-clean air system, with or without body exhaust suits or a surgical isolator system (290). However, ultra-clean air systems probably have marginal additional benefit in reducing infection rates when prophylactic antibiotics are used (291).

Prophylactic administration of systemic antibiotics has been shown to lower the incidence of infection following cardiac surgery (292) and implantation of prosthetic devices such as total joint replacements (270,293) and synthetic vascular grafts (294). Although prophylactic antibiotics are often given at the time of CSF shunt placement, there is no consensus regarding their efficacy in this setting (295). For open-heart surgery, first- or second-generation cephalosporins are the agents most widely used for prophylaxis in this country. Cefazolin is still considered a good choice for perioperative prophylaxis during total joint replacement and implantation of vascular grafts (293,296). In facilities where methicillin-resistant staphylococci are a common cause of infections following cardiovascular surgery, it may be acceptable to give a short course of prophylactic vancomycin to patients undergoing placement of a prosthetic valve or vascular graft, or to those who have recently received broad-spectrum antibiotic therapy and require other forms of cardiovascular surgery (171,297). However, wide-scale use of vancomycin for perioperative prophylaxis should be discouraged since this practice is likely to favor the emergence of vancomycin-resistant enterococci (298). Antibiotics such as gentamicin or cefuroxime are incorporated into the cement used in total hip replacement surgery at some centers, particularly for surgical revision of a prosthetic hip joint (181,293,294). Bonding antibiotics to prosthetic vascular grafts is another potential method of administering prophylactic antibiotics locally during implant surgery, but this approach requires additional studies to determine its efficacy (175, 294). Irrigating the operative field with antibiotic-containing solutions is performed during many different types of surgery, but careful studies of its efficacy are lacking. Further studies are warranted to establish the efficacy of many of the above measures in reducing the incidence of nosocomial coagulase-negative staphylococcal infections.

REFERENCES

1. Koiwai EK, Nahas HC. Subacute bacterial endocarditis following cardiac surgery. *Arch Surg* 1956;73:272–278.
2. Denton C, Pappas EG, Uricchio JF, et al. Bacterial endocarditis following cardiac surgery. *Circulation* 1957;15:525–531.
3. Smith IM, Beals PD, Kingsbury KR, et al. Observations on *Staphylococcus albus* septicemia in mice and men. *Arch Intern Med* 1958;102: 375–388.
4. Callaghan RP, Cohen SJ, Stewart GT. Septicaemia due to colonization of Spitz-Holter valves by staphylococci. *Br Med J* 1961;1: 860–863.
5. Forse RA, Dixon C, Bernard K, et al. *Staphylococcus epidermidis*: an important pathogen. *Surgery* 1979;86:507–514.
6. Sitges-Serra A, Puig P, Jaurrieta E, et al. Catheter sepsis due to *Staphylococcus epidermidis* during parenteral nutrition. *Surg Gynecol Obstet* 1980;151:481–483.
7. Goldmann DA, Durbin WA Jr, Freeman J. Nosocomial infections in a neonatal intensive care unit. *J Infect Dis* 1981;144:449–459.
8. Centers for Disease Control. *National Nosocomial Infections Study Report, annual summary 1979.* Atlanta: CDC, 1982.
9. Richards MJ, Edwards JR, Culver DH, et al. Nosocomial infections in combined medical-surgical intensive care units in the United States. *Infect Control Hosp Epidemiol* 2000;21:510–515.
10. Kloos WE, Bannerman TL. Staphylococcus and Micrococcus. In: Murray PR, Baron EJ, Pfaller MA, et al., eds. *Manual of clinical microbiology.* Washington, DC: ASM Press, 1995:282–298.
11. Kloos WE, Lambe DW Jr. Staphylococcus. In: Balows A, Hausler WJ Jr, Herrmann KL, et al., eds. *Manual of clinical microbiology.* Washington, DC: American Society for Microbiology, 1991: 222–237.
12. Kloos WE, Bannerman TL. Update on clinical significance of coagulase-negative staphylococci. *Clin Microbiol Rev* 1994;7:117–140.
13. Ponce de Leon S, Guenthner SH, Wenzel RP. Microbiologic studies of coagulase-negative staphylococci isolated from patients with nosocomial bacteraemias. *J Hosp Infect* 1986;7:121–129.
14. Refsahl K, Andersen BM. Clinically significant coagulase-negative staphylococci: identification and resistance patterns. *J Hosp Infect* 1992;22:19–31.
15. Schnitzler N, Meilicke R, Conrads G, et al. Staphylococcus lugdunensis: report of a case of peritonitis and an easy-to-perform screening strategy. *J Clin Microbiol* 1998;36:812–813.
16. Leung MJ, Nuttall N, Pryce TM, et al. Colony variation in Staphylococcus lugdunensis. *J Clin Microbiol* 1998;36:3096–3098.
17. Kloos WE. Ecology of human skin. In: Mardh PA, Schleifer KH, eds. *Coagulase-negative staphylococci.* Stockholm, Sweden: Almquist and Wiksell International, 1986:37–50.
18. Berke A, Tilton RC. Evaluation of rapid coagulase methods for the identification of *Staphylococcus aureus*. *J Clin Microbiol* 1986;23: 916–919.
19. Fournier JM, Bouvet A, Mathieu D, et al. New latex reagent using monoclonal antibodies to capsular polysaccharide for reliable identification of both oxacillin-susceptible and oxacillin-resistant *Staphylococcus aureus*. *J Clin Microbiol* 1993;31:1342–1344.
20. Gregson DB, Low DE, Skulnick M, et al. Problems with rapid agglutination methods for identification of *Staphylococcus aureus* when *Staphylococcus saprophyticus* is being tested. *J Clin Microbiol* 1988;26: 1398–1399.
21. Kleeman KT, Bannerman TL, Kloos WE. Species distribution of coagulase-negative staphylococcal isolates at a community hospital and implications for selection of staphylococcal identification procedures. *J Clin Microbiol* 1993;31:1318–1321.
22. Woolfrey BF, Lally RT, Ederer MN. An evaluation of three rapid coagglutination tests: sero STAT, Accu-Staph, and Staphyloslide, for differentiating *Staphylococcus aureus* from other species of staphylococci. *Am J Clin Pathol* 1984;81:345–348.
23. Aldridge KE, Kogos C, Sanders CV, et al. Comparison of rapid identification assays for *Staphylococcus aureus*. *J Clin Microbiol* 1984;19: 703–704.
24. Pfaller MA, Herwaldt LA. Laboratory, clinical, and epidemiological aspects of coagulase-negative staphylococci. *Clin Microbiol Rev* 1988; 1:281–299.
25. Hebert GA, Crowder CG, Hancock GA, et al. Characteristics of coagulase-negative staphylococci that help differentiate these species and other members of the family Micrococcaceae. *J Clin Microbiol* 1988; 26:1939–1949.
26. Thornsberry C. Methicillin-resistant staphylococci. *Clin Lab Med* 1989;9:255–267.
27. Hackbarth CJ, Chambers HF. Methicillin-resistant staphylococci: de-

tection methods and treatment of infections. *Antimicrob Agents Chemother* 1989;33:995–999.

28. Horstkotte MA, Knobloch JKM, Rohde H, et al. Rapid detection of methicillin resistance in coagulase-negative staphylococci with the VITEK 2 system. *J Clin Microbiol* 2002;40:3291–3295.
29. Ramotar K, Woods W, Toye B. Oxacillin susceptibility testing of Staphylococcus saprophyticus using disk diffusion, agar dilution, broth microdilution, and the Vitek GPS-105 card. *Diagn Microbiol Infect Dis* 2001;40:203–205.
30. Louie L, Majury A, Goodfellow J, et al. Evaluation of a latex agglutination test (MRSA-Screen) for detection of oxacillin resistance in coagulase-negative staphylococci. *J Clin Microbiol* 2001;39:4149–4151.
31. Elek SD, Fleming PC. A new technique for the control of hospital cross-infection. Experience with BRL.1241 in a maternity unit. *Lancet* 1960;2:569–572.
32. Stewart GT. Changes in sensitivity of staphylococci to methicillin. *Br Med J* 1961;1:863–866.
33. Kjellander JO, Klein JO, Finland M. *In vitro* activity of penicillins against *Staphylococcus albus. Proc Soc Exp Biol Med* 1963;113: 1023–1031.
34. Archer GL. Antimicrobial susceptibility and selection of resistance among *Staphylococcus epidermidis* isolates recovered from patients with infections of indwelling foreign devices. *Antimicrob Agents Chemother* 1978;14:353–359.
35. Archer GL, Tenenbaum MJ. Antibiotic-resistant Staphylococcus epidermidis in patients undergoing cardiac surgery. *Antimicrob Agents Chemother* 1980;17:269–272.
36. Christensen GD, Bisno AL, Parisi JT, et al. Nosocomial septicemia due to multiply antibiotic-resistant *Staphylococcus epidermidis. Ann Intern Med* 1982;96:1–10.
37. Karchmer AW, Archer GL, Dismukes WE. *Staphylococcus epidermidis* causing prosthetic valve endocarditis: microbiologic and clinical observations as guides to therapy. *Ann Intern Med* 1983;98:447–455.
38. Schaberg DR, Culver DH, Gaynes RP. Major trends in the microbial etiology of nosocomial infection. *Am J Med* 1991;91:72S–75S.
39. Emori TG, Gaynes RP. An overview of nosocomial infections, including the role for the microbiology laboratory. *Clin Microbiol Rev* 1993; 6:428–442.
40. Centers for Disease Control and Prevention. National Nosocomial Infections Surveillance (NNIS) system report, data summary from January 1992–June 2001, Issued August 2001. *Am J Infect Control* 2001;29:404–421.
41. Ubukata K, Yamashita N, Konno M. Occurrence of a beta-lactam-inducible penicillin-binding protein in methicillin-resistant staphylococci. *Antimicrob Agents Chemother* 1985;27:851–857.
42. Chambers HF. Coagulase-negative staphylococci resistant to β-lactam antibiotics in vivo produce penicillin-binding protein 2a. *Antimicrob Agents Chemother* 1987;31:1919–1924.
43. Froggatt JW, Johnston JL, Galetto DW, et al. Antimicrobial resistance in nosocomial isolates of Staphylococcus haemolyticus. *Antimicrob Agents Chemother* 1989;33:460–466.
44. Murakami K, Minamide W, Wada K, et al. Identification of methicillin-resistant strains of staphylococci by polymerase chain reaction. *J Clin Microbiol* 1991;29:2240–2244.
45. Suzuki E, Hiramatsu K, Yokota T. Survey of methicillin-resistant clinical strains of coagulase-negative staphylococci for *mecA* gene distribution. *Antimicrob Agents Chemother* 1992;36:429–434.
46. Ubukata K, Nonoguchi R, Song MD, et al. Homology of mecA gene in methicillin-resistant Staphylococcus haemolyticus and Staphylococcus simulans to that of Staphylococcus aureus. *Antimicrob Agents Chemother* 1990;34:170–172.
47. Archer GL, Vazquez GJ, Johnston JL. Antibiotic prophylaxis of experimental endocarditis due to methicillin-resistant *Staphylococcus epidermidis. J Infect Dis* 1980;142:725.
48. Blouse LE, Lathrop GD, Kolonel LN, et al. Epidemiologic features and phage types associated with nosocomial infections caused by Staphylococcus epidermidis. Zentralbl Bakteriol Hyg 1978;241: 119–135.
49. Archer GL, Dietrick DR, Johnston JL. Molecular epidemiology of transmissible gentamicin resistance among coagulase-negative staphylococci in a cardiac surgery unit. *J Infect Dis* 1985;151:243–251.
50. Houang ET, Marples RR, Weir I, et al. Problems in the investigation of an apparent outbreak of coagulase-negative staphylococcal septicaemia following cardiac surgery. *J Hosp Infect* 1986;8:224–232.
51. Archer GL. Molecular epidemiology of multiresistant Staphylococcus epidermidis. *J Antimicrob Chemother* 1988;21(suppl C):133–138.
52. Galetto DW, Johnston JL, Archer GL. Molecular epidemiology of trimethoprim resistance among coagulase-negative staphylococci. *Antimicrob Agents Chemother* 1987;31:1683–1688.
53. Jaffe HW, Sweeney HM, Nathan C, et al. Identify and interspecific transfer of gentamicin-resistance plasmids in *Staphylococcus aureus* and *Staphylococcus epidermidis. J Infect Dis* 1980;141:738–747.
54. Forbes BA, Schaberg DR. Transfer of resistance plasmids from *Staphylococcus epidermidis* to *Staphylococcus aureus*: evidence for conjugative exchange of resistance. *J Bacteriol* 1983;153:627–634.
55. Cohen ML, Wong ES, Falkow S. Common R-plasmids in *Staphylococcus aureus* and *Staphylococcus epidermidis* during a nosocomial *Staphylococcus aureus* outbreak. *Antimicrob Agents Chemother* 1982;21: 210–215.
56. McDonnell RW, Sweeney HM, Cohen S. Conjugational transfer of gentamicin resistance plasmids intra- and interspecifically in *Staphylococcus aureus* and *Staphylococcus epidermidis. Antimicrob Agents Chemother* 1983;23:151–160.
57. Oppenheim BA, Hartley JW, Lee W, et al. Outbreak of coagulase negative staphylococcus highly resistant to ciprofloxacin in a leukaemia unit. *Br Med J* 1989;299:294–297.
58. Schwalbe RS, Stapleton JT, Gilligan PH. Emergence of vancomycin resistance in coagulase-negative staphylococci. *N Engl J Med* 1987; 316:927–931.
59. Goldstein FW, Coutrot A, Sieffer A, et al. Percentages and distributions of teicoplanin- and vancomycin-resistant strains among coagulase-negative staphylococci. *Antimicrob Agents Chemother* 1990;34: 899–900.
60. Maugein J, Pellegrin JL, Brossard G, et al. In vitro activities of vancomycin and teicoplanin against coagulase-negative staphylococci isolated from neutropenic patients. *Antimicrob Agents Chemother* 1990; 34:901–903.
61. Johnson AP, Henwood C, Mushtaq S, et al. Susceptibility of gram-positive bacteria from ICU patients in US hospitals to antimicrobial agents. *J Hosp Infect* 2003;54:179–187.
62. Pagano L, Tacconelli E, Tumbarello M, et al. Teicoplanin-resistant coagulase-negative staphylococcal bacteraemia in patients with haematological malignancies: a problem of increasing importance. *J Antimicrob Chemother* 1997;40:738–740.
63. Schwalbe RS, Ritz WJ, Verma PR, et al. Selection for vancomycin resistance in clinical isolates Staphylococcus haemolyticus. *J Infect Dis* 1990;161:45–51.
64. Veach LA, Pfaller MA, Barrett M, et al. Vancomycin resistance in *Staphylococcus haemolyticus* causing colonization and bloodstream infection. *J Clin Microbiol* 1990;28:2064–2068.
65. Sieradzki K, Villari P, Tomasz A. Decreased susceptibilities to teicoplanin and vancomycin among coagulase-negative methicillin-resistant clinical isolates of staphylococci. *Antimicrob Agents Chemother* 1998;42:100–107.
66. Van Der Zwet WC, Debets-Ossenkopp YJ, Reinders E, et al. Nosocomial spread of a *Staphylococcus capitis* strain with heteroresistance to vancomycin in a neonatal intensive care unit. *J Clin Microbiol* 2002; 40:2520–2525.
67. Blouse LE, Kolonel LN, Watkins CA, et al. Efficacy of phage typing epidemiologically related *Staphylococcus epidermidis* strains. *J Clin Microbiol* 1975;2:318–321.
68. Christensen GD, Parisi JT, Bisno AL, et al. Characterization of clinically significant strains of coagulase-negative staphylococci. *J Clin Microbiol* 1983;18:258–269.
69. Van Den Broek PJ, Lampe AS, Berbee GAM, et al. Epidemic of prosthetic valve endocarditis caused by *Staphylococcus epidermidis. Br Med J* 1985;291:949–950.
70. Parisi JT, Lampson BC, Hoover DL, et al. Comparison of epidemio-

logic markers for *Staphylococcus epidermidis. J Clin Microbiol* 1986; 24:56–60.

71. Renaud F, Freney J, Etienne J, et al. Restriction endonuclease analysis of Staphylococcus epidermidis DNA may be a useful epidemiological marker. *J Clin Microbiol* 1988;26:1729–1734.
72. Herwaldt LA, Boyken LD, Pfaller MA. Biotyping of coagulase-negative staphylococci. 108 isolates from nosocomial bloodstream infections. *Diagn Microbiol Infect Dis* 1990;13:461–466.
73. Etienne J, Renaud F, Bes M, et al. Instability of characteristics amongst coagulase-negative staphylococci causing endocarditis. *J Med Microbiol* 1990;32:115–122.
74. Bialkowska-Hobrzanska H, Jaskot D, Hammergerg O. Evaluation of restriction endonuclease fingerprinting of chromosomal DNA and plasmid profile analysis for characterization of multiresistant coagulase-negative staphylococci in bacteremic neonates. *J Clin Microbiol* 1990;28:269–275.
75. Walcher-Salesse S, Monzon-Moreno C, Aubert S, et al. An epidemiological assessment of coagulase-negative staphylococci from an intensive care unit. *J Med Microbiol* 1992;36:321–331.
76. Thomson-Carter FM, Pennington TH. Characterization of coagulase-negative staphylococci by sodium dodecyl sulfate-polyacrylamide gel electrophoresis and immunoblot analyses. *J Clin Microbiol* 1989; 27:2199–2203.
77. Kotilainen P, Huovinen P, Eerola E. Application of gas-liquid chromatographic analysis of cellular fatty acids for species identification and typing of coagulase-negative staphylococci. *J Clin Microbiol* 1991; 29:315–322.
78. Marples RR, Hone R, Notley CM, et al. Investigation of coagulase-negative staphylococci from infections in surgical patients. *Zentralbl Bakteriol Hyg* 1978;241:140–156.
79. Mickelsen PA, Plorde JJ, Gordon KP, et al. Instability of antibiotic resistance in a strain of *Staphylococcus epidermidis* isolated from an outbreak of prosthetic valve endocarditis. *J Infect Dis* 1985;152: 50–58.
80. Boyce JM, Potter-Bynoe G, Opal SM, et al. A common-source outbreak of *Staphylococcus epidermidis* infections among patients undergoing cardiac surgery. *J Infect Dis* 1990;161:493–499.
81. Hartstein AI, Valvano MA, Morthland VH, et al. Antimicrobic susceptibility and plasmid profile analysis as identity tests for multiple blood isolates of coagulase-negative staphylococci. *J Clin Microbiol* 1987;25:589–593.
82. Shayegani M, Parsons LM, Waring AL, et al. Molecular relatedness of *Staphylococcus epidermidis* isolates obtained during a platelet transfusion-associated episode of sepsis. *J Clin Microbiol* 1991;29: 2768–2773.
83. Archer GL, Vishniavsky N, Johnston JL. Plasmid-pattern analysis for the differentiation of infecting from noninfecting *Staphylococcus epidermidis. J Infect Dis* 1984;149:913–920.
84. Archer GL, Vishniavsky N, Stiver HG. Plasmid pattern analysis of *Staphylococcus epidermidis* isolates from patients with prosthetic valve endocarditis. *Infect Immun* 1982;35:627–632.
85. Parisi JT, Hecht DW. Plasmid profiles in epidemiologic studies of infections by *Staphylococcus epidermidis. J Infect Dis* 1980;141: 637–643.
86. Herwaldt LA, Hollis RJ, Boyken LD, et al. Molecular epidemiology of coagulase-negative staphylococci isolated from immunocompromised patients. *Infect Control Hosp Epidemiol* 1992;13:86–92.
87. Wilton J, Jung K, Vedin I, et al. Comparative evaluation of a new molecular method for typing *Staphylococcus epidermidis. Eur J Clin Microbiol Infect Dis* 1992;11:515–521.
88. Goering RV, Duensing TD. Rapid field inversion gel electrophoresis in combination with an rRNA gene probe in the epidemiological evaluation of staphylococci. *J Clin Microbiol* 1990;28:426–429.
89. Burnie JP, Naderi-Nasab M, Loudon KW, et al. An epidemiological study of blood culture isolates of coagulase-negative staphylococci demonstrating hospital-acquired infection. *J Clin Microbiol* 1997;35: 1746–1750.
90. Kluytmans J, Berg H, Steegh P, et al. Outbreak of Staphylococcus schleiferi wound infections: strain characterization by randomly amplified polymorphic DNA analysis, PCR ribotyping, conventional ribotyping, and pulsed-field gel electrophoresis. *J Clin Microbiol* 1998; 36:2214–2219.
91. Nouwen JL, vanBelkum A, deMarie S, et al. Clonal expansion of Staphylococcus epidermidis strains causing Hickman catheter-related infections in a hemato-oncologic department. *J Clin Microbiol* 1998; 36:2696–2702.
92. Maslow RN, Mulligan ME, Arbeit RD. Molecular epidemiology: application of contemporary techniques to the typing of microorganisms. *Clin Infect Dis* 1993;17:153–164.
93. Wade JC, Schimpff SC, Newman KA, et al. Staphylococcus epidermidis: an increasing cause of infection in patients with granulocytopenia. *Ann Intern Med* 1982;97:503–508.
94. Winston DJ, Dudnick DV, Chapin M, et al. Coagulase-negative staphylococcal bacteremia in patients receiving immunosuppressive therapy. *Arch Intern Med* 1983;143:32–36.
95. Fleer A, Gerards LJ, Aerts P, et al. Opsonic defense to *Staphylococcus epidermidis* in the premature neonate. *J Infect Dis* 1985;152:930–937.
96. Keane WF, Comty CM, Verbrugh HA, et al. Opsonic deficiency of peritoneal dialysis effluent in continuous ambulatory peritoneal dialysis. *Kidney Int* 1984;25:539–543.
97. Freeman J, Goldmann DA, Smith NE, et al. Association of intravenous lipid emulsion and coagulase-negative staphylococcal bacteremia in neonatal intensive care units [see comments]. *N Engl J Med* 1990; 323:301–308.
98. Archer GL, Armstrong BC. Alteration of staphylococcal flora in cardiac surgery patients receiving antibiotic prophylaxis. *J Infect Dis* 1983;147:642–649.
99. Peters G, Locci R, Pulverer G. Adherence and growth of coagulase-negative staphylococci on surfaces of intravenous catheters. *J Infect Dis* 1982;146:479–482.
100. Sattler FR, Foderaro JB, Aber RC. Staphylococcus epidermidis bacteremia associated with vascular catheters: an important cause of febrile morbidity in hospitalized patients. *Infect Control* 1984;5:279–283.
101. Corman LC, Levisin ME. Sustained bacteremia and transvenous cardiac pacemakers. *JAMA* 1975;233:264–266.
102. Peters G, Saborowski F, Locci R, et al. Investigations on staphylococcal infection of transvenous endocardial pacemaker electrodes. *Am Heart J* 1984;108:359–365.
103. Gruer LD, Bartlett R, Ayliffe GAJ. Species identification and antibiotic sensitivity of coagulase-negative staphylococci from CAPD peritonitis. *J Antimicrob Chemother* 1984;13:577–583.
104. Rubin J, Rogers WA, Taylor HM, et al. Peritonitis during continuous ambulatory peritoneal dialysis. *Ann Intern Med* 1980;92:7–13.
105. Bandyk DF, Berni GA, Thiele BL, et al. Aortofemoral graft infection due to *Staphylococcus epidermidis. Arch Surg* 1984;119:102–108.
106. Schimke RT, Black PH, Mark VH, et al. Indolent *Staphylococcus albus* or *aureus* bacteremia after ventriculoatriostomy. *N Engl J Med* 1961; 264:264–270.
107. Schoenbaum SC, Gardner P, Shillito J. Infections of cerebrospinal fluid shunts: epidemiology, clinical manifestations, and therapy. *J Infect Dis* 1975;131:543–552.
108. Patterson FP, Brown CS. The McKee-Farrar total hip replacement. *J Bone Joint Surg* 1972;54A:257–275.
109. Brause BD. Infections associated with prosthetic joints. *Clin Rheum Dis* 1986;12:523–536.
110. Freedman AM, Jackson IT. Infections in breast implants. *Infect Dis Clin North Am* 1989;3:275–287.
111. Weber DJ, Hoffman KL, Thoft RA, et al. Endophthalmitis following intraocular lens implantation: report of 30 cases and review of the literature. *Rev Infect Dis* 1986;8:12–20.
112. Driebe WT Jr, Mandelbaum S, Forster RK, et al. Pseudophakic endophthalmitis. *Ophthalmology* 1986;93:442–448.
113. Davis JL, Koidou-Tsiligianni A, Pflugfelder SC, et al. Coagulase-negative staphylococcal endophthalmitis. *Ophthalmology* 1988;95: 1404–1410.
114. Gordon SM, Schmitt SK, Jacobs M, et al. Nosocomial bloodstream infections in patients with implantable left ventricular assist devices. *Ann Thorac Surg* 2001;72:725–730.
115. Blum MD. Infections of genitourinary prostheses. *Infect Dis Clin North Am* 1989;3:259–274.

116. Bayston R, Penny SR. Excessive production of mucoid substance in Staphylococcus SIIA: a possible factor in colonization of Hotter shunts. *Dev Med Child Neurol* 1972;27 (suppl):25–28.
117. Peters G, Locci R, Pulverer G. Microbial colonization of prosthetic devices. II. Scanning electron microscopy of naturally infected intravenous catheters. *Zentralbl Bakteriol Mikrobiol Hyg [B]* 1981;173: 293–299.
118. Locci R, Peters G, Pulverer G. Microbial colonization of prosthetic devices. III. Adhesion of staphylococci to lumina of intravenous catheters perfused with bacterial suspensions. *Zentralbl Bakteriol Mikrobiol Hyg[A]* 1981;173:300–307.
119. Christensen GD, Simpson WA, Bisno AL, et al. Adherence of slime-producing strains of *Staphylococcus epidermidis* to smooth surfaces. *Infect Immun* 1982;37:318–326.
120. von Eiff C, Peter G, Heilmann C. Pathogenesis of infections due to coagulase-negative staphylococci. *Lancet Infect Dis* 2002;2:677–685.
121. Tojo M, Yamashita N, Goldmann DA, et al. Isolation and characterization of a capsular polysaccharide adhesin from *Staphylococcus epidermidis. J Infect Dis* 1988;157:713.
122. Christensen GD, Barker LP, Mawhinney TP, et al. Identification of an antigenic marker of slime production for *Staphylococcus epidermidis. Infect Immun* 1990;58:2906–2911.
123. Mack D, Siemssen N, Laufs R. Parallel induction by glucose of adherence and a polysaccharide antigen specific for plastic-adherent *Staphylococcus epidermidis*: evidence for functional relation to intercellular adhesion. *Infect Immun* 1992;60:2048–2057.
124. McKenney D, Hubner J, Muller E, et al. The ica locus of Staphylococcus epidermidis encodes production of the capsular polysaccharide/adhesin. *Infect Immun* 1998;66:4711–4720.
125. Herrmann M, Vaudaux PE, Pittet D, et al. Fibronectin, fibrinogen, and laminin act as mediators of adherence of clinical staphylococcal isolates to foreign material. *J Infect Dis* 1988;158:693–701.
126. Mack D, Fischer W, Krokotsch A, et al. The intercellular adhesin involved in biofilm accumulation of Staphylococcus epidermidis is a linear beta-1,6-linked glucosaminoglycan: purification and structural analysis. *J Bacteriol* 1996;178:175–183.
127. Shiro H, Muller E, Gutierrez N, et al. Transposon mutants of Staphylococcus epidermidis deficient in elaboration of capsular polysaccharide/adhesin and slime are avirulent in a rabbit model of endocarditis. *J Infect Dis* 1994;169:1042–1049.
128. Shiro H, Meluleni G, Groll A, et al. The pathogenic role of Staphylococcus epidermidis capsular polysaccharide/adhesin in a low-inoculum rabbit model of prosthetic valve endocarditis. *Circulation* 1995; 92:2715–2722.
129. Peters G. Pathogenesis of S epidermidis foreign body infections. *Br J Clin Pract Symp Suppl* 1988;57:62–65.
130. Noble MA, Grant SK, Hajen E. Characterization of a neutrophil-inhibitory factor from clinically significant Staphylococcus epidermidis. *J Infect Dis* 1990;162:909–913.
131. Johnson GM, Lee DA, Regelmann WE, et al. Interference with granulocyte function by *Staphylococcus epidermidis* slime. *Infect Immun* 1986;54:13–20.
132. Farber BF, Kaplan MH, Clogston AG. Staphylococcus epidermidis extracted slime inhibits the antimicrobial action of glycopeptide antibiotics. *J Infect Dis* 1990;161:37–40.
133. Vergeres P, Blaser J. Amikacin, ceftazidime, and flucloxacillin against suspended and adherent *Pseudomonas aeruginosa* and *Staphylococcus epidermidis* in an in vitro model of infection. *J Infect Dis* 1992;165: 281–289.
134. Gemmell CG. Virulence characteristics of *Staphylococcus epidermidis. J Med Microbiol* 1986;22:287–289.
135. von Eiff C, Vaudaux P, Kahl BC, et al. Bloodstream infections caused by small-colony variants of coagulase-negative staphylococci following pacemaker implantation. *Clin Infect Dis* 1999;29:932–934.
136. Banerjee SN, Emori TG, Culver DH, et al. Secular trends in nosocomial primary bloodstream infections in the United States, 1980–1989. National Nosocomial Infections Surveillance System. *Am J Med* 1991;91:86S–89S.
137. National Nosocomial Infections Surveillance System. National Nosocomial Infections Surveillance (NNIS). Report, data summary from October 1986–April 1996, issued May 1996. *Am J Infect Control* 1996;24:380–388.
138. Mayhall CG. Diagnosis and management of infections of implantable devices used for prolonged venous access. In: Remington JS, Swartz MN, eds. *Current clinical topics in infectious diseases.* Boston: Blackwell Scientific, 1992:83–110.
139. Arnow PM, Quimosing EM, Beach M. Consequences of intravascular catheter sepsis. *Clin Infect Dis* 1993;16:778–784.
140. Sitges-Serra A, Puig P, Linares J, et al. Hub colonization as the initial step in an outbreak of catheter-related sepsis due to coagulase negative staphylococci during parenteral nutrition. *JPEN J Parenter Enteral Nutr* 1984;8:668–672.
141. Martin MA, Pfaller MA, Wenzel RP. Coagulase-negative staphylococcal bacteremia. Mortality and hospital stay [see comments]. *Ann Intern Med* 1989;110:9–16.
142. Shuttleworth R, Behme RJ, McNabb A, et al. Human isolates of Staphylococcus caprae: association with bone and joint infections. *J Clin Microbiol* 1997;35:2537–2541.
143. Pittet D, Davis CS, Li N, et al. Identifying the hospitalized patient at risk for nosocomial bloodstream infection: a population-based study. *Proc Assoc Am Physicians* 1997;109:58–67.
144. Rupp ME. Infections of intravascular catheters and vascular devices. In: Crossley KB, Archer GL, eds. *The staphylococci in human disease.* New York: Churchill Livingstone, 1997:379–399.
145. Raad II, Hohn DC, Gilbreath BJ, et al. Prevention of central venous catheter-related infections by using maximal sterile barrier precautions during insertion. *Infect Control Hosp Epidemiol* 1994;15:231–238.
146. Danzig LE, Short LJ, Collins K, et al. Bloodstream infections associated with a needleless intravenous infusion system in patients receiving home infusion therapy. *JAMA* 1995;273:1862–1864.
147. McDonald LC, Banerjee SN, Jarvis WR. Line-associated bloodstream infections in pediatric intensive-care-unit patients associated with a needleless device and intermittent intravenous therapy. *Infect Control Hosp Epidemiol* 1998;19:772–777.
148. Safdar N, Kluger DM, Maki DG. A review of risk factors for catheter-related bloodstream infection caused by percutaneously inserted, noncuffed central venous catheters. *Medicine* 2002;81:466–479.
149. Ponce de Leon S, Wenzel RP. Hospital-acquired bloodstream infections with *Staphylococcus epidermidis. Am J Med* 1984;77:639–644.
150. Bender JW, Hughes WT. Fatal *Staphylococcus epidermidis* sepsis following bone marrow transplantation. *Johns Hopkins Med J* 1980;146: 13–15.
151. Eykyn SJ. Staphylococcal sepsis. The changing pattern of disease and therapy. *Lancet* 1988;1:100–104.
152. Society for Hospital Epidemiology of America, Association for Practitioners in Infection Control, Centers for Disease Control, Surgical Infection Society. Consensus paper on the surveillance of surgical wound infections. *Infect Control Hosp Epidemiol* 1992;13:599–605.
153. Horan TC, Gaynes RP, Martone WJ, et al. CDC definitions of nosocomial surgical site infections, 1992: a modification of CDC definitions of surgical wound infections. *Infect Control Hosp Epidemiol* 1992; 13:606–608.
154. Horan TC, Culver DH, Gaynes RP, et al. Nosocomial infections in surgical patients in the United States, January 1986–June 1992. *Infect Control Hosp Epidemiol* 1993;14:73–80.
155. Bannerman TL, Rhoden DL, McAllister SK, et al., Endophthalmitis Vitrectomy Study Group. The source of coagulase-negative staphylococci in the endophthalmitis vitrectomy study. *Arch Ophthalmol* 1997; 115:357–361.
156. Horan T, Culver D, Jarvis W, et al. et al. Pathogens causing nosocomial infections. Preliminary data from the National Nosocomial Infections Surveillance System. *Antimicrobic Newslett* 1988;5:65–67.
157. Culliford AT, Cunningham JN Jr, Zeff RH, et al. Sternal and costochondral infections following open-heart surgery. *J Thorac Cardiovasc Surg* 1976;72:714–726.
158. Bor DH, Rose RM, Modlin JF, et al. Mediastinitis after cardiovascular surgery. *Rev Infect Dis* 1983;5:885–897.
159. Culver DH, Horan TC, Gaynes RP, et al. Surgical wound infection rates by wound class, operative procedure, and patient risk index. *Am J Med* 1991;91(suppl B):152S–157S.

160. Finland M, Barnes MW. Changing etiology of bacterial endocarditis in the antibacterial era. *Ann Intern Med* 1970;72:341–348.
161. Brandt L, Swahn B. Subacute bacterial endocarditis due to coagulase-negative Staphylococcus albus. *Acta Med Scand* 1960;166:125–132.
162. Dismukes WE, Karchmer AW, Buckley MJ, et al. Prosthetic valve endocarditis. Analysis of 38 cases. *Circulation* 1973;48:365–377.
163. Karchmer AW, Dismukes WE, Buckley MJ, et al. Late prosthetic valve endocarditis. *Am J Med* 1978;64:199–206.
164. Ivert TSA, Dismukes WE, Cobbs CG, et al. Prosthetic valve endocarditis. *Circulation* 1984;69:223–232.
165. Calderwood SB, Swinski LA, Karchmer AW, et al. Prosthetic valve endocarditis. Analysis of factors affecting outcome of therapy. *J Thorac Cardiovasc Surg* 1986;92:776–783.
166. Whitener C, Caputo GM, Weitekamp MR, et al. Endocarditis due to coagulase-negative staphylococci. *Infect Dis Clin North Am* 1993; 7:81–96.
167. Hammond GW, Stiver HG. Combination antibiotic therapy in an outbreak of prosthetic endocarditis caused by *Staphylococcus epidermidis*. *CMA* 1978;118:524–530.
168. Liekweg WG Jr, Greenfield LJ. Vascular prosthetic infections: collected experience and results of treatment. *Surgery* 1977;81:335–342.
169. Bunt TJ. Synthetic vascular graft infections. I. Graft infections. *Surgery* 1983;93:733–746.
170. Lorentzen JE, Nielsen OM, Arendrup H, et al. Vascular graft infection: an analysis of sixty-two graft infections in 2411 consecutively implanted synthetic vascular grafts. *Surgery* 1985;98:81–86.
171. O'Brien T, Collin J. Prosthetic vascular graft infection. *Br J Surg* 1992;79:1262–1267.
172. Richet HM, Chidiac C, Prat A, et al. Analysis of risk factors for surgical wound infections following vascular surgery. *Am J Med* 1991; 91(suppl 3B):170S–172S.
173. Kaebnick HW, Bandyk DF, Bergamini TW, et al. The microbiology of explanted vascular prostheses. *Surgery* 1987;102:756–762.
174. Tollefson DF, Bandyk DF, Kaebnick HW, et al. Surface biofilm disruption. *Arch Surg* 1987;122:38–43.
175. Golan JF. Vascular graft infection. *Infect Dis Clin North Am* 1989; 3:247–258.
176. Charnley J. Postoperative infection after total hip replacement with special reference to air contamination in the operating room. *Clin Orthop* 1972;87:167–187.
177. Fitzgerald RH Jr, Nolan DR, Ilstrup DM, et al. Deep wound sepsis following total hip arthroplasty. *J Bone Joint Surg* 1977;59A:847–855.
178. Buchholz HW, Elson RA, Engelbrecht E, et al. Management of deep infection of total hip replacement. *J Bone Joint Surg* 1981;63B: 342–353.
179. Fitzgerald RH Jr. Infections of hip prostheses and artificial joints. *Infect Dis Clin North Am* 1989;3:329–338.
180. Sampathkumar P, Osmon DR, Cockerill FR III. Prosthetic joint infection due to Staphylococcus lugdunensis. *Mayo Clin Proc* 2000;75: 511–512.
181. Gillespie WJ. Infection in total joint replacement. *Infect Dis Clin North Am* 1990;4:465–484.
182. Rand JA, Fitzgerald RH Jr. Diagnosis and management of the infected total knee arthroplasty. *Orthop Clin North Am* 1989;20:201–210.
183. Morrey BF, Bryan RS, Dobyns JH, et al. Total elbow arthroplasty. A five-year experience at the Mayo Clinic. *J Bone Joint Surg* 1981; 63A:1050–1063.
184. Berbari EF, Hanssen AD, Duffy MC, et al. Risk factors for prosthetic joint infection: case-control study. *Clin Infect Dis* 1998;27: 1247–1254.
185. Perdreau-Remington F, Stefanik D, Peters G, et al. A four-year prospective study on microbial ecology of explanted prosthetic hips in 52 patients with "aseptic" prosthetic joint loosening. *Eur J Clin Microbiol Infect Dis* 1996;15:160–165.
186. Renier D, Lacombe J, Pierre-Kahn A, et al. Factors causing acute shunt infection. Computer analysis of 1174 operations. *J Neurosurg* 1984;61:1072–1078.
187. Blomstedt GC. Infections in Neurosurgery: a retrospective study of 1143 patients and 1517 operations. *Acta Neurochir* 1985;78:81–90.
188. Stromblad M-G, Schalen C, Steen A, et al. Bacterial contamination in cerebrospinal fluid shunt surgery. Scand *J Infect Dis* 1987;19: 211–214.
189. Younger JJ, Simmons JCH, Barrett FF. Operative related infection rates for ventriculoperitoneal shunt procedures in a children's hospital. *Infect Control* 1987;8:67–70.
190. Mayhall CG, Archer NH, Lamb AV, et al. Ventriculostomy-related infections. *N Engl J Med* 1984;310:553–559.
191. Vas SI. Infections of continuous ambulatory peritoneal dialysis catheters. *Infect Dis Clin North Am* 1989;3:301–328.
192. Bernardini J, Holley JL, Johnston JR, et al. An analysis of ten-year trends in infections in adults on continuous ambulatory peritoneal dialysis (CAPD). *Clin Nephrol* 1991;36:29–34.
193. Working party of the British Society for Antimicrobial Chemotherapy. Diagnosis and management of peritonitis in continuous ambulatory peritoneal dialysis. *Lancet* 1987;i:845–848.
194. Piraino B, Bernardini J, Sorkin M. A five-year study of the microbiologic results of exit site infections and peritonitis in continuous ambulatory peritoneal dialysis. *Am J Kidney Dis* 1987;10:281–286.
195. Beard-Pegler MA, Gabelish CL, Stubbs E, et al. Prevalence of peritonitis-associated coagulase-negative staphylococci on the skin of continuous ambulatory peritoneal dialysis patients. *Epidemiol Infect* 1989; 102:365–378.
196. Eisenberg ES, Ambalu M, Szylagi G, et al. Colonization of skin and development of peritonitis due to coagulase-negative staphylococci in patients undergoing peritoneal dialysis. *J Infect Dis* 1987;156: 478–482.
197. Carozzi S, Lamperi S. Peritonitis prevention in CAPD. *Clin Nephrol* 1988;30(suppl 1):45–48.
198. Battisti O, Mitchison R, Davies PA. Changing blood culture isolates in a referral neonatal intensive care unit. *Arch Dis Child* 1981;56: 775–778.
199. Munson DP, Thompson TR, Johnson DE, et al. Coagulase-negative staphylococcal septicemia: experience in a newborn intensive care unit. *J Pediatr* 1982;101:602–605.
200. Fleer A, Senders RC, Visser MR, et al. Septicemia due to coagulase-negative staphylococci in a neonatal intensive care unit: clinical and bacteriological features and contaminated parenteral fluids as a source of sepsis. *Pediatr Infect Dis J* 1983;2:426–431.
201. Donowitz LG, Haley CE, Gregory WW, et al. Neonatal intensive care unit bacteremia: emergence of gram-positive bacteria as major pathogens. *Am J Infect Control* 1987;15:141–147.
202. Schmidt BK, Kirpalani HM, Corey M, et al. Coagulase-negative staphylococci as true pathogens in newborn infants: a cohort study. *Pediatr Infect Dis J* 1987;6:1026–1031.
203. Jarvis WR. Epidemiology of nosocomial infections in pediatric patients. *Pediatr Infect Dis J* 1987;6:344–351.
204. Noel GJ, Edelson PJ. *Staphylococcus epidermidis* bacteremia in neonates: further observations and the occurrence of focal infection. *Pediatrics* 1984;74:832–837.
205. Simpson RA, Spencer AF, Speller DC, et al. Colonization by gentamicin-resistant Staphylococcus epidermidis in a special care baby unit. *J Hosp Infect* 1986;7:108–120.
206. Freeman J, Platt R, Sidebottom DG, et al. Coagulase-negative staphylococcal bacteremia in the changing neonatal intensive care unit population. Is there an epidemic? *JAMA* 1987;258:2548–2552.
207. Carlos CC, Ringertz S, Rylander M, et al. Nosocomial Staphylococcus epidermidis septicaemia among very low birth weight neonates in an intensive care unit. *J Hosp Infect* 1991;19:201–207.
208. Sidebottom DG, Freeman J, Platt R, et al. Fifteen-year experience with bloodstream isolates of coagulase-negative staphylococci in neonatal intensive care. *J Clin Microbiol* 1988;26:713–718.
209. Freeman J, Platt R, Epstein MF, et al. Birth weight and length of stay as determinants of nosocomial coagulase-negative staphylococcal bacteremia in neonatal intensive care unit populations: potential for confounding. *Am J Epidemiol* 1990;132:1130–1140.
210. Goldmann DA, Leclair J, Macone A. Bacterial colonization of neonates admitted to an intensive care environment. *J Pediatr* 1978;93: 288–293.
211. Low DE, Schmidt BK, Kirpalani HM, et al. An endemic strain of

Staphylococcus haemolyticus colonizing and causing bacteremia in neonatal intensive care unit patients. *Pediatrics* 1992;89:696–700.
212. Nystrom B, Ransjo U, Ringertz S, et al. Colonization with coagulase-negative staphylococci in two neonatal units. *J Hosp Infect* 1992;22: 287–298.
213. Raimundo O, Huessler H, Bruhn JB, et al. Molecular epidemiology of coagulase-negative staphylococcal bacteraemia in a newborn intensive care unit. *J Hosp Infect* 2002;51:33–42.
214. Patrick CC, Kaplan SL, Baker CJ, et al. Persistent bacteremia due to coagulase-negative staphylococci in low birth weight neonates. *Pediatrics* 1989;84:977–985.
215. Powell DA, Aungst J, Snedden S, et al. Broviac catheter-related *Malassezia furfur* sepsis in five infants receiving intravenous fat emulsions. *J Pediatr* 1984;105:987–990.
216. Freeman J, Epstein MF, Smith NE, et al. Extra hospital stay and antibiotic usage with nosocomial coagulase-negative staphylococcal bacteremia in two neonatal intensive care unit populations. *Am J Dis Child* 1990;144:324–329.
217. Hall SL. Coagulase-negative staphylococcal infections in neonates. *Pediatr Infect Dis J* 1991;10:57–67.
218. Davies HD, Jones EL, Sheng RY, et al. Nosocomial urinary tract infections at a pediatric hospital. *Pediatr Infect Dis J* 1992;11: 349–354.
219. Gruskay J, Harris MC, Costarino AT, et al. Neonatal *Staphylococcus epidermidis* meningitis with unremarkable CSF examination results. *Am J Dis Child* 1989;143:580–582.
220. Grushkay JA, Abbasi S, Anday E, et al. *Staphylococcus epidermidis* associated enterocolitis. *J Pediatr* 1986;109:520–524.
221. Brand KG. Infection of mammary prostheses: a survey and the question of prevention. *Ann Plast Surg* 1993;30:289–295.
222. Virden CP, Dobke MK, Stein P, et al. Subclinical infection of the silicone breast implant surface as a possible cause of capsular contracture. *Aesthet Plast Surg* 1992;16:173–179.
223. Carlson AN, Tetz MR, Apple DJ. Infectious complications of modern cataract surgery and intraocular lens implantation. *Infect Dis Clin North Am* 1989;3:339–355.
224. Carson CC. Infections in genitourinary prostheses. *Urol Clin North Am* 1989;16:139–147.
225. Montague DK. Periprosthetic infections. *J Urol* 1987;138:68–69.
226. Hedin G, Hambraeus A. Multiply antibiotic-resistant Staphylococcus epidermidis in patients, staff and environment—a one-week survey in a bone marrow transplant unit. *J Hosp Infect* 1991;17:95–106.
227. Richards JM, Gilewski TA, Vogelzang NJ. Association of interleukin-2 therapy with staphylococcal bacteremia. *Cancer* 1991;67: 1570–1575.
228. Counihan PJ, Yelland A, de Belder MA, et al. Infective endocarditis in a heart transplant recipient. *J Heart Lung Transplant* 1991;10: 275–279.
229. Kunin CM, Dobbins JJ, Melo JC, et al. Infectious complications in four long-term recipients of the Jarvik-7 artificial heart. *JAMA* 1988; 259:860–864.
230. Dobbins JJ, Johnson S, Kunin CM, et al. Postmortem microbiological findings of two total artificial heart recipients. *JAMA* 1988;259: 865–869.
231. Safdar N, Maki DG. Inflammation at the insertion site is not predictive of catheter-related bloodstream infection with short-term, non-cuffed central venous catheters. *Crit Care Med* 2002;30:2632–2635.
232. Maki DG, Weise CE, Sarafin HW. A semiquantitative culture method for identifying intravenous-catheter-related infection. *N Engl J Med* 1977;296:1305–1309.
233. Cooper GL, Hopkins CC. Rapid diagnosis of intravascular catheter-associated infection by direct gram staining of catheter segments. *N Engl J Med* 1985;312:1142–1147.
234. Zufferey J, Rime B, Francioli P, et al. Simple method for rapid diagnosis of catheter-associated infection by direct acridine orange staining of catheter tips. *J Clin Microbiol* 1988;26:175–177.
235. Armstrong CW, Mayhall CG, Miller KB, et al. Clinical predictors of infection of central venous catheters used for total parenteral nutrition. *Infect Control Hosp Epidemiol* 1990;11:71–78.
236. Cleri DJ, Corrado ML, Seligman SJ. Quantitative culture of intravenous catheters and other intravascular inserts. *J Infect Dis* 1980;141: 781–786.
237. Linares J, Sitges-Serra A, Garau J, et al. Pathogenesis of catheter sepsis: a prospective study with quantitative and semiquantitative cultures of catheter hub and segments. *J Clin Microbiol* 1985;21:357–360.
238. Brun-Buisson C, Abrouk F, Legrand P, et al. Diagnosis of central venous catheter-related sepsis. *Arch Intern Med* 1987;147:873–877.
239. Sherertz RJ, Raad II, Belani A, et al. Three-year experience with sonicated vascular catheter cultures in a clinical microbiology laboratory. *J Clin Microbiol* 1990;28:76–82.
240. Mosca R, Curtas S, Forbes B, et al. The benefits of isolator cultures in the management of suspected catheter sepsis. *Surgery* 1987;102: 718–723.
241. Capdevila JA, Planes AM, Palomar M, et al. Value of differential quantitative blood cultures in the diagnosis of catheter-related sepsis. *Eur J Clin Microbiol Infect Dis* 1992;11:403–407.
242. Sherertz RJ, Heard SO, Raad II. Diagnosis of triple-lumen catheter infection: comparison of roll plate, sonication, and flushing methodologies. *J Clin Microbiol* 1997;35:641–646.
243. Raad II, Baba M, Bodey GP. Diagnosis of catheter-related infections: the role of surveillance and targeted quantitative skin cultures. *Clin Infect Dis* 1995;20:593–597.
244. Mermel LA, Farr BM, Sherertz RJ, et al. Guidelines for the management of intravascular catheter-related infections. *Clin Infect Dis* 2001; 32:1249.
245. Mermel LA, McCormick RD, Springman SR, et al. The pathogenesis and epidemiology of catheter-related infection with pulmonary artery Swan-Ganz catheters: a prospective study utilizing molecular subtyping. *Am J Med* 1991;91(suppl 3B):197S–205S.
246. Bates DW, Goldman L, Lee TH. Contaminant blood cultures and resource utilization. *JAMA* 1991;265:365–369.
247. Bates DW, Lee TH. Rapid classification of positive blood cultures. *JAMA* 1992;267:1962–1966.
248. Calderwood SB, Swinski LA, Waternaux CM, et al. Risk factors for the development of prosthetic valve endocarditis. *Circulation* 1985; 72:31–37.
249. Heimberger TS, Duma RJ. Infections of prosthetic heart valves and cardiac pacemakers. *Infect Dis Clin North Am* 1989;3:221–245.
250. Lukes AS, Bright DK, Durack DT. Diagnosis of infective endocarditis. *Infect Dis Clin North Am* 1993;7:1–8.
251. Wade JS, Cobbs CG. Infections in cardiac pacemakers. In: Remington JS, Swartz MN, eds. *Current clinical topics in infectious diseases.* New York: McGraw-Hill, 1989:44–61.
252. Chua JD, Wilkoff BL, Lee I, et al. Diagnosis and management of infections involving implantable electrophysiologic cardiac devices. *Ann Intern Med* 2000;133:604–608.
253. Bergamini TM, Bandyk DF, Govostis D, et al. Identification of Staphylococcus epidermidis vascular graft infections: a comparison of culture techniques. *J Vasc Surg* 1989;9:665–670.
254. Venes JL. Infections of CSF shunt and intracranial pressure monitoring devices. *Infect Dis Clin North Am* 1989;3:289–299.
255. Sanchez-Mora D, Mermel L, Parenteau S, et al. Epidural catheter infection: epidemiology and pathogenesis. Presented at the 33rd Interscience Conference on Antimicrobial Agents and Chemotherapy, New Orleans, LA, Abstr. 517. 1993.
256. Ludlam HA, Price TNC, Berry J, et al. Laboratory diagnosis of peritonitis in patients on continuous ambulatory peritoneal dialysis. *J Clin Microbiol* 1988;26:1757–1762.
257. Haley RW, Culver DH, White JW, et al. The nation-wide nosocomial infection rate: a new need for vital statistics. *Am J Epidemiol* 1985; 121:159.
258. Scheckler WE, Scheibel W, Kresge D. Temporal trends in septicemia in a community hospital. *Am J Med* 1991;91(suppl B):90S–94S.
259. Gaynes RP, Martone WJ, Culver DH, et al. Comparison of rates of nosocomial infections in neonatal intensive care units in the United States. *Am J Med* 1991;91(suppl 3B):192–196.
260. Parisi JT. Epidemiologic markers in *Staphylococcus epidermidis* infections. In: Leive L, ed. *Microbiology—1986.* Washington DC: American Society for Microbiology, 1986:139–144.
261. Lark RL, VanderHyde K, Deeb GM, et al. An outbreak of coagulase-

negative staphylococcal surgical-site infections following aortic valve replacement. *Infect Control Hosp Epidemiol* 2001;22:618–623.
262. Cove JH, Eady EA, Cunliffe WJ. Skin carriage of antibiotic-resistant coagulase-negative staphylococci in untreated subjects. *J Antimicrob Chemother* 1990;25:459–469.
263. Kernodle DS, Barg NL, Kaiser AB. Low-level colonization of hospitalized patients with methicillin-resistant coagulase-negative staphylococci and emergence of the organisms during surgical antimicrobial prophylaxis. *Antimicrob Agents Chemother* 1988;32:202–208.
264. McLauchlan J, Smylie HG, Logie JRC, et al. A study of the wound environment during total hip arthroplasty. *Postgrad Med J* 1976;52: 550–557.
265. Shapiro S, Boaz J, Kleiman M, et al. Origin of organisms infecting ventricular shunts. *Neurosurgery* 1988;22:868–872.
266. Ludlam HA, Noble NC, Marples RR, et al. The epidemiology of peritonitis caused by coagulase-negative staphylococci in continuous ambulatory peritoneal dialysis. *J Med Microbiol* 1989;30:167–174.
267. Dryden MS, Talsania H, McCann M, et al. The epidemiology of ciprofloxacin resistance in coagulase-negative staphylococci in CAPD patients. *Epidemiol Infect* 1992;109:97–112.
268. Perl TM, Sanford L, Bale M, et al. Coagulase-negative staphylococcal (CNS) infections: the role of endogenous flora in sternal wound infections. Program and Abstracts of the 33rd ICAAC (abstr. 1442), 1993: 383.
269. Bunt TJ. Sources of *Staphylococcus epidermidis* at the inguinal incision during peripheral revascularization. *Am Surg* 1986;52:472–473.
270. Lidwell OM, Lowbury EJL, Whyte W, et al. Effect of ultraclean air in operating rooms on deep sepsis in the joint after total hip or knee replacement: a randomised study. *Br Med J* 1982;285:10–14.
271. Fishman IJ. Complicated implantations of inflatable penile prostheses. *Urol Clin North Am* 1987;14:217–239.
272. Bayston R, Lari J. A study of the sources of infection in colonized shunts. *Dev Med Child Neurol* 1974;16:16–22.
273. Duhaime AC, Bonner K, McGowan KL, et al. Distribution of bacteria in the operating room environment and its relation to ventricular shunt infections: a prospective study. *Childs Nerv Syst* 1991;7: 211–214.
274. Kotilainen P, Nikoskelainen J, Huovinen P. Emergence fo ciprofloxacin-resistant coagulase-negative staphylococcal skin flora in immunocompromised patients receiving ciprofloxacin. *J Infect Dis* 1990;161: 41–44.
275. Hall SL, Hall RT, Barnes WG, et al. Relationship of maternal to neonatal colonization with coagulase-negative staphylococci. *Am J Perinatol* 1990;7:384–388.
276. Ayliffe GAJ. Role of the environment of the operating suite in surgical wound infection. *Rev Infect Dis* 1991;13(suppl 10):S800–S804.
277. Walter CW, Kundsin RB. The bacteriologic study of surgical gloves from 250 operations. *Surg Gynecol Obstet* 1969;949–952.
278. Blakemore WS, McGarrity GJ, Thurer RJ, et al. Infection by airborne bacteria with cardiopulmonary bypass. *Surgery* 1971;70: 830–838.
279. Ankeney JL, Parker RF. Staphylococcal endocarditis following open heart surgery related to positive intraoperative blood cultures. In: Brewer LAI, Cooley DA, Davila JC, et al., eds. *Prosthetic heart valves.* Springfield, IL: Charles C. Thomas, 1969:719–731.
280. Boyce JM, Pittet D, Healthcare Infection Control Practices Advisory Committee and the HICPAC/SHEA/APIC/IDSA Hand Hygiene Task Force. Guideline for hand hygiene in health-care settings. *MMWR* 2002;51(RR-16):1–45.
281. O'Grady NP, Alexander M, Dellinger EP, et al. Guidelines for the prevention of intravascular catheter-related infections. *MMWR* 2002; 51(RR-10):1–36.
282. Maki DG, Stolz SM, Wheeler S, et al. Prevention of central venous catheter-related bloodstream infection with an antiseptic-impregnated catheter. A prospective randomized controlled trial. *Ann Intern Med* 1997;127:257–266.
283. Raad I, Darouiche R, Dupuis J, et al. Central venous catheters coated with minocycline and rifampin for the prevention of catheter-related colonization and bloodstream infections. A randomized, double-blind trial. *Ann Intern Med* 1997;127:267–274.
284. McConnell SA, Gubbins PO, Anaissie EJ. Do antimicrobial-impregnated central venous catheters prevent catheter-related bloodstream infection? *Clin Infect Dis* 2003;37:65–72.
285. Shorr AF, Humphreys CW, Helman DL. New choices for central venous catheters. Potential financial implications. *Chest* 2003;124: 275–284.
286. Walder B, Pittet D, Tramer MR. Prevention of bloodstream infections with central venous catheters treated with anti-infective agents depends on catheter type and insertion time: evidence from a meta-analysis. *Infect Control Hosp Epidemiol* 2002;23:748–756.
287. Marciante KD, Veenstra DL, Lipsky RA, et al. Which antimicrobial impregnated central venous catheter should we use? Modeling the costs and outcomes of antimicrobial catheter use. *Am J Infect Control* 2003;31:1–8.
288. Mangram AJ, Horan TC, Pearson ML, et al., and the Hospital Infection Control Practices Advisory Committee. Guideline for prevention of surgical site infection, 1999. *Infect Control Hosp Epidemiol* 1999; 20:247–280.
289. Parienti JJ, Thibon P, Heller R, et al. Hand-rubbing with an aqueous alcohol solution vs traditional surgical hand-scrubbing and 30-day surgical site infection rates: randomized equivalence study. *JAMA* 2002;288:722–727.
290. Persson U, Montgomery F, Carlsson A, et al. How far does prophylaxis against infection in total joint replacement offset its cost? *Br Med J* 1988;296:99–102.
291. Gillespie WJ. Prevention and management of infection after total joint replacement. *Clin Infect Dis* 1997;25:1310–1317.
292. Kreter B, Woods M. Antibiotic prophylaxis for cardiothoracic operations. Metaanalysis of thirty years of clinical trials. *J Thorac Cardiovasc Surg* 1992;104:590–599.
293. Norden CW. Antibiotic prophylaxis in orthopedic surgery. *Rev Infect Dis* 1991;13(suppl 10):842–846.
294. Strachan CJL. Antibiotic prophylaxis in peripheral vascular and orthopaedic prosthetic surgery. *J Antimicrob Chemother* 1993;31(suppl B): 65–78.
295. Brown EM. Antimicrobial prophylaxis in neurosurgery. *J Antimicrob Chemother* 1993;31(suppl B):49–63.
296. Edwards WH Jr, Kaiser AB, Kernodle DS, et al. Cefuroxime versus cefazolin as prophylaxis in vascular surgery. *J Vasc Surg* 1992;15: 35–42.
297. Maki DG, Bohn MJ, Stolz SM, et al. Comparative study of cefazolin, cefamandole, and vancomycin for surgical prophylaxis in cardiac and vascular operations. *J Thorac Cardiovasc Surg* 1992;104:1423–1434.
298. Hospital Infection Control Practices Advisory Committee (HICPAC). Recommendations for preventing the spread of vancomycin resistance. *Infect Control Hosp Epidemiol* 1995;16:105–113.

31

STREPTOCOCCI

KENT B. CROSSLEY

Microorganisms of the genus *Streptococcus* were a major cause of nosocomial infection in the preantibiotic era. During the last half-century, they have been associated with occasional outbreaks of infection in hospitals. Although no recent comparable data are available from the National Nosocomial Infection Surveillance (NNIS) system, streptococci accounted for 2% of all nosocomial infections between 1986 and 1989 (1).

The major streptococcal species encountered are group A β-hemolytic streptococci *(Streptococcus pyogenes)* (GABHS), group B β-hemolytic streptococci *(Streptococcus agalactiae)* (GBS) and *Streptococcus pneumoniae.* This chapter discusses nosocomial infections caused by these microorganisms. It concludes with an overview of streptococci less commonly associated with nosocomial infection (e.g., group C and G streptococci). Nosocomial infections caused by enterococci are considered in Chapter 32.

Streptococci were first described in material recovered from wound infections by Billroth in 1874 and 5 years later by Pasteur in the blood of a patient with puerperal sepsis (2). Until the introduction of sulfonamides, streptococci (particularly GABHS) were common causes of nosocomial infection. Puerperal sepsis was a major concern in the first third of the twentieth century (3). The mortality rate from bacteremic group A streptococcal infections at Boston City Hospital in the 1930s was 72% (4).

Although antimicrobials have markedly reduced the frequency of these infections, streptococci continue to cause nosocomial disease. In a recent study of nosocomial bacteremia, 5.9% of cases were caused by streptococci. Viridans streptococci accounted for half, followed by GBS, GABHS, and pneumococci in decreasing frequency (5).

GROUP A β-HEMOLYTIC STREPTOCOCCI

GABHS are relatively uncommon causes of nosocomial infection (1). Of bacteremias caused by this microorganism, two recent American studies suggest that less than 10% are hospital-acquired (6,7). However, in a Danish study, 38% of GABHS bacteremias from 1981 to 1993 were nosocomial (8). GABHS tend to cause outbreaks of burn wound, puerperal, and neonatal infection that persist and that are difficult to evaluate and control.

GABHS may be serogrouped on the basis of protein antigens, designated as M and T antigens. Although M protein is primarily related to virulence, typing of strains to determine their M and T antigens followed by DNA restriction enzyme analysis is the best way to demonstrate identity of strains. Polymerase chain reaction (PCR) of amplified nucleotide sequences of the *emm* gene, which specifies filamentous M protein, is also useful (9).

Surgical Site Infection and the Epidemiology of GABHS Infection

GABHS are common causes of community-acquired pharyngitis and skin infection. These microorganisms may also be carried in the throat, on the skin, and in the rectum and vagina of asymptomatic people (10–13). Wu et al. (10) reported that 12.3% to 18.4% of hospital employees with pharyngitis had throat cultures positive for GABHS. It is curious that, despite frequent carriage of this microorganism in the respiratory tract of healthcare workers, very little nosocomial transmission from this source has been documented. Only five small outbreaks of infections appear to be directly the result of pharyngeal carriage of GABHS (14–18). In one of these outbreaks, the same strain that infected the patients and an anesthesiologist was also recovered from a member of the physician's family (14).

Although GABHS may be carried on unbroken skin (13), outbreaks resulting from cutaneous sources in healthcare workers have primarily been traced to individuals with clinically evident infection. Bisno et al. (19) described a patient who developed GABHS bacteremia from an intravascular catheter inserted by a physician who had an identical *Streptococcus* isolated from a healing wound on the dorsum of his hand (19). Mastro et al. (20) reported an outbreak of 20 postoperative surgical site infections that occurred over 40 months. This outbreak was eventually traced to an operating room technician who had the identical type of GABHS cultured from psoriatic lesions on his scalp. This individual worked in the operating rooms only before operations were performed.

Asymptomatic rectal or vaginal carriage of GABHS is the most commonly reported source of outbreaks of nosocomial surgical site infection. Schaffner et al. (21) described an outbreak that resulted from anal carriage of streptococci by an anesthesiologist. His throat culture was negative, but an M nontypable group A *Streptococcus* similar to that recovered from nine patients with infection was cultured from an anal swab. McKee et al. (22) reported an outbreak of 11 cases of infection associated with a medical attendant who was a rectal carrier. The same microorganism was also cultured from two of four family members. In this study, after the carrier exercised in an 8-ft by 11-ft examining room, settling plates yielded GABHS. A similar outbreak involving four patients was reported by Richman et al. (23) and resulted from carriage by a surgeon. Kolmos et al. (18), in a review of surgical site infections causally tied to healthcare workers, noted that anal carriage appeared to be associated with rectal ulcers, hemorrhoids, and other rectal pathology.

Viglionese et al. (24) described an outbreak of postpartum infections traced to an obstetrician who was an anal carrier of GABHS. Of 34 patients delivered vaginally by this physician, 6 (18%) were infected. The obstetrician was treated with penicillin, rifampin, and hexachlorophene; surveillance cultures were negative 1 week, 1 month, and 3 months later. Subsequently, however, four additional cases occurred 14 months after the end of his treatment, and he was again found to be colonized with the same microorganism. One additional case occurred during the next 19 months. This is the only published report that suggests that recurrent outbreaks might be caused by one healthcare worker who continues to carry or becomes recolonized with the same GABHS. We have had a similar experience with a vaginal carrier of GABHS. After treatment with erythromycin and rifampin, additional infections occurred, and she was found again to be colonized.

Vaginal carriage has been documented as a source of surgical site infections less often than has rectal carriage. Berkelman et al. (25) reported postoperative surgical site infections that occurred on two occasions, 5 months apart, associated with a nurse with both vaginal and rectal carriage of GABHS. (In this case, the two outbreaks involved serologically different streptococci.) Stamm et al. (26) reported another outbreak involving 18 patients. The source was a nurse with vaginal colonization with GABHS.

Somewhat less than 1% of normal individuals have positive anal or vaginal cultures for group A streptococci (12,26). Anal carriage in children with group A β-hemolytic streptococcal pharyngitis appears to be somewhat more frequent; in one study, 6% of children with documented GABHS pharyngitis had the same microorganisms recovered from anal swabs (11).

Based on evidence presented by Berkelman et al. (25) and Mastro et al. (20), it seems most likely that aerosolization of GABHS with motion or activity followed by contamination of the surgical site is the usual mode of transmission. In the outbreaks described by Stamm et al. (26) and Schaffner et al. (21), cases occurred in operating rooms adjacent to the one in which the source employee worked. Rutishauser et al. (27) reported two patients who developed streptococcal toxic shock after exposure to a surgeon who had nasal (but not pharyngeal) GABHS colonization. An outbreak involving three patients (two of whom died) was reported to be associated with a surgeon believed to be colonized with GABHS (28).

GABHS may also be recovered from dust in the environment, and it is possible (but unlikely) that microorganisms disseminated by a rectal carrier could contaminate hands or other surfaces and then be transmitted to a patient.

There are several reported outbreaks in which clusters of employees have acquired GABHS in an outbreak. Ramage et al. (29) reported three patients and six nurses who had developed infection; the nurses (three of whom were not cultured) all had developed pharyngitis. Kakis et al. (30) described transmission of an identical GABHS strain to 24 healthcare workers. All 24 developed symptoms of pharyngitis within 4 days of contact with the source patient, and transmission occurred within 25 hours following exposure to this individual.

Nearly all of the approximately 20 reported outbreaks of GABHS surgical site infection have been small, relatively chronic, and associated with an infected or colonized healthcare worker who is not immediately identified as the source. Occasional outbreaks not associated with an identified source have been reported. Webster et al. (31) described an outbreak of infection in seven patients on a plastic and maxillofacial surgery ward and in one patient on an adjacent psychiatric ward in London. The source of the outbreak was unclear, and it ended with the closure of the unit before its move to a new building.

Burn Wound Infection

GABHS were important pathogens in burn units before the introduction of routine penicillin prophylaxis for patients with thermal injuries. They continue to cause episodic burn wound infections and occasional outbreaks.

Three relatively recent outbreaks of streptococcal burn wound infection have been described. In 1984, Whitby et al. (32) reported an outbreak that began in a burn center and eventually spread to involve an intensive care unit in an associated hospital. Of the eight patients in the burn unit who were colonized with GABHS, two developed clinical evidence of infection and one additional patient became bacteremic. The outbreak apparently resulted from admission of a patient who carried GABHS in his pharynx.

Burnett et al. (33) described an outbreak involving four patients, six relatives of the index case, and four staff members in Sheffield. The source was a child with burns who had streptococcal pharyngitis. GABHS infection developed in four nurses (cellulitis in two, a facial pustule and an infected whitlow in one each). The outbreak was controlled by treatment with penicillin V. In the index case, the burn wounds did not clear with oral antibiotic therapy alone but were cured after mupirocin was applied to the burn wounds. The authors believed that the use of short-sleeved isolation gowns was related to the occurrence of the lesions on the forearms of two of the nurses.

Allen and Ridgway (34) reported a small outbreak of *S. pyogenes* infection in a burn unit in Liverpool. The source was apparently GABHS pharyngeal colonization in a patient admitted to the burn unit. The outbreak appeared to persist despite treatment of cases and careful hand washing. Prophylaxis of all uninfected patients on the unit and all new admissions with penicillin V, 500 mg each day, terminated the outbreak.

Puerperal and Neonatal Infection

The communicable nature of puerperal fever was well understood by 1840 (35,36). The careful observations of Semmelweis made prevention possible. Semmelweis noted that an obstetric service staffed by midwives had little puerperal infection. On an adjacent ward, the service run by physicians (who also participated in autopsies on patients who had died) experienced three to five times the number of infections. He also observed that, in hospitals in which obstetric units were distant from autopsy rooms (and here he compared Dublin and Vienna), puerperal infection was uncommon. In May 1847, he introduced chlorine water hand rinses to the first obstetric clinic in Vienna and documented a dramatic decrease in the frequency of puerperal infections (37).

Despite the significant reduction in the occurrence of these infections through hand washing, major outbreaks were relatively common until effective antimicrobials became available (3). Isolated outbreaks of puerperal infection caused by GABHS have continued to occur. Small outbreaks of infections in newly delivered neonates are also well recognized. Studies published in the last 30 years include an outbreak caused by a tetracycline-resistant strain of GABHS that was isolated from both adults and neonates (38). The outbreak was terminated by closing the implicated ward and administering penicillin prophylaxis or treatment to all of the mothers and infants. Tancer et al. (39) reported an outbreak involving 11 infants, 2 postpartum mothers, 3 nurses, and another hospital employee. This outbreak was temporally related to episodes of pharyngitis in a newly delivered mother and an elevator operator in the maternity wing of the hospital. Neither of these individuals was cultured. Ogden and Amstey (40) described five patients with puerperal GABHS infection in 1978. These cases were characteristic of the clinical presentation of puerperal GABHS infection. All of the mothers experienced uterine tenderness and then developed fever spikes associated with recovery of these microorganisms from the lochia. McGregor et al. (41) reported a similar-sized outbreak. A labor room nurse had mild eczema on her hands, and these lesions grew GABHS and *Staphylococcus aureus.* The microorganism was serologically identical to that recovered from the patients. An outbreak of postpartum GABHS involving seven patients was recently reported. The source was a healthcare worker with a positive rectal isolate (30). In two studies, evidence has suggested that outbreaks were related to contamination of inanimate objects. In one, a handheld shower head was seen as a possible route of transmission; in the other, use of a communal bidet was implicated (42,43). GABHS were shown by Claesson and Claesson (42) to remain viable on a metal surface for more than 9 days.

Outbreaks of GABHS infection also have involved neonates. In these episodes, microorganisms have primarily contaminated the umbilicus. Transmission between infants has apparently occurred with nursing care. In the two outbreaks described by Geil et al. (44), penicillin was administered to all of the infants in the nursery on both occasions. This regimen was successful in the first of their two outbreaks. However, in the second outbreak it was not successful without the additional application of bacitracin ointment to the umbilical stumps of the infants. Bygdeman et al. (45) reported an outbreak in Stockholm in which 67% of infants had umbilical colonization with GABHS. Pharyngitis was documented among family members of neonates. Five of 69 mothers who had nose and throat cultures for GABHS yielded this microorganism. Presumably, this outbreak resulted from introduction of an epidemiologically virulent strain by a mother or healthcare worker. Transmission at the time of delivery could also have been responsible, although the authors did not perform vaginal or rectal cultures.

An outbreak was described by Isenberg et al. (46) in 1984 that involved 10 newborn infants over a 2-month period. Nineteen percent of the infants in the nursery were found to be carriers of streptococci. Again, umbilical infection was most frequent. Only 1 of the 10 infected infants had GABHS isolated from throat cultures.

Infections Associated with Nursing Homes

GABHS has been reported over the last 30 years to cause outbreaks of infection in various healthcare settings (including facilities for the elderly) (47–49). Over the last 15 years, a number of outbreaks of GABHS infections have been reported in long-term care units in the United States. These reports have occurred during a period in which GABHS disease has been caused by strains of apparent increasing virulence (50,51).

The Centers for Disease Control and Prevention (CDC) described outbreaks in four nursing homes during the winter of 1989 to 1990, each in a different state (52). Infection occurred in 18 residents, with slightly over half [(10 of 18 (56%)] of the residents dying. Pneumonia and cutaneous infection were most common. Culture surveys to identify pharyngeal carriage in each of the four nursing homes revealed that 11 of 312 residents (4%) and 4 of 297 staff members (1%) had asymptomatic pharyngeal carriage of GABHS. These isolates were found to be the same serotype as the strains causing infection in each of the homes. The outbreaks were controlled following antimicrobial prophylaxis or therapy.

Auerbach et al. (53) described one of these clusters in more detail. This outbreak, in a North Carolina nursing home of 50 beds, involved 16 of 80 residents (20%) and 3 of 45 staff members (7%). Cases were spatially clustered within the nursing home (Fig. 31.1). The outbreak was ended after improvement in infection control practices and antibiotic prophylaxis.

Outbreaks were described in 1992 in two different nursing homes in Rochester, New York. In one, 14 residents of a large intermediate-care facility developed infection over a period of 4 months (54). Cellulitis was the most frequent manifestation in these patients. Two sequential outbreaks were reported by McNutt et al. (55) in another facility in Rochester; these were notable for the absence of severe disease. None of the patients died; wound infection and conjunctivitis were most common. No clear source was documented. A second outbreak involved six patients on floors above the ward of the original outbreak.

Schwartz and Ussery (56) reviewed reports to the CDC of invasive GABHS infections in nursing homes and described five other outbreaks (including the two described by McNutt et al.) that were primarily associated with noninvasive infection. Outbreaks of noninvasive disease tended to last longer, were associated with more cases, and characteristically involved patients who were more physically impaired than those infected in the invasive outbreaks.

In all of these nursing home outbreaks, there was no clear proof that healthcare workers were sources of the microorganism. (The positive pharyngeal cultures in the initial CDC study

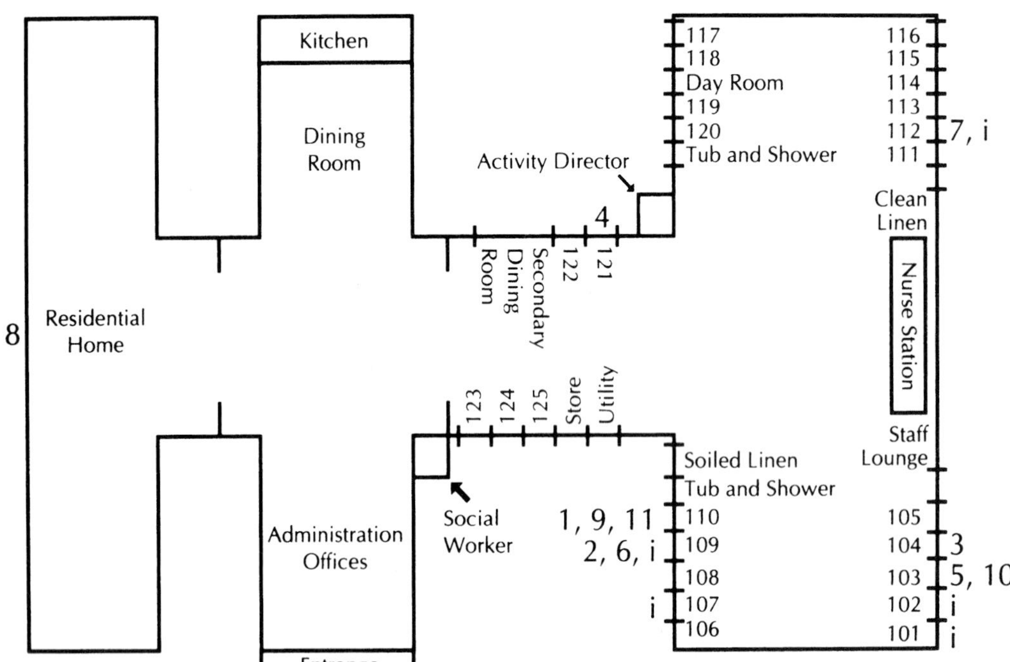

Figure 31.1. Distribution of cases of group A β-hemolytic streptococci (GABHS) infection in a North Carolina nursing home. Spatial clustering of infections in one wing of the nursing home is evident. (From Auerbach SB, Schwartz B, Williams D, et al. Outbreak of invasive group A streptococcal infections in a nursing home. Lessons on prevention and control. *Arch Intern Med* 1992;152:1017–1022, with permission.)

suggest possible introduction of these microorganisms, but obviously the healthcare workers might have been colonized by exposure to the nursing home patients.) In two of the nursing home outbreaks investigated by the CDC, extensive environmental culturing yielded only one positive culture for GABHS. This would suggest that these microorganisms are uncommonly transmitted by fomites.

Critical Care Units

Several outbreaks of GABHS have been described in intensive care units in teaching hospitals. In a review of clusters of GABHS, Schwartz et al. (57) describe family and nosocomial clusters and outbreaks within nursing homes. All five nosocomial clusters reported to the CDC occurred in intensive care units. The index patient in each had streptococcal toxic shock syndrome. Types of infections included cellulitis, paronychia, and pharyngitis. In three of the four outbreaks in which the causal microorganisms were typed, a serotype M1 strain was identified. This serotype has often been associated with invasive infection and the streptococcal toxic shock syndrome (58,59).

Lannigan et al. (60) described a cluster of five cases that followed the admission of a patient with necrotizing fasciitis to a Canadian hospital. The microorganism was serotype M1. Two nurses developed cellulitis (superimposed on underlying dermatitis), and three patients had GABHS isolated from endotracheal secretions. Both of the isolates from the nurses and one of the three isolates from endotracheal secretions were the same M and T type as the index patient's microorganism; in two of the patients, sputum isolates were not typed. Transmission by contamination of the nurses' hands seemed most likely. A similar outbreak, involving two patients with isolates of the same M and T type, occurred following admission of a patient with facial cellulitis to an intensive care unit (61). The two patients who acquired the microorganism had endotracheal tubes in place and developed pneumonia and bacteremia.

Control of Infections in Hospitals and Long-Term Care

Outbreaks of infection caused by GABHS in healthcare centers are difficult to control. Several of the reported outbreaks have lasted for relatively long periods. Because of the need to serotype GABHS and the difficulty of causally associating an infected or colonized patient or healthcare worker with an outbreak, the epidemiology of many of these infections has not been well understood. It is possible that outbreaks of invasive GABHS disease may be characterized by higher attack rates, more obvious infection, and shorter duration than has been typical of GABHS outbreaks in the past. Too few of these clusters have been documented to determine that they are epidemiologically distinct or to draw such conclusions.

Whether a GABHS outbreak occurs in an acute care hospital or a nursing home (and no matter the types of infection), much of the process of evaluation and control is the same (Table 31.1). Most outbreaks of GABHS are small; a single case that is apparently nosocomial should warrant an investigation.

After developing appropriate case definitions, determining

TABLE 31.1. STEPS IN THE MANAGEMENT OF AN OUTBREAK OF GROUP A β-HEMOLYTIC STREPTOCOCCAL (GABHS) INFECTION

More than one case of apparent institutionally acquired infection should initiate an outbreak investigation
Develop case definitions (*definite* infection if culture positive for GABHS, *probable* if symptoms and signs compatible with streptococcal infection but no culture done)
Examine susceptibility of isolates and treat cases appropriately
Make an effort to determine likely sources for the outbreak by examining data about contacts between patients and healthcare workers
Attempt to identify healthcare workers and patients who might be sources (by examining for dermatitis and by asking about skin infections and sore throat)
Do vaginal, rectal, and pharyngeal cultures (and cultures of areas of dermatitis) of healthcare workers or patients who may be potential sources
Arrange for M and T serotyping of isolates
Isolate apparent sources and patients until appropriately treated (see text)
Reculture source of outbreak at 1 week and at 1 and 3 months after treatment

the time course of the outbreak, and examining basic epidemiologic data, it is appropriate to look for patients or healthcare workers who might be carrying GABHS. Rectal and/or vaginal carriage is at least as frequent as pharyngeal carriage. Penicillin alone has not been effective in eliminating pharyngeal, rectal, or vaginal colonization in a number of carriers. Recently published recommendations for chemoprophylaxis from CDC are summarized in Table 31.2 (62).

Prompt culturing and treatment of individuals who have clinical manifestations of streptococcal infection is appropriate. Although penicillin remains uniformly effective against GABHS, resistance to alternative agents (e.g., the macrolides or tetracycline) occurs in 10% to 15% of isolates. Before erythromycin is used in place of penicillin to treat a carrier or for prophylaxis, susceptibility of the isolate to this drug should be determined. In some settings, antibiotic treatment has been given to all of the patients on a ward or a unit. Although this has not been done in a controlled fashion, outbreaks have usually ended after this intervention (56).

In settings other than operating rooms, GABHS infections are occasionally spread by the respiratory route or, more often, by contamination of hands of healthcare workers. Appropriate infection control intervention will, therefore, require emphasis on careful hand washing. Interruption of respiratory spread (by use of a mask) in individuals who are known or suspected to be infected or colonized with GABHS before antibiotic administration is also necessary. In acute care hospitals, these are relatively easy interventions, but in nursing homes, limited hand-washing facilities and infection control resources may make it difficult to take appropriate control steps. Most homes do not pay employees when they are ill. Thus, workers with streptococcal pharyngitis may often be providing care while they are infectious.

Especially when patients are infected with large numbers of microorganisms (e.g., burn wound infections), control may require awareness of the potential of airborne transmission and the possible (although unlikely) role of fomites. GABHS are very resistant to desiccation, and reports of infections in operating rooms adjacent to those in which colonized surgeons or anesthe-

TABLE 31.2. RECOMMENDED REGIMENS FOR ELIMINATION OF ASYMPTOMATIC GROUP A STREPTOCOCCAL COLONIZATION

Drug	Dosage(s)	Comment(s)
BPG plus rifampin	BPG. 600,000 U im in 1 dose for patients weighing <27 kg or 1,200,000 U im in 1 dose for patients weighing ≥27 kg; rifampin; 20 mg/kg/day po (max. daily dose, 600 mg) in 2 divided doses for 4 days	Not recommended for pregnant women because rifampin is teratogenic in laboratory animals. Because the reliability of oral contraceptives may be affected by rifampin therapy, alternative contraceptive measures should be considered while rifampin is being administered
Clindamycin	20 mg/kg/day po (max. daily dose, 900 mg) in 3 divided doses for 10 days	Preferred for healthcare workers who are rectal carriers of GAS[a]
Azithromycin	12 mg/kg/day po (max. daily dose, 500 mg/day) in a single dose for 5 days	Pregnancy category B: human data reassuring (animal positive) or animal studies show no risk[a]

All regimens are acceptable for nonpregnant persons who are not allergic to penicillin, BPG, benzathine penicillin G; GAS, group A streptococci; max., maximum.
[a] Clindamycin or azithromycin is acceptable for persons allergic to penicillin. If administered to healthcare workers implicated in an outbreak or to their colonized household contacts, susceptibility testing should be performed.
From The Prevention of Invasive Group & A Streptococcal Infections Workshop Participants. Prevention of invasive Group A Streptococcal disease among household contacts of case patients and among post partum and postsurgical patients; recommendations from the Centers for Disease Central and Prevention. *Clin Infect Dis* 2002; 35:950–959, with permission.

siologists have worked indicate that airborne transmission may occur (21,23,25).

GROUP B β-HEMOLYTIC STREPTOCOCCI

S. agalactiae (β-hemolytic streptococci belonging to Lancefield group B) was originally described as a cause of mastitis in cattle (63). Since the mid-1960s, GBS have become a common cause of puerperal and neonatal infections, some of which are nosocomially acquired (64). In one recent population-based study, 22% of GBS infection were nosocomial (65). GBS also has been recognized as a cause of other types of nosocomial infections. Dessau (66) reviewed all of the bacteremias in residents of Funen County in Denmark between 1978 and 1988. Twenty-two cases of GBS bacteremia in adults among the 450,000 inhabitants of the county were documented. Ten of these were nosocomial, with onset from 3 to 30 days following hospital admission. Four infections were urogenital, and one each involved a surgical site, an intravenous catheter, a bridge graft, and a prosthetic aortic valve. In two cases, the site could not be determined. These findings are similar to those of other studies that suggest that between 46% and 70% of *S. agalactiae* bacteremias are nosocomial (67–69).

Group B streptococci may be subdivided into three types on the basis of immunospecific carbohydrates (70). Type I may be further divided into Ia, Ib, and Ic. Type II is most commonly associated with early-onset disease (usually characterized by meningitis occurring shortly after birth). Type III has been isolated largely from blood cultures of infants taken more than 10 days after birth (71,72). Use of this type of identification (along with phage typing) has been of help in documenting nosocomial transmission of these microorganisms.

Epidemiology and Transmission in the Hospital

Group B streptococci are carried within the gastrointestinal tract (73,74) and may colonize the urinary tract and the vagina. Rates of colonization vary depending on the number of cultures, the sites sampled, and whether an enrichment medium is used. In keeping with other authors, Easmon (75) suggests that 20% to 25% of women carry GBS genitally during pregnancy. Among infants, Ferrieri et al. (76) showed that the external ear was the most commonly colonized site, with nose, umbilicus, and rectum also often yielding GBS.

It has been repeatedly demonstrated that a significant proportion of infants who are colonized with group B streptococci acquire their microorganisms by nosocomial transmission and not from their mothers (77). Easmon et al. (78) reported that 36% of infants who acquired GBS did so through nosocomial routes. (The other 64% of infants who were colonized in this study acquired infection from their mothers.) These authors and others have noted that nosocomial acquisition of this microorganism is associated with colonization at fewer sites and by smaller numbers of microorganisms (79). Presumably, infants contaminated by maternal routes may, thus, be at greater risk for development of infection. Easmon et al. showed that at 6 weeks after discharge from the hospital, colonization was present in only 10% of babies who were colonized with GBS during their hospitalization but whose mothers were not. In contrast, infants who were positive for GABHS and whose mothers were also culture-positive with the same microorganism during hospitalization were five times as likely to be carriers at 6 weeks (52% vs. 10%).

Easmon et al. (78) compared the frequency of transmission in an obstetric unit with that of a neonatal intensive care unit (NICU). In the obstetric unit, 38 of 107 (36%) colonized babies acquired the microorganism from a nonmaternal source versus only 2 of 23 (9%) in the NICU (78). This suggests that more careful attention to infection control measures in the intensive care unit may be associated with a reduction in the frequency of nosocomial transmission of GBS (80).

Group B streptococcal carriage among healthcare workers is relatively common (81). In one study, the carriage rate ranged from 6% to 50% in serial prevalence surveys of NICU staff (78). Eighty-eight percent of the carriers had the microorganism recovered from perianal swabs; pharyngeal carriage (or simultaneous carriage at both sites) accounted for the remainder. Despite rather frequent colonization of healthcare workers, documented transmission of identifiable strains of GBS to patients is rare. Easmon et al. (78) reported that a pediatrician apparently transmitted a group III phage type 11 strain to four babies on whom he did well-child examinations.

The bulk of cases of group B streptococcal infection acquired in the hospital appear to have occurred because of transient hand contamination of healthcare workers (82). GBS have also been reported to contaminate devices and cause infection in this manner. Davis et al. (83) found group B streptococci in pressure transducer domes. The authors were able to correlate colonization with use of intrauterine transducers and documented a reduction in colonization following sterilization of domes after each maternal use.

Puerperal and Neonatal Infections

GBS are relatively common causes of nosocomial infections in neonates. Gaynes et al. (84) reported data about 13,179 nosocomial infections in 10,296 neonates in high-risk nurseries of the 99 NNIS system hospitals for the period of October 1986 to September 1994. GBS accounted for 7.9% of the bloodstream infections and was the second most frequent isolate (after coagulase-negative staphylococci, which accounted for 51% of bacteremias). Although less common than a number of other microorganisms, GBS caused 5.7% of pneumonias. Interestingly, maternally acquired GBS accounted for 46.4% of bloodstream infections versus 0.9% of bacteremias that were not maternally acquired.

Only a small proportion of newborns colonized with GBS will develop clinical infection. Two syndromes in neonates have been associated with GBS infection. One is an infection of sudden onset developing within the first few days of life (early onset) and characterized by meningitis or pneumonia, often with bacteremia. The mortality rate is high, and serious sequelae in survivors of central nervous system disease are common. All three of the major serogroups are recovered with approximately equal frequency. Major risk factors associated with this syndrome include premature labor and prolonged rupture of membranes (85).

The other type of neonatal infection occurs characteristically 3 to 4 weeks after birth (late onset) and is associated with a lower mortality rate. Meningitis is the most common manifestation, and sequelae are often frequent and serious. Approximately 90% of cases of late-onset disease are caused by type III microorganisms.

Although GBS neonatal infection is relatively common, recognizable outbreaks are not often described. In part, this must be because of the difficulties in distinguishing maternally acquired from nosocomial disease. Noya et al. (86) described an epidemic of late-onset infection occurring in five infants in an NICU. Two nursery personnel carried the same type as was recovered from the patients (Ib/c). In this outbreak, transmission apparently occurred from infant to infant on the hands of hospital personnel (see Chapter 52).

In adults, GBS infections may be encountered in women following delivery. Surgical site infections in women who have had a cesarean section and endometritis are most common. Evidence suggests that these infections are particularly common in immunocompromised women (87).

Group B streptococci may also be encountered as causes of nosocomial urinary tract infection, pneumonia, or meningitis. GBS have been associated with intravenous line infection and have been described as the cause of a small outbreak of infections associated with arthroscopy (88). The exact route of infection in this outbreak is unclear. GBS infection has been reported following cardiac catheterization and, in the one case reported, was felt to be associated with multiple puncture sites made to gain vascular access (89). Burn wound infection has also occurred (90).

The most serious group B streptococcal infections are acquired maternally. For this reason, extensive efforts have been made during the past 25 years to reduce or eliminate acquisition of GBS at the time of delivery. The most popular strategy employs screening cultures and subsequent administration of antibiotics such as ampicillin during labor. Antibiotic administration is especially indicated in women who are at high risk for serious GBS infection or for delivering a child who is likely to be infected (81). Data from the CDC suggests that a significant decline in early onset GBS disease has occurred in recent years (91).

Nosocomial acquisition of GBS infection is primarily a result of transmission on the hands of healthcare workers, enabling microorganisms to be spread between infected mothers or infants and other mothers or neonates. Thus, hand washing is perhaps the most important mechanism for preventing transmission of this microorganism within the hospital.

OTHER NOSOCOMIAL (NONENTEROCOCCAL) STREPTOCOCCAL INFECTIONS

Pneumococci

S. pneumoniae is a well-recognized cause of nosocomial infection. The first probable outbreak was described in 1903 (92). In the study of nosocomial pneumonia by Bartlett et al. (93), this microorganism was the predominant isolate in 26% of cases. Alvarez et al. (94) described 56 episodes of pneumococcal bacteremia; 23 (41%) were nosocomial. Patients with nosocomial *S. pneumoniae* bacteremia were of poor functional status and were more likely to die than were bacteremic patients who acquired their infection in the community. Only 1 of the 56 patients had received pneumococcal polysaccharide vaccine although most of the infections were caused by strains included in the vaccine. More recently, Lääveri et al. (95) noted that only 11/94 adults with *S. pneumoniae* bacteremia had nosocomial infection; these patients were significantly older than those with community-acquired infection. Nosocomial pneumococcal bacteremia has also been described in elderly men (96) and in adults infected with the human immunodeficiency virus (HIV) (97).

A case-control study of 37 patients with nosocomial pneumococcal bacteremia (first positive blood culture performed >72 hours after admission in a patient who did not have a clinical syndrome compatible with infection on admission) were compared with controls. Respiratory and hematologic malignancy, anemia, chronic obstructive pulmonary disease, and coronary artery disease were significantly associated with nosocomial pneumococcal bacteremia. There was also a strong association with death within the 7 days of the date of the initial blood culture; the mortality rate was 40.5% compared with 1.2% for members of the control population (98). In a study that examined patients with levofloxacin-resistant *S. pneumoniae,* two thirds were hospital-acquired. Age, nursing home residence, chronic obstructive pulmonary disease (COPD), number of hospitalizations, and exposure to fluoroquinolones correlated with infection or colonization with the resistant pneumococcal strains (99).

Multiply antibiotic-resistant isolates of *S. pneumoniae* were initially reported from hospitalized children in South Africa. Although there is only limited data about the nasal carriage of antibiotic-resistant strains of *S. pneumoniae,* in one recent study 43/103 (41.7%) children hospitalized in Sofia, Bulgaria, had these microorganisms recovered from nasopharyngeal swabs (100). In a nursing home outbreak of multidrug-resistant pneumococci, 17/74 (23%) of asymptomatic residents and 2/69 (3%) employees had nasopharyngeal carriage of these microorganisms (101). Recent use of antibiotics was associated with both nasopharyngeal colonization and the development of clinical disease. In another study, more than 5 days of therapy with an oral β-lactam antibiotic in low dose has been found to be significantly associated with nasal carriage of resistant pneumococci (102).

Nosocomial transmission of these strains has been documented in South Africa (103,104), Britain (105–107), and The Netherlands (108,109). In the largest of these studies in an acute care hospital, 36 patients had the same strain of antibiotic-resistant *S. pneumoniae* cultured in an outbreak that persisted for 2 years. The patients were elderly and 89% had chronic obstructive pulmonary disease. The outbreak ended after patients were treated with ceftriaxone and rifampin (109).

Nursing home outbreaks caused by both antibiotic-susceptible and multidrug-resistant strains of *S. pneumoniae* are well documented (101,110). Immunization programs and use of prophylactic antibiotics have effectively terminated these episodes. In each of these outbreaks, fewer than 5% of residents had received pneumococcal vaccine. This reinforces the need for widespread routine immunization with pneumococcal vaccine among the institutionalized elderly.

Primary methods of prevention of nosocomial pneumococcal infection should include immunization of susceptible individuals (111). Careful hand washing is also appropriate. Transmission of pneumococci by contaminated respiratory therapy equipment has been documented, and appropriate disinfection is needed (112). A nosocomial central venous line infection in an infant also has been described (113).

Miscellaneous Microorganisms

Group C and G Streptococci

Streptococci belonging to Lancefield group C and group G may be associated with pharyngitis, pneumonia, and cellulitis. The microorganisms are often β-hemolytic and may be confused with Lancefield group A streptococci (114,115). Efstratiou (116) has reported on identification of T antigens in these strains; this is a useful technique for evaluating possible nosocomial outbreaks.

Group C streptococci have been recognized as causes of puerperal infection and of surgical site infection (117). In an outbreak of two postoperative surgical site infections, a surgeon was found to carry the microorganism in his nose and rectum. Administration of topical bacitracin and orally administered penicillin and vancomycin ended the carrier state. This outbreak shares many characteristics with outbreaks of group A streptococcal infection. Teare et al. (118) described an outbreak of 33 cases of puerperal infection in three hospitals in Britain caused by group C streptococci. Environmental contamination was documented. The outbreak strain carried M protein antigen.

Efstratiou (119) reported outbreaks of infections noted in a laboratory-based study of 749 strains of group C streptococci *(Streptococcus equisimilis)* and 2,348 strains of group G streptococci that were referred to the public health laboratory at Colindale, United Kingdom, over a 6-year period. Ten outbreaks were reported (Table 31.3). These included pharyngitis, cutaneous infection, and puerperal sepsis. Except for pharyngitis, all of these clusters were in hospitals or nursing homes (most pharyngitis outbreaks occurred in schools).

Group G streptococci were much more frequent causes of outbreaks. Forty-one institutions in Great Britain reported outbreaks in the 6-year period. Group G streptococci were associated with outbreaks in three burn units, where they were found to occasionally colonize the nose and pharynx of staff members and were isolated from the environment. Most outbreaks of group G streptococci reported in this study involved skin and soft tissue. Twelve puerperal outbreaks were reported; in two hospitals, the implicated serotype was isolated from bath water, toilet seats, and showers in the maternity ward. In each of the reports of puerperal fever caused by group G streptococci, none of the babies born to infected mothers had invasive disease. Haynes et al. (120) reported an outbreak of puerperal fever among 15 mothers that was associated with contamination of automated douches. Although group G streptococci may be recovered from the pharynx of up to 25% of normal individuals (114), group C streptococci also may be recovered from a few normal individuals (3%) (121).

Streptococcus viridans

Streptococcus milleri and other viridans streptococci have become important causes of infection in immunocompromised patients in recent years. These microorganisms have been associated with bacteremia, endocarditis, cellulitis, abscesses (subcutaneous, intraabdominal, and intracranial), and other infections (122). Seven of 18 bacteremias with *S. milleri* in one recent

TABLE 31.3. PRESUMPTIVE NOSOCOMIAL OUTBREAKS OF GROUP C AND GROUP G STREPTOCOCCI IN A 6-YEAR PERIOD[a]

Location	Source	Number of isolates	T-type
Group C			
Pharyngitis			
Hospital A	Throat (staff)		
	Foodborne	146	204
Skin sepsis			
Hospital B—ward	Skin	4	PT1058
Hospital C—geriatric ward	Pressure sores	3	305
Hospital D—burn unit patients	Skin	13	21
—burn unit staff	Throat	3	
Puerperal sepsis			
Hospital E—maternity unit patients	Vagina	29	204
—maternity unit staff	Throat	8	204
Group G			
Skin sepsis			
22 outbreaks	Skin, wounds, ulcers	119	Varied
Puerperal infection			
12 outbreaks	Perineum, throat, vagina	104	Varied

[a] Outbreaks are presumptive, and no detailed epidemiologic data are provided. From Esfstration A. Outbreaks of human infection caused by pyogenic streptococci of Lance groups C and G. *J Med Microbiol* 1989; 29: 207–219, with permission.

study were nosocomial (123). Other studies do not report the proportion of cases that were nosocomial. Two recent papers stress a relationship to the presence of a central venous line and to the administration of cytosine arabinoside (124,125).

Two additional points about this microorganism should be made. It is noteworthy that isolates of *S. viridans* recovered from hospital workers in wards on which penicillin is extensively used commonly are penicillin resistant (126). Thus, healthcare workers who need prophylaxis for bacterial endocarditis and who work in units in which antibiotics are extensively used might be advised to obtain an antibiogram of their oral *S. viridans* or be given erythromycin.

S. viridans has been reported to cause pseudobacteremia. Church and Bryant (127) reported an outbreak in which a phlebotomist did not wear gloves but had eczema involving her hands. Skin scrapings from her hands and fingernails grew this microorganism and contaminated blood cultures.

REFERENCES

1. Schaberg DR, Culver DH, Gaynes RP. Major trends in the microbial etiology of nosocomial infection. *Am J Med* 1991;91(Suppl B): 72S–75S.
2. Dubos RJ, Hirsch JG, eds. *Bacterial and mycotic infections of man,* 4th ed. Philadelphia: JB Lippincott, 1965.
3. Williams JT. Epidemic puerperal sepsis. *N Engl J Med* 1936;215: 1022–1027.
4. Keefer CS, Ingelfinger FJ, Spink WW. Significance of hemolytic streptococcal bacteremia. *Arch Intern Med* 1937;60:1084–1097.
5. Pfaller MA, Jones RN, Doern GV, et al. Bacterial pathogens isolated from patients with bloodstream infection: frequencies of occurrence and antimicrobial susceptibility patterns from the SENTRY Antimicrobial Surveillance Program (United States and Canada, 1997). *Antimicrob Agents Chemother* 1998;42:1762–1770.
6. Zurawski CA, Bardsley MS, Beall, B, et al. Invasive group A streptococcal disease in metropolitan Atlanta: a population-based assessment. *Clin Infect Dis* 1998;27:150–157.
7. Burkert T, Watanakunakorn C. Group A streptococcal bacteremia in a community teaching hospital—1980–1989. *Clin Infect Dis* 1992; 14:29–37.
8. Kristensen B, Schonheyder HC. A 13-year survey of bacteraemia due to β-haemolytic streptococci in a Danish county. *J Med Microbiol* 1995;43:63–67.
9. Stanley J, Desai M, Efstratiou A, et al. High-resolution genotyping of *Streptococcus pyrogenes:* Application to outbreak studies and population genetics. In: Horaud T, Bouvet A, Leclercq R, de Montclos H, Sicard M, eds. *Streptococci and the host.* New York: Plenum Press, 1997.
10. Wu AF, Wojcik D, Kupchik SC, et al. Group A streptococcal pharyngitis in hospital personnel. *Infect Control* 1985;6:389–390.
11. Asnes RS, Vail D. Anal carrier rate of group A beta-hemolytic streptococci in children with streptococcal pharyngitis. *Pediatrics* 1973;52: 438–441.
12. Schoenknecht FD, Batjer JD, Sherris JC. Anal streptococci. *N Engl J Med* 1969;281:220–221.
13. Dudding BA, Burnett JW, Chapman SS, et al. The role of normal skin in the spread of streptococcal pyoderma. *J Hyg* 1970;68:19–28.
14. Quinn RW, Hillman JW. An epidemic of streptococcal wound infections. *Arch Environ Health* 1965;11:28–33.
15. Zimmerman RA, Sciple GW. Streptococcal wound infections. *Rocky Mt Med J* 1966;63:63–65.
16. Paul SM, Genese C, Spitalny K. Postoperative group A beta-hemolytic *Streptococcus* outbreak with the pathogen traced to a member of a healthcare worker's household. *Infect Control Hosp Epidemiol* 1990; 11:643–646.
17. Campbell JR, Arango CA, Garcia-Prats JA, et al. An outbreak of M serotype 1 group A *Streptococcus* in a neonatal intensive care unit. *J Pediatr* 1996;129:396–402.
18. Kolmos HJ, Svendsen RN, Nielsen SV. The surgical team as a source of postoperative wound infections caused by *Streptococcus pyogenes. J Hosp Infect* 1997;35:207–214.
19. Bisno AL, Turpin P, Ledes CP. Pyoderma streptococci as a cause of nosocomial sepsis. *South Med J* 1973;66:1071–1072.
20. Mastro TD, Farley TA, Elliott JA, et al. An outbreak of surgical wound infections due to group A *Streptococcus* carried on the scalp. *N Engl J Med* 1990;323:968–972.
21. Schaffner W, Lefkowitz LB, Goodman JS, et al. Hospital outbreak of infections with group A streptococci traced to an asymptomatic anal carrier. *N Engl J Med* 1969;280:1224–1225.
22. McKee WM, Di Caprio JM, Roberts CE Jr, et al. Anal carriage as the probable source of a streptococcal epidemic. *Lancet* 1966;2: 1007–1009.
23. Richman DD, Breton SJ, Goldmann DA. Scarlet fever and group A streptococcal surgical wound infection traced to an anal carrier. *J Pediatr* 1977;90:387–390.
24. Viglionese A, Nottebart VF, Bodman HA, et al. Recurrent group A streptococcal carriage in a health care worker associated with widely separated nosocomial outbreaks. *Am J Med* 1991;91(Suppl 3B): 329S–333S.
25. Berkelman RL, Martin D, Graham DR, et al. Streptococcal wound infections caused by a vaginal carrier. *JAMA* 1982;247:2680–2682.
26. Stamm WE, Feeley JC, Facklam RR. Wound infections due to group A *Streptococcus* traced to a vaginal carrier. *J Infect Dis* 1978;138: 287–292.
27. Rutishauser J, Funke G, Lütticken R, Ruef C. Streptococcal toxic shock syndrome in two patients infected by a colonized surgeon. *Infection* 1999;27:259–260.
28. Centers for Disease Control and Prevention. Nosocomial group A streptococcal infections associated with asymptomatic health-care workers—Maryland and California, 1997. *MMWR Morb Mortal Wkly Rep* 1999;48:163–165.
29. Ramage L, Green K, Pyskir D, et al. An outbreak of fatal nosocomial infections due to group A streptococcus on a medical ward. *Infect Control Hosp Epidemiol* 1996;17:429–431.
30. Kakis A, Gibbs L, Eguia J, et al. An outbreak of group A streptococcal infection among health care workers. *Clin Infect Dis* 2002;35: 1353–1359.
31. Webster A, Scott GMS, Ridgway GL, et al. An outbreak of group A streptococcal skin infection: control by source isolation and teicoplanin therapy. *Scand J Infect Dis* 1987;19:205–209.
32. Whitby M, Sleigh JD, Reid W, et al. Streptococcal infection in a regional burns centre and a plastic surgery unit. *J Hosp Infect* 1984; 5:63–69.
33. Burnett IA, Norman P. *Streptococcus pyogenes:* an outbreak on a burns unit. *J Hosp Infect* 1990;15:173–176.
34. Allen KD, Ridgway EJ. *Streptococcus pyogenes:* an outbreak on a burns unit. *J Hosp Infect* 1990;16:178–179.
35. Moore G. *An inquiry into the pathology, causes and treatment of puerperal fever.* London: S. Highley, 1836.
36. Holmes OW. *The contagiousness of puerperal fever in medical essays, 1842–1882.* Boston: Houghton Mifflin, 1896:103–172.
37. Semmelweis IF. *The etiology, the concept and the prophylaxis of childbed fever.* Birmingham: Classics of Medicine Library, 1981.
38. Nash FW, Mann TP, Haydu IW. An outbreak of streptococcal infection in a maternity unit. *Postgrad Med J* 1965;41:182–184.
39. Tancer ML, McManus JE, Bellotti G. Group A, type 33, beta-hemolytic streptococcal outbreak on a maternity and newborn service. *Am J Obstet Gynecol* 1969;103:1028–1033.
40. Ogden E, Amstey M. Puerperal infection due to group A beta hemolytic *Streptococcus. Obstet Gynecol* 1978;52:53–55.
41. McGregor J, Ott A, Villard M. An epidemic of childbed fever. *Am J Obstet Gynecol* 1984;150:385–388.
42. Claesson BEB, Claesson ULE. An outbreak of endometritis in a maternity unit caused by spread of group A streptococci from a showerhead. *J Hosp Infect* 1985;6:304–311.

43. Gordon G, Dale BAS, Lochhead D. An outbreak of group A haemolytic streptococcal puerperal sepsis spread by the communal use of bidets. *Br J Obstet Gynaecol* 1994;101:447–448.
44. Geil CC, Castle WK, Mortimer EA Jr. Group A streptococcal infections in newborn nurseries. *Pediatrics* 1970;46:849–854.
45. Bygdeman S, Jacobsson E, Myrback K-E, et al. Hemolytic streptococci among infants in a maternity department. Report of an outbreak. *Scand J Infect Dis* 1978;10:45–49.
46. Isenberg HD, Tucci V, Lipsitz P, et al. Clinical laboratory and epidemiological investigations of a *Streptococcus pyogenes* cluster epidemic in a newborn nursery. *J Clin Microbiol* 1984;19:366–370.
47. Ruben FL, Norden CW, Heisler B, et al. An outbreak of *Streptococcus pyogenes. Ann Intern Med* 1984;101:494–496.
48. Rahman M. Outbreak of *Streptococcus pyogenes* in a geriatric hospital and control by mass treatment. *J Hosp Infect* 1981;2:63–69.
49. Reid RI, Briggs RS, Seal DV, et al. Virulent *Streptococcus pyogenes:* outbreak and spread within a geriatric unit. *J Infect* 1983;6:219–225.
50. Centers for Disease Control and Prevention. Group A beta-hemolytic streptococcal bacteremia: Colorado, 1989. *MMWR Morb Mortal Wkly Rep* 1990;39:3–6, 11.
51. Gaworzewska E, Colman G. Changes in the pattern of infection caused by *Streptococcus pyogenes. Epidemiol Infect* 1988;100:257–269.
52. Centers for Disease Control and Prevention. Nursing home outbreaks of invasive group A streptococcal infections—Illinois, Kansas, North Carolina, and Texas. *MMWR Morb Mortal Wkly Rep* 1990;39: 577–579.
53. Auerbach SB, Schwartz B, Williams D, et al. Outbreak of invasive group A streptococcal infections in a nursing home. Lessons on prevention and control. *Arch Intern Med* 1992;152:1017–1022.
54. Harkness GA, Bentley DW, Mottley M, et al. *Streptococcus pyogenes* outbreak in a long-term care facility. *Am J Infect Control* 1992;20: 142–148.
55. McNutt LA, Casiano-Colon AE, Coles FB, et al. Two outbreaks of primarily noninvasive group A streptococcal disease in the same nursing home, New York, 1991. *Infect Control Hosp Epidemiol* 1992;13: 748–751.
56. Schwartz B, Ussery XT. Group A streptococcal outbreaks in nursing homes. *Infect Control Hosp Epidemiol* 1992;13:742–747.
57. Schwartz B, Elliott JA, Butler JC, et al. Clusters of invasive group A streptococcal infections in family, hospital, and nursing home settings. *Clin Infect Dis* 1992;15:277–284.
58. Schwartz B, Facklam RR, Breiman RF. Changing epidemiology of group A streptococcal infection in the USA. *Lancet* 1990;336: 1167–1171.
59. Talkington DF, Schwartz B, Elliott JA, et al. Analysis of streptococcal pyrogenic exotoxin A and B, and M-type, among invasive group A streptococcal strains [Abstract B271]. In: *Abstracts of the 91st general meeting of the American Society for Microbiology.* Washington, DC: American Society for Microbiology, 1991.
60. Lannigan R, Hussain Z, Austin TW. *Streptococcus pyogenes* as a cause of nosocomial infection in a critical care unit. *Diagn Microbiol Infect Dis* 1985;3:337–341.
61. Nicolle LE, Hume K, Sims H, et al. An outbreak of group A streptococcal bacteremia in an intensive care unit. *Infect Control* 1986;7: 177–180.
62. The Prevention of Invasive Group A Streptococcal Infections Workshop Participants. Prevention of invasive group A streptococcal disease among household contacts of case patients and among postpartum and postsurgical patients: recommendations from the Centers for Disease Control and Prevention. *Clin Infect Dis* 2002;35:950–959.
63. Nocard EIE, Mollereau H. Sur une mammite contagieuse des vaches laitières. *Ann Institut Pasteur* 1887;1:109–126.
64. Eickhoff TC, Kelin JO, Daly AK, et al. Neonatal sepsis and other infections due to group B beta-hemolytic streptococci. *N Engl J Med* 1964;271:1221–1228.
65. Jackson LA, Hilsdon R, Farley MM, et al. Risk factors for group B streptococcal disease in adults. *Ann Intern Med* 1995;123:415–420.
66. Dessau RB. Serious infections with *Streptococcus agalactiae* in adults: how often is it a nosocomial infection? *J Hosp Infect* 1989;14: 269–271.
67. Verghese A, Mireault K, Arbeit RD. Group B streptococcal bacteremia in men. *Rev Infect Dis* 1986;8:912–917.
68. Opal SM, Cross A, Palmer M, et al. Group B streptococcal sepsis in adults and infants. *Arch Intern Med* 1988;148:641–645.
69. Gallagher PG, Watanakunakorn C. Group B streptococcal bacteremia in a community teaching hospital. *Am J Med* 1985;78:795–800.
70. Klein NC, Schoch PE, Cunha BA. Nosocomial group B streptococcal infections. *Infect Control Hosp Epidemiol* 1989;10:475–479.
71. Wilkinson HW. Analysis of group B streptococcal types associated with disease in human infants and adults. *J Clin Microbiol* 1978;7: 176–179.
72. Anthony BF, Concepcion NF. Group B *Streptococcus* in a general hospital. *J Infect Dis* 1975;132:561–567.
73. Dillon HC Jr, Gray E, Pass MA, et al. Anorectal and vaginal carriage of group B streptococci during pregnancy. *J Infect Dis* 1982;145: 794–799.
74. Anthony BF, Eisenstadt R, Carter J, et al. Genital and intestinal carriage of group B streptococci during pregnancy. *J Infect Dis* 1981; 143:761–766.
75. Easmon CSF. The carrier state: group B *Streptococcus. J Antimicrob Chemother* 1986;18(Suppl A):59–65.
76. Ferrieri P, Cleary PP, Seeds AE. Epidemiology of group B streptococci in pregnant women and newborn infants. *J Med Microbiol* 1977;10: 103–114.
77. Paredes A, Wong P, Mason EO Jr, et al. Nosocomial transmission of group B streptococci in a newborn nursery. *Pediatrics* 1977;59: 679–682.
78. Easmon CSF, Hastings MJG, Blowers A, et al. Epidemiology of group B streptococci: one year's experience in an obstetric and special care baby unit. *Br J Obstet Gynaecol* 1983;90:241–246.
79. Anthony BF, Okada DM, Hobel CJ. Epidemiology of the group B *Streptococcus*: maternal and nosocomial sources for infant acquisitions. *J Pediatr* 1979;95:431–436.
80. Easmon CSF, Hastings MJG, Clare AJ, et al. Nosocomial transmission of group B streptococci. *BMJ* 1981;283:459–461.
81. Steere AC, Aber RC, Warford LR, et al. Possible nosocomial transmission of group B streptococci in a newborn nursery. *J Pediatr* 1975; 87:784–787.
82. Boyer KM, Vogel LC, Gotoff SP, et al. Nosocomial transmission of bacteriophage type 7/11/12 group B streptococci in a special care nursery. *Am J Dis Child* 1980;134:964–966.
83. Davis JP, Gutman LT, Higgins MV, et al. Nasal colonization of infants with group B *Streptococcus* associated with intrauterine pressure transducers. *J Infect Dis* 1978;138:804–810.
84. Gaynes R, Edwards JR, Jarvis WR, et al. Nosocomial infections among neonates in high-risk nurseries in the United States. *Pediatrics* 1996; 98:357–361.
85. Wilkinson HW. Group B streptococcal infections in humans. *Annu Rev Microbiol* 1978;32:41–57.
86. Noya FJD, Rench MA, Metzger TG, et al. Unusual occurrence of an epidemic of type Ib/c group B streptococcal sepsis in a neonatal intensive care unit. *J Infect Dis* 1987;155:1135–1144.
87. Sweet RL, Gibbs RS. Group B streptococci. In: *Infectious diseases of the female genital tract,* 2nd ed. Baltimore: Williams & Wilkins, 1990: 22–37.
88. Ajemian E, Andrews L, Hryb K, et al. Hospital-acquired infections after arthroscopic knee surgery: a probable environmental source. *Am J Infect Control* 1987;15:159–162.
89. Strampfer MJ, Ullman RF, Sacks-Berg A, et al. Group B streptococcal bacteremia after cardiac catheterization. *Crit Care Med* 1987;15: 625–626.
90. Smith RF, Dayton SL, Chipps DD. Autograft rejection in acutely burned patients: relation to colonization by *Streptococcus agalactiae. Appl Microbiol* 1973;25:493–495.
91. Centers for Disease Control and Prevention. Decreasing incidence of perinatal Group B streptococcal disease—United States, 1993–1995. *MMWR Morb Mortal Wkly Rep* 1997;46:473–477.
92. Sinigar H. The variability in virulence of the pneumococcus. *Lancet* 1903;1:169–170.

93. Bartlett JG, O'Keefe P, Tally FP, et al. Bacteriology of hospital-acquired pneumonia. *Arch Intern Med* 1986;146:868–871.
94. Alvarez S, Guarderas J, Shell CG, et al. Nosocomial pneumococcal bacteremia. *Arch Intern Med* 1986;146:1509–1512.
95. Lääveri T, Nikoskelaine J, Meurman O, et al. Bacteraemic pneumococcal disease in a teaching hospital in Finland. *Scand J Infect Dis* 1996;28:41–46.
96. Chang JI, Mylotte JM. Pneumococcal bacteremia. Update from an adult hospital with a high rate of nosocomial cases. *J Am Geriatr Soc* 1987;35:747–754.
97. Garcia-Leoni ME, Moreno S, Rodeno P, et al. Pneumococcal pneumonia in adult hospitalized patients infected with the human immunodeficiency virus. *Arch Intern Med* 1992;152:1808–1812.
98. Rubins JB, Cheung S, Carson P, et al. Identification of clinical risk factors for nosocomial pneumococcal bacteremia. *Clin Infect Dis* 1999;29:178–183.
99. Ho PL, Tse WS, Tsang KWT, et al. Risk factors for acquisition of levofloxacin-resistant *Streptococcus pneumoniae*: a case-control study. *Clin Infect Dis* 2001;32:701–707.
100. Setchanova L. Clinical isolates and nasopharyngeal carriage of antibiotic-resistant *Streptococcus pneumoniae* in hospital for infectious diseases, Sofia, Bulgaria, 1991–1993. *Microb Drug Resist* 1995;1:79–84.
101. Nuorti JP, Butler JC, Crutcher JM, et al. An outbreak of multidrug-resistant pneumococcal pneumonia and bacteremia among unvaccinated nursing home residents. *N Engl J Med* 1998;338:1861–1868.
102. Guillemot D, Carbon C, Balkau B, et al. Low dosage and long treatment duration of beta-lactam: risk factors for carriage of penicillin-resistant *Streptococcus pneumoniae*. *JAMA* 1998;279:365–370.
103. Jacobs MR, Koornhof HJ, Robins-Browne RM, et al. Emergence of multiply resistant pneumococci. *N Engl J Med* 1978;299:735–740.
104. Friedland IR, Klugman KP. Antibiotic-resistant pneumococcal disease in South African children. *Am J Dis Child* 1992;146:920–923.
105. Moore EP, Williams EW. Hospital transmission of multiply antibiotic-resistant *Streptococcus pneumoniae*. *J Infect* 1988;16:199–208.
106. Cartmill TDI, Panigrahi H. Hospital outbreak of multiresistant *Streptococcus pneumoniae*. *J Hosp Infect* 1992;20:130–132.
107. Gillespie SH, McHugh TD, Hughes JE, et al. An outbreak of penicillin resistant *Streptococcus pneumoniae* investigated by a polymerase chain reaction based genotyping method. *J Clin Pathol* 1997;50: 847–851.
108. Mandigers CMPW, Diepersloot RJA, Dessens M, et al. A hospital outbreak of penicillin-resistant pneumococci in the Netherlands. *Eur Respir J* 1994;7:1635–1639.
109. de Galan BE, van Tilburg PMB, Sluijter M, et al. Hospital-related outbreak of infection with multidrug-resistant *Streptococcus pneumoniae* in the Netherlands. *J Hosp Infect* 1999;42:185–192.
110. Centers for Disease Control and Prevention. Outbreaks of pneumococcal pneumonia among unvaccinated residents in chronic-care facilities—Massachusetts, October 1995, Oklahoma, February 1996, and Maryland, May–June 1996. *MMWR Morb Mortal Wkly Rep* 1997; 46:60–62.
111. Centers for Disease Control and Prevention. Pneumococcal polysaccharide vaccine. *MMWR Morb Mortal Wkly Rep* 1989;38:64–68, 73–76.
112. Mehtar S, Drabu YJ, Vijeratnam S, et al. Cross infection with *Streptococcus pneumoniae* through a resuscitaire. *BMJ* 1986;292:25–26.
113. Rabinovitch RA, Chusid MJ, Nathan R. A nosocomial pneumococcal wound infection. *Wis Med J* 1984;83:27–28.
114. Hill HR, Caldwell GC, Wilson E, et al. Epidemic of pharyngitis due to streptococci of Lancefield group G. *Lancet* 1969;2:371–374.
115. Maxted WR, Potter EV. The presence of type 12M-protein antigen in group G streptococci. *J Gen Microbiol* 1967;49:119–125.
116. Efstratiou A. The serotyping of hospital strains of streptococci belonging to Lancefield group C and group G. *J Hyg* 1983;90:71–80.
117. Goldmann DA, Breton RN. Group C streptococcal surgical wound infections transmitted by an anorectal and nasal carrier. *Pediatrics* 1978;61:235–237.
118. Teare EL, Smithson RD, Efstratiou A, et al. An outbreak of puerperal fever caused by group C streptococci. *J Hosp Infect* 1989;13:337–347.
119. Efstratiou A. Outbreaks of human infection caused by pyogenic streptococci of Lancefield groups C and G. *J Med Microbiol* 1989;29: 207–219.
120. Haynes J, Anderson AW, Spence WN. An outbreak of puerperal fever caused by group G streptococci. *J Hosp Infect* 1987;9:120–125.
121. Hare R. Sources of haemolytic streptococcal infection of wounds in war and in civil life. *Lancet* 1940;1:109–112.
122. Molina JM, Leport C, Bure A, et al. Clinical and bacterial features of infections caused by *Streptococcus milleri. Scand J Infect Dis* 1991; 23:659–666.
123. Sánchez-Porto A, Torres-Tortosa M, Canueto J, et al. Bacteriemias por el grupo streptococcus milleri. Análisis de 18 episodios. *Rev Clin Esp* 1997;197:393–397.
124. Rieske K, Handrick W, Spencker FB, et al. Sepsis durch vergrünende Streptokokken bein Kindern mit malignen hämatologischen Erkrankungen. *Klin Pädiatr* 1997;209:364–372.
125. Engelhard D, Elishoov H, Or R, et al. Cytosine arabinoside as a major risk factor for *Streptococcus viridans* septicemia following bone marrow transplantation: a 5-year prospective study. *Bone Marrow Transplant* 1995;16:565–570.
126. Leviner E, Tzukert A, Wolf A, et al. Hospital personnel with penicillin-resistant *Streptococcus viridans. Oral Surg* 1984;58:394–396.
127. Church DL, Bryant HE. Investigation of a *Streptococcus viridans* pseudobacteremia epidemic at a University teaching hospital. *Infect Control Hosp Epidemiol* 1989;10:416–421.

32

ENTEROCOCCUS SPECIES

CAROL E. CHENOWETH

Compared with other gram-positive cocci such as *Staphylococcus aureus* and *Streptococcus pyogenes,* enterococci were viewed as relatively avirulent, endogenous flora with little potential for human infection. Despite their apparent lack of virulence, enterococci have emerged as important nosocomial pathogens (1–3). The enterococci possess several characteristics that allow them to survive and cause serious infections in hospitalized patients. They are intrinsically resistant to many antimicrobial agents commonly used in hospitalized patients, and they have considerable ability to acquire antibiotic resistance through exchange of genetic elements with other gram-positive cocci. They are hardy microorganisms and can survive in the environment and on the hands of hospital personnel. These factors have allowed the enterococci to flourish, spread from patient to patient on hospital wards, and emerge as a major nosocomial pathogen (1–3).

ETIOLOGIES

Microbiologic Features and Taxonomy of Enterococci

Enterococci are catalase-negative, gram-positive, facultative anaerobic cocci that have classically belonged to the Lancefield group D streptococci. In the mid-1980s they were officially classified, based on DNA-DNA and DNA-RNA homology, into their own genus (2–5). Their characteristic biochemical features include the ability to grow in the presence of 6.5% NaCl and at extremes of temperature (range of 10° to 45°C) and pH (up to 9.6). They share the ability to hydrolyze esculin in the presence of 40% bile with the remaining members of the group D streptococci. The ability of enterococci to hydrolyze L-pyrrolidonyl β-naphthylamide has been used also as part of a rapid screening method for enterococci in the laboratory (2,3). Although other strains of gram-positive microorganisms (e.g., *Lactococcus, Aerococcus, Gemella, Leuconostoc, Lactobacillus*) may show one or more of the previously listed characteristics, these microorganisms are rarely isolated from clinical infections. Therefore, these classic physiologic tests are still useful for initial identification of enterococci in clinical laboratories (2–5).

There are five recognized groups of enterococci, with a total of 21 species. Most species can be identified with conventional techniques using a combination of biochemical and morphologic characteristics, such as motility and pigmentation (2,4,5). The most clinically important species of enterococci are listed with their distinguishing biochemical features in Table 32.1. *Enterococcus faecalis* remains the major human pathogen, accounting for 60% to 90% of clinical isolates of enterococci. *Enterococcus faecium* is the second most commonly isolated species, historically accounting for 5% to 16% of enterococcal clinical isolates (2,5). With the emergence of vancomycin resistance, the relative proportion of *E. faecium* in clinical isolates has been increasing. In recent studies, *E. faecium* represented 20% of enterococcal isolates from serious infections (6). Two motile strains of enterococcus, *Enterococcus gallinarum* and *Enterococcus casseliflavus,* which also exhibit intrinsic vancomycin resistance, can be identified using special media (7,8).

Typing Methods

Early epidemiologic studies of nosocomial enterococcal infections were limited by a lack of typing methods. Biochemical tests and antibiograms were insufficient because enterococci rarely exhibit enough variation to allow for adequate strain differentiation. Total plasmid DNA analysis, with or without restriction enzyme digestion, was used in many studies to type enterococci (9–11). Problems associated with plasmid analysis include the difficulty of extracting plasmid DNA from enterococci and the lack of plasmids in some clinical isolates. Clinical strains of enterococci also acquire or recombine plasmid DNA, which may result in changing plasmid banding patterns in a single strain over time. These techniques have been uniformly replaced by newer methods for bacterial typing.

Pulsed-field gel electrophoresis (PFGE) or contour-clamped homogeneous electric field (CHEF) electrophoresis of restriction enzyme digested genomic DNA has been the dominant method used for typing enterococci (12–15). Enterococci have a relatively low guanine plus cytosine content of DNA, which, when digested with *sma*1 (a restriction enzyme seeking G-plus C-rich sequences), yields diverse, easily interpreted patterns. These techniques produce high-resolution, reproducible bands, which allow confident interpretation (12,14,15).

Newer methods of typing for enterococci have recently been applied. Ribotyping is a reproducible means of differentiating enterococcal strains, and automated systems have been developed for rapid typing. However, the reliability of the automated systems in comparison to other typing systems for enterococci has not been determined (15). Amplified fragment length polymorphism (AFLP) has been used as a new method of typing

TABLE 32.1. PHENOTYPIC CHARACTERISTICS OF CLINICALLY SIGNIFICANT *ENTEROCOCCUS* SPECIES

	Mannose	Sorbose	Arginine	Arabinose	Motility	Yellow Pigment
E. faecalis	+	−	+	−	−	−
E. faecium	+	−	+	+	−	−
E. avium	+	+	−	+	−	−
E. durans	−	−	+	−	−	−
E. gallinarium	+	−	+	+	+	−
E. casseliflavus	+	−	+	+	+	+
E. mundtii	+	−	+	+	−	+
E. pseudoavium	+	+	−	−	−	−
E. raffinosus	+	+	−	+	−	−
E. malodoratus	+	+	−	−	−	−

From Teixeira LM, Carvalho MG, Merquior VL et al. Recent approaches on the taxonomy of the enterococci and some related microorganisms. *Adv Exp Med Biol* 1997; 418: 379–400; Facklam RR, Sahm DF, Teixeira LM, Enteroccus. In: Murray PR, ed. Manual of Clinical Microbiology, Washington DC: American Society for Microbiology, 1999: 297–305, with permission.

enterococci. This method is fast, reproducible, and appears to discriminate enterococcal strains well enough for the recognition of hospital outbreaks (16). Recently, a multilocus sequence typing scheme has been developed and compared with PFGE. This method appears promising for use in global epidemiologic analysis of *E. faecalis* and *E. faecium,* in addition to use in local outbreak investigations (14).

ANTIBIOTIC RESISTANCE IN ENTEROCOCCI

Enterococcal infections are a therapeutic challenge because of the intrinsic resistance of enterococci to many antibiotics. In addition to their intrinsic resistance, enterococci have a remarkable ability to acquire antibiotic resistance genes (2,17). Enterococci with high-level resistance (HLR) to multiple antibiotics have become endemic in many institutions; infections resulting from these microorganisms may be untreatable with currently available antimicrobials (18–20). As humans enter an era of decreased antibiotic effectiveness, it becomes imperative to develop appropriate infection control procedures to decrease the transmission of these microorganisms in the hospital setting.

Intrinsic Resistance

Most enterococci are inherently resistant to many antibiotics, as shown in Table 32.2. The gene coding for intrinsic resistance resides on the chromosome and confers resistance to cephalosporins and penicillinase-resistant penicillins, clindamycin, low-levels of aminoglycosides, and trimethoprim-sulfamethoxazole (TMP-SMX) (1–3). Most clinical isolates of enterococci are inherently tolerant to all β-lactams and glycopeptides and are typically not killed by concentrations of antibiotics many times higher than the minimum inhibitory concentration (MIC). The relative resistance to β-lactam antibiotics is due to low affinity of the penicillin-binding proteins for these antibiotics. The MICs of *E. faecalis* to penicillin average 2 to 8 μg/mL, which is approximately 10 to 100 times greater than those for most streptococci (2,21). *E. faecium* strains are even more resistant, with MICs of 16 to 32 μg/mL and higher (2,21).

In addition, all enterococci exhibit resistance to low concentrations of aminoglycosides (MIC = 8 to 64 μg/mL for gentamicin). This resistance trait appears to be due to a decreased uptake of the drug. Even in the presence of low-level aminogly-

TABLE 32.2. CHARACTERISTICS OF ANTIMICROBIAL RESISTANCE IN ENTEROCOCCI

Antimicrobial	Characteristic
Intrinsic resistance	
Penicillins	Relative resistance, tolerance
Cephalosporins	Diminished affinity for PBPs 4, 5, 6
Clindamycin	Low-level resistance
Aminoglycosides	Low-level resistance
Trimethoprim/sulfamethoxazole	*In vivo* resistance
Quinupristin/dalfopristin (*E. faecalis*)	Possible efflux
Acquired resistance	
Macrolides	Transposon, plasmid-mediated
Tetracyclines	Transposon, plasmid-mediated
Lincosamides	High-level; plasmid or transposon
Chloramphenicol	Transferable acetyltransferase activity
Aminoglycosides	High-level; plasmid or transposon
Penicillin (without β-lactamase)	Altered penicillin-binding proteins
Penicillin (with β-lactamase)	Transposon, plasmid-mediated
Vancomycin	Plasmid- or chromosome-mediated
Quinolones	Plasmid-mediated
Quinupristin/dalfopristin (*E. faecium*)	Drug inactivation, ribosomal mutation, efflux
Linezolid	Ribosomal mutation

PBP, penicillin-binding protein.
Data from references 2, 18, 72.

coside resistance, however, aminoglycosides may be used in combination with a cell-wall active agent (i.e., a penicillin or vancomycin) to achieve synergistic killing (3,22,23). The combination of an aminoglycoside with a penicillin or vancomycin is required for reliable bactericidal therapy for the treatment of serious enterococcal infections (3,22,23).

Enterococci are intrinsically resistant to TMP-SMX, because they are able to use exogenous folates to bypass the inhibitory effects of TMP-SMX. *In vitro* susceptibility testing is unreliable in enterococci, because media used in these tests do not contain thymidine or folates (2). Animal studies confirm that TMP-SMX is ineffective *in vivo* despite apparent *in vitro* susceptibility (24,25).

Acquired Resistance

High-Level Aminoglycoside Resistance

HLR to streptomycin and gentamicin were first identified in the 1970s (2,26). Over the next decade, the prevalence of these resistant strains increased dramatically in diverse geographic areas (26,27). HLR (MICs >2,000 μg/mL) confers resistance to the synergistic killing normally observed with combinations of cell-wall active agents and an aminoglycoside (23,26).

HLR to aminoglycosides in enterococci occurs primarily through acquisition of genes encoding aminoglycoside-modifying enzymes; these resistance genes are usually found on a transferable plasmid. Streptomycin is inactivated by an enzyme that adenylates the 6-hydroxyl position of streptomycin (26). A second mechanism of streptomycin resistance confers HLR (MICs up to 128,000 /mL) through ribosomal resistance (26).

HLR to gentamicin, in most clinical isolates, is mediated by a bifunctional aminoglycoside-modifying enzyme with 6′-acetyltransferase and 2″-phosphotransferase activity. The presence of this enzyme confers HLR to gentamicin, tobramycin, kanamycin, amikacin, sisomicin, and netilmicin (2,26). The gene encoding for HLR to gentamicin has a DNA sequence homologous to the gene conferring gentamicin resistance in *S. aureus* (28), and has been localized to transposons found on conjugative plasmids and chromosomes, which has allowed spread to multiple unrelated strains of enterococci (11,29,30). New gentamicin resistance genes encoding other 2″-phosphorylating enzymes have been identified in clinical isolates (26,31). Arbekacin, an investigational aminoglycoside, may have synergistic activity against enterococci with HLR to aminoglycosides (32).

HLR to gentamicin does not always correlate with HLR to streptomycin; therefore, screening for HLR to both streptomycin and gentamicin is important (26). There are several screening methods currently available, but the disk method and the single-concentration agar plate method are most reliable for detecting high-level aminoglycoside resistance in enterococci and are recommended by the National Committee for Clinical Laboratory Standards (NCCLS) (2,7). Disks containing 120 μg of gentamicin generate a zone of 15 mm or less in strains with HLR to gentamicin. For streptomycin, disks containing 300 μg give rise to zones of 12 mm or less in HLR strains (7). These screening methods may not be adequate for detection of the less clinically important newer gentamicin HLR genes (26).

β-Lactam Resistance

Penicillin resistance in enterococci occurs through two distinct mechanisms (21,33–35). The most common mechanism of penicillin resistance occurs primarily in *E. faecium* and correlates with increased amounts of a low affinity penicillin-binding protein (21,33,34). A large, multicenter study of enterococcal bloodstream isolates recently reported that only 12.5% of *E. faecium* isolates were susceptible to penicillin (36). In the United States, ampicillin resistance is highly associated with vancomycin resistance in *E. faecium* (36–38), but in Sweden an outbreak of ampicillin- and quinolone-resistant *E. faecium* was identified (39). *In vitro* penicillin or ampicillin susceptibility generally predicts susceptibility to imipenem (40). However, imipenem-resistant, ampicillin-sensitive *E. faecium* have been identified (41).

Since 1981, numerous centers have reported β-lactamase–producing strains of enterococci (10,35,42). The β-lactamase gene has been localized to transferable plasmids or to the chromosome in some isolates (35). The β-lactamase gene in enterococci is homologous with the *S. aureus* β-lactamase gene and has features suggesting that it resides on a transposon similar to *S. aureus* transposon Tn4201 (43). Routine susceptibility tests may not reliably detect β-lactamase–producing strains (42). Several β-lactamase tests, including nitrocefin disks, have been used to successfully identify β-lactamase production (35).

Vancomycin Resistance

Vancomycin-resistant enterococci (VRE), first detected in Europe in 1986, have increased in prevalence dramatically in the United States (1,44–47) and worldwide (48,49). There are several phenotypes and genotypes for vancomycin resistance in the enterococcus, and some of these phenotypes have been studied in detail (Table 32.3). *vanA* and *vanB* are the most predominant phenotypes in clinical isolates of VRE (1,44,45). All phenotypes code for alternate biosynthetic pathways that alter the D-ala-D-ala cell wall precursors that normally bind vancomycin. *vanA, vanB,* and *vanD* genes code for D-ala-D-lac ligases (50, 51), whereas *vanC* and *vanE* genes code for D-ala-D-ser ligases (52).

vanA strains exhibit high-level, inducible resistance (MICs >64 μg/mL) to both vancomycin and teicoplanin (53). The *vanA* trait is carried by a gene cluster located in a transposon, Tn*1546* (54). The transposon is usually found on a plasmid, which is transferable to other gram-positive cocci. This accounts for the presence of *vanA* genes in widely heterogeneous strains of enterococci (37,55). Although *vanA* is usually found in *E. faecium* and *E. faecalis,* it has recently been identified in *E. gallinarum* and other enterococcal species (44). In addition, the *vanA* gene cluster recently has been found in two separate isolates of methicillin-resistant *S. aureus* in the United States. (56).

vanB strains have variable resistance to vancomycin (MICs 16 to >1,000 μg/mL) but in general remain susceptible to teicoplanin. The genes that code for *vanB* trait are very similar to *vanA* genes, are usually found within large mobile elements lo-

TABLE 32.3. CHARACTERISTICS OF PHENOTYPES OF GLYCOPEPTIDE-RESISTANT ENTEROCOCCI

	Phenotype					
Characteristic	*vanA*	*vanB*	*vanC*	*vanD*	*vanE*	*vanG*
Min. inhibitory concentration (μg/mL)						
Vancomycin	64–>1000	4–>1000	2–32	16–64	16	12–16
Teicoplanin	16–512	0.5–>32	0.5–1	2–4	0.5	0.5
Ligase activity	D-ala-D-lac	D-ala-D-lac	D-ala-D-ser	D-ala-D-lac	D-ala-D-ser	ND
Genetic characteristics	Acquired	Acquired	Intrinsic, chromosomal	Acquired	Acquired	ND
Major *Enterococcus* species	*E. faecium* *E. faecalis* *E. durans* *E. mundtii* *E. avium* *E. gallinarium* *E. casseliflavus*	*E. faecalis* *E. faecium*	*E. casseliflavus* *E. gallinarium*	*E. faecium*	*E. faecalis*	*E. faecalis*

ND, not done.

cated on the chromosome, and can be transferred to other enterococci. The *vanC* phenotype is typically found intrinsically on the chromosome of motile species of enterococci, *E. gallinarum (vanC-1)* and *E. casseliflavus* (*vanC-2* and *vanC-3*) (57–59). These strains are moderately resistant to vancomycin (MICs 8 to 16 μg/mL) but remain susceptible to teicoplanin. The resistance in these isolates is not inducible or transferable (57,58).

The *vanD* phenotype has constitutive intermediate resistance to vancomycin and low level resistance to teicoplanin (51,60). *vanE* resistance is nontransferable and confers a low-level resistance phenotype (61,62). A new phenotype, *vanG,* has moderate level resistance to vancomycin (MIC = 16 μg/mL), has no resistance to teicoplanin, and is negative by polymerase chain reaction (PCR) for *vanA, vanB, vanC,* or *vanE* (63). Vancomycin-resistant strains that are dependent on vancomycin for growth have been identified from clinical isolates (64–66).

Many laboratories have difficulty detecting vancomycin resistance when the MICs are less than 64 μg/mL (67); however, HLR can be detected more readily (68). The agar screen test using 6 μg/mL of vancomycin in brain-heart infusion agar is a simple, sensitive, confirmatory test and is recommended by NCCLS (7,67). Heteroresistance to vancomycin, confirmed by presence of the *vanA* gene by PCR, has been identified recently in a clinical isolate (69). PCR assays have been developed for identification of VRE isolates and may be commonly used in the future (70).

Resistance to Newer Antimicrobials

E. faecalis is inherently resistant to the new combination antimicrobial, quinupristin/dalfopristin, with MICs of 4 to 32 μg/mL (71,72). This is thought to be a species characteristic and may be related to an efflux mechanism (72). *E. faecium* does not have inherent resistance, and most strains of *E. faecium* remain susceptible to quinupristin/dalfopristin (73). Mechanisms of resistance to quinupristin/dalfopristin in *E. faecium* include inactivation by enzymes, structural or conformational alterations in ribosomal target binding sites, and efflux of antibiotic out of cells (72,74).

Linezolid, a new oxazolidinone, has activity against most enterococci, including VRE (75). However, linezolid resistance was reported in isolates from 9 of 501 patients treated with linezolid during the manufacturer's compassionate use program and was related to ribosomal mutations (76). Although large prevalence studies reveal near universal susceptibility of enterococci to linezolid (75), nosocomial outbreaks of linezolid-resistant strains of VRE have occurred (18,20).

Evernimicin, an investigational oligosaccharide antimicrobial, has antimicrobial activity against most enterococci (77). However, HLR to evernimicin, conferred by rRNA methyltransferase, has been identified in *E. faecium* strains from animal sources (78). It is unclear how rapidly this resistance gene will emerge and spread in human isolates.

EPIDEMIOLOGY OF NOSOCOMIAL INFECTIONS

Descriptive Epidemiology

The prevalence of enterococci in nosocomial infections has increased in the past 3 decades. Whiteside et al. (79) noted an increase in enterococcal bacteremia of approximately 20% between 1976 and 1981. Maki and Agger (80) also reported a threefold increase in hospital-acquired cases of enterococcal bacteremia between 1970 and 1983, with no change in the number of community-acquired bacteremias. During the same time period (1975 to 1984), another institution noted that nosocomial urinary tract infections (UTIs) resulting from enterococci increased from 12.3 to 32.3 cases per 10,000 patient discharges (81).

In current reports from the National Nosocomial Infections Surveillance (NNIS) system at the Centers for Disease Control and Prevention, enterococci rank as one of the most common causes of all nosocomial infections hospital-wide (82,83). In data analyzed from 1990 to June, 1999, enterococci accounted for 13.5% and 13.8% of all nosocomial bloodstream infections (BSIs) and UTIs, respectively (82). Other national surveys confirm these findings. In 1996, enterococci accounted for 11.7% of nosocomial BSI in the Surveillance and Control of Pathogens of Epidemiologic Importance (SCOPE) program (36). Enterococci made up 9% of all BSI isolates from North America between 1997 to 1999. (6) The increased prevalence of enterococci in nosocomial infections is more apparent in the intensive care unit (ICU) setting (84).

At the same time their prevalence was increasing, the enterococci were also developing increased antibiotic resistance. One institution reported their first clinical isolate of high-level gentamicin-resistant enterococci in 1981, but, by 1989, 20% of clinical isolates were high-level gentamicin-resistant and, by 1992, 23% of nonurinary isolates were highly resistant to gentamicin (85). Other institutions noted a similar increase in prevalence of high-level gentamicin-resistant isolates; some centers reported that 50% to 55% of clinical isolates exhibited HLR (9,86). In a recent survey of more than 4,998 enterococcal isolates, 14% to 40% of enterococcal strains were gentamicin-resistant, and 30% to 45% were streptomycin-resistant, with variations reflected by geographic area (6).

Even more dramatic has been the continued increase in the prevalence of VRE in the United States (48,49,83,87–89). Between 1998 and June of 2002, the NNIS system reported that 12.8% of ICU enterococcal isolates were vancomycin resistant, compared with 12% in non-ICU and 4.7% in outpatient isolates (83). *E. faecium* are more frequently vancomycin resistant (47%) compared with *E. faecalis* (88). Rates of VRE vary between geographic areas (6) and institutions (87), with some centers reporting 31% of enterococcal blood isolates resistant to vancomycin (89). However, other areas of the world report lower prevalence rates of VRE than the United States (6,48,49). Canada and Latin America report 0% to 2% VRE, whereas Europe reports 1% to 3% VRE (6,48,49).

Reservoirs

Enterococci are normal inhabitants of the human gastrointestinal tract. *E. faecalis* are found in concentrations of 10^5 to 10^7 colony-forming units (CFUs)/g of feces in 80% of hospitalized patients. *E. faecium* is recovered in smaller amounts in 30% of adult patients (2,3,85). Other parts of the gastrointestinal tract such as the oropharynx and hepatobiliary tract may also harbor enterococci (85,90). The gastrointestinal tract of hospitalized patients is the major reservoir for resistant enterococci (10, 91–96). Rectal colonization was found in 100% of patients with VRE bacteremia (93) and may persist for years after identification (97–99). Prolonged colonization has been associated with prolonged hospitalization, ICU care, and antibiotic use (92,98). In addition, the higher density colonization by VRE has been associated with use of antianaerobic antibiotic regimens (91).

Enterococci may also colonize the gastrointestinal tract of hospital personnel, as illustrated by an outbreak of a β-lactamase–producing enterococcus on an infant/toddler ward, where the resistant strain was isolated from 8 of 33 employees (10). Healthcare worker colonization with VRE is uncommon, but a recent study showed that 12 of 228 healthcare workers carried VRE (100). In addition, identical strains of VRE were identified in household members of two colonized healthcare workers (100). Antibiotic therapy may place healthcare workers at risk for colonization with VRE (101). The significance of colonization of healthcare workers with VRE in the transmission of VRE has not been defined.

Other major sites of colonization that are reservoirs for enterococci in hospitalized patients include skin, wounds, and chronic decubital ulcers (93,102). In patients with VRE bacteremia, 86% were found to have VRE colonizing their skin in the inguinal or antecubital fossa areas (93). Enterococci, when present in wounds, are usually found in mixed culture (2,85). Asymptomatic women may also carry enterococci in high numbers in their vagina, and more than 60% of men in hospital may carry enterococci in their perineal or meatal areas (2,85,103).

Enterococci are also hardy microorganisms, which allows them to survive well on environmental surfaces (13,104). Resistant enterococci have been cultured from environmental surroundings of infected or colonized patients in many studies (9, 10,96,104–108). Heavy contamination of the surrounding environment is more likely to occur when the patient has diarrhea or is incontinent (96,108). Medical equipment may also become contaminated with resistant enterococci and serve as a reservoir for these microorganisms. In one notable outbreak of infection resulting from VRE, the epidemic strain was cultured from electronic thermometers within the ICU (109). VRE has since been found to contaminate electronic ear thermometers, blood pressure cuffs, patient gowns and linen, fabric seat cushions, beds, bed rails, bedside tables, and commodes (13,96,105,108,110). Although the transmission of resistant enterococci from environmental surfaces to patients is possible (106,111), the role of environment as a source of spread of enterococci requires further evaluation.

Residents of long-term care facilities may serve as a reservoir for introduction of resistant enterococci into the hospital (13, 87,102,112). Recently, rectal VRE colonization of patients in a single long-term care facility increased from 9% in December 1994 to 22% in January 1996 (13). In another hospital where VRE has become endemic, it was found that 45% of patients admitted to the hospital from long-term care facilities were colonized with VRE (102). VRE colonization at admission was associated with the presence of a decubitus ulcer and prior use of antibiotics (102).

In Europe, VRE colonization of nonhospitalized people was identified in the early 1990s. Evidence suggested that foodborne VRE may lead to human colonization in the community setting (113,114). Avoparcin, a glycopeptide used as a food supplement in animals, was identified as an important factor in the emergence of VRE in the community setting (113,114). A recent study confirms that persons ingesting meat products contaminated with antibiotic-resistant enterococci will develop transient intestinal colonization (115). In the United States, avoparcin has not been approved for use as a food additive; however, resistant enterococci have been found in the community (116,117). In 200 patients admitted to a community hospital, ten patients were colonized with enterococci with HLR to aminoglycosides and two patients were colonized with ampicillin-resistant enterococci (116). VRE colonization of outpatients without hospital exposures is rare in the United States (116–118), but person-to-person transmission of VRE has been reported in the household setting (119,120). Virginiamycin, a streptogramin similar to quinupristin/dalfopristin, has been used in animal feed since 1974 in the United States. A large proportion of chicken sold in the United States was contaminated with quinupristin/dalfopristin-resistant enterococci (121). At this point, persons living in the community are not a major reservoir for VRE or other resistant enterococci, but the potential for increased dissemination in the community is concerning.

Modes of Transmission

Early studies suggested that enterococci isolated from sites of infection were from the host's own gastrointestinal tract (122). Since the emergence of antibiotic resistance and more sophisticated molecular typing tools, numerous studies have shown that person-to-person spread of enterococci is a significant mode of transmission of nosocomial enterococci (9,10,38,42,86,108, 123). Zervos et al. (86) used total plasmid content and a high-level gentamicin-resistance marker, which was uncommon at that time, to show exogenous acquisition of enterococci. Since the emergence of VRE, the understanding of the spread of enterococci within a hospital has become more complete. The most important method of spread of VRE and other resistant enterococci is through transient carriage on the hands of healthcare personnel (10,13,103,108). Regional dissemination of VRE has resulted from interfacility transfer of colonized patients (124, 125).

Recent studies suggest that the environment may have a role in the transmission of resistant enterococci (96,104–106). Electronic thermometers, including ear thermometers, have been implicated as a vehicle of transmission (109,110). Other medical equipment used on multiple patients should be considered a possible route of patient-to-patient transmission. Resistant enterococci have been found to heavily contaminate environmental surfaces in both acute care and extended care facilities (10,13, 86,96). Whether the environment becomes passively colonized with patients' fecal flora or plays an active role in the person-to-person dissemination of these resistant microorganisms is unclear. More studies addressing the interactions of patients, staff, medical equipment, and environment are needed to clearly understand the transmission of these resistant microorganisms.

Risk Factors for Enterococcal Infections

Early studies examining risk factors for the development of enterococcal UTIs identified urinary tract instrumentation or catheterization; other genitourinary pathology; and the previous use of antibiotics, especially cephalosporins, as significant risk factors (81,122). Most patients who became colonized with resistant enterococci had serious underlying illnesses, as indicated by the Acute Physiology and Chronic Health Evaluation (APACHE) system score, being bedridden, or having had prior surgery (9,85,86).

TABLE 32.4. MAJOR RISK FACTORS FOR COLONIZATION WITH VANCOMYCIN-RESISTANT ENTEROCOCCI

Risk Factor	References
Underlying disease or debilitation	(126, 127)
Organ transplantation	(128–133, 139)
Renal failure	(126, 127, 134)
Malignancy	(135, 136)
Prolonged hospital stay	(135, 137–139)
Intrahospital transfers	(137)
Diarrhea	(111)
Enteral feedings	(125, 140, 141)
Colonization pressure	(95, 140, 141, 143)
Antibiotic use	
Multiple antibiotics	(127)
Antianacrobic antibiotics	(94, 141, 143, 147, 148)
Vancomycin	(126, 137, 144)
Cephalosporin	(92, 136, 137, 139, 140, 147)

Risk factors for acquisition of VRE include serious underlying disease or debilitation (126,127), organ transplantation (128–133), renal failure (126,127,134), malignancy (135,136), prolonged hospital stay (135,137–139), intrahospital transfers (137), diarrhea (111), and enteral feedings (125,140,141). Residence in an ICU setting has been a major risk factor for acquisition of VRE (125,135,139,142). However, VRE has increased steadily in frequency in non-ICU settings (83). Recent studies highlight the importance of colonization pressure (defined as the proportion of other patients colonized) or proximity to VRE-colonized patients as significant risk factors for acquisition of VRE (95,140,141,143). Changes in gastrointestinal function, resulting from either oral medication or gastrointestinal bleeding, may affect the risk of colonization with VRE. A recent retrospective case-control study on the effect of oral medication on acquisition of VRE identified presence of central venous lines and use of vancomycin or antacids as independent risk factors for VRE colonization. Interestingly, gastrointestinal bleeding or use of hydrocodone with acetaminophen protected against colonization (144) (Table 32.4).

Previous antibiotic therapy is the most consistent risk factor for colonization with resistant enterococci (91,127,135–138, 140,144,145). The acquisition of gentamicin-resistant enterococci has been associated with previous treatment with cephalosporins or aminoglycosides (9,86). Imipenem was found to significantly predispose to acquisition of ampicillin-resistant enterococci (146). VRE colonization has been associated with use of multiple antibiotics (127), antianaerobic antibiotics (94, 141,143,147,148), vancomycin (126,137,144), and cephalosporin (92,136,137,139,140,149).

PATHOGENESIS OF NOSOCOMIAL INFECTIONS CAUSED BY ENTEROCOCCI

Little is known about virulence factors in enterococci. Generally, enterococci are normal human commensals and have minimal pathogenic potential in the normal host. However, in the immunocompromised patient or when invasive procedures are performed, enterococci are common opportunistic pathogens. The increase in prevalence of enterococci in healthcare-related infections is more related to the accumulation of antimicrobial resistance than to inherent pathogenicity in the enterococci (17, 88,150).

Hemolysin has been identified as a potential virulence factor in enterococci (151). Patients with bacteremia caused by hemolytic, gentamicin-resistant *E. faecalis* were shown to have a fivefold increased risk of death compared with patients with nonhemolytic, gentamicin-susceptible strains (151). It is unclear from this study whether the increased mortality was due to the presence of hemolysin or an aminoglycoside-resistant phenotype. Other potential virulence factors include production of enterococcal surface protein (Esp), aggregation substances (asa1 or asa373), or gelatinase (17,150,152,153). One study noted that hemolysin and *asa1* were found more frequently in blood isolates and isolates from liver transplant recipients, whereas Esp was found more frequently in fecal isolates. The authors speculated that hemolysin and aggregation factor may be associated with infection, whereas Esp is associated with colonization and spread (153). Recently, however, among 398 enterococcal bacteremia isolates, 64% of isolates produced gelatinase, 32% carried the *esp* gene, and 11% produced hemolysin. There was no association of these putative virulence markers with 14-day mortality (152). More studies will be necessary to further define true virulence factors in the enterococcus.

CLINICAL MANIFESTATIONS OF NOSOCOMIAL INFECTIONS CAUSED BY ENTEROCOCCI

Urinary Tract Infection

In young healthy women, enterococci cause less than 5% of UTIs. However, in persons who have had urinary catheterization or instrumentation, have urinary tract pathology, or have received antibiotics, the proportion of UTIs associated with enterococci increases dramatically (81,84,154,155). Morrison and Wenzel (81) found an increase in the rate of UTIs caused by enterococci from 12.3 to 32.2 cases per 10,000 patient discharges. Between January 1990 and March 1996, the NNIS system ranked the enterococcus as the second most common cause of nosocomial UTI hospital-wide, accounting for 16% of nosocomial UTIs (156).

Risk factors for enterococcal UTI are urinary tract instrumentation, catheterization, and genitourinary tract pathology (81, 122,155). The previous use of antibiotics, especially cephalosporins, has also been associated with enterococcal UTI (81,155). One study showed a parallel rise in nosocomial enterococcal UTI and in cephalosporin use in a single hospital (81). Prior antibiotic use was found to be more frequent in patients with enterococcal UTI than in controls in a rehabilitation facility with a high rate of enterococcal UTI (155). Little has been published about specific risk factors for VRE UTI.

Early studies suggested that enterococci associated with UTIs were predominantly from the patients' own gastrointestinal flora. Patients found to be colonized with enterococci later developed enterococcal UTI with microorganisms identical to their previously cultured enterococci (122). More recent studies suggest that direct cross-infection is not the predominant source of enterococci in UTIs (155). However, fecal flora of hospitalized patients may be altered through the acquisition or selection of hospital-specific strains (93,154).

The clinical manifestations of UTI caused by enterococci are indistinguishable from those of UTIs caused by other microorganisms. The spectrum of disease ranges from asymptomatic bacteriuria to bacteremic pyelonephritis. Mortality resulting from enterococcal UTI in the absence of bacteremia is low (see Chapter 20) (81,122,154,155). In a recent study of 97 evaluable patients with VRE bacteriuria, 37 patients were colonized with VRE, 21 had asymptomatic bacteriuria, and 13 patients had symptomatic UTI. The status of 27 patients was not ascertainable (154). Patients with UTI were more likely to have malignancy (154).

Bacteremia

The incidence of bacteremia resulting from enterococci has increased over the past 2 decades (6,80,84,87,156). Maki and Agger (80) cited a threefold increase in nosocomial enterococcal bacteremia in their hospital between 1970 and 1983. In their study, hospital-acquired bacteremias accounted for 77% to 78% of enterococcal bacteremias (80). Between 1990 and 1996, enterococci were associated with 9% of cases of nosocomial BSI reported through NNIS; the proportion of BSIs was greater (12.8%) in ICUs (84,156). Other recent surveys found enterococci as a cause of bacteremia in 9% to 30.6% of cases (6,36, 157).

Enterococcal bacteremia is associated with prolonged hospitalization, malignancy, neutropenia, urethral catheterization, intravascular lines, recent surgery, biliary tree complications, and major burns (see Chapter 25) (80,130,158,159). Prior antimicrobial therapy is also associated with enterococcal bacteremia. In particular, use of a cephalosporin, imipenem, aztreonam, or ciprofloxacin have been shown to predispose to bacteremia (80, 159,160). In children, the most common predisposing factors for enterococcal bacteremia are indwelling central venous catheters, gastrointestinal lesions, and pulmonary infiltrates (161).

As the prevalence of VRE has increased, bacteremia with VRE has increased (6,36,87,162,163). VRE account for 14.4% to 19% of enterococci isolated from BSIs (6,36). Bacteremia resulting from VRE have been associated with severity of illness (164,165), underlying disease (especially hematologic malignancy) (162,165), human immunodeficiency virus (HIV) infection (166), liver transplantation (166), prolonged hospitalization (157,158,167), corticosteroid use (164), drug abuse (166), renal failure (162,168), central venous catheterization (158), indwelling bladder catheter (169), hyperalimentation (158), and previous gastrointestinal colonization with VRE (170). Prior exposure to antibiotics, especially vancomycin, has been a consistent risk factor for VRE bacteremia (157,164–166,168,169,171). Antimicrobials that disrupt the anaerobic flora of the intestinal tract (e.g., clindamycin, metronidazole, and imipenem) and *Clostridium difficile* colitis have also been associated with increased risk of VRE bacteremia (158,170,172).

Risk factors for VRE bacteremia in high-risk patient populations have been assessed. In patients undergoing liver transplantation, VRE bacteremia was associated with co-infections with other pathogens and biliary complications requiring repeat laparotomy (129,130). VRE bacteremia in patients with malignancy has been associated with vancomycin use (168,173), neutropenia (173), *C. difficile* infection (172), diabetes mellitus (168), or gastrointestinal procedures (168). Recurrence of VRE bacteremia in patients with cancer has been associated with prolonged gastrointestinal colonization (99,174).

In secondary enterococcal bacteremia without endocarditis, the urinary tract is the most common source of bacteremia, accounting for 19% to 43% of cases (80,159). Other major sources of enterococcal bacteremia include the hepatobiliary tract and intraabdominal infections (80,85,159). Soft tissue infections are another major source of bacteremia, with 15% to 30% of bacteremias arising from these sites (80,159). It is not surprising, given the nature of common sources of bacteremia, that enterococcal bacteremia is frequently polymicrobial. Enterococci are associated with other bacteria in 25% to 46% of bacteremia cases (2,80,85,159).

The clinical manifestations of enterococcal bacteremia are influenced by whether enterococci are isolated alone or as part of a polymicrobial bacteremia. When caused solely by enterococci, bacteremia is typically an indolent disease, frequently characterized by fever only. Signs of local infection may be minimal. Bacteremia is rarely associated with disseminated intravascular coagulation or shock. VRE are more likely than vancomycin-susceptible enterococci to occur as the sole isolated blood pathogen (158,167). Polymicrobial bacteremia and VRE bacteremia are much more likely to be associated with the development of shock (50%), thrombocytopenia, or disseminated intravascular coagulation (30%) (80). Recent studies have indicated higher rates of sepsis and shock, refractory infection and serious morbidity, and increased length of stay and hospital costs in patients with VRE bacteremia (157,162,166,167,169,175–177).

Overall mortality of enterococcal bacteremia has been estimated to be 30% to 76% (80,157,159,164,166,167,169, 175–178), with an attributable mortality of 7% to 37% (167, 178). Mortality resulting from polymicrobial bacteremia was two times higher than mortality associated with bacteremia resulting from enterococci alone (80).

Whether vancomycin-resistance increases mortality resulting from enterococcal bacteremia is still unclear. Some studies show no increased mortality with VRE bacteremia when compared with bacteremia caused by vancomycin-susceptible enterococci (157,165,177). However, a growing number of studies have found that vancomycin resistance is an independent risk factor for death in enterococcal bacteremia (164,166,167,169,176, 178). Mortality resulting from VRE bacteremia is associated with severe underlying disease, hematologic malignancy, presence of shock, and liver failure (164,167,175). Treatment with effective antimicrobial agents within 48 hours independently predicts survival from VRE bacteremia (164).

Endocarditis

Enterococci are the third most common cause of endocarditis, accounting for 5% to 20% of cases of native valve endocarditis (179,180). Patients with enterococcal endocarditis are predominantly men, with an average age of 56 to 59 years. In women, enterococcal endocarditis occurs during the childbearing years. A source of enterococci is usually not found; however, in many cases the genitourinary tract is implicated. Mandell et al. (179) found that 50% of men with enterococcal endocarditis had a previous history of enterococcal UTI or genitourinary tract instrumentation and that 43% of women had a history of childbirth or a genitourinary tract procedure in the preceding 3 months. Patients with underlying valvular heart disease are at greatest risk for developing enterococcal endocarditis (179,180); however, 42% of patients in the Mandell et al. (179) series had no underlying heart disease.

Although endocarditis resulting from enterococci occurs more commonly in the community setting, hospital-acquired endocarditis also occurs (80). Antibiotic resistance in hospital strains of enterococci has decreased therapeutic options for the treatment of enterococcal endocarditis. As the prevalence of these resistant strains increased, it is not surprising that endocarditis resulting from resistant enterococci has been reported (181–183).

Intraabdominal and Pelvic Infections

The clinical manifestations of enterococcal intraabdominal infections are similar to infections caused by other microorganisms. Enterococci are found in intraabdominal infections, usually in mixed culture (184). Nichols and Muzik (184) found that enterococci were rarely isolated in postoperative infections after penetrating abdominal trauma unless there was gastrointestinal perforation and the patient received broad-spectrum cephalosporins. Others have found an increased prevalence of enterococci in intraabdominal infections from a hepatobiliary source (85,131). In reviews of enterococcal bacteremia, intraabdominal sites are often the source of bacteremia (80,159). When enterococcal bacteremia arises from an intraabdominal site, the mortality is high with rates more than 40% (80,159).

Patients undergoing orthotopic liver transplantation (OLT) are at particular risk of developing intraabdominal infections resulting from enterococci, in particular VRE (128–133). Enterococcal bacteremia, including VRE bacteremia, are more likely to occur following OLT if hepatobiliary surgical complications and infection occur (129,130,132). In one series, 14 of 34 patients with VRE infection following OLT had an intraabdominal site of infection (129). In another study, 23 of 27 infections with VRE had an intraabdominal site. Risk factors for VRE infection in this patient population include biliary complications requiring reexploration (91%), prolonged intensive care stay, and administration of vancomycin preoperatively (132).

Skin and Soft Tissue Infections

Enterococci are rarely isolated in pure culture from skin and soft tissue infections. However, they are identified frequently in mixed surgical site infections, diabetic foot ulcers, decubitus wounds, and burns (2). Enterococci were associated with 12% to 19% of wound or surgical site infections (185,186). In several studies of enterococcal bacteremia, skin and soft tissue infections were identified as the source of bacteremia in 15% to 30% of cases (80,85,159). Infected burn wounds have been found to be a significant source of enterococcal bacteremia; bacteremia secondary to burn wounds is associated with a high mortality rate (80,159).

Neonatal and Pediatric Infections

Neonatal bacteremia and sepsis resulting from enterococci account for approximately 13% of bacteriologically confirmed cases of neonatal sepsis and meningitis (187). Risk factors for enterococcal sepsis included low birth weight (mean birth weight of 913 g), prolonged nonumbilical central venous catheterization, bowel resection or other abdominal surgery, prolonged hospitalization, and treatment with cephalosporins (187,188). The development of meningitis in neonates and older children has been associated with anatomic central nervous system defects or prior neurologic procedures, especially ventriculoperitoneal shunts, with particular predisposition to enterococcal meningitis (see Chapter 27) (189,190).

Although VRE colonization and infection are less common in children than in adults, outbreaks of VRE have been described in neonatal and pediatric patients (188,191–193). Risk factors for VRE colonization and infection have included neutropenia, vancomycin use, and broad-spectrum antimicrobial use (191–193). Overall, prospective prevalence studies have shown wide variability in colonization rates in pediatric populations, ranging from 0% to 50% (194–196).

Other Miscellaneous Infections

Outside the neonatal setting, enterococci are a rare cause of meningitis. Risk factors for enterococcal meningitis include prior neurologic procedures, especially ventriculoperitoneal shunts (190,197,198). Other risk factors include enterococcal UTI, endocarditis, and the immunocompromised state (197). A recent report describes a case of community-acquired meningitis, associated *Strongyloides stercoralis* hyperinfection (198). Other unusual infections associated with enterococci include endogenous endophthalmitis, arthritis, or osteomyelitis (199,200). Enterococci are rarely implicated as the cause of lower respiratory tract infections, although there have been reports of pneumonia occurring in patients receiving topical antimicrobial prophylaxis (201).

Impact of Vancomycin Resistance on Patient Outcome

Recent matched case-control studies confirm that infections with VRE decrease survival, increase length of stay, and significantly increase costs of hospitalization (149,202,203). In one institution, hospital costs for a patient with VRE were $52,449 compared with $31,915 for controls (149). Similarly, VRE infection was associated with an attributable ICU cost of $33,251 and increased length of hospital stay of 22 days (204). In addition, patients identified as carrying VRE waited significantly longer for placement into long-term care facilities when compared with matched controls, requiring an average of 2.5 requests for placement (205).

PREVENTION AND CONTROL OF NOSOCOMIAL INFECTIONS CAUSED BY ENTEROCOCCI

As antibiotic resistance in the enterococcus increases in prevalence and therapeutic options become more limited, the prevention of emergence and spread of resistant enterococci is imperative. Although most outbreaks of VRE have been controlled with strict application of barrier precautions, a multidisciplinary approach is recommended for continued prevention and control of multiresistant enterococci.

Decreasing Risk of Colonization

Numerous studies have emphasized the role of previous antibiotics as a risk factor for colonization and infection resulting from enterococcal species (206–210). Therefore, a key element for decreasing the risk of colonization with resistant enterococci is to limit the injudicious use of antimicrobials that select for their growth (148,206,210,211). Some hospitals have effectively used restriction of vancomycin to help control outbreaks of VRE (206,210). Vancomycin use has been closely linked to central venous catheter infection rate and prevalence of methicillin-resistant *S. aureus* (212). Feedback of specific prescriber use of vancomycin with benchmarking data has resulted in decreased vancomycin use and decreased VRE prevalence (208).

In addition, formulary restriction of cephalosporins may be important in decreasing the risk of colonization with enterococci, including VRE (210). However, one institution had an increase in VRE colonization while restricting vancomycin and cephalosporins and noted that clindamycin restriction may be an important component of an antibiotic restriction program for controlling VRE (148). Although recommendations for antimicrobial control have been outlined, most hospitals do not have restriction programs that fully meet the recommendations (213).

Along with selective use of antimicrobials, another necessary measure to decrease infection resulting from enterococci is to reduce the use of invasive devices whenever possible. Urinary catheterization predisposes to enterococcal UTIs (81,122). In addition, central vascular catheterization has been recognized as a risk factor for the development of enterococcal bacteremia (80). Finally, attempts should be made to eliminate the modifiable risk factors for colonization and infection with resistant enterococci as mentioned previously (Table 32.4).

Interruption of Transmission

Early identification of patients infected and colonized with antibiotic-resistant enterococci is an important step in interrupting transmission of these microorganisms (143,211,214,215). Active screening for VRE colonization, when used with other infection control measures, has been found to be effective in decreasing prevalence of VRE colonization (143,215). In addition, active surveillance and control has been shown to be cost-effective for hospitals (214,216). For active surveillance for gastrointestinal VRE colonization, perirectal swabs have been effective in most studies (143,214,217–219); however, false-negative results may occur in patients with low-density colonization (220). Others have effectively used passive surveillance through routine laboratory culturing or culturing stool samples sent for *C. difficile* studies to identify and control VRE colonization (107,221,222). Passive reporting may underestimate the prevalence of VRE (223). It is essential that hospital microbiology laboratories use accurate screening methods for VRE and have a system for quickly reporting these microorganisms so that appropriate precautions may be instituted (7,211).

Private rooms, gowns, and gloves have been used and recommended for the prevention of transmission and control of VRE (108,211). However, in a hospital with a high rate of endemic VRE, the addition of gown use did not decrease acquisition of VRE when compared with glove use alone (224). Two new studies support the HICPAC guidelines for control of VRE and indicate that gowns have an added benefit to the use of gloves in the ICU setting (225,226). Cohorting of colonized patients, in addition to contact precautions, have been used in outbreak situations to help control transmission of VRE (227).

Hand washing is a key element in controlling spread of resistant enterococci (211,228). Gloves reduce hand carriage of VRE but do not completely prevent contamination of hands (229). In one study, 5 of 17 healthcare workers were found to have VRE on the hands after glove removal, emphasizing the importance of hand washing after removal of gloves (211,228,229). Wade et al. (230) showed that washing with alcoholic chlorhexidine was more reliable at removing resistant *E. faecium* than was washing with soap and water. After a 15-second scrub with disinfectant scrub, VRE could still be recovered from the hands of 3 of 60 (5%) healthcare providers (13).

Barrier precautions have been successful, for the most part, in ending epidemics as long as all reservoirs have been identified and eradicated. Barrier precautions were unsuccessful in one outbreak in which a nurse disseminated resistant enterococci to patients on an infant/toddler ward (10). Contact precautions were also unsuccessful in outbreaks in which environmental reservoirs, such as electronic thermometers or electrocardiogram (ECG) leads, were a persistent reservoir and vehicle of transmission (109–111).

Elimination of Reservoirs

Patients harboring resistant enterococci in their gastrointestinal tract are the major reservoirs for transmission within hospitals, but healthcare workers may also carry enterococci. Eradication of enterococci from human carriers has been problematic (97,231,232). During an outbreak of β-lactamase–producing gentamicin-resistant enterococci, a 14-day course of oral vancomycin and rifampin, based on the isolate's antibiotic susceptibilities, was used to eradicate carriage in a nurse (10). Eradication of VRE from the intestinal tract has been attempted with several oral antimicrobial regimens with little success (97,231–233). Ramoplanin, a nonabsorbable glycolipopeptide with bactericidal activity against VRE, was successful in temporarily suppressing VRE in the gastrointestinal tract of colonized patients. However, the suppressive effects were lost by 3 weeks after discontinuing treatment (232). In this study, repopulation of the intestinal tract with VRE within 7 days of discontinuing ramoplanin represented relapse with a genotypically similar isolate of VRE (94).

In many studies, the environment surrounding infected patients had become heavily contaminated with enterococci (10, 86,96,234). Noncritical medical equipment, such as thermometers, stethoscopes, and blood pressure cuffs, should be dedicated to a single VRE colonized patient (211). If equipment must be used on multiple patients, it should be disinfected after each use (211). Other authors have incorporated a thorough cleaning of the environment into control measures during an epidemic (227). Enterococci, including VRE, appear to be susceptible to disinfectants routinely used in hospitals (235). Screening for environmental contamination may be performed, when applicable, through use of Rodac imprints or use of swabs with enrichment broth (107,218).

REFERENCES

1. Moellering RJ. Vancomycin-resistant enterococci. *Clin Infect Dis* 1998; 26:1196–1199.
2. Murray B. The life and times of the *Enterococcus. Clin Microbiol Rev* 1990;3:46–65.
3. Murray BE, Weinstock GM. Enterococci: new aspects of an old organism. *Proc Assoc Am Physicians* 1999;111:328–334.
4. Teixeira LM, Carvalho MG, Merquior VL, et al. Recent approaches on the taxonomy of the enterococci and some related microorganisms. *Adv Exp Med Biol* 1997;418:397–400.
5. Facklam RR, Sahm DF, Teixeira LM. Enterococcus. In: Murray PR, ed. *Manual of clinical microbiology.* Washington DC: American Society for Microbiology, 1999:297–305.
6. Low DE, Keller N, Barth A, et al. Clinical prevalence, antimicrobial susceptibility, and geographic resistance patterns of enterococci: results from the SENTRY Antimicrobial Surveillance Program, 1997–1999. *Clin Infect Dis* 2001;32:S133–145.
7. Jorgensen JH, Ferraro MJ. Antimicrobial susceptibility testing: special needs for fastidious organisms and difficult-to-detect resistance mechanisms. *Clin Infect Dis* 2000;30:799–808.
8. Van Horn K, Toth C, Kariyama R, et al. Evaluation of 15 motility media and a direct microscopic method for detection of motility in enterococci. *J Clin Microbiol* 2002;40:2476–2479.
9. Zervos M, Kauffman C, Therasse P, et al. Nosocomial infection by gentamicin-resistant *Streptococcus faecalis.* An epidemiologic study. *Ann Intern Med* 1987;106:687–691.
10. Rhinehart E, Smith N, Wennersten C, et al. Rapid dissemination of beta-lactamase-producing, aminoglycoside-resistant *Enterococcus faecalis* among patients and staff on an infant-toddler surgical ward. *N Engl J Med* 1990;323:1814–1818.
11. Chenoweth C, Bradley S, Terpenning M, et al. Colonization and transmission of high-level gentamicin-resistant enterococci in a long-term care facility. *Infect Control Hosp Epidemiol* 1994;15:703–709.
12. Green M, Barbadora K, Donabedian S, et al. Comparison of field inversion gel electrophoresis with contour-clamped homogeneous electric field electrophoresis as a typing method for *Enterococcus faecium. J Clin Microbiol* 1995;33:1554–1557.
13. Bonilla H, Zervos M, Lyons M, et al. Colonization with vancomycin-resistant *Enterococcus faecium*: comparison of a long term care unit with an acute care hospital. *Infect Control Hosp Epidemiol* 1997;18: 333–339.
14. Nallapareddy SR, Duh RW, Singh KV, et al. Molecular typing of selected *Enterococcus faecalis* isolates: pilot study using multilocus sequence typing and pulsed-field gel electrophoresis. *J Clin Microbiol* 2002;40:868–876.
15. Price CS, Huynh H, Paule S, et al. Comparison of an automated

ribotyping system to restriction endonuclease analysis and pulsed-field gel electrophoresis for differentiating vancomycin-resistant Enterococcus faecium isolates. *J Clin Microbiol* 2002;40:1858–1861.
16. Antonishyn NA, McDonald RR, Chan EL, et al. Evaluation of fluorescence-based amplified fragment length polymorphism analysis for molecular typing in hospital epidemiology: comparison with pulsed-field gel electrophoresis for typing strains of vancomycin-resistant *Enterococcus faecium. J Clin Microbiol* 2000;38:4058–4065.
17. Mundy LM, Sahm DF, Gilmore M. Relationships between enterococcal virulence and antimicrobial resistance. *Clin Microbiol Rev* 2000; 13:513–522.
18. Herrero IA, Issa NC, Patel R. Nosocomial spread of linezolid-resistant, vancomycin-resistant *Enterococcus faecium. N Engl J Med* 2002; 346:867–869.
19. Morris JJ, Shay D, Hebden J, et al. Enterococci resistant to multiple antimicrobial agents, including vancomycin. Establishment of endemicity in a university medical center. *Ann Intern Med* 1995;123: 250–259.
20. Pai MP, Rodvold KA, Schreckenberger PC, et al. Risk factors associated with the development of infection with linezolid- and vancomycin-resistant *Enterococcus faecium. Clin Infect Dis* 2002;35: 1269–1272.
21. Rybkine T, Mainardi J, Sougakoff W, et al. Penicillin-binding protein 5 sequence alterations in clinical isolates of *Enterococcus faecium* with different levels of beta-lactam resistance. *J Infect Dis* 1998;178: 159–163.
22. Murray B, Singh K, Heath J, et al. Comparison of genomic DNAs of different enterococcal isolates using restriction endonucleases with infrequent recognition sites. *J Clin Microbiol* 1990;28:2059–2063.
23. Dressel DC, Tornatore-Reuscher MA, Boschman CR, et al. Synergistic effect of gentamicin plus ampicillin on enterococci with differing sensitivity to gentamicin: a phenotypic assessment of NCCLS guidelines. *Diagn Microbiol Infect Dis* 1999;35:219–225.
24. Chenoweth C, Robinson K, Schaberg D. Efficacy of ampicillin versus trimethoprim-sulfamethoxazole in a mouse model of lethal enterococcal peritonitis. *Antimicrob Agents Chemother* 1990;34:1800–1802.
25. Grayson M, Thauvin-Eliopoulos C, Eliopoulos G, et al. Failure of trimethoprim-sulfamethoxazole therapy in experimental enterococcal endocarditis. *Antimicrob Agents Chemother* 1990;34:1792–1794.
26. Chow JW. Aminoglycoside resistance in enterococci. *Clin Infect Dis* 2000;31:586–589.
27. Schmitz FJ, Verhoef J, Fluit AC. Prevalence of aminoglycoside resistance in 20 European university hospitals participating in the European SENTRY Antimicrobial Surveillance Programme. *Eur J Clin Microbiol Infect Dis* 1999;18:414–421.
28. Ounissi H, Derlot E, Carlier C, et al. Gene homogeneity for aminoglycoside-modifying enzymes in gram-positive cocci. *Antimicrob Agents Chemother* 1990;34:2164–2168.
29. Hodel-Christian S, Murray B. Mobilization of the gentamicin resistance gene in *Enterococcus faecalis. Antimicrob Agents Chemother* 1990; 34:1278–1280.
30. Thal L, Chow J, Clewell D, et al. Tn924, a chromosome-borne transposon encoding high-level gentamicin resistance in *Enterococcus faecalis. Antimicrob Agents Chemother* 1994;38:1152–1156.
31. Chow JW, Kak V, You I, et al. Aminoglycoside resistance genes aph(2″)-Ib and aac(6′)-Im detected together in strains of both *Escherichia coli* and *Enterococcus faecium. Antimicrob Agents Chemother* 2001;45:2691–2694.
32. Kak V, Donabedian SM, Zervos MJ, et al. Efficacy of ampicillin plus arbekacin in experimental rabbit endocarditis caused by an *Enterococcus faecalis* strain with high-level gentamicin resistance. *Antimicrob Agents Chemother* 2000;44:2545–2546.
33. Rice LB, Carias LL, Hutton-Thomas R, et al. Penicillin-binding protein 5 and expression of ampicillin resistance in *Enterococcus faecium. Antimicrob Agents Chemother* 2001;45:1480–1486.
34. Sifaoui F, Arthur M, Rice L, et al. Role of penicillin-binding protein 5 in expression of ampicillin resistance and peptidoglycan structure in *Enterococcus faecium. Antimicrob Agents Chemother* 2001;45: 2594–2597.
35. Murray B. Beta-lactamase-producing enterococci. *Antimicrob Agents Chemother* 1992;36:2355–2359.
36. Jones R, Marshall S, Pfaller M, et al. Nosocomial enterococcal blood stream infections in the SCOPE Program: antimicrobial resistance, species occurrence, molecular testing results, and laboratory testing accuracy. SCOPE Hospital Study Group. *Diagn Microbiol Infect Dis* 1997;29:95–102.
37. Hanrahan J, Hoyen C, Rice LB. Geographic distribution of a large mobile element that transfers ampicillin and vancomycin resistance between *Enterococcus faecium strains. Antimicrob Agents Chemother* 2000;44:1349–1351.
38. Montecalvo M, Horowitz H, Gedris C, et al. Outbreak of vancomycin-, ampicillin-, and aminoglycoside-resistant *Enterococcus faecium* bacteremia in an adult oncology unit. *Antimicrob Agents Chemother* 1994;38:1363–1367.
39. Torell E, Cars O, Olsson-Liljequist B, et al. Near absence of vancomycin-resistant enterococci but high carriage rates of quinolone-resistant ampicillin-resistant enterococci among hospitalized patients and nonhospitalized individuals in Sweden. *J Clin Microbiol* 1999;37: 3509–3513.
40. Weinstein MP. Comparative evaluation of penicillin, ampicillin, and imipenem MICs and susceptibility breakpoints for vancomycin-susceptible and vancomycin-resistant Enterococcus faecalis and *Enterococcus faecium* [comment]. *J Clin Microbiol* 2001;39:2729–2731.
41. El Amin N, Lund B, Tjernlund A, et al. Mechanisms of resistance to imipenem in imipenem-resistant, ampicillin-sensitive *Enterococcus faecium. APMIS* 2001;109:791–796.
42. Wells V, Wong E, Murray B, et al. Infections due to beta-lactamase-producing, high-level gentamicin-resistant *Enterococcus faecalis. Ann Intern Med* 1992;116:285–292.
43. Smith M, Murray B. Comparison of enterococcal and staphylococcal beta-lactamase-encoding fragments. *Antimicrob Agents Chemother* 1992;36:273–276.
44. Cetinkaya Y, Falk P, Mayhall CG. Vancomycin-resistant enterococci. *Clin Microbiol Rev* 2000;13:686–707.
45. Gold HS. Vancomycin-resistant enterococci: mechanisms and clinical observations. *Clin Infect Dis* 2001;33:210–219.
46. Murray BE. Vancomycin-resistant enterococcal infections. *N Engl J Med* 2000;342:710–721.
47. Perl TM. The threat of vancomycin resistance. *Am J Med* 1999;106: 26S–37S, discussion 48S–52S.
48. Harbarth S, Albrich W, Goldmann DA, et al. Control of multiply resistant cocci: do international comparisons help? *Lancet Infect Dis* 2001;1:251–261.
49. Schouten MA, Hoogkamp-Korstanje JA, Meis JF, et al. Prevalence of vancomycin-resistant enterococci in Europe. *Eur J Clin Microbiol Infect Dis* 2000;19:816–822.
50. Roper DI, Huyton T, Vagin A, et al. The molecular basis of vancomycin resistance in clinically relevant enterococci: crystal structure of D-alanyl-D-lactate ligase (VanA). *Proc Nat Acad Sci U S A* 2000;97: 8921–8925.
51. Perichon B, Casadewall B, Reynolds P, et al. Glycopeptide-resistant *Enterococcus faecium* BM4416 is a VanD-type strain with an impaired D-Alanine:D-Alanine ligase. *Antimicrob Agents Chemother* 2000;44: 1346–1348.
52. Boyd DA, Conly J, Dedier H, et al. Molecular characterization of the vanD gene cluster and a novel insertion element in a vancomycin-resistant *Enterococcus* isolated in Canada. *J Clin Microbiol* 2000;38: 2392–2394.
53. Arthur M, Courvalin P. Genetics and mechanisms of glycopeptide resistance in enterococci. *Antimicrob Agents Chemother* 1993;37: 1563–1571.
54. Arthur M, Molinas C, Depardieu F, et al. Characterization of Tn1546, a Tn3-related transposon conferring glycopeptide resistance by synthesis of depsipeptide peptidoglycan precursors in Enterococcus faecium BM4147. *J Bacteriol* 1993;175:117–127.
55. Schouten MA, Willems RJ, Kraak WA, et al. Molecular analysis of Tn1546-like elements in vancomycin-resistant enterococci isolated from patients in Europe shows geographic transposon type clustering. *Antimicrob Agents Chemother* 2001;45:986–989.

56. Anonymous. Public health dispatch: vancomycin-resistant *Staphylococcus aureus*—Pennsylvania, 2002. *MMWR Morb Mortal Wkly Rep* 2002;51:902.
57. Clark NC, Teixeira LM, Facklam RR, et al. Detection and differentiation of vanC-1, vanC-2, and vanC-3 glycopeptide resistance genes in enterococci. *J Clin Microbiol* 1998;36:2294–2297.
58. Arias CA, Courvalin P, Reynolds PE. vanC cluster of vancomycin-resistant *Enterococcus gallinarum* BM4174. *Antimicrob Agents Chemother* 2000;44:1660–1666.
59. Toye B, Shymanski J, Bobrowska M, et al. Clinical and epidemiological significance of enterococci intrinsically resistant to vancomycin (possessing the vanC genotype). *J Clin Microbiol* 1997;35:3166–3170.
60. Ostrowsky BE, Clark NC, Thauvin-Eliopoulos C, et al. A cluster of VanD vancomycin-resistant *Enterococcus faecium*: molecular characterization and clinical epidemiology. *J Infect Dis* 1999;180:1177–1185.
61. Boyd DA, Cabral T, Van Caeseele P, et al. Molecular characterization of the vanE gene cluster in vancomycin-resistant *Enterococcus faecalis* N00-410 isolated in Canada. *Antimicrob Agents Chemother* 2002;46:1977–1979.
62. Fines M, Perichon B, Reynolds P, et al. VanE, a new type of acquired glycopeptide resistance in *Enterococcus faecalis* BM4405. *Antimicrob Agents Chemother* 1999;43:2161–2164.
63. McKessar SJ, Berry AM, Bell JM, et al. Genetic characterization of vanG, a novel vancomycin resistance locus of *Enterococcus faecalis. Antimicrob Agents Chemother* 2000;44:3224–3228.
64. Kirkpatrick BD, Harrington SM, Smith D, et al. An outbreak of vancomycin-dependent *Enterococcus faecium* in a bone marrow transplant unit. *Clin Infect Dis* 1999;29:1268–1273.
65. Green M, Shlaes J, Barbadora K, et al. Bacteremia due to vancomycin-dependent *Enterococcus faecium. Clin Infect Dis* 1995;20:712–714.
66. Fraimow H, Jungkind D, Lander D, et al. Urinary tract infection with an *Enterococcus faecalis* isolate that requires vancomycin for growth. *Ann Intern Med* 1994;121:22–26.
67. Rosenberg J, Tenover F, Wong J, et al. Are clinical laboratories in California accurately reporting vancomycin-resistant enterococci? *J Clin Microbiol* 1997;35:2526–2530.
68. Steward CD, Wallace D, Hubert SK, et al. Ability of laboratories to detect emerging antimicrobial resistance in nosocomial pathogens: a survey of project ICARE laboratories. *Diagn Microbiol Infect Dis* 2000;38:59–67.
69. Alam MR, Donabedian S, Brown W, et al. Heteroresistance to vancomycin in *Enterococcus faecium. J Clin Microbiol* 2001;39:3379–3381.
70. Sahm D, Free L, Smith C, et al. Rapid characterization schemes for surveillance isolates of vancomycin-resistant enterococci. *J Clin Microbiol* 1997;35:2026–2030.
71. Chow JW, Davidson A, Sanford E, 3rd, et al. Superinfection with *Enterococcus faecalis* during quinupristin/dalfopristin therapy. *Clin Infect Dis* 1997;24:91–92.
72. Singh KV, Weinstock GM, Murray BE. An *Enterococcus faecalis* ABC homologue (Lsa) is required for the resistance of this species to clindamycin and quinupristin-dalfopristin. *Antimicrob Agents Chemother* 2002;46:1845–1850.
73. Eliopoulos GM, Wennersten CB, Gold HS, et al. Characterization of vancomycin-resistant *Enterococcus faecium* isolates from the United States and their susceptibility in vitro to dalfopristin-quinupristin. *Antimicrob Agents Chemother* 1998;42:1088–1092.
74. Chow J, Donabedian S, Zervos M. Emergence of increased resistance to quinupristin/dalfopristin during therapy for *Enterococcus faecium* bacteremia. *Clin Infect Dis* 1997;24:90–91.
75. Ballow CH, Jones RN, Biedenbach DJ, et al. A multicenter evaluation of linezolid antimicrobial activity in North America. *Diagn Microbiol Infect Dis* 2002;43:75–83.
76. Prystowsky J, Siddiqui F, Chosay J, et al. Resistance to linezolid: characterization of mutations in rRNA and comparison of their occurrences in vancomycin-resistant enterococci. *Antimicrob Agents Chemother* 2001;45:2154–2156.
77. Jones RN, Hare RS, Sabatelli FJ, et al. In vitro Gram-positive antimicrobial activity of evernimicin (SCH 27899), a novel oligosaccharide, compared with other antimicrobials: a multicentre international trial. *J Antimicrob Chemother* 2001;47:15–25.
78. Mann PA, Xiong L, Mankin AS, et al. EmtA, a rRNA methyltransferase conferring high-level evernimicin resistance. *Mol Microbiol* 2001;41:1349–1356.
79. Whiteside M, Moore J, Ratzan K. An investigation of enterococcal bacteremia. *Am J Infect Control* 1983;11:125–129.
80. Maki D, Agger W. Enterococcal bacteremia: clinical features, the risk of endocarditis, and management. *Medicine* 1988;67:248–269.
81. Morrison AJ, Wenzel R. Nosocomial urinary tract infections due to enterococcus. Ten years' experience at a university hospital. *Arch Intern Med* 1986;146:1549–1551.
82. Anonymous. National Nosocomial Infections Surveillance (NNIS) system report, data summary from January 1990–May 1999, Issued June 1999. *Am J Infect Control* 1999;27:520–532.
83. National Nosocomial Infections Surveillance. National Nosocomial Infections Surveillance (NNIS) system report, data summary from January 1992 to June 2002, issued August 2002. *Am J Infect Control* 2002;30:458–475.
84. Anonymous. National Nosocomial Infections Surveillance (NNIS) report, data summary from October 1986–April 1997, issued May 1997. A report from the NNIS System. *Am J Infect Control* 1997;25:477–487.
85. Chenoweth C, Schaberg D. The epidemiology of enterococci. *Eur J Clin Microbiol Infect Dis* 1990;9:80–89.
86. Zervos M, Dembinski S, Mikesell T, et al. High-level resistance to gentamicin in *Streptococcus faecalis*: risk factors and evidence for exogenous acquisition of infection. *J Infect Dis* 1986;153:1075–1083.
87. Huang SS, Labus BJ, Samuel MC, et al. Antibiotic resistance patterns of bacterial isolates from blood in San Francisco County, California, 1996–1999. *Emerg Infect Dis* 2002;8:195–201.
88. Jones RN. Resistance patterns among nosocomial pathogens: trends over the past few years. *Chest* 2001;119:397S–404S.
89. Lautenbach E, Patel JB, Bilker WB, et al. Trends in antimicrobial susceptibility patterns among inpatient enterococcal isolates (1990 to 1999): implications for therapeutic options. *Infect Control Hosp Epidemiol* 2002;23:416–418.
90. Bonten MJ, Gaillard CA, van der Geest S, et al. The role of intragastric acidity and stress ulcus prophylaxis on colonization and infection in mechanically ventilated ICU patients. A stratified, randomized, double-blind study of sucralfate versus antacids. *Am J Respir Crit Care Med* 1995;152:1825–1834.
91. Donskey CJ, Chowdhry TK, Hecker MT, et al. Effect of antibiotic therapy on the density of vancomycin-resistant enterococci in the stool of colonized patients.[comment]. *N Engl J Med* 2000;343:1925–1932.
92. Loeb M, Salama S, Armstrong-Evans M, et al. A case-control study to detect modifiable risk factors for colonization with vancomycin-resistant enterococci. *Infect Control Hosp Epidemiol* 1999;20:760–763.
93. Beezhold D, Slaughter S, Hayden M, et al. Skin colonization with vancomycin-resistant enterococci among hospitalized patients with bacteremia. *Clin Infect Dis* 1997;24:704–706.
94. Baden LR, Critchley IA, Sahm DF, et al. Molecular characterization of vancomycin-resistant enterococci repopulating the gastrointestinal tract following treatment with a novel glycolipodepsipeptide, ramoplanin. *J Clin Microbiol* 2002;40:1160–1163.
95. D'Agata EM, Horn MA, Webb GF. The impact of persistent gastrointestinal colonization on the transmission dynamics of vancomycin-resistant enterococci. *J Infect Dis* 2002;185:766–773.
96. Trick WE, Temple RS, Chen D, et al. Patient colonization and environmental contamination by vancomycin-resistant enterococci in a rehabilitation facility. *Arch Phys Med Rehabil* 2002;83:899–902.
97. Baden LR, Thiemke W, Skolnik A, et al. Prolonged colonization with vancomycin-resistant *Enterococcus faecium* in long-term care patients and the significance of "clearance". *Clin Infect Dis* 2001;33:1654–1660.
98. Byers KE, Anglim AM, Anneski CJ, et al. Duration of colonization with vancomycin-resistant *Enterococcus. Infect Control Hosp Epidemiol* 2002;23:207–211.

99. Roghmann M, Qaiyumi S, Johnson J, et al. Recurrent vancomycin-resistant Enterococcus faecium bacteremia in a leukemia patient who was persistently colonized with vancomycin-resistant enterococci for two years. *Clin Infect Dis* 1997;24:514–515.
100. Baran J Jr, Ramanathan J, Riederer KM, et al. Stool colonization with vancomycin-resistant enterococci in healthcare workers and their households. *Infect Control Hosp Epidemiol* 2002;23:23–26.
101. Ray AJ, Donskey CJ. Clostridium difficile infection and concurrent vancomycin-resistant Enterococcus stool colonization in a health care worker: case report and review of the literature. *Am J Infect Control* 2003;31:54–56.
102. Elizaga ML, Weinstein RA, Hayden MK. Patients in long-term care facilities: a reservoir for vancomycin-resistant enterococci. *Clin Infect Dis* 2002;34:441–446.
103. Gross PA, Messinger Harkavy L, Barden GE, et al. The epidemiology of nosocomial enterococcal urinary tract infection. *Am J Med Sci* 1976;272:75–81.
104. Neely AN, Maley MP. Survival of enterococci and staphylococci on hospital fabrics and plastic.[comment]. *J Clin Microbiol* 2000;38:724–726.
105. Noskin GA, Bednarz P, Suriano T, et al. Persistent contamination of fabric-covered furniture by vancomycin-resistant enterococci: implications for upholstery selection in hospitals. *Am J Infect Control* 2000;28:311–313.
106. Ray AJ, Hoyen CK, Taub TF, et al. Nosocomial transmission of vancomycin-resistant enterococci from surfaces. *JAMA* 2002;287:1400–1401.
107. Hacek DM, Trick WE, Collins SM, et al. Comparison of the Rodac imprint method to selective enrichment broth for recovery of vancomycin-resistant enterococci and drug-resistant Enterobacteriaceae from environmental surfaces. *J Clin Microbiol* 2000;38:4646–4648.
108. Boyce J, Opal S, Chow J, et al. Outbreak of multidrug-resistant *Enterococcus faecium* with transferable vanB class vancomycin resistance. *J Clin Microbiol* 1994;32:1148–1153.
109. Livornese LJ, Dias S, Samel C, et al. Hospital-acquired infection with vancomycin-resistant *Enterococcus faecium* transmitted by electronic thermometers. *Ann Intern Med* 1992;117:112–116.
110. Porwancher R, Sheth A, Remphrey S, et al. Epidemiological study of hospital-acquired infection with vancomycin-resistant *Enterococcus faecium*: possible transmission by an electronic ear-probe thermometer. *Infect Control Hosp Epidemiol* 1997;18:771–773.
111. Falk PS, Winnike J, Woodmansee C, et al. Outbreak of vancomycin-resistant enterococci in a burn unit. *Infect Control Hosp Epidemiol* 2000;21:575–582.
112. Tokars J, Satake S, Rimland D, et al. The prevalence of colonization with vancomycin-resistant *Enterococcus* at a Veterans' Affairs institution. *Infect Control Hosp Epidemiol* 1999;20:171–175.
113. McDonald L, Kuehnert M, Tenover F, et al. Vancomycin-resistant enterococci outside the health-care setting: prevalence, sources, and public health implications. *Emerg Infect Dis* 1997;3:311–317.
114. Wegener HC, Aarestrup FM, Jensen LB, et al. Use of antimicrobial growth promoters in food animals and *Enterococcus faecium* resistance to therapeutic antimicrobial drugs in Europe.[erratum appears in *Emerg Infect Dis* 1999;5:844]. *Emerg Infect Dis* 1999;5:329–335.
115. Sorensen TL, Blom M, Monnet DL, et al. Transient intestinal carriage after ingestion of antibiotic-resistant *Enterococcus faecium* from chicken and pork.[comment]. *N Engl J Med* 2001;345:1161–1166.
116. Silverman J, Thal L, Perri M, et al. Epidemiologic evaluation of antimicrobial resistance in community-acquired enterococci. *J Clin Microbiol* 1998;36:830–832.
117. Coque T, Tomayko J, Ricke S, et al. Vancomycin-resistant enterococci from nosocomial, community and animal sources in the United States. *Antimicrob Agents Chemother* 1996;40:2605–2609.
118. D'Agata EM, Jirjis J, Gouldin C, et al. Community dissemination of vancomycin-resistant *Enterococcus faecium. Am J Infect Control* 2001;29:316–320.
119. Baran J Jr, Paruchuri R, Ramanathan J, et al. Unrecognized cross-infection with vancomycin-resistant *Enterococcus faecium* and *faecalis* detected by molecular typing of blood isolates. *Infect Control Hosp Epidemiol* 2002;23:172–173.
120. Shekar R, Chico G, Bass S, et al. Household transmission of vancomycin-resistant *Enterococcus faecium. Clin Infect Dis* 1995;21:1511–1512.
121. McDonald LC, Rossiter S, Mackinson C, et al. Quinupristin-dalfopristin-resistant *Enterococcus faecium* on chicken and in human stool specimens.[comment]. *N Engl J Med* 2001;345:1155–1160.
122. Gross P, Harkavy L, Barden G, et al. The epidemiology of nosocomial enterococcal urinary tract infection. *Am J Med Sci* 1976;272:75–81.
123. Karanfil L, Murphy M, Josephson A, et al. A cluster of vancomycin-resistant *Enterococcus faecium* in an intensive care unit. *Infect Control Hosp Epidemiol* 1992;13:195–200.
124. Trick WE, Kuehnert MJ, Quirk SB, et al. Regional dissemination of vancomycin-resistant enterococci resulting from interfacility transfer of colonized patients. *J Infect Dis* 1999;180:391–396.
125. Gardiner D, Murphey S, Ossman E, et al. Prevalence and acquisition of vancomycin-resistant enterococci in a medical intensive care unit. *Infect Control Hosp Epidemiol* 2002;23:466–468.
126. D'Agata EM, Green WK, Schulman G, et al. Vancomycin-resistant enterococci among chronic hemodialysis patients: a prospective study of acquisition. *Clin Infect Dis* 2001;32:23–29.
127. Beltrami EM, Singer DA, Fish L, et al. Risk factors for acquisition of vancomycin-resistant enterococci among patients on a renal ward during a community hospital outbreak. *Am J Infect Control* 2000;28:282–285.
128. Bakir M, Bova JL, Newell KA, et al. Epidemiology and clinical consequences of vancomycin-resistant enterococci in liver transplant patients. *Transplantation* 2001;72:1032–1037.
129. Newell K, Millis J, Arnow P, et al. Incidence and outcome of infection by vancomycin-resistant *Enterococcus* following orthotopic liver transplantation. *Transplantation*1998;65:439–442.
130. Patel R, Badley A, Larson-Keller J, et al. Relevance and risk factors of enterococcal bacteremia following liver transplantation. *Transplantation* 1996;61:1192–1197.
131. Patel R, Allen SL, Manahan JM, et al. Natural history of vancomycin-resistant enterococcal colonization in liver and kidney transplant recipients. *Liver Transpl* 2001;7:27–31.
132. Papanicolaou G, Meyers B, Meyers J, et al. Nosocomial infections with vancomycin-resistant *Enterococcus faecium* in liver transplant recipients: risk factors for acquisition and mortality. *Clin Infect Dis* 1996;23:760–766.
133. Singh N, Gayowski T, Rihs JD, et al. Evolving trends in multiple-antibiotic-resistant bacteria in liver transplant recipients: a longitudinal study of antimicrobial susceptibility patterns.[erratum appears in *Liver Transpl* 2001;7:471]. *Liver Transpl* 2001;7:22–26.
134. Tokars JI, Gehr T, Jarvis WR, et al. Vancomycin-resistant enterococci colonization in patients at seven hemodialysis centers. *Kidney Int* 2001;60:1511–1516.
135. Suntharam N, Lankford MG, Trick WE, et al. Risk factors for acquisition of vancomycin-resistant enterococci among hematology-oncology patients. *Diagn Microbiol Infect Dis* 2002;43:183–188.
136. Suppola J, Volin L, Valtonen V, et al. Overgrowth of *Enterococcus faecium* in the feces of patients with hematologic malignancies. *Clin Infect Dis* 1996;23:694–697.
137. Tornieporth N, Roberts R, John J, et al. Risk factors associated with vancomycin-resistant *Enterococcus faecium* infection or colonization in 145 matched case patients and control patients. *Clin Infect Dis* 1996;23:767–772.
138. Pegues D, Pegues C, Hibberd P, et al. Emergence and dissemination of a highly vancomycin-resistant vanA strain of *Enterococcus faecium* at a large teaching hospital. *J Clin Microbiol* 1997;35:1565–1570.
139. Ostrowsky BE, Venkataraman L, D'Agata EM, et al. Vancomycin-resistant enterococci in intensive care units: high frequency of stool carriage during a non-outbreak period. *Arch Intern Med* 1999;159:1467–1472.
140. Bonten M, Slaughter S, Ambergen A, et al. The role of "colonization pressure" in the spread of vancomycin-resistant enterococci: an important infection control variable. *Arch Intern Med* 1998;158:1127–1132.
141. Puzniak LA, Mayfield J, Leet T, et al. Acquisition of vancomycin-

resistant enterococci during scheduled antimicrobial rotation in an intensive care unit. *Clin Infect Dis* 2001;33:151–157.
142. Anonymous. Nosocomial enterococci resistant to vancomycin—United States, 1989–1993. *MMWR Morb Mortal Wkly Rep* 1993; 42:597–599.
143. Byers KE, Anglim AM, Anneski CJ, et al. A hospital epidemic of vancomycin-resistant *Enterococcus*: risk factors and control. *Infect Control Hosp Epidemiol* 2001;22:140–147.
144. Cetinkaya Y, Falk PS, Mayhall CG. Effect of gastrointestinal bleeding and oral medications on acquisition of vancomycin-resistant *Enterococcus faecium* in hospitalized patients. *Clin Infect Dis* 2002;35: 935–942.
145. Garbutt JM, Littenberg B, Evanoff BA, et al. Enteric carriage of vancomycin-resistant *Enterococcus faecium* in patients tested for *Clostridium difficile* [comment]. *Infect Control Hosp Epidemiol* 1999;20:664–670.
146. Boyce J, Opal S, Potter-Bynoe G, et al. Emergence and nosocomial transmission of ampicillin-resistant enterococci. *Antimicrob Agents Chemother* 1992;36:1032–1039.
147. Carmeli Y, Eliopoulos GM, Samore MH. Antecedent treatment with different antibiotic agents as a risk factor for vancomycin-resistant *Enterococcus. Emerg Infect Dis* 2002;8:802–807.
148. Lautenbach E, LaRosa LA, Marr AM, et al. Changes in the prevalence of vancomycin-resistant enterococci in response to antimicrobial formulary interventions: impact of progressive restrictions on use of vancomycin and third-generation cephalosporins. *Clin Infect Dis* 2003; 36:440–446.
149. Carmeli Y, Eliopoulos G, Mozaffari E, et al. Health and economic outcomes of vancomycin-resistant enterococci. *Arch Intern Med* 2002; 162:2223–2228.
150. Jett B, Huycke M, Gilmore M. Virulence of enterococci. *Clin Microbiol Rev* 1994;7:462–478.
151. Huycke M, Spiegel C, Gilmore M. Bacteremia caused by hemolytic, high-level gentamicin-resistant *Enterococcus faecalis. Antimicrob Agents Chemother* 1991;35:1626–1634.
152. Vergis EN, Shankar N, Chow JW, et al. Association between the presence of enterococcal virulence factors gelatinase, hemolysin, and enterococcal surface protein and mortality among patients with bacteremia due to *Enterococcus faecalis. Clin Infect Dis* 2002;35:570–575.
153. Waar K, Muscholl-Silberhorn AB, Willems RJ, et al. Genogrouping and incidence of virulence factors of *Enterococcus faecalis* in liver transplant patients differ from blood culture and fecal isolates. *J Infect Dis* 2002;185:1121–1127.
154. Wong AH, Wenzel RP, Edmond MB. Epidemiology of bacteriuria caused by vancomycin-resistant enterococci—a retrospective study. *Am J Infect Control* 2000;28:277–281.
155. Lloyd S, Zervos M, Mahayni R, et al. Risk factors for enterococcal urinary tract infection and colonization in a rehabilitation facility. *Am J Infect Control* 1998;26:35–39.
156. Anonymous. National Nosocomial Infections Surveillance (NNIS) report, data summary from October 1986–April 1996, issued May 1996. A report from the National Nosocomial Infections Surveillance (NNIS) System. *Am J Infect Control* 1996;24:380–388.
157. Mainous M, Lipsett P, O'Brien M. Enterococcal bacteremia in the surgical intensive care unit. Does vancomycin resistance affect mortality? The Johns Hopkins SICU Study Group. *Arch Surg* 1997;132: 76–81.
158. Lucas G, Lechtzin N, Puryear D, et al. Vancomycin-resistant and vancomycin-susceptible enterococcal bacteremia: comparison of clinical features and outcomes. *Clin Infect Dis* 1998;26:1127–1133.
159. Graninger W, Ragette R. Nosocomial bacteremia due to *Enterococcus faecalis* without endocarditis. *Clin Infect Dis* 1992;15:49–57.
160. Pallares R, Pujol M, Pena C, et al. Cephalosporins as risk factor for nosocomial *Enterococcus faecalis* bacteremia. A matched case-control study. *Arch Intern Med* 1993;153:1581–1586.
161. Bonadio W. Group D streptococcal bacteremia in children: a review of 72 cases in 12 years. *Clin Pediatr* 1993;32:20–24.
162. Montecalvo M, Shay D, Patel P, et al. Bloodstream infections with vancomycin-resistant enterococci. *Arch Intern Med* 1996;156: 1458–1462.
163. Iwen P, Kelly D, Linder J, et al. Change in prevalence and antibiotic resistance of *Enterococcus* species isolated from blood cultures over an 8-year period. *Antimicrob Agents Chemother* 1997;41:494–495.
164. Vergis EN, Hayden MK, Chow JW, et al. Determinants of vancomycin resistance and mortality rates in enterococcal bacteremia. a prospective multicenter study. *Ann Intern Med* 2001;135:484–492.
165. Shay D, Maloney S, Montecalvo M, et al. Epidemiology and mortality risk of vancomycin-resistant enterococcal bloodstream infections. *J Infect Dis* 1995;172:993–1000.
166. Bhavnani SM, Drake JA, Forrest A, et al. A nationwide, multicenter, case-control study comparing risk factors, treatment, and outcome for vancomycin-resistant and -susceptible enterococcal bacteremia. *Diagn Microbiol Infect Dis* 2000;36:145–158.
167. Linden P, Pasculle A, Manez R, et al. Differences in outcomes for patients with bacteremia due to vancomycin-resistant *Enterococcus faecium* or vancomycin-susceptible *E. faecium. Clin Infect Dis* 1996;22: 663–670.
168. Zaas AK, Song X, Tucker P, et al. Risk factors for development of vancomycin-resistant enterococcal bloodstream infection in patients with cancer who are colonized with vancomycin-resistant enterococci. *Clin Infect Dis* 2002;35:1139–1146.
169. Stosor V, Peterson L, Postelnick M, et al. Enterococcus faecium bacteremia: does vancomycin resistance make a difference? *Arch Intern Med* 1998;158:522–527.
170. Edmond M, Ober J, Weinbaum D, et al. Vancomycin-resistant *Enterococcus faecium* bacteremia: risk factors for infection. *Clin Infect Dis* 1995;20:1126–1133.
171. Krcmery V, Bilikova E, Svetlansky I, et al. Is vancomycin resistance in enterococci predictive of inferior outcome of enterococcal bacteremia?[comment]. *Clin Infect Dis* 2001;32:1110–1112.
172. Roghmann M, McCarter RJ, Brewrink J, et al. Clostridium difficile infection is a risk factor for bacteremia due to vancomycin-resistant enterococci (VRE) in VRE-colonized patients with acute leukemia. *Clin Infect Dis* 1997;25:1056–1059.
173. Husni R, Hachem R, Hanna H, et al. Risk factors for vancomycin-resistant *Enterococcus* (VRE) infection in colonized patients with cancer. *Infect Control Hosp Epidemiol* 2002;23:102–103.
174. Noskin G, Cooper I, Peterson L. Vancomycin-resistant *Enterococcus faecium* sepsis following persistent colonization. *Arch Intern Med* 1995;155:1445–1447.
175. Stroud L, Edwards J, Danzing L, et al. Risk factors for mortality associated with enterococcal bloodstream infections. *Infect Control Hosp Epidemiol* 1996;17:576–580.
176. Lodise TP, McKinnon PS, Tam VH, et al. Clinical outcomes for patients with bacteremia caused by vancomycin-resistant enterococcus in a level 1 trauma center. *Clin Infect Dis* 2002;34:922–929.
177. Garbutt JM, Ventrapragada M, Littenberg B, et al. Association between resistance to vancomycin and death in cases of Enterococcus faecium bacteremia [comment]. *Clin Infect Dis* 2000;30:466–472.
178. Edmond M, Ober J, Dawson J, et al. Vancomycin-resistant enterococcal bacteremia: natural history and attributable mortality. *Clin Infect Dis* 1996;23:1234–1239.
179. Mandell G, Kaye D, Levison M, et al. Enterococcal endocarditis. An analysis of 38 patients observed at the New York Hospital-Cornell Medical Center. *Arch Intern Med* 1970;125:258–264.
180. Olaison L, Schadewitz K, Swedish Society of Infectious Diseases Quality Assurance Study Group for E. Enterococcal endocarditis in Sweden, 1995–1999: can shorter therapy with aminoglycosides be used? *Clin Infect Dis* 2002;34:159–166.
181. Babcock HM, Ritchie DJ, Christiansen E, et al. Successful treatment of vancomycin-resistant *Enterococcus* endocarditis with oral linezolid. *Clin Infect Dis* 2001;32:1373–1375.
182. Matsumura S, Simor AE. Treatment of endocarditis due to vancomycin-resistant *Enterococcus faecium* with quinupristin/dalfopristin, doxycycline, and rifampin: a synergistic drug combination. *Clin Infect Dis* 1998;27:1554–1556.
183. Rao N, White GJ. Successful treatment of *Enterococcus faecalis* prosthetic valve endocarditis with linezolid. *Clin Infect Dis* 2002;35: 902–904.
184. Nichols R, Muzik A. Enterococcal infections in surgical patients: the mystery continues. *Clin Infect Dis* 1992;15:72–76.

185. Anonymous. National Nosocomial Infections Surveillance (NNIS) report, data summary from October 1986–April 1996, issued May 1996. *Am J Infect Control* 1996;24:380–388.
186. Mylotte JM, Kahler L, Graham R, et al. Prospective surveillance for antibiotic-resistant organisms in patients with spinal cord injury admitted to an acute rehabilitation unit. *Am J Infect Control* 2000;28: 291–297.
187. Dobson S, Baker C. Enterococcal sepsis in neonates: features by age at onset and occurrence of focal infection. *Pediatrics* 1990;85:165–171.
188. Green M. Vancomycin resistant enterococci: impact and management in pediatrics. *Adv Pediatr Infect Dis* 1997;13:257–277.
189. Graham PL, Ampofo K, Saiman L. Linezolid treatment of vancomycin-resistant *Enterococcus faecium* ventriculitis. *Pediatr Infect Dis J* 2002;21:798–800.
190. Jang TN, Fung CP, Liu CY, et al. Enterococcal meningitis: analysis of twelve cases. *J Formos Med Assoc* 1995;94:391–395.
191. McNeeley DF, Brown AE, Noel GJ, et al. An investigation of vancomycin-resistant *Enterococcus faecium* within the pediatric service of a large urban medical center. *Pediatr Infect Dis J* 1998;17:184–188.
192. Nourse C, Murphy H, Byrne C, et al. Control of a nosocomial outbreak of vancomycin resistant *Enterococcus faecium* in a paediatric oncology unit: risk factors for colonisation. *Eur J Pediatr* 1998;157: 20–27.
193. Rupp ME, Marion N, Fey PD, et al. Outbreak of vancomycin-resistant *Enterococcus faecium* in a neonatal intensive care unit. *Infect Control Hosp Epidemiol* 2001;22:301–303.
194. Bratcher DF. Vancomycin-resistant enterococci in the pediatric patient. *Pediatr Infect Dis J* 2001;20:621–622.
195. Christenson J, Korgenski E, Jenkins E, et al. Detection of vancomycin-resistant enterococci colonization in a children's hospital. *Am J Infect Control* 1998;26:569–571.
196. von Baum H, Schehl J, Geiss HK, et al. Prevalence of vancomycin-resistant enterococci among children with end-stage renal failure. Mid-European Pediatric Peritoneal Dialysis Study Group. *Clin Infect Dis* 1999;29:912–916.
197. Stevenson K, Murray E, Sarubbi F. Enterococcal meningitis: report of four cases and review. *Clin Infect Dis* 1994;18:233–239.
198. Zeana C, Kubin CJ, Della-Latta P, et al. Vancomycin-resistant *Enterococcus faecium* meningitis successfully managed with linezolid: case report and review of the literature. *Clin Infect Dis* 2001;33:477–482.
199. Uchio E, Inamura M, Okada K, et al. A case of endogenous *Enterococcus faecalis* endophthalmitis. *Jpn J Ophthalmol* 1992;36:215–221.
200. Raymond NJ, Henry J, Workowski KA. Enterococcal arthritis: case report and review [comment]. *Clin Infect Dis* 1995;21:516–522.
201. Bonten M, van Tiel F, van der Geest S, et al. *Enterococcus faecalis* pneumonia complicating topical antimicrobial prophylaxis. *N Engl J Med* 1993; 328:209–210.
202. Bach PB, Malak SF, Jurcic J, et al. Impact of infection by vancomycin-resistant *Enterococcus* on survival and resource utilization for patients with leukemia. *Infect Control Hosp Epidemiol* 2002;23:471–474.
203. Webb M, Riley LW, Roberts RB. Cost of hospitalization for and risk factors associated with vancomycin-resistant *Enterococcus faecium* infection and colonization. *Clin Infect Dis* 2001;33:445–452.
204. Pelz RK, Lipsett PA, Swoboda SM, et al. Vancomycin-sensitive and vancomycin-resistant enterococcal infections in the ICU: attributable costs and outcomes. *Intensive Care Med* 2002;28:692–697.
205. Bryce EA, Tiffin SM, Isaac-Renton JL, et al. Evidence of delays in transferring patients with methicillin-resistant *Staphylococcus aureus* or vancomycin-resistant *Enterococcus* to long-term-care facilities. *Infect Control Hosp Epidemiol* 2000;21:270–271.
206. Anglim A, Klym B, Byers K, et al. Effect of a vancomycin restriction policy on ordering practices during an outbreak of vancomycin-resistant *Enterococcus faecium. Arch Intern Med* 1997;157:1132–1136.
207. Fridkin SK, Edwards JR, Courval JM, et al. The effect of vancomycin and third-generation cephalosporins on prevalence of vancomycin-resistant enterococci in 126 U.S. adult intensive care units. *Ann Intern Med* 2001;135:175–183.
208. Fridkin SK, Lawton R, Edwards JR, et al. Monitoring antimicrobial use and resistance: comparison with a national benchmark on reducing vancomycin use and vancomycin-resistant enterococci. *Emerg Infect Dis* 2002;8:702–707.
209. Harbarth S, Cosgrove S, Carmeli Y. Effects of antibiotics on nosocomial epidemiology of vancomycin-resistant enterococci. *Antimicrob Agents Chemother* 2002;46:1619–1628.
210. Quale J, Landman D, Saurina G, et al. Manipulation of a hospital antimicrobial formulary to control an outbreak of vancomycin-resistant enterococci. *Clin Infect Dis* 1996;23:1020–1025.
211. Anonymous. Recommendations for preventing the spread of vancomycin resistance. Recommendations of the Hospital Infection Control Practices Advisory Committee (HICPAC). *MMWR Morb Mortal Wkly Rep* 1995;44:1–13.
212. Fridkin S, Edwards J, Pichette S, et al. Determinants of vancomycin use in adult intensive care units in 41 United States hospitals. *Clin Infect Dis* 1999;28:1119–1125.
213. Lawton RM, Fridkin SK, Gaynes RP, et al. Practices to improve antimicrobial use at 47 US hospitals: the status of the 1997 SHEA/IDSA position paper recommendations. Society for Healthcare Epidemiology of America/Infectious Diseases Society of America. *Infect Control Hosp Epidemiol* 2000;21:256–259.
214. Muto CA, Giannetta ET, Durbin LJ, et al. Cost-effectiveness of perirectal surveillance cultures for controlling vancomycin-resistant *Enterococcus. Infect Control Hosp Epidemiol* 2002;23:429–435.
215. Siddiqui AH, Harris AD, Hebden J, et al. The effect of active surveillance for vancomycin-resistant enterococci in high-risk units on vancomycin-resistant enterococci incidence hospital-wide. *Am J Infect Control* 2002;30:40–43.
216. Montecalvo MA, Jarvis WR, Uman J, et al. Costs and savings associated with infection control measures that reduced transmission of vancomycin-resistant enterococci in an endemic setting. *Infect Control Hosp Epidemiol* 2001;22:437–442.
217. Ostrowsky BE, Trick WE, Sohn AH, et al. Control of vancomycin-resistant enterococcus in health care facilities in a region. *N Engl J Med* 2001;344:1427–1433.
218. Reisner BS, Shaw S, Huber ME, et al. Comparison of three methods to recover vancomycin-resistant enterococci (VRE) from perianal and environmental samples collected during a hospital outbreak of VRE. *Infect Control Hosp Epidemiol* 2000;21:775–779.
219. Hendrix CW, Hammond JM, Swoboda SM, et al. Surveillance strategies and impact of vancomycin-resistant enterococcal colonization and infection in critically ill patients. *Ann Surg* 2001;233:259–265.
220. D'Agata EM, Gautam S, Green WK, et al. High rate of false-negative results of the rectal swab culture method in detection of gastrointestinal colonization with vancomycin-resistant enterococci. *Clin Infect Dis* 2002;34:167–172.
221. Leber AL, Hindler JF, Kato EO, et al. Laboratory-based surveillance for vancomycin-resistant enterococci: utility of screening stool specimens submitted for *Clostridium difficile* toxin assay. *Infect Control Hosp Epidemiol* 2001;22:160–164.
222. Ray AJ, Hoyen CK, Das SM, et al. Undetected vancomycin-resistant Enterococcus stool colonization in a Veterans Affairs Hospital using a *Clostridium difficile*-focused surveillance strategy. *Infect Control Hosp Epidemiol* 2002;23:474–477.
223. Dembek ZF, Kellerman SE, Ganley L, et al. Reporting of vancomycin-resistant enterococci in Connecticut: implementation and validation of a state-based surveillance system. *Infect Control Hospital Epidemiol* 1999;20:671–675.
224. Slaughter S, Hayden M, Nathan C, et al. A comparison of the effect of universal use of gloves and gowns with that of glove use alone on acquisition of vancomycin-resistant enterococci in a medical intensive care unit. *Ann Intern Med* 1996;125:448–456.
225. Srinivasan A, Song X, Ross T, et al. A prospective study to determine whether cover gowns in addition to gloves decrease nosocomial transmission of vancomycin-resistant enterococci in an intensive care unit. *Infect Control Hosp Epidemiol* 2002;23:424–428.
226. Puzniak LA, Leet T, Mayfield J, et al. To gown or not to gown: the effect on acquisition of vancomycin-resistant enterococci. *Clin Infect Dis* 2002;35:18–25.
227. Sample ML, Gravel D, Oxley C, et al. An outbreak of vancomycin-resistant enterococci in a hematology-oncology unit: control by pa-

tient cohorting and terminal cleaning of the environment. *Infect Control Hosp Epidemiol* 2002;23:468–470.

228. Boyce JM, Pittet D, Healthcare Infection Control Practices Advisory Committee. Society for Healthcare Epidemiology of America. Association for Professionals in Infection Control. Infectious Diseases Society of America. Hand Hygiene Task Force. Guideline for hand hygiene in health-care settings: recommendations of the Healthcare Infection Control Practices Advisory Committee and the HICPAC/SHEA/APIC/IDSA Hand Hygiene Task Force. *Infect Control Hosp Epidemiol* 2002;23:S3–S40.
229. Tenorio AR, Badri SM, Sahgal NB, et al. Effectiveness of gloves in the prevention of hand carriage of vancomycin-resistant *Enterococcus* species by health care workers after patient care. *Clin Infect Dis* 2001; 32:826–829.
230. Wade J, Desai N, Casewell M. Hygienic hand disinfection for the removal of epidemic vancomycin-resistant *Enterococcus faecium* and gentamicin-resistant *Enterobacter cloacae. J Hosp Infect* 1991;18: 211–218.
231. Hachem R, Raad I. Failure of oral antimicrobial agents in eradicating gastrointestinal colonization with vancomycin-resistant enterococci. *Infect Control Hosp Epidemiol* 2002;23:43–44.
232. Wong MT, Kauffman CA, Standiford HC, et al. Effective suppression of vancomycin-resistant *Enterococcus* species in asymptomatic gastrointestinal carriers by a novel glycolipodepsipeptide, ramoplanin. *Clin Infect Dis* 2001;33:1476–1482.
233. Weinstein MR, Dedier H, Brunton J, et al. Lack of efficacy of oral bacitracin plus doxycycline for the eradication of stool colonization with vancomycin-resistant *Enterococcus faecium. Clin Infect Dis* 1999; 29:361–366.
234. Weber D, Rutala W. Role of environmental contamination in the transmission of vancomycin-resistant enterococci. *Infect Control Hosp Epidemiol* 1997;18:306–309.
235. Anderson R, Carr J, Bond W, et al. Susceptibility of vancomycin-resistant enterococci to environmental disinfectants. *Infect Control Hosp Epidemiol* 1997;18:195–199.

33

ENTEROBACTERIACEAE

STEPHANIE R. BLACK
MARC J. M. BONTEN
ROBERT A. WEINSTEIN

The family Enterobacteriaceae comprises a wide array of gram-negative bacilli whose reservoirs include soil, water, plants, and the gastrointestinal tracts of humans and animals. As a group, Enterobacteriaceae are the most frequent bacterial isolates recovered from inpatient and outpatient clinical specimens (1). In 1990 to 1996, Enterobacteriaceae accounted for 30% and 34% of pathogens isolated from all infection sites in the Centers for Disease Control and Prevention (CDC) National Nosocomial Infections Surveillance (NNIS) system and the European Prevalence of Infection in Intensive Care Study (2,3), respectively. As the use of invasive devices, broad-spectrum antibiotics, and immunosuppressive agents has increased in hospitals, the Enterobacteriaceae, particularly *Escherichia coli,* have become somewhat less prevalent, and gram-positive microorganisms, especially staphylococci and enterococci, more prevalent as causes of nosocomial infection. Nevertheless, increasing antibiotic resistance among Enterobacteriaceae has continued to make infections due to them a major cause of concern in hospitals. Data from the Intensive Care Antimicrobial Resistance Epidemiology (ICARE) Project and the NNIS Antimicrobial Use and Resistance (AUR) component from 1998–2002 demonstrate that resistant gram-positive species represent the top three, *Pseudomonas aeruginosa* resistant to fluoroquinolones the fourth, and *Enterobacter* spp. resistant to third-generation cephalosporins the fifth most common antibiotic-resistant pathogens recovered from intensive care unit (ICU) patients (4).

OVERVIEW

Microbiologically, all members of the Enterobacteriaceae are facultative anaerobes that, with few exceptions, ferment glucose, reduce nitrate to nitrite, and are oxidase negative (5). Several approaches to classifying the Enterobacteriaceae have been used over the years, including phenotypic subgroupings (6), DNA relatedness studies (7), and a combination of the two methods (8). A summary of a current classification is presented in Table 33.1 (9).

For identification of aerobic gram-negative bacilli, many hospital microbiology laboratories now use automated rapid identification systems rather than conventional biochemical testing (5). Of particular importance to infection control is the ability to determine in the microbiology laboratory whether nosocomial infections are due to the spread of a single species. This requires the ability to type strains by classic or newer molecular methods (Table 33.2). Pulsed-field gel electrophoresis (PFGE) is the most widely used method of genotyping, and for small sets of isolates empiric guidelines have been formulated to interpret chromosomal DNA restriction patterns produced by this method (11) (see Chapter 102). These guidelines have been validated for some species (12).

To illustrate the changing overall role of Enterobacteriaceae in the pathogenesis of nosocomial infections, Table 33.3 presents NNIS data from 1980–1982 and 1990–1996. The percentage of pathogens recovered from nosocomial infections that were Enterobacteriaceae declined from 42% in 1980–1982 to 29% in 1990–1996, primarily because of less frequent recovery of *E. coli.* This trend is apparent and continues in all major infection sites. For example, Enterobacteriaceae accounted for 18% of the 14,424 isolates causing bloodstream infections (BSIs) in the 1990–1996 NNIS data, but accounted for only 10% of the 21,942 isolates causing BSIs in the 1992–1999 data (13). Selected data from other, more recent multicenter nosocomial surveillance systems are shown in Table 33.4.

Although the overall percentage of nosocomial infections due to the Enterobacteriaceae has declined, Enterobacteriaceae remain important nosocomial pathogens. They have been implicated in almost half (46%) of all nosocomial urinary tract infections (UTIs), in nearly a quarter (24%) of all surgical site infections, in up to 18% of all bloodstream infections, and in 30% of all nosocomial pneumonias. Overall, *E. coli, Klebsiella pneumoniae, Enterobacter* spp., and *Proteus mirabilis* were the most common nosocomial pathogens in the family Enterobacteriaceae and together accounted for about one quarter of all nosocomial isolates in 1990–1996. Enterobacteriaceae continue to cause a decreasing but significant percentage of nosocomial infections. Enterobacteriaceae represented almost a third (29%) of nosocomial UTIs, 10% of nosocomial BSIs, and 22% of nosocomial pneumonias in 1992–1999 (13).

PATHOGENESIS OF NOSOCOMIAL INFECTIONS CAUSED BY ENTEROBACTERIACEAE

Multiple factors are involved in the pathogenesis of infection caused by Enterobacteriaceae. As discussed below, a variety of pathogen-specific factors, device-related factors, and host factors act together to determine the likelihood of infection. The viru-

TABLE 33.1. AEROBIC GRAM-NEGATIVE BACILLI: ENTEROBACTERIACEAE (PERTINENT CHARACTERISTICS: FERMENT SUGARS; OXIDASE NEGATIVE; MOST REDUCE NITRATE TO NITRITE)

Current Name	Synonym
Budvicia aquatica	
Buttiauxella noackiae	CDC enteric group 59
Cedecea davisae	CDC enteric group 15
Cedecea lapagei	
Cedecea neteri	*Cedecea* sp. 4
Cedecea sp. 3	
Cedecea sp. 5	
Citrobacter amalonaticus	*Levinea amalonatica*
Citrobacter braakii	*Citrobacter freundii*
Citrobacter diversus	
Citrobacter farmeri	*Citrobacter amalonaticus* biogroup 1
Citrobacter freundii	*Colobactrum freundii*
Citrobacter gillenii	*Citrobacter* genomospecies 10 *Citrobacter freundii*
Citrobacter koseri	*Citrobacter diversus* *Levinea malonatica*
Citrobacter murliniae	*Citrobacter* genomospecies 11 *Citrobacter freundii*
Citrobacter rodentium	*Citrobacter* genomospecies 9 *Citrobacter freundii*
Citrobacter sedlakii	*Citrobacter* genomospecies 8 *Citrobacter freundii*
Citrobacter werkmanii	Citrobacter genomospecies 7 *Citrobacter freundii*
Citrobacter youngae	*Citrobacter* genomospecies 5 *Citrobacter freundii*
Edwardsiella hoshinae	
Edwardsiella tarda	
Enterobacter aerogenes	*Aerobacter aerogenes*
Enterobacter agglomerans group	
Enterobacter amnigenus	
Enterobacter asburiae	CDC enteric group 17
Enterobacter cancerogenus	*Enterobacter taylorae* *Erwinia cancerogena* CDC enteric group 19
Enterobacter cloacae	
Enterobacter gergoviae	
Enterobacter hormaechei	CDC enteric group 75
Enterobacter intermedius	*Enterobacter intermedium*
Enterobacter kobei	
Enterobacter sakazakii	
Erwinia persicinus	
Escherichia blattae	
Escherichia coli	
Escherichia fergusonii	CDC enteric group 10
Escherichia hermannii	CDC enteric group 11
Escherichia vulneris	CDC enteric group 1
Ewingella americana	CDC enteric group 40
Hafnia alvei	*Enterobacter hafniae*
Klebsiella ornithinolytica	*Klebsiella oxytoca* ornithine positive
Klebsiella oxytoca	
Klebsiella planticola	*Klebsiella travisanii*
Klebsiella pneumoniae ssp. *ozaenae*	*Klebsiella ozaenae*
Klebsiella pneumoniae ssp. *pneumoniae*	*Klebsiella pneumoniae*
Klebsiella pneumoniae ssp. *rhinoscleromatis*	*Klebsiella rhinoscleromatis*
Klebsiella terrigena	
Kluyvera ascorbata	CDC enteric group 8
Kluyvera cryocrescens	
Kluyvera georgiana	CDC enteric group 36/37 *Kluyvera* species group 3
Leclercia adecarboxylata	*Escherichia adecarboxylata* CDC enteric group 41
Leminorella grimontii	CDC enteric group 57
Leminorella richardii	
Moellerella wisconsensis	CDC enteric group 46
Morganella morganii ssp. *morganii*	*Proteus morganii*
Morganella morganii ssp. *sibonii*	*Proteus morganii*
Pantoea agglomerans	*Enterobacter agglomerans*
Pantoea dispersa	
Photorhabdus luminescens	*Xenorhabdus luminescens*
Pragia fontium	
Proteus mirabilis	
Proteus penneri	*Proteus vulgaris* biogroup 1
Proteus vulgaris	*Proteus vulgaris* biogroup 1
Providencia alcalifaciens	*Proteus inconstans*
Providencia rettgeri	*Proteus rettgeri*
Providencia rustigianii	*Providencia alcalifaciens* biogroup 3
Providencia stuartii	*Proteus inconstans*
Rahnella aquatilis	
Salmonella bongori	*Salmonella* subgroup 5
Salmonella choleraesuis ssp. *arizonae*	*Salmonella* subgroup 3a
Salmonella choleraesuis ssp. *choleraesius*	*Salmonella* subgroup 1
Salmonella choleraesuis ssp. *diarizonae*	*Salmonella* subgroup 3b
Salmonella choleraesuis ssp. *houtenae*	*Salmonella* subgroup 4
Salmonella choleraesuis ssp. *indica*	*Salmonella* subgroup 6
Salmonella choleraesuis ssp. *salamae*	*Salmonella* subgroup 2
Serratia ficaria	
Serratia fonticola	
Serratia grimesii	*Serratia liquefaciens*
Serratia liquefaciens	*Enterobacter liquefaciens*
Serratia marcescens	
Serratia odoriferae	
Serrattia plymuthica	
Serratia proteamaculans ssp. *proteamaculans*	*Serratia liquefaciens*
Serratia proteamaculans ssp. *quinovora*	*Serratia liquefaciens*
Serratia rubidaea	
Shigella boydii	*Shigella* biogroup C
Shigella dysenteriae	*Shigella* biogroup A
Shigella flexneri	*Shigella* biogroup B
Shigella sonnei	*Shigella* biogroup D
Tatumella ptyseos	CDC group EF-9
Trabulsiella guamensis	CDC enteric group 90
Yersinia aldovae	
Yersinia bercovieri	*Yersinia enterocolitica* biogroup 3b
Yersinia enterocolitica	*Pasteurella enterocolitica*
Yersinia frederiksenii	
Yersinia intermedia	
Yersinia kristensenii	
Yersinia mollaretii	*Yersinia enterocolitica* biogroup 3a
Yersinia pestis	*Pasteurella pestis*
Yersinia pseudotuberculosis	*Pasteurella pseudotuberculosis*
Yersinia rohdei	
Yokenella regensburgei	*Koserella trabulsii* CDC enteric group 45

Note: Diagnostic laboratories may report *Salmonella* serovars by name, e.g., *Salmonella typhi* or *Salmonella* serovar *typhi*.
CDC, Centers for Disease Control and Prevention.
Adapted from Bruckner DA, Colonna P, Bearson BL. Nomenclature for aerobic and facultative bacteria. *Clin Infect Dis* 1999;29:713–723.

TABLE 33.2. CHARACTERISTICS OF BACTERIAL TYPING SYSTEMS

Typing System	Proportion of Strains Typeable	Reproducibility	Discriminatory Power
Phenotypic methods			
Biotyping	All	Fair	Poor
Antimicrobial susceptibility testing	All	Fair	Poor
Serotyping	Most	Good	Fair
Bacteriophage typing	Most	Fair	Poor
Immunoblotting	All	Excellent	Good
Multilocus enzyme electrophoresis	All	Excellent	Good
Genotypic methods			
Plasmid profile analysis	Most	Fair	Fair
Restriction endonuclease analysis	All	Good	Fair
Ribotyping	All	Excellent	Fair
Pulsed-field gel electrophoresis	All	Excellent	Excellent
Polymerase chain reaction restriction digests	All	Excellent	Good
Arbitrarily primed polymerase chain reaction	All	Good	Good
Nucleotide sequence analysis	All	Excellent	Excellent

Note: These judgments represent the views of Maslow et al. (10); many systems remain incompletely evaluated, and characteristics may vary when the systems are applied to different species.
Modified from Maslow JN, Mulligan ME, Arbeit RD. Molecular epidemiology: application of contemporary techniques to the typing of microorganisms. *Clin Infect Dis* 1993;17:153–164.

lence of the microorganism (i.e., the ability to invade and cause disease) relates to both pathogen factors and to the immune status of the patient.

Pathogen-Specific Factors

Adhesion

Bacterial adhesion is a highly specific phenomenon that leads to attachment of bacteria to mucosal surfaces and, thus, to colonization and potentially to bacterial overgrowth and to tissue invasion. Adhesins may also function as invasins, promote biofilm formation, and transmit signals to epithelial cells leading to inflammation (18,19). Among Enterobacteriaceae, adhesion is mediated by both fimbrial and nonfimbrial adhesins (Table 33.5) that are encoded on plasmids and on the bacterial genome, forming "pathogenicity islands" (43). The locus for enterocyte effacement (LEE) on the chromosome encodes the virulence types necessary for attachment and ef-

TABLE 33.3. DISTRIBUTION OF SELECTED ENTEROBACTERIACEAE AND OTHER PATHOGENS ISOLATED FROM ALL MAJOR INFECTION SITES, NATIONAL NOSOCOMIAL INFECTIONS SURVEILLANCE (NNIS) SYSTEM

	Percentage (*n*)		Rank	
Pathogen	1980–1982	1990–1996	1980–1982	1990–1996
Selected Enterobacteriaceae				
Citrobacter spp.	1	1	12	11
Enterobacter spp.	5	6	6	6
E. coli	20	12	1	2
K. pneumoniae	6	5	5	8
Klebsiella spp. (other)	2	1	10	12
P. mirabilis	5	3	7	9
Proteus spp. (other)	1	0	13	13
S. marcescens	2	1	11	10
Serratia spp. (other)	0	0	14	14
Total	42	29		
Other pathogens				
P. aeruginosa	10	9	4	5
S. aureus	11	13	2	1
Coagulase-negative staphylococci	5	11	8	3
Enterococci	10	10	3	4
C. albicans	3	5	9	7
Other	19	23		
Total	100 (132, 686)	100 (101, 821)		

Data from Centers for Disease Control and Prevention and ref. 3.

TABLE 33.4. EXAMPLES OF MULTICENTER SURVEILLANCE STUDIES OF NOSOCOMIAL ENTEROBACTERERIACEAE

Year	Ref.	Study Eponym	No. of Centers	Countries	Type of Units	Source of Isolates	Total Bacterial Isolates	No. (%) of Isolates that Were Entero-bactereriaceae	Percent of Total Isolates						
									Escherichia	*Klebsiella*	*Enterobacter*	*Serratia*	*Proteus*	*Morganella*	*Citrolbacter*
1997–1998	14	SENTRY	24	Europe (14 countries)	Hospital-wide	Pneumonia	2,052	650 (32)	7	8	8	4	2	1	2
1997	15	SENTRY	37	U.S. and Canada	Hospital-wide	Pneumonia	2,757	698 (25)	5	9	7	3	1	—	1
1999–2000	16	N/A	16	Italy	Hospital-wide	Bloodstream	1,352	483 (36)	17	8	7	2	2	—	—
1999	17	ESGNI	228	Europe (29 countries)	Hospital-wide, one day point prevalence	Urinary tract	607	316 (52)	36	8	—	—	8	—	—

ESGNI, European Study Group on Nosocomial Infections.

TABLE 33.5. EXAMPLES OF PATHOGEN-SPECIFIC VIRULENCE FACTORS IN ENTEROBACTERIACEAE

Virulence Factor	Pathogen (Reference)	Infection
Bacterial adhesins		
Fimbrial adhesins		
P fimbriae	*E. coli* (20,21)	UTI/pyelonephritis
Type I fimbriae	*E. coli* (20,21), *K. pneumoniae* (22)	Cystitis
S fimbriae	*E. coli* (20,21)	Neonatal sepsis/meningitis
Colonization factor Ag (CFAI, CFAII)	*E. coli* (20,21)	Diarrhea
K88, K89	*E. coli* (10,21)	Diarrhea
Type 3 fimbriae	*K. pneumoniae* (22)	Cystitis/UTI
Type 6 fimbriae	*K. pneumoniae* (22)	?
MR-K hemagglutinin	*P. stuartii* (23)	LT catheter UTI
Cell adhesin	*P. mirabilis* (24–27)	UTI (?)
Type IV pili	*E. coli* (28)	Diarrhea
Nonfimbrial adhesins		
R-plasmid–encoded adhesive factor	*K. pneumoniae* (29,30)	UTI, CSF shunt infection
Bacterial toxins		
Hemolysin (α,β)	*E. coli* (31)	UTI/pyelonephritis
Enterotoxin	*E. coli* (31)	Diarrhea
Verotoxin	*E. coli* (31)	HUS, HC, diarrhea
Endotoxin	*E. coli* (31)	Sepsis
Bacterial capsules		
K antigens	*E. coli* (32–34)	Extraintestinal/invasive disease
	K. pneumoniae (35–37)	?
Bacterial siderophores		
Aerobactin	*E. coli* (38)	Pyelonephritis, cystitis
	K. pneumoniae (39,40)	Pyelonephritis
Urease production	*Proteus* (41)	LT catheter UTI
Outer membrane proteins	*C. diversus* (40,42)	Brain abscess
	Yersinia spp. (37)	Increased virulence

CFAI, II, colonization factor antigen I, II; HC, hemorrhagic colitis; HUS, hemolytic-uremic syndrome; LT, long-term; MR-K, mannose-resistant *Klebsiella*-like hemagglutinin; UTI, urinary tract infection.

facement of *E. coli* to enterocytes (44). The *E. coli* fimbrial adhesins are among the most studied and best characterized of the bacterial adhesins.

P fimbriae anchor bacteria to uroepithelial cells (20) and are found in strains that cause pyelonephritis in adults and children (45–47). The symbol P was chosen because P-fimbriated *E. coli* were a frequent cause of pyelonephritis and because glycolipids were receptors for P fimbriae and antigens in the P blood group system (48). Compared to non–P-fimbriated strains of *E. coli*, isolates with P fimbriae can adhere to specific receptors on human colonic epithelial cells (leading to colonization), spread more easily to the urinary tract, have a better ability to persist in kidneys and bladders, and enhance a more pronounced inflammatory response (48).

A relationship between adherence and virulence has been demonstrated. Among *E. coli* strains from patients with different forms of UTIs, *in vitro* adherence to uroepithelial cells was found in 80% of the patients with pyelonephritis, 40% to 50% of the patients with acute cystitis, and 20% of the patients with asymptomatic bacteriuria (48). Studies of bacteremia secondary to urosepsis have shown that *E. coli* strains that cause urosepsis in healthy patients almost always have P fimbriae, whereas *E. coli* urosepsis in immunocompromised patients is less often due to such P-fimbriated strains (45–47). In a study of fimbrial types found in respiratory isolates from ICU patients with presumed nosocomial pneumonia, P fimbriae were found in approximately half of the *E. coli* respiratory isolates (49). This rate is higher than the rate of P fimbriation commonly found in fecal isolates (14–16%) and, thus, raises the question of how the presence of this adhesin may be advantageous to strains causing pulmonary infection (49). Another study looked at the role of the *papG* class II gene, a P-fimbrial structural allele causing uroepithelial attachment of *E. coli*, and the pathogenesis of *E. coli* bacteremia in upper UTIs and ascending cholangitis. The authors found a significant difference between the presence of the virulence factor, *papG* class II, in bacteremic patients with upper UTI compared to bacteremic patients with ascending cholangitis and to controls (50).

Cranberry juice consumption may offer protection against P-fimbriated strains of *E. coli* by the action of cranberry proanthocyanidin (condensed tannin), which inhibits P-fimbriated *E. coli* from adhering to uroepithelial cells (51). A randomized controlled study with 50 women per arm compared drinking 50 mL of cranberry juice concentrate daily for 6 months to drinking 100 mL of lactobacillus GG 5 days a week for 1 year, compared to controls. The authors found an absolute risk reduction for recurrent UTI of 20% in the group that drank cranberry juice (52). Cranberry juice consumption, as an alternative to antimicrobial prophylaxis of UTIs, warrants further evaluation.

S fimbriae are present on many *E. coli* strains that cause infant meningitis. The presence of binding sites for S fimbriae on blood vessels in the central nervous system (CNS) and on epithelial cells of the choroid plexus and of the ventricle of the infant rat brain provides a model for the pathogenesis of neonatal *E. coli* meningitis (53). Binding affinity of S fimbriae for vascular endothelium and epithelium of the choroid plexus and ventricles decreases after the neonatal period in rats, paralleling the decrease in susceptibility to *E. coli* meningitis (54). S fimbriae also allow *E. coli* to bind to intact endothelial cells (53,55) and thus may be an important virulence factor for septicemia. When isolates of *E. coli* that caused a variety of invasive bacterial infections were compared to fecal isolates in healthy children, P fimbriae and S fimbriae were predominant in *E. coli* isolates causing invasive disease (56).

Type I pili have been associated with uropathogenic *E. coli* (UPEC). Type I pili facilitate entry of UPEC into bladder epithelial cells, with subsequent exfoliation (57). The ability of UPEC to invade and persist in bladder epithelial cells has been suggested as an explanation of recurrent UTIs.

Type IV pili have been identified in enteropathogenic *E. coli,* which frequently cause childhood diarrhea in developing countries. Type IV pili are known as bundle-forming pili (BFP) and are critical to the full virulence of these bacteria (28). Mutants without these pili could not attach to epithelial cells *in vitro,* and were relatively benign when fed to human volunteers. These pili facilitate bacterial bundling into ropelike filaments that attach to epithelial cells; subsequently the clumped bacteria disperse to cause infection (28).

The role of adhesins in the pathogenesis of infection caused by other Enterobacteriaceae is not well characterized. Types 1, 3, and 6 fimbriae have been found in *Klebsiella,* but their function as virulence factors remains largely unknown (22,58). The majority of respiratory isolates of *K. pneumoniae* and *K. oxytoca* from ICU patients with presumed nosocomial pneumonia have been shown to express type 3 fimbriae and a mannose-resistant, *Klebsiella*-like (MR-K) hemagglutinin (49). Multidrug-resistant *K. pneumoniae* strains from a variety of nosocomial infections have been found to colonize the human intestinal tract through a plasmid-encoded 29,000-dalton surface protein (22) that facilitates adherence to gastrointestinal epithelium. Type 3 fimbriae also are commonly found in *Klebsiella* isolates associated with human UTIs (22). An MR-K fimbria has been isolated in *Providencia stuartii* and appears to be related to adherence to genitourinary catheters (23). Cell adhesins that allow attachment to exfoliated uroepithelium (24–26) have been found in *Proteus* spp. as well. Nonfimbrial adhesive factors also are being characterized in the Enterobacteriaceae (29,30). An R-plasmid encoded nonfimbrial adhesive factor has been isolated from strains of *K. pneumoniae* responsible for a variety of nosocomial infections (29).

Capsules

The bacterial capsule, which is well characterized for *Klebsiella* spp. and *E. coli,* and *Salmonella typhi* can partly protect the microorganisms against the bactericidal effect of serum and against phagocytosis (29,36,59). However, most of the Enterobacteriaceae do not possess a substantial bacterial capsule and do not have serum resistance. In a prospective observational study from six United States university teaching hospitals evaluating the incidence and risk factors for the development of endocarditis in bacteremic patients with prosthetic cardiac valves, a significant proportion of cases of new endocarditis were due to gram-negative aerobic bacilli, often when a portal of entry was found (60). This study suggests that the previous hypothesis that endocarditis was unlikely in the presence of gram-negative bacteremia, presumably because gram-negative bacilli are serum-susceptible or if a portal of entry is identified, may not be correct.

A capsule, when present, can also directly suppress the host immune response (35). In invasive *E. coli* disease in children, K1 and K5 capsules are found most commonly (56). It has been suggested that these capsules are more virulent, because they are structurally similar to human antigens, and therefore may be spared by or elude specific host defense mechanisms. The size of the capsule and the rate of capsule polysaccharide production appear to influence bacterial virulence (35).

Iron Chelators

The ability of some gram-negative bacteria to acquire iron for growth becomes an important factor in many gram-negative infections. Almost all the iron in the human body is bound to various proteins such as hemoglobin, myoglobin, and transferrin, thereby limiting the availability of free iron for utilization by bacteria. Some Enterobacteriaceae contain low molecular weight, high-affinity iron chelators called siderophores. The chelator permits the bacteria to scavenge iron from the host for growth purposes.

Aerobactin is an iron-chelating bacterial siderophore associated with increased virulence in *E. coli* (38) and *Klebsiella* (39, 58). In Enterobacteriaceae, the catechol enterobactin is the most commonly occurring iron-chelating siderophore but does not appear to be associated with increased bacterial virulence (39, 61) possibly because enterobactin is more antigenic than aerobactin and causes a strong antibody response in the host that diminishes enterobactin's ability to take up iron (61).

Yersinia enterocolitica 1B, *Y. pseudotuberculosis,* and *Y. pestis* have been found to contain chromosomal gene sets designated high-pathogenicity islands (HPIs) that are involved in the synthesis, transport, and regulation of the siderophore yersiniabactin. This HPI has also been found in other genera including *E. coli, Klebsiella, Citrobacter,* and Enterobacter (62–64). *Y. enterocolitica* has increased virulence in patients receiving desferrioxamine therapy, presumably because *Yersinia* can use desferrioxamine to meet some of its growth requirements more effectively in these patients (65,66).

Another method by which bacteria may acquire iron is hemolysis. Hemolysins are cytotoxic proteins encoded by chromosomal or plasmid genes. The chromosomal localization seems to be predominant for *E. coli* causing extraintestinal infections, whereas hemolysins are usually carried on plasmid genes in *E. coli* strains from veterinary sources. Hemolysins are cytotoxic for erythrocytes, and *in vitro* for polymorphonuclear leukocytes, monocytes, and isolated renal tubular cells. These proteins contribute to virulence in intraperitoneal infection models, but their role in ascending UTIs is uncertain. Hemolysin production is frequent in pyelonephritic clones of *E. coli*, but does not enhance bacterial persistence in kidneys and bladders (48,56).

Other Pathogen Factors and Tropisms

Other virulence factors, such as bacterial motility (67); the ability to grow in alkaline pH; the ability to colonize skin (especially hands) of healthcare workers; the ability to produce urease, which catalyzes hydrolysis of urea in the urine and increases urinary pH (68); and the ability to produce biofilms (69) contribute to the ability of various members of the Enterobacteriaceae to produce disease. Enterobacteriaceae liberate numerous toxins, endotoxin being one of the most lethal, that contribute to bacterial virulence (Table 33.5). The role of endotoxins in nosocomial infection is no different from their role in community-acquired infection. Finally, some virulence factors have been associated with worsened patient outcome, although precise mechanisms of tissue injury are unknown. For example, a minor outer membrane protein (molecular weight of 32,000) is found more often in strains of *Citrobacter diversus* causing neonatal meningitis and abscess than in strains of *C. diversus* from other body sites (42). Evidence from an infant rat model suggests that strains of *C. diversus* with this outer membrane protein can produce more extensive histopathologic changes within the brain (33).

Infection by several species of Enterobacteriaceae have been associated with specific devices, materials, and/or procedures because of increased device affinity or specific tropisms. For example, *P. mirabilis* is a urease-producing bacteria that has been associated with bacteriuria and obstructed urinary catheters in patients with long-term indwelling bladder catheters (41). Urease catalyzes the hydrolysis of urea in the urine, thus alkalinizing it; this permits the formation of struvite and carbonate-apatite stones or sludge or concretions within the catheter lumen, leading to catheter obstruction. Other members of the Enterobacteriaceae family, including *Morganella morganii, K. pneumoniae, Proteus vulgaris,* and *P. stuartii,* also produce urease. Although no association between bacteriuria and catheter obstruction has been demonstrated for these microorganisms (41), some, such as *P. stuartii,* are very commonly associated with long-term urinary catheterization. An MR-K hemagglutinin has been identified in *P. stuartii* that increases adherence to catheter material (23).

The cell-surface characteristics of *K. pneumoniae* may also play a role in increased adherence to ventriculoperitoneal shunts. For example, when a multiresistant strain of *K. pneumoniae* was compared to its spontaneous *in vitro* antibiotic-susceptible derivative, the derivative was more adherent to the surface of ventriculoperitoneal catheters (30). Genetic studies suggested that the absence of a plasmid-mediated outer membrane protein led to increased adherence to the ventriculoperitoneal shunt surface.

Enterobacter sakazakii has been associated with several neonatal outbreaks and sporadic cases of sepsis, meningitis, and diarrhea (70–74). No environmental source for *E. sakazakii* has been identified (74). Most outbreaks have been associated with either intrinsic or extrinsic contamination of powdered milk substitute. *E. sakazakii* has been isolated from powdered infant formula produced in 13 different countries by multiple manufacturers (72), suggesting that this microorganism has the propensity to contaminate such products. *In vitro* studies show that *E. sakazakii* survives better than *E. cloacae* in infant formula (70).

Y. enterocolitica has been associated with several series of blood transfusion–related sepsis (75,76). Apparently, blood donors with asymptomatic gastrointestinal infection with *Y. enterocolitica* and transient bacteremia at the time of blood donation are the most common source of such cases (77). The environment of cold stored red blood cells favors the growth of *Y. enterocolitica* more than the growth of other, more likely contaminants (e.g., skin flora from donors) since *Y. enterocolitica* survives better than most bacteria at refrigeration temperatures. In addition, progressive hemolysis of stored blood may provide an ongoing supply of iron for *Yersinia's* growth. Virulent strains of *Yersinia* can also grow in calcium-free media such as that produced by citrate chelation of red blood cells for storage. Serotype 0:3 has accounted for the majority of cases of transfusion-related *Yersinia* sepsis. This serotype shows a persistent resistance to the bactericidal effect of serum at cold temperatures and has a growth-response curve that is directly related to the iron content of the culture medium (78).

Enterobacter spp. and *Citrobacter* spp. thrive in aqueous environments and may cause nosocomial bacteremia by their ability to grow in infusion fluids (79). *Enterobacter* spp. can fix nitrogen, allowing for replication in nitrogen-deficient fluids, and has been shown to have more rapid replication than *E. coli, Klebsiella, Pseudomonas,* or *Proteus* (80) in dextrose-containing solutions.

Examples of Genetics of Some Virulence Factors

R-plasmids, commonly found in Enterobacteriaceae, are also associated with bacterial virulence. They carry genes encoding virulence factors, such as adhesive factors (29), enterotoxins, and hemolysins (81). Plasmids code for outer membrane proteins for various Enterobacteriaceae. In *Y. enterocolitica,* a 70-kb plasmid codes proteins of the outer membrane that are associated with resistance to complement-mediated opsonization, to neutrophil phagocytosis, and to bactericidal activity of human serum (37). Similar plasmids have been isolated in *Y. pseudotuberculosis* and *Y. pestis.* Two soluble plasmid-mediated antigens, V and W, have been isolated from virulent strains of *Y. pestis, Y. pseudotuberculosis,* and *Y. enterocolitica* (37). Because plasmids are also important determinants of antimicrobial resistance, they may allow pathogens to link drug resistance and virulence determinants, which may be transferred together to other species.

Examples of Development of Antibiotic Resistance

In January 1999 the hospital-wide component of NNIS was eliminated; NNIS data from 1998–2002 focus on antimicrobial resistance and pooled mean rates in the ICU compared to non-ICU inpatient areas (Table 33.6) (4).

The increasing prevalence of antibiotic-resistant Enterobacteriaceae has contributed to the difficulty in treating nosocomial infections. Antibiotic resistance often is related to excessive or widespread use of a particular antibiotic (82). For example, aminoglycoside and cephalosporin resistance in *Klebsiella* has been correlated with exposure to and intensity of use of these drugs

TABLE 33.6. POOLED MEANS OF NOSOCOMIAL ANTIMICROBIAL RESISTANCE RATES[a] FOR SELECTED ENTEROBACTERIACEAE AND OTHER PATHOGENS BY ALL ICUS COMBINED AND NON-ICU INPATIENT AREAS, ICARE/AUR, JANUARY 1998 TO JUNE 2002

	ICUs		Non-ICUs	
Antimicrobial-Resistant Pathogens	No. Tested	Pooled Mean	No. Tested	Pooled Mean
Selected Enterobacteriaceae				
Cef3-resistant *Enterobacter* spp.	4,061	26.3	5,534	19.8
Cef3-resistant *Klebsiella pneumoniae*	6,101	6.1	10,733	5.7
Quinolone-resistant *Escherichia coli*	9,696	5.8	30,557	5.3
Cef3-resistant *Escherichia coli*	9,891	1.2	30,585	1.1
Carbapenem-resistant *Enterobacter* spp.	3,477	0.8	4,180	1.1
Other pathogens				
Methicillin-resistant coagulase-negative staphylococci	11,262	75.7	18,191	64.0
MRSA	18,397	51.3	30,850	41.4
Levofloxacin-resistant *P. aeruginosa*	3,921	37.8	6,084	28.9
Ciprofloxacin/ofloxacin-resistant *P. aeruginosa*	11,232	36.3	16,824	27.0
Imipenem-resistant *P. aeruginosa*	9,850	19.6	13,037	12.7
Piperacillin-resistant *P. aeruginosa*	9,553	17.5	12,977	11.5
Ceftazidime-resistant *P. aeruginosa*	10,538	13.9	15,149	8.3
Vancomycin-resistant *Enterococcus* spp.	11,623	12.8	24,491	12.0

Cef3, ceftazidime, cefotaxime, or ceftriaxone; quinolone, ciprofloxacin, ofloxacin, or levofloxacin; carbapenem, imipenem or meropenem; MRSA, methicillin-resistant *Staphylococcus aureus*.

[a] For each antimicrobial agent and pathogen combination, resistance rates were calculated as follows: Number of resistant isolates/Number of isolates tested × 100.

Adapted from National Nosocomial Infections Surveillance (NNIS) System Report, data summary from January 1992 to June 2002, Issued August 2002. *Am J Infect Control* 2002;30:458–475.

(83,84). Mechanisms of antibiotic resistance in the Enterobacteriaceae include enzyme production that can inactivate or modify the drug (e.g., β-lactamase production), diminished permeability of antibiotics, and altered antibiotic target sites. Bacteria may acquire these mechanisms of resistance spontaneously via chromosomal mutation or via transfer of plasmids or transposable genetic elements from other bacteria (85). Genes that determine resistance to different classes of antibiotics may occur on a single plasmid so that use of one antimicrobial can lead to resistance to other classes of antibiotics.

Common mechanisms of β-lactam antibiotic resistance include chromosomal mutation, which is frequent and offers a bacterial survival advantage during antibiotic therapy. This is the mechanism of resistance found in Enterobacteriaceae, such as *Enterobacter, Serratia,* indole-positive *Proteus,* and *Citrobacter,* that carry chromosomal genes that encode a type 1 β-lactamase (85,86). These bacteria can undergo single-step mutations to constitutive high-level β-lactamase production. Thus, initially susceptible strains of *Enterobacter* and other Enterobacteriaceae may develop spontaneous resistant mutants to broad-spectrum cephalosporins during 20% to 50% of courses of therapy (87).

Plasmid-mediated β-lactamases also are present in the Enterobacteriaceae. Enterobacteriaceae have responded to the widespread use of β-lactam antibiotics with inactivation of these drugs by β-lactamases (such as TEM-1, TEM-2 and SHV-1 β-lactamases), which are typically plasmid encoded (85). These resistances were overcome by the development of second- and third-generation cephalosporins and combinations of β-lactam antibiotics with β-lactamase inhibitors. However, in 1982 the first Enterobacteriaceae with resistance to broad-spectrum cephalosporins, such as cefuroxime, cefotaxime, and ceftazidime, were isolated in Europe (88,89). These extended-spectrum β-lactamases (ESBLs) arose by point mutations, probably under pressure of widespread use of antibiotics. ESBLs differ in only one or a few amino acids from the original TEM-1, TEM-2, and SHV-1 β-lactamases and are also plasmid mediated (85). By now, more than 150 different ESBLs have been described (90–92). Although the first ESBLs were reported from Europe, they have spread to most continents during the last decade (93). In the U.S., resistance rates of *K. pneumoniae* to ceftazidime in ICUs rose from 3.6% in 1990 to 14.4% in 1993 (94). NNIS data from January to December 1999 compared with 1994 to 1998 suggest that rates of *K. pneumoniae* resistance to third-generation cephalosporins have stabilized or declined to 10% (NNIS Selected Antimicrobial Resistant Pathogens at *www.cdc.gov/ncidid/hip/NNIS/ar_surv99.htm*) (95). This decline may be due to pharmacy restriction of third-generation cephalosporins or a shift to more frequent use of fluoroquinolones rather than ceftazidime. Hospital outbreaks with ceftazidime-resistant *E. coli* and *K. pneumoniae* have been frequent (96–98). These strains that produce β-lactamases with an extended spectrum of resistance may remain susceptible to the cephamycins and have variable resistance to combination therapy with a β-lactamase inhibitor such as clavulanic acid or sulbactam.

Spread of resistant strains in institutions may be extensive. Approximately 40% of *Enterobacter* spp. from one study of U.S. ICUs were resistant to extended-spectrum cephalosporins (99). In another study, 60% of patients had acquired their resistant pathogens before hospital admission; the majority of these patients (82%) came from nursing homes (96). Patients from large skilled-care nursing homes have been shown to harbor multiply resistant gram-negative bacilli significantly more often than patients from small nursing homes. In one outbreak of ceftazidime-resistant Enterobacteriaceae (primarily *Klebsiella*) in a chronic care facility, resistant isolates continued to be recovered 7 months after empiric use of ceftazidime was discontinued (98).

Spread of multidrug-resistant *E. coli* clonal group A (CGA), was described initially in London, England, in 1986 (100) and has now been reported in cohorts of women with UTIs in California, Minnesota, and Michigan. This CGA *E. coli* accounted for almost 50% of community acquired UTIs that were resistant to trimethoprim-sulfamethoxazole (101). This clone also has been associated with the development of pyelonephritis (102) and anecdotally in a renal transplant patient from Buffalo, New York, with pneumonia and bacteremia who had taken trimethoprim-sulfamethoxazole prophylactic therapy (103).

A surveillance study of 35,790 isolates (more than 50% of which were respiratory) from U.S. ICUs in 43 states and the District of Columbia demonstrated decreasing susceptibility of gram-negative bacilli (including *Enterobacter* spp. and *Klebsiella*) to ciprofloxacin from 86% in 1994 to 76% in 2000 (104). This decline coincided with increased national use of fluoroquinolones measured by sales of pharmaceuticals to retail stores and healthcare facilities. Resistance to ciprofloxacin was associated with cross-resistance to other classes of broad-spectrum antimicrobial agents, including aminoglycosides, carbapenems, and third-generation cephalosporins (104).

Chapters 90 and 91 discuss antibiotic resistance in more detail.

Host Factors

Host factors are important in controlling the extent of colonization with Enterobacteriaceae, as discussed below. Host factors are also important in determining the susceptibility of the host to developing disease. Bacterial virulence factors tend to be associated with disease in patients with normal immunity, whereas bacteria without these virulence factors often can only cause disease in patients with diminished immunity (e.g., the very young and very old), in patients with abnormal anatomy (e.g., hydronephrosis), or in patients whose mucosal barriers are breached by invasive devices. Site-specific infections and host factors are discussed briefly here and in the site-specific chapters.

EPIDEMIOLOGY OF NOSOCOMIAL INFECTIONS CAUSED BY ENTEROBACTERIACEAE

Reservoirs/Sources

The primary reservoirs for the Enterobacteriaceae are water, soil, and the human gastrointestinal tract (5). Oropharyngeal and gastrointestinal colonization of hospital patients is common. Intestinal carriage of Enterobacteriaceae is associated with increased risk of infection. For example, the gastrointestinal tract is an important reservoir in outbreaks of nosocomial *K. pneumoniae* UTIs. A prospective study examining the role of intestinal colonization with multiply resistant *K. pneumoniae* demonstrated that 14 of 31 patients who became intestinal carriers of *K. pneumoniae* developed clinical infections with the same serotype, whereas only 11 of 101 patients who were not intestinal carriers developed clinical disease (105).

In outbreaks of multidrug-resistant *P. mirabilis*, gastrointestinal carriage of the epidemic strain by susceptible patients has been shown to be an important reservoir for outbreak development and propagation (106). In one study, approximately 75% of patients with nosocomial *Proteus* infections were intestinal carriers of the microorganism (107). In contrast, the major reservoir of *Providencia rettgeri* has been the urinary tract (108), and in one study of 2,693 fecal isolates tested, no *P. stuartii* microorganisms were isolated (109).

Many of the members of the family Enterobacteriaceae have a propensity for certain environments and reservoirs. *Serratia* thrives in moist environments. It frequently contaminates solutions and hospital equipment (110,111). Its human reservoirs are the urinary and respiratory tracts, primarily in patients subjected to devices such as indwelling bladder catheters (110) or endotracheal tubes (112). The gastrointestinal tract may be the primary reservoir in infants and children but is an uncommon reservoir of *Serratia* in adults.

Enterobacter spp. thrive in moist environments and have been found contaminating the environment (113), distilled water and humidifiers (114), and infusion fluids (115,116). *Enterobacter* also may be found in low numbers in the intestinal flora of 40% to 80% of healthy outpatients (117). Multiple studies have shown increased rates of rectal colonization by *Enterobacter* after patient use of cephalosporin antibiotics (117–119). *E. cloacae* is found more frequently than *E. aerogenes* and more often leads to clinical disease (117).

Citrobacter freundii is the most prevalent *Citrobacter* microorganism found in stool and is an occasional cause of gastrointestinal disease (gallbladder, peritonitis) (120,121).

Factors Controlling Colonization

A number of studies have shown that the patient's endogenous oropharyngeal flora is a common source of Enterobacteriaceae that cause infection in the hospitalized patient (122–124). Oropharyngeal colonization with these bacteria is uncommon in healthy subjects, but increases with severity of underlying diseases or the presence of other risk factors for infection (125). Many patients are colonized with potentially pathogenic Enterobacteriaceae before admission to the hospital (126–128). These bacteria may increase in colony counts under selective pressures of antibiotic use in the ICU (126,129) or with increased duration of hospitalization (130,131).

Oropharyngeal colonization with gram-negative bacteria is an important risk factor for the development of nosocomial pneumonia. In the early 1970s, 23% of patients with oropharyngeal colonization developed nosocomial pneumonia as compared to only 3% of the patients without colonization (132). Similar findings were reported 25 years later; in multivariate risk factor analysis, oropharyngeal colonization with Enterobacteriaceae was the most important risk factor for the development of ventilator-associated pneumonia (130), and the risk of gram-negative pneumonia was estimated to be approximately eight times greater in patients with gram-negative bacillary oropharyngeal colonization (125).

In contrast to oropharyngeal colonization, intestinal colonization with Enterobacteriaceae is universal in healthy subjects and hospitalized patients. However, intestinal colonization with resistant *E. coli* strains has been shown to increase with length of hospital stay. Approximately 30% to 40% of patients admitted to the hospital become colonized with hospital flora, including antibiotic-resistant Enterobacteriaceae, within 48 hours of admission. This rate of colonization increases in critically ill patients (125).

Gastric pH

The stomach is usually not colonized with gram-negative bacteria. However, in critically ill patients gastric colonization frequently occurs and its incidence increases with time. Among mechanically ventilated patients, gastric colonization with gram-negative bacteria was found in 25% on admission to the ICU, and another 40% acquired colonization during the ICU stay (133). In ICU patients receiving enteral feeding, 20% to 40% of the patients had gastric colonization when enteral feeding was started, and this proportion increased to 80% after 1 week (134). Gastric colonization with gram-negative bacteria has been assumed to be an important risk factor for the development of ventilator-associated pneumonia (VAP). According to the hypothesis of the gastropulmonary route of infection, bacteria colonizing the stomach will subsequently colonize the oropharynx and be aspirated into the lower respiratory tract (135,136). The relevance of the gastropulmonary hypothesis has been debated recently, since several studies failed to show an important role of gastric colonization in the pathogenesis of VAP (137,138). The concept of the gastropulmonary route of infection was addressed in a double-blind randomized trial on oropharyngeal decontamination. Eradication of oropharyngeal colonization in mechanically ventilated patients without disturbing gastric and intestinal flora was associated with a 63% relative risk reduction of VAP (139).

The role of patients' gastric pH has been studied extensively in relation to the pathogenesis and epidemiology of gastric colonization and nosocomial pneumonia. The stomach is normally sterile, and colonization with gram-negative bacilli correlates with increase of gastric pH above 4 (140). Gastric colonization with Enterobacteriaceae was demonstrated in 30% of the patients with median intragastric pH <4 and in 56% when intragastric pH was >4 (133). Host factors such as increased age, malnutrition, achlorhydria, and abnormally slow gastric peristalsis and gastroduodenal reflux have been associated with gastric colonization (141,142). In addition, treatment with antacids and histamine type 2 receptor blockers has been associated with increased intragastric pH levels and increased risk of gastric colonization with gram-negative bacilli (141). Based on these findings, sucralfate has been advocated as an alternative for stress ulcer prophylaxis. In contrast to antacids and histamine type 2 blockers, sucralfate offers protection against stress ulcers without influencing intragastric acidity. The net result should be that patients receiving sucralfate should have lower intragastric pH levels, lower gastric colonization rates, and lower incidences of nosocomial pneumonia. Fourteen studies addressed this issue, and protective effects of sucralfate on the incidence of VAP were found in 5 (137). Only three studies used a double-blind study design, and all three failed to show benefits from the use of sucralfate on the incidence of VAP (133,143,144). In one study, intragastric acidity was monitored continuously with a computerized intragastric pH measuring instrument, and gastric pH levels were similar in patients receiving high dosages of antacids or sucralfate. Median pH values were >4 in both groups, demonstrating that critically ill patients have elevated pH levels even without antacids or histamine type 2 blockers (133). In another study, sucralfate proved to be inferior to histamine type 2 blockers with regard to protection against gastric bleeding (143). Administration of acidified enteral feeding (pH = 3.5) was associated with substantially decreased colonization rates with gram-negative bacteria in the stomach but not in the respiratory tract (145). Intragastric acidity, therefore, influences gastric colonization, but whether this influences respiratory tract colonization and infection remains uncertain.

Fibronectin

In normal hosts, fibronectin, a glycoprotein, is present on oral epithelial cells and facilitates adherence of gram-positive bacteria. It has been observed that loss of fibronectin uncovers cellular binding sites and leads to increased rates of oropharyngeal colonization by gram-negative bacilli. One hypothesis to explain the loss of fibronectin is that salivary protease secretion, which degrades fibronectin, is increased in critically ill patients (146,147).

Hormonal Modulation of Colonization

Very little is known about the relationship between hormones and colonization. It has been observed that recurrent UTIs occur in many postmenopausal women. Investigators have hypothesized that lack of estrogen leads to diminished colonization of the vagina by lactobacilli. Normally, lactobacilli adhere to uroepithelial cells and have been shown to exclude the adherence of *E. coli, K. pneumoniae,* and *P. aeruginosa* (148). The absence of lactobacilli appears to result in increased vaginal pH (>4) and increased rates of colonization by Enterobacteriaceae, especially *E. coli.* In one study intravaginal estriol administration resulted in increased colonization by lactobacilli, decreased vaginal pH, decreased Enterobacteriaceae colonization, and significantly reduced incidence of recurrent UTI in postmenopausal women (149).

Biliary Tract and Urinary Tract Obstruction

Colonization and stasis facilitate the development of acute cholangitis and UTI. Wang et al. (50) examined the role of *E. coli* virulence factors and host factors in patients with *E. coli* bacteremia who met clinical and radiographic criteria for acute cholangitis or upper UTI. The authors found that obstruction was an important host factor leading to bacteremia (100% of those with acute cholangitis and bacteremia were obstructed; 31% of those with upper UTI were obstructed). The most common causes of biliary obstruction included choledocholithiasis, cholangiocarcinoma, ampullary carcinoma, and pancreatic head tumor and the causes of urinary tract obstruction included nephrolithiasis, ureteral tumor, neurogenic bladder, benign prostatic hypertrophy, and uterine tumor.

Neutrophil Elastase

Neutrophil elastase (NE) is the first neutrophil factor that targets bacterial virulence proteins. In neutrophils with inactivated NE, *Shigella* escapes from phagosomes, increasing bacterial survival. NE cleaves virulence factors in *Shigella, Salmonella,* and *Yersinia* (150).

Modes of Transmission and Outbreaks of Enterobacteriaceae

Enterobacteriaceae are primarily spread in the hospital from person to person via the hands of hospital personnel or from environmental reservoirs to patients (Fig. 33.1). These modes of transmission have been documented in multiple outbreaks of nosocomial UTIs due to *Klebsiella, P. rettgeri,* and *Serratia,* as well as in multiple neonatal ICU (NICU) outbreaks due to the Enterobacteriaceae. The majority of studies commonly cited in discussions of the epidemiology of nosocomial infections caused by the Enterobacteriaceae are analyses of common source (Table 33.7) or person-to-person (Table 33.8) outbreaks. Thus, much of the data characterizing the epidemiology of Enterobacteriaceae are derived from retrospective studies of epidemic strains.

Many nosocomial outbreaks caused by Enterobacteriaceae that produce ESBLs have been reported (97,98,196–208), and several examples with documented infection control measures and their effects are listed in Table 33.9. Most outbreaks occurred in special care wards such as ICUs and oncology wards; *K. pneumoniae* was involved in almost all outbreaks; and extensive use of third-generation cephalosporins, mostly as monotherapy, frequently was a risk factor (97,98,198,205). Some outbreaks were caused by the spread of a single ESBL gene among multiple genotypes of Enterobacteriaceae (97,200,205), although horizontal spread of bacteria with ESBLs has been described as well (199,203). As with methicillin-resistant *Staphylococcus aureus* (MRSA) and vancomycin-resistant enterococci (VRE), environmental contamination may contribute to the epidemiology of Enterobacteriaceae containing ESBLs (203,206). Situations of endemicity of colonization with ESBL-producing Enterobacteriaceae have been reported (210–213). For example, in Chicago, ceftazidime resistance due to TEM-10 is now endemic among multiple strains of *K. pneumoniae* and *E. coli*; the prevalence of these strains was especially high in nursing home patients (210). In addition, ESBL-producing Enterobacteriaceae were already endemic in a French ICU in 1990; the risk for patients to acquire these bacteria was 4.2% in the first week in the ICU and increased to 24% in the fourth week, and most cases of colonization were caused by the same strain type (211).

TYPES OF NOSOCOMIAL INFECTIONS CAUSED BY ENTEROBACTERIACEAE

Urinary Tract

UTIs are the most common hospital-acquired infection in the U.S. Approximately 50% of the pathogens associated with nosocomial UTIs are members of the family Enterobacteriaceae. *E. coli* is the leading pathogen, implicated in 24% of all nosocomial UTIs (NNIS data, 1990–1996) (5). *K. pneumoniae* is the fifth leading cause of nosocomial UTIs and is recovered from 8% of cases. *Enterobacter* spp. and *P. mirabilis* are ranked sixth, and are recovered from 5% of cases (Table 33.10). The European Study Group on Nosocomial Infections published a point-prevalence study conducted in 1999 in 228 hospitals in 29 European countries. *E. coli* was the most commonly isolated microorganism (35.6%) followed by enterococci (15.8%), *Candida* sp. (9.4%), *Klebsiella* sp. (8.3%), *Proteus* sp. (7.9%), and *P. aeruginosa* (6.9%) (17).

Risk factors for hospital-acquired UTIs usually are host and device related rather than pathogen related, with the presence of a urinary catheter being most important. The catheter predisposes to UTIs in several ways. It offers a possibility for bacteria to enter the bladder along external or internal surfaces of the catheter and for development of a biofilm that can protect bacteria from antibiotics and host defenses; adhesion to mucosal surfaces will be facilitated; the catheter may blunt adequate antibac-

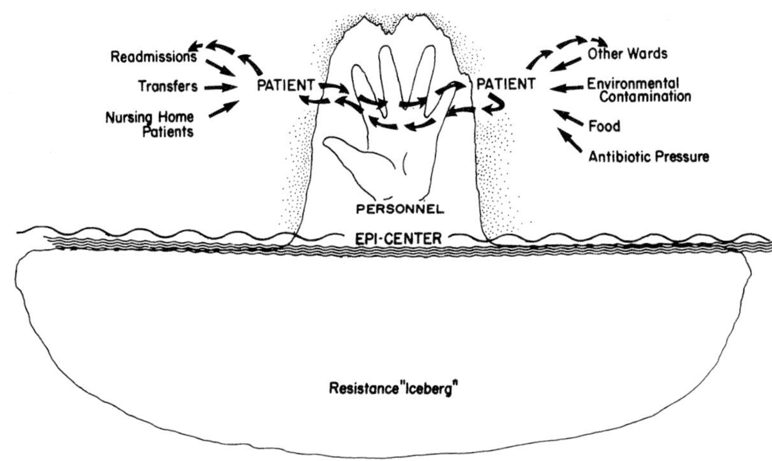

Figure 33.1. Infection control "iceberg," depicting the epidemiology of infections in hospitals, emphasizing the often unrecognizable colonization of patients with antibiotic-resistant Enterobacteriaceae and other potential pathogens (e.g., other gram-negative bacilli, methicillin-resistant *Staphylococcus aureus,* vancomycin-resistant enterococci). (From Weinstein RA, Kabins SA. Strategies for prevention and control of multiple drug resistant nosocomial infection. *Am J Med* 1981;70:449–454, with permission.)

TABLE 33.7. EXAMPLES OF COMMON-SOURCE OUTBREAKS DUE TO ENTEROBACTERIACEAE

Species (Ref.)	Sites	Number of Cases (Attack Rate per 100 Discharges)	Source	Risk Factors	Antibiotic Resistance
P. rettgeri, *P. stuartii* (152)	Urine	48	Urinary leg bag	Chronic indwelling urinary catheter	Gentamicin
P. stuartii (153)	Urine, blood	4	Urinals, patients with condom catheters	NA	Sensitive to amikacin, carbenicillin, cefoxitin only
S. liquifaciens (154)	Blood	12	Pooled epoetin alpha	Hemodialysis	NA
S. marcescens (155)	No clinical infection	30 (colonized)	Breast pump	Infants receiving pumped human milk	NA
S. marcescens (156)	Eye	3	Eye dropper	Keratoplasty	NA
S. marcescens (157)	Urine	32	Urometers and urine-measuring containers	Exposure to ICU Indwelling urinary catheter Antibiotics Exposure to urine measuring devices	Sensitive to nalidixic acid and/or amikacin only
S. marcescens (158)	Blood	6	Mean arterial pressure monitor	ICU hospitalization with arterial line	NA
S. marcescens (159)	Blood, wound	6	Quatenary ammonium disinfectant	Use of cardiopulmonary bypass with extracorporeal circulation	NA
S. marcescens (160)	Blood	7	Pressure transducer	Use of intraarterial balloon pump and pulmonary artery pressure measurement	NA
S. marcescens (161)	Blood	21	Dialyzer	Hemodialysis	Ampicillin, tetracycline
S. marcescens (162)	Knee/shoulder joints	10	Aqueous benzalkonium chloride	Joint infection in same physician	NA
S. marcescens (163)	Lung, wound, blood, urine	14	Reusable 12-lead electrocardiogram bulb	Open heart surgery Severity of underlying disease	NA
S. marcescens (164)	Wound	4	Extrinsically contaminated saline solution	Volume of saline injected into mammary implant	Ampicillin, cefazolin
S. marcescens (165)	Urine	10	Urinary tract of asymptomatic catheterized patients	Increased length of hospital stay, >3 UTIs in previous 6 months	Ampicillin, cephalothin, cefoxitin, gentamicin, tobramycin, ticarcillin, nitrofurantoin
S. marcescens (116)	Lung, blood, CSF, urine	6	Graduated cylinder to measure urine output	NA	Gentamicin, tobramycin
E. sakazakii (70)	Blood, stool, urine	4	Powdered infant formula	Receiving implicated formula	NA
C. freundii (166)	Blood	3	Intrinsically contaminated 5% dextrose in lactated Ringer's solution	Receiving intravenous fluid	NA
E. agglomerans, *E. cloacae*, (167)	Blood	378	Elastomer disk within screw cap of intravenous fluid bottle	Receiving intravenous fluid manufactured by one company	*E. cloacae*—ampicillin, cephalothin *E. agglomerans*—nitrofurantoin
E. cloacae (114)	Blood	4	Distilled water containers, (respiratory) humidifiers	NA	Gentamicin, tobramycin, kanamycin, piperacillin, chloramphenicol
E. cloacae (168)	Blood	15	Hydrotherapy water (bum unit)	Extent of burn, severity of underlying diseases	Streptomycin, chloramphenicol carbenicillin, ampicillin, cephalothin
S. typhimurium (169)	Stool	18	Eggs	Consumed fresh egg nog	NA
S. typhimurium (170)	Stool	7	Fiberoptic endoscope	Upper endoscopy	NA
S. enteritidis (171)	Blood, stool	4	Refrigerator and sink in hemodialysis unit	Hemodialysis	NA
S. enteritidis (172) (serotype drypool)	Stool	11	Luncheon food	NA	NA
S. enteritidis (173) (serotype drypool)	Stool	404	Eggs	Eating hospital-prepared mayonnaise	NA
S. emsobuettal (174)	Stool	25	Rectal thermometer	Newborn infants receiving rectal thermometers, mothers, staff	NA
S. worthington (175)	CSF, stool, blood	18	Rubber tubing of oropharyngeal suctioning apparatus	Oropharyngeal suctioning in NICU	

CSF, cerebrospinal fluid; ICU, intensive care unit; NA, not available.

TABLE 33.8. EXAMPLES OF PERSON-TO-PERSON OUTBREAKS DUE TO ENTEROBACTERIACEAE

Species (Ref.)	Sites	Number of Cases (Attack Rate per 100 Discharges)	Risk Factors	Antibiotic Resistance
K. pneumoniae (176)	Urine	(2.5)	Urinary catheterization, broad-spectrum antibiotics, bladder irrigation	NA
K. pneumoniae (176)	Urine	(2.9)	Urinary catheterization, bladder irrigation, broad-spectrum antibiotics	NA
K. pneumoniae (176)	Urine	(1.4)	Urinary catheterization, bladder irrigation, broad-spectrum antibiotics	NA
K. pneumoniae (177)	Urine, wound, lung	60	Urinary catheterization, bladder irrigation, broad-spectrum antibiotics	Gentamicin, tobramycin, kanamycin, cephalothin, chloramphenicol, ampicillin
K. pneumoniae (178)	Blood	6	Presence in premature nursery	Kanamycin, ampicillin, sulfisoxazole
K. pneumoniae (179)	Urine, blood, wound, abdomen, lungs	24	Bag resuscitation, oropharyngeal suction, nasogastric feeding tubes	Gentamicin
K. pneumoniae (180)	Blood	10	Infants in NICU	Kanamycin
P. mirabilis (181)	Wound, urine, lungs, blood	15	Number of operations, proximity to another case	Ampicillin, cephalothin, gentamicin, carbenicillin, colistin, trimethoprim, sulfisoxazole
P. mirabilis (182)	Blood, wound, CSF, bone	11	Umbilical cord manipulation by nurse carrier	NA
M. morganii (183)	Blood, wound, urine	11	NK	Ampicillin, cephalothin, colistin
S. marcescens (176)	Urine	NA	Urinary catheter, broad-spectrum antibiotics	NA
S. marcescens (176)	Urine	(1.75)	Urinary catheter, broad-spectrum antibiotics	NA
C. diversus (184)	Blood, CSF	2	Infants in NICU	Ampicillin, carbenicillin
C. diversus (185)	Blood, CSF	3	Infants in NICU	NA
C. diversus (186)	CSF	5	NICU care, gavage feeding, prenatal intrauterine monitoring	Ampicillin, kanamycin, carbenicillin
E. coli (187) (enterotoxigenic)	CSF	3	NK	NA
E. coli (188)	Stool	18	Oral formula	Ampicillin, carbenicillin, kamaycin, chloramphenicol
Y. enterocolitica (189)	Stool	6	NK	NA
Y. enterocolitica (190)	Stool	9	NK	NA
S. indiana (191)	Stool	46	NK	Ampicillin
S. typhimurium (192)	Stool	488	Current or prior antibiotics	Ampicillin, carbenicillin, cefamandole, cefuroxime, sulfamethoxazole, chloramphenicol, trimethoprim
S. typhimurium (116)	Stool	14	Contact with culture-positive patient	NA
P. rettgeri (176)	Urine	(3.2)	Broad-spectrum antibiotics, urinary catheter, genitourinary instrumentation	NA
P. rettgeri (176)	Urine	(4.4)	Broad-spectrum antibiotics, urinary catheter, genitourinary instrumentation	NA
P. rettgeri (193)	Urine	11	Broad-spectrum antibiotics, urinary catheter	Ampicillin, carbenicillin, cephalothin, gentamicin, kanamycin, chloramphenicol, sulfonamide, nalidixic acid, nitrofurantoin
P. rettgeri (194)	Urine	10	Broad-spectrum antibiotics, urinary catheter, genitourinary instrumentation	Ampicillin, carbenicillin, tetracycline, chloramphenicol, polymyxin, rifampin, gentamicin, kanamycin, tobramycin
P. stuartii (195)	Urine	NA	Urinary catheter	Ampicillin, cephalexin, carbenicillin, sulfisoxazole, sulfamethoxazole, nitrofurantoin, chloramphenicol

CSF, cerebrospinal fluid; NA, not available; NICU, neonatal intensive care unit; NK, not known.

TABLE 33.9. EXAMPLES OF OUTBREAKS OF ENTEROBACTERIACEAE WITH EXTENDED-SPECTRUM β-LACTAMASES

First Author (Reference), Year	Setting, Country (No. of Patients)	Bacterial Species (No.)	β-Lactamase	Resistant to	Risk Factors Identified	Infection Control Measures
Brun-Buisson (196), 1987	3 ICUs, France (?)	*K. pneumoniae* (62)	SVH-2	CEP, CFA[b], AZT[b], CTX[b], CFX[b]	Urinary tract catherization	Reinforcement of hand washing, and use of disposable gloves decreased spread
Rice (98), 1990	Chronic care ward, U.S. (29)	*K. pneumoniae* (22) *E. cloacae* (3) Others[a]	TEM-12 TEM-26	CFA, AZT, CFO, CFX	CFA therapy	Discontinuation of empiric CFA use resulted in a decline of CFA-resistant isolates, but not eradication
Naumovski (97), 1992	Pediatric cancer ward, U.S. (13)	*K. pneumoniae* (12) *E. coli* (2)	TEM-26	CFA, AZT	CFA monotherapy	No further cases were detected after changing empirical therapy from CFA to amikacin, azlocillin, and nafcillin
Coovadia (202), 1992	Neonatal nursery, South Africa (9)	*K. pneumoniae* (12)	Not determined	CTX	Not analyzed	Outbreak was controlled by cohorting of patients, reemphasizing infection control measures and extensive disinfection of environmental surfaces and using gowns
Bauernfeind (203), 1993	Five hospital wards, Germany (22)	*K. pneumoniae* (22)	SHV-5	CFA, AZT	Not analyzed	Intensified infection control procedures failed to eradicate strain
Meyer (204), 1993	Teaching hospital, U.S. (155)	*K. pneumoniae* (432)	TEM-10 TEM-26	CFA	CFA therapy	Reduction in ceftazidime use and barrier precautions reduced incidence of colonization and infection
Prodinger (205), 1996	3 ICUs, Austria (32)	*K. pneumoniae* (30) *K. oxytoca* (1) *E. coli* (1)	SHV-5	CFA, AZT, CFO	Not analyzed	Incidence of infections decreased after facilitating appropriate room disinfection
Hobson (206), 1996	Several hospitals, U.K. (283)	*K. pneumoniae* (628)	Not determined	CFU	Not analyzed	Outbreak declined after reemphasis of standard infection control procedures and addressing environmental contamination

[a] *Enterobacter agglomerans* (1), *Citrobacter diversus* (1), *E. coli* (1), *Serratia* spp. (1).
[b] Decreased susceptibility.
CEP, cephalothin; *CFA*, ceftazidime; *AZT*, aztreonam; *CTX*, cefotaxime, *CFX*, ceftriaxone; *CFO*, cefoxitin; *CFU*, cefuroxime.
From Denessen PJW, Bonten MJM, Weinstein RA. Multiresistant bacteria as a hospital epidemic problem. *Ann Med* 1998; 30:176–185.

terial polymorphonuclear leukocyte function; and catheter drainage is frequently imperfect, leading to residual urine volumes in the bladder (214). In multivariate analysis nine independent risk factors for catheter-associated bacteriuria were found: duration of urinary catheterization, absence of use of a urinometer, microbial colonization of the drainage bag, diabetes mellitus, absence of antibiotic use, female gender, indications for other than surgery or output measurement, abnormal serum creatinine, and errors in catheter care (215). Other risk factors reported include any urinary tract or catheter obstruction to flow (e.g., prostatic hypertrophy or stones) and periurethral colonization (214,216). In the presence of urinary catheters with or without obstruction, relatively nonvirulent microorganisms can cause infection (45–47). For instance, P fimbriae, the most important virulence factor in non–catheter-associated UTIs, were found in only 10% of *E. coli* strains recovered during febrile episodes of catheter-associated UTIs (214). The incidence of new-onset bacteriuria is approximately 5% to 10% per day during the first week of catheterization. The prevalence of bacteriuria increases during the first month of catheterization until virtually all patients have bacteriuria (217).

Routes of entry of bacteria into the bladder vary for catheter-

TABLE 33.10. MOST FREQUENTLY REPORTED ENTEROBACTERIACEAE AND SELECTED OTHER PATHOGENS ASSOCIATED WITH NOSOCOMIAL URINARY TRACT INFECTION (UTI) (NNIS)

	Percentage (*n*)			Rank		
	Hospital-wide		ICUs	Hospital-wide		ICUs
Pathogen	1980–82	1990–96	1992–99	1980–82	1990–96	1992–99
Enterobacteriaceae						
Citrobacter spp.	2	2	NA	11	8	NA
Enterobacter spp.	4	5	5	6	6	6
E. coli	32	24	18	1	1	1
K. pneumoniae	7	8	6	4	4	5
Klebsiella spp. (other)	2	1	NA	9	10	NA
P. mirabilis	7	5	NA	5	6	NA
Proteus spp. (other)	1	0	NA	13	12	NA
S. marcescens	1	1	NA	12	10	NA
Serratia spp. (other)	0	0	NA	14	12	NA
Total	56	46	29			
Other pathogens						
P. aeruginosa	12	11	11	3	3	4
S. aureus	2	2	2	10	8	8
Coagulase-negative staphylococci	3	4	3	7	7	7
Enterococci	14	16	14	2	2	3
C. albicans	3	8	16	8	4	2
Other	10	13	26			
Total	100 (56,316)	100 (35, 079)	100 (30, 701)			

NA, not available.
Data from refs. 3 and 13; data from 1980–1982 and 1990–1996 represent the hospital-wide component, and data from 1992–99 the ICU component, of the National Nosoconial Infections Surveillance (NNIS) system.

ized men and women. Approximately 70% of bacteriuria cases in women occur as a result of periurethral entry of Enterobacteriaceae that have colonized the perineum (218,219). In men, because the urethral passage is longer, the primary route of bacterial entry presumably is through the catheter lumen (216,219). Although periurethral colonization in men does occur, transient hand carriage of pathogens by personnel leading to cross-infection may have a greater role in nosocomial UTIs in men (216).

Broad-spectrum antibiotics alter flora, increasing colonization with resistant Enterobacteriaceae and thus increasing the likelihood of UTI with these strains. In two studies, *E. coli* and *Proteus* accounted for a progressively smaller, and *Serratia* and *Pseudomonas* a progressively greater, proportion of nosocomial UTIs as length of hospitalization and catheterization increased (220,221) (see also Chapter 20).

Pulmonary

The second most common site of hospital-acquired infection (222) is the lungs. However, respiratory tract infections outnumber symptomatic UTIs in the ICU. In the European Prevalence of Infection in Intensive Care Study, a 1-day point prevalence study in April 1992 including 10,038 patients in 1,417 ICUs, 2,064 patients had at least one ICU-acquired infection. Pneumonia accounted for 47% and other respiratory tract infections for 18% of all infections. Eighteen percent of infected patients had UTI (2). In studies using expectorated sputum or endotracheal secretions from intubated patients, up to 30% of the pathogens involved in nosocomial pneumonia are Enterobacteriaceae (NNIS, 1990–1996). *Enterobacter* spp. and *K. pneumoniae* are the third and fourth (11% and 8%) leading causes of nosocomial pneumonia after *S. aureus* and *P. aeruginosa* (19% and 17%) (Table 33.11) (3). These proportions do not change significantly when care is taken to exclude contamination of respiratory specimens by upper airway and oropharyngeal secretions. For individual pathogens, highest percentages are found for *S. aureus* and *P. aeruginosa,* but as a group Enterobacteriaceae still represent an important proportion of pathogens, especially when nosocomial pneumonia is diagnosed after 4 days of mechanical ventilation (late-onset pneumonia). At that time, most patients have respiratory tract colonization with these pathogens. In contrast, early-onset pneumonia (i.e., diagnosed within 4 days of ventilation) is more frequently caused by streptococci and *Haemophilus influenzae.* These community-acquired bacteria colonize the upper respiratory tract at the time of intubation. However, in a comparison of patients with early-onset pneumonia, defined as occurring within 96 hours of ICU admission [n = 235 patients (56%)] to late-onset pneumonia [n = 185 patients (44%)] in a medical ICU and a surgical ICU from a teaching hospital, *Enterobacter* spp. represented 10% of isolates from both groups, *K. pneumoniae* represented 5.5% and 6.5%, respectively, *E. coli* was found in 2.6% and 1.6%, respectively, and *Citrobacter* represented approximately 1% of each (223).

The pathogenesis of nosocomial pneumonia most often involves the patient's aspiration of oropharyngeal contents, or inoculation of contaminated material directly into an endotracheal tube (224). Duration of ventilation and oropharyngeal colonization with Enterobacteriaceae are important risk factors for pneumonia (130). Oropharyngeal colonization with Enterobacteriaceae can also occur via exogenous contamination from

TABLE 33.11. MOST FREQUENTLY REPORTED ENTEROBACTERIACEAE AND SELECTED OTHER PATHOGENS ASSOCIATED WITH NOSOCOMIAL PNEUMONIA (NNIS)

	Percentage (n)			Rank		
	Hospital-wide		ICUs	Hospital-wide		ICUs
Pathogen	1980–82	1990–96	1992–99	1980–82	1990–96	1992–99
Enterobacteriaceae						
Citrobacter spp.	1	1	NA	11	11	NA
Enterobacter spp.	9	11	11	4	3	3
E. coli	8	4	4	5	6	6
K. pneumoniae	10	8	7	3	4	4
Klebsiella spp. (other)	4	1	NA	8	11	NA
P. mirabilis	5	2	NA	6	8	NA
Proteus spp. (other)	0	0	NA	14	13	NA
S. marcescens	4	3	NA	7	7	NA
Serratia spp. (other)	1	0	NA	12	13	NA
Total	42	30	22			
Other pathogens						
P. aeruginosa	13	17	17	2	2	2
S. aureus	13	19	18	1	1	1
Coagulase-negative staphylococci	1	2	NA	13	8	NA
Enterococci	2	2	2	10	8	7
C. albicans	3	5	5	9	5	5
Other	26	25	32			
Total	100 (15, 331)	100 (13, 433)	100 (39, 810)			

NA, not available.
Data from refs. 3 and 13; data from 1980–1982 and 1990–1996 represent the hospital-wide component, and data from 1992–99 the ICU component, of NNIS.

respiratory therapy equipment and from patient-to-patient spread of bacteria on the unlearned hands of personnel (see also Chapter 22).

Surgical Site Infections

Approximately a quarter of incisional surgical site infections involve Enterobacteriaceae (NNIS, 1990–1996) (3). *E. coli* accounts for 8% and *Enterobacter* spp. account for 7% of pathogens recovered from incisional surgical site infections (Table 33.12). The pathogens isolated from surgical site infections vary primarily with the type of surgery performed. In surgical procedures involving clean-contaminated, contaminated, and dirty fields, the pathogens isolated reflect the normal endogenous flora of the resected organ (225,226). Antibiotic prophylaxis may permit selective overgrowth of Enterobacteriaceae that are resistant to the prophylactic agent.

Enterobacteriaceae have been associated with extrinsic contamination of devices and solutions used perioperatively, leading to surgical site infections. For example, *Serratia marcescens* has contaminated saline solutions, leading to surgical site infection after breast reconstruction with silicone mammary prostheses (164), and has contaminated reusable electrocardiogram bulbs, leading to postoperative sternal and leg incision infections in cardiac surgery patients (163) (see also Chapter 21).

Diarrhea

Although *Salmonella, Shigella, Yersinia, E. coli, Citrobacter,* and *Enterobacter* all have been implicated as nosocomial diarrheal pathogens, the Enterobacteriaceae are uncommon causes of nosocomial diarrhea. Nosocomial infectious diarrhea due to Enterobacteriaceae usually represents exogenously acquired disease. The mode of transmission is either the fecal-oral route by cross-infection or common source infection secondary to contaminated food or medicine. Patients may have indirect contact with an infectious patient either by sharing a room or bathroom or via the hands of hospital personnel (116,191,192).

Salmonella infections are the most common of the nosocomial diarrheal diseases due to the Enterobacteriaceae. Between 10% and 30% of the reported cases of *Salmonella* infection in the U.S. occur in institutions (hospitals, nursing homes, custodial facilities) (227,228). Nosocomial infection with *Salmonella* is more common in developing countries (229,230). Fifty percent of nosocomial cases of salmonellosis in the U.S. occur in newborn nurseries and pediatric wards (228,231).

Sources of *Salmonella* in nosocomial outbreaks include other patients and contaminated foods, especially eggs, and devices. In the past, contaminated egg products, hospital eggnog (169), and raw eggs used in the preparation of mayonnaise (173) have led to large outbreaks of nosocomial diarrhea. The routine availability of pasteurized egg products should eliminate this problem in U.S. hospitals. The mayonnaise outbreak that occurred in 1989 was the largest nosocomial outbreak of *S. enteritidis* in U.S. history, with 404 (42%) of 965 inpatients in a single hospital affected, resulting in nine deaths (173).

Contaminated devices, rectal thermometers (174), gastroscopes (170), and rubber tubing of oropharyngeal suction devices (175) all have been associated with nosocomial *Salmonella* infection. Soiled linens have been reported as a source of nosocomial *Salmonella* infection in laundry workers in both hospital

TABLE 33.12. MOST FREQUENTLY REPORTED ENTEROBACTERIACEAE AND SELECTED OTHER PATHOGENS ASSOCIATED WITH NOSOCOMIAL SURGICAL SITE INFECTION (NNIS)

	Percentage (*n*)		Rank	
Pathogen	**1980–1982**	**1990–1996**	**1980–1982**	**1990–1996**
Enterobacteriaceae				
Citrobacter spp.	1	1	11	10
Enterobacter spp.	6	7	6	6
E. coli	13	8	2	4
K. pneumoniae	4	3	8	7
Klebsiella spp. (other)	1	1	9	10
P. mirabilis	5	3	7	7
Proteus spp. (other)	1	0	13	13
S. marcescens	1	1	10	10
Serratia spp. (other)	0	0	14	13
Total	32	24		
Other pathogens				
P. aeruginosa	7	8	4	4
S. aureus	18	20	1	1
Coagulase-negative staphylococci	6	14	5	2
Enterococci	11	12	3	3
C. albicans	1	3	12	7
Other	25	20		
Total	100 (28,906)	100 (17,871)		

Data from ref. 3.

and nursing home outbreaks of *Salmonella* gastroenteritis (232–234).

Neonatal outbreaks generally are associated with infant-to-infant spread, presumably on the hands of hospital personnel, from an index patient who acquired the infection at delivery from the mother.

The correlation of specific serotypes and sources should be considered when *Salmonella* is isolated in the hospital. For example, *S. choleraesuis* has been associated with pork products, *S. cubana* with carmine dye, *S. dublin* with beef products, and *S. pullorum* with poultry products.

Nosocomial transmission of *Shigella* has been reported (235, 236), and termed "asylum dysentery" in the early 1900s (237). An outbreak of *Shigella* dysenteriae type 1 occurred at a chronic care psychiatric facility in Durban, South Africa, involving ten patients, four of whom died. The infection in the index case was thought to be community acquired. Strict adherence to infection control measures (cohorting, hand hygiene, and restriction of food supplies brought in from outside the hospital) resulted in control of the outbreak. The high mortality rate was attributed to late recognition of the etiologic agent and failure to treat with appropriate antimicrobials (236).

E. coli is a serious nosocomial enteric pathogen for newborn infants and young children. The commonest scenario is cross-infection and environmental contamination from an infected child with diarrhea due to an enteropathogenic *E. coli*. Asymptomatic carriers also are an important cause of epidemics. Although most nosocomial enteric disease is due to enteropathogenic *E. coli*, there has been one large hospital nursery outbreak due to enterotoxigenic *E. coli* (188). Enterohemorrhagic *E. coli* has been reported in several nosocomial outbreaks (238–242). Transmission has been attributed to person-to-person spread, to environmental contamination, and contaminated lettuce (243).

There have been at least four reports of nosocomial transmission of *Y. enterocolitica* diarrhea (189,190,244,245). The mode of transmission is similar to that of the other enteric pathogens, with indirect contact spread from patient to patient via shared fomites and via the hands of personnel. A retrospective analysis of *Yersinia* infections in one hospital revealed 18 infections over 4 years; five infections appeared to be hospital-acquired (245). In most of these cases, a patient admitted with *Y. enterocolitica* gastroenteritis appeared to be the source of cross-infection. *Y. enterocolitica* is a rarely recognized enteric nosocomial pathogen, perhaps because it is difficult to isolate in the laboratory, because clinicians do not have a high index of suspicion for *Yersinia* as a pathogen, and because many patients may not be symptomatic (246). The outbreaks that have been reported to date have been small, and it is likely that such outbreaks may be missed easily (see also Chapter 24).

Bacteremia

The Enterobacteriaceae are not major causes of hospital-acquired bacteremia. As a group, they account for approximately 18% of bloodstream infections (NNIS, 1990–1996) (3). *E. coli, Enterobacter* spp., and *K. pneumoniae* are the Enterobacteriaceae most often associated with bacteremia (Table 33.13). In a Spanish multicenter study, *K. pneumoniae, E. cloacae,* and *E. coli* accounted for 5.6%, 1.9%, and 2.5%, respectively, of 590 cases of nosocomial bacteremia (247). Approximately half of *E. coli* bacteremias are acquired nosocomially. The most common portal of entry of infection for both community-acquired and nosocomial *E. coli* bacteremia is the urinary tract (248). The overall mortality rate from *E. coli* bacteremia is approximately 20% (247,248). Bacteremias that originate outside the urinary tract tend to have a worse outcome.

TABLE 33.13. MOST FREQUENTLY REPORTED ENTEROBACTERIACEAE AND SELECTED OTHER PATHOGENS ASSOCIATED WITH NOSOCOMIAL BLOODSTREAM INFECTION (NNIS)

	Percentage (n)			Rank		
	Hospital-wide		ICUs	Hospital-wide		ICUs
Pathogen	1980–82	1990–96	1992–99	1980–82	1990–96	1992–99
Enterobacteriaceae						
Citrobacter spp.	1	1	NA	12	9	NA
Enterobacter spp.	6	4	5	6	7	4
E. coli	13	5	2	2	4	8
K. pneumoniae	8	5	3	4	4	7
Klebsiella spp. (other)	2	1	NA	10	9	NA
P. mirabilis	2	1	NA	11	9	NA
Proteus spp. (other)	0	0	NA	14	13	NA
S. marcescens	3	1	NA	8	9	NA
Serratia spp. (other)	1	0	NA	13	13	NA
Total	36	18	10			
Other pathogens						
P. aeruginosa	6	3	4	7	8	6
S. aureus	13	16	13	1	2	3
Coagulase-negative staphylococci	11	31	37	3	1	1
Enterococci	7	9	14	5	3	2
C. albicans	3	5	5	9	4	5
Other	24	18	17			
Total	100 (7,815)	100 (14,424)	100 (21,943)			

NA, not available.
Data from refs. 3 and 13; data from 1980–1982 and 1990–1996 represent the hospital-wide component, and data from 1992–99 the ICU component, of NNIS.

The majority of bacteremias due to *Enterobacter* spp., primarily *E. cloacae* and *E. aerogenes,* are nosocomial. Several large series of cases of bacteremia due to *Enterobacter* spp. report that 67% to 84% of the bacteremias were acquired nosocomially (248–252). Approximately one third of these cases are polymicrobial. Major portals of entry for *Enterobacter* spp. in bacteremic patients include the lung, surgical sites/skin wounds, the urinary tract, and central venous lines, in descending order of frequency (249–254). The use of devices (e.g., endotracheal tubes, Foley catheters) and the prior use of antibiotics appeared to be associated with increased risk of *Enterobacter* bacteremia. Mortality rates of 24% to 69% have been reported (247,249–252).

Large series that describe *Klebsiella* bacteremia report that approximately one half to three quarters of these bacteremias are acquired nosocomially (255–259); up to 25% of these cases are polymicrobial (255,256). Major portals of entry include the urinary tract and lung, although in some series the gastrointestinal tract and intravenous catheters were major sites of primary infection (255,256,259). Patients with pneumonia as a primary source of bacteremia tend to have a worse outcome (255,257, 259). In children, *Klebsiella* bacteremia has been reported in outbreaks in the NICU (180). Widespread colonization of the gastrointestinal tract and respiratory tract with *Klebsiella* has been documented in these outbreaks, as has hand carriage of these strains by hospital personnel. Overall mortality rates for nosocomial *Klebsiella* bacteremia vary from 21% to 55% (247, 255,258–260). Increasingly, ESBL-producing *Klebsiella* are causing bacteremia (261,262). In a retrospective study of 162 *K. pneumoniae* isolates, 44 (27.2%) were ESBL-producing. In a multivariate analysis, risk-factors for ESBL-producing *Klebsiella* bacteremia, compared to non-ESBL producing strains, included presence of a biliary drainage catheter, prior antibiotic therapy, and nosocomial acquisition of bacteremia. Mortality attributable to *Klebsiella* bacteremia did not differ significantly between the two groups (23.3 vs. 20% in ESBL-producers vs. nonproducers, respectively) (261).

Bacteremia due to *Citrobacter* spp. is primarily a nosocomial infection (263,264). It occurs most frequently in elderly or very young patients, with initial sites of infection in the urinary tract, gastrointestinal tract, and wounds, in decreasing frequency of occurrence. *C. diversus* is frequently associated with genitourinary or intraabdominal disease, and *C. freundii,* the most prevalent *Citrobacter* spp. found in stool (120,264,265), is associated with gallbladder disease and peritonitis. Bacteremia with *Citrobacter* is commonly preceded by instrumentation at the site of the primary infection. Mortality rates from *Citrobacter* bacteremia are high (approximately 50%) and are related to severity of the patient's underlying medical condition.

One series of bacteremias due to *Serratia* reported that 82% were acquired nosocomially; 23% had polymicrobial bacteremia. The portal of entry was unknown in 64% of patients. Clinical syndromes included primary bacteremia (in two thirds of patients), pneumonia, UTI, thrombophlebitis, and surgical site infection. The mortality rate attributable to *Serratia* bacteremia was 32% (266) (see also Chapter 19).

Central Nervous System Infections

Nosocomial CNS infections occur primarily in neurosurgical patients, neonates, and patients undergoing procedures that penetrate the CNS (267). A review of gram-negative bacillary meningitis showed that 69% of the cases occurred in postneurosurgical patients, with the majority (70%) of infections due to *E. coli* (268). In a review of acute bacterial meningitis (118), approximately 50% of the cases of nosocomial meningitis were due to gram-negative bacilli, with approximately 50% of these cases due to infection with *E. coli* or *K. pneumoniae.* A descriptive review of 55 adult cases of *Klebsiella* meningitis over 13 years found that "spontaneous" meningitis occurred in 80% and post-neurosurgical meningitis occurred in 20% of patients. Underlying conditions in the patients with spontaneous meningitis included diabetes mellitus (70%), alcoholism (30%) and chronic otitis media (17%). Other less common underlying diseases included neoplasm, stroke, nasopharyngeal carcinoma, and end-stage renal disease (269).

In neonates, the most common etiologic agent of gram-negative bacillary meningitis remains *E. coli.* The K1 strains are the etiologic agents in most cases (33). Unusual pathogens associated with outbreaks of neonatal meningitis include *C. diversus, S. marcescens,* and *E. sakazakii. C. diversus* has been reported to cause meningitis and CNS abscess in both preterm and full-term infants. One cluster of nosocomial neonatal *C. diversus* meningitis cases was found to be due to hand carriage of this strain by a nurse with dermatitis. Removal of the nurse from the unit resulted in decreased rates of neonatal colonization with *C. diversus* and no further clinical cases of *C. diversus* sepsis and meningitis (184). During reported outbreaks of *C. diversus* infections in nurseries, rates of fecal and umbilical carriage are high (50% to nearly 100%), yet few infants acquire clinical disease (185). One case of *C. diversus* brain abscess has been reported in an adult following a community-acquired *C. diversus* UTI (270). A case of multiple brain abscesses in association with bacteremia has been reported with *Salmonella paratyphi* B in an infant (271).

S. marcescens meningitis occurs primarily in neonates, particularly in premature infants requiring ICU care. Most of these infants have multiple invasive catheters and have received a prior course of antibiotics (272). Notable features of *Serratia* meningitis in infants include a propensity for progression to ventriculitis, a frequent lack of cerebrospinal fluid pleocytosis and of hypoglycorrhachia (present in only 50% of cases), the development of *Serratia* meningitis despite receiving therapy for *Serratia* bacteremia, concurrent soft tissue infection or UTI with *Serratia,* and a high mortality rate (>45%) (272) (see also Chapters 27, 49, and 52).

PREVENTION AND CONTROL OF NOSOCOMIAL INFECTIONS DUE TO ENTEROBACTERIACEAE TABLE 33.14

Hand Hygiene

The importance of hand hygiene cannot be overemphasized. Hand transfer of the Enterobacteriaceae between patients by healthcare personnel has been implicated in numerous outbreaks of nosocomial infection (Table 33.8). It is felt that most endemic infections also are transmitted by the hands of healthcare workers (273). In most studies, the Enterobacteriaceae are only transient hand flora; *Acinetobacter* is usually the only gram-negative bacillus found consistently in hand cultures. For example, *Klebsiella* has been shown to survive on the hands for about 2 hours (274). In one study, however, approximately 60% of people demonstrated endemic hand carriage of gram-negative bacilli, primarily the Enterobacteriaceae (275). In that study, healthcare workers with hand dermatitis carried gram-negative bacilli more frequently and in greater numbers than other healthcare workers (276). The investigators also found that continuous hand carriage (over 3–6 weeks) was common. In an epidemic in an NICU, a nurse with hand dermatitis was found to be the reservoir for the epidemic strain of *C. diversus* (184).

TABLE 33.14. EXAMPLES OF CONVENTIONAL INFECTION CONTROL POLICIES[a]

- Identify reservoirs
  - Colonized and infected patients
  - Environmental contamination; common sources
- Halt transmission among patients
  - Improve hand washing and asepsis
  - Barrier precautions (gloves, gowns) for colonized and infected patients
  - Eliminate any common source; disinfect environment
  - Separate susceptible patients
  - Close unit to new admissions if necessary
- Halt progression from colonization to infection—examples of site-specific measures
  - Rotate intravenous catheter sites
  - Discontinue bladder catheters as clinically indicated
  - Extubate and remove nasogastric tube
  - Position patients to decrease risk of aspiration
  - 48-hour (or less frequent) ventilator circuit tubing changes
  - Proper removal of ventilator tubing condensate
  - Proper endotracheal suctioning technique
- Modify host risk
  - Treat underlying disease and complications
  - Control antibiotic use

[a] See Chapters 17 to 27 for more detailed site-specific control measures.
Adapted from Baine WB, Gangerosa EJ, Bonnet JV, et al. CDC news. Institutional salmnellosis. *J Infect Dis* 1973;128:357.

Observations of hand washing behavior in university hospital ICUs have found compliance rates ranging from 28% to 41% (277). Strategies such as increasing the number of sinks and installing automated sinks have not been shown to improve hand-washing compliance and have had little effect on infection rates (278–282). Efficacy of specific hand-cleansing agents in preventing horizontal pathogen-transmission has not been studied extensively. Based on efficacy of hand degerming, ease of use, and salutary effect on the condition of the hands of healthcare workers, alcohol-based hand rubs are now recommended for hand hygiene between patient contacts (283) (see Chapter 96).

Other Conventional Methods of Infection Control

Barrier precautions, when used aggressively, have successfully prevented the nosocomial spread of multiply resistant Enterobacteriaceae and have reduced ICU infection rates (151,284). The institution of barrier precautions (primarily gloving) resulted in a sustained 87% reduction in gentamicin-resistant Enterobacteriaceae in one hospital (151). Even with the use of gloves, hand washing should be emphasized, as studies have shown that up to 50% of hands were contaminated after glove removal (285). Use of gloves and gowns has been shown to reduce the incidence of nosocomial infections in the pediatric ICU as well (286,287).

Elimination of common reservoirs of infection and proper care of invasive monitoring equipment are also important in prevention of nosocomial infection due to the Enterobacteriaceae. A variety of invasive devices have been implicated as sources of epidemic infections (Table 33.7). Care of all invasive devices should include removal of the device as soon as a patient's clinical condition permits and careful asepsis during use.

The environment is usually not a major source or vector in infections with Enterobacteriaceae. Contamination from environmental reservoirs that may come into contact with patients has been the cause of nosocomial outbreaks. These outbreaks have called attention to reservoirs that may warrant special care (Table 33.7).

Because broad-spectrum antibiotic therapy alters patients' microflora and may lead to colonization and to infection with multiply resistant microorganisms, restriction of broad-spectrum antibiotics has been cited as an important infection control measure (82,288). Resistance rates generally diminish with antibiotic restriction, although most studies introduce several control measures simultaneously, making assignment of causality difficult.

With regard to infection control, two aspects are instrumental when attempting to control outbreaks of ESBL-containing Enterobacteriaceae or to prevent nosocomial epidemics (82,288). First, as for all other nosocomial pathogens, enforcement of compliance with infection control measures is of key importance. Reinforcement of hand hygiene compliance (196,289), glove use (196), barrier precautions (204,289), and appropriate room disinfection (205) have reduced the spread of resistant bacteria. A limited and rational use of broad-spectrum antibiotics, such as third-generation cephalosporins, is the second strategy to prevent and control outbreaks with these bacteria. ESBL genes can be transferred easily to other bacteria and even other bacterial species, especially in the presence of antibiotic pressure. In three studies the use of ceftazidime was a risk factor for infection with ESBL-containing microorganisms (97,98,204). Discontinuation of empiric ceftazidime and reduction of ceftazidime use in combination with barrier precautions resulted in a decline of resistant isolates, but they were not completely eradicated (98, 205). In a smaller outbreak in a pediatric cancer ward, no further cases of infection with resistant strains were detected after a change of empirical therapy from ceftazidime to a combination of amikacin, azlocillin, and nafcillin (97). An outbreak of gentamicin-resistant Enterobacteriaceae (85 isolates comprising eight species) on neurology and neurosurgery wards was controlled following restriction of broad-spectrum beta-lactams, cephalosporins, gentamicin, tobramycin, quinolones, and cotrimoxazole. Only after addition of the antibiotic restriction policy to infection control measures already in place (barrier precautions, educational sessions, and new hand hygiene products) did the incidence of multidrug resistant Enterobacteriaceae decrease to half of the preintervention phase (290). An experimental approach would be to use intestinal decontamination by nonabsorbable antibiotics, as a temporary adjunct to strict hygienic and antimicrobial control measures, to eradicate colonization with multiresistant bacteria (291).

Efficacy of screening for multidrug-resistant Enterobacteriaceae in the absence of an outbreak was studied in patients admitted for organ transplantation. Of 287 patients (75% of whom underwent liver or kidney transplant), 69 (24%) were colonized with multidrug resistant Enterobacteriaceae; six (9%) of 69 colonized patients developed clinical infections. These six isolates were all unique by PFGE. Of 995 other transplant ward patients who underwent passive clinical culture surveillance for multidrug-resistant Enterobacteriaceae, 12 (1.2%) were noted to be colonized; no clinical infections were detected in these patients. Typing of isolates included PFGE, plasmid, and integron analysis. There was no patient-to-patient transmission detected. The authors demonstrated a large cost for surveillance cultures and concluded that in a setting where multidrug-resistant Enterobacteriaceae are endemic, surveillance of clinical isolates was adequate for infection control purposes (292).

Control and/or Eradication of Colonization

Conventional approaches to control of nosocomial infection due to the Enterobacteriaceae as outlined above are not always successful, in part because of lack of compliance. But even when compliance is total, endogenous oropharyngeal or rectal carriage of Enterobacteriaceae may create an "iceberg" effect (Fig. 33.1). Thus, conventional infection control methods aimed at reducing cross-infection may not work, because many patients arrive at the hospital already colonized. Studies have shown that isolation, barrier nursing, and strict antibiotic policies reduce rates of cross-infection and cross-colonization, but overall rates of infection, especially pneumonia, may be unchanged (293). Thus, antibiotic prophylaxis has been studied repeatedly since the 1950s as a method to decrease rates of nosocomial infection, particularly pneumonia.

Early trials of systemic antibiotics in the 1950s showed no decrease in the risk of pneumonia and, furthermore, showed increased risk of gram-negative bacilli overgrowth and increased risk of pneumonia, skin infection, and bacteremia (294,295). Two later studies addressed the issue of systemic intravenous prophylaxis to prevent early-onset VAP. In one study, 570 patients were randomized to receive either 24 hours of penicillin G, cefoxitin, or no antibiotics, and the incidences of early-onset VAP were 6% in patients with and 7% in patients without antibiotics (296). In the other study, two dosages of intravenous cefuroxime 12 hours apart after intubation resulted in a reduction in the incidence of early-onset VAP from 36% to 16% in comatose ICU patients (297).

In the 1970s, use of topical antibiotics, either aerosolized polymyxin or endotracheal aminoglycosides, delivered directly to the site of potential infection, was studied as prophylaxis of gram-negative pneumonia. Use of polymyxin led to decreased rates of pneumonia but to increased rates of colonization with polymyxin-resistant *Serratia, Proteus,* and *Flavobacterium* (298, 299). Use of an endotracheal aminoglycoside, gentamicin, was also associated with decreased rates of pneumonia but with increased rates of colonization by gentamicin-resistant *Providencia*

components of SDD should be evaluated. Moreover, more studies should determine the relative benefits of SDD in specific patient populations (i.e., medical, surgical, or trauma) or subgroups of patients with different levels of illness. Nevertheless, SDD may increase the risk of colonization and infection with antibiotic-resistant gram-positive microorganisms, such as staphylococci and enterococci, in some ICUs, so that units having problems with such strains should avoid SDD. SDD has contributed to outbreak control in a few ICUs with epidemics of multiply resistant Enterobacteriaceae that had not been controlled by conventional methods.

Other Strategies

Immunoprophylaxis has also been studied as an alternative approach to infection prevention in the ICU. Clinical studies have suggested that immunization of high-risk ICU patients with plasma from volunteers immunized with *E. coli* J5, a mutant in which core lipid A determinants are exposed (320), failed to lower the infection rate but did prevent gram-negative shock.

Intravenously administered immunoglobulin reduced the infection rate when given prophylactically to selected high-risk patients in a surgical ICU in one study (321), but did not reduce patient mortality. Prophylactic intravenous administration of immunoglobulin has been shown not to reduce the nosocomial infection rate in very low birth weight infants (322). Passive immunization with intravenous hyperimmune globulin, derived from donors immunized with a 24-valent *Klebsiella* capsular polysaccharide plus an eight-valent *P. aeruginosa* O-polysaccharide–toxin A conjugate vaccine, was tested in 725 ICU patients and compared to albumin administered to 667 patients. Although there was some evidence that passive immunization decreased the incidence and severity of vaccine-specific *Klebsiella* infections (from 2.7% to 1.2% and from 1.0% to 0.3%, respectively), the reductions were not statistically significant. Moreover, patients receiving hyperimmunoglobulin had more adverse reactions (323).

Passive systemic vaccination with immune sera to bacteria-specific adhesins may be another approach for the future. Sera from animals vaccinated with adhesins from type 1 pili (FimH) inhibited uropathogenic *E. coli* from binding to human bladder cells *in vitro*. Immunization with FimH almost completely reduced *in vivo* colonization of the bladder in a murine cystitis model, and levels of immunoglobulin G to FimH could be detected in the urine samples of these mice (324).

Less invasive and colonization-resistant devices are needed. These may very well be the most useful aids in controlling nosocomial infection by Enterobacteriaceae (325,326).

CONCLUSION

The incidence of nosocomial gram-negative infection due to the Enterobacteriaceae appears to be decreasing as infections with gram-positive bacteria become more common. This may very well be a circular evolution, and the Enterobacteriaceae may reemerge as leading pathogens for nosocomial infection later in this decade. Regardless, the Enterobacteriaceae remain a continuing clinical problem because of the prevalence of chromosomal- and plasmid-mediated antibiotic-resistant strains. As new devices and procedures continue to be developed, propagation of serious gram-negative infection assuredly will continue.

The control of nosocomial infections due to the Enterobacteriaceae is based on our understanding of the basic epidemiology of the pathogen. Whether the push for use of sinkless alcohol rubs will improve healthcare worker adherence to hand hygiene remains to be seen. However, strides are being made in the development of safer and less invasive devices and approaches to surgery and in our understanding of colonization and in ways to control colonization and prevent invasive disease.

REFERENCES

1. Kelley MT, Brenner DJ, Farmer JJ III. Enterobacteriaceae. In: Lennette EH, Balaws A, Hausler WJ Jr, et al., eds. *Manual of clinical microbiology,* 4th ed. Washington, DC: American Society of Microbiology, 1985:263–277.
2. Vincent JL, Bihari DJ, Suter PM, et al. The prevalence of nosocomial infection in intensive care units in Europe. Results of the European prevalence of infection in intensive care (EPIC) study. *JAMA* 1995; 274:639–644.
3. Hospital Infections Program National Center for Infectious Diseases, Centers for Disease Control and Prevention. National Nosocomial Infections Surveillance (NNIS) Report, data summary from October 1986–April 1996, issued May 1996. *Am J Infect Control* 1996;24: 380–388.
4. National Nosocomial Infections Surveillance (NNIS) System Report, data summary from January 1992 to June 2002, issued August 2002. *Am J Infect Control* 2002;30:458–475.
5. Enterobacteriaceae. In: Koneman EW, Allen SD, Janda WM, et al, eds. *Color atlas and textbook of diagnostic microbiology,* 4th ed. Philadelphia: JB Lippincott, 1992:103–184.
6. Ewing WH. *Identification of Enterobacteriaceae,* 4th ed. New York: Elsevier, 1986.
7. Brenner DJ. Enterobacteriaceae. In: Krieg NR, Holt JG, eds. *Bergey's manual of systemic bacteriology,* vol 1. Baltimore: Williams & Wilkins, 1984:408–420.
8. Farmer JJ III, Davis BR, Hickman-Brenner FW, et al. Biochemical identification of new species and biogroups of Enterobacteriaceal isolated from clinical specimens. *J Clin Microbiol* 1985;21:46–76.
9. Bruckner DA, Colonna P, Bearson BL. Nomenclature for aerobic and facultative bacteria. *Clin Infect Dis* 1999;29:713–23.
10. Maslow JN, Mulligan ME, Arbeit RD. Molecular epidemiology: application of contemporary techniques to the typing of microorganisms. *Clin Infect Dis* 1993;17:153–164.
11. Tenover FC, Arbeit RD, Goering RV, et al. Interpreting chromosomal DNA restriction patterns produced by pulsed-field gel electrophoresis: criteria for bacterial strain typing. *J Clin Microbiol* 1995;33: 2233–2239.
12. Bonten MJM, Hayden MK, Nathan C, et al. Stability of vancomycin-resistant enterococcal genotypes isolated from long-term-colonized patients. *J Infect Dis* 1998;177:378–382.
13. National Nosocomial Infections Surveillance (NNIS) System Report, data summary from January 1990–May 1999, issued June 1999. *Am J Infect Control* 1999;27:520–532.
14. Fluit AC, Schmitz FJ, Verhoef J. Frequency of isolation of pathogens from bloodstream, nosocomial pneumonia, skin and soft tissue, and urinary tract infections occurring in European patients. *Eur J Clin Microbiol Infect Dis* 2001;20(3):188–191.
15. Jones RN, Croco MA, Kugler KC, et al. Respiratory tract pathogens isolated from patients hospitalized with suspected pneumonia: frequency of occurrence and antimicrobial susceptibility patterns from the SENTRY Antimicrobial Surveillance Program (United States and Canada, 1997). *Diagn Microbiol Infect Dis* 2000;37(2):115–125.

16. Luzzaro F, Vigano EF, Fossati D, et al. Prevalence and drug susceptibility of pathogens causing bloodstream infections in northern Italy: a two-year study in 16 hospitals. *Eur J Clin Microbiol Infect Dis* 2002; 21(12):849–855.
17. Bouza E, San Juan R, Munoz P, et al. A European perspective on nosocomial urinary tract infections I. Report on the microbiology workload, etiology and antimicrobial susceptibility (ESGNI-003 study). European Study Group on Nosocomial Infections. *Clin Microbiol Infect* 2001;7(10):523–531.
18. Oelschlaeger TA, Dobrindt U, Hacker J. Virulence factors of uropathogens. *Curr Opin Urol* 2002;12(1):33–38.
19. Baumler AJ, Tsolis RM, Heffron F. Fimbrial adhesins of *Salmonella typhimurium.* Role in bacterial interactions with epithelial cells. *Adv Exp Med Biol* 1997;412:149–158.
20. Hacker J. Role of fimbrial adhesins in the pathogenesis of *Escherichia coli* infections. *Can J Microbiol* 1992;38:720–727.
21. Krogfelt KA. Bacterial adhesion: genetics, biogenesis, and role in pathogenesis of fimbrial adhesins of *Escherichia coli. Rev Infect Dis* 1991; 13:721–735.
22. Tarkkanen AM, Allen BL, Williams PH, et al. Fimbriation, capsulation, and iron-scavenging systems of *Klebsiella* strains associated with human urinary tract infections. *Infect Immun* 1992;60:1187–1192.
23. Mobley HLT, Chippendale GR, Tenney JH, et al. MR/K hemagglutination of *Providencia stuartii* correlates with adherence to catheters and with persistence in catheter-associated bacteriuria. *J Infect Dis* 1988;157:264–271.
24. Lomberg H, Larsson P, Leffler H, et al. Different binding specificities of *P. mirabilis* compared to *E. coli. Scand J Infect Dis* 1982;33(suppl): 37–42.
25. Svanborg Eden C, Larsson P, et al. Attachment of *Proteus mirabilis* to human urinary sediment epithelial cells in vitro is different from that of *Escherichia coli. Infect Immun* 1980;27:804–807.
26. Wray SK, Hull SI, Cook RG, et al. Identification and characterization of a uroepithelial cell adhesin from a uropathogenic isolate of *Proteus mirabilis. Infect Immun* 1986;54:43–49.
27. Senior BW. The special affinity of particular types of *Proteus mirabilis* for the urinary tract. *J Med Microbiol* 1979;12:1–8.
28. Bieber D, Ramer SW, Wu C-Y, et al. Type IV pili, transient bacterial aggregates, and virulence of enteropathogenic *Escherichia coli. Science* 1998;280:2114–2118.
29. Darfeuille-Michaud A, Jallat C, Aubel D, et al. R-plasmid-encoded adhesive factor in *Klebsiella pneumoniae* strains responsible for human nosocomial infections. *Infect Immun* 1992;60:44–55.
30. Denoya CD, Trevisan AR, Zorzopulos J. Adherence of multiresistant strains of *Klebsiella pneumoniae* to cerebrospinal fluid shunts: correlation with plasmid content. *J Med Microbiol* 1986;21:225–231.
31. Gyles CL. *Escherichia coli* cytotoxins and enterotoxins. *Can J Microbiol* 1992;38:734–746.
32. Jann K, Jann B. Capsules of *Escherichia coli*, expression and biological significance. *Can J Microbiol* 1992;38:705–710.
33. Cross AS, Gemski P, Sadoff JC, et al. The importance of the K1 capsule in invasive infections caused by *Escherichia coli. J Infect Dis* 1984;149:184–193.
34. Sarff LD, McCracken GH, Schiffer MS, et al. Epidemiology of *Escherichia coli* K1 in healthy and diseased newborns. *Lancet* 1975; 1099–1104.
35. Highsmith K, Jarvis WR. *Klebsiella pneumoniae:* selected virulence factors that contribute to pathogenicity. *Infect Control* 1985;6:75–77.
36. Simoons-Smit AM, Verweij-Van Vught JJ, Maclaren DM. The role of K antigens as virulence factors in *Klebsiella. J Med Microbiol* 1986; 21:133–137.
37. Cornelis G, Laroche Y, Balligand G, et al. *Yersinia enterocolitica,* a primary model for bacterial invasiveness. *Rev Infect Dis* 1987;9:64–87.
38. Johnson JR, Moseley SL, Roberts PL, et al. Aerobactin and other virulence factor genes among strains of *Escherichia coli* causing urosepsis: association with patient characteristics. *Infect Immun* 1988;56: 405–412.
39. Nassif X, Sansonetti PJ. Correlation of the virulence of *Klebsiella pneumoniae* K1 and K2 with the presence of a plasmid encoding aerobactin. *Infect Immun* 1986;54:603–608.
40. Kline MW, Kaplan SL, Hawkins EP, et al. Pathogenesis of brain abscess formation in an infant rat model of *Citrobacter diversus* bacteremia and meningitis. *J Infect Dis* 1988;157:106–112.
41. Mobley HLT, Warren JW. Urease-positive bacteriuria and obstruction of long-term urinary catheters. *J Clin Microbiol* 1987;2: 2216–2217.
42. Kline MW, Mason EO, Kaplan SL. Characterization of *Citrobacter diversus* strains causing neonatal meningitis. *J Infect Dis* 1988;157: 101–105.
43. Kuhnert P, Boerlin P, Frey J. Target genes for virulence assessment of *Escherichia coli* isolates from water, food and the environment. *FEMS Microbiol Rev* 2000;24(1):107–117.
44. Noel JM, Boedeker EC. Enterohemorrhagic *Escherichia coli:* a family of emerging pathogens. *Dig Dis* 1997;15(1–2):67–91.
45. Brauner A, Leissner M, Wretlind B, et al. Occurrence of P-fimbriated *Escherichia coli* in patients with bacteremia. *Eur J Clin Microbiol* 1985; 4:566–569.
46. Tullus K, Brauner A, Fryklund B, et al. Host factors versus virulence-associated bacterial characteristics in neonatal and infantile bacteraemia and meningitis caused by *Escherichia coli. J Med Microbiol* 1992; 36:203–208.
47. Johnson JR, Roberts PL, Stamm WE. P fimbriae and other virulence factors in *Escherichia coli* urosepsis: association with patients' characteristics. *J Infect Dis* 1987;156:225–229.
48. Svanborg C, Godaly G. Bacterial virulence in urinary tract infection. *Infect Dis Clin North Am* 1997;11(3):513–529.
49. Hornick DB, Allen BL, Horn MA, et al. Fimbrial types among respiratory isolates belonging to the family Enterobacteriaceae. *J Clin Microbiol* 1991;29:1795–1800.
50. Wang MC, Tseng CC, Chen CY, et al. The role of bacterial virulence and host factors in patients with *Escherichia coli* bacteremia who have acute cholangitis or upper urinary tract infection. *Clin Infect Dis* 2002; 35(10):1161–1166.
51. Howell AB, Foxman B. Cranberry juice and adhesion of antibiotic-resistant uropathogens. *JAMA* 2002;287(23):3082–3083.
52. Kontiokari T, Sundqvist K, Nuutinen M, et al. Randomised trial of cranberry-lingonberry juice and lactobacillus GG drink for the prevention of urinary tract infections in women. *BMJ* 2001; 322(7302):1571–1575.
53. Saukkonen KMJ, Nowicki B, Leinonen M. Role of type 1 and S fimbriae in the pathogenesis of *Escherichia coli* 018:K1 bacteremia and meningitis in the infant rat. *Infect Immun* 1988;56:892–897.
54. Parkkinen J, Korhonen TK, Pere A, et al. Binding sites in the rat brain for *Escherichia coli* S fimbriae associated with neonatal meningitis. *J Clin Invest* 1988;81:860–865.
55. Parkkinen J, Ristimaki A, Westerlund B. Binding of *Escherichia coli* S fimbriae to cultured human endothelial cells. *Infect Immun* 1989; 57:2256–2259.
56. Siitonen A, Takala A, Ratiner YA, et al. Invasive *Escherichia coli* infections in children: bacterial characteristics in different age groups and clinical entities. *Pediatr Infect Dis J* 1993;12:606–612.
57. Schilling JD, Mulvey MA, Hultgren SJ. Structure and function of *Escherichia coli* type 1 pili: new insight into the pathogenesis of urinary tract infections. *J Infect Dis* 2001;183(suppl 1):S36–40.
58. Podschum R, Sievers D, Fischer A, et al. Serotypes, hemagglutinins, siderophore synthesis, serum resistance of Klebsiella isolates causing human urinary tract infections. *J Infect Dis* 1993;168:1415–1421.
59. Lindberg AA. Polyosides (encapsulated bacteria). *C R Acad Sci III* 1999;322(11):925–932.
60. Fang G, Keys TF, Gentry LO, et al. Prosthetic valve endocarditis resulting from nosocomial bacteremia. *Ann Intern Med* 1993;119: 560–567.
61. Moore DG, Yancey RJ, Lankford CE, et al. Bacteriostatic enterocholin-specific immunoglobulin from normal human serum. *Infect Immun* 1980;27:418–423.
62. Carniel E. The *Yersinia* high-pathogenicity island. *Int Microbiol* 1999; 2(3):161–167.
63. Schubert S, Cuenca S, Fischer D, et al. High-pathogenicity island of *Yersinia pestis* in Enterobacteriaceae isolated from blood cultures and

urine samples: prevalence and functional expression. *J Infect Dis* 2000; 182(4):1268–1271.

64. Schubert S, Picard B, Gouriou S, et al. *Yersinia* high-pathogenicity island contributes to virulence in *Escherichia coli* causing extraintestinal infections. *Infect Immun* 2002;70(9):5335–5337.
65. Foberg U, Fryden A, Kihlstrom E, et al. *Yersinia enterocolitica* septicemia: clinical and microbiological aspects. *Scand J Infect Dis* 1986;18: 269–279.
66. Robins-Browne RM, Prpic JK. Desferrioxamine and systemic yersiniosis. *Lancet* 1983;2:1372.
67. Pazin GJ, Braude A. 1. Immobilizing antibodies in urine. 2. Prevention of ascending spread of *Proteus mirabilis. Invest Urol* 1974;12: 129–133.
68. Griffith DP, Musher DM, Itin C. Urease: the preliminary cause of infection-induced urinary stones. *Invest Urol* 1976;13:340–346.
69. Prouty AM, Schwesinger WH, Gunn JS. Biofilm formation and interaction with the surfaces of gallstones by *Salmonella* spp. *Infect Immun* 2002;70(5):2640–2649.
70. Simmons BP, Gelfand MS, Haas M, et al. *Enterobacter sakazakii* infections in neonates associated with intrinsic contamination of a powdered infant formula. *Infect Control Hosp Epidemiol* 1989;10: 398–401.
71. Muytjens HL, Roelofs-Willemse H, Jaspar GHJ. Quality of powdered substitutes for breast milk with regard to members of the family Enterobacteriaceae. *J Clin Microbiol* 1988;26:743–746.
72. Biering G, Karlsson S, Clark NC, et al. Three cases of neonatal meningitis caused by *Enterobacter sakazakii* in powdered milk. *J Clin Microbiol* 1989;27:2054–2056.
73. Bar-Oz B, Preminger A, Peleg O, et al. *Enterobacter sakazakii* infection in the newborn. *Acta Paediatr* 2001;90(3):356–358.
74. Nazarowec-White M, Farber JM. *Enterobacter sakazakii*: a review. *Int J Food Microbiol* 1997;34(2):103–113.
75. Wright DC, Selss IF, Vinton KJ, et al. Fatal *Yersinia enterocolitica* sepsis after blood transfusion. *Arch Pathol Lab Med* 1985;109: 1040–1042.
76. *Yersinia enterocolitica* bacteremia and endotoxin shock associated with red blood cell transfusion—United States, 1987–1988. *MMWR* 1988;37:577–578.
77. Tipple MA, Bland LA, Murphy JJ, et al. Sepsis associated with transfusion of red cells contaminated with *Yersinia enterocolitica. Transfusion* 1990;30:207–213.
78. Bufill JA, Ritch PS. *Yersinia enterocolitica* serotype 0:3 sepsis after blood transfusion. *N Engl J Med* 1989;320:810.
79. Maki DG, Martin WT. Nationwide epidemic of septicemia caused by contaminated infusion products. IV. Growth of microbial pathogens in fluids for intravenous infusion. *J Infect Dis* 1975;131: 267–272.
80. Ristuccia PA, Cunha BA. Enterobacter. *Top Clin Microbiol* 1985;6: 124–128.
81. Timmis KN, Gonzalez-Carrero MI, Sekizaki T, et al. Biological activity specified by antibiotic resistance plasmids. *J Antimicrob Chemother* 1986;18(suppl C):1–12.
82. Weinstein RA. Controlling antimicrobial resistance in hospitals: infection control and use of antibiotics. *Emerg Infect Dis* 2001;7(2): 188–192.
83. Flynn DM, Weinstein RA, Kabins SA. Infections with gram-negative bacilli in a cardiac surgery intensive care unit: the relative role of enterobacter. *J Hosp Infect* 1988;11(suppl A):367–373.
84. Bryan CS, John JF, Pai MS, et al. Gentamicin vs cefotaxime for therapy of neonatal sepsis. *Am J Dis Child* 1985;139:1086–1089.
85. Jacoby GA, Archer GL. New mechanisms of bacterial resistance to antimicrobial agents. *N Engl J Med* 1991;324:601–612.
86. Lodge JM, Piddock LJV. The control of class I β-lactamase expression in Enterobacteriaceae and *Pseudomonas aeruginosa. J Antimicrob Chemother* 1991;28:167–172.
87. Weinstein RA. Endemic emergence of cephalosporin-resistant enterobacter: relation to prior therapy. *Infect Control* 1986;7:120–123.
88. Knothe H, Shah P, Krcmery V, et al. Transferable resistance to cefotaxime, cefoxitin, cefamandole and cefuroxime in clinical isolates of *Klebsiella pneumoniae* and *Serratia marcescens. Infection* 1983;11: 315–317.
89. Payne DJ, Marriott MS, Amyes SGB. Mutants of the TEM-1 betalactamase conferring resistance to ceftazidime. *J Antimicrob Chemother* 1989;24:103–110.
90. Bush K, Jacoby G. Nomenclature of TEM beta-lactamases. *J Antimicrob Chemother* 1997;39:1–3.
91. Medeiros AA. Evolution and dissemination of beta-lactamases accelerated by generations of beta-lactam antibiotics. *Clin Infect Dis* 1997; 24(suppl 1):S19–S45.
92. Bradford PA. Extended-spectrum beta-lactamases in the 21st century: characterization, epidemiology, and detection of this important resistance threat. *Clin Microbiol Rev* 2001 Oct;14(4):933–951.
93. Paterson DL, Ko WC, Mohapatra S, et al. *Klebsiella pneumoniae* bacteremia: impact of extended spectrum beta-lactamases production in a global study of 216 patients. In: Proceedings of the 37th Interscience Conference on Antimicrobial Agents and Chemotherapy, Toronto, 1997:328.
94. Itokazu GS, Quinn JP, Bell-Dixon C, et al. Antimicrobial resistance rates among aerobic gram-negative bacilli recovered from patients in intensive care units: evaluation of a national postmarketing surveillance program. *Clin Infect Dis* 1996;23:779–784.
95. NNIS system selected antimicrobial resistant pathogens associated with nosocomial infections in ICU patients. Available at *www.cdc.gov/ncidod/hip/NNIS/ar__surv99.htm.*
96. Rasmussen BA, Bradford PA, Quinn JP, et al. Genetically diverse ceftazidime-resistant isolates from a single center: biochemical and genetic characterization of TEM-10 β-lactamases encoded by different nucleotide sequences. *Antimicrob Agents Chemother* 1993;37: 1989–1992.
97. Naumovski L, Quinn JP, Miyashiro D, et al. Outbreak of ceftazidime resistance due to a novel extended-spectrum β-lactamase in isolates from cancer patients. *Antimicrob Agents Chemother* 1992;36: 1991–1996.
98. Rice LB, Willey SH, Papanicolaou GA, et al. Outbreak of ceftazidime resistance caused by extended-spectrum β-lactamases at a Massachusetts chronic-care facility. *Antimicrob Agents Chemother* 1990;34: 2193–2199.
99. Gaynes RP, Weinstein RA, Chamberlin W, et al. Antibiotic-resistant flora in nursing home patients admitted to the hospital. *Arch Intern Med* 1985;145:1804–1807.
100. Phillips I, Eykyn S, King A, et al. Epidemic multiresistant *Escherichia coli* infection in West Lambeth Health District. *Lancet* 1988;1(8593): 1038–1041.
101. Manges AR, Johnson JR, Foxman B, et al. Widespread distribution of urinary tract infections caused by a multidrug-resistant *Escherichia coli* clonal group. *N Engl J Med* 2001;345(14):1007–1013.
102. Johnson JR, Manges AR, O'Bryan TT, et al. A disseminated multidrug-resistant clonal group of uropathogenic *Escherichia coli* in pyelonephritis. *Lancet* 2002;359(9325):2249–2251.
103. Johnson JR, Russo TA. Uropathogenic *Escherichia coli* as agents of diverse non-urinary tract extraintestinal infections. *J Infect Dis* 2002; 186(6):859–864.
104. Neuhauser MM, Weinstein RA, Rydman R, et al. Antibiotic resistance among gram-negative bacilli in US intensive care units: implications for fluoroquinolone use. *JAMA* 2003;289(7):885–888.
105. Selden R, Lee S, Wang WLL, et al. Nosocomial *Klebsiella* infections: intestinal colonization as a reservoir. *Ann Intern Med* 1971;74: 657–664.
106. DeLouvois J. Serotyping and the Dienes reaction on *Proteus mirabilis* from hospital infections. *J Clin Pathol* 1969;22:263–268.
107. Story P. *Proteus* infections in hospital. *J Pathol Bacteriol* 1954;68: 55–62.
108. Kaslow RA, Lindsey JO, Bisno AL, et al. Nosocomial infection with highly resistant *Proteus rettgeri*—report of an epidemic. *Am J Epidemiol* 1976;104:218–284.
109. Muller HE. Occurrence and pathogenic role of *Morganella Proteus Providencia* group bacteria in human feces. *J Clin Microbiol* 1986;23: 404–405.

110. Farmer JJ, Davis BR, Hickman FW, et al. Detection of serratia outbreaks in hospital. *Lancet* 1976;2:455–459.
111. Mermel LA, Maki DJ. Epidemic bloodstream infections from hemodynamic pressure monitoring: signs of the times. *Infect Control Hosp Epidemiol* 1989;10(2):47.
112. Yu, VL. Serratia marcescens. Historical perspective and clinical review. *N Engl J Med* 1979;300:887–893.
113. Andersen BM, Sorlie D, Hotvedt R, et al. Multiply beta-lactam resistant *Enterobacter cloacae* infections linked to the environmental flora in a unit for cardiothoracic and vascular surgery. *Scand J Infect Dis* 1989;21:181–191.
114. Wang CC, Chu ML, Ho LJ, et al. Analysis of plasmid pattern in paediatric intensive care unit outbreaks of nosocomial infection due to *Enterobacter cloacae. J Hosp Infect* 1991;19:33–40.
115. Felts SK, Schaffner W, Melly MA, et al. Sepsis caused by contaminated intravenous fluids. *Ann Intern Med* 1972;77:881–890.
116. Geiseler PJ, Harris B, Andersen BR. Nosocomial outbreak of nitrate-negative *Serratia marcescens* infections. *J Clin Microbiol* 1982;15:728–730.
117. Flynn DM, Weinstein RA, Nathan C, et al. Patients' endogenous flora as the source of "nosocomial" *Enterobacter* in cardiac surgery. *J Infect Dis* 1987;156:363–368.
118. Johnson MP, Ramphal R. β-Lactam-resistant *Enterobacter* bacteremia in febrile neutropenic patients receiving monotherapy. *J Infect Dis* 1990;162:981–983.
119. Rose HD, Schreier J. The effect of hospitalization and antibiotic therapy on the gram-negative fecal flora. *Am J Med Sci* 1968;255:228–236.
120. Hodges GR, Degener CE, Barnes WG. Clinical significance of *Citrobacter* isolates. *Am J Clin Pathol* 1978;70:37–40.
121. Lew PD, Baker AS, Kunz LJ, et al. Intra-abdominal *Citrobacter* infections: association with biliary or upper gastrointestinal source. *Surgery* 1984;95:398–402.
122. Ashbaugh DC, Petty TL. Sepsis complicating the acute respiratory distress syndrome. *Surg Gynecol Obstet* 1972;135:865–868.
123. Lepper MH. Opportunistic gram-negative rod pulmonary infections. *Dis Chest* 1963;44:18–26.
124. Johanson WG, Pierce AK, Sanford JP. Changing pharyngeal bacterial flora of hospitalized patients. Emergence of gram-negative bacilli. *N Engl J Med* 1969;281:1137–1140.
125. Mason CM, Nelson S, Summer WR. Bacterial colonization. Pathogenesis and clinical significance. *Immunol Allergy Clin North Am* 1993;13:93–108.
126. Rosenthal S, Tager IB. Prevalence of gram-negative rods in the normal pharyngeal flora. *Ann Intern Med* 1975;83:355–357.
127. Sveinbjornsdottir S, Gudmundsson S, Briem H. Oropharyngeal colonization in the elderly. *Eur J Clin Microbiol Infect Dis* 1991;10:959–963.
128. Fuxench-Lopez Z, Ramirez-Ronda CH. Pharyngeal flora in ambulatory alcoholic patients. Prevalence of gram negative bacilli. *Arch Intern Med* 1978;138:1815–1816.
129. Sprunt K, Redman W. Evidence suggesting importance of role of interbacterial inhibition in maintaining balance of normal flora. *Ann Intern Med* 1968;68:579–590.
130. Bonten MJM, Bergmans DCJJ, Ambergen AW, et al. Risk factors for pneumonia, and colonization of respiratory tract and stomach in mechanically ventilated ICU patients. *Am J Respir Crit Care Med* 1996;154:1339–1346.
131. LeFrock JL, Ellis CA, Weinstein L. The relation between aerobic fecal and oropharyngeal microflora in hospitalized patients. *Am J Med Sci* 1979;277:275–280.
132. Johanson WG, Pierce AK, Sanford JP, et al. Nosocomial respiratory infections with gram-negative bacilli: the significance of colonization of the respiratory tract. *Ann Intern Med* 1972;77:701–706.
133. Bonten MJM, Gaillard CA, van der Geest S, et al. The role of intragastric acidity and stress ulcer prophylaxis on colonization and infection in mechanically ventilated patients. A stratified, randomized, double blind study of sucralfate versus antacids. *Am J Respir Crit Care Med* 1995;152:1825–1834.
134. Bonten MJM, Gaillard CA, van der Hulst R, et al. Intermittent enteral feeding: the influence on respiratory and digestive tract colonization in mechanically ventilated intensive-care-unit patients. *Am J Respir Crit Care Med* 1996;154:394–399.
135. Daschner F, Kapstein I, Engels I, et al. Stress ulcer prophylaxis and ventilation pneumonia: prevention by antibacterial cytoprotective agents. *Infect Control* 1988;9:59–65.
136. Goularte TA, Lichtenberg OA, Craven DE. Gastric colonization in patients receiving antacids and mechanical ventilation: a mechanism for pharyngeal colonization. *Am J Infect Control* 1986;14:88.
137. Bonten MJM, Gaillard CA, de Leeuw PW, et al. Role of colonization of the upper intestinal tract in the pathogenesis of ventilator-associated pneumonia. *Clin Infect Dis* 1997;24:309–319.
138. Niederman MS, Craven DE. Editorial response: devising strategies for preventing nosocomial pneumonia—should we ignore the stomach? *Clin Infect Dis* 1997;24:320–323.
139. Bergmans DCJJ, Bonten MJM, Gaillard CA, et al. Prevention of ventilator-associated pneumonia by oral decontamination—a prospective, randomized, double-blind, placebo-controlled study. *Am J Respir Crit Care Med* 2001;164(3):382–388.
140. duMoulin GC, Paterson DG, Hedley-Whyte J, et al. Aspiration of gastric bacteria in antacid-treated patients: a frequent cause of postoperative colonization of the airway. *Lancet* 1982;1:242–245.
141. Craven DE, Steger KA. Nosocomial pneumonia in the intubated patient: new concepts on pathogenesis and prevention. *Infect Dis Clin North Am* 1989;3:843–866.
142. Inglis TJJ, Sherratt MJ, Sproat LJ, et al. Gastroduodenal dysfunction and bacterial colonisation of the ventilated lung. *Lancet* 1993;341:911–913.
143. Cook D, Guyatt G, Marshall J, et al. A comparison of sucralfate and ranitidine for the prevention of upper gastrointestinal bleeding in patients requiring mechanical ventilation. *N Engl J Med* 1998;338:791–797.
144. Artigas A, Campillo M, Cardona A, et al., Collaborative LAMG Working Group. Nosocomial pneumonia and gastrointestinal bleeding in mechanically ventilated patients receiving ranitidine or sucralfate. *Am J Respir Crit Care Med* 1995;151:A721.
145. Heyland DK, Cook DJ, Schoenfeld PS, et al. The effect of acidified enteral feeds on gastric colonization in critically ill patients: results of a multicenter randomized trial. Canadian Critical Care Trials Group. *Crit Care Med* 1999;27(11):2399–2406.
146. Dal Nogare AR, Toews GB, Pierce AK. Increased salivary elastase precedes gram-negative bacillary colonization in postoperative patients. *Am Rev Respir Dis* 1987;135:671–675.
147. Woods DE, Straus DC, Johanson WG, et al. Role of salivary protease activity in adherence of gram-negative bacilli to mammalian buccal epithelial cells in vivo. *J Clin Invest* 1981;68:1435–1440.
148. Chan RC, Reid G, Irvin RT, et al. Competitive exclusion of uropathogens from human uro-epithelial cells by lactobacillus whole cells and cell wall fragments. *Infect Immun* 1985;47:84–89.
149. Raz R, Stamm WE. A controlled trial of intravaginal estriol in postmenopausal women with recurrent urinary tract infections. *N Engl J Med* 1993;329:753–756.
150. Weinrauch Y, Drujan D, Shapiro SD, et al. Neutrophil elastase targets virulence factors of enterobacteria. *Nature* 2002;417(6884):91–94.
151. Weinstein RA, Kabins SA. Strategies for prevention and control of multiple drug resistant nosocomial infection. *Am J Med* 1981;70:449–454.
152. Washington JA, Senjem DH, Haldorson A, et al. Nosocomially acquired bacteriuria due to *Proteus rettgeri* and *Providencia stuartii. Am J Clin Pathol* 1973;60:836–838.
153. Fierer J, Ekstrom M. An outbreak of *Providencia stuartii* urinary tract infections. *JAMA* 1981;245:1553–1555.
154. Grohskopf LA, Roth VR, Feikin DR, et al. Serratia liquefaciens bloodstream infections from contamination of epoetin alfa at a hemodialysis center. *N Engl J Med* 2001;344(20):1491–1497.
155. Gransden WR, Webster M, French GL, et al. An outbreak of *Serratia marcescens* transmitted by contaminated breast pumps in a special care baby unit. *J Hosp Infect* 1986;7:149–154.
156. Templeton WC, Eiferman RA, Snyder JW, et al. *Serratia* keratitis

transmitted by contaminated eyedroppers. *Am J Ophthalmol* 1982; 93:723–726.

157. Rutala WA, Kennedy VA, Loflin HB, et al. *Serratia marcescens* nosocomial infections of the urinary tract associated with urine measuring containers and urinometers. *Am J Med* 1981;70:659–663.
158. Walton JR, Shapiro BA, Harrison RA, et al. *Serratia* bacteremia from mean arterial pressure monitors. *Anesthesiology* 1975;43:113–114.
159. Ehrenkranz NJ, Bolyard EA, Wiener M, et al. Antibiotic-sensitive *Serratia marcescens* infections complicating cardiopulmonary operations: contaminated disinfectant as a reservoir. *Lancet* 1980;2: 1289–1292.
160. Villarino ME, Jarvis WR, O'Hara C, et al. Epidemic of *Serratia marcescens* bacteremia in a cardiac intensive care unit. *J Clin Microbiol* 1989;27:2433–2436.
161. Krishnan PU, Pereira B, Macaden R. Epidemiological study of an outbreak of *Serratia marcescens* in a haemodialysis unit. *J Hosp Infect* 1991;18:57–61.
162. Nakashima AK, McCarthy MA, Martone WJ, et al. Epidemic septic arthritis caused by *Serratia marcescens* and associated with a benzalkonium chloride antiseptic. *J Clin Microbiol* 1987;25:1014–1018.
163. Sokalski SJ, Jewell MA, Asmus-Shillington AC, et al. An outbreak of *Serratia marcescens* in 14 adult cardiac surgical patients associated with 12-lead electrocardiogram bulbs. *Arch Intern Med* 1992;152: 841–844.
164. Pegues DA, Shireley LA, Riddle CF, et al. *Serratia marcescens* surgical wound infection following breast reconstruction. *Am J Med* 1991; 91(suppl 3):173S–178S.
165. Simor AE, Ramage L, Wilcox L, et al. Molecular and epidemiologic study of multiresistant *Serratia marcescens* infections in a spinal cord injury rehabilitation unit. *Infect Control Hosp Epidemiol* 1988;9: 20–27.
166. Centers for Disease Control and Prevention. Septicemias associated with contaminated intravenous fluids. *MMWR* 1973;22(11,12,1): 99,115,124.
167. Maki DG, Rhame FS, Mackel DC, et al. Nationwide epidemic of septicemia caused by contaminated intravenous products. *Am J Med* 1976;60:471–485.
168. Mayhall CG, Lamb VA, Gayle WE, et al. *Enterobacter cloacae* septicemia in a burn center: epidemiology and control of an outbreak. *J Infect Dis* 1979;139:166–171.
169. Steere AC, Craven PJ, Hall WJ, et al. Person-to-person spread of *Salmonella typhimurium* after a hospital common-source outbreak. *Lancet* 1975;1:319–322.
170. Beecham HJ, Cohen ML, Parkin WE. *Salmonella typhimurium.* Transmission by fiberoptic upper gastrointestinal endoscopy. *JAMA* 1979;241:1013–1015.
171. Lockyer WA, Feinfeld DA, Cherubin CE, et al. An outbreak of *Salmonella* enteritis and septicemia in a population of uremic patients. *Arch Intern Med* 1980;140:943–945.
172. Linnemann CC, Cannon CG, Staneck JL, et al. Prolonged hospital epidemic of salmonellosis: use of trimethoprim-sulfamethoxazole for control. *Infect Control* 1985;6:221–225.
173. Telzak EE, Budnick LD, Greenberg MSZ, et al. A nosocomial outbreak of *Salmonella* enteritidis infection due to the consumption of raw eggs. *N Engl J Med* 1990;323:394–397.
174. McAllister TA, Roud JA, Marshall A, et al. Outbreak of *Salmonella eimsbuettel* in newborn infants spread by rectal thermometers. *Lancet* 1986;2:1262–1264.
175. Khan MA, Abdur-Rab M, Israr N, et al. Transmission of *Salmonella worthington* by oropharyngeal suction in hospital neonatal unit. *Pediatr Infect Dis J* 1991;10:668–672.
176. Centers for Disease Control and Prevention. Epidemics of nosocomial urinary tract infection caused by multiply resistant gram-negative bacilli: epidemiology and control. *J Infect Dis* 1976;133:363–366.
177. Gerding DN, Buxton AE, Hughes RA, et al. Nosocomial multiply resistant *Klebsiella pneumoniae*: epidemiology of an outbreak of apparent index case origin. *Antimicrob Agents Chemother* 1979;15:608–615.
178. Adler JL, Shulman JA, Terry PM, et al. Nosocomial colonization with kanamycin-resistant *Klebsiella pneumoniae* types 2 and 11, in a premature nursery. *J Pediatr* 1970;77:376–385.
179. Mayhall CG, Lamb VA, Bitar CM, et al. Nosocomial Klebsiella infection in a neonatal unit: identification of risk factors for gastrointestinal colonization. *Infect Control* 1980;1:239–246.
180. Hable KA, Matsen JM, Wheeler DJ, et al. *Klebsiella* type 33 septicemia in an infant intensive care unit. *J Pediatr* 1972;80:920–924.
181. Chow AW, Taylor PR, Yoshikawa TT, et al. A nosocomial outbreak of infections due to multiply resistant *Proteus mirabilis:* role of intestinal colonization as a major reservoir. *J Infect Dis* 1979;139:621–627.
182. Burke JP, Ingall D, Klein JO, et al. *Proteus mirabilis* infections in a hospital nursery traced to a human carrier. *N Engl J Med* 1971;284: 115–121.
183. Tucci V, Isenberg HD. Hospital cluster epidemic with *Morganella morganii. J Clin Microbiol* 1981;14:563–566.
184. Parry MF, Hutchinson JH, Brown NA, et al. Gram-negative sepsis in neonates: a nursery outbreak due to hand carriage of *Citrobacter diversus. Pediatrics* 1980;65:1105–1109.
185. Ribeiro CD, Davis P, Jones DM. *Citrobacter koseri* meningitis in a special care baby unit. *J Clin Pathol* 1976;29:1094–1096.
186. Graham DR, Anderson RL, Ariel FE, et al. Epidemic nosocomial meningitis due to *Citrobacter diversus* in neonates. *J Infect Dis* 1981; 144:203–209.
187. Headings DL, Overall JC. Outbreak of meningitis in a newborn intensive care unit caused by a single *Escherichia coli* K1 serotype. *J Pediatr* 1977;90:99–102.
188. Ryder RW, Wachsmuth IK, Buxton AE, et al. Infantile diarrhea produced by heat-stable enterotoxigenic *Escherichia coli. N Engl J Med* 1976;295:849–853.
189. Toivaneen P, Olkkonen L, Toivanen A, et al. Hospital outbreak of *Yersinia enterocolitica* infection. *Lancet* 1973;2:801–803.
190. Ratnam S, Mercer E, Picco B, et al. A nosocomial outbreak of diarrheal disease due to *Yersinia enterocolitica* serotype 0:5, biotype 1. *J Infect Dis* 1982;145:242–247.
191. Adler JI, Anderson RL, Boring JR, et al. A protracted hospital-associated outbreak of salmonellosis due to a multiple-antibiotic resistant strain of *Salmonella indiana. J Pediatr* 1970;77:970–975.
192. Robins-Browne RM, Rowe B, Ramsaroop R, et al. A hospital outbreak of multiresistant *Salmonella typhimurium* belonging to phage type 193. *J Infect Dis* 1983;147:210–216.
193. Lindsey JO, Martin WT, Sonnenwirth AC, et al. An outbreak of nosocomial *Proteus rettgeri* urinary tract infection. *Am J Epidemiol* 1976;103:261–269.
194. Edwards LD, Cross A, Levin S, et al. Outbreak of a nosocomial infection with a strain of *Proteus rettgeri* resistant to many antimicrobials. *Am J Clin Pathol* 1974;61:41–46.
195. Whiteley GR, Penner JL, Stewart IO, et al. Nosocomial urinary tract infections caused by two 0 serotypes of *Providencia stuartii* in one hospital. *J Clin Microbiol* 1977;6:551–554.
196. Brun-Buisson C, Legrand P, Philippon A, et al. Transferable enzymatic resistance to third-generation cephalosporins during nosocomial outbreak of multiresistant *Klebsiella pneumoniae. Lancet* 1987;2: 302–306.
197. Jarlier V, Nicolas MH, Fournier G, et al. Extended broad-spectrum beta-lactamases conferring transferable resistance to newer beta-lactam agents in Enterobacteriaceae: hospital prevalence and susceptibility patterns. *Rev Infect Dis* 1988;10:867–878.
198. Sirot J, Chanal C, Petit A, et al. *Klebsiella pneumoniae* and other Enterobacteriaceae producing novel plasmid-mediated beta-lactamases markedly active against third-generation cephalosporins: epidemiologic studies. *Rev Infect Dis* 1988;10:850–859.
199. Arlet G, Sanson-le Pors MJ, Rouveau M, et al. Outbreak of nosocomial infections due to *Klebsiella pneumoniae* producing SHV-4 beta-lactamase. *Eur J Clin Microbiol Infect Dis* 1990;9:797–803.
200. Papanicolaou GA, Medeiros AA, Jacoby GA. Novel plasmid-mediated beta-lactamase (MIR-1) conferring resistance to oxyimino- and beta-methoxy beta-lactams in clinical isolates of *Klebsiella pneumoniae. Antimicrob Agents Chemother* 1990;34:2200–2209.
201. de Champs C, Rouby D, Guelon D, et al. A case-control study of an outbreak of infections caused by *Klebsiella pneumoniae* strains producing CTX-1 (TEM-3) beta-lactamase. *J Hosp Infect* 1991;18:5–13.
202. Coovadia YM, Johnson AP, Bhana RH, et al. Multiresistant *Klebsiella*

pneumoniae in a neonatal nursery: the importance of maintenance of infection control policies and procedures in the prevention of outbreaks. *J Hosp Infect* 1992;22:197–205.
203. Bauernfeind A, Rosenthal E, Eberlein E, et al. Spread of *Klebsiella pneumoniae* producing SHV-5 beta-lactamase among hospitalized patients. *Infection* 1993;21:18–22.
204. Meyer KS, Urban C, Eagan JA, et al. Nosocomial outbreak of *Klebsiella* infection resistant to late-generation cephalosporins. *Ann Intern Med* 1993;119:353–358.
205. Prodinger WM, Fille M, Bauernfeind A, et al. Molecular epidemiology of *Klebsiella pneumoniae* producing SHV-5 beta-lactamase: parallel outbreaks due to multiple plasmid transfer. *J Clin Microbiol* 1996; 34:564–568.
206. Hobson RP, MacKenzie FM, Gould IM. An outbreak of multiply-resistant *Klebsiella pneumoniae* in the Grampian region of Scotland. *J Hosp Infect* 1996;33:249–262.
207. Pegues DA, Pegues CF, Hibberd PL, et al. Emergence and dissemination of a highly vancomycin-resistant vanA strain of *Enterococcus faecium* at a large teaching hospital. *J Clin Microbiol* 1997;35: 1565–1570.
208. Dunne WM, Wang W. Clonal dissemination and colony morphotype variation of vancomycin-resistant *Enterococcus faecium* isolates in metropolitan Detroit, Michigan. *J Clin Microbiol* 1997;35:388–392.
209. Denessen PJW, Bonten MJM, Weinstein RA. Multiresistant bacteria as a hospital epidemic problem. *Ann Med* 1998;30:176–185.
210. Schiappa DA, Hayden MK, Matushek MG, et al. Ceftazidime-resistant *Klebsiella pneumoniae* and *Escherichia coli* bloodstream infection: a case-control and molecular epidemiologic investigation. *J Infect Dis* 1996;174:529–536.
211. Lucet J-C, Chevret S, Decré D, et al. Outbreak of multiply resistant Enterobacteriaceae in an intensive care unit: epidemiology and risk factors for acquisition. *Clin Infect Dis* 1996;22:430–436.
212. Coudron PE, Moland ES, Sanders C. Occurrence and detection of extended-spectrum beta-lactamases in members of the family Enterobacteriaceae at a veterans medical center: seek and you may find. *J Clin Microbiol* 1997;35:2593–2597.
213. D'Agata E, Venkataraman L, DeGirolami P, et al. Molecular epidemiology of acquisition of ceftazidime-resistant gram-negative bacilli in a nonoutbreak setting. *J Clin Microbiol* 1997;35:2602–2605.
214. Warren JW. Catheter-associated urinary tract infections. *Infect Dis Clin North Am* 1997;11(3):609–622.
215. Platt R, Polk BF, Murdock B, et al. Risk factors for nosocomial urinary tract infection. *Am J Epidemiol* 1986;124:977–985.
216. Stamm WE. Catheter-associated urinary tract infections: epidemiology, pathogenesis, prevention. *Am J Med* 1991;91(suppl 3):65S–71S.
217. Warren JW, Tenney JH, Hoopes JM, et al. A prospective microbiologic study of bacteriuria in patients with chronic indwelling urethral catheters. *J Infect Dis* 1982;146:719–723.
218. Stamm WE, Hooten TM, Johnson JR, et al. Urinary tract infections from pathogenesis to treatment. *J Infect Dis* 1989;159:400–406.
219. Daifuku R, Stamm WE. Association of rectal and urethral colonization with urinary tract infection in patients with indwelling catheters. *JAMA* 1984;252:2028–2030.
220. Krieger JN, Kaiser DL, Wenzel RP. Urinary tract etiology of bloodstream infections in hospitalized patients. *J Infect Dis* 1983;148: 57–62.
221. Stamm WE, Martin SM, Bennett JV. Epidemiology of nosocomial infections due to gram-negative bacilli: aspects relevant to development and use of vaccines. *J Infect Dis* 1977;136(suppl):S151–S160.
222. Craven DE, Steger KA, Barber TW. Preventing nosocomial pneumonia: state of the art and perspectives for the 1990s. *Am J Med* 1991; 91(suppl 3):44S–53S.
223. Ibrahim EH, Ward S, Sherman G, et al. A comparative analysis of patients with early-onset vs late-onset nosocomial pneumonia in the ICU setting. *Chest* 2000;117(5):1434–1442.
224. Donowitz LG, Page MC, Mileur GL, et al. Alteration of normal gastric flora in critical care patients receiving antacid and cimetidine therapy. *Infect Control* 1986;7:23–26.
225. The Society for Hospital Epidemiology of America, the Association for Practitioners in Infection Control, the Centers for Disease Control, the Surgical Infection Society. Consensus paper on the surveillance of surgical wound infections. *Infect Control Hosp Epidemiol* 1992;13:599–605.
226. Nichols RL. Surgical wound infection. *Am J Med* 1991;91(suppl 3): 64S.
227. Baine WB, Gangerosa EJ, Bonnett JV, et al. CDC News. Institutional salmonellosis. *J Infect Dis* 1973;128:357.
228. DuPont HL. Nosocomial salmonella and shigellosis. *Infect Control Hosp Epidemiol* 1991;12:707–709.
229. Riley LW, Ceballos BSO, Trabulsi LR, et al. The significance of hospitals as reservoirs for endemic multiresistant *Salmonella typhimurium* causing infection in urban Brazilian children. *J Infect Dis* 1984; 150:236–241.
230. Paton S, Nicolle L, Mwongera M, et al. *Salmonella* and *Shigella* gastroenteritis at a public teaching hospital in Nairobi, Kenya. *Infect Control Hosp Epidemiol* 1991;12:710–717.
231. Werkel CS, Guerrant RL. Nosocomial salmonellosis. *Infect Control* 1985;6:218–220.
232. Standaert SM, Hutcheson RH, Schaffner W. Nosocomial transmission of *Salmonella* gastroenteritis to laundry workers in a nursing home. *Infect Control Hosp Epidemiol* 1994;15:22–26.
233. Smart MR. *Salmonella typhi. Can Epidemiol Bull* 1972;16:128–129.
234. Datta N, Pridie RB, Anderson ES. An outbreak of infection with *Salmonella typhimurium* in a general hospital. *J Hyg* 1960;58: 229–241.
235. Weissman JB, Hutcheson RH. Shigellosis transmitted by nurses. *South Med J* 1976;69(10):1341–1346.
236. Pillay DG, Karas JA, Pillay A, et al. Nosocomial transmission of *Shigella dysenteriae* type 1. *J Hosp Infect* 1997;37(3):199–205.
237. Eyre JWH. Asylum dysentery in relation to *B. dysenteriae. BMJ* 1904; 1:1002–1004.
238. Karmali MA, Arbus GS, Petric M, et al. Hospital-acquired *Escherichia coli* O157:H7 associated haemolytic uraemic syndrome in a nurse. *Lancet* 1988;1(8584):526.
239. Kohli HS, Chaudhuri AK, Todd WT, et al. A severe outbreak of *E. coli* O157:H7 in two psychogeriatric wards. *J Public Health Med* 1994; 16(1):11–15.
240. Preston M, Borczyk A, Davidson R. Hospital outbreak of *Escherichia coli* O157:H7 associated with a rare phage type—Ontario. *Can Commun Dis Rep* 1997;23(5):33–36; discussion 36–37.
241. Cheasty T, Robertson R, Chart H, et al. The use of serodiagnosis in the retrospective investigation of a nursery outbreak associated with *Escherichia coli* O157:H7. *J Clin Pathol* 1998;51(7):498–501.
242. Weightman NC, Kirby PJ. Nosocomial *Escherichia coli* O157 infection. *J Hosp Infect* 2000;44(2):107–111.
243. Weber DJ, Rutala WA. The emerging nosocomial pathogens Cryptosporidium, *Escherichia coli* O157:H7, *Helicobacter pylori,* and hepatitis C: epidemiology, environmental survival, efficacy of disinfection, and control measures. *Infect Control Hosp Epidemiol* 2001;22(5): 306–315.
244. McIntyre M, Unochiri E. A case of hospital-acquired *Yersinia enterocolitica* gastroenteritis. *J Hosp Infect* 1986;7:299–301.
245. Cannon CG, Linnemann CC. *Yersinia enterocolitica* infections in hospitalized patients: the problem of hospital-acquired infections. *Infect Control Hosp Epidemiol* 1992;13:139–143.
246. Jarvis WR. *Yersinia enterocolitica:* a new or unrecognized nosocomial pathogen? *Infect Control Hosp Epidemiol* 1992;13:137–138.
247. Vallés J, Leon C, Alvarez-Lerma F. Nosocomial bacteremia in critically ill patients: a multicenter study evaluating epidemiology and prognosis. *Clin Infect Dis* 1997;24:387–395.
248. Gransden WR, Elykyn SJ, Phillips I, et al. Bacteremia due to *Escherichia coli:* a study of 861 episodes. *Rev Infect Dis* 1990;12: 1008–1018.
249. Watanakunakorn C, Weber J. *Enterobacter* bacteremia: a review of 58 episodes. *Scand J Infect Dis* 1989;21:1–8.
250. Bouza E, Garcia de la Toree M, Erice A, et al. *Enterobacter* bacteremia. An analysis of 50 episodes. *Arch Intern Med* 1985;145:1024–1027.
251. Chow JW, Fine MJ, Shlaes DM, et al. *Enterobacter* bacteremia: clinical features and emergence of antibiotic resistance during therapy. *Ann Intern Med* 1991;115:585–590.

252. Gallagher PG. *Enterobacter* bacteremia in pediatric patients. *Rev Infect Dis* 1990;12:808–812.
253. Burchard KW, Barrall DT, Reed M, et al. *Enterobacter* bacteremia in surgical patients. *Surgery* 1986;100:857–861.
254. Weischer M, Kolmos HJ. Retrospective 6-year study of *Enterobacter* bacteraemia in a Danish university hospital. *J Hosp Infect* 1992;20: 15–24.
255. Garcia de la Torre MG, Romero-Vivas J, Martinez-Beltran J, et al. *Klebsiella* bacteremia: an analysis of 100 episodes. *Rev Infect Dis* 1985; 7:143–150.
256. Watanakunakorn C, Jura J. *Klebsiella* bacteremia: a review of 196 episodes during a decade (1980–1989). *Scand J Infect Dis* 1991;23: 399–405.
257. Bodey GP, Elting LS, Rodriguez S, et al. *Klebsiella* bacteremia. A 10 year review in a cancer institution. *Cancer* 1989;64:2368–2376.
258. Feldman C, Smith C, Levy H, et al. *Klebsiella pneumoniae* bacteraemia at an urban general hospital. *J Infect* 1990;20:21–31.
259. Montgomerie JZ, Ota JK. *Klebsiella* bacteremia. *Arch Intern Med* 1980;140:525–527.
260. Tsay RW, Siu LK, Fung CP, et al. Characteristics of bacteremia between community-acquired and nosocomial *Klebsiella pneumoniae* infection: risk factor for mortality and the impact of capsular serotypes as a herald for community-acquired infection. *Arch Intern Med* 2002; 162(9):1021–1027.
261. Kim BN, Woo JH, Kim MN, et al. Clinical implications of extended-spectrum beta-lactamase-producing *Klebsiella pneumoniae* bacteraemia. *J Hosp Infect* 2002;52(2):99–106.
262. Siu LK, Lu PL, Hsueh PR, et al. Bacteremia due to extended-spectrum beta-lactamase-producing *Escherichia coli* and *Klebsiella pneumoniae* in a pediatric oncology ward: clinical features and identification of different plasmids carrying both SHV-5 and TEM-1 genes. *J Clin Microbiol* 1999;37(12):4020–4027.
263. Drelichman V, Band JD. Bacteremias due to *Citrobacter diversus* and *Citrobacter freundii.* Incidence, risk factors, clinical outcome. *Arch Intern Med* 1985;145:1808–1810.
264. Samonis G, Anaissie E, Elting L, et al. Review of *Citrobacter* bacteremia in cancer patients over a sixteen-year period. *Eur J Clin Microbiol Infect Dis* 1991;10:479–485.
265. Chen YS, Wong WW, Fung CP, et al. Clinical features and antimicrobial susceptibility trends in *Citrobacter freundii* bacteremia. *J Microbiol Immunol Infect* 2002;35(2):109–114.
266. Yu WL, Lin CW, Wang DY. *Serratia marcescens* bacteremia: clinical features and antimicrobial susceptibilities of the isolates. *J Microbiol Immunol Infect* 1998;31(3):171–179.
267. Durand ML, Calderwood SB, Weber DJ, et al. Acute bacterial meningitis in adults. A review of 493 episodes. *N Engl J Med* 1993;328: 21–28.
268. Mangi RJ, Quintiani R, Andriole VT. Gram-negative bacillary meningitis. *Am J Med* 1975;59:829–836.
269. Lu CH, Chang WN, Chang HW. *Klebsiella* meningitis in adults: clinical features, prognostic factors and therapeutic outcomes. *J Clin Neurosci* 2002;9(5):533–538.
270. Booth LV, Palmer JD, Pateman J, et al. *Citrobacter diversus* ventriculitis and brain abscesses in an adult. *J Infect* 1993;26:207–209.
271. Yildiran A, Siga E, Baykal S, et al. Sepsis and multiple brain abscesses caused by *Salmonella paratyphi* B in an infant: successful treatment with sulbactam-ampicillin and surgical drainage. *Turk J Pediatr* 2001; 43(1):85–87.
272. Campbell JR, Diacovo T, Baker CJ. *Serratia marcescens* meningitis in neonates. *Pediatr Infect Dis J* 1992;11:881–886.
273. Bauer TM, Ofner E, Just HM, et al. An epidemiological study assessing the relative importance of airborne and direct contact transmission of microorganisms in a medical intensive care unit. *J Hosp Infect* 1990; 15:301–309.
274. Casewell M, Phillips I. Hands as transmission for *Klebsiella* species. *Br Med J* 1977;2:1315–1317.
275. Adams BG, Marrie TJ. Hand carriage of aerobic gram-negative rods by health care personnel. *J Hyg* 1982;89:23–31.
276. Adams BG, Marrie TJ. Hand carriage of aerobic gram-negative rods may not be transient. *J Hyg* 1982;89:33–46.
277. Albert RK, Condie F. Handwashing patterns in medical intensive care units. *N Engl J Med* 1981;304:1465–1466.
278. Preston MA, Larson E, Stamm WE. The effect of private isolation rooms on patient care practices, colonization and infection in an intensive care unit. *Am J Med* 1981;70:641–645.
279. Larson E, McGeer A, Quroshi ZA, et al. Effect of an automated sink on handwashing practices and attitudes in high-risk units. *Infect Control Hosp Epidemiol* 1991;12:422–428.
280. Flaherty JP, Weinstein RA. Infection control and pneumonia prophylaxis strategies in the intensive care unit. *Semin Respir Infect* 1990;5: 191–203.
281. Boyce JM, Larson EL, Weinstein RA. Alcohol-based hand gels and hand hygiene in hospitals. *Lancet* 2002;360(9344):1509–1510.
282. Harbarth S, Pittet D, Grady L, et al. Interventional study to evaluate the impact of an alcohol-based hand gel in improving hand hygiene compliance. *Pediatr Infect Dis J* 2002;21(6):489–495.
283. Boyce JM, Pittet D. Guideline for hand hygiene in health-care settings. Recommendations of the Healthcare Infection Control Practices Advisory Committee and the HICPAC/SHEA/APIC/IDSA Hand Hygiene Task Force. *MMWR Recomm Rep* 2002;51(RR-16): 1–45.
284. Weinstein RA, Nathan C, Gruensfelder R, et al. Endemic aminoglycoside resistant in gram-negative bacilli: epidemiology and mechanisms. *J Infect Dis* 1980;141:338–349.
285. Doebbeling BN, Pfaller MA, Houston AK, et al. Removal of nosocomial pathogens from the contaminated glove implications for glove reuse and handwashing. *Ann Intern Med* 1988;109:394–398.
286. Klein BS, Perloff WH, Maki DG. Reduction of nosocomial infection during pediatric intensive care by protective isolation. *N Engl J Med* 1989;320:1714–1721.
287. Leclair JM, Freeman J, Sullivan BF, et al. Prevention of nosocomial respiratory syncytial virus infections through compliance with glove and gown isolation precautions. *N Engl J Med* 1987;317:329–334.
288. Bonten MJ, Weinstein RA. Infection control in intensive care units and prevention of ventilator-associated pneumonia. *Semin Respir Infect* 2000;15(4):327–335.
289. French GL, Shannon KP, Simmons N. Hospital outbreak of *Klebsiella pneumoniae* resistant to broad-spectrum cephalosporins and beta-lactam-beta-lactamase inhibitor combinations by hyperproduction of SHV-5 beta-lactamase. *J Clin Microbiol* 1996;34:358–363.
290. Leverstein-van Hall MA, Fluit AC, Blok HE, et al. Control of nosocomial multiresistant Enterobacteriaceae using a temporary restrictive antibiotic agent policy. *Eur J Clin Microbiol Infect Dis* 2001;20(11): 785–791.
291. Brun-Buisson C, Legrand P, Rauss A, et al. Intestinal decontamination for control of nosocomial multiresistant gram-negative bacilli: study of an outbreak in an intensive care unit. *Ann Intern Med* 1989; 110:873–881.
292. Gardam MA, Burrows LL, Kus JV, et al. Is surveillance for multidrug-resistant Enterobacteriaceae an effective infection control strategy in the absence of an outbreak? *J Infect Dis* 2002;186(12):1754–1760.
293. Nystrom B, Frederici H, van Euler C. Bacterial colonization and infection in an intensive care unit. *Intensive Care Med* 1988;14:34–38.
294. Petersdorf RG, Custin JA, Hoeprich PD, et al. A study of antibiotic prophylaxis in unconscious patients. *N Engl J Med* 1957;257: 1001–1009.
295. Petersdorf RG, Merchant RK. A study of antibiotic prophylaxis in patients with acute heart failure. *N Engl J Med* 1959;260:565–575.
296. Mandelli M, Mosconi P, Langer M, et al. Prevention of pneumonia in an intensive care unit: a randomized multicenter clinical trial. *Crit Care Med* 1989;17:501–505.
297. Sirvent JM, Torres A, El-Ebiary M, et al. Protective effect of intravenously administered cefuroxime against nosocomial pneumonia in patients with structural coma. *Am J Respir Crit Care Med* 1997;155: 1729–1734.
298. Klick JM, du Moulin GC, Hedley-Whyte J, et al. Prevention of gram-negative bacillary pneumonia using polymyxin aerosol as prophylaxis. *J Clin Invest* 1975;55:514–519.
299. Feeley TW, duMoulin GC, Hedley-Whyte J, et al. Aerosol polymyxin

and pneumonia in seriously ill patients. *N Engl J Med* 1975;293: 471–475.

300. Klastersky J, Huysmans G, Weerts D, et al. Endotracheally administered gentamicin for the prevention of infections of the respiratory tract in patients with tracheostomy: a double-blind study. *Chest* 1974; 65:650–654.
301. D'Amico R, Pifferi S, Leonetti C, et al. Effectiveness of antibiotic prophylaxis in critically ill adult patients: systemic review of randomised controlled trials. *Br Med J* 1998;316:1275–1285.
302. Selective Decontamination of the Digestive Tract Trialists' Collaborative Group. Meta-analysis of randomised controlled trials of selective decontamination of the digestive tract. *Br Med J* 1993;307:525–532.
303. Vandenbroucke-Grauls CMJE, Vandenbroucke JP. Effect of selective decontamination of the digestive tract on respiratory tract infections and mortality in the intensive care unit. *Lancet* 1991;338:859–862.
304. Kollef MH. The role of selective digestive tract decontamination on mortality and respiratory tract infections: a meta-analysis. *Chest* 1994; 105:1101–1108.
305. Heyland DK, Cook DJ, Jaeschke R, et al. Selective decontamination of the digestive tract. *Chest* 1994;105:1221–1129.
306. Nathens AB, Marshall JC. Selective decontamination of the digestive tract in surgical patients: a systematic review of the evidence. *Arch Surg* 1999;134(2):170–176.
307. van Nieuwenhoven CA, Buskens E, van Tiel FH, et al. Relationship between methodological trial quality and the effects of selective digestive decontamination on pneumonia and mortality in critically ill patients. *JAMA* 2001;286(3):335–340.
308. Villar J, Carroli G, Beliz JM. Predictive ability of meta-analyses of randomised controlled trials. *Lancet* 1995;345:772–776.
309. Borzak S, Ridker PM. Discordance between meta-analyses and large-scale randomized, controlled trials. Examples from the management of acute myocardial infarction. *Ann Intern Med* 1995;123:873–877.
310. Sun X, Wagner DP, Knaus WA. Does selective decontamination of the digestive tract reduce mortality for severely ill patients? *Crit Care Med* 1996;24:753–755.
311. Jacobs S, Foweraker JE, Roberts SE. Effectiveness of selective decontamination of the digestive tract in an ICU with a policy encouraging a low gastric pH. *Clin Intensive Care* 1992;3:52–58.
312. Blair P, Rowlands BJ, Lowry K, et al. Selective decontamination of the digestive tract: a stratified, randomized, prospective study in a mixed intensive care unit. *Surgery* 1991;110:303–310.
313. Krueger WA, Lenhart FP, Neeser G, et al. Influence of combined intravenous and topical antibiotic prophylaxis on the incidence of infections, organ dysfunctions, and mortality in critically ill surgical patients: a prospective, stratified, randomized, double-blind, placebo-controlled clinical trial. *Am J Respir Crit Care Med* 2002;166(8): 1029–1037.
314. Hammond JMJ, Potgieter PD, Saunders GL, et al. Double-blind study of selective decontamination of the digestive tract in intensive care. *Lancet* 1992;340:5–9.
315. Hamer DH, Barza M. Prevention of hospital-acquired pneumonia in critically ill patients. *Antimicrob Agents Chemother* 1993;37:931–938.
316. Webb CH. Antibiotic resistance associated with selective decontamination of the digestive tract. *J Hosp Infect* 1992;22:1–5.
317. Daschner F. Emergence of resistance during selective decontamination of the digestive tract. *Eur J Clin Microbiol Infect Dis* 1992;11: 1–3.
318. Lingnau W, Berger J, Javorsky F, et al. Changing bacterial ecology during a five-year period of selective intestinal decontamination. *J Hosp Infect* 1998;39(3):195–206.
319. Taylor ME, Oppenheim BA. Selective decontamination of the gastrointestinal tract as an infection control measure. *J Hosp Infect* 1991; 17:271.
320. Baumgartner JD, McCutchan JA, van Melle G. Prevention of gram-negative shock and death in surgical patients by antibody to endotoxin core glycolipid. *Lancet* 1985;1:59–62.
321. The Intravenous Immunoglobulin Collaborative Study Group. Prophylactic intravenous administration of standard immune globulin as compared with core-lipopolysaccharide immune globulin in patients at high risk of postsurgical infection. *N Engl J Med* 1992;327: 234–240.
322. Fanaroff AA, Korones SB, Wright LL, et al. A controlled trial of intravenous immune globulin to reduce nosocomial infections in very low birth weight infants. *N Engl J Med* 1994;330:1107–1113.
323. Donta ST, Peduzzi P, Cross AS, et al. Immunoprophylaxis against *Klebsiella* and *Pseudomonas aeruginosa* infections. *J Infect Dis* 1996; 174:537–543.
324. Langermann S, Palaszynski S, Barnhart M, et al. Prevention of mucosal *Escherichia coli* infection by FimH-adhesin-based systemic vaccination. *Science* 1997;276:607–611.
325. Maki DG, Cobb L, Garman JK, et al. An attachable silver-impregnated cuff for prevention of infection with central venous catheters: a prospective randomized multicenter trial. *Am J Med* 1988;85: 307–314.
326. Adair CG, Gorman SP, Feron BM, et al. Implications of endotracheal tube biofilm for ventilator-associated pneumonia. *Intensive Care Med* 1999;25(10):1072–1076.

34

NONFERMENTATIVE GRAM-NEGATIVE BACILLI

JOHN P. FLAHERTY
VALENTINA STOSOR

Nonfermentative gram-negative bacilli are a diverse array of microorganisms that have evolved in aquatic environments, have minimal growth requirements, and differ substantially in virulence. Included in this category are *Pseudomonas aeruginosa,* other *Pseudomonas* species, and genera such as *Stenotrophomonas, Acinetobacter, Burkholderia, Flavobacterium,* and *Achromobacter.* During the past half-century, nonfermentative gram-negative bacilli have become significant nosocomial pathogens because of the many reservoirs they inhabit in hospitals and the resistance of these microorganisms to commonly used antibiotics. Furthermore, the virulence of *P. aeruginosa* and its frequency as a nosocomial pathogen have been important factors impelling increased use of antipseudomonal β-lactam antibiotics and quinolones as presumptive therapy where *P. aeruginosa* is a potential pathogen.

MICROORGANISM CHARACTERISTICS

Pathogenicity

The pathogenicity of nonfermentative gram-negative bacilli depends on several capabilities, most notably attachment to host cells, production of extracellular polysaccharide (biofilm matrix) and extracellular toxins (exotoxins), resistance to serum bactericidal factors, and the presence of a lipopolysaccharide cell wall (endotoxin). These features have been studied most extensively in *P. aeruginosa* (formerly *P. pyocyanea*), which is the most virulent of the nonfermentative gram-negative bacilli. Healthy individuals are repeatedly exposed to this bacterium, which is ubiquitous in our environment. When host epithelial cell barriers are intact, *P. aeruginosa* is not a significant pathogen. But when skin and mucosal surfaces are disrupted by mechanical ventilation, burn wounds, corneal abrasion, indwelling catheters, or cytotoxic chemotherapy in the setting of a compromised immune system, *P. aeruginosa* infection may result. Bacterial attachment to host epithelial cells typically precedes infection at many sites, and patients whose epithelial cells permit greater *P. aeruginosa* attachment more often become colonized by *P. aeruginosa* than do other patients (1). Attachment of *P. aeruginosa* is achieved primarily by pili, or fimbriae, which project outward from the bacterial cell surface, are associated with virulence (2), and have specific molecular sequences that act as ligands for host cell receptors (3). It has been shown in animal models that adherence of *P. aeruginosa* to tracheal and corneal epithelium is enhanced by epithelial cell injury due to viral infection or trauma that may expose additional binding sites (4,5), such as laminin (6). Attachment of *P. aeruginosa* is inhibited by fibronectin (7), and diminished levels of fibronectin are associated with increased adherence of *P. aeruginosa* to epithelial cells (8).

Biofilms are communities of microbes embedded in an organic polymer matrix adherent to an inert or living surface. Biofilm formation by *P. aeruginosa* may play an important role in the pathogenesis of central venous catheter–related infection, urinary catheter cystitis, contact lens–associated corneal infection, lung infection in cystic fibrosis, and ventilator-associated pneumonia (9). A recent study reports that the extracellular matrix of the biofilm produced by *P. aeruginosa* is extracellular DNA rather than glycocalyx (10). This extracellular matrix appears to facilitate adherence (11,12), and it confers partial resistance by inhibiting antibody coating, phagocytosis, and intracellular killing by leukocytes (9,13–15). Even in individuals with normal cellular and humoral immune function, biofilm-related infections are rarely resolved by the host defense mechanisms (9). Antibiotic therapy typically eliminates the symptoms caused by the planktonic cells released from the biofilm but fails to kill the biofilm. As a result, biofilm infections typically show recurring symptoms, until the sessile population of bacteria is surgically removed from the host. The most intuitive explanation for the diminished activity of antibiotics in biofilms is that polymeric substances like those that make up the matrix of biofilms retard the diffusion of antibiotics. Aminoglycosides, in particular, have been reported to diffuse slowly, perhaps because they bind to extracellular polymers. A second hypothesis is that nutrient limitation leads to slow growth or stationary phase existence for many of the cells in a biofilm, reducing their antibiotic susceptibility. For example, in one *P. aeruginosa* biofilm system, ciprofloxacin and tobramycin penetrated biofilm but failed to kill the bacteria (16). Oxygen limitation and low metabolic activity in the interior of the biofilm, not poor antibiotic penetration, were correlated with antibiotic failure.

Exotoxins of *P. aeruginosa* contribute significantly to virulence, and the most potent of these is exotoxin A. Exotoxin A is a secreted adenosine ribosyltransferase that inhibits protein synthesis in eukaryotic cells by modifying the structure of elongation factor-2 (17). Exotoxin A is produced by most clinical isolates of *P. aeruginosa* and has potent local and systemic effects. These include necrosis of soft tissues into which sublethal doses are injected (18), and shock and hepatocellular necrosis following systemic administration (19). Although experimental models of local infection have not consistently shown enhanced virulence of *P. aeruginosa* isolates that produce exotoxin A (20,21), studies of bacteremic infection in humans indicate an important role (22,23). Exoenzyme S is another extracellular enzyme of *P. aeruginosa* that causes tissue injury and increases virulence (24, 25).

Extracellular proteases of *P. aeruginosa*, most notably elastase and alkaline protease, contribute to adherence (11,26) and probably to virulence. Although there is no clear association of these enzymes with a worse outcome of bacteremic infection (27), purified preparations of these enzymes cause necrosis of connective tissues, apparently by breaking down elastin, laminin, and collagen (28,29). In animal models, strains of *P. aeruginosa* that produce elastase have an enhanced ability to cause soft tissue infection compared to elastase-deficient mutants (20). These proteases can also inactivate complement components and cleave immunoglobulin G (IgG) and IgA, particularly in patients with cystic fibrosis (30,31). Finally, *in vitro* studies have shown that elastase and alkaline protease degrade cytokines, including interleukin-2, interferon-γ, and tumor necrosis factor-α (32–34).

Other extracellular protein enzymes with demonstrated toxicity against eukaryotic cells are phospholipase C, a heat-stable hemolysin, and a cytotoxin (35–37). The first two degrade phospholipids and lecithin, hemolyze erythrocytes, and cause tissue destruction. The cytotoxin damages most eukaryotic cell membranes and has a cytopathic effect on polymorphonuclear leukocytes (38).

The pathogenicity of *P. aeruginosa* also is enhanced by its lipopolysaccharide cell wall, which, like that of other gram-negative bacilli, is composed of a long-chain polysaccharide, a core polysaccharide, and lipid A. Lipid A has been shown to produce most of the effects of endotoxin, which include release of interleukin-1 and tumor necrosis factor, complement activation, initiation of disseminated intravascular coagulation, and activation or release of mediators of vascular tone. Antibodies directed against *P. aeruginosa* lipopolysaccharide have been shown to enhance phagocytosis and improve survival in experimental models of *P. aeruginosa* infection (39–41). In humans, these antibodies appear to protect against a lethal outcome of *P. aeruginosa* sepsis (22,42).

Quorum sensing allows bacteria to detect the density of their own species and alter their metabolism to take advantage of this density. *Pseudomonas* utilizes quorum sensing systems to control expression of virulence factors, including biofilm formation and exoenzyme and toxin production. Quorum sensing systems regulate gene expression in a population-dependent manner. Small diffusible signal molecules called acyl-homoserine lactones are secreted by *P. aeruginosa*. At a specific cell density, the concentration of these molecules becomes sufficient to activate transcriptional regulator proteins and induce gene transcription. At least 39 quorum sensing-regulated genes have been identified in *P. aeruginosa* (43). At least two quorum sensing systems have been identified in *P. aeruginosa*: the *las* and *rhl* systems. The autoinducer molecule PAI-1 activates the LasR protein, which enhances the transcription of extracellular virulence factors including alkaline protease, toxin A, and two different elastases. The formation of a normal, dense biofilm is also dependent on the synthesis of PAI-1 (44,45). The autoinducer molecule PAI-2 binds RhlR and initiates transcription of several different genes involved in a variety of adaptations including biofilm formation. *P. aeruginosa* strains with inactivated quorum sensing systems demonstrate significantly diminished virulence in animal models of infection (46).

Some *P. aeruginosa* isolates harbor the type III secretion system. The type III secretion system uses a complex secretion/translocation mechanism to inject effector proteins directly into adjacent host cells (47). These effector proteins are postulated to interrupt eukaryotic signal transduction and cause apoptotic cell death. Infection with type-III–secreting isolates of *P. aeruginosa* has been associated with worse clinical outcomes in patients with ventilator-associated pneumonia and bloodstream infection (48,49).

The pathogenesis of *P. aeruginosa* infection is complex, involving an interaction of bacterial pathogenicity factors with the host's immune system (50,51). Key components of immunity to invasive infection are polymorphonuclear leukocytes (52,53) and antibodies against the lipopolysaccharide cell wall (54,55). A role for cellular immunity also is suggested by reports of invasive pseudomonal infection in patients with cellular immune impairment (56,57) and is supported by experimental findings involving T cells (58–60).

By most measures, *Stenotrophomonas maltophilia* (formerly *Pseudomonas maltophilia* and then *Xanthomonas maltophilia*) is not particularly virulent. In the burned mouse model, inocula of 3×10^7 colony-forming units (CFU)/mL of *S. maltophilia* failed to establish lethal infection (61). In contrast, only 2×10^2 CFU/mL of *P. aeruginosa* caused fatal infection in all of the animals studied. Nevertheless, *S. maltophilia* can cause serious infection in compromised hosts. The majority of *S. maltophilia* strains produce protease, elastase, DNase, lipase and fibrinolysin, and these extracellular enzymes are potential virulence factors (62–64). Particularly significant protease and elastase production was identified in a clinical isolate of *S. maltophilia* from a leukemic patient with bacteremia and ecthyma gangrenosum mimicking both the clinical and virulence properties of *P. aeruginosa* (65). Non-*aeruginosa* pseudomonads do not appear to produce exotoxin A (61,66).

Burkholderia cepacia, originally described in 1950 as a cause of soft rot in onions (Latin: *coepa*) and previously named eugonic oxidizer group 1 (EO-1), *Pseudomonas kingii, Pseudomonas multivorans, Pseudomonas alcaligenes* IVc, and *Pseudomonas cepacia,* is an extremely versatile bacterium capable of utilizing a wide variety of nutrients for growth. It thrives in natural water sources and can proliferate in tap or distilled water, presumably by utilizing trace elements and low concentrations of organic materials (67–71). The term *genomovar* has been used to denote phenotypically similar but genotypically distinct groups of *B. cepacia* strains. The *B. cepacia* complex includes nine genomovars: *B. cepacia* genomovars I, III, and VI, *Burkholderia multivorans* (formerly genomovar II), *Burkholderia stabilis* (formerly genomovar IV), *Burkholderia vietnamiensis* (formerly genomovar V), *Burkholderia ambifaria*, *Burkholderia anthina*, and *Burkholderia pyrrocinia* (72). Strains representing each genomovar have been associated with opportunistic infections in humans (73). In animal models, *B. cepacia* is not pathogenic except in extremely large inocula (61,70). Even direct injection of contaminated fluids into immunocompetent patients may result in only transient fever or colonization (71,74). *B. cepacia* is considerably less virulent than *P. aeruginosa* in the burned mouse model (61). Like *S. maltophilia, B. cepacia* can produce significant disease in the compromised patient. In an assessment of nosocomial *B. cepacia* infections reported to the Centers for Disease Control and Prevention's National Nosocomial Infections Surveillance (NNIS) system between 1980 and 1985, infection was judged to have caused or contributed to death in 11% of cases (75). Virulence properties are not well understood, but *B. cepacia* is known to produce a number of extracellular products, including hemolysins, proteases, and lipases (76). However, the role these play in disease is uncertain. The ability of *B. cepacia* to acquire iron is a virulence factor that may play a role in colonization and contribute to severity in lung infection (77). *B. cepacia* produces at least four iron-binding siderophores, including salicylic acid, ornibactin, pyochelin, and cepabactin. Mutant strains with attenuated ornibactin synthesis demonstrate attenuated virulence in both acute and chronic animal models of infection (77). *B. cepacia* can enter and survive intracellularly in cultured macrophages and pulmonary epithelial cells, which may provide a protected niche, allowing persistent infection (78). Like *P. aeruginosa, B. cepacia* utilizes quorum sensing or autoinduction to regulate extracellular virulence factor production (79). The quorum sensing system of *B. cepacia* may also respond to interspecies signals from *P. aeruginosa* (80).

Acinetobacter, formerly classified as *Mima, Herellea, Moraxella, Neisseria, Bacterium, Alcaligenes, Achromobacter,* and *Pseudomonas,* is widely distributed in nature and is part of the normal flora of many animal species and humans (81,82). By DNA hybridization, there may be as many as 17 genomic species (83). *Acinetobacter* is an uncommon pathogen (84,85) that usually infects immunocompromised or debilitated hosts and sometimes causes outbreaks in intensive care units (ICU) (86–88). Outcome of bloodstream and respiratory infection has correlated more consistently with underlying illness and manifestations of infection than with the strain of *Acinetobacter* or the appropriateness of antibiotic therapy (85–87,89). Isolation of *Acinetobacter* is of uncertain significance in most nosocomial settings. In contrast, community-acquired *Acinetobacter* pneumonia has been associated with a fulminant course and high infection-related mortality (90). The factors that explain this disparity remain to be determined; little is known regarding the pathogenesis of *Acinetobacter* infection or the elaboration of specific virulence factors.

Similarly, the pathogenesis or virulence properties of other nonfermenters have not been fully elucidated. *Sphingomonas paucimobilis* appears to have limited inherent virulence, but it does have endotoxin activity and produces alkaline and acid phosphatases and several esterases (91,92). A report of *Shewanella putrefaciens* causing refractory ulcerative cellulitis and septic shock suggested possible exotoxin production (93).

Resistance to Antimicrobial Agents

P. aeruginosa and other nonfermentative gram-negative bacilli are resistant to many common antibiotics, including first- and second-generation cephalosporins. Only advanced-generation cephalosporins, extended-spectrum penicillins, carbapenems, aminoglycosides, and fluoroquinolones generally offer any useful activity (84,94–97). Increased resistance across many classes of antimicrobial agents is a concerning trend exhibited by all of the clinically important nonfermentative gram-negative bacteria (98,99). Mechanisms of resistance to each class of antibiotics are diverse, and more than one mechanism may contribute to resistance to some antibiotics (100). Antimicrobial resistance exhibited by the clinically important nonfermentative gram-negative pathogens is discussed below. Other nonfermenters that are less commonly encountered have varying antimicrobial susceptibility patterns (95,101–103). Treatment of infections caused by these pathogens is typically guided by susceptibility testing of individual isolates.

For *P. aeruginosa*, inherent mechanisms such as outer cell membrane permeability factors and active drug efflux systems result in reduced susceptibility to many antimicrobial agents (100,104). Efflux pumps (100,104,105) play a role in reduced susceptibility to sulfonamides, tetracycline, macrolides, fluoroquinolones (106), penicillins (107), cephalosporins (107), meropenem (108), and even the aminoglycosides (109). All *P. aeruginosa* inherently produce the AmpC β-lactamase that hydrolyzes penicillins and cephalosporins (105). Additionally, acquired β-lactamases are responsible for penicillin, and first- and second-generation cephalosporin resistance (104,105). Production of a number of extended-spectrum β-lactamases is reported with increasing frequency, resulting in resistance to advanced-generation cephalosporins, monobactams, and extended-spectrum penicillins, depending on the enzyme(s) present (104,105). Changes in penicillin binding proteins are a relatively uncommon mechanism of β-lactam resistance in *P. aeruginosa* (100, 110). Reduced activity of carbapenems, when present, is mainly attributed to reduced accumulation of the drug via downregulation of carbapenem-specific porin production (108,111,112); however, carbapenemase production is reported with increasing frequency (113,114). Aminoglycosides are inactivated by enzymatic modification via the acquisition of plasmids carrying any of a number of such enzymes. The rise in fluoroquinolone resistance among *P. aeruginosa* is remarkable (98,99); mutations in the topoisomerase genes, *gyrA* and *parC*, are the genetic basis for such resistance (115–118), in addition to resistance caused by active efflux and membrane impermeability. Based on recent surveillance studies, amikacin, tobramycin, carbapenems, piperacillin/tazobactam, piperacillin, ceftazidime, and cefepime remain the most active antipseudomonal agents (95,98,99,119, 120).

S. maltophilia demonstrates high-level resistance to many antimicrobial agent classes including the β-lactams, tetracyclines, and aminoglycosides (64,121,122). Fluoroquinolone agents have unreliable activity against this pathogen (64,95). As a rule, the carbapenems are hydrolyzed by a chromosomally encoded zinc-dependent β-lactamase possessed by most strains, thus rendering these agents ineffective for the treatment of *S. maltophilia* infections. The most reliable agents include trimethoprim/sulfamethoxazole and ticarcillin/clavulanate (64,95,123,124).

B. cepacia complex strains are resistant to most antibiotics commonly used for treatment of gram-negative bacterial infections, including the extended-spectrum penicillins and aminoglycosides (95,97,125). The most active antimicrobial agents are ceftazidime, the carbapenems, and the fluoroquinolones (64). Antimicrobial resistance is more common among isolates recovered from patients with cystic fibrosis (97). Effective therapy is further limited by the fact that *in vitro* susceptibility does not necessarily predict clinical response to antimicrobials in this patient population (126). Typically, serious infections are treated with combinations of antimicrobial agents.

Acinetobacter varies substantially in its susceptibility to specific antibiotics, and resistance has steadily increased over the past three decades (84,127). Multiple drug resistance has emerged (64), and alarmingly, outbreaks caused by *Acinetobacter* strains that are resistant to imipenem, ceftazidime, amikacin, and all other routinely tested antibiotics have been reported (128–131). Appropriate therapy in such circumstances is unclear. A variety of antibiotic combinations appear to be synergistic *in vitro* (132,133), and combination therapy or alternative agents such as minocycline or ampicillin-sulbactam may be useful in selected cases (83,128,134,135). The polymyxins, such as polymyxin B, colistin, and similar investigational peptides, demonstrate activity *in vitro* against *Acinetobacter* and *Pseudomonas* and offer a potential therapy for infections caused by strains that are resistant to all other agents (128,133,136–138).

Antimicrobial resistance exhibited by the nonfermentative gram-negative bacilli creates an epidemiologic niche for these pathogens that facilitates colonization and superinfection in antibiotic-treated patients. For example, multiple studies demonstrate that patients who receive antibiotics not active against *P. aeruginosa* are at risk for intestinal colonization (139–142) and bloodstream infections (143) caused by this bacterium. Similarly, for the other nonfermentative gram-negative bacilli, including *Acinetobacter* and *S. maltophilia*, administration of broad-spectrum antibiotics lacking activity against these pathogens predisposes toward colonization and infection (144–148).

Resistance to Antiseptics and Disinfectants

Partial resistance to antiseptics is a feature of some nonfermentative gram-negative bacilli, most notably *P. aeruginosa* and *B. cepacia*. This problem initially was recognized in the 1950s when *Pseudomonas* contamination of dilute aqueous benzalkonium chloride was reported at several hospitals (149,150). At these hospitals, use of contaminated aqueous benzalkonium chloride to disinfect intravascular catheters and needles caused outbreaks of *Pseudomonas* bacteremia. The continued use of aqueous benzalkonium chloride alone or with other agents for antiseptic preparation of the skin or urethral meatus before catheter insertion resulted in further cases of bloodstream or urinary tract infection (151–156). Most outbreaks involved aqueous benzalkonium chloride diluted in hospitals to an in-use concentration of 1:1,000; however, in several instances, *B. cepacia* was an intrinsic contaminant of commercially prepared swabs containing a 1:500 concentration of aqueous benzalkonium chloride (154,157).

Other antiseptic preparations, such as chlorhexidine (158–160), chlorhexidine and cetrimide (161,162), cetrimide (163), hexachlorophene (164), and green soap (165), have become contaminated with *Pseudomonas, Burkholderia, Ralstonia,* or *Stenotrophomonas.* While the presence of organic materials enhances survival of bacteria in these antiseptics (149,163,166), *Pseudomonas* and related nonfermenters may proliferate substantially in antiseptics in the absence of such contaminants (163, 166). These bacteria may also contaminate phenolic disinfectants (166–168). Even commercial preparations of poloxamer-iodine and povidone-iodine have become contaminated with *P. aeruginosa* (169) and *B. cepacia* (170–172); in such reports, products from different manufacturers were implicated, and concentrations of free iodine, when tested, were sometimes in the same range as uncontaminated products (171,172).

The susceptibility of *P. aeruginosa* and *B. cepacia* to commonly used antiseptics and disinfectants varies. Some strains are resistant to in-use dilutions of benzalkonium chloride, chlorhexidine, cetrimide, phenolic disinfectant, iodophor disinfectant, or quaternary ammonium disinfectant (173–179).

Although the biologic basis is not completely understood, gram-negative bacteria may possess multiple intrinsic and acquired mechanisms for antiseptic and disinfectant resistance (180). *P. aeruginosa* and *B. cepacia* within biofilms are more resistant to biocides of all types, including antibiotics, than their free-living counterparts (9,181–184). Studies of iodophor contamination by *P. aeruginosa* and *B. cepacia* demonstrate this potential protective role of biofilm matrix (185–187). The ways in which bacteria within a biofilm evade the actions of antimicrobials and disinfectants remain under investigation but appear identical to the mechanisms by which biofilms inhibit antibiotic activity. First, biofilms act as a permeability barrier to biocides (9,181,188). For example, *in vitro* resistance to povidone-iodine is mediated by the protective layering of *Pseudomonas* bacterial cells within a biofilm (189). *In vitro,* higher concentrations of biocides can overcome this type of resistance (190). Second, bacteria within a biofilm have slower growth rates that result in reduced efficacy of antimicrobials such as β-lactams. Third, within biofilms, expression of a "resistance phenotype" is a way that bacteria evade the effects of biocides; the expression of multidrug efflux pumps and alteration of bacterial outer membrane proteins are proposed mechanisms of biocide resistance (182, 188).

Resistance of *Pseudomonas* species to other compounds, such as phenols, may be mediated by catabolic enzymes (191–193). Plasmid-mediated resistance to silver has occurred in *Pseudomonas stutzeri* (194) (see also Chapter 85).

Replication and Survival

Species of *Pseudomonas* and *B. cepacia* replicate in a wide range of moist environments because of their ability to obtain carbon and nitrogen from diverse substrates. Aliphatic amides or amino acids provide the source of both carbon and nitrogen.

Alternatively, carbon may be derived from organic acids or esters of organic acids, whereas nitrogen is extracted from ammonium or nitrate. The range of substrates includes both antibiotics and germicides. For example, penicillin has served as a carbon source for *B. cepacia* (195) and *Pseudomonas fluorescens* (196), chlorinated phenols were utilized by an isolate designated *Pseudomonas* species B 13 (197), and chlorhexidine and cetrimide were utilized by *B. cepacia* (161). Additionally, ammonium acetate buffered benzalkonium chloride has supported the growth of *P. aeruginosa* (198).

The minimal nutrient requirements of *P. aeruginosa* and *B. cepacia* permit their growth in tap water and distilled or deionized water up to concentrations of 10^5 to 10^7 CFU/mL (199–202). Presumably, organic compounds absorbed in water from plumbing and storage systems are utilized as substrates. Naturally occurring pseudomonads in these minimal medium environments are more resistant to chemical inactivation by agents such as chlorine or iodine than are bacteria grown in enriched media (161,171,199,203).

Pseudomonads are capable of prolonged survival in moist or dry environments. In laboratory studies, *P. aeruginosa* can survive in water for more than 300 days, on dry filter paper disks for up to 150 days, on hardened plaster of Paris bandages for at least 20 days, and in dried sputum for at least 5 days (204–206). In the hospital environment, *P. aeruginosa* was recovered from a dry floor 5 weeks after the ward was closed and from burn eschar tissue samples excised 8 weeks earlier (207).

Acinetobacter demonstrates even better survival than *P. aeruginosa* under some dry conditions (208–213). For example, *Acinetobacter calcoaceticus* survived an average of 9 days on a dry Formica surface compared to less than 1 day for *P. aeruginosa* (210). Survival of *A. baumannii* at high colony counts for at least 16 weeks on dry surfaces has been shown using a strain initially isolated from dry environmental surfaces (211). Additionally, strains of *A. baumannii* survived on glass coverslips for an average of 27 days when incubated under conditions mimicking the hospital environment (213).

B. cepacia achieved concentrations of 10^6 to 10^8 CFU/mL when inoculated into sterile 5% dextrose and normal saline solutions but appeared to exhaust its nutrient supply after 21 days of incubation (214). *B. cepacia* did not multiply in 50% dextrose, 3% saline, or hyperalimentation solutions (69). After prolonged storage of a contaminated solution of minimal inorganic salts containing benzalkonium chloride and ammonium acetate, cultures demonstrated viable *B. cepacia* after 14 years (215).

CLINICAL AND EPIDEMIOLOGIC MANIFESTATIONS

Bacteremia

Bacteria may enter the bloodstream either because of microorganism virulence or because direct access is provided by contaminated intravascular devices or fluids. *P. aeruginosa* bacteremia usually arises by the former mechanism, whereas the latter mechanism accounts for most cases of bacteremia by other nonfermentative gram-negative bacilli.

The frequency of *P. aeruginosa* bacteremia largely depends on the population of patients studied. At university teaching hospitals, the overall incidence has been about one case per 1,000 admissions (216,217). In patients with burn injuries or cancer, the incidence has been about five cases per 1,000 admissions (218,219), and the incidence has exceeded 50 cases per 1,000 admissions in patients with acute leukemia (219,220). The great majority of cases of *P. aeruginosa* bacteremia appear to be hospital acquired.

The usual clinical picture of *P. aeruginosa* bacteremia is the same as that of bacteremia caused by other gram-negative bacilli. Fever is almost always present, except in infants, and tachycardia and hypotension are common findings (219,221–223). Necrotizing skin lesions, called ecthyma gangrenosum, are considered pathognomonic of *P. aeruginosa* bacteremia (224,225) but occasionally are seen in bloodstream infections by other pathogens, including *S. maltophilia* (65,226,227) and *B. cepacia* (228). Ecthyma and other skin lesions were not uncommon in infected cancer patients treated in the 1950s and 1960s (229,230) but are rare in later series (219,222,223).

When present in the bloodstream of cancer patients, *P. aeruginosa* is virtually always the sole pathogen, and bacteremia is thought to arise from the alimentary tract. Gut colonization with *P. aeruginosa* has been associated with a risk of *P. aeruginosa* bacteremia exceeding 40% during neutropenia (231–233). In other settings, about 20% of the cases of *P. aeruginosa* bacteremia are polymicrobial (216,222,234). The most common primary sites of infection from which bacteremia arises are the urinary tract and respiratory tract (216,217,222,234).

The outcome of *P. aeruginosa* bacteremia is poor, especially in neutropenic cancer patients. The mortality rate for these patients was about 90% until the 1970s, when it became common practice to administer combination therapy with gentamicin and carbenicillin presumptively for neutropenic fever (220,229,235). Subsequently, the timely administration of more potent antipseudomonal antibiotics has lowered mortality rates below 40% (236). In unselected patients at teaching hospitals, the mortality rate of *P. aeruginosa* bacteremia has remained about 40% to 50% (227,237) and has exceeded that for other bacteria (238). Some of this mortality can be attributed to the severity of underlying disease in patients with *P. aeruginosa* bacteremia. A matched cohort study of ICU patients with *P. aeruginosa* bacteremia reported an overall mortality of 62%, but an attributable mortality of only 15% (239). Improved outcomes have been associated with resolution of neutropenia, prompt administration of an effective antibiotic, and use of synergistic combinations of antibiotics (229,235–237,240). In striking contrast to the life-threatening nature of most cases of nosocomial *P. aeruginosa* bacteremia, there are occasional examples of asymptomatic *P. aeruginosa* bacteremia (241) and of symptomatic intravenous catheter sepsis that resolved without specific antibiotic therapy (242,243).

Cases of primary *P. aeruginosa* bacteremia occasionally have been linked to intravenous devices or infusion products that became contaminated during preparation in hospitals (150,244, 245). Bacteremia arising from contaminated endoscopes has been a more frequent problem (246–248), especially if endoscopic retrograde cholangiopancreatography was performed (249–252) (see Chapter 63). In these cases, the onset of symptoms usually was a few hours to a few days after the procedure. Hemodialysis treatment also has been a source of *P. aeruginosa* bacteremia and has been associated with inadequate reprocessing of hemodialyzers with benzalkonium chloride (241,253), incorrectly diluted formaldehyde (254), or contaminated dialysate waste drainage ports (255).

In some centers treating neutropenic cancer patients, the overall incidence of *P. aeruginosa* bacteremia has declined during the past decade (256). However, other centers have reported outbreak or hyperendemic problems apparently linked to contamination of a mouthwash (257), environmental contamination (233), and cross-transmission from patients (141).

Pseudobacteremia due to *P. aeruginosa* contamination of blood culture specimens rarely has been reported (258) (see Chapter 8).

Although *P. aeruginosa* bacteremia is almost always life threatening, bacteremia caused by other nonfermenting gram-negative bacilli is frequently self-limited. Outbreaks of *B. cepacia* bacteremia associated with common source exposure to contaminated fluids (71,259–262), disinfectants (157,172,263), or medical devices (253–262,264–266) sometimes have been associated with significant morbidity, but there has been little or no mortality. Most reported cases of *B. cepacia* bacteremia have in common the direct introduction of contaminated material into the bloodstream. Pseudobacteremia due to *B. cepacia* rarely has occurred (267).

S. maltophilia bacteremia generally is secondary to respiratory tract or intravenous catheter–related infection in immunocompromised patients receiving broad-spectrum antibiotics. *S. maltophilia* bacteremia often occurs as a breakthrough infection (268). Unlike *B. cepacia, S. maltophilia* bacteremia is often associated with signs and symptoms of sepsis and carries a mortality rate of 25% to 57% (269–271). One case-control study identified an attributable mortality rate of 27% in *S. maltophilia* bacteremia (272). Mortality is increased when the patient is immunocompromised, the primary source is the lung, or antibiotic therapy is inappropriate (268–271).

Acinetobacter species accounted for 1.5% of all nosocomial bloodstream infections in a survey of 49 U.S. hospitals from 1995 to 1998 (126). *A. baumannii* accounted for 86% of *Acinetobacter* isolates. *A. baumannii* bacteremia was more frequently observed in the ICU than bloodstream infections with other gram-negative bacilli (69% vs. 47%, respectively). *Acinetobacter* bacteremia has the dual potential to present as very low grade infection or as septic shock. Early reports emphasized the transient or benign nature of *Acinetobacter* bacteremia (271, 273–277). Bacteremia often cleared with removal of the associated intravenous catheter with or without antibiotic therapy. A report of catheter-related *Acinetobacter johnsonii* bacteremia described a similarly benign clinical course (278). In other series, high fever, leukocytosis, and septic shock were present in 37% to 78% of cases, mortality rates ranged from 15% to 32%, and metastatic complications including endocarditis, septic thrombophlebitis, and intraabdominal abscess were detected (84,126, 279–281). A case-control study of ICU patients with *Acinetobacter baumannii* bacteremia found an overall mortality of 42%, but an attributable mortality of only 8%, reflecting the severity of illness in patients with *Acinetobacter* bacteremia (282). *Acinetobacter* infection tends to occur in patients with impaired host defenses. Almost all have intravenous catheters and are receiving broad-spectrum antibiotics (84,258–284).

Pseudomonas fluorescens is an important cause of transfusion-associated infection. This microorganism is psychrophilic (grows at 4°C) and utilizes citrate as a carbon source. Refrigerated citrate anticoagulated red blood cell units serve as an ideal growth medium. *P. fluorescens* can achieve peak concentrations of 10^6 to 10^7 CFU/mL within 1 week of storage at 4°C. Transfusion-related infection has been associated with severe illness and mortality rates exceeding 50% (285–288). These infections are characterized by the sudden onset of fever, chills, and hypotension during red blood cell transfusion, and the source of infection has been confirmed by positive culture of untransfused blood.

Bacteremia caused by *Ralstonia pickettii* (160,280–293), *S. paucimobilis* (92,294–298), *Ochrobactrum anthropi* (299), or *Pseudomonas stutzeri* (300) almost always results from either infusion of contaminated solutions or direct contact with contaminated ventilators or dialysis equipment. These infections generally have produced few symptoms, and many episodes of bacteremia have cleared without antibiotic therapy. Complications such as hematogenous infection of central nervous system or bone rarely have been reported (294), and catheter removal to resolve intravascular catheter-related bacteremia sometimes has been necessary (301). Other *Ralstonia* species (302,303), *Pseudomonas* (formerly *Flavimonas) oryzihabitans* (101), and *Agrobacterium* species (304) rarely have been reported to cause bacteremia in severely immunocompromised patients.

Pneumonia

Prior to the 1980s, *P. aeruginosa* usually was isolated from fewer than 10% of patients with nosocomial pneumonia (305–307). Thereafter, the proportion of cases attributed to *P. aeruginosa* nearly doubled, and *P. aeruginosa* has been the most common pathogen or the most common gram-negative bacterium isolated from patients with nosocomial pneumonia (306, 308–310). It remains uncertain whether detection of *P. aeruginosa* in sputum obtained by expectoration or tracheal aspiration necessarily indicates a causative role in lower respiratory tract infection since tracheal colonization may be present without causing pneumonia (311). Nonetheless, *P. aeruginosa* has been the leading gram-negative pathogen in several studies in which selected patients underwent bronchial lavage or protected brush sampling (312–315).

Factors that predispose to *P. aeruginosa* pneumonia include cystic fibrosis (316–318), other underlying chronic pulmonary diseases (311,317–320), mechanical ventilation (319–321), and hematologic malignancies (317,321). The pathogenesis of infection can involve microaspiration of microorganisms colonizing the hypopharynx but more often appears to be due to direct contamination of the trachea with microorganisms from environmental or patient reservoirs (322–325). Once initiated, *P. aeruginosa* infection of the lungs may progress to a necrotizing bronchopneumonia. Cavitation sometimes occurs radiographically (320,326), and pathologic features include diffuse small necrotic nodules, areas of hemorrhage, and pseudomonal vasculitis of small arteries (319,320,327).

Survival of patients with *P. aeruginosa* pneumonia was infrequent prior to the 1980s, when potent antipseudomonal antibiotics became available (317,321,328,329). Bacteremic pneumonia had an especially dismal prognosis. In later studies, survival rates have reached about 50% (319,330,331). However, in patients with severe pneumonia, the prognosis remains poorest when *P. aeruginosa* is the bacterial pathogen isolated from initial respiratory tract cultures or blood cultures (329–331). Ventilator-associated pneumonia also appears to have a worse prognosis when *P. aeruginosa* is the pathogen (332–334). Specific problems in the treatment of *P. aeruginosa* pneumonia are recurrence, even after treatment for several weeks (319), and emergence of resistance to the antibiotics used during treatment (330,331). Even when potent antibiotics such as ciprofloxacin or imipenem have been used, resistance has emerged in more than one fourth of cases (331).

During the 1960s and early 1970s, respiratory therapy equipment was recognized to be a potential source from which nonfermentative gram-negative bacilli could be introduced into the respiratory tract (335–338). Contaminated nebulizers were the major problem and were shown in an experimental model to cause *P. aeruginosa* pneumonia in mechanically ventilated dogs (339). Other devices that produce respirable aerosols, such as room humidifiers (340) and oxygen humidifiers (341,342), also have been identified as potential sources of pseudomonal respiratory infection (see also Chapter 68). Investigations in specialized care units have shown that tracheal acquisition of *P. aeruginosa* sometimes is preceded by gastrointestinal tract colonization, and that sources of *P. aeruginosa* include the inanimate environment and other patients (325,343–349).

In cystic fibrosis centers, cross-transmission of *P. aeruginosa* is a significant concern. Contamination of the environment has been detected in some clinics (205) but not in others (348,350). Where environmental contamination is minimized by routine or contact isolation precautions, cross-transmission is infrequent (350–352).

P. aeruginosa is a rare cause of community-acquired pneumonia. The clinical presentation is nonspecific, but the disease may be rapidly fatal. Patients with previous hospitalization or antimicrobial therapy and underlying pulmonary disease seem to be at highest risk (353) In previously healthy persons with community-acquired pneumonia, *P. aeruginosa* should be considered in the differential diagnosis for anyone with a smoking history who presents with rapidly progressive pneumonia (354).

B. cepacia is a rare pulmonary pathogen except in patients with cystic fibrosis or chronic granulomatous disease (355). Epidemic recovery of *B. cepacia* from respiratory specimens has been reported when contaminated lidocaine, tetracaine, or cocaine was used in bronchoscopy or otolaryngology procedures, but pneumonia did not occur (356–358). In one outbreak, there was no reported evidence of clinical illness among 18 patients with *B. cepacia* respiratory tract colonization despite instillation into the respiratory tract of 10 mL of contaminated anesthetic containing up to 10^{10} CFU/mL (356).

B. cepacia is an important respiratory pathogen in individuals with cystic fibrosis. Persistent infection with *B. cepacia* has been associated with worsening pulmonary status and increased mortality when compared with noninfected controls (125, 359–361). The response to acquisition of *B. cepacia* appears to take one of two forms: about 25% of patients develop fulminant infection characterized by high fever, leukocytosis, and severe progressive respiratory failure, whereas the remaining patients, usually those with mild cystic fibrosis, have persistent colonization without evidence of significant adverse effect (125,360). Risk factors associated with acquisition of *B. cepacia* include older age, more advanced pulmonary disease, and exposure to *B. cepacia* from previous hospitalization or a sibling with *B. cepacia* colonization (359).

B. cepacia pneumonia is a serious illness in individuals with chronic granulomatous disease (362). Of note, six of ten cases reported in the literature were not known to have chronic granulomatous disease before the occurrence of *B. cepacia* pneumonia (362). Isolation of this unusual pathogen from patients with community-acquired pneumonia should prompt an evaluation of phagocyte function and screening for cystic fibrosis.

S. maltophilia typically occurs as a late-onset nosocomial infection. *S. maltophilia* pneumonia has been associated with previous antibiotic therapy, in particular, imipenem and cefepime, tracheostomy, and severity of illness (363,364). *S. maltophilia* has been associated with increased morbidity, but the attributable mortality is uncertain.

The respiratory tract is the most frequent site of *Acinetobacter* infection. Nosocomial pneumonia usually occurs in debilitated ICU patients receiving prolonged mechanical ventilation and broad-spectrum antibiotics (83,282,365,366). Distinguishing colonization from infection in these patients can be very difficult. Although some investigators have reported very low morbidity associated with *Acinetobacter* recovery from ventilated patients (367), others have described severe illness with mortality rates of 36% due to infection (83,365). These latter patients present with fever, purulent sputum, leukocytosis, and a multilobar patchy infiltrate on chest radiograph. Studies utilizing quantitative cultures of bronchoscopy specimens in ventilated patients support the role of *Acinetobacter* as an important pathogen in ventilator-associated pneumonia (332,368).

Acinetobacter demonstrates a unique seasonal variation in the U.S. with infection rates twice as high during July to October than during November to June (369). In contrast, rates of *P. aeruginosa* show little seasonal variation. The cause of seasonal variation in *Acinetobacter* infection rates is uncertain and may be important for the design of prevention measures.

Acinetobacter occasionally causes severe community-acquired pneumonia, especially in individuals with underlying alcoholism and chronic obstructive pulmonary disease (89,370,371). The illness manifests as an acute, fulminant pneumonia and has a mortality rate of about 50%. Mortality is strongly associated with inappropriate antibiotic therapy (89,370), which has been linked to misidentification of the bipolar gram-negative rods of *Acinetobacter* as over-decolorized pneumococci.

Other nonfermenters have been associated with respiratory tract colonization but cause little morbidity and little or no mortality (160,355,372–375). (For more information on nosocomial pneumonia, see Chapter 22.)

Urinary Tract Infection

P. aeruginosa adheres well to bladder uroepithelial cells but is not a common cause of urinary tract infection (376,377). It accounts for only about 12% of nosocomial urinary tract infections and ranks third in frequency at this site behind *Escherichia coli* and *Enterococcus* (308,309). The pathogenesis of infection, as elucidated from case clusters, involves primarily retrograde introduction of microorganisms into the bladder via urinary drainage catheters or contaminated urologic instruments (378–380). Colonization of the rectum, perineum, or urethra may precede *P. aeruginosa* urinary tract infection (381,382).

P. aeruginosa bacteruria in catheterized patients often resolves spontaneously within 2 to 3 months (383). Necrotizing infection of the bladder or kidney is extremely rare, and pyelonephritis as a complication of bacteruria is uncommon (379). Rates of secondary bacteremia in patients with *P. aeruginosa* urinary tract infection were 3.1% in an endemic setting and 4.5% in an epidemic setting (379,384). Urologic procedures have induced *P. aeruginosa* bacteremia, but there is no evidence that the procedure-related risk is greater than for other uropathogens (385).

P. aeruginosa has been reported to be the most common cause of clustered cases of urinary tract infection (386). Case clusters have been linked to contaminated urologic instruments (378, 380,387), urine collection or measuring devices (379,388–390), and cross-transmission due to contamination of the hands of personnel (391). Where infected urine is not well contained, *P. aeruginosa* contamination of the perineum and hands of infected patients and of bed linen has been noted (391).

Efforts to prevent catheter-related urinary tract infection by instilling a disinfectant into the drainage system or by using a silver oxide–coated catheter have not clearly helped against *P. aeruginosa* (392,393).

Urinary tract infection with nonfermenters other than *P. aeruginosa* is notable for the lack of significant morbidity. All episodes occur in patients who have undergone urologic procedures or bladder catheterization, and most infections are asymptomatic and resolve spontaneously with catheter removal (73,83,156, 394,395). (See Chapter 20 for more information on nosocomial urinary tract infections.)

Burn Wound Infections

P. aeruginosa is one of the most common burn wound pathogens, and it has colonized or infected more than one fourth of patients in several series (396–399). Increased extent of burn has been associated with an increased risk of both colonization and burn wound sepsis (396,398). *P. aeruginosa* colonization or infection is almost always hospital-acquired (206,396,400,401). Culture surveys to identify reservoirs of *P. aeruginosa* in burn units have yielded positive cultures from sinks and hydrotherapy equipment (397,400,401). Only hydrotherapy equipment has been compellingly linked to cases. Strains of *P. aeruginosa* acquired during hospitalization have been matched to those in hydrotherapy equipment, and disinfection of the equipment or suspension of its use has been associated with outbreak termination (400,401) (see Chapter 66). Dispersal of *P. aeruginosa*, presumably from colonized or infected patients, has resulted in contamination of air (396,402), the hands of personnel (396), and surfaces such as bed rails (397), counters (397), food trays (396), and transport equipment (400).

Measures to control *P. aeruginosa* in burn units have included topical treatment of burn wounds, aseptic practices to prevent acquisition, and aggressive systemic antibiotic treatment of infections (399–401). Use of selective bowel decontamination regimens to suppress aerobic gram-negative bacilli in the alimentary tract has been proposed (403) but may be of limited benefit against microorganisms such as *P. aeruginosa*, which multiply primarily in the burn wound. (See Chapter 25 for more information on burn wound infections.)

Eye Infections

P. aeruginosa is a highly destructive ocular pathogen (22,404, 405), and it has been reported to account for about 8% of postoperative ocular infections at one center (406). Superficial infection may rapidly lead to corneal or scleral perforation, and endophthalmitis can cause complete loss of vision. Keratitis typically presents as an acute, rapidly progressive corneal ulcer with greenish pus and hypopyon (407). Extension from cornea to sclera may occur and is associated with a poor outcome (408). Postoperative endophthalmitis usually becomes clinically evident within 1 to 2 days but may evolve over 5 to 10 days (409, 410).

Several risk factors for *P. aeruginosa* ocular infection have been identified, and most apply to nosocomial cases. Keratitis may be a consequence of corneal trauma, corneal surgery, or treatment with multidose eyedrops or eyewash solutions that became contaminated during use (407,409,411,412). Scleral irradiation has preceded scleral and corneal infection (413), and neutropenia has been associated with blepharoconjunctivitis (414). Endophthalmitis usually has been a consequence of surgery, and case clusters have been traced to contaminated solutions or implants (409,410,415).

Sporadic cases and clusters of cases of *P. aeruginosa* conjunctivitis have been recognized in patients receiving respiratory care (416–420). Almost all of the patients were intubated, had *P. aeruginosa* in their respiratory secretions, and had frequent suctioning to remove respiratory secretions. Impaired consciousness was noted in some patients. Strikingly, infection involved primarily the left eye in almost all adult cases (415,416). Hilton et al. (416) explained the left eye predominance by showing that *P. aeruginosa* in respiratory secretions was dispersed during suctioning and that nurses usually withdrew suction catheters diagonally across the left side of patients' faces. Cases of nosocomial conjunctivitis in newborn infants also have been reported and were traced to contaminated incubators (421).

S. maltophilia is a rare cause of postoperative endophthalmitis after cataract surgery (422,423). Other nonfermenters are occasionally isolated from conjunctival swabs but are rare causes of infection (419,424,425). (For more information on nosocomial ocular infections, see Chapter 26.)

Meningitis

Nosocomial meningitis caused by nonfermentative gram-negative bacilli is almost always a complication of neurosurgical procedures other than shunt operations. *Pseudomonas* and *Acinetobacter* have been the predominant nonfermenters, accounting for about one fourth to one half of cases of postneurosurgical gram-negative meningitis in adults (426–429). *P. aeruginosa* also is an important cause of meningitis in burn unit patients (430) and has caused nosocomial meningitis in patients hospitalized for cranial trauma (431).

Investigations of cases of *P. aeruginosa* meningitis several decades ago implicated contaminated medications that had been injected intrathecally (432,433) and a contaminated shaving brush used in neurosurgical patients to prepare the site for incision (434). The sources of *P. aeruginosa* causing recent cases have not been reported.

The first reported cases of *Acinetobacter* meningitis were community acquired (435,436), and the early genus name *Mima* ("mimic") arose from the frequent misidentification on Gram stain of the bipolar-staining rod as *Neisseria meningitidis* (437). *Acinetobacter* meningitis was later reported almost exclusively in association with neurosurgical procedures or cranial trauma (437,438). Occasional cases have occurred in neonates in the absence of invasive procedures (439). Patients with *Acinetobacter* meningitis usually are receiving antibiotic therapy at the onset, and clinical features include fever (95%), mental status changes (50%), neck stiffness (25%), cerebrospinal fluid pleocytosis (100%), and low cerebrospinal fluid glucose (60%) (438). Half of the recent cases have been polymicrobial. The overall mortality rate is about 20%, and survival is associated with prompt appropriate therapy. Sources of *Acinetobacter* causing nosocomial meningitis have not been identified. Other nonfermentative gram-negative bacilli have caused sporadic cases of meningitis (440–445). (For more information on nosocomial central nervous system infections, see Chapter 27.)

Surgical Site Infection, Osteomyelitis

Overall, *P. aeruginosa* has been isolated from about 9% of surgical site infections (309). The relative frequency of *P. aeruginosa* as a pathogen is high at some sites, such as sternotomy for cardiac surgery (446–448), whereas *P. aeruginosa* accounts for only a few percent of infections following implantation of prosthetic joints (449,450). Because of its virulence, the presence of *P. aeruginosa* in an incisional surgical site at the time of closure has been associated with a risk of subsequent surgical site infection exceeding 30% (451,452). Administration of perioperative antibiotics directed against *P. aeruginosa* appears to diminish the risk (452). Although an uncommon cause of osteomyelitis, *P. aeruginosa* was associated with more than a twofold risk of recurrence compared with infection with *Staphylococcus aureus* (453).

The source of *P. aeruginosa* causing infection after intraabdominal operations generally is considered to be the patient (451,452). Exogenous sources in the operating theater have been sought to explain infections following other types of surgery, and positive cultures have been reported from a water bath (244), a scrub sink faucet (454), suction pumps for chest tubes (454), and an arterial pressure monitoring system (455). One cluster of cases of *P. aeruginosa* surgical site infections was attributed to preparation of the skin incision site with a dilute solution of chlorhexidine contaminated with *P. aeruginosa* (158), and another cluster, involving orthopedic patients, was traced to contaminated plaster-of-Paris bandages (456).

Acinetobacter is a frequent isolate from skin, and recovery of the microorganism from surgical sites is not surprising. *S. maltophilia* and *B. cepacia* also have been recovered from surgical sites, but typically in mixed culture (457,458). The clinical significance of these microorganisms in surgical site cultures is often uncertain. (For more information on surgical site infections, see Chapter 21.)

EPIDEMIOLOGY

Rates of Nosocomial Infection

The frequency of nonfermentative aerobic gram-negative bacilli as nosocomial pathogens has been characterized each year through the NNIS system. During 1987–1997, nonfermenters were isolated from about 13% of the reported nosocomial infections (Table 34.1). *P. aeruginosa* was isolated from about three fourths of the infections attributed to nonfermenters, and the only other nonfermenters identified on average at least once per

TABLE 34.1. FREQUENCY OF ISOLATION OF NONFERMENTATIVE GRAM-NEGATIVE BACILLI (NFGNB) FROM NOSOCOMIAL INFECTIONS, NNIS HOSPITALS, 1987–1997

Year	No. of Infections	No. (%) from which NFGNB Isolated	No. (%) of Nosocomial Infections from which Specified Microorganism Was Isolated			
			Pseudomonas aeruginosa	*Burkholderia cepacia*[a]	*Acinetobacter* species	*Stenotrophomonas maltophilia*[b]
1987	32,151	4,472 (13.9)	3,725 (11.6)	37 (0.1)	80 (0.3)	115 (0.4)
1988	36,068	4,885 (13.5)	3,938 (10.9)	67 (0.2)	93 (0.3)	224 (0.6)
1989	39,226	5,405 (13.8)	4,137 (10.5)	87 (0.2)	144 (0.4)	317 (0.8)
1990	39,541	5,145 (13.0)	3,955 (10.0)	32 (0.1)	134 (0.3)	283 (0.7)
1991	37,792	4,914 (13.0)	3,618 (9.6)	63 (0.2)	104 (0.3)	271 (0.7)
1992	37,848	5,000 (13.2)	3,603 (9.5)	52 (0.1)	134 (0.4)	201 (0.5)
1993	39,824	5,025 (12.6)	3,752 (9.4)	33 (0.1)	119 (0.3)	198 (0.5)
1994	39,520	5,111 (12.9)	3,774 (9.5)	56 (0.1)	122 (0.3)	336 (0.9)
1995	43,361	5,806 (13.4)	4,180 (9.6)	72 (0.2)	97 (0.2)	487 (1.1)
1996	45,763	6,157 (13.5)	4,449 (9.7)	87 (0.2)	115 (0.3)	498 (1.1)
1997	46,724	6,022 (12.9)	4,348 (9.3)	40 (0.1)	95 (0.2)	478 (1.0)

[a] Includes microorganisms previously classified as *Pseudomonas cepacia*.
[b] Includes microorganisms previously classified as *Pseudomonas maltophilia* or *Xanthomonas* species. NNIS, National Nosocomial Infections Surveillance.

TABLE 34.2. MAJOR SITES FROM WHICH NONFERMENTATIVE GRAM-NEGATIVE BACILLI (NFGNB) WERE ISOLATED, NNIS HOSPITALS, 1987–1997

Year	Urinary Tract Infection[a]	Pneumonia	Surgical Site Infection	Bloodstream Infection
1987	1,614 (1,490)	1,267 (905)	735 (621)	309 (203)
1988	1,695 (1,554)	1,494 (996)	711 (584)	370 (244)
1989	1,675 (1,483)	1,740 (1,104)	813 (639)	436 (235)
1990	1,624 (1,463)	1,573 (1,024)	785 (626)	431 (221)
1991	1,535 (1,329)	1,519 (925)	751 (550)	429 (236)
1992	1,366 (1,163)	1,690 (1,041)	779 (580)	436 (221)
1993	1,216 (1,052)	1,883 (1,258)	715 (571)	428 (234)
1994	1,132 (1,004)	2,039 (1,294)	760 (586)	428 (251)
1995	1,127 (1,015)	2,450 (1,484)	802 (639)	550 (309)
1996	1,108 (981)	2,705 (1,656)	877 (718)	533 (274)
1997	1,061 (913)	2,563 (1,622)	878 (702)	565 (318)

[a] First number indicates infections culture-positive for NFGNB; number in parentheses indicates infections positive for *Pseudomonas aeruginosa*.

hospital each year were *Acinetobacter* species and *S. maltophilia*. The most common site of isolation of nonfermenters was the urinary tract through 1992 and the respiratory tract thereafter (Table 34.2).

During 1987–1997, *P. aeruginosa* was the fifth most common nosocomial pathogen and accounted for about 10% of reported nosocomial infections. In the urinary tract, *P. aeruginosa* was the second most common pathogen, whereas in cases of pneumonia it was the leading pathogen. Nonfermenters other than *P. aeruginosa* were recovered from only 1% of nosocomial infections. The most common site of isolation was the respiratory tract, which yielded about half of these isolates.

Inanimate Reservoirs

Extensive culture studies have been conducted, mostly during the 1950s and 1960s, to identify hospital sources of nonfermentative gram-negative bacilli. As summarized in Table 34.3, these microorganisms have been found in virtually every moist area of the hospital, many fluids, and an array of equipment and surfaces that were exposed to the hands, secretions, and excretions of patients. Recognition that these microorganisms are ubiquitous has prompted increased attention to aseptic practices, particularly in the use of respiratory equipment (531). Nonetheless, nonfermentative gram-negative bacilli continue to test the adequacy of aseptic practices and to find deficiencies in product manufacturing (154,157,169,171,186,248,293,478,512) and in disinfection of medical devices for reuse (150,246–254,415,475, 511).

The major vehicles by which *P. aeruginosa* is conveyed into hospitals are food and tap water. Vegetables are the most commonly contaminated foods, and rates of positive cultures of salads have ranged from 11% to 44% (143,537–541). The concentration of *P. aeruginosa* in individual vegetables or in salads has ranged up to 10^3 CFU/g (143,539–541). The concentration of *P. aeruginosa* in hot and cold tap water systems in hospitals appears to be extremely low, as evidenced by frequent negative cultures in most settings.

Studies to ascertain whether environmental isolates of *P. aeruginosa* cause colonization or infection of patients have implicated most of the potential sources listed in Table 34.3. The major exceptions are sinks, drains, and suction apparatus. Typing of isolates from serial cultures of patients and sinks has shown that patients typically become culture-positive first and that there are at most a few occasions when the sink or drain might have been the source of patient colonization (141,485,500,502,506).

Animate Reservoirs

Colonization of patients by *P. aeruginosa* constitutes an important reservoir, particularly in specialty care units where patients are exposed to broad-spectrum antibiotics, medical devices, and the hands of healthcare personnel. Culture studies have shown colonization rates of 4% to 58% in hematology-oncology patients (141,143,557,558), 13% to 39% in ICU patients (483,487,501,559–561), 19% to 43% in surgery patients (480,560), and 2% to 51% in special care baby units (562,563). Factors in individual studies that are associated with an increased risk of colonization include ileostomy or colostomy (480), tracheal intubation (480), tracheostomy (561), mechanical ventilation (342), broad-spectrum antibiotic therapy (483,561), prior hospitalization (480,487), age over 65 years (521), previous gastrointestinal surgery (560), and anemia (560). *P. aeruginosa* often is acquired after admission, and the proportion of patients with positive cultures usually increases by at least 50% during hospitalization (143,480,483,487,560,562). The most common site from which *P. aeruginosa* is recovered is the rectum, and in most studies at least 80% of colonized patients can be detected by cultures of that site (143,483,487,564). The pharynx is usually the second most common culture-positive site (487,558,560, 564), although higher carriage rates occasionally have been reported for the perineum or urine (141,563). In a culture study of intestinal contents of 100 cadavers, Stoodley and Thom (565) demonstrated that when *P. aeruginosa* was present, it usually could be recovered from both the small intestine and colon and that rates of isolation were about half as high in the jejunum as in lower segments of the gut. The concentration of *P. aeruginosa* has reached 10^6 to 10^7 CFU/g of feces in a patient receiving broad-spectrum, orally administered, nonabsorbable antibiotics

TABLE 34.3. HOSPITAL SOURCES OF NONFERMENTATIVE GRAM-NEGATIVE BACILLI

Source	Microorganism	References
Tap water supply	*Pseudomonas aeruginosa*	233,237,257
	Pseudomonas fluorescens	459
	Stenotrophomonas maltophilia	460
Water for humidification	*Pseudomonas aeruginosa*	231,461–464,469
	Acinetobacter species	465–467
	Sphingomonas paucimobilis	468
	Pseudomonas fluorescens	374
Distilled water	*Pseudomonas aeruginosa*	341,469
	Burkholderia cepacia	468,470
	Acinetobacter species	471
	Pseudomonas fluorescens	374
	Ralstonia pickettii	475
Sterile water or saline	*Pseudomonas aeruginosa*	409,461,476
	Burkholderia cepacia	259,262
	Acinetobacter species	477
	Ralstonia pickettii	291,372,373,478
	Sphingomonas paucimobilis	479
Nonsterile water	*Pseudomonas aeruginosa*	245,476,480,481
	Burkholderia cepacia	159
	Acinetobacter species	482
Suction apparatus	*Pseudomonas aeruginosa*	325,344,461,483–488
Ventilator	*Pseudomonas aeruginosa*	325,336,337,343,483
	Burkholderia cepacia	202,355,470,490,492
	Stenotrophomonas maltophilia	491
	Acinetobacter species	365,367,477,489,493–497
	Sphingomonas paucimobilis	471,498
	Pseudomonas fluorescens	459
Faucet aerator	*Pseudomonas aeruginosa*	499,461
Sink or wash basin	*Pseudomonas aeruginosa*	141,143,325
	Stenotrophomonas maltophilia	480,483,500–502
	Acinetobacter species	503,504
Sink drain	*Pseudomonas aeruginosa*	346,347,462,483–485, 500,505,506
Showerhead	*Pseudomonas aeruginosa*	507
Water fountain or ice machine	*Pseudomonas aeruginosa*	508
Whirlpool or hydrotherapy tank	*Pseudomonas aeruginosa*	290,400,508,509
Urine collection or measuring device	*Pseudomonas aeruginosa*	379,388,390
Endoscope, cystoscope, or bronchoscope	*Pseudomonas aeruginosa*	246–252,378,380,510–514
Endoscope washer	*Pseudomonas aeruginosa*	512,513
Miscellaneous equipment	*Acinetobacter* species	472
	Sphingomonas paucimobilis	473,474
	Pseudomonas aeruginosa	387,415,421,434,487,515
	Burkholderia cepacia	266,455,516,517
	Stenotrophomonas maltophilia	518–520
Hemodialyzers or dialysis machines	*Pseudomonas aeruginosa*	255
	Burkholderia cepacia	264,265
	Stenotrophomonas maltophilia	264,521
	Acinetobacter species	255,264
	Pseudomonas stutzeri	299
Injected medication	*Pseudomonas aeruginosa*	244,432,433
	Burkholderia cepacia	260,490,522–524
	Acinetobacter species	525
	Ralstonia pickettii	289,293
Topical medications	*Burkholderia cepacia*	356–358,517,521,526,527

(continued)

TABLE 34.3. *(continued)*

Source	Microorganism	References
Inhaled medication	*Burkholderia cepacia*	528
Linen, bedclothes, or mattresses	*Pseudomonas aeruginosa*	391,396,480
	Acinetobacter species	529,530
Objects or surfaces	*Pseudomonas aeruginosa*	206,325,400,484,531,532
	Stenotrophomonas maltophilia	491
	Acinetobacter species	494,530,533,534
	Pseudomonas fluorescens	459
Pericardial allograft	*Ochrobactrum anthropi*	535
Organ allograft	*Pseudomonas aeruginosa*	536
Blood products	*Burkholderia cepacia*	259,261
	Acinetobacter species	533
	Pseudomonas fluorescens	285–288
Foods (salads)	*Pseudomonas aeruginosa*	143,508,537–541
Enteral formula	*Pseudomonas aeruginosa*	481,542
	Acinetobacter species	543
Food dye	*Pseudomonas aeruginosa*	349
Mouth wash	*Pseudomonas aeruginosa*	257,485,537
	Burkholderia cepacia	544–545
Skin cream	*Pseudomonas aeruginosa*	546,547
	Burkholderia cepacia	548
Soap or detergent	*Pseudomonas aeruginosa*	206,325,461,481,484,549
	Burkholderia cepacia	455
	Acinetobacter species	550
	Pseudomonas stutzeri	551
Bath sponge	*Pseudomonas oryzihabitans*	552
Antiseptic or disinfectant	*Pseudomonas aeruginosa*	150,158,169,499,508,547
	Burkholderia cepacia	74,157,161,166,170–172, 263,490,553–555
	Stenotrophomonas maltophilia	162
	Ralstonia pickettii	160,556

for total digestive decontamination (564). In that patient, colonization persisted for at least 5 months.

Hospital personnel infrequently are a reservoir for *P. aeruginosa*. Rates of positive cultures from stool have been less than 13% (434,483), and the concentration of microorganisms may be too low to be detected by rectal swab (483). Other sites, such as nose, throat, or skin, may be culture-positive in up to 5% of personnel caring for colonized patients (396). Hand colonization for at least 4 weeks has been reported in a nurse (487).

Acinetobacter is present on the skin in up to one fourth of normal individuals and about one third of hospitalized patients (566,567). Sites that are most frequently culture-positive are intertriginous areas such as the toe web and groin. Oropharyngeal or rectal carriage is uncommon, except in patients in ICUs (568,569). The hands of hospital personnel have been sampled for *Acinetobacter*, and the proportion of individuals with at least one positive specimen from serial cultures is about one third (566,570). Persistent colonization of the hands of a respiratory therapist has been reported (570). The frequency of hand colonization by *S. maltophilia* has not been investigated other than in response to outbreaks of infection. During an ICU epidemic, half of the hand cultures from nurses and respiratory therapists were positive (491). *S. maltophilia* rarely is present in stool of outpatients with diarrhea but has been detected in feces of one third of hematologic malignancy patients (227). *B. cepacia* rarely is recovered from sites other than the respiratory tract of patients with cystic fibrosis (561,571). Prior broad-spectrum antibiotic therapy appears to be an important risk factor for colonization or infection by *S. maltophilia* or *Acinetobacter* (270,282,283, 491,572).

Transmission

Nosocomial transmission of *P. aeruginosa* almost always results either from contact with environmental sources or from patient-to-patient spread via personnel. Possible transmission from environmental sources usually has been examined in response to case clusters or unusual clinical events. Even though many of the early studies did not utilize rigorous epidemiologic methods or *P. aeruginosa* typing systems, plausible circumstantial evidence was provided for transmission from most of the sources listed in Table 34.3. Later studies, in which patients and environmental isolates were typed, confirmed that contaminated items, such as water (257,400), food (143), antiseptics (169), endoscopes (249,250,252), and bronchoscopes (248,512), can transmit *P. aeruginosa* to patients. Such transmission occurs infrequently when standard aseptic practices are followed (141,487).

Patient-to-patient transmission of *P. aeruginosa* is documented by prospective studies in which periodic surveillance cultures of patients, personnel, and the environment were performed. Patient-to-patient transmission was considered to occur when a patient acquired a strain of *P. aeruginosa* that matched that of another patient and that was not present in any likely environmental source. Instances of apparent cross-transmission have been noted in increased-risk settings, such as ICUs (345, 487,560,573), hematology-oncology units (143,564), and pediatric units (344,505,506). Contaminated hands of personnel are the likely vehicle of cross-transmission, and numerous investigations have demonstrated frequent (325,347,396,487,505,574) or occasional (346,575–577) positive cultures of hands. During routine care and in designed experiments (344), the hands of personnel have become contaminated, especially after contact with heavily colonized patients (487), exudates (396), secretions (325,487), or excretions (462,575). The frequency of patient-to-patient transmission by personnel probably reflects the inadequacy of staffing, availability of gloves and hand-washing sinks, and attention to hand washing and other aseptic practices.

There now is compelling evidence that when proper aseptic practices are observed, most of the apparent acquisitions of *P. aeruginosa* represent the emergence of strains carried in the alimentary tract at concentrations below the threshold of detection. Careful long-term studies in ICUs (505,578) and an oncology ward (143) showed that "acquisitions" usually represent an array of *P. aeruginosa* types that do not match those isolated from environmental or patient reservoirs.

Clusters of cases of colonization or infection with other nonfermenters are usually caused by direct exposure to contaminated fluids or medical devices. Infection is facilitated by breaches in the normal host defenses by endotracheal tubes, intravenous catheters, hemodialyzers, peritoneal dialysis catheters, ventriculostomy tubes, or indwelling urinary catheters. For *S. maltophilia*, culture studies and epidemiologic findings sometimes suggest patient-to-patient transmission via the hands of personnel (366,491,572). Investigations of ICU outbreaks of colonization and infection by *Acinetobacter* have demonstrated multiple likely modes of transmission involving the environment and the hands of personnel. Cultures of surfaces (87,504,529,530,534,568, 579–581), equipment (87,503,530,568,581,582), hands of personnel (87,530,581), and latex gloves worn by personnel (568, 582) are commonly positive. Barrier or contact isolation precautions have been at least partly effective in controlling outbreaks (568,580–582); additionally, closure of units temporarily for cleaning, disinfection, and/or repainting also has been useful in some (530,579,580) but not all (569) settings. Air samples taken near culture-positive patients have yielded *Acinetobacter* (530, 580), but airborne transmission has not been proven. Conflicting findings about a possible summer peak in the incidence of *Acinetobacter* infections have been reported (90,282,366,438, 530,583,584).

DETECTION AND TYPING

P. aeruginosa grows readily on most standard laboratory media. For isolation from specimens or sources with mixed flora, media that are selective for gram-negative bacilli, such as MacConkey and eosin-methylene blue agars, are utilized (585). When culture surveillance of body sites or the environment is warranted, the detection of *P. aeruginosa* is facilitated by the use of selective media, and agar containing cetyltrimethylammonium bromide (cetrimide) is the most widely employed (564, 586–588). Other agents selective for *P. aeruginosa* include acetamide (589), nitrofurantoin (590), 9-chloro-9-(4-diethylaminophenyl)-10-phenylacridan (C-390) (591–593), 1,10-phenanthroline (594), C-390 and phenanthroline (595), and 2,4,4-trichloro-2-hydroxydiphenyl ether (Irgasan) (588). Before embarking on a culture survey with a selective medium, it is worthwhile to first confirm that the chosen medium inhibits competing species but not the strain(s) of interest. After isolation of bacteria on agar, characteristics that distinguish *P. aeruginosa* include a grape-like odor and production of a blue-green pigment (pyocyanin). Bacterial colonies exhibiting these features are definitively identified as *P. aeruginosa* by standard laboratory methods (585).

Most nonfermenters also grow well on nonselective media and MacConkey agar (596,597). For patients with cystic fibrosis, the isolation of *B. cepacia* from culture is significantly enhanced by the use of selective media. *Pseudomonas cepacia* agar (PCA) and oxidation-fermentation polymyxin-bacitracin-lactose (OFPBL) medium increase the yield of *B. cepacia* to three to four times that of MacConkey agar (598,599) and demonstrate evidence of growth 24 to 48 hours earlier (600). *B. cepacia* selective agar (BCSA), containing 1% lactose, 1% sucrose, polymyxin, gentamicin, and vancomycin, achieves better suppression of other respiratory tract pathogens than PCA or OFPBL while allowing the isolation of *B. cepacia* (601,602). *S. maltophilia* has been misidentified as *B. cepacia* based on a false-negative DNase reaction. Because of the important clinical and prognostic implications in patients with cystic fibrosis, careful interpretation of such laboratory assays is essential (603). Selective and differential media for the detection of *Acinetobacter* species, such as Leeds *Acinetobacter* medium (LAM), *Herellea* agar, and Holton's agar, were developed for use with clinical specimens and environmental testing (597,604,605).

Because strain typing systems have become more sophisticated and accessible, epidemiologic investigations of *P. aeruginosa* are now more efficient and provide increasingly meaningful information. Early typing systems relied on phenotypic characteristics such as biochemical reactions, antibiotic susceptibility patterns, bacteriophage susceptibility, pyocin susceptibility, pyocin production, O-serotype, and enzyme electrophoretic mobility. Because of the limited discriminatory power and sometimes cumbersome nature of such methods, these approaches largely have been replaced by DNA-based techniques (606,607). Only serotyping, based on antigenic determinants on cell wall lipopolysaccharide (International Antigenic Typing System), remains a useful, widely available system (606,608,609).

Plasmid profile analysis was among the first nucleic acid-based techniques applied to strain typing. This technique has been used infrequently (610), and its interpretation is limited by the absence of plasmids in some strains and by potential transfer or spontaneous loss of plasmid(s) in others. Newer techniques have focused on chromosomal DNA (genotyping) to demonstrate genetic relatedness. Restriction endonuclease analysis (REA) of genomic DNA is the simplest approach and is useful as a screening tool (609,611,612). Ribotyping has been employed successfully in epidemiologic investigations but is the least discriminatory of molecular methods (401,488,611, 613–615). A more precise approach is Southern blot analysis of chromosomal DNA, in which restriction endonuclease fragments carrying a specific sequence are detected by a DNA probe. Probes encoding the exotoxin A gene have proven useful (327, 401,545,611,616,617), but not all strains carry this gene. Probes encoding for phospholipase C or the pilin polypeptide also have been used alone or in combination with exotoxin A gene probes (327,616,618). REA of genomic DNA using enzymes with infrequent recognition sites followed by pulsed-field gel electrophoresis (PFGE) has proven highly discriminatory in epidemiologic investigations involving *P. aeruginosa* (564,611,619–622). This method is now considered the typing method of choice for *P. aeruginosa. P. aeruginosa* genotyping is also feasible by polymerase chain reaction (PCR) methodology such as random amplified polymorphic DNA analysis (RAPD) or enterobacterial repetitive intergenic consensus PCR (ERIC-PCR) (613,618, 623).

Similarly, for *B. cepacia*, the phenotypic typing methods (624) employed in the past are now considered unreliable (625). Ribotyping has documented patient-to-patient transmission (626–628); however, PFGE and RAPD are now the most commonly employed genotypic methods in epidemiologic investigations (625–630). Genotyping by repetitive extrapalindromic PCR (REP-PCR) is also reported (631). Multilocus restriction typing is under investigation as a tool to examine the molecular epidemiology of geographically remote clusters of *B. cepacia* (632).

For other nonfermenters, older methods such as serotyping (491,633) and plasmid DNA electrophoresis (634,635) are sometimes helpful. However, PFGE of digested genomic or total DNA is most commonly used, especially for *Acinetobacter* (84, 87,584,586,633,636–639) and *Stenotrophomonas* (640–644). Molecular epidemiologic investigations of the nonfermenters have been performed using a variety of other techniques, including ribotyping (645) and PCR-based systems (504,641, 646–651). (For more details on typing systems, see Chapter 102.)

PREVENTION AND CONTROL

Prevention and control of infections caused by nonfermenting gram-negative bacilli requires attention to many aspects of patient care and the hospital environment. Important measures are the following:

1. Tap water, especially after storage and/or treatment in the hospital, must be ensured to have minimal contamination. Systems such as those used to prepare and distribute water for hemodialysis should be monitored, because they may permit increased bacterial growth due to removal of chlorine and to stagnation.
2. Nonsterile (tap) water should not be allowed to stand in patient-care areas or areas where medical equipment or supplies are prepared or stored. For example, water baths and cut flowers in water are potentially hazardous. Tap water does collect in sink drains, but this has not been a significant hazard.
3. Whenever feasible, sterile water should be used in humidification devices. This is especially important for patients receiving mechanical ventilation and for neonates.
4. Antiseptics and disinfectants should be mixed to adequate concentrations, and the agents should be active against nonfermentative gram-negative bacilli. There is little justification for use of aqueous benzalkonium chloride antiseptics.
5. Medical equipment should be adequately sterilized or disinfected between patient uses. Problems usually have involved endoscopes, hemodialyzers, or reusable components of respiratory devices.
6. Avoid use of multidose vials of medications whenever possible.
7. Routine aseptic practices (glove removal and hand disinfection after each patient contact) should be emphasized throughout the hospital to reduce the potential for patient-to-patient transmission of microorganisms via the hands of healthcare workers. Strict adherence to these practices is particularly important in burn units, other ICUs, and settings for the care of persons with cystic fibrosis.
8. During contact with individual patients, care should be taken to avoid transfer of microorganisms from colonized sites to noncolonized sites susceptible to infection. Examples include the transfer of microorganisms from stool or the perineum to the respiratory tract or from the respiratory tract to a sternotomy wound or conjunctivae.
9. For established infections, utilize appropriate antibiotic therapy, including full doses and combination regimens, when indicated. This is especially important for *P. aeruginosa* sepsis and pneumonia and possibly for serious infections caused by *Acinetobacter*. When the emergence of resistance is likely (e.g., *P. aeruginosa* pneumonia), bacteriologic monitoring during therapy is warranted.
10. Judicious use of antibiotics should help to prevent the acquisition or emergence of highly resistant microorganisms such as *Acinetobacter, S. maltophilia*, and multiple-resistant *P. aeruginosa*.
11. In high-risk settings, surveillance should be conducted at least periodically to detect an increased incidence of sporadic cases or the occurrence of case clusters due to nonfermenters. Case clusters should be investigated to identify potentially preventable causes such as cross-transmission or transmission from environmental sources.
12. When outbreaks are caused by patient-to-patient cross-transmission, increased attention to aseptic practices is the primary control measure. Selective bowel decontamination can be considered an ancillary measure if enteric colonization constitutes a significant reservoir and the pathogen is fully susceptible to the regimen.
13. Because enteric colonization by *P. aeruginosa* poses a substantial risk of bacteremia during periods of neutropenia, it is advisable to exclude potentially contaminated foods, such

as uncooked vegetables, from the diet of neutropenic cancer patients.

REFERENCES

1. Johanson WG Jr, Higuchi JH, Chaudhuri TR, et al. Bacterial adherence to epithelial cells in bacillary colonization of the respiratory tract. *Am Rev Respir Dis* 1980;121:55–63.
2. Hahn HP. The type-4 pilus is the major virulence-associated adhesin of *Pseudomonas aeruginosa*—a review. *Gene* 1997;192:99–108.
3. Woods DE, Straus DC, Johnson WG Jr, et al. Role of pili in adherence of *Pseudomonas aeruginosa* to mammalian buccal epithelial cells. *Infect Immun* 1980;29:1146–1151.
4. Ramphal R, Small PM, Shands JW Jr, et al. Adherence of *Pseudomonas aeruginosa* to tracheal cells injured by influenza infection or by endotracheal intubation. *Infect Immun* 1980;27:614–619.
5. Ramphal R, McNiece MT, Polack FM. Adherence of *Pseudomonas aeruginosa* to the injured cornea: a step in the pathogenesis of corneal infections. *Ann Ophthalmol* 1981;13:421–425.
6. Plotkowski MC, Tournier JM, Puchelle E. *Pseudomonas aeruginosa* strains possess specific adhesins for laminin. *Infect Immun* 1996;64: 600–605.
7. Woods DE, Straus DC, Johanson WG Jr, et al. Role of fibronectin in the prevention of adherence of *Pseudomonas aeruginosa* to buccal cells. *J Infect Dis* 1981;143:784–790.
8. Woods DE, Straus DC, Johanson WG Jr, et al. Role of salivary protease activity in adherence of gram-negative bacilli to mammalian buccal epithelial cells in vivo. *J Clin Invest* 1981;68:1435–1440.
9. Costerton JW, Stewart PS, Greenberg EP. Bacterial biofilms: a common cause of persistent infections. *Science* 1999;284:1318–1322.
10. Whitchurch CB, Tolker-Nielsen T, Ragas PC, et al. Extracellular DNA required for bacterial biofilm formation. *Science* 2002;295: 1487.
11. Ramphal R, Pier GB. Role of *Pseudomonas aeruginosa* mucoid exopolysaccharide in adherence to tracheal cells. *Infect Immun* 1985;47: 1–4.
12. Hata JS, Fick RB. Airway adherence of *Pseudomonas aeruginosa*: mucoexopolysaccharide binding to human and bovine airway proteins. *J Lab Clin Med* 1991;117:410–422.
13. Marrie TJ, Harding GKM, Ronald AR, et al. Influence of mucoidy on antibody coating of *Pseudomonas aeruginosa. J Infect Dis* 1979; 139:357–361.
14. Simpson JA, Smith SF, Dean RT. Alginate inhibition of the uptake of *Pseudomonas aeruginosa* by macrophages. *J Gen Microbiol* 1988; 34:29–36.
15. Schwarzmann S, Boring JR III. Antiphagocytic effect of slime from a mucoid strain of *Pseudomonas aeruginosa. Infect Immun* 1971;3: 762–767.
16. Walters MC III, Roe F, Bugnicourt A, et al. Contributions of antibiotic penetration, oxygen limitation, and low metabolic activity to tolerance of *Pseudomonas aeruginosa* biofilms to ciprofloxacin and tobramycin. *Antimicrob Agents Chemother* 2003;47:317–323.
17. Iglewski BH, Liu PV, Kabat D. Mechanism of action of *Pseudomonas aeruginosa* exotoxin A: adenosine diphosphate-ribosylation of mammalian elongation factor 2 in vitro and in vivo. *Infect Immun* 1977; 15:138–144.
18. Pollack M, Taylor NS, Callahan LT III. Exotoxin production by clinical isolates of *Pseudomonas aeruginosa. Infect Immun* 1977;15: 446–480.
19. Pollack M. The role of exotoxin A in *Pseudomonas* disease and immunity. *Rev Infect Dis* 1983;5(suppl 5):5979–5984.
20. Blackwood LL, Stone RM, Iglewski BH, et al. Evaluation of *Pseudomonas aeruginosa* exotoxin A and elastase as virulence factors in acute lung infection. *Infect Immun* 1983;39:198–201.
21. Woods DE, Cryz SJ, Friedman RL, et al. Contribution of toxin A and elastase to virulence of *Pseudomonas aeruginosa* in chronic lung infection of rats. *Infect Immun* 1982;36:1223–1228.
22. Pollack M, Young LS. Protective activity of antibodies to exotoxin A and lipopolysaccharide at the onset of *Pseudomonas aeruginosa* septicemia in man. *J Clin Invest* 1979;63:276–286.
23. Cross AS, Sadoff JC, Iglewski BH, et al. Evidence for the role of toxin A in the pathogenesis of infection with *Pseudomonas aeruginosa* in humans. *J Infect Dis* 1980;142:538–546.
24. Woods DE, Que JU. Purification of *Pseudomonas aeruginosa* exoenzyme S. *Infect Immun* 1987;55:579–586.
25. Nicas TI, Bradley J, Lochner JE, et al. The role of exoenzyme S in infections with *Pseudomonas aeruginosa. J Infect Dis* 1985;152: 716–721.
26. Saiman L, Ishimoto K, Lory S, et al. The effects of piliation and exoproduct expression on the adherence of *Pseudomonas aeruginosa* to respiratory epithelial monolayers. *J Infect Dis* 1990;161:541–548.
27. Baltch AL, Griffen PE, Hammer M. *Pseudomonas aeruginosa* bacteremia: relationship of bacterial enzyme production and piocine types with clinical prognosis in 100 patients. *J Lab Clin Med* 1979;93: 600–606.
28. Mull JD, Callahan WS. The role of elastase of *Pseudomonas aeruginosa* in experimental infection. *Exp Mol Pathol* 1965;4:567–575.
29. Heck LW, Morihara K, Abrahamson DR. Degradation of soluble laminin and depletion of tissue-associated basement membrane laminin by *Pseudomonas aeruginosa* elastase and alkaline protease. *Infect Immun* 1986;54:149–153.
30. Schultz DR, Miller KD. Elastase of *Pseudomonas aeruginosa*: inactivation of complement components and complement derived chemotactic and phagocytic factors. *Infect Immun* 1974:10:128–135.
31. Fick RB, Baltimore RS, Squier SU, et al. IgG proteolytic activity of *Pseudomonas aeruginosa* in cystic fibrosis. *J Infect Dis* 1985;151: 589–598.
32. Theander TG, Kharazmi A, Pedersen BK, et al. Inhibition of human lymphocyte proliferation and cleavage of interleukin-2 by *Pseudomonas aeruginosa* proteases. *Infect Immun* 1988;56:1673–1677.
33. Horvat RT, Parmely ML. *Pseudomonas aeruginosa* alkaline protease degrades human gamma interferon and inhibits its bioactivity. *Infect Immun* 1988;56:2925–2932.
34. Parmely M, Gale A, Calbaugh M, et al. Proteolytic inactivation of cytokines by *Pseudomonas aeruginosa. Infect Immun* 1990;58: 3009–3014.
35. Becka RM, Vasil ML. Phospholipase C (heat-labile hemolysin) of *Pseudomonas aeruginosa*: purification and preliminary characterization. *J Bacteriol* 1981;152:239–245.
36. Johnson MK, Boese-Marrazzo D. Production and properties of heat-stable extracellular hemolysin from *Pseudomonas aeruginosa. Infect Immun* 1980;29:1028–1033.
37. Bishop MB, Baltch Al, Hill LA, et al. The effect of *Pseudomonas aeruginosa* cytotoxin and toxin A on human polymorphonuclear leukocytes. *J Med Microbiol* 1987;24:315–324.
38. Scharmann W. Purification and characterization of leucocidin from *Pseudomonas aeruginosa. J Gen Microbiol* 1976;93:292–302.
39. Young LS. Human immunity to *Pseudomonas aeruginosa*. II. Relationship between heat-stable opsonins and type-specific lipopolysaccharides. *J Infect Dis* 1972;126:277–287.
40. Pennington JE. Lipopolysaccharide pseudomonas vaccine: efficacy against pulmonary infection with *Pseudomonas aeruginosa. J Infect Dis* 1979;140:73–80.
41. Ziegler EJ, McCutchan JA, Doublas H, et al. Prevention of lethal *Pseudomonas* bacteremia with epimerase-deficient *E. coli* antiserum. *Trans Assoc Am Phys* 1975;88:101–108.
42. Pollack M, Huang AI, Prescott RK, et al. Enhanced survival in *Pseudomonas aeruginosa* septicemia associated with high levels of circulating antibody to *Escherichia coli* endotoxin core. *J Clin Invest* 1983; 72:1874–1881.
43. Whiteley M, Lee KM, Greenberg EP. Identification of genes controlled by quorum sensing in *Pseudomonas aeruginosa. Proc Natl Acad Sci USA* 1999;96:13904–13909.
44. Davies DG, Parsek MR, Pearson JP, et al. The involvement of cell-to-cell signals in the development of a bacterial biofilm. *Science* 1998; 280:295–298.
45. Singh PK, Schaefer AL, Parsek MR, et al. Quorum-sensing signals

indicate that cystic fibrosis lungs are infected with bacterial biofilms. *Nature* 2000;407:762–764.

46. Donabedian H. Quorum sensing and its relevance to infectious diseases. *J Infect* 2003;46:207–214.
47. Galán JE, Collmer A. Type III secretion machines: bacterial devices for protein delivery into host cell. *Science* 1999;284:1322–1328.
48. Hauser AR, Cobb E, Bodí M, et al. Type III protein secretion is associated with poor clinical outcomes in patients with ventilator-associated pneumonia caused by *Pseudomonas aeruginosa. Crit Care Med* 2002;30:521–528.
49. Roy-Burman A, Savel RH, Racine S, et al. Type III protein secretion is associated with death in lower respiratory and systemic *Pseudomonas aeruginosa* infections. *J Infect Dis* 2001;183:1767–1774.
50. Pollack M. The virulence of *Pseudomonas aeruginosa. Rev Infect Dis* 1984;6(suppl 3):S617–S626.
51. Buret A, Cripps AW. The immunoevasive activities of *Pseudomonas aeruginosa*. Relevance for cystic fibrosis. *Am Rev Respir Dis* 1993;148:793–805.
52. Brownstein DG, Johnson E. Experimental nasal infection of normal and leukopenic mice with *Pseudomonas aeruginosa. Vet Pathol* 1982;19:169–178.
53. Whimbey E, Kiehn TE, Brannon P, et al. Bacteremia and fungemia in patients with neoplastic disease. *Am J Med* 1987;82:723–730.
54. Jones RJ, Roe EA, Gupta JL. Controlled trial of *Pseudomonas* immunoglobulin and vaccine in burn patients. *Lancet* 1980;2:1263–1265.
55. Pennington JE. *Pseudomonas aeruginosa*. Vaccines and immunotherapy. *Infect Dis Clin North Am* 1990;4:259–270.
56. Korvick JA, Marsh JW, Starzl TE, et al. *Pseudomonas aeruginosa* bacteremia in patients undergoing liver transplantation: an emerging problem. *Surgery* 1991;109:62–68.
57. Kielhofner M, Atmar RL, Hamill RJ, et al. Life-threatening *Pseudomonas aeruginosa* infections in patients with human immunodeficiency virus infection. *Clin Infect Dis* 1992;14:403–411.
58. Markham RB, Pier GB, Goellner JJ, et al. In vitro T cell-mediated killing of *Pseudomonas aeruginosa*. II. The role of macrophages and T cell subsets in T cell killing. *J Immunol* 1985;134:4112–4117.
59. Powderly WG, Pier GB, Markham RB. T lymphocyte mediated protection against *Pseudomonas aeruginosa* infection in granulocytopenic mice. *J Clin Invest* 1986;78:375–380.
60. Nieuwenhuis ES, Matsumoto T, Exley M, et al. CD1d-dependent macrophage-mediated clearance of *Pseudomonas aeruginosa* from lung. *Nature Med* 2002;8:588–593.
61. Stover GB, Drake DR, Montie TC. Virulence of different *Pseudomonas* species in a burned mouse model: tissue colonization by *Pseudomonas cepacia. Infect Immun* 1983;41:1099–1104.
62. Gilardi GL. *Pseudomonas maltophilia* infections in man. *Am J Clin Pathol* 1969;51:58–61.
63. O'Brien M, Davis GHG. Enzymatic profile of *Pseudomonas maltophilia. J Clin Microbiol* 1982;16:417–421.
64. Denton M, Kerr KG. Microbiological and clinical aspects of infection associated with *Stenotrophomonas maltophilia. Clin Microbiol Rev* 1998;11:57–80.
65. Bottone EJ, Reitano M, Janda JM, et al. *Pseudomonas maltophilia* exoenzyme activity as correlate in pathogenesis of ecthyma gangrenosum. *J Clin Microbiol* 1986;24:995–997.
66. McKevitt AI, Woods DE. Characterization of *Pseudomonas cepacia* isolates from patients with cystic fibrosis. *J Clin Microbiol* 1984;19:291–293.
67. Moffet HL, Allan D, Williams T. Survival and dissemination of bacteria in nebulizers and incubators. *Am J Dis Child* 1967;114:13–20.
68. Carson LA, Favero MS, Bond WW, et al. Morphological, biochemical, and growth characteristics of *Pseudomonas cepacia* from distilled water. *Appl Microbiol* 1973;25:476–483.
69. Gelbart SM, Reinhardt GF, Greenlee HB. *Pseudomonas cepacia* strains isolated from water reservoirs of unheated nebulizers. *J Clin Microbiol* 1976;3:62–66.
70. Jonsson V. Proposal of a new species *Pseudomonas kingii. Int J Systemic Bacteriol* 1970;20:255–257.
71. Pegues DA, Carson LA, Anderson RL, et al. Outbreak of *Pseudomonas cepacia* bacteremia in oncology patients. *Clin Infect Dis* 1993;16:407–411.
72. Coenye T, Vandamme P, Govan JRW, et al. Taxonomy and identification of *Burkholderia cepacia* complex. *J Clin Microbiol* 2001;39:3427–3436.
73. Bevivino A, Dalmastri C, Tabacchioni S, et al. *Burkholderia cepacia* complex bacteria from clinical and environmental sources in Italy: genomovar status and distribution of traits related to virulence and transmissibility. *J Clin Microbiol* 2002;40:846–851.
74. Speller DCE, Stephens ME, Viant AC. Hospital infection by *Pseudomonas cepacia. Lancet* 1971;1:798–799.
75. Jarvis WR, Olson D, Tablan O, et al. The epidemiology of nosocomial *Pseudomonas cepacia* infections: endemic infections. *Eur J Epidemiol* 1987;3:233–236.
76. Mohr CD, Tomich M, Herfst CA. Cellular aspects of *Burkholderia cepacia* infection. *Microbes Infect* 2001;3:425–435.
77. Sokol PA, Darling P, Woods DE, et al. Role of ornibactin biosynthesis in virulence of *Burkholderia cepacia*: characterization of *pvdA*, the gene encoding L-ornithine N^5-oxygenase. *Infect Immun* 1999;67:4443–4455.
78. Martin DW, Mohr CD. Invasion and intracellular survival of *Burkholderia cepacia. Infect Immun* 2000;68:24–29.
79. Lewenza S, Conway B, Greenberg EP, et al. Quorum sensing in *Burkholderia cepacia*: identification of the LuxRI homologs CepRI. *J Bacteriol* 1999;181:748–756.
80. McKenney D, Brown KE, Allison DG. Influence of *Pseudomonas aeruginosa* exoproducts on virulence factor production in *Burkholderia cepacia*: evidence of interspecies communication. *J Bacteriol* 1995;177:6989–6992.
81. Henriksen SD. *Moraxella, Acinetobacter*, and the *Mimeae. Bacteriol Rev* 1973;37:522–561.
82. Ristuccia RA, Cunha BA. *Acinetobacter. Infect Control* 1983;4:226–229.
83. Bouvet PJM, Grimont PAD. Taxonomy of the genus *Acinetobacter* with the recognition of *Acinetobacter baumannii* sp. nov., *Acinetobacter haemolyticus* sp. nov., *Acinetobacter johnsonii* sp. nov., and *Acinetobacter junii* sp. nov. and emended descriptions of *Acinetobacter calcoaceticus* and *Acinetobacter wolffii. Int J Sys Bacteriol* 1986;36:228–240.
84. Bergogne-Bérézin E, Towner KJ. *Acinetobacter* spp. as nosocomial pathogens: microbiological, clinical, and epidemiological features. *Clin Microbiol Rev* 1996;9:148–165.
85. Tilley PAG, Roberts FJ. Bacteremia with *Acinetobacter* species: risk factors and prognosis in different clinical settings. *Clin Infect Dis* 1994;18:896–900.
86. Cisneros JM, Reyes MJ, Pachon J, et al. Bacteremia due to *Acinetobacter baumannii:* epidemiology, clinical findings and prognostic features. *Clin Infect Dis* 1996;22:1026–1032.
87. Kaul R, Burt JA, Cork L, et al. Investigation of a multiyear multiple critical care unit outbreak due to relatively drug-sensitive *Acinetobacter baumannii:* risk factors and attributable mortality. *J Infect Dis* 1996;174:1279–1287.
88. Villers D, Espaze E, Costa-Bure M, et al. Nosocomial *Acinetobacter baumannii* infections: microbiological and clinical epidemiology. *Ann Intern Med* 1998;129:182–189.
89. Fagon J-Y, Chastre J, Domart Y, et al. Mortality due to ventilator-associated pneumonia or colonization with *Pseudomonas* or *Acinetobacter* species: assessment by quantitative culture of samples obtained by a protected specimen brush. *Clin Infect Dis* 1996;23:538–542.
90. Austery NM, Currie BJ, Withnall KM. Community-acquired *Acinetobacter* pneumonia in the northern territory of Australia. *Clin Infect Dis* 1992;14:83–91.
91. Smalley DL. Endotoxin-like activity in *Pseudomonas paucimobilis* (group IIK biotype 1) and *Flavobacterium multivorium* (group IIK biotype 2). *Experientia* 1982;38:1483–1484.
92. Morrison AJ Jr, Shulman JA. Community-acquired bloodstream infection caused by *Pseudomonas paucimobilis:* case report and review of the literature. *J Clin Microbiol* 1986;24:853–855.
93. Chen SCA, Lawrence RH, Packham DR, et al. Cellulitis due to *Pseu-*

domonas putrefaciens: possible production of exotoxins. *Rev Infect Dis* 1991;13:642–643.
94. Visalli MA, Jacobs MR, Appelbaum PC. Activities of three quinolones, alone and in combination with extended-spectrum cephalosporins or gentamicin, against *Stenotrophomonas maltophilia. Antimicrob Agents Chemother* 1998;42:2002–2005.
95. Fass RJ, Barnishan J, Solomon MC, et al. In vitro activities of quinolones, β-lactams, tobramycin, and trimethoprim-sulfamethoxazole against nonfermentative gram-negative bacilli. *Antimicrob Agents Chemother* 1996;40:1412–1418.
96. Jones RN, Pfaller MA, Marshall SA, et al. Antimicrobial activity of 12 broad spectrum-spectrum agents tested against 270 nosocomial blood stream infection isolates caused by non-enteric gram-negative bacilli: occurrence of resistance, molecular epidemiology, and screening for metallo-enzymes. *Diagn Microbiol Infect Dis* 1997;29: 187–192.
97. Quinn JP. Clinical problems posed by multiresistant nonfermenting gram-negative pathogens. *Clin Infect Dis* 1998;27(suppl 1): S117–124.
98. Karlowsky JA, Draghi DC, Jones ME, et al. Surveillance for antimicrobial susceptibility among clinical isolates of *Pseudomonas aeruginosa* and *Acinetobacter baumannii* from hospitalized patients in the United States, 1998 to 2001. *Antimicrob Agents Chemother* 2003;47: 1681–1688.
99. Friedland I, Stinson L, Ikaiddi M, et al. Phenotypic antimicrobial resistance patterns in *Pseudomonas aeruginosa* and *Acinetobacter*: results of a multicenter intensive care unit surveillance study, 1995–2000. *Diagn Microbiol Infect Dis* 2003;45:245–250.
100. Hancock REW. Resistance mechanisms in *Pseudomonas aeruginosa* and other nonfermentative gram-negative bacteria. *Clin Infect Dis* 1998;27(suppl 1):S93–S99.
101. Lin RD, Hsueh PR, Chang JC, et al. *Flavimonas oryzihabitans* bacteremia: clinical features and microbiological characteristics of isolates. *Clin Infect Dis* 1997;24:867–873.
102. Rolston KVI, Ho DH, LeBlance B, et al. In vitro activities of antimicrobial agents against clinical isolates of *Flavimonas oryzihabitans* obtained from patients with cancer. *Antimicrob Agents Chemother* 1993; 37:2504–2505.
103. Saiman L, Chen Y, tabibi S, et al. Identification and antimicrobial susceptibility of *Alcaligenes xylosoxidans* isolated from patients with cystic fibrosis. *J Clin Microbiol* 2001;39:3942–3945.
104. Livermore DM. Multiple mechanisms of antimicrobial resistance in *Pseudomonas aeruginosa*: our worst nightmare? *Clin Infect Dis* 2002; 34:634–640.
105. Lambert PA. Mechanisms of antibiotic resistance in *Pseudomonas aeruginosa. J R Soc Med* 2002;95(suppl 41):22–26.
106. Zhang L, Li X, Poole K. Fluoroquinolone susceptibilities of efflux-mediated multidrug-resistant *Pseudomonas aeruginosa, Stenotrophomonas maltophilia* and *Burkholderia cepacia. J Antimicrob Chemother* 2001;48:549–552.
107. Pitout JD, Sanders C, Sanders WE Jr. Antimicrobial resistance with focus on β-lactam resistance in gram-negative bacilli. *Am J Med* 1997; 103:51–59.
108. Livermore DM. Of *Pseudomonas* porins, pumps, and carbapenems. *J Antimicrob Chemother* 2001;47:247–250.
109. Li X, Poole K, Nikaido H. Contributions of MexAB-OprM and an EmrE homolog to intrinsic resistance of *Pseudomonas aeruginosa* to aminoglycosides and dyes. *Antimicrob Agents Chemother* 2003;47: 27–33.
110. Godrey AJ, Bryan LE, Rabin HR. β-lactam resistant *Pseudomonas aeruginosa* with modified penicillin binding proteins emerging during cystic fibrosis treatment. *Antimicrob Agents Chemother* 1981;19: 705–711.
111. Vurma-Rapp U, Kayser FH, Hadorn K, et al. Mechanism of imipenem resistance acquired by three *Pseudomonas aeruginosa* strains during imipenem therapy. *Eur J Clin Microbiol Infect Dis* 1990;9: 580–587.
112. Quinn JP, Studemeister AE, DiVincenzo CA, et al. Resistance to imipenem in *Pseudomonas aeruginosa*: clinical experience and biochemical mechanisms. *Rev Infect Dis* 1988;10:892–898.
113. Woodford N, Palepou MFI, Babini GS, et al. Carbapenemase-producing *Pseudomonas aeruginosa* in UK. *Lancet* 1998;352:546–547.
114. Pournaras S, Maiati M, Petinaki E, et al. Hospital outbreak of multiple clones of *Pseudomonas aeruginosa* carrying the unrelated metallo-β-lactamase gene variants bla_{VIM-2} and bla_{VIM-4}. *J Antimicrob Chemother* 2002;51:1409–1414.
115. Mouneimné H, Robert J, Jarlier V, et al. Type II topoisomerase mutations in ciprofloxacin-resistant strains of *Pseudomonas aeruginosa. Antimicrob Agents Chemother* 1999;43:62–66.
116. Takenouchi T, Sakagawa E, Sugawara M. Detection of gyrA mutations among 335 *Pseudomonas aeruginosa* strains isolated in Japan and their susceptibilities to fluoroquinolones. *Antimicrob Agents Chemother* 1999;43:406–409.
117. Akasaka T, Tanaka M, Yamaguchi A, et al. Type II topoisomerase mutations in fluoroquinolone-resistant clinical strains of *Pseudomonas aeruginosa* isolated in 1998 and 1999: role of target enzyme in mechanism of fluoroquinolone resistance. *Antimicrob Agents Chemother* 2001;45:2263–2268.
118. Higgins PG, Fluit AC, Milatovic M, et al. Mutations in GyrA, ParC, MexR and NfxB in clinical isolates of *Pseudomonas aeruginosa. Int J Antimicrob Agents* 2003;21:409–413.
119. Hoban DJ, Biedenbach DJ, Mutnick AH, et al. Pathogen of occurrence and susceptibility patterns associated with pneumonia in hospitalized patients in North America: results of the SENTRY Antimicrobial Surveillance Study (2000). *Diagn Microbiol Infect Dis* 2003;45: 279–285
120. Jones RN, Kirby JT, Beach ML, et al. Geographic variations in activity of broad-spectrum β-lactams against *Pseudomonas aeruginosa*: summary of the worldwide SENTRY Antimicrobial Surveillance Program (1997–2000). *Diagn Microbiol Infect Dis* 2002;43:239–243.
121. Gales AC, Jones RN, Forward KR, et al. Emerging importance of multi-drug resistant *Acinetobacter* species and *Stenotrophomonas maltophilia* as pathogens in seriously ill patients: geographic patterns, epidemiological features, and trends in the SENTRY Antimicrobial Surveillance Program (1997–1999). *Clin Infect Dis* 2001;32(suppl 2):104–113.
122. Micozzi A, Venditti M, Monaco M, et al. Bacteremia due to *Stenotrophomonas maltophilia* in patients with hematologic malignancies. *Clin Infect Dis* 2000;31:705–711.
123. Betriu C, Sánchez A, Palau ML, et al. Correspondence. Antibiotic resistance surveillance of *Stenotrophomonas maltophilia*, 1993–1999. *J Antimicrob Chemother* 2001;48:141–156.
124. Cohn ML, Waites KB. Antimicrobial activities of gatifloxacin against nosocomial isolates of *Stenotrophomonas maltophilia* measured by MIC and time-kill studies. *Antimicrob Agents Chemother* 2001;45: 2126–2128.
125. Speert DP. Advances in *Burkholderia cepacia* complex. *Pediatr Respir Rev* 2002;3:230–235.
126. Isles A, Maclusky I, Corey M, et al. *Pseudomonas cepacia* infection in cystic fibrosis: an emerging problem. *J Pediatr* 1984;104:206–210.
127. Wisplinghoff H, Edmond MB, Pfaller MA, et al. Nosocomial bloodstream infections caused by *Acinetobacter* species in United States hospitals: clinical features, molecular epidemiology, and antimicrobial susceptibility. *Clin Infect Dis* 2000;31:690–697.
128. Urban C, Segal-Maurer S, Rahal JJ. Considerations in control and treatment of nosocomial infections due to multidrug-resistant *Acinetobacter baumannii. Clin Infect Dis* 2003;36:1268–1274.
129. Landman D, Quale JM, Mayora D, et al. Citywide clonal outbreak of multiresistant *Acinetobacter baumannii* and *Pseudomonas aeruginosa* in Brooklyn, NY: the preantibiotic era has returned. *Arch Intern Med* 2002;162:1515–1520.
130. Corbella X, Montero A, Pujol M, et al. Emergence and rapid spread of carbapenem resistance during a large and sustained hospital outbreak of multiresistant *Acinetobacter baumannii. J Clin Microbiol* 2000;38:4086–4095.
131. Das I, Lambert P, Hill D, et al. Carbapenem-resistant *Acinetobacter* and role of curtains in an outbreak in intensive care units. *J Hosp Infect* 2002;50:110–114.
132. Chow AW, Wong J, Bartlett KH. Synergistic interactions of ciprofloxacin and extended spectrum beta-lactams or aminoglycosides against

Acinetobacter calcoaceticus ss. anitratus. *Diagn Microbiol Infect Dis* 1988;9:213–217.
133. Traub WH, Spohr M, Bauer D. Susceptibility of *Acinetobacter calcoaceticus* to antimicrobial drugs, alone and combined, with and without defibrinated human blood. *Chemotherapy* 1989;35:95–104.
134. Wood CG, Hanes SD, Croce MA, et al. Comparison of ampicillin-sulbactam and imipenem-cilastatin for the treatment of *Acinetobacter* ventilator-associated pneumonia. *Clin Infect Dis* 2002;34: 1425–1430.
135. Crues JV III, Murray BE, Moellering RC Jr. In vitro activity of three tetracycline antibiotics against *Acinetobacter calcoaceticus* subsp. anitratus. *Antimicrob Agents Chemother* 1979;16:690–692.
136. Gales AC, Reis AO, Jones RN. Contemporary assessment of antimicrobial susceptibility testing methods for polymyxin B and colistin: review of available interpretative criteria and quality control guidelines. *J Clin Microbiol* 2001;39:183–190.
137. Saugar JM, Alarcón T, López-Hernández S, et al. Activities of polymyxin B and cecropin A-melittin peptide CA(1–8)M(1–18) against a multiresistant strain of *Acinetobacter baumannii. Antimicrob Agents Chemother* 2002;56:875–878.
138. Levin AS, Barone AA, Penco J, et al. Intravenous colisitin as therapy for nosocomial infections caused by multi-drug-resistant *Pseudomonas aeruginosa* and *Acinetobacter baumannii. Clin Infect Dis* 1999;28: 1008–1011.
139. Rose HD, Schreier J. The effect of hospitalization and antibiotic therapy on the gram-negative fecal flora. *Am J Med Sci* 1968;255: 228–236.
140. Buck AC, Cooke EM. The fate of ingested *Pseudomonas aeruginosa* in normal persons. *J Med Microbiol* 1969;2:521–525.
141. Richet H, Escande MC, Marie JP, et al. Epidemic *Pseudomonas aeruginosa* serotype 016 bacteremia in hematology-oncology patients. *J Clin Microbiol* 1989;27:1992–1996.
142. Gaya H, Adnitt PI, Turner P. Changes in gut flora after cephalexin treatment. *Br Med J* 1970;3:624–625.
143. Griffith SJ, Nathan C, Selander RK, et al. The epidemiology of *Pseudomonas aeruginosa* in oncology patients in general hospital. *J Infect Dis* 1989;160:1030–1036.
144. Villarino ME, Stevens LE, Schable B, et al. Risk factors for epidemic *Xanthomonas maltophilia* infection/colonization in intensive care unit patients. *Infect Control Hosp Epidemiol* 1992;13:201–206.
145. Carmeli Y, Samore MH. Comparison of treatment with imipenem vs. ceftazidime as a predisposing factor for nosocomial acquisition of *Stenotrophomonas maltophilia*: a historical cohort study. *Clin Infect Dis* 1997;24:1131–1134.
146. Peacock JE, Sorrell L, Sottile FD, et al. Nosocomial respiratory tract colonization and infection with aminoglycoside-resistant *Acinetobacter calcoaceticus* var anitratus: epidemiologic characteristics and clinical significance. *Infect Control Hosp Epidemiol* 1988;9:302–308.
147. Elting LS, Bodey GP. Septicemia due to *Xanthomonas* species and non-*aeruginosa Pseudomonas* species: increasing incidence of catheter-related infections. *Medicine* 1990;69:296–306.
148. Lortholary O, Fagon J-Y, Hoi AB, et al. Nosocomial acquisition of multiresistant *Acinetobacter baumannii:* risk factors and prognosis. *Clin Infect Dis* 1995;20:790–796.
149. Plotkin SA, Austrian R. Bacteremia caused by Pseudomonas sp. following the use of materials stored in solutions of a catonic surface-active agent. *Am J Med Sci* 1958;235:621–627.
150. Shickman MD, Guze LB, Pearce ML. Bacteremia following cardiac catheterization. Report of a case and studies on the source. *N Engl J Med* 1959;260:1164–1166.
151. Lee JC, Fialkow PJ. Benzalkonium chloride source of hospital infection with gram-negative bacteria. *JAMA* 1961;177:708–710.
152. Frank MJ, Schaffner W. Contaminated aqueous benzalkonium chloride. An unnecessary hospital infection hazard. *JAMA* 1976;236: 2418–2419.
153. Kaslow RA, Mackel DC, Mallison GF. Nosocomial pseudobacteremia. Positive blood cultures due to contaminated benzalkonium antiseptic. *JAMA* 1976;236:2407–2409.
154. Dixon RE, Kaslow RA, Mackel DC, et al. Aqueous quaternary ammonium antiseptics and disinfectants. Use and misuse. *JAMA* 1976;236: 2415–2417.
155. Guinness M, Levey J. Contamination of aqueous dilutions of resiguard disinfectant with *Pseudomonas. Med J Aust* 1976;2:392.
156. Levey JM, Guinness MDG. Hospital microbial environment. Need for continual surveillance. *Med J Aust* 1981;1:590–592.
157. Hardy PC, Ederer GM, Matsen JM. Contamination of commercially packaged urinary catheter kits with the pseudomonad EO-1. *N Engl J Med* 1970;282:33–35.
158. Anyiwo CE, Coker AO, Daniel SO. *Pseudomonas aeruginosa* in post-operative wounds from chlorhexidine solutions. *J Hosp Infect* 1982; 3:189–191.
159. Sobel JC, Hashman N, Reinherz G, et al. Nosocomial *Pseudomonas cepacia* infection associated with chlorhexidine contamination. *Am J Med* 1982;73:183–186.
160. Kahan A, Philippon A, Paul G, et al. Nosocomial infections by chlorhexidine solution contaminated with *Pseudomonas pickettii* (Biovar VA-1). *J Infect* 1983;7:256–263.
161. Bassett DCJ, Stokes KJ, Thomas WRG. Wound infection with *Pseudomonas multivorans.* A water-borne contaminant of disinfectant solutions. *Lancet* 1970;1:1188–1191.
162. Wishart MM, Riley TV. Infection with *Pseudomonas maltophilia* hospital outbreak due to contaminated disinfectant. *Med J Aust* 1976;2: 710–712.
163. Lowbury EJL. Contamination of cetrimide and other fluids with *Pseudomonas pyocyanea. Br J Ind Med* 1951;8:22–25.
164. Anderson K. The contamination of hexachlorophene soap with *Pseudomonas pyocyanea. Med J Aust* 1962;2:463.
165. Keys TF, Melton LJ, Maker MD, et al. A suspected hospital outbreak of pseudobacteremia due to *Pseudomonas stutzeri. J Infect Dis* 1983; 147:489–493.
166. Burdon DW, Whitby JL. Contamination of hospital disinfectants with *Pseudomonas* species. *Br Med J* 1967;2:153–155.
167. Elliott B, Masters P. *Pseudomonas* contamination of antiseptic/disinfectant solutions. *Med J Aust* 1977;1:155–156.
168. Newman KA, Tenney JH, Oken HA, et al. Persistent isolation of an unusual *Pseudomonas* species from a phenolic disinfectant system. *Infect Control* 1984;5:219–222.
169. Parrott PL, Terry PM, Whitworth EN, et al. *Pseudomonas aeruginosa* peritonitis associated with contaminated polaxamer-iodine solution. *Lancet* 1982;2:683–685.
170. Craven DE, Moody B, Connolly MG, et al. Pseudobacteremia caused by povidone-iodine solution contaminated with *Pseudomonas cepacia. N Engl J Med* 1981;305:621–623.
171. Berkelman RL, Lewin S, Allen JR, et al. Pseudobacteremia attributed to contamination of povidone-iodine with *Pseudomonas cepacia. Ann Intern Med* 1981;95:32–36.
172. Panlilo AL, Beck-Sague CM, Siegel JD, et al. Infections and pseudoinfections due to povidone-iodine solution contaminated with *Pseudomonas cepacia. Clin Infect Dis* 1992;14:1078–1083.
173. Parker RH, Hoeprich PD. In vitro effect of buffered solutions of acetic acid, triclobisonium chloride, chlorhexidine diacetate, and chlorhexidine digluconate on urinary tract pathogens. *Antimicrob Agents Chemother* 1962;2:26–34.
174. Richards RME, Richards JM. *Pseudomonas cepacia* resistance to antibacterials. *J Pharm Sci* 1979;68:1436–1438.
175. Stickler DJ, Thomas B, Chawla JC. Antiseptic and antibiotic resistance in gram-negative bacteria causing urinary tract infection in spinal cord injured patients. *Paralegia* 1981;19:50–58.
176. Shiraishi T, Nakagawa Y. Review of disinfectant susceptibility of bacteria isolated in hospital to commonly used disinfectants. *Postgrad Med J* 1993;69(suppl 3):S70–S77.
177. Rutala WA, Cole EC. Ineffectiveness of hospital disinfectants against bacteria: a collaborative study. *Infect Contr* 1987;8:501–506.
178. Prince HN, Nonemaker WS, Norguard RC, et al. Drug resistance studies with topical antiseptics. *J Pharm Sci* 1978;67:1629–1631.
179. Higgins CS, Murtough SM, Williamson E, et al. Resistance to antibiotics and biocides among non-fermenting gram-negative bacteria. *Clin Microbiol Infect* 2001;7:308–315.

180. McDonnell G, Russell AD. Antiseptics and disinfectants: activity, action, and resistance. *Clin Microbiol Rev* 1999;12:147–179.
181. Stewart PS, Costerton JW. Antibiotic resistance of bacteria in biofilms. *Lancet* 2001;358:135–188.
182. Mah TFC, O'Toole GA. Mechanisms of biofilm resistance to antimicrobial agents. *Trends Microbiol* 2001;9:34–39.
183. Donlon RM, Costerton RM. Biofilms: survival mechanisms of clinically relevant microorganisms. *Clin Microbiol Rev* 2002;167–193.
184. Cochran WL, McFeters GA, Stewart PS. Reduced susceptibility of thin *Pseudomonas aeruginosa* biofilms to hydrogen peroxide and monochloramine. *J Appl Microbiol* 2000;88:22–30.
185. Vess RW, Anderson RL, Carr JH, et al. The colonization of solid PVC surfaces and the acquisition of resistance to germicides by water micro-organisms. *J Appl Bacteriol* 1993;74:215–221.
186. Anderson RL, Holland BW, Carr JK, et al. Effect of disinfectants on pseudomonads colonized on the interior surface of PVC pipes. *Am J Public Health* 1990;80:17–21.
187. Anderson RL, Vess RW, Carr JH, et al. Investigations of intrinsic *Pseudomonas cepacia* contamination in commercially manufactured povidone-iodine. *Infect Control Hosp Epidemiol* 1991;12:297–302.
188. Poole K. Mechanisms of bacterial biocide and antibiotic resistance. *J Appl Microbiol Symp Suppl* 2002;92:55S–64S.
189. Brown ML, Aldrich HC, Gauthier JJ. Relationship between glycocalyx and povidone-iodine resistance in *Pseudomonas aeruginosa* (ATCC 27853) biofilms. *Appl Environ Microbiol* 1995;61:187–193.
190. Grobe KJ, Zahller J, Stewart PS. Role of dose concentration in biocide efficacy against *Pseudomonas aeruginosa* biofilms. *J Ind Microbiol Biotechnol* 2002;29:10–15.
191. Tyler JE, Finn RK. Growth rates of a pseudomonad on 2,4-dichlorophenoxyacetic acid and 2,4-dichlorophenol. *Appl Microbiol* 1974;28: 181–184.
192. Hopper DJ, Taylor DG. Pathways for the degradation of m-cresol and p-cresol by *Pseudomonas putida. J Bacteriol* 1975;122:1–6.
193. Wong CL, Dunn NW. Combined chromosomal and plasmid encoded control for the degradation of phenol in *Pseudomonas putida. Genet Res* 1976;27:405–412.
194. Haefeli C, Franklin, C, Hardy K. Plasmid-determined silver resistance in *Pseudomonas stutzeri* isolated from a silver mine. *J Bacteriol* 1984; 158:389–392.
195. Beckman W, Lessie TG. Response of *Pseudomonas cepacia* to β-lactam antibiotics: utilization of penicillin G as the carbon source. *J Bacteriol* 1979;140:1126–1128.
196. Johnsen J. Utilization of benzylpenicillin as carbon, nitrogen and energy source by a *Pseudomonas fluorescens* strain. *Arch Microbiol* 1977; 115:271–275.
197. Knackmuss H, Hellwig M. Utilization and cooxidation of chlorinated phenols by *Pseudomonas* sp. B 13. *Arch Microbiol* 1978;117:1–7.
198. Adair FW, Geftic SG, Gelzer J. Resistance of *Pseudomonas* to quaternary ammonium compounds. *Appl Microbiol* 1969;18:299–302.
199. Price D, Ahearn DG. Incidence and persistence of *Pseudomonas aeruginosa* in whirlpools. *J Clin Microbiol* 1988;26:1650–1654.
200. Favero MS, Carson LA, Bond WW, et al. *Pseudomonas aeruginosa*: growth in distilled water from hospitals. *Science* 1971;173:836–838.
201. Levey JM, Guinness MDG. Hospital microbial environment. Need for continual surveillance. *Med J Aust* 1981;1:590–592.
202. Gelbart SM, Reinhardt GF, Greenlee HB. *Pseudomonas cepacia* strains isolated from water reservoirs of unheated nebulizers. *J Clin Microbiol* 1976;3:62–66.
203. Favero MS, Drake CH. Factors influencing the occurrence of high numbers of iodine-resistant bacteria in iodinated swimming pools. *Appl Microbiol* 1966;14:627–635.
204. Emmanouilidou-Arseni A, Koumentakou I. Viability of *Pseudomonas aeruginosa. J Bacteriol* 1964;87:1253.
205. Houang ET, Buckley R, Smith M, et al. Survival of *Pseudomonas aeruginosa* in plaster of Paris. *J Hosp Infect* 1981;2:231–235.
206. Zimakoff J, Hoiby N, Rosendal K, et al. Epidemiology of *Pseudomonas aeruginosa* infection and the role of contamination of the environment in a cystic fibrosis clinic. *J Hosp Infect* 1983;4:31–40.
207. Hurst V, Sutter VL. Survival of *Pseudomonas aeruginosa* in the hospital environment. *J Infect Dis* 1966;116:151–154.
208. Rosenthal SL. Sources of *Pseudomonas* and *Acinetobacter* species found in human culture materials. *Am J Clin Pathol* 1974;62:807–811.
209. Getchell-White SI, Donowitz LG, Gröschel DHM. The inanimate environment of an intensive care unit as a potential source of nosocomial bacteria: evidence for long survival of *Acinetobacter calcoaceticus. Infect Control Hosp Epidemiol* 1989;10:402–407.
210. Hirai Y. Survival of bacteria under dry conditions; from a viewpoint of nosocomial infection. *J Hosp Infect* 1991;19:191–200.
211. Musa EK, Desai N, Casewell MW. The survival of *Acinetobacter* calcoaceticus inoculated on fingertips and on formica. *J Hosp Infect* 1990; 15:219–227.
212. Wendt C, Dietze B, Dietz E, et al. Survival of *Acinetobacter baumannii* on dry surfaces. *J Clin Microbiol* 1997;35:1394–1397.
213. Jawad A, Seifert H, Snelling AM, et al. Survival of *Acinetobacter baumannii* on dry surfaces: comparison of outbreak and sporadic isolates. *J Clin Microbiol* 1998;36:1938–1941.
214. Meyer GW. *Pseudomonas cepacia* septicemia associated with intravenous therapy. *Calif Med* 1973;119:15–18.
215. Geftic SG, Heymann H, Adair FW. Fourteen-year survival of *Pseudomonas cepacia* in a salts solution preserved with benzalkonium chloride. *Appl Environ Microbiol* 1979;37:505–510.
216. Kreger BE, Craven DE, Carling PC, et al. Gram-negative bacteremia. III. Reassessment of etiology, epidemiology, and ecology in 612 patients. *Am J Med* 1980;68:332–343.
217. Sherertz RJ, Sarubbi FA. Three year study of nosocomial infections associated with *Pseudomonas aeruginosa. J Clin Microbiol* 1983;18: 160–164.
218. McManus AT, Mason AD Jr, McManus WF, et al. Twenty-five year review of *Pseudomonas aeruginosa* bacteremia in a burn center. *Eur J Clin Microbiol* 1985;4:219–223.
219. Bodey GP, Jadeja L, Elting L. *Pseudomonas* bacteremia: retrospective analysis of 410 episodes. *Arch Intern Med* 1985;145:1621–1629.
220. Schimpff SC, Greene WH, Young VM, et al. Significance of *Pseudomonas aeruginosa* in the patient with leukemia or lymphoma. *J Infect Dis* 1974;130(suppl):S24–S31.
221. Curtin JA, Petersdorf RG, Bennett IL Jr. *Pseudomonas* bacteremia: review of ninety-one cases. *Ann Intern Med* 1961;54:1077–1107.
222. Baltch AL, Griffin PE. *Pseudomonas aeruginosa* bacteremia: a clinical study of 75 patients. *Am J Med Sci* 1977;274:119–129.
223. McKendrick MW, Geddes AM. *Pseudomonas* septicemia in a general hospital—seven years experience. *Q J Med* 1981;series L:331–344.
224. Dorff GJ, Geimer NF, Rosenthal DR, et al. *Pseudomonas* septicemia: illustrated evolution of its skin lesion. *Arch Intern Med* 1971;128: 591–595.
225. Teplitz C. Pathogenesis of *Pseudomonas* vasculitis and septic lesions. *Arch Pathol* 1965;80:297–307.
226. Muder RR, Yu VL, Dummer JS, et al. Infections caused by *Pseudomonas maltophilia:* expanding clinical spectrum. *Arch Intern Med* 1987; 147:1672–1674.
227. Kerr KG, Corps CM, Hawkey PM. Infections due to *Xanthomonas maltophilia* in patients with hematologic malignancy. *Rev Infect Dis* 1991;13:762.
228. Mandell IN, Feiner HD, Price NM, et al. *Pseudomonas cepacia* endocarditis and ecthyma gangrenosum. *Arch Dermatol* 1977;113: 199–202.
229. Fishman LS, Armstrong D. *Pseudomonas aeruginosa* bacteremia in patients with neoplastic disease. *Cancer* 1972;30:764–773.
230. Forkner CE, Frei E III, Edgcomb JH, et al. *Pseudomonas* septicemia. *Am J Med* 1958;25:877–889.
231. Schimpff SC, Young VM, Greene WH, et al. Origin of infection in acute nonlymphocytic leukemia: significance of hospital acquisition of potential pathogens. *Ann Intern Med* 1972;77:707–714.
232. Schimpff SC, Moody M, Young VM. Relationship of colonization with *Pseudomonas aeruginosa* to development of *Pseudomonas* bacteremia in cancer patients. *Antimicrob Agents Chemother* 1970;10: 240–244.
233. Grigis A, Goglio A, Parea M, et al. Nosocomial outbreak of severe *Pseudomonas aeruginosa* infections in haematological patients. *Eur J Epidemiol* 1993;9:390–395.
234. Gallagher PG, Watanakunakorn C. *Pseudomonas* bacteremia in a com-

munity teaching hospital, 1980–1984. *Rev Infect Dis* 1989;11: 846–852.

235. Tapper ML, Armstrong D. Bacteremia due to *Pseudomonas aeruginosa* complicating neoplastic disease: a progress report. *J Infect Dis* 1974; 130(suppl):S14–S23.
236. Fergie JE, Shema SJ, Lott L, et al. *Pseudomonas aeruginosa* bacteremia in immunocompromised children: analysis of factors associated with a poor outcome. *Clin Infect Dis* 1994;18:390–394.
237. Hilf M, Yu VL, Sharp J, et al. Antibiotic therapy for *Pseudomonas aeruginosa* bacteremia: outcome correlations in a prospective study of 200 patients. *Am J Med* 1989;87:540–546.
238. Miller PJ, Wenzel RP. Etiologic organisms as independent predictors of death and morbidity associated with bloodstream infections. *J Infect Dis* 1987;156:471–477.
239. Blot S, Vandewoude K, Hoste E, et al. Reappraisal of attributable mortality in critically ill patients with nosocomial bacteremia involving *Pseudomonas aeruginosa*. *J Hosp Infect* 2003;53:18–24.
240. Bisbe J, Gatell JM, Puig J, et al. *Pseudomonas aeruginosa* bacteremia: univariate and multivariate analysis of factors influencing the prognosis in 133 episodes. *Rev Infect Dis* 1988;10:629–635.
241. Wagnild JP, McDonald P, Craig WA. *Pseudomonas aeruginosa* bacteremia in a dialysis unit. II. Relationship to reuse of coils. *Am J Med* 1977;62:672–676.
242. Collins RN, Braun PA, Zinner SH, et al. Risk of local and systemic infection with polyethylene intravenous catheters: a prospective study of 213 catheterizations. *N Engl J Med* 1968;279:340–343.
243. Collignon PJ, Munro R, Sorrell TC. Systemic sepsis and intravenous devices: a prospective survey. *Med J Aust* 1984;141:345–348.
244. Sarubbi FA, Wilson B, Lee M, et al. Nosocomial meningitis and bacteremia due to contaminated amphotericin B. *JAMA* 1978;239: 416–418.
245. Casewell MW, Slater NGP, Cooper JE. Operating theatre water-baths as a cause of *Pseudomonas* septicaemia. *J Hosp Infect* 1981;2:237–240.
246. Alvarado CJ, Stolz SM, Maki DG. Nosocomial infections from contaminated endoscopes: a flawed automated endoscope washer. An investigation using molecular epidemiology. *Am J Med* 1991;91(suppl 3B):272S–280S.
247. Greene WH, Moody M, Hartley R, et al. Esophagoscopy as a source of *Pseudomonas aeruginosa* sepsis in patients with active leukemia: the need for sterilization of endoscopes. *Gastroenterology* 1974;67: 912–919.
248. Srinivasan A, Wolfenden LL, Song X, et al. An outbreak of *Pseudomonas aeruginosa* infections associated with flexible bronchoscopes. *N Engl J Med* 2003;348:221–227.
249. Cryan EMJ, Falkiner FR, Mulvihill TE, et al. *Pseudomonas aeruginosa* cross-infection following endoscopic retrograde cholangiopancreatography. *J Hosp Infect* 1984;5:371–376.
250. Earnshaw JJ, Clark AW, Thom BT. Outbreak of *Pseudomonas aeruginosa* following endoscopic retrograde cholangiopancreatography. *J Hosp Infect* 1985;6:95–97.
251. Doherty DE, Falko JM, Lefkovitz N, et al. *Pseudomonas aeruginosa* sepsis following retrograde cholangiopancreatography (ERCP). *Dig Dis Sci* 1982;27:169–170.
252. Classen DC, Jacobson JA, Burke JP, et al. Serious *Pseudomonas* infections associated with endoscopic retrograde cholangiopancreatography. *Am J Med* 1988;84:590–596.
253. Uman SJ, Johnson CE, Beirne GJ, et al. *Pseudomonas aeruginosa* bacteremia in a dialysis unit. I. Recognition of cases, epidemiologic studies and attempts at control. *Am J Med* 1977;62:667–671.
254. Vanholder R, Vanhaecke E, Ringoir S. *Pseudomonas* septicemia due to deficient disinfectant mixing during reuse. *Int J Artif Organs* 1992; 15:19–24.
255. Arnow PA, Garcia-Houchins S, Neagle MB, et al. An outbreak of bloodstream infections arising form hemodialysis equipment. *J Infect Dis* 1998;178:783–791.
256. Pizzo PA. Management of fever in patients with cancer and treatment-induced neutropenia. *N Engl J Med* 1993;328:1323–1332.
257. Stephenson JR, Heard SR, Richards MA, et al. Gastrointestinal colonization and septicemia with *Pseudomonas aeruginosa* due to contaminated thymol mouthwash in immunocompromised patients. *J Hosp Infect* 1985;6:369–378.
258. Farmer JJ III, Weinstein RA, Zierdt CH, et al. Hospital outbreaks caused by *Pseudomonas aeruginosa*: importance of serogroup 011. *J Clin Microbiol* 1982;16:266–270.
259. Cabrera HA, Drake MA. An epidemic in a coronary care unit caused by *Pseudomonas* species. *Am Soc Clin Pathol* 1975;64:700–704.
260. Siboni K, Olsen H, Ravn E, et al. *Pseudomonas cepacia* in 16 non-fatal cases of postoperative bacteremia derived from intrinsic contamination of the anaesthetic fentanyl. *Scand J Infect Dis* 1979;11:39–45.
261. Steere AC, Tenney JH, Mackel DC, et al. *Pseudomonas* species bacteremia caused by contaminated normal human serum albumin. *J Infect Dis* 1977;135:729–735.
262. van Laer F, Raes D, Vandamme P, et al. An outbreak of *Burkholderia cepacia* with septicemia on a cardiology ward. *Infect Control Hosp Epidemiol* 1998;19:112–113.
263. Kaitwatcharachai C, Silpapojakul K, Jitsurong S, et al. An outbreak of *Burkholderia cepacia* bacteremia in hemodialysis patients: an epidemiological and molecular study. *Am J Kidney Dis* 2000;36:199–204.
264. Flaherty JP, Garcia-Houchins S, Chudy R, et al. An outbreak of gram-negative bacteremia traced to contaminated o-rings in reprocessed dialyzer. *Ann Intern Med* 1993;119:1072–1078.
265. Kuehnel E, Lundh H. Outbreak of *Pseudomonas cepacia* bacteremia related to contaminated reused coils. *Dialysis Transplant* 1976;5: 44–47.
266. Rutala WA, Weber DJ, Thomann CA, et al. An outbreak of *Pseudomonas cepacia* bacteremia associated with a contaminated intra-aortic balloon pump. *J Thorac Cardiovasc Surg* 1988;96:157–161.
267. Gravel-Tropper D, Sample ML, Oxley C, et al. Three-year outbreak of pseudobacteremia with *Burkholderia cepacia* traced to a contaminated blood gas analyzer. *Infect Control Hosp Epidemiol* 1996;17: 737–740.
268. Micozzi A, Venditti M, Monaco M, et al. Bacteremia due to *Stenotrophomonas maltophilia* in patients with hematologic malignancies. *Clin Infect Dis* 2000;31:705–711.
269. Morrison AJ, Hoffmann KK, Wenzel RP. Associated mortality and clinical characteristics of nosocomial *Pseudomonas maltophilia* in a university hospital. *J Clin Microbiol* 1986;24:52–55.
270. Noskin GA, Grohmann SM. *Xanthomonas maltophilia* bacteremia: an analysis of factors influencing outcome. *Infect Dis Clin Pract* 1992; 1:230–236.
271. Muder RR, Harris AP, Muller S, et al. Bacteremia due to *Stenotrophomonas (Xanthomonas) maltophilia:* a prospective, multicenter study of 91 episodes. *Clin Infect* 1996;22:508–512.
272. Senol E, DesJardin J, Stark PC, et al. Attributable mortality of *Stenotrophomonas maltophilia* bacteremia. *CID* 2002;34:1653–1656.
273. Green GS, Johnson RH, Shively JA. Mimae: opportunistic pathogens. A review of infections in a cancer hospital. *JAMA* 1965;194:163–166.
274. Gardner P, Griffen WB, Swartz MN, et al. Nonfermentative gram-negative bacilli of nosocomial interest. *Am J Med* 1970;48:735–749.
275. Robinson RG, Garison RG, Brown RW. Evaluation of the clinical significance of the genus *Herellea. Ann Intern Med* 1964;60:19–27.
276. Reynolds RC, Cluff LE. Infection of man with *Mimeae. Ann Intern Med* 1963;58:759–767.
277. Daly AK, Postic B, Kass EH. Infections due to organisms of the genus *Herellea. Arch Intern Med* 1962;110:86–97.
278. Seifert H, Strate A, Schulze A, et al. Vascular catheter-related bloodstream infection due to *Acinetobacter johnsonii* (formerly *Acinetobacter calcoaceticus* var. lwoffii): report of 13 cases. *Clin Infect Dis* 1993;17: 632–636.
279. Smego RA Jr. Endemic nosocomial *Acinetobacter calcoaceticus* bacteremia. *Arch Intern Med* 1985;145:2174–2179.
280. Inclan AP, Massey LC, Crook BG, et al. Organisms of the tribe *Mimeae:* incidence of isolation and clinical correlation at the city of Memphis hospitals. *South Med J* 1965;58:1261–1266.
281. Seifert H, Strate A, Pulverer G. Nosocomial bacteremia due to *Acinetobacter baumannii:* clinical features, epidemiology, and predictors of mortality. *Medicine* 1995;74:340–349.
282. Blot S, Vandewoude K, Colardyn F. Nosocomial bacteremia involving

Acinteobacter baumannii in critically ill patients: a matched cohort study. *Intensive Care Med* 2003;29:471–475.

283. Ramphal R, Kluge RM. *Acinetobacter calcoaceticus* variety anitratus: an increasing nosocomial problem. *Am J Med Sci* 1979;277:57–66.
284. García-Garmendia J-L, Ortiz-Leyba C, Garnacho-Montero J, et al. Risk factors for *Acinetobacter baumannii* nosocomial bacteremia in critically ill patients: a cohort study. *Clin Infect Dis* 2001;33:939–946.
285. Tabor E, Gerety RJ. Five cases of *Pseudomonas* sepsis transmitted by blood transfusions. *Lancet* 1984;1:1403.
286. Phillips P, Grayson L, Stockman K, et al. Transfusion-related *Pseudomonas* sepsis. *Lancet* 1984;2:879.
287. Khabbaz RF, Arnow PM, Highsmith AK, et al. *Pseudomonas fluorescens* bacteremia from blood transfusion. *Am J Med* 1984;76: 62–68.
288. Morduchowicz G, Pitlik SD, Huminer D, et al. Transfusion reactions due to bacterial contamination of blood and blood products. *Rev Infect Dis* 1991;13:307–314.
289. Maki DG, Klein BS, McCormick RD, et al. Nosocomial *Pseudomonas pickettii* bacteremias traced to narcotic tampering. *JAMA* 1991;265: 981–986.
290. Roberts LA, Collignon PJ, Cramp VB et al. An Australia-wide epidemic of *Pseudomonas pickettii* bacteremia due to contaminated sterile water for injection. *Med J Aust* 1990;152:652–655.
291. Lacey S, Want SV. *Pseudomonas pickettii* infections in a paediatric oncology unit. *J Hosp Infect* 1991;17:45–51.
292. Raveh D, Simhon A, Gimmon Z, et al. Infections caused by *Pseudomonas pickettii* in association with permanent indwelling intravenous devices: four cases and a review. *Clin Infect Dis* 1993;17:877–880.
293. Fernandez C, Wilhelmi I, Andradas E, et al. Nosocomial outbreak of *Burkholderia pickettii* infection due to a manufactured intravenous product used in three hospitals. *Clin Infect Dis* 1996;22:1092–1095.
294. Wertheim WA, Markovitz DM. Osteomyelitis and intervertebral discitis caused by *Pseudomonas pickettii. J Clin Microbiol* 1992;30: 2506–2508.
295. Studemeister AE, Beilke MA, Kirmani N. Splenic abscess due to *Clostridium difficile* and *Pseudomonas paucimobilis. Am J Gastroenterol* 1987;82:389–390.
296. Reina J, Bassa A, Llompart I, et al. Infections with *Pseudomonas paucimobilis:* report of four cases and review. *Rev Infect Dis* 1991;13: 1072–1075.
297. Slotnick IJ, Hall J, Sacks H. Septicemia caused by *Pseudomonas paucimobilis. Am Soc Clin Pathol* 1978;72:882–884.
298. Southern PM Jr, Kutscher AE. *Pseudomonas paucimobilis* bacteremia. *J Clin Microbiol* 1981;13:1070–1073.
299. Chertow GM. *Ochrobacterum anthropi* bacteremia in a patient on hemodialysis. *Am J Kidney Dis* 2000;35:E30.
300. Goetz A, Yu VL, Hanchett JE, et al. *Pseudomonas stutzeri* bacteremia associated with hemodialyzers. *Arch Intern Med* 1983;143: 1909–1912.
301. Hsueh P-R, Teng L-J, Yang P-C, et al. Nosocomial infections caused by *Sphingomonas paucimobilis:* clinical features and microbiological characteristics. *Clin Infect Dis* 1998;26:676–681.
302. Wauters G, Claeys G, Verschraegen G, et al. Case of catheter sepsis with *Ralstonia gilardii* in a child with acute lymphoblastic leukemia. *J Clin Microbiol* 2001;39:4583–4584.
303. Vaneechoutee M, de Baere T, Wauters G, et al. One case each of recurrent meningitis and hemoperitoneum infection with *Ralstonia mannitolilytica. J Clin Microbiol* 2001;39:4588–4590.
304. Chalandon Y, Roscoe DL, Nantel SH. *Agrobacterium* yellow group: bacteremia and possible septic arthritis following peripheral blood stem cell transplantation. *Bone Marrow Transplant* 2000;20:101–104.
305. Bartlett JG, O'Keefe P, Talley FP, et al. Bacteriology of hospital-acquired pneumonia. *Arch Intern Med* 1986;146:868–871.
306. Botzenhart K, Ruden H. Hospital infections caused by *Pseudomonas aeruginosa. Antibiot Chemother* 1987;39:1–15.
307. Cross A, Allen JR, Burke J, et al. Nosocomial infections due to *Pseudomonas aeruginosa*: review of recent trends. *Rev Infect Dis* 1983; 5(suppl 5):S837–S845.
308. Jarvis WR, Martone WJ. Predominant pathogens in hospital infections. *J Antimicrob Chemother* 1992;29(suppl A):19–24.
309. Centers for Disease Control. Nosocomial infection surveillance, 1984. In: *CDC Surveillance Summaries.* 1984;33(3SS):17SS–29SS.
310. National Nosocomial Infections Surveillance System. National nosocomial infections surveillance (NNIS) report, data summary from October 1986–April 1996, issued May 1996. *Am J Infect Control* 1996;24:380–388.
311. Talon D, Mulin B, Rouget C, et al. Risks and routes for ventilator-associated pneumonia with *Pseudomonas aeruginosa. Am J Respir Crit Care Med* 1998;157:978–984.
312. A'Court CHD, Garrard CS, Crook D, et al. Microbiological lung surveillance in mechanically ventilated patients, using non-directed bronchial lavage and quantitative culture. *Q J Med* 1993;86:635–648.
313. Papazian L, Martin C, Albanese J, et al. Comparison of two methods of bacteriologic sampling of the lower respiratory tract: a study in ventilated patients with nosocomial bronchopneumonia. *Crit Care Med* 1989;17:461–464.
314. Rello J, Quintana E, Ausina V, et al. Incidence, etiology, and outcome of nosocomial pneumonia in mechanically ventilated patients. *Chest* 1991;100:439–444.
315. Kulczycki LL, Murphy TM, Bellanti JA. *Pseudomonas* colonization in cystic fibrosis: a study of 160 patients. *JAMA* 1978;240:30–34.
316. Bregeon F, Papazian L, Visconti A, et al. Relationship of microbiologic diagnostic criteria to morbidity and mortality in patients with ventilator-associated pneumonia. *JAMA* 1997;277:655–662.
317. Pennington JE, Reynolds AY, Carbone PP. *Pseudomonas* pneumonia: a retrospective study of 36 cases. *Am J Med* 1973;55:155–160.
318. Cheng K, Smyth RL, Govan JRW, et al. Spread of β-lactam-resistant *Pseudomonas aeruginosa* in a cystic fibrosis clinic. *Lancet* 1996;348: 639–642.
319. Silver DR, Cohen IL, Weinberg PF. Recurrent *Pseudomonas aeruginosa* pneumonia in an intensive care unit. *Chest* 1992;101:194–198.
320. Tillotson JR, Lerner AM. Characteristics of nonbacteremic *Pseudomonas* pneumonia. *Ann Intern Med* 1968;68:295–307.
321. Ianni PB, Claffey T, Quintiliani R. Bacteremic *Pseudomonas* pneumonia. *JAMA* 1974;230:558–561.
322. Tillotson JR, Finland M. Bacterial colonization and clinical superinfection of the respiratory tract complicating treatment of pneumonia. *J Infect Dis* 1969;119:597–624.
323. Schwartz SN, Dowling JN, Benkovic C, et al. Sources of gram-negative bacilli colonizing the trachea of intubated patients. *J Infect Dis* 1978;138:227–231.
324. Pierce AK, Sanford JP, Thomas GD, et al. Long-term evaluation of decontamination of inhalation-therapy equipment and the occurrence of necrotizing pneumonia. *N Engl J Med* 1970;282:528–531.
325. Lowbury EJL, Thom BT, Lilly HA, et al. Sources of infection with *Pseudomonas aeruginosa* in patients with tracheostomy. *J Med Microbiol* 1970;3:39–56.
326. Valdivieso M, Gil-Extremera B, Zornoza J, et al. Gram-negative bacillary pneumonia in the compromised host. *Medicine* 1977;56: 241–254.
327. Fetzer AE, Werner AS, Hagstrom JWC. Pathologic features of pseudomonal pneumonia. *Am Rev Respir Dis* 1967;96:1121–1130.
328. Phair JP, Bassaris HP, Williams JE, et al. Bacteremic pneumonia due to gram-negative bacilli. *Arch Intern Med* 1983;143:2147–2149.
329. Bryan CS, Reynolds KL. Bacteremic nosocomial pneumonia: analysis of 172 episodes from a single metropolitan area. *Am Rev Respir Dis* 1984;129:668–671.
330. Malangoni MA, Crafton R, Mocek FC. Pneumonia in the surgical intensive care unit: factors determining successful outcome. *Am J Surg* 1994;167:250–255.
331. Fink MP, Snydman DR, Niederman MS, et al. Treatment of severe pneumonia in hospitalized patients: results of a multicenter, randomized, double-blind trial comparing intravenous ciprofloxacin with imipenem-cilastatin. *Antimicrob Agents Chemother* 1994;38:547–557.
332. Rello J, Jubert P, Valles J, et al. Evaluation of outcome for intubated patients with pneumonia due to *Pseudomonas aeruginosa. Clin Infect Dis* 1996;23:973–978.
333. Rello J, Rue M, Jubert P, et al. Survival in patients with nosocomial pneumonia: impact of the severity of illness and the etiologic agent. *Crit Care Med* 1997;25:1862–1867.

334. Reinarz JA, Pierce AK, Mays BB, et al. The potential role of inhalation therapy equipment in nosocomial pulmonary infection. *J Clin Invest* 1965;44:831–839.
335. Phillips I, Spencer G. *Pseudomonas aeruginosa* cross-infection: due to contaminated respiratory apparatus. *Lancet* 1965;2:1325–1327.
336. Olds JW, Kisch AL, Eberle BJ, et al. *Pseudomonas aeruginosa* respiratory tract infection acquired from a contaminated anesthesia machine. *Am Rev Respir Dis* 1972;105:628–632.
337. Morris AH. Nebulizer contamination in a burn unit. *Am Rev Respir Dis* 1973;107:802–808.
338. Christopher KL, Saravolatz LD, Bush TL, et al. The potential role of respiratory therapy equipment in cross infection: a study using a canine model for pneumonia. *Am Rev Respir Dis* 1983;128:271–275.
339. Grieble HG, Colton R, Bird TJ, et al. Fine-particle humidifiers: source of *Pseudomonas aeruginosa* infections in a respiratory-disease unit. *N Engl J Med* 1970;282:531–535.
340. Macpherson CR. Oxygen therapy an unsuspected source of hospital infections? *JAMA* 1958;167:1083–1086.
341. Rhame FS, Streifel A, McComb C, et al. Bubbling humidifiers produce microaerosols which can carry bacteria. *Infect Control* 1986;7: 403–407.
342. Labarca JA, Pegues DA, Wagar EA, et al. Something's rotten: a nosocomial outbreak of malodorous *Pseudomonas aeruginosa. Clin Infect Dis* 1998;26:1440–1446.
343. Craven DE, Goularte TA, Make BJ. Contaminated condensate in mechanical ventilator circuits: a risk factor for nosocomial pneumonia. *Am Rev Respir Dis* 1984;128:625–628.
344. Morehead CD, Houck PW. Epidemiology of *Pseudomonas* infections in a pediatric intensive care unit. *Am J Dis Child* 1972;124:564–570.
345. Widmer AF, Wenzel RP, Trilla A, et al. Outbreak of *Pseudomonas aeruginosa* infections in a surgical intensive care unit: probable transmission via hands of a health care worker. *Clin Infect Dis* 1993;16: 372–376.
346. Teres D, Schweers P, Bushnell LS, et al. Sources of *Pseudomonas aeruginosa* infection in a respiratory/surgical intensive-therapy unit. *Lancet* 1973;1:415–417.
347. Noone MR, Pitt TL, Bedder M, et al. *Pseudomonas aeruginosa* colonisation in an intensive therapy unit: role of cross infection and host factors. *Br Med J* 1983;286:341–344.
348. Speert DP, Campbell ME. Hospital epidemiology of *Pseudomonas aeruginosa* from patients with cystic fibrosis. *J Hosp Infect* 1987;9: 11–21.
349. File TM, Tan JS, Thomson, RB, et al. An outbreak of *Pseudomonas aeruginosa* ventilator-associated respiratory infections due to contaminated food coloring dye-further evidence of the significance of gastric colonization preceding nosocomial pneumonia. *Infect Control Hosp Epidemiol* 1995;16:417–418.
350. Wolz C, Kiosz G, Ogle JW, et al. *Pseudomonas aeruginosa* cross-colonization and persistence in patients with cystic fibrosis. Use of a DNA probe. *Epidemiol Infect* 1989;102:205–214.
351. Pedersen SS, Koch C, Hoiby N, et al. An epidemic spread of multiresistant *Pseudomonas aeruginosa* in a cystic fibrosis center. *J Antimicrob Chemother* 1986;17:505–516.
352. Tummler B, Koopman U, Grothues D, et al. Nosocomial acquisition of *Pseudomonas aeruginosa* by cystic fibrosis patients. *J Clin Microbiol* 1991;29:1265–1267.
353. Arancibia F, Bauer T, Ewig S, et al. Community-acquired pneumonia due to gram-negative bacteria and *Pseudomonas aeruginosa. Arch Intern Med* 2002;162:1849–1858.
354. Hatchette TF, Gupta R, Marrie TJ. *Pseudomonas aeruginosa* community-acquired pneumonia in previously healthy adults: case report and review of literature. *Clin Infect Dis* 2000;31:1349–1356.
355. Poe RH, Marcus HR, Emerson GL. Lung abscess due to *Pseudomonas cepacia. Am Rev Respir Dis* 1977;115:861–865.
356. Schaffner W, Reisig G, Verrall RA. Outbreak of *Pseudomonas cepacia* infection due to contaminated anaesthetics. *Lancet* 1973;1: 1050–1051.
357. Casewell MW, Dalton MT. Forrester laryngeal sprays as a source of *Pseudomonas* respiratory tract infection. *Br Med J* 1977;2:680–681.
358. Centers for Disease Control. *Pseudomonas cepacia* colonization—Minnesota. *MMWR* 1981;30:610–611.
359. Gilligan PH. Microbiology of airway disease in patients with cystic fibrosis. *Clin Microbiol Rev* 1991;4:35–51.
360. Lewin LO, Byard PJ, Davis PB. Effect of *Pseudomonas cepacia* colonization on survival and pulmonary function of cystic fibrosis patients. *J Clin Epidemiol* 1990;43:125–131.
361. Tablan OC, Martone WJ, Doershuk CF, et al. Colonization of the respiratory tract with *Pseudomonas cepacia* in cystic fibrosis: risk factors and outcomes. *Chest* 1987;91:527–532.
362. O'Neil KM, Herman JH, Modlin JF, et al. *Pseudomonas cepacia:* an emerging pathogen in chronic granulomatous disease. *J Pediatr* 1986; 108:940–942.
363. Hanes SD, Demirkan K, Tolley E, et al. Risk factors for late-onset nosocomial pneumonia caused by *Stenotrophomonas maltophilia* in critically ill trauma patients. *Clin Infect Dis* 2002;35:228–234.
364. Gopalakrishnan R, Hawley HB, Czachor JS, et al. *Stenotrophomonas maltophilia* infection and colonization in the intensive care units of two community hospitals: a study of 143 patients. *Heart Lung* 1999; 28:134–141.
365. Cunha BA, Klimek JJ, Gracewski J, et al. A common source outbreak of *Acinetobacter* pulmonary infections traced to Wright respirometers. *Postgrad Med J* 1980;56:169–172.
366. Gerner-Smidt P. Endemic occurrence of *Acinetobacter calcoaceticus* biovar anitratus in an intensive care unit. *J Hosp Infect* 1987;10: 265–272.
367. Hartstein AI, Rashad AL, Liebler JM, et al. Multiple intensive care unit outbreak of *Acinetobacter calcoaceticus* subspecies antitratus respiratory infection and colonization associated with contaminated, reusable ventilator circuits and resuscitation bags. *Am J Med* 1988;85: 624–631.
368. Fagon JY, Chastre J, Domart Y, et al. Nosocomial pneumonia in patients receiving continuous mechanical ventilation. *Am Rev Respir Dis* 1989;139:877–883.
369. McDonald LC, Banerjee SN, Jarvis WR, National Nosocomial Infections Surveillance System. Seasonal variation of Acinetobacter infections: 1987–1996. *Clin Infect Dis* 199;29:1133–1137.
370. Barnes DJ, Naraqi S, Igo JD. Community-acquired *Acinetobacter* pneumonia in adults in Papua New Guinea. *Rev Infect Dis* 1988;10: 636–639.
371. Gottlieb T, Barnes DJ. Community-acquired *Acinetobacter* pneumonia. *Aust N Z J Med* 1989;19:259–260.
372. McNeil MM, Solomon SL, Anderson RL, et al. Nosocomial *Pseudomonas pickettii* colonization associated with a contaminated respiratory therapy solution in a special care nursery. *J Clin Microbiol* 1985;22: 903–907.
373. Gardner S, Shulman ST. A nosocomial common source outbreak caused by *Pseudomonas pickettii. Pediatr Infect Dis* 1984;3:420–422.
374. Redding PJ, McWalter PW. *Pseudomonas fluorescens* cross-infection due to contaminated humidifier water. *Br Med J* 1980;281:275.
375. Crane LR, Tagle LC, Palutke WA. Outbreak of *Pseudomonas paucimobilis* in an intensive care facility. *JAMA* 1981;246:985–987.
376. Bruce AW, Chan RCY, Pickerton D, et al. Adherence of gram-negative uropathogens to human uroepithelial cells. *J Urol* 1983;130: 293–298.
377. Daifuku R, Stamm WE. Bacterial adherence to bladder uroepithelial cells in catheter-associated urinary tract infection. *N Engl J Med* 1986; 314:1208–1213.
378. Moore B, Forman A. An outbreak of urinary *Pseudomonas aeruginosa* infection acquired during urological operations. *Lancet* 1966;2: 929–931.
379. Marrie TJ, Major H, Gurwith M, et al. Prolonged outbreak of nosocomial urinary tract infection with a single strain of *Pseudomonas aeruginosa. Can Med Assoc J* 1978;119:593–596.
380. Strand CL, Bryant JK, Morgan JW, et al. Nosocomial *Pseudomonas aeruginosa* urinary tract infections. *JAMA* 1982;248:1615–1618.
381. Montgomerie JZ, Morrow JW. Long-term *Pseudomonas* colonization in spinal cord injury patients. *Am J Epidemiol* 1980;112:508–517.
382. Bultitude MI, Eykyn S. The relationship between the urethral flora

and urinary infection in the catheterised male. *Br J Urol* 1973;45: 678–683.

383. Warren JW, Tenney JH, Hoopes JM, et al. A prospective microbiologic study of bacteriuria in patients with chronic indwelling urethral catheters. *J Infect Dis* 1982;146:719–723.
384. Krieger JN, Kaiser DL, Wenzel RP. Urinary tract etiology of bloodstream infections in hospitalized patients. *J Infect Dis* 1983;148: 57–62.
385. Sullivan NM, Sutter VL, Mims MM, et al. Clinical aspects of bacteremia after manipulation of the genitourinary tract. *J Infect Dis* 1978; 127:49–55.
386. Schaberg DR, Haley RW, Highsmith AK, et al. Nosocomial bacteriuria: a prospective study of case clustering and antimicrobial resistance. *Ann Intern Med* 1980;93:420–424.
387. Talbot GH, Doorley M, Banner MP. Urosepsis associated with videourodynamic studies. *Am J Infect Control* 1984;12:266–270.
388. Kocka FE, Roemisch E, Causey WA, et al. The urometer as a reservoir of infectious organisms. *Am J Clin Pathol* 1977;67:106–107.
389. Murray SA, Snydman DR. Investigation of an epidemic of multidrug resistant *Pseudomonas aeruginosa. Infect Control* 1982;3: 456–460.
390. Pyrah LN, Goldie W, Parsons FM, et al. Control of *Pseudomonas pyocyanea* infection in a urological ward. *Lancet* 1955;2:314–317.
391. Montgomerie JZ, Morrow JW. *Pseudomonas* colonization in patients with spinal cord injury. *Am J Epidemiol* 1978;108:328–336.
392. Thompson RL, Haley CE, Searcy MA, et al. Catheter associated bacteriuria: failure to reduce attack rates using periodic instillations of a disinfectant into urinary drainage systems. *JAMA* 1984;251:747–751.
393. Johnson JR, Roberts PL, Olsen RJ, et al. Prevention of catheter associated urinary tract infection with a silver oxide-coated urinary catheter: clinical and microbiological correlates. *J Infect Dis* 1990;162: 1145–1150.
394. French GL, Casewell MW, Roncoroni AJ, et al. A hospital outbreak of antibiotic-resistant *Acinetobacter anitratus:* epidemiology and control. *J Hosp Infect* 1980;1:125–131.
395. Zuravleff JJ, Yu VL. Infections caused by *Pseudomonas maltophilia* with emphasis on bacteremia: case reports and review of the literature. *Rev Infect Dis* 1982;4:1236–1246.
396. Lowbury EJL, Fox J. The epidemiology of infection with *Pseudomonas pyocyanea* in a burns unit. *J Hyg* 1954;52:403–416.
397. MacMillan BG, Edmonds P, Hummel RP, et al. Epidemiology of *Pseudomonas* in a burn intensive care unit. *J Trauma* 1973;13: 627–638.
398. Pruitt BA Jr. Infections caused by *Pseudomonas* species in patients with burns and in other surgical patients. *J Infect Dis* 1974;130(suppl): S8–S13.
399. MacMillan BG. Infections following burn injury. *Surg Clin North Am* 1980;60:185–196.
400. Tredget EE, Shankowsky HA, Joffe AM. Epidemiology of infections with *Pseudomonas aeruginosa* in burn patients: the role of hydrotherapy. *Clin Infect Dis* 1992;15:941–949.
401. Richard P, LeFloch R, Chamoux C, et al. *Pseudomonas aeruginosa* outbreak in a burn unit: role of antimicrobials in the emergence of multiply resistant strains. *J Infect Dis* 1994;170:377–383.
402. Ransjo U. Attempts to control clothes-borne infection in a burn unit. 2. Clothing routines in clinical use, and the epidemiology of cross-colonization. *J Hyg* 1979;82:369–384.
403. van Saene HKF, Nicolai JPA. The prevention of wound infections in burn patients. *Scand J Plast Reconstr Surg* 1979;13:63–67.
404. Kreger AS, Gray LD. Purification of *Pseudomonas aeruginosa* proteases and microscopic characterization of pseudomonal protease-induced rabbit corneal damage. *Infect Immun* 1978;19:630–648.
405. Iglewski BH, Burns RP, Gipson IK. Pathogenesis of corneal damage from pseudomonas exotoxin A. *Invest Ophthalmol Vis Sci* 1977;16: 73–76.
406. Mahajan VM. Postoperative ocular infections: an analysis of laboratory data on 750 cases. *Ann Ophthalmol* 1984;16:847–848.
407. Burns RP. *Pseudomonas aeruginosa* keratitis: mixed infections of the eye. *Am J Ophthalmol* 1969;67:257–262.
408. Raber IM, Laibson PR, Kurz GH, et al. *Pseudomonas* corneoscleral ulcers. *Am J Ophthalmol* 1981;92:353–362.
409. Ayliffe GAJ, Barry DR, Lowbury EJL, et al. Postoperative infection with *Pseudomonas aeruginosa* in an eye hospital. *Lancet* 1966;1: 1113–1117.
410. Gerding DN, Poley BJ, Hall WH, et al. Treatment of *Pseudomonas* endophthalmitis associated with prosthetic intraocular lens implantation. *Am J Ophthalmol* 1979;88:902–908.
411. Reid FR, Wood TO. *Pseudomonas* corneal ulcer: the causative role of contaminated eye cosmetics. *Arch Ophthalmol* 1979;97:1640–1641.
412. Schein OD, Wasson PJ, Boruchoff SA, et al. Microbial keratitis associated with contaminated ocular medications. *Am J Ophthalmol* 1988; 105:361–365.
413. Tarr KH, Constable IJ. *Pseudomonas* endophthalmitis associated with scleral necrosis. *Br J Ophthalmol* 1980;64:676–679.
414. Rosenoff SH, Wolf ML, Chabner BA. *Pseudomonas* blepharoconjunctivitis. *Arch Ophthalmol* 1974;91:490–491.
415. Cruciani M, Malena M, Amalfitano G, et al. Molecular epidemiology in a cluster of cases of postoperative *Pseudomonas aeruginosa* endophthalmitis. *Clin Infect Dis* 1998;26:330–333.
416. Hilton E, Adams AA, Uliss A, et al. Nosocomial bacterial eye infections in intensive care units. *Lancet* 1983;1:1318–1320.
417. Hutton WL, Sexton RR. Atypical *Pseudomonas* corneal ulcers in semicomatose patients. *Am J Ophthalmol* 1972;73:37–39.
418. King S, Devi SP, Mindorff C, et al. Nosocomial *Pseudomonas aeruginosa* conjunctivitis in a pediatric hospital. *Infect Control Hosp Epidemiol* 1988;9:77–80.
419. Kirwan JF, Potamitis T, El-Kasaby H, et al. Microbial keratitis in intensive care. *Br Med J* 1997;314:433–434.
420. Parkin B, Turner A, Moore E, et al. Bacterial keratitis in the critically ill. *Br J Ophthalmol* 1997;81:1060–1063.
421. Barrie D. Incubator-borne *Pseudomonas pyocyanea* infection in a newborn nursery. *Arch Dis Child* 1965;40:555–559.
422. Chaudhry NA, Flynn HW, Smiddy WE, et al. *Xanthomonas maltophilia* endophthalmitis after cataract surgery. *Arch Ophthalmol* 2000;118: 572–575.
423. Kaiser GM, Tso PC, Morris R, et al. *Xanthomonas maltophilia* endophthalmitis after cataract extraction. *Am J Ophthalmol* 1997;123: 410–411.
424. Sutter VL. Identification of *Pseudomonas* species isolated from hospital environment and human sources. *Appl Microbiol* 1968;16: 1532–1538.
425. Khater TT, Jones DB, Wilhelmus KR. Infectious crystalline keratopathy caused by gram-negative bacteria. *Am J Ophthalmol* 1997;124: 19–23.
426. Hodges GR, Perkins RL. Hospital-associated bacterial meningitis. *Am J Med Sci* 1976;271:335–341.
427. Buckwold FJ, Hand R, Hansebout RR. Hospital acquired bacterial meningitis in neurosurgical patients. *J Neurosurg* 1977;46:494–500.
428. Berk SL, McCabe WR. Meningitis caused by gram-negative bacilli. *Ann Intern Med* 1980;93:253–260.
429. Mancebo J, Domingo P, Blanch L, et al. Post-neurosurgical and spontaneous gram-negative bacillary meningitis in adults. *Scand J Infect Dis* 1986;18:533–538.
430. Winkelman MD, Galloway PG. Central nervous system complications of thermal burns: a postmortem study of 139 patients. *Medicine* 1992;71:271–283.
431. Jones SR, Luby JP, Sanford JP. Bacterial meningitis complicating cranial-spinal trauma. *J Trauma* 1973;13:895–900.
432. Botterell EH, Magner D. Meningitis due to *Ps. pyocyanea:* penetrating wounds of the head. *Lancet* 1945;1:112–115.
433. Harris RC, Buxbaum L, Appelbaum E. Secondary *Bacillus pyocyanues* infection in meningitis following intrathecal penicillin therapy. *J Lab Clin Med* 1946;31:1113–1120.
434. Ayliffe GAJ, Lowbury EJL, Hamilton JG, et al. Hospital infection with *Pseudomonas aeruginosa* in neurosurgery. *Lancet* 1965;2: 365–368.
435. Olafsson M, Lee YC, Abernethy TJ. Mima polymorpha meningitis. *N Engl J Med* 1958;258:465–470.

436. Sprecace GA, Dunkelberg WE Jr. Mima polymorpha—causative agent in acute and chronic meningitis. *JAMA* 1961;177:706–708.
437. Berk SL, McCabe WR. Meningitis caused by *Acinetobacter calcoaceticus* var anitratus. *Arch Neurol* 1981;38:95–98.
438. Siegman-Igra Y, Bar-Yosef S, Gorea A, et al. Nosocomial *Acinetobacter* meningitis secondary to invasive procedures: report of 25 cases and review. *Clin Infect Dis* 1993;17:843–849.
439. Morgan MEI, Hart CA. *Acinetobacter* meningitis: acquired infection in a neonatal intensive care unit. *Arch Dis Child* 1982;57:557–559.
440. Nguyen MH, Muder RR. Meningitis due to *Xanthomonas maltophilia:* case report and review. *Clin Infect Dis* 1994;19:325–326.
441. Trump DL, Grossman SA, Thompson G, et al. CSF infections complicating the management of neoplastic meningitis: clinical features and results of therapy. *Arch Intern Med* 1982;142:583–586.
442. Patrick S, Hindmarch JM, Hague RV, et al. Meningitis caused by *Pseudomonas maltophilia. J Clin Pathol* 1975;28:741–743.
443. Fass RJ, Barnishan J. Acute meningitis due to a *Pseudomonas*-like group va-1-bacillus. *Ann Intern Med* 1976;84:51.
444. Hajiroussou V, Holmes B, Bullas J, et al. Meningitis caused by *Pseudomonas paucimobilis. J Clin Pathol* 1979;32:953–955.
445. Papadakis KA, Vartivarian SE, Vassilaki ME, et al. *Stenotrophomonas maltophilia* meningitis: report of two cases and review of literature. *J Neurosurg* 1997;87:106–108.
446. Ottino G, DePaulis R, Pansini S, et al. Major sternal wound infection after open-heart surgery: a multivariate analysis of risk factors in 2,579 consecutive operative procedures. *Ann Thorac Surg* 1987;44: 173–179.
447. Selick JA Jr, Stelmach M, Mylotte JM. Surveillance of surgical wound infections following open heart surgery. *Infect Control Hosp Epidemiol* 1991;12:591–596.
448. Siegman-Igra Y, Shafir R, Weiss J, et al. Serious infectious complications of midsternotomy: a review of bacteriology and antimicrobial therapy. *Scand J Infect Dis* 1990;22:633–643.
449. Fitzgerald RH, Nolan DR, Ilstrup DM, et al. Deep wound sepsis following total hip arthroplasty. *J Bone Joint Surg* 1977;59A:847–855.
450. Inman RD, Gallegos KV, Brause BD, et al. Clinical and microbial features of prosthetic joint infection. *Am J Med* 1984;77:47–53.
451. Stone HH, Hester TR Jr. Incisional and peritoneal infection after emergency celiotomy. *Ann Surg* 1973;177:669–678.
452. Heseltine PNR, Yellin AE, Appleman MD, et al. Perforated and gangrenous appendicitis: an analysis of antibiotic failures. *J Infect Dis* 1983;148:322–329.
453. Tice AD, Hoaglund PA, Shoultz DA. Risk factors and treatment outcomes in osteomyelitis. *J Antimicrob Chemother* 2003;51: 1261–1268.
454. Stiver HG, Clark J, Kennedy J, et al. *Pseudomonas* sternotomy wound infection and sternal osteomyelitis: complications after open heart surgery. *JAMA* 1979;241:1034–1036.
455. Weinstein RA, Stamm WE, Kramer L, et al. Pressure monitoring devices: overlooked source of nosocomial infection. *JAMA* 1976;236: 936–938.
456. Sussman H, Stevens J. *Pseudomonas pyocyanea* wound infection: an outbreak in an orthopedic unit. *Lancet* 1960;2:734–736.
457. Gilardi GL. Infrequently encountered *Pseudomonas* species causing infection in humans. *Ann Intern Med* 1972;77:211–215.
458. Dyte PH, Gillians JA. *Pseudomonas maltophilia* infection in an abattoir worker. *Med J Aust* 1977;1:444–445.
459. Simor AE, Ricci J, Lau A, et al. Pseudobacteremia due to *Pseudomonas fluorescens. Pediatr Infect Dis* 1985;4:508–512.
460. Rosenthal SL. Sources of *Pseudomonas* and *Acinetobacter* species found in human cultures. *Am J Clin Pathol* 1974;62:807–811.
461. Kresky B. Control of gram-negative bacilli in a hospital nursery. *Am J Dis Child* 1964;107:363–369.
462. Fierer J, Taylor PM, Gezon HM. *Pseudomonas aeruginosa* epidemic traced to delivery-room resuscitators. *N Engl J Med* 1967;276: 991–996.
463. Grieble HG, Colton FR, Bird TI, et al. Fine-particle humidifiers: source of *Pseudomonas aeruginosa* infections in a respiratory-disease unit. *N Engl J Med* 1970;282:531–535.
464. Morris AH. Nebulizer contamination in a burn unit. *Am Rev Respir Dis* 1973;107:802–808.
465. Gervich DH, Grout CS. An outbreak of nosocomial *Acinetobacter* infections from humidifiers. *Am J Infect Control* 1985;13:210–215.
466. Smith PW, Massanari RM. Room humidifiers as the source of *Acinetobacter* infections. *JAMA* 1977;237:795–797.
467. Snydman DR, Maloy MF, Brock SM, et al. Pseudobacteremia: false-positive blood cultures from mist tent contamination. *Am J Epidemiol* 1977;106:154–159.
468. Buxton AE, Highsmith AK, Garner JS, et al. Contamination of intravenous infusion fluid: effects of changing administration sets. *Ann Intern Med* 1979;90:764–768.
469. Sever JL. Possible role of humidifying equipment in spread of infections from the newborn nursery. *Pediatrics* 1959;24:50–53.
470. Rapkin RH. *Pseudomonas cepacia* in an intensive care nursery. *Pediatrics* 1976;57:239–243.
471. Reyes MP, Ganguly S, Fowler M, et al. Pyrogenic reactions after inadvertent infusion of endotoxin during cardiac catheterizations. *Ann Intern Med* 1980;93:32–35.
472. Beck-Sague CM, Jarvis WR, Brook JH, et al. Epidemic bacteremia due to *Acinetobacter baumannii* in five intensive care units. *Am J Epidemiol* 1990;132:723–733.
473. Holmes B, Owen RJ, Evans A, et al. *Pseudomonas paucimobilis,* a new species isolated from human clinical specimens, the hospital environment, and other sources. *Int J System Bacteriol* 1977;27:133–146.
474. Glupczynski Y, Hansen W, Dratwa M, et al. *Pseudomonas paucimobilis* peritonitis in patients treated by peritoneal dialysis. *J Clin Microbiol* 1984;20:1225–1226.
475. Yoneyama A, Yano H, Hitomi S, et al. *Ralstonia pickettii* colonization of patients in an obstetric ward caused by a contaminated irrigation system. *J Hosp Infect* 2000;46:79–80.
476. Corbett JJ, Rosenstein BJ. *Pseudomonas* meningitis related to spinal anesthesia. *Neurology* 1971;21:946–950.
477. Castle M, Tenney JH, Weinstein MP, et al. Outbreak of a multiply resistant *Acinetobacter* in a surgical intensive care unit: epidemiology and control. *Heart Lung* 1978;7:641–644.
478. Labarca J, Peterson C, Benadana N, et al. Nosocomial *Ralstonia pickettii* colonization associated with intrinsically contaminated saline solution—Los Angeles, California, 1998. *MMWR* 1998;47:285–286.
479. Faden H, Britt M, Epstein B. Sinus contamination with *Pseudomonas paucimobilis:* a pseudoepidemic due to contaminated irrigation fluid. *Infect Control* 1981;2:233–235.
480. Shooter RA, Walker KA, Williams VR, et al. Faecal carriage of *Pseudomonas aeruginosa* in hospital patients. *Lancet* 1966;2:1331–1334.
481. Victorin L. An epidemic of otitis in newborns due to infection with *Pseudomonas aeruginosa. Acta Paediatr Scand* 1967;56:344–348.
482. Abrutyn E, Goodhart GL, Roos K, et al. *Acinetobacter calcoaceticus* outbreak associated with peritoneal dialysis. *Am J Epidemiol* 1978; 107:328–335.
483. Allen KD, Bartzokas R, Graham MF, et al. Acquisition of endemic *Pseudomonas aeruginosa* on an intensive therapy unit. *J Hosp Infect* 1987;10:156–164.
484. Whitby JL, Rampling A. *Pseudomonas aeruginosa* contamination in domestic and hospital environments. *Lancet* 1972;1:15–17.
485. Millership SE, Patel N, Chattopadhyay B. The colonization of patients in an intensive treatment unit with gram-negative flora: the significance of the oral route. *J Hosp Infect* 1986;7:226–235.
486. Bassett DCJ, Thompson SAS, Page B. Neonatal infections with *Pseudomonas aeruginosa* associated with contaminated resuscitation equipment. *Lancet* 1965;1:781–784.
487. Olson B, Weinstein RA, Nathan C, et al. Epidemiology of endemic *Pseudomonas aeruginosa*: why infection control efforts have failed. *J Infect Dis* 1984;150:808–816.
488. Anon. Infected suction apparatus. *Br Med J* 1973;1:810–811.
489. Buxton AE, Anderson RL, Werdegar D, et al. Nosocomial respiratory tract infection and colonization with *Acinetobacter calcoaceticus. Am J Med* 1978;65:507–513.
490. Phillips I, Eykyn S. *Pseudomonas cepacia (multivorans)* septicaemia in an intensive-care unit. *Lancet* 1971;1:375–377.
491. Villarino ME, Stevens LE, Schable B, et al. Risk factors for epidemic

Xanthomonas maltophilia infection/colonization in intensive care unit patients. *Infect Control Hosp Epidemiol* 1992;13:201–206.
492. Burdge DR, Nakielna EM, Noble MA. Case-control and vector studies of nosocomial acquisition of *Pseudomonas cepacia* in adult patients with cystic fibrosis. *Infect Control* 1993;14:127–130.
493. Vandenbroucke-Grauls CMJE, Kerver AJH, Rommes JH, et al. Endemic *Acinetobacter anitratus* in a surgical intensive care unit: mechanical ventilators as reservoir. *Eur J Clin Microbiol* 1988;7:485–489.
494. Patterson JE, Vecchio J, Pantelick EL, et al. Association of contaminated gloves with transmission of *Acinetobacter calcoaceticus* var. antitratus in an intensive care unit. *Am J Med* 1991;91:479–483.
495. Stone JW, Das BC. Investigation of an outbreak of infection with *Acinetobacter calcoaceticus* in a special care baby unit. *J Hosp Infect* 1985;6:42–48.
496. Cefai C, Richards J, Gould FK, et al. An outbreak of *Acinetobacter* respiratory tract infection resulting from incomplete disinfection of ventilatory equipment. *J Hosp Infect* 1990;15:177–182.
497. Craven DE, Lichtenberg DA, Goularte TA, et al. Contaminated medication nebulizers in mechanical ventilator circuits: source of bacterial aerosols. *Am J Med* 1984;77:834–838.
498. Lemaitre D, Elaichoun A, Hundausen M, et al. Tracheal colonization with *Sphingomonas paucimobilis* in mechanically ventilated neonates due to contaminated ventilator temperature probes. *J Hosp Infect* 1996;32:199–206.
499. Wilson MG, Nelson RC, Phillips LH, et al. New sources of *Pseudomonas aeruginosa* in a nursery. *JAMA* 1961;175:1146–1148.
500. Ayliffe GAJ, Babb JR, Collins BJ, et al. *Pseudomonas aeruginosa* in hospital sinks. *Lancet* 1974;2:578–581.
501. Stoddard JC, Airey IL, Al-Jumaili IJ, et al. *Pseudomonas aeruginosa* in the intensive care unit. *Intensive Care Med* 1982;8:279–282.
502. Chadwick P. The epidemiological significance of *Pseudomonas aeruginosa* in hospital sinks. *Can J Public Health* 1976;67:323–328.
503. Sakata H, Fujita K, Maruyama S, et al. *Acinetobacter calcoaceticus* biovar anitratus septicemia in a neonatal intensive care unit: epidemiology and control. *J Hosp Infect* 1989;14:15–22.
504. Debast SB, Meis JFGM, Melcherws WJG, et al. Use of interrupt PCR fingerprinting to investigate an *Acinetobacter baumannii* outbreak in an intensive care unit. *Scand J Infect Dis* 1996;28:577–581.
505. Brown DG, Baublis J. Reservoirs of *Pseudomonas* in an intensive care unit for newborn infants: mechanisms of control. *J Pediatr* 1977;90: 453–457.
506. Levin MH, Olson B, Nathan C, et al. *Pseudomonas* in the sinks in an intensive care unit: relation to patients. *J Clin Pathol* 1984;37: 424–427.
507. Lyytikainen O, Golovanova V, Kolho E, et al. Outbreak caused by tobramycin-resistant *Pseudomonas aeruginosa* in a bone marrow transplant unit. *Scand J Infect Dis* 2001;33:445–449.
508. Bruun JN, McGarrity GJ, Blakemore WS, et al. Epidemiology of *Pseudomonas aeruginosa* infections: determination by pyocin typing. *J Clin Microbiol* 1976;3:264–271.
509. Schlech WF, Simonsen N, Sumarah R, et al. Nosocomial outbreak of *Pseudomonas aeruginosa* folliculitis associated with a physiotherapy pool. *Can Med Assoc J* 1986;134:909–913.
510. Cand MS, Carter A, Sheppard PS. Endoscopic retrograde cholangiopancreatography: related nosocomial infections. *N Z Med J* 1980;92: 275–277.
511. Sorin M, Segal-Maurer S, Mariano N, et al. Nosocomial transmission of imipenem-resistant *Pseudomonas aeruginosa* following bronchoscopy associated with improper connection to the Steris System 1 processor. *Infect Control Hosp Epidemiol* 2001;22:409–413.
512. Kirschke DL, Hones TF, Craig AS, et al. *Pseudomonas aerguinosa* and *Serratia marcescens* contamination associated with a manufacturing defect in bronchoscopes. *N Engl J Med* 2003;348:214–220.
513. Alvarado CA, Stolz SM, Maki DM. Nosocomial infections from contaminated endoscopes: a flawed automated endoscope washer. An investigation using molecular epidemiology. *Am J Med* 1991;91(suppl 3B):272S–280S.
514. Blanc DS, Parret T, Janin B, et al. Nosocomial infections and pseudoinfections from contaminated bronchoscopes: two-year follow up using molecular markers. *Infect Control Hosp Epidemiol* 1997;18: 134–136.
515. Thom AR, Cole AP, Watrasiewicz K. *Pseudomonas aeruginosa* infection in a neonatal nursery, possibly transmitted by a breast-milk pump. *Lancet* 1970;1:560–561.
516. Henderson DK, Baptiste R, Parrillo J, et al. Indolent epidemic of *Pseudomonas cepacia* bacteremia and pseudobacteremia in an intensive care unit traced to a contaminated blood gas analyzer. *Am J Med* 1988;84:75–81.
517. Berkelman RL, Godley J, Weber JA, et al. *Pseudomonas cepacia* peritonitis associated with contamination of automatic peritoneal dialysis machines. *Ann Intern Med* 1982;96:456–458.
518. Hamill RJ, Houston ED, Georghiou PR, et al. An outbreak of *Burkholderia* (formerly *Pseudomonas*) *cepacia* respiratory tract colonization and infection associated with nebulized albuterol therapy. *Ann Intern Med* 1995;122:762–766.
519. Semel JD, Trenholme GM, Harris AA, et al. *Pseudomonas maltophila* pseudosepticemia. *Am J Med* 1978;64:403–406.
520. Rogues AM, Maugein J, Allety A, et al. Electronic ventilator temperature sensors as a potential source of respiratory tract colonization with *Stenotrophomonas maltophilia*. *J Hosp Infect* 2001;49:289–292.
521. Centers for Disease Control. Bacteremia associated with reuse of disposable hollow-fiber hemodialyzers. *MMWR* 1986;35:417–418.
522. Kothari T, Reyes MP, Brooks N, et al. *Pseudomonas cepacia* septic arthritis due to intra-articular injections of methylprednisolone. *Can Med Assoc J* 1977;115:1230–1231.
523. Fisher MC, Long SS, Roberts EM, et al. *Pseudomonas maltophilia* bacteremia in children undergoing open heart surgery. *JAMA* 1981; 246:1571–1574.
524. van Laer F, Raes D, Andamme P, et al. An outbreak of *Burkholderia cepacia* with septicemia on a cardiology ward. *Infect Control Hosp Epidemiol* 1998;19:112–113.
525. Kantor RJ, Carson LA, Graham DR, et al. Outbreak of pyrogenic reactions at a dialysis center: association with infusion of heparinized saline solution. *Am J Med* 1983;74:449–456.
526. DeCicco BT, Lee EC, Sorrentino JV. Factors affecting survival of *Pseudomonas cepacia* in decongestant nasal sprays containing thimerosal as preservative. *J Pharm Sci* 1982;71:1231–1234.
527. Tablan OC, Anderson LJ, Arden NH, et al. Guideline for prevention of nosocomial pneumonia. *Infect Control Hosp Epidemiol* 1994;9: 587–627.
528. Ramsey AH, Skonieczny P, Coolidge DT, et al. *Burkholderia cepacia* lower respiratory tract infection associated with exposure to a respiratory therapist. *Infect Control Hosp Epidemiol* 2001;22:423–426.
529. Sherertz RJ, Sullivan ML. An outbreak of infections with *Acinetobacter calcoaceticus* in burn patients: contamination of patients' mattresses. *J Infect Dis* 1985;151:252–258.
530. Allen KD, Green HT. Hospital outbreak of multi-resistant *Acinetobacter anitratus*: an airborne mode of spread? *J Hosp Infect* 1987;9: 110–119.
531. Berkowitz DM, Lee W, Pazin GJ, et al. Adhesive tape: potential source of nosocomial bacteria. *Appl Microbiol* 1974;28:651–654.
532. Vanhegan RI, Mitchell RG. *Pseudomonas* infection associated with contamination of wick-type air freshener. *Br Med J* 1975;3:685.
533. Harvey K, Schuck S. *Acinetobacter* septicaemia following prolonged intravenous therapy. *Med J Aust* 1977;6:121–124.
534. Das I, Lambert P, Hill D, et al. Carbapenem-resistant *Acinetobacter* and role of curtains in an outbreak in intensive care units. *J Hosp Infect* 2000;50:110–114.
535. Chang HJ, Christenson JC, Paria AT, et al. *Ochrobactrum anthropi* meningitis in pediatric pericardial allograft transplant recipients. *J Infect Dis* 1996;173:656–660.
536. Kumar D, Cattral MS, Robiscek A, et al. Outbreak of *Pseudomonas aeruginosa* by multiple organ transplantation from a common donor. *Transplantation* 2003;75:1053–1055.
537. Shooter RA, Cooke EM, Gaya H, et al. Food and medicaments as possible sources of hospital strains of *Pseudomonas aeruginosa*. *Lancet* 1969;1:1227–1229.
538. Shooter RA, Faiers MC, Cooke EM, et al. Isolation of *Escherichia*

coli, Pseudomonas aeruginosa, and *Klebsiella* from food in hospitals, canteens, and schools. *Lancet* 1971;2:390–392.

539. Wright C, Kominos SD, Yee RB. Enterobacteriaceae and *Pseudomonas aeruginosa* recovered from vegetable salads. *Appl Environ Microbiol* 1976;31:453–454.
540. Correa CMC, Tibana A, Gonitijo-Filho PP. Vegetables as a source of infection with *Pseudomonas aeruginosa* in a university and oncology hospital of Rio de Janeiro. *J Hosp Infect* 1991;18:301–306.
541. Kominos SD, Copeland CE, Grosiak B, et al. Introduction of *Pseudomonas aeruginosa* into a hospital via vegetables. *Appl Microbiol* 1972; 24:567–570.
542. Ayliffe GAJ, Collins BJ, Pettit F. Contamination of infant feeds in a Milton milk kitchen. *Lancet* 1970;1:559–561.
543. Thurn J, Crossley K, Gerdts A, et al. Enteral hyperalimentation as a cause of nosocomial infection. *J Hosp Infect* 1990;15:203–217.
544. Centers for Disease Control. Nosocomial *Burkholderia cepacia* infection and colonization associated with intrinsically contaminated mouthwash—Arizona, 1998. *MMWR* 1998;47:926–928.
545. Matrician L, Ange G, Burns S, et al. Outbreak of nosocomial *Burkholderia cepacia* infection and colonization associated with intrinsically contaminated mouthwash. *Infect Control Hosp Epidemiol* 2000;21: 739–741.
546. Noble WC, Savin JA. Steroid cream contaminated with *Pseudomonas aeruginosa. Lancet* 1966;1:347–351.
547. Baird RM, Shooter RA. *Pseudomonas aeruginosa* infections associated with use of contaminated medicaments. *Br Med J* 1976;2:349–350.
548. Stirland RM, Tooth JA. *Pseudomonas cepacia* as contaminant of propamidine disinfectants. *Br Med J* 1976;1505.
549. Cooke EM, Shooter RA, O'Farrell SM, et al. Faecal carriage of *Pseudomonas aeruginosa* by newborn babies. *Lancet* 1970;2:1045–1046.
550. Billing E. Studies on a soap organism: a new variety of *Bacterium anitratum. J Gen Microbiol* 1955;13:226–252.
551. Keys TF, Melton IJ III, Maker MD, et al. A suspected hospital outbreak of pseudobacteremia due to *Pseudomonas stutzeri. J Infect Dis* 1983;3:489–493.
552. Marin M, de Viedma DG, Martin-Rabadan P, et al. Infection of Hickman catheter by *Pseudomonas* (formerly *Flavimonas*) *oryzihabitans* traced to a synthetic bath sponge. *J Clin Microbiol* 2000;38: 4577–4579.
553. Mackel DC. Contamination of disposable catheter kits with EO-1. *N Engl J Med* 1970;282:752–753.
554. Mitchell RG, Oxon BM, Hayward AC. Postoperative urinary-tract infections caused by contaminated irrigating fluid. *Lancet* 1966;1: 793–795.
555. Morris S, Gibbs M, Hansman D, et al. Contamination of aqueous dilutions of resiguard disinfectant with *Pseudomonas. Med J Aust* 1976: 110–111.
556. Verschraegen G, Claeys G, Meeus G, et al. *Pseudomonas pickettii* as a cause of pseudobacteremia. *J Clin Microbiol* 1985;21:278–279.
557. Bodey GP. Epidemiological studies of *Pseudomonas* species in patients with leukemia. *Am J Med Sci* 1970;260:82–89.
558. Murthy SK, Baltch AL, Smith RP, et al. Oropharyngeal and fecal carriage of *Pseudomonas aeruginosa* in hospital patients. *J Clin Microbiol* 1989;27:35–40.
559. Freeman R, McPeake PK. Acquisition, spread, and control of *Pseudomonas aeruginosa* in a cardiothoracic unit. *Thorax* 1982;37: 732–736.
560. Kropec A, Huebner J, Riffel M, et al. Exogenous or endogenous reservoirs of nosocomial *Pseudomonas aeruginosa* and *Staphylococcus aureus* infections. *Intensive Care Med* 1993;19:161–165.
561. Grogan JB. *Pseudomonas aeruginosa* carriage in patients. *J Trauma* 1966;6:639–643.
562. Davies AJ, Bullock DW. *Pseudomonas aeruginosa* in two special care baby units patterns of colonization and infection. *J Hosp Infect* 1981; 2:241–247.
563. Neter E, Weintraub DH. An epidemiologic study on *Pseudomonas aeruginosa (Bacillus pyocyaneus)* in premature infants in the presence and absence of infection. *J Pediatr* 1955;46:280–287.
564. Boukadida J, de Montalembert M, Gaillard J-L. Outbreak of gut colonization by *Pseudomonas aeruginosa* in immunocompromised children undergoing total digestive decontamination: analysis by pulsed-field electrophoresis. *J Clin Microbiol* 1991;29:2068–2071.
565. Stoodley BJ, Thom BT. Observations on the intestinal carriage of *Pseudomonas aeruginosa. J Med Microbiol* 1970;3:367–375.
566. Maysoon SA, Darrell JH. The skin as the source of *Acinetobacter* and *Moraxella* species occurring in blood cultures. *J Clin Pathol* 1979;32: 497–499.
567. Taplin D, Rebell G, Zaias N. The human skin as a source of Mima-Herella infections. *JAMA* 1963;186:952–955.
568. Corbella X, Pujal M, Ayats J, et al. Relevance of digestive tract colonization in the epidemiology of nosocomial infections due to multiresistant *Acinetobacter baumannii. Clin Infect Dis* 1996;23:329–334.
569. Timsit JF, Gattait V, Misset B, et al. The digestive tract is a major site for *Acinetobacter baumannii* colonization in intensive care unit patients. *J Infect Dis* 1993;168:1336–1337.
570. Buxton AE, Anderson RL, Werdegar D, et al. Nosocomial respiratory tract infection and colonization with *Acinetobacter calcoaceticus. Am J Med* 1978;65:507–513.
571. Thomassen MJ, Demdo CA, Doershuk CF, et al. *Pseudomonas cepacia:* decrease in colonization in patients with cystic fibrosis. *Am Rev Respir Dis* 1986;134:669–671.
572. Elting LS, Khardori N, Bodey GP, et al. Nosocomial infection caused by *Xanthomonas maltophilia*: a case control study for predisposing factors. *Infect Control Hosp Epidemiol* 1990;11:134–138.
573. Chetchotisakd P, Phelps CL, Hartstein AI. Assessment of bacterial cross-transmission as a cause of infections in intensive care units. *Clin Infect Dis* 1994;18:929–937.
574. Bauer TM, Ofner E, Just HM, et al. An epidemiological study assessing the relative importance of airborne and direct contact transmission of microorganisms in a medical intensive care unit. *J Hosp Infect* 1990; 15:301–309.
575. Florman AL, Schifrin N. Observations on a small outbreak of infantile diarrhea associated with *Pseudomonas aeruginosa. J Pediatr* 1950;36: 758–766.
576. MacArthur RD, Lehman MH, Currie-McCumber CA, et al. The epidemiology of gentamicin-resistant *Pseudomonas aeruginosa* on an intermediate care unit. *Am J Epidemiol* 1988;128:821–827.
577. Adams BG, Marrie TJ. Hand carriage of aerobic gram-negative rods by health care personnel. *J Hyg* 1982;89:23–31.
578. Gruner E, Kropec A, Huebner J, et al. Ribotyping of *Pseudomonas aeruginosa* strains isolated from surgical intensive care patients. *J Infect Dis* 1993;167:1216–1220.
579. Tankovic J, Legrand P, DeGatines G, et al. Characterization of a hospital outbreak of imipenem-resistant *Acinetobacter baumannii* by phenotypic and genotypic typing methods. *J Clin Microbiol* 1994;32: 2677–2681.
580. Crowe M, Towner KJ, Humphreys H. Clinical and epidemiological features of an outbreak of *Acinetobacter* infection in an intensive therapy unit. *J Med Microbiol* 1995;43:55–62.
581. Go ES, Urban C, Burns J, et al. Clinical and molecular epidemiology of *Acinetobacter* infections sensitive only to polymyxin B and sulbactam. *Lancet* 1994;344:1329–1332.
582. Patterson JE, Vecchio J, Pantelick EL, et al. Association of contaminated gloves with transmission of *Acinetobacter calcoaceticus* var. anitratus in an intensive care unit. *Am J Med* 1991;91:479–483.
583. Gilardi GL. Pseudomonas and related genera. In: Ballows A, Hausler WJ Jr, Herrmann KL, et al., eds. *Manual of clinical microbiology,* 5th ed. Washington, DC: American Society for Microbiology, 1991: 429–441.
584. Christie C, Mazon D, Hierholzer W, et al. Molecular heterogeneity of *Acinetobacter baumannii* isolates during seasonal increase in prevalence. *Infect Control Hosp Epidemiol* 1995;16:590–594.
585. Kiska DL, Gilligan PH. *Pseudomonas.* In: Murray PR, Baron EJ, Jorgensen JH, et al., eds. *Manual of clinical microbiology,* 8th ed. Washington, DC: American Society for Microbiology, 2003:719–728.
586. Brown VI, Lowbury EJ. Use of an improved cetrimide agar medium and other culture methods for *Pseudomonas aeruginosa. J Clin Pathol* 1965;18:752–756.
587. Lambe DW Jr, Stewart P. Evaluation of Pseudosel agar as an aid in

the identification of *Pseudomonas aeruginosa. Appl Microbiol* 1972; 23:377–381.
588. Fonseca K, MacDougall J, Pitt TL. Inhibition of *Pseudomonas aeruginosa* from cystic fibrosis by selective media. *J Clin Pathol* 1986;39: 220–222.
589. Hedberg M. Acetamide agar medium selective for *Pseudomonas aeruginosa. Appl Microbiol* 1969;17:481.
590. Krueger CL, Sheikh W. A new selective medium for isolating *Pseudomonas* spp. from water. *Appl Environ Microbiol* 1987;53:895–897.
591. Araj GF. Use of 9-chloro-9-(4-diethylaminophenyl)-10-phenylacridan as a primary medium for recovery of *Pseudomonas aeruginosa* from clinical specimens. *J Clin Microbiol* 1984;20:330–333.
592. Fader RC, Latimer J, Bannister E, et al. Evaluation of 9-chloro-9-[4-(diethylamino)phenyl]-9, 10-dihydro-10-phenylacridine hydrochloride (C-390) in broth and agar media for identification of *Pseudomonas aeruginosa. J Clin Microbiol* 1988;26:1901–1903.
593. Marold LM, Freedman R, Chamberlain RE, et al. New selective agent for isolation of *Pseudomonas aeruginosa. Appl Environ Microbiol* 1981; 41:977–980.
594. Keeven JK, DeCicco BT. Selective medium for *Pseudomonas aeruginosa* that uses 1,10-phenanthroline as the selective agent. *Appl Environ Microbiol* 1989;55:3231–3233.
595. Campbell ME, Farmer SW, Speert DP. New selective medium for *Pseudomonas aeruginosa* with phenanthroline and 9-chloro-9-[4-(diethylamino)phenyl]-9,10-dihydro-10-phenylacridine hydrochloride (3–390). *J Clin Microbiol* 1988;26:1910–1912.
596. Gilligan PH, Lum G, Vandamme PAR, et al. *Burkholderia, Stenotrophomonas, Ralstonia, Brevundimonas, Comamonas, Delftia, Pandoraea,* and *Acidovorax.* In: Murray PR, Baron EJ, Jorgensen JH, et al., eds. *Manual of clinical microbiology,* 8th ed. Washington, DC: American Society for Microbiology, 2003:729–748.
597. Schreckenberger PC, Daneshvar MI, Weyant RS, et al. *Acinetobacter, Achromobacter, Chryseobacterium, Moraxella,* and other nonfermentative gram-negative rods. In: Murray PR, Baron EJ, Jorgensen JH, et al., eds. *Manual of clinical microbiology,* 8th ed. Washington, DC: American Society for Microbiology, 2003:749–779.
598. Tablon OC, Carson LA, Cusick LB, et al. Laboratory proficiency test results on use of selective media for isolating *Pseudomonas cepacia* from simulated sputum specimens of patients with cystic fibrosis. *J Clin Microbiol* 1987;25:485–487.
599. Welch DF, Muszynski MJ, Pai CH, et al. Selective and differential medium for recovery of *Pseudomonas cepacia* from the respiratory tracts of patients with cystic fibrosis. *J Clin Microbiol* 1987;25: 1730–1734.
600. Gilligan PH, Gage PA, Bradshaw LM, et al. Isolation medium for the recovery of *Pseudomonas cepacia* from respiratory secretions of patients with cystic fibrosis. *J Clin Microbiol* 1985;22:5–8.
601. Henry DA, Campbell ME, LiPuma JJ, et al. Identification of *Burkholderia cepacia* isolates from patients with cystic fibrosis and use of a simple new selective medium. *J Clin Microbiol* 1997;35:614–619.
602. Henry D, Campbell M, McGimpsey C, et al. Comparison of isolation media for recovery of *Burkholderia cepacia* complex from respiratory secretions of patients with cystic fibrosis. *J Clin Microbiol* 1999;37: 1004–1007.
603. Burdge DR, Noble MA, Campbell MC, et al. *Xanthomonas maltophilia* misidentified as *Pseudomonas cepacia* in cultures of sputum from patients with cystic fibrosis: a diagnostic pitfall with major clinical implications. *Clin Infect Dis* 1995;20:445–448.
604. Holton J. A note on the preparation and use of a selective differential medium for the isolation of *Acinetobacter* spp. from clinical sources. *J Appl Bacteriol* 1983;54:141–142.
605. Jawad A, Hawkey PM, Heritage J, et al. Description of Leeds *Acinetobacter* Medium, a new selective and differential medium for isolation of clinically important *Acinetobacter* spp., and comparison with Herellea agar and Holton's agar. *J Clin Microbiol* 1994;32:2353–2358.
606. Speert DP. Molecular epidemiology of *Pseudomonas aeruginosa. Front Biosci* 2002;7:354–361.
607. Tenover FC, Arbeit RD, Goering RV, Molecular Typing Working Group of the Society for Healthcare Epidemiology of America. SHEA position paper. How to select and interpret molecular strain typing methods for epidemiological studies of bacterial infections: a review for healthcare epidemiologists. *Infect Control Hosp Epidemiol* 1997; 18:426–439.
608. The International *Pseudomonas aeruginosa* Typing Study Group. A multicenter comparison of methods for typing strains of *Pseudomonas aeruginosa* predominantly from patients with cystic fibrosis. *J Infect Dis* 1994;169:134–142.
609. Bergmans D, Bonten M, van Tiel F, et al. Value of phenotyping methods as a initial screening of *Pseudomonas aeruginosa* in epidemiological studies. *Infection* 1997;6:350–354.
610. John JF Jr, Twitty JA. Plasmids as epidemiologic markers in nosocomial gram-negative bacilli: experience at a university and review of the literature. *Rev Infect Dis* 1985;8:693–704.
611. Grundmann H, Schneider C, Hartung D, et al. Discriminatory power of three DNA-based typing techniques for *Pseudomonas aeruginosa. J Clin Microbiol* 1995;33:528–534.
612. Maher WE, Kobe M, Fass RJ. Restriction endonuclease analysis of clinical *Pseudomonas aeruginosa* strains: useful epidemiologic data from a simple and rapid method. *J Clin Microbiol* 1993;31: 1426–1429.
613. Pujana I, Gallego L, Canduela MJ, et al. Specific and rapid identification of multiple-antibiotic resistant *Pseudomonas aeruginosa* clones isolated in an intensive care unit. *Diagn Microbiol Infect Dis* 2000;35: 65–68.
614. Bingen EH, Denamur E, Elion J. Use of ribotyping in epidemiological surveillance of nosocomial outbreaks. Clin Microbiol Rev 1667;7: 311–327.
615. Denamur E, Picard B, Goullet P, et al. Complexity of *Pseudomonas aeruginosa* infection in cystic fibrosis: combined results from esterase electrophoresis and rDNA restriction fragment length polymorphism analysis. *Epidemiol Infect* 1991;106:531.
616. Ogle JW, Janda JM, Woods DE, et al. Characterization and use of a DNA probe as an epidemiologic marker for *Pseudomonas aeruginosa. J Infect Dis* 1987;155:119–126.
617. Samadpour M, Moseley SL, Lory S. Biotinylated DNA probes for exotoxin A and pilin genes in the differentiation of *Pseudomonas aeruginosa* strains. *J Clin Microbiol* 1988;26:2319–2323.
618. Speert DP, Campbell ME, Farmer SW, et al. Use of a pilin gene probe to study molecular epidemiology of *Pseudomonas aeruginosa. J Clin Microbiol* 1989;27:2589–2593.
619. Grothues D, Koopmann U, von der Hardt H, et al. Genome fingerprinting of *Pseudomonas aeruginosa* indicates colonization of cystic fibrosis sibling with closely related strains. *J Clin Microbiol* 1988;26: 1973–1977.
620. Talon D, Cailleaux V, Thouverez M, et al. Discriminatory power and usefulness of pulsed-field gel electrophoresis in epidemiological studies of *Pseudomonas aeruginosa. J Hosp Infect* 1996 32:135–145.
621. Talon D, Capellier G, Boillot A, et al. Use of pulsed-field gel electrophoresis as an epidemiologic tool during an outbreak of *Pseudomonas aeruginosa* lung infections in an intensive care unit. *Intensive Care Med* 1995;21:996–1002.
622. Speijer H, Savelkoul PHM, Bonten MJ, et al. Application of different genotyping methods for *Pseudomonas aeruginosa* in a setting of endemnicity in an intensive care unit. *J Clin Microbiol* 1999;37:3654–3661.
623. Lau YJ, Liu PY, Hu BS, et al. DNA fingerprinting of *Pseudomonas aeruginosa* serotype 011 by enterobacterial repetitive intergenic consensus-polymerase chain reaction and pulsed-field gel electrophoresis. *J Hosp Infect* 1995;31:61–66.
624. Rabkin CS, Jarvis WR, Anderson RL, et al. *Pseudomonas cepacia* typing systems: collaborative study to assess their potential in epidemiologic investigations. *Rev Infect Dis* 1989;11:600–607.
625. Speert DP. Advances in *Burkholderia cepacia* complex. *Paediatr Respir Rev* 2002;3:230–235.
626. Sun L, Jiang RZ, Steinbach S, et al. The emergence of a highly transmissible lineage of *cbl+ Pseudomonas (Burkholderia) cepacia* causing CF centre epidemics in North America and Britain. *Nature Med* 1995; 1:661–666.
627. Anderson DJ, Kuhns JS, Vasil ML, et al. DNA fingerprinting by pulsed field gel electrophoresis and ribotyping to distinguish *Pseudom-*

onas cepacia isolates from a nosocomial outbreak. *J Clin Microbiol* 1991;29:648–649.

628. Holmes A, Nolan R, Taylor R, et al. An epidemic of *Burkholderia cepacia* transmitted between patients with and without cystic fibrosis. *J Infect Dis* 1999;179:1197–1205.
629. Pegues CF, Pegues DA, Ford DS, et al. *Burkholderia cepacia* respiratory tract acquisition: epidemiology and molecular characterization of large nosocomial outbreak. *Epidemiol Infect* 1996;116:309–317.
630. Mahenthiralingam E, Campbell ME, Henry DA, et al. Epidemiology of *Burkholderia cepacia* infection in patients with cystic fibrosis: analysis by randomly amplified polymorphic DNA fingerprinting. *J Clin Microbiol* 1996;34:2914–2920.
631. Hamill RJ, Houston ED, Georghiou PR, et al. An outbreak of *Burkholderia* (formerly *Pseudomonas*) *cepacia* respiratory tract colonization and infection associated with nebulized albuterol therapy. *Ann Intern Med* 1995;122:762–766.
632. Coenye T, LiPuma JJ. Multilocus restriction typing: a novel tool for studying global epidemiology of *Burkholderia cepacia* complex infection in cystic fibrosis. *J Infect Dis* 2002;185:1454–1462.
633. Schable B, Rhoden DL, Hugh R, et al. Serological classification of *Xanthomonas maltophilia (Pseudomonas maltophilia)* based on heat-stable O antigens. *J Clin Microbiol* 1989;27:1011–1014.
634. Seifert H, Boullion B, Schulze A, et al. Plasmid DNA profiles of *Acinetobacter baumannii:* clinical applications in a complex endemic setting. *Infect Control Hosp Epidemiol* 1994;15:520–528.
635. Traub WH. *Acinetobacter baumannii* serotyping for delineation of outbreaks of nosocomial cross-infection. *J Clin Microbiol* 1989;27: 2713–2716.
636. Tankovic J, Legrand P, De Gatines G, et al. Characterization of a hospital outbreak of imipenem-resistant *Acinetobacter* baumannii by phenotypic and genotypic typing methods. *J Clin Microbiol* 1994;32: 2677–2681.
637. Scerpella EG, Wanger AR, Armitage L, et al. Nosocomial outbreak caused by a multiresistant clone of *Acinetobacter baumannii:* results of the case-control and molecular investigations. *Infect Control Hosp Epidemiol* 1995;16:92–97.
638. D'Agata EMC, Thayer V, Schaffner W. An outbreak of *Acinetobacter baumannii*: the importance of cross transmission. *Infect Control Hosp Epidemiol* 2000;21:588–591.
639. Christie C, Mazon D, Hierholzer W Jr, et al. Molecular heterogeneity of *Acinetobacter baumannii* isolates during seasonal increase in prevalence. *Infect Control Hosp Epidemiol* 1995;16:590–594.
640. Laing FP, Ramotar K, Read R, et al. Molecular epidemiology of *Xanthomonas maltophilia* colonization and infection in the hospital environment. *J Clin Microbiol* 1995;33:513–518.
641. Yao JDC, Conly JM, Krajden M. Molecular typing of *Stenotrophomonas (Xanthomonas) maltophilia* by DNA macrorestriction analysis and random amplified polymorphic DNA analysis. *J Clin Microbiol* 1995; 33:2195–2198.
642. Denton M, Todd NJ, Kerr KG, et al. Molecular epidemiology of *Stenotrophomonas maltophilia* isolated from clinical specimens from patients with cystic fibrosis and associated environmental samples. *J Clin Microbiol* 1998;36:1953–1958.
643. Alfieri N, Ramotar K, Armstrong P, et al. Two consecutive outbreaks of *Stenotrophomonas maltophilia* (*Xanthomonas maltophilia*) in an intensive-care unit defined by restriction fragment-length polymorphism typing. *Infect Control Hosp Epidemiol* 1999;20:553–556.
644. Berg G, Roskot N, Smalla K. Genotypic and phenotypic relationships between clinical and environmental isolates of *Stenotrophomonas maltophilia. J Clin Microbiol* 1999;37:3594–3600.
645. Chetoui H, Melin P, Struelens MJ, et al. Comparison of biotyping, ribotyping, and pulsed-field gel electrophoresis for investigation of a common-source outbreak of *Burkholderia pickettii* bacteremia. *J Clin Microbiol* 1997;35:1398–1403.
646. Reboli AC, Houston ED, Monteforte JS, et al. Discrimination of epidemic and sporadic isolates of *Acinetobacter baumannii* by repetitive element PCR-mediated DNA fingerprinting. *J Clin Microbiol* 1994;32:2635–2640.
647. Webster CA, Crow M, Humphreys H, et al. Surveillance of an adult intensive care unit for long-term persistence of multi-resistant strain of *Acinetobacter baumannii. Eur J Clin Microbiol* Infect Dis 1998;17: 171–176.
648. Ehrenstein B, Bernards AT, Dijkshoorn L, et al. *Acinetobacter* species identification by using tRNA spacer fingerprinting. *J Clin Microbiol* 1996;34:2414–2420.
649. Liu PYF, Shi ZY, Lau YJ, et al. Epidemiological typing of *Flavimonas oryzihabitans* by PCR and pulsed-field gel electrophoresis. *J Clin Microbiol* 1996;34:68–70.
650. Maroye P, Doermann HP, Rogues AM, et al. Investigation of an outbreak of Ralstonia pickettii in a paediatric hospital by RAPD. *J Hosp Infect* 2000;44:267–272.
651. Krzewinski JW, Nguyen CD, Foster JM, et al. Use of random amplified polymorphic DNA PCR to examine epidemiology of *Stenotrophomonas maltophilia* and *Achromobacter* (Alcaligenes) *xylosoxidans* from patients with cystic fibrosis. *J Clin Microbiol* 2001;39:3597–3602.

35

NOSOCOMIAL *LEGIONELLA* INFECTION

JANET E. STOUT
VICTOR L. YU

HISTORY

Legionnaires' disease made its debut in July 1976 as an explosive outbreak of community-acquired pneumonia. The outbreak of pneumonia was among attendees of the American Legion Convention at a hotel in Philadelphia, Pennsylvania (1). Six months later, the causative agent was isolated from the lung tissue of Legionnaires' cases by workers at the Centers for Disease Control and Prevention (CDC), Atlanta, Georgia (2). The microorganism, an aerobic gram-negative bacterium, was named *Legionella pneumophila.* The first known epidemic of nosocomial *Legionella* pneumonia was in July 1965 at St. Elizabeth's Hospital, a psychiatric institution in Washington, D.C. (3). In this outbreak, 81 patients were afflicted, with an attack rate of 1.4%. It was not until 1980 that hospital water distribution systems were first implicated as the source for nosocomial Legionnaires' disease. Tobin (4) isolated *Legionella* from showerheads in the hospital room of a patient with nosocomial Legionnaires' disease (4). Shortly thereafter, the microorganism was isolated from potable water distribution systems of numerous hospitals experiencing outbreaks of Legionnaires' disease (5–9).

Among cases of Legionnaires' disease reported annually to the CDC from 1980 to 1998, the proportion of cases identified as nosocomial Legionnaires' disease varied from 25% to as high as 45% (10). Twenty-eight percent of these cases were associated with an outbreak of nosocomial Legionnaires' disease.

MICROBIOLOGY

The Legionellaceae family has been characterized as one monophyletic family belonging to the gamma subdivision of the class Proteobacteria (11,12). Although a single genus and species (*Legionella pneumophila*) was originally proposed for the family Legionellaceae (13), the Legionellaceae family now contains more than 48 species and 70 serogroups in the genus *Legionella* (14,15). Approximately half of these *Legionella* species have been implicated in human disease. Among the species, *L. pneumophila* is responsible for 90% of infections (Table 35.1) (14). These microorganisms are saprophytic water bacteria that can become opportunistic pathogens. Most cases of Legionellosis are caused by *L. pneumophila* serogroups 1, 4, and 6 (16).

Other species implicated in human infection include *L. micdadei* (the Pittsburgh Pneumonia Agent), *L. bozemanii, L. dumoffii, L. tucsonensis, L. cincinnatiensis, L. feeleii, L. longbeachae,* and *L. oakridgensis* (17–20). Most patients with nonpneumophila *Legionella* species infections have been severely immunocompromised due to corticosteroid therapy, organ transplantation, or malignancy (21,22).

Legionella species are small (0.3 to 0.9 μm in width and approximately 2 μm in length) faintly staining gram-negative rods with polar flagella (except *L. oakridgensis*). They generally appear as small coccobacilli in infected tissue or secretions, whereas long filamentous forms (up to 20 μm in length) can be seen when they are grown in culture media. Legionellaceae are obligately aerobic slow-growing nonfermentative bacteria. They are distinguished from other saccharolytic bacteria by their requirement for L-cysteine and iron salts for primary isolation on solid media and by their unique cellular fatty acids and ubiquinones. Differences among species have been assessed by phenotypic (23,24) and chemotaxonomic tests. Phenotypic tests include composition of lipopolysaccharides (LPS) (24), electrophoretic protein profiles (25), monoclonal antibodies (26), fatty acid composition (27), and cellular carbohydrates (28). Genotypic tests include random amplified polymorphic DNA profiles (RAPD) (29,30), heteroduplex analysis of 5S ribosomal RNA (rRNA) gene sequences (31), and computer-assisted matching of transfer DNA (tDNA)-intergenic length polymorphism (ILP) patterns (32).

The microorganism can be visualized, with some difficulty, with Gram stains of clinical specimens taken from normally sterile sites (e.g., pleural fluid). Both the Gram and Gimenez stains can be used for clinical specimens, whereas silver impregnation stains, including the Dieterle and Warthin-Starry stains, can be used for paraffin-fixed tissue sections. *L. micdadei* (Pittsburgh pneumonia agent) can stain weakly acid-fast in tissue with Kinyoun and Fite stains and on smears with a modified acid-fast stain in tissue or sputum specimens. These microorganisms are nutritionally fastidious and do not grow on standard bacteri-

TABLE 35.1. *LEGIONELLA PNEUMOPHILA* IS RESPONSIBLE FOR THE MAJORITY OF INFECTIONS DUE TO LEGIONELLACEAE

	Percentage of cases			
		Serogroups		
First Author, Year (Reference)	L. pneumophila	1	Other	Other Species
Benin, 2002 (10)	91	51	9	9
Yu, 2002 (243)	92	84	7	9
Marston, 1994 (61)	91	57	13	9
Reingold, 1984 (244)	85	52	24	15

ologic media, which explains why the microorganism was so difficult to isolate in the original American Legion outbreak.

PATHOGENESIS

Pneumonia is the presenting clinical syndrome in almost all cases of nosocomial legionellosis. Although rare, extrapulmonary *Legionella* infection has been documented (33) Legionnaires' disease can be acquired by the inhalation of aerosols containing *Legionella* or by aspiration of water or respiratory secretions containing *Legionella* (34,35). Other possible modes of transmission include direct inhalation or hematogenous dissemination from other foci of infection.

Cigarette smokers, patients with chronic pulmonary disease, and alcoholics—all conditions in which mucociliary clearance is impaired—are at increased risk for Legionnaires' disease. This barrier to entry can be overcome by adherence of the microorganism to respiratory epithelial cells. *Legionella* does possess pili that are known to mediate adherence to epithelial cells (36). Symbiosis has also been shown *in vitro* between oropharyngeal flora and *Legionella* (37).

Legionella is an intracellular pathogen both in humans and in aquatic environments (38). *Legionella* survives and multiplies as parasites of single-celled protozoa in fresh water and moist soil (39). Virulence may be increased by replication in amebae (40). In humans, *Legionella* replicates within mononuclear phagocytes, primarily monocytes, and alveolar macrophages (41,42). Cell-mediated immunity plays the central role in host defense against *L. pneumophila* as it does against other intracellular pathogens. Although the resident alveolar macrophage normally degrades most microorganisms, *Legionella* is able to subvert this host defense. The macrophage readily phagocytoses *Legionella,* a process that is more avid in the presence of specific opsonizing antibody. Attachment of *Legionella* to epithelial cells or macrophages may be related to the expression of pili. A pilin mutant showed a 50% decrease in attachment to human macrophages and epithelial cells (36). Once inside the cell, the microorganism evades phagosome-lysosome fusion, converts to a replicative form that is acid-tolerant, and multiplies until the cell ruptures (38,43,44). Presumably, the liberated bacteria are phagocytosed by newly recruited cells, and the cycle of ingestion, multiplication, and liberation with cell lysis begins anew.

Intracellular multiplication of *Legionella* within human monocytes depends on the availability of iron (45). The lymphokine interferon-γ (IFN-γ) stimulates human alveolar macrophages and monocytes to resist *Legionella* infection by upregulating reactive oxygen production and downregulating cellular iron content. Other cytokines and hemopoietic growth factors, such as interleukin-10 (IL-10) and granulocyte-macrophage colony-stimulating factor (GM-CSF), have not been shown to enhance anti-*Legionella* activity (46,47). Significant rises in the Th-1 cytokines IFN-γ and IL-12 were detected in the serum of patients with Legionnaires' disease, supporting the importance of cellular immunity in this disease (48). Neutrophils are less important, and neutropenic patients are not at undue risk for Legionnaires' disease. Nevertheless, *L. pneumophila* is susceptible to oxygen-dependent microbicidal systems *in vitro.* Neutrophils inhibit *Legionella* growth but lack the capacity to kill *L. pneumophila.* Lysis of infected macrophages by lymphokine-activated killer (LAK) cells or natural killer (NK) cells may also be an important cell-mediated immune function for eliminating intracellular *Legionella.*

Humoral immunity is also important. For patients with Legionnaires' disease, type-specific antibodies are measurable within several weeks of infection. Moreover, immunized animals and patients develop a specific antibody response with subsequent resistance to *Legionella* challenge.

A number of factors have been postulated to contribute to the virulence of *L. pneumophila*(38): type I and type II secretion systems, a pore-forming toxin, type IV pili, flagella, a *Legionella* toxin (49), a 24-kd protein called Mip (50), a zinc metalloprotease (51–53), and proteases (54,55) including enzymes that scavenge reduced-oxygenated metabolites (56).

Strains of *L. pneumophila* differ in virulence. *L. pneumophila,* serogroup 1, is known to cause most cases of Legionnaires' disease. Although multiple strains of *L. pneumophila* serogroup 1 may colonize water distribution systems, only a few strains are likely to cause disease in patients exposed to the water (8,57,58). Monoclonal antibody subtyping of strains of *L. pneumophila,* serogroup 1, have shown that a surface epitope recognized by one particular monoclonal antibody (MAB-2) may be associated with virulence. The immunodominant part of this virulence-associated epitope has been identified as the 8-0-acetyl group of the 0-specific polysaccharide chain of the LPS (59).

Legionella species other than *L. pneumophila* appear to be less virulent and occur almost exclusively among immunocompromised hosts. They also respond more readily to antibiotic therapy (20,60).

EPIDEMIOLOGY

Although legionellosis is a reportable disease in many countries including the United States, the extent of this infection is still uncertain. Underestimates are likely due to cases that are overlooked because of the persistent lack of availability of specialized laboratory tests. From 1980 through 1998, the median number of cases reported per year to the CDC was 360 (10,61, 62). If the incidence of Legionnaires' disease is estimated to be a minimum of 8,000 to 14,500 cases, then less than 5% of cases are being reported. Approximately 35% of the reported cases met the definition for nosocomial infection (10).

Nosocomial legionellosis has been classified as "endemic" and "hyperendemic." These terms have become less useful with the recognition that they merely designate different prevalences of the disease over a spectrum. Thus, although hospitals may be labeled as experiencing sporadic disease (implying frequent cases of Legionnaires' disease scattered over a long period), the possibility is that only a proportion of actual cases are diagnosed. These cases surface because of a combination of circumstances: improved diagnostic methods, clinical suspicion of Legionnaires' disease by an individual physician, or isolation of the microorganism from open lung biopsy or postmortem lung culture (22). The introduction of a diagnostic test for Legionnaires' disease, the urine antigen test, was responsible for the detection of a recurrent outbreak of nosocomial Legionnaires' disease at a hospital in Connecticut (63). From 1987 to 1996, routine testing for Legionnaires' disease at autopsy identified eight cases of nosocomial Legionnaires' disease at a regional transplant center in the southwestern U.S. (64). The occurrence of three cases in early 1996 led to a retrospective review, which suggested that nosocomial transmission had occurred for more than 17 years. An additional 14 cases were identified for a total of 25 culture-confirmed cases of nosocomial Legionnaires' disease. Thus, situations labeled as sporadic or nonepidemic may merely represent chance discovery of disease occurring at a low endemic level. Likewise, situations labeled as "epidemic" may merely represent a cyclical peak at a hospital with endemic but previously undiscovered disease.

The reported nosocomial *Legionella* infection rates vary widely from 1% to 40% (65–68). This variable infection rate reflects a dependence on multiple variables. These include a contaminated potable water system with *Legionella*, exposure of the host to the contaminated water, susceptibility of the patient exposed, and recognition of the disease by the physician.

Consistently identified risk factors for Legionnaires' disease include advanced age, male gender, smoking, alcohol abuse, chronic pulmonary disease, and immunosuppression (malignancy, corticosteroid use). Males are affected at two to three times the rate of women; this may be related to cigarette smoking or underlying medical conditions (e.g., chronic obstructive pulmonary disease). Attributable mortality for Legionnaires' disease is approximately 20%; however, the likelihood of death from *Legionella* infection increases in patients who are elderly or male, with nosocomial infection, renal disease, malignancy, or immunosuppression (61,64). Mortality can be as high as 40% for hospital-acquired cases (61).

Nosocomial infections due to *Legionella* occur most frequently in immunosuppressed hosts. The patients at highest risk are organ transplant recipients (69). During an outbreak in an acute care hospital, 55% (5/9) of all patients undergoing kidney transplantation developed Legionnaires' disease over a 5-month period (70). Nosocomial *Legionella* infection has been reported in transplant recipients of kidneys (70,71), hearts (64,72), livers (73,74), and bone marrow (64,74,75). Corticosteroids are an important independent risk factor. Neoplastic disease, diabetes, and renal failure are often cited as risk factors. The broader use of diagnostic testing may result in more patients being identified without these classic risk factors. A retrospective review of over 400 cases of Legionnaires' disease in the Pittsburgh area showed that 25% of reported cases did not have the classic risk factors (76).

There is a striking association of Legionnaires' disease with surgery. Up to 40% of cases reported in the literature occurred in surgical patients (77). Nosocomial *Legionella* infection increased with use of general anesthesia and endotracheal intubation (64, 66,78,79).

Surprisingly, neutropenic or leukemic hosts appear to have an attack rate no higher than that of the general population. The exception are patients with hairy cell leukemia (80,81). Likewise, the risk of *Legionella* infection in the HIV-infected patient appears to be no greater than other high-risk populations, with reports of less than 1% to 4%. However, these patients are prone to extrapulmonary manifestations, bacteremia, and lung abscesses.

Increasing use of diagnostic tests for *Legionella* has led to new risk groups of patients being discovered as susceptible victims for Legionnaires' disease. They include immunocompromised children in pediatric hospitals colonized with *Legionella* and elderly patients residing in long-term-care facilities and rehabilitation centers colonized by *Legionella.*

Nosocomial cases have been reported in immunosuppressed children (74,82–87) and children with underlying pulmonary disease (88,89). In three hospitals in which epidemiologic investigations were conducted (82,88,90), a link to the hospital water supply was made.

At least three outbreaks of Legionnaires' disease have been reported in long-term-care facilities (91–93). The investigation identified *Legionella* in the potable water supply as the source for two of the outbreaks. In a third outbreak, only limited environmental sampling was performed. Aspiration was presumed to be the mode of transmission for most of these outbreaks. In one outbreak, eating pureed food was a significant risk factor for *Legionella*, consistent with aspiration originating from a swallowing disorder (93). In another prospective study, *L. pneumophila* serogroup 1 was isolated from a newly constructed long-term-care facility (94). Six cases of Legionnaires' disease were diagnosed over 2 years. DNA subtyping established that the patient isolates were identical to the environmental isolates from the water supply.

Reservoir

The environmental ecology of *Legionella* is particularly pertinent in that Legionnaires' disease is a pneumonia that theoretically could be prevented with eradication of the microorganism from its reservoir. The natural habitat for *Legionella* appears to be aquatic bodies including rivers, streams, and thermally polluted waters, although *L. longbeachae* has been isolated from moist soil in Australia (95). Natural aquatic bodies contain only small numbers of *Legionella*. Since *Legionella* tolerates chlorine, the microorganism easily survives the water treatment process and passes into water distribution systems but, again, only in small numbers (96–98).

Subsequent growth and proliferation occur in man-made habitats, especially water distribution systems, which provide favorable water temperatures (25° to 42°C), physical protection (biofilm), and nutrients (99). The single most important factor appears to be temperature. The microorganism is most readily found at the bottom of hot water tanks—a relation that parallels its propensity for colonization in thermally polluted rivers. Interestingly, bacteria populating hot water tanks were more likely to demonstrate a symbiotic relationship with *L. pneumophila* than bacteria populating cold water tanks (100). Bacteria, protozoa, and amoeba also colonize water pipe surfaces, some of which have been shown to promote *Legionella* replication (100–102). *Legionella* and other microorganisms attach to surfaces and form biofilms on pipes throughout the water distribution system (103). Water pressure changes that disturb the biofilm may dramatically increase the concentration of *Legionella* (104).

Hospitals with hot water distribution systems colonized with *L. pneumophila* were significantly more likely to have lower water temperatures (<140°F), have a vertical configuration, be older, and have elevated calcium and magnesium concentrations in the water (105,106). Cold-water sources, such as ice machines, have also been implicated as a source of nosocomial infection (97, 107,108).

The role of *Legionella*-contaminated potable water distribution systems as a source for nosocomial Legionnaires' disease has been well established. The British Communicable Disease Surveillance Centre reported that 19 of 20 hospital outbreaks of Legionnaires' disease in the United Kingdom from 1980 to 1992 were attributed to such systems (109,110).

Cooling towers and, to a lesser degree, evaporative condensers were implicated in the earlier outbreaks prior to recognition of potable water as a reservoir. Surprisingly, air conditioners have never been directly implicated as a source of Legionnaires' disease, despite widespread belief that they are. The role of cooling towers in the dissemination of *Legionella* has been challenged (111). Following the recognition in 1982 that potable water distribution systems were a source (6), reports of cooling towers as reservoirs for nosocomial legionellosis have essentially disappeared. One exception was a report published in 1985 of a Rhode Island hospital in which cooling towers were cited as the source (112); this now appears to be a typical scenario of water distribution system contamination in which the original epidemiologic investigation was flawed (104).

Subtyping of *L. pneumophila* with molecular methods has proven invaluable in elucidating environmental sources, permitting application of rational methods for prevention (113). In fact, application of subtyping provided the first concrete evidence that water distribution systems rather than cooling towers were the actual sources of infection (9,114). The subtype of *Legionella* isolates taken from patients were identical to the isolates taken from putative environmental reservoirs. Both phenotypic and genotypic methods have been used to demonstrate identity among strains of *Legionella pneumophila* in epidemiologic investigations. These methods include serotyping, monoclonal antibody subtyping, isoenzyme analysis, protein and carbohydrate profiling, plasmid analysis, restriction endonuclease analysis, restriction fragment length polymorphism (RFLP) of rRNA (ribotyping) or chromosomal DNA, amplified fragment length polymorphism (AFLP), restriction endonuclease analysis of whole-cell DNA with or without pulsed-field gel electrophoresis (PFGE), and DNA fingerprinting using polymerase chain reaction (PCR) (113,115–119). However, PFGE has been the most widely applied (117,120–122). Maximum discrimination among isolates is achieved by combining both monoclonal antibody subtyping and PFGE (117,123).

Modes of Transmission

Multiple modes have been identified for transmission of *Legionella* to humans; there is evidence for aerosolization, aspiration, or even instillation into the lung during respiratory tract manipulation. Aspiration of contaminated water or oropharyngeal secretions appears to be the major mode of transmission in the hospital setting (35). Colonization of oropharyngeal flora by *L. pneumophila* is a theoretical possibility (124–128). The evidence for aspiration is impressive. *Legionella* was found to be the most common cause of nosocomial pneumonia in a population of oncologic head and neck surgery patients (65); these patients had a propensity for aspiration as a result of their oral surgery and extensive cigarette smoking. Nasogastric tube placement has been shown to be a significant risk factor for nosocomial legionellosis in intubated patients in three studies; microaspiration of contaminated water was the presumed mode of entry (34, 129,130). It should be noted that, in the original 1976 outbreak, consumption of water at the implicated hotel was associated with acquisition of disease—an association that has been generally overlooked (1). Contaminated ice and water from an ice machine have been implicated as the source of nosocomial infection (97,108,131).

Healthcare personnel frequently use tap water to rinse respiratory apparatus and tubing for use in mechanical ventilation machines. If the tap water is contaminated with *L. pneumophila*, the microorganism can be instilled directly into the lung (132–134). In numerous studies, patients with Legionnaires' disease underwent endotracheal tube placement significantly more often or had a significantly longer duration of intubation than patients who had other causes of pneumonia (64,66,78, 135,136). The use of a nasogastric tube, the presence of immunosuppression, and ventilator use were highly correlated with the acquisition of nosocomial Legionnaires' disease in a hospital in Halifax, Nova Scotia (129). Use of sterile water for all nasogastric suspensions and for flushing tubes has been recommended to prevent nosocomial Legionnaires' disease. Intermittent positive pressure ventilators have been associated with nosocomial legionellosis, or more likely, the tubing attached to these ventilators. The use of such equipment was epidemiologically linked to Legionnaires' disease in 18 hospital patients over a 2-year period; again, it was noted that the equipment was rinsed with tap water between treatments (34). Three cases of nosocomial *L. pneumophila* pneumonia were acquired from contaminated transesophageal echocardiography (TEE) probes (137). Again, contaminated tap water had been used to rinse the probes.

Investigators from the CDC presented the first evidence to support the aerosolization theory when reporting the Legionnaires' disease outbreak in Memphis (138). Tracer smoke studies indicated that aerosols from an auxiliary air conditioning tower could have reached an air intake supplying certain patient rooms. However, the attack rate for patients occupying rooms supplied with air from the air intake was not higher than the attack rate for patients occupying rooms in the same wing but receiving air from other sources (111). Cases also occurred in hospital wings having no relationship to the cooling towers. Water was not cultured since this investigation antedated the discovery that drinking water could be the source for Legionnaires' disease.

Because the first environmental isolation of *L. pneumophila* was from a showerhead (4), it has been widely thought that aerosols from showers may be an important means for dissemination of this microorganism. However, simulation studies show that only small numbers of *Legionella* are aerosolized and only for short distances (132,139). Although a few retrospective studies have suggested showers as a potential source (140,141), an epidemiologic link between showering and acquisition of disease has never been shown in prospective studies; in fact, prospective studies have consistently shown that showers are not a risk factor (34,64,142–145).

Aerosolization by respiratory tract devices including the humidifier of oxygen therapy equipment, nebulizers, and room humidifiers has been documented (146,147). Humidifiers are water-filled devices that add water vapor to air, oxygen, or other gases without producing particulate water. Guinea pigs exposed to a room humidifier contaminated with*Legionella* experienced subclinical infection as demonstrated by seroconversion. In a hospital setting, a portable room humidifier filled with *Legionella*-contaminated tap water disseminated the microorganism up to distances of 300 cm. Furthermore, recovery of aerosolized *Legionella* increased with proximity to the humidifier, and seroconversion of exposed animals was directly proportional to the concentration of *Legionella* in humidifier water. Humidifiers have been implicated in transmission of Legionnaires' disease in humans. Five of eight patients with nosocomial Legionnaires' disease in an Italian hospital had been exposed to bubble diffuser humidifiers filled with water containing *L. pneumophila* (148). An immunosuppressed patient at the University of Chicago Hospital acquired Legionnaires' disease after exposure to a room humidifier that had been filled with contaminated tap water for 15 days (149). The statistical association between disease and humidifier exposure was highly significant. Use of a room humidifier was also associated with 18 cases of nosocomial Legionnaires' disease in a 2-year period in a limited retrospective study (150). In all three of these studies, the humidifiers had been filled with tap water (148–150).

A postlaryngectomy patient died from pneumonia following exposure to a room humidifier. *L. pneumophila* serogroups 4 and 5 were isolated from the patient's lung and from the tap water and containers used to fill the humidifier reservoir (133). Distilled water in humidifiers has also been linked to hospital outbreaks of *Legionella* infection; one patient with *L. dumoffii* was exposed to a room humidifier presumably filled with contaminated distilled water (151). Nosocomial pneumonia in a neonate was linked to the presence of *Legionella* in the humidifier of the incubator (152). In one French hospital, the use of contaminated tap water to fill the humidifier of oxygen therapy equipment and for aerosol delivery of drugs led to five cases of Legionnaires' disease caused by *L. pneumophila*, serogroup 1 (147).

Nebulizers are devices that generate aerosols of uniform particulate size. Ultrasonic nebulizers can produce water particles ranging in size from 0.9 to 10 μm; water droplets of 1 to 2 μm in diameter can reach the alveoli. Medication jet nebulizers have been shown to aerosolize water particles containing *L. pneumophila* when the nebulizer water was seeded with the microorganism (153); these particles were less than 5 μm in diameter, so it is likely they could bypass the pulmonary defenses and reach the alveoli. Jet nebulizers have been epidemiologically linked to nosocomial Legionnaires' disease (149). Inhalation of contaminated tap water aerosols from jet nebulizers was found to be a highly significant risk factor for four patients who acquired nosocomial Legionnaires' disease.

In addition to filling nebulizers with tap water, rinsing the chambers of hand-held medication nebulizers has been suggested as a source of contamination. In one study of 13 patients with nosocomial Legionnaires' disease due to *L. pneumophila*, serogroup 3, there was a trend toward more frequent use of nebulizer medications in patients with Legionnaires' disease. It was subsequently established that jet nebulizers were often rinsed with tap water (153). Medication nebulizers have also been implicated in one of the few reports of pediatric nosocomial Legionella infection (82). Two children with Legionnaires' disease received nebulizer treatments using equipment likely to have been rinsed under tap water.

Aerosolization via excavated soil was suggested as a possible mode of transmission for the outbreaks at the Wadsworth Veterans Administration (VA) Medical Center and St. Elizabeth's Hospital; in retrospect, contaminated water distribution systems were probably the actual reservoirs. Finally, person-to-person transmission has not been demonstrated (154).

CLINICAL MANIFESTATIONS

Legionella infection presents as two clinical entities: Pontiac fever and pneumonia (Legionnaires' disease). Pontiac fever is an acute, self-limiting illness. Chills, high fever, headache, and myalgias are typical. Pneumonia is not seen, and nosocomial cases of Pontiac fever have not been reported.

Pneumonia is the predominant clinical syndrome in Legionnaires' disease. The incubation period for Legionnaires' disease usually ranges from 2 to 10 days. One report demonstrated the onset of disease 63 days after discharge from the hospital, and molecular typing linked the hospital water supply as the source. This led to the speculation that oropharyngeal colonization with *Legionella* had occurred (127). Subsequent studies have not been successful in demonstrating oropharyngeal colonization with *Legionella* (125,155).

Legionnaires' disease encompasses a broad spectrum of illnesses ranging from mild cough and low-grade fever to stupor, rapidly progressive pneumonia, and multiorgan system failure. Nonspecific symptoms including malaise, myalgias, anorexia, and headache are common in the first 48 hours. Fever is virtually always present, and temperatures in excess of 40°C should lead to the consideration of Legionnaires' disease. Relative bradycardia has been emphasized by some investigators in earlier studies, but we have found this to be a nonspecific finding (156).

Initially, the cough is mild and only slightly productive. The character of the sputum is often nonpurulent. Although the sputum may be streaked with blood, gross hemoptysis is rare. Chest pain, often pleuritic, is common, and when coupled with hemoptysis, can masquerade as pulmonary infarction.

Gastrointestinal symptoms are more prominent in community-acquired pneumonia, but less so in nosocomial pneumonia; diarrhea, nausea, vomiting, and abdominal pain are common. The most common neurologic finding in Legionnaires' disease is change in mental status, although a wide variety of findings, including encephalopathy, have been reported (157,158).

L. pneumophila microorganisms can disseminate from their pulmonary niche to various extrapulmonary sites including spleen, liver, kidney, bone marrow, myocardium, and lymph nodes. Dissemination apparently occurs via the hematogenous or lymphatic system. Extrapulmonary nosocomial *Legionella* infections occurred in cardiothoracic surgical patients at Stanford University (33,79,159). Seven patients presented with *Legionella* prosthetic valve endocarditis, three had sternal surgical site infections, and one patient manifested both infections. *L. pneumophila*, serogroup 1, and *L. dumoffii* were isolated from clinical samples as well as from the potable water system of the hospital. The origin of the sternal surgical site infections was contaminated tap water used to remove the povidone-iodine solution from the operative site.

Other reports have implicated tap water as the source for extrapulmonary *Legionella* infections. In one patient, an open hip wound infection due to *L. pneumophila* was linked to colonized water from a Hubbard tank used for rehabilitation (160). Nosocomial extrapulmonary legionellosis involving hemodialysis fistula infections (two cases) (161) and a perirectal abscess (162) were probably secondary to hematogenous seeding from confirmed *Legionella* pneumonia; however, direct inoculation by contaminated water or equipment could not be excluded. Detection of the microorganism at extrapulmonary sites is problematic. Since selective media must be used to isolate the microorganism, the clinician must think of the possibility of *Legionella* as the cause of the infection. Other bacteria may also be isolated, thereby confounding the diagnosis.

LABORATORY DIAGNOSIS

The prompt diagnosis of Legionnaires' disease in the hospital setting can save lives. Not only has early initiation of appropriate therapy been associated with improved outcome, but the diagnosis of a single case of hospital-acquired Legionnaires' disease can prompt the recognition of endemic Legionnaires' disease at the facility (63,163). For patients with severe pneumonia, the Infectious Diseases Society of America recommends diagnostic tests for *Legionella* (164).

The diagnosis of Legionnaires' disease based on a syndromic approach has been suggested (158); however, most studies have shown that the clinical manifestations of Legionnaires' disease are nonspecific (156). Laboratory abnormalities including abnormal liver function tests, elevated creatinine phosphokinase, hypophosphatemia, hematuria, hemolytic anemia, and thrombocytopenia have been reported. Hyponatremia with a serum sodium of less than 130 mEq/L occurs significantly more often in Legionnaires' disease than in other pneumonias; it appears to be more common in nosocomial Legionnaires' disease than in the community-acquired disease. This syndrome probably is caused by salt and water loss rather than inappropriate antidiuretic hormonal secretion (V. L. Yu, unpublished data).

Specialized diagnostic laboratory tests are the key feature for diagnosing Legionnaires' disease, because the clinical presentation is nonspecific. Most hospitals, including university and tertiary care hospitals, often do not have the most sensitive tests available, namely culture on selective media and urinary antigen (110), and up to 40% of hospitals send samples off-site for testing (165). Data from a CDC survey showed that hospitals where *Legionella* diagnostic tests were available on-site were more likely to identify nosocomial Legionnaires' disease (165).

Urinary Antigen

Among case reports of Legionnaires' disease submitted to the CDC, there has been a significant increase in the proportion of patients reported with a positive urine antigen test result (10). The *Legionella* urine antigen test has a high sensitivity (90%), high specificity (99%), and relatively low cost, and the results can be available within hours of submission of the test (166–168). The urine antigen test is available as an enzyme immunoassay (EIA) or an immunochromatographic (ICT) test. The EIA test is available commercially from two U.S. suppliers (Wampole Laboratories, a division of Carter-Wallace Inc., Cranbury, NJ; and Bartels, Issaquah, WA) and includes the Binax *Legionella* Urinary Antigen EIA and the Bartels *Legionella* Urinary Antigen EIA (Intracel, Frederick, MD). The Binax NOW *Legionella* urinary antigen test is a rapid ICT membrane assay for the qualitative detection of *L. pneumophila* serogroup-1 antigen (Binax, Inc., Portland, Maine). A swab is dipped in urine and inserted into the test device, and the reagent is added. The reaction is read after 15 minutes as the presence or absence of a visually detectable pink-purple colored line that results from the antigen-antibody reaction giving the result (Fig. 35.1) (169). The EIA and ICT tests have been shown to have comparable sensitivity and specificity (166,170).

The fact that test positivity can persist for days, even during administration of antibiotic therapy, makes it useful in those patients who receive empiric anti-*Legionella* therapy (171). A shortcoming of the test is that it can detect only serogroup 1 of *L. pneumophila* (172). Since the other serogroups of *L. pneumophila* and other *Legionella* species are less common, this test is still extremely useful. There has been some evidence that the urine antigen test can detect other serogroups and species; however, this requires further validation (172). In addition, it is

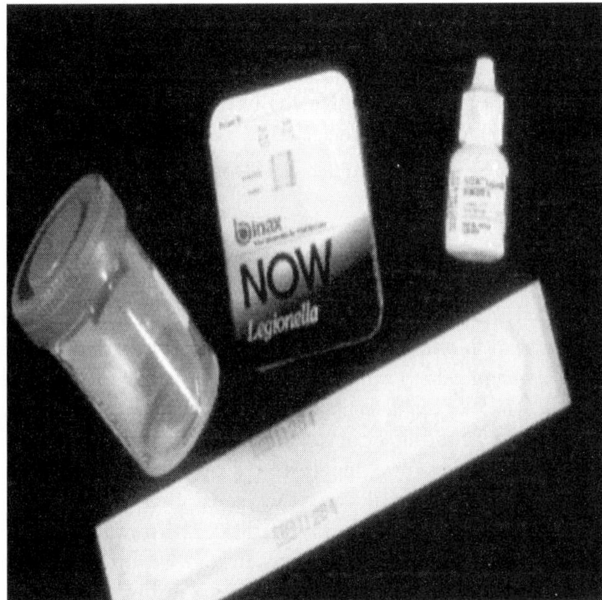

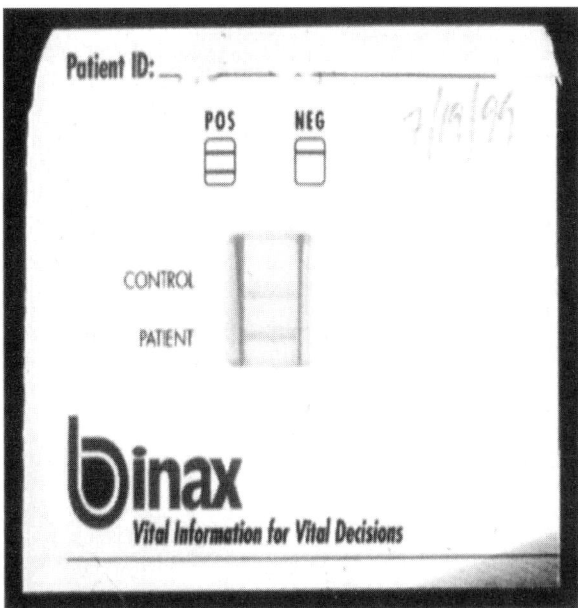

Figure 35.1. The NOW immunochromatographic (ICT) test is performed by dipping a swab in urine and inserting it into the test device. Two drops of a reagent are added and the card is closed and allowed to react for 15 minutes. A positive result is the presence of a visually detectable pink-purple colored line (next to the "Patient" line) resulting from the antigen-antibody reaction.

often easier to obtain a urine specimen than an adequate sputum specimen. A positive urinary antigen test, along with culture positivity and seroconversion, is now one of the criteria for a definitive diagnosis of Legionnaires' disease (173).

Early diagnosis and treatment has resulted from the increased use of the rapid urinary antigen test. This, in combination with the increasing empiric use of quinolones for hospital-acquired pneumonia, may explain the decline in Legionnaires' disease-related mortality in the U.S. The case-fatality rate for nosocomial Legionnaires' disease has decreased from 46% in 1982 to 14% in 1998 (10).

Culture on Selective Media

When Legionnaires' disease is suspected, both a urinary antigen test and *Legionella* culture of a respiratory specimen should be ordered. The single most important diagnostic test for Legionnaires' disease is isolation of the microorganism by culture. The availability of the clinical isolate from culture can be critical for subsequent epidemiologic investigations (174). Another reason not to rely exclusively on the urine antigen test is that the urinary antigen test may be negative if the infecting strain is not serogroup 1 or when the infecting strain is serogroup 1 but MAB-2 negative (Dresden Panel MAB-3/1 negative). Among 317 culture-proven cases of Legionnaires' disease, 67 (21%) were nosocomial cases. Only 45% of these cases were urine antigen positive, because 22% of the cases were caused by the MAB-2 negative serotype (175).

To achieve a high yield from sputum, multiple media containing antibiotics and dyes are required (169,176–178). Buffered charcoal yeast extract (BCYE) agar is the primary medium used for isolation of these microorganisms. The culture media can be made more selective by incorporating antibacterial agents (cefamandole, polymyxin B, vancomycin, aztreonam), antifungal agents (anisomycin), and inhibitors (glycine) into the media to suppress competing microflora. Pretreatment with acid is extremely useful for respiratory tract and environmental specimens, because *Legionella* microorganisms are acid-resistant, whereas most other bacteria are not. The addition of dyes to the media enhances the visibility of the colonies, because *Legionella* takes up the dye preferentially. The dye-containing media are especially important in detection of the nonpneumophila species (178). The microorganism grows slowly, taking up to 5 days for visible colonies to develop. Under a dissecting stereomicroscope, the colony surface shows a characteristic ground glass appearance.

Legionella culture is performed only when specifically requested. A physician often orders a *Legionella* urinary antigen test, and only a routine microbiology culture. As a result, when the urine antigen test is positive, no sputum is available for *Legionella* culture. We refrigerate all respiratory specimens for 7 days by placing them in bins marked by the days of the week. This practice allows for subsequent retrieval of the specimen for *Legionella* culture if a urine test is positive. The isolate from the patient is now available if an epidemiologic investigation is performed to determine the source of the infection.

Transtracheal aspirate specimens that bypass contaminating oropharyngeal flora can achieve a sensitivity as high as 90% (176). Sputum obtained by bronchoscopy can be useful but does not provide any higher yield than a good sputum specimen. If sputum is not available, however, bronchoalveolar lavage can yield the microorganism. Bronchial washings, in which the volume of fluid instilled is notably lower than that of lavage, appear to be less sensitive. Transbronchial biopsy can yield the microorganism in tissue by direct fluorescent antibody stains and culture and has been successful in identifying *Legionella* when sputum and bronchial washings were unrevealing. Percutaneous needle aspiration of a lung abscess has yielded the microorganism in culture from a patient who had negative sputum and bronchoscopy cultures.

Bacteremia is actually common in severely ill patients. The microorganism can be isolated from blood by biphasic BCYE agar bottles, a radiometric system (Bactec, Johnston Laboratories, Towson, MD), or VACUTAINER tube (Becton Dickinson, Rutherford, NJ). In one study, 38% of cases of Legionnaires' disease had positive blood cultures when subcultures from Bactec bottles were plated onto buffered charcoal yeast extract agar (179). At the Pittsburgh VA Medical Center, an aliquot (0.1 mL) from all negative blood culture bottles is plated to BCYE prior to being discarded.

Direct Fluorescent Antibody (DFA) Stain

The reported sensitivity of direct fluorescent antibody stains has ranged from 25% to 75% (180). It is highly specific, and the monoclonal antibody test (MONOFLUO, Bio-Rad Laboratories, Redmond, WA) has eliminated the rare occurrence of cross-reactivity with other gram-negative bacilli. Due to low sensitivity compared to culture, we do not perform the DFA on a specimen unless the direct culture is overgrown with competing flora and acid pretreatment of the specimen is required. Polyclonal DFA reagents are available from a number of suppliers for definitive identification of isolates of *Legionella* (Monoclonal Technologies, Atlanta, GA; Meridian Diagnostics, Inc., Cincinnati, OH; Zeus Technologies, Raritan, NJ).

Serology

Antibody tests have become less important with the advent of rapid diagnostic tests. Because the definitive criterion for diagnosis is a fourfold rise in antibody titer, repeat serology is required 4 to 6 weeks after onset of infection. Sensitivity in the 1976 outbreak was 91% (181), but sensitivity in studies of nosocomial pneumonia has been less than 50% (34,182,183). Maximal sensitivity requires detection of both immunoglobulin G (IgG) and IgM antibody (14). Effective antibiotics and suboptimal timing of specimen collection are possible reasons for the decrease in sensitivity. Diagnosis of Legionnaires' disease by serologic testing has decreased significantly from 1980 to 1998 (10).

Polymerase Chain Reaction (PCR)

DNA amplification by PCR of *Legionella* has been reported from patients with pneumonia using throat swab specimens, bronchoalveolar lavage (BAL), urine, and serum (79,184–186). Primer sequences of the macrophage infectivity potentiator *(mip)* gene of *L. pneumophila* and the 5S rRNA or 16S rRNA have been utilized in PCR assays. A real-time quantitative PCR assay has been used to detect *L. pneumophila* in respiratory tract secretions (187). One PCR kit was used successfully to detect *Legionella* in both clinical and environmental samples (188,189), but it is no longer commercially available. Although *Legionella* DNA has been detected in urine and serum samples from patients with legionellosis (190), clinical experience has not shown PCR to be more sensitive than culture. Therefore, the CDC does not recommend the routine use of genetic probes or PCR for detection of *Legionella* in clinical samples (180,191).

PREVENTION

It is now well established that there is a direct relationship between colonization of hospital water systems with *L. pneumophila* and the occurrence of nosocomial Legionnaires' disease (192–195). *Legionella* species have been shown to colonize between 12% and 85% of hospital water systems (193,196). Prospective studies have demonstrated cases of nosocomial Legionnaires' disease in colonized hospitals after environmental and clinical surveillance were initiated (193). Knowledge of this relationship is the first step to prevention. Unfortunately, there is a lack of consensus with respect to the utility of environmental monitoring for *Legionella* as part of a prevention strategy (193).

There are essentially two approaches to prevention of hospital-acquired Legionnaires' disease. One approach suggests maintaining a high index of suspicion for Legionellosis with the use of diagnostic testing in patients with healthcare-associated pneumonia (191,197). Routine culturing of the hospital water system for *Legionella* is *not* initiated unless one case of definite or two cases of possible hospital-acquired pneumonia have been identified. We consider this approach to be "re-active," and it is favored by many public health authorities including the CDC.

An alternate and "proactive" approach has been advocated by Pittsburgh investigators and the Allegheny County Health Department in Pittsburgh, Pennsylvania, for many years (193). This approach recommends proactively culturing the hospital water system as the initial step in making a risk assessment of the facility. Guidelines for *Legionella* prevention from the Allegheny County Health Department and from the state of Maryland specifically recommend routine environmental monitoring of the hospital water system (198,199) (Table 35.2). If any outlets yield *L. pneumophila*, diagnostic tests for *Legionella* are made available in-house. The presence of *L. pneumophila* serogroup 1 in the water supply necessitates the on-site availability of the urinary antigen test. If greater than 30% of outlets are culture-positive for *L. pneumophila*, the Allegheny County guidelines recommend that the facility consider disinfection of the water system (198).

The Texas Department of Health has also issued guidelines that recommend environmental surveillance for *Legionella* only if a risk assessment indicates that the facility has a significant risk of legionellosis transmission (200). For example, a high-risk facility could be a multistory facility with multiple water distribution systems, supplied with water treated with chlorine, stored hot water at 51°C (124° F) and delivered at 43°C (110°F), and housing bone marrow or solid organ transplant recipients or cancer patients undergoing chemotherapy.

Proactive approaches mandating routine environmental cultures within hospitals have now been adopted in Denmark, the Netherlands, France, and Taiwan.

TABLE 35.2. GUIDELINES FOR CONTROL OF *LEGIONELLA* IN HEALTHCARE FACILITIES IN PENNSYLVANIA AND MARYLAND RECOMMEND ROUTINE ENVIRONMENTAL CULTURING OF THE HOSPITAL WATER SYSTEM FOR *LEGIONELLA*

Organization (Reference)	Diagnostic Testing	Clinical Surveillance	Routine Environmental Testing	Approach to Prevention
Allegheny County Health Department 1993/1997 (245)	Active: In-house urinary antigen (UA) testing	If environ positive, active clinical surveillance	Yes: annually; transplant hospital, more often	Consider disinfection if >30% sites positive; empiric antimicrobial therapy with a macrolide or quinolone
Maryland Health Department (199)	Acute care: UA in-house/if transplant hospital, culture on site	Test pneumonia cases for *Legionella*	Yes: routine culture	If cases identified, disinfection recommended
Texas Department of Health (200)	Acute and long-term: UA in-house/if transplant hospital, culture on site	Active case detection after case identified	Routine: no; if high risk of cases: Yes	Enhanced clinical surveillance and remediation if cases identified
Centers for Disease Control and Prevention (191)	Routinely test without knowledge of environmental status	Educate re: diagnosis/400+beds = UA/culture in-house	No: unless cases identified or transplant unit	Disinfect only if source identified

From Stout JE, Yu VL. Hospital-acquired Legionnaires' disease: new developments. *Clin Infect Dis* 2003;16:337–341.

The "Guideline for Prevention of Nosocomial Pneumonia" from the CDC's Healthcare Infection Control Practices Advisory Committee (HICPAC) (201) is under revision and cites a number of important issues that remain unresolved, including the role of routine culturing of water systems for *Legionella* species in healthcare facilities. Opposition to routine environmental cultures in the absence of documented disease is often based on the premise that *Legionella* colonization is ubiquitous, that *Legionella* can colonize water distribution systems without causing disease, and that environmental culturing is expensive (191, 202,203). However, these assertions have been refuted based on studies in both the U.S. and the U.K. (193,204,205).

As part of a comprehensive strategy to prevent Legionnaires' disease in transplant units, HICPAC recommends that facilities with solid organ transplant programs or hematopoietic stem cell transplant recipients perform periodic culturing for *Legionella* in the transplant unit's potable water supply. This recommendation also appears in the "Guidelines for Prevention of Opportunistic Infections in Bone Marrow Transplant Recipients" (206). If *Legionella* species are detected in the unit's water system, corrective measures (disinfection) should be performed until no *Legionella* is cultured. No such recommendation is made for healthcare facilities treating nontransplant patients, or for disinfection of areas serving these patients.

One problem with this approach is that many cases of hospital-acquired Legionnaires' disease occur in nontransplant patients. In fact, not a single one of the patients in our original report of endemic hospital-acquired Legionnaires' disease were transplant recipients, and Legionnaires' disease constituted 22.5% (32/142) of the cases of hospital-acquired pneumonia (67). In a Swedish hospital, 31 patients with hospital-acquired Legionnaires' disease were diagnosed over a 14-month period; eight were from surgical wards, 16 from internal medicine or geriatric wards, three each from psychiatric and physiotherapy units, and one was from the maintenance department (207).

Environmental Culturing

Culture of hospital hot water tanks and selected showerheads and faucets (especially in transplant wards or intensive care units) is performed by collection of either swab and/or water samples from water outlets throughout the facility. Swabs of distal sites are used because the yield is higher than for water specimens (208) (Fig. 35.2). If a water sample is collected, at least 100 mL should be collected, and it should be from the hot water system. The sample should be collected immediately after turning on the faucet or shower. A minimum of ten outlets plus the hot water storage tank should be cultured for the average 250-bed hospital (198). If *Legionella* is isolated, specialized laboratory

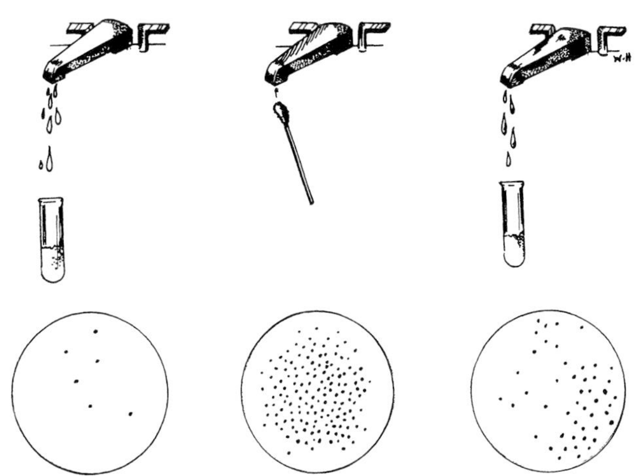

Figure 35.2. Environmental cultures obtained by swabbing distal sites yield considerably more *Legionella* microorganisms than culturing water does. Culture of water only yields few *Legionella* microorganisms on the selective culture plate *(left)*. Rotating a swab upward about the circumference of the faucet yields many *Legionella* microorganisms *(middle)*. Culture of the water after the sediment within the faucet has been dislodged by the swab yields moderate numbers of *Legionella* microorganisms *(right)*.

tests are made available in-house. The urinary antigen is especially recommended as a cost-effective test if the *Legionella* isolated is serogroup 1. The infection control professional then begins prospective surveillance of all nosocomial pneumonias (198,209,210). It has been well documented that, unless the hospital laboratory can isolate *Legionella,* nosocomial cases can be overlooked (193). It has also been suggested that surveillance for nosocomial legionellosis can be targeted to select high-risk patients for cost-effectiveness (68,209); high-risk patients include transplant recipients, immunosuppressed patients, patients with underlying pulmonary disease, and intensive care unit patients. Surveillance could be expanded to all patients with nosocomial pneumonia if cases of legionellosis were uncovered in the high-risk group. It is important to point out that if the frequency of contaminated sites is low, disinfection of the water supply is not necessarily required. Legionnaires' disease is readily treatable; macrolides and quinolones can be used effectively to treat hospital-acquired pneumonias of uncertain etiology. Antibiotic prophylaxis of transplant patients with macrolides or quinolones has even been used to stem outbreaks (211). If the level of contamination increases, the option to disinfect the water supply can be exercised.

Contaminated Respiratory Devices

The use of sterile water for filling and rinsing humidifiers, nebulizers, and all other respiratory equipment is recommended. We have banned portable room humidifiers from our hospital. Even rinsing respiratory device tubing with tap water may create a secondary reservoir for *Legionella.* Subsequently, reattachment of the device to the patient could directly instill *Legionella*-containing respirable droplets into the respiratory tract. Devices such as medication nebulizers may retain water 12 hours after rinsing (153).

DISINFECTION OF WATER DISTRIBUTION SYSTEMS

Nosocomial legionellosis has been effectively controlled by disinfection of hospital water distribution systems that are colonized by *Legionella.* There are two basic types of disinfection systems: focal and systemic. Focal disinfection is directed at only a portion of the water distribution system, usually the incoming water or individual outlets, but not at the entire water distribution system. Systemic disinfection is directed at the entire water distribution system and the biofilm throughout the system.

Focal disinfection modalities are modular and easy to install, but are notably less effective if the water distribution system is extensive or if the plumbing is heavily colonized with *Legionella* (212). Focal modalities include ultraviolet light, instantaneous heating systems, and ozone (213). Focal modalities are not effective if the water distribution system has preexisting *Legionella* colonization, because the *Legionella* in the water distribution system remains unaffected. Focal modalities may work best in a virgin water distribution system (e.g., in a new hospital) (214). For maximal effectiveness, a heat and flush sterilization or shock chlorination prior to activation and intermittently thereafter is advisable. Localized disinfection of faucets or showers by physical cleaning and or chlorination has a short-lived effect and is not effective (215).

Systemic modalities provide a disinfectant residual that is bacteriostatic or bacteriocidal throughout the water distribution system; these modalities include hyperchlorination, copper/silver ionization, and chlorine dioxide (216–219). Superheat and flush is a systemic modality that cannot be applied continuously; however, maintaining hot water temperatures at 140°F (60°C) minimizes recolonization (145,213,220,221).

In some hospitals with endemic legionellosis and a high-risk population (especially transplantation patients), multiple disinfection modalities may be needed so that, if one modality fails because of human error or mechanical failure, the other modality can serve as a safety net (75,216). Furthermore, a focal modality (ultraviolet light) can be combined with two systemic modalities (superheat and flush, copper-silver) to ensure maximal kill of *Legionella.* Routine continual surveillance with environmental cultures is critical, since mechanical failures and human error are expected with any system. Cultures performed at 2-month intervals are recommended. The endpoints for disinfection should be realistic and clinically relevant. Total sterility is extremely difficult to achieve with any disinfection modality, and zero positivity is not required to prevent nosocomial Legionnaires' disease (222,223).

The efficacy of some modalities may vary depending on water use. For example, if superheated water or water containing metallic ions or chlorine cannot reach a site because the faucet is unused, disinfection cannot occur. Although the disinfection modality may remove the larger portion of the biomass of *Legionella,* small pockets of *Legionella* in protected niches may still be present but in insufficient amounts to cause infection. At our institution, *Legionella* infections in the hospital setting did not occur until the percentage of colonized sites exceed 30% (7). The cut point of 30% distal site positivity as an indicator of increased risk of transmission of *Legionella* has not been universally applicable to all hospitals. However, it does demonstrate that the concept of correlating environmental monitoring with predicting increased risk of disease is valid for Legionnaires' disease. In a study by the CDC, increased risk was associated with the extent of colonization (percentage of outlets positive) and not the concentration of *Legionella* recovered from a given outlet (224). The precise figure depends not only on the extent of *Legionella* colonization, but also on the susceptibility of patient populations to *Legionella* infection. For example, patients on a transplant ward may become infected with *Legionella* with a much smaller inoculum of *Legionella* in the water than would ambulatory patients on a psychiatric ward. This may be the basis for the more stringent recommendations from the CDC for monitoring and disinfection of bone marrow transplant units (206).

Options for Disinfection

It is important to apply a scientific method to the evaluation of disinfection methods. We have proposed that any disinfection method should be subjected to a standardized evaluation with the following steps: (a) demonstrated efficacy *in vitro* against

TABLE 35.3. *LEGIONELLA* DISINFECTION METHODS: A COST COMPARISON

Method	Startup Cost	Annual Operating Cost
Copper-silver ionization	$20,000–$40,000	$2,000–$4,000
Thermal disinfection	$5,000–$20,000	Repeating costs
Chlorine dioxide	$15,000–$20,000	$2,000–$10,000
Hyperchlorination (includes silicate injection)	$50,000–$80,000	$10,000–$20,000
Ultraviolet light units	$10,000–$20,000	$1,000–2,000

Estimates based on a 250 to 500-bed hospital.

Legionella microorganisms; (b) anecdotal experience of efficacy in controlling *Legionella* contamination in individual hospitals; (c) controlled studies of prolonged duration (years, not months) of efficacy in controlling *Legionella* growth and in preventing cases of hospital-acquired Legionnaires disease in individual hospitals; and (d) confirmatory reports from *multiple* hospitals with prolonged duration of follow-up (validation step) (222). Given the current reality of economic constraints, disinfection modalities should also be selected with the long-term goals of sustained efficacy at reasonable costs (Table 35.3). Important factors include the area requiring disinfection (one building or multiple buildings, number of floors), the number of hot water heating systems in place (one vs. multiple), the extent of colonization, and the age of the facility. Older hospitals generally pose a more formidable task in disinfection than newer hospitals because of accumulation of scale and *Legionella* within biofilms (106). Disinfection efforts that target the hot water system have been effective in controlling *Legionella.* This would suggest that treating the cold water supply may not be necessary. Given the public health implications, any commercial vendor's history of experience and service commitment in *Legionella* disinfection should be reviewed. It would be prudent to obtain assessments from other hospitals that have used the vendor's product.

It should be emphasized that appearance, degree of cleanliness, and regular preventive maintenance of the system have not been shown to minimize *Legionella* contamination (106). Plumbing modifications including "dead-leg" removal and cleaning or replacing showerheads have been overemphasized. Nevertheless, many engineering guidelines have advocated such unvalidated approaches despite evidence that they are tedious and ineffective (106,213,225). The only way to be certain that a system is free of *Legionella* is to obtain samples for environmental cultures.

Finally, a strong infection control program is critical if the approach is to be cost-effective and scientifically valid. We advise that each hospital evaluate the utility of its modality scientifically. Baseline cultures prior to disinfection over an adequate period is critical, so that the efficacy of a new disinfection modality can be adequately evaluated.

Copper-Silver Ionization

Ionization is the only disinfection method that has fulfilled all four evaluation criteria (222). The systems (Tarn-Pure, T.P. Technology, Buckinghamshire, UK; Liqui-Tech, Bolingbrook, IL; Enrich Products, Pittsburgh, PA) use copper/silver electrodes that generate ions when an electrical current is applied. The positively charged ions form electrostatic bonds with negatively hypercharged sites on bacterial cell walls. The distorted cellular permeability coupled with protein denaturation leads to cell lysis and death. Copper-silver ionization provides residual protection throughout the system. Theoretically, microorganisms are killed rather than suppressed, which should minimize the possibility of recolonization. Controlled studies have shown that this modality is highly effective in eradicating *Legionella* (217,218,223, 226). This system can be used in concert with ultraviolet light and chlorine (216). Two hospitals that switched from thermal eradication (superheat-and-flush) to copper-silver ionization reported that ionization was more effective for reducing the recovery of *Legionella* from the hospital water system (218,223).

Among the first 16 hospitals to use ionization for *Legionella* disinfection, 75% had attempted disinfection with other methods (222) (Fig. 35.3). All 16 hospitals were successful in preventing nosocomial Legionnaires' disease after installation of ionization systems. Although elevated pH can adversely effect the action of copper (227) and there has been speculation of ion resistance (228,229), these hospitals reported satisfactory control of *Legionella* within the hospital hot water supply. The systems had been in place from 5 to 11 years. Cost depended on the number of systems installed, but the average cost was $20,000 to $40,000 (Table 35.3).

Chlorine Dioxide

Although this technology has been used to control *Legionella* in European hospital water systems for many years, it has only recently been introduced into the U.S. healthcare market for this application (219,230,231). New technology now allows for the safe generation of chlorine dioxide on a small scale. This generation unit utilizes an electrical source and membrane technology to directly oxidize sodium chlorite (Halox, Inc., Bridgeport, CT, a unit of IDEX, Corp.) (Fig. 35.4). These generators typically provide 5 g/hour to 2.4 kg/day of chlorine dioxide. The chlorine dioxide can be fed into the water system at various points (cold water supply, hot water supply, reservoir) depending on where disinfection is desired. The required maintenance involves changing the membrane-containing cartridges. As chlorine dioxide is generated, these cartridges slowly lose their oxidizing ability and require replacement (typically after 2,000 operating hours). Preventative maintenance includes replacing various filters and tubing.

There are minimum allowable levels of chlorine dioxide and its by-product chlorite. The U.S. Environmental Protection Agency (EPA) requirements are set forth in the National Primary Drinking Water Standards. The maximum residual disinfectant level for chlorine dioxide is 0.8 mg/L, and the maximum contaminant level for chlorite is 1.0 mg/L (232). Installations using chlorine dioxide as a supplemental disinfectant may be required to implement the same monitoring programs as primary water treatment operators. Potential users should check with their local environmental protection agency for regulatory requirements.

Two controlled evaluations of chlorine dioxide have been

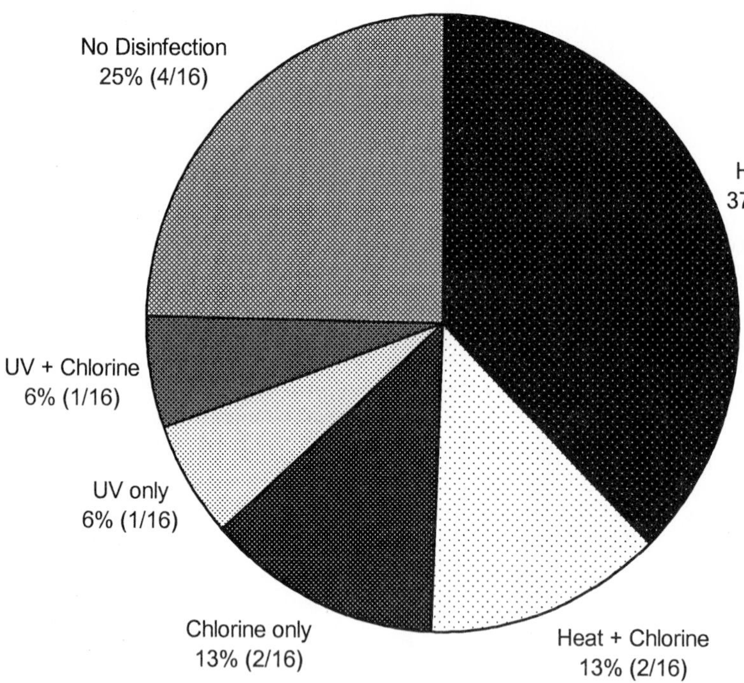

Figure 35.3. Among 16 hospitals that implemented *Legionella* water system disinfection practices, various methods were attempted and failed prior to installation of copper-silver ionization systems. All 16 hospitals reported no cases of nosocomial Legionnaires' disease after installation of the ionization system. (From Stout JE, Yu VL. Experiences of the first 16 hospitals using copper-silver ionization for *Legionella* control: implications for the evaluation of other disinfection modalities. *Infect Control Hosp Epidemiol* 2003;24:563–568, with permission.)

performed in the U.S. (219,230), and both have shown that chlorine dioxide at a concentration of <0.8 mg/L was effective in reducing *Legionella* species in the hospital water system. In both studies there was a significant reduction in the percentage of positive outlets; however, *Legionella* persisted at a low level in the treated systems and months were required to reach these levels. Difficulties were encountered in maintaining an adequate chlorine dioxide residual in the hot water system; the residual in the hot water was often <0.1 mg/L (230). This was attributed to a combination of loss of residual with increased distance from the injection point and increased decay of chlorine dioxide at higher water temperatures. Prospective studies of sufficient duration from different institutions are required to validate these results. Cost depends on the number of systems installed, but the average cost was $15,000 to $20,000 plus installation costs (Table 35.3).

Superheat and Flush

If *Legionella* must be eradicated from the water distribution system immediately, the superheat and flush method warrants primary consideration. The basic method requires that hot water tank temperatures be elevated to greater than 70°C (158°F) followed by flushing of all faucets and showerheads to kill *L. pneumophila* colonizing these sites (7,213).

All hot water tanks are shut down, drained, descaled with high-pressure steam, and then chlorinated to 100 parts per million (ppm) for 12 to 14 hours. The chlorinated water is drained and the tank flushed with water to remove the residual chlorine. The tanks are then placed back on line and the temperature is elevated to 70° to 80°C (158° to 176°F) for 72 hours. All distal water sites in patient care wards are flushed once a day for 2 days, whereas those sites located on patient units housing high-risk patients (intensive care units and transplant wards) are flushed once a day for 3 consecutive days. The outlets are flushed for 30 minutes. It is critical that temperatures of the flushed water be monitored to ensure that the temperature exceeds 60°C (140°F) distally. On the fourth day, selected distal sites are recultured; if no *Legionella* microorganisms are recovered, the procedure is considered completed. If *Legionella* is still isolated, the entire heat and flush protocol is repeated. Both maximum temperature and duration of the flush are important for successful decontamination. Hospitals that have used shorter flush times have failed to eradicate *Legionella* (233). Unfortunately, a minimum flush time of 5 to 10 minutes has been erroneously recommended by HICPAC (191); although the 30-minute flush is tedious, it will be more successful than the 5- to 10-minute flush.

Recolonization can be delayed and minimized by maintaining hot water tank temperatures at 60°C (140°F). At the Pittsburgh VA Medical Center, the heat and flush method was required only once every 2 to 3 years, making this method a cost-effective one. The costs are low except for personnel time; if overtime is required, the costs can quickly escalate. We used volunteers, when possible, for the flushing process. One hospital reported overtime costs of approximately $20,000 (Table 35.3) (205). Ultimately, we abandoned this method of control in favor of the less labor-intensive copper-silver ionization system (223).

The main disadvantage is that numerous personnel are involved to monitor distal sites, water tank temperatures, and flushing times. Scalding can occur, although such incidents have not been reported in numerous hospitals using this method. It should be noted that the Joint Commission on Accreditation of Healthcare Organizations has rescinded its earlier standard for a maximum water temperature of 110°F and allows each hospital to establish its own maximum temperature. However, many

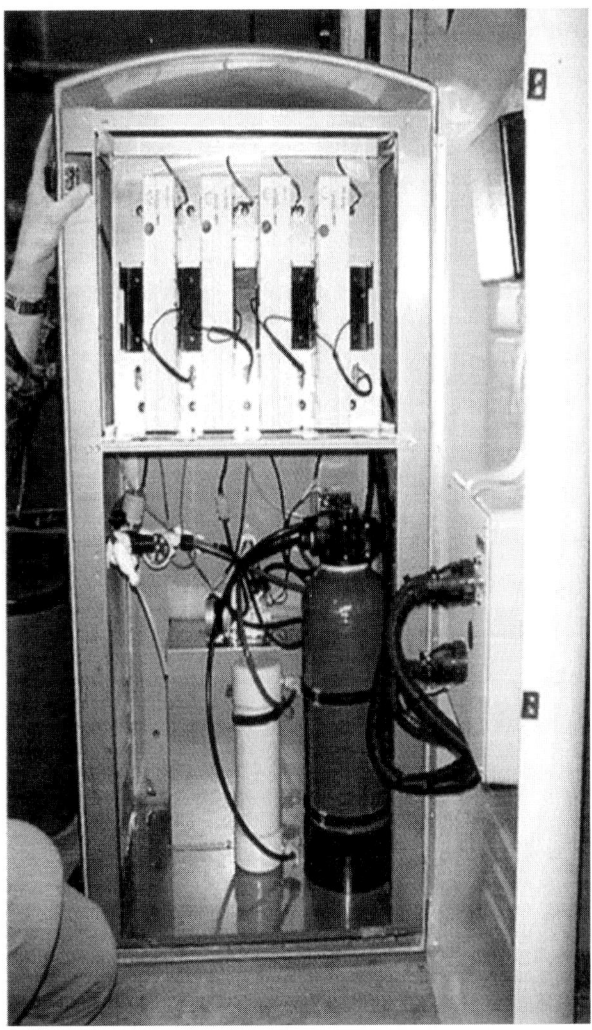

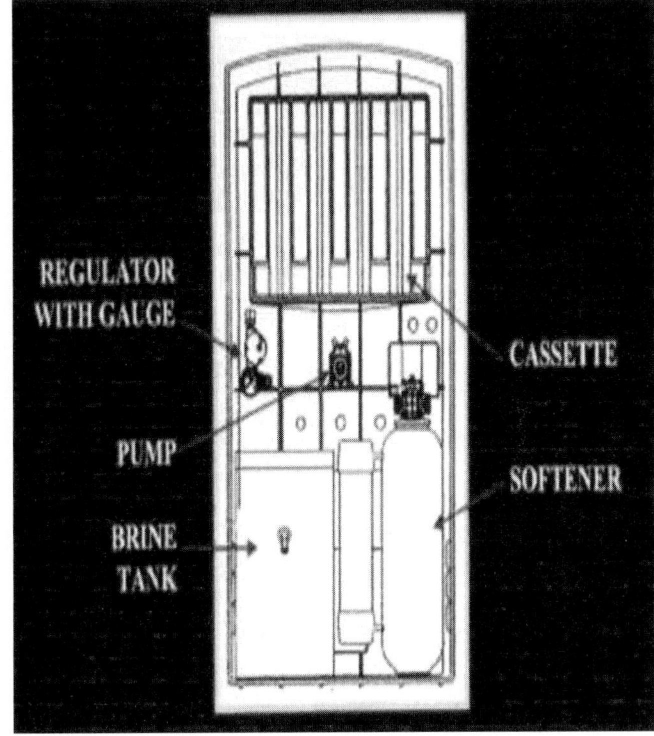

Figure 35.4. Chlorine dioxide is a *Legionella* disinfection option that has been used extensively in Europe, but has recently been under evaluation in the United States. Chlorine dioxide is generated electrochemically from a sodium chlorite precursor within a self-contained unit. The electrochemical reaction occurs within removable cassettes. The unit generates a solution of concentrated chlorine dioxide (approx. 500 mg/L), which is injected into the water stream to achieve a 0.5 mg/L target concentration.

states have regulations for rehabilitation and long-term-care institutions that prohibit temperature in excess of 43°C (110°F) at the tap (234).

Hyperchlorination

Hyperchlorination has proven disappointing as a long-term solution due to high expense, pipe corrosion (235,236), introduction of carcinogenic by-products into the drinking water (237–239), and difficulty in maintaining high concentrations (2–4 ppm) of chlorine to sustain efficacy. The EPA instituted stricter standards on January 1, 2002, because of concern about chlorination by-products.

Ultraviolet Light

Ultraviolet light kills *Legionella* by disrupting cellular DNA. These systems have proven to be effective if disinfection can be localized—for example, to a transplant or an intensive care unit (75,143,240,241). Because ultraviolet sterilization provides no residual protection, areas distal to the sterilizer must be disinfected following installation and startup. One effective approach is to use superheat and flush to disinfect most of the system and then to introduce chemical disinfection (metallic ion or chlorine) as an adjunct. Prefiltration is necessary to prevent the accumulation of scale on the ultraviolet lamps. One hospital reported successful control of *Legionella* in the water system after installation of ultraviolet units on the main water supply to a newly constructed hospital (214).

GUIDELINES

The control and prevention of Legionnaires' disease crosses many disciplines, and as such there are numerous guidance documents and resources for physicians, infection control profession-

TABLE 35.4. INTERNET WEB SITES ARE VALUABLE RESOURCES FOR INFORMATION ON ALL ASPECTS OF LEGIONNAIRES' DISEASE

Web Address (http://)	Publisher	Focus
www.cdc.gov/ncidod/dbmd/diseaseinfo/legionellosis_g.htm	Centers for Disease Control and Prevention (CDC)	Medical
www.legionella.org	Pittsburgh Legionella Group	General information for laypersons as well as information for MDs, ICPs and engineers
www.osha-slc.gov/dts/osta/otm/otm_iii/otm_iii_7.html	Department of Labor and Occupational Safety and Health Administration	Laypersons, industrial hygiene, workplace investigations
www.ashrae.org	American Society of Heating, Refrigerating, and Air-Conditioning Engineers (ASHRAE)	ASHRAE guideline 12: engineering and general information

Adapted from Bassetti S, Widmer AF. Legionella resources on the World Wide Web. *Clin Infect Dis* 2002;34: 1633–1640.

als (ICPs), engineers, and industrial hygienists. Unfortunately, many recommendations including those that emphasize maintenance by engineers and prohibition of showering are not evidence-based, leading to adoption of ineffective methods that are tedious and expensive. Many of these documents are available via the World Wide Web (Table 35.4). The quality of *Legionella*-related Web sites maintained by private and state institutions, universities, professional organizations, and individuals has been reviewed (242).

REFERENCES

1. Fraser DW, Tsai T, Ornstein W, et al. Legionnaires' disease: description of an epidemic of pneumonia. *N Engl J Med* 1977;297: 1189–1197.
2. McDade J, Shepard C, Fraser D, et al. Legionnaires' disease: isolation of a bacterium and demonstration of its role in other respiratory disease. *N Engl J Med* 1977;297:1197–1203.
3. Thacker SB, Bennet JV, Tsai T. An outbreak in 1965 of severe respiratory illness caused by Legionaires' disease bacterium. *J Infect Dis* 1978; 138:512–519.
4. Tobin JO. Legionnaires' disease in a transplant unit: isolation of the causative agent from shower baths. *Lancet* 1980;2:118–121.
5. Fisher-Hoch SP, Tobin JO, Belson AM. Investigation and control of an outbreak of Legionnaires' disease in a district hospital. *Lancet* 1981; 1:932–936.
6. Stout JE, Yu VL, Vickers RM, et al. Ubiquitousness of *Legionella pneumophila* in the water supply of a hospital with endemic Legionnaires' disease. *N Engl J Med* 1982;36:466–468.
7. Best M, Yu VL, Stout J, et al. Legionellaceae in the hospital water supply—epidemiological link with disease and evaluation of a method of control of nosocomial Legionnaires' disease and Pittsburgh pneumonia. *Lancet* 1983;2:307–310.
8. Plouffe JR, Para MF, Maher WE, et al. Subtypes of Legionella pneumophila serogroup 1 associated with different attack rates. *Lancet* 1983;2:649–650.
9. Nolte FS, Conlin C, Roisin A. Plasmids as epidemiological markers in nosocomial Legionnaires' disease. *J Infect Dis* 1984;149:251–256.
10. Benin AL, Benson RF, Beser RE. Trends in Legionnaires' disease, 1980–1998: declining mortality and new patterns of diagnosis. *Clin Infect Dis* 2002;35:1039–1046.
11. Hookey JV, Saunders NA, Fry NK, et al. Phylogeny of Legionellaceae based on small-subunit ribosomal DNA sequences and proposal of *Legionella lytica* comb. nov. for *Legionella*-like amoebal pathogens. *Int J Syst Bacteriol* 1996;46:526–531.
12. Fry NK, Warwick S, Saunders NA, et al. The use of 16S ribosomal RNA analysis to investigate the phylogeny of the family Legionellaceae. *J Gen Microbiol* 1991;137:1215–1222.
13. Brenner DJ, Steigerwalt AG, McDade JE. Classification of the Legionnaires' disease bacterium: *Legionella pneumophila*, genus novum, species nova, of the family *Legionellaceae. Ann Intern Med* 1979;90: 656–658.
14. Fields BS, Benson RF, Besser RE. *Legionella* and Legionnaires' disease: 25 years of investigation. *Clin Microbiol Rev* 2003;15:506–526.
15. Adeleke AA, Fields BS, Benson RF, et al. Legionella drozanskii sp. nov., Legionella rowbothamii sp. nov. and Legionella fallonii sp. nov.: three unusual new Legionella species. *Int J Syst Evol Microbiol* 2001; 51(3):1151–1160.
16. Benson RF, Fields BS. Classification of the genus *Legionella. Semin Respir Infect* 1998;13:90–99.
17. Schousboe M, Gibbons S, Chereshsky A. Community-acquired pneumonia due to *Legionella feeleii* serogroup 2. *N Z Med J* 1995;108: 279.
18. Harris A, Lally M, Albrecht M. *Legionella bozemanii* pneumonia in three patients with AIDS. *Clin Infect Dis* 1998;27:97–99.
19. McNally C, Hackman B, Fields BS, et al. Potential importance of *Legionella* species as etiologies in community acquired pneumonia (CAP). *Diagn Microbiol Infect Dis* 2000;38:79–82.
20. Muder RR, Yu VL. Infection due to *Legionella* species other than *L. pneumophlla. Clin Infect Dis* 2002;35:990–998.
21. Fang GD, Yu VL, Vickers RM. Disease due to Legionellaceae (other

than *Legionella pneumophila*): historical, microbiological, clinical and epidemiological review. *Medicine* 1989;68:116–139.

22. Knirsch CA, Jakob K, Schoonmaker D, et al. An outbreak of *Legionella micdadei* pneumonia in transplant patients: education, molecular epidemiology, and control. *Am J Med* 2000;108:290–295.
23. Waite R. Confirmation of identity of legionellae by whole cell fatty-acid and isoprenoid quinone profiles. In: Harrison TG, Taylor AG, eds. *A laboratory manual for Legionella*. Chichester, UK: John Wiley, 1988:69–101.
24. Sonesson A, Jantzen E, Bryn K, et al. Composition of 2, 3-dihdroxy fatty acid-containing lipopolysaccharides from *Legionella israelensis, Legionella maceachernii*, and *Legionella micdadei*. *Microbiol* 1994;140: 1261–1271.
25. Lema M, Brown A. Electrophoretic characterization of soluble protein extracts of *Legionella pneumophila* and other members of the family Legionellaceae. *J Clin Microbiol* 1983;17:1132–1140.
26. Brindle RJ, Bryant TN, Draper PW. Taxonomic investigation of *Legionella pneumophila* using monoclonal antibodies. *J Clin Microbiol* 1989;27:536–539.
27. Diogo A, Verissimo A, Nobre MF, et al. Usefulness of fatty acid composition for differentiation of *Legionella* species. *J Clin Microbiol* 1999;37:2248–2254.
28. Fox A, Lau PY, Brown A, et al. Capillary gas chromatographic analysis of carbohydrates of *Legionella pneumophila* and other members of the family Legionellaceae. *J Clin Microbiol* 1984;19:326–332.
29. Lo Presti F, Riffard S, Vandenesch F, et al. Identification of *Legionella* species by random amplified polymorphic DNA profiles. *J Clin Microbiol* 1998;36:3193–3197.
30. Bansal NS, McDonell F. Identification and DNA fingerprinting of *Legionella* strains by randomly amplified polymorphic DNA analysis. *J Clin Microbiol* 1997;35(9):2310–2314.
31. Pinar A, Ahkee S, Miller RD, et al. Use of heteroduplex analysis to classify legionellae on the basis of 5S rRNA gene sequences. *J Clin Microbiol* 1997;35(6):1609–1611.
32. Gheldre YD, Maes N, Lo Presti F, et al. Rapid identification of clinically relevant *Legionella* spp. by analysis of transfer DNA intergenic spacer length polymorphism. *J Clin Microbiol* 2001;39(1):162–169.
33. Lowry PW, Tompkins LS. Nosocomial legionellosis: a review of pulmonary and extrapulmonary syndromes. *Am J Infect Cont* 1993;21: 21–27.
34. Blatt SP, Parkinson MD, Pace E, et al. Nosocomial Legionnaires' disease: aspiration as a primary mode of transmission. *Am J Med* 1993; 95:16–22.
35. Yu VL. Could aspiration be the major mode of transmission for *Legionella? Am J Med* 1993;95:13–15.
36. Stone BJ, Kwaik YA. Expression of multiple pili by *Legionella pneumophila*: identification and characterization of a type IV pilin gene and its role in adherence to mammalian and protozoan cells. *Infect Immun* 1998;66:1768–1775.
37. Stout JE, Best M, Yu VL, et al. A note on symbiosis of *Legionella pneumophila* and *Tatlockia micdadei* with human respiratory flora. *J Appl Bacteriol* 1986;60:297–299.
38. Swanson MS, Hammer BK. *Legionella pneumophila* pathogenesis: a fateful journey from amoebae to macrophages. *Annu Rev Microbiol* 2000;54:567–613.
39. Fields BS. The molecular ecology of legionellae. *Trends Microbiol* 1996;4:286–290.
40. Cirillo JD, Falkow S, Tompkins LS. Legionella pneumophila in Acanthamoeba castellani enhances invasion. *Infect Immun* 1994;62: 3254–3261.
41. Shuman HA, Purcell M, Segal G, et al. Intracellular multiplication of *Legionella pneumophila*: human pathogen or accidental tourist? *Curr Top Microbiol Immunol* 1998;225:99–112.
42. Horwitz MA. Toward an understanding of host and bacterial molecules mediating *L. pneumophila* pathogenesis. In: Barbaree JM, Breiman RF, Dufour AP, eds. *Legionella: current status and emerging perspectives.* Washington, DC: American Society of Microbiology, 1993: 55–62.
43. Swanson MS, Fernandez-Moreia E. A microbial strategy to multiply in macrophages: the pregnant pause. *Traffic* 2002;3:170–177.
44. Hammer BK, Tateda ES, Swanson MS. A two-component regulator induces the transmission phenotype of stationary-phase *Legionella pneumophila. Mol Microbiol* 2002;44:107–118.
45. Byrd TF, Horwitz MA. Lactoferrin inhibits or promotes *Legionella pneumophila* intracellular multiplication in nonactivated and interferon gamma activated human monocytes depending upon its degree of iron saturation. Iron-lactoferrin and nonphysiologic iron chelates reverse monocyte activation against *Legionella pneumophila. J Clin Invest* 1991;88:1103–1112.
46. Yamamoto Y, Klein TW, Tomioka M, et al. Differential effects of granulocyte/macrophage colony-stimulating factor (GM CSF) in enhancing macrophage resistance to *Legionella pneumophila* vs. *Candida albicans. Cell Immunol* 1997;176:75–81.
47. Park DR, Skerrett SJ. IL-10 enhances the growth of *Legionella pneumophila* in human mononuclear phagocytes and reverses to protective effect of IFN-γ. *J Immonol* 1996;157:2528–2538.
48. Tateda K, Matsumoto T, Ishii Y, et al. Direct evidence of interleukin-12 as a critical mediator in patients with *Legionella pneumonia* (G-38). 37th Interscience Conference on Antimicrobial Agents and Chemotherapy, Toronto, Ontario, Canada, 1997.
49. Lochner TC, Bigley R, Iglewski BH. Defective triggering of polymorphonuclear leukocyte oxidative metabolism by L. pneumophila toxin. *J Infect Dis* 1985;151:42–46.
50. Cianciotto NP, Eisenstein BI, Mody CH, et al. A mutation in the mip gene results in an attenuation of *Legionella pneumophila* virulence. *J Infect Dis* 1990;162:121–126.
51. Williams A, Rechnitzer C, Lever MS et al. Intracellular production of *Legionella pneumophila* destructive protease in alveolar macrophage. In: Barbaree JM, Breiman RF, Dufour AP, eds. *Legionella—current status and emerging perspectives.* Washington, DC: American Society for Microbiology, 1993:88–90.
52. Conlan JW, Williams A, Ashworth L. In vivo production of a tissue-destructive protease by *Legionella pneumophila* in the lungs of experimentally infected guinea pigs. *J Gen Microbiol* 1988;134:143–149.
53. Black WJ, Quinn FD, Tompkins LS. *Legionella pneumophila* zinc metalloprotease is structurally and functionally homologous to *Pseudomonas aeruginosa* elastase. *J Bacteriol* 1990;172:2608–2613.
54. Muller HE. Proteolytic action of *Legionella pneumophila* on human serum proteins. *Infect Immun* 1980;27:51–53.
55. Nolte FS, Hollick GE, Robertson RG. Enzymatic activities of *Legionella pneumophila* and Legionella-like organisms. *J Clin Microbiol* 1982;15:175–177.
56. Pine L, Hoffman PS, Malcolm GB, et al. Determination of catalase peroxidase, and superoxide dismutase within the genus of Legionella. *J Clin Microbiol* 1984;20:421–429.
57. Dournon E, Bibb WF, Rajagopalan P, et al. Monoclonal antibody reactivity as a virulence marker for Legionella pneumophila serogroup 1 strains. *J Infect Dis* 1988;157:496–501.
58. Stout JE, Joly J, Para M, et al. Comparison of molecular methods for subtyping patients and epidemiologically-linked environmental isolates of L. pneumophila. *J Infect Dis* 1988;157:486–494.
59. Helbig JH, Luck PC, Knirel YA, et al. Molecular characterization of a virulence-associated epitope on lipopolysaccharide of *Legionella pneumophila* serogroup 1. *Epidemiol Infect* 1995;115:71–78.
60. Alli OA, Zink S, von Lackum NK, et al. Comparative assessment of virulence traits in *Legionella* spp. *Microbiol* 2003;149:631–641.
61. Marston BJ, Lipman HB, Breiman RF. Surveillance for Legionnaires' disease. Risk factors for morbidity and mortality. *Arch Intern Med* 1994;154:2417–2422.
62. Hoge CW, Breiman RF. Advances in the epidemiology and control of Legionella infections. *Epidemiol Rev* 1991;13:329–340.
63. Lepine LA, Jernigan DB, Butler JC, et al. A recurrent outbreak of nosocomial Legionnaire's disease detected by urinary antigen testing: evidence for long-term colonization of a hospital plumbing system. *Infect Control Hosp Epidemiol* 1998;19:905–910.
64. Kool JL, Fiore AE, Kioski CM, et al. More than ten years of unrecognized nosocomial transmission of Legionnaires' disease among transplant patients. *Infect Control Hosp Epidemiol* 1998;19:898–904.
65. Johnson JT, Yu VL, Best M, et al. Nosocomial legionellosis uncovered in surgical patients with head and neck cancer: implications for epide-

miologic reservoir and mode of transmission. *Lancet* 1985;2: 298–300.
66. Muder RR, Yu VL, McClure J, et al. Nosocomial Legionnaires' disease uncovered in a prospective pneumonia study: Implications for underdiagnosis. *JAMA* 1983;249:3184–3188.
67. Yu VL, Kroboth FJ, Shonnard J, et al. Legionnaires' disease: new clinical perspective from a prospective pneumonia study. *Am J Med* 1982;73:357–361.
68. Marrie TJ, Macdonald S, Clarke K, et al. Nosocomial Legionnaires' disease: lessons from a four year prospective study. *Am J Infect Control* 1991;19:79–85.
69. Chow J, Yu VL. *Legionella*: a major opportunistic pathogen in transplant recipients. *Semin Respir Infect* 1998;13:132–139.
70. Bock B, Edelstein P, Snyder K, et al. Legionnaires' disease in renal transplant recipients. *Lancet* 1978;1:410–413.
71. Prodinger WM, Bonatti H, Allerberger F, et al. *Legionella* pneumonia in transplant recipients: a cluster of cases of eight years duration. *J Hosp Infect* 1994;26:191–202.
72. Fuller J, Levinson MD, Kline JR, et al. Legionnaires' disease after heart transplantation. *Ann Thoracic Surg* 1985;39:308–311.
73. Singh N, Muder RR, Yu VL, et al. Legionella infection in liver transplant recipients: implications for management. *Transplantation* 1993; 56:1549–1551.
74. Kugler JW, Armitage JO, Helms CM, et al. Nosocomial Legionnaires' disease: occurrence in recipients of bone marrow transplants. *Am J Med* 1983;74:218–228.
75. Matulonis U, Rosenfeld CS, Shadduck RK. Prevention of Legionella infections in a bone marrow transplant unit: multifaceted approach to decontamination of a water system. *Infect Control Hosp Epidemiol* 1993;14:571–575.
76. Squier C, Krystofiak S, McMahon J, et al. Decrease in nosocomial Legionnaires' disease in Allegheny County: guidelines for prevention work (abstract). Association of Practitioners of Infection Control, Seattle, WA, 2001.
77. Korvick J, Yu VL. Legionnaires' disease: an emerging surgical problem. *Ann Thorac Surg* 1987;43:341–347.
78. Strebel P, Ramos J, Eidelman I, et al. Legionnaires' disease in a Johannesburg teaching hospital. Investigation and control of an outbreak. *S Afr Med J* 1988;19:329–333.
79. Tompkins LS, Roessler BJ, Redd SC, et al. Legionella prosthetic-valve endocarditis. *N Engl J Med* 1988;318:530–535.
80. Cordonnier C, Farcet JP, Desforges L. Legionnaires' disease and hairy-cell leukemia. *Arch Intern Med* 1984;144:2373–2375.
81. Voirot P, Melet M, Aymand J, et al. Legionnaires' disease in hairy cell leukemia. Two new cases. *Ann Med Interne (Paris)* 1987;138: 287–288.
82. Brady M. Nosocomial Legionnaires' disease in a children's hospital. *J Pediatr* 1989;115:46–50.
83. Gutzeit M, Laver S, Dunne WM, et al. Fatal Legionella pneumonitis in a neutropenic leukemic child. *Pediatr Infect Dis J* 1987;6:68–69.
84. Hervas J, Lopez P, de la Fuente A, et al. Multiple organ system failure in an infant with Legionella infection. *Pediatr Infect Dis J* 1988;7: 671–673.
85. Dobranowski J, Stringer D. Diagnosis of Legionella lung abscess by percutaneous needle aspiration. *Can Assoc Radiol J* 1989;40:43–44.
86. Trubel HKF, Meyer HGW, Jahn B, et al. Complicated nosocomial pneumonia due to *Legionella pneumophila* in an immunocompromised child. *Scand J Infect Dis* 2002;34:219–221.
87. Franzin L, Scolfaro C, Cabodi D, et al. *L. pneumophila* pneumonia in a newborn after water birth: a new mode of transmission. *Clin Infect Dis* 2001;33:103–104.
88. Carlson NC, Kuskie MR, Dobyns EL, et al. Legionellosis in children: an expanding spectrum. *Infect Dis J* 1990;9:133–137.
89. Qin X, Abe PM, Weissman SJ, et al. Extrapulmonary *Legionella micdadei* infection in a previously healthy child. *Pediatr Infect Dis J* 2002; 21:1174–1176.
90. Aubert G, Bornstein N, Rayet, et al. Nosocomial infection with *Legionella pneumophila*, serogroup 1 and 8 in a neonate. *Scand J Infect Dis* 1990;22:367–370.
91. Loeb M, Simor AE, Mandell L, et al. Two nursing home outbreaks of respiratory infections with *Legionella sainthelensi*. *J Am Geriatr Soc* 1999;47:547–552.
92. Maesaki S, Kohno S, Kog H, et al. An outbreak of Legionnaires' pneumonia in a nursing home. *Intern Med* 1992;31:508–512.
93. Nechwatal R, Ehret W, Klatte OJ, et al. Nosocomial outbreak of legionellosis in a rehabilitation center. Demonstration of potable water as a source. *Infection* 1993;21(4):235–240.
94. Stout JE, Brennen C, Muder RR. Legionnaires' disease in a newly constructed long-term care facility. *Soc Healthcare Epidemiol Am* 1997;154.
95. Steele TW, Lanser J, Sangster N. Isolation of L. longbeachae serogroup 1 from potting mixes. *Appl Environ Microbiol* 1990;56:49–53.
96. Hsu C, Martin R, Wentworth BB. Isolation of Legionella species from drinking water. *Appl Environ Microbiol* 1984;48:830–832.
97. Stout J, Yu VL, Muraca P. Isolation of *Legionella pneumophila* from the cold water of hospital ice machines: implications for its origin and transmission. *Infect Control* 1985;6:141–146.
98. Witherall LE, Duncan R, Store K, et al. Investigation of *L. pneumophila* in drinking water. *J Am Water Works Assoc* 1988;80:87–93.
99. Steinert M, Hentschel U, Hacker J. *Legionella pneumophila*: an aquatic microbe goes astray. *Microbiol Rev* 2002;26:149–162.
100. Stout JE, Yu VL, Best M. Ecology of *Legionella pneumophila* within water distribution systems. *Appl Env Microbiol* 1985;49:221–228.
101. Wadowsky RM, Yee RB. Effect of non-Legionellaceae bacteria on the multiplication of *Legionella pneumophila* in potable water. *Appl Env Microbiol* 1985;49:1206–1210.
102. Fields BS. Legionella and protozoa: interaction of a pathogen and its natural host. In: Barbaree JM, Breiman RF, Dufour AP, eds. *Legionella: current status and emerging perspectives.* Washington, DC: American Society for Microbiology, 1993:129–136.
103. Wright JB, Ruseska I, Athar M, et al. *Legionella pneumophila* grows adherent to surfaces in vitro and in situ. *Infect Cont Hosp Epidemiol* 1989;10:408–415.
104. Mermel LA, Josephson SL, Girogio CH, et al. Association of Legionnaires' disease with construction: contamination of potable water. *Infect Control Hosp Epidemiol* 1995;16:76–81.
105. Alary M, Joly JR. Factors contributing to the contamination of hospital water distribution systems. *J Infect Dis* 1992;165:565–569.
106. Vickers RM, Yu VL, Hanna SS, et al. Determinants of *Legionella pneumophila* contamination of water distribution systems: 15 hospital prospective study. *Infect Control* 1987;8:357–363.
107. Hung LL, Copperthite DC, Yang CS, et al. Environmental Legionella assessment in office buildings of continental United States. *Indoor Air* 1993;349:353.
108. Graman PS, Quinlan GA, Rank JA. Nosocomial legionellosis traced to a contaminated ice machine. *Infect Control Hosp Epidemiol* 1998; 18:637–640.
109. Joseph CA, Watson JM, Harrison TG, et al. Nosocomial Legionnaires' disease in England and Wales. *Epidemiol Infect* 1994;112: 329–345.
110. Stout JE, Yu VL. Current concepts: legionellosis. *N Engl J Med* 1997; 337:682–687.
111. Muder RR, Yu VL, Woo A. Mode of transmission of Legionella pneumophila: a critical review. *Arch Intern Med* 1986;146: 1607–1612.
112. Garbe P, David B, Weisfeld J, et al. Nosocomial Legionnaires' disease—epidemiologic demonstration of cooling towers as a source. *JAMA* 1985;254:521–524.
113. Barbaree JM. Selecting a subtyping technique for use in investigations of Legionellosis epidemics. In: Barbaree JM, Brieman RF, Dufour AP, eds. *Legionella: current status and emerging perspectives.* Washington, DC: American Society for Microbiology, 1993:169–172.
114. Struelens MJ, Maes N, Rost F, et al. Genotypic and phenotypic methods for the investigation of a hospital-acquired *Legionella pneumophila* outbreak and efficacy of control measures. *J Infect Dis* 1992;166: 22–30.
115. Bangsborg JM, Gerner-Smidt P, Colding H, et al. Restriction fragment length polymorphism of rRNA genes for molecular typing of members of the family *Legionellaceae*. *J Clin Microbiol* 1995;33: 402–406.

116. Georghiou PR, Doggett AM, Kielhofner MA, et al. Molecular fingerprinting of *Legionella* species by repetitive element PCR. *J Clin Microbiol* 1994;32:2989–2994.
117. Pruckler JM, Mermel LA, Benson RF. Comparison of *Legionella pneumophila* isolates by arbitrarily primed PCR and pulsed-field gel electrophoresis: analysis from seven epidemic investigations. *J Clin Microbiol* 1995;33:2872–2875.
118. Martone WJ, Jarvis WR, Culver DH, et al. Incidence and nature of endemic and epidemic nosocomial infections. In: Bennet JV, Brachman PS, eds. *Hospital infections.* Boston: Little, Brown, 1992.
119. Riffard S, Presti FL, Vandenesch F, et al. Comparative analysis of infrequent-restriction-site PCR and pulsed-field gel electrophoresis for epidemiological typing of *Legionella pneumophila* serogroup 1 strains. *J Clin Microbiol* 1998;36:161–167.
120. Marrie TJ, Johnson W, Tyler S, et al. Potable water and nosocomial Legionnaires disease—check water from all rooms in which patient has stayed. *Epidemiol Infect* 1995;114:267–276.
121. Marrie TJ, Tyler S, Bezanson G, et al. Analysis of *Legionella pneumophila* serogroup 1 isolates by pulsed-field gel electrophoresis. *J Clin Microbiol* 1999;37:251–254.
122. Schoonmaker DJ, Kondracki ST. Investigation of nosocomial legionellosis using restriction enzyme analysis by pulsed field gel electrophoresis. In: Barbaree JM, Breiman RF, Dufour AP, eds. *Legionella—current status and emerging perspectives.* Washington, DC: American Society for Microbiology, 1993:189–194.
123. Drenning SD, Stout JE, Joly JR, et al. Unexpected similarity of pulsed-field gel electrophoresis patterns of unrelated clinical isolates of *Legionella pneumophila*, serogroup 1. *J Infect Dis* 2001;183:628–632.
124. Saravolatz L, Pohlod D, Helzer K, et al. Legionella infections in renal transplant recipients. In: Thornsberry C, Balows A, Feeley JC, et al., eds. *Proceedings of the 2nd International Symposium.* Washington, DC: American Society of Microbiology, 1984:231–233.
125. Bridge JA, Edelstein PH. Oropharyngeal colonization with *Legionella pneumophila. J Clin Microbiol* 1983;18:1108–1112.
126. Muder RR, Stout JE, Yee YC. Isolation of *Legionella pneumophila* serogroup 5 from empyema following esophageal perforation: source of the organism and mode of transmission. *Chest* 1992;102: 1601–1603.
127. Marrie TJ, Bezanson G, Haldane DJM, et al. Colonization of the respiratory tract with *Legionella pneumophila* for 63 days before onset of pneumonia. *J Infect* 1992;24:81–86.
128. Finkelstein R, Palutke WA, Wentworth BB, et al. Colonization of the respiratory tract with Legionella species. *Isr J Med Sci* 1993;29: 277–279.
129. Marrie TJ, Haldane D, Macdonald S. Control of endemic nosocomial Legionnaires' disease by using sterile potable water for high risk patients. *Epidemiol Infect* 1991;107:591–605.
130. Venezia RA, Agresta MD, Hanley EM, et al. Nosocomial legionellosis associated with aspiration of nasogastric feedings diluted in tap water. *Infect Control Hosp Epidemiol* 1994;15:529–533.
131. Brennen C, Stout JE, Muder RR. *Legionella* on ice: ice as a source for nosocomial Legionnaires' disease. *Soc Healthcare Epidemiol Am* 1999;70(Abstract).
132. Woo AH, Yu VL, Goetz A. Potential in-hospital mode of transmission for *Legionella pneumophila*: demonstration experiments for dissemination by showers, humidifiers, and rinsing of ventilation bag apparatus. *Am J Med* 1986;80:567–573.
133. Kaan J, Simoons-Smit AM, MacLaren D. Another source of aerosol causing nosocomial Legionnaires' disease. *J Infect* 1985;11:145–148.
134. Bouvet A, deFenoyl O, Desplaces N. Maladie des Legionnaires' due au serogroup Legionella pneumophila—contamination of a domicile par canule de tracheostomie. *Presse Med* 1986;15:15–35.
135. Seu P, Winston DJ, Olthoft KM, et al. Legionnaires' disease in liver transplant recipients. *Infect Dis Clin Pract* 1993;2:109–113.
136. Markowitz L, Tompkins L, Wilkinson H, et al. Transmission of nosocomial Legionnaires' disease in heart transplant patients. In: *Program and Abstracts of the 24th Interscience Conference of Antimicrobial Agents and Chemotherapy of the American Society of Microbiology, Washington, DC,* 1984.
137. Levy P-Y, Teysseire N, Etienne J, et al. A nosocomial outbreak of*Legionella pneumophila* caused by contaminated transesophageal echocardiography probes. *Infect Control Hosp Epidemiol* 2003;24:619–622.
138. Dondero TJ Jr, Rendtorff RC, Mallison GF, et al. An outbreak of Legionnaires' disease associated with a contaminated air-conditioning cooling tower. *N Engl J Med* 1980;302:365–370.
139. Bollin GE, Plouffe JF, Para MF, et al. Legionella pneumophila generated by shower heads and hot water faucets. *Appl Environ Microbiol* 1986;50:1128–1131.
140. Cordes LG, Wiesenthal AM, Gorman GW, et al. Isolation of *Legionella pneumophila* from hospital showerheads. *Ann Intern Med* 1981; 94:195–197.
141. Breiman R, Fields B, Sanden G, et al. Association of shower use with Legionnaires' disease: possible role of amoebae. *JAMA* 1990; 263:2924–2926.
142. Helms CM, Massanari R, Zeiter S, et al. Legionnaires' disease associated with a hospital water system: a cluster of 24 nosocomial cases. *Ann Intern Med* 1983;99:172–178.
143. Farr BM, Gratz J, Tartaglino J, et al. Evaluation of ultraviolet light for disinfection of hospital water contaminated with Legionella. *Lancet* 1988;2:669–672.
144. Shands K, Ho J, Meyer R, et al. Potable water as a source of Legionnaires' disease. *JAMA* 1985;253:1412–1416.
145. Ezzedine H, VanOssel C, Delmee M, et al. *Legionella* spp. in a hospital hot water system: effect of control measures. *J Hosp Infect* 1989;13: 121–131.
146. Woo AH, Goetz A, Yu VL. Transmission of *Legionella* by respiratory equipment aerosol generating devices. *Chest* 1992;102:1586–1590.
147. Berthelot P, Grattard F, Ros A, et al. Nosocomial legionellosis outbreak over a three-year period: investigation and control. *Clin Microbiol Infect* 1998;4:385–391.
148. Moriaghi A, Castellani Pastoris M, Barral C, et al. Nosocomial legionellosis associated with use of oxygen bubble humidifiers and underwater chest drain. *J Hosp Infect* 1987;10:47–50.
149. Arnow P, Chou T, Weil D, et al. Nosocomial Legionnaires' disease caused by aerosolized tap water from respiratory devices. *J Infect Dis* 1982;146:460–467.
150. Jones E, Checko P, Dalton A, et al. Nosocomial Legionnaires' disease associated with exposure to respiratory therapy equipment, Connecticut. In: Thornsberry C, Balonos A, Feeley JC, Jakubowski W, eds. *Proceedings of the 2nd International Symposium.* Washington, DC: American Society of Microbiology, 1984:225–227.
151. Joly JR, Diery P, Gauvrau L, et al. Legionnaires' disease caused by *Legionella dumoffi* in distilled water. *Can Med Assoc J* 1986;135: 1273–1277.
152. Luck PC, Dinger D, Helbig JH, et al. Analysis of Legionella pneumophila strains associated with nosocomial pneumonia in a neonatal intensive care unit. *Eur J Clin Microbiol Infect Dis* 1994;13:565–571.
153. Mastro TD, Fields BS, Breiman RF, et al. Nosocomial Legionnaires' disease and use of medication nebulizers. *J Infect Dis* 1991;163: 667–671.
154. Yu VL, Zuravleff JJ, Gavlik L, et al. Lack of evidence for person-to-person transmission of Legionnaires' disease. *J Infect Dis* 1983;147: 362.
155. Pedro-Botet ML, Sabria M, Sopena N, et al. Environmental Legionellosis and oropharyngeal colonization by *Legionella* in immunosuppressed patients. *Infect Cont Hospital Epidemiol* 2002;23(5):279–281.
156. Mulazimoglu L, Yu VL. Can Legionnaires' disease be diagnosed by clinical criteria: a critical review. *Chest* 2001;120:1049–1953.
157. Johnson JT, Raff M, VanArsdall J. Neurologic manifestations of Legionnaires' disease. *Medicine* 1984;63:303–310.
158. Cunha BA. Clinical features of Legionnaires' disease. *Semin Respir Infect* 1998;13:116–127.
159. Lowry PW, Blankenship RJ, Gridley W, et al. A cluster of *Legionella* sternal wound infections due to postoperative topical exposure of contaminated tap water. *N Engl J Med* 1991;324:109–112.
160. Brabender W, Hinthorn DR, Asher M. *Legionella pneumophila* wound infection. *JAMA* 1983;250:3091–3095.
161. Kalweit W, Winn WC, Racco T, et al. Hemodialysis fistula infections caused by Legionella pneumophila. *Ann Intern Med* 1982;96: 173–175.

162. Arnow P, Boyko E, Friedman E. Perirectal abscess caused by *Legionella pneumophila* and mixed anaerobic bacteria. *Ann Intern Med* 1983;98: 184–185.
163. Heath CH, Grove DI, Looke DFM. Delay in appropriate therapy of *Legionella* pneumonia associated with increased mortality. *Eur J Clin Microbiol Infect Dis* 1996;15:286–290.
164. Bartlett JG, Dowell SF, Mandell LA, et al. Practice guidelines for management of community-acquired pneumonia. *Clin Infect Dis* 2000;31:347–382.
165. Fiore AE, Butler JC, Emori TG, et al. A survey of methods to detect nosocomial legionellosis among participants in the National Nosocomial Infectious Surveillance System. *Infect Control Hosp Epidemiol* 1999;20:412–416.
166. Yzerman EP, den Boer JW, Lettinga KD, et al. Sensitivity of three urinary antigen tests associated with clinical severity in a large outbreak of Legionnaires' disease in the Netherlands. *J Clin Microbiol* 2002; 40:3232–3236.
167. Dominguez J, Gail N, Matas L, et al. Evaluation of a rapid immunochromatographic assay for the detection of *Legionella* antigen in urine samples. *Eur J Clin Microbiol Infect Dis* 1999;18:896–898.
168. Stout JE. Laboratory diagnosis of Legionnaires' disease: the expanding role of the *Legionella* urinary antigen test. *Clin Microbiol Newsletter* 2000;22:62–64.
169. Stout JE, Rihs JD, Yu VL. *Legionella.* In: Murray PR, Baron EJ, Jorgensen JH, et al., eds. *Manual of clinical microbiology.* Washington, DC: ASM Press, 2003:809–823.
170. Wever P, Yzerman EP, Kuijper EJ, et al. Rapid diagnosis of Legionnaires' disease using an immunochromatographic assay for *Legionella pneumophila* serogroup 1 antigen in urine during an outbreak in the Netherlands. *J Clin Microbiol* 2000;38:2738–1739.
171. Sopena N, Sabria M, Pedro-Botet ML, et al. Factors related to persistence of *Legionella* urinary antigen excretion in patients with Legionnaires' disease. *Eur J Clin Microbiol Infect Dis* 2002;21:845–848.
172. Benson RF, Tang PW, Fields BS. Evaluation of the Binax and Biotest urinary antigen kits for detection of Legionnaires' disease due to multiple serogroups and species of *Legionella. J Clin Microbiol* 2000;38(7): 2763–2765.
173. Plouffe JF, File TM, Breiman RF, et al. Reevaluation of the definition of Legionnaires' disease: use of the urinary antigen assay. *Clin Infect Dis* 1995;20:1286–1291.
174. Marrie TJ. Diagnosis of Legionellaceae as a cause of community-acquired pneumonia—continue to treat first and not both to ask questions later: not a good idea. *Am J Med* 2001;110:73–75.
175. Helbig JH, Uldman SA, Bernander S, et al. Clinical utility of urinary antigen detection for diagnosis of community-acquired, travel-associated, and nosocomial Legionnaires' disease. *J Clin Microbiol* 2003; 41:838–840.
176. Zuravleff JJ, Yu VL, Shonnard J, et al. Diagnosis of Legionnaires' disease: an update of laboratory methods with new emphasis on isolation by culture. *JAMA* 1983;250:1981–1985.
177. Stout JE. Culture methodology for Legionella species. In: Freije MR, ed. Fallbrook, CA: HC Information Resources, 1998.
178. Muder RR, Stout JE, Yu VL. Nosocomial *Legionella micdadei* infection in transplant patients: fortune favors the prepared mind. *Am J Med* 2000;108:346–348.
179. Rihs JD, Yu VL, Zuravleff JJ, et al. Isolation of *Legionella pneumophila* from blood with the BACTEC system: a prospective study yielding positive results. *J Clin Microbiol* 1985;22:422–424.
180. Fiore AE, Butler JC. Detecting nosocomial Legionnaires' disease. *Infect Med* 1998;15:625–630.
181. Wilkinson H, Cruce D, Brome C. Validation of Legionella pneumophila indirect immunofluorescence assay with epidemic sera. *J Clin Microbiol* 1981;13:139–146.
182. Ruf B, Schurmann D, Horbach I, et al. Frequency and diagnosis of Legionella pneumonia: a 3 year prospective study with emphasis on application of urinary antigen detection. *J Infect Dis* 1990;62: 1341–1347.
183. Vickers RM, Yee YC, Rihs JD, et al. Prospective assessment of sensitivity, quantitation, and timing of urinary antigen, serology, direct immunofluorescence (DFA) for diagnosis of Legionnaires' disease (LD) (C-17). In: *Abstracts of the annual meeting of the American Society for Microbiology.* 1994:493.
184. Ramirez JA, Ahkee S, Tolentino A, et al. Diagnosis of *Legionella pneumophila, Mycoplasma pneumoniae,* or *Chlamydia pneumoniae* lower respiratory infection using the polymerase chain reaction on a single throat swab specimen. *Diagn Microbiol Infect Dis* 1996;24: 7–14.
185. Jonas D, Rosenbaum A, Weyrich S, et al. Enzyme-linked immunoassay for detection of PCR-amplified DNA of legionellae in bronchoalveolar fluid. *J Clin Microbiol* 1995;33:1247–1252.
186. Murdoch DR, Walford EJ, Jennings LC, et al. Use of polymerase chain reaction to detect *Legionella* DNA in urine and serum samples from patients with pneumonia. *Clin Infect Dis* 1996;23:475–480.
187. Welti M, Jaton K, Altwegg M, et al. Development of multiplex real-time quantitative PCR assay to detect *Chlamydia pneumoniae, Legionella pneumophila* and *Mycoplasma pneumoniae* in respiratory tract secretions. *Diagn Microbiol Infect Dis* 2003;45:85–95.
188. Matsiota-Bernard P, Pitsouni E, Legakis N, et al. Evaluation of commercial amplification kit for detection of *Legionella pneumophila* in clinical samples. *J Clin Microbiol* 1994;32:1503–1505.
189. Martin WT, Fields BS, Hutwagoner LC. Comparison of culture and polymerase chain reaction to detect legionellae in environmental samples. In: Barbaree JM, Breiman RF, Dufour AP, eds. *Legionella: current status and emerging perspectives.* Washington, DC: American Society for Microbiology, 1993:175.
190. Murdoch DR. Nucleic acid amplification tests for the diagnosis of pneumonia. *Clin Infect Dis* 2003;36:1162–1170.
191. Centers for Disease Control. Guidelines for prevention of nosocomial pneumonia. *MMWR* 1997;46(RR-1):1–79.
192. Sabria M, Yu VL. Hospital-acquired legionellosis: solutions for a preventable disease. *Lancet Infect Dis* 2002;2:368–373.
193. Yu VL. Resolving the controversy on environmental cultures for *Legionella. Infect Control Hosp Epidemiol* 1998;19:893–897.
194. Roig J, Domingo C, Morera J. Legionnaires' disease. *Chest* 1994;105: 1817–1825.
195. Yu VL. Nosocomial legionellosis. *Curr Opin Infect Dis* 2000;13: 385–388.
196. Sabria M, Garcia-Nunez M, Pedro-Botet ML, et al. Presence and chromosomal subtyping of *Legionella* spp in potable water systems in 20 hospitals of Catalonia, Spain. *Infect Control Hosp Epidemiol* 2002; 22:673–676.
197. Centers for Disease Control and the Healthcare Infection Control Practices Advisory Committee (HICPAC). Guidelines for Environmental Infection Control in Health-Care Facilities. *MMWR* 2003; 52(RR-10):1–12.
198. Allegheny County Health Department. *Approaches to prevention and control of Legionella infection in Allegheny County health care facilities,* 1st ed. Pittsburgh, PA: Allegheny County Health Department, 1993: 1–15.
199. State of Maryland Department of Health and Mental Hygiene. Report of the Maryland Scientific Working Group to study *Legionella* in water systems in healthcare institutions, June 2000.
200. Texas Department of Health. Report of the Legionnaires' disease task force. *www.tdh.state.tx.us.* Austin, TX: 2002.
201. Centers for Disease Control and Prevention. Guidelines for Prevention of Nosocomial Pneumonia. *MMWR* 1997;46:31–34.
202. Redd SC, Cohen ML. Legionella in water: what should be done? *JAMA* 1999;257:1221–1222.
203. Butler JC, Fields BS, Breiman RF. Prevention and control of legionellosis. *Infect Dis Clin Pract* 1997;6:458–464.
204. Liu Z, Stout JE, Boldin M, et al. Intermittent use of copper-silver ionization for Legionella control in water distribution systems: a potential option in buildings housing individuals at low risk of infection. *Clin Infect Dis* 1998;26:138–140.
205. Lin YE, Vidic RD, Stout JE, et al. *Legionella* in water distribution systems. *J Am Water Works Assoc* 1998;90:112–121.
206. Centers for Disease Control. Guidelines for prevention of opportunistic infections among hematopoietic stem cell transplant recipients. *MMWR* 2000;49:1–128.

207. Darelid J, Bengtsson L, Gastrin B, et al. An outbreak of Legionnaires' disease in a Swedish hospital. *Scand J Infect Dis* 1994;26:417–425.
208. Ta AC, Stout JE, Yu VL, et al. Comparison of culture methods for monitoring Legionella species in hospital potable water systems and recommendations for standardization of such methods. *J Clin Microbiol* 1995;33:2118–2123.
209. Goetz A, Yu VL. Screening for nosocomial legionellosis by culture of the water supply and targeting of high-risk patients for specialized laboratory testing. *Am J Infect Control* 1991;19:63–66.
210. Yu VL, Beam TR, Lumish RM, et al. Routine culturing for Legionella in the hospital environment may be a good idea: a three-hospital prospective study. *Am J Med Sci* 1987;294:97–99.
211. Oren I, Zuckerman T, Aviv I, et al. Nosocomial outbreak of *Legionella pneumophila* serogroup 3 pneumonia in a new bone marrow transplant unit: evaluation, treatment and control. *Bone Marrow Transplant* 2002;30:175–179.
212. Yu VL, Liu Z, Stout JE, et al. Legionella disinfection of water distribution systems: principles, problems, and practice. *Infect Control Hosp Epidemiol* 1993;14:567–570.
213. Lin YE, Stout JE, Yu VL. Disinfection of water distribution systems for *Legionella. Semin Respir Infect* 1998;13:147–159.
214. Hall KK, Giannetta ET, Gretchell-White SI, et al. Ultraviolet light disinfection of hospital water for preventing nosocomial *Legionella*infection: a 13-year follow-up. *Infect Control Hosp Epidemiol* 2003;24: 580–583.
215. Kusnetsov J, Torvinen E, Perola O, et al. Colonization of hospital water systems by legionellae, mycobacteria and other heterotrophic bacteria potentially hazardous to risk group patients. *APMIS* 2003; 111:546–556.
216. Baker RL, Stevens J, Fish L, et al. Nosocomial Legionnaires' disease controlled by UV light and low level silver/copper ions (abstract 72). Third International Conference on Nosocomial Infections, Atlanta, 1990.
217. Liu Z, Stout JE, Tedesco L, et al. Controlled evaluation of copper-silver ionization in eradicating *Legionella pneumophila* from a hospital water distribution system. *J Infect Dis* 1994;169:919–922.
218. Mietzner S, Schwille RC, Farley A, et al. Efficacy of thermal treatment and copper-silver ionization for controlling *Legionella pneumophila* in high-volume hot water. *Am J Infect Control* 1997;25:452–457.
219. Srinivasan A, Bova G, Ross T, et al. A 17-month evaluation of a chlorine dioxide water treatment system to control *Legionella* species in a hospital water supply. *Infect Control Hosp Epidemiol* 2003;24: 575–579.
220. Farrell ID, Barker JE, Miles EP, et al. A field study of the survival of *Legionella pneumophila* in a hospital hot-water system. *Epidemiol Infect* 1990;104:381–387.
221. Darelid J, Lôfgren S, Malmvall B-E. Control of nosocomial Legionnaires' disease by keeping the circulating hot water temperature above 55°C: experience from a 10-year surveillance programme in a district general hospital. *J Hosp Infect* 2002;50:213–219.
222. Stout JE, Yu VL. Experiences of the first 16 hospitals using copper-silver ionization for *Legionella* control: implications for the evaluation of other disinfection modalities. *Infect Control Hosp Epidemiol* 2003; 24:563–568.
223. Stout JE, Lin YSE, Goetz AM, et al. Controlling *Legionella* in hospital water systems: experience with the superheat-and-flush method and copper-silver ionization. *Infect Contr Hosp Epidemiol* 1998;19: 911–914.
224. Kool JL, Bergmire-Sweat D, Butler JC, et al. Hospital characteristics associated with colonization of water systems by *Legionella* and risk of nosocomial Legionnaires' disease: a cohort study of 15 hospitals. *Infect Control Hosp Epidemiol* 1999;20:798–805.
225. Liu WK, Healing DE, Yeomans JT, et al. Monitoring of hospital water supplies for Legionella. *J Hosp Infect* 1993;24:1–9.
226. Kusnetsov J, Ilvanainen E, Elomaa N, et al. Copper and silver ions more effective against legionellae than against mycobacteria in a hospital warm water system. *Water Res* 2001;35:4217–4225.
227. Lin YE, Vidic RD, Stout JE, et al. Negative effect of high pH on biocidal efficacy of copper and silver ions in controlling *Legionella pneumophila. J Appl Environ Microbiol* 2002;68(6):2711–2715.
228. Rohr U, Senger M, Selenka F, et al. Four years of experience with silver-copper ionization for control of *Legionella* in a German University Hospital hot water plumbing system. *Clin Infect Dis* 1999;29: 1507–1511.
229. Lin YE. Ionization failure not due to resistance. *Clin Infect Dis* 2000; 31:1315–1316.
230. Sidari FP, Stout JE, VanBriesen JM, et al. Chlorine dioxide as a disinfection method for *Legionella* control. *Journal Am Water Works Assoc.* 2003 *(accepted for publication).*
231. Hamilton E, Seal DV, Hay J. Comparison of chlorine and chlorine dioxide disinfection for control of Legionella in a hospital water supply. *J Hosp Infect* 1996;32(2):156–160.
232. U.S. Environmental Protection Agency. National primary drinking water rules: disinfectants-disinfection by-products. Final rule. *Federal Register* 1998;63:241.
233. Stout JE, Yu VL. Eradicating *Legionella* from hospital water. *JAMA* 1997;278:1404.
234. Mandel AS, Sprauer MA, Sniadack DH, et al. State regulation of hospital water temperatures. *Infect Control Hosp Epidemiol* 1993;14: 642–645.
235. Grosserode M, Helms C, Pfaller M, et al. Continuous hyperchlorination for control of nosocomial Legionnaires' disease: a ten year follow-up of efficacy, environmental effects, and cost. In: Barbaree JM, Breiman RF, Dufour AP, eds. *Legionella—current status and emerging perspectives.* Washington, DC: American Society for Microbiology, 1993:226–229.
236. Snyder MB, Siwicki M, Wireman J. Reduction in *Legionella pneumophila* through heat flushing followed by continuous supplemental chlorination of hospital hot water. *J Infect Dis* 1990;162:127–132.
237. Vickers R, Stout JE, Yu VL. Failure of a diagnostic monoclonal immunofluorescent reagent to detect *Legionella pneumophila* in environmental samples. *Appl Environ Microbiol* 1990;56:2912–2914.
238. Morris RD, Audet AM, Angelillo IF, et al. Chlorination, chlorination by-products, and cancer: a meta-analysis. *Am J Public Health* 1993; 82:955–963.
239. Swan SH, Waller K, Hopkins B, et al. A prospective study of spontaneous abortion: relation to amount and source of drinking water consumed in early pregnancy. *Epidemiology* 1998;9:126–133.
240. Liu Z, Stout JE, Tedesco L. Efficacy of ultraviolet light in preventing Legionella colonization of a hospital water system. *Water Res* 1995; 29:2275–2280.
241. Franzin L, Dal Conte I, Cabodi D, et al. Culture proven *Legionella pneumophila* pneumonia in a HIV infected patient: case report and review. *J Infect* 2002;45:199–201.
242. Bassetti S, Widmer AF. Legionella resources on the World Wide Web. *Clin Infect Dis* 2002;34:1633–1640.
243. Yu VL, Plouffe JF, Castellani-Pastoris M, et al. Distribution of *Legionella* species and serogroups isolated by culture in consecutive patients with community acquired pneumonia: an international collaborative survey. *J Infect Dis* 2002;186:127–128.
244. Reingold A, Thompson B, Brake B, et al. Legionella pneumonia in the U.S.: the distribution of serogroups and species causing human illness. *J Infect Dis* 1984;149:819–824.
245. Allegheny County Health Department. *Approaches to prevention and control of Legionella infection in Allegheny County health care facilities,* 2nd ed. Pittsburgh, PA: Allegheny County Health Department, 1997: 1–15. *www.legionella.org.*
246. Stout JE, Yu VL. Hospital-acquired Legionnaires' disease: new developments. *Clin Infect Dis* 2003;16:337–341.

36

CLOSTRIDIUM DIFFICILE

STUART JOHNSON
DALE N. GERDING

Clostridium difficile was identified as the etiologic agent of antibiotic-associated pseudomembranous colitis in 1978 (1,2) and is now recognized as the most important identifiable cause of nosocomial infectious diarrhea. *C. difficile* may be the only pathogen sufficiently prevalent to warrant testing on a routine basis during the evaluation of nosocomial diarrhea (3,4). It is estimated that each case of nosocomial *C. difficile*–associated diarrhea (CDAD) costs $3,669 and results in 3.6 excess hospital days (5). Readmission for CDAD costs $128,200 per hospital per year (6). A conservative annual cost estimate for CDAD in the United States is $1.1 billion (5). Our present understanding of the pathogenesis of *C. difficile* disease and rationale for preventive and interventive measures is supported by (a) observations on antimicrobial use in patients who acquire this pathogen, (b) potential infectious reservoirs, (c) modes of *C. difficile* transmission, and (d) host risk factors.

PATHOGENESIS

The manifestation of enteric disease due to *C. difficile* depends on at least three critical events: disruption of the normal colonic microflora, exposure to a toxigenic *C. difficile* strain, and the presence of one or more host factors. Epidemiologic evidence also supports the order of these events in that with most cases exposure to antimicrobials with subsequent compromise of host colonization resistance is followed by *C. difficile* acquisition from exogenous sources (rather than reactivation from an endogenous source).

The normal colonic flora provides a profound resistance to infection with *C. difficile.* It appears that the host is susceptible to infection with this pathogen only after disruption of the colonic flora by antimicrobial therapy or, in some cases, by antineoplastic agents (7). The next critical event, exposure to toxigenic *C. difficile,* occurs most often in hospitals and chronic-care facilities, which serve as the main reservoirs for this infection. With the recognition that asymptomatic carriage of *C. difficile* is very common among hospitalized patients, it might seem intuitive that these carriers are at high risk of subsequent CDAD (Fig. 36.1A). However, a meta-analysis of four prospective studies that included 810 patients followed for 1,348 weeks with weekly surveillance cultures indicated that asymptomatic carriers were, conversely, at decreased risk of subsequent CDAD (pooled risk difference −2.3% [95% confidence interval (CI) 0.3–4.3] $p =$ .021) (8,9).

In our revised hypothesis (Fig. 36.1B) a patient is admitted to the hospital and, although exposed intermittently to *C. difficile,* is susceptible to colonization or disease only following antimicrobial therapy. The subsequent clinical outcome is determined shortly after acquisition (within a few days) and, like other enteric and infectious diseases, the majority of patients remain asymptomatic. These asymptomatic carriers are then at decreased risk for CDAD when compared with noncolonized patients. Host risk factors comprise the third critical component to the pathogenesis of CDAD and are discussed later in this chapter.

C. difficile elaborates two major toxins: toxin B, a potent cytotoxin; and toxin A, a potent enterotoxin that is also cytotoxic (10). Although measurement of cytotoxicity in stool specimens is used to diagnose CDAD, the enterotoxic effect of toxin A has been presumed to be critical in the pathogenesis of the disease. The evidence implicating toxin A includes the observation that disease severity correlates more closely with toxin A production *in vivo* (11), and that hamsters immunized with toxoid A but not toxoid B are protected against *C. difficile*–induced disease (12). Toxin A alone, but not toxin B, given intragastrically reproduces the pathology of *C. difficile* cecitis in hamsters (13). However, toxin B acts synergistically with toxin A in this model, and new data support virulence for variant strains that produce toxin B, but not toxin A.

Toxin A is a unique enterotoxin unrelated to cholera toxin or the *Escherichia coli* heat-labile toxin and causes extensive mucosal damage with hemorrhagic fluid response (14). The receptor for toxin A involves a trisaccharide moiety, Gala1–3Galb1–4GlcNAc (15), which is present on antigens within the brush border of human and hamster intestinal epithelium (16). Subsequent toxic cellular events involve internalization of toxin A by receptor-mediated endocytosis and disruption of the cellular cytoskeleton. Toxin A (and B) induce glycosylation of small guanosine triphosphate (GTP)-binding proteins named Rho, important regulators of actin polymerization (17).

Variant strains of *C. difficile* that do not produce toxin A have been recovered from clinical specimens around the world. These toxin A−/B+ strains were initially recovered from asymptomatic children and were not thought to be pathogenic. Recently, a particular toxin A−/B+ variant that has a 1.8-

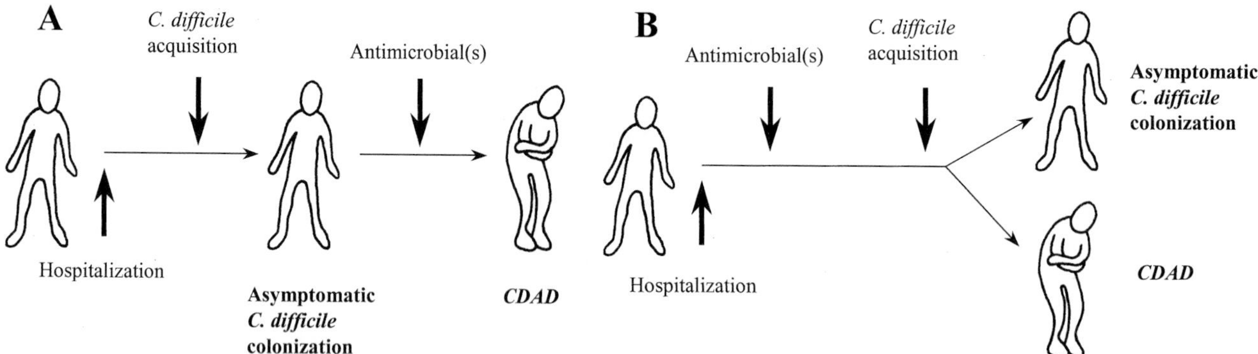

Figure 36.1. **A:** Hypothesis A (rejected) of the pathogenesis of *Clostridium difficile* infection. An intuitive hypothesis that includes the two major known risk factors for *C. difficile*–associated diarrhea (CDAD) (antimicrobial therapy and hospitalization) supposes that a patient acquires *C. difficile* after some period of hospitalization and is subsequently at risk for CDAD when exposed to antimicrobial therapy. If this hypothesis were true, these asymptomatic carriers would be a potential target for infection control interventions to prevent CDAD. **B:** Hypothesis B (revised) of the pathogenesis of *C. difficile* infection. Although patients are likely exposed to *C. difficile* throughout their hospitalization, we hypothesize that they are at negligible risk for *C. difficile* infection until exposed to an antimicrobial agent. Following antimicrobial exposure, the patient is now susceptible to infection and when exposed to *C. difficile* one of three outcomes ensue: the patient becomes colonized but remains asymptomatic, the patient develops CDAD, or potentially the patient does not develop any detectable infection. Once the patient is established as an asymptomatic carrier, data indicate that the patient is at decreased risk for subsequent CDAD (7). (From Johnson S, Gerding DN. *Clostridium difficile*–associated diarrhea. *Clin Infect Dis* 1998; 26:1027–1036.)

kilobase (kb) deletion in the toxin A gene [referred to as toxinotype VIII, serogroup F, restriction endonuclease analysis (REA) group CF] (18) has been recovered from multiple CDAD cases, including a fatal case of pseudomembranous colitis (PMC) (19). In addition, two well-documented hospital outbreaks with this A−/B+ variant (20,21) suggest that toxin B or some virulence determinant other than toxin A in these strains is sufficient to cause *C. difficile* disease. In addition to toxins A and B, some strains of *C. difficile* (but not toxinotype VIII stratins) also produce an adenosine diphosphate (ADP)-ribosyltransferase (referred to as binary toxin) (22). The role of binary toxin in the pathogenesis of CDAD has not yet been determined.

The other important aspect of *C. difficile* pathogenesis lies within the apparent host resistance of some patients to *C. difficile* disease. Newborn infants frequently carry *C. difficile* in high numbers with high levels of both toxins in their stools (23), yet *C. difficile* disease is rare in this group. Age-dependent expression of the epithelial cell receptor for toxin A may explain this apparent resistance in young infants (24). Additionally, during outbreaks in adult settings, asymptomatic carriage is a more frequent outcome of *C. difficile* infection than is symptomatic infection (8,25). Disease manifestation and severity is not solely a strain-specific phenomenon (26); although the mechanism of this apparent host resistance in adult asymptomatic fecal excretors is not completely known, host antibody response to toxin A has been one factor implicated.

CLINICAL DISEASE SPECTRUM

Although the most common clinical manifestation of *C. difficile* infection is diarrhea, the disease spectrum ranges from asymptomatic colonization or fecal excretion to PMC to toxic megacolon, which may present with signs of an acute abdomen but without diarrhea (27). As with other enteric infections, asymptomatic colonization is two to five times more common than clinical disease associated with *C. difficile* (8,25). Even though such patients may carry epidemic strains responsible for illness in other patients, they are not at increased risk of CDAD (9), they are not at risk for subclinical protein-losing enteropathy (28), and treatment of these patients with metronidazole or vancomycin is not advised (29). Asymptomatic colonization is also very common in neonates, and it has been difficult to attribute any disease manifestation in neonates to *C. difficile.* However, the pathogenic role of *C. difficile* in children cannot be completely ignored, particularly in older children and children with hypogammaglobulinemia (30).

Diarrhea with or without demonstrable pseudomembranes in the colon is the most common manifestation of *C. difficile* disease. Although *C. difficile* is the most common recognized cause of antibiotic-associated diarrhea, *C. difficile* accounts for only 15% to 25% of these cases (31). CDAD may occur during antimicrobial administration or several weeks after discontinuation of the antimicrobial. In a prospective study of clindamycin therapy, one third of the patients developed diarrhea or colitis several days to 3 weeks after completion of clindamycin treatment (32). This marked variability of time between onset of diarrhea and antimicrobial exposure also supports exogenous acquisition as the major source of *C. difficile* infection. The incubation period for diarrhea after acquisition of *C. difficile* is less than 1 week, with a median onset of 2 days following acquisition (8,25).

The severity and chronicity of diarrhea is also variable. In some cases symptoms may be mild and respond to simply withdrawing the offending antimicrobial. CDAD resolved spontaneously within 48 to 72 hours in 25% of patients in one series

(33). More commonly, the diarrhea becomes chronic and severe if not diagnosed and treated with specific therapy. At presentation, symptoms may consist of only a few loose stools per day or multiple, large-volume, watery stools and signs of dehydration (31). Stools may have mucus or evidence of occult blood, but are rarely associated with visible blood (34). In addition, a distinct fecal odor is often recognized by personnel caring for these patients. Other findings commonly associated with CDAD include abdominal pain (22%), ileus (21%), fever (28%), and leukocytosis (50%) (34). CDAD should be considered in any hospitalized patient with leukocytosis, particularly those with white blood cell counts >30,000 cells/mm^3, even without the presence of diarrhea (35). Complications of severe disease include dehydration, electrolyte imbalance, hypotension, hypoalbuminemia with anasarca, toxic megacolon, colonic perforation, and sepsis, and in 1% to 2% of cases death can result (31). Another characteristic of CDAD is the high rate of clinical relapse following successful therapy, which may result from either reactivation with the same strain or reinfection with a new strain (36,37).

In distinction from antibiotic-associated diarrhea in general, *C. difficile* is responsible for nearly all cases of PMC that have been reported since 1978 (31). The pseudomembranous intestinal lesions associated with *C. difficile* have a characteristic gross and histologic appearance (38). Early in the disease course, small (1- to 2-mm), raised, yellowish-white plaques are noted, which may enlarge and coalesce (39). These lesions, which are composed of fibrin, mucus, necrotic epithelial cells, and leukocytes, are restricted to the colon; therefore, this disease should be referred to as PMC rather than enterocolitis. Although PMC can be visualized by the sigmoidoscope in 90% of patients who have PMC, some patients have disease limited to the right colon, and the presentation may mimic appendicitis or Crohn's disease (40, 41).

Fulminant *C. difficile* colitis and toxic megacolon are less common manifestations, but important syndromes to recognize, as they are associated with a high mortality rate and frequently require surgical intervention (41–43). It is ironic that this most severe manifestation of *C. difficile* infection often occurs without diarrhea and as a result the diagnosis is frequently missed or delayed (27). Risk factors for severe disease in one study included immunosuppression, prior CDAD, and prior surgical procedures (43). A rapidly increasing peripheral white blood cell count with a left shift may be an important clue to impending fulminant disease.

Extraintestinal *C. difficile* infections are uncommon, but include splenic abscess, bacteremia, wound infections, osteomyelitis, pleuritis, peritonitis, and urogenital tract infections (44). As with other enteric infections, *C. difficile* infection has been associated with reactive arthritis (45).

DIAGNOSIS

The diagnosis of nosocomial CDAD depends first on establishing the presence of clinical diarrhea or other gastrointestinal symptoms compatible with *C. difficile* disease such as abdominal pain or, rarely, ileus without diarrhea. Two major avenues are available to establish the diagnosis in a clinically ill patient: endoscopic procedures to detect the presence of PMC and laboratory studies to document the presence of *C. difficile* or its toxins in the stool. The latter tests include (a) stool culture, antigen tests, and the polymerase chain reaction (PCR) to detect the microorganism; (b) the cell cytotoxin test for toxin B; and (c) a variety of immunoassay tests for the presence of toxin A or toxins A and B in stool. The best way to establish the diagnosis of CDAD remains controversial, because no single test achieves the desired level of both sensitivity and specificity (46–50); however, clinical information such as prior antibiotic use can improve the efficiency of the diagnosis (51,52). Advantages and disadvantages of each of the diagnostic modalities are discussed below. Sensitivity and specificity are summarized in Table 36.1.

Endoscopic Procedures

Endoscopic procedures indirectly indicate *C. difficile* disease by demonstrating PMC. The procedure may be performed with a rigid proctoscope, a flexible fiberoptic sigmoidoscope, or a fiberoptic colonoscope. The latter is the only device that permits visualization of the entire colon, but it is not routinely used for this diagnosis because of the need for extensive colon preparation and the high cost of the procedure. Flexible sigmoidoscopy is

TABLE 36.1. SENSITIVITY AND SPECIFICITY[a] OF DIAGNOSTIC TESTS FOR *C. DIFFICILE*–ASSOCIATED DISEASE

Test	Sensitivity	Specificity	Comment
Pseudomembrane detection			
Flexible sigmoidoscopy	+	+++++	Biopsy often required
Microorganism detection			
C. difficile culture	+++++	+++	Most sensitive test available
C. difficile latex test	++	+++	Detects glutamate dehydrogenase (GDH)
PCR for *C. difficile*	?	?	Potentially very high sensitivity
Toxin detection			
Cell cytotoxicity	++++	+++++	Most specific test available
Immunoassay for toxins A and B	+++	+++++	Less sensitive than cell cytotoxicity
Immunoassay for toxin A	++	+++++	Less sensitive than immunoassay for toxins A and B

[a] Relative sensitivity and specificity: +++++, highest; +, lowest. PCR, polymerase chain reaction.

the most frequently employed of these procedures and allows visualization of the distal 60 cm of the colon. The diagnosis can be made by direct visualization of the pseudomembranes; biopsy may be required if the lesions are small (39). The major deficiency of endoscopy is that it is highly insensitive. Pseudomembranes were seen in only 51% of patients who had diarrhea, a positive stool cytotoxin assay, and positive stool culture for *C. difficile* (34). It is probable that PMC is a late manifestation of *C. difficile* disease that is more likely to occur in the proximal colon first, accounting for the low sensitivity of endoscopy for the diagnosis of CDAD (40).

Clinically, the major advantage of endoscopy is the rapidity with which a diagnosis can be made. This is particularly important in critically ill patients in whom the diagnosis of a surgical abdominal process is being considered. These patients often have symptoms of ileus or obstruction, which can be caused infrequently by *C. difficile.* Visualization of PMC by endoscopy can avert emergency abdominal surgery and permit confident initiation of *C. difficile*–specific treatment. However, the vast majority of *C. difficile*–infected patients are not critically ill, and endoscopy has been supplanted by laboratory tests for the diagnosis of CDAD.

Laboratory Diagnosis

Stool Toxin Tests

Cell Cytotoxin Assay

The most specific laboratory test for CDAD is the cell cytotoxin assay (53,54). A wide variety of cell types may be used for testing, but the test requires that laboratories maintain their own cell lines or purchase them in commercially available kits. For the test to be diagnostic, the cytopathic effect of the specimen (primarily due to the effects of toxin B) must be neutralized by specific *C. difficile* or *C. sordellii* antitoxin. Appropriate specimen dilution is critical to achieving test sensitivity and specificity (46). Sensitivity of the cell cytotoxin assay has ranged from 67% to 100% (46) when used to detect *C. difficile* disease in patients with clinically significant diarrhea (six or more unformed stools in 36 hours). Low sensitivity is thought to be due to the inactivation of toxins by proteases or other inactivating substances in stool, an occurrence that is more likely if the specimen remains at room temperature for a long period (48). Despite its relative insensitivity, stool testing for cytotoxin remains one of the gold standards against which newer *C. difficile* laboratory tests are evaluated. A major drawback of this test is the long (48-hour) turnaround time for results in most laboratories.

Immunoassay for Toxins A and B

A variety of immunoassays are available that detect *C. difficile* toxin A, or toxins A and B. These tests have now been widely adopted by clinical laboratories (and are often the only tests offered) because of the rapid turnaround time and decreased workload compared to cytotoxin assays. A review of the published literature in 1993 showed that sensitivity of toxin immunoassays ranged from 63% to 85% compared to culture and cytotoxin testing, and specificity ranged from 75% to 100% in patients with diarrhea (Table 36.1). When compared only to cytotoxin testing, the sensitivity was 71% to 88% and the specificity was 95% to 100%. Subsequent studies have confirmed the relative insensitivity of toxin immunoassays compared to cytotoxin testing (55) and to culture with confirmation of toxin-producing isolates (56). In general, the detection limit for immunoassays is 10- to 100-fold lower than for cytotoxin assays (57) and the titer of the cell cytotoxin assay correlates with the likelihood of toxin A immunoassay positivity (58,59). Immunoassays that detect both toxins (A/B) may be more sensitive than assays that just detect toxin A (55). Toxin A/B immunoassays also detect variant strains of *C. difficile* that are not detected by toxin A immunoassays (60). The frequency of toxin A−/B+ variant strains has been low (0.2% to 3%) in most surveys (60–63), but may be higher in other settings (64) and hospital outbreaks have been reported (20,21). Infections due to these A−/B+ variants are important to recognize clinically (19,65); however, many laboratories still rely on toxin A immunoassays, which fail to detect these strains, as their sole test for *C. difficile* (19). Advantages of the toxin immunoassays are the high specificity and rapid turnaround time (if the tests are not batched).

Tests for the Detection of the Microorganism in Stool

Stool Culture

Stool culture for *C. difficile* on selective media [cycloserine-cefoxitin-fructose agar (CCFA)] has proven to be one of the most sensitive tests for CDAD (53,54). Special transport of stool specimens is not required for culture; however, CCFA media should be anaerobically reduced prior to inoculation for optimal culture results (46). Clinical laboratories must exercise diligent quality control of commercially purchased media, as recovery rates have been shown to vary widely among manufacturers (66, 67). Culture is the critical diagnostic test if epidemiologic investigation employing microorganism typing (including molecular techniques) is desired. The major criticism of culture as a diagnostic test for CDAD is that it lacks specificity when compared with the cytotoxin assay, and is explained by high rates of asymptomatic *C. difficile* carriage in many hospital settings (8,68). When culture and cell cytotoxin assay are both performed for CDAD diagnosis, both tests yield positive results in approximately two thirds of patients, but stools are culture-positive and cytotoxin-negative in one third of patients (69). About 75% of the *C. difficile* isolates recovered from this latter group produce toxins *in vitro.* Patients with culture-positive, cytotoxin-negative stool specimens should be considered presumptive CDAD cases (33,70). Testing of the recovered *C. difficile* isolate for toxin production *in vitro* increases the specificity of the test (56), but also increases the turnaround time.

Antigen Tests

The latex agglutination test is a commercially available stool test that was originally thought to detect toxin A but was subsequently shown to detect a different *C. difficile* protein, glutamate dehydrogenase (71,72). The test is rapid, simple to use, and relatively inexpensive but lacks both sensitivity and specificity and does not distinguish toxigenic from nontoxigenic strains of *C. difficile* (53,54) (Table 36.1). The ImmunoCard *C. difficile* test is an enzyme-linked immunosorbent-based assay for detection of *C. difficile* antigens (73). The predominant antigen detected by the ImmunoCard test is a 43,000-dalton subunit of *C. difficile* glutamate dehydrogenase; the test does not distinguish between toxigenic and nontoxigenic strains of *C. difficile.* It is recommended that this test be used in conjunction with a toxin-based assay for *C. difficile.* One commercially available test, the Triage *C. difficile* Panel, combines antigen testing ("common antigen") with a toxin A immunoassay that is reported to have a high negative predictive value (59).

Polymerase Chain Reaction

The use of PCR to detect *C. difficile* in stool is still an experimental procedure but one that, with the selection of appropriate primers, can be used to detect toxigenic and nontoxigenic strains of *C. difficile* with a degree of sensitivity 100 times greater than that of culture (74,75). Data on the use of PCR for clinical diagnosis in large numbers of patients are lacking, as are considerations of cost, test turnaround time, and specificity.

Diagnostic Summary

Testing of stools for fecal leukocytes (34,51,58) and examination by Gram stain for gram-positive bacilli (76) are of questionable utility as screening tests for CDAD because of low sensitivity and low specificity. Of the available laboratory tests, the cell cytotoxin assay is the most specific, whereas culture is the most sensitive. For epidemiologic purposes, there is no substitute for stool culture in the diagnosis and epidemiologic management of nosocomial *C. difficile* infections. Because most clinical laboratories have abandoned culture and cytotoxin testing in favor of toxin immunoassays, additional testing or empiric treatment should be considered in patients with negative test results and high pretest probability for CDAD (e.g., recent hospitalization and antibiotic exposure).

EPIDEMIOLOGY

Infection Rates and Epidemic Characteristics

Rates of *C. difficile* diarrhea and colonization vary markedly from one setting to another. The incidence of CDAD in acute care hospitals has ranged from 0.3 cases per 1,000 patient admissions (77) to 78 cases per 1,000 patient admissions (25). An extraordinary incidence of diarrhea (21%) and PMC (10%) was documented at one hospital in patients receiving clindamycin (32), whereas CDAD is only infrequently recognized at other hospitals. CDAD has also been documented in chronic care facilities and nursing homes at the somewhat lower rate of 0.08 cases per 1,000 resident days (78). Although CDAD is rare in newborn infants, up to 60% of neonates are colonized, albeit at markedly different rates on different wards within the same hospital (23). These differences in disease rates may reflect different diagnostic criteria and, particularly in regard to neonates, different clinical settings, but also likely reflect the endemic or epidemic status of *C. difficile* in different institutions, emphasizing the importance of nosocomial acquisition over endogenous activation in the pathogenesis of this disease.

Even before the development of reliable typing schemes for *C. difficile,* the nosocomial nature of this disease was suspected. *C. difficile* is only infrequently cultured from stools of healthy adults who have not had recent exposure to antimicrobial agents (79,80), and institutional outbreaks of CDAD with time–space clustering frequently have been recognized. Development and application of various typing schemes has demonstrated the importance of nosocomial acquisition and has clarified many aspects of *C. difficile* transmission within hospitals (8,25,81,82).

Among the numerous phenotypic and genotypic typing schemes that have been employed, serogrouping, PCR ribotyping, and REA of total genomic DNA may be the best characterized and most useful methods available (83). Pulse-field gel electrophoresis (PFGE) and arbitrary primed PCR (AP-PCR) methods have been used, but are limited by the inability of some strains to be typed by PFGE and the differing banding patterns with AP-PCR when used in different laboratories (82). We have used the high discrimination of REA to demonstrate the marked genetic diversity of *C. difficile.* Over 200 unique REA types were identified among *C. difficile* isolates from one hospital over a 10-year period (84). This diversity has been interpreted as evidence for endogenous carriage when unique types have been detected in different asymptomatic patients without evidence of cross-infection (78). However, many outbreaks caused by multiple different REA types have been documented within the same institution (68). In addition, silent clusters of *C. difficile* acquisitions occur in which few or no patients develop symptoms related to acquisition of that particular strain (68). Even among clinical relapses of CDAD in the same patient that occur within the hospital setting, half of the cases involve acquisition of new strains (36,37). Prospective studies have also shown that patients already colonized on admission to the hospital are more likely than are noncolonized patients to have been recently hospitalized (68). Thus, nosocomial acquisition appears to be the most important source of *C. difficile* infections.

Antimicrobial Use

Nearly all antibacterial agents given by either oral or parenteral routes have been associated with CDAD. The most commonly implicated agents have been clindamycin, ampicillin, and cephalosporins (7). A meta-analysis of risk factors for *C. difficile* infection allowed ranking of individual agents and found that four of the five agents with the greatest relative risk were cephalosporins. Until recently, it was accepted that susceptibility of *C. difficile* to the antimicrobial agent does not predict the likelihood of CDAD following exposure to that agent. Ampicillin frequently precipitates CDAD despite susceptibility of most *C. difficile* isolates to this agent. Although more cases of CDAD have probably resulted from ampicillin and cephalosporin use, the unique predisposition of patients treated with clindamycin has been repeatedly documented (32,34,85,86). The mechanism of this unique propensity may be partially explained by the marked activity of clindamycin against anaerobic bacteria and a prolonged effect on the colonic flora. Clindamycin resistance has been a marker for *C. difficile* strains implicated in several epidemics (85–87). It is now recognized that clindamycin use is a specific risk factor for diarrhea due to a widely disseminated clindamycin-resistant *C. difficile* strain, and this finding may also explain the unique predisposition of clindamycin to precipitate CDAD (88). Third-generation cephalosporins have been repeatedly associated with CDAD (89), and studies have demonstrated a lower risk of CDAD following treatment with ticarcillin/clavulanate or piperacillin/tazobactam than with ceftazidime or ceftriaxone (90,91). Antimicrobial agents that are infrequently implicated include tetracycline, erythromycin, chloramphenicol, vancomycin, parenteral aminoglycosides, and metronidazole (92). In addition, CDAD can occur during or following antimicrobial therapy at any dosage, and cases have occurred after a few doses given for surgical prophylaxis (93,94). However, prophylactic antimicrobials were not significantly associated with CDAD in a prospective case-controlled study (34).

Reservoirs and Modes of Transmission

Environmental Contamination

Environmental surfaces contaminated with *C. difficile* spores are a potentially important source of nosocomial *C. difficile* infections. The environment of patients with CDAD is more frequently contaminated than the environment of other patients, and the degree of contamination has correlated with *C. difficile* outbreaks (25,95,96). Floors and bathroom sites tend to be most heavily contaminated (97). In addition, commode chairs, sigmoidoscopes, bed pans, nursery baby baths, patient phones, and electronic thermometers have been found to be contaminated and can serve as reservoirs for nosocomial transmission of *C. difficile* (98–100). There is still controversy as to whether the environment is a source of patient infections or whether the environment is merely contaminated as a result of occupancy by a *C. difficile*–infected patient.

Asymptomatic Patient Carriers

Whenever patients with nosocomial CDAD are identified, it can be assumed that higher numbers of asymptomatic *C. difficile* carriers (fecal excretors) are also on the same ward or in the same room (8,25). Although these asymptomatic carriers are not at an increased risk for diarrhea themselves, they are potential reservoirs for infection in other susceptible patients (8). Acquisition of *C. difficile* has been documented more frequently and earlier among patients exposed to roommates with positive cultures (25). In one 9-month prospective surveillance study, nosocomial patient acquisitions of *C. difficile* were preceded by a documented introduction to that same ward of the identical REA type strain by a newly admitted patient (68). This sequence of events occurred in 16 (84%) of the 19 instances in which a specific *C. difficile* REA type strain was isolated from more than one patient. These data suggest that asymptomatic carriers are an important source of nosocomial *C. difficile* infections.

Personnel Hand Carriage

If either the environment or asymptomatic carriers are important sources of infections, *C. difficile* could be transmitted from those sources by direct contact or indirectly by the hands of patient care personnel. Hands are frequently contaminated with *C. difficile* (25,96), and hand colonization rates as high as 59% after patient contact, that, in some instances, amounted to mere patient assessment and charting, have been documented (25). Vinyl glove use by hospital personnel when handling body substances was also associated with a significant reduction in the incidence of CDAD on acute care wards (101). Thus, direct and indirect evidence supports transient hand carriage by patient care personnel as a mode of *C. difficile* transmission.

Host Risk Factors

Before the etiology of PMC was elucidated, this disease was postulated to be an idiosyncratic host reaction to clindamycin. Since the role of *C. difficile* in antibiotic-associated diarrhea and colitis has been clarified, it is clear that *C. difficile* infections frequently occur as outbreaks associated with unique strains (8, 91). However, the clinical manifestations and severity of *C. difficile* infections are not solely attributable to specific *C. difficile* strains (26) but also depend on specific host factors.

Risks of Acquisition

Asymptomatic fecal excretion is a more common outcome of infection with *C. difficile* than is diarrhea, and although antimicrobial exposure, the classic risk factor for CDAD, has been associated with asymptomatic carriage (8,34,102), this association is not as strong as it is with CDAD (103). Risk factors consistently associated with acquisition include advanced age, more severe underlying illnesses, and length of hospital stay (8, 103). Acquisition of *C. difficile* is highly correlated with the duration of hospital stay so that, by 4 weeks of hospitalization, 50% of previously uninfected patients may be culture-positive (68,103). Patients with cystic fibrosis have high rates of *C. difficile* colonization (104) that may reflect their high rates of antimicrobial use, but as with newborn infants, associated disease is rare. Stool softener and antacid use may also be risk factors for asymptomatic carriage (103).

Risks of Illness

Increased age, severe underlying illness, and length of hospital stay are also associated with CDAD (25,34). As the names for CDAD and colitis often indicate, antimicrobials are highly associated with *C. difficile* disease. Clindamycin, multiple antimicrobials, and antimicrobials given for therapy rather than for prophylaxis have been significantly associated with CDAD (34). Cephalosporin and penicillin use have also been significantly associated with illness (103). Failure to develop an amnestic response to toxin A is a recognized risk factor for CDAD (105, 106). Shortly after exposure, serum anti–toxin A immunoglobulin G (IgG) levels predict subsequent clinical outcome (105). Asymptomatic carriers have higher levels than those who develop CDAD, which may partially explain our previous observation that asymptomatic carriers are at decreased risk for subsequent CDAD (9). These antibody responses shortly after exposure also influence the risk of subsequent relapse among those who develop CDAD (106).

Another repeated association with *C. difficile* disease has been the manipulation of the gastrointestinal tract by enemas, insertion of nasogastric and gastrostomy tubes, motility altering drugs such as atropine sulfate-diphenoxylate hydrochloride and codeine, and gastrointestinal surgery (8,98,103). A well-controlled prospective cohort study has demonstrated tube-feeding and, in particular, postpyloric administration, as a risk factor for acquiring *C. difficile* and developing CDAD (107). Insertion of nasogastric and gastrostomy tubes and enema administration may reflect increased contact with hospital personnel and with their potentially contaminated hands, which may be a partial explanation for these risk factors (78).

CDAD has also been reported in association with cancer chemotherapy, chronic renal disorders, HIV infection, and inflammatory bowel disease (98,108). *C. difficile* has not been implicated as a cause of inflammatory bowel disease but may be responsible for some of the symptomatic relapses in patients with established inflammatory bowel disease (109). Also, for unknown reasons, women may have a higher rate of *C. difficile* disease than do men (80).

PREVENTION AND CONTROL

No single infection control practice has effectively prevented and controlled nosocomial *C. difficile* infection. We postulate that CDAD is at least a "three-hit" process that begins with (a) administration of antimicrobial or chemotherapeutic agents, (b) acquisition of the *C. difficile* microorganism, and (c) other factors such as the interaction with the host immune response that result in clinical illness in a minority of the large number of patients who both receive antimicrobials and acquire *C. difficile.* Prevention and control measures have focused largely on (a) interruption of the process of nosocomial microorganism acquisition and (b) measures to reduce the likelihood of clinical illness if a patient acquires *C. difficile.* The various interventive measures have been critiqued in terms of established evidence of benefit (Table 36.2). Two sets of practice guidelines for prevention and control of *C. difficile* infection have also been published by the American College of Gastroenterology (ACG) and Society for Healthcare Epidemiology of America (SHEA) (110,111).

Prevention of Acquisition of *C. difficile*

Barrier Precautions

Cohorting, patient isolation, hand washing, and glove use are included under barrier techniques. A number of studies indirectly suggest that person-to-person spread of *C. difficile* occurs in the hospital, either from patient to patient or from personnel to patient. Hands of personnel are frequently contaminated with *C. difficile* (25,34,101,112) and a prospective controlled trial has shown that vinyl glove use by hospital personnel when contacting patient body substances was effective in interrupting transmission (101). CDAD rates declined from 7.7/1,000 patient discharges to 1.5/1,000 (p = .015) after glove use was instituted, whereas control wards in the same institution showed no significant change in rates. Hand washing following patient or body substance contact should also be an effective way to interrupt transmission via the hands of personnel, although the efficacy of soap in removing *C. difficile* from hands was questioned in one study, whereas chlorhexidine appeared effective (25). Both agents were equally effective in removing seeded *C. difficile* from the hands of volunteers (113). The efficacy of waterless alcohol–based hand hygiene products (that are not sporicidal) in removing spores of *C. difficile* from the hands of healthcare workers has not been clinically evaluated.

The difficulty in implementing isolation techniques (private rooms, enteric isolation, cohorting) in the control of *C. difficile* transmission is that they cannot be employed rapidly (unless patients are isolated before infection is identified). Assessment of efficacy is difficult, because isolation methods frequently are not employed alone as control measures (114–116). Whereas hand washing and glove use can be employed in the care of all patients, isolation techniques are directed at those patients who have been identified as infected. These patients are almost always symptomatic with diarrhea and have been diagnosed with CDAD prior to being isolated. Aggressive patient identification and rapid isolation was employed by Struelens et al. (77) and was associated with a reduction in the rate of *C. difficile* cases from 1.5/1,000 to 0.3/1,000 admissions. However, patients were treated early with vancomycin and the environment was disinfected with formaldehyde and glutaraldehyde, making the contribution of isolation impossible to discern. Isolation of patients with CDAD has been recommended by a number of authors (95,96,117,118). A modified approach in which patients are placed in private rooms only if they are incontinent and unable to maintain good bowel hygiene has also been used (8, 34,68).

Environmental Cleaning and Disinfection

Numerous environmental sites and devices have been shown to be contaminated with *C. difficile* (95,96,117). The rate of room contamination is proportional to the status of the patient in the room: highest for patients with CDAD, intermediate for patients with asymptomatic *C. difficile* colonization, and lowest for patients without the microorganism (25). Spread of *C. difficile* has been linked to contaminated environmental devices including commodes, electronic rectal thermometer handles, and baby baths (23,119,120). Replacement of contaminated electronic thermometers with disposable thermometers (100) and subsequent replacement of all disposable thermometers (rectal and oral) with tympanic thermometers (121) showed a reduced incidence of *C. difficile* infections. Flexible sigmoidoscopes and colonoscopes are frequently contaminated by *C. difficile* microorganisms following endoscopy in patients with CDAD (122). The potential for spread of *C. difficile* by contaminated endoscopes is real but has not been documented. The presently recommended regimen of endoscopic cleaning and disinfection with 2% glutaraldehyde immersion for as short a time as 10 minutes is sporicidal for *C. difficile* (122,123) and should adequately prevent transmission via endoscopes, provided the procedures are reliably followed (see Chapter 63).

Contamination of the patient's environment can be reduced significantly by employing a sporicidal disinfectant such as un-

TABLE 36.2. INFECTION CONTROL PRACTICES TO PREVENT NOSOCOMIAL *C. DIFFICILE*–ASSOCIATED DISEASE

Practice	Efficacy	Reference
Barrier precautions		
Glove use when handling body substances	Proven	101
Hand washing before treating each patient	Probable	113
Isolation precautions and cohorting	Probable	77,114–116
Environmental cleaning and disinfection		
Rectal thermometers		
Substitution of disposables	Proven	100
Switch to tympanic thermometers	Proven	121
Gastrointestinal endoscopes	Accepted	122,123
Patient rooms and bathrooms	Possible	77,97
Hypochlorite disinfection	Probable	124,125
Bedside commodes	Untested	
Identification and management of asymptomatic carriers		
Vancomycin treatment of asymptomatic carriers	Possible	29,126
Metronidazole treatment of asymptomatic carriers	Ineffective	29,115
Isolation or cohorting of asymptomatic carriers	Untested	
Measures to reduce the risk of symptomatic disease		
Antimicrobial use restriction		
Clindamycin	Proven	85,86,116
Cefotaxime (switch to P/T)	Probable	91
Prophylactic agents for patients receiving antimicrobials		
Saccharomyces boulardii	Possible	129
Lactobacillus species	Untested	
C. difficile bovine antibodies	Untested	130
Colonization with nontoxigenic *C. difficil*	Untested	132

P/T, piperacillin-tazobactam.

buffered hypochlorite solution [500 parts per million (ppm) available chloride], phosphate buffered hypochlorite (1,600 ppm chloride), or a combination of 0.04% formaldehyde and 0.03% glutaraldehyde (97,116). Two recent studies have documented reduced CDAD rates on wards where hypochlorite environmental disinfection was introduced, but the effectiveness of this intervention may be confounded by additional factors (124,125).

Identification and Treatment of Asymptomatic C. difficile Carriers

Asymptomatic patient carriers of *C. difficile* are a potential source of spread of the microorganism to other susceptible patients via contamination of the environment or the hands of personnel (68,126). Although there is a decreased risk of CDAD in the carriers themselves, they may be a source of transmission to other patients (8). Identification of asymptomatic carriers requires extensive stool and/or rectal swab culturing, which is labor intensive for both infection control and laboratory personnel. The appropriate action following carrier identification is unknown (68). No one has attempted a study of carrier isolation or cohorting. Intervention studies that involved treatment of asymptomatic colonized patients with metronidazole or vancomycin were ineffective (115), inconclusive (127), or the potential effect was confounded by other simultaneous interventions (126). A randomized study that attempted to eradicate colonization found that whereas vancomycin was temporarily effective, treated patients were more likely to be colonized at the end of follow-up than were placebo-treated control patients (29). Metronidazole treatment results were no different that placebo. Thus, how to address the asymptomatic colonized patient remains unresolved.

Reducing Risk of Clinical Illness

Antimicrobial Restriction

Prior exposure to antimicrobials is virtually universal in patients who develop symptomatic *C. difficile* disease. Risk of CDAD is increased for specific antimicrobials such as ampicillin, amoxicillin, clindamycin, and cephalosporins (34,128). Risk is higher if multiple antibiotics are administered, if the number of doses or days of therapy is higher, and if antimicrobials are administered to treat an infection rather than for prophylaxis (34,85,103,116). These observations suggest the opportunity to reduce *C. difficile* disease risk by reducing exposure and duration of antimicrobial therapy. There are three examples of a restricted clindamycin use policy that have reduced CDAD rates (85,86, 116). In one instance, this intervention stopped an extended outbreak within a month of implementation (85). Subsequent investigation showed that this outbreak was due to a highly clindamycin-resistant epidemic strain and that clindamycin use was a risk factor (88). The most convincing intervention strategy for cephalosporin restriction was a prospective, ward-based, crossover study replacing empiric cefotaxime therapy with piperacillin/tazobactam (91). Piperacillin/tazobactam use was associated with a lower incidence of colonization and CDAD; rates increased when cefotaxime was reintroduced. More environmental contamination was also documented during cefotaxime use.

Prophylactic Measures for Patients Receiving Antimicrobials

Although as yet unproven, the hypothesis that patients receiving antimicrobials can be treated effectively with a prophylactic agent that will prevent CDAD is an attractive one. The yeast *Saccharomyces boulardii,* several strains of lactobacilli, and orally administered *C. difficile* antibodies have been proposed as preventive agents (129,130). *S. boulardii* has been used in humans and was found to reduce antibiotic-associated diarrhea significantly (p = .038) when given during and for 2 weeks after antibiotic administration. CDAD was also reduced, but this was not statistically significant (p = .07) (129). A subsequent study failed to show efficacy of *S. boulardii* in elderly hospitalized patients receiving antibiotics (131). *C. difficile* antibodies extracted from the colostrum of immunized cattle have been used successfully in the hamster model to prevent *C. difficile* disease, but no data are available for use in humans (130). Lactobacilli in yogurt and acidophilus milk have been used to reduce diarrheal side effects of antibiotics and to treat relapsing CDAD, but efficacy remains questionable. No data are available for use in prevention of CDAD. A novel approach that has been highly successful in the hamster model but has not yet been studied in humans involves colonization with nontoxigenic strains of *C. difficile* to prevent CDAD (132).

REFERENCES

1. Bartlett JG, Chang TW, Gurwith M, et al. Antibiotic-associated pseudomembranous colitis due to toxin-producing clostridia. *N Engl J Med* 1978;298:531–534.
2. Larson HE, Price AB, Honour P, et al. *Clostridium difficile* and the aetiology of pseudomembranous colitis. *Lancet* 1978;1:1063–1066.
3. Yannelli B, Gurevich I, Schoch PE, et al. Yield of stool cultures, ova and parasite tests, and *Clostridium difficile* determinations in nosocomial diarrheas. *Am J Infect Control* 1988;16:246–249.
4. Siegel DL, Edelstein PH, Nachamkin I. Inappropriate testing for diarrheal diseases in the hospital. *JAMA* 1990;263:979–982.
5. Kyne L, Hamel MB, Polavaram R, et al. Health care costs and mortality associated with nosocomial diarrhea due to *Clostridium difficile. Clin Infect Dis* 2002;34:346–53.
6. Miller M, Hyland M, Ofner-Agostini M, et al. Morbidity, mortality, and healthcare burden of nosocomial *Clostridium difficile*-associated diarrhea in Canadian hospitals. *Infect Cont Hosp Epidemiol* 2002;23: 137–140.
7. Bartlett JG. Antimicrobial agents implicated in *Clostridium difficile* toxin associated diarrhea or colitis. *Johns Hopkins Med J* 1981;149: 6–9.
8. Johnson S, Clabots CR, Linn FV, et al. Nosocomial *Clostridium difficile* colonization and disease. *Lancet* 1990;336:97–100.
9. Shim JK, Johnson S, Samore MH, et al. Primary symptomless colonisation by *Clostridium difficile* and decreased risk of subsequent diarrhoea. *Lancet* 1998;351:633–636.
10. Tucker KD, Carrig PE, Wilkins TD. Toxin A of *Clostridium difficile* is a potent cytotoxin. *J Clin Microbiol* 1990;28:869–871.
11. Borriello SP, Barclay FE, Welch AR, et al. Host and microbial determinants of the spectrum of *Clostridium difficile* mediated gastrointestinal disorders. *Microecol Ther* 1985;15:231–236.
12. Kim P-H, Iaconis JP, Rolfe RD. Immunization of adult hamsters against *Clostridium difficile* associated ileocecitis and transfer of protection to infant hamsters. *Infect Immun* 1987;55:2984–2992.
13. Lyerly DM, Saum KE, MacDonald DK, et al. Effects of *Clostridium difficile* toxins given intragastrically to animals. *Infect Immun* 1985; 47:349–352.
14. Lima AAM, Lyerly DM, Wilkins TD, et al. Effects of *Clostridium difficile* toxins A and B in rabbit small and large intestine in vivo and on cultured cells in vitro. *Infect Immun* 1988;56:582–588.
15. Krivan HC, Clark GF, Smith DF, et al. Cell surface binding site for *Clostridium difficile* enterotoxin: evidence for a glycoconjugate containing the sequence Gala1–3Galb1–4GlcNAc. *Infect Immun* 1986;53:573–581.
16. Tucker KD, Wilkins TD. Toxin A of *Clostridium difficile* binds to the human carbohydrate antigens I, X, and Y. *Infect Immun* 1991; 59:73–78.
17. von Eichel-Streiber C, Boquet P, Sauerborn M, et al. Large clostridial toxins—a family of glycosyltransferases modifying small GTP-binding proteins. *Trends Microbiol* 1996;4:375–382.
18. Johnson S, Sambol SP, Brazier JS, et al. International typing study of toxin A-negative, B-positive *Clostridium difficile* variants. *J Clin Microbiol* 2003;41:1543–1547.
19. Johnson S, Kent SA, O'Leary KJ, et al. Fatal pseudomembranous colitis associated with a variant *Clostridium difficile* strain not detected by toxin A immunoassay. *Ann Intern Med* 2001;135:434–438.
20. Alfa MJ, Kabani A, Lyerly D, et al. Characterization of a toxin A-negative, toxin B-positive strain of *Clostridium difficile* responsible for a nosocomial outbreak of *Clostridium difficile*-associated diarrhea. *J Clin Microbiol* 2000;38:2706–2714.
21. Kuijper EJ, de Weerdt J, Kato H, et al. Nosocomial outbreak of *Clostridium difficile*-associated diarrhea due to a clindamycin-resistant enterotoxin A-negative strain. *Eur J Clin Microbiol Infect Dis* 2001; 20:528–534.
22. Stubbs S, Rupnik M, Gibert M, et al. Production of actin-specific ADP-ribosyltransferase (binary toxin) by strains of *C. difficile. FEMS Microbiol Lett* 2000;186:307–312.
23. Larson HE, Barclay FE, Honour P, et al. Epidemiology of *Clostridium difficile* in infants. *J Infect Dis* 1982;146:727–733.
24. Eglow R, Pothoulakis C, Itzkowitz S, et al. Diminished *Clostridium difficile* toxin A sensitivity in newborn rabbit ileum is associated with decreased toxin A receptor. *J Clin Invest* 1992;90:822–829.
25. McFarland LV, Mulligan ME, Kwok RYY, et al. Nosocomial acquisition of *Clostridium difficile* infection. *N Engl J Med* 1989;320: 204–210.
26. McFarland LV, Elmer GW, Stamm WE, et al. Correlation of immunoblot type, enterotoxin production, and cytotoxin production with clinical manifestations of *Clostridium difficile* infection in a cohort of hospitalized patients. *Infect Immun* 1991;59:2456–2462.
27. Burke GW, Wilson ME, Mehrez IO. Absence of diarrhea in toxic megacolon complicating *Clostridium difficile* pseudomembranous colitis. *Am J Gastroenterol* 1988;83:304–307.
28. Dansinger ML, Johnson S, Jansen PC, et al. Protein-losing enteropathy is associated with *Clostridium difficile* diarrhea, but not asymptomatic colonization: a prospective, case-controlled study. *Clin Infect Dis* 1996;22:932–937.
29. Johnson S, Homann SR, Bettin KM, et al. Treatment of asymptomatic *Clostridium difficile* carriers (fecal excretors) with vancomycin or metronidazole: a randomized, placebo-controlled trial. *Ann Intern Med* 1992;117:297–302.
30. Gryboski JD, Pellerano R, Young N, et al. Positive role of *Clostridium difficile* infection in diarrhea in infants and children. *Am J Gastroenterol* 1991;86:685–689.
31. Bartlett JG. *Clostridium difficile*: clinical considerations. *Rev Infect Dis* 1990;12(suppl 2):S243–S251.
32. Tedesco FJ, Barton RW, Alpers DH. Clindamycin-associated colitis: a prospective study. *Ann Intern Med* 1974;81:429–433.
33. Teasley DG, Olson MM, Gebhard RL, et al. Prospective randomized trial of metronidazole versus vancomycin for *Clostridium difficile* associated diarrhea and colitis. *Lancet* 1983;2:1043–1046.
34. Gerding DN, Olson MM, Peterson LR, et al. *Clostridium difficile*

associated diarrhea and colitis in adults: a prospective case-controlled epidemiologic study. *Arch Intern Med* 1986;146:95–100.

35. Wanahita A, Goldsmith EA, Musher DM. Conditions associated with leukocytosis in a tertiary care hospital, with particular attention to the role of infection caused by *Clostridium difficile. Clin Infect Dis* 2002:34:1585–92.
36. Johnson S, Adelmann A, Clabots CR, et al. Recurrences of *Clostridium difficile* diarrhea not caused by the original infecting organism. *J Infect Dis* 1989;159:340–343.
37. O'Neill GL, Beaman MH, Riley TV. Relapse versus reinfection with *Clostridium difficile. Epidemiol Infect* 1991;107:627–635.
38. Price AB, Davies DR. Pseudomembranous colitis. *J Clin Pathol* 1977; 30:1–12.
39. Gebhard RL, Gerding DN, Olson MM, et al. Clinical and endoscopic findings in patients early in the course of *Clostridium difficile* associated pseudomembranous colitis. *Am J Med* 1985;78:45–48.
40. Tedesco FJ, Corless JK, Brownstein RE. Rectal sparing in antibiotic-associated pseudomembranous colitis: a prospective study. *Gastroenterology* 1982;83:1259–1260.
41. Morris JB, Zollinger RM Jr, Stellato TA. Role of surgery in antibiotic-associated pseudomembranous enterocolitis. *Am J Surg* 1990;160: 535–539.
42. Cone JB, Wetzel W. Toxic megacolon secondary to pseudomembranous colitis. *Dis Colon Rectum* 1982;25:478–482.
43. Dallal RM, Harbrecht BG, Boujoukas AJ, et al. Fulminant *Clostridium difficile*: an underappreciated and increasing cause of death and complications. *Ann Surg* 2002;235:363–372.
44. Levett PN. *Clostridium difficile* in habitats other than the human gastrointestinal tract. *J Infect* 1986;12:253–263.
45. Lofgren RP, Tadlock LM, Soltis RD. Acute oligoarthritis associated with *Clostridium difficile* pseudomembranous colitis. *Arch Intern Med* 1984;144:617–619.
46. Peterson LR, Kelly PJ. The role of the clinical microbiology laboratory in the management of *Clostridium difficile* associated diarrhea. *Infect Dis Clin North Am* 1993;7:277–293.
47. Gerding DN, Brazier JS. Optimal methods for identifying *Clostridium difficile* infections. *Clin Infect Dis* 1993;16(suppl 4):S439–S442.
48. Brazier JS. The role of the laboratory in investigations of *Clostridium difficile* diarrhea. *Clin Infect Dis* 1993;16(suppl 4):S228–S233.
49. Barbut F, Kajzer C, Planas N, et al. Comparison of three enzyme immunoassays, a cytotoxicity assay and toxigenic culture for the diagnosis of *Clostridium difficile* associated diarrhea. *J Clin Microbiol* 1993; 31:963–967.
50. Fekety R, Shah AB. Diagnosis and treatment of *Clostridium difficile* colitis. *JAMA* 1993;269:71–75.
51. Manabe YC, Vinetz JM, Moore RD, et al. *Clostridium difficile* colitis: an efficient clinical approach to diagnosis. *Ann Intern Med* 1995;123: 835–840.
52. Katz DA, Lynch ME, Littenberg B. Clinical prediction rules to optimize cytotoxin testing for *Clostridium difficile* in hospitalized patients with diarrhea. *Am J Med* 1996;100:487–495.
53. Shanholtzer CJ, Willard KE, Holter JJ, et al. Comparison of the VIDAS *Clostridium difficile* toxic A immunoassay with *C. difficile* culture and cytotoxin and latex tests. *J Clin Microbiol* 1992;30: 1837–1840.
54. Peterson LR, Olson MM, Shanholtzer CJ, et al. Results of a prospective, 18-month clinical evaluation of culture, cytotoxin testing, and culturette brand (CDT) latex testing in the diagnosis of *Clostridium difficile* associated diarrhea. *Diagn Microbiol Infect Dis* 1988;10: 85–91.
55. O'Connor D, Hynes P, Cormican M, et al. Evaluation of methods for detection of toxins in specimens of feces submitted for diagnosis of *Clostridium difficile*-associated diarrhea. *J Clin Microbiol* 2001;39: 2846–2849.
56. Lozniewski A, Rabaud C, Dotto E, et al. Laboratory diagnosis of *Clostridium difficile*-associated diarrhea and colitis: usefulness of premier Cytoclone A + B enzyme immunoassay for combined detection of stool toxins and toxigenic *C. difficile* strains. *J Clin Microbiol* 2001; 39:1996–1998.
57. Bartlett JG. Antibiotic-Associated Diarrhea. *N Engl J Med* 2002;346: 334–339.
58. Schleupner MA, Garner DC, Sosnowski KM, et al. Concurrence of *Clostridium difficile* toxin A enzyme-linked immunosorbent assay, fecal lactoferrin assay, and clinical criteria with *C. difficile* cytotoxin titer in two patient cohorts. *J Clin Microbiol* 1995;33:1755–1759.
59. Landry ML, Topal J, Ferguson D, et al. Evaluation of Biosite triage *Clostridium difficile* panel for rapid detection of *Clostridium difficile* in stool specimens. *J Clin Microbiol* 2001;39:1855–1858.
60. Lyerly DM, Neville LM, Evans DT, et al. Multicenter evaluation of the *Clostridium difficile* Tox A/B Test. *J Clin Microbiol* 1998;36: 184–190.
61. Brazier JS, Stubbs SL, Duerden BI. Prevalence of toxin A negative/ B positive *Clostridium difficile* strains. *J Hosp Infect* 1999;42:248–249.
62. Merrigan M, Kelly PJ, Sambol SP, et al. Endemic toxin A-negative, B-positive *Clostridium difficile* infections in a large U.S. hospital: 2½ years of prospective surveillance (abstract 413). Infectious Diseases Society of America 40th annual meeting, Chicago, October 24–27, 2002.
63. Barbut F, Lalande V, Burghoffer B, et al. Prevalence and genetic characterization of toxin A variant strains of *Clostridium difficile* among adults and children with diarrhea in France. *J Clin Microbiol* 2002;40:2079–2083.
64. Kato H, Kato N, Watanabe K, et al. Identification of toxin A-negative, toxin B-positive *Clostridium difficile* by PCR. *J Clin Microbiol* 1998; 36:2178–2182.
65. Sambol SP, Merrigan MM, Lyerly DM, et al. Toxin gene analysis of a variant strain of *Clostridium difficile* that causes human clinical disease. *Infect Immun* 2000;68:5480–5487.
66. Marler LM, Siders JA, Wolters LC, et al. Comparison of five cultural procedures for isolation of *Clostridium difficile* from stools. *J Clin Microbiol* 1992;30:514–516.
67. Shanholtzer CJ, Peterson LR. Laboratory quality assurance testing of microbiologic media from commercial sources. *Am J Clin Pathol* 1987;88:210–215.
68. Clabots CR, Johnson S, Olson MM, et al. Acquisition of *Clostridium difficile* by hospitalized patients: evidence for colonized new admissions as a source of infection. *J Infect Dis* 1992;166:561–567.
69. Clabots CR, Johnson S, Olson MM, et al. *Clostridium difficile* associated diarrhea diagnosis in patients with positive stool culture and negative stool cytotoxin assays (abstract 1567). Program and abstracts, 33rd Interscience Conference on Antimicrobial Agents and Chemotherapy, New Orleans, October 17–20, 1993.
70. Lashner BA, Todorczuk J, Sahm DF, et al. *Clostridium difficile* culture-positive toxin-negative diarrhea. *Am J Gastroenterol* 1986;81: 940–943.
71. Lyerly DM, Barroso LA, Wilkins TD. Identification of the latex test-reactive protein of *Clostridium difficile* as glutamate dehydrogenase. *J Clin Microbiol* 1991;29:2639–2642.
72. Willis DH, Kraft JA, Lyerly DM, et al. Confirmation that the latex-reactive protein of *Clostridium difficile* is a glutamate dehydrogenase. *J Clin Microbiol* 1992;30:1363–1364.
73. Staneck JL, Weckbach LS, Allen SD, et al. Multicenter evaluation of four methods for *Clostridium difficile* detection: ImmunoCard *C. difficile*, cytotoxin assay, culture, and latex agglutination. *J Clin Microbiol* 1996;34:2718–2721.
74. Kuhl SJ, Tang YJ, Navarro L, et al. Diagnosis and monitoring of *Clostridium difficile* infections with the polymerase chain reaction. *Clin Infect Dis* 1993;16(suppl 4):S234–S238.
75. Gumerlock PH, Tang YJ, Weiss JB, et al. Specific detection of toxigenic strains of *Clostridium difficile* in stool specimens. *J Clin Microbiol* 1993;31:507–511.
76. Shanholtzer CJ, Peterson LR, Olson MM, et al. Selective study of gram-stained stool smears in diagnosis of *Clostridium difficile* colitis. *J Clin Microbiol* 1983;17:906–908.
77. Struelens MJ, Maas A, Nonhoff C, et al. Control of nosocomial transmission of *Clostridium difficile* based on sporadic case surveillance. *Am J Med* 1991;91(suppl 3B):1385–1445.
78. Simor AE, Yake SL, Tsimidis K. Infection due to *Clostridium difficile*

among elderly residents of a long-term-care facility. *Clin Infect Dis* 1993;17:672–678.

79. Viscidi R, Willey S, Bartlett JG. Isolation rates and toxigenic potential of *Clostridium difficile* isolates from various patient populations. *Gastroenterology* 1981;81:5–9.
80. Aronsson B, Möllby R, Nord C-E. Antimicrobial agents and *Clostridium difficile* in acute enteric disease: epidemiologic data from Sweden, 1980–1982. *J Infect Dis* 1985;151:476–481.
81. Tabaqchali S, Holland D, O'Farrell S, et al. Typing scheme for *Clostridium difficile*: its application in clinical and epidemiological studies. *Lancet* 1984;1:935–938.
82. Samore M, Killgore G, Johnson S, et al. Multicenter typing comparison of sporadic and outbreak *Clostridium difficile* isolates from geographically diverse hospitals. *J Infect Dis* 1997;176:1233–1238.
83. Johnson S, Sambol SP, Brazier JS, et al. International typing study of toxin A-negative, B-positive *Clostridium difficile* variants. *J Clin Microbiol* 2003;41:1543–1547.
84. Clabots CR, Johnson S, Bettin KM, et al. Development of a rapid and efficient restriction endonuclease analysis typing system for *Clostridium difficile* and correlation with other typing systems. *J Clin Microbiol* 1993;31:1870–1875.
85. Pear S, Williamson T, Bettin K, et al. Reduction in nosocomial *Clostridium difficile* associated diarrhea by control of clindamycin usage. *Ann Intern Med* 1994;120:272–277.
86. Climo MW, Israel DS, Wong ES, et al. Hospital-wide restriction of clindamycin: effect on the incidence of *Clostridium difficile*-associated diarrhea and cost. *Ann Intern Med* 1998;128:989–995.
87. Clabots CR, Peterson LR, Gerding DN. Characterization of a nosocomial *Clostridium difficile* outbreak by using plasmid profile typing and clindamycin testing. *J Infect Dis* 1988;158:731–736.
88. Johnson S, Samore MH, Farrow KA, et al. Epidemics of diarrhea caused by a clindamycin-resistant strain of *Clostridium difficile* in four hospitals. *N Engl J Med* 1999;341:1645–1651.
89. Anonymous. *C. difficile* and cephalosporins: an unholy alliance. *Infect Dis Clin Pract* 1996;5:144.
90. Anand A, Bashey B, Mir T, et al. Epidemiology, clinical manifestations, and outcome of *Clostridium difficile*-associated diarrhea. *Am J Gastroenterol* 1994;89:519–523.
91. Settle CD, Wilcox MH, Fawley WN, et al. Prospective study of the risk of *Clostridium difficile* diarrhea in elderly patients following treatment with cefotaxime or piperacillin-tazobactam. *Aliment Pharmacol Ther* 1998;12:1217–1223.
92. Gerding DN, Olson MM, Johnson S, et al. *Clostridium difficile* diarrhea and colonization after treatment with abdominal infection regimens containing clindamycin or metronidazole. *Am J Surg* 1990;159:212–217.
93. Privitera G, Scarpellini P, Ortisi G, et al. Prospective study of *Clostridium difficile* intestinal colonization and disease following single dose antibiotic prophylaxis in surgery. *Antimicrob Agents Chemother* 1991;35:208–210.
94. Yee J, Dixon CM, McLean APH, et al. *Clostridium difficile* disease in a department of surgery: the significance of prophylactic antibiotics. *Arch Surg* 1991;126:241–246.
95. Mulligan ME, Rolfe RD, Finegold SM, et al. Contamination of a hospital environment by *Clostridium difficile. Curr Microbiol* 1979;3:173–175.
96. Kim KH, Fekety R, Batts DH, et al. Isolation of *Clostridium difficile* from the environment and contacts of patients with antibiotic-associated colitis. *J Infect Dis* 1981;143:42–50.
97. Kaatz GW, Gitlin SD, Schaberg DR, et al. Acquisition of *Clostridium difficile* from the hospital environment. *Am J Epidemiol* 1988;127:1289–1294.
98. McFarland LV, Stamm WE. Review of *Clostridium difficile* associated diseases. *Am J Infect Control* 1986;14:99–109.
99. Kuijper ED, Oudbier JH, Stuifbergen WNHM, et al. Application of whole-cell DNA restriction endonuclease profiles to the epidemiology of *Clostridium difficile* induced diarrhea. *J Clin Microbiol* 1987;25:751–753.
100. Brooks SE, Veal RO, Kramer M, et al. Reduction in the incidence of *Clostridium difficile* associated diarrhea in an acute care hospital and a skilled nursing facility following replacement of electronic thermometers with single-use disposables. *Infect Control Hosp Epidemiol* 1992;13:98–103.
101. Johnson S, Gerding DN, Olson MM, et al. Prospective, controlled study of vinyl glove use to interrupt *Clostridium difficile* nosocomial transmission. *Am J Med* 1990;88:137–140.
102. Bignardi GE. Risk factors for *Clostridium difficile* infection. *J Hosp Infect* 1998;40:1–15.
103. McFarland LV, Surawicz CM, Stamm WE. Risk factors for *Clostridium difficile* carriage and *C. difficile* associated diarrhea in a cohort of hospitalized patients. *J Infect Dis* 1990;162:678–684.
104. Wu TC, McCarthy VP, Gill VJ. Isolation rate and toxigenic potential of *Clostridium difficile* isolates from patients with cystic fibrosis. *J Infect Dis* 1983;148:176.
105. Kyne L, Warny M, Qamar A, et al. Asymptomatic carriage of *Clostridium difficile* and serum levels of IgG antibody against toxin A. *N Engl J Med* 2000;342:390–397.
106. Kyne L, Warny M, Qamar A, et al. Association between antibody response to toxin A and protection against recurrent *Clostridium difficile* diarrhea. *Lancet* 2001;357:189–93.
107. Bliss DZ, Johnson S, Savik K, et al. Acquisition of *Clostridium difficile* and *Clostridium difficile*-associated diarrhea in hospitalized patients receiving tube feeding. *Ann Intern Med* 1998;129:1012–1019.
108. Tumbarello M, Tacconelli E, Leone F, et al. *Clostridium difficile*-associated diarrhoea in patients with human immunodeficiency virus infection: a case-control study. *Eur J Gastroenterol Hepatol* 1995;7:259–263.
109. Trnka YM, Lamont JT. Association of *Clostridium difficile* toxin with symptomatic relapse of chronic inflammatory bowel disease. *Gastroenterology* 1981;80:693–696.
110. Gerding DN, Johnson S, Peterson LR, et al. Society for Healthcare Epidemiology of America position paper on *Clostridium difficile*-associated diarrhea and colitis. *Infect Control Hosp Epidemiol* 1995;16:459–477.
111. Fekety R. Guidelines for the diagnosis and management of *Clostridium difficile*-associated diarrhea and colitis. *Am J Gastroenterol* 1997;92:739–750.
112. Fekety R, Kim KH, Brown D, et al. Epidemiology of antibiotic-associated colitis: isolation of *Clostridium difficile* from the hospital environment. *Am J Med* 1981;70:906–908.
113. Bettin KM, Clabots CR, Mathie P, et al. Effectiveness of liquid soap vs. chlorhexidine gluconate for the removal of *Clostridium difficile* from bare hands and gloved hands. *Infect Cont Hosp Epidemiol* 1994;15:697–702.
114. Nolan NPM, Kelly CP, Humphreys JFH, et al. An epidemic of pseudomembranous colitis: importance of person-to-person spread. *Gut* 1987;28:1467–1473.
115. Bender BS, Bennett R, Laughon BE, et al. Is *Clostridium difficile* endemic in chronic-care facilities? *Lancet* 1986;2:11–13.
116. Brown E, Talbot GM, Axelrod P, et al. Risk factors for *Clostridium difficile* toxin-associated diarrhea. *Infect Control Hosp Epidemiol* 1990;11:283–290.
117. Malamou-Ladas H, Farrell SO, Nash JO, et al. Isolation of *Clostridium difficile* from patients and the environment of hospital wards. *J Clin Pathol* 1983;6:88–92.
118. Burdon DW. *Clostridium difficile*: the epidemiology and prevention of hospital-acquired infection. *Infection* 1982;10:203–204.
119. Savage AM, Alford RH. Nosocomial spread of *Clostridium difficile. Infect Control* 1983;4:31–33.
120. Brooks S, Real R, Kramer M, et al. *Clostridium difficile* associated diarrhea. *Infect Control Hosp Epidemiol* 1990;11:574.
121. Brooks S, Khan A, Stoica D, et al. Reduction in vancomycin-resistant *Enterococcus* and *Clostridium difficile* infections following change to tympanic thermometers. *Infect Control Hosp Epidemiol* 1998;19:333–336.
122. Hughes CE, Gebhard RL, Peterson LR, et al. Efficacy of routine fiberoptic endoscope cleaning and disinfection for killing *Clostridium difficile. Gastrointest Endosc* 1986;32:7–9.

123. Rutala WA, Gergen MF, Weber DJ. Inactivation of spores by disinfectants. *Infect Control Hosp Epidemiol* 1993;14:36–39.
124. Mayfield JL, Leet T, Miller J, et al. Environmental control to reduce transmission of *Clostridium difficile. Clin Infect Dis* 2000;31: 995–1000.
125. Wilcox MH, Fawley WN, Wigglesworth N, et al. Comparison of the effect of detergent versus hypochlorite cleaning on environmental contamination and incidence of *Clostridium difficile* infection. *J Hosp Infect* 2003;54:109–114.
126. Delmee M, Vandercam B, Avesani V, et al. Epidemiology and prevention of *Clostridium difficile* infections in a leukemia unit. *Eur J Clin Microbiol* 1987;6:623–627.
127. Kerr RB, McLaughlin DI, Sonnenberg LW. Control of *Clostridium difficile* colitis outbreak by treating asymptomatic carriers with metronidazole. *Am J Infect Control* 1990;18:332–333.
128. Thibault A, Miller MA, Gaese C. Risk factors for the development of *Clostridium difficile* associated diarrhea during a hospital outbreak. *Infect Control Hosp Epidemiol* 1991;12:345–348.
129. Surawicz CM, Elmer GW, Speelman P, et al. Prevention of antibiotic-associated diarrhea by *Saccharomyces boulardii:* a prospective study. *Gastroenterology* 1989;96:981–988.
130. Lyerly DM, Bostwick EF, Binion SB, et al. Passive immunization of hamsters against disease caused by *Clostridium difficile* by use of bovine immunoglobulin G concentrate. *Infect Immun* 1991;59:2215–2218.
131. Lewis SJ, Potts LF, Barry RE. The lack of therapeutic effect of *Saccharomyces boulardii* in the prevention of antibiotic-related diarrhoea in elderly patients. *J Infect* 1998;36:171–174.
132. Sambol SP, Merrigan MM, Tang JK, et al. Colonization for the prevention of *Clostridium difficile* disease in hamsters. *J Infect Dis* 2002; 186:1781–1789.
133. Johnson S, Gerding DN. *Clostridium difficile*–associated diarrhea. *Clin Infect Dis* 1998;26:1027–1036.

B

Mycobacterial Infections

37

MYCOBACTERIUM TUBERCULOSIS

KELLY L. MOORE
SAMUEL W. DOOLEY
WILLIAM R. JARVIS

Tuberculosis (TB) is a major global health problem. Worldwide, an estimated 8 million new cases occur each year and 2 million deaths are attributed to this disease annually (1). TB case rates in the United States have been decreasing since the most recent peak in cases in 1992, but an increasing number of TB outbreaks in institutional settings, including hospitals, has been noted. Of greatest concern are outbreaks due to microorganisms resistant to multiple anti-TB drugs (2).

THE ETIOLOGIC AGENT

Tuberculosis is caused by bacteria of the *Mycobacterium tuberculosis* complex, which includes *M. tuberculosis, M. bovis, M. bovis* [bacille Calmette Guérin (BCG)], *M. africanum,* and *M. microti. M. tuberculosis* is by far the most frequent and most important pathogen in this complex. It grows slowly and is usually identified by its rough, nonpigmented, corded colonies on oleic acid albumin agar; a positive niacin test; generally weak catalase activity, which is lost completely by heating to 68°C; and a positive nitrate reduction test. *M. bovis* is indistinguishable from *M. tuberculosis* except by culture followed by *in vitro* tests, restriction fragment length polymorphism (RFLP), or phage typing (3,4).

MODE OF TRANSMISSION

M. tuberculosis is carried in airborne droplet nuclei, which are produced when persons with pulmonary or laryngeal TB cough, sneeze, speak, or sing. The nuclei also can be produced by irrigation or manipulation of tuberculous lesions or processing of tissue or secretions in the hospital or laboratory. Droplet nuclei are so small (1 to 5 μm) and light that ambient air currents can keep them airborne for long periods of time and carry them for substantial distances. Persons who breathe air contaminated with infectious droplet nuclei (i.e., droplet nuclei that contain tubercle bacilli) may inhale microorganisms into the alveoli of the lungs and become infected. The risk of infection is correlated with the concentration of infectious droplet nuclei in the air and the duration of exposure to the contaminated air. Airborne transmission of *M. bovis* also can occur.

PATHOGENESIS OF TUBERCULOSIS

Once tubercle bacilli become implanted in a respiratory bronchiole or alveolus, they are engulfed by macrophages, but they can remain viable and even multiply within the cells. The tubercle bacilli are spread via the lymphatic channels to regional lymph nodes and via the bloodstream to more distant sites. A specific cell-mediated immune response, which usually develops several weeks after infection, usually limits further multiplication of the bacilli; the lesions heal, although the tubercle bacilli may remain viable. This condition, which is referred to as latent *M. tuberculosis* infection (LTBI), is asymptomatic and noncontagious. Bacilli deposited in some sites, such as the upper lung zones, kidneys, bones, and brain, may find an environment favorable for growth before specific immunity develops and limits multiplication. Hypersensitivity to components of the microorganism, as demonstrated by the development of a positive reaction to the tuberculin skin test, develops 2 to 10 weeks after the initial infection.

At any point after the first infection, tubercle bacilli that have spread through the body may begin to replicate and produce active disease. In approximately 5% of all infected persons, disease occurs within 1 year of infection. In another 5%, containment of the infection fails at a later time and disease results. The most common site for this reactivation of infection is the upper lung zone, but foci anywhere in the body can be the sites of disease. The ability of the host to contain the infection is reduced by certain diseases, especially human immunodeficiency virus (HIV) infection, silicosis, and diabetes mellitus, as well as by treatment with corticosteroids or other immunosuppressive drugs. In these circumstances, the likelihood of TB developing can be greater than 10% per year (5). For persons with LTBI, the risk of progressing to active disease is greatly reduced in persons with drug susceptible strains by preventive therapy with isoniazid (or rifampin).

CLINICAL FEATURES

Early symptoms of TB include fatigue, anorexia, weight loss, or low-grade fevers. However, a few patients may present with an acute febrile illness. Erythema nodosum may occur with the acute onset of TB.

Pulmonary TB is the most common form of the disease, and the most important from the perspective of hospital infection control. In pulmonary TB, there is insidious onset of cough, which usually progresses slowly over weeks or months to become more frequent and associated with the production of mucoid or mucopurulent sputum. Hemoptysis also may occur. Some patients present with the acute onset of productive cough, fever, chills, myalgia, and sweating similar to the signs and symptoms of influenza, acute bronchitis, or pneumonia. Hoarseness or a sore throat may suggest tuberculous laryngitis. Laryngeal involvement with TB is usually associated with extensive pulmonary involvement, a large number of microorganisms in the sputum, and a very high degree of contagiousness. Physical findings of pulmonary TB may include crackles or signs of lung consolidation.

The infectiousness of a TB patient correlates with the number of microorganisms expelled into the air; this correlates with the site of disease (pulmonary, laryngeal, tracheal, or endobronchial TB being the most infectious), the presence of cough (or performance of cough inducing procedures), the presence of acid-fast bacilli (AFB) on sputum smears, the presence of cavitation on chest radiograph, the duration of adequate chemotherapy, and the ability or willingness of the patient to cover his or her mouth when coughing.

Other clinical manifestations of the disease include tuberculous pleuritis, hematogenous dissemination (miliary TB), genitourinary tract TB, TB of the lymph nodes, skeletal TB, tuberculous meningitis, tuberculous peritonitis, or tuberculous pericarditis.

In addition to these sites, there are many other potential body sites where TB may occur less commonly. TB in most of these extrapulmonary sites, without pulmonary or laryngeal involvement, usually is not contagious. However, irrigation or other manipulation of tuberculous lesions can produce infectious droplet nuclei and result in transmission of *M. tuberculosis*, as can laboratory processing of specimens that contain *M. tuberculosis*. Standard textbooks can be consulted for information on disease at these sites.

DIAGNOSIS

Radiography

In patients who have signs or symptoms suggesting pulmonary or pleural TB, standard posterior-anterior and lateral radiographs of the chest should be obtained. Special imaging techniques, such as computed tomography or magnetic resonance imaging, may be of value in defining nodules, cavities, cysts, calcifications, contours of large bronchi, or vascular details in lung parenchyma.

The radiographic manifestation of initial infection in the lung, whether in a child or an adult, is usually parenchymal infiltration accompanied by ipsilateral lymph node enlargement. The parenchymal lesion may be detected at any stage of development and in any portion of the lung, or it may be too small to be seen on the radiograph.

In adults with progression to disease from LTBI, the common presentation is lesions in the apical and posterior segments of the upper lobes or in the superior segments of the lower lobes. However, lesions may appear in any segment. Cavitation is common except in immunocompromised patients. Other findings include atelectasis and fibrotic scarring with retraction of the hilus and deviation of the trachea. Rarely, patients may present with normal chest radiographs, particularly patients with HIV infection or other conditions associated with severe cell-mediated immunosuppression and endobronchial TB.

Hematogenous TB is characterized by diffuse, finely nodular, uniformly distributed lesions on the chest radiograph. The word *miliary* is applied to this appearance, because the nodules are about the size of millet seeds (approximately 2 mm in diameter). Unilateral or, rarely, bilateral pleural effusion usually is the only radiographic abnormality evident with pleural TB.

Laboratory Procedures

The identification of *M. tuberculosis* microorganisms is of great importance for diagnosing TB. Therefore, careful attention should be given to the collection and handling of specimens. Specimens should be transported to the laboratory and processed as soon as possible after collection.

Because TB may occur in almost any body site, a variety of specimens may be appropriate to collect, including sputum (natural or induced), bronchial washings or biopsy material, gastric aspirates, urine, cerebrospinal fluid, pleural fluid, pus, endometrial scrapings, bone marrow biopsy, or other biopsy or resected tissue. All of these materials should be stained and examined by microscopy for the presence of AFB and should be cultured for mycobacteria.

The detection of AFB in stained smears is the easiest and quickest procedure that can be performed, and it provides preliminary support for the diagnosis. Also, the smear is of importance in assessing the patient's degree of infectiousness. The use of fluorescence microscopy allows the smears to be read much more rapidly than does standard microscopy. If necessary for confirmation, smears stained for fluorescence microscopy can be over-stained and examined by standard light microscopy under an oil immersion lens.

All specimens from patients suspected of having *M. tuberculo-*

sis disease should be inoculated (after appropriate digestion and decontamination, if required) onto appropriate culture media such as Lowenstein-Jensen or Middlebrook 7H10.

Genotyping, or DNA fingerprinting, of *M. tuberculosis* is used to determine the clonality of bacterial cultures. Because this technology is useful for studying the molecular epidemiology of *M. tuberculosis* and investigating outbreaks, the Centers for Disease Control and Prevention (CDC) established a National TB Genotyping and Surveillance Network in the 1990s. This diagnostic technique in conjunction with traditional epidemiologic methods has enhanced TB surveillance and control programs (6) and has been instrumental in the identification of several pseudo-outbreaks of active TB caused by laboratory cross-contamination of sputum samples from patients without clinical signs of TB (7–10).

Drug Susceptibility Testing

The initial isolate from all patients with positive cultures for *M. tuberculosis* should be tested for susceptibility to anti-TB drugs. Drug susceptibility tests for *M. tuberculosis* are important for choosing the most effective treatment regimen. The laboratory should report to the clinician the amount of growth on drug-containing medium as compared with growth on drug-free control medium. By counting the colonies on the drug-containing medium and on the control medium, the proportion of resistant cells in the total population can be calculated and expressed as a percentage. Generally, when 1% or more of a bacillary population become resistant to the critical concentration of a drug, then that agent is not, or soon will not be, useful for continued therapy, because the resistant population will soon predominate. If broth culture is used, results are reported as resistant or susceptible, and no colony percentage is reported.

Newer Diagnostic Techniques

Radiometric Technology

Compared with standard culture methods using solid media, radiometric culture methods, which employ a ^{14}C-labeled substrate medium that is almost specific for mycobacteria, provide much more rapid detection of growth and rapid drug susceptibility testing. These automated broth culture systems using Middlebrook 7H12 media with added material for detection of mycobacteria can detect growth in 1 to 3 weeks, compared to 3 to 8 weeks for solid media. However, at least one container of solid culture media should be used in conjunction with broth culture systems (11). Combining radiometric culture with techniques for rapid species identification (e.g., genetic probes, high-performance liquid chromatography, or monoclonal antibodies) can further shorten the time required for species identification.

Genetic Probes

Genetic probes offer tremendous promise for providing rapid identification. One such probe, a nucleic acid amplification (NAA) test (Gen-Probe, San Diego, CA), has been approved by the U.S. Food and Drug Administration (FDA) for detection of *M. tuberculosis* in AFB smear-positive or smear-negative respiratory specimens in patients suspected of having TB. Another NAA test (Amplicor, Roche Diagnostic Systems, Branchburg, NJ) is approved by the FDA only for use on AFB smear-positive respiratory specimens. Patients with AFB-positive sputum smears and positive NAA tests may be presumed and are likely to have TB. An AFB smear-positive specimen with a negative NAA test must be tested further for the presence of inhibitors; if none are present, the patient can be presumed to have nontuberculous mycobacterial infection and is unlikely to have TB. If two of no more than four sputum specimens are AFB smear negative but NAA test positive, the patient can be presumed to have TB (12). Probes specific for the genus *Mycobacterium,* the *M. tuberculosis* complex, and the two species *M. avium* and *M. intracellulare* are available.

Diagnosis of Latent Tuberculosis Infection

Tuberculin Skin Test

The tuberculin skin test (TST) is the standard method available for identifying persons infected with *M. tuberculosis* (11,13). Currently available TSTs remain substantially less than 100% sensitive and specific for detection of infection with *M. tuberculosis.* Some causes of false-negative reactions are shown in Table 37.1. False-positive reactions can be due to prior infection with other mycobacteria, BCG vaccination, or problems with the an-

TABLE 37.1. FACTORS CAUSING DECREASED ABILITY TO RESPOND TO TUBERCULIN SKIN TESTS

Factors related to the person being tested
Infections
Viral (measles, mumps, chicken pox, HIV)
Bacterial (typhoid fever, brucellosis, typhus, leprosy, pertussis, overwhelming tuberculosis, tuberculous pleurisy)
Fungal (South American blastomycosis)
Live virus vaccination (measles, mumps, polio, varicella)
Metabolic derangements (chronic renal failure)
Low protein states (severe protein depletion, afibrinogenemia)
Diseases affecting lymphoid organs (Hodgkin's disease, lymphoma, chronic leukemia, sarcoidosis)
Drugs (corticosteroids and many other immunosuppressive agents)
Age (newborns, elderly patients)
Stress (surgery, burns, mental illness, graft-versus-host reactions)
Factors related to the tuberculin used
Improper storage (exposure to light and heat)
Improper dilutions
Chemical denaturation
Contamination
Adsorption (partially controlled by adding Tween 80)
Factors related to the method of administration
Injection of too little antigen
Subcutaneous injection
Delayed administration after drawing into syringe
Injection too close to other skin tests
Factors related to reading the test and recording results
Inexperienced reader
Conscious or unconscious bias
Error in recording

From American Thoracic Society/CDC. Diagnostic standards and classification of tuberculosis in adults and children. *Am J Respir Crit Care Med* 2000; 161: 1376–1395.

tigen. Anecdotal reports also have raised concern that different commercially available reagents produce different degrees of induration (14); however, a large scale study of the two reagents available in the U.S. revealed comparable specificity in people at low risk for tuberculous infection (15).

The intradermal administration of 0.1 mL purified protein derivative (PPD) tuberculin into the skin of the volar surface of the forearm (Mantoux technique) is the preferred method of performing the TST. Tests should be read by a trained health professional between 48 and 72 hours after injection. The basis of reading is the presence or absence of induration, which should be measured transversely to the long axis of the forearm and recorded in millimeters.

The positive predictive value of the TST varies widely in relation to the prevalence of true *M. tuberculosis* infection in any given population; furthermore, as already noted, the risk of progression to disease from LTBI varies according to the characteristics of the infected person (11,13). Thus, to increase the likelihood that a positive test represents true infection with *M. tuberculosis* and to improve the benefit-to-risk ratio of preventive therapy, the cut point used for defining a positive TST is varied in different populations. A reaction ≥5 mm is considered positive in persons with HIV infection or severe immunosuppression, persons with close contacts of infectious TB cases, and persons with abnormal chest radiographs consistent with TB.

A reaction ≥10 mm is classified as positive in persons who do not meet the above criteria but who have other risk factors for TB. These would include (a) recent (≤5 years) immigrants from countries with a high prevalence of TB; (b) intravenous drug users; (c) residents and employees of high-risk congregate settings (e.g., correctional institutions, nursing homes, healthcare facilities, homeless shelters, or mental institutions); (d) persons with medical conditions that have been reported to increase the risk of TB (e.g., silicosis, gastrectomy, jejunoileal bypass, being 10% or more below ideal body weight, chronic renal failure, diabetes mellitus, some hematologic disorders such as leukemias and lymphomas, and carcinomas of the head, neck or lung); (e) mycobacteriology laboratory personnel; (f) children <4 years of age or infants, children, and adolescents exposed to adults in high-risk categories; and (g) other high-risk populations identified locally as having a relatively high incidence of TB.

A reaction of 15 mm is classified as positive in persons with no risk factors for TB.

The tuberculin test can be valuable for identifying persons newly infected with *M. tuberculosis* when repeated periodically in surveillance of tuberculin-negative persons likely to be exposed to TB (e.g., healthcare workers) (13). However, there are special considerations in identifying newly infected persons.

First, there are unavoidable errors in even the most carefully performed tests. For this reason, small increases in reaction size may not be meaningful. For persons whose previous reaction was negative, an increase in reaction size of 10 mm or more in diameter within a period of 2 years should be considered a skin test conversion. Healthcare workers with some degree of TST induration as a result of nontuberculous mycobacterial infection or previous vaccination with BCG have converted if induration increases by at least 10 mm over previous tests. For healthcare workers at low risk of exposure with a history of a negative TST, an increase of 15 mm within a 2-year period may be more appropriate for defining a recent conversion. Converters should be considered newly infected with *M. tuberculosis* and strongly considered for preventive therapy (11,16).

A second problem in identifying newly infected persons is the so-called booster phenomenon (17). Repeated testing of uninfected persons does not sensitize them to tuberculin. However, delayed hypersensitivity to tuberculin, once it has been established by infection with any species of mycobacteria or by BCG vaccination, may gradually wane over the years, resulting in a TST reaction that is negative. The stimulus of this test may recall the immune reaction, which results in an increase in the size of the reaction to a subsequent test, sometimes causing an apparent conversion that is then interpreted as indicating new infection. The booster effect can be seen on a second test done as soon as a week after the initial stimulating test and the booster effect can persist for a year and perhaps longer.

When tuberculin skin testing of adults is to be repeated periodically, the initial use of a two-step testing procedure can reduce the likelihood of interpreting a boosted reaction as representing recent infection (18). In two-step testing, an initial TST is performed. If the reaction to the first test is negative, a second test should be given from 1 to 3 weeks later. If the reaction to the second of the initial two tests reaches the appropriate cut point for a positive result in the patient, this probably represents a boosted reaction. On the basis of this second test result, the person should be classified as being previously infected and managed accordingly. If the second test result remains below the appropriate cut point, the person is classified as being uninfected. A positive reaction to a third test (with an appropriate increase) in such a person, within the next 2 years, is likely to represent the occurrence of new infection with *M. tuberculosis* in the interval.

Whole-Blood Interferon-γ Test

In 2001, a whole-blood interferon-γ test was approved by the FDA as an aid in detecting LTBI in addition to the TST. The test results are based on the quantity of interferon-γ released from sensitized lymphocytes in whole blood after incubation with tuberculin PPD and control antigens. It is less likely to be concordant with the TST in persons with a history of BCG vaccination and in persons with immune reactivity to nontuberculous mycobacteria (19). The advantages of this test are that it requires only one patient visit, does not boost immune response like the TST, and is less subject to reader bias and error. Its disadvantages are that it requires phlebotomy and processing within 12 hours. Its use can be considered for people who otherwise qualify for screening for LTBI, with some exceptions. The test should not be used for patients with suspected active TB, children aged <17 years, or patients with HIV or other conditions who may not mount an immune response. The test also is not indicated for contact tracing and evaluation because the length of time between exposure and a positive test is not yet established. The TST can be used to confirm the results of a positive interferon-γ test for persons at increased risk for LTBI. When the probability of LTBI is low, confirmation of a positive interferon-γ test is recommended. Negative interferon-γ test results do not require confirmation. The interferon-γ test should

TABLE 37.2. INTERIM RECOMMENDATIONS FOR APPLYING AND INTERPRETING QUANTIFERON TB (QFT)[a]

Reason for Testing	Population	Initial Screening	Positive Results	Evaluation
Suspect tuberculosis (TB)	Persons with symptoms of active TB	Tuberculin skin testing (TST) might be useful; QFT not recommended	Induration ≥5 mm	Chest radiograph, smears, and cultures, regardless of test results
Increased risk for progression to active TB, if infected	Persons with recent contact with TB, changes on chest radiograph consistent with prior TB, organ transplants, or human immuncodeficiency virus infection, and those receiving imumnosuppresaing drugs equivalent of ≥15 mg/day of prednisone for ≥1 month[b]	TST; QFT not recommended	Induration ≥5 mm	Chest radiograph if TST is positive; treat for latent TB infection (LTBI) after active TB disease is ruled out
	Persons with diabetes, silicosis, chronic renal failure, leukemia, lymphoma, carcinoma of the head, neck, or lung, and persons with weight loss of ≥10% of ideal body weight, gastrectomy, or jejunoileal bypass[b]	TST; QFT not recommended	Induration ≥10 mm	
Increased risk for LTBI	Recent immigrants, injection-drug users, and residents and employees of high-risk congregate settings (e.g., prisons, jails, homeless shelters, and certain healthcare facilities)[c]	TST or QFT	Induration ≥10 mm; percentage tuberculin response ≥15[d]	Chest radiograph if either test is positive; confirmatory TST is optional if QFT is positive; treat for LTBI after active TB disease is ruled out; LTBI treatment when only QFT is positive should be based on clinical judgment and estimated risk
Other reasons for testing among persons at low risk for LTBI	Military personnal, hospital staff, and healthcare workers whose risk of prior exposure to TB patients is low, and U.S. born students at certain colleges and universities[c]	TST or QFT	Induration ≥15 mm; percentage tuberculin response ≥30[d]	Chest radiograph if either test is positive; confirmatory TST if QFT is positive; treatment for LTBI (if QFT and TST are positive and after active TB disease is ruled out) on the basis of assessment of risk for drug toxicity, TB transmission, and patient preference

[a] QFT is available from Cellestis Ltd, Carnegie, Victoria, Australia.
[b] QFT has not been adequately evaluated among persons with these conditions; it is not recommended for such populations.
[c] QFT has not been adequately evaluated among persons aged <17 years, or among pregnant women; it is not recommended for such populations.
[d] The following additional conditions are required for QFT to indicate *Mycobacterlum tuberculosis* infection: (1) mitogen–nil and tuberculin–nil are both >1.5 IU. and (2) percentage avian difference is ≤10.
From Centers for Disease Control and Prevention. Guidelines for using the QuantiFERON® -TB test for diagnosis of latest Mycobacterium tuberculosis infection. *MMWR* ____; 51 : 1–5.

not be used to confirm a positive TST, as the TST may boost the immune response. The CDC guidelines for use and interpretation of the interferon-γ test are listed in Table 37.2 (20).

GENERAL EPIDEMIOLOGY OF TUBERCULOSIS IN THE UNITED STATES

In the U.S., TB affects certain segments of the population disproportionately, because the factors that affect the likelihood of exposure to and infection with *M. tuberculosis* and the likelihood of progression to disease from LTBI are not homogeneously distributed throughout the population.

For 2002, 15,078 episodes of TB were reported to the CDC, reflecting a rate of 5.2 cases per 100,000 population (21). This represents the tenth consecutive year that TB cases declined and a 5.7% decrease in the number of cases from 2001. Six percent of TB cases in 2001 were reported in children under 15 years of age, 10% in persons aged 15 to 24 years, 35% in persons aged 25 to 44 years, 28% in persons aged 45 to 64 years, and 21% in persons aged 65 years and older. Overall, 62% were males and 38% females (22).

The overall national trend reflects the impact of changes within population subgroups. During 1992 to 2002, there was a 62% decline in TB cases among U.S.-born persons of all age groups; 19,225 reported in 1992 versus 7,252 in 2002. In contrast, the number of cases among foreign-born persons increased 4%, from 7,270 in 1992 to 7,865 in 2001. U.S.-born non-Hispanic blacks comprised the largest number of TB cases among U.S.-born and foreign-born populations combined, representing 47% of TB cases in U.S.-born persons and approximately 25% of all cases.

The geographic distribution of TB in the U.S. also is not homogeneous. In 2002, seven states (California, Florida, Illinois, Georgia, New Jersey, New York, and Texas) reported 60% of all TB cases. However, by 2002, 23 of 50 states had met the Advisory Council for TB Elimination interim goal of ≤3.5 cases/100,000 population. Cases of TB remained concentrated in urban areas: in 2001, 39% of TB cases were reported from 64 major cities (23).

The proportion of isolates from persons with no history of TB resistant to at least isoniazid dropped from 8.4% to 7.1% during 1993 to 2001 (22). More than 85% of isolates were tested for drug susceptibility in these years. Ninety-two percent (11,787) of culture positive cases had drug susceptibility testing performed. Of these, 870 (7.4%) isolates were resistant to at least isoniazid, and 145 (1.2%) were multidrug resistant (MDR) TB (i.e., resistant to at least isoniazid and rifampin). Thirty-seven percent of all MDR-TB cases were reported from New York City (n = 26) and California (n = 27).

Data on the HIV status of persons with TB reported to the national TB surveillance system at the CDC is limited. Reporting of HIV status has improved slowly since 1993, the year such information was first included on TB case reports submitted to the CDC. In 2001, 3,254 (58%) of 5,630 TB case reports for persons aged 25 to 44 years included information about HIV status (22). In 2001, 26 states reported HIV test results for at least 75% of cases in persons in this age group. Of these 26 states, the percentage of TB cases in persons aged 25 to 44 years who were co-infected with HIV ranged from 0% (New Hampshire, South Dakota, and Wyoming) to >39% (District of Columbia and Florida). To help estimate the proportion of reported TB cases co-infected with HIV, state health departments have compared TB and acquired immunodeficiency syndrome (AIDS) registries. During 1993 to 1994, 14% of all TB cases (27% of cases in persons aged 25 to 44 years) had a match in the AIDS registry (24).

From 1953, when national reporting of incident TB cases was first fully implemented in the U.S., through 1984, the number of cases reported to the CDC decreased from 84,304 to 22,255. This average annual decline of 5% to 6% was interrupted only by a transient increase in 1980, which was attributed to cases arising from a large influx of refugees from Southeast Asia (25). Between 1984 and 1992, there was a dramatic reversal of the longstanding decline in the number of TB cases. From 1985 through 1992, reported cases increased 20.1%, from 22,201 to 26,673. Based on an extrapolation of the trend in cases observed from 1980 through 1984, approximately 52,000 excess cases of TB were reported to the CDC from 1985 through 1992 (26).

Increases in the number of cases in the late 1980s were mainly due to the HIV/AIDS epidemic and the emergence of MDR TB. Other contributing factors include (a) an increase in the number of cases occurring in persons who immigrate to the U.S. from areas of the world that have a high prevalence of TB; and (b) an increase in active transmission of *M. tuberculosis* caused largely by adverse social conditions and an inadequate healthcare infrastructure (26).

The decline in the overall number of reported TB cases and in the level of MDR TB since 1992 has been attributed to stronger TB controls that emphasize prompt identification of persons with TB, initiation of appropriate therapy, and ensuring completion of therapy. The declining TB trend among U.S.-born persons reflects the reduction of community transmission of *M. tuberculosis*, particularly in areas with a high incidence of HIV (27). In comparison, the relatively stable number of reported cases of TB among foreign-born persons indicate that most cases of active TB disease among foreign-born persons residing in the U.S. results from infection with *M. tuberculosis* in the person's country of birth (28). The CDC, in collaboration with state and local health departments, continues to focus on its comprehensive plan to reduce active TB disease among foreign-born persons residing in the U.S. This plan includes strategies to (a) improve case finding and completion of therapy, (b) conduct contact investigations, (c) screen those at high risk for infection, and (d) ensure completion of preventive therapy in eligible candidates (29).

EPIDEMIOLOGY OF NOSOCOMIAL TUBERCULOSIS IN THE UNITED STATES

Factors Influencing the Epidemiology of Nosocomial Tuberculosis

The factors that influence the epidemiology of nosocomial TB are the joint probabilities that exposure to *M. tuberculosis* will occur, exposure will result in infection, and infection will lead to active TB (Fig. 37.1). In a healthcare facility, the likelihood of exposure to *M. tuberculosis* may be affected by factors such as the prevalence of infectious TB in the population served by the facility; the degree of crowding in the facility; the effectiveness of the facility's TB infection control program in rapidly

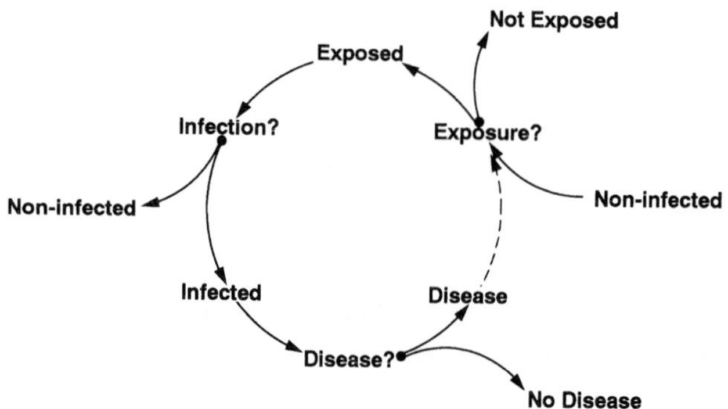

Figure 37.1. Schematic illustration of the steps involved in the acquisition of tuberculous infection and the development of active tuberculosis.

identifying, isolating, and treating persons with infectious TB; and the effectiveness of engineering controls, such as directional airflow and booths for cough-inducing procedures, in preventing the spread of contaminated air throughout the facility.

Factors that may affect the likelihood that exposure to *M. tuberculosis* will result in infection are largely related to the effectiveness of the facility's infection control program. These factors include the effectiveness of the program in identifying and successfully treating persons with infectious TB, thereby rendering them noninfectious; the effectiveness of engineering controls, such as ventilation and ultraviolet germicidal irradiation, in reducing the concentration of infectious droplet nuclei in the air; and the effectiveness of the respiratory protection program in preventing the inhalation of infectious droplet nuclei. Additionally, although supporting data are lacking, it is possible that medical conditions that cause severe suppression of cell-mediated immunity may increase susceptibility to infection with *M. tuberculosis*; thus, the prevalence of such conditions, either in patients or healthcare workers, may affect the likelihood that exposure of these persons will result in infection.

Factors that are likely to influence the risk that infection with *M. tuberculosis* will result in progression to active TB probably include the prevalence in the facility's patient and healthcare worker population of medical conditions that increase the likelihood of progression from LTBI to active disease (e.g., HIV infection). In addition, the infection control program's effectiveness in identifying persons who have been exposed and infected and providing them with appropriate preventive therapy is likely to influence the likelihood of progression to active disease. Events or conditions that alter any of these probabilities (the probability of exposure, infection, or progression to active TB) may result in changes in the epidemiology of TB in a healthcare facility.

Several types of information may be considered in describing the epidemiology of nosocomial TB. These include surveillance for active TB in healthcare workers, surveillance for TST conversions in healthcare workers, and reports of episodes of nosocomial *M. tuberculosis* transmission (such as reports of outbreaks).

Surveillance for Active Tuberculosis in Healthcare Workers

There are very few national data on the recent or current risk of active TB in healthcare workers. Information on the occupation of persons with TB was not collected in the national TB surveillance system until 1993, at which time limited variables on occupation were added to the data collection forms. However, without appropriate denominators, it is not possible to calculate incidence rates or relative risks for healthcare workers. In 2001, 50 of the reporting areas in the U.S. reported information on occupation for at least 75% of TB cases. There were 414 reported TB cases among healthcare workers in 2001, a slight decline when compared to the 427 cases reported in 2000 (22,30). The percentage of cases occurring among healthcare workers in 2001 ranged from 0% in the District of Columbia, Idaho, Indiana, Nevada, North Dakota, South Dakota, Utah, Vermont, West Virginia, and Wyoming to 6.6% in Massachusetts and 15.8% in New Hampshire.

In a questionnaire survey of medical school–affiliated physicians in California, Barrett-Connor (31) found that 3.5% had been treated for active TB. Seventy-five percent of cases of active disease began when the physicians were within 10 years of beginning medical school; 62% of cases of active disease followed infection acquired after beginning medical school. In the cohort of those who graduated between 1966 and 1975, disease rates after beginning medical school were 0% (0/54) among those who were tuberculin positive at entry; 1.0% (7/669) among those who were tuberculin negative at entry; and 10.0% (7/69) among those who became tuberculin positive after entry.

A questionnaire survey of 1938 to 1981 graduates of the University of Illinois Medical School found that, for most years, the incidence of TB in the cohort of graduates was higher than that in the general population (32). More than two thirds of all cases of TB occurred during medical school or within 6 years of graduation.

Finally, a review of the recorded occupations of persons with TB reported to the North Carolina TB control program found that TB case rates in hospital personnel in 1983 and 1984 were similar to or lower than rates in the general population (33). However, these data were not adjusted for age or race, nor was a definition of the term *hospital employee* provided.

In summary, data concerning the recent or current risk of active TB in healthcare workers in the U.S. are limited. Two questionnaire surveys suggest an increased risk among physicians, whereas a third study suggests that the risk for hospital employees in general is similar to that for the general population. The data from Barrett-Connor's survey suggest a protective effect of a previous positive TST. The incidence of TB is a relatively insensitive measure of the actual risk posed to healthcare workers by occupational exposure to *M. tuberculosis*. A more sensitive measure of this risk is the rate of TST conversions among healthcare workers.

Surveillance for TST Conversions in Healthcare Workers

The annual rate of TST conversions in healthcare workers is the best potential indicator of the risk of becoming infected with *M. tuberculosis* through occupational exposure in the healthcare setting. However, there is no systematic national surveillance for TST conversions in U.S. healthcare workers. In 1995, the CDC, in collaboration with selected state and local health departments, began a prospective TST surveillance project to estimate the incidence of occupational transmission of *M. tuberculosis* to healthcare workers. Participating sites (Florida, Massachusetts, Mississippi, New Jersey, New York City, San Francisco, and San Diego) were required to implement TST programs consistent with current CDC guidelines and to pilot test a CDC developed microcomputer software system, staffTrakTB, to assist with collection, tracking, management, and analysis of data (34). The project areas enrolled 26 facilities: eight hospitals, five health departments, two long-term-care facilities, three correctional facilities, and eight other facilities (including a state laboratory). From 1995 to 1997, a total of 29,004 healthcare workers were enrolled in the project; 9,088 (31.3%) were included in the analysis. TST conversions (i.e., $\geq$10 mm increase in reaction size on follow-up TST) were documented in 1.1% (104 of 9,

088) of healthcare workers (35). Conversion rates varied by project area, ranging from 0% in Florida to 4.2% in New York City, and by facility (correctional, 2.1%; health departments, 1.3%; hospitals, 1.0%; or nursing homes, 0.8%). TST conversion rates also varied by occupation of the healthcare worker (outreach worker, 4.2%; scientist, 2.7%; technician, 2.2%; nurse, 1.2%; housekeeper, 1.2%; clerical worker, 1.0%; administrator, 0.8%; attending physician, 0.6%; and social worker, 0.3%). TST conversion rates among nurses were highest in New York City (4.2%) and San Francisco (2.2%) and lowest in Mississippi (0.1%) and Florida (0%), probably reflecting an elevated risk of *M. tuberculosis* transmission in areas with high TB incidence such as New York City and San Francisco. Healthcare workers who were outreach workers, nonwhite, non–U.S.-born, or BCG-vaccinated were at a significantly higher risk of conversion. These data suggest that foreign-born status and certain occupations may be associated with an elevated risk of *M. tuberculosis* transmission, possibly reflecting more exposure to infectious individuals in the healthcare worker's household or community, and in certain healthcare settings.

There are several reports in the literature of the risk of TST conversion among U.S. healthcare workers (Table 37.3) (18,31, 33–59). These reports suggest that, since 1980, the risk of TST conversion among hospital employees in general has been about 1% or less.

One recently published prospective study followed workers at an urban hospital in a high TB-incidence area where TST screening was required of all eligible employees every 6 months (59). This study found an overall TST conversion rate of 0.38% per year. TST conversion was not associated with the degree of patient contact, but was associated with BCG vaccination, low annual salary, and increasing age. The researchers concluded that, in a hospital with an effective TB infection control program, TST conversion rates were low and that the most important risk factors for TST conversion among workers were not occupational.

At least two other studies have found a higher risk for TST conversion with increasing age of the workers (40,43). A third study that examined age as a risk factor for TST conversion found an association with increasing age when two-step skin testing was not used to establish the employees' baseline skin test status; however, when two-step testing was used to eliminate apparent conversions caused by the booster phenomenon, there was no longer any correlation between age and the risk of conversion (18). This finding suggests that the higher rate of apparent conversion sometimes observed in older workers may

TABLE 37.3. TUBERCULIN SKIN TEST CONVERSION RATES IN HEALTHCARE WORKERS UNITED STATES, 1960–1998

First Author (Reference)	Institution Location	Time Period	Population	Annual Conversion Rate (%)[a]
Levine (36)	Kings County Hospital Brooklyn, New York	1960–1967	Student nurses	1.05
Weiss (37)	Philadelphia General Hospital Philadelphia, Pennsylvania	1962–1971	Student nurses	4.20
Atuk (38)	University of Virginia Hospital Charlottesville, Virginia	1968–1969	Hospital employees	1.92
Gregg (39)	State Park Health Center South Carolina	1969–1973	Hospital employees	4.08
Berman (40)	Sinai Hospital of Baltimore Baltimore, Maryland	1971–1976	Hospital employees	1.41
Craven (41)	University of Virginia Hospital Charlottesville, Virginia	1972–1973	Hospital employees	0.52
Vogeler (42)	LDS Hospital Salt Lake City, Utah	1972–1975	Hospital employees	0.16
Ruben (43)	Montefiore Hospital Pittsburgh, Pennsylvania	1973–1975	Hospital employees	3.07
Ktsanes (44)	Charity Hospital New Orleans, Louisiana	1972–1981	Hospital employees	1.04
Barrett-Connor (31)	Multiple institutions California	1974–1975	Medical school-affiliated physicians	0.4–1.8
Weinstein (45)	Mount Sinai School of Medicine New York City	1974–1982	Medical students	0.13
Chan (46)	Jackson Memorial Hospital Miami, Florida	1978–1981	House staff	3.96
Bass (18)	University of South Alabama Medical Center Mobile, Alabama	1979	Hospital employees	2.9
Thompson (47)	10 hospitals 9 states[b]	1979	Hospital employees	2.9
Kantor (43)	Veterans Administration Medical Center Chicago, Illinois	1979–1986	Hospital employees	0.94
Price (33)	167 hospitals North Carolina	1980–1984	Hospital employees	1.14
Aitken (49)	114 hospitals Washington	1982–1984	Hospital employees	0.87
Malasky (50)	Multiple Institutions Multiple U.S. cities	1984–1986	Pulmonary fellows	5.65
Raad (51)	Shands Hospital Gainesville, Florida	1984–1987	Hospital employees	0.13
Raad (51)	Florida State Psychiatric Hospital Chattahoochee, Florida	1985–1987	Hospital employees	0.42
Ramirez (52)	Humana Hospital University of Louisville Louisville, Kentucky	1986–1991	Hospital employees	0.68
Ikeda (53)	Health Science Center State University of New York Syracuse, New York	1989–1990	Hospital employees	0.84
Ramaswamy (54)	Bronx, New York	1990–1993	Hospital employees	1.40
Zahnow (55)	Multiple institutions providing HIV-related healthcare	1992–1993	House staff	3.00
Christie (56)	Children's Hospital Medical Center Cincinnati, Ohio	1986–1994	Hospital employees	0.03–0.28
Panlilio (57)	5 hospitals New York City, Boston, Massachusetts	1994–1995	Hospital employees	1.61
Manangan (58)	Multiple institutions multiple cities	1996	Hospital employees	0.27[a]
Larsen (59)	Grady Memorial Hospital Atlanta, Georgia	1994–1998	Hospital employees	0.38

[a] In some cases, the annual conversion rate has been recalculated from data provided in the article referenced.
[b] The nine states are Pennsylvania, Colorado, Maryland, Texas, New Mexico, Ohio, Montana, New Hampshire, and Georgia.

actually be the result of an increased level of boosting in older persons.

Race has been found to correlate with risk of TST conversion in two studies. One of these reported a higher risk among nonwhites compared with whites, as well as a higher risk among employees in the lowest socioeconomic quintile (40). The other found a higher risk of TST conversion among black employees than among nonblacks; however, among blacks, the risk was higher among nurses than among persons in other job categories (44). In the one study that examined gender as a potential risk factor, no association was found between gender and the risk of TST conversion (40). A survey that included multiple institutions throughout North Carolina found that the risk of conversion varied according to geographic region within the state (33).

Few reported studies have examined the relationship between job category and risk of TST conversions. One study found a higher risk of conversion among persons in laundry, housekeeping, and engineering and maintenance departments than among persons in other departments (40). A second study found a higher conversion rate among nurses than among persons in other job categories (44). A third study found higher conversion rates among admissions clerks, phlebotomists, and nurse technicians than among respiratory therapists, environmental services workers, or registered nurses (52). A survey of self-reported TST conversions among medical fellows at multiple institutions found a higher reported rate of conversion among pulmonary fellows than among infectious diseases fellows (50). Finally, a survey of self-reported TST conversions among medical school–affiliated physicians in California found that physicians in the major clinical specialties reported comparable infection rates before and during medical school, but that rates after medical school were highest in medicine, pediatrics, and surgery; intermediate in obstetrics and gynecology and orthopedics; and lowest in radiology and psychiatry (31). In this survey, the cumulative percentage of tuberculin-positive physicians was at least twice the estimated age-specific infection rate for the general U.S. population.

Several studies have found higher conversion rates among workers with a higher likelihood of exposure to patients with TB than among those with a relatively lower likelihood of such exposure (38,39,41,42,57,58). In contrast, in a hospital in Pennsylvania, the reported conversion rates for groups with high or low degrees of exposure to patients with TB were not significantly different (43). Similarly, in a multi-institution survey in Washington, reported conversion rates were not significantly different in hospitals that had admitted no patients with TB compared with hospitals that had admitted patients with AFB smear-negative TB or hospitals that had admitted patients with AFB smear-positive TB (49). In this study, however, postexposure conversions were excluded from analysis, and there was no analysis by risk of exposure within the hospitals that did admit TB patients. A study from Florida reported a higher conversion rate among employees in a psychiatric hospital, in which there was presumably a low risk of exposure, than in a general hospital in which the risk of exposure was presumably higher (51). Again, this study did not examine the risk of TST conversion according to the likelihood of exposure within each hospital. Finally, a prospective study to assess the prevalence of TST positivity among healthcare workers providing service to HIV-infected persons found no association between the amount or type of contact with HIV-infected individuals and the risk of TB infection (55). Therefore, according to this study, caring for HIV-infected patients was not related to an increased rate of TB infections among healthcare workers in these settings.

These studies, in addition to being few in number, have substantial limitations. With the exception of one study (59), most are retrospective; the populations being studied often are not well defined; participation rates are not consistently reported but are variable and often quite low; the methods of applying and reading the tests are variable and often rely on employees' self-reporting of results; two-step testing to establish a baseline is rarely used; the definitions of positive skin tests and of TST conversions are not always specified and are variable; the classification of job categories and definitions of exposure are inconsistent; there are essentially no data on background risk in the community or on the performance of serial tuberculin testing in the general population from which to make estimates of attributable risk; the analyses often are insufficiently detailed to allow an estimation of relative risks for different job categories; and problems with the specificity and positive predictive value of the TST rarely are addressed adequately. Furthermore, the antigens used often are not described and appear to vary between, and possibly within, studies. It has been noted that a change in products can result in an increase in the conversion rate or pseudo-outbreak (14). For these reasons, interpretation of the data is difficult, and comparison of data from different studies is problematic. In spite of all these limitations, it is interesting that the overall risk among hospital employees in general seems to be fairly consistent.

In summary, available data suggest that the risk of TST conversion among hospital employees in general is approximately 1% or less. The data, although conflicting, also suggest that there may be substantial variation in risk according to the type of hospital, geographic location, occupational category, and a priori likelihood of exposure. Interpretation of the data is made difficult by methodologic limitations, by the lack of specificity and positive predictive value of the TST, by the difficulty of differentiating occupational risk from exposure in the community, and by an inadequate understanding of serial TSTs reflected in some studies.

Nosocomial Outbreaks of Tuberculosis

A nosocomial outbreak of TB may be defined as transmission of *M. tuberculosis* in a healthcare setting, resulting in the acquisition of LTBI or development of TB among exposed persons. There is no systematic national surveillance for nosocomial TB outbreaks; therefore, data on such outbreaks are limited to reports in the literature. Since 1960, at least 40 nosocomial outbreaks occurring in the U.S. have been reported in the literature (Table 37.4) (48,53–55,60–96).

The reported outbreaks have occurred in a wide variety of geographic areas. Most have occurred in general medical-surgical hospitals; one occurred in a health department clinic, one in an outpatient methadone treatment program, one in an outpatient hemodialysis unit, one in a pediatric office, one in two nursing

TABLE 37.4. REPORTED NOSOCOMIAL OUTBREAKS OF TUBERCULOSIS (TB), UNITED STATES, 1960–1999

Type of Facility, First Author (Reference)	Setting	Patients (Including Source)		Healthcare Workers (Including Source)		Contributing Factors
		Infection	Active Disease	Infection	Active Disease	
Medical school/medical center, northeastern U.S. 1962–1964	—	—	—	—	27	Undiagnosed, untreated pulmonary TB
Alpert (60) Municipal general hospital Miami, Florida 1969 Ehrenkranz (61)	Emergency department; inpatient medical ward; intensive care unit	—	1[a]	23/100 (23%)	2	Undiagnosed, untreated pulmonary TB Positive pressure ventilation Endotracheal inlubation Nasotracheal suctioning Air recirculation
University-affiliated hospital, San Diego, California 1980 Catanzaro (62)	Intensive care unit	—	1[a]	14/45 (31%)	—	Undiagnosed, untreated pulmonary TB Bronchoscopy Endotracheal intubation and suctioning Inadequate ventilation rate
General hospital, Dallas, Texas 1983–1984 Haley (63)	Emergency department; intensive care unit; radiology suite	—	3[a]	26/160 (16.3%)	7	Newly diagnosed, untreated pulmonary TB Endotracheal intubation and suctioning Air recirculation Inadequate respiratory protection
Community hospital, Arkansas (rural) 1985 Hutton (64)	Surgical suite; Inpatient medical ward; Intensive care unit	0%–67%	3[a]	59/492 (12%)	5	Undiagnosed, untreated tuberculous abscess Positive pressure ventilation Surgical drainage of abscess Irrigation of abscess
Veterans Administration Medical Center, Chicago, Illinois 1985 Kantor (48)	Inpatient medical ward; radiology suite; autopsy room	—	1[a]	8/55 (14.5%)	3	Undiagnosed, untreated pulmonary TB No control of directional airflow Nasotracheal suctioning Inadequate ventilation rate Autopsy
Municipal general hospital, San Juan, Puerto Rico 1987–1989 Dooley (65)	Inpatient HIV ward	—	8[a]	—	—	Undiagnosed, untreated pulmonary TB Delayed isolation Positive pressure ventilation Immunocompromised patients (HIV)
Health department clinic, West Palm Beach 1988 Calder (66)	Outpatient clinic	—	1[a]	17/63 (27%)	—	Positive pressure ventilation Aerosolized pentamidine treatments Inadequate ventilation rate Air recirculation
Community general hospital, Amarillo, Texas 1989 Pierce (67)	Inpatient medical ward; hospice	—	1[a]	30/158 (19%)	1	Undiagnosed, untreated pulmonary TB
University-affiliated hospital, Pittsburgh, Pennsylvania 1990–1991 Jereb (68) Sundberg (69)	Inpatient medical ward (renal transpiant unit)	7	11[a]	2	0	Undiagnosed, untreated pulmonary TB Positive pressure ventilation Bronchoscopy Endotracheal intubation Inadequate ventilation rate Immunocompromised patients (renal transplant)

(continued)

TABLE 37.4. *(continued)*

Type of Facility, First Author (Reference)	Setting	Patients (Including Source)		Healthcare Workers (Including Source)		Contributing Factors
		Infection	Active Disease	Infection	Active Disease	
Urban general hospital, Atlanta, Georgia 1991–1992 Zaza (70)	Inpatient medical ward	—	3	50/131 (38%)	8[b]	Undiagnosed, untreated pulmonary TB Positive pressure ventilation Inadequate ventilation rate
Community hospital, Rochester, New York 1992 Frampton (71)	Inpatient medical-surgical ward	—	1[a]	12/59 (20%)	2	Undiagnosed, untreated tuberculous ulcer Surgical debridement of ulcer Dressing changes
Multidrug-resistant outbreaks						
Municipal general hospital, Miami, Florida 1988–1990 Beck-Sagué (72)	Inpatient HIV ward; outpatient HIV clinic	—	29[a]	13/39 (33%)	—	Undiagnosed, untreated pulmonary TB Unrecognized drug resistance Lapses in isolation practices Positive pressure ventilation Aerosolized pentamidlne treatments Air recirculation Immunocompromised patients (HIV)
Urban voluntary hospital, New York City 1989–1990 Edlin (73)	Inpatient medical ward	—	18[a]	—	1	Undiagnosed, untreated pulmonary TB Positive pressure ventilation Immunocompromised patients (HIV)
Urban voluntary hospital, New York City 1989–1991 CDC (74)	Inpatient HIV ward; Inpatient prison ward	—	17[c]	—	—	Undiagnosed, untreated pulmonary TB Unrecognized drug resistance No control of directional air flow Lapses in isolation practices Inadequate ventilation rate Immunocompromised patients (HIV)
Urban teaching hospital, New York City 1989–1991 Pearson (75)	Inpatient HIV ward; inpatient medical ward	—	23[a]	11/32 (34%)	—	Undiagnosed, untreated pulmonary TB Lapses in isolation practices Positive pressure ventilation Immunocompromised patients (HIV)
General teaching hospital, Upstate New York 1991 Ikeda (53)	Inpatient medical wards	—	6[a]	46/696 (6.6%)	—	Positive pressure ventilation Prolonged infectiousness Immunocompromised patients (HIV)
Urban tertiary care hospital, New York City 1990–1991 Coronado (76)	Inpatient medical wards	—	15[a]	—	1	No control of directional air flow Lapses in isolation practices Inadequate ventilation rate Immunocompromised patients (HIV)
Veterans Administration Medical Center, New Jersey 1990–1992 Coronado (77)	Inpatient infectious diseases ward	—	13[a]	5/10 (50%)	—	Positive pressure ventilation Lapses in isolation practices Inadequate ventilation rate Inadequate use of respiratory protection by workers Immunocompromised patients (HIV)

(continued)

TABLE 37.4. *(continued)*

Type of Facility, First Author (Reference)	Setting	Patients (Including Source)		Healthcare Workers (Including Source)		Contributing Factors
		Infection	Active Disease	Infection	Active Disease	
Urban general hospital, New York City 1991–1992 CDC (78)	Inpatient HIV ward	—	37	—	—[a]	Undiagnosed, untreated pulmonary TB Lapses in isolation practices Positive pressure ventilation Immunocompromised patients (HIV)
Teaching hospital, New York City 1989–1992 Jereb (79)	Inpatient medical ward	—	—	88/352 (25%)	6	Lapses in isolation practices
Multiple hospitals, New York City 1990–1993 Frieden (80)	—	—	256	—	15[b]	Lapses in isolation practices
Community hospital, La Mirada, California 1992 Griffith (81)	Emergency room; medical intensive care unit	—	1	13/20 (65%)	3	Undiagnosed TB Positive pressure ventilation Lack of respiratory protection by workers
Urban hospital, New York City 1993–1994 Nivin (82)	Nursery; medical ward	— —	4 17[b]	— —	3 —	Undiagnosed TB Lapses in isolation practices
Community hospital, South Carolina 1994 Luby (83)	Inpatient medical ward	—	1	12/28 (43%)	—	Unrecognized TB
Private hospital, Chicago, IL 1994–1995 Kenyon (84)	Inpatient medical ward	—	6	11/74 (15%)	1	Immunocompromised patients (HIV)
General hospital, South Carolina 1995 Agerton (85)	Bronchoscopy room	—	4[b]	—	—	Contaminated bronchoscope
Teaching hospital, Baltimore, MD 1996 Michele (86)	Bronchoscopy room	—	4	—	—	Contaminated bronchoscope
Urban teaching hospital, Tennessee 1992 Haas (87)	Inpatient medical ward	—	2	35/172 (20.3%)	1	Undiagnosed pulmonary tuberculosis, immunocompromised patients (HIV)
Outpatient clinic, New Jersey 1992–1993 Askew (88)	Pediatric office	3	—	2	1	Undiagnosed TB
General hospital, New York 1996–1997 Lee (89)	Neonatal intensive care unit	—[e]	1	2/260 (0.8%)	—	Undiagnosed TB, positive pressure ventilation, suctioning
Community hospital, Arizona 1996 Spark (90)	Nursery	—	1	1/119 (0.8%)	—	Undiagnosed TB, inadequate use of respiratory protection during endotracheal intubation
Nursing homes, community hospital, Arkansas 1995–1998 Ijaz (91)	Two nursing homes; one community hospital ward	24/98 (24%)	2	48/320 (15%)	2	Undiagnosed TB

(continued)

TABLE 37.4. *(continued)*

Type of Facility, First Author (Reference)	Setting	Patients (Including Source)		Healthcare Workers (Including Source)		Contributing Factors
		Infection	Active Disease	Infection	Active Disease	
Community hospital, California 1998 Linquist (92)	Outpatient hemodialysis unit	12/89 (13%) no prior TST	—	1/23 (4%)	1	Anergy of case patient
Community hospital, Wisconsin 1999 Ramsey (93)	Bronchoscopy suite	10	2/10 (20 %)	1	—	Contamination of bronchoscope in procedure on TB patient, inadequate bronchoscope reprocessing procedure, inadequate use of respiratory protection by worker
HIV dental clinic, New York City 1990–1991 Cleveland (94)	Clinic	—	—	—	2[b]	Undiagnosed TB, inadequate use of respiratory protection by workers, immunocompromised patients and workers (HIV), lack of screening program for workers
Urban hospital Chicago 1994–1995 Kenyon (95)	Inpatient medical ward	—	6[b]	11/74 (15%)	1[b]	Immunocompromised patients (HIV), lapses in isolation practices, undiagnosed TB
Outpatient clinic Chicago 1994–1995 Conover (96)	Methadone treatment program	51/302 (17%)	13	5/29 (17%)	—	Undiagnosed TB, immunocompromised patients (HIV)

[a]Includes source(s) of outbreak.
[b]See also Table 37.5.
[c]For multidrug-resistant outbreaks, the number of cases in patients and the number of healthcare workers listed in this table include only those identified in the initial investigation.
[d]Although the Initial report of this outbreak notes several "skin test conversions" in healthcare workers, the criteria used to define a skin test conversion in that report did not meet the general accepted definition.
[e]All exposed neonates presumptively treated with isoniazid for 6 months.

homes and a community hospital, and one involved both a general hospital and a hospice. Outbreak settings within the hospitals have included emergency departments, inpatient medical wards, adult or neonatal intensive care units, a surgical suite, radiology suites, inpatient HIV wards and an outpatient HIV clinic, an inpatient renal transplant unit, an inpatient prison ward, an autopsy suite, a nursery, a maternity ward, and bronchoscopy rooms.

The earlier reports of outbreaks in this series primarily focused on transmission of *M. tuberculosis* from patients to healthcare workers, with an occasional secondary case identified in another patient. The apparent infrequency of transmission to other patients in these outbreaks may be artifactual because of the difficulty often encountered in obtaining follow-up information on exposed patients and the natural history of TB. Because the interval from infection to disease is highly variable (ranging from weeks to decades) the occurrence of active TB is not likely to be attributed to a hospitalization in the more remote past. Thus, in the absence of temporal clustering of TB cases or the appearance of strains of *M. tuberculosis* with distinctive drug resistance or DNA fingerprint patterns, transmission to patients in a hospital may go unrecognized (2). In contrast to the earlier reports, many of the more recently reported outbreaks have occurred in settings where many of the persons exposed were severely immunocompromised patients. These outbreaks have involved rapid propagation of active TB among relatively large numbers of patients.

A variety of factors have been identified as possibly contributing to the reported nosocomial TB outbreaks. In many cases, these factors represent empiric observations, and the actual contribution of any given factor cannot be calculated. In some instances, the analysis presented has allowed an estimate of the relative contribution of a specific factor. In general, potential contributing factors can be categorized into those that increase the likelihood of exposure to *M. tuberculosis*, those that increase the likelihood of infection occurring among persons who are exposed, and those that increase the likelihood of active disease in persons who become infected.

Factors that Affect the Likelihood of Exposure

A major factor increasing the likelihood of exposure to *M. tuberculosis* has been failure to promptly identify and isolate a potential source of transmission, usually a patient with undiagnosed and untreated, or inadequately treated, TB (Table 37.4). In at least three outbreaks, healthcare workers also have been implicated as sources of transmission (70,88,94); in one, transmission only occurred from healthcare worker to healthcare worker in a setting where routine employee screening did not take place (94). Failure to identify persons with infectious TB has resulted in these persons not being isolated and appropriately treated, thus increasing the number of persons exposed.

In most instances, transmission has occurred from patients with pulmonary TB. However, in two outbreaks, transmission occurred as a result of irrigation or manipulation of an undiagnosed tuberculous abscess or skin ulcer (64,71). The presence of drug-resistant microorganisms that are inadequately treated also may lead to prolonged infectiousness and an increased likelihood of exposure.

In recent outbreaks, there often have been multiple sources, resulting in a web of possible transmissions, rather than a clearly defined single chain of transmission. In at least three recent outbreaks, DNA fingerprinting using RFLP has demonstrated the presence of more than one chain of transmission involving different strains of *M. tuberculosis*, when epidemiologic evidence seemed to suggest a single chain of transmission (68,72,92).

Inadequate ventilation also has increased the likelihood of exposure to *M. tuberculosis*. In some instances, the presence of positive air pressure in isolation rooms has allowed potentially contaminated air to escape from the isolation rooms into other areas of the facility. In most situations, the presence of other potentially contributing factors has made it difficult to assess the effect of positive air pressure alone; however, in one outbreak in which other aspects of the infection control program were adequately implemented, the role of positive air pressure was clearly demonstrated (53). In other instances, recirculation of potentially contaminated air from sputum induction or isolation rooms into other areas of the facility has been implicated as a factor in transmission (61,63,66,72).

Lapses in isolation practices have increased the likelihood of exposure in several outbreaks. Such lapses have included not keeping isolation room doors closed, thereby allowing efflux of potentially contaminated air from the room into adjacent areas; not keeping patients with infectious TB confined to their rooms; not enforcing the use of masks by patients with infectious TB when they are out of their rooms; and not maintaining isolation for a period long enough to ensure that the patient is no longer infectious. Additionally, inadequate cleaning, disinfection, or leak testing of bronchoscopes after performing bronchoscopy in pulmonary TB patients led to transmission of infection and active TB disease (86,94) (see also Chapter 63).

Factors that Affect the Likelihood of Infection

In general, factors that are likely to produce a relatively high concentration of infectious droplet nuclei in the air also are likely to increase the likelihood that an exposed person will inhale tubercle bacilli and become infected. Thus, patients identified as outbreak sources often have had chest radiographs showing extensive cavitary disease and sputum smears that were positive for AFB—factors suggesting a high bacterial burden. However, in outbreaks among immunocompromised persons, extensive cavitary disease has been relatively infrequent (67,68,72,73,75,77,87,95,96). Furthermore, in rare cases, high rates of transmission from persons with sputum smears that were negative for AFB have been documented (48,62).

Inadequate ventilation rates and recirculation of potentially contaminated air within closed environments can lead to increased concentrations of infectious droplet nuclei in the air and have been implicated in several outbreaks (48,61–63,66,68,70,72,74,76,77). Patients in rooms in close proximity to a room housing a patient with infectious TB have been shown to be at increased risk when the isolation room is not under appropriate negative pressure (64,73,76).

Performing procedures that stimulate cough or generate aerosols in persons with TB also may lead to an increased concentration of infectious droplet nuclei in the air. A number of such procedures have been reported in association with outbreaks. These procedures have included endotracheal intubation and suctioning (61–63,68,90); bronchoscopy (62,68,93); surgical drainage and irrigation of a tuberculous abscess, and surgical debridement of a tuberculous skin ulcer (64,71); administration of aerosolized pentamidine (66,72); and autopsy (48). Finally, lack of or inappropriate use of respiratory protection also has been reported in some outbreaks (63,68,76,77,90,93,94).

Whether or not underlying HIV infection causes increased susceptibility to infection with *M. tuberculosis* is not yet clearly established. In an MDR TB outbreak in the New York state prison system, HIV infection was not found to be associated with an increased risk of becoming infected with *M. tuberculosis*; however, the small numbers included in this analysis limited the power of the analysis to detect such a risk (97). In two studies, patients with HIV hospitalized for active TB caused by drug-susceptible microorganisms developed secondary infection with a hospital-acquired MDR TB (98,99).

Factors that Affect the Likelihood of Active Tuberculosis

Although, hypothetically, the virulence of the infecting microorganism may increase the likelihood of progression from infection to active TB, this issue remains unresolved (100). Profound suppression of cell-mediated immunity in the infected host is the only factor that has been definitively identified in the outbreaks as increasing the likelihood of active TB. In most cases, immunosuppression has resulted from co-infection with HIV (Table 37.4). In one outbreak, the cause was pharmacologic immunosuppression in renal transplant recipients (68). In each of these cases, immunosuppression has increased both the risk of developing active disease and the rate at which it developed, leading to rapid and widespread propagation of the outbreak.

In summary, at least 40 nosocomial outbreaks of TB among adults in the U.S. have been reported in the literature since 1960. Because there is no systematic national surveillance of such outbreaks, it is unknown how many other outbreaks may have occurred but have not been reported, nor is it known whether those that have been reported are representative of all outbreaks. A multiplicity of factors potentially contributing to the reported outbreaks has been identified. Although it is difficult to estimate the quantitative contribution of each of these factors to the outbreaks, it is clear that failure to identify and appropriately isolate and treat persons with infectious TB is one of the most important factors.

Nosocomial Outbreaks of Multidrug-Resistant Tuberculosis

In the 1990s, several large, nosocomial outbreaks of MDR TB were reported (Tables 37.4 and 37.5) (2). Outbreaks of MDR TB are not a new phenomenon, having been reported in at least three communities, a residential substance-abuse treatment center, and a homeless shelter since 1976 (82,85,94–96, 101–105). However, in contrast to these earlier outbreaks, which were relatively small and propagated slowly, the nosocomial outbreaks of the early to mid-1990s involved large numbers of patients in institutional settings and propagated rapidly.

From 1990 through 1992, the CDC collaborated with officials from state and local health departments, hospitals, and prisons to investigate eight outbreaks of MDR TB in hospitals and in the New York state prison system (53,72–97,106–110). In addition to the initial investigations, follow-up investigations have been conducted in some of the hospitals to evaluate the effectiveness of infection control interventions that were initiated after the outbreaks were detected (111–114). The total number of cases identified in each of the outbreaks has ranged from approximately 8 to 70, with the total for all the outbreaks combined exceeding 300 cases.

All of these outbreaks involved the transmission of MDR *M. tuberculosis* from person to person, including from patient to patient, patient to healthcare worker, and healthcare worker to healthcare worker. In each instance, the epidemiologic evidence of nosocomial transmission has been compelling. For patients, factors associated with an increased risk of MDR TB have included previous hospitalization in the associated outbreak hospital, previous hospitalization on the same ward as a patient with infectious MDR TB, physical proximity to a patient with infectious MDR TB during a previous hospitalization, or previous exposure to patients with infectious MDR TB in an outpatient clinic. For healthcare workers, exposure to patients with MDR TB has been associated with a higher risk of tuberculin skin test conversion than has exposure to patients with drug-susceptible TB (72). This is probably explained by prolonged infectiousness of patients with inadequately treated drug-resistant TB rather than by increased infectiousness of such patients. In all of the outbreaks, the epidemiologic evidence of nosocomial transmission has been corroborated by laboratory evidence in the form of DNA fingerprinting using RFLP.

Nearly all patients in these outbreaks have had *M. tuberculosis* isolates resistant to both isoniazid and rifampin, the two most effective anti-TB drugs available. Most isolates have been resistant to other drugs as well. In four hospitals and the New York state prison system, the outbreak strain was resistant to seven anti-TB drugs. Mortality among patients with MDR TB in these outbreaks has been extraordinarily high (43% to 93%) and has been associated with rapid progression from diagnosis of TB to death (range of median intervals: 4 to 16 weeks). The high mortality rates observed in these outbreaks are probably explained by the severe degree of immunosuppression in many of the patients combined with ineffective treatment for unrecognized drug-resistant disease.

In all but two of these outbreaks, over 85% of cases have occurred in persons infected with HIV. This high proportion of HIV infection can be explained in two ways. First, the outbreaks have occurred predominantly in settings, such as HIV wards and clinics, in which most of the persons exposed to and infected with *M. tuberculosis* have been HIV infected. Second, once infected with *M. tuberculosis*, HIV-infected persons are highly likely to develop active TB, especially when they are profoundly immunosuppressed, as often has been true of the persons exposed in these outbreaks.

Healthcare workers at hospitals experiencing outbreaks of

TABLE 37.5. REPORTED NOSOCOMIAL OUTBREAKS OF MULTIDRUG-RESISTANT TUBERCULOSIS, UNITED STATES, 1988–1995

Facility First Author (Reference)	Location and Year(s)	Total Cases[a]	Drug Resistance Pattern[b,c]	Prevalence of HIV[d] Infection (%[a])	Mortality Rate (%)[e]	Median Interval from TB Diagnosis to Death (Weeks)
Hospital A Beck-Sagué (72) CDC (106) CDC (74) Wenger (111) Fischl (107) Fischl (108)	Miami 1988–1991	65	INH, RIF (EMB, ETA, SM, CYC)	93	72	7
Hospital B Edlin (73) CDC (74) Stroud (112)	New York City 1989–1991	51	INH, SM (RIF, EMB)	100[f]	89	16
Hospital C CDC (74) Jereb (109)	New York City 1989–1992	70	INH, RIF, SM (EMB, ETA, KM, RBT)	95	77	4
Hospital D Pearson (75) CDC (74) Maloney (113)	New York City 1990–1991	40	INH, RIF (EMB, ETA, SM, PZA, KM, RBT)	91	83	4
Hospital E Ikeda (53)	New York City 1991	8	INH, RIF, SM (EMB, ETA, KM, RBT)	63	43	4
Hospital F Coronado (76)	New York City 1990–1991	16	INH, RIF, SM (EMB, ETA, KM, RBT)	88	88	8
Hospital I Coronado (77)	New Jersey 1990–1992	13	INH, RIF (EMB)	100	85	4
Hospital J CDC (78)	New York City 1991–1992	37	INH, RIF (SM, EMB, ETA, KM)	96	93	4
Prison system Valway (97) Valway (110)	New York State 1990–1992	42[g]	INH, RIF (SM, EMB, ETA, KM, RBT)	98	79	4
Hospital K Nivin (82)	New York City 1993–1994	24	INH, RIF, SM	—	—	—
Hospital L Agerton (85)	South Carolina 1995	4	INH, RIF, SM (EMB, ETA, KM, RBT)	—	—	—
Hospital M Cleveland (94)	New York City 1990–1991	2	INH, RIF	100	100	—
Hospital N Kenyon (95)	Chicago 1994–1995	7	INH, RIF	100	—	—
Clinic O Conover (96)	Chicago 1994–1995	13	INH, RIF	85	69	—

[a]Includes cases identified during initial investigation and cases identified during subsequent follow-up.
[b]All cases resistant to drugs listed outside of parentheses; some cases resistant to drugs listed in parentheses.
[c]INH, isoniezid; RIF, rifampin; EMB, ethambutol; ETA, ethionamide; SM, streptomycin; CYC, cycloserine; KM, Kanamycin; RBT, rifabutin; PZA, pyrazinamide.
[d]HIV, human immunodeficiency virus.
[e]Includes only cases for which outcome information has been ascertained.
[f]HIV infection was part of the case definition in this outbreak.
[g]Includes 24 cases also counted with Hospital C.

MDR TB also have been affected. In some instances, it has been difficult to document infection of healthcare workers, because results of baseline TSTs were not available. However, in several of the facilities, it has been possible to document TST conversions in healthcare workers in association with exposure to patients with MDR TB (Table 37.4) (53,72,75,77,95,96,109). At least 23 healthcare workers at these facilities have developed active MDR TB; at least 11 of these workers have died with MDR TB.

The factors contributing to the MDR-TB outbreaks are essentially the same as already described for other outbreaks, including delayed diagnosis and isolation of patients with TB. Of particular importance has been delayed recognition of drug resistance leading to delays in initiating effective therapy that, in turn, resulted in prolonged periods of infectiousness. In several instances, the delays that have occurred in identifying persons with TB and recognizing drug resistance have been exacerbated by delays in performing and reporting the results of laboratory tests.

Also of particular importance is the observation that each of the MDR TB outbreaks occurred in a setting where many HIV-infected and often profoundly immunosuppressed patients were exposed. In one outbreak, 21 (6.1%) of 346 patients with AIDS hospitalized on the same ward as one or more patients with infectious MDR TB were subsequently diagnosed with active MDR TB, demonstrating the very high disease attack rate that can occur in such a setting (73). In several of the outbreaks, the interval from exposure to onset of active TB (that is, the incubation period) has been estimated (72,73,76,77,97). Although different methodologies used in these calculations make summary and comparison difficult, all have documented that the incubation period can be remarkably short, possibly as short as 3 to 4 weeks. As a result of the short incubation period, as many as three complete generations of transmission and onset of clinical TB have been observed in one outbreak in a 12-month period (CDC, unpublished data). Thus, the amplifying and accelerating effect that HIV has on the pathogenesis of TB has contributed substantially to the propagation of these outbreaks.

Nosocomial MDR TB outbreaks also have been reported from countries other than the U.S. (99,115–122). Clinically and epidemiologically, these outbreaks are similar to those reported in the U.S. Many episodes occurred in HIV-infected patients with short onset of active TB after exposure, and high mortality rates (99,115–122).

In summary, MDR-TB outbreaks in hospitals and correctional facilities illustrate the tremendous rapidity and extent of spread that can occur when persons who have undiagnosed or untreated (or inadequately treated) TB, caused by drug-resistant microorganisms, are brought together with highly vulnerable, immunosuppressed persons in an enclosed and relatively densely populated environment in the absence of adequate infection control precautions.

Special Settings

Pediatric Settings

Nosocomial transmission of *M. tuberculosis* in the pediatric setting usually has involved exposure of hospitalized infants or children to hospital employees or adult visitors with active TB (88,123–129). Transmission from infants and young children is generally regarded as unlikely because an infant's microorganism load is low, cavitary disease is usually absent (indeed, many cases of TB in children involve primary disease with minimal pulmonary involvement), and infants have a reduced ability to expectorate (130–132). However, TST conversion occurred in two healthcare workers who cared for an infant on a ventilator with widely disseminated congenital TB diagnosed at autopsy (89). In another case, possible transmission to healthcare workers from a 5-year-old child with cavitary TB was reported (133). In a third case, TST conversions occurred in 3.7% (5/134) of hospital employees identified as contacts of a 7-year-old child with cystic fibrosis who was hospitalized for 2 months with undiagnosed, disseminated pulmonary TB (38). In a fourth case, TST conversion occurred in one healthcare worker not using respiratory protection who intubated a neonate with congenital TB (90). Thus, although transmission of *M. tuberculosis* from infants and young children probably is uncommon, there are circumstances in which it may occur.

Nursing Homes and Chronic Care Facilities

Transmission of *M. tuberculosis* in nursing homes and chronic care facilities has been well documented. Several outbreaks of TB in such facilities have been reported (91,134–139). These outbreaks have involved transmission both to residents of the facilities and to staff. In each case, the source of the outbreak was a resident with pulmonary TB in whom the diagnosis was delayed by 2 to 12 months or was only made postmortem. In some instances, the outbreaks were discovered as a result of a routine TST screening program for staff or residents (134,137, 139); in other instances, the outbreaks were discovered in the course of conducting a contact investigation (135,136,138) (see also Chapter 106).

Dental Settings

An outbreak of TB in dental patients following tooth extractions has been reported (140). The source of the outbreak was a dentist with undiagnosed pulmonary TB. Of 15 secondary cases, 13 involved tuberculous lesions in the mouth with involvement of regional lymph nodes, one involved both the mouth and the lungs, and one involved a pleural effusion with associated erythema nodosum. The investigators postulated that the tooth sockets became infected at the time of extraction, presumably by mycobacteria on the dentist's fingers. In another outbreak, transmission occurred from one dental worker to another in an HIV patient dental clinic without evidence of transmission to dental patients (94). The source of the index worker's infection was not determined. Both workers were HIV positive and the clinic had no routine screening program for employees. There are no reported episodes of *M. tuberculosis* transmission from a patient with TB to dental workers as a result of performing dental procedures.

One prospective study has been conducted on the TST conversion rates of dental healthcare workers in Texas counties along the Mexican border with a high prevalence rate of TB in the population. Although the study size was small ($n = 240$), the authors reported a 1.7% conversion rate after 12 months (141).

International Settings

Tuberculosis is increasing in the developing world (142). Since TB infection control programs in most low-income countries are nonexistent or ineffective, there is concern about the risk of *M. tuberculosis* transmission to healthcare workers in those settings. There are several reports suggesting that healthcare workers caring for infectious TB patients in low-income countries are at increased risk of *M. tuberculosis* infection and disease. During 1993 to 1994, a study of the incidence of TB disease in nurses working at a hospital in Malawi showed that 12 (4%) of 310 nurses had been diagnosed and treated for TB (143). The number of nurses acquiring TB while working on the medical and TB wards was significantly higher (13%) than among nurses working in other areas of the hospital (3%). Rates of TB among the nurses working on medical or TB wards was five times higher than rates among nurses working in other hospital areas (143).

In 1996, a TST cross-sectional evaluation of 512 healthcare workers working in a hospital in Abidjan, Ivory Coast, was conducted to assess the risk of TST positivity and to identify risk factors for occupational *M. tuberculosis* acquisition (144). Seventy-nine percent of the healthcare workers had positive TST at the 10-mm cutoff. The duration of employment in areas where TB patients were admitted and the level of patient care influenced levels of positive TST reactions. Healthcare workers working 1 year or longer in areas where TB patients were admitted and those involved in patient care (physicians, nurses, and midwives) had a significantly higher rate of TST positivity than those working in the same areas for less than 1 year or those who did not have patient contact. Five healthcare workers had radiographic abnormalities suggestive of TB. Two of those, both working in areas with high TB prevalence, were diagnosed with active TB.

In 1996, a similar TST survey was conducted among 911 healthcare workers in a hospital in Chiang Rai, Thailand (145). Sixty-nine percent of healthcare workers had an initial positive TST at the 10-mm cutoff. Risk factors for TST positivity included working in the hospital 1 year and having contact with patients. Eleven healthcare workers had an abnormal chest radiograph compatible with TB; of these, seven (64%) were determined to have active TB.

The increased risk of active TB among healthcare workers is not limited to nations with high rates of HIV. For example, the rate of active TB among healthcare workers in Estonia was 1.5 to 3 times that of the general population from 1994 through 1998 (146). Reported rates were 30 to 90 times higher among workers in a regional chest hospital. MDR TB accounted for 38% of disease among healthcare workers, but was 10% to 14% of TB in the general population. A lack of infection control strategies for protecting workers from infectious patients was cited as the cause of the high rates of active disease.

An increased risk of nosocomial acquisition of *M. tuberculosis* infection also was shown among Brazilian healthcare workers (147). In 1997, 542 healthcare workers in a large urban hospital in Belo Horizonte, Brazil, completed an exposure questionnaire and received a two-step TST. Of those, 48% had TST reactions ≥10 mm. Having a positive TST was associated with working in areas of the hospital where TB patients were admitted and with prolonged employment duration. A study in Rio de Janeiro, performed during 1994 to 1997, evaluated the risk of TST conversion among 351 healthcare workers in a large urban hospital (A. L. Kritski, personal communication). TST conversion was defined as an increase of ≥10 mm for BCG negative healthcare workers and an increase of ≥15 mm for healthcare workers who had a previous history of BCG vaccination. TST conversion rates among healthcare workers were significantly higher than in the general population (8% vs. 1%). Also, TST conversion rates were significantly higher among medical, technical, and nursing personnel (14%, 13%, and 11%, respectively) compared to administrative and maintenance personnel (1%). An additional study in Rio de Janeiro, evaluated the risk of TST conversion after 1 year among 414 junior and senior medical students with negative two-step TST in 1998. The 1-year TST conversion rate was 3.9%, and the degree of patient contact in the teaching hospital was independently associated with TST conversion (148).

In 1997, teams from the CDC composed of industrial engineers and medical epidemiologists visited several healthcare facilities in five developing countries (Malawi, Brazil, Thailand, Ivory Coast, and Latvia) to develop simple, cost-effective, and feasible TB control interventions to be implemented in these settings. During these visits, a number of factors contributing to the spread of nosocomial *M. tuberculosis* were identified. The main factors contributing to the nosocomial spread of *M. tuberculosis* in low-income countries are delays in diagnosis, usually due to the lack of suspicion of TB by healthcare providers, slow laboratory turnaround of sputum AFB smears, and atypical clinical manifestations in HIV-infected patients. Inadequate isolation of infectious TB patients, underestimation of risk due to BCG coverage leading to a false sense of security, and the lack of personal protection during high-risk procedures (i.e., bronchoscopy, sputum induction, or autopsies) are additional factors contributing to the spread of nosocomial *M. tuberculosis* in low-income countries. TB control guidelines for hospitals in resource-limited countries have been published by the World Health Organization (149).

Other Modes of Transmission

Although nosocomial transmission of *M. tuberculosis* nearly always occurs via the airborne route, there are occasional reports of transmission by other routes. Primary cutaneous inoculation TB has been reported in medical students, autopsy students, or laboratory workers as a result of accidental self-inoculation during postmortem examinations (150,151) and during injection of laboratory animals with *M. tuberculosis* (152,153). A case of primary cutaneous inoculation TB was reported in a nurse who was lacerated with a needle that had been inserted in the port of a central-line catheter of a patient who had disseminated TB with positive blood cultures for *M. tuberculosis* (154).

Transmission of *M. tuberculosis* to patients via bronchoscopes that have been used on patients with TB have been reported (93,155). In one case, the bronchoscope had been inadequately disinfected with a detergent soap solution, wiped with alcohol, and soaked for 30 minutes in a solution of povidone-iodine, ethanol, and sterile water (155) (see also Chapter 63). In the other, an undetected leak in the distal end of a bronchoscope used on a patient with cavitary TB created a reservoir for bacteria and apparently inoculated nine subsequent patients, two of whom developed active disease with the same strain as the index patient (93).

Finally, transmission of *M. tuberculosis* via organ transplantation has been reported (156). In this incident, active TB developed in two patients, each of whom received a kidney from the same cadaver donor, whose cerebrospinal fluid cultures grew *M. tuberculosis*.

PREVENTION AND CONTROL OF NOSOCOMIAL TRANSMISSION OF *M. TUBERCULOSIS*

Because *M. tuberculosis* is transmitted by the airborne route, its control is complex and requires multiple interventions. Therefore, prevention of nosocomial transmission of *M. tuberculosis* requires the complete implementation of an appropriately designed TB infection control program that ensures the early identification, isolation, and treatment of persons who have active TB (157). In each of the nosocomial TB outbreaks previously described, the CDC guidelines for preventing the transmission of *M. tuberculosis* were incompletely implemented (79,82, 84,86,97,101–103,112,124–126). Follow-up studies at several of these hospitals have documented termination of patient-to-patient and/or patient-to–healthcare worker *M. tuberculosis* transmission after implementation of the recommended guidelines (111–114).

The TB infection control program should be based on the hierarchy of control measures recommended to prevent nosocomial *M. tuberculosis* transmission. This hierarchy includes (a) administrative procedures to reduce the risk of exposure to persons with infectious TB, (b) engineering controls to reduce the concentration of infectious droplet nuclei and prevent their spread, and (c) a respiratory protection program to protect healthcare workers and other persons in settings where administrative and engineering controls alone may not provide adequate protection (e.g., TB isolation rooms).

Specific measures to reduce the risk of nosocomial *M. tuberculosis* transmission (Table 37.6) include (a) clearly assigning to

TABLE 37.6. CHARACTERISTICS OF AN EFFECTIVE TUBERCULOSIS (TB) INFECTION CONTROL PROGRAM[a]

I. Assignment of responsibility
   A. Assign responsibility for the TB infection control program to qualified person(s).
   B. Ensure that persons with expertise in infection control, occupational health, and engineering are identified and included.

II. Risk assessment, TB infection control plan, and periodic reassessment
   A. Initial risk assessments
      1. Obtain information concerning TB in the community.
      2. Evaluate data concerning TB patients in the facility.
      3. Evaluate data concerning purified protein derivative (PPD) tuberculin skin test conversions among healthcare workers (HCWs) in the facility.
      4. Rule out evidence of person-to-person transmission.
   B. Written TB infection control program
      1. Select initial risk protocol(s).
      2. Develop written TB infection control protocols.
   C. Repeat risk assessment at appropriate intervals.
      1. Review current community and facility surveillance data and PPD-tuberculin skin test results.
      2. Review records of TB patients.
      3. Observe HCW infection-control practices.
      4. Evaluate maintenance of engineering controls.

III. Identification, evaluation, and treatment of patients who have TB
   A. Screen patients for signs and symptoms of active TB.
      1. On initial encounter in emergency department or ambulatory care setting.
      2. Before or at the time of admission.
   B. Perform radiologic and bacteriologic evaluation of patients who have signs and symptoms suggestive of TB.
   C. Promptly initiate treatment.

IV. Managing outpatients who have possible infectious TB
   A. Promptly initiate TB precautions.
   B. Place patients in separate waiting areas or TB isolation rooms.
   C. Give patients a surgical mask, a box of tissues, and instructions regarding the use of these items.

V. Managing inpatients who have possible infectious TB
   A. Promptly isolate patients who have suspected or known infectious TB.
   B. Monitor the response to treatment.
   C. Follow appropriate criteria for discontinuing isolation.

VI. Engineering recommendations
   A. Design local exhaust and general ventilation in collaboration with persons who have expertise in ventilation engineering.
   B. Use a single-pass air system or air recirculation after high-efficiency particulate air (HEPA) filtration in areas where infectious TB patients receive care.
   C. Use additional measures, if needed, in areas where TB patients may receive care.
   D. Design TB isolation rooms in healthcare facilities to achieve >6 air changes per hour (ACH) for existing facilities and >12 ACH for new or renovated facilities.
   E. Regularly monitor and maintain engineering controls.
   F. TB isolation rooms that are being used should be monitored daily to ensure they maintain negative pressure relative to the hallway and all surrounding areas.
   G. Exhaust TB isolation room air to outside or, if absolutely unavoidable, recirculate after HEPA filtration.

VII. Respiratory protection
   A. Respiratory protective devices should meet recommended performance criteria.
   B. Respiratory protection should be used by persons entering rooms in which patients with known or suspected infectious TB are being isolated, by HCWs when performing cough-inducing or aerosol-generating procedures on such patients, and by persons in other settings where administrative and engineering controls are not likely to protect them from inhaling infectious airborne droplet nuclei.
   C. A respiratory protection program is required at all facilities in which respiratory protection is used.

VIII. Cough-inducing procedures
   A. Do not perform such procedures on TB patients unless absolutely necessary.
   B. Perform such procedures in areas that have local exhaust ventilation devices (e.g., booths or special enclosures) or, if this is not feasible, in a room that meets the ventilation requirements for TB isolation.
   C. After completion of procedures, TB patients should remain in the booth or special enclosure until their coughing subsides.

IX. HCW TB training and education
   A. All HCWs should receive periodic TB education appropriate for their work responsibilities and duties.
   B. Training should include the epidemiology of TB in the facility.
   C. TB education should emphasize concepts of the pathogenesis of and occupational risk for TB.
   D. Training should describe work practices that reduce the likelihood of transmitting *M. tuberculosis*.

X. HCW counseling and screening
   A. Counsel all HCWs regarding TB and TB infection.
   B. Counsel all HCWs about the increased risk to immunocompromised persons for developing active TB.
   C. Perform PPD skin tests on HCWs at the beginning of their employment, and repeat PPD tests at periodic intervals.
   D. Evaluate symptomatic HCWs for active TB.

XI. Evaluate HCW PPD test conversions and possible nosocomial transmission of *M. tuberculosis*.

XII. Coordinate efforts with public health department(s).

[a] A program such as this is appropriate for healthcare facilities in which there is a high risk for transmission of *Mycobacterium tuberculosis*.
From Centers for Disease Control. Guidelines for preventing the transmission of *Mycobacterium tuberculosis* in healthcare facilities, 1994. *MMWR* 1994; 43(RR-13): 1–132.

specific persons the responsibility for the TB infection control program; (b) conducting a risk assessment, and developing a written program based on this assessment; (c) developing protocols to facilitate the early identification of persons who may have infectious TB, and promptly initiating and maintaining isolation for such persons; (d) using ventilation and other engineering controls to reduce the potential for airborne exposure to *M. tuberculosis*; (e) maintaining an appropriate healthcare worker respiratory protection program; (f) educating and training healthcare workers about TB; (g) maintaining a program for routine periodic counseling and screening of healthcare workers for LTBI and TB; (h) evaluating possible episodes of *M. tuberculosis* transmission in the facility; (i) coordinating activities with the appropriate public health department; and (j) periodically evaluating the effectiveness of the control program and modifying it, if necessary.

Administrative Controls

To ensure the appropriate design, implementation, and evaluation of the TB infection control program, one person should be assigned supervisory responsibility. This person should have expertise in infection control and occupational health and should work with a multidisciplinary team, including persons with experience in infection control, infectious diseases, pulmonary medicine, microbiology, occupational health, engineering, administration, and employee representation.

The first step in the development of the TB control program is to assess the risk of *M. tuberculosis* transmission in each area of the healthcare facility and in certain occupational groups (Table 37.7 and Fig. 37.2). The risk assessment should be based on the incidence of TB in the community, the number and location of TB patients in the facility, the likelihood of healthcare worker exposure to a patient with infectious TB, the incidence of healthcare worker TST conversions in each area and job category, and evaluation of possible person-to-person transmission of *M. tuberculosis*. Based on the results of the risk assessment, a written TB infection control plan with explicit policies and procedures should be developed. Systematic, periodic reassessment of these data will allow estimation of the number of TB isolation rooms needed, facilitate identification of nosocomial *M. tuberculosis* transmission and outbreaks, allow estimation of the risk of occupational *M. tuberculosis* exposure, and suggest ways in which the infection control program can be made more effective and efficient.

Information on the incidence of TB in the community can be obtained from the public health department. To determine the hospital areas where TB exposures are most likely to occur, microbiology and infection control records should be reviewed to identify all TB patients seen in the facility and the locations in which they were evaluated or treated. These data should be examined to identify the degree of risk in various locations within the hospital. Examination of these data, including evaluation of drug susceptibility test results, also may lead to recognition of possible nosocomial transmission from patient to patient and to recognition of the need to enhance the initial treatment regimen that is used empirically until drug susceptibility results are available. These data should be collected prospectively and analyzed periodically to identify changes in the distribution of infectious TB patients by location, possible clusters of patient infection, and changes in *M. tuberculosis* antimicrobial resistance patterns by location.

TABLE 37.7. ELEMENTS OF A RISK ASSESSMENT OF TUBERCULOSIS IN HEALTHCARE FACILITIES

1. Review the community TB profile (from public health department data).
2. Review the number of TB patients who were treated in each area of the facility (both inpatient and outpatient). (This information can be obtained by analyzing laboratory surveillance data and by reviewing discharge diagnoses or medical and infection control records.)
3. Review the drug-susceptibility patterns of TB isolates of patients who were treated at the facility.
4. Analyze purified protein derivative (PPD) tuberculin skin test results of healthcare workers (HCWs), by area or by occupational group for HCWs not assigned to a specific area (e.g., respiratory therapists).
5. To evaluate infection control parameters, review medical records of a sample of TB patients seen at the facility:

Calculate intervals from:

- Admission until TB suspected
- Admission until TB evaluation performed
- Admission until acid-fast bacilli (AFB) specimens ordered
- AFB specimens ordered until AFB specimens collected
- AFB specimens collected until AFB smears performed and reported
- AFB specimens collected until cultures performed and reported
- AFB specimens collected until species identification conducted and reported
- AFB specimens collected until drug-susceptibility tests performed and reported
- Admission until TB isolation initiated
- Admission until TB treatment initiated
- Duration of TB isolation

Obtain the following additional information:

- Were appropriate criteria used for discontinuing isolation?
- Did the patient have a history of prior admission to the facility?
- Was the TB treatment regimen adequate?
- Were follow-up sputum specimens collected properly?
- Was appropriate discharge planning conducted?

6. Perform an observational review of TB infection control practices.
7. Review the most recent environmental evaluation and maintenance procedures.

From Centers for Disease Control. Guidelines for preventing the transmission of Mycobacterium tuberculosis in healthcare facilities, 1994. *MMWR* 1994; 43(RR-13): 1–132.

To determine the risk of acquiring *M. tuberculosis* infection or active disease from occupational exposure and to assess the effectiveness of the infection control program, employee health records should be maintained to identify all healthcare workers who have developed active TB or those who have had TST conversions and to facilitate analysis of this information. At the time of hire, all healthcare workers should be screened for a history of TB or receipt of BCG and should receive a TST using the two-step Mantoux method. (If analysis of the data indicates a very low level of boosting, for example, $<1\%$, two-step testing may not be needed.)

The TSTs should be applied and read by trained personnel responsible for maintaining healthcare worker TST records, not

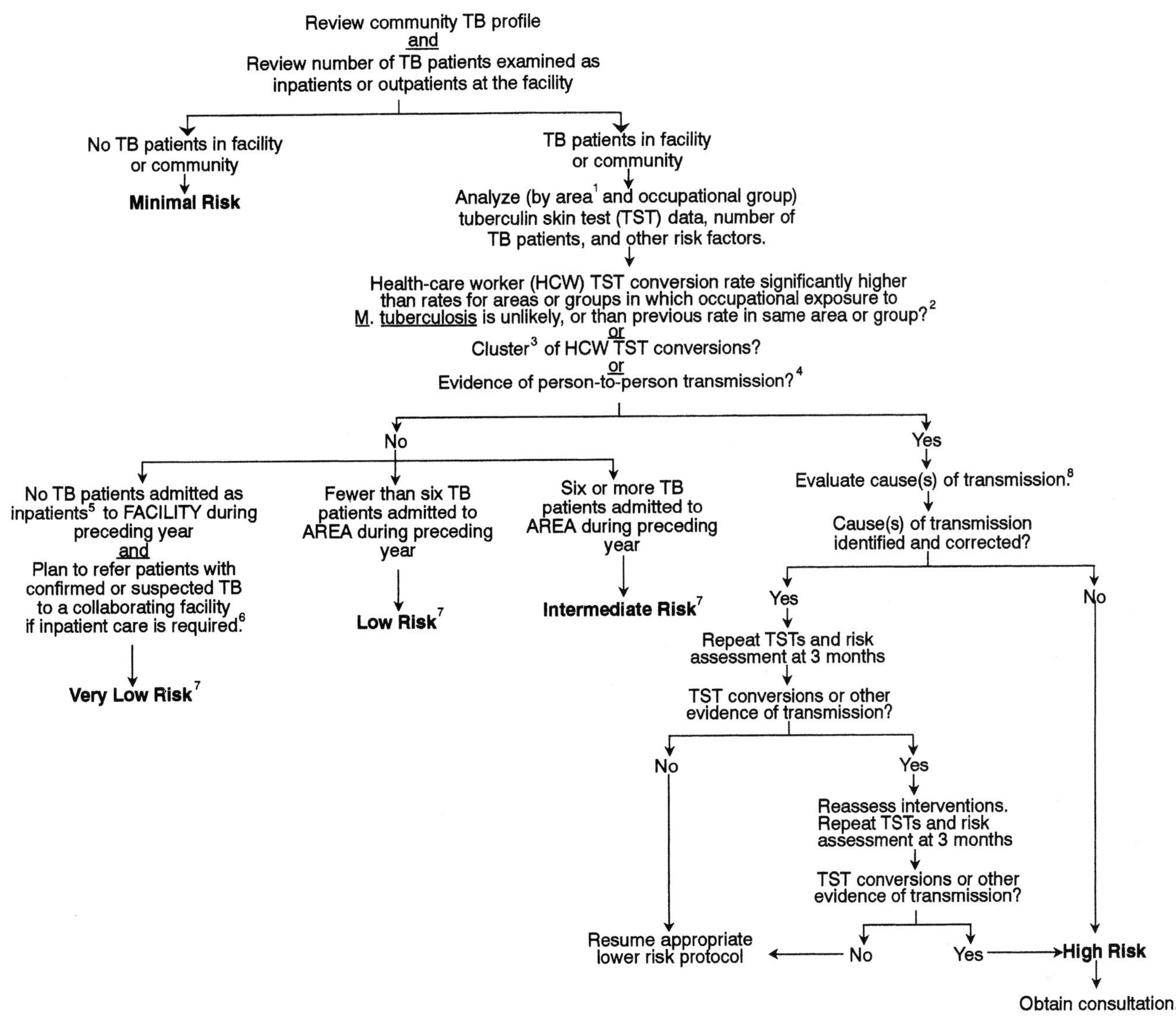

Figure 37.2. Example of an algorithm for conducting a tuberculosis risk assessment in a healthcare facility.

by the healthcare workers who are being tested. Individual results should be recorded in the employee's health record and a retrievable aggregate database. Persons with positive TSTs or TST conversions should be evaluated for preventive therapy. All tuberculin-negative healthcare workers (paid and unpaid) with the potential for exposure to infectious TB patients or *M. tuberculosis*–contaminated air should be included in the facility's ongoing TST program. The frequency of repeat testing should be based on the risk in each area or occupational group (157). Initial and then periodic review of these data will allow identification of areas where healthcare workers are at increased risk for *M. tuberculosis* infection or disease and permit classification of these areas by degree of risk. This permits focusing of infection control and educational efforts to areas where they are most needed.

Healthcare worker TST conversion rates (i.e., the number of healthcare workers who have converted to positive divided by the number of healthcare workers tested) should be calculated during the initial risk assessment and then periodically during reassessments for healthcare workers in each area of the hospital and for healthcare workers in job categories that involve work in multiple areas of the facility (e.g., respiratory therapists). Overall hospital TST conversion rates may dilute high rates in specific units or occupational categories and fail to detect problem areas; therefore, ward or unit-specific rates should be calculated (113). If a cluster of TST conversions is identified [i.e., two or more TST conversions occurring within a 3-month period among healthcare workers in a specific area or occupational group, with epidemiologic evidence suggesting occupational (nosocomial) transmission], additional control measures should be immediately implemented and further evaluation conducted to identify factors that may be leading to transmission (Fig. 37.3).

The most important element of the TB control program is early identification, treatment, and triage of patients with suspected or confirmed infectious TB. To prevent nosocomial *M. tuberculosis* transmission, it is essential that all potentially infectious TB patients be rapidly identified on first contact with the

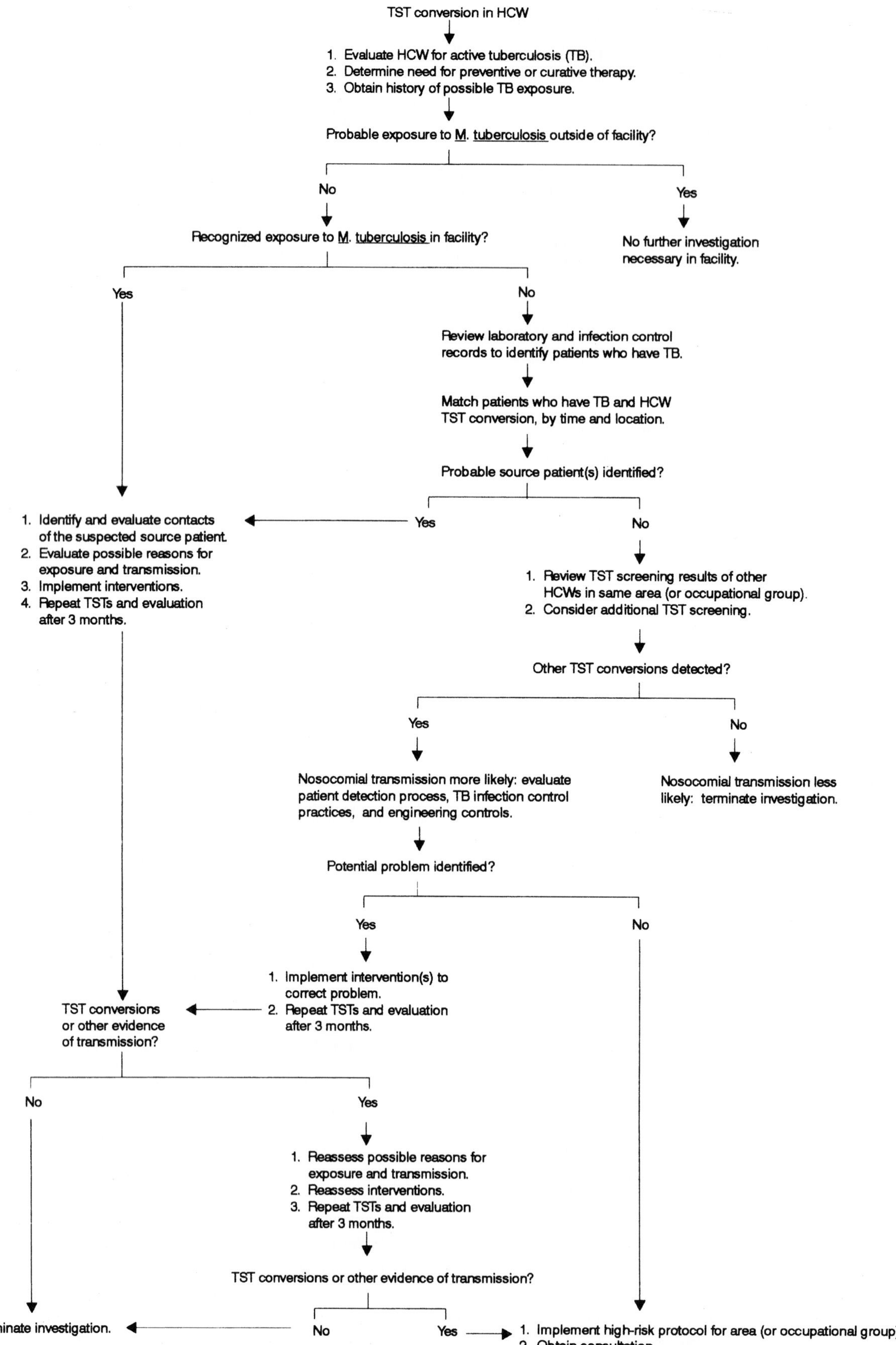

Figure 37.3. Example of an algorithm for investigating tuberculin skin test (TST) conversions in healthcare workers (HCWs).

healthcare facility. This requires that physicians, nurses, and other triage personnel who perform initial patient evaluations understand the signs and symptoms of TB, the populations at greatest risk of TB, and the appropriate approach to the evaluation and initial management of patients with TB. In addition, written protocols to facilitate the early identification of persons who have infectious TB should be developed. These protocols may vary in different facilities, depending on the incidence of TB in the area and the characteristics of the TB patients treated in the facility.

Previously, most nosocomial *M. tuberculosis* transmission was associated with exposure to an unknown or unsuspected TB patient (158). Often these patients were either unsuspected or unknown, were not receiving anti-TB therapy, or were receiving inadequate therapy. Clinicians should be alert to the possibility of concomitant infection with other pathogens. In particular, HIV-infected patients may be co-infected with *M. tuberculosis* and *Pneumocystis carinii* or *M. avium* (67,159). For these reasons, HIV-infected patients with signs and symptoms of TB and AFB-positive sputum smears should be assumed to have TB until proven otherwise. In recent MDR TB outbreak settings, early identification, treatment, and triage of infectious TB patients significantly reduced or terminated patient-to-patient and patient-to–healthcare worker transmission (111–113).

Patients suspected of having TB should be immediately triaged to an appropriate isolation room. In the outpatient setting (e.g., emergency room or clinic), such patients should not be placed in common waiting rooms or in areas where air is recirculated to other patient areas without high-efficiency particulate air (HEPA) filtration. They should either be masked (surgical masks) or instructed to cover their mouth and nose with tissues when coughing or sneezing while they are waiting or being evaluated. Ambulatory care settings in which patients with TB are frequently examined or treated should have a room that is equipped for TB isolation.

Inpatients should be placed in TB isolation rooms and promptly evaluated for TB by appropriate history, physical examination, TST, and appropriate laboratory (smears and cultures) and radiologic tests. Healthcare facilities in which TB patients are evaluated should have the capability to provide AFB sputum smear results to clinicians within 24 hours. To reduce the time from specimen collection until smear, culture, and antimicrobial susceptibility results are available, more rapid methods such as fluorescence staining of smears and use of radiometric culture and susceptibility testing and genetic probes are recommended (160,161).

Prompt treatment with appropriate antimicrobial agents significantly reduces the period of infectiousness. Because of the relatively high proportion of adult patients with TB caused by organisms that are resistant to isoniazid, four drugs are necessary in the initial phase for the 6-month regimen to be maximally effective (162).

Patients in TB isolation should remain in their rooms with the door closed, unless a medically essential procedure is necessary and cannot be performed in the room. Persons entering isolation rooms should wear appropriate respiratory protective devices (see below). Patients with suspected or confirmed TB should remain in isolation until the diagnosis of TB has been ruled out or until they are no longer infectious (i.e., they have clinical improvement and negative AFB sputum smears on three separate days). Patients with MDR TB are at risk of relapse and thus should be considered for isolation during their entire hospitalization. When infectious TB patients are kept in appropriate isolation rooms, the risk of nosocomial *M. tuberculosis* transmission from patient to patient is significantly reduced (111–123). When TB patients are to be discharged, continuation of therapy should be ensured by coordinating with the public health department and local healthcare providers prior to the time of discharge. The patient's treatment strategy should always emphasize directly observed therapy.

The last element of administrative controls is providing healthcare workers with education and training about TB. All healthcare workers should be educated about the epidemiology and pathogenesis of TB, the risk of occupational *M. tuberculosis* transmission, the infection control measures needed to reduce *M. tuberculosis* transmission, the increased risk of disease in immunocompromised healthcare workers, the importance of adhering to infection control recommendations, the importance of the healthcare worker TST program, and the importance of prompt evaluation of healthcare workers with symptoms consistent with TB.

Environmental Controls

The most important environmental control measures include engineering controls via ventilation and the use of ultraviolet germicidal irradiation (UVGI). There are a variety of methods that can be used to reduce the concentration of airborne droplet nuclei and achieve appropriate directional airflow (i.e., negative pressure) (Table 37.8). Ventilation controls can be divided into local exhaust, general exhaust, and air cleaning.

Local Exhaust Ventilation

Local exhaust captures infectious droplet nuclei at the source and removes them before dispersion into the air. This is the safest and most efficient type of control, since it prevents infectious *M. tuberculosis* particles from ever getting into the air circulation system. This method is primarily used during medical procedures, such as sputum induction, bronchoscopy, or aerosolized pentamidine administration. Local exhaust hoods can be of the enclosing type, where the hood totally or partially encloses the source, or the exterior type, where the source is near but not inside the hood. The enclosing type of hood, booth, or tent is preferable (163). Booths or other enclosing type devices should have sufficient air flow capacity to remove nearly 100% of airborne particles between patient uses. The time required to remove airborne particles depends on the number of air changes per hour, the rate at which air enters the device, the location of the air inlet and outlet, and the rate of air exhaust. To minimize the possible escape of infectious *M. tuberculosis* droplet nuclei, the exhaust fan should be located on the discharge side of the filter at the booth discharge. For exterior devices, the patient should face directly into the opening and air flow should be sufficient (200 ft/min) across the patient's breathing zone to prevent crosscurrents near the patient's face.

TABLE 37.8. HIERARCHY OF VENTILATION METHODS FOR TUBERCULOSIS ISOLATION ROOMS AND TREATMENT ROOMS

Reducing concentration of airborne tubercle bacilli[a]
- Facility heating, ventilation, and air-conditioning system
- Fixed room-air high-efficiency particulate air (HEPA) recirculation system
- Wall or ceiling-mounted room-air HEPA recirculation system
- Portable room-air HEPA recirculation unit[b]

Achieving directional airflow using negative pressure[c]
- Facility HVAC system
- Bleed air[d] from fixed room-air HEPA recirculation system
- Bleed air from wall- or ceiling-mounted room-air HEPA recirculation system
- Bleed air from portable room-air HEPA recirculation unit
- Exhaust air from room through window-mounted fan[e]

[a] Ventilation methods are used to reduce the concentration of airborne tubercle bacilli. If the facility HVAC system cannot achieve the recommended ventilation rate, auxiliary room-air recirculation cleaning methods may be used. These methods are listed in order from the most desirable to the least desirable. Ultraviolet germicidal irradiation may be used as a supplement to any of the ventilation methods for air cleaning.
[b] The effectiveness of portable room-air HEPA recirculation units can vary depending on the room's configuration, the furniture and persons in the room, the placement of the unit, the supply and exhaust grilles, and the achievable ventilation rates and air mixing. Units should be designed and operated to ensure that persons in the room cannot interfere with or otherwise compromise the function of the unit. Fixed recirculating systems are preferred over portable units in TB isolation rooms of facilities in which services are provided regularly to TB patients.
[c] Directional airflow using negative pressure can be achieved with the facility HVAC system and/or the auxiliary air recirculation cleaning systems. These methods are listed in order from the most desirable to the least desirable.
[d] To remove the amount of return air necessary to achieve negative pressure.
[e] This method simply achieves negative pressure and should be used only as a temporary measure.
From Centers for Disease Control. Guidelines for preventing the transmission of Mycobacterium tuberculosis in healthcare facilities, 1994. *MMWR* 1994; 43(RR-13): 1–132.

Air from booths, tents, and hoods may be discharged into the room in which the device is located or it may be exhausted to the outside. If the air is discharged into the room, a HEPA filter should be incorporated at the discharge duct or vent of the device. The exhaust fan should be located on the discharge side of the HEPA filter to ensure that the air pressure in the filter housing and booth is negative with respect to adjacent areas. If the device does not incorporate a HEPA filter, the air from the device should be exhausted directly to the outside.

General Exhaust Ventilation

General ventilation reduces airborne contaminants by dilution and removal and can be achieved by either single-pass or recirculating systems. In single-pass systems, the supply air is either outside air or air from a central system that supplies a number of areas. After air passes through the room or area, 100% of that air is exhausted directly to the outside. This type of ventilation system is preferred in areas where infectious airborne contaminants exist, since it prevents contaminated air from being recirculated to other areas of the facility. In recirculating systems, a small portion of the exhaust air is discharged to the outside and is replaced with fresh air, which mixes with the portion of exhaust air that was not discharged to the outside. The resulting mixture, which can contain a large proportion of contaminated air, then is recirculated to the areas serviced by the system. If the air mixture is recirculated into the general ventilation, airborne contaminants could be carried from contaminated to uncontaminated areas. Alternatively, the air mixture could be recirculated only within a specific room or area in which case other areas of the facility will not be affected.

Recommended general ventilation rates for healthcare facilities are based on comfort and odor control rather than infection control considerations. For facilities built or renovated before 2001, the American Society of Heating, Refrigerating, and Air Conditioning Engineers (ASHRAE) and the American Institute of Architects (AIA) recommend six air changes per hour for isolation and treatment rooms (164,165) to reduce the concentration of droplet nuclei. Where feasible, this airflow should be increased to 12 air changes per hour by adjusting or modifying the ventilation system or by using auxiliary means (e.g., recirculation of air through fixed HEPA filtration units or portable air cleaners or use of ultraviolet germicidal irradiation). Since 2001, the AIA has recommended 12 air changes per hour for renovated or newly constructed isolation and treatment rooms (166), a recommendation now endorsed by the CDC and the Healthcare Infection Control Practices Advisory Committee (HICPAC) (167).

The number of air changes per hour is equal to the ratio of the volume of air entering the room per hour to the room volume and is equal to the exhaust flow divided by the room volume multiplied by 60. Because air mixing within a room usually is not perfect, this calculated ventilation rate should be multiplied by a mixing factor to estimate the effective ventilation rate (157). Although ventilation rates higher than six air changes per hour probably improve dilution and removal of airborne particles, few if any studies have been done assessing the efficacy of this or any other level of air flow in reducing transmission of *M. tuberculosis*. Airflow patterns should be from more clean to less clean areas. For example, in emergency departments or TB isolation rooms, air should flow inward to prevent spread of airborne infectious droplet nuclei.

Tuberculosis isolation rooms should be designed to have negative pressure with respect to the hallway or adjacent rooms. The airflow direction in isolation rooms should be checked with smoke tubes on a periodic basis, preferably each day that an infectious TB patient is in the room. An anteroom outside the TB isolation room is not essential, but may serve as an extra measure of protection to prevent the escape of droplet nuclei during opening and closing of the isolation room door.

Air from TB isolation rooms and treatment rooms used for patients with TB should be exhausted directly to the outside of the building and away from air-intake vents, persons, and animals in accordance with applicable laws and regulations. If recirculation of air from such rooms into the general ventilation system is unavoidable, the air should be passed through a HEPA filter before recirculation.

Air Cleaning: High-Efficiency Particulate Air Filtration

High-efficiency particulate air filtration can be used as a method of air cleaning to supplement other ventilation measures. HEPA filters can be used in a number of ways to reduce the concentration of infectious droplet nuclei in the air. These methods include placement of HEPA filters (a) in exhaust ducts to remove droplet nuclei from air being discharged from a room or booth to the outside or into the general ventilation system; (b) in fixed room-air cleaners, which may be built into a room or may be mounted on the wall or ceiling; and (c) in portable room-air cleaners. With wall or ceiling-mounted or portable HEPA filter units, the effectiveness of the unit is dependent on all the air in the room circulating through the HEPA filter, which can be difficult to achieve. The effectiveness also is dependent on the room configuration, unit placement, and location of furniture and people. Thus, the effectiveness of the unit may vary considerably in rooms with different configurations or in the same room if moved from one location to another within the room. Portable HEPA filtration units have been evaluated for their ability to remove aerosolized particles in the size range of *M. tuberculosis* (168). Although this study indicates that portable filtration units reduce levels of airborne particles similar in size to infectious droplet nuclei, studies are needed to confirm that these units reduce *M. tuberculosis* exposure risk. If HEPA filtration units are used, they must be installed, maintained, and monitored properly.

Ultraviolet Germicidal Irradiation

Ultraviolet germicidal irradiation is effective in killing *M. tuberculosis* under experimental conditions (169–172). UVGI is another method of air cleaning that can be used to supplement other TB control measures. UVGI can be installed in the ventilation duct, as was the case in the experiments of Riley et al. (169–172), or can be placed in the upper part of the room. Duct UVGI, in which UV lamps are placed inside the ducts that remove air from the room, has two advantages: high levels of UV irradiation may be produced; and since the UVGI is inside the duct, the risk of human exposure is reduced or eliminated. Duct UVGI is dependent on adequate air flow from the room into the duct. Duct UVGI may be particularly useful in isolation rooms and other patient areas, such as waiting rooms and emergency departments. Most of the experimental data on UVGI are derived from studies using duct irradiation.

In upper room air irradiation, UVGI lamps are suspended from the ceilings or mounted on walls. The lamp must be shielded so that radiation is directed upward rather than down toward patients or healthcare workers. The UVGI disinfects the upper air; thus adequate air mixing in the room is essential. Contact time is very important; thus, increased ventilation rates actually may decrease the efficacy of UVGI. The effectiveness of upper room UVGI depends on the room configuration, lamp placement, air flow pattern and mixing, intensity of the UVGI, relative humidity, and contact time.

Appropriate installation, regular maintenance, and monitoring are essential if UVGI is used. Short-term exposure to UV irradiation can cause keratoconjunctivitis and erythema of the skin (173). UVC radiation is classified by the International Agency for Research on Cancer as "probably carcinogenic to humans" (174). Recommended exposure limits for occupational exposure to UV radiation have been published (173). If UVGI is used, workers should be educated about how UVGI works and its limitations, the potentially hazardous effects of overexposure, the potential for photosensitivity, and the principles of maintenance of UVGI fixtures.

Respiratory Protection

The precise level of effectiveness of respiratory protective devices in protecting healthcare workers against inhaling *M. tuberculosis* is unknown. Numerous studies have been conducted on the efficacy of respiratory protection for other hazardous airborne materials, but not *M. tuberculosis*. Information concerning the transmission of *M. tuberculosis* is incomplete; for example, neither the smallest infectious dose of *M. tuberculosis* nor the highest level of exposure to *M. tuberculosis* at which transmission will not occur has been defined. The size distribution of droplet nuclei and the number or concentration of viable *M. tuberculosis* particles generated by infectious TB patients have not been adequately defined. Nevertheless, personal respiratory protection should be used by (a) persons entering rooms where patients with known or suspected TB are being isolated, (b) persons present when cough-inducing or aerosol-generating procedures are performed on such patients, and (c) persons in other settings where administrative and engineering controls are not likely to protect them from inhaling infectious airborne droplet nuclei. These other settings should be identified on the basis of the facility's risk assessment. Respiratory protective devices used in these settings should have characteristics that are suitable for the microorganism they are protecting against and the settings in which they are used.

In 1990, the CDC first recommended that particulate respirators be used by healthcare workers for protection against inhalation of *M. tuberculosis* (175). In 1994, the CDC's TB guidelines enhanced its recommendations to include specific performance criteria (157). In 1995, the National Institute for Occupational Safety and Health (NIOSH) developed a new set of regulations, 42 CFR 84, for testing and certifying nonpowered, air purifying, particulate-filter respirators (176). The new regulation provides for nine classes of filters (three levels of filter efficiency, each with three categories of resistance to filter efficiency degradation). The three levels of filter efficiency are 95%, 99%, and 99.97% (referred to as 95, 99, 100). The three categories of resistance to filter efficiency degradation are as follows: not resistant to oil, resistant to oil, and oil proof (labeled as N, R, and P). For example, a filter labeled N95 would mean an N-series respirator (not resistant to oil) that is at least 95% efficient. All nine classes of nonpowered, air-purifying, particulate-filter respirators certified under 42 CFR 84 meet or exceed the CDC filtration efficiency performance criteria set forth in the 1994 CDC Guidelines. Current Occupational Safety and Health Administration (OSHA) policy permits the use of any 42 CFR 84 particulate filter for protection against TB (177).

To understand the complex nature of arriving at an appropriate respirator recommendation for healthcare workers to prevent occupational acquisition of TB, it is important to understand the relationship between OSHA and NIOSH. OSHA requires that any respiratory protective device used to protect workers must be NIOSH certified. NIOSH certifies respirator filtration in two ways. N100, R100, and P100 particulate-filter respirators are challenged with the most penetrating aerosol size (approximately 0.3 μm) particles; 99.97% of particles must be collected in a filter (i.e., the instantaneous penetration must be less than 0.03%). N99, R99, and P99 are challenged with the same size aerosol, with 99% of the particles collected (less than 1% penetration). N95, R95, and P95 are challenged with the same size aerosol, with 95% of the particles collected (less than 5% penetration). No certification test uses a biologic particle or a particle size similar to that of *M. tuberculosis*, nor is there evidence to indicate that a biologic particle acts any differently than a nonbiologic particle.

Based on all of the above considerations, the CDC recommends that respiratory protective devices used in healthcare settings for protection against inhaling *M. tuberculosis* should meet the following standard criteria: (a) the ability to filter particles 1 μm in size in the unloaded state with a filter efficiency of 95% at flow rates of up to 50 L/min; (b) the ability to be qualitatively or quantitatively fit-tested in a reliable way to obtain a face-seal leakage of ≤10%; (c) the ability to fit different facial sizes and characteristics of healthcare workers, which can usually be met by making the respirators available in at least three sizes; and (d) the ability to be checked for face-piece fit by healthcare workers each time they put on their respirator. The facility's risk assessment may identify a limited number of selected settings (e.g., bronchoscopy performed on patients suspected of having TB) where the estimated risk for transmission of *M. tuberculosis* may be such that a level of protection exceeding the standard criteria is appropriate. The N95 respirators meet the above criteria.

Follow-up data from several of the MDR-TB outbreak hospitals show that use of submicron surgical masks or dust-mist respirators that meet the CDC filtration criteria, when used with a fully implemented CDC TB control program, prevents patient-to–healthcare worker *M. tuberculosis* transmission (111–113). Furthermore, *in vitro* studies of particulate respirators show that some dust-mist and dust-fume-mist respirators filter >95% of particles with a mean size of 0.8 μm, smaller than the estimated size of droplet nuclei that contain *M. tuberculosis*.

Factors used to determine the efficacy of respirators include face-seal and filter efficacy. Face-seal leakage may compromise the ability of particulate respirators to protect the healthcare worker from airborne droplet nuclei. Face-seal leakage may result from incorrect face-piece size or shape, defective face-piece or sealing lip, beard growth, moisture (i.e., perspiration, facial oils), failure to use the head straps properly, improper maintenance, or damage. Filter leakage through the respirator is dependent on filter filtration characteristics, size of the aerosol, velocity through the filter, filter loading, and electrostatic charge. All healthcare workers with potential exposure to infectious TB patients should be fit-tested and trained in the proper use and maintenance of respirators and should fit-check the respirator before each use in accordance with the OSHA regulations, which require that a respiratory protection program be in place whenever a respirator is used to prevent exposure of the healthcare worker, regardless of class of respirator. The OSHA-mandated program includes written standard operating procedures, selection of respirators based on the hazard, respirator use instruction and training, cleaning and disinfection of the respirators, storage of the respirators, inspection of the respirators, surveillance of work area conditions, evaluation of the respirator protection program, medical evaluation of the user's ability to wear a respirator, and the use of NIOSH-certified respirators.

BCG Vaccination

Because of the risk of occupational acquisition of TB, some have advocated the BCG vaccination of healthcare workers. Over the years, there has been considerable debate about the efficacy of BCG. A large number of studies of BCG vaccination of infants have been conducted. These studies provide widely disparate results, with vaccine efficacy ranging from 0% to 100% (178). Differences in vaccine efficacy may be due to different BCG products used, different populations studied (e.g., rural vs. urban, high risk vs. low risk, geography), differences in the prevalence of TB and nontuberculous mycobacteria, or the intensity of follow-up. These studies suggest that when BCG is efficacious, it does not prevent infection but rather prevents disseminated disease or mortality, especially in infants and young children. Few data exist assessing the efficacy of BCG given for the first time in adulthood. This would be the situation with healthcare workers in most U.S. hospitals, since BCG is not given in infancy in the U.S.

Potential advantages of using BCG are that it is inexpensive and that, even with 50% efficacy, it might reduce the risk of TB disease in some healthcare workers. The disadvantages are that, once given, it will hinder the interpretation of the TST as a measure of *M. tuberculosis* infection, thus halting the use of preventive therapy, an intervention with a known and predictable effectiveness. TST studies among healthcare workers in the Ivory Coast, Thailand, and Brazil showed that having a BCG scar was associated with a positive TST when considering the 10-mm cutoff (144,145,147). No association between having a BCG scar and a positive TST was seen when using the 15-mm cutoff. Furthermore, BCG is unlikely to be protective (and may even be harmful) in the highest risk healthcare worker group, those who are infected with HIV or are otherwise severely immunocompromised.

Transmission of *M. tuberculosis* in healthcare facilities poses a risk not only to healthcare workers, but also to patients, volunteers, and visitors. Therefore, BCG vaccination of healthcare workers cannot substitute for a comprehensive TB infection control program. In the U.S., BCG vaccination of healthcare workers may be considered on an individual basis in high-risk settings where (a) a high proportion of *M. tuberculosis* isolates are resistant to both isoniazid and rifampin, (b) there is a strong likelihood of transmission and infection with such drug-resistant microorganisms, and (c) comprehensive TB infection control precautions have been implemented but have proved inadequate. BCG vaccination is not recommended for HIV-infected persons. BCG vaccination is not recommended for healthcare workers in settings in which there is a relatively high risk of *M. tuberculosis* transmission but most isolates are susceptible to isoniazid or rifampin, nor is it recommended in settings in which there is a low risk of transmission (179).

Special Considerations in Pediatric Hospitals

It is a widely held belief that pediatric TB patients usually are not infectious. Unfortunately, this is the result of historical belief rather than extensive published scientific data. Several factors are given for assuming that pediatric patients are less infectious. First, pediatric patients usually present with primary disease, whereas adults usually present with disease resulting from progression of LTBI. For this reason, it is believed that the bacterial burden is less in pediatric TB patients. Second, pediatric TB patients, particularly those younger than 10 years of age, usually do not produce sputum with coughing. Most pediatric TB patients are diagnosed as a result of contact investigation of an adult, and less than 50% of pediatric patients with active disease have a positive culture. In contrast, adults often have cavitary, endobronchial, or laryngeal TB and cough and have AFB-positive sputum smears.

Despite these facts, there is no documentation that pediatric patients always are noninfectious, and markers to identify infectious pediatric TB patients have not been developed. In contact investigations, an adult with TB is usually present, and any secondarily infected patients are thought to have acquired the infection from the adult rather than the pediatric patient. Although one study reports TST conversion rates between 0.03% and 0.40% from 1986 to 1994 among workers in a pediatric hospital in Ohio with mandatory annual TST screening (56), most children's hospitals have not maintained active healthcare worker TST programs (particularly including house staff or attending physicians), so that documentation of TST negativity after pediatric TB patient exposures is lacking. An observational study of adherence to TB control guidelines was conducted during 1996–1997 in two pediatric hospitals (178). Investigators noted that despite frequent lapses in respiratory protection and isolation, neither institution had documented any health care worker skin test conversions in the previous 2 years. These studies suggest that the risk to workers in pediatric hospitals is low, but no separate guidelines for pediatric hospitals exist. The TB infection control program in a pediatric hospital should be designed with consideration of the epidemiology of TB in its catchment area and with awareness that teenage patients with active TB may be as infectious as adults.

Because pediatric patients with suspected or confirmed TB may transmit *M. tuberculosis*, such patients should be evaluated for potential infectiousness using the same criteria as adults (i.e., on the basis of symptoms, radiologic findings, sputum AFB smears, treatment status, and performance of cough-inducing or aerosol-generating procedures). Children who may be infectious should be placed in isolation until the diagnosis of TB is ruled out or they are determined to be noninfectious. Pediatric patients who may be infectious include those with laryngeal or extensive pulmonary involvement (especially with pulmonary cavitation), pronounced cough, or AFB-positive sputum smears, or those for whom cough-inducing procedures are being performed. Because the source of infection for a child with TB often is a member of the child's family, parents and other visitors of all pediatric TB patients should themselves be evaluated for TB as soon as possible.

Regulation of Tuberculosis Infection Control

The Occupational Safety and Health Administration has been concerned about the safety of healthcare workers from the threat of occupationally acquired TB infection. In 1997, OSHA published a draft standard for the protection of healthcare workers from TB in hospitals, but to date no standard has been adopted (179). Concern expressed from the medical community over the necessity and cost of such regulation and potential compromise of patient care has halted implementation of these proposed regulations indefinitely. Even without regulation, hospitals have improved their application of TB infection control guidelines (114,180), although institutions still exhibit problems with the inclusion of attending physicians and house officers in mandatory employee TB screening programs, consistent use of appropriate respiratory protection by healthcare workers, or testing of engineering controls in isolation rooms (114,178, 180–182). Despite these lapses, these studies did not find evidence of ongoing transmission of TB to healthcare workers. In hospitals that apply the CDC guidelines, the risk of exposure to *M. tuberculosis* in the workplace can be minimized effectively in both low- and high-transmission areas (56,59). In light of hospitals' continued improvement in the application of CDC guidelines, OSHA will continue to regulate TB infection control under its general duty clause for employee protection from hazards in the workplace, rather than under separate and specific TB infection control regulations.

The OSHA general duty clause states in section 5(a) (1) of the Occupational Safety and Health Act of 1970 that the employer "shall furnish . . . a place of employment which is free from recognized hazards that are causing or are likely to cause death or serious harm to his employees." Every hospital that may treat a patient with active TB should maintain a TB protection program addressing five abatement methods outlined by OSHA's 1993 enforcement policy (183): (a) a protocol for early identification of patients with active TB, (b) a program of medical surveillance of employees, (c) evaluation and management of employees with a positive TST or active TB, (d) isolation of persons with suspected or confirmed TB, and (e) appropriate training of employees. The implementation of these methods may be tailored to the specific needs of the institution; OSHA expects institutions to follow the 1994 CDC guidelines in selecting these methods (157). In the states and territories where OSHA has direct jurisdiction, citations for failure to protect healthcare workers may be issued only where exposure of workers to *M. tuberculosis* occurs and where every known feasible and useful method to correct the hazard has not been implemented. Hospitals are in compliance with OSHA as long as the methods they select for TB control ensure that no exposure occurs (184, 185).

REFERENCES

1. World Health Organization. *http://www.who.int/mediacentre/factsheets/who104/en/index.html.*
2. Dooley SW, Jarvis WR, Martone WJ, et al. Multidrug-resistant tuberculosis [editorial]. *Ann Intern Med* 1992;117:257–258.
3. Niemann S, Harmsen D, Rusch-Gerdes S, et al. Differentiation of

clinical *Mycobacterium tuberculosis* complex isolates by *gyrB* DNA sequence polymorphism analysis. *J Clin Microbiol* 2000;38:3231–3234.
4. Huard RC, Lazzarini LC, Butler WR, et al. PCR-based method to differentiate the subspecies of the *Mycobacterium tuberculosis* complex on the basis of genomic deletions. *J Clin Microbiol* 2003;41: 1637–1650.
5. Selwyn PA, Hartel D, Lewis VA, et al. A prospective study of the risk of tuberculosis among intravenous drug users with human immunodeficiency virus infection. *N Engl J Med* 1989;320:545–550.
6. Centers for Disease Control and Prevention. *Status of tuberculosis epidemic in United States: 1997 data point to number of warning signals.* Atlanta: CDC, April 1998.
7. Wurtz R, Demarais R, Trainor W, et al. Specimen contamination in mycobacteriology laboratory detected by pseudo-outbreak of multidrug-resistant tuberculosis: analysis by routine epidemiology and confirmation by molecular technique. *J Clin Microbiol* 1996;34(4): 1017–1019.
8. Centers for Disease Control and Prevention. Misdiagnoses of tuberculosis resulting from laboratory cross-contamination of *Mycobacterium tuberculosis* cultures—New Jersey, 1998. *MMWR* 2000;49:413.
9. Cronin W, Rodriguez E, Valway S, et al. Pseudo-outbreak of tuberculosis in an acute-care general hospital: epidemiology and clinical considerations. *Infect Control Hosp Epidemiol* 1998;19:345–347.
10. Segal-Maurer S, Kreiswirth BN, Burns JM, et al. *Mycobacterium tuberculosis* specimen contamination revisited: the role of laboratory environmental control in a pseudo-outbreak. *Infect Control Hosp Epidemiol* 1998;19:101–105.
11. American Thoracic Society/CDC. Diagnostic standards and classification of tuberculosis in adults and children. *Am J Respir Crit Care Med* 2000;161:1376–1395.
12. Centers for Disease Control and Prevention. Update: nucleic acid amplification tests for tuberculosis. *MMWR* 2000;49:593.
13. Huebner RE, Schein MF, Bass JB Jr. The tuberculin skin test. *Clin Infect Dis* 1993;17:968–975.
14. Blumberg HM, White N, Parrott P, et al. False positive tuberculin skin test results among health care workers. *JAMA* 2000;283:2793.
15. Villarino ME, Brennan MJ, Nolan CM, et al. Comparable specificity of 2 commercial tuberculin reagents in persons at low risk for tuberculous infection. *JAMA* 1999;281:169–171.
16. Centers for Disease Control and Prevention. Targeted tuberculin testing and treatment of latent tuberculosis infection. *MMWR* 2000; 49(RR-6):1–54.
17. Snider DE Jr, Cauthen GM. Tuberculin skin testing of hospital employees: infection, boosting, and two-step testing. *Am J Infect Control* 1984;12:305–311.
18. Bass JB Jr, Serio RA. The use of repeat skin tests to eliminate the booster phenomenon in serial tuberculin testing. *Am Rev Respir Dis* 1981;123:394–396.
19. Mazurek GH, LoBue PA, Daley CL, et al. Comparison of a whole-blood interferon gamma assay with tuberculin skin testing for detecting latent *Mycobacterium tuberculosis* infection. *JAMA* 2001;286: 1740–1747.
20. Centers for Disease Control and Prevention. Guidelines for using the QuantiFERON® -TB test for diagnosis of latent *Mycobacterium tuberculosis* infection. *MMWR* 2003;52(RR02):15–18.
21. Centers for Disease Control and Prevention. Trends in tuberculosis mortality. *MMWR* 2003;52:217–222.
22. Centers for Disease Control and Prevention. Reported Tuberculosis in the United States, 2001. *http://www.cdc.gov/nchstp/tb/surv/surv2001/default.htm.*
23. Centers for Disease Control and Prevention. Progressing toward tuberculosis elimination in low-incidence areas of the United States: recommendations of the Advisory Council for the Elimination of Tuberculosis. *MMWR* 2002;51(RR05):1–16.
24. Moore M, McGray E, Onorato IM. The proportion of U.S. TB cases with a match in the AIDS registry. *Am J Respir Crit Care Med* 1997; 155:123.
25. Rieder HL, Cauthen GM, Kelly GD, et al. Tuberculosis in the United States. *JAMA* 1989;262:385–389.
26. Cantwell MF, Snider DE Jr, Cauthen GM, et al. Epidemiology of tuberculosis in the United States, 1985 through 1992. *JAMA* 1994; 272:535–539.
27. Mckenna MT, McGray E, Jones JL, et al. The fall after the rise: tuberculosis in the United States, 1991 to 1994. *Am J Public Health* 1998;88:1059–1063.
28. Zuber PLF, McKenna MT, Binkin NJ, et al. Long-term risk of tuberculosis among foreign-born persons in the United States. *JAMA* 1997; 278:304–307.
29. Centers for Disease Control and Prevention. Recommendations for prevention and control of tuberculosis among foreign-born persons. *MMWR* 1998;47(RR16):1–26.
30. Centers for Disease Control and Prevention. Reported tuberculosis in the United States, 2000. *http://www.cdc.gov/nchstp/tb/surv/surv2000/default.htm.*
31. Barrett-Connor E. The epidemiology of tuberculosis in physicians. *JAMA* 1979;241:33–38.
32. Geisler PJ, Nelson KE, Crispen RJ, et al. Tuberculosis in physicians: a continuing problem. *Am Rev Respir Dis* 1986;133:773–778.
33. Price LE, Rutala WA, Samsa GP. Tuberculosis in hospital personnel. *Infect Control* 1987;8:97–101.
34. Lambert LA, Davis YM, McCray E. Implementing tuberculosis skin testing programs in health departments and hospitals (abstract). American Lung Association/American Thoracic Society International Conference, San Francisco, May, 1997.
35. Davis YM, McCray E, Lambert LA, et al. Tuberculosis skin testing surveillance of health care workers (abstract). International Union Against Tuberculosis and Lung Disease Meeting, Chicago, February, 1997.
36. Levine I. Tuberculosis risk in students of nursing. *Arch Intern Med* 1968;121:545–548.
37. Weiss W. Tuberculosis in student nurses at Philadelphia General Hospital. *Am Rev Respir Dis* 1973;107:136–139.
38. Atuk NO, Hunt EH. Serial tuberculin testing and isoniazid therapy in general hospital employees. *JAMA* 1971;218:1795–1798.
39. Gregg D, Gibson M. Employee TB control in a predominantly tuberculosis hospital. *J SC Med Assoc* 1975;71:160–165.
40. Berman J, Levin ML, Orr ST, et al. Tuberculosis risk for hospital employees: analysis of a five-year tuberculin skin testing program. *Am J Public Health* 1981;71:1217–1222.
41. Craven RB, Wenzel RP, Atuk NO. Minimizing tuberculosis risk to hospital personnel and students exposed to unsuspected disease. *Ann Intern Med* 1975;82:628–632.
42. Vogeler DM, Burke JP. Tuberculosis screening for hospital employees. A five year experience in a large community hospital. *Am Rev Respir Dis* 1978;117:227–232.
43. Ruben FL, Norden CW, Schuster N. Analysis of a community hospital employee tuberculosis screening program 31 months after its inception. *Am Rev Respir Dis* 1977;115:23–28.
44. Ktsanes VK, Williams WL, Boudreaux VV. The cumulative risk of tuberculin skin test conversion for five years of hospital employment. *Am J Public Health* 1986;76:65–67.
45. Weinstein RS, Oshins J, Sacks HS. Tuberculosis infection in Mount Sinai medical students: 1974–1982. *Mt Sinai J Med* 1984;51: 283–286.
46. Chan JC, Tabak JI. Risk of tuberculous infection among house staff in an urban teaching hospital. *South Med J* 1985;78:1061–1064.
47. Thompson NJ, Glassroth JL, Snider DE Jr, et al. The booster phenomenon in serial tuberculin testing. *Am Rev Respir Dis* 1979;119: 587–597.
48. Kantor HS, Poblete R, Pusateri SL. Nosocomial transmission of tuberculosis from unsuspected disease. *Am J Med* 1988;84:833–838.
49. Aitken ML, Anderson KM, Albert RK. Is the tuberculosis screening program of hospital employees still required? *Am Rev Respir Dis* 1987; 136:805–807.
50. Malasky C, Jordan T, Potulski F, et al. Occupational tuberculosis infections among pulmonary physicians in training. *Am Rev Respir Dis* 1990;142:505–507.
51. Raad I, Cusick J, Sherertz RJ, et al. Annual tuberculin skin testing of employees at a university hospital: a cost-benefit analysis. *Infect Control Hosp Epidemiol* 1989;10:465–469.

52. Ramirez JA, Anderson P, Herp S, et al. Increased rate of tuberculin skin test conversion among workers at a university hospital. *Infect Control Hosp Epidemiol* 1992;13:579–581.
53. Ikeda RM, Birkhead GS, DiFerdinando GT, et al. Nosocomial tuberculosis: an outbreak of a strain resistant to seven drugs. *Infect Control Hosp Epidemiol* 1995;16:152–159.
54. Ramaswamy R, Corpuz M, Hewlett D. Tuberculosis surveillance of community hospital employees. A recommended strategy. *Arch Intern Med* 1995;155(15):1637–1639.
55. Zahnow K, Matts JP, Hillman D, et al., at the Terry Beirn Community Programs for Clinical Research on AIDS. Rates of tuberculosis infection in health care workers providing services to HIV-infected populations. *Infect Control Hosp Epidemiol* 1998;19(11):829–835.
56. Christie CDC, Constantinou P, Marx ML, et al. Low risk for tuberculosis in a regional pediatric hospital: nine-year study of community rates and the mandatory employee tuberculin skin-test program. *Infect Control Hosp Epidemiol* 1998;19:168–174.
57. Panlilio AL, Burwen DR, Curtis AB, et al. Tuberculin skin testing surveillance of health care personnel. *Clin Infect Dis* 2002;35:219–227.
58. Manangan LP, Bennett CL, Tablan N, et al. Nosocomial tuberculosis prevention measures among two groups of U.S. hospitals, 1992–1996. *Chest* 2000;117:380–384.
59. Larsen NM, Biddle CL, Sotir MJ, et al. Risk of tuberculin skin test conversion among health care workers: occupational versus community exposure and infection. *Clin Infect Dis* 2002;35:796–801.
60. Alpert ME, Levison ME. An epidemic of tuberculosis in a medical school. *N Engl J Med* 1965;272:718–721.
61. Ehrenkranz NJ, Kicklighter JL. Tuberculosis outbreak in a general hospital: evidence for airborne spread of infection. *Ann Intern Med* 1972;77:377–382.
62. Catanzaro A. Nosocomial tuberculosis. *Am Rev Respir Dis* 1982;125:559–562.
63. Haley CE, McDonald RC, Rossi L, et al. Tuberculosis epidemic among hospital personnel. *Infect Control Hosp Epidemiol* 1989;10:204–210.
64. Hutton MD, Stead WS, Cauthen GM, et al. Nosocomial transmission of tuberculosis associated with a draining abscess. *J Infect Dis* 1990;161:286–295.
65. Dooley SW, Villarino ME, Lawrence M, et al. Nosocomial transmission of tuberculosis in a hospital unit for HIV-infected patients. *JAMA* 1992;267:2632–2635.
66. Calder RA, Duclos P, Wilder MH, et al. *Mycobacterium tuberculosis* transmission in a health clinic. *Bull Int Union Tuberc Lung Dis* 1991;66:103–106.
67. Pierce JR Jr, Sims SL, Holman GH. Transmission of tuberculosis to hospital workers by a patient with AIDS. *Chest* 1992;101:581–582.
68. Jereb JA, Burwen DR, Dooley SW, et al. Nosocomial outbreak of tuberculosis in a renal transplant unit: application of a new technique for restriction fragment length polymorphism analysis of *Mycobacterium tuberculosis* isolates. *J Infect Dis* 1993;168:1219–1224.
69. Sundberg R, Shapiro R, Darras F, et al. A tuberculosis outbreak in a renal transplant program. *Transplant Proc* 1991;23:3091–3092.
70. Zaza S, Blumberg HM, Beck-Sagué C, et al. Nosocomial transmission of *Mycobacterium tuberculosis*: role of health care workers in outbreak propagation. *J Infect Dis* 1995;172:1542–1549.
71. Frampton MW. An outbreak of tuberculosis among hospital personnel caring for a patient with a skin ulcer. *Ann Intern Med* 1992;117:312–313.
72. Beck-Sagué C, Dooley SW, Hutton MD, et al. Hospital outbreak of multidrug-resistant *Mycobacterium tuberculosis* infections: factors in transmission to staff and HIV-infected patients. *JAMA* 1992;268:1280–1286.
73. Edlin BR, Tokars JI, Grieco MH, et al. An outbreak of multidrug-resistant tuberculosis among hospitalized patients with the acquired immunodeficiency syndrome. *N Engl J Med* 1992;326:1514–521.
74. Centers for Disease Control. Nosocomial transmission of multidrug-resistant tuberculosis among HIV-infected persons Florida and New York, 1988–1991. *MMWR* 1991;40:585–591.
75. Pearson ML, Jereb JA, Frieden TR, et al. Nosocomial transmission of multidrug-resistant *Mycobacterium tuberculosis.* A risk to patients and health care workers. *Ann Intern Med* 1992;117:191–196.
76. Coronado VG, Beck-Sagué CM, Hutton MD, et al. Transmission of multidrug-resistant *Mycobacterium tuberculosis* among persons with human immunodeficiency virus infection in an urban hospital: epidemiologic and restriction fragment length polymorphism analysis. *J Infect Dis* 1993;168:1052–1055.
77. Coronado VG, Valway S, Finelli L, et al. Nosocomial transmission of multidrug-resistant *Mycobacterium tuberculosis* among intravenous drug users with human immunodeficiency virus infection (Abstract S50). In: *Abstracts of the Third Annual Meeting of the Society for Hospital Epidemiology of America,* Chicago, April 18–20, 1993.
78. Centers for Disease Control. Outbreak of multidrug-resistant tuberculosis at a hospital: New York City, 1991. *MMWR* 1993;42:427–434.
79. Jereb JA, Klevens RM, Privett TD, et al. Tuberculosis in health care workers at a hospital with an outbreak of multidrug-resistant *Mycobacterium tuberculosis. Arch Intern Med* 1995;155(8):854–859.
80. Frieden TR, Sherman LF, Maw KL, et al. A multi-institutional outbreak of highly drug-resistant tuberculosis. Epidemiology and clinical outcomes. *JAMA* 1996;276(15):1229–1235.
81. Griffith DE, Hardeman JL, Zhang Y, et al. Tuberculosis outbreak among healthcare workers in a community hospital. *Am J Respir Crit Care Med* 1995;152:801–811.
82. Nivin B, Nicholas P, Gayer M, et al. A continuing outbreak of multidrug-resistant tuberculosis, with transmission in a hospital nursery. *Clin Infect Dis* 1998;26:303–307.
83. Luby S, Carmichael S, Shaw G, et al. A nosocomial outbreak of *Mycobacterium tuberculosis. J Fam Pract* 1994;39(1):21–25.
84. Kenyon TA, Ridzon R, LuskinHawk R, et al. A nosocomial outbreak of multidrug-resistant tuberculosis. *Ann Intern Med* 1997;127(1):32–33.
85. Agerton T, Valway S, Gore B, et al. Transmission of a highly drug-resistant strain (strain W) of *Mycobacterium tuberculosis. JAMA* 1997;278(13):1073–1077.
86. Michele TM, Cronin WA, Graham NMH, et al. Transmission of *Mycobacterium tuberculosis* by a fiber-optic bronchoscope. Identification by DNA fingerprinting. *JAMA* 1997;278(13):1093–1095.
87. Haas DW, Milton S, Kreiswirth BN, et al. Nosocomial transmission of a drug-sensitive W-variant *Mycobacterium tuberculosis* strain among patients with acquired immune deficiency syndrome in Tennessee. *Infect Control Hosp Epidemiol* 1998;19:635–639.
88. Askew GL, Finelli L, Hutton M, et al. *Mycobacterium tuberculosis* transmission from a pediatrician to patients. *Pediatrics* 1997;100:19–23.
89. Lee LH, LeVea CM, Graman PS. Congenital tuberculosis in a neonatal intensive care unit: case report, epidemiological investigation, and management of exposures. *Clin Infect Dis* 1998;27:474–477.
90. Spark RP, Pock NA, Pedron SL, et al. Perinatal tuberculosis and its public health impact: a case report. *Texas Med* 1996;92:50–53.
91. Ijaz K, Dillaha JA, Yang Z, et al. Unrecognized tuberculosis in a nursing home causing death with spread of tuberculosis to the community. *J Am Geriatr Soc* 2002;50:1213–1218.
92. Linquist JA, Rosaia CM, Riemer B, et al. Tuberculosis exposure of patients and staff in an outpatient hemodialysis unit. *Am J Infect Control* 2002;30:307–310.
93. Ramsey AH, Oemig TV, Davis JP, et al. An outbreak of bronchoscopy-related *Mycobacterium tuberculosis* infections due to lack of bronchoscope leak testing. *Chest* 2002;121:976–981
94. Cleveland JL, Kent J, Gooch BF, et al. Multidrug-resistant *Mycobacterium tuberculosis* in an HIV dental clinic. *Infect Control Hosp Epidemiol* 1995;16:7–11.
95. Kenyon TA, Ridzon R, Luskin-Hawk R, et al. A nosocomial outbreak of multidrug-resistant tuberculosis. *Ann Intern Med* 1997;127:32–36.
96. Conover C, Ridzon R, Valway S, et al. Outbreak of multidrug-resistant tuberculosis at a methadone treatment program. *Int J Tuberc Lung Dis* 2001;5:59–64.
97. Valway SE, Greifinger RB, Papania M, et al. Multidrug-resistant tuberculosis in the New York State prison system, 1990–1991. *J Infect Dis* 1994;170:151–156.
98. Small PM, Shafer RW, Hopewell PC, et al. Exogenous reinfection

with multidrug-resistant *Mycobacterium tuberculosis* in patients with advanced HIV infection. *N Engl J Med* 1993;328:1137–1144.

99. Sacks LV, Pendle S, Orlovic D, et al. A comparison of outbreak- and nonoutbreak-related multidrug-resistant tuberculosis among human immunodeficiency virus-infected patients in a South African hospital. *Clin Infect Dis* 1999;29:96–101.
100. Murray M, Nardell E. Molecular epidemiology of tuberculosis: achievements and challenges to current knowledge. *Bull World Health Organ* 2002;80:477–482.
101. Reves R, Blakey D, Snider DE, et al. Transmission of multiple drug-resistant tuberculosis: report of a school and community outbreak. *Am J Epidemiol* 1981;113:423–435.
102. Centers for Disease Control. Multidrug-resistant tuberculosis: North Carolina. *MMWR* 1987;35:785–787.
103. Centers for Disease Control. Outbreak of multidrug-resistant tuberculosis: Texas, California, and Pennsylvania. *MMWR* 1990;39: 369–372.
104. Nardell E, McInnis B, Thomas B, et al. Exogenous reinfection with tuberculosis in a shelter for the homeless. *N Engl J Med* 1986;315: 1570–1575.
105. Centers for Disease Control. Transmission of multidrug-resistant tuberculosis from an HIV-positive client in a residential substance-abuse treatment facility: Michigan. *MMWR* 1991;40:129–131.
106. Centers for Disease Control. Nosocomial transmission of multidrug-resistant TB to healthcare workers and HIV-infected patients in an urban hospital Florida. *MMWR* 1990;39:718–722.
107. Fischl MA, Uttamchandani RB, Daikos GL, et al. An outbreak of tuberculosis caused by multiple-drug-resistant tubercle bacilli among patients with HIV infection. *Ann Intern Med* 1992;117:177–183.
108. Fischl MA, Daikos GL, Uttamchandani RB, et al. Clinical presentation and outcome of patients with HIV infection and tuberculosis caused by multiple-drug-resistant bacilli. *Ann Intern Med* 1992;117: 184–190.
109. Jereb JA, Dooley SW, Klevens R, et al. Nosocomial transmission of multidrug-resistant tuberculosis to health care workers, New York City (abstract 51A). In: *Program and abstracts of the 1992 World Congress on Tuberculosis,* Bethesda, MD, November 16–19 1992.
110. Valway SE, Richards SB, Kovacovich J, et al. Outbreak of multidrug-resistant tuberculosis in a New York State prison, 1991. *Am J Epidemiol* 1994;140:113–122.
111. Wenger PN, Beck-Sagué CM, Otten J, et al. Efficacy of control measures in preventing nosocomial transmission of multidrug-resistant *Mycobacterium tuberculosis* among healthcare workers and HIV-infected patients. *Lancet* 1995;345:235–240.
112. Stroud C, Tokars J, Grieco M, et al. Evaluation of infection control measures in preventing the nosocomial transmission of multidrug-resistant *Mycobacterium tuberculosis* in a New York City hospital (Abstract A1–3). Third Annual Meeting of the Society for Hospital Epidemiologists of America, Chicago, April 18–20, 1993.
113. Maloney S, Pearson M, Gordon M, et al. Nosocomial multidrug-resistant tuberculosis revisited: assessing the efficacy of recommended control measures in preventing transmission to patients and health care workers. *Ann Intern Med* 1995;122:90–95.
114. Tokars JI, McKinley GF, Otten J, et al. Use and efficacy of tuberculosis infection control practices at hospitals with previous outbreaks of multidrug-resistant tuberculosis. *Infect Control Hosp Epidemiol* 2001; 22:449–455.
115. Moro ML, Errante I, Infuso A, et al. An outbreak of multidrug-resistant tuberculosis involving HIV-infected patients of two hospitals in Milan, Italy. Italian multidrug-resistant tuberculosis outbreak study group. *AIDS* 1998;12(9):1095–1102.
116. Centers for Disease Control. Multidrug-resistant tuberculosis outbreak on an HIV ward: Madrid, Spain, 1991–1995. *MMWR* 1996; 45(16):330–333.
117. Aita J, Barrera L, Reniero A, et al. Hospital transmission of multidrug-resistant *Mycobacterium tuberculosis* in Rosario, Argentina. *Medicina* 1996;56:48–50.
118. Ritacco V, Lonardo MD, Reniero A, et al. Nosocomial spread of human immunodeficiency virus-related multidrug-resistant tuberculosis in Buenos Aires. *J Infect Dis* 1997;176:637–642.
119. Gutierrez MC, Galan JC, Blazquez J, et al. Molecular markers demonstrate that the first described multidrug-resistant *Mycobacterium bovis* outbreak was due to *Mycobacterium tuberculosis. J Clin Microbiol* 1999; 37:971–975.
120. Breathnach AS, de Ruiter A, Holdsworth GMC, et al. An outbreak of multi-drug-resistant tuberculosis in a London teaching hospital. *J Hosp Infect* 1998;39:111–117.
121. Hannan MM, Peres H, Maltez F, et al. Investigation and control of a large outbreak of multi-drug resistant tuberculosis at a central Lisbon hospital. *J Hosp Infect* 2001;47:91–97.
122. Alonso-Echanove J, Granich RM, Laszlo A, et al. Occupational transmission of Mycobacterium tuberculosis to health care workers in a university hospital in Lima, Peru. *Clin Infect Dis* 2001;33:589–596.
123. Steward CJ. Tuberculous infection in a paediatric department. *Br Med J* 1976;1:30–32.
124. Steiner P, Rao M, Victoria MS, et al. Miliary tuberculosis in two infants after nursery exposure: epidemiologic, clinical, and laboratory findings. *Am Rev Respir Dis* 1976;113:267–271.
125. Light IJ, Saidleman M, Sutherland JM. Management of newborns after nursery exposure to tuberculosis. *Am Rev Respir Dis* 1974;109: 415–419.
126. Burk JR, Bahar D, Wolf FS, et al. Nursery exposure of 528 newborns to a nurse with pulmonary tuberculosis. *South Med J* 1978;71:7–10.
127. George RH, Gully PR, Gill ON, et al. An outbreak of tuberculosis in a children's hospital. *J Hosp Infect* 1986;8:129–142.
128. Beddall AC, Hill FG, George RH, et al. Unusually high incidence of tuberculosis among boys with haemophilia during an outbreak of the disease in hospital. *J Clin Pathol* 1985;38:1163–1165.
129. Muñoz FM, Ong LT, Seavey D, et al. Tuberculosis among adult visitors of children with suspected tuberculosis and employees at a children's hospital. *Infect Control Hosp Epidemiol* 2002;23:568–572.
130. Wallgren A. On contagiousness of childhood tuberculosis. *Acta Paediatr Scand* 1937;22:229–234.
131. Starke JR. Modern approaches to the diagnosis and treatment of tuberculosis in children. *Pediatr Clin North Am* 1988;35:441–464.
132. Smith MHD. Tuberculosis in children and adolescents. *Clin Chest Med* 1989;10:381–395.
133. Varteresian-Karanfil L, Josephson A, Fikrig S, et al. Pulmonary infection and cavity formation caused by *Mycobacterium tuberculosis* in a child with AIDS. *N Engl J Med* 1988;319:1018–1019.
134. Narain JP, Lofgren JP, Warren E, et al. Epidemic tuberculosis in a nursing home: a retrospective cohort study. *J Am Geriatr Soc* 1985; 33:258–263.
135. Centers for Disease Control. Tuberculosis North Dakota. *MMWR* 1979;27:523–525.
136. Centers for Disease Control. Tuberculosis in a nursing home Oklahoma. *MMWR* 1980;29:465–467.
137. Stead WW. Tuberculosis among elderly persons: an outbreak in a nursing home. *Ann Intern Med* 1981;94:606–610.
138. Centers for Disease Control. Tuberculosis in a nursing care facility: Washington. *MMWR* 1983;32:121–122,128.
139. Brennen C, Muder RR, Muraca PW. Occult endemic tuberculosis in a chronic care facility. *Infect Control Hosp Epidemiol* 1988;9: 548–552.
140. Smith WHR, Mason KD, Davies D, et al. Intraoral and pulmonary tuberculosis following dental treatment. *Lancet* 1982;1:842–844.
141. Porteous NB, Brown JP. Tuberculin skin test conversion rate in dental health care workers—results of a prospective study. *Am J Infect Control* 1999;27:385–387.
142. Raviglione MC, Snider DE, Kochi A. Global epidemiology of tuberculosis; morbidity and mortality of a worldwide epidemic. *JAMA* 1995;273:220–222.
143. Harries AD, Karnenya A, Namarika D, et al. Delays in diagnosis in treatment of smear-positive tuberculosis and the incidence of tuberculosis in hospital nurses in Blantyre, Malawi. *Trans R Soc Trop Med Hyg* 1997;91:15–17.
144. Kassim S, Zuber P, Wiktor SZ, et al. Tuberculin skin test reactivity among health care workers and level of exposure to tuberculosis patients in Abidjan, Cote d'Ivoire. In: *International Union Against Tuberculosis and Lung Disease,* vol 1(5), October 1997, suppl 1:S103.

145. Do A, Limpakarnjarat K, Uthaivoravit W, et al. Increased risk of *Mycobacterium tuberculosis* infection related to the occupational exposures of health care workers in Chiang Rai, Thailand. *Int J Tuberc Lung Dis* 1999;3:377–381.
146. Kruuner A, Danilovitsh M, Pehme L, et al. Tuberculosis as an occupational hazard for health care workers in Estonia. *Int J Tuberc Lung Dis* 2001;5:170–176.
147. Garrett DO, Laserson K, Almeida FF, et al. Risk of nosocomial acquisition of *Mycobacterium tuberculosis* infection among health care workers at a Brazilian hospital. 38th Interscience Conference on Antimicrobial Agents and Chemotherapy, San Diego, CA, September 1998.
148. Silva VM, Cunha AJ, Kritski AL. Tuberculin skin test conversion among medical students at a teaching hospital in Rio de Janeiro, Brazil. *Infect Control Hosp Epidemiol* 2002;23:591–594.
149. Granich R, Binkin NJ, Jarvis WR, et al. *Guidelines for the prevention of tuberculosis in health care facilities in resource-limited settings.* Geneva: World Health Organization, 1999.
150. Rytel MW, Davis ES, Prebil KJ. Primary cutaneous inoculation tuberculosis. *Am Rev Respir Dis* 1974;102:264–267.
151. Goette DK, Jacobson KW, Doty RD. Primary inoculation tuberculosis of the skin. *Arch Dermatol* 1978;114:567–569.
152. Sahn SA, Pierson DJ. Primary cutaneous inoculation of drug resistant tuberculosis. *Am J Med* 1974;57:676–678.
153. Sharma VK, Kumar B, Radotra BD, et al. Cutaneous inoculation tuberculosis in laboratory personnel. *Int J Dermatol* 1990;29: 293–294.
154. Kramer F, Sasse SA, Simms JC, et al. Primary cutaneous tuberculosis after a needlestick injury from a patient with AIDS and undiagnosed tuberculosis. *Ann Intern Med* 1993;119:594–595.
155. Nelson KE, Larson PA, Schraufnagel DE, et al. Transmission of tuberculosis by flexible fiber-bronchoscopes. *Am Rev Respir Dis* 1983;127: 97–100.
156. Peters TG, Reiter CG, Boswell RL. Transmission of tuberculosis by kidney transplantation. *Transplantation* 1984;38:514–526.
157. Centers for Disease Control. Guidelines for preventing the transmission of *Mycobacterium tuberculosis* in healthcare facilities, 1994. *MMWR* 1994;43(RR-13):1–132.
158. Hutton MD, Dooley SW, Cauthen GM. Nosocomial TB Transmission: characteristics of source-patients in reported outbreaks, 1970–1991. First World Congress on Tuberculosis, Rockville, Maryland, November 15–18, 1992.
159. Coronado VG, Beck-Sagué CM, Pearson ML, et al. Clinical and epidemiologic characteristics of multidrug-resistant *Mycobacterium tuberculosis* among patients with human immunodeficiency virus (HIV) infection. *Infect Dis Clin Pract* 1993;2:297–302.
160. Huebner RE, Good RC, Tokars JI. Current practices in mycobacteriology: results of a survey of state public health laboratories. *J Clin Microbiol* 1993;31:771–775.
161. Tenover FC, Crawford JT, Huebner RE, et al. Guest commentary. The resurgence of tuberculosis: is your laboratory ready? *J Clin Microbiol* 1993;31:767–770.
162. Blumberg HM, Burman WJ, Chaisson RE, et al. American Thoracic Society/Centers for Disease Control and Prevention/Infectious Diseases Society of America: treatment of tuberculosis. *Am J Respir Crit Care Med* 2003;167:603–662.
163. American Conference of Governmental Industrial Hygienists. *Industrial ventilation: a manual of recommended practice.* Cincinnati: American Conference of Governmental Hygienists, 1992.
164. American Society of Heating, Refrigerating, and Air-Conditioning Engineers. Health facilities. In: *1991 application handbook.* Atlanta: American Society of Heating, Refrigerating, and Air-Conditioning Engineers, 1991.
165. American Institute of Architects, Committee on Architecture for Health. General hospital. In: *Guidelines for construction and equipment of hospital and medical facilities.* Washington, DC: American Institute of Architects Press, 1996.
166. American Institute of Architects, Committee on Architecture for Health. General hospital. In: *Guidelines for construction and equipment of hospital and medical facilities.* Washington, DC: American Institute of Architects Press, 2001.
167. Centers for Disease Control and Prevention. CDC/HICPAC Guideline for Environmental Infection Control in Healthcare Facilities. *MMWR* 2003;52 *(in press).*
168. Rutala WA, Jones SM, Worthington JM, et al. Efficacy of portable filtration units in reducing aerosolized particles in the size range of *Mycobacterium tuberculosis. Infect Control Hosp Epidemiol* 1995;16: 391–398.
169. Riley RL, Mills CC, O'Grady F, et al. Infectiousness of air from a tuberculosis ward. *Am Rev Respir Dis* 1962;85:511–525.
170. Riley RL, Wells WF, Mills CC, et al. Air hygiene in tuberculosis: quantitative studies of the infectivity and control in a pilot ward. *Am Rev Tuberc* 1957;75;420–431.
171. Riley RL, Nardell EA. Clearing the air: the theory and application of UV air disinfection. *Am Rev Respir Dis* 1989;139:1286–1294.
172. Riley RL. Ultraviolet air disinfection for control of respiratory contagion. In: Kundsin RB, ed. *Architectural design and indoor microbial pollution.* New York: Oxford University Press, 1988:175–197.
173. National Institute for Occupational Safety and Health. *Criteria for a recommended standard . . . occupational exposure to ultraviolet radiation.* Publication no. (HSM) 73110009. Washington, DC: National Institute for Occupational Safety and Health, 1972.
174. International Agency for Research on Cancer. *IARC monographs on the evaluation of carcinogenic risks to humans: solar and ultraviolet radiation,* vol 55. Lyon, France: World Health Organization, International Agency for Research on Cancer, 1992.
175. Centers for Disease Control. Guidelines for preventing the transmission of tuberculosis in healthcare settings, with special focus on HIV-related issues. *MMWR* 1990;39(RR-17):1–29.
176. Title 42 Code of Federal Regulations Part 84, Washington, DC: United States Government Printing Office, 1995.
177. Miles JB Jr. Memorandum of September 6, 1995, from John B. Miles, Jr. Occupational Safety and Health Administration, to Regional Administrators, National Office Directorates, and Area Directors. Occupational Safety and Health Administration, U.S. Department of Labor, 1995.
178. Fine PE, Carneiro IA, Milstien JB, et al. *Issues relating to the use of BCG in immunization programmes.* WHO/V&B/99.23. Geneva: World Health Organization, 1999.
179. Centers for Disease Control and Prevention. The role of BCG vaccine in the prevention and control of tuberculosis in the United States: a joint statement by the Advisory Council for the Elimination of Tuberculosis and the Advisory Committee on Immunization Practices. *MMWR* 1996;45(RR-04).
180. Kellerman SE, Saiman L, San Gabriel P, et al. Observational study of the use of infection control interventions for *Mycobacterium tuberculosis* in pediatric facilities. *Pediatr Infect Dis J* 2001;20:566–570.
181. Department of Labor. Occupational Safety and Health Administration. Occupational exposure to tuberculosis; proposed rule. *Fed Reg* 1997;62:54160–54307.
182. Manangan LP, Bennett CL, Tablan N, et al. Nosocomial tuberculosis prevention measures among two groups of U.S. hospitals, 1992–1996. *Chest* 2000;117:380–384.
183. Sutton PM, Nicas M, Reinisch F, et al. Evaluating the control of tuberculosis among healthcare workers: adherence to CDC guidelines of three urban hospitals in California. *Infect Control Hosp Epidemiol* 1998;19:487–493.
184. Bratcher DF, Stover BH, Lane NE, et al. Compliance with national recommendations for tuberculosis screening and immunization of healthcare workers in a children's hospital. *Infect Control Hosp Epidemiol* 2000;21:338–340.
185. Clark RA. *Enforcement policy and procedures for occupational exposure to tuberculosis.* Washington, DC: U.S. Department of Labor, 1993.

38

NONTUBERCULOUS MYCOBACTERIA

RICHARD J. WALLACE, JR.
VENKATARAMA R. KOPPAKA

Although the existence of nontuberculous mycobacteria was recognized over a century ago, the microorganisms were originally thought to be contaminants or harmless colonizers. Increases in numbers of severely immunosuppressed patients, extensive utilization of invasive procedures, and more sensitive diagnostic tests have contributed to an increase in the isolation of the nontuberculous mycobacteria from clinical samples (1–7). As a consequence, over the past four decades the recognition and relative importance of nontuberculous mycobacteria as causes of human disease have increased dramatically. Nontuberculous mycobacteria are ubiquitous in nature, having been isolated from a variety of environmental sources, including dust, water, soil, domestic and wild animals, milk, and food (5,8–17). More than 90 species are currently recognized. Although many of these species are nonpathogenic, an increasing number, including *Mycobacterium avium-intracellulare, M. kansasii, M. chelonae, M. fortuitum, M. xenopi, M. lentiflavum, M. marinum, M. simiae, M. haemophilum,* and *M. genavense,* have been associated with disease in normal and immunosuppressed hosts (1,2,4,18–30). A select number of these species have also been linked to healthcare-associated disease, including *M. fortuitum* complex (including *M. chelonae, M. abscessus, M. fortuitum,* and *M. immunogenum*), *M. kansasii, M. avium* complex, and *M. xenopi.*

MICROBIOLOGY

The slow-growing nontuberculous mycobacteria, including those species usually associated with healthcare-associated diseases, grow well on the same types of media used for cultivation of *M. tuberculosis.* With some exceptions, they grow best at 37°C in an atmosphere supplemented with carbon dioxide.

M. xenopi grows optimally at 42° to 43°C, but with prolonged incubation will grow at 37°C. Some species, especially those associated with cutaneous disease such as *M. haemophilum, M. chelonae,* and *M. marinum* grow best at 28° to 32°C, especially on primary isolation. Most species produce visible colonies on solid agar within 7 to 14 days. More than 20 species of rapidly growing mycobacteria are recognized, with this number increasing rapidly with the primary use and availability of 16S ribosomal RNA (rRNA) gene sequencing for identification. The rapidly growing mycobacteria are susceptible to the NaOH decontamination process performed on sputum to facilitate isolation of *M. tuberculosis.* They are nonfastidious microorganisms that produce visible colonies on solid agar in 3 to 7 days. The microorganisms grow well at 35°C on standard bacterial media, including 5% sheep's blood and chocolate agar. Isolation of *M. chelonae* may take as long as 4 to 6 weeks at 37°C compared with 7 days at 28° to 32°C, its optimal growth temperature range.

IDENTIFICATION

The recent reemergence of tuberculosis as well as heightened awareness of nontuberculous mycobacteria as human pathogens has fueled an intense effort to develop rapid and accurate methods of identifying and speciating mycobacteria. Traditional identification schemes for slow-growing species utilize growth rates, pigment production, and biochemicals such as niacin production, urease, and catalase. Biochemical tests used in identifying the pathogenic rapidly growing mycobacteria include the rapid (3-day) arylsulfatase reaction, iron uptake, nitrate reduction, and the ability to utilize mannitol, inositol, and/or citrate as carbon sources (31–34). Although the rapidly growing mycobacteria can be identified by these methods, many laboratories do not identify these microorganisms to the species level, instead reporting them as *M. chelonae/M. abscessus* or just *M. chelonae.*

More recently, identification has utilized high-performance liquid chromatography (HPLC) and multiple molecular-based tests, including commercial DNA probes, polymerase chain reaction (PCR) amplification followed by restriction enzyme analysis (PRA), and 16S rRNA gene sequencing (35–39). HPLC methods for separation of mycolic acids has allowed the identification of most slowly growing mycobacterial species and some rapidly growing groups or complexes, with a greater specificity and speed than traditional methods (40,41). Nonradioactive commercial probes are available (Accu-Probe, Gen-Probe) and are routinely utilized for identifying isolates of *M. tuberculosis, M. avium* complex, *M. kansasii,* and *M. gordonae.* These probes offer excellent sensitivity and specificity, and because they can be used directly on broth cultures (usually the first medium to show growth), they have significantly reduced the time for final reporting of results (42,43). Currently no commercial probes are available for identification of the rapidly growing mycobacteria. Newest among the modern identification methods are adaptations of

PCR technology for detection and identification of mycobacteria in clinical samples (44,45). Two different nucleic acid amplification techniques for assaying directly from sputum are now commercially available (Amplicor, Roche Diagnostics, Indianapolis, Ind; and MTD test, Gen-Probe, San Diego, CA) and are approved for detection of *M. tuberculosis* (45,46). Currently, no systems are commercially available for direct detection of nontuberculous mycobacteria from clinical specimens or for species identification of pure cultures, although several novel approaches have been published. One approach utilizes PCR to amplify the gene encoding the 16S rRNA. The amplified fragment is then analyzed by species-specific probes (47,48) or partial nucleotide sequencing (49) for speciation. A second approach capitalizes on species-specific restriction fragment length polymorphisms in a PCR-amplified segment of the 65-kd heat shock protein gene (50,51).

TYPING SYSTEMS

Typing systems for rapidly growing mycobacteria have utilized a number of phenotypic and genotypic methods, including detailed species identification, heavy metal and antimicrobial susceptibility patterns, plasmid profiles, multilocus enzyme electrophoresis (MEE), pulsed-field gel electrophoresis (PFGE), and, more recently, random amplified polymorphic DNA (RAPD) PCR. PFGE has proven to be a highly useful tool for typing rapidly growing mycobacteria. This method utilizes restriction endonucleases with rare recognition sites such as *Dra*I and *Asn*I to generate a small series of large genomic restriction fragments (LRFs), the pattern of which is strain specific. Wallace's group (38,52) described the use of PFGE to type *M. chelonae* and *M. abscessus* with three reference strains, 28 sporadic isolates, and 62 healthcare-associated isolates from ten healthcare-associated outbreaks. LRF patterns satisfactory for comparison were achieved in 54% of *M. abscessus* and 90% of *M. chelonae* isolates by using the restriction endonucleases *Dra*I, *Asn*I, *Xba*I, and *Spe*I. The sporadic isolates were all highly variable. Isolates from five of ten outbreaks that gave satisfactory LRF patterns were identical. Strains that had been repetitively isolated from patients over periods of time ranging from 2 to 11 years demonstrated that LRF patterns were highly stable. Previous studies with *M. fortuitum* with this technique showed similar results, except that satisfactory LRF patterns were obtained with all strains studied (38,53). Environmental water isolates were identical (clonal) to some outbreak strains, indicating that water was the likely source of these past outbreaks. No human carrier or environmental nonwater sources have been identified as an outbreak source by this technique. PFGE is currently the most definitive epidemiologic tool available for comparing suspected outbreak strains of most isolates and species of rapidly growing mycobacteria.

More recently, methods have been introduced for DNA stabilization, which prevent the DNA denaturation seen with PFGE with select strains of bacterial species. Application of one of these methods, the use of hydroxyurea in the running buffer, allows for quality PFGE patterns with the approximate 50% of *M. abscessus* strains that produced broken DNA (54).

A nucleic acid amplification technique, termed RAPD-PCR or arbitrary primer (AP)-PCR, has also been applied to the investigation of outbreaks of *M. abscessus* (55,56). This technique offered the advantage of being simpler and unaffected by spontaneous lysis of the DNA sample during preparation for PFGE, as has occurred with 50% of isolates of *M. abscessus* (52). Its major disadvantage is that fewer patterns are produced with each primer; hence, at least three primers that produce quality patterns are needed, a finding that likely reflects the closely related character of these strains (56). Numerous outbreaks due to *M. abscessus* that produced broken DNA have taken advantage of this technically easier approach to determining strain relatedness.

PFGE has also been used to study clustering or pseudo-outbreaks of slow-growing mycobacteria, including *M. tuberculosis, M. xenopi* (57,58), *M. kansasii* (59,60), *M. simiae*, (61–63), and *M. avium* complex (64,65). Other fingerprint techniques used for slow-growing species include serotyping with *M. avium* complex (66), MEE with *M. fortuitum* (32), *M. abscessus* (67), and *M. simiae* (68), and the use of hybridization with repetitive insertional elements for *M. xenopi* (57), *M. kansasii* (59), and *M. avium* (64).

EPIDEMIOLOGY

Nontuberculous mycobacteria are not reportable by law in most states, and thus precise estimates of their incidence and prevalence are not available. Most nontuberculous species, with the exception of *M. avium* complex, are found in specific geographic areas. Overall, *M. avium-intracellulare* is the most common nontuberculous mycobacterial species recovered in the United States, followed by *M. kansasii* and the rapidly growing mycobacteria, *M. abscessus* and *M. fortuitum* (1). *M. xenopi* is the second most commonly isolated nontuberculous mycobacterium in England and Canada (69), whereas in the U.S. it is much less common. In some areas of northern Europe, *M. malmoense* is second only to *M. avium* complex (7). Again, this species is rare in the U.S. *M. simiae* is second to *M. avium* complex in some cities in the southwestern U.S. (61,70). Tap water and biofilms in the pipes appear to be the major reservoirs for *M. kansasii, M. xenopi,* and *M. simiae*, and a reservoir for *M. avium* and *M. intracellulare* (71).

In contrast to surveys done in the late 1970s and early 1980s, current studies show that there are now more laboratory isolates of nontuberculous mycobacteria, especially *M. avium* complex, than isolates of *M. tuberculosis* (1,69,72). The epidemiology of disease due to nontuberculous mycobacteria has changed because of the improvement in laboratory recovery and identification of these species and the increased awareness of the clinician of these species as potential pathogens. The emergence of better antiretroviral therapies for human immunodeficiency virus (HIV) infection and the acquired immunodeficiency syndrome (AIDS) has resulted in a dramatic decline in the incidence of nontuberculous mycobacterial disease in patients with far advanced disease. Among AIDS patients, *M. avium* complex had been a common mycobacterial cause of opportunistic infection and a frequent cause of disseminated disease.

The rapidly growing mycobacteria are the most commonly described and the most significant nontuberculous mycobacteria for healthcare-associated epidemiology (73). Of the human diseases attributable to this group of microorganisms, over 90% are due to *M. fortuitum, M. abscessus*, and *M. chelonae* (2,13,21, 73). These species readily survive nutritional deprivation and extremes of temperature. For example, most pathogenic species have been shown to grow and survive in distilled water, and they have been identified from soil, dust, domestic animals, and marine life (3,5,31,71,74,75). Multiple water sources have been identified, including tap water, municipal water, and aquariums (2,3,5,10). Mycobacteria have also been found in high numbers in biofilms on water delivery devices, such as dental handpieces (76). Similar biofilms may exist within bronchoscope channels, endoscope washers, ice machines, and water tanks, explaining the tendency of these devices to become colonized with mycobacteria. Biofilms are important not only because they enable bacteria to adhere and persist on artificial surfaces, but also because they provide protection from the action of disinfectants (77,78).

PATHOGENESIS AND CLINICAL MANIFESTATIONS

The pathology of nontuberculous mycobacterial infection can be identical to that of *M. tuberculosis*. Chronic inflammation, acute suppuration, nonnecrotic epithelioid tubercles, and caseation are all seen on histopathology. The coexistence of granulomatous and acute inflammation (so-called dimorphic inflammatory response) is not seen with tuberculosis but is commonly seen in cervical lymph nodes (79) and cutaneous disease (2,21, 80) due to the nontuberculous mycobacteria. Animal models to study the pathology of nontuberculous mycobacteria have been difficult to develop, even when the animals are immunosuppressed (81,82).

Isolation of nontuberculous mycobacteria in the laboratory may represent an environmental or laboratory contaminant, transient patient colonization, or true disease. In the absence of known environmental contamination, isolation of any nontuberculous mycobacteria from a normally sterile site should be considered significant. Contamination of a skin wound with these microorganisms is rare, and even a single positive culture from this site generally indicates disease. Similarly, recovery of these microorganisms from cultures of lymph node specimens or blood is sufficient for establishing the diagnosis of nontuberculous lymphadenitis or disseminated disease, respectively. In contrast, isolation of nontuberculous mycobacteria from pulmonary specimens can be particularly difficult to evaluate. The American Thoracic Society last published criteria for the diagnosis of nontuberculous mycobacterial pulmonary disease in 1997 (7). According to these criteria, a definitive diagnosis requires compatible clinical symptoms along with characteristic radiographic abnormalities, which are not attributable to any other cause. Multiple cultures of respiratory specimens are required to demonstrate persistent culture positivity. The microorganism must be grown from three acid-fast bacilli (AFB) smear-negative specimens of sputum, from two specimens of which at least one is AFB smear positive, or from at least one specimen obtained from a normally sterile site such as bronchial wash or broncho-

TABLE 38.1. CLINICAL PRESENTATIONS OF NONTUBERCULOUS MYCOBACTERIA

Clinical Syndrome	Common Causes	Less Common Causes
Bronchopulmonary infection	*M. avium* complex *M. kansasii* *M. abscessus*	*M. xenopi* *M. fortuitum* *M. malmoense* *M. szulgai* *M. simiae* *M. asiaticum*
Lymphadenitis	*M. avium* complex	*M. malmoense* *M. abscessus* *M. fortuitum*
Disseminated disease	*M. avium* complex *M. chelonae*	*M. abscessus* *M. haemophilum* *M. genavense* *M. kansasii*
Skeletal and joint infection	*M. marinum* *M. avium* complex *M. fortuitum* *M. abscessus*	*M. kansasii* *M. chelonae* *M. haemophilum*
Skin and soft tissue infection	*M. marinum* *M. fortuitum* *M. chelonae* *M. abscessus* *M. ulcerans*	*M. haemophilum* *M. smegmatis* group

pulmonary tissue. The clinical syndromes most commonly associated with nontuberculous mycobacterial infections and the microorganisms usually responsible are summarized in Table 38.1.

DESCRIPTION OF COMMUNITY-ACQUIRED INFECTIONS

Rapidly Growing Mycobacteria

Cutaneous Disease

Rapidly growing mycobacteria most commonly cause posttraumatic and postsurgical skin and soft tissue infections but can also cause lymphadenitis, keratitis, suppurative arthritis, osteomyelitis, endocarditis, peritonitis, bacteremia, and disseminated disease (21,55,83–90). In a review of 125 cases of infection due to rapidly growing mycobacteria (2), 60% presented with cutaneous manifestations, half of which were due to penetrating trauma (85). The usual pathogens in this setting are *M. fortuitum, M. abscessus*, and *M. fortuitum* third biovariant complex (2). Infections are typically chronic and may heal spontaneously or after surgical debridement. Even without medical intervention, the lesions usually remain well localized. Infections typically present as cellulitis with acute and chronic inflammation, which may form ulcers or sinus tracts with serous, watery drainage (2,55,80,91,92).

Disseminated Disease

Disseminated disease due to the rapidly growing species is intimately related to immunosuppression, particularly with corticosteroid therapy. Dissemination primarily occurs with *M. chelonae* and to a lesser degree with *M. abscessus*. These patients typically have no history of prior trauma but present with multiple draining skin lesions. Infections with *M. chelonae* and *M. abscessus* have been described in solid organ transplant patients, including renal, heart, and lung transplant patients as well as patients with rheumatoid arthritis or other autoimmune disorders on long-term, low-dose corticosteroids (2,21,85,93). In one series of renal transplant patients, ten patients with *M. chelonae* infections (including both *M. chelonae* and *M. abscessus*) were identified over a 6-year period from four hospitals (94).

Pulmonary Disease

The rapidly growing mycobacteria also cause pulmonary disease, with *M. abscessus* accounting for the majority of cases. Pulmonary infection is usually chronic, insidious, and slowly progressive. Patients may have minimal symptoms of cough or fatigue for many years, and subtle changes on high-resolution computed tomography (CT) scanning or subtle deterioration in pulmonary function may be the only markers of disease progression. Clinically, these patients are older and typically present with bilateral nodular interstitial disease associated with cylindrical bronchiectasis (2,21,73,95). Their presentation appears identical to that in women with *M. avium* complex lung disease.

Slow-Growing Nontuberculous Mycobacteria

M. malmoense, M. kansasii, M. avium complex, *M. xenopi*, and *M. simiae* can all occasionally cause community-acquired pulmonary or extrapulmonary disease in HIV-negative patients (4,7). *M. avium* complex, *M. kansasii, M. haemophilum,* and *M. genavense* are the usual causes of infections including disseminated disease in HIV-infected persons. All the slow-growing species are infrequent causes of healthcare-associated disease (4,7). Detailed descriptions of the clinical disease associated with these microorganisms are reported elsewhere (4,7,13).

DESCRIPTION OF HEALTHCARE-ASSOCIATED INFECTIONS

Healthcare-associated mycobacterial infections (almost exclusively due to rapidly growing mycobacteria) have been recognized for 25 years and remain relatively common. They have been most often recognized as causes of surgical site infections and postinjection abscesses; however, they have also been reported to cause catheter-related infections, dialysis-related infections, and, most recently, bronchoscope and endoscope contamination. For outbreaks and sporadic reports of infections due to rapidly growing mycobacteria, there is a strong geographic relationship to the Gulf Coast and the southeastern U.S. Figure 38.1 demonstrates the focal geography of some of the early outbreaks reported in the U.S.

Surgical Site Infections

Outbreaks of mycobacterial surgical site infections were first recognized in 1975 to 1976 with the report of four such out-

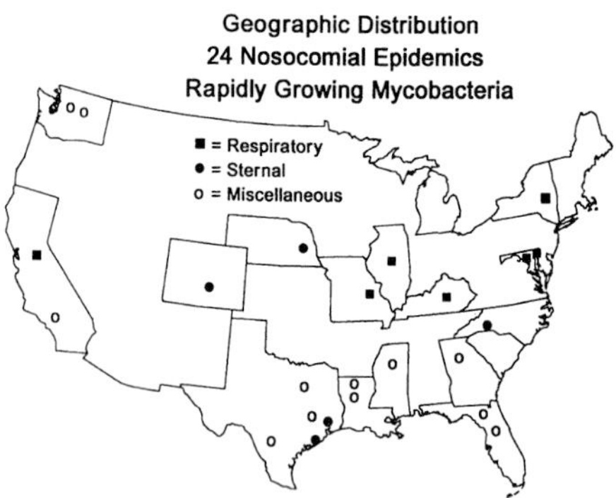

Figure 38.1. The geographic focality of nosocomial outbreaks due to the rapidly growing mycobacteria.

breaks (96–98). These reports were followed in the 1980s by at least 14 additional outbreaks (99–104). Outbreaks have been described involving cardiothoracic surgery, plastic surgery, augmentation mammaplasty, and arthroplasty (96–104). A summary of the major healthcare-associated outbreaks due to the rapidly growing mycobacteria is given in Table 38.2. Following recognition of epidemic surgical site infections, it became apparent that most surgical site infections due to rapidly growing mycobacteria are sporadic (21,32,99,105–117). Such infections with rapidly growing mycobacteria have been described following vascular surgery, oophorectomy, neurosurgery, corneal surgery, the insertion of middle ear tubes, biopsy procedures, and plastic surgery, including procedures such as face lifts and liposuction (86,88,110,111,113,114,117–124). It is unclear whether there is a predisposition for certain types of surgery; however, more than 60% of surgical site infections due to rapidly growing mycobacteria reported in the 1980s were reported after cardiac surgery (96,100,103,108) or augmentation mammaplasty (99,111,119).

Cardiothoracic Surgery

A review of rapidly growing mycobacterial isolates associated with cardiac surgery was published in 1989 (32). This study evaluated isolates from eight cardiac surgery outbreaks, as well as 45 sporadic isolates. Disease isolates were recovered from sternal wounds, donor vein graft sites, blood, and artificial valves. The isolates included *M. fortuitum, M. abscessus,* and the *M. smegmatis* group (32). The development several years later of DNA fingerprinting for *M. fortuitum* and *M. abscessus* permitted better evaluation of these outbreaks (52–56). The first reported cardiac surgery–associated outbreak occurred in 1976 in North Carolina. Nineteen cases of disease due to *M. abscessus* occurred over a 10-week period, but no source was identified. Five (26%) patients died of their disease. In a second similar outbreak in Colorado, 10 of 75 cardiac surgery patients developed infections with *M. fortuitum. M. fortuitum* was recovered from a settling plate in the operating room (96), but subsequent molecular studies using PFGE showed that it differed from the disease strain (38).

The best clue to the potential reservoir for these outbreaks was provided in a later outbreak from Texas involving both *M.*

TABLE 38.2. OUTBREAKS DUE TO RAPIDLY GROWING MYCOBACTERIA

Disease	Year of Outbreak	Location	Microorganism
Surgical site infections			
Cardiac surgey	1977	Hungary	*M. abscessus*
	1987–1989	Hong Kong	*M. fortuitum* and *M. perigrinum*
	1987	Texas	*M. abscessus*
	1976	N. Carolina	*M. abscessus*
	1976	Colorado	*M. fortuitum*
	1976	Multistate	*M. abscessus*
	1981	Nebraska	*M. fortuitum*
	1981	Texas	*M. fortuitum* and *M. abscessus*
Plastic surgery			
Augmentation mammaplasty	1985	Florida	*M. abscessus*
Vascular (vein stripping)	1974	Spain	*M. abscessus*
Nasal surgery	1987–1988	Mexico	*M. abscessus?*[a]
Liposuction	1996–1997	California	*M. chelonae*
Ocular surgery	1991	Taiwan	*M. fortuitum* and *M. chelonae*
Injection abscesses	1961	Belgium	*M. fortuitum?*[a]
	1962	Congo	*M. fortuitum?*[a]
	1963	Texas	*M. fortuitum?*[a]
	1966–1968	England	*M. chelonae*
	1969	Netherlands	*M. chelonae*
	1977	Texas	*M. abscessus*
	1989	Georgia	*M. chelonae*
	1993	Colombia, South America	*M. abscessus*
	1995–6	Colorado/Wyoming	*M. abscessus*
	1999	Texas	*M. abscessus*
EMG needles	1985	Washington	*M. fortuitum*
Podiatry jet injector	1988	Florida	*M. abscessus*
Dialysis-related	1982	Louisiana	*M. abscessus*
Bronchoscopy/endoscopy	1987	California	*M. abscessus*
	1987	Washington	*M. mucogenicum*[b]
	1981	Illinois	*M. chelonae*?[a]
	1989	Missouri	*M. immunogenum*
	1989	England	*M. immunogenum*
	1989	Switzerland	*M. immunogenum*
	1991	Missouri	*M. immunogenum*
	1991–1992	England	*M. fortuitum* and *M. chelonae*
	1992	Maryland	*M. immunogenum*
	1992	Ireland	*M. chelonae*
	1992	Australia	*M. chelonae*
	1992	Kentucky	*M. immunogenum*
	1992	Taiwan	*M. chelonae*
	1993	Florida	*M. chelonae*
	1999	Scotland	*M. chelonae*
Respiratory	1985	New York	*M. peregrinum*
	1988–1989	California	*M. fortuitum*
	1989–1990	Washington, DC	*M. fortuitum*
Other			
Laparoscopy	1986	Mississippi	*M. abscessus*
Bone Marrow Biopsy	1987	Texas	*M. fortuitum*
Middle ear irrigation	1988	Louisiana	*M. abscessus*

[a] Species of the microorganism by current taxonomy has not been confirmed.
[b] Formerly known as *M. chelonae*-like organism (MCLO).
EMG, electromyography.

fortuitum and *M. abscessus. M. fortuitum* with a DNA fingerprint identical to that of the outbreak strain was isolated from the tap water in the operating room, ice water used to cool the cardioplegia solution, ice machines, and municipal water coming into the hospital. An identical strain was recovered from patients with several types of noncardiac surgical site infections. In this same outbreak, *M. abscessus*, which was found by RAPD-PCR to be identical to some disease isolates (56), was isolated from hospital ice water used to cool the cardioplegia solution and a pair of surgical scissors (2,32,38,100). This investigation was the first major study to identify water (in this case as ice used for surgical purposes) as the major reservoir for the microorganism. Another

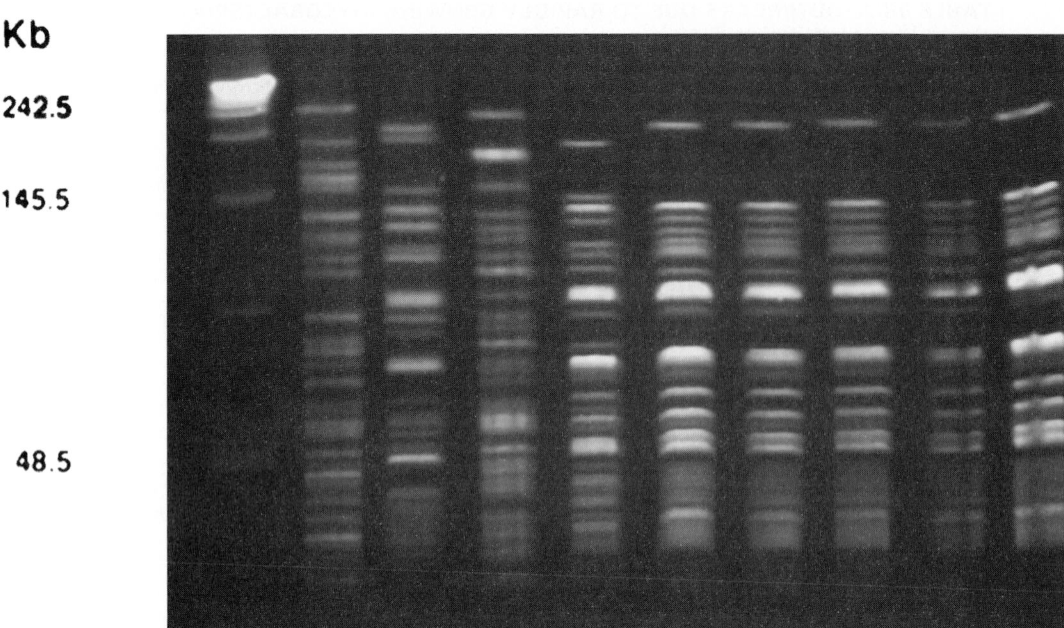

Figure 38.2. Pulsed-field gel electrophoresis of *M. abscessus* from a surgical site infection outbreak in Texas using *Xba I*. Lanes 1 to 5 are genomic DNA and control strains. Lanes 6 and 10 are isolates obtained from tap water, and lanes 7 to 9 are case isolates from infected patients.

unreported outbreak from Texas also helped to clarify the role of water as a reservoir for rapidly growing mycobacteria. In this outbreak, PFGE demonstrated the clonality of tap water and case isolates (Fig. 38.2). Several cases of perivalvular infection occurred following contamination of commercial porcine valves with *M. chelonae* (125,126).

Outbreaks of sternal wound disease have not been limited to the U.S. An outbreak of sternal infections due to *M. abscessus* following cardiac surgery in Budapest was described in 1976, but the source was not identified (98). An outbreak of sternal surgical site infections caused by *M. fortuitum* and *M. peregrinum* occurred in Hong Kong among patients who had undergone cardiothoracic surgery at a single hospital during 1987–1989 (104). Investigators used rRNA gene restriction fragment-length polymorphisms to determine that, in most cases, the microorganism belonged to one of two groups. The source of contamination could not be identified and was presumed to be environmental in origin. No additional outbreaks have been reported in the past 14 years, presumably because of avoidance of contaminated tap water and ice in the operating room.

In addition to these outbreaks, numerous sporadic infections due to rapidly growing mycobacteria have been reported following cardiac surgery (2,108,113,127–130), including a case of subacute bacterial endocarditis for which a source was never documented. When 89 isolates from cardiac surgical site infections were analyzed, 45 were sporadic; these were more likely to be due to *M. fortuitum* or the *M. smegmatis* group. Eighty percent were from southern coastal states (52). Sporadic cases of disease continue to be seen.

Cardiac surgery patients with surgical site infections due to rapid growers have presented with failure of surgical site healing or breakdown of healed surgical sites with drainage of serous fluid. Endocarditis patients presented with fever and cutaneous and embolic phenomena, along with positive blood cultures 4 to 12 weeks after surgery (2,131). In the outbreak related to contaminated porcine valves, patients presented with pericardial effusions and aortic abscesses.

Plastic Surgery/Augmentation Mammaplasty

Infections due to rapid growers following plastic surgery for breast augmentation are well described (99,101,109,111,116, 119) and, along with cardiac surgery infections, were the most common surgical site infections due to these microorganisms. However, with the exception of one outbreak, the pathogenesis of these infections has yet to be defined (99,101,132). The one outbreak in which a well-defined source was identified included infections following both augmentation mammaplasty and blepharoplasty (101). During April to October 1985, an outbreak of *M. abscessus* was identified affecting eight patients. *M. abscessus* was recovered from the gentian violet in the office and the stock solution in the pharmacy, which had been using distilled water to reconstitute the gentian violet crystals instead of 10% alcohol, thus allowing *M. abscessus* to replicate. Previous studies have shown that *M. abscessus* grows well in potable and distilled water (8,74,100). No source has been identified for any of the cases of sporadic mammaplasty wound infections, although the tendency for more than one case to occur in a plastic surgeon's practice makes environmental sources highly likely (99,116,132). Almost 90% of sporadic cases of surgical site infections following augmentation mammaplasty have been reported from three states—Texas, North Carolina, and Florida (99,116) (see also Chapter 67). Sporadic surgical site infections after other types of breast surgery as well as spontaneous breast infections have also been reported (116).

Outbreaks and/or sporadic surgical site infections have been described after other types of plastic surgery procedures, including face lifts (115), blepharoplasty (110), and liposuction (133). In a liposuction-associated outbreak reported in 2001 involving an outpatient clinic, tap water was used for flushing and rinsing suction tubing, and inadequate sterilization procedures were in place. *M. chelonae* recovered from patient wounds and the tap water system were found to be clonal when studied by PFGE (133).

Miscellaneous Surgery

Although outbreaks of surgical site infections were first reported after cardiac surgery and augmentation mammaplasty, outbreaks have been described after general surgical procedures as well. In one outbreak, a cluster of *M. abscessus* surgical site infections occurred in a Mississippi hospital in 1985 in women who had undergone laparoscopy. In this outbreak, four cases confirmed by culture and 12 probable cases were identified. *M. abscessus* with the same antimicrobial susceptibility profile as the patient isolates was identified from the mineral oil used to lubricate the laparoscope and from multiple specimens of tap water throughout the hospital. The outbreak stopped when a sterile aqueous-based solution was substituted for mineral oil as a lubricant and when laparoscopes received high-level disinfection without exposure to tap water [Centers for Disease Control and Prevention (CDC) investigation no. 91-01].

Postinjection Abscesses

The first description of *M. fortuitum* as a pathogen in 1936 involved an abscess that resulted from a vitamin injection (134). Since that time, a number of sporadic cases as well as outbreaks of localized cutaneous abscesses have been reported involving injections with needles (55,80,135–144). Unlike other healthcare-associated infections, outbreaks of postinjection abscesses are most often due to *M. chelonae*, although outbreaks involving *M. fortuitum* and *M. abscessus* have also been reported. Some outbreaks, especially those before the 1980s, relate to reuse or inadequate sterilization of needles (135,142). Other outbreaks appear to relate to contaminated biologics, especially the use of multidose vials or materials. An outbreak among student nurses occurred when a single liter bottle of saline was used repetitively to practice injection techniques (136). An outbreak of *M. abscessus* (identified then as *M. chelonae* subspecies *abscessus*) was identified from a podiatry practice in which jet injectors were placed in distilled water for rinsing between patients. *M. abscessus* was identified in the container of distilled water. A similar outbreak of *M. fortuitum* infections occurred in patients who had undergone electromyography. This office was using reusable needle electrodes that were disinfected with 2% glutaraldehyde and then rinsed with tap water. The outbreak stopped when the needles were routinely autoclaved between patients. Tap water was considered the likely source of infection, but no environmental cultures were positive (143).

Even though these infections have been described for more than four decades, they continue to occur. In 1995 to 1996, an outbreak of abscesses occurred in 47 patients in Colorado and Wyoming (139). All had received intramuscular injections of a preparation alleged to be adrenal cortex extract provided by a single physician as part of a weight loss regimen. The extract, which had not been approved by the U.S. Food and Drug Administration (FDA), was found to be contaminated with *M. abscessus*. The largest single outbreak of postinjection abscesses due to rapidly growing mycobacteria occurred in Colombia, South America (55,80,140). Of 2,000 patients treated by a single physician from November 1992 to April 1993, 350 developed skin abscesses due to *M. abscessus*. Five representative isolates from the epidemic were identical by RAPD-PCR (55). The outbreak was associated with local injections of lidocaine administered by the physician, and the microorganism was recovered from one of the reusable multidose vials (140). The latest reported outbreak of postinjection abscesses occurred in 1999 and involved the use of contaminated benzalkonium chloride used for skin disinfection. Clinical and environmental isolates of *M. abscessus* were indistinguishable by RAPD-PCR (145).

Single sporadic cases of postinjection abscesses likely occur in the same way as epidemic disease (144). Focal abscesses, especially of the arm or hip, therefore should be investigated for any relationship to injections, and if a relationship is identified, infection control policies and procedures should be reviewed to prevent recurrences and outbreaks.

Dialysis-Related Infections

Hemodialysis

The risk of infection due to rapidly growing mycobacteria in patients undergoing hemodialysis was first reported in 1982, when 27 cases of nontuberculous mycobacterial infection were identified in a group of patients from two Louisiana hemodialysis centers. *M. abscessus* was identified in 24 patients, and one had *M. mucogenicum*. The attack rate in one dialysis unit was 19%. Bacteremia occurred in 18 patients, and four had localized infections. There were 13 deaths, for an overall mortality rate of 48%. Nontuberculous mycobacteria were identified throughout the water system in two dialysis centers. *M. abscessus* (later shown by PFGE to be identical to disease isolates) (52) was identified in the water of the reverse osmosis room, the reverse osmosis tank, and the formaldehyde used to reprocess dialyzers, and from the blood compartment side of five of 31 dialyzers. The outbreak stopped when the reuse of dialyzers was discontinued.

A number of important lessons were learned from this outbreak. Tap water is not sterile and allows good growth of rapidly growing mycobacteria. These microorganisms are relatively resistant to chlorine and glutaraldehyde, and decontamination of dialyzers and dialysis machines may be difficult. Protocols for disinfection and reprocessing of dialyzers must therefore be rigorously followed. Finally, cultures of dialysis patients should be held for a minimum of 14 days to facilitate identification of fastidious or unusual water microorganisms (146,147).

From 1987 to 1988, another outbreak of *M. abscessus* disease occurred, this one involving a hemodialysis unit in California. Infection occurred in five patients; four of five had arteriovenous graft infections and two died. *M. abscessus* was subsequently identified from municipal water and the hose of the water spray device used for reprocessing the high-flux but not the regular dialyzers. High-flux dialysis had been instituted in this center in 1986, and in 1987 Renalin (hydrogen peroxide/peracetic acid–based disinfectant) was substituted for 4% formaldehyde to reprocess dialyzers. A number of infection control issues were identified that may have contributed to the outbreak (147–150). These types of infections may increase with widespread use of high-flux dialysis, reprocessed dialyzers, and increasing use of Renalin. The effectiveness of dialyzer disinfection is critical to providing patients with safe dialysis (147,150). No major outbreak of mycobacterial infection involving hemodialysis has been reported in the past 15 years (see also Chapter 64).

Peritoneal Dialysis

Peritonitis is a common complication of chronic ambulatory peritoneal dialysis (CAPD). After beginning peritoneal dialysis, 60% of patients develop peritonitis in the first year and 80% develop peritonitis within 2 years. Most episodes are due to staphylococci (40–70%) and aerobic gram-negative bacilli (15–30%). Culture-negative peritonitis represents 8% to 27% of reported episodes of CAPD-related peritonitis. Mycobacteria account for <3% of cases but may be more common and simply underrecognized. Hakim et al. (151) reviewed 31 cases of peritonitis in CAPD patients due to nontuberculous mycobacteria. Most of the cases reported in the literature have been due to rapidly growing mycobacteria (86%), mostly *M. fortuitum*, although other mycobacteria have also been implicated (87, 152–154). In one outbreak involving 17 cases due to rapidly growing mycobacteria (155), most patients presented with fever, abdominal pain, and cloudy dialysis fluid. Catheter dysfunction, vomiting, diarrhea, and weight loss were also described. However, the illness may be more insidious in onset, signaled only by increases in cell counts in the dialysis fluid, particularly with polymorphonuclear leukocytes. Diagnosis is usually made by culture, since AFB smears are generally negative. The unexpected staining and growth characteristics of the rapidly growing mycobacteria may result in misidentification as diphtheroids or debris due to fragmentation and beading on Gram stain. When gram-positive rods resembling corynebacteria are isolated from peritoneal fluid, a smear stained for AFB should be examined (155–159). Peritoneal biopsies may be helpful in some cases, particularly if they show mixed acute and chronic granulomatous inflammation with pyogenic abscesses or sinus tracts (2). Management consists of catheter removal along with multidrug chemotherapy, based on *in vitro* susceptibility (7,33,87). Catheter removal improves the success rate (160). Treatment in the past has been with aminoglycosides, although the fluoroquinolones, clarithromycin, and imipenem have also shown potential utility (87,155,160,161) (see also Chapter 65).

Catheter-Related Infections

Catheter-related infections due to rapidly growing mycobacteria are well-described complications of intravenous catheters, arteriovenous catheters, peritoneal dialysis catheters, and even lacrimal duct catheters. Exit-site infections, tunnel infections, and bacteremias have all been reported (2,86,162–168). Catheter-related infections are currently the most common healthcare-associated infections caused by the rapidly growing mycobacteria. The largest single series of infections was reported by Raad et al. (164), who described intravenous catheter–related infections due to rapid growers in 15 cancer patients over 12 years at the University of Texas M. D. Anderson Cancer Center. These authors also reviewed the literature through 1991 and described an additional 14 cases. Among the M. D. Anderson cases, 60% had cancer as an underlying disease. There were 11 bacteremias and four catheter site infections with nine due to *M. fortuitum* and six to the *M. chelonae/abscessus* group (the authors did not discriminate between *M. chelonae* and *M. abscessus*). All of the patients who had their catheter removed recovered. Treatment failed in seven bacteremic patients who had their central line left in place. After catheter removal, six of the seven infections subsequently responded. Foreign bodies and devices appear to play a significant role in facilitating and perpetuating such infections (105,116,126,165,166,168). An unusual syndrome of cholestatic hepatitis associated with fever, right upper quadrant pain, and marked elevation of alkaline phosphatase has been observed in some patients with central venous catheter sepsis due to mycobacteria. The patients have granulomas with positive cultures on liver biopsies. The syndrome presumably results from seeding of the liver at the time of bacteremia (169).

Rarely, catheter sepsis has been reported due to slow-growing mycobacteria (170–173). This probably occurs more often than has been reported but goes undetected because of failure to use culture media that will grow mycobacteria and/or too short an incubation time.

Infections Related to Foreign Bodies/ Prosthetic Devices

Healthcare-associated infections due to the rapidly growing mycobacteria have been described after the insertion of a variety of prosthetic devices other than catheters and silicone breast implants, including prosthetic hips, prosthetic knees, pacemakers, defibrillators, and myringotomy tubes. Although most cases have been sporadic, disease outbreaks have been reported. Seventeen cases of otitis media due to *M. abscessus* (identified then as *M. chelonae,* subspecies *abscessus*) identified in Louisiana in 1987 were related to an outbreak in an ear, nose, and throat (ENT) practice (174). All of the patients involved in the outbreak had myringotomy tubes and developed chronic otorrhea. The most important risk factors for infection were presence of a perforation or myringotomy tube, suctioning of the ears, and an increasing number of ear examinations. Pathology showed abundant granulation tissue and multiple granulomas with positive AFB smears. In outbreak cases, the suction catheters used to wash out patients' ears had been rinsed with tap water. Instruments were not disinfected or sterilized properly. Ear specula were never sterilized. *M. abscessus* was identified in the water supply (174). However, the epidemic isolate seen in 13 of 14 cases had high-level aminoglycoside resistance (including amikacin), subsequently shown to result from an acquired point mutation in the 16S rRNA gene (175) that occurs only with prior aminoglycoside therapy

(86,175–177). This finding suggests that the epidemic strain originated from an infected patient rather than the tap water in the physician's office and spread because of improper sterilization of instruments between patients.

Subsequently, 21 sporadic cases of chronic otitis media due to rapidly growing mycobacteria were reported. All the patients with available histories had prior myringotomy tubes, and more than 90% of cases were due to *M. abscessus* (86). In a survey of infection control practices in ENT offices, 70% of ENT physicians were using tap water on their instruments, and 52% used tap water to rinse suction catheter tips between patients. Eighty-six percent reported performing high-level disinfection on their instruments between patients, but only 67% used adequate time to actually achieve high-level disinfection (30 minutes in a 2% glutaraldehyde solution, boiling for 5 minutes, and autoclaving for 20 minutes) (174). Epidemic disease potentially could occur with high-level tap water colonization or spread from an already infected patient. In addition to these infections due to the rapidly growing mycobacteria, foreign body–associated and healthcare-associated infections with other nontuberculous mycobacteria have also been reported sporadically (170,171). These have included meningitis in a baby with a ventriculoperitoneal shunt (172), peritonitis in patients undergoing peritoneal dialysis (153,154,173), and endocarditis in a patient with a prosthetic aortic valve (178).

PSEUDOINFECTIONS AND PSEUDO-OUTBREAKS

Equipment Related

Bronchoscopes

Since the early 1980s, mycobacteria have been the major pathogens transmitted via the bronchoscope, resulting in both pseudoinfections and true infections. Mycobacterial contamination of bronchoscopes and other endoscopes has previously been reported most commonly with *M. abscessus* and *M. chelonae.* A recent study has shown, however, that these isolates of *M. chelonae/abscessus* recovered in this setting are actually a new species called *M. immunogenum* (179). Contamination has also occurred with *M. xenopi* and *M. avium-intracellulare* (180–192) and has been linked to suction valves, suction channels, and biopsy forceps (193). Contamination has also been linked to automated endoscope washers, use of tap water to rinse endoscopes after manual disinfection, and failure to disinfect endoscopes adequately between patients (58,180,182,186,190,194). Bronchoscopes and other endoscopes as well as automated washers are difficult to disinfect, in part due to the propensity for formation of biofilms, which can serve as a sanctuary from the actions of chemical disinfectants (193). Colonization of some automated endoscope disinfection machines with nontuberculous mycobacteria has been associated with contamination of bronchoscopic and other endoscopic equipment due to problems with product design that facilitated the formation of biofilms in the automated washers (180,181,186,189,191). One such outbreak occurred in St. Louis, Missouri, from December 1989 to September 1990, when 14 patients were identified with *M. abscessus* (later correctly identified as *M. immunogenum*) in their bronchoscopic washings in a hospital using an automated disinfection machine to reprocess bronchoscopes. All specimens were smear negative and no patients developed disease. The patient isolates had the same DNA fingerprint pattern by PFGE (180). This same isolate (with the same fingerprint pattern) was identified from the rinse water in the endoscope disinfecting machine. The PFGE patterns from this outbreak are shown in Fig. 38.3. To determine the mechanism of bronchoscope contamination, ex-

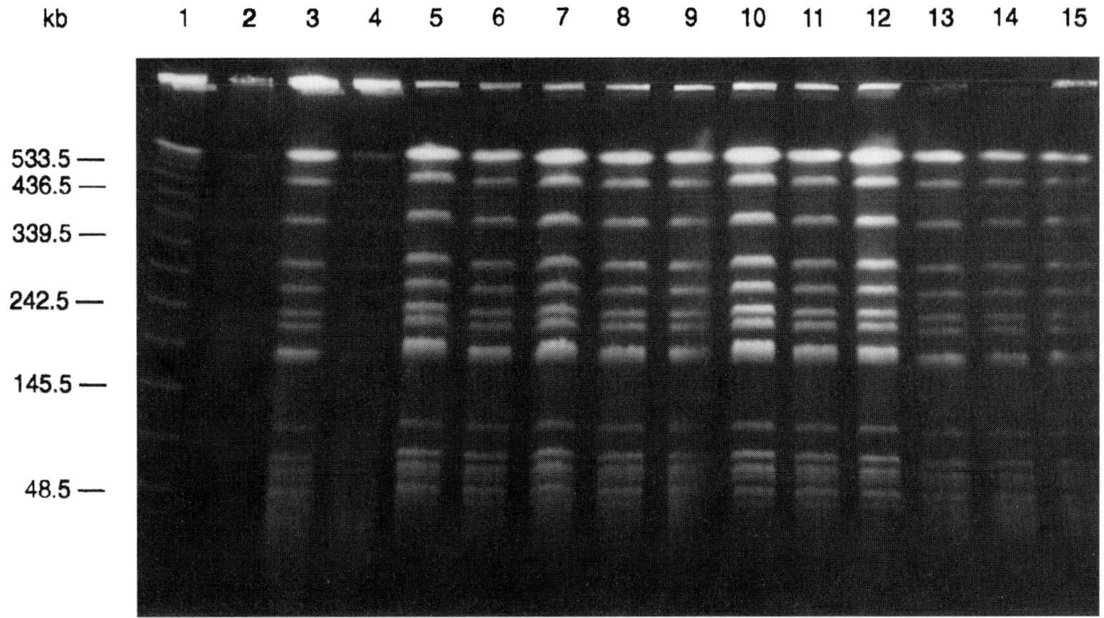

Figure 38.3. Pulsed-field gel electrophoresis of *M. immunogenum* (originally identified as *M. abscessus)* associated with bronchoscope contamination from St. Louis, Missouri. Lane 1 is genomic DNA, lane 6 is an isolate from the rinse water, and lane 7 is the isolate identified from the endoscope washing machine. All other lanes are patient isolates of *M. immunogenum* obtained from bronchoalveolar lavage.

periments were performed to evaluate the mycobactericidal activity of the glutaraldehyde solution being used to disinfect the bronchoscopes. The microorganisms were susceptible to glutaraldehyde. However, a 2% concentration of glutaraldehyde less than 14 days old was required to kill *M. chelonae* (180).

Outbreaks of endoscope contamination have been described with the Olympus EW 10 and EW 20 and the Keymed auto disinfector II. In 1990, because of these reports, the FDA issued a class II recall prohibiting further sale of the Olympus EW 10 and EW 20 washers in the U.S. The manufacturer was also required to modify the machines in use in U.S. hospitals to try to eliminate the problem. A product alert was also issued, recommending that all users institute a terminal rinse of endoscopes or bronchoscopes with 70% alcohol after disinfection in one of these automated washers.

However, pseudoinfection and contamination of endoscopes have been reported from automated washers that have undergone modifications (186). Maloney et al. (186) reported 15 patients with *M. abscessus* (later identified as *M. immunogenum*) (179) pseudoinfection due to bronchoscopes contaminated by an automated endoscope washer. *M. immunogenum*–positive cultures were more likely to have been obtained from bronchoscopes than gastroscopes (p = .002) and from bronchoscopes that had been processed by an automated washer rather than manual disinfection (p = .001). *M. immunogenum* was cultured from the inlet water, a flexible bronchoscope, and the automated washer. Environmental and case isolates had identical large restriction fragment patterns of genomic DNA separated by PFGE (186).

Several similar outbreaks have been reported from outside the U.S. (188–192). In another pseudo-outbreak from England, bronchoscopes became contaminated with rapidly growing mycobacteria when the endoscopes were rinsed with tap water after they had undergone manual high-level disinfection with glutaraldehyde. *M. chelonae* (details were not provided as to whether the causative agent was *M. immunogenum*) was identified from the detergent dispensers and the water in the room used to reprocess the bronchoscopes. The contamination was impossible to eradicate until the bronchoscopes were sterilized with ethylene oxide and the use of tap water for rinsing was discontinued (188).

Although this issue has been reported numerous times, the problem is probably still underrecognized. Rapidly growing mycobacteria survive well in adverse conditions and are resistant to antibiotics and disinfectants. Since they are present in tap water, use of tap water has been associated with contamination of instruments and specimens. *M. fortuitum* and *M. abscessus* can also multiply to levels of 10^4 to 10^6 colony-forming units (CFU)/mL in commercially distilled water and retain viability with only a slight decline in 1 year (74). Tap water should not be used to rinse bronchoscopes or critical or semicritical instruments. If tap water must be used, it should be followed by a 70% alcohol rinse (180,186,188,191,195). (For additional information on cleaning and disinfection of endoscopes, see Chapter 63.)

Ice Machines

In several healthcare-associated outbreaks due to rapidly growing mycobacteria, ice made in the hospital was found to be contaminated. These outbreaks have included cardiac surgery infections (100) and a pseudo-outbreak involving bone marrow aspirates (196). It has not always been determined whether the machine was contaminated or the contaminated ice reflected contamination of the hospital water supply. In one outbreak, a single ice machine was at fault. This outbreak occurred in 1987 when 30 patients in a New York hospital became colonized with *M. peregrinum* (identified at the time as *M. fortuitum* biovariant *peregrinum*). *M. peregrinum* was identified in a single ice machine and in the ice produced by the machine. Contamination of sputum samples in these patients was associated with consumption of tap water, melted ice, and ice chips, as well as showering and bathing immediately before obtaining the sputum samples (102). Pseudoinfections due to contamination of bone marrow specimens were reported from a Texas hospital where *M. fortuitum* was cultured from bone marrow aspirates in four patients. Only syringes chilled with ice from contaminated ice machines were involved. Both the ice and the ice machine were found to be contaminated (196).

Outbreaks and Pseudo-Outbreaks Directly Related to Contaminated Hospital Water Supplies

The prior sections discussed contaminated equipment, but these pseudo-outbreaks were almost certainly due to the hospital and/or municipal water supply being contaminated with the same microorganism that contaminated the equipment. Direct contamination of culture specimens or colonization or transient contamination of the respiratory tract with nontuberculous mycobacteria has been a major healthcare-associated problem related to contaminated hospital water systems. Healthcare-associated respiratory tract infections due to these microorganisms have been rare and have been limited to occasional single cases. This, presumably, reflects the fact that, despite frequent exposure from the environment, the lungs are relatively resistant to infection.

Mycobacterium gordonae, M. avium complex, *M. scrofulaceum, M. fortuitum, M. abscessus, M. chelonei, M. mucogenicum, M. terrae* complex, *M. kansasii, M. simiae,* and *M. xenopi* have all been identified from hospital water systems (53,58,65,194, 197–200). Some of these microorganisms have been associated with hospital outbreaks/pseudo-outbreaks, and thus are of significance for the hospital epidemiologist and infection control professional. A number of these pseudo-outbreaks have been reported.

Mycobacterium xenopi has been associated with four healthcare-associated outbreaks in the U.S. The first of these occurred in a Los Angeles hospital in 1983; *M. xenopi* was identified in 43 specimens from 34 patients. Fewer than five colonies were recovered from cultures in 70% of these cases. None of the patients had a clinical picture compatible with mycobacterial disease, except a 76-year-old woman whose isolate was obtained from a lung biopsy that showed caseating granulomas with AFB, from which *M. xenopi* was identified on culture. Cultures yielded *M. xenopi* throughout the hospital water system. Case-control studies suggested that patients acquired *M. xenopi* from exposure to hospital water in various ways, including showering (CDC investigation 84-78-1).

A second outbreak occurred in a Connecticut hospital where 608 patients over a 7-year period had positive respiratory cultures for *M. xenopi* due to heavy contamination of the hospital water supply. The water was maintained at 110°F, and *M. xenopi* grows in water at temperatures as high as 115°F. By 1981, 19 patients had developed healthcare-associated pulmonary disease (201,202) (CDC investigation 92-01).

The third outbreak occurred over a 3-year period from 1988 to 1991 in a Michigan hospital (58). Seventeen isolates of *M. xenopi* were identified, of which 13 were bronchoscopy specimens. *M. xenopi* was isolated from warm tap water samples taken from various parts of the hospital, including the bronchoscopy unit. Tap water had been used to rinse the bronchoscopes following disinfection.

A fourth outbreak was identified in 1993 when the CDC investigated a hospital that had recovered 13 of the 20 isolates of *M. xenopi* isolated in Indiana (194). All the specimens were smear negative and yielded rare or few colonies on culture. Only one isolate was identified from each of 13 patients. None of the patients met the American Thoracic Society criteria for pulmonary disease; however, 38% of the patients were treated with antituberculous therapy for a mean of 3 months. The investigation found frequent use of tap water throughout the hospital, including use of tap water to rinse bronchoscopes and bedpans as well as use of tap water gargles before sputum induction. *M. xenopi* was isolated from 17 of 19 (89%) water samples in patient care areas, and heavy growth of *M. xenopi* was observed on cultures from the hospital water mixing tank. This pseudo-outbreak was terminated by improving culture techniques and by eliminating the use of tap water to rinse bronchoscopes (194).

Although *M. xenopi* has been identified in hot water taps in hospitals (194,197), it has generally not been identified in city water. The microorganism can replicate between 43° and 45°C; thus, small numbers of microorganisms may enter hospital water tanks and multiply, resulting in colonization of the water systems. The pseudo-outbreak in the Indiana hospital was thought to have occurred after the hospital decreased its baseline water temperature in the tanks from 130° to 120°F. Overgrowth or contamination may be eradicated from hospital water systems by mechanically cleaning the holding tanks, increasing the water temperature to 180°F for 1 hour, flushing the system, and then increasing the baseline hot water temperature to 130°F. Routine surveillance cultures may be indicated in certain areas to detect overgrowth (58,194,197,198,202). In another similar outbreak, *M. terrae* was identified from 163 patients in a hospital that had recently renovated one wing (199). The source of contamination was the new water system. No *M. terrae* was cultured from patients after the water system was flushed and hyperchlorinated.

M. simiae has been a problem in several hospitals in the southwestern U.S. (61–63). A New Mexico hospital reported an outbreak of *M. simiae* involving 56 patients over a 3-year period. *M. simiae* was identified from sputum, stool, and gastric biopsy specimens. None of the patients had clinical disease due to *M. simiae*. Although environmental cultures have been negative to date, MEE was performed on 23 isolates and demonstrated three electrophoretic types. Eighteen (78%) were type 1, four were type 2, and there was a single isolate of a third type, implying a likely common environmental source (68). (For more information on pseudo-outbreaks, see Chapter 8.) A similar cluster of 33 isolates, identified over 12 months, was reported from a single clinical laboratory in Tucson, Arizona. It was the third most common nontuberculous mycobacterium to be recovered during this time period. Isolates studied by PFGE were either the same or highly related (clonal), suggesting a common source (61). It is unclear whether these represented hospital pseudo-outbreaks or most samples were contaminated from another source.

Recently, two pseudo-outbreaks involving *M. simiae* have been reported from Texas, with identical strains recovered from the hospital water systems. El Sahly et al. (62) reported recovery of 65 isolates of *M. simiae* from 62 patients in a single hospital in Houston. This represented 90% of *M. simiae* isolates recovered in the city. *M. simiae* was recovered from multiple sites in the hospital water system, with identical or highly related genomic DNA restriction patterns by PFGE. Conger et al. (63) reported recovery of seven patient isolates over a 5-month period from a single hospital in San Antonio, with identical DNA patterns by PFGE that also matched the pattern of microorganisms from the hospital water supply. The latter two pseudo-outbreaks represent the first recovery of *M. simiae* from the environment.

Contaminated Biologics

There have been numerous reports of pseudoinfections with nontuberculous mycobacteria due to contaminated biologics. In one hospital, pseudoinfection of the urinary tract with *M. avium-intracellulare* was related to contamination of urine specimens by contaminated phenol red (66). In another report, a cluster of *M. gordonae* was identified in bronchoscopy specimens due to a contaminated dye used in the topical anesthetic (203). Multiple pseudo-outbreaks due to rapidly growing mycobacteria have been linked to the BACTEC blood culture system. In one report, pseudoinfection with *M. gordonae* was traced to the BACTEC Panta Plus antimicrobial solution and enrichment broth added by the user to the BACTEC vials (204,205). Pseudoinfection with *M. gordonae* has also been described in association with the BACTEC TB system and a contaminated antimicrobial additive. In this pseudo-outbreak, *M. gordonae* was recovered from 46 specimens submitted for culture for mycobacteria over 8 weeks in a single Northeastern laboratory. Two lots (B9k1 and C9k1) of BACTEC Panta Plus were found to be contaminated with *M. gordonae.* The additive had been shipped to 173 laboratories. The contamination was due to failure to sterilize the water used in processing. This was the first report of mycobacterial pseudoinfection due to a commercially distributed product. Twenty other laboratories also reported contamination (203). In a later report, 23 blood cultures from HIV-positive patients grew *M. abscessus*, which was ultimately traced to a multidose supplement vial used with the BBL Septi-check AFB culturing system (67).

Laboratory Cross-Contamination

A number of pseudo-outbreaks have resulted from laboratory cross-contamination involving the BACTEC system or related to specimen contamination at the time of digestion or processing. In one case, *M. chelonae* was identified due to contamination of the BACTEC system during automated reading (204). Similar pseudo-outbreaks, attributed to inadequate heating of the needle probe of the BACTEC system, have been reported (206,207). Given the large numbers of specimens processed in many laboratories and the close proximity of the specimens, it is not surprising that cross-contamination occurs. As molecular typing techniques become more widely available, more precise confirmation of this phenomenon will be possible. Laboratories should be aware of this potential problem and take steps to limit the possibility of cross-contamination.

PREVENTION AND CONTROL OF DISEASE DUE TO NONTUBERCULOUS MYCOBACTERIA

Surveillance plays an important role in early recognition and identification of outbreaks and pseudo-outbreaks due to nontuberculous mycobacteria. Surveillance should identify and facilitate investigation of any increase in isolation of nontuberculous mycobacteria above thresholds. In addition, given the strong association with healthcare-associated disease, infection control professionals should evaluate every patient with a nontuberculous mycobacterial infection, particularly rapidly growing mycobacteria isolated from surgical patients, dialysis patients, bronchoscopy specimens, or sterile sites. Active surveillance should facilitate early identification of healthcare-associated infections or pseudoinfections and thereby limit the extent of the problem. In addition, personnel in areas in which immunosuppressed, high-risk patients are hospitalized or where diagnostic or therapeutic procedures that require high-level disinfection of instruments are performed should receive intensive education about the relationship between nontuberculous mycobacteria and water and the role of nontuberculous mycobacteria as healthcare-associated pathogens.

Education on the appropriate disinfection procedures for critical and semicritical instruments may help prevent healthcare-associated infections and pseudoinfections. Special attention must be given to meticulous cleaning and disinfection of items that are particularly difficult to disinfect, including bronchoscopes and other endoscopes. Use of ethylene oxide to sterilize endoscopes or other instruments between patients can eliminate contamination due to nontuberculous mycobacteria, but processing with ethylene oxide is expensive and requires extended periods of time for sterilization and aeration following sterilization. Glutaraldehyde disinfection using an automated system has been shown to be effective, provided appropriate safeguards are taken to guard against contamination (208).

Personnel should be reminded that tap water should not be used to rinse instruments or for preparing specimens for culture. Some problems with instrument disinfection have been associated with slowly progressive dilution of glutaraldehyde during multiple uses, and rapidly growing mycobacteria have been demonstrated to survive in 2% glutaraldehyde (180,209). Personnel using glutaraldehyde must be aware of the necessity for monitoring its concentration, the duration of its activity after activation, and the immersion time required for high-level disinfection (195,210).

Active surveillance, periodic review of cleaning and disinfection procedures for equipment, and use of sterile water to rinse critical and semicritical items after disinfection are recommended as infection control measures to prevent both true outbreaks and pseudo-outbreaks due to nontuberculous mycobacteria. A recent study has shown that disinfecting bronchoscopes with 70% alcohol prior to the use of automated washers, increasing the glutaraldehyde concentration to 3%, and recirculation of used disinfectant were effective in the elimination of established contamination (211). Use of in-line filters may help reduce water contamination. Ice should be considered potentially contaminated, and its use should be limited in operating rooms. Dialysis units should be aware that water may be a source of nontuberculous mycobacteria. Dialysis units need to be meticulous when they disinfect and reuse dialyzers, and they must perform careful surveillance for infections. Water cultures are routinely performed as a quality assurance measure in many dialysis units; these data should be evaluated to determine whether excessive contamination or colonization is developing. Elimination of colonization above established thresholds before any patients develop infections should be the goal of performing such cultures. In addition, Renalin may be a less effective disinfectant than formaldehyde or glutaraldehyde, and so its use must be monitored closely. Dialysis centers that reuse dialyzers or perform high-flux dialysis should be particularly meticulous in their disinfection practices and their surveillance.

If increases in the isolation of nontuberculous mycobacteria are detected, a chart review should be performed to determine whether patients are infected and to obtain demographic information, medical history, information on inpatient or outpatient procedures, and other possible risk factors. A case definition should be developed and microbiology and pathology records reviewed to find additional cases. The laboratory should be notified to save all isolates so that case and environmental isolates may be typed. Investigations should focus on the key issues described above, including the relationship of nontuberculous mycobacteria to tap and distilled water, ice, ice machines, and improperly or inadequately sterilized instruments. Policies and procedures for obtaining and processing specimens and for disinfecting equipment should be reviewed. Frequently, direct observation of the process is often more enlightening than reviewing the written procedure. The written policy and procedure may be technically correct, but observing the performance of the procedure may provide evidence to suggest the route of contamination. Selected environmental cultures may be useful to identify the source of the contamination. Patients who have been exposed to contaminated bronchoscopes or other critical or semicritical instruments should be followed closely for the development of disease.

Increasing recognition of the role of nontuberculous mycobacteria in healthcare-associated pseudoinfections and infections should facilitate early identification of clusters and outbreaks. Prevention and control of these infections relies on active surveillance and rigorous attention to aseptic technique, appropriate disinfection and sterilization of instruments, and awareness that water is frequently contaminated with nontuberculous mycobacteria. Recent improvements in culture, identification, and molecular typing methods will also facilitate more rapid identification of the source of the problem so that prevention and control can be achieved.

REFERENCES

1. O'Brien RJ, Geiter LJ, Snider DE Jr. The epidemiology of nontuberculous mycobacterial diseases in the United States. Results from a national survey. *Am Rev Respir Dis* 1987;135:1007–1014.
2. Wallace RJ Jr, Swenson JM, Silcox VA, et al. Spectrum of disease due to rapidly growing mycobacteria. *Rev Infect Dis* 1983;5:657–679.
3. Wallace RJ Jr. Nontuberculous mycobacteria and water: a love affair with increasing clinical importance. *Infect Dis Clin North Am* 1987; 1:677–686.
4. Diagnosis and treatment of disease caused by nontuberculous mycobacteria. *Am Rev Respir Dis* 1990;142:940–953.
5. Portaels F. Epidemiology of mycobacterial diseases. *Clin Dermatol* 1995;13:207–222.
6. Roy V, Weisdorf D. Mycobacterial infections following bone marrow transplantation: a 20 year retrospective review. *Bone Marrow Transplant* 1997;19:467–470.
7. Diagnosis and treatment of disease caused by nontuberculous mycobacteria. *Am J Respir Crit Care Med* 1997;156:S1–25.
8. Goslee S, Wolinsky E. Water as a source of potentially pathogenic mycobacteria. *Am Rev Respir Dis* 1976;113:287–292.
9. Gruft H, Falkinham JO 3rd, Parker BC. Recent experience in the epidemiology of disease caused by atypical mycobacteria. *Rev Infect Dis* 1981;3:990–996.
10. Wolinsky E, Rynearson TK. Mycobacteria in soil and their relation to disease-associated strains. *Am Rev Respir Dis* 1968;97:1032–1037.
11. Harrington R, Korston AG. Destruction of various kinds of mycobacteria in milk by pasteurization. *Appl Microbiol* 1965;13:394–395.
12. Chapman JS, Speight M. Isolation of atypical mycobacteria from pasteurized milk. *Am Rev Respir Dis* 1968;98:1052–1054.
13. Wolinsky E. Nontuberculous mycobacteria and associated diseases. *Am Rev Respir Dis* 1979;119:107–159.
14. Chapman JS. The ecology of the atypical mycobacteria. *Arch Environ Health* 1971;22:41–46.
15. Reznikov M, Leggo JH, Dawson DJ. Investigation by seroagglutination of strains of the *Mycobacterium intracellulare–M. scrofulaceum* group from house dusts and sputum in Southeastern Queensland. *Am Rev Respir Dis* 1971;104:951–953.
16. Kirschner RA Jr, Parker BC, Falkinham JO 3rd. Epidemiology of infection by nontuberculous mycobacteria. *Mycobacterium avium, Mycobacterium intracellulare*, and *Mycobacterium scrofulaceum* in acid, brown-water swamps of the southeastern United States and their association with environmental variables. *Am Rev Respir Dis* 1992;145: 271–275.
17. Holland J, Smith C, Childs PA, et al. Surgical management of cutaneous infection caused by atypical mycobacteria after penetrating injury: the hidden dangers of horticulture. *J Trauma* 1997;42:337–340.
18. Weinberger M, Berg SL, Feuerstein IM, et al. Disseminated infection with *Mycobacterium gordonae*: report of a case and critical review of the literature. *Clin Infect Dis* 1992;14:1229–1239.
19. Clark R, Cardona L, Valainis G, et al. Genitourinary infections caused by mycobacteria other than *Mycobacterium tuberculosis. Tubercle* 1989;70:297–300.
20. de Haller R, Fritschi D, Kobel T. Infections due to *Mycobacterium chelonae. Bull Int Union Tuberc Lung Dis* 1988;63:23.
21. Wallace RJ Jr. The clinical presentation, diagnosis, and therapy of cutaneous and pulmonary infections due to the rapidly growing mycobacteria, *M. fortuitum* and *M. chelonae. Clin Chest Med* 1989;10: 419–429.
22. Kristjansson M, Bieluch VM, Byeff PD. *Mycobacterium haemophilum* infection in immunocompromised patients: case report and review of the literature. *Rev Infect Dis* 1991;13:906–910.
23. Dever LL, Martin JW, Seaworth B, et al. Varied presentations and responses to treatment of infections caused by *Mycobacterium haemophilum* in patients with AIDS. *Clin Infect Dis* 1992;14:1195–1200.
24. Shafer RW, Sierra MF. *Mycobacterium xenopi, Mycobacterium fortuitum, Mycobacterium kansasii*, and other nontuberculous mycobacteria in an area of endemicity for AIDS. *Clin Infect Dis* 1992;15:161–162.
25. Correa AG, Starke JR. Nontuberculous mycobacterial disease in children. *Semin Respir Infect* 1996;11:262–271.
26. Griffith DE, Wallace RJ Jr. Pulmonary disease due to rapidly growing mycobacteria. *Semin Respir Infect* 1988;9:505–513.
27. Bottger EC. *Mycobacterium genavense*: an emerging pathogen. *Eur J Clin Microbiol Infect Dis* 1994;13:932–936.
28. Stewart MG, Starke JR, Coker NJ. Nontuberculous mycobacterial infections of the head and neck. *Arch Otolaryngol Head Neck Surg* 1994;120:873–876.
29. Harth M, Ralph ED, Faraawi R. Septic arthritis due to *Mycobacterium marinum. J Rheumatol* 1994;21:957–960.
30. Wright JE. Non-tuberculous mycobacterial lymphadenitis. *Aust N Z J Surg* 1996;66:225–228.
31. Silcox VA, Good RC, Floyd MM. Identification of clinically significant *Mycobacterium fortuitum* complex isolates. *J Clin Microbiol* 1981; 14:686–691.
32. Wallace RJ Jr, Musser JM, Hull SI, et al. Diversity and sources of rapidly growing mycobacteria associated with infections following cardiac surgery. *J Infect Dis* 1989;159:708–716.
33. Swenson JM, Wallace RJ Jr, Silcox VA, et al. Antimicrobial susceptibility of five subgroups of *Mycobacterium fortuitum* and *Mycobacterium chelonae. Antimicrob Agents Chemother* 1985;28:807–811.
34. Wallace RJ Jr, Dalovisio JR, Pankey GA. Disk diffusion testing of susceptibility of *Mycobacterium fortuitum* and *Mycobacterium chelonei* to antibacterial agents. *Antimicrob Agents Chemother* 1979;16: 611–614.
35. Jenkins PA, Marks J, Schaefer WB. Lipid chromatography and seroagglutination in the classification of rapidly growing mycobacteria. *Am Rev Respir Dis* 1971;103:179–187.
36. Pattyn SR, Magnusson M, Stanford JL, et al. A study of *Mycobacterium fortuitum (ranae). J Med Microbiol* 1974;7:67–76.
37. Rogall T, Wolters J, Flohr T, et al. Towards a phylogeny and definition of species at the molecular level within the genus Mycobacterium. *Int J Syst Bacteriol* 1990;40:323–330.
38. Hector JS, Pang Y, Mazurek GH, et al. Large restriction fragment patterns of genomic *Mycobacterium fortuitum* DNA as strain-specific markers and their use in epidemiologic investigation of four nosocomial outbreaks. *J Clin Microbiol* 1992;30:1250–1255.
39. Kirschner P, Kiekenbeck M, Meissner D, et al. Genetic heterogeneity within *Mycobacterium fortuitum* complex species: genotypic criteria for identification. *J Clin Microbiol* 1992;30:2772–2775.
40. Glickman SE, Kilburn JO, Butler WR, et al. Rapid identification of mycolic acid patterns of mycobacteria by high-performance liquid chromatography using pattern recognition software and a *Mycobacterium* library. *J Clin Microbiol* 1994;32:740–745.
41. Thibert L, Lapierre S. Routine application of high-performance liquid chromatography for identification of mycobacteria. *J Clin Microbiol* 1993;31:1759–1763.
42. Telenti M, de Quiros JF, Alvarez M, et al. The diagnostic usefulness of a DNA probe for *Mycobacterium tuberculosis* complex (Gen-Probe) in Bactec cultures versus other diagnostic methods. *Infection* 1994; 22:18–23.
43. Metchock B, Diem L. Algorithm for use of nucleic acid probes for identifying *Mycobacterium tuberculosis* from BACTEC 12B bottles. *J Clin Microbiol* 1995;33:1934–1937.
44. Soini H, Viljanen MK. Gene amplification in the diagnosis of mycobacterial infections. *APMIS* 1997;105:345–353.
45. Ichiyama S, Iinuma Y, Tawada Y, et al. Evaluation of Gen-Probe Amplified Mycobacterium Tuberculosis Direct Test and Roche PCR-microwell plate hybridization method (AMPLICOR MYCOBACTERIUM) for direct detection of mycobacteria. *J Clin Microbiol* 1996; 34:130–133.
46. Rapid diagnostic tests for tuberculosis: what is the appropriate use? American Thoracic Society Workshop. *Am J Respir Crit Care Med* 1997;155:1804–1814.

47. Kirschner P, Rosenau J, Springer B, et al. Diagnosis of mycobacterial infections by nucleic acid amplification: 18-month prospective study. *J Clin Microbiol* 1996;34:304–312.
48. Kox LF, Jansen HM, Kuijper S, et al. Multiplex PCR assay for immediate identification of the infecting species in patients with mycobacterial disease. *J Clin Microbiol* 1997;35:1492–1498.
49. Springer B, Stockman L, Teschner K, et al. Two-laboratory collaborative study on identification of mycobacteria: molecular versus phenotypic methods. *J Clin Microbiol* 1996;34:296–303.
50. Taylor TB, Patterson C, Hale Y, et al. Routine use of PCR-restriction fragment length polymorphism analysis for identification of mycobacteria growing in liquid media. *J Clin Microbiol* 1997;35:79–85.
51. Yakrus MA, Hernandez SM, Floyd MM, et al. Comparison of methods for identification of *Mycobacterium abscessus* and *M. chelonae* isolates. *J Clin Microbiol* 2001;39:4103–4110.
52. Wallace RJ Jr, Zhang Y, Brown BA, et al. DNA large restriction fragment patterns of sporadic and epidemic nosocomial strains of *Mycobacterium chelonae* and *Mycobacterium abscessus. J Clin Microbiol* 1993;31:2697–2701.
53. Burns DN, Wallace RJ Jr, Schultz ME, et al. Nosocomial outbreak of respiratory tract colonization with *Mycobacterium fortuitum*: demonstration of the usefulness of pulsed-field gel electrophoresis in an epidemiologic investigation. *Am Rev Respir Dis* 1991;144:1153–1159.
54. Zhang Y, Yakrus MA, Wallace Jr RJ. An improved technique for pulsed-field gel electrophoresis (PFGE) of *Mycobacterium abscessus* isolates affected by DNA degradation (abstract U-025). In: *103rd General Meeting of the American Society for Microbiology,* Washington, DC, May 18–22, 2003:636.
55. Villanueva A, Calderon RV, Vargas BA, et al. Report on an outbreak of postinjection abscesses due to *Mycobacterium abscessus,* including management with surgery and clarithromycin therapy and comparison of strains by random amplified polymorphic DNA polymerase chain reaction. *Clin Infect Dis* 1997;24:1147–1153.
56. Zhang Y, Rajagopalan M, Brown BA, et al. Randomly amplified polymorphic DNA PCR for comparison of *Mycobacterium abscessus* strains from nosocomial outbreaks. *J Clin Microbiol* 1997;35:3132–3139.
57. Desplaces N, Picardeau M, Dinh V, et al. Spinal infections due to *Mycobacterium xenopi* after discectomies (abstract J162). 35th General Meeting of Interscience Conference on Antimicrobial Agents and Chemotherapy, San Francisco, CA, 1995.
58. Bennett SN, Peterson DE, Johnson DR, et al. Bronchoscopy-associated *Mycobacterium xenopi* pseudoinfections. *Am J Respir Crit Care Med* 1994;150:245–250.
59. Picardeau M, Prod'Hom G, Raskine L, et al. Genotypic characterization of five subspecies of *Mycobacterium kansasii. J Clin Microbiol* 1997;35:25–32.
60. Iinuma Y, Ichiyama S, Hasegawa Y, et al. Large-restriction-fragment analysis of *Mycobacterium kansasii* genomic DNA and its application in molecular typing. *J Clin Microbiol* 1997;35:596–599.
61. Rynkiewicz DL, Cage GD, Butler WR, et al. Clinical and microbiological assessment of *Mycobacterium simiae* isolates from a single laboratory in southern Arizona. *Clin Infect Dis* 1998;26:625–630.
62. El Sahly HM, Septimus E, Soini H, et al. *Mycobacterium simiae* pseudo-outbreak resulting from a contaminated hospital water supply in Houston, Texas. *Clin Infect Dis* 2002;35:802–807.
63. Conger NG, Laurel V, Olivier K, et al. *Mycobacterium simiae* pseudo-outbreak among hospitalized patients (abstract 422). In: *40th Annual Meeting of the Infectious Diseases Society of America,* Chicago IL, October 24–27, 2002:118.
64. Picardeau M, Varnerot A, Lecompte T, et al. Use of different molecular typing techniques for bacteriological follow-up in a clinical trial with AIDS patients with Mycobacterium avium bacteremia. *J Clin Microbiol* 1997;35:2503–2510.
65. von Reyn CF, Maslow JN, Barber TW, et al. Persistent colonisation of potable water as a source of *Mycobacterium avium* infection in AIDS. *Lancet* 1994;343:1137–1141.
66. Graham L Jr, Warren NG, Tsang AY, et al. *Mycobacterium avium* complex pseudobacteriuria from a hospital water supply. *J Clin Microbiol* 1988;26:1034–1036.
67. Ashford DA, Kellerman S, Yakrus M, et al. Pseudo-outbreak of septicemia due to rapidly growing mycobacteria associated with extrinsic contamination of culture supplement. *J Clin Microbiol* 1997;35:2040–2042.
68. Crosey MJ, Yakrus MA, Cook MB, et al. Isolation of *Mycobacterium simiae* in a southwestern hospital and typing by multilocus enzyme electrophoresis (abstract U-38). 94th Annual Meeting of the American Society of Microbiology, Las Vegas, NE.
69. Yates MD, Grange JM, Collins CH. The nature of mycobacterial disease in south east England, 1977–84. *J Epidemiol Community Health* 1986;40:295–300.
70. Valero G, Peters J, Jorgensen JH, et al. Clinical isolates of *Mycobacterium simiae* in San Antonio, Texas. An 11-year review. *Am J Respir Crit Care Med* 1995;152:1555–1557.
71. Falkinham JO 3rd. Nontuberculous mycobacteria in the environment. *Clin Chest Med* 2002;23:529–551.
72. Good RC, Snider DE Jr. Isolation of nontuberculous mycobacteria in the United States, 1980. *J Infect Dis* 1982;146:829–833.
73. Wallace RJ Jr. Recent changes in taxonomy and disease manifestations of the rapidly growing mycobacteria. *Eur J Clin Microbiol Infect Dis* 1994;13:953–960.
74. Carson LA, Petersen NJ, Favero MS, et al. Growth characteristics of atypical mycobacteria in water and their comparative resistance to disinfectants. *Appl Environ Microbiol* 1978;36:839–846.
75. Collins CH, Grange JM, Yates MD. Mycobacteria in water. *J Appl Bacteriol* 1984;57:193–211.
76. Schulze-Robbecke R, Feldmann C, Fischeder R, et al. Dental units: an environmental study of sources of potentially pathogenic mycobacteria. *Tuber Lung Dis* 1995;76:318–323.
77. Gander S. Bacterial biofilms: resistance to antimicrobial agents. *J Antimicrob Chemother* 1996;37:1047–1050.
78. Reid G, Bailey RR. Biofilm infections: implications for diagnosis and treatment. *N Z Med J* 1996;109:41–42.
79. Reid JD, Wolinsky E. Histopathology of lymphadenitis caused by atypical mycobacteria. *Am Rev Respir Dis* 1969;99:8–12.
80. Rodriguez G, Ortegon M, Camargo D, et al. Iatrogenic *Mycobacterium abscessus* infection: histopathology of 71 patients. *Br J Dermatol* 1997;137:214–218.
81. Meissner G. The value of animal models for study of infection due to atypical mycobacteria. *Rev Infect Dis* 1981;3:953–959.
82. Gangadharam PR, Pratt PF, Davidson PT. Experimental infections with *Mycobacterium intracellulare. Rev Infect Dis* 1981;3:973–978.
83. Wolinsky E. Mycobacterial diseases other than tuberculosis. *Clin Infect Dis* 1992;15:1–10.
84. Nelson BR, Rapini RP, Wallace RJ Jr, et al. Disseminated *Mycobacterium chelonae* ssp. *abscessus* in an immunocompetent host and with a known portal of entry. *J Am Acad Dermatol* 1989;20:909–912.
85. Ingram CW, Tanner DC, Durack DT, et al. Disseminated infection with rapidly growing mycobacteria. *Clin Infect Dis* 1993;16:463–471.
86. Franklin DJ, Starke JR, Brady MT, et al. Chronic otitis media after tympanostomy tube placement caused by *Mycobacterium abscessus*: a new clinical entity? *Am J Otol* 1994;15:313–320.
87. White R, Abreo K, Flanagan R, et al. Nontuberculous mycobacterial infections in continuous ambulatory peritoneal dialysis patients. *Am J Kidney Dis* 1993;22:581–587.
88. Huang SC, Soong HK, Chang JS, et al. Non-tuberculous mycobacterial keratitis: a study of 22 cases. *Br J Ophthalmol* 1996;80:962–968.
89. Artenstein AW, Eiseman AS, Campbell GC. Chronic dacryocystitis caused by *Mycobacterium fortuitum. Ophthalmology* 1993;100:666–668.
90. Pruitt TC, Hughes LO, Blasier RD, et al. Atypical mycobacterial vertebral osteomyelitis in a steroid-dependent adolescent. A case report. *Spine* 1993;18:2553–2555.
91. Baldi S, Rapellino M, Ruffini E, et al. Atypical mycobacteriosis in a lung transplant recipient. *Eur Respir J* 1997;10:952–954.
92. Kelley LC, Deering KC, Kaye ET. Cutaneous *Mycobacterium chelonei* presenting in an immunocompetent host: case report and review of the literature. *Cutis* 1995;56:293–295.
93. Wallace RJ Jr, Brown BA, Onyi GO. Skin, soft tissue, and bone infections due to *Mycobacterium chelonae chelonae*: importance of prior corticosteroid therapy, frequency of disseminated infections, and resis-

tance to oral antimicrobials other than clarithromycin. *J Infect Dis* 1992;166:405–412.
94. Cooper JF, Lichtenstein MJ, Graham BS, et al. *Mycobacterium chelonae*: a cause of nodular skin lesions with a proclivity for renal transplant recipients. *Am J Med* 1989;86:173–177.
95. Griffith DE, Girard WM, Wallace RJ Jr. Clinical features of pulmonary disease caused by rapidly growing mycobacteria. An analysis of 154 patients. *Am Rev Respir Dis* 1993;147:1271–1278.
96. Hoffman PC, Fraser DW, Robicsek F, et al. Two outbreaks of sternal wound infection due to organisms of the *Mycobacterium fortuitum* complex. *J Infect Dis* 1981;143:533–542.
97. Foz A, Roy C, Jurado J, et al. *Mycobacterium chelonei* iatrogenic infections. *J Clin Microbiol* 1978;7:319–321.
98. Szabo I, Szrkozi K. *Mycobacterium chelonei* endemy after heart surgery with fatal consequences [letter]. *Am Rev Respir Dis* 1980;121:607.
99. Clegg HW, Foster MT, Sanders WE Jr, et al. Infection due to organisms of the *Mycobacterium fortuitum* complex after augmentation mammaplasty: clinical and epidemiologic features. *J Infect Dis* 1983; 147:427–433.
100. Kuritsky JN, Bullen MG, Broome CV, et al. Sternal wound infections and endocarditis due to organisms of the *Mycobacterium fortuitum* complex. *Ann Intern Med* 1983;98:938–939.
101. Safranek TJ, Jarvis WR, Carson LA, et al. *Mycobacterium chelonae* wound infections after plastic surgery employing contaminated gentian violet skin-marking solution. *N Engl J Med* 1987;317:197–201.
102. Laussucq S, Baltch AL, Smith RP, et al. Nosocomial *Mycobacterium fortuitum* colonization from a contaminated ice machine. *Am Rev Respir Dis* 1988;138:891–894.
103. Robicsek F, Daugherty HK, Cook JW, et al. *Mycobacterium fortuitum* epidemics after open-heart surgery. *J Thorac Cardiovasc Surg* 1978; 75:91–96.
104. Yew WW, Wong PC, Woo HS, et al. Characterization of *Mycobacterium fortuitum* isolates from sternotomy wounds by antimicrobial susceptibilities, plasmid profiles, and ribosomal ribonucleic acid gene restriction patterns. *Diagn Microbiol Infect Dis* 1993;17:111–117.
105. Repath F, Seabury JH, Sanders CV, et al. Prosthetic valve endocarditis due to *Mycobacterium chelonei. South Med J* 1976;69:1244–1246.
106. Horadam VW, Smilack JD, Smith EC. *Mycobacterium fortuitum* infection after total hip replacement. *South Med J* 1982;75:244–246.
107. Weinstein RA, Jones EL, Schwarzmann SW, et al. Sternal osteomyelitis and mediastinitis after open-heart operation: pathogenesis and prevention. *Ann Thorac Surg* 1976;21:442–444.
108. Grange JM. Mycobacterial infections following heart valve replacement. *J Heart Valve Dis* 1992;1:102–109.
109. Wolfe JM, Moore DF. Isolation of *Mycobacterium thermoresistible* following augmentation mammaplasty. *J Clin Microbiol* 1992;30: 1036–1038.
110. Moorthy RS, Rao NA. Atypical mycobacterial wound infection after blepharoplasty. *Br J Ophthalmol* 1995;79:93.
111. Widgerow AD, Brink AJ, Koornhof HJ. Atypical Mycobacterium and breast surgery. *Ann Plast Surg* 1995;35:204–207.
112. Krishnan S, Haglund L, Ashfaq A, et al. Iatrogenically induced spondylodiskitis due to *Mycobacterium xenopi* in an immunocompetent patient. *Clin Infect Dis* 1996;22:723.
113. Samuels LE, Sharma S, Morris RJ, et al. *Mycobacterium fortuitum* infection of the sternum. Review of the literature and case illustration. *Arch Surg* 1996;131:1344–1346.
114. Saluja A, Peters NT, Lowe L, et al. A surgical wound infection due to *Mycobacterium chelonae* successfully treated with clarithromycin. *Dermatol Surg* 1997;23:539–543.
115. Pennekamp A, Pfyffer GE, Wuest J, et al. *Mycobacterium smegmatis* infection in a healthy woman following a facelift: case report and review of the literature. *Ann Plast Surg* 1997;39:80–83.
116. Wallace RJ Jr, Steele LC, Labidi A, et al. Heterogeneity among isolates of rapidly growing mycobacteria responsible for infections following augmentation mammaplasty despite case clustering in Texas and other southern coastal states. *J Infect Dis* 1989;160:281–288.
117. Pope J Jr, Sternberg P Jr, McLane NJ, et al. *Mycobacterium chelonae* scleral abscess after removal of a scleral buckle. *Am J Ophthalmol* 1989; 107:557–558.
118. Soto LE, Bobadilla M, Villalobos Y, et al. Post-surgical nasal cellulitis outbreak due to *Mycobacterium chelonae. J Hosp Infect* 1991;19: 99–106.
119. Centers for Disease Control. Mycobacterial infections associated with augmentation mammoplasty. *MMWR* 1978;27:513–516.
120. Roussel TJ, Stern WH, Goodman DF, et al. Postoperative mycobacterial endophthalmitis. *Am J Ophthalmol* 1989;107:403–406.
121. Grigg J, Hirst LW, Whitby M, et al. Atypical mycobacterium keratitis. *Aust N Z J Ophthalmol* 1992;20:257–261.
122. Bullington RH Jr, Lanier JD, Font RL. Nontuberculous mycobacterial keratitis. Report of two cases and review of the literature. *Arch Ophthalmol* 1992;110:519–524.
123. Rootman DS, Insler MS, Wolfley DE. Canaliculitis caused by *Mycobacterium chelonae* after lacrimal intubation with silicone tubes. *Can J Ophthalmol* 1989;24:221–222.
124. Lois N, Perez del Molino ML. *Mycobacterium chelonae* keratitis: resolution after debridement and presoaked collagen shields. *Cornea* 1995; 14:536–539.
125. Centers for Disease Control. Follow-up on mycobacterial contamination of porcine heart valve prosthesis—US. *MMWR* 1978;27:97–98.
126. Laskowski LF, Marr JJ, Spernoga JF, et al. Fastidious mycobacteria grown from porcine prosthetic-heart-valve cultures. *N Engl J Med* 1977;297:101–102.
127. Altmann G, Horowitz A, Kaplinsky N, et al. Prosthetic valve endocarditis due to *Mycobacterium chelonei. J Clin Microbiol* 1975;1:531–533.
128. Narasimhan SL, Austin TW. Prosthetic valve endocarditis due to *Mycobacterium fortuitum. Can Med Assoc J* 1978;119:154–155.
129. Kuhn AW. *Mycobacterium fortuitum* infection following coronary bypass surgery. *Clin Microbiol News* 1983;5:145–146.
130. Jauregui L, Arbulu A, Wilson F. Osteomyelitis, pericarditis, mediastinitis, and vasculitis due to *Mycobacterium chelonei. Am Rev Respir Dis* 1977;115:699–703.
131. Woods GL, Washington JA 2nd. Mycobacteria other than *Mycobacterium tuberculosis*: review of microbiologic and clinical aspects. *Rev Infect Dis* 1987;9:275–294.
132. Clegg HW, Bertagnoll P, Hightower AW, et al. Mammaplasty-associated mycobacterial infection: a survey of plastic surgeons. *Plast Reconstr Surg* 1983;72:165–169.
133. Meyers H, Brown-Elliott BA, Moore D, et al. An outbreak of *Mycobacterium chelonae* infection following liposuction. *Clin Infect Dis* 2002;34:1500–1507.
134. da Costa-Cruz J. *Mycobacterium fortuitum* um novo bacilo acidoresistente patogenico para ohomen. *Acta Med (Rio de Janeiro)* 1938; 1:298–301.
135. Owen M, Smith A, Coultras J. Granulomatous lesions occurring at site of injections of vaccines and antibiotics. *South Med J* 1963;56: 949–952.
136. Gremillion DH, Mursch SB, Lerner CJ. Injection site abscesses caused by *Mycobacterium chelonei. Infect Control* 1983;4:25–28.
137. Borghans JG, Stanford JL. *Mycobacterium chelonei* in abscesses after injection of diphtheria-pertussis-tetanus-polio vaccine. *Am Rev Respir Dis* 1973;107:1–8.
138. Petrini B, Hellstrand P, Eriksson M. Infection with *Mycobacterium cheloni* following injections. *Scand J Infect Dis* 1980;12:237–238.
139. Centers for Disease Control. Infection with *Mycobacterium abscessus* associated with intramuscular injection of adrenal cortex extract—Colorado and Wyoming, 1995–1996. *MMWR* 1996;45: 713–715.
140. Camargo D, Saad C, Ruiz F, et al. Iatrogenic outbreak of *M. chelonae* skin abscesses. *Epidemiol Infect* 1996;117:113–119.
141. Buckley R, Cobb MW, Ghurani S, et al. *Mycobacterium fortuitum* infection occurring after a punch biopsy procedure. *Pediatr Dermatol* 1997;14:290–292.
142. Vandepitte J, Desmyter J, Gatti F. Mycobacteria, skins, and needles. *Lancet* 1969;2:691.
143. Nolan CM, Hashisaki PA, Dundas DF. An outbreak of soft-tissue infections due to *Mycobacterium fortuitum* associated with electromyography. *J Infect Dis* 1991;163:1150–1153.
144. Torres JRR, Rios-Fabra A, Murillo J, et al. Injection site abscess due

to the *Mycobacterium fortuitum-chelonei* complex in the immunocompetent host. *Infect Dis Clin Pract* 1998;7:56–60.
145. Tiwari TSP, Ray B, Jost KC Jr, et al. Forty years of disinfectant failure: outbreak of postinjection *Mycobacterium abcessus* infection caused by contamination of benzalkonium chloride. *Clin Infect Dis* 2003;36.
146. Bolan G, Reingold AL, Carson LA, et al. Infections with *Mycobacterium chelonei* in patients receiving dialysis and using processed hemodialyzers. *J Infect Dis* 1985;152:1013–1019.
147. Lowry PW, Beck-Sague CM, Bland LA, et al. *Mycobacterium chelonae* infection among patients receiving high-flux dialysis in a hemodialysis clinic in California. *J Infect Dis* 1990;161:85–90.
148. Carson LA, Bland LA, Cusick LB, et al. Prevalence of nontuberculous mycobacteria in water supplies of hemodialysis centers. *Appl Environ Microbiol* 1988;54:3122–3125.
149. *Renin dialyzer reprocessing concentrate: instructions for use and technical notes.* Minneapolis: Renal Systems, 1983.
150. Bauer H, Brunner H, Franz HE. Experience with the disinfectant peroxyacetic acid (PES) for hemodialyzer reuse. *Trans Am Soc Artif Intern Organs* 1983;29:662–665.
151. Hakim A, Hisam N, Reuman PD. Environmental mycobacterial peritonitis complicating peritoneal dialysis: three cases and review. *Clin Infect Dis* 1993;16:426–431.
152. Giladi M, Lee BE, Berlin OG, et al. Peritonitis caused by *Mycobacterium kansasii* in a patient undergoing continuous ambulatory peritoneal dialysis. *Am J Kidney Dis* 1992;19:597–599.
153. Perlino CA. *Mycobacterium avium* complex: an unusual cause of peritonitis in patients undergoing continuous ambulatory peritoneal dialysis. *Clin Infect Dis* 1993;17:1083–1084.
154. Harro C, Braden GL, Morris AB, et al. Failure to cure *Mycobacterium gordonae* peritonitis associated with continuous ambulatory peritoneal dialysis. *Clin Infect Dis* 1997;24:955–957.
155. Band JD, Ward JI, Fraser DW, et al. Peritonitis due to a *Mycobacterium chelonei*-like organism associated with intermittent chronic peritoneal dialysis. *J Infect Dis* 1982;145:9–17.
156. Pulliam JP, Vernon DD, Alexander SR, et al. Nontuberculous mycobacterial peritonitis associated with continuous ambulatory peritoneal dialysis. *Am J Kidney Dis* 1983;2:610–614.
157. Selgas R, Munoz J, Aquella A, et al. *Mycobacterium chelonei* peritonitis due to hematogenous dissemination in a continuous ambulatory peritoneal dialysis patient. *Am J Kidney Dis* 1987;10:144–146.
158. Merlin TL, Tzamaloukas AH. *Mycobacterium chelonae* peritonitis associated with continuous ambulatory peritoneal dialysis. *Am J Clin Pathol* 1989;91:717–720.
159. Kolmos HJ, Brahm M, Bruun B. Peritonitis with *Mycobacterium fortuitum* in a patient on continuous ambulatory peritoneal dialysis. *Scand J Infect Dis* 1992;24:801–803.
160. Wallace RJ Jr, Swenson JM, Silcox VA, et al. Treatment of nonpulmonary infections due to *Mycobacterium fortuitum* and *Mycobacterium chelonei* on the basis of in vitro susceptibilities. *J Infect Dis* 1985;152: 500–514.
161. Wallace RJ Jr, Brown BA, Onyi GO. Susceptibilities of *Mycobacterium fortuitum* biovar. *fortuitum* and the two subgroups of *Mycobacterium chelonae* to imipenem, cefmetazole, cefoxitin, and amoxicillin-clavulanic acid. *Antimicrob Agents Chemother* 1991;35:773–775.
162. Flynn PM, Van Hooser B, Gigliotti F. Atypical mycobacterial infections of Hickman catheter exit sites. *Pediatr Infect Dis J* 1988;7: 510–513.
163. Hoy JF, Rolston KV, Hopfer RL, et al. *Mycobacterium fortuitum* bacteremia in patients with cancer and long-term venous catheters. *Am J Med* 1987;83:213–217.
164. Raad II, Vartivarian S, Khan A, et al. Catheter-related infections caused by the *Mycobacterium fortuitum* complex: 15 cases and review. *Rev Infect Dis* 1991;13:1120–1125.
165. Gehr TW, Walters BA. Catheter-related *Mycobacterium chelonei* infection in a CAPD patient. *Perit Dial Int* 1994;14:278–279.
166. Rodgers GL, Mortensen JE, Blecker-Shelly D, et al. Two case reports and review of vascular catheter-associated bacteremia caused by nontuberculous Mycobacterium species. *Pediatr Infect Dis J* 1996;15: 260–264.
167. Holland DJ, Chen SC, Chew WW, et al. *Mycobacterium neoaurum* infection of a Hickman catheter in an immunosuppressed patient. *Clin Infect Dis* 1994;18:1002–1003.
168. Moreno A, Llanos M, Gonzalez A, et al. *Mycobacterium fortuitum* bacteremia in an immunocompromised patient with a long-term venous catheter. *Eur J Clin Microbiol Infect Dis* 1996;15:423–424.
169. Brannan DP, DuBois RE, Ramirez MJ, et al. Cefoxitin therapy for *Mycobacterium fortuitum* bacteremia with associated granulomatous hepatitis. *South Med J* 1984;77:381–384.
170. Schelonka RL, Ascher DP, McMahon DP, et al. Catheter-related sepsis caused by *Mycobacterium avium* complex. *Pediatr Infect Dis J* 1994;13:236–238.
171. Dube MP, Sattler FR. Catheter-related bacteremia due to *Mycobacterium avium* complex. *Clin Infect Dis* 1996;23:405–406.
172. Gonzales EP, Crosby RM, Walker SH. *Mycobacterium aquae* infection in a hydrocephalic child (*Mycobacterium aquae* meningitis). *Pediatrics* 1971;48:974–977.
173. Kurnik PB, Padmanabh U, Bonatsos C, et al. *Mycobacterium gordonae* as a human hepato-peritoneal pathogen, with a review of the literature. *Am J Med Sci* 1983;285:45–48.
174. Lowry PW, Jarvis WR, Oberle AD, et al. *Mycobacterium chelonae* causing otitis media in an ear-nose-and-throat practice. *N Engl J Med* 1988;319:978–982.
175. Prammananan T, Sander P, Brown BA, et al. A single 16S ribosomal RNA substitution is responsible for resistance to amikacin and other 2-deoxystreptamine aminoglycosides in *Mycobacterium abscessus* and *Mycobacterium chelonae. J Infect Dis* 1998;177:1573–1581.
176. Austin WK, Lockey MW. *Mycobacterium fortuitum* mastoiditis. *Arch Otolaryngol* 1976;102:558–560.
177. Neitch SM, Sydnor JB, Schleupner CJ. *Mycobacterium fortuitum* as a cause of mastoiditis and wound infection. *Arch Otolaryngol* 1982; 108:11–14.
178. Lohr DC, Goeken JA, Doty DB, et al. *Mycobacterium gordonae* infection of a prosthetic aortic valve. *JAMA* 1978;239:1528–1530.
179. Wilson RW, Steingrube VA, Bottger EC, et al. *Mycobacterium immunogenum* sp. nov., a novel species related to *Mycobacterium abscessus* and associated with clinical disease, pseudo-outbreaks and contaminated metalworking fluids: an international cooperative study on mycobacterial taxonomy. *Int J Syst Evol Microbiol* 2001;51:1751–1764.
180. Fraser VJ, Jones M, Murray PR, et al. Contamination of flexible fiberoptic bronchoscopes with *Mycobacterium chelonae* linked to an automated bronchoscope disinfection machine. *Am Rev Respir Dis* 1992;145:853–855.
181. Gubler JG, Salfinger M, von Graevenitz A. Pseudoepidemic of nontuberculous mycobacteria due to a contaminated bronchoscope cleaning machine. Report of an outbreak and review of the literature. *Chest* 1992;101:1245–1249.
182. Elston RA, Hay AJ. Acid-fast bacillus contamination of a bronchoscope washing machine. *J Hosp Infect* 1991;19:72–73.
183. Nosocomial infection and pseudoinfection from contaminated endoscopes and bronchoscopes—Wisconsin and Missouri. *MMWR* 1991; 40:675–678.
184. Spach DH, Silverstein FE, Stamm WE. Transmission of infection by gastrointestinal endoscopy and bronchoscopy. *Ann Intern Med* 1993; 118:117–128.
185. Alvarado CJ, Stolz SM, Maki DG. Nosocomial infections from contaminated endoscopes: a flawed automated endoscope washer. An investigation using molecular epidemiology. *Am J Med* 1991;91:272S-280S.
186. Maloney S, Welbel S, Daves B, et al. *Mycobacterium abscessus* pseudoinfection traced to an automated endoscope washer: utility of epidemiologic and laboratory investigation. *J Infect Dis* 1994;169: 1166–1169.
187. Pappas SA, Schaaff DM, DiCostanzo MB, et al. Contamination of flexible fiberoptic bronchoscopes. *Am Rev Respir Dis* 1983;127: 391–392.
188. Nye K, Chadha DK, Hodgkin P, et al. *Mycobacterium chelonei* isolation from broncho-alveolar lavage fluid and its practical implications. *J Hosp Infect* 1990;16:257–261.
189. Brown NM, Hellyar EA, Harvey JE, et al. Mycobacterial contamination of fiberoptic bronchoscopes. *Thorax* 1993;48:1283–1285.

190. Campagnaro RL, Teichtahl H, Dwyer B. A pseudoepidemic of *Mycobacterium chelonae*: contamination of a bronchoscope and autocleaner. *Aust N Z J Med* 1994;24:693–695.
191. Wang HC, Liaw YS, Yang PC, et al. A pseudoepidemic of *Mycobacterium chelonae* infection caused by contamination of a fibreoptic bronchoscope suction channel. *Eur Respir J* 1995;8:1259–1262.
192. Cox R, deBorja K, Bach MC. A pseudo-outbreak of *Mycobacterium chelonae* infections related to bronchoscopy. *Infect Control Hosp Epidemiol* 1997;18:136–137.
193. Uttley AH, Simpson RA. Audit of bronchoscope disinfection: a survey of procedures in England and Wales and incidents of mycobacterial contamination. *J Hosp Infect* 1994;26:301–308.
194. Sniadack DH, Ostroff SM, Karlix MA, et al. A nosocomial pseudo-outbreak of *Mycobacterium xenopi* due to a contaminated potable water supply: lessons in prevention. *Infect Control Hosp Epidemiol* 1993;14:636–641.
195. Takigawa K, Fujita J, Negayama K, et al. Eradication of contaminating *Mycobacterium chelonae* from bronchofibrescopes and an automated bronchoscope disinfection machine. *Respir Med* 1995;89: 423–427.
196. Hoy J, Rolston K, Hopfer RL. Pseudoepidemic of *Mycobacterium fortuitum* in bone marrow cultures. *Am J Infect Control* 1987;15: 268–271.
197. McSwiggan DA, Collins CH. The isolation of *M. kansasii* and *M. xenopi* from water systems. *Tubercle* 1974;55:291–297.
198. du Moulin GC, Stottmeier KD, Pelletier PA, et al. Concentration of *Mycobacterium avium* by hospital hot water systems. *JAMA* 1988;260: 1599–1601.
199. Lockwood WW, Friedman C, Bus N, et al. An outbreak of *Mycobacterium terrae* in clinical specimens associated with a hospital potable water supply. *Am Rev Respir Dis* 1989;140:1614–1617.
200. Stine TM, Harris AA, Levin S, et al. A pseudoepidemic due to atypical mycobacteria in a hospital water supply. *JAMA* 1987;258:809–811.
201. Costrini AM, Mahler DA, Gross WM, et al. Clinical and roentgenographic features of nosocomial pulmonary disease due to *Mycobacterium xenopi. Am Rev Respir Dis* 1981;123:104–109.
202. Gross WM, Hawkins JE, Murphy DB. Origin and significance of mycobacterium xenopi in clinical specimens. I. Water as a source of contamination. *Bull Int Union Tuberc* 1976;51:267–269.
203. Tokars JI, McNeil MM, Tablan OC, et al. Mycobacterium gordonae pseudoinfection associated with a contaminated antimicrobial solution. *J Clin Microbiol* 1990;28:2765–2769.
204. Vannier AM, Tarrand JJ, Murray PR. Mycobacterial cross contamination during radiometric culturing. *J Clin Microbiol* 1988;26: 1867–1868.
205. Siddiqi SH, Hwangbo CC, Silcox V, et al. Rapid radiometric methods to detect and differentiate *Mycobacterium tuberculosis/M. bovis* from other mycobacterial species. *Am Rev Respir Dis* 1984;130:634–640.
206. Mehta JB, Kefri M, Soike DR. Pseudoepidemic of nontuberculous mycobacteria in a community hospital. *Infect Control Hosp Epidemiol* 1995;16:633–634.
207. Bignardi GE, Barrett SP, Hinkins R, et al. False-positive *Mycobacterium avium-intracellulare* cultures with the Bactec 460 TB system. *J Hosp Infect* 1994;26:203–210.
208. Fraser VJ, Zuckerman G, Clouse RE, et al. A prospective randomized trial comparing manual and automated endoscope disinfection methods. *Infect Control Hosp Epidemiol* 1993;14:383–389.
209. Griffiths PA, Babb JR, Bradley CR, et al. Glutaraldehyde-resistant *Mycobacterium chelonae* from endoscope washer disinfectors. *J Appl Microbiol* 1997;82:519–526.
210. Akamatsu T, Tabata K, Hironaga M, et al. Evaluation of the efficacy of a 3.2% glutaraldehyde product for disinfection of fibreoptic endoscopes with an automatic machine. *J Hosp Infect* 1997;35:47–57.
211. Kiely JL, Sheehan S, Cryan B, et al. Isolation of *Mycobacterium chelonae* in a bronchoscopy unit and its subsequent eradication. *Tuber Lung Dis* 1995;76:163–167.

C

Fungal Infections

39

CANDIDA

MICHAEL M. MCNEIL

Medical and surgical advances in the areas of medical technology, chemotherapeutics, cancer therapy, and organ transplantation have markedly altered the hospitalized patient population. Widespread use of these advances has considerably lessened the morbidity and mortality associated with a wide spectrum of severe life-threatening medical and surgical conditions and enabled the survival of a greater number of hospitalized patients who are severely ill. Consequently, there has been a dramatic increase in the number of severely immunocompromised hospitalized patients. Frequently, these patients are in medical and surgical intensive care units (ICUs) that care for neonatal, pediatric, and adult patients. These patients are at increased risk for infections with relatively avirulent microorganisms, particularly opportunistic fungal infections caused by *Candida* species. Increasingly, nosocomial *Candida* species infections have been recognized to cause serious morbidity and mortality, in particular in immunocompromised hospitalized patients, and they have caused several well-documented nosocomial infection outbreaks.

This chapter reviews current knowledge of the epidemiology of nosocomial *Candida* species infections, placing special emphasis on newer clinical syndromes that have been associated with *Candida* species among hospitalized adult and pediatric patients, pathogenesis of these infections, newer laboratory methods for their diagnosis, risk factors for the development of nosocomial *Candida* infections, application of molecular typing techniques for *Candida* microorganisms, and current strategies and control measures for preventing both superficial and invasive *Candida* species infections.

ETIOLOGY

Among the many different *Candida* species described in the mycologic literature, relatively few have been identified as potential human pathogens and isolated from clinical specimens. In humans, *C. albicans* has been recognized as the most common *Candida* species causing both colonization and infection. In general, the spectrums of disease caused by *C. albicans* and by non–*C. albicans* species have been similar. However, notable differences exist between *C. albicans* and pathogenic non–*C. albicans* species with respect to some important nosocomial epidemiologic associations, their prevalence in surveillance cultures, virulence potential, and innate resistance to antifungal drugs.

The only major natural reservoirs for *Candida* species microorganisms are humans and animals. Although there have been reports of nosocomial *Candida* species outbreaks in which the microorganism was isolated from hospital environmental sources, these are usually not implicated as causes of *Candida* species outbreaks. *C. albicans* is the most common *Candida* species to be implicated in nosocomial fungal infections. Other medically important *Candida* species include *C. tropicalis, C. parapsilosis, C. krusei, C. lusitaniae, C. guillermondii*, and *C. dubliniensis.* Infections may also be caused by *C. glabrata*, and with the implementation of azole drug prophylaxis and therapy, infections caused by this *Candida* species are becoming more common. Because of the emergence of pathogenic non–*C. albicans* species that have variable resistance to antifungal drugs and their widely variable interinstitutional occurrence, the accurate identification of bloodstream and other invasive *Candida* isolates to species level has become an infection control priority. In addition, the newly available standardized method for antifungal susceptibility testing for yeasts now makes it possible to incorporate the ongoing surveillance of antifungal susceptibility patterns for *Candida* species into an institution's infection control program for these nosocomial fungal infections.

Candida albicans

C. albicans is the most frequently identified *Candida* species in the clinical laboratory and is the major pathogenic *Candida* species of humans. Two serotypes of *C. albicans* have been recognized and designated serotypes A and B (1). Numerous methods are now available for determining the serotype of clinical isolates, including agglutination titers, slide agglutination tests, Iatron

IF6 serotyping, indirect fluorescent antibody tests using anti-A antiserum, and monoclonal antibodies. Several reports have described serotype distributions of clinical *C. albicans* isolates in different countries and in particular population groups, most recently human immunodeficiency virus (HIV)-infected patients; however, the interpretation of the results of these serotyping studies depends on the particular method used for determining serotypes (2).

C. albicans is a part of the normal microbial flora of the human respiratory, enteric, and female genital tracts. Acquisition in most persons probably results soon after birth, presumably from the maternal vaginal flora; thereafter, carriage of this species in normal healthy persons, particularly in the gastrointestinal tract, is extremely common. Superficial *C. albicans* infections often affect the oropharynx (oral thrush), esophagus, skin, nails, and vagina. Oral thrush especially occurs in neonates. However, adult patients may also be affected, especially denture wearers, diabetics, women taking oral contraceptives, pregnant women in the third trimester, and HIV-infected patients. These superficial infections are usually self-limited except in rare, often immunocompromised, individuals who may develop chronic mucosal involvement.

Importantly, *C. albicans* may exploit any deficiency in the host's cell-mediated immune defenses. This is evidenced by the development of unusually severe, chronic, and intractable superficial *Candida* infection of cutaneous and mucosal sites in HIV-infected patients and patients with chronic mucocutaneous candidiasis. In HIV-infected patients, progression to full-blown acquired immunodeficiency syndrome (AIDS) is accompanied by a drop in CD4 T-helper cell levels to less than $400/mm^3$; coincident with this, these patients almost invariably demonstrate severe mucosal involvement with *C. albicans.* The most common AIDS-related *Candida* species infections are chronic or recurrent oral candidiasis, candidal esophagitis, and vulvovaginitis. Patients with chronic mucocutaneous candidiasis have a rare genetic condition that results from a specific alteration in cell-mediated immunity to *Candida.* Despite chronic and occasionally dramatic clinical involvement of mucosal and superficial sites with *Candida* species, candidemia and invasive candidiasis is a relatively rare complication in these patients and in HIV-infected patients; in the latter, it has usually been associated with the presence of other risk factors such as intravenous catheters.

Severely immunocompromised, usually granulocytopenic patients are the major population at high risk for the development of invasive *C. albicans* infection, and infection in these patients may involve multiple deep organ systems. Invasive infections caused by *C. albicans* may include fungemia, meningitis, brain abscess, ocular infection, pneumonia, endocarditis, peritonitis, enteritis, pyelonephritis, cystitis, arthritis, and osteomyelitis. Important additional factors that may affect the normal host defenses and predispose patients to invasive candidiasis include prematurity, surgery, parenteral drug abuse, the administration of broad-spectrum antimicrobial agents and total parenteral nutrition, and the use of indwelling central venous catheters.

Candida tropicalis

C. tropicalis has been identified much less commonly than *C. albicans* as a commensal fungal microorganism and has been an infrequent isolate from cultures of the urine, oropharynx, and stools of hospitalized patients. However, in certain hospitals, *C. tropicalis* may be the predominant *Candida* species identified in clinical specimens. *C. tropicalis* is an important opportunistic *Candida* species that has been implicated in invasive candidiasis, in particular in acute leukemia patients. No specific risk factors for invasive *C. tropicalis* infections have been identified that differ from those for invasive *C. albicans.* However, a clinical triad of fever, rash, and myalgias has been suggested as characteristic of the clinical presentation of *C. tropicalis* infection (3).

Candida parapsilosis

C. parapsilosis is a component of the normal human skin flora and has been found particularly in cultures of the healthy subungual space. Rarely, this species causes onychomycosis. *C. parapsilosis* has also rarely been found colonizing the human gastrointestinal tract and female genital mucosal surfaces and may be an infrequent cause of vulvovaginitis or oral candidiasis. Additional specific sites of isolation of *C. parapsilosis* may include the oropharynx of healthy neonates and asymptomatic diabetics and the feces of malnourished patients. *C. parapsilosis* is most often isolated from the bloodstream, in particular from hospitalized patients. However, studies reporting the prevalence of *C. parapsilosis* bloodstream infections have shown that this varies among institutions; in a review of reported series of *C. parapsilosis* fungemia from large hospitals, Weems (4) found that the prevalence of this infection ranged between 3% and 27%.

In contrast with fungemia caused by *C. albicans* and *C. tropicalis, C. parapsilosis* may more often be an important hospital environmental contaminant and gain access to the bloodstream from environmental sources. Nosocomial *C. parapsilosis* infections have been associated with both implanted prosthetic devices and invasive procedures. Several reports of nosocomial outbreaks of *C. parapsilosis* fungemia and endophthalmitis have implicated contaminated hyperalimentation solutions, intravascular pressure-monitoring devices, and ophthalmic irrigating solutions, respectively (Table 39.1). In a report of an investigation of a cluster of *C. parapsilosis* prosthetic valve endocarditis infections in a hospital, results of an epidemiologic investigation, together with molecular subtyping of isolates obtained from patients, the environment, and healthcare workers' hands, suggested that the most likely mechanism for transmission was frequent surgical glove tears occurring during a surgical procedure (25). Horizontal transmission of *C. parapsilosis* was also postulated to have occurred in a hospital's neonatal ICU when a premature infant with progeria who was not colonized on admission developed conjunctivitis and a bloodstream infection, and molecular subtyping found that *C. parapsilosis* isolates from the hands of two of the neonatal ICU nurses and from both the conjunctiva and blood of the infected infant were identical (26).

Extravascular involvement caused by *C. parapsilosis* is relatively uncommon. Endophthalmitis is the most important ocular infection and usually arises following cataract extraction and intraocular lens implantation procedures (see Chapter 26). Rarely, this infection also occurs in patients as a complication of primary fungemia. *C. parapsilosis* may also cause arthritis and has a predilection for involvement of the large joints. In such

TABLE 39.1. NOSOCOMIAL FUNGAL OUTBREAKS INVESTIGATED BY THE CENTERS FOR DISEASE CONTROL AND PREVENTION 1981–2003

Year (Reference)	Fungi	Infection	No. of Patients	Unit/Service	Source	Control Measures
1981 (5)	*C. parapsilosis*	Fungemia	5	Medical and surgical	Contaminated PN	Discontinue use of pharmacy PN pump
1983 (6)	*C. parapsilosis*	Fungemia	8	NICU	Contaminated PN	General infection control
1984 (7)	*Aspergillus* species; *Mucor* species	Systemic infections	5	Hematology-oncology	Construction activity	Environmental control
1984 (8)	*C. parapsilosis*	Endophthalmitis	13	Ophthalmic surgery	Contaminated solution[a]	Discontinue product
1985 (9)	*A. flavus* and *A. fumigatus*	Systemic infection and pseudoinfection	39	BMTU	Laboratory storage of blood culture bottles[b]	Discontinue storing blood culture bottles
1985 (10)	*C. parapsilosis*	Fungemia	12	ICU	Contaminated PN	General infection control
1987 (11)	*Malassezia furfur*	Systemic infection	3	NICU	Endogenous and personnel hand carriage	Identify high-risk patients General infection control
1987 (12)	*A. flavus*	Pseudoinfection	–	BMTU	Construction activity	Environmental control
1988 (13)	*Candida* species	Fungemia	24	Hematology-oncology	Endogenous	General infection control
1988 (14)	*A. fumigatus*	Sternal wound infection	6	Cardiac surgery	Endogenous	Identify high-risk patients
1989 (15)	*C. albicans*	Sternal wound infection	15	Cardiac surgery	OR scrub nurse carrier	Removal from OR of implicated personnel
1990 (16)	*C. albicans*	Fungemia and endophthalmitis	4	Ophthalmic surgery and general surgery	Contaminated IV anesthetic agent[c]	Discontinue product General infection control
1991 (17)	*A. flavus*	Systemic infection	7	Hematology-oncology	Construction activity	Environmental control
1991 (18)	*A. flavus*	Systemic infection	5	NICU	Construction activity	Environmental control
1991 (19)	*C. parapsilosis*	Fungemia	5	NICU	Contaminated liquid glycerin[c]	Discontinue product General infection control
1991 (20)	*M. pachydermatis*	Fungemia	5	NICU	Endogenous and personnel hand carriage	General infection control
1992 (CDC)[d]	*A. fumigatus*	Systemic infection	4	Cardiac transplantation	Severe immunosuppression	Monitor immunosuppression General infection control
1994 (21)	*Acremonium kiliense*	Endophthalmitis	6	Eye surgery clinic	Humidifier	Environmental control
1995 (22)	*M. pachydermatis*	Fungemia, UTI, meningitis and asymptomatic colonization	15	NICU	Personnel hand carriage from pet dogs	General infection control
1996 (23)	*Aspergillus* species	Systemic infection	5	Rheumatology service	Severe immunosuppression and construction activity	Monitor immunosuppression Environmental control
1998 (CDC)	*M. pachydermatis*	UTI, fungemia, skin infection	17	NICU	Personnel hand carriage	General infection, control
1999 (CDC)	*C. parapsilosis*	Fungemia	5	Outpatients on home hyperalimentation	Possibly endogenous and caregiver hand carriage	General infection control
2000 (24)	*A. fumigatus*	Systemic infection	4	Renal transplantation	Severe immunosuppression and construction activity	Monitor immunosuppression Environmental control
2002 (CDC)	*C. parapsilosis*	Fungemia	22	ICU	Personnel hand carriage	General infection control
2002 (CDC)	*C. parapsilosis*	Fungemia	9	ICU	Possibly personnel hand carriage	General infection control
2003 (CDC)	*Phialemonium*	Fungemia and systemic infection	4	Hemodialysis	Unknown, possibly environmental	General infection control

[a] Intrinsic contamination.
[b] Source of pseudo-outbreak.
[c] Extrinsic contamination.
[d] Unpublished data.
UTI, urinary tract infection; NICU, neonatal intensive care unit; BMTU, bone marrow transplantation unit; ICU, intensive care unit; PN, parenteral nutrition fluid; OR, operating room.

patients, development of the infection often is preceded by prior joint surgery (e.g., placement of a joint prosthesis, intraarticular injection, or arthrocentesis). Peritonitis caused by *C. parapsilosis* has been reported among patients undergoing long-term ambulatory peritoneal dialysis or patients who have undergone abdominal surgery for intestinal perforation or other procedures involving peritoneal lavage. These patients may have a history of intraperitoneal and systemic antimicrobial therapy for bacterial peritonitis.

Other Candida Species (*C. krusei, C. glabrata, C. lusitaniae, C. guillermondii, C. dubliniensis*)

C. krusei has been identified as a colonizing yeast in the gastrointestinal, respiratory, and urinary tracts of severely granulocytopenic patients, particularly patients with underlying hematologic malignancies, and has been associated with invasive opportunistic infections in these patients. Local gastrointestinal mucosal deterioration secondary to cytotoxic chemotherapy or radiation has been suggested as a risk factor for *C. krusei* fungemia (27). In granulocytopenic patients, *C. krusei* fungemia is associated with a high mortality. A shift to non–*C. albicans* species, predominantly *C. krusei* and *C. glabrata*, has been well documented in bone marrow transplant patients exposed to fluconazole prophylaxis.

C. glabrata has been documented as an important emerging nosocomial pathogen. In a national survey in the United States of nosocomial bloodstream infections, *C. glabrata* was identified as the most common non–*C. albicans* species causing these infections (28). In addition, this survey found that of the non–*C. albicans* species causing bloodstream infections, *C. glabrata* was associated with the highest complication rate. It has also been suggested that increased utilization of fluconazole may be responsible for the increased frequency of this and other non–*C. albicans* species bloodstream infections (29). Molecular subtyping methods for *C. glabrata* have also been reported (30,31). Management of patients infected with *C. glabrata* and *C. krusei* may be more difficult because of the inherent reduced susceptibility of these species to azole drugs.

C. lusitaniae is an unusual *Candida* species that has been recognized as a nosocomial pathogen. In the laboratory, *C. lusitaniae* may be misidentified as *C. parapsilosis* (both are germ tube negative and form blastoconidia and pseudohyphae on corn meal agar) (32). Rarely, *C. lusitaniae* colonizes the gastrointestinal, respiratory, and urinary tracts of hospitalized patients. In addition, *C. lusitaniae* has caused invasive infections similar to *C. albicans* infections in immunocompromised patients. There have also been reports that clinical *C. lusitaniae* isolates may possess natural and sometimes acquired resistance to amphotericin B, a finding that may complicate the outcome of infected patients.

C. guillermondii is a rare, potentially pathogenic yeast that may colonize skin and has been described to cause invasive candidiasis in intravenous drug abusers (endocarditis), postsurgical patients, and severely immunocompromised patients. A pseudo-outbreak in a neonatal ICU has also been reported (33).

C. dubliniensis is a species that shares many phenotypic characteristics with *C. albicans*, including the ability to form germ tubes and chlamydospores. Isolates have been recovered mainly from HIV-infected patients' oropharyngeal cultures, most often patients with recurrent oropharyngeal candidiasis following antifungal treatment. This species has been associated with invasive disease. Although preliminary studies indicate that most strains of *C. dubliniensis* are susceptible to antifungal agents, fluconazole resistant strains have been detected. It has been suggested that *C. dubliniensis* may develop azole resistance faster than other *Candida* species (34). The clinical importance and role of drug resistance in its epidemiology have yet to be determined (34).

PATHOGENESIS

Candida species have been identified as saprophytes in the human respiratory tract, gastrointestinal tract, and vagina. Therefore, in the clinical laboratory, isolation of these microorganisms from specimens from these sites and the skin may be considered a normal finding. In addition, epidemiologic evidence suggests that in severely immunocompromised hospitalized patients, commensal yeast microorganisms are the major source of subsequent invasive infections. The pathogenesis of *Candida* species infections is multifactorial. Invasion by these colonizing *Candida* strains may be facilitated when there is disruption of local barriers, interference with the cellular host defenses, or both.

The cell wall of *Candida* species has long been considered very important in the pathogenesis of candidal infections. The chemical components of the cell wall of *C. albicans* have been reviewed (35). There are wall components that act as immunodeterminants and immunomodulators, and the cell wall itself is a potential target for new antifungal agents. Considerable research effort has been made to elucidate the role of *Candida*-specific virulence factors in the pathogenesis of these infections. Putative virulence factors for *Candida* species microorganisms have included hypha formation, selective adhesion, secreted aspartyl proteases and phospholipases, and phenotypic switching. However, the exact role of each of these factors is unclear, and other unknown factors may also be involved. Such virulence factors, both individually or collectively, may aid *C. albicans* colonization at multiple sites and enable tissue invasion. The ability of *C. albicans* to adhere to a variety of host tissues and implanted prosthetic devices may be an important prerequisite in the colonization and pathogenesis of candidiasis. Biofilm formation is a potential virulence factor that has been studied *in vitro* on catheter materials. It provides a protective niche from antifungal treatment for these microorganisms and thus may be the source of persistent infection. Relative to noninvasive *Candida* strains and species, invasive ones appear to be superior at forming biofilms and unique biofilm morphology of *C. albicans* has been demonstrated compared to *C. parapsilosis*.

The intact skin is an effective barrier to invasion by *Candida* species. However, local disruption resulting from wounds (including intravascular catheters, burns, and ulceration) may permit skin penetration by these yeast microorganisms. Excessive moisture, as occurs in the perineum (in diapered infants), hands, intertriginous regions (in workers whose hands are frequently immersed in water), and vulvovaginal area (from wearing occlusive undergarments), may be another important local factor in determining sites of cutaneous or mucosal involvement.

Similarly, the intact gastrointestinal mucosa serves as a mechanical barrier preventing bloodstream invasion by *Candida* species. However, the passage of some *Candida* species microorganisms across the gastrointestinal tract wall may occur normally. Sites of injury may greatly facilitate passage of these yeast microorganisms across the gastrointestinal barrier. *Candida* species have been shown to be attracted to and colonize peptic ulcers. *Candida* colonization and invasive infection also occur in patients with marked disruption of the gastrointestinal wall, often in patients with severe burns or those receiving cytotoxic chemotherapeutic drugs.

Another locally protective mechanism in the gastrointestinal tract is the normal bacterial gut flora, which competes with colonizing *Candida* species microorganisms and prevents their overgrowth and subsequent bloodstream invasion. Antimicrobial agents that eliminate the gastrointestinal tract bacterial microflora and permit selective overgrowth of yeasts may be another cause of invasive disease in hospitalized patients.

The host's cell-mediated immunity is a very effective second line of defense against tissue invasion by these *Candida* species microorganisms. *Candida* species microorganisms that enter the bloodstream by traversing the gastrointestinal tract barrier are phagocytosed and thereby eliminated by various cellular components of the normal host defenses. The occurrence of invasive candidiasis in patients with disease- or therapy-induced severe granulocytopenia supports an important role for granulocytes in this defense.

In addition, certain disorders affecting the host's cell-mediated immunity to *Candida* species, such as chronic mucocutaneous candidiasis and AIDS, indicate that an intact cell-mediated immune system also defends against the development of mucositis and mucosal invasion. Precise mechanisms whereby the host is afforded this protection, however, remain incompletely understood. A poorly defined *Candida* antigen-specific deficiency in cell-mediated immunity is responsible for the rare childhood disease chronic mucocutaneous candidiasis (36). Patients with this disorder develop severe, chronic, and intractable mucocutaneous infection and may have associated endocrine disorders. Also, severe virus-induced CD4 T-cell lymphopenia is the cause of severe mucosal disease affecting the oropharynx and esophagus in AIDS patients. Despite the obvious marked superficial candidal involvement in both of these patient groups, neither demonstrates an increased risk for candidemia or disseminated candidiasis, which suggests that other components of the host immune defense system (e.g., an intact humoral and phagocytic system) are also necessary for protection from *Candida* species invasion.

The role of humoral immunity in defense against *Candida* species infections remains largely undefined (37). No specific function has been postulated for immunoglobulin A (IgA) in host defense against candidiasis, and this is supported by the absence of serious yeast infection in patients with IgA deficiency or hypogammaglobulinemia. Also, there is a paucity of published data on the role of cytokines in the pathogenesis of *Candida* species infections.

The results of pathogenicity studies have suggested that *C. parapsilosis* isolates may be less virulent than those of other *Candida* species (*C. albicans* or *C. tropicalis*). Studies of adherence by *C. parapsilosis* isolates to buccal and vaginal epithelial cells, vascular endothelial cells, and fibrin clots have found this to be less marked than the adherence of the other *Candida* species (4). Alternatively, isolates from patients with *C. parapsilosis* vaginitis have been shown to secrete more aspartyl proteinase and appear to be more pathogenic in an animal model compared with isolates from asymptomatic patients (4). Other potentially important findings are the enhanced growth of *C. parapsilosis* isolates in solutions with high glucose concentration and an apparent selective growth advantage of the yeast in hyperalimentation solutions. The results of antifungal susceptibility tests of *C. parapsilosis* clinical isolates (given the limitations of current methods) have generally shown them to be susceptible to amphotericin B.

There is some evidence that *C. krusei* might represent a less virulent *Candida* species, including a decreased ability of *C. krusei* isolates to adhere to human mucosal epithelial cells *in vitro* and their decreased ability to cause cell death in mouse kidney tissue cultures (38,39). In addition, when compared with other *Candida* species, higher inocula of *C. krusei* are required to infect animals in experimental disease models. However, in the severely immunocompromised patient population where fluconazole prophylaxis or therapy has been instituted, *C. krusei* has been problematic (39). Also, studies have emphasized this species' innate resistance to fluconazole, and clinical *C. krusei* isolates have demonstrated relative *in vitro* resistance to both fluconazole and amphotericin B compared with *C. albicans* isolates from similar populations (38,39).

TYPES OF NOSOCOMIAL INFECTIONS CAUSED BY *CANDIDA* SPECIES

Invasive Infections

Of the nosocomial infections caused by *Candida* species, bloodstream infection has been reported most frequently. As previously mentioned, *C. parapsilosis* candidemia has commonly been associated with the use of contaminated intravascular catheters or pressure-monitoring devices. An outbreak of *C. albicans* candidemias in postsurgical patients was also traced to use of a contaminated intravenously administered anesthetic agent (16). Clusters of nosocomial *C. albicans* and *C. tropicalis* sternal surgical site infections have also been reported (15,40).

Mucocutaneous Infections

Outbreaks of *Candida* species infections affecting mucocutaneous sites have rarely been described. However, one outbreak of oral thrush has been reported in the neonatal ICU (NICU) of a hospital in the United Kingdom (41). The source of these infections was traced to a bowl contaminated with *C. albicans, C. glabrata*, and *C. tropicalis* that was used for soaking rubber teats from infants' feeding bottles. In addition, investigation of an outbreak of superficial groin candidiasis in a team of college athletes identified use of a communal ointment container (42).

CLINICAL MANIFESTATIONS

In severely immunocompromised patients, *Candida* infections usually have no specific symptoms and signs, and the only indication of underlying fungal infection may be fever that is unresponsive to antibacterial therapy. All too often, the diagnosis is not made until the patient undergoes postmortem examination. Nonetheless, clinical suspicion for the infection should be high in the management of predisposed severely ill patients. For patients predisposed to the infection, a careful search should be instituted for evidence of candidemia. For infected patients, establishing the diagnosis rapidly avoids an excessive and potentially life-threatening delay in instituting specific antifungal treatment.

The clinical presentation associated with candidemia may be variable. Some patients may have an acute onset of sepsis accompanied by high fever, chills, tachycardia, tachypnea, and hypotension with rapid progression to septic shock; alternatively, a chronic low-grade febrile illness may develop without any specific clinical findings. Development of septic shock in nonimmunocompromised patients with candidemia is rare, more often occurs in patients who have demonstrable renal failure, and is associated with a very high mortality (43). In patients in whom candidemia is associated with a colonized intravascular catheter, spontaneous resolution of the infection may follow removal of the catheter. Alternatively, patients with candidemia may progress to develop disseminated disease with eventual widespread involvement of multiple deep organs.

Cutaneous lesions may develop in patients with candidemia, especially those with acute leukemia. Although these lesions may be extremely variable in number and appearance, they are usually described as firm, erythematous, raised nodules. A definitive diagnosis is provided only by histopathologic examination of a skin biopsy specimen that demonstrates the presence of *Candida* species microorganisms in the dermis. Distinctive skin lesions also occur in premature neonates with congenital cutaneous candidiasis. This rare disorder results from prenatally acquired *Candida* species infection and is often associated with the presence of an intrauterine foreign body. The spectrum of involvement in these neonates ranges from diffuse skin eruption (macules, papules, and/or pustules that may evolve into vesicles and bullae) in the absence of systemic infection, which usually affects infants weighing more than 1,000 g, to widespread desquamating and/or erosive dermatitis predominately, which affects infants who weigh under 1,000 g and is associated with frequent development of invasive candidiasis and high mortality (44). In addition, candidemic patients frequently have evidence of muscle tenderness, particularly of the lower extremities. This may be the only clinical indication that the patient has an associated *Candida* myositis, and the diagnosis requires a muscle biopsy that shows histopathologic evidence of invasion of muscle tissue by *Candida* species.

Ocular candidiasis is common in patients with other clinical evidence of candidemia or invasive candidiasis. Ocular infection with *Candida* species is usually unilateral and often is asymptomatic. Patients with *Candida* species infection and ocular involvement demonstrate visual impairment, which may range from scotomata to complete blindness. Two prospective studies reported 9% and 26% candidemic patients, respectively, developed ocular candidiasis and emphasized the funduscopic finding of chorioretinitis (a focal white chorioretinal lesion with or without overlying vitreal haze) and less frequently the classic white fluffy mass with extension from the retina to the vitreous or a vitreal abscess (endophthalmitis) (45,46). It has been proposed that the less common occurrence of endophthalmitis in candidemic patients may result from more of these patients receiving prophylactic antifungal therapy. In a postmortem study by Edwards et al. (47), 22 of 26 patients (85%) had tissue candidiasis if hematogenous ocular candidiasis was present. Between 10% and 15% of surgical patients who were prospectively studied and received parenteral nutrition were found to demonstrate these same lesions (48). The diagnosis of *Candida* endophthalmitis usually relies on characteristic intraocular findings in a patient with risk factors for invasive candidiasis along with positive blood or vitreous fluid cultures (45). Krishna et al. (46) have recommended ophthalmologic follow-up for development of ocular candidiasis be done in patients for at least 2 weeks after an initial negative eye examination. The treatment of choice for this infection is usually systemic and intraocular amphotericin B therapy in conjunction with appropriate surgical management; however, there is evidence that fluconazole following short course amphotericin B ($\sim$200 mg total dose) or possibly as sole therapy may be effective. Removal of a lens implant, if present in the infected eye, is considered critical for the resolution of the infection (49). The outlook regarding the patient's vision is usually guarded.

Dissemination of *Candida* infection to the central nervous system as a result of hematogenous spread has been increasingly recognized and may often be accompanied by invasive *Candida* species infection at other sites. Characteristic involvement of the central nervous system by candidiasis may include meningitis, diffuse cerebritis with microabscesses, mycotic aneurysms, fungus ball formation, and parenchymal hemorrhage. In infected patients, the diagnostic usefulness of cerebrospinal fluid (CSF) examination may vary; involvement of specific anatomic central nervous system sites determines whether fungal microorganisms are in the CSF and the nature of the cellular content. Meningitis caused by *Candida* species has been most frequently reported to affect newborns (50). Intravenous amphotericin B with or without flucytosine is usually effective and intrathecal amphotericin B may be added to this regimen in some patients.

Chronic disseminated candidiasis (also called hepatosplenic candidiasis) is a form of localized invasive candidiasis that, as the name implies, most commonly involves the liver and/or spleen. As with other forms of invasive candidiasis, blood cultures are frequently negative in these patients, and the diagnosis may not be made until postmortem examination. The most common histopathologic findings are hepatic granulomas and microabscesses. This form of the disease predominantly affects severely granulocytopenic patients, in particular patients receiving chemotherapy with cytosine arabinoside for underlying acute myeloblastic leukemia. The disease usually coincides with recovery of the patient's granulocyte count following a course of ablative chemotherapy. In these patients, gastrointestinal tract ulceration complicates receipt of this and other chemotherapeutic agents and allows gut-colonizing *Candida* species to gain direct access to the portal venous system. It has been suggested that this diagnosis should be suspected in any immunocompromised patient with unexplained fever with or without elevation of serum alkaline phosphatase or bilirubin. Magnetic resonance imaging is a technique that has also been shown to have high diagnostic accuracy for the acute, subacute-treated, and chronic-healed lesions of hepatosplenic fungal disease (51). Optimal antifungal therapy for the infection is unclear; however, during the last decade its incidence has decreased dramatically at large leukemia and bone marrow transplant centers where fluconazole prophylaxis has been extensively used.

Endocarditis caused by *Candida* species often has been associated with disseminated infection in patients with malignancies. It can originate from intravenous catheters and affect high-risk infants, patients receiving parenteral nutrition, parenteral drug abusers, and cardiac surgical patients, particularly as a complication of prosthetic heart valve implantation (52). This infection may be an uncommon cause of persistent candidemia. However, only 50% of patients diagnosed postmortem with *Candida* endocarditis have positive premortem blood cultures for *Candida* species. Natural heart valves appear to be rarely affected; the infection usually is associated with implanted prosthetic heart valves. In their review of the Cleveland Clinic experience, Nasser et al. (53) found that patients with prosthetic heart valves who develop nosocomial candidemia are at significant risk of having or developing *Candida* prosthetic valve endocarditis even months or years later. These investigators also suggested that late-onset candidemia and lack of an identifiable portal of entry should heighten concern about *Candida* prosthetic valve endocarditis in such patients. Of ten of their 11 patients with *Candida* prosthetic valve endocarditis treated with amphotericin B and valve replacement, two patients had a total of three documented relapses. Endocarditis may also occur as a secondary complication of an indwelling transvenous pacemaker, and surgical removal of the infected device and prolonged systemic antifungal therapy are required (54).

Suppurative peripheral thrombophlebitis caused by *Candida* species has been reported to be a distinct clinical entity that may uncommonly cause persistent candidemia. Walsh et al. (55) reported seven patients with this infection over a 15-month period. Factors implicated by these authors as important in the occurrence of these infections were catheter insertion techniques and suboptimal care of the catheter insertion site. Therapy usually comprises removal of the catheter, surgical intervention, and a short course of systemic antifungal therapy. Rarely, *Candida* species may infect arteriovenous dialysis fistulas, and effective treatment in these patients includes removal of the fistula and systemic antifungal therapy (56).

Peritonitis caused by *Candida* species has been reported as a complication in patients receiving long-term ambulatory peritoneal dialysis (see Chapter 65). Also, *Candida* species peritonitis may occur secondary to a perforated ulcer or postoperative anastomotic leakage following colonic surgery (as part of a polymicrobial infection) and may be complicated by the formation of intraperitoneal abscesses or subsequent candidemia. In patients with *Candida* species peritonitis, both an early diagnosis of the infection and prompt institution of specific systemic antifungal therapy are essential. In addition, appropriate surgical intervention in these patients to repair an underlying bowel perforation or to drain peritoneal abscesses may also be required.

Invasive renal candidiasis is most frequently the result of hematogenous dissemination and complicates candidemia or disseminated candidiasis. The kidney is the most commonly involved organ in invasive candidiasis (90%) (57). Rarely, usually only when there is coexistent obstruction, renal parenchymal infection and pyelonephritis are the result of retrograde renal tract infection.

DIAGNOSIS

Diagnosis of mucocutaneous *Candida* species infections usually depends on examination and identification of typical morphologic forms in a potassium hydroxide-stained smear preparation. Walsh and Pizzo (58) have summarized methods for the direct examination of clinical specimens for detection of *Candida* species. The yield from direct microscopic examination of these specimens may be significantly improved by use of calcifluor white stain and subsequent examination by fluorescence microscopy. Use of commercial agar with chromogenic substrates may aid in rapid presumptive identification of *C. albicans, C. tropicalis,* and *C. krusei* in cultures.

In patients with invasive candidiasis, the diagnosis is often extremely difficult to establish. Frequently, a high index of clinical suspicion, the use of blood cultures and diagnostic imaging techniques (computed tomography and magnetic resonance imaging), and invasive biopsy procedures are required. The combination of histopathologic demonstration of morphologically compatible yeasts and hyphal forms together with a positive culture is considered to be the gold standard for diagnosing invasive *Candida* species infection.

The sensitivity of routine blood culture methods is low (<50%); in granulocytopenic patients, this insensitivity may be further exaggerated (<20%) (59). Advances reported to improve the recovery of *Candida* species from the bloodstream of infected patients include the lysis centrifugation (Isolator system, Dupont, Wilmington, DE), agitated biphasic blood culture systems, and automated, continuous monitoring, broth-based systems. Automated broth-based systems have equal sensitivity for detecting *Candida* species to lysis-centrifugation methods (60). However, despite these advances in blood culture technology, recovery of *Candida* species from blood remains an insensitive marker of invasive infections. In patients with postmortem-confirmed candidiasis Berenguer et al. (61) found a direct relationship between the number of visceral organs involved and the frequency with which lysis centrifugation blood cultures detected *Candida* species. Using this modern method, only 28% patients with single visceral organ involvement (excluding gastrointestinal tract) and only 58% of patients with involvement of two or more visceral organs were fungemic.

False-positive *Candida* species blood cultures (positive culture in the absence of candidemia or invasive infection in the patient) may occur; this is particularly likely when blood for culture is drawn via an intravascular catheter that itself has become colonized with *Candida* species. Another important mechanism of contamination of blood culture specimens is inoculation with extrinsic yeasts from sources such as the skin of the patient or personnel. This can occur because of improper techniques of specimen collection and handling or laboratory manipulation.

Although a single positive blood culture for *Candida* species may indicate contamination, this is an important finding in the severely granulocytopenic patient. The finding of a single blood culture positive for *Candida* species, even when possibly caused by an indwelling intravascular line, should prompt further clinical evaluation of the patient for evidence of invasive infection (62).

Intravascular catheters may not only serve as the portal of entry for *Candida* species and be an important primary source of candidemia but also provide a secondary site of attachment for *Candida* species that invade the bloodstream from other sites, most frequently the gastrointestinal tract. A semiquantitative method developed principally for detecting catheter-associated bacteremia also is applicable to the evaluation of catheter-associated candidemia. Following removal from the patient, the distal (5-cm) intravascular segment of the catheter is rolled four times across the surface of a sheep's blood agar plate and immediately afterward is placed into a tube of broth medium for additional culturing. Growth of 15 or more colony-forming units (CFU) on the solid medium has been used to identify bacteria as the cause of catheter-associated bacteremia (58) (see Chapter 17). However, it has been suggested that the recovery of *Candida* species in any amount from either the solid or liquid media cultures of a vascular catheter tip should prompt a thorough clinical reevaluation of the patient for invasive candidiasis (62).

Candida species in urine is an abnormal finding in clean-voided specimens or specimens obtained by suprapubic aspiration from normal individuals. However, the incidence of candiduria is high in ICU patients. The most commonly identified risk factor for the development of candiduria is an indwelling Foley catheter. Additional important factors that may coexist with an indwelling urinary catheter in seriously ill patients include diabetes mellitus, administration of antimicrobial agents, urinary tract instrumentation, and prior bacteriuria.

The presence of candiduria in an ICU patient may indicate extrinsic contamination of the urine specimen, innocuous lower urinary tract colonization from an indwelling Foley catheter, or, most importantly, invasive upper or lower urinary tract infection. Quantitative urine yeast colony counts are an unreliable method both for distinguishing active infection due to *Candida* species from colonization and for localizing the source of candiduria; although a level of less than 10^4 CFU/mL argues against renal candidiasis (63), levels above 10^5 CFU/mL may be associated with a colonized indwelling Foley catheter. Microscopic examination of a Gram-stained urine specimen may not be helpful; however, the presence of hyaline renal tubular casts containing *Candida* species, particularly with pseudohyphae, may correlate with renal infection.

In patients following neurosurgery, the clinical significance of a single CSF sample culture positive for *Candida* species when obtained via an indwelling device (shunt) is difficult to assess, and a definitive diagnosis may require repeated cultures of CSF samples obtained by lumbar puncture (64).

Conventional serologic techniques for detecting serum anti-*Candida* antibodies have not been useful for diagnosing invasive candidiasis, because most normal individuals have circulating antibodies to this microorganism and, in immunocompromised patients, antibody production is variable.

Several prototype antigen/metabolite tests and polymerase chain reaction methods for the diagnosis of invasive candidiasis have been described; however, none can currently be recommended for routine use in clinical laboratories.

EPIDEMIOLOGY

Descriptive Epidemiology

Data from the Centers for Disease Control and Prevention's (CDC) National Nosocomial Infections Surveillance (NNIS) system indicate that in the U.S. during 1980 to 1990 there was an approximate doubling of the nosocomial fungal infection rate from 2 to 3.8 per 1,000 discharges. During the same period, the proportion of reported nosocomial infections from fungal pathogens also increased approximately twofold from 6.0% to 10.4% at all major sites of infection (65). *Candida* species commonly cause nosocomial bloodstream infections among patients in ICUs. During 1990 to 1999, NNIS system data have shown that risk-adjusted nosocomial infection rates have decreased for all three body sites (i.e., respiratory tract, urinary tract, and bloodstream) monitored in ICUs (66). In particular rates for nosocomial bloodstream infections have decreased markedly in medical (nonsurgical) ICUs (44%), coronary ICUs (43%), pediatric ICUs (32%), and surgical ICUs (31%) (66).

The NNIS system data also showed that the most common fungi causing nosocomial infections were *Candida* species (predominantly *C. albicans*), followed by *C. glabrata* and *Aspergillus* species (Fig. 39.1). In addition, in the 1980s, the proportion of nosocomial fungal infections caused by *C. albicans* showed a relative increase (52% in 1980 to 63% in 1990) versus a relative decline in the proportion of *C. tropicalis* and other *Candida* species infections (21% in 1980 to 16% in 1990) (65). However, a recent review of NNIS system data during 1989 through 1999, found a significant decrease in the incidence of *C. albicans* bloodstream infections and a significant increase in the incidence of *C. glabrata* bloodstream infections (67). It has been postulated that these trends have likely occurred in association with a national increase in fluconazole use, which received U.S. Food and Drug Administration (FDA) approval in 1990. The introduction and widespread use of fluconazole may have also contributed to the trend in multiple cause mortality rate in the U.S. for the period 1980 to 1997 due to candidiasis, which showed a markedly steady increase to a peak in 1989 followed by a gradual decline (68). The changing epidemiology of *Candida* species nosocomial infections has also been reflected in several surveys that have demonstrated an increase in non–*C. albicans* species nosocomial bloodstream infections (see below). Nosocomial fungal infections are an important cause of morbidity and mortality. The direct (attributable) mortality of nosocomial candidemia, which accounts for approximately 10% of all hospital-acquired bloodstream infections, has been estimated to be approximately 50% (69,70). The significant impact of nosocomial candidemia on a hospitalized patient's outcome has also been assessed in relation to increased length of hospital stay, and an

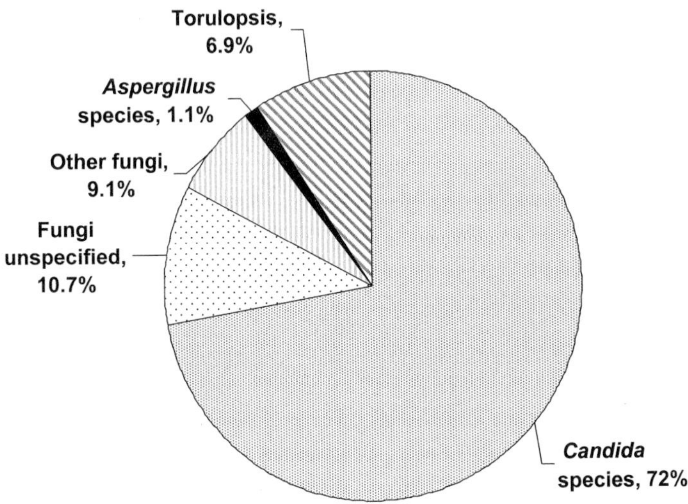

Figure 39.1. Distribution of nosocomial fungal infections by species, National Nosocomial Infections Surveillance (NNIS) system, 1980–1990.

episode of care for candidemia has been estimated to cost between $34,123 and $44,536 (71).

According to NNIS system data, primary nosocomial candidemia rates ranged from 2.8 per 10,000 discharges in nonteaching hospitals to 6.1 per 10,000 discharges in large teaching hospitals in 1989 (72); this represented a fivefold increase in the rates from 1980 to 1989 at large teaching institutions. During 1989 through 1999 data for all ICU categories indicated that 85% of bloodstream infections associated with *Candida* species were monomicrobial and their incidence was 4.8 cases per 10,000 central venous catheter (CVC) days (66). Horn et al. (73) previously observed that the total number of episodes of fungemia increased 31% in a large cancer hospital from 1974–1977 to 1978–1982. The most common fungal pathogen at their hospital was *C. albicans*, which accounted for 45% of the total. Most of the episodes were preceded by colonization of some other body site by the same fungal species. This observation had been reported in an earlier 4-year study of systemic candidiasis (n = 188) in another large cancer center (74). One fourth of the patients with disseminated infection had previously documented site colonization. Reports of candidemia during the 1990s from each of these centers have emphasized the emergence of *C. parapsilosis* and *C. glabrata*, respectively (75,76).

During the 1980s, *Candida* species were estimated to account for 72.2% of U.S. nosocomial fungal infections reported to the NNIS system; the three most common pathogenic species identified were *C. albicans* (76% of infections), *C. tropicalis* (7.3%), and *C. parapsilosis* (2.5%) (77). The distribution of *Candida* species reported to the NNIS system during 1989 through 1999 for all ICUs was *C. albicans* (59% of all *Candida* bloodstream infections), *C. glabrata* (12%), *C. parapsilosis* (11%), *C. tropicalis* (10%), and *C. krusei* (1.2%) (Fig. 39.2) (67). In addition, the NNIS system data for the 1980s showed that the urinary tract, respiratory tract, bloodstream, and surgical sites were the four most common *Candida* species infection sites (Fig. 39.3). However, colonization with *Candida* species occurs normally throughout the human gastrointestinal tract and on skin surfaces, and since the criteria used by the NNIS system to report

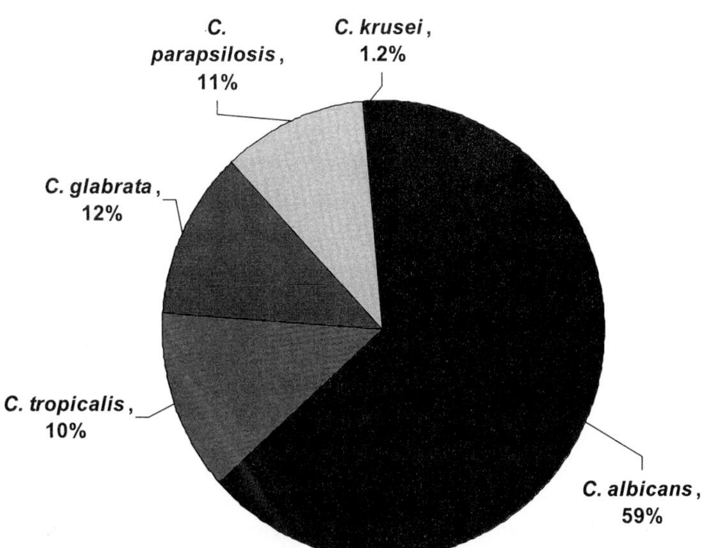

Figure 39.2. Distribution of nosocomial *Candida* bloodstream infections in intensive care units by species, NNIS system, 1989–1999.

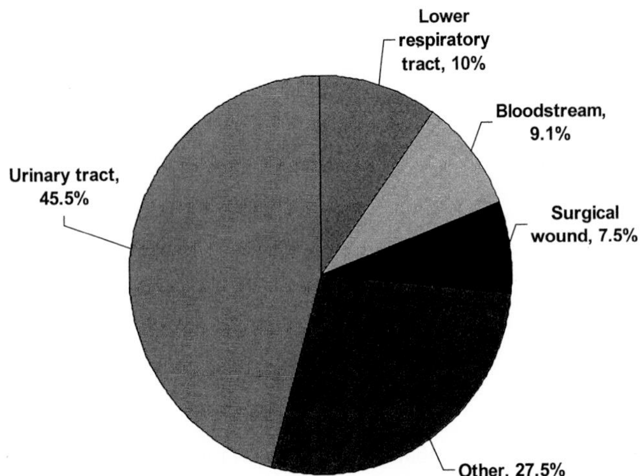

Figure 39.3. Distribution of nosocomial *Candida* species infections by site, NNIS system, 1980–1990.

cases consist of a combination of clinical and laboratory findings and do not require confirmatory histopathologic evidence of fungal tissue invasion, these data may include patients who are colonized with fungi. Nevertheless, despite this limitation, NNIS system data for the 1980s showed that the greatest increase in incidence occurred for bloodstream infections (from 0.1 to 0.5 per 10,000 discharges); infection at this site has also been associated with the greatest number of illnesses and deaths (77). Analysis of patients with nosocomial bloodstream infections reported to the NNIS system has further shown a significant association of fungemia with the presence of a central intravascular catheter and a higher risk of death with bloodstream infection during hospitalization. In a review of three national hospital discharge data sources during the period 1980 to 1989, Fisher-Hoch and Hutwanger (78) found rates of oropharyngeal candidiasis increased 4.7-fold. Although the highest rates were among pediatric patients, the greatest rate increases occurred in males in the 15- to 44-year age group with a very marked increase in rates among patients with HIV infection/AIDS. In the same study, rates of disseminated candidiasis increased 11-fold; this increase was predominantly among patients with HIV infection/AIDS or patients who had a diagnosis of malignancy or who had undergone a transplant procedure (78).

National surveillance of nosocomial bloodstream infections conducted prospectively in 49 hospitals in the U.S. by the SCOPE group (Surveillance and Control of Pathogens of Epidemiologic Importance) between April 1995 and April 1998 found *Candida* was the fourth leading cause of nosocomial bloodstream infections, accounting for 7.6% of all infections (79). Of 934 episodes of candidemia, 46.8% were due to the non–*C. albicans* species identified as *C. glabrata* (42.3%), *C. tropicalis* (26.1%), *C. parapsilosis* (21.1%), *C. krusei* (3%), and other *Candida* species (2%) (79). The proportion of non–*C. albicans* species isolates varied with geographic region and ranged from 30.2% in the Southwest to 54.5% in the Northeast (79). A suggested important factor responsible for this increased trend in fungemias caused by non–*C. albicans* species is widespread use of fluconazole for prophylaxis and therapy (28). A recent report from this group on 22,631 episodes of bloodstream infections during March 1995 through February 2001 observed that despite *Candida* species accounting for 9% and 8% of isolates recovered from all neutropenic and nonneutropenic patients with bloodstream infections, respectively, *Candida* species was notably isolated latest during the patient's hospital stay (mean, 18 days) and monomicrobial *Candida* species bloodstream infections were associated with the worst outcome (crude mortality rate, 45%), and this did not differ according to the patient's neutropenic status (70).

The National Epidemiology of Mycoses Survey (NEMIS) prospectively identified *Candida* species isolated from blood and other normally sterile sites during October 1993 to November 1995 from patients hospitalized in surgical and neonatal ICUs of six academic medical centers located in Oregon, Iowa, California, Texas, Georgia, and New York (80,81). The incidence reported for nosocomial bloodstream infections due to *Candida* species was 0.99/1,000 patient days for surgical ICU patients and 0.64/1,000 patient days for neonatal ICU patients. Of the patients surveyed (4,276 surgical ICU patients and 2,847 babies), 30% to 50% developed incidental stool colonization, 23% of surgical ICU patients developed incidental urine colonization, and one third of surgical ICU healthcare workers' hands were positive for *Candida* species. In addition to a marked interinstitutional variation in rates of bloodstream infections due to *Candida* species, there was variation found in antifungal susceptibility to fluconazole (81). Analysis of patient isolates using a DNA subtyping method enabled investigators to identify 13 clusters of suggested cross-infection occurring in five of the study centers. Nine (69%) of these clusters involved non–*C. albicans* species. The conclusions from this analysis were that the possible mechanisms of *Candida* species transmission that occurred were from patient to patient *(C. albicans, C. glabrata, C. tropicalis, C. parapsilosis)* and from healthcare worker to patient *(C. albicans, C. parapsilosis, C. krusei)* (80). A comprehensive molecular subtyping study of *C. albicans* isolates from patients with bloodstream infections and surgical ICU and neonatal ICU healthcare workers from four hospitals participating in the NEMIS study demonstrated that for the majority of patients (90%), isolates collected from commensal sites before and after collection of a bloodstream infection isolate were highly similar or identical to the bloodstream infection isolate (82). The study also suggested that multiple endemic strains rather than a single, dominant endemic strain were more often responsible for nosocomial bloodstream infections in surgical ICUs and neonatal ICUs and that cross-contamination occurs between patients and healthcare workers and between healthcare workers in the same ICU and in different ICUs (82).

The SENTRY Antifungal Surveillance Program has been operational since January 1997 and prospectively collects nosocomial bloodstream isolates from 72 participating hospitals in the U.S., Canada, Latin America, and Europe (83). This system has confirmed the rank order of *Candida* species causing fungemia in U.S. hospitals recently reported by the NNIS system and its stability year to year (67). Eighty percent of bloodstream infections reported to this system were nosocomial (versus community-acquired) and 50% occurred in patients in an ICU. In addition, this system has noted differences in species distribution, with U.S. medical centers having higher rates of bloodstream infections due to *Candida* species, such as *C. glabrata* and *C. krusei*, which are less susceptible to the triazoles compared with Canada and South America (83). Data from this system have also demonstrated differences in antifungal resistance among isolates from pediatric and adult patients, which likely reflect differences in the distributions of infecting *Candida* species between these age groups (i.e., predominance of *C. albicans* and *C. parapsilosis* in age groups ≤1 year and 2 to 15 years of age and fewer *C. albicans* and significantly more *C. glabrata* infections in persons ≥65 years) (84). A further report from this system has shown variation in antifungal susceptibility to fluconazole among *C. glabrata* bloodstream isolates according to geographic location and age group (i.e., lowest in Pacific [44%] and East South Central [47%] regions and highest in West South Central region [82%], and isolates from pediatric patients were virtually all susceptible to fluconazole, whereas the highest frequency of resistance was observed in isolates from patients 16 to 64 years of age) (85).

Recent reports of surveillance for candidemia conducted in other countries have broadened our understanding of the epidemiology of the condition. In a representative sample of French hospitals in 1995, Richet et al. (86) reported an overall incidence rate of 0.29 per 1,000 admissions, ranging from 0.71 per 1,000 admissions in cancer referral centers to 0.17 per 1,000 admissions in general hospitals. In this study *C. albicans* (53%) was the predominant species isolated, a central venous catheter (26%) was the most common portal of entry, and 50% of the candidemic patients had a neoplasm. Prospective candidemia surveillance conducted in 1992 to 1994 in 14 Canadian medical centers found a 4:1 adult to child ratio, more frequent occurrence of *C. parapsilosis* (second only to *C. albicans* and associated with lower mortality), and age greater than 60 and stay in an ICU as the two most significant risk factors for overall mortality (87). In a retrospective review of *Candida* species bloodstream infections in nine Australian tertiary referral hospitals during 1995 to 1998, Slavin's group (88) reported a rate for candidemia of 0.1 to 0.27 per 1,000 discharges and demonstrated a decreasing trend in the proportion of *C. albicans* to non–*C. albicans* species. In a review of candidemia from Finland, Poikonen et al. (89) found the annual incidence increased from 1.7 per 100,000 population in 1995 to 2.2 per 100,000 in 1999; however, the proportion of non–*C. albicans* species cases (30%) did not increase during the study period. In addition, the highest annual incidence (24.4/100,000 population) occurred in 1999 in infants <1 year of age, which was primarily caused by *C. albicans* (11 cases, five of which occurred in one tertiary hospital).

Rees et al. (90) reported results of population-based active laboratory surveillance conducted for invasive mycotic infections during 1992 and 1993 in three California counties in the San Francisco Bay Area; they found the cumulative incidence for these infections was 178.3 per million per year and *Candida* (72.8 per million per year) was the most common infection. The case fatality ratio was 33.9%. The *Candida* species they identified in order of frequency were *C. albicans* (50.9%), *C. parapsilosis* (22.2%), *C. glabrata* (11.7%), and *C. tropicalis* (7.9%). Species-specific case fatality ratios were *C. tropicalis* (44.1%), *C. albicans* (38.1%), *C. glabrata* (34.7%), and *C. parapsilosis* (16.8%). Major underlying conditions among all patients with invasive candidal infections were nonhematologic malignancies (18.2%), HIV infection (15.3%), diabetes mellitus (13.6%), and chronic lung disease (13.6%) (90). Recent abdominal or cardiac surgery had been performed on 17.9% of patients with invasive candidiasis and was particularly associated with *C. tropicalis* and *C. glabrata* infections. *C. parapsilosis* was the most frequently isolated invasive fungal pathogen in children under 10 years of age (cumulative incidence 33.3 per million per year) followed by *C. albicans* (29.6 per million per year), and for both these species race-specific cumulative incidence rates among blacks were more than double those of other racial groups. The majority of infections with *C. parapsilosis* and *C. albicans* in children <10 years occurred in those <1 year. No cases of invasive *C. glabrata* infection occurred in patients under 20 years of age (90). In a later study, Kao et al. (91) reported results of a prospective, active population-based surveillance for candidemia in Atlanta and San Francisco during 1992 to 1993. The average annual incidence of candidemia at both sites was 8 per 100,000 population; the highest incidence (75 per 100,000) occurred among infants ≤1 year old. In 19% patients, candidemia developed prior to or on the day of admission. Underlying medical conditions included cancer (26%), abdominal surgery (14%), diabetes mellitus (13%), and HIV infection (10%). In 47% of cases, non–*C. albicans* species were isolated, most commonly *C. parapsilosis, C. glabrata*, and *C. tropicalis*. Antifungal susceptibility testing of 394 isolates revealed minimal levels of azole resistance among *C. albicans, C. tropicalis* and *C. parapsilosis.*

Reservoirs and Sources of Infection

Candida species may enter the blood via several routes; the major routes are intubation, intravenous catheterization, and intestinal translocation. The last route becomes important when the burden of yeast microorganisms exceeds a certain but as yet undetermined threshold in humans. A prospective study involving biweekly quantitative stool cultures from very low birth weight (≤1,500 g) infants during the first 6 weeks of life revealed a threshold (8×10^6 *Candida* species CFU/g of stool) beyond which 50% of the patients developed gastrointestinal symptoms (92). More than half of these same patients also developed invasive infection within the following weeks. These results may be of particular importance, because they provide a basis for developing and evaluating effective interventions for the prevention of candidemia originating from the gut in these high-risk pediatric patients.

In most hospitalized *Candida*-infected patients, the likely source of the infecting strains is *Candida* species from the patient's own endogenous fungal flora of the gastrointestinal tract and skin. Clinical studies using newer molecular typing techniques have confirmed that patients' endogenous colonizing *Candida* species strain(s) may be the cause of invasive disease (93–95). Long-term indwelling intravascular catheters, in particular central venous catheters, provide another portal of entry for endogenous pathogenic *Candida* species. Finally, despite the isolation of *Candida* species from a variety of hospital environmental sources, including air, food, fomites, and environmental surfaces, these have not been implicated as sources for nosocomial *Candida* species infections.

Modes of Transmission of Infection

Nosocomial transmission of *Candida* species may result from either extrinsic or intrinsic contamination of solutions or devices. Carriage of *Candida* species on the hands of hospital personnel may cause extrinsic contamination of central lines and devices, parenteral hyperalimentation fluids, and other intravenous solutions and medications. Outbreaks of nosocomial *Candida* species infections have been reported often in special care units and attributed to cross-infection (Table 39.1). Outbreaks of nosocomial *C. parapsilosis* fungemia, in particular, have been traced to contaminated intravascular lines and pressure-monitoring devices and/or parenteral hyperalimentation fluids (Table 39.1). Extrinsic contamination of a new intravenous anesthetic agent without a preservative was also responsible for an outbreak of postsurgical *C. albicans* fungemia and endophthalmitis (16) (see Chapter 61). In a multistate outbreak of *C. parapsilosis* endophthalmitis, the vehicle identified was an intrinsically contaminated ophthalmic irrigating solution (8). Antifungal susceptibilities of outbreak isolates found them to have a uniform pattern that differed from those of control isolates (96). In the outbreak of candidemia in an NICU reported by Sherertz et al. (97), infants' bloodstream infections were traced to the administration of *Candida* species–contaminated retrograde medication syringe fluid. Pertowski et al. (15) investigated an outbreak of sternal wound infections in patients following cardiac surgery, and found that exposure to a particular scrub nurse in the operating room with a history of recurrent vulvovaginal candidiasis was significantly associated with case-patients. Molecular subtyping of case patients' isolates was performed and these results suggested a common source; however, no isolates from the scrub nurse were available. Following reassignment of the scrub nurse outside the operating room, the outbreak ceased. Also, a distinctly unusual source, a multidose bottle of liquid glycerin used for per-rectal administration, was identified by Welbel et al. (19) in an outbreak of *C. parapsilosis* bloodstream infections in neonates.

More specific evidence regarding nosocomial *Candida* species transmission has been provided by several investigators who have used new molecular typing methods to study isolates from infected patients, hospital personnel, and the hospital environment. In an outbreak of *C. tropicalis* sternal surgical site infections in patients undergoing cardiac surgery, a staff member carrier was identified who had contact with all the case-patients and who was colonized (nares and hand) by a *C. tropicalis* strain with a DNA type identical to that of the case-patient isolates and different from those of control *C. tropicalis* isolates (40). In another report, three of four infants infected over a 3-month period from an unspecified source in a neonatal ICU acquired the same strain of *C. albicans* (98). In a third report, five of 98 bone marrow transplantation unit (BMTU) patients studied prospectively acquired *C. parapsilosis* exogenously during their admission; although isolates of a single DNA type were isolated from four patients, the hands of three hospital staff members, and two environmental surfaces in the BMTU, no common source could be identified, and a total of three different DNA types were demonstrated for the outbreak isolates (99). In a prospective study of 98 patients admitted to a university hospital's medical ICU and BMTUs, prolonged stay in the unit and prior antimicrobial use were each identified as significant risk factors for nosocomial *C. glabrata* colonization (31). Molecular subtyping analysis of *C. glabrata* isolates obtained from patients, healthcare workers' hands, and the environment further suggested that exogenous nosocomial acquisition of these isolates may have occurred from sources in the hospital environment, and indirect contact may have been important in their transmission (31). Application of these newer methods of molecular typing to the study of *Candida* species infection should enhance our understanding of the epidemiology of this important nosocomial pathogen.

Risk Factors for Infection

Factors that have increased the number of severely immunocompromised hospitalized patients who are at highest risk for nosocomial fungal infections include modern pharmacologic treatments for hematologic and other malignancies, including intensive ablative and immunosuppressive chemotherapeutic regimens, broad-spectrum antimicrobial agents, parenteral hyperalimentation, and prolonged treatment of patients in adult and neonatal ICUs, frequently with invasive devices such as CVCs. Other important factors contributing to the number of highly immunocompromised hospitalized patients include the AIDS epidemic and an increase in the number of patients with solid organ (kidney, heart, liver) or bone marrow transplants.

Few well-controlled studies have properly assessed predisposing factors for the development of nosocomial invasive candidiasis. Karabinis et al. (100) studied candidemia in cancer patients and, in a multivariable analysis of a matched case-control study, found that positive peripheral cultures for *Candida* species, central catheterization, and neutropenia were significant independent risk factors for infection in these patients. In a matched case-control study by Wey et al. (101), the stepwise logistic regression analysis identified four independent variables that together predicted the acquisition of nosocomial candidemia: the number of antibiotics received before infection, prior hemodialysis, prior use of a Hickman catheter, and isolation of *Candida* species from nonblood body sites. A third matched case-control study by Bross et al. (102) drew similar conclusions concerning the use of central lines and antibiotics; moreover, the presence of a urinary catheter, azotemia, diarrhea, candiduria, and the transfer of the patient from another hospital also were associated with an increased risk of candidemia. These studies will help determine high-risk populations and preventive approaches that may reduce the incidence of nosocomial candidemia.

In another study, Richet et al. (13) showed that significantly granulocytopenic patients with acute lymphocytic leukemia were predisposed to candidemia following administration of vancomycin and/or imipenem. This study also found that, in these patients, proliferation of *Candida* species in the gastrointestinal tract as a result of vancomycin therapy was associated with an increased risk for candidemia, and that concurrent prophylactic oral amphotericin B therapy was protective. Thus, in granulocytopenic patients, receipt of specific antimicrobial agents for prophylaxis of bacterial infections may itself predispose these patients to invasive candidiasis. A better understanding of the risk factors for invasive candidiasis will await future studies.

Turner et al. (103) examined nosocomial candidemia in pediatric patients at two university hospitals over a 5-year period. Forty percent of the patients with candidemia were premature infants, 38% had gastrointestinal and hepatic disorders, and 15% had underlying malignancies. The infection was related to intravenous lines in 90% of cases.

A few studies have examined the role of preexisting colonizing *Candida* species strains in patients who subsequently develop invasive candidiasis. Solomkin et al. (104) reported that, in patients undergoing elective abdominal surgical procedures, there was evidence of sequential spread of colonizing yeasts from the abdominal cavity to the bloodstream and other body sites. Pittet et al. (105) used electrophoretic karyotyping to delineate *Candida* species strains isolated from critical care unit patients. In this study, *Candida* species carriage was found to be patient specific rather than site specific; each patient was colonized with *Candida* species with identical karyotype patterns. Colonization always preceded infection that occurred a mean of 25 days after initial surveillance cultures grew yeast. These investigators further determined that, among surgical patients heavily colonized with *Candida* species, the three significant risk factors for candidemia were the length of previous antibiotic therapy, an Acute Physiology and Chronic Health Evaluation (APACHE II) score greater than 20, and the degree of *Candida* colonization (105). In another study, Reagan et al. (106) used restriction endonuclease digests of chromosomal DNA and a DNA probe to demonstrate the sequence of initial colonization of patients with *Candida* species followed by their infection with strains considered identical with these techniques. These studies highlight the importance of using molecular epidemiologic tools for further understanding of the pathogenesis and mode of transmission of candidal infections.

Infections with *Candida* species that are resistant to new antifungal agents used in prophylaxis for severely immunocompromised patients were initially identified with the widespread use of fluconazole in the therapy of nonhospitalized AIDS patients, which was associated with the emergence of *Candida* species strains resistant to the drug. As early as 1991, a report of a significant association of fluconazole prophylaxis and *C. krusei* opportunistic infections was documented among patients in the Johns Hopkins University's Hospital BMTU (39). These *C. krusei* isolates demonstrated innate resistance to fluconazole. In a follow-up study from this institution, the administration of early empiric amphotericin B plus flucytosine therapy to febrile neutropenic BMTU patients colonized with *C. krusei* was associated with a reduction in the proportion of *C. krusei* fungemias in patients receiving fluconazole (107). However, in the same study, a higher proportion of fungemias attributable to fluconazole-resistant *C. glabrata* was noted among patients receiving fluconazole. Since these preliminary studies, several epidemiologic reports have shown that the widespread use of fluconazole-suppressive therapy for patients at high risk for disseminated *Candida* species infections in these and other hospital critical care units has presaged the emergence of infections caused by less pathogenic but innately resistant *Candida* species.

PREVENTION AND CONTROL

Until the pathogenicity of specific fungal microorganisms is better understood, effective control and prevention strategies for nosocomial *Candida* species infections must use available epidemiologic information, be targeted at patients who are at highest risk for these infections, and aim at interrupting or preventing transmission of infection. Additional strategies now include the development of new, rapid, sensitive diagnostic tests and the development of newer, more effective therapies.

Proper implementation and strict adherence to established infection control guidelines remain the best means to prevent nosocomial candidiasis. Perhaps the single most effective infection control intervention is emphasis of the need for hand washing and aseptic technique in routine patient care. Additional specific measures to prevent intravascular fungal infections include strict aseptic technique in the insertion and maintenance of intravenous lines. In high-risk patients and patients in whom the diagnosis of invasive candidiasis is suspected or confirmed, the administration of antifungal drugs may be for prophylactic, empiric, or specific therapy. A more aggressive approach to the management of candidal infections with antifungal agents has become the standard because of the potentially high mortality and morbidity associated with these infections and the wide availability of azole anticandidal agents, which are less toxic than amphotericin B.

Antifungal prophylactic strategies using the oral azole drugs have been extensively studied, mostly in patients with hematologic malignancies or AIDS. In high-risk granulocytopenic or bone marrow transplant patients, fluconazole has been shown to be effective not only for the prevention of superficial and/or invasive candidal infections (see below), but also for prolonging overall patient survival (108); however, this therapy may also select for less susceptible or resistant *Candida* species.

For patients who have persistent severe granulocytopenia, remain febrile despite broad-spectrum antibiotic therapy, and have no identifiable source of fever after a thorough evaluation for a nonfungal (bacterial or viral) infection, empiric antifungal therapy has been recommended. Marr (109) summarized several recently published randomized trials in support of empirical antifungal therapy in febrile granulocytopenic patients that have found equivalence in composite efficacy endpoints for conventional amphotericin B versus fluconazole, conventional amphotericin B versus selected lipid formulations of amphotericin B, conventional amphotericin B versus itraconazole, and voriconazole and a lipid formulation of amphotericin B (liposomal amphotericin B). However, the results of the last of these studies, a large, multicenter, randomized trial (110), have been controversial because the voriconazole treatment group did not meet the predefined composite primary endpoint for noninferiority and because of this voriconazole did not gain FDA approval for empirical treatment of febrile granulocytopenic patients (111). Furthermore, although fewer associated toxic effects were evident with fluconazole and itraconazole, these agents may be inappropriate therapy for patients who have been heavily treated with prophylactic triazoles or for those at high risk of mold infections because of long-term granulocytopenia. For such patients, acceptable alternatives now include lipid formulations of amphotericin B and voriconazole, and to these, possibly new antifungal drug regimens (see below) may be added (109).

Treatment guidelines for invasive candidiasis have clarified the indications and use of fluconazole and lipid formulations of amphotericin B, each of which provides a safer alternative to conventional amphotericin B therapy with its associated toxicities (112). Supporting these recommendations are data from two randomized controlled trials in nonneutropenic patients (113, 114) and two large observational studies that included granulocytopenic and immunocompromised patients (115,116), which documented that fluconazole in a dosage of 400 mg per day was comparable in efficacy with amphotericin B for the therapy of candidemia. The choice of antifungal agent depends on the clinical status of the patient, the *Candida* species detected (or antifungal susceptibility, if known), and whether the patient had previously been treated or had received prophylaxis with an azole. In patients who are clinically stable (i.e., do not have hypotension and whose overall condition is not considered to be worsening), initial therapy with fluconazole is reasonable (112). In clinically unstable patients and those who may have previously received the azole, amphotericin B at a dose of ≥0.7 mg/kg per day should be considered until the pathogenic species is known (112). Speciation of a patient's pathogenic *Candida* species may guide subsequent antifungal drug treatment. Amphotericin B is the drug of choice for the treatment of *C. krusei* infections and stable patients infected with *C. glabrata*; however, invasive *C. lusitaniae* infection warrants fluconazole. *C. albicans, C. tropicalis* and *C. parapsilosis* are generally susceptible to fluconazole; treatment with either fluconazole or amphotericin B is considered acceptable. At present, the lipid formulations of amphotericin B should be reserved for the treatment of candidemia in patients intolerant or refractory to the aforementioned antifungal agents. New antifungal compounds, such as broad-spectrum triazoles and echinocandins, are being developed and may be used against fluconazole–resistant oropharyngeal candidiasis and to treat invasive *Candida* infections. Of the former drugs, voriconazole, a synthetic derivative of fluconazole, has expanded antifungal activity, including *C. krusei, C. glabrata* that are inherently fluconazole-resistant, and strains of *C. albicans* that have acquired resistance to fluconazole (111). A multicenter, randomized, study comparing voriconazole with fluconazole for the treatment of esophageal candidiasis in 391 immunocompromised patients, most of whom had AIDS, found no difference between the treatment groups with respect to cure as determined by esophagoscopy (117).

The increasing importance of antifungal resistance in *Candida* has underscored the need for development of antifungal agents with alternative mechanisms of action and lesser toxicity. Of drugs currently in trials, echinocandins have unique characteristics that render them potentially suitable drugs against *Candida* species, including azole-resistant candidiasis. These drugs impair glucan synthesis and are fungicidal against a number of pathogenic fungi including *Candida* species. The efficacy and safety of caspofungin has been demonstrated in comparative studies with both fluconazole (118) and amphotericin B (119) for treatment of esophageal candidiasis, and in a recent report it was shown to be as effective as amphotericin B for the treatment of invasive candidiasis and more specifically candidemia (120). Additional novel classes of antifungals (pradimicins, sordarins) with activity against a wide range of pathogenic fungi including *Candida* species are currently under development. Combination therapy of infected patients is another benefit of the development of antifungal agents with alternative mechanisms of action.

The experimental prophylactic therapies such as the cytokines, including granulocyte colony-stimulating factor (G-CSF) and granulocyte-macrophage colony-stimulating factor (GM-CSF), may lessen the extent and duration of the patient's chemotherapy-induced immunosuppression (granulocytopenia). Cytokine administration to patients together with antifungal agents, as well as transfusion of cytokine-upgraded phagocytes, are promising immunotherapeutic modalities for further research. The widespread use of highly active antiretroviral therapy for HIV-infected patients may also be expected to significantly reduce the incidence of opportunistic fungal infections including mucosal candidiasis in these patients (121).

Routine surveillance cultures have also been suggested to aid in determining which high-risk patients will develop invasive candidiasis. Sandford et al. (122) assessed the usefulness of surveillance colonization cultures for predicting the development of systemic fungal infection in patients with prolonged granulocytopenia. These researchers found that, despite the frequent occurrence of stool colonization with *Candida* species (80% of study patients), this finding was not a reliable predictor for the development of invasive candidiasis in these patients. The data also suggested that any benefit conferred by surveillance cultures applied only to *C. tropicalis*–infected patients and not to *C. albicans*–infected patients. Future studies are needed to better elucidate the role of these cultures.

NOSOCOMIAL *CANDIDA* SPECIES INFECTIONS IN SPECIAL PATIENT POPULATIONS

Neonatal Candidiasis

Prenatally acquired *Candida* species infection resulting in congenital cutaneous candidiasis in premature neonates has been discussed (see above), and the condition must be distinguished from neonatal invasive candidiasis.

Colonization with *Candida* species in hospitalized neonates is thought to result most commonly from acquisition of microorganisms that are part of the maternal vaginal flora. The infant's gastrointestinal tract then becomes the predominant site of colonization with these fungal microorganisms. Alternatively, hospital personnel may be colonized with *Candida* species on their hands; transmission of these yeasts from personnel to infant and from infant to infant via the hands of NICU personnel may be important. In a prospective study of *Candida* species colonization of hospitalized infants, Reef et al. (123), using molecular typing techniques, found evidence that acquisition of *Candida* species was nosocomial rather than maternally derived. Another unusual mode of acquisition of *Candida* species was demonstrated in an NICU outbreak of *C. parapsilosis* fungemias that was traced to probable extrinsic contamination of a multiuse bottle of liquid glycerin (19).

Neonatal invasive candidiasis is predominantly a disease of

low birth weight infants, in particular, very low birth weight infants. Because of modern advances in medical technology since the 1960s, NICUs have proliferated and have contributed to the prolonged survival of more critically ill infants. *C. albicans* is the most frequently identified fungal species to cause disseminated disease in neonates; however, potentially fatal infection may also be due to *C. tropicalis* and *C. parapsilosis,* and rarely *C. glabrata, C. guillermondii,* and *C. lusitaniae.* In a review of 111 cases of candidemia in their NICU during 1981 to 1995, Kossoff et al. (124) noted a more than 11-fold increase; a shift in the prevalent *Candida* species from *C. albicans* to *C. parapsilosis,* and a significantly higher mortality associated with *C. albicans* than with *C. parapsilosis.*

Prior colonization with *Candida* species and these infants' degree of underlying immunologic immaturity are both important in the subsequent development of fungal infection. Oral thrush and perineal rash are the most frequent clinical presentations of *Candida* species involvement in this population. Invasive disease, which is usually fungemia, occurs in approximately 1% to 3% of neonatal ICU infants. Risk factors identified as important for the development of fungemia in this population include intravascular catheters, total parenteral nutrition, prior receipt of antimicrobial agents, necrotizing enterocolitis and surgery specific for this condition, and medications such as steroids and aminophylline (125). Recently, pulmonary hemorrhage and intrauterine growth restriction were identified as independent risk factors for fungemia in neonates (126).

Invasive candidiasis in infants usually has a nonspecific clinical presentation (127). Signs of respiratory deterioration and apnea predominate (70%); however, other manifestations include temperature instability, irritability, lethargy, carbohydrate intolerance, abdominal distention, and rash. Despite the tendency for blood cultures in these infants to be only intermittently positive, the rate of positivity may be higher than that seen for adults; thus, a single positive blood culture is important for instituting therapy. Also, although there is some evidence that, in infants with candidemia associated with catheters, removal of the catheter alone may clear the infection, these infants should probably receive a course of systemic amphotericin B therapy following removal of the catheter (127). Meningitis in neonates is a well-recognized complication of *Candida* species sepsis, with an incidence ranging from 27% to 59% (126). Therefore, a critical requirement for all fungemic infants is the performance of a CSF tap to examine CSF; these cultures may be positive without positive blood cultures (127).

Evidence of *Candida* species meningitis requires early institution of antifungal therapy and may affect both the choice and duration of antifungal therapy and the infant's prognosis and follow-up. In addition, positive urine cultures may be found in 50% of infants with disseminated candidiasis and may be the initial indicator of disseminated infection (127). However, in infants, the presence of yeast skin contamination may invalidate a urine specimen collected in a bag as a diagnostic tool for *Candida* species urinary tract infection, and suprapubic aspiration may be needed. When such an aspirate is culture-positive for *Candida* species, antifungal therapy may be indicated (127). The importance of a screening ophthalmologic examination for infants with suspected *Candida* species fungemia is underscored by the finding that endophthalmitis occurs in as many as 50% of these infants (128). In infected infants, the classic ophthalmologic lesion is described as a yellow-white, fluffy patch of retinitis with indistinct margins that may develop more gradually than lesions caused by bacterial sepsis. Resolution of the infection usually follows the introduction of systemic amphotericin B therapy; however, prolonged therapy is needed to prevent recurrences (127).

The hematologic profile in infants with invasive candidiasis may also be nonspecific. Thrombocytopenia ($\leq$100,000/mm^3) may occur in up to 70% of infants with fungemia (127), and the leukocyte count may be variable. Abnormal liver function test results may suggest hepatic involvement in infected infants (127).

Reports of nosocomial outbreaks of *Candida* species infections have identified various sources for these infections in infants. In an investigation of a cluster of *C. albicans* fungemias involving seven preterm infants in a Canadian neonatal ICU, Vaudry et al. (129) failed to identify any significant risk factors for these infections in a case-control study, and further laboratory evaluation of the case-patient isolates using DNA restriction enzyme digests identified two different strains. A small outbreak of fungemias caused by *C. parapsilosis* in an Albany, New York, hospital was traced to defective filters for hyperalimentation fluids, and outbreak strains showed a single electrophoretic karyotype (130). A pseudo-outbreak caused by *C. guillermondii* resulted from flushing needles with a contaminated heparin solution (33). Contaminated retrograde intravenous medication was found to be the cause of an outbreak of *Candida* species fungemia involving five infants in an NICU, and molecular typing revealed identical *C. albicans* strains from patients and medication syringe fluid (97). A report by Fowler et al. (131) of an outbreak of *C. lusitaniae* infections used molecular subtyping methods to establish that person-to-person transmission of the yeast had occurred among neonates in their NICU. Roiloides et al. (132) reported a 4-year trend with increased isolation of non–*C. albicans* species as causes of fungemia in the absence of routine use of antifungal drug prophylaxis in their NICU. When these investigators studied a cluster of *C. tropicalis* colonization and fungemia cases using molecular subtyping methods, they concluded that cross-colonization was the likely mechanism for transmission possibly via transient hand colonization of personnel (see also Chapter 52).

Postsurgical Infections

Patients demonstrating a variety of postsurgical invasive infections caused by *Candida* species have been described by several investigators. In most reported patients, these infections have been associated with surgical procedures involving all levels of the gastrointestinal tract. However, there have also been reports of unusual outbreaks of postsurgical *Candida* species endophthalmitis and candidemia traced to intrinsically contaminated ophthalmologic irrigating solution and extrinsic contamination of an intravenous anesthetic agent without preservative (see Chapter 26) (Table 39.1). Localized infections caused by *Candida* species in postsurgical patients have included sternal surgical site infections, abdominal abscesses, peritonitis, anastomotic breakdown, and intestinal necrosis; however, candidemia and disseminated candidiasis may also occur. Cultures of blood and deep incisional or organ/space surgical sites may be positive for *Candida* species in infected postsurgical patients. However, postoperative patients tend to be a heterogeneous population that is often critically ill with underlying medical conditions, which often makes it difficult to ascribe a specific role to the surgical procedure in the development of invasive candidiasis. Important underlying conditions in these patients may include malignancies and gastrointestinal, cardiac, and renal system disease; such patients may also have multiple exposures to risk factors for candidemia and invasive *Candida* species infections (e.g., vascular catheters, hemodialysis, total parenteral nutrition, and broad-spectrum antimicrobial agents and corticosteroids). *Candida* species has been isolated from CSF in patients following neurosurgery, most commonly in association with shunts. Pancreatic surgery may also be associated with an apparent increased likelihood of *Candida* infection. Hospitalized patients with burn wounds demonstrate frequent wound colonization with *Candida* species and are at particularly high risk for candidemia and potentially fatal disseminated candidiasis (see Chapter 25). During the 1990s, azole (fluconazole) usage in ICUs, particularly surgical ICUs, has steadily increased. This trend has raised considerable concern since a majority of azole utilization in this setting is as prophylaxis or empirical therapy and not for the treatment of documented infection. There is an urgent need for prospective, randomized trials to confirm a protective role for azole therapy in this setting. In the meantime, known untoward effects of azole overuse include both a selection for less susceptible non–*C. albicans* species and induction of azole-class resistance.

CONCLUSION

Nosocomial *Candida* species infections continue to present clinicians with considerable diagnostic and therapeutic challenges. Few well-controlled studies have determined risk factors for these infections; standardized methods for antifungal susceptibility testing of clinical isolates have been developed but are yet to be readily available, and more therapeutic options are needed for the effective management of infected patients. However, laboratory and therapeutic advances have included rapid and specific diagnostic tests for invasive fungal infections in severely immunocompromised patients, successful application of molecular techniques to type common nosocomial *Candida* species pathogens, and several promising antifungal agents. New molecular typing methods in outbreak investigations have improved documentation of modes of transmission of nosocomial *Candida* species pathogens, and, together with new diagnostic and therapeutic advances, they may aid considerably in the development of effective prevention strategies for these important infections.

AUTHOR'S NOTE

Use of trade names and commercial sources is for identification purposes only and does not imply endorsement by the Public Health Service or the U.S. Department of Health and Human Services.

REFERENCES

1. Hasenclever HF, Mitchell WO. Antigenic studies of *Candida*. I. Observation of two antigenic groups of *Candida albicans*. *Br Med J* 1961; 82:570–573.
2. Brawner DL. Comparison between methods for serotyping of *Candida albicans* produced discrepancies in results. *J Clin Microbiol* 1991; 29:1020–1025.
3. Jarowski CI, Fialk MA, Murray HW, et al. Fever, rash, and muscle tenderness: a distinctive clinical presentation of disseminated candidiasis. *Arch Intern Med* 1978;138;544–546.
4. Weems JJ Jr. *Candida parapsilosis*: epidemiology, pathogenicity, clinical manifestations, and antimicrobial susceptibility. *Clin Infect Dis* 1992;14:756–766.
5. Solomon SL, Khabbaz RF, Parker RH, et al. An outbreak of *Candida parapsilosis* bloodstream infections in patients receiving parenteral nutrition. *J Infect Dis* 1984;149:98–102.
6. Solomon S, Alexander H, Eley J, et al. Nosocomial fungemia in neonates associated with intravascular pressure-monitoring devices. *Pediatr Infect Dis J* 1986;5:680–685.
7. Weems JJ Jr, Davis BJ, Tablan OC, et al. Construction activity: an independent risk factor for invasive aspergillosis and zygomycosis in patients with hematologic malignancy. *Infect Control* 1987;8:71–75.
8. McCray E, Rampell N, Solomon SL, et al. Outbreak of *Candida parapsilosis* endophthalmitis after cataract extraction and intraocular lens implantation. *J Clin Microbiol* 1986;24:625–628.
9. Weems JJ Jr, Andremont A, Davis BJ, et al. Pseudoepidemic of aspergillosis after development of pulmonary infiltrates in a group of bone marrow transplant patients. *J Clin Microbiol* 1987;25:1459–1462.
10. Weems JJ Jr, Chamberland ME, Ward J, et al. *Candida parapsilosis* fungemia associated with parenteral nutrition and contaminated blood pressure transducers. *J Clin Microbiol* 1987;25:1029–1032.
11. Richet HM, McNeil MM, Edwards M, et al. Cluster of *Malassezia furfur* pulmonary infections in infants in a neonatal intensive care unit. *J Clin Microbiol* 1989;27:1197–1200.
12. Richet H, McNeil M, Peters W, et al. *Aspergillus flavus* in a bone marrow transplant unit: pseudofungemia traced to hallway carpeting (abstract F-23). In: *Abstracts of the 89th General Meeting of the American Society of Microbiology,* New Orleans, 1989:462.
13. Richet HM, Andremont A, Tancrede C, et al. Risk factors for candidemia in patients with acute lymphocytic leukemia. *Rev Infect Dis* 1991; 13:211–215.
14. Richet HM, McNeil MM, Davis BJ, et al. *Aspergillus fumigatus* sternal wound infections in patients undergoing open heart surgery. *Am J Epidemiol* 1992;136:48–58.
15. Pertowski CA, Baron RC, Lasker BA, et al. Nosocomial outbreak of *Candida albicans* sternal wound infections following cardiac surgery traced to a scrub nurse. *J Infect Dis* 1995;172:817–822.
16. McNeil MM, Lasker BA, Lott TJ, et al. Postsurgical *Candida albicans* infections associated with an extrinsically contaminated intravenous anesthetic agent. *J Clin Microbiol* 1999;37:1398–1403.
17. Buffington J, Reporter R, Lasker BA, et al. Investigation of an epidemic of invasive aspergillosis: utility of molecular typing with the use of random amplified polymorphic DNA probes. *Pediatr Infect Dis J* 1994;13:386–393.
18. Burwen D, Durry E, Rao N, et al. Host-related risk factors for invasive filamentous fungal infection (abstract L-9). In: *Abstracts of the 92nd General Meeting of the American Society of Microbiology,* New Orleans, 1992:519.
19. Welbel SF, McNeil MM, Kuykendall RJ, et al. *Candida parapsilosis* bloodstream infections in neonatal intensive care unit patients: epidemiologic and laboratory confirmation of a common source outbreak. *Pediatr Infect Dis J* 1996;15:998–1002.
20. Welbel SF, McNeil MM, Pramanik A, et al. Nosocomial *Malassezia pachydermatis* bloodstream infections in a neonatal intensive care unit. *Pediatr Infect Dis J* 1994;13:104–108.

21. Fridkin SK, Kremer FB, Bland LA, et al. *Acremonium kiliense* endophthalmitis after cataract extraction in an ambulatory surgical center traced to an environmental reservoir. *Clin Infect Dis* 1996;22: 222–227.
22. Chang HJ, Miller HL, Watkins N, et al. An epidemic of *Malassezia pachydermatis* in an intensive care nursery associated with colonization of health care workers' pet dogs. *N Engl J Med* 1998;338:706–711.
23. Garrett DO, Jochimsen E, Jarvis W. Invasive *Aspergillus* species infections in rheumatology patients. *J Rheumatol* 1999;26:146–149.
24. Panackal AA, Dahlman A, Keil KT, et al. Outbreak of invasive aspergillosis among renal transplant recipients. *Transplantation* 2003;75: 1050–1053.
25. Diekema DJ, Messer SA, Hollis RJ, et al. An outbreak of *Candida parapsilosis* prosthetic valve endocarditis. *Diagn Microbiol Infect Dis* 1997;29:147–153.
26. Lupetti A, Tavanti A, Davini P, et al. Horizontal transmission of *Candida parapsilosis* candidemia in a neonatal intensive care unit. *J Clin Microbiol* 2002;40:2363–2369.
27. Goldman M, Pottage JC, Weaver DC. *Candida krusei* fungemia. Report of 4 cases and review of the literature. *Medicine (Baltimore)* 1993; 72:143–150.
28. Pfaller MA, Jones RN, Messer SA, et al. National surveillance of nosocomial bloodstream infection due to species of *Candida* other than *Candida albicans*: frequency of occurrence and antifungal susceptibility in the SCOPE program. *Diagn Microbiol Infect Dis* 1998;30: 121–129.
29. Nguyen MH, Peacock JE, Morris AJ, et al. The changing face of candidemia: emergence of non–*Candida albicans* species and antifungal resistance. *Am J Med* 1996;100:617–623.
30. Schwab U, Chernomas F, Larcom L, et al. Molecular typing and fluconazole susceptibility of urinary *Candida glabrata* isolates from hospitalized patients. *Diagn Microbiol infect Dis* 1997;29:11–17.
31. Vasquez JA, Dembry LM, Sanchez V, et al. Nosocomial *Candida glabrata* colonization: an epidemiologic study. *J Clin Microbiol* 1998; 36:421–426.
32. Christenson JC, Guruswamy A, Mukwaya G, et al. *Candida lusitaniae:* an emerging human pathogen. *Pediatr Infect Dis J* 1987;6:755–757.
33. Yagupsky P, Dagan R, Chipman M, et al. Pseudooutbreak of *Candida guillermondii* fungemia in a neonatal intensive care unit. *Pediatr Infect Dis J* 1991;10:928–932.
34. Sullivan D, Coleman D. *Candida dubliniensis:* characteristics and identification. *J Clin Microbiol* 1998;36:329–334.
35. Shepherd MG, Gopal PK. *Candida albicans*: cell wall physiology and metabolism. In: Tumbay E, Seeliger HPR, Ang O, eds. *Candida and candidamycosis.* New York: Plenum Press, 1991:21–33.
36. Edwards JE Jr, Lehrer RI, Stiehm ER, et al. Severe candidal infections: clinical perspective, immune defense mechanisms, and current concepts of theory. *Ann Intern Med* 1978;89:91–106.
37. Vartivarian S, Smith CB. Pathogenesis, host resistance, and predisposing factors. In: Bodey GP, ed. *Candidiasis: pathogenesis, diagnosis, and treatment,* 2nd ed. New York: Raven Press, 1993:59–84.
38. Merz WG, Karp JE, Schron D, et al. Increased incidence of fungemia caused by *Candida krusei. J Clin Microbiol* 1986;24:581–584.
39. Wingard JR, Merz WG, Rinaldi MG, et al. Increase in *Candida krusei* infection among patients with bone marrow transplantation and neutropenia treated prophylactically with fluconazole. *N Engl J Med* 1991; 325:1274–1277.
40. Doebbeling BN, Hollis RJ, Isenberg HD, et al. Restriction fragment analysis of a *Candida tropicalis* outbreak of sternal wound infections. *J Clin Microbiol* 1991;29:1268–1270.
41. Cremer G, de Groot W. An epidemic of thrush in a premature nursery. *Dermatologica* 1967;135:107–114.
42. Malamatinis JE, Mattmiller ED, Westfall JN. Cutaneous moniliasis affecting varsity athletes. *J Am Coll Health Assoc* 1968;16:294–295.
43. Hadley S, Lee WW, Ruthazer R, et al. Candidemia as a cause of septic shock and multiple organ failure in nonimmunocompromised patients. *Crit Care Med* 2002;30:1808–1814.
44. Darmstadt GL, Dinulos JG, Miller Z. Congenital cutaneous candidiasis: clinical presentation, pathogenesis, and management guidelines. *Pediatrics* 2000;105:438–444.
45. Donahue SP, Greven CM, Zuravelff JJ, et al. Intraocular candidiasis in patients with candidemia: clinical implications derived from a prospective multicenter study. *Ophthalmology* 1994;101:1302–1309.
46. Krishna R, Amuh D, Lowder CY, et al. Should all patients with candidaemia have an ophthalmic examination to rule out ocular candidiasis? *Eye* 2000,14:30–34.
47. Edwards JE Jr, Foos RY, Montgomerie JZ, et al. Ocular manifestations of *Candida* septicemia: review of seventy-six cases of hematogenous *Candida* endophthalmitis. *Medicine* 1974;53:47–75.
48. Moyer DV, Edwards JE Jr. *Candida* endophthalmitis and central nervous system infection. In: Bodey GP, ed. *Candidiasis: pathogenesis, diagnosis, and treatment,* 2nd ed. New York: Raven Press, 1993: 331–355.
49. Kauffman CA, Bradley SF, Vine AK. *Candida* endophthalmitis associated with intraocular lens implantation: efficacy of fluconazole therapy. *Mycoses* 1993;36:13–17.
50. Fernandez M, Moylett EH, Noyola DE, et al. Candidal meningitis in neonates: a 10-year review. *Clin Infect Dis* 2000;31:458–463.
51. Semelka RC, Kelekis NL, Sallah S, et al. Hepatosplenic fungal disease: diagnostic accuracy and spectrum of appearances on MR imaging. *Am J Roentgenol* 1997;169:1311–1316.
52. Hallum JL, Williams TW Jr. *Candida* endocarditis. In: Bodey GP, ed. *Candidiasis: pathogenesis, diagnosis, and treatment,* 2nd ed. New York: Raven Press, 1993:357–369.
53. Nasser RM, Melgar GR, Longworth DL, et al. Incidence and risk of developing fungal prosthetic valve endocarditis after nosocomial candidemia. *Am J Med* 1997;103:25–32.
54. Joly V, Belmatoug N, Leperre A, et al. Pacemaker endocarditis due to *Candida albicans*: case report and review. *Clin Infect Dis* 1997;25: 1359–1362.
55. Walsh TJ, Bustamente CI, Vlahov D, et al. Candidal suppurative peripheral thrombophlebitis: recognition, prevention, and management. *Infect Control Hosp Epidemiol* 1986;7:16–22.
56. Nguyen MH, Yu VL, Morris AJ. *Candida* infection of the arteriovenous fistula used for hemodialysis. *Am J Kidney Dis* 1996;27: 596–598.
57. Edwards JE Jr. *Candida* species. In: Mandell GL, Bennett JE, Dolin R, eds. *Principles and practice of infectious diseases,* 5th ed. Philadelphia: Churchill Livingstone, 2000:2656–2674.
58. Walsh TJ, Pizzo PA. Laboratory diagnosis of candidiasis. In: Bodey GP, ed. *Candidiasis: pathogenesis, diagnosis, and treatment,* 2nd ed. New York: Raven Press, 1993:109–135.
59. Dupont B. Clinical manifestations and management of candidosis in the compromised patient. In: Warnock DW, Richardson MD, eds. *Fungal infections in the compromised patient.* New York: Wiley, 1991: 55–83.
60. Stevens DA. Diagnosis of fungal infections: current status. *J Antimicrob Chemother* 2002;49(suppl):11–19.
61. Berenguer J, Buck M, Witebsky F, et al. Lysis-centrifugation blood cultures in the detection of tissue-proven invasive candidiasis: disseminated versus single organ infection. *Diagn Microbiol Infect Dis* 1993; 17:103–109.
62. Walsh T, Pizzo P. Nosocomial fungal infections: a classification for hospital-acquired fungal infections and mycoses arising from endogenous flora or reactivation. *Annu Rev Microbiol* 1988;42:517–545.
63. Goldberg PK, Kozinn PJ, Wise GJ, et al. Incidence and significance of candiduria. *JAMA* 1979;241:582–584.
64. Geers TA, Gordon SM. Clinical significance of *Candida* species isolated from cerebrospinal fluid following neurosurgery. *Clin Infect Dis* 1999;28:1139–1147.
65. Beck-Sague CM, Jarvis WR, National Nosocomial Infections Surveillance System. Secular trends in the epidemiology of nosocomial fungal infections in the United States, 1980–1990. *J Infect Dis* 1993;167: 1247–1251.
66. Monitoring hospital-acquired infections to promote patient safety—United States, 1990–1999. *MMWR* 2000;49:149–153.
67. Trick WE, Fridkin SK, Edwards JR, et al., and the National Nosocomial Infections Surveillance System Hospitals. Secular trend of hospital-acquired candidemia among intensive care unit patients in the United States during 1989–1999. *Clin Infect Dis* 2002;35:627–630.

68. McNeil MM, Nash SL, Hajjeh RA, et al. Trends in mortality due to invasive mycotic diseases in the United States, 1980–1997. *Clin Infect Dis* 2001:33:641–647.
69. Wenzel R, Pfaller M. *Candida* species: emerging hospital bloodstream pathogens [editorial]. *Infect Control Hosp Epidemiol* 1991;12: 523–524.
70. Wisplinghoff H, Seifert H, Wenzel RP, et al. Current trends in the epidemiology of nosocomial bloodstream infections in patients with hematological malignancies and solid neoplasms in hospitals in the United States. *Clin Infect Dis* 2003;36:1103–1110.
71. Rentz AM, Halpern MT, Bowden R. The impact of candidemia on length of hospital stay, outcome, and overall cost of illness. *Clin Infect Dis* 1998;27:781–788.
72. Banerjee SN, Emori TG, Culver DH, et al. Secular trends in nosocomial primary bloodstream infections in the United States, 1980–1989. National Nosocomial Infections Surveillance System. *Am J Med* 1991;91:86S–89S.
73. Horn R, Wong B, Kiehn TE, et al. Fungemia in a cancer hospital: changing frequency, earlier onset, and results of therapy. *Rev Infect Dis* 1985;7:646–655.
74. Maksymiuk AW, Thongprasert S, Hopfer R, et al. Systemic candidiasis in cancer patients. *Am J Med* 1984;77:20–27.
75. Safdar A, Perlin DS, Armstrong DA. Hematogenous infections due to *Candida parapsilosis*: changing trends in fungemic patients at a comprehensive cancer center during the last four decades. *Diagn Microbiol Infect Dis* 2002;44:11–16.
76. Bodey GP, Mardani M, Hanna HA, et al. The epidemiology of *Candida glabrata* and *Candida albicans* fungemia in immunocompromised patients with cancer. *Am J Med* 2002;112:380–385.
77. Beck-Sague CM, Jarvis WR, Banerjee SN, et al., National Nosocomial Infections Surveillance System. Nosocomial fungal infections in U.S. hospitals, 1980–1990 (abstract 1129). In: *Program and abstracts of the 30th Interscience Conference on Antimicrobial Agents and Chemotherapy,* Atlanta, 1990:274.
78. Fisher-Hoch SP, Hutwanger LC. Opportunistic candidiasis: an epidemic of the 1990s. *Clin Infect Dis* 1995;21:897–904.
79. Edmond MB, Wallace SE, McClish DK, et al. Nosocomial bloodstream infections in United States hospitals: a three-year analysis. *Clin Infect Dis* 1999;29:239–244.
80. Pfaller MA, Messer SA, Houston A, et al. National epidemiology of mycoses survey: a multicenter study of strain variation and antifungal susceptibility among isolates of *Candida* species. *Diagn Microbiol Infect Dis* 1998;31:289–296.
81. Rangel-Frausto MS, Wiblin T, Blumberg HM, et al. National epidemiology of mycoses survey (NEMIS): variations in rates of bloodstream infections due to *Candida* species in seven surgical intensive care units and six neonatal intensive care units. *Clin Infect Dis* 1999; 29:253–258.
82. Marco F, Lockhart S, Pfaller M, et al. Elucidating the origins of nosocomial infections with *Candida albicans* by DNA fingerprinting with the complex probe Ca3. *J Clin Microbiol* 1999;37:2817–2828.
83. Pfaller MA, Lockhart SR, Pujol C, et al. Hospital specificity, region specificity, and fluconazole resistance of *Candida albicans* bloodstream isolates. *J Clin Microbiol* 1998;36:1518–1529.
84. Pfaller MA, Diekema DJ, Jones RN, et al., and the SENTRY Participants Group. Trends in antifungal susceptibility of *Candida* species isolated from pediatric and adult patients with bloodstream infections: SENTRY Antimicrobial Surveillance Program, 1997 to 2000. *J Clin Microbiol* 2002;40:852–856.
85. Pfaller MA, Messer SA, Boyken L, et al. Variation in susceptibility of bloodstream isolates of *Candida glabrata* to fluconazole according to patient age and geographic location. *J Clin Microbiol* 2003;41: 2176–2179.
86. Richet H, Roux P, Des Champs C, et al., French Candidemia Study Group. Candidemia in French hospitals: incidence rates and characteristics. *Clin Microbiol Infect* 2002;8:405–412.
87. Yamamura DL, Rotstein C, Nicolle LE, et al. Candidemia at selected Canadian sites: results from the Fungal Disease Registry of the Canadian Infectious Disease Society. *Can Med Assoc J* 1999;160:493–499.
88. Slavin MA, Australian Mycology Interest Group. The epidemiology of candidaemia and mould infections in Australia. *J Antimicrob Chemother* 2002;49(suppl S1):3–6.
89. Poikonen E, Lyytikainen O, Veli-Jukka A, et al. Candidemia in Finland, 1995–1999. *Emerg Infect Dis* 2003;9:985–990.
90. Rees JR, Pinner RW, Hajjeh RA, et al. The epidemiological features of invasive mycotic infections in the San Francisco Bay Area, 1992–1993: results of population-based laboratory active surveillance. *Clin Infect Dis* 1998;27:1138–1147.
91. Kao AS, Brandt ME, Pruitt WR, et al. The epidemiology of candidemia in two United States cities: results of a population-based active surveillance. *Clin Infect Dis* 1999;29:1164–1170.
92. Pappu-Katikaneni LD, Rao KP, Bannister E. Gastrointestinal colonization with yeast species and *Candida* septicemia in very low birth weight infants. *Mycoses* 1990;33:20–23.
93. Merz WG, Connelly C, Hieter P. Variation in electrophoretic karyotypes among clinical isolates of *Candida albicans*. *J Clin Microbiol* 1988;26:842–845.
94. Katib R, Thirumoorthi MC, Riederer KM, et al. Clustering of *Candida* infections in the neonatal intensive care unit: concurrent emergence of multiple strains simulating intermittent outbreaks. *Pediatr Infect Dis J* 1998;17:130–134.
95. Ruiz-Diez B, Martinez V, Alvarez M, et al. Molecular tracking of *Candida albicans* in a neonatal intensive care unit: long-term colonizations versus catheter-related infections. *J Clin Microbiol* 1997;35: 3032–3036.
96. O'Day DM, Head WS, Robinson RD. An outbreak of *Candida parapsilosis* endophthalmitis: analysis of strains by enzyme profile and antifungal susceptibility. *Br J Ophthalmol* 1987;71:126–129.
97. Sherertz RJ, Gledhill KS, Hampton KD, et al. Outbreak of *Candida* bloodstream infections associated with retrograde medication administration in a neonatal intensive care unit. *J Pediatr* 1992;120: 455–461.
98. Reagan DR, Pfaller MA, Hollis RJ, et al. Evidence of nosocomial spread of *Candida albicans* causing bloodstream infection in a neonatal intensive care unit. *Diagn Microbiol Infect Dis* 1995;21:191–194.
99. Sanchez V, Vasquez JA, Barth-Jones D, et al. Nosocomial acquisition of *Candida parapsilosis*: an epidemiologic study. *Am J Med* 1993;94: 577–582.
100. Karabinis A, Hill C, Leclercq B, et al. Risk factors for candidemia in cancer patients: a case-control study. *J Clin Microbiol* 1988;26: 429–432.
101. Wey SB, Mori M, Pfaller MA, et al. Risk factors for hospital-acquired candidemia. A matched case-control study. *Arch Intern Med* 1989; 149:2349–2353.
102. Bross J, Talbot GH, Maislin G, et al. Risk factors for nosocomial candidemia: a case-control study in adults without leukemia. *Am J Med* 1989;87:614–620.
103. Turner RB, Donowitz LG, Hendley JO. Consequences of candidemia for pediatric patients. *Am J Dis Child* 1985;139:178–180.
104. Solomkin JS, Flohr AB, Quie PG, et al. The role of *Candida* in intraperitoneal infections. *Surgery* 1980;88:524–530.
105. Pittet D, Monod M, Filthuth I, et al. Contour-clamped homogeneous electric field gel electrophoresis as a powerful epidemiologic tool in yeast infections. *Am J Med* 1991;91:256S–263S.
106. Reagan DR, Pfaller MA, Hollis RJ, et al. Characterization of the sequence of colonization and nosocomial candidemia using DNA fingerprinting and a DNA probe. *J Clin Microbiol* 1990;28:2733–2738.
107. Wingard JR, Merz WG, Rinaldi MG, et al. Association of *Torulopsis glabrata* infections with fluconazole prophylaxis in neutropenic bone marrow transplant patients. *Antimicrob Agents Chemother* 1993;37: 1847–1849.
108. Marr KA, Seidel K, Slavin MA, et al. Prolonged fluconazole prophylaxis is associated with persistent protection against candidiasis-related death in allogeneic marrow transplant recipients: long-term follow-up of a randomized, placebo-controlled trial. *Blood* 2000;96:2055–2061.
109. Marr KA. Empirical antifungal therapy—new options, new tradeoffs [editorial]. *N Engl J Med* 2002;346:278–280.
110. Walsh TJ, Pappas P, Winston DJ, et al. Voriconazole compared with liposomal amphotericin B for empirical antifungal therapy in patients

with neutropenia and persistent fever. *N Engl J Med* 2002;346: 225–234.

111. Johnson LB, Kauffman CA. Voriconazole: a new triazole antifungal agent. *Clin Infect Dis* 2003;36:630–637.
112. Rex JH, Walsh TJ, Sobel JD, et al. Practice guidelines for the treatment of candidiasis. *Clin Infect Dis* 2000;30:662–678.
113. Phillips P, Shafran S, Garber G, et al. Multicenter randomized trial of fluconazole versus amphotericin B for treatment of candidemia in non-neutropenic patients. *Eur J Clin Microbiol Infect Dis* 1997;16: 337–345.
114. Rex JH, Bennett JE, Sugar AN, et al. A randomized trial comparing fluconazole with amphotericin B for the treatment of candidemia in patients without neutropenia. *N Engl J Med* 1994;331:1325–1330.
115. Anaissie EJ, Rex JH, Uzun O, et al. Predictors of adverse outcome in cancer patients with candidemia. *Am J Med* 1998;104:238–245.
116. Nguyen MH, Peacock JE Jr, Tanner DC, et al. Therapeutic approaches in patients with candidemia. Evaluation in a multicenter, prospective observational study. *Arch Intern Med* 1995;155: 2429–2435.
117. Ally R, Schurmann D, Kreisel W, et al. A randomized, double-blind, double-dummy, multicenter trial of voriconazole and fluconazole in the treatment of esophageal candidiasis in immunocompromised patients. *Clin Infect Dis* 2001;33:1447–1454.
118. Villanueva A, Gotuzzo E, Arathoon EG, et al. A randomized double-blind study of caspofungin versus fluconazole for the treatment of esophageal candidiasis. *Am J Med* 2002;113:294–299.
119. Villanueva A, Arathoon EG, Gotuzzo E, et al. A randomized double-blind study of caspofungin versus amphotericin for the treatment of candidal esophagitis. *Clin Infect Dis* 2001;33:1529–1535.
120. Mora-Duarte J, Betts R, Rotstein C, et al. Comparison of caspofungin and amphotericin B for invasive candidiasis. *N Engl J Med* 2002;347: 2020–2029.
121. Fichtenbaum CJ, Powderley WG. Refractory mucosal candidiasis in patients with human immunodeficiency virus infection. *Clin Infect Dis* 1998;26:556–565.
122. Sandford GR, Merz WG, Wingard JR, et al. The value of fungal surveillance cultures as predictors of systemic fungal infections. *J Infect Dis* 1980;142:503–509.
123. Reef SE, Lasker BA, Butcher DS, et al. Nonperinatal nosocomial transmission of *Candida albicans* in a neonatal intensive care unit: prospective study. *J Clin Microbiol* 1998;36:1255–1259.
124. Kossoff E, Buescher S, Karlowicz G. Candidemia in a neonatal intensive care unit: trends during fifteen years and clinical features of 111 cases. *Pediatr Infect Dis J* 1998;17:504–508.
125. Baley JE, Kliegman RM, Faranoff AA. Disseminated fungal infections in very low birth weight infants: clinical manifestations and epidemiology. *Pediatrics* 1984;73:144–152.
126. El-Masry F, Neal TJ, Subhedar NV. Risk factors for invasive fungal infection in neonates. *Acta Paediatr* 2002;91:198–202.
127. Hughes PA, Lepow ML, Hill HR. Neonatal candidiasis. In: Bodey GP, ed. *Candidiasis: pathogenesis, diagnosis, and treatment,* 2nd ed. New York: Raven Press, 1993:261–277.
128. Baley JE, Annable WL, Kliegman RM. *Candida* endophthalmitis in the premature infant. *J Pediatr* 1981;98:458–461.
129. Vaudry WL, Tierney AJ, Wenman WM. Investigation of a cluster of systemic *Candida albicans* infections in a neonatal intensive care unit. *J Infect Dis* 1988;158:1375–1379.
130. Hughes PA, Venezia RA, Yocum DM, et al. *Candida parapsilosis* (CP) fungemia in a neonatal intensive care unit (NICU) (abstract 543). *Pediatr Res* 1992;31:93A.
131. Fowler SL, Rhoton B, Springer SC, et al. Evidence for person-to-person transmission of *Candida lusitaniae* in a neonatal intensive-care-unit. *Infect Control Hosp Epidemiol* 1998;19:343–345.
132. Roilides E, Farmaki E, Evdoridou J, et al. *Candida tropicalis* in a neonatal intensive care unit: epidemiologic and molecular analysis of an outbreak of infection with an uncommon neonatal pathogen. *J Clin Microbiol* 2003;41:735–741.

40

FILAMENTOUS FUNGI

LUIS OSTROSKY-ZEICHNER
JOHN H. REX

INTRODUCTION

Nosocomial infection by filamentous fungi was a minor issue for infection control until the frequency of these diseases began to increase in the 1970s (1–3). This increased incidence is attributed to a larger immunocompromised population in relation to advances in invasive medical technology and highly immunosuppressive therapies (1,3). These infections have very high mortality rates and are also associated with significant morbidity in the hospital in relation to therapy and diagnostic procedures. The increased incidence, high mortality, and recent advances in diagnosis and therapy have made these infections a more attractive and "surveillance-worthy" target for infection control programs. Important observations have been made regarding the incidence of these diseases and the presence of their causative agents in the hospital environment. This chapter focuses on the cause, epidemiology, and prevention of these infections while addressing infection control considerations.

CAUSE AND FORMS OF DISEASE

Although there are many reports of virtually any fungal species causing some form of nosocomial disease in humans, the most often encountered diseases caused by filamentous fungi are invasive aspergillosis and zygomycosis (1,4,5). There are also numerous reports of agents of hyalohyphomycosis such as *Acremonium* spp. and *Fusarium* spp. (1,6–9), but these are usually associated with an outbreak related to the use of contaminated patient-care materials or in the case of *Fusarium* with environmental sources and dissemination from sites of onychomycosis (10). Their frequency is much lower than *Aspergillus* and the Zygomycetes; thus, this chapter concentrates on the latter.

Aspergillus spp. are the most often encountered filamentous fungi in clinical practice, causing invasive, allergic, and toxic diseases. They are ubiquitous filamentous fungi found in soil, plant debris, and air. There are over 180 described species, although only 20 or so have been reported to be pathogenic for humans (1,2). Table 40.1 summarizes the *Aspergillus* spp. that are most commonly isolated from clinical specimens. Invasive disease can be found in almost any organ, but the most commonly affected are lungs, brain, paranasal sinuses, heart, and bones. *Aspergillus* fungemia is very rare, even in the setting of disseminated disease (11). Aspergillosis can also be related to medical devices such as intravenous or peritoneal catheters and prosthetic materials (12–16). Invasive aspergillosis occurs almost exclusively in patients with a high degree of immunosuppression, such as that seen in leukemia and in bone marrow and solid organ transplantation. Its incidence has been on a steady rise, as evidence by epidemiologic and postmortem studies. Mortality is very high, reaching nearly 90% in some series, and therapy often requires intensive medical treatment with amphotericin B (or its lipid formulations), caspofungin, or voriconazole, alone or in combination, in addition to aggressive surgical debridement when appropriate (2).

The term *zygomycosis* comprises a class of filamentous fungi that cause highly invasive disease in humans. The Class Zygomycetes includes three orders: Mucorales, Entomophthorales and Mortierellales. The term *mucormycosis* has been used to describe these infections, but this term has fallen from favor because (a) the term could be taken to imply that only fungi from Order Mucorales cause disease and (b) *Mucor* spp. are one of the less

TABLE 40.1. ASPERGILLUS SPP. AND ZYGOMYCETES AS CAUSES OF NOSOCOMIAL INFECTION

Aspergillus spp.	Zygomycetes
Common	**Mucorales**
Aspergillus fumigatus	*Absidia* spp.
Aspergillus flavus	*Apophysomyces* spp.
Aspergillus terreus	*Cokeromyces* spp.
Aspergillus niger	*Cunninghamella* spp.
Aspergillus nidulans	*Mucor* spp.
	Rhizomucor spp.
Rare	*Rhizopus* spp.
Aspergillus oryzae	*Saksenaea* spp.
Aspergillus ustus	*Syncephalastrum* spp.
Aspergillus amstelodami	
Aspergillus avenaceous	**Entomophthorales**
Aspergillus candidus	*Basidiobolus* spp.
Aspergillus carneus	*Conidiobolus* spp.
Aspergillus caesiellus	
Aspergillus clavatus	**Mortiellerales**
Aspergillus quadrilineatus	*Mortierella* spp.
Aspergillus restrictus	
Aspergillus sydowi	
Aspergillus versicolor	

common causes of zygomycosis. The most often encountered clinical pathogens fall in the order Mucorales, and their species are shown in Table 40.1. They are all ubiquitous fungi found in soil and decaying fruits, vegetables, and food. These microorganisms affect immunocompromised patients, such as those with: diabetic ketoacidosis, malnourishment, and burns. They are also seen in patients with hematologic malignancies, patients with acquired immunodeficiency syndrome (AIDS), and patients receiving immunosuppressive therapies such as corticosteroids (1,4,5). Although they can affect almost any organ or body system, the most common forms of invasive disease are rhinocerebral, pulmonary, cutaneous, and gastrointestinal. They have also been associated with medical devices such as intravascular and peritoneal catheters. Mortality is very high and prognosis is poor, even in the face of aggressive treatment, which includes prompt and extensive surgical debridement and intensive therapy with high doses of amphotericin B or its lipid preparations (17).

FILAMENTOUS FUNGI IN THE HOSPITAL: ECOLOGY AND EPIDEMIOLOGY

The body of information on nosocomial reservoirs, transmission, and infection by filamentous fungi is constantly growing. Although the early years of studying this problem were characterized by debate, today there is little question that these microorganisms are present and can be transmitted in the hospital. Nosocomial acquisition of infection by filamentous fungi is extremely important for centers that have a large immunocompromised population, such as cancer or transplant centers, and great efforts and advances have been undertaken to control them.

Acquisition of these diseases is a function of a susceptible host and the presence of a pathogenic microorganism in the environment. Table 40.2 summarizes host risk factors for invasive aspergillosis and zygomycosis. As seen in the table varying degrees of immunosuppression and underlying illness are required for the host to be susceptible.

As for the presence of the microorganisms in the hospital environment, it is now know that the main source for them is environmental contamination, which can include various surfaces, air, and water (1,4,5,12,15,18–21). Disturbances in the hospital environment, such as construction, can cause wide dissemination of the microorganisms and even outbreaks. Much of the evidence linking aspergillosis to the nosocomial environment comes from outbreak investigations (7,22–26).

TABLE 40.2. RISK FACTORS FOR INVASIVE ASPERGILLOSIS AND ZYGOMYCOSES

Aspergillosis	Zygomycoses
• Prolonged neutropenia • Neutrophil/macrophage dysfunction • Cytotoxic chemotherapy • Bone marrow transplantation • Organ transplantation • Congenital or acquired immunodeficiency	• Hematologic malignancy • Myelosuppression • Renal failure • Diabetes mellitus (particularly in acidosis) • Broad-spectrum antibiotics • Severity of underlying illness (high APACHE II score)

APACHE, Acute Physiology and Chronic Health Evaluation.

Patterson et al. (27) defined nosocomial aspergillosis as that occurring more than 1 week after admission or less than 2 weeks after discharge. Setting those temporal limits allows for community-acquired cases to be excluded from any analysis. Most cases are pneumonias; thus, the most likely route of infection is by direct inhalation of spores by a susceptible host. Although the primary source of *Aspergillus* spp. spores is soil and decaying vegetation, its main form of nosocomial spread is through hospital air (12,15,19–21,28). The spore concentration in outdoor air ranges from 0.2 to 15.0 spores/m^3, and the density of spores in hospital air is a direct function of the level of filtration that is used in a particular unit (1,3,14,21,22,29). High-efficiency particulate air (HEPA) filtration and laminar air flow (LAF) are highly effective methods to reduce spore content in hospital air (3,20,29), but the quality of output air is a function of the quality of the input air and the filtration system cannot effectively control spores generated within the hospital environment. Assessment of hospital air for fungal contaminations is often done using two methods: particles counts and air cultures. Particle counts are very sensitive for *Aspergillus* spores (2 to 5 micron diameter) but not very specific. Air culture using fungal culture media at 35°C is very useful for identifying real pathogens, but it is more expensive and time consuming and results are not available for several weeks. Thus, one often uses particle counts initially and reserves air cultures for special situations. The relationship between hospital air spore burden and development of aspergillosis is controversial. However, most of the research indicates that there may be a direct relationship between spore density and disease. Although no firm threshold value has been established, spore concentrations greater than 1/m^3 are thought to be associated with an increased incidence of disease in susceptible immunocompromised hosts (1,21,23,29). Extensive molecular epidemiology studies have linked the strains isolated from the patients to those found in the hospital environment (1,13, 19,22). Other sources of *Aspergillus* in the hospital may include food, plants, and flowers. A recent source of concern has been hospital water. Anaissie et al. (10,18,30–33) have reported isolation of spores in hospital water and showers identical to those isolated from the patients, both for *Aspergillus* and *Fusarium* spp.

The reservoir and modes of transmission for the Zygomycetes are similar to those of *Aspergillus* (1). Nevertheless, there are numerous reports of infection by direct inoculation from contaminated materials, such as bandages, intravenous or peritoneal catheters, and even tongue depressors. Because outbreaks of zygomycosis from these sources have been reported, such sources should be considered when a cluster of infections resulting from Zygomycetes occurs in a hospital (1,4,5,17).

PREVENTION: ENVIRONMENTAL AND PHARMACOLOGIC INTERVENTIONS

Preventive strategies work best when the hosts at highest risk are protected with the interventions that have shown the best

TABLE 40.3. PREVENTIVE MEASURES IN HIGH-RISK HOSTS FOR NOSOCOMIAL INFECTIONS CAUSED BY FILAMENTOUS FUNGI

Aspergillosis	Mucormycoses
• High-efficiency particulate air (HEPA) filtration • Laminar airflow (LAF) rooms • Limitation or containment of hospital construction • Use of plain surgical masks or high-efficiency masks when traveling outside protected environments, particularly through construction areas • Mold remediation for air ducts, carpets, wall panels, showers, etc. • Antifungal prophylaxis	• Control of diabetes and/or acidosis • Limitation of duration of neutropenia with less immunosuppressive regimens

efficacy and safety. This is as true for nosocomial filamentous fungal infections as for any other area of medicine. Interventions that protect against these infections can be classified in two categories: environmental and pharmacologic. Table 40.3 summarizes current preventive strategies for nosocomial acquisition of filamentous fungal infections. Environmental measures are safe and generally presumed effective in preventing these types of infections, although their cost can range from very affordable (e.g., plain surgical masks) to highly expensive (e.g., modifications in hospital infrastructure and physical plant). Pharmacologic measures have been extensively studied, and they do not necessarily pertain to the specific prevention of nosocomial acquisition of these diseases but to general prophylaxis of fungal infection in susceptible hosts.

As discussed previously, *Aspergillus* is ubiquitous in the environment, but there are certain conditions that may cause it to overgrow or disseminate: humidity and construction. Environmental control measures are designed to avoid these two phenomena and minimize patient exposures to spores. The simpler measures include avoiding, limiting, or containing construction in patient care areas; using plain surgical masks or high-efficiency masks (there are no clear data to support one over the other) when patients are transported through construction areas (34); prohibiting live plants and flowers in patient rooms; disinfecting showers and wet surfaces; and repairing faulty air handlers (32). The more sophisticated and highly effective measures include HEPA air filtration and LAF for the rooms of high-risk patients. These measures have data to support their use, but their high cost makes them only worthwhile for programs or facilities with a high volume of high-risk patients, such as cancer and transplant centers (3,20,23).

Pharmacologic prophylaxis has also been shown to be effective and safe in selected populations at high risk. Again, these interventions are not specific to nosocomial transmission, but they are becoming the standard of care for selected immunocompromised populations, which include induction chemotherapy, patients with prolonged neutropenia, organ transplant recipients, and hematopoietic stem cell transplant recipients (35). Current prophylaxis options relevant to filamentous fungi include amphotericin B (intravenous, low dose at 0.1 mg/kg daily, or full doses at 0.7 to 1.0 mg/kg weekly) and itraconazole (intravenous or cyclodextrin-based oral solution at 400 mg per day). Prophylaxis with itraconazole is highly dependent on achieving a blood level of approximately 500 ng/mL (36–38). Intense research is now concentrating on other options such as nebulized amphotericin B and its lipid-based preparations (39–41) and the use of new agents such as voriconazole (42,43) and the echinocandins (44).

INFECTION CONTROL CONSIDERATIONS

As stated previously, the frequency of these infections is on the rise, and the problem becomes relevant for centers that handle large volumes of immunocompromised patients. These centers should organize active surveillance programs to detect clusters of filamentous fungal infection, which may indicate environmental contamination. Such centers should consider HEPA filtration and LAF units and have construction, environmental sampling and cleaning, and patient transport policies designed to minimize exposure. It is also helpful to have prophylaxis protocols in place for the patients at highest risk.

Environmental sampling is not routinely recommended but may be indicated during investigations of suspected clusters or outbreaks of infection. There are no standards for indoor quality of air in hospitals. As noted previously, particle counts and air cultures for molds are useful tools in those selected situations in which one must identify and remediate contaminated areas. The principal goal of testing is to ensure that the hospital's air filtration equipment is functioning correctly and, thus, delivering the cleanest air possible for the system.

For general acute-care hospitals, appropriate general nosocomial infection surveillance should be enough to detect clusters of fungal infections. Investigation of such clusters of infection should include a search for possible reservoirs for the filamentous fungus, evaluation of the hospital ventilation system, and sites where outside air may be infiltrating the inside air. (See also Chapter 89.)

As medical technology and interventions advance and patients live longer, these filamentous fungal infections will become more common. Infection control programs will increasingly acknowledge their relevance as infections of nosocomial acquisition.

REFERENCES

1. Fridkin SK, Jarvis WR. Epidemiology of nosocomial fungal infections. *Clin Microbiol Rev* 1996;9:499–511.
2. Stevens DA, et al. Practice guidelines for diseases caused by *Aspergillus.* Infectious Diseases Society of America. *Clin Infect Dis* 2000;30:696–709.
3. Warnock DW, Hajjeh RA, Lasker BA. Epidemiology and prevention of invasive aspergillosis. *Curr Infect Dis Rep* 2001;3:507–516.
4. Carlisle PS, Gucalp R, Wiernik PH. Nosocomial infections in neutropenic cancer patients. *Infect Control Hosp Epidemiol* 1993;14:320–324.
5. Dykewicz CA. Hospital infection control in hematopoietic stem cell transplant recipients. *Emerg Infect Dis* 2001;7:263–267.

6. Feldman DL, et al. Nosocomial phaeomycotic cyst of the hand. *Ann Plast Surg* 1995;35:113–115.
7. Krasinski K, et al. Nosocomial fungal infection during hospital renovation. *Infect Control* 1985;6:278–282.
8. Orth B, et al. Outbreak of invasive mycoses caused by *Paecilomyces lilacinus* from a contaminated skin lotion. *Ann Intern Med* 1996;125: 799–806.
9. Warris A, et al. Recovery of filamentous fungi from water in a paediatric bone marrow transplantation unit. *J Hosp Infect* 2001;47:143–148.
10. Anaissie EJ, et al. Fusariosis associated with pathogenic *Fusarium* species colonization of a hospital water system: a new paradigm for the epidemiology of opportunistic mold infections. *Clin Infect Dis* 2001; 33:1871–1878.
11. Duthie R, Denning DW. *Aspergillus* fungemia: report of two cases and review. *Clin Infect Dis* 1995;20:598–605.
12. Alberti C, et al. Relationship between environmental fungal contamination and the incidence of invasive aspergillosis in haematology patients. *J Hosp Infect* 2001;48:198–206.
13. Diaz-Guerra TM, et al. Genetic similarity among one *Aspergillus flavus* strain isolated from a patient who underwent heart surgery and two environmental strains obtained from the operating room. *J Clin Microbiol* 2000;38:2419–2422.
14. Girardin H, et al. Molecular epidemiology of nosocomial invasive aspergillosis. *J Clin Microbiol* 1994;32:684–690.
15. Hajjeh RA, Warnock DW. Counterpoint: invasive aspergillosis and the environment—rethinking our approach to prevention. *Clin Infect Dis* 2001;33:1549–1552.
16. Pla, M.P, et al. Surgical wound infection by *Aspergillus fumigatus* in liver transplant recipients. *Diagn Microbiol Infect Dis* 1992;15:703–706.
17. Patterson JE, Barden GE, Bia FJ. Hospital-acquired gangrenous mucormycosis. *Yale J Biol Med* 1986;59:453–459.
18. Anaissie EJ, Penzak SR, Dignani MC. The hospital water supply as a source of nosocomial infections: a plea for action. *Arch Intern Med* 2002;162:1483–1492.
19. Chazalet V, et al. Molecular typing of environmental and patient isolates of *Aspergillus fumigatus* from various hospital settings. *J Clin Microbiol* 1998;36:1494–1500.
20. Hahn T, et al. Efficacy of high-efficiency particulate air filtration in preventing aspergillosis in immunocompromised patients with hematologic malignancies. *Infect Control Hosp Epidemiol* 2002;23:525–531.
21. Leenders AC, et al. Density and molecular epidemiology of *Aspergillus* in air and relationship to outbreaks of *Aspergillus* infection. *J Clin Microbiol* 1999;37:1752–1757.
22. Walsh TJ, Dixon DM. Nosocomial aspergillosis: environmental microbiology, hospital epidemiology, diagnosis and treatment. *Eur J Epidemiol* 1989;5:131–142.
23. VandenBergh MF, Verweij PE, Voss A. Epidemiology of nosocomial fungal infections: invasive aspergillosis and the environment. *Diagn Microbiol Infect Dis* 1999;34:221–227.
24. Streifel AJ, et al. *Aspergillus fumigatus* and other thermotolerant fungi generated by hospital building demolition. *Appl Environ Microbiol* 1983;46:375–378.
25. Sessa A, et al. Nosocomial outbreak of *Aspergillus fumigatus* infection among patients in a renal unit? *Nephrol Dial Transplant* 1996;11: 1322–1324.
26. Oren I, et al. Invasive pulmonary aspergillosis in neutropenic patients during hospital construction: before and after chemoprophylaxis and institution of HEPA filters. *Am J Hematol* 2001;66:257–262.
27. Patterson JE, et al. Hospital epidemiologic surveillance for invasive aspergillosis: patient demographics and the utility of antigen detection. *Infect Control Hosp Epidemiol* 1997;18:104–108.
28. Arnow PM, et al. Pulmonary aspergillosis during hospital renovation. *Am Rev Respir Dis* 1978;118:49–53.
29. Rose HD, Hirsch SR. Filtering hospital air decreases *Aspergillus* spore counts. *Am Rev Respir Dis* 1979;119:511–513.
30. Anaissie EJ, Costa SF. Nosocomial aspergillosis is waterborne. *Clin Infect Dis* 2001;33:1546–1548.
31. Anaissie EJ, et al. Pathogenic moulds (including *Aspergillus* spp.) in hospital water distribution systems: a three-year prospective study and clinical implications for patients with hematological malignancies. *Blood* 2002;5:5.
32. Anaissie EJ, et al. Cleaning patient shower facilities: a novel approach to reducing patient exposure to aerosolized *Aspergillus* species and other opportunistic molds. *Clin Infect Dis* 2002;35:E86–88.
33. Anaissie EJ, et al. Pathogenic *Aspergillus* species recovered from a hospital water system: a 3-year prospective study. *Clin Infect Dis* 2002;34: 780–789.
34. Raad I, et al. Masking of neutropenic patients on transport from hospital rooms is associated with a decrease in nosocomial aspergillosis during construction. *Infect Control Hosp Epidemiol* 2002;23:41–43.
35. Dykewicz CA. Summary of the guidelines for preventing opportunistic infections among hematopoietic stem cell transplant recipients. *Clin Infect Dis* 2001;33:139–144.
36. Boyle BM, McCann SR. The use of itraconazole as prophylaxis against invasive fungal infection in blood and marrow transplant recipients. *Transpl Infect Dis* 2000;2:72–79.
37. Harousseau JL, et al. Itraconazole oral solution for primary prophylaxis of fungal infections in patients with hematological malignancy and profound neutropenia: a randomized, double-blind, double-placebo, multicenter trial comparing itraconazole and amphotericin B. *Antimicrob Agents Chemother* 2000;44:1887–1893.
38. Glasmacher A, et al. Antifungal prophylaxis with itraconazole in neutropenic patients with acute leukaemia. *Leukemia* 1998;12:1338–1343.
39. Klepser ME. Amphotericin B in lung transplant recipients. *Ann Pharmacother* 2002;36:167–169.
40. Monforte V, et al. Nebulized amphotericin B prophylaxis for *Aspergillus* infection in lung transplantation: study of risk factors. *J Heart Lung Transplant* 2001;20:1274–1281.
41. Allen SD, et al. Prophylactic efficacy of aerosolized liposomal (AmBisome) and non-liposomal (Fungizone) amphotericin B in murine pulmonary aspergillosis. *J Antimicrob Chemother* 1994;34:1001–1013.
42. Pound MW, Drew RW, Perfect JR. Recent advances in the epidemiology, prevention, diagnosis, and treatment of fungal pneumonia. *Curr Opin Infect Dis* 2002;15:183—194.
43. Hoffman HL, Ernst EJ, Klepser ME. Novel triazole antifungal agents. *Expert Opin Investig Drugs* 2000;9:593–605.
44. Denning DW. Echinocandins: a new class of antifungal. *J Antimicrob Chemother* 2002;49:889–891.

D

Viral Infections

41

INFLUENZA VIRUSES

WILLIAM M. VALENTI

Influenza continues to be an important cause of morbidity and mortality in hospitalized and long-term care patients, particularly among the elderly and those with chronic underlying cardiac and pulmonary diseases. Effective strategies for influenza prevention must be multifaceted because of the uniqueness of the influenza viruses, including their seasonal nature, antigenic drift, and antigenic shift. Because all known influenza A subtypes exist in the aquatic bird reservoir, influenza is not an eradicable disease (1). Prevention and control are the most realistic public health strategies for influenza. Continued surveillance of influenza in humans and in animal reservoirs is an important part of these prevention and control strategies (1). In healthcare settings, the best approach to influenza prevention involves a vaccination program starting in the fall of each year. Limitations for prevention by vaccination include inconsistent use and underuse of vaccines and problems with incomplete immunity despite vaccination, especially in the elderly, people with human immunodeficiency virus (HIV) and acquired immunodeficiency syndrome (AIDS), and young children (2).

BACKGROUND

The subtypes of influenza A virus are classified on the basis of their surface antigens, which are called hemagglutinins (H) and neuraminidases (N). There are three hemagglutinins (H1, H2, H3) and two neuraminidases (N1, N2). Immunity to these antigens reduces the likelihood of infection and reduces the severity of illness if it does occur. However, antigenic drift and antigenic shift (i.e., subtle and marked changes, respectively, within a subtype) make long-lasting immunity difficult to achieve. Of the two antigenic changes, antigenic drift is the more gradual, with the H and N subtypes retaining some similarity as each changes from one to the other. Antigenic shift is a more abrupt change in H or N subtype that occurs at longer intervals (e.g., every 10 years). When the marked changes of antigenic shift occur, infection or vaccination with one strain may not necessarily induce immunity to distant strains even though they are of the same subtype. Influenza B is more antigenically stable than influenza A and undergoes antigenic drift but not the major structural changes of antigenic shift.

Effectiveness of influenza vaccine is determined by the closeness of the vaccine-induced antibody to the H and N surface antigens of influenza A and B. Influenza vaccine loses its protective effects as more major shifts of influenza H and N surface antigens or subtypes occur.

The nomenclature for influenza strains is a useful way to learn more about that particular strain. The standard way of describing strains includes the serotype, host of origin (human unless otherwise specified), geographic origin, strain number, year of isolation, and the H and N designation.

For 2002 to 2003, the U.S. Food and Drug Administration's (FDA) Vaccines and Related Biological Products Advisory Committee (VRBPAC) recommended that trivalent influenza vaccine for the United States contain A/New Caledonia/20/99-like (H1N1), A/Moscow/10/99-like (H3N2), and B/Hong Kong/330/01-like viruses (3). This recommendation was based on antigenic analyses of influenza viruses isolated recently, epidemiologic data, and postvaccination serologic studies in humans (2,3).

VACCINATION AND INFLUENZA-RELATED VIRUS MORBIDITY AND MORTALITY

The so-called high-risk groups for influenza include older persons (i.e., 65 years of age and older); very young children; and persons of any age with certain underlying health conditions who are at increased risk for hospitalization, death, and other complications of influenza infection. During major epidemics, hospitalization rates for high-risk persons may increase two- to fivefold. Despite this, only about 30% of people aged 65 or older are vaccinated with influenza vaccine every year (2). Most outbreaks are reported from nursing homes and chronic care facilities (4–6), in part because of underuse of vaccine in these closed populations (see Chapter 106). In addition to underuse of vaccine, many high-risk individuals fail to develop a protective antibody response to vaccination (2,5,6). Outbreaks have also occurred in general hospitals, psychiatric units, and medical and pediatric services (7,8). This underuse of vaccine is a major contributing factor in outbreaks of influenza in healthcare facilities with associated morbidity and, on occasion, mortality.

As the population ages, the risk of influenza death increases. Thompson et al. (9) reported that the death rate from influenza rose markedly in the 1990s, and in 2001 it exceeded the number of deaths resulting from AIDS. Annual estimates of influenza-associated deaths increased significantly between the 1976 to 1977 and 1998 to 1999 seasons with a mean of 20,000 and 36,000 deaths, respectively. Ninety percent of respiratory and circulatory deaths occurred in persons 65 years old or older. Since its emergence in the 1960s, type A (H3N2) epidemics have caused approximately 400,000 deaths in the United States alone, and more than 90% of these deaths have occurred in people older than age 65. Of the influenza viruses currently in worldwide circulation, A (H3N2) still has the most severe overall impact (2).

Gross et al. (4) characterized a typical nursing home outbreak that began in November, peaked in February, and ended in April. The outbreak progressed slowly from November through April and was complicated by concurrent infections with respiratory syncytial virus, parainfluenza virus, and *Mycoplasma pneumoniae.* The patient population in this case had an immunization rate of 59%, affording it some degree of herd immunity. The authors contrast the pattern of slow spread in this closed, partially immunized population to the more explosive outbreaks described in open, unimmunized populations (e.g., acute care settings and on psychiatric services) (2,7).

In another nursing home outbreak, Gross et al. (5) found that influenza illness was significantly more common in the unvaccinated group, as was mortality (17.7% in the unvaccinated group and 7.2% in the vaccinated group). When controlled for sex and severity of illness, influenza vaccine reduced mortality by 59% in this closed, partially vaccinated population.

Patriarca et al. (6) developed an interesting model to project morbidity, mortality, and costs associated with type A influenza illness in nursing homes. The model used demographics similar to the real world of long-term care: 100 residents and a 60% rate of vaccination in the fall of the prior year. In this model, the combination of previous vaccination and amantadine during outbreaks was associated with significantly fewer cases compared with vaccine alone. This difference is probably due to the less than 100% efficacy of vaccine in inducing protective antibody. The authors predicted an increase in herd immunity as more patients were vaccinated beyond the 60% receiving it initially. They concluded appropriately that influenza control programs in nursing homes are beneficial, cost effective, and clinically sound. There was only a modest increase in program costs with the addition of amantadine, and, overall, indices of cost-effectiveness used by the researchers justified vaccination. When vaccine use reached 70%, the risk of an outbreak approached zero supporting the Advisory Committee on Immunization Practices' (ACIP) target of 80% vaccine use in populations at risk (2,6).

CLINICAL MANIFESTATIONS

Typical influenza illness in the adult is characterized by sudden onset of fever, myalgia, sore throat, headache, retroorbital pain, and nonproductive cough. Unlike most other viral respiratory infections, influenza causes myalgias and other constitutional symptoms that can last a week or more.

Some patients with influenza A may develop additional complications of primary influenza pneumonia or secondary bacterial pneumonia most often resulting from *Streptococcus pneumoniae* or *Staphylococcus aureus.* These complications are not associated with influenza B infection, which is usually a milder illness.

The disease in children has been described as clinically different from that in adults. The illness in children may have a major gastrointestinal component or may mimic sepsis (10,11). In an influenza A outbreak on a pediatrics ward, 7 of 12 infected children (58%) developed pulmonary infiltrates, and 5 of the 7 went on to develop a secondary bacterial pneumonia. In the young infant, influenza may mimic sepsis with fever and no localizing findings (11). In contrast to the disease in children, influenza in adults is first and foremost a respiratory disease and not a gastrointestinal illness (2,10). The term *intestinal flu* in adults is generally a misnomer.

DIAGNOSIS

Diagnostic tests available for influenza include viral isolation (culture), rapid antigen testing, polymerase chain reaction (PCR), and immunofluorescence (2,12). The latter tests are the most useful laboratory techniques for prospective, real-time diagnosis of influenza. Sensitivity and specificity of any test for influenza might vary by the laboratory that performs the test, the type of test used, and the type of specimen tested. Among respiratory specimens for viral isolation or rapid detection, nasopharyngeal specimens are typically more effective than throat swab specimens (2,12). As with any diagnostic test, results should be evaluated in the context of other clinical information available to the provider.

The value of a rapid diagnostic testing allows for more timely institution of therapy and infection control precautions. However, the specificity and, in particular, the sensitivity of rapid tests are lower than for viral culture and vary by test. Because of the lower sensitivity of the rapid tests, providers should consider confirming negative tests with viral culture. The additional advantage of viral culture over rapid tests is the ability to provide specific information regarding circulating influenza subtypes and strains. If virus isolation facilities are not readily available locally or via reference laboratory, they may be available on a regional level as part of the global surveillance network described later.

Acute- and convalescent-phase serologies (antibody determination) are a helpful epidemiologic tool retrospectively but are not particularly useful clinically or for prospective surveillance.

Diagnosis of influenza can also be made using epidemiologic parameters in combination with clinical and laboratory parameters, In the past, when influenza was prevalent in the community, adult patients with acute febrile respiratory illness were assumed to have influenza virus infection (2,7,8,13). However, with the availability of rapid diagnostic tests and viral culture, the epidemiologic method is less specific because other respiratory viral illnesses can overlap with influenza disease (2).

EPIDEMIOLOGY

Surveillance and Monitoring

The Centers for Disease Control and Prevention (CDC) conducts influenza surveillance in the United States yearly from October through May to monitor influenza infections and any antigenic changes in the circulating strains of virus. This is part of a worldwide collaborative surveillance system that ultimately leads to recommendations for future vaccine formulations (2,3). The CDC monitors a variety of state and local health departments, university and hospital laboratories, a small number of so-called sentinel physician practices, and reports of pneumonia and influenza deaths from a sampling of vital statistics offices throughout the United States.

Once influenza infection establishes itself in the community, sporadic cases of influenza may be seen in both healthcare workers and patients. In the healthcare setting, employee absenteeism for influenza-like illness often precedes an outbreak by several weeks, suggesting transmission from healthcare worker to patients (2,13). The introduction of influenza by patients has been reported also (14–16). Either way, nosocomial influenza increase hospital days and costs of hospitalization. In one study, costs of hospitalization increased by $3,798 per infected patient (14).

In healthcare settings, prospective monitoring and surveillance of influenza-like respiratory illness are of debatable value, unless accompanied by an influenza vaccination program. Traditionally, influenza and respiratory virus surveillance are done to varying degrees by hospitals and/or local public health departments. It is important to be aware of the results of ongoing influenza surveillance locally as one part of a healthcare facility's plan to prevent nosocomial influenza.

Influenza as an Emerging Infectious Disease

Novel influenza viruses have the potential to initiate global pandemics if they are sufficiently transmissible among humans (1). Recent experience in Asia supports continued public health surveillance. From May 1997 to January 1998, a total of 16 confirmed and three suspected cases of human infection with avian influenza A (H5N1) viruses were identified in Hong Kong (17). The first known case of human infection with influenza A (H5N1) occurred in a 3-year-old boy who died from respiratory failure in May 1997. The cases reported in Hong Kong represent the first identified instances of human illness associated with infection with influenza A (H5N1) viruses. Except for a cluster of two confirmed and two suspected cases in one family, case-patients were not known to have had contact with each other or a common source of exposure and were geographically distributed throughout Hong Kong. All cases of infection occurred among residents of Hong Kong, and no cases of infection with influenza A (H5N1) viruses have been identified among persons residing outside Hong Kong (17).

Serologic data obtained as part of the investigation of the initial case confirmed that persons with high levels of exposure to infected poultry or direct exposure to the virus in the laboratory were at increased risk for infection with influenza A (H5N1) virus (17). However, the investigation did not rule out the possibility of person-to-person transmission from exposure to ill and infectious persons; two seropositive persons who had contact with the first case-patient included a child care center classmate and a healthcare worker, and the classmate had contact with both the ill child and the same potential environmental source of exposure to ill chickens at the school as the ill child. However, the healthcare worker reported no history of exposure to the virus in the laboratory or any recent exposure to poultry, and a history of exposure to the child or to poultry was unknown for a seropositive elderly neighbor. This strain's unusual pattern of spread, from birds to humans, has not been documented previously. However, based on the overall low rates of infection among contacts and controls and the lack of seropositivity among family members, the virus probably is not transmitted efficiently among humans (17).

This outbreak demonstrates that influenza is still a serious public health issue and that global epidemiologic surveillance is an important public health tool for prevention and control of influenza. Early detection by this global surveillance system probably played a role in containing the outbreak. Additional measures taken by the Hong Kong health authorities included destroying all poultry in Hong Kong and surrounding areas, with a significant adverse economic impact in the region (1,17). In April 1999, isolation of avian influenza A (H9N2) viruses from humans was confirmed for the first time. H9N2 viruses were isolated from nasopharyngeal aspirate specimens collected from two children who were hospitalized with uncomplicated, febrile, upper respiratory tract illnesses in Hong Kong during March 1999 (17).

Public health authorities conducted four retrospective cohort studies of persons exposed to these two H9N2 patients to assess whether human-to-human transmission of avian H9N2 viruses had occurred. No serologic evidence of H9N2 infection was found in family members or healthcare workers who had close contact with the H9N2-infected children, suggesting that these H9N2 viruses were not easily transmitted from person to person (18).

Modes of Transmission

Influenza A and B viruses are among the most communicable viruses of man and have produced explosive epidemics. Nosocomial transmission of both influenza A and B is well documented. Humans are reservoirs of infection, and person-to-person transmission is thought to be airborne. Infection also may occur on occasion via fomites (droplet spread) and hands contaminated with virus (13). In most cases, small-particle aerosols (less than 10 μm median diameter) containing infectious virus particles are produced and disseminated by coughing or sneezing. These small-diameter infectious virus particles can be transmitted over long distances (>6 feet).

Larger droplets require closer person-to-person contact for virus transmission, generally less than 3 feet separating two persons (8,13). These large droplets are produced by coughing or sneezing and can infect the susceptible host directly or indirectly. Direct transmission involves direct inoculation of mucous membranes of the eye or nose. Indirect transmission refers to contamination of the donor's hands, which spread infectious material to the skin or mucous membranes of a susceptible host.

The aerosol mode of transmission may be responsible for the explosive nature of influenza transmission, with one infected person shedding large numbers of infectious virus particles and subsequently infecting a large number of susceptible people (2, 4,7,8,13).

In healthcare settings, a reservoir of infection can be a healthcare worker, a patient, or a visitor. Once infection is established and infection is being transmitted, infection control interventions, especially vaccination, need to include all three groups when developing an outbreak control plan.

CONTROL AND PREVENTION OF INFLUENZA

Control of influenza requires herd immunity, which requires that large numbers of people in a particular group at risk be immune to infection (2,5). There are two approaches to reduce the impact of influenza infection: inactivated influenza vaccine (immunoprophylaxis) and antiviral drugs (chemoprophylaxis). Antiviral drugs are a useful adjunct when herd immunity is not present because of underuse of vaccine and/or inadequate protective antibody response to vaccination (2,5) (Table 41.1).

Vaccination

As influenza viruses continue to evolve through antigenic shift and antigenic drift, new strains emerge to which the population is susceptible. Therefore, annual vaccination is recommended using the current trivalent vaccine for that year, even if the current vaccine has one or more antigens administered in the previous year's formulation (2,3). This is because immunity declines over a year's time, and patients require an annual booster dose to maintain immunity to influenza strains that appear in the general population each year.

There are a number of strategies for prevention and control of nosocomial influenza. The most important is vaccination in the fall of each year before the onset of influenza infection. Vaccine efficacy (i.e., the rate of reducing influenza infections in those who receive it) ranges from 80% to 90% in healthy individuals (2) to 50% in some nursing home populations (2, 6). The problem for healthcare facilities involves unacceptably low rates of vaccination of both healthcare workers (including physicians) and patients.

In recent years, the ACIP has expanded and clarified its definition of high risk to better reflect the epidemiology of influenza. In addition to patients 65 years of age and older and those with chronic illnesses, strong emphasis is given to vaccination of those who also might infect elderly and chronically ill patients. Healthcare workers in traditional inpatient and outpatient settings constitute only one of several groups in this category. For the purpose of identifying healthcare workers, the best definition of healthcare worker is a broad one: workers who might transmit infection to patients. This approach means that vaccine programs in healthcare settings need not be limited only to employees who are direct caregivers (2). Others in the group who might infect high-risk patients include employees of chronic care facilities, home health providers, and family members of elderly and chronically ill patients. Equally broad is the ACIP's category of other groups which includes pregnant women, people with HIV infection anywhere within the HIV continuum, otherwise healthy children aged 6 to 23 months because of their increased risk for influenza-related hospitalization, and persons who wish to reduce their chances of acquiring influenza infection (2). Because vaccine is not recommended for infants younger than 6 months, vaccine is recommended for their household contacts to reduce the risk for these infants. This broader approach to influenza vaccination can help achieve the necessary herd immunity that may reduce transmission to and within high-risk groups by increasing the numbers of immune individuals in each of the groups (2).

In a recent study of healthy, working adults, those who received influenza vaccine reported 25% fewer episodes of upper respiratory illness than those who received the placebo, 43% fewer days of sick leave from work because of upper respiratory illness, and 44% fewer visits to physicians' offices for upper respiratory illness (19). Therefore, influenza vaccine is an essential, inexpensive component of an infection control program for healthcare workers. Because of the benefits to patients and the additional implications for increased employee productivity, healthcare settings of any type should offer influenza vaccine to all employees, regardless of their degree of patient contact.

Healthcare workers and the general public alike have misconceptions that the vaccine can cause illness. The most common are that vaccine can cause the flu and that the vaccine can cause the Guillain-Barré syndrome similar to that seen during the nationwide swine influenza vaccination program in 1976. Influenza vaccines are made from egg-grown viruses that are rendered inactive as part of the vaccine manufacturing process and cannot cause influenza or any other disease (2). Employee education programs should include a reminder that influenza vaccine provides immunity to influenza only and that it does not provide protection from other respiratory viruses such as respiratory syncytial virus or the rhinoviruses (2,8,13). As for Guillain-Barré, that complication was unique to the swine influenza vaccine program for unclear reasons. However, vaccine preparations used in years subsequent to the 1976 vaccine program have not been associated with vaccine-associated Guillain-Barré syndrome (2).

One group of investigators has reviewed vaccine use in healthcare workers systematically by comparing responses to questionnaires from vaccine recipients and nonrecipients. Vaccine recipients were significantly more likely to believe that influenza disease and its complications were more serious to high-risk patients, that influenza vaccine was effective and uncommonly associated with side effects, and that influenza vaccination was important for healthcare workers to decrease transmission to high-risk patients. They concluded that these issues were the major educational components of a vaccination program for healthcare workers (20). However, another study in Europe showed that even educational interventions targeted to specific healthcare workers' misinformation or misunderstandings only increased vaccine use by healthcare workers in three targeted departments from 13% to 37% (21).

TABLE 41.1. RECOMMENDED DAILY DOSAGE OF INFLUENZA ANTIVIRAL MEDICATIONS FOR TREATMENT AND PROPHYLAXIS

	Age Group (Yrs)				
Antiviral Agent	1–6	7–9	10–12	13–64	≥65
Amantadine*					
Treatment, Influenza A	5 mg/kg/day up to 150 mg in two divided doses†	5 mg/kg/day up to 150 mg in two divided doses†	100 mg twice daily§	100 mg twice daily§	≤100 mg/day
Prophylaxis, Influenza A	5 mg/kg/day up to 150 mg in two divided doses†	5 mg/kg/day up to 150 mg in two divided doses†	100 mg twice daily§	100 mg twice daily§	≤100 mg/day
Rimantadine¶					
Treatment,** Influenza A	NA††	NA	NA	100 mg twice daily§§	100 mg/day
Prophylaxis, Influenza A	5 mg/kg/day up to 150 mg in two divided doses§	5 mg/kg/day up to 150 mg in two divided doses†	100 mg twice daily§	100 mg twice daily§	100 mg/day¶
Zanamivir* †††**					
Treatment, Influenza A and B	NA	10 mg twice daily	10 mg twice daily	10 mg twice daily	10 mg twice daily
Oseltamivir§§§					
Treatment, Influenza A and B	Dose varies by child's weight†††	Dose varies by child's weight¶¶¶	Dose varies by child's weight¶¶¶	75 mg twice daily	75 mg twice daily
Prophylaxis, Influenza A and B	NA	NA	NA	75 mg/day	75 mg/day

Amantadine manufacturers include Endo Pharmaceuticals (Symmetre—tablet and syrup); Geneva Pharms Tech and Rosemont (Amantadine HCL—capsule); and Alpharma, Copley Pharmaceutical HiTech Pharma, Mikart Morton Grove, and Pharmaceutical Associates (Amantadine HCL—syrup). Rimantadine is manufactured by Forest Laboratories (Flumadine—tablet and syrup) and Corepharma (Rimantadine HCL—tablet). Zanamivir is manufactured by GalxoSmithKline (Relenza—inhaled powder). Oseltamivir is manufactured by Hoffman-LaRoche, Inc. (Tamilflu—tablet). This information is based on data published by the Food and Drug Administration (FDA), which is available at www.fda.gov.

* The drug package insert should be consulted for dosage recommendations for administering amantandine to persons with creatinine clearance ≤50 mL/min/1.73 m^2.

† 5 mg/kg of amantadine or rimantadine syrup = 1 tsp/22 lbs.

§ Children aged ≥10 years who weigh <40 kg should be administered amantadine or rimantadine at a dosage of 5 mg/kg/day.

¶ A reduction in dosage to 100 mg/day of rimantadine is recommended for persons who have severe hepatic dysfunction or those with creatinine clearance ≤10 mL/min. Other persons with less severe hepatic or renal dysfunction taking 100 mg/day of rimantadine should be observed closely, and the dosage should be reduced or the drug discontinued, if necessary.

** Only approved by FDA for treatment among adults.

†† Not applicable.

§§ Rimantadine is approved by FDA for treatment among adults. However, certain specialists in the management of Influenza consider rimantadine appropriate for treatment among children (see American Academy of Pediatrics. 2000 red book: report of the Committee on Infectious Diseases, 25th ed. Elk Grove Village, IL: American Academy of Pediatrics, 2000).

¶¶ Older nursing-home residents should be administered only 100 mg/day of rimantadine. A reduction in dosage to 100 mg/day should be considered for all persons aged ≥65 years, if they experience possible side effects when taking 200 mg/day.

*** Zanamivir is administered through inhalation by using a plastic device included in the medication package. Patients will benefit from instruction and demonstration of correct use of the device.

††† Zanamivir is not approved for prophylaxis.

§§§ A reduction in the dose of oseltamivir is recommended for persons with creatinine clearance <30 mL/min.

¶¶¶ The dose recommendation for children who weigh ≤15 kg is 30 mg twice a day. For children who weigh >15–23 kg, the dose is 45 mg twice a day. For children who weigh >23–40 kg, the dose is 60 mg twice a day. For children who weigh >40 kg, the dose is 75 mg twice a day.

From Centers for Disease Control and Prevention. Prevention and control of influenza: recommendations of the Advisory Committee on Immunization Practices (ACIP). *MMWR Morb Mortal Wkly Rep* 2002;51(RR03):1–31, with permission. Available at http://www.cdc.gov/mmwr/preview/mmwrhtml/rr5103al.htm

With underuse of vaccine in major populations at risk (i.e., healthcare workers, the elderly and chronically ill, and persons likely to spread influenza to high-risk people), influenza prevention programs in many healthcare facilities are haphazard and incomplete and must react when clusters or outbreaks of infection occur. Even though a substantial number of healthcare workers and patients have not been vaccinated at the time of the first report of influenza, the arrival of influenza in the community and/or hospital is still a good time to try to vaccinate these groups, keeping in mind that the time from vaccination to protective antibody response is about 2 weeks.

Strategies to Improve Vaccination Rates

Despite the efficacy of vaccine and a public health commitment to childhood and adult immunization, fewer than 30% of persons aged 65 and older receive the influenza vaccine each year (2), although vaccination rates are reported to be higher in closed populations (e.g., nursing homes) (2,6). The collective experience of public health and infection control experts is that promoting influenza vaccination, or any other kind of vaccination, requires more than just posters announcing the availability of vaccine (2,20,21). A recent review of strategies for management of influenza in the elderly provides a comprehensive review of this important subject (22).

Strategies are evolving to increase influenza vaccination rates and reduce influenza-related morbidity and mortality. In addition to broadening the definition of high risk for influenza, the ACIP adopted a resolution expanding the group of children eligible for influenza vaccine coverage under the Vaccines for Children (VFC) program (23). The resolution extends VFC coverage for influenza vaccine to all VFC-eligible children aged 6 to 23 months and VFC-eligible children aged 2 to 18 years who are household contacts of children younger than 2 years. The resolution became effective on March 1, 2003, for vaccine to be administered during the 2003 to 2004 influenza vaccination season and subsequent seasons. ACIP is expanding VFC influenza coverage because children younger than 23 months are at substantially increased risk for influenza-related hospitalizations (2,23). Other elements of a successful vaccination program are education for healthcare workers, a plan for identifying people at risk (often by review of medical records), and efforts to remove administrative and financial barriers that prevent people from receiving vaccine (2,21,24). Efforts should be made to administer vaccine where various high-risk populations receive their medical care. The ACIP also recommends a staggered approach to vaccination. The optimal time to receive influenza vaccine is during October and November. However, because of vaccine distribution delays during the past 2 years, ACIP recommends that vaccination efforts in October focus on persons at greatest risk followed by other high-risk people starting in November (2, 22).

In the case of healthcare workers, vaccine should be administered in the workplace (e.g., patient units in hospitals, ambulatory clinics, physician private offices, etc.) to maximize participation. Making influenza vaccine available to employees is no guarantee of acceptance. However, offering free vaccine, addressing employee concerns about vaccine side effects (24) and making vaccination more convenient and accessible to employees (25) reduce some of the barriers to an effective program for healthcare workers.

In primary care settings, innovative, computer-generated reminders to physicians have been effective (26). Physicians who received such reminders as a part of a study were twice as likely to vaccinate their patients as those physicians who did not receive the reminders.

Simultaneous use of other vaccines with influenza vaccine is generally not a problem. Influenza vaccine can be included as part of any healthcare encounter that includes other adult or childhood vaccinations. Because the target groups for influenza and pneumococcal vaccines overlap, both vaccines can be administered at the same time at different sites without increasing side effects of either vaccine (2). Children at high risk for influenza may receive influenza vaccine at the same time as measles-mumps-rubella, *Haemophilus influenzae* B, pneumococcal, and oral polio vaccines. Vaccines should be administered at different sites on the body, and influenza vaccine should not be given within 3 days of administration of pertussis vaccine (2).

Innovative Methods of Vaccine Administration

Intranasal influenza vaccine spray is currently under review of the U.S. FDA (2). There are no reports of its use in either adults or healthcare workers. However, this newer delivery technology may lend itself to faster, more convenient vaccination of adults, including healthcare workers. In a study of 1,602 children in a randomized double-blind efficacy study of a trivalent cold-adapted live-attenuated influenza vaccine given by nasal spray, children aged 15 to 72 months were randomized to receive either two doses of vaccine or placebo (1,314 children) or one dose of vaccine or placebo (288 children) (27). Immunogenicity studies were performed in a subset of the children. One dose of vaccine stimulated a fourfold antibody rise to H3 (92%), B (88%), and H1 (16%) among seronegative children, and these rates increased to 96%, 96%, and 61%, respectively, after dose 2. During the 1996 to 1997 winter season, the overall efficacy for prevention of influenza was 93% [95% confidence interval (CI) = 87% to 96%]. The authors conclude that the ease of administration, safety, and high efficacy make this vaccine suitable for use in children to prevent influenza (27).

Use of Antiviral Agents for Influenza

Antiviral drugs for influenza are an adjunct to influenza vaccine for controlling and preventing influenza (28,29). However, these agents are not a substitute for vaccination. Four licensed influenza antiviral agents are available in the United States: amantadine, rimantadine, zanamivir (Relenza), and oseltamivir (Tamiflu). The dosages and indications for each drug are summarized in Table 41.1.

Amantadine hydrochloride and rimantadine hydrochloride are effective against influenza A. Neither drug is effective against influenza B. Zanamivir and oseltamivir are neuraminidase inhibitors, which inhibit neuraminidase and have activity against both influenza A and B viruses. Both zanamivir and oseltamivir were approved in 1999 for treating uncomplicated influenza infections. Zanamivir is approved for treating persons older than 7 years, and oseltamivir is approved for treatment for persons older than 1 years. In 2000, oseltamivir was approved for chemoprophylaxis of influenza among persons aged older than 13 years (29).

TREATMENT

When administered within 2 days of illness onset to otherwise healthy adults, amantadine and rimantadine can reduce the duration of uncomplicated influenza A illness, and zanamivir and oseltamivir can reduce the duration of uncomplicated influenza A and B illness by approximately 1 day compared with placebo (27). More clinical data are available concerning the efficacy of zanamivir and oseltamivir for treatment of influenza A infection than for treatment of influenza B infection (27). However, *in vitro* data and studies of treatment among mice and ferrets, in addition to clinical studies, have documented that zanamivir and oseltamivir have activity against influenza B viruses (2,29).

To reduce the emergence of antiviral drug-resistant viruses, amantadine or rimantadine therapy for persons with influenza A illness should be discontinued as soon as clinically warranted, typically after 3 to 5 days of treatment or within 24 to 48 hours after the disappearance of signs and symptoms (29,30,31). The recommended duration of treatment with either zanamivir or oseltamivir is 5 days (29).

PROPHYLAXIS

Prophylactic drugs are not a substitute for vaccination, although they are critical adjuncts in the prevention and control of influenza (Table 41.1). Both amantadine and rimantadine are indicated for the chemoprophylaxis of influenza A infection but not influenza B. Both drugs are approximately 70% to 90% effective in preventing illness from influenza A infection (2,29). When used as prophylaxis, these antiviral agents can prevent illness and still permit subclinical infection and the development of protective antibody against circulating influenza viruses. Therefore, certain persons who take these drugs develop protective immune responses to circulating influenza viruses. Amantadine and rimantadine do not interfere with the antibody response to the vaccine (2). Both drugs have been studied extensively among nursing home populations as a component of influenza outbreak control programs, which can limit the spread of influenza within chronic care institutions (2,28).

Of the neuraminidase inhibitor antivirals, zanamivir and oseltamivir, only oseltamivir has been approved for prophylaxis, but community studies of healthy adults indicate that both drugs are similarly effective in preventing febrile, laboratory-confirmed influenza illness (efficacy: zanamivir, 84%; oseltamivir, 82%) (32). Both antiviral agents have also been reported to prevent influenza illness among persons given chemoprophylaxis after a household member was diagnosed with influenza (33). Experience with prophylactic use of these agents in institutional settings or among patients with chronic medical conditions is limited in comparison with the adamantanes (amantadine rimantadine) (2,32).

To be maximally effective as prophylaxis, the drug must be taken each day for the duration of influenza activity in the community. However, to be most cost-effective, one study of amantadine or rimantadine prophylaxis reported that the drugs should be taken only during the period of peak influenza activity in a community (29,32). Persons for whom prophylaxis is indicated are high-risk persons vaccinated after influenza activity has begun, unvaccinated persons or persons vaccinated after influenza activity has begun who provide care to high-risk patients, immunodeficient persons who may not respond to vaccination, and persons for whom vaccine is contraindicated (e.g., persons with allergy to egg protein) (2).

None of the four antiviral agents has been demonstrated to be effective in preventing serious influenza-related complications (e.g., bacterial or viral pneumonia or exacerbation of chronic diseases). Evidence for the effectiveness of these four antiviral drugs is based principally on studies of patients with uncomplicated influenza (27). Data are limited and inconclusive concerning the effectiveness of amantadine, rimantadine, zanamivir, and oseltamivir for treatment of influenza among persons at high risk for serious complications of influenza (2,29). Fewer studies of the efficacy of influenza antivirals have been conducted among pediatric populations compared with adults (29). One study of oseltamivir treatment documented a decreased incidence of otitis media among children (2).

OUTBREAK CONTROL

Antiviral administration remains an appropriate outbreak control measure (2) but requires considerable coordination to implement successfully with a minimum of delays (33–35). For outbreak control, however, it is also recommended that, in closed populations such as nursing homes, patients with influenza taking one of these drugs for treatment be isolated or cohorted from the asymptomatic patients who are taking amantadine, rimantadine, or oseltamivir for prophylaxis (2,28,29,35).

High-risk individuals can still be vaccinated after an outbreak of influenza A has begun. Because the development of antibodies in adults after vaccination takes 2 weeks, prophylaxis should be administered during the 2 weeks following vaccination while waiting for maximum vaccine antibody production (2,29).

Children being vaccinated for the first time may need 6 weeks for antibody development after vaccination or 2 weeks after the second vaccine dose. In either case, influenza antivirals do not interfere with antibody response after vaccination (2).

LIMITATIONS ON ANTIVIRAL USE

Outbreak-initiated use of amantadine or rimantadine is usually problematic. Often, the spread of influenza among patients and healthcare workers can outpace the best intentions and efforts to provide prophylaxis and treatment to those who might benefit from it (2,13,34). Additional problems involve drug distribution, staff education, compliance, and financial considerations.

It is not known whether these drugs are effective if they are given more than 48 hours after the onset of illness. This means that, unless rapid diagnostic techniques are readily available, treatment will be based on clinical and/or epidemiologic diagnosis of influenza, because it may take several days to weeks to establish a laboratory diagnosis of influenza A.

Side effects, which tend to be less severe in young healthy adults at the usual adult doses , include mild central nervous system symptoms (nervousness, anxiety, insomnia, difficulty in concentrating) or gastrointestinal symptoms (anorexia and nausea). These side effects often improve after a week on the drug or can be reduced by an appropriate dosage adjustment (2,27). Dosage adjustments are needed for these drugs in patients with renal or hepatic failure (2,27). The recommended dose for patients aged 65 years and older is 100 mg/day because of the potential for the drugs to accumulate in patients with decreased renal clearance (2,29).

In recent years, there have been reports of amantadine-resistant influenza virus emerging during hospital outbreaks (2,29, 30). Amantadine and rimantadine are cross-resistant because of their structural similarity. Although amantadine and rimantadine resistance can appear in up to one third of patients when these drugs are used for treatment, there is no evidence that amantadine- and rimantadine-resistant viruses are more easily transmitted or more virulent than sensitive isolates. Development of viral resistance to zanamivir and oseltamivir during treatment has been identified but appears to be infrequent (2).

To reduce the risk of developing antiviral resistance, it is recommended that, when used for treatment, these drugs be discontinued as soon as clinically warranted (2,29,30), usually after 3 to 5 days or 24 to 48 hours after the disappearance of symptoms. The recommended duration of treatment with either zanamivir or oseltamivir is 5 days (2,29).

ISOLATION PRECAUTIONS AND INFECTION CONTROL

The components of a comprehensive approach to prevent nosocomial influenza infection include immunization of healthcare workers and patients at high risk in the fall of each year, early identification, isolation and/or cohorting of infected patients and personnel, and the flexibility to offer vaccine later in the year when influenza is first identified in the community or hospital (2). In addition, isolation in private rooms with negative pressure, if possible, is best for known or suspected cases of influenza.

The infection control isolation strategy of cohort isolation (cohorting) may be useful when larger numbers of patients or personnel are infected with influenza (2,36). Cohort isolation attempts to separate different groups of people in an effort to reduce disease transmission (2,36,37). In this case, cohorts of infected and uninfected individuals are identified and separated as a means of reducing spread of influenza. Because most facilities have only a limited supply of private rooms or rooms equipped with negative pressure, more than one patient with proven influenza may be cohorted or isolated together. Depending on the severity of the outbreak, it may also be necessary to restrict ill healthcare workers from work, curtail visitation, and reschedule some elective admissions and surgical procedures (2, 36,37).

Droplet precautions, which require the use of a mask for direct patient contact (i.e., within 3 feet of the patient) are recommended (2,37). Precautions for patients with influenza should be maintained for 7 days or the duration of clinical illness, whichever is longer. Because the duration of clinical illness in antiviral-treated patients is shortened if the drug is given in a timely fashion (i.e., within 48 hours of onset of illness), the period of isolation precautions, especially the use of a mask, may be shortened accordingly.

CONCLUSION

The approach to prevention and control of influenza in healthcare settings relies heavily on vaccine use as the cornerstone of an infection control program for influenza. This is in conjunction with early identification, isolation, and/or cohort isolation. To reduce the risk of an outbreak, vaccine use must be high enough to yield some degree of herd immunity. Therefore, the ACIP recommendation of 80% vaccine use is appropriate when one considers the scientific basis from outbreak experience and sophisticated projection models.

Antiviral drugs are a necessary adjunct to vaccine during outbreak periods to increase the potential for developing herd immunity, especially when vaccine use is less than the 80% threshold. When vaccine use is low and/or influenza infection occurs, additional measures such as restriction of personnel, visitors, and certain procedures may also be indicated.

The ACIP continues to broaden its recommendations for vaccine use, which will probably lead to universal vaccination recommendations over the next several years. In the meantime, the use of innovative federal and local programs that promote healthcare provider education and awareness will help increase vaccine use. These vaccination programs will require an additional administrative and financial commitment in healthcare and community settings. The real payback will come later in the form of reductions in morbidity, mortality, and hospital use and the added benefit of more appropriate use of healthcare resources.

REFERENCES

1. Webster RG. Influenza: an emerging disease. *Emerg Infect Dis* 1998; 4:436–441.
2. Centers for Disease Control and Prevention. Prevention and control of influenza: recommendations of the advisory committee on immunization practices (ACIP). *MMWR Morb Mortal Wkly Rep* 2002; 51(RR03):1–31. Available at http://www.cdc.gov/mmwr/preview/mmwrhtml/rr5103a1.htm (accessed 1/12/2004).
3. Update: influenza activity—United States and worldwide, 2001–02 season, and composition of the 2002–03 influenza vaccine. *MMWR Morb Mortal Wkly Rep* 2002;51:503–506. Available at http://www.cdc.gov/mmwr/preview/mmwrhtml/mm5123a3.htm (accessed).
4. Gross PA, Rodstein M, LaMontagne JR, et al. Epidemiology of acute respiratory illness during an influenza outbreak in a nursing home. *Arch Intern Med* 1988;148:559–561.
5. Gross PA, Quinnan GV, Rodstein M, et al. Association of influenza immunization with reduction in mortality in an elderly population. *Arch Intern Med* 1988;148:562–565.
6. Patriarca PA, Arden NH, Koplan JP, et al. Prevention and control of type A influenza infections in nursing homes. *Ann Intern Med* 1987; 107:732–740.
7. Valenti WM, Menegus MA, Hall CB, et al. Nosocomial virus infections: I. epidemiology and significance. *Infect Control* 1980;1:33–37.
8. Valenti WM, Betts RF, Hall CB, et al. Nosocomial viral infections: II. guidelines for prevention and control of respiratory viruses, herpes viruses, and hepatitis viruses. *Infect Control* 1980;1:38–49.
9. Thompson WW, Shay, DK, Weintraub E, et al. Mortality associated with influenza and respiratory syncytial virus in the United States. *JAMA* 2003;289:179–186.
10. Glezen WP, Cherry JD. Influenza viruses. In: Feigin RD, Cherry JD, eds. *Pediatric infectious diseases,* 4th ed. Philadelphia: WB Saunders, 1998:1688–1704.
11. Hall CB. Nosocomial influenza as a cause of intercurrent fevers in infants. *Pediatrics* 1975;55:673–677.
12. Schmid ML, Kudesia G, Wake S, et al. Prospective comparative study of culture specimens and methods in diagnosing influenza in adults. *BMJ* 1998;316:275.
13. Graman PS, Hall CB. Epidemiology and control of nosocomial virus infections in nosocomial infections. *Infect Dis Clin North Am* 1989;3: 4–12.
14. Sartor, C, Zandotti C, Romain F, et al. Disruption of services in an internal medicine unit due to a nosocomial influenza outbreak. *Infect Control Hosp Epidemiol* 2002;23:615–619.
15. Berlinberg CD, Weingarten SR, Bolton LB, et al. Occupational exposure to influenza-introduction of an index case to a hospital. *Infect Control Hosp Epidemiol* 1989;10:70–73.
16. Nichol KL, Pachuki CT, Pappas SA, et al. Influenza A among hospital personnel and patients. Implications for recognition, prevention, and control. *Arch Intern Med* 1989;149:77–80.
17. Class ECJ, Osterhaus AD, van Beek R, et al. Human influenza A H5N1 virus related to a highly pathogenic avian influenza virus. *Lancet* 1998; 351:472–477.
18. Uyeki, TM, Chong YH, Katz JM, et al. Evidence for human-to-human transmission of avian influenza A (H9N2) viruses in Hong Kong, China 1999. *Emerg Infect Dis* 2002;8:154–159. Available at http://www.cdc.gov/ncidod/eid/vol8no2/01-0148.htm (accessed 1/12/2004).
19. Nichol KL, Lind A, Margolis KL, et al. The effectiveness of vaccination against influenza in healthy, working adults. *N Engl J Med* 1995;333: 889–893.

20. Nichol KL, Hauge M. Influenza vaccination of health care workers. *Infect Control Hosp Epidemiol* 1997;18:189–194.
21. Harbarth S, Siegrist C, Schira J, et al. Influenza immunization: improving compliance of health care workers. *Infect Control Hosp Epidemiol* 1998;19:337–342.
22. Gravenstein S, Davidson HE. Current strategies for management of influenza in the elderly population. *Clinical Infect Dis* 2002;35: 729–737.
23. Centers for Disease Control and Prevention. Notice to readers: expansion of eligibility for influenza vaccine through the vaccines for children program. *MMWR Morb Mortal Wkly Rep* 2002;51:864,875.
24. Begue RE, Gee SQ. Improving influenza immunization among healthcare workers. *Infect Control Hosp Epidemiol* 1998;19:518–520.
25. Cooper E, O'Reilly M. A novel staff vaccination strategy. *Infect Control Hospital Epidemiol* 2002;23:232–233.
26. Barton MB, Schoenbaum SC. Improving influenza vaccination performance in an HMO setting: the use of computer generated reminders. *Am J Public Health* 1990;80:534–536.
27. Belshe RB, Mendelman PM, Treanor J, et al. Efficacy of live attenuated, cold-adapted, trivalent, intranasal influenza virus vaccine in children. *N Engl J Med* 1998;338:1405–1412.
28. Centers for Disease Control and Prevention. Control of influenza A outbreaks in nursing homes—amantadine as adjunct to vaccine, 1989–1990. *MMWR Morb Mortal Wkly Rep* 1991;40:841–844.
29. Jackson HC, Roberts N, Wang M, et al. Management of influenza: use of new antivirals an d resistance in perspective. *Clin Drug Invest* 2000;20:447–454.
30. Degelau J, Somani SK, Cooper SL, et al. Amantadine-resistant influenza A in a nursing facility. *Arch Intern Med* 1992;152:390–392.
31. Hayden FG, Belshe RB, Clover RD, et al. Emergence and apparent transmission of rimantadine-resistant influenza A virus in families. *N Engl J Med* 1989;321:1696–702.
32. Hayden FG, Atmar RL, Schilling M, et al. Use of the selective oral neuraminidase inhibitor oseltamivir to prevent influenza. *N Engl J Med* 1999;341:1336–1343.
33. Hayden FG, Gubareva LV, Monto AS, et al. Inhaled zanamivir for the prevention of influenza in families: Zanamivir Family Study Group. *N Engl J Med* 2000;343:1282–1289.
34. Drinka PJ, Krause P, Nest L, et al. Delays in application of outbreak control prophylaxis for influenza A in a nursing home. *Infect Control Hosp Epidemiol* 2002; 23: 600–603.
35. Hirji Z, O'Grady S, Bonham J, et al. Utility of Zanamivir for chemoprophylaxis of concomitant influenza A and B in a complex continuing care population. *Infect Control Hosp Epidemiol* 2003;23:604–608.
36. Valenti WM, Menegus MM. Nosocomial virus infections IV: guidelines for cohort isolation, communicable disease survey, collection and transport of specimens for virus isolation. *Infect Control* 1981;2: 236–245.
37. Garner JS, for the Hospital Infection Control Practices Advisory Committee. Guideline for isolation precautions in hospitals. *Infect Control Hosp Epidemiol* 1996;17:53–80.

42

VARICELLA-ZOSTER VIRUS

JOHN A. ZAIA

HISTORICAL BACKGROUND AND CURRENT SCOPE OF THE PROBLEM

Varicella is a vesicular exanthema caused by primary infection with varicella-zoster virus (VZV) and is commonly termed chickenpox in English because of the itching observed, derived from the Old English word *gican,* to scratch (1). Herpes zoster is the clinical syndrome of segmental vesicular exanthema and pain associated with reactivation of latent VZV infection in a dorsal nerve ganglion. This is commonly called "shingles" in English because of the way the rash encircles the body, derived from the Latin *cingulum,* a girdle (2). Varicella had been known for centuries as a relatively benign infection of childhood. It was first differentiated from smallpox in recorded medical texts in the ninth century A.D. by the Persian physician Rhazes, who noted that the mild pustular skin eruption was not protective against smallpox (2,3). From an epidemiologic standpoint, much of what clinicians know and practice regarding management of disease prevention derives from the clinical descriptions that linked varicella and herpes zoster (4).

These two entities have taken on new significance in modern medicine. With the advent of immunosuppression, severe VZV infection with visceral dissemination after both primary and reactivated infection was common (5,6). Because of the resultant morbidity and mortality associated with VZV infection, immunologic and chemotherapeutic antiviral methods were developed to minimize this outcome in high-risk individuals. Today, the availability of VZV immune globulin, anti-VZV chemotherapy, and VZV vaccination assist in minimizing or preventing the complications of this important nosocomial infection. It is important that persons involved in the control of nosocomial infections remain knowledgeable about these methods of intervention and about the vast informational background on which many of the recommendations are based.

DISTINCTION BETWEEN VARICELLA AND HERPES ZOSTER

Before the modern methods for virologic diagnosis, clinical observation had suggested that the causative agents of varicella and herpes zoster were related (7,8). Varicella was observed to occur not only following exposure to zoster but also after vesicle fluid was purposely inoculated into susceptible children (9). In addition, the pathologic description of the two clinical entities was similar (10,11). The major significant advance in understanding the nature of these agents was contributed by Weller et al. (12–14), who demonstrated the method for isolation and serial propagation of VZV. These investigators demonstrated that virus isolates made from persons with chickenpox or zoster were identical in terms of cytopathic effect (CPE) in tissue culture (13) and antigenic analysis (14,15). Subsequently, others demonstrated that the VZV strains isolated from these two clinical syndromes were identical by morphology (16,17) and by DNA analysis (18,19).

NATURE OF VZV

Structure and Replication of VZV

Like the other members of the herpesvirus family, VZV is an enveloped virus that contains double-stranded DNA within its protein core. The viral particle is an icosahedron, and the complete enveloped virion measures between 150 and 200 nm in diameter, whereas the naked particle is about 95 nm in diameter. The VZV genome has been sequenced (20) and contains 124,884 base pairs (20), with 71 open reading frames, among which are at least five that encode VZV glycoproteins. These glycoprotein genes have been designated gpI through gpV (21).

Similar to herpes simplex virus (HSV) (22), the VZV replication cycle consists of three phases, designated immediate early, early, and late. The synthesis of proteins in each phase is coordinately regulated and ordered in a sequential cascade such that groups of viral peptides appear in an infected cell in a predictable pattern with the later appearing structural proteins dependent on the prior synthesis of the earlier proteins necessary for DNA replication. VZV antiviral agents inhibit DNA replication by blocking the early protein functions necessary for virus growth.

The CPE of VZV infection produces syncytial cells with intranuclear inclusion bodies (13). In clinical disease, a similar inclusion body is observed in infected tissue, and, as noted, this CPE is identical for both chickenpox and herpes zoster (12). Electron micrographic analysis of vesicle fluid from children with chickenpox demonstrates cell-free enveloped virions (16). It is presumed that VZV acquires an envelope by budding out of the nucleus and into a cytoplasmic Golgi vesicle (23). The membrane of these Golgi vesicles contains viral glycoproteins, and, thus, the virus obtains the surface glycoproteins to which the immune system will be targeted. The molecular aspects of VZV replication have recently been reviewed (24).

IMMUNE RESPONSE TO VZV INFECTION

The antibody response to VZV has been measured by several methods with varying degrees of sensitivity since the initial isolation of the virus. In the 1950s and 1960s, the usual procedure was the complement fixation (CF) test. When sera from individuals with chickenpox were assayed for CF antibody, it was observed that almost all children developed VZV antibody by the second week of illness. However, CF antibody is present in only approximately 80% of adult populations in which the serostatus would be expected to be greater than 90% positive, indicating that CF antibody is lost over time (25). Thus, the CF test is a poor assay to determine humoral immune status in the general population.

The method of anti-VZV antibody detection was greatly improved in the 1970s by the development of an indirect fluorescence antibody for membrane antigen (FAMA) method that used VZV-infected cells as a substrate (26,27). With this test, it became possible to determine the humoral immune status in high-risk populations (28) and to develop more effective approaches to control of nosocomial VZV infection. In addition, there are VZV-specific antibody assays based on neutralization, indirect hemagglutination, immune adherence hemagglutination, radioimmunoassay (RIA), and enzyme-linked immunosorbent assay (ELISA) (29–32). Of these, the RIA and ELISA are more sensitive than immunofluorescence assays (30).

Humoral immune responses to the individual VZV glycoprotein antigens can be assessed by immunoprecipitation reactions between crude radiolabeled VZV antigens (33), by ELISA (34, 35), and by latex agglutination (LA) (36). Using these methods, antibody to at least one of the major VZV glycoproteins is easily demonstrable within 1 week after onset of chickenpox. By 2 weeks, antibodies to two more viral glycoproteins are present. The amount of glycoprotein antibody reaches a peak by 4 to 8 weeks, before a gradual decline occurs over the years after the episode of chickenpox (33). The LA assay has a sensitivity and specificity similar to the FAMA assay, and, because it can be performed in minutes and is commercially available, this assay can be particularly helpful to the hospital epidemiologist (36, 37).

Cellular Immunity to VZV

It is well recognized that iatrogenic or natural reduction in cellular immunity is associated with both severe varicella and increased reactivation of latent VZV (38–43). Cellular immunity to VZV has been classically measured by VZV-specific lymphocyte proliferation assays (44,45) and by measures of inducibility of cytotoxic T lymphocytes (46,47). Susceptible individuals fail to have an *in vitro* response to either crude VZV antigens or to individual VZV protein, but those with prior history of chickenpox develop a cell-mediated immune response to the individual VZV glycoproteins (45). Analyses suggest that VZV proteins gI (ORF68) and IE62 (ORF62) are important for induction of a protective immune response to VZV (47). More recently, with the development of quantitative assays of T-cell immune function, the frequency of VZV-specific immune memory has been described (48–50).

CLINICAL MANIFESTATIONS OF VZV INFECTION

Primary Infection: Varicella

In healthy children, the clinical features of VZV infection present as a mild exanthema, often associated with prodromal malaise, pharyngitis, and rhinitis, appearing at a median time of 15 days after exposure (51,52). The rash is characterized as a vesicular eruption that emerges in successive crops over the first 3 to 4 days of illness, usually with concomitant exanthema. Each skin vesicle appears on an erythematous base, thereby giving rise to the descriptive "dewdrop on a rose petal." It can be difficult to see this stage of infection because of the rapid progression of the skin changes. A quick progression from stage to stage is characteristic of varicella in the otherwise healthy child and allows it to be distinguished from certain other vesicular eruptions and from varicella in the immunosuppressed person. Within 12 hours, the initial lesion becomes an umbilicated papule, and the crusted area then undergoes leukocyte infiltration and develops into a pustule. This then evolves into a hardened, crusted papule. The exanthema usually begins on the head and quickly progresses to the trunk and arms and finally appears on the legs. Because of the rapid progression of individual lesions, it is common to see all stages of the exanthema, including macules, vesicles, papules, and crusts, in the same region of the skin. Fever can be expected to be elevated for the first 4 days of the exanthema, and much of the morbidity is associated with the extent of the cutaneous exanthema (52).

Reactivation Infection: Herpes Zoster

In 1900, Head and Campbell (53) described the anatomic pathology of this syndrome and its precise localization to sites of single dermatomes, which permitted a mapping of the cutaneous distribution of the spinal nerves. The clinical morbidity of herpes zoster is determined in large part by the spinal ganglion involved. The most common area of involvement is the trunk, presumably because this is the area of greatest VZV infection during the primary infection, followed by cranial dermatomes, and then by cervical and lumbar dermatomes (53–55). The involvement of cranial nerves is usually associated with the most clinically severe syndromes.

The pain associated with this disease is usually its major complication, although motor incapacitation can also be significant in the symptom complex. The pain of herpes zoster is called postherpetic neuralgia and occurs with increasing frequency in older persons; it can be a significant problem, lasting for many months (55–58). This is presumably due to the fact that virus reactivation occurs in the dorsal spinal ganglion, which becomes a site of intense inflammation, often with hemorrhagic necrosis of nerve cells and eventual destruction of portions of the ganglion and with poliomyelitis of posterior spinal columns and leptomeningitis (59). This intense inflammation results in nerve damage manifested clinically by meningitis and myelitis, with or without paresis of limbs, face, gut, or urinary bladder (57, 59–65). In addition, there can be considerable inflammation and scarring of the involved epidermis, resulting in loss of epidermal appendages, corneal clouding, and vascularization of ophthalmic structures (63).

Historical Complication and Mortality Rates for VZV Infection

Before the licensure of VZV vaccine in the United States in March 1995, there were an estimated 9,300 VZV-related hospitalizations annually in the United States, 80% of which occurred in otherwise healthy children (66). The rate of complications was highest for persons younger than 1 year old and older than 15 years old. Hospitalization rates relating to varicella, calculated from the Michigan Inpatient Database from 1983 to 1987, were 10 per 1,000 cases below age 1, 2 per 1,000 for ages 1 to 14, 5 per 1,000 for ages 15 to 19, and 8 per 1,000 for age 20 and above. The types of complications that lead to hospitalization in VZV infection have been reviewed (4,66–68) and consist of bacterial superinfection of skin, dehydration, pneumonia, encephalitis, and hepatitis. Bacterial skin infections and bacterial pneumonias occur in the youngest groups; before the antibiotic era, severe bacterial infections, including osteomyelitis, were not uncommon in association with varicella. With the development of antibiotics, but before the recognition of an association between aspirin and Reye's syndrome (69), the major fatal complications of VZV infection in childhood were encephalitis and Reye's syndrome. Encephalitis occurred in approximately 1 in 11,000 cases in the age group 5 to 14 years and is described later. Reye's syndrome was associated with varicella and formerly occurred at a rate as high as 1 in 6,600 cases in certain regions of the United States (70). With the reduction in occurrence of Reye's syndrome after varicella, VZV-associated mortality decreased from an average of 106 deaths per year in 1973 to 1979, to 57 per year for the period 1982 to 1986 (71), and 43 per year in 1990 to 1994 (72). This reduction also coincided with the availability of acyclovir and of varicella-zoster immune globulin (VZIG), and undoubtedly each contributed to this reduced mortality. The pre-VZV vaccine age-specific case-fatality ratios were reported as 6.23 per 100,000 at ages younger than 1 year, 0.75 per 100,000 at ages 1 to 14 years, 2.72 per 100,000 at ages 15 to 19 years, and 25.2 per 100,000 for ages 30 to 49 years (71). Mortality rates in the postvaccine era have fallen dramatically (see the section on VZV vaccine).

Bacterial Infections

Clusters of severe, occasionally fatal, group A streptococcal infection have historically been associated with varicella, and, therefore, aggressive management of bacterial infection is warranted (72,73). Although not usually considered a nosocomial infection, pyoderma, the most often observed bacterial complication of varicella (4,67), should be considered a nosocomial infection if it complicates the course of the hospitalized patient with VZV infection. This problem can be minimized by attention to good hygiene, including daily bathing with bacteriostatic soap, trimming of children's fingernails to minimize excoriation of itchy skin, and early recognition and treatment of superinfection.

Respiratory Tract Infection

In addition to the occasional laryngitis and laryngotracheobronchitis that can occur during varicella, bacterial superinfection can also involve the lower respiratory tract, producing pneumonia and bronchitis. Treatment should be directed toward the usual respiratory pathogens, including *Streptococcus pneumoniae, Haemophilus influenzae,* and *Staphylococcus aureus* (67). Viral pneumonia is more likely to be a problem in older persons with varicella. In persons ages 15 to 19, varicella-related pneumonia occurred in 1 in 3,000 cases, but in adults clinically significant disease has been reported in 1 in 375 cases of varicella (70). Asymptomatic pulmonary disease with radiographic changes has been reported to occur in 16% of adults (74).

Mucositis

Varicella is a generalized infection involving all epithelial areas, including mucosal surfaces of respiratory, alimentary, and genitourinary systems. Involvement of the bladder and urethra can result in severe dysuria with functional bladder obstruction. Urinary analgesics and bladder drainage may be required.

Gastrointestinal Complications and Reye's Syndrome

When death occurs during VZV infection, the gastrointestinal system is often involved. Bleeding requires specific attention, particularly in the immunosuppressed person. In addition, vomiting is not a usual part of the clinical course of this infection, and this symptom should alert the physician to look for abdominal or central nervous system (CNS) complications. As with other viral infections, surgical emergencies such as appendicitis and intussusception can occur during varicella. Mild hepatic involvement is seen in most children with varicella and is usually manifested by asymptomatic elevation of hepatic enzymes, for which no treatment is necessary (75). As noted previously, Reye's syndrome was described in association with varicella, often with concomitant use of aspirin in the child older than 5 years (69, 76,77). Reye's syndrome and other metabolic diseases must be excluded in any child with varicella in whom there is vomiting and changes in mental status (78).

Encephalitis/Myelitis

VZV appears to be trophic for epithelial tissue, and the CNS is not spared from this trophism, with encephalitis and myelitis appearing as important complications of VZV infection. It is important to note that, with both varicella and herpes zoster, neurologic disease can occur either before or after the acute infection (79,80) and can even occur with VZV reactivation in the absence of skin eruption, an entity called *zoster sine herpete* (81). Several CNS syndromes, including aseptic meningitis, polyneuropathy, myelitis, and encephalitis, have been observed in normal persons in association with otherwise occult VZV infection (82). VZV infection involving the CNS is of two types: cerebellar or cerebral complications during varicella, and cranial or peripheral nerve complications during herpes zoster. Cerebral complications present equally as either cerebral or cerebellar abnormalities, the latter being more benign (62,79,80). Cerebellar ataxia is the most common syndrome associated with varicella encephalitis in children and is generally a benign entity that is thought to be due to postinfectious demyelination (79,80,83). In older teenagers and adults, encephalitis occurred in approximately 1 in 3,000 cases of varicella (70). Rarer CNS syndromes, such as granulomatous angiitis, have been observed following herpes zoster, but these are poorly understood syndromes that have not been etiologically related to reactivation of VZV infection. As with varicella, CNS disease in immunodeficient persons is an important problem in herpes zoster, and progressive CNS disease can occur in persons with human immunodeficiency virus (HIV) infection (84–87).

Bleeding Disorders

Bleeding disorders can occur during varicella and are due to disseminated intravascular coagulation, vasculitis, or idiopathic thrombocytopenic purpura (ITP). The syndrome of purpura fulminans must be treated with supportive therapy and with antibiotic therapy until bacterial sepsis is ruled out. Anaphylactoid purpura can follow an otherwise uncomplicated course of varicella and must be managed with appropriate attention to the status of renal function and the possibility of occult intraabdominal hemorrhage. ITP can occur during active infection or during convalescence and responds to treatment with intravenously administered immune globulin (88).

Infection in the Immunocompromised Host

The era of aggressive anticancer chemotherapy and acquired immunodeficiency syndrome (AIDS) has been associated with progressive VZV infection (5,6,84–87,89,90). VZV infection in the immunosuppressed individual is associated with progression of infection from skin to internal organs. Severe skin eruption occurs with or without hemorrhage; there is high fever and spread of virus to visceral organs, producing hepatitis, pneumonitis, pancreatitis, small bowel obstruction, and encephalitis (90, 91). A major manifestation of visceral dissemination in addition to fever is severe abdominal and/or back pain (91,92). In the pre-antiviral era, visceral dissemination occurred in 30% of children who had chickenpox while on active cancer therapy (90). Pneumonitis occurred between 3 and 7 days after onset of varicella in 25% of such patients; without antiviral therapy, the overall mortality rate in such patients was approximately 7%. In the placebo-controlled trials of antiviral agents in similar patients, a fatal outcome occurred in 17% and visceral dissemination occurred in 52% of the placebo groups (93–95). In addition to viral dissemination, bacterial superinfection was a problem in these patients, and bacteremia accounted for significant morbidity during VZV dissemination (90).

The severity of herpes zoster is less predictable in patients receiving immunosuppressive agents. Historically, VZV reactivates in 35% to 50% of persons with Hodgkin's disease and in those undergoing bone marrow transplantation during the first year of treatment (96,97), and persons undergoing other forms of chemotherapy are at increased risk for zoster (98,99). The rates have not changed with intensive anticancer chemotherapy, and antiviral therapy significantly reduces this morbidity. When used early in reactivation, acyclovir can usually eliminate mortality (94,100,101).

PATHOGENESIS OF VZV INFECTION AND DISEASE

Pathogenesis of Chickenpox

The events that lead to the clinical syndrome of varicella are thought to be similar to those that were first proposed by Fenner to explain an animal model of viral exanthem (102). In this schema, virus enters the host from an exogenous source and spreads locally to a site of initial augmentation and then, by a primary viremia, to a location of subsequent viral growth. After several days of replication, the virus then spreads by means of a second viremia to the skin and mucosal surfaces, where the exanthema and exanthema occur (102). The entire time course for such virus replication and spread varies from 10 to 21 days, the range observed for the incubation period of varicella (51, 52,103). The existence of the primary viremia has not been documented, but the secondary viremia is well described (104). Virus spreads to endothelial cells of the skin and then infects the basal and deep malpighian layers of the epidermis. Here, ballooning degeneration of these cells occurs, and local collection of extracellular edema results in unilocular and multilocular vesicles (2,10). In addition to swelling of infected cells, multinucleation occurs, forming the basis for the Tzanck assay, and condensation of viral proteins within the nuclei results in intranuclear inclusions.

Pathogenesis of Herpes Zoster

The two important events in the pathogenesis of herpes zoster are the development of latent VZV infection in dorsal spinal ganglia following primary VZV infection (17,105,106) and subsequent reactivation of latent VZV with disruption of ganglionic structure and spread to the areas distributed by this spinal nerve (60,107). Additional factors involved in controlling this reactivation event are not understood. The virus is thought to reactivate in either the ganglion cell or the perineuronal cells (108); when reactivation occurs, the virus then spreads within the ganglion and within the distribution of that spinal nerve. Because of VZV tropism for nervous tissue, in persons with profound immunodeficiency VZV can spread trans-synaptically within specific neuronal systems, producing necrosis of brain (109). Before this can happen, however, the immune system usually generates intense inflammation at the initial site of virus reactivation (59), and the resultant tissue reaction leads to nerve damage with pain syndrome and to damage in the epidermal structures with the functional abnormalities noted previously. Of concern for nosocomial infection control, a generalized vesicular rash appears during the first week of herpes zoster in approximately 10% of normal adults (54,55,110), suggesting that failure to control the virus at the initial site of reactivation permits spread of virus, much as in varicella. This rash consists of a single crop of vesicles that lacks the polymorphism of varicella, unless continued dissemination occurs (111). Furthermore, in recipients of marrow transplantation, disseminated vesicular exanthema without primary dermatomal skin eruption can follow reactivation (97).

DIAGNOSIS OF VZV INFECTION AND IMMUNITY

Diagnosis by Direct Antigen or by DNA Detection

VZV infection can be diagnosed reliably on clinical grounds alone when there is a history of close exposure to chickenpox or herpes zoster in the past 10 to 21 days and a vesicular eruption consistent with chickenpox (Table 42.1). However, in many situations, particularly those involving immunocompromised persons, no clear historical data support the diagnosis. In this situation, because treatment is of paramount importance, laboratory diagnosis is necessary.

The earliest method for diagnosis was light microscopic examination of the vesicle contents to demonstrate multinucleated giant cells when stained with Wright-Giemsa stain. This method, called a Tzanck prep, has now been superseded by a fluorescent antigen detection assay, which is available in a commercial kit for confirmation of the diagnosis. This assay consists of a direct fluorescent antigen stain of samples of cells that are scraped from the base of a vesicle and dried onto a glass slide. Rapid diagnosis by antigen detection can also be performed on punch biopsy specimens of vesicular lesions. The test takes only 1 to 2 hours and can quickly differentiate between vesicular rashes caused by VZV or HSV infection.

The specific diagnosis of VZV infection can also be made by DNA hybridization techniques or by polymerase chain reaction (PCR) (112). PCR is the more sensitive assay and can discriminate between vaccine and wild strains of VZV, but, for the hospital epidemiologist, it can be more tedious and less practical than rapid antigen detection using VZV-specific monoclonal antibodies.

TABLE 42.1. DIAGNOSIS OF VARICELLA-ZOSTER VIRUS (VZV) INFECTION

History of exposure to varicella or herpes zoster in past 3 weeks
Physical examination of rash indicates
- For varicella: lesions in all stages of development from vesicle on red base to umbilicated pustule to crusted lesion
- For zoster: dermatome distribution of lesions

VZV-antigen detection using lesion scraping
Culture of vesicle or PCR for VZV (optional if antigen-positive)
Antibody assay on acute/convalescent paired sera (optional if antigen-, culture-, or PCR-positive)

PCR, Polymerase chain reaction.

Viral Culture for Isolation of VZV

For confirmation of laboratory diagnosis or to obtain the virus strain for determination of epidemiologic analysis or antibiotic resistance testing, VZV infection is isolated in cell culture (13). Vesicular fluid is collected in sterile capillary tubes or tuberculin syringes, which are subsequently evacuated into culture medium. The medium is then layered over cultured cells, and, in 3 to 5 days, CPE is visible in the monolayer. In human fibroblast cells, the CPE consists of multiple foci of swollen, rounded refractile cells. A definitive diagnosis of VZV infection is made by immunostaining of the infected monolayer with a VZV-specific monoclonal antibody.

Detection of Susceptibility to VZV

The simplest method for reliably determining susceptibility to varicella is to take a history for previous chickenpox. A positive history from adults correlates with serologic confirmation 97% to 99% of the time (113–115). A positive history of previous chickenpox in a child with recent household VZV exposure is associated with subsequent disease in only 7% (52). Conversely, a negative history from an adult does not correlate with serostatus in 72% to 93% (113–116). Thus, serologic tests of immunity are most useful in adults with a negative history of chickenpox. The FAMA, RIA, ELISA, LA, and hemagglutination antibody (HA) assays, because they are sufficiently sensitive, are reliable methods for demonstration of prior infection with VZV (30,32,35). For this reason, these tests are widely used as presumptive evidence of immunity following exposure to chickenpox, for preemployment evaluation, or for follow-up after vaccination. It should be noted that these assays are not reliable in persons who have received blood products and who might have acquired passive antibody. As mentioned previously, the CF test, because it is an insensitive test for antibody, should not be used for determination of prior infection. The immediate availability of the RIA, ELISA, or FAMA assays can be problematic when the question of susceptibility must be determined quickly, as is usually the case in matters relating to nosocomial infection. The LA assay is commercially available (36) and reliably determines immune status to VZV (36,37).

EPIDEMIOLOGY OF VZV INFECTIONS

Transmission and Communicability of VZV

Early observations suggested that chickenpox was an airborne disease (117,118), and this was subsequently confirmed using sophisticated methods of air-flow analysis (119,120). The spread of infectious VZV from a person with chickenpox is by air droplets from nasopharyngeal secretions, which usually requires face-to-face exposure but can also occur via air currents to susceptible individuals without direct contact (119,120).

The period of infectivity is generally considered to be between 48 hours before exanthema and 4 days after exanthema, a range derived from published observations of varicella in cohorts of children quarantined for other infections. In this setting, it was rare to observe spread of varicella from a child who exposed other ward-mates more than 2 days before the onset of rash (51, 121). Although there is a single report that infectivity could occur 4 days before exanthema (122), this case is suspect and would be the exception to the common experience, which suggests that exposure more than 1 day before exanthema is unlikely to be infectious (51,121). The usual recommendation is to consider the period of infectivity as 48 hours before rash until the skin lesions are crusted.

Herpes zoster is spread by direct contact or by exposure to airborne infectious material (103,123). The incubation period for chickenpox following exposure to zoster (103) is the same as that following exposure to varicella (51) (median time = 15 days, range 10 to 21 days). The clinical varicella attack rate, following household zoster, however, is only 25% among history-negative children (103), compared with an attack rate of 87% following exposure to household chickenpox (52).

Age-Specific Incidence of VZV Infection

Postvaccine era incidence of varicella in the United States is not know with certainty, but, using index counties as representative, the number of cases and the complications requiring hospitalization have been reduced by 80% (124). Historically, the estimated incidence of chickenpox in the United States in the prevaccine era was based on the size of the birth cohort and on the assumption that nearly everyone developed chickenpox over a lifetime. Thus, for example, with approximately 4 million births in the United States annually, approximately 3.7 million cases of varicella occurred each year (66). More than 90% of all cases of varicella occurred in persons younger than 15 years, and nearly half of all cases in children occurred between the ages of 5 and 9 years. Age-specific incidence data were reported for the years 1980 to 1990 from the National Health Interview Survey, indicating that 33% of cases occurred in preschool children ages 1 to 4 years, in whom the incidence was 82.2 per 1,000 per year (66,71). In the age group 5 to 9 years, the incidence was estimated to be 91.1 per 1,000 per year (66).

There are approximately 300,000 cases of herpes zoster in the United States per year (68). Based on public records, the incidence of herpes zoster is constant for each age group through mid-adulthood. Thereafter, the incidence of zoster increases with age such that persons in their 80s have a 1 in 100 chance per year of developing zoster (56). When adjusted for prior occurrence of varicella, younger children also have a higher incidence of zoster, a known association in children who have acquired varicella before their first year of life (125).

VARICELLA-ZOSTER VACCINE

Background

The VZV vaccine is the single most important tool in prevention and control of nosocomial VZV infection. The live attenuated VZV vaccine was developed by Takahashi et al. (126) in 1974; and was prepared by attenuation of a VZV isolate (Oka strain) in human embryonic cells and then in human diploid fibroblasts (127). The vaccine virus is biologically different from wild VZV in its growth characteristics and DNA restriction enzyme profile (128,129). This vaccine was used extensively in Japan in healthy children and was effective for the prevention of varicella after exposure and for curtailment of outbreaks of VZV infection (126,130).

Recommended Use of VZV Vaccine

A live attenuated VZV vaccine (Varivax) was approved in the United States in 1995 (131). Vaccine should be administered at any routine visit at or after age 12 months for susceptible children (i.e., those without prior history of prior chickenpox); susceptible persons 13 years old should receive two doses at least 4 weeks apart. The vaccine is particularly important in chickenpox history-negative teens and adults, especially college students, healthcare and daycare workers, prisoners, military recruits, nonpregnant women of childbearing age, and international travelers. For adolescent and adult patients serologic testing for VZV antibody is usually cost effective before vaccination (132,133). The vaccine is not recommended for infants younger than 1 year; for immunosuppressed persons; for those receiving salicylate therapy; for pregnant women; or for persons allergic to components of the vaccine, including neomycin, gelatin, and monosodium glutamate. Severe infection resulting from VZV vaccine has been observed in immunodeficient children (85–87). Despite this, VZV vaccine can be administered to HIV-infected children (134), and, because of the likely severity of chickenpox in children with AIDS, the vaccine is recommended for consideration on a case-by-case basis for asymptomatic or mildly symptomatic patients with age-specific CD4 T-lymphocyte percentages of 25% or more. Other immunosuppressed individuals such as solid organ transplant recipients who are on continuous iatrogenic immunosuppression are not recommended for receipt of VZV vaccine, and it is unlikely that these patients will have an effective immune response to the vaccine (135). However, in children with leukemia studied in the United States, vaccination given to those in remission produced a 5-year seropositivity of 70% and an attack rate of chickenpox after household exposure to VZV of only 14% (136,137).

The protection of at-risk patients from varicella exposure requires use of VZV vaccine in healthcare workers, and the safe use of this vaccine in this population has been described (138). For healthcare workers, screening for prior VZV infection should be done at the time of employment, and seronegative persons should receive the two-dose VZV vaccine immunization schedule. For patients about to undergo intensive immunosuppression, the healthy family members who have no history of VZV infection or who are seronegative for VZV antibody should be vaccinated. For severely immunocompromised patients (e.g., hematopoietic cell transplant recipients) the recommendation states that ideally patients should not have contact with vaccinees at times of severe immunosuppression until 4 weeks after completion of vaccine doses (139). However, in practice, the more important concern is that the patient should not have contact with any vaccinee who experiences a rash after vaccination. At present, transmission from a healthcare worker to a patient has not been documented, and vaccine virus is susceptible to acyclovir, which many immunosuppressed patients receive during intense immunosuppression. Thus, most centers allow the employee to start work before the completion of VZV immunization, but with the caution that any rash must be reported and that patient care must stop until the rash resolves.

The effectiveness of the VZV vaccine has been reported in long-term follow-up studies. (130,140,141). A single dose of vaccine results in seroconversion in 97% of susceptible children 1 to 12 years old, in 79% of children 13 to 17 years old, and in 82% of adults. Two doses of vaccine result in seroconversion in 94% of adults (130,140,141). Vaccine effectiveness in preventing chickenpox is approximately 85%, and the effectiveness for preventing severe disease is approximately 97%. As noted previously, the number of chickenpox cases and hospitalizations have decreased between 1995 to 2000 by approximately 80%, based on analysis of representative counties in the United States (124). Breakthrough varicella occurs in approximately 20% of vaccinees after household exposure, and the risk factors for such breakthrough are close contact with varicella, age 14 months or younger at vaccination, and receipt of low-titer vaccine (136). In this regard, subjects with low serologic immune response to the vaccine appear to reactivate the vaccine virus resulting in persistent increasing serum antibody titers suggesting that the vaccine virus persisted *in vivo* and reactivates in the presence of low antibody titers (137). If this is true, the vaccination should result in long-term immunity.

Herpes zoster resulting from vaccine strain virus is very rare but does occur (86,142). Chickenpox has been contracted from a sibling who developed zoster 5 months after immunization with VZV vaccine (143). The inadvertent exposure of susceptible women to VZV vaccine during pregnancy has been monitored since 1995 in the United States, and, to date, there has been no congenital varicella syndrome or other VZV-specific birth defects in this group (144). Other aspects of VZV vaccine have recently been reviewed (145).

PREVENTION AND CONTROL OF NOSOCOMIAL VZV INFECTION

Employee Policy Regarding VZV Infection

The control of nosocomial VZV infection begins with the development of a rational employment policy for the healthcare worker (Table 42.2). It cannot be overemphasized that healthcare workers are a significant source of exposure to primary nosocomial VZV infection (113,116,146–148); therefore, one of the first lines of protection of susceptible patient populations is to minimize spread of infection from hospital workers. This begins with the initial employment history and physical examination, which should include history regarding prior chickenpox (116). If this history is negative, appropriate serologic testing should be performed to confirm antibody status if the employee will be involved in interactions with patients. VZV seropositive employees will not be at risk for primary VZV infection. VZV history-negative/seronegative employees who receive VZV vaccine should be restricted from patient responsibilities involving VZV-infected individuals and should be counseled to recognize VZV infection and the appropriate isolation methods (Figs. 42.1 and 42.2).

In the past, the practice of furloughing healthcare workers known to be susceptible to VZV, after exposure to this virus, was less than satisfactory, because of both cost to the healthcare institution (74) and lost time for the employee. With the approval of the VZV vaccine in the United States, there is an opportunity to reduce the potential for employee-mediated nosocomial VZV infection. Healthcare institutions are advised to consider the use of the VZV vaccine for control of employee-related nosocomial infection (71). In addition to healthy children aged 12 months to 12 years, the vaccine is recommended for healthy adolescents and adults with no prior history of chickenpox (Table 42.3). Before age 13 years, the vaccine is given as a single, 0.5-mL subcutaneous dose; thereafter, a vaccinee should receive two 0.5-mL doses of vaccine given subcutaneously 4 to 8 weeks apart. It is recommended for all such healthcare workers, especially those having contact with susceptible children, pregnant women, and immunocompromised individuals.

In the policy recommendation, it is noted that individual institutional policies should be developed in regard to the use of the VZV vaccine, and these policies must consider certain factors about which there is imprecise information. For example, the question of whether to furlough or to reassign vaccinated personnel after exposure is unclear because the occurrence rate of breakthrough varicella is not accurately known. In addition, 5.5% of adolescents and adults develop a rash after the first injection, and there is the rare instance of transmission of virus from healthy vaccinee to susceptible household contact. Hence, it is recommended that recent vaccinees who develop a rash following vaccination avoid patient contact. Recent vaccinees with or without a rash should avoid contact with high-risk persons (e.g., newborns, pregnant women, and immunocompromised persons). In addition, testing for seroconversion at the completion of immunization is not recommended, because approximately 99% will be seropositive; however, consideration should be given to testing vaccinated healthcare workers at the time of a subsequent exposure, because detection of antibody could become a method for identifying employees who are at

TABLE 42.2. VZV POLICY FOR HEALTHCARE WORKERS

- Determine history of prior varicella at initial intake interview
- Obtain serologic information of immune status for persons with negative or unknown history of varicella and consider such workers susceptible
- Seronegative healthcare workers should receive VZV vaccine (alternatively, vaccinate all persons with negative or unknown history of varicella)
- Unvaccinated susceptible employees should avoid contact with patients having varicella or herpes zoster
- Susceptible or recently vaccinated healthcare workers must report any VZV exposure to the infection control department
- After valid exposure:
  - Susceptible, unvaccinated workers must be furloughed away from direct patient care from days 10 to 21 after exposure; consider administration of VZIG or VZV vaccine
  - Recently vaccinated workers can be assigned to patient care responsibility if VZV-seropositive on retesting; seronegative workers can be retested 5 to 6 days later and, if still seronegative, furloughed away from direct patient care from days 10 to 21 after exposure

VZIG, varicella-zoster immune globulin; VZV, varicella-zoster virus.

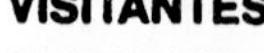
VISITORS
Report to nurse before visiting patient
VISITANTES
FAVOR DE ANUNCIARSE A LA ENFERMERA DE PISO ANTES DE ENTRAR AL CUARTO
VISITEURS
VEUILLEZ VOUS ADRESSER AU BUREAU DES INFIRMIERES AVANT D'ENTRER DANS LA CHAMBRE

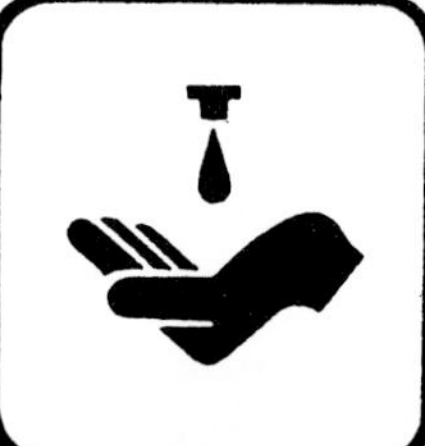
WASH
Hands must be washed after touching the patient or potentially contaminated articles and before taking care of another patient.

MASK
Masks are indicated for all persons entering room.

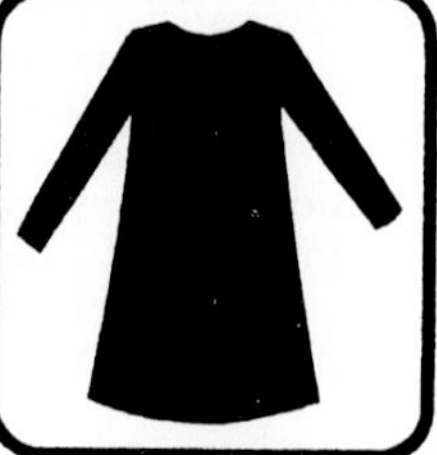
GOWN
Gowns are indicated when substantial contact with patient, enviromental surfaces, or items in the patient's room is anticipated

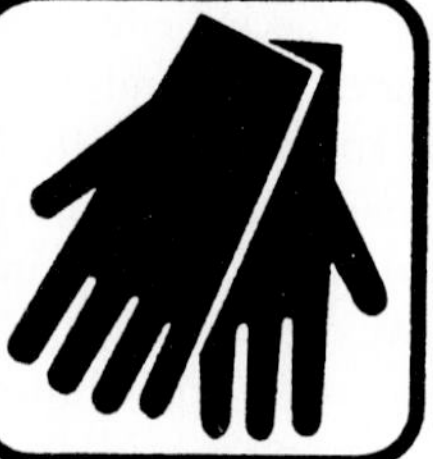
GLOVE
Gloves are indicated for all persons entering room.

WASTE
Articles contaminated with infective material should be discarded or bagged and labeled before being sent for decontamination and reprocessing.

Figure 42.1. Notice to hospital visitors and staff regarding precautions for isolation of patients with varicella or disseminated zoster. (Courtesy of Brevis Corp.)

minimum risk for breakthrough infection. It should be noted that breakthrough cases of varicella in vaccinated persons are mild, but the rate of transmission of disease from vaccinees who develop varicella is not well studied (71). For this reason, daily monitoring while employees continue at work is suggested for vaccinated healthcare workers following VZV exposure (71). In addition, VZV-serostatus should be determined by LA assay, and seronegative workers should be retested 5 to 6 days later, before the tenth day postexposure; if the worker is still seronegative, he or she should be furloughed away from direct patient care during days 10 to 21 postexposure. VZV-seropositive healthcare workers can be assigned patient-care duties but should be monitored daily for rash and removed from such duties if rash appears (71). For susceptible healthcare workers who have been exposed to varicella, removal from patient contact is recommended beginning on the tenth day following initial exposure and continuing until day 21 after the last exposure. Although postexposure vaccination has been shown to have a 90% protective effect in children vaccinated within 3 days of close exposure, vaccination is not recommended as a means of limiting nosocomial VZV infection after healthcare worker exposure (71) (see also Chapter 99).

GLOVE

IF YOU NEVER HAD CHICKEN POX
DO NOT ENTER

Figure 42.2. Notice to hospital visitors and staff regarding contact precautions for patients with herpes zoster. (Modified courtesy of Brevis Corp.)

Infection Control of VZV Infection in Hospitalized Patients

Initial Containment Response: Isolation Precautions

Before the VZV vaccine, pediatric patients, especially those younger than 5 years, formed a population in which most were susceptible to chickenpox, and VZV infections spread and endured over many months within an institution (122). When immunocompromised pediatric patients existed in the same setting, the need was heightened for control of such nosocomial infections (149,150). Guidelines for prevention and control of such infections have been published, and there is advice for

TABLE 42.3. INDICATION FOR VZV VACCINATION[a]

Healthy children aged 12 months to 12 years
Healthcare workers
Persons working in day care or pediatric institutions
College students
Prisoners
Military recruits
Nonpregnant women of childbearing age
International travelers

[a] Vaccine (Varivax, Merck) recommended for healthy children older than 12 months and for healthy adolescents and adults with no prior history of varicella.

VZV, varicella-zoster virus.

managing such problems (71,151–153). However, with the use of VZV vaccine, the pediatric inpatient population older than 1 year should be immune to VZV, and such institutional outbreaks could be a thing of the past.

If the exposure is from a patient, he or she should be discharged if possible. If this is not possible, then for patients with either varicella or disseminated zoster, or for immunosuppressed patients with localized zoster, isolation precautions designed to prevent spread of infection by both air and direct contact are recommended. Optimally, this consists of a private room with negative air pressure relative to the corridor (152). Immunocompromised individuals with zoster are unlikely to disseminate infection after 24 hours of treatment with acyclovir (100), and, for that reason, continued strict isolation is not necessary for this subgroup. The precaution guidelines should be posted on the door to restrict entry to susceptible persons (Figs. 42.1 and 42.2). Immunocompetent patients with localized zoster should be placed on precautions to prevent transmission by direct or indirect contact with infectious material or drainage from an infected body site. For varicella and disseminated zoster, isolation should remain in effect until all skin lesions are crusted. For localized zoster, contact precautions should continue until all drainage from the lesions has ceased.

Secondary Response: Control of Extended Infection

After initiating control of the source of VZV infection, the problem then is to quickly access three types of information: (a) the nature of the VZV exposure and whether this exposure is likely to result in secondary infections, (b) information on the susceptibility of each of the exposed patients, and (c) a list of patients at risk for life-threatening VZV-related complications. The type of exposures that are likely to lead to varicella transmission are those involving close contact. A close contact is defined as one in which there is more than 1 hour in the same area indoors with the infected source (e.g., exposure in the same two to four bed hospital room or indoor play area). However, even less than 1 hour of exposure should be taken seriously when exposure is direct face-to-face contact with the infectious person (71). As noted earlier (see the section on detection of susceptibility to VZV), positive or negative history of prior varicella can be highly reliable in the first assessment of who is susceptible. Pediatric admission records should indicate whether the exposed patients have received the VZV vaccine. Serologic tools can be used to clarify the status of those with ambiguous history. Thus, the initial step is to define the hospital area(s) in which a definite VZV exposure occurred and then to focus on which patients in this area are at risk for infection. Finally, among these exposed patients, immunosuppressed individuals are considered to be at high risk for VZV-related complications, and these persons should be given separate attention (see later discussion).

Once this information is available, those susceptible patients who are exposed should be discharged if possible. Those who cannot be discharged should be isolated beginning 10 days from initial exposure through 21 days from last exposure. Those who must remain in the hospital who were not exposed to varicella should be placed in a cohort to keep them away from the VZV-exposed susceptible patients to prevent further spread of infection. It has been shown that the use of the VZV vaccination in this situation can stop an extended round of varicella in a pediatric setting (154). At present, however, except for use in children with leukemia under a special protocol, the vaccine is only recommended for use in healthy individuals, and, hence, this modality is not recommended for nosocomial control of VZV in U.S. institutions.

Approach to Protection of Immunocompromised Persons

An institution's policy regarding nosocomial spread of VZV infection is designed in large part to minimize the possibility of immunocompromised persons becoming infected with VZV in the hospital. Those at risk are defined as patients who have primary and acquired immunodeficiency disorders, have neoplastic diseases, have recently received immunosuppressive treatment, are premature newborns of varicella-susceptible mothers, or are premature infants born at less than 28 weeks gestation or weighing less than 1,000 g (71). As noted previously, these individuals should receive special attention in the form of antiviral prevention. This type of prevention should begin before there is a known problem. The clinic staff and inpatient personnel should become familiar with and enforce visiting policy that minimizes the exogenous introduction of infection into the patient areas. As mentioned, the employee policy should serve to protect the patients from exposure to VZV infection. In addition to employee vaccination, the children with acute leukemia should have access to VZV vaccine, and the infection control office should work with the pediatric hematology clinic to provide vaccination for appropriate clinic patients. Information can be obtained regarding eligibility for the VZV vaccine from the Varivax Coordinating Center (IBAH Inc., 4 Valley Square, Blue Bell, PA 19422, telephone 215-283-0897).

Of greatest concern, of course, are those who are both susceptible and immunocompromised. As noted, these children should be provided exogenous antibody to VZV in the form of VZIG (Table 42.4). VZIG is an immune globulin prepared from pooled blood plasma containing high antibody titers to VZV (25). VZIG is given intramuscularly and will modify varicella but does not always prevent infection and disease. The median incubation period of immunosuppressed children who receive VZIG is 15 days, similar to that of natural infection, but the range is increased to at least 28 days (155). Proper dosage is based on weight and is provided with the particular lot available. In addition, discontinuation of immunosuppressive therapy should be instituted if possible. Again, these children should be isolated on day 10 following initial exposure and should be kept in isolation through day 28.

Management of Adult Patients with VZV Exposure

More than 95% of all adults have been infected with VZV, and these persons do not develop disease after repeat exposure to the virus (113–115). Nevertheless, it has been shown by Arvin et al. (156) that normal adults often are reinfected by VZV after exposure to chickenpox. However, despite this finding, recurrent varicella is sufficiently rare that, for practical purposes, it need not be considered in the construction of guidelines for management of nosocomial VZV. Susceptible adults do develop chickenpox, provide the source for unexpected epidemics, and are at increased risk for life-threatening complications. The susceptible individual must be identified and appropriately managed. One population that is at risk for varicella are adults from subtropical climates, where, it has been reported, varicella occurs well into adult life (157,158). Because immigrants from these areas can be found in health-related employment, attention should be addressed to any such person to confirm varicella immunity and provide VZV vaccine before that person has contact with high-risk patients.

With the availability of the VZV vaccine, vaccination is recommended for all healthy persons after 12 years of age who do not have a reliable history of chickenpox at the time of any routine healthcare visit (Table 42.3). As noted for healthcare workers, the vaccine is given to adolescents and adults in two doses, subcutaneously, 4 to 8 weeks apart. Vaccination is particularly recommended for susceptible persons: (a) who live or work in settings with high transmission of VZV, including day care and institutional settings; (b) who live or work in environments in which VZV transmission might occur, including college dormitories, correctional institutions, and the military; (c) who are nonpregnant women of childbearing age and who will avoid pregnancy for 1 month following each dose of vaccine; and (d) who are international travelers likely to have close contact with local populations (71). The vaccine should not be given to persons with neomycin allergy or to individuals with blood dyscrasias, leukemia (except childhood leukemia in remission for 12 months when selected clinical criteria are met), lymphomas or other malignant neoplasms, HIV infection, or AIDS or to anyone receiving immunosuppressive medication or having a first-degree relative with a congenital immunodeficiency.

It is important to recognize the need for passive immunization of persons encountered during an evaluation of nosocomial VZV exposure. VZIG is recommended not only for immunosuppressed infants and children but also for certain susceptible, unvaccinated, healthy adults following close exposure to VZV. This is because of the morbidity that can occur in such individuals during chickenpox. This decision, however, should be made individually, taking into consideration the person's health status, the type of exposure, and the likelihood of previous varicella. VZV vaccination should be considered beginning 5 months after VZIG administration.

TABLE 42.4. INDICATIONS FOR VARICELLA-ZOSTER IMMUNE GLOBULIN[a]

Immunocompromised children
- Primary and acquired immune deficiency disorder
- HIV infection
- Neoplastic disease
- Treatment with immunosuppressive agent

Newborns
- Newborns exposed to maternal varicella 5 days before and up to 2 days after delivery
- Newborns weighing <1,000 g at birth
- Premature neonates born to varicella-susceptible mothers

Adults
- Immunocompromised adults based on individual evaluation[b]
- Healthy adults based on individual evaluation[b]
- Pregnant women

[a] Situations in which varicella-zoster immune globulin (VZIG) is indicated following exposure to varicella-zoster virus.
[b] Evaluation should consider the type of exposure, the likelihood of prior infection, and the health status of the individual.
HIV, human immunodeficiency virus.

Management of the Pregnant Woman after VZV Exposure

Congenital Varicella Syndrome

The congenital varicella syndrome was first described in 1947, and less than 100 cases have been described (159–163). The syndrome consists of low birth weight, cutaneous scarring, limb hypoplasia, microcephaly, cortical atrophy of brain, chorioretinitis, and cataracts. Intrauterine VZV infection can occur following maternal varicella in all trimesters of gestation, but teratogenic or developmental damage results from infection before the third trimester (164,165). The rate of transplacental infection is 24%, but clinically apparent disease occurs in only about 2% to 3% after maternal varicella in early pregnancy (162–164).

Perinatal VZV Infection

Perinatal infection can develop when chickenpox occurs late in the third trimester, and newborns are considered at risk if chickenpox occurs in the mother from 5 days before to 2 days after delivery (71,164,166). The precise risk of severe disease is not known, and the initial report (166), which showed a mortality rate of 31%, probably is inflated compared with the risk in a modern neonatal intensive care unit. The risk of severe VZV infection appears to be a function of the presence of transplacental maternal antibody to VZV in the baby (165,167). VZIG is recommended in any neonate with maternal chickenpox occurring 5 days before to 2 days after delivery or in any VZV-exposed neonate born to a susceptible mother or born weighing less than 1,000 g. With such use of VZIG in neonates exposed to maternal chickenpox, the death rate from VZV infection has been reported to have decreased from 7% to 0% (168). Contrary to varicella exposure, maternal herpes zoster occurs only in the setting of prior maternal antibody, and this presents no significant risk to the baby (164).

Approach to the Pregnant Woman Exposed to VZV

A pregnant woman with significant exposure to VZV infection should be evaluated for susceptibility to VZV with an appropriate antibody assay, if she has a negative or unknown history of varicella as a child. But congenital infection is rare, and the woman should be reassured. The most significant risk is to the health of the mother rather than to the infant (164), and the susceptible seronegative pregnant women should receive passive immunization with VZIG (71).

USE OF ACYCLOVIR TO PREVENT VZV INFECTION

It has long been recognized that acyclovir, and other drugs having anti-VZV activity, can prevent or modify chickenpox after primary exposure (169) and can prevent zoster in immunocompromised patients at risk reactivation of VZV (170,171). The use of acyclovir and valacyclovir after organ transplantation lessens the incidence of VZV infection (172), and acyclovir can be used to supplement VZIG in prevention of chickenpox in high-risk children (173,174). Thus, although not approved for these indications, for prevention of primary VZV infection, some physicians now use acyclovir (600 mg/m^2 by mouth 4-times daily for susceptible children less than age 12 years, or valacyclovir 1 gm 3-times daily (500 mg 3-times daily if less than 40 kg) from days 3–22 post-VZV exposure (3–28 days if used with VZIG). For prevention of zoster in the chronically immunosuppressed adult patient with normal renal function, valacyclovir 500 mg 2-times daily by mouth can be used, although the cost-benefit of this approach is unknown.

ACKNOWLEDGMENT

I acknowledge the assistance of Ms. Michael Hill in the preparation of this manuscript.

REFERENCES

1. Scott-Wilson JH. Why "chicken" pox? *Lancet* 1978;1:1152.
2. Taylor-Robinson D, Caunt AE. *Varicella virus.* Vienna: Springer-Verlag, 1972.
3. Bett W. *A short history of some common diseases.* London: Oxford University Press, 1934.
4. Gordon J. Chickenpox: an epidemiologic review. *Am J Med Sci* 1962; 244:362–389.
5. Dolin R. Herpes zoster-varicella infections in immunosuppressed patients. *Ann Intern Med* 1978;89:375–378.
6. Zaia JA, Grose C. Varicella and herpes zoster. In: Gorbach SL, Bartlett JG, Blacklow NR, eds. *Infectious diseases,* 2nd ed. Philadelphia: WB Saunders, 1998:1311–1323.
7. Shelmire J. Concurrent herpes zoster and varicella. *Arch Dermatol Syph* 1928;17:687–700.
8. Blatt M. Chickenpox following contact with herpes zoster: report of two minor epidemics. *J Lab Clin Med* 1940;25:951–954.
9. Lipschutz B. Uber die aetiologie des zoster und uber seine beziehungen zu varizellen. *Wein Klin Wochenschr* 1925;38:499.
10. Tyzzer EE. The histology of the skin lesions in varicella. *J Med Res* 1906;14:361.
11. Taniguchi T. Cultivation of chickenpox on the chorio-allantoic membrane and vaccine studies. *Jpn J Exp Med* 1935;13:19.
12. Weller T. Serial propagation in vitro of agents producing inclusion bodies derived from varicella and herpes zoster. *Proc Soc Exp Biol Med* 1953;83:340.
13. Weller T. The etiologic agents of varicella and herpes zoster isolation, propagation, and cultural characteristics in vitro. *J Exp Med* 1958; 108:843.
14. Weller T. Fluorescent antibody studies with agents of varicella and herpes zoster propagated in vitro. *Proc Soc Exp Biol Med* 1954;86: 789–794.
15. Weigle KA, Grose C. Common expression of varicella-zoster viral glycoprotein antigens in vitro and in chickenpox and zoster vesicles. *J Infect Dis* 1983;148:630–638.
16. Kimura A, Tosaka K, Nakao T. An electron microscopic study of varicella skin lesions. *Arch Gesamte Virusforsch* 1972;36:1–12.
17. Esiri MM, Tomlinson AH. Herpes Zoster. Demonstration of virus in trigeminal nerve and ganglion by immunofluorescence and electron microscopy. *J Neurol Sci* 1972;15:35–48.
18. Iltis JP, Oakes JE, Hyman RW, et al. Comparison of the DNAs of varicella-zoster viruses isolated from clinical cases of varicella and herpes zoster. *Virology* 1977;82:345–352.
19. Richards JC, Hyman RW, Rapp F. Analysis of the DNAs from seven varicella-zoster virus isolates. *J Virol* 1979;32:812–21.
20. Davison AJ, Scott JE. The complete DNA sequence of varicella-zoster virus. *J Gen Virol* 1986;67(Pt 9):1759–1816.
21. Davison AJ, Edson CM, Ellis RW, et al. New common nomenclature for glycoprotein genes of varicella-zoster virus and their glycosylated products. *J Virol* 1986;57:1195–1197.
22. Honess RW, Roizman B. Regulation of herpesvirus macromolecular synthesis. I. Cascade regulation of the synthesis of three groups of viral proteins. *J Virol* 1974;14:8–19.
23. Jones F, Grose C. Role of cytoplasmic vacuoles in varicella-zoster virus glycoprotein trafficking and virion envelopment. *J Virol* 1988; 62:2701–2711.
24. Arvin AM. Varicella-zoster virus: molecular virology and virus-host interactions. *Curr Opin Microbiol* 2001;4:442–449.
25. Zaia JA, Levin MJ, Wright GG, et al. A practical method for preparation of varicella-zoster immune globulin. *J Infect Dis* 1978;137: 601–604.
26. Williams V. Serologic response to varicella-zoster membrane antigens measured by indirect immunofluorescence. *J Infect Dis* 1971;130: 669–672.
27. Zaia JA, Oxman MN. Antibody to varicella-zoster virus-induced membrane antigen: immunofluorescence assay using monodisperse glutaraldehyde-fixed target cells. *J Infect Dis* 1977;136:519–530.
28. Gershon AA, Steinberg SP. Antibody responses to varicella-zoster virus and the role of antibody in host defense. *Am J Med Sci* 1981; 282:12–17.
29. Furukawa T, Plotkin SA. Indirect hemagglutination test for varicella-zoster infection. *Infect Immun* 1972;5:835–839.
30. Wreghitt TG, Tedder RS, Nagington J, et al. Antibody assays for varicella-zoster virus: comparison of competitive enzyme-linked immunosorbent assay (ELISA), competitive radioimmunoassay (RIA), complement fixation, and indirect immunofluorescence assays. *J Med Virol* 1984;13:361–370.
31. Demmler GJ, Steinberg SP, Blum G, et al. Rapid enzyme-linked immunosorbent assay for detecting antibody to varicella-zoster virus. *J Infect Dis* 1988;157:211–212.
32. Larussa P, Steinberg S, Waithe E, et al. Comparison of five assays for antibody to varicella-zoster virus and the fluorescent-antibody-to-membrane-antigen test. *J Clin Microbiol* 1987;25:2059–2062.
33. Grose C, Litwin V. Immunology of the varicella-zoster virus glycoproteins. *J Infect Dis* 1988;157:877–881.
34. Diaz PS, Smith S, Hunter E, et al. Immunity to whole varicella-zoster virus antigen and glycoproteins I and p170: relation to the immunizing regimen of live attenuated varicella vaccine. *J Infect Dis* 1988;158:1245–1252.
35. Provost PJ, Krah DL, Kuter BJ, et al. Antibody assays suitable for assessing immune responses to live varicella vaccine. *Vaccine* 1991;9: 111–116.
36. Steinberg SP, Gershon AA. Measurement of antibodies to varicella-zoster virus by using a latex agglutination test. *J Clin Microbiol* 1991; 29:1527–1529.
37. Bendig, J, Meurisse J, Chambers S. Severe chickenpox during treatment with corticosteroids. *BMJ* 1995;310:327–328.
38. Arvin AM. Cellular and humoral immunity in the pathogenesis of recurrent herpes viral infections in patients with lymphoma. *J Clin Invest* 1980;65:869.
39. Sorensen OS, Haahr S, Moller-Larsen A, et al. Cell-mediated and humoral immunity to herpesviruses during and after herpes zoster infections. *Infect Immun* 1980;29:369–375.
40. Hayes FA, Feldman S. Cell-mediated immunity to varicella zoster virus in children being treated for cancer. *Cancer* 1978;42:159–163.

41. Meyers JD, Flournoy N, Thomas ED. Cell-mediated immunity to varicella-zoster virus after allogeneic marrow transplant. *J Infect Dis* 1980;141:479–487.
42. Giller RH, Bowden RA, Levin MJ, et al. Reduced cellular immunity to varicella zoster virus during treatment for acute lymphoblastic leukemia of childhood: in vitro studies of possible mechanisms. *J Clin Immunol* 1986;6:472–480.
43. Hayward AR, Herberger M. Lymphocyte responses to varicella zoster virus in the elderly. *J Clin Immunol* 1987;7:174–178.
44. Zaia JA, Leary PL, Levin MJ. Specificity of the blastogenic response of human mononuclear cells to herpesvirus antigens. *Infect Immun* 1978;20:646–651.
45. Giller RH, Winistorfer S, Grose C. Cellular and humoral immunity to varicella zoster virus glycoproteins in immune and susceptible human subjects. *J Infect Dis* 1989;160:919–928.
46. Arvin AM, Koropchak CM, Williams BR, et al. Early immune response in healthy and immunocompromised subjects with primary varicella-zoster virus infection. *J Infect Dis* 1986;154:422–429.
47. Arvin AM, Sharp M, Smith S, et al. Equivalent recognition of a varicella-zoster virus immediate early protein (IE62) and glycoprotein I by cytotoxic T lymphocytes of either CD4+ or CD8+ phenotype. *J Immunol* 1991;146:257–264.
48. Asanuma H, Sharp M, Maecker HT, et al. Frequencies of memory T cells specific for varicella-zoster virus, herpes simplex virus, and cytomegalovirus by intracellular detection of cytokine expression. *J Infect Dis* 2000;181:859–866.
49. Smith JG, Liu X, Kaufhold RM, et al. Development and validation of a gamma interferon ELISPOT assay for quantitation of cellular immune responses to varicella-zoster virus. *Clin Diagn Lab Immunol* 2001;8:871–879.
50. Arvin AM, Sharp M, Moir M, et al. Memory cytotoxic T cell responses to viral tegument and regulatory proteins encoded by open reading frames 4, 10, 29, and 62 of varicella-zoster virus. *Viral Immunol* 2002; 15:507–516.
51. Gordon J. The period of infectivity and serum prevention of chickenpox. *JAMA* 1929;93:2013–2015.
52. Ross AH. Modification of chickenpox in family contacts by administration of gamma globulin. *N Engl J Med* 1962;267:369–376.
53. Head H, Campbell AW. The pathology of herpes zoster and its bearing on sensory localization. *Brain* 1900;23:353–523.
54. Hope-Simpson R. The nature of herpes zoster: a long-term study and a new hypothesis. *Proc R Soc Med* 1965;58:9–20.
55. Burgoon D Jr. The natural history of herpes zoster. *JAMA* 1957;164: 265–269.
56. Hope-Simpson R. Herpes zoster in the elderly. *Geriatrics* 1967;22: 151–159.
57. Ragozzino MW, Melton LJ 3rd, Kurland LT, et al. Population-based study of herpes zoster and its sequelae. *Medicine (Baltimore)* 1982; 61:310–316.
58. Gilden DH. Herpes zoster with postherpetic neuralgia—persisting pain and frustration. *N Engl J Med* 1994;330:932–934.
59. Denny-Brown D. Pathologic features of herpes zoster - a note on geniculate herpes. *Arch Neurol Psychol* 1944;51:216–231.
60. Gold E. Serologic and virus-isolation studies of patients with varicella or herpes-zoster infection. *N Engl J Med* 1966;274:181–185.
61. Jellinek EH, Tulloch WS. Herpes zoster with dysfunction of bladder and anus. *Lancet* 1976;2:1219–1222.
62. Jemsek J, Greenberg SB, Taber L, et al. Herpes zoster-associated encephalitis: clinicopathologic report of 12 cases and review of the literature. *Medicine (Baltimore)* 1983;62:81–97.
63. Womack LW, Liesegang TJ. Complications of herpes zoster ophthalmicus. *Arch Ophthalmol* 1983;101:42–45.
64. Winkelmann R. Herpes zoster in children. *JAMA* 1959;171: 376–380.
65. Guess HA, Broughton DD, Melton LJ 3rd, et al. Epidemiology of herpes zoster in children and adolescents: a population-based study. *Pediatrics* 1985;76:512–517.
66. Wharton M. Health impact of varicella in the 1980's [abstract no. 1138]. 30th Interscience Conference on Antimicrobial Agents and Chemotherapy, Atlanta, October 21–24, 1990.
67. Bullowa J. Complications of varicella: I. their occurrence among 2,534 patients. *Am J Dis Child* 1935;49:923–926.
68. Preblud SR. Varicella: complications and costs. *Pediatrics* 1986;78: 728–735.
69. Barrett MJ, Hurwitz ES, Schonberger LB, et al. Changing epidemiology of Reye syndrome in the United States. *Pediatrics* 1986;77: 598–602.
70. Guess HA, Broughton DD, Melton LJ 3rd, et al. Population-based studies of varicella complications. *Pediatrics* 1986;78:723–727.
71. Centers for Disease Control and Prevention. ACIP issues recommendations on the prevention of varicella. *Am Fam Physician* 1996;54: 2578–2581.
72. Centers for Disease Control and Prevention. Varicella-related deaths among children—United States, 1997. *MMWR Morb Mortal Wkly Rep* 1998;47:365–368.
73. Centers for Disease Control and Prevention. Outbreak of invasive group A Streptococcus associated with varicella in a childcare center—Boston, Massachusetts. *MMWR Morb Mortal Wkly Rep* 1997; 46:944–948.
74. Weber D. Varicella pneumonia: study of prevalence in adult men. *JAMA* 1965;192:572–573.
75. Pitel PA, McCormick KL, Fitzgerald E, et al. Subclinical hepatic changes in varicella infection. *Pediatrics* 1980;65:631–633.
76. Hurwitz ES, Nelson DB, Davis C, et al. National surveillance for Reye syndrome: a five-year review. *Pediatrics* 1982;70:895–900.
77. Hurwitz ES, Barrett MJ, Bregman D, et al. Public Health Service study of Reye's syndrome and medications. Report of the main study. *JAMA* 1987;257:1905–1911.
78. Rowe PC, Valle D, Brusilow SW. Inborn errors of metabolism in children referred with Reye's syndrome. A changing pattern. *JAMA* 1988;260:3167–3170.
79. Underwood E. The neurological complications of varicella—a clinical and epidemiologic study. *Br J Child Dis* 1935;32:83–107, 177–196, 241–263.
80. Johnson R, Milbourn PE. Central nervous system manifestations of chickenpox. *Can Med Assoc J* 1970;102:831–834.
81. Lewis G. Zoster sine herpete. *BMJ* 1958;2:418.
82. Mayo DR, Booss J. Varicella zoster-associated neurologic disease without skin lesions. *Arch Neurol* 1989;46:313–315.
83. McCormick WF, Rodnitzky RL, Schochet SS Jr, et al. Varicella-Zoster encephalomyelitis. A morphologic and virologic study. *Arch Neurol* 1969;21:559–570.
84. Gilden DH, Murray RS, Wellish M, et al. Chronic progressive varicella-zoster virus encephalitis in an AIDS patient. *Neurology* 1988; 38:1150–1153.
85. Ghaffar F, Carrick K, Rogers BB, et al. Disseminated infection with varicella-zoster virus vaccine strain presenting as hepatitis in a child with adenosine deaminase deficiency. *Pediatr Infect Dis J* 2000;19: 764–766.
86. Sharrar RG, LaRussa P, Galea SA, et al. The postmarketing safety profile of varicella vaccine. *Vaccine* 2000;19:916–923.
87. Kramer JM, LaRussa P, Tsai WC, et al. Disseminated vaccine strain varicella as the acquired immunodeficiency syndrome-defining illness in a previously undiagnosed child. *Pediatrics* 2001;108:E39.
88. Wright JF, Blanchette VS, Wang H, et al. Characterization of platelet-reactive antibodies in children with varicella-associated acute immune thrombocytopenic purpura (ITP). *Br J Haematol* 1996;95:145–152.
89. Cheatham WJ, Weller TH, Dolan TF Jr. Varicella: report of 2 fatal cases with necroscopy, virus isolation, and serologic studies. *Am J Pathol* 1956;32:1015.
90. Feldman S, Hughes WT, Daniel CB. Varicella in children with cancer: seventy-seven cases. *Pediatrics* 1975;56:388–397.
91. Chang AE, Young NA, Reddick RL, et al. Small bowel obstruction as a complication of disseminated varicella-zoster infection. *Surgery* 1978;83:371–374.
92. Simmons RL, Balfour HH. Complication of disseminated varicella-zoster infection. *Surgery* 1978;83:486–487.
93. Arvin AM, Kushner JH, Feldman S, et al. Human leukocyte interferon for the treatment of varicella in children with cancer. *N Engl J Med* 1982;306:761–765.

94. Prober CG, Kirk LE, Keeney RE. Acyclovir therapy of chickenpox in immunosuppressed children—a collaborative study. *J Pediatr* 1982;101:622–625.
95. Whitley R, Hilty M, Haynes R, et al. Vidarabine therapy of varicella in immunosuppressed patients. *J Pediatr* 1982;101:125–131.
96. Sokol J. Varicella-zoster infection in Hodgkin's disease. *Am J Med* 1965;39:452–463.
97. Locksley RM, Flournoy N, Sullivan KM, et al. Infection with varicella-zoster virus after marrow transplantation. *J Infect Dis* 1985;152: 1172–1181.
98. Schimpff S, Serpick A, Stoler B, et al. Varicella-Zoster infection in patients with cancer. *Ann Intern Med* 1972;76:241–254.
99. Feldman S, Hughes WT, Kim HY. Herpes zoster in children with cancer. *Am J Dis Child* 1973;126:178–184.
100. Balfour HH Jr, Bean B, Laskin OL, et al. Acyclovir halts progression of herpes zoster in immunocompromised patients. *N Engl J Med* 1983; 308:1448–1453.
101. Shepp DH, Dandliker PS, Meyers JD. Treatment of varicella-zoster virus infection in severely immunocompromised patients. A randomized comparison of acyclovir and vidarabine. *N Engl J Med* 1986; 314:208–212.
102. Grose C. Variation on a theme by Fenner: the pathogenesis of chickenpox. *Pediatrics* 1981;68:735–737.
103. Seiler HE. A study of herpes zoster particularly in its relationship to chickenpox. *J Hyg* 1949;47:253–262.
104. Ozaki T, Ichikawa T, Matsui Y, et al. Viremic phase in non-immunocompromised children with varicella. *J Pediatr* 1984;104:85–87.
105. Hyman RW, Ecker JR, Tenser RB. Varicella-zoster virus RNA in human trigeminal ganglia. *Lancet* 1983;2:814–816.
106. Gilden DH, Rozenman Y, Murray R, et al. Detection of varicella-zoster virus nucleic acid in neurons of normal human thoracic ganglia. *Ann Neurol* 1987;22:377–380.
107. Pichini B, Ecker JR, Grose C, et al. DNA mapping of paired varicella-zoster virus isolates from patients with shingles. *Lancet* 1983;2: 1223–1225.
108. Croen KD, Ostrove JM, Dragovic LJ, et al. Patterns of gene expression and sites of latency in human nerve ganglia are different for varicella-zoster and herpes simplex viruses. *Proc Natl Acad Sci U S A* 1988; 85:9773–9777.
109. Rostad SW, Olson K, McDougall J, et al. Transsynaptic spread of varicella zoster virus through the visual system: a mechanism of viral dissemination in the central nervous system. *Hum Pathol* 1989;20: 174–179.
110. Oberg G, Svedmyr A. Varicelliform eruptions in herpes zoster—some clinical and serological observations. *Scand J Infect Dis* 1969;1:47–49.
111. Hutton P. Bilateral zoster and zoster varicellosus. *Lancet* 1935;2:302.
112. Lassker U, Harder TC, Hufnagel M, et al. Rapid molecular discrimination between infection with wild-type varicella-zoster virus and varicella vaccine virus. *Infection* 2002;30:320–322.
113. Alter SJ, Hammond JA, McVey CJ, et al. Susceptibility to varicella-zoster virus among adults at high risk for exposure. *Infect Control* 1986;7:448–451.
114. McKinney WP, Horowitz MM, Battiola RJ. Susceptibility of hospital-based health care personnel to varicella-zoster virus infections. *Am J Infect Control* 1989;17:26–30.
115. Kelley PW, Petruccelli BP, Stehr-Green P, et al. The susceptibility of young adult Americans to vaccine-preventable infections. A national serosurvey of US Army recruits. *JAMA* 1991;266:2724–2729.
116. Ferson MJ, Bell SM, Robertson PW. Determination and importance of varicella immune status of nursing staff in a children's hospital. *J Hosp Infect* 1990;15:347–351.
117. Habel K. Mumps and chickenpox as airborne diseases. *Am J Med Sci* 1945;209:75–78.
118. Nelson A. On the respiratory spread of varicella-zoster virus. *Pediatrics* 1966;37:1007–1009.
119. Leclair JM, Zaia JA, Levin MJ, et al. Airborne transmission of chickenpox in a hospital. *N Engl J Med* 1980;302:450–453.
120. Gustafson TL, Lavely GB, Brawner ER Jr, et al. An outbreak of airborne nosocomial varicella. *Pediatrics* 1982;70:550–556.
121. Thomson F. The aerial conveyance of infection. *Lancet* 1916;1: 341–344.
122. Evans P. An epidemic of chickenpox. *Lancet* 1940;2:339–340.
123. Josephson A, Gombert ME. Airborne transmission of nosocomial varicella from localized zoster. *J Infect Dis* 1988;158:238–241.
124. Seward JF, Watson BM, Peterson CL, et al. Varicella disease after introduction of varicella vaccine in the United States, 1995–2000. *JAMA* 2002;287:606–611.
125. Brunell PA, Kotchmar GS Jr. Zoster in infancy: failure to maintain virus latency following intrauterine infection. *J Pediatr* 1981;98: 71–73.
126. Takahashi M. Clinical overview of varicella vaccine: development and early studies. *Pedatrics* 1986;78:736.
127. Takahashi M. Development of a live attenuated varicella vaccine. *Biken J* 1975;18:25.
128. Loparev V. Improved identification and differentiation of varicella-zoster virus (VZV) wild-type strains and an attenuated varicella vaccine strain using a VZV open reading frame 62-based PCR. *J Clin Microbiol* 2000;38:3156–3160.
129. Gomi Y, Sunamachi H, Mori Y, et al. Comparison of the complete DNA sequences of the Oka varicella vaccine and its parental virus. *J Virol* 2002;76:11447–11459.
130. Ozaki T. Experience with live attenuated varicella vaccine (Oka strain) in healthy Japanese subjects; 10-year survey at pediatric clinic. *Vaccine* 2000;18:2375–2380.
131. Prevention of varicella. Update recommendations of the Advisory Committee on Immunization Practices (ACIP). *MMWR Morb Mortal Wkly Rep* 1999;48:1–5.
132. Harel Z, Ipp L, Riggs S, et al. Serotesting versus presumptive varicella vaccination of adolescents with a negative or uncertain history of chickenpox. *J Adolesc Health* 2001;28:26–29.
133. Smith K. Cost effectiveness of vaccination strategies in adults without a history of chickenpox. *Am J Med* 2000;108:723–729.
134. Levin MJ, Gershon AA, Weinberg A, et al. Immunization of HIV-infected children with varicella vaccine. *J Pediatr* 2001;139:305–310.
135. Donati M, Zuckerman M, Dhawan A, et al. Response to varicella immunization in pediatric liver transplant recipients. *Transplantation* 2000;70:1401–1404.
136. Lim Y. Risk factors for breakthrough varicella in healthy children. *Arch Dis Child* 1998;79:478–480.
137. Krause PR, Klinman DM. Varicella vaccination: evidence for frequent reactivation of the vaccine strain in healthy children. *Nat Med* 2000; 6:451–454.
138. Burgess M. Varicella vaccination of health-care workers. *Vaccine* 1999; 17:765–769.
139. Dykewicz CA. Summary of the guidelines for preventing opportunistic infections among hematopoietic stem cell transplant recipients. *Clin Infect Dis* 2001;33:139–144.
140. Vazquez M, LaRussa PS, Gershon AA, et al. The effectiveness of the varicella vaccine in clinical practice. *N Engl J Med* 2001;344:955–960.
141. Vessey SJ. The effectiveness of the varicella vaccine in clinical practice. *N Engl J Med* 2001;344:955–960.
142. Liang M. Herpes zoster after varicella immunization. *J Am Acad Dermatol* 1998;38:761–763.
143. Brunell PA. Chickenpox attributable to a vaccine virus contracted from a vaccinee with zoster. *Pedatrics* 2000;106:E28.
144. Shields KE, Galil K, Seward J, et al. Varicella vaccine exposure during pregnancy: data from the first 5 years of the pregnancy registry. *Obstet Gynecol* 2001;98:14–19.
145. Gershon AA. Live-attenuated varicella vaccine. *Infect Dis Clin North Am* 2001;15:65–81, viii.
146. Hyams PJ, Stuewe MC, Heitzer V. Herpes zoster causing varicella (chickenpox) in hospital employees: cost of a casual attitude. *Am J Infect Control* 1984;12:2–5.
147. Shehab ZM, Brunell PA. Susceptibility of hospital personnel to varicella-zoster virus. *J Infect Dis* 1984;150:786.
148. Haiduven-Griffiths D, Fecko H. Varicella in hospital personnel: a challenge for the infection control practitioner. *Am J Infect Control* 1987;15:207–211.

149. Meyers JD, MacQuarrie MB, Merigan TC, et al. Nosocomial varicella. Part I: outbreak in oncology patients at a children's hospital. *West J Med* 1979;130:196–199.
150. Morens DM, Bregman DJ, West CM, et al. An outbreak of varicella-zoster virus infection among cancer patients. *Ann Intern Med* 1980; 93:414–419.
151. Myers MG, Rasley DA, Hierholzer WJ. Hospital infection control for varicella zoster virus infection. *Pediatrics* 1982;70:199–202.
152. Garner JS, Simmons BP. Guideline for isolation precautions in hospitals. *Infect Control* 1983;4:245–325.
153. Weitekamp MR, Schan P, Aber RC. An algorithm for the control of nosocomial varicella-zoster virus infection. *Am J Infect Control* 1985; 13:193–198.
154. Takahashi M, Otsuka T, Okuno Y, et al. Live vaccine used to prevent the spread of varicella in children in hospital. *Lancet* 1974;2: 1288–1290.
155. Zaia JA. Clinical spectrum of varicella-zoster virus infection. In: Nahmias A, ed. *The human herpesviruses.* New York: Elsevier North-Holland, 1981.
156. Arvin AM, Koropchak CM, Wittek AE. Immunologic evidence of reinfection with varicella-zoster virus. *J Infect Dis* 1983;148:200–205.
157. Maretic Z. Comparisons between chickenpox in a tropical and a European country. *J Trop Med Hyg* 1963;66:311–315.
158. Sinha DP. Chickenpox—a disease predominantly affecting adults in rural West Bengal, India. *Int J Epidemiol* 1976;5:367–374.
159. Laforet E. Multiple congenital defects following maternal varicella. *N Engl J Med* 1947;236:534–537.
160. Siegel M. Congenital malformations following chickenpox, measles, mumps, and hepatitis. Results of a cohort study. *JAMA* 1973;226: 1521–1524.
161. Enders G. Varicella-zoster virus infection in pregnancy. *Prog Med Virol* 1984;29:166–196.
162. Preblud SR. Varicella-zoster infection in pregnancy. *N Engl J Med* 1986;315:1416.
163. Balducci J, Rodis JF, Rosengren S, et al. Pregnancy outcome following first-trimester varicella infection. *Obstet Gynecol* 1992;79:5–6.
164. Paryani SG, Arvin AM. Intrauterine infection with varicella-zoster virus after maternal varicella. *N Engl J Med* 1986;314:1542–1546.
165. Grose C, Itani O. Pathogenesis of congenital infection with three diverse viruses: varicella-zoster virus, human parvovirus, and human immunodeficiency virus. *Semin Perinatol* 1989;13:278–293.
166. Meyers JD. Congenital varicella in term infants: risk reconsidered. *J Infect Dis* 1974;129:215–217.
167. Gershon AA, Raker R, Steinberg S, et al. Antibody to Varicella-Zoster virus in parturient women and their offspring during the first year of life. *Pediatrics* 1976;58:692–696.
168. Miller E, Cradock-Watson JE, Ridehalgh MK. Outcome in newborn babies given anti-varicella-zoster immunoglobulin after perinatal maternal infection with varicella-zoster virus. *Lancet* 1989;2:371–373.
169. Asano Y, Yoshikawa T, Suga S, et al. Postexposure prophylaxis of varicella in family contact by oral acyclovir. *Pediatrics* 1993;92: 219–222.
170. Lundgren G, Wilczek H, Lonnqvist B, et al. Acyclovir prophylaxis in bone marrow transplant recipients. *Scand J Infect Dis Suppl* 1985; 47:137–44.
171. Steer CB, Szer J, Sasadeusz J, et al. Varicella-zoster infection after allogeneic bone marrow transplantation: incidence, risk factors and prevention with low-dose aciclovir and ganciclovir. *Bone Marrow Transplant* 2000;25:657–664.
172. Fiddian P, Sabin CA, Griffiths PD. Valacyclovir provides optimum acyclovir exposure for prevention of cytomegalovirus and related outcomes after organ transplantation. *J Infect Dis* 2002;186[Suppl 1]: S110–115.
173. Goldstein SL, Somers MJ, Lande MB, Acyclovir prophylaxis of varicella in children with renal disease receiving steroids. *Pediatr Nephrol* 2000;14:305–308.
174. Huang YC, Lin TY, Lin YJ, et al. Prophylaxis of intravenous immunoglobulin and acyclovir in perinatal varicella. *Eur J Pediatr* 2001;160: 91–94.

43

HERPES SIMPLEX VIRUS

STUART P. ADLER

Herpes simplex virus (HSV), a common cause of morbidity among humans, has two distinct serotypes, HSV-1 and HSV-2. HSV-1 primarily causes cold sores; oral or labial lesions are the most common manifestation. HSV-1 is presumably transmitted by contact with infected saliva or cutaneous lesions. HSV-2 is found predominantly in the genital areas and causes vesicular lesions with red borders that often appear in crops or clusters with satellite lesions. Both oral and genital lesions are often swollen and painful but eventually crust over and heal. HSV-2 transmission can be reduced with the use of condoms.

Newborns younger than 1 month are especially susceptible, because infection of the skin and mucous membranes by HSV leads to viremia with viral dissemination to multiple organs, including the central nervous system. Newborns usually become infected at birth via contact with maternal cervical-vaginal secretions infected with HSV-2, but occasionally they become infected via contact with infected personnel or contaminated equipment in the nursery.

In adults, HSV usually causes an asymptomatic infection but occasionally HSV-1, or less commonly HSV-2, invades the central nervous system, causing encephalitis. This occurs when virus in the upper respiratory tract migrates along the olfactory nerve through the cribriform plate, most typically into the frontal or temporal lobes. The most common manifestations of herpes infection, however, are cutaneous, mucocutaneous, or oculocutaneous lesions.

BIOLOGY OF HERPES SIMPLEX VIRUS

HSV particles contain a double-stranded DNA genome enclosed in a nucleocapsid surrounded by enveloped glycoprotein. HSV may survive in humans for decades despite circulating neutralizing antibodies. After a primary infection, the virus usually remains latent in neuroganglion cells. Reactivation from these cells, with or without symptoms, is the hallmark of HSV infection. Reactivation of HSV may occur frequently over time and can be induced by stimuli noxious to the skin, such as ultraviolet radiation.

EPIDEMIOLOGY OF HERPES SIMPLEX VIRUS

The prevalence of HSV infections among humans has been determined by virologic and seroepidemiologic surveys. Based on serologic surveys of adults (antibodies to HSV-1, HSV-2, or both), seroprevalence ranges from 15% to 100% (1–5). Seroprevalence is associated with many variables including socioeconomic status, crowded living conditions, age, geographic location, and sexual practices. Surveys using viral isolation from healthy individuals without HSV disease, to determine prevalence of HSV infection, have found that between 1% and 20% of asymptomatic children and adults are shedding HSV-1 in saliva at any given time. However, in populations in which individuals are cared for or live together for a long time, the prevalence may increase to more than 30% (6).

Immunocompromised patients, particularly those with acquired immunodeficiency syndrome (AIDS) or those who have received a bone marrow or solid organ transplant, will shed HSV either symptomatically or asymptomatically following infection. Estimates of the frequency of asymptomatic infection and seropositive patients after transplantation range up to 80%.

Between 0.1% and 7.3% of men attending sexually transmissible diseases clinics have HSV-2 infections (7). For pregnant women from lower socioeconomic groups, the cumulative incidence of asymptomatic shedding varies between 1% and 4% (8). The cumulative incidence is significantly higher in high-risk populations such as prostitutes, who may have a cumulative incidence up to 12% (9). Asymptomatic genital shedding of HSV-2 is intermittent, and serial studies have found that the virus is not persistently present and varies from individual to individual.

HSV TRANSMISSION IN HOSPITALS

Prevalence of Herpes Simplex Virus Shedding among Hospital Personnel and Adult and Pediatric Patients

No studies have addressed the prevalence of asymptomatic shedding of HSV among hospitalized adults or children. Among institutionalized children, however, one 6-year study that used serologic testing and viral isolation at a children's home found that, of 70 initially seronegative children, eight (11.4%) had a primary infection while at the home and six were symptomatic (6). In another study in Australia, in a home for children younger than 3 years, 29 of 43 seronegative children developed HSV antibodies over 1 year (10). The prevalence of HSV infections among any hospitalized group will depend highly on whether the patients are immunocompromised and on socioeconomic background, the presence of risk factors for HSV, and the history of previous HSV infection. Hence, for practical purposes, hospital personnel should assume that all patients are potentially infectious for HSV.

In 1980, Hatherley et al. (11) studied the frequency of asymptomatic HSV excretion in the saliva of 384 asymptomatic members of the staff of an obstetric hospital. HSV was isolated from 10% of the employees.

Nosocomial HSV Transmission

HSV transmission in the hospital is an infrequent but serious problem when it occurs. Documented hospital transmission of HSV has been confirmed in numerous studies; the virus is transmitted from patient to patient, from personnel to patient, and from patient to personnel.

The patients at highest risk for nosocomial acquisition of HSV are infants younger than 30 days (see Chapter 52). Several studies have documented acquisition of HSV by hospitalized infants, occasionally with fatal outcomes. The first cluster of cases was reported in 1975 by Francis et al. (12), who identified four fatal infections that occurred over a 2-month period in a pediatric intensive care unit. Each patient was infected with HSV-2.

In the late 1970s, DNA fingerprinting for HSV became possible using restriction endonuclease. Halperin et al. (13) first determined that each epidemiologically unrelated strain had a different endonuclease pattern and that strains epidemiologically related had identical DNA fingerprints. This technique has been applied to a number of outbreaks of HSV infection in the hospital and is a potent epidemiologic tool to confirm HSV transmission.

Infants who acquire HSV infection during the first month of life always do so postnatally. The usual source of acquisition is the maternal genital tract, although infants may acquire HSV-1 from labial lesions of either parent; occasionally, infections have been acquired by nursing infants from breast lesions. In 1978, Linnemann et al. (14) observed two infants in a nursery infected within 1 month with HSV-1. The two isolates had identical DNA fingerprints. The source of infection for one child was the father's labial lesion, implying that the second child had acquired HSV virus via horizontal transmission in the nursery.

In 1983, Hammerberg et al. (15) described an HSV outbreak in a nursery in which four infants acquired HSV-1 infection over 10 days. Endonuclease patterns of each of the four isolates were identical, indicating the strong possibility of horizontal transmission. In 1984, Van Dyke and Spector (16) reported a case of apparent transmission of HSV-1 from a physician with a labial lesion to an infant who had received endotracheal suctioning for meconium aspiration. This was the first reported case of transmission of HSV from hospital staff to a patient.

In 1986, Sakaoka et al. (17) reported an unusual outbreak in Japan. They identified three infants who were infected with the same HSV-1 isolate, although the three cases occurred over 2.5 years. None of the mothers of these infants had a history of any genital herpes, and HSV could not be obtained from the genital tract of the mothers. All three infants were infected with a strain with the same restriction endonuclease pattern. This suggested that a single individual in the nursery with recurrent asymptomatic HSV may have infected infants intermittently in the nursery. In a second outbreak, the same authors isolated HSV-1 from three infants in the same room of a hospital within 1 month (17). The mother of one of the infants had herpetic lesions at a genital site at delivery. The infant of this infected mother was the source of infection for the other two infants. The three infants had occupied a common radiant warmer, which was thought to be a potential source of HSV transmission.

The DNA technique has also been used to exclude horizontal transmission. Halperin et al. (13) reported two infants who were cared for side by side in a hospital nursery who both developed HSV infections with HSV-2. Restriction endonuclease patterns of the two isolates were different, indicating that nosocomial transmission had not occurred. Similarly genotyping of the hypervariable region of the HSV-1 genome was used to exclude horizontal transmission of a acyclovir-resistant HSV among four bone marrow recipients in a French hospital (18).

In addition to hospitalized newborns, other patients at risk include surgical patients, particularly burn patients (see Chapter 25). Any patient with a breakdown in the skin has an increased risk for serious HSV infection, because it is easy for HSV to enter the wound and, thus, the bloodstream. In 1985, Brandt et al. (19) used restriction endonuclease patterns to determine that three HSV wound infections that occurred on a burn unit over 6 weeks were caused by unrelated isolates, although temporarily there appeared to be an outbreak in the unit. In 1981, Adams et al. (20) described two outbreaks of HSV-1 infection in a pediatric intensive care unit, one in early summer and one in late summer. In one outbreak, three nurses had herpetic whitlow (cutaneous infection of the fingertip and/or nail bed). The husband of one of the nurses had an acute HSV gingival stomatitis, and a fourth nurse had acute recurrent oral ulcers associated with HSV infection. Restriction endonuclease analysis of the DNA showed that each nurse was infected with the same isolate. In the second outbreak, two different isolates were transmitted in the intensive care unit. In both outbreaks, a patient was identified as the possible source of infection.

In 1992, Perl et al. (21) described an outbreak in a hospital unit caring for adults with cancer. The index patient was a 64-year-old man immunocompromised by lymphoma. He developed perioral HSV-1 infection. He subsequently required intubation, and the physician who intubated him developed herpetic keratoconjunctivitis. The nurse caring for the patient and a family member visiting the man both developed HSV infections with the same strain as the one found in the infected patient. At least once, HSV-1 has also been transmitted via a needlestick. A physician developed vesicles on the hand at the penetration site of a needle used to aspirate oral vesicles of a 2 year old with labial HSV-1 lesions (22).

Thus, there is little doubt that HSV infection is a potentially serious problem for both patients and personnel. Personnel are more likely to acquire HSV from immunocompromised patients who shed high titers of HSV for long periods.

PREVENTION AND CONTROL

Prevention and control of HSV infections in the hospital is easily accomplished by rigorous adherence to standard hygienic practices. Of nine adults with HSV labialis, Turner et al. (23) found HSV in the oral secretions of seven and on the hands of six. HSV survives for as long as 2 hours on skin, 3 hours on cloth, and 4 hours on plastics. HSV is an enveloped virus and, therefore, is easily inactivated by standard denaturing agents such as alcohol, soaps, and detergents. Its survival on fomites and on hands means that rigorous care must be taken to protect personnel and patients from infection from both environmental surfaces and hands (24,25).

Currently, there is no evidence that hospital personnel with genital infections pose a high risk to patients if infected personnel follow good patient care practices. The risk to patients by personnel with oral labial herpes is unknown. Personnel with oral infections, however, can reduce the risk of infecting patients by wearing an appropriate barrier such as a mask over the lesions and avoiding hand contact with the lesions. Hand washing is absolutely essential to prevent transmission from personnel to patients. Personnel with either oral lesions or active cutaneous lesions on the hands should not care for high-risk patients such as neonates and patients with severe malnutrition, burns, or immunodeficiencies.

Personnel who have exposed active lesions of herpes simplex should not work with newborn infants (term or preterm), burn patients, or immunocompromised hosts until all lesions have dried and crusted. Personnel with herpetic whitlow may be more likely to transmit infection by contact (26–28). For personnel with herpetic whitlow, the effectiveness of gloves in preventing transmission is unknown; in general, personnel with herpetic whitlow should not work with patients while they have active lesions. There is no evidence that the treatment of infected personnel with oral antiviral agents such as acyclovir, famciclovir, or valacyclovir, although they may reduce the titer of virus shed, will eliminate the risk of transmission (24,29,30).

Several guidelines for preventing infection of personnel by infected patients have been published. Personnel can prevent infection by avoiding contact with contaminated oral secretions. Such exposure is a hazard for nurses, anesthesiologists, dentists, respiratory personnel, and others who usually have hand contact with the respiratory secretions from patients. Patients in an immunodeficiency state with active HSV infections are more likely to be infectious over a longer period than are immunocompetent individuals. Personnel can protect themselves from such infections by (a) avoiding direct contact with active lesions, (b) wearing gloves on both hands or using no-touch techniques when handling oral and vaginal secretions, and (c) thorough hand washing after patient contact.

Management of Needlesticks

Regarding puncture wounds with needles likely to be contaminated with HSV, there are no available guidelines or controlled trials in humans regarding the efficacy of postexposure prophylaxis using antiviral agents such as famciclovir or valacyclovir. In animal experiments, however, postexposure treatment with these agents inhibited peripheral replication of HSV, reducing the incidence of latent infection but not completely eliminating it (31). Given that orally administered famciclovir and valacyclovir are well absorbed, have minimal toxicity, and are effective in treating HSV, it seems reasonable to use them to prevent latent infection, particularly if antiviral therapy can be started promptly after inoculation. There is one report of the apparent success of famciclovir prophylaxis (500 mg three times daily for 4 days) started within 1 hour after confirmed needlestick inoculation of HSV (32).

Management of Obstetric Patients with HSV Infections

Women on an obstetric ward with proven or suspected genital herpes should be assigned to a private room with a private bath (33). Standard precautions should be taken by personnel who have contact with such women. Meticulous hand washing is important. The infant of a woman who has an active HSV infection or who is asymptomatic but HSV culture positive may be allowed to visit the mother provided the mother washes her hands and wears a clean gown before handling the child. The patient should sit in a chair while holding the infant, and the neonate should not be placed in a bed with the mother; the mother should wear gloves as well. The patient may walk in the hall if she wears a clean gown but may not visit the nursery. Mothers with active genital HSV infections should be treated with acyclovir. These precautionary measures should be maintained for at least 7 days. Also, linens from patients with HSV infections should be considered contaminated and promptly and appropriately bagged for transport to the laundry.

Management of Neonates with Active or Suspected HSV Infection

Infants born of mothers with active HSV infections should be cultured for HSV 48 hours after birth and should be kept in special care under close observation in a nursery unit. The infant should be placed in isolation, which includes gown and glove precautions along with proper disposal and containment of all articles coming in contact with the infant. The infant should be kept in isolation until at least 96 hours have passed since birth and until cultures for HSV including conjunctivae, urine, blood, skin, posterior pharynx, and nose are negative. The infant may go home with the mother and should be followed closely for the first 30 days of life. Prophylactic use of acyclovir in infants exposed to HSV at birth has no known benefit.

Pregnant personnel may care for patients with HSV infections but must observe strict hand-washing techniques (34).

CONCLUSION

HSV infections in the hospital are uncommon, but transmission from patient to patient, patient to personnel, or personnel to patient may occur. In a survey done by Perl et al. (21), the annual rates of nosocomial HSV-1 infection at a large hospital were between 9 and 15 per 10,000 admissions. When clusters of cases occur temporarily within a given unit, transmission should be suspected and isolates gathered and typed by restriction endonuclease digestion to determine the source of the infection. This is important, because occasionally the source is an asymptomatic patient or staff member. HSV transmission is easily prevented by appropriate barrier methods and decontamination of surfaces with standard soaps, detergents, and alcohols. HSV is very labile and easily eliminated from both hands and inanimate surfaces.

REFERENCES

1. Nahmias AJ, Josey WE, Naib ZM, et al. Antibodies to herpesvirus hominis types 1 and 2 in humans. I. Patients with genital herpetic infections. *Am J Epidemiol* 1970;91:539–546.
2. Rawls WE, Campione-Piccardo J. Epidemiology of herpes simplex virus type 1 and type 2. In: Nahmias A, Dowdle W, Schinazi R, eds. *The human herpesviruses: an interdisciplinary perspective.* New York: Elsevier-North Holland, 1981:137–152.
3. Buddingh GJ, Schrum DI, Lanier JC, et al. Studies of the natural history of herpes simplex infections. *Pediatrics* 1953;11:595–610.
4. Guinan ME, Wolinsky SM, Reichman RC. Epidemiology of genital herpes simplex virus infection [Revision]. *Epidemiology* 1985;7: 127–146.
5. Lindgren KM, Douglas RG Jr, Crouch RB. Significance of herpesvirus hominis in respiratory secretions of man. *N Engl J Med* 1968;278: 517–523.
6. Cesario TC, Poland JD, Wulff H. Six years experience with herpes simplex virus in a children's home. *Am J Epidemiol* 1969;90:416–422.
7. Centers for Disease Control and Prevention. Non-reported sexually transmitted diseases in the United States. *MMWR Morb Mortal Wkly Rep* 1979;28:61–63.
8. Tejani N, Klein SW, Kaplan M. Subclinical herpes simplex genitalis infections in the perinatal period. *J Obstet Gynecol* 1979;135:547.
9. Duenas A, Adam E, Melnick JL, et al. Herpesvirus type 2 in a prostitute population. *Am J Epidemiol* 1972;95:483–489.
10. Anderson SG, Hamilton J. The epidemiology of primary herpes simplex infection. *Med J Aust* 1949;1:308–311.
11. Hatherley LI, Hayes K, Jack I. Herpes virus in an obstetric hospital. II: asymptomatic virus excretion in staff members. *Med J Aust* 1980; 2:273–275.
12. Francis DP, Herrmann KL, MacMahon JR, et al. Nosocomial and maternally acquired herpesvirus hominis infections. A report of four fetal cases in neonates. *Am J Dis Child* 1975;129:889–893.
13. Halperin SA, Hendley JO, Nosal C, et al. DNA fingerprinting in investigation of apparent nosocomial acquisition of neonatal herpes simplex. *J Pediatr* 1980;97:91–93.
14. Linnemann CC Jr, Buchman TG, Light IJ, et al. Transmission of herpes-simplex virus type 1 in a nursery for newborn. Identification of viral isolates by D.N.A. fingerprinting. *Lancet* 1978;1:964–966.
15. Hammerberg O, Watts J, Chernesky M, et al. An outbreak of herpes simplex virus type 1 in an intensive care nursery. *Pediatr Infect Dis* 1983;2:290–294.
16. Van Dyke RB, Spector SA. Transmission of herpes simplex virus type 1 to a newborn infant during endotracheal suctioning for meconium aspiration. *Pediatr Infect Dis* 1984;3:153–156.
17. Sakaoka H, Saheki Y, Uzuki K, et al. Two outbreaks of herpes simplex virus type 1 nosocomial infection among newborns. *J Clin Microbiol* 1986;24:36–40.
18. Venard V, Dauendorffer JN, Carret AS, et al. Investigation of acyclovir-resistant herpes simplex virus I infection in a bone marrow transplantation unit: genotyping shows that different strains are involved. *J Hosp Infect* 2001;47:161–167.
19. Brandt SJ, Tribble CG, Lakeman AD, et al. Herpes simplex burn wound infections: epidemiology of a case cluster and responses to acyclovir therapy. *Surgery* 1985;98:238–243.
20. Adams G, Stover BH, Keenlyside RA, et al. Nosocomial herpetic infections in a pediatric intensive care unit. *Am J Epidemiol* 1981;113: 126–132.
21. Perl TM, Haugen TH, Pfaller MA, et al. Transmission of herpes simplex virus type 1 infection in an intensive care unit. *Ann Intern Med* 1992;117:584–586.
22. Douglas MW, Walters JL, Currie BJ. Occupational infection with herpes simplex virus type I after a needlestick injury. *Med J Aust* 2002; 176:240.
23. Turner R, Shehab Z, Osborne K, et al. Shedding and survival of herpes simplex virus from fever blisters. *Pediatrics* 1982;70:547–549.
24. Valenti WM, Betts RF, Hall CB, et al. Nosocomial viral infections: II. guidelines for prevention and control of respiratory viruses, herpesviruses, and hepatitis viruses. *Infect Control* 1980;1:165–178.
25. Valenti WM, Mengus MA, Hall CB, et al. Nosocomial viral infections: I. epidemiology and significance. *Infect Control* 1980;1:33–37.
26. Louis DS, Silva J Jr. Herpetic whitlow: herpetic infections of the digits. *J Hand Surg* 1979;4:90–94.
27. Lucey J, Baroni M. Herpetic whitlow. *Am J Nurs* 1984;84:60–61.
28. Dunbar C. Herpetic whitlow: an occupational hazard for nursing personnel. *Heart Lung* 1978;7:645–646.
29. Williams WW. CDC guidelines for the prevention and control of nosocomial infections. Guideline for infection control in hospital personnel. *Am J Infect Control* 1984;12:34–63.
30. Simmons BP, Gelfand MS. Herpes simplex virus. *Infect Control* 1986; 7:380–383.
31. Thackray AM, Field HJ. Comparison of the effects of famciclovir and valaciclovir on pathogenesis of herpes simplex virus type 2 in a murine infection model. *Antimicrob Agents Chemother* 1996;40:846–851.
32. Manian FA. Potential role of famciclovir for prevention of herpetic whitlow in the health care setting. *Clin Infect Dis* 2000;31:E18–E19.
33. Gibbs RS. Infection control of herpes simplex virus infections in obstetrics and gynecology. *J Reprod Med* 1986;31(Suppl 5):395–398.
34. Valenti WM. Infection control and the pregnant health care worker. *Am J Infect Control* 1986;14:20–27.

44

CYTOMEGALOVIRUS

STUART P. ADLER

During pregnancy, if a woman acquires a primary infection with cytomegalovirus (CMV), the fetus is placed at highest risk for symptomatic congenital disease. Because of this risk and because acquisition of a primary CMV infection is often associated with morbidity and mortality in very low birth weight infants, immunocompromised patients, and transplant recipients, concern has been raised about the possible transmission of CMV within hospitals. Several studies of the hospital transmission of CMV have been completed. To accurately interpret these studies and understand the hospital transmission of CMV, one must first have a basic understanding of the virus and the way that it is transmitted within the general population.

BIOLOGY, DIAGNOSIS, AND CLINICAL FEATURES

Human CMV and the other human herpesviruses share certain common features. All human herpesviruses contain large DNA genomes, and CMV has the largest with a DNA molecular weight of 150 million. In addition, they all feature a nucleic acid core, a nucleocapsid, and an envelope glycoprotein derived primarily from the cell membrane when mature virions bud from within one cell to another. This cell membrane makes the virus very susceptible to inactivation by common disinfectants.

A transient viremia is produced by a primary infection with CMV. For immunocompetent individuals, primary CMV infections are almost always asymptomatic, although CMV occasionally causes an infectious mononucleosis syndrome in adults. For immunocompromised patients, particularly those immunosuppressed because of the acquired immunodeficiency syndrome (AIDS) or bone marrow transplantation, CMV infections may cause severe disease in almost any organ system. CMV appears to be able to replicate in all tissues and organs, and when immunity, particularly cell-mediated immunity, is deficient, reactivation of latent CMV infections is common. The severity and location of tissue inflammation associated with CMV depends on the degree of immunosuppression. Among transplant recipients of solid organs, those who are seronegative before transplantation and acquire CMV via a donor organ or infected blood have the most severe CMV disease after transplantation. This disease is often associated with fever, neutropenia, and, occasionally, organ rejection.

CMV infections are best diagnosed by recovery of the virus from infected tissues or organs. In tissues with high titers of virus, histopathologic examination may reveal the presence of CMV inclusion cells. In immunocompromised patients, viremia is very common. In immunocompetent individuals, viremia occurs only transiently during a primary infection. The viremia clears with the appearance of neutralizing antibodies. However, the virus eludes antibody neutralization within tissues when it buds from cell to cell, thus causing, in most cases, a focal infection. Viral excretion of the original infecting strain may resume at any time; therefore, CMV apparently becomes latent. Such latency is most often noted in individuals with severely impaired cellular immunity; in these individuals, a secondary viremia may disseminate the virus to all organs and tissues. A latent infection can recur, and reinfection with a second strain of CMV may occur in both immunocompetent and immunocompromised individuals. To date, no studies have revealed the frequency of naturally occurring reinfection (1–6).

EPIDEMIOLOGY

Because CMV is ubiquitous in the human population, nearly all individuals eventually become infected. The percentage of seropositive individuals in central Virginia increases with age approximately 1% or 2% per year, and a mean of about 50% of the population possesses antibodies to the virus (7). Nearly 100% of these individuals are seropositive by age 70. Around the world, the mean seropositivity rate for particular populations varies with location, race, and socioeconomic status; regardless of location, however, nearly all individuals eventually become seropositive (8–13).

One can also examine the prevalence of CMV infection within a particular population by determining the frequency of viral excretion. The rate of excretion for any age group depends on many factors, including geographic location, and is extremely variable. The congenital infection rate worldwide, however, is remarkably constant; in any population, between 0.5% and 2% of newborns excrete CMV (14–18).

For the most part, CMV produces no disease when acquired postnatally. A few adults with CMV may develop an infectious mononucleosis syndrome. Viremia persists for a few days or weeks following a primary infection, and prolonged viral excretion in saliva and urine may persist for weeks or months. After infection, young children excrete CMV in saliva and urine for a period of 12 to 40 months, significantly longer than adults do (1). Immunoglobulin G (IgG) antibodies to CMV appear 2 to 3 weeks following a primary infection and persist for life in both children and adults.

When, where, and how is CMV transmitted? In up to 2% of all pregnancies, transplacental transmission may occur. In most cases of transmission, the mother is seropositive before becoming pregnant, and the infants become congenitally infected *in utero* following a recurrence of the mother's infection. Although primary maternal infection during pregnancy is responsible for only a small percentage of the total number of congenitally infected newborns, it is responsible for the majority of the symptomatic infections and severe handicaps caused by congenital infection (14–18). Perinatal transmission rather than transplacental transmission accounts for most CMV infections acquired by infants. Breast milk is the most common form of transmission of CMV from seropositive mothers and accounts for up to 50% of transmitted infections; 10% to 20% transmit the infection via cervical and vaginal secretions (19). Also, CMV can be acquired postnatally from other children, such as in a day care setting; intrafamilial transmission is frequent following a primary infection in a single family member, with a rate of transmission of about 50% (20).

CMV is often excreted in semen and cervical secretions. In addition, CMV infections are more prevalent among those who have multiple sex partners. However, the frequency of sexual transmission of CMV is problematic, because the virus can be transmitted orally or by close and frequent contact.

There is clear evidence of how slowly CMV is transmitted, even under optimal circumstances, which has been documented in studies of CMV transmission among children in day care. Children initially shed CMV at a concentration of about 10^4 plaque-forming units per milliliter (PFUs/mL) of urine following a primary infection; this titer declines slowly thereafter (21). Those younger than 2 years shed CMV for between 6 and 40 months with a mean of about 2 years (1).

Our group monitored three day care centers in Richmond for 3 years (1). At the three centers, 14%, 27%, and 45% of the children became infected, with most becoming infected in the second year of life. The most significant data indicate that, even at the center with the highest rate of infection, on average only one child per month acquired a primary CMV infection. Therefore, even under ideal transmission conditions of close, intimate daily contact (i.e., children playing daily together in the same room), the virus is transmitted slowly.

The period for CMV transmission from infected children to their mothers or caregivers is also very slow and depends on the age of an infected child (22). We observed that, among the seronegative mothers of infected children, 16 (57%) of 28 mothers with infected children 20 months of age or younger acquired CMV from their children, whereas only 3 (14%) of 22 mothers with infected children older than 20 months acquired the infection ($p < .007$). In the group of mothers with infected children younger than 20 months, the average interval between identification of the child's infection and transmission to the mother was 8 months (SD = ± 6 months).

Caregivers can also be infected with CMV through transmission from children (23–25). We studied 614 caregivers in Richmond, and the rate of CMV infections among caregivers was independently associated with the age and race of the caregiver and the ages of children for whom they cared. The highest rate of CMV infections occurred in women caring for children younger than 2 years, independent of age and race (23,24). For the caregivers in our study, the annual seroconversion rate was 11% for a group of 202 initially seronegative women, compared with a 2% rate for hospital employees during the same period.

CMV TRANSMISSION IN HOSPITALS

Prevalence of CMV Excretion among Hospitalized Adults and Children

The previous short review of CMV transmission outside the hospital describes the relative rates of transmission and indicates why nearly all the hospital transmission studies have been conducted in pediatric units.

In general, children have higher excretion rates than adults as indicated by published reports on the prevalence of CMV excretion among hospitalized adults and children. In a home care setting, 8% of children younger than 5 years excrete CMV (26–29). This rate increases to between 9% and 75% for children in day care depending on the day care center (1,21,30–39). Between 1% and 7% of hospitalized children beyond the newborn period shed CMV (28,29,40–45). From 1% to 3% of infants in newborn nurseries shed CMV at any time (44,46,47).

Viremia is rare among healthy adults, and less than 1% are viruric. Likewise, in a study completed on a general oncology ward in Richmond, less than 1% of adult patients excreted CMV (48). Published data suggest that up to 45% of bone marrow recipients may excrete CMV, but at present this percentage may be decreasing because of blood and marrow donor selection and the frequent use of ganciclovir (49–51). Among AIDS patients, rates of CMV excretion vary widely, but it is probable that at least 25% of symptomatic patients shed CMV (52). In the 1970s, between 38% and 96% of kidney recipients excreted CMV (53–59). Again, current rates are probably lower, because cyclosporine is less immunosuppressive than previously used drugs were. Finally, 8% to 35% of pregnant women excrete CMV in the third trimester (60,61).

An examination of CMV infection at eight different hospital units in two children's hospitals was completed by Demmler et al. (44) in Houston, Texas. The group surveyed each unit at least three times and surveyed the chronic care unit 18 times. Infection rates in the units ranged from 3% to 6%, but the chronic care units had much higher rates of CMV infection (15%). In these units, the children were together for many months, were chronically ill, and had multiple blood transfusions. Overall, infection rates among hospitalized children in Houston were similar to those observed in an earlier study of hospitalized children in Richmond.

CMV on Surfaces

Where is CMV found in a hospital setting, in addition to the presence of CMV in the urine and saliva of infected patients? In Houston the Demmler group (44) obtained numerous environmental samples and surface swabs for CMV culture including toys, Ambu bags, scales, intravenous tubing, crib rails, and thermometers. The swabs did not recover CMV from any inanimate object. However, the virus was isolated on the hands of a patient, a nurse, and a laboratory worker. Hands are a known reservoir for CMV. In Birmingham, Alabama, a similar survey done in day care centers recovered CMV from the hands of children and caregivers (62).

It is easy to deactivate CMV with such products as soaps, detergents, and alcohol; CMV also washes off surfaces with plain water (63). The virus is not very stable in the environment (64). CMV has a half life of 2 to 6 hours on surfaces, but low titers of virus may persist for 24 hours.

Transmission from Patients to Personnel—Published Rates of CMV Infection among Pediatric Nurses and Controls

Table 44.1 (44,46,47,65–69) lists the published rates of CMV infection among pediatric nurses and control subjects (women without patient contact). Relatively low numbers of primary CMV infections and low numbers of total subjects have affected the results of each survey. In the early 1970s, Yeager (65) first reported data that suggested a nosocomial infection risk for pediatric nurses. Her group observed infection in 3 of 31 ward nurses, 2 of 34 nursery nurses, and 0 of 27 control subjects. Studies in Sweden and Philadelphia showed similar results, but low rates of CMV infection were found in studies in Richmond, Birmingham, Houston, and Minneapolis (see Table 44.1).

One observation that has been consistent among all the studies is a relatively low infection rate among the control subjects. When the infection rates (number of persons infected per 100 person-years observed) for each of the studies listed in Table 44.1 were averaged, a higher annual infection rate was found among those who worked in pediatric hospitals than among the control subjects. Ward nurses display an annual average infection rate of 3.1 infections/100 person-years (24 infections for 778 person-years); this does not differ statistically from the 2.1 infections/100 person-years (45 infections for 2,126 person-years) observed for the control group. In nursery nurses the average annual infection rate is 3.9 infections/100 person-years (21 infections for 534 person-years), which is a significantly higher rate than that observed in the control group ($p < .05$, chi-square $= 4.8$, 1 degree of freedom).

The previous analysis should be approached with skepticism for several reasons. First, the statistical analysis depends on the large group of pregnant women who served as controls in the Birmingham study. If this control group had not been available, the analysis would lack sufficient statistical power to detect small differences among groups. Second, in three of the studies, nursery nurses did not acquire CMV from infected infants in their care, according to restriction enzyme analysis data. This was true of one woman in the Richmond study, of two in the Birmingham study, and of two in the Houston study. Third, one may be comparing very dissimilar groups when combining studies, because nurses engage in many different activities, and these activities and their relative frequencies may vary widely among hospitals. For example, a recent French study after adjusting CMV seroprevalence for age and parity, found that nurses aides caring for children and immunocompromised adults, who worked in close contact with patients, had a rate of CMV seroprevalence higher than that observed among nurses with more technical skills caring for similar patients (57.3% vs. 34.5%, $p < 0.01$), suggesting that nurses with prolonged close contact may have the greatest risk for CMV acquisition from patients (70). Fourth, the highest rate of infection occurs in nursery nurses, and these nurses care for children with the lowest rate of CMV excretion. Summarizing the data in Table 44.1, under

TABLE 44.1. RATES OF PRIMARY CYTOMEGALOVIRUS (CMV) INFECTION AMONG PEDIATRIC NURSES AND CONTROL SUBJECTS

		Ward nurses		Nursery nurses		Controls (women without patient contact)	
Authors	Location (reference)	Annual seroconversion rate[a]	No. of nurses studied	Annual seroconversion rate	No. of nurses studied	Annual seroconversion rate	No. of women studied
Yeager, et al.	Denver, CO (65)	7.7 (3/39)[b]	31	4.1 (2/49)	34	0	27[c]
Ahlfors, et al.	Malmo, Sweden (66)	6.9 (2/29)	29	—	—	3.0 (1/33)	52
Dworsky, et al.	Birmingham, AL (46)	—	—	3.4 (4/118)	61	2.3 (23/1,000)	1,549
Friedman, et al.	Philadelphia, PA (67)	6.0 (7/117)	115	13 (3/23)	23	2.9 (1/35)	35
Adler, et al.	Richmond, VA (47)	4.4 (2/45)	31	1.8 (1/55)	40	—	—
Demmler, et al.	Houston, TX (44)	0	48[c]	6.5 (7/107)	70	—	—
Balfour, et al.	Minneapolis, MN (68)	1 (2/200)[d]	117	2.2 (4/182)	96	1.8 (16/867)	519
Balcarek, et al.	Birmingham, AL (69)	2.3 (8/348)[e]	183	—	—	2.1 (4/191)	105
All studies		3.1 (24/778)[f]	506	3.9 (21/534)	324	2.1 (45/2,126)	2,260

[a] Seroconversions per 100 person-years observed.
[b] Numbers in parentheses are the number of women seroconverting per total number of person-years observed. Not all women were monitored for 1 year.
[c] Not included in the total number of nurses per women studied or in the summary of all studies, because the person-years per subject could not be calculated.
[d] Renal transplantation/dialysis nurses.
[e] A mixture of nurses and other women with patient contact.
[f] See text for statistical comparisons.

the worst circumstances, the rate of CMV infection for nursery nurses is probably no more than three times higher than the rate for control subjects (relative risk = 1.83; 95% confidence interval = 1.01 to 3.04).

Patient-to-Patient Transmission

A powerful tool for studying CMV transmission is analysis of viral DNA. Table 44.2 lists the results of studies that applied this technique to epidemiologic studies of CMV in the hospital. Between 1982 and 1985, my colleagues and I monitored the number of children in the newborn nursery in Richmond who were shedding CMV virus and the periods they were viruric while hospitalized (47). We monitored 40 seronegative women over the course of this study. One of this group seroconverted, but she shed an isolate that had a DNA pattern different from 34 of the isolates excreted by the children in the nursery for that period. Also, no infant-to-infant transmission occurred.

In Durham, it was believed that a house officer had acquired CMV from a child in her care, but the DNA of her isolate differed from that of the isolate shed by the child (71). Surveys revealed similar observations for nurses in Houston and Birmingham (46,72).

In 1983, Spector (73) used DNA analysis of viral isolates to conclude that two babies in a neonatal nursery in Oakland had probably acquired CMV from another infected infant in that nursery. The infants became infected after being located side by side for approximately 6 weeks. They received care from common caregivers but did not receive blood from common donors.

In another study in Houston, Demmler et al. (44) studied the DNA patterns of 27 viral isolates, 24 from children and 3 from nurses, derived from 18 sets of samples obtained for culture from children and staff on a pediatric chronic care unit. Four children produced two pairs of identical isolates. Because one pair of children had shared a common blood donor, it is uncertain whether the CMV was acquired from the blood donor or via horizontal transmission. The second pair of children who shed identical isolates had been given care for 20 weeks or more side by side in the same unit, and they had not received blood from a common donor. One nurse had cared for both children for 3 weeks. Therefore, it is reasonable to assume that these children shed isolates with identical DNA patterns because patient-to-patient transmission occurred.

Based on analysis of viral DNA, there have been no documented instances of CMV transmission from patients to hospital caregivers, but, at least in the two reports cited previously, patient-to-patient transmission probably did occur. In both cases, patient-to-patient transmission occurred in chronic care units with children crowded side by side for long periods; this is an institutional setting similar to that of day care.

PREVENTION AND CONTROL

According to published data, CMV transmission from patients to hospital personnel occurs rarely, if at all, and has never been documented. An analysis of the seroconversion data shows that there may be an annual infection rate 1% to 4% greater for nursery nurses than for the general population, but, as noted previously, there are many problems with this type of analysis of published data.

CMV may be transmitted between hospitalized patients, but transmission is easily prevented. Soap and water readily inactivate the virus, and simple hand-washing techniques should prevent transmission.

If strictly adhered to, standard precautions will protect both patients and personnel (74,75). One should not be concerned about patient-to-patient transmission unless dealing with immunocompromised patients or premature infants. In either of those situations, one should be very careful about the kinds of contact these patients have with other patients and personnel; one should adhere to frequent and adequate hand-washing techniques and to standard precautions.

It is not necessary to test hospital personnel for CMV immunity either before or during pregnancy because of the low incidence of infection, the high cost of testing, the difficulty in establishing a diagnosis of primary infection during pregnancy, and the extreme uncertainties involved in counseling a woman who acquires CMV during pregnancy. Pregnant women also should not be furloughed or transferred with the idea that their exposure frequency would decrease on different units. They should instead assume that all patients may be infectious and are best advised to practice frequent hand washing and strictly adhere to standard precautions. Standard precautions apply to all body fluids, secretions, and excretions except sweat, regardless of whether or not they contain visible blood; thus, pregnant

TABLE 44.2. CYTOMEGALOVIRUS (CMV) TRANSMISSION STUDIES USING ANALYSIS OF VIRAL DNA

			Number of isolates studied		Number of isolates	
Authors	Location (reference)	Type of unit	Children	Nurses	Different	Identical
Wilfert, et al.	Durham, NC (71)	NICU	1	1	2	0
Yow, et al.	Houston, TX (72)	NICU	1	1	2	0
Spector	Oakland, CA (73)	NICU	7	0	4	3
Dworsky, et al.	Birmingham, AL (46)	NICU	1	1	2	0
Adler, et al.	Richmond, VA (47)	NICU	34	1	35	0
Demmler, et al.	Houston, TX (44)	Chronic care	24	3	25	2

NICU, neonatal intensive care unit.

hospital personnel should assume that all body fluids are possibly infectious. As stated previously, they should practice frequent hand washing after patient contact. When they perceive that they are most likely to be exposed to body fluids or when they are handling urine and respiratory secretions, they should wear gowns and gloves.

Although CMV is seldom, if ever, transmitted via respiratory droplets, the polymerase chain reaction, a very sensitive method for detecting minute quantities of DNA, has detected CMV DNA in the filtered air near immunosuppressed patients with CMV pneumonia and other respiratory infections (76). Because the infectivity of aerosols from such patients is unknown, use of a mask by pregnant women is appropriate when prolonged or frequent exposure to aerosolized urine or respiratory secretions is likely to occur.

REFERENCES

1. Adler SP. Molecular epidemiology of cytomegalovirus: a study of factors affecting transmission among children at three day-care centers. *Pediatr Infect Dis J* 1991;10:584–590.
2. Collier AC, Chandler SH, Handsfield HH, et al. Identification of multiple strains of cytomegalovirus in homosexual men. *J Infect Dis* 1989;159:123–126.
3. Chandler SH, Handsfield HH, McDougall JK. Isolation of multiple strains of cytomegalovirus from women attending a clinic for sexually transmitted diseases. *J Infect Dis* 1987;155:655–660.
4. Spector SA, Hirata KK, Neuman TR. Identification of multiple cytomegalovirus strains in homosexual men with acquired immunodeficiency syndrome. *J Infect Dis* 1984;150:953–956.
5. Drew WL, Sweet ES, Miner RC, et al. Multiple infections by cytomegalovirus in patients with acquired immunodeficiency syndrome: documentation by Southern blot hybridization. *J Infect Dis* 1984;150: 952–953.
6. Chou S. Acquisition of donor strains of cytomegalovirus by renal-transplant recipients. *N Engl J Med* 1986;134:1418–1423.
7. Bodurtha J, Adler SP, Nance WE. Seroepidemiology of cytomegalovirus and herpes simplex virus in twins and their families. *Am J Epidemiol* 1988;128:268–276.
8. Evans AS, Cook J, Kapikian AZ, et al. A serological survey of St. Lucia. *Int J Epidemiol* 1979;8:327–332.
9. Krech UH, Jung M. Age distribution of complement-fixing antibodies in Tanzania, 1970. In: Krech UH, Jung M, Jung F, eds. *Cytomegalovirus infections of man.* New York: S. Karger, 1971:27–28.
10. Evans A, Cox F, Nankervis G, et al. A health and seroepidemiological survey of a community in Barbados. *Int J Epidemiol* 1974;3:167–175.
11. Palacios O, Cavau N, Horaud F, et al. Serologic survey of antibodies to cytomegalovirus in women and infants in Lima, Peru. *J Infect Dis* 1983;147:777.
12. Williams JO, Fagbami AH, Omilabu SA. Cytomegalovirus antibodies in Nigeria. *Trans R Soc Trop Med Hyg* 1989;83:260.
13. Liu Z, Wang E, Taylor W, et al. Prevalence survey of cytomegalovirus infection in children in Chengdu. *Am J Epidemiol* 1990;131:143–150.
14. Stagno S, Pass RF, Cloud G, et al. Primary cytomegalovirus infection in pregnancy, incidence, transmission to fetus, and clinical outcome. *JAMA* 1986;256:1904–1908.
15. Grant S, Edmond JE, Syme J. A prospective study of cytomegalovirus infection in pregnancy. I. Laboratory evidence of congenital infection following maternal primary and reactivated infection. *J Infect* 1981;3: 24–31.
16. Griffiths PD, Baboonian C. A prospective study of primary cytomegalovirus infection during pregnancy: final report. *Br J Obstet Gynaecol* 1984;91:307–315.
17. Ahlfors K, Ivarsson SA, Harris S, et al. Congenital cytomegalovirus infection and disease in Sweden and the relative importance of primary and secondary maternal infections: preliminary findings from a prospective study. *Scand J Infect Dis* 1984;16:129–137.
18. Nankervis GA, Kumar ML, Cox FE, et al. A prospective study of maternal cytomegalovirus infection and its effect on the fetus. *Am J Obstet Gynecol* 1984;149:435–440.
19. Dworsky M, Yow M, Stagno S, et al. Cytomegalovirus infection of breast milk and transmission in infancy. *Pediatrics* 1983;72:295–299.
20. Taber LH, Frank AL, Yow MD, et al. Acquisition of cytomegaloviral infections in families with young children: a serological study. *J Infect Dis* 1985;151:948–952.
21. Murph JR, Bale JF. The natural history of acquired cytomegalovirus infection among children in group day care. *Am J Dis Child* 1988;142: 843–846.
22. Adler SP. Cytomegalovirus and child day care: risk factors for maternal infection. *Pediatr Infect Dis J* 1991;10:590–594.
23. Adler SP. Cytomegalovirus and child day care: evidence for an increased infection rate among day-care workers. *N Engl J Med* 1989;321: 1290–1296.
24. Pass RF, Hutto C, Lyon MD, et al. Increased rate of cytomegalovirus infection among day care center workers. *Pediatr Infect Dis J* 1990;9: 465–470.
25. Murph JR, Baron JC, Brown CK, et al. The occupational risk of cytomegalovirus infection among day-care providers. *JAMA* 1991;265: 603–608.
26. Levinsohn EM, Foy HM, Kenny GE, et al. Isolation of cytomegalovirus from a cohort of 100 infants throughout the first year of life. *Proc Soc Exp Biol Med* 1969;132:957–962.
27. Hutto C, Ricks R, Garvie M, et al. Epidemiology of cytomegalovirus infections in young children: day care vs. home care. *Pediatr Infect Dis* 1985;4:149–152.
28. Hanshaw JB, Betts RF, Simon G, et al. Acquired cytomegalovirus infection: association with hepatomegaly and abnormal liver-function tests. *N Engl J Med* 1965;272:602–609.
29. Adler SP. The molecular epidemiology of cytomegalovirus transmission among children attending a day care center. *J Infect Dis* 1985;152: 760–768.
30. Pass RF, August AM, Dworsky M, et al. Cytomegalovirus infection in a day-care center. *N Engl J Med* 1982;307:477–479.
31. Jones LA, Duke-Duncan PM. Cytomegaloviral infections in infant-toddler centers: centers for the developmentally delayed versus regular day care. *J Infect Dis* 1985;151:953–955.
32. Murph JR, Bale JF, Murray JC, et al. Cytomegalovirus transmission in a midwest day care center: possible relationship to child care practices. *J Pediatr* 1986;109:35–39.
33. Adler SP. Molecular epidemiology of cytomegalovirus: viral transmission among children attending a day care center, their parents, and caretakers. *J Pediatr* 1988;112:366–372.
34. Prevalence of cytomegalovirus excretion from children in five day-care centers: Alabama. *MMWR* 1985;34:49–51.
35. Volpi A, Pica F, Cauletti A, et al. Cytomegalovirus infection in day care centers in Rome, Italy: viral excretion in children and occupational risk among workers. *J Med Virol* 1988;26:119–125.
36. Grillner L, Strangert K. A prospective molecular epidemiological study of cytomegalovirus infections in two day care centers in Sweden: no evidence for horizontal transmission within the centers. *J Infect Dis* 1988;157:1080–1083.
37. Nelson DB, Peckham CS, Pearl KN, et al. Cytomegalovirus infection in day nurseries. *Arch Dis Child* 1987;62:329–332.
38. Adler SP. Cytomegalovirus transmission among children in day care, their mothers and caretakers. *Pediatr Infect Dis* 1988;7:279–285.
39. Grillner L, Strangert K. Restriction endonuclease analysis of cytomegalovirus DNA from strains isolated in day care centers. *Pediatr Infect Dis* 1986;5:184– 187.
40. MacDonald H, Tobin JO. Congenital cytomegalovirus infection: a collaborative study on epidemiological, clinical and laboratory findings. *Dev Med Child Neurol* 1978;20:471–482.
41. Stern H. Isolation of cytomegalovirus and clinical manifestations of infection at different ages. *BMJ* 1968;1:665–669.
42. Ahlfors K. Ivarsson SA, Johnsson T, et al. Congenital and acquired

cytomegalovirus infections. Virological and clinical studies on a Swedish infant population. *Acta Paediatr Scand* 1978;67:321–328.
43. Brady, MT, Demmler GJ, Seavy D, et al. Method of blood processing affects the prevalence of cytomegalovirus excretion in newborn nurseries. *Am J Infect Control* 1987;15:245–248.
44. Demmler GJ, Yow MD, Spector SA, et al. Nosocomial cytomegalovirus infections within two hospitals caring for infants and children. *J Infect Dis* 1987;156:9– 16.
45. Brady MT, Demmler GJ, Reis S. Factors associated with cytomegalovirus excretion in hospitalized children. *Am J Infect Control* 1988;16: 41–45.
46. Dworsky ME, Welch K, Cassady G, et al. Occupational risk for primary cytomegalovirus infection among pediatric health-care workers. *N Engl J Med* 1983;309:950–953.
47. Adler SP, Baggett J, Wilson M, et al. Molecular epidemiology of cytomegalovirus transmission in a nursery: lack of evidence for nosocomial transmission. *J Pediatr* 1986;108:117–123.
48. McVoy MA, Adler SP. Immunologic evidence for frequent age related cytomegalovirus reactivation in seropositive immunocompetent individuals. *J Infect Dis* 1989;160:1–10.
49. Neiman PE, Reeves W, Ray G, et al. A prospective analysis of interstitial pneumonia and opportunistic viral infection among recipients of allogeneic bone marrow grafts. *J Infect Dis* 1977;136:754–767.
50. Winston DJ, Gale RP, Meyer DV, et al., and the UCLA Bone Marrow Transplantation Group. Infectious complications of human bone marrow transplantation. *Medicine* 1979;58:1–31.
51. Meyers JD, Flournoy N, Thomas ED. Nonbacterial pneumonia after allogeneic marrow transplantation: a review of ten years' experience. *Rev Infect Dis* 1982;4:1119–1132.
52. Rodgers MF, Morens DM, Stewart JA, et al. National case-control study of Kaposi's sarcoma and *Pneumocystis carinii* pneumonia in homosexual men. Part 2. Laboratory results. *Ann Intern Med* 1983;99: 151–158.
53. Armstrong JA, Evans AS, Rao N, et al. Viral infections in renal transplant recipients. *Infect Immun* 1976;14:970–975.
54. Fiala M, Payne JE, Berne TV, et al. Epidemiology of cytomegalovirus infection after transplantation and immunosuppression. *J Infect Dis* 1975;132:421– 433.
55. Gadler H, Tillegard A, Groth CG. Studies of cytomegalovirus infection in renal allograft recipients. I. Virus isolation. *Scand J Infect Dis* 1982; 14:81–87.
56. Rubin RH, Wolfson JS, Cosimi AB, et al. Infection in the renal transplant recipient. *Am J Med* 1981;70:405–411.
57. Ramos E, Karmi S, Alogi SV, et al. Infectious complications in renal transplant recipients. *South Med J* 1980;73:751–754.
58. Rubin RH, Cosimi AB, Tolkoff-Rubin NE, et al. Infectious disease syndromes attributable to cytomegalovirus and their significance among renal transplant recipients. *Transplantation* 1977;24:458–464.
59. Glenn J. Cytomegalovirus infections following renal transplantation. *Rev Infect Dis* 1981;3:1151–1178.
60. Stagno S, Pass RF, Dworsky ME, et al. Maternal cytomegalovirus infection and prenatal transmission. *Clin Obstet Gynecol* 1982;25:563–576.
61. Chandler SH, Alexander ER, Holmes KK. Epidemiology of cytomegalovirus infection in a heterogeneous population of pregnant women. *J Infect Dis* 1985;152:249–256.
62. Hutto C, Little EA, Ricks R. Isolation of cytomegalovirus from toys and hands in a day care center. *J Infect Dis* 1986;154:527–530.
63. Faiz RG. Comparative efficacy of handwashing agents against cytomegalovirus. *Pediatr Res* 1986;20:227A.
64. Faix RG. Survival of cytomegalovirus on environmental surfaces. *J Pediatr* 1985;106:649–652.
65. Yeager AS. Longitudinal, serological study of cytomegalovirus infections in nurses and in personnel without patient contact. *J Clin Microbiol* 1975;2:448– 452.
66. Ahlfors K, Ivarsson SA, Johnsson T, et al. Risk of cytomegalovirus infection in nurses and congenital infection in their offspring. *Acta Paediatr Scand* 1981;70:819–823.
67. Friedman HM, Lewis MR, Nemerofsky DM, et al. Acquisition of cytomegalovirus infection among female employees at a pediatric hospital. *Pediatr Infect Dis* 1984;3:233–235.
68. Balfour CL, Balfour HH. Cytomegalovirus is not an occupational risk for nurses in renal transplant and neonatal units. *JAMA* 1986;256: 1909–1914.
69. Balcarek KB, Bagley R, Cloud GA, et al. Cytomegalovirus infection among employees of a children's hospital. *JAMA* 1990;263:840–844.
70. Sobaszek A, Fantoni-Quiton S, Frimat P, et al. Prevalence of cytomegalovirus infection among health care workers in pediatric and immunocompromised adult units. *J Occup Environ Med* 2000;42:1109–1114.
71. Wilfert CM, Huang EA, Stagno S, et al. Restriction endonuclease analysis of cytomegalovirus deoxyribonucleic acid as an epidemiologic tool. *Pediatrics* 1982;70:717–721.
72. Yow MD, Lakeman AD, Stagno S, et al. Use of restriction enzymes to investigate the source of a primary cytomegalovirus infection in a pediatric nurse. *Pediatrics* 1982;70:713–716.
73. Spector SA. Transmission of cytomegalovirus among infants in hospital documented by restriction-endonuclease-digestion analyses. *Lancet* 1983;1:378–380.
74. Centers for Disease Control. Guidelines for the prevention of transmission of human immunodeficiency virus and hepatitis B to healthcare and public safety workers. *MMWR Morb Mortal Wkly Rep* 1989; 38(Suppl 6):3–37.
75. Garner JS, Simmons BP. Guideline for isolation precautions in hospitals. *Infect Control* 1983;4:245–325.
76. McCluskey R, Sandin R, Greene J. Detection of airborne cytomegalovirus in hospital rooms of immunocompromised patients. *J Virol Methods* 1996;56:115–118.

45

HEPATITIS VIRUSES

ADELISA L. PANLILIO
IAN T. WILLIAMS
DENISE M. CARDO

Three hepatitis viruses are of clinical significance in healthcare settings in the United States: hepatitis A virus (HAV), hepatitis B virus (HBV), and hepatitis C virus (HCV). This chapter discusses the epidemiology, clinical presentation, diagnosis, and prevention of transmission of these viruses, focusing on transmission from patient to patient in healthcare settings. Transmission in dialysis settings and transmission to and from healthcare personnel are covered in Chapters 64 and 78, respectively.

Patient-to-patient transmission of HAV, HBV, and HCV has been detected in a variety of healthcare settings, both in developed and less-developed countries (1–6). Such transmission occurs indirectly through inappropriate infection control practices of caregivers, and almost all of the transmissions reported were preventable through adherence to recommended practices for infection control.

Worldwide, exposures associated with healthcare delivery account for many HBV and HCV infections. Therapeutic injections, which are commonly overused and administered in an unsafe manner in developing and transitional countries, are estimated to account for over 21 million new HBV infections and 2 million new HCV infections each year (7). In the U.S., surveillance data suggest that transmission of viral hepatitis related to healthcare procedures is unusual (8).

HEPATITIS A

Epidemiology

Hepatitis A is caused by HAV, an RNA virus, classified as a picornavirus. HAV infection can cause both acute disease and asymptomatic infection but does not cause chronic infection, and confers lifelong immunity from future HAV infection (9). HAV is transmitted primarily by the fecal-oral route, by either person-to-person contact or ingestion of contaminated food or water.

Hepatitis A occurs worldwide, but major geographic differences exist in endemicity and resulting epidemiologic features. The degree of endemicity is closely related to sanitary and living conditions and other indicators of the level of development. Most U.S. cases of hepatitis A result from person-to-person transmission, and infection often occurs in the context of community-wide and child day-care center outbreaks (10). The most frequently reported source of infection (12% to 26%) is either household or sexual contact with a person with hepatitis A (8, 10,11). Less than 5% of cases report being part of a recognized food-borne outbreak. More than half of persons with hepatitis A cannot identify a risk factor for their infection (8,10,11).

Hepatitis A is the most frequently reported viral hepatitis in the U.S., with 10,615 cases reported in 2001 (8). However, incidence models indicate that the majority of infections are not detected in national surveillance systems that collect data on symptomatic cases. One such analysis estimated that the number of HAV infections were, on average, 10.4 times the reported number of cases (12).

On rare occasions, HAV infection has been transmitted by transfusion of blood or blood products collected from donors during the viremic phase of their infection, before they are symptomatic or jaundiced (1,13–20). Transmission has not been reported to occur after inadvertent needlesticks or other contact with blood.

Depending on conditions, HAV can be stable in the environment for months (21). Heating foods at temperatures greater than 185°F (85°C) for 1 minute or disinfecting surfaces with a 1:100 dilution of sodium hypochlorite (i.e., household bleach) in tap water is necessary to inactivate HAV (22).

Clinical Illness

The average incubation period for hepatitis A is 28 days (range 15–50 days) (23). Typically, acute hepatitis A starts abruptly with symptoms that can include fever, malaise, anorexia, nausea, abdominal discomfort, dark urine, and jaundice. The severity of clinical disease associated with HAV infection increases with age. In children <6 years of age, most (70%) infections are asymptomatic; if illness does occur, it is usually anicteric (24). Among older children and adults, infection is usually symptomatic, with jaundice occurring in >70% of patients (25). Signs and symptoms usually last <2 months, although 10% to 15% of symptomatic persons have prolonged or relapsing disease lasting up to 6 months (26).

Fulminant hepatitis is a rare complication of hepatitis A; the case-fatality rate can be greater than 50%. Other complications include cholestatic hepatitis, with very high bilirubin levels that can persist for months, and relapsing hepatitis, in which exacerbations can occur weeks to months after apparent recovery. Chronic infection does not occur following HAV infection.

In infected persons, HAV replicates in the liver, is excreted in bile, and is shed in the stool. Feces can contain up to 10^8 infectious virions per milliliter and are the primary source of HAV (27,28). Fecal excretion of HAV, and hence, peak infectivity, is greatest during the incubation period of disease before the onset of jaundice or elevation of liver enzymes (27,28). The concentration of virus in stool declines after jaundice appears; once disease is clinically obvious, the risk of transmitting infection is decreased. However, some patients admitted to the hospital with HAV, particularly immunocompromised patients, may still be shedding virus because of prolonged or relapsing disease, and such patients are potentially infective (29). Fecal shedding of HAV, formerly believed to continue only as long as 2 weeks after onset of dark urine, has been shown to occur as late as 6 months after diagnosis of infection in premature infants (who are more likely to be anicteric). Children and infants can shed HAV for longer periods than adults, up to several months after the onset of clinical illness (20). Viremia occurs soon after infection and persists through the period of liver enzyme elevation (30,31). Viremia is several orders of magnitude lower than in stool (30–32).

Although virus has also been found in saliva during the incubation period in experimentally infected animals, transmission by saliva has not been reported (32).

Diagnosis

Hepatitis A cannot be differentiated from other types of viral hepatitis on the basis of clinical or epidemiologic features alone. The diagnosis of acute HAV infection is confirmed during the acute or early convalescent phase of infection by the presence of immunoglobulin M (IgM) anti-HAV. In most persons, IgM anti-HAV becomes detectable 5 to 10 days before the onset of symptoms and can persist for up to 6 months after infection (31,33). Immunoglobulin G (IgG) anti-HAV, which also appears early in the course of infection, remains detectable for the lifetime of the individual and confers lifelong protection against infection (9). Commercial tests are available for the detection of IgM and total (IgM and IgG) anti-HAV in serum.

HAV RNA can be detected in the blood and stool of most persons during the acute phase of infection by using nucleic acid amplification methods, and nucleic acid sequencing has been used to determine the relatedness of HAV isolates (34). However, these methods are available in only a limited number of research laboratories and generally are not used for diagnostic purposes.

HAV Transmission in Healthcare Settings

Transmission of HAV from patient to patient in healthcare settings has been reported infrequently and usually occurred when the source patient had unrecognized hepatitis and was fecally incontinent or had diarrhea. Other risk factors for HAV transmission include activities that increase the risk of fecal-oral contamination, such as eating or drinking in patient care areas, not washing hands after handling an infected infant, and sharing food, beverages, or cigarettes with patients, their families, or other staff members.

Several outbreaks have occurred in neonatal intensive care units (NICUs) involving transfusion of neonates with infected blood, with subsequent transmission of HAV infection to other infants and staff (16,18,20). The first reported outbreak resulted from transfusion of blood from a single infected donor to 11 neonates (16). (The donor became ill 1 week after donation.) A multistate outbreak of 55 cases of hepatitis A resulted. HAV infection was acquired by parents and relatives of the neonates as well as by nurses and physicians having direct contact with the neonates. Three neonates who had not received transfusions with the infected blood also acquired hepatitis A. All neonates with hepatitis A were asymptomatic. A second outbreak resulted from transfusion of blood to six neonates in an NICU. Four of the six showed serologic evidence of acute hepatitis A (IgM anti-HAV) (18). Subsequently, four more neonates who had not received blood from the infected donor and five nurses developed hepatitis A. These four infants had been in beds adjacent to those who became infected after transfusion. The third outbreak involved two infants in an NICU who had received blood transfusions from a single donor with HAV infection (20). Their infection was transmitted to 13 NICU patients, 22 NICU nurses, and eight other staff caring for NICU infants, as well as four household contacts. Breaks in technique observed during the outbreak investigation included smoking, eating and drinking in patient-care areas, and not wearing gloves when taping intravenous lines and endotracheal tubes.

Investigation of a multinursery outbreak involving seven neonates and 15 secondary cases did not identify a common source of infection. However, it was suggested that the index infection might have resulted from transfusion of a blood product from a donor who was viremic at the time of donation (35).

Another outbreak of hepatitis A in an NICU was traced to a neonate who acquired his infection from his mother before or during birth (36). HAV was subsequently transmitted from him to three infants and ten staff through breaks in infection control. Infants who became infected shared the same nurse as the index case during several shifts. Staff who reported not washing hands routinely after treating the infant for his frequent episodes of apnea and bradycardia had a greater risk for infection.

The index case in an outbreak of hepatitis A in Sweden received an exchange transfusion as a newborn from a donor in the prodrome of hepatitis (13). The infant's mother became clinically ill, but the infant remained asymptomatic. After the index case was readmitted for treatment of a bacterial infection, apparently still shedding HAV fecally, her infection was transmitted to another patient and three nurses.

As described in these outbreaks, NICUs provide a setting that has been conducive to further spread of HAV once it is introduced. The combination of frequent contact with soiled diapers, asymptomatic infection in neonates, and prolonged HAV excretion among preterm infants may facilitate HAV transmission.

Most patients hospitalized for symptomatic hepatitis A are admitted after onset of jaundice, when they are beyond the point of peak infectivity (1,37). Consequently, source patients for outbreaks of hepatitis A usually involve patients who are incubating

HAV infection and develop hepatitis after hospitalization. Patient-to-healthcare worker and patient-to-patient transmission of HAV in such situations are usually associated with fecal incontinence. An adult hospitalized for elective cholecystectomy developed fever, abdominal pain, vomiting, and diarrhea postoperatively (38). She had several episodes of incontinence with gross contamination of her bed linen and floor. The index patient was not diagnosed as having hepatitis A until after discharge. The hospital roommate who assisted the index patient in the bathroom developed clinical illness as did six staff. Another outbreak involving 11 nurses and one patient was traced to a mentally handicapped patient who was incontinent (39). The patient was hospitalized for malaria 4 days after returning from a trip to India. Acute HAV infection was not suspected. Another outbreak involved 19 hospital staff and one inpatient (40). Transmission was from a pediatric patient with diarrhea so profuse that there was gross fecal contamination of her environment. Factors causing this outbreak included prolonged viral excretion by the source patient (likely related to her transient immunodeficiency), the severity of her diarrhea and resultant environmental contamination, a lengthy hospitalization, and possible breaks in infection control, such as inconsistent use of gloves and handwashing. A 1-year-old child developed unrecognized hepatitis A while recovering from cardiac surgery (41). Her infection was transmitted to another patient from whom infection was subsequently transmitted to two other patients, 12 nurses, three physicians, and two medical students.

Prevention of Healthcare-Related HAV Transmission

The primary means of preventing HAV transmission in healthcare settings is by observing contact precautions with patients with acute hepatitis A who are in diapers and/or incontinent and by avoiding fecal-oral contact (42). Continent patients can be managed with standard precautions alone (42). Meticulous hand hygiene after touching the patient, the patient's feces, or the environment around the patient and not eating, drinking, or smoking in patient-care areas are essential to preventing HAV transmission in healthcare settings (43).

Inactivated hepatitis A vaccines are now available for prevention of hepatitis A (44,45). These vaccines are both highly immunogenic as well as highly effective in the prevention of clinical hepatitis A (46,47). Immune globulin (IG) is also available for preexposure and postexposure prophylaxis.

Because serologic surveys among healthcare personnel have not shown greater prevalence of HAV infection than in control populations, routine administration of vaccine in healthcare personnel is not recommended (44,48,49). Vaccine may be useful for personnel working or living in areas where HAV is highly endemic and is indicated for personnel who handle HAV-infected primates or are exposed to HAV in a research laboratory (44). Hepatitis A vaccine is also recommended for persons at increased risk of infection, such as those traveling or working in countries with high or intermediate endemicity of infection, men who have sex with men, illegal-drug users, persons with clotting factor disorders, and persons with chronic liver disease (44). The role of hepatitis A vaccine in controlling outbreaks has not been adequately investigated to make recommendations for its use in this manner in the U.S.

Immune globulin (IG) provides protection against hepatitis A through passive transfer of antibody. IG is 80% to 90% effective in preventing clinical hepatitis A when administered before exposure or early in the incubation period after exposure, i.e., within 14 days (44). The primary routine indication for postexposure prophylaxis is for household or other intimate contacts of persons with hepatitis A. In addition, postexposure prophylaxis might be indicated when hepatitis A cases occur in some institutional settings (e.g., child day-care centers) and after some common source exposures (e.g., persons who ate food prepared by an infected food handler). Local and/or state health departments should be consulted regarding the use of IG for postexposure prophylaxis in these settings (45).

IG is not routinely indicated when a single case occurs in an elementary or secondary school, an office, or in other work settings, and the source of infection is outside the school or work setting (44). Similarly, when a person who has hepatitis A is admitted to a hospital, staff should not routinely be administered IG; instead, careful hygienic practices should be emphasized. IG should be administered to persons who have close contact with index patients if an epidemiologic investigation indicates HAV transmission has occurred among students in a school or among patients or between patients and staff in a hospital. When outbreaks occur in hospitals, use of IG for persons in close contact with infected patients is recommended (44).

HEPATITIS B

Epidemiology

HBV belongs to the family Hepadnaviridae, a group of DNA viruses. The only known hosts for HBV are humans, although some nonhuman primates can be infected under laboratory conditions (50). HBV infection can cause both acute disease and asymptomatic infection and may result in chronic infection. Worldwide, HBV is the most common cause of chronic viremia; there are an estimated 200 to 300 million chronic carriers worldwide (50). HBV causes up to 80% of hepatocellular carcinomas and more than 250,000 deaths each year due to acute and chronic liver disease (50). In the U.S., approximately 0.4% of the general population is chronically infected with HBV and provides a reservoir for maintenance of the disease in the population (51).

HBV is transmitted by percutaneous or mucosal exposure to blood and other body fluids from infected persons. Blood contains the highest HBV titers of all body fluids and is the most important vehicle of transmission in the healthcare setting. Hepatitis B surface antigen (HBsAg) is also found in several other body fluids, including breast milk, bile, cerebrospinal fluid, feces, nasopharyngeal washings, saliva, semen, sweat, and synovial fluid (52). However, the concentration of HBsAg in body fluids can be 100- to 1,000-fold higher than the concentration of infectious HBV particles. Therefore, most body fluids are not efficient vehicles of transmission because they contain low quantities of infectious HBV, despite the presence of HBsAg.

Children born to infected mothers are at high risk for perinatally acquired HBV infection. Persons parenterally exposed to blood, particularly injection drug users, also are at significant risk. Sexual contact with infected partners is another efficient mode of HBV spread. In most industrialized countries, adult infections usually are acquired sexually or by injection drug use (8,10,53).

HBV is a relatively hardy virus, resistant to drying, ambient temperatures, simple detergents, and alcohol. It has been found to be stable on environmental surfaces for at least 7 days (54, 55). Thus, indirect inoculation can occur through inanimate objects (e.g., contaminated medical equipment or environmental surfaces). Transmission in households is well documented, and in part may be attributable to mucosal contact with fomites contaminated with secretions or blood from infected persons. HBV also has been shown to be inactivated by several intermediate-level disinfectants, including 0.1% glutaraldehyde and 500 parts per million (ppm) free chlorine from sodium hypochlorite (i.e., household bleach) (56,57). Heating to 98°C for 2 minutes also inactivates HBV (58).

Clinical Illness

Hepatitis B has an incubation period of 40 to 180 days (50). The period of infectivity precedes the development of jaundice by 2 to 7 weeks and correlates with the presence of HBsAg in the serum. The risk of developing chronic HBV infection varies inversely with the age of infection. Chronic infection occurs in 90% of infants infected at birth, 25% to 50% of children infected at 1 to 5 years of age, and about 5% to 10% of people infected as older children and adults (59). However, only 10% of children and 30% to 50% of adults with acute HBV infection have icteric disease.

Clinical hepatitis may be preceded by a prodrome of fever, malaise, urticarial or maculopapular rash, and arthralgias for several days. Fever usually resolves before the onset of jaundice. Jaundice, dark urine, and scleral icterus usually are present by the time patients seek medical attention.

Fulminant liver involvement occurs in about 1% of adults. Hepatic encephalopathy, hepatorenal syndrome, and bleeding diatheses are life-threatening complications seen in these patients. An estimated 15% to 25% of persons with chronic HBV infection will die prematurely of either cirrhosis or primary hepatocellular carcinoma (HCC) (60).

Diagnosis

Hepatitis B is differentiated from other causes of hepatitis by serologic assays. Several well-defined antigen-antibody systems are associated with HBV infection, including HBsAg and antibody to hepatitis B surface antigen (anti-HBs); hepatitis B core antigen (HBcAg) and anti-HBc; and hepatitis B early antigen (HBeAg) and antibody to HBeAg (anti-HBe). Serologic assays are commercially available for all of these except HBcAg, because no free HBcAg circulates in blood. These markers of HBV infection change over time, with different patterns seen in patients with acute infection that resolves and patients with chronic infection (Table 45.1) (61).

The presence of HBsAg is indicative of ongoing HBV infection and potential infectiousness. In newly infected persons, HBsAg is present in serum 30 to 60 days after exposure to HBV and persists for variable periods. Transient HBsAg positivity (lasting ≤18 days) can be detected in some patients during vaccination (62,63). Anti-HBc develops in all HBV infections, appearing at onset of symptoms or liver test abnormalities in acute HBV infection, rising rapidly to high levels, and persisting for life. Acute or recently acquired infection can be distinguished by presence of the IgM class of anti-HBc, which persists for approximately 6 months.

TABLE 45.1. INTERPRETATION OF PATTERNS OF HEPATITIS B VIRUS SEROLOGIC MARKERS

Serologic Markers				
HbsAg*	Total Anti-HBc[H]	IgM′ Anti-HBc	Anti-HBs¶	Interpretation
−	−	−	−	Susceptible, never infected
+	−	−	−	Acute infection, early incubation**
+	+	+	−	Acute resolving infection
−	+	+	−	Acute resolving infection
−	+	−	+	Past infection, recovered and immune
+	+	−	−	Chronic infection
−	+	−	−	False positive (i.e., susceptible), past infection, or "low-level" chronic infection
−	−	−	+	Immune if titer is ≥10 mIU/mL

* HBsAg – Hepatitis B surface antigen.
[H] Anti-HBc – Antibody to hepatitis B core antigen. The total anti-HBc assay detects both IgM and IgG antibody.
′ Immunoglobulin M
¶ Anti-HBs – Antibody to hepatitis B surface antigen.
** Transient HbsAg positivity (lasting ≤18 days) might be detected in some patients during vaccination.
+ = Positive − = Negative
Adapted from Table 1 Centers for Disease Control and Prevention. Recommendations for preventing transmission of infections among chronic hemodialysis patients. *Morb Mortal Wkly Rep* 2001;50(No. RR-5):1–43.

In persons who recover from HBV infection, HBsAg is eliminated from the blood, usually in 2 to 3 months, and anti-HBs develops during convalescence. The presence of anti-HBs indicates immunity from HBV infection. After recovery from natural infection, most persons will be positive for both anti-HBs and anti-HBc, whereas only anti-HBs develops in persons who are successfully vaccinated against hepatitis B. Persons who do not recover from HBV infection and become chronically infected remain positive for HBsAg (and anti-HBc), although a small proportion (0.3% per year) eventually clear HBsAg and might develop anti-HBs (64). The persistence of HBsAg for 6 months after the diagnosis of acute HBV is indicative of progression to chronic HBV infection.

HBeAg can be detected in serum of persons with acute or chronic HBV infection. The presence of HBeAg correlates with viral replication and high levels of virus (i.e., high infectivity). Anti-HBe correlates with the loss of replicating virus and with lower levels of virus. However, all HBsAg-positive persons should be considered potentially infectious, regardless of their HBeAg or anti-HBe status.

HBV infection can be detected using qualitative or quantitative tests for HBV DNA. These tests are not Food and Drug Administration (FDA) approved and are most commonly used for patients being managed with antiviral therapy.

Transmission of HBV in Healthcare Settings

The delivery of healthcare has the potential to transmit HBV to patients. Settings in which HBV transmission from patient to patient has occurred include hospitals, outpatient clinics, private offices, and hemodialysis centers. Incidents of HBV transmission can be grouped by the presumed mechanism of transmission.

Contamination of Blood Sampling Equipment

Several episodes of HBV transmission to patients through contamination of equipment used during blood sampling have been reported. These episodes, which occurred in hospitals and a nursing home, were associated with the use of spring-loaded fingerstick devices and other blood sampling systems in which components of the systems and/or gloves used by healthcare personnel had been contaminated with blood. In two outbreaks in which a reusable spring-loaded fingerstick device was used for several patients, the platform used to stabilize the patient's finger during the procedure was either not changed or not cleaned between uses (65,66). During the investigations, visible blood contamination was observed on the platform and was believed to be the probable mechanism of transmission.

In three outbreaks, reusable pen-like devices that included both disposable and reusable components were implicated in transmission (67,68). In two of these outbreaks the device used had a separate lancet and end cap (67,68). The end cap rested on the skin during the procedure and could have become contaminated after the lancet retracted. Both the lancets and end caps were disposable and should have been replaced after each use. However, only the lancet was routinely replaced, suggesting that exposure of subsequent patients to residual blood in the end cap contributed to transmission. In the third outbreak, the lancet and end cap formed a single unit that was changed between patients (67). However, the reusable pen-like component was not cleaned between patients and may have contributed to transmission. Other possible transmission factors in these outbreaks were blood contamination of gloves that were not routinely changed between patients and contamination of unused caps and other supplies. These same opportunities for cross-contamination were found during the investigation of an outbreak in a drug trials unit where visible blood contamination of hands or gloves and lack of hand hygiene between individual blood sampling were recalled by staff and volunteers (69).

Multidose Vials and Injection Equipment

Contamination of multidose vials containing heparin, saline flush solution, and bupivacaine also has been implicated in HBV transmission in hospitals and an outpatient clinic (70–73). Evidence suggesting a common-source outbreak and an epidemiologic association among infected patients receiving medication from multidose vials implicated these devices as a mechanism of transmission. Multidose vials can be contaminated by a needle/syringe previously used in an infected patient/source.

Improperly Cleaned, Disinfected, or Sterilized Equipment

Inadequate cleaning, disinfection, or sterilization of equipment has been linked to HBV transmission. Endoscopy equipment in which either biopsy or air/water channels were inadequately cleaned, the immersion time in a high-level disinfectant was inadequate, or biopsy forceps were not sterilized between patients contributed to HBV transmission (74) (see also Chapter 63).

One outbreak of HBV was associated with a jet injection gun used to administer daily injections in a weight reduction clinic and resulted in 31 cases of clinical hepatitis (75). In this instance, problems with device design most likely contributed to transmission. Although swabbing the exterior nozzle with alcohol between patients was practiced routinely, interior surfaces of the device were inaccessible and therefore could not be reached for cleaning.

The use of needles for acupuncture has been associated with at least three outbreaks of HBV. This ancient Chinese practice is commonly used in Western cultures to manage a variety of medical ailments, including pain, smoking cessation, and the control of allergies and hypertension. In the episodes reported, improperly sterilized or unsterilized acupuncture needles and opportunities for cross-contamination during the procedures contributed to transmission (76–78).

Other or Undetermined Breaches in Infection Control

In two outbreaks of HBV infections associated with endomyocardial biopsy (EMB), droplets of blood generated when inserting and withdrawing biopsy forceps were believed to contaminate unwrapped biopsy forceps, introducer sets, and opened medication vials to be used on subsequent patients. Simulation of EMB subsequently showed viral contamination and supported the hypothesized mechanism of transmission. Cross-contamination by staff was not believed to be involved (79–81).

In other reports, the mechanism of transmission has remained obscure. In a large outbreak of HBV involving at least 72 patients in a dermatology practice, several possible vehicles for transmission were implicated, exemplifying how breaches of infection control can involve several areas of practice (82). In this instance, the dermatologist operated without gloves, his hands were often blood contaminated, and he did not routinely wash them between patients. Furthermore, large multidose volumes of injectable anesthetic were routinely used and there was evidence of possible contamination. Only one 5-mL syringe was used per patient and used syringes were refilled through a needle that remained in the vial. Electrocautery tips were neither changed nor cleaned between patients and cotton-tipped nitrogen applicators were returned to their reservoir. Any of these breaches could have contributed to HBV transmission.

A large outbreak of HBV (and HCV) infections in a pediatric oncology ward involved 106 patients, infected from 1996 to 2000 (83). Epidemiologic investigation excluded a common source infection and indicated that transmission of infection was most likely due to inappropriate infection control measures, such as poor staff compliance with routine hand hygiene and changing gloves. Multidose vials of isotonic solution were used for flushing of intravenous catheters and preparation of parenteral injections, although staff denied reusing syringes.

Case-control studies conducted in Moldova suggested injections as a major route of HBV transmission (84). Adult patients were more likely to report having received injections while receiving medical or dental care in the 6 months before illness. In this study by Hutin et al. (84), it was estimated that 52% of acute hepatitis B cases in adults and 21% of such cases in children might be attributable to injections. Similar associations between hepatitis B and injections have been reported in India, Taiwan, Egypt, and the Sudan (85–89).

The most recently reported large outbreak of HBV infection in a U.S. healthcare setting involved unsafe injection practices in a single private physician's office (90). A total of 38 case-patients were identified who developed acute HBV infection during a 25-month period. HBV DNA genetic sequences of 24 patients with acute and four patients with chronic infection were identical in the 1,500 base pair region examined. No HCV or HIV infections associated with this office were identified. Most case patients received multiple injections, consisting of doses of atropine, dexamethasone, and/or vitamin B_{12} drawn from multidose vials into one syringe. The same workspace was used to prepare, dismantle, and dispose of injection equipment. Administration of unnecessary injections combined with failure to separate clean from contaminated areas and follow safe injection practices likely resulted in patient-to-patient HBV transmission.

Prevention of Healthcare-Related HBV Transmission

The outbreaks described above could have been prevented by various practices including using disposable lancets, assigning dedicated reusable spring-loaded devices to individual patients, changing gloves and performing hand hygiene between patients, and preventing blood contamination of clean equipment. Prevention of these events must focus on minimizing the use of multidose vials and ensuring that healthcare personnel understand and use aseptic technique when preparing injectables for patient administration (Table 45.2).

HBV infection is largely preventable through vaccination. Hepatitis B vaccine provides both preexposure and postexposure

TABLE 45.2. RECOMMENDED INFECTION CONTROL AND SAFE INJECTION PRACTICES TO PREVENT PATIENT-TO-PATIENT TRANSMISSION OF BLOODBORNE PATHOGENS

1. Injection safety
   a. Use a sterile, single-use, disposable needle and syringe for each injection and dispose intact in an appropriate sharps container after use.
   b. Use single-dose medication vials, prefilled syringes, and ampules when possible. Do not administer medications from single-dose vials to multiple patients or combine leftover contents for later use.
   c. If multidose vials are used, restrict them to a centralized medication area or for single patient use. Never re-enter a vial with a needle or syringe used on one patient if that vial will subsequently be used to withdraw medication for use on another patient. Store vials in accordance with manufacturer's recommendations and discard if sterility is compromised.
   d. Do not use bags or bottles of intravenous solution as a common source of supply for multiple patients.
   e. Use aseptic technique to avoid contamination of sterile injection equipment and medications.
2. Patient-care equipment
   a. Handle patient-care equipment that may be contaminated with blood in a way that prevents skin and mucous membrane exposures, contamination of clothing, and transfer of microorganisms to other patients and surfaces.
   b. Evaluate equipment and devices for potential cross-contamination of blood. Establish procedures for safe handling during and after use, including cleaning and disinfection or sterilization as indicated.
3. Work environment
   a. Dispose of used syringes and needles at the point of use in a sharps container that is puncture-resistant and leak-proof and that can be sealed before completely full.
   b. Maintain physical separation between clean and contaminated equipment and supplies.
   c. Prepare medications in areas physically separate from those with potential blood contamination.
   d. Use barriers to protect surfaces from blood contamination during blood sampling.
   e. Clean and disinfect blood-contaminated equipment and surfaces in accordance with recommended guidelines.
4. Hand hygiene and gloves
   a. Perform hand hygiene (i.e., handwashing with soap and water or use of an alcohol-based hand rub) before preparing and administering an injection, before and after donning gloves for performing blood sampling, after inadvertent blood contamination, and between patients.
   b. Wear gloves for procedures that may involve contact with blood and change gloves between patients.

Adapted from Centers for Disease Control and Prevention. Transmission of hepatitis B and C viruses in outpatient settings — New York, Oklahoma, and Nebraska, 2000–2002. *Morb Mortal Wkly Rep* 2003;52:901–6.

protection against HBV infection. The currently available vaccines in the U.S. are produced by recombinant DNA technology. Three intramuscular doses of hepatitis B vaccine induce a protective antibody response in >90% of healthy recipients. Adults who develop a protective antibody response are protected from clinical disease and chronic infection. The duration of vaccine protection is under investigation. Most data suggest that protection persists even when anti-HBs concentrations fall below the level of detection, and routine screening and boosting are not currently recommended (50).

HEPATITIS C

Epidemiology

HCV is an RNA virus of the Flaviviridae family. There are six HCV genotypes and more than 50 subtypes. Genotype 1 accounts for 70% to 75% of all HCV infections in the U.S.; subtype 1a predominates over subtype 1b (91).

HCV infection is the most common chronic blood-borne infection in the U.S., affecting an estimated 1.3% of the U.S. population (92). HCV-associated end-stage liver disease is the most frequent indication for liver transplantation among U.S. adults (93).

The highest prevalence of HCV infection (70% to 90%) is reported among those persons with substantial or repeated direct percutaneous exposures to blood [e.g., injecting drug users (IDUs), persons with hemophilia treated with clotting factor concentrates that did not undergo viral inactivation, and recipients of transfusions from HCV-positive donors]. Risk factors associated with acquiring HCV infection in the U.S. have included transfusion of blood and blood products and transplantation of solid organs from infected donors, occupational exposure to blood (primarily contaminated needlesticks), birth to an infected mother, sex with an infected partner, and multiple heterosexual partners. Although the incidence of acute hepatitis C in the U.S. has declined by >80% since 1989, primarily as a result of a decrease in cases among IDUs, the major risk factor for HCV infection remains injection-drug use, which accounts for 60% of newly acquired cases (94,95).

Degradation of HCV occurs when serum containing HCV is left at room temperature. Specific animal infectivity studies have shown survival up to 16 hours but not longer than 4 days (96). The potential for environmental survival of HCV suggests that environmental contamination with blood containing HCV could pose a risk for transmission in the healthcare setting. The risk for transmission from exposure to fluids or tissues other than HCV-infected blood has not been quantified but is expected to be low. HCV is not known to be transmissible through the airborne route, through casual contact in the workplace, or by fomites.

Clinical Illness

The incubation period for acute HCV infection ranges from 2 to 24 weeks (averaging 6 to 7 weeks). HCV infection produces a spectrum of clinical illness similar to that of HBV infection and is indistinguishable from other forms of viral hepatitis based on clinical symptoms alone. Most adults acutely infected with HCV are asymptomatic. The course of acute hepatitis C is variable, although elevations in serum alanine aminotransferase (ALT) levels, often in a fluctuating pattern, are its most characteristic feature. Normalization of ALT levels might occur and suggests full recovery, but this is frequently followed by ALT elevations that indicate progression to chronic disease (97). Fulminant hepatic failure following acute hepatitis C is rare (98, 99). After acute infection, 15% to 25% of persons appear to resolve their infection without sequelae as defined by sustained absence of HCV RNA in serum and normalization of ALT levels (100).

The lack of a vigorous T-lymphocyte response and the high propensity of the virus to mutate appear to promote a high rate of chronic infection (91). HCV preferentially replicates in hepatocytes but is not directly cytopathic, resulting in persistent infection. During chronic infection, HCV RNA reaches high levels, generally ranging from 10^5 to 10^7 international units (IU)/mL, but the levels can fluctuate widely. Within the same individual, however, RNA levels are generally relatively stable.

Chronic HCV infection develops in most (75% to 85%) persons; 60% to 70% of these chronically infected persons have persistent or fluctuating ALT elevations, indicating active liver disease. The course of chronic liver disease is usually insidious, progressing slowly without symptoms or physical signs in the majority of patients during the first two or more decades after infection. Chronic hepatitis C frequently is not recognized until asymptomatic persons are identified as HCV-positive during blood-donor screening, or elevated ALT levels are detected during routine physical examinations. Most studies have reported that cirrhosis develops in 10% to 20% of persons with chronic hepatitis C over 20 to 30 years, and HCC in 1% to 5%, with striking geographic variations in rates of this disease (101–105). However, when cirrhosis is established, the rate of development of HCC might be as high as 1% to 4% per year. Longer follow-up studies are needed to assess lifetime consequences of chronic hepatitis C, particularly among those who acquired infection at young ages.

Diagnosis

As with other types of viral hepatitis, laboratory testing is necessary to establish a specific diagnosis of hepatitis C (61,106, 107). The two major types of tests available for the laboratory diagnosis of HCV infections are serologic assays for anti-HCV and the nucleic acid test (NAT) to detect HCV RNA. Testing for anti-HCV is recommended for initially identifying persons with HCV infection and includes initial screening with an immunoassay, and if positive, confirmation by an additional more specific assay (106). Assays for anti-HCV detect only IgG antibody; no IgM assays are available. Within 15 weeks after exposure and within 5 to 6 weeks after the onset of hepatitis, 80% of patients will have positive test results for serum HCV antibody. False-negative results early in the course of acute infection are due to the prolonged interval between exposure and seroconversion.

There are several FDA-licensed diagnostic NATs for qualitative detection of HCV RNA. HCV RNA can be detected in serum or plasma within 1 to 2 weeks after exposure to the virus and weeks before onset of liver enzyme abnormalities or appearance of anti-HCV. NATs for HCV RNA are used commonly in clinical practice in the early diagnosis of infection, for determining the presence of chronic infection, and for monitoring patients receiving antiviral therapy. However, false-positive and false-negative results can occur from improper handling, storage, and contamination of the test specimens. Viral RNA may be detected intermittently, and thus, a single negative assay result is not conclusive. Genotype determination is used in clinical management to determine the appropriate antiviral therapy regimen.

HCV Transmission in Healthcare Settings

Nosocomial transmission of HCV is possible if infection control techniques or disinfection procedures are inadequate and contaminated equipment is shared among patients. Mechanisms similar to those involved in HBV transmission have been implicated or suspected in outbreaks of HCV transmission in healthcare settings.

Contamination of Blood Sampling Equipment

Sharing spring-loaded devices for self-monitoring of capillary blood glucose among patients in a ward for cystic fibrosis and diabetes led to transmission of HCV to 18 patients with cystic fibrosis and 12 with diabetes during 1986–1988 (108). Transmission was stopped when the sharing of spring-loaded devices was banned in early 1992, following report of HBV transmission involving the use of a similar device (65).

Multidose Vials and Injection Equipment

Several reports of HCV transmission have implicated either contaminated multidose vials and/or injection equipment as the mechanism of transmission (109–112). Two cases of acute HCV infection after medical procedures (arthroscopy and colonoscopy) were traced to contamination of intravenous anesthetic ampules used on multiple patients (109). Contamination of multidose vials used for flushing of intravenous catheters or treatment has been reported as the most likely mode of HCV transmission in three separate outbreaks of acute HCV infection on a pediatric oncology service in Sweden, a Swedish cardiology ward, and a U.S. medical ward (110–112).

Investigation of an outbreak of HCV infection in the emergency ward of a Spanish municipal hospital presumptively identified a multidose vial of heparin as the most likely source of infection (113). Nine patients became acutely infected on a single day. A patient with chronic HCV infection had been seen earlier the same day. All patients had intravenous catheters that had been flushed with heparin solution from a multidose vial.

A cluster of four patients who developed primary HCV infection after undergoing gynecologic surgery on the same day was identified (114). It was determined that these four patients had undergone surgery following surgery on a patient with chronic HCV infection. The only risk factor identified for transmission was the use of propofol from multidose vials.

Two separate instances of transmission of HCV to participants in research studies were reported from Canada and Sweden (115,116). The suspected mode of transmission was the possible use of common syringes to flush intravenous cannulae from the participants who required frequent blood sampling as part of the research protocols.

Three outbreaks of HCV infections that occurred in outpatient healthcare settings in the U.S. were recently reported (90). In each, it is likely that unsafe injection practices, primarily reuse of syringes and needles or contamination of multidose medication vials, led to patient-to-patient transmission of bloodborne pathogens. One outbreak involved patients who had undergone endoscopic procedures in a private physician's office. The investigation indicated that the probable route of transmission was contamination of multidose anesthesia medication vials through the introduction of contaminated needles into the vials.

A second cluster of HCV cases resulted from reuse of needles and syringes by a registered nurse anesthetist working in a pain remediation clinic (90). This nurse used a single needle/syringe to administer each of three sedation medications [Versed (midazolam HCl), fentanyl, and propofol] to up to 24 sequentially treated patients at each clinic session. These medications were administered through heparin locks that were connected directly to intravenous cannulas.

The last cluster of HCV cases was among patients who had received chemotherapy at the same hematology/oncology clinic (90). The healthcare worker responsible for medication infusions routinely used a syringe to draw blood from patients' central venous catheters and subsequently reused the same syringe to draw catheter-flushing solution from 500-cc saline bags that were used for multiple patients. A patient known to have chronic HCV genotype 3a infection began attending the clinic at the beginning of the 22-month period investigated. Of the six patients for whom HCV genotype was available, all were genotype 3a, which is rare in the U.S. (117). After the reuse of syringes and the use of common bags of saline for catheter flushing were halted and changes made in clinic staff and infection control practices, no further HCV transmission was found.

These last three outbreaks are among the largest healthcare-related viral hepatitis outbreaks reported in the U.S. and share several common characteristics. All occurred in outpatient settings. Transmission most likely occurred indirectly from patient to patient following exposure to injection equipment that was contaminated with the blood of one or more source patients. All of the outbreaks involving unsafe injection practices could have been prevented by adherence of staff to basic principles of aseptic technique for the preparation and administration of parenteral medications (Table 45.2) (118,119).

Improperly Cleaned/Sterilized Equipment

Transmission of HCV to two patients who underwent colonoscopy following colonoscopy on a patient known to be HCV positive has been reported (120). The same colonoscope was used for all three procedures, and biopsies were obtained from all three patients. The method of cleaning and disinfecting the endoscopes between patients was not as stringent as that recommended by professional societies concerned with transmission of infections through endoscopy (121,122). The biopsy-suction channel was not cleaned with a brush as part of the reprocessing procedure in the clinic. Furthermore, diathermic loop and biopsy forceps were disinfected but not autoclaved after each use.

Other or Undetermined Breaches in Infection Control

Five clusters (totaling 37 patients) of HCV infection were found among patients admitted to a hematology ward (123). Each cluster had patients with genotypically identical virus. HCV transmission through transfusion was ruled out. These patients' admissions to the ward during overlapping time periods suggested that HCV transmission occurred. Although no specific mode of transmission was identified, mistakes in percutaneous, diagnostic, or therapeutic procedures may have caused HCV transmission.

A large outbreak of both HBV and HCV transmission on a pediatric oncology ward was believed due to breaches in infection control practices such as poor compliance with hand hygiene and glove use (83). The use of multidose saline vials for flushing intravenous catheters also may have contributed to these transmissions. Investigation of HCV transmission in another hematology ward also did not identify the origin of the outbreak (124). However, adoption of measures including discontinuation of use of multidose vial medications and screening for HCV and isolation of HCV-positive patients ended transmission.

Two separate instances of patient-to-patient transmission of HCV during surgery have been reported (125,126). They suggested that the transmission was related to a reusable part of the anesthetic respiratory circuit that may have been contaminated by blood or infected respiratory secretions.

Transmission of HCV to a blood donor was detected by nucleic acid testing (127). The donor had received parenteral antibiotic therapy at an outpatient clinic over a 9-day period in the month before the donation when his HCV positivity was discovered. The donor's clinic visits overlapped with a visit to the same clinic of an HCV-infected patient. Genomic sequencing of HCV isolates from the blood donor and the putative source demonstrated a high degree of relatedness. The specific mechanism by which transmission occurred was not determined but may have involved the reuse of intravenous bag and tubing for administration of antimicrobials on multiple visits to the clinic. The bag intended for use in the index patient may have been mistakenly used by/connected to the putative source patient, may have become contaminated, and may have been subsequently used by the index patient.

Two transmissions of HCV during ancillary procedures for assisted conception have been described (128). The two patients developed acute HCV infection after undergoing follicular puncture immediately after puncture performed on an HCV-infected patient. Although the exact nature of transmission was not identified, it was surmised that the contamination occurred outside the direct practice of in vitro fertilization (IVF) and possibly through procedures practiced by ancillary staff. The authors recommended against inclusion of HCV-positive patients in assisted reproduction programs unless the patients are HCV RNA negative at the beginning of the IVF cycle.

Multiple breaches in infection control practices have been implicated as the cause of HCV transmission in a renal transplantation center (129). These breaches included not changing gloves between patients and inadequate sterilization of reusable equipment (not specified).

Prevention of Healthcare-Related HCV Transmission

Because HBV and HCV have similar modes of transmission in healthcare settings, the same infection control principles apply to preventing their transmission. Care must be exercised in preparation of parenteral medications and blood drawing. Aseptic technique is essential to prevent contamination of sterile injection equipment and solutions. Single-use needles and syringes should not be reused. Multidose vials should be restricted for use only on a single patient or in a centralized medication area. Each time such a vial is entered, a new sterile needle and syringe should be used to withdraw solution. There should be physically separate areas for handling clean versus contaminated equipment and supplies. All of the outbreaks involving unsafe injection practices could have been prevented by adherence of staff to basic principles of aseptic technique for the preparation and administration of parenteral medications (Table 45.2) (118, 119).

Standard sterilization and disinfection procedures recommended for patient-care equipment are adequate to sterilize or disinfect items contaminated with blood or other body fluids from people infected with blood-borne pathogens, including HBV and HCV. Because foreign material may interfere with the sterilization or disinfection procedure, devices must first be adequately cleaned. This is particularly important for devices such as endoscopes that may become heavily soiled and cannot tolerate heat sterilization (121,122).

All spills of blood and blood-contaminated body fluids should be promptly cleaned by a person wearing gloves and using an Environmental Protection Agency–approved disinfectant or a 1:10 to 1:100 solution of household bleach. Visibly bloody material should first be removed with disposable towels or other means to prevent direct contact with blood. The area should then be decontaminated with an appropriate disinfectant (130, 131).

There is currently no vaccine against HCV, and postexposure prophylaxis is not recommended for exposures to HCV (132).

CONCLUSION

Hepatitis A, B, and C viruses have different routes of transmission and all have been involved in healthcare-related transmissions, largely due to breaches in infection control practices. Transmissions of HBV and HCV have frequently involved unsafe injection practices. Preventing transmission of these viruses in the healthcare setting requires strict adherence to infection control practices, especially hand hygiene, appropriate use of gloves, and careful attention to aseptic technique during injections and blood drawing.

Since a large proportion of patients with acute HAV, HBV,

or HCV infection are asymptomatic, newly acquired infections may not come to the attention of healthcare providers, and clusters of infected patients with common risk factors may not be recognized and reported to public health authorities. In addition, when cases do occur, they may not be reported or adequately investigated. Healthcare-related transmission should be suspected when cases without traditional risk factors for infection are detected.

In some of the outbreaks reported above, healthcare workers violated fundamental principles related to safe injection practices, which suggests that they failed to understand the potential of their actions to lead to disease transmission. In two of these outbreaks (90), the relevant healthcare worker reported performing the implicated practices routinely over a period of years.

Awareness of fundamental infection control principles, aseptic techniques, and safe injection practices is essential to prevent healthcare-related transmission of hepatitis viruses. These principles, techniques, and practices need to be reinforced in training programs; added to institutional policies and in-service education for healthcare staff, including those in outpatient settings; and monitored as part of the oversight process. Episodes of such transmission should be viewed as sentinel events for the detection of breaches in infection control practice. They are reminders that such lapses have important public health and patient safety implications.

REFERENCES

1. Goodman RA. Nosocomial hepatitis A. *Ann Intern Med* 1985;103:452–454.
2. Maynard J. Nosocomial viral hepatitis. *Am J Med* 1981;70:439–444.
3. Knoll A, Helmig M, Peters Ö, et al. Hepatitis C virus transmission in a pediatric oncology ward: analysis of an outbreak and review of the literature. *Lab Invest* 2001;81:251–262.
4. Sanchez-Tapias JM. Nosocomial transmission of hepatitis C virus. *J Hepatol* 1999;31(suppl):107–112.
5. Chiarello LA. Prevention of patient-to-patient transmission of bloodborne viruses. *Semin Infect Control* 2001;1:44–48.
6. Alter MJ. Epidemiology and prevention of hepatitis B. *Semin Liver Dis* 2003;23:39–46.
7. Ezzati M, Lopez AD, Rodgers A, et al. Selected major risk factors and global and regional burden of disease. *Lancet* 2002;360:1347–1360.
8. Centers for Disease Control and Prevention. *Hepatitis surveillance report,* no. 58. Atlanta: U.S. Department of Health and Human Services, Public Health Service, CDC, 2001.
9. Stapleton JT. Host immune response to hepatitis A virus. *J Infect Dis* 1995;171(suppl 1):S9–14.
10. Bell BP, Shapiro CN, Alter MJ, et al. The diverse patterns of hepatitis A epidemiology in the United States—implications for vaccination strategies. *J Infect Dis* 1998;178:1579–1584.
11. Staes CJ, Schlenker TL, Risk I, et al. Sources of infection among persons with acute hepatitis A and no identified risk factors during a sustained community-wide outbreak. *Pediatrics* 2000;106(4):E54.
12. Armstrong GL, Bell BP. Hepatitis A virus infections in the United States: model-based estimates and implications for childhood immunization. *Pediatrics* 2002;109:839–845.
13. Seeberg S, Brandberg Å, Hermodsson S, et al. Hospital outbreak of hepatitis A secondary to blood exchange in a baby. *Lancet* 1981;1:1155–1156.
14. Skidmore SJ, Boxall EH, Ala F. A case report of post-transfusion hepatitis A. *J Med Virol* 1982;10:223.
15. Hollinger FB, Khan NC, Oefinger PE, et al. Posttransfusion hepatitis type A. *JAMA* 1983;250:;2323–2327.
16. Noble RC, Kane MA, Reeves SA, et al. Posttransfusion hepatitis A in a neonatal intensive care unit. *JAMA* 1984;252:2711–2715.
17. Sheretz RJ, Russell BA, Reumann PD. Transmission of hepatitis A by transfusion of blood products. *Arch Intern Med* 1984;144:1579–1580.
18. Giacoia GP, Kasprisin DO. Transfusion-acquired hepatitis A. *South Med J* 1989;82:1357–1360.
19. Azimi PH, Roberto RR, Guralnik J, et al. Transfusion-acquired hepatitis A in a premature infant with secondary nosocomial spread in an intensive care nursery. *Am J Dis Child* 1986;140:23–27.
20. Rosenblum LS, Villarino ME, Nainan OV, et al. Hepatitis A outbreak in a neonatal intensive care unit: risk factors for transmission and evidence of prolonged viral excretion among preterm infants. *J Infect Dis* 1991;164:476–482.
21. McCaustland KA, Bond WW, Bradley DW, et al. Survival of hepatitis A virus in feces after drying and storage for 1 month. *J Clin Microbiol* 1982;16:957–958.
22. Favero MS, Bond WW. Disinfection and sterilization. In: Zuckerman AJ, Thomas HC, eds. *Viral hepatitis, scientific basis and clinical management.* New York: Churchill Livingstone, 1993:565–575.
23. Krugman S, Giles JP. Viral hepatitis: new light on an old disease. *JAMA* 1970;212:1019–1029.
24. Hadler SC, Webster HM, Erben JJ, et al. Hepatitis A in day-care centers: a community-wide assessment. *N Engl J Med* 1980;302:1222–1227.
25. Lednar WM, Lemon SM, Kirkpatrick JW, et al. Frequency of illness associated with epidemic hepatitis A virus infection in adults. *Am J Epidemiol* 1985;122:226–233.
26. Glikson M, Galun E, Oren R, et al. Relapsing hepatitis A. Review of 14 cases and literature survey. *Medicine* 1992;71:14–23.
27. Skinhpj P, Mathiesen LR, Kryger P, et al. Faecal excretion of hepatitis A virus in patients with symptomatic hepatitis A infection. *Scand J Gastroenterol* 1981;16:1057–1059.
28. Tassopoulos NC, Papaevangelou GJ, Ticehurst JR, et al. Fecal excretion of Greek strains of hepatitis A virus in patients with hepatitis A and in experimentally infected chimpanzees. *J Infect Dis* 1986;154:231–237.
29. Sjogren MH, Tanno H, Fay O, et al. Hepatitis A virus in stool during clinical relapse. *Ann Intern Med* 1987;106:221–226.
30. Lemon SM. The natural history of hepatitis A: the potential for transmission by transfusion of blood or blood products. *Vox Sang* 1994;67(suppl 4):19–23.
31. Bower WA, Nainan OV, Han X, et al. Duration of viremia in hepatitis A virus infection. *J Infect Dis* 2000;182(1):12–17.
32. Cohen JI, Feinstone S, Purcell RH. Hepatitis A virus infection in a chimpanzee: duration of viremia and detection of virus in saliva and throat swabs. *J Infect Dis* 1989;160:887–890.
33. Liaw YF, Yang CY, Chu CM, et al. Appearance and persistence of hepatitis A IgM antibody in acute clinical hepatitis A observed in an outbreak. *Infection* 1986;14:156–158.
34. Hutin YJF, Pool V, Cramer EH, et al. A multistate, foodborne outbreak of hepatitis A. *N Engl J Med* 1999;340:595–602.
35. Klein BS, Michaels JA, Rytel MW, et al. Nosocomial hepatitis A: a multinursery outbreak in Wisconsin. *JAMA* 1984;252:2716–2721.
36. Watson JC, Fleming DW, Borella AJ, et al. Vertical transmission of hepatitis A resulting in an outbreak in a neonatal intensive care unit. *J Infect Dis* 1993;167:567–571.
37. Papaevangelou GJ, Roumeliotou-Karayannis AJ, Contoyannis PC. The risk of nosocomial hepatitis A and B virus infections from patients under care without isolation precaution. *J Med Virol* 1981;7:143–148.
38. Goodman RA, Carder CC, Allen JR, et al. Nosocomial hepatitis A transmission by an adult patient with diarrhea. *Am J Med* 1982;73:220–226.
39. Skidmore SJ, Gully PR, Middleton JD, et al. An outbreak of hepatitis A on a hospital ward. *J Med Virol* 1985;1:175–177.
40. Burkholder BT, Coronado VG, Brown J, et al. Nosocomial transmission of hepatitis A in a pediatric hospital traced to an anti-hepatitis A virus-negative patient with immunodeficiency. *Pediatr Infect Dis J* 1995;14:261–266.

41. Reed CM, Gustafson TL, Siegel J, et al. Nosocomial transmission of hepatitis A from a hospital-acquired case. *Pediatr Infect Dis* 1984;3: 300–303.
42. Garner JS. Guideline for isolation precautions in hospitals. The Hospital Infection Control Practices Advisory Committee. *Infect Control Hosp Epidemiol* 1996;17:53–80.
43. Centers for Disease Control and Prevention. Guideline for hand hygiene in health-care settings: recommendations of the Healthcare Infection Control Practices Advisory Committee and the HICPAC/SHEA/APIC/IDSA Hand Hygiene Task Force. *MMWR* 2002; 51(RR-16):1–45.
44. Centers for Disease Control and Prevention. Prevention of hepatitis A through active or passive immunization: recommendations of the Advisory Committee on Immunization Practices (ACIP). *MMWR* 1999;48(RR-12):1–37.
45. Hepatitis A. In: Atkinson W, Wolfe C, eds. *Epidemiology and prevention of vaccine-preventable diseases.* Atlanta: U.S. Department of Health and Human Services, CDC, 2002.
46. Clemens R, Safary A, Hepburn A, et al. Clinical experience with an inactivated hepatitis A vaccine. *J Infect Dis* 1995;171(suppl 1): S44–49.
47. Nalin DR. VAQTA, hepatitis A vaccine, purified inactivated. *Drugs Future* 1995;20:24–29.
48. Kashiwagi S, Hayashi J, Ikematsu H, et al. Prevalence of immunologic markers of hepatitis A and B infection in hospital personnel in Miyazaki Prefecture, Japan. *Am J Epidemiol* 1985;122:960–969.
49. Gibas A, Blewett DR, Schoenfield DA, et al. Prevalence and incidence of viral hepatitis in health workers in the prehepatitis B vaccination era. *Am J Epidemiol* 1992;136:603–610.
50. Hepatitis B. In: Atkinson W, Wolfe C, eds. *Epidemiology and prevention of vaccine-preventable diseases.* Atlanta: U.S. Department of Health and Human Services, CDC, 2002.
51. McQuillan GM, Coleman PJ, Kruszon-Moran D, et al. Prevalence of hepatitis B virus infection in the United States: the National Health and Nutrition Examination Surveys, 1976 through 1994. *Am J Public Health* 1999;89:14–18.
52. Favero MS. Sterilization, disinfection and antisepsis in the hospital. In: Lennett EH, Ballows A, Hausler WJ, et al., eds. *Manual of clinical microbiology,* 4th ed. Washington, DC: American Society of Microbiology, 1985:129–137.
53. Goldstein ST, Alter MJ, Williams IT, et al. Incidence and risk factors for acute hepatitis B in the United States, 1982–1998: implications for vaccination programs. *J Infect Dis* 2002;185:713–719.
54. Pattison CP, Boyer KM, Maynard JE, et al. Epidemic hepatitis in a clinical laboratory: possible association with computer card handling. *JAMA* 1974;230:854–857.
55. Bond WW, Favero MS, Petersen NJ, et al. Inactivation of hepatitis B virus by intermediate-to-high level disinfectant chemicals. *J Clin Microbiol* 1983;18:535–538.
56. Favero MS, Bond WW. Disinfection and sterilization. In: Zuckerman AJ, Thomas HC, ed. *Viral hepatitis: scientific basis and clinical management.* New York: Churchill Livingstone, 1993:565–575.
57. Kobayashi H, Tsuzuki M, Koshimizu K, et al. Susceptibility of hepatitis B virus to disinfectants and heat. *J Clin Microbiol* 1984;20: 214–216.
58. Bond WW, Petersen NJ, Favero MS. Viral hepatitis B: aspects of environmental control. *Health Lab Sci* 1977;14:235–252.
59. McMahon BJ, Alward WL, Hall DB, et al. Acute hepatitis B virus infection: relation of age to the clinical expression of disease and subsequent development of the carrier state. *J Infect Dis* 1985;151(4): 599–603.
60. Margolis HS, Alter MJ, Hadler SC. Hepatitis B: evolving epidemiology and implications for control. *Semin Liver Dis* 1991;11(2):84–92.
61. Centers for Disease Control and Prevention. Recommendations for preventing transmission of infections among chronic hemodialysis patients. *MMWR* 2001;50(RR-5):1–43.
62. Kloster B, Kramer R, Eastlund T, et al. Hepatitis B surface antigenemia in blood donors following vaccination. *Transfusion* 1995;35: 475–477.
63. Lunn ER, Hoggarth BJ, Cook WJ. Prolonged hepatitis B surface antigenemia after vaccination. *Pediatrics* 2000;105:E81.
64. McMahon BJ, Alberts SR, Wainwright RB, et al. Hepatitis B-related sequelae: prospective study in 1400 hepatitis B surface antigen-positive Alaska Native carriers. *Arch Intern Med* 1990;150:1051–1054.
65. Douvin C, Simon D, Zinelabidine H, et al. An outbreak of hepatitis B in an endocrinology unit traced to a capillary-blood sampling device. *N Engl J Med* 1990;322:57–58.
66. Polish LB, Shapiro CN, Bauer F, et al. Nosocomial transmission of hepatitis B virus associated with the use of a spring-loaded fingerstick device. *N Engl J Med* 1992;326:721–725.
67. Centers for Disease Control and Prevention. Nosocomial hepatitis B virus associated with spring-loaded fingerstick blood sampling devices—Ohio and New York City, 1996. *MMWR* 1997;46:217–221.
68. Quale JM, Landman D, Wallace B, et al. Déja vu: nosocomial hepatitis B virus transmission and finger-stick monitoring. *Am J Med* 1998; 105:296–301.
69. Vickers J, Painter MJ, Heptonstall J, et al. Hepatitis B outbreak in a drug trials unit: investigation and recommendations. *Commun Dis Rep* 1994;4:R1–5.
70. Kidd-Ljunggren K, Broman E, Ekvall H, et al. Nosocomial transmission of hepatitis B virus infection through multiple-dose vials. *J Hosp Infect* 1999;43:57–62.
71. Oren I, Hershow RC, Ben-Porath E, et al. A common-source outbreak of fulminant hepatitis B in a hospital. *Ann Intern Med* 1989;110: 691–698.
72. Liang TJ, Hasegawa K, Rimon N, et al. A hepatitis B virus mutant associated with an epidemic of fulminant hepatitis. *N Engl Med* 1991; 324:1705–1709.
73. Petrosillo N, Ippolito G, Solforosi G, et al. Molecular epidemiology of an outbreak of fulminant hepatitis B. *J Clin Microbiol* 2000;38: 2975–2981.
74. Birnie GG, Quigley EM, Clements GB, et al. Endoscopic transmission of hepatitis B virus. *Gut* 1983;24:171–174.
75. Canter J, Mackey K, Good LS, et al. An outbreak of hepatitis B associated with jet injections in a weight reduction clinic. *Arch Intern Med* 1990;150:1923–1927.
76. Kent GP, Brondum J, Keenlyside RA, et al. A large outbreak of acupuncture-associated hepatitis B. *Am J Epidemiol* 1988;127:591–598.
77. Slater PE, Ten-Ishai P, Leventhal A, et al. An acupuncture-associated outbreak of hepatitis B in Jerusalem. *Eur J Epidemiol* 1988;4: 322–325.
78. Stryker WS, Gunn RA, Francis DP. Outbreak of hepatitis B associated with acupuncture. *J Fam Pract* 1986;22:155–158.
79. Drescher J, Wagner D, Haverich A, et al. Nosocomial hepatitis B virus infections in cardiac transplant recipients transmitted during transvenous endomyocardial biopsy. *J Hosp Infect* 1994;26:81–92.
80. Petzold DR, Tautz B, Wolf F, et al. Infection chains and evolution rates of hepatitis B virus in cardiac transplant recipients infected nosocomially. *J Med Virol* 1999;58(1):1–10.
81. Stuyver L, De Gendt S, Cadranel JF, et al. Three cases of severe subfulminant hepatitis in heart-transplanted patients after nosocomial transmission of a mutant hepatitis B virus. *Hepatology* 1999;29(6): 1876–1883.
82. Hlady WG, Hopkins RS, Ogilby TE, et al. Patient-to-patient transmission of hepatitis B in a dermatology practice. *Am J Public Health* 1993;83:1689–1693.
83. Dumpis U, Kovalova Z, Jansons J, et al. An outbreak of HBV and HCV infection in a paediatric oncology ward: epidemiological investigations and prevention of further spread. *J Med Virol* 2003;69(3): 331–338.
84. Hutin YJ, Harpaz R, Drobeniuc J, et al. Injections given in healthcare settings as a major source of acute hepatitis B in Moldova. *Int J Epidemiol* 1999;28(4):782–786.
85. Narendranathan M, Philip M. Reusable needles—a major risk factor for acute virus B hepatitis. *Trop Doct* 1993;23:54–56.
86. Singh J, Bhatia R, Gandhi JC, et al. Outbreak of viral hepatitis B in a rural community in India linked to inadequately sterilized needles and syringes. *Bull WHO* 1998;76:93–98.
87. Ko YC, Li SC, Yen YY, et al. Horizontal transmission of hepatitis

B virus from siblings and intramuscular injection among preschool children in a familial cohort. *Am J Epidemiol* 1991;133:1015–1023.
88. Hyams KC, Mansour MM, Massoud A, et al. Parenteral anti-schistosomal therapy: a potential risk factor for hepatitis B infection. *J Med Virol* 1987;23:109–114.
89. McCarthy MC, Hyams KC, el-Tigani el Hag A, et al. HIV-1 and hepatitis B transmission in Sudan. *AIDS* 1989;3:725–729.
90. Centers for Disease Control and Prevention. Transmission of hepatitis B and C viruses in outpatient settings—New York, Oklahoma, and Nebraska, 2000–2002. *MMWR* 2003;52:901–906.
91. National Institutes of Health. National Institutes of Health Consensus Development Conference Panel Statement: management of hepatitis C. *Hepatology* 2002;36:S3–20.
92. Centers for Disease Control and Prevention. Prevention and control of hepatitis viruses in correctional settings. *MMWR* 2003;52(RR-1): 1–44.
93. Centers for Disease Control and Prevention. Recommendations for prevention and control of hepatitis C virus (HCV) infection and HCV-related chronic disease. *MMWR* 1998;47(RR-19):1–39.
94. Alter MJ. Epidemiology of hepatitis C. *Hepatology* 1997;26(suppl 1): 62S–65S.
95. Williams IT, Fleenor M, Judson F, et al. Risk factors for hepatitis C virus (HCV) transmission in the USA: 1991–1998 (abstract 114). Presented at the 10th International Symposium on Viral Hepatitis and Liver Disease, Atlanta, 2000.
96. Krawczynski K, Alter MJ, Robertson BH, et al. Environmental stability of hepatitis c virus (HCV): viability of dried/stored HCV in chimpanzee infectivity studies (abstract 556). *Hepatology* 2003;38:S428A.
97. Alter MJ, Margolis HS, Krawczynski K, et al. The natural history of community-acquired hepatitis C in the United States. *N Engl J Med* 1992;327:1899–1905.
98. Liang TJ, Jeffers L, Reddy RK, et al. Fulminant or subfulminant non-A, non-B viral hepatitis: the role of hepatitis C and E viruses. *Gastroenterology* 1993;104:556–562.
99. Wright TL. Etiology of fulminant hepatic failure: is another virus involved? *Gastroenterology* 1993;104:640–643.
100. Shakil AO, Conry-Cantilena C, Alter HJ, et al. Volunteer blood donors with antibody to hepatitis C virus: clinical, biochemical, virologic, and histologic features. *Ann Intern Med* 1995;123:330–337.
101. Seeff LB, Buskell-Bales Z, Wright EC, et al. Long-term mortality after transfusion-associated non-A, non-B hepatitis. *N Engl J Med* 1992;327:1906–1911.
102. Kiyosawa K, Sodeyama T, Tanaka E, et al. Interrelationship of blood transfusion, non-A, non-B hepatitis and hepatocellular carcinoma: analysis by detection of antibody to hepatitis C virus. *Hepatology* 1990; 12:671–675.
103. Di Bisceglie AM, Order SE, Klein JL, et al. The role of chronic viral hepatitis in hepatocellular carcinoma in the United States. *Am J Gastroenterol* 1991;86:335–338.
104. Fattovich G, Giustina G, Degos F, et al. Morbidity and mortality in compensated cirrhosis type C: a retrospective follow-up study of 384 patients. *Gastroenterology* 1997;112:463–472.
105. Di Bisceglie AM, Goodman ZD, Ishak KG, et al. Long-term clinical and histopathological follow-up of chronic posttransfusion hepatitis. *Hepatology* 1991;14:969–974.
106. Centers for Disease Control and Prevention. Guidelines for laboratory testing and result reporting of antibody to hepatitis C virus. *MMWR* 2003;52(RR-3):1–15.
107. Pawlotsky JM. Use and interpretation of virological tests for hepatitis C. *Hepatology* 2002;36:S65–73.
108. Desenclos JC, Bourdiol-Razes M, Rolin B, et al. Hepatitis C in a ward for cystic fibrosis and diabetic patients: possible transmission by spring-loaded finger-stick devices for self-monitoring of capillary blood glucose. *Infect Control Hosp Epidemiol* 2001;22(11):701–707.
109. Tallis GF, Ryan GM, Lambert SB, et al. Evidence of patient-to-patient transmission of hepatitis C virus through contaminated intravenous anaesthetic ampoules. *J Viral Hepat* 2003;10(3):234–239.
110. Widell A, Christensson B, Wiebe T, et al. Epidemiologic and molecular investigation of outbreaks of hepatitis C virus infection on a pediatric oncology service. *Ann Intern Med* 1999;13:130–134.
111. Lagging LM, Åneman C, Nenonen N, et al. Nosocomial transmission of HCV in a cardiology ward during the window phase of infection: an epidemiological and molecular investigation. *Scand J Infect Dis* 2002;34(8):580–582.
112. Krause G, Trepka MJ, Whisenhunt RS, et al. Nosocomial transmission of hepatitis C virus associated with the use of multidose saline vials. *Infect Control Hosp Epidemiol* 2003;24:122–127.
113. Bruguera M, Saiz JC, Franco S, et al. Outbreak of nosocomial hepatitis C virus infection resolved by genetic analysis of HCV RNA. *J Clin Microbiol* 2002;40:4363–4366.
114. Massari M, Petrosillo N, Ippolito G, et al. Transmission of hepatitis C virus in a gynecological surgery setting. *J Clin Microbiol* 2001;39: 2860–2863.
115. Schvarcz R, Johansson B, Nyström B, et al. Nosocomial transmission of hepatitis C virus. *Infection* 1997;25:74–77.
116. Saginur R, Nixon J, Devries B, et al. Transmission of hepatitis C in a pharmacologic study. *Infect Control Hosp Epidemiol* 2001;22: 697–700.
117. Alter MJ, Kruszon-Moran D, Nainan OV, et al. The prevalence of hepatitis C virus infection in the United States, 1988 through 1994. *N Engl J Med* 1999;341(8):556–562.
118. Alter MJ. Prevention of spread of hepatitis C. *Hepatology* 2002;36: S93–98.
119. Centers for Disease Control and Prevention. Guidelines for the prevention of intravascular catheter-related infections. *MMWR* 2002; 51(RR-10):1–26.
120. Bronowicki JP, Venard V, Botté C, et al. Patient-to-patient transmission of hepatitis C virus during colonoscopy. *N Engl J Med* 1997; 337:237–240.
121. Spach DH, Silverstein FE, Stamm WE. Transmission of infection by gastrointestinal endoscopy and bronchoscopy. *Ann Intern Med* 1993; 118:117–128.
122. Alvarado C, Reichelderfer M, Association for Professionals in Infection Control and Epidemiology, Inc. APIC guideline for infection prevention and control in flexible endoscopy. *Am J Infect Control* 2000;28:138–155.
123. Allander T, Gruber A, Naghavi M, et al. Frequent patient-to-patient transmission of hepatitis C virus in a haematology ward. *Lancet* 1995; 345:603–607.
124. Silini E, Locasciulli A, Santoleri L, et al. Hepatitis C virus infection in a hematology ward: evidence for nosocomial transmission and impact on hematologic disease outcome. *Haematologica* 2002;87: 1200–1208.
125. Chant K, Kociuba K, Munro R, et al. Investigation of possible patient-to-patient transmission of hepatitis C in a hospital. *NSW Public Health Bull* 1994;5:47–51.
126. Heinsen A, Bendtsen F, Fomsgaard A. A phylogenetic analysis elucidating a case of patient-to-patient transmission of hepatitis C virus during surgery. *J Hosp Infect* 2000;46(4):309–313.
127. Larke B, Hu YW, Krajden M, et al. Acute nosocomial HCV infection detected by NAT of a regular blood donor. *Transfusion* 2002;42: 759–765.
128. Lesourd F, Izopet J, Mervan C, et al. Transmissions of hepatitis C virus during the ancillary procedures for assisted conception. *Human Reprod* 2000;15:1083–1085.
129. Zeytinoglu A, Erensoy S, Abacioglu H, et al. Nosocomial hepatitis C virus infection in a renal transplantation center. *Clin Microbiol Infect* 2002;8:741–744.
130. Centers for Disease Control. Recommendations for prevention of HIV transmission in health-care settings. *MMWR* 1987;36(2S): 1S–18S.
131. Centers for Disease Control and Prevention. Guideline for environmental control in healthcare facilities. *MMWR* 2003;52(RR-10): 1–44.
132. Centers for Disease Control and Prevention. Updated U.S. Public Health Service guidelines for the management of occupational exposure to HBV, HCV, and HIV and recommendations for postexposure prophylaxis. *MMWR* 2001;50(RR-11):1–52.

E

Other Pathogens

46

ECTOPARASITES

SUSIE J. SARGENT

Infestations with ectoparasites are common in the community and among hospitalized patients. Nosocomial transmission has been reported with scabies, lice, maggots, and pigeon mites. These ectoparasites tend to be more troublesome to infection control professionals than detrimental to patients; however, in immunosuppressed patients, they can be a source of serious morbidity.

SCABIES

Etiology and Pathogenesis

Cutaneous infestation with the human itch mite, *Sarcoptes scabiei* var. hominis, causes the highly contagious condition known as scabies. The mite is a tiny arthropod with four pairs of short legs and an oval translucent sac-like body with transverse corrugations and brown spines (Fig. 46.1). The female is larger than the male, measuring 0.3 to 0.4 mm in length, whereas the male is approximately 0.15 to 0.2 mm long. The mite is an obligate human parasite, completing its entire life cycle on human skin, and is generally able to survive only 2 to 3 days off the body. It often causes mini-epidemics in families, hospitals, and institutions. After direct contact with an infested person or possibly fomites, the gravid female mite rapidly traverses the human body, quickly attaches itself, and burrows into the stratum corneum of the skin. As the female continues to burrow, it deposits about two or three eggs per day along the tunnel before completing its life cycle in approximately 30 days. The eggs hatch into larvae in 3 to 4 days, migrate to the skin surface, subsequently molt into nymphs, and develop into adults in 10 to 17 days. The adults live for 4 to 5 weeks and then mate; the newly fertilized female then burrows into the cuticle to complete the cycle. Most patients harbor about 10 to 15 burrowing female mites. As the population builds up over 2 to 4 months, the females feed on cells of the stratum corneum, thereby producing excretions that sensitize the host and create intense pruritus. Once sensitization occurs, a generalized rash develops with eosinophilic infiltrates around the burrows.

Epidemiology

Although not a reportable disease, the prevalence of scabies has increased in the United States since the mid-1970s (1–3). Worldwide, outbreaks have generally occurred in association with conditions of crowding, poor hygiene, and malnutrition (4,5). However, the current nationwide resurgence has affected persons from all socioeconomic levels without regard to age, sex, or cleanliness (4,6). Scabies is spread by close personal contact despite good personal hygiene; therefore, it is often seen among families and sexual partners. One study showed a 38% attack rate among family contacts (7). Transmission can also occur in institutional settings (8), nursing homes (6,9), and day care centers (10) via skin-to-skin contact with an infested person. By contrast, although scabies is common among schoolchildren, there is little evidence that transmission occurs within the classroom. In hospitals, personnel can acquire and transmit infestation during direct hands-on contact with infested patients while performing patient care activities such as sponge-bathing or applying lotions. An attack rate of 30% has been noted among hospital personnel caring for undiagnosed cases. Transmission is especially likely when personnel are exposed to patients with large mite populations such as in Norwegian or crusted scabies, because the exfoliated scales contain numerous mites. (11) Although the role of fomite transmission via infested clothes, bedding, or linens is controversial, several reports have indicated that fomites may be important when large numbers of mites are present (12,13).

Clinical Manifestations

Scabies is often misdiagnosed, because it may mimic several other cutaneous disorders such as eczema, atopic dermatitis, con-

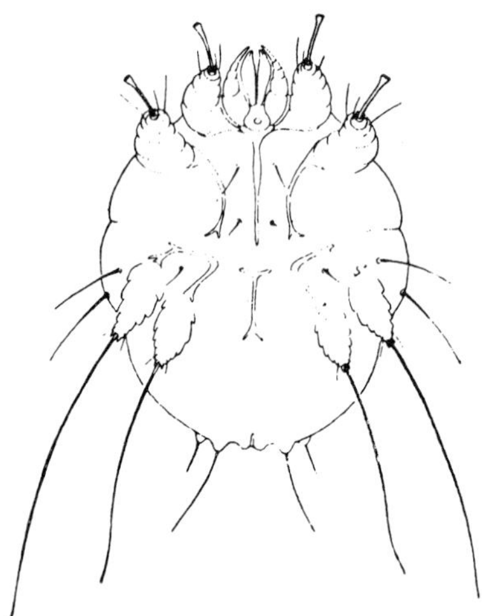

Figure 46.1. The itch mite, *Sarcoptes scabiei.* (Reprinted from Harwood RF, Maurice JT. *Entomology in human and animal health,* 7th ed. New York: Simon & Schuster, Macmillan, 1979:361, with permission.)

tact dermatitis, insect bites, urticaria, or impetigo. However, it should be suspected in patients with pruritic excoriations and pleomorphic lesions with a characteristic distribution. There is usually a slow onset of pruritus and cutaneous eruption, because the incubation period in a previously unexposed individual may be 4 weeks or more until the onset of symptoms. Shorter incubation periods of 1 to 2 weeks may be seen with reinfestations (14). The pathognomonic feature is the burrow, which is a short (1 to 10 mm), wavy, elevated linear eruption that may be capped with a small vesicle. Occasionally, brown-black material composed of feces, eggs, or mites may be visible in the burrow. Different types of lesions in varying stages may also be present, such as papules, crusts, pustules, bullae, excoriations, and, occasionally, nodules. In classic scabies, the lesions are symmetric, involving the finger webs, hands, wrists, elbows, axillae, umbilicus, female breasts, and male genitals. The histopathology of the lesions is compatible with a hypersensitivity reaction probably involving both humoral and cell-mediated immunity. Sensitization to mite antigens occurs 4 to 6 weeks after infestation, gradually causing a generalized rash with intense pruritus, especially at night. The nocturnal pruritus may be so prominent that patients develop hemorrhagic excoriations, which are less common in other dermatoses. This typically symmetric, pruritic rash does not correspond to the sites of the burrows but usually affects the hands, arms, legs, inner thighs, and waist. Scabies generally does not involve the face, scalp, neck, chest, or back except in children younger than 12 months or in immunosuppressed persons. Infants and children usually have fewer burrows and may have eczematous involvement of the head, neck, palms, and soles.

Variations from the typical presentation of scabies may be caused by host differences or other factors (15). Burrows may be less prevalent in persons with better personal hygiene, possibly because of frequent bathing (16). Persons using topical or systemic steroids may not have signs or symptoms of inflammation, despite being able to readily transmit the infestation. Bedridden patients in nursing homes or chronic care facilities may have scabies limited to sites in constant contact with sheets (17). A persistent pruritic nodular form of scabies may develop despite treatment in 5% to 7% of scabietic patients. The reddish-brown nodules are thought to represent a continued hypersensitivity reaction. They usually occur in the intertriginous areas such as the groin, genitals, or axilla, but rarely contain mites, and eventually clear after several months. Scabies may also be seen in patients attending sexually transmitted disease clinics in association with other venereal diseases.

A special form of scabies known as Norwegian or crusted scabies was originally described among Norwegians with leprosy in 1848 (18). Instead of the usual small number of mites on the skin of an infested person, patients with crusted scabies may harbor thousands of mites. Although less common, this condition is highly contagious, and has contributed to several nosocomial outbreaks (3,19–24). Because the presentation is not classic, diagnosis is often delayed, increasing the risk of transmission. Clinically, patients present with atypical crusted or hyperkeratotic plaques that may become generalized but are minimally pruritic. Erythroderma and nail dystrophy may also be present. Usually seen in persons who are physically debilitated or immunologically deficient, the mites are able to proliferate to enormous numbers. Norwegian scabies has been described in patients affected by leprosy (18), Down syndrome (25,26), renal dialysis (27), infection with the human immunodeficiency virus or human T-lymphotrophic virus-1 (28–43), diabetes (9,44–46), transplantation (47–49), hematologic malignancy (50,51), nutritional deficiency (52), connective tissue disorders (53,54), and steroid use (55,56). Because the exfoliated scales sloughed by patients with crusted scabies contain numerous mites, these scabietic patients are extremely contagious via contact and may heavily contaminate their environment (6,57). One study estimated that 7,640 mites were shed into the environment from a single patient over 2 days (52).

A common complication of scabietic patients is pyoderma. Scratching may disrupt the normal cutaneous barrier, allowing for colonization and proliferation of bacteria in the abraded skin. This also contributes to misdiagnosis, because physicians may attribute the inflammation and skin lesions to pyoderma alone, as opposed to a secondary bacterial infection associated with scabies. Norwegian scabies, when complicated by bacterial sepsis, can be life threatening (58–60). Scalded skin syndrome has been reported in patients whose scabietic lesions were colonized or infected with staphylococci, as has poststreptococcal glomerulonephritis in patients with a virulent nephritogenic strain of streptococci on their skin (17,61).

All patients develop a hypersensitivity reaction to mite antigens and their excretions, but many also experience a postscabietic pruritus, dermatitis, or urticaria even after adequate treatment. Dead mites, eggs, and feces remain in the stratum corneum, causing continued pruritus until naturally sloughed in 2 weeks to 3 months. Therefore, persistent pruritus does not necessarily indicate treatment failure, although resistance to scabicides has been reported (62–64).

Diagnosis

The definitive diagnosis depends on identification of a scabies mite, egg, or fecal pellet (scybala) from a burrow on the skin.

Most commonly, a drop of mineral oil is applied to an unexcoriated papule or burrow of recent onset, which is then scraped with a scalpel or curette to unroof the burrow. The scrapings are transferred to a glass slide, a coverslip is applied, and the specimen is examined under low power. False-negative scrapings may occur if the scraping is performed by inexperienced personnel or if the specimen is taken from severely excoriated lesions. Because the sensitivity of this procedure varies from 10% to 60%, several specimens may be needed before evidence of mites is found. Alternatively, the burrow ink test may be performed by applying a felt-tipped ink pen to the burrow and wiping off the excess ink with alcohol, thereby allowing the ink to penetrate the burrow and become visible (65,66). Skin biopsy specimens may also detect the parasite (67). Other possible methods of diagnosis include videodermatoscopy (68,69) and epiluminescence microscopy (69,70), but these require special diagnostic equipment and have not been shown to be more sensitive than skin scrapings.

Other supporting features of infestation include nocturnal or intense pruritus, burrows, or suggestive skin lesions in the characteristic distribution or a history of contact with a case.

Prevention and Control

Personnel can help prevent exposure to scabies by having a high index of suspicion for any rash of unknown cause and practicing appropriate infection control precautions until a diagnosis is made. Once infestation is suspected or identified, special precautions should be instituted, depending on whether the patient is classified as having conventional or crusted scabies (71). Adequate treatment with permethrin, 1% lindane lotion, ivermectin (69,72–79), or other appropriate scabicide should be instituted as soon as possible for the patient and for all close personal contacts. Crusted scabies or severe disease may require repeat dosing or a combination of oral ivermectin and a topical scabicide (63,69,77,78,80–82). Skin-to-skin contact with the patient should be avoided for 8 hours after the application of a scabicide. Routine disinfection procedures are adequate for room cleaning (83).

A single case of conventional scabies requires only contact precautions with careful gloving and hand washing. Crusted scabies, however, is associated with increased transmissibility because of the large mite population and requires more extensive controls and environmental decontamination. Gloves, long-sleeved gowns with the wrist area covered, and shoe covers are indicated when touching the patient or his or her clothing or bed linens. Hands should be washed after removal of gloves. Barrier protection may be enhanced with insecticide sprays. Protective items should be removed before leaving the room. Furniture containing textiles should be removed and replaced with vinyl furniture. Special bagging of infested laundry (i.e., plastic bags) may be necessary, because outbreaks in hospital laundry workers have been reported (20,84). Bagged laundry should not be sorted before washing. Laundry workers should wear gowns and gloves if handling contaminated linen. Clothing and linens used before treatment must be washed at a temperature in excess of 50°C for at least 10 minutes to kill mites and eggs. Personal articles such as shoes or toys should be sealed in a plastic bag for 10 days. These precautionary measures should remain in effect until skin scrapings have been negative for 3 consecutive days. Terminal cleaning of the room involves thorough vacuuming with insecticide spraying or fogging before reassignment (14, 83). Hospital staff, relatives, or friends who may have had contact with a scabietic patient before precautions were instituted should be identified and treated. All infested persons should be treated at the same time, if possible.

If hospital personnel are infested with scabies, they should be allowed to return to work the day after completing treatment. Gloves may be used for 2 to 3 days after symptomatic staff members have been treated if extensive hands-on care is required.

PEDICULOSIS

Etiology and Pathogenesis

Pediculosis implies infestation with one of three clinically important species of lice from the family Pediculidae. Humans are the only reservoir for these parasites, which usually localize to a specific area of the body. The species parasitic to humans are *Pediculus humanus* var. *capitis* (the human head louse), *Pediculus humanus* var. *corporis* (the human body louse), and *Phthirus pubis* (the pubic or crab louse).

P. capitis and *P. corporis* are nearly identical in appearance; the latter probably evolved from the head louse after humans became clothed (85). They are small (2 to 4 mm), elongated, grayish, flat, wingless parasites. They have three pairs of lateral jointed legs extending from the thorax with terminal crab-like claws (Fig. 46.2). The pubic louse is more rounded in shape, resembling a crab (Fig. 46.3). The life cycles are similar; eggs are deposited by fertilized adult females on body hairs close to the scalp or on cloth fibers in oval protrusions called nits. Generally, only one viable egg is attached to each hair (Fig. 46.4). After 7 to 10 days, small nymphs emerge leaving an empty shell or nit; the nymphs must have a human blood meal within 24 hours to survive. The nymphs molt a total of three times before becoming mature adults, feeding frequently on blood and maintaining close body contact for warmth, which is required for

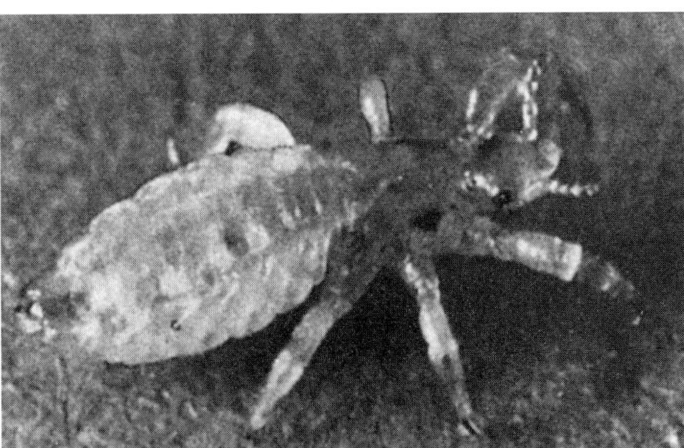

Figure 46.2. The human body louse, *Pediculus humanus.* (Reprinted from Harwood RF, Maurice JT. *Entomology in human and animal health,* 7th ed. New York: Simon & Schuster, Macmillan, 1979:132, with permission.)

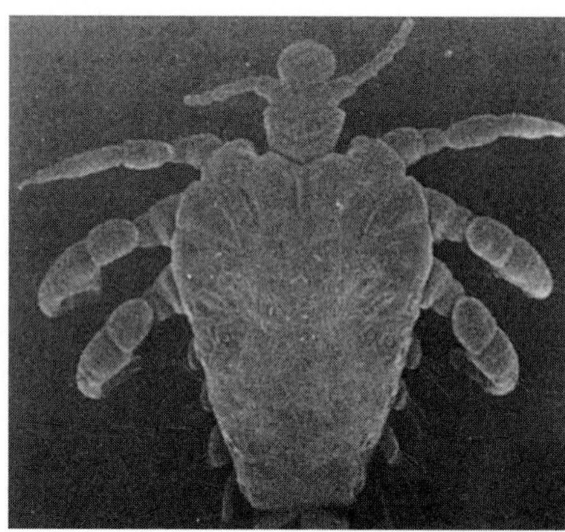

Figure 46.3. The crab louse, *Phthirus pubis.* (Reprinted from Harwood RF, Maurice JT. *Entomology in human and animal health,* 7th ed. New York: Simon & Schuster, Macmillan, 1979:130, with permission.)

hatching. Once fertilized, the female produces 250 to 300 eggs during her lifetime of approximately 30 days.

Epidemiology

The incidence of infestation with lice is increasing worldwide and in the United States. All socioeconomic classes are affected, but conditions of crowding, poor hygiene, communal living, and sexual freedom are contributory. Infestation tends to be higher among children, among whom close proximity to each other and their clothing may be important.

Pediculus capitis

The head louse is transmitted primarily through direct head-to-head contact (86). Transmission by indirect contact with shared hats, caps, brushes, combs, or bedding is less well documented and somewhat controversial (87–89). Head lice are seen more commonly among school-aged children, especially young girls. Although lice climb easily from hair to hair when it is dry, combing can disrupt them, often causing the loss of a leg, which is usually fatal. Away from the host, eggs can live only about 10 days but cannot hatch at room temperature or below. However, the head louse can survive prolonged immersion in water by closing off its breathing apertures and locking its legs around the hair shaft (89). Nosocomial transmission is infrequent but has been reported in pediatric and adolescent institutions (14).

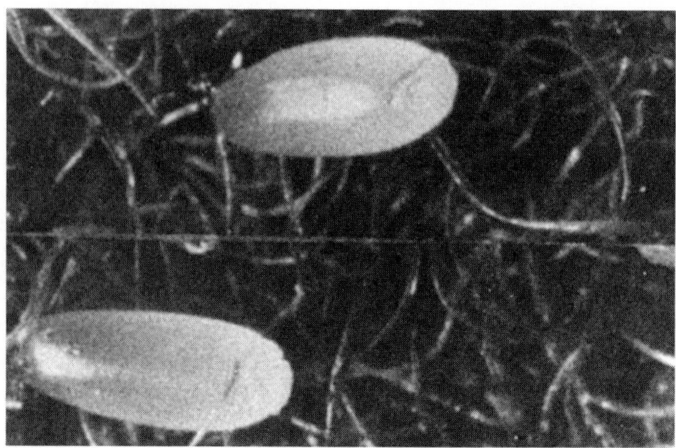

Figure 46.4. *Pediculus humanus* eggs. (Reprinted from Harwood RF, Maurice JT. *Entomology in human and animal health,* 7th ed. New York: Simon & Schuster, Macmillan, 1979:132, with permission.)

Pediculus corporis

The body louse surfaces primarily in conditions of crowding, poor personal hygiene, poverty, or inadequate sanitation; thus, it is also called vagabond's disease. It is transmitted by direct contact with the body or, more commonly, through contact with infested clothing or bedding. The parasite resides and lays its eggs primarily in the inner seams of clothes that are in close contact with the skin. It is usually absent from the body except while feeding. Nosocomial transmission is uncommon, because infested clothing is the primary mode of transmission, and the louse only transfers from clothing to skin in the dark (90). The human body louse has also been an important vector in the transmission of epidemic typhus, trench fever, and louse-borne relapsing fever. In contrast, head lice and pubic lice are not known to transmit other diseases.

Phthirus pubis

The pubic louse is spread primarily through close physical or sexual contact; about 95% of sexual contacts become infested (14). It is uncommonly transmitted through clothing, toilet seats, or bedding because of its short survival time and decreased mobility off the host. The pubic louse resides predominately in the pubic hair but rarely is found in the axilla, eyelashes, eyebrows, or other areas of the body with hair. Because the role of fomites is limited, nosocomial transmission is unlikely.

Clinical Manifestations

Pediculus capitis

Head lice are generally confined to the temporal and occipital areas of the scalp but may involve the entire scalp and beard. The egg is firmly attached to the base of a hair via the nit composed of cement-like secretions, which also allows for a steady temperature of greater than 22°C as required for hatching. The nits are readily visible on the hair shaft but are not removed by washing. Pruritus of the scalp, which may be intense, is generally the presenting symptom. Excoriations resulting from scratching may become secondarily infected, causing weeping or crusting scalp lesions with related cervical or occipital adenopathy. Some patients may develop a hypersensitivity or "id" reaction to the inflammation, manifested by a symmetric, pruritic, morbilliform truncal eruption.

Pediculus corporis

The body louse causes pruritus with small erythematous, maculopapular lesions primarily located on the trunk and around the waist. Excoriations are often present and, if chronic, may cause generalized hyperpigmentation with thickening and scarring. Pruritus and other secondary id reactions are caused by host reactions to salivary antigens.

Phthirus pubis

Intense pruritus involving primarily the pubic hair or other affected areas is usually the presenting complaint with infestation by the pubic or crab louse. Nits may be visualized at the base of the hairs. If the eyelashes are involved, crusting may be observed along the eyelids. Small bluish-gray macules (maculae caeruleae) may be seen on the trunk, thighs, abdomen, or upper arms and are caused by an anticoagulant injected by the louse. Excoriated macules and papules with secondary bacterial infection are seen less often with the pubic louse than with head or body lice.

Diagnosis

In general, the diagnosis of pediculosis requires the identification of live lice or viable nits on the infested individual. Body lice are often found on clothing. Because eggs are deposited on the hair close to skin and cannot hatch at temperatures lower than 22°C, any nits located more than 1 cm away from the skin are probably empty. Because hair grows at a rate of about 1 cm per month, the age of an infestation can be estimated by measuring the number of centimeters to the most distant nit (91). With the head louse, few adult lice are generally found, but many nits firmly attached to the hair shaft can be seen. These nits must be differentiated from dandruff or hair casts, which slide freely along the hair. Infested hair fluoresces under a Wood's lamp (ultraviolet light).

Prevention and Control

Control of pediculosis involves treatment of the infested individual with an appropriate topical pediculicide such as permethrin, lindane, γ-benzene hexachloride, malathion, pyrethrin, or oral ivermectin (92–95). Only permethrins are ovicidal; if other topical agents are used, therapy should be repeated in 7 to 10 days to kill newly hatched lice. Family members and other personal contacts should also be examined. If they are infested, they should be treated. Sexual contacts of patients with pubic lice may be treated empirically because of the high rate of transmission.

The potential for fomite spread is greatest with body lice, because the parasite survives off the host longer than with head or pubic lice. Methods of decontamination for clothing or bedding include dry cleaning, machine washing, drying, or ironing. Heating to 60°C for 5 to 10 minutes kills all lice and eggs. Nonwashable items may be decontaminated by storage in plastic bags for 7 days for crab lice or 10 to 14 days for head lice. This is not as effective for body lice, because the eggs may survive for up to 30 days in plastic (96). However, eggs do not hatch in the inanimate environment at room temperature. Combs and brushes in contact with head lice may be soaked in 2% Lysol for 1 hour (14).

Hospitalized patients need not be isolated as long as bedding and clothing are disinfected and are not shared. Hospital personnel with patient contact do not require treatment unless infestation is evident. Routine terminal room cleaning and vacuuming are sufficient, because the adult parasite from all these species cannot survive without frequent blood meals. Fumigation and insecticide sprays are not necessary.

MYIASIS

Etiology and Pathogenesis

Myiasis is defined as the infestation of living or necrotic tissue of humans or animals by the larvae (maggots) of various two-winged fly species. Over 50 different species have been reported to cause human myiasis (97). There are three general patterns of myiasis that depend on the larvae conditions required for development. In obligatory or primary myiasis, larvae must develop or pass a stage of their life cycle within living tissue. They are able to avoid the host's immune system and often produce nodules or furuncles. The life cycle usually involves a mosquito; the fly eggs are attached to the mosquito's abdomen. While the mosquito is feeding on a warm-blooded host, the temperature change is detected, causing the eggs to hatch and allowing the larvae to penetrate the host's skin. A small nodule with a central pore develops. In 6 to 12 weeks, the maggot will emerge through the central pore.

Larvae of species that cause facultative or secondary myiasis are able to develop on surfaces and invade healthy or necrotic tissue, and they are often involved in nosocomial infections. Blood and body tissue fluids provide an olfactory stimulant for gravid flies. Hundreds of eggs are deposited on skin, wounds, body orifices, or dead tissue; the larvae emerge within a few days. Most infestations occur in patients who are debilitated, have altered levels of consciousness, or are unable to protect themselves from flies.

In intestinal myiasis, eggs or larvae are accidentally ingested but are not killed within the intestine. Although occasionally gastrointestinal complaints are noted, most patients are asymptomatic (98).

Maggots are variable in appearance but generally are small (3 to 7 mm), white, soft, segmented, and worm-like; some have hooks or spines (Fig. 46.5). Historically, maggots have been used to debride wounds and treat chronic osteomyelitis (99).

Epidemiology

Myiasis occurs more commonly in tropical areas but has been reported worldwide, especially during the summer months when fly populations are the largest. It is more prevalent in areas with inadequate sanitation and poor personal hygiene.

Because myiasis is not a reportable disease, the number of cases occurring in the United States is probably underreported for aesthetic or medicolegal reasons. In one report, 111 cases were identified from 1952 to 1962 in North America (100); 137 cases of U.S.-acquired myiasis have been published from 1960 to 1995 (101). Worldwide, at least 25 cases of nosocomial myiasis have been reported in the literature (14,102,103). In-

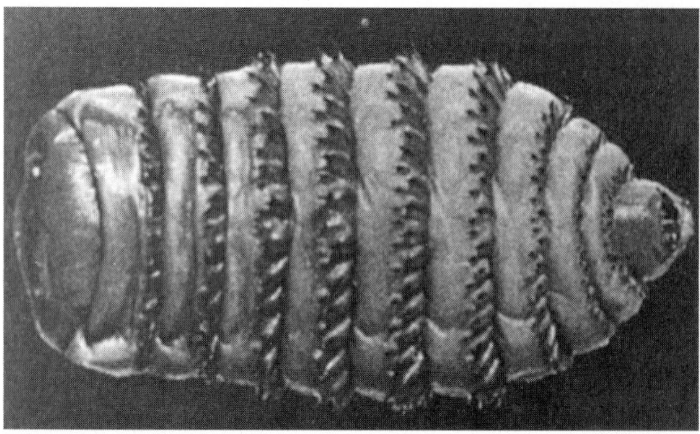

Figure 46.5. Botfly larva. (Reprinted from Harwood RF, Maurice JT. *Entomology in human and animal health,* 7th ed. New York: Simon & Schuster, Macmillan, 1979:306, with permission.)

volved sites have been the nose, nasopharynx, eye, ear, wound, urogenital tract, and intestines. Most infested patients have had altered mental status.

Clinical Manifestations

The larvae may remain superficial and produce little systemic reaction; colonize body orifices; or become invasive, burrowing into normal skin. Some species attack cutaneous tissue, causing furuncles known as subcutaneous myiasis. Once the skin has been invaded by the larvae, a furuncle or abscess may form, draining purulent material or releasing the maggot. Larvae may also burrow through the dermis as a creeping eruption known as dermal myiasis; these larvae are unable to develop fully in humans and produce dermatitis. Secondary bacterial infections are possible with wound myiasis or with myiasis involving necrotic tissue. Other species invade body cavities such as the nasal passages, mouth, ears, anus, vagina, or the orbit of the eye (104). In intestinal myiasis, accidentally ingested eggs or larvae pass intact through the bowel and emerge in the stool. Pseudomyiasis can also occur when dead larvae are passed in the stool, unable to survive the gastrointestinal environment (98).

Diagnosis

The diagnosis of myiasis depends on identifying the larvae from a suspicious lesion. Alternatively, larvae can be reared on sheep blood agar and identified as adults. They can be defined by the tissues affected or the type of lesion produced. Burrowing species may require a tissue biopsy. Larvae may be obtained for examination by application of occlusive salves, chloroform, vegetable oil (98), or bacon fat (105).

Prevention and Control

Nosocomial myiasis can be prevented by controlling flies in the environment. This can be accomplished by good sanitation and appropriate disposal of hospital waste and food-related garbage. This should be supplemented with an adequate insect control program that uses insecticide repellents to decrease fly populations. Physical barriers to fly entry are also important, such as screens or sealed windows. Equally important is an educated staff who have been made aware of the possibility of such infestations; special attention should be paid to good patient hygiene and wound care.

PIGEON MITES

Etiology and Pathogenesis

The chicken or pigeon mite, *Dermanyssus gallinae,* is a blood-sucking arthropod with four pairs of legs averaging 0.5 to 1.0 mm in size (Fig. 46.6). It prefers avian hosts (e.g., pigeons, parakeets, or chickens), but, in their absence, it feeds on the blood of humans, horses, and other mammals, including pet gerbils (106). However, pigeon mites cannot reproduce on humans. Unlike the scabies mite, it is unable to burrow or lay eggs in human skin. In 1828, de Saint-Vincent (107) observed the parasite on the skin of an infested individual; however, it was not until 1958 that Williams (108) demonstrated its ability to feed on human blood. The parasite's small size, rapid movement, and pattern of leaving the host as soon as it has bitten makes it difficult to implicate in an outbreak (109). Its color is yellow-brown when unfed but red-black when gorged with blood.

Epidemiology

The ectoparasite is found worldwide and prefers warm environments. The mite is hardy and can survive 4 to 6 months without a blood meal. It is a nocturnal parasite that hides in cracks, crevices, and shaded areas during the day.

At least four outbreaks involving nosocomial infestations have been reported, involving up to 10 patients each (109–112). Most outbreaks have been linked to pigeon roosts located near vents, windows, or outside air conditioners of healthcare facilities. The mites gain access via cracks around doors, windows, or ventilation ducts.

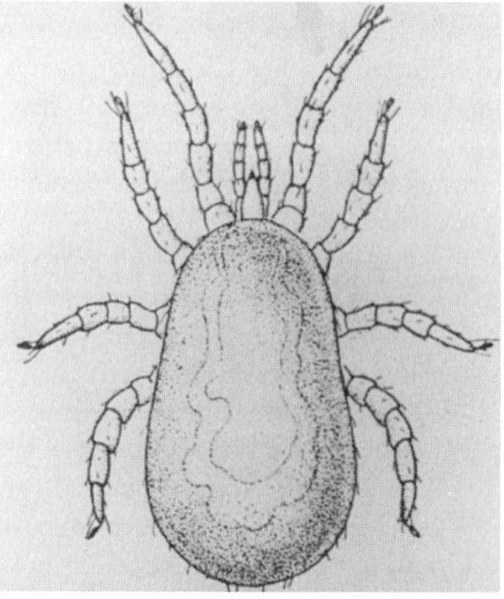

Figure 46.6. The pigeon mite, *Dermanyssus gallinae.* (Reprinted from Harwood RF, Maurice JT. *Entomology in human and animal health,* 7th ed. New York: Simon & Schuster, Macmillan, 1979:347, with permission.)

Although probably an inefficient vector, this mite has been reported to carry the viruses of eastern and western equine encephalitis and St. Louis encephalitis (113).

Clinical Manifestations

The bite is painful, with the subsequent development of a pruritic, macular, papular, vesicular, or urticarial rash. The face, finger webs, and genitalia are usually spared. The rash may last 1 to 3 weeks, but no impetigo or burrows are seen. Nocturnal pruritus is a prominent feature.

Diagnosis

Because the mites are small and only remain on the host while feeding, the diagnosis may be delayed or the infestation may be misdiagnosed as scabies or pediculosis. However, large numbers of mites may be present on the bedding or in the environment. Once the mite is found and identified, the source of mites should be investigated and removed.

Prevention and Control

Preventive measures include removing pigeon roosts from around healthcare facilities and not allowing the feeding of pigeons. Thorough cleaning and spraying with insecticides may also be beneficial. Treatment of patients with scabicides is ineffective. Because the ectoparasite does not burrow, the organism can be easily removed by showering. Practitioners should be aware that mites may be the cause of any chronic or recurrent pruritic dermatitis unresponsive to scabicides in patients or employees.

REFERENCES

1. Shaw PK, Juranek DD. Recent trends in scabies in the United States. *J Infect Dis* 1976;134:414–416.
2. Centers for Disease Control and Prevention. Scabies in health-care facilities—Iowa. *MMWR Morb Mortal Wkly Rep* 1988;37:178–179.
3. Gooch JJ, Strasius ST, Bearmer B, et al. Nosocomial outbreak of scabies. *Arch Dermatol* 1978;114:897–898.
4. Burkhart CG. Scabies: an epidemiologic reassessment. *Ann Intern Med* 1983;98:498–503.
5. Orkin M. Resurgence of scabies. *JAMA* 1979;217:593–597.
6. Arlian LG, Estes SA, Vyszenski-Moher DL. Prevalence of *Sarcoptes scabiei* in the homes and nursing homes of scabietic patients. *J Am Acad Dermatol* 1988;19:806–811.
7. Church RE, Knoweldon J. Scabies in Sheffield: a family infestation. *BMJ* 1978;1:761–763.
8. Holness DL, Dekoven JF, Nethercott JR. Scabies in chronic health care institutions. *Arch Dermatol* 1992;128:1257–1260.
9. Hopper AH, Salisbury J, Jegadeva AN, et al. Epidemic Norwegian scabies in a geriatric unit. *Age Ageing* 1990;19:125–127.
10. Sargent SJ, Martin JT. Scabies outbreak in a day care center. *Pediatrics* 1994;94(Suppl):1012–1013.
11. Voss A, Wallrauch C. Occupational scabies in healthcare workers [Letter]. *Infect Control Hosp Epidemiol* 1995;16:4.
12. Estes SA. Diagnosis and management of scabies. *Med Clin North Am* 1982;66:955–963.
13. McRae ME. Scabies. *Cutis* 1977;20:90–92.
14. Lettau LA. Nosocomial transmission and infection control aspects of parasitic and ectoparasitic diseases. Part III. Ectoparasites/summary and conclusions. *Infect Control Hosp Epidemiol* 1991;12:179–185.
15. Orkin M. Today's scabies [Editorial]. *Arch Dermatol* 1975;111: 1431–1432.
16. Tschen EH. What treatment for skin infestations in the elderly? *Geriatrics* 1982;37:38–44.
17. Orkin M, Maibach HI. Scabies, a current pandemic. *Postgrad Med J* 1979;66:52–62.
18. Danielssen DG, Boeck W. *Traité de la spedalkshet ou éléphantiasis des Grècs.* Paris: JB Ballière, 1848.
19. Blatchley D. Scabies in a spinal injuries ward. *BMJ* 1975;2:617.
20. Thomas MC, Giedinghagen DH, Hoff GL. Brief report: an outbreak of scabies among employees in a hospital-associated commercial laundry. *Infect Control* 1987;8:427–429.
21. Cooper CL, Jackson MM. Outbreak of scabies in a small community hospital. *Am J Infect Control* 1986;14:173–179.
22. Centers for Disease Control and Prevention. Patient-source scabies among hospital personnel Pennsylvania. *MMWR Morb Mortal Wkly Rep* 1983;32:489–490.
23. Lam S, Brennessel D. Norwegian scabies and HIV infection—case report and literature review. *Infect Dis Clin Pract* 1993;3:169–173.
24. Jimenez-Lucho V, Fallon F, Caputo C, et al. Role of prolonged surveillance in the eradication of nosocomial scabies in an extended care Veterans Affairs medical center. *Am J Infect Control* 1995;23:44–49.
25. Hayden JF, Caplan RM. Epidemic scabies. *Arch Dermatol* 1971;103: 168–173.
26. Hubler WR, Clabaugh W. Epidemic Norwegian scabies. *Arch Dermatol* 1976;112:179–181.
27. Lempert KD, Baltz PS, Welton WA, et al. Pseudouremic pruritus: a scabies epidemic in a dialysis unit. *Am J Kidney Dis* 1985;5:117–119.
28. Clar J, Friesen DL, Williams WA. Management of an outbreak of Norwegian scabies. *Am J Infect Control* 1992;20:217–220.
29. Rostami G, Sorg TB. Nosocomial outbreak of scabies associated with Norwegian scabies in an AIDS patient. *Int J STD AIDS* 1990;1: 209–210.
30. Sirera G, Rius F, Romeu J, et al. Hospital outbreak of scabies stemming from two AIDS patients with Norwegian scabies. *Lancet* 1990; 335:1227.
31. Lee, WY. An unusual scabies epidemic in an urban hospital. *Am J Infect Control* 1989;17:95.
32. Sadick N, Kaplan MH, Pahwa SG, et al. Unusual features of scabies complicating human T-lymphotropic virus type III infection. *J Am Acad Dermatol* 1986;15:482–486.
33. Rau RC, Baird IM. Crusted scabies in a patient with acquired immunodeficiency syndrome. *J Am Acad Dermatol* 1986;15:1058–1059.
34. Jucowics P, Ramon ME, Don PC, et al. Norwegian scabies in an infant with acquired immunodeficiency syndrome. *Arch Dermatol* 1989;125:1670–1671.
35. Donabedian H, Khazan U. Norwegian scabies in a patient with AIDS. *Clin Infect Dis* 1992;14:162–164.
36. Kelly A, Fry C. Outbreak of Norwegian scabies among health care workers [Abstract MBP308]. Fifth International Conference on AIDS/III STD World Congress, Montreal, June 1989.
37. Ardo M, Noto G, La Rocca E, et al. Localized Norwegian scabies as an opportunistic infestation in AIDS [Abstract MB 2297]. Seventh International Conference on AIDS/III STD World Congress, Florence, June 16–21, 1991.
38. Jessurun J, Romo-Garcia J, Lopez-Denis O, et al. Crusted scabies in a patient with acquired immunodeficiency syndrome. *Virchows Arch [A]* 1990;416:461–463.
39. Drabick JJ, Lupton GP, Tompkins K. Crusted scabies in human immunodeficiency virus. *J Am Acad Dermatol* 1987;17:142.
40. Moss VA, Salisbury J. Scabies in an AIDS hospice unit. *Br J Clin Pract* 1991;45:35–36.
41. Orkin M. Scabies in AIDS. *Semin Dermatol* 1993;12:9–14.
42. Portu JJ. A typical scabies in HIV-positive patients. *J Am Acad Dermatol* 1996;34(5 Part 2):915–917.
43. Brites C, Weyll M, Pedroso C, et al. Severe and Norwegian scabies are strongly associated with retroviral (HIV-1,HTLV-1) infection in Bahia, Brazil. *AIDS* 2002;16:1292–1293.

44. Yarbrough GK, Iriondo M. Diabetic patient with crusted plaques: crusted (Norwegian) scabies. *Arch Dermatol* 1987;123:811, 814.
45. Lerche NW, Currier RW, Juranek DD, et al. Atypical crusted Norwegian scabies: report of nosocomial transmission in a community hospital and an approach to control. *Cutis* 1983;13:127–131.
46. Centers for Disease Control and Prevention. Patient-source scabies among hospital personnel—Pennsylvania. *MMWR Morb Mortal Wkly Rep* 1983;32:489–490.
47. Barnes L, McCallister RE, Lucky AW. Crusted (Norwegian) scabies: occurrence in a child undergoing bone marrow transplant. *Arch Dermatol* 1987;123:95–97.
48. Peterson WD, Allen BR, Beveridge GW. Norwegian scabies during immunosuppressive therapy. *BMJ* 1973;4:211–212.
49. Wolf R, Wolf D, Viskoper RJ, et al. Norwegian-type scabies mimicking contact dermatitis in an immunosuppressed patient. *Postgrad Med J* 1985;78:228–30.
50. Egawa K, Johno M, Hayashibara T, et al. Familial occurrence of crusted (Norwegian) scabies with adult T-cell leukemia. *Br J Dermatol* 1992;127:57–59.
51. Tibbs CJ, Wilcox DJ. Norwegian scabies and herpes simplex in a patient with chronic lymphatic leukemia and hypogammaglobulinemia. *Br J Dermatol* 1992;126:523–524.
52. Estes SA, Estes J. Therapy of scabies: nursing homes, hospitals, and the homeless. *Semin Dermatol* 1993;12:26–33.
53. Bernstein B, Mihan R. Hospital epidemic of scabies. *J Pediatr* 1973; 83:1086–1087.
54. Ting HC, Wang F. Scabies and systemic lupus erythematosus. *Int J Dermatol* 1983;22:473–476.
55. Lipitz R, Tur E, Brenner S, et al. Norwegian scabies following topical corticosteroid therapy. *Isr J Med Sci* 1981;17:1165–1168.
56. Jaramillo-Ayerbe F, Berrio-Munoz J. Ivermectin for crusted Norwegian scabies induced by use of topical steroids. *Arch Dermatol* 1998; 134:143–145.
57. Carslaw RW, Dobson RM, Hood AJK, et al. Mites in the environment of cases of Norwegian scabies. *Br J Dermatol* 1975;92:333–337.
58. Glover R, Young L, Goltz RW. Norwegian scabies in acquired immunodeficiency syndrome: report of a case resulting in death from associated sepsis. *J Am Acad Dermatol* 1987;16:396–399.
59. Hall JD, Brewere J, Brad A. Norwegian scabies in a patient with acquired immune deficiency syndrome. *Cutis* 1989;43:325–329.
60. Hulbert TV, Larson RA. Hyperkeratotic (Norwegian) scabies with gram-negative bacteremia as the initial presentation of AIDS [Letter]. *Clin Infect Dis* 1992;14:1164–1165.
61. Svartman M, Potter EV, Finklea JF, et al. Epidemic scabies and acute glomerulonephritis in Trinidad. *Lancet* 1972;1:249–251.
62. Boix V, Sanchez-Paya J, Portilla J, et al. Nosocomial outbreak of scabies clinically resistant to lindane. *Infect Control Hosp Epidemiol* 1997;18:677.
63. Cook AM, Romanelli F. Ivermectin for the treatment of resistant scabies. *Ann Pharmacother* 2003;37:279–281.
64. Chosidow O. Scabies and pediculosis. *Lancet* 2000;355:819–826.
65. Taplin D, Meinking TL. Scabies, lice, and fungal infections. *Primary Care* 1989;16:551–576.
66. Woodley D, Saurat JH. The burrow ink test and the scabies mite. *J Am Acad Dermatol* 1981;4:715–722.
67. Martin WE, Wheeler CE. Diagnosis of human scabies by epidermal shave biopsy. *J Am Acad Dermatol* 1979;1:335–337.
68. Micali G, Lacarrubba F, Lo GG. Scraping versus videodermatoscopy for the diagnosis of scabies: a comparative study. *Acta Derm Venereol* 1999;79:396.
69. Wendel K, Rompalo A, Scabies and pediculosis pubis: an update of treatment regimens and general review. *Clin Infect Dis* 2002;35(Suppl 2):S146–151.
70. Argenziano G, Fabbrocini G, Delfino M. Epiluminescence microscopy: a new approach to in vivo detection of *Sarcoptes scabiei. Arch Dermatol* 1997;133:751–753.
71. Haag ML, Brozena SJ, Fenske NA. Attack of the scabies: what to do when an outbreak occurs. *Geriatrics* 1993;48(10):45–46, 51–53.
72. Meinking T, Taplin D, Herminda J, et al. The treatment of scabies with ivermectin. *N Engl J Med* 1995;333:26–30.
73. Chouela E, Albeldano A, Pellerano G, et al. Equivalent therapeutic efficacy and safety of ivermectin and lindane in the treatment of human scabies. *Arch Dermatol* 1999;135:651–655.
74. Elmogy M, Fayed H, Marzok H, et al. Oral ivermectin in the treatment of scabies. *Int J Dermatol* 1999;38:926–928.
75. Conti Diaz IA, Amaro J. Treatment of human scabies with oral ivermectin. *Rev Inst Med Trop Sao Paulo* 1999;41:259–261.
76. Usha V, Gopalakrishnan Nair TV. A comparative study of oral ivermectin and topical permethrin cream in the treatment of scabies. *J Am Acad Dermatol* 2000;42:236–240.
77. del Giudice P. Ivermectin in scabies. *Curr Opin Infect Dis* 2002;15: 123–126.
78. Centers for Disease Control and Prevention. Sexually transmitted diseases treatment guidelines, 2002. *MMWR Morb Mortal Wkly Rep* 2002;51(RR-6):132–136.
79. Victoria J, Trujillo R. Topical ivermectin: a new successful treatment for scabies. *Pediatr Dermatol* 2001;18:63–65.
80. Corbett E, Crossley I, Holton J, et al. Crusted ("Norwegian") scabies in a specialist HIV unit: successful use of ivermectin and failure to prevent nosocomial transmission.*Genitourin Med* 1996;72:115–117.
81. Huffam SE, Currie BJ. Ivermectin for *Sarcoptes scabiei* hyperinfestation. *Int J Infect Dis* 1998;2:152–154.
82. Alberici F, Pagani L, Ratti G, et al. Ivermectin alone or in combination with benzyl benzoate in the treatment of human immunodeficiency virus-associated scabies. *Br J Dermatol* 2000;142:969–972.
83. Juranek DD, Currier RW, Millikan LE. Scabies control in institutions. In: Orkin M, Maibach HI, eds. *Cutaneous infestations and insect bites.* New York: Marcel Dekker, 1985:139–156.
84. Pasternak J, Richtmann R, Gamme APP, et al. Scabies epidemic: price and prejudice. *Infect Control Hosp Epidemiol* 1994;15:540–542.
85. Rook A, Wilkinson DJ, Ebling FJG, eds. *Textbook of dermatology,* 3rd ed. Oxford: Blackwell Scientific, 1979:935–938.
86. Juranek DD. *Pediculus capitis* in school children. In: Orkin M, Maibach HI, eds. *Cutaneous infestation and insect bites.* New York: Marcel Dekker, 1985:199– 211.
87. Altachuler DZ, Kenney LR. More on pediculosis capitis. *N Engl J Med* 1984;310:1668.
88. Fine BC. Controversy about pediculosis capitis [Letter]. *N Engl J Med* 1984;311:801.
89. Maunder JW. Human lice—biology and control. *R Soc Health J* 1977; 97:29– 32.
90. Ward K. The management of skin infestations. *Nurs Stand* 1992;6: 28–30.
91. Fine BC. *Pediculosis capitis* [Letter]. *N Engl J Med* 1983;309:1461.
92. Abramowicz M, ed. Drugs for head lice. *Med Lett Drugs Ther* 1997; 39:6–7.
93. Glaziou P, Nyguyen LN, Moulia-Pelat JP, et al. Efficacy of ivermectin for the treatment of head lice *(Pediculosis capitis). Trop Med Parasitol* 1994;45:253–254.
94. Frankowski BL, Weiner LB, Head Committee on School Health the Committee on Infectious Diseases. American Academy of Pediatrics. *Pediatrics* 2002;110:638–643.
95. Mazurek CM, Lee NP. How to manage head lice. *West J Med* 2000; 172:342–345.
96. Soule BM, ed. *The APIC curriculum for infection control practice,* vol 1. Dubuque, IA: Kendall/Hunt, 1983:339–348.
97. James MT. *Flies that cause myiasis in man.* Misc. publication no. 631. Washington DC: U.S. Department of Agriculture, 1947:134–137.
98. Centers for Disease Control and Prevention. Intestinal myiasis—Washington. *MMWR Morb Mortal Wkly Rep* 1985;34:141–142.
99. Chernin E. Surgical maggots. *South Med J* 1986;79:1143–1145.
100. Scott HG. Human myiasis in North America (1952–1962 inclusive). *Fla Entomologist* 1964;47:255–261.
101. Sherman RA. Wound myiasis in urban and suburban United States. *Arch Intern Med* 2000;160:2004–2014.
102. Mielke U. Nosocomial myiasis. *J Hosp Infect* 1997;37:1–5.
103. Beckendorf R, Klotz SA, Hinkle N, et al. Nasal myiasis in an intensive care unit linked to hospital-wide mouse infestation. *Arch Intern Med* 2002;162:638–640.
104. Chodosh J, Clarridge JE, Matoba A. Nosocomial conjunctival oph-

thalmomyiasis with *Cochliomyia macellaria. Am J Ophthalmol* 1991; 111:520–521.

105. Brewer TF, Wilson ME, Gonazlez E, et al. Bacon therapy and furuncular myiasis. *JAMA* 1993;270:2087–2088.
106. Lucky AW, Sayers CP, Argus JD, et al. Avian mite bites acquired from a new source—pet gerbils: report of 2 cases and review of the literature. *Arch Derm* 2001;137:168–170.
107. Sulzberger MB, Kaminstein I. Avian itch mites as a cause of human dermatoses; canary birds' mites responsible for 2 groups of cases in New York. *Arch Dermatol Syphilol* 1936;33:60.
108. Williams RW. An infestation of a human habitation by *Dermanyssus gallinae* (de Geer, 1778) (Acarina: Dermanyssidae) in New York resulting in sanguisugent attacks upon the occupants. *Am J Trop Med Hyg* 1958;7:627.
109. Auger P, Natel J, Meunier N, et al. Skin acariasis caused by *Dermanyssus gallinae* (de Geer): an in-hospital outbreak. *Can Med Assoc J* 1979; 120:700–703.
110. Vargo JA, Ginsbery MM, Mizrahi M. Human infestation by the pigeon mite: a case report. *Assoc Pract Infect Control* 1983;11: 2425.
111. Sexton DJ, Haynes B. Bird-mite infestation in a university hospital. *Lancet* 1975;1:445.
112. Regan AM, Metersky ML, Craven DE. Nosocomial dermatitis and pruritus caused by pigeon mite infestation. *Arch Intern Med* 1987; 147:2185–2187.
113. Wisseman CL, Sulikn SE. Observations on laboratory case, life cycle, and hosts of chicken mite, *Dermanyssus gallinae. Am J Trop Med* 1947; 27:463.

47

UNCOMMON CAUSES OF NOSOCOMIAL INFECTIONS

BRYAN P. SIMMONS
MICHAEL S. GELFAND

Some community-acquired infections are seen infrequently in hospitals either because they are rare (e.g., rabies) or because they are not endemic to the United States (e.g., hemorrhagic fever virus infections). Some of these infections are potentially lethal and have been transmitted in hospitals. Thus, the diagnosis of these infections can cause great concern and even panic among healthcare workers and infection control personnel. This chapter discusses such uncommon nosocomial infections.

RABIES

Etiology and Pathogenesis

Rabies is a severe encephalitis caused by the rabies virus, a rhabdovirus, that infects mammals, including humans. In most areas of the world, rabies is almost always transmitted by the bite of an infected mammal. In the United States most cases are now cryptic, that is, they occur without a clear exposure to the rabies virus (1–4). Nearly 90% of the 28 cases of rabies documented since 1980 had no documented bite from a rabid animal. Many of these are believed to result from inapparent bites from bats or from rabies virus that comes into contact with a break in the skin or mucous membranes (2,4). The virus is believed to multiply at the inoculation site and then spread via peripheral nerves to the spinal cord and central nervous system. By the time systemic symptoms develop, the virus has traveled peripherally down efferent nerves to nearly every organ and tissue including, most importantly for the life cycle of the virus, the salivary glands (1). The incubation period is usually 20 to 90 days but has varied from 5 days to many years (3,4). Antigenic and genetic analyses have demonstrated different viral strains that are endemic to different areas of the world and even to different animal species (3,4).

Epidemiology

Human rabies has been acquired on all continents except the Antarctic. The epidemiology of rabies reflects that of local animal rabies. Dogs are the most important rabies reservoir for humans in underdeveloped countries. In the United States, wild carnivorous animals such as skunks, raccoons, bats, coyotes, and foxes are the most important reservoirs for rabies (3). Hawaii is the only state that remains rabies-free.

In the United States, rabies in humans has decreased from an average of 22 cases per year in 1946 to 1950 to 0 to 5 cases per year since 1960. The number of rabies cases among domestic animals has decreased similarly. However, approximately 16,000 to 39,000 persons receive rabies prophylaxis every year because of animal exposures, about half of which are nonbite exposures (5). The risk of rabies from nonbite exposures is extremely low. Scratches, abrasions, open wounds, or mucous membranes contaminated with saliva or other potentially infectious material (such as brain tissue) from a rabid animal are the usual nonbite exposures requiring prophylaxis. If the material containing the virus is dry, the virus can be considered noninfectious. Since 1980 an increasing number of human rabies cases have been associated with a rabies variant that circulates in bats; only one of these cases has been associated with any known exposure, such as a bite or scratch (2–4). The nonbite exposures of highest risk appear to be exposures to large amounts of aerosolized rabies virus or to organs or tissues (i.e., corneas) transplanted from patients who died of rabies and to scratches from rabid animals (6). Two cases of rabies have been attributed to airborne exposures in laboratories, and two cases of rabies have been attributed to probable airborne exposures in a bat-infested cave in Texas (6).

Human-to-human transmission of rabies occurred among eight recipients of transplanted corneas. Investigations revealed that each of the donors had died of an illness compatible with or proven to be rabies (6). Stringent guidelines for acceptance of donor corneas have reduced this risk (6).

The risk for rabies transmission to healthcare workers is low (7,8). Apart from corneal transplants, bite and nonbite exposures inflicted by infected humans could theoretically transmit rabies, but no laboratory-diagnosed cases occurring under such situations have been documented (9). Two human-to-human transmissions of rabies by saliva (a bite and a kiss) are not laboratory confirmed (6).

Clinical Manifestations

The early manifestations of rabies are usually nonspecific and can be difficult to differentiate from other encephalitic diseases. These consist of malaise, fatigue, headache, anorexia, and fever.

Rabies progresses to one of two distinct presentations: the most common is the furious form characterized by hydrophobia, aerophobia, or episodic agitation and anxiety; the least common is the paralytic form. Rabies should be considered in any patient with rapidly progressive encephalitis of unknown etiology, particularly in patients who have lived in an area with enzootic canine rabies.

Diagnosis

In the United States, the rapid fluorescent focus inhibition test is the standard test for measuring rabies neutralizing antibody. The results from this *in vitro* cell culture neutralization test are available within 24 hours. In one study of antibody titers of rabies patients who did not receive postexposure treatment, 50% had serum antibodies by the eighth day and 100% by the fifteenth day of illness (10). Rabies virus may be demonstrated by immunofluorescent antibody staining of brain and skin tissue. The most reliable and reproducible of the direct immunofluorescent studies that can aid in patient diagnosis is that performed on neck skin obtained by biopsy (1). In this test, a 6- to 8-mm full-thickness wedge or punch biopsy specimen containing as many hair follicles as possible is obtained from the posterior aspect of the neck above the hair line. Histologic examination of brain tissue from human rabies cases typically shows perivascular inflammation of the gray matter, various amounts of neuronal degeneration, and, in many cases, characteristic cytoplasmic inclusion bodies (Negri bodies). A reverse transcriptase-polymerase chain reaction test may be the diagnostic procedure of choice for suspected rabies (4).

Prevention and Control

Patients who have suspected rabies should be placed on Contact Precautions (see Chapter 95) to minimize the number of possible healthcare worker exposures and to minimize anxiety,

TABLE 47.1. TYPE OF TREATMENT AND REGIMEN FOR RABIES POSTEXPOSURE PROPHYLAXIS, BY VACCINATION STATUS

Vaccination status	Treatment	Regimen[a]
Not previously vaccinated	Wound cleansing	All postexposure treatment should begin with immediate thorough cleansing of all wounds with soap and water. If available, a virucidal agent such as a povidone-iodine solution should be used to irrigate the wounds.
	RIG	Administer 20 IU per kg body weight. If anatomically feasible, **the full dose** should be infiltrated around the wounds(s) and any remaining volume should be administered IM at an anatomic site distant from vaccine administration. Also, RIG should not be administered in the same syringe as vaccine. Because RIG might partially suppress active production of antibody, no more than the recommended dose should be given.
	Vaccine	HDCV, RVA, or PCEC 1.0 mL, IM (deltoid area[b]), one each on days 0[c], 3, 7, 14, and 28.
Previously vaccinated[d]	Wound cleansing	All postexposure treatment should begin with immediate through cleansing of all wounds with soap and water. If available, a virucidal agent such as a povidone-iodine solution should be used to irrigate the wounds.
	RIG	RIG should **not** be administered.
	Vaccine	HDCV, RVA, or PCEC 1.0 mL, IM (deltoid area[b]), one each on days 0[c] and 3.

HDCV, human diploid cell vaccine; IM, Intramuscular; PCEC, purified chick embryo cell vaccine; RIG, rabies immune golbulin; RVA, rabies vaccine adsorbed.

[a] These regimens are applicable for all age groups, including children.

[b] The deltoid area is the only acceptable site of vaccination for adults and older children. For younger children, the outer aspect of the thigh may be used. Vaccine should never be administered in the gluteal area.

[c] Day 0 is the day the first dose of vaccine is administered.

[d] Any person with a history of preexposure vaccination with HDCV, RVA, or PCEC; prior postexposure prophylaxis with HDCV, RVA, or PCED; or previous vaccination with any other type of rabies vaccine and a documented history of antibody response to the prior vaccination.

From Centers for Disease Control and Prevention. Rabies prevention—United States, 1999: recommendations of Immunization Practices Advisory Committee (ACIP). *MMWE Morb Mortal Wkly Rep* 1999;48(RR-1):1–21, with permission.

although standard precautions are adequate (11). Possible cases should be reported to public health officials immediately so that they can assist with an epidemiologic and diagnostic workup. Healthcare workers who have had a significant exposure should receive postexposure prophylaxis (6) (Table 47.1). Casual contact with a person with rabies (i.e., touching the patient) or contact with noninfectious fluid or tissue (e.g., blood or feces) does not constitute an exposure and is not an indication for prophylaxis (6). Postexposure prophylaxis is recommended after contact with human rabies only if a bite or nonbite exposure (e.g., contamination of abraded skin or mucous membranes with saliva, nerve tissue, urine sediments, or other potentially infectious material) can be documented. Because postexposure prophylaxis after the onset of disease is of no known benefit, such treatment for patients after onset of clinical rabies is not recommended.

CREUTZFELDT-JAKOB DISEASE/ TRANSMISSABLE SPONGIFORM ENCEPHALOPATHIES

Etiology

Creutzfeldt-Jakob disease (CJD) is an uncommon dementing illness caused by a transmissible pathogen often called CJD agent. It is not yet clear whether CJD agent is a virus or prion, but it has the characteristics of extremely small size, great resistance to chemical and physical agents (e.g., sterilization procedures), failure to induce either an inflammatory or an immune response, and lack of demonstrable nucleic acid or nonhost protein (12). Gajdusek (13) has called CJD agent and other related transmissible spongiform encephalopathy agents [e.g., kuru, scrapie, and bovine spongiform encephalopathy (BSE)] unconventional viruses. Although CJD agent is clearly transmissible to animals and humans (14,15), CJD is also a genetic disorder inherited as a familial dominant trait (16).

A new form of CJD in humans, called variant CJD (vCJD), emerged in the 1990s and is believed to be related to BSE (15, 17,18). BSE is also known as "mad cow disease" and may be transmitted to humans by consumption of beef products contaminated by central nervous system tissue. An outbreak of BSE in cattle in the United Kingdom occurred from the early 1980s to the late 1990s (15). As of October 2002, a total of 138 cases of vCJD have occurred in humans, most of them in the United Kingdom (17). Strong laboratory and epidemiologic evidence indicates that vCJD is linked causally with BSE. The epidemics of BSE and vCJD in the United Kingdom have prompted blood collection agencies in the United States to refuse donors who have lived or traveled in Europe for an extended period of time. Variant CJD occurs at an unusually young age compared with classic CJD (median age 26 years versus 68 years) (17).

Pathogenesis

Infection by CJD agent causes central nervous system degeneration with spongiform degeneration of gray matter, severe loss of neurons, vacuolization of neuronal cytoplasm, marked proliferation of astrocytes, and little inflammation. The actual mechanisms by which the agent causes neurologic disease are unknown. There is no significant humoral or cell-mediated immune response to any known infectious agent. However, a characteristic brain protein can sometimes be detected in spinal fluid and used for diagnosis (19,20). CJD agent has been found in lymph nodes, liver, kidney, spleen, lung, cornea, and cerebrospinal fluid, although less regularly and in far lower titers than in the brain and spinal cord. The brain may contain at least 10^8 infectious units per gram (21).

Epidemiology

CJD is found in the United States in an incidence of about one case per million persons per year (22). This incidence appears stable, or at least has been for the last 10 years. The age-specific incidence peaks at 65 to 69 years, but occasional cases occur as early as the second decade and as late as the ninth decade of life. Variant CJD cases occur at a younger age (17).

More than 250 iatrogenic cases of CJD have been reported worldwide (23). Most of these have been associated with use of cadaveric dura mater grafts, growth hormone, and corneal grafts. Six cases are linked to contaminated invasive equipment, four with neurosurgical instruments and two with stereotactic electroencephalographic (EEG) depth electrodes. All of these equipment-related cases occurred before the routine implementation of sterilization procedures currently used in healthcare facilities. No such cases have been reported since 1976. There is no evidence of occupational transmission to healthcare workers (23).

Clinical Manifestations

Patients with CJD usually present with progressive mental deterioration. In about half the patients, cerebellar or visual signs dominate the clinical presentation with only moderate to minimal mental deterioration. Abnormal movements, usually including myoclonus, are found late in the illness. The progression of disease is usually relentless. Most patients die within 6 months. There are no verified recoveries.

Diagnosis

Diagnosis can often be inferred by clinical features of the illness and by an immunoassay for protein 14-3-3 in the cerebrospinal fluid of patients with rapidly progressive dementias accompanied by myoclonus or ataxia (19). A magnetic resonance imaging study may show characteristic findings for vCJD (17). However, a brain biopsy or autopsy may be needed to confirm the diagnosis (12,18).

Prevention and Control

Any program to prevent transmission of CJD and transmissible spongiform encephalopathies from patients in hospitals should first seek to detect all such patients before brain or other high-risk tissues (dura mater, spinal cord, and eyes) are biopsied. Such patients can be identified by screening patients for "unexplained dementia without a detectable brain mass." Any patient

TABLE 47.2. DECONTAMINATION OF CONTAMINATED MEDICAL DEVICES USED ON PATIENTS WITH KNOWN OR SUSPECTED CREUTZFELDT-JAKOB DISEASE (CJD)

High-risk tissues [defined as brain (including dura mater), spinal cord, and eyes] from high-risk patients (e.g., those with known or suspected CJD or who have dementia without a brain mass). For use with critical[a] or semicritical[b] items:

1. Those devices that are constructed so that cleaning procedures result in effective tissue removal (e.g., surgical instruments) can be cleaned and then sterilized by autoclaving either at 134°C for ≥18 min in a prevacuum sterilizer or at 121°C–132°C for 1 hr in a gravity displacement sterilizer.
2. Those devices that are impossible or difficult to clean could be discarded. Alternatively, one should place the contaminated items in a container filled with a liquid (e.g., saline, water, or phenolic solution) to retard adherence of material to the medical device. This should be followed by initial decontamination done by autoclaving at 134°C for 18 min in a prevacuum sterilizer (liquids must be removed before sterilization) or at 121°C–132°C for 1 hr in a gravity displacement sterilizer or by soaking in 1/N NaOH for 1 hr. Finally, terminal cleaning, wrapping, and sterilization can be done by conventional means.
3. To minimize drying of tissues and body fluids on the object, instruments should be kept moist until cleaned and decontaminated.
4. Flash sterilization should not be used for reprocessing.
5. Items that permit only low-temperature sterilization (e.g., ethylene oxide or hydrogen peroxide gas plasma) should be discarded.
6. If a patient is diagnosed with CJD but the CJD protocol was not used, all contaminated items should be recalled and discarded or appropriately reprocessed by the CJD protocol. The preoperative CJD screening protocol should then be reviewed such that there is a heightened awareness of the need to detect CJD patients before high-risk tissues are biopsied.
7. Equipment that requires special CJD reprocessing should be tagged after use. Clinicians and reprocessing technicians should be thoroughly trained on how to properly tag the equipment and follow the special CJD reprocessing protocols.
8. Noncritical[c] equipment contaminated with high-risk tissue should be cleaned and then disinfected with a 1:10 dilution of sodium hypochlorite or 1 N NaOH, depending on material compatibility. All contaminated surfaces must be exposed to the disinfectant.
9. Environmental surfaces (noncritical[c]) contaminated with high-risk tissues (e.g., laboratory surface in contact with brain tissue of a person infected with CJD) should be cleaned and then spot-decontaminated with a 1:10 dilution of sodium hypochlorite (i.e., bleach). To minimize environmental contamination, disposable cover sheets could be used on work surfaces.
10. For ease of cleaning and to minimize percutaneous injury and generation of aerosols, use nonpowered instruments (e.g., drills or saws) or ensure that disposable protective equipment covers are available for powered instruments.

Low-risk tissues (defined as the CSF, kidney, liver, spleen, lung, and lymph nodes) from a high-risk patient. For use with critical[a] or semicritical[b] medical devices:

1. These devices can be cleaned and either disinfected or sterilized by use of conventional protocols of heat or chemical sterilization or high-level disinfection.
2. Environmental surfaces contaminated with low-risk tissues require only standard disinfection. Use disinfectants recommended by OSHA for disinfection of blood-contaminated surfaces.

No-risk tissues (defined as peripheral nerve, intestine, bone marrow, blood leukocytes, serum, thyroid gland, adrenal gland, heart, skeletal muscle, adipose tissue, gingiva, prostate, testis, placenta, tears, nasal mucus, saliva, sputum, urine, feces, semen, vaginal secretions, and milk) from a high-risk patient. For use with critical[a] or semicritical[b] medical devices:

1. These devices can be cleaned and either disinfected or sterilized by means of conventional protocols of heat or chemical sterilization or by means of high-level disinfection.
2. Endoscopes (except neurosurgical endoscopes) would be contaminated only with no-risk materials, and, thus, standard cleaning and high-level disinfection protocols would be adequate for reprocessing.
3. Environmental surfaces (noncritical[c]) contaminated with no-risk tissues or fluids require only standard disinfection (use disinfectants recommended by OSHA for decontamination of blood-contaminated surfaces [e.g., 1:10 to 1:100 dilution of 5.25% sodium hypochlorite]). To minimize environmental contamination, disposable cover sheets could be used on work surfaces.

OSHA, Occupational Safety and Health Administration.
[a] Critical items are those that enter sterile tissue or the vascular system.
[b] Semicritical items are those that contact mucous membranes or skin that is not intact (e.g., endoscopes).
[c] Noncritical items are those that come in contact with intact skin but not mucous membranes (e.g., floors and walls).
Adapted from Rutala WA, Weber DJ. Creutzfeldt-Jakob disease: recommendations for disinfection and sterilization. *Clin Infect Dis* 2001;32:1348–1356, with permission.

meeting this description should be considered to have CJD until proven otherwise even if another diagnosis such as vasculitis is being considered. The neurosurgeons, pathologists, and others in the operating room and pathology department and the infection control department should be alerted about such a patient if a biopsy of high-risk tissue is being considered. Some neurosurgeons may elect not to biopsy potential CJD patients unless an alternate, treatable diagnosis is also under consideration. Hospitals should develop a CJD protocol for brain biopsies done on such patients (Table 47.2) (23,24). Disposable surgical instruments should be used when possible. Reusable instruments should be discarded or sterilized according to a CJD protocol or the instruments should be quarantined until another diagnosis is made. Powered instruments, such as drills and saws, should be avoided or covered by a disposable protective shield. Brain and other high-risk tissues should be labeled as "suspected CJD" before being sent to pathology. The pathology department should have a plan to track such tissue and quarantine and disinfect instruments, such as microtomes, that contact CJD tissue. It is important to note that formalin- and glutaraldehyde-fixed tissues may be infectious indefinitely (24). Confirmed CJD tissue can be managed as regulated medical waste per state regulations. No one suspected of having CJD should serve as a blood or tissue donor even though transmission of CJD has never been linked to blood (25). Blood or blood products from such patients should be disposed of per state regulations for regulated medical waste.

CJD patients should be cared for using Standard Precautions (11). Sharps injuries involving spinal fluid or high-risk tissues can be cleansed using 0.5% sodium hypochlorite or 1 N sodium hydroxide (23,24). During an operation or autopsy, disposable surgical caps, water-repellant gowns, aprons, double gloves, and face visors (covering eyes, nose, and mouth) should be worn (24). Autopsies should be done only if the pathologist is aware of the potential diagnosis of CJD and uses the precautions mentioned previously for the autopsy suite and pathology laboratory (24). When the patient dies, the morgue and funeral home should be notified that the patient had suspected or confirmed CJD.

VIRAL HEMORRHAGIC FEVER

The term *viral hemorrhagic fever* (VHF) refers to the illness associated with a number of geographically restricted viruses. This illness is characterized by fever and, in the most severe cases, shock and hemorrhage (26). Although a number of other febrile viral infections may produce hemorrhage, only the agents of Lassa, Marburg, Ebola, and Crimean-Congo hemorrhagic fevers are known to have caused significant outbreaks of diseases with person-to-person transmission.

None of these viruses are endemic to the United States (Table 47.3). However, increasing levels of international travel result in rare cases of VHF imported into the United States, and there is concern that these viruses may be used for bioterrorism (26–28). When cases are hospitalized, there is often concern about the potential for nosocomial transmission. However, evidence shows that transmission of these viruses does not occur through casual contact and is rare in hospitals if adequate universal precautions are used (26,27,29). Hantaviruses can cause hemorrhagic fever and are endemic in the United States but are not spread person-to-person or in hospitals (30).

TABLE 47.3. VIRAL HEMORRHAGIC FEVER VIRUSES

Disease	Viral family	Distribution	Mode of transmission
Lassa fever	Arenaviridae	West Africa	Rodent
Marburg hemorrhagic fever	Filoviridae	Sub-Saharan Africa	Unknown
Ebola hemorrhagic fever	Filoviridae	Sub-Saharan Africa	Unknown
Crimean-Congo hemorrhagic fever	Bunyaviridae	Africa, Asia, southern parts of former USSR	Tick

Lassa Fever Virus

Lassa fever virus is spread in Africa by a rodent not present in the United States. Person-to-person spread requires close personal contact or contact with blood or excreta. Careful follow-up of household and other close contacts of cases imported into Western Europe and North America has shown no evidence of secondary transmission from casual contact, in stark contrast to earlier reports from African hospitals (26,27). The clinical spectrum of Lassa fever is wide, and the likelihood ratio of illness to infection is 9% to 26% (31). After an incubation period of 1 to 3 weeks, illness begins insidiously with fever, sore throat, weakness, and malaise. The long incubation period increases the likelihood that asymptomatic cases will be imported into the United States. The infection often progresses over several days to a generalized toxic syndrome with pharyngitis (often severe and exudative); retrosternal pain; vomiting; abdominal tenderness; and signs of vascular instability and capillary leakage including hypotension, bleeding, and edema of tissues. High levels of viremia and aminotransferase concentrations are associated with mortality and probably infectiousness of body fluids. The virus is present in blood and, sporadically, the throat and urine of patients (29). Overall, the case-fatality rate is about 1% to 2% (31). Diagnosis can be made by viral isolation or by demonstrating immunoglobulin M (IgM) antibodies to Lassa fever virus or a fourfold rise in titer of IgG antibody between acute- and convalescent-phase serum specimens (26). Treatment with ribavirin effectively reduces mortality (32).

Marburg and Ebola Viruses

Marburg and Ebola hemorrhagic fever viruses are closely related, as is their endemic geographic area (see Table 47.3). The mode of acquiring natural infection is unknown. Secondary person-to-person transmission results from close personal contact. Nosocomial transmission has occurred with both viruses and appears to depend on contact with blood, secretions, and excretions (26,33). There is no evidence of spread by casual contact or aerosol. The onset of illness is abrupt, and clinical manifestations include fever, headache, general malaise, myalgia, arthralgia, and sore throat. These symptoms are often followed by diarrhea, abdominal pain, a desquamating morbilliform rash, and hemorrhagic manifestations including petechiae and frank bleeding. Diagnosis requires isolating the virus from blood or demonstrating IgM or rising IgG antibodies. Treatment is supportive. In one epidemic of Marburg hemorrhagic fever in Europe related to an imported African green monkey, the case-fatality rate was 23% for primary cases, but no deaths were reported among the six secondary cases (34). The incubation period ranges from 3 to 10 days for Marburg hemorrhagic fever. For Ebola hemorrhagic fever, the case-fatality rate is even higher, generally greater than 50% in reported epidemics. The incubation period ranges from 2 to 21 days and averages about 7 days (26).

Crimean-Congo Hemorrhagic Fever Virus

Crimean-Congo hemorrhagic fever (CCHF) virus is present in many wild and domestic animals in the endemic areas (see Table 47.3). Ticks act as both a reservoir and a vector for CCHF; ground-feeding birds may disseminate infected ticks (26). Humans become infected by being bitten by ticks or crushing them. Contact with blood, secretions, or excretions of infected animals or humans may also transmit infection. Nosocomial transmission is well described (26). Evidence suggests that blood and other body fluids are highly infectious and that airborne transmission is unlikely. Initial symptoms include fever, headache, myalgia, arthralgia, abdominal pain, and vomiting. Sore throat, conjunctivitis, jaundice, photophobia, and various sensory and mood alterations may develop. A petechial rash is common and may precede a hemorrhagic diathesis including hemorrhage from multiple sites. The case-fatality rate is estimated to range from 15% to 70%, but more than 15% of cases may be asymptomatic. The incubation period is 2 to 9 days. Diagnosis requires isolating the virus from blood or detecting rising IgG antibody. Treatment is supportive.

Diagnosis

The patient's travel history, symptoms, and physical signs provide the most important clues to the diagnosis of any of the causes of VHF. Travel exclusively to urban zones in endemic areas or an interval of greater than 3 weeks from travel in an endemic area to onset of symptoms make VHF unlikely (26). Other patients at risk for VHF include those who, within 3 weeks before onset of fever, have had direct contact with blood or other body fluids, secretions, or excretions of a person or animal with VHF or who worked in a laboratory or animal facility that handles hemorrhagic fever viruses. A single case of any VHF from Table 47.3 in the United States should suggest bioterrorism unless there is an appropriate travel history (33).

Initial symptoms are flu-like and nonspecific. The differential diagnosis includes influenza, arboviral, and other viral infections; bacterial infections such as typhoid fever, toxic shock, streptococcal pharyngitis, and rickettsial diseases; and parasitic infections such as malaria. Symptoms and signs supporting the diagnosis of VHF are pharyngitis, conjunctivitis, a skin rash, and, later, hemorrhage and shock.

Prevention and Control

If clinicians feel that VHF is likely, they should take two immediate steps: (a) notify local and state health departments and the Centers for Disease Control and Prevention (CDC) and (b) institute special precautions, including the use of a private room and use of gloves for all patient and specimen contact. The CDC in 1988 recommended precautions for VHF that were updated in 1995 (26,35). Blood, urine, feces, vomitus, and respiratory droplets should be considered infectious. Gloves, gowns, face shields, and goggles should be used as necessary to prevent exposures to these body fluids. Patients should be placed on Contact Precautions (see Chapter 95) (11). In addition, the following measures should also be implemented: (a) eye covering (goggles or shields) for all contact within 3 feet, (b) a negative pressure room and use of a high-efficiency particulate air respirator (mask) if aerosolization of virus is likely (e.g., patients who have a prominent cough), (c) use of class II biologic safety cabinet following biosafety level 3 practices for laboratory specimens, and (d) pretreatment of serum specimens with polyethylene glycol p-tert-octylphenyl ether (10 μL of 10% triton x-100 per mL of serum) for 1 hour (35). All specimens should be marked with the biohazard symbol so that all persons handling these specimens will be alerted to use proper precautions, including gloves. If a patient with any VHF dies, all unnecessary handling of the body, including embalming and autopsy, should be avoided. The corpse should be placed in an airtight bag and cremated or buried immediately.

Patients who likely have Lassa fever should be treated with ribavirin, as should all individuals who have had unprotected contact with the patient's body fluids or excretions (32). Examples of unprotected contact include sexual intercourse, shared use of eating or drinking utensils, and failure to use gloves to handle items known to be contaminated with the patient's blood or secretions.

MENINGOCOCCAL INFECTIONS, INCLUDING PNEUMONIA

Infections caused by *Neisseria meningitidis* are endemic throughout the world but also occur in epidemics. Among civilians in the United States, meningococcal disease occurs primarily as single isolated cases or, infrequently, in small localized clusters. One third of all cases of meningococcal disease occur among patients 20 years of age or older. Nosocomial spread of the meningococcus is rare, but hospitalization of a case of invasive meningococcal disease is often associated with severe anxiety among healthcare workers caring for the patient.

Etiology

N. meningitidis is a gram-negative diplococcus that produces a polysaccharide capsule that forms the basis for the serogroup typing system. There are at least 13 serogroups, but serogroups B and C cause most cases of meningococcal disease in the United States, with serogroups Y and W135 accounting for most of the rest (36).

Epidemiology

Carriage of meningococci in the pharynx is common. One study found a 4.9% to 10.6% prevalence of carriage in a nonepi-

TABLE 47.4. SCHEDULE FOR ADMINISTERING CHEMOPROPHYLAXIS AGAINST MENINGOCOCCAL DISEASE

Drug	Age group	Dosage	Duration and routine of administration[a]
Rifampin[b]	children <1 month	5 mg/kg every 12 hours	2 days
	children ≥1 month	10 mg/kg every 12 hours	2 days
	Adults	600 mg every 12 hours	2 days
Ciprofloxacin[c]	Adults	500 mg	Single dose
Ceftriaxone	children <15 years	125 mg	Single intramuscular dose
Ceftriaxone	Adults	250 mg	Single intramuscular dose

[a] Oral administration unless indicated otherwise.
[b] Not recommended for pregnant women, because the drug is teratogenic in laboratory animals. Because the reliability of oral contraceptives may be affected by rifampin therapy, consideration should be given to using alternative contraceptive measures while rifampin is being administered.
[c] Not generally recommended for persons aged <18 years or for pregnant and lactating women, because the drug causes cartilage damage in immature laboratory animals. However, ciprofloxacin can be used for chemoprophylaxis of children when no acceptable alternative therapy is available.

demic situation involving crowded living conditions (37). No disease was noted in this population. The median duration of carriage was 9.6 months, and a 5.7% to 12.5% yearly incidence of acquisition was noted. Crowding appears to be one important factor influencing the prevalence of meningococcal carriage. The risk of acquisition of carriage is also increased if the index carrier is ill rather than asymptomatic (38,39). Acquisition of a new meningococcal serotype can result in asymptomatic colonization (the carrier state), local infection, or, rarely, invasive disease. The recent acquisition of carriage, rather than chronic carriage, may be the factor associated with the greatest risk of disease, because carriage longer than 2 weeks results in the development of apparently protective type-specific antibody (40). Transmission is believed to occur by direct contact, including contact with large droplets from the nose and throat of infected or colonized carriers. Generally, close live-in or intimate contact (e.g., mouth-to-mouth contact) is required to transmit meningococci effectively, especially if the index carrier is asymptomatic (37).

Risk to hospital personnel and patients from casual contact with an infected patient appears to be small. Epidemics of disease and colonization related to meningococcal pneumonia have been reported (41). However, most *N. meningitidis* pulmonary infections apparently are not associated with serious illness or transmission. Transmission from patients who have meningococcemia or meningitis to hospital personnel is rare but can occur to personnel who have intimate contact with respiratory secretions from infected patients (42–45). Laboratory workers are also at risk for meningococcal disease (46). Laboratory workers should follow biosafety procedures and consider meningococcal vaccination (46) (see also Chapter 82). It is not clear why transmission of meningococcal disease in hospitals is so rare compared with community transmission. Perhaps, transmission is limited because of the rapid institution of barrier precautions, treatment of the patient, and prophylaxis of exposed persons. The incubation period for disease varies from 2 to 14 days and is commonly 3 to 4 days.

Clinical Manifestations and Diagnosis

Meningococcal disease includes bacteremia without sepsis, meningococcemia without meningitis, meningitis with or without meningococcemia, and the meningoencephalitic presentation. A petechial rash is often present in invasive disease. Diagnosis is made by appropriate cultures and detection of antigen in spinal fluid, blood, or urine (47).

Prevention and Control

Droplet Precautions should be used to minimize transmission from patients with invasive meningococcal disease (see Chapter 95). Confirmed cases should be promptly reported to public health authorities to limit illness in prehospital contacts.

In addition, antibiotic prophylaxis should be considered for those with intimate contact with an untreated patient. This group potentially includes (a) community contacts, including family; (b) rarely, hospital personnel; and (c) possibly, hospitalized patients who are close contacts of a patient with untreated meningococcal pneumonia. When prophylaxis is necessary, it is important to begin it immediately, often before results of antimicrobial susceptibility testing are available (Table 47.4) (47,48). Ceftriaxone can be used for pregnant women. In the absence of a known exposure to meningococcal illness, personnel found to be colonized with meningococci should not be treated or removed from patient care activities.

Laboratory scientists with percutaneous exposure to an invasive *N. meningitidis* isolate from a sterile site should receive treatment with penicillin; those with known mucosal exposure should receive antimicrobial chemoprophylaxis (Table 47.4) (46). Microbiologists who manipulate invasive *N. meningitidis* isolates in a manner that could induce aerosolization or droplet formation (including plating, subculturing, and serogrouping) on an open bench top and in the absence of effective protection from droplets or aerosols also should consider antimicrobial chemoprophylaxis (see also Chapter 82).

PLAGUE

Etiology

Plague is a zoonotic infection caused by *Yersinia pestis* (49). *Y. pestis* is a gram-negative, facultatively anaerobic, asporogenous bacillus that belongs to the bacterial family Enterobacteriaceae. It grows aerobically on most culture media, including blood agar and MacConkey's agar (49). *Y. pestis* produces several essential virulence factors, including V and W antigens and endotoxin (49,50).

Pathogenesis

Plague bacteria are inoculated by the bite of an infected flea and migrate by cutaneous lymphatics to the regional lymph nodes. *Y. pestis* resists destruction within mononuclear phagocytes and multiplies intracellularly. Acute necrotizing suppurative lymphadenitis develops in the involved lymph nodes (the bubo) (50). Transient bacteremia is common in bubonic plague and may result in metastatic lesions (liver, spleen, meninges) and endotoxemia with hypotension, oliguria, altered mental status, and subclinical disseminated intravascular coagulation.

Epidemiology

Plague is an ancient disease. Epidemics of plague brought devastation to many societies, including medieval Europe, with a massive loss of population. Humans, however, are an accidental host and have no role in the maintenance or propagation of plague in nature. Rats, which were the reservoir of epidemic plague, no longer are subject to epizootics of plague as they were in the past. Now, infected sylvatic rodents are the primary reservoir in the southwestern United States and have become entrenched in rural areas of many countries (49,50). Plague occurs worldwide, with most of the human cases reported from developing countries of Asia, Africa, and South America. Several hundred cases are reported annually to the World Health Organization (WHO) (49–51). From 1980 through 1994, 18,739 cases of plague and 1,853 deaths (10%) were reported to the WHO by 24 countries in Africa, the Americas, and Asia (52).

In the United States most of the human plague (except for rare laboratory accidents and imported cases) is contracted in nonurban sylvatic foci in the states of New Mexico, Arizona, Colorado, Utah, and California. Ten to 40 cases per year are reported in the United States (49–51,53,54). From 1980 through 1994, 229 cases of plague were reported in the United States (a mean of 15 cases per year), with 33 deaths (14%) (52). Cases in travelers, acquired in endemic areas but manifested elsewhere, have been reported (55). A delay in diagnosis and poor outcome may result if travel history is not ascertained. Most of the cases are diagnosed during the months of May to October. A disproportionately large number of cases occur in American Indians (56).

Plague is primarily a zoonotic infection. It is perpetuated in the natural animal reservoirs of urban and sylvatic rodents by flea bites or by ingestion of infected animal tissues. Worldwide, rats are the most important reservoirs of plague bacillus. In sylvatic foci of plague, such as in the southwestern United States, the important reservoirs are the ground squirrel, rock squirrel, and prairie dog. Humans become infected when bitten by rodent fleas and occasionally by handling of contaminated animal tissues (57). Transmission from domestic cats has been reported in the United States (58–60). Direct person-to-person spread of plague is rare and occurs during epidemics of pneumonic plague.

Clinical Manifestations

Bubonic plague is the most common clinical presentation. The incubation period is 2 to 7 days following the bite of an infected flea. Patients present with a sudden onset of high fever; chills; weakness; headache; and, at the same time or shortly thereafter, a swollen and intensely painful regional group of lymph nodes (the bubo) usually in the groin, axilla, or neck (49–51). Hematogenous spread may result in secondary pneumonia characterized by a rapid course and high mortality. The sputum is purulent and contains plague bacilli. Plague pneumonia is highly contagious by airborne transmission. Primary inhalation pneumonia is rare, but it is always a potential threat following exposure to a patient or a cat with plague pneumonia (58,59). Any patient with plague and cough should be suspected of having pneumonia until proven otherwise.

Other clinical syndromes include septicemia, meningitis, pharyngitis, and cutaneous plague. Gastrointestinal symptoms (nausea, vomiting, diarrhea) may dominate the clinical picture and lead to diagnostic confusion.

Diagnosis

Diagnosis of plague should be suspected in febrile patients with a history of exposure to rodents or to other mammals in endemic areas. The aspirate from the bubo should be stained with Gram and Wayson (or Giemsa or Wright) stains and also cultured. Several blood cultures should be obtained. Blood smears may be positive in patients with septicemia. Smears and cultures of the sputum, cerebrospinal fluid, and skin lesions should be done when appropriate. Rapid diagnostic tests, such as antigen detection, IgM enzyme immunoassay, immunostaining, and polymerase chain reaction are available only at some state health departments, the CDC, and military laboratories (49). Chest radiography should be done in every patient with suspected plague. Testing of clinical specimens and isolates from suspected plague patients should be coordinated through state health departments and sent to CDC's Diagnostic and Reference Laboratory Section, Division of Vector-Borne Infectious Diseases, National Center for Infectious Diseases (telephone 970-221-6400) (61). The CDC, Plague Branch, P.O. Box 2087, Fort Collins, Colorado 80522 (telephone: 303-221-6450) can perform the fluorescent antibody stain, the definitive culture identification (mail in double containers), and serologic testing on acute- and convalescent-phase sera (49).

Prevention and Control

No nosocomial transmission of plague has occurred in the United States in modern times, but the potential danger demands prompt institution of infection control measures any time the disease is suspected. Plague is an internationally quarantinable disease. All patients with suspected plague must be immediately reported to the health department.

All patients with plague must be placed on Droplet Precautions for the first 72 hours after start of effective treatment because of the possibility that pneumonia may supervene (11,62). Standard Precautions are then adequate for the duration of hospitalization. In patients with pharyngitis or a positive throat culture, droplet precautions should continue until a negative throat culture is obtained. For patients who have plague and have a cough or pneumonia, droplet precautions plus eye protection should be continued for at least 72 hours after the initiation of effective antimicrobial therapy. All contacts of plague pneumonia patients should be rapidly identified. Individuals with a direct face-to-face contact (less than 2 m) should be given prophylactic or abortive treatment (63). Tetracycline 2 g/day or doxycycline 200 mg/day for 5 to 10 days is recommended in nonpregnant adults. Streptomycin, gentamicin, chloramphenicol, sulfadiazine, ciprofloxacin, or, in pregnant women, trimethoprim-sulfamethoxazole may also be used for abortive therapy (63–65). All contacts should be instructed to have their temperature taken twice daily and to report fever, cough, or other symptoms. Surveillance may terminate 7 days after the last contact with the case-patient. All laboratory specimens should be handled with gloves. Laboratory personnel should be alerted to the possibility of plague to avoid skin contact with and aerosolization of cultures. A previously used formalin-killed vaccine was discontinued in 1999 by its manufacturers and is no longer available (49).

Bioterrorism Potential

Plague outbreaks following a use of an aerosolized plague bacillus as a biologic weapon are a plausible threat (see Chapter 112) (63). The occurrence of cases and clusters of cases of primary pneumonic plague in locations not known to have enzootic infection or in persons without risk factors should lead to a suspicion of bioterrorism. Recommendations on the management of bioterrorism-related plague outbreaks have been published (63) (see also Chapter 111).

PSITTACOSIS

Etiology

Psittacosis (ornithosis) is a disease of birds caused by *Chlamydia psittaci* and is transmissible to humans. *C. psittaci* is an obligate intracellular parasite and is considered a specialized bacterium (66).

Pathogenesis

C. psittaci enters the body via the upper respiratory tract after the inhalation of infectious material. The microorganism spreads to the reticuloendothelial cells of the liver and spleen and, after replication, invades the lungs and other organs by hematogenous dissemination (66). Psittacosis is a systemic illness with predominantly pulmonary involvement.

Epidemiology

Dried excreta of birds is the main source of infection. Human-to-human transmission is rarely reported but may result in more severe disease. Human-to-human transmission has also been reported with the related species *Chlamydia pneumoniae* (TWAR) (66–68). Clusters of possible nosocomial transmission of *C. psittaci* have been reported, but possible serologic cross-reactivity with *C. pneumoniae* complicates the evaluation of these reports (69–71).

Psittacosis is reported worldwide and is associated with exposure to infected birds and other animals (66–72). There has been a recent decline in psittacosis cases in the United States associated with effective control of the disease in domestic and imported birds, but 100 to 250 cases are reported annually, and small outbreaks continue to occur (66,73,74). Psittacosis is an occupational hazard for people working with birds, including veterinarians, and poultry processing plant employees and bird fanciers are also at risk for infection (75,76). A minority of patients have no history of bird contact and may have had only an exposure to a contaminated environment or to an infected human (77).

Clinical Manifestations

The incubation period is 6 to 20 days. The severity of illness ranges from a mild flu-like illness to an overwhelming lethal infection. In the preantibiotic era the mortality rate was 20%. Chills, fever, headache (often severe), malaise, anorexia, myalgias, and persistent cough are the usual symptoms (78–80). Pneumonia is the major clinical manifestation. Hepatosplenomegaly is common and should lead to a consideration of psittacosis in a patient with pneumonia. Asymptomatic seroconversion can occur.

Diagnosis

A compatible clinical illness in a patient with a history of exposure to birds should lead to a suspicion of psittacosis. Chest radiography usually shows a pulmonary infiltrate but is nonspecific. A fourfold rise in titer of complement-fixing antibodies to *Chlamydia* antigen to at least 1:32 between acute and convalescent specimens is diagnostic. A single titer of 1:32 in a compatible clinical setting is presumptive evidence of psittacosis (66). Effective antibiotic therapy may blunt the antibody response. The isolation of *C. psittaci* by culture of respiratory secretions is possible but not routinely available except in reference laboratories (66).

Prevention and Control

Prevention of psittacosis consists of control of avian infection and prevention of bird-to-human transmission (81). Human respiratory secretions may be infectious, but human-to-human transmission is very rare, and nosocomial psittacosis is only a remote possibility. CDC guidelines do not recommend isolation of hospitalized patients with psittacosis or the use of a private room, masks, gowns, or gloves (11). Pet-assisted therapy in healthcare facilities is gaining in popularity in the United States. The introduction of birds as pets into hospitals is undesirable (see Chapter 101). Psittacosis is a notifiable disease, and cases should be reported to the local health department (67). The mortality rate in treated patients is low (<1%) (66).

TETANUS

Tetanus (lockjaw) is a disease caused by a neurotoxin tetanospasmin produced by *Clostridium tetani*. Tetanus is manifested by uncontrolled muscle spasms, results in high mortality, and is preventable by immunization. It is more common in developing countries but continues to occur in the United States, especially in unimmunized or inadequately immunized elderly persons (82).

Etiology

C. tetani is a motile, gram-positive, strictly anaerobic, nonencapsulated, spore-forming rod. The drumstick-shaped spores are highly resistant to chemical disinfection and heat but are destroyed by autoclaving. *C. tetani* can be found in human and animal feces, and the spores can survive in dry soil for years. *C. tetani* is a noninvasive microorganism and depends on the introduction of its spores into damaged or devitalized tissue to provide the anaerobic conditions favorable for its growth.

Pathogenesis

The potent neurotoxin tetanospasmin is produced by vegetative *C. tetani* in a localized site of infection and enters the nervous system at myoneural junctions of motor neurons either locally or after hematogenous and/or lymphatic spread. Tetanospasmin is carried by retrograde axonal transport to the neuraxis, where it binds to the presynaptic terminals of the inhibitory synapses, preventing transmitter release. The absence of inhibition results in increased muscle tone, rigidity, and simultaneous spasms of both agonist and antagonist muscles (82).

Epidemiology

C. tetani resides harmlessly in the intestines of horses and other animals, including humans. Soil or fomites contaminated with human or animal feces serve as a source of infection. *C. tetani* spores are ubiquitous, and essentially any wound or infected area with an anaerobic environment can serve as a nidus for the disease (82). The incidence of tetanus in a population is related to the prevalence of immunity and the frequency of trauma. In the United States the incidence of tetanus has been between 0.02 and 0.04 cases per 100,000 in recent years. Fifty to 70 cases are reported annually (82–89). The disease in the United States occurs predominantly in older adults who are either unimmunized or inadequately immunized. Women and Mexican-Americans have a significantly lower rate of immunity than non-Hispanic white males (90). Neonatal tetanus is very rare in the United States. Tetanus is a major problem in developing countries, where the prevalence of immunity is low. Common predisposing factors in developing countries include wounds, contamination of umbilical stumps in neonates, postpartum manipulation of the placenta, chronic ear infections, nonsterile injections, unskilled abortions, ear piercing, scarification rituals, and female circumcision (82,83).

Most of the cases are secondary to acute wounds. Other predisposing conditions include chronic wounds, skin ulcers, abscesses, burns, gangrene, parenteral drug abuse, and surgery. Tetanus occasionally follows surgical procedures (82,91,92). Several small outbreaks of postoperative tetanus have been reported. Both exogenous surgical site contamination in the operating room and endogenous sources (intestinal flora of the patient) of *C. tetani* have been implicated. Rarely, the patient has no recognizable tetanus-prone wound.

Clinical Manifestations

The incubation period usually is within 2 weeks but may range from 2 days to months. Early manifestations include localized or generalized weakness, stiffness or cramping, difficulty in chewing and swallowing food, and trismus resulting from increased masseter muscle tone (lockjaw). The disease progresses to generalized muscle rigidity and reflex spasms. Tonic contractions of muscles may result in painful opisthotonos, abdominal rigidity, and the characteristic facial expression called risus sardonicus. Laryngospasm and/or respiratory muscle involvement may interfere with ventilation. Aspiration may result from difficulty in swallowing. Reflex tetanic spasms may be precipitated by stimuli such as noise, light, or touch and may result in opisthotonos, apnea, fractures, tendon separations, and rhabdomyolysis. The autonomic dysfunction with excessive catecholamine release is common and may result in labile hypertension, tachycardia, cardiac arrhythmias, peripheral vasoconstriction, sweating, elevated temperature, toxic myocarditis, and cardiac arrest (82,85). The mortality rate is high in severe tetanus, especially in infants and the elderly, and may exceed 40% (82,87).

Diagnosis

The diagnosis of tetanus is primarily clinical and is based on history and examination. *C. tetani* is rarely seen in Gram stains from a wound or recovered on culture. A definite history of having received a complete immunization series and/or a serum antitoxin level of 0.01 units/mL or higher makes the diagnosis very unlikely (82). The differential diagnosis of tetanus includes meningitis, dental abscess, peritonitis, rabies, hypocalcemic tetany, epilepsy, decerebrate posturing, alcohol and drug withdrawal, dystonic reactions to antipsychotic drugs, and strychnine poisoning.

Prevention and Control

Antibody to tetanospasmin is protective. Serum antitoxin levels of 0.01 units/mL or above are considered protective, although mild tetanus cases have been reported in patients with titers in the range of 0.01 to 1.0 units/mL (82,85). Tetanus is a disease with no naturally acquired immunity but is preventable with appropriate immunization and wound care. Tetanus toxoid is an effective immunizing agent and is administered via intramus-

TABLE 47.5. ROUTINE DIPHTHERIA, TETANUS, AND PERTUSSIS VACCINATION SCHEDULE SUMMARY FOR CHILDREN—UNITED STATES, 1991

Dose	Customary age	Age/interval	Product
Age <7 years			
Primary 1	2 months	6 weeks old or older	DTP[b,c]
Primary 2	4 months	4–8 weeks after first dose[a]	DTP[b,c]
Primary 3	6 months	4–8 weeks after second dose[a]	DTP[b,c]
Primary 4	15 months	6–12 months after third dose[a]	DTP[b,c]
Booster	4–6 years old, before entering kindergarten or elementary school (not necessary if fourth primary vaccinating dose administered after fourth birthday)		DTP[b,c]
Additional boosters	Every 10 years after last dose		Td[d]
Age ≥7 years			
Primary 1	7 years and older	First dose	Td[d]
Primary 2	7 years and older	4–8 weeks after first dose[a]	Td[d]
Primary 3	7 years and older	6–12 months after second dose[a]	Td[d]
Booster	Every 10 years after last dose		Td[d]

[a] Prolonging the interval does not require restarting series.
[b] Use DT if pertussis vaccine is contraindicated. If the child is ≥1 year of age at the time that primary dose three is due, a third dose 6–12 months after the second completes primary vaccination with DT.
[c] Diphtheria-tetanus toxoids and pertussis.
[d] Tetanus-diphtheria toxoids.
From Centers for Disease Control and Prevention. Diphtheria, tetanus and pertussis: guidelines for vaccine use and other preventive measures: recommendations of the Immunization Practices Advisory Committee (ACIP). *MMWR Morb Mortal Wkly Rep* 1991;40(RR-10):1–28, with permission.

cular injections. Current recommendations for active immunization are given in Table 47.5 (93). Completion of the primary series confers immunity to tetanus for at least 10 years in 95% or more of vaccinees. Booster vaccinations are recommended every 10 years to maintain protective antitoxin levels. Healthcare employees can be immunized or given booster injections as part of the preemployment screening process.

Appropriate management of wounds is very important in preventing tetanus. Tetanus-prone wounds include those contaminated with dirt, feces, or saliva; puncture wounds (including accidental needle punctures); avulsions; and wounds resulting from missiles, crushing, burns, and frostbite. However, any wound can result in tetanus, including surgical sites and decubitus ulcers. Careful cleansing, drainage, and debridement of the wound and removal of foreign bodies and necrotic tissue can reduce the likelihood of tetanus. Recommendations for specific immunoprophylaxis depend on the patient's prior immunization history and the nature of the wound (Table 47.6) (93). Patients who have received a full immunization series but who have not received a dose for more than 10 years should be given a booster vaccination with (or without) any type of wound. This is especially important in preoperative patients, pregnant women (to protect both mother and child), nursing home residents and paraplegics (risk of decubitus ulcer), intravenous drug abusers, and healthcare personnel sustaining accidental needle punctures. If the patient is uncertain about prior vaccinations or knows that the full tetanus series has not been received, tetanus vaccine should be given for any type of wound (with arrangements made to complete the series), and additional passive immunization with tetanus immune globulin (TIG) should be given for tetanus-prone wounds. When vaccine and TIG are given concurrently, separate syringes and separate sites of administration should be used. One study demonstrated that the antitetanus prophylaxis given in hospital emergency rooms is often inadequate (94).

Tetanus is not directly transmissible from person to person, and no isolation precautions are indicated for the management of a patient with tetanus. Cases of tetanus must be reported to

TABLE 47.6. SUMMARY OF RECOMMENDATIONS OF ADVISORY COMMITTEE ON IMMUNIZATION PRACTICES FOR TETANUS PROPHYLAXIS IN ROUTINE WOUND MANAGEMENT—UNITED STATES, 1991

History of absorbed tetanus toxoid (doses)	Clean, minor wounds		All other wounds[a]	
	Td[b]	TIG	Td[b]	TIG
Unknown or <3	Yes	No	Yes	Yes
≥3[c]	No[d]	No	No[e]	No

[a] Such as, but not limited to, wounds contaminated with dirt, feces, soil, saliva; puncture wounds; avulsions; and wounds resulting from missiles, crushing, burns, and frostbite.
[b] For children <7 years old; DTP (DT, if pertussis vaccine is contraindicated) is preferred to tetanus toxoid alone. For persons ≥7 years of age, Td is preferred to tetanus toxoid alone. Diphtheria and tetanus toxoids and acellular pertussis vaccine (DTaP) may be used instead of DTP for the fourth and fifth doses.
[c] If only three doses of fluid toxoid have been received, then a fourth dose of toxoid, preferably an adsorbed toxoid, should be given.
[d] Yes, if more than 10 years since last dose.
[e] Yes, if more than 5 years since last dose. (More frequent boosters are not needed and can accentuate side effects.)
From Centers for Disease Control and Prevention. Diphtheria, tetanus, pertussis: guidelines for vaccine use and other preventive measures: recommendations of the Immunization Practices Advisory Committee (ACIP). *MMWR Morb Mortal Wkly Rep* 1991;40(RR-10):1–28, with permission.

the health department. Hospitalization or a visit to an emergency room may be the only contact of an unimmunized or inadequately immunized individual with the healthcare system, and routine review of tetanus immunity status should be considered for all hospitalized patients but especially for the elderly, children, pregnant women, preoperative patients, patients with wounds (including burns and decubitus ulcers), and parenteral drug abusers.

BOTULISM

Etiology

Botulism is a disease caused by *Clostridium botulinum* exotoxin. *C. botulinum* is a gram-positive spore-forming anaerobic bacillus. The neurotoxin produced by the microorganism causes a paralytic illness.

Pathogenesis

The toxin can cause the disease by (a) being preformed in the food (botulism food poisoning), (b) being produced in a traumatic wound contaminated by *C. botulinum* (wound botulism), and (c) being produced by *C. botulinum* in the gastrointestinal tract of infants (infant botulism) (95–97). A potent neurotoxin is released after spores germinate and bacterial growth and autolysis occur under appropriate conditions. These conditions include an appropriate pH (greater than 4.6), a temperature generally greater than 10°C, sufficient availability of water, and a relatively anaerobic environment (96). Eight toxin types have been described (A, B, C_a, C_b, D, E, F, and G). Types A, B, and E are the most common causes of disease in humans. Botulinum neurotoxins are the most potent known poison. The toxins interfere with neurotransmission at peripheral cholinergic synapses by binding tightly to the presynaptic membrane and preventing the release of the neurotransmitter acetylcholine.

Epidemiology

Twenty to 50 cases of foodborne botulism have occurred annually in the United States since 1981 (98). The toxin, when ingested with food, is absorbed from the stomach, the small intestine, and, slowly, the colon. Food items contaminated by botulinum toxin may have a completely normal appearance and taste. If *C. botulinum* microorganisms or spores are ingested and reach the colon, toxin production and absorption can occur in the human gastrointestinal tract as in infant botulism (95,99). The spores of *C. botulinum* are heat resistant, but the toxins are heat labile and are destroyed by boiling for 10 minutes or by heating at 80°C for 30 minutes. Thus, terminal heating of toxin-containing food can prevent botulism (95).

Wound botulism occurs when *C. botulinum* contaminates a traumatic wound and produces toxin *in situ* (100–102). The toxin is then absorbed systemically. The incubation period is 4 to 14 days from the time of injury. The wound may appear clean, but antibiotic therapy may not prevent intoxication. The clinical picture is similar to foodborne botulism but without gastrointestinal symptoms; fever may occur secondary to wound infection. Wound botulism is rare, with only a few cases reported annually (98). Compound fractures and crush injuries to the extremity are the major types of associated wounds (100). Postoperative cases have been reported (102). Parenteral and/or intranasal illicit drug use has been reported as a risk factor for wound botulism (103,104).

Infant botulism is the most common form of botulism in the United States, with 50 to 100 cases reported annually (97,98, 105). The infant gastrointestinal tract becomes colonized with *C. botulinum* (often from honey contaminated with spores), and toxin is produced *in vivo*. Infants younger than 1 year are usually affected. The illness typically begins with constipation followed by lethargy, listlessness, poor feeding, ptosis, difficulty in swallowing, loss of head control, hypotonia and generalized weakness (the floppy baby), and, in some cases, respiratory arrest. Occasionally, infant-type botulism can occur in adults with altered gastrointestinal anatomy or microbial flora that permits the proliferation of ingested *C. botulinum* and production of toxin *in vivo* (106). With the availability of botulinum toxin for therapeutic use in muscle spasm disorders, the possibility of inadvertent, surreptitious, or criminal misuse of the toxin should be considered in patients with an otherwise unexplained clinical syndrome consistent with botulism (107).

C. botulinum spores are found in soil and marine sediment worldwide and, therefore, may easily contaminate food products. In the United States, type A spores predominate west of the Mississippi River, and type B spores predominate in the eastern states. Type E disease is usually associated with fish products (95,96).

Most cases of botulism food poisoning occur singly or in small clusters and are due to home-canned or home-prepared foods; commercial products and restaurant-prepared foods are implicated in some instances (108,109).

Clinical Manifestations

The incubation period is 12 to 36 hours, with a range of 6 hours to 8 days. Early symptoms include weakness and dizziness. Nausea and vomiting are uncommon. The picture of cholinergic inhibition is manifested by diminished salivation, extreme dryness of the mouth and throat, ileus, constipation, and urinary retention. Cranial nerve involvement is manifested by diplopia, blurred vision, photophobia, dysphonia, dysarthria, and dysphagia. Symmetric descending weakness of the extremities and respiratory muscle weakness occur. The patient characteristically is alert, oriented, and afebrile. Orthostatic hypotension may be present. Ptosis, extraocular muscle palsies, and dilated fixed pupils usually (but not always) are present on eye examination. Oral mucous membranes are dry. Variable degrees of muscle weakness and deep tendon reflex abnormalities are observed. Sensory examination is normal. Respiratory failure may develop secondary to respiratory muscle weakness. The clinical course is often prolonged, and the recovery is gradual (110,111).

Diagnosis

A characteristic clinical picture and history of exposure should lead to suspicion of botulism. Characteristic abnormalities are observed on electromyographic studies in patients with botulism (95). The diagnosis is confirmed by detecting *C. botulinum* toxin (by bioassay in mice) in the blood, stool, gastric contents, or suspected food or by culturing *C. botulinum* from the food, stool, gastric contents, or wounds (in patients with wound botulism) (112). These tests usually are performed by reference laboratories.

Prevention and Control

The health department should be promptly notified of all suspected cases of botulism. The source food should be identified, and all potentially exposed individuals should be informed. The disease is not communicable, and isolation is not indicated. The mortality rate for adult botulism is 10% to 25% with modern supportive care and is as low as 2% in infant botulism.

Bioterrorism Potential

An aerosolized or foodborne botulinum toxin weapon potential exists (Chapter 112). Botulinum toxin has been weaponized, and terrorists have tried to use botulinum toxin as a weapon (113). Hospital personnel should be alert to a possibility of a deliberate attack with botulinum toxin when an outbreak of flaccid paralysis is detected. (See also Chapter 111.)

REFERENCES

1. Bleck TP, Rupprecht CE. Rabies virus. In: Mandel GL, Bennett JE, Dolin R, eds. *Principles and practice of infectious diseases,* 5th ed. Philadelphia: Churchill Livingstone, 2000:1811–1820.
2. Messenger SL, Smith JS, Rupprecht CE. Emerging epidemiology of bat-associated cryptic cases of rabies in humans in the United States. *Clin Infect Dis* 2002;35:738–747.
3. Plotkin SA. Rabies. *Clin Infect Dis* 2000;30:4–12.
4. Noah DL, Drenzek CL, Smith JS, et al. Epidemiology of human rabies in the United States, 1980 to 1996. *Ann Intern Med* 1998; 128:922–930.
5. Krebs JW, Long-Marin SC, Childs JE. Causes, costs and estimates of rabies postexposure prophylaxis treatments in the United States. *J Public Health Pract* 1998;4:57–63.
6. Centers for Disease Control and Prevention. Rabies prevention—United States, 1999: recommendations of Immunization Practices Advisory Committee (ACIP). *MMWR Morb Mortal Wkly Rep* 1999;48(RR-1):1–21.
7. Anderson LJ, Winkler WG, Vernon AA, et al. Prophylaxis for persons in contact with patients who have rabies. *N Engl J Med* 1980;302: 967–968.
8. Centers for Disease Control and Prevention. Human rabies diagnosed 2 months postmortem—Texas. *MMWR Morb Mortal Wkly Rep* 1985; 34:700, 705–707.
9. Helmick CG, Tauxe RV, Vernon AA. Is there a risk to contacts of patients with rabies? *Rev Infect Dis* 1987;9:511–518.
10. Anderson LJ, Nicholson KG, Tauxe RV, et al. Human rabies in the United States, 1960–1979: epidemiology, diagnosis, and prevention. *Ann Intern Med* 1984;100:728–735.
11. Garner JS, Hospital Infection Control Practices Advisory Committee. Guideline for isolation precautions in hospitals. *Infect Control Hosp Epidemiol* 1996;17:54–80.
12. Tyler KL. Prions and prion diseases of the central nervous system (transmissible neurodegenerative diseases). In: Mandell GL, Bennett JE, Dolin R., eds. *Principles and practice of infectious diseases,* 5th ed. Philadelphia: Churchill Livingstone, 2000:1971–1985.
13. Gajdusek DC. Unconventional viruses and the origin and disappearance of kuru. *Science* 1977;197:943–960.
14. Brown P, Preece MA, Well RG. "Friendly fire" in medicine: hormones, homografts, and Creutzfeldt-Jakob disease. *Lancet* 1992;340: 24–27.
15. Brown P, Will RG, Bradley R, et al. Bovine spongiform encephalopathy and variant Creutzfeldt-Jakob disease: background, evolution and current concerns. *Emerg Infect Dis* 2001;7:6–16.
16. Hsiao KH, Meiner Z, Kahana E, et al. Mutation of the prion protein in Libyan Jews with Creutzfeldt-Jakob disease. *N Engl J Med* 1991; 324:1091–1097.
17. Centers for Disease Control and Prevention. Probable variant Creutzfeldt-Jakob disease in a U.S. resident—Florida, 2002. *MMWR Morb Mortal Wkly Rep* 2002;51:927–929.
18. Roos RP. Controlling prion diseases. *N Engl J Med* 2001:344; 1548–1551.
19. Hsick G, Kenney K, Gibbs CJ, et al. The 14-3-3 brain protein in cerebrospinal fluid as a marker for transmissible spongiform encephalopathies. *N Engl J Med* 1996;335:924--930.
20. Collinge J. New diagnostic tests for prion diseases [Editorial]. *N Engl J Med* 1996;335:963–965.
21. Gajdusek DC. *Unconventional viruses and the origin and disappearance of kuru.* Les Prix Nobel en 1976. Stockholm: Nobel Foundation, 1977:167–216.
22. Holman RC, Khan AS, Belay ED, et al. Creutzfeldt-Jakob disease in the United States, 1979–1994: using national mortality data to assess the possible occurrence of variant cases. *Emerging Infect Dis* 1996;4: 333–337.
23. Rutala WA, Weber DJ. Creutzfeldt-Jakob disease: recommendations for disinfection and sterilization. *Clin Infect Dis* 2001;32:1348–1356.
24. World Health Organization. WHO infection control guidelines for transmissible spongiform encephalopathies. Available at *http://www.WHO/cds/csr/aph/2000.3.*
25. Ricketts MN, Cashman NR, Stratton EE, et al. Is Creutzfeldt-Jakob disease transmitted by blood? *Emerging Infect Dis* 1997;3:155–163.
26. Centers for Disease Control and Prevention. Management of patients with suspected viral hemorrhagic fever. *MMWR Morb Mortal Wkly Rep* 1988;37:1–6.
27. Holmes GP, McCormick JB, Trock SC, et al. Lassa fever in the United States: investigation of a case and new guidelines for management. *N Engl J Med* 1990;323:1120–1123.
28. Borio L, Inglesby T, Peters CJ, et al. Hemorrhagic fever viruses as biological weapons: medical and public health management. *JAMA* 2002;287;2391–2405.
29. Johnson KM, Monath TP. Imported Lassa fever—reexamining the algorithms. *N Engl J Med* 1990;323:1139–1141.
30. Wenzel RP. A new hantavirus infection in North America [Editorial]. *N Engl J Med* 1994;330:1004–1005.
31. McCormick JB, Webb PA, Krebs JW, et al. A prospective study of the epidemiology and ecology of Lassa fever. *J Infect Dis* 1987;155: 437–444.
32. McCormick JB, King IJ, Webb PA, et al. Lassa fever: effective therapy with ribavirin. *N Engl J Med* 1986:314:20–26.
33. Tomori O, Bertolli J, Rollin PE, et al. Serologic survey among hospital and health care workers during the Ebola hemorrhagic fever outbreak in Kikwit, Democratic Republic of the Congo, 1995. *J Infect Dis* 1999;179(Suppl 1);S98–101.
34. Martini GA, Siegert R, eds. *Marburg virus disease.* Berlin: Springer-Verlag, 1971.
35. Centers for Disease Control and Prevention. Update: management of patients with suspected viral hemorrhagic fever—United States. *MMWR Morb Mortal Wkly Rep* 1995;44:475–479.
36. Centers for Disease Control and Prevention. Laboratory-based surveillance for meningococcal disease in selected areas, United States, 1989–1991. *MMWR Morb Mortal Wkly Rep* 1993;42:21–30.
37. Greenfield S, Sheehe PR, Feldman HA. Meningococcal carriage in a population of "normal" families. *J Infect Dis* 1971;123:67–73
38. Foster MT, Sanders E, Ginter M. Epidemiology of sulfonamide-resistant meningococcal infections in a civilian population. *Am J Epidemiol* 1971;93:346–353.

39. Munford RS, de E Tauney A, de Morais JS, et al. Spread of meningococcal infection within households. *Lancet* 1974;1:1275–1278.
40. Goldschneider I, Gotschlich EC, Artenstein MS. Human immunity to the meningococcus. II. Development of natural immunity. *J Exp Med* 1969;129:1327–1348.
41. Winstead JM, McKinsey DS, Tasker S, et al. Meningococcal pneumonia: characterization and review of cases seen over the past 25 years. *Clin Infect Dis* 2000;30:87–94.
42. Centers for Disease Control and Prevention. Nosocomial meningococcemia—Wisconsin. *MMWR Morb Mortal Wkly Rep* 1979;27:358, 363.
43. Feldman HA. Some recollections of the meningococcal diseases. *JAMA* 1972;220:1107–1112.
44. Gehanno J-F, Kohen-Couderc L, Lemeland J-F, et al. Nosocomial meningococcemia in a physician. *Infect Control Hosp Epidemiol* 1999; 20:564–565.
45. Gilmore A, Stuart J. Risk of secondary meningococcal disease in health-care workers. *Lancet* 2000;356:1654–1655.
46. Centers for Disease Control and Prevention. Laboratory-acquired meningococcal disease—United States, 2000. *MMWR Morb Mortal Wkly Rep* 2002;51:141–144.
47. Apicella MA. *Neisseria meningitidis.* In: Mandell GL, Bennett JE, Dolin R, eds. *Principles and practice of infectious diseases,* 5th ed. Philadelphia: Churchill Livingstone, 2000:2228–2239.
48. Schwartz B. Chemoprophylaxis for bacterial infections: principles of and application to meningococcal infection. *Rev Infect Dis* 1991; 13(Suppl):S170.
49. Butler T. *Yersinia* species (including plague). In: Mandell GL, Bennett JE, Dolin R, eds. *Principles and practice of infectious diseases,* 5th ed. New York: Churchill Livingstone, 2000:2406–2414.
50. Butler T. *Plague and other Yersinia infections.* New York: Plenum Press, 1983.
51. Palmer D. Plague. In: Gorbach SL, Bartlett JG, Blacklow NR, eds. *Infectious diseases,* 2nd ed. Philadelphia: WB Saunders, 1998: 1568–1575.
52. Dennis DT, Hughes JM. Multidrug resistance in plague. *N Engl J Med* 1997;337:702–704.
53. Reed WP, Palmer DL, Williams RC, et al. Bubonic plague in the southwestern United States. *Medicine* 1970,49:465–486.
54. Centers for Disease Control and Prevention. Plague. Summary of notifiable diseases, United States 2000. *MMWR Morb Mortal Wkly Rep* 2002;49:55.
55. Mann JM, Schmid GP, Stoesz PA, et al. Peripatetic plague. *JAMA* 1982;247:47–48.
56. Mann JM, Martone WJ, Boyce JM, et al. Endemic human plague in New Mexico; risk factors associated with infection. *J Infect Dis* 1979;140:397–401.
57. Centers for Disease Control and Prevention. Plague—United States, 1992. *MMWR Morb Mortal Wkly Rep* 1992;41:787–790.
58. Werner SB, Weidmer CE, Nelson BC, et al. Primary plague pneumonia contracted from a domestic cat at South Lake Tahoe, Calif. *JAMA* 1984;251:929–931.
59. Centers for Disease Control and Prevention. Pneumonic plague—Arizona, 1992. *MMWR Morb Mortal Wkly Rep* 1992;41:737–739.
60. Weniger BG, Warren AJ, Forseth V, et al. Human bubonic plague transmitted by a domestic cat scratch. *JAMA* 1984;251:927–928.
61. Centers for Disease Control and Prevention. Fatal human plague—Arizona and Colorado, 1996. *MMWR Morb Mortal Wkly Rep* 1997;46:617–620.
62. White ME, Gordon D, Poland JD, et al. Recommendation for the control of *Yersinia pestis* infections. *Infect Control* 1980;1:324–329.
63. Inglesby TV, Dennis DT, Henderson DA, et al. Plague as a biological weapon. *JAMA* 2000;283:2282–2290.
64. Crook LD, Tempest B. Plague a clinical review of 27 cases. *Arch Intern Med* 1992;152:1253–1256.
65. Centers for Disease Control and Prevention. Prevention of plague. Recommendations of the Advisory Committee on Immunization Practices (ACIP). *MMWR Morb Mortal Wkly Rep* 1996;45(RR-14): 1–15.
66. Schlossberg D. *Chlamydia psittaci* (psittacosis). In: Mandell GL, Douglas RG, Bennett JE, eds. *Principles and practice of infectious diseases,* 5th ed. New York: Churchill Livingstone, 2000:2004–2007.
67. Psittacosis. In: Benenson AS. *Control of communicable diseases in man,* 15th ed. Washington, DC: American Public Health Association, 1990:347–349.
68. Schachter J. *Chlamydia psittaci*—reemergence of a forgotten pathogen. *N Engl J Med* 1986;315:189–191.
69. Broholm K-A, Bottiger M, Jermelius H, et al. Ornithosis as a nosocomial infection. *Scand J Infect Dis* 1977;9:263–267.
70. Hughes C, Maharg P, Rosario P, et al. Possible nosocomial transmission of psittacosis. *Infect Control Hosp Epidemiol* 1997;18:165–168.
71. Schaffner W. Birds of a feather—do they flock together? *Infect Control Hosp Epidemiol* 1997;9:18:162–164. 72. Anonymous. Psittacosis of non-avian origin. *Lancet* 1984;1:442–443.
73. Centers for Disease Control and Prevention. Psittacosis. Summary of notifiable diseases. United States 2000. *MMWR Morb Mortal Wkly Rep* 2002;49:57.
74. Centers for Disease Control and Prevention. Human psittacosis linked to a bird distributor in Mississippi, Massachusetts and Tennessee, 1992. *MMWR Morb Mortal Wkly Rep* 1992;41:794–797.
75. Andrews BE, Major R, Palmer SR. Ornithosis in poultry workers. *Lancet* 1981;1:632–634.
76. Palmer SR, Andrews BE, Major R. A common-source outbreak of ornithosis in veterinary surgeons. *Lancet* 1981;1:798–799.
77. Byrom NP, Walls J, Mair HJ. Fulminant psittacosis. *Lancet* 1979;1: 353–356.
78. Seibert RH, Jordan WS, Dingle JH. Clinical variations in the diagnosis of psittacosis. *N Engl J Med* 1956;254:925–930.
79. Schaffner W, Drutz DJ, Duncan GW, et al. The clinical spectrum of endemic psittacosis. *Arch Intern Med* 1967;119:433–443.
80. Yung AP, Grayson ML. Psittacosis—a review of 135 cases. *Med J Aust* 1988;148:228–233.
81. Centers for Disease Control and Prevention. Compendium of measures to control *Chlamydia psittaci* infection among humans (psittacosis) and pet birds (avian chlamydiosis). *MMWR Morb Mortal Wkly Rep* 2000;49(RR8).
82. Bleck TP. *Clostridium tetani.* In: Mandell GL, Bennett JE, Dolin R, eds. *Principles and practice of infectious diseases,* 5th ed. New York: Churchill Livingstone, 2000:2173–2178.
83. Wyszynski DR, Kechichian M. Outbreak of tetanus among elderly women treated with sheep cell therapy. *Clin Infect Dis* 1997;24:738.
84. Centers for Disease Control and Prevention. Tetanus. Summary of notifiable diseases, United States 2000. *MMWR Morb Mortal Wkly Rep* 2002;49:72.
85. Furste W, Aguirre A, Knoepfler DJ. Tetanus. In: Finegold SM, George W, eds. *Anaerobic infections in humans.* San Diego: Academic Press, 1989:611–627.
86. Centers for Disease Control and Prevention. Pertussis surveillance—United States, 1989–1991. *MMWR Morb Mortal Wkly Rep* 1992;41(SS-8):11–19.
87. Tetanus. In: Benenson AS. *Control of communicable diseases in man,* 15th ed. Washington, DC: American Public Health Association, 1990:430–434.
88. Centers for Disease Control and Prevention. Tetanus surveillance—United States, 1989–1990. *MMWR Morb Mortal Wkly Rep* 1992;41(SS-8):1–9.
89. Anonymous. Postoperative tetanus. *Lancet* 1984;2:964–965.
90. Geryan DT, McQuillan GM, Kielyn, et al. A population based serologic survey of immunity to tetanus in the United States. *N Engl J Med* 1995;332:761–766.
91. Simonsen O, Block AV, Klaerke A, et al. Immunity against tetanus and response to revaccination in surgical patients more than 50 years of age. *Surg Gynecol Obstet* 1987;164:329–334.
92. Bardenheier B, Prevots DR, Khetsuriani N, et al. Tetanus surveillance-United States, 1995-1997. *MMWR Morb Mortal Wkly Rep* 1998;47: (SS-2)1–13.
93. Centers for Disease Control and Prevention. Diphtheria, tetanus, and pertussis: guidelines for vaccine use and other preventive measures: recommendations of the Immunization Practices Advisory Committee (ACIP). *MMWR Morb Mortal Wkly Rep* 1991;40(RR-10):1–28.

94. Brand DA, Acampora D, Gottlier LD, et al. Adequacy of antitetanus prophylaxis in six hospital emergency rooms. *N Engl J Med* 1983; 309:634–640.
95. Bleck TP. *Clostridium botulinum.* In: Mandell GL, Bennett JE, Dolin R, eds. *Principles and practice of infectious diseases,* 5th ed. New York: Churchill Livingstone, 2000:2543–2548.
96. MacDonald KL. Botulism in adults. In: Finegold SM, George WL, eds. *Anerobic infections in humans.* San Diego: Academic Press, 1989: 591–600.
97. Arnon SS. Infants botulism. In: Finegold SM, George WL, eds. *Anerobic infections in humans.* San Diego: Academic Press, 1989:601–609.
98. Centers for Disease Control and Prevention. Botulism. Summary of notifiable diseases, United States 2000. *MMWR Morb Mortal Wkly Rep* 2002;49:22–24.
99. Botulism. In: Benenson AS, ed. *Control of communicable diseases in man,* 15th ed. Washington, DC: American Public Health Association, 1990:61–66.
100. Merson MH, Dowell VR. Epidemiologic, clinical and laboratory aspects of wound botulism. *N Engl J Med* 1973;289:1005–1010.
101. Elston HR, Wang M, Loo LK. Arm abscesses caused by *Clostridium botulinum. J Clin Microbiol* 1991;29:2678–2679.
102. Weber JT, Goodpasture HC, Alexander H, et al. Wound botulism in a patient with a tooth abscess: case report and review. *Clin Infect Dis* 1993;16:635–639.
103. MacDonald KL, Rutherford GW, Friedman SM, et al. Botulism and botulism-like illness in chronic drug abusers. *Ann Intern Med* 1985; 102:616–618.
104. Kudrow DB, Henry DA, Haake DA, et al. Botulism associated with *Clostridium botulinum* sinusitis after intranasal cocaine abuse. *Ann Intern Med* 1988;109:984–985.
105. Hatheway CL, McCroskey LM. Examination of feces and serum for diagnosis of infant botulism in 336 patients. *J Clin Microbiol* 1987; 25:2334–2338.
106. Chia JK, Clark JB, Ryan CA, et al. Botulism in an adult associated with food-borne intestinal infection with *Clostridium botulinum. N Engl J Med* 1986;315:239–241.
107. Jankovic J, Brin MF. Therapeutic uses of botulinum toxin. *N Engl J Med* 1991;324:1186–1194.
108. MacDonald KL, Spengler RF, Hatheway CL, et al. Type A botulism from sauteed onions. *JAMA* 1985;253:1275–1278.
109. Rigau-Perez JG, Hatheway CL, Valentin V. Botulism from acidic food; first cases of botulinic paralysis in Puerto Rico. *J Infect Dis* 1982; 145:783–785.
110. Hughes JM, Blumenthal JR, Merson MH, et al. Clinical features of types A and B food-borne botulism. *Ann Intern Med* 1981;95: 442–445.
111. Woodruff BA, Griffin PM, McCroskey LM, et al. Clinical and laboratory comparison of botulism from toxin types A, B, and E in the United States, 1975–1988. *J Infect Dis* 1992:166:1281–1286.
112. Dowell VR, McCroskey LM, Hatheway CL, et al. Coproexamination for botulinal toxin and *Clostridium botulinum. JAMA* 1977;238: 1829–1832.
113. Arnon SS, Schechter R, Inglesby TV, et al. Botulinum toxin as a biological weapon. *JAMA* 2001;285:1059–1070.

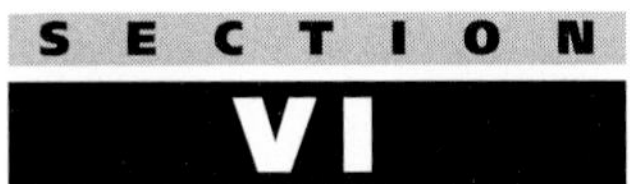

SECTION VI

EPIDEMIOLOGY AND PREVENTION OF NOSOCOMIAL INFECTIONS IN PEDIATRIC PATIENTS

48

NOSOCOMIAL VIRAL RESPIRATORY INFECTIONS IN PEDIATRIC PATIENTS

RONALD B. TURNER

Nosocomial viral respiratory infection is an important cause of morbidity in pediatric patients. In a general hospital population with active surveillance for nosocomial infections and high-quality diagnostic virology services, viral infections accounted for 5.3% of all nosocomial infections over a 17-month study period, an incidence of 0.19 per 100 patients (1). In contrast, in pediatric patients, viral pathogens cause 23% to 35% of all nosocomial infections, and the incidence of nosocomial viral infections in this population ranges from 0.59 to 0.72 per 100 patients (1–3).

The viral pathogens that have been most commonly associated with nosocomial respiratory infections in pediatric patients include respiratory syncytial virus (RSV), parainfluenza virus, adenovirus, rhinovirus, and influenza virus. Viruses that are spread via the respiratory tract but that produce more prominent symptoms in other organ systems (i.e., measles, varicella-zoster, and parvovirus B19) are not considered in this chapter (see Chapters 42 and 51). A new viral respiratory pathogen, human metapneumovirus, has recently been described (4). The epidemiology and clinical manifestations of this virus appear to be similar to those of RSV, but the role of human metapneumovirus in nosocomial infection has not been defined (4–10).

VIRAL PATHOGENS

Respiratory Syncytial Virus

RSV is an enveloped virus with a genome composed of a single negative strand of RNA. The virus has a diameter of 150 to 300 nm. The nucleocapsid, 12 to 15 nm in diameter, is smaller than that of the other members of the paramyxovirus family; thus, the virus has been placed in the separate genus Pneumovirus.

RSV is relatively quickly inactivated after exposure to different environmental conditions. In studies using partially purified virus, virus survival decreased as the temperature at which the virus was stored was increased over the range from 55° to 65°C (11). Virus survival was best at a pH of 7.5 with decreasing infectivity as pH was raised or lowered. RSV is rapidly inactivated by ether, chloroform, and detergents (12,13). Studies of virus survival using nasal secretions from infected infants revealed that infectious virus could be recovered for approximately 0.5 hours on skin, 1 hour on porous surfaces, and 7 hours on nonporous surfaces (14).

On the basis of neutralization with human sera, only a single serotype of RSV can be detected. Studies employing monoclonal antibody analysis, however, have identified two distinct subtypes (usually identified as group A and group B), which arise primarily from differences in the structure of the G glycoprotein (15). The clinical and immunologic significance of these antigenic differences has not been clarified; however, the detection of different viral strains by monoclonal antibody testing and/or nucleic acid analysis is useful in epidemiologic studies (16,17).

RSV infection is the most common cause of lower respiratory infection in young infants. Fifty percent to 70% of all infants are infected during the first year of life, and by the age of 4 virtually all infants have had at least one infection (18,19). Reinfection with RSV is common and, despite the nearly universal experience with this infection, the attack rate is approximately 40% for exposed individuals in all age groups (18,20).

The seasonal occurrence of RSV infections is well defined. Epidemics of RSV occur annually in the winter or spring (21). These epidemics are consistently associated with increased hospital admissions for pediatric respiratory infection, although the severity of the epidemic varies from year to year. RSV is transmitted by contact with infected respiratory secretions. A study of RSV transmission found that close contact with an infected infant, when virus may be transmitted directly or by large-particle aerosols, or contact with virus-contaminated fomites could transmit infectious RSV to volunteer recipients (22). Transmission of virus by small-particle aerosols was not detected in this study. The role of environmental contamination in the transmission of RSV is not clear, although RSV can survive on environmental surfaces for hours (14) and can be recovered from the environment of infected infants (22). Infection with RSV requires that the virus reach the respiratory mucosa. Inoculation of infectious virus into either the nose or the eye is equally efficient for initiation of infection and much more efficient than oral inoculation (23). The incubation period of RSV infection is 2 to 8 days with an average of about 5 days (24–26). Once virus infects the upper respiratory mucosa, it may spread to the lower respiratory tract. RSV infection is limited to the respiratory tract, and respiratory secretions are the only body fluids that contain infectious virus. Shedding of RSV can be detected for a few days before onset of symptoms and generally continues for approximately 1 week (27). Shedding is detected for more than 2 weeks in approximately 10% of patients.

The immune response to RSV is not well defined. Some studies have reported an association between high titers of serum antibody and partial protection from infection (18,28). Similarly, an association has been reported between high levels of passively transferred maternal antibody and delay in acquisition of primary infection in infants (29,30). A role for cell-mediated immune responses in the termination of RSV infection is suggested by the observation that children with deficiencies of T-cell immunity have unusually severe infections and prolonged shedding of virus (31).

RSV infection may result in clinical illness involving any level of the respiratory tract. The most severe manifestations of RSV infection are bronchiolitis or pneumonia. The incidence of lower respiratory symptoms is greatest during primary infections in young infants (18,19). Both increasing age and recurrences of infection are associated with an increasing proportion of infections that are asymptomatic or limited to the upper respiratory tract. Hospitalization for RSV infection is generally due to lower respiratory tract infection or apnea. However, during the RSV season, many infants admitted to the hospital have an incidental, community-acquired, RSV infection.

Parainfluenza Virus

The parainfluenza viruses are enveloped RNA viruses that are members of the genus Paramyxovirus in the family Paramyxoviridae. These viruses are susceptible to a variety of chemical disinfectants (32,33). There are four different serotypes of parainfluenza, types 1 to 4, which can be differentiated by antibody to complement-fixing and hemagglutinating antigens. No antigenic variation in these serotypes has been recognized over many years of observation.

Early studies of the parainfluenza viruses reported that both parainfluenza type 1 and type 3 were endemic with infections reported in virtually all months of the year (34). Since the mid-1960s, parainfluenza virus infections caused by serotypes 1 and 2 have been reported to occur in epidemics each fall (21). The specific serotype associated with the annual epidemic tends to alternate each year, so that infection associated with each serotype occurs in 2-year cycles. Infections with parainfluenza virus types 1 and 2 are most common in children between 6 months and 6 years of age. By 5 years of age, most children have been infected with both serotypes of virus (34).

In contrast to the behavior of serotypes 1 and 2, infection with serotype 3 has continued to be endemic (21), although an epidemic pattern similar to that of the other serotypes has been reported in some geographic areas (35). It remains to be seen whether parainfluenza virus type 3 will develop an epidemic pattern similar to the other parainfluenza serotypes. Parainfluenza virus type 3 is a common cause of infection in young infants. A serologic survey reported that 60% of infants were seropositive by 1 year of age and 80% were positive by the time they were 4 years old (34). The actual incidence of infection may be somewhat higher because reinfection, which would not be detected by serology, occurs often in young infants (36). Parainfluenza type 3 often produces illness in the first 6 months of life despite the presence of maternal antibody. The peak incidence of illness is in the second year of life. Primary infections occurring in the second year of life are more likely to be associated with lower respiratory tract infection than those that occur earlier or later. Reinfections with parainfluenza type 3 occur commonly but are generally associated with mild upper respiratory illness.

The parainfluenza viruses have an apparent incubation period of 2 to 8 days (37,38). Viral shedding from the upper respiratory tract occurs 1 to 4 days before the onset of symptoms and continues for 7 to 10 days in most patients with primary infection (27). Some patients with primary infection continue to have intermittent shedding of virus for 3 to 4 weeks. The duration of shedding following reinfection is generally shorter than after primary infection; however, reinfected patients occasionally shed virus for longer than 2 weeks (27). The mechanism of transmission of the parainfluenza viruses is not known; however, the route of spread is presumed to be by large droplets or direct person-to-person contact.

The serotype of the virus and the presence of preexisting homotypic antibody appear to affect the clinical manifestations of parainfluenza virus infection. Infection with parainfluenza type 1 is most commonly associated with a febrile upper respiratory infection. The most common lower respiratory tract manifestation of type 1 infection is croup. Parainfluenza type 2 is associated with similar clinical manifestations, although the illnesses are generally less severe. Preexisting nasal secretory antibody appears to offer some protection against infection (37). Parainfluenza virus type 3 is associated with disease at all levels of the respiratory tract and is not associated with a predominant clinical syndrome (39). This virus is second only to RSV as a cause of bronchiolitis and pneumonia in young infants.

Adenovirus

The adenoviruses are nonenveloped viruses with a genome of double-stranded DNA. These viruses are not inactivated by ether or chloroform and are stable at temperatures of 4° to 36°C and pH of 5.0 to 9.0 (40). Adenovirus is inactivated by sodium dodecylsulfate, chlorine, ultraviolet (UV) radiation, or formalin (41). There are more than 40 distinct serotypes of adenovirus; types 1 to 7 are the most important in pediatric respiratory disease.

Adenovirus infections are an important cause of illness in childhood. Antibody to serotypes 1 and 2 is detected in the serum of 60% to 80% of children by 5 years of age, and approximately 40% also have antibody to serotypes 3 and 5 (42,43). About one half of the adenovirus infections in these infants are associated with illness. The peak incidence of adenovirus-related illness occurs between 6 months and 2 years of age (44), and adenovirus causes 5% to 10% of all febrile respiratory illnesses in children younger than 7 years (43,44). Adenovirus is a much less common cause of respiratory illness in older children or adults. Adenovirus infections are endemic and cause illness in all months of the year (21); an increased incidence of infection has been noted between December and July in some studies (42, 43).

The most likely route of transmission of adenovirus between young children is fecal-oral. Transmission of infection has been documented in families following experimentally induced fecal excretion of adenovirus type 4 (45). During adenovirus infections, fecal excretion of virus occurs in more than 75% of children (43). Transmission of infection is relatively efficient; 46% to 67% of susceptible household and day care contacts were infected after exposure to adenovirus (43,44). The incubation period of adenovirus in children is not known. However, in adults challenged by the aerosol route, the incubation period was 6 to 13 days (46), and, in a hospital outbreak, the apparent incubation period was 2 to 18 days (47). A unique feature of adenovirus among the pediatric respiratory viruses is that intermittent shedding of the virus may continue for years after infection. Approximately one half of adenovirus infections are associated with only a single day of virus shedding. One fourth of the infections, however, result in intermittent shedding of virus for more than 3 months, and almost 10% continue to shed virus for more than 1 year (43). Homotypic antibody, whether actively acquired by previous infection or passively acquired by maternal transmission, is partially protective for both infection and illness. Heterotypic antibody is not protective (43).

The most common clinical manifestation of adenovirus infection in young infants is a febrile upper respiratory syndrome (44,48,49). Although conjunctivitis is widely recognized as a manifestation of adenovirus infection, only 12% of outpatients (44) and 4% of hospitalized patients (49) have this finding. Hospitalized patients with adenovirus infection often have high and prolonged fevers (48,49). Gastrointestinal symptoms are the primary manifestation of about 10% of infections in hospitalized infants.

Rhinovirus

The rhinoviruses are small, nonenveloped, single-stranded RNA viruses in the picornavirus family. The human rhinoviruses are stable at a pH of 6 to 8 and are not inactivated by chloroform, ether, or detergents (50–52). These viruses are rapidly inactivated at a pH of 3 and by UV irradiation. Rhinovirus survives well under environmental conditions. Virus was recovered after 1 hour on porous surfaces, 3 hours on nonporous surfaces, and 3 hours on human skin (53). There are more than 100 distinct rhinovirus serotypes that all appear to have similar epidemiologic characteristics and produce a similar clinical syndrome.

In contrast to other viral respiratory pathogens of childhood, the incidence of rhinovirus infection varies little with age. Approximately two thirds of children experience a rhinovirus infection each year (54,55); about 60% of these infections are associated with illness. Rhinoviruses cause illness in all months of the year, but there are distinct epidemic peaks of illness in the early fall and in the late spring (54–56).

The mechanism of transmission of rhinovirus has been studied extensively. In experimental models, rhinovirus is transmitted most efficiently by direct person-to-person contact (57), although transmission by large-particle aerosols has also been documented (58). A study of natural colds found that treatment of the hands with a virucidal compound prevented transmission of rhinovirus infection, suggesting that hand-to-hand transmission may be important in a natural setting (59). Once virus is transmitted, the incubation period is generally short, with onset of symptoms in 2 to 3 days (60), although, in a family setting, rhinovirus was cultured from 15% of specimens collected 7 to 10 days before onset of symptoms (54). Rhinovirus is shed exclusively from the upper respiratory tract. Shedding is most efficient from nasal secretions, although lower titers of virus can be detected in saliva and pharyngeal secretions (61). Virus can also be recovered from the hands of a high proportion of infected volunteers (53). Shedding of virus from infected individuals continues for 2 to 3 weeks after the onset of illness (54,62). Homotypic serum neutralizing antibody correlates with resistance to rhinovirus infection (55,63,64). The only clinical syndrome that has been clearly associated with rhinovirus infection is the common cold. These infections are generally not associated with fever.

Influenza

The influenza viruses are discussed in detail in Chapter 41. These viruses are enveloped RNA viruses classified in the family of Orthomyxovirus. The virus is classified as type A, B, or C according to the antigenicity of the nucleoprotein of the viral nucleocapsid. Heat (56°C), lipid solvents, acid, formaldehyde, and UV irradiation all inactivate influenza viruses (65). Influenza is capable of prolonged survival on fomites. On nonporous surfaces, the virus was detectable for more than 48 hours, and, on porous surfaces, virus was detectable for 8 to 12 hours (66). The protective immune response to the viruses is directed at the hemagglutinin and neuraminidase antigens on the surface of the virion. The epidemic behavior of the influenza viruses is a result of variation in the antigenicity of these surface antigens.

The incidence of influenza infections is highest in preschool and school-aged children, with infection rates of 20% to 50% per year (67–69); 60% to 80% of influenza infections in the pediatric age group are associated with illness (68,69). The seasonal epidemiology of influenza virus infection is well established, with annual midwinter and spring epidemics (67,68). Transmission of influenza is most likely by small-particle aerosols (70,71), although direct contact or large-particle aerosols may also contribute to spread of the virus. The incubation period for influenza is 24 to 48 hours (72). Virus shedding is exclusively from the respiratory tract, and most patients shed virus for less than 1 week after the onset of illness (70), although shedding may last somewhat longer in young children (73,74). The clinical manifestations of influenza in children differ from adult infections in that children are much less likely to have lower respiratory infection and tend to have higher fevers (67,69).

NOSOCOMIAL VIRAL RESPIRATORY INFECTION

Respiratory viruses contribute significantly to the incidence of nosocomial infection in pediatric patients. In one report, respiratory viruses were implicated in 61% of the nosocomial respiratory infections for which an etiologic diagnosis was established (2). Wenzel et al. (75) reported that 17% of preschool children who were hospitalized for at least 1 week during the winter or spring seasons developed a nosocomial viral respiratory infection.

Nosocomial viral respiratory infections have important implications for the patient. The development of a febrile illness in a hospitalized patient may result in unnecessary diagnostic studies and/or administration of antibiotics. Nosocomial viral respiratory infection is associated with an average increase of 5 to 6 days in the length of hospitalization (1,76,77). A study of nosocomial influenza infections reported that hospitalization was extended by 4 to 14 days in 6 of 11 patients (78). In addition to the increased length of stay, most patients underwent additional diagnostic studies or administration of unnecessary antibiotics.

Although nosocomial viral respiratory infections are not generally associated with increased mortality, some specific patient populations are at risk for serious illness and increased mortality when they acquire a respiratory infection. Patients with congenital heart disease, premature infants, and patients with compromised immune function are at increased risk from nosocomial viral infections. In 1982, MacDonald et al. (79) reported that nosocomial RSV infection was associated with a mortality rate of 44% in patients with congenital heart disease, compared with 5% in other patients. A more recent study reported a mortality rate of 8% associated with nosocomial RSV infection in patients with heart disease (80). The authors of the latter study suggested that improvements in intensive care management and pediatric cardiac surgery account for the reduction in the mortality in this population. No controlled studies have assessed the impact of antiviral therapy on the mortality of RSV infections in these high-risk populations. A high mortality rate has been associated with nosocomial adenovirus infections in patients with underlying pulmonary or cardiac disease in two studies (81,82).

The impact of nosocomial viral respiratory infections in neonatal intensive care nurseries is inconsistent from study to study. RSV and adenovirus infections in these patients have been associated with a high, 18% to 22% mortality rate in some reports (83,84). In contrast, other studies have reported no mortality (85–92), and in many of these studies a large proportion of patients were asymptomatic. Most studies, however, have reported significant morbidity associated with nosocomial viral infections in neonates. (See Chapter 52 for additional information on nosocomial viral respiratory infections in neonates.)

Patients who are immunosuppressed, particularly those who have undergone bone marrow or solid organ transplantation, are also at increased risk of mortality if they acquire a nosocomial viral respiratory infection (93–97). Mortality rates in these patients range from 5% to 40%.

Nosocomial respiratory infections with a particular virus are temporally related to the presence of the virus in the community (73,74,98–100). Thus, the incidence of hospital-acquired viral respiratory disease is seasonal, and the risk of infection is greatest during community epidemics. Virtually all patients, visitors, and hospital personnel are at risk for infection with nosocomial viral respiratory pathogens and may serve as a source of infection in the hospital. A respiratory viral pathogen or *Mycoplasma* was detected in 61% of symptomatic pediatric patients admitted to the hospital during the respiratory virus season (77). Furthermore, a viral pathogen was detected in almost 50% of patients in whom respiratory symptoms were initially overlooked or who were asymptomatic. Thus, 57% of all pediatric patients admitted to medical services during the respiratory season were shedding virus or *Mycoplasma* from the upper respiratory tract. The incidence of RSV infection in hospital personnel during community outbreaks has been reported to range from 5% to 61% depending on the infection control measures used (101,102). In one study, 18% of the infections were asymptomatic, and an additional 36% were associated only with mild illness (103). Consistent with the multiple potential sources of virus, detailed studies of nosocomial outbreaks of viral respiratory pathogens have found that these outbreaks are usually caused by different strains of virus (16,104–107).

In contrast to other nosocomial infections, specific risk factors, such as intravascular lines or immunosuppression, appear to contribute little to the overall incidence of viral respiratory infection. A few risk factors, however, have been identified. Children with immunosuppression resulting from cancer have been found to have a higher incidence of influenza infection than children with normal immunity (108). This increased incidence appeared to be related to a failure of preexisting antibody to protect from disease in immunocompromised patients. Specific procedures and devices have been associated with an increased risk of nosocomial viral respiratory infection in some outbreaks. Orotracheal and orogastric intubation have both been associated with an increased risk of acquisition of infection in neonates (89,90). Despite these reports, targeting high-risk patients for specific preventive measures would have little impact on the overall incidence of nosocomial viral respiratory infection.

DIAGNOSIS

Epidemiologic and clinical information can provide important clues to the specific etiology of viral respiratory infections. The occurrence of viral respiratory disease in a community is the result of sequential and relatively discrete epidemics of individual pathogens (109,110). The etiologic diagnosis of an individual patient is aided by knowledge of which viruses are prevalent in the community at a given time. Furthermore, although any of the viral respiratory syndromes may be caused by any of the pathogens, specific pathogens are often associated with particular clinical syndromes as described previously. A clinical syndrome characteristic of a virus known to be present in the community provides a reasonably reliable prediction of the etiologic diagnosis.

Laboratory Tests for Diagnosis

Laboratory confirmation of the etiologic diagnosis is usually not necessary for management of viral respiratory infections or for the institution of appropriate infection control measures. When it is necessary to know the specific etiology of an infection, the methods available for viral diagnosis are virus isolation, viral antigen detection in respiratory secretions, polymerase chain reaction (PCR), and detection of specific antiviral antibodies in acute and convalescent sera.

Virus isolation in cell cultures remains the standard method for diagnosis of the respiratory pathogens. Isolation of these viruses in cell culture, however, generally requires several days and, in some cases, may take more than 2 weeks (111,112). Specimens for virus isolation should be obtained as early as possible in the course of the patient's illness. Although some individuals may shed virus for weeks (27,62), virus is most consistently recovered in the first few days after the onset of symptoms. Nasal wash specimens are better than swab specimens for detection of respiratory pathogens (113–115).

Detection of viral antigen in respiratory secretions or detection of virus by PCR, which allow a diagnosis within hours, has been reported for many of the respiratory viruses. Enzyme-linked immunosorbent assay (ELISA) reagents are commercially available as kit technologies for RSV and influenza. Many laboratories offer antigen detection by fluorescent antibody methods; however, the accuracy of these techniques depends on the technical expertise of the laboratory and the quality of the specimen submitted for testing. Commercial PCR assays for the detection of the parainfluenza viruses, RSV, and the influenza viruses are also available. Specimens collected for virus isolation are generally also suitable for antigen detection or PCR methods; however, because specimen requirements may vary for some methods, the laboratory should be consulted before collection of specimens.

Serologic assays are available for most of the respiratory pathogens; however, the need for a convalescent serum limits the usefulness of the serologic tests in the clinical setting. Acute serum specimens should be obtained as soon as possible after onset of symptoms, and convalescent sera should be collected 2 to 3 weeks later. Sera may be stored at 4°C for short periods and may be stored at −20°C indefinitely. Hemolyzed specimens may not be acceptable for some serologic assays.

Interpretation of Laboratory Results

Virus Isolation

The isolation of a viral pathogen from the upper respiratory tract of a patient with respiratory symptoms is generally considered diagnostic. Virus isolation is absolutely specific if the laboratory confirms the identity of the virus by immunologic methods.

Virus isolation has traditionally been considered the "gold standard" for detection of viral respiratory pathogens. Recent studies of RSV, influenza, and rhinovirus have found that virus isolation has a sensitivity of 75% to 85% compared with detection of virus by PCR (116–118). The time of collection in relation to onset of symptoms, the method of specimen collection, and the handling of the specimen before inoculation into cell culture all affect the recovery of virus from infected individuals.

Viral Antigen Detection and PCR

Detection of viral antigen in respiratory secretions allows rapid diagnosis of viral infection. The commercially available reagents for detection of RSV infection generally have a sensitivity and specificity of 85% to 95% compared with virus isolation, although individual studies have reported markedly lower sensitivities (119,120). When antigen detection methods are compared with PCR, the sensitivity of antigen detection appears to be 65% to 75% (118,121).

PCR is more sensitive than other methods for detection of viral respiratory pathogens. The sensitivity of PCR relative to virus isolation and antigen detection is consistently greater than 90% (116–118, 122). The exquisite sensitivity of PCR can lead to false-positive results if meticulous care is not taken to prevent contamination of the assay.

Viral Serology

Interpretation of serologic results depends on comparison of antibody levels in acute and convalescent sera. Antibody levels in a single serum specimen are generally not helpful for diagnosis of viral infection. A fourfold increase in antibody titer in a convalescent serum specimen compared with the titer in an acute serum specimen drawn early in the illness is evidence of infection with the virus.

PREVENTION AND CONTROL OF NOSOCOMIAL INFECTIONS

Active Immunization

The influenza vaccine is the only vaccine available for the prevention of infection by the respiratory viruses. The influenza vaccine usually contains one or more type A strains and one type B strain selected to provide immunity to the virus expected in the following influenza season. The strains of virus in the vaccine are changed, as necessary, in response to the changing epidemiology of the influenza viruses. The vaccine viruses are cultured in eggs and then inactivated and purified so that the vaccine contains no infectious material. Some vaccines are treated with lipid solvents, which produces a split-virus vaccine. These preparations produce fewer side effects than whole-virus vaccine and are the recommended vaccine for children younger than 12 years. Pediatric patients older than 12 years may be given either the whole-virus or the split-virus vaccine. The efficacy of the influenza vaccine is generally between 70% and 90%.

Patients for whom the influenza vaccine is indicated include patients with chronic cardiac or pulmonary disease, diabetes mellitus, chronic renal disease, compromised immune function, or patients who are receiving long-term aspirin therapy (123). Family members and healthcare workers who are in contact with patients in these high-risk groups should also be immunized. Immunization is encouraged when feasible for all children between 6 and 23 months of age (123). Immunization of these target groups would be expected to reduce the morbidity associated with infection in high-risk patients (124) and to reduce the nosocomial acquisition of influenza by these patients from infected healthcare workers. Immunization is not effective for intervention in nosocomial outbreaks of influenza (125) unless antiviral therapy is given for 2 weeks following vaccination to prevent infection while one waits for antibody titers to rise to a protective level (see also Chapter 41).

The side effects of the vaccine are generally mild, although some patients develop influenza-like symptoms such as fever, myalgia, and headache. These symptoms are readily controlled with analgesics and generally persist for less than 48 hours. The vaccine contains small amounts of egg protein and should not be given to patients who are allergic to eggs.

Passive Immunization

Palivizumab, a humanized monoclonal antibody to RSV, reduces the severity of illness in premature infants but has no effect on the incidence of infection (126). The role of this preparation for the prevention of nosocomial infection has not been studied. Because of the lack of effect on RSV infection, it is unlikely that passive immunization will be useful for prevention of transmission of virus. The use of palivizumab to protect appropriate high-risk patients during nosocomial outbreaks of RSV infection is a potential approach that should be evaluated.

Antivirals

Effective antiviral therapy is available for the treatment or prevention of influenza infection. Amantadine and rimantadine are approved for prophylaxis of influenza A infections (127–130) in children older than 1 year, and oseltamivir is approved for prevention of influenza A and B infections in children 13 years of age or older. These drugs are not a substitute for immunization but can be used for short-term prophylaxis in patients who are immunized after influenza is already present in the community to prevent infection before development of a protective antibody response. These agents may also be used to prevent infections in immunocompromised patients who may have an impaired antibody response to the vaccine (123). These antiviral agents are generally safe and well tolerated in children. Antiviral prophylaxis with amantadine has been found to be effective for prevention of nosocomial influenza infections (131); however, there is little information on the use of zanamivir or oseltamivir in this setting. Patients who are at high risk from influenza infections should be immunized or treated prophylactically before hospitalization; the cost-benefit ratio of prophylaxis for low-risk patients has not been established. Prophylaxis with antivirals in the setting of a nosocomial outbreak may be of use; however, detection of the outbreak in time to institute effective prophylaxis may be difficult (125) (see also Chapter 41).

Isolation

Respiratory viruses can be transmitted from person to person by aerosols or by hand contact with the virus followed by self-inoculation. Aerosols are readily produced by coughing, sneezing, and nose blowing (132,133). Some aerosolized particles have also been detected during normal speech (132).

Small-particle aerosols, composed of droplet nuclei 2 to 3 μm in diameter, account for approximately 95% of the total number of particles and 25% of the total volume of coughs and sneezes (132). The small-particle aerosol fraction is slightly higher for coughs than for sneezes. These particles remain suspended in the air and can be transmitted over extended distances. Once a virus suspended in a small-particle aerosol contaminates an air space, only the circulation of the air and the ability of the virus to survive in the environment limit the time during which infection can be transmitted. Small-particle aerosols are not filtered by the nose and are inhaled into the lungs.

Large-particle aerosols are composed of particles larger than 10 μm in diameter. These particles settle quickly and are transmitted only a few feet. For this reason, transmission of infection by a large-particle aerosol requires relatively close contact between infected and susceptible individuals. Large-particle aerosols are effectively filtered in the nose and do not reach the lower respiratory tract.

Transmission of viral respiratory infections by direct contact requires that susceptible individuals contaminate their hands with virus by contact with either an infected individual or contaminated objects in the environment. The virus is then inoculated onto the mucous membranes by hand-to-nose or hand-to-eye contact. Respiratory viruses can conceivably be spread from infected to susceptible individuals by an uninfected intermediate person, but this has not been demonstrated. Spread of infection by direct contact is limited only by the ability of viruses to survive on skin and environmental surfaces.

Information about the mechanisms of spread of different viral pathogens under natural conditions is limited. Although it is likely that any of the different mechanisms of transmission may be involved in the spread of respiratory infection, studies in controlled settings suggest that for some viruses one route may be more efficient than another (22,59,70,71).

The viruses associated with nosocomial respiratory infections in children, with the exception of influenza, appear to require relatively close contact for transmission from person to person (22,59,70,71). Given the role of direct person-to-person contact in the transmission of these pathogens, strict compliance with good hand hygiene should theoretically be sufficient to control nosocomial spread. The alcohol-based hand cleaners recommended in recent guidelines (134) rapidly inactivate viral respiratory pathogens (135–137), but the effectiveness of these preparations for prevention of nosocomial viral respiratory infections has not been studied. The efficacy of various other interventions for prevention of transmission of respiratory viruses, particularly RSV, in the hospital setting has been examined in a number of studies. The intensity of the interventions studied has ranged from the use of gloves to cohorting of patients based on universal preadmission testing for viral antigen. The use of gowns and masks does not appear to effectively interrupt transmission of RSV (138,139). Cohorting of symptomatic infants also appears to contribute little to the control of nosocomial RSV (101,103, 140). Demonstration of self-inoculation of personnel by transfer of RSV from contaminated hands to the eyes (22) suggested the potential for the use of face shields as a control measure for prevention of these infections. Two studies have reported a significant reduction in infections in personnel when goggles were used (101,102), and in one study this was associated with a decrease in nosocomial infections in patients (101). Gloves might also be expected to reduce hand-to-face contact, and in one study strict enforcement of gloving effectively prevented nosocomial transmission of RSV (141). A more recent study found that gloves were ineffective (140); however, the mechanism by which compliance with glove use was enforced was not described. Two studies have shown that diagnostic viral testing of infants at the time of admission with subsequent cohorting to infected and uninfected cohorts effectively controls nosocomial RSV (140,142), but this is not feasible as a routine infection control measure.

Several issues specific to the respiratory viruses present obstacles to the success of interventions for the prevention of nosocomial infections: (a) nosocomial infections with these agents occur when there are large numbers of infected individuals in the community providing an opportunity for new introductions of the virus not only by patients but also by personnel and visitors; (b) a large proportion of the patient population is susceptible to infection; (c) many infected individuals will be asymptomatic; and (d) diagnostic testing for most of the viral pathogens of concern is either not sufficiently rapid or not sufficiently accurate to guide decisions for isolation. With these limitations in mind, all patients with symptoms consistent with viral respiratory illness should be placed on contact precautions and droplet precautions (143). If a nosocomial outbreak of viral respiratory disease occurs, cohorting of infected infants (based on diagnostic testing if possible), cohorting of uninfected high-risk patients, and heightened surveillance of staff and visitors for symptomatic infections should be instituted.

Isolation for Prevention of Influenza

Transmission of influenza may occur by small-particle aerosols (70,71). Respiratory isolation using a negative pressure airflow room interrupts spread of infection by small-particle aerosols, although the efficacy of this intervention has never been established for the prevention of nosocomial influenza. Furthermore, an attempt to isolate all influenza-infected patients in negative pressure rooms is not feasible in most hospitals. It is recommended that Contact and Droplet Precautions be used when caring for patients with known or suspected influenza, but the usefulness of these measures is not known. UV radiation has been reported to reduce the incidence of influenza infections in the hospital setting (144). However, carefully controlled studies of UV radiation for disinfection in the general hospital setting have not been done, and it is likely that this modality would be effective only under very limited conditions (145) (see also Chapter 95).

REFERENCES

1. Valenti WM, Menegus MA, Hall CB, et al. Nosocomial viral infections: I. epidemiology and significance. *Infect Control* 1980;1:33–37.
2. Welliver RC, McLaughlin S. Unique epidemiology of nosocomial infection in a children's hospital. *Am J Dis Child* 1984;138:131–135.
3. Moore DL, Rodrigues R. Surveillance for nosocomial infections in a pediatric teaching hospital: a five year study [Abstract M36]. The Second Annual Meeting of the Society for Hospital Epidemiology of America, April 12–14, Baltimore, 1992.
4. van den Hoogen BG, de Jong JC, Groen J, et al. A newly discovered human pneumovirus isolated from young children with respiratory tract disease. *Nat Med* 2001;7:719–724.
5. Falsey AR, Erdman D, Anderson LJ, et al. Human metapneumovirus infections in young and elderly adults. *J Infect Dis* 2003;187:785–790.
6. Nissen MD, Siebert DJ, Mackay IM, et al. Evidence of human metapneumovirus in Australian children. *Med J Aust* 2002;176:188.
7. Peret TC, Boivin G, Li Y, et al. Characterization of human metapneumoviruses isolated from patients in North America. *J Infect Dis* 2002; 185:1660–1663.
8. Stockton J, Stephenson I, Fleming D, et al. Human metapneumovirus as a cause of community-acquired respiratory illness. *Emerg Infect Dis* 2002;8:897–901.
9. Boivin G, Abed Y, Pelletier G, et al. Virological features and clinical manifestations associated with human metapneumovirus: a new paramyxovirus responsible for acute respiratory-tract infections in all age groups. *J Infect Dis* 2002;186:1330–1334.
10. Freymouth F, Vabret A, Legrand L, et al. Presence o the new human metapneumovirus in French children with bronchiolitis. *Pediatr Infect Dis J* 2003;22:92–94.
11. Hambling MH. Survival of the respiratory syncytial virus during storage under various conditions. *Br J Exp Pathol* 1964;45:647–655.
12. Chanock R, Roizman B, Myers R. Recovery from infants with respiratory illness of a virus related to chimpanzee coryza agent (CCA). I. Isolation, properties, and characterization. *Am J Hyg* 1957;66: 281–290.
13. Krilov LR, Harkness SH. Inactivation of respiratory syncytial virus by detergents and disinfectants. *Pediatr Infect Dis J* 1993;12:582–584.
14. Hall CB, Douglas RG Jr, Geiman JM. Possible transmission by fomites of respiratory syncytial virus. *J Infect Dis* 1980;141:98–102.
15. Mufson MA, Orvell C, Rafnar B, et al. Two distinct subtypes of human respiratory syncytial virus. *J Gen Virol* 1985;66:2111–2124.
16. Storch GA, Hall CB, Anderson LJ, et al. Antigenic and nucleic acid analysis of nosocomial isolates of respiratory syncytial virus. *J Infect Dis* 1993;167:562–566.
17. Taylor GS, Vipond IB, Caul EO. Molecular epidemiology of outbreak of respiratory syncytial virus within bone marrow transplantation unit. *J Clin Microbiol* 2001;39:801–803.
18. Glezen WP, Taber LH, Frank AL, et al. Risk of primary infection and reinfection with respiratory syncytial virus. *Am J Dis Child* 1986; 140:543–546.
19. Henderson FW, Collier AM, Clyde WA Jr, et al. Respiratory-syncytial-virus infections, reinfections, and immunity: a prospective, longitudinal study in young children. *N Engl J Med* 1979;300:530–534.
20. Hall CB, Geiman JM, Biggar R, et al. Respiratory syncytial virus infections within families. *N Engl J Med* 1976;294:414–419.
21. Denny FW, Clyde WA Jr. Acute lower respiratory tract infections in nonhospitalized children. *J Pediatr* 1986;108:635–646.
22. Hall CB, Douglas RG Jr. Modes of transmission of respiratory syncytial virus. *J Pediatr* 1981;99:100–103.
23. Hall CB, Douglas RG Jr, Schnabel KC, et al. Infectivity of respiratory syncytial virus by various routes of inoculation. *Infect Immun* 1981; 33:779–783.
24. Johnson KM, Chanock RM, Rifkind D, et al. Respiratory syncytial virus. IV. Correlation of virus shedding, serologic response, and illness in adult volunteers. *JAMA* 1961;176:663–667.
25. Kravetz HM, Knight V, Chanock RM, et al. Respiratory syncytial virus: III. production of illness and clinical observations in adult volunteers. *JAMA* 1961;176:657–663.
26. Jordan WS Jr. Acute respiratory diseases of viral etiology: I. ecology of respiratory viruses–1961. *Am J Public Health* 1962;52:897–902.
27. Frank AL, Taber LH, Wells CR, et al. Patterns of shedding myxoviruses and paramyxoviruses in children. *J Infect Dis* 1981;144: 433–441.
28. Glezen WP. Pathogenesis of bronchiolitis epidemiologic considerations. *Pediatr Res* 1977;11:239–243.
29. Glezen WP, Paredes A, Allison JE, et al. Risk of respiratory syncytial virus infection for infants from low-income families in relationship to age, sex, ethnic group, and maternal antibody level. *J Pediatr* 1981; 98:708–715.
30. Olgilvie MM, Vathenen AS, Radford M, et al. Maternal antibody and respiratory syncytial virus infection in infancy. *J Med Virol* 1981; 7:263–271.
31. Fishaut M, Tubergen D, McIntosh K. Cellular response to respiratory viruses with particular reference to children with disorders of cell-mediated immunity. *J Pediatr* 1980;96:179–186.
32. Brady MT, Evans J, Cuartas J. Survival and disinfection of parainfluenza viruses on environmental surfaces. *Am J Infect Control* 1990;18: 18–23.
33. Sattar SA, Springthorpe VS, Karim Y, et al. Chemical disinfection of non-porous inanimate surfaces experimentally contaminated with four human pathogenic viruses. *Epidemiol Infect* 1989;102:493–505.
34. Parrott RH, Vargosko AJ, Kim HW, et al. Myxoviruses: parainfluenza. *Am J Public Health* 1962;52:907–917.
35. Glezen WP, Frank AL, Taber LH, et al. Parainfluenza virus type 3: seasonality and risk of infection and reinfection in young children. *J Infect Dis* 1984;150:851–857.

36. Welliver R, Wong DT, Choi TS, et al. Natural history of parainfluenza virus infection in childhood. *J Pediatr* 1982;101:180–187.
37. Smith CB, Purcell RH, Bellanti JA, et al. Protective effect of antibody to parainfluenza virus type 1. *N Engl J Med* 1966;275:1145–1152.
38. Chanock RM, Parrott RH, Johnson KM, et al. Myxoviruses: parainfluenza. *Am Rev Respir Dis* 1963;88:152–166.
39. Glezen WP, Denny FW. Epidemiology of acute lower respiratory disease in children. *N Engl J Med* 1973;288:498–505.
40. Foy HM, Grayston JT. Adenoviruses. In: Evans AS, ed. *Viral infections of humans: epidemiology and control,* 2nd ed. New York: Plenum, 1982: 67–84.
41. Hierholzer JC. Adenoviruses. In: Schmidt NJ, Emmons RW, eds. *Diagnostic procedures for viral, rickettsial and chlamydial infections,* 6th ed. Washington DC: American Public Health Association, 1989: 219–264.
42. Brandt CD, Kim HW, Jeffries BC, et al. Infections in 18,000 infants and children in a controlled study of respiratory tract disease. II. Variation in adenovirus infections by year and season. *Am J Epidemiol* 1972;95:218–227.
43. Fox JP, Hall CE, Cooney MK. The Seattle virus watch. VII. Observations of adenovirus infections. *Am J Epidemiol* 1977;105:362–386.
44. Edwards KM, Thompson J, Paolini J, et al. Adenovirus infections in young children. *Pediatrics* 1985;76:420–424.
45. Mueller RE, Muldoon RL, Jackson GG. Communicability of enteric live adenovirus type 4 vaccine in families. *J Infect Dis* 1969;119: 60–66.
46. Couch RB, Cate TR, Douglas RG Jr, et al. Effect of route of inoculation on experimental respiratory viral disease in volunteers and evidence for airborne transmission. *Bacteriol Rev* 1966;30:517–529.
47. Brummitt CF, Cherrington JM, Katzenstein DA, et al. Nosocomial adenovirus infections: molecular epidemiology of an outbreak due to adenovirus 3a. *J Infect Dis* 1988;158:423–432.
48. Ruuskanen O, Meurman O, Sarkkinen H. Adenoviral diseases of children: a study of 105 hospital cases. *Pediatrics* 1985;76:79–83.
49. Van Leirde S, Corbeel L, Eggermont E. Clinical and laboratory findings in children with adenovirus infections. *Eur J Pediatr* 1989;148: 423–425.
50. Dimmock NJ, Tyrrell DAJ. Some physico-chemical properties of rhinoviruses. *Br J Exp Pathol* 1964;45:271–280.
51. Stott EJ, Killington RA. Rhinoviruses. *Annu Rev Microbiol* 1972;26: 503–524.
52. Hughes JH, Mitchell M, Hamparian VV. Rhinoviruses: kinetics of ultraviolet inactivation and effects of UV and heat on immunogenicity. *Arch Virol* 1979;61:313–319.
53. Hendley JO, Wenzel RP, Gwaltney JM Jr. Transmission of rhinovirus colds by self-inoculation. *N Engl J Med* 1973;288:1361–1364.
54. Fox JP, Cooney MK, Hall CE. The Seattle virus watch V. Epidemiologic observations of rhinovirus infections, 1965–1969, in families with young children. *Am J Epidemiol* 1975;101:122–143.
55. Fox JP, Cooney MK, Hall CE, et al. Rhinoviruses in Seattle families, 1975–1979. *Am J Epidemiol* 1985;122:830–846.
56. Gwaltney JM Jr, Hendley JO, Simon G, et al. Rhinovirus infections in an industrial population. I. The occurrence of illness. *N Engl J Med* 1966;275:1261–1268.
57. Gwaltney JM Jr, Moskalski PB, Hendley JO. Hand-to-hand transmission of rhinovirus colds. *Ann Intern Med* 1978;88:463–467.
58. Dick EC, Jennings LC, Mink KA, et al. Aerosol transmission of rhinovirus colds. *J Infect Dis* 1987;156:442–448.
59. Hendley JO, Gwaltney JM Jr. Mechanisms of transmission of rhinovirus infections. *Epidemiol Rev* 1988;10:242–258.
60. Gwaltney JM Jr. Rhinoviruses. In: Evans AS, ed. *Viral infections of humans: epidemiology and control,* 2nd ed. New York: Plenum, 1982: 491–517.
61. Gwaltney JM Jr. Epidemiology of the common cold. *Ann N Y Acad Sci* 1980;353:54–60.
62. Winther B, Gwaltney JM Jr, Mygind N, et al. Sites of rhinovirus recovery after point inoculation of the upper airway. *JAMA* 1986; 256:1763–1767.
63. Hendley JO, Edmondson WP Jr, Gwaltney JM Jr. Relation between naturally acquired immunity and infectivity of two rhinoviruses in volunteers. *J Infect Dis* 1972;125:243–248.
64. Hendley JO, Gwaltney JM Jr, Jordan WS Jr. Rhinovirus infections in an industrial population. IV. Infections within families of employees during two fall peaks of respiratory illness. *Am J Epidemiol* 1969;89: 184–196.
65. Harmon MW, Kendal AP. Influenza viruses. In: Schmidt NJ, Emmons RW, eds. *Diagnostic procedures for viral, rickettsial and chlamydial infections,* 6th ed. Washington DC: American Public Health Association, 1989:631–668.
66. Bean B, Moore BM, Sterner B, et al. Survival of influenza viruses on environmental surfaces. *J Infect Dis* 1982;146:47–51.
67. Monto AS, Koopman JS, Longini IM Jr. Tecumseh study of illness. XIII. Influenza infection and disease, 1976–1981. *Am J Epidemiol* 1985;121:811–822.
68. Frank AL, Taber LH, Glezen WP, et al. Influenza B virus infections in the community and the family. *Am J Epidemiol* 1983;118:313–325.
69. Wright PF, Ross KB, Thompson J, et al. Influenza A infections in young children. *N Engl J Med* 1977;296:829–834.
70. Douglas RG Jr. Influenza in man. In: Kilbourne ED, ed. *The influenza viruses and influenza.* New York: Academic Press, 1975:395–447.
71. Moser MR, Bender TR, Margolis HS, et al. An outbreak of influenza aboard a commercial airliner. *Am J Epidemiol* 1979;110:1–6.
72. Davenport FM. Influenza viruses. In: Evans AS, ed. *Viral infections of humans: epidemiology and control,* 2nd ed. New York: Plenum, 1982: 373–396.
73. Hall CB, Douglas RG Jr. Nosocomial influenza infection as a cause of intercurrent fevers in infants. *Pediatrics* 1975;55:673–677.
74. Brocklebank JT, Court SDM, McQuillin J, et al. Influenza—an infection in children. *Lancet* 1972;2:497–500.
75. Wenzel RP, Deal EC, Hendley JO. Hospital-acquired viral respiratory illness on a pediatric ward. *Pediatrics* 1977;60:367–371.
76. Roy TE, McDonald S, Patrick ML, et al. A survey of hospital infection in a pediatric hospital. II. The distribution of hospital infections in different areas of the hospital, postoperative wound infections, and the consequences of infection. *Can Med Assoc J* 1962;87:592–599.
77. Goldwater PN, Martin AJ, Ryan B, et al. A survey of nosocomial respiratory viral infections in a children's hospital: occult respiratory infection in patients admitted during an epidemic season. *Infect Control Hosp Epidemiol* 1991;12:231–238.
78. Serwint JR, Miller RM. Why diagnose influenza infections in hospitalized pediatric patients? *Pediatr Infect Dis J* 1993;12:200–204.
79. MacDonald NE, Hall CB, Suffin SC, et al. Respiratory syncytial viral infection in infants with congenital heart disease. *N Engl J Med* 1982; 307:397–400.
80. Moler FW, Khan AS, Meliones JN, et al. Respiratory syncytial virus morbidity and mortality estimates in congenital heart disease patients: a recent experience. *Crit Care Med* 1992;20:1406–1413.
81. Straube RC, Thompson MA, Van Dyke RB, et al. Adenovirus type 7b in a children's hospital. *J Infect Dis* 1983;147:814–819.
82. Alpert G, Charney E, Fee M, et al. Outbreak of fatal adenovirus type 7a respiratory disease in a children's long-term care inpatient facility. *Am J Infect Control* 1986;14:188–190.
83. Hall CB, Kopelman AE, Douglas RG Jr, et al. Neonatal respiratory syncytial virus infection. *N Engl J Med* 1979;300:393–396.
84. Finn A, Anday E, Talbot GH. An epidemic of adenovirus 7a infection in a neonatal nursery: course, morbidity, and management. *Infect Control Hosp Epidemiol* 1988;9:398–404.
85. Meibalane R, Sedmak GV, Sasidharan P, et al. Outbreak of influenza in a neonatal intensive care unit. *J Pediatr* 1977:91:974–976.
86. Wilson CW, Stevenson DK, Arvin AM. A concurrent epidemic of respiratory syncytial virus and echovirus 7 infections in an intensive care nursery. *Pediatr Infect Dis J* 1989;8:24–29.
87. Mintz L, Ballard RA, Sniderman SH, et al. Nosocomial respiratory syncytial virus infections in an intensive care nursery: rapid diagnosis by direct immunofluorescence. *Pediatrics* 1979;64:149–153.
88. Singh-Naz N, Willy M, Riggs N. Outbreak of parainfluenza virus type 3 in a neonatal nursery. *Pediatr Infect Dis J* 1990;931–933.
89. Meissner HC, Murray SA, Kiernan MA, et al. A simultaneous out-

break of respiratory syncytial virus and parainfluenza virus type 3 in a newborn nursery. *J Pediatr* 1984;104:680–684.

90. Valenti WM, Clarke TA, Hall CB, et al. Concurrent outbreaks of rhinovirus and respiratory syncytial virus in an intensive care nursery: epidemiology and associated risk factors. *J Pediatr* 1982;100: 722–726.
91. Sagrera X, Ginovart G, Raspall F, et al. Outbreaks of influenza A virus infection in neonatal intensive care units. *Pediatr Infect Dis J* 2002;21:196–200.
92. Ng W, Rajadurai VS, Pradeepkumar VK, et al. Parainfluenza type 3 viral outbreak in a neonatal nursery. *Ann Acad Med Singapore* 1999; 28:471–475.
93. Hall CB, Powell KR, MacDonald NE, et al. Respiratory syncytial viral infection in children with compromised immune function. *N Engl J Med* 1986;315:77–81.
94. Pohl C, Green M, Wald ER, et al. Respiratory syncytial virus infections in pediatric liver transplant recipients. *J Infect Dis* 1992;165: 166–169.
95. Wendt CH, Weisdorf DJ, Jordan MC, et al. Parainfluenza virus respiratory infection after bone marrow transplantation. *N Engl J Med* 1992;326:921–926.
96. Shields AF, Hackman RC, Fife KH, et al. Adenovirus infections in patients undergoing bone-marrow transplantation. *N Engl J Med* 1985;312:529–533.
97. Michaels MG, Green M, Wald ER, et al. Adenovirus infection in pediatric liver transplant recipients. *J Infect Dis* 1992;165:170–174.
98. Gardner PS, Court SDM, Brocklebank JT, et al. Virus cross-infection in paediatric wards. *BMJ* 1973;2:571–575.
99. Hall CB, Douglas RG Jr, Geiman JM, et al. Nosocomial respiratory syncytial virus infections. *N Engl J Med* 1975;293:1343–1346.
100. Ditchburn RK, McQuillin J, Gardner PS, et al. Respiratory syncytial virus in hospital cross-infection. *BMJ* 1971;3:671–673.
101. Gala CL, Hall CB, Schnabel KC, et al. The use of eye-nose goggles to control nosocomial respiratory syncytial virus infection. *JAMA* 1986;256:2706–2708.
102. Agah R, Cherry JD, Garakian AJ, et al. Respiratory syncytial virus (RSV) infection rate in personnel caring for children with RSV infections. *Am J Dis Child* 1987;141:695–697.
103. Hall CB, Geiman JM, Douglas RG Jr, et al. Control of nosocomial respiratory syncytial viral infections. *Pediatrics* 1978;62:728–732.
104. Karron RA, O'Brien KL, Froehlich JL, et al. Molecular epidemiology of a parainfluenza type 3 virus outbreak on a pediatric ward. *J Infect Dis* 1993;167:1441–1445.
105. Singh-Naz N, Brown M, Ganeshananthan M. Nosocomial adenovirus infection: molecular epidemiology of an outbreak. *Pediatr Infect Dis J* 1993;12:922–925.
106. Harrington RD, Hooton TM, Hackman RC, et al. An outbreak of respiratory syncytial virus in a bone marrow transplant center. *J Infect Dis* 1992;165:987–993.
107. Brummitt CF, Cherrington JM, Katzenstein DA, et al. Nosocomial adenovirus infections: molecular epidemiology of an outbreak due to adenovirus 3a. *J Infect Dis* 1988;158:423–432.
108. Kempe A, Hall CB, MacDonald NE, et al. Influenza in children with cancer. *J Pediatr* 1989;115:33–39.
109. Monto AS, Cavallaro JJ. The Tecumseh study of respiratory illness. II. Patterns of occurrence of infection with respiratory pathogens, 1965–1969. *Am J Epidemiol* 1971;94:280–289.
110. Johnston SL, Pattemore PK, Sanderson G, et al. Community study of role of viral infections in exacerbations of asthma in 9-11 year old children [see comments]. *BMJ* 1995;310:1225–1229.
111. Herrmann EC Jr. Experience in providing a viral diagnostic laboratory compatible with medical practice. *Mayo Clin Proc* 1967;42:112–123.
112. Menegus MA, Douglas RG Jr. Viruses, rickettsiae, chlamydiae, and mycoplasmas. In: Mandell GL, Douglas RG Jr, Bennett JE, eds. *Principles and practice of infectious diseases,* 3rd ed. New York: Wiley, 1990: 193–205.
113. Cate TR, Couch RB, Johnson KM. Studies with rhinoviruses in volunteers: production of illness, effect of naturally acquired antibody, and demonstration of a protective effect not associated with serum antibody. *J Clin Invest* 1964;43:56–67.
114. Hall CB, Douglas RG Jr. Clinically useful method for the isolation of respiratory syncytial virus. *J Infect Dis* 1975;131:1–5.
115. Masters H, Weber K, Groothuis J, et al. Comparison of nasopharyngeal washings and swab specimens for diagnosis of respiratory syncytial virus by EIA, FAT and cell culture. *Diagn Microbiol Infect Dis* 1987; 8:101–105.
116. Makela MJ, Puhakka T, Ruuskanen O, et al. Viruses and bacteria in the etiology of the common cold. *J Clin Microbiol* 1998;36:539–542.
117. Arruda E, Pitkaranta A, Witek TJ Jr, et al. Frequency and natural history of rhinovirus infections in adults during autumn. *J Clin Microbiol* 1997;35:2864–2868.
118. Kehl SC, Henrickson KJ, Hua W, et al. Evaluation of the Hexaplex assay for detection of respiratory viruses in children. *J Clin Microbiol* 2001;39:1696–1701.
119. Halstead DC, Todd S, Fritch G. Evaluation of five methods for respiratory syncytial virus detection. *J Clin Microbiol* 1990;28:1021–1025.
120. Lipson SM, Popiolek D, Hu QZ, et al. Efficacy of Directigen RSV testing in patient management following admission from a paediatric emergency department. *J Hosp Infect* 1999;41:323–329.
121. Abels S, Nadal D, Stroehle A, et al. Reliable detection of respiratory syncytial virus infection in children for adequate hospital infection control management. *J Clin Microbiol* 2001;39:3135–3139.
122. Hindiyeh M, Hillyard DR, Carroll KC. Evaluation of the Prodesse Hexaplex multiplex PCR assay for direct detection of seven respiratory viruses in clinical specimens. *Am J Clin Pathol* 2001;116:218–224.
123. Bridges CB, Fukuda K, Uyeki TM, et al. Prevention and control of influenza: recommendations of the Advisory Committee on Immunization Practices (ACIP). *MMWR Morb Mortal Wkly Rep* 2002; 51(RR03):1–31.
124. Serwint JR, Miller RM, Korsch BM. Influenza type A and B infections in hospitalized pediatric patients: who should be immunized? *Am J Dis Child* 1991;145:623–626.
125. Pachucki CT, Pappas SAW, Fuller GF, et al. Influenza A among hospital personnel and patients: implications for recognition, prevention, and control. *Arch Intern Med* 1989;149:77–80.
126. The Impact-RSV Study Group. Palivizumab, a humanized respiratory syncytial virus monoclonal antibody, reduces hospitalization from respiratory syncytial virus infection in high-risk infants. *Pediatrics* 1998; 102:531–537.
127. LaMontagne JR, Galasso GJ. Report of a workshop on clinical studies of the efficacy of amantadine and rimantadine against influenza virus. *J Infect Dis* 1978;138:928–931.
128. Stanley ED, Muldoon RE, Akers LW, et al. Evaluation of antiviral drugs: the effect of amantadine on influenza in volunteers. *Ann N Y Acad Sci* 1965;130:44–51.
129. Togo Y, Hornick RB, Dawkins AT Jr. Studies on induced influenza in man. 1. Double-blind studies designed to assess prophylactic efficacy of amantadine hydrochloride against A2/Rockville/1/65–strain. *JAMA* 1968;203:1089–1094.
130. Clover RD, Crawford SA, Abell TD, et al. Effectiveness of rimantadine prophylaxis of children within families. *Am J Dis Child* 1986; 140:706–709.
131. O'Donoghue JM, Ray GC, Terry DW Jr, et al. Prevention of nosocomial influenza infection with amantadine. *Am J Epidemiol* 1973;97: 276–282.
132. Buckland FE, Tyrrell DAJ. Experiments on the spread of colds. I. Laboratory studies on the dispersal of nasal secretion. *J Hyg (Cambridge)* 1964;62:365–377.
133. Gerone PJ, Couch RB, Keefer GV, et al. Assessment of experimental and natural viral aerosols. *Bacteriol Rev* 1966;30:576–584.
134. Boyce JM, Pittet D. Guideline for hand hygiene in health-care settings. *MMWR Morb Mortal Wkly Rep* 2002;51(RR16):1–44.
135. Platt J, Bucknall RA. The disinfection of respiratory syncytial virus by isopropanol and a chlorhexidine-detergent handwash. *J Hosp Infect* 1985;6:89–94.
136. Sattar SA, Abebe M, Bueti AJ, et al. Activity of an alcohol-based hand gel against human adeno-, rhino-, and rotaviruses using the fingerpad method. *Infect Control Hosp Epidemiol* 2000;21:516–519.
137. Schurmann W, Eggers HJ. Antiviral activity of an alcoholic hand disinfectant. Comparison of the in vitro suspension test with in vivo

experiments on hands, and on individual fingertips. *Antiviral Res* 1983;3:25–41.
138. Murphy D, Todd JK, Chao RK, et al. The use of gowns and masks to control respiratory illness in pediatric hospital personnel. *J Pediatr* 1981;99:746–750.
139. Hall CB, Douglas RG Jr. Nosocomial respiratory syncytial viral infections: should gowns and masks be used? *Am J Dis Child* 1981;135: 512–515.
140. Madge P, Paton JY, McColl JH, et al. Prospective controlled study of four infection-control procedures to prevent nosocomial infection with respiratory syncytial virus. *Lancet* 1992;340:1079–1083.
141. Leclair JM, Freeman J, Sullivan BF, et al. Prevention of nosocomial respiratory syncytial virus infections through compliance with glove and gown isolation precautions. *N Engl J Med* 1987;317:329–334.
142. Krasinski K, LaCouture R, Holzman RS, et al. Screening for respiratory syncytial virus and assignment to a cohort at admission to reduce nosocomial transmission. *J Pediatr* 1990;116:894–898.
143. Garner JS, Hospital Infection Control Practices Advisory Committee. Guideline for isolation precautions in hospitals. *Infect Control Hosp Epidemiol* 1996;17:53–80.
144. McLean RL. General discussion of the mechanism of spread of Asian influenza. *Am Rev Respir Dis* 1960;83(part 2):36–38.
145. Riley RL, Nardell EA. Clearing the air: the theory and application of ultraviolet air disinfection. *Am Rev Respir Dis* 1989;139:1286–1294.

49

NOSOCOMIAL BACTERIAL INFECTIONS OF THE CENTRAL NERVOUS SYSTEM, UPPER AND LOWER RESPIRATORY TRACTS, AND SKIN IN PEDIATRIC PATIENTS

TERRY YAMAUCHI
GORDON E. SCHUTZE

Clinicians involved in the care of children must be alert for signs or symptoms of nosocomial infections in their pediatric patients. Infections involving the central nervous system, respiratory tract, and skin can occur even under optimal conditions. Clinicians must be aware of the potential infecting microorganisms and should understand the pathogenesis of these illnesses. An understanding of these factors allows for appropriate therapy and infection control measures.

CENTRAL NERVOUS SYSTEM INFECTIONS

Nosocomial infections of the central nervous system include intracranial infections, meningitis or ventriculitis, and shunt infections. Central nervous system infections account for 2% to 17% of all nosocomial infections in infants in intensive care units (1–7). Most of these infections involve surgical procedures and/or manipulation/trauma within the central nervous system. Information concerning pediatric intensive care units is less readily available; although some investigators have demonstrated a central nervous system infection rate of 25% in their pediatric intensive care units, others have had no occurrences (8,9).

Intracranial Infections

Pathogenesis

Intracranial infections, such as brain abscesses, are not commonly encountered and should meet the criteria from the Centers for Disease Control and Prevention (CDC) in Table 49.1 for diagnosis (10). Brain abscesses commonly form via direct spread from a contiguous source or via hematogenous spread from a distant source. In approximately one third of situations, however, no predisposing factors are identified. Respiratory diseases such as chronic sinusitis, otitis media, and mastoiditis account for the majority of sites from which microorganisms can extend directly into the brain (11,12). Patients who develop abscesses resulting from contiguous spread usually have a single abscess in the proximity of the infected region. Abscesses acquired through the hematogenous route tend to follow the course of the middle cerebral artery and cause abscesses in the frontal and parietal regions. Cyanotic congenital heart disease with right-to-left shunts or pulmonary arteriovenous fistulas predispose patients to brain abscess formation (13,14). The most common lesion encountered in such patients is tetralogy of Fallot (15). A nosocomial brain abscess is especially likely in patients who have suffered head trauma or who have undergone neurosurgical procedures. Approximately 6% to 11% of abscesses are in patients with head trauma or neurosurgical procedures, and their symptoms usually develop within 10 days to 2 months following the inciting episode (13,14,16,17).

Etiology

Brain abscesses are often polymicrobial in origin, but, when they occur in patients who have had head injuries or neurosurgical procedures, *Staphylococcus aureus* followed by the viridans streptococci and *Streptococcus pneumoniae* are the most common microorganisms isolated (13–17). Abscesses in patients with complex congenital heart disease include anaerobes, viridans streptococci, microaerophilic streptococci, enterococci, and *Haemophilus* species. The etiologic agents in patients with a history of chronic sinusitis or otitis media are anaerobes, gram-negative rods *(Proteus, Pseudomonas, Haemophilus)*, and *S. aureus.*

Clinical Manifestations

Symptoms associated with a brain abscess include fever (68%), headache (66%), vomiting (59%), focal neurologic deficits (46%), seizures (44%), papilledema (39%), and meningeal signs (36%). Papilledema and meningeal signs may not be pres-

TABLE 49.1. DEFINITIONS FOR CENTRAL NERVOUS SYSTEM INFECTIONS IN PEDIATRIC PATIENTS

Intracranial infection
- The microorganism must be cultured from the brain tissue or dura
- Evidence of infection at surgery or by histopathologic examination
- Two or more of the following without another recognizable cause: headache, dizziness, fever (>38°C), localizing neurologic signs, change in mental status; these symptoms must be followed by institution of appropriate antimicrobial therapy with the microorganism seen on microscopic examination, or there must be a positive antigen test, radiographic evidence of infection, or a diagnostic antibody test
- Criteria are similar for patients younger than 12 months with the inclusion of hypothermia (<37°C), apnea, or bradycardia

Meningitis/ventriculitis
- Isolation of the microorganism from the cerebrospinal fluid
- Institution of appropriate antimicrobial therapy and the patient has one or more of the following: fever (>38°C), headache, stiff neck, meningeal signs, cranial nerve signs, irritability; *and* one of the following laboratory abnormalities: increased white cells, elevated protein, and/or decreased glucose in the cerebrospinal fluid; positive Gram stain; positive blood culture; positive antigen detection; or a diagnostic antibody test
- Criteria are similar for patients younger than 12 months with the inclusion of hypothermia (<37°C), apnea, and bradycardia

Adapted from Garner JS, Jarvis WR, Emori TG, et al. CDC definitions for nosocomial infections, 1988. *Am J Infect Control* 1988; 16: 128–140, with permission.

TABLE 49.2. BACTERIAL PROPHYLAXIS FOR PATIENTS WITH COMPLEX CONGENITAL HEART DISEASE

Dental, oral, upper respiratory tract procedures

Oral prophylaxis
- Amoxicillin 50 mg/kg (2 g maximum) 1 hour before procedure
- *or*
- Clindamycin 20 mg/kg (600 mg maximum) or cephalexin or cefadroxil 50 mg/kg (2 g maximum) or azithromycin or clarithromycin 15 mg/kg (500 mg maximum) 1 hour before procedure

Intravenous/intramuscular prophylaxis
- Ampicillin 50 mg/kg (2 g maximum) or cefazolin 25 mg/kg (1 g maximum) or clindamycin 20 mg/kg (600 mg maximum) within 30 minutes before procedure

Genitourinary/gastrointestinal procedures

High-risk patients
- Ampicillin 50 mg/kg IM or IV (2 g maximum) plus gentamicin 1.5 mg/kg (120 mg maximum) within 30 minutes of starting the procedure; 6 hours later, ampicillin 25 mg/kg (1 g maximum) IM/IV or amoxicillin 25 mg/kg (1 g maximum) orally

Moderate-risk patients
- Amoxicillin 50 mg/kg (2 g maximum) orally 1 hour before procedure or ampicillin 50 mg/kg (2 g maximum) IM/IV within 30 minutes of starting the procedure

High-risk patients allergic to ampicillin/amoxicillin
- Vancomycin 20 mg/kg (1 g maximum) IV over 1–2 hours and gentamicin 1.5 mg/kg (120 mg maximum) IV/IM; complete injection/infusion within 30 minutes of starting the procedure

Moderate-risk patients allergic to ampicillin/amoxicillin
- Vancomycin 20 mg/kg (1 g maximum) IV over 1–2 hours; complete the infusion within 30 minutes of starting the procedure.

Adapted from Dajani AS, Taubert KA, Wilson W, et al. Prevention of bacterial endocarditis: recommendations by the American Heart Association. *JAMA* 1997;277:1794–1801, with permission.

ent in patients younger than 2 years (13,14). The classic triad of symptoms (headache, fever, and focal neurologic deficits) is demonstrated in less than 30% of patients (14).

Diagnosis

The diagnosis of a brain abscess can be established by cerebral imaging using cranial ultrasonography, computed tomography, or magnetic resonance imaging.

Prevention

Prophylactic antimicrobial agents may prevent the development of brain abscesses in certain situations. For patients with cyanotic congenital heart disease who are at high or moderate risk for endocarditis, antimicrobial prophylaxis is indicated in patients before dental, genitourinary, and gastrointestinal procedures. Procedures requiring prophylaxis include those that children might undergo, such as dental procedures known to induce gingival bleeding (teeth cleaning), tonsillectomy/adenoidectomy, surgical procedures involving intestinal and respiratory mucosa, bronchoscopy with a rigid bronchoscope, urethral catheterization or urinary tract surgery if a urinary tract infection is present, and incision and drainage of infected tissue (18). Recommended prophylaxis regimens are outlined in Table 49.2.

Antimicrobial prophylaxis for neurosurgical procedures has been demonstrated to be effective for clean and clean-contaminated procedures (19–24). Multiple regimens have been used involving vancomycin (22), vancomycin/gentamicin (20), cefazolin/gentamicin (21), piperacillin (23), cloxacillin (24), and cefuroxime (25). Despite the multiple combinations that have been used, all the regimens are delivered for only a short time (<24 hours) and are active against staphylococci. In light of these studies, it is recommended that patients undergoing clean or clean-contaminated neurosurgical procedures undergo prophylaxis beginning preoperatively and continuing during the procedure, with vancomycin/gentamicin or cloxacillin alone as the drugs of choice (19). In hospitals with high rates of nosocomial gram-negative infections, consideration should be given to including antimicrobial agents in the regimen that is active against the prominent gram-negative microorganisms as well.

Meningitis and Ventriculitis

Pathogenesis

Meningitis or ventriculitis is usually the result of a bacteremia. The bacteria gain access to the central nervous system from the blood in the region of the choroid plexus. Meningitis less commonly develops as a complication of endocarditis, pneumonia, or thrombophlebitis. There may also be direct extension from a chronic respiratory source (i.e., mastoiditis) or as a complication of trauma (i.e., basilar skull fracture), an anatomic defect of the cribriform plate, or a direct communication between the skin and meninges (meningomyelocele) (26). Some degree of ventriculitis can be demonstrated in most cases of bacterial meningitis, but ventriculitis is more common as an infectious complication of ventricular shunting. The predominant microorganisms involved in nosocomial meningitis or ventriculitis are different from those involved in community-acquired disease. Factors contributing to this include the age and immune status of the patient. The diagnostic criteria for nosocomial meningitis or ventriculitis are outlined in Table 49.1.

Etiology

In children older than 3 months, the common pathogens causing meningitis have traditionally included *Haemophilus influenzae* type b, *S. pneumoniae,* and *Neisseria meningitidis.* Because of the efficiency of the *Haemophilus* vaccines, however, this microorganism is no longer the predominant pathogen (27). For children younger than 3 months, group B β-hemolytic streptococci (GBS), *Escherichia coli, Klebsiella pneumoniae,* and *Listeria monocytogenes* are the most frequent causes of meningitis. Newborns become colonized with these microorganisms from passage through the birth canal and may develop illness within hours after birth. If illness occurs within the first 5 days of life, it is considered an early-onset illness. Those that develop after 5 days of life are considered late-onset illnesses. Early-onset illnesses are due to microorganisms harbored in the mother's birth canal. Microorganisms that cause late-onset disease may have been transmitted from the mother or may have also been acquired from caregivers or the environment.

Most nosocomial cases of meningitis in children older than 3 months are due to the staphylococci, although enterococcal and gram-negative enteric *(E. coli, Klebsiella, Enterobacter, Proteus)* infections do occur (3,28). When staphylococcal meningitis occurs, there is an associated defect in the central nervous system resulting from surgery or trauma in approximately 75% of cases (29,30). Therefore, most cases are due to direct extension of the microorganism instead of hematogenous spread. Spread of the more traditional microorganisms such as *N. meningitidis* and *H. influenzae* occurs via the respiratory route, and, therefore, respiratory spread is a potential hazard for nosocomial transmission. These microorganisms are responsible for secondary diseases in family members but only rarely have been associated with nosocomial infections of the central nervous system (31).

Early-onset GBS disease usually manifests itself as respiratory distress with bacteremia. Most early-onset disease, regardless of the microorganism, usually lacks meningeal involvement. Meningeal involvement is a common manifestation in late-onset disease (32) (see also Chapter 31). Most newborns that develop meningitis while hospitalized are in neonatal intensive care units. Therefore, clinicians should be concerned about the bacteria that are known to be present in each nursery. Outbreaks of meningitis in neonatal intensive care units have been attributed to many microorganisms, both gram-positive and gram-negative including *S. aureus, Staphylococcus epidermidis, Serratia, Klebsiella,* and *Citrobacter* (2,33–35) (see also Chapter 52).

Clinical Manifestations

Children with meningitis usually have signs and symptoms relating to their central nervous system, whereas infants may not. The diagnosis of meningitis must be considered in any patient with fever, altered mental status, and meningismus.

Diagnosis

A lumbar puncture is the method of choice for establishing this diagnosis. An increased number of white blood cells with a polymorphonuclear predominance, an elevated cerebrospinal fluid (CSF) protein, and decreased glucose are found with bacterial meningitis. The CSF should be sent for Gram staining, and CSF and blood should be cultured for bacteria to aid in finding the etiologic agent. Bacterial antigens are less helpful, because the more common nosocomial pathogens are not included in such panels.

Prevention

To aid in the prevention of nosocomial disease, patients admitted to the hospital with meningitis resulting from *N. meningitidis* or *S. pneumoniae* should be placed into respiratory isolation for the first 24 hours of hospitalization, and all contacts of the patient should observe strict hand washing (36). Prophylaxis of family members or hospital personnel may also be indicated. Rifampin, 10 mg/kg (maximum of 600 mg), every 12 hours for 2 days is indicated for persons 1 month of age or older who are household members or school or day care contacts of patients with *N. meningitidis* infection. Contacts who are younger than 1 month should receive 5 mg/kg every 12 hours for 2 days. Hospital personnel who deliver mouth-to-mouth resuscitation, intubate the patient, or examine the oropharynx should also receive prophylaxis (see Chapter 81). Affected individuals should be alerted to potential side effects of the medication. Urine and other secretions are discolored (orange or red). Contact lenses can become permanently discolored, and rifampin may alter the activity of birth control pills. Pregnant women should be excluded from rifampin prophylaxis (37). Options for rifampin-sensitive individuals or individuals unable to take rifampin include ceftriaxone or ciprofloxacin (38). Ceftriaxone given in a single intramuscular injection at a dose of 125 mg for children younger than 15 years and 250 mg for others has been demonstrated to effectively eradicate the meningococcal carrier state with group A *N. meningitidis* (39). A single oral dose of ciprofloxacin (500 to 750 mg) has been demonstrated to be effective in adults but cannot be used in children or in pregnant or lactating mothers (40). Ceftriaxone should be used in pregnant women. These options should only be considered in circumstances in which rifampin cannot be used. Meningococcal vaccine can be considered a possible adjunct to chemoprophylaxis but should not be used as the single agent. The vaccine is a serogroup-specific quadrivalent vaccine against groups A, C, 4, and W-135 N. meningitides. Serogroup B is not contained in the vaccine. The quadrivalent vaccine has been used in children younger than 18 months; however, two doses 3 months apart have been given for control of outbreaks.

For trauma patients with basilar skull fractures, antimicrobial prophylaxis for the prevention of meningitis is controversial (41). Many encourage the use of antimicrobial prophylaxis in basilar skull fractures, because the CSF is exposed to the poten-

TABLE 49.3. MATERNAL RISK FACTORS FOR EARLY-ONSET MENINGITIS

Preterm labor (<37 weeks' gestation)
Premature rupture of membranes (<37 weeks' gestation)
Fever during labor (≥38°C)
Multiple births
Prolonged rupture of membranes (≥18 hours)

tially pathogenic microorganisms of the upper airway. Opponents argue that the use of such antimicrobial agents only risks a life-threatening illness with a resistant microorganism. Currently, antimicrobial prophylaxis does not appear to decrease the incidence of meningitis after a basilar skull fracture (41). Surgical intervention should be performed when there is no evidence of healing and/or repeated infection occurs.

The prevention of early-onset meningitis begins with good prenatal care and intervention strategies to prevent transmission of potentially harmful microorganisms to the newborn infant (42). Regardless of the preventive strategy used, women found to have symptomatic or asymptomatic GBS bacteriuria during pregnancy should be treated at the time of diagnosis. Intrapartum prophylaxis should be administered to all women who have had a previous infant with invasive GBS disease. Two strategies are now acceptable for the evaluation and treatment of pregnant mothers (43). One option is to screen all pregnant women at 35 to 37 weeks of gestation and offer intrapartum prophylaxis to GBS carriers even if no sepsis risk factors (e.g., gestation of <37 weeks, prolonged rupture of membranes ≥18 hours, intrapartum temperature ≥38°C) are present (Table 49.3). If the results of the GBS screen are not known at the onset of labor or rupture of membranes, intrapartum antimicrobial prophylaxis should be administered if any of the previously mentioned risk factors are present. A second preventive strategy is based on the presence of sepsis risk factors without culture screening. If any risk factors are present, the mother should receive intrapartum chemoprophylaxis. The antimicrobial agent of choice is penicillin G (5 million U initially then 2.5 million U every 4 hours) given intravenously until delivery. Intravenous ampicillin (2 g initially followed by 1 g every 4 hours until delivery) can be used, but penicillin is preferred because of its narrow spectrum. Intravenous clindamycin or erythromycin can be used for penicillin-allergic patients. The management of infants born to mothers that have received chemoprophylaxis should be based on the gestational age of the infant, the number of doses of the prophylactic agent received, and the clinical findings of the infant (43).

Shunt Infections

Pathogenesis

Approximately 4.5% to 25% of patients who have undergone CSF shunting procedures develop infectious complications (44–46). Risk factors for infection include young age of the patient (<3 months), inexperienced surgeons, prolonged shunting procedures, and distal catheter tip location (47–50). Shunt infections usually occur within 2 months after placement; most are caused by transient or permanent bacterial inhabitants of the skin. The latter observations suggest that direct inoculation in the perioperative period is probably the pathogenesis of this infection (51).

Etiology

The staphylococci are responsible for approximately 75% of infections; *S. epidermidis* is the primary agent in 50% and *S. aureus* in 25% (44,45). Infections with gram-negative enteric microorganisms *(E. coli, Klebsiella, Proteus)* and *Pseudomonas* account for approximately 20%; the remainder of infections are caused by less common microorganisms such as *Enterococcus,* viridans streptococci, *N. meningitidis,* micrococcus, *H. influenzae,* diphtheroids, *Propionibacterium,* and *Corynebacterium* (44, 45,52–55).

Clinical Manifestations

The most common symptoms of shunt infections are usually symptoms of shunt malfunction. Headache, irritability, lethargy, nausea, and change of mental status are quite common. Although fever is usually present, approximately 10% to 20% of children are afebrile (44,45). In most shunt infections, signs of meningeal irritation are absent because there is no communication between the infected ventricle and the CSF.

Diagnosis

Shunt infections should be suspected in any patient who has a ventricular shunt with complaints of malfunction. Fluid from the shunt or ventricle is needed to secure the diagnosis, and the fluid usually displays an increase in the white blood cell count (>10 cells/mm^3). CSF should be cultured aerobically and anaerobically and also plated on media for isolation of fungi. Extreme care should be used when obtaining a CSF specimen from a ventricular shunt bubble. Neurosurgical consultation should be considered before attempting to violate the shunt. The area should be cleaned before penetration with a needle to avoid contaminating the shunt. If patients have concomitant complaints of abdominal distention, peritonitis, shunt wound infection, erythema, or swelling along the shunt tract or if they appear toxic, the shunt should be assumed to be infected.

Prevention

The role of prophylactic antimicrobial agents for the prevention of shunt infections is not well understood. The protective efficacy has been demonstrated to vary widely (5% to 84%) (19). In a meta-analysis of five randomized studies reviewing the use of prophylaxis, it was demonstrated that no single study was large enough to detect a statistical difference (56). Although the evidence supports the need for prophylaxis in shunt operations, the benefit of this procedure is still in question. It is not unreasonable, however, to use prophylaxis with an antistaphylococcal agent (i.e., nafcillin, cephalothin, vancomycin) beginning before the procedure and continuing for 24 to 48 hours after the procedure if the endemic rate of infection exceeds 3% (19) (see also Chapters 27 and 67).

Occasionally, patients require external ventricular drains. These drains may be placed for limited periods after surgery or trauma or when the release of ventricular fluid is required to combat increased intracranial pressure. Catheters are placed directly into the ventricle and drain into an external receptacle. Patients who require these drains are at an increased risk for infectious complications; therefore, CSF specimens should be carefully extracted when these devices are entered. These drain sites should be rotated every 5 to 7 days to avoid infections, and prophylaxis with antimicrobial agents active against staphylococci should be given to the patient for as long as the drains are required.

RESPIRATORY TRACT INFECTIONS

Upper Respiratory Tract Infections

Most nosocomial upper respiratory tract infections are nonbacterial and appear approximately 2 weeks after admission (1,3). Respiratory syncytial virus, adenovirus, and influenza virus account for most of these infections (57) (see Chapter 48). The role of bacteria in nosocomial upper respiratory tract infections is manifested predominately in sinusitis and otitis media. Less commonly encountered problems include pharyngitis, bacterial tracheitis, and diphtheria.

Pharyngitis

Group A *Streptococcus* is a common cause of community-acquired pharyngitis but not nosocomial disease. Patients are rarely admitted to the hospital for a streptococcal throat infection but may be admitted for complications of this infection, such as a peritonsillar abscess. Secondary cases of disease resulting from *Streptococcus pyogenes* are higher among siblings than among adult contacts. Rates of infection may be as high as 50% for sibling contacts, compared with 20% for adult contacts. Asymptomatic, culture-positive individuals (children and adults) are well documented and may be the source for some infections (58). The most important means of controlling group A streptococcal infections, therefore, is early identification and treatment of disease. Although many contacts develop illness, asymptomatic contacts should not be cultured or treated. Symptomatic contacts should undergo a throat culture and be treated if group A *Streptococcus* is isolated (58).

Bacterial Tracheitis

Bacterial tracheitis is a bacterial infection thought to be secondary to a primary viral respiratory infection, usually parainfluenza virus. The viral infection may cause local mucosal damage, alter the patient's immune response, or both, thus leading to a secondary bacterial infection (59,60). The most common microorganisms involved are *S. aureus* and *H. influenzae.* Before the availability of *H. influenzae* conjugate vaccines, this disorder was as common as epiglottitis, but, because of a dramatic decrease of invasive *H. influenzae* disease, bacterial tracheitis may now be more common. The patient with bacterial tracheitis usually has a waning viral respiratory illness when the fever rises and stridor begins or worsens. The patient assumes any position that maximizes his or her air flow, not just the sniffing position as demonstrated with epiglottitis. Endoscopic examination reveals copious tenacious purulent secretions above the subcricoid trachea. No isolation is required, and early recognition and treatment is the only method to prevent life-threatening illness.

Diphtheria

Diphtheria is a disease that usually manifests itself as a membranous nasopharyngitis and/or an obstructive laryngotracheitis resulting from *Corynebacterium diphtheriae.* This disease has been uncommon since the advent of the diphtheria vaccine. Specimens for culture should be obtained from the nose and throat; culture requires special media from the clinical laboratory. Once the culture has been obtained, the laboratory should be alerted to facilitate the evaluation. Patients with pharyngeal diphtheria should be placed in strict isolation until two cultures from both the nose and throat are negative. Communicability is usually less than 4 days once effective antimicrobial treatment has started. Patients with cutaneous forms of diphtheria should be placed in contact isolation until two cultures of the skin are negative (61). (Note, these recommendations for isolation of patients with pharyngeal diphtheria differ from those in the CDC's "Guideline for Isolation Precautions in Hospitals"; see Chapter 95.) Close contacts of the patient should be cultured irrespective of their immunization status and should be given antimicrobial prophylaxis with orally administered erythromycin or intramuscularly administered penicillin. The efficacy of antimicrobial prophylaxis is presumed but not proven; therefore, these patients should be kept under surveillance for 7 days. Asymptomatic contacts should receive a booster of diphtheria toxoid if they have not received a booster in the preceding 5 years. Series should be started for unimmunized individuals. Diphtheria antitoxin for unimmunized close contacts is not generally recommended (61). However, in the rapidly deteriorating patient with the presumptive diagnosis of diphtheria, a dose of equine antitoxin administered intravenously may be needed. Tests for sensitivity to horse serum should be performed before the antitoxin is given.

Sinusitis

Most cases of acute sinusitis in children are due to *S. pneumoniae, H. influenzae,* and *Moraxella catarrhalis* (62). These agents are also recovered from patients with chronic sinusitis, but *S. aureus* and anaerobic bacteria *(Peptococcus, Peptostreptococcus, Bacteroides)* are recovered more often from children with sinus symptoms that have lasted longer than 1 year (63–65). Nosocomial sinusitis may be due to the major agents of acute or chronic sinusitis but also include pathogens endemic to the hospital such as *Pseudomonus aeruginosa, E. coli, K. pneumoniae, Enterobacter,* and *Proteus* (66). *Aspergillus* species have also been recovered from hospitalized patients with sinusitis, in which the most likely source of the fungus was hospital construction or a faulty ventilation system (see the section on lower respiratory tract infections in this chapter).

The major predisposing factor for the development of nosocomial sinusitis is the use of obstructive devices in the nasal cavity. The paranasal sinuses are inflamed or infected because of the trapping of sinus secretions in closed spaces. Nasogastric and nasotracheal tubes are the most common instruments noted to predispose patients to sinusitis (66–70). This may occur in up to 40% of patients who have undergone nasotracheal intubation (71). Other forms of instrumentation of the oropharynx, such as oropharyngeal intubation and tracheostomy, also contribute to this disease process. Nasal packing, high-dose corticosteroid therapy, prior antimicrobial treatment, and facial or cranial fractures have also been described as risk factors for this disease.

The symptoms are nonspecific. Most patients develop illness during the first 2 weeks of intubation. Fever is usually the only complaint, although purulent rhinitis may be demonstrated (67). Radiographic studies are usually needed to establish a diagnosis. The demonstration of sinus thickening or air fluid levels on plain radiographs of the sinuses is consistent with an inflammatory process. In selected patients, however, computed tomography of the sinuses may be indicated to delineate the extent of disease, because this method has been demonstrated to be superior to plain roentgenographs (72).

Prevention of sinusitis includes good oral hygiene while patients are mechanically intubated. Nasogastric and nasotracheal tubes can still be used but should be promptly removed when they are no longer indicated. Although patients are predisposed to sinusitis with nasotracheal intubation, this technique should still be used, because there are fewer airway complications with nasotracheal intubation than with oropharyngeal intubation (68) (see also Chapter 23).

Otitis Media

Otitis media is one of the most common illnesses of infants and children. Particularly high rates of otitis media are demonstrated among Eskimos, American Indians, and children with cleft palates. Other predisposing factors include lower socioeconomic groups, bottle-feeding, day care attendance, and atopy. The most common microorganisms involved in acute otitis media are *S. pneumoniae, M. catarrhalis,* and *H. influenzae* (73). Microorganisms that have been associated with chronic suppurative otitis media include *P. aeruginosa* and *S. aureus* (74). Nosocomial otitis media is a common entity, especially in intensive care units. The bacteriology usually reflects that of the hospital environment and not that of the community (75).

Nosocomial otitis media is usually due to prolonged dysfunction of the eustachian tubes. Like sinusitis, it is most commonly demonstrated with the use of devices that occlude the airways (75). This dysfunction of the eustachian tube leads to the stasis of fluid and bacteria in the middle ear and allows infection. Fever is the most common symptom associated with otitis media. Older children may be able to verbalize a complaint of ear pain, and, occasionally, there may be purulent otorrhea. The diagnosis can be established by physical examination. An absent light reflex, decreased tympanic motility, a retracted or bulging tympanic membrane, or purulence behind the tympanic membrane can be demonstrated by otoscopy. In severely ill or immunocompromised patients, a diagnostic myringotomy may be indicated to direct therapy.

Many children who are admitted to the hospital have a recent history of antimicrobial therapy for otitis media. If the child develops this complication while hospitalized, there is always a question of whether this represents disease that was resistant to initial therapy or a new infection. Currently, it is believed that children presenting with symptoms of otitis media within 1 month after therapy have an infection caused by a new microorganism (76). The bacteria that cause most recurrences are also sensitive to the antimicrobial agent just completed (77). Therefore, children who develop otitis media while hospitalized usually have a nosocomial infection rather than a relapse from a previously treated case of otitis media.

Using devices that obstruct the oropharynx such as nasogastric or nasotracheal tubes for as short a time as possible may aid in the prevention of nosocomial otitis media. For infants and children with a history of repeated ear infections maintained on antimicrobial prophylaxis at home, these medications should be continued while patients are mechanically ventilated. Long-term prophylaxis with medications such as sulfisoxazole has effectively prevented cases of otitis media (78). Antimicrobial prophylaxis reduces the occurrence of otitis media, presumably by providing antimicrobial agents in the tissues of the nasopharynx, eustachian tube, and middle ear at concentrations high enough to keep the number of pathogenic bacteria below the levels needed to initiate infection (79).

Lower Respiratory Tract Infections

Nosocomial lower respiratory tract infections (LRTIs) account for approximately 15% to 20% of nosocomial infections of infants and children (1–3,8). These infections constitute a common but potential life-threatening complication of hospitalization. It has been estimated that the mortality rate associated with nosocomial LRTIs ranges from 20% to 50% and that 15% of all deaths occurring in hospitalized patients of all ages are directly related to these infections (80). The increased risk of poor outcome with nosocomial LRTI has become more obvious because of the modern intensive care facilities. Intensive care units can support critically ill patients for prolonged periods with invasive life support techniques. Many of the patients undergoing prolonged support are very low birth weight infants, premature infants, or immunocompromised patients; these conditions enhance the risk of nosocomial LRTI with subsequent increased morbidity and mortality.

Pathophysiology

The pathophysiology of nosocomial LRTI is thought to involve the altered or circumvented pulmonary antimicrobial defenses of the upper and lower respiratory tract (81). Although a few infections represent hematogenous seeding of the lungs from a distant suppurative focus (i.e., endocarditis, meningitis), most patients suffer from subclinical aspiration of oropharyngeal secretions containing bacteria that have colonized the upper airway of the patient. This flora includes aerobic gram-positive and gram-negative microorganisms commonly identified in the hospital where the patient is located (82). Flora commonly found in the oropharynx of children admitted to the hospital includes both gram-positive (i.e., staphylococci, streptococci) and gram-negative microorganisms (i.e., *Neisseria* species). In colder months, many healthy infants and children are commonly colonized with microorganisms considered to be pathogens (i.e., *S. pneumoniae, S. pyogenes)* (80). The flora commonly demonstrated on admission changes within 1 to 4 days after admission to those microorganisms commonly found in the hospital. The risk factors for colonization include acidosis, endotracheal intubation, hypotension, and broad-spectrum antimicrobial therapy (82,83). Turbulence in the nasal airways normally prevents deposition of large particles in the lower respiratory tract. Nasotracheal, orotracheal, or tracheostomy tubes bypass this defense mechanism and allow colonization of the upper respiratory tract with hospital-acquired microorganisms. Without colonization of the upper airways, only a few patients develop nosocomial LRTI as compared with colonized patients (3% vs. 23%) (84).

Most nosocomial LRTIs are caused by gram-negative microorganisms (3,8,80). A fecal-oral route for bacterial contamination of the upper airways has always been suspected but has never explained the frequency of colonization with microorganisms such as *P. aeruginosa* or *Acinetobacter* species. These microorganisms are not the usual inhabitants of the human gastrointestinal tract. In studies addressing this, members of the Enterobacteriaceae family (i.e., *E. coli, Klebsiella*) were isolated from the hypopharynx and rectum before they were isolated from the trachea in patients undergoing prolonged intubation in whom daily cultures were monitored from rectal, hypopharyngeal, and tracheal sites. In contrast, non-Enterobacteriaceae (i.e., *P. aeruginosa, Acinetobacter*) were rarely demonstrated before their appearance in the trachea (80). This suggests that non-Enterobacteriaceae microorganisms have environmental sources and that colonization with Enterobacteriaceae occurs from the patient's endogenous flora. The hands of the healthcare worker and certain components of the respiratory therapy equipment, therefore, may be important factors in the transmission of disease.

A nosocomial LRTI results when the colonizing microorganisms evade the mucociliary and cellular defenses of the lower respiratory tract. Microorganisms can then attack the respiratory epithelium and cause disease. The most important factor predisposing infants and children to the development of nosocomial LRTI is endotracheal intubation. Nosocomial LRTIs have been shown to occur four times more often in intubated patients than in nonintubated patients (80). Rates for patients with tracheostomy tubes appear to be even higher. Although the critically ill patient requiring prolonged hospitalization in intensive care units is at increased risk for nosocomial infections, the endotracheal tube eliminates the most effective natural host defense mechanism of the upper airway. The filtration system of the upper airway and the mucociliary system of the large airways is bypassed during intubation. The loss of the mucociliary transport system is accentuated by mechanical irritation and damage to the respiratory epithelium, which predisposes the patient to colonization with potential pathogens. Other risk factors for nosocomial LRTI in infants and children are premature and low birth weight infants, poor nutrition, underlying pulmonary disease, length of hospitalization, general anesthesia, and respiratory therapy.

Any infant or child admitted to the hospital should be considered at risk for nosocomial LRTI. However, patients who have problems with acidosis, hypotension, hypoperfusion, or altered mental status or who have tubes (nasotracheal, orotracheal, nasogastric) are at increased risk for these infections (84,85). Infants and children with symptomatic or asymptomatic aspiration are also at risk (80). Patients with tracheoesophageal fistulae, swallowing dyscoordination, gastroesophageal reflux, facial burns, cardiac disease (i.e., shunt lesions with pulmonary hypertension), pulmonary disease, malnutrition, or immunodeficiencies or who have undergone surgery with unprotected airways also risk aspirating the resident flora in the hypopharynx.

Etiology

The specific etiologic microorganisms for nosocomial LRTI vary from institution to institution. The clinician, therefore, must be familiar with the common microorganisms and antimicrobial susceptibility of these microorganisms at his or her institution. Gram-negative rods are the most common bacterial cause of a nosocomial LRTI in infants and children (86) (Table 49.4). The predominance of gram-negative microorganisms has been demonstrated in community and teaching hospitals. This raises concern because the mortality associated with gram-negative LRTI is often estimated at 50%. Among gram-positive microorganisms, staphylococci are the predominant microorganisms encountered, with methicillin-resistant *S. aureus* increasing in occurrence, and less common microorganisms include *Legionella* spp. (87,88). In pediatric hospitals, community-acquired microorganisms such as *S. pneumoniae* and *N. meningitidis* may also be encountered. If these microorganisms are identified, however, a septic metastasis or direct respiratory tract spread should be considered, because these microorganisms are an uncommon cause of nosocomial LRTI.

Pertussis is caused by the microorganism *Bordetella pertussis* and has been an important respiratory pathogen with high infectivity in children, which sometimes results in death. More recently, the disease has had an increased incidence in older pa-

TABLE 49.4. COMMON ETIOLOGIC AGENTS CAUSING LOWER RESPIRATORY TRACT INFECTIONS IN HOSPITALIZED CHILDREN

Escherichia coli
Klebsiella pneumoniae
Pseudomonas aeruginosa
Moraxella catarrhalis
Staphylococcus aureus
Staphylococcus epidermidis
Enterococcus species
Other gram-negative bacilli

tients, specifically adolescents and adults (89). Outbreaks of pertussis in the hospital setting have also been recently reported (90). Because of decreasing immunity, the incidence of clinical disease has increased in certain populations, especially in medical personnel. Adults are more effective disseminators and, therefore, serve as major reservoirs for disease. Even when pertussis is present in a community in epidemic proportions, it is rarely transmitted within the hospital if the proper precautions are taken (91). (Nosocomial pertussis is also covered in Chapter 81.)

Children with pulmonary infections resulting from *Mycobacterium tuberculosis* rarely transmit this microorganism to other individuals. Children are generally ineffective coughers, and, in most cases, pulmonary involvement in infants and children is manifested by closed caseous lesions that have lower numbers of acid-fast bacilli compared with the cavitary lesions commonly demonstrated in adults with pulmonary disease (92).

In neonatal intensive care units, coagulase-negative staphylococci (i.e., *S. epidermidis*) have emerged as a major cause of nosocomial infections, and patients infected with this microorganism should be treated aggressively (7,93). In hospitals undergoing renovation or nearby construction of ventilation changes, *Aspergillus* may cause LRTI in the hospitalized patient. Other agents that can present a problem for premature infants include *Chlamydia trachomatis, Ureaplasma urealyticum,* and *Mycoplasma hominis* (94–96) (see also Chapter 52).

TABLE 49.5. DEFINITIONS FOR NOSOCOMIAL LOWER RESPIRATORY TRACT INFECTIONS

Rales or dullness to percussion on physical examination of the chest and *any* of the following: new onset of purulent sputum; microorganism isolated from a blood culture; isolation of a microorganism from transtracheal aspirate, bronchial brushing, or biopsy
Chest radiograph demonstrates new or progressive infiltrate, consolidation, cavitation, or pleural effusion and *any* of the following: new onset of purulent sputum; microorganism isolated from a blood culture; isolation of the microorganism by transtracheal aspirate, bronchial brushing, or biopsy; isolation of virus or detection of viral antigen in respiratory secretions; diagnostic antibody titer
A patient <12 months of age must have *two* of the following: apnea, tachypnea, bradycardia, wheezing, rhonchi, or cough with *any* of the following: increased production of respiratory secretions; new onset of purulent sputum; microorganism isolated from a blood culture; isolation of a pathogen from transtracheal aspirate, bronchial brushings, or biopsy; isolation of virus or detection of viral antigen in respiratory secretions; diagnostic antibody titer; histopathologic evidence of pneumonia
A patient <12 months of age has chest radiographic examination that demonstrates new or progressive infiltrate, cavitation, consolidation, or pleural effusion and *any* of the following: increased production of respiratory secretions; new onset of purulent sputum; microorganism isolated from the blood culture; isolation of a pathogen from transtracheal aspirate, bronchial brushing, or biopsy; isolation of virus or detection of viral antigen in respiratory secretions; diagnostic antibody titer; histopathologic evidence of pneumonia

Adapted from Garner JS, Jarvis WR, Emori; TG, et al. CDC definitions for nosocomial infections, 1988. *Am J Infect Control* 1988; 16:128–140, with permission.

Diagnosis

The optimal method for diagnosing nosocomial LRTI remains controversial. Historically, clinical presentation, chest radiograph, Gram stain, and culture of respiratory secretions have established the diagnosis. Unfortunately, this method of detection has probably overestimated the true incidence of disease, because other entities can be easily confused with LRTI in critically ill patients. Entities such as chemical aspiration, respiratory distress syndrome, pulmonary hemorrhage, lung contusion, atelectasis, congestive heart failure, pulmonary edema, pleural effusion, pulmonary emboli, or tumor may be confused with LRTI (97). Other conditions that can be confused with LRTI in infants and children include congenital heart disease, bronchopulmonary dysplasia, and cancer chemotherapy effects (80). Because of such controversy, the CDC has provided clinicians with guidelines for the definition of a nosocomial LRTI (10) (Table 49.5).

Culture results from specimens obtained from endotracheal tubes correlate poorly with those obtained from sterile sites such as lung, blood, or pleural fluid. Qualitative culture of specimens obtained from endotracheal tubes has failed to predict the causative agent of respiratory deterioration in infants and children (98). Quantitative culture of specimens obtained from endotracheal tubes using a diagnostic threshold of 10^6 colony-forming units (CFU)/mL, however, has been demonstrated to be superior to qualitative culture of endotracheal secretions and may be as useful as many of the invasive procedures (99,100). The difficulty in interpreting cultures of endotracheal secretions is accentuated by the fact that patients in intensive care units generally have abnormal chest radiographs regardless of whether infection is present (Fig. 49.1). Likewise, fever and leukocytosis are often present irrespective of the presence of an LRTI. Cough and sputum production are infrequently diagnostic of LRTI in intubated infants and children. If tracheal secretions are purulent, the differentiation between tracheobronchitis and LRTI may be difficult. Clinical suspicion, therefore, is needed to diagnose nosocomial LRTI.

A change in clinical status that is unexplained by other events is helpful in diagnosing nosocomial LRTI. Changes such as a drop in oxygenation, increased requirements for supplemental oxygen, fever or metabolic acidosis, or increasing ventilator requirements may be manifestations of nosocomial disease. These factors, combined with a new or progressive infiltrate on chest radiograph, should alert the clinician to a possible nosocomial LRTI. Although these criteria may lack sensitivity and specificity, they may be the only available parameters for the clinician.

Once a nosocomial LRTI is suspected, an attempt should be made to identify the specific etiologic agent. Microscopic examination of a Gram-stained smear of upper airway secretions may reveal the presence of polymorphonuclear cells and bacteria. As mentioned previously, however, cultures of these specimens, unless performed quantitatively, does not help to identify the etiologic agent. Although rarely positive, blood cultures may help in identifying the etiologic microorganism; culture of pleural fluid may also yield the etiologic agent. Transtracheal aspiration in nonintubated patients, percutaneous thin needle lung aspiration, and protected bronchoscopic sampling of the lower airways have all been suggested as methods to prevent

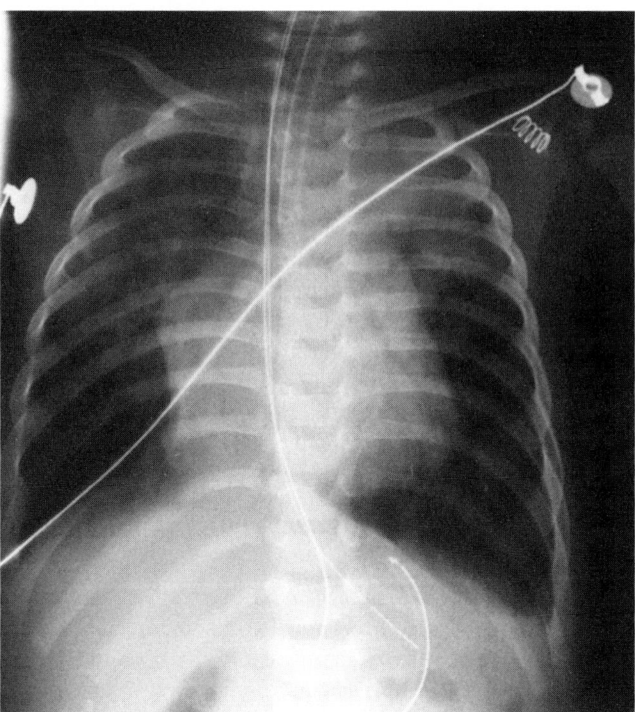

Figure 49.1. A chest radiograph demonstrating the difficulty in diagnosing a nosocomial lower respiratory tract infection in a child with respiratory distress syndrome.

contamination of lower respiratory tract secretions with upper airway flora. Transtracheal aspirations are difficult to perform, and bronchoscopic equipment for protected specimen collection cannot be used in infants and small children because of the small airways size. Percutaneous thin-needle aspiration is contraindicated in patients on mechanical ventilation because of an increased risk of complications. Therefore, the use of such techniques is severely limited in infants and children. Urine bacterial antigens can be helpful in diagnosing community-acquired LRTI, but their use in diagnosing nosocomial infections is limited because antigen tests are not available for the microorganisms that usually cause these infections. *Legionella* can be diagnosed through the use of special respiratory cultures, direct immunofluorescence of respiratory secretions, or indirect immunofluorescent antibody assay. Pertussis can be suspected in the unimmunized patient with a history of coughing to the point of vomiting, exposure to a known case, and lymphocytosis. Pertussis can also be diagnosed by the examination of nasopharyngeal secretions using direct immunofluorescence. Culture of *B. pertussis* requires inoculation of nasopharyngeal mucus onto special media (Regan-Lowe or Bordet-Gengou).

Prevention

The goal in preventing nosocomial LRTI is to reduce the colonization of the upper airways by potential pathogens; this reduces the potential for aspiration of microorganisms into the lower respiratory tract. To attain this goal, the problem may need to be approached in several different ways. The most important factor is strict compliance by healthcare workers with hand washing between patients. It has been demonstrated that approximately 50% of physicians and nurses fail to wash their hands after patient contact (101). Effective hand washing can prevent nosocomial LRTI, particularly in areas such as intensive care units. Various agents have been used for hand washing, including chlorhexidine, iodophors, quaternary ammonium compounds, and alcohols. Of these agents, chlorhexidine appears to reduce the nosocomial infection rate more effectively than others, but large field trials are lacking (102) (see Chapter 96). The volume and number of times that these chemicals are used may be an important determinant of the efficacy of hand washing in reducing the number of microorganisms on the hands (103). In addition to hand washing, employees should strictly comply with hospital infection control policies and isolation techniques. Patients infected or colonized with antibiotic-resistant microorganisms should be selectively grouped or isolated (cohorted).

Proper cleaning and disinfection of ventilator equipment is always important. Contaminated equipment has been incriminated in numerous outbreaks of respiratory infections (104). Such reports have pointed out that many respiratory devices are capable of harboring and spreading pathogenic microorganisms, including in-line medication nebulizers, ventilator tubing (particularly when condensate is present), bedside resuscitation bags, and endotracheal tubes. Only sterile fluids should be nebulized or used in a humidifier, disposable equipment should not be reused, personnel who have contact with respiratory secretions or intubated patients should wash their hands after delivering care, and ventilator circuit tubing should be changed no more often than every 48 hours. Although endotracheal suctioning may dislodge bacterial aggregates often found in the lumina of endotracheal tubes, endotracheal suctioning should be performed, as needed, to remove secretions (105).

The use of isolation techniques for high-risk patients hospitalized in intensive care units is controversial. Opponents of their use have demonstrated less patient interaction during isolation. In addition to lack of patient contact, hospital personnel were no more likely to wash their hands after patient contact. Isolation was felt to be an expensive and ineffective method of preventing nosocomial infections (106). Proponents of isolation, however, have demonstrated that colonization of the upper airways occurred later (12 vs. 7 days), there was a longer interval until the first infection (20 vs. 8 days), there was a lower daily infection rate, and there were fewer days with fever. The benefit of isolation was most notable after 7 days of intensive care and did not predispose patients to less contact with hospital personnel (107). Certain illnesses, however, always require isolation.

Patients admitted to the hospital with pertussis should be placed on droplet precautions for the first 5 days of antimicrobial therapy. This therapy does not change the course of the disease but renders the patient noninfectious. For hospital personnel exposed to the patient before the diagnosis of pertussis, chemoprophylaxis with erythromycin (40 to 50 mg/kg/day in four divided doses; maximum of 2 g) is indicated. If patients cannot take erythromycin, trimethoprim-sulfamethoxazole, azithromycin, or clarithromycin can be used. Therapies such as azithromycin have been well tolerated in treating hospital employees during hospital outbreaks (90,108). Prompt erythromycin chemoprophylaxis effectively limits secondary cases and is recommended regardless of age or immunization status, because pertussis immunity is not absolute. In addition to chemoprophylaxis, children younger than 7 years of age who are not immunized or have had fewer than four doses of vaccine should undergo initiation or continuation of pertussis immunization according to schedule. If a child received the third dose of vaccine 6 months or more before exposure, the fourth dose should be given as soon as possible after the exposure (109) (see also Chapter 81). Patients admitted with *Legionella* infection do not need to be isolated.

The role of the gastrointestinal tract as a source for endogenous upper airway colonization cannot be overlooked. Much of the attention has centered around the stomach, and it is quite clear that this organ can serve as a reservoir for pathogenic microorganisms; the esophagus may serve as a conduit for transmission of these microorganisms to the upper respiratory tract. The use of enteral feeding, antacids, and H_2-blockers in critically ill patients can elevate the gastric pH and facilitate gastric microbial colonization and growth (110,111). These medications are used in intensive care patients for prophylaxis against upper gastrointestinal bleeding. If these medications are indicated, it is important to choose an agent that does not elevate the gastric pH (103). In patients who have received prophylaxis with sucralfate, for example, a lower gastric pH and fewer nosocomial LRTIs have been demonstrated (112).

Reports have suggested that selective decontamination of the digestive tract with nonabsorbable antimicrobial agents can prevent the development of nosocomial infections in patients receiving mechanical ventilation. Recent reports about the use of selective decontamination however, have demonstrated that it adds substantially to the cost of hospitalization, increases the potential for infections with resistant microorganisms, and has not been well accepted among clinicians (113–116). Many antimicrobial agents have been used, including colistin, tobramycin, gentamicin, polymyxin, nystatin, and amphotericin B. Although many of the preliminary studies were encouraging, such procedures are not currently the standard of care (105). Furthermore, data concerning selective decontamination in preventing nosocomial LRTI in infants and children are lacking at this time. (Pneumonia in adult patients is covered in Chapter 22.)

SKIN INFECTIONS

Cutaneous infections of infants and children have been reported to occur in 5% to 74% of nosocomial infections, with the highest rates occurring in neonatal intensive care units (1–9). Although most reported infections are associated with intravenous catheter sites, there is always a concern for the development of more invasive disease (i.e., bacteremia). Most of these infections are due to microorganisms already colonizing the patient or are transmitted to the patient via the hands of hospital personnel. In addition to poor hand washing, overcrowding and understaffing lead to an increase in infections. These infections commonly present as an intravenous catheter-site infection; impetigo; cellulitis; or, less commonly, a life-threatening infection such as necrotizing fasciitis.

Catheter-Site Infections

Hospitalized infants and children usually require venous access while receiving medical therapy. Most venous access is obtained by cannulation of peripheral veins. Occasionally, more critically ill patients require cannulation of larger vessels. Phlebitis is the most common complication associated with peripheral vein cannulation (117,118). Catheters in the antecubital fossa, the arm, or the leg and those used for hyperalimentation are among those most often complicated by phlebitis. Colonization rates of between 4% and 13% occur after these catheters have been in place for 48 hours and increases to more than 30% if left in for longer than 6 days (117–121). The coagulase-negative staphylococci (i.e., *S. epidermidis, Staphylococcus hominis, Staphylococcus warnerii*) are the most common microorganisms isolated, but colonization may occur with other microorganisms from the hospital flora. These colonized catheters then become a nidus for infection that may result in cutaneous infection or bacteremia.

Materials used for venous catheters may affect colonization rates as well. It has been proposed that some microorganisms can actually metabolize components of the plastic catheters in the absence of other nutrients and use them to sustain growth on the surface of biomaterials (122). Polyvinyl chloride and siliconized latex catheters have been demonstrated to have higher colonization rates than polyurethane, Vialon, or Teflon catheters (123). Antibiotic and chlorhexidine-sliver sulfadiazine coating of catheters may be antiinfective and prevent colonization for short periods of time (up to 1 week) (124). Pediatric scalp vein needles, however, have been associated with a marked decrease in colonization and infections (125). This may be true, because these needles cause less trauma to the vein, are shorter, and tend to stay in place for a shorter period.

To avoid catheter-related infections, the skin should be disinfected before catheter insertion. Skin may be disinfected with chlorhexidine, an iodophor, or alcohol (126). Quaternary ammonium compounds should not be used. The catheter site and cannulated vein should be inspected daily for signs of inflammation and the catheter removed promptly if they occur. The date and time of insertion should be labeled on the dressing of catheters to ensure removal after 72 hours. If phlebitis or a local abscess should develop, the entire infusion system, including the bag of intravenous fluid, tubing, and needle or catheter should be removed. If purulent material is present, it should be Gram stained and cultured.

Suppurative thrombophlebitis is a life-threatening complication of intravenous catheter placement. When catheter-associated bacteremia does not respond to catheter removal and appropriate antimicrobial therapy, this diagnosis should be considered. The diagnosis may be established by examination of the catheter site. In suppurative thrombophlebitis, purulent material can sometimes be expressed from the catheter site. Occasionally, an exploratory venotomy is needed to locate the purulence. Most responsible microorganisms tend to be gram-positive agents; *S. aureus* is often encountered (127).

Semipermanent indwelling catheters [e.g., Infuse-a-ports, Broviac, peripherally inserted catheter (PIC) lines] are now widely used in children undergoing chemotherapy or long-term parenteral nutrition. Approximately 5% to 30% of these central venous catheters develop infectious complications. Local infections such as exit-site infections or tunnel infections may develop. Microorganisms may gain access to the space between the catheter and the subcutaneous tissue during catheter insertion or migrate into the catheter tract after insertion. *S. aureus* or coagulase-negative staphylococci (i.e., *S. epidermidis*) cause the majority of these infections. The entrance site (point at which the catheter enters the vein) or intravascular portion of the catheter may also became infected. These latter infections are often associated with bacteremia (see also Chapters 17 and 18).

Prevention

Prevention of such complications requires effective disinfection of the skin before insertion of the catheter. There is little information on the relationship of infection and the type of antiseptic used to decontaminate the skin before insertion of the catheter. In one trial, however, preparation of the skin with chlorhexidine was associated with fewer infections than when alcohol or iodophor preparations were used to disinfect the skin (128). Once the central venous catheters have been inserted, investigators have demonstrated that application of iodophor ointments to the site are ineffective in decreasing catheter-related infections and that polyantibiotic ointments decrease the incidence of bacterial colonization but increase the risk of fungal colonization (129). Infections are associated with the type of dressings used as well. Transparent dressings have been associated with increased colonization and infection rates as compared to gauze dressings (130). Although these dressings adhere well and are transparent and easy to use, they are not perfectly semipermeable. Moisture becomes trapped under the dressing, which increases the colonization of the site. These dressings can be used safely, however, it they are changed every 48 hours or three times weekly (131).

Impetigo

Impetigo contagiosa is a contagious superficial infection of the skin. The causative agent is usually *S. pyogenes* alone or in combination with *S. aureus.* Bullous impetigo is caused almost exclusively by *S. aureus.* Although this disorder is seen commonly in the community, impetiginous lesions often develop while patients are hospitalized and reflect the flora of the hospital. This infection occurs most often in the diaper region as a complication of diaper dermatitis. Usually, local care with soap and water or antimicrobial cream effectively eradicates the infection. Occasionally, parenteral therapy is indicated, and the agents chosen should be active against *Staphylococcus* species and *Streptococcus* species. Close attention to hand washing among hospital personnel and routine baths for the patients help alleviate this problem. Patients with impetigo should be placed on contact precautions.

Staphylococcal scalded skin syndrome is an unusual skin infection caused by exfoliative toxin-producing strains of *S. aureus.* The syndrome starts as a bullous lesion and may spread to involve the entire body. The microorganism enters the skin through an area of trauma, such as a circumcision or other surgical procedure. It is generally spread on the hands of healthcare personnel or a family member. The microorganism is more likely to be recovered from the nares than the lesion itself. Preferred treatment is a semisynthetic penicillin. Isolates should be saved for typing if an outbreak is suspected (132).

Cellulitis

Cellulitis is an acute inflammation of the skin and subcutaneous tissues that may be associated with fever, warmth, erythema, edema, tenderness, lymphadenopathy, and an elevated peripheral leukocyte count (133). This illness may represent a primary infection of the skin or may be secondary to bacteremia. *S. aureus* or *S. pyogenes* most commonly causes cellulitis of the extremities. In infants, in addition to *S. aureus,* GBS is a predominant microorganism. With facial involvement, *S. pneumoniae* is currently the most common cause, but *H. influenzae* type B should be considered as a potential pathogen in infants younger than 1 year who are not completely immunized. Nosocomial cellulitis most commonly involves microorganisms endemic to the hospital or endogenous to the patient. The diagnosis of cellulitis is based on physical examination. Aspiration of the leading edge or the area most intensely involved by the cellulitis may aid in identifying a microorganism. Most patients are not bacteremic unless they appear toxic.

Omphalitis is a severe form of cellulitis affecting the newborn infant. This usually results from colonization of the umbilical cord by *S. pyogenes.* In more recent years, gram-negative microorganisms have become more prominent causes of omphalitis because of the use of prophylactic agents on the umbilical cord (134). Funisitis usually begins as a wet, malodorous umbilical stump with minimal inflammation. Inflammation may continue to develop and may spread to involve the wall of the abdomen. Patients with severe forms of omphalitis may develop necrotizing fasciitis. The infants become irritable, and a cellulitis surrounding the umbilical cord is noted on physical examination. Dissemination into the bloodstream is uncommon but may occur.

Adequate cord care is the key to preventing complications such as omphalitis. A single application of triple dye to the cord results in significant reduction of all bacteria, including staphylococci, streptococcal species, and coliforms. Triple dye, however, has only limited effectiveness in preventing colonization with methicillin-resistant *S. aureus* (135). After the application of triple dye, the umbilical cord should be kept clean with soap and water. If the cord becomes wet or malodorous, it can be routinely cleaned with alcohol. Good hand-washing technique should always be used, and immediate isolation of a single infant who develops omphalitis from *S. pyogenes* should be instituted. Infection control measures for identification and segregation of all colonized infants is necessary.

Necrotizing Fasciitis

Necrotizing fasciitis is a rapidly progressive soft tissue infection involving the skin, subcutaneous tissue, and superficial fascia. It is a rare but life-threatening complication following surgery or trauma in the infant or child. The infection may begin in an operative site or at the site of an injury, or it may develop without apparent cause. The infection spreads rapidly along fas-

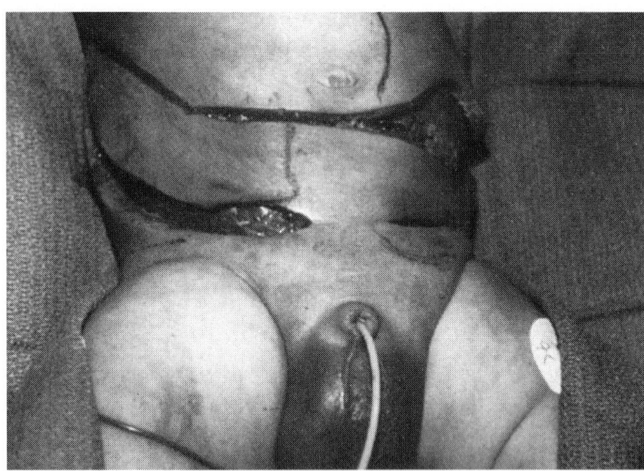

Figure 49.2. A patient has undergone the wide surgical debridement needed for treatment of necrotizing fasciitis.

cial planes, producing thrombosis of nutrient vessels, which results in necrosis of overlying subcutaneous tissue and skin. Although *S. pyogenes* was initially described as the causative microorganism for this disorder, the infection in most individuals is polymicrobial (136). This disorder has been described in postoperative cases after appendectomy, inguinal herniorrhaphy, and circumcision.

The diagnosis of necrotizing fasciitis is based on clinical findings. Adults usually demonstrate a triad of cellulitis, crepitus, and the presence of gas in tissues on a radiograph. Children usually do not manifest these findings. In infants and children, the diagnosis should be considered when a patient develops a new case of cellulitis with an area of induration that far exceeds the area of erythema. The patient appears toxic out of proportion to the area of cellulitis (137). Gas or crepitus is uncommon in infants and children. The treatment for necrotizing fasciitis demands early wide surgical debridement and broad-spectrum antimicrobial agents (Fig. 49.2). To prevent necrotizing fasciitis, good hand washing and meticulous wound care are needed.

REFERENCES

1. Jarvis WR. Epidemiology of nosocomial infections in pediatric patients. *Pediatr Infect Dis* 1987;6:344–351.
2. Maguire GC, Nordin J, Myers MG, et al. Infections acquired by young infants. *Am J Dis Child* 1981;135:693–698.
3. Ford-Jones EL, Mindorff CM, Langley JM, et al. Epidemiologic study of 4684 hospital-acquired infections in pediatric patients. *Pediatr Infect Dis* 1989;8:668–675.
4. Hemming VG, Overall JC Jr, Britt MR. Nosocomial infections in a newborn intensive-care unit: results of forty-one months of surveillance. *N Engl J Med* 1976;294:1310–1316.
5. Daschner F. Analysis of bacterial infections in a neonatal intensive care unit. *J Hosp Infect* 1983:4:90–91.
6. Goldmann DA, Durbin WA Jr, Freeman J. Nosocomial infections in a neonatal intensive care unit. *J Infect Dis* 1981;144:449–459.
7. Gaynes RP, Edwards JR, Jarvis WR, et al. Nosocomial infections among neonates in high risk nurseries in the United States. *Pediatrics* 1996;98:357–361.
8. Brown RB, Hosmer D, Chen HC, et al. A comparison of infections in different ICUs within the same hospital. *Crit Care Med* 1985,13:472–476.
9. Milliken J, Tait GA, Ford-Jones EL, et al. Nosocomial infections in a pediatric intensive care unit. *Crit Care Med* 1988;16:233–237.
10. Garner JS, Jarvis WR, Emori TG, et al. CDC definitions for nosocomial infections, 1988. *Am J Infect Control* 1988;16:128–140.
11. Brook I. Brain abscess in children: microbiology and management. *J Child Neurol* 1995;10:283–288.
12. Johnson DL, Markle BM, Wiedermann BL, et al. Treatment of intracranial abscesses associated with sinusitis in children and adolescents. *J Pediatr* 1988;113:15–23.
13. Jadavji T, Humphreys RP, Prober CG. Brain abscesses in infants and children. *Pediatr Infect Dis* 1985;4:394–398.
14. Saez-Llorens XJ, Umana MA, Odio CM, et al. Brain abscess in infants and children. *Pediatr Infect Dis* 1989;8:449–458.
15. Patrick CC, Kaplan SL. Current concepts in the pathogenesis and management of brain abscesses in children. *Pediatr Clin North Am* 1988;35:625–636.
16. Idriss ZH, Gutman LT, Kronfol NM. Brain abscesses in infants and children: current status of clinical findings, management and prognosis. *Clin Pediatr* 1978;17:738–746.
17. Fischer EG, McLennan JE, Suzuki Y. Cerebral abscess in children. *Am J Dis Child* 1981;135:746–749.
18. Dajani AS, Taubert KA, Wilson W, et al. Prevention of bacterial endocarditis: recommendations by the American Heart Association. *JAMA* 1997;277:1794–1801.
19. Shapiro M. Prophylaxis in otolaryngologic surgery and neurosurgery: a critical review. *Rev Infect Dis* 1991;13:S858–S868.
20. Shapiro M, Wald U, Simchen E, et al. Randomized clinical trial of intra-operative antimicrobial prophylaxis of infection after neurosurgical procedures. *J Hosp Infect* 1986;8:283–295.
21. Young RF, Lawner PM. Perioperative antibiotic prophylaxis for prevention of postoperative neurosurgical infections: a randomized clinical trial. *J Neurosurg* 1987;66:701–705.
22. Blomstedt GC, Kytta J. Results of a randomized trial of vancomycin prophylaxis in craniotomy. *J Neurosurg* 1988;69:216–220.
23. Bullock R, van Dellen JR, Ketelbey W, et al. A double-blind placebo-controlled trial of perioperative prophylactic antibiotics for elective neurosurgery. *J Neurosurg* 1988;69:687–691.
24. Van Ek B, Dijkmans BAC, van Dulken H, et al. Antibiotic prophylaxis in craniotomy: a prospective double-blind placebo-controlled study. *Scand J Infect Dis* 1988;20:633–639.
25. Holloway KL, Smith EW, Wilberger JE Jr, et al. Antibiotic prophylaxis during clean neurosurgery: a large multicenter study using cefuroxime. *Clin Ther* 1996;18:84–94.
26. Feigin RD, McCracken GH, Klein JO. Diagnosis and management of meningitis. *Pediatr Infect Dis* 1992;11:785–814.
27. Broadhurst LE, Erickson RL, Kelley PW. Decreases in invasive *Hemophilus influenzae* diseases in the US army children, 1984 through 1991. *JAMA* 1993;269:227–231.
28. Spanjaard L, Bol P, Zanen HC. Non-neonatal meningitis due to less common bacterial pathogens, the Netherlands, 1975–1983. *J Hyg (Cambridge)* 1986;97:219–228.
29. Kim JH, van der Horst C, Mulrow CD, et al. *Staphylococcus aureus* meningitis: review of 28 cases. *Rev Infect Dis* 1989;11:698–705.
30. Givner LB, Kaplan SL. Meningitis due to *Staphylococcus aureus* in children. *Clin Infect Dis* 1993;16:766–771.
31. Barton LL, Granoff DM, Barenkamp SJ. Nosocomial spread of *Hemophilus influenzae* type b infection documented by outer membrane protein subtype analysis. *J Pediatr* 1983;102:820–824.
32. Klein JO, Marcy SM. Bacterial sepsis and meningitis. In: Remington JS, Klein JO, eds. *Infectious diseases of the fetus and newborn infant,* 4th ed. Philadelphia: WB Saunders, 1995:835–890.
33. Campbell JR, Diacovo T, Baker CJ. *Serratia marcescens* meningitis in neonates. *Pediatr Infect Dis* 1992;11:881–886.
34. Cichon MJ, Craig CP, Sargent J, et al. Nosocomial *Klebsiella* infections in an intensive care nursery. *South Med J* 1977;70:33–35.
35. Graham DR, Anderson RL, Ariel FE, et al. Epidemic nosocomial meningitis due to *Citrobacter diversus* in neonates. *J Infect Dis* 1981; 144:203–209.
36. American Academy of Pediatrics, Committee on Infectious Diseases.

Report of the Committee on Infectious Diseases, 23rd ed. Elk Grove Village, IL: American Academy of Pediatrics, 1997:357–362.

37. Hart CA, Rogers TRF. Meningococcal disease. *J Med Microbiol* 1993; 39:3–25.
38. Centers for Disease Control and Prevention. Control and prevention of meningococcal disease and control and prevention of serogroup C meningococcal disease: evaluation and management of suspected outbreaks. *MMWR Morb Mortal Wkly Rep* 1997;46(RR-5):1–21.
39. Schwartz B, Al-Tobaiqi A, Al-Ruwais, et al. Comparative efficacy of ceftriaxone and rifampin in eradicating pharyngeal carriage of group A *Neisseria meningitidis. Lancet* 1988;1:1239–1242.
40. Pugsley MP, Dworzack DL, Roccaforte JS, et al. An open study of the efficacy of a single dose of ciprofloxacin in eliminating the chronic nasopharyngeal carriage of *Neisseria meningitidis. J Infect Dis* 1988; 157:852–853.
41. Rathore MH. Do prophylactic antibiotics prevent meningitis after basilar skull fracture? *Pediatr Infect Dis J* 1991;10:87–88.
42. Mohle-Boetani JC, Schuchat A, Plikaytis BD, et al. Comparison of prevention strategies for neonatal group B streptococcal infection: a population-based economic analysis. *JAMA* 1993;270:1442–1448.
43. Committee on Infectious Diseases and Committee on Fetus and Newborn, American Academy of Pediatrics. Revised guidelines for prevention of early-onset group B streptococcal (GBS) infection. *Pediatrics* 1997;99:489–496.
44. Schoenbaum SC, Gardner P, Shillito J. Infections of cerebrospinal fluid shunts: epidemiology, clinical manifestations, and therapy. *J Infect Dis* 1975;131:543–552.
45. Odio C, McCracken GH, Nelson JD. CSF shunt infections in pediatrics: a seven-year experience. *Am J Dis Child* 1984;138:1103–1108.
46. Ronan A, Hogg GG, Klug GL. Cerebrospinal fluid shunt infections in children. *Pediatr Infect Dis J* 1995;14:782–786.
47. Haines SJ, Taylor F. Prophylactic methicillin for shunt operations: effects on incidence of shunt malfunction and infection. *Childs Brain* 1982;9:10–22.
48. Sekhar LN, Moossy J, Guthkelch AN. Malfunctioning ventriculoperitoneal shunts: clinical and pathological features. *J Neurosurg* 1982; 56:411–416.
49. Yogev R, Davis AT. Neurosurgical shunt infections: a review. *Childs Brain* 1980:6:74–81.
50. Pudenz RH. The ventriculo-atrial shunt. *J Neurosurg* 1966;25: 602–608.
51. Schimke RT, Black PH, Mark VH, et al. Indolent *Staphylococcus albus* or *aureus* bacteremia after ventriculoatriostomy: role of foreign body in its initiation and perpetuation. *N Engl J Med* 1961;264:264–270.
52. Lerman SJ. *Hemophilus influenzae* infections of cerebrospinal fluid shunts: report of two cases. *J Neurosurg* 1981;54:261–263.
53. Rekate HL, Ruch T, Nulsen FE. Diphtheroid infections of cerebrospinal fluid shunts: the changing pattern of shunt infection in Cleveland. *J Neurosurg* 1980;52:553–556.
54. Skinner PR, Taylor AJ, Coakham H. Propionibacteria as a cause of shunt and postneurosurgical infections. *J Clin Pathol* 1978;31: 1085–1090.
55. Riebel W, Frantz N, Adelstein D, et al. *Corynebacterium* JK: a cause of nosocomial device-related infection. *Rev Infect Dis* 1986;8:42–49.
56. Rieder MJ, Frewen TC, Del Maestro RF, et al. The effect of cephalothin prophylaxis on postoperative ventriculoperitoneal shunt infections. *Can Med Assoc J* 1987;136:935–938.
57. Graman PS, Hall CB. Nosocomial viral respiratory infections. *Semin Respir Infect* 1989;4:253–260.
58. American Academy of Pediatrics, Committee on Infectious Diseases. *Report of the Committee on Infectious Diseases,* 23rd ed. Elk Grove Village, IL: American Academy of Pediatrics, 1997:483–494.
59. Donnelly BW, McMillan JA, Weiner LB. Bacterial tracheitis: report of eight new cases and review. *Rev Infect Dis* 1990;12:729–735.
60. Brook I. Aerobic and anaerobic microbiology of bacterial tracheitis in children. *Pediatr Emerg Care* 1997;13:16–18.
61. American Academy of Pediatrics, Committee on Infectious Diseases. *Report of the Committee on Infectious Diseases,* 26th ed. Elk Grove Village, IL: American Academy of Pediatrics, 2003:265.
62. Wald ER. Sinusitis in children. *N Engl J Med* 1992;326:319–323.
63. Tinkelman DG, Silk HJ. Clinical and bacteriologic features of chronic sinusitis in children. *Am J Dis Child* 1989;143:938–941.
64. Wald ER. Chronic sinusitis in children. *J Pediatr* 1995;127:339–347.
65. Muntz HR, Lusk RP. Bacteriology of the ethmoid bullae in children with chronic sinusitis. *Arch Otolaryngol Head Neck Surg* 1991;117: 179–181.
66. Brook I. Microbiology of nosocomial sinusitis in mechanically ventilated children. *Arch Otolaryngol Head Neck Surg* 1998;124:35–38.
67. Desmond P, Raman R, Idikula J. Effect of nasogastric tubes on the nose and maxillary sinus. *Crit Care Med* 1991;19:509–511.
68. Bach A, Boehrer H, Schmidt H, et al. Nosocomial sinusitis in ventilated patients. Nasotracheal versus orotracheal intubation. *Anaesthesiology* 1992;47:335–339.
69. Grindlinger GA, Niehoff J, Hughes SL, et al. Acute paranasal sinusitis related to nasotracheal intubation of head injured patients. *Crit Care Med* 1987;15:214–217.
70. Hansen M, Poulsen MR, Bendixen DK, et al. Incidence of sinusitis in patients with nasotracheal intubation. *Br J Anaesth* 1988;61:231–232.
71. Boles JM. Upper respiratory tract infections in patients with tracheal intubation. *Rev Praticien* 1990;40:2341–2343.
72. McAlister WH, Lusk R, Muntz HR. Comparison of plain radiographs and coronal CT scans in infants and children with recurrent sinusitis. *Am J Roentgenol* 1989;153:1259–1264.
73. Klein JO. Otitis media. *Clin Infect Dis* 1994;19:823–833.
74. Kenna MA, Bluestone CD. Microbiology of chronic suppurative otitis media in children. *Pediatr Infect Dis J* 1986;5:223–225.
75. Derkay CS, Bluestone CD, Thompson AE, et al. Otitis media in the pediatric intensive care unit: a prospective study. *Otolaryngol Head Neck Surg* 1989;100:292–299.
76. Carlin SA, Marchant CD, Shurin PA, et al. Early recurrences of otitis media: reinfection or relapse? *J Pediatr* 1987;110:20–25.
77. Harrison CJ, Marks MI, Welch DF. Microbiology of recently treated acute otitis media compared with previously untreated acute otitis media. *Pediatr Infect Dis* 1985;4:641–646.
78. Bernard PAM, Stenstrom RJ, Feldman W, et al. Randomized, controlled trial comparing long-term sulfonamide therapy to ventilation tubes for otitis media with effusion. *Pediatrics* 1991;88:215–222.
79. Paradise JL. Antimicrobial drugs and surgical procedures in the prevention of otitis media. *Pediatr Infect Dis J* 1989;8:S35–37.
80. Jacobs RF. Nosocomial pneumonia in children. *Infection* 1991;19: 64–72.
81. Busse WW. Pathogenesis and sequelae of respiratory infections. *Rev Infect Dis* 1991;13:S477–485.
82. Schwartz SN, Dowling JN, Benkovic C, et al. Sources of gram-negative bacilli colonizing the trachea of intubated patients. *J Infect Dis* 1978;138:227–231.
83. Crouch TN, Higuchi JH, Coalson JJ, et al. Pathogenesis and prevention of nosocomial pneumonia in a nonhuman primate model of acute respiratory failure. *Am Rev Respir Dis* 1984;130:502–504.
84. Craven DE, Kunches LM, Kilinsky V, et al. Risk factors for pneumonia and fatality in patients receiving continuous mechanical ventilation. *Am Rev Respir Dis* 1986;133:792–796.
85. Graybill JR, Marshall LW, Charache P, et al. Nosocomial pneumonia: a continuing major problem. *Am Rev Respir Dis* 1973;108: 1130–1140.
86. National Nosocomial Infections Surveillance Systems. National Nosocomial Infections Surveillance (NNIS) report, data summary from October 1986–April 1997, issued May 1997. *Am J Infect Control* 1997;25:477–487.
87. Brady MT. Nosocomial legionnaires disease in a children's hospital. *J Pediatr* 1989;115:46–50.
88. Carlson NC, Kuskie MR, Dobyns EL, et al. Legionellosis in children: an expanding spectrum. *Pediatr Infect Dis J* 1990;9:133–137.
89. Aoyama T, Takeuchi Y, Goto A, et al. Pertussis in adults. *Am J Dis Child* 1992;146:163–166.
90. Martines SM, Kemper CA, Haiduven D, et al. Azithromycin prophylaxis during a hospitalwide outbreak of a pertussis-like illness. *Infect Control Hosp Epid* 2002;22:781–783.
91. Christie CD, Glover AM, Wilke MJ, et al. Containment of pertussis

in the regional pediatric hospital during the Greater Cincinnati epidemic of 1993. *Infect Control Hosp Epidemiol* 1995;16:556–563.
92. Starke JR, Jacobs RF, Jereb J. Resurgence of tuberculosis in children. *J Pediatr* 1992;120:839–855.
93. Hall SL. Coagulase-negative staphylococcal infections in neonates. *Pediatr Infect Dis* 1991;10:57–67.
94. Rettig PJ. Infections due to *Chlamydia trachomatis* from infancy to adolescence. *Pediatr Infect Dis J* 1986;5:449–457.
95. Ollikainen J, Hiekkaniemi H, Korppi M, et al. Ureaplasma urealyticum infection associated with acute respiratory insufficiency and death in premature infants. *J Pediatr* 1993;122:756–760.
96. Valencia GB, Banzon F, Cummings M, et al. *Mycoplasma hominis* and *Ureaplasma urealyticum* in neonates with suspected infection. *Pediatr Infect Dis J* 1993;12:571–573.
97. Meduri GU. Ventilator-associated pneumonia in patients with respiratory failure: a diagnostic approach. *Chest* 1990;97:1208–1219.
98. Thureen PJ, Moreland S, Rodden DJ, et al. Failure of tracheal aspirate cultures to define the cause of respiratory deteriorations in neonates. *Pediatr Infect Dis J* 1993;12:560–564.
99. Torres A, Martos A, De La Bellacasa JP, et al. Specificity of endotracheal aspiration, protected specimen brush, and bronchoalveolar lavage in mechanically ventilated patients. *Am Rev Respir Dis* 1993; 147:952–957.
100. Marquette CH, Georges H, Wallet F, et al. Diagnostic efficiency of endotracheal aspirates with quantitative bacterial cultures in intubated patients with suspected pneumonia: comparison with the protected specimen brush. *Am Rev Respir Dis* 1993;148:138–144.
101. De Carvalho M, Lopes JMA, Pellitteri M. Frequency and duration of handwashing in a neonatal intensive care unit. *Pediatr Infect Dis J* 1989;8:179–180.
102. Doebbeling BN, Stanley GL, Sheetz CT, et al. Comparative efficacy of alternative hand-washing agents in reducing nosocomial infections in intensive care units. *N Engl J Med* 1992;327:88–93.
103. Larson E. A causal link between handwashing and risk of infection? Examination of the evidence. *Infect Control Hosp Epidemiol* 1988;9: 28–36.
104. Centers for Disease Control and Prevention. Guidelines for prevention of nosocomial pneumonia. *MMWR Morb Mortal Wkly Rep* 1997; 46(RR-1):1–79.
105. Nelson S, Chidiac C, Summer WR. New strategies for preventing nosocomial pneumonia: which common interventions leave patients at increased risk? *J Crit Illness* 1988;3:12–24.
106. Donowitz LG. Failure of the overgown to prevent nosocomial infection in a pediatric intensive care unit. *Pediatrics* 1986;77:35–38.
107. Klein BS, Perloff WH, Maki DG. Reduction of nosocomial infection during pediatric intensive care by protective isolation. *N Engl J Med* 1989;320:1714–1720.
108. Weber DJ, Rutala WA. Pertussis: a continuing hazard for healthcare facilities. *Infect Control Hosp Epid* 2002;22:736–739.
109. American Academy of Pediatrics, Committee on Infectious Diseases. *Report of the Committee on Infectious Diseases,* 26th ed. Elk Grove Village, IL: American Academy of Pediatrics, 2003:475–486.
110. Pingleton SK, Hinthorn DR, Liu C. Enteral nutrition in patients receiving mechanical ventilation: multiple sources of tracheal colonization includes the stomach. *Am J Med* 1986;80:827–832.
111. Du Moulin GC, Hedley-Whyte J, Paterson DG, et al. Aspiration of gastric bacteria in antacid-treated patients: a frequent cause of postoperative colonization of the airway. *Lancet* 1982;1:242–245.
112. Driks MR, Craven DE, Celli BR, et al. Nosocomial pneumonia in intubated patients given sucralfate as compared with antacids or histamine type 2 blockers: the role of gastric colonization. *N Engl J Med* 1987;317:1376–1382.
113. Wiener J, Itokazu G, Nathan C, et al. A randomized, doubled-blind, placebo controlled trial of selective digestive decontamination in a medical-surgical intensive care unit. *Clin Infect Dis* 1995;20:861–867.
114. Verwaest C, Verhaegen J, Ferdinande P, et al. Randomized, controlled trial of selective digestive decontamination in 600 mechanically ventilated patients in a multidisciplinary intensive care unit. *Crit Care Med* 1997;25:63–71.
115. Misset B, Aritgas A, Bihari D, et al. Short term impact of the European Consensus Conference on the use of selective decontamination of the digestive tract with antibiotics in ICU patients. *Intensive Care Med* 1996;22:981–984.
116. Flaherty J, Nathan C, Kabins SA, et al. Pilot trial of selective decontamination for prevention of bacterial infection in an intensive care unit. *J Infect Dis* 1990;162:1393–1397.
117. Garland JS, Dunne WM Jr, Havens P, et al. Peripheral intravenous catheter complications in critically ill children: a prospective study. *Pediatrics* 1992;89:1145–1150.
118. Pearson ML, Hierholzer WJ Jr, Garner JS, et al. Guideline for prevention of intravascular device-related infections. Part I. Intravascular device-related infections: an overview. *Am J Infect Control* 1996;24: 262–277.
119. Garland JS, Nelson DB, Cheah TE, et al. Infectious complications during peripheral intravenous therapy with Teflon7 catheters: a prospective study. *Pediatr Infect Dis J* 1987;6:918–921.
120. Batton DG, Maisels M, Appelbaum P. Use of peripheral intravenous cannulas in premature infants: a controlled study. *Pediatrics* 1982; 70:487–490.
121. Cronin WA, Germanson TP, Donowitz LG. Intravascular catheter colonization and related bloodstream infection in critically ill neonates. *Infect Control Hosp Epidemiol* 1990;11:301–308.
122. Franson TR, Sheth NK, Menon L, et al. Persistent in vitro survival of coagulase-negative staphylococci adherent to intravascular catheters in the absence of conventional nutrients. *J Clin Microbiol* 1986;24: 559–561.
123. Lopez-Lopez G, Pascual A, Perea EJ. Effect of plastic catheter material on bacterial adherence and viability. *J Med Microbiol* 1991;34: 349–353.
124. Walder B, Pittet D, Tramier MR. Prevention of bloodstream infections with central venous catheters treated with anti-infective agents depends on catheter type and insertion time: evidence from a meta-analysis. *Infection Control Hosp Epidemiol* 2002;23:748–756.
125. Peter G, Lloyd-Still JD, Lovejoy FH. Local infection and bacteremia from scalp vein needles and polyethylene catheters in children. *J Pediatr* 1972;80:78– 83.
126. Hospital Infection Control Practices Advisory Committee. Part II. Recommendations for the prevention of nosocomial intravascular device-related infections. *Am J Infect Control* 1996;24:277–293.
127. Khan EA, Correa AG, Baker CJ. Suppurative thrombophlebitis in children: a ten-year experience. *Pediatr Infect Dis J* 1997;16:63–67.
128. Maki DG, Ringer M, Alvarado CJ. Prospective randomised trial of povidone-iodine, alcohol, and chlorhexidine for prevention of infection associated with central venous and arterial catheters. *Lancet* 1991; 338:339–343.
129. Flowers RH, Schwenzer KJ, Kopel RF, et al. Efficacy of an attachable subcutaneous cuff for the prevention of intravascular catheter-related infections: a randomized controlled trial. *JAMA* 1989;261:878–883.
130. Conly JM, Grieves K, Peters B. A prospective, randomized study comparing transparent and dry gauze dressings for central venous catheters. *J Infect Dis* 1989;159:310–319.
131. Curchoe RM, Powers J, El-Daher N. Weekly transparent dressing changes linked to increased bacteremia rates. *Infect Control Hosp Epidemiol* 2002;23:730–732.
132. Darmstadt GL. The skin: cutaneous bacterial infections. In: Behrman RE, Kliegman RM, Jenson HB, eds. *Nelson textbook of pediatrics,* 16th ed. Philadelphia: WB Saunders, 2000:2028–2036.
133. Magee JS, Schutze GE. Bacterial infections of the skin. *Semin Pediatr Infect Dis* 1997;8:215–219.
134. Mason WH, Andrews R, Ross LA, et al. Omphalitis in the newborn infant. *Pediatr Infect Dis J* 1989;8:521–525.
135. Rosenfeld CR, Laptook AR, Jeffery J. Limited effectiveness of triple dye in preventing colonization with methicillin-resistant *Staphylococcus aureus* in a special care nursery. *Pediatr Infect Dis J* 1990;9: 290–291.
136. Quinonez JM, Steele RW. Necrotizing fasciitis. *Semin Pediatr Infect Dis* 1997;8:207–214.
137. Farrell LD, Karl SR, Davis PK, et al. Postoperative necrotizing fasciitis in children. *Pediatrics* 1988;82:874–879.

50

NOSOCOMIAL GASTROINTESTINAL TRACT INFECTIONS IN PEDIATRIC PATIENTS

DOUGLAS K. MITCHELL

Gastrointestinal tract infections are a major cause of morbidity and mortality in children worldwide. Data from a group of private hospitals showed that gastroenteritis was the leading reason for hospital admission of children in their population (1). Children can develop diarrhea as the result of infections acquired before hospital admission or during hospitalization. Either mode of acquisition may result in significant complications including dehydration, chronic diarrhea, prolonged hospitalization, and death. Each child infected with an enteropathogen may then become a potential source of further spread within the hospital population.

The Centers for Disease Control and Prevention (CDC) defines nosocomial gastrointestinal system infections, as "gastroenteritis, hepatitis, necrotizing enterocolitis, gastrointestinal tract infections, and intra-abdominal infections not specified elsewhere." In this chapter, we address nosocomial gastroenteritis as defined by the CDC (2):

Gastroenteritis must meet either of the following criteria:

1. Acute onset of diarrhea (liquid stools for more than 12 hours) with or without vomiting or fever (>38°C) AND no likely noninfectious cause (e.g., diagnostic tests, therapeutic regimen, acute exacerbation of a chronic condition, psychologic stress)
2. Two of the following with no other recognized cause: nausea, vomiting, abdominal pain, or headache AND any of the following:
   a. Enteric pathogen isolated from stool or rectal swab culture
   b. Enteric pathogen detected by routine or electron microscopy (EM) examination
   c. Enteric pathogen detected by antigen or antibody assay on feces or blood
   d. Evidence of enteric pathogen detected by cytopathic changes in tissue culture (toxin assay)
   e. Diagnostic single antibody titer [immunoglobulin M (IgM)] or fourfold increase in paired serum samples (IgG) for pathogen.

For an episode of diarrhea to be considered nosocomial, the onset of disease must occur during hospitalization or shortly after discharge, and the infection should not be present or incubating at the time of the patient's admission. This assessment of nosocomial versus community-acquired infection also should consider the expected incubation period for each possible enteropathogen.

A review of 26 pediatric wards in 1949 revealed a cross-infection (nosocomial infection) rate of 7%, 21% of which was gastroenteritis (3). Subsequent reports have described gastroenteritis as the first to the fifth most frequent type of nosocomial infection in children (4,5). Gastroenteritis has been reported as the cause of 13% to 35% of nosocomial infections in pediatric hospitals (6–11). In addition, 5% to 14% of pediatric patients developed nosocomial gastroenteritis (6,9). A Canadian pediatric hospital reported nosocomial viral gastrointestinal infections in 1.2% of hospitalizations, and nurse understaffing was a significant risk factor (12). The overall nosocomial gastrointestinal tract infection attack rate in one study was 0.68 infections per 100 discharges, and another study reported a rate of 1.1 episodes per 100 hospital days (6,13).

A 9-year period of surveillance in a children's hospital identified diarrhea as the third most common nosocomial infection (15%) with 0.5 to 1.0 episodes per 1,000 patient-days (5). A pathogen was identified in 56% of episodes including *Clostridium difficile* (32%), rotavirus (31%), adenovirus (30%), and other viral etiologies (7%). The median age was 1.3 years, 0.8 years for viral diarrhea and 3.9 years for *C. difficile* diarrhea. Of the children with nosocomial diarrhea, 75% were diapered at the time of the episode.

Reports by the CDC as part of the National Nosocomial Infections Surveillance (NNIS) system have included the incidence of nosocomial diarrhea in participating hospitals. The NNIS system data from 1985 to 1991 demonstrated that nosocomial diarrhea occurred in general pediatric care units at a rate of 11 per 10,000 discharges and in newborn nurseries at a rate of 3 per 10,000 discharges. This rate is higher in high-risk nurseries, wherein the rate is 20 per 10,000 discharges. The NNIS system also reported that gastrointestinal tract infections make up 8% of all nosocomial infections in high-risk nurseries (14). More recently (1992 to 1997), the NNIS system reported that gastrointestinal tract infections compose 5% of nosocomial infections in pediatric intensive care units (15). *C. difficile* was implicated in 52% and viruses in 44%. Rotaviruses were the etiology in 74% of viral cases and enteroviruses in 13%.

Data describing the ultimate economic or medical impact of pediatric nosocomial gastrointestinal tract infections in the United States are lacking. Two reports from developing countries indicated that nosocomial gastroenteritis increased the mean length of hospital stay by 7 and by 20 days, respectively. Nosocomial rotavirus infection increased length of hospital stay by 8 days in a French hospital (16). An Austrian study estimated annual costs of 6.2 million EUR resulting from nosocomial rotavirus infections (17,18). Many reports have described outbreaks of nosocomial gastrointestinal tract infections resulting from specific enteropathogens. These specific pathogens and their relative importance are discussed in the following sections (7,8).

ETIOLOGY

Many viral, bacterial, and parasitic enteropathogens have been associated with nosocomial infections (Table 50.1). The NNIS system reports for 1985 to 1991 indicated that an etiologic agent was identified in 97% of the adult and pediatric cases of nosocomial gastroenteritis and that bacteria accounted for 93% of the reported enteropathogens. *C. difficile* was the most frequent pathogen, but because this report included adults and children, it is not a true reflection of nosocomial gastroenteritis in children. In addition, most of the NNIS system participating hospitals lack diagnostic virology laboratories, so the relative importance of enteric viruses was underestimated. Rotavirus ranked second, accounting for 5% of all nosocomial infections. Studies limited to the pediatric population have identified viral agents as the most frequent nosocomial enteropathogens; rotavirus is the agent most often identified (13). In one study in a pediatric hospital, the following nosocomial enteropathogens were detected: rotavirus, 43%; calicivirus, 16%; astrovirus, 14%; mini-reovirus, 12%; adenovirus, 8%; *Salmonella* species, 4%; and parvovirus/picornavirus, 3% (19).

TABLE 50.1. ENTEROPATHOGENS AND OTHER MICROORGANISMS ASSOCIATED WITH NOSOCOMIAL GASTROENTERITIS

Bacteria
Campylobacter jejuni
Clostridium difficile
Escherichia coli
Enteroaggregative (EAEC)
Enterohemorrhagic (EHEC)
Enteroinvasive (EIEC)
Enteropathogenic (EPEC)
Enterotoxigenic (ETEC)
Salmonella species
Shigella species
Vibrio cholerae
Yersinia enterocolitica
Viral
Enteric adenovirus
Astrovirus
Human calicivirus including noroviruses and sapoviruses
Rotavirus
Parasites
Cryptosporidium parvum
Cyclospora cayetanensis
Entamoeba histolytica
Giardia lamblia
Strongyloides stercoralis
Other
Candida species
Agents possibly associated with necrotizing enterocolitis
Potential nosocomial gastrointestinal tract pathogens
Aeromonas species
Klebsiella species
Plesiomonas shigelloides
Pseudomonas aeruginosa
Known gastrointestinal tract pathogens (that are potential nosocomial pathogens)
Campylobacter upsaliensis
Vibrio parahaemolyticus
Isospora belli
Encephalitozoon intestinalis
Enterocytozoon bieneusi

Viruses

Viruses are recognized as important nosocomial enteropathogens spread via person-to-person transmission or point-source infection through food or water. Studies show that enteric viruses have caused 86% of nosocomial gastroenteritis in infants and children (9,19–21).

Enteric Adenoviruses

Enteric adenoviruses consist of two serotypes, 40 and 41, which are members of group F adenoviruses (22). These agents primarily infect children younger than 2 years and occur year-round (23,24). Adenoviruses cause a spectrum of conditions ranging from asymptomatic infection in 40% of infected children to diarrhea and vomiting lasting for 7 to 10 days. The incubation period is 3 to 10 days. Illness often is associated with fever and respiratory tract symptoms (25). Transmission is by the fecal-oral route and readily occurs from person to person (23). Treatment is nonspecific, and fluid replacement is dictated by the patient's condition. The frequency of dehydration and fever resulting from enteric adenovirus gastroenteritis appears to be similar to that of other enteric viruses (26). In several reports, enteric adenovirus was the third most frequent cause of viral gastroenteritis in hospitalized infants and young children (25–29). In one study, 54% of 127 enteric adenovirus infections were nosocomial (28). These viruses have been shown to be a major cause of morbidity in hospitalized infants who have undergone ileostomy or colostomy procedures for necrotizing enterocolitis (NEC) (30). The nosocomial infection rate in these patients was higher than other nursery patients, and infection resulted in a prolonged hospital stay. Diagnosis of enteric adenovirus-associated gastroenteritis can be made by evaluation of stool specimens using either EM or a commercially available enzyme immunosorbent assay (EIA).

Astrovirus

Eight antigenic types of human astrovirus have been identified. Gastroenteritis from astrovirus occurs worldwide and has been associated with outbreaks of mild diarrhea in schools (31, 32), child care centers (33,34), nursing homes (35,36), and pediatric hospital wards (37–39). Astroviruses are responsible for approximately 3% to 5% of hospital admissions for gastroenteritis. Illness occurs mainly in children younger than 2 years and often causes asymptomatic infection (40). The illness lasts 1 to 4 days following an incubation period of 24 to 36 hours. Gastrointestinal tract symptoms are nonspecific, consisting of vomiting, diarrhea, fever, and abdominal pain. Transmission is person to person among children. Astrovirus has been reported to be responsible for 5% to 7% of nosocomial gastroenteritis in children's hospitals (37,39,41–44). An attack rate of between 7% and 62% was reported during an outbreak of nosocomial infection in a children's ward (39). Astrovirus caused a prolonged outbreak of diarrhea among immunocompromised patients in a pediatric bone marrow transplant unit (45). Astrovirus-associated gastroenteritis is diagnosed by examination of a stool specimen by EM, EIA, or reverse transcription polymerase chain reaction (RT-PCR) (33,45,46). Commercial EIAs for the detection of human astroviruses are not available in the United States, but may be used in other countries.

Caliciviruses

Four genera of the family Caliciviridae have been described including noroviruses (formerly known as Norwalk-like viruses) and sapoviruses (formerly known as Sapporo-like viruses) (47). Human calicivirus infections occur year-round, although some studies suggest a seasonal predominance. The incubation period is 12 hours to 4 days, and the clinical symptoms include vomiting and diarrhea, which last for 1 to 4 days. The severity of symptoms caused by caliciviruses is indistinguishable from that of symptoms caused by other enteric viruses (48,49). Persistent excretion may occur in immunocompromised hosts. Caliciviruses have been identified in stools for up to 2 weeks after the onset of symptoms (50). Calicivirus is transmitted by the fecal-oral route, and foodborne and water-borne transmission have also been described (51). Calicivirus can be detected in stool specimens of 0.2% to 6% of children hospitalized for gastroenteritis. When calicivirus was detected in hospitalized children, it was nosocomially acquired in approximately 40% of cases (42,49,52). Caliciviruses have tremendous antigenic and genetic diversity, which makes detection assays insensitive. It is apparent that most studies have certainly underreported the significance of calicivirus infections because of these insensitive assays. Caliciviruses can be detected in stool specimens by EM, immune EM, RT-PCR, or EIA, but these tests are available only in research laboratories (22). A new commercial EIA is not available in the United States.

Two of these genera, the noroviruses (Norwalk-like viruses) and sapoviruses (Sapporo-like viruses), infect humans. Many of the noroviruses are known only from a single outbreak and have been named after the sites at which the outbreaks occurred. They include Norwalk, Hawaii, Snow Mountain, Mexico (MX), and Lordsdale (47,53,54). Norwalk virus is the best studied member of the genus. Norwalk virus illness follows an incubation period of 18 to 48 hours and is characterized by vomiting, diarrhea, abdominal pain, and low-grade fever lasting 1 to 2 days (55). Epidemics of noroviruses have been reported in nursing homes, schools, recreational areas, cruise ships, and hospitals (56–62). Water-borne (51), foodborne (63,64), and person-to-person transmission have all been implicated in epidemics (53,65,66), and results of volunteer studies suggest fecal-oral transmission. Aerosolization of vomitus also has been implicated as a mode of transmission. In one hospital outbreak, 55% of elderly patients and 61% of the healthcare workers on one floor became ill (67). The healthcare workers most likely spread infection from patient to patient. Another reported outbreak affected 57 patients and 69 staff members over a 26-day period. The index case was a patient hospitalized with acute abdominal pain and diarrhea 2 days before the outbreak. The epidemic curve indicated person-to-person transmission (68). In another report of an outbreak in a children's ward, 15 children had Norwalk virus in stool specimens, and the ward had to be closed to control the outbreak (56).

The sapoviruses also have been associated with sporadic outbreaks and have been named after the location of the outbreak. They include Sapporo, Houston, London, Manchester, and Parkville (69–71). Illnesses resulting from sapoviruses are similar to illnesses associated with the noroviruses.

Rotavirus

Rotavirus is the most thoroughly investigated and described cause of nosocomial viral gastroenteritis and is one of the most important enteric pathogens worldwide. There are six distinct rotavirus groups, three of which infect humans. Group A rotavirus is the most common cause of diarrhea in infants and children throughout the world including the United States. Groups B and C cause human disease in the Far East (22,24,72).

Rotavirus has an incubation period of 1 to 3 days. Excretion of rotavirus in stool can precede the onset of illness by several days and can persist for 8 to 10 days after symptoms of illness have abated (73). The illness usually has an abrupt onset characterized by explosive, watery diarrhea and is often associated with vomiting either before or after onset of diarrhea. Dehydration occurs in 40% to 80% of patients and usually is mild, but severe dehydration and death have been reported in children and adults (74). Rotaviruses are transmitted principally by the fecal-oral route. They are found in nearly 50% of stool specimens from children admitted to the hospital with gastroenteritis. Most patients with rotavirus infection are between 6 and 24 months of age (75). In North America, the annual rotavirus season begins in late fall in Mexico and moves across the continental United States from southwest to northeast, resulting in a peak of rotavirus activity in March and April in eastern Canada and the northeastern United States (76).

Nosocomial transmission of rotavirus has been well documented on pediatric hospital wards; 2% to 24% of children admitted to the hospital with other diagnoses acquire rotavirus in the hospital (17,27,77–83). In several reports, up to 70% of infants in a nursery have acquired rotavirus nosocomially (84–87). Hospital surveillance for rotavirus using molecular methods has detected newly emerging strains and nosocomial transmission of those new strains (86–90). Immunocompromised children acquire rotavirus in the hospital with an infection rate of 12% to 25%. Immunocompromised children have an extended period of virus excretion and may be a source of virus for transmission to others (91,92). Community-acquired symptomatic rotaviral infection in children admitted to the hospital and asymptomatic rotavirus shedding by neonates and other hospitalized infants appear to be the primary reservoirs for nosocomial rotavirus infection in susceptible children (93–95). Fomites may play a role in rotavirus transmission. Rotavirus contamination was detected by polymerase chain reaction (PCR) in 19% of inanimate objects in a child care center during an outbreak (96,97). Nosocomial rotavirus infection may cause both outbreaks and endemic diarrheal disease in newborn nurseries; however, infection usually is asymptomatic (84,95,98–105). Asymptomatic rotavirus infection also occurs in older children, with evidence of asymptomatic rotavirus infection occurring in 24% to 50% of infants younger than 2 years during rotavirus season (106–108). The role of asymptomatic excreters in nosocomial rotavirus infection is not known (109). The incidence of confirmed nosocomial rotavirus diarrhea in a large pediatric hospital was found to be 0.5 to 0.9 per 1,000 admissions (110,111).

In one hospital, the incidence of nosocomial rotavirus infection among infants was 28%. The incidence of symptomatic infections was 17%, and the incidence of asymptomatic infections was 11%. Breast-feeding was protective against both infection and symptoms; 32% of formula-fed and 11% of breast-fed infants acquired rotavirus in the hospital ($p < .005$). No breast-fed infant had symptomatic infection (112).

Rotavirus is detected in stool specimens by EIA, latex agglutination, EM, polyacrylamide gel electrophoresis, and PCR (113–116). Several EIA and latex agglutination assays are commercially available. Detection rates depend on which assay is used, because of their varying sensitivities.

Bacteria

Nosocomial bacterial gastroenteritis is less common than viral gastroenteritis. In the United States, most information about nosocomial bacterial gastroenteritis consists of reports of outbreaks, many of which are foodborne or water borne. Several prospective studies of nosocomial diarrhea in children failed to demonstrate any bacterial causes (13,19), although *C. difficile* is common in adults. Bacterial infections are much more significant in less developed countries. A patient with poor nutritional status or an immunocompromised patient is at particularly high risk for nosocomial bacterial gastroenteritis.

Campylobacter Species

Twenty-one species have been identified in the family Campylobacteraceae, but only 12 cause disease in humans. *Campylobacter jejuni, Campylobacter coli, Campylobacter upsaliensis,* and *Campylobacter jejuni* subspecies *doylei* are the most common species isolated from children. *Campylobacter fetus* is a rare cause of bloodstream and systemic infections occurring mostly in immunocompromised and debilitated hosts and as a cause of perinatal infection and abortion. Because *C. jejuni* is the species that usually causes intestinal illness, many laboratories place stool specimens on selective media with incubation temperatures of 42°C to isolate this species. With this method, several other *Campylobacter* species will be missed as a cause of diarrhea. Therefore, the extent of nosocomial infection by many of the *Campylobacter* species is not known. Isolation of *Campylobacter* species from blood and other sterile body sites does not present the same isolation problem as isolation from feces does (117).

Predominant symptoms are diarrhea, abdominal pain, malaise, and fever. Stools may contain blood. *C. jejuni* has been reported as a cause of severe infection in neonates following vertical transmission (118). Vertical transmission of a microorganism is considered a nosocomial infection in the nursery for purposes of surveillance reporting. Postnatal person-to-person transmission also has been documented with reports of nursery epidemics of *Campylobacter* species diarrhea and meningitis (118). The incubation period is 1 to 7 days.

Nosocomial transmission of *Campylobacter* species is not common. The gastrointestinal tract of domestic and wild birds and animals is the reservoir of infection. A Finnish hospital reported a water-borne nosocomial outbreak of *C. jejuni* gastroenteritis in both patients and hospital staff (119). Several community-acquired outbreaks caused by *C. jejuni* have been reported, usually resulting from ingestion of contaminated raw milk, water, or food. In addition, infection can occur through person-to-person transmission or contact with infected animals (120). For example, an outbreak involving two very closely related strains of *C. upsaliensis* in four child care centers implicated person-to-person transmission (121).

Clostridium difficile

Nosocomial gastrointestinal tract infection caused by *C. difficile* in adults and children is discussed in Chapter 36. The role of *C. difficile* in antibiotic-associated diarrhea has been more difficult to establish in infants and young children than in adults, because *C. difficile* commonly is recovered from stools of asymptomatic infants and young children.

The reported incidence of neonatal colonization varies, with isolation rates as high as 90% in neonatal intensive care units (NICUs) and 2% to 30% in healthy newborn infants. *C. difficile* toxin has been detected in up to 36% of sick neonates without gastrointestinal tract symptoms (118). The incidence of *C. difficile* toxin detection in stool specimens declines with age and approaches 1% to 3% in healthy adults (122). Pseudomembranous colitis has been reported in infants and children, but the incidence is difficult to assess. *C. difficile* was described as the cause of 13% to 16% of nosocomial gastrointestinal tract infections (8,123). Outbreaks of diarrhea associated with *C. difficile* have been reported in child care centers (124). The incubation period is unknown.

C. difficile may be isolated from stool using a selective cycloserine-cefoxitin-fructose agar in an anaerobic environment. *C. difficile* produces two toxins. The *C. difficile* cytotoxin B may be detected by cell culture cytotoxicity assay or EIA. Some commercially available EIAs detect both toxins A and B (125). There have been reports of toxin A negative, toxin B positive *C. difficile* antibiotic-associated diarrhea in adults (126). Arbitrarily primed

PCR has been used for genotypic differentiation of strains in hospital outbreaks (127).

Escherichia coli

E. coli strains that cause acute diarrheal disease may be classified into five groups: enterotoxigenic (ETEC), enteroaggregative (EAEC), enteroinvasive (EIEC), enteropathogenic (EPEC), and enterohemorrhagic (EHEC) (128). ETEC usually infects infants and children in developing countries or adults following travel in developing countries. EAEC produces acute or chronic diarrhea in all age groups but predominantly in infants by attachment to and effacement of the intestinal mucosa. EIEC infects all ages and causes diarrhea containing blood and mucus as a result of tissue invasion. These infections occasionally may be foodborne or may occur as the result of travel to developing countries. EPEC produces acute and chronic diarrhea generally in infants younger than 2 years in developing countries (129). EHEC causes abdominal pain and bloody diarrhea in children and adults, mostly in developed countries. The illness may be complicated by the hemolytic-uremic syndrome (HUS) in children or thrombotic thrombocytopenic purpura in adults. It is most often spread by undercooked contaminated meat, but many other vehicles of transmission have been described.

The reported incidence of nosocomial gastroenteritis caused by these five groups of *E. coli* is low. This may be a reflection of the unavailability of detection methods in most clinical microbiology laboratories. The incubation periods range from 10 hours to 6 days.

Reports of nosocomial ETEC-associated diarrheal outbreaks in special care nurseries resulting from heat-stable enterotoxin (STa)-producing strains include one report from Spain with six ETEC-associated neonatal diarrheal outbreaks (130). In another report, ETEC was cultured from infants, nurses, family members, infant formula, and surfaces in the nursery (131). This report implicated person-to-person transmission and foodborne transmission by formula. In another report of a hospital outbreak, a rare phage type further differentiated the infected strain (132). *E. coli* also has been reported as a contaminant of expressed human milk, which caused both asymptomatic infections and gastroenteritis in a nursery (133).

A single report described person-to-person transmission of EIEC in students and staff of a school for mentally retarded adults and children; 48% of the students and 28% of the staff were ill. Control of the outbreak was achieved by cohorting and an emphasis on hand washing (134).

Community-acquired foodborne outbreaks of EHEC serotype 0157:H7 are well documented. *E. coli* O157:H7 Phage type 8 caused a hospital outbreak by food brought to a party from the outside (135). Many outbreaks have occurred in nursing homes, and a report of an outbreak in an institution for mentally retarded children and adults demonstrated the devastating effects of this microorganism in an outbreak. Eight of 20 infected residents developed HUS, and four died of complications (136). Twenty-nine children with *E. coli* 0157:H7 in nine child care centers were reported. There was evidence of person-to-person transmission in all nine facilities (137). Spread of *E. coli* 0157:H7 from a patient to a nurse in the hospital setting has been reported (138,139).

EPEC is the strain most commonly associated with nosocomial infections. It was the cause of 1.3% of gastrointestinal tract infections in a children's hospital in the United States (9) and of 6 of 10 nosocomial bacterial gastrointestinal tract infections in a South African hospital (8). Many studies of outbreaks of diarrhea in NICUs have demonstrated person-to-person transmission by hands of hospital personnel. Premature infants are the most susceptible to severe morbidity and to mortality resulting from these infections (140–145). Detection of EPEC requires a high level of suspicion. Colonies of *E. coli* from a routine bacterial culture must be screened by type-specific antisera. Research methods for identifying related serotypes include adherence of microorganisms in HEp-2 cells, DNA probes, and PCR to detect EPEC strains with the enteroadherence plasmid.

Salmonella Species

The genus *Salmonella* is now considered to comprise a single species named *Salmonella enterica* based on DNA structure and biochemical properties. Within this species are seven subspecies with almost all serotypes pathogenic for humans classified into subgroup I (*S. enterica* subspecies *enterica*). The subspecies can be divided into serotypes based on their somatic (O) and flagellar (H) antigens. Two main clinical syndromes are associated with *Salmonella.* The first is the protracted bacteremia of typhoid *(Salmonella typhi)* and paratyphoid *(Salmonella paratyphi)* fevers. The second is the predominantly gastrointestinal tract illness caused by animal-adapted *Salmonella* strains. *Salmonella typhimurium* is the serotype most commonly reported as the cause of human *Salmonella* infections in the United States. Many outbreaks of *Salmonella* gastroenteritis in hospitalized patients resulting from a variety of serotypes have occurred through various methods of transmission. Person-to-person transmission may occur among patients or from healthcare personnel. Common-source outbreaks also have been traced to diagnostic agents and medications (146–148). *Salmonella* infections have been acquired from reptiles, highlighting the importance of avoiding exposure to pet reptiles in a hospital setting (149). The incubation period for gastroenteritis is from 6 to 12 hours. For enteric fever, the incubation period is from 3 to 60 days but is usually 7 to 14 days.

Foodborne *Salmonella* outbreaks simultaneously may affect patients in multiple hospitals. In 1962 and 1963, a large outbreak of nosocomial gastroenteritis caused by *Salmonella derby* occurred among patients, medical staff, and employees of 53 hospitals in 13 states (150). Contaminated eggs, which were eaten raw or undercooked, were responsible for this and many other outbreaks (151–154). Person-to-person transmission to hospital staff and to other patients has been documented (153, 155,156). Foodborne outbreaks also have occurred following ingestion of improperly cooked and stored poultry (157,158). Foodborne outbreaks may originate in hospital personnel or in patients (159–162). An epidemic caused by *Salmonella kottbus* was traced to contaminated pooled human milk (163,164).

Common-source *Salmonella* outbreaks also have been traced to contaminated diagnostic reagents and medications. These types of outbreaks generally do not present as typical common-source outbreaks and, therefore, may be difficult to recognize. An interstate outbreak of *Salmonella cubana* infection occurred in 1966 because of contaminated carmine dye used as a marker of gastrointestinal tract transit (146–148). Nosocomial outbreaks of salmonellosis also have been traced to bile salts, gelatin, pancreatin, pepsin, vitamins, and extracts of various endocrine glands (165,166). These outbreaks appeared to be sporadic and, therefore, required a high index of suspicion to document their association with a common vehicle.

Outbreaks of *Salmonella* gastroenteritis also have been associated with a variety of medical instruments or procedures, including upper gastrointestinal tract endoscopy (167), fiberoptic colonoscopy (168), rubber tubing attached to a suction apparatus (169–171), rectal thermometers (172), and contaminated mattresses (173). Nosocomial *Salmonella hadar* infection occurred in laundry personnel at a nursing home following a foodborne outbreak in the nursing home residents. This report implicated handling of the soiled laundry in the absence of person-to-person contact (174).

Outbreaks of *Salmonella* infection have been reported in nurseries. The microorganism generally is introduced into the nursery by an infant recently born to a mother with clinical or asymptomatic salmonellosis (175) or a child with community-acquired *Salmonella* infection. *Salmonella* is transmitted among the staff and patients by person-to-person contact. Acquisition of multiresistant microorganisms by premature infants in special care nurseries results in increased rates of morbidity and mortality (176,177). A case control study of an outbreak of *Salmonella infantis* in a neonatal care unit in Brazil demonstrated protection by increased birth weight, and peripheral intravenous (IV) catheter use was a risk factor. Overcrowding and understaffing were associated with the outbreak (178).

Salmonella can be cultured from stool, rectal swabs, blood, urine, bone marrow aspirates, and other foci of infection. Serotyping with specific antisera provides further identification for epidemiologic investigation. Determining serotypes remains a useful epidemiologic tool for investigations of outbreaks in both the hospital and the community setting. Plasmid pattern analysis (PPA) and pulsed-field gel electrophoresis (PFGE) are useful methods for determining the relatedness of infecting strains during an outbreak (158,179,180).

Shigella Species

Shigellosis occurs worldwide, although its prevalence differs by location. It is largely a disease associated with poverty, crowding, poor levels of personal hygiene, inadequate water supplies, and malnutrition (181). There are four species of *Shigella* (*Shigella dysenteriae, Shigella flexneri, Shigella boydii,* and *Shigella sonnei*), which are differentiated by group-specific polysaccharide antigens of lipopolysaccharides (LPS), designated A, B, C, and D, respectively; biochemical properties; and phage or colicin susceptibility. *S. sonnei* is the most common cause of bacillary dysentery in the United States, with *S. flexneri* responsible for most of the remaining cases. *S. dysenteriae* type 1 and *S. flexneri* are the most common species causing disease in developing countries. Direct fecal-oral transmission can contribute to endemic shigellosis in institutional environments such as mental hospitals, child care centers, nursing homes, and prisons and at outdoor gatherings (182,183). The incubation period is 1 to 7 days. Nosocomial outbreaks have seldom been reported despite the low inoculum necessary to cause infection (184). *Shigella* was the cause of 3% of nosocomial gastrointestinal tract infections among patients in a hospital in a developing country and also caused nosocomial infections among staff of the clinical microbiology laboratory of a large university-affiliated hospital (185,186).

In one large nosocomial outbreak, hospital workers had dysentery caused by *S. dysenteriae* type 2 after eating at the salad bar in the hospital cafeteria. Ninety-five workers were ill, but only three hospital inpatients became ill following person-to-person transmission (187).

Both *S. flexneri* and *S. sonnei* have been reported in newborn infants who acquired the microorganism from an infected mother during labor and delivery. Bacteremia in neonates has been reported but is uncommon (188,189). In one report, 3 of 32 healthcare providers caring for an infected neonate acquired shigellosis (190). *Shigella* is detected by routine microbiologic culture of stool specimens; ribotyping and plasmid profile analysis have been used to differentiate strains.

Vibrio Species

Vibrio cholerae 01, the etiologic agent of cholera, and *V. cholerae* non-01 strains including *V. cholerae* 0139 are recognized as important causes of acute, often severe, diarrheal disease in developing countries. A number of other *Vibrio* species have been identified and associated with gastroenteritis including (191,192): *Vibrio parahaemolyticus, Vibrio mimicus, Vibrio fluvialis* (193), *Vibrio furnissii* (194), and *Vibrio hollisae* (195). *V. parahaemolyticus* is a common marine isolate that has been found in water, shellfish, fish, and plankton. *V. parahaemolyticus* has caused foodborne outbreaks in the United States, but there have been no reports of nosocomial gastroenteritis (191,192). Foodborne nosocomial *V. parahaemolyticus* has been reported in Asia (196). In countries with endemic cholera, all ages are affected, although children older than 1 year are disproportionately involved. *V. cholerae* 01 is primarily a problem in Asia, Africa, and South America, although there is a focus in the Gulf Coast of the United States, where the microorganism has been associated with undercooked shellfish consumption (197). Since 1992, *V. cholerae* 0139 has been reported in several countries in southeast Asia in epidemic proportions (198). The incubation period of cholera is usually 1 to 3 days.

Nosocomial transmission of cholera has been described in developing countries but not in the United States. Close person-to-person contact and sharing of food was implicated in these outbreaks (199–202). In one hospital in Thailand, the microorganism was isolated from water used for bathing on a pediatric ward (203).

Vibrio species may be isolated from stool specimens on thiosulfate-citrate bile salts sucrose agar (TCBS). Serotyping is performed to distinguish 01 and non-01 strains. Enterotoxins may be detected by animal or tissue culture assays, EIA, and DNA probes (191).

Yersinia enterocolitica

Y. enterocolitica is associated with a wide spectrum of clinical and immunologic manifestations. The clinical illness caused by this pathogen ranges from self-limited enterocolitis to potentially fatal systemic infection; postinfection manifestations include erythema nodosum and reactive arthritis. *Y. enterocolitica* enterocolitis is characterized by diarrhea with blood-streaked stools, fever, vomiting, and abdominal pain (204,205). Serogroups 0: 3, 0:8, and 0:9 are most commonly implicated as a cause of enterocolitis in the United States. *Y. enterocolitica* has been isolated from a variety of animate reservoirs, including birds, frogs, fish, flies, fleas, snails, crabs, oysters, and a wide array of mammals with swine the major reservoir for human pathogens (206). Animal products including raw milk, whipped cream, ice cream, beef, lamb, and poultry also may harbor the microorganism. Other reservoirs include lakes, streams, well water, soil, and vegetables (207). The most frequent outbreaks in the United States have been associated with preparation of chitterlings for holiday meals in the South (208,209).

Several mechanisms of nosocomial transmission have been described. Transfusion-related yersiniosis has been reported in several countries including the United States and in Europe. In 1987 through 1991, seven deaths occurred among the ten reported patients with transfusion-associated *Y. enterocolitica* (210). Blood donors apparently had low-grade *Y. enterocolitica* bacteremia at the time of donation, and the microorganism replicated at the storage conditions provided for units of red blood cells (211,212). Children and adults with hematologic conditions resulting in iron overload are at greater risk of yersiniosis (206).

There is a report of an 11-day-old infant with *Y. enterocolitica* enterocolitis acquired either during delivery from an infected mother or postnatally during routine care (213). The incubation period in single-source outbreaks is 1 to 14 days, so either method of transmission was possible in this case. Acquisition and excretion of *Yersinia* species has been associated with consumption of pasteurized milk on a pediatric ward (214). The same serotype of *Y. enterocolitica* was isolated from the patients and the pasteurized milk.

Person-to-person spread to both patients and staff within adult and pediatric inpatient populations also has been reported (215,216). In one study, 28% of *Y. enterocolitica*-infected patients acquired the microorganism in the hospital (217).

The detection of *Y. enterocolitica* requires isolation on selective media. Cold enrichment techniques may increase the rate of recovery from stool cultures. Serotyping is performed to identify the most common serotypes in human disease and may be used for outbreak investigation. Chromosomal DNA restriction fragment length polymorphism (RFLP) (208), plasmid profile analysis, and phage typing have been used to evaluate the relatedness of serotypes during outbreaks.

Parasites

Cryptosporidium

Cryptosporidia are small coccidian parasites that infect the microvillous region of epithelial cells lining the digestive and respiratory organs. Since 1982, these microorganisms have been recognized as an important cause of widespread diarrheal illness in humans and some domesticated animals. In immunocompetent persons, *Cryptosporidium parvum* may cause a short-term (3 to 20 days) diarrheal illness that resolves spontaneously. However, in the immunocompromised patient, cryptosporidiosis usually presents as a life-threatening, prolonged, cholera-like illness (218,219). Nitazoxanide was recently approved for the treatment of cryptosporidiosis in children (220). Newer approaches to therapy for human immunodeficiency virus (HIV)-infected persons, such as highly active antiretroviral therapy (HAART), have reduced the frequency and severity of cryptosporidiosis in patients with acquired immunodeficiency syndrome (AIDS). Person-to-person transmission is common, and outbreaks of cryptosporidiosis among children in child care centers have been reported, hospital-acquired infections have been investigated, water-borne outbreaks have been documented, and *Cryptosporidium* is recognized as a cause of traveler's diarrhea. The incubation period is estimated to be 2 to 14 days.

Nosocomial *Cryptosporidium* infections have occurred by person-to-person transmission, particularly among immunocompromised patients. Outbreaks have been reported among patients with AIDS, patients on a bone marrow transplant unit, and severely malnourished children in a developing country (221–224). Transmission among patients with AIDS also has occurred following contamination of an ice machine on a nursing unit by a patient infected with *Cryptosporidium* (225). There also has been a report of transmission to hospital workers after caring for a patient with chronic cryptosporidiosis (226).

The detection of *Cryptosporidium* is accomplished by microscopic examination of fresh or concentrated stool specimens followed by staining with a modified Kinyoun acid-fast stain (227). The microorganism also can be seen on intestinal biopsy. A monoclonal antibody-based fluorescein conjugated stain for detecting oocysts in stool and an EIA for detecting antigen in stool are available commercially (228). PCR may be a useful tool for use in the diagnosis and study of the molecular epidemiology of *Cryptosporidium* infections (229). Outbreak control has been achieved by intensified enteric precautions and cleaning (221).

Cyclospora

Cyclospora cayetanensis has been associated with diarrhea. It has been reported as a cause of foodborne diarrhea outbreaks; fresh berries are most commonly implicated. Watery diarrhea, abdominal cramping, decreased appetite, and low-grade fever characterize the illness. Symptoms can occur in cycles of remission and exacerbation lasting up to several weeks. A hospital-associated outbreak among staff persons was associated with stagnant water in a storage tank (230).

Cyclospora are detected by identifying the 8- to 10-μm spherical bodies that autofluoresce or by acid-fast staining (231,232). Direct person-to-person transmission is unlikely, because *Cyclospora* oocysts require time and favorable conditions to become infectious.

Entamoeba histolytica

Amebiasis is a major health problem in Asia, Latin America, and Africa. Childhood intestinal amebiasis generally presents with diarrhea containing blood and mucus and no fever. Diarrhea without blood, fever, fulminating colitis, appendicitis, and ameboma occur infrequently in children. The cyst form is resistant to environmental stresses and is the infective stage. Transmission is by the fecal-oral route. The incubation period is variable, ranging from a few days to months or years; commonly, it is 2 to 4 weeks. Nosocomial infection is rare but has been reported in hospitalized adults in a developing country (233). A colonic irrigation machine was implicated in an outbreak of amebiasis in adults after therapy at a chiropractic clinic (234).

E. histolytica is detected by direct examination of fresh stool specimens. *E. histolytica* actually comprises two genetically distinct but morphologically indistinguishable species. *E. histolytica* is pathogenic and causes invasive amebiasis, and *Entamoeba dispar* is probably nonpathogenic and is often reported as *E. histolytica* because of the microscopic resemblance of the two species. *E. histolytica* and *E. dispar* have been differentiated using restriction fragment analysis of DNA amplified by PCR, PCR, isoenzyme analysis, and antigen detection (235,236).

Giardia lamblia

G. lamblia is transmitted directly from person to person by fecal-oral transmission of cysts or indirectly by transmission in water and occasionally food (237). Travelers often become infected when they ingest contaminated ground water or surface water. The cyst is highly infectious for humans, and infections can occur following ingestion of as few as 10 to 100 cysts (238). Infection by *G. lamblia* may produce flatulence, foul-smelling stools, abdominal cramps, abdominal distention, anorexia, nausea, and weight loss (239). Outbreaks of infection and endemic infections occur in child care centers and other institutional settings and among family members of infected children (240, 241). The incubation period is usually 1 to 4 weeks. Nosocomial hospital outbreaks are uncommon, but outbreaks among children in child care centers are well documented (242,243). An outbreak of giardiasis with person-to-person and foodborne transmission in nursing home residents, employees, and children in a combined child care center with an adopted grandparent program has been reported (244).

G. lamblia may be detected by microscopic examination of fresh or formalin-preserved concentrated stool or by use of a commercially available EIA. Specific DNA probes for *Giardia* may assist in the diagnosis in the future.

Strongyloides stercoralis

S. stercoralis is a nematode that infects humans and sometimes other animals. It has a complicated life cycle that may have both parasitic and free-living phases. Strongyloidiasis has a worldwide distribution. The prevalence of infection varies inversely with socioeconomic level and is highest in warm, moist regions where sanitary practices are poor. The parasite is endemic in certain southern areas of the United States including eastern Kentucky, Tennessee, and elsewhere in southern Appalachia. Most human infections are acquired outdoors when polluted soil containing filariform larvae comes in contact with skin. The filariform larvae then penetrate intact skin of the new host, travel through blood vessels to the lungs, penetrate alveoli, are coughed up and swallowed, and then establish infection in the mucosa of the small intestine (245,246). There have been no reports of nosocomial infection within a hospital, but human-to-human transmission of *S. stercoralis* has been reported in residents of homes for the mentally retarded (247–249). The incubation period is not known.

Disseminated strongyloidiasis has been reported in two recipients of kidney allografts from a single cadaver donor (250). Neither recipient had previous evidence of parasitic infection or risk factors for strongyloidiasis. Disseminated strongyloidiasis also has been reported as a complication of immunosuppression. Patients with a history of exposure to *S. stercoralis* many years previously have experienced hyperinfection with the parasite during immunosuppression following renal transplantation (251,252).

S. stercoralis is detected by microscopic examination of fresh stool to identify the rhabditiform larvae. The method of placing stool in an agar plate and observing worms and worm tracks on the agar is an efficient method of detecting the parasite (253). Several immunoassays for detection of serum antibodies against filarial larvae or larval antigens are available (254).

Isospora belli

I. belli is an obligate, intracellular protozoan. Humans are the only known host for *I. belli,* and transmission is believed to occur by ingestion of oocysts contaminating food, water, or environmental surfaces. *I. belli* infection usually has an acute onset with fever, diarrhea, and colicky abdominal pain. The illness may be self-limiting with spontaneous resolution in the healthy host. Prolonged watery diarrhea accompanied by malabsorption, weight loss, and asthenia may occur in immunocompromised patients. The incubation period is 8 to 14 days. Isosporiasis has been encountered in 15% of patients with AIDS in Haiti, but it is much less frequent in the United States (255, 256). There have been no reports of nosocomial isosporiasis; in fact, 170 healthy siblings, friends, and spouses of patients with AIDS did not have *I. belli* in their stool specimens (256).

Diagnosis is made by demonstration of oocysts in feces or duodenal aspirates or by finding developmental stages of the parasite in biopsy specimens of the small intestine. Oocysts can be detected by a modified Kinyoun acid-fast stain and by auramine-rhodamine stains.

Microsporidia

Microsporidia are ubiquitous, spore-forming, intracellular protozoal parasites that cause disease in a wide range of vertebrate and invertebrate animals. Manifestations of disease in humans range from asymptomatic infections to fulminant cerebritis and/or nephritis; ocular infections are recognized infrequently. Since 1985, enteric microsporidial infections have been reported with increasing frequency in patients with AIDS and chronic diarrhea. *Enterocytozoon bieneusi* and *Encephalitozoon intestinalis* are the species associated with diarrhea (257). Common epidemiologic characteristics have not been identified and the mode of transmission in humans is not known for certain. Fecal-oral transmission is the likely route of infection in humans with intestinal microsporidiosis, but the source of ocular infections is not clear. To date, there have been no reports of nosocomial infections with this microorganism.

Routine histopathologic studies can provide presumptive identification, but diagnostic confirmation requires EM visualization of the microorganism's characteristic ultrastructure (258). Microsporidia have been detected from formalin-fixed stool specimens following staining by a chromotrope-based technique and light microscopy (259). PCR also has been used for detection from stools or from small intestine biopsy (260).

Other Causes

Candida Species

Candida species have been associated with gastroenteritis in two settings: noninvasive enteritis in healthy persons (261,262) and invasive enteritis in patients with underlying diseases (263, 264). *Candida* is a saprophyte in healthy humans and is present in approximately 60% of stool specimens (265). Because *Candida* species often can be isolated from the gastrointestinal tract of healthy individuals, their presence does not necessarily signify disease. Gastroenteritis associated with *Candida* species is characterized by intermittent, watery, explosive diarrhea that is not bloody and rarely is accompanied by fever, nausea, anorexia, or vomiting. These symptoms can be chronic and have been reported for up to 3 months (266).

A prospective study of nosocomial diarrhea in newborns and infants isolated *Candida* species from 5% of stool specimens. *Candida* was the third most common cause (267) and appeared most often in premature infants. The causative role of *Candida* in diarrhea was not clear in this study. Healthy patients who develop *Candida* gastroenteritis generally do not develop candidemia and usually respond to either nystatin or clotrimazole within 72 hours (266). Nosocomial diarrhea associated with *Candida albicans* is especially prevalent in immunocompromised or malnourished patients (268,269) and in patients receiving antibiotic or antineoplastic drugs (233,270). *Candida* is detected by routine microscopy of stool specimens or by growth on agar plates.

Necrotizing Enterocolitis

NNIS system data showed that NEC occurred in 6 of 10,000 discharges: 8.7 per 100,000 patients overall and 60 per 10,000 infants in high-risk nurseries. Microorganisms associated were *C. difficile* (28%), *E. coli* (19%), *Klebsiella pneumoniae* (15%), coagulase-negative staphylococci (5%), *Enterobacter cloacae* (7%), and enterococci (6%). Gerber and others did not identify a cause in an outbreak of NEC, but nurses caring for infants involved in the outbreak also became ill (104,271,272). A review of several outbreaks included the previously mentioned causes and added viral enteropathogens including coronavirus, adenovirus, rotaviruses, and echovirus type 22 as isolates during outbreaks (273,274). Further discussion of NEC can be found in Chapters 24 and 52.

Potential Nosocomial Gastrointestinal Tract Pathogens

Aeromonas Species

Species of *Aeromonas*, including *Aeromonas caviae, Aeromonas hydrophila,* and *Aeromonas sobria* have been associated with acute gastroenteritis (275–280), but other studies do not support this finding (281). *Aeromonas* species have been implicated in nosocomial diarrhea, but this association is debated. *A. hydrophila* has been described as the cause of an acute diarrheal outbreak in a geriatric long-term care facility (282). In a study in child care centers, *Aeromonas* was identified in the stool specimens of 25% of children during an outbreak of diarrheal illness (283). These outbreaks of diarrhea were unusual in that several different *Aeromonas* species were involved in each outbreak. In another study, *Aeromonas* species were recovered from stool specimens of 15 hospitalized children, but all were community acquired (284). Surveillance in a French hospital revealed a seasonal variation in nosocomial *A. hydrophila* infection that was correlated with the number of *Aeromonas* microorganisms in the hospital water supply (285,286).

Aeromonas species are recovered by culture and identified by biotyping. DNA hybridization has been used to investigate the relatedness of strains in hospital outbreaks (283,287,288). PFGE was useful in the investigation of outbreaks in child care centers (283).

Klebsiella Species

Klebsiella species are members of the Enterobacteriaceae family. They can cause a wide variety of clinical infections including urinary tract infections, pneumonia, and bacteremia. *Klebsiella* species have not been proven to cause enteritis. *Klebsiella* is mentioned here because of a report of an outbreak of *Klebsiella* species bacteremia following nasoduodenal feeding of premature infants with human milk contaminated with *Klebsiella* (289). None of the bacteremic infants had diarrhea. Diarrhea was reported in preterm infants who had *Klebsiella* isolated from stool specimens, but a causal association was not established (141,290).

EPIDEMIOLOGY

Descriptive Epidemiology

The behavior of infants and children places them at increased risk of nosocomial acquisition of enteropathogens. The close, frequent contact among children facilitates person-to-person transmission. Infants and children do not wash their hands and often place their fingers, toys, and other items in their mouths. Children cared for in child care centers have a threefold greater risk of acquiring diarrhea than children cared for at home (291, 292). Hospitalized children display these same behavior patterns, which place them at an increased risk of fecal-oral transmission of enteropathogens. This is especially true of infants and toddlers who are not toilet trained.

Reservoirs and Sources of Infection

The pattern and timing of an outbreak of diarrhea in a hospital may provide clues about the reservoir or source and mode

TABLE 50.2. FACTORS IMPORTANT IN THE INTRODUCTION OF NOSOCOMIAL INFECTIOUS GASTROENTERITIS

Short-term, asymptomatic carriers of enteropathogens
Colonized, asymptomatic prolonged carriers of enteropathogens
Patient-to-patient transmission via hands of hospital personnel, generally after contact with a child with diarrhea
Contaminated medications, food, or medical instruments
Hospital crowding
Lack of adherence to infection control procedures

of transmission. The possible reservoirs and sources of these microorganisms are considered first (Table 50.2). Patients may act as a reservoir for enteropathogens. As described previously, many potential enteropathogens often are excreted asymptomatically. If an asymptomatic patient is not isolated because the infection is not suspected, microorganisms may be introduced into the hospital environment. The second scenario of the patient as the reservoir is a child admitted for management of an acute gastrointestinal tract infection. Enteropathogens may be transmitted to other patients, to hospital personnel, or to hospital visitors. Immunosuppressed patients may become infected with enteric microorganisms that are part of their own normal flora.

Hospital personnel may act as a reservoir of infection. The same conditions occur as with patients. An employee may be an unknown chronic carrier of an enteropathogen or may be present in the hospital with an acute illness. The enteropathogen may then be transmitted to patients or co-workers by direct person-to-person contact or indirectly through fomites.

Food products may serve as a point source for nosocomial infections. Patients, hospital personnel, visitors, or all three groups eat the implicated food items. The food reservoir may originate outside or within the hospital. Several *Salmonella* species outbreaks have been traced to intact and properly stored eggs (151). Improperly stored foods have been implicated in several foodborne diarrheal outbreaks among both patients and employees (157,293). Norwalk virus has been described as a cause of foodborne outbreaks in the hospital setting (63). In addition to prepared foods, enteral feedings and infant formulas have become contaminated during storage (161).

The definition of water-borne disease outbreaks by the CDC for surveillance purposes is restricted to illness that occurs after consumption or use of water intended for drinking. Outbreaks have been associated with private wells, small water systems, and community water systems (294). Reservoirs for water-borne outbreaks also may include drinking water contaminated at the faucet, as occurs with *Aeromonas*, or ice (285,286). The contamination may occur away from the hospital, as has been reported in outbreaks resulting from *G. lamblia, Cryptosporidium, Cyclospora,* Microsporidia, and viruses (294). Various reservoirs exist within the hospital where water-holding units such as whirlpools, storage tanks, or common bathing tanks may be contaminated (203). *C. difficile* spores remain on surfaces in patient rooms after cleaning (295).

All hospital devices should be considered potential reservoirs. The reservoir may exist as the result of inadequate cleaning and sterilization, as occurred with endoscope-transmitted infections (167,168); lack of proper cleaning, as in the use of common suction traps and tubing (169–171); or inadequate sterilization, as occurred when a breast pump used by several mothers in an NICU became contaminated (170).

Blood products are a well-known risk factor for nosocomial infections such as hepatitis B and C, HIV, and cytomegalovirus. The contamination of whole blood units with *Y. enterocolitica* resulted in bacteremia in recipients. It is thought that the blood donors had a mild bacteremia at the time of their donation and that the refrigerated storage supported growth of *Y. enterocolitica* (210–212).

Other reservoirs may include animals outside the hospital or pets used in pet therapy programs within the hospital (see Chapter 101). There have been no reports of gastrointestinal tract disease resulting from pet therapy, but immunosuppressed patients may be particularly at risk. The association of salmonellosis with reptiles warrants restriction of reptiles from the hospital setting. Vectors have not been implicated in gastrointestinal tract infections in this country.

Modes of Transmission of Infection

The mode of transmission describes how the enteropathogen gets from the reservoir to the host. The pattern and timing of an outbreak may provide clues about transmission. Several cases occurring in a short period may be easy to recognize and trace to a point source such as food or a specific patient or employee. Other point sources such as an endoscope may be more difficult to recognize, because the number of infections may be few and may appear sporadic. Routine surveillance is an important tool in the recognition of these sources.

Person-to-person transmission may occur as the result of many practices. Poor hand washing by personnel results in direct spread to patients or self-inoculation. The patients may secondarily infect (3) other family members either as hospital visitors or after returning home. Fomites play a role in patient-to-patient transmission. Many items within a room or within common areas may become contaminated by enteropathogens. Subsequent contact with these items results in transmission. This is particularly important for microorganisms for which transmission of infection is associated with a low inoculum, such as rotavirus, *Shigella, Giardia,* enteric adenovirus, astrovirus, calicivirus, *E. coli* O157:H7, and *Cryptosporidium.* Person-to-person spread also occurs through vertical transmission of a microorganism from a mother to her newborn child at the time of delivery. Several enteropathogens, such as *S. sonnei* (188), *S. flexneri* (189), *C. fetus,* and *C. jejuni* (118) have been transmitted to neonates in this manner.

Foodborne transmission results from ingesting contaminated foods, poorly cleaned fresh foods, or nasoduodenal infusion of contaminated nutritional supplements or infant formulas. Nasoduodenal feedings may be a greater risk than nasogastric feedings, because the feeding tube bypasses the normal protective acidic environment of the stomach. Infections have resulted from *Salmonella* species (164), *Campylobacter* species (120,296), *Klebsiella* species (289), and ETEC contamination of milk (131) and *Campylobacter* species (120) contamination of poorly cleaned vegetables. *Salmonella* (150–152,155,161), *Staphylococcus aureus, E. coli* (138), and Norwalk virus (63) have all been described in foodborne nosocomial infections in the hospital setting.

A gastroduodenal endoscope transmitted *Helicobacter pylori* in adults (297,298). *Salmonella newport* was transmitted by fiberoptic colonoscopy in 8 of 28 patients who underwent the procedure after the colonoscope had been used in a patient with acute disease resulting from *S. newport* (297). Transmission resulted from inadequate cleaning and sterilization of the biopsy forceps. Chapter 63 describes nosocomial infections associated with endoscopic procedures.

Transmission of enteric pathogens by hospital instruments occurs most often in NICUs. Nursery isolettes have been implicated in transmission of ETEC and *C. difficile.* Common use suction tubing and an overflow reservoir were reported to transmit *Salmonella worthington* in an NICU (170). *Klebsiella* was cultured from tubing of a breast milk pump following an outbreak of bacteremia in preterm infants receiving donor human milk by nasoduodenal feedings (289). Rectal thermometers have been reported to spread *Salmonella eimsbuettel* among newborn infants (172).

Risk Factors for Infection

The most severely ill patients are at greatest risk for nosocomial gastrointestinal tract infections for several reasons. The patients may be immunocompromised by the severity of illness, by poor nutritional status, and/or by therapeutic modalities. The use of antacids and H_2-blockers in intensive care units may decrease the protective effect of gastric acidity. Children in intensive care units require frequent manipulation by multiple hospital personnel, which increases the risk of person-to-person transmission.

Neonates, especially premature infants, are unique in that they are immunocompromised. The incidence of nosocomial gastrointestinal tract infection is twice as high in the high-risk nursery as in the general pediatric population (9). The types of nosocomial infections of the gastrointestinal tract that occur in the nursery include NEC, rotavirus, *Klebsiella* species, *C. difficile,* EPEC, and *Salmonella.* See Chapter 52 for a review of nosocomial infections in hospital nurseries.

Immunocompromised patients constitute a special high-risk group. Malnourished persons are at high risk for severe gastrointestinal tract disease. This is particularly evident in the reports of nosocomial gastroenteritis from developing countries. Patients infected with HIV have an increased risk of infection with microorganisms previously not shown to be enteropathogens. *C. parvum* and Microsporidia species have been described as enteropathogens in this population. There have been no reports of nosocomial transmission, but such events may occur. Patients with severe combined immunodeficiency disease acquire enteropathogens nosocomially and suffer prolonged disease with significant morbidity and often a fatal outcome (91,299).

Patients receiving chemotherapy for malignancies or persons who are immunosuppressed after organ transplantation are at an increased risk for infection by microorganisms that are part of their normal flora. *C. difficile* and *Candida,* in particular, have been reported to cause gastroenteritis under these conditions (300). Forty percent of bone marrow transplant patients developed nosocomial gastroenteritis in one study, and another unit had a prolonged nosocomial astrovirus outbreak (45,301).

Prolonged hospital stay is another risk factor for nosocomial gastroenteritis. These children are at risk both because of their underlying medical condition and their continued exposure to a variety of enteropathogens. Children in long-term care facilities have an increased risk of foodborne, water-borne, and person-to-person transmission of enteropathogens (14,302–304). In one study, 10% of children with an infected roommate developed nosocomial diarrhea. The risk was directly proportional to the number of roommates. Younger hospitalized children were at a greater risk: 10% of diapered children developed nosocomial diarrhea, compared with only 2% of nondiapered children (19). The viral nosocomial diarrhea rate decreases with age. The rate at 0 to 11 months was 9%; at 12 to 35 months, 4%; and at 36 months or more, 0.6%. The rate does not significantly increase with length of hospital stay (9,19–21,305).

PATHOGENESIS

Viral enteropathogens are transmitted by the fecal-oral route. Enteric viruses tend to infect the small intestine, with replication occurring in epithelial cells at the tips of the villi; infection is confined primarily to these cells. The changes include shortening and blunting of villi and increased infiltration of the lamina propria with mononuclear cells. Mucosal damage is repaired rapidly, as early as 3 weeks after onset. Many children with acute viral gastroenteritis have lactose malabsorption and intolerance. Loss of fluids and electrolytes in viral gastroenteritis can lead to severe dehydration and even death and requires fluid and electrolyte replacement therapy. The severity of intestinal mucosal injury varies among the enteric viruses.

The major virulence properties of bacterial enteropathogens include adherence, enterotoxin production, cytotoxin production, epithelial cell invasion, and translocation. Certain enteropathogens may produce diarrhea by other mechanisms, and enteric pathogens may possess one or several of these virulence properties. Enterotoxins are bacterial products that act on the mucosal epithelium of the small intestine causing fluid secretion and profuse watery diarrhea without damage to intestinal mucosa. Functionally similar enterotoxins are produced by *V. cholerae,* ETEC, *Aeromonas, C. difficile, C. jejuni, Salmonella,* and *Y. enterocolitica.* Presumptive evidence indicates that rotavirus nonstructural glycoprotein (NSP4) functions as an enterotoxin (306,307). Cytotoxins kill mammalian cells, usually by inhibition of protein synthesis. *In vivo,* they cause damage to intestinal epithelial cells and destruction of normal absorptive mechanisms, which results in diarrhea containing blood. Fluid loss probably is related to impaired absorption resulting from intestinal damage; unlike enterotoxins, cytotoxins do not cause active fluid secretion by the gut. Microorganisms such as *Shigella,* EIEC, *C. jejuni, Salmonella,* and *Y. enterocolitica* can invade the mucosa of the colon or small intestine and result in an inflammatory host response. This invasion is characterized clinically by fever; abdominal pain; tenesmus; and stools containing blood, mucus, and fecal leukocytes. Adherence, the ability of microorganisms to attach and colonize gut epithelium, is the least specific virulence property in terms of related clinical findings. The ability of ETEC to adhere to and colonize the upper small intestine, where it causes disease by production of enterotoxin, has been well described.

Parasitic enteropathogens possess a variety of pathogenetic mechanisms. The spore-forming protozoa (cryptosporidia, microsporidia, *Isospora,* and *Cyclospora*) produce abnormalities in absorption, secretion, and motility of the small bowel and are associated with inflammatory infiltrates. This may be associated with villus blunting and crypt hyperplasia but not mucosal invasion. Gastrointestinal tract function and morphology relate to the number of microorganisms present. *Giardia* produce disease and malabsorption by producing varying degrees of mucosal injury and by influencing conditions in the intestinal lumen, which may impair digestion and absorption. *Strongyloides* is acquired by penetration of intact skin by the filariform larvae. All other parasitic enteropathogens are acquired by fecal-oral transmission through ingestion of cysts or oocysts that are resistant to physical destruction.

CLINICAL MANIFESTATIONS

Localized

The approach to hospitalized patients with acute infectious diarrhea begins with a carefully obtained medical history including epidemiologic considerations and a physical examination. Acute diarrhea can be caused by one of the many microorganisms discussed previously. Clinical manifestations occurring in patients with diarrhea reflect either localized involvement of the gastrointestinal tract or systemic involvement, manifested by generalized symptoms or signs. The presence of a specific clinical manifestation is not pathognomonic of any causative agent; however, some clinical features occur more often as a result of infection by certain microorganisms. The most common localized manifestations may occur with varying degrees of severity. These include diarrhea, nausea, anorexia, vomiting, and abdominal discomfort or cramping. The character of the diarrhea may provide a clue as to the associated enteropathogen. Bacterial microorganisms that invade intestinal mucosa often cause abdominal cramps, tenesmus, fecal urgency, and passage of stools containing blood and mucus and fecal leukocytes. Patients with secretory diarrhea have abdominal cramps and pass a low to moderate number of large volume watery stools that, when passed, may be associated with temporary relief. Patients infected with *E. coli* O157:H7 and *E. histolytica* may have bloody diarrhea without fecal leukocytes and severe cramps. Patients with giardiasis or cryptosporidiosis often have watery, foul-smelling stools associated with nausea and flatulence or chronic diarrhea with malabsorption and abdominal distention. Diarrhea resulting from viral enteropathogens generally occurs in infants who present with low-grade fever, vomiting, and watery diarrhea.

Generalized

Many enteropathogens present with systemic manifestations of illness. Fever is a common, but not universal, manifestation of these infections. The parasitic enteropathogens that involve the small intestine rarely cause febrile illness, whereas acute infection with many of the enteric viruses and bacteria may result in fever. Dehydration is the most common reason for hospitalization of children with gastroenteritis in the United States. Dehydration occurs as the result of increased fluid losses from vomiting, diarrhea, and increased insensible losses associated with fever. Dehydration may result in shock if not recognized or corrected early. Shock may lead to multiple organ system involvement. Mild to moderate dehydration is most appropriately treated with an oral rehydration solution (308,309). This has been demonstrated to be effective in developing countries and is the mainstay of therapy in cholera.

Enteric pathogens have extraintestinal manifestations. These include cutaneous involvement by *S. typhi* and strongyloidiasis; bacteremia and other organ system involvement by bacterial and parasitic enteropathogens; the complications of HUS with *E. coli* O157:H7, other EHEC, and *S. dysenteriae* type 1; and pulmonary compromise in immunosuppressed patients with strongyloidiasis. A wasting syndrome of malnutrition occurs in HIV-infected patients with microsporidiosis or cryptosporidiosis. In addition, several immune-mediated conditions can occur following enteric infections including reactive arthritis, Reiter's syndrome, Guillain-Barré syndrome, glomerulonephritis, erythema nodosum, and hemolytic anemia. These manifestations have been associated with *Salmonella, Shigella, Yersinia, Campylobacter, Giardia,* or *Cryptosporidium.*

DIAGNOSIS AND EVALUATION OF OUTBREAKS

The evaluation of either endemic infections or outbreaks of nosocomial gastroenteritis has two purposes. The first is to identify the enteropathogen and determine the method of transmission. The second is to evaluate isolated strains of the enteropathogens for relatedness. For epidemiologic purposes, the more closely related the strains of microorganisms, the stronger the proof that an outbreak is due to a common epidemic strain. Merely proving that several patients are infected with the same species does not substantiate the occurrence of an outbreak. Many techniques are available to evaluate genetic relatedness (see Chapter 102). The identification of microorganisms may be approached in a stepwise fashion. First, nonspecific tests are used to support infection and identify the type of enteropathogens (viral, bacterial, or parasitic). Next, phenotypic techniques are used to identify the microorganism based on characteristics expressed by the microorganism. Finally, genotypic techniques that involve direct DNA-based analyses of chromosomal or extrachromosomal genetic elements are used for molecular fingerprinting. In general, these three steps to diagnosis move from evaluation at the bedside, to routine laboratory evaluation, to testing in research or referral laboratories (310–313). See Table 50.3 for a list of methods and Chapter 7 for further information about outbreak investigations. I briefly describe the techniques generally available, but more detailed descriptions may be found in listed references.

The timing of the onset of diarrhea in relationship to the

TABLE 50.3. LABORATORY TESTS USED TO EVALUATE NOSOCOMIAL OUTBREAKS OF INFECTIOUS GASTROENTERITIS

Nonspecific tests
Stool fecal leukocytes
Microscopy
Stool occult blood
Complete blood count
Stool culture
Electron microscopy
Immunoelectron microscopy
Phenotypic techniques
Biotyping
Antibiograms (antimicrobial susceptibility patterns)
Serotyping
Bacteriophage typing
Immunoblotting
Enzyme immunoassay (EIA)
Multilocus enzyme electrophoresis (MEE)
Genotypic techniques
Electropherotyping
Plasmid profile analysis (PPA)
Restriction endonuclease analysis (REA)
Southern hybridization analysis (SHA) using specific DNA probes
Ribotyping
DNA profiling using pulsed-field gel electrophoresis (PFGE)
Polymerase chain reaction (PCR)
Nucleotide sequence analysis

admission to the hospital should be used to guide the evaluation. Diarrhea occurring more than 3 days after admission is unlikely to be caused by either bacterial or parasitic etiologies. Viral or *C. difficile*-associated diarrhea are more likely. Therefore, routine bacterial cultures and studies for ova and parasites are not cost-effective for the initial testing of diarrhea occurring more than 3 days after admission (314–317).

The utility of the age-old technique of microscopy permits evaluation of fresh stool specimens for the presence of fecal leukocytes. This single procedure differentiates inflammatory diarrhea from noninflammatory diarrhea, thereby narrowing the differential diagnosis considerably. Microscopic examination of either fresh or concentrated stool specimens is the mainstay in the diagnosis of parasitic diseases. Trophozoites, cysts, oocysts, or worms can be identified in stool specimens (256,259). Gram stain of a stool specimen may not be useful to identify a specific enteric gram-negative bacterium, but yeast cells can be identified in this manner, as can the spiral-shaped *Campylobacter* microorganisms. Testing a stool sample for occult blood is a simple, inexpensive, and rapid method for evaluating the presence of gastrointestinal tract inflammation or mucosal damage.

The interpretation of a complete blood count and differential cell count also provides nonspecific evidence as to the cause. Anemia or hemolysis may occur, particularly with HUS. Leukocytosis is more often seen with a bacterial gastrointestinal tract infection. Eosinophilia supports further investigation for a parasitic infection.

Several phenotypic methods are used to characterize microorganisms including biotyping, antimicrobial susceptibility testing, serotyping, bacteriophage typing, immunoblotting, EIA, and multilocus enzyme electrophoresis. The mainstay of the diagnosis of bacterial diarrheal illness is the stool culture. Many of the microorganisms discussed in this chapter are not detected with routine stool culture methods. Selective media and special conditions for growth may be necessary for isolation of many microorganisms. Communication with the clinical microbiology laboratory is essential for identification of these enteropathogens. The microbiologist should be notified about the suspected microorganisms so that appropriate media and techniques may be used for identification. *C. jejuni* and other *Campylobacter* species, *Y. enterocolitica, V. cholerae* and other *Vibrio* species, pathogenic *E. coli,* and *C. difficile* all require special procedures for isolation (309).

EIA is a relatively rapid technique to identify many of the microorganisms and toxins described previously. Commercially produced EIAs are available for detection of *Cryptosporidium, G. lamblia,* rotavirus, enteric adenovirus, astrovirus, calicivirus, cholera toxin, and *C. difficile* toxins. Other EIAs for detection of other enteropathogens are available in reference or research laboratories.

Evaluation of the molecular structure of enteropathogens is useful for analysis of different strains of the same microorganism. These methods add nothing to the identification of a specific microorganism but are used for comparison of strains based on genetic similarities or dissimilarities. Application of one or more of these methods to various collections of nosocomial pathogens has shown that DNA-based typing methods are useful in studying the relationship between colonizing and infecting isolates in an individual patient, distinguishing contaminating from infecting strains, documenting cross-infection among hospitalized patients, and evaluating reinfection versus relapse in patients being treated for an infectious process. Examples of genotypic methods include electropherotyping, plasmid profile analysis, restriction endonuclease analysis, Southern hybridization analysis, ribotyping, PFGE, PCR, random amplified polymorphism of DNA, and nucleotide sequence analysis (318–325).

Biopsy may be the only possible method to identify some of the microorganisms mentioned in this chapter. Microsporidia are identified on EM of intestinal biopsy specimens. Microscopic examination of biopsy material may accurately identify *Giardia, Strongyloides, E. histolytica,* EPEC, and EAEC.

PREVENTION AND CONTROL

Nosocomial gastrointestinal tract infections are best prevented by surveillance and identification of methods to improve hospital procedures. It is important that infection control methods be based on scientific data not just on speculation. It is difficult to know how many nosocomial enteric infections can be prevented. The CDC's Study of the Efficacy of Nosocomial Infection Control project noted that surveillance by infection control professionals decreased nosocomial infections by 32%, but in this study gastrointestinal tract infections and pediatric hospital infections were not addressed specifically (326). One study of pediatric nosocomial gastrointestinal tract infections indicated that educational intervention programs decreased the incidence of nosocomial rotavirus infection (327). It is accepted universally that effective hand washing is the mainstay of prevention of nosocomial infections including gastroenteritis (328). Observational studies have noted that physicians wash their hands before only 30% to 85% of patient contacts, indicating the need for continuing education for healthcare providers about appropriate infection control procedures including hand washing (111,329,330). Alcohol-based products reduce rotavirus on hands by approximately 99% in reported studies (331). No antiseptic agents are effective against spore-forming microorganisms such as *C. difficile*; therefore the use of gloves is recommended (331). For more information on hand hygiene, see Chapter 96.

Cohorting or grouping neonates and their nursing staff was not effective for prevention of nosocomial infections in an NICU (332). In another study, Klein et al. (333) demonstrated that protective isolation of patients in a pediatric intensive care unit using gowns and gloves decreased the nosocomial infection rate in that environment. Unfortunately, this study did not address gastrointestinal tract infection rates.

Appropriate isolation of patients that are excreting enteropathogens is a necessary part of prevention. Table 50.4 shows diseases transmitted by the fecal-oral route. All patients are to be managed using standard precautions. Those patients with acute diarrhea with a likely infectious cause or diarrhea in an adult with a history of recent antibiotic use should be managed using additional Contact Precautions (Table 50.5) (334). (See Chapter 95 for more details.) Patients in the same room as an index patient should be managed with the same precautions. Exposed patients may be incubating the enteropathogen, and they should not be transferred into a room with unexposed children. In addition, gloves should be considered for diaper changing of all hospitalized children. A uniform hospital policy rather than unit-specific guidelines is advantageous. The incidence of *C. difficile*-associated diarrhea was decreased among adult bone marrow transplant patients by cleaning the rooms with sodium hypochlorite rather than with quaternary ammonium products (335).

TABLE 50.4. DISEASES TRANSMITTED BY THE FECAL-ORAL ROUTE

Amebic dysentery
Cholera
Coxsackie virus disease
Diarrhea, acute illness with suspected infectious etiology
Echovirus disease
Encephalitis (unless known not to be caused by enteroviruses)
Enterocolitis caused by *Clostridium difficile*
Enteroviral infection
Gastroenteritis caused by:
- *Campylobacter* species
- *Cryptosporidium*
- *Dientamoeba fragilis*
- *Escherichia coli* (EAEC, ETEC, EPEC, EIEC, or EHEC)
- *Giardia lamblia*
- *Isospora belli*
- *Salmonella* species
- *Shigella* species
- *Vibrio cholerae*
- *Vibrio parahaemolyticus*
- Viruses, including rotavirus, astrovirus, calicivirus (including noroviruses), and enteric adenovirus
- *Yersinia enterocolitica*
- Unknown etiology but presumed to be an infectious agent

Hand, foot, and mouth disease
Hepatitis, viral, type A
Herpangina
Meningitis, viral (unless known not to be caused by enteroviruses)
Necrotizing enterocolitis
Pleurodynia
Poliomyelitis
Typhoid fever (*Salmonella typhi*)
Viral pericarditis, myocarditis, or meningitis (unless known not to be caused by enteroviruses)

EAEC, enteroaggregative *E. coli*; EHEC, enterohemorrhagic *E. coli*; EIEC, enteroinvasive *E. coli*; EPEC, enteropathogenic *E. coli*; ETEC, enterotoxigenic *E. coli*.

TABLE 50.5. CONTACT PRECAUTIONS

Use Standard Precautions for all patients

Masks are not indicated
Gowns are indicated
Gloves are indicated
Hands must be washed after touching the patient or potentially contaminated articles and before taking care of another patient
Single room is indicated if possible

Surveillance is integral for identification of nosocomial infections and for identification of the source and mode of transmission. If the source and mode of transmission are not identified, control of an outbreak will be difficult, if not impossible.

Employee health plays an important role in the prevention of nosocomial gastroenteritis. Any staff member with symptoms that suggest infection should be excluded from contact with potentially susceptible persons for at least 2 days after resolution of illness (75) (see Chapter 99).

Appropriate antimicrobial agents may be given to patients known to be infected with an enteropathogen. This therapy may shorten the time that a patient excretes the microorganism, although there is concern that treatment of salmonellosis may increase the period of excretion. Table 50.6 lists enteropathogens for which antimicrobial therapy may be useful. Conversely, limiting antibiotic use for other infections may decrease *C. difficile*-associated diarrhea (336).

Immunizations may play a role in prevention and control of nosocomial infections by some enteropathogens, but commercially available enteric vaccines are limited. Typhoid and cholera vaccines are available and may be useful for prevention of disease in developing countries.

Human milk decreases the frequency and severity of diarrhea in infants. Therefore, all providers should encourage the initiation and continuation of breast-feeding during the first year of life.

There is increasing support for the use of probiotics for the prevention and treatment of gastrointestinal tract infections. These live culture "good" bacteria may be beneficial in both prevention and treatment of diarrhea. *Lactobacillus* GG was effective in preventing symptomatic infections from rotavirus in hospitalized infants in a randomized, double-blinded study (337).

Gastrointestinal tract decontamination by giving enteral antibiotics to modify the gut flora and delay gastrointestinal tract colonization has had mixed success. Studies in adults in intensive

TABLE 50.6. POTENTIAL BENEFIT FOR ANTIMICROBIAL THERAPY FOR ENTEROPATHOGENS

Potential benefit	Enteropathogen or disease
No therapy available	Enteric viruses
Established benefit	Necrotizing enterocolitis
	Antimicrobial-associated colitis (*Clostridium difficile*)
	Cholera
	Cryptosporidium parvum
	Cyclospora cayetanensis
	Entamoeba histolytica
	Enterotoxigenic *Escherichia coli*
	Giardia lamblia
	Isospora belli
	Shigella species
	Strongyloidiasis
Absolute	Any bacterium that produces bacteremia (e.g., typhoid fever)
Questionable or unknown	*Aeromonas* species
	Campylobacter jejuni
	Candida species
	Enterohemorrhagic *E. coli*
	Intestinal salmonellosis
	Microsporidi
	Yersinia enterocolitica

care units have shown both decreased infection rates and no difference in infection rates (338,339). The studies reported to date have evaluated invasive infections and did not comment on prevention of diarrheal illness.

The CDC lists the following items as necessary steps for the control of an outbreak of viral gastroenteritis: (a) common sources should be identified and eliminated; (b) employee transmission of illness should be prevented by use of appropriate gowns and gloves when handling infectious materials; (c) soiled linens and clothing should be handled as little as possible; and (d) because environmental surfaces in some settings have been implicated in the transmission of enteric viruses, bathrooms and rooms occupied by ill persons should be kept visibly clean on a routine basis.

REFERENCES

1. Grossman M, Applebaum MN. Demographics of community-acquired bacterial infection in hospitalized children. *Pediatr Infect Dis J* 1992;11:139–142.
2. Garner JS, Jarvis WR, Emori TG, et al. CDC definitions for nosocomial infections, 1988. *Am J Infect Control* 1988;16:128–140.
3. Watkins AG, Lewis-Fanning E. Incidence of cross-infection in children's wards. *BMJ* 1949;2:616–619.
4. Gardner P, Carles DG. Infections acquired in a pediatric hospital. *J Pediatr* 1972;81:1205–1210.
5. Langley JM, LeBlanc JC, Hanakowski M, et al. The role of *Clostridium difficile* and viruses as causes of nosocomial diarrhea in children. *Infect Control Hosp Epidemiol* 2002;23:660–664.
6. Bennet R, Hedlund KO, Ehrnst A, et al. Nosocomial gastroenteritis in two infant wards over 26 months. *Acta Paediatr* 1995;84:667–671.
7. Bowen-Jones J. Infection and cross-infection in paediatric gastroenteritis unit. *Curationis* 1989;12:30–33.
8. Cotton MF, Berkowitz FE, Berkowitz Z, et al. Nosocomial infection in black South African children. *Pediatr Infect Dis J* 1989;8:676–683.
9. Ford Jones EL, Mindorff CM, Langley JM, et al. Epidemiologic study of 4684 hospital-acquired infections in pediatric patients. *Pediatr Infect Dis J* 1989;8:668–675.
10. Grassano Morin A, de Champs C, Lafeuille H, et al. [Nosocomial intestinal infections in an infant ward. The importance of phone inquiries of the families]. *Arch Pediatr* 2000;7:1059–1063.
11. Kamalaratnam CN, Kang G, Kirubakaran C, et al. A prospective study of nosocomial enteric pathogen acquisition in hospitalized children in South India. *J Trop Pediatr* 2001;47:46–49.
12. Stegenga J, Bell E, Matlow A, et al. The role of nurse understaffing in nosocomial viral gastrointestinal infections on a general pediatrics ward. *Infect Control Hosp Epidemiol* 2002;23:133–136.
13. Welliver RC, MacLaughlin S. Unique epidemiology of nosocomial infection in a children's hospital. *Am J Dis Child* 1984;138:131–135.
14. Gaynes RP, Martone WJ, Culver DH, et al. Comparison of rates of nosocomial infections in neonatal intensive care units in the United States. National Nosocomial Infections Surveillance System. *Am J Med* 1991;91:192s–196s.
15. Richards MJ, Edwards JR, Culver DH, et al. Nosocomial infections in pediatric intensive care units in the United States. National Nosocomial Infections Surveillance System. *Pediatrics* 1999;103:e39.
16. Maille L, Beby-Defaux A, Bourgoin A, et al. [Nosocomial infections due to rotavirus and respiratory syncytial virus in pediatric wards: a 2-year study]. *Ann Biol Clin (Paris)* 2000;58:601–606.
17. Fruhwirth M, Heininger U, Ehlken B, et al. International variation in disease burden of rotavirus gastroenteritis in children with community- and nosocomially acquired infection. *Pediatr Infect Dis J* 2001; 20:784–791.
18. Fruhwirth M, Berger K, Ehlken B, et al. Economic impact of community- and nosocomially acquired rotavirus gastroenteritis in Austria. *Pediatr Infect Dis J* 2001;20:184–188.
19. Ford Jones EL, Mindorff CM, Gold R, et al. The incidence of viral-associated diarrhea after admission to a pediatric hospital. *Am J Epidemiol* 1990;131:711–718.
20. Anderson LJ. Major trends in nosocomial viral infections. *Am J Med* 1991;91:107–111.
21. Brady MT, Pacini DL, Budde CT, et al. Diagnostic studies of nosocomial diarrhea in children: assessing their use and value. *Am J Infect Control* 1989;17:77–82.
22. Christensen ML. Human viral gastroenteritis. *Clin Microbiol Rev* 1989;2:51–89.
23. Van R, Wun CC, O'Ryan ML, et al. Outbreaks of human enteric adenovirus types 40 and 41 in Houston day care centers. *J Pediatr* 1992;120:516–521.
24. Rodriguez WJ. Viral enteritis in the 1980s: perspective, diagnosis and outlook for prevention. *Pediatr Infect Dis J* 1989;8:570–578.
25. Yolken RH, Lawrence F, Leister F, et al. Gastroenteritis associated with enteric type adenovirus in hospitalized infants. *J Pediatr* 1982; 101:21–26.
26. Kotloff KL, Losonsky GA, Morris JG, et al. Enteric adenovirus infection and childhood diarrhea: an epidemiologic study in three clinical settings. *Pediatrics* 1989;84:219–225.
27. Ushijima H, Shinozaki T, Araki K, et al. Nosocomial infection by rotavirus and adenovirus within one month. *Acta Paediatr Jpn* 1988; 30:13–16.
28. Krajden M, Brown M, Petrasek A, et al. Clinical features of adenovirus enteritis: a review of 127 cases. *Pediatr Infect Dis J* 1990;9:636–641.
29. Pena MJ, Elcuaz R, Suarez J, et al. Gastroenteritis caused by adenovirus 40/41: epidemiological and clinical aspects. *Inferm Infecc Microbiol Clin* 1992;10:481–485.
30. Yolken RH, Franklin CC. Gastrointestinal adenovirus: an important cause of morbidity in patients with necrotizing enterocolitis and gastrointestinal surgery. *Pediatr Infect Dis J* 1985;4:42–47.
31. Utagawa ET, Nishizawa S, Sekine S, et al. Astrovirus as a cause of gastroenteritis in Japan. *J Clin Microbiol* 1994;32:1841–1845.
32. Oishi I, Yamazaki K, Kimoto T, et al. A large outbreak of acute gastroenteritis associated with astrovirus among students and teachers in Osaka Japan. *J Infect Dis* 1994;170:439–443.
33. Mitchell DK, Monroe SS, Jiang X, et al. Virologic features of an astrovirus diarrhea outbreak in a day care center revealed by reverse

transcriptase-polymerase chain reaction. *J Infect Dis* 1995;172: 1437–1444.

34. Taylor MB, Marx FE, Grabow WO. Rotavirus, astrovirus and adenovirus associated with an outbreak of gastroenteritis in a South African child care centre. *Epidemiol Infect* 1997;119:227–230.
35. Lewis DC, Lightfoot NF, Cubitt WD, et al. Outbreaks of astrovirus type 1 and rotavirus gastroenteritis in a geriatric in-patient population. *J Hosp Infect* 1989;14:9–14.
36. Gray JJ, Wreghitt TG, Cubitt WD, et al. An outbreak of gastroenteritis in a home for the elderly associated with astrovirus type 1 and human calicivirus. *J Med Virol* 1987;23:377–381.
37. Kurtz JB, Lee TW, Pickering D. Astrovirus associated gastroenteritis in a children's ward. *J Clin Pathol* 1977;30:948–952.
38. Ashley CR, Caul EO, Paver WK. Astrovirus-associated gastroenteritis in children. *J Clin Pathol* 1978;31:939–943.
39. Esahli H, Breback K, Bennet R, et al. Astroviruses as a cause of nosocomial outbreaks of infant diarrhea. *Pediatr Infect Dis J* 1991;10: 511–515.
40. Mitchell DK, Van R, Morrow AL, et al. Outbreaks of astrovirus gastroenteritis in day care centers. *J Pediatr* 1993;123:725–732.
41. Kotloff KL, Herrmann JE, Blacklow NR, et al. The frequency of astrovirus as a cause of diarrhea in Baltimore children. *Pediatr Infect Dis J* 1992;11:587–589.
42. Traore O, Belliot G, Mollat C, et al. RT-PCR identification and typing of astroviruses and Norwalk-like viruses in hospitalized patients with gastroenteritis: evidence of nosocomial infections. *J Clin Virol* 2000;17:151–158.
43. Rodriguez-Baez N, O'Brien R, Qiu SQ, et al. Astrovirus, adenovirus, and rotavirus in hospitalized children: prevalence and association with gastroenteritis. *J Pediatr Gastroenterol Nutr* 2002;35:64–68.
44. Dennehy PH, Nelson SM, Spangenberger S, et al. A prospective case-control study of the role of astrovirus in acute diarrhea among hospitalized young children. *J Infect Dis* 2001;184:10–15.
45. Cubitt WD, Mitchell DK, Carter MJ, et al. Application of electromicroscopy, enzyme immunoassay, and RT-PCR to monitor an outbreak of astrovirus type 1 in a paediatric bone marrow transplant unit. *J Med Virol* 1999;57:313–321.
46. Glass RI, Noel J, Mitchell D, et al. The changing epidemiology of astrovirus-associated gastroenteritis: a review. *Arch Virol Suppl* 1996; 12:287–300.
47. Berke T, Golding B, Jiang X, et al. Phylogenetic analysis of the Caliciviruses. *J Med Virol* 1997;52:419–424.
48. Cubitt WD, McSwiggan DA, Moore W. Winter vomiting disease caused by calicivirus. *J Clin Pathol* 1979;32:786–793.
49. Cubitt WD, McSwiggan DA. Calicivirus gastroenteritis in North West London. *Lancet* 1981;2:975–977.
50. Matson DO, Estes MK, Tanaka T, et al. Asymptomatic human calicivirus infection in a day care center. *Pediatr Infect Dis J* 1990;9: 190–196.
51. Khan AS, Moe CL, Glass RI, et al. Norwalk virus-associated gastroenteritis traced to ice consumption aboard a cruise ship in Hawaii: comparison and application of molecular method-based assays. *J Clin Microbiol* 1994;32:318–322.
52. Spratt HC, Marks MI, Gomersall M, et al. Nosocomial infantile gastroenteritis associated with minirotavirus and calicivirus. *J Pediatr* 1978;93:922–926.
53. Lewis DC, Hale A, Jiang X, et al. Epidemiology of Mexico virus, a small round-structured virus in Yorkshire, United Kingdom, between January 1992 and March 1995. *J Infect Dis* 1997;175:951–954.
54. Jiang X, Cubitt D, Hu J, et al. Development of an ELISA to detect MX virus, a human calicivirus in the Snow Mountain Agent genogroup. *J Gen Virol* 1995;76:2739–2747.
55. Kaplan JE, Gary GW, Baron RC, et al. Epidemiology of Norwalk gastroenteritis and the role of Norwalk virus in outbreaks of acute nonbacterial gastroenteritis. *Ann Intern Med* 1982;96:756–761.
56. Spender QW, Lewis D, Price EH. Norwalk like viruses: study of an outbreak. *Arch Dis Child* 1986;61:142–147.
57. Storr J, Rice S, Phillips AD, et al. Clinical associations of Norwalk-like virus in the stools of children. *J Pediatr Gastroenterol Nutr* 1986; 5:576–580.
58. Riordan T, Wills A. An outbreak of gastroenteritis in a psycho-geriatric hospital associated with a small round structured virus. *J Hosp Infect* 1986;8:296–299.
59. Vinje J, Altena SA, Koopmans MPG. The incidence and genetic variability of small round-structured viruses in outbreaks of gastroenteritis in The Netherlands. *J Infect Dis* 1997;176:1374–1378.
60. Russo PL, Spelman DW, Harrington GA, et al. Hospital outbreak of Norwalk-like virus. *Infect Control Hosp Epidemiol* 1997;18:576–579.
61. Jiang X, Turf E, Hu J, et al. Outbreaks of gastroenteritis in elderly nursing homes and retirement facilities associated with human caliciviruses. *J Med Virol* 1996;50:335–341.
62. Cubitt WD, Jiang X. Study on occurrence of human calicivirus (Mexico strain) as cause of sporadic cases and outbreaks of calicivirus-associated diarrhoea in the United Kingdom, 1983–1995. *J Med Virol* 1996;48:273–277.
63. Pether JV, Caul EO. An outbreak of food-borne gastroenteritis in two hospitals associated with a Norwalk-like virus. *J Hyg Lond* 1983; 91:343–350.
64. Kilgore PE, Belay ED, Hamlin DM, et al. A university outbreak of gastroenteritis due to a small round-structured virus: application of molecular diagnostics to identify the etiologic agent and patterns of transmission. *J Infect Dis* 1996;173:787–793.
65. Morse DL, Guzewich JJ, Hanrahan JP, et al. Widespread outbreaks of clam- and oyster-associated gastroenteritis. Role of Norwalk virus. *N Engl J Med* 1986;314:678–681.
66. Sharp TW, Hyams KC, Watts D, et al. Epidemiology of Norwalk virus during an outbreak of acute gastroenteritis aboard a US aircraft carrier. *J Med Virol* 1995;45:61–67.
67. Gustafson TL, Kobylik B, Hutcheson RH, et al. Protective effect of anticholinergic drugs and psyllium in a nosocomial outbreak of Norwalk gastroenteritis. *J Hosp Infect* 1983;4:367–374.
68. Leers WD, Kasupski G, Fralick R, et al. Norwalk-like gastroenteritis epidemic in a Toronto hospital. *Am J Public Health* 1987;77: 291–295.
69. Noel JS, Liu BL, Humphrey CD, et al. Parkville virus: a novel genetic variant of human calicivirus in the Sapporo virus clade, associated with an outbreak of gastroenteritis in adults. *J Med Virol* 1997;52: 173–178.
70. Numata K, Hardy ME, Nakata S, et al. Molecular characterization of morphologically typical human calicivirus Sapporo. *Arch Virol* 1997;142:1537–1552.
71. Jiang X, Cubitt WD, Berke T, et al. Sapporo-like human caliciviruses are genetically and antigenically diverse. *Arch Virol* 1997;142: 1813–1827.
72. Taterka JA, Cuff CF, Rubin DH. Viral gastrointestinal infections. *Gastroenterol Clin North Am* 1992;21:303–330.
73. Pickering LK, Bartlett AV, Reves RR, et al. Asymptomatic excretion of rotavirus before and after rotavirus diarrhea in children in day care centers. *J Pediatr* 1988;112:361–365.
74. Glass RI, Kilgore PE, Holman RC, et al. The epidemiology of rotavirus diarrhea in the United States: surveillance and estimates of disease burden. *J Infect Dis* 1996;174(Suppl 1):S5–11.
75. Lebaron CW, Furutan NP, Lew JF, et al. Viral agents of gastroenteritis. Public health importance and outbreak management. *MMWR Morb Mortal Wkly Rep* 1990;39:1–24.
76. CDC. Laboratory-based surveillance for rotavirus—United States, July 1996–June 1997. *MMWR Morb Mortal Wkly Rep* 1997;46: 1092–1094.
77. Dennehy PH, Peter G. Risk factors associated with nosocomial rotavirus infection. *Am J Dis Child* 1985;139:935–939.
78. Cone R, Mohan K, Thouless M, et al. Nosocomial transmission of rotavirus infection. *Pediatr Infect Dis J* 1988;7:103–109.
79. Hjelt K, Krasilnikoff PA, Grauballe PC, et al. Nosocomial acute gastroenteritis in a pediatric department, with special reference to rotavirus infections. *Acta Paediatr Scand* 1985;74:89–95.
80. Pacini DL, Brady MT, Budde CT, et al. Nosocomial rotaviral diarrhea: pattern of spread on wards in a children's hospital. *J Med Virol* 1987;23:359–366.
81. Steel HM, Garnham S, Beards GM, et al. Investigation of an outbreak

of rotavirus infection in geriatric patients by serotyping and polyacrylamide gel electrophoresis (PAGE). *J Med Virol* 1992;37:132–136.
82. Raad, II, Sherertz RJ, Russell BA, et al. Uncontrolled nosocomial rotavirus transmission during a community outbreak. *Am J Infect Control* 1990;18:24–28.
83. Gaggero A, Avendano LF, Fernandez J, et al. Nosocomial transmission of rotavirus from patients admitted with diarrhea. *J Clin Microbiol* 1992;30:3294–3297.
84. Jayashree S, Bhan MK, Raj P, et al. Neonatal rotavirus infection and its relation to cord blood antibodies. *Scand J Infect Dis* 1988;20: 249–253.
85. Kilgore PE, Unicomb LE, Gentsch JR, et al. Neonatal rotavirus infection in Bangladesh: strain characterization and risk factors for nosocomial infection. *Pediatr Infect Dis J* 1996;15:672–677.
86. Linhares AC, Mascarenhas JD, Gusmao RH, et al. Neonatal rotavirus infection in Belem, northern Brazil: nosocomial transmission of a P[6] G2 strain. *J Med Virol* 2002;67:418–426.
87. Widdowson MA, van Doornum GJ, van der Poel WH, et al. Emerging group-A rotavirus and a nosocomial outbreak of diarrhoea. *Lancet* 2000;356:1161–1162.
88. Gusmao RH, Mascarenhas JD, Gabbay YB, et al. Rotavirus subgroups, G serotypes, and electrophoretypes in cases of nosocomial infantile diarrhoea in Belem, Brazil. *J Trop Pediatr* 1999;45:81–86.
89. Fruhwirth M, Brosl S, Ellemunter H, et al. Distribution of rotavirus VP4 genotypes and VP7 serotypes among nonhospitalized and hospitalized patients with gastroenteritis and patients with nosocomially acquired gastroenteritis in Austria. *J Clin Microbiol* 2000;38: 1804–1806.
90. Widdowson MA, van Doornum GJ, van der Poel WH, et al. An outbreak of diarrhea in a neonatal medium care unit caused by a novel strain of rotavirus: investigation using both epidemiologic and microbiological methods. *Infect Control Hosp Epidemiol* 2002;23: 665–670.
91. Saulsbury FT, Winkelstein JA, Yolken RH. Chronic rotavirus infection in immunodeficiency. *J Pediatr* 1980;97:61–65.
92. Fitts SW, Green M, Reyes J, et al. Clinical features of nosocomial rotavirus infection in pediatric liver transplant recipients. *Clin Transplant* 1995;9:201–204.
93. Eiden JJ, Verleur DG, Vonderfecht SL, et al. Duration and pattern of asymptomatic rotavirus shedding by hospitalized children. *Pediatr Infect Dis J* 1988;7:564–569.
94. Chrystie IL, Totterdell BM, Banatvala JE. Asymptomatic endemic rotavirus infections in the newborn. *Lancet* 1978;1:1176–1178.
95. Dearlove J, Latham P, Dearlove B, et al. Clinical range of neonatal rotavirus gastroenteritis. *Br Med J Clin Res Ed* 1983;286:1473–1475.
96. Butz AM, Fosarelli P, Dick J, et al. Prevalence of rotavirus on high-risk fomites in day-care facilities. *Pediatrics* 1993;92:202–205.
97. Wilde J, Van R, Pickering L, et al. Detection of rotaviruses in the day care environment by reverse transcriptase polymerase chain reaction. *J Infect Dis* 1992;166:507–511.
98. Berger R, Hadziselimovic F, Just M, et al. Influence of breast milk on nosocomial rotavirus infections in infants. *Infection* 1984;12: 171–174.
99. Oelofsen MJ, Venter EH, Smith MS. Nosocomial rotavirus infections in a South African hospital nursery for white infants. *S Afr Med J* 1985;68:394–396.
100. Rodriguez WJ, Kim HW, Brandt CD, et al. Rotavirus: a cause of nosocomial infection in the nursery. *J Pediatr*1982;101:274–277.
101. Rodriguez WJ, Kim HW, Brandt CD, et al. Use of electrophoresis of RNA from human rotavirus to establish the identity of strains involved in outbreaks in a tertiary care nursery. *J Infect Dis* 1983; 148:34–40.
102. Tufvesson B, Polberger S, Svanberg L, et al. A prospective study of rotavirus infections in neonatal and maternity wards. *Acta Paediatr Scand* 1986;75:211–215.
103. Vial PA, Kotloff KL, Losonsky GA. Molecular epidemiology of rotavirus infection in a room for convalescing newborns. *J Infect Dis* 1988; 157:668–673.
104. Rotbart HA, Levin MJ, Yolken RH, et al. An outbreak of rotavirus-associated neonatal necrotizing enterocolitis. *J Pediatr* 1983;103: 454–459.
105. Chen HN, Dennehy PH, Oh W, et al. Outbreak and control of a rotaviral infection in a nursery. *J Formos Med Assoc* 1997;96:884–889.
106. Champsaur H, Questiaux E, Prevot J, et al. Rotavirus carriage, asymptomatic infection, and disease in the first two years of life. I. Virus shedding. *J Infect Dis* 1984;149:667–674.
107. O'Ryan ML, Matson DO, Estes MK, et al. Molecular epidemiology of rotavirus in children attending day care centers in Houston. *J Infect Dis* 1990;162:810–816.
108. Velazquez FR, Matson DO, Calva JJ, et al. Rotavirus infections in infants as protection against subsequent infections. *N Engl J Med* 1996;335:1022–1028.
109. Nakata S, Adachi N, Ukae S, et al. Outbreaks of nosocomial rotavirus gastro-enteritis in a paediatric ward. *Eur J Pediatr* 1996;155:954–958.
110. Matson DO, Estes MK. Impact of rotavirus infection at a large pediatric hospital. *J Infect Dis* 1990;162:598–604.
111. Valenti WM, Menegus MA, Hall CB, et al. Nosocomial viral infections: I. Epidemiology and significance. *Infect Control* 1980;1:33–37.
112. Gianino P, Mastretta E, Longo P, et al. Incidence of nosocomial rotavirus infections, symptomatic and asymptomatic, in breast-fed and non-breast-fed infants. *J Hosp Infect* 2002;50:13–17.
113. Flewett TH, Bryden AS, Davies H, et al. Epidemic viral enteritis in a long stay children's ward. *Lancet* 1975;1:4.
114. Dennehy PH, Tente WE, Fisher DJ, et al. Lack of impact of rapid identification of rotavirus-infected patients on nosocomial rotavirus infections. *Pediatr Infect Dis J* 1989;8:290–296.
115. Wilde J, Yolken R, Willoughby R, et al. Improved detection of rotavirus shedding by polymerase chain reaction. *Lancet* 1991;337: 323–326.
116. Gerna G, Forster J, Parea M, et al. Nosocomial outbreak of neonatal gastroenteritis caused by a new serotype 4, subtype 4B human rotavirus. *J Med Virol* 1990;31:175–182.
117. Pigrau C, Bartolome R, Almirante B, et al. Bacteremia due to *Campylobacter* species: clinical findings and antimicrobial susceptibility patterns. *Clin Infect Dis* 1997;25:1414–1420.
118. Pickering LK, Cleary TG, Guerrant R. Microorganisms responsible for neonatal diarrhea. In: Remington JS, Klein JO, eds. *Infectious diseases of the fetus and newborn infant,* 4th ed. Philadelphia: WB Saunders, 1995:1142–1222.
119. Rautelin H, Koota K, von Essen R, et al. Waterborne *Campylobacter jejuni* epidemic in a Finnish hospital for rheumatic diseases. *Scand J Infect Dis* 1990;22:321–326.
120. Allos BM, Blaser MJ. *Campylobacter jejuni* and the expanding spectrum of related infections. *Clin Infect Dis* 1995;20:1092–1099.
121. Goossens H, Giesendorf AJ, Vandamme P, et al. Investigation of an outbreak of *Campylobacter upsaliensis* in day care centers in Brussels: analysis of relationships among isolates by phenotypic and genotypic typing methods. *J Infect Dis* 1995;172:1298–1303.
122. Bartlett JG. *Clostridium difficile*: history of its role as an enteric pathogen and the current state of knowledge about the organism. *Clin Infect Dis* 1994;18:S265–S272.
123. Oguz F, Uysal G, Dasdemir S, et al. The role of *Clostridium difficile* in childhood nosocomial diarrhea. *Scand J Infect Dis* 2001;33:731–733.
124. Kim K, DuPont HL, Pickering LK. Outbreaks of diarrhea associated with *Clostridium difficile* and its toxin in day-care centers: evidence of person-to-person spread. *J Pediatr* 1983;102:376–382.
125. Lyerly DM, Krivan HC, Wilkins TD. *Clostridium difficile*: its disease and toxins. *Clin Microbiol Rev* 1988;1:1–18.
126. Alfa MJ, Kabani A, Lyerly D, et al. Characterization of a toxin A-negative, toxin B-positive strain of *Clostridium difficile* responsible for a nosocomial outbreak of *Clostridium difficile*-associated diarrhea. *J Clin Microbiol* 2000;38:2706–2714.
127. Lemann F, Chambon C, Barbut F, et al. Arbitrary primed PCR rules out *Clostridium difficile* cross-infection among patients in a haematology unit. *J Hosp Infect* 1997;35:107–115.
128. Nataro JP, Kaper JB. Diarrheagenic *Escherichia coli. Clin Microbiol Rev* 1998;11:142–201.
129. Robins-Browne RM. Traditional enteropathogenic *Escherichia coli* of infantile diarrhea. *Rev Infect Dis* 1987;9:28–53.

130. Blanco J, Gonzalez EA, Espinosa P, et al. Enterotoxigenic and necrotizing *Escherichia coli* in human diarrhoea in Spain. *Eur J Epidemiol* 1992;8:548–552.
131. Ryder RW, Wachsmuth IK, Buxton AE, et al. Infantile diarrhea produced by heat-stable enterotoxigenic *Escherichia coli. N Engl J Med* 1976;295:849–853.
132. Preston M, Borczyk A, Davidson R. Hospital outbreak of *Escherichia coli* O157:H7 associated with a rare phage type—Ontario. *Can Commun Dis Rep* 1997;23:33–36.
133. Stiver HG, Albritton WL, Clark J, et al. Nosocomial colonization and infection due to *E. coli* 0125:K70 epidemiologically linked to expressed breast-milk feedings. *Can J Public Health* 1977;68: 479–482.
134. Harris JR, Mariano J, Wells JG, et al. Person-to-person transmission in an outbreak of enteroinvasive *Escherichia coli. Am J Epidemiol* 1985; 122:245–252.
135. O'Brien SJ, Murdoch PS, Riley AH, et al. A foodborne outbreak of Vero cytotoxin-producing *Escherichia coli* O157:H-phage type 8 in hospital. *J Hosp Infect* 2001;49:167–172.
136. Pavia AT, Nichols CR, Green DP, et al. Hemolytic-uremic syndrome during an outbreak of *Escherichia coli* O157:H7 infections in institutions for mentally retarded persons: clinical and epidemiologic observations. *J Pediatr* 1990;116:544–551.
137. Belongia EA, Osterholm MT, Soler JT, et al. Transmission of *Escherichia coli* O157:H7 infection in Minnnesota child day-care facilities. *JAMA* 1993;269:883–888.
138. Karmali MA, Arbus GS, Petric M, et al. Hospital-acquired *Escherichia coli* O157:H7 associated haemolytic uraemic syndrome in a nurse. *Lancet* 1988;1:526.
139. Weightman NC, Kirby PJ. Nosocomial *Escherichia coli* O157 infection. *J Hosp Infect* 2000;44:107–111.
140. Kaslow RA, Taylor A Jr, Dweck HS, et al. Enteropathogenic *Escherichia coli* infection in a newborn nursery. *Am J Dis Child* 1974;128: 797–801.
141. Senerwa D, Olsvik O, Mutanda LN, et al. Enteropathogenic *Escherichia coli* serotype O111:HNT isolated from preterm neonates in Nairobi, Kenya. *J Clin Microbiol* 1989;27:1307–1311.
142. Senerwa D, Olsvik O, Mutanda LN, et al. Colonization of neonates in a nursery ward with enteropathogenic *Escherichia coli* and correlation to the clinical histories of the children. *J Clin Microbiol* 1989; 27:2539–2543.
143. Boyer KM, Petersen NJ, Farzaneh I, et al. An outbreak of gastroenteritis due to *E. coli* 0142 in a neonatal nursery. *J Pediatr* 1975;86: 919–927.
144. Wu SX, Peng RQ. Studies on an outbreak of neonatal diarrhea caused by EPEC 0127:H6 with plasmid analysis restriction analysis and outer membrane protein determination. *Acta Paediatr* 1992;81:217–221.
145. Senerwa D, Mutanda LN, Gathuma JM, et al. Antimicrobial resistance of enteropathogenic *Escherichia coli* strains from a nosocomial outbreak in Kenya. *Apmis* 1991;99:728–734.
146. Lang DJ, Kunz LJ, Martin AR, et al. Carmine as a source of nosocomial salmonellosis. *N Engl J Med* 1967;276:829–832.
147. Komarmy LE, Oxley ME, Brecher G. Hospital-acquired salmonellosis traced to carmine dye capsules. *N Engl J Med* 1967;276:850–852.
148. Eickhoff TC. Nosocomial salmonellosis due to carmine. *Ann Intern Med* 1967;66:813–814.
149. Mermin J, Hoar B, Angulo FJ. Iguanas and *Salmonella marina* infection in children: a reflection of the increasing incidence of reptile-associated salmonellosis in the United States. *Pediatrics* 1997;99: 399–402.
150. Sanders E, Sweeney FJ Jr, Friedman EA, et al. An outbreak of hospital-acquired infections due to *Salmonella derby. JAMA* 1963;186: 984–986.
151. Telzak EE, Budnick LD, Greenberg MS, et al. A nosocomial outbreak of *Salmonella enteritidis* infection due to the consumption of raw eggs. *N Engl J Med* 1990;323:394–397.
152. Neill MA, Opal SM, Heelan J, et al. Failure of ciprofloxacin to eradicate convalescent fecal excretion after acute salmonellosis: experience during an outbreak in health care workers. *Ann Intern Med* 1991; 114:195–199.
153. Mishu B, Koehler J, Lee LA, et al. Outbreaks of *Salmonella enteritidis* infections in the United States, 1985-1991. *J Infect Dis* 1994;169: 547–552.
154. Hennessy TW, Hedberg CW, Slutsker L, et al. A national outbreak of *Salmonella enteritidis* infections from ice cream. *N Engl J Med* 1996; 334:1281–1286.
155. Steere AC, Hall WJd, Wells JG, et al. Person-to-person spread of *Salmonella typhimurium* after a hospital common-source outbreak. *Lancet* 1975;1:319–322.
156. Goh KT, Teo SH, Tay L, et al. Epidemiology and control of an outbreak of typhoid in a psychiatric institution. *Epidemiol Infect* 1992; 108:221–229.
157. CDC. Foodborne nosocomial outbreak of *Salmonella reading*—Connecticut. *MMWR Morb Mortal Wkly Rep* 1991;40:804–806.
158. L'Ecuyer PB, Diego J, Murphy D, et al. Nosocomial outbreak of gastroenteritis due to *Salmonella senftenberg. Clin Infect Dis* 1996;23: 734–742.
159. Molina Gamboa JD, Ponce de Leon Rosales S, Guerrero Almeida ML, et al. *Salmonella* gastroenteritis outbreak among workers from a tertiary care hospital in Mexico City. *Rev Invest Clin* 1997;49: 349–353.
160. Maguire H, Pharoah P, Walsh B, et al. Hospital outbreak of *Salmonella virchow* possibly associated with a food handler. *J Hosp Infect* 2000;44:261–266.
161. Bornemann R, Zerr DM, Heath J, et al. An outbreak of *Salmonella*serotype Saintpaul in a children's hospital. *Infect Control Hosp Epidemiol* 2002;23:671–676.
162. Kistemann T, Dangendorf F, Krizek L, et al. GIS-supported investigation of a nosocomial Salmonella outbreak. *Int J Hyg Environ Health* 2000;203:117–126.
163. CDC. *Salmonella kottbus* meningitis-associated with contaminated milk. *MMWR Morb Mortal Wkly Rep* 1971;20:154.
164. Ryder RW, Crosby Ritchie A, McDonough B, et al. Human milk contaminated with *Salmonella kottbus.* A cause of nosocomial illness in infants. *JAMA* 1977;238:1533–1534.
165. Baine WB, Gangarosa EJ, Bennett JV, et al. Institutional salmonellosis. *J Infect Dis* 1973;128:357–360.
166. Glencross EJ. Pancreatin as a source of hospital-acquired salmonellosis. *BMJ* 1972;2:376–378.
167. Chmel H, Armstrong D. *Salmonella oslo.* A focal outbreak in a hospital. *Am J Med* 1976;60:203–208.
168. Dwyer DM, Klein EG, Istre GR, et al. *Salmonella newport* infections transmitted by fiberoptic colonoscopy. *Gastrointest Endosc* 1987;33: 84–87.
169. Ip HMH, Sin WK, Chau PY, et al. Neonatal infection due to *Salmonella worthington* transmitted by a delivery room suction apparatus. *J Hyg* 1976;77:307–314.
170. Khan MA, Abdur Rab M, Israr N, et al. Transmission of *Salmonella worthington* by oropharyngeal suction in hospital neonatal unit. *Pediatr Infect Dis J* 1991;10:668–672.
171. Aber RC, Banks WV. An outbreak of nosocomial *Salmonella typhimurium* infection linked to environmental reservoir. *Infect Control* 1980; 1:386–390.
172. McAllister TA, Roud JA, Marshall A, et al. Outbreak of *Salmonella eimsbuettel* in newborn infants spread by rectal thermometers. *Lancet* 1986;1:1262–1264.
173. Newman MJ. Multiple-resistant *Salmonella* group G outbreak in a neonatal intensive care unit. *West Afr J Med* 1996;15:165–169.
174. Standaer SM, Hutcheson RH, Schaffer W. Nosocomial transmission of Salmonella gastroenteritis to laundry workers in a nursing home. *Infect Control Hosp Epidemiol* 1994;15:22–26.
175. Kostiala AA, Westerstrahle M, Muttilainen M. Neonatal *Salmonella panama* infection with meningitis. *Acta Paediatr* 1992;81:856–858.
176. Lamb VA, Mayhall CG, Spadora AC, et al. Outbreak of *Salmonella typhimurium* gastroenteritis due to an imported strain resistant to ampicillin, chloramphenicol, and trimethoprim-sulfamethoxazole in a nursery. *J Clin Microbiol* 1984;20:1076–1079.
177. Smith SM, Palumbo PE, Edelson PJ. *Salmonella* strains resistant to multiple antibiotics: therapeutic implications. *Pediatr Infect Dis J* 1984;3:455–460.

178. Pessoa-Silva CL, Toscano CM, Moreira BM, et al. Infection due to extended-spectrum beta-lactamase-producing *Salmonella enterica*-subsp. enterica serotype infantis in a neonatal unit. *J Pediatr* 2002; 141:381–387.
179. Riley LW, Ceballos BS, Trabulsi LR, et al. The significance of hospitals as reservoirs for endemic multiresistant *Salmonella typhimurium* causing infection in urban Brazilian children. *J Infect Dis* 1984;150: 236–241.
180. Rushdy AA, Wall R, Seng C, et al. Application of molecular methods to a nosocomial outbreak of *Salmonella enteritidis* phage type 4. *J Hosp Infect* 1997;36:123–131.
181. Keusch GT, Bennish ML. Shigellosis: recent progress, persisting problems and research issues. *Pediatr Infect Dis J* 1989;8:713–719.
182. Pillay DG, Karas JA, Pillay A, et al. Nosocomial transmission of *Shigella dysenteriae* type 1. *J Hosp Infect* 1997;37:199–205.
183. Brian MJ, Van R, Townsend I, et al. Evaluation of the molecular epidemiology of an outbreak of multiply resistant *Shigella sonnei* in a day-care center by using pulsed-field gel electrophoresis and plasmid DNA analysis. *J Clin Microbiol* 1993;31:2152–2156.
184. Hale TL. Genetic basis of virulence in *Shigella* species. *Microbiol Rev* 1991;55:206–224.
185. Paton S, Nicolle L, Mwongera M, et al. *Salmonella* and *Shigella* gastroenteritis at a public teaching hospital in Nairobi, Kenya. *Infect Control Hosp Epidemiol* 1991;12:710–717.
186. Mermel LA, Josephson SL, Dempsey J, et al. Outbreak of *Shigella sonnei* in a clinical microbiology laboratory. *J Clin Microbiol* 1997; 35:3163–3165.
187. Centers for Disease Control and Prevention. Hospital-associated outbreak of *Shigella dysenteriae* type 2-Maryland. *MMWR Morb Mortal Wkly Rep* 1983;32:250.
188. Ruderman JW, Stoller KP, Pomerance JJ. Bloodstream invasion with *Shigella sonnei* in an asymptomatic newborn infant. *Pediatr Infect Dis J* 1986;5:379–380.
189. Starke JR, Baker CJ. Neonatal shigellosis with bowel perforation. *Pediatr Infect Dis J* 1985;4:405–407.
190. Beers LM, Burke TL, Martin DB. Shigellosis occurring in newborn nursery staff. *Infect Control Hosp Epidemiol* 1989;10:147–149.
191. Janda JM, Powers C, Bryant RG, et al. Current perspectives on the epidemiology and pathogenesis of clinically significant *Vibrio* spp. *Clin Microbiol Rev* 1988;1:245–267.
192. Morris JG Jr, Black RE. Cholera and other vibrioses in the United States. *N Engl J Med* 1985;312:343–350.
193. Tacket CO, Hickman F, Pierce GV, et al. Diarrhea associated with *Vibrio fluvialis* in the United States. *J Clin Microbiol* 1982;16: 991–992.
194. Brenner DJ, Hickman Brenner FW, Lee JV, et al. *Vibrio furnissii* (formerly aerogenic biogroup of *Vibrio fluvialis*), a new species isolated from human feces and the environment. *J Clin Microbiol* 1983;18: 816–824.
195. Hickman FW, Farmer JJ, Hollis DG, et al. Identification of *Vibrio hollisae* sp. nov. from patients with diarrhea. *J Clin Microbiol* 1982; 15:395–401.
196. Lu PL, Chang SC, Pan HJ, et al. Application of pulsed-field gel electrophoresis to the investigation of a nosocomial outbreak of Vibrio parahaemolyticus. *J Microbiol Immunol Infect* 2000;33:29–33.
197. Swerdlow DL, Ries AA. Cholera in the Americas. Guidelines for the clinician. *JAMA* 1992;267:1495–1499.
198. Nair GB, Ramamurthy T, Bhattacharya SK, et al. Spread of *Vibrio cholerae* 0139 Bengal in India. *J Infect Dis* 1994;169:1029–1034.
199. Mhalu FS, Mtango FD, Msengi AE. Hospital outbreaks of cholera transmitted through close person-to-person contact. *Lancet* 1984;2: 82–84.
200. Swaddiwudhipong W, Kunasol P. An outbreak of nosocomial cholera in a 755-bed hospital. *Trans R Soc Trop Med Hyg* 1989;83:279–281.
201. Cliff JL, Zinkin P, Martelli A. A hospital outbreak of cholera in Maputo, Mozambique. *Trans R Soc Trop Med Hyg* 1986;80:473–476.
202. Hernandez JE, Mejia CR, Cazali IL, et al. Nosocomial infection due to *Vibrio cholerae* in two referral hospitals in Guatemala. *Infect Control Hosp Epidemiol* 1996;17:371–372.
203. Tabtieng R, Wattanasri S, Echeverria P, et al. An epidemic of *Vibrio cholerae* el tor Inaba resistant to several antibiotics with a conjugative group C plasmid coding for type II dihydrofolate reductase in Thailand. *Am J Trop Med Hyg* 1989;41:680–686.
204. Bergstrand CG, Winblad S. Clinical manifestations of infection with *Yersinia enterocolitica* in children. *Acta Paediatr Scand* 1974;63: 875–877.
205. Rodriquez WJ, Controni G, Cohen GJ, et al. *Yersinia enterocolitica* enteritis in children. *JAMA* 1979;242:1978–1980.
206. Bottone EJ. *Yersinia enterocolitica*: the charisma continues. *Clin Microbiol Rev* 1997;10:257–276.
207. Cover TL, Aber RC. *Yersinia enterocolitica. N Engl J Med* 1989;321: 16–24.
208. Blumberg HM, Kiehlbauch JA, Wachsmuth IK. Molecular epidemiology of *Yersinia enterocolitica* O:3 infections: use of chromosomal DNA restriction fragment length polymorphisms of rRNA genes. *J Clin Microbiol* 1991;29:2368–2374.
209. Lee LA, Taylor J, Carter GP, et al. *Yersinia enterocolitica* O:3: an emerging cause of pediatric gastroenteritis in the United States. The *Yersinia enterocolitica* Collaborative Study Group. *J Infect Dis* 1991; 163:660–663.
210. Update: *Yersinia enterocolitica* bacteremia and endotoxin shock associated with red blood cell transfusions—United States, 1991. *MMWR Morb Mortal Wkly Rep* 1991;40:176–178.
211. Jacobs J, Jamaer D, Vandeven J, et al. *Yersinia enterocolitica* in donor blood: a case report and review. *J Clin Microbiol* 1989;27:1119–1121.
212. Wright DC, Selss IF, Vinton KJ, et al. Fatal *Yersinia enterocolitica* sepsis after blood transfusion. *Arch Pathol Lab Med* 1985;109: 1040–1042.
213. Paisley JW, Lauer BA. Neonatal *Yersinia enterocolitica* enteritis. *Pediatr Infect Dis J* 1992;11:331–332.
214. Greenwood MH, Hooper WL. Excretion of *Yersinia* spp. associated with consumption of pasteurized milk. *Epidemiol Infect* 1990;104: 345–350.
215. Kist M, Langmaack H, Just M. [Spread of *Yersinia enterocolitica* infection within a hospital]. *Dtsch Med Wochenschr* 1980;105:185–189.
216. Ratnam S, Mercer E, Picco B, et al. A nosocomial outbreak of diarrheal disease due to *Yersinia enterocolitica* serotype 0:5, biotype 1. *J Infect Dis* 1982;145:242–247.
217. Cannon CG, Linnemann CC Jr. *Yersinia enterocolitica* infections in hospitalized patients: the problem of hospital-acquired infections. *Infect Control Hosp Epidemiol* 1992;13:139–143.
218. Miller RA, Holmberg RE Jr, Clausen CR. Life-threatening diarrhea caused by *Cryptosporidium* in a child undergoing therapy for acute lymphocytic leukemia. *J Pediatr* 1983;103:256–259.
219. Chen XM, Keithly JS, Paya CV, et al. Cryptosporidiosis. *N Engl J Med* 2002;346:1723–1731.
220. Amadi B, Mwiya M, Musuku J, et al. Effect of nitazoxanide on morbidity and mortality in Zambian children with cryptosporidiosis: a randomised controlled trial. *Lancet* 2002;360:1375–1380.
221. Martino P, Gentile G, Caprioli A, et al. Hospital-acquired cryptosporidiosis in a bone marrow transplantation unit. *J Infect Dis* 1988;158: 647–648.
222. Sarabia Arce S, Salazar Lindo E, Gilman RH, et al. Case-control study of *Cryptosporidium parvum* infection in Peruvian children hospitalized for diarrhea: possible association with malnutrition and nosocomial infection. *Pediatr Infect Dis J* 1990;9:627–631.
223. Farias P, Duffau G. [Intestinal cryptosporidiosis: a case of hospital infection]. *Rev Chil Pediatr* 1989;60:44–46.
224. Weber DJ, Rutala WA. The emerging nosocomial pathogens *Cryptosporidium,* Escherichia coli O157:H7, *Helicobacter pylori,* and hepatitis C: epidemiology, environmental survival, efficacy of disinfection, and control measures. *Infect Control Hosp Epidemiol* 2001;22: 306–315.
225. Ravn P, Lundgren JD, Kjaeldgaard P, et al. Nosocomial outbreak of cryptosporidiosis in AIDS patients. *BMJ* 1991;302:277–280.
226. Koch KL, Phillips DJ, Aber RC, et al. Cryptosporidiosis in hospital personnel. Evidence for person-to-person transmission. *Ann Intern Med* 1985;102:593–596.
227. Current WL, Garcia LS. Cryptosporidiosis. *Clin Microbiol Rev* 1991; 4:325–358.

228. Ungar BL. Enzyme-linked immunoassay for detection of *Cryptosporidium* antigens in fecal specimens. *J Clin Microbiol* 1990;28:2491–2495.
229. Morgan UM, Pallant L, Dwyer BW, et al. Comparison of PCR and microscopy for detection of *Cryptosporidium parvum* in human fecal specimens: clinical trial. *J Clin Microbiol* 1998;36:995–998.
230. Huang P, Weber JT, Sosin DM, et al. The first reported outbreak of diarrheal illness associated with Cyclospora in the United States. *Ann Intern Med* 1995;123:409–414.
231. Eberhard ML, Pieniazek NJ, Arrowood MJ. Laboratory diagnosis of Cyclospora infections. *Arch Pathol Lab Med* 1997;121:792–797.
232. Soave R, Herwaldt BL, Relman DA. Cyclospora. *Infect Dis Clin North Am* 1998;12:1–12.
233. Zaidi M, Ponce de Leon S, Ortiz RM, et al. Hospital-acquired diarrhea in adults: a prospective case-controlled study in Mexico. *Infect Control Hosp Epidemiol* 1991;12:349–355.
234. Istre GR, Kreiss K, Hopkins RS, et al. An outbreak of amebiasis spread by colonic irrigation at a chiropractic clinic. *N Engl J Med* 1982;307:339–342.
235. Tachibana H, Kobayashi S, Kato Y, et al. Identification of a pathogenic isolate-specific 30,000-Mr antigen of *Entamoeba histolytica* by using a monoclonal antibody. *Infect Immun* 1990;58:955–960.
236. Tannich E, Burchard GD. Differentiation of pathogenic from nonpathogenic *Entamoeba histolytica* by restriction fragment analysis of a single gene amplified in vitro. *J Clin Microbiol* 1991;29:250–255.
237. Petersen LR, Carter ML, Hadler JL. A foodborne outbreak of *Giardia lamblia. J Infect Dis* 1988;157:846–848.
238. Adam RD. The biology of *Giardia* spp. *Microbiol Rev* 1991;55:706–732.
239. Hopkins RS, Juranek DD. Acute giardiasis: an improved clinical case definition for epidemiologic studies. *Am J Epidemiol* 1991;133:402–407.
240. Wolfe MS. Giardiasis. *Clin Microbiol Rev* 1992;5:93–100.
241. Lengerich EJ, Addiss DG, Juranek DD. Severe giardiasis in the United States. *Clin Infect Dis* 1994;18:760–763.
242. Pickering LK, Engelkirk PG. *Giardia lamblia. Pediatr Clin North Am* 1988;35:565–567.
243. Rauch AM, Van R, Bartlett AV, et al. Longitudinal study of *Giardia lamblia* infection in a day care center population. *Pediatr Infect Dis J* 1990;9:186–189.
244. White KE, Hedberg CW, Edmonson LM, et al. An outbreak of giardiasis in a nursing home with evidence for multiple modes of transmission. *J Infect Dis* 1989;160:298–304.
245. Burke JA. Strongyloidiasis in childhood. *Am J Dis Child* 1978;132:1130–1136.
246. Smith SB, Schwartzman M, Mencia LF, et al. Fatal disseminated strongyloidiasis presenting as acute abdominal distress in an urban child. *J Pediatr* 1977;91:607–609.
247. Yoeli M, Most H, Berman HH, et al. The problem of strongyloidiasis among the mentally retarded in institutions. *Trans R Soc Trop Med Hyg* 1963;57:336–345.
248. Proctor EM, Muth HA, Proudfoot DL, et al. Endemic institutional strongyloidiasis in British Columbia. *Can Med Assoc J* 1987;136:1173–1176.
249. Braun TI, Fekete T, Lynch A. Strongyloidiasis in an institution for mentally retarded adults. *Arch Intern Med* 1988;148:634–636.
250. Hoy WE, Roberts NJ Jr, Bryson MF, et al. Transmission of strongyloidiasis by kidney transplant? Disseminated strongyloidiasis in both recipients of kidney allografts from a single cadaver donor. *JAMA* 1981;246:1937–1939.
251. DeVault GA Jr, King JW, Rohr MS, et al. Opportunistic infections with *Strongyloides stercoralis* in renal transplantation. *Rev Infect Dis* 1990;12:653–671.
252. Igra Siegman Y, Kapila R, Sen P, et al. Syndrome of hyperinfection with *Strongyloides stercoralis. Rev Infect Dis* 1981;3:397–407.
253. Koga K, Kasuya S, Khamboonruang C, et al. A modified agar plate method for detection of *Strongyloides stercoralis. Am J Trop Med Hyg* 1991;45:518–521.
254. Mahmoud AA. Strongyloidiasis. *Clin Infect Dis* 1996;23:949–952.
255. Pape JW, Verdier RI, Johnson WD Jr. Treatment and prophylaxis of *Isospora belli* infection in patients with the acquired immunodeficiency syndrome. *N Engl J Med* 1989;320:1044–1047.
256. DeHovitz JA, Pape JW, Boncy M, et al. Clinical manifestations and therapy of *Isospora belli* infection in patients with the acquired immunodeficiency syndrome. *N Engl J Med* 1986;315:87–90.
257. Didier ES. Microsporidiosis. *Clin Infect Dis* 1998;27:1–8.
258. Rijpstra AC, Canning EU, Van Ketel RJ, et al. Use of light microscopy to diagnose small-intestinal microsporidiosis in patients with AIDS. *J Infect Dis* 1988;157:827–831.
259. Weber R, Bryan RT, Owen RL, et al. Improved light-microscopical detection of microsporidia spores in stool and duodenal aspirates. The Enteric Opportunistic Infections Working Group. *N Engl J Med* 1992;326:161–166.
260. David F, Schuitema ARJ, Sarfati C, et al. Detection and species identification of intestinal microsporidia by polymerase chain reaction in duodenal biopsies from human immunodeficiency virus-infected patients. *J Infect Dis* 1996;174:874–877.
261. Siregar CD, Sinuhaji AB, Sutanto AH. Spectrum of digestive tract diseases 1985–1987 at the Pediatric Gastroenterology Outpatient Clinic of Dr. Pirngadi General Hospital, Medan. *Paediatr Indones* 1990;30:133–138.
262. Talwar P, Chakrabarti A, Chawla A, et al. Fungal diarrhoea: association of different fungi and seasonal variation in their incidence. *Mycopathologia* 1990;110:101–105.
263. Guerrant RL, Bobak DA. Bacterial and protozoal gastroenteritis. *N Engl J Med* 1991;325:327–340.
264. Diebel LN, Liberati DM, Diglio CA, et al. Synergistic effects of *Candida* and *Escherichia coli* on gut barrier function. *J Trauma* 1999;47:1045–1050.
265. Cohen R, Roth FJ, Delgado E, et al. Fungal flora of the normal human small and large intestine. *N Engl J Med* 1989;280:638-641.
266. Kane JG, Chretien JH, Garagusi VF. Diarrhoea caused by *Candida. Lancet* 1976;1:335–336.
267. Forster J, Knoop U. [Nosocomial dyspepsia in newborn and young infants. A 15-month prospective study with continuous Rotavirus surveillance]. *Monatsschr Kinderheilkd* 1983;131:441–447.
268. Gupta TP, Ehrinpreis MN. *Candida*-associated diarrhea in hospitalized patients. *Gastroenterology* 1990;98:780–785.
269. Ullrich R, Heise W, Bergs C, et al. Gastrointestinal symptoms in patients infected with human immunodeficiency virus: relevance of infective agents isolated from gastrointestinal tract. *Gut* 1992;33:1080–1084.
270. Danna PL, Urban C, Bellin E, et al. Role of *Candida* in pathogenesis of antibiotic-associated diarrhoea in elderly inpatients. *Lancet* 1991;337:511–514.
271. Gerber AR, Hopkins RS, Lauer BA, et al. Increased risk of illness among nursery staff caring for neonates with necrotizing enterocolitis. *Pediatr Infect Dis J* 1985;4:246–249.
272. Han VK, Sayed H, Chance GW, et al. An outbreak of *Clostridium difficile* necrotizing enterocolitis: a case for oral vancomycin therapy? *Pediatrics* 1983;71:935–941.
273. Boccia D, Stolfi I, Lana S, et al. Nosocomial necrotising enterocolitis outbreaks: epidemiology and control measures. *Eur J Pediatr* 2001;160:385–391.
274. Birenbaum E, Handsher R, Kuint J, et al. Echovirus type 22 outbreak associated with gastro-intestinal disease in a neonatal intensive care unit. *Am J Perinatol* 1997;14:469–473.
275. Deodhar LP, Saraswathi K, Varudkar A. *Aeromonas* spp. and their association with human diarrheal disease. *J Clin Microbiol* 1991;29:853–856.
276. Namdari H, Bottone EJ. Microbiologic and clinical evidence supporting the role of *Aeromonas caviae* as a pediatric enteric pathogen. *J Clin Microbiol* 1990;28:837–840.
277. San Joaquin VHS, Pickett DA. *Aeromonas*-associated gastroenteritis in children. *Pediatr Infect Dis J* 1988;7:53–57.
278. Agger WA. Diarrhea associated with *Aeromonas hydrophila. Pediatr Infect Dis* 1986;5:S106–108.
279. Challapalli M, Tess BR, Cunningham DG, et al. *Aeromonas*-associated diarrhea in children. *Pediatr Infect Dis J* 1988;7:693–698.
280. Burke V, Gracey M, Robinson J, et al. The microbiology of childhood

gastroenteritis: *Aeromonas* species and other infective agents. *J Infect Dis* 1983;148:68–74.

281. Figura N, Marri L, Verdiani S, et al. Prevalence, species differentiation, and toxigenicity of *Aeromonas* strains in cases of childhood gastroenteritis and in controls. *J Clin Microbiol* 1986;23:595–599.
282. Bloom HG, Bottone EJ. *Aeromonas hydrophila* diarrhea in a long-term care setting. *J Am Geriatr Soc* 1990;38:804–806.
283. de la Morena ML, Van R, Singh K, et al. Diarrhea associated with *Aeromonas* species in children in day care centers. *J Infect Dis* 1993; 168:215–218.
284. Janda JM, Bottone EJ, Reitano M. *Aeromonas* species in clinical microbiology: significance, epidemiology, and speciation. *Diagn Microbiol Infect Dis* 1983;1:221–228.
285. Picard B, Goullet P. Seasonal prevalence of nosocomial *Aeromonas hydrophila* infection related to *Aeromonas* in hospital water. *J Hosp Infect* 1987;10:152–155.
286. Picard B, Goullet P. Epidemiological complexity of hospital *Aeromonas* infections revealed by electrophoretic typing of esterases. *Epidemiol Infect* 1987;98:5–14.
287. Carnahan AM, Chakraborty T, Fanning GR, et al. *Aeromonas trota* sp. nov., an ampicillin-susceptible species isolated from clinical specimens. *J Clin Microbiol* 1991;29:1206–1210.
288. Janda JM. Recent advances in the study of the taxonomy, pathogenicity, and infectious syndromes associated with the genus *Aeromonas. Clin Microbiol Rev* 1991;4:397–410.
289. Donowitz LG, Marsik FJ, Fisher KA, et al. Contaminated breast milk: a source of *Klebsiella* bacteremia in a newborn intensive care unit. *Rev Infect Dis* 1981;3:716–720.
290. Guerrant RL, Dickens MD, Wenzel RP, et al. Toxigenic bacterial diarrhea: nursery outbreak involving multiple bacterial strains. *J Pediatr* 1976;89:885–891.
291. Alexander CS, Zinzeleta EM, Mackenzie EJ, et al. Acute gastrointestinal illness and child care arrangements. *Am J Epidemiol* 1990;131: 124–131.
292. Reves RR, Morrow AL, Bartlett AV, et al. Child day care increases the risk of clinic visits for acute diarrhea and diarrhea due to rotavirus. *Am J Epidemiol* 1993;137:97–107.
293. Tauxe RV, Hassan LF, Findeisen KO, et al. Salmonellosis in nurses: lack of transmission to patients. *J Infect Dis* 1988;157:370–373.
294. Hedberg CW, Osterholm MT. Outbreaks of foodborne and waterborne viral gastroenteritis. *Clin Microbiol Rev* 1993;6:199–210.
295. Kim KH, Fekety R, Batts DH, et al. Isolation of *Clostridium difficile* from the environment and contacts of patients with antibiotic-associated colitis. *J Infect Dis* 1981;143:42–50.
296. Walker RI, Caldwell MB, Lee EC, et al. Pathophysiology of *Campylobacter* enteritis. *Microbiol Rev* 1986;50:81–94.
297. Karim QN, Rao GG, Taylor M, et al. Routine cleaning and the elimination of *Campylobacter pylori* from endoscopic biopsy forceps. *J Hosp Infect* 1989;13:87–90.
298. Langenberg W, Rauws EA, Oudbier JH, et al. Patient-to-patient transmission of *Campylobacter pylori* infection by fiberoptic gastroduodenoscopy and biopsy. *J Infect Dis* 1990;161:507–511.
299. Jarvis WR, Middleton PJ, Gelfand EW. Significance of viral infections in severe combined immunodeficiency disease. *Pediatr Infect Dis J* 1983;2:187–192.
300. Heard SR, Wren B, Barnett MJ, et al. *Clostridium difficile* infection in patients with haematological malignant disease. Risk factors, faecal toxins and pathogenic strains. *Epidemiol Infect* 1988;100:63–72.
301. Yolken RH, Bishop CA, Townsend TR, et al. Infectious gastroenteritis in bone-marrow-transplant recipients. *N Engl J Med* 1982;306: 1010–1012.
302. Josephson A, Karanfil L, Alonso H, et al. Risk-specific nosocomial infection rates. *Am J Med* 1991;91:131s–137s.
303. Jarvis WR, Edwards JR, Culver DH, et al. Nosocomial infection rates in adult and pediatric intensive care units in the United States. National Nosocomial Infections Surveillance System. *Am J Med* 1991; 91:185s–191s.
304. Brown RB, Stechenberg B, Sands M, et al. Infections in a pediatric intensive care unit. *Am J Dis Child* 1987;141:267–270.
305. Lam BC, Tam J, Ng MH, et al. Nosocomial gastroenteritis in paediatric patients. *J Hosp Infect* 1989;14:351–355.
306. Ball JM, Tian P, Zeng CQY, et al. Age-dependent diarrhea induced by a rotaviral nonstructural glycoprotein. *Science* 1996;272:101–104.
307. Dong Y, Zeng CQY, Ball JM, et al. The rotavirus enterotoxin NSP4 mobilizes intracellular calcium in human intestinal cells by stimulating phospholipase C-mediated inositol 1,4,5-trisphosphate production. *Proc Natl Acad Sci* 1997;94:3960–3965.
308. Centers for Disease Control and Prevention. The management of acute diarrhea in children: oral rehydration, maintenance, and nutritional therapy. *MMWR Morb Mortal Wkly Rep* 1992;41:1–20.
309. Pickering LK. Approach to diagnosis and management of gastrointestinal tract infections. In: Long SS, Pickering LK, Prober CG, eds. *Principles and practice of pediatric infectious diseases.* New York: Churchill-Livingstone, 1997:410–418.
310. Goldmann DA, Macone AB. A microbiologic approach to the investigation of bacterial nosocomial infection outbreaks. *Infect Control* 1980;1:391–400.
311. McGowan JE Jr. New laboratory techniques for hospital infection control. *Am J Med* 1991;91:245s–251s.
312. Maslow JN, Mulligan ME, Arbeit RD. Molecular epidemiology: application of contemporary techniques to the typing of microorganisms. *Clin Infect Dis* 1993;17:153–162.
313. Weber S, Pfaller MA, Herwaldt LA. Role of molecular epidemiology in infection control. *Infect Dis Clin North Am* 1997;11:257–278.
314. Meropol SB, Luberti AA, De Jong AR. Yield from stool testing of pediatric inpatients. *Arch Pediatr Adolesc Med* 1997;151:142–145.
315. Chitkara YK, McCasland KA, Kenefic L. Development and implementation of cost-effective guidelines in the laboratory investigation of diarrhea in a community hospital. *Arch Intern Med* 1996;156: 1445–1448.
316. Bauer TM, Lalvani A, Fehrenbach J, et al. Derivation and validation of guidelines for stool cultures for enteropathogenic bacteria other than *Clostridium difficile* in hospitalized adults. *JAMA* 2001;285: 313–319.
317. Gorschluter M, Hahn C, Ziske C, et al. Low frequency of enteric infections by *Salmonella, Shigella, Yersinia* and *Campylobacter* in patients with acute leukemia. *Infection* 2002;30:22–25.
318. Rivera MJ, Rivera N, Castillo J, et al. Molecular and epidemiological study of *Salmonella* clinical isolates. *J Clin Microbiol* 1991;29: 927–932.
319. Estes MK, Graham DY, Dimitrov DH. The molecular epidemiology of rotavirus gastroenteritis. *Prog Med Virol* 1984;29:1–22.
320. Clark JD, Hill SM, Phillips AD. Investigation of hospital-acquired rotavirus gastroenteritis using RNA electrophoresis. *J Med Virol* 1988; 26:289–299.
321. Scholl DR, Kaufmann C, Jollick JD, et al. Clinical application of novel sample processing technology for the identification of salmonellae by using DNA probes. *J Clin Microbiol* 1990;28:237–241.
322. Bracha R, Diamond LS, Ackers JP, et al. Differentiation of clinical isolates of *Entamoeba histolytica* by using specific DNA probes. *J Clin Microbiol* 1990;28:680–684.
323. Gordillo ME, Reeve GR, Pappas J, et al. Molecular characterization of strains of enteroinvasive *Escherichia coli* O143, including isolates from a large outbreak in Houston, Texas. *J Clin Microbiol* 1992;30: 889–893.
324. Samore M, Killgore G, Johnson S, et al. Multicenter typing comparison of sporadic and outbreak *Clostridium difficile* isolates from geographically diverse hospitals. *J Infect Dis* 1997;176:1233–1238.
325. Mereghetti L, Tayoro J, Watt S, et al. Genetic relationship between *Escherichia coli* strains isolated from the intestinal flora and those responsible for infectious diseases among patients hospitalized in intensive care units. *J Hosp Infect* 2002;52:43–51.
326. Haley RW, Culver DH, White JW, et al. The efficacy of infection surveillance and control programs in preventing nosocomial infections in US hospitals. *Am J Epidemiol* 1985;121:182–205.
327. Rouget F, Chomienne F, Laurens E, et al. [Evaluation of a prevention program against nosocomial rotavirus infections in a pediatric ward]. *Arch Pediatr* 2000;7:948–954.
328. Gibson LL, Rose JB, Haas CN, et al. Quantitative assessment of risk

reduction from hand washing with antibacterial soaps. *J Appl Microbiol* 2002;92(Suppl):136S–143S.

329. Donowitz LG. Handwashing technique in a pediatric intensive care unit. *Am J Dis Child* 1987;141:683–685.
330. DeCarvalho M, Lopes JMA, Pellitteri M. Frequency and duration of handwashing in a neonatal intensive care unit. *Pediatric Infect Dis J* 1989;8:179–180.
331. Boyce JM, Pittet D. Guideline for hand hygiene in health-care settings. Recommendations of the Healthcare Infection Control Practices Advisory Committee and the HICPAC/SHEA/APIC/IDSA Hand Hygiene Task Force. Society for Healthcare Epidemiology of America/Association for Professionals in Infection Control/Infectious Diseases Society of America. *MMWR Recomm Rep* 2002;51:1–45.
332. Ehrenkranz NJ, Sanders CC, Eckert Schollenberger D, et al. Lack of evidence of efficacy of cohorting nursing personnel in a neonatal intensive care unit to prevent contact spread of bacteria: an experimental study. *Pediatr Infect Dis J* 1992;11:105–113.
333. Klein BS, Perloff WH, Maki DG. Reduction of nosocomial infection during pediatric intensive care by protective isolation. *N Engl J Med* 1989;320:1714–1721.
334. The revised CDC guidelines for isolation precautions in hospitals: implications for pediatrics. *Pediatrics* 1998;101:e13.
335. Mayfield JL, Leet T, Miller J, et al. Environmental control to reduce transmission of *Clostridium difficile. Clin Infect Dis* 2000;31: 995–1000.
336. McNulty C, Logan M, Donald IP, et al. Successful control of *Clostridium difficile* infection in an elderly care unit through use of a restrictive antibiotic policy. *J Antimicrob Chemother* 1997;40:707–711.
337. Szajewska H, Kotowska M, Mrukowicz JZ, et al. Efficacy of *Lactobacillus* GG in prevention of nosocomial diarrhea in infants. *J Pediatr* 2001;138:361–365.
338. Ledingham IM, Alcock SR, Eastaway AT, et al. Triple regimen of selective decontamination of the digestive tract, systemic cefotaxime, and microbiological surveillance for prevention of acquired infection in intensive care. *Lancet* 1988;1:785–790.
339. Brun Buisson C, Legrand P, Rauss A, et al. Intestinal decontamination for control of nosocomial multiresistant gram-negative bacilli. Study of an outbreak in an intensive care unit. *Ann Intern Med* 1989;110: 873–881.

51

NOSOCOMIAL MEASLES, MUMPS, RUBELLA, AND OTHER VIRAL INFECTIONS

MARK PAPANIA
SUSAN REEF
AISHA JUMAAN
JAIRAM LINGAPPA
WALTER W. WILLIAMS

Nosocomial measles, mumps, rubella, and varicella are well recognized and have been the cause of substantial morbidity among both patients and hospital workers. Immunocompromised patients and healthcare workers (HCWs) are especially vulnerable to severe infections and even death with some of these diseases. The transmission and impact of parvovirus B19 in hospital settings are less well understood. Pediatric patients are at risk, as may be adults—particularly older persons and those with chronic illnesses. HCWs are at risk for exposure to each of these diseases, and have played an important role in transmitting these infections in healthcare settings. This draws attention to the critical need for comprehensive prevention and control programs. One important component of such programs is providing basic education to HCWs on the modes of transmission of these nosocomial pathogens and methods of prevention and control.

Integral to any prevention and control efforts are systematic vaccination programs for HCWs, prompt diagnosis and management of potentially transmissible illnesses or exposures among hospital workers, and implementation of patient management techniques that decrease the risks of transmission.

All medical institutions (inpatient and outpatient, private and public) should ensure that all HCWs who work within their facilities (i.e., medical or nonmedical, paid staff, student or volunteer, full time or part time, with or without patient care responsibility) are immune to measles, rubella, and varicella. Immunity to mumps is also highly desirable. A comprehensive program of HCW immunization should include systematic evaluation of the immune status of existing staff as well as routine evaluation of incoming staff (see also Chapter 80).

All hospitals should have standard guidelines and procedures for identifying HCWs with infectious diseases or susceptible HCWs exposed to infectious diseases and for managing situations in which personnel may be infectious. For situations involving measles, rubella, mumps, and varicella, these procedures are greatly simplified if the personnel already have documentation of immunity.

Promptly instituting and complying with proper isolation precautions for patients with known or suspected communicable infections protects personnel and patients. In addition, hospital-acquired infections have been demonstrated to spread from patients and hospital personnel to their community contacts, as well as from the community to hospital settings. Transmission of infectious diseases is theoretically possible anywhere in hospitals where individuals, including HCWs, patients, volunteers, trainees, and visitors, may come into contact. This includes waiting areas, cafeterias, playrooms, and other locations. Because visitors and friends and relatives of hospital staff (including small children) may be infected or incubating infections, the important relationship between hospitals and their communities must be considered in developing prevention and control programs. Visitors, particularly children, may need to be screened for present or incubating infectious diseases before they are allowed to enter all or some patient care areas.

MEASLES

Epidemiology

Prior to the availability of measles vaccine, approximately 95% of persons living in urban areas of the United States were infected by age 15 years (1,2). From 1950 to 1959, an annual average of 549,000 cases and 495 deaths were reported. The licensure of live-virus vaccine in 1963 and its widespread use led to a greater than 99% reduction in the reported incidence of measles. Following a resurgence of measles from 1989 to 1991 (3,4), efforts were made to increase vaccination coverage among preschool children, which emphasized vaccination as close to the recommended age as possible (5–7). These efforts, coupled with ongoing implementation of the two-dose measles-mumps-rubella (MMR) recommendation (8–10), decreased the number of measles cases to the record low levels reported from 1997 to 2001, when less than 150 measles cases were reported annually, an incidence of <1 case/million population (11).

In addition to a reduction in total reported cases, the epidemiology of measles changed after introduction of the vaccine. One of the largest changes has been the variation in the age distribution of cases. Although measles incidence has decreased dramatically in all age groups, the intensive focus of vaccination efforts on preschool and school-age children caused relatively greater decreases in incidence in these age groups. The decrease in incidence has been less pronounced in adults, resulting in an increase in the proportion of measles cases occurring among adults (12). In 1997 to 2001 for the first time in reporting history, adults accounted for the largest proportion of cases (39%) of this "childhood disease," compared to 36% in preschool children and 25% in the school-age group (11).

Another significant change in the epidemiology of measles in the U.S. is the increase in the proportion of cases that are internationally imported. From 1997 to 2001, 36% of measles cases occurred in persons infected outside of the U.S. and an additional 25% were epidemiologically linked to internationally imported cases (11). Although a small number of cases occur every year for which a link to importation cannot be detected, measles is no longer an endemic disease in the U.S. Maintenance of this status will require continued vigorous immunization programs, including sustaining high coverage among HCWs.

Measles in Medical Settings

Measles transmission in medical settings has been well described (13,14), and descriptions of many measles outbreaks in the medical setting have been published (15–21). According to reports from state health departments to the Centers for Disease Control and Prevention (CDC) from 1985 through 1991, medical facilities were identified as the most likely setting of transmission for 2,997 reported measles cases (4% of all cases) (22). Almost half of these cases in the medical setting were acquired in hospital inpatient units. The remaining cases were equally divided between physician's offices and hospital emergency departments (22).

Two-thirds of persons who acquired measles in medical settings from 1985 to 1989 were patients, and 75% of these patients were children younger than 5 years (14). Measles was commonly transmitted to and among patients in emergency departments and hospital outpatient waiting areas. Visiting a hospital emergency room was identified as a risk factor for measles infection during community measles outbreaks in Houston and Los Angeles in 1989 (23). In addition, medical facilities can contribute to the propagation and amplification of community measles outbreaks (15,23,24).

From 1985 to 1991, HCWs accounted for 25% of measles cases acquired in the medical setting (22). The largest groups of HCWs who acquired measles at work were nurses (29%), physicians (15%), laboratory and radiology technicians (11%), clerks (11%), nursing assistants (4%), and medical and nursing students (4%). However, cases of measles were reported in persons of virtually all occupations who provided patient services or ancillary support (22). Transmission has been reported between patients, between HCWs, from patient to HCW, and from HCW to patient. In many instances, the patient contact that led to measles in the HCW did not qualify as direct patient care, which illustrates the extreme transmissibility of measles virus. Visitors were rarely identified as the source for measles transmitted in these settings. In a study of a measles outbreak in Clark County Oregon in 1996, HCWs were 18 times more likely to be infected with measles than the general adult population of the county (25).

Measles incidence declined after the 1989 to 1991 resurgence (11). However, in 24 (20%) of the 120 measles outbreaks reported during 1993 to 2001, the predominant setting of transmission was healthcare facilities (26). These outbreaks included more than 422 cases of measles; at least 37 measles cases occurred among persons working in healthcare facilities (CDC, unpublished data).

Clinical Description

Measles is a viral infection characterized by a generalized maculopapular rash and high fever. Following an incubation period of 10 to 12 days, the patient typically develops a prodrome consisting of fever and malaise, followed by cough, coryza, and conjunctivitis. The fever may exceed 40°C (104°F), and the patient may appear toxic. An enanthem, characterized by small bluish-white spots on a red background (Koplik's spots), may be seen on the buccal mucosa from 2 days before to 2 days after onset of rash. The characteristic rash of measles usually appears 2 to 4 days after onset of the prodromal symptoms. The rash first appears on the face, usually at the hairline, and then spreads to the trunk and extremities. It is initially maculopapular, but becomes confluent, particularly on the face. The rash lasts 5 to 7 days and fades in order of appearance.

Measles is typically mild and self-limited but may be associated with serious complications. The most common complications of measles are otitis media, diarrhea, and pneumonia. Pneumonia is the most common cause of death, and may be caused by measles virus itself or by secondary bacterial or viral infection. Severe diarrhea may also occur. Measles encephalitis is reported once in every 1,000 cases and can result in permanent neurologic sequelae or death. Measles can be severe in immunocompromised patients, particularly those with abnormalities of cellular immunity. From 1997 to 2001, 23% of reported measles cases in the U.S. required hospitalization (CDC, unpublished data). In the U.S., measles infection results in death in 2 to 3 of every 1,000 cases (27).

The age-specific rates of complications of measles are highest among infants, children 1 to 4 years of age, and adults over 20 years of age, and lowest in children 5 to 19 years of age (28).

Pathogenesis

Measles is an acute viral illness caused by a single-stranded RNA virus of the Paramyxovirus family. Infection with measles virus usually confers lifelong immunity. Measles is transmitted by respiratory droplets and usually requires relatively close contact between infected and susceptible persons. However, measles virus can survive for at least 2 hours in fine droplets, and airborne spread in medical settings has been documented (29,30). Secondary attack rates of over 90% have been documented among susceptible populations into which measles virus was introduced

(31,32). Neither a long-term infectious carrier state nor an animal reservoir is known to exist.

Measles is a systemic viral infection. The primary site of infection is the respiratory epithelium of the nasopharynx. Two to three days after invasion and replication in the respiratory epithelium, a primary viremia with infection of the reticuloendothelial system occurs. Following further viral replication in regional and distal reticuloendothelial sites, there is a second viremia, which occurs 5 to 7 days after initial infection. During this viremia, there may be infection of the respiratory tract and other organs. The characteristic pathologic feature of measles infection is the presence of multinucleated giant cells, which are found in the reticuloendothelial (Warthin-Finkeldey cells) or in the respiratory epithelium. In an immunocompetent person, measles virus is shed from the nasopharynx beginning with the prodrome until 3 to 4 days after rash onset.

Diagnosis

Measles is a rare disease in the U.S., and few clinicians have ever seen a case of measles. Cases that occur in vaccinated persons can have a milder clinical presentation. The key to diagnosing measles is suspecting measles in any patient with a generalized rash and fever and performing the appropriate laboratory tests. Recent international travel or exposure to persons who have recently traveled internationally should increase the diagnostic suspicion of measles. A history of vaccination, even with multiple doses of measles vaccine, does not preclude a diagnosis of measles. Measles is usually confirmed by the presence of immunoglobulin M (IgM) antibodies in a single serum specimen. Enzyme immunoassay (EIA) is the most common assay currently in use and is commercially available. IgM antibodies appear with or soon after rash onset, peak 1 to 2 weeks later, and fall to nondetectable levels 1 to 2 months after appearance of the rash. Serum specimens for IgM testing should be collected at the first clinical contact with a person with suspected measles. Measles may also be diagnosed by documenting a significant rise in immunoglobulin G (IgG) antibody titer in paired sera, with an acute specimen collected within 1 week after rash onset and a convalescent specimen collected 2 weeks later. Measles virus can be cultured from urine, nasal or throat swabs, or whole blood. Because viral isolation takes several weeks and is not sensitive enough to exclude the diagnosis of measles, it is not often used for laboratory diagnosis. However, virus isolation is very useful in identifying the measles virus strains occurring in the U.S., and clinicians are encouraged to collect specimens for virus isolation at the first clinical contact with a person with suspected measles.

Prevention and Control

Because of the ease of transmission of measles, and because measles cases are frequently misdiagnosed, especially during the prodrome, prevention of nosocomial measles transmission is difficult. However, a number of strategies will lower the risk. These include strategies to (a) maintain a high awareness among staff that a measles case could enter the facility; (b) maintain high vaccine coverage in the health facility staff; (c) exclude potentially infectious HCWs from duty in the healthcare facility; (d) promptly identify and isolate individuals with fever and rash; (e) observe appropriate procedures for airborne isolation in separate waiting areas (33); (f) inform health authorities of cases of this reportable disease; (g) ensure measles immunity in the patient population through routine vaccination programs that eliminate missed vaccination opportunities; (h) identify and vaccinate potentially exposed patients; and (i) administer immune globulin as needed to selected immunocompromised patients and HCWs where live viral vaccines, such as measles vaccine, are contraindicated (34,35).

Patients with suspected or confirmed measles should be placed on Airborne Precautions to prevent small droplet transmission until 4 days after the onset of rash (33). Immunocompromised persons with measles (e.g., persons with acquired immunodeficiency syndrome) may shed virus for extended periods, and should be kept on Airborne Precautions for the duration of their hospitalization for the acute illness.

Ideally, all healthcare personnel should have documented immunity to measles prior to possible exposure in the work setting. Measles immunity is defined as (a) documentation of receipt of at least two doses of measles containing vaccine after the first birthday, or (b) serologic evidence of measles immunity, or (c) history of physician-diagnosed measles, or (d) birth prior to 1957 (8,9). During a measles outbreak in the community served by a hospital or within a hospital, all personnel who cannot document immunity to measles should receive a dose of measles vaccine (9,36) or be excluded from duty.

Exposed personnel whose measles immunity is unknown should undergo serum sampling as soon as possible for measles IgG antibody testing. If less than 72 hours have elapsed since the exposure, a dose of measles vaccine may be given while awaiting the results of the antibody testing. If more than 72 hours but fewer than 6 days have elapsed since exposure, immune globulin may be given (8,9). If the antibody test indicates measles immunity, the exposed employee may return to work. If antibody testing indicates that the exposed worker is susceptible, the worker should be relieved from direct patient care from the fifth day after the first exposure to the 21st day after the last exposure, regardless of whether postexposure vaccine or immune globulin was given. Personnel who develop measles should be relieved from patient contact for at least 4 days after a rash develops (9,37).

Measles vaccine is a live attenuated viral vaccine, usually administered in the U.S. as combined MMR vaccine. Measles vaccine induces seroconversion in over 95% of susceptible persons with a single dose. The majority of persons who do not respond to the first dose of measles vaccine seroconvert following the second dose (38–40).

In 1997, the Advisory Committee on Immunization Practices (ACIP) recommended that any HCW (as defined above) who works within medical facilities (e.g., inpatient and outpatient, public and private) be required to provide evidence of appropriate vaccination against measles (e.g., two doses of live measles vaccine separated by ≥28 days on or after the first birthday), documentation of physician-diagnosed measles, or laboratory evidence of measles immunity (persons who have an indeterminate level of immunity upon testing should be considered nonimmune) (9,41).

Almost 30% of HCWs who acquired measles in medical settings from 1985 to 1991 were born before 1957 (i.e., they were older than the age for routine vaccination) (22). This observation is consistent with studies among hospital personnel indicating that up to 5% of hospital workers born before 1957 are susceptible to measles (21,40,42–47). The ACIP recommends that although birth before 1957 generally is considered acceptable evidence of measles immunity, healthcare facilities should consider recommending a dose of MMR vaccine to unvaccinated workers born before 1957 who do not have physician-diagnosed measles disease or laboratory evidence of measles immunity, or do not have laboratory evidence of rubella immunity (9,41).

There are two approaches to ensuring that HCWs without prior evidence of immunity are immune to measles: (a) serologic screening programs, in which employees are serologically tested for measles immunity with subsequent vaccination of persons without serologic evidence of immunity; and (b) vaccination without prior screening. The targeted approach to measles vaccination has been shown to be cost-effective in some settings (48–51), since more than 90% of adults can be expected to be immune to measles, either from previous vaccination or from disease, and vaccination of immune persons is of no proven benefit. However, three important points should be considered while developing a systematic measles immunity policy for a healthcare facility. First, if a screen-and-vaccinate approach is chosen, the facility must develop a recall system that can ensure that seronegative persons are vaccinated. Second, the cost savings from a screen-and-vaccinate program depend on the cost of the screening test, cost of the vaccine, and expected seroprevalence of measles antibody (49,50). Since both expected seroprevalence of measles antibody (90–95%) and vaccine cost are relatively constant, the key variable is the cost of screening. In-house testing is usually inexpensive, but sera sent to outside reference laboratories may be so expensive as to remove any economic advantage to this approach. Third, a screen-and-vaccinate approach does not consider immunity to rubella and mumps. Although hospital outbreaks of rubella and mumps are reported less frequently than measles outbreaks, a 1991 study among U.S. Army recruits suggested that as many as 16% to 21% of young adults were susceptible to these diseases (52). Considering the potential impact of these diseases, particularly the devastating effect of rubella infection of a pregnant woman, the opportunity to ensure immunity to these viruses should not be overlooked. The additional cost of screening for immunity to rubella and mumps would probably eliminate the cost savings of a screen-and-vaccinate approach, and would favor an MMR vaccination program of all employees without documented immunity.

MMR or its component vaccines should not be administered to women known to be pregnant. However, receipt of MMR or its component vaccines is not a reason to consider termination of pregnancy. A theoretical risk to the fetus from administration of live virus vaccines cannot be excluded; however, no actual risk of measles vaccination has ever been documented. Women should be counseled to avoid pregnancy for 30 days after administration of measles vaccines or MMR vaccine. However, termination of pregnancy is not recommended for pregnant women who have received measles vaccine or MMR (9,41). Measles-containing vaccine is recommended for all asymptomatic HIV-infected HCWs who do not have evidence of severe immunosuppression. Vaccine-associated measles infection has been associated with deaths in persons with severe immunosuppression (41, 53), and measles vaccine is not recommended for persons with severe immunosuppression from human immunodeficiency virus (HIV) or other diseases (9).

Tuberculin testing is not a prerequisite for vaccination with MMR or any of its component vaccines. MMR vaccine may interfere with the response to a tuberculin test (9). Therefore, tuberculin testing, if otherwise indicated, can be done either on the same day that the MMR is administered or 4 to 6 weeks later. Although some reports have suggested that tuberculosis may be exacerbated by natural measles infection, MMR and other measles-containing vaccines have not been demonstrated to have such an effect (9).

MUMPS

Epidemiology

The reported occurrence of mumps cases in the U.S. has decreased steadily since the introduction of live mumps-virus vaccine. In 2001, a record low of 274 cases was reported; this number represented a greater than 99% decline from the 152,209 cases reported in 1968, the year after live-mumps vaccine was licensed. Prior to vaccine licensure and during the early years of vaccine use, most reported cases occurred in the 5- to 9-year age group. In the late 1980s, there was a shift in the age-specific incidence to older children, but the overall risk for infection in all age groups declined by more than 90%. Between 1985 and 1987, a relative resurgence of mumps occurred, particularly among 10- to 14-year-olds (sevenfold increase) and 15- to 19-year-olds (more than an eightfold increase), probably because of suboptimal vaccination coverage of these children in the early years of mumps vaccination. Reported mumps has generally continued to decline since 1987 and throughout the 1990s, and currently cases no longer follow a seasonal pattern. As most mumps cases are not confirmed by laboratory testing, it is likely that many reflect parotitis caused by other infectious or noninfectious causes. However, these agents do not produce parotitis on an epidemic scale. Outbreaks have been observed wherever children or young adults congregate.

Although most cases of mumps in HCWs may be community-acquired, sporadic transmission of mumps within hospitals to patients and staff is well documented (54). Cases of mumps in HCWs and patients have been reported following nosocomial exposure, particularly in long-term-care facilities housing adolescents and young adults. Outbreaks of mumps within hospitals, however, have only rarely been reported (55). Presumably, the rare occurrence of nosocomial mumps outbreaks is because mumps virus is less communicable than measles and many other viruses. The level of mumps transmission in the surrounding community may also affect the risk for introduction into hospitals (54).

Clinical Description

Mumps is generally a mild, self-limited illness, but it may be moderately debilitating. The incubation period varies from 12 to 25 days and is usually 16 to 18 days. Onset of the disease usually occurs with nonspecific prodromal symptoms lasting up to several days, including anorexia, myalgia, malaise, headache, and low-grade fever. Up to one third of infected persons have minimal or no manifestations of disease. Parotitis is the most common manifestation, and data from longitudinal studies indicate that mumps virus infection produces typical parotitis in 15% to 20% of mumps infections. This may be unilateral or bilateral, be associated with earache and pain on chewing, and involve other salivary glands, including the submaxillary and sublingual glands. Parotitis is usually accompanied by moderate fever, but temperature may range from normal up to 40°C (104°F). Parotitis usually peaks in 1 to 3 days. Symptoms tend to decrease after 1 week and are usually gone by 2 weeks.

Two common complications are epididymo-orchitis, affecting 20% to 30% of postpubertal males, and mastitis, affecting up to 31% of females older than 15 years. Although some testicular atrophy occurs in about 35% of cases of mumps orchitis, sterility is a rare sequela. Oophoritis occurs in 5% of postpubertal females. Meningeal signs may appear in up to 15% of cases. Reported rates of mumps encephalitis range as high as 5 cases per 1,000 reported mumps cases. Permanent sequelae are rare, but the reported encephalitis case-fatality rate has averaged 1.4%. Sensorineural deafness occurs at a rate of 1 case per 15,000 to 20,000 cases of mumps. Mumps infection during the first trimester of pregnancy may increase the rate of spontaneous abortion (reported to be as high as 27%).

Pathogenesis

Mumps virus is a member of the Paramyxovirus family. Mumps virus is transmitted in saliva and respiratory secretions (56–58). Mumps is acquired through the nose or mouth by direct contact with infected droplets, saliva, or contaminated fomites. Primary viral replication occurs in the epithelium of the respiratory tract and possibly in regional lymph nodes. This is followed by viremia, which persists for 3 to 5 days, disseminates mumps virus throughout the body with localization in glandular tissue, and terminates with the development of humoral antibody (59). Virus may be present in saliva for 6 to 10 days before parotitis and persists for 5 to 9 days after onset of disease, ending with the appearance of virus-specific secretory IgA (56–58,60, 61). During viremia, virus may be disseminated to the salivary glands, meninges, kidneys, testes, and other organs. Viruria is frequent and may last 10 days or more. Virus can be isolated from breast milk of infected women. Parotitis accounts for most of the observed elevation of serum and urine amylase. About a week after onset of parotitis, orchitis and other complications may occur. Development of measurable neutralizing antibody correlates best with immunity to mumps.

Diagnosis

When parotitis is present, the clinical diagnosis of mumps is generally apparent. Parotitis, however, may be caused by other agents, such as parainfluenza and coxsackievirus, bacterial infections, systemic diseases such as lupus and sarcoid, and certain drugs. Because mumps is now a rare infection in the U.S., diagnostic testing for children with parotitis has been recommended (62). Laboratory diagnosis of mumps requires either detection of mumps IgM antibodies, a fourfold rise between acute and convalescent-phase titers in serum IgG antibody level, isolation of mumps virus, or detection of virus by reverse-transcriptase polymerase chain reaction (RT-PCR). Sera for IgM testing should be collected as soon as possible after onset of parotitis or as the acute specimen for examining seroconversion. The convalescent specimen for IgG detection should be collected about 2 to 4 weeks later. Virus may be isolated from saliva for up to 5 days after onset of symptoms, from urine for about 14 days, and from cerebrospinal fluid when tested within 8 to 9 days of the onset of central nervous system disease. EIA is a specific test for diagnosing acute mumps infection and mumps immunity. The complement fixation (CF) and hemagglutination inhibition (HI) antibody tests for mumps immunity may be unreliable, because they are relatively insensitive and cross-react with other viral antigens.

Prevention and Control

Preventing mumps through an effective vaccination program is the best approach to controlling this disease. The relatively long period of virus shedding before clinical symptoms begin and the high incidence of asymptomatic infections render other methods to control mumps unreliable. Vaccination with the live, attenuated Jeryl-Lynn strain mumps virus vaccine is recommended for all those who are susceptible unless otherwise contraindicated (9,41,63,64). Combined MMR vaccine is the vaccine of choice for routine administration and always should be used when recipients are also likely to be susceptible to measles and/or rubella. The favorable benefit-cost ratio for routine mumps vaccination is increased when vaccine is administered as MMR (65). Persons should be considered susceptible to mumps unless they have documentation of physician-diagnosed mumps, adequate immunization with live mumps vaccine on or after the first birthday, or laboratory evidence of immunity (41). Most persons born before 1957 are likely to have been infected naturally, and generally may be considered to be immune even if they may not have had clinically recognizable mumps. This arbitrary cutoff date, however, does not preclude vaccinating possibly susceptible persons born before 1957 who may be exposed in outbreak settings. Revaccination with MMR is recommended under certain circumstances for measles and may also be important for mumps, because studies have shown that mumps can occur in highly vaccinated populations, presumably because of primary vaccine failure (66–68). Persons who are unsure about their history of mumps disease or vaccination should be vaccinated.

Susceptible personnel who are exposed to or develop mumps should be relieved from direct patient contact from the 12th day after the first exposure through the 26th day after the last exposure or until 9 days after the onset of parotitis (69). Droplet precautions to prevent transmission are recommended for patients with mumps, including a private room and use of masks for those close to the patient (33). These precautions should be maintained for 9 days after onset of parotitis.

During mumps outbreaks, exclusion of susceptible persons from affected institutions should be considered. Although protection from mumps vaccination does not develop for at least 2 weeks after vaccination, during outbreaks in schools excluded students can be readmitted immediately after vaccination (9). Policies in healthcare settings should be more stringent to decrease the risk for transmission. Persons who have been exempted from vaccination because of medical, religious, or other reasons should be excluded until at least 26 days after the onset of parotitis in the last person with mumps in the affected institution (9).

RUBELLA

Epidemiology

The number of reported rubella cases has decreased steadily from over 56,000 cases in 1969, the year rubella vaccine was licensed, to 176 cases in 2000, and 23 cases in 2001. Until the mid-1970s, the strategy was to vaccinate all children; this strategy dramatically reduced the incidence of rubella but had less impact on older age groups, resulting in an increased proportion of cases in adolescents and adults. Enhanced efforts to vaccinate susceptible adults, especially through premarital-screening and postpartum vaccination, resulted in decreased rubella in these age groups in the 1980s. During the 1990s, the epidemiology of rubella changed significantly. The incidence of rubella in children younger than 15 years decreased (0.63 vs. 0.06 per 100, 000) whereas the incidence in adults aged 15 to 44 years increased (0.13 vs. 0.24 per 100,000). Furthermore, the incidence among Hispanics increased from 0.06 per 100,000 population in 1992 to a high of 0.97 per 100,000 population in 1998. During the mid 1990s to 2000, the majority of cases in rubella outbreaks were among foreign-born Hispanic adults. These changes reflect the growing number of rubella cases among adults from countries without a history of routine rubella vaccination programs (70). Still, an estimated 10% to 15% of young U.S.-born adults remain susceptible to rubella. Although not as infectious as measles, rubella can be transmitted effectively whenever a large number of susceptible persons congregate in one place, and outbreaks continue to be a possibility in these settings, including hospitals.

The number of reported congenital rubella syndrome (CRS) cases has also declined significantly in the U.S., from 77 cases in 1970 to 8 cases in 2000. However, in the U.S., surveillance for CRS relies on a passive system. Consequently, the reported annual totals of CRS are regarded as minimum figures, representing an estimated 40% to 70% of the cases that occur (9). All eight of the infants with CRS born in 2000 were born to foreign-born, Hispanic women.

Rubella in Medical Settings

Nosocomial rubella has involved both personnel and patients (71–79). Outbreaks have resulted in serious consequences, including therapeutic abortions, disruption of hospital routine, time loss from work, costly control or containment measures, adverse publicity, and the potential for legal action. Although vaccination has decreased the overall risk for rubella transmission in all age groups in the U.S. by ≥95%, the potential for transmission in hospital and similar settings persists because 10% to 15% of young adults are still susceptible (41,80). In an ongoing study of rubella vaccination in a health maintenance organization, 7,890 of 92,070 (8.6%) women 29 years of age or older were susceptible to rubella (41; CDC, unpublished data). Persons born before 1957 generally are considered to be immune to rubella. However, findings of seroepidemiologic studies indicate that about 6% of HCWs (including persons born in 1957 or earlier) do not have detectable rubella antibody (CDC, unpublished data).

Transmission of rubella has occurred both from male and female HCWs to susceptible co-workers and patients and from patients to healthcare personnel and other patients. Medical and dental students have been sources of infection and vectors in rubella outbreaks (74,75; CDC, unpublished data).

In 1996, rubella was reported in an HCW who worked in a hospital with no policy requiring rubella immunity; this case was linked to a community rubella outbreak. In 1997, rubella transmission occurred in two healthcare settings. In the first, an HCW working in a hospital with no policy requiring rubella immunity was diagnosed with rubella disease. The HCW had claimed to be fully vaccinated, but had no documentation of vaccination or serologic evidence of rubella immunity; 100 hospital employees were vaccinated as a result of this case. The other healthcare setting involved rubella transmission among four patients who lived in one wing of a hospital; over 500 persons (about 80% were patients) were vaccinated as a result of this outbreak. This hospital did have a policy that required immunity to rubella; on investigation, most of the staff members were considered immune (CDC, unpublished data). Between 1997 and 1998, one state reported six rubella cases in HCWs.

Clinical Description

Rubella in adults is usually a mild disease, lasting only a few days (81–84); 30% to 50% of cases may be subclinical or inapparent. The incubation period is variable but may range from 12 to 23 days, with most persons developing a rash 14 to 16 days after exposure. In adults, about the time virus appears in the blood a prodrome frequently occurs. It precedes the rash, lasts 1 to 5 days, and consists of malaise; low-grade fever; postauricular, occipital, and posterior cervical adenopathy; and upper respiratory infection. At the end of the incubation period, a maculopapular erythematous rash begins on the face and spreads rapidly to the chest, abdomen, and extremities. Cell-free viremia ends with the onset of rash, but mononuclear cell–borne viremia continues for a week or more after the rash subsides. Lymphadenopathy is a major clinical manifestation of rubella, and in addition to the characteristic suboccipital and postauricular nodes, there can be generalized involvement as well. Transient polyarthralgia and polyarthritis sometimes accompany or follow rubella. Among adults, particularly women, acute joint manifestations are common (up to 70%). Rubella virus has been recovered from synovial fluid of patients with acute disease (85) and in some instances from individuals with chronic arthritis in the absence of clinical rubella (86,87), although the overall risk of persistent arthritis appears to be low. Central nervous system complications (encephalopathy or encephalomyelitis) and thrombocytopenia have been reported at rates of 1 per 6,000 cases and 1 per 3,000 cases, respectively. Hemorrhagic manifestations occur with an approximate incidence of 1 per 3,000 cases, occurring more often in children than in adults.

By far, the most important consequences of rubella are the abortions, miscarriages, stillbirths, and multiple anomalies in infants that result from maternal infection in early pregnancy, especially in the first trimester. The most commonly described anomalies associated with CRS are auditory (sensorineural hearing impairment), ophthalmic (cataracts, microphthalmia, glaucoma, chorioretinitis), cardiac (patent ductus arteriosus, pulmonary artery stenosis, atrial or ventricular septal defects), and neurologic (microcephaly, meningoencephalitis, developmental delay). Preventing fetal infection and the consequent congenital rubella syndrome is the objective of rubella vaccination programs.

Pathogenesis

Transmission of rubella virus, an RNA virus in the Togavirus family, is from person to person via droplets shed from the respiratory secretions of infected persons. The disease is most contagious when the rash is erupting, but virus may be shed from 1 week before to 5 to 7 days after the rash onset. The mucosa of the upper respiratory tract and the nasopharyngeal lymphoid tissue are the primary portals for virus entry and the initial sites of viral replication. Virus spreads via the lymphatic system, or viremia may seed regional lymph nodes. The appearance of the rubella rash coincides with the detection of rubella-specific antibody. Cell-mediated immunity is also induced. Immunity is generally long lasting, but reinfection may occur following either naturally acquired rubella or vaccine-induced immunity (88,89). Although some individuals have antibody levels that are not detectable by HI antibody testing following previous vaccination or infection, the clinical significance of such low-level antibody has not been well documented. Limited data suggest that reinfection with the rubella virus may occur in persons with low antibody levels. During reinfection, there is limited viral replication in the nasopharynx, and viremia and systemic manifestations are uncommon. CRS following reinfection has been documented, although such instances have been rare (90).

In fetal infection, transmission occurs during maternal viremia when the placenta is seeded with virus followed by development of inflammatory foci in the chorionic villi, granulomatous changes, and necrosis (91,92). Ascending infection from the female genital tract has also been postulated (83).

Diagnosis

Clinical diagnosis of rubella is difficult and may be inaccurate without laboratory investigation. Although suboccipital and postauricular lymphadenopathy are characteristic, enlargement of these nodes can occur in adults with other conditions such as infectious mononucleosis, acquired toxoplasmosis, and *Mycoplasma pneumoniae* infection. Because rubella virus grows slowly in tissue culture, viral isolation is often omitted for serologic diagnosis, although virus can be recovered from the blood, urine, and the nasopharynx during the prodromal period and from the nasopharynx for a week or more after onset of rash. Serologic diagnosis can be made by demonstrating a fourfold rise in antibody titer between acute and convalescent serum samples or demonstrating IgM antibody in an acute specimen. The HI test was once the most commonly used technique. It is no longer used for routine testing but serves as a reference method for other tests that are more rapid and easier to use, including enzyme-linked immunosorbent assay (ELISA), immunofluorescent antibody assays (IFAs), and latex agglutination (LA). For these assays, the criteria for a significant rise in antibody level vary by type of assay. The ELISA is used most frequently for IgM testing, and results may be positive for up to 6 weeks after acute infection.

Prevention and Control

To minimize introduction and transmission of rubella in medical facilities, all personnel (e.g., volunteers, trainees, nurses, physicians), both male and female, who might transmit rubella to pregnant patients or other rubella susceptible patients or personnel should be immune to rubella (93–97). Persons should be considered susceptible to rubella unless they have documentation of (a) vaccination on or after the first birthday or (b) laboratory evidence of immunity, or were born before 1957 (except women who could become pregnant) (9,98). A history of past rubella infection is unreliable and should not be accepted as a criterion of immunity. Routine serologic screening before vaccination is not necessary unless the facility considers it cost-effective (41). Serologic testing is not necessary for persons who have documentation of appropriate vaccination or other acceptable evidence of immunity to rubella. Serologic testing before vaccination is appropriate only if tested persons identified as nonimmune are subsequently vaccinated in a timely manner (41). During outbreaks of rubella, serologic screening before vaccination is not generally recommended, because rapid vaccination is necessary to halt disease transmission (9,41).

Rubella vaccination or laboratory evidence of rubella immunity is important for all HCWs, particularly for female HCWs who could become pregnant, including those born before 1957. Although no evidence indicates that administration of rubella-containing vaccine virus (e.g., MMR) to a pregnant woman presents a risk for her fetus, such a risk cannot be excluded on theoretical grounds. Therefore, women of childbearing age should receive rubella-containing vaccines only if they state that they are not pregnant and only if they are counseled not to become pregnant for 1 month after vaccination (99). If a pregnant woman is vaccinated or if she becomes pregnant within 1 month after vaccination, she should be counseled about the theoretical risk of congenital rubella syndrome for the fetus, but MMR vaccination during pregnancy should not ordinarily be a reason to consider termination of pregnancy (9). Rubella-susceptible women from whom vaccine is withheld because they state they are or may be pregnant should be counseled about the potential risk for congenital rubella syndrome and the importance of being vaccinated as soon as they are no longer pregnant

(41). Published data indicate that the risk for adverse events is not increased in persons already immune from either previous infection or vaccination (100).

Ideally, all personnel should be immune, but highest priority should be given to personnel who are at increased risk for exposure to rubella or who are in direct contact with pregnant patients. To maximize compliance, mandatory programs should be considered; voluntary programs may be inadequate (98,101). MMR trivalent vaccine is the vaccine of choice.

Susceptible personnel who are exposed to or develop rubella should be relieved of direct patient contact from the seventh day after the first exposure through the 21st day after the last exposure or until 5 days after rash appears (33). Isolation precautions to prevent spread by close or direct contact are recommended for infants with congenital rubella, including placement in a private room and use of gowns and gloves when soiling is likely or for touching infective material. These precautions should be maintained during any admission for the first year after birth unless nasopharyngeal and urine cultures, obtained at least 1 month apart, after 3 months of age are negative for rubella virus. Similar precautions are also recommended for other patients with rubella for 7 days after onset of rash. Susceptible patients who have been exposed to rubella should be isolated for 21 days after exposure or, if they develop clinical rubella, for 5 days after the onset of rash.

Although methods for controlling rubella outbreaks are evolving, the primary strategy should be to ensure that susceptible persons are vaccinated rapidly (or excluded from exposure if a contraindication exists) and maintain active surveillance to permit modification of control measures as needed (96). Mandatory exclusion and vaccination of HCWs who cannot document rubella immunity is recommended in medical settings, because pregnant women may be exposed. Persons who have an equivocal serologic test result should be considered susceptible to rubella unless they have evidence of adequate vaccination or a subsequent serologic test result indicates rubella immunity (9).

Occasionally, persons with documented histories of rubella vaccination are found to have rubella serum IgG levels that are not clearly positive by ELISA. Such persons can be administered a dose of MMR vaccine and need not be retested for serologic evidence of rubella immunity (9).

VARICELLA

Epidemiology

Before the licensure of the varicella vaccine (VARVAX) in 1995, almost everyone developed varicella (chickenpox) during their lifetime, resulting in an estimated 4 million cases (birth cohort, 1994), 11,000 hospitalizations, and 100 deaths annually (102–104). Currently, varicella disease surveillance is limited; in 2002, only 18 states and territories reported cases to the CDC's National Notifiable Disease Surveillance System (NNDSS), and reporting within states is incomplete. In the prevaccine era, reporting efficiency was estimated at approximately 5% (105), which is adequate for surveillance purposes to monitor trends in reported diseases. In 2002, only seven states reported over 5% of their expected cases to NNDSS. Varicella deaths have been nationally notifiable since 1999 and varicella cases will become nationally notifiable in 2003 (106).

In the prevaccine era in the U.S., about 90% of varicella disease occurred among children less than 15 years of age (102), with the highest incidence occurring among children 1 to 9 years of age. Serologic data from a nationally representative population survey in the U.S. from 1988 to 1994 confirmed that about 99% of individuals older than 30 years of age were immune, and that the likelihood of immunity increased with age, ranging from 86% for persons 6 to 11 years of age to >99% for those 40 years of age or older (52,107). In tropical or subtropical climates, cases occur at older ages resulting in a higher susceptibility rates among adults (102,108–110). A positive history of varicella is a good predictor of immunity, but a negative history is not a good predictor of susceptibility. Most persons (95–98%) with a positive history have varicella zoster virus (VZV) IgG antibodies and are likely to be immune (52,111–115), and the majority (range: 48–96%) with negative or unknown histories are also likely to be immune (111–114,116–122). Nevertheless, without varicella vaccination, studies of HCWs in the U.S. have documented susceptibility to varicella ranging from 1% to 7% (112,113,116–118,120–125).

The varicella vaccine, licensed in March 1995, is a live attenuated cell-free preparation of the Oka strain of VZV. Routine vaccination of all children at 12 to 18 months, with catch-up vaccination of all susceptible children before the 13th birthday, is recommended (126). The varicella vaccine is also recommended for susceptible persons with close contact to persons at high risk for serious complications (e.g., HCWs and susceptible household contacts of immunocompromised persons) (41,114, 126–129), susceptible persons at high risk for exposure or transmission, postexposure (within 3 to 5 days), for outbreak control, and for day care and school entry requirements (130). The vaccine should be considered for HIV-positive children with the percentage of CD4 cells >25% (two doses, 3 months apart), and is desirable for other susceptible adolescents and adults (130). Persons <13 years of age receive one dose, whereas those ≥13 years receive two doses, 4 to 8 weeks apart.

In the U.S., before implementation of the varicella vaccination program, children less than 10 years of age accounted for 61% of an estimated 11,000 varicella-related hospitalizations, and healthy persons, without severe underlying conditions, accounted for 89% of all hospitalizations per year from 1988 through 1995 (103). Many of the hospitalized cases had one or more complications, and 64% of the complications occurred among children <5 years of age and adults ≥20 years of age. The most common complications of varicella that result in hospitalizations include pneumonia, dehydration, secondary bacterial infection, and encephalitis. Adults hospitalized for varicella are more likely to have encephalitis than children, who experience more secondary bacterial infection of the skin (103,131). The risk of varicella death increases with increasing age, except for infants <1 year of age where the rate is 3.7 per 100,000 cases (104). The fatality rate per 100,000 cases in the prevaccine era, 1990 to 1994 ranged from 0.8 per 100,000 cases among persons 1 to 4 years of age to 21.3 per 100,000 cases among persons aged 20 years of age or older (104). Although prenatal infection is uncommon because most women of childbearing age are immune (132), chickenpox in pregnant women in the first trimester is associated with a risk of transmission of VZV infection to the fetus or newborn. Intrauterine infection may result in the congenital varicella syndrome (characterized by low birth weight, cutaneous scarring and limb hypoplasia, microcephaly, cortical atrophy, chorioretinitis, cataract, and other anomalies), clinical varicella in the newborn, or clinical zoster in infancy.

The clinical presentation in the infant is determined by the time during pregnancy when the mother is infected. Results from several studies (133–136) estimated a 2% risk of congenital varicella syndrome in infants born to mothers with chickenpox in the first 20 weeks of their pregnancy. In the largest of these studies (136), risk for congenital varicella syndrome was 0.4% when maternal infection occurred from 1 to 12 weeks of gestation, and was 2% when maternal infection occurred at 13 to 20 weeks of gestation. Intrauterine infection after 20 weeks of gestation is associated with an increased risk of zoster in infancy (137,138). The onset of chickenpox in pregnant women from 5 days before to 2 days after delivery may result in severe varicella infection in an estimated 17 to 30% of their newborn infants, because they are exposed to VZV without the benefit of maternal antibody (139,140). However, severe infections can be avoided with prompt prophylactic use of VZV immunoglobulin (VZIG) and acyclovir (ACV) (140,141).

Nosocomial transmission of VZV infection is well recognized (111–112,114,116,117,119,120,124,125,142–154). Sources of nosocomial exposure of patients and staff have included other patients, hospital staff, and visitors (including the children of staff members) with either varicella or herpes zoster. Airborne transmission of varicella in hospitals has been demonstrated (143–146,155), with nosocomial varicella occurring in staff members who had no direct contact with the index case (144, 146,155). Varicella may be transmitted to susceptible individuals from generalized herpes zoster or localized herpes zoster in immunocompromised patients via the airborne route. The occurrence of chickenpox in a hospital can be disruptive and potentially life-threatening to certain patients. Although all susceptible hospitalized patients are at risk for severe disease and complications, patients with certain conditions are at a higher risk for severe disease and complications. These patients include premature infants born to susceptible mothers and infants born before 28 weeks' gestation or weighing 1,000 g or less, regardless of the mother's immune status, and immunocompromised patients of all ages, including persons undergoing immunosuppressive therapy, persons with malignant disease, and those with immunodeficiencies.

Clinical Description

Varicella, or chickenpox, in adults is often a more severe disease than it is in children (156–158). In adults, varicella commonly begins with a prodrome characterized by several days of fever, chills, malaise, headache, and irritability. Varicella is characterized by a generalized rash that appears in crops. Each crop begins as small macules and progresses within 24 hours to papules, vesicles, pustules, and finally crusts. The vesicles initially contain clear fluid that rapidly becomes purulent, and then dries beginning centrally to form an umbilicated appearance before crusting. Virus generally can be isolated from skin lesions, but it is hard to isolate from respiratory secretions. New successive crops of lesions occur in the next 5 to 6 days at various stages of development in any one part of the body. Lesions have a central distribution, appearing first and with the greatest number of lesions on the scalp, face, and trunk, with fewer lesions on the extremities. Vesicles may develop on mucosal surfaces, including the mucous membranes of the mouth, the pharynx, larynx, trachea, rectal and vaginal mucosa, and conjunctiva. The most marked symptom of varicella is pruritus, which lasts throughout the vesicular stage. Varicella can vary in intensity, being inapparent in less than 5% of cases (159), and severe with primary varicella pneumonia requiring hospitalization in 1% to 3% of cases (103,160,161). Secondary bacterial infection of skin lesions is the most common complication of varicella; varicella is a risk factor for invasive group A *Streptococcus* infection (103, 162–165). Increased severity and other complications are common in immunocompromised persons (particularly leukemics) and in adults, including varicella pneumonia, central nervous system involvement, and visceral spread (103,166). Cutaneous complications (e.g., purpura fulminans, bullous varicella) are common in persons with underlying skin disorders. Rare complications include myocarditis, hepatitis, nephritis, orchitis, pancreatitis, arthritis, and iritis (166).

Pathogenesis

VZV, a member of the herpesvirus family (Alphaherpesvirinae), spreads from person to person via direct contact with vesicular fluid or droplets from respiratory secretions, or via aerosolized droplet nuclei. The virus apparently enters through the mucosa of the upper respiratory tract or the conjunctiva. During the incubation period, the virus replicates locally in lymph nodes and 4 to 6 days later, a small primary viremia disseminates virus to sites of secondary viral replication, the reticuloendothelial cells in the spleen, liver, and other organs (156,158), where there is further replication until 10 to 12 days after inoculation. Prodromal symptoms begin with a more significant secondary viremia, spreading the virus to the skin, 14 to 16 days (range 10 to 21 days) after inoculation resulting in cutaneous and mucosal lesions. Cyclic viremia accounts for successive crops of lesions and terminates after several days in immunocompetent hosts as a result of specific humoral and cellular immune responses (167, 168). Rises in VZV-specific IgG, and IgA can be demonstrated within 3 days of onset of clinical disease (156,167); the timing and duration of the IgM response in both varicella and herpes zoster remains poorly defined. Several small studies show that rises in IgM are detectable for days to weeks (169,170). Complications of varicella reflect a failure to limit the virus replication (156). During infection, VZV is thought to pass from skin and mucosal lesions to the corresponding sensory ganglia via the contiguous sensory nerve endings and fibers, or, alternatively, VZV may seed the ganglia hematogenously (156). Zoster results when latent virus in the neuronal cells reactivates. Although the mechanism of reactivation is unclear, known risk factors relate to the state of cell-mediated immunity to VZV (aging, immunosuppression, primary VZV infection *in utero* or early infancy) (171).

Diagnosis

Diagnosis of acute varicella or herpes zoster is generally based on the distinctive rash. Rapid detection of VZV in clinical specimens may be needed in severe or unusual cases, to identify patients for antiviral therapy or institute appropriate isolation procedures. The direct fluorescent antibody (DFA) test and polymerase chain reactions (PCR) test are currently the preferred method for rapid laboratory diagnosis of VZV infections (172). Tzanck smears may also be useful in hospital settings, though, if positive, they indicate an alpha herpes virus infection, which may be due to either VZV or herpes simplex virus infection.

Numerous methods have been used to detect IgG antibody to VZV, including CF, IFA, fluorescent antibody to membrane antigen (FAMA), neutralization, indirect hemagglutination (IHA), immune adherence hemagglutination (IAHA), radioimmunoassay (RIA), latex agglutination (LA), and ELISA (173). The IFA, FAMA, neutralization, and RIA methods are sensitive tests, but they are time-consuming and have requirements that make them unsuitable for use in general diagnostic laboratories. The CF test has been widely used but is the least sensitive; antibody may reach levels that are undetectable by CF several months after natural varicella infection. The RIA and ELISA have been shown to be equal in sensitivity (174). Commercially available ELISA tests have sensitivity in the range of 86% to 97% and specificity in the range of 82% to 99% for the detection of antibodies following natural varicella infection, which is substantially higher than antibody produced by immunization (175, 176). The ELISA may not be sufficiently sensitive to detect seroconversion in all individuals following vaccination, and thus, a glycoprotein ELISA (gpELISA) using purified viral glycoproteins as antigens has been used in clinical trials for the large-scale testing of immunogenicity of varicella vaccine; however, this assay is not commercially available (177–179). An LA test using latex particles coated with VZV glycoprotein antigens, which can be completed in 15 minutes and does not require special equipment, is now commercially available (180). The sensitivity and specificity of the LA test is comparable to that of the FAMA test for the detection of antibody responses to natural varicella infection, more sensitive than ELISA for detection of antibody responses after vaccination, and has detected antibody as long as 11 years after varicella vaccination (181). Experience in reading the test is needed, since the identification of agglutination is subjective and occasional false positives and false negatives have been reported (182).

Prevention and Control

Even though healthcare personnel who are susceptible to varicella may be few, it is important to identify such persons when they begin employment in a healthcare field. It is advisable to allow only personnel who are immune to varicella to take care of patients with known or suspected varicella or zoster. Adults with a history of varicella can be assumed to be immune, although some hospital-based screening programs have elected to test all employees irrespective of disease history since seronegative adults with a positive varicella history have been documented, albeit rarely. Those without a history or with uncertain history of varicella may be considered susceptible or may be tested serologically to determine susceptibility or immunity. Those vaccinated with two doses of the varicella vaccine can be assumed to be immune. As the vaccination program progresses, a positive disease history may become a less reliable indicator of immunity.

Universal vaccination of children is expected to reduce varicella exposure in the healthcare setting. Since the vaccine licensure in 1995, more than 30 million doses have been distributed. In 2001, the national varicella vaccine coverage among children 19 to 35 months increased to 76%, with varying state estimates ranging from 53% in South Dakota to 90% in Rhode Island (183). Moreover, by September 2003, 38 states will have established a requirement for varicella vaccination for child care or school entry.

Despite availability of the vaccine, varicella-related deaths among unvaccinated children and adults still occur (184,185; CDC unpublished data). Herpes zoster will continue to be a significant source of VZV exposure in healthcare settings (186).

Serologic screening of adults with a negative or equivocal history of varicella is likely to be cost-saving compared to vaccinating all those without a definitive history of varicella (187). In healthcare institutions, serologic screening of those with negative or uncertain varicella history and vaccination of those testing susceptible should be cost-saving compared to not instituting any varicella vaccination program at all; key factors determining cost-effectiveness include sensitivity and specificity of serologic tests, cost of serology testing, the nosocomial transmission rate, seroprevalence of VZV antibody in the worker population, and policies for managing vaccine recipients developing postvaccination rash or who are subsequently exposed to VZV (188–190). Varicella vaccination should help control the spread of VZV to and from hospital workers, but may not eliminate nosocomial transmission (191,192). Varicella vaccination programs may not be as simple as those for measles, mumps, and rubella. Two doses of vaccine are required to achieve high seroconversion rates in adults (191,193), and the need for and response to booster doses of vaccine are unknown. In adults followed for 7 to 21 years after vaccination, antibodies to VZV persisted in over 60%, and breakthrough varicella developed in 9% to 10% of these exposed (176,194,195). Breakthrough infection was mild, and severity did not increase with time since vaccination. The role of boosting from exposure to wild VZV in maintaining vaccine-induced immunity remains unclear. Some experience with the vaccine will be required to optimize varicella prevention and control strategies.

Several options for management of vaccinated HCWs who may be exposed to varicella are available. Testing for varicella immunity following two doses of vaccine in HCWs is not currently recommended because 99% of persons are seropositive after the second dose using the gpELISA (the most sensitive, but not commercially available, antibody test), and because sensitive tests for validating postvaccine immunity are not commercially available. Moreover, seroconversion does not always result in full protection against disease. However, results of a 10-year prospective follow-up of varicella vaccination of children found that breakthrough cases of varicella never developed in children with a FAMA titer >1:16 in the preceding 1 to 2 years, and that the FAMA response to vaccination was predictive of breakthrough varicella risk (196). However, studies among adults are needed to identify correlates of protection. A potentially effective strategy for identifying individuals who remain at risk for varicella is to test vaccinees for seropositivity immediately after they are exposed to VZV (126). Persons with detectable antibody are unlikely to develop varicella. Persons without antibody can be retested in 5 to 6 days to determine if an anamnestic response is present, in which case they are unlikely to develop disease; those who remain susceptible may be furloughed. An alternative to furloughing vaccinated persons without detectable antibody following exposure to varicella is daily monitoring of their clinical status. Institutional guidelines will be needed for management of exposed vaccinees without detectable antibody, as well as for those who develop clinical varicella.

Vaccination is recommended for unvaccinated HCWs without documented immunity who are exposed to varicella. However, staff members should be managed as previously recommended for unvaccinated persons.

Although over 30 million doses of the varicella vaccine have been distributed, only three cases of secondary transmission from healthy vaccinees with vesicular lesions to healthy close contacts have been documented (197). This transmission occurred only when vaccinees developed a rash after vaccination (198–201). In one study of leukemic vaccine recipients, transmission occurred in 17% of susceptible siblings; however, transmission did not occur in the absence of a rash, and risk of transmission increased as the number of lesions appearing on the vaccinee increased (199). Transmission of vaccine virus was assessed in the household setting (during the 8-week postvaccination period) in 416 susceptible placebo recipients who were household contacts of 445 vaccine recipients (202). Of the 416 placebo recipients, three developed chickenpox during months of high incidence (December to June) and seroconverted, nine reported a varicella-like rash and did not seroconvert, and six had no rash but seroconverted. These cases may represent either natural varicella from community contacts or a low incidence of transmission of vaccine virus from vaccinated contacts. If vaccine virus was transmitted, it happened at a very low rate and possibly without recognizable clinical disease in contacts. Vaccine virus has been cultured from vesicular fluid following vaccination (191). As a precaution, some institutions may wish to temporarily furlough or curtail the duties of personnel who develop a rash following vaccination, and consider precautions for other vaccine recipients, including avoiding close association with susceptible high-risk persons (e.g., newborns, pregnant women, immunocompromised persons). In addition, since breakthrough infections can occur in persons who have previously seroconverted, reporting rash illness suspected of being varicella, especially after a known exposure, will have to be emphasized.

Strategies for managing varicella clusters in hospitals have generally involved rapid serologic testing for susceptibility, when necessary; furlough of susceptible personnel, usually at substantial cost; and isolation of patients with varicella or disseminated herpes zoster, or exposed susceptible patients (33,41,114,117, 118,203–205). Control of airflow has been employed (147), and in lieu of furloughing, daily screening of exposed susceptible personnel for skin lesions, fever, or constitutional symptoms, and temporary reassignment of susceptible personnel to locations remote from patient care areas (111,120,121,192,203–205). Ideally, susceptible personnel who are exposed to or develop varicella should be relieved from direct patient contact from the eighth or tenth day after the first exposure through the 21st day after the last exposure, or if varicella occurs, until all lesions dry and crust (37,41,69,127). Susceptible personnel who are exposed to herpes zoster should be restricted from patient contact (41). Because of the possibility of transmission and development of severe illness in high-risk patients, personnel with localized zoster should not take care of these patients until all lesions dry and crust. Personnel with localized zoster may not pose a special risk to other patients if the lesions can be covered; however, some institutions may wish to institute stricter precautions for all patients, including furlough of personnel with zoster until all lesions dry and crust (114).

After exposure, hospital personnel with absence of VZV antibodies and no history of vaccination can be offered varicella vaccine or VZIG (126). The major effect of the vaccine, if given within 3 to 5 days postexposure, and VZIG, if given <96 hours of exposure, is to modify or prevent varicella disease, and prevent serious complications. Postexposure effectiveness studies have been mainly done in children (206–209); few data are available on the effectiveness of one dose of varicella vaccine administered postexposure in adults. Susceptible personnel who receive the varicella vaccine still need to be reassigned or furloughed for 21 days after exposure; those who receive VZIG should be reassigned or furloughed for 28 days or more after exposure since VZIG prolongs the varicella incubation period. Personnel developing varicella should receive acyclovir within 24 hours of rash onset (unless pregnant) to reduce duration and severity of clinical illness; personnel with herpes zoster should receive acyclovir, famciclovir, or valacyclovir as soon as possible after rash onset to accelerate the rate of cutaneous healing (114,126,127). Healthy patients with varicella or disseminated zoster and immunocompromised patients with localized zoster should be placed on airborne precautions and contact precautions designed to prevent spread by both air and contact, including a private room with special ventilation, if available (33). Susceptible persons should stay out of the room. Neonates born to mothers with active varicella should be placed on similar contact precautions at birth. Immunocompetent patients with localized zoster may be placed on contact precautions to prevent transmission by direct or indirect contact with purulent material or drainage from an infected body site, although some also recommend Airborne Precautions to prevent airborne transmission for these patients (114). Exposed susceptible patients should be placed on airborne precautions to prevent airborne spread beginning 8 to 10 days after the first exposure until 21 days after the last exposure. (See Chapter 42 for more information on VZV and Chapter 95 for more information on isolation precautions.)

HUMAN PARVOVIRUS B19

Overview

Parvoviruses are small nonenveloped, single-stranded DNA viruses in the family Parvoviridae (210). Although many parvoviruses are known to infect other vertebrates, only two groups are known to infect humans: adeno-associated viruses (AAVs) and parvovirus B19 (B19). AAVs are defective parvoviruses that replicate in the presence of helper viruses like adenovirus and herpesvirus; however, these viruses are believed to be nonpathogenic in humans. B19 is the only parvovirus known to be a pathogen in humans. Human bone marrow and other tissue explants (211) can be used for B19 growth *in vitro,* and some human leukemic cell lines (UT-7, MB-02, JK-1, and KU812) have been used to support low levels of B19 replication (212); however these approaches are not generally used for clinical studies. Other members of the Parvoviridae family, such as canine and porcine parvovirus, are important veterinary pathogens but are not closely related to B19 or human AAVs by nucleotide or amino acid sequence.

There is only one serotype of B19, but there is genetic and antigenic variability within this serotype (213,214). B19 binds to the blood group P-antigen (globoside) (215) and productively infects and replicates in erythroid progenitor cells (216). Bone marrow is the primary tissue for viral replication, but as a result of extensive extramedullary hematopoiesis, fetal liver is also an important site of infection *in utero* (211).

Clinical manifestations of B19 infection include asymptomatic infection, the rash-illness erythema infectiosum, aplastic anemia, hydrops fetalis, and chronic B19 infection.

Epidemiology

Prevalence

B19 infections are common worldwide, occurring as sporadic cases or community-wide outbreaks (210,217). School outbreaks of erythema infectiosum (fifth disease) may be protracted, often beginning in winter or spring and frequently lasting until the school year ends months later (218). Prevalence of B19-specific antibodies rise steeply during childhood from 2% to 15% among children 1 to 5 years of age to 35% to 60% at 11 to 19 years of age (219–221). This rise in prevalence is consistent with the fact that B19 infection is most commonly diagnosed in school-age children. The seroprevalence of anti-B19 IgG antibodies continues to increase during adulthood, reaching 75% to 90% among persons over 50 years of age. In the absence of community outbreaks, the annual incidence of B19 infection in HCWs is about 1% (222).

Transmission

The primary route of transmission for the virus has not been determined. Respiratory secretions are known to contain B19 DNA, suggesting that they are likely important in B19 circulation. However, the slow spread of virus through schools indicates aerosol transmission is not efficient; close contact, fomite, and droplet transmission are more likely to be important modes of transmission (223–225). The importance of fomites for communicating B19 infection is underscored by the environmental stability of parvoviruses and the presence of B19 DNA on environmental surfaces (226).

Transmission is very effective in household settings, in which 50% of susceptible exposed household members can become infected (223,224,227). Although 25% to 50% of students in a school outbreak can have clinical or serologic evidence of infection, adult staff in schools and child-care settings generally have less pronounced seroconversion rates of 5% annually (222); however, in one outbreak 20% of staff had serologic evidence of infection (218).

Nosocomial transmission of parvovirus B19 among hospitalized patients and hospital staff has been described (228–232), but in such cases an index viremic patient is often not identified (228,233–235). The capacity to transmit B19 virus varies by the clinical syndrome of the index patient: patients with erythema infectiosum are likely to be infectious before, and not after, the onset of illness, based on B19 DNA levels in blood and presence in respiratory secretions (223–225); however, patients with transient aplastic crisis can be infectious a week after onset of illness (229,236), and immunocompromised patients with chronic B19 infection can be infectious for very prolonged periods (237,238). Some outbreaks of B19 infection that were initially presumed to be of nosocomial origin were, on careful evaluation, more likely to have been manifestations of community outbreaks (226, 239). Therefore, the possibility of a community-based outbreak should be evaluated before attributing hospital-associated cases of B19 to nosocomial transmission.

B19 viral transmission has also been documented in other settings. As determined by serologic testing, vertical transmission of B19 infection occurs in 25% to 50% of infants born to mothers with B19 infection during pregnancy (240–242), and fetal B19 infection occurs in an estimated 5% to 20% of autopsy-confirmed nonimmune hydrops (243–245). Laboratory workers have also become infected following exposure to specimens from viremic patients (246,247).

B19 antigen has been found in 1 of 20,000 units of blood for transfusion, and B19 DNA has been found in 1 of 100 to 1 of 3,000 units, depending on the detection assay used (248–250). However, units positive by DNA assays frequently are also positive for anti-B19 antibodies, presumably reducing the likelihood of transmitting infection. B19 also can contaminate a variety of plasma products (251). Transmission of B19 infection to recipients of heat or solvent-treated blood products has been described (252–255); and the seroprevalence of anti-B19 is also higher among persons receiving plasma products (244–248,252,256).

Pathogenesis

The natural history of B19 infection has been evaluated through human volunteer studies (225,257). Viremia is usually detectable at day 6 after intranasal inoculation, peaks between 6 to 12 days, and resolves by 11 to 16 days. Viremia is associated with cessation of new red cell production and reticulocytopenia along with nonspecific signs and symptoms, including fever, headache, myalgia, and chills. During the peak of the viremia, B19 DNA can be detected in respiratory secretions. IgM antibody response is first detectable at 10 to 14 days after infection and correlates with clearing infection and onset of erythema infectiosum and arthralgias. An anti-B19 IgG response persists long-term and presumably confers protection against disease.

The importance of anti-B19 IgG in protection is emphasized by the efficacy of intravenous immunoglobulin (IVIG) in controlling and sometimes curing infection in immunocompromised patients (237).

Lytic infection of red cell progenitors and arrest of hematopoiesis lead to the anemia commonly associated with B19 infection. Anemia is not clinically significant in persons without underlying illness. However, among persons with underlying medical problems, including sickle cell disease, hereditary spherocytosis, thalassemia, and acquired hemolytic anemias, B19 infection can lead to a transient aplastic crisis, with hemoglobin levels falling 30% or more. In such cases, a hypoplastic or aplastic erythroid and normal myeloid series are seen in the patient's bone marrow. A brisk reticulocytosis is seen with the onset of host immune response and termination of viremia at 7 to 10 days after onset of illness. Some patients with an impaired immune response cannot control infection and develop chronic hypoplasia or aplasia of the erythroid series in the bone marrow.

Clinical Description

In outbreaks of erythema infectiosum, the incubation period before the onset of rash is most commonly 1 to 2 weeks but can be as long as 3 weeks. Outbreak investigations have shown nearly half of exposed persons do not report a rash and one quarter do not report symptoms (222,223,258). When illness does occur, it is often biphasic. An initial phase of nonspecific systemic symptoms (fever, malaise, and myalgias) develops at 1 to 2 weeks and correlates with the onset of viremia at 5 to 7 days (225). The second phase of illness begins 2 to 5 days after viremia is cleared and is associated with the onset of rash and arthralgias, the classic symptoms of B19 infection.

The most commonly recognized clinical condition associated with B19 infection, the rash illness erythema infectiosum, was well characterized (as fifth disease) centuries before the discovery of the etiologic agent (236). This illness is defined by bilateral, intensely erythematous, maculopapular facial rash affecting the cheeks but sparing the bridge of the nose and circumoral region. Patients with this rash are often described as having a "slapped-cheek" appearance. In addition, a lace-like rash can concurrently affect the trunk and extremities but usually spares the palms and soles. Vesicles, papules, purpura, and desquamation have also been reported in some cases. The rash normally fades over a period of 2 weeks, but for several weeks afterward, the rash may reappear transiently following nonspecific stimuli, such as changes in ambient temperature, exposure to sunlight, exercise, or stress. Fever, if noted, is usually low grade; other symptoms may include sore throat, headache, and pruritus. Because there is variability between individuals in the intensity and distribution of the rash, sporadic cases of erythema infectiosum cannot be distinguished on the basis of clinical criteria alone from other exanthemas caused by rubella, enteroviruses, and other viruses or from some drug rashes. Adults may also develop erythema infectiosum, but the facial rash is usually less prominent; consequently, the diagnosis of B19 in adults is difficult to make if there is no laboratory confirmation or epidemiologic link to a child with typical erythema infectiosum.

A self-limited symmetric peripheral polyarthropathy particularly affecting the hands, wrists, and knees has been reported with B19 infection of children and adults, but it is most often found in adult women. The arthropathy can occur with or without a rash. Joint manifestations frequently include arthralgias or stiffness and less commonly include swelling or other signs of inflammation. These signs and symptoms usually improve within a few days or weeks, but occasionally last for months and rarely for years and can mimic rheumatoid arthritis.

Persons with underlying hematologic disorders characterized by decreased red cell production (e.g., thalassemia) or increased red cell destruction (e.g., sickle cell disease, hereditary spherocytosis) can acutely develop severe symptomatic anemia (i.e., fatigue, pallor, tachycardia, congestive heart failure) because of the red blood cell aplasia. This transient aplastic crisis can be complicated by bone marrow necrosis or stroke, and can lead to death. Hematologic recovery generally occurs within 7 to 10 days of presentation. Medical management of the patient may necessitate hospitalization and supportive care including red cell transfusions. Prior to hematologic recovery, the patient is viremic and should be considered infectious. Erythema infectiosum and arthropathy are usually not observed in persons with transient aplastic crisis. In some cases, by precipitating transient aplastic crisis, B19 infection may serve to unmask a previously undiagnosed, preexisting condition, such as autoimmune hemolytic anemia.

Immunocompromised patients may develop chronic B19 infection and chronic anemia. This complication of B19 infection has been identified most often in children undergoing treatment for leukemia, in persons infected with human immunodeficiency virus type 1 (HIV-1), and in some cases, following solid organ transplantation. The clinical course varies. In leukemic patients, completion, modification, or interruption of chemotherapy may lead to spontaneous viral clearance. In persons with HIV-1 infection, viral clearance can be achieved by administering intravenous immunoglobulins, but relapse is common. Chronic B19 infection has rarely been documented in patients without recognized immunodeficiency.

Maternal B19 infection during pregnancy is associated with an increased risk of fetal anemia, hydrops, and death (217). The fetus is particularly susceptible to severe anemia with B19 infection owing to its expanding red cell volume, increased erythrocyte turnover, and immature immune system that often cannot control infection. Vertical transmission of B19 infection from mother to fetus can lead to chronic fetal anemia with high-output congestive heart failure with fetal death (242,259,260). However, the natural history of fetal B19 infection is varied: 30% to 50% of maternal infections lead to fetal infection (238, 242), and 2% to 10% of maternal infections are associated with fetal death (240,241,261,262). Fetal death appears to be highest in association with infection between the 10th and 20th weeks of gestation (210). This may be due to increased transplacental transfer of maternal antibody during the second trimester. Chronic red cell aplasia in infancy has been reported as a complication of intrauterine B19 infection in a few cases (263). Case reports have also noted B19 infection in infants with birth defects (264,265). However, infants born to women with B19 infection during pregnancy do not have a significantly increased incidence of birth defects, suggesting that the magnitude of the risk is small (217,261,262,266).

In addition to the well-established disease associations described above, acute and chronic B19 infections have been reported in sporadic cases of hemophagocytic syndrome, peripheral and central neurologic disorders, myocarditis, systemic vasculitis, and a variety of other conditions that are reviewed elsewhere (210,267). Etiologic links between B19 and many of these conditions have not been confirmed in controlled studies or by histopathologic criteria, and for some of these conditions B19 infection may be coincidental or represent an opportunistic pathogen in an abnormal host.

Diagnosis

Clinical Diagnosis

The diagnosis of erythema infectiosum on clinical grounds is not reliable, because other viral infections and drug reactions may produce a similar rash illness (210). Likewise, sudden onset of symmetric polyarthropathy is suggestive of acute B19 infection, but B19-associated joint disease cannot be distinguished clinically from other arthropathies without B19-specific laboratory testing.

Virus Isolation

Although erythroid cell lines have been developed that support B19 cultivation (212,268), these are not efficient virus isolation tools and therefore have not been used for clinical diagnosis.

Antibody Detection

Antibody assays are currently the cornerstone of clinical diagnosis for most B19 infections. Acute B19 infection in the immunologically normal patient can be diagnosed by detection of anti-B19 IgM antibodies that develop within 10 to 12 days after infection and can remain present for months. Anti-B19 IgG antibodies usually become detectable several days after the appearance of IgM; IgG can persist for years and perhaps for life. Over 90% of patients with erythema infectiosum or arthropathy will have both anti-B19 IgM and IgG antibodies at the time of presentation with acute onset of rash. IgM antibody is present in 80% of patients with transient aplastic crisis (219,269); however, serologic studies can be misleading for persons presenting in the early stages of anemia prior to the rise of B19-specific antibody. Serologic studies of mother and infant can also be of use in diagnosing acute B19 fetal infections.

Since high levels of B19-specific IgG will compete and block detection of IgM antibodies and since rheumatoid factors or nonspecific binding of IgM antibodies can yield false-positive reactions, indirect IgM assays tend to have lower sensitivity and specificity than IgM capture assays. Acute infection can also be evaluated using non–IgM-based assays designed to detect either a high frequency of low-avidity antibodies (270) or antibodies recognizing antigens indicative of acute or early convalescent infection (271–273). Antibody assays are not useful for detecting B19 infection in immunodeficient patients who may not have a normal antibody response to the infection. In such situations, immunohistology and nucleic acid detection are more appropriate diagnostic tools.

Antigen Detection

Current antigen detection assays (enzyme-linked and radioimmune assay) are not sensitive enough to reliably diagnose acute infection (219,269). Immunohistologic techniques have been useful for detection of B19 antigen in fetal tissues and bone marrow samples (273,274)

Nucleic Acid Detection

Both probe hybridization and PCR assays have become important diagnostic tools for B19 detection. Probe hybridization assays require high titers of virus but can be used to detect virus in patients presenting with transient aplastic crisis or to screen blood for high-titer viremia. Hybridization assays have been developed that use a variety of probes labeled with radioisotopes, digoxigenin, or biotin in conjunction with chemiluminescence, colorimetric, or radiographic detection (275–278).

Nucleic acid amplification technologies (NAT) for B19 have been developed that use a variety of primers and amplification parameters. Sensitivity and specificity of these assays can vary greatly between laboratories (279); international standards for B19 NAT assays have been developed recently (280). The most sensitive assays use a nested PCR approach (two successive amplification reactions) or a sensitive detection method (e.g., hybridization or enzyme immunoassay) to detect viral DNA (281–283). Quantitative PCR assays have also been described recently (284–286); these may offer sensitivities similar to those of earlier PCR methods but with shorter processing times.

Prevention and Control

B19 infection is most likely transmitted through respiratory secretions and close contact (fomite and perhaps droplet transmission). Attention to hand washing and not sharing food or drinks therefore should be effective for preventing spread of the virus. However, since the classic signs and symptoms of B19 infection (rash and arthralgias) are not apparent until after the patient has been viremic, good hygienic practices particularly during outbreaks, need to be universally applied to be effective at prevention.

Parvoviruses, in general, are highly resistant to disinfection procedures and can remain infectious in the environment for prolonged periods of time; the virus is stable in lipid solvents, such as ether and chloroform. There are no specific data about the viability of B19 in the environment, but on the basis of properties exhibited by other members of the Parvoviridae family, surfaces contaminated with bodily fluids containing B19 should be considered infectious. In one case, vaginal delivery of a B19-infected fetus resulted in widespread contamination of environmental surfaces in the patient's room with B19 DNA (226).

Patients and staff with erythema infectiosum or B19-associated arthropathy are past the infectious period and therefore do not require special precautions (33,37,287). Patients with transient aplastic crisis and patients with chronic B19 infection may be viremic for up to a week after presentation and do pose a risk of nosocomial transmission. Little is known about the risk for transmission from immunodeficient patients. The CDC recommends that patients with transient aplastic crisis be placed on Droplet Precautions for 7 days or for the duration of illness (33). Most patients with transient aplastic crisis will mount an effective immune response that cures the infection; isolation precautions can be removed after hematologic recovery, which usually occurs 7 to 10 days after presentation. Immunodeficient patients with chronic B19 infection should be placed on Droplet Precautions for the duration of their hospitalization (33). For chronically infected patients treated with immunoglobulins, isolation precautions can be removed if hematologic recovery occurs and if available virologic surveillance (e.g., PCR test) demonstrates that the B19 viremia has been cleared. In pregnant women with suspected or proven intrauterine B19 infection, amniotic fluid and fetal tissues should be considered infectious, and Contact Precautions should be used in addition to Standard Precautions if exposure is likely (226).

B19 community outbreaks particularly those associated with schools and day-care centers are often associated with heightened concern about infection of persons at risk for complications, particularly pregnant women. Depending on the community and on the assay used, 40% to 60% of women of childbearing age test positive for anti-B19 IgG antibodies and therefore are not thought to be susceptible to infection. The risk of fetal death in pregnancy can be estimated to be 0.4% to 3% after exposure to B19 in the household and 0.16% to 1.2% after exposures associated with working in a school or child-care setting with a B19 disease outbreak. The CDC recommends that persons be informed of potential exposures to B19 and that efforts to decrease the risk of exposures (e.g., avoiding the workplace or school environment) be made on an individual basis after consultation with family members, healthcare providers, public health officials, and employers or school officials (287).

Many HCWs already have anti-B19 IgG antibodies from prior infection and are believed to be at low risk of becoming reinfected or of transmitting B19 to patients or other staff (37). Serologic screening of asymptomatic HCWs to identify susceptible staff is not currently recommended by the CDC. HCWs should be advised that they are at risk of B19 infection after exposure in the hospital or in the community and that there may be a risk for further transmission to patients. Routine infection control practices, particularly hand washing, should minimize the risk for transmission. Pregnant personnel should be advised about potential risks of B19 infection to the fetus and advised to consult with their healthcare providers; the CDC does not recommend that pregnant personnel routinely be excluded from caring for patients with B19 infection.

Treatment

Most cases of erythema infectiosum or B19-associated arthropathy are mild and self-limited and require no treatment other than supportive care with antipruritis medications or nonsteroidal antiinflammatory agents, respectively. Transient aplastic crisis can be a life-threatening event, but if diagnosed early, it can be managed with red cell transfusions to relieve signs and symptoms associated with anemia. Chronic B19 infections in immunosuppressed patients have been successfully controlled and sometimes cured with IVIG. Successful treatment has been reported using IVIG doses of 400 mg/kg for 5 or 10 days or 1 g/kg for 3 days (288,289). Recurrent anemia and viremia have been successfully treated with additional IVIG doses; however, IVIG may be less effective in treating chronic B19 infection that is not associated with anemia. Use of immunoglobulins to prevent or treat other types of B19 disease has not been studied. There are no established guidelines for clinical management of pregnancies complicated by intrauterine B19 infection and fetal hydrops (217). Limited data suggest that B19 infected fetuses can be ultrasonographically monitored for hydrops; intrauterine blood transfusions can be considered for treatment of B19-associated hydrops. However, since fetuses can survive and be normal without treatment and since transfusions can be associated with fetal death, it is not possible to determine when the benefits of this procedure outweigh the risks.

REFERENCES

1. Centers for Disease Control. *Measles surveillance report,* no. 11, 1977–1981. Atlanta: Centers for Disease Control and Prevention, 1982.
2. Langmuir A. The medical importance of measles. *Am J Dis Child* 1962;103:54–56.
3. Atkinson WL, Orenstein WA, Krugman S. Resurgence of measles in the United States, 1989–1990. *Annu Rev Med* 1992;43:451–463.
4. Gindler JG, Atkinson WL, Markowitz LE, et al. Epidemiology of measles in the United States in 1989 and 1990. *Pediatr Infect Dis J* 1992;11:841–846.
5. National Vaccine Advisory Committee. The measles epidemic: the problems, barriers and recommendations. *JAMA* 1991;266: 1547–1552.
6. Centers for Disease Control and Prevention. Reported vaccine-preventable diseases—United States, 1993, and the Childhood Immunization Initiative. *MMWR* 1994;43:57–60.
7. Centers for Disease Control and Prevention. Status report on the Childhood Immunization Initiative: reported cases of selected vaccine-preventable diseases—United States, 1996. *MMWR* 1997; 46(29):665–671.
8. Centers for Disease Control. Measles prevention: recommendations of the Immunization Practices Advisory Committee (ACIP). *MMWR* 1989;38(S-9):1–18.
9. Centers for Disease Control and Prevention. Measles, mumps, and rubella—vaccine use and strategies for elimination of measles, rubella, and congenital rubella syndrome and control of mumps: recommendations of the Advisory Committee on Immunization Practices (ACIP). *MMWR* 1998;47(RR-8):1–57.
10. Kolasa M, Klemperer-Johnson S, Papania MJ. Second dose measles immunization requirements for school children—progress toward implementation for all school children in all states. *J Infect Dis* 2003 *(in press).*
11. Papania MJ, Seward J, Redd S, et al. Measles Epidemiology, United States 1997–2001. *J Infect Dis* 2003 *(in press).*
12. Miller M, Williams WW, Redd SC. Measles among adults, United States, 1985–1995. *Am J Prev Med*1999;17:114–119.
13. Davis RM, Orenstein WA, Frank JA, et al. Transmission of measles in medical settings, 1980 through 1984. *JAMA* 1986;255:1295–1298.
14. Atkinson WL, Markowitz LE, Adams NC, et al. Transmission of measles in medical settings—United States, 1985–1989. *Am J Med 1991;*91(suppl 3):320S–324S.

15. Raad II, Shererty RJ, Rains CS, et al. The importance of nosocomial transmission of measles in the propagation of a community outbreak. *Infect Control Hosp Epidemiol* 1989;10:161–166.
16. Istre GR, McKee PA, West GR, et al. Measles spread in medical settings: an important focus of disease transmission? *Pediatrics* 1987; 79:356–358.
17. Dales LG, Kizer KW. Measles transmission in medical facilities. *West J Med* 1985;142:415–416.
18. Sienko DG, Friedman C, McGee HB, et al. A measles outbreak at university medical settings involving health care providers. *Am J Public Health* 1987;77:1222–1224.
19. Rivera ME, Mason WH, Ross LA, et al. Nosocomial measles infection in a pediatric hospital during a community-wide epidemic. *J Pediatr* 1991;119:183–186.
20. Rank EL, Brettman L, Katz-Pollack H, et al. Chronology of a hospital-wide measles outbreak: lessons learned and shared from an extraordinary week in late March 1989. *Am J Infect Control* 1992;20:315–318.
21. Watkins NM, Smith RP, St Germain DL, et al. Measles (rubeola) infection in a hospital setting. *Am J Infect Control* 1987;15:201–206.
22. Atkinson WL. Measles and health care workers. *Infect Control Hosp Epidemiol* 1994;15:5–7.
23. Farizo KM, Stehr-Green PA, Simpson DM, et al. Pediatric emergency room visits: a risk factor for acquiring measles. *Pediatrics* 1991;87: 74–79.
24. Cowan V, Huggins-Martin V, Brindle P, et al. Control of a community-wide outbreak of measles. Abstract 263. The Eighth Annual Meeting of the Society for Healthcare Epidemiology of America, April 1998:41.
25. Steingart KR, Thomas AR, Dykewicz CA, et al. Transmission of measles virus in healthcare settings during a communitywide outbreak. *Infect Control Hosp Epidemiol* 1999;20(2):115–119.
26. Yip FY, Papania MJ, Redd SB. Measles outbreak epidemiology in the United States, 1993–2001. *J Infect Dis* 2003 *(in press).*
27. Gindler JG, Tinker S, Markowitz LE, et al. Acute measles mortality in the United States, 1987–2002. *J Infect Dis* 2003 *(in press).*
28. Perry RT, Halsey NA. The clinical significance of measles: A Review *J Infect Dis* 2003 *(in press).*
29. Bloch AB, Orenstein WA, Ewing WM. Measles outbreak in a pediatric practice: airborne transmission in an office setting. *Pediatrics* 1985; 75:676–683.
30. Remington PL, Hall WN, Davis IH, et al. Airborne transmission of measles in a physician's office. *JAMA* 1985;253:1574–1577.
31. Sutter RW, Markowitz LE, Bennetch JM, et al. Measles among the Amish: a comparative study of measles severity in primary and secondary cases in households. *J Infect Dis* 1991;163:12–16.
32. Rogers DV, Gindler JS, Atkinson WL, et al. High attack rates and case fatality during a measles outbreak in groups with religious exemption to vaccination. *Pediatr Infect Dis J* 1993;12:288–292.
33. Garner JS. The Hospital Infection Control Practices Advisory Committee. Guideline for isolation precautions in hospitals. *Infect Control Hosp Epidemiol* 1996;17:53–80.
34. Krause PJ, Gross PA, Barrett TL, et al. Quality standard for assurance of measles immunity among health care workers. Infectious Diseases Society of America. *Clin Infect Dis* 1994;18(3):431–436.
35. Biellik RJ, Clements CJ. Strategies for minimizing nosocomial measles transmission [review]. *Bull WHO* 1997;75(4):367–375.
36. Kessler ER. Vaccine-preventable diseases in health care [review]. *Occup Med* 1997;12(4):731–739.
37. Bolyard EA, Tablan OC, Williams WW, et al. Guideline for infection control in hospital personnel, 1998. Hospital Infection Control Practices Advisory Committee. *Am J Infect Control* 1998;26:289–354.
38. Watson JC, Pearson JA, Markowitz LE, et al. Evaluation of measles revaccination among school-entry-aged children. *Pediatrics* 1996;97: 613–618.
39. Coté TR, Sivertson D, Horan JM, et al. Evaluation of a two-dose measles, mumps, and rubella vaccination schedule in a cohort of college athletes. *Public Health Rep* 1993;4:431–435.
40. Willy ME, Koziol DE, Fleisher T, et al. Measles immunity in a population of healthcare workers. *Infect Control Hosp Epidemiol* 1994;14: 14–19.
41. Centers for Disease Control and Prevention. Immunization of health-care workers: recommendations of the Advisory Committee on Immunization Practices (ACIP) and the Hospital Infection Control Practices Advisory Committee (HICPAC). *MMWR* 1997;46(RR-18): 1–42.
42. Wright LJ, Carlquist JF. Measles immunity in employees of a multi-hospital health care provider. *Infect Control Hosp Epidemiol* 1994;15: 10–13.
43. Braunstein H, Thomas S, Ito R. Immunity to measles in a large population of varying age. *Am J Dis Child* 1990;144:296–298.
44. Chou T, Weil D, Arnow PM. Prevalence of measles antibodies in hospital personnel. *Infect Control* 1986;7:309–311.
45. Houck P, Scott-Johnson G, Krebs L. Measles immunity among community hospital employees. *Infect Control Hosp Epidemiol* 1991;12: 663–668.
46. Schwarcz S, McCaw B, Fukushima P. Prevalence of measles susceptibility in hospital staff. Evidence to support expanding the recommendations of the Immunization Practices Advisory Committee. *Arch Intern Med* 1992;152:1481–1483.
47. Enguidanos R, Mascola L, Frederick P. A survey of hospital infection control policies and employee measles cases during Los Angeles County's measles epidemic, 1987–1989. *Am J Infect Control* 1992;20(6): 301–304.
48. Sellick J, Longbine D, Schiffeling R, et al. Screening hospital employees for measles is more cost-effective than blind immunization. *Ann Intern Med* 1992;116:982–984.
49. Subbarao EK, Amin S, Kumar ML. Prevaccination serologic screening for measles in health care workers. *J Infect Dis* 1991;163:876–878.
50. Grabowsky M, Markowitz LE. Serologic screening, mass immunization, and implications for immunization programs. *J Infect Dis* 1991; 164:1237–1238.
51. Stover BH, Kuebler CA, Cost KM, et al. Measles-mumps-rubella immunization of susceptible hospital employees during a community measles outbreak: cost-effectiveness and protective efficacy. *Infect Control Hosp Epidemiol* 1994;15:20–23.
52. Kelley PW, Petrucelli BP, Stehr-Green P, et al. The susceptibility of young adult Americans to vaccine-preventable infections. *JAMA* 1991;266:2724–2729.
53. Institute of Medicine. Measles and mumps vaccines. In: Stratton KR, Howe CJ, Johnston RB, eds. *Adverse events associated with childhood vaccines. Evidence bearing on causality.* Washington, DC: National Academy Press 1994:118–116.
54. Wharton M, Cochi SL, Hutcheson RH, et al. Mumps transmission in hospitals. *Arch Intern Med* 1990;150:47–49.
55. Fischer PR, Brunetti C, Welch V, et al. Nosocomial mumps: report of an outbreak and its control. *Am J Infect Control* 1996;24:13–18.
56. Cochi SL, Wharton M, Plotkin SA. Mumps vaccine. In: Plotkin SA, Mortimer EA Jr, eds. *Vaccines.* Philadelphia: WB Saunders, 1994: 277–301.
57. Wolinsky JS, Mumps virus. In: Fields BN, Knipe DM, Howley PM, eds. *Fields' virology,* 3rd ed. Philadelphia: Lippincott-Raven, 1996: 1243–1265.
58. Holmes SJ. Mumps. In: Evans AS, Kaslow RA, eds. *Viral infections of humans: epidemiology and control,* 4th ed. New York: Plenum, 1997: 531–550.
59. Overman JR. Viremia in human mumps virus infections. *Arch Intern Med* 1958;102:354–356.
60. Ennis FA, Jackson D. Isolation of virus during the incubation period of mumps infection. *J Pediatr* 1968;72:536–537.
61. Chiba Y, Horino K, Umetsu M, et al. Virus excretion and antibody responses in saliva in natural mumps. *Tohoku J Exp Med* 1973;11: 229–238.
62. American Academy of Pediatrics. Summaries of infectious diseases: mumps. In: Peter G, ed. *1997 red book: report of the Committee on Infectious Diseases,* 24th ed. Elk Grove Village, IL: American Academy of Pediatrics, 1997:366–369.
63. Centers for Disease Control and Prevention. Mumps prevention. Recommendations of the Immunization Practices Advisory Committee (ACIP). *MMWR* 1989;38:388–392,397–400.
64. Centers for Disease Control and Prevention. Update on adult immu-

nization. Recommendations of the Immunization Practices Advisory Committee (ACIP). *MMWR* 1991;40(RR-12):1–94.
65. Koplan JP, Preblud SR. A benefit-cost analysis of mumps vaccine. *Am J Dis Child* 1982;136:362–364.
66. Hersh BS, Fine PEM, Kent WK, et al. Mumps outbreak in a highly vaccinated population. *J Pediatr* 1991;119:187–193.
67. Briss PA, Fehrs LJ, Parker RA, et al. Sustained transmission of mumps in a highly vaccinated population: assessment of primary vaccine failure and waning vaccine-induced immunity. *J Infect Dis* 1994;169: 77–82.
68. Cheek JE, Baron R, Atlas H, et al. Mumps outbreak in a highly vaccinated school population. *Arch Pediatr Adolesc Med* 1995;149: 774–778.
69. Polder JA, Tablan OC, Williams WW. Personnel health services. In: Bennett JV, Brachman PS, eds. *Hospital infections,* 3rd ed. Boston: Little, Brown, 1992:31–61.
70. Reef S, Frey TK, Theall K, et al. The changing epidemiology of rubella in the 1990s: on the verge of elimination and new challenges for control and prevention. *JAMA* 2002;287:464–472.
71. Polk FB, White JA, DeGirolami PC, et al. An outbreak of rubella among hospital personnel. *N Engl J Med* 1980;303:541–545.
72. Greaves WL, Orenstein WA, Stetler HC, et al. Prevention of rubella transmission in medical facilities. *JAMA* 1982;248:861–864.
73. Centers for Disease Control and Prevention. Rubella in hospitals—California. *MMWR* 1983;32:37–39.
74. Poland GA, Nichol KL. Medical students as sources of rubella and measles outbreaks. *Arch Intern Med* 1990;150:44–46.
75. Storch GA, Gruber C, Benz B, et al. A rubella outbreak among dental students: description of the outbreak and analysis of control measures. *Infect Control* 1985;6:150–156.
76. Strassburg MA, Stephenson TG, Habel LA, et al. Rubella in hospital employees. *Infect Control* 1984;5:123–126.
77. Fliegel PE, Weinstein WM. Rubella outbreak in a prenatal clinic: management and prevention. *Am J Infect Control* 1982;10:29–33.
78. Strassburg MA, Imagawa DT, Fannin SL, et al. Rubella outbreak among hospital personnel. *Obstet Gynecol* 1981;57:283–288.
79. Gladstone JL, Millian SJ. Rubella exposure in an obstetric clinic. *Obstet Gynecol* 1981;57:182–186.
80. Fraser V, Spitznagel E, Medoff G, et al. Results of a rubella screening program for hospital employees: a five-year review (1986–1990). *Am J Epidemiol* 1993;138(9):756–764.
81. Plotkin SA. Rubella vaccine. In: Plotkin SA, Mortimer EA Jr, eds. *Vaccines.* Philadelphia: WB Saunders, 1988:235–262.
82. Wolinsky JS. Rubella. In: Fields BN, Knipe DM, eds. *Fields' virology,* 2nd ed. New York: Raven Press, 1990:815–838.
83. Horstmann DM. Rubella. In: Evans AS, ed. *Viral infections of humans: epidemiology and control,* 3rd ed. New York: Plenum, 1989:617–631.
84. Cherry JD. Rubella. In: Feigin RD, Cherry JD, eds. *Textbook of pediatric infectious diseases,* 2nd ed. Philadelphia: WB Saunders, 1987: 1810–1841.
85. Fraser JR, Cunningham AL, Hayes K, et al. Rubella arthritis in adults. Isolation of virus, cytology and other aspects of the synovial reaction. *Clin Exp Rheumatol* 1983;1:287–293.
86. Chantler JK, Ford DK, Tingle AJ, et al. Persistent rubella infection associated with chronic arthritis in children. *N Engl J Med* 1985;313: 1117–1123.
87. Grahame R, Armstrong R, Simmons N, et al. Chronic arthritis associated with the presence of intrasynovial rubella virus. *Ann Rheum Dis* 1983;42:2–13.
88. Horstman DM, Liebhaber H, LeBouvier GL, et al. Rubella: reinfection of vaccinated and naturally immune persons exposed in an epidemic. *N Engl J Med* 1970;283:771–778.
89. Wilkens J, Leedom JM, Salvatore MA, et al. Clinical rubella with arthritis resulting from reinfection. *Ann Intern Med* 1972;77: 930–932.
90. Plotkin SA, Farquhar JD, Ogra PL. Immunologic properties of RA 27/3 rubella virus vaccine. A comparison with strains presently licensed in the U.S. *JAMA* 1973;225:585–590.
91. Driscoll SG. Histopathology of gestational rubella. *Am J Dis Child* 1969;118:49–53.
92. Esterly JR, Oppenheimer EH. Pathological reactions due to congenital rubella. *Arch Pathol* 1969;87:380–388.
93. Williams WW, Preblud SR, Reichelderfer PS, et al. Vaccines of importance in the hospital setting. *Infect Dis Clin North Am* 1989;3: 701–722.
94. Polder JA, Tablan OC, Williams WW. Personnel health services. In: Bennett JV, Brachman PS, eds. *Hospital infections,* 3rd ed. Boston: Little, Brown, 1992:31–61.
95. Centers for Disease Control and Prevention. Update on adult immunization. Recommendations of the Immunization Practices Advisory Committee (ACIP). *MMWR* 1991;40(RR-12):1–94.
96. Centers for Disease Control and Prevention. Rubella prevention. Recommendations of the Immunization Practices Advisory Committee (ACIP). *MMWR* 1990;39(RR-15):1–18.
97. Valenti WM. Selected viruses of nosocomial importance. In: Bennett JV, Brachman PS, eds. *Hospital infections,* 3rd ed. Boston: Little, Brown, 1992:789–821.
98. Heseltine PN, Ripper M, Wohlford P. Nosocomial rubella—consequences of an outbreak and efficacy of a mandatory immunization program. *Infect Control* 1985;6:371–374.
99. Centers for Disease Control and Prevention. Notice to readers: revised ACIP recommendations for avoiding pregnancy after receiving a rubella-containing vaccine. *MMWR* 2001;50:1117.
100. Preblud SR. Some current issues related to rubella vaccine. *JAMA* 1985;254:253–256.
101. Sacks JJ, Olson B, Soter J, et al. Employee rubella screening programs in Arizona hospitals. *JAMA* 1983;249:2675–2678.
102. Wharton M. The epidemiology of varicella-zoster virus infections. *Infect Dis Clin North Am* 1996;10:571–581.
103. Galil K, Brown C, Lin F, et al. Hospitalizations for varicella in the United States, 1988 to 1999. *Pediatr Infect Dis J* 2002;21:931–934.
104. Meyer PA, Seward JF, Jumaan AO, et al. Varicella mortality: trends before vaccine licensure in the United States, 1970–1994. *J Infect Dis* 2000;182:383–390.
105. Centers for Disease Control and Prevention. Evaluation of varicella reporting to the National Notifiable Disease Surveillance System—United States, 1972–1997. *MMWR* 1999;48(3):55–58.
106. Centers for Disease Control and Prevention. National vaccination coverage levels among children aged 19–35 months— United States, 2001. *MMWR* 2002;51(30):664–666.
107. Kilgore PE, Kruszon-Moran D, Seward J, et al. Varicella in Americans from NAHNES III: implications for control through routine immunization. *J Med Virol* 2003;70:S111–S118.
108. Garnett GP, Cox MJ, Bundy DAP, et al. The age of infection with varicella-zoster virus in St. Lucia, West Indies. *Epidemiol Infect* 1993; 110:361–372.
109. Lolekha S, Tanthiphabha W, Sornchai P, et al. Effect of climatic factors and population density on varicella zoster virus epidemiology within a tropical country. *Am J Trop Med Hyg* 2001;64:131–136.
110. Mandal BK, Mukherjee PP, Murphy C, et al. Adult susceptibility to varicella in the tropics is a rural phenomenon due to the lack of previous exposure. *J Infect Dis* 1998;178(suppl):S52–S54.
111. Myers MG, Rasley DA, Hierholzer WJ. Hospital infection control for varicella zoster virus infection. *Pediatrics* 1982;70:199–202.
112. Shehab ZM, Brunell PA. Susceptibility of hospital personnel to varicella-zoster virus. *J Infect Dis* 1984;150:786.
113. McKinney WP, Horowitz MM, Battiola RJ. Susceptibility of hospital-based health care personnel to varicella-zoster virus infections. *Am J Infect Control* 1989;17:26–30.
114. Weber DJ, Rutala WA, Hamilton H. Prevention and control of varicella-zoster infections in healthcare facilities. *Infect Control Hosp Epidemiol* 1996;17:694–705.
115. Wallace MR, Chamberlin CJ, Zerboni L, et al. Reliability of a history of previous varicella infection in adults. *JAMA* 1997;278:1520–1522.
116. Alter SJ, Hammond JA, McVey CJ, et al. Susceptibility to varicella-zoster virus among adults at high risk for exposure. *Infect Control* 1986;7:448–451.
117. Krasinski K, Holzman RS, LaCouture R, et al. Hospital experience with varicella-zoster virus. *Infect Control* 1986;7:312–316.
118. Haiduven-Griffiths D, Fecko H. Varicella in hospital personnel: a

challenge for the infection control practitioner. *Am J Infect Control* 1987;15:207–211.
119. Weber DJ, Rutala WA, Parham C. Impact and costs of varicella prevention in a university hospital. *Am J Public Health* 1988;78:19–23.
120. Stover BH, Cost KM, Hamm C, et al. Varicella exposure in a neonatal intensive care unit: case report and control measures. *Am J Infect Control* 1988;16:167–172.
121. Ferson MJ, Bell SM, Robertson PW. Determination and importance of varicella immune status of nursing staff in a children's hospital. *J Hosp Infect* 1990;15:347–351.
122. Haiduven DJ, Hench CP, Stevens DA. Postexposure varicella management of nonimmune personnel: an alternative approach. *Infect Control Hosp Epidemiol* 1994;15:329–334.
123. Gallagher J, Quaid B, Cryan B. Susceptibility to varicella zoster virus infection in health care workers. *Occup Med* 1996;46(4):289–292.
124. Gustafson TL, Shehab Z, Brunell PA. Outbreak of varicella in a new born intensive care nursery. *Am J Dis Child* 1984;138:548–550.
125. Morens DM, Bregman DJ, West CM, et al. An outbreak of varicella-zoster virus infection among cancer patients. *Ann Intern Med* 1980; 93:414–419.
126. Centers for Disease Control and Prevention. Prevention of varicella. Recommendations of the Advisory Committee on Immunization Practices. *MMWR* 1996;45(RR-11):1–36.
127. American Academy of Pediatrics. Summaries of Infectious Diseases: Varicella-zoster infections. In: Peter G, ed. *1997 red book: report of the Committee on Infectious Diseases,* 24th ed. Elk Grove Village, IL: American Academy of Pediatrics, 1997:573–585.
128. Gardner P, Eickhoff T, Poland GA, et al. Adult immunization. *Ann Intern Med* 1996;124:35–40.
129. American Medical Association. *Immunization of health care workers with varicella vaccine.* Chicago: American Medical Association, Council on Scientific Affairs Report 2, June 22–26, 1997.
130. Centers for Disease Control and Prevention. Prevention of varicella: updated recommendations of the Advisory Committee on Immunization Practices. *MMWR* 1999;48(RR-6).
131. Ratner AJ. Varicella-related hospitalizations in the vaccine era. *Pediatr Infect Dis J* 2002;21:927–930.
132. Gershon AA, Raker R, Steinberg S, et al. Antibody of varicella-zoster virus in parturient women and their offspring during the first year of life. *Pediatrics* 1976;58:692–696.
133. Paryani SG, Arvin AM. Intrauterine infection with varicella-zoster virus after maternal varicella. *N Engl J Med* 1986;314:1542–1546.
134. Balducci J, Rodis JF, Rosengren S, et al. Pregnancy outcome following first-trimester varicella zoster virus infections. *Obstet Gynecol* 1992; 79:5–6.
135. Pastuszak AL, Levy M, Shick B, et al. Outcome after maternal varicella infection in the first 20 weeks of pregnancy. *N Engl J Med* 1994;330: 901–905.
136. Enders G, Miller E, Craddock-Watson J, et al. Consequences of varicella and herpes zoster in pregnancy: prospective study of 1739 cases. *Lancet* 1994;343:1548–1550.
137. Brunell PA, Kotchmar GS. Zoster in infancy: failure to maintain virus latency following intrauterine infection. *J Pediatr* 1981:98:71–73.
138. Dworsky M, Whitely R, Alford C. Herpes zoster in early infancy. *Am J Dis Child* 1980;134:618–619.
139. Gershon A. Chickenpox, measles, and mumps. In: Remington J, Klein J, eds. *Infections of the fetus and newborn infant,* 5th ed. Philadelphia: Saunders, 2001:683–732.
140. Meyers J. Congenital varicella in term infants: risk reconsidered. *J Infect Dis* 1974;129:215–217.
141. Hanngren K, Grandien M, Granstrom G. Effect of zoster immunoglobulin for varicella prophylaxis in the newborn. *Scand J Infect Dis* 1985;17:343–347.
142. Meyers JD, MacQuarrie MB, Merigan TC, et al. Nosocomial varicella. Part 1: outbreak in oncology patients at a children's hospital. *West J Med* 1979;130:196–199.
143. Asano Y, Iwayama S, Miyata T, et al. Spread of varicella in hospitalized children having no direct contact with an indicator zoster case and its prevention by a live vaccine. *Biken J* 1980;23:157–161.
144. Gustafson TL, Lavely GB, Brawner ER, et al. An outbreak of airborne nosocomial varicella. *Pediatrics* 1982;70:550–556.
145. Josephson A, Herring L, Gombert M, et al. Airborne transmission of chicken pox from localized zoster [abstract 140]. *J Infect Dis* 1988; 158:238–241.
146. Thomson FH, Aberd CM. The serial conveyance of infection. *Lancet* 1916;1:341–344.
147. Anderson JD, Bonner M, Scheifele DW, et al. Lack of nosocomial spread of varicella in a pediatric hospital with negative pressure ventilated patient rooms. *Infect Control* 1985;6:120–121.
148. Evans P. An epidemic of chicken pox. *Lancet* 1940;2:339–340.
149. Faizallah R, Green HT, Krasner N, et al. Outbreak of chicken pox from a patient with immunosuppressed herpes zoster in hospital. *Br Med J* 1982;285:1022–1023.
150. Hyams PJ, Stuewe MCS, Heitzer V. Herpes zoster causing varicella (chicken pox) in hospital employees: cost of a casual attitude. *Infect Control* 1984;12:2–5.
151. McKendrick GDW, Emond RTD. Investigation of cross-infection in isolation wards of different design. *J Hyg (Cambridge)* 1976;76:23–31.
152. Wreghitt TG, Whipp PJ, Bagnall J. Transmission of chickenpox to two intensive care unit nurses from a liver transplant patient with zoster [letter]. *J Hosp Infect* 1992;20:125–126.
153. Friedman CA, Temple DM, Robbins KK, et al. Outbreak and control of varicella in a neonatal intensive care unit. *Pediatr Infect Dis J* 1994; 13:152–154.
154. Faoagali JL, Darcy D. Chickenpox outbreak among the staff of a large, urban adult hospital: costs of monitoring and control. *Am J Infect Control* 1995;23:247–250.
155. Leclair JM, Zaia JA, Levine MJ, et al. Airborne transmission of chickenpox in a hospital. *N Engl J Med* 1980;302:450–453.
156. Arvin AM. Varicella-zoster virus. In: Fields BN, Knipe DM, Howley PM, eds. *Fields' virology,* 3rd ed. Philadelphia: Lippincott-Raven, 1996:2547–2585.
157. Gershon AA. Varicella-zoster virus. In: Feigin RD, Cherry JD, eds. *Textbook of pediatric infectious diseases,* 4th ed. Philadelphia: WB Saunders, 1998:1769–1777.
158. Gershon AA, Takahashi M, White CJ. Varicella vaccine. In: Plotkin SA, Mortimer EA Jr, eds. *Vaccines,* 3rd ed. Philadelphia: WB Saunders, 1999:457–507.
159. Ross AH. Modification of chicken pox in family contacts by administration of gamma globulin. *N Engl J Med* 1962;267:369–376.
160. Triebwasser JH, Harris RE, Bryant RE, et al. Varicella pneumonia in adults. Report of seven cases and a review of the literature. *Medicine* 1967;46:409–423.
161. Choo PW, Donahue JG, Manson JE, et al. The epidemiology of varicella and its complications. *J Infect Dis* 1995;172:706–712.
162. Centers for Disease Control and Prevention. Outbreak of invasive group A streptococcus associated with varicella in a childcare center—Boston, Massachusetts, 1997. *MMWR* 1997;46:944–948.
163. Caroline Quach C, Tapiero B, Noya F. Group A streptococcus spinal epidural abscess during varicella. *Pediatrics* 2002; 109:1–3
164. Wallace MR, Woelfl I, Bowler WA, et al. Tumor necrosis factor, interleukin-2, and interferon-gamma in adult varicella. *J Med Virol* 1994;43:69–71.
165. Wallace MR, Chamberlin CJ, Sawyer MH, et al. Treatment of adult varicella with sorivudine: a randomized, placebo controlled trial. *J Infect Dis* 1996;174:249–255.
166. Guess HA. Population-based studies of varicella complications. *Pediatrics* 1986;78:723–727.
167. Arvin AM, Koropchak CM, Williams BRG, et al. Early immune response in healthy and immunocompromised subjects with primary varicella-zoster virus infection. *J Infect Dis* 1986;154:422–429.
168. Asano Y, Itakura N, Hiroishi Y, et al. Viral replication and immunologic responses in children naturally infected with varicella-zoster virus and in varicella vaccine recipients. *J Infect Dis* 1985;152:863–868.
169. Gershon A, Steinberg S, Borkowsky W, et al. IgM to varicella-zoster virus: demonstration in patients with and without clinical zoster. *Pediatr Infect Dis* 1982;1:164–167.
170. Gershon A, LaRussa P, Steinberg S. Varicella-zoster virus. In: Murray

PR, ed. *Manual of clinical microbiology,* 7th ed. Washington, DC: American Society for Microbiology, 1999:900–918.

171. Levin MJ, Hayward AR. Prevention of herpes zoster. *Infect Dis Clin North Am* 1996;10:657–675.
172. Gershon AA, Forghani B. Varicella-zoster virus. In: Lennette EH, Lennette DA, Lennette ET, eds. *Diagnostic procedures for viral, rickettsial, and chlamydial infections,* 7th ed. Washington, DC: American Public Health Association, 1995:601–613.
173. Krah DL. Assays for antibodies to varicella-zoster virus. *Infect Dis Clin North Am* 1996;10:507–527.
174. Wreghitt TG, Tedder RS, Naginton J, et al. Antibody assays for varicella virus: comparison of competitive enzyme-linked immunosorbent assay (ELISA), competitive radioimmunoassay (RIA), complement fixation, and indirect fluorescence assays. *J Med Virol* 1984;13: 361–370.
175. Bogger-Goren S, Baba K, Hurley P, et al. Antibody response to varicella-zoster virus after natural or vaccine-induced infection. *J Infect Dis* 1982;146:260–265.
176. Saiman L, LaRussa P, Steinberg S, et al. Persistence of immunity to varicella-zoster virus vaccination among health care workers. *Inf Control Hosp Epidemiol* 2001;22:279–283.
177. Provost PJ, Krah DL, Kuter BJ, et al. Antibody assays suitable for assessing immune responses to live varicella vaccine. *Vaccine* 1991;9: 111–116.
178. Krah DL, Cho I, Schofield T, et al. Comparison of gpELISA and neutralizing antibody responses to Oka/Merck live varicella vaccine (Varivax) in children and adults. *Vaccine* 1997;15:61–64.
179. Wasmuth EH, Miller WJ. Sensitive enzyme-linked immunosorbent assay for antibody to varicella-zoster virus using purified VZV glycoprotein antigen. *J Med Virol* 1990;32:189–193.
180. Steinberg SP, Gershon AA. Measurement of antibodies to varicella-zoster virus by using a latex agglutination test. *J Clin Microbiol* 1991; 29:1527–1529.
181. Gershon AA, LaRussa PS, Steinberg SP. Detection of antibody to varicella zoster virus using the latex agglutination assay. *Clin Diag Virol* 1994;2:271–278.
182. Landry ML, Ferguson D. Comparison of latex agglutination test with enzyme-linked immunosorbent assay for detection of antibody to varicella-zoster virus. *J Clin Microbiol* 1993;31:3031–3033.
183. Centers for Disease Control and Prevention. National Vaccination Coverage Levels Among Children Aged 19–35 Months—United States, 2001. *MMWR* 2002;51(30):664–666.
184. Centers for Disease Control and Prevention. Varicella-related deaths among children—United States, 1997. *MMWR* 1998;47:365–368.
185. Centers for Disease Control and Prevention. Varicella-related deaths among adults—United States, 1997. *MMWR* 1997;46:409–412.
186. Wreghitt TG, Whipp J, Redpath C, et al. An analysis of infection control of varicella-zoster virus infections in Addenbrooke's Hospital Cambridge over a 5-year period, 1987–92. *Epidemiol Infect* 1996; 117:165–171.
187. Smith KJ, Roberts MS. Cost effectiveness of vaccination strategies in adults without a history of chickenpox. *Am J Med* 2000;108: 723–729.
188. Nettleman MD, Schmid M. Controlling varicella in the healthcare setting: the cost effectiveness of using varicella vaccine in healthcare workers. *Infect Control Hosp Epidemiol* 1997;18:504–508.
189. Hamilton HA. A cost minimization analysis of varicella vaccine in healthcare workers [thesis]. Chapel Hill, NC: University of North Carolina School of Public Health, 1996.
190. Tennenberg AM, Brassard JE, Van Lieu J, et al. Varicella vaccination for healthcare workers at a university hospital: an analysis of costs and benefits. *Infect Control Hosp Epidemiol* 1997;18:405–411.
191. Gershon AA, Steinberg SP, LaRussa P, et al. Immunization of healthy adults with live attenuated varicella vaccine. *J Infect Dis* 1988;158: 132–137.
192. Preblud SR. Nosocomial varicella: worth preventing but how? *Am J Public Health* 1988;78:13–15.
193. Kuter BJ, Ngai A, Patterson CM, et al. Safety, tolerability, and immunogenicity of two regimens of Oka/Merck varicella vaccine (Varivax) in healthy adolescents and adults. *Vaccine* 1995;13:967–972.
194. Gershon AA. Varicella-zoster virus: prospects for control. *Adv Pediatr Infect Dis* 1995;10:93–124.
195. Ampofo K, Saiman L, LaRussa P, et al. Persistence of immunity to live attenuated varicella vaccine in healthy adults. *Clin Infect Dis* 2002; 34:774–779.
196. Johnson CE, Stancin T, Fattlar D, et al. A long-term prospective study of varicella vaccine in healthy children. *Pediatrics* 1997;100: 761–766.
197. Sharrar RG, LaRussa P, Galea S, et al. The postmarketing safety profile of varicella vaccine. *Vaccine* 2000;19:916–923.
198. Asano Y, et al. Contact infection from live varicella vaccine recipients. *Lancet* 1976;1:965.
199. Tsolia M, Gershon AA, Steinberg SP, et al. Live attenuated varicella vaccine: evidence that the virus is attenuated and the importance of skin lesions in transmission of the varicella-zoster virus. *J Pediatr* 1990; 116:184–189.
200. Salzman MB, Sharrar RG, Steinberg S, et al. Transmission of varicella-vaccine virus from a healthy 12-month-old child to his pregnant mother. *J Pediatr* 1997;131:151–154.
201. LaRussa P, Steinberg S, Meurice F, et al. Transmission of vaccine strain varicella-zoster virus from a healthy adult with vaccine-associated rash to susceptible household contacts. *J Infect Dis* 1997;176: 1072–1075.
202. Weibel RE, Neff BJ, Kuter BH, et al. Live attenuated varicella virus vaccine: efficacy trial in healthy children. *N Engl J Med* 1984;310: 1409–1415.
203. Josephson A, Karanfil L, Gombert ME. Strategies for the management of varicella-susceptible healthcare workers after a known exposure. *Infect Control Hosp Epidemiol* 1990;11:309–313.
204. Lipton SV, Brunell PA. Management of varicella exposure in a neonatal intensive care unit. *JAMA* 1989;261:1782–1784.
205. Sayre MR, Lucid EJ. Management of varicella-zoster virus-exposed hospital employees. *Ann Emerg Med* 1987;16:421–424.
206. Asano Y, Hirose S, Iwayama S, et al. Protective effect of immediate inoculation of a live varicella vaccine in household contacts in relation to the viral dose and interval between exposure and vaccination. *Biken J* 1982;25:43–45.
207. Arbeter A, Starr SE, Plotkin SA. Varicella vaccine studies in healthy children and adults. *Pediatrics* 1986;78(suppl):748–756.
208. Salzman MB, Garcia C. Postexposure varicella vaccination in siblings of children with active varicella. *Pediatr Infect Dis J* 1998;17:256–257.
209. Watson B, Seward J, Yang A, et al. Post exposure effectiveness of varicella vaccine. *Pediatrics* 2000;105:84–88.
210. Anderson LJ, Young NS, eds. *Human parvovirus B19.* Monographs in virology, vol 20. New York: Karger, 1997.
211. Morey AL, Porter HJ, Keeling JW, et al. Non-isotopic in situ hybridisation and immunophenotyping of infected cells in the investigation of human fetal parvovirus infection. *J Clin Pathol* 1992;45:673–678.
212. Ozawa K, Kurtzman G, Young N. Replication of the B19 parvovirus in human bone marrow cell cultures. *Science* 1986;233:883–886.
213. Erdman DD, Durigon EL, Wang QY, et al. Genetic diversity of human parvovirus B19: sequence analysis of the VP1/VP2 gene from multiple isolates. *J Gen Virol* 1996;77:2767–2774.
214. Nguyen QT, Sifer C, Schneider V, et al. Novel human erythrovirus associated with transient aplastic anemia. *J Clin Microbiol* 1999;37: 2483–2487.
215. Brown KE, Anderson SM, Young NS. Erythrocyte P antigen: cellular receptor for B19 parvovirus. *Science* 1993;262:114–117.
216. Morey AL, Ferguson DJ, Leslie KO, et al. Intracellular localization of parvovirus B19 nucleic acid at the ultrastructural level by in situ hybridization with digoxigenin-labelled probes. *Histochem J* 1993;25: 421–429.
217. Török TJ. Human parvovirus B19. In: Remington JS, Klein JO, eds. *Infectious diseases of the fetus and newborn infant,* 4th ed. Philadelphia: WB Saunders; 1995:668–702.
218. Gillespie SM, Cartter ML, Asch S, et al. Occupational risk of human parvovirus B19 infection for school and day-care personnel during an outbreak of erythema infectiosum. *JAMA* 1990;263:2061–2065.
219. Anderson LJ, Tsou C, Parker RA, et al. Detection of antibodies and

antigens of human parvovirus B19 by enzyme-linked immunosorbent assay. *J Clin Microbiol* 1986;24:522–526.
220. Cohen BJ, Buckley MM. The prevalence of antibody to human parvovirus B19 in England and Wales. *J Med Microbiol* 1988;25: 151–153.
221. Kelly HA, Siebert D, Hammond R, et al. The age-specific prevalence of human parvovirus immunity in Victoria, Australia compared with other parts of the world. *Epidemiol Infect* 2000;124:449–457.
222. Adler SP, Manganello AMA, Koch WC, et al. Risk of human parvovirus B19 infections among school and hospital employees during endemic periods. *J Infect Dis* 1993;168:361–368.
223. Chorba T, Coccia P, Holman RC, et al. The role of parvovirus B19 in aplastic crisis and erythema infectiosum (fifth disease). *J Infect Dis* 1986;154(3):383–393.
224. Plummer FA, Hammond GW, Forward K, et al. An erythema infectiosum-like illness caused by human parvovirus infection. *N Engl J Med* 1985;313(2):74–79.
225. Anderson MJ, Higgins PG, Davis LR, et al. Experimental parvoviral infection in humans. *J Infect Dis* 1985;152:257–265.
226. Dowell SF, Török TJ, Thorp JA, et al. Parvovirus B19 infection in hospital workers: community or hospital acquisition? *J Infect Dis* 1995;172:1076–1079.
227. Tuckerman JG, Brown T, Cohen BJ. Erythema infectiosum in a village primary school: clinical and virological studies. *J R Coll Gen Pract* 1986;36:267–270.
228. Seng C, Watkins P, Morse D, et al. Parovirus B19 outbreak on an adult ward. *Epidemiol Infect* 1994;113:345–353.
229. Evans JPM, Rossiter MA, Kumaran TO, et al. Human parvovirus aplasia: case due to cross infection in a ward. *Br Med J* 1984;288: 681.
230. Bell LM, Naides SJ, Stoffman P, et al. Human parvovirus B19 infection among hospital staff members after contact with infected patients. *N Engl J Med* 1989;321:485–491.
231. Koziol DE, Kurtzman G, Ayub JA, et al. Nosocomial human parvovirus B19 infection: lack of transmission from a chronically infected patient to hospital staff. *Infect Control Hosp Epidemiol* 1992;13: 343–348.
232. Miyamoto K, Ogami M, Takahashi Y, et al. Outbreak of human parvovirus B19 in hospital workers. *J Hosp Infect* 2000;45:238–241.
233. Farr RW, Hutzel D, D'Aurora R, et al. Parvovirus B19 outbreak in a rehabilitation hospital. *Arch Phys Med Rehabil* 1996;77:208–210.
234. Harrison J, Jones CE. Human parvovirus B19 infection in healthcare workers. *Occup Med* 1995;45:93–96.
235. Lohiya GS, Stewart K, Perot K, et al. Parvovirus B19 outbreak in a developmental center. *Am J Infect Control* 1995;23:373–376.
236. Saarinen UM, Chorba TL, Tattersall P, et al. Human parvovirus B19-induced epidemic acute red cell aplasia in patients with hereditary hemolytic anemia. *Blood* 1986;67:1411–1417.
237. Kurtzman G, Frickhofen N, Kimball J, et al. Pure red-cell aplasia of 10 years' duration due to persistent parvovirus B19 infection and its cure with immunoglobulin therapy. *N Engl J Med* 1989;321: 519–523.
238. Moudgil A, Shidban H, Nast CC, et al. Parvovirus B19 infection-related complications in renal transplant recipients: treatment with intravenous immunoglobulin. *Transplantation* 1997;64:1847–1850.
239. Ray SM, Erdman DD, Berschling JD, et al. Nosocomial exposure to parvovirus B19: low risk of transmission to healthcare workers. *Infect Control Hosp Epidemiol* 1997;18:109–114.
240. Gratacos E, Torres PJ, Vidal J, et al. The incidence of human parvovirus B19 infection during pregnancy and its impact on perinatal outcome. *J Infect Dis* 1995;171:1360–1363.
241. Koch WC, Harger JH, Barnstein B, et al. Serologic and virologic evidence for frequent intrauterine transmission of human parvovirus B19 with a primary maternal infection during pregnancy. *Pediatr Infect Dis J* 1998;17:489–494.
242. Public Health Laboratory Service Working Party on Fifth Disease, Prospective study of human parvovirus (B19) infection in pregnancy. *Br Med J* 1990;300:1166–1170.
243. Essary LR, Vnencak-Jones CL, Manning SS, et al. Frequency of parvovirus B19 infection in nonimmune hydrops fetalis and utility of three diagnostic methods. *Hum Pathol* 1998;29:696–701.
244. Jordan JA. Identification of human parvovirus B19 infection in idiopathic nonimmune hydrops fetalis. *Am J Obstet Gynecol* 1996;174(1 pt 1):37–42.
245. Mark Y, Rogers BB, Oyer CE. Diagnosis and incidence of fetal parvovirus infection in an autopsy series: II. DNA amplification. *Pediatr Pathol* 1993;13:381–386.
246. Cohen BJ, Courouce AM, Schwarz TF, et al. Laboratory infection with parvovirus B19 [letter]. *J Clin Pathol* 1988;41:1027–1028.
247. Shiraishi H, Sasaki T, Nakamura M, et al. Laboratory infection with human parvovirus B19 [letter]. *J Infect* 1991;22:308–310.
248. Cohen BJ, Field AM, Gudnadottir S, et al. Blood donor screening for parvovirus B19. *J Virol Methods* 1990;30:233–238.
249. Jordan J, Tiangco B, Kiss J, et al. Human parvovirus B19: prevalence of viral DNA in volunteer blood donors and clinical outcomes of transfusion recipients. *Vox Sang* 1998;75:97–102.
250. Yoto Y, Kudoh T, Haseyama K, et al. Large-scale screening for human parvovirus B19 DNA in clinical specimens by dot blot hybridization and polymerase chain reaction. *J Med Virol* 1995;47:438–441.
251. Saldanha J, Minor P. Detection of human parvovirus B19 DNA in plasma pools and blood products derived from these pools: implications for efficiency and consistency of removal of B19 DNA during manufacture. *Br J Haematol* 1996;93:714–719.
252. Bartolomei Corsi O, Azzi A, Morfini M, et al. Human parvovirus infection in haemophiliacs first infused with treated clotting factor concentrates. *J Med Virol* 1988;25:165–170.
253. Azzi A, Ciappi S, Zakvrzewska K, et al. Human parvovirus B19 infection in hemophiliacs first infused with two high-purity, virally attenuated factor VIII concentrates. *Am J Hematol* 1992;39:228–230.
254. Williams MD, Cohen BJ, Beddall AC, et al. Transmission of human parvovirus B19 by coagulation factor concentrates. *Vox Sang* 1990; 58:177–181.
255. Lyon DJ, Chapman CS, Martin C, et al. Symptomatic parvovirus B19 infection and heat-treated factor IX concentrate. *Lancet* 1989; 1(8646):1085.
256. Brojer E, Grabarczyk P, Lopaciuk S, et al. Prevalence of human parvovirus B19 DNA and IgG/IgM antibodies in Polish haemophilia patients. *Vox Sang* 1999;779(2):107.
257. Potter CG, Potter AC, Hatton CSR, et al. Variation of erythroid and myeloid precursors in the marrow of volunteer subjects infected with human parvovirus (B19). *J Clin Invest* 1987;79:1486–1492.
258. Woolf AD, Campion GV, Chishick A, et al. Clinical manifestations of human parvovirus B19 in adults. *Arch Intern Med* 1989;149: 1153–1156.
259. Forestier F, Tissot JD, Vial Y, et al. Haematological parameters of parvovirus B19 infection in 13 fetuses with hydrops foetalis. *Br J Haematol* 1999;104:925–927.
260. Torok TJ, Wang QY, Gary GW Jr, et al. Prenatal diagnosis of intrauterine infection with parvovirus B19 by the polymerase chain reaction technique. *Clin Infect Dis* 1992;14:149–155.
261. Miller E, Fairley CK, Cohen BJ, et al. Immediate and long term outcome of human parvovirus B19 infection in pregnancy. *Br J Obstet Gynaecol* 1998;105:174–178.
262. Jensen IP, Thorsen P, Jeune B, et al. An epidemic of parvovirus B19 in a population of 3,596 pregnant women: a study of sociodemographic and medical risk factors. *Br J Obstet Gynaecol* 2000;107: 637–643.
263. Miniero R, Dalponte S, Linari A, et al. Severe Shwachman-Diamond syndrome and invasive parvovirus B19 infection. *Pediatr Hematol Oncol* 1996;13:555–561.
264. Katz VL, McCoy MC, Kuller JA, et al. An association between fetal parvovirus B19 infection and fetal anomalies: a report of two cases. *Am J Perinatol* 1996;13:43–45.
265. Van Elsacker-Niele AM, Salimans MM, Weiland HT, et al. Fetal pathology in human parvovirus B19 infection. *Br J Obstet Gynaecol* 1989;96:768–775.
266. Rodis JF, Rodner C, Hansen AA, et al. Long-term outcome of children following maternal human parvovirus B19 infection. *Obstet Gynecol* 1998;91:125–128.

267. Torok TJ. Unusual clinical manifestations reported in patients with parvovirus B19 infection. In: Anderson LJ, Young NS, eds. *Monographs in virology,* vol 20, New York: Karger, 1997:61–92.
268. Miyagawa E, Yoshida T, Takahashi H, et al. Infection of the erythroid cell line, KU812Ep6 with human parvovirus B19 and its application to titration of B19 infectivity. *J Virol Methods* 1999;83:45–54.
269. Cohen BJ, Mortimer PP, Pereira MS. Diagnostic assays with monoclonal antibodies for the human serum parvovirus-like virus (SPLV). *J Hyg (Lond)* 1983;91:113–130.
270. Kaikkonen L, Lankinen H, Harjunpaa I, et al. Acute-phase-specific heptapeptide epitope for diagnosis of parvovirus B19 infection. *J Clin Microbiol* 1999;37:3952–3956.
271. Manaresi E, Gallinella G, Zerbini M, et al. IgG immune response to B19 parvovirus VP1 and VP2 linear epitopes by immunoblot assay. *J Med Virol* 1999;57:174–178.
272. Soderlund M, Brown CS, Spaan WJ, et al. Epitope type-specific IgG responses to capsid proteins VP1 and VP2 of human parvovirus B19. *J Infect Dis* 1995;172:1431–1436.
273. Moore L, Chambers HM, Foreman AR, et al. A report of human parvovirus B19 infection in hydrops fetalis. First Australian cases confirmed by serology and immunohistology. *Med J Aust* 1993;159: 344–345.
274. Anderson LJ, Tsou C, Parker RA, et al. Detection of antibodies and antigens of human parvovirus B19 by enzyme-linked immunosorbent assay. *J Clin Microbiol* 1986;24:522–526.
275. Kim EC, Durigon EL, Erdman DD, et al. Chemiluminescent microwell hybridization assay for direct detection of human parvovirus B19 DNA. *J Virol Methods* 1994;50:349–354.
276. Mori J, Field AM, Clewley JP, et al. Dot blot hybridization assay of B19 virus DNA in clinical specimens. *J Clin Microbiol* 1989;27: 459–464.
277. Musiani M, Zerbini M, Gibellini D, et al. Chemiluminescence dot blot hybridization assay for detection of B19 parvovirus DNA in human sera. *J Clin Microbiol* 1991;29:2047–2050.
278. Zerbini M, Musiani M, Gibellini D, et al. Evaluation of strand-specific RNA probes visualized by colorimetric and chemiluminescent reactions for the detection of B19 parvovirus DNA. *J Virol Methods* 1993;45:169–178.
279. Saldanha J, Minor P. Collaborative study to assess the suitability of a proposed working reagent for human parvovirus B19 DNA detection in plasma pools by gene amplification techniques. B19 Collaborative Study Group. *Vox Sang* 1997;73:207–211.
280. Saldanha J, Lelie N, Yu MW, Heath A. Establishment of the first World Health Organization International Standard for human parvovirus B19 DNA nucleic acid amplification techniques. *Vox Sang* 2002;82:24–31.
281. Patou G, Pillay D, Myint S, et al. Characterization of a nested polymerase chain reaction assay for detection of parvovirus B19. *J Clin Microbiol* 1993;31:540–546.
282. Durigon EL, Erdman DD, Gary GW, et al. Multiple primer pairs for polymerase chain reaction (PCR) amplification of human parvovirus B19 DNA. *J Virol Methods* 1993;44:155–165.
283. Erdman DD, Durigon EL, Wang QY, et al. Genetic diversity of human parvovirus B19: sequence analysis of the VP1/VP2 gene from multiple isolates. *J Gen Virol* 1996;77:2767–2774.
284. Aberham C, Pendl C, Gross P, et al. A quantitative, internally controlled real-time PCR assay for the detection of parvovirus B19 DNA. *J Virol Methods* 2001;92:183–191.
285. Knoll A, Louwen F, Kochanowski B, et al. Parvovirus B19 infection in pregnancy: quantitative viral DNA analysis using a kinetic fluorescence detection system (TaqMan PCR). *J Med Virol* 2002;67: 259–266.
286. Manaresi E, Gallinella G, Zuffi E, et al. Diagnosis and quantitative evaluation of parvovirus B19 infections by real-time PCR in the clinical laboratory. *J Med Virol* 2002;67:275–281.
287. CDC. Risks associated with human parvovirus B19 infection. *MMWR* 1989;38:81–88,93–97.
288. Koch WC, Massey G, Russell CE, et al. Manifestations and treatment of human parvovirus B19 infection in immunocompromised patients. *J Pediatr* 1990;116(3):355–359.
289. Koduri PR, Kumapley R, Valladares J, et al. Chronic pure red cell aplasia caused by parvovirus B19 in AIDS: use of intravenous immunoglobulin—a report of eight patients. *Am J Hematol* 1999;61(1): 16–20.

52

NOSOCOMIAL INFECTIONS IN NEWBORN NURSERIES AND NEONATAL INTENSIVE CARE UNITS

DOROTHY L. MOORE

Infections are an important cause of neonatal morbidity and mortality worldwide. Although most neonatal infections are of maternal or community origin, an increasing proportion are acquired in the nursery. Advances in newborn intensive care have permitted the survival of low-birth-weight and sick infants and have simultaneously created risks for nosocomial infection, which are themselves a significant cause of mortality in these infants (1–3). Prevention of infection in the premature infant who starts life in an intensive care unit and whose immature defenses are further depleted by illness and invasive procedures is a major challenge.

DESCRIPTIVE EPIDEMIOLOGY

Surveillance

The newborn may acquire infection from the mother *in utero* or during delivery or postpartum from maternal, hospital, or community sources. Many infections transmitted from mother to infant during delivery, such as group B β-hemolytic streptococci (GBS), *Listeria,* hepatitis B virus (HBV), or herpes simplex virus (HSV), have not traditionally been considered nosocomial. On the other hand, infections classified as nosocomial are often caused by microorganisms acquired from the mother that become part of the flora of the newborn and subsequently invade because of immature or impaired defenses.

Difficulty in distinguishing between maternal and hospital sources makes identification of newborn nosocomial infections imprecise. Because of this difficulty, the Centers for Disease Control and Prevention (CDC) has defined all neonatal infections, whether acquired during delivery or during hospitalization, as nosocomial unless evidence indicates transplacental acquisition (4). Most published reports of nosocomial infections have included only those infections with onset within a specified period after admission to the nursery, whereas some have attempted to separately define infections from maternal and hospital sources.

The need to distinguish between maternal and hospital sources is more than semantic. Infection control measures designed to prevent acquisition of microorganisms within the nursery will not affect pathogens acquired perinatally, for which control measures involve prevention, diagnosis, and treatment of infection in the pregnant woman; intrapartum antibiotic prophylaxis; postpartum antibiotic or immune prophylaxis for the infant; and prevention of obstetric complications known to be associated with increased intrapartum transmission.

Nosocomial infections may become manifest only after discharge from the hospital, especially in normal newborns whose short hospital stay is within the incubation period for many infections (5). Such infections may be brought to the attention of the infant's primary physician rather than the nursery. Surveillance for nosocomial infection in normal newborns requires close communication between community physicians and the nursery; otherwise, recognition of hospital-based outbreaks may be delayed. Programs for active postdischarge surveillance have been developed (6) but may not be cost effective in the absence of an outbreak, because most sporadic infections in normal newborns are benign.

CDC definitions of nosocomial infections in the newborn are based on those for older children and adults with certain modifications for children younger than 12 months (4). Methods of case finding vary and may include prospective daily clinical case review and/or review of laboratory results or retrospective chart review. Laboratory-based surveillance, although very sensitive for bloodstream, urinary tract, and central nervous system (CNS) infections, is less sensitive for infections at other sites and depends on the availability of laboratory facilities and the intensity of testing. Not all centers have ready access to virology cultures. Surveillance may include all infections or infections at specific sites such as bacteremia. The high-risk nursery component of the CDC's National Nosocomial Infections Surveillance (NNIS) system collects data on all infections at all sites (7).

An overall newborn nosocomial infection rate is of limited use, because it is influenced by the type of hospital or nursery, the patient mix, referral patterns, whether or not newborn surgery is performed, the type of surveillance, and the denominator used (5,8,9). Also, total infections must be distinguished from the numbers of infected patients, because many patients have more than one infection. The denominators most often reported are infections per 100 admissions or discharges or, for maternity hospitals, infections per 1,000 deliveries or live births. For the

TABLE 52.1. NOSOCOMIAL INFECTION RATES IN THE *NICU*

Infections per 100 admissions or discharges	Infections per 1,000 patient-days	Year	Location	Reference
14.0	—	1984–1987	Toronto	26
30.0	—	1987–1989	Curitiba, Brazil	27
14.5	—	1988–1989	Brooklyn	28
3.2	—	1989	Nice	29
28.4	—	1992–1995	Trinidad	30
27.1	21.9	1991	Freiburg[a]	31
6.2	4.8	1994–1995	New South Wales, Australia[a]	32
19.1	11.6	1996	Italy (mulicenter)	33
7.0	—	1996	European (multicenter)[b]	34
19.0	9.9	1987–1997	Montreal	35
18.9	23.8	1993–1997	Sao Paulo, Brazil[a]	36
—	4.6–18.1 (median 8.9)	1997	USA (multicenter)	37

NICU, neonatal intensive care unit.
[a] Stated that maternally acquired are included.
[b] Major infections only.

neonatal intensive care unit (NICU), where infection risk is related to duration of stay, patient-days is a more appropriate denominator (9) (see Chapter 94).

Infection rates expressed per admission or per patient-day may be useful for following infection rates in a specific NICU over time or for interhospital comparison, provided that the rates are adjusted for severity of illness or are expressed by risk group. Severity of illness scores (10–13) and a measure of the intensity of care required (14) have been used to control for differences in severity of illness in recent reports.

Birth weight has been used as a marker for severity of underlying illness in the NICU. Goldmann et al. (15) found a strong correlation between infection and low birth weight, with a mean birth weight of 1,581 g for infants with major nosocomial infections versus 2,607 g for those without. The NNIS system stratifies data by birth-weight groups (16).

Use of invasive devices may be a more relevant marker for average severity of illness and for the type of NICU. NICU infection rates vary with intensity of device use. In a study of 35 hospitals using NNIS protocols, assessment of device use (central or umbilical lines and ventilators) by total device-days and calculation of device-associated infection rates by device-days controlled for this variation. Stratification by birth weight did not eliminate the need to control for device use (9).

With infants staying in the NICU for longer periods, the need for another classification, the "late, late onset" infection or infection onset after 30 days of age, has arisen. Risk factors and the predominant microorganisms involved differ from those of the short-stay NICU patient (17).

Where a system of continuing surveillance has not been established or is not feasible, cross-sectional prevalence studies provide information on the spectrum of nosocomial infections and may help in allocation of resources. In addition, prevalence studies may permit collection of more detailed patient data. National prevalence studies from Spain (18), Norway (19), and the United States (20) have reported NICU infection rates of 16.7%, 14%, and 11%, respectively.

Reported Infection Rates

There are few data on infection rates in normal nurseries, where the infant is healthy and the hospital stay short. Reported rates are low, from 0.3 to 1.7 per 100 newborns (21–23). NNIS rates for all newborn nurseries reporting in 1984 were 0.9 and 1.7 per 100 discharges for nonteaching and large teaching hospitals, respectively (24). Similar rates for a small number of hospitals surveyed in Canada in 1984 were 1.4 and 3.1 per 100 discharges (25).

Reported infection rates in the NICU in the last 20 years vary from 3.2 to 30 per 100 admissions or discharges, illustrating the wide variability among centers (Table 52.1)(26–37). The low rate from Nice was attributed to minimal use of invasive procedures and antibiotics, rapid enteral feeding, and the limited number of personnel to which each infant was exposed (29). NICUs that admit surgery patients may have higher rates. A rate of 58 per 100 admissions was reported in one small series from a newborn surgery unit (38). Rates controlled for length of stay are 4.6 to 23.8 infections per 1,000 patient-days (Table 52.1).

Infection rates in infants of birth weights less than 1,500 g, 1,501 to 2,500 g, and more than 2,500 g were 63%, 8.2%, and 6%, respectively, in a study from Brooklyn (28) and 74%, 28%, and 13%, respectively, in a study from Brazil (39). The association of birth weight with infection rate may be lost if length of stay is considered (Table 52.2).

ACQUISITION OF INFECTION IN THE NEWBORN NURSERY AND NEONATAL INTENSIVE CARE UNIT

Bacterial Colonization of the Newborn

The fetus is relatively protected from acquisition of microorganisms, although infections may occur transplacentally or by direct extension from the maternal genital tract. Initial exposure to maternal microbial flora usually occurs during passage

TABLE 52.2. NOSOCOMIAL INFECTION RATES IN THE *NICU*: RELATION TO BIRTH WEIGHT

	Freiburg 1991 (31) Infections per		Montreal 1992–1997 (35) Infections per	
Birth weight (g)	100 admissions	1,000 patient-days	100 admissions	1,000 patient-days
<1,000	70.4	22.8	25.7	9.9
1,001–1,500	31.9	18.5	39.4	9.6
1,501–2,500	21.4	23.8	19.4	9.0
>2,500	13.6	23.5	9.6	7.1

NICU, neonatal intensive care unit.

through the birth canal. Colonization proceeds more slowly after delivery by cesarean section (40). Postnatally, colonization continues with new microbes acquired from mother, other family members, hospital personnel, and, occasionally, inanimate objects.

Healthy newborns establish normal flora within a few days of birth. Gram-positive microorganisms predominate in the pharynx (41,42), and coagulase-negative staphylococci (CONS) predominate at the umbilicus (41). Gastrointestinal colonization is more complex. Anaerobic bifidobacteria are found in very high concentrations, with smaller numbers of *Bacteroides,* other anaerobes, and *Escherichia coli* in stools of breast-fed infants. With formula feeding, Enterobacteriaceae predominate, and there are more *Bacteroides* microorganisms and other anaerobes and fewer bifidobacteria (40–44). The lower pH in the gastrointestinal tract of breast-fed infants may permit preferential growth of bifidobacteria (43).

The normal newborn with a short hospital stay has little opportunity to acquire nursery flora with the exception of *Staphylococcus aureus* and some viruses. However, in a report from nurseries in Japan wherein mothers and infants were separated for up to 72 hours after birth, 85% of healthy newborns acquired *E. coli* strains of nonmaternal, presumably nursery, origin (45).

Colonization of the infant in the NICU follows a different pattern as a result of limited maternal contact, delayed feeding, antibiotic treatment, and exposure to NICU flora. Each NICU has its unique endemic flora with colonized infants serving as reservoirs for transmission to newly admitted infants. The pattern of antibiotic use influences NICU flora (5). Colonization occurs later, especially when antibiotics are used or feeding is delayed (46), and gram-negative aerobic bacilli are prominent at multiple sites (41,42,46,47). Graham et al. (41) found that low-birth-weight and ill infants acquired fewer gram-positive and more gram-negative microorganisms in the mouth and umbilicus and more gram-negative aerobic rods and fewer anaerobes in the rectum than did healthy newborns. *Klebsiella, Enterobacter, Serratia,* and *Pseudomonas* were more frequent in those receiving antibiotics. *Klebsiella, Enterobacter,* and *Citrobacter* were often isolated from stool, nose, throat, or umbilicus of NICU infants studied by Goldmann et al. (47). Risk of acquisition of these microorganisms was increased in infants receiving antibiotics for more than 3 days and with increased duration of stay in the NICU. Antibiotics suppress stool anaerobic flora and favor growth of aerobic gram-negative rods (46,48).

NICU strains are often antibiotic resistant (5,49–52). The NICU offers ideal conditions for emergence of resistance: intense antibiotic pressure in a population with high bacterial loads. The high risk of severe infection and the difficulty in making a definitive diagnosis of infection or of identifying the causative microorganisms result in widespread empiric use of broad-spectrum antibiotics. Reports indicate that 50% to 81% of infants admitted to NICU receive antibiotics (47,53–55). Resistance appears to occur more rapidly with routine use of broad-spectrum cephalosporins than with penicillins and aminoglycosides (52,56–58).

CONS were the predominant flora of stool, skin, and mucous membranes in a series of premature infants delivered by cesarean section and not treated with antibiotics (59). Gram-negative bacilli were rare even in the stool. Antibiotic resistance patterns suggested that these CONS were acquired from the nursery. Although strains of CONS are normal flora, infants in the NICU may acquire unique nursery strains characterized by antibiotic resistance and enhanced slime production (60,61).

Acquisition of abnormal flora does not necessarily lead to infection, although the risk of infection may be increased. Sprunt (62) reported nosocomial infections in 0.5% of infants with normal pharyngeal flora and in 15% of those with abnormal flora. She considered normal flora to be protective against colonization with potential pathogens and showed that artificial implantation of α-hemolytic streptococci interfered with the growth of gram-negative rods in the pharynx. A more recent study showed that neonates colonized with viridans group streptococci were less likely to acquire methicillin-resistant *S. aureus* (MRSA) (63). Experimental evidence in animals suggests that the normal intestinal flora also has a protective effect (64).

Sources of Infectious Agents and Modes of Transmission

The usual mode of transmission of microbes in the nursery is by contact, either direct physical contact with an infected or colonized person or, more often, transfer from one infant to another on the hands of personnel. The classic experiments of Rammelkamp and colleagues (65,66) during the 1960s demonstrated hand transfer as the predominant mode of transmission of *S. aureus.* Hands have been implicated in several nursery outbreaks with various gram-negative bacilli, *S. aureus, Enterococcus,* and viruses (5,67–74). Goldmann et al. (47) documented the presence of gram-negative bacilli on the hands of 75% of NICU personnel. Usually, hands are transiently contaminated, and hand washing removes the microorganisms and interrupts transmission (75). Less often, personnel who are persistent carriers have been implicated in nursery outbreaks (76–78). Artificial fingernails have been associated with transmission of *Pseudomonas aeruginosa.* (68,69) Hand washing may itself perpetuate outbreaks if hand-washing agents become contaminated (79,80).

Transmission by indirect contact may also occur through patient care equipment that is not adequately decontaminated between patients or through equipment, solutions, and topical preparations contaminated from hands. Infections have been related to contamination of such items as resuscitation equipment (81–85), suction devices (86–88), ventilator circuits (89), rectal thermometers (90), and feeding bottles (91,92) and to application of contaminated eyewash (93), umbilical cord wash (94), mineral oil (95), ultrasound gel (96,97), glycerine (98), and antiseptic soap (99).

Water sources are additional potential hazards in the NICU (100,101). Microorganisms such as *Pseudomonas, Serratia, Stenotrophomonas,* and *Flavobacterium* are prevalent in the inanimate environment and grow readily at room temperature in water and moist environments such as incubators, humidifier reservoirs, and respirator nebulizers and tubing. *Pseudomonas* infection has been associated with a water bath used to thaw plasma (102) and *Stenotrophomonas* with tap water used to bathe premature babies (103).

Intravenous fluids, especially those used for parenteral nutrition (PN), were frequent sources of infection in the past (104, 105). With current standards of preparation, intravenous fluids are rarely intrinsically contaminated (106) but may become extrinsically contaminated by handling during use (107–112).

Blood transfusions may be a source of viruses such as cytomegalovirus (CMV) (113) hepatitis A virus (HAV) (114), HBV (115), hepatitis C virus (HCV) (116), and human immunodeficiency virus (HIV) (117). Neonatal transfusion-acquired malaria has also been reported (118,119) (see Chapters 44 and 69).

Breast milk is another source of blood-borne viruses (120). Approximately one third of CMV-seropositive women excrete CMV in their breast milk, and two thirds of these women were found to transmit CMV to their newborns by breast-feeding (121). HIV is transmitted from mother to newborn by breast milk, and breast-feeding may be the major means of acquisition of human T-cell leukemia virus type I (HTLV-I) (120). Breast milk may contain bacteria if the mother is bacteremic or has mastitis but is more likely to be contaminated with bacteria during collection or handling. One study reported growth of gram-negative bacilli in 36% of samples of unpasteurized human milk (122). Outbreaks of *Klebsiella* (123) and *Serratia* (122,124) have been associated with contaminated breast milk pumps. Contamination of banked breast milk with *Salmonella* (125), enteropathogenic *E. coli* (126), and MRSA (127) has been reported.

Formula feeds may also become contaminated during preparation or handling (128). Contaminated blenders have been identified as a source of infection (129,130). Bacteremia and meningitis have been associated with powdered infant formula intrinsically contaminated with *Enterobacter sakazakii* (131).

Infected personnel and visitors may introduce pathogens into the nursery, especially during community outbreaks of viral infections. Most respiratory viruses are spread by large droplets expelled from the respiratory tract that travel distances of less than a meter and settle on surfaces close to the infected person. Infection is acquired by close contact with the infected person or with contaminated objects (132). This is probably not an important means of transmission between newborns, because they do not cough vigorously and are inefficient generators of droplets. However, it can be an important means of transmission to newborns from infected personnel or visitors (133).

True airborne transmission, in which microorganisms remain suspended in aerosols for significant periods and are carried by air currents over considerable distances, occurs infrequently in the nursery. Diseases transmitted in this manner include varicella, measles, and tuberculosis, all of which are rare in newborns. Airborne fungal spores are rare causes of infection in NICUs, but such infections may be devastating (5).

Risk Factors for Infection

The Newborn

The newborn is at risk for infection because of immaturity of the normal structural barriers and the immune system. The defenses of the premature newborn are particularly inadequate. Before 32 weeks' gestation, the stratum corneum is poorly developed and the skin is fragile, easily traumatized, and very permeable. The skin matures rapidly postnatally and, by 2 weeks of life, is well developed in most newborns regardless of gestational age (134).

Immune function in the newborn has been extensively reviewed by Lewis and Wilson (135) Although the fetus is capable of early antibody production, there is little antibody synthesis *in utero,* and the newborn initially depends on passively transferred maternal antibody. The repertoire of antibodies received depends on maternal exposure. The newborn of less than 34 weeks' gestation may not receive protective levels of antibody. Premature newborns respond adequately to most protein antigens, but response to polysaccharide antigens is poor in the first 2 years of life. Opsonization activity of the alternate complement system and serum fibronectin levels are deficient in the term infant. These deficiencies put the newborn at risk for overwhelming bacterial and fungal infections.

T-cell function is important for control of intracellular pathogens such as *Listeria, Toxoplasma,* and *Salmonella.* The newborn has a high total T-lymphocyte count, but phenotypic surface markers differ from those in the older child. Cytotoxic T-cell activity is decreased as is T-cell helper function. T-cell dependent antigen specific response is delayed, and there is limited production of several cytokines. Natural killer cell activity, important in control of herpes group viral infections, is also decreased.

The newborn has a decreased granulocyte storage pool and defective neutrophil and monocyte chemotaxis. Under optimal conditions, phagocytosis and microbial killing by neonatal granulocytes are normal, but these functions are impaired if opsonization is deficient.

Environment

Infection rates in the NICU increase with overcrowding and understaffing. Haley and Bregman (136) reported a 16-fold increase in outbreaks of *S. aureus* infection when the infant-to-nurse ratio exceeded 7 and a sevenfold increase when the nursery was crowded. More recently, they reported increasing rates of endemic MRSA linked to overcrowding and understaffing, with eradication of MRSA when these conditions improved (14). An outbreak of *Enterobacter cloacae* infection was associated with understaffing and overcrowding in another report (137). Goldmann et al. (15) observed a decrease in percentage of nosocomial infections from 5.8 to 1.8 after a move to a new NICU with more nurses and space per infant, more accessible sinks, and improved ventilation.

Invasive Procedures

Any procedure that disrupts the normal barriers to infection is likely to present a higher risk of infection in the newborn than later in life. The normal newborn escapes most invasive procedures but may be subjected to scalp electrodes or percutaneous punctures for blood sampling. Scalp electrodes provide a portal of entry for maternal genital microorganisms. Infectious complications occur in less than 1% of infants and most are benign abscesses, but severe cellulitis, bacteremia, osteomyelitis, and disseminated HSV infection have been reported (138,139). Osteomyelitis has resulted from infected toe and heel punctures (140).

Premature and ill newborns often require feeding by nasogastric tubes, which provide a portal of entry and potentiate overgrowth of microbes in the upper gastrointestinal tract (74, 141–143). Breast milk (122) and formula feeds (128) administered by continuous infusion remain at room temperature for several hours, allowing microbes to proliferate in the reservoir or tubing during infusion. Botsford et al. (122) found that colony counts of enteric gram-negative rods in milk samples taken from connecting tubings changed after 24 hours of use were often greater than 10^6/mL. Counts of 10^3/mL or higher were associated with feeding intolerance. Counts of 10^6/mL or higher were associated with symptoms of sepsis and necrotizing enterocolitis (NEC) in some infants. In another study, formula contamination with 10^6/mL of gram-negative bacteria was associated with NEC (143).

Bacterial colonization of intravascular catheters, including peripheral lines, occurs more often in neonates than in older children (144). Infections are rare with radial artery and scalp vein needles (145), although the latter did serve as significant portals of entry in an outbreak of *Serratia* infection (146). Catheter-associated bloodstream infection (BSI) rates compiled from several studies were 3.7% for umbilical vein and 1.2% for umbilical artery catheters and 3% to 8% for central venous lines (CVLs) used for PN (145). BSI was associated with 5% of umbilical artery and 3% of umbilical vein catheters in one report (147) and with 17.6% of umbilical artery and 13.2% of umbilical vein catheters in another. Umbilical catheterization for more than 5 days was an independent risk factor for sepsis (33). Rates of BSI associated with Broviac cuffed silicone catheters are 2.9 to 5.4 per 1,000 catheter-days (148). These are higher than in older children and are particularly elevated in low-birth-weight infants (149). Peripherally inserted, noncuffed, silicone CVLs are being increasingly used in newborns because of ease of insertion and decreased trauma to small central vessels. Infection rates of 1 to 5.7 per 1,000 catheter-days are reported (148,150,151). In a recent multicenter study, rates of BSI for umbilical, percutaneous central, and tunneled catheters were 7.2, 13.1, and 12.1 per 1,000 catheter-days, respectively (152). Risk factors for catheter-associated BSI include catheter disconnection, blood sampling, and colonization of the catheter hub (153). Contamination of intravascular pressure-monitoring devices has resulted in neonatal infections (154,155). Extracorporeal membrane oxygenation was associated with a BSI rate of 3.4%; duration of bypass was the major risk factor (156).

Other invasive devices associated with infection in the newborn include endotracheal tubes, urinary catheters, and ventriculoperitoneal shunts (see later discussion). Infants have higher rates of catheter-associated urinary tract infections (UTIs) (157) and ventriculoperitoneal shunt infections (158) than older children. However, NNIS data suggest a lower rate of ventilator-associated pneumonia in NICUs than in other intensive care units (16).

INFECTIONS AT SPECIFIC SITES

In the normal nursery, most infections are superficial infections of the skin, mouth, and eyes. Outbreaks of infections with common viral pathogens also occur (5,22). These outbreaks may represent admission of large numbers of maternally infected infants or the introduction of a microbe by one or a few maternally infected infants and subsequent transmission in the nursery.

In the NICU, skin and mucous membrane infections predominate in most early reports (8). More recently, BSIs have been more common (Table 52.3). In general, BSIs are more common and surgical site infections and UTIs are less common than in older children and adults (7,8,24). NNIS data of infection site by birth-weight group are summarized in Table 52.4 (7). Approximately 15% of BSIs and pneumonia and less than 8% of the other infections were maternally acquired.

Skin, Subcutaneous Tissues, Mouth, and Eyes

Pustules, cellulitis, subcutaneous abscesses, lymphadenitis, and infections at sites of percutaneous punctures are most often due to *S. aureus*, although streptococci may also be involved. Infections resulting from gram-negative bacilli and other microorganisms may occur in the NICU (159). Microbes causing infections at scalp monitor sites are more diverse and include maternal genital microorganisms such as HSV (138,139), *Mycoplasma hominis* (160), and *Gardnerella* (161). *Candida* infections of the skin and mouth are frequent in infants in NICUs (162).

Omphalitis is uncommon; it occurred in 0.5% of term and 2% of preterm infants in one report (163). The presentation varies from mild erythema or serous drainage to purulent discharge, cellulitis, and acute necrotizing fasciitis of the abdominal

TABLE 52.3. NOSOCOMIAL INFECTIONS IN THE *NICU*: PERCENTAGE OF INFECTION BY SITE IN SELECTED STUDIES

Site of infection	Toronto 1984–1987 (26)	Freiburg 1991 (31)[a]	Montreal 1987–1997 (35)	São Paulo 1993–1995 (36)[a]	USA multicenter 1999 (20)[b]
Skin, mucous membranes	15	11	19	17.5	8.6
Pneumonia	7	32	6	42.1	Not specified
Upper respiratory tract	4	2	9	0.3	Not specified
Respiratory tract unspecified	—	—	—	—	12.9
Blood	45	27	27	29.1	52.6
Urinary tract	5	3	14	2.4	8.6
Surgical site	2	11	5	1.4	Not specified
Gastrointestinal tract	16	2	19	6.5	Not specified
Other	7	2	6	—	17.2

NICU, neonatal intensive care unit.
[a] Includes maternally acquired.
[b] Prevalence study.

wall. *S. aureus* is most often isolated, but group A *Streptococcus,* CONS, enterococci, gram-negative rods, and anaerobes may also be involved (164,165). A mortality rate of 7% was reported in a series of hospitalized patients. All deaths were in infants presenting with rapidly progressing cellulitis or necrotizing fasciitis (165). Tetanus secondary to umbilical infection is common when conditions of delivery and cord care are not hygienic and mothers are nonimmune (166) (see Chapter 47).

Circumcision is the most common surgical procedure performed in the newborn. For CDC surveillance purposes, circumcision infections are classified with skin and soft tissue infections and not with surgical site infections. Reported infection rates are low, at 0.06% to 0.4% (167,168). Most are simple site infections, but bullous impetigo, staphylococcal scalded skin syndrome, necrotizing fasciitis, and bacteremia have been reported (159).

Infectious conjunctivitis in the normal newborn is most often due to *Chlamydia* and presents after discharge from hospital (159). Gonococcal infections, which are rare, may present earlier. *S. aureus* infection is next in frequency to *Chlamydia* and may be of nursery origin with outbreaks occurring in normal nurseries and NICUs (71). In the NICU, conjunctivitis is a frequent finding in outbreaks of *Serratia* (80,87). *P. aeruginosa* conjunctivitis has been associated with contaminated resuscitation equipment (86), and infection in intubated patients has been related to endotracheal tube colonization and eye contamination during suctioning (169). *P. aeruginosa* eye infection is particularly severe in premature infants, in whom it may progress rapidly to destruction of the cornea by proteolytic enzymes, invasion of the eye, and secondary bacteremia (170). Endophthalmitis secondary to BSI occurs with disseminated *Candida* infection (171). Ophthalmologic examination was a common factor in an outbreak of adenoviral conjunctivitis (172).

Bloodstream Infections

Neonatal BSI is reported in one to eight newborns per 1,000 live births (173). Early-onset BSI, occurring shortly after birth as a result of infection in the birth canal, is characterized by fulminant multisystem disease with a high mortality rate. Risk

TABLE 52.4. NOSOCOMIAL INFECTIONS BY SITE OF INFECTION AND BIRTH WEIGHT

	Birth weight (g)			
	<1,000 (*n* = 3,987) %	1,001–1,500 (*n* = 1,881) %	1,501–2,500 (*n* = 3,547) %	>2,500 (*n* = 3,764) %
Blood	43	38	26	28
Pneumonia	16	12	13	18
Gastrointestinal tract	7	10	11	5
Conjunctivitis	4	10	16	9
Ear, nose, throat	4	4	5	4
Skin, soft tissue	6	7	10	9
Surgical site	1	1	3	7
Clinical sepsis	6	7	6	8
Other	13	11	10	12

Data from the National Nosocomial Infections Surveillance, 1986–1994. From Gaynes RP, Edwards JR, Jarvis WR, et al. Nosocomial infections among neonates in high-risk nurseries in the United States. *Pediatrics* 1996;98: 357–361, with permission.

factors are prematurity, low birth weight, prolonged rupture of membranes, maternal chorioamnionitis, and maternal fever. Predominant causes are GBS and *E. coli.* Pathogens generally seen in older infants, such as *Haemophilus influenzae* and *Streptococcus pneumoniae,* are now encountered in increasing numbers in newborns (17,54,173,174).

Late-onset BSI, usually occurring after the first week of life, is also often due to maternal microorganisms but shows less relation to obstetric complications, occurs more often in term infants, and is often associated with focal infection, especially meningitis. Late-onset BSI acquired in the nursery is more often due to CONS, *S. aureus,* enterococci, or gram-negative rods (17, 175). In BSI occurring after more than 30 days in the NICU, CONS and *Candida* are prominent (17).

Microorganisms isolated in neonatal sepsis have been monitored at Yale-New Haven Hospital since 1928 (17). Changes over time are presented in Table 52.5. Beta-hemolytic streptococci, *S. aureus,* and *E. coli* were the main microorganisms encountered during the first 20 years. With increasing use of antibiotics, *E. coli, P. aeruginosa,* and *Klebsiella-Enterobacter* became more important, reaching a peak in the period 1958 to 1965. GBS became prominent in the 1970s. In the 1980s, GBS and *E. coli* remained the most frequent isolates, but CONS became more prominent. There were increasing rates of late, late onset infections related to increasing admission and survival of infants of birth weight less than 1,000 g. In 1979 to 1988, the overall rate of BSI was 2.7 per 1,000 live births for newborns less than 30 days of age and 3.8 per 1,000 if those remaining in the NICU for more than 30 days were included. Of these infections, 46% were of early onset, 27% had onset at 5 to 30 days, and 28% had onset after 30 days of life.

A 1993 review from Spain reported that sepsis and/or meningitis occurred in 4.9 per 1,000 live births, again with increasing GBS and CONS infections and decreasing gram-negative bacillary infections over time (176). A similar pattern has been reported in many centers in North America and Europe (173). In developing countries, GBS is less common and gram-negative rods and *S. aureus* are more prominent (177)

In data reported to NNIS from 1986 to 1994, GBS accounted for 46% of maternally acquired BSI, followed by CONS (12%) and *E. coli* (10%). CONS were associated with 58% of BSI acquired in the NICU, followed by *Candida* (9%), *S. aureus* (8%), and enterococci (7%) (7). Anaerobes are an uncommon cause of neonatal bacteremia, accounting for only 2.2% of infections over an 18-year period in a series from New York. Those occurring in the first 48 hours of life were usually penicillin-sensitive gram-positive microorganisms associated with chorioamnionitis. Gram-negative anaerobes were more common after 48 hours and were often associated with NEC and gastrointestinal perforation (178).

Intrapartum prophylaxis for early-onset GBS sepsis has resulted in a shift in predominant pathogens. At Yale-New Haven Hospital, an increasing incidence of gram negative rod bacteremia was noted in 1995 to 1997; maternal intrapartum antibiotic prophylaxis was an independent risk factor (179). However, another study in Connecticut showed a decrease in incidence of early-onset GBS sepsis from 0.61 to 0.23 per 1,000 live births but no increase in early-onset non-GBS sepsis (180). A multicenter study in the United States showed no increase in rate of gram-negative sepsis but an increasing proportion of *E. coli* infections that were resistant to ampicillin (181). In Australia, de-

TABLE 52.5. MICROBIOLOGY OF NEONATAL SEPSIS IN INFANTS BORN AT YALE-NEW HAVEN HOSPITAL, 1928 TO 1988

	Percentage in each study					
	1928–1932	1933–1943	1944–1957	1958–1965	1966–1978	1979–1988
Gram-positive aerobic bacteria						
Staphylococcus aureus	28	9	13	3	5	3
Coagulase-negative staphylococci	—	—	—	1	1	8
β-Hemolytic streptococci						
Group B	—	5	6	1	32	37
Group D	—	—	2	10	4	8
Nongrouped and other	38	36	10	—	—	—
Viridans streptococci	—	2	—	3	1	3
Streptococcus pneumoniae	5	11	5	3	1	1
Listeria monocytogenes	—	2	2	—	1	1
Gram-negative aerobic bacteria						
Escherichia coli	26	25	37	45	32	20
Klebsiella-Enterobacter	—	—	—	11	12	3
Pseudomonas	3	—	21	15	2	3
Haemophilus	—	—	—	1	4	5
Salmonella	—	—	2	—	1	1
Gram-negative anaerobic bacteria	—	—	—	—	1	3
Fungi	—	—	—	—	2	1
Other	—	9	3	5	5	1
n	39	44	62	73	239	147

From Gladstone IM, Ehrenkranz RA, Edberg SC, Baltimore RS. A ten-year review of neonatal sepsis and comparison with the previous fifty-year experience. *Pediatr Infect Dis J* 1990;9:819–825, with permission.

creased rates of early-onset GBS sepsis and also non-GBS sepsis were reported (182).

Low birth weight is a major risk factor for BSI, with very-low-birth-weight (VLBW) infants at especially high risk. A multicenter study of sepsis in VLBW infants was carried out by the U.S. National Institute of Child Health and Human Development (NICHD) from 1991 to 1993 (54,175). Early-onset BSI (within 72 hours of birth) was uncommon, occurring in 1.9% of infants. The predominant microorganisms were GBS (31%), *E. coli* (16%), and *H. influenzae* (12%). In contrast, late-onset BSI occurred in 25% of infants. The microorganisms most often isolated were CONS (55%), *S. aureus* (9%), enterococcus (5%), and *Candida* (7%), with enteric gram-negative rods accounting for 12%. Early- or late-onset infection increased length of hospitalization, but only late-onset disease increased risk of death. Infants infected with gram-negative bacteria or *Candida* were more likely to die. BSI rates by birth weight reported from the Yale-New Haven Hospital (17), the Vermont-Oxford Trials Network Database (183), and the NICHD study (54,175) are presented in Table 52.6.

In a NICHD report from 1998 to 2000, the rate of early-onset sepsis in VLBW infants was 1.5%, similar to the previous rate. However, the rate of GBS sepsis decreased from 5.9 to 1.7, whereas the rate of *E. coli* sepsis increased from 3.2 to 6.8 per 1,000 live births (184). Rate of late-onset sepsis and the microorganisms isolated were similar to those reported earlier (185).

The effect of birth weight on risk of BSI remains when CVL use is taken into account. NNIS data for 1995 to 2002 showed median rates of CVL-associated BSI of 10.3, 6.6, 3.9, and 2.7 per 1,000 CVL-days for infants of birth weights below 1,000 g, 1,001 to 1,500 g, 1,501 to 2,500 g, and more than 2,500 g, respectively (16).

Although low birth weight and use of CVL and PN are interrelated, CVL and PN are independent risk factors for BSI. Donowitz et al. (186) reported Broviac catheters, PN, and surgery as risk factors; catheters were the major risk in infants weighing less than 1,500 g, and surgery was the major risk in those weighing more than 3,000 g. Administration of lipid is an independent risk factor for CONS bacteremia (12,187). Low birth weight; admission for respiratory illness; and treatment with H_2-blockers (11), mechanical ventilation (33,36), and dexamethasone (188) were independently associated with BSI in other studies.

Neonatal bowel resection was a risk factor for late, late onset nosocomial gram-negative bacteremia; a report showed that 39% of infants developed infection at a mean of 17 weeks after surgery (189). Enteral feeding was associated with an increased risk of gram-negative bacteremia in infants with short bowel syndrome, possibly resulting from an effect of enteral feeding on bacterial translocation across the gut wall (190).

Central Nervous System Infections

The microorganisms isolated and risk factors identified for BSI also apply to neonatal meningitis, which occurs in approximately 25% of bacteremic newborns (173). In a review of neonatal meningitis from Parkland Memorial Hospital, Dallas from the period 1969 to 1989, microorganisms isolated were GBS (53%), gram-negative enteric bacilli (31%), *Listeria* (7%), and other gram-positive cocci (6%). *E. coli, Klebsiella, Enterobacter,* and *Citrobacter* were the principal enteric bacilli; *Klebsiella* and *Enterobacter* were more frequent in premature infants (191).

In contrast, gram-negative bacteria, predominantly *Klebsiella* and *E. coli,* accounted for 64% of cases of neonatal meningitis in a report from Panama. CONS and *S. aureus* were the most common gram-positive isolates (192).

Outbreaks of nosocomial CNS infections in NICUs are usually due to gram-negative bacilli (91,93,96,109,193–197), although *Listeria* (82,95), group A streptococci (198,199), and *S. aureus* (200) have also been involved. *Citrobacter diversus,* a cause of sporadic meningitis of maternal origin in normal newborns, has also caused clusters of hospital-acquired CNS infections in normal nurseries and in NICUs (201,202). Meningitis is complicated by focal brain lesions in 77% of cases (203). Outbreaks of meningitis from *Campylobacter fetus* (204) and *Campylobacter jejuni* (205) have been reported. Viruses causing maternally or nursery-acquired CNS infection are discussed later.

Neural tube defects (173,191) and ventricular drains and shunts (158) are risk factors for CNS infection. In a study of shunt placement for hydrocephalus in newborns of less than 2,000 g, the shunt infection rate was 25% after primary placement and 36% after revision (206). Pople et al. (158) found that contamination during surgery correlated with a high preoperative skin bacterial density, which was found in younger infants. CONS was the most frequent etiology, and CONS strains with high adherence were more common in the newborn. The role of perioperative antibiotic prophylaxis in the newborn has

TABLE 52.6. BACTEREMIA RATES IN RELATION TO BIRTH WEIGHT

Yale-New Haven Hospital (17)			Vermont-Oxford Trials Network (183)	NICHD (54,184)	
Birth weight (g)	Bacteremia[a]	Birth weight (g)	Bacteremia[b]	Bacteremia[b] Early onset	Late onset
<1,000	17.2	≤750	26	2.4	50
1,000–1,499	6.1	751–1,000	22	2.3	33
1,500–2,499	1.5	1,001–1,250	15	1.6	21
≥2,500	0.11	1,251–1,500	8	1.7	10

[a] Bacteremias per 100 births.
[b] Bacteremic infants per 100 births.

not been established, but preoperative antiseptic bathing and use of intraoperative topical antiseptics may be beneficial (158). (For additional information on CNS infections in newborns, see Chapters 27 and 49.)

Respiratory Tract Infection

Early-onset pneumonia is usually related to intrapartum infection and is most often due to GBS (7,207). Maternally transmitted *Chlamydia* (208) and *Ureaplasma* infection (209) may cause pneumonia, usually mild, with onset at 1 to 3 months of age. *Ureaplasma* may cause earlier more severe infection in the very premature infant. Respiratory viruses may be acquired postnatally from the mother or from nursery sources (see later discussion). *S. aureus* and gram-negative enteric bacilli are important causes of nosocomial pneumonia in NICUs (7,15). CONS is also implicated (207,210,211). In the 1986 to 1994 NNIS data, the predominant etiologic agents reported were *S. aureus* (16.7%), CONS (16.5%), *P. aeruginosa* (11.7%), and *Enterobacter* (8.2%) (7). Gram-negative microorganisms have often been reported in outbreaks, which have occurred after exposure to contaminated resuscitation and respiratory therapy equipment (83,86,87).

Endotracheal intubation is a major risk factor; pneumonia developed in 10% of intubated neonates in one report (207) and 16% in another (211). The pathogenesis of ventilator-associated pneumonia in the newborn has been less well studied than in the adult, but mechanisms are expected to be similar (212). Colonization of the gastrointestinal tract precedes colonization of the respiratory tract (213). The mean rates of NICU ventilator-associated pneumonia in NNIS hospitals reported for 2002 were 2.4, 1.7, 2.0, and 0.7 infections per 1,000 ventilator-days in birth-weight groups of less than 1,000 g, 1,001 to 1,500 g, 1,501 to 2,500 g, and greater than 2,500 g, respectively. These rates are lower than those reported for any other intensive care units (16). However, diagnosis of pneumonia in the intubated newborn is difficult, and many infants are treated empirically for presumed lung infection. Underlying lung disease complicates interpretation of radiographic changes, and procedures used to diagnose pneumonia in the older patient, such as bronchoscopy and lung biopsy, are rarely performed. Specific microbiologic diagnosis is rarely obtained unless there is secondary bacteremia. Endotracheal cultures are useful in predicting the etiology of perinatal pneumonia (214). However, the respiratory tract of the intubated newborn rapidly becomes colonized, and, subsequently, such cultures are not helpful in determining the cause of invasive infection or diagnosing pneumonia (207,215,216). Intubated newborns are also at risk for otitis media (217) and tracheitis (218).

Surfactant is now used in many premature infants to prevent or treat respiratory distress syndrome. There has been no report of an increased infection rate with surfactant use; in fact, decreasing the need for ventilation would be expected to reduce the risk of infection (5). However, two infants receiving surfactant developed rapidly progressive necrotizing pneumonia resulting from *Bacillus cereus,* an unusual pathogen in the newborn. Surfactant was not found to be contaminated, but it was postulated that it might have served as a growth factor for this lecithinase-producing microorganism, which is commonly found in the environment (219).

Gastrointestinal Infections

The newborn is at increased risk for infections with gastrointestinal pathogens, because local gastrointestinal immunity and normal flora have not yet developed and the high gastric pH and short gastric emptying time allow ingested microorganisms to survive and to be passed to the intestine. Normal newborns and those in the NICU are susceptible. When outbreaks have occurred, the index case has often been infected by vertical transmission, and subsequent transmission has occurred by way of the contaminated hands of personnel or contaminated equipment. Infected personnel have rarely been involved (5,220). Epidemic nosocomial diarrhea is especially a problem in developing countries, where outbreaks of *Salmonella* and enteropathogenic or enterotoxigenic *E. coli* occur often (88,166,220,221).

Nursery outbreaks of enteropathogenic *E. coli* infection were common in developed countries in the past but are now unusual. Outbreaks may be explosive, with rapid progression and symptomatic infection of most newborns at risk, or more indolent, with occasional clinical infections and many carriers. *Salmonella* outbreaks are often protracted and recognized late because of delayed onset of symptoms and prolonged carriage in the newborn (220,222). The newborn is at high risk for *Salmonella* bacteremia, and focal infections are also common. Although *Shigella* has a low infective dose and spreads very rapidly in older children, symptomatic infection in the newborn is surprisingly rare and transmission to other newborns is unusual; transmission to nursery personnel has been reported (223). *C. jejuni* is an uncommon newborn pathogen and is usually of maternal origin, but nosocomial outbreaks have been described (220,224,225). Rotavirus is the gastrointestinal pathogen most often identified in nurseries in developed countries. Infections may be epidemic or endemic and are often asymptomatic (220,226) (see later discussion). There is little information on the role of other viruses in neonatal gastrointestinal disease. (For additional information on nosocomial gastrointestinal infections, see Chapters 24 and 50.)

Necrotizing Enterocolitis

NEC is a disease of multifactorial origin involving an immature gastrointestinal tract, ischemia, overgrowth of gastrointestinal bacteria, oral feeding that provides substrate for bacterial growth or production of toxins, and local production of inflammatory mediators (227,228). Although not strictly an infectious process, microbes are involved in the pathogenesis. It is included in the CDC definitions of nosocomial infections; therefore, data on NEC are found in most surveillance reports. Cases often occur in clusters, suggesting a transmissible agent. It is likely that any microbe capable of causing damage to the gastrointestinal tract can contribute to this disease; thus, NEC may accompany any outbreak of gastrointestinal infection in a population at risk. Microorganisms isolated from stool often reflect those predominant in the NICU at the time, and isolates from blood and peritoneal fluid are those that have invaded through the damaged gut wall and are not necessarily causative.

NEC is mainly a disease of the convalescing premature infant, occurring in up to 10% to 15% of VLBW infants. Term infants are also affected, making up 5% to 10% of cases (159). Microbes temporally associated with outbreaks of NEC include *Klebsiella; Clostridia; E. coli; Serratia; Pseudomonas; Staphylococcus epidermidis;* and enteric pathogens such as *Salmonella*, toxigenic *E. coli*, and *S. aureus* (227–229). Delta toxin produced by *S. epidermidis* and *S. aureus* is enteropathogenic, and many of the other microorganisms encountered are toxin producers. Free cytotoxins have been detected in stools in some outbreaks (229). The role of *Clostridium difficile* toxin, which is often found in the stools of asymptomatic infants, is not clear. Rotavirus has also been associated with outbreaks of NEC (230). When compared with other infants with NEC, those with rotavirus were of older gestational age at birth, had been fed at an earlier age, were older at onset of symptoms, and had less severe disease (231).

Prophylactic oral vancomycin protected VLBW infants against NEC and may be indicated in specific situations, but routine use may increase the risk of colonization with resistant microorganisms. (232). Breast milk is protective (233). In one study, oral immunoglobulin containing IgA and IgG was protective when fed to low-birth-weight infants for whom breast milk was not available (234). Feeding neonates with *Lactobacillus* and *Bifidobacterium* reduced the incidence of NEC when compared with historical controls (235) (see also Chapter 24).

Urinary Tract Infection

Neonatal UTI has been reported in approximately 0.7% of term infants and 1.9% to 2.9% of high-risk and premature infants (236,237). In a study of nosocomial UTIs in a children's hospital, the highest rate of infection was observed on the neonatal surgery unit at 4.8 UTIs per 100 admissions. The NICU rate was 1.9 per 100 admissions. Seventeen percent of the NICU and 44% of the neonatal surgery infections were catheter-related. One third of the infections were due to CONS, followed in frequency by *Candida*, enterococci, and *Klebsiella* (238). Another hospital reported an infection rate of 0.79 UTIs per 100 NICU admissions. Two thirds of these were catheter-associated, and one third was due to CONS (239). In another pediatric study, the rate of catheter-associated UTI was highest in neonates, at 10.2 per 1,000 patient-days (240). Catheters are not often used in newborns, but when they are the risk of infection is high, possibly because of the use of feeding tubes, which are not well stabilized, rather than the balloon-tipped catheters used in older children (157).

Bacteria acquired in the nursery may also cause pyelonephritis later in infancy. Tullus (241) found an association between pyelonephritis resulting from a nephritogenic strain of *E. coli* in children younger than 2 years and previous admission to a particular neonatal ward. Similar strains were found in stools of personnel and newborns on the ward. UTI rates over several years correlated with the bed occupancy rate on the ward at the time of admission there.

Surgical Site Infections

Neonates are also at elevated risk for surgical site infections (242,243). Reported infection rates are presented in Table 52.7. Small-for-date infants undergoing major procedures had an increased risk of infection compared with premature and term infants. Use of prophylactic antibiotics was associated with a lower infection rate after potentially contaminated surgery but not after clean surgery (244). In the largest study reported to date involving 1,433 operations over 12 years, infection rates increased over time. Risk factors for infection were increased incision length, increased duration of surgery, and contamination of the operative site, but there was no relation to gestational or chronologic age or birth weight (245). Data from our institution (246) show neonates to have higher infection rates than older children, but rates were lower than those reported in earlier publications (Table 52.7).

In contrast to these reports is one of a lower infection rate in newborns than older children, with only 1 of 137 neonatal surgical sites becoming infected (247) and another showing no difference in infection rates by age (248). The reason for these discrepancies is not apparent, but differences in patient population and types of surgical procedures must be considered. Infection rates classified by surgical site infection risk, severity of illness, and duration of operation are now used for surgical site infection surveillance (16), and a classification system is needed for newborn surgery.

S. aureus, CONS, and *E. coli* are the microorganisms most often reported (7,242,244,245). Despite the high risk of surgery-

TABLE 52.7. SURGICAL SITE INFECTION RATES AFTER NEONATAL SURGERY: PERCENTAGE OF SURGICAL SITES INFECTED

	Location and year(s) of study (reference)				
Surgical site classification	United Kingdom 1973 (242)	United Kingdom 1975–1987 (245)	United Kingdom 1989[a] (244)	India 1986[a] (243)	Montreal 1992–1997 (246)
Clean	18.5	11.1	3.9	5.3	4.6
Potentially contaminated	45	20.9	11.2	21.2	5.0
Contaminated/dirty	55.5	20.5	16.7	42.9	1.9
Total	38	16.6	—	13.7	4.5

[a] Year of report.

related infection, there are few data on the efficacy of antibiotic prophylaxis for surgical procedures in the newborn (245), and there are no precise guidelines. The American Academy of Pediatrics (AAP) includes "body cavity exploration in neonates" in a statement concerning circumstances in which prophylaxis in clean surgical site procedures may be justified (249). (For additional information on surgical site infections, see Chapter 21.)

Bone and Joint Infections

Neonatal osteomyelitis and septic arthritis are usually secondary to bacteremia or fungemia and, as such, may be of maternal or nursery origin. Osteomyelitis may also occur from local infection at sites of invasive procedures (140).

INFECTIONS CAUSED BY SPECIFIC MICROORGANISMS

Microorganisms causing infections in the normal nursery are usually true pathogens, acquired either from the mother (e.g., GBS, *Listeria,* HSV) or in the nursery (*S. aureus*, group A *Streptococcus,* bacterial enteric pathogens, and respiratory and enteric viruses). In the NICU, additional causes of infection are microorganisms that are not usually pathogenic in the healthy newborn, including gram-negative enteric bacilli, other gram-negative bacilli from water sources, and commensal microorganisms such as CONS and *Candida.*

With the development of neonatal intensive care and widespread use of antibiotics and respirator therapy, *Pseudomonas* replaced *S. aureus* as the microorganism of main concern in the nursery. With better control of environmental sources of infection, gram-negative enteric bacilli such as *Klebsiella, Enterobacter,* and *Serratia* became more prominent. Increased survival of VLBW infants and increasing use of invasive procedures have resulted in the increasing prevalence of CONS and *Candida.* Gram-positive cocci predominate in infections reported to the NNIS system in recent years (7). Viruses, not included in the earlier reports, are recognized as important causes of infection in NICU.

Staphylococcus aureus

S. aureus was recognized as a cause of newborn infection in the nineteenth century. Investigations of nursery outbreaks during the pandemic in the 1950s and 1960s contributed significantly to the understanding of nosocomial infections and the development of infection control policies. In the 1970s, less virulent strains became prominent, but *S. aureus* remains an important cause of newborn infections (250,251).

Newborns become colonized with *S. aureus* within the first few days of life at rates of 40% to 90%. The microorganism may be acquired from the mother but is more often of nursery origin (250). Mortimer and co-workers (65,66) demonstrated that transfer of infection between infants was by the hands of personnel rather than airborne. Infants rarely became infected with nursery strains unless cared for by the same personnel, even when bassinets were in close proximity. Transmission may be reduced by hand washing (65). When nurses who were staphylococcal carriers handled infants through the portholes of incubators for 10 minutes, 20 of 37 infants (54%) became colonized, yet a carrier nurse sitting between two bassinets for 8 hours a day did not transmit the microorganism (66). In most instances, personnel are transiently colonized, but outbreaks have occasionally been linked to true staphylococcal carriers (77,252).

Rates of endemic *S. aureus* disease are usually in the range of three to six infants with mild skin infection per 1,000 live births. Overall rates of colonization do not correlate with outbreaks of disease (253), which occur when more virulent strains are introduced (250). During epidemic periods, attempts were made to reduce colonization and infection by bathing infants with hexachlorophene. Concern about neurotoxicity (254) led to a discontinuation of this practice and a subsequent increase in rates of infection (255,256). Because colonization usually begins at the umbilicus, application of various antiseptic and antimicrobial agents to the umbilical stump has been used as a control measure with varying degrees of success (250). Artificial colonization with an avirulent strain of *S. aureus* has been used successfully to prevent colonization with virulent strains (257).

Infections occur in normal newborns, usually after discharge, and in infants in the NICU. Risk factors for infection include skin abrasions and invasive procedures. Most infections are benign skin pustules, but bullous impetigo, cellulitis, scalded skin syndrome, staphylococcal toxic shock, omphalitis, breast abscess, conjunctivitis, and infections of surgical sites and puncture sites occur, as do occasional cases of bacteremia, pneumonia, osteomyelitis, and enterocolitis. *S. aureus* is an important cause of infections of ventricular drains and shunts (250) (see also Chapters 27 and 49).

MRSA infections have become a problem in newborn nurseries. Most outbreaks have been described in NICUs, but outbreaks occur in normal newborn nurseries as well, where large numbers of mothers and infants may become infected because of delayed recognition (258). Infection may become endemic with persistent newborn colonization rates of more than 30% (259) and may involve multiple strains (200). The major reservoir in the nursery is the infected newborn, although infected staff are occasionally involved (78,260). MRSA strains are not necessarily more virulent but are more difficult to treat when infection does occur, which has led to renewed attempts to eliminate colonization. Cohorting and hand washing have been successful in some outbreaks (200,261). Contact Precautions were effective in another (262). Other measures used have been replacement of chlorhexidine hand wash with hexachlorophene (72,200) or triclosan (263) and application of mupirocin to the cord and nares of newborns (264). Mild skin infection is the most common manifestation, but outbreaks of severe disease have occurred (200,265) (see also Chapters 28 and 29).

Coagulase-negative Staphylococci

CONS are normal inhabitants of the newborn skin and nose and rarely cause disease in the healthy infant (210). They can colonize prosthetic materials, especially intravascular catheters and endotracheal tubes, and they produce large amounts of extracellular matrix or slime and other adherence factors (104).

The increasing prominence of CONS infections in NICUs is due to increasing numbers of infants at risk, namely, small premature infants with invasive devices. Low birth weight and prolonged NICU stay are major determinants of CONS bacteremia (266). Intravenous lipids and intravascular catheters are significant independent risk factors (12,187). It is suggested that lipids enhance the rate of bacterial growth in colonized catheters (187).

Indolent bacteremia without focal findings is the most frequent manifestation of infection. Endocarditis, abscesses, omphalitis, surgical site infections, and meningitis occur occasionally, and a mild form of NEC has been described. Pulmonary infiltrates on chest radiograph are frequent with CONS bacteremia. CONS are also the major cause of ventricular shunt and drain infections (210). Freeman et al. (267) reported that CONS infection in the newborn was associated with extra hospital stay but not with excess mortality.

Control measures involve limiting the use of invasive devices and aseptic technique for insertion and handling of intravascular and other prosthetic devices. Addition of vancomycin to intravenous fluids has been shown to reduce the incidence of CONS bacteremia in neonates but is not recommended for routine use because of potential for inducing vancomycin resistance (250). Transmission of CONS with heteroresistance to vancomycin in NICU has been reported (268). In view of increasing indications for invasive devices and the ubiquitous nature of CONS, infection rates probably will not be reduced until materials used for prosthetic devices are improved (104) (see also Chapter 30).

Streptococci

Group B Streptococci

GBS is a leading cause of neonatal sepsis and meningitis in most centers in North America and Europe. The mother is the most important source of infection with this microorganism. Approximately 20% to 35% of pregnant women are colonized with GBS, and 50% to 75% of these women will transmit the microorganism to their newborns. Only 1% to 2% of colonized newborns develop disease. Early-onset disease usually presents on the first day of life with septic shock, pneumonia, and severe multiorgan failure. Risk factors include premature labor, premature rupture of membranes, multiple births, maternal bacteremia or bacteriuria, and low maternal levels of type-specific antibody to GBS capsular polysaccharide. Several serotypes are involved. Late-onset disease, occurring after 7 days of age, usually presents as meningitis, although other focal infections and bacteremia without an identified focus may occur. Lack of maternal antibody is a risk factor, but obstetric complications are not. Most late-onset infections and meningeal infections are due to serotype III. Late-onset disease may be due to microorganisms acquired from the mother at delivery or acquired postnatally (269). Transmission in the nursery is uncommon but has been reported, especially in crowded nurseries with a high rate of maternal colonization (270).

The risk of early-onset GBS disease is reduced by maternal intrapartum antibiotic prophylaxis. The AAP in 1992 recommended screening of all pregnant women for GBS carriage and intrapartum prophylaxis for selected culture-positive women at high risk of delivering infected infants. Revisions in 1996 included alternative strategies based on screening and intrapartum treatment of all women with positive cultures or no screening and intrapartum treatment of all women with risk factors (271). Prophylaxis led to a 70% decline in the incidence of early-onset disease. However, screening was found to be more effective than the risk-based strategy (272). Current recommendations are to screen all women at 35 to 37 weeks' gestation and offer intrapartum prophylaxis to all with positive cultures except those undergoing planned cesarean section before rupture of membranes. All women with GBS bacteriuria during pregnancy or previous delivery of an infant with invasive GBS disease should be receive intrapartum treatment. If GBS status is not known at delivery, prophylaxis is indicated if gestation is less than 37 weeks, duration of amniotic membrane rupture is 18 hours or longer, or there is intrapartum fever (271). Active immunization of pregnant women is a promising approach if effective vaccines can be developed (269,271) (see also Chapter 31).

Enterococci

Newborn enterococcal infections are occasionally acquired from the mother, but there is an increasing incidence of nursery-acquired infection in low-birth-weight infants (273,274). NICU outbreaks of *S. faecium* (73) and *S. faecalis* (275) have been reported. Infants who have undergone bowel resection or CVL placement and those with prolonged hospitalization are at risk (274,275). Bacteremia is often associated with focal infection such as NEC, soft tissue abscesses, pneumonia, and meningitis (273) and is often polymicrobial (274). Vancomycin-resistant enterococcus may cause widespread colonization and occasional invasive infection in the NICU and poses a therapeutic challenge (274,276) (see also Chapter 32).

Group A Streptococci

Infection with group A *Streptococcus,* a prominent cause of newborn sepsis in the past, is now rare. Most infections were of nursery origin, introduced by the infant of an infected mother or by infected personnel and then transmitted from infant to infant. In normal newborns, infection may become manifest only after discharge (198,277). Disease is usually mild, with most infants presenting with omphalitis, but sepsis and meningitis may occur (198,199,277–279). Administration of prophylactic penicillin to all exposed infants has been successful in terminating some outbreaks but not others (198,199,277). Cohorting (199) and application of bacitracin (277), triple dye (199), or chlorhexidine (278) to the umbilical stump have been used successfully in some outbreaks (see also Chapter 31).

Other Gram-positive Bacteria

Listeria is usually maternally acquired (280). Maternal infection is foodborne, and clusters of infection in newborns usually indicate community outbreaks. Early-onset disease, often associated with maternal symptoms, presents with pneumonia and rash and multisystem disease. Meningitis is the major form of late-onset disease. Control measures include advising pregnant women to avoid unpasteurized milk products and foods epidemiologically associated with an outbreak and diagnosing and treating infection in pregnancy. Nursery transmission is reported but rare. Contaminated resuscitation equipment (82) and mineral oil used to bathe infants (95) have been implicated (see Chapter 24).

S. pneumoniae is an unusual cause of neonatal sepsis. Early-onset infection may be associated with maternal sepsis and has a poor prognosis (174). Nosocomial transmission has been reported (281).

The role of *C. difficile* as a pathogen in the newborn is questionable, although it has been associated with outbreaks of NEC. Cultures are usually negative at birth. A high incidence of asymptomatic postnatal colonization has been detected in the normal nursery and in NICUs (159,220,229) (see Chapter 36).

Enterobacteriaceae

Members of Enterobacteriaceae include normal stool flora transmitted to the newborn at birth or acquired in the nursery. These microorganisms are common causes of nosocomial bacteremia, meningitis, pneumonia, and UTI. *E. coli, Enterobacter,* and *Klebsiella* are encountered most often (7). Transmission is usually person to person via hands, although contaminated patient care items have also been involved. The Enterobacteriaceae that are normally enteric pathogens are discussed in the section on gastrointestinal infections.

E. coli, the second most frequent cause of sepsis and meningitis in the newborn, is usually of maternal origin. Newborns are particularly susceptible to strains bearing the K1 capsular antigen (173). Risk factors for infection are similar to those for GBS, although infants with *E. coli* infection tend to be of lower birth weight (17). Newborns may also acquire nursery strains of *E. coli* (51).

Klebsiella may also be transmitted from the mother but is an unusual cause of sepsis in healthy newborns. It is an important cause of epidemic and endemic infections in the NICU and was the major cause of infection in many NICUs in the 1970s and 1980s. Newborns in NICU readily become colonized; the gastrointestinal tract is the major reservoir (49). *Klebsiella* survives well on skin and is more resistant to desiccation than other Enterobacteriaceae (282). Outbreaks have been associated with enteral feeding (141) and infusion therapy practices (283) and may result in ward closure (284).Control was achieved in one outbreak after introduction of alcohol hand rinses (285).

Enterobacter species are frequent components of NICU flora and may now be more common than *Klebsiella* as causes of neonatal infections (7,67,286). Outbreaks have been associated with contaminated infant formula (130,131) and intravenous fluids (105,106,111). Sepsis may be accompanied by meningitis and focal brain lesions (194).

C. diversus infections in newborns have become increasingly prominent in recent years. This microorganism is part of the normal gastrointestinal flora and may be transmitted vertically to the newborn, occasionally causing serious infection (287,288). *Citrobacter* strains may also be endemic in NICUs (5). Outbreaks affect normal newborns and those in NICUs (76,201, 202,287) and are characterized by large numbers of colonized infants with small numbers of symptomatic infants over extended periods (201,202). Single strains differing from one hospital to another may be implicated (201), or several strains may be present in one outbreak, suggesting multiple introductions (287). Infection may be manifested as meningitis with focal brain lesions (203).

Serratia, once considered a benign commensal, is now known to cause serious endemic and epidemic infection in NICUs. Outbreaks are characterized by widespread newborn gastrointestinal colonization with the infants serving as reservoirs (87,213, 289). Contaminated intravenous fluids (109), delivery room equipment (87), breast pumps (124), and soap (80) have been implicated. Sepsis, meningitis, pneumonia, and UTIs are often associated with invasive procedures (87,109,146,289), and low-birth-weight infants are especially at risk (80,213). Conjunctivitis is often described (80,87). Resistance to antibiotics is common and may arise during treatment (196) (see also Chapter 33).

Other Gram-negative Bacilli

P. aeruginosa was a major NICU pathogen in the past but has become less prominent. It is ubiquitous in the environment and proliferates in water (101). Outbreaks have been associated with contaminated equipment (81,86). It readily colonizes skin and gastrointestinal and respiratory tracts, especially when antibiotics are used. *P. aeruginosa* causes sepsis and pneumonia (68, 81). Low-birth-weight infants are particularly at risk, and the case fatality rate is high (290). It is also an important cause of nosocomial conjunctivitis (86,169) and the leading cause of neonatal endophthalmitis (170). *Burkholderia cepacia* (291), *Ralstonia pickettii* (292), and *Stenotrophomonas maltophilia* (103) may also be acquired from environmental water sources. Outbreaks of neonatal meningitis resulting from *B. cepacia* (195) and sepsis and meningitis with *S. maltophilia* (96,293) have been described.

Flavobacterium meningosepticum is another microorganism of environmental origin that occasionally causes nosocomial infections, usually meningitis, in newborns. Outbreaks of meningitis have been related to contaminated water sources (91,93,193).

Acinetobacter calcoaceticus is often isolated from the hospital environment and skin and is usually considered a commensal microorganism. Outbreaks of bacteremia (70,112,294), meningitis, (197), and pneumonia (83) have been described. Low birth weight was a risk factor for infection.

C. fetus is an uncommon cause of stillbirths, prematurity, and severe early-onset sepsis and is usually of maternal origin (295). An outbreak of nosocomial meningitis in an NICU has been described (204). *C. jejuni* has been responsible for an outbreak of nosocomial meningitis in a normal nursery (205).

H. influenzae is found with increasing frequency in newborns with early-onset sepsis associated with prematurity and maternal complications. Infections are usually due to nonencapsulated nontypable strains (296).

Pertussis is unusual in the newborn but when it occurs is often severe. Newborns may acquire the disease from visitors (297) or personnel (298) with atypical unrecognized infection (see also Chapters 34 and 81).

Legionella infections have rarely been described in the newborn but sporadic cases occur. Infection has been linked to water used in an oxygen nebulizer and for heating feeding bottles and to postoperative contamination of a sternal incision with tap water (299). Pneumonia has been reported after water birth (300) (see also Chapters 35 and 55).

Other Bacteria

Colonization from vertical transmission of *Ureaplasma urealyticum* occurs in 22% to 58% of infants of colonized mothers, but neonatal disease is rare. *U. urealyticum* has been found in the lungs of premature infants with severe pneumonia (208, 209,301). *M. hominis* is also transmitted vertically (209). Both microorganisms have been isolated from cerebrospinal fluid and from blood of ill newborns. Nosocomial transmission has not been reported.

The infant of a mother with *Chlamydia trachomatis* infection has a 50% risk of becoming colonized. Conjunctivitis occurs in 25% to 50% of colonized infants, and 5% to 20% develop pneumonia. Infections in normal newborns become evident only after discharge from hospital. Transmission in the nursery has not been reported. Prevention involves diagnosis and treatment of the mother before delivery (208).

Congenital or perinatal tuberculosis may be acquired from an infected mother. It is rare, and diagnosis may be delayed. Infants are unlikely to transmit infection by coughing but suctioning may generate infectious aerosols. Tuberculin skin test conversions have occurred in healthcare workers exposed to infected neonates (302,303).

Candida

Newborns often acquire *Candida* at birth; 10% are colonized in the first 5 days of life. Many normal newborns develop oral thrush or diaper dermatitis, usually after discharge from hospital. *Candida* may also be acquired postnatally in the NICU (171). Common-source outbreaks have been associated with contaminated pressure transducers (154,155), syringes (110), and glycerine suppositories (98).

Systemic *Candida* infection, a disease of sick or VLBW infants, is increasing in frequency because of increased survival of infants at risk (171,304). Antibiotic therapy suppresses normal flora and allows overgrowth of *Candida,* invasive procedures provide portals of entry, PN provides growth medium, and the immature defense system of the newborn permits invasion. In a multicenter study, risk factors for colonization included use of third-generation cephalosporins, central venous catheters, intravenous lipid, and H_2-blockers (305). In one series, 27% of infants of birth weight less than 1,500 g became colonized; of those, 30% developed mucocutaneous disease and 8% developed systemic infection. Rates of systemic candidiasis in VLBW infants are 2% to 4%. Sick term infants requiring invasive procedures, especially after abdominal surgery, are also at risk. (171, 304).

Duration of antibiotic therapy was the most strongly associated independent variable identified in a case-control study of risk factors for invasive candidiasis (306). Duration of hyperalimentation, lipid infusion, and endotracheal intubation were also significantly associated with infection. In another series, prolonged antibiotic therapy and endotracheal intubation were significant risks (162). The presence of CVLs and duration of use were less important than the infusate used (306), and in one series, most infected infants received PN through peripheral lines (307). Administration of intravenous hydrocortisone was associated with dissemination in another study (308). Endotracheal colonization and colonization in the first week of life identified VLBW infants at high risk to develop systemic disease (309). Petrolatum ointment skin care increased risk of invasive disease in neonates with birth weight of less than 1,000 g (310). Systemic disease is more frequent in newborns hospitalized for more than 4 weeks (17,171).

Infection may be limited to fungemia in association with intravenous lines or to the urinary tract in association with urinary catheters. Disseminated infection may involve the lungs, kidneys, CNS, eyes, gastrointestinal tract, or skin. Symptoms are often nonspecific and suggestive of bacterial sepsis with respiratory deterioration, hypotension, and gastric distension. Diagnosis is difficult and requires a high index of suspicion, because cultures may be negative despite extensive disease (171).

Candida albicans and *Candida parapsilosis* are now the species most often involved in North American series, followed by *Candida glabrata* and *Candida tropicalis* (304,305). *C. parapsilosis* is more often associated with vascular catheters and appears to be less invasive than *C. albicans* (304,311). *C. glabrata* may be relatively resistant to fluconazole (312). Newborn infections with *Candida lusitaniae,* which may be resistant to amphotericin B, have been reported (313).

Prevention of *Candida* infection in the NICU is a challenge. Antibiotic therapy is the major risk factor for invasion, yet it is often impossible to withhold empiric antibiotic therapy in sick premature infants when bacterial infection cannot be ruled out. Attempts to prevent invasive disease with prophylactic nystatin have been unsuccessful (162,307). Administration of fluconazole prophylaxis was successful in terminating a prolonged NICU outbreak of *C. parapsilosis* (314) and reduced risk of invasive disease in VLBW babies (315). Fluconazole reduces but does not prevent colonization, and, although it may be beneficial in selected risk groups, widespread use may select for resistant *Candida* species (316) (see also Chapter 39).

Other Fungi

Yeasts

Malassezia furfur, a dimorphic lipophilic yeast causing tinea versicolor in older children, is a cause of fungemia in the NICU (317). Cultures of infants in a normal nursery were negative, whereas skin (318) and rectal (319) colonization were frequent in the NICU. The increased humidity in the incubator and the moist macerated skin of the premature infant may enhance fungus replication. Skin colonization was correlated with younger gestational age, lower birth weight, and longer NICU stay (318). Rectal colonization was increased in infants receiving antibiotics (319). Fungemia occurred exclusively in infants receiving lipids intravenously; lipids serve as a growth factor (317). Symptoms were apnea, bradycardia, interstitial pneumonitis, and thrombocytopenia (317). Although most infants recovered with removal of intravenous lines, three infants with severe pneumonia were described, two of whom died (320). Isolation of the fungus is enhanced by the use of lipid-supplemented media (317).

Malassezia pachydermatis, an animal pathogen, can also colonize infants in NICU and cause fungemia in association with intravenous administration of lipids. Disease is generally mild (321), but meningitis has been reported (322). One NICU outbreak was associated with healthcare workers' pet dogs (322).

Clusters of invasive infections with *Trichosporon asahii (beigelii),* a yeast found in the soil and water, have been described in NICUs. Infection is often fatal (323). Outbreaks of *Pichia anomala* fungemia have recently been reported in NICUs in Brazil and India (324,325).

Filamentous Fungi

Invasive infections with filamentous fungi are rare in the newborn, but sporadic cases of aspergillosis and zygomycosis have been reported (5,326–328). They occur as a result of environmental contamination with dust containing fungal spores such as may occur during hospital renovation (327) or with faulty cleaning practices. Contamination of adhesive tape has been implicated (5,326). An outbreak of *Rhizopus* infections was associated with contamination of wooden tongue depressors used to support intravascular cannulation sites (328). Spores may be inhaled or may infect puncture sites or wounds. Extreme prematurity, acidosis, renal failure, and treatment with steroids are risk factors. Infection usually progresses rapidly to death, and diagnosis is often made only at autopsy.

Neonatal infection with dermatophytes is also rare. Nurses with unrecognized infections were the sources of two nursery outbreaks of *Microsporum canis* skin infection (329). In another outbreak, nurses were infected by contact with an infected newborn (330).

Respiratory Viruses

Nosocomial respiratory virus infections reflect virus activity in the community. Because of their incubation periods, these infections are rarely recognized in normal nurseries, but respiratory viruses, especially respiratory syncytial virus (RSV), are important causes of infection in the NICU. The newborn may acquire infection from the mother, other family members or hospital staff, or other infants in the nursery. Most respiratory viruses are spread by direct, indirect, and respiratory droplet contact (132). Newborns shed viruses for prolonged periods after symptoms cease, and their surroundings become contaminated. RSV, parainfluenza, and influenza viruses survive on hands or contaminated surfaces or equipment long enough to permit transfer between patients (132,331). Hospital personnel often become infected and play an important role in nosocomial transmission (133). Newborns are likely to present with atypical features such as apnea, lethargy, and feeding difficulties, and pulmonary infiltrates on chest radiograph are common.

RSV outbreaks are most common and may include large numbers of infants (133,332–335). In one outbreak, 35% of newborns in the NICU for more than 6 days and 34% of the staff were infected (133), whereas, in another outbreak, infections occurred in 84% of newborns in the NICU for more than 3 weeks (335). Clinical manifestations range from nonspecific symptoms or mild upper respiratory tract disease to severe respiratory compromise and death. Maternal antibody may decrease the risk or modify the severity of disease (133). Disease is more severe in premature infants (335).

Concurrent outbreaks of RSV and rhinovirus (332) and parainfluenza 3 virus (334) have been described. Symptoms with rhinovirus and parainfluenza 3 virus infections were similar to those with RSV infection. Risk factors for transmission included contiguous bed space, nasogastric tubes, and tracheal intubation (332,334). Outbreaks of parainfluenza 3 infection have occurred at times of crowding and understaffing (336,337), with attack rates of 63% in infants and 25% in personnel (337). Nosocomial influenza infections in neonates have been described less often. Symptoms may be mild or may resemble bacterial sepsis. In two recent outbreaks, attack rates in neonates were 35% and 32% (338,339). Most nursery personnel had not received influenza vaccine, and 16% were symptomatic in one outbreak (338).

Nosocomial adenovirus infections may present as mild respiratory tract infections and conjunctivitis or as severe pneumonia, sepsis syndrome, and death (340,341). Severe neonatal disease may result from symptomatic maternal infection, presumably resulting from lack of passive immunity in the newborn (340). An outbreak of conjunctivitis and pulmonary disease was associated with ophthalmologic examination (172). Nosocomial respiratory adenoviral infections may contribute to the development of bronchopulmonary dysplasia in premature infants (341) (see also Chapter 48).

Enteroviruses

Neonatal enteroviral infections are commonly associated with community outbreaks. Perinatal echovirus and Coxsackie B virus infections are most frequent (342). Infants are usually infected at birth. During a community outbreak, 3.4% of mothers were found to have enterovirus in the stool at delivery. Transmission rates from mother to infant of 29% and 57% have been reported. Horizontal transmission occurs in the nursery by fecal-oral contamination.

Infants may be symptomatic within the first day of life, and outbreaks occur in normal newborn nurseries and NICUs with attack rates of 22% to 54%. Personnel may also become infected. Risk factors for infection include mouth care, gavage feeding, proximity to an infected child, and care by the same nurse (74, 343). Mild febrile illness and aseptic meningitis are the most frequent presentations, but disease may resemble bacterial sepsis. Severe hepatic necrosis may occur with echovirus infection. Coxsackie B viruses may cause myocarditis and, less often, hepatitis. Infection acquired from the mother tends to be most severe, probably because of lack of maternal antibody. Coxsackie A infections are rare in the newborn, although outbreaks of herpangina (344) and aseptic meningitis (345) have been reported.

Rotavirus

Rotavirus is endemic in many normal newborn nurseries and NICUs, and epidemics have often been described (220,226). Unlike respiratory viruses and enteroviruses, nursery rotavirus infections tend to be unrelated to community outbreaks and are usually acquired from nursery rather than maternal sources. Infection rates vary considerably from 3.5% to 15% in endemic periods to 50% during nursery outbreaks. Transmission is fecal-oral via contaminated hands or equipment. The virus survives on environmental surfaces for prolonged periods (142).

Many neonatal rotavirus infections are asymptomatic. Clinical disease occurs in up to 28% of those with positive stools and is often mild, although occasional severe disease with dehydration, bloody diarrhea, or NEC has been reported (220). Abdominal distension and bloody mucoid stools may be more prominent than watery diarrhea in premature infants (346). Enzymatic cleavage of the rotavirus outer capsid protein enhances infectivity *in vitro.* Immaturity of proteolytic enzymes in the newborn gut, the presence of antibody or trypsin inhibitors in breast milk, or immaturity of receptor sites on enterocytes have been suggested as explanations for the paucity of symptoms in newborns (220, 226). An alternative explanation may be attenuation of endemic nursery strains (226) (see also Chapter 50).

Hepatitis A

HAV may be introduced into the nursery by an infant infected by blood transfusion (114) (see Chapter 69) or by vertical transmission from a mother with acute infection (347). The virus is readily transmitted to other infants, staff members, and parents by fecal-oral contact. In one outbreak, 20% of exposed infants and 24% of exposed nurses became infected. Newborns excreted the virus for prolonged periods of up to 4 to 5 months (114). Because infection is usually asymptomatic in the newborn, outbreaks may be recognized late, only after staff members or parents become ill. Infection has spread to other nurseries when infants were transferred (348). Administration of immune globulin to all exposed contacts may be necessary to bring the outbreak to a halt (114) (see also Chapter 45).

Herpes Simplex Virus

Neonatal HSV infections are usually acquired from the mother. The infant is especially at risk if the mother has primary HSV in pregnancy. Approximately 33% to 50% of mothers with primary genital lesions transmit infection to the infant perinatally. These infants are exposed to a high virus load and lack protective maternal antibody. Risk of transmission from mothers with reactivation at delivery is low, at less than 2% to 5% (208, 349). Scalp monitors may increase the risk of infection by providing a portal of entry for the virus (138,139).

Infected infants may present with mucocutaneous lesions, encephalitis with or without mucocutaneous lesions, or disseminated multisystem disease. Despite antiviral therapy, morbidity and mortality remain significant (350). Management of HSV infection in pregnancy has been a controversial issue. Cesarian section reduces risk of transmission (351). Current recommendations are to assess the parturient for lesions at the onset of labor and consider cesarean section if lesions are present (349). The risks and benefits of cesarean section should be considered if membranes have been ruptured for more than 6 hours (208). Scalp monitors should not be used. An infant exposed during vaginal delivery should have specimens obtained for culture at 24 to 48 hours of life and be carefully observed for signs compatible with HSV infection. Prophylactic acyclovir may be indicated for exposed high-risk infants (208,349). Acyclovir suppression in late pregnancy reduces the rate of recurrent infection at delivery and may have a role in reducing the need for cesarean section (349,350,352).

Transmission of HSV in the nursery is rare, but small outbreaks have been described (353,354). Infection has been transmitted to an infant suctioned by a healthcare worker with orolabial lesions (355) (see also Chapter 43).

Varicella-Zoster Virus

Varicella is readily transmitted by the airborne route, and transmission may occur before onset of the rash. Nevertheless, varicella is rare in the newborn nursery, because most adults are immune and most infants are protected by maternal antibody. The newborn is at risk for severe perinatal disease acquired from a mother who has onset of varicella lesions from 5 days before to 2 days after delivery, presumably because virus but no antibody is transmitted to the fetus (208,349). Prophylactic varicella-zoster immune globulin (VZIG) is recommended for these newborns. Varicella may be introduced into the nursery by mothers, employees, or visitors with unrecognized infection (356,357) or by an infant with perinatal varicella (358). Hospitalized premature infants of seronegative mothers and those born before 28 weeks of gestation are at risk for more severe disease and should receive prophylactic VZIG after postnatal exposure (208,349). Severe varicella may occur despite VZIG prophylaxis; acyclovir prophylaxis may be more effective and warrants further evaluation (359) (see also Chapter 42).

Cytomegalovirus

Intrauterine and perinatal CMV infection is common and usually benign. Approximately 1% of all newborns are infected *in utero.* In most cases, the mother has reactivation of a past CMV infection, and the infant is protected from severe illness by passive transfer of antibody. Severe disease occurs when the mother has primary CMV infection in pregnancy.

Perinatal CMV acquisition during delivery or postnatal acquisition from breast milk is usually asymptomatic but may present as mild self-limited pneumonia or hepatitis at 1 to 4 months of age (360). Premature infants of birth weight less than 1,500 g who receive little maternal antibody may have severe disease (361,362).

Transfusion-acquired CMV infection has been a problem in NICUs, especially for low-birth-weight infants of seronegative mothers (113) (see Chapter 69). A sepsis-like syndrome with hepatomegaly, respiratory deterioration, and atypical lymphocytosis was described in low-birth-weight infants. Some infants died with severe multisystem involvement (113). Transmission of CMV between infants in the NICU has been reported (363) but is extremely rare (364).

The evidence suggests that nursery personnel are not at increased risk of acquisition of CMV despite widespread concern (113). Transmission of CMV requires direct inoculation of mucous membranes with fresh secretions and can be prevented by the normal nursery routine of hand washing after handling respiratory secretions or diapers (365). For the protection of both neonates and personnel, personnel should not kiss the newborns in their care (see also Chapter 44).

Human Immunodeficiency Virus

The usual source of neonatal HIV infection is the mother. Transfusion-acquired infection occurred in newborns before routine screening of blood donors for HIV (117). Vertical transmission may occur *in utero,* at delivery, or postnatally through breast milk. Zidovudine treatment during pregnancy and delivery followed by postnatal treatment of the newborn reduced the rate of HIV transmission from 25% to 8% (349). More aggressive measures such as combination antiretroviral therapy, monitoring of viral suppression, and cesarean section for women with elevated viral load at delivery reduce the risk of transmission to less than 2 % (366). In countries with resources for antiretroviral treatment, screening for HIV should be part of routine prenatal care, and all pregnant women with HIV infection should be offered antiretroviral therapy. It is recommended that the HIV-infected mother should not breast-feed if a safer alternative source of feeding is available (208,349,366).

Hepatitis B and C

The newborn may acquire HBV from a mother with chronic or acute infection in pregnancy. Infection is almost always asymptomatic in the infant, but neonatal acquisition carries a high risk of lifetime chronic infection and consequent serious liver disease in adulthood. Transmission usually occurs at delivery, and administration of hepatitis B hyperimmune globulin and vaccine at birth prevents infection in the newborn (208, 349). Transfusion-acquired HBV infection in the newborn has rarely been reported (115), even in the era before universal screening of blood donors, probably because infections were asymptomatic and not recognized (see also Chapter 45).

Approximately 5% of infants of seropositive mothers acquire HCV vertically. Whether transmission occurs *in utero* or intrapartum is not known. Breast-feeding does not appear to increase risk of transmission. Transmission risk correlates with maternal serum virus concentration and is higher in women co-infected with HIV. Infection in the newborn is usually asymptomatic but chronic. The AAP recommends screening of infants born to HCV-infected mothers and mothers at high risk. There is no prophylaxis available at present (208,349). Neonates have also acquired HCV from transfusions before universal screening of blood (116)

PREVENTION AND CONTROL OF INFECTIONS

Policies for prevention of infection in nurseries have evolved over the years from a combination of custom, common sense, and epidemiologic study. Many procedures that have been considered important are little more than rituals (5,367) carried out because of tradition and have little bearing on transmission of infection. They were based on the assumption that the sources of infection in the nursery are extrinsic and that preventing entry of microorganisms from outside will keep the nursery infection-free. The available evidence indicates that the initial source for microbial colonization of the newborn is the mother and that, subsequently, within the nursery the infants themselves are the major reservoirs. Transmission of microbes between infants is not affected by rituals performed at entry to the nursery. Thus, it makes little sense to perform surgical scrubs and don gowns or other protective apparel at entry to the nursery if similar precautions are not taken between infants. The emphasis is shifting from consideration of the nursery as a unit to consideration of each infant as a potential source and recipient of microorganisms. The AAP states that "Neonates should be approached as though they harbored colonies of unique flora that should not be transmitted to any other neonate" (365).

Infection control strategies can have an impact on NICU endemic infection rates. A multidisciplinary quality improvement model was developed by the Vermont Oxford Perinatal Network and implemented in selected NICUs. Rates of CONS bacteremia decreased in the project NICUs in comparison with control NICUs (368). In an NICU in Argentina, implementation of locally developed guidelines resulted in a decrease in bacteremia rate from 20.0 to 7.7 per 1,000 patient-days (369).

Nursery Design and Personnel

Design

Nursery design should provide adequate space for appropriate care of the infant and for the necessary equipment and sufficient numbers of strategically placed sinks. Specific recommendations have been published by the AAP in collaboration with the American College of Obstetricians and Gynecologists (ACOG) (370) and by others (371,372). A space of 30 net square feet per neonate with at least 3 feet between bassinets is recommended in the normal newborn nursery. For continuing care of low-birth-weight infants who are not ill but require more nursing hours than term infants, 50 square feet per infant with 4 feet between bassinets is recommended. Intermediate-care nurseries should have 100 to 120 square feet per patient station if subspecialty care is required, with at least 4 feet between incubators or bassinets and 5-foot-wide aisles. NICUs should have 150 square feet per infant with at least 6 feet between incubators and 8-foot aisles (370). There should be one sink for every six to eight patients in the normal newborn nursery and one sink for every three or four patients in intermediate- and intensive-care nurseries (370).

Central ventilation should be equipped with filters with efficiency of at least 90% (370). The AAP-ACOG guidelines recommend a minimum of six air exchanges per hour (370). A higher rate of 10 to 15 air exchanges per hour has been suggested (5). Canadian guidelines recommend positive pressure airflow with air passing from a ceiling entry to a floor exhaust, pulling dust downward and out (371). Each nursery should have access to at least one negative pressure isolation room, with exhaust air vented to the outside, to accommodate newborns with airborne infections (365,371,372).

During construction or renovation, including dust-generating activities such as breaking into or drilling holes in walls or ceilings or removal of ceiling tiles, newborns and patient care equipment should be protected from exposure to dust and debris that may contain fungal spores (327,371). Newborns should be moved to a separate hospital area unless impermeable barriers can be set up to prevent influx of air into the nursery from the construction zone.

With the trend toward encouraging early contacts between newborns and their families, rooming-in programs for healthy newborns and early discharge from the hospital have become prevalent in North America (370,371). Both practices reduce the risk of exposure of the newborn to flora of other infants. Studies suggest that infection rates are lower for infants rooming with their mothers than for those in communal nurseries (373, 374).

Staffing

Staffing should be sufficient to allow for adequate care of infants with sufficient time for hand washing between patient contacts. For normal newborn nurseries, recommendations are one nurse for every six to eight infants or for every three to four mother-infant pairs. A ratio of one nurse for every two to three patients is recommended in intermediate-care units and of one nurse for every one to two patients in NICUs (370,371).

Employee Health

Personnel should be immune to rubella, measles, mumps, varicella, HBV (375), and polio (208) and should receive influenza vaccine annually (365,375). Tuberculin reactivity should be determined on employment and periodically (365,375). Acellular pertussis vaccine should be considered if an adult formulation is available (376).

It is important that employees understand the risks of transmission of contagious diseases to newborns and report acute infections for assessment. It is rarely feasible to remove all persons with communicable infection from the nursery, and decisions should be made on an individual basis, taking into consideration the mode of transmission of the particular infection and the ability of the employee to comply with preventive measures. Employees with exudative or herpetic hand lesions should not have direct patient contact or handle patient care equipment. Personnel with herpes labialis are unlikely to transmit infection but should avoid touching the lesions during patient care and cover any external lesions (365).

Nonimmune persons exposed to varicella, measles, or rubella should not work during the latter part of the incubation period, because these diseases may be transmitted for a few days before eruption of the rash (208) (see Chapter 99).

Personnel should take precautions to minimize the risk of potential infection with blood-borne viruses and should be familiar with hospital protocols for postexposure prophylaxis after occupational exposures to blood (365) (see also Chapters 78 and 79).

Routine Procedures

Hand Washing

Hand washing has been recognized as an important means of prevention of transmission of infection since the experiments of Semmelweiss (75,377); however, it is difficult to monitor or enforce, and studies show poor compliance with this procedure in the NICU (367,378–380) and in other hospital areas (367).

It is recommended that, before handling neonates for the first time on a work shift, personnel wash hands and arms to above the elbows, with care to clean all parts of the hands and beneath the nails. Watches, rings, and bracelets should be removed. Nails should be trimmed short, and no false fingernails should be worn (365,381). The optimal duration of hand washing has not been established, but sufficient time should be taken to thoroughly wash and rinse all parts of the hands. Two- (371) or 3-minute (365) scrubs have been suggested. However, performance of a prolonged scrub on entry to the nursery is likely of less benefit than careful hand washing between patients (5). A hand wash of 10 to 15 seconds before and after patient contacts should be sufficient to remove transient flora unless hands are heavily contaminated. Whether this should be with soap or antiseptic is controversial. Some recommend an antiseptic hand wash for certain specified activities only (365), and others recommend antiseptic hand wash for all hand washing in the nursery (5,371).

Antiseptic agents commonly used for hand washing are chlorhexidine and iodophors. Chlorhexidine has the advantage of being tightly bound to skin and leaving a residual antibacterial effect. It is less irritating than iodophors. In outbreaks of *S. aureus* infection, the more potent antistaphylococcal agent hexachlorophene may be indicated; however, it is less effective against gram-negative microorganisms than the former agents and, therefore, should not be used routinely. (365). Triclosan and chloroxylenol are more recently introduced hand-washing agents and less is known about their effectiveness; further evaluation is needed (381). Alcohol-based antimicrobial hand rinses are as effective as soap or water-based antiseptics, are well tolerated and convenient to use, and are especially useful when water is not available or access to sinks is limited. Hand rinses may be less effective on heavily soiled skin (381) (see also Chapter 96).

Special Attire

The requirement for special attire for persons entering the nursery has caused much controversy and needless expenditure. Unlike hand washing, this ritual is easily monitored and enforced, and compliance is good (367). Unfortunately, the donning of special attire often replaces hand washing as the entrance ritual to the nursery, and, once garbed, personnel may consider themselves to be incapable of transmitting infection. Over the years, routine use of caps, masks, and beard bags has been dropped. Most nurseries provide scrub suits or dresses that are laundered by the hospital for personnel spending most of the day in the nursery. This practice may prevent soiling of personal clothing and may be reassuring to parents in providing easy recognition of personnel but should not be considered an infection control measure.

The routine use of gowns by persons entering the nursery is of no proven value in infection control. A gown protects the infant from contact with the wearer's forearms and clothing. In practice, most contact occurs via the hands of personnel and is not prevented by use of gowns. Several studies have shown that gowns have no effect on colonization or infection rates in the newborn nursery or the NICU (379,382–385). In one report, there was a decrease in NEC during the period of gown use but no effect on other infections (386). Because NEC often occurs in clusters, this may have been coincidental.

Although it is sometimes argued that gowns serve as reminders for hand washing, this has not been shown to be so. Studies in NICU showed no difference in hand washing frequency or in traffic through the NICU when gowns were or were not used (379,385).

Current recommendations are for a long-sleeved gown to be worn by personnel holding newborns outside of the bassinet or incubator. A separate gown should be used for each infant and discarded after use or maintained exclusively for the care of that neonate and changed regularly (365), such as at the end of a shift or if wet or soiled (387).

Visitors

The advantages to the family of allowing siblings to visit newborns has been stressed (388). Limited data suggest that neonatal colonization and infection are not increased with such visits (389,390). However, introduction of highly contagious diseases such as varicella, pertussis, or RSV into a nursery has the potential for serious results.

In the normal newborn nursery, visiting in the mother's room or a special visiting room reduces the exposure of other newborns. Visiting in the NICU requires clearly defined policies. Visitors should be screened for infection and individually assessed as to potential for transmission of infection and ability to comply with instructions. The visitor should not have been recently exposed to varicella or measles (unless already immune); should not have fever or acute respiratory, gastrointestinal, or skin infection; and should be prepared in advance for the visit. The visiting child's hands should be washed before contact with the newborn, and parents should ensure adult supervision of the child during the visit. The visiting child should not have contact with newborns other than the sibling and should not handle patient care equipment (371,388,391).

Limiting the number of visitors per visiting period and the duration of visits is advisable. It may be prudent to restrict visiting during community epidemics of respiratory tract infection (333).

Decontamination and Cleaning

Examples of outbreaks of infection related to contaminated equipment were given earlier. It is important that all equipment in direct contact with skin or mucous membranes of newborns be decontaminated with a high-level disinfectant or sterilized between patients. Examining equipment such as stethoscopes should be reserved for use with one patient or decontaminated with alcohol or iodophor between uses (365,371). Respiratory support equipment such as resuscitation bags, masks, and laryngoscope blades should be in sufficient supply to permit decontamination between patients.

The nursery should be kept clean and dust free by daily cleaning using cleaning methods that minimize dust dispersal. Quaternary ammonium, chlorine, and phenolic compounds are satisfactory low-level disinfectants for nursery cleaning (365). These do not sterilize but reduce the concentration of microbes to an acceptable level. Phenolic compounds should be used with caution, because inappropriate use has been associated with absorption by the newborn resulting in hyperbilirubinemia (392) (see also Chapter 85).

It is important that NICU equipment be kept dust free, because fungal spores from dust may result in serious infections. Responsibility for the cleaning of delicate equipment, especially monitoring equipment, radiant heaters, or infant care units in constant use, must be clearly assigned, because these items are often not handled by the regular cleaning personnel (5). Incubators, open care units, and bassinets should be cleaned between infants and changed and cleaned periodically for those infants with prolonged stay (365).

Humidifier reservoirs in incubators are potential sources of *Pseudomonas, Legionella,* and other water-borne microorganisms and should not be used in nurseries in which central humidification provides sufficient humidity. If used, the reservoir should be drained, cleaned, and refilled with sterile water every 24 hours. Nebulizers and attached tubing and water traps should be replaced regularly with equipment that is sterile or has undergone high-level disinfection. Sterile water should be used in nebulizers and humidifiers (365,371). Ventilator tubing, bags, and masks should be replaced and decontaminated according to hospital protocol periodically and between patients (see Chapter 68).

Linen for newborns does not need to be autoclaved. There is no evidence of infection related to linen, and cultures of NICU linen yielded small numbers of normal skin flora only (393). Clean linen should be stored in closed cabinets to prevent dust contamination. Used linen should be handled as little as possible to avoid hand contamination and aerosolization of microorganisms (365).

Skin and Cord Care

Once the newborn's temperature has stabilized, blood and meconium should be removed with sterile cotton sponges and warm water. If soap is used it should be supplied in a single-use container or reserved for use with one infant. Because of potential exposure to blood-borne viruses, personnel should wear gloves when handling the neonate until this has been done (365). Localized skin care using warm water and a mild soap for the diaper area and other soiled areas may be sufficient throughout the nursery stay (388,371,394). Whole-body bathing and antiseptic agents are not necessary for routine newborn care but may be indicated in outbreaks.

Antiseptic agents should be used only if the benefit outweighs the risk of toxicity. When nursery *S. aureus* infections were rampant, it was common practice to bathe newborns daily with hexachlorophene. This practice was discontinued when reports of neurotoxicity in premature infants appeared (254,395). Bathing with hexachlorophene reduced *S. aureus* colonization and infection, and many nurseries reported increasing infection rates when it was discontinued (255,256,396). Hexachlorophene is useful in control of *S. aureus* outbreaks but should be used only for term infants, for no more than two baths, and at a concentration of no more than 3%; hexachlorophene should be carefully rinsed off (250). A safer alternative, although possibly less effective against *S. aureus*, is chlorhexidine. It is less toxic, and unlike hexachlorophene, cutaneous absorption is negligible (381,394). No absorption was detected when 4% chlorhexidine solution was used to bathe term infants (397) or for cord care (398). Minimal blood levels were detected in some premature infants bathed with 4% solution (399) and when 1% chlorhexidine in ethanol was used for cord care (400). No significant toxicity has been reported. Iodophors may not be safe for bathing newborns because of absorption of iodine, and isopropyl alcohol has caused skin necrosis in premature infants (394). Triclosan has been used to bathe neonates (263) but should be used with caution because there is little information about safety and efficacy (381).

Care should be taken to avoid damage to the newborn skin from excessive drying, manipulation, exposure to irritating chemicals, or other trauma (388,394,401). The skin of the premature infant is especially fragile, and minor trauma such as removal of adhesive tapes or oxygen probes may remove the outer layer of the epidermis (134,394,401). Application of topical ointment to the skin of VLBW infants decreased skin damage, intensity of skin colonization, and nosocomial bacteremia in one study (402). To prevent contamination of the product, unit dose containers are advised (394).

The cord should be cut and tied under aseptic conditions. Subsequent procedures for cord care vary, and none is clearly superior. Local applications of triple dye or bacitracin delay or reduce cord colonization in comparison to dry cord care. Alcohol hastens drying but may not affect colonization (388,371,403). Triple dye delayed, but did not prevent, eventual MRSA colonization in NICU patients in one report (259). Chlorhexidine cord care has been effective in reducing colonization and infection (404) and may be the most effective product with the least toxicity (394). Any agent used should be provided in single-dose containers or reserved for use with a single patient.

Eye Care

The eyes of the neonate should be cleaned with sterile cotton to remove secretions and debris. Topical prophylaxis against gonococcal eye infection has been routine for many years; the agents used are 1% silver nitrate drops, 0.5% erythromycin or 1% tetracycline ointment, or 2.5% povidone-iodine solution (249,388). Single-dose containers should be provided. Topical prophylaxis appears to be ineffective against neonatal *Chlamydia* conjunctivitis. Diagnosis and treatment of *Chlamydia* infection in the mother before delivery is a more effective strategy (249).

Nosocomial conjunctivitis is a frequent occurrence in the NICU. Eyes may become infected with water-borne microorganisms or from infected respiratory tract secretions. Care should be taken to avoid contaminating the eyes with secretions dripped from catheters used to suction the nasopharynx or endotracheal tube (169).

Infant Feeding

Natural breast-feeding is the optimal method of infant feeding. Human milk provides immunologic and nutritional benefits and has been reported to reduce the risk of sepsis in premature infants (405,406). When the sick newborn cannot suck, the mother may express and store breast milk. This should be done aseptically to minimize bacterial contamination. Hands should be washed with an antiseptic, and milk should be expressed into sterile containers. If a breast pump is used, all pump components in contact with milk should be washed with hot soapy water after each use (388) and sterilized or disinfected daily. Expressed milk stored in the refrigerator showed no significant growth in 48 hours (407). It is recommended that milk be stored in the refrigerator for a maximum of 48 hours or frozen for up to 6 months. Frozen milk should be thawed in the refrigerator or quickly under running or fresh warm water, because standing water may become contaminated. Milk should not be subjected to excessive heat from hot water or a microwave oven. After thawing, milk should be used promptly or stored in the refrigerator for up to 24 hours (388,408). When breast milk is stored in hospital, protocols should be established to ensure proper identification to prevent infants inadvertently being fed milk from mothers other than their own (409).

Routine microbiologic monitoring of expressed milk is not recommended (388), but screening may be advisable if there is concern about collection technique or if gastrointestinal intolerance or sepsis is suspected. The presence of gram-negative bacilli suggests contamination during collection. (122,371).

Human milk banking is an established practice in many countries (120,405), but concerns over transmission of infection have led to a decline in this practice (388). Milk donors require careful screening (371,388,391,405). They should be (a) able to carry out aseptic technique, (b) healthy and without acute or chronic infections, and (c) screened for use of drugs and medications and other factors that might impair the quality of their milk. Donors should be serologically negative for hepatitis B surface antigen (HBsAg), HIV-1, HIV-2, HCV, HTLV-I, HTLV-II, and syphilis (391) and should not have active untreated tuberculosis (388,405). Screening for CMV has also been recommended (371) but may not be indicated if milk is heated to 62.5°C (391). To ensure microbiologic safety, especially against blood-borne viruses, it is recommended that all donor milk be pasteurized at 56°C or 62.5°C for 30 minutes, even though this process results in loss of some immunologic factors (120,371, 391,388,405). The higher temperature results in more destruction of protective components (405) but may be more effective in inactivation of CMV (391). Contamination may occur after pasteurization if appropriate care is not taken during handling (126,127). The Human Milk Banking Association of North America recommends that donor milk should be used only if it contains no pathogenic bacteria and less than 10^4 nonpathogenic bacteria per milliliter (391,405). The Canadian Paediatric Society does not recommend the use of donor milk, considering that the potential risks and costs outweigh the benefits (408).

Most hospitals in North America use sterile commercial formula prepared ready to feed. This should be used within 4 hours of uncapping (388). Commercial liquid concentrates are sterile. Powdered formulas are not sterile but undergo microbiologic testing to ensure that the level of contamination meets safety requirements. These should be used only if there is no alternative (131). Formula made from liquid concentrates or powders must be prepared using aseptic technique. Detailed guidelines for aseptic preparation of infant formula have been published by the American Dietetic Association (410). Water should be sterile or boiled for 5 minutes. Utensils and containers should be sterilized or undergo decontamination to remove vegetative forms of microorganisms. Boiling for 5 minutes and cooling before use may suffice. Blenders should be cleaned after each use and sterilized daily (129). Formula should be bottled in quantities for individual feeds or for 4 hours continuous feeding, refrigerated for a maximum of 24 hours, and used within 4 hours of opening. Routine microbiologic testing is not recommended but may be indicated if problems occur.

Nasogastric feeding administration sets should be changed every 24 hours (371). Continuous infusion tube feeding should be set up with the same aseptic precautions as used for intravenous fluids. Syringes and tubing used for continuous feeding should be changed at 4 to 6 hours (388) because bacteria may multiply to high levels in small volumes held at room temperature (122).

Special Procedures

Invasive Devices

Technologic advancements in neonatal care have given rise to new and sometimes unexpected infection risks. As a general principle, whenever a new invasive procedure or device is introduced, the potential risk for nosocomial infection should be considered, protocols established to minimize this risk, and surveillance set up to monitor for infection. The need for any invasive device should be assessed daily, and use should be discontinued promptly when no longer essential.

Infection control recommendations for the insertion and maintenance of intravascular catheters, endotracheal tubes, and urinary catheters in the newborn are not different from those in other patients and are discussed elsewhere in this book and not repeated here (see Chapters 17 to 20, 22, and 49). Umbilical vessel catheters warrant special mention. Although now replaced by central lines for infants requiring long-term vascular access, they are still often used in initial management of the sick newborn. These lines should be inserted and maintained with aseptic technique, but the nonsterile insertion site and devitalized cord tissue increase the potential for colonization. It is recommended that umbilical arterial catheters be removed before 5 days and venous catheters before 14 days of use (411). A chlorhexidine-impregnated dressing reduced colonization of intravascular catheters in neonates. Local skin reactions occurred in some low-birth-weight infants (412), precluding use of the dressing for infants younger than 7 days, especially if gestational age is less than 26 weeks (411). Central vascular catheters coated with antiseptics or antibiotics have a lower risk of infection but have not been evaluated in neonates.

Blood

Indications for transfusions of newborns have become more stringent in recent years; nevertheless, many premature or ill newborns receive blood products (413,414). In many countries, blood donors are routinely screened for HBV, HIV-1, HIV-2, HTLV-I, HTLV-II, HCV, and syphilis (391,414). All cellular blood products given to low-birth-weight infants should be from CMV-seronegative donors or treated to remove CMV (113,391, 414). Some centers use these products for all newborns. Fatal disseminated CMV infection was reported in a term infant of a CMV-seronegative mother after exposure to large volumes of unscreened blood and blood products during extracorporeal membrane oxygenation (415). If CMV-negative blood is not used for all newborns, it should be considered for seronegative infants receiving large volumes of blood and others at elevated risk of CMV disease (see also Chapter 44).

Surveillance

Surveillance for nosocomial infections in nurseries permits early detection of infection trends and clusters and identification of new risks, provides information on which to base empiric antibiotic therapy, and is a measure of quality of care. The intensity of surveillance varies with the type of nursery and the facilities available. Development of a surveillance program involves selection of definitions and determination of the types of infections to be monitored, the methods of case finding, and the denominator data to be collected (births, admissions, patient-days, birth weights, device-days).

For the NICU, infections at all sites should be monitored if this is feasible (7). If resources are limited, targeted surveillance with collection of appropriate denominators such as birth weight and device use will be more useful than total surveillance without relevant denominators. Surveillance in the normal newborn nursery should concentrate on infections likely to be associated with nursery outbreaks such as staphylococcal or streptococcal skin infections, gastroenteritis, and viral infections. Because many of these infections manifest only after discharge, coordination with community healthcare providers is essential.

Routine surveillance cultures are generally not recommended, because colonization is not a good positive predictor of infection and correlation of isolates from surveillance cultures and invasive infections has been poor (215,416–418). In outbreaks, surveillance cultures may be indicated to identify colonized infants for purposes of cohorting or isolation or for assessment of risk factors for acquisition of the microorganism (5,365,371). (For more details on the surveillance of nosocomial infections, see Chapter 94.)

Isolation Procedures

Revised guidelines for isolation precautions for hospitalized patients were published by CDC in 1996 (419) and Health

Canada in 1999 (387). CDC Standard Precautions refer to barrier precautions to be taken with all patients to reduce transmission from recognized and unrecognized sources. This principle embodies the concept that the flora of neonatal patients should not be shared. Standard Precautions include (a) hand washing between patient contacts and after removal of gloves; (b) use of gloves for touching the patient's mucous membranes or nonintact skin and for all contact with blood, body fluids, secretions, excretions, and contaminated items; (c) removal of gloves promptly after use and before going to another patient; (d) use of masks, protective eyewear, and gowns to protect the healthcare worker's mucous membranes and uncovered skin during procedures that are likely to generate splashes or sprays of body substances; (e) care in handling patient care equipment and linen to avoid contamination of skin and mucous membranes; (f) provision of resuscitation bags, mouthpieces, and mechanical suctioning equipment to eliminate the need for emergency procedures involving oral suctioning; and (g) taking precautions to reduce the risk of injury from needles and other sharp instruments.

Standard Precautions should be sufficient to prevent transmission of most infections encountered in nurseries. Extensive use of gloves may not be indicated if appropriate hand washing is performed. The AAP suggests that gloving is not mandatory for diapering of infants (391). Additional transmission-based precautions (Airborne, Droplet, or Contact) are recommended for certain clinical conditions and infectious agents based on modes of transmission of the microbes known or suspected to be involved (387,419).

Prevention of airborne transmission, such as occurs with varicella, measles, or tuberculosis, requires a single room with negative pressure ventilation. The infant of a mother with perinatal varicella or measles requires similar isolation. Fortunately, these infections are rare in the nursery. Forced-air incubators cannot be substituted for isolation rooms, because they discharge unfiltered air into the nursery (391). High-efficiency filtration masks should be worn by nonimmune healthcare workers who must enter the room. Droplet Precautions require that a mask is worn when within 3 feet of the patient. For Contact Precautions, gloves are recommended for entry into the room or the patient's designated bed space in a shared room and gowns for substantial contact with the patient, environmental surfaces, or items in the room.

Although single rooms are recommended with Droplet and Contact Precautions, they are not mandatory and may be inadequate for the care of the critically ill child needing close observation. Newborns are nonmobile, so transmission by direct contact is not a problem, and they do not grossly contaminate their environments. Separate isolation rooms are not considered to be necessary for newborns if the following conditions are met: (a) the infection is not transmitted by the airborne route, (b) there is sufficient space for a 4- to 6-foot aisle between infant stations, (c) there are an adequate number of nursing and medical personnel and they have sufficient time for hand washing, (d) an adequate number of sinks are available for hand washing, and (e) continuing instruction is given to personnel about the ways that infections are spread (365,391).

Isolation requirements are determined by the number of infected or colonized newborns in the nursery and the care required by the newborn. In the normal newborn nursery, the most feasible policy may be to isolate the occasional newborn with gastroenteritis, respiratory tract infection, or infectious skin lesions in a single room or to have the newborn room with the mother. When multiple cases of infection occur, as is common during community outbreaks of viral infection, cohorting in a communal nursery is more feasible than use of isolation rooms. An isolation area can be defined in the nursery or NICU by curtains, partitions, or other markers. A closed incubator may be helpful in maintaining barrier precautions, but because incubator surfaces and entry ports readily become contaminated with the microorganisms carried by the infant, the outside of the incubator should be considered contaminated and the boundaries of the isolation area should extend beyond the incubator itself. Where droplet precautions are required, infected infants should be separated from other patients by a distance sufficient to prevent transmission of large droplets (at least 3 feet). Newborns are unlikely to generate large-droplet aerosols, but aerosolization may be a problem with infected infants on respirators.

Respiratory viral infections are a significant problem in NICU. Most respiratory viral infections are spread by large droplets and by contact with respiratory secretions. Healthcare workers are at high risk for nosocomial respiratory viral infections (133,336–338) and should take precautions to prevent inoculation of their eyes or mucous membranes with infectious respiratory secretions. Gloves reduce the risk of accidental inoculation (420). Masks alone are of little value, but goggles and face shields may give added protection against inoculation (421).

The Infected Mother

Infection control precautions for the mother with peripartum communicable infection are similar to those for other patients (387,419). Transmission of maternal infection to the newborn usually occurs during delivery, and postpartum separation of mother and newborn is rarely necessary. Most maternal postpartum infections are urinary or gynecologic from endogenous flora. The mother with a communicable infection should wash her hands before handling the infant and take measures to prevent contact of the infant with potentially contaminated clothing, bedclothes, tissues, and other fomites (365).

Untreated active pulmonary tuberculosis in the mother is an indication for separation of the newborn until the mother is considered noninfectious (see Chapter 37). The newborn who has received VZIG may remain with the mother (349). Separation should be considered if a mother has extensive *S. aureus* infection with drainage not contained by dressings (371) or if a mother has a group A *Streptococcus* infection until she has received antibiotic therapy and the infection is no longer communicable (365).

Mothers with HIV infection should not breast-feed. Those with active untreated tuberculosis should not breast-feed until they have received adequate therapy. Otherwise, breast-feeding by the infected mother is rarely dangerous for her infant. HSV lesions around the nipples are a contraindication. AAP suggests that mothers with antibody to HTLV-I or HTLV-II should not breast-feed, pending further knowledge about transmission of these agents. For mothers with primary CMV infection who are seronegative at delivery and CMV-seropositive mothers who deliver VLBW infants, potential risks and benefits of breast-feeding should be weighed; pasteurization of milk may be considered (362,388,391).

Antibiotic therapy per se is not a contraindication but depends on the choice of antibiotic, because many are harmless to the newborn or are excreted in minimal amounts in breast milk (388,391). Breast-feeding is not contraindicated for mothers with simple mastitis on antibiotic therapy but is contraindicated for those with breast abscesses because of the risk of transmission of large doses of bacteria to the newborn (391).

Outbreak Control

A significant change over background rate in infections at a certain site or with a particular microbe should be considered an outbreak, and measures should be taken to identify the microorganisms involved, the reservoir, and the risk factors for transmission or acquisition of infection (422). Suspicion of an outbreak should lead to review of general infection control procedures, with emphasis on compliance with hand washing between infants and review of practices for sterilization and decontamination of equipment, preparation of infant formula, and aseptic techniques for invasive procedures. In many instances, such review alone has ended an outbreak before or without identification of a specific point source or problem in procedure.

Increased infection rates involving a number of different microbes or strains of the same microbe are likely to be related to (a) breakdown in infection control procedures such as occurs with crowding, understaffing, or other major disruption of the routine functioning of the unit; (b) defective sterilization or disinfection technique; or (c) a change in the use of invasive procedures.

If an epidemic microbe is suspected, attempts should be made to identify and isolate or cohort infected or colonized patients using rapid microbiologic testing. If this is not possible, infants who are symptomatic, infants who are asymptomatic but exposed, and infants who are not exposed (including new admissions) should be cohorted. Cohorts should be kept in separate rooms or in well-demarcated areas of a large room (365). Cohorting of personnel has also been recommended, but the efficacy of this has been questioned (423). It may be counterproductive if it results in understaffing and disruption of nursery routine. Enhanced attention to hand washing and barrier precautions may be more productive. Surveillance should be instituted for infants recently discharged. Potential environmental sources or personnel should be cultured only if preliminary epidemiologic investigation suggests an association with infection (371). If an outbreak is not brought under control by these measures, it may be necessary to close the unit to new admissions until all exposed infants have been discharged.

If the microorganism implicated is endemic to nursery populations, such as *S. epidermidis, E. coli,* or *Candida,* further typing by molecular techniques may be necessary to determine if a true common-source outbreak exists or if several strains are involved (61,287,424). Outbreak investigation is discussed in detail in Chapter 7.

Enhancement of Neonatal Defenses

Bacterial Interference

The principle of using one strain of bacteria to prevent colonization with another was used during the *S. aureus* pandemic, when Shinefield implanted the avirulent *S. aureus* strain 502A into the nose and umbilicus of newborns and found protection against colonization with virulent strains. This approach was used successfully to control outbreaks of *S. aureus* infections in several nurseries (250,257).

Artificial colonization of the pharynx with α-hemolytic *Streptococcus* strain 215 protected infants in NICUs from pharyngeal colonization with gram-negative microorganisms (425). Pharyngeal implantation of this strain was used, along with other infection control measures, to control an NICU outbreak of infections caused by antibiotic-resistant Enterobacteriaceae (426).

More recently, attempts to control fecal colonization with gram-negative aerobes by feeding premature infants *Lactobacillus* were unsuccessful (427,428). In other reports, antibiotic-sensitive *E. coli* strains were used successfully to suppress gastrointestinal colonization with resistant enteric microorganisms (429), and infants artificially colonized with an avirulent *E. coli* strain had fewer nosocomial infections than control infants (430).

Postexposure Prophylaxis

Postexposure antibiotic prophylaxis is recommended for the newborn of a mother with untreated gonorrhea, syphilis, infectious tuberculosis, or pertussis (208,371). Antiretroviral prophylaxis is recommended for infants born to HIV-infected mothers (366). There may be an indication for antibiotic or acyclovir prophylaxis in selected high-risk newborns with intrapartum exposure to GBS or HSV (271,208,349). Newborns exposed postnatally to pertussis or to invasive *H. influenzae* or meningococcal infection should receive prophylaxis (208).

Postexposure immunoprophylaxis for HBV and varicella were discussed earlier. Immune globulin is recommended for nonimmune newborns exposed to measles (208). Immune globulin has been administered to newborns and nursery staff to control outbreaks of HAV (114) and has been used in nursery outbreaks of enteroviral infections with variable results (342).

Immunizations

Premature infants respond well to protein antigens, including diphtheria and tetanus toxoids (431). Newborns remaining in the NICU should receive diphtheria, tetanus, acellular pertussis, *H. influenzae* B conjugate, and inactivated polio vaccines at full dose at the usual chronologic age (375). Failure to vaccinate newborns who remain in the hospital leaves them at risk for pertussis from in-hospital exposure (432). Vaccination with live polio vaccine should be deferred until discharge because of the risk of transmission of the vaccine virus to immunocompromised patients. VLBW infants respond to HBV vaccine given at birth, but response is suboptimal (433). Those born to HBsAg-positive mothers should be vaccinated at birth. Otherwise, HBV vaccination of premature infants of less than 2-kg birth weight should be deferred until weight is 2 kg or until age 2 months (375).

Conjugated pneumococcal vaccine is immunogenic in preterm infants and should also be given at the usual chronologic age (434). Neonates with chronic pulmonary disease, congenital heart disease, or other specified high-risk conditions should receive influenza vaccine at age 6 months (208,375). Influenza vaccine is recommended for pregnant women who will be in the second or third trimester during influenza season (375). Immunization during pregnancy to protect the newborn against other pathogens is an approach that is being explored (435).

Immunotherapeutic Agents

Attempts to prevent infections in premature newborns by intravenous administration of γ-globulin have had conflicting results, but recent analyses suggest there is no benefit (436,437). Effective prophylaxis probably awaits the development of immunoglobulin preparations with sufficient concentrations of antibodies against common neonatal pathogens. Immunoglobulin with high antibody titer to RSV and monoclonal anti-RSV antibody (palivizumab) are protective against RSV disease and recommended for selected high-risk infants (208).

Neutrophil transfusions may be useful as adjunctive therapy in sepsis but are not a practical prophylactic measure. Granulocyte colony-stimulating factor and granulocyte-monocyte colony-stimulating factor enhance neutrophil production and function in newborns and may have potential for prophylaxis, but data to date are inconclusive (436,438). Further advances in the understanding of immune function in the newborn may lead to new strategies to strengthen neonatal defenses.

REFERENCES

1. Goldmann DA, Freeman J, Durbin WA. Nosocomial infection and death in a neonatal intensive care unit. *J Infect Dis* 1983;147: 635–641.
2. La Gamma EF, Drusin LM, Mackles AW, et al. Neonatal infections. An important determinant of late NICU mortality in infants less than 1000 g at birth. *Am J Dis Child* 1983;137:838–841.
3. Zafar N, Wallace CM, Kieffer P, et al. Improving survival of vulnerable infants increases neonatal intensive care unit nosocomial infection rate. *Arch Pediatr Adolesc Med* 2001;155:1098–1104.
4. Garner JS, Jarvis WR, Emori TG, et al. CDC definitions for nosocomial infections, 1988. *Am J Infect Control* 1988;15:128–140.
5. Goldmann DA. Prevention and management of neonatal infections. *Infect Dis Clin North Am* 1989;3:779–813.
6. Holbrook KF, Nottebart VF, Hameed SR, et al. Automated postdischarge surveillance for postpartum and neonatal nosocomial infections. *Am J Med* 1991;91(Suppl 3B):125S–130S.
7. Gaynes RP, Edwards JR, Jarvis WR, et al. Nosocomial infections among neonates in high-risk nurseries in the United States. *Pediatrics* 1996;98:357–361.
8. Jarvis WR. Epidemiology of nosocomial infections in pediatric patients. *Pediatr Infect Dis J* 1987;6:344–351.
9. Gaynes RP, Martone WJ, Culver DH, et al. Comparison of rates of nosocomial infections in neonatal intensive care units in the United States. *Am J Med* 1991:91(Suppl 3B):192S–196S.
10. Gray JE, Richardson DK, McCormick MC, et al. Coagulase-negative staphylococcal bacteremia among very low birth weight infants: relation to admission illness severity, resource use and outcome. *Pediatrics* 1995;95:225–230.
11. Beck-Sague CM, Azimi P, Fonesca SN, et al. Bloodstream infections in neonatal intensive care unit patients: results of a multicenter study. *Pediatr Infect Dis J* 1994;13:1110–1116.
12. Avila-Figueroa C, Goldmann DA, Richardson DK, et al. Intravenous lipid emulsions are the major determinant of coagulase-negative staphylococcal bacteremia in very low birth weight newborns. *Pediatr Infect Dis J* 1998:17:10–17.
13. Auriti C, Maccallini A, Di Liso G, et al. Risk factors for nosocomial infections in a neonatal intensive-care unit. *J Hosp Infect* 2003;53: 25–30.
14. Haley RW, Cushion NB, Tenover FC, et al. Eradication of endemic methicillin-resistant *Staphylcoccus aureus* infections from a neonatal intensive care unit. *J Infect Dis* 1995;171:614–624.
15. Goldmann DA, Durbin WA, Freeman J. Nosocomial infections in a neonatal intensive care unit. *J Infect Dis* 1981;144:449–459.
16. CDC NNIS System. National Nosocomial Infections Surveillance (NNIS) System report, data summary from January 1992 to June 2002, issued August 2002. *Am J Infect Control* 2002;30:458–75.
17. Gladstone IM, Ehrenkranz RA, Edberg SC, et al. A ten year review of neonatal sepsis and comparison with the previous fifty-year experience. *Pediatr Infect Dis J* 1990;9:819–825.
18. Campins M, Vaqué J, Rosselló, et al. Nosocomial infections in pediatric patients: a prevalence study in Spanish hospitals. *Am J Infect Control* 1993;21:58–63.
19. Aavitsland P, Stormark M, Lystad A. Hospital-acquired infections in Norway: a national prevalence survey in 1991. *Scand J Infect Dis* 1992;24:477–483.
20. Sohn AH, Garrett DO, Sinkowitz-Cochran RL, et al. Prevalence of nosocomial infections in neonatal intensive care unit patients: results from the first national point-prevalence survey. *J Pediatr* 2001;139: 821-7.
21. Scheckler WE, Peterson PJ. Nosocomial infections in 15 rural Wisconsin hospitals—results and conclusions from 6 months of comprehensive surveillance. *Infect Control* 1986;7:397–402.
22. Maguire GC, Nordin J, Myers MG, et al. Infections acquired by young infants. *Am J Dis Child* 1981;135:693–698.
23. Welliver RC, McLaughlin S. Unique epidemiology of nosocomial infection in a children's hospital. *Am J Dis Child* 1984;138:131–135.
24. Horan TC, White JW, Jarvis WR, et al. Nosocomial infection surveillance, 1984. *MMWR CDC Surveill Summ* 1986;35:17SS–29SS.
25. Bureau of Communicable Disease Epidemiology, Laboratory Centre for Disease Control, Health and Welfare Canada. Canadian Nosocomial Infection Surveillance Program. Annual summary June 1984–May 1985. *Can Dis Wkly Rep* 1986;12:S1.
26. Ford-Jones EL, Mindorff CM, Langley JM, et al. Epidemiologic study of 4684 hospital-acquired infections in pediatric patients. *Pediatr Infect Dis J* 1989;8:668–675.
27. Flenik LT, Bagatin AC, Castro ME, et al. Hospital infections in a high-risk nursery: 2-year analysis. *Rev Soc Bras Med Trop* 1990;23: 91–95.
28. Josephson A, Karanfil L, Alonso H, et al. Risk-specific nosocomial infection rates. *Am J Med* 1991;91(Suppl 3B):131S–137S.
29. Boutte P, Berard E, Haas H, et al. L'infection néonatale nosocomiale dans une unité de réanimation pédiatrique et une unité d'élevage. *Pédiatrie* 1990;45:889–893.
30. Orrett FA, Brooks PJ, Richardson EG. Nosocomial infections in a rural regional hospital in a developing country: incidence rates by site, service, cost and infection control practices. *Infect Control Hosp Epidemiol* 1998;19:136–140.
31. Drews MB, Ludwig AC, Leititis JU, et al. Low birth weight and nosocomial infection of neonates in a neonatal intensive care unit. *J Hosp Infect* 1995;30:65–72.
32. Ferguson JK, Gill A. Risk-stratified nosocomial infection surveillance in a neonatal intensive care unit: report on 24 months of surveillance. *J Paediatr Child Health* 1996;32:525–531.
33. Moro ML, De Toni A, Stolfi I, et al. Risk factors for nosocomial sepsis in newborn intensive care and intermediate care units. *Eur J Pediatr* 1996;155:315–322.
34. Raymond J, Aujard Y, the European Study Group. Nosocomial infections in pediatric patients: a European, multicenter prospective study. *Infect Control Hosp Epidemiol* 2000;21:260–263.
35. Moore DL, Rodrigues R. Surveillance for nosocomial infections in a neonatal intensive care unit—a ten year perspective. *Abstracts of the*

37th Interscience Conference on Antimicrobial Agents and Chemotherapy. Washington DC: American Society for Microbiology, 1997:312.

36. Kawagoe JY, Segre CA, Pereira CR, et al. Risk factors for nosocomial infections in critically ill newborns: a 5-year prospective cohort study. *Am J Infect Control* 2001;29:109–114.
37. Stover BH, Shulman ST, Bratcher DF, et al. Nosocomial infection rates in US children's hospitals' neonatal and pediatric intensive care units. *Am J Infect Control* 2001;29:152–157.
38. Leonard EM, van Saene HK, Shears P, et al. Pathogenesis of colonization and infection in a neonatal surgical unit. *Crit Care Med* 1990; 18:264–269.
39. Khuri-Bulos NA, Shennak M, Agabi S, et al. Nosocomial infections in the intensive care units at a university hospital in a developing country: comparison with National Nosocomial Infections Surveillance intensive care unit rates. *Am J Infect Control* 1999; 27:547–552.
40. Long SS, Swenson RM. Development of anaerobic fecal flora in healthy newborn infants. *J Pediatr* 1977;91:298–301.
41. Graham JM, Taylor J, Davies PA. Some aspects of bacterial colonization in ill, low-birth-weight, and normal newborns. In: Stern L, Friis-Hansen B, Kildeberg P, eds. *Intensive care in the newborn.* New York: Masson, 1976:59–72.
42. Sprunt K, Leidy G, Redman W. Abnormal colonization of neonates in an intensive care unit: means of identifying neonates at risk of infection. *Pediatr Res* 1978;12:998–1002.
43. Bullen CL, Tearle PV, Willis AT. Bifidobacteria in the intestinal tract of infants: an in-vivo study. *J Med Microbiol* 1976;9:325–333.
44. Yoshioka H, Iseki K, Fujita K. Development and differences of intestinal flora in the neonatal period in breast-fed and bottle-fed infants. *Pediatrics* 1983;72:317–321.
45. Murono K, Fujita K, Yoshikawa M, et al. Acquisition of nonmaternal Enterobacteriaceae by infants delivered in hospitals. *J Pediatr* 1993; 122:120–125.
46. Blakey JL, Lubitz L, Barnes GL, et al. Development of gut colonization in pre-term neonates. *J Med Virol* 1982;15:519–529.
47. Goldmann DA, Leclair J, Macone A. Bacterial colonization of neonates admitted to an intensive care environment. *J Pediatr* 1978;93: 288–293.
48. Bennet R, Eriksson M, Nord C-E, et al. Fecal bacterial microflora of newborn infants during intensive care management and treatment with five antibiotic regimens. *Pediatr Infect Dis J* 1986;5:533–539.
49. Jarvis WR, Munn VP, Highsmith AK, et al. The epidemiology of nosocomial infections caused by *Klebsiella pneumoniae. Infect Control* 1985;6:68–74.
50. Toltzis P, Dul MJ, Hoyen C, et al. Molecular epidemiology of antibiotic-resistant gram-negative bacilli in a neonatal intensive care unit during a nonoutbreak period. *Pediatrics* 2001;108:1143–1148.
51. Almuneef MA, Baltimore RS, Farrel PA, et al. Molecular typing demonstrating transmission of gram-negative rods in a neonatal intensive care unit in the absence of a recognized epidemic. *Clin Infect Dis* 2001;32:220–227.
52. Singh N, Patel KM, Leger MM, et al. Risk of resistant infections with Enterobacteriaceae in hospitalized neonates. *Pediatr Infect Dis J* 2002;21:1029–1033.
53. Fonesca SN, Ehrenkrantz RA, Baltimore RS. Epidemiology of antibiotic use in a neonatal intensive care unit. *Infect Control Hosp Epidemiol* 1994;15:156–162.
54. Stoll BJ, Gordon T, Korones SB, et al. Early-onset sepsis in very low birth weight neonates: a report from the National Institute of Child Health and Human Development Neonatal Research Network. *J Pediatr* 1996;129:72–80.
55. Lee SK, McMillan DD, Ohlsson A, et al. Variations in practice and outcomes in the Canadian NICU network: 1996–1997. *Pediatrics* 2000;106:1070–1079.
56. Cordero L, Sananes M, Ayers LW. Bloodstream infections in a neonatal intensive-care unit: 12 years' experience with an antibiotic control program. *Infect Control Hosp Epidemiol* 1999;20:242–246.
57. de Man P, Verhoeven BA, Verbrugh HA, et al. An antibiotic policy to prevent emergence of resistant bacilli. *Lancet* 2000;355:973–978.
58. Calil R, Marba ST, von Nowakonski A, et al. Reduction in colonization and nosocomial infection by multiresistant bacteria in a neonatal unit after institution of educational measures and restriction in the use of cephalosporins. *Am J Infect Control* 2001;29:133–138.
59. Savey A, Fleurette J, Salle BL. An analysis of the microbial flora of premature neonates. *J Hosp Infect* 1992 21:275–289.
60. D'Angio CT, McGowan KL, Baumgart S, et al. Surface colonization with coagulase-negative staphylococci in premature neonates. *J Pediatr* 1989;114:1029–1034.
61. Huebner J, Pier GB, Maslow JN et al. Endemic nosocomial transmission of *Staphylococcus epidermidis* bacteremia isolates in a neonatal intensive care unit over 10 years. *J Infect Dis* 1994;169;526–531.
62. Sprunt K. Practical use of surveillance for prevention of nosocomial infection. *Semin Perinatol* 1985;9:47–50.
63. Uehara Y, Kikuchi K, Nakamura T, et al. Inhibition of methicillin-resistant *Staphylococcus aureus* colonization of oral cavities in newborns by viridans group streptococci. *Clin Infect Dis* 2001;32:1399–1407.
64. Hentges DJ. The anaerobic microflora of the human body. *Clin Infect Dis* 1993;16(Suppl 4):S175–180.
65. Mortimer EA, Lipsitz PJ, Wolinsky E, et al. Transmission of staphylococci between newborns. Importance of the hands of personnel. *Am J Dis Child* 1962;104:289–295.
66. Rammelkamp CH, Mortimer EA, Wolinksy E. Transmission of streptococcal and staphylococcal infections. *Ann Intern Med* 1964;60: 753–758.
67. Yu WL, Cheng HS, Lin HC, et al. Outbreak investigation of nosocomial *Enterobacter cloacae* bacteraemia in a neonatal intensive care unit. *Scand J Infect Dis* 2000;32:293–298.
68. Moolenaar RL, Crutcher JM, San Joaquin VH, et al. A prolonged outbreak of *Pseudomonas aeruginosa* in a neonatal intensive care unit: did staff fingernails play a role in disease transmission? *Infect Control Hosp Epidemiol* 2000;21:80–85.
69. Foca M, Jakob K, Whittier S, et al. Endemic *Pseudomonas aeruginosa* infection in a neonatal intensive care unit. *N Engl J Med* 2000;343: 695–700.
70. Huang YC, Su LH, Wu TL, et al. Outbreak of *Acinetobacter baumannii* bacteremia in a neonatal intensive care unit: clinical implications and genotyping analysis. *Pediatr Infect Dis J* 2002;21:1105–1109.
71. Hedberg K, Ristinen TL, Soler JT, et al. Outbreak of erythromycin-resistant staphylococcal conjunctivitis in a newborn nursery. *Pediatr Infect Dis J* 1990;9:268–273.
72. Reboli AC, John JF, Levkoff AH. Epidemic methicillin-gentamicin-resistant *Staphylococcus aureus* in a neonatal intensive care unit. *Am J Dis Child* 1989;143:34–39.
73. Coudron PE, Mayhall CG, Facklam RR, et al. *Streptococcus faecium* outbreak in a neonatal intensive care unit. *J Clin Microbiol* 1984;20: 1044–1048.
74. Kinney JS, McCray E, Kaplan JE, et al. Risk factors associated with echovirus 11 infection in a hospital nursery. *Pediatr Infect Dis J* 1986; 5:192–197.
75. Steere AC, Mallison GF. Handwashing practices for the prevention of nosocomial infections. *Ann Intern Med* 1975;83:683–690.
76. Parry MF, Hutchinson JH, Brown NA, et al. Gram-negative sepsis in neonates: a nursery outbreak due to hand carriage of *Citrobacter diversus. Pediatrics* 1980;65:1105–1109.
77. Belani A, Sherertz RJ, Sullivan ML, et al. Outbreak of staphylococcal infection in two hospital nurseries traced to a single nasal carrier. *Infect Control* 1986;7:487–490.
78. Coovadia YM, Bhana RH, Johnson AP, et al. A laboratory-confirmed outbreak of rifampicin-methicillin resistant *Staphylococcus aureus* (RMRSA) in a newborn nursery. *J Hosp Infect* 1989;14:303–312.
79. Anagnostakis D, Fitsialos J, Koutsia C, et al. A nursery outbreak of *Serratia marcescens* infection. *Am J Dis Child* 1981;135:413–414.
80. Archibald LK, Corl A, Shah B, et al. *Serratia marcescens* outbreak associated with extrinsic contamination of 1% chloroxylenol soap. *Infect Control Hosp Epidemiol* 1997;18:704–709.
81. Bobo RA, Newton EJ, Jones LF, et al. Nursery outbreak of *Pseudomonas aeruginosa*: epidemiologic conclusions from five different typing methods. *Appl Microbiol* 1973;25:414–420.
82. Nelson KE, Warren D, Tomasi AM, et al. Transmission of neonatal listeriosis in a delivery room. *Am J Dis Child* 1985;139:903–905.

83. Hartstein AI, Rashad AL, Liebler JM, et al. Multiple intensive care unit outbreak of *Acinetobacter calcoaceticus* subspecies anitratus respiratory tract infection and colonization associated with contaminated reusable ventilator circuits and resuscitation bags. *Am J Med* 1988; 85:624–631.
84. Neal TJ, Hughes CR, Rothburn MM, et al. The neonatal laryngoscope as a potential source of cross-infection. *J Hosp Infect* 1995;30: 315–321.
85. Van Der Zwet WC, Parlevliet GA, Savelkoul PH, et al. Outbreak of *Bacillus cereus* infections in a neonatal intensive care unit traced to balloons used in manual ventilation. *J Clin Microbiol* 2000;38: 4131–4136.
86. Drewett SE, Payne DJH, Tuke W, et al. Eradication of *Pseudomonas aeruginosa* infection from a special-care nursery. *Lancet* 1972;1: 946–948.
87. Montanaro D, Grasso GM, Annino I, et al. Epidemiological and bacteriological investigation of *Serratia marcescens* epidemic in a nursery and in a neonatal intensive care unit. *J Hyg (Camb)* 1984;93: 67–78.
88. Khan MA, Abdur-Rab M, Israr N, et al. Transmission of *Salmonella worthington* by oropharyngeal suction in hospital neonatal unit. *Pediatr Infect Dis J* 1991;10:668–672.
89. Gray J, George RH, Durbin GM, et al. An outbreak of *Bacillus cereus* respiratory tract infections on a neonatal unit due to contaminated ventilator circuits. *J Hosp Infect* 1999;41:19–22.
90. McAllister TA, Roud JA, Marshall A, et al. Outbreak of *Salmonella eimsbuettel* in newborn infants spread by rectal thermometers. *Lancet* 1986;1:1262–1264.
91. Abrahamsen TG, Finne PH, Lingaas E. *Flavobacterium meningosepticum* infections in a neonatal intensive care unit. *Acta Paediatr Scand* 1989;78:51–55.
92. Fleisch F, Zimmermann-Baer U, Zbinden R, et al. Three consecutive outbreaks of *Serratia marcescens* in a neonatal intensive care unit. *Clin Infect Dis* 2002;34:767–773.
93. Plotkin SA, McKitrick JC. Nosocomial meningitis of the newborn caused by a flavobacterium. *JAMA* 1966;198:194–196.
94. McCormack RC, Kunin CM. Control of a single source nursery epidemic due to *Serratia marcescens. Pediatrics* 1966;37:750–755.
95. Schuchat A, Lizano C, Broome CV, et al. Outbreak of neonatal listeriosis associated with mineral oil. *Pediatr Infect Dis J* 1991;10:183–189.
96. Mumford F, Hindes R, Given L. Nosocomial Xanthomonas meningitis/ventriculitis. *Am J Infect Control* 1993;21:85(abst).
97. Weist K, Wendt C, Petersen LR, et al. An outbreak of pyodermas among neonates caused by ultrasound gel contaminated with methicillin-susceptible *Staphylococcus aureus. Infect Control Hosp Epidemiol* 2000;21:761–764.
98. Welbel SF, McNeil MM, Kuykendall RJ, et al. *Candida parapsilosis* bloodstream infections in neonatal intensive care unit patients: epidemiologic and laboratory confirmation of a common source outbreak. *Pediatr Infect Dis J* 1996;15:998–1002.
99. McNaughton M, Mazinke N, Thomas E. Newborn conjunctivitis associated with triclosan 0.5% antiseptic intrinsically contaminated with Serratia marcescens. *Can J Infect Control* 1995;10:7–8.
100. Anonymous. Water bugs in the bassinet [Editorial]. *Am J Dis Child* 1961;101:273–277.
101. Moffet HL, Allan D, Williams T. Survival and dissemination of bacteria in nebulizers and incubators. *Am J Dis Child* 1967;114:13–20.
102. Muyldermans G, Desmet F, Pierard D, et al. Neonatal infections with *Pseudomonas aeruginosa* associated with a water-bath used to thaw fresh frozen plasma. *J Hosp Infect* 1998;39:309–314.
103. Verweij PE, Meis JF, Christmann V, et al. Nosocomial outbreak of colonization and infection with *Stenotrophomonas maltophilia* in preterm infants associated with contaminated tap water. *Epidemiol Infect* 1998;120:251–256.
104. Goldmann DA, Pier GB. Pathogenesis of infections related to intravascular catheterization. *Clin Microbiol Rev* 1993;6:176–192.
105. Matsaniotis NS, Syriopoulou VP, Theodoridou MC, et al. *Enterobacter* sepsis in infants and children due to contaminated intravenous fluids. *Infect Control* 1984;5:471–477.
106. Tresoldi AT, Padoveze MC, Trabasso P, et al. *Enterobacter cloacae* sepsis outbreak in a newborn unit caused by contaminated total parenteral nutrition solution. *Am J Infect Control* 2000;28:258–261.
107. Jarvis WR, Highsmith AK, Allen JR, et al. Polymicrobial bacteremia associated with lipid emulsion in a neonatal intensive care unit. *Pediatr Infect Dis J* 1983;2:203–208.
108. Fleer A, Senders RC, Visser MR, et al. Septicemia due to coagulase-negative staphylococci in a neonatal intensive care unit: clinical and bacteriological features and contaminated parenteral fluids as a source of sepsis. *Pediatr Infect Dis J* 1983;2:426–431.
109. Zaidi M, Sifuentes J, Bobadilla M, et al. Epidemic of *Serratia marcescens* bacteremia and meningitis in a neonatal unit in Mexico City. *Infect Control Hosp Epidemiol* 1989;10:14–20.
110. Sherertz RJ, Gledhill KS, Hampton KD, et al. Outbreak of *Candida* bloodstream infections associated with retrograde medication administration in a neonatal intensive care unit. *J Pediatr* 1992;120: 455–461.
111. Archibald LK, Ramos M, Arduino MJ, et al. *Enterobacter cloacae* and *Pseudomonas aeruginosa* polymicrobial bloodstream infections traced to extrinsic contamination of a dextrose multidose vial. *J Pediatr* 1998; 133:640–644.
112. de Beaufort AJ, Bernards AT, Dijkshoorn L, et al. *Acinetobacter junii* causes life-threatening sepsis in preterm infants. *Acta Paediatr* 1999; 88:772–775.
113. Adler SP. Nosocomial transmission of cytomegalovirus. *Pediatr Infect Dis J* 1986;5:239–246.
114. Rosenblum LS, Villarino ME, Nainan OV, et al. Hepatitis A outbreak in a neonatal intensive care unit: risk factors for transmission and evidence of prolonged viral excretion among preterm infants. *J Infect Dis* 1991;164:476–482.
115. King EA, Alter AA, Schwartz O, et al. Postexchange transfusion hepatitis in the newborn infant. *J Pediatr* 1973;83:341–342.
116. Aach RD, Yomtovian RA, Hack M. Neonatal and pediatric posttransfusion hepatitis C: a look back and a look forward. *Pediatrics* 2000; 105:836–842.
117. Saulsbury FT, Wykoff RF, Boyle RJ. Transfusion-acquired human immunodeficiency virus in twelve neonates: epidemiologic, clinical and immunological features. *Pediatr Infect Dis J* 1987;6:544–549.
118. Shulman IA, Saxena S, Nelson JM, et al. Neonatal exchange transfusions complicated by transfusion-induced malaria. *Pediatrics* 1984; 73:330–332.
119. Piccoli DA, Perlman S, Ephros M. Transfusion-acquired *Plasmodium malariae* infection in two premature infants. *Pediatrics* 1983;72: 560–562.
120. Oxtoby MJ. Human immunodeficiency virus and other viruses inhuman milk: placing the issues in broader perspective. *Pediatr Infect Dis J* 1988;7:825–835.
121. Dworsky M, Yow M, Stagno S, et al. Cytomegalovirus infection of breast milk and transmission in infancy. *Pediatrics* 1983;72:295–299.
122. Botsford KB, Weinstein RA, Boyer KB, et al. Gram-negative bacilli in human milk feedings: quantitation and clinical consequences for premature infants. *J Pediatr* 1986;109:707–710.
123. Donowitz LG, Marsik FJ, Fisher KA, et al. Contaminated breast milk: a source of *Klebsiella* bacteremia in a newborn intensive care unit. *Rev Infect Dis* 1981;3:716–720.
124. Gransden WR, Webster M, French GL, et al. An outbreak of *Serratia marcescens* transmitted by contaminated breast pumps in a special care baby unit. *J Hosp Infect* 1986;7:149–154.
125. Ryder RW, Crosby-Ritchie A, McDonough B, et al. Human milk contaminated with *Salmonella kottbus.* A cause of nosocomial illness in infants. *JAMA* 1977;238:1533–1534.
126. Stiver HG, Albritton WL, Clark J, et al. Nosocomial colonization and infection due to *E. coli* 0125:K70 epidemiologically linked to expressed breast-milk feedings. *Can J Public Health* 1977;68: 479–482.
127. Parks YA, Noy MF, Aukett MA, et al. Methicillin resistant *Staphylococcus aureus* in milk. *Arch Dis Child* 1987;62:82–83.
128. Schreiner RL, Eitzen H, Gfell MA, et al. Environmental contamination of continuous drip feedings. *Pediatrics* 1979;63:232–237.
129. Noriega FR, Kotloff KL, Martin MA, et al. Nosocomial bacteremia caused by *Enterobacter sakazakii* and *Leuconostoc mesenteroides* result-

ing from extrinsic contamination of infant formula. *Pediatr Infect Dis J* 1990;9:447–449.
130. Block C, Peleg O, Minster N, et al. Cluster of neonatal infections in Jerusalem due to unusual biochemical variant of *Enterobacter sakazakii. Eur J Clin Microbiol Infect Dis* 2002;21:613–616.
131. Himelright I, Harris E, Lorch V, et al. *Enterobacter sakazakii* infections associated with the use of powdered infant formula—Tennessee, 2001. *MMWR Mortal Morb Wkly Rep* 2002;51:298–300.
132. Graman PS, Hall CB. Epidemiology and control of nosocomial viral infections. *Infect Dis Clin North Am* 1989;3:815–841.
133. Hall CB, Kopelman AE, Douglas G, et al. Neonatal respiratory syncytial virus infection. *N Engl J Med* 1979;300:393–396.
134. Harpin VA, Rutter N. Barrier properties of the newborn infant's skin. *J Pediatr* 1983;102:419–425.
135. Lewis DB, Wilson CB. Developmental immunology and role of host defenses in fetal and neonatal susceptibility to infection. In: Remington JS, Klein JO, eds. *Infectious diseases of the fetus and newborn infant,* 5th ed. Philadelphia: WB Saunders, 2001:25–138.
136. Haley RW, Bregman DA. The role of understaffing and overcrowding in recurrent outbreaks of staphylococcal infection in a neonatal special-care unit. *J Infect Dis* 1982;145:875–885.
137. Harbarth S, Sudre P, Dharan S, et al. Outbreak of *Enterobacter cloacae* related to understaffing, overcrowding, and poor hygiene practices. *Infect Control Hosp Epidemiol* 1999;20:598–603.
138. Cordero L, Anderson CW, Zuspan FP. Scalp abscess: a benign and infrequent complication of fetal monitoring. *Am J Obstet Gynecol* 1983;146:126–130.
139. Parvey LS, Ch'ien LT. Neonatal herpes simplex virus infection introduced by fetal-monitor scalp electrodes. *Pediatrics* 1980;65: 1150–1153.
140. Asmar BI. Osteomyelitis in the neonate. *Infect Dis Clin North Am* 1992;6:117–132.
141. Berthelot P, Grattard F, Patural H, et al. Nosocomial colonization of premature babies with *Klebsiella oxytoca*: probable role of enteral feeding procedure in transmission and control of the outbreak with the use of gloves. *Infect Control Hosp Epidemiol* 2001;22:148–151.
142. Widdowson MA, van Doornum GJ, van der Poel WH, et al. Emerging group-A rotavirus and a nosocomial outbreak of diarrhoea. *Lancet* 2000;356:1161–1162.
143. Mehall JR, Kite CA, Gilliam CH, et al. Enteral feeding tubes are a reservoir for nosocomial antibiotic-resistant pathogens. *J Pediatr Surg* 2002;37:1011–1012.
144. Cronin WA, Germanson TP, Donowitz LG. Intravascular catheter colonization and related bloodstream infection in critically ill neonates. *Infect Control Hosp Epidemiol* 1990;11:301–308.
145. Nelson JD. The neonate. In: Donowitz LG, ed. *Hospital-acquired infection in the pediatric patient.* Baltimore: Williams & Wilkins, 1988: 273–294.
146. Stamm WE, Kolff CA, Dones EM, et al. A nursery outbreak caused by *Serratia marcescens*—scalp-vein needles as a portal of entry. *J Pediatr* 1976;89:96–99.
147. Landers S, Moise AA, Fraley JK, et al. Factors associated with umbilical catheter-related sepsis in neonates. *Am J Dis Child* 1991;145: 675–680.
148. Decker MD, Edwards KM. Central venous catheter infections. *Pediatr Clin North Am* 1988;35:579–612.
149. Sadiq HF, Devaskar S, Keenan WJ, et al. Broviac catheterization in low birth weight infants: incidence and treatment of associated complications. *Crit Care Med* 1987;15:47–50.
150. Chathas MK, Paton JB, Fisher DE. Percutaneous central venous catheterization. *Am J Dis Child* 1990;144:1246–1250.
151. Polberger S, Jirwe M, Svenningsen NW. Silastic central venous catheters for blood sampling and infusions in newborn infants. *Prenat Neonat Med* 1998;3:340–345.
152. Chien LY, Macnab Y, Aziz K, et al. Variations in central venous catheter-related infection risks among Canadian neonatal intensive care units. *Pediatr Infect Dis J* 2002;21:505–511.
153. Mahieu LM, De Dooy JJ, Lenaerts AE, et al. Catheter manipulations and the risk of catheter-associated bloodstream infection in neonatal intensive care unit patients. *J Hosp Infect* 2001;48:20–26.
154. Solomon SL, Alexander H, Eley JW, et al. Nosocomial fungemia in neonates associated with intravascular pressure-monitoring devices. *Pediatr Infect Dis J* 1986;5:680–685.
155. Weems JJ Jr, Chamberland ME, Ward J, et al. *Candida parapsilosis* fungemia associated with parenteral nutrition and contaminated blood pressure transducers. *J Clin Microbiol* 1987;25:1029–1032.
156. Steiner CK, Stewart DL, Bond SJ, et al. Predictors of acquiring a nosocomial bloodstream infection on extracorporeal membrane oxygenation. *J Pediatr Surg* 2001;36:487–492.
157. Kaisan GF, Elash JH, Tan LK. Bacteriologic surveillance of indwelling urinary catheters in pediatric intensive care unit patients. *Crit Care Med* 1988;16:679–682.
158. Pople IK, Bayston R, Hayward RD. Infection of cerebrospinal fluid shunts in infants: a study of etiological factors. *J Neurosurg* 1992;77: 29–36.
159. Overturf GD, Marcy SM. Focal bacterial infections. In: Remington JS, Klein JO, eds. *Infectious diseases of the fetus and newborn infant,* 5th ed. Philadelphia: WB Saunders, 2001:1047–1089.
160. Glaser JB, Engelberg M, Hammerschlag M. Scalp abscess associated with *Mycoplasma hominis* infection complicating intrapartum monitoring. *Pediatr Infect Dis J* 1983;2:468–470.
161. Nightingale LM, Eaton CB, Fruehan AE, et al. Cephalohematoma complicated by osteomyelitis due to *Gardnerella vaginalis. JAMA* 1986;256:1936–1937.
162. Faix RG, Kovarik SM, Shaw TR, et al. Mucocutaneous and invasive candidiasis among very low birth weight (<1500 grams) infants in intensive care nurseries: a prospective study. *Pediatrics* 1989;83: 101–107.
163. McKenna H, Johnson D. Bacteria in neonatal omphalitis. *Pathology* 1977;9:111–113.
164. Cushing AH. Omphalitis: a review. *Pediatr Infect Dis* 1985;4: 282–285.
165. Mason WH, Andrews R, Ross LA, et al. Omphalitis in the newborn infant. *Pediatr Infect Dis J* 1989;8:521–525.
166. Stoll BJ. The global impact of infection. *Clin Perinatology* 1997;24: 1–21.
167. Gee WF, Ansell JS. Neonatal circumcision: a ten-year overview: with comparison of the Gomco clamp and the Plastibell device. *Pediatrics* 1976;58:824–827.
168. Wiswell TE, Geschke DW. Risks from circumcision during the first month of life compared with those for uncircumcised boys. *Pediatrics* 1989;83:1011–1015.
169. King S, Devi SP, Mindorff C, et al. Nosocomial *Pseudomonas aeruginosa* conjunctivitis in a pediatric hospital. *Infect Control Hosp Epidemiol* 1988;9:77–80.
170. Lohrer R, Belohradsky BH, Bacterial endophthalmitis in neonates. *Eur J Pediatr* 1987;146:354–359.
171. Baley JE. Neonatal candidiasis: the current challenge. *Clin Perinatol* 1991;18:263–280.
172. Birenbaum E, Linder N, Varsano N, et al. Adenovirus type 8 conjunctivitis outbreak in a neonatal intensive care unit. *Arch Dis Child* 1993; 68:610–611.
173. Klein JO. Bacterial sepsis and meningitis. In: Remington JS, Klein JO, eds. *Infectious diseases of the fetus and newborn infant,* 5th ed. Philadelphia: WB Saunders, 2001:943–998.
174. Gomez M, Alter S, Kumar ML, et al. Neonatal *Streptococcus pneumoniae* infection: case reports and review of the literature. *Pediatr Infect Dis J* 1999;18:1014–1018.
175. Stoll BJ, Gordon T, Korones SB, et al. Late-onset sepsis in very low birth weight neonates: a report from the National Institute of Child Health and Human Development Neonatal Research Network. *J Pediatr* 1996;129:63–71.
176. Hervás JA, Alomar A, Salvá F, et al. Neonatal sepsis and meningitis in Mallorca, Spain, 1977–91. *Clin Infect Dis* 1993;16:719–724.
177. The WHO Young Infants Study Group. Serious infections in young infants in developing countries: rationale for a multicenter study. *Pediatr Infect Dis J* 1999;18(10 Suppl):S4–7.
178. Noel GJ, Laufer DA, Edelson PJ. Anaerobic bacteremia in a neonatal intensive care unit: an eighteen-year experience. *Pediatr Infect Dis J* 1988;7:858–862.

179. Shah SS, Ehrenkranz RA, Gallagher PG. Increasing incidence of gram-negative rod bacteremia in a newborn intensive care unit. *Pediatr Infect Dis J* 1999;18:591–595.
180. Baltimore RS, Huie SM, Meek JI, et al. Early-onset neonatal sepsis in the era of group B streptococcal prevention. *Pediatrics* 2001;108: 1094–1098.
181. Hyde TB, Hilger TM, Reingold A, et al. Trends in incidence and antimicrobial resistance of early-onset sepsis: population-based surveillance in San Francisco and Atlanta. *Pediatrics* 2002;110:690–695.
182. Isaacs D, Royle JA, Australasian Study Group for Neonatal Infections. Intrapartum antibiotics and early onset neonatal sepsis caused by group B *Streptococcus* and by other organisms in Australia. *Pediatr Infect Dis J* 1999;18:524–528.
183. The Investigators of the Vermont-Oxford Trials Network Database project. The Vermont-Oxford trials network: very low birth weight outcomes for 1990. *Pediatrics* 1993;91:540–545.
184. Stoll BJ, Hansen N, Fanaroff AA, et al. Changes in pathogens causing early-onset sepsis in very-low-birth-weight infants. *N Engl J Med* 2002;347:240–247.
185. Stoll BJ, Hansen N, Fanaroff AA, et al. Late-onset sepsis in very low birth weight neonates: the experience of the NICHD Neonatal Research Network. *Pediatrics* 2002;110:285–291.
186. Donowitz LG, Haley CE, Gregory WW, et al. Neonatal intensive care unit bacteremia: emergence of gram-positive bacteria as major pathogens. *Am J Infect Control* 1987;15:141–147.
187. Freeman J, Goldmann DA, Smith NE, et al. Association of intravenous lipid emulsion and coagulase-negative staphylococcal bacteremia in neonatal intensive care units. *N Engl J Med* 1990;323:301–308.
188. Stoll BJ, Temprosa M, Tyson JE, et al. Dexamethasone therapy increases infection in very low birth weight infants. *Pediatrics* 1999; 104:e63.
189. Walsh MC, Simpser EF, Kliegman RM. Late onset of sepsis in infants with bowel resection in the neonatal period. *J Pediatr* 1988;112: 468–471.
190. Weber TR. Enteral feeding increases sepsis in infants with short bowel syndrome. *J Pediatr Surg* 1995;30:1086–1089.
191. Unhanand M, Mustafa MM, McCracken GH, et al. Gram-negative enteric bacillary meningitis: a twenty-one-year experience. *J Pediatr* 1993;122:15–21.
192. Moreno MT, Vargas S, Poveda R, et al. Neonatal sepsis and meningitis in a developing Latin American country. *Pediatr Infect Dis J* 1994; 13:516–520.
193. Cabrera HA, Davis GH. Epidemic meningitis of the newborn caused by *Flavobacterium. Am J Dis Child* 1961;101:289–295.
194. Willis J, Robinson JE. *Enterobacter sakazakii* meningitis in neonates. *Pediatr Infect Dis J* 1988;7:196–199.
195. Krcméry V, Havlik J, Vicianová L. Nosocomial meningitis caused by multiply resistant *Pseudomonas cepacia. Pediatr Infect Dis J* 1987;6: 769.
196. Campbell JR, Diacovo T, Baker, CJ. *Serratia marcescens* meningitis in neonates. *Pediatr Infect Dis J* 1992;11:881–886.
197. Morgan MEI, Hart CA. *Acinetobacter* meningitis: acquired infection in a neonatal intensive care unit. *Arch Dis Child* 1982:57:557–559.
198. Dillon HC. 1966 Group A type 12 streptococcal infections in a newborn nursery. *Am J Dis Child* 1966;112:177–184.
199. Nelson JD, Dillon HC, Howard JB. A prolonged nursery epidemic associated with a newly recognized type of group A streptococcus. *J Pediatr* 1976;89:792–796.
200. Noel GJ, Kreiswirth BN, Edelson PJ, et al. Multiple methicillin-resistant *Staphylococcus aureus* strains as a cause for a single outbreak of severe disease in hospitalized neonates. *Pediatr Infect Dis J* 1992; 11:184–188.
201. Morris JG, Lin F-YC, Morrison CB, et al. Molecular epidemiology of neonatal meningitis due to Citrobacter diversus: a study of isolates from hospitals in Maryland. *J Infect Dis* 1986;154:409–414.
202. Lin FC, Devoe WF, Morrison C, et al. Outbreak of neonatal *Citrobacter diversus* meningitis in a suburban hospital. *Pediatr Infect Dis J* 1987;6:50–55.
203. Graham DR, Band JD. *Citrobacter diversus* brain abscess and meningitis in neonates. *JAMA* 1981;245:1923–1925.
204. Morooka T, Takeo H, Yasumoto S, et al. Nosocomial meningitis due to *Campylobacter fetus* subspecies fetus in a neonatal intensive care unit. *Acta Paediatr Jpn* 1992;34:530–533.
205. Goossens H, Henocque G, Kremp L, et al. Nosocomial outbreak of *Campylobacter jejuni* meningitis in newborn infants. *Lancet* 1986;2: 146–149.
206. James HE, Bejar R, Gluck L, et al. Ventriculoperitoneal shunts in high risk newborns weighing under 2000 grams: a clinical report. *Neurosurgery* 1984;15:198–202.
207. Webber S, Wilkinson AR, Lindsell D, et al. Neonatal pneumonia. *Arch Dis Child* 1990;65:207–211.
208. American Academy of Pediatrics. Summaries of infectious diseases. In: Pickering LK, ed. *2003 red book: report of the Committee on Infectious Diseases,* 26th ed. Elk Grove Village, IL: American Academy of Pediatrics, 2003:189–692.
209. Taylor-Robinson D. Infections due to species of *Mycoplasma* and *Ureaplasma*: an update. *Clin Infect Dis* 1996;23:671–684.
210. Hall SL. Coagulase-negative staphylococcal infections in neonates. *Pediatr Infect Dis J* 1991;10:57–67.
211. Mas-Muñoz RL, Udaeta-Mora E, Rivera-Rueda MA, et al. Infección nosocomial en recién nacidos con ventilación mecanica. *Bol Med Hosp Infant Mex* 1992;49:839–844.
212. Craven DE, Steger KA. Nosocomial pneumonia in the intubated patient. New concepts on pathogenesis and prevention. *Infect Dis Clin North Am* 1989;3:843–866.
213. Newport MT, John JF, Michel YM, Levkoff AH. Endemic *Serratia marcescens* infection in a neonatal intensive care nursery associated with gastrointestinal colonization. *Pediatr Infect Dis J* 1985;4: 160–167.
214. Sherman MP, Goetzman BW, Ahlfors CE, et al. Tracheal aspiration and its clinical correlates in the diagnosis of congenital pneumonia. *Pediatrics* 1980;65:258–263.
215. Slagle TA, Bifano EM, Wolf JW, et al. Routine endotracheal cultures for the prediction of sepsis in ventilated babies. *Arch Dis Child* 1989; 64:34–38.
216. Cordero L, Sananes M, Dedhiya P, et al. Purulence and gram-negative bacilli in tracheal aspirates of mechanically ventilated very low birth weight infants. *J Perinatol* 2001;21:376–381.
217. Berman SA, Balkany TJ, Simmons MA. Otitis media in the neonatal intensive care unit. *Pediatrics* 1978;62:198–201.
218. Rojas J, Flanigan TH. Postintubation tracheitis in the newborn. *Pediatr Infect Dis* 1986;5:714–715.
219. Jevon GP, Dunne WM, Hicks MJ, et al. *Bacillus cereus* pneumonia in premature neonates: a report of two cases. *Pediatr Infect Dis J* 1993; 12:251–253.
220. Cleary TG, Guerrant RL, Pickering LK. Microorganisms responsible for neonatal diarrhea. In: Remington JS, Klein JO, eds. *Infectious diseases of the fetus and newborn infant,* 5th ed. Philadelphia: WB Saunders, 2001:1249–1326.
221. Yankauer A. Epidemic diarrhea of the newborn, a nosocomial problem in developing countries [Editorial]. *Am J Public Health* 1991;81: 415–417.
222. Seals JE, Parrott PL, McGowan JE, et al. Nursery salmonellosis: delayed recognition due to unusually long incubation period. *Infect Control* 1983;4:205–208.
223. Beers LM, Burke TL, Martin DB. Shigellosis occurring in newborn nursery staff. *Infect Control Hosp Epidemiol* 1989;10:147–149.
224. Terrier A, Altwegg M, Bader P, et al. Hospital epidemic of neonatal *Campylobacter jejuni* infection. *Lancet* 1985;2:1182.
225. Hershkowici S, Barak M, Cohen A, et al. An outbreak of *Campylobacter jejuni* infection in a neonatal intensive care unit. *J Hosp Infect* 1987;9:54–59.
226. Haffejee IE. Neonatal rotavirus infections. *Rev Infect Dis* 1991;13: 957–962.
227. Kosloske AM. A unifying hypothesis for pathogenesis and prevention of necrotizing enterocolitis. *J Pediatr* 1990:117:S68–S74.
228. Caplan MS, Jilling T. New concepts in necrotizing enterocolitis. *Curr Opin Pediatr* 2001;13:111–115.
229. Scheifele DW. Role of bacterial toxins in neonatal necrotizing enterocolitis. *J Pediatr* 1990;117:S44–S46.

230. Rotbart HA, Nelson WL, Glode MP, et al. Neonatal rotavirus-associated necrotizing enterocolitis: case control study and prospective surveillance during an outbreak. *J Pediatr* 1988;112:87–93.
231. Keller KM, Schmidt H, Wirth S, et al. Differences in the clinical and radiological pattern of rotavirus and non-rotavirus necrotizing enterocolitis. *Pediatr Infect Dis J* 1991;10:734–738.
232. Siu YK, Ng PC, Fung SC, et al. Double blind, randomised, placebo controlled study of oral vancomycin in prevention of necrotising enterocolitis in preterm, very low birthweight infants. *Arch Dis Child Fetal Neonatal Med* 1998;79:F105–109.
233. Lucas A, Cole TJ. Breast milk and necrotising enterocolitis. *Lancet* 1990:336;1519–1523.
234. Eibl MM, Wolf HM, Fürnkranz H, et al. Prevention of necrotizing enterocolitis in low-birth-weight infants by IgA-IgG feeding. *N Engl J Med* 1988;319:1–7.
235. Hoyos AB. Reduced incidence of necrotizing enterocolitis associated with enteral administration of *Lactobacillus acidophilus* and *Bifidobacterium infantis* to neonates in an intensive care unit. *Int J Infect Dis* 1999;3:197–202.
236. Edelmann CM, Ogwo JE, Fine BP, et al. The prevalence of bacteriuria in full-term and premature infants. *J Pediatr* 1973;82:125–132.
237. Maherzi M, Guignard J-P, Torrada A. Urinary tract infection in high-risk newborn infants. *Pediatrics* 1978;62:521–523.
238. Davies HD, Ford-Jones EL, Sheng RY, et al. Nosocomial urinary tract infections at a pediatric hospital. *Pediatr Infect Dis J* 1992;11: 349–354.
239. Lohr JA, Donowitz LG, Sadler JE III. Hospital-acquired urinary tract infection. *Pediatrics* 1989;83:193–199.
240. Langley JM, Hanakowski M, Leblanc JC. Unique epidemiology of nosocomial urinary tract infection in children. *Am J Infect Control* 2001;29:94–98.
241. Tullus K. Fecal colonization with P-fimbriated *Escherichia coli* in newborn children and relation to development of extraintestinal *E. coli* infections. *Acta Paediatr Scand* 1987;334(Suppl):1–35.
242. Doig CM, Wilkinson AW. Wound infection in a children's hospital. *Br J Surg* 1976;63:647–650.
243. Sharma LK, Sharma PK. Postoperative wound infection in a pediatric surgical service. *J Pediatr Surg* 1986;21:889–891.
244. Madden NP, Levinsky RJ, Bayston R, et al. Surgery, sepsis, and nonspecific immune function in neonates. *J Pediatr Surg* 1989:24: 562–566.
245. Davenport M, Doig CM. Wound infection in pediatric surgery: a study of 1094 neonates. *J Pediatr Surg* 1993;28:26–30.
246. Moore D, Rodrigues R. Surgical site and other nosocomial infections after newborn surgery. *J Hosp Infect* 1998;40(Suppl A):Abstract p 2.2.1.15.
247. Bhattacharyya N, Kosloske AM. Postoperative wound infection in pediatric surgical patients: a study of 676 infants and children. *J Pediatr Surg* 1990;25:125–129.
248. Horwitz JR, Chawls WJ, Doski JJ, et al. Pediatric wound infections: a prospective mulicenter study. *Ann Surgery* 1998;227:553–558.
249. American Academy of Pediatrics. Antimicrobial prophylaxis. In: Pickering LK, ed. *2003 red book: report of the Committee on Infectious Diseases,* 26th ed. Elk Grove Village, IL: American Academy of Pediatrics, 2003:773–787.
250. Shinefield HR, St. Geme JW. Staphylococcal infections. In: Remington JS, Klein JO, eds. *Infectious diseases of the fetus and newborn infant,* 5th ed. Philadelphia: WB Saunders, 2001:1217–1247.
251. Wise RI, Ossman EA, Littlefield DR. Personal reflections on nosocomial staphylococcal infections and the development of hospital surveillance. *Rev Infect Dis* 1989;11:1005–1019.
252. Back NA, Linnemann CC, Pfaller MA, et al. Recurrent epidemics caused by a single strain of erythromycin-resistant *Staphylococcus aureus. JAMA* 1993;270:1329–1333.
253. Gooch JJ, Britt EM. *Staphylococcus aureus* colonization and infections in newborn nursery patients. *Am J Dis Child* 1978;132:893–896.
254. Lockhart JD. How toxic is hexachlorophene? *Pediatrics* 1972:50: 229–235.
255. Kaslow RA, Dixon RE, Martin SM, et al. Staphylococcal disease related to hospital nursery bathing practices—a nationwide epidemiologic investigation. *Pediatrics* 1973;51:418–429.
256. Johnson JD, Malachowski NC, Vosti KL, et al. A sequential study of various modes of skin and umbilical care and the incidence of staphylococcal colonization and infection in the neonate. *Pediatrics* 1976;58:354–361.
257. Shinefield HR, Ribble JC, Boris M. Bacterial interference between strains of *Staphylococcus aureus,* 1960 to 1970. *Am J Dis Child* 1971; 121:148–152.
258. Moore EP, Williams EW. A maternity hospital outbreak of methicillin-resistant *Staphylococcus aureus. J Hosp Infect* 1991;19:5–16.
259. Rosenfeld CR, Laptook AR, Jeffery J. Limited effectiveness of triple dye in preventing colonization with methicillin-resistant *Staphylococcus aureus* in a special care nursery. *Pediatr Infect Dis J* 1990;9: 290–291.
260. Farrington M, Ling J, Ling T, et al. Outbreaks of infection with methicillin-resistant *Staphylococcus aureus* on neonatal and burn units of a new hospital. *Epidemiol Infect* 1990;105:215–228.
261. Millar MR, Keyworth N, Lincoln C, et al. Methicillin-resistant *Staphylococcus aureus* in a regional neonatal unit. *J Hosp Infect* 1987;10: 187–197.
262. Jernigan JA, Titus MG, Gröschel DHM, et al. Effectiveness of contact isolation during a hospital outbreak of methicillin-resistant *Stapylococcus aureus. Am J Epidemiol* 1996:143;496–504.
263. Zafar AB, Butler RC, Reese DJ, et al. Use of 0.3% triclosan (Bacti-Stat) to eradicate an outbreak of methicillin-resistant *Stahylococcus aureus* in a neonatal nursery. *Am J Infect Control* 1995;23:200–208.
264. Hitomi S, Kubota M, Mori N, et al. Control of a methicillin-resistant *Staphylococcus aureus* outbreak in a neonatal intensive care unit by unselective use of nasal mupirocin ointment. *J Hosp Infect* 2000;46: 123–129.
265. Ish-Horowicz MR, McIntyre P, Nade S. Bone and joint infections caused by multiply resistant *Staphylococcus aureus* in a neonatal intensive care unit. *Pediatr Infect Dis J* 1992;11:82–87.
266. Freeman J, Platt R, Epstein MF, et al. Birth weight and length of stay as determinants of nosocomial coagulase-negative staphylococcal bacteremia in neonatal intensive care unit populations: potential for confounding. *Am J Epidemiol* 1990;132:1130–1140.
267. Freeman J, Epstein MF, Smith NE, et al. Extra hospital stay and antibiotic usage with nosocomial coagulase-negative staphylococcal bacteremia in two neonatal intensive care unit populations. *Am J Dis Child* 1990;144:324–329.
268. Van Der Zwet WC, Debets-Ossenkopp YJ, Reinders E, et al. Nosocomial spread of a *Staphylococcus capitis* strain with heteroresistance to vancomycin in a neonatal intensive care unit. *J Clin Microbiol* 2002; 40:2520–2525.
269. Noya FJD, Baker CJ. Prevention of group B streptococcal infection. *Infect Dis Clin North Am* 1992;6:41–55.
270. Noya FJ, Rench MA, Metzger TG, et al. Unusual occurrence of an epidemic of type Ib/c group B streptococcal sepsis in a neonatal intensive care unit. *J Infect Dis* 1987;155:1135–1144.
271. Centers for Disease Control and Prevention. Prevention of perinatal group B streptococcal disease. *MMWR Mortal Morb Wkly Rep* 2002; 51(no. RR-11):1–24
272. Schrag SJ, Zell ER, Lynfield R, et al. A population-based comparison of strategies to prevent early-onset group B streptococcal disease in neonates. *N Engl J Med* 2002;347:233–239.
273. Dobson SR, Baker CJ. Enterococcal sepsis in neonates: features by age at onset and occurrence of focal infection. *Pediatrics* 1990;85: 165–171.
274. McNeeley DF, Saint-Louis F, Noel GJ. Neonatal enterococcal bacteremia: an increasingly frequent event with potentially untreatable pathogens. *Pediatr Infect Dis J* 1996;15:800–805.
275. Luginbuhl LM, Rotbart HA, Facklam RR, et al. Neonatal enterococcal sepsis: case-control study and description of an outbreak. *Pediatr Infect Dis J* 1987;6:1022–1026.
276. Malik RK, Montecalvo MA, Reale MR, et al. Epidemiology and control of vancomycin-resistant enterococci in a regional neonatal intensive care unit. *Pediatr Infect Dis J* 1999;18:352–526.

277. Geil CG, Castle WK, Mortimer EA. Group A streptococcal infections in newborn nurseries. *Pediatrics* 1970;46:849–854.
278. Lehtonen OP, Kero P, Ruuskanen O, et al. A nursery outbreak of group A streptococcal infection. *J Infect* 1987;14:263–270.
279. Campbell JR, Arango CA, Garcia-Prats JA, et al. An outbreak of M serotype group A *Streptococcus* in a neonatal intensive care unit. *J Pediatr* 1996;129:396–402.
280. Bortolussi R. Neonatal listeriosis. *Semin Perinatol* 1990;14(Suppl 1): 44–48.
281. Melamed R, Greenberg D, Landau D, et al. Neonatal nosocomial pneumococcal infections acquired by patient-to-patient transmission. *Scand J Infect Dis* 2002;34:385–386.
282. Hart CA. *Klebsiella* and neonates. *J Hosp Infect* 1993;23:83–86.
283. Al-Rabea AA, Burwen DR, Eldeen MA, et al. *Klebsiella pneumoniae* bloodstream infections in neonates in a hospital in the Kingdom of Saudi Arabia. *Infect Control Hosp Epidemiol* 1998;19:674–679.
284. Macrae MB, Shannon KP, Rayner DM, et al. A simultaneous outbreak on a neonatal unit of two strains of multiply antibiotic resistant *Klebsiella pneumoniae* controllable only by ward closure. *J Hosp Infect* 2001;49:183–192.
285. Herruzo-Cabrera R, Garcia-Caballero J, Martin-Moreno JM, et al. Clinical assay of N-duopropenide alcohol solution on hand application in newborn and pediatric intensive care units: control of an outbreak of multiresistant *Klebsiella pneumoniae* in a newborn intensive care unit with this measure. *Am J Infect Control* 2001;29: 162–167.
286. Hervas JA, Ballesteros F, Alomar A, et al. Increase of *Enterobacter* in neonatal sepsis: a twenty-two-year study. *Pediatr Infect Dis J* 2001; 20:134–140.
287. Goering RV, Ehrenkranz J, Sanders CC, et al. Long term epidemiological analysis of *Citrobacter diversus* in a neonatal intensive care unit. *Pediatr Infect Dis J* 1992;11:99–104.
288. Finn A, Talbot GH, Anday E, et al. Vertical transmission of *Citrobacter diversus* from mother to infant. *Pediatr Infect Dis J* 1988;7: 293–294.
289. Villari P, Crispino M, Salvadori A, et al. Molecular epidemiology of an outbreak of *Serratia marcescens* in a neonatal intensive care unit. *Infect Control Hosp Epidemiol* 2001;22:630–634.
290. Leigh L, Stoll BJ, Rahman M, et al. *Pseudomonas aeruginosa* infection in very low birth weight infants: a case-control study. *Pediatr Infect Dis J* 1995;14:367–371.
291. Rapkin RH. *Pseudomonas cepacia* in an intensive care nursery. *Pediatrics* 1976;57:239–243.
292. Labarca JA, Trick WE, Peterson CL, et al. A multistate nosocomial outbreak of *Ralstonia pickettii* colonization associated with an intrinsically contaminated respiratory care solution. *Clin Infect Dis* 1999;29: 1281–1286.
293. VanCowenbergh C, Cohen S. Analysis of epidemic and endemic isolates of *Xanthomonas maltophilia* by contour-clamped homogenous electric field gel electrophoresis. *Infect Control Hosp Epidemiol* 1994; 15:691–696.
294. McDonald LC, Walker M, Carson L, et al. Outbreak of *Acinetobacter* spp. bloodstream infections in a nursery associated with contaminated aerosols and air conditioners. *Pediatr Infect Dis J* 1998;17:716–722.
295. Simor AE, Karmali MA, Jadavji T, et al. Abortion and perinatal sepsis associated with *Campylobacter* infection. *Rev Infect Dis* 1986;8: 397–402.
296. Falla TJ, Dobson SRM, Crook DWM, et al. Population-based study of non-typable *Haemophilus influenzae* invasive disease in children and neonates. *Lancet* 1993;341:851–854.
297. Valenti WM, Pincus PH, Messner MK. Nosocomial pertussis: possible spread by a hospital visitor. *Am J Dis Child* 1980;134:520–521.
298. Linnemann CC, Ramundo N, Perlstein PH, et al. Use of pertussis vaccine in an epidemic involving hospital staff. *Lancet* 1975;2: 540–543.
299. Levy I, Rubin LG. *Legionella* pneumonia in neonates: a literature review. *J Perinatol* 1998;18:287–290.
300. Franzin L, Scolfaro C, Cabodi D, et al. *Legionella pneumophila* pneumonia in a newborn after water birth: a new mode of transmission. *Clin Infect Dis* 2001;33:e103–e104.
301. Heggie AD, Bar-Shain D, Boxerbaum B, et al. Identification and quantification of ureaplasmas colonizing the respiratory tract and assessment of their role in the development of chronic lung disease in preterm infants. *Pediatr Infect Dis J* 2001;20:854–859.
302. Lee LH, LeVea CM, Graman PS. Congenital tuberculosis in a neonatal intensive care unit: case report, epidemiological investigation, and management of exposures. *Clin Infect Dis* 1998;27:474–477.
303. Saitoh M, Ichiba H, Fujioka H, et al. Connatal tuberculosis in an extremely low birth weight infant: case report and management of exposure to tuberculosis in a neonatal intensive care unit. *Eur J Pediatr* 2001;160:88–90.
304. Kossoff EH, Buescher ES, Karlowicz MG. Candidemia in a neonatal intensive care unit: trends during fifteen years and clinical features of 111 cases. *Pediatr Infect Dis J* 1998;17:504–508.
305. Saiman L, Ludington E, Dawson JD, et al. Risk factors for *Candida* species colonization of neonatal intensive care unit patients. *Pediatr Infect Dis J* 2001;20:1119–1124.
306. Weese-Mayer DE, Fondriest DW, Brouillette RT, et al. Risk factors associated with candidemia in the neonatal intensive care unit: a case-control study. *Pediatr Infect Dis J* 1987;6:190–196.
307. Leibovitz E, Iuster-Reicher A, Amitai M, et al. Systemic candidal infections associated with use of peripheral venous catheters in neonates: a 9-year experience. *Clin Infect Dis* 1992;14:485–491.
308. Botas CM, Kurlat I, Young SM, et al. Disseminated candidal infections and intravenous hydrocortisone in preterm infants. *Pediatrics* 1995;95:883–887.
309. Rowen JL, Rench MA, Kozinetz CA, et al. Endotracheal colonization with *Candida* enhances risk of systemic candidiasis in very low birth weight neonates. *J Pediatr* 1994;124:789–794.
310. Campbell JR, Zaccaria E, Baker CJ. Systemic candidiasis in extremely low birth weight infants receiving topical petrolatum ointment for skin care: a case-control study. *Pediatrics* 2000;105:1041–1045.
311. Faix RG. Invasive neonatal candidiasis: comparison of albicans and parapsilosis infections. *Pediatr Infect Dis J* 1992;11:88–93.
312. Fairchild KD, Tomkoria S, Sharp EC, et al. Neonatal C*andida glabrata* sepsis: clinical and laboratory features compared with other *Candida* species. *Pediatr Infect Dis J* 2002;21:39–43.
313. Yinnon AM, Woodin KA, Powell KR. *Candida lusitaniae* infection in the newborn: case report and review of the literature. *Pediatr Infect Dis J* 1992;11:878–880.
314. Saxen H, Virtanen M, Carlson P, et al. Neonatal *Candida parapsilosis* outbreak with a high case fatality rate. *Pediatr Infect Dis J* 1995;14: 776–781.
315. Kaufman D, Boyle R, Hazen KC, et al. Fluconazole prophylaxis against fungal colonization and infection in preterm infants. *N Engl J Med* 2001;345:1660–1666.
316. Neely MN, Schreiber JR. Fluconazole prophylaxis in the very low birth weight infant: not ready for prime time. *Pediatrics* 2001;107: 404–405.
317. Dankner WM, Spector SA, Fierer J, et al. *Malassezia fungemia* in neonates and adults: complication of hyperalimentation. *Rev Infect Dis* 1987;9:743–753.
318. Powell DA, Hayes J, Durrell DE, et al. *Malassezia furfur* skin colonization of infants hospitalized in intensive care units. *J Pediatr* 1987; 111:217–220.
319. Gross GJ, MacDonald NE, Mackenzie AMR. Neonatal rectal colonization with *Malassezia furfur*. *Can J Infect Dis* 1992;3:9–13.
320. Richet HM, McNeil MM, Edwards MC, et al. Cluster of *Malassezia furfur* pulmonary infections in infants in a neonatal intensive-care unit. *J Clin Microbiol* 1989;27:1197–1200.
321. Welbel SF, McNeil MM, Pramanik A, et al. Nosocomial *Malassezia pachydermatis* bloodstream infections in a neonatal intensive care unit. *Pediatr Infect Dis J* 1994;13:104–108.
322. Chang HJ, Miller HL, Watkins N, et al. An epidemic of *Malassezia pachydermatis* in an intensive care nursery associated with colonization of health care workers' pet dogs. *N Engl J Med* 1998;338:706–711.
323. Salazar GE, Campbell JR. Trichosporonosis, an unusual fungal infection in neonates. *Pediatr Infect Dis J* 2002;21:161–165.
324. Aragao PA, Oshiro IC, Manrique EI, et al. *Pichia anomala* outbreak in a nursery: exogenous source? *Pediatr Infect Dis J* 2001;20:843–848.

325. Chakrabarti A, Singh K, Narang A, et al. Outbreak of *Pichia anomala* infection in the pediatric service of a tertiary-care center in Northern India. *J Clin Microbiol* 2001;39:1702–1706.
326. Groll AH, Jaeger G, Allendorf A, et al. Invasive pulmonary aspergillosis in a critically ill neonate: case report and review of invasive aspergillosis during the first 3 months of life. *Clin Infect Dis* 1998;27: 437–452.
327. Krasinski K, Holzman RS, Hanna B, et al. Nosocomial fungal infection during hospital renovation. *Infect Control* 1985;6:278–282.
328. Mitchell SJ, Gray J, Morgan MEI, et al. Nosocomial infection with *Rhizopus microsporus* in preterm infants: association with wooden tongue depressors. *Lancet* 1996;348:441–443.
329. Drusin LM, Ross BG, Rhodes KH, et al. Nosocomial ringworm in a neonatal intensive care unit: a nurse and her cat. *Infect Control Hosp Epidemiol* 2000;21:605–607.
330. Mossovitch M, Mossovitch B, Alkan M. Nosocomial dermatophytosis caused by *Microsporum canis* in a newborn department. *Infect Control* 1986;7:593–595.
331. Brady MT, Evans J, Cuartas J. Survival and disinfection of parainfluenza viruses on environmental surfaces. *Am J Infect Control* 1990;18: 18–23.
332. Valenti WM, Clarke TA, Hall CB, et al. Concurrent outbreaks of rhinovirus and respiratory syncytial virus in an intensive care nursery: epidemiology and associated risk factors. *J Pediatr* 1982;100: 722–726.
333. Snydman DR, Greer C, Meissner HC, et al. Prevention of nosocomial transmission of respiratory syncytial virus in a newborn nursery. *Infect Control Hosp Epidemiol* 1988;9:105–108.
334. Meissner HC, Murray SA, Kiernan MA, et al. A simultaneous outbreak of respiratory syncytial virus and parainfluenza virus type 3 in a newborn nursery. *J Pediatr* 1984;104:680–684.
335. Wilson CW, Stevenson DK, Arvin AM. A concurrent epidemic of respiratory syncytial virus and echovirus 7 infections in an intensive care nursery. *Pediatr Infect Dis J* 1989;8:24–29.
336. Singh-Naz N, Willy M, Riggs N. Outbreak of parainfluenza virus type 3 in a neonatal nursery. *Pediatr Infect Dis J* 1990;9:31–33.
337. Moisiuk SE, Robson D, Klass L, et al. Outbreak of parainfluenza virus type 3 in an intermediate care neonatal nursery. *Pediatr Infect Dis J* 1998;17:49–53.
338. Cunney RJ, Bialachowski A, Thornley D, et al. An outbreak of influenza A in a neonatal intensive care unit. *Infect Control Hosp Epidemiol* 2000;21:449–454.
339. Sagrera X, Ginovart G, Raspall F, et al. Outbreaks of influenza A virus infection in neonatal intensive care units.*Pediatr Infect Dis J* 2002;1:196–200.
340. Abzug MJ, Levin MJ. Neonatal adenovirus infection: four patients and review of the literature. *Pediatrics* 1991;87:890–896.
341. Piedra PA, Kasel JA, Norton HJ, et al. Description of an adenovirus type 8 outbreak in hospitalized neonates born prematurely. *Pediatr Infect Dis J* 1992;11:460–465.
342. Modlin JF. Perinatal echovirus and group B coxsackievirus infections. *Clin Perinatol* 1988;15:233–246.
343. Rabkin CS, Telzak EE, Ho MS, et al. Outbreak of echovirus 11 infection in hospitalized neonates. *Pediatr Infect Dis J* 1988;7: 186–190.
344. Chawareewong S, Kiangsiri S, Lokaphadhana K, et al. Neonatal herpangina caused by coxsackie A-5 virus. *J Pediatr* 1978;93:492–494.
345. Helin I, Widell A, Borulf S, et al. Outbreak of coxsackievirus A-14 meningitis among newborns in a maternity hospital ward. *Acta Paediatr Scand* 1987;76:234–238.
346. Sharma R, Hudak ML, Premachandra BR, et al. Clinical manifestations of rotavirus infection in the neonatal intensive care unit. *Pediatr Infect Dis J* 2002;21:1099–1105.
347. Watson JC, Fleming DW, Borella AJ, et al. Vertical transmission of hepatitis A resulting in an outbreak in a neonatal intensive care unit. *J Infect Dis* 1993;167:567–571.
348. Klein BS, Michaels JA, Rytel MW, et al. Nosocomial hepatitis A. A multinursery outbreak in Wisconsin. *JAMA* 1984;252:2716–2721.
349. American Academy of Pediatrics and American College of Obstetricians and Gynecologists. Perinatal infection. In: Gilstrap LC, Oh W, eds. *Guidelines for perinatal care,* 5th ed. Elk Grove Village, IL: American Academy of Pediatrics, 2002:285–329.
350. Whitley RJ, Kimberlin DW. Treatment of viral infections during pregnancy and the neonatal period. *Clin Perinatol* 1997;24:267–283.
351. Brown ZA, Wald A, Morrow RA, et al. Effect of serologic status and cesarean delivery on transmission rates of herpes simplex virus from mother to infant. *JAMA* 2003;289:203–209.
352. Scott LL, Hollier LM, McIntyre D, et al. Acyclovir suppression to prevent clinical recurrences at delivery after first episode genital herpes in pregnancy: an open label trial. *Infect Dis Obstet Gynecol* 2001;9: 75–80.
353. Hammerberg O, Watts J, Chernesky M, et al. An outbreak of herpes simplex virus type 1 in an intensive care nursery. *Pediatr Infect Dis J* 1983;2:290–294.
354. Sakaoka H, Saheki Y, Uzuki K, et al. Two outbreaks of herpes simplex virus type 1 nosocomial infection among newborns. *J Clin Microbiol* 1986;24:36–40.
355. Van Dyke RB, Spector SA. Transmission of herpes simplex virus type 1 to a newborn infant during endotracheal suctioning for meconium aspiration. *Pediatr Infect Dis* 1984;3:153–156.
356. Gershon AA, Raker R, Steinberg S, et al. Antibody to varicella-zoster virus in parturient women and their offspring during the first year of life. *Pediatrics* 1976;58:692–696.
357. Gustafson TL, Shehab Z, Brunell PA. Outbreak of varicella in a newborn intensive care nursery. *Am J Dis Child* 1984;138:548–550.
358. Friedman CA, Temple DM, Robbins KK, et al. Outbreak and control of varicella in a neonatal intensive care unit. *Pediatr Infect Dis J* 1994; 13:152–154.
359. Huang YC, Lin TY, Lin YJ, et al. Prophylaxis of intravenous immunoglobulin and acyclovir in perinatal varicella. *Eur J Pediatr* 2001;160: 91–94.
360. Demmler GJ. Summary of a workshop on surveillance for congenital cytomegalovirus disease. *Rev Infect Dis* 1991;13:315–329.
361. Yeager AS, Palumbo PE, Malachowski N, et al. Sequelae of maternally derived cytomegalovirus infections in premature infants. *J Pediatr* 1983;102:918–922.
362. Maschmann J, Hamprecht K, Dietz K, et al. Cytomegalovirus infection of extremely low-birth weight infants via breast milk.*Clin Infect Dis* 2001;33:1998–2003.
363. Spector SA. Transmission of cytomegalovirus among infants in hospital documented by restriction-endonuclease-digestion analysis. *Lancet* 1983;1:378–381.
364. Adler SP, Baggett J, Wilson M, et al. Molecular epidemiology of cytomegalovirus in a nursery: lack of evidence for nosocomial transmission. *J Pediatr* 1986;108:117–123.
365. American Academy of Pediatrics and American College of Obstetricians and Gynecologists. Infection control. In: Gilstrap LC, Oh W, eds. *Guidelines for perinatal care,* 5th ed. Elk Grove Village, IL: American Academy of Pediatrics, 2002:331–353.
366. Centers for Disease Control and Prevention. U.S. Public Health Service Task Force recommendations for the use of antiretroviral drugs in pregnant HIV-1-infected women for maternal health and interventions to reduce perinatal HIV-1 transmission in the United States. *MMWR Mortal Morb Wkly Rep* 2002;51(no. RR-18):1–38.
367. Larson E. Rituals in infection control: what works in the newborn nursery? *J Obstet Gynecol Neonatal Nurs* 1987;16:411–416.
368. Horbar JD, Rogowski J, Plsek PE, et al. Collaborative quality improvement for neonatal intensive care. NIC/Q Project Investigators of the Vermont Oxford Network. *Pediatrics* 2001;107:14–22.
369. Kurlat I, Corral G, Oliveira F, et al. Infection control strategies in a neonatal intensive care unit in Argentina. *J Hosp Infect* 1998;40: 149–154.
370. American Academy of Pediatrics and American College of Obstetricians and Gynecologists. Inpatient perinatal care services. In: Gilstrap LC, Oh W, eds. *Guidelines for perinatal care,* 5th ed. Elk Grove Village, IL: American Academy of Pediatrics, 2002:17–55.
371. Bureau of Communicable Disease Epidemiology, Health Protection Branch and Health Services Directorate, Health Services and Promotion Branch. *Infection control guidelines for perinatal care.* Ottawa, Canada: Health and Welfare Canada, 1988.

372. American Institute of Architects Academy of Architecture for Health. *Guidelines for design and construction of hospital and health care facilities.* Washington, DC: American Institute of Architects, 2001.
373. Bishop RF, Cameron DJS, Veenstra AA, et al. Diarrhea and rotavirus infection associated with differing regimens for postnatal care of newborn babies. *J Clin Microbiol* 1979;9:525–529.
374. Daschner F. Infectious hazards in rooming-in systems. *J Perinatal Med* 1984;12:3–6.
375. American Academy of Pediatrics. Active and passive immunization. In: Pickering LK, ed. *2003 red book: report of the Committee on Infectious Diseases,* 26th ed. Elk Grove Village, IL: American Academy of Pediatrics, 2003:1–98.
376. Campins-Marti M, Cheng HK, Forsyth K, et al. Recommendations are needed for adolescent and adult pertussis immunisation: rationale and strategies for consideration. *Vaccine* 2001;20:641–646.
377. Larson E. A causal link between handwashing and risk of infection? Examination of the evidence. *Infect Control Hosp Epidemiol* 1988;9: 28–36.
378. De Carvalho M, Lopes JMA, Pellitteri M. Frequency and duration of handwashing in a neonatal intensive care unit. *Pediatr Infect Dis J* 1989;8:179–180.
379. Haque KN, Chagla AH. Do gowns prevent infection in neonatal intensive care units? *J Hosp Infect* 1989;14:159–162.
380. Brown J, Froese-Fretz A, Luckey D, et al. High rate of hand contamination and low rate of hand washing before infant contact in a neonatal intensive care unit. *Pediatr Infect Dis J* 1996;15:908–910.
381. Centers for Disease Control and Prevention. Guideline for hand hygiene in health-care settings: recommendations of the Healthcare Infection Control Practices Advisory Committee and the HICPAC/SHEA/APIC/IDSA Hand Hygiene Task Force. *MMWR Mortal Morb Wkly Rep* 2002;51(no. RR-16):8–15.
382. Cloney DL, Donowitz LG. Overgown use for infection control in nurseries and neonatal intensive care units. *Am J Dis Child* 1986;140: 680–683.
383. Birenbaum HJ, Glorioso L, Rosenberger C, et al. Gowning on a postpartum ward fails to decrease colonization in the newborn infant. *Am J Dis Child* 1990;144:1031–1033.
384. Rush J, Fiorino-Chiovitti R, Kaufman K, et al. A randomized controlled trial of a nursery ritual: wearing covergowns to care for healthy newborns. *Birth* 1990;17:25–30.
385. Pelke S, Ching D, Easa D, et al. Gowning does not affect colonization or infection rates in a neonatal intensive care unit. *Arch Pediatr Adolesc Med* 1994;148:1016–1020.
386. Agbayani M, Rosenfeld W, Evans H, et al. Evaluation of modified gowning procedures in a neonatal intensive care unit. *Am J Dis Child* 1981;135:650–652.
387. Health Canada, Steering Committee on Infection Control Guidelines. Infection control guidelines. Routine practices and additional precautions for preventing the transmission of infection in health care. *Can Commun Dis Rep* 1999;25S4:1–142.
388. American Academy of Pediatrics and American College of Obstetricians and Gynecologists. Care of the neonate. In: Gilstrap LC, Oh W, eds. *Guidelines for perinatal care,* 5th ed. Elk Grove Village, IL: American Academy of Pediatrics, 2002:187–235.
389. Schwab F, Tolbert B, Bagnato S, et al. Sibling visiting in a neonatal intensive care unit. *Pediatrics* 1983;71:835–838.
390. Maloney MJ, Ballard JL, Hollister L, et al. A prospective controlled study of scheduled sibling visits to a newborn intensive care unit. *J Am Acad Child Psychiatry* 1983;22:565–570.
391. American Academy of Pediatrics. Recommendations for care of children in special circumstances. In: Pickering LK, ed. *2003 red book: report of the Committee on Infectious Diseases,* 26th ed. Elk Grove Village, IL: American Academy of Pediatrics, 2003:99–188.
392. Rutala WA. APIC guideline for selection and use of disinfectants. *Am J Infect Control* 1996;24:313–342.
393. Meyer CL, Eitzen HE, Schreiner RL, et al. Should linen in newborn intensive care units be autoclaved? *Pediatrics* 1981;67:362–364.
394. Darmstadt GL, Dinulos JG. Neonatal skin care. *Pediatr Clin North Am* 2000;47:757–782.
395. Shuman RM, Leech RW, Alvord EC. Neurotoxicity of hexachlorophene in the human. I. A clinicopathologic study of 248 children. *Pediatrics* 1974;54:689–695.
396. Dixon RE, Kaslow RA, Mallison GF, et al. Staphylococcal disease outbreaks in hospital nurseries in the United States-December 1971 through March 1972. *Pediatrics* 1973;51:413–417.
397. Husak M, Wiltshire J, Carr H, et al. Effect of Hibiclens bathing on neonatal bactericidal colonization [Abstract 714]. Twenty-first Interscience Conference on Antimicrobial Agents and Chemotherapy, Chicago, 1981.
398. Johnsson J, Seeberg S, Kjellmer I. Blood concentrations of chlorhexidine in neonates undergoing routine cord care with 4% chlorhexidine gluconate solution. *Acta Paediatr Scand* 1987;76:675–676.
399. Cowen J, Ellis SH, McAinsh J. Absorption of chlorhexidine from the intact skin of newborn infants. *Arch Dis Child* 1979;54:379–383.
400. Aggett PJ, Cooper LV, Ellis SH, et al. Percutaneous absorption of chlorhexidine in neonatal cord care. *Arch Dis Child* 1981;56: 878–891.
401. Lund CH, Osborne JW, Kuller J, et al. Neonatal skin care: clinical outcomes of the AWHONN/NANN evidence-based clinical practice guideline. *J Obstet Gynecol Neonatal Nurs* 2001;30:41–51.
402. Nopper AJ, Horii KA, Sookdeo-Drost S, et al. Topical ointment therapy benefits premature infants. *J Pediatr* 1996;128:660–669.
403. Janssen PA, Selwood BL, Dobson SR, et al. To dye or not to dye: a randomized, clinical trial of a triple dye/alcohol regime versus dry cord care. *Pediatrics* 2003;111;15–20.
404. Smales O. A comparison of umbilical cord treatment in the control of superficial infections. *N Z Med J* 1988;101:453–455.
405. Arnold LDW, Larson E. Immunologic benefits of breast milk in relation to human milk banking. *Am J Infect Control* 1993;21:235–242.
406. Furman L, Taylor G, Minich N, et al. The effect of maternal milk on neonatal morbidity of very low-birth-weight infants. *Arch Pediatr Adolesc Med* 2003;157:66–71.
407. Larson E, Zuill R, Zier V, Berg B. Storage of human breast milk. *Infect Control* 1984;5:127–130.
408. Canadian Paediatric Society. Human milk banking and storage. *Paediatr Child Health 1996*;1:141–145.
409. Barry C, Verncombe M. Is the right breast milk being fed to infants? *Can J Infect Control* 1998;13:16–19.
410. American Dietetic Association. *Preparation of formula for infants: guidelines for health care facilities.* Chicago: American Dietetic Association, 1991.
411. Garland JS, Henrickson K, Maki DG. The 2002 Hospital Infection Control Practices Advisory Committee Centers for Disease Control and Prevention guideline for prevention of intravascular device-related infection. *Pediatrics* 2002;110:1009–1013.
412. Garland JS, Alex CP, Mueller CD, et al. A randomized trial comparing povidone-iodine to a chlorhexidine gluconate-impregnated dressing for prevention of central venous catheter infections in neonates. *Pediatrics* 2001;107:1431–1436.
413. Levy GJ, Strauss RG, Hume H, et al. National survey of neonatal transfusion practices. I. Red blood cell therapy. *Pediatrics* 1993;91: 523–529.
414. Canadian Paediatric Society. Red blood cell transfusions in newborn infants: revised guidelines. *Paediatr Child Health* 2002;7:553–558.
415. Tierney AJ, Higa TE, Finer NN. Disseminated cytomegalovirus infection after extracorporeal membrane oxygenation. *Pediatr Infect Dis J* 1992;11:241–243.
416. Evans ME, Schaffner W, Federspiel CF, et al. Sensitivity, specificity, and positive predictive value of body surface cultures in a neonatal intensive care unit. *JAMA* 1988;259:248–252.
417. Fulginiti VA. Ray CG. Body surface cultures in the newborn infant. An exercise in futility, wastefulness, and inappropriate practice. *Am J Dis Child* 1988;142:19–20.
418. Lau YL, Hey E. Sensitivity and specificity of daily tracheal aspirate cultures in predicting organisms causing bacteremia in ventilated neonates. *Pediatr Infect Dis J* 1991;10:290–294.
419. Garner JS, Hospital Infection Control Practices Advisory Committee. Guideline for isolation precautions in hospitals. *Infect Control Hosp Epidemiol* 1996;17:53–80.
420. Leclair JM, Freeman J, Sullivan BF, et al. Prevention of nosocomial

respiratory syncytial virus infections through compliance with glove and gown isolation precautions. *N Engl J Med* 1987;317:329–334.

421. Gala CL, Hall CB, Schnabel KC, et al. The use of eye-nose goggles to control nosocomial respiratory syncytial virus infection. *JAMA* 1986;256:2706–2708.
422. Haas JP, Trezza LA. Outbreak investigation in a neonatal intensive care unit. *Semin Perinatol* 2002;26:367–378.
423. Ehrenkrantz NJ, Sanders CG, Eckert-Schollenberger D, et al. Lack of evidence of efficacy of cohorting nursing personnel in a neonatal intensive care unit to prevent contact spread of bacteria: an experimental study. *Pediatr Infect Dis J* 1992;11:105–113.
424. Wu F, Della-Latta P. Molecular typing strategies. *Semin Perinatol* 2002;26:357–366.
425. Sprunt K, Leidy G, Redman W. Abnormal colonization of neonates in an ICU: conversion to normal colonization by pharyngeal implantation of alpha hemolytic streptococcus strain 215. *Pediatr Res* 1980; 14:308–313.
426. Cook LN, Davis RS, Stover, BH. Outbreak of amikacin-resistant Enterobacteriaceae in an intensive care nursery. *Pediatrics* 1980;65: 264–268.
427. Reuman PD, Duckworth DH, Smith KL, et al. Lack of effect of *Lactobacillus* on gastrointestinal bacterial colonization in premature infants. *Pediatr Infect Dis J* 1986;5:663–668.
428. Millar MR, Bacon C, Smith SL, et al. Enteral feeding of premature infants with *Lactobacillus* GG. *Arch Dis Child* 1993;69:483–487.
429. Rastegar Lari A, Gold F, Borderon JC, et al. Implantation and in vivo antagonistic effects of antibiotic-susceptible *Escherichia coli* strains administered to premature newborns. *Biol Neonate* 1990;58: 73–78.
430. Lodinová-Zádníková R, Tlaskalová H, Bartáková Z. The antibody response in infants after colonization of the intestine with *E. coli* O83. Artificial colonization used as a prevention against nosocomial infections. *Adv Exp Med Biol* 1991;310:329–335.
431. Khalak R, Pichichero ME, D'Angio CT. Three-year follow-up of vaccine response in extremely premature infants. *Pediatrics* 1998;101: 597–603.
432. Blake KD, Jellinek DC. Visiting and immunization policies in a regional neonatal unit. *Lancet* 1990;336:308–309.
433. Patel DM, Butler J, Feldman S, et al. Immunogenicity of hepatitis B vaccine in healthy very low birth weight infants. *J Pediatr* 1997; 131:641–643.
434. Shinefield H, Black S, Ray P, et al. Efficacy, immunogenicity and safety of heptavalent pneumococcal conjugate vaccine in low birth weight and preterm infants. *Pediatr Infect Dis J* 2002;21:182–186.
435. Munoz FM, Englund JA. A step ahead. Infant protection through maternal immunization. *Pediatr Clin North Am* 2000;47:449–463.
436. Perez EM, Weisman LE. Novel approaches to the prevention and therapy of neonatal bacterial sepsis. *Clin Perinatol* 1997;24:213–229.
437. Hill HR. Additional confirmation of the lack of effect of intravenous immunoglobulin in the prevention of neonatal infection. *J Pediatr* 2000;137:595–597.
438. Parravicini E, van de Ven C, Anderson L, et al. Myeloid hematopoietic growth factors and their role in prevention and/or treatment of neonatal sepsis. *Transfus Med Rev* 2002;16:11–24.

53

INFECTIONS ACQUIRED IN CHILD CARE FACILITIES

RALPH L. CORDELL
STEVEN L. SOLOMON

Out-of-home child care has gone from being the exception to being the rule for many families in the United States. According to the Bureau of Labor Statistics, in 2001 more than 9 million families included working mothers with children younger than 6 years (1). Census Bureau statistics suggest that in 1999, out-of-home child care was the primary child care arrangement for 39% of 10.5 million children younger than 5 years in households with employed mothers (2). The 1990 National Child Care Survey reported that unemployed mothers of more than 1.5 million preschool children used child care centers or family day care as their primary source of child care (3). Children in out-of-home child care tend to have higher rates of infectious diseases and antimicrobial use than children cared for at home, and their illnesses often spread to their caretakers and family members. As a result, the recent social and demographic trends have resulted in new challenges in infectious diseases prevention and control and influenced the epidemiology of many common childhood infectious diseases (4–10).

Trends and research activities noted in recent years have continued (11). Antimicrobial resistance and inappropriate use of antimicrobials for children in child care facilities continue to be a cause for concern (12–21) as are low immunization levels (22, 23). The effectiveness of influenza vaccine (24–26), pneumococcal vaccine (27), and more recently available varicella vaccine (28–31) in preventing illness and reducing absenteeism is being evaluated. Increased risks of illness that have been associated with various types of child care continue to be studied (32,33). However, recent work suggests that there may be a negative association between early child care and illness later in life (34, 35).

The national interest in promoting better child care has been augmented by publication of the second edition of *Caring for Our Children: National Health and Safety Performance Standards: Guidelines for Out-of-Home Child Care* published by the American Academy of Pediatrics (36). As with the first edition, this comprehensive document is a compendium of best practices and policies developed by committees of experts in child care and child care health and safety. The new edition includes many revised standards and addresses a number of new issues including those surrounding ill-child care.

TYPES OF CHILD CARE SETTINGS

Broadly defined, short-term child care is provided in a variety of settings, including bowling alleys, health clubs, shopping malls, and restaurants; many religious institutions provide some form of child care while parents attend services and other events. However, most studies on illness incidence and prevention have focused on more formal settings. These have been categorized into the following groups by the American Academy of Pediatrics (36). *Child care centers* (also known as day care centers) are free-standing facilities enrolling more than 12 children. Children are often grouped into two or more classrooms, usually on the basis of age, during much of the day. *Family child care homes* (also known as group homes or child care homes) are in residential settings, usually the provider's home, and provide care for up to 12 children. A further distinction has been made between small family child care homes, which care for up to 6 children, and large family child care homes, which care for 7 to 12 children. Unfortunately, these terms have not been used uniformly in research reports. In this discussion, terms that most accurately represent the study populations are used. *Home care* refers to care for children who are not in out-of-home child care, whereas *center care* and *family child care* refer to care provided by child care centers and family child care homes, respectively. The terms *caregiver* and *child care provider* are used interchangeably to identify persons providing direct care to children.

MAGNITUDE OF CHILD CARE HEALTH ISSUES

Children attending out-of-home child care generally have higher rates of infectious diseases and antibiotic use than children in home care. Among preschool children in the United States, 9% to 11% of all upper respiratory tract infections, 10% to 14% of all otitis media cases, and 19% of all clinic visits for diarrheal disease are attributable to child care attendance (37–39). The results of several studies comparing the incidence of illness among children in different categories of child care facilities are summarized in Table 53.1. Despite variations in study methods and definitions, the increased burden of illness associated with child care compared with that among children

TABLE 53.1. MAGNITUDE OF INFECTIOUS DISEASE BURDEN ON CHILDREN IN CHILD CARE SETTINGS

Study	Outcome examined	Settings studied	Age group(s)	Result
Fleming 1987 (37)	Respiratory illness	OHCC, HC	<5 yr	32% of children in OHCC had URI in preceding 2 wk compared with 21% of HC children; 12% of children in full-time OHCC had OM in preceding 2 wk compared with 5% of HC children.
Hurwitz 1991 (38)	Respiratory illness	OHCC, HC	<5 yr	38% of children 18–35 mo old and 34% of children ≤17 mo old in OHCC had URI in preceding 2 wk vs. 30% (18–35 mo old) and 27% (≤17 mo old) of children in HC.
Strangert 1976 (110)	Respiratory illness	CCC, FCCH, HC	6–18 mo	Febrile illness/child/9 mo: CCC = 4, HC = 1.
			6–24 mo	Mean no. of antibiotic Rx/child/8 mo: CCC 2.3, FCCH 1.9, HC 1.5.
				Mean no. of cases of OM/child/8 mo: CCC 2.3, FCCH 2.0, HC 1.3.
Loda 1972 (123)	Respiratory illness	CCC	<5 yr	8.4 total illnesses/child-yr; 3.2 febrile illnesses/child-yr.
Johansen 1988 (44)	Bed-days	CCC, FCCH, HC		Bed-days per child per yr:
			6–30 mo	CCC 5.0, FCCH 5.0, HC 3.7
			30–60 mo	CCC 3.8, FCCH 3.0, HC 2.7
Bell 1989 (40)	Physician-diagnosed illnesses per month	CCC, FCCH, HC	≤36 mo	URI without OM: CCC 1.03, FCCH 0.88, HC 0.79
				OM: CCC 1.40, FCCH 1.21, HC 0.84
				Total infections: CCC 2.95, FCCH 2.54, HC 2.03
				Adjusted excess no. of infections/mo/child, CCC vs. HC: OM 0.66; Total infections, 0.79.
Agre 1985 (316)	Physician-diagnosed infections	OHCC, HC	≤12 mo	Infections/child/yr: OHCC 3.8, HC 2.8
Doyle 1976 (43)	Symptom-wk/child	CCC, FCCH, HC	≤30 mo	Vomiting, diarrhea: CCC 0.42, HC 0.12
				All symptoms: CCC 2.70, HC 1.50
Wald 1988 (48)	Parent-reported illness/yr	CCC, FCCH, HC	≤18 mo	All illness: CCC 7.1, FCCH 6.0, HC 4.7
				Respiratory: CCC 6.3, FCCH 5.1, HC 3.9
				Days of illness: CCC 96, FCCH 78, HC 41
Cordell 1997 (50)	Illness	CCC, FCCH	All attendees (most ≤5)	Illness episodes/100 child-wk: CCC 6.7, FCCH 10.4
	Days absent due to illness			Days absent/100 child-wk: CCC 4.5, FCCH 2.3 (above rates are age-adjusted).
Cordell 1999 (51)	Illness	CCC, LCCH, SCCH	All attendees (most ≤5)	Illness episodes/child-yr: SCCH 9.7, LCCH 7.4, CCC 6.6
	Days absent due to illness			Days absent/child-yr: SCCH 2.5, LCCH 2.4, CCC 4.5
Strangert 1977 (47)	OM	CCC, FCCH, HC	6–24 mo	OM episodes/child/8 mo: CCC 0.8, FCCH 0.9, HC 0.3
Etzel 1992 (162)	OM with effusion	CCC	≤3 yr	2.9 episodes/yr/child
Black 1981 (232)	Diarrhea incidence	CCC	6–17 mo	3.5–19.3 episodes/100 child-wk
			18–29 mo	2.6–13.9 episodes/100 child-wk
Sullivan 1984 (231)	Diarrhea incidence	CCC	0–2 yr	1.24 episodes/child/yr
			3–5 yr	0.07 episodes/child/yr
Lemp 1984 (67)	Diarrhea incidence	CCC	≤36 mo	2.90 cases/100 child-wk
			>36 mo	0.26 cases/100 child-wk
Bartlett 1985 (66)	Diarrhea incidence	CCC	≤36 mo	1.02 cases/child-yr
Bartlett 1985 (42)	Diarrhea incidence	CCC, FCCH, HC	≤36 mo	Cases/100 child-mo: CCC 42, FCCH 23, HC 27
Bartlett 1988 (233)	Diarrhea incidence	CCC	≤36 mo	0.70–0.78 cases per child-yr
Staat 1991 (230)	Diarrhea incidence	CCC	≤24 mo	2.8 cases/child-yr
Bartlett 1988 (191)	Diarrhea incidence	CCC	≤24 mo	2.82 cases/child-yr
Laborde 1993 (317)	Diarrhea incidence	CCC	≤36 mo	2.0 cases/child-yr

CCC, child care center; FCCH, family child care homes; LCCH, large family child care home; SCCH, small family child care homes; HC, home care; OHCC, out-of-home child care (includes care in centers and/or family child care homes); URI, upper respiratory infection; OM, otitis media.

in home care has been demonstrated fairly consistently. In a study of children enrolled in a Memphis health maintenance organization, for example, children in out-of-home child care had 2.5 to 3.1 physician-diagnosed infections during a 7-month study period compared with 2.0 infections among children in home care (40). These differences were statistically significant. Results from the recent National Institute of Child Health and Human Development Study of Early Child Care suggest that these differences still exist for children younger than 2 years but that, by age 3 years, illness experiences among children in out-of-home child care are comparable to those of children cared for at home (32).

The risk of illness associated with family child care has usually, although not uniformly, been found to be intermediate between the risks associated with center care and those associated with home care or no different than the risk associated with home care (32,40–49). However, some studies have indicated that provider-reported illness rates in children attending child care homes were greater than those among children in centers (50,51). Because many previous studies obtained data through retrospective telephone interviews with parents, these differences in results suggest that comparisons of illness rates from various types of child care facilities may be influenced by the information source.

Child care-associated illness has been estimated to cost the U.S. economy at least $1.8 billion per year (52). Two thirds of that cost is due to time off work because of illness or care for an ill child. Hofferth et al. (3) reported that almost 18% of mothers interviewed had missed an average of 2.2 days of work during the month before their interview because of care for an ill child. In the Memphis studies, the mean monthly costs of medical care for children in home care and center care were $19.78 and $32.94, respectively (40). After including lost income for parents who missed work, the mean monthly cost of illnesses ranged from $29.50 for families with children in home care to $61.64 for those with children in center care. Total parent and societal adjusted average costs for illness among toddlers in Quebec child care facilities over a 6-month period was U.S. $260.70 (53). The authors pointed out that they may have underestimated the costs of medical care ($47.47 for medication and $49.10 consultation). However, they included an estimate of $35.68 for the previously overlooked cost of care by family members.

By amplifying the prevalence of pathogens already present in the community, child care patterns have influenced the epidemiology of a number of illnesses, including cytomegalovirus (CMV) infection, hepatitis A, shigellosis, giardiasis, and cryptosporidiosis. Perhaps one of the most disturbing issues is the widespread use of antimicrobials among children attending child care and the increased likelihood of isolation of antibiotic-resistant bacteria from children in out-of-home child care (12–21, 54–59).

INFECTION CONTROL CONSIDERATIONS

The concept of infection control, as applied in the hospital or other healthcare setting, can serve as a model for understanding the epidemiology of infectious diseases in the child care setting. Although the differences between the child care and hospital settings are significant, some common elements can be found. Very young children, like hospitalized patients, have an increased susceptibility to infections. Like many patients in hospitals and nursing homes, young children depend on caregivers for even the most basic functions, including eating and personal hygiene. Caregivers inadvertently transmit infections between children and are themselves at risk for contracting infections through occupational exposures. Prevention methods focus on increased recognition of the risks of transmission and on interrupting the chain of transmission within the institutional setting (4–6,10,60–62).

EPIDEMIOLOGY OF INFECTIOUS DISEASES IN CHILD CARE

The incidence of illness within a child care facility is determined by factors influencing both the rate of introduction of pathogens into a facility and the rate of transmission once a pathogen has been introduced (63). Factors influencing the rate of introduction are often beyond the control of the facility and include such factors as the prevalence of the illness in the community, the age and health status of children served by the facility, and facility size (usually expressed as the total number of children enrolled). One model suggests that the geographic distribution of the homes of children attending the facility may influence morbidity and that facilities with more widely distributed homes of attendees were less likely to experience major epidemics than those with clustering of homes (63,64).

Factors influencing the rate of transmission once a pathogen has been introduced can often be addressed and modified. These include practices and policies concerning hygiene and disinfection, staffing patterns, isolation or exclusion of ill children, mixing of children of various ages in the same classroom, and diaper type and use of overclothing with diapers. Ekanem et al. (62) presented a simple scheme depicting the mode of spread of enteric bacteria within day care centers. This scheme has been developed further (65) and probably applies, with some modification, to nonenteric pathogens as well.

Factors Related to Increased Transmission among Children

Young children have an increased susceptibility and high age-specific attack rates for numerous infections. Infections in child care settings are transmitted primarily by person-to-person spread of pathogens through body substances, including feces, saliva, nasal secretions, and urine; through direct contact; or by children's and caregivers' hands. Children, especially toddlers, in child care have frequent person-to-person contact and often have poor personal hygiene with regard to contact with and disposal of potentially infectious body substances (4,7,8,10). Frequent hands-on contact by staff, often under hectic circumstances, provides additional opportunity for person-to-person spread via the caregivers' hands both to other children and to the caregivers themselves (62,65–67). The lack of fecal continence in children who are not toilet trained and the tendency for children to explore their environment with their hands and mouths lead to frequent sharing of oral secretions and fecal-oral spread of infection (8,10,65,68–70).

Children also share secretions and excretions via fomites; contaminated toys and environmental surfaces are important in the epidemiology of child care-associated infections. Environmental surfaces, especially those in classrooms for non–toilet-trained children, are often contaminated with fecal bacteria (65,70–74). Many microorganisms associated with child care-related infections can survive on environmental surfaces for considerable periods. Some, including CMV, rotavirus, and *Giardia,* have been isolated from environmental surfaces in child care facilities (69, 75–77). The concentration of microorganisms recovered from surfaces and air samples in child care center classrooms is inversely related to the age of the children in the room (78), and environmental levels of fecal coliforms in child care classrooms often increase during outbreaks of diarrheal illness (62). Group A *Streptococcus* (GAS) was isolated from plastic toy food during an investigation of two cases of invasive GAS infections in a child care facility (79). Although mouthing behavior is uncommon among children aged 3 and 4 years, such as those involved in this outbreak, these toys encourage this behavior and are examples of the types of fomites that contribute to transmission.

Airborne transmission also contributes to the spread of pathogens. Respiratory infections, transmitted through respiratory aerosols and droplets, are the most common infections associated with child care attendance (32,48,50,51,61,80). Studies in crowded homes and child care settings have shown that the risk of respiratory infections, including otitis media, increases as the number of children per room increases (37,81,82). Results from a series of longitudinal studies suggest that a positive association between frequency of respiratory illness and child care among preschool children. These results also suggest that this association is related to the number of children in the group, may be moderated by length of time in child care, and is reversed to a protective effect in school-aged children, with the difference disappearing by age 13 years (32,34).

Common source and foodborne transmission are rarely reported causes of outbreaks in child care settings (83–87). However, nonhygienic food-handling practices have been shown to be a risk factor for illness spread by fecal-oral transmission in child care facilities (42,66), and clinicians probably have not fully recognized the significance of foodborne transmission in this setting.

Other Persons and Groups at Risk

Child Care Providers

Child care providers, like healthcare providers, are at risk of acquiring infectious diseases in the workplace (88,89). Most child care providers are women; many are of child-bearing age (90–93). Child care providers have an increased endemic risk of a number of infections including those from CMV, parvovirus B19, and *Giardia* and an increased epidemic risk for infections with other agents such as *Shigella,* hepatitis A, and *Cryptosporidium.*

Infections caused by pathogens, such as varicella, parvovirus B19, and CMV, which are common in child care settings, pose a significant risk of adverse consequences for pregnancy outcomes. However, few studies have focused on infections among child care workers, and the actual risk of maternal or fetal infection or of specific adverse pregnancy outcomes as a result of these likely exposures has not been well defined. Women who worked in Scandinavian day nurseries between their fourth and sixteenth weeks of pregnancy had higher rates of spontaneous abortions than child care providers who did not work during the same period of pregnancy (94). Seroepidemiologic studies among Seattle child care workers found that antibody to the hepatitis A virus was uncommon under nonoutbreak circumstances. However, among these women, changing diapers 3 or more days per week was associated with an increased seroprevalence of antibody to CMV (95).

Family Members

Family members of both providers and children may be infected by pathogens transmitted in child care settings. Preschool children often introduce infections into their families (8,38, 96–101). Secondary attack rates among family contacts are often high (7,84,89,102,103), especially for highly communicable diseases such as shigellosis. In the case of hepatitis A, clinical illness among older household contacts may be the first indication of transmission within a child care facility (99). Mothers of children in child care are at increased risk of acquiring child care-associated infections (96,99,100,102,104). Older siblings, secondarily infected at home, may spread infections to other children through school and play contact (105).

The Community

Child care-associated infections generally reflect agents circulating in the community. Transmission within child care facilities amplifies the prevalence of pathogens in the community. This amplification can have a significant impact on the incidence of infection and has influenced the epidemiology of a number of pathogens, including *Giardia, Cryptosporidium, Shigella,* hepatitis A, and CMV. Interrupting disease transmission in child care settings may lead to a reduction in the disease burden within the community. This strategy has been used successfully in community-wide outbreaks of shigellosis and hepatitis A infections (106–109).

Antimicrobial Resistance and Antimicrobial Use

The frequent and often inappropriate use of antimicrobials among children in child care and the resulting emergence of antimicrobial-resistant strains of bacteria are among the most serious public health consequences of the increasing use of out-of-home child care. Children in child care generally receive more antimicrobial treatments than children in home care (19,45, 58,110). During an 8-week study period at a Houston health maintenance organization, 35.7% of children in center care received antimicrobials compared with 7.1% in family child care homes and 8.2% of children in home care (58). The average duration of therapy was more than four times longer for children in center care (19.9 days) than for children in family child care homes (4.0 days) or home care (4.6 days). The increased use of antimicrobials by children in center care may have been due to a number of factors, including an increased frequency of bacterial and parasitic infections. Parents of children in center care may also have been more likely to seek medical attention for mild or moderate illnesses than parents of children not enrolled in center care, reflecting the parents' need for rapid resolution of any illness lest the child be unable to attend child care and the parent be forced to miss work. Although child care providers may also apply pressure to use antimicrobials inappropriately (18), the influence of parental knowledge on demand may be a more important factor (21).

Children attending child care have been shown to harbor strains of resistant *Escherichia coli, Streptococcus pneumoniae, Streptococcus pyogenes, Haemophilus influenzae, Shigella sonnei,* and *Staphylococcus aureus* (16,17,57–59,111–116). Among Houston children younger than 2 years, resistant strains of *E. coli* were more likely to be isolated from diapered children attending child care centers than from those attending well-baby clinics (59). The association between the likelihood of infection among children in center care and the number of diapered children enrolled was positive. In a second study, trimethoprim-resistant strains of *E. coli* spread efficiently to family members of children in center care. Resistant isolates were identified in stools of 13 of 23 children (57%) and in stools of 13 of 50 (26%) of these children's household contacts (117). Resistant strains of *H. influenzae* and *S. sonnei* have been isolated during investigations of outbreaks. Evidence suggests a relationship between carriage of resistant *H. influenzae* in nonoutbreak settings and prior receipt of antimicrobials (58). A recent report suggesting transmission of methicillin-resistant *S. aureus* in a Canadian child care center makes this the latest of what will undoubtedly be a growing list of antimicrobial-resistant pathogens in child care (17). Infection with resistant *S. pneumoniae* has been studied in both outbreak and nonoutbreak settings and is discussed later in this chapter.

Ill-Child Care

The shortage of out-of-home care for children with mild or moderate illness is a major factor in the inappropriate use of antimicrobials among children in child care. Parents of children in out-of-home child care must often find care for children with mild or moderate illnesses who are excluded from their normal child care setting or they must take time off work to care for their children themselves. Mildly ill children are more likely to be excluded from child care centers than from family child care homes (50,51,118). Several different solutions have been developed to provide care for mildly ill children outside of their usual child care arrangement (119). These include specially designated areas in the same centers, different facilities set up especially to care for ill children, informal settings outside the children's homes, or the child's own home with care provided by parents or other caregivers. Each option has advantages and disadvantages. The second edition of the National Health and Safety Performance Standards addresses a number of issues involving the care of mildly ill children and includes a classification of various levels of severity of illness, types of services needed, and appropriate activities for each (36).

Considerations affecting the choice of an appropriate alternative include the need to ensure the child's health and well-being, increased costs of alternative arrangements, the desire to reduce parental absenteeism from work, disruption of the child's routine, and the potential for spread of infection to children or adults in the alternative setting (119).

Although ill-child care raises concerns about children's emotional and medical needs and the risk of transmission among children in such settings (120), few studies have addressed these issues. A comparison of 118 children who attended a center providing short-term care for children with mild illnesses with an age-matched cohort of ill children who received care from a home care provider in their own homes indicated no increased risk of subsequent illness in the former group (121).

EPIDEMIOLOGY OF DISEASE SYNDROMES

Respiratory Tract Infections

Upper and Lower Respiratory Infections

Infections of the upper respiratory tract are the most common illnesses experienced by children in both home and child care settings (97,122). Selected studies that have assessed the child care setting as a risk for upper respiratory infections are listed in Table 53.2.

Respiratory symptoms were involved in 45% of illness episodes reported among children attending Seattle child care facilities (50), and 52% of illnesses among children in San Diego child care facilities involved rhinitis (51). Respiratory infections accounted for 85% of illnesses in children younger than 18 months in Pittsburgh child care centers and 89% of children in group care (48).

Although usually considered minor, respiratory infections contribute to the burden of otitis media, antibiotic use, and absenteeism experienced by children in out-of-home child care. Approximately 29% of respiratory infections among young children are complicated by otitis (49). Respiratory infections (excluding otitis) accounted for 28% of antibiotic use among children in Seattle child care facilities (Centers for Disease Control and Prevention, unpublished data, 1996). Because most respiratory illnesses in this age group are due to viral infections, much of this antibiotic use was probably unnecessary. Children with respiratory infections in Seattle child care facilities were absent for an average of 0.9 days per illness episode; these infections accounted for 3,558 days of absence, almost half of the 7,635 days of absence because of illness among these children (50). Among children in San Diego child care facilities, illness episodes involving rhinitis accounted for 2,335 days of absence (1.6 days per child-year), an average of 0.3 days absent per illness episode (51).

The incidence of respiratory infection is inversely associated with age. Children younger than 18 months have the greatest risk of illness (48,49,123). Among children in a North Carolina day care center, the incidence of respiratory illness peaked among those 6 to 12 months of age (5). At younger ages, children in child care have a somewhat greater risk of upper respiratory illness than those in home care. A 1984 survey found that 9% to 14% of upper respiratory illness in Atlanta preschool children was related to child care (37). Children younger than 18 months in Pittsburgh child care centers experienced 6.3 respiratory infections per year, whereas those in group care experienced 5.1 and those in home care experienced 3.9 infections per year, respectively (48). Results of a nationwide telephone survey in the United States indicated that child care was associated with an increased risk of respiratory illness among children younger than 5 years. However, the association was statistically significant only for children aged between 6 weeks and 17 months and for those aged 18 to 35 months who had no older siblings (38). Children aged 6 to 17 months in Swedish child care centers had more febrile illness, coughing, and rhinitis than did children not in child care; differences were not statistically significant for children older than 17 months (110).

Early research suggested that children who have been in child

TABLE 53.2. SELECTED STUDIES ASSESSING CHILD CARE AS A RISK FACTOR FOR RESPIRATORY DISEASE

Study	Location	No. in sample	Settings studied	Results
Strangert 1976 (110)	Sweden			
	a	82	CCC, HC	Children 6–18 mo old in OHCC had more symptoms during study period, no difference for older children; children in CCC had more lower respiratory tract disease and more antibiotic Rx.
	b	108	CCC	Among children in CCC, incidence of OM, LRI, and antibiotic Rx decreased with age; slight or no decrease with age in other symptoms; rhinitis was the only symptom to increase with number of other children in the setting.
	c	207	CCC, FCCH, HC	No difference in disease incidence between FCCH and CCC; both have increased incidence vs. HC.
Wald 1991 (161)	Pennsylvania	244	CCC, FCCH, HC	Children in OHCC more likely to have OM complicating URI: children $<$1 yr, CCC $>$ HC ($p < .01$); age 1–2 yr, FCCH $>$ HC ($p < .01$); age 2–3 yr, NSD between settings Children in CCC have prolonged symptoms ($>$15 days) twice as often as HC children.
Fleming 1987 (37)	Georgia	575	CCC, FCCH, HC	Children in OHCC had more URI than HC children (OR = 1.6).
Stahlberg 1980 (45)	Finland	69	CCC, FCCH, HC	Children in CCC had more rhinitis, cough, and fever than those in FCCH or HC; NSD between FCCH and HC; children in CCC had more antibiotic Rx than those in HC.
Hurwitz 1991 (38)	United States	2137	OHCC, HC	Children in OHCC more likely to have URI, antibiotic Rx, and visits to health care providers. Increased risk of URI by age $<$18 mo, OR = 1.6; 18–35 mo: with older sibling, OR = 1.0; 18–35 mo: without older sib, OR = 3.4; = 36 mo, OR = 1.3. No difference in risk for part-time vs. full-time OHCC; longer duration of prior enrollment was protective; increased risk with exposure to larger group settings.
Wald 1991 (49)	Pennsylvania	244	CCC, FCCH, HC	Three-year follow-up study of birth cohort. Comparison in mean no. of URI/child by year of study: Yr 1 and Yr 3: CCC and FCCH $>$ HC ($p < 0.1$); Yr 2: CCC $>$ FCCH and HC ($p < .01$). Likelihood of having URI sx for $>$60 days/yr; yr 1 and yr 2: CCC and FCCH $>$ HC ($p < .05$); yr 3 NSD between settings.
Louhiala 1995 (318)	Finland	2568	CCC, FCCH, HC	Overall incidence common cold in CCC = 2.74/child-yr, FCCH = 2.64/child-yr, HC = 2.64/child-yr; for children 1 yr CCC = 5.06/child-yr, FCCH = 2.97/child-yr, HC = 3.07/child-yr.
Cordell 1997 (50)	Washington	41 CCC, 91 FCCH	CCC, FCCH	Provider reported incidence in FCCH = 6.0 cases/100 child-wk CCC = 3.4 cases/100 child-wk.
National Institutes of Health 2001 (33)	United States	1364	CCC, FCCH, HC	OR – age 12 mo CCC = 1.92, FCCH = 1.42 – age 24 mo CCC = 1.62, FCCH = 1.26 – age 36 mo CCC = 1.36, FCCH = 1.11

CCC, child care center; FCCH, family child care home; OHCC, out-of-home child care (includes care in child care centers and/or family child care homes); HC, home care (children not in out-of-home child care); URI, upper respiratory tract infection; LRI, lower respiratory tract infection; OM, otitis media; NSD, no significant difference; OR, odds ratio.

care for some time may have no greater risk, or even a decreased risk, of respiratory infections than their same-aged peers who stay at home (5,38,124). Results from the National Institute of Child Health and Human Development Study of Early Child Care support this finding and suggest that, although child care was associated with increased illness in children younger than 2 years, the difference was negligible by age 3 years (32). Children who first entered out-of-home child care after age 3 years experience more illness than their classmates who were in child care before age 3 years (33). Also, the excess respiratory illness among children in day care centers does appear to protect those children against respiratory infections during the early school years although this advantage largely disappears by age 13 (34).

Although the results of those few studies assessing the impact of child care attendance on lower respiratory infections are not definitive, they suggest an increased risk among children in child care (123,125–128). After other risk factors were controlled, children hospitalized with lower respiratory tract infections at one of four Atlanta-area hospitals were more likely than control patients to have been in out-of-home child care (125). Center care posed a greater risk for hospitalization than care in a child care home. However, other studies have found no association between lower respiratory illnesses and child care (110,128).

Relatively little information is available on the types and frequency distribution of various pathogens in child care-associated respiratory infections. Studies at Atlanta hospitals of children with lower respiratory infections demonstrated that the most common causative agent associated with illness was respiratory syncytial virus, followed by other respiratory viruses (including parainfluenza viruses), *H. influenzae,* and *S. pneumoniae* (125).

Most information on agents involved in child care-associated respiratory infections has come from studies at the Frank Porter Graham Child Development Center in North Carolina (5,123, 129) or from outbreak investigations. Viruses were isolated from

31% of respiratory infections among children in the North Carolina studies (5); respiratory syncytial viruses, parainfluenza viruses, adenoviruses, enteroviruses, and rhinoviruses were common isolates. Although viruses were rarely isolated from well children, bacteria were commonly isolated from these children. Common isolates included *S. pneumoniae,* nontypable *H. influenzae,* and *S. pyogenes.* Carriage rates were generally greater than 10% and 40% for nontypable *H. influenzae* and *S. pneumoniae,* respectively.

Outbreaks of respiratory illnesses have been associated with influenza type B (130) and GAS (131,132).

Invasive Bacterial Infections

Invasive bacterial infections, especially meningitis caused by *H. influenzae* type b (Hib), *Neisseria meningitidis,* and *S. pneumoniae,* are some of the most serious problems encountered in child care facilities. The widespread use of vaccines for Hib has had a dramatic impact on the epidemiology of this disease. The subsequent reduction in the incidence of invasive Hib infections is a public health success story of considerable gratification to those who worked in this area in the prevaccine era. In 1985, polysaccharide vaccines were licensed in the United States for use in children older than 18 months (133,134). Conjugate vaccines, with superior immunogenicity, were introduced in 1987. The age of recommended first immunization against Hib was lowered to 15 months in April 1990 and to 2 months in October 1990 (133,134). The average annual rate of invasive Hib infections for 1998 to 2000 (0.3 cases per 100,000 children younger than 5 years) represents a 99% decline from the 1990 rate (2.3 cases per 100,000) (135). As new vaccines became available, marked decreases in incidence were noted among children in age cohorts younger than those for which the vaccine was recommended (136). These decreases have been ascribed to reduced colonization among children immunized with conjugate vaccines (137). The prevention of invasive Hib infections in child care settings today requires ensuring appropriate immunization of all enrolled children, complete reporting to allow the characterization of suspect vaccine failures, standardized serotyping procedures, and serotype tracking for all invasive *H. influenzae* infections (135).

Although household contacts of *N. meningitidis* infections are at increased risk of disease, the magnitude of risk for child care contacts has not been studied extensively and is uncertain (138). Reports from outbreaks suggest that child care contacts of cases are at increased risk (139–141). During a period of increased incidence of *N. meningitidis* in Belgium, children younger than 3 years in day care nurseries had a relative risk of secondary infection 76 times greater than the baseline age-specific incidence; children aged 2 to 5 years in preprimary schools had a relative risk 23 times the age-specific baseline incidence (138).

Colonization with *S. pneumoniae* is endemic among child care populations. In a prospective study of 81 children in a North Carolina day care center, this microorganism was recovered from 43.3% of well children and 51.5% of ill children (5). The prevalence was greatest among children younger than 3 years. Swedish investigators reported that *S. pneumoniae* was isolated from 31.9% of cultures from children younger than 5 years and in center care (142). Carriage rates were highest in facilities with 45 or more children and among children younger than 2 years. Child care attendance was shown to be a risk factor for invasive pneumococcal disease among Finnish children (143). Outbreaks of invasive pneumococcal infections have been reported in child care homes (144) and centers (145).

The emergence of antibiotic-resistant strains of pneumococci is a matter of both clinical and public health concern. Israeli investigators reported that the risk of resistant pneumococcal infections in children who attended child care centers and who had received at least one course of antimicrobial treatment in the previous 3 months was 12.9 times that of children who had neither of these risk factors (146). In studies among children attending four Houston child care centers, *S. pneumoniae* was recovered from 40% of 140 children younger than 3 years (147). Intermediate penicillin resistance was found in 11% of isolates; none was highly resistant. During a 7-year prospective study, upper respiratory tract cultures were collected monthly from 72 children (56). Each child had an average of 2.1 episodes of *S. pneumoniae* colonization; 68% had resistant pneumococci isolated at least once. In another study, multiply resistant strains were isolated from nasopharyngeal cultures from 9 of 47 children in a center attended by two toddlers hospitalized with invasive pneumococcal infections (57). After isolation of resistant *S. pneumoniae* from the middle ear fluid of a child with otitis media, Reichler et al. (114) found that 52 of 250 exposed children were carriers of a resistant pneumococcus. Carriage was associated with receipt of antimicrobials, especially at prophylactic doses. This association has been demonstrated elsewhere (148,149). Conversely, studies in an Omaha child care center suggest that decreasing antibiotic use may control the spread of resistant pneumococci (148). Resistant pneumococci may persist among children in centers. Although treatment with rifampin or rifampin and clindamycin can reduce the prevalence of carriage temporarily (145), it may not eliminate carriage or reduce spread (57,147).

Although more commonly in upper respiratory tract infections, GAS has been associated with invasive infections (79,150), including one cluster of two cases in a Boston child care center (79).

Tuberculosis

The principal risk of tuberculosis in the child care setting is transmission from infected adults to children (151). In three of four reports of outbreaks in family child care settings, the source case was an adult relative of the caregiver (152–154); in the fourth report, a source case was not identified, but children most likely acquired their infection from an infected caregiver (155).

Transmission in child care generally results in multiple cases; in two outbreaks, 4 children were found to be infected (153, 154), 5 children were infected in another (155), and 11 were infected in the last (152). In England, a community outbreak involving 12 children in a play group was traced to 1 child's infected mother (156). Investigators were unable to identify a source of infection for two infected children in a Kentucky child care center (157).

Otitis Media

Otitis media is associated with viral respiratory infections and respiratory tract colonization or infection with bacteria such as *H. influenzae* or *S. pneumoniae* (158,159). Thus, child care attendance, with increased risks of both respiratory infections and exposure to pathogenic bacteria, is also associated with an increased incidence of otitis media (158,160). Selected studies that have assessed the child care setting as a risk factor for otitis media are listed in Table 53.3.

Children aged 6 to 24 months in Swedish child care centers and family child care homes (caring for one to four children) had 2.5 to 3 times the mean number of episodes of otitis media per child compared with children in home care (47). Older children in child care were not at increased risk of otitis. Neither the facility's policy concerning exclusion of ill children nor the number of children enrolled in the facility influenced the risk of illness. A telephone survey of families of 575 children in Atlanta found that children in full-time child care (more than 40 hours per week) had 3.8 times the risk of developing an ear infection compared with children in home care (37). The risk was greatest among children younger than 36 months. Wald et al. (161) showed that, for children younger than 2 years with upper respiratory tract infections, attending child care for at least 20 hours per week resulted in a 1.6- to 1.7-times higher likelihood that the upper respiratory infection would be complicated by an episode of otitis media. The risk was not increased significantly among children older than 2 years.

Other studies have suggested that the incidence of otitis media among children in out-of-home child care increases as the number of children present in that setting increases (e.g., in a child care center rather than family child care home) and decreases with increasing age at entry into child care (40,82, 162–164). Results from the Child Health Survey of the National Health Interview Survey suggest that children in child care have 1.5 times the risk of repeated ear infections compared with children in home care (82). Attending a facility with more than

TABLE 53.3. SELECTED STUDIES ASSESSING CHILD CARE AS A RISK FACTOR FOR OM

Study	Location	No. in sample	Settings studied	Results
Fleming 1987 (37)	Georgia	575	CCC, FCCH, HC	Increased incidence in children ≤35 mo in OHCC (OR = 3.2); increased incidence in children with preceding URI (OR = 6); increased incidence in children attending CCC or FCCH full time.
Vinther 1984 (164)	Denmark	681	CCC, HC	Children starting OHCC at age <6 mo more likely ($p < .05$) to have OM; abnormal tympanometry more likely in children in OHCC ($p < .05$); adenoidectomy more likely in children in OHCC.
Strangert 1977 (47)	Sweden	207	CCC, FCCH, HC	Children in CCC more likely to have OM ($p < .01$); no effect of exclusion policies, size of enrollment in center, or length of child's enrollment; no difference in risk for children attending CCC vs. FCCH.
Hardy 1993 (82)	United States	5818	CCC, FCCH, HC	Children in OHCC were more likely to have repeated ear infections (OR = 1.5); risk increased for children <3 yr old; no difference in risk between HC and care in FCCH.
Stahlberg 1986 (163)	Finland	438	CCC, FCCH, HC	Children hospitalized for adenoidectomy to prevent recurrent otitis more likely to be enrolled in large CCC settings than controls.
Daly 1988 (165)	Minnesota	386	OHCC, HC	Children attending CCC more likely to have chronic OM with effusion ($p = .06$).
Froom 1991 (166)	International	1335	OHCC, HC	Children in child care more likely to have OM (1.7 times), recurrent OM (1.8 times), poor hearing (2.0 times), and ear tubes (2.5 times) compared with children not in child care.
Alho 1993 (319)	Finland	1956	CCC, FCCH, HC	Increased risk of OM for children in FCCH (OR = 1.5) and children in day nurseries.
Marx 1995 (320)	United States	2179	CCC, FCCH, HC	After adjusting for group size, OR for OM children ,12 mo NSD for both CCC and FCCH; children 12–23 mo CCC = 2.05, FCCH = 1.6.
Alho 1996 (321)	Finland	2512	CCC, FCCH, HC	Children <2 yr OR for unplanned visits for OM CCC = 1.13, FCCH = 1.16.
Louhiala 1995 (318)	Finland	2,568	CCC, FCCH, HC	Overall incidence OM CCC = 1.04/child-yr, FCCH = 0.91/child-yr, HC = 1.01/child-yr; for children 1 yr CCC = 2.53/child-yr, FCCH = 1.81/child-yr, HC = 1.60/child-yr.
Cordell 1997 (50)	Washington	41 CCC, 91 FCCH	CCC, FCCH	Provider reported incidence in FCCH = 1.1 cases/100 child-wk CCC = 0.8 cases/100 child-wk.
National Institutes of Health 2001 (33)	United States	1364	CCC, FCCH, HC	OR – age 12 mo CCC = 2.37, FCCH = 1.26 – age 24 mo CCC = 1.70, FCCH = 1.07 – age 36 mo CCC = 1.22, FCCH = 0.90

CCC, child care center; FCCH, family child care home; OHCC, out-of-home child care (includes care in child care centers and/or family child care homes); HC, home care (children not in out-of-home child care); URI, upper respiratory tract infection; LRI, lower respiratory tract infection; OM, otitis media; NSD, no significant difference; OR, odds ratio.

six children significantly increases the risk of repeated otitis in children younger than 3 years. Child care attendance is also associated with an increased risk of recurrent and more severe otitis media, including persistent effusion and complications such as a need for tympanotomy tube placement (82,163–166).

Enteric Diseases

Diarrheal Disease

The child care setting has been associated with infection caused by a wide variety of enteric pathogens, including *Shigella* (42,66,116,167–173), *Salmonella* (85,86,174,175), *E. coli* (176–185), *Campylobacter* (66,169,170,186–188), *Clostridium difficile* (189), *Aeromonas* (189,190), rotavirus (66,169, 191–200), coxsackievirus (201,202), calicivirus (203–205), astrovirus (206–210), adenovirus (207,211,212), *Giardia* (213–224), *Cryptosporidium* (202,225–228), *Dientamoeba fragilis* (219), and *Blastocystis hominis* (229). A study of child care-associated diarrhea in Maricopa County, Arizona, showed that specific pathogens could be identified from stools of 18% of sporadic cases and 26% of outbreak-associated cases (66). Other investigators have obtained comparable results (84,215,230). During outbreak investigations, multiple pathogens are frequently recovered from stools (66,172,173,221,222), suggesting that diarrhea caused by one agent may facilitate transmission of other pathogens.

The risk of diarrhea among children in child care centers is 1.6 to 3.5 times that of children taken care of at home (41,66). The risk may be much greater for certain pathogens such as *Giardia* and among subgroups of children, such as infants or toddlers in diapers (84,231) or those recently enrolled in the facility (66,230,232). Studies based on clinic visits or information from parents have suggested that children in child care homes have a lower risk of diarrhea than those in centers (39, 41,42). However, results of studies comparing illness incidence in child care homes and centers may be biased by the source of information. Data obtained from child care providers in Seattle and San Diego showed that the incidence of illness (including diarrhea) among children in child care homes was greater than that among children in centers (50,51). Selected studies assessing the child care setting as a risk factor for diarrheal diseases are listed in Table 53.4.

Rotavirus, *Giardia, Cryptosporidium,* and *Shigella* appear to be the most common causes of diarrhea in child care settings. Rotavirus appears to cause disease more commonly in infants, and *Giardia* and *Cryptosporidium* appear to cause disease more commonly in toddlers (66,169,230). *Shigella* infections generally

TABLE 53.4. SELECTED STUDIES ASSESSING CHILD CARE AS A RISK FACTOR FOR DIARRHEAL DISEASE IN PRESCHOOL CHILDREN

Study	Location	No. in sample	Settings studied	Results
Alexander 1990 (41)	United States	4,845	CCC, FCCH, HC	CCC attendance .10 hr/wk associated with increased risk of acute GI illness (OR = 3.5 for children age <3 yr old, OR = 1.8 for children aged 3–5 yr); FCCH attendance not associated with increased risk.
Sullivan 1984 (231)	Texas	3,800	CCC	Increased risk in CCC that accepted children who weren't bowel-trained and in CCC in which staff who worked with infants also prepared food.
Lemp 1984 (67)	Texas	60 CCC	CCC	Increased risk in: CCC that accepted children <2 yr of age (RR = 3.6); CCC wherein staff changed diapers and prepared and/or served food (RR = 1.7–3.3).
Barlett 1985 (66)	Arizona	22 CCC	CCC	Children enrolled for a shorter time more likely to be ill; increased risk of diarrhea in centers with low scores on observational study of hand washing and food-handling practices.
Bartlett 1985 (42)	Arizona	6 CCC, 30 FCCH 102 households	CCC, FCCH, HC	Information from parents indicated that children in CCC had more diarrhea than children in FCCH or HC; no difference between FCCH and HC; provider data indicated that FCCH > CCC > HC.
Reves 1993 (39)	Texas	702 children	CCC	Increased incidence during first 4 wk enrollment vs. later attendance (rate ratio = 1.6); incidence decreased with increasing age; risk did not change with size of CCC or with child's history of prior OHCC.
Staat 1991 (230)	Texas	442 children	CCC	Increased incidence during first 4 wk enrollment vs. later attendance (rate ratio = 1.6); incidence decreased with increasing age; risk did not change with size of CCC or with child's history or prior OHCC.
Cordell 1997 (50)	Washington	41 CCC, 91 FCCH	CCC, FCCH	Provider reported incidence in FCCH = 0.5 cases/100 child-wk CCC = 0.3 cases/100 child-wk.
National Institutes of Health 2001 (33)	United States	1364	CCC, FCCH, HC	OR – age 12 mo CCC = 1.15, FCCH = 1.05 (NS) – age 24 mo CCC = 1.04, FCCH = 1.05 (NS) – age 36 mo CCC = 0.95, FCCH = 1.05 (NS)

CCC, child care center; FCCH, family child care home; OHCC, out-of-home child care (includes care in child care centers and/or family child care homes); HC, home care (children not in out-of-home child care); GI, gastrointestinal; OR, odds ratio; RR, relative risk.

occur in outbreaks and are more likely to involve adults and children older than those at greatest risk for the other three common infections (169,170,172). *Giardia, Cryptosporidium,* rotavirus, and *Shigella* are more frequent causes of infectious diarrhea in child care settings because of their low infectious dose (84,170). Outbreaks of these infections are often associated with high rates of asymptomatic infection and prolonged excretion of enteropathogens by both asymptomatic persons and convalescent cases who no longer have diarrhea (172,173,191,221, 222). This may pose difficulties in management and making decisions regarding excluding and/or cohorting infected persons.

Secondary attack rates are often quite high among family members of children with child care-associated diarrheal illness. These rates have ranged from 12% to 47% for *Giardia,* 24% to 62% for *Cryptosporidium,* 17% to 79% for rotavirus, and 22% to 29% for *Shigella* (84,169,170,172,215,225,227). Child care-associated outbreaks, especially cases of shigellosis, may spread to the community (116,167,168,172) and play an important role in the epidemiology of community-acquired infections (223).

Outbreaks of diarrheal disease occur primarily among children in diapers. Other risk factors associated with an increased incidence of diarrheal disease in child care settings include age of child, duration of attendance in a particular child care facility, type of setting, and levels of environmental sanitation and adherence to good hygienic practices (e.g., hand washing) (62,66,67, 232).

Children in diapers generally have the highest attack rates during child care center outbreaks of many diarrheal agents, including *Cryptosporidium* (103), *Giardia* (169), and rotavirus. In a 2-year prospective study of diarrheal illness among children in Houston child care facilities, the risk of diarrheal illness in children younger than 3 years was 17 times that of children aged 3 to 5 years; the mean incidence of diarrheal illness in facilities that accepted children in diapers was significantly greater than in facilities that did not (231).

The principal means by which enteric diseases spread in child care facilities is by the fecal-oral route, direct interactions between toddlers, or contamination of caregiver hands or the environment (4,61,84). Low scores on assessments of hygiene and environmental sanitation in Maricopa County, Arizona, child care facilities were associated with an increased risk of outbreaks of diarrheal illness (66). Practices particularly linked to the occurrence of outbreaks included failing to observe proper hand washing protocols and having staff both changing diapers and preparing or serving food (66,67,231). Studies in Atlanta child care centers have shown that a rigorously monitored hand washing program can reduce the incidence of diarrheal illness, especially among children aged 6 to 18 months (232). However, training of child care staff, without monitoring compliance with hand washing protocols, has been shown to be ineffective in reducing diarrheal incidence (233). The impact of even subtle reinforcement of hand washing protocols is suggested by decreases in both diarrhea and environmental contamination rates among facilities participating in research projects (72,233).

Levels of environmental contamination with fecal coliforms are associated with the incidence of diarrheal illness (62,65). The proportion of cultures from hands and environmental surfaces positive for fecal coliforms increases when cases of diarrhea occur in a classroom (62,65,73). One study demonstrated an association between the incidence of diarrhea and the recovery of fecal coliforms from hands of children and staff and from moist environmental surfaces, including sinks and faucet handles (65). Because many enteric pathogens are relatively stable in the environment and some, such as *Cryptosporidium,* are resistant to many commonly used disinfectants, addressing this potential environmental link in the transmission of enteric diseases will require careful adherence to cleaning and disinfection protocols (69,70, 234).

The types of diapers used in facilities may also influence environmental contamination levels. Having children wear clothing over diapers has been shown to reduce levels of environmental contamination with fecal coliforms in classrooms (73). Wearing disposable diapers with absorbent gelling was also associated with lower levels of environmental coliforms than wearing reusable cloth diapers was (73). Another study showed no significant differences in either the frequency or intensity of environmental contamination between facilities using disposable diapers with gelling and those using all-in-one design reusable diapers with front closures (72).

Children newly enrolled in child care centers have a greater incidence of diarrheal illness than those who have attended for at least 3 months (66,230,232). This was first recognized during a hand washing intervention study by Black et al. (232), who noticed a peak incidence in diarrhea among children enrolled in centers for 2 to 4 weeks. Although the peak was somewhat smaller in intervention facilities with hand-washing programs than in control facilities, it was present in both groups. Children enrolled in Phoenix child care centers for less than 3 weeks not only had an increased risk of sporadic diarrhea but also were significantly more likely to be ill during an outbreak of diarrhea than other children (66). Children with a previous history of day care attendance who were newly enrolled in Houston child care centers had an incidence of diarrheal illness comparable to that of newly enrolled children with no previous history of day care attendance (230). This phenomenon, coupled with the large influx of children into child care facilities in the early fall, may explain the increased incidence of *Giardia* and *Cryptosporidium* infections during the late fall and winter months. (For more information on nosocomial gastrointestinal infections in children, see Chapter 50.)

Hepatitis A

Because hepatitis A is spread principally by the fecal-oral route, child care settings offer many opportunities to spread this virus. Several child care-associated outbreaks of hepatitis A have been reported; some of these may have led to community-wide epidemics (99,107,108,235–238). The early recognition of outbreaks in child care facilities is complicated by the high proportion of asymptomatic or mild infections among young children. In a follow-up study of 28 outbreaks of hepatitis A in Maricopa County child care centers, 84% of cases in children aged 1 to 2 years were asymptomatic, compared with 50% of cases in children aged 3 and 4 years and 20% in older children (238). Children with hepatitis A infections who are symptomatic may be only mildly ill and these infections may not be accurately diagnosed; fewer than 10% show evidence of jaundice (239, 240). Outbreaks are usually recognized when cases begin to appear among the children's adult contacts (99). In one study of a community-wide outbreak, household contacts of children in Maricopa County child care facilities accounted for the largest number of outbreak-associated hepatitis A cases (204 of 342 cases) reported to the health department (99). The attack rate among child care workers (12%) was greater than that among household contacts (4%). The remainder of reported cases involved the children themselves and other adult contacts such as babysitters. Similar patterns have been reported in other outbreaks associated with child care facilities (240,241).

The distinction between factors influencing the introduction of pathogens into a facility and those influencing transmission within the facility after introduction was first applied to hepatitis A by Hadler and associates (63, 241). They found that the more hours each day a center is open and the more children it provides care for, the greater its risk of hepatitis A introduction. Once hepatitis A is introduced, its transmission is more likely in centers that enroll younger children in diapers.

Infection appears to be spread by contact between children and possibly by contamination of caregivers' hands (63,238,240, 241). Fomites and environmental contamination may also play a role; the virus is relatively stable and can survive on environmental surfaces for as long as 1 month (234).

Blood-borne Infections

Hepatitis B

The transmission of hepatitis B virus (HBV) between persons in close daily contact, such as in households and facilities for the developmentally disabled, has raised concern about transmission in child care settings (238,241,242). Suspected potential routes of transmission include bites and inoculation of infectious blood or body fluids onto mucous membranes or broken skin (238,241,243).

Reports of HBV transmission in child care settings in the United States are rare (238). A case of apparent child-to-child transmission in a center has been reported; no specific exposure episode could be identified in that case (243). In another report, a child care provider was infected after exposure to the blood of an infected child (244). Other cases of apparent transmission related to child care have been reported from outside the United States. In Japan, where HBV is endemic, 15 of 269 children younger than 5 years who attended a nursery school were hepatitis B surface antigen (HBsAg) positive in the absence of any apparent household exposure, suggesting that transmission may have occurred in the school (245). However, two different studies of separate instances in which an HBsAg-positive and hepatitis B e antigen-positive child was attending a child care facility showed that the mere attendance of such children does not necessarily result in transmission of infection (243,246). In each instance, the child had been in the facility for more than a year before the infection was recognized and no special infection control precautions had been taken. Contact screening showed no transmission to other children or staff. Reviews of national surveillance data have not demonstrated an excess proportion of cases that could be linked to child care exposure (238,243). Although HBV transmission can occur in child care settings and appropriate precautions must be observed, the risk appears to be very low.

Widespread compliance with recommendations for universal infant HBV immunization would significantly reduce any current risk (247).

Human Immunodeficiency Virus (HIV)

Principal concerns regarding the presence of children and providers with HIV in child care facilities include the possibility that they are particularly susceptible to, or have more severe illness as a result of, infections transmitted in that setting, and that they may transmit HIV infection to others (248,249). Immunosuppressed children are at increased risk for severe complications from infections, such as those caused by varicella, herpes simplex, CMV, *H. influenzae, Mycobacterium tuberculosis, Cryptosporidium,* and measles (248–250). Information is limited on the risk that any one child with HIV will acquire a specific infection. However, the prevalence of intestinal parasites in a hospital-affiliated child care center for HIV-infected children was lower than the prevalence typically reported in other child care facilities (251). Rigorous infection control procedures were followed, and it should be noted that the infection control resources available to this center were probably greater than those available to most child care facilities.

Although HIV transmission in out-of-home child care settings has not been reported (248,252), surveys of both parents and providers indicate a reluctance, largely because of fear of HIV transmission, to admit HIV-infected children into child care settings (253,254). Although HIV has been isolated from several body fluids, including saliva, urine, and tears, only blood, semen, cervicovaginal secretions, and human milk have been implicated in the transmission of infection (248,250). Extensive studies of household contacts of HIV-infected children and adults indicate a very low risk of transmission other than through sexual contact, needle sharing, or vertical transmission from mothers to children (248,255). Only a single case of child-to-child transmission (not involving percutaneous or intravenous exposure) among preschool-aged children living in the same home has been reported (248,255–257).

Biting is often proposed as a possible means of HIV transmission in child care settings. Transmission via this route is rare and probably involves exposure to blood from either the biter or bitten person rather than saliva (258). Recommendations for healthcare workers call for postexposure follow-up of both parties when biting results in blood exposure (259). Concern has also been raised about transmission of HIV to staff or children through accidental exposure to breast milk.

Recommendations have been made concerning follow-up in the event a child is inadvertently fed expressed breast milk intended for another child (260,261). Skin exposure resulting from spills of breast milk or vomitus is unlikely to result in transmission.

Vaccine-Preventable Diseases

Routine immunization is recommended for nine infectious diseases: measles, mumps, rubella, diphtheria, pertussis, tetanus, poliomyelitis, Hib, and hepatitis B (247,262–265).

Preschool-aged children continue to have the highest age-specific attack rates of measles, rubella, pertussis, and Hib infections and can suffer more severe sequelae than older children if they become infected (8,263). Most states require immunization before attendance in licensed child care facilities, and children in this setting have more complete immunizations than children not in licensed child care establishments (263) (Centers for Disease Control and Prevention, unpublished data, 1995). The Public Health Service's Year 2000 Health Objectives for the Nation called for 95% of all children in licensed child care facilities to be up to date with age-appropriate vaccination (266). Although the 1997 to 1998 baseline immunization level for measles, mumps, and rubella was only 89%, the objective was exceeded for polio (96%) and diphtheria-tetanus-acellular pertussis (96%). The Year 2010 objectives call for maintaining very high immunization levels for children in licensed day care facilities and children in kindergarten through the first grade (267).

Children's attendance in out-of-home child care offers healthcare providers and the public health system an opportunity to ensure that children have received appropriate immunization (265).

Other Infections

Cytomegalovirus (CMV)

CMV infection is the most common congenital infectious disease in the United States (267,268). Most congenitally infected infants are asymptomatic at birth, but, within the first few years of life, 10% to 20% of these children will suffer severe long-term sequelae, including mental retardation, sensorineural hearing loss, cerebral palsy, and visual impairment from chorioretinitis or optic atrophy (267–269). Contact with children in child care is a well-documented risk factor for adult infection with CMV; child care workers and family members of children in child care are particularly at risk (90,92,93,100,102,104, 269–274). When the exposed adult is pregnant, the fetus may be at risk for congenital infection.

Transmission of CMV among children in out-of-home child care is common; virus excretion rates as high as 69% have been reported (93,269,271,272,275–279). Children in home care have significantly lower excretion rates, around 8% (93,275, 276). Restriction endonuclease patterns of CMV DNA have demonstrated transmission between children in child care settings; infected children in the same child care facility have been shown to share identical CMV strains (102,275).

Children enrolled in child care before their first birthday are more likely to be infected; mixing children younger than 18 months with children older than 18 months also appears to increase the risk of transmission. The likelihood of excretion is age dependent, with the highest excretion rates in children aged between 1 and 3 years (102,268,275,276,278). Pass et al. (93) found that 78% of children aged 12 to 18 months were excreting virus in saliva or urine. Viral shedding may last for more than 2 years in children (102,269,278). One cohort of uninfected children experienced an annual acquisition rate of 12.6% per year (278). Excretion began between 11 and 59 months after entering child care; the duration of excretion ranged from 3 to 28 months, with excretion in the urine lasting longer than excretion in the saliva (278).

The high rates of transmission and excretion among children in out-of-home child care pose an infection risk for pregnant women in contact with these children. Baseline rates of seropositivity of CMV antibody among child care providers range from 38% to 63%; annual seroconversion rates among initially seronegative workers are from 8% to 20% (90,92,93). The annual seroconversion rate in a comparison group of 229 seronegative female hospital workers was 2% (90). Seropositivity is associated with a history of contact with children younger than age 2 years (90,93); seroconversion is associated with providing care for children younger than age 3 years (90).

Children in out-of-home child care play a significant role in introducing CMV into their homes (100,102,104,269–272, 274). Taber et al. (274) showed an annual seroconversion rate of 10.6% for mothers with young children in child care. An index case for intrafamilial spread could be identified for 14 families in that study; in 10 of those instances, a child introduced the infection into the family. In another study, 14 of 67 seronegative parents of children in child care and none of 31 control subjects seroconverted to CMV (280). All seroconversions occurred among parents whose children were actively excreting virus. Restriction endonuclease techniques have shown that identical virus strains can be recovered from children in child care and from their parents and from congenitally infected siblings (100,104,270). (For more information on the epidemiology of CMV infections, see Chapter 44.)

Parvovirus B19

Parvovirus B19, the etiologic agent of erythema infectiosum (fifth disease), has been linked with several conditions, including fetal hydrops and fetal death if a pregnant woman becomes infected and transmits the infection to her fetus (281). As with CMV, concern exists regarding the risk of exposure and infection of pregnant child care providers and transmission from children attending child care to their mothers. The seroprevalence of immunoglobulin G (IgG) antibodies to parvovirus B19 among 122 child care workers in Virginia was 25%, whereas that among 68 mothers of children in child care was 29% (105). The annual seroconversion rate among providers and parents of children in child care was 1.5%. Higher prevalence and incidence rates were reported from studies during a large outbreak in Connecticut in 1988 (96,282). Gillespie et al. (282) studied teachers and child care workers using serum IgG as a marker for preoutbreak seroprevalence and IgM as an indicator of recent infection. The preoutbreak seroprevalence among 50 child care workers was 68%; 5 of 16 susceptible workers (31%) exposed to children with erythema infectiosum showed evidence of recent infection. The number of classroom exposures to children with a rash was significantly correlated with risk of infection. In a second study during the same outbreak, the highest rates of seroconversion were among teachers (16% of susceptible persons), child care workers (9%), and homemakers (9%) (96). Teachers and child care workers who were exposed to erythema infectiosum at work and who also had children living in their homes had higher infection rates (13%) than occupationally exposed teachers and child care providers who did not live with children (10%) (see also Chapter 51).

Herpes Simplex Virus

According to one study, by 5 years of age, 42 of 115 children (37%) at a North Carolina child care center had evidence of primary infection with herpes simplex virus (283). Children aged 1 year had the highest incidence; 20.5 infections occurred per 100 children per year. During the 12-year study, most primary viral isolates (55%) were recovered during outbreaks. (For more information on the epidemiology of infections caused by herpes simplex virus, see Chapter 43.)

INFECTION CONTROL IN CHILD CARE FACILITIES

Several excellent sources of detailed recommendations on health and safety practices in out-of-home child care include publications from the American Academy of Pediatrics (AAP) (283) and the National Association for Education of Young Children (284), books specifically addressing the topic of infection control in child care (285), and publications from state and local health departments (286,287). In 1992, the American Public Health Association (APHA) and AAP jointly published a detailed compendium of guidelines and recommendations for health, safety, nutrition, and sanitation for child care facilities. A revised version was issued in 2002 (36,283). The Maternal and Child Health Bureau of the U.S. Department of Health and Human Services recently released *Stepping Stones to Using Caring for Our Children,* a collection of the most critical recommendations from these standards.

In addition to these reference materials, child care facilities should have access to a health consultant—usually a physician or nurse with expertise in children's health—to whom caregivers can turn for advice and assistance when making decisions on health issues (36,288). Public health authorities are often relied on to fulfill this role (289). Infection control professionals (ICPs) also frequently serve as health consultants to child care facilities in the community and to those facilities managed by the ICPs' healthcare institution.

General Recommendations

Many general principles of infection control in child care settings are similar to those in healthcare settings: interruption of transmission through hand washing and proper handling of contaminated material, management of the environment, surveillance, and limitation of the potential for exposure of susceptible persons. As in healthcare settings, hand washing is generally considered the single most important step in preventing and controlling infectious diseases in child care settings (4,36,60,61, 68,232,264). Careful attention by providers to hand-washing practices, both their own and those of the children, can reduce the incidence of infectious diseases (66,68,232). Guidelines stress both frequency and timing of hand washing and use of proper technique (36,260). Although the use of alcohol gels has been promoted for use in healthcare settings (290), these products have not been recommended for use in child care settings because of differences in the overall level of hygiene, common endemic and epidemic pathogens, groups served, and care provided.

Attention to environmental sanitation is also important to infection control in child care settings, especially in facilities with non–toilet-trained children. Younger children often explore their environment by crawling on the floor and mouthing; environmental contamination with feces, saliva, and other body fluids is common. Several of the most common pathogens causing disease among children and providers have been found on environmental surfaces and objects in child care settings (36,59, 65,69,70,72,194,289,291).

Meals are often prepared and served in child care settings. Care should be taken in the storage, handling, and preparation of all food items and in sanitizing food-handling areas. Hands of caregivers who change diapers often become contaminated with feces; staff who prepare or serve food should not change diapers (36,264). Where staff constraints make it impossible to follow this recommendation, the importance of hand washing before preparing and serving food must be stressed in training and reinforced and monitored to ensure compliance (36).

Surveillance of Child Care Infections

As in the hospital setting, effective surveillance is central to preventing and controlling communicable diseases in child care facilities. Although the major purpose of surveillance is to detect potential problems or outbreaks within facilities, surveillance data can also contribute to the understanding of specific risk factors for infection. It can also help in designing and evaluating prevention and control measures and in developing and conducting training programs for child care providers and parents (4,292,293). Implementation of surveillance has been associated with decreases in diarrheal illness in child care facilities (233), and surveillance can serve as a sentinel system for illness in the community (289,292).

However, a number of obstacles exist to surveillance in child care facilities. Perhaps the greatest obstacle is that child care providers may not fully appreciate the need to monitor illness levels or may not be willing to devote resources to surveillance activities. They are often concerned about confidentiality and understandably hesitant to report information about children in their care to health officials. The large number of, and rapid turnover in, both child care personnel and the facilities themselves and the administrative separation of public health and licensing responsibilities within governmental agencies make it difficult for health officials to ensure that all child care facilities in a given jurisdiction are familiar with the requirements and mechanisms for notifiable disease reporting. As a result, many child care providers are unaware of reporting requirements (294). Also, these requirements are often described in technical jargon or contain vague criteria, such as "unusual occurrences," for reporting.

Many obstacles can be addressed. Although it may be unrealistic to expect all providers to differentiate between type B viral influenza and Hib or to welcome teams of public health workers to their facilities during outbreaks, studies in Seattle and San Diego indicate that providers are able and willing to monitor and report well-defined sentinel events and readily recognizable symptoms to local health authorities (51,293).

Frequent positive interactions between public health officials and the child care community in the form of training sessions and educational materials may reduce concerns about confidentiality and encourage a collaborative response to potential problems. Maintenance of current lists of licensed providers by public health authorities not only allows notification of reporting requirements but also is invaluable in rapidly disseminating information to child care facilities during public health emergencies, such as the 1993 outbreak of cryptosporidiosis in Milwaukee (118). Although several groups have recommended routine monitoring of illness in child care settings and provided models for these programs (36), the experience in Seattle and San Diego suggests that monitoring still has not been routinely accepted as an integral part of the child care process (51,293). Although health consultants with expertise in infection control can help, surveillance is not likely to be optimally effective until child care providers recognize its importance (295).

Role of the Health Department

State and local health departments play an important role in monitoring the health status of children in child care. For example, they routinely ask about child care contact in case investigations of notifiable diseases and generally intervene quickly to interrupt transmission when they learn of an outbreak (36,289, 295,296). Health departments are often a principal resource for information, training, and education for child care providers and parents. Public health officials often serve as consultants to child care licensing and regulatory agencies. Some communities have model programs in which health departments serve as a focus for developing community-wide programs for child health and safety (36,289,295,296).

Training and Education

Staff Training

Successful child care infection control programs require high levels of staff training and education. Child care workers are less likely to receive infection control training than healthcare workers; however, when child care workers understand the rationale behind guidelines and recommendations they appear to increase compliance and cooperation (297). Studies have shown that caregivers need and are interested in receiving training, independent of licensing requirements (91,298). Training for child care providers should cover basic infection control principles, and providers should understand the potential risks, to themselves and to the children, of infections that may be acquired in child care settings (89,90). Additional topics to address include techniques to control those risks, including hand washing, environmental sanitation, avoidance of exposures to blood and body fluids, and steps to protect personal health such as immunizations (66,72,91,264,269,297).

Health Education for Parents

The child care setting offers opportunities to provide health education to parents and to caregivers (124,299,300). Current standards call for such opportunities to be provided even by family child care home providers (36). Such programs could provide information about various health topics, such as immunization, signs of illness requiring medical consultation, fluid replacement for diarrheal disease, and proper use of antipyretics (299).

Exclusion and Cohorting

Among the more difficult problems in the child care setting is establishing and implementing appropriate criteria for excluding ill children from the facility (301). Parents of excluded children must either seek alternative forms of child care or miss work to stay home with the sick child. Much of the economic burden of child care-associated illness is due to missed work. Parents of ill children frequently pressure physicians to prescribe antimicrobials for conditions for which antimicrobial therapy is not indicated.

Overly strict exclusion policies can create tension between parents and caregivers and encourage parents to enroll, or "drop in," an ill child at other facilities without notifying the new facility of the child's health status; this may introduce an infection into a new group of susceptible children (4). However, failure to exclude ill children when it is appropriate to do so may increase the risk of spreading infection to other children in the facility, child care providers, children's household contacts, and thus the community at large.

In the event of an illness outbreak, the benefits of closing a facility to prevent additional spread of disease should be weighed against the possibility of infected children being sent to other facilities (5,116,173) and difficulties in communicating with and monitoring a now dispersed group of households. Cohorting—separating infected and uninfected children into different groups—has been proposed as an alternative to excluding children who are well enough to attend child care but who may have a transmissible infectious disease. Although this strategy can work, it requires careful monitoring to determine which children are and are not infected and to ensure that cohorts are maintained. Cohorting is also very resource intensive, because it often requires additional staffing and rearrangements of or finding additional physical space. These factors make this strategy impractical for many facilities (4,167,173,299).

Specific exclusion criteria for a number of conditions have been published (Table 53.5). These guidelines take into consideration the fact that mild illness is common among children, that infection is often transmitted before onset of symptoms, and that infected children may be asymptomatic (4,89,124,302). Most children do not need to be excluded from child care when they have mild respiratory illness. However, children in obvious

TABLE 53.5. CRITERIA FOR EXCLUDING AN ILL OR INFECTED CHILD FROM AN OUT-OF-HOME CHILD CARE PROGRAM[a]

Fever, defined by the child's age as follows:
- Infants 4 mo of age and younger: temperature ≥101°F rectal or ≥100°F axillary
- Children aged 4–48 mo: temperature ≥102°F rectal or ≥100°F axillary
- Children older than 48 mo: as for younger children, or oral temperature ≥101°F

Signs of possible severe illness, including unusual lethargy, irritability, persistent crying, difficult breathing, uncontrolled coughing

Diarrhea, defined as increased number of stools compared with the child's normal pattern, with increased stool water and/or decreased form

Blood in stools not explained by dietary change, medication or hard stools

Vomiting two or more times in the previous 24 hr unless the vomiting is determined to be due to a noncommunicable condition and the child is not in danger of dehydration

Persistent abdominal pain continuing for more than 2 hrs or intermittent pain associated with fever or other signs or symptoms

Mouth sores associated with an inability of the child to control his or her saliva, unless the child's physician or local health officer states the child is noninfectious

Rash with fever or behavior change until a physician has determined the rash to be noncommunicable

Purulent conjunctivitis, defined as pink or red conjunctiva with white or yellow eye discharge, often with matted eyelids after sleep, and including a child with eye pain or redness of the eyelids or skin surrounding the eye

Infestation (e.g., scabies, head lice), until 24 hr after treatment has been initiated (head lice) or completed (scabies)

Tuberculosis, until the child's physician or local health authority states the child is noninfectious

Impetigo, until 24 hr after treatment has been initiated

Streptococcal pharyngitis, until 24 hr after treatment has been initiated, and until the child has been afebrile for 24 hr

Varicella, until 6 days after onset of rash or until all lesions have dried and crusted

Pertussis, laboratory-confirmed or suspected because of symptoms of the illness or because of cough onset within 14 days after face-to-face contact with a laboratory-confirmed case of pertussis in a household or classroom, until 5 days of appropriate chemoprophylaxis (currently erythromycin) has been completed

Mumps, until 9 days after onset of parotid gland swelling

Measles, until 4 days after onset of rash

Rubella, until 6 days after onset of rash

Hepatitis A virus infection, until 1 wk after onset of illness or until after passive immunoprophylaxis (currently, immune serum globulin) has been administered to appropriate children and staff in the program, as directed by the responsible health department

Child is unable to participate comfortably in program

Care for the child requires greater attention than staff can provide without compromising the health and safety of other children

[a] Local public health laws and child care licensing codes address many of the above conditions and take precedence over these recommendations.

discomfort, those whose symptoms interfere with their ability to participate comfortably in child care activities, and those whose illness requires a level of attention by staff that may interfere with the care of other children should be sent home (36,264).

Most states have regulations requiring isolation for persons with various types of communicable diseases, including those common among child care attendees. These vary by state and take precedence over recommendations from other groups. Local or state health departments should be contacted for information about these regulations and their interpretation and enforcement.

Environmental Control

Disinfection

An overriding principle in environmental control of infectious diseases is good physical cleaning using a detergent or detergent-germicide solution. Many difficulties in recommending the use of specific products or formulations for hospital disinfection also apply to the child care environment (302). In addition, because they crawl on the floor and mouth inanimate objects or furnishings, children in child care, unlike hospitalized patients, are at risk for exposure to toxic substances used for cleaning and disinfection. Thus, disinfectants may need to be assessed in ways not always relevant to the hospital setting (e.g., the potential for chemical residue to remain on environmental surfaces such as floors, walls, and furniture and the risk that chemical agents may be accidentally ingested). The U.S. Environmental Protection Agency registers specific products as detergent-disinfectants for cleaning and disinfecting specific settings and materials. The APHA/AAP standards specifically recommend a diluted bleach solution for disinfection in child care settings (36) (also see Chapter 85).

Physical Facilities

The design of the environment in and around the facility can directly affect the risk of infectious diseases (78). Ideally, areas for different activities that may affect health risks—diaper changing, play, and food preparation and handling—should be separated.

Diaper-changing areas, accessories, and receptacles should be arranged to facilitate appropriate hygiene while changing, handling, and disposing of soiled diapers (36,302). Sinks should be easily accessible, preferably within arm's reach. Children of different age groups should be separated to decrease exposure of older children to environmental fecal contamination.

Environmental surfaces, including furnishings and other objects in child care facilities, should be easy to clean and disinfect (36,78). Toys that are shared by children, especially children in diapers who frequently mouth objects, should be cleaned and disinfected daily and removed for cleaning when obviously contaminated with saliva or other body fluids (36,302).

Personnel Health Issues

All staff should have a health appraisal before or within 1 month after starting work (36). This appraisal should include assurance of appropriate immunizations and screening (and follow-up as needed) for tuberculosis (36). Caregivers should have documented evidence of immunity to tetanus, diphtheria, measles, mumps, rubella, and poliomyelitis, either through vaccination or prior infection (4,36). The potential for adverse consequences of exposure to infections that commonly occur among children in child care should be considered and discussed with the employee; this is particularly true for infections such as CMV, parvovirus B19, and varicella that could affect a fetus if a pregnant woman became infected (4,36,89). (See also Chapters 42, 44, 51, and 80.)

Recommendations for Prevention of Specific Infections

The spread of infectious diseases in child care settings is best prevented by careful adherence to routinely recommended precautions: hand washing; good hygiene; environmental sanitation; and care in handling potentially contaminated material such as tissues, eating utensils, and mouthed toys (4,36,61,302). Special care should be observed in dealing with exposures to blood or blood-containing body fluids (302,303). Children and caregivers should be appropriately immunized, and immunization records should be kept by the facility operator or director (4,36,302). Public health officials and parents should be notified if a child or caregiver is exposed to a communicable disease; exposed persons should be referred, as appropriate, to both the health department and healthcare providers for chemoprophylaxis or immunoprophylaxis (4,36,264,302). Persons who could transmit infection may need to be excluded from the child care setting (4,36,302). Some of these considerations are summarized in Table 53.6. More detailed discussion and recommendations are available elsewhere (4,36,264,301,302).

Respiratory Tract Infections

Most authorities agree that children with mild to moderate symptoms of viral upper respiratory infection, such as rhinitis, cough, pharyngitis, or otitis media, may continue in their usual child care arrangement unless they meet other criteria for exclusion (4,36,264,302). Care should be taken to clean objects, including toys, and surfaces contaminated with oral or nasal secretions. Tissues, towels, or other material used to wipe children's noses and mouths should be handled as contaminated items (4, 36,61,304). Hand washing protocols must be carefully followed (4,36,61,264).

Influenza

Immunization of healthy children aged 6 to 24 months with influenza vaccine is encouraged to reduce the impact of influenza on the health of both the children and public (264). Immunization of high-risk children older than 6 months, including those with chronic pulmonary disease, hemodynamically significant cardiac disease, immunosuppressive disorders (including HIV infection), sickle cell disease, conditions requiring long-term salicylate therapy, chronic renal disfunction, and chronic metabolic disease, is recommended (264). Influenza and other respiratory infections predispose children to otitis media. Immunization against influenza may provide some protection against otitis among vaccinees and may even reduce respiratory illness among household contacts (25,26,305,306). (See also Chapter 41.)

Neisseria meningitidis

In the event of a case of invasive *N. meningitidis* disease in a facility, rifampin prophylaxis should generally be given to child care contacts (both children and adults) (4,36,138,264). It is often not necessary to administer rifampin to all center attendees as they may not have had at-risk contact with the case. Public health authorities and healthcare providers should be involved in evaluating the significance of exposure on an individual basis. Routine immunization is not recommended (264,307). The current vaccine is not as immunogenic in infants and very young children as it is in older children and adults. It also does not provide protection against *N. meningitidis* group B, which is responsible for more than half of the meningococcal disease in the United States. However, the vaccine may be indicated in high-risk children older than 2 years (e.g., those with asplenia and terminal complement deficiencies) and may be useful in controlling outbreaks caused by serogroups to which it does confer immunity (264,307).

Group A Streptococcal Infections

A program of aggressive intervention that involves culturing and treating symptomatic contacts and environmental sanitation measures has been recommended for outbreaks of symptomatic

TABLE 53.6. RECOMMENDATIONS FOR PREVENTING SELECTED INFECTIOUS DISEASES IN CHILD CARE

Infection	Immunization required or commonly available	Postexposure immuno/ chemoprophylaxis available	Notification of parents/ health department if case occurs[a]	May require exclusion from child care (see Table 53.5)
H. influenzae type b	Yes	Yes	Yes	Yes
N. meningitidis	A	Yes	Yes	Yes
Group A streptococcus	No	A	Yes	Yes
M. tuberculosis	No	Yes	Yes	Yes
Pertussis	Yes	Yes	Yes	Yes
Varicella-zoster	Yes	B	Yes	Yes
Hepatitis A	Yes	Yes	Yes	Yes
Hepatitis B	Yes	Yes	Yes	*See text*
Measles	Yes	B	Yes	Yes
Rubella	Yes	B	Yes	Yes

[a] The responsible health department and parents of exposed children should be notified promptly.
A, may be appropriate in an outbreak; B, may be appropriate for persons at high risk of serious adverse outcomes of infection. From refs. 21, 129, 287.

GAS disease with a high attack rate (132). However, the relative benefits of this approach in comparison to less aggressive interventions has not been evaluated (4,131,132).

Varicella-Zoster Virus

Although the licensure of an effective vaccine against varicella will undoubtedly have an impact on risk of outbreaks of chickenpox in child care facilities, recommendations for managing outbreaks have not yet changed. Children with chickenpox should generally be excluded from attendance. State health laws vary in the duration of required exclusion, which may not be exactly the same as that recommended by the AAP (264) or other groups. Immunization may not prevent disease in recently exposed children and has not been approved for use in postexposure prophylaxis (264,308). However, consideration may be given to immunizing children with no history of immunization or clinical illness; parents of such children should be informed of the possibility of clinical illness from preimmunization exposure still exists. All staff members and parents should be informed of the potential for serious infection in susceptible adults and older children and of the potential for fetal damage if infection occurs during pregnancy (264,302,309). Susceptible pregnant staff should be referred to qualified physicians or other health professionals within 24 hours of exposure (4,36,302) (also see Chapter 42).

Herpes Simplex Virus

Children with mild herpes simplex virus disease and good control of oral secretions may be admitted to child care after consultation with their healthcare providers and after staff have been reminded of the importance of limiting contact with infected secretions (36).

Tuberculosis

Current recommendations call for preemployment screening of all child care providers with the five tuberculin units intradermal purified protein derivative skin test and chest radiograph follow-up of all positive reactors (36,302). Because the risk of transmission from infected children to other children is low, children do not need routine screening before entry into child care (4,36,61,264).

Caregivers or children with active disease who are infectious should be excluded from child care and treated in accordance with the appropriate protocols. After initiation of therapy, public health authorities should determine that the patient is noninfectious before the caregiver or child is readmitted (4,36,61,264).

Diarrheal Diseases

Strategies for controlling diarrheal illness focus on preventing fecal-oral transmission (4,61). Child care providers should ensure that their own hands and the child's hands are washed after diapers are changed (36,74,264). Diapers should be of a type that contain feces without leaking; clothing should be worn over diapers (36,74,264). Appropriate environmental sanitation must be maintained, especially in places likely to be contaminated with feces, such as diaper-changing areas. Proper handling of soiled diapers and other contaminated items such as disposable wipes must be ensured (4,36).

Exclusion of children with diarrhea is somewhat controversial. Some authorities maintain that only children with uncontrollable diarrhea, that is, leaking of feces from the diaper, need to be excluded (36,264). Others recommend that any non–toilet-trained child with diarrhea should be excluded rather than risk the occurrence of leaks (282,301). Readmission criteria for asymptomatic persons excreting enteropathogens depend on the pathogen (9,36,173,264,299,302). Because public health laws frequently call for isolation of persons with enteric diseases, local health authorities should be contacted regarding criteria for readmission.

Hepatitis A

The principles for preventing hepatitis A infections in child care facilities are similar to those for other infections transmitted through the fecal-oral route—hand washing, environmental sanitation and hygiene, and exclusion of ill children (4,238). Immune globulin administered within 2 weeks of exposure can prevent symptomatic disease and may be useful in controlling an outbreak (36,238,264,310). Several factors should be considered in determining how extensively to use immune globulin once a case of hepatitis A is recognized in a child or caregiver in a child care facility. These include the presence of diapered children in the facility, delays in recognizing the outbreak after onset of illness in the index case, and evidence of spread among families of children attending the facility (238). Decisions to administer immune globulin should be made in conjunction with local health authorities and the children's and caregivers' physicians (4,36).

Cytomegalovirus

The risk of long-term sequelae from congenital CMV infection should be communicated as part of employee counseling and education to all providers who may be at risk (4,36,89,302). Caregivers should be given information regarding preventing infection through the use of appropriate hygienic precautions (4,36,264). This is especially important for women of childbearing age.

Hepatitis B

Current guidelines recommend that children who are chronic HBV carriers may be admitted to a child care facility if they have no behavioral or medical conditions that could facilitate transmission of HBV (36,264), including aggressive behavior (e.g., biting or scratching), dermatitis, bleeding problems, or open skin lesions that cannot be appropriately covered (36,238, 264).

The decision to admit or not admit a child with the previously mentioned risk factors who is a chronic carrier of HBV should be made in conjunction with the child's healthcare provider, the facility's health consultant, and local public health authorities (36,238,302). Information regarding a child's HBV carrier status should be available to caregivers who regularly provide care to the child; however, the confidentiality of the child and the child's family must be respected and this information must be appropriately limited to those persons who need to know to protect the child's health and the health of others (36,238). The child should be observed for the development of any behaviors that could increase the likelihood of transmission. If a bite or other exposure places a susceptible staff member or child at risk, the exposed person should be promptly referred to his or her healthcare provider and to the health department for evaluation of the need for postexposure prophylaxis (36,238,264).

Because symptomatic undiagnosed HBV carriers may be enrolled in child care, all staff members should be appropriately trained and educated regarding specific precautions to avoid exposure to potentially contaminated blood and body fluids (247, 302,303). Asymptomatic staff members infected with HBV may be allowed to work as long as they have no conditions (e.g., dermatitis) that may facilitate transmission, have received necessary training, and are compliant with methods to prevent transmission of HBV (36,247).

The Advisory Committee on Immunization Practices (ACIP) recommends universal immunization of infants with hepatitis B vaccine (247). The potential benefits of hepatitis B vaccination for older nonimmune children and caregivers in the child care setting should be considered (264).

Human Immunodeficiency Virus

Decisions regarding the attendance of an HIV-infected child should be made on a case-by-case basis by knowledgeable individuals, including the child's physician, the child's parents or guardian, public health authorities, and the child care facility operator or director (36,249,264,311–314). Criteria to address include whether the child poses a risk to others in that particular setting and whether the facility can provide an appropriate level of care for the child. Assessment of these risks should include consideration of the child's neurologic development, behavior, and health status, including the level of the child's immune system dysfunction (36,315). Immunization protocols for HIV-infected children have been published by the ACIP; compliance with these protocols should be ensured (309).

Many precautions that apply to the prevention of hepatitis B are relevant to the discussion of the HIV-infected child or caregiver. Child care settings may contain children or caregivers with unrecognized HIV infection (314). Thus, precautions, including careful attention to the handling of potentially contaminated body fluids in both everyday care and as a result of less common events (e.g., blood spills or injuries) should be implemented routinely (36,234,303,314).

Privacy and confidentiality must be considered when an HIV-infected child is enrolled in a child care facility (36,314). Knowledge of the child's status should be restricted to those persons who need to know to ensure proper care of the child, to be aware of situations that place the infected child at risk for other infections, and to detect situations in which the potential for transmission may increase (36,314). Involvement of the parents or legal guardians of the infected child in the process of determining which staff need to know the child's status can be a positive experience for all parties. As is true for any child exposed to a potentially serious infection, the child's parents or guardian should be notified promptly of exposure to communicable illnesses (36). Ongoing involvement of parents, child care providers, the child's healthcare provider, and local health officials will help to ensure appropriate care.

In general, asymptomatic HIV-infected caregivers may be allowed to work if they have no conditions (e.g., open sores or weeping dermatitis that cannot be adequately contained) that would facilitate contact between potentially contaminated body fluids and children or other adults (36,302,314). The potential for and management of exposures of such caregivers to other infectious diseases should be addressed as recommended for HIV-infected children (36,302).

Vaccine-preventable Diseases

All children enrolling in child care should have written documentation of age-appropriate immunizations (36). Depending on local public health and licensing regulations, unimmunized children may be allowed to attend child care if the appropriate immunization series are started within 1 month and completed according to recommended schedules.

Unimmunized children or those who are exempt from routine childhood immunizations for medical or other reasons should be excluded if the facility has cases of a vaccine-preventable disease. These children may be allowed to return to the center only after the risk of exposure no longer exists or they have been appropriately immunized.

REFERENCES

1. U.S. Bureau of Labor Statistics. Employment characteristics of families: table 4. Families with own children: employment status of parents by age of youngest child and family type, 2000-01 annual averages. US Bureau of Labor Statistics, 2003. Available at *www.bls.gov/news.release/famee.t04.htm* (accessed).
2. U.S. Census Bureau, Population Division Fertility & Family Statistics Branch. Who's minding the kids? Child care arrangements: spring 1999 detailed tables (PPL-168). Available at *http://www.census.gov/population/www/socdemo/child/ppl-168.html* (accessed 1-27-2003).
3. Hofferth SL, Brayfield A, Deich S, et al. National Child Care Survey, 1990, 1991. Washington DC: The Urban Institute.
4. The Child Day Care Infectious Disease Study Group. Public health considerations of infectious diseases in child day care centers. *J Pediatr* 1984;105:683–701.
5. Denny FW, Collier AM, Henderson FW. Acute respiratory infections in day care. *Rev Infect Dis* 1986;8:527–332.
6. Goodman RA, Osterholm MT, Granoff DM, et al. Infectious diseases and child day care. *Pediatrics* 1984;74:134–139.
7. Holmes SJ, Morrow AL, Pickering LK. Child-care practices: effects of social change on the epidemiology of infectious diseases and antibiotic resistance. *Epidemiol Rev*1996;18:10–28.
8. Klein JO. Infectious diseases and day care. *Rev Infect Dis* 1986;8: 521–526.
9. Osterholm MT, Reves RR, Murph JR, et al. Infectious diseases and child day care. *Pediatr Infect Dis J* 1992;11:S31–S41.
10. Pickering LK. Infections in day care. *Pediatr Infect Dis J* 1987;6: 614–617.

11. Cordell RL, Solomon SL. Infections acquired in child care centers. In: Mayhall CG, ed. *Hospital epidemiology and infection control.* Philadelphia: Lippincott Williams & Wilkins, 1999:695–718.
12. Chiou CC, Liu YC, Huang TS, et al. Extremely high prevalence of nasopharyngeal carriage of penicillin-resistant *Streptococcus pneumoniae* among children in Kaohsiung, Taiwan. *J Clin Microbiol* 1998;36: 1933–1937.
13. Dellamonica P, Pradier C, Dunais B, et al. New perspectives offered by a French study of antibiotic resistance in day-care centers. *Chemother* 1998;44(Suppl 1):10–14.
14. Givon-Lavi N, Dagan R, Fraser D, et al. Marked differences in pneumococcal carriage and resistance patterns between day care centers located within a small area. *Clin Infect Dis* 1999;29:1274–1280.
15. Kellner JD, Ford-Jones EL, Toronto Child Care Centre Study Group. *Streptococcus pneumoniae* carriage in children attending 59 Canadian child care centers. *Arch Pediatr Adolesc Med* 1999;153:495–502.
16. Mainous AG III, Evans ME, Hueston WJ, et al. Patterns of antibiotic-resistant *Streptococcus pneumoniae* in children in a day-care setting. *J Family Pract* 1998;46:142–146.
17. Shahin R, Johnson IL, Jamieson F, et al, Toronto Child Care Center Study Group. Methicillin-resistant *Staphylococcus aureus* carriage in a child care center following a case of disease. *Arch Pediatr Adolesc Med* 1999;153:864–868.
18. Skull SA, Ford-Jones EL, Kulin NA, et al. Child care center staff contribute to physician visits and pressure for antibiotic prescription. *Arch Pediatr Adolesc Med* 2000;154:180–183.
19. Thrane N, Olesen C, Sondergaard C, et al. Influence of day care attendance on the use of systemic antibiotics in 0- to 2-year-old children. *Pediatrics* 2001;107:E76.
20. Belongia EA, Sullivan BJ, Chyou PH, et al. A community intervention trial to promote judicious antibiotic use and reduce penicillin-resistant *Streptococcus pneumoniae* carriage in children. *Pediatrics* 2001;108: 575–583.
21. Friedman JF, Lee GM, Kleinman KP, et al. Acute care and antibiotic seeking for upper respiratory tract infections for children in day care: parental knowledge and day care center policies. *Arch Pediatr Adolesc Med* 2003;157:369–374.
22. Jiles RB, Fuchs C, Klevens RM. Vaccination coverage among children enrolled in Head Start programs or day care facilities or entering school. *MMWR CDC Surveillance Summaries* 2000;49:27–38.
23. Centers for Disease Control and Prevention. Vaccination coverage among children enrolled in Head Start programs, licensed child care facilities, and entering school—United States, 2000–01 school year. *MMWR Morb Mortal Wkly Rep* 2003;52:175–180.
24. Clements DA, Langdon L, Bland C, et al. Influenza A vaccine decreases the incidence of otitis media in 6- to 30-month-old children in day care. *Arch Pediatr Adolesc Med* 1995;149:1113–1117.
25. Hurwitz ES, Haber M, Chang A, et al. Studies of the 1996–1997 inactivated influenza vaccine among children attending day care: immunologic response, protection against infection, and clinical effectiveness. *J Infect Dis* 2000;182:1218–1221.
26. Hurwitz ES, Haber M, Chang A, et al. Effectiveness of influenza vaccination of day care children in reducing influenza-related morbidity among household contacts. *JAMA* 2000;284:1677–1682.
27. Dagan R, Sikuler-Cohen M, Zamir O, et al. Effect of a conjugate pneumococcal vaccine on the occurrence of respiratory infections and antibiotic use in day-care center attendees. *Pediatr Infect Dis J* 2001; 20:951–958.
28. Buchholz U, Moolenaar R, Peterson C, et al. Varicella outbreaks after vaccine licensure: should they make you chicken? *Pediatrics* 1999; 104:561–563.
29. Clements DA, Moreira SP, Coplan PM, et al. Postlicensure study of varicella vaccine effectiveness in a day-care setting. *Pediatr Infect Dis J* 1999;18:1047–1050.
30. Clements DA, Zaref JI, Bland CL, et al. Partial uptake of varicella vaccine and the epidemiological effect on varicella disease in 11 day-care centers in North Carolina. *Arch Pediatr Adolesc Med* 2001;155: 455–461.
31. Galil K, Lee B, Strine T, et al. Outbreak of varicella at a day-care center despite vaccination. *N Engl J Med* 2002;347:1909–1915.
32. National Institute of Child Health and Human Development Early Child Care Research Network. Child care and common communicable illnesses: results from the National Institute of Child Health and Human Development Study of Early Child Care. *Arch Pediatr Adolesc Med* 2001;155:481–488.
33. Bradley RH, National Institute of Child Health and Human Development (NICHD) Early Child Care Research Network. Child care and common communicable illnesses in children aged 37 to 54 months. *Arch Pediatr Adolesc Med* 2003;157:196–200.
34. Ball TM, Holberg CJ, Aldous MB, et al. Influence of attendance at day care on the common cold from birth through 13 years of age. *Arch Pediatr Adolesc Med* 2002;156:121–126.
35. Svanes C, Jarvis D, Chinn S, et al. Early exposure to children in family and day care as related to adult asthma and hay fever: results from the European Community Respiratory Health Survey. *Thorax* 2002;57:945–950.
36. American Academy of Pediatrics, American Public Health Association. *Caring for our children: national health and safety performance standards: guidelines for out-of-home child care,* 2nd ed. Elk Grove Village, IL: American Academy of Pediatrics, 2002.
37. Fleming DW, Cochi SL, Hightower AW, et al. Childhood upper respiratory tract infections: to what degree is incidence affected by day-care attendance? *Pediatrics* 1987;79:55–60.
38. Hurwitz ES, Gunn WJ, Pinsky PF, et al. Risk of respiratory illness associated with day-care attendance: a nationwide study. *Pediatrics* 1991;87:62–69.
39. Reves RR, Morrow AL, Bartlett AV, et al. Child day care increases the risk of clinic visits for acute diarrhea and diarrhea due to rotavirus. *Am J Epidemiol* 1993;137:97–107.
40. Bell DM, Gleiber DW, Mercer AA, et al. Illness associated with child day care: a study of incidence and cost. *Am J Public Health* 1989;79: 479–484.
41. Alexander CS, Zinzeleta EM, Mackenzie EJ, et al. Acute gastrointestinal illness and child care arrangements. *Am J Epidemiol* 1990;131: 124–131.
42. Bartlett AV, Moore M, Gary GW, et al. Diarrheal illness among infants and toddlers in day care centers. II. Comparison with day care homes and households. *J Pediatr* 1985;107:503–509.
43. Doyle AB. Incidence of illness in early group and family day-care. *Pediatrics* 1976;58:607–613.
44. Johansen AS, Leibowitz A, Waite LJ. Child care and children's illness. *Am J Public Health* 1988;78:1175–1177.
45. Stahlberg MR. The influence of form of day care on occurrence of acute respiratory tract infections among young children. *Acta Paediatr Scand* 1980;282:1–84.
46. Strangert K, Carlstrom G, Jeansson S, et al. Infections in preschool children in group day care. *Acta Paediatr Scand* 1976; 65:455–463.
47. Strangert K. Otitis media in young children in different types of day-care. *Scand J Infect Dis* 1977;9:119–123.
48. Wald ER, Dashefsky B, Byers C, et al. Frequency and severity of infections in day care. *J Pediatr* 1988;112:540–546.
49. Wald ER, Guerra N, Byers C. Frequency and severity of infections in day care: three-year follow-up. *J Pediatr* 1991;118:509–514.
50. Cordell RL, MacDonald JK, Solomon SL, et al. Illnesses and absence due to illness among children attending child care facilities in Seattle-King County, Washington. *Pediatrics* 1997;100:850–855.
51. Cordell RL, Waterman SH, Chang A, et al. Provider-reported illness and absence due to illness among children attending child-care homes and centers in San Diego, Calif. *Arch Pediatr Adolesc Med* 1999;153: 275–280.
52. Haskins R. Acute illness in day care: how much does it cost?. *Bull N Y Acad Med* 1989;65:319–343.
53. Carabin H, Gyorkos TW, Soto JC, et al. Estimation of direct and indirect costs because of common infections in toddlers attending day care centers. *Pediatrics* 1999;103:556–564.
54. Adcock PM, Pastor P, Medley F, et al. Methicillin-resistant *Staphylococcus aureus* in two child care centers. *J Infect Dis* 1998;178:577–580.
55. Campos J, Garcia-Tornel S, Musser JM, et al. Molecular epidemiology of multiply resistant *Haemophilus influenzae* type b in day care centers. *J Infect Dis* 1987;156:483–489.

56. Henderson FW, Gilligan PH, Wait K, et al. Nasopharyngeal carriage of antibiotic-resistant pneumococci by children in group day care. *J Infect Dis* 1988;157:256–263.
57. Rauch AM, O'Ryan M, Van R, et al. Invasive disease due to multiply resistant *Streptococcus pneumoniae* in a Houston, Tex, day-care center. *Am J Dis Child* 1990;144:923–927.
58. Reves RR, Jones JA. Antibiotic use and resistance patterns in day care centers. In: Pickering LK, ed. *Seminars in pediatric infectious diseases.* Philadelphia: WB Saunders, 1990:212–221.
59. Reves RR, Fong M, Pickering LK, et al. Risk factors for fecal colonization with trimethoprim-resistant and multiresistant *Escherichia coli* among children in day-care centers in Houston, Texas. *Antimicrob Agents Chemother* 1990;34:1429–1434.
60. The Child Day Care Infectious Disease Study Group. Considerations of infectious diseases in day care centers. *Pediatr Infect Dis* 1985;4: 124–136.
61. Thacker SB, Addiss DG, Goodman RA, et al. Infectious diseases and injuries in child day care. Opportunities for healthier children. *JAMA* 1992;268:1720–1726.
62. Ekanem EE, DuPont HL, Pickering LK, et al. Transmission dynamics of enteric bacteria in day-care centers. *Am J Epidemiol* 1983;18: 562–572.
63. Hadler SC, Erben JJ, Francis DP, et al. Risk factors for hepatitis A in day-care centers. *J Infect Dis* 1982;145:255–261.
64. Sattenspiel L. Epidemics in nonrandomly mixing populations: a simulation. *Am J Physical Anthropol* 1987;73:251–265.
65. Laborde DJ, Weigle KA, Weber DJ, et al. Effect of fecal contamination on diarrheal illness rates in day-care centers. *Am J Epidemiol* 1993;138:243–255.
66. Bartlett AV, Moore M, Gary GW, et al. Diarrheal illness among infants and toddlers in day care centers. I. Epidemiology and pathogens. *J Pediatr* 1985;107:495–502.
67. Lemp GF, Woodward WE, Pickering LK, et al. The relationship of staff to the incidence of diarrhea in day-care centers. *Am J Epidemiol* 1984;120:750–758.
68. Butz AM, Larson E, Fosarelli P, et al. Occurrence of infectious symptoms in children in day care homes. *Am J Infect Control* 1990;18: 347–353.
69. Hutto C, Little EA, Ricks R, et al. Isolation of cytomegalovirus from toys and hands in a day care center. *J Infect Dis* 1986;154:527–530.
70. Weniger BG, Ruttenber AJ, Goodman RA, et al. Fecal coliforms on environmental surfaces in two day care centers. *Appl Environ Microbiol* 1983;45:733–735.
71. Holaday B, Pantell R, Lewis C, et al. Patterns of fecal coliform contamination in day-care centers. *Public Health Nursing* 1990;7: 224–228.
72. Holaday B, Waugh G, Moukaddem VE, et al. Fecal contamination in child day care centers: cloth vs paper diapers. *Am J Public Health* 1995;85:30–33.
73. Van R, Wun CC, Morrow AL, et al. The effect of diaper type and overclothing on fecal contamination in day-care centers. *JAMA* 1991; 265:1840–1844.
74. Van R, Morrow AL, Reves RR, et al. Environmental contamination in child day-care centers. *Am J Epidemiol* 1991;133:460–470.
75. Cody MM, Sottnek HM, O'Leary VS. Recovery of *Giardia lamblia* cysts from chairs and tables in child day-care centers. *Pediatrics* 1994; 94:1006–1008.
76. Keswick BH, Pickering LK, DuPont HL, et al. Survival and detection of rotaviruses on environmental surfaces in day care centers. *Appl Environ Microbiol* 1983;46:813–816.
77. Wilde J, Van R, Pickering L, et al. Detection of rotaviruses in the day care environment by reverse transcriptase polymerase chain reaction. *J Infect Dis* 1992;166:507–611.
78. Petersen NJ, Bressler GK. Design and modification of the day care environment. *Rev Infect Dis* 1986;8:618–621.
79. Centers for Disease Control and Prevention. Outbreak of invasive group A *Streptococcus* associated with varicella in a childcare center—Boston, Massachusetts, 1997. *MMWR Morb Mortal Wkly Rep* 1997;46:944–948.
80. Huskins WC. Transmission and control of infections in out-of-home child care. *Pediatr Infect Dis J* 2000;19:S106–S110.
81. Cochi SL, Fleming DW, Hightower AW, et al. Primary invasive *Haemophilus influenzae* type b disease: a population-based assessment of risk factors. *J Pediatr* 1986;108:887–896.
82. Hardy AM, Fowler MG. Child care arrangements and repeated ear infections in young children. *Am J Public Health* 1993;83: 1321–1325.
83. Centers for Disease Control and Prevention. *Bacillus cereus* food poisoning associated with fried rice at two child day care centers—Virginia, 1993. *MMWR Morb Mortal Wkly Rep* 1994;43:177–178.
84. Pickering LK. Bacterial and parasitic enteropathogens in day care. In: Pickering LK, ed. *Seminars in pediatric infectious diseases.* Philadelphia: WB Saunders, 1990:263–269.
85. Chorba TL, Meriwether RA, Jenkins BR, et al. Control of a non-foodborne outbreak of salmonellosis: day care in isolation. *Am J Public Health* 1987;77:979–981.
86. Newcomb S, Broadhurst L, Kissane K. *Salmonella* outbreak in an American child development center in Germany. *Military Med* 1997; 162:783–787.
87. Gotz H, de JB, Lindback J, et al. Epidemiological investigation of a food-borne gastroenteritis outbreak caused by Norwalk-like virus in 30 day-care centres. *Scand J Infect Dis* 2002;34:115–121.
88. Cordell RL. The risk of infectious diseases among child care providers. *J Am Med Womens Assoc* 2001;56:109–112.
89. Reves RR, Pickering LK. Impact of child day care on infectious diseases in adults. *Infect Dis Clin North Am* 1992;6:239–250.
90. Adler SP. Cytomegalovirus and child day care. Evidence for an increased infection rate among day-care workers. *N Engl J Med* 1989; 321:1290–1296.
91. Kendall ED, Aronson SS, Goldberg S, et al. Training for child day care staff and for licensing and regulatory personnel in the prevention of infectious disease transmission. *Rev Infect Dis* 1986;8:651–656.
92. Murph JR, Baron JC, Brown CK, et al. The occupational risk of cytomegalovirus infection among day-care providers. *JAMA* 1991; 265:603–608.
93. Pass RF, Hutto SC, Reynolds DW, et al. Increased frequency of cytomegalovirus infection in children in group day care. *Pediatrics* 1984;74:121–126.
94. Gothe CJ, Hillert L. Spontaneous abortions and work in day nurseries. *Acta Obstet Gynecol Scand* 1992;71:284–292.
95. Jackson LA, Stewart LK, Solomon SL, et al. Risk of infection with hepatitis A, B or C, cytomegalovirus, varicella or measles among child care providers. *Pediatr Infect Dis J* 1996;15:584–589.
96. Cartter ML, Farley TA, Rosengren S, et al. Occupational risk factors for infection with parvovirus B19 among pregnant women. *J Infect Dis* 1991;163:282–285.
97. Dingle J, Badger G, Jordan WS Jr. *Illness in the home.* Cleveland: Western Reserve University, 1964.
98. Fox J, Hall C. *Viruses in families: surveillance of families as a key to epidemiology of virus infections.* Littleton, MA: PSC Publishing Co, 1981.
99. Hadler SC, Webster HM, Erben JJ, et al. Hepatitis A in day-care centers. A community-wide assessment. *N Engl J Med* 1980;302: 1222–1227.
100. Pass RF, Little EA, Stagno S, et al. Young children as a probable source of maternal and congenital cytomegalovirus infection. *N Engl J Med* 1987;316:1366–1370.
101. Polis MA, Tuazon CU, Alling DW, et al. Transmission of *Giardia lamblia* from a day care center to the community. *Am J Public Health* 1986;76:1142–1144.
102. Adler SP. Cytomegalovirus transmission and child day care. *Adv Pediatr Infect Dis* 1992;7:109–122.
103. Cordell RL, Addiss DG. Cryptosporidiosis in child care settings: a review of the literature and recommendations for prevention and control.. *Pediatr Infect Dis J* 1994;13:310–317.
104. Adler SP. Molecular epidemiology of cytomegalovirus: viral transmission among children attending a day care center, their parents, and caretakers. *J Pediatr* 1988;112:366–372.
105. Koch WC, Adler SP. Human parvovirus B19 infections in women

of childbearing age and within their families. *Pediatr Infect Dis J* 1989; 8:83–97.
106. Mohle-Boetani JC, Stapleton M, Finger R, et al. Communitywide shigellosis: control of an outbreak and risk factors in child day-care centers. *Am J Public Health* 1995;85:812–816.
107. Skinner JT. Community-wide epidemic of hepatitis A-Shelby County, Tennessee. *J Tenn Med Assoc* 1995;88:468–469.
108. Smith PF, Grabau JC, Werzberger A, et al. The role of young children in a community-wide outbreak of hepatitis A. *Epidemiol Infect* 1997; 118:243–252.
109. Venczel LV, Desai MM, Vertz PD, et al. The role of child care in a community-wide outbreak of hepatitis A. *Pediatrics* 2001;108:E78.
110. Strangert K. Respiratory illness in preschool children with different forms of day care. *Pediatrics* 1976;57:191–196.
111. Gomez-Barreto D, Calderon-Jaimes E, Rodriguez RS, et al. Carriage of antibiotic-resistant pneumococci in a cohort of a daycare center. *Salud Publica de Mexico* 2002;44:26–32.
112. Monteros L, Bustos I, Flores L, et al. Outbreak of scarlet fever caused by an erythromycin-resistant *Streptococcus pyogenes* emm22 genotype strain in a day-care center. *Pediatr Infect Dis J* 2003;20:807–809.
113. Nilsson P, Laurell MH. Carriage of penicillin-resistant *Streptococcus pneumoniae* by children in day-care centers during an intervention program in Malmo, Sweden. *Pediatr Infect Dis J* 2001;20:1144–1149.
114. Reichler MR, Allphin AA, Breiman RF, et al. The spread of multiply resistant *Streptococcus pneumoniae* at a day care center in Ohio. *J Infect Dis* 1992;166:1346–1353.
115. Reves RR, Murray BE, Pickering LK, et al. Children with trimethoprim- and ampicillin-resistant fecal *Escherichia coli* in day care centers. *J Infect Dis* 1987;156:758–762.
116. Tacket CO, Cohen ML. Shigellosis in day care centers: use of plasmid analysis to assess control measures. *Pediatr Infect Dis* 1983;2:127–130.
117. Fornasini M, Reves RR, Murray BE, et al. Trimethoprim-resistant *Escherichia coli* in households of children attending day care centers. *J Infect Dis* 1992;166:326–330.
118. Cordell RL, Thor PM, Addiss DG, et al. Impact of a massive waterborne cryptosporidiosis outbreak on child care facilities in metropolitan Milwaukee, Wisconsin. *Pediatr Infect Dis J* 1997;16:639–644.
119. Landis SE, Chang A. Child care options for ill children. *Pediatrics* 1991;88:705–718.
120. Furman L. Infirmary-style sick-child day care: do we need more information? *Pediatrics* 1991;88:290–293.
121. MacDonald KL, White KA, Heiser J, et al. Evaluation of a sick child day care program: lack of detected increased risk of subsequent infections. *Pediatr Infect Dis J* 1990;9:15–20.
122. Schwartz B, Giebink GS, Henderson FW, et al. Respiratory infections in day care. *Pediatrics* 1994;94:1018–1020.
123. Loda FA, Glezen WP, Clyde WA Jr. Respiratory disease in group day care. *Pediatrics* 1972;49:428–437.
124. Haskins R, Kotch J. Day care and illness: evidence, cost, and public policy. *Pediatrics* 1986;77:951–982.
125. Anderson LJ, Parker RA, Strikas RA, et al. Day-care center attendance and hospitalization for lower respiratory tract illness. *Pediatrics* 1988; 82:300–308.
126. Gardner G, Frank AL, Taber LH. Effects of social and family factors on viral respiratory infection and illness in the first year of life. *J Epidemiol Comm Health* 1984;38:42–48.
127. Holberg CJ, Wright AL, Martinez FD, et al. Child day care, smoking by caregivers, and lower respiratory tract illness in the first 3 years of life. Group Health Medical Associates. *Pediatrics* 1993;91:885–892.
128. Margolis PA, Greenberg RA, Keyes LL, et al. Lower respiratory illness in infants and low socioeconomic status. *Am J Public Health* 1992; 82:1119–1126.
129. Pacini DL, Collier AM, Henderson FW. Adenovirus infections and respiratory illnesses in children in group day care. *J Infect Dis* 1987; 156:920–927.
130. Klein JD, Collier AM, Glezen WP. An influenza B epidemic among children in day-care. *Pediatrics* 1976;58:340–345.
131. Falck G, Kjellander J. Outbreak of group A streptococcal infection in a day-care center. *Pediatr Infect Dis J* 1992;11:914–919.
132. Smith TD, Wilkinson V, Kaplan EL. Group A streptococcus-associated upper respiratory tract infections in a day-care center. *Pediatrics* 1989;83:380–384.
133. Centers for Disease Control and prevention. Haemophilus b conjugate vaccines for prevention of *Haemophilus influenzae* type b disease among infants and children two months of age and older. Recommendations of the immunization practices advisory committee (ACIP). *MMWR Recommend Rep* 1991;40:1–7.
134. Adams WG, Deaver KA, Cochi SL, et al. Decline of childhood *Haemophilus influenzae* type b (Hib) disease in the Hib vaccine era. *JAMA* 1993;269:221–226.
135. Centers for Disease Control and Prevention. Progress toward elimination of *Haemophilus influenzae* type b invasive disease among infants and children—United States, 1998–2000. *MMWR Morb Mortal Wkly Rep* 2002;51:234.
136. Murphy TV, White KE, Pastor P, et al. Declining incidence of *Haemophilus influenzae* type b disease since introduction of vaccination. *JAMA* 1993;269:246–248.
137. Murphy TV, Pastor P, Medley F, et al. Decreased *Haemophilus* colonization in children vaccinated with *Haemophilus influenzae* type b conjugate vaccine. *J Pediatr* 1993;122:517–523.
138. Osterholm MT. Invasive bacterial diseases and child day care. In: Pickering LK, ed. *Seminars in pediatric diseases.* Philadelphia: WB Saunders, 1990:222–223.
139. Jacobson JA, Filice GA, Holloway JT. Meningococcal disease in day-care centers. *Pediatrics* 1977;59:299–300.
140. Leggiadro RJ, Baddour LM, Frasch CE, et al. Invasive meningococcal disease: secondary spread in a day-care center. *South Med J* 1989;82: 511–513.
141. Saez-Nieto JA, Perucha M, Casamayor H, et al. Outbreak of infection caused by *Neisseria meningitidis* group C type 2 in a nursery. *J Infect* 1984;8:49–55.
142. Rosen C, Christensen P, Hovelius B, et al. A longitudinal study of the nasopharyngeal carriage of pneumococci as related to pneumococcal vaccination in children attending day-care centres. *Acta Oto Laryngologica* 1984;98:524–532.
143. Takala AK, Jero J, Kela E, et al. Risk factors for primary invasive pneumococcal disease among children in Finland. *JAMA* 1995;273: 859–864.
144. Cherian T, Steinhoff MC, Harrison LH, et al. A cluster of invasive pneumococcal disease in young children in child care. *JAMA* 1994; 271:695–697.
145. Craig AS, Erwin PC, Schaffner W, et al. Carriage of multidrug-resistant *Streptococcus pneumoniae* and impact of chemoprophylaxis during an outbreak of meningitis at a day care center. *Clin Infect Dis* 1999; 29:1257–1264.
146. Regev-Yochay G, Raz M, Shainberg B, et al. Independent risk factors for carriage of penicillin-non-susceptible *Streptococcus pneumoniae. Scand J Infect Dis* 2003;35:219–222.
147. Doyle MG, Morrow AL, Van R, Pickering LK. Intermediate resistance of *Streptococcus pneumoniae* to penicillin in children in day-care centers. *Pediatr Infect Dis J* 1992;11:831–835.
148. Boken DJ, Chartrand SA, Goering RV, et al. Colonization with penicillin-resistant *Streptococcus pneumoniae* in a child-care center. *Pediatr Infect Dis J* 1995;14:879–884.
149. Radetsky MS, Istre GR, Johansen TL, et al. Multiply resistant pneumococcus causing meningitis: its epidemiology within a day-care centre. *Lancet* 1981;2:771–773.
150. Engelgau MM, Woernle CH, Schwartz B, et al. Invasive group A streptococcus carriage in a child care centre after a fatal case. *Arch Dis Child* 1994;71:318–322.
151. Starke JR, Jacobs RF, Jereb J. Resurgence of tuberculosis in children. *J Pediatr* 1992;120:839–855.
152. Kaupas V. Tuberculosis in a family day-care home. Report of an outbreak and recommendations for prevention. *JAMA* 1974;228: 851–854.
153. Leggiadro RJ, Callery B, Dowdy S, et al. An outbreak of tuberculosis in a family day care home. *Pediatr Infect Dis J* 1989;8:52–54.
154. Nolan CM, Barr H, Elarth AM, et al. Tuberculosis in a day-care home. *Pediatrics* 1987;79:630–632.

155. Gross TP, Silverman PR, Bloch AB, et al. An outbreak of tuberculosis in rural Delaware. *Am J Epidemiol* 1989;129:362–371.
156. Bosley AR, George G , Eorge M. Outbreak of pulmonary tuberculosis in children. *Lancet* 1986;1:1141–1143.
157. Driver CR, Jones JS, Cavitt L, et al. Tuberculosis in a day-care center, Kentucky, 1993. *Pediatr Infect Dis J* 1995;14:612–616.
158. Frenck RW, Glezen WP. Respiratory infections in children in day care. In: Pickering LK, ed. *Seminars in pediatric infectious diseases.* Philadelphia: WB Saunders, 1990:234–244.
159. Henderson FW, Collier AM, Sanyal MA, et al. A longitudinal study of respiratory viruses and bacteria in the etiology of acute otitis media with effusion. *N Engl J Med* 1982;306:1377–1383.
160. Henderson FW, Giebink GS. Otitis media among children in day care: epidemiology and pathogenesis. *Rev Infect Dis* 1986;8:533–538.
161. Wald ER, Guerra N, Byers C. Upper respiratory tract infections in young children: duration of and frequency of complications. *Pediatrics* 1991;87:129–133.
162. Etzel RA, Pattishall EN, Haley NJ, et al. Passive smoking and middle ear effusion among children in day care. *Pediatrics* 1992;90:228–232.
163. Stahlberg MR, Ruuskanen O, Virolainen E. Risk factors for recurrent otitis media. *Pediatr Infect Dis* 1986;5:30–32.
164. Vinther B, Brahe PC, Elbrond O. Otitis media in childhood. Sociomedical aspects with special reference to day-care conditions. *Clin Otolaryngol Allied Sci* 1984;9:3–8.
165. Daly K, Giebink GS, Le CT, et al. Determining risk for chronic otitis media with effusion. *Pediatr Infect Dis J* 1988;7:471–475.
166. Froom J, Culpepper L. Otitis media in day-care children. A report from the International Primary Care Network. *J Fam Pract* 1991;32: 289–294.
167. Centers for Disease Control and Prevention. Shigellosis in child day care centers—Lexington-Fayette County, Kentucky, 1991. *MMWR Morb Mortal Wkly Rep* 1992;41:440–442.
168. Pelletier AR, Finger RF, Sosin DM. Shigellosis in Kentucky, 1986 through 1989. *South Med J* 1991;84:818–821.
169. Pickering LK, Evans DG, DuPont HL, et al. Diarrhea caused by *Shigella,* rotavirus, and *Giardia* in day-care centers: prospective study. *J Pediatr* 1981;99:51–56.
170. Pickering LK, Bartlett AV, Woodward WE. Acute infectious diarrhea among children in day care: epidemiology and control. *Rev Infect Dis* 1986;8:539–547.
171. Tauxe RV, Johnson KE, Boase JC, et al. Control of day care shigellosis: a trial of convalescent day care in isolation. *Am J Public Health* 1986;76:627–630.
172. Weissman JB, Schmerler A, Weiler P, et al. The role of preschool children and day-care centers in the spread of shigellosis in urban communities. *J Pediatr* 1974;84:797–802.
173. Weissman JB, Gangorosa EJ, Schmerler A, et al. Shigellosis in day-care centres. *Lancet* 1975;1:88–90.
174. Lieb S, Gunn RA, Taylor DN. Salmonellosis in a day-care center. *J Pediatr* 1982;100:1004–1005.
175. Oberhelman RA, Flores-Abuxapqui J, Suarez-Hoil G, et al. Asymptomatic salmonellosis among children in day-care centers in Merida, Yucatan, Mexico. *Pediatr Infect Dis J* 2001;20:792–797.
176. Allaby MA, Mayon-White R. *Escherichia coli* O 157: outbreak in a day nursery. *Comm Dis Rep CDR Rev* 1995;5:R4–R6.
177. Belongia EA, Osterholm MT, Soler JT, et al. Transmission of *Escherichia coli* O157:H7 infection in Minnesota child day-care facilities. *JAMA* 1993;269:883–888.
178. Bower JR, Congeni BL, Cleary TG, et al. *Escherichia coli* O114:nonmotile as a pathogen in an outbreak of severe diarrhea associated with a day care center. *J Infect Dis* 1989;160:243–247.
179. Lerman Y, Cohen D, Gluck A, et al. A cluster of cases of *Escherichia coli* O157 infection in a day-care center in a communal settlement (Kibbutz) in Israel. *J Clin Microbiol* 1992;30:520–521.
180. Paulozzi LJ, Johnson KE, Kamahele LM, et al. Diarrhea associated with adherent enteropathogenic *Escherichia coli* in an infant and toddler center, Seattle, Washington. *Pediatrics* 1986;77:296–300.
181. Samadpour M, Grimm LM, Desai B, et al. Molecular epidemiology of *Escherichia coli* O157:H7 strains by bacteriophage lambda restriction fragment length polymorphism analysis: application to a multistate foodborne outbreak and a day-care center cluster. *J Clin Microbiol* 1993;31:3179–3183.
182. Spika JS, Parsons JE, Nordenberg D, et al. Hemolytic uremic syndrome and diarrhea associated with *Escherichia coli* O157:H7 in a day care center. *J Pediatr* 1986;109:287–291.
183. Oberhelman RA, Laborde D, Mera R, et al. Colonization with enteroadherent, enterotoxigenic and enterohemorrhagic *Escherichia coli* among day-care center attendees in New Orleans, Louisiana. *Pediatr Infect Dis J* 1998;17:1159–1162.
184. Galanis E, Longmore K, Hasselback P, et al. Investigation of an *E. coli* O157:H7 outbreak in Brooks, Alberta, June–July 2002: the role of occult cases in the spread of infection within a daycare setting. *Can Comm Dis Rep* 2003;29:21–28.
185. O'Donnell JM, Thornton L, McNamara EB, et al. Outbreak of Vero cytotoxin-producing *Escherichia coli* O157 in a child day care facility. *Comm Dis Public Health* 2002;5:54–58.
186. Goossens H, Giesendorf BA, Vandamme P, et al. Investigation of an outbreak of *Campylobacter upsaliensis* in day care centers in Brussels: analysis of relationships among isolates by phenotypic and genotypic typing methods. *J Infect Dis* 1995;172:1298–1305.
187. Itoh T, Saito K, Maruyama T, et al. An outbreak of acute enteritis due to *Campylobacter fetus* subspecies *jejuni* at a nursery school of Tokyo. *Microbiol Immunol* 1980;24:371–379.
188. Riordan T, Humphrey TJ, Fowles A. A point source outbreak of *Campylobacter* infection related to bird-pecked milk. *Epidemiol Infect* 1993;110:261–265.
189. Kim K, DuPont HL, Pickering LK. Outbreaks of diarrhea associated with *Clostridium difficile* and its toxin in day-care centers: evidence of person-to-person spread. *J Pediatr* 1983;102:376–382.
190. de la Morena ML, Van R, Singh K, Brian M, et al. Diarrhea associated with *Aeromonas* species in children in day care centers. *J Infect Dis* 1993;168:215–218.
191. Bartlett AV III, Reves RR, Pickering LK. Rotavirus in infant-toddler day care centers: epidemiology relevant to disease control strategies. *J Pediatr* 1988;113:435–441.
192. Ferson MJ, Stringfellow S, McPhie K, et al. Longitudinal study of rotavirus infection in child-care centres. *J Paediatr Child Health* 1997; 33:157–160.
193. Hjelt K, Paerregaard A, Nielsen OH, et al. Acute gastroenteritis in children attending day-care centres with special reference to rotavirus infections. I. Aetiology and epidemiologic aspects. *Acta Paediatr Scand* 1987;76:754–762.
194. Keswick BH, Pickering LK, DuPont HL, et al. Prevalence of rotavirus in children in day care centers. *J Pediatr* 1983;103:85–86.
195. Matson DO, O'Ryan ML, Herrera I, et al. Fecal antibody responses to symptomatic and asymptomatic rotavirus infections. *J Infect Dis* 1993;167:577–583.
196. O'Ryan M, Matson DO. Viral gastroenteritis in the day care setting. In: Pickering LK, ed. *Seminars in pediatric infectious diseases.* Philadelphia: WB Saunders, 1990:252–262.
197. O'Ryan ML, Matson DO, Estes MK, et al. Molecular epidemiology of rotavirus in children attending day care centers in Houston. *J Infect Dis* 1990;162:810–816.
198. Pickering LK, Bartlett AV III, Reves RR, et al. Asymptomatic excretion of rotavirus before and after rotavirus diarrhea in children in day care centers. *J Pediatr* 1988;112:361–365.
199. Rodriguez WJ, Kim HW, Brandt CD, et al. Common exposure outbreak of gastroenteritis due to type 2 rotavirus with high secondary attack rate within families. *J Infect Dis* 1979;140:353–357.
200. Waters V, Ford-Jones EL, Petric M, et al. Etiology of community-acquired pediatric viral diarrhea: a prospective longitudinal study in hospitals, emergency departments, pediatric practices and child care centers during the winter rotavirus outbreak, 1997 to 1998. The Pediatric Rotavirus Epidemiology Study for Immunization Study Group. *Pediatr Infect Dis J* 2000;19:843–848.
201. Ferson MJ, Bell SM. Outbreak of coxsackievirus A16 hand, foot, and mouth disease in a child day-care center. *Am J Public Health* 1991; 81:1675–1676.
202. Ferson MJ, Young LC. Cryptosporidium and coxsackievirus B5 caus-

ing epidemic diarrhoea in a child-care centre. *Med J Aust* 1992;156: 813.
203. Grohmann G, Glass RI, Gold J, et al. Outbreak of human calicivirus gastroenteritis in a day-care center in Sydney, Australia. *J Clin Microbiol* 1991;29:544–550.
204. Matson DO, Estes MK, Glass RI, et al. Human calicivirus-associated diarrhea in children attending day care centers. *J Infect Dis* 1989;159: 71–78.
205. Matson DO, Estes MK, Tanaka T, et al. Asymptomatic human calicivirus infection in a day care center. *Pediatr Infect Dis J* 1990;9: 190–196.
206. Lew JF, Glass RI, Petric M, et al. Six-year retrospective surveillance of gastroenteritis viruses identified at ten electron microscopy centers in the United States and Canada. *Pediatr Infect Dis J* 1990;9:714.
207. Lew JF, Moe CL, Monroe SS, et al. Astrovirus and adenovirus associated with diarrhea in children in day care settings. *J Infect Dis* 1991; 164:673–678.
208. Mitchell DK, Van R, Morrow AL, et al. Outbreaks of astrovirus gastroenteritis in day care centers. *J Pediatr* 1993;123:725–732.
209. Mitchell DK, Monroe SS, Jiang X, et al. Virologic features of an astrovirus diarrhea outbreak in a day care center revealed by reverse transcriptase-polymerase chain reaction. *J Infect Dis* 1995;172: 1437–1444.
210. Mitchell DK, Matson DO, Jiang X, et al. Molecular epidemiology of childhood astrovirus infection in child care centers. *J Infect Dis* 1999;80:514–517.
211. Paerregaard A, Hjelt K, Genner J, et al. Role of enteric adenoviruses in acute gastroenteritis in children attending day-care centres. *Acta Paediatr Scand* 1990;79:370–371.
212. Van R, Wun CC, O'Ryan ML, et al. Outbreaks of human enteric adenovirus types 40 and 41 in Houston day care centers. *J Pediatr* 1992;120:516–521.
213. Addiss DG, Stewart JM, Finton RJ, et al. *Giardia lamblia* and *Cryptosporidium* infections in child day-care centers in Fulton County, Georgia. *Pediatr Infect Dis J* 1991;10:907–911.
214. Bartlett AV, Englender SJ, Jarvis BA, et al. Controlled trial of *Giardia lamblia*: control strategies in day care centers. *Am J Public Health* 1991;81:1001–1006.
215. Black RE, Dykes AC, Sinclair SP, et al. Giardiasis in day-care centers: evidence of person-to-person transmission. *Pediatrics* 1977;60: 486–491.
216. Chute CG, Smith RP, Baron JA. Risk factors for endemic giardiasis. *Am J Public Health* 1987;77:585–587.
217. Crawford FG, Vermund SH. Parasitic infections in day care centers. *Pediatr Infect Dis J* 1987;6:744–749.
218. Keystone JS, Krajden S, Warren MR. Person-to-person transmission of *Giardia lamblia* in day-care nurseries. *Can Med Assoc J* 247;119: 241–242.
219. Keystone JS, Yang J, Grisdale D, et al. Intestinal parasites in metropolitan Toronto day-care centres. *Can Med Assoc J* 1984;131:733–735.
220. Novotny TE, Hopkins RS, Shillam P, et al. Prevalence of *Giardia lamblia* and risk factors for infection among children attending daycare facilities in Denver. *Public Health Rep* 1990;105:72–75.
221. Pickering LK, Woodward WE, DuPont HL, et al. Occurrence of *Giardia lamblia* in children in day care centers. *J Pediatr* 1984;104: 522–526.
222. Rauch AM, Van R, Bartlett AV, et al. Longitudinal study of *Giardia lamblia* infection in a day care center population. *Pediatr Infect Dis J* 1990;9:186–189.
223. Sealy DP, Schuman SH. Endemic giardiasis and day care. *Pediatrics* 1983;72:154–158.
224. Steketee RW, Reid S, Cheng T, et al. Recurrent outbreaks of giardiasis in a child day care center, Wisconsin. *Am J Public Health* 1989;79: 485–490.
225. Alpert G, Bell LM, Kirkpatrick CE, et al. Cryptosporidiosis in a daycare center. *N Engl J Med* 1984;311:860–861.
226. Alpert G, Bell LM, Kirkpatrick CE, et al. Outbreak of cryptosporidiosis in a day-care center. *Pediatrics* 1986;77:152–157.
227. Combee CL, Collinge ML, Britt EM. Cryptosporidiosis in a hospital-associated day care center. *Pediatr Infect Dis* 1986;5:528–532.
228. Taylor JP, Perdue JN, Dingley D, et al. Cryptosporidiosis outbreak in a day-care center. *Am J Dis Child* 1985;139:1023–1025.
229. Koutsavlis AT, Valiquette L, Allard R, et al. *Blastocystis hominis*: a new pathogen in day-care centres? *Can Comm Dis Rep* 2001;27:76–84.
230. Staat MA, Morrow AL, Reves RR, et al. Diarrhea in children newly enrolled in day-care centers in Houston. *Pediatr Infect Dis J* 1991; 10:282–286.
231. Sullivan P, Woodward WE, Pickering LK, et al. Longitudinal study of occurrence of diarrheal disease in day care centers. *Am J Public Health* 1984;74:987–991.
232. Black RE, Dykes AC, Anderson KE, et al. Handwashing to prevent diarrhea in day-care centers. *Am J Epidemiol* 1981;113:445–451.
233. Bartlett AV, Jarvis BA, Ross V, et al. Diarrheal illness among infants and toddlers in day care centers: effects of active surveillance and staff training without subsequent monitoring. *Am J Epidemiol* 1988;127: 808–817.
234. Rutala WA. APIC guideline for selection and use of disinfectants. *Am J Infect Control* 1990;18:99–117.
235. Benenson MW, Takafuji ET, Bancroft WH, et al. A military community outbreak of hepatitis type A related to transmission in a child care facility. *Am J Epidemiol* 1980;112:471–481.
236. Sagliocca L, Mele A, Gill ON, et al. A village outbreak of hepatitis A: acquaintance network and inapparent pre-school transmission compared. *Eur J Epidemiol* 1988;4:470–472.
237. Sagliocca L, Mele A, Ferrigno L, et al. Case control study of risk factors for hepatitis A: Naples 1990–1991. Hepatitis Collaborating Group. *Ital J Gastroenterol* 1995;27:181–184.
238. Shapiro C. Significance of hepatitis in children in day care. In: Pickering LK, ed. *Seminars in pediatric infectious diseases.* Philadelphia: WB Saunders, 1990:270–279.
239. Gingrich GA, Hadler SC, Elder HA, et al. Serologic investigation of an outbreak of hepatitis A in a rural day-care center. *Am J Public Health* 1983;73:1190–1193.
240. Storch G, McFarland LM, Kelso K, et al. Viral hepatitis associated with day-care centers. *JAMA* 1979;242:1514–1518.
241. Hadler SC, McFarland L. Hepatitis in day care centers: epidemiology and prevention. *Rev Infect Dis* 1986;8:548–557.
242. Hershow RC, Hadler SC, Kane MA. Adoption of children from countries with endemic hepatitis B: transmission risks and medical issues. *Pediatr Infect Dis J* 1987;6:421–437.
243. Shapiro CN, McCaig LF, Gensheimer KF, et al. Hepatitis B virus transmission between children in day care. *Pediatr Infect Dis J* 1989; 8:870–875.
244. Deseda CC, Shapiro CN, Carroll K, et al. Hepatitis B virus transmission between a child and staff member at a day-care center. *Pediatr Infect Dis J* 1994;13:828–830.
245. Hayashi J, Kashiwagi S, Nomura H, et al. Hepatitis B virus transmission in nursery schools. *Am J Epidemiol* 1987;125:492–498.
246. Shapiro ED. Lack of transmission of hepatitis B in a day care center. *J Pediatr* 1987;110:90–92.
247. Centers for Disease Control and Prevention. Hepatitis B virus: a comprehensive strategy for eliminating transmission in the United States through universal childhood vaccination. Recommendations of the Immunization Practices Advisory Committee (ACIP). *MMWR Recommend Rep* 1991;40:1–19.
248. Jones DS, Rogers MF. Human immunodeficiency virus infection in children in day care. *Pediatrics* 1990;85:280–286.
249. MacDonald KL, Danila RN, Osterholm MT. Infection with human T-lymphotropic virus type III/lymphadenopathy-associated virus: considerations for transmission in the child day care setting. *Rev Infect Dis* 1986;8:606–612.
250. Anonymous. American Academy of Pediatrics Committee on Infectious Diseases: health guidelines for the attendance in day-care and foster care settings of children infected with human immunodeficiency virus. *Pediatrics* 1987;79:466–471.
251. Stoller JS, Adam HM, Weiss B, et al. Incidence of intestinal parasitic disease in an acquired immunodeficiency syndrome day-care center. *Pediatr Infect Dis J* 1991;10:654–658.
252. Heagarty MC. Day care for the child with acquired immunodeficiency

syndrome and the child of the drug-abusing mother. *Pediatrics* 1993; 91:199–201.
253. Morrow AL, Benton M, Reves RR, et al. Knowledge and attitudes of day care center parents and care providers regarding children infected with human immunodeficiency virus. *Pediatrics* 1991;87: 876–883.
254. Renaud A, Ryan B, Cloutier D, et al. Knowledge and attitude assessment of Quebec daycare workers and parents regarding HIV/AIDS and hepatitis B. *Can J Public Health* 1997;88:23–26.
255. Rogers MF, White CR, Sanders R, et al. Lack of transmission of human immunodeficiency virus from infected children to their household contacts. *Pediatrics* 1990;85:210–214.
256. Fitzgibbon JE, Gaur S, Frenkel LD, et al. Transmission from one child to another of human immunodeficiency virus type 1 with a zidovudine-resistance mutation. *N Engl J Med* 1993;329:1835–1841.
257. Simonds RJ, Rogers MF. HIV prevention—bringing the message home. *N Engl J Med* 1993;329:1883–1885.
258. Centers for Disease Control and Prevention. Fact sheet: HIV and its transmission. Centers for Disease Control and Prevention, 2003. Available at *http://www.cdc.gov/hiv/pubs/facts/transmission.htm* (accessed).
259. Centers for Disease Control and Prevention. Public Health Service guidelines for the management of health-care worker exposures to HIV and recommendations for postexposure prophylaxis. *MMWR Recommend Rep* 1998;47:1–33.
260. Hale CM, Polder JA. *The ABCs of safe and healthy child care.* Atlanta: Centers for Disease Control and Prevention, 1996.
261. American Academy of Pediatrics, American Public Health Association. Standard 3.027. Feeding of human milk to another mother's child. In: *Caring for our children: national health and safety performance standards: guidelines for out-of-home child care.* Elk Grove Village, IL: American Academy of Pediatrics, 2002:103–104.
262. Atkinson WL, Pickering LK, Schwartz B, et al. General recommendations on immunization. Recommendations of the Advisory Committee on Immunization Practices (ACIP) and the American Academy of Family Physicians (AAFP). *MMWR Recommend Rep* 2002;51:1–35.
263. Cochi SL. New policies of vaccine use affecting children in day care. In: Pickering LK, ed. *Seminars in infectious diseases.* Philadelphia: WB Saunders, 1990:287–292.
264. Committee on Infectious Diseases American Academy of Pediatrics. *Red book: 2003 Report of the Committee on Infectious Diseases.* Elk Grove Village, IL: American Academy of Pediatrics, 2003.
265. Hinman AR. Vaccine-preventable diseases and child day care. *Rev Infect Dis* 1986;8:573–583.
266. National Center for Health Statistics. *Healthy people 2000 final review.* Hyattsville, MD: Public Health Service, 2001:279–293
267. U.S. Department of Health and Human Services. *Healthy People 2010,* 2nd ed. Washington, DC: U.S. Government Printing Office, 2000:14-1–14-53.
268. Stagno S, Pass RF, Cloud G, et al. Primary cytomegalovirus infection in pregnancy. Incidence, transmission to fetus, and clinical outcome. *JAMA* 1986;256:1904–1908.
269. Pass RF. Day care centers and transmission of cytomegalovirus: new insight into an old problem. In: Pickering LK, ed. *Seminars in infectious diseases.* Philadelphia: WB Saunders, 1990:245–251.
270. Adler SP. Molecular epidemiology of cytomegalovirus: evidence for viral transmission to parents from children infected at a day care center. *Pediatr Infect Dis* 1986;5:315–318.
271. Adler SP. Cytomegalovirus transmission among children in day care, their mothers and caretakers. *Pediatr Infect Dis J* 1988;7:279–285.
272. Pass RF, Hutto C, Ricks R, et al. Increased rate of cytomegalovirus infection among parents of children attending day-care centers. *N Engl J Med* 1986;314:1414–1418.
273. Pass RF, Hutto C. Group day care and cytomegaloviral infections of mothers and children. *Rev Infect Dis* 1986;8:599–605.
274. Taber LH, Frank AL, Yow MD, et al. Acquisition of cytomegalovirus infections in families with young children. *J Infect Dis* 1985;151: 948–952.
275. Adler SP. The molecular epidemiology of cytomegalovirus transmission among children attending a day care center. *J Infect Dis* 1985; 152:760–768.
276. Hutto C, Ricks R, Garvie M, et al. Epidemiology of cytomegalovirus infections in young children: day care vs. home care. *Pediatr Infect Dis* 1985;4:149–152.
277. Murph JR, Bale JF Jr, Murray JC, et al. Cytomegalovirus transmission in a Midwest day care center: possible relationship to child care practices. *J Pediatr* 1986;109:35–39.
278. Murph JR, Bale JF Jr. The natural history of acquired cytomegalovirus infection among children in group day care. *Am J Dis Child* 1988; 142:843–846.
279. Pass RF, August AM, Dworsky M, et al. Cytomegalovirus infection in day-care center. *N Engl J Med* 1982;307:477–479.
280. Pass RF, Hutto C, Lyon MD, et al. Increased rate of cytomegalovirus infection among day care center workers. *Pediatr Infect Dis J* 1990; 9:465–470.
281. Chorba T, Coccia P, Holman RC, et al. The role of parvovirus B19 in aplastic crisis and erythema infectiosum (fifth disease). *J Infect Dis* 1986;154:383–393.
282. Gillespie SM, Cartter ML, Asch S, et al. Occupational risk of human parvovirus B19 infection for school and day-care personnel during an outbreak of erythema infectiosum. *JAMA* 1990;263:2061–2065.
283. Schmitt DL, Johnson DW, Henderson FW. Herpes simplex type 1 infections in group day care. *Pediatr Infect Dis J* 1991;10:729–734.
284. Aronson SS. *Healthy young children: a manual for programs.* Washington, DC: National Association for the Education of Young Children, 2002.
285. Grossman LB. *Infection control in child care center and preschool.* Baltimore: Williams & Wilkins, 2002.
286. Seattle-King County Department of Public Health. *Child care health handbook.* Seattle, WA: Seattle-King County Department of Public Health, 2001.
287. Hooker C, Fritz MJ, Grimm MB. *Infectious diseases in child care settings: information for directors, caregivers, and parents or guardians.* Hopkins, MN: Hennepin County Community Health Department, 1998.
288. Aronson SS. Role of the pediatrician in setting and using standards for child care. *Pediatrics* 1993;91:239–243.
289. Goodman RA, Glode MP, Pfeiffer JA, et al. A role for the infection control specialist in child day care? *Rev Infect Dis* 1986;8:631–633.
290. Boyce JM, Pittet D. Guideline for hand hygiene in health-care settings. Recommendations of the Healthcare Infection Control Practices Advisory Committee and the HICPAC/SHEA/APIC/IDSA Hand Hygiene Task Force. *MMWR Recommend Rep* 2002;51:1–44.
291. Butz AM, Fosarelli P, Dick J, et al. Prevalence of rotavirus on high-risk fomites in day-care facilities. *Pediatrics* 1993;92:202–205.
292. Davis JP, Pfeiffer JA. Surveillance of communicable diseases in child day care settings. *Rev Infect Dis* 1986;8:613–617.
293. MacDonald JK, Boase J, Stewart LK, et al. Active and passive surveillance for communicable diseases in child care facilities, Seattle-King County, Washington. *Am J Public Health* 1997;87:1951–1955.
294. Addiss DG, Sacks JJ, Kresnow MJ, et al. The compliance of licensed US child care centers with national health and safety performance standards. *Am J Public Health* 1994;84:1161–1164.
295. Sherman IL, Langmuir AD. Usefulness of communicable disease reports. *Public Health Rep* 1952; 67:1249–1257.
296. Morgan GG, Stevenson CS, Fiene R, et al. Gaps and excesses in the regulation of child day care: report of a panel. *Rev Infect Dis* 1986; 8:634–643.
297. Aronson SS, Aiken LS. Compliance of child care programs with health and safety standards: impact of program evaluation and advocate training. *Pediatrics* 1980;65:318–325.
298. Bassoff BZ, Willis WO. Requiring formal training in preventive health practices for child day care providers. *Public Health Rep* 1991; 106:523–529.
299. Hoffman RE, Shillam PJ. The use of hygiene, cohorting, and antimicrobial therapy to control an outbreak of shigellosis. *Am J Dis Child* 1990;144:219–221.
300. Sterne GG, Hinman A, Schmid S. Potential health benefits of child day care attendance. *Rev Infect Dis* 1986;8:660–662.

301. Cordell RL, Solomon SL, Hale CM. Exclusion of mildly ill children from out-of-home child care facilities. *Infect Med* 1996;13:41–48.
302. Giebink GS. National standards for infection control in out of home child care. In: Pickering LK, ed. *Seminars in infectious diseases.* Philadelphia: WB Saunders, 1990:184–194.
303. Centers for Disease Control and Prevention. Update: universal precautions for prevention of transmission of human immunodeficiency virus, hepatitis B virus, and other bloodborne pathogens in health-care settings. *MMWR Morb Mortal Wkly Rep* 1988;37:377–382, 387–388.
304. Wenger JD, Harrison LH, Hightower A, et al. Day care characteristics associated with *Haemophilus influenzae* disease. *Haemophilus influenzae* Study Group. *Am J Public Health* 1990;80:1455–1458.
305. Clements DA, Langdon L, Bland C, et al. Influenza A vaccine decreases the incidence of otitis media in 6- to 30-month-old children in day care. *Arch Pediatr Adolesc Med* 1995;149:1113–1117.
306. Heikkinen T, Ruuskanen O, Waris M, et al. Influenza vaccination in the prevention of acute otitis media in children. *Am J Dis Child* 1991;145:445–448.
307. Centers for Disease Control and Prevention. Control and prevention of meningococcal disease: recommendations of the Advisory Committee on Immunization Practices (ACIP). *MMWR Recommend Rep* 1997;46:1–8.
308. Centers for Disease Control and Prevention. Prevention of varicella. Update recommendations of the Advisory Committee on Immunization Practices (ACIP). *MMWR Recommend Rep* 1996;45:1–36.
309. Centers for Disease Control and Prevention. Recommendations of the Advisory Committee on Immunization Practices (ACIP): use of vaccines and immune globulins for persons with altered immunocompetence. *MMWR Recommend Rep* 1993;43:1–18.
310. Hadler SC, Erben JJ, Matthews D, et al. Effect of immunoglobulin on hepatitis A in day-care centers. *JAMA* 1983;249:48–53.
311. American Academy of Pediatrics Committee on Infectious Diseases. Health guidelines for the attendance in day-care and foster care settings of children infected with human immunodeficiency virus. *Pediatrics* 2003;79:466–471.
312. Blackman JA, Appel BR. Epidemiologic and legal considerations in the exclusion of children with acquired immunodeficiency syndrome, cytomegalovirus or herpes simplex virus infection from group care. *Pediatr Infect Dis J* 1987;6:1011–1015.
313. Rubinstein A. Schooling for children with acquired immune deficiency syndrome. *J Pediatr* 1986;109:242–244.
314. Simonds RJ, Chanock S. Medical issues related to caring for human immunodeficiency virus-infected children in and out of the home. *Pediatr Infect Dis J* 1993;12:845–852.
315. Centers for Disease Control and Prevention. Education and foster care of children infected with human T-lymphotropic virus type III/lymphadenopathy-associated virus. *MMWR Morb Mortal Wkly Rep* 1985;34:517–521.
316. Agre F. The relationship of mode of infant feeding and location of care to frequency of infection. *Am J Dis Child* 1985;139:809–811.
317. Laborde DJ, Weigle KA, Weber DJ, et al. The frequency, level, and distribution of fecal contamination in day-care center classrooms. *Pediatrics* 1994;94:1008–1011.
318. Louhiala PJ, Jaakkola N, Ruotsalainen R, et al. Form of day care and respiratory infections among Finnish children. *Am J Public Health* 1995;85:1109–1112.
319. Alho OP, Kilkku O, Oja H, et al. Control of the temporal aspect when considering risk factors for acute otitis media. *Arch Otolaryngol Head Neck Surg* 1993;19:444–449.
320. Marx J, Osguthorpe JD, Parsons G. Day care and the incidence of otitis media in young children. *Otolaryngol Head Neck Surg* 1995; 112:695–699.
321. Alho OP, Laara E, Oja H. Public health impact of various risk factors for acute otitis media in northern Finland. *Am J Epidemiol* 1996;143: 1149–1156.

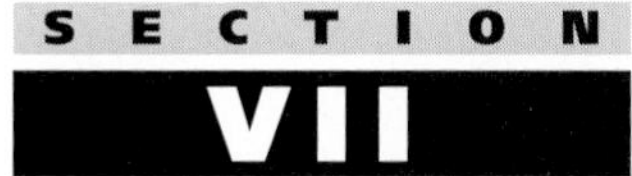

EPIDEMIOLOGY AND PREVENTION OF NOSOCOMIAL INFECTIONS IN SPECIAL PATIENT POPULATIONS

54

NOSOCOMIAL INFECTIONS IN DENTAL, ORAL, AND MAXILLOFACIAL SURGERY

CYNTHIA J. WHITENER
BRUCE H. HAMORY

Dental and oral surgical procedures are some of the most frequently performed minor surgical procedures in the United States. Because these procedures rarely occasion admission to hospital, either for the initial procedure or for the care of a complication, data on incidence rates for procedure-related infections in this setting are scanty. Maxillofacial surgery is more commonly performed in an inpatient setting, especially surgery for reconstructive purposes after trauma or that involving major restructuring of bones for cosmetic surgical reasons. Therefore, more information exists concerning risks of procedure-related infection for maxillofacial procedures. Because of the recognition of human immunodeficiency virus (HIV) transmission in one dentist's practice, national attention has been focused on infection control practices in dentistry (1). This chapter discusses the infections seen in these settings, their recognition, and measures for their prevention.

ETIOLOGY

Infections after surgery to the gums or teeth or involving mucosal incisions made in the mouth are caused by a combination of the aerobic, facultatively anaerobic, and anaerobic microorganisms found in the saliva and the gingival crevices (2,3).

The number and variety of bacteria found in the oral cavity of each person increases as he or she matures, the dentition erupts, and the flora of the gingival crevice establishes itself. Cross-sectional surveys have suggested that a few anaerobes are present in the mouth of young children before the eruption of their first deciduous teeth (4,5). Older children have a microbial flora closely approximating that of the mature dentulous adult. This includes the presence of *Prevotella* and spirochetal microorganisms. *Actinomyces naeslundii* can be recovered from the mouths of most infants but is replaced by *Actinomyces viscosus* when the teeth erupt (4).

The bacteriology of the saliva is somewhat different from that of the gingival crevice. The gingival crevice has approximately 100 times more microorganisms per gram than saliva does and 70% of these microorganisms are anaerobic, whereas most salivary flora are aerobic and facultatively anaerobic. As an illustration of this difference, *Streptococcus salivarius* accounts for approximately 47% of facultative microorganisms in saliva but less than 1% of those found in the gingival crevice. There appears to be no relationship between the appearance of the tongue (presence of white coating or not) and salivary bacterial load (6). Table 54.1 lists the microorganisms in the saliva and gingival crevice of adults (7–9).

A study of the short-term effect of full-mouth tooth extractions (in eight patients with severe periodontitis) on periodontal pathogens colonizing the oral mucous membranes revealed that many *Prevotella* species still colonized the oral mucous membranes of edentulous patients. However, it was unlikely that these patients would continue to be reservoirs for *Actinobacillus actinomycetemcomitans* or *Prevotella gingivalis* (10).

Although no studies have documented transmission of oral flora from one patient to another in the dental operatory, Genco and Loos (11) reviewed several studies using molecular epidemiologic techniques to demonstrate the transmission of *Streptococcus mutans* by vertical transmission from mother to infant (but not from father to infant) and intrafamilial transmission of *A. actinomycetemcomitans.* These studies are the first to document the spread of oral microorganisms and raise the possibility of whether oral bacteria can be transferred in a medical setting from one patient to another.

Many aerobic bacteria transiently colonize or infect the pharynx and posterior nasopharynx. Recognition of these agents depends either on characteristic clinical symptoms, such as the chancre of syphilis or the adherent membrane of diphtheria, or on culture to demonstrate the presence of group A β-hemolytic streptococci or *Neisseria meningitidis.*

The viruses often present in saliva are those agents causing latent infection, particularly the herpes group and less commonly hepatitis B virus (HBV), hepatitis C virus (HCV), or HIV (12). Herpes simplex virus (HSV) has been recovered from the saliva of approximately 1% of asymptomatic children and between 0.75% and 5% of asymptomatic adults. Serial sampling of the saliva from normal adults over time has demonstrated that HSV can be recovered from oral secretions in more than 50% of adults in the absence of clinical lesions. More than 50% of seropositive

TABLE 54.1. NORMAL FLORA OF THE ORAL CAVITY

Saliva	Gingival crevice/plaque
Streptococci	Streptococci
S. salivarius	*S. sanguis*
S. faecalis	*S. mutans*
	S. milleri
	Peptostreptococcus
Staphylococcus aureus	
Veillonellae	Veillonellae
Neisseria	*Neisseria*
Branhamella	*Branhamella*
	Actinomyces
Candida albicans	*A. naeslundii*
Herpes simplex	*A. odontolyticus*
	A. viscosus
	A. israellii
Entamoeba gingivalis	*Bacterionema matruchotii*
Trichomonas tenax	*Bacteroides* species
	Porphyromonas species
	Prevotella species
	Capnocytophaga
	Eikenella corrodens
	Fusobacterium nucleatum
	Actinobacillus actinomycetemcomitans
	Treponema
	T. macrodentium
	T. denticola
	T. orale

patients undergoing organ transplantation shed oral HSV asymptomatically (13). HSV is a recognized occupational hazard for dentists, oral surgeons, and dental technicians.

Cytomegalovirus (CMV) has been isolated from salivary glands, adenoid tissue, and pharyngeal secretions. The prevalence of antibody to CMV increases with age and is further increased among people from lower socioeconomic groups. In seroprevalence studies performed in the 1970s, between 40% and 80% of adults had serologic evidence of infection with CMV by the age of 40 (14). CMV excretion is increased in the presence of transplantation and immunosuppression. No transmission to dental workers or medical staff has been shown (15).

Epstein-Barr virus (EBV) is another herpesvirus that causes acute infectious mononucleosis followed by a chronic infection of lymphocytes. The prevalence of infection as indicated by the presence of antibody is higher at early ages in the tropics and in underdeveloped countries. Prevalence progressively increases with age in developed countries (16). No transmission to dental workers or medical staff has been demonstrated.

Herpesvirus 6 (HHV-6), herpesvirus 7 (HHV-7), and herpesvirus 8 (HHV-8) have been identified in up to 29% of gingival biopsies of HIV-seronegative adults with periodontitis suggesting that the periodontium might constitute a reservoir for these viruses (17).

The blood-borne viruses, including HBV, HCV, and HIV, may be present in the saliva of persons with chronic infection. Small cuts and abrasions in the oral cavity, especially when made acutely during dental or intraoral surgery, serve as the primary sources for seeding the saliva with virus. These viruses are addressed in the epidemiology section of this chapter.

Many other viral agents can be recovered from oropharyngeal secretions during or after acute infection. These agents include polioviruses, coxsackieviruses and echoviruses, influenza viruses A and B, rhinoviruses, and coronaviruses. Despite the occasional isolation from saliva and nasal secretions of these viruses and the childhood respiratory pathogens rubeola (measles), mumps, and rubella, no occupationally related transmission of any of these viral agents to a dental worker has been documented except for one case of coxsackievirus infection (12). Dental procedures should be avoided in patients suspected of having active severe acute respiratory syndrome (SARS), which is caused by a newly discovered coronavirus and is likely transmitted by droplet and contact routes.

Yeasts and fungi also are part of the normal flora of the oral cavity. *Candida albicans* can be isolated from the mouths of approximately 55% of healthy people. Many other species of *Candida* are found less often. The dorsum of the tongue has the greatest density of yeast. Carriage rates for yeast are increased among hospitalized patients, people with dentures, persons who are blood type O or nonsecretors, and people who are in the HIV-positive population (18–20). Transient carriage of filamentous soil fungi from the genera *Penicillium, Aspergillus, Geotrichum,* and others can be shown.

Protozoa are also normal inhabitants of the healthy mouth. *Entamoeba gingivalis* and *Trichomonas tenax* can be demonstrated in more than 50% of the healthy population.

TYPES OF INFECTIONS

Infections of the oral cavity and maxillofacial regions can be grouped loosely into the categories of localized infection, infection by direct extension, and distant infection.

Localized infections can be classified as dentoalveolar, periodontal, infections of the salivary glands or tonsils, and cellulitis from tissue injury. Dentoalveolar infections are also known as odontogenic infections and include carious teeth with resulting infections of the dental pulp and periapical dental abscess. Infections involving the gingiva, periodontal ligament, and other tissues supporting the teeth are known as periodontal infections. These infections include gingivitis and acute necrotizing ulcerative gingivitis (ANUG). Parotitis and sialoadenitis are infections of glands.

Infections resulting from the direct extension of one or more of these localized infections include osteomyelitis of the mandible or maxilla, infection of the deep fascial spaces (e.g., submandibular, canine, retropharyngeal), maxillary sinusitis, noma (necrotizing infection of the cheek), posterior mediastinal infection, and anaerobic pulmonary infection. The anatomy of the deep fascial spaces is beyond the scope of this discussion but is well treated in standard texts (2,4,21).

Distant infections that may develop secondary to oral infection include brain and liver abscesses and septic arthritis (22–26). Distant spread of bacteria from the oral cavity to implanted prosthetic devices via the bloodstream is well documented (27,28). The risk of bacteremia may increase with increasing severity of gingival inflammation.

PATHOGENESIS OF INFECTION

Localized Infection

Infection of the dental pulp may result from microbial penetration directly through the dentin secondary to dental caries, dental drilling, or tooth fracture or by hematogenous spread. The most common cause of pulpal infection is from dental caries that begins with the formation of dental plaque. Plaque is composed of a large number of bacteria (>10^8 CFU/mm^3), including *S. mutans,* which firmly adhere to the enamel of the tooth. These bacteria secrete enzymes that progressively dissolve away the tooth enamel and dentin, permitting the bacteria to access the pulp (29). Microbial infection of the pulp (pulpitis) results and manifests clinically with pain and temperature sensitivity in the tooth. If the infection is not recognized and treated, the bacteria may then migrate through the pulpal foramen at the apex of the tooth into the alveolar bone at the root of the tooth, forming a periapical abscess, or extend beyond into the medullary space of the mandible, resulting in osteomyelitis. Needle aspiration and appropriate culture of pus from dentoalveolar abscesses reveal a polymicrobial flora (>2.4 isolates per specimen) with a predominance of facultatively anaerobic streptococci together with obligately anaerobic gram-positive cocci and gram-negative rods (30). More than 60% of these infections include aerobic microorganisms, whereas approximately one third have purely anaerobic isolates.

Gingivitis is a periodontal process. Mild inflammation of the gums is present in almost all adolescents and in most American adults (31). Acute and chronic gingivitis begin with the formation of plaque below the gumline. Swelling and hyperemia of the free gum margin occurs, and the gums may bleed easily with brushing. Gingivitis is increased in frequency or severity in certain patient groups such as HIV-positive patients (up to 20% incidence), cancer patients undergoing chemotherapy, and young patients with type I diabetes mellitus (32). The healthy gingival sulcus has few microorganisms. Cessation of dental oral hygiene results in the appearance of dental plaque and gingivitis within 10 to 21 days.

The most extreme form of gingivitis is ANUG. ANUG represents tissue invasion and destruction by mixed anaerobes and facultatively anaerobic bacteria. Data suggest an important role for spirochetes and for *Fusobacterium* species (33). In HIV-seropositive patients, yeasts and herpesviruses may also contribute (34). ANUG manifests as a loss of the papillae between adjacent teeth and results in exposure of the roots of the tooth. It is accompanied by systemic symptoms. The disease is characterized by the sudden onset of pain and tenderness of the gums associated with increased salivation and a peculiar metallic taste. Physical examination demonstrates bleeding of the gingivae with blunting and necrotic punched-out lesions of the interdental papillae. ANUG most often occurs in adolescents and young adults. Risk factors include poor oral hygiene, infrequent dental care, poor nutrition, and possibly diabetes (35). Prevalence studies have demonstrated that 4% of students using dental services at Harvard University, and 6.7% of 9,203 adolescents in Chile have this condition (35,36).

Periodontal infections usually begin with gingivitis. As the infection becomes chronic, it extends deeper into the junction between the tooth and gingiva. This leads to loss of the connective tissue attaching the tooth to the bone (the periodontal ligament) and resorption of the bone. The resulting periodontitis causes a pocket to form between the tooth and the gingiva. This space is ideal for the growth of anaerobes because of the very low reduction oxidation potential. Spirochetes of many morphotypes, some uncultivable, appear to be the most predominant bacteria in advanced lesions (37,38). The chronic infection that occurs causes loosening and then loss of teeth. Periodontal abscesses result from infection of deep periodontal gingival pockets (39,40).

Acute suppurative parotitis is a nosocomial infection that occurs after surgery or in patients who are predisposed because of malnutrition, immunosuppression, or dehydration or in whom drugs have been used that decrease salivary flow (41). Such drugs include anticholinergic agents, antihistamines, and tranquilizers. The condition is unilateral in 80% to 90% of cases and presents clinically as the acute onset of unilateral facial swelling with pain. Physical examination demonstrates purulent fluid, which can be expressed from the parotid duct. The microbial causes reported in the older literature were *Staphylococcus aureus* in most patients, occasionally *Streptococcus viridans,* and rarely *Actinomyces* (41). Newer studies using proper anaerobic culture methods demonstrate anaerobes in most patients (42). The microorganisms are the same as those recovered from the gingival sulcus. Methicillin-resistant *S. aureus* has been reported as the cause of one outbreak in a nursing home (43). The pathogenesis of this infection is presumed to be retrograde movement of mouth microorganisms up the parotid duct in patients with diminished rates of salivary flow. Some authors report a correlation between increased numbers of bacteria in saliva and decreased rates of salivary flow (44).

Acute tonsillitis is rarely an institutionally related infection unless an outbreak of acute group A β-hemolytic streptococcal infection is spreading through the population. Although group A β-hemolytic *Streptococcus* is the most commonly recognized cause of tonsillitis, the significance of recovery of other microorganisms such as *Mycoplasma* and *Chlamydia* from inflamed tonsils has been debated (45–48). The pathogenetic role of these bacteria is not known. Microbiologic studies of the core of tonsils removed from 150 children with recurrent tonsillitis resulting from group A β-hemolytic streptococci during three periods beginning in 1977 and ending in 1993 revealed mixed flora (8.1 microorganisms per tonsil) in all tonsils and an increased rate of recovery of β-lactamase–producing bacteria with time (49).

Erysipelas, a soft tissue infection of the cheek resulting from direct extension of bacteria from the mouth, often is due to group A or C streptococci. This rare complication follows 2 to 3 days after oral surgery and represents bacterial entry into soft tissues injured by instrumentation.

Noma (gangrenous stomatitis) is an acute, fulminant, necrotizing infection of the cheek and facial tissue that destroys the oral and para-oral structures and is found predominantly in malnourished children, particularly in sub-Saharan Africa. Certain groups of adult patients may develop noma-like lesions that are slowly progressive. These adults have chronic lymphocytic leukemia, are receiving cytotoxic chemotherapy, or are neutropenic. The antecedent lesions to noma are believed to be oral herpetic ulcers, necrotizing gingivitis, or a buccal abrasion resulting from the rubbing of a tooth or from surgery (50,51). Infection of these precursor lesions with synergistic bacteria, such as *Fusobacterium* and *Prevotella,* causes progressive full-thickness necrosis of the cheek, leaving a large open defect through which the mandible and tongue can be seen. Fusospirochetal infection with a mixed flora is the cause (51,52).

Cervicofacial actinomycosis is a rare disease most commonly caused by *Actinomyces israelii.* Healthy individuals are affected most often, although the incidence of infection is decreasing with time. This decline is possibly related to more frequent antibiotic use, better oral hygiene, and water fluoridation. The portal of entry is through disrupted mucosal barriers after trauma, dental manipulations, or oral and maxillofacial surgery (53,54). The infection often appears as a chronic, slowly progressive induration or soft tissue mass in the mandibular-preauricular area and is sometimes accompanied by fistulous tracts to the skin that release sulfur-like granules. Systemic signs usually are absent (55).

Primary oral tuberculous lesions are seen rarely (56,57). Primary lesions occur in younger patients, are painless, and are associated with cervical lymphadenopathy. Secondary oral tuberculous lesions are more common and are seen mainly in older persons. Although the lesions are variable in appearance, the ulcerative form is the most usual, occurring on the tongue base or gingiva. These lesions are often painful. Most of these patients have accompanying active pulmonary tuberculosis (58–60).

There are many oral complications from cancer therapy; one of the most prominent is infection. As a result of treatment effects on the mouth and immunosuppression, the oral cavity has the potential to become a reservoir for opportunistic microorganisms. *Candida* microorganisms are the primary cause of opportunistic fungal disease in patients who are immunocompromised. As many as 60% of cases of fungal septicemia in cancer patients are associated with prior oral infections (61). The most common oral manifestation of a candidal infection is pseudomembranous candidiasis, manifested by removable white curd-like plaques over an inflamed mucosa. Other forms include leukoplakia-like white plaques that are not removable, referred to as chronic hyperplastic candidiasis and chronic erythematous candidiasis that appears as patchy or diffuse mucosal erythema. Oral infections can extend to involve the esophagus. Candidiasis can be diagnosed by microscopic examination of a potassium hydroxide preparation of mucosal scrapings or a Gram-stained smear of mucosal scrapings or by culture.

Aspergillosis is the second most frequent fungal infection in cancer patients, particularly in patients with hematologic malignancies (62). The paranasal sinuses are the most common sites of *Aspergillus* infection in the facial region, but there have been a few reports of primary oral aspergillosis (62–67). The oral lesions initially manifest on the gingiva and then develop into necrotic ulcers covered by a pseudomembrane. Spread to the alveolar bone and facial muscles may occur rapidly.

HSV is the most common viral pathogen in patients receiving cytotoxic agents or bone marrow transplants. The vesicular lesions on an erythematous base may appear anywhere on the mucosa and in addition to the mouth can involve the respiratory and gastrointestinal tracts. In immunocompromised patients, the oral mucositis associated with HSV may be particularly painful, severe, and prolonged. The oral HSV ulcerations may act as portals of entry for bacterial and fungal microorganisms.

The most frequent viral infection following solid organ transplants is CMV. This infection can develop in high-risk transplant recipients despite ganciclovir or valganciclovir prophylaxis (68). Oral manifestations, when they occur, are nonspecific and require biopsy to confirm the cause. The infection often consists of a single, large, shallow ulceration (69).

Infections by Direct Extension

An epidemiologic retrospective study of hospitalized patients with maxillofacial infections noted differences between pediatric and adult patients. Upper face infections predominate in children (81%), whereas in adults, lower face infections, mainly odontogenic or peritonsillar, are more common (66%) (70).

Osteomyelitis of the jaw (usually the mandible) most often results from chronic infection of a tooth, either from periapical abscess or from gingivitis. Other risk factors for osteomyelitis of the jaw include compound jaw fractures, diabetes mellitus, treatment with steroids, and surgery (50). Infection is particularly likely to occur when surgery is performed after irradiation of the mandible for tumor removal or after compound fracture of the mandible through the socket of a molar tooth. The causative microorganisms are *S. aureus* or anaerobes.

Peritonsillar abscesses arise by direct extension from infected tonsils and tonsillar remnants and are rarely nosocomial in nature. It is critical to recognize and treat this infection to avoid respiratory compromise and other serious complications (71, 72).

Maxillary sinusitis caused by mixed aerobes and anaerobes is recognized as a complication of periapical dental abscesses in the upper teeth (73–75). Sinusitis sometimes complicates extraction of the premolars and first molar on the upper side, because the root tips of these teeth almost touch the lower border of the maxillary sinuses.

Retropharyngeal abscesses arise by direct extension from uncontrolled tonsillar infection or after perforation of the posterior pharyngeal wall by a foreign body. The foreign body may be a bone or another sharp object carried in the mouth. A retropharyngeal abscess presents initially with pharyngeal discomfort, limited neck motion, and nonspecific constitutional symptoms, including fever and chills (76). In its later stages, the abscess can be recognized by forward displacement of the posterior pharyngeal wall (77). A lateral soft tissue film of the neck or computed tomography of the neck is required for diagnosis and will demonstrate air fluid levels or pockets of air in the retropharyngeal space. Clinical differentiation between a retropharyngeal abscess and cellulitis of the retropharyngeal space is difficult and may be accomplished by performing needle aspiration of the area. A return of pus signifies an abscess (78). Prompt recognition and urgent surgical management by incision and drainage is the standard treatment because the retropharyngeal space directly communicates with the posterior mediastinum and life-threatening complications may occur rapidly (79–82). However, there are recent reports of children being treated successfully without surgical intervention (76).

Anaerobic pulmonary infection ("aspiration pneumonia") resulting from mixed anaerobes and facultatively anaerobic microorganisms occurs after aspiration of oral contents. Clinical evidence suggests that the presence of severe gingivitis and/or oral surgery on the gums is associated with subsequent development of aspiration pneumonia. Clearly, the very large numbers of microorganisms ($>10^{10}$ microorganisms per gram of tissue) found in gingival material provide a large inoculum if aspirated into the lungs. The interplay of local host defense and the frequency of dental procedures on patients with gingivitis suggests that local host defense usually overcomes this inoculum. As an extreme example of the aspiration of oral flora, pulmonary actinomycosis has been reported to follow partial full-mouth dental extractions by 4 years (83).

Deep fascial space infections in the upper neck and underneath the jaw usually result from direct extension of odontogenic or oropharyngeal infection. Ludwig's angina is a diffuse fasciitis and cellulitis involving the submandibular and submental spaces. It is the result of a polymicrobial infection, often originating in the periodontal region (gingivitis, periapical abscess) or after injury to the gums or soft tissues (84). The fascial space involved secondary to infection of the maxillary or mandibular bicuspid and molar teeth depends on the relation of the root apex to the mylohyoid and buccinator muscles. Progression of infection upward may involve the whole side of the face, including the eyelids and orbit, whereas downward movement of infection can lead to necrotizing cervical fasciitis or mediastinitis (85–88). The anatomic parameters influencing the spread of infection in these areas is beyond the scope of this chapter but is covered in other works (21,31).

Distant Infection

Many distant abscesses have been reported as complications of dental and periodontal infection, including brain abscess, meningitis, paraspinal abscess, liver abscess, suppurative jugular thrombophlebitis, septic cavernous sinus thrombosis, septic arthritis, cellulitis, and necrotizing cavernositis of the penis (22–26,89–93). The route of migration is held to be bacteremia. Hematogenous seeding of oral flora to native heart valves and prosthetic material is discussed in Chapter 67.

EPIDEMIOLOGY

The accuracy of published rates of infection for common dental procedures is limited generally by small numbers in the denominator. Even with limited data, infection rates for some common procedures appear to be very low. For example, one 1992 review of the complications of oral surgical procedures commented that of approximately 50 million intraoral injections of local anesthetic each year, a literature search turned up only two case reports of injection-associated infection (94). Even if this represents underreporting by 100 times, the rate is still 1 infection per 10,000 injections. Table 54.2 summarizes available data concerning the frequency of procedure-related infections (95–108).

Dental caries and periapical abscess usually are not considered nosocomial infections because of their long incubation period and their association with poor oral hygiene and dental plaque formation. However, as noted previously, the periodontal flora begins to change within 10 days of stopping aggressive oral hygiene. Therefore, these complications may occur in head trauma, burns, and other patients with prolonged periods of unconsciousness or intubation. Fourrier et al. (109) studied the relationship between dental status and colonization of dental plaque by aerobic pathogens and the occurrence of nosocomial infections in 57 intensive care unit (ICU) patients in France. The amount of dental plaque increased during the ICU stay. Colonization of dental plaque was present in 40% of patients, either acquired or present on admission. A positive dental plaque culture was associated with the occurrence of nosocomial pneumonia and bacteremia. In 6 of 15 cases of ICU-related nosocomial infection, the pathogen isolated from dental plaque was the first identified source of the nosocomial pneumonia or bacteremia. The results from this study, and others, suggest dental plaque colonization and oral flora may be a source of nosocomial infection (110,111).

Several prophylactic oral measures have been tried to decrease nosocomial pneumonia. One prospective, randomized, double-blind, placebo-controlled trial in a cardiovascular ICU in a tertiary care center studied oropharyngeal decontamination with 0.12% chlorhexidine gluconate oral rinse (112). The nosocomial respiratory infection rate and the use of nonprophylactic systemic antibiotics in patients undergoing heart surgery were reduced. More recent studies have also demonstrated lower rates

TABLE 54.2. NOSOCOMIAL INFECTION RATES FOR ORAL AND DENTAL OPERATIONS

Reference	Procedure/condition	Rate (%)
95	After third molar extraction	5.8
	After partial bony impaction	4.4
	After complete bony impaction	10.1
	After cyst or tumor	17.0
96	After extraction of impacted third molar[a]	20–30
97–99	After dental implant[b]	1.2
	Periapical infection in implant	
	If edentulous	1–2
	If partial teeth	3–6
100, 101	With comminuted fracture of mandible	8
	If using fixed rigid internal device	2–9
102	Mandibular fracture involving third molar	24
103	After orthognathic surgery	10–25
	After compound maxillofacial fracture	50
	With antibiotic prophylaxis	10
104	After extraoral osteotomy	1–5
105	After transoral osteotomy	4–15
	After sagittal split osteotomy	1.3
106	After temporomandibular joint (TMJ) surgery	16
107	After TMJ arthroscopy	
	Surgical site infection	2.5
	Ear infection	2.2
108	ENT surgery (clean)	<1
	(Clean-contaminated)	18–87

ENT, ear-nose-throat.
[a] Alveolar osteitis.
[b] Surgical site dehiscence.

of nosocomial pneumonia in ventilated ICU patients treated with chlorhexidine oral decontamination when compared with control groups (113,114) (see also Chapter 22).

Acute suppurative parotitis was often reported in the past among patients undergoing general anesthesia for surgery. With better attention to adequate hydration and oral care and the widespread use of antibiotics in surgery, it is now reported to occur less than 0.5% of the time after use of a general anesthetic (94).

Placement of dental implants is usually accompanied by the administration of prophylactic penicillin. When antibiotic prophylaxis was used, Larsen (97) reported five instances of wound dehiscence in 445 implants but without any evidence of inflammation or infection. The relationship between the preoperative administration of antibiotics and the success of 2,641 endosseous implants was investigated as part of the comprehensive Dental Implant Clinical Research Group clinical implant study (115). Overall implant failure rate was very low. When preoperative antibiotics were not used, the risk of implant failure increased two to three times, suggesting that antibiotic prophylaxis may be helpful.

Osteotomy for correction of maxillary or mandibular deformities is occasionally followed by surgical site infection. One series recorded eight infections among 600 cases of sagittal split osteotomy, for a rate of 1.8%. Another retrospective analysis of 2,049 patients who underwent maxillofacial orthopedic surgery over a 21-year period reported only eight severe infections requiring incision and drainage, with no results compromised because of infection (116). Maxillary sinusitis after osteotomy of the maxilla is reported to be rare (105).

The risk of bacteremia with dental manipulation has been quantified. One such study reported bacteremia in 72% of 183 patients undergoing one or more tooth extractions, and it occurred most often when teeth were extracted for inflammatory conditions (117). Seventy-one percent of isolates were anaerobes. Even minor oral manipulation such as periodontal probing leads to bacteremia in as many as 43% of patients and is more frequent in patients with periodontitis than in patients with chronic gingivitis (118,119). Some authors suggest using antibacterial mouthwashes preprocedure to reduce gingival bacterial counts and the incidence of procedure-related bacteremias. Flood et al. (120) examined the frequency of bacteremia during routine incision and drainage of dentoalveolar abscesses. They demonstrated bacteremia during incision and drainage in 25% of such abscesses (3 of 12 patients). Bacteremia was found only during the drainage procedure in two of three patients, although, in the third instance, bacteremia was also demonstrated 5 minutes after the procedure ended. When abscesses were aspirated with a needle before incision and drainage, no blood cultures were positive. The authors suggested that the risk of bacteremia may be significantly reduced by needle aspiration of the abscess contents before incision and drainage.

Oral infections may be an important cause of septicemia in patients with hematologic malignancies. Dens et al. (121) noted a marked reduction of salivary flow rate in patients after bone marrow transplant that was more pronounced if total body irradiation had been included in the pretransplant therapy. A higher concentration of cariogenic microorganisms and a shift toward a lower buffering capacity in saliva were found. These changes may lead to an increased risk of caries and oral complications posttransplant.

Bergmann (122) prospectively followed 46 patients with hematologic malignancies through 78 febrile episodes. He estimated that a probable oral focus for septicemia was demonstrable in 10.5% of these individuals and that an oral origin was possible in an additional 21.1%. Other authors have sought a relationship between the mucositis that often follows chemotherapy for leukemia or bone marrow transplantation and the oral microbial flora as a way to explain the infections seen in these settings. Dreizen et al. (123) prospectively studied patients undergoing treatment for acute leukemia and found that 34.2% developed chemotherapy-related oral infection and 16.3% developed chemotherapy-related oral mucositis. In patients with mucositis, the viridans group of streptococci seems to be the most frequent cause of septicemia. *Staphylococcus epidermidis,* typically thought of as a skin bacterium, has been suggested to have an oral origin in a bone marrow transplant patient with bacteremia (124).

Ferretti et al. (125) demonstrated that antimicrobial mouthwashes such as 0.12% chlorhexidine gluconate protected against these oral complications. Barker et al. (126) showed a possible reduction in incidence of α-hemolytic streptococcal sepsis among children receiving myelosuppressive chemotherapy who received prophylactic oral vancomycin paste. Various oral protocols for preventing oral sequelae in immunocompromised patients have been suggested (127–131).

Not all studies show a correlation between the oral cavity and sepsis in patients with hematologic malignancies. A recent retrospective study of 77 patients after hematopoietic stem cell and bone marrow transplant showed no relationship between advanced periodontal disease and septicemia within the initial 100 days after transplant (132).

Fortunately, the frequency of fungal and viral oral infections in cancer and transplant patients has been reduced dramatically by the institution of prophylactic agents. However, one of the unfortunate potential consequences of this practice is the emergence of resistant microorganisms.

Oral candidiasis and hairy leukoplakia are conditions that should trigger an assessment of HIV infection risk factors. Many oral diseases in persons with HIV infection appear to be modified presentations of conventional disorders, such as gingivitis, necrotizing periodontal diseases, and exacerbated periodontitis (133, 134). Lower frequencies of oral disease have been seen in those on HIV therapy and in those who receive regular oral healthcare (135,136). There are insufficient studies on the complication risks for HIV-positive patients undergoing invasive dental procedures (137).

Literature on the complications of tongue piercing is beginning to emerge. Adverse outcomes have occasionally been life threatening. The reported complications include pain; tongue swelling; tongue abscess; airway problems; profuse bleeding; mucosal or gingival trauma or recession; chipped or fractured teeth; and interference with speech, mastication, and swallowing (138–141). In addition, there have been reports of endocarditis resulting from *Neisseria mucosa, Haemophilus aphrophilus,* and methicillin-resistant *S. aureus* following tongue piercing (142–144). Polymicrobial cerebellar brain abscess subsequent to tongue piercing has also been noted (145). There appears to be fewer problems associated with lip piercing, although gingival recession of previously healthy tissue has been seen (146).

Viral Agents

HSV is the latent herpesvirus in the oral cavity most commonly expressed during hospitalization. The virus is latent in the trigeminal ganglion and is secreted in saliva from the parotid gland. Reactivation of labial lesions in a patient is triggered by oral surgical procedures, trauma, ultraviolet light, and major injuries such as burns. Because of the frequency of asymptomatic excretion of the virus in saliva (virus can be recovered at intervals from the saliva of more than 50% of adults in the United States), the unprotected hands of dental surgeons, dental hygienists, and oral surgeons, which are bathed in saliva, are exposed to HSV. A common result of such exposure has been herpetic whitlow, which is a painful infection localized to the periungual region of the fingernail. This is recognized as an occupational hazard for dental workers (147). Because acquisition of HSV infection depends on direct contact between saliva or active lesions and an opening in skin, the frequency of herpetic whitlow possibly has been reduced by the use of gloves for blood-borne disease precautions (also see Chapters 43 and 81). Latex and vinyl gloves have been shown to be impermeable to HSV and to protect against HSV infection (148).

Despite their recovery from saliva and associated oral tissues, EBV and CMV have not been recognized as nosocomially important pathogens in the dental or oral surgery setting, either for spread to other patients or for spread to staff. However, a seroprevalence study done in the United Kingdom suggests possible occupational risk of infection with EBV in dentists based on a higher seroprevalence to EBV among clinical dental students and qualified dentists than among preclinical dental students (149). Another seroprevalence study done in England showed a greater prevalence of antibodies to influenza A and B viruses and respiratory syncytial virus in dental surgeons compared with control subjects, suggesting occupational risk for respiratory virus infections (150). Based on questionnaire results, reported donning of masks did not reduce seroprevalence with these viruses.

Blood-borne Pathogens

HBV may be transmitted both from patients to dentists and oral surgeons and from oral surgeons and dentists to patients (151–154). HBV can cause a chronic latent infection of the liver and is associated with large numbers of virus particles circulating in the blood of chronically infected persons. Because all intraoral surgery and many dental procedures cause breaks in the mucosa of the oral cavity or gums that result in bleeding, the risk of spread of HBV from the patient to the operator is substantial (155). In prevaccine surveys, the annual incidence of HBV was five to ten times higher among physicians and dentists than among blood donors (154,156). Infections occur when blood from the patient enters the body of the dentist through small breaks in the skin. In recent years, gloves have been used routinely as part of Standard/Universal Precautions. However, exposures of breaks in the skin to blood still occur because of glove perforation. Glove puncture occurs in 2.1% to 16% of oral surgery procedures (157,158). Aerosol transmission from high-speed drills used in dentistry with resulting aerosolization of saliva and blood has never been documented to result in occupationally related infections. Transmission of HBV via a human bite has been reported (159,160).

Several outbreaks of HBV infection have been reported among patients who underwent surgery by oral surgeons chronically infected with HBV (12,152,155). The precise mechanism(s) resulting in transmission of infection has not been determined, but infection was likely transmitted from dental workers to patients rather than from one patient to another. These outbreaks usually have been terminated after the involved surgeon began to wear gloves when performing procedures. The authors are unaware of any reports of transmission of HBV from dentists to patients since 1987. This may be due to increased adherence to universal precautions/standard precautions, higher levels of immunity resulting from use of hepatitis B vaccine, incomplete reporting, or isolated sporadic cases that are difficult to associate with a dental worker (161).

HCV was identified in 1989 and is recognized as the main agent of what was previously termed non-A, non-B viral hepatitis. The virus causes chronic latent infection of the liver in most infected persons. In the U.S. general population it is estimated that 3.9 million people have been infected with HCV, of whom 2.7 million have chronic infection. The prevalence of antibody to HCV in the homeless and incarcerated may be as high as 40% (162). In the United States, injecting drug users account for one half of all newly infected persons (163). HCV RNA is variably detected in the saliva of infected persons (164–166). Oral surgery appears to increase the occurrence of HCV in saliva (167). Transmission of HCV through a human bite has been reported (168,169).

Like HBV, HCV is a known occupational hazard for healthcare personnel by contact with contaminated blood, although HCV seems to be transmitted in the occupational setting less efficiently than HBV. To date, no dental worker is known to have acquired HCV occupationally, but the high frequency of sharps injuries occurring in the dental setting places the dental worker at risk of HCV acquisition (170). Despite this risk, the prevalence of HCV infection among dental workers appears to be similar to that of the general population. Anti-HCV may be more common in dental workers who are older, have more years of practice, and have serologic markers of HBV infection (171). A review of self-reported and observational studies of occupational blood exposures among U.S. dental workers between 1986 and 1995 suggested that percutaneous injuries steadily declined to an average of three injuries per year (172).

The data on the frequency of transmission of HCV during dental care are very limited. Gingivectomy performed by a dental surgeon of unknown HCV status was identified as the only risk factor for the seroconversion of one patient (173). A case-control study found an association between dental treatment and HCV positivity (174).

HIV infection causes a chronic infection of human lymphocytes and many other cell types and has a latency period of at least several years before onset of symptoms. The epidemiology of HIV in the medical setting likely is the same as that of HBV (175). As of December 2001, the Centers for Disease Control and Prevention received reports of 57 U.S. healthcare workers with documented HIV conversion temporally associated with an occupational HIV exposure. An additional 138 cases are considered to have possibly been acquired occupationally, but the source of infection cannot be documented with certainty. No dental personnel are among any of the documented cases, but six dental workers are in the group of possible occupational transmissions (176). Occupationally acquired HIV infection recognized among healthcare workers most commonly resulted from blood transmitted by hollow-bore needles (176). Because hollow-bore needles are used less often in dental practice, the risk of occupationally acquired HIV infection for dental workers may be slightly lower than that for some other groups of healthcare workers. A serosurvey combined with a questionnaire administered to 321 oral and maxillofacial surgeons revealed no HIV-seropositive participants despite a mean number of recalled percutaneous injuries within the previous year of 2.4 (most commonly associated with wire) (177). The results imply a low occupational risk for HIV infection.

In the United States, the only documented transmission of HIV from an operating surgeon to a patient occurred with one cluster of six cases related to a single dentist in Florida (178). The events that resulted in the infection of these patients remain unknown, although the evidence suggests that HIV was transmitted from dentist to patient rather than from patient to patient (179).

PREVENTION AND CONTROL

Infections may be transmitted in the dental operatory through direct contact with blood, oral fluids, or other secretions; via indirect contact with contaminated instruments, equipment, or environmental surfaces; or by contact with airborne contaminants present in either droplet splatter or aerosols of oral and respiratory fluids (161). Strategies to prevent dental patient infections have focused on four areas.

The first is sterilization of all instruments used in intraoral procedures and disinfection of related equipment. The second is use of good infection control practices in the dental operatory (161). These measures are aimed at preventing the spread of an infectious agent on instruments or dental apparatus from one patient to another. The third is rigid asepsis during intraoral procedures, including the use of preprocedure mouthwashes to reduce the burden of intraoral flora. Local antisepsis with topically applied antiseptic agents must be used particularly for root canal work, endodontic procedures, and gum surgery. The fourth is antibiotic prophylaxis or treatment of infected areas in which work is performed. These measures are directed at preventing the entry of the patient's own resident oral and gingival flora into the operative site in numbers great enough to cause infection.

Instruments used to penetrate soft tissue or bone (forceps, scalpels, bone chisels, etc.) are classified as critical and should be sterilized after each use. Instruments that are not intended to penetrate oral soft tissues or bone such as mirrors and amalgam condensers but may come in contact with oral tissues are classified as semicritical and also should be sterilized after each use. If a semicritical item will be damaged by heat sterilization, the instrument should receive, at a minimum, high-level disinfection. Instruments or devices that come into contact only with intact skin such as external components of x-ray heads are classified as noncritical. These items may be reprocessed between patients with intermediate-level or low-level disinfection or detergent and water washing, depending on the type of surface and the degree and nature of the contamination (161).

Before sterilization or high-level disinfection, instruments should be cleaned thoroughly to remove debris. They should be placed into a presoak solution immediately after use to prevent the drying of saliva or blood on the instruments and to make cleaning easier. The soak contains an antimicrobial agent to reduce the levels of bacteria and viruses. Cleaning is accomplished by scrubbing in a detergent solution or, preferably, to minimize handling and the exposure of workers to sharps injuries, by placing the instruments into a mechanical device (an ultrasonic cleaner). After cleansing, the instruments should be thoroughly rinsed with water while they are still in the cleaning basket, inspected carefully to make sure all visible debris has been removed, and then allowed to dry. Critical and semicritical instruments then should be sterilized. The most common forms of sterilization used in a dental office include steam (autoclaving) and dry heat. Sterilization processes must be monitored and periodically tested for efficacy using bacterial spores (see Chapter 86).

The use of liquid chemical germicides for high-level disinfection of heat-sensitive semicritical instruments may require up to 10 hours of exposure. Indications for wet sterilization are very limited, and manufacturers' directions regarding the correct concentration and exposure time should be followed closely. The process should be followed by aseptic rinsing with sterile water, drying, and, if not used immediately, placing in a sterile container (161) (see Chapter 85).

Because of the transmission of both HIV and HBV in the dental setting, much concern has been expressed over the dental handpieces used to transmit rotary energy to dental drills (180, 181). These handpieces are composed of a number of moving parts and typically have many cracks and crevices, which make them difficult to clean. They cannot be adequately disinfected by wet disinfectants (i.e., glutaraldehyde) because the agent cannot penetrate into the crevices. Studies have shown that residual live bacteria are recoverable from handpieces even after cleaning and wet chemical disinfection. Because all currently manufactured high-speed handpieces and most low-speed handpieces are heat tolerant, these items should be cleaned and lubricated, followed by sterilization between successive patients. Handpieces that are not heat tolerant should be modified to make them tolerant to heat. Those that cannot be heat sterilized should not be used (161,182).

Another potential concern is of dental unit water systems supplying dental handpieces and air water syringes becoming contaminated with microorganisms from the incoming water supply and, less often, with oral flora (183,184). Methods to minimize this risk include use of various flushing techniques (183,185).

Good infection control practices in the dental operatory are directed at the use of hand washing, appropriate barrier precautions, and attention to reducing the contamination of environmental surfaces by saliva and blood. These measures include the use of impervious paper or plastic covers to protect surfaces that may become contaminated during use and that are difficult to disinfect. Such surfaces include x-ray unit heads and light handles. Between patients, the coverings should be removed and replaced and all flat surfaces potentially soiled with patient material should be wiped off with an Environmental Protection Agency-approved hospital disinfectant, also labeled as "tuberculocidal." These intermediate-level disinfectants are effective against most bacteria and viruses (161). Other methods to reduce salivary contamination of the operatory include patient use of a mouthrinse before the procedure, use of a rubber dam, and use of a high-speed air evacuator during high-speed drilling.

Creutzfeldt-Jakob disease, one of the transmissible spongiform encephalopathies (TSEs), is a rapidly progressive, invariably fatal neurodegenerative disorder believed to be caused by an abnormal isoform of a cellular glycoprotein known as the prion protein. Although epidemiologic investigation has not revealed any evidence that dental procedures lead to increased risk of iatrogenic transmission of TSEs among humans, studies have shown that infected animals develop infectivity in gingival and dental pulp tissues. Transmission to healthy animals can occur by exposing root canals and gingival abrasions to infectious brain homogenate. The World Health Organization guidelines suggest that the usual infection control guidelines are sufficient when treating patients with TSEs during procedures not involving neurovascular tissue (186). Extra precautions should be considered for major dental procedures (186) (see also Chapter 47).

Local antiseptics reduce bacterial contamination of the operative site. They are applied to the prepared sites of dental fillings for caries, crowns, and root canals before closing the defect. Topical disinfection of the gingiva with H_2O_2 or chlorhexidine mouthwashes before elective gingival surgery reduces the rates of soft tissue infection.

Marten and van Saene (131) discussed methods to prevent each of the seven major oral infectious complications of cancer therapy. Four of these complications (caries, osteomyelitis, periodontal disease, and mucositis) can be prevented by strict application of local measures in the mouth. These measures include good oral hygiene to prevent caries and periodontal disease and to reduce the likelihood of osteomyelitis and topically applied antimicrobials to prevent osteomyelitis and mucositis.

Systemic antibiotics have a more limited role in reducing the rate of infectious complications. Converse and McCarthy (187) list the following indications for the use of prophylactic antibiotics for surgery on the jaw (mandible): (a) use of an intraoral approach, (b) previous irradiation of the operative field, (c) use of a bone graft, (d) use of an alloplastic implant, and (e) surgery in a patient prone to infection (diabetes patient).

As demonstrated in Table 54.2, the rate of surgical site infection is increased when a transmucosal or intraoral approach is used or when the socket of a tooth is involved in a fracture. This risk rises because of the large number of bacteria in the gingival sulcuses. In addition to the situations listed by Converse and McCarthy, systemic antibiotic administration is of proven benefit for transoral procedures more than 3 hours in length and for orthognathic or other major maxillofacial surgery.

In addition, patients may require antibiotics to protect heart valves or other distant foci from bacteremia originating in the mouth. Routine antibiotic prophylaxis to prevent hematogenous prosthetic joint infections is not recommended, although premedication may be warranted in some patients (188).

SAFETY FOR DENTAL HEALTHCARE WORKERS

Worker safety is provided by the following measures (161):

1. Every dentist, oral surgeon, or assistant who is exposed to blood or blood products or who handles needles or sharp instruments within the office should be offered and encouraged to accept hepatitis B vaccination.
2. Standard/universal precautions for handling all patient-related and derived substances should be rigorously used. These include the use of gloves for any work done in or around the mouth and for handling any instruments, surfaces, or substances contaminated with saliva or blood. Goggles and a mask or a face shield should be worn during all procedures. Any visible wounds suffered from sharp instruments should be immediately cleansed and assessed. The assessment should include informed consent for testing the patient for HBV, HCV, and HIV according to applicable state and federal laws. In addition, a postexposure prophylaxis protocol should be followed (189,190).
3. In addition to glove use, hands should be washed after removing gloves.
4. Gowns or dental clinic jackets should be worn in the office and operatory setting. These items should be removed on leaving work and laundered separately from personal clothing.
5. Because many studies have shown widespread salivary contamination of surfaces in the operatory, barrier protection of commonly touched surfaces such as radiographic handles and controls, bucket handles, and light switches should be provided.
6. The bacterial content of saliva can be reduced by rinsing the patient's mouth with water before any dental examination. Additional reductions can be accomplished by use of a mouthwash.
7. A careful general medical history should be completed for all new patients and at periodic intervals to look for symptoms or signs of pulmonary tuberculosis. Patients with signs or symptoms suggestive of tuberculosis should not undergo elective dental or oral procedures until they have been evaluated by a physician. All dental office workers should receive a yearly test for tuberculosis (191).

These measures are the minimum for providing reasonable protection to dental staff and patients against communicable diseases. Numerous studies demonstrate improved compliance by dental and oral surgery personnel with recommended infection control practices in recent years (192–197). However, the results of these studies suggest that further education and encouragement are needed to attain a more desirable level of understanding and adherence to the recommended practices.

REFERENCES

1. Ciesielski C, Marianos D, Chin-Yiu OU, et al. Transmission of human immunodeficiency virus in a dental practice. *Ann Intern Med* 1992;116:798–805.
2. Krizek TJ, Arigar S. Infection. In: Conley JJ, ed. *Complications of head and neck surgery.* Philadelphia: WB Saunders, 1979:55.
3. Heimdahl A, Nord CE. Antimicrobial prophylaxis in oral surgery. *Scand J Infect Dis Suppl* 1990;70:91–101.
4. Schuster GS. Microbiology of oral and maxillofacial infections. In: Topazian RG, Goldberg MH, eds. *Oral and maxillofacial infections,* 3rd ed. Philadelphia: WB Saunders, 1994.
5. Long SS, Swenson RM. Determinants of the developing oral flora in normal newborns. *Appl Environ Microbiol* 1976;32:494.
6. Mantilla GS, Danser MM, Sipos PM, et al. Tongue coating and salivary bacterial counts in healthy/gingivitis subjects and periodontitis patients. *J Clin Periodontol* 2001;28:970–978.
7. Mackiowak PA. The normal microbial flora. *N Engl J Med* 1983; 307:83.
8. Schuster GS, ed. *Oral microbiology and infectious disease,* 3rd ed. St. Louis: CV Mosby, 1990.
9. Chen CK, Wilson ME. *Eikenella corrodens* in human oral and non-oral infections: a review. *J Periodontol* 1992;63:941–953.
10. Danser MM, van Winkelhoff AJ, de Graaff J, et al. Short-term effect of full-mouth extraction on periodontal pathogens colonizing the oral mucous membranes. *J Clin Periodontol* 1994;21:484–489.
11. Genco RJ, Loos BG. The use of genomic DNA fingerprinting in studies of the epidemiology of bacteria in periodontitis. *J Clin Periodontol* 1991;18:396–405.
12. Dolan MM, Yankell SL. Transmissible infections in dentistry. In: Slots J, Taubman MA, eds. *Contemporary oral microbiology and immunology.* St. Louis: Mosby Year Book, 1992.
13. Corey L, Spear PG. Infections with herpes simplex virus. *N Engl J Med* 1986;314:686–691, 749–757.
14. Gold E, Nankervis GA. Cytomegalovirus. In: Evans AS, ed. *Viral infections of humans: epidemiology and control,* 3rd ed. New York: Plenum, 1991.
15. Pomeroy C, Englund JA. Cytomegalovirus: epidemiology and infection control. *Am J Infect Control* 1987;15:107–119.
16. Evans AS, Niederman JC. Epstein-Barr virus. In: Evans AS, ed. *Viral infections of humans: epidemiology and control,* 3rd ed. New York: Plenum, 1991.
17. Mardirossian A, Contreras A, Navazesh M, et al. Herpesviruses 6, 7, and 8 in HIV- and non-HIV-associated periodontitis. *J Periodontal Res* 2000;35:278–284.
18. Stenderup A. Oral mycology. *Acta Odontol Scand* 1990;48:3–10.
19. Hunter KD, Gibson J, Lockhart P, et al. Fluconazole-resistant *Candida* species in the oral flora of fluconazole-exposed HIV-positive patients. *Oral Surg Oral Med Oral Pathol Oral Radiol Endod* 1998; 85:558–564.
20. Korting HC, Ollert M, Georgii A, et al. In vitro susceptibilities and biotypes of *Candida albicans* isolates from the oral cavities of patients infected with human immunodeficiency virus. *J Clin Microbiol* 1989; 26:2626–2631.
21. Chow AW. Infections of the oral cavity, head and neck. In: Mandell G, Douglas RG, Bennett JE, eds. *Principles and practice of infectious diseases,* 4th ed. New York: Churchill Livingstone, 1995:593–606.
22. Saal CJ, Mason JC, Cheuk SL, et al. Brain abscess from chronic odontogenic cause: report of case. *J Am Dent Assoc* 1988;117: 453–455.
23. Andersen WC, Horton HL. Parietal lobe abscess after routine periodontal recall therapy. Report of a case. *J Periodontal* 1990;61: 243–247.
24. Crippin JS, Wang KK. An unrecognized etiology for pyogenic hepatic abscesses in normal hosts: dental disease. *Am J Gastroenterol* 1992; 87:1740–1743.
25. Kawamata T, Takeshita M, Ishizuka N, et al. Patent foramen ovale as a possible risk factor for cryptogenic brain abscess: report of two cases. *Neurosurgery* 2001;49:204–206.
26. Edson RS, Osmon DR, Berry DJ. Septic arthritis due to *Streptococcus sanguis. Mayo Clin Proc* 2002;77:709–710.
27. Field EA, Martin MV. Prophylactic antibiotics for patients with artificial joint undergoing oral and dental surgery: necessary or not? *Br J Oral Maxillofacial Surg* 1991;29:341–346.
28. van Winkelhoff AJ, Overbeek BP, Pavicic MJAMP, et al. Long-standing bacteremia caused by oral *Actinobacillus actinomycetemcomitans* in a patient with a pacemaker. *Clin Infect Dis* 1993;16:216–218.
29. Thoden van Velzen SK, Abraham-Inpijn L, Moorer WR. Plaque and systemic disease: a reappraisal of the focal infection concept. *J Clin Periodontol* 1984;11:209–220.
30. Lewis MA, MacFarlane TW, McGowan DA. A microbiological and clinical review of the acute dentoalveolar abscess. *Br J Oral Maxillofac Surg* 1990;28:359–366.
31. Trummel CL. Periodontal infections. In: Topazian RG, Goldberg MH, eds. *Oral and maxillofacial infection,* 3rd ed. Philadelphia: WB Saunders, 1994.
32. Slots J, Rams TE. New views on periodontal microbiota in special patient categories. *J Clin Periodontol* 1991;18:411–420.
33. Tanner A. Microbial etiology of periodontal diseases. Where are we? Where are we going? *Curr Opin Dent* 1992;2:12–24.
34. Cobb CM, Ferguson BL, Keselyak NT, et al. A TEM/SEM study of the microbial plaque overlying the necrotic gingival papillae of HIV-seropositive, necrotizing ulcerative periodontitis. *J Periodontal Res* 2003;38:147–155.
35. Lopez R, Fernandez O, Jara G, et al. Epidemiology of necrotizing ulcerative gingival lesions in adolescents. *J Periodontal Res* 2002;37: 439–444.
36. Burket LW, Greenberg MS. Gingival diseases. In: Lynch MA, ed. *Oral medicine diagnosis and treatment,* 7th ed. Philadelphia: JB Lippincott, 1977.
37. Moter A, Hoenig C, Choi BK, et al. Molecular epidemiology of oral treponemes associated with periodontal disease. *J Clin Microbiol* 1998; 36:1399–1403.
38. Sela MN. Role of *Treponema denticola* in periodontal diseases. *Crit Rev Oral Biol Med* 2001;12:399–413.
39. Hirsch RS, Clarke NG. Infection and periodontal diseases. *Rev Infect Dis* 1989;11:707–715.
40. Kerkes K, Olsen I. Similarities in the microflora of root canals and deep periodontal pockets. *Endodontics Dent Traumatol* 1990;6:1–5.
41. Brook I. Diagnosis and management of parotitis. *Arch Otolaryngol* 1992;118:469–471.
42. Brook I. Acute bacterial suppurative parotitis: microbiology and management. *J Craniofac Surg* 2003;14:37–40.
43. Raad II, Sabbagh MF, Caranasos GJ. Acute bacterial sialadenitis: a study of 29 cases and review. *Rev Infect Dis* 1990;12:591–601.
44. Fox PC. Bacterial infection of salivary glands. *Curr Opin Dent* 1991; 1:411–414.
45. Huminer D, Levy R, Pitlik S, et al. Mycoplasma and chlamydia in adenoids and tonsils of children undergoing adenoidectomy or tonsillectomy. *Ann Otol Rhinol Laryngol* 1994;103:135–138.
46. Charnock DR, Chapman GD, Taylor RE, et al. Recurrent tonsillitis. *Arch Otolaryngol Head Neck Surg* 1992;118:507–508.
47. Hone SW, Moore J, Fenton J, et al. The role of *Chlamydia pneumoniae* in severe acute tonsillitis. *J Laryngol Otol* 1994;108:135–137.
48. Kobayashi S, Tamura N, Ichikawa G, et al. Infection related arthritis induced by tonsillar *Chlamydia trachomatis* and streptococcal infection. *Clin Exp Rheumatol* 2002;20:732.
49. Brook I, Yocum P, Foote PA. Changes in the core tonsillar bacteriology of recurrent tonsillitis: 1977–1993. *CID* 1995;21:171–176.
50. Topazian RG. Uncommon infections of the oral and maxillofacial regions. In: Topazian RG, Goldberg MH, eds. *Oral and maxillofacial infections,* 3rd ed. Philadelphia: WB Saunders, 1994.
51. Enwonwu CO, Falkler WA, Idigbe EO. Oro-facial gangrene (noma/ cancrum oris): pathogenetic mechanisms. *Crit Rev Oral Biol Med* 2000;11:159–171.
52. Paster BJ, Falkler WA Jr, Enwonwu CO, et al. Prevalent bacterial

species and novel phylotypes in advanced noma lesions. *J Clin Microbiol* 2002;40:2187–2191.
53. Alderson G, Aufdemorte TB, Jones AC, et al. Oral and maxillofacial pathology case of the month. Actinomycosis. *Tex Dent J* 2000;117: 54, 92–93.
54. Maurer P, Otto C, Eckert AW, et al. Actinomycosis as a rare complication of orthognathic surgery. *Int J Adult Orthodon Orthognath Surg* 2002;17:230–233.
55. Miller M, Haddad AJ. Cervicofacial actinomycosis. *Oral Surg Oral Med Oral Pathol Oral Radiol Endod* 1998;85:496–508.
56. Carnelio S, Rodrigues G. Primary lingual tuberculosis: a case report with review of literature. *J Oral Sci* 2002;44:55–57.
57. Rivera H, Correa MF, Castillo-Castillo S, et al. Primary oral tuberculosis: a report of a case diagnosed by polymerase chain reaction. *Oral Dis* 2003;9:46–48.
58. Eng HL, Lu SY, Yang CH, et al. Oral tuberculosis. *Oral Surg Oral Med Oral Pathol Oral Radiol Endod* 1996;81:415–420.
59. Hashimoto Y, Tanioko H. Primary tuberculosis of the tongue: report of a case. *J Oral Maxillofacial Surg* 1989;47:744–746.
60. Smith WHR, Davis D, Mason KD, et al. Intraoral and pulmonary tuberculosis following dental manipulation. *Lancet* 1982;1:842–843.
61. Greenberg MS, Cohen SG, McKitrick JC, et al. The oral flora as a source of septicemia in patients with acute leukemia. *Oral Surg Oral Med Oral Pathol Oral Radiol Endod* 1982;53:32–35.
62. Dreizen S, Keating MJ, Beran M. Orofacial fungal infections: nine pathogens that may invade during chemotherapy. *Postgrad Med* 1992; 91:349–364.
63. Talbot SH, Huang A, Provencher M. Invasive aspergillus rhinosinusitis in patients with acute leukemia. *Rev Infect Dis* 1991;13:219–232.
64. Sugata T, Myoken Y, Kyo T, et al. Invasive oral aspergillosis in immunocompromised patients with leukemia. *J Oral Maxillofac Surg* 1994; 52:382–386.
65. Sugata T, Myoken Y, Kyo T, et al. Oral aspergillosis in compromised patients. *Oral Surg Oral Med Oral Pathol Oral Radiol Endod* 1996; 81:632.
66. Myoken Y, Sugata T, Fujita Y, et al. Molecular epidemiology of invasive stomatitis due to *Aspergillus flavus* in patients with acute leukemia. *J Oral Pathol Med* 2003;32:215–218.
67. Khoury H, Poh CF, Williams M, et al. Acute myelogenous leukemia complicated by acute necrotizing ulcerative gingivitis due to Aspergillus terreus. *Leuk Lymphoma* 2003;44:709–713.
68. Akalin E, Sehgal V, Ames S, et al. Cytomegalovirus disease in high-risk transplant recipients despite ganciclovir or valganciclovir prophylaxis. *Am J Transplant* 2003;3:731–735.
69. Epstein JB, Sherlock CH, Wolber RA. Oral manifestations of cytomegalovirus infection. *Oral Surg Oral Med Oral Pathol Oral Radiol Endod* 1993;75:443–451.
70. Scutari P, Dodson TB. Epidemiologic review of pediatric and adult maxillofacial infections in hospitalized patients. *Oral Surg Oral Med Oral Pathol Oral Radiol Endod* 1996;81:270–274.
71. Maharaj D, Rajah V, Hemsley S. Management of peritonsillar abscess. *J Laryngol Otol* 1991;105:743–745.
72. Stevens NE. Vascular complication of neck space infection: case report and literature review. *J Otolaryngol* 1990;19:206–210.
73. Randall CJ, Jefferis AF. Quinsy following tonsillectomy (five case reports). *J Laryngol Otol* 1984;98:367–369.
74. Brook I, Frazier EH, Gher ME Jr. Microbiology of periapical abscesses and associated maxillary sinusitis. *J Periodontol* 1996;67:608–610.
75. Paju S, Bernstein JM, Haase EM, et al. Molecular analysis of bacterial flora associated with chronically inflamed maxillary sinuses. *J Med Microbiol* 2003;52:591–597.
76. Craig FW, Schunk JE. Retropharyngeal abscess in children: clinical presentation, utility of imaging, and current management. *Pediatrics* 2003;111:1394–1398.
77. Cottrell DA, Bankoff M, Norris LH. Computed-tomography guided percutaneous drainage of a head and neck infection. *J Oral Maxillofac Surg* 1992;50:1119.
78. Herzon FS. Needle aspiration of nonperitonsillar head and neck abscesses. *Arch Otolaryngol Head Neck Surg* 1988;114:1312.
79. Levine TM, Wurster CF, Krespi YP. Mediastinitis occurring as a complication of odontogenic infections. *Laryngoscope* 1986;96: 747–750.
80. Wenig BL, Shikowitz MJ, Abramson AL. Necrotizing fasciitis as a lethal complication of peritonsillar abscess. *Laryngoscope* 1984;94: 1576-1579.
81. Waggie Z, Hatherill M, Millar A, et al. Retropharyngeal abscess complicated by carotid artery rupture. *Pediatr Crit Care Med* 2002;3: 303–304.
82. Hari MS, Nirvala KD. Retropharyngeal abscess presenting with upper airway obstruction. *Anaesthesia* 2003;58:714–715.
83. Suzuki JB, Delisle AL. Pulmonary actinomycosis of periodontal origin. *J Periodontol* 1984;55:581–584.
84. Balcerak RJ, Sisto JM, Bosack RC. Cervicofacial necrotizing fasciitis: report of three cases and literature review. *J Oral Maxillofac Surg* 1988;46:450.
85. Thakar M, Thakar A. Odontogenic orbital cellulitis. Report of a case and considerations on route of spread. *Acta Ophthalmol Scand* 1995; 73:470–471.
86. Chan CH, McGurk M. Cervical necrotising fasciitis—a rare complication of periodontal disease. *Br Dent J* 1997;183:293–296.
87. Newton CL, deLemos D, Abramo TJ, et al. Cervical necrotizing fasciitis caused by Serratia marcescens in a 2 year old. *Pediatr Emerg Care* 2002;18:433–435.
88. Haraden BM, Zwemer FL. Descending necrotizing mediastinitis: complication of a simple dental infection. *Ann Emerg Med* 1997;29: 683–686.
89. Weesner CL, Cisek JE. Lemierre syndrome: the forgotten disease. *Ann Emerg Med* 1993;22:256–258.
90. Pearle MS, Wendel EF. Necrotizing cavernositis secondary to periodontal abscess. *J Urol* 1993;149:1137–1138.
91. Montejo M, Aguirrebengoe K. *Streptococcus oralis* meningitis after dental manipulation. *Oral Surg Oral Med Oral Pathol Oral Radiol Endod* 1998;85;126–127.
92. Larkin EB, Scott SD. Metastatic paraspinal abscess and paraplegia secondary to dental extraction. *Br Dent J* 1994;177:340–342.
93. Manian FA. Cellulitis associated with an oral source of infection in breast cancer patients: report of two cases. *Scand J Infect Dis* 1997; 29:421–422.
94. Malamed SF, Sykes P, Kubota Y, et al. Local anesthetic: a review. *Anesth Pain Control Dent* 1992;1:11–24.
95. Osbourne TP, Fredericksen G, Small IA, et al. A prospective study of complications related to mandibular third molar surgery. *J Oral Maxillofac Surg* 1985;43:7671769.
96. Larsen PE. Role of antimicrobials for dentoalveolar surgery. *J Oral Maxillofac Surg* 1993;51(Suppl 3):155.
97. Larsen PE. Antibiotic prophylaxis for placement of dental implants. *J Oral Maxillofac Surg* 1993;51(Suppl 3):194.
98. Buser D, Ingimarsson S, Dula K, et al. Long-term stability of osseointegrated implants in augmented bone: a 5-year prospective study in partially edentulous patients. *Int J Periodontics Restorative Dent* 2002; 22:109–117.
99. Romeo E, Chiapasco M, Ghisolfi M, et al. Long-term clinical effectiveness of oral implants in the treatment of partial edentulism. Seven-year life table analysis of a prospective study with ITI dental implants system used for single-tooth restorations. *Clin Oral Implants Res* 2002; 13:133–143.
100. Islamoglu K, Coskunfirat OK, Tetik G, et al. Complications and removal rates of miniplates and screws used for maxillofacial fractures. *Ann Plast Surg* 2002;48:265–268.
101. Assael L, Hamman K. A comparison of rigid internal fixation with wire osteosynthesis of mandibular fracture. Case reports and outlines of scientific sessions. *J Oral Maxillofac Surg* 1987;45:M5–M6.
102. Assael LA. Infection in the maxillofacial trauma patient. In: Topazian RG, Goldberg MH, eds. *Oral and maxillofacial infections,* 3rd ed. Philadelphia: WB Saunders, 1994.
103. Peterson LJ. Antibiotic prophylaxis against wound infections in oral and maxillofacial surgery. *J Oral Maxillofacial Surg* 1990;48:617–620.
104. Peterson LJ. Principles of antibiotics. In: Topazian RG, Goldberg MH, eds. *Oral and maxillofacial infections,* 3rd ed. Philadelphia: WB Saunders, 1994.

105. Hinds EC, Kent JN. *Surgical treatment of developmental jaw deformities.* St. Louis: CV Mosby, 1972.
106. Dingaman RO, Dingaman DL, Lawrence DA. Surgical correction of lesions in the temporomandibular joint. *Plastic Reconstruct Surg* 1978; 55:335.
107. Tarro AW. Arthroscopic treatment of anterior disc displacement: a preliminary report. *J Oral Maxillofacial Surg* 1989;47:353.
108. Sanders B, Buoncristiani R. Diagnostic and surgical arthroscopy of the temporomandibular joint: clinical experience with 137 procedures over a two year period. *J Craniomandib Dis* 1987;1:202.
109. Fourrier F, Duvivier B, Boutigny H, et al. Colonization of dental plaque: a source of nosocomial infections in intensive care unit patients. *Crit Care Med* 1998;26:301–308.
110. Sole ML, Poalillo FE, Byers JF, et al. Bacterial growth in secretions and on suctioning equipment of orally intubated patients: a pilot study. *Am J Crit Care* 2002;11:141–149.
111. Imsand M, Janssens JP, Auckenthaler R, et al. Bronchopneumonia and oral health in hospitalized older patients. A pilot study. *Gerodontology* 2002;19:66–72.
112. DeRiso AJ, Ladowski JS, Dillon TA, et al. Chlorhexidine gluconate 0.12% oral rinse reduces the incidence of total nosocomial respiratory infection and nonprophylactic systemic antibiotic use in patients undergoing heart surgery. *Chest* 1996;109:1556–1561.
113. Fourrier F, Cau-Pottier E, Boutigny H, et al. Effects of dental plaque antiseptic decontamination on bacterial colonization and nosocomial infections in critically ill patients. *Intensive Care Med* 2000;26: 1239–1247.
114. Houston S, Hougland P, Anderson JJ, et al. Effectiveness of 0.12% chlorhexidine gluconate oral rinse in reducing prevalence of nosocomial pneumonia in patients undergoing heart surgery. *Am J Crit Care* 2002;11:567–570.
115. Dent CD, Olson JW, Farish SE, et al. The influence of preoperative antibiotics on success of endosseous implants up to and including stage II surgery: a study of 2,641 implants. *J Oral Maxillofac Surg* 1997;55:19–24.
116. Van de Perre JPA, Stoelinga PJW, Blijdorp PA, et al. Perioperative morbidity in maxillofacial orthopaedic surgery: a retrospective study. *J Craniomaxillofac Surg* 1996;24:263–270.
117. Okabe K, Nakagawa K, Yamamoto E. Factors affecting the occurrence of bacteremia associated with tooth extraction. *Int J Oral Maxillofac Surg* 1995;24:239–242.
118. Daly C, Mitchell D, Grossberg D, et al. Bacteraemia caused by periodontal probing. *Aust Dent J* 1997;42:77–80.
119. Daly CG, Mitchell DH, Highfield JE, et al. Bacteremia due to periodontal probing: a clinical and microbiological investigation. *J Periodontol* 2001;72:210–214.
120. Flood TR, Samaranayake LP, McFarlane TW, et al. Bacteraemia following incision and drainage of dentoalveolar abscesses. *Br Dent J* 1990;169:51–53.
121. Dens F, Boogaerts M, Boute P, et al. Caries-related salivary microorganisms and salivary flow rate in bone marrow recipients. *Oral Surg Oral Med Oral Pathol Oral Radiol Endod* 1996;81:38–43.
122. Bergmann OJ. Oral infections and septicemia in immunocompromised patients with hematologic malignancies. *J Clin Microbiol* 1988; 26:2105–2109.
123. Dreizen S, McCredie KB, Bodey GP, et al. Quantitative analysis of the oral complications of antileukemia therapy. *J Oral Surg Oral Med Oral Pathol* 1986;62:650–653.
124. Kennedy HF, Morrison D, Kaufmann ME, et al. Origins of *Staphylococcus epidermidis* and *Streptococcus oralis* causing bacteraemia in a bone marrow transplant patient. *J Med Microbiol* 2000;49:367–370.
125. Ferretti GA, Ash RC, Brown AT, et al. Chlorhexidine for prophylaxis against oral infections and associated complications in patients receiving bone marrow transplant. *J Am Dent Assoc* 1987;114:461–467.
126. Barker GJ, Call SK, Gamis AS. Oral care with vancomycin paste for reduction in incidence of α-hemolytic streptococcal sepsis. *J Pediatr Hematol Oncol* 1995;17:151–155.
127. Jansma J, Vissink A, Spijkervet FK, et al. Protocol for the prevention and treatment of oral sequelae resulting from head and neck radiation therapy. *Cancer* 1992;70:2171–2180.
128. Solomon CS, Shaikh AB, Arendorf TM. An efficacious oral health care protocol for immunocompromised patients. *Special Care Dentistry* 1995;15:228–233.
129. Meurman JH, Pyrhonen S, Teerenhovi L, et al. Oral sources of septicaemia in patients with malignancies. *Oral Oncol* 1997;33:389–397.
130. Anonymous. Periodontal considerations in the management of the cancer patient. Committee on Research, Science and Therapy of the American Academy of Periodontology. *J Periodontol* 1997;68: 791–801.
131. Marten MV, van Saene HKF. The role of oral micro-organisms in cancer therapy. *Oral Maxillofac Surg Infect* 1992;11:81–84.
132. Akintoye SO, Brennan MT, Graber CJ, et al. A retrospective investigation of advanced periodontal disease as a risk factor for septicemia in hematopoietic stem cell and bone marrow transplant recipients. *Oral Surg Oral Med Oral Pathol Oral Radiol Endod* 2002;94:581–588.
133. Robinson PG, Adegboye A, Rowland RW, et al. Periodontal diseases and HIV infection. *Oral Dis* 2002;8(Suppl 2):144–150.
134. Robinson PG. The significance and management of periodontal lesions in HIV infection. *Oral Dis* 2002;8(Suppl 2):91–97.
135. Tappuni AR, Fleming GJ. The effect of antiretroviral therapy on the prevalence of oral manifestations in HIV-infected patients: a UK study. *Oral Surg Oral Med Oral Pathol Oral Radiol Endod* 2001;92: 623–628.
136. Hastreiter RJ, Jiang P. Do regular dental visits affect the oral health care provided to people with HIV? *J Am Dent Assoc* 2002;133: 1343–1350.
137. Patton LL, Shugars DA, Bonito AJ. A systematic review of complication risks for HIV-positive patients undergoing invasive dental procedures. *J Am Dent Assoc* 2002;133:195–203.
138. Farah CS, Harmon DM. Tongue piercing: case report and review of current practice. *Aust Dent J* 1998;43:387–389.
139. Stroud R. Tongue piercing. *Br Dent J* 2002;193:3.
140. Campbell A, Moore A, Williams E, et al. Tongue piercing: impact of time and barbell stem length on lingual gingival recession and tooth chipping. *J Periodontol* 2002;73:289–297.
141. Hardee PS, Mallya LR, Hutchison IL. Tongue piercing resulting in hypotensive collapse. *Br Dent J* 2000;188:657–658.
142. Tronel H, Chaudemanche H, Pechier N, et al. Endocarditis due to *Neisseria mucosa* after tongue piercing. *Clin Microbiol Infect* 2001;7: 275–276.
143. Akhondi H, Rahimi AR. *Haemophilus aphrophilus* endocarditis after tongue piercing. *Emerg Infect Dis* 2002;8:850–851.
144. Harding PR, Yerkey MW, Deye G, et al. Methicillin resistant *Staphylococcus aureus* (MRSA) endocarditis secondary to tongue piercing. *J Miss State Med Assoc* 2002;43:109.
145. Martinello RA, Cooney EL. Cerebellar brain abscess associated with tongue piercing. *Clin Infect Dis* 2003;36:e32–34.
146. OíDwyer JJ, Holmes A. Gingival recession due to trauma caused by a lower lip stud. *Br Dent J* 2002;192:615–616.
147. Straus SE. Herpes simplex virus infections: biology, treatment and prevention. *Ann Intern Med* 1985;103:404.
148. Kotilainen HR, Brinker JP, Avato JL, et al. Latex and vinyl examination gloves. Quality control procedures and implications for health care workers. *Arch Intern Med* 1989;149:2749–2753.
149. Herbert AM, Bagg J, Walker DM, et al. Seroepidemiology of herpes virus infections among dental personnel. *J Dentistry* 1995;23: 339–342.
150. Davies KJ, Herbert AM, Westmoreland D, et al. Seroepidemiological study of respiratory virus infections among dental surgeons. *Br Dent J* 1994;176:262–265.
151. Siew C, Gruninger SE, Mitchell EW, et al. Survey of hepatitis B exposure and vaccination in volunteer dentists. *J Am Dent Assoc* 1987; 114:457–459.
152. Ahtone J, Goodman RA. Hepatitis B and dental personnel: transmission to patients and prevention issues. *J Am Dent Assoc* 1983;106: 219–222.
153. Mast EE, Alter MJ. Prevention of hepatitis B virus infection among health-care workers. In: Ellis RW, ed. *Hepatitis B vaccines in clinical practice.* New York: Marcel Dekker, 1993:295–307.

154. West DJ. The risk of hepatitis B infection among health professionals in the United States: a review. *Am J Med Sci* 1984;287:26–33.
155. Hu DI, Kane MA, Heymann DL. Transmission of HIV, hepatitis B virus and other bloodborne pathogens in healthcare settings: a review of risk factors and guidelines for prevention. *Bull WHO* 1991;69: 623–630.
156. Gibas A, Blewett DR, Schoenfeld DA, et al. Prevalence and incidence of viral hepatitis in health workers in the prehepatitis B vaccination era. *Am J Epidemiol* 1992;136:603–610.
157. Burke FJT, Baggett FJ, Lomax AM. Assessment of the risk of glove puncture during oral surgery procedures. *Oral Surg Oral Med Oral Pathol Oral Radiol Endod* 1996;82:18–21.
158. Avery CME, Hjort A, Walsh S, et al. Glove perforation during surgical extraction of wisdom teeth. *Oral Surg Oral Med Oral Pathol Oral Radiol Endod* 1998;86:23–25.
159. Cancio-Bello TP, de Medina M, Shorey J, et al. An institutional outbreak of hepatitis B related to a human biting carrier. *J Infect Dis* 1982;146:652–656.
160. Stornello C. Transmission of hepatitis B via human bite. *Lancet* 1991; 338:1024–1025.
161. Centers for Disease Control and Prevention. Recommended infection-control practices for dentistry. *MMWR Mortal Morb Wkly Rep* 1993;41:1–12.
162. Kim WR. The burden of hepatitis C in the United States. *Hepatology* 2002;36(5 Suppl 1):S30–34.
163. Marwick C. Hepatitis C is focus of NIH consensus panel. *JAMA* 1997;277:1268–1269.
164. Hsu HH, Wright TL, Luba D, et al. Failure to detect hepatitis C virus genome in human secretions with the polymerase chain reaction. *Hepatology* 1991;14:763–767.
165. Couzigous P, Richard L, Dumas F, et al. Detection of HCV-RNA in saliva of patients with chronic hepatitis C. *Gut* 1993;34:559–560.
166. Wang JT, Wang TH, Lin JT, et al. Hepatitis C virus RNA in saliva of patients with post-transfusion hepatitis C infection. *Lancet* 1991; 337:48.
167. Chen M, Yun ZB, Sailberg M, et al. Detection of hepatitis C virus RNA in the cell fraction of saliva before and after oral surgery. *J Med Virol* 1995;45:223–226.
168. Dusheiko GM, Smith M, Scheuer PJ. Hepatitis C virus transmitted by human bite. *Lancet* 1990;336:503–504.
169. Figueiredo JF, Borges AS, Martinez R, et al. Transmission of hepatitis C virus but not human immunodeficiency virus type I by a human bite. *Clin Infect Dis* 1994;19:546–547.
170. Siew C, Gruninger SE, Miaw CL, et al. Percutaneous injuries in practicing dentists: a prospective study using a 20-day diary. *J Am Dent Assoc* 1995;126:1227–1234.
171. Thomas DL, Gruninger SE, Siew C, et al. Occupational risk of hepatitis C infections among general dentists and oral surgeons in North America. *Am J Med* 1996;100:41–45.
172. Cleveland JL, Gooch BF, Lockwood SA. Occupational blood exposures in dentistry: a decade in review. *Infect Control Hosp Epidemiol* 1997;18:717–721.
173. Prati D, Capelli C, Silvani C, et al. The incidence and risk factors of community-acquired hepatitis C in a cohort of Italian blood donors. *Hepatology* 1997;25:702–704.
174. Mele A, Sagliocca L, Manzillo G, et al. Risk factors for acute non-A, non-B hepatitis and their relationship to antibodies for hepatitis C virus: a case-control study. *Am J Public Health* 1994;84: 1640–1643.
175. Bell DM. Human immunodeficiency virus transmission in healthcare settings: risk and risk reduction. *Am J Med* 1991;91(Suppl 3B): 294–300.
176. Do AN, Ciesielski CA, Metler RP, et al. Occupationally acquired human immunodeficiency virus (HIV) infection: national case surveillance data during 20 years of the HIV epidemic in the United States. *Infect Control Hosp Epidemiol* 2003;24:86–96.
177. Gooch BF, Siew C, Cleveland JL, et al. Occupational blood exposure and HIV infection among oral and maxillofacial surgeons. *Oral Surg Oral Med Oral Pathol Oral Radiol Endod* 1998;85:128–134.
178. Centers for Disease Control and Prevention. Possible transmission of human immunodeficiency virus to a patient during an invasive dental procedure. *MMWR Mortal Morb Wkly Rep* 1990;39:489–493.
179. Gooch B, Marianos D, Ciesielski C, et al. Lack of evidence for patient-to-patient transmission of HIV in a dental practice. *J Am Dent Assoc* 1993;124:38–44.
180. Lewis DL, Boe RK. Cross infection risks associated with current procedures for using high-speed dental handpieces. *J Clin Microbiol* 1992; 30:401–406.
181. Lewis DL, Arens M, Appleton SS, et al. Cross-contamination potential with dental equipment. *Lancet* 1992;340:1252–1254.
182. Rutala WA. APIC guideline for selection and use of disinfectants. *Am J Infect Control* 1996;24:313–342.
183. Fayle SA, Pollard MA. Decontamination of dental unit water systems: a review of current recommendations. *Br Dent J* 1996;181:369–372.
184. Jensen ET, Giwercman B, Ojeniyi B, et al. Epidemiology of *Pseudomonas aeruginosa* in cystic fibrosis and the possible role of contamination by dental equipment. *J Hosp Infect* 1997;36:117–122.
185. Matsuyama M, Usami T, Masuda K, et al. Prevention of infection in dental procedures. *J Hosp Infect* 1997;35:17–25.
186. WHO infection control guidelines for transmissible spongiform encephalopathies. Report of a WHO consultation, Geneva, Switzerland, 23–26 March 1999. Available at *http://www.who.int/emc-documents/tse/whocdscsraph2003c.html* (accessed 12/29/2003).
187. Converse JM, McCarthy JG. Infection in plastic surgery. *Surg Clin North Am* 1972;52:1459.
188. Anonymous. Advisory statement. Antibiotic prophylaxis for dental patients with total joint replacements. American Dental Association: American Academy of Orthopaedic Surgeons. *J Am Dent Assoc* 1997; 128:1004–1008.
189. Younai FS. Postexposure protocol. *Dental Clin North Am* 1996;40: 457–486.
190. Cleveland JL, Barker L, Gooch BF, et al. Use of HIV postexposure prophylaxis by dental health care personnel: an overview and updated recommendations. *J Am Dent Assoc* 2002;133:1619–1626.
191. Centers for Disease Control and Prevention. Guidelines for preventing the transmission of *Mycobacterium tuberculosis* in health-care facilities, 1994. In: Abrutyn E, Goldman DA, Scheckler WE, eds. *Saunders infection control reference service.* Philadelphia: WB Saunders, 1998; 1041–1042.
192. McCarthy GM, MacDonald JK. Improved compliance with recommended infection control practices in the dental office between 1994 and 1995. *Am J Infect Control* 1998;26:24–28.
193. Gershon RRM, Karkashian C, Vlahov D, et al. Correlates of infection control practices in dentistry. *Am J Infect Control* 1998;26:29–34.
194. McCarthy GM, Koval JJ, MacDonald JK. Compliance with recommended infection control procedures among Canadian dentists: results of a national survey. *Am J Infect Control* 1999;27:377–384.
195. McCarthy GM, MacDonald JK. A comparison of infection control practices of different groups of oral specialists and general dental practitioners. *Oral Surg Oral Med Oral Pathol Oral Radiol Endod* 1998; 85:47–54.
196. DePaola LG. Managing the care of patients infected with bloodborne diseases. *J Am Dent Assoc* 2003;134:350–358.
197. Williams HN, Singh R, Romberg E. Surface decontamination in the dental operatory: a comparison over two decades. *J Am Dent Assoc* 2003;134:325–330.

55

NOSOCOMIAL INFECTIONS IN OBSTETRICAL PATIENTS

AMY BETH KRESSEL
CALVIN C. LINNEMANN JR.

The obstetric unit in a hospital is one of the first examples of a characteristic of the modern hospital—a specialized patient population in a specialized hospital unit. "Lying-in" or obstetric hospitals were introduced in the eighteenth century, and some of the first significant studies on the epidemiology of hospital-acquired infections were made on obstetric services (1). Today's hospital is increasingly becoming a collection of specialized units containing unique patient populations characterized by specific disease entities and undergoing specialized treatments that either make the host more vulnerable to infection or facilitate transmission of infections. Obstetric care differs from other hospital infection problems in that both the primary patient and the newborn infant are at risk.

A recent survey of postpartum infections reported an overall infection rate of 6%, as shown in Table 55.1 (2). Ledger (3) pointed out that the frequent empiric use of antibiotics for febrile patients on the obstetric service probably leads to lower reported infection rates and obscures the true frequency of hospital-acquired infections. The most important change in obstetric care in recent decades has been the increasingly shorter hospital stays mandated by cost concerns in managed care systems. Shortened hospital stays may decrease some risk factors for hospital-acquired infections, such as the use of catheters and intravenous lines, and may result in further decreases in infection rates. Unfortunately, shortened hospital stays also make surveillance of infections more difficult; thus, changes in infection rates cannot be confirmed by current data.

HISTORY OF HOSPITAL-ACQUIRED OBSTETRIC INFECTIONS

The establishment of obstetric hospitals in the mid-eighteenth century created the setting for epidemics of puerperal infections (1). The epidemics in turn provided the opportunity to demonstrate that the infections were contagious and to develop prevention methods. Alexander Gordon was one of the first to document this (4) and, later, so did Oliver Wendell Holmes (5), but the most famous was Ignaz Semmelweis in Vienna because of his extensive and carefully detailed observations (6).

The "great free Vienna Lying-in Hospital" created a natural epidemiologic experiment that Semmelweis had the insight to appreciate. The hospital had two separate divisions: the First Division for teaching medical students and the Second Division for teaching midwives. The mortality was so much greater in the First Division that even the patients knew about it and tried to be admitted to the Second Division if at all possible. Semmelweis took advantage of this natural experiment to carefully collect data to document and determine the cause of the epidemics. Not only did he evaluate the data on hospital-acquired infections but also he made anecdotal observations that supported his conclusions, such as the low infection rate in women who delivered in the street on the way to the hospital as compared with those who delivered in the hospital.

To explain the increased mortality in the First Division, he noted the similarity of the fatal illness in a pathologist who had been stuck in the finger by a medical student during an autopsy and the fatal infections in the obstetric patients. He concluded that material from the autopsies was being transmitted back to the patients and causing their illnesses. Hand washing with soap was done after autopsies, and thus he concluded that this was inadequate to remove all "cadaveric particles." He added hand rinsing with chlorinated lime water after performing autopsies and after each patient contact (7). The result was a dramatic decrease in mortality in the First Division to rates similar to that of the Second Division.

It took decades before Semmelweis' ideas became standard

TABLE 55.1. INFECTION RATES (CASES/100 DELIVERIES) ON OBSTETRIC SERVICES BY SITE OF INFECTION, 1993–1995

Type of delivery	Site of infection					
	UTI	SSI	Epi	End	Mast	All sites
Cesarean	1.1	3.4	NA	0.8	1.7	7.4
Vaginal	2.0	NA	0.3	0.2	3.0	5.5

End, endometritis; EPI, episiotomy; Mast, mastitis; SSI, surgical site infection (excluding endometritis); UTI, urinary tract infection.
From Yokre DS, Christiansen CL, Johnson R, et al. Epidemiology of and surveillance for post partum infections. *Emerg Infect Dis* 2001;7:837–841, with permission

practice, stimulated by Lister's concept of antisepsis. Even then, obstetric infections and maternal mortality remained major problems into the 1930s. The appearance of the first antimicrobial agents and improvements in other aspects of obstetric care resulted in a major decrease in maternal mortality (8). Presumably, the reason for the persistence of high obstetric infection rates into the 1900s was that even though epidemics of puerperal fever transmitted by cross-infections were prevented by hand washing and antiseptic techniques, infection from patients' endogenous flora remained a problem.

PATHOGENESIS OF OBSTETRIC INFECTIONS

Most obstetric infections are caused by maternal vaginal and cervical flora, and, thus, increases in infections usually relate to risk factors other than the introduction of exogenous pathogens. Hospital pathogens are seldom problems on obstetric services. This is because obstetric patients have short stays, and obstetric units are separated from other hospital units.

As Bartlett et al. (9,10) pointed out, vaginal flora is a dynamic ecosystem, with some differences between vaginal and cervical flora. Anaerobic bacteria usually outnumber aerobes, with anaerobic and facultative lactobacilli predominating. Other anaerobes include *Peptostreptococcus* species, *Bacteroides* species, and *Prevotella* species. The aerobic gram-positive flora include coagulase-negative staphylococci, with varying amounts of streptococci, enterococci, and *Staphylococcus aureus,* and the gram-negative flora include *Escherichia coli, Gardnerella vaginalis, Enterobacter* species, *Klebsiella pneumoniae,* and *Proteus mirabilis* (11,12). Both *Mycoplasma* and *Ureaplasma* are also found in the vagina. Sexually transmitted diseases may add *Neisseria gonorrhoeae, Chlamydia trachomatis,* or herpes simplex virus (HSV) to this flora. Vaginal flora may change during pregnancy. Some studies suggested that lactobacilli increase in pregnancy and that other anaerobes decrease (13). Antibiotics also change the flora, and the use of multiple doses of cephalosporins for prophylaxis has been reported to increase enterococci and perhaps *Enterobacter* species (14).

As would be expected, most obstetric intrauterine infections are polymicrobial, representing contiguous spread from the vagina (15). Ascending infection is demonstrated both by the presence of routine cervicovaginal flora in endometritis and surgical site infections (SSIs) and the ability to predict postcesarean infections by intraoperative lower uterine cultures (16). Although a significant proportion of postcesarean SSIs is caused by staphylococci, as in other SSIs, most postcesarean infections are caused by endometrial contamination (17).

Many risk factors have been proven or suggested to be associated with endometrial infection, including those that increase entry of vaginal flora such as prolonged rupture of the membranes, frequent vaginal and rectal examinations, or intrauterine monitoring; those that result in tissue injury such as soft tissue trauma, midforceps delivery, or inexperienced surgeons; and host factors that are associated with increased infections such as maternal age, lower socioeconomic status, or obesity. Understanding these risk factors may become important in evaluating infection rates on specific obstetric units.

OBSTETRIC INFECTIONS (INFECTIONS RELATED TO PREGNANCY AND DELIVERY)

Postpartum Endometritis

The classic obstetric infection is postpartum endometritis. The postpartum patient develops fever that may be associated with abdominal pain, uterine tenderness, or foul-smelling discharge and in most cases is started on antibiotics without obtaining cultures (15). Endometritis can occur after either vaginal delivery or cesarean section but is diagnosed most often after cesarean section. Infection has been reported to occur after fewer than 3% of vaginal deliveries and 5% to 95% of cesarean sections (2,15,18). The variation in infection rates results from the prevalence of risk factors in the population studied and the way that patients are managed. Endometritis after cesarean section occurs earlier than after vaginal delivery, as shown by hospital readmissions for postpartum endometritis. Most women who were readmitted for endometritis had delivered vaginally (19).

Infections may be caused by a single bacterial species but are often polymicrobial (20). Common etiologic agents include the gram-positive cocci such as streptococci and enterococci; gram-negative bacilli such as *E. coli, K. Pneumoniae,* and *P. mirabilis*; and anaerobes such as *Bacteroides bivius* and peptostreptococci (15,20,21). Some studies have distinguished between early and late postpartum endometritis; late infection is a milder disease that occurs after vaginal delivery (22,23). It has been suggested that genital mycoplasma and *Chlamydia* are important etiologic agents in late endometritis and that erythromycin may be effective therapy.

The most important risk factor for postpartum endometritis is cesarean section, and the risk of infection is greatest when it is a nonelective procedure after rupture of the membranes and the onset of labor (15,18,24). General anesthesia, long duration of surgery, intraoperative problems, and poor surgical technique may all be risk factors. Patients undergoing nonelective cesarean sections are routinely given prophylactic antibiotics, because this has been shown to reduce infection rates by 50% or more (24). In vaginal deliveries, prolonged rupture of the membranes, midforceps delivery, and soft tissue trauma increase the risk. With many other risk factors for postpartum endometritis, it is difficult to separate out relative risks, because the factors are interrelated. This applies to risk factors such as prolonged labor, frequent vaginal examinations, and internal monitoring. Host factors that increase risk include bacterial vaginosis, human immunodeficiency virus (HIV) infection, anemia, low socioeconomic status, maternal age, and obesity (24–26).

Infection of the endometrium may extend into the myometrium and parametrial tissue, with abscess formation or sepsis. One clinical complication that should be suspected in a patient who does not respond to antibiotic therapy is septic pelvic thrombophlebitis (27). If the workup fails to identify another infection, computed tomography should be performed and a therapeutic trial of anticoagulation considered. In such cases, antibiotics would be continued in addition to heparinization, and a rapid defervescence may be observed.

Laboratory evaluation of the febrile postpartum patient should include a complete blood count, chest x-ray, urine culture, and blood cultures. Leukocytosis is usually present but may also be seen in the noninfected postpartum patient. Uterine cultures are often not done because of the difficulty in interpreting the results. Because the microorganisms recovered are usually part of the normal maternal flora, these may either represent contamination during specimen collection or may be the cause of endometritis. Unless a blood culture is positive, there is no way to confirm that the isolates are significant. However, good aerobic and anaerobic cultures do show the range of potential pathogens and detect infections caused by unusual pathogens such as the rare group A β-hemolytic streptococci (GABHS) infection. Uterine cultures can be collected with a cotton swab (28).

Historically, GABHS has been a significant cause of postpartum endometritis but now is uncommon (3). These infections occur in previously colonized mothers or can be acquired by cross-infection from healthcare workers, other patients, or colonized infants. GABHS endometritis may differ from endometritis caused by the usual maternal vaginal flora, with an abrupt onset of high spiking fevers and diffuse tenderness. Diagnosis can be made by Gram stain and cultures of uterine discharge. The streptococcal toxic shock syndrome caused by GABHS has been reported in postpartum patients (29).

Surgical Site Infections

Episiotomy infections are uncommon and usually not serious, but severe complications such as necrotizing fasciitis can develop (30,31). Episiotomy sites should be examined carefully to detect infection early and infections should be treated to prevent complications.

A more serious problem is infection of the surgical site of a cesarean section. SSIs are reported to occur in about 3% to 4% of cesarean section patients, including both incisional and organ and space infections (2,32). SSIs are usually caused by maternal flora in the endometrium but, as with any other surgical sites, can be caused by organisms from exogenous sources (17,33). In the latter cases, *S. aureus* is the most frequent cause of infection. Although the pathogenicity of genital mycoplasma in SSIs has not been proved, a recent study reported these to be the most common bacteria isolated in infected postcesarean surgical sites (33). SSIs should be cultured before antibiotic therapy is begun.

Urinary Tract Infection

Urinary tract infections are a common problem in pregnancy and during the postpartum period (34). Risk factors for postpartum infections include urinary retention from anesthesia, trauma during delivery, and the need for catheterization. Urine cultures of the febrile patient should always be collected, although midstream samples may be contaminated by vaginal discharge. In those cases, the results are interpreted in the context of the clinical findings and the response to empiric antibiotic therapy. The major preventable risk factor in the postpartum period is catheterization. This is necessary with urinary retention but should be done only as needed. Another risk factor for postpartum urinary tract infection is bacteriuria during pregnancy. Detection and treatment of bacteriuria in pregnant women may decrease postpartum urinary tract infections.

Chorioamnionitis (Intraamniotic Infection)

Intrauterine infection during pregnancy, like postpartum endometritis, is usually caused by ascending infection from vaginal flora and is caused by similar bacteria (15,35,36). Most infections are also polymicrobial, and the major risk factor is prolonged rupture of the membranes. Infection is rare in women with intact membranes. Other risk factors are similar to those for postpartum endometritis, including duration of labor, number of vaginal examinations, internal monitoring, and possibly bacterial vaginosis. A variety of other obstetric procedures may introduce infection such as amniocentesis, chorionic villus sampling, and percutaneous umbilical blood sampling.

Initially, the diagnosis may be difficult, because fever can be the only presenting sign. Specific diagnosis requires examination of amniotic fluid by Gram stain, culture, and amniotic fluid glucose level (37). Hospital-acquired chorioamnionitis can be suspected in patients who become febrile after vaginal examinations, internal fetal monitoring, or other such procedures, but there is no standardized definition for nosocomial infection. Once the diagnosis is suspected, the patient should be started on antibiotic therapy and delivered as soon as possible.

Mastitis

In a study of obstetric patients who were contacted after discharge from the hospital, mastitis was the most common infection reported (38). Very few breast infections were seen during hospitalization, because mastitis and breast abscess usually occur several weeks into the postpartum period. A slight fever can develop early with breast engorgement, but it is transient. Later in the postpartum period, infectious mastitis must be distinguished from milk stasis and noninfectious inflammation (39). Infection is associated with higher fevers and erythema and is usually unilateral.

The most common cause of breast infection is *S. aureus* (40). Epidemics of staphylococcal mastitis occurred in the past but have not been reported in recent years. Therefore, the traditional classification of infectious mastitis into sporadic and epidemic forms is seldom useful. Both types are usually caused by *S. aureus*. Predisposing factors include the lack of nipple care, poor feeding technique, and inadequate emptying of the breasts. Infection can be confirmed by Gram stain and culture and responds to antistaphylococcal antibiotics and, if needed, surgical drainage. Continued breast drainage is important and can be accomplished by continued nursing, if appropriate, or pumping and discarding milk.

NONOBSTETRIC INFECTIONS IN THE OBSTETRIC PATIENT

There are many nonobstetric infections that must be considered in the evaluation and management of obstetric patients, not only for the sake of the patient but also for the safety of the fetus or neonate and the protection of others on the obstetric service. Selected infections of particular importance in the obstetric patient are described.

Listeria

Listeria monocytogenes causes a febrile illness in obstetric patients and may rarely result in severe diseases such as meningitis (41). It can be transmitted to the neonate and cause severe disease. Contaminated food, particularly soft cheeses and cold meats, can infect the obstetric patient. Transmission of *Listeria* to neonates in the delivery room has been reported on several occasions (42,43). The collection of routine blood cultures during the evaluation of fever provides a diagnosis, allowing directed antibiotic therapy.

Group B Streptococcal Infection

Group B β-hemolytic streptococci (GBS) are normal flora in the gastrointestinal and genitourinary tract and occasionally cause obstetric infections, including chorioamnionitis, endometritis, urinary tract infections, or SSIs (44). More often, the colonized mother may transmit GBS to the neonate, sometimes causing neonatal sepsis. The Centers for Disease Control and Prevention (CDC) recommends universal prenatal screening of pregnant women for GBS colonization of vagina and rectum (45). Antibiotic prophylaxis is recommended for colonized women delivering vaginally or who have had rupture of membranes (45). (See also Chapter 31.)

Human Immunodeficiency Virus Infection

One of the most important infections to identify in the pregnant patient is HIV, because prepartum diagnosis allows preventive treatment with antiretroviral drugs and possibly delivery by cesarean section (46). HIV antibody testing is offered to all pregnant patients, and if positive they should be treated according to current Public Health Service Task Force guidelines (46), which are frequently updated. HIV-infected mothers should not breast-feed their children.

Hepatitis B Virus Infections

All pregnant women should be tested for hepatitis B virus (HBV) surface antigen [and for hepatitis C virus (HCV) antibody if liver function tests are abnormal] to prevent transmission of HBV infection to neonates. If HBV infection is identified in the obstetric patient, the neonate can be treated with HBV immunoglobulin and vaccine (47).

Healthcare workers with HBV also pose a risk to uninfected obstetric patients during high-risk procedures. Obstetricians with HBV have been reported to infect their patients during cesarean section and forceps deliveries (48). Every obstetrician should know his or her HBV status, including tests for HBV surface antigen, e antigen and antibody, and core antibody. If susceptible to HBV, obstetricians should be immunized (see also Chapters 45 and 78).

Hepatitis C Virus Infection

No prophylaxis is currently available to prevent transmission of HCV from infected mother to neonate.

Herpes Simplex Virus Infection

Genital HSV, both primary and recurrent infection, occurs in obstetric patients and on rare occasion may result in disseminated disease (49). HSV can be transmitted from mother to neonate intrapartum. Cesarean section is indicated for women with active HSV lesions at the time of delivery (50). Internal fetal monitoring should not be done if HSV is suspected (50).

Postpartum, the mother with HSV lesions should be advised of potential risks of transmission to her newborn and educated about appropriate measures to limit contact transmission. (50) If healthcare workers with active lesions are allowed to continue working with patients, similar measures should be taken (51) (see also Chapter 43).

Chickenpox (Varicella Zoster Virus Infection)

Chickenpox in the obstetric patient may result in severe pneumonia, requiring hospitalization and antiviral therapy (52). The obstetric patient with chickenpox who is not in labor should be admitted to a nonobstetric unit and placed in a negative pressure room, because airborne transmission can occur (53,54). A patient admitted to our obstetric unit and placed in a regular hospital room with the door closed still infected a susceptible nurse who walked past the closed door (54). After delivery of a pregnant patient with chickenpox, the mother and infant should be separated until all of the mother's lesions have crusted over (see also Chapters 42, 51, and 52).

Smallpox Vaccine (Vaccinia Virus)

The United States began smallpox vaccination of healthcare workers in 2003. Hospitals will need to ensure that vaccinated healthcare workers do not transmit vaccinia to pregnant women, because fetal vaccinia can occur (55).

Rubella Virus

Despite the availability of an effective vaccine, rubella outbreaks and congenital rubella continue to occur. Pregnant women should be screened for rubella antibody. If not immune, they should be advised and monitored for signs and symptoms of rubella (56) (see also Chapter 51).

INFECTION CONTROL PROGRAM FOR OBSTETRICS

Surveillance

There are limited surveillance data available on hospital-acquired infections on obstetric units. The National Nosocomial Infections Surveillance (NNIS) system and other organizations do provide some data that are useful to hospitals doing surveillance on obstetric services (32). As would be expected, these reports show that SSIs are the major nosocomial infection problem in obstetrics, with urinary tract infections the next most frequent. However, the reported infection rates on obstetric services are lower than on medical and surgical services. The infection rates vary by the size and type of hospital, and the SSIs vary by the number of risk factors. More recent NNIS reports are limited to data on SSIs from in-hospital surveillance of patients who have had cesarean sections (32). None of these data provides a basis for comparing infection rates observed in routine surveillance with data from other hospitals (57). The best comparison is with rates in the same hospital at previous times. The CDC does provide standardized definitions for surveillance (Table 55.2) (58,59). As discussed previously, many risk factors have been identified for obstetric infections. However, for most surveillance purposes it is sufficient to relate infections to the type of delivery, vaginal or cesarean, and to distinguish between elective and nonelective cesarean sections.

The general value of surveillance and infection control programs in hospitals has been documented by the CDC Study on the Efficacy of Nosocomial Infection Control, and the effective use of surveillance data on an obstetrics and gynecology service has been demonstrated by a study at a Swedish hospital (60,61). In the Swedish report, data collected on patients having cesarean sections showed that 15% of them were infected (urinary tract infections excluded). The infection rates decreased to 9% after the introduction of quarterly surveillance reports to obstetric personnel. These reports included surgeon-specific infection rates. This decrease was mainly in postpartum endometritis. Despite this success with surveillance of postcesarean infections, developing an overall obstetric surveillance program may be difficult.

A traditional method of surveillance on obstetric services is to monitor fevers in all patients. Most infected patients will be detected by this approach, and a routine fever workup in the postpartum patient will identify many infectious causes. The limitation of fever surveillance is that half of the fevers are either due to noninfectious causes or the specific infection cannot be identified (62). Despite this limitation, fever surveillance on an obstetric unit is a good screening technique and can indicate the development of potential problems.

Mead et al. (63) reported the use of a "sentinel list" technique on an obstetric unit, where the bedside nurse is involved in collecting information including fever and antimicrobial therapy and the collected information is reviewed for continuous surveillance. This method may be implemented and maintained by the obstetric staff, who would report to infection control when problems develop. Another technique to identify infections is to link computer data on patients who have cesarean sections with antibiotic utilization records and admission and discharge diagnoses (64).

Short hospital stays and outpatient management of most postdischarge infections limit hospital-based surveillance of obstetric patients. Supplemental postdischarge surveillance systems are needed to provide an accurate picture of obstetric infections.

Several different approaches to postdischarge surveillance have been tried, involving either the patients directly or their physicians. The gold standard of postdischarge surveillance is direct observation of patients after hospital discharge. Couto et al. (65) did this at a Brazilian hospital by having postcesarean patients return on the tenth to the fifteenth postoperative day (65). While in the hospital, 1.6% of the patients had SSIs, and this increased to 9.6% with postdischarge examination.

A more practical approach was used by Holbrook et al. (38) who mailed one-page questionnaires to 19,650 women who delivered at their hospital. They received responses from only 36% of them (38). Ten percent of the patients who responded reported infections after discharge, including mastitis (6%), urinary tract infections (3%), and endometritis (1%). Postdischarge surveillance detected twice as many infections as in-hospital surveillance. The additional infections that were identified were mostly mastitis and urinary tract infections. Most cases of endometritis were reported by in-hospital surveillance, but an additional 1% of women reported endometritis after discharge. A major limitation of this approach is the poor response rate by the patients.

Postdischarge surveillance using physician questionnaires to identify infections after cesarean section has been reported to be more successful (66). In a study by Hulton et al. (66), 90% of physicians completed questionnaires about their patients. These questionnaires indicated an infection rate of 6.3% compared with 1.6% observed by in-hospital surveillance before the intro-

TABLE 55.2. DEFINITIONS FOR SURVEILLANCE OF NOSOCOMIAL INFECTIONS ON OBSTETRIC UNITS: CENTERS FOR DISEASES CONTROL AND PREVENTION

Endometritis must meet either of the following criteria:
- Microorganism isolated from culture of fluid or tissue from endometrium obtained during surgery, by needle aspiration, or by brush biopsy
- Purulent drainage from uterus *and* two of the following: fever (>38°C), abdominal pain, or uterine tenderness

Episiotomy site infection must meet either of the following criteria:
- Purulent drainage from episiotomy
- Episiotomy abscess

Other infections (excluding surgical site infections) must meet one of the following criteria:
- Microorganism isolated from culture of tissue or fluid from affected site
- Abscess or other evidence of infection seen during surgery or by histopathologic examination
- Two of the following: fever (>38°C), nausea, vomiting, pain, tenderness, dysuria, *and* either of the following:
- Microorganism isolated from blood culture
- Physician's diagnosis

Postcesarean surgical site infections must meet the definitions used for all surgical site infections and are classified into the following categories:
- **Superficial incisional:** involves only skin or subcutaneous tissue and excludes stitch abscess or an episiotomy infection
- **Deep incisional:** involves deep tissues, e.g., fascial or muscle layers
- **Organ/space:** involves any part of the anatomy, other than an incision, opened or manipulated during surgery and includes postoperative endometritis

From Garner JS, Jarvis WR, Emori TG, et al. CDC definitions for nosocomial infections, 1988. *Am J Infect Control* 1988;16:128–140; Horan TC, Gaynes RP, Martone WJ, et al. CDC definitions of nosocomial Surgical site infection, 1992; a modification of CDC definitions of surgical wound infections. *Am J Infect Control* 1992;20:271–274, with permission.

duction of the postdischarge system. The increase occurred in incisional SSIs (0.3% to 3.9%) and endometritis (1.3% to 2.5%). Despite the success of this study, maintaining physician cooperation over a long period of time may be difficult. The low infection rates in obstetric patients may not warrant the resources needed for postdischarge surveillance. A reasonable approach is to do postdischarge surveillance for a limited period each year (67).

Data mining of computerized records can augment traditional surveillance. Yokoe et al. (2) have used this method to determine postpartum infection rates among women in a large managed care organization (see also Chapter 94).

Facilities on an Obstetric Unit

Obstetric units vary greatly in design, ranging from birthing centers designed for low-risk deliveries to standard labor and delivery units including operating rooms for cesarean sections. The design needs are similar to other patient care areas in the hospital, including conveniently placed alcohol hand rubs and sinks for hand disinfection by staff, easily cleaned surfaces, and, in the case of complicated deliveries, a fully equipped operating room. The American College of Obstetricians and Gynecologists outlined basic standards for obstetric facilities (68). An isolation facility should be available for the rare delivery of an obstetric patient with airborne infectious diseases such as chickenpox or tuberculosis. A pregnant patient with such an infection who is not in labor can be isolated in a room with negative air pressure on other hospital units.

The use of hydrotherapy to assist in labor raises additional environmental infection control concerns (69). Some obstetric units use baths, whirlpools, or Jacuzzi showers as an aid in delivery. This practice raises the same concerns about bacterial contamination as hydrotherapy in physical therapy (see Chapter 66). Very few studies have been reported that evaluate the potential infectious risks of obstetric hydrotherapy. In one nonrandomized study of 1,385 women with prelabor rupture of the membranes, 538 chose to use a warm tub bath during labor and 847 did not (70). Of those who used the bath, 1.1% developed chorioamnionitis and 0.6% developed endometritis. Of those who did not, 0.2% developed chorioamnionitis and 0.4% developed endometritis, suggesting no infectious risk. However, in a small study of 32 women, one infant developed a *Pseudomonas* infection that was isolated from the prelabor bath water (71). Presumably, this resulted from a lapse in cleaning technique and indicates a potential infectious risk. Whirlpool baths present even more complex maintenance problems. In a randomized controlled trial of whirlpool baths, 785 patients were studied (72). Benefits in regard to analgesics, instrumentation, and perineal conditions were reported, but no difference was observed in maternal and neonatal infections.

These studies provide limited guidance in making an infection control decision regarding maternal hydrotherapy. If a facility decides to use hydrotherapy, a detailed protocol must be developed that includes both a procedure and a cleaning or maintenance protocol. Women with complicated pregnancies should be excluded, and many facilities require that the patient sign a consent form. Cleaning and maintenance protocols depend on the type of equipment used. To avoid these problems, some facilities use inflatable single-use tubs.

Prevention

Antepartum

The goal of good medical care during pregnancy is to ensure that a healthy patient presents for delivery. Conditions that place the pregnant patient at risk for postpartum infection, including urinary tract infection and perhaps bacterial vaginosis, should be identified and treated during routine prenatal care (34,73). Routine screening for infections, including sexually transmitted and blood-borne diseases such as HIV, HBV, syphilis, chlamydia, and gonorrhea should identify other infections in the pregnant patient. Dietary restrictions are appropriate to avoid infection with *Listeria* (74).

Intrapartum

Semmelweis' (6,7) original observations on the value of good hand washing with an antibacterial agent remain the cornerstone of good obstetric infection control. The number of vaginal examinations should be limited, and internal monitoring with pressure catheters and scalp electrodes should be used only when necessary and should be introduced with aseptic technique. Fetal electrodes should be avoided in women with HSV, HIV, or HBV. Despite the effectiveness of traditional preventive measures, infection control measures will not prevent many intrapartum infections (35).

Studies during obstetric procedures have clearly shown the high risk of exposure of the obstetric team to blood and body fluids during deliveries (75–78). In one study, observers were placed in delivery rooms and directly recorded how often blood or amniotic fluid exposures were occurring (75). In 230 deliveries observed, blood or amniotic fluid exposure occurred in 39% of 202 vaginal deliveries and 50% of 28 cesarean sections. The highest rates of exposure occurred in obstetricians and midwives. Another study comparing different surgical procedures showed that the frequency of blood exposures during cesarean sections was exceeded only by cardiothoracic and trauma surgery (76). Tichenor et al. (77) demonstrated the need for good eye protection. They collected eye shields attached to surgical masks worn during deliveries and counted the visible splashes. This study found that 54% of the eye shields from the primary obstetricians had been splashed, including 30 of 68 shields from vaginal deliveries and 30 of 44 from cesarean sections. Perforation of surgical gloves is also common during deliveries and often goes unrecognized. Serrano et al. (78) collected 754 surgical gloves used by obstetricians during vaginal and cesarean deliveries and postpartum ligations. The gloves were examined for perforations by an air inflation-water submersion technique, and 13% of the gloves had been perforated. They noted that 62% of the perforations were not recognized during the surgical procedure; thus, the obstetricians were unaware of the potential exposure to blood or body fluids.

Because all deliveries are associated with the splatter of blood and body fluids and exposures are common, the delivery team never knows for sure when they will be exposed. Also, they cannot be certain that any specific patient does not have a blood-borne disease at the time of delivery, even if screening was done during prenatal care. Therefore, appropriate protective equipment should always be worn, including gloves, long-sleeved impervious gowns, shoe covers, masks, and eye protection, and the obstetrician should always be aware of the possibility of glove perforation.

Prophylactic antibiotics are given for all nonelective cesarean sections and will prevent 50% or more of postpartum endometritis (24). Despite this, as always, good surgical technique is critical to the prevention of surgical infections (79).

Postpartum

Good perineal, surgical site, and breast care is important in the postpartum period. Mother and newborn should be separated in the case of infections like tuberculosis or chickenpox. Masks should be worn during minor respiratory infections. The patient should be monitored for urinary retention, with urinary catheterization used only as needed.

Epidemic Investigations

The most common epidemic problem on obstetric units is an increase in postcesarean fevers, which is easy to investigate, because it is usually related to procedures in the surgical suite. One of the first things to review is the use of prophylactic antibiotics. Failure to give antibiotics or failure to give them appropriately can result in an increase in postpartum infections that is easily correctable. In a teaching hospital, another potential cause of increased infection rates is the presence of a resident with poor surgical technique. We appreciated this phenomenon on our own obstetric unit only when the increase in fevers disappeared at the end of the month when a resident rotated off service and reappeared when the same resident came back on service.

The classic epidemic problems on obstetric units are outbreaks of streptococcal or staphylococcal infections.

Streptococcus pyogenes (Group A β-Hemolytic Streptococcal Infections)

Despite good infection control practices, GABHS epidemics can still occur if a member of the obstetric team is a streptococcal carrier. The problem of the carrier is dramatically illustrated by an outbreak reported from a hospital in Washington state in the 1960s (80,81). Eleven patients, nine obstetric and two gynecologic, developed GABHS infections and one died. Eight of nine obstetric patients developed signs of endometritis within 30 to 60 hours of delivery, and the ninth patient was readmitted on the sixth postpartum day. Although nasopharyngeal cultures were negative from all staff who had contact with the patients, epidemiologic investigation identified the only staff member who had contact with all infected patients. When he stopped practicing, the infections disappeared, and when he returned to practice, the infections reappeared. This pattern was seen on three separate occasions, despite empiric antibiotic treatment with penicillin. Finally, the physician was hospitalized for clinical and microbiologic studies and was found to be an anal carrier of GABHS. It was demonstrated that he disseminated streptococci when he was moving about, including undressing and exercising. Antibiotic treatment of the physician and his family cleared the carrier state and ended the epidemic.

Such outbreaks of GABHS infections continue to be a problem, although rare, and must be recognized quickly because of the potential for severe disease (3,82). The diagnosis of postpartum GABHS infection on an obstetric service should always be an infection control priority and should be investigated immediately (see also Chapter 31).

Staphylococcus aureus

Outbreaks of staphylococcal infections are also uncommon on the modern obstetric unit. Exceptions occur, which are of concern mainly because of the risk of introduction of methicillin-resistant *S. aureus* (MRSA) into other hospital units such as neonatal intensive care units. An outbreak of MRSA at a large regional maternity unit in England identified 37 patients who had MRSA and noted that perineal colonization was common in postpartum women but not in staff members (83). This was attributed to perineal injury from delivery that created a favorable site for colonization. The wards in this hospital differed from most American hospitals in that common toilet facilities with baths were provided for each ward rather than private bathrooms. Contamination of baths and bidets with MRSA was documented. Mattress covers were also contaminated and remained contaminated even after cleaning with detergent. Most mattress covers were found to be porous, and the core of some mattresses contained MRSA. The relative contribution of environmental transmission cannot be determined from this study because, as in most MRSA outbreaks, transient carriage by staff members was demonstrated. MRSA was eradicated from the maternity wards with infection control measures, including replacement of all mattresses.

Staphylococcal infections do not present the same urgency as GABHS infections, but clustering of infections should be investigated thoroughly both for staphylococcal carriers and for breaks in technique that facilitate cross-infection on the obstetric ward (see also Chapters 28 and 29).

CONCLUSIONS

Hospital-acquired infections in obstetric patients have a long and dramatic history, but modern obstetric practices have produced low infection rates and extremely low maternal mortality. Good surveillance data on obstetric infection are limited because of difficulties in establishing specific diagnosis and the short hospital stays of most obstetric patients. It is important to appreciate that these infections still occur, produce significant maternal and neonatal morbidity, and require careful monitoring. Also, nonobstetric infections in the obstetric patient and infections in newborns remain a major concern for hospital staff, requiring good infection control practice and careful patient management.

REFERENCES

1. Bridson EY. Iatrogenic epidemics of puerperal fever in the 18th and 19th centuries. *Br J Biomed Sci* 1996;53:134–139.
2. Yokoe DS, Christiansen CL, Johnson R, et al. Epidemiology of and surveillance for postpartum infections. *Emerg Infect Dis* 2001;7: 837–841.
3. Ledger WJ. Puerperal endometritis. In: Bennet JV, Brachman PS eds. *Hospital infections,* 4th ed. Philadelphia: Lippincott-Raven Publishers, 1998:551–561.
4. Lowis GW. Epidemiology of puerperal fever: the contributions of Alexander Gordon. *Med Hist* 1993;37:399–410.
5. Holmes OW. The contagiousness of puerperal fever. *N Engl Q J Med Surg* 1843;1:503–530.
6. Semmelweis IP. Childbed fever. *Rev Infect Dis* 1981;3:808–811.
7. Semmelweis I. The etiology of childbed fever. In: *The classics of medicine library.* Birmingham: Gryphon Editions, 1981.
8. Loudon I. Puerperal fever, the streptococcus, and the sulphonamides, 1911–1945. *BMJ* 1987;295:485–490.
9. Bartlett JG, Onderdonk AB, Drude E, et al. Quantitative bacteriology of the vaginal flora. *J Infect Dis* 1977;136:271–277.
10. Bartlett JG, Moon NE, Goldstein PR, et al. Cervical and vaginal microflora: ecologic niches in the female lower genital tract. *Am J Obstet Gynecol* 1978;130:658–661.
11. Gibbs RS. Microbiology of the female genital tract. *Am J Obstet Gynecol* 1987;156:491–495.
12. Hammill HA. Normal vaginal flora in relation to vaginitis. *Obstet Gynecol Clin North Am* 1989;16:329–336.
13. Larsen B, Galask RP. Vaginal microbial flora: practical and theoretical relevance. *Obstet Gynecol* 1980;55(Suppl 5):100s–113s.
14. Faro S, Cox S, Phillips L, et al. Influence of antibiotic prophylaxis on vaginal microflora. *J Obstet Gynecol* 1986;6(Suppl 1):S4–S6.
15. Casey BM, Cox SM. Chorioamnionitis and endometritis. *Infect Dis Clin North Am* 1997;11:203–222.
16. Awadalla SG, Perkins RP, Mercer LJ. Significance of endometrial cultures performed at cesarean section. *Obstet Gynecol* 1986;68:220–225.
17. Emmons SL, Krohn M, Jackson M, et al. Development of wound infections among women undergoing cesarean section. *Obstet Gynecol* 1988;72:559–564.
18. Gibbs RS. Infection after cesarean section. *Clin Obstet Gynecol* 1985; 28:697–710.
19. Atterbury JL, Groome LJ, Baker SL, et al. Hospital readmission for postpartum endometritis. *J Matern Fetal Med* 1998;7:250–254.
20. Faro S, Phillips LE, Martens MG. Perspectives on the bacteriology of postoperative obstetric-gynecologic infections. *Am J Obstet Gynecol* 1988;158:694–700.
21. Gibbs RS, Blanco JD, Bernstein S. Role of aerobic gram-negative bacilli in endometritis after cesarean section. *Rev Infect Dis* 1985;7(Suppl 4): S690–S695.
22. Watts DH. Eschenbach DA, Kenny GE. Early postpartum endometritis: the role of bacteria, genital mycoplasma and *Chlamydia trachomatis. Obstet Gynecol* 1989;73:52–60.
23. Hoyme UB, Kiviat N, Eschenbach DA. Microbiology and treatment of late postpartum endometritis. *Obstet Gynecol* 1986;68:226–232.
24. Hemsell DL. Prophylactic antibiotics in gynecologic and obstetrical surgery. *Rev Infect Dis* 1991;13(Suppl 10):S821–S841.
25. Newton ER, Prihoda TJ, Gibbs RS. A clinical and microbiologic analysis of risk factors for puerperal endometritis. *Obstet Gynecol* 1990;75: 402–406.
26. Semprini AE, Castagna C, Ravizza M, et al. The incidence of complications after cesarean section in 156 HIV-positive women. *AIDS* 1995; 9:913–917.
27. Calhoun BC, Brost B. Emergency management of sudden puerperal fever. *Obstet Gynecol Clin North Am* 1995;22:357–367.
28. Martens MG, Faro S, Hammill HA, et al. Transcervical uterine cultures with a new endometrial suction curette: a comparison of three sampling methods in postpartum endometritis. *Obstet Gynecol* 1989;74: 273–276.
29. Noronha S, Yue CT, Sekosan M. Puerperal group A beta-hemolytic streptococcal toxic shock-like syndrome. *Obstet Gynecol* 1996;88:728.
30. Larsson PG, Platz-Christensen J, Bergman B, et al. Advantage or disadvantage of episiotomy compared with spontaneous perineal laceration. *Gynecol Obstet Invest* 1991;31:213–216.
31. Shy KK, Eschenbach DA. Fatal perineal cellulitis from an episiotomy site. *Obstet Gynecol* 1979;54:292–298.
32. CDC NNIS System. National Nosocomial Infections Surveillance (NNIS) system report, data summary from January 1992–June 2001, issued August 2001. *Am J Infect Control* 2001;29:404–421.
33. Roberts S, Maccato M, Faro S, et al. The microbiology of post-cesarean wound morbidity. *Obstet Gynecol* 1993;81:383–386.
34. Millar LK, Cox SM. Urinary tract infections complicating pregnancy. *Infect Dis Clin North Am* 1997;11:13–26.
35. Soper DE, Mayhall CG, Froggatt JW. Characterization and control of intraamniotic infection in an urban teaching hospital. *Am J Obstet Gynecol* 1996;175:304–309.
36. Riggs JW, Blanco JD. Pathophysiology, diagnosis, and management of intraamniotic infection. *Semin Perinatol* 1998;22:251–259.
37. Hussey MJ, Levy ES, Pombar X, et al. Evaluating rapid diagnostic tests of intraamniotic infection: gram stain, amniotic fluid glucose level, and amniotic fluid to serum glucose level ratio. *Am J Obstet Gynecol* 1998; 179:650–656.
38. Holbrook KF, Nottebart VF, Hameed SR, et al. Automated postdischarge surveillance for postpartum and neonatal nosocomial infections. *Am J Med* 1991;91(Suppl 3B):S125–S130.
39. Marchant DJ. Inflammation of the breast. *Obstet Gynecol Clin North Am* 2002;29:89–102.
40. Marshall BR, Hepper JK, Zirbel CC. Sporadic puerperal mastitis: an infection that need not interrupt lactation. *JAMA* 1975;233: 1377–1379.
41. Lorber B. State of the art clinical article: listeriosis. *J Infect Dis* 1997; 24:1–11.
42. Campbell AN, Sill PR, Wardle JK. Listeria meningitis acquired by cross infection in a delivery suite. *Lancet* 1981:2:752–753.
43. Simmons MD, Cockcroft PM, Okubadejo OA. Neonatal listeriosis due to cross-infection in an obstetric theatre. *J Infect* 1986;13:235–239.
44. McKenna DS, Iams JD. Group B streptococcal infections. *Semin Perinatol* 1998;22:267–276.
45. Centers for Disease Control and Prevention. Prevention of perinatal group B streptococcal disease: revised guidelines from the CDC. *MMWR Mortal Morb Wkly Rep* 2002;51(RR11):1–22. Available at *http://www.cdc.gov/mmwr/preview/mmwrhtml/rr5111a1.htm* (accessed).
46. Public Health Service Task Force. Recommendations for use of antiretroviral drugs in pregnant HIV-1-infected women for maternal health and interventions to reduce perinatal HIV-1 transmission in the United States, 2002. Available at *http://www.aidsinfo.nih.gov/guidelines/perinatal/perinatal/perinatal.pdf* (accessed).
47. ACOG Educational Bulletin. Viral hepatitis in pregnancy. *Int J Gynaecol Obstet* 1998;63:195–202.
48. Weber DJ, Hoffmann KK, Rutala WA. Management of the healthcare worker with human immunodeficiency virus: lessons from nosocomial transmission of hepatitis B virus. *Infect Control Hosp Epidemiol* 1991; 12:625–630.
49. Young EJ, Chafizadeh E, Oliveira VL, et al. Disseminated herpesvirus infection during pregnancy. *Clin Infect Dis* 1996;22:51–58.
50. ACOG Practice Bulletin. Management of herpes in pregnancy. *Int J Gynaecol Obstet* 2000; 68:165–174.
51. Bolyard EA, Tablan OC, Williams WW, et al. Guideline for infection control in healthcare personnel. *Infect Control Hosp Epidemiol* 1998; 19:407–463.
52. Chandra PC, Patel H, Schiavello HJ, et al. Successful pregnancy outcome after complicated varicella pneumonia. *Obstet Gynecol* 1998;92: 680–682.
53. Nathwani D, Maclean A, Conway S, et al. Varicella infections in pregnancy and the newborn. *J Infect* 1998;36(Suppl 1):59–71.

54. Menkhaus NA, Lanphear B, Linnemann CC. Airborne transmission of varicella-zoster virus in hospitals [Letter]. *Lancet* 1990;336:1315.
55. Centers for Disease Control and Prevention. Vaccinia (smallpox) vaccine: recommendations of the Advisory Committee on Immunization Practices (ACIP), 2001. *MMWR Mortal Morb Wkly Rep* 2001; 50(RR10):1–26.
56. Centers for Disease Control and Prevention. Control and prevention of rubella: evaluation and management of suspected outbreaks, rubella in pregnant women, and surveillance for congenital rubella syndrome. *MMWR Mortal Morb Wkly Rep* 2001;50(RR12):1–23.
57. Nosocomial infection rates for interhospital comparison: limitations and possible solutions. *Infect Control Hosp Epidemiol* 1991;12: 609–621.
58. Garner JS, Jarvis WR, Emori TG, et al. CDC definitions for nosocomial infections, 1988. *Am J Infect Control* 1988;16:128–140.
59. Horan TC, Gaynes RP, Martone WJ, et al. CDC definitions of nosocomial surgical site infection, 1992: a modification of CDC definitions of surgical wound infections. *Am J Infect Control* 1992;20:271–274.
60. Haley RW, Culver DH, White JW, et al. The efficacy of infection surveillance and control programs in preventing nosocomial infections in US hospitals. *Am J Epidemiol* 1985;121:182–205.
61. Evaldson GR, Frederici H, Jullig C, et al. Hospital-associated infections in obstetrics and gynecology: effects of surveillance. *Acta Obstet Gynaecol Scand* 1992;71:54–58.
62. Klimek JJ, Ajemian ER, Gracewski J, et al. A prospective analysis of hospital-acquired fever in obstetric and gynecologic patients. *JAMA* 1982;247:3340–3343.
63. Mead PB, Hess SM, Page SD. Prevention and control of nosocomial infection in obstetrics and gynecology. In: Wenzel RP, ed. *Prevention and control of nosocomial infections,* 3rd ed. Baltimore: Williams & Wilkins, 1997:995–1016.
64. Baker C, Luce J, Chemoweth C, et al. Comparison of case-finding methodologies for endometritis after cesarean section. *Am J Infect Control* 1995;23:27–33.
65. Couto RC, Pedrosa TMG, Nogueria JM, et al. Post-discharge surveillance and infection rates in obstetric patients. *Int J Gynaecol Obstet* 1998;61:227–231.
66. Hulton LJ, Olmsted RN, Treston-Aurand J, et al. Effect of postdischarge surveillance on rates of infectious complications after cesarean section. *Am J Infect Control* 1992;20:198–201.
67. Gravel-Tropper D, Oxley C, Memish Z, et al. Underestimation of surgical site infection rates in obstetrics and gynecology. *Am J Infect Control* 1995;23:22–26.
68. Inpatient perinatal care services. In: American Academy of Pediatrics and American College of Obstetricians and Gynecologists: guidelines for perinatal care, 5th ed. Washington DC: American College of Obstetricians and Gynecologists, 2002:17–55.
69. McCandlish R, Renfrew M. Immersion in water during labor and birth: the need for evaluation. *Birth* 1993;20:79–85.
70. Eriksson M, Ladfors L, Mattsson LA, et al. Warm tub bath during labor. A study of 1385 women with prelabor rupture of the membranes after 34 weeks of gestation. *Acta Obstet Gynaecol Scand* 1996;75: 642–644.
71. Hawkins S. Water vs conventional births: infection rates compared. *Nursing Times* 1995;91:38–40.
72. Rush J, Burlock S, Lambert K, et al. The effects of whirlpool baths in labor: a randomized controlled trial. *Birth* 1996;23:136–143.
73. ACOG Educational Bulletin. Antimicrobial therapy for obstetrical patients. *Int J Gynaecol Obstet* 1998;61:299–308.
74. Centers for Disease Control and Prevention. Foodborne listeriosis—United States, 1988–1990. *JAMA* 1992;267:2446–2448.
75. Panlilio AL, Welch BA, Bell DM, et al. Blood and amniotic fluid contact sustained by obstetric personnel during deliveries. *Am J Obstet Gynecol* 1992;167:703–708.
76. Popejoy SL, Fry DE. Blood contract and exposure in the operating room. *Surg Gynecol Obstet* 1991;172:480–483.
77. Tichenor JR, Miller RC, Wolf EJ. Risk of eye splash in obstetric procedures. *Am J Perinatol* 1994;11:359–361.
78. Serrano CW, Wright JW, Newton ER. Surgical glove perforation in obstetrics. *Obstet Gynecol* 1991;77:525–528.
79. Lyon JB, Richardson AC. Careful surgical technique can reduce infectious morbidity after cesarean section. *Am J Obstet Gynecol* 1987;157: 557–562.
80. McIntyre DM. An epidemic of *Streptococcus pyogenes* puerperal and postoperative sepsis with an unusual carrier site the anus. *Am J Obstet Gynecol* 1968;101:308–314.
81. McKee WM, Di Caprio JM, Roberts CE Jr, et al. Anal carriage as the probable source of a streptococcal epidemic. *Lancet* 1966;2: 1007–1009.
82. Mastro TD, Farley TA, Elliott JA, et al. An outbreak of surgical-wound infections due to group A streptococcus carried on the scalp. *N Engl J Med* 1990;323:968–972.
83. Moore EP, Williams EW. A maternity hospital outbreak of methicillin-resistant *Staphylococcus aureus. J Hosp Infect* 1991;19:5–16.

56

NOSOCOMIAL INFECTIONS IN PATIENTS WITH SPINAL CORD INJURY

RABIH O. DAROUICHE

BACKGROUND

Patients with spinal cord injury constitute a unique population with distinct multidisciplinary problems. According to a consensus statement by the National Institute on Disability and Rehabilitation Research, at least 8,000 new cases of spinal cord injury accrue each year in the United States and about 200,000 Americans suffer from the consequences of such an injury (1). The number of patients living with spinal cord injury is expected to continue to rise owing to the increase in their life expectancy. Most cases of spinal cord injury are traumatic, most notably due to motor vehicle accidents, gunshot wounds, and falls.

Nosocomial infections are a major cause of morbidity and mortality in this population of patients (2,3). The three most common infections in patients with spinal cord injury are urinary tract infections, infections of pressure sores and underlying bone, and respiratory tract infections. These three infections have certain characteristics when they occur in patients with spinal cord injury as compared with the able-bodied population. This chapter discusses the factors that predispose to nosocomial infections in relation to time of injury; delineates the interrelated pathogenesis and microbiology, unusual clinical manifestations, problematic diagnosis, and difficult prevention of infections involving the urinary tract, pressure sores and underlying bone, and respiratory tract; and addresses the issue of colonization and infection by multiresistant microorganisms.

FACTORS THAT PREDISPOSE TO NOSOCOMIAL INFECTIONS IN RELATION TO TIME OF INJURY

Patients with spinal cord injury are predisposed to nosocomial infections both in the acute and chronic settings after injury (Table 56.1). Immediately after the injury, patients are admitted to the hospital for management of injuries to the spinal cord and possibly other organs, and usually remain hospitalized for about 2 to 3 months for initial rehabilitation. Patients with spinal cord injury frequently have wounds of the chest, abdomen, and neck that may require surgical intervention, thereby imposing additional risks for postoperative infections. Critically ill patients have a particularly high risk of developing infections with resistant microorganisms, including multiresistant gram-negative bacilli, methicillin-resistant *Staphylococcus aureus* (MRSA), and vancomycin-resistant *Enterococcus* (VRE). Large doses of glucocorticosteroids, given immediately after traumatic injury, may also predispose these patients to infection. The majority of patients during the period of spinal cord shock suffer from neurogenic bladder that necessitates catheter drainage, often leading to development of urinary tract infection. Patients with high cervical injury usually require mechanical ventilation and can develop ventilator-associated pneumonia.

Although the likelihood of developing infection per hospital day appears to be the highest in the acute postinjury period, the vast majority of infections occur long after the injury. This is due to the fact that most such patients sustain spinal cord injury when still young and have an almost normal life expectancy. Since most patients with spinal cord injury chronically rely on bladder catheters for urinary drainage, urinary tract infection is the most common infection long after the injury. Second in frequency are infections associated with pressure ulcers. Patients with high cervical lesions are predisposed to tracheostomy- and endotracheal tube–related respiratory tract infections. Surgical management of the chronic sequelae of spinal cord injury can be complicated by surgical site infections.

TABLE 56.1. FACTORS THAT PREDISPOSE TO NOSOCOMIAL INFECTIONS IN RELATION TO TIME OF INJURY

Soon after the injury
Prolonged initial hospitalization
Surgical management of injuries to the spinal cord and possibly other organs
Admission to the intensive care unit
Administration of glucorticosteroids after the injury
Bladder catheterization
Mechanical ventilation
Long after the injury
Bladder catheterization
Pressure ulcers
Tracheostomy in patients with high cervical lesions
Surgical interventions for chronic complications of the injury

URINARY TRACT INFECTIONS

Pathogenesis and Epidemiology

Urinary tract infection is the most common infection in patients with spinal cord injury. Unique factors that predispose this population to urinary tract infection include bladder catheterization and urinary stasis (4). Although the sterile technique of bladder catheterization can theoretically be safer, at least in hospitalized patients, than the clean technique, both catheterization techniques can introduce microorganisms into the urinary tract. Urinary stasis impairs the naturally occurring mechanisms that protect the urinary tract from infection, including the washout effect of voiding and the phagocytic capacity of bladder epithelial cells. Multiplication of bacteria in the urine and invasion of host tissues are promoted in the presence of reduced bladder emptying, increased residual urine, and high bladder pressure (5).

Although more than 90% of episodes of urinary tract infection in this population appear to involve only the lower urinary tract, serious complications can still arise secondary to such infections. Ascending infection of the urinary tract may evolve in the presence of vesicoureteral reflux or as a consequence of manipulations used to empty the bladder. Kidney infection with loss of renal function is particularly worrisome, because renal failure was once the leading cause of death in patients with spinal cord injury. Additionally, urinary tract infection can be associated with a number of anatomic changes, such as renal calculi (occupying the bladder, ureters, or kidneys), bladder diverticula and fibrosis, penile and scrotal fistulas, epididymoorchitis, and abscesses. The frequency of these anatomic changes depends on the type and duration of bladder drainage; these changes are most commonly detected in patients with indwelling bladder catheters.

The vast majority of episodes of urinary tract infection in patients with spinal cord injury are caused by commensal bowel flora, primarily gram-negative bacilli and enterococci. The microbiology of microorganisms residing in the bladder can be affected by patients' gender, the place where pathogens are acquired (i.e., nosocomial vs. community acquisition), and the method of urinary drainage. For instance, *Klebsiella pneumoniae* is a very common cause of urinary tract infection in hospitalized patients (6,7). In contrast, *Escherichia coli* and *Enterococcus* species cause more than two thirds of cases of urinary tract infection in female patients undergoing intermittent bladder catheterization (8). The presence of condom catheters increases the likelihood of colonizing the urethra and perineal skin with *Pseudomonas, Klebsiella*, and other Gram-negative bacilli. Although the virulence of *Pseudomonas aeruginosa* when isolated from the urinary tract of patients with spinal cord injury has been questioned (9), tissue invasion and bacteremia due to this microorganism can still occur (10,11). As in able-bodied subjects, the presence of renal calculi in patients with spinal cord injury suggests etiology by urease-producing bacteria (12). Spinal cord injury units are no different from other types of specialized care units as to the occurrence of outbreaks of urinary tract infection due to multiresistant gram-negative bacilli (13). Polymicrobial growth is detected in almost half of positive urine cultures obtained from patients with spinal cord injury, particularly those with chronic indwelling urethral catheters (14).

Clinical Manifestations

Urinary tract infection may manifest differently in patients with spinal cord injury than in the general population. For instance, infected patients with spinal cord injury may not complain of dysuria, frequency, and urgency, which usually exist in able-bodied patients with urinary tract infection. Furthermore, suprapubic and flank pain or tenderness are not felt in insensate patients. More common manifestations of urinary tract infection in patients with spinal cord injury include worsening spasm, increasing dysreflexia, and change in voiding habits. Fever is usually, but not always, present.

Diagnosis

Diagnosis of urinary tract infection in patients with spinal cord injury can be problematic for several reasons. First, by masking urinary-specific symptoms, absent sensations constitute the single most important obstacle in the diagnosis of urinary tract infection in this population. Second, the unusual manifestations of urinary tract infection in these patients are nonspecific and may be caused by a variety of other infectious or noninfectious conditions, including osteomyelitis beneath pressure ulcers, ingrown toe nails, and heterotopic bone ossification. Third, bacteriuria, the cornerstone for diagnosing urinary tract infection, is nonspecifically prevalent in this population. Bacteriuria is most frequent in patients who have chronic indwelling bladder catheters, as cultures of randomly obtained urine samples yield bacterial growth in about 98% of instances (15). Even patients who undergo intermittent bladder catheterization have a 70% likelihood of being bacteriuric (16). Most cases of bacteriuria in patients with spinal cord injury represent asymptomatic bladder colonization. Although asymptomatic bladder colonization can progress to symptomatic infection, often it does not. Fourth, the finding of pyuria, which can reflect inflammation of the uromucosal lining and signal the transition from bladder colonization to symptomatic urinary tract infection is not specific for infection. Pyuria can be caused by a variety of noninfectious conditions, including catheter-induced trauma, renal stone, recent urologic procedure, and interstitial nephritis.

Because of these potential problems in establishing a diagnosis, there exists no universally accepted definition of symptomatic urinary tract infection in patients with spinal cord injury. A commonly used definition of symptomatic urinary tract infection in these patients requires the presence of significant bacteriuria [$\geq 10^5$ colony-forming units (CFU)/mL], pyuria [$>10^4$ white blood cells (WBC)/mL of uncentrifuged urine or >10 WBC/high power field (hpf) for spun urine], and fever (>100°F) plus more than one of the following signs and symptoms—(a) suprapubic or flank discomfort, (b) bladder spasm, (c) change in voiding habits, (d) increased spasticity, and (e) worsening dysreflexia—provided that no other potential etiologies for these clinical manifestations could be identified (6). Most healthcare providers tend to distinguish upper from lower urinary tract infection based on clinical manifestations and laboratory data rather than imaging findings. For example, the presence of high fever (>102°F), chills, systemic toxicity, high grade leukocytosis (>20 thousands per mm^3), and/or leukocyte casts in urinary sediment supports the presence of pyelonephritis.

Prevention

Mechanical Approaches

Since the indwelling transurethral and suprapubic catheters pose a higher risk of infection than intermittent bladder catheterization, the latter method of bladder drainage should always be considered, barring any anatomic or functional constraints. Increasing the frequency of intermittent bladder catheterization can decrease the risk of urinary tract infection. Although the technique of clean nonsterile intermittent self-catheterization is considered rather safe for use by outpatients, sterile intermittent catheterization is implemented by most hospitals owing to the fear of nosocomial introduction of multiresistant and virulent mircroorganisms into the urinary tract. In patients with persistent or recurrent urinary tract infections, the urinary tract should be investigated for anatomic abnormalities (including abscess, stone, obstruction, and stricture) and functional alterations (such as vesicoureteral reflux, high residual volume of urine in bladder, and elevated bladder pressure). The use of drugs and surgical procedures to reduce bladder pressure and aid bladder emptying can help alleviate the risk of urinary tract infection.

Antimicrobial Approaches

Since asymptomatic bacteriuria can progress to symptomatic infection, it is theoretically possible that prevention or eradication of asymptomatic bacteriuria may decrease the rate of symptomatic urinary tract infection (6). Although instillation of antibiotic solutions, such as kanamycin-colistin, into the bladder at the time of intermittent catheterization may alleviate bacteriuria at the expense of a switch in the microbiology of clinical isolates (17), there exists no evidence that this practice prevents urinary tract infection. Studies that examined the administration of systemic antimicrobial agents in patients with spinal cord injury (18,19) have yielded either conflicting or disappointing results. For example, the administration of trimethoprim-sulfamethoxazole has been shown in some studies (19), but not others (20), to significantly reduce the overall rate of asymptomatic bacteriuria and symptomatic urinary tract infection. This approach, however, was associated with relatively common adverse effects (19) and antibiotic resistance (20,21). Therefore, systemic antimicrobial use is generally discouraged for prevention of asymptomatic bacteriuria in patients with spinal cord injury. Exceptions may include patients with (a) enlarging struvite stones associated with urea-splitting microorganisms, such as *Proteus mirabilis* and *Providentia stuartii*; (b) conditions that enhance the likelihood of developing significant complications from having asymptomatic bacteriuria, such as premature birth in pregnant women; and (c) recurrent episodes of upper urinary tract infection that are complicated by sepsis or other clinical complications, particularly if the recurrent infections are caused by the same microorganism. Based on the results of a recent study (22), antimicrobial treatment of asymptomatic bacteriuria in women with diabetes mellitus is probably not warranted.

Bacterial Interference

The limited success of traditional antimicrobial prophylaxis prompted interest in exploring the novel approach of bacterial interference (23). This approach is based on the principle that nonpathogenic microorganisms may prevent colonization of the urinary tract by pathogenic microorganisms. A preliminary nonrandomized, open-label clinical trial in patients with spinal cord injury who had suffered from frequent episodes of infection (24–27) indicated that intentional colonization of the neurogenic bladder by a nonpathogenic strain of *Escherichia coli* 83972 reduced the rate of symptomatic urinary tract infection. The efficacy and safety of this approach is currently being investigated in a prospective, randomized clinical trial.

INFECTIONS OF PRESSURE SORES AND UNDERLYING BONE

Pathogenesis and Epidemiology

Although the incidence of pressure ulcers varies among medical centers and is affected by the level and completeness of spinal cord injury, about one third of patients develop clinically relevant pressure ulcers at one time or another after the injury. Pressure sores delay rehabilitation, prolong hospital stay, and incur excessive costs, particularly when infected. Although pressure sores may develop either at home or while residing at a medical institution, most patients get admitted for management of the infectious complications of the ulcers. Factors that contribute to skin and soft tissue infection in the vicinity of pressure sores include break in skin integrity and bacterial contamination due to soiling of the ulcer by stools or urine. The former factor predisposes to infection by skin microorganisms including staphylococci and streptococci, whereas the latter factor promotes infection by gram-negative bacilli and anaerobic bacteria (28). Infected pressure sores involve mostly the ischial tuberosities, trochanters, and sacrum—areas that are anatomically exposed to high pressure and likely to be exposed to fecal or urinary microorganisms.

Pressure sores often harbor multiple aerobes and anaerobes. The type of microbes colonizing the pressure sores was shown to be affected by the presence of devitalized tissue (29). Pressure sores with tissue necrosis had comparably high concentrations (>10^5 CFU/g) of both aerobes and anaerobes in deep tissues. However, upon excision of the necrotic tissue and healing of the infected pressure sores, the bacterial density dropped to less than 10^4 CFU/g of tissue, accompanied by disappearance of anaerobes. *Bacteroides* species, *Peptostreptococcus, E. coli, Proteus* species, and enterococci were the most prominent microorganisms isolated from necrotic pressure sores. In contrast, *P. aeruginosa* and *S. aureus* were the two microorganisms that were most frequently isolated from healing pressure sores. There exists some variability in the culture results of deep tissue obtained from different parts of the pressure sore, and the value of obtaining repeated cultures of pressure ulcers remains in question. The polymicrobial spectrum of flora in pressure ulcers in children is rather similar to that in adults, but, additionally, includes *Haemophilus influenzae* (30). *Candida* infection of pressure sores in patients with spinal cord injury is unusual.

In patients with spinal cord injury, most cases of osteomyelitis occur beneath pressure sores. Most such cases are caused by two or more bacterial species, including gram-positive cocci (particularly *S. aureus* and *Streptococcus* species), gram-negative bacilli (including the Enterobacteriaceae group and *P. aeruginosa*), and anaerobic bacteria (mainly *Bacteroides* species) (31). Vertebral and cranial osteomyelitis may also occur in association with spinal hardware and cervical halos, respectively.

Clinical Manifestations

Infection of pressure sores can be associated with cellulitis, abscess formation, osteomyelitis of underlying bone, septic arthritis, infected bursae, and septicemia. Local signs of infection include erythema, drainage, and foul-smelling or purulent drainage. Systemic manifestations of fever and leukocytosis commonly, but not invariably, occur. Septicemia is much rarer in the context of osteomyelitis beneath pressure ulcers in patients with spinal cord injury than in able-bodied adult patients with spinal osteomyelitis or children with long bone osteomyelitis. Clinically relevant blood cultures in patients with infected pressure ulcers suggests the presence of soft tissue abscess (28) or, less commonly, an infected hematoma.

Diagnosis

A number of factors can impede making a proper diagnosis of infection of pressure sores with or without underlying osteomyelitis in patients with spinal cord injury:

Inadequate History

Patients with spinal cord injury usually have no or altered sensations in the area of the pressure ulcers. Since most pressure ulcers occur in the trochanteric, ischial, and sacral regions, immobile patients cannot directly visualize the ulcers. Furthermore, such patients often complain of neurogenic or referred pain that may have no relation to the infection. These factors result in frequently obtaining an incomplete or inaccurate history from patients and help underscore the diagnostic importance of performing comprehensive physical examination by healthcare providers.

Microbiologic Uncertainties

Since pressure sores are universally colonized by bacteria, swab cultures of open ulcers should not be obtained unless infection is clinically evident. Sinus tract cultures are also usually unreliable. Cultures of material obtained by needle aspiration tend to overestimate the number of bacterial isolates (32). Although cellulitis adjacent to a pressure sore can theoretically be caused by a microorganism(s) present in the pressure sore, there is no evidence that skin biopsy in patients with spinal cord injury yields clinically relevant results. Cultures of biopsied deep soft tissue remains the most accurate means for determining the microbiologic cause of soft tissue infection.

In patients with underlying osteomyelitis, swab cultures of pressure sores do not accurately predict the microorganisms causing bone infection (31). Moreover, since fibrotic tissue adherent to bone is usually colonized with bacteria, bone cultures are positive in at least two thirds of patients in whom histopathologic examination of bone tissue is incompatible with osteomyelitis (31). Therefore, osteomyelitis should not be diagnosed solely by positive cultures of biopsied bone.

Radiologic Limitations

Another diagnostic problem in patients with spinal cord injury arises from the limited ability to delineate the extent and depth of infection in association with pressure sores. Deep soft tissue abscesses can exist beneath apparently healed pressure sores. Although highly sensitive for detecting soft tissue abscesses, radionuclide scans can yield false-positive results in patients with spinal cord injury who have an infected pressure sore without an associated abscess (33). Computed tomography (CT) and magnetic resonance imaging (MRI) can detect abscesses in both soft tissue and muscle, as is the case with the infrequently diagnosed iliopsoas abscess (34).

Since pressure necrosis affects subcutaneous and muscular tissues more than skin, the visualized skin opening of a sinus tract may seem deceptively small. Probing of the sinus tract, although generally helpful, may still not reveal the full depth of the sinus tract. Sinography can better delineate the full depth of the sinus tract and reveal potential communications with bone, joint, visceral organs, or deep-seated abscesses. In patients with nonhealing pressure sores who have persistent or recurrent infection, injection of dye into the bladder or intestines may help establish the presence of fistulous communications.

Misinterpretation of the findings of imaging studies is particularly prominent when attempting to diagnose bone infection beneath pressure ulcers. Bone scan is very sensitive (almost 100%) but poorly specific (<33%) for diagnosing osteomyelitis beneath pressure sores (35). The low specificity of bone scan is attributed to the aggregation of technetium in areas of bone that are affected by pressure-induced changes and in foci of heterotopic bone ossification. Therefore, bone scan should be used primarily for its high negative predictive value (i.e., in an attempt to rule out osteomyelitis and, therefore, obviate the need for bone biopsy) rather than its low positive predictive value (i.e., to diagnose osteomyelitis). Neither clinical evaluation (duration of ulcer, bone exposure, purulent drainage, fever, peripheral WBC count, and erythrocyte sedimentation rate) nor radiologic examination (plain roentgenogram and bone scan) correlates well with the likelihood of finding histopathologic evidence for bone infection (31,35,36). Although the finding of bone changes by CT scan or MRI can be very helpful in supporting the diagnosis of osteomyelitis, there are no studies in patients with spinal cord injury that correlate the abnormal findings of these imaging studies with bone biopsy results.

Multiple Sores

Patients with spinal cord injury often have multiple pressure sores. In such patients, infection of soft tissue and/or bone may exist at some sites but not others. Furthermore, different sites may be infected by different microorganisms.

Because of the above-described diagnostic limitations, definitive diagnosis of osteomyelitis beneath pressure sores requires histopathologic examination of bone tissue (35,36). Percutaneous needle bone biopsy yields histopathologic evidence for infection of bone beneath nonhealing pressure sores in only one fifth to one third of cases (31,35,36). These findings support the clinical observation that nonhealing of pressure sores is much less likely to result from underlying osteomyelitis than from noninfectious conditions, such as pressure-related changes, malnutrition, anemia, heterotopic bone ossification, and spasticity.

Prevention

The process of preventing infection of pressure sores and underlying bone starts with preventing the development of pressure sores. This consists of quality nursing care, frequent turning of the patient for pressure relief, careful attention to bony prominences, avoidance of friction and shear forces, correction of anemia, adequate nutrition, and training patients and their attendants in skin care. The relationship between bacterial counts in wounds and delayed healing remains controversial, and their exists no evidence from prospective randomized studies that local or systemic antimicrobial agents enhance wound healing or prevent infection in patients with spinal cord injury. Systemic antibiotics, however, ought to be given perioperatively in patients undergoing myocutaneous flap surgery (37,38). Although perioperatively administered antibiotics are typically active against the gram-positive skin flora, a broader spectrum regimen that provides additional coverage against gram-negative bacilli and anaerobes may be warranted if supported by the results of preoperative or intraoperative wound cultures. There exists no convincing evidence to support the prevailing practice of continuing perioperative antibiotics until wound drains are removed, usually 10 to 14 days after myocutaneous flap surgery.

RESPIRATORY TRACT INFECTIONS

Pathogenesis and Epidemiology

The most serious respiratory tract infection is pneumonia, which constitutes the leading cause of death due to infection in this population (2). Pneumonia is the most common pulmonary complication in the immediate postinjury period (39), and is particularly likely to occur in the first few months after cervical or high thoracic injury and among quadriplegics and persons older than 55 years (2). A five-center study of respiratory complications following spinal cord injury found that almost one third of patients developed pneumonia while undergoing initial rehabilitation in the hospital (40).

Factors that predispose patients with spinal cord injury to develop pneumonia or tracheitis include (a) weakness of the diaphragmatic and intercostal muscles in patients with cervical or high thoracic spinal cord injury, which would impair the capacity to clear respiratory secretions; (b) indwelling respiratory devices, such as endotracheal or tracheostomy tubes; and (c) aspiration that is promoted either by an abnormal state of consciousness due to illicit drug ingestion or associated head injury or by paralytic ileus that often occurs soon after spinal cord injury (40).

The microbiology of nosocomial respiratory tract infections in this population is affected by the type of predisposing factor(s). For example, *S. aureus* (particularly MRSA) and *P. aeruginosa* are the two most common causes of pneumonia and tracheitis in patients with respiratory devices, whereas aspiration pneumonia is mostly caused by gram-negative and anaerobic bacteria.

Clinical Manifestations

Patients with cervical or thoracic spinal cord injury can have absent or altered sensations of chest pain and dyspnea. Infected patients with weakness of the diaphragmatic and intercostal muscles may also have no or minimal cough, and are unlikely to spontaneously produce sputum. In such patients, the only clinical manifestations of pneumonia may consist of physical findings (distressed appearance, fever, tachypnea, and tachycardia) and abnormal test results (leukocytosis, hypoxemia, and infiltrates on chest radiographs).

Diagnosis

Because of ineffective cough, patients with cervical or high thoracic lesions may not be able to provide adequate sputum samples for Gram stain and cultures. If tracheal secretions cannot be adequately suctioned, bronchoscopy may be required for both diagnostic and therapeutic purposes. The most prominent impediment to diagnosing pneumonia in patients with spinal cord injury arises from the limited ability to clinically distinguish pneumonia from a number of noninfectious pulmonary complications, including atelectasis, chemical pneumonitis, pulmonary embolism, and fat embolism (41). For instance, atelectasis, like pneumonia, commonly occurs in patients with cervical or high thoracic spinal cord injury who retain pulmonary secretions and can also manifest with fever. Furthermore, the site of pulmonary involvement may not help differentiate atelectasis from pneumonia since both conditions predominantly affect the left lung. Chemical pneumonitis due to aspiration can also mimic bacterial pneumonia. When adequate samples of respiratory secretions are available, microbiologic examination may help distinguish between these two clinical entities by showing a plethora of microorganisms (along with WBCs) in samples obtained from patients with bacterial pneumonia. Pulmonary embolism can also be clinically confused with pneumonia (42). This is partially attributed to the fact that the majority of patients with spinal cord injury disclose no thrombotic source for pulmonary embolism (43). Furthermore, since patients with spinal cord injury commonly display baseline roentgenographic changes in the lungs due to atelectasis or other causes that make it difficult to interpret ventilation-perfusion lung scans, a definitive diagnosis of pulmonary embolism often requires pulmonary angiography.

Fat embolism, which can occur acutely after spinal cord injury in association with fracture of long bones, may be suspected if petechiae and cerebral dysfunction are present.

Prevention

Potential approaches for preventing pneumonia in patients with spinal cord injury include some that center around control of predisposing conditions and others that provide antimicrobial activity. The first group of approaches is intended to augment cough and lessen retention of secretions. Cough can be assisted by using abdominal binders or corsets. Adequate hydration, chest physical therapy, and postural drainage can enhance drainage of secretions, although it may be difficult to achieve certain optimal positions during the acute period following spinal cord injury.

Antimicrobial approaches include antibiotics and immunization. In general, the use of systemic antibiotics for prevention of pneumonia in high-risk patients with spinal cord injury is not advocated. Because pneumonia can either occur more frequently or result in more serious complications in patients with spinal cord injury than in the general population, eligible patients should be immunized against potentially preventable causes of pneumonia. Almost two thirds of patients with spinal cord injury are eligible for vaccination against *Streptococcus pneumoniae* and influenza virus by virtue of old age, chronic respiratory disease, and/or residence in chronic-care facilities. The antibody response to pneumococcal (44) and influenza vaccination of patients with spinal cord injury appears adequate. Although there have been no prospective studies of the clinical efficacy of these vaccinations in patients with spinal cord injury, it is generally recommended that patients at risk receive influenza vaccine every year and pneumococcal vaccine every 5 years.

COLONIZATION AND INFECTION BY MULTIRESISTANT MICROORGANISMS

Patients in spinal cord injury units may acquire multiresistant microorganisms while residing at a referring institution (hospital or nursing home) or another unit (particularly the intensive care unit) within the same hospital. Alternatively, patients may acquire multiresistant microorganisms while hospitalized at the spinal cord injury unit either directly from already colonized patients or indirectly via the hands of healthcare providers (who care for colonized persons) or contaminated inanimate surfaces (in patients' rooms, rehabilitation areas, and whirlpools). Fortunately, most cases of growth of multiresistant microorganisms in clinical specimens represent colonization rather than clinical infection.

The most commonly studied multiresistant microorganism in spinal cord injury units is MRSA, which accounts for at least half of all clinical isolates of *S. aureus*. The generally problematic diagnosis of infection in these insensate patients makes it sometimes difficult to distinguish between clinical infection and colonization. This microorganism most frequently infects the urinary tract, wounds, lungs, and blood. The sites that are most commonly colonized by MRSA include the anterior nares, wounds, urine, perineum, and stools (45). Patients may remain colonized with MRSA for months or years. Although the combination of an oral regimen of minocycline and rifampin and topical mupirocin was found to be effective in eradicating MRSA colonization, it is unwise to routinely attempt to eradicate MRSA colonization in this population of patients (46). Unfortunately, transfer of hospitalized patients to nursing homes may be delayed until MRSA colonization is eradicated.

The prevalence of VRE in spinal cord injury units appears to have increased in recent years. For instance, preliminary findings from our center indicated that the gastrointestinal tract of one third to one half of patients residing in the spinal cord injury unit is colonized with VRE (47). In the vast majority of instances, isolation of VRE from stools was not associated with clinical infection. Molecular typing demonstrated that the majority of VRE isolates had distinctly different patterns, even in the case of patients sharing bedrooms. These findings suggested that nosocomial transmission of VRE within the spinal cord injury unit was rather unusual.

Patients with spinal cord injury often harbor multiresistant gram-negative bacilli that produce extended spectrum β-lactamases (ESBL). Such microorganisms are isolated mostly from the urine, wounds, and respiratory secretions. Most urinary ESBL-producing isolates belong to the *Klebsiella–Enterobacter* group of microorganisms that are fully susceptible only to carbapenems; some isolates are also susceptible to aminoglycosides.

REFERENCES

1. National Institute on Disability and Rehabilitation Research (NIDRR) Consensus Statement. The prevention and management of urinary tract infection among people with spinal cord injuries. *J Am Paraplegia Soc* 1992;15:194–207.
2. DeVivo MJ, Kartus PL, Stover SL, et al. Cause of death for patients with spinal cord injuries. *Arch Intern Med* 1989;149:1761–1766.
3. Sugarman B, Brown D, Musher D. Fever and infection in spinal cord injury patients. *JAMA* 1982;248:66–70.
4. Stover SL, Lloyd LK, Waites KB, et al. Urinary tract infection in spinal cord injury. *Arch Phys Med Rehabil* 1989;70:47–54.
5. Merritt JL. Residual urine volume: correlate of urinary tract infection in patients with spinal cord injury. *Arch Phys Med Rehabil* 1981;62:558–561.
6. Darouiche R, Cadle R, Zenon G, et al. Progression from asymptomatic to symptomatic urinary tract infection in patients with SCI: a preliminary study. *J Am Paraplegia Soc* 1993:16:221–226.
7. Kil KS, Darouiche RO, Hull RA, et al. Identification of a *Klebsiella pneumoniae* strain associated with nosocomial urinary tract infection. *J Clin Microbiol* 1997;35:2370–2374.
8. Bennett CJ, Young MN, Darrington H. Differences in urinary tract infection in male and female spinal cord injury patients on intermittent catheterization. *Paraplegia* 1995;33:69–72.
9. Lindan R, Joiner E. A prospective study of the efficacy of low dose nitrofurantoin in preventing urinary tract infections in spinal cord injury patients with comments on the role of pseudomonads. *Paraplegia* 1984;22:61–65.
10. Montgomerie JZ, Guerra DA, Schick DG, et al. *Pseudomonas* urinary tract infection in patients with spinal cord injury. *J Am Paraplegia Soc* 1989;12:8–10.
11. Montgomerie JZ, Chan E, Gilmore DS, et al. Low mortality among patients with spinal cord injury and bacteremia. *Rev Infect Dis* 1991; 13:867–871.
12. DeVivo MJ, Fine PR. Predicting renal calculus occurrence in spinal cord injury patients. *Arch Phys Med Rehabil* 1986;67:722–725.

13. Simor AE, Ramage L, Wilcox L, et al. Molecular and epidemiologic study of multiresistant *Serratia marcescens* infections in a spinal cord injury rehabilitation unit. *Infect Control Hosp Epidemiol* 1988;9:20–27.
14. Darouiche RO, Priebe M, Clarridge JE. Limited vs full microbiological investigation for the management of symptomatic polymicrobial urinary tract infection in adult spinal cord-injured patients. *Spinal Cord* 1997;35:534–539.
15. Warren JW, Tenney JH, Hoopes JM, et al. A prospective microbiologic study of bacteriuria in patients with chronic indwelling urethral catheters. *J Infect Dis* 1982;146:719–723.
16. McGuire EJ, Savastano JA. Long-term followup of spinal cord injury patients managed by intermittent catheterization. *J Urol* 1983;129: 775–776.
17. Pearman JW. The value of kanamycin-colistin bladder instillations in reducing bacteriuria during intermittent catheterization of patients with acute spinal cord injury. *J Urol* 1979;51:367–374.
18. Mohler JL, Cowen DL, Flanigan RC. Suppression and treatment of urinary tract infection in patients with an intermittently catheterized neurogenic bladder. *J Urol* 1987;138:336–340.
19. Gribble MJ, Puterman ML. Prophylaxis of urinary tract infection in persons with recent spinal cord injury: a prospective, randomized, double-blind, placebo-controlled study of trimethoprim-sulfamethoxazole. *Am J Med* 1993;95:141–152.
20. Sandock DS, Gothe BG, Bodner DR. Trimethoprim-sulfamethoxazole prophylaxis against urinary tract infection in the chronic spinal cord injury patient. *Paraplegia* 1995;33:156–160.
21. Jiminez EM, Schick DG, Canawati HN, et al. *Klebsiella pneumoniae* colonization of the bowel associated with the use of trimethoprim-sulfamethoxazole. *Eur J Clin Microbiol* 1982;1:253–254.
22. Harding GKM, Zhanel GG, Nicolle LE, et al. Antimicrobial treatment in diabetic women with asymptomatic bacteriuria. *N Engl J Med* 2002; 347:1576–1583.
23. Darouiche RO, Hull RA. Bacterial interference for prevention of urinary tract infection: an overview. *J Spinal Cord Med* 2000;23:136–141.
24. Hull RA, Rudy DC, Donovan WH, et al. Virulence properties of *Escherichia coli* 83972, a prototype strain associated with asymptomatic bacteriuria. *Infect Immun* 1999;67:429–432.
25. Hull RA, Rudy DC, Donovan WH, et al. Urinary tract infection prophylaxis using *Escherichia coli* 83972 in spinal cord injured patients. *J Urol* 2000;163:872–877.
26. Hull RA, Donovan WH, del Terzo M, et al. Role of type 1 fimbria- and P fimbria-specific adherence in colonization of the neurogenic human bladder by *Escherichia coli*. *Infect Immun* 2002;70:6481–6484.
27. Darouiche RO, Donovan WH, del Terzo M, et al. Pilot trial of bacterial interference for preventing urinary tract infection. *Urology* 2001;58: 2339–2344.
28. Sugarman B. Infection and pressure sores. *Arch Phys Med Rehabil* 1985; 66:177–179.
29. Sapico FL, Ginunas VJ, Thornhill-Joynes M, et al. Quantitative microbiology of pressure sores in different stages of healing. *Diagn Microbiol Infect Dis* 1986;5:31–38.
30. Brook I. Microbiological studies of decubitus ulcers in children. *J Pediatr Surg* 1991;26:207–209.
31. Thornhill-Joynes M, Gonzales F, Stewart CA, et al. Osteomyelitis associated with pressure ulcers. *Arch Phys Med Rehabil* 1986;67:314–318.
32. Rudensky B, Lipschits M, Isaacsohn M, et al. Infected pressure sores: comparison of methods for bacterial identification. *South Med J* 1992; 85:901–903.
33. Firooznia H, Rafii M, Golimbu C, et al. Computerized tomography of pelvic osteomyelitis in patients with spinal cord injuries. *Clin Orthop* 1983;126–131.
34. Rubayi S, Soma C, Wang A. Diagnosis and treatment of iliopsoas abscess in spinal cord injury patients. *Arch Phys Med Rehabil* 1993;74: 1186–1191.
35. Sugarman B. Pressure sores and underlying bone infection. *Arch Intern Med* 1987;147:553–555.
36. Darouiche RO, Landon GC, Klima M, et al. Osteomyelitis associated with pressure sores. *Arch Intern Med* 1994;154:753–758.
37. Salzberg CA, Gray BC, Petro JA, et al. The perioperative antimicrobial management of pressure ulcers. *Decubitus* 1990;3:24–26.
38. Garg M, Rubayi S, Montgomerie JZ. Postoperative wound infections following mycocutaneous flap surgery in spinal injury patients. *Paraplegia* 1992;30:734–739.
39. Fishburn MJ, Marino RJ, Ditunno JF Jr. Atelectasis and pneumonia in acute spinal cord injury. *Arch Phys Med Rehabil* 1990;71:197–200.
40. Jackson AB, Groomes TE. Incidence of respiratory complications following spinal cord injury. *Arch Phys Med Rehabil* 1994;75:270–275.
41. Reines HD, Harris RC. Pulmonary complications of acute spinal cord injuries. *Neurosurgery* 1987;21:193–196.
42. Dee PM, Suratt PM, Bray ST, et al. Mucous plugging simulating pulmonary embolism in patients with quadriplegia. *Chest* 1984;85: 363–366.
43. Waring WP, Karunas RS. Acute spinal cord injuries and the incidence of clinically occurring thromboembolic disease. *Paraplegia* 1991;29: 8–16.
44. Darouiche RO, Groover J, Rowland J, et al. Pneumococcal vaccination for patients with spinal cord injury. *Arch Phys Med Rehabil* 1993;74: 1354–1357.
45. Darouiche R, Wright C, Hamill R, et al. Eradication of methicillin-resistant *Staphylococcus aureus* by using oral minocycline-rifampin and topical mupirocin. *Antimicrob Agents Chemother* 1991;35:1612–1615.
46. Maeder K, Ginunas VJ, Montgomerie JZ, et al. Methicillin-resistant *Staphylococcus aureus* (MRSA) colonization in patients with spinal cord injury (SCI). *Paraplegia* 1993;31:639–644.
47. Byers PA, Koza MA, Abraham FP, et al. Prevalence of vancomycin resistant *Enterococcus* (VRE) in spinal cord injury patients. The 42nd Interscience Conference on Antimicrobial Agents and Chemotherapy (abstract K-1951), San Diego, CA, 2002.

57

HEALTHCARE-ASSOCIATED INFECTIONS IN ADULTS INFECTED WITH HUMAN IMMUNODEFICIENCY VIRUS

DONALD E. CRAVEN
KATHLEEN A. STEGER CRAVEN
FRANCESCO G. DE ROSA

Nosocomial or hospital-acquired infections are a major source of patient morbidity and mortality in the United States (1). Nosocomial infections represent the fourth leading cause of mortality in the U.S., and a large portion of these infections are preventable (*www.chicagotribune.com/news/specials/chi0207210272jul21.story*). A number of factors underscore the need for the broader term "healthcare-associated" infections: the aging population in the U.S., shortened hospital stays, greater colonization with multidrug-resistant (MDR) bacterial pathogens, widespread use of invasive devices in the outpatient setting, and recycling of patients from chronic care facilities and nursing homes.

Traditional risk factors for healthcare-associated infections include severity of the patient's acute and chronic underlying disease, presence of invasive devices, and treatment with medications that increase colonization and the risk of infection (1). Acquired immune deficiency syndrome (AIDS) caused by human immunodeficiency virus (HIV) is a major cause of immunosuppression in the U.S., and is also a significant contributing factor to healthcare-associated infections (2–5). Widespread use of antibiotics for prophylaxis and treatment of AIDS-related opportunistic infections also contributes to the pathogenesis of healthcare-associated infections (6). After 1995–1996, the use of highly active antiretroviral therapy (HAART) in the U.S. has dramatically reduced the incidence of opportunistic and bacterial infections requiring hospitalization and improved patient's nutritional status, survival, and quality of life (7–9). By comparison, for HIV-infected patients in countries where HAART is not widely available, for those with undiagnosed HIV disease, and for patients who fail to respond to HAART or are infected with a MDR strain of HIV, the risk of healthcare-associated infections has remained unchanged.

This chapter reviews the state of the art of the impact of HIV/AIDS on development and outcome of healthcare-associated infections in adults. Changes in the epidemiology and natural history of HIV from the pre-HAART to post-HAART era are reviewed with an emphasis on the more common healthcare–associated infections and pathogens in adults. Due to the magnitude of this topic, we focus on issues in the more industrialized countries, realizing that this represents only the tip of the iceberg.

CHANGING EPIDEMIOLOGY OF HIV

International HIV/AIDS

As we enter the third decade of the HIV/AIDS pandemic, the statistics on the growth of the pandemic are overwhelming and the number of new AIDS cases continues to grow at an alarming rate (*www.cdc.gov/HIV/AIDS*). The epidemiology of HIV disease is changing worldwide and the economic and social impact in many countries cannot be calculated. In addition, the high cost and disparity in the availability of HAART has been recognized and continues to be a world health crisis (*www.UNAIDS.org/hivaidsinfo*).

In December 2002, UNAIDS at the World Health Organization estimated that more than 42 million people worldwide are living with HIV/AIDS, of whom 38.6 million are adults and 19.2 million are women. UNAIDS estimates 5 million people are newly infected annually and that there were 3.1 million AIDS deaths in 2002. In some countries in sub-Saharan Africa, the prevalence of HIV infection is nearly 30% and rates of infection are rapidly increasing in different parts of Asia. Heterosexual transmission is the most common source of infection and rates of perinatal transmission are highest in women who are not known to be HIV infected, have high rates of plasma viremia or those who do not receive prophylaxis (*www.UNAIDS.org/hivaidsinfo*). In many areas of the world HIV/AIDS disease is causing economic and social devastation, overwhelming the healthcare delivery systems and contributing to the spread of endemic diseases.

HIV/AIDS in the United States

Cumulative data from the Centers for Disease Control and Prevention (CDC) in the U.S. through December 2001 indicate that 816,149 cases of AIDS have been reported, of which 82% have been males. Total cumulative deaths of persons reported with AIDS is 467,910. It is estimated that between 800,000 and 900,000 people are currently living with HIV in the U.S. (*www.cdc.gov/HIV/AIDS*).

The epidemiology of HIV disease has changed over the last decade in the U.S. Perinatal transmission is now rare, reducing the number of new pediatric cases. HIV disease disproportionately affects people of color and is increasing in women and adolescents. Estimates of new HIV infections by gender are approximately 70% men and 30% women. Of these, 54% are black, 19% Hispanic, and 26% white, whereas blacks represent only 13% and Hispanics only about 12% of the population in the U.S. Of these new cases, men who have sex with men account for 42% of new cases, heterosexually acquired cases 33%, and transmission by injection drug use 25% (*www.cdc.gov/HIV/AIDS*).

Risk behavior estimates for new HIV infections vary by race and gender. For men, 50% are black, 30% are white, and 20% are Hispanic; 60% are men who have sex with men, 25% are injection drug users, and only 15% are heterosexual. By comparison, women are 64% black, 18% white, and 18% Hispanic; 75% acquired HIV by heterosexual exposure and 25% by injection drug use (*www.cdc.gov/HIV/AIDS*).

During the first 15 years of the epidemic, healthcare-associated infections from HIV were primarily related to profound and chronic immunosuppressive effects of the virus, hospitalization with AIDS-associated opportunistic infections or other underlying diseases in the patient, use of invasive devices such as chronic intravenous catheters, and treatment with medications that increased or altered host colonization (1–5,10–12).

HAART therapy, which was introduced in 1995 and led to a dramatic reduction in numbers of patients with advanced immunosuppression, decreased numbers of opportunistic infections, hospitalizations, deaths, and patients with device-related healthcare-associated infections, but increased the number of persons living with HIV/AIDS (Figs. 57.1 and 57.2) (7,8,12). However, HAART has also increased the impact of chronic hepatitis C disease, induced new issues of HIV-drug resistance, and increased the risk for metabolic complications, such as diabetes mellitus, hyperlipidemia, osteoporosis, lactic acidosis, hepatitis and hepatic steatosis, and unusual lipodystrophy syndromes (Fig. 57.3). Thus, the increased survival of HIV/AIDS patients on HAART will translate into an older population of HIV-infected patients, who will be at greater risk for traditional chronic diseases, such as diabetes mellitus, coronary artery disease, hepatitis, cirrhosis, and neoplastic diseases. (9) Over the next decade, the aging of the HIV-infected population may result in greater hospitalization rates, chronic care, and increased risk for healthcare-associated infections. In addition, the rapid emergence and spread of primary and secondary resistance to the spectrum of antiretroviral agents in the U.S., coupled with greater complications related to chronic hepatitis C infection, and the metabolic consequences of HAART outlined above will need continued surveillance as potential risk factors to healthcare-associated infections (9). By comparison, HIV patients in countries lacking resources for HAART will continue to be at greater risk for overall mortality, as well as the HIV-

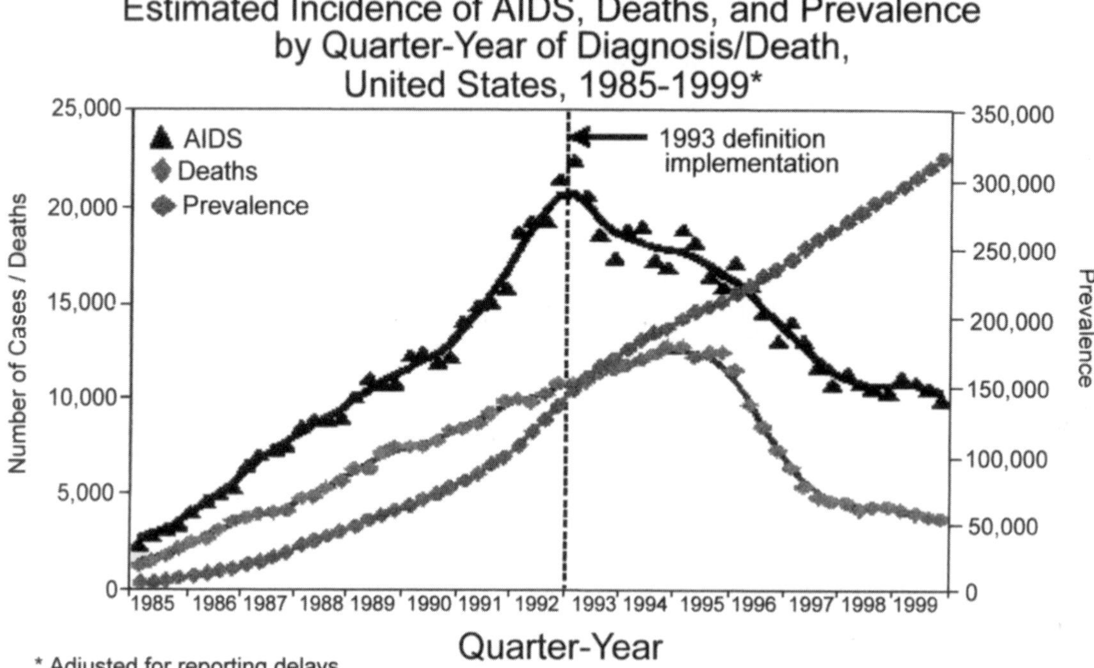

Figure 57.1. Reduction in patient mortality in acquired immune deficiency syndrome (AIDS) cases following the widespread use of highly active antiretroviral therapy (HAART) in the United States from January 1985 to June 2000. Increasing prevalence of human immunodeficiency virus (HIV) means that more patients live with HIV/AIDS. (From the Centers for Disease Control and Prevention, with permission; *www.cdc/gov/hiv/graphics/surveill.*)

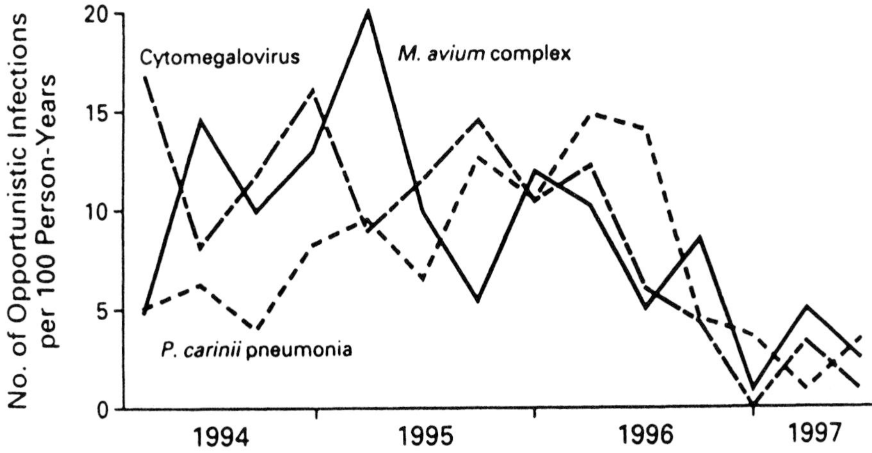

Figure 57.2. Changing rates of AIDS-related opportunistic infections following the widespread use of HAART in the United States. CMV, cytomegalovirus infection; PCP, *Pneumocystis carinii* pneumonia; MAC, *Mycobacterium avium* complex disease among human immunodeficiency virus-infected patients with fewer than 100 CD4 lymphocytes/mL. (From the Centers for Disease Control and Prevention, with permission; *www.cdc/gov/hiv/graphics/surveill.*)

related infections associated with chronic immunosuppression, hospitalization, and use of invasive medical devices. The dynamic landscape of healthcare-associated infections in this population underscores the need for timely epidemiologic studies to improve our understanding of the present and future impact of HAART on specific patient populations.

HIV PATHOGENESIS AND CLINICAL FEATURES

HIV Pathogenesis

Since the isolation and identification of HIV in 1983, there is a greater knowledge about its genome, structure, functions, and pathogenic interactions with the host (Fig. 57.4) (13). Of the core HIV gag proteins, p24 antigen is a marker of HIV replication, and antibody to p24 can be detected in enzyme assays to detect HIV infection in adults and older children. The env portion of the HIV genome produces the envelope glycoprotein, gp120, which is important for initial attachment to the CD4 receptor on the T-helper lymphocyte. The gp41 attaches to the HIV co-receptor and is critical for entry of the HIV into the T-helper lymphocyte (14). Those who lack the genes that code for this co-receptor appear to be more resistant to infection with HIV (14). The pol region of the HIV genome produces the enzyme reverse transcriptase that allows the HIV-RNA to convert to a DNA provirus and interact with integrase to enter the genome DNA of the CD4 T-helper lymphocyte.

HIV infection is characterized by rapid production of large numbers of viral particles with a half-life of less than 24 hours and by rapid turnover of CD4 cells (<2 days) (15). Untreated, HIV-infected adults may produce several billion viral particles per day depending on the viral strain, stage of disease, and host

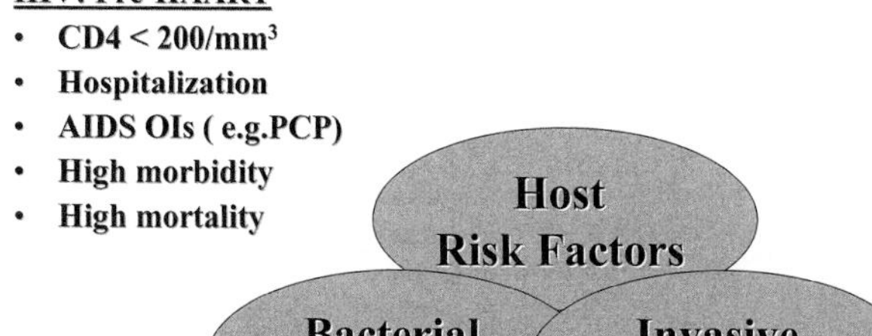

HIV: Post-HAART
- **CD4 < 200/mm^3**
- **Aging & comorbidity**
- **HAART complications**
- **HIV drug resistance**
- **Hepatitis C**
- **Immune reconstitution**

Figure 57.3. Traditional risk factors for healthcare-associated infections in patients: host risk factors (e.g., age, underlying disease), bacterial colonization (related to prior hospitalization, use of antibiotics, and needles), and invasive devices (e.g., intravenous or urinary catheters, endotracheal or nasogastric tubes). For HIV-infected patients, serum CD4 counts <200/mm^3 was a marker of immunosuppression and a major predictor of bacterial and other opportunistic infections. Note the different influences of HIV risk factors in the era before highly active antiretroviral therapy (Pre-HAART) and after HAART therapy (Post-HAART).

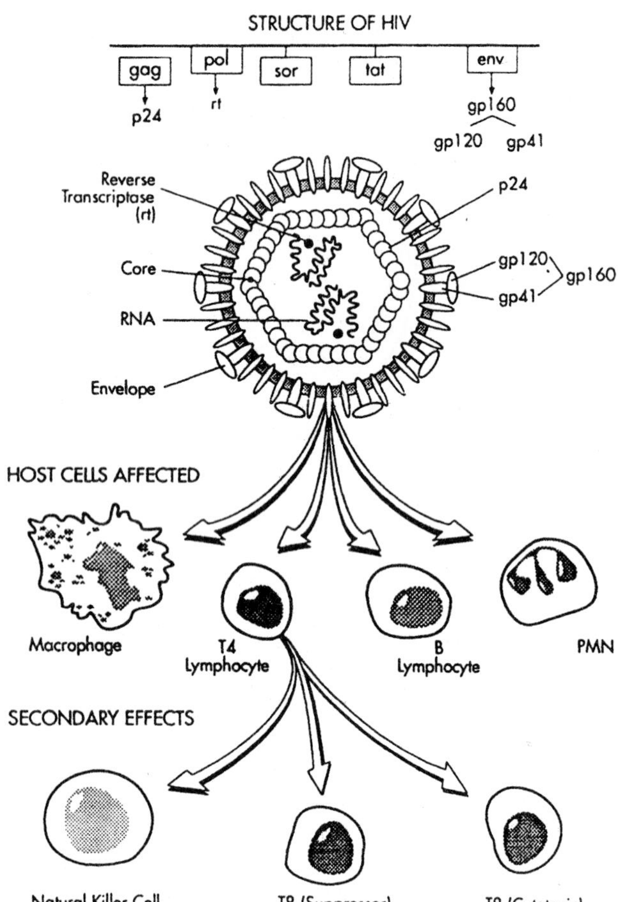

Figure 57.4. Structure of HIV and the effect of the virus on $CD4^+$ and $CD8^+$ cells and macrophages, and indirectly on natural killer (NK) cells and polymorphonuclear leukocytes (PMNs).

response to infection (15). Progression of HIV disease is related to HIV viral load, measured by quantitative plasma RNA (pRNA) levels (HIV-RNA), and degree of immunosuppression is related to level of CD4 lymphocytes depletion (13,16).

After seroconversion, patients establish a "set-point" pRNA level that reflects the equilibrium between viral replication and host response to HIV infection. Higher set-points predict a more rapid progression of HIV disease to death. Levels of pRNA are also used to assess the need for and response to combination antiretroviral therapy (16–18).

CD4 or T-helper lymphocytes, a central component of the host immune system, are involved in the induction of cytotoxic T-cell activity, natural killer cell function, activation of macrophages, and induction of B cells (13). Patients with advanced HIV disease, characterized by depletion of CD4 lymphocytes <200 cells/mL, have an increased risk of infections caused by bacteria, fungi, protozoa, and other viruses. Most infections requiring admission to the hospital and subsequent healthcare-associated infections occur in patients with CD4 counts <200 cells/mL and increase when CD4 counts are <100 and <50 cells/mm^3 (19,20).

Quantitative levels of CD4 lymphocytes are a widely used test to assess the severity of immunosuppression in individuals with HIV disease, eligibility for antiretroviral therapy, and to assist in the diagnosis and prevention of opportunistic infections (13). The recommendations for prophylaxis against opportunistic infections have been published, but the impact of HAART on these recommendations is currently under investigation, particularly in patients whose immune systems appear to have been reconstituted (6).

Important abnormalities of B-cell function also exist in patients with HIV infection that may be secondary to T-lymphocyte regulation or to a direct polyclonal stimulatory effect on the B lymphocyte. Thus, even though patients infected with HIV have high levels of immunoglobulins, they often have difficulty mounting specific antibody responses to vaccines or pathogens causing healthcare-associated infections (21,22). Peripheral-blood macrophages may ingest HIV or immune complexes that may contain HIV, and although the viral burden appears to be lower than reported for CD4 lymphocytes, macrophage function is impaired (23). Polymorphonuclear leukocyte function may also be impaired in HIV-infected persons, and these defects appear to increase susceptibility to bacterial infections.

HIV Diagnosis and Therapy

Chronic HIV infection can be diagnosed by antibody response to the core and envelope antigens using enzyme immunoassay (EIA) with Western blot (WB) confirmation. EIA for HIV is highly sensitive, specific, inexpensive, and easy to perform but may not detect early or acute HIV infection. Confirmation of HIV infection is critical, because false-positive tests may occur and some patients with low CD4 counts and opportunistic infection may have the idiopathic lymphocyte depletion syndrome rather than AIDS (24,25).

During seroconversion or in patients with suspected acute retroviral syndrome, both the HIV antibody and HIV-RNA levels should be measured. The HIV antibody test may be negative (not yet positive), but the presence of a positive qualitative or high quantitative HIV viral load (HIV-RNA) in plasma, using the polymerase chain reaction or branched-DNA assay, is diagnostic of acute infection (26).

Drugs commonly used for treatment of HIV infection inhibit reverse transcriptase and are called reverse transcriptase inhibitors (RTI). Of this group, there are nucleoside reverse transcriptase inhibitors (NRTIs), such as zidovudine or azidothymidine (ZDV or AZT, Retrovir), dideoxyinosine (ddI, Videx) and dideoxycytidine (ddC, Zalcitabine), stavudine (D4T, Zerit), and lamivudine (3TC, Epivir), tenofovir (TFV, Viread), and nonnucleoside reverse transcriptase inhibitors (NNRTIs), such as efavirenz (EFV, Sustiva), nevirapine (NVP, Viramune), and delaviradine (DLV, Rescriptor) (9). The other class of drugs commonly used for HAART is the HIV protease inhibitors (PIs), such as indinavir (IDV, Crixivan), nelfinavir (NFV, Viracept), saquinavir (SQV, Fortavase), or ritonavir (RTV, Norvir), lopinavir/ritonavir (LPV/RTV, Kaletra), and amprenavir (APV, Agenerase). These potent antiretroviral agents target the assembly and release of HIV after integration into the nucleus of the CD4 lymphocyte. HAART is based on the use of combinations of at least three antiviral agents, such as two NRTIs combined with an NNRTI or a PI (9). New agents in each of these classes, as well as HIV integrases and agents to prevent HIV entry into the CD4 lymphocyte, such as T-20 (enfuvirtide, Fuzeon) are scheduled for release in 2003.

Emergence and Spread of HIV Drug Resistance

Several complications post–HAART therapy have been identified since 1996. Primary and secondary resistance to all HIV medications has emerged as a significant problem in the U.S. (9). This has been related to a variety of factors, such as poor adherence to medications, inappropriate therapy, and resistance mutations on therapy. Selection and transmission of resistant strains resulting in HAART failures may result in progression of HIV disease and associated complications, such as infection.

Metabolic Complications of HAART

The widespread use of HAART has been associated with several notable metabolic complications (9). The use of certain protease inhibitors has been associated with increased risk of diabetes mellitus, insulin resistance, osteoporosis, and hyperlipidemia syndromes. Physical changes related to fat redistribution may include a buffalo hump, increased breast tissue or development of abdominal fat pads ("protease paunch"). Some patients on chronic combination therapy have developed hepatic steatosis, wasting syndromes, and severe lactic acidosis syndrome due to mitochondrial toxicity. The increased risk of diabetes and hyperlipidemia associated with the use of PIs has raised concerns of greater risk of coronary artery and cardiovascular complications in patients on long-term HAART. Clearly, these metabolic complications may add to the HIV-infected person's chronic disease burden, and increase the risk of future infectious complications.

Immune Reconstitution Inflammatory Syndrome

The immune reconstitution syndrome, immune restoration disease, or more precisely immune reconstitution inflammatory syndrome (IRIS), stands to describe the unique set of complications that arise in a small proportion of patients after treatment with HAART (27). This syndrome is characterized by the discrepancy between the immune response to HAART, with increase in $CD4^+$ T lymphocytes, decrease in viral load (HIV-RNA), and a paradoxical inflammatory response associated with clinical deterioration. The pathogenetic basis of IRIS is consistent with a restoration of the host immune response against an infectious agent and/or noninfectious antigens and release of different inflammatory mediators (27,28). IRIS has been associated with infections caused by *M. tuberculosis, Mycobacterium avium* complex (MAC), *Bartonella henselae, Cryptococcus neoformans, Pneumocystis carinii*, viruses such as cytomegalovirus (CMV), *Herpes simplex* virus (HSV), *Herpes zoster* virus (VZV), hepatitis C virus (HCV), hepatitis B virus (HBV), progressive multifocal leukoencephalopathy (JK virus), Kaposi sarcoma or human herpes virus, type 8 (HHV-8). It is important to recognize IRIS, and not to confuse it with drug toxicity, clinical deterioration due to HIV-disease, or failure of HAART. IRIS usually resolves spontaneously or responds to corticosteroid therapy (29). Rare fatal cases have also been reported (30).

Emergence of Hepatitis C Virus (HCV) and HIV Co-Infection

HCV infection has emerged as a significant HIV-related infection and is estimated to be present in 15% to 30% of patients with HIV disease in the U.S. HCV is primarily transmitted through contact with contaminated blood, and therefore is more common in HIV patients with a history of injection drug use or hemophilia (31–35). Approximately 85% of patients with acute HCV infection develop chronic infection, of whom nearly 30% may develop cirrhosis. HIV accelerates the progression of HCV disease, particularly in patients with low CD4 counts or AIDS (32,36). Genotype 1 accounts for approximately 75% of HCV disease in the U.S. and response rates to pegylated interferon (p-IFN) plus ribavirin (RBV) are substantially lower for patients infected with genotype 1 compared to other genotypes. Treatment with p-IFN plus RBV has greatly increased cure rates for genotype 1 in co-infected individuals, particularly those with CD4 counts $>200/mm^3$.

Greub et al. (32) studied the HCV serostatus of 3,111 Swiss HIV-infected patients starting HAART, of whom 87.7% were co-infected, and most of the patients had a history of injection drug use. The data from the Swiss cohort study indicated that co-infected patients receiving HAART were more likely to progress to a new AIDS-defining event or death and was associated with impaired CD4 recovery (32). Data from De Luca et al. (37) confirmed these findings in a prospective study. By comparison, Sulkowski et al. (38) collected data from 1,955 patients from 1995 to 2001, and suggested that HCV infection did not substantially alter the risk of dying, developing AIDS, or the response to HAART even when stratified by CD4 counts. Differences in results between these studies may be related to differences in the use of HAART, incidence of hepatotoxicity, and rate of active drug use.

HIV/HCV co-infected patients are also probably at greater risk for healthcare-associated infections caused by MDR pathogens, due to increased risk of hospitalization, greater exposure to antibiotics, and complications related to cirrhosis, end-stage liver disease, or increased hepatotoxicity from HAART. Injection drug users may be at risk for greater colonization and infections due to *Staphylococcus aureus.* The increased incidence rates of diabetes mellitus and hyperlipidemia in HIV- and HCV-infected patients are also potential risk factors (9,39).

Thus, in the era of HAART therapy, persons with HIV/AIDS have a greater risk of developing traditional chronic diseases as they age, such as diabetes mellitus or coronary artery disease, as well as complications related to chronic HCV infection, which in the future may result in more morbidity, risk for healthcare-related infections, and poorer outcomes (Fig. 57.3) (33–35,40).

HIV AND HEALTHCARE-ASSOCIATED INFECTIONS

Incidence and Prevalence Rates

Data on HIV infection rates and their relation to healthcare-associated infections have been limited by laws preventing HIV testing without informed consent, the time the study was conducted, epidemiologic methods, patient population studied, and type and geographic location of the hospital.

HIV seroprevalence rates in the U.S. among hospitalized patients in the pre-HAART era ranged between 0.3% and 6.0% (41,42). In a CDC HIV seroprevalence survey of patients hospitalized in the U.S., the overall HIV infection rate was 4.7% with a range from 0.2% to 14.2% depending on the site and type of hospital surveyed (43). In one study, the overall incidence rate of nosocomial infections was 5.1 per 1,000 patient-days [95% confidence interval (CI), 5.5 to 6.7] (11). Frank et al. (10) reported a rate of 8.7% per patients discharged.

In 19 Italian acute-care infectious diseases wards, Petrosillo et al. (44) reported an incidence of 3.6/1,000 patient-days in the HIV-infected patients; rates of infection correlated with traditional risk factors and a CD4 count $<200/mm^3$. A later study in a Brazilian infectious diseases unit by Padoveze et al. (45) reported that patients with HIV disease had a nosocomial infection rate of 8.16/1000 patient-days compared to a rate of 3.94 for patients without HIV disease ($p < .01$).

Although there was a steady growth in AIDS cases in the U.S. from 1980 to 1994, the use of HAART redefined the course of the HIV epidemic. For example, from 1995 to the second quarter of 1997, mortality rates among patients in the U.S. declined from 29.4 per 100 person-years to 8.8 per 100 person-years (7). These reductions were independent of gender, race, age, and risk factors for transmission of HIV and were directly related to the use of HAART (Fig. 57.1). The use of prophylaxis and HAART during this period also reduced the incidence of serious opportunistic infections (6,7). As shown in Fig. 57.2, rates of opportunistic infections due to *P. carinii* pneumonia (PCP), MAC disease, and CMV retinitis declined from 21.9 per 100 person-years in 1994 to 3.7 per 100 person-years by mid-1997 (7). As the result of the impact of HAART, the numbers of HIV-infected patients admitted to the hospital has decreased, whereas numbers of outpatients with HIV disease has increased significantly (8).

With the continued use of HAART in the U.S., it is likely that the decrease in AIDS-related mortality and morbidity will continue, but at a slower rate. HIV-infected patients will be living longer with greater risks for healthcare-associated infection that will parallel other at risk populations (7,25,46). These data emphasize the need for case finding of HIV-infected persons who come into contact with the healthcare system as inpatients or outpatients to prevent a later presentation with AIDS and the risk of healthcare-associated infection (2).

Importance of HIV Case Finding

It is estimated that there are over 300,000 people in the U.S. who remain unaware of their HIV infection (47). Since HIV infection is often asymptomatic, undiagnosed HIV infection may be a major problem in some hospitals. Based on previous data from 1990, only a third of HIV-infected patients were admitted due to their HIV infection, which emphasizes the need for improved case finding for at-risk inpatients and outpatients in endemic areas (43). Data from the inpatient medical service at Boston Medical Center in 1999 by Walensky et al. (47) found an estimated prevalence of HIV of 3.8% in patients who were part of a routine, voluntary, inpatient HIV-testing program that probably would not have been otherwise diagnosed. These types of data suggest that we may be underestimating healthcare-associated infections in HIV-infected persons.

Rapid HIV-testing of at-risk inpatients and outpatients is an important consideration for case finding, which has been limited in part because of the time to obtain HIV-antibody results. In 2002, a new rapid test for HIV antibody testing (OraQuick Rapid HIV-1 Antibody Test), performed on blood from a fingerstick, was approved, which can provide results in less than 20 minutes (48). The sensitivity of OraQuick is 99.6% and specificity is 100%. For patients with recent exposure, retesting is recommended in 3 months and all reactive (positive) tests should be confirmed by supplemental testing, such as a WB or immunofluorescence assay.

In summary, changes in the HIV epidemic since HAART have reduced the numbers of HIV-related healthcare-associated infections. However, there may be a rebound effect over the next several years as the HIV-infected population ages, and many HIV-infected patients are suboptimally adherent to HAART or become infected with MDR HIV strains. The changing demographics of HIV-infected patients in the U.S. are also of note. HIV disease now involves fewer white homosexual men and potentially more complicated populations, such as those with a history of injection drug use, indigent minorities, and homeless persons (4). Case finding should be an important strategy in the inpatient and outpatient setting.

Changing Survival Rates of HIV-Infected Intensive Care Unit (ICU) Patients

Over the past two decades, there has been discussion about outcomes and life support for HIV-infected patients in the ICU, a subject that J. Randall Curtis (49) appropriately called in his editorial "a moving target." Before 1986, Curtis points out, several studies reported that only 13% to 18% of patients with PCP and respiratory failure survived to hospital discharge. HAART and better prevention and treatment of opportunistic infections, such as PCP, have increased survival rates of HIV/AIDS patients.

Casalino et al. (50) evaluated the short- and long-term survival of HIV-infected patients admitted to an ICU in France in 1994. Of the 1,258 admissions to the ICU, 421 (33%) were HIV related, and for 354 patients it was their first admission. Respiratory failure accounted for 49% of the admissions, followed by neurologic disorders (27%), and sepsis (10%). Univariate and multivariable analysis of risk factors for survival were performed. In-hospital outcome was significantly associated with functional status ($p < .05$), time since AIDS diagnosis ($p = .04$), stage of HIV disease ($p < .02$), simplified acute physiology score (SAPS) ($p = .06$), need for mechanical ventilation ($p < .000001$) and its duration ($p < .0001$). Of the 281 patients who were discharged from the ICU alive, cumulative survival rates were 51% at 6 months, 28% at 12 months, and 18% at 24 months. Thus, short-term survival in the ICU was associated with severity of the acute illness, cause of admission, functional status, and duration of mechanical ventilation. Of note is that

HIV variables had little impact on in-ICU outcome but were closely related to in-hospital outcome. The authors suggest that ICU support for HIV-infected patients should not be considered futile. Clearly, more studies on outcomes of HIV-infected patients, similar to the data of Casalino et al., are needed as the HIV epidemic continues to evolve. The question is, Will these predictors of short- and long-term survival stand the test of time? Rosenberg et al. (51) reported on an observational cohort and retrospective chart review of 129 consecutive ICU admissions for patients with AIDS from 1993 to 1996. Of these, 102 (79%) were admitted for infections, 45% of which were bacterial (51). *P. aeruginosa* and *S. aureus* were the most common pathogens isolated. Pneumonia accounted for 65% of the admissions. Overall hospital mortality was 54% and 68% for those with bacterial infections. Neutropenia, but not CD4 count, was associated with survival and hospital mortality, which correlated well with the acute physiology score and severity of the sepsis. Independent predictors of mortality by multivariable analysis included admission Acute Physiology and Chronic Health Evaluation (APACHE III) score, bacterial cause of infection, and pneumonia (all $p < 0.001$). Possible causes of increased bacterial infection include neutropenia, decreased cytokines, and specific antibody production (52). Therefore, if the etiology of infection is uncertain, broad-spectrum empiric antibacterial therapy is recommended.

Many of the patients who are admitted to hospitals and ICUs in the third decade of HIV/AIDS disease are critically ill and may have a MDR strain of HIV, severe immune suppression, serious opportunistic infections, or end-stage liver disease due to HCV. Thus, with time, the variables keep changing, and the target keeps moving (Fig 57.4).

BLOODSTREAM INFECTION

Of the 35 million patients admitted annually to hospitals in the U.S., nearly 250,000 will experience bloodstream infection (BSI), and rates of BSI have varied from 1.2 to 13.9 per 1,000 hospital admissions (53). Primary BSIs are often attributed to intravascular catheters, and secondary BSIs are equally dispersed among surgical wounds, respiratory, and genitourinary tract sources. Crude mortality for nosocomial BSI has ranged from 20% to 50% depending on the underlying disease of the patient; attributable mortality has ranged from 14% to 38%.

Bloodstream Infection in HIV-Infected Patients

Nosocomial BSI in HIV-infected patients includes traditional risk factors and is related to level of immune suppression (Table 57.1). In a prospective multicenter surveillance study of nosocomial infections at five Veterans Administration Medical Centers (VAMCs), 2,541 HIV-infected patients studied from 1989 to March 1995 had 530 nosocomial infections of which primary BSI accounted for 31% (11) (Fig. 57.5). Of these, central line–associated BSI accounted for 6.5/1,000 central line days with a range of 2.3 to 8.3 at different hospitals. *S. aureus* was isolated in 35% of cases, coagulase-negative staphylococci in 22%, *Enterococcus* species in 14%, and gram-negative bacilli, including *P. aeruginosa*, in 18% of cases (Table 57.2). Devices were clearly a major risk factor for HIV-infected patients in and out of the ICU (Table 57.3). There was a trend toward more infections in patients with CD4 counts <200 cells/mm^3 (p = .08), and there was a significant association with the use of temporary rather than permanent central venous catheters (CVCs) ($p < .001$). Data on bacteremia and other nosocomial infections in HIV-infected patients in this study were compared with data for non–HIV-infected patients followed in the National Nosocomial Infections Surveillance (NNIS) system (Table 57.3).

A multicenter, prospective study of nosocomial infections in consecutive HIV-infected patients admitted to 19 Italian acute care infectious diseases wards was performed during 1998 by Petrosillo et al. (44). There were 344 nosocomial infections identified in 4,330 admissions (7.9%) for an incidence of 3.6/1,000 patient days. Overall distribution of major infections by site was 37% bloodstream, 31% urinary tract, 18% pneumonia, and 2% surgical wounds. Of the 126 BSI, 55 (44%) were related to CVCs for a rate of 7/1,000 device days. The most common pathogens were coagulase-negative staphylococci (31%) and *S. aureus* (24%). Multivariable analysis identified CD4 count $<200 \times 10^6$/L, odds ratio (OR) = 2.21, (95% CI, 1.28–3.62), Karnofsky performance status <40, OR = 1.89 (1.28–2.78), corticosteroids OR = 1.78 (1.29–2.45), CVC OR = 3.24 (2.41–4.35), urinary catheter OR = 6.53 (4.81–8.86), and surgery OR = 3.13 (1.90–5.15) as independent risk factors for nosocomial infection.

A study on incidence and risk factors for nosocomial BSI in HIV-infected patients was carried out in 1999 in a multicenter study of 17 Italian infectious diseases wards by Petrosillo et al. (54). BSIs were identified in 65 of 1,379 admissions (4.7%) for an incidence rate of 2.45/1,000 patient days. The catheter-associated BSI infection rate was 9.6/1,000 device days (96% CI = 6.5–13.9). Of the 29 catheter-related BSIs, 15 were related to short-term catheters and 14 to long-term catheters. *S. aureus* was isolated in 30% of BSI and 32% of CVC-BSI cases, coagulase-negative staphylococci in 28% of BSI and 29% of CVC-BSI cases, and *Candida* species in 15% of BSI and 19% of CVC-BSI cases. Independent risk factors identified by multivariable analysis included active injection drug use, Karnofsky performance status scores of <40, presence of a CVC, and length of hospital stay. Mortality rates were 25% in patients with BSIs versus 7.2% for those without BSIs ($p < .00001$); the attributable mortality was 18% for gram-positive microorganisms, 30% for gram-negative bacilli, and 63% for *Candida* species. The authors concluded that nosocomial BSIs occur frequently and remain a severe and life-threatening infection in the era of HAART therapy. The authors emphasize that HIV-infected patients in this series were likely to be more immunocompromised and malnourished and have a history of injection drug use with greater skin colonization and carriage, poor peripheral access, greater skin colonization, and more advanced HIV disease. Common factors for catheter-related BSI were the use of invasive devices, and having greater access to and use of CVC lines.

Studies on the risk of bacteremia in HIV-infected inpatients initially focused on community-acquired pathogens. Krumholz et al. (55) reported 44 episodes of community-acquired bacteremia in 38 hospitalized patients with AIDS over a 14-month

TABLE 57.1. SUMMARY OF RISK FACTORS AND SPECIAL CONSIDERATIONS FOR HEALTHCARE-ASSOCIATED INFECTIONS IN HIV-INFECTED PERSONS

Type of Infection	Traditional Risk Factors/Rates	HIV-Specific Risk Factors/Rates	Special Considerations
Bloodstream infection			
Staphylococcus aureus	IV catheters, injection drug use, valvular disease, skin disease, burns, prior hospitalization	Low CD4 count, AIDS, neutropenia, injection drug use	Patient education, substance abuse treatment, catheter care, HAART
Pseudomonas aeruginosa	Disruption of natural barriers, presence of invasive devices, prior antibiotic use	Low CD4 count (<100/mm^3), AIDS patients, prior antibiotics, prior infection	Patients may become colonized in the healthcare facility, HAART
Pneumonia			
Streptococcus pneumoniae	Rates 1 to 2/1,000 persons Risk factors: age, underlying cardiopulmonary disease, sickle cell disease, smoking alcoholism	Rates 5- to 15-fold higher in HIV-infected persons; (range 9.5–45/1,000 persons) Recurrent episodes AIDS, low CD4 count	Response to the pneumococcal vaccine impaired in HIV-infected persons Person-to-person spread suspected in healthcare facilities May be presenting sign of HIV disease
Haemophilus influenzae	Rates 1–2/1000 persons Increased rates in household contacts	Rates 79/100,000 One third on invasive cases are due to type b microorganisms Person-to-person important in pathogenesis	Immune response to the vaccine is impaired in advanced HIV disease Potential misclassification as community acquired
Pneumocystis carinii	Numerous hospital outbreaks, most likely due to airborne spread	Risk may be increased by use of spututm induction, bronchoscopy, or aerosolized pentamidine treatment	Healthcare-associated transmission difficult to document Focused prevention strategies for at-risk patients
Mycobacterium tuberculosis	The rate increased paralleling the HIV epidemic Lifetime risk of reactivation of latent tuberculosis 10%	Incubation period shorter, and attack rates as high as 44%; significant healthcare-associated spread Reactivation risk 10%/year Recently acquired infection was responsible for two thirds of cases in some series	Diagnosis is complicated by anergy, atypical presentations and decreased sensitivity of sputum smears in advanced HIV disease High level of suspicion needed Multidrug-resistant strains associated with significant mortality
Gastrointestinal disease			
Clostridium difficile	Most common cause of healthcare-associated diarrhea Increased length of hospitalization, frequent antibiotic exposure, and ?decreased gastric acidity	Low CD4 count	Strategies for prevention are important Definitions, study design and assays for *C. difficile* vary
Salmonella species	Implicated in a number of nosocomial outbreaks Contaminated food, medication, and possibly person-to-person-spread	HIV-infected patients are at increased risk of secondary bloodstream infection and recurrent bacteremia	Patient education regarding proper food preparation and hygiene May be presenting sign of HIV disease
Mycobacterium avium complex	Underlying heart disease, hairy cell leukemia, chronic steroid use	Common in AIDS and when CD4 count <100/mm^3	Data on nosocomial spread are sparse Persistent colonization of H_2O supplies (heated) documented
Cryptosporidium	Described in immunocompromised hosts Outbreaks due to contaminated H_2O supplies or person-to-person transmission	Low CD4 count Increased risk in AIDS patients on oral sulfonamide treatment or exposed to contaminated water	Bottled H_2O may be indicated High associated morbidity and mortality in AIDS Body substance precautions should be implemented Boiled, filtered, or bottled H_2O implicated in outbreaks

IV, intravenous; CD4, CD4$^+$ T lymphocytes; AIDS, acquired immune deficiency syndrome; HIV, human immunodeficiency virus; H_2O, water; HAART, highly active antiretroviral therapy.

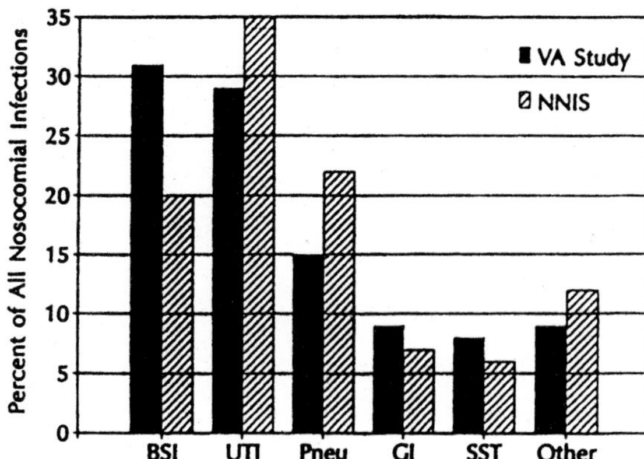

Figure 57.5. Distribution of major nosocomial infection sites for all HIV-seropositive adult medical patients 1989 through 1995 in the Veterans Affairs Hospital (VAH) study of all adult male medical patients 1989 through 1994 versus the National Nosocomial Infections Surveillance (NNIS) system. BSI, primary bloodstream infection; UTI, urinary tract infection; Pneu, pneumonia; SST, skin and soft tissue infection. (From Stroud L, Srivastava P, Culver D, et al. Nosocomial infections in HIV-infected patients: preliminary results from a multicenter surveillance system (1989–1995). *Infect Control Hosp Epidemiol* 1997;18:479–485, with permission.)

period. Central lines and soft tissue infection were the most common sources identified, but no source could be established in 14 patients (37%). *S. aureus, Streptococcus pneumoniae*, and *Escherichia coli* were the most common microorganisms isolated. Other sources of secondary BSI in HIV-infected patients included pneumonia (pneumococcus and *Haemophilus influenzae*) and gastrointestinal (GI) tract infections (*Salmonella, Shigella,* or *Listeria*). BSI due to unusual bacterial, mycobacterial, and fungal pathogens may also occur in patients with AIDS (56,57). As HIV-associated morbidity and mortality and related hospitalization rates decline, it may be expected that the incidence of nosocomial BSI will decrease in parallel (7,58).

Bloodstream Infection Due to *Staphylococcus aureus*

S. aureus BSIs are common in HIV-infected patients and may be associated with a higher incidence of metastatic complications (Table 57.1) (59). In most cases of community-acquired *S. aureus* bacteremia, a history of intravenous drug use, nasal colonization, lymphatic obstruction, skin disease, or colonization have been implicated. However, Jacobson et al. (59) reported 22 cases of *S. aureus* bacteremia in AIDS/AIDS-related complex patients who lacked the above risk factors. Fifty percent of the infections were nosocomial and 73% were secondary to intravenous catheters (eight central and eight peripheral). In a multicenter cohort study of nosocomial infections in HIV-infected patients, *S. aureus* was the most frequent cause of BSI, accounting for 35% of cases, with coagulase-negative staphylococci accounting for 22% (11). In this study, two thirds of nosocomial BSI were associated with an indwelling central line. The observed incidence of central line–associated BSI was 6.5/1,000 device-days with a significantly higher rate in ICU patients than in non-ICU patients (12.1 vs. 5.9). Interestingly, although the per-day risk of central line–associated bacteremia did not increase with duration of catheter placement, the per-day risk for temporary central lines significantly exceeded that of permanent devices. These results suggested that HIV-infected patients are more susceptible to central line infections than other hospitalized patients.

Raviglione et al. (60) also found high rates of intravenous (Hickman) catheter infection in 44 patients with AIDS versus 25 control subjects who required chemotherapy, with *S. aureus* the most frequently isolated microorganism. Rates of catheter infection were 0.47/100 catheter-days in persons with AIDS versus 0.09 for the control group, but the frequency with which the catheters were accessed may have been different in the two study groups. In a retrospective review of 75 central venous lines placed for treatment of CMV retinitis, Moore et al. (61) determined that use of a Port-a-Cath was associated with a significantly lower rate of line infection than use of a Hickman line (0.39/100 vs. 0.97/100 line-days, $p < .05$). The effect of reduced hospitalization of HIV-infected patients on *S. aureus* BSI and catheter infections remains to be seen; however, it is reasonable to assume that future studies will show decreased rates of infection (7).

Rates of nosocomial BSI have also been reported in the

TABLE 57.2. NOSOCOMIAL PATHOGEN DISTRIBUTION FOR SELECTED SITES OF INFECTION

	BSI		UTI		Pneu	
Pathogen	No. (%)					
Staphylococcus aureus	63	(35)	11	(6)	15	(33)
Coagulase-negative staphylococci	40	(22)	4	(3)	0	(0)
Enterococcus species	25	(14)	32	(18)	0	(0)
Pseudomonas aeruginosa	14	(8)	24	(14)	17	(37)
Klebsiella pneumoniae	11	(6)	21	(13)	6	(13)
Escherichia coli	5	(3)	32	(18)	3	(7)
Enterobacter species	2	(1)	14	(8)	5	(11)
Other	18	(10)	38	(22)	—	—
Total	178	(100)	176	(100)	46	(100)

BSI, bloodstream infection; UTI, urinary tract infection; Pneu, pneumonia.
From Stroud L, Srivastava P, Culver D, et al. Nosocomial infections in HIV-infected patients: preliminary results from a multicenter surveillance system (1989–1995). *Infect Control Hosp Epidemiol* 1997;18:479–485.

TABLE 57.3. DEVICE-ASSOCIATED INFECTION RATES[a] AMONG HOSPITALIZED HUMAN IMMUNODEFICIENCY VIRUS-INFECTED PATIENTS, 1989–1995

	All Patients Rate	Non-ICU Patients	Device Days Rate	ICU Patients	Device Days Rate	NNIS ICU Rate[b]
Ventilator-associated Pneu	9.3	196	5.1	1,308	9.9	9.7
Catheter-associated UTIs	8.8	2,248	11.1	1,603	5.6	9.4
Central line-associated BSIs	6.5	14,165	5.9	1,573	12.1	6.8

[a]Number of device-associated infections per 1,000 device days.
[b]For comparison, the pooled mean rates for all patients in medical ICUs of NNIS hospitals, January 1990 through December 1994.
ICU, intensive care unit; NNIS, National Nosocomial Infections Surveillance system; PNEU, pneumonia; UTI, urinary tract infection; BSI, bloodstream infection.
Data from Stroud L, Srivastava P, Culver D, et al. Nosocomial infections in HIV-infected patients: preliminary results from a multicenter surveillance system (1989–1995). *Infect Control Hosp Epidemiol* 1997;18:479–485.

HAART era by Petrosillo et al. (54). *S. aureus* accounted for 30% of the BSIs and 32% of the catheter-related BSIs. Independent risk factors for BSI included active injection drug use, Karnofsky score <40, the presence of a CVC, and greater length of hospital stay. The authors cite level of immunosuppression, injection drug use, colonization with *S. aureus*, poor peripheral access, and the use of the CVCs for obtaining blood samples as contributing risk factors. No association with co-trimoxazole use was observed in this study.

The predominance of *S. aureus* in BSI in HIV-infected patients has not been fully explained. It is known that patients with a history of intravenous drug use have high rates of *S. aureus* BSI (59,60,62–65). In addition, *S. aureus* nasal colonization has been reported in approximately 50% of HIV-infected patients, with colonization rates increasing in advanced HIV disease and correlating with rates of invasive infection (65). Nasal colonization and past intravenous drug use may serve as a marker for *S. aureus* skin colonization shown to be associated with an increased incidence of staphylococcal infections (65). Stroud et al. (11) found that chronic renal failure was the only factor significantly associated with the occurrence of catheter-related BSI, possibly reflecting impaired host defenses, increased colonization, and poor catheter care. Patients with a CD4 count greater than 200 cells/mm^3 tended to have a higher incidence of catheter-related BSI than those with lower CD4 counts, perhaps reflecting the use of prophylactic trimethoprim-sulfamethoxazole in the latter group (11,65). This is consistent with previous observations that trimethoprim-sulfamethoxazole prophylaxis against PCP significantly reduced colonization rates (65,66). Thus, antibiotics such as trimethoprim-sulfamethoxazole, ciprofloxacin, and rifampin may reduce *S. aureus* colonization and infection, particularly in patients with advanced HIV disease. The most dramatic reduction in *S. aureus* infections may result from the use of HAART, fewer hospitalizations, and the reduced need for central line placement (7). However, with the spread and emergence of MDR stains of HIV and the increased age and metabolic complications of HIV-infected patients on HAART therapy, more patients need hospitalization or care in chronic care facilities.

Despite the widespread emergence of methicillin-resistant *S. aureus* (MRSA) in the U.S., few reports have provided detailed data on MRSA in HIV-infected patients. In the report of nosocomial infections in HIV-infected patients in Brazil by Padoveze et al. (45), infections due to *S. aureus* were significantly higher for HIV-infected patients compared to controls, and MRSA isolates accounted for 24% of the BSIs. We suspect that infections due to MRSA will be increasing over the next decade. In addition, based on the rapid emergence of antibiotic resistance in strains of *S. aureus*, reports of vancomycin-resistant *S. aureus* (VRSA) in 2002 require vigilance for spread among injection drug users who may be infected with HIV (67).

Bloodstream Infection Due to Gram-Negative Bacilli

Several studies have suggested an increased risk of nosocomial BSI due to aerobic gram-negative bacilli in patients with AIDS, many of whom have invasive devices in place. Yamaguchi and Chaisson (68) reported 30 episodes of gram-negative bacteremia that occurred in 5% of patients admitted to their AIDS unit; the associated mortality was 38%. The most common microorganisms isolated were *P. aeruginosa* (13), *E. coli* (10), *Salmonella* (10), and *Klebsiella pneumoniae* (4). Sources of bacteremia were indwelling central venous lines (8), respiratory tract (10), gastrointestinal tract (4), genitourinary tract (3), and no established source (7). In a prospective study of nosocomial infections in HIV-infected adults, gram-negative bacilli accounted for 18% of BSI, with *P. aeruginosa* being the most frequently identified gram-negative bacterium (11).

The occurrence of pseudomonal infections in HIV-infected patients has been well documented. Nelson's group (61) reported that 19 of 584 HIV-infected patients (3.3%) with septicemia had *Pseudomonas* species isolated from blood. *P. aeruginosa* was isolated in 12 episodes; CVCs (Hickman) were the source of infection in 14 patients, and four patients were neutropenic with an absolute neutrophil count (ANC) less than 750/mm^3. Unfortunately, no information was provided on the number of patients with CVCs or the length of time the devices were in place. Seven patients (37%) died; mortality was associated with the isolation of *P. aeruginosa* but not with neutropenia, low CD4 count, p24 antigenemia, or whether acquisition of the infection was in the community or hospital.

Of the seven HIV-infected patients with serious *P. aeruginosa* infection reported by Kielhofner et al. (69), all had CD4 counts less than 200/mm^3; one had neutropenia and two infections were hospital-acquired. The lung was the source in five patients, two had relapsing infection, and two patients died. Similar findings were reported by Mendelson et al. (70). Of 21 primary episodes of pseudomonal bacteremia, 12 were community-acquired, 12 were associated with pneumonia, and nine were associated with intravenous devices. Of note, a relapse rate of 33% was reported in those who survived the primary episode of bacteremia, and overall mortality from pseudomonal bacteremia was 53%. Additional studies have also identified the two most important sources of pseudomonal bacteremia as central line infections and pneumonia (71,72). Risk factors for pseudomonal infections include advanced HIV disease, the use of CVCs, urinary catheterization, and steroid therapy (71).

BSI due to gram-negative bacilli occurred in 12 (18%) of the 67 patients, but in only four (13%) of the 31 patients with catheter-related BSI reported by Petrosillo et al. (54). *E. coli* and *P. aeruginosa* were the most common gram-negative bacilli isolated.

Although there are limited data on the rates of nosocomial BSI in HIV-infected patients, particularly since the advent of HAART, indwelling central lines appear to be a significant risk factor. Although some studies have cited advanced HIV disease as an independent risk factor for BSI, Stroud et al. (11) reported that the risk of central line–associated bacteremia was higher in those with CD4 counts greater than 200 cells/mm^3, possibly reflecting trimethoprim-sulfamethoxazole prophylaxis in those with lower counts. Despite recent advances in therapy, it is likely that a small proportion of HIV-infected patients will continue to require central line placement. To reduce colonization and prevent infection, intravascular catheters should be inserted and maintained using careful aseptic technique.

Although infections with *P. aeruginosa* are uncommon in HIV/AIDS patients, mortality and recurrence rates are high (73). Using a case-control design, independent predictors of infection due to *P. aeruginosa* (60% were nosocomial) were AIDS and a CD4 count <50/mm^3 (OR 13.2; 95% CI, 1.4–129), trimethoprim sulfamethoxazole (Bactrim) (OR 5.5; 1.1–26.9), penicillin (OR 5.2; 1.1–25.3), and steroids (OR 5.5; 1.2–25.5).

Bloodstream Infection Due to *Mycobacterium avium* Complex (MAC)

Infection due to *M. avium* and *M. intracellulare*, now grouped as MAC, typically occurs in persons with underlying pulmonary disease, hairy cell leukemia, chronic steroid use, and AIDS (74). MAC bacteremia and associated infections in HIV-infected persons invariably occurs late in the course of the disease when CD4 counts are less than 100/mm^3. MAC usually presents as disseminated disease with nonspecific symptoms such as fever, weight loss, and lymphadenopathy. In patients with disseminated disease, MAC is often isolated from blood, bone marrow, and liver tissue. As shown in Fig. 57.2, rates of MAC infection have dropped precipitously over the past decade with the use of HAART and primary prophylaxis (6,7).

The source of MAC is environmental, including water and food, with infection probably following mucosal exposure via the gastrointestinal tract (74). Data on nosocomial transmission are sparse; however, colonization of water supplies in outpatient clinics and inpatient facilities may serve as a potential source of nosocomial transmission (75). Von Reyn et al. (76), using pulsed-field gel electrophoretic analysis, studied the molecular epidemiology of MAC isolates from AIDS patients (76). They found persistent colonization of two hospital water systems with single strains of *M. avium*. The molecular analysis implicated these hospital water supplies as the sources for MAC infection in five of 47 patients studied, strongly suggesting nosocomial acquisition. With better data on the epidemiology and pathogenesis of MAC, the need for intervention strategies to prevent nosocomial transmission can be more accurately assessed.

PNEUMONIA

Nosocomial pneumonia occurs at a rate of six to ten episodes per 1,000 hospitalizations and is 10- to 20-fold higher in patients who are intubated or hospitalized in an ICU (77,78). Crude mortality rates for nosocomial pneumonia range from 20% to 60%, with an attributable mortality of 33% (79).

Because there is no gold standard for the diagnosis of nosocomial pneumonia, most cases are diagnosed clinically. Although the sensitivity of clinical diagnosis is high, the specificity is often low, but the specificity of diagnosis for ventilator-associated pneumonia may be increased with the use of bronchoscopy with bronchoalveolar lavage or protected specimen brush (80).

Aspiration of bacteria from the oropharynx is the major route of entry of bacteria into the lung, and anaerobic bacteria are common except in intubated patients. Nosocomial pneumonia that occurs during the first 4 days of the hospital stay is more commonly caused by *S. pneumoniae, Moraxella catarrhalis*, or *H. influenzae*; thereafter, aerobic gram-negative bacilli, such as *K. pneumoniae, Enterobacter* species, *Serratia* species, or *P. aeruginosa* and *S. aureus* become more likely. Nosocomial pneumonia is frequently caused by more than one microorganism (80).

Pneumonia in HIV-Infected Patients

HIV-infected adults and children are at high risk for community-acquired pneumococcal and *H. influenzae* pneumonia and secondary bacteremia (Table 57.1) (62,63,66,81–84).

Morbidity and mortality have been low, except in cases of misdiagnosis, more severe underlying disease, or co-infection with opportunistic pathogens such as *P. carinii* (62,63,83). Rates of pneumococcal infections are estimated to be increased 5- to 15-fold in HIV-infected persons and have occurred at rates ranging from 9.5 to 45 in 1,000 compared with 1 to 2 in 1,000 in control subjects (62,82,83). Recurrent episodes of pneumococcal pneumonia are common in persons with HIV disease (62, 63,83).

HIV-infected adults also appear to be at increased risk for *H. influenzae* pneumonia and bacteremia, with rates in men with AIDS estimated to be 79.2 per 100,000 compared with 1 to 2 per 100,000 in healthy adults (22,85). Approximately 33% of the cases of invasive *H. influenzae* disease were due to type b microorganisms, for which there is a protein-polysaccharide vaccine available. Unfortunately, as with pneumococcal vaccine, the immune response after vaccination is impaired in persons with advanced HIV disease (21,22). With the use of trimethoprim-sulfamethoxazole for prophylaxis against PCP and the use of macrolides for MAC prophylaxis, there have been significant decreases in the rates of pneumococcal and *H. influenzae* pneumonia (12,66). In addition, HAART has substantially reduced the rates of bacterial infections among AIDS patients in the U.S. (8).

Nosocomial transmission of the pneumococcus is an increasing concern given the emergence of clinically significant penicillin resistance. Numerous studies have found higher colonization rates of HIV-infected patients with penicillin-resistant *S. pneumoniae*, possibly related to the use of prophylactic trimethoprim-sulfamethoxazole. An investigation of risk factors for transmission of penicillin-resistant pneumococci implicated hospitalization within the prior 3 months, use of beta-lactam antibiotics, and diagnosis of nosocomial pneumonia as risk factors (86). In-hospital person-to-person spread of MDR pneumococcus has been described (87). Of note, an affected patient developed clinical infection 20 days after discharge, illustrating the potential for misclassification of nosocomial infections and underestimation of the significance of in-hospital transmission of respiratory pathogens.

The CDC multicenter surveillance study from 1989 to 1995 reported that pneumonia was responsible for 15% of the 530 nosocomial infections identified in 2,541 HIV-infected patients (11). Rates of ventilator-associated pneumonia were 9.3 in 1,000 device-days with a range of 4.3 to 14.3 for the different VAMCs studied. Lower than expected rates of infection for the HIV-infected patients compared with patients in the NNIS system (9.7/1,000 device days) may be related to the use of antibiotic prophylaxis for PCP and MAC. Cofactors may contribute to the high rates of bacterial pneumonia and secondary BSI reported in HIV-infected persons (64,83). These include injection drug use, neutropenia, and prior exposure to antibiotics, including prophylaxis for opportunistic infections (64). Although trimethoprim-sulfamethoxazole when taken for PCP prophylaxis may decrease the risk of bacterial pneumonia, it may also increase colonization and infection with resistant bacteria, notably pneumococcus (66).

In a study by Frank et al. (10), respiratory tract infections accounted for 16 of 39 nosocomial infections identified in 405 patients, and rates were estimated to be 2.7% per discharge. Gram-negative bacilli were most commonly isolated, and HIV-infected patients with nosocomial infections had longer lengths of hospital stay. *S. aureus* and *P. aeruginosa* together accounted for 47% of the nosocomial pneumonias reported by Stroud et al. (11), with pseudomonal infections occurring slightly more frequently. As discussed above, these microorganisms have a high propensity to infect HIV-infected patients, and empiric therapy of nosocomial pneumonia should include adequate coverage for both. There have been several reports of nosocomial transmission of a number of respiratory pathogens that may pose a risk to HIV-infected patients. Transmission of encapsulated bacteria between persons has been described in shelters and in the hospital setting (87). Rates of *H. influenzae*, type b disease, are also higher in household contacts of cases, providing further evidence of person-to person spread (85,88).

From 1994 to 1998, Tumbarello et al. (89) studied the incidence, risk factors, and outcome of nosocomial bacterial pneumonia in 42 HIV-infected persons versus 84 controls matched by age, gender, and cause of hospital admission. The incidence of nosocomial pneumonia in the HIV group was 10.8/10,000 hospital patient days and decreased significantly during 1997–1998 compared to 1994–1996. Predictors for developing bacterial nosocomial pneumonia were increasing APACHE III score and presence of AIDS-related central nervous system (CNS) disease. The length of stay was increased 15 days in the HIV group and the attributable mortality was estimated to be 29%.

Bacterial pneumonia may be superimposed on coexisting opportunistic respiratory infection. Franzetti et al. (90) reported 16 episodes of bacterial nosocomial pneumonia in 36 patients admitted with AIDS/AIDS-related complex, 14 of whom had opportunistic pulmonary infections. In contrast, Peruzzi et al. (91) reported that concurrent bacterial lung infection in ICU patients with AIDS and PCP was lower than HIV-uninfected control subjects, possibly because trimethoprim-sulfamethoxazole was used in the HIV-infected group for the treatment of PCP. However, as rates of hospitalization of HIV-infected patients for opportunistic infections decrease, the occurrence of nosocomial pneumonia should also decline (8). At the same time, with the emergence of MDR bacteria, nosocomial pneumonia is likely to remain a significant problem in HIV-infected patients receiving intensive care.

Afessa and Green (20) studied the impact and outcomes of patients with bacterial pneumonia who were hospitalized patients with HIV infection from 1995 to 1998 at a university-affiliated medical center. Of the 1,225 consecutive admissions studied, bacterial pneumonia was diagnosed in 111 (9%) of admissions, of which 80 (72%) were community acquired. Compared to HIV-infected patients without pneumonia, patients with bacterial pneumonia had lower CD4 counts (median 38 vs. 66 /mm^3, $p < .003$), higher APACHE II scores (17 vs. 13, $p < .0001$), longer length of hospital stay (6 vs. 4 days, $p < .0001$), ICU admission (28 vs. 9%, $p < .0001$), and a higher case fatality rate (21% vs. 4%, $p < .0001$). The most common pathogens were *P. aeruginosa* (32 admissions), *S. aureus* (16 admissions) and *H. influenzae* (11 admissions). Bacteremia was present in 30% of the pneumonias. Pneumococcal bacteremia was more common in patients with pneumococcal pneumonia (95%) versus *Pseudomonas* pneumonia (9%). Of note is that compared to patients with pneumococcal pneumonia, patients with *Pseudomonas* pneumonia had lower CD4 counts and a longer hospital stay, but no difference in case fatality rate. The authors concluded that HIV patients with low leukocyte and CD4 counts who have pneumonia should receive coverage for *P. aeruginosa* in either the community or nosocomial setting.

HIV and Bacterial Pneumonia at Autopsy

Bacterial infection has been identified in 30% to 86% of patients who die of HIV infection. In the autopsy study by Nichols et al. (92), bacterial infection was documented in 83%

of 46 AIDS patients and contributed to death in 36% of cases. Pneumonia was the most common bacterial infection identified, occurring in more than 50% of the patients. Niedt and Schinella (56) found bacterial infection in more than 50% of 56 autopsies, and the lung was again the most common site of infection. *S. aureus, P. aeruginosa, K. pneumoniae,* and *Enterobacter cloacae* were the most common pathogens isolated, and multiple pathogens were commonly observed. These data suggest that hospitalized terminally ill AIDS patients become infected with traditional nosocomial pathogens that may contribute significantly to mortality. However, as mortality rates decline, the relative importance of pneumonia as an end-stage event may also be expected to decrease (7,8).

Healthcare-Associated *Pneumocystis carinii* Pneumonia (PCP)

Outbreaks of PCP were reported as early as 1968. Current epidemiologic and animal studies suggest that airborne droplets are the most likely source of transmission (93–97). Several clusters of cases of PCP among HIV-infected individuals suggest that *P. carinii* may be acquired from patients in the healthcare setting. Implicated procedures include sputum induction, bronchoscopy, or aerosolized pentamidine treatment (Table 57.1).

Hoover et al. (98) found temporal and geographic relationships suggesting person-to-person spread of *P. carinii* in HIV-infected men compared with seronegative control subjects. Haron et al. (93) correlated increases in PCP among their cancer patients from 1980 to 1987 to increasing numbers of cases of AIDS admitted to their institution. No specific epidemiologic routes of transmission could be determined, although the AIDS clinic and leukemia outpatient clinics were contiguous and the two patient populations mingled freely. In addition, Chave et al. (94) identified PCP in five of 144 renal transplant recipients over a 22-month period. All five patients attended the same outpatient facility where they shared waiting and treatment rooms and had multiple encounters with AIDS patients who later developed PCP. Four patients had previously received methylprednisolone. Rates of PCP decreased after the two patient populations were separated.

Helweg-Larsen et al. (99) have studied person-to-person transmission using genotyping in eight patients with hematologic malignancies and six patients with HIV infection. Common sequences were observed in two patients with hematologic malignancies who shared the same room and two patients with HIV disease who had prolonged close contact on the ward. These data suggest that nosocomial transmission may occur, but person-to-person transmission of *P. carinii* may be relatively infrequent and may depend on the susceptibility of the host (99).

Because carriage is difficult to detect and cultures and antibody tests are not available, nosocomial transmission of PCP between HIV-infected patients is difficult to prove. Although these data on nosocomial transmission are not conclusive, the circumstantial evidence should not be ignored, and consideration should be given to preventing the spread of *P. carinii* among immunosuppressed patients.

Healthcare-Associated Viral Pneumonia

Nosocomial viral infections due to influenza, adenovirus, and respiratory syncytial virus can prolong hospitalization and are associated with serious complications (100). Respiratory syncytial virus has been the most extensively studied of the nosocomial respiratory viruses, and numerous outbreaks have been reported on pediatric and neonatal units. Because hospital personnel may transfer respiratory syncytial virus passively between patients or by self-inoculation followed by infection and secondary spread to patients, prevention and control measures include hand washing, isolation or cohorting of patients and personnel, gowning for close contact, and possibly protective isolation of high-risk patients.

Nosocomial outbreaks of influenza in hospitals and chronic care facilities are not unusual occurrences, particularly when the virus is present in the community (100). Although some studies have suggested that influenza vaccination may increase plasma HIV RNA levels, the effect appears to be uncommon, transient, and probably will have little impact with the widespread use of HAART (101,102). Persons with influenza may have a higher prevalence of hypoxia or prolonged duration of illness, but this observation requires confirmation in larger studies with appropriate control subjects. Because persons with HIV infection may have limited protection from influenza vaccine and a higher risk of secondary bacterial infection, prophylaxis and treatment of influenza A with amantadine should be considered. Efforts should also be directed at controlling influenza among hospital staff by the use of vaccine or chemoprophylaxis and limiting visitors during outbreaks (see Chapter 41).

TUBERCULOSIS

Changing Epidemiology of Tuberculosis (TB) in HIV

The number of reported cases of TB in the U.S. declined steadily between 1953 and 1984, but there was a dramatic reversal of this trend beginning in 1986 (103). The HIV epidemic was largely responsible for this resurgence, which persisted to the early 1990s, fueled by cutbacks in the public health infrastructure during President Reagan's administration (104). Moreover, the emergence of MDR TB was implicated in numerous hospital outbreaks described in Table 57.4 (105). Thereafter, TB control measures were intensified and the rates of TB and clustered TB cases decreased overall and among high-risk groups (106,107).

Of all opportunistic infections associated with HIV, TB is of particular interest from a public health perspective, because it is contagious by the respiratory route and is relatively easy to treat and prevent (107). Control of TB requires early recognition and proper management, including isolation of cases, adherence to effective therapy, and identification and proper prophylaxis of exposed individuals (103). Directly observed therapy has been used in special areas or in special at-risk populations, and has been a useful tool in decreasing the rate of TB transmission (106). The increased knowledge of the risk of reactivation of latent TB in HIV-positive patients, improved TB control efforts,

TABLE 57.4. SUMMARY OF SELECTED REPORTS OF OUTBREAKS OF DRUG-SENSITIVE AND DRUG-RESISTANT TUBERCULOSIS INVOLVING HIV-INFECTED INDIVIDUALS

First Author (Reference)	Location	Number of Cases of TB	Attack Rate (%)	Incubation Period for TB (Days)	Survival (Weeks)	Risk Factors for TB	Transmission to Healthcare Workers	Comments
Drug-sensitive TB								
Di Perri (122)	Inpatient ward	8	44	All <60	NA	Lower CD4 count (mean, 143) PPD or anergic	Four of six volunteers had conversion of PPD; one possibly related case of TB in a nurse	High attack rate of TB documented; strong evidence of nosocomial transmission of TB
Dooley (109)	Inpatient HIV unit	12	5[a]	80 (median)	NA	Hospitalization in same room as active TB case	Increased rate of PPD positivity in nurses on HIV unit	Fifty percent of TB cases spent time in nonprivate room prior to diagnosis
Daley (111)	Residential care facility for HIV-positive persons	11	37	28–106	NA	NA	Six of 28 staff with documented PPD conversion	Fifty percent of exposed residents developed TB infection or active disease; RFLP results linked all 11 cases
Multidrug-resistant TB[b]								
Fischl (119)	Hospital and HIV clinic	62[c]	NA	22–182	8	Contact with HIV clinic; AP or IV therapy in clinic; AIDS (median CD4 = 78)	NA	Outpatient clinic implicated as major TB exposure site; results of susceptibility tests delayed
Pearson (128)	Hospital	23 (21 HIV positive)	NA	NA	4	Hospitalization in 7 months prior to TB diagnosis; HIV infection	PPD conversion rates of 22–50% on wards with TB case	Controls in study were HIV-positive and HIV-negative patients with drug-sensitive TB; 14 of 16 cases tested infected with same strain by RFLP analysis; only six of 23 cases ever in isolation rooms
Beck-Sague (137)	HIV ward and outpatient clinic	25	NA	<97 (median)	7	Advanced HIV; exposure to smear-positive MDR-TB case; clinic visit during AP treatment of MDR-TB case; history of "failure" of prior TB treatment	PPD conversion rates increased in HIV clinic or ward; PPD conversion rates increased with exposure to smear-positive TB case	Transmission associated with AP administration and AFB smear positivity; 13 of 13 cases tested were infected with 1 of 2 strains by RFLP
CDC (126)	Prison system	17 (15 HIV positive)	NA	NA	4	NA	Transmission of MDR-TB to a correctional worker guarding TB cases[d]	PPD conversion in at least 55 inmates; significant delay in availability of drug resistance testing; 7 of 7 infected with same strain by RFLP

Note: Mortality rates attributable to tuberculosis ranged from 52% to 70%.
[a]Attack rate of 17% among patients exposed to a roommate with active TB.
[b]Risk factors for acquisition of MDR-TB were analyzed in comparison with HIV-infected patients with drug-sensitive TB, unless otherwise noted.
[c]Forty-six of 62 cases (74%) had contact with the medical center before their diagnosis of TB.
[d]Correctional worker was immunocompromised due to malignancy, had CD4 <110/mm^3, and died from TB.
TB, tuberculosis; NA, not available from published report; PPD, skin test for TB using purified protein derivative; HIV, human immunodeficiency virus; RFLP, restriction fragment length polymorphism; AP, aerosolized pentamidine; AIDS, acquired immunodeficiency syndrome; MDR-TB, multidrug-resistant tuberculosis, defined as resistance to two or more standard antituberculosis drugs.

early identification, and appropriate treatment of cases resulted in a decline of rates of TB in the last 10 years (107,108). In San Francisco, annual TB case rates peaked in 1992, and decreased significantly in 1997 (106).

Despite these improvements in case finding, treatment, and prevention, outbreaks of TB have persisted in healthcare settings, prisons, shelters for the homeless, and other settings (109–113). Kenyon et al. (112) described an outbreak of seven cases of MDR TB that occurred in six patients and one healthcare worker, all of whom had AIDS. The authors suggested that respirator-fit test programs may not protect healthcare workers in the absence of appropriate isolation rooms.

Data suggest that transmission, virulence, and susceptibility rates of TB may vary widely (114,115). Valway et al. (114) suggested that extensive transmission of *M. tuberculosis* in a small rural community was due to a virulent strain rather than to environmental or patient characteristics. Among people exposed to the three patients infected with this strain, over 70% developed tuberculin positivity, three to four times the expected rate. However, host factors also clearly influence the epidemiology of TB. Bellamy et al. (115) demonstrated a genetic predilection to the development of TB in a case-control study completed among West Africans. Racial variations in the susceptibility to TB and studies in twins provide evidence that genetic factors are important in susceptibility to this disease (116,117).

Natural History of Tuberculosis in HIV Infection

The association between HIV infection and the rising rate of infection due to *M. tuberculosis* in the U.S. has been well documented (109,118). Pulmonary involvement occurs in 70% to 93% of cases of TB in HIV-infected patients, but concurrent involvement at other sites is common (104,119–121). The diagnosis of pulmonary TB may be obscured by other pulmonary complications of HIV (104,122,123), such as a negative tuberculin skin test (124), atypical presentations, and decreased sensitivity of sputum acid-fast bacillus smears in patients with advanced HIV disease (104,118,119,121).

After recent infection with *M. tuberculosis*, primary TB occurs at an increased rate and is characterized by an incubation period as short as 4 weeks (111). Two studies using analysis of restriction fragment length polymorphisms (RFLP) have shown that recently transmitted *M. tuberculosis* was responsible for two thirds of TB cases in HIV-infected individuals in two urban centers, compared with up to one third of TB cases overall in the cities studied (110,125). In addition, based on the results of the RFLP analysis, Small et al. (110) were able to show transmission in both inpatient and outpatient hospital settings. The molecular epidemiology of TB spread among residents of an AIDS housing unit was not only part of the study by Small et al. but was also summarized in detail by Daley et al. (111). This study illustrates the use of molecular epidemiologic techniques to confirm person-to-person spread of TB among AIDS patients in a closed facility (Fig. 57.6). Others have reported person-to-person spread of other respiratory pathogens such as *H. influenzae*, *S. pneumoniae*, and *P. carinii* in hospitals, nursing homes, or possibly in outpatient clinics.

Reactivation of latent TB secondary to HIV disease accounts for the majority of cases, and occurs at a rate of 5% to 10% per year compared with a similar rate over a lifetime in persons without HIV infection (104). The response to therapy is excellent in patients who adhere to treatment regimens and who have drug-sensitive *M. tuberculosis* and are early in the course of HIV disease, but high failure rates and mortality have characterized treatment of MDR TB (126–128).

Two new issues have complicated the management of HIV-infected patients with *M. tuberculosis*: (a) drug–drug interactions between rifamycins and PIs and NNRTIs, and (b) IRIS. The former are due to induction or inhibition of the cytochrome P450 isoenzymes, which are involved in the metabolism of these drugs (103,107,129). Existing guidelines have suggested the substitution of rifabutin for rifampin, although conclusive evidence is still lacking (103,130). Spradling et al. (130) recently reported on the administration of a rifabutin-containing regimen and on rifabutin drug concentrations, toxicity, and clinical outcomes, and they concluded that the rifabutin concentrations were highly unpredictable, regardless of the dosage. This report highlights the current need to understand these drug–drug interactions and the possible use of therapeutic drug monitoring (TDM), keeping in mind that conclusive evidence should be provided before doing formal recommendations.

IRIS has been reported in patients undergoing HAART and TB treatment, manifesting with fever, respiratory symptoms, and a variety of other findings such as lymphadenopathy, abdominal complaints, and ascites (27,131,132). A review of the literature was included in a recent report of two cases (133). A total of 31 patients were reported: IRIS was suspected in the majority of cases for radiographic worsening of chest x-rays, or for enlargement of lymph nodes or appearance of new lymphadenopathy. The authors concluded that clinicians should recognize these findings as inflammatory responses to treatment, and not interpret them as drug resistance or inadequate response to treatment (134).

A recent review on the treatment of latent TB highlighted the current standard in HIV-positive patients (135). Among the different options, it should be remembered that the rifampin-pyrazinamide (PZA) combination is associated with higher rates of liver disease, so that patients on this regimen should be carefully monitored, and perhaps this combination should not be used in HIV-infected patients on HAART or in patients with HCV or HBV infection (136).

Hospital-Associated Tuberculosis in HIV-Infected Patients

The nosocomial outbreaks of TB involving HIV-infected persons described earlier have been characterized by attack rates that range from 5% to 44%, rapid progression from infection to active disease, and evidence of significant nosocomial spread to both patients and healthcare workers (Table 57.4) (127). These outbreaks have occurred in healthcare settings and in residential and correctional facilities (105,111). The conclusion that these outbreaks occurred by nosocomial transmission was based on strong epidemiologic data and supported in a number of outbreaks by RFLP analysis of the *M. tuberculosis* isolates (105,

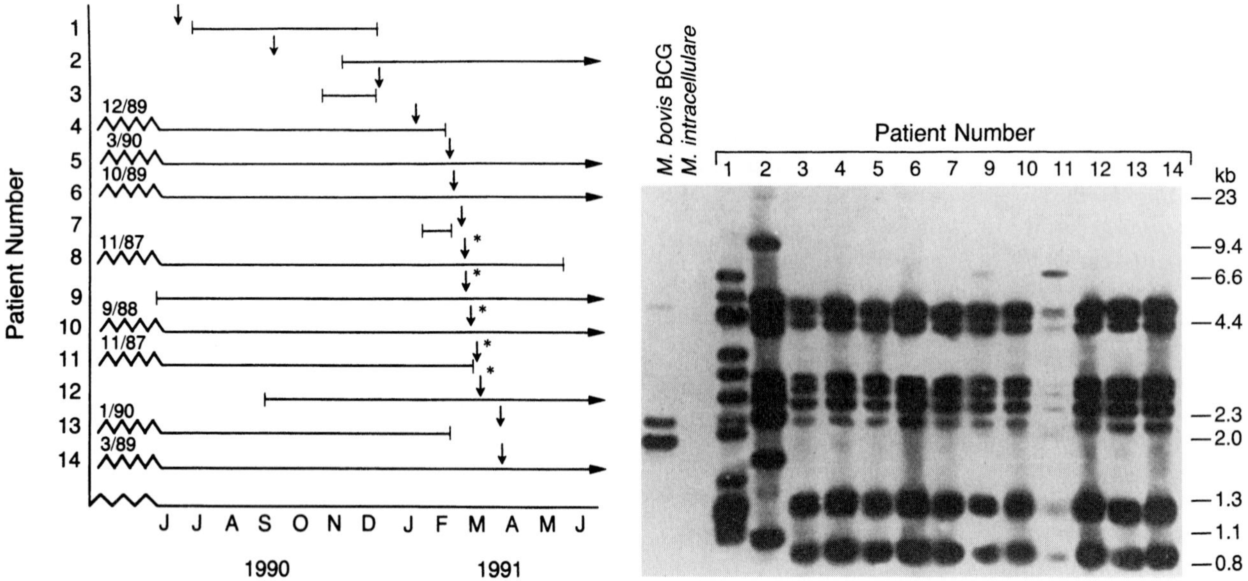

Figure 57.6. **A:** Person-to-person spread of tuberculosis in a residential facility for HIV-infected patients. **B:** Molecular analysis demonstrating similarity between resident strains from the outbreak (lanes 3–14) vs. patients in lanes 1 and 2 who were on therapy for tuberculosis before they entered the facility. (From Daley CL, Small PM, Schecter GF, et al. An outbreak of tuberculosis with accelerated progression among persons infected with the human immunodeficiency virus. An analysis using restriction-fragment-length polymorphisms. *N Engl J Med* 1992;326:231–235, with permission.)

111,137). Nosocomial outbreaks of MDR TB are of greater concern (105,109). These outbreaks have primarily involved HIV-infected patients with advanced disease who have demonstrated rapid progression from exposure to active MDR TB and poor response to therapy (105,127,137). Mortality attributed to TB has ranged from 52% to 70% (105,127).

Factors that have contributed to TB outbreaks include an increasing number of HIV-infected patients exposed to TB; delays in proper isolation, diagnosis, and treatment of TB; and delays in availability of drug susceptibility results (103,105,109, 127,138). In addition, inadequate ventilation, lack of isolation rooms with negative air pressure, and inadequate precautions for cough-inducing procedures such as aerosolized pentamidine and bronchoscopy have contributed to transmission.

Tuberculosis outbreaks have been notable for increasing evidence of transmission of both drug-sensitive and drug-resistant TB to healthcare workers. Beck-Sague et al. (137) reported increased skin test conversion rates in healthcare workers on the HIV ward or clinic and increased risk associated with working during the presence of a smear-positive MDR TB case. In one survey the risk of tuberculin skin conversion was greater among healthcare workers in hospitals that specialized in care for HIV-positive patients (139).

In response to the growing number of TB outbreaks, the CDC published a set of guidelines for preventing TB transmission in healthcare settings (103). These guidelines stress early identification of active disease and prompt isolation and early initiation of effective therapy. In addition, routine skin testing for TB exposure among healthcare workers is advocated and contact investigation is coupled with the use of appropriate preventive therapy after an exposure.

Recent improvements in TB control need to be maintained to prevent future nosocomial outbreaks of TB (103). New technology such as fluorescence microscopy, RFLP analysis, and radiometric culture systems should be routinely incorporated into standard diagnostic evaluations to facilitate rapid identification of *M. tuberculosis*, drug susceptibility patterns, and early detection of outbreaks and ongoing transmission. There is a need for appropriate prophylaxis or treatment guided by drug-resistance surveillance data, with careful monitoring of the clinical and bacteriologic response and directly observed therapy as warranted (140). In addition, isolation of suspected cases of TB in properly functioning isolation rooms and continuous staff education are necessary to reduce potential exposures (112) (see also Chapter 37). A survey was made in 1992 and 1996 in U.S. hospitals with and without patients with PCP to compare trends in nosocomial TB prevention measures and healthcare worker tuberculin skin test seroconversion (139). Almost 100% of the hospitals studied had rooms meeting the CDC criteria for acid-fast bacilli isolation in 1996, compared to only 63% in 1992. There was a significant decreasing trend in tuberculin skin test conversion rates among healthcare workers in both hospitals, although healthcare workers of hospitals with PCP had a higher risk of tuberculin skin test conversion.

GASTROINTESTINAL INFECTIONS

Healthcare-associated gastroenteritis has been estimated to occur at a rate of 10.5 per 10,000 discharges but may vary by hospital service, type, and size (141). Identified risk factors for gastrointestinal (GI) infection include impaired host immunity, abnormal gastric motility, decreased gastric acidity, prior antibiotic exposure, and hospitalization in the intensive care unit (141,142).

Gastrointestinal Infections in HIV-Infected Patients

Diarrhea occurred in 30% to 50% of AIDS patients in the U.S., but the use of HAART and prophylaxis with trimethoprim-sulfamethoxazole and macrolides have reduced the rates of GI infections (Table 57.1) (143,144). In a multicenter study by Stroud et al. (11), the incidence of GI nosocomial infections in HIV-infected patients was similar to those of the NNIS system, but AIDS patients may have a reduced gastric acid barrier and increased susceptibility to nosocomial infection if they are immunosuppressed. Potential GI pathogens include *Salmonella* species (143,145), *Shigella flexneri* (146), *Campylobacter jejuni* (147), toxin-producing *Clostridium difficile* (148), MAC (74), CMV (149), *Cryptosporidium, Isospora belli* (150), and *Enterocytozoan bieneusi* (microsporidia) (151); these pathogens usually occurred in patients in the pre-HAART era and in patients with more advanced HIV disease or CD4 counts less than 200/mm^3. GI infections in HIV-infected persons can be complicated by prolonged disease, recurrent infection, and BSI (144). Increased host susceptibility is attributed to HIV-mediated defects in humoral and mucosal immunity coupled with a high rate of decreased gastric acidity in HIV-infected persons (144,152).

Clostridium difficile

C. difficile–associated diarrhea and colitis, the most common cause of hospital-acquired diarrhea, is an increasing problem in many hospitals and long-term-care facilities (153). Although HIV-infected patients may have an increased risk of colonization and infection with *C. difficile*, traditional risk factors such as increased length of hospital stay, frequent antibiotic exposure, and decreased gastric acidity also contribute substantially to risk (152). DeMarais et al. (2) reported that *C. difficile*–associated diarrhea was one of the most common nosocomial infections in HIV-infected patients in a long-term-care setting. Infections were associated with low CD4 counts, poor functional status, and length of stay at the facility.

Pulvirenti et al. (154) reported on the incidence of *C. difficile* among patients infected with HIV admitted to a public hospital compared to a private hospital. Patients admitted to the public hospital were significantly more likely to be colonized on admission (14.7% vs. 2.9%, p <.001) and that the acquisition rate at the public hospital was also sevenfold higher than the private hospital. Risk factors for *C. difficile* acquisition were more severe HIV disease, use of acyclovir or H2-blockers, and longer hospital stay. Public hospital HIV patients were also taking more antibiotics, had longer hospital stays and more frequently had a history of *C. difficile* infection. Mortality rates for HIV patients with and without HIV infection were similar. During the study, two strains of *C. difficile* contaminated the environment. Both strains were clindamycin-resistant and toxin-positive, but only one strain, typed by pulsed-field gel electrophoresis, caused the outbreak. The authors postulated that *C. difficile* transmission occurred between patients in common areas, such as common toilets, showers, or the communal television room.

Barbut et al. (155) conducted a retrospective analysis of all *C. difficile*–associated diarrhea in hospitalized patients with HIV over a 52-month period. *C. difficile*–associated diarrhea was defined as patients with diarrhea and a positive cytotoxin B assay. Annual incidence ranged from 1.7 to 6.4 per 100 HIV-infected patients. Of the 67 cases identified, 72% were first episodes and 28% were relapses. To identify risk factors, 34 patients with first episodes were compared to 66 HIV-infected controls matched for length of hospital stay. Three independent risk factors were identified in the HIV-infected group: CD4 counts <50/mm^3 (OR = 5.2; 95% CI, 1.4–19.3; p = .01) penicillin use (OR = 4.6; 1.1–188; p = .03), and clindamycin use (OR = 5.0; 1.3–18.3; p = .02). These data suggest that nosocomial diarrhea in HIV-infected patients should be suspected in individuals with a low CD4 count and use of prior penicillin or clindamycin. No association was observed between *C. difficile*–associated diarrhea and age, gender, HIV risk behavior, Karnofsky score, gastrointestinal procedures, or use of antacids. Most of the isolates in this study were serogroup C, which has been associated with multidrug resistance, especially clindamycin. It is not clear whether *C. difficile* infection is more severe in HIV-infected individuals. These investigators found strong time-space clustering of cases infected with the outbreak strain.

Tumbarello et al. (156) studied *C. difficile*–associated diarrhea in patients with HIV using another case-control design that compared 31 HIV-infected patients with *C. difficile*–associated diarrhea (group A) to 31 HIV-seronegative patients (group B) and 62 HIV-infected patients without *C. difficile* disease (group C). On univariate analysis, risk factors in group A versus group C were antibiotic use in the 4 weeks prior to onset (p <.03), prolonged hospitalization >20 days (p <.04), low CD4 counts (p <.03), and the use of antacids (p <.04), but prior antibiotic use was the only independent predictor after univariate analysis. Antibiotics significantly associated (p <.05) with *C. difficile*–associated diarrhea were trimethoprim-sulfamethoxazole, cephalosporins, and clindamycin. Clinical symptoms were more severe in HIV-infected persons, but the outcome was not influenced by circulating CD4 counts.

Both HIV-infected and HIV-negative patients may benefit from preventive measures for *C. difficile*, which have been recently summarized and are outlined in more detail in Chapter 36 (153).

Salmonella Species

Salmonella have been implicated in a large number of diarrheal outbreaks in hospitals and long-term-care facilities that were attributed to contaminated food (particularly raw eggs), medications, and possible person-to-person spread (157). High rates of antibiotic usage and decreased gastric acidity may increase susceptibility of HIV-infected patients to acute and recurrent infection. This infection poses a serious threat to HIV-infected patients because of increased rates of secondary BSI and recurrent bacteremia. A number of other bacteria, including *Shigella* species, *Yersinia enterocolitica*, and *E. coli*, are less common causes of hospital outbreaks. Although HIV-infected persons may be more susceptible to infection by these pathogens, an increased risk during a nosocomial outbreak has not been documented.

Gastrointestinal Viruses

Rotaviruses are a common cause of nosocomial infection, particularly in the pediatric population, with outbreaks also described in elderly patients and in long-term-care facilities (158). Potential transmission of rotavirus to HIV-infected patients in such facilities may occur, and prolonged shedding and chronic infection may result (158,159).

Gastrointestinal Protozoa

Cryptosporidium has been recognized as a cause of diarrhea in persons with HIV infection or other immunocompromised hosts (150,160,161). The use of HAART and macrolide prophylaxis against MAC have substantially reduced rates of cryptosporidiosis in HIV-infected persons (162,163).

Outbreaks of cryptosporidiosis have resulted from contaminated water supplies or transfer from infected persons with HIV and other immunocompromised patients at increased risk of infection (150,160,161). During an outbreak of *Cryptosporidium* infections traced to a contaminated ice machine, 73 seronegative subjects and 60 HIV-infected patients were exposed. Patients with AIDS or those receiving oral sulfonamide therapy had the highest risk of infection (164). Of 18 patients with symptomatic HIV-infection who developed cryptosporidiosis, two became chronic carriers and eight died after prolonged diarrhea. These data indicate that HIV-infected patients are at high risk for infection and associated morbidity and mortality. The use of body-substance precautions should reduce person-to-person transmission, and immunocompromised patients may benefit from boiled, filtered, or bottled water in outbreak settings such as an outbreak involving the water supply in Milwaukee (161).

SURGICAL SITE INFECTIONS

Surgical site infection (SSI) rates in the NNIS system ranged from 0 to 2.5 per 100 patient discharges and varied by type of surgery and surgical service (165). Risk factors for SSI include the likelihood of microbial contamination, duration of surgery, length of preoperative hospitalization, type of preoperative skin preparation, and host factors.

SSIs are primarily caused by the patient's endogenous flora. Common etiologic agents include *S. aureus*, streptococci, and, less commonly, gram-negative bacilli and other microorganisms. Data suggest that certain anesthetic and operative procedures may cause a reversible decrease in CD4 cell count, impairment of neutrophil function, and alterations in lymphokine function, but correlation with SSI has not been demonstrated.

Surgical Site Infections in HIV-Infected Patients

Although early studies reported a high 30-day postoperative mortality rate for HIV-infected patients, most deaths resulted from progression of their HIV disease rather than SSI (166, 167). Studies have demonstrated more favorable outcomes (167, 168). In a retrospective case-control study, Buehrer et al. (169) reported only two SSIs in 83 patients undergoing 108 surgical procedures, with no difference related to HIV status. In a retrospective review of 56 consecutive HIV-infected trauma patients, development of infectious complications was associated with severity of injury but not with degree of immunosuppression (170). Although other investigators have also reported no increase in SSI in HIV-infected patients (167,171), in a report of 28 AIDS patients with appendicitis, six patients (21%) had postoperative complications (168).

HIV-mediated immune defects, debilitation, and malnutrition, coupled with increased colonization by *S. aureus*, may increase the risk of SSI in HIV-infected patients (172). More data are needed to assess the risk of SSI by stage of HIV disease and the contributions of HIV-mediated immune defects and *S. aureus* colonization in the pathogenesis of SSI.

URINARY TRACT INFECTIONS

Urinary tract infections (UTIs) comprise 40% of nosocomial infections in the U.S. and are a significant problem for both acute care hospitals and long-term-care settings (1). Risk factors for UTIs include presence of an indwelling urinary catheter, increased age, debilitation, and abnormal bladder function.

Urinary Tract Infections in HIV-Infected Patients

Although HIV infection may cause proteinuria, microscopic hematuria, and HIV-related nephropathy, it is unknown if HIV infection is also a risk factor for the development of community-acquired or nosocomial UTI (173,174). UTIs in HIV-infected patients are usually caused by enteric gram-negative bacilli or *P. aeruginosa*, but more unusual microorganisms have also been reported (175).

DeMarais et al. (2) reported nosocomial infections in 65 HIV-infected persons in a long-term-care facility in which there were 24 episodes of UTIs in 16 patients, accounting for 3.8 episodes per 1,000 long-term-care days. Nine of 16 patients had urinary catheters, and 70% of the episodes were polymicrobial. In the multicenter study of Stroud et al. (11), 28% of the nosocomial infections in HIV-infected patients were UTIs, but this percent was lower than for the NNIS system data.

As increasing numbers of debilitated HIV-infected patients are cared for in long-term-care facilities, and as this population ages there will probably be increased numbers of UTIs, especially when urinary catheters are used or abnormalities in bladder function develop. Careful attention to infection control procedures, including hand washing and prudent use and care of urinary catheters, will be needed.

CENTRAL NERVOUS SYSTEM INFECTIONS

Nosocomial CNS infections are serious, infrequent, and primarily affect postsurgical and pediatric patients (176). Infections in nonsurgical patients generally occur in patients who are immunocompromised, have had head trauma, after an invasive procedure, or by direct extension from a parameningeal focus.

Central Nervous System Infection in HIV-Infected Patients

HIV commonly involves the CNS and increases susceptibility to meningitis with *Cryptococcus neoformans* and encephalitis due to *Toxoplasma gondii* (177). There is also a potential risk of secondary meningitis with CNS pathogens, such as *S. pneumoniae* (81), *H. influenzae* (85), and *Listeria monocytogenes* (178, 179). Nosocomial infections caused by these pathogens have been previously reported in immunocompromised hosts (179–181).

Other potential risk factors for CNS infections in HIV-infected patients include increased rates of sinusitis, endocarditis in patients with active injection drug use or line infections, and increased rates of nasopharyngeal colonization by *S. aureus*. Studies evaluating these risk factors are lacking. Despite the high number of sources of bacterial CNS infection, overall prevalence in this population is surprisingly low, and healthcare-associated transmission is rare.

More prospective studies are needed to assess the risk of nosocomial CNS infection before formulating policies for prophylaxis and surveillance cultures in HIV-infected persons. In the meantime, appropriate infection control procedures should be followed and efforts should be directed at proper diagnosis of opportunistic pathogens that may mimic nosocomial infection.

SINUSITIS

Sinusitis in hospitalized patients is primarily a disease associated with prolonged nasotracheal intubation and use of nasogastric feeding tubes (182,183). Sinusitis may be clinically silent or present solely with fever and leukocytosis. Treatment includes appropriate antibiotics and, in some cases, surgical drainage.

Sinusitis in HIV-Infected Patients

The risk of sinusitis in hospitalized HIV-infected patients is unknown. Because HIV-infected persons with advanced disease appear to be at increased risk for sinusitis, efforts are needed to reduce the risk of nosocomial sinusitis and to establish early diagnosis and treatment. Sinusitis is also a common complication of HIV disease. The predisposition to sinusitis may be related to defects in humoral immunity, infections in the oropharynx, or possibly an increased rate of allergic conditions (184).

In a prospective study of HIV-infected patients admitted to a hospital, Godofsky et al. (184) diagnosed sinusitis either radiographically or clinically in 11% of 667 patients. Disease was most common in patients with advanced HIV disease (median CD4 count 38/mm^3). Most patients had classic symptoms of fever, headache, and nasal congestion. Bacteriologic evaluation revealed a wide spectrum of pathogens, with a high rate of *P. aeruginosa* isolated from patients who had antral punctures. Although a high percentage of individuals had a partial response to treatment, sinusitis was often extensive and chronic. Other studies also indicate that HIV-infected patients with low CD4 counts have high rates of sinusitis and increased relapse rates after antimicrobial therapy (184,185).

FEVER AND NEUTROPENIA

Bacterial and fungal infections may result from neutropenia in patients with malignancies treated with chemotherapy (186). Bacterial infections are often due to gram-negative bacilli but in the presence of indwelling venous catheters may involve *Staphylococcus* species. Neutropenic patients, particularly those hospitalized, are also at risk for infection with various other bacterial species, *Candida* species, and *Aspergillus* species.

Neutropenia in HIV-Infected Patients

HIV-infected persons may have neutropenia as a result of HIV, chronic infections, or treatment with drugs such as zidovudine, ganciclovir, and chemotherapy (187). The risk of infection in HIV-infected patients with neutropenia is unknown at this time and probably varies depending on the patient population, acuity, degree, and etiology of the neutropenia (188). Before HAART, several studies produced inconsistent results to suggest that neutropenia (ANC less than 1,000/mL) was associated with an increased risk of bacteremia (189). In a case-control study by Keiser et al. (189) in symptomatic HIV-infected patients with ANC less than 1,000/mL, bacteremia occurred at a rate of 12.6 per 100 patient-months in HIV-infected patients versus 0.87 for matched control subjects [relative risk (RR) = 14.9, p = .003] (189). Multivariate analysis demonstrated that neutropenia (p <.03) and the presence of a CVC (p <.03) were associated with an increased risk of bacteremia. Jacobson et al. (190) reported a significant increase in the incidence of hospitalization for serious bacterial infections in HIV-infected persons with an ANC less than 750 cells/mL, and multivariate analysis demonstrated that severity and duration of the neutropenia and black race were significant predictors of hospitalization for severe bacterial infections.

Moore et al. (191) found no association between neutropenia (ANC less than 1,000/mL) and severe individual bacterial infections, but when analyzed as a group, there was a significantly (p = .05) increased risk of bacterial infection in patients with advanced HIV disease (191). By comparison, Farber et al. (192) found infection rates that were considerably lower than a control population of neutropenic oncology patients. Furthermore, infection rates were no different for these HIV-infected patients when neutropenia was absent.

Neutropenia in HIV-infected patients has been implicated as a risk factor for the development of other complications such as invasive aspergillosis and neutropenic enterocolitis (193–195). However, despite a high prevalence of mucosal disease with *Candida* species, candidemia in HIV-infected patients is surprisingly low.

As the survival from infectious complications of HIV increases, there will be greater numbers of patients with HIV-related malignancies requiring chemotherapy (196,197). Until further data are available, HIV-infected neutropenic patients should be treated with standard infection control practices, appropriate antibiotics, and granulocyte-stimulating factors as indicated (186).

NOSOCOMIAL VIRAL INFECTIONS

Nosocomial viral infections are an often-unrecognized source of hospital-acquired morbidity and mortality, accounting for 5% of all nosocomial infections and 34% of pediatric infections in one hospital (198). Infants, the elderly, and immunocompromised patients, including HIV-infected persons, are particularly susceptible to infection. Because a number of these viruses are reviewed elsewhere in this book, only VZV and CMV are discussed here.

Nosocomial transmission of VZV from primary varicella and disseminated and local zoster has been documented among immunocompromised patients and nonimmune immunocompetent patients and healthcare workers (199). Persons with HIV infection reactivate VZV at a relatively high rate, which may be complicated by dissemination and atypical appearance (200, 201). HIV-infected persons pose a potential problem in healthcare settings both for acquisition and transmission of disease. Adherence to recommended isolation procedures and high levels of suspicion for even atypical rashes are needed to prevent outbreaks (see Chapter 42).

CMV infection is most common in HIV disease when CD4 counts fall below 100/mm^3, with retinitis and GI disease as the most frequent manifestations (202). Parenteral transmission by blood products or transplanted organs is the most common mode of nosocomial infection, particularly in CMV-seronegative patients. Transfusion-associated infection can be prevented in seronegative patients by the use of CMV-seronegative products or the use of blood cells that are washed before transfusion. Nonparenteral spread in hospitals is rare, and the risk to healthcare workers, even from individuals excreting large amounts of virus, is believed to be small (also see Chapter 44).

More data are needed to assess the risk and impact of nosocomial viral infections in HIV-infected persons. Increasing awareness of nosocomial viral infection is indicated, along with the use of appropriate infection control and intervention measures to reduce exposure and limit the spread of viruses in the hospital setting.

CONCLUSION AND FUTURE DIRECTIONS

Healthcare-associated infections in HIV-infected patients have decreased with the widespread use of HAART and use of chemoprophylaxis against common opportunistic infections in industrialized nations but remain a significant problem in the less developed countries. As the AIDS population ages and more patients experience HAART failure, the risk of nosocomial infection is likely to increase. Existing data suggest that those with advanced HIV disease are at greater risk of nosocomial infection due to immunosuppression, increased hospitalizations with longer lengths of stay, and greater exposure to invasive devices such as intravenous or urinary catheters. These data underscore the need to examine rates of infection in different healthcare settings and in specific subsets of patients, such as HIV-infected patients with HIV disease or co-infection with HCV.

Diagnosis and management of nosocomial infections in HIV-infected persons may be complicated by atypical presentations, increased rates of relapse after treatment, and earlier discharge. Accurate assessment of nosocomial outbreaks in the hospital are complicated by limited data on the risk of transmission of both traditional and unusual pathogens in this population and lack of data using molecular techniques. In addition, these data may also be compromised by the accuracy of the HIV case finding that may be poor for inpatients, and there are limited data on nosocomial transmission in the outpatient setting. Furthermore, some patients may acquire nosocomial pathogens during their hospitalization and present later with infections that would normally be classified as community acquired. For this reason, "hospital-associated" infection is a better term than nosocomial or hospital-acquired infection. Prospective studies with appropriate control groups, molecular techniques, and adequate length of follow-up are needed to more clearly define the incidence of healthcare-associated infections in HIV-infected persons in the current era of HAART therapy and primary prophylaxis of opportunistic infections.

REFERENCES

1. Haley RW, Culver DH, White JW, et al. The nationwide nosocomial infection rate. A new need for vital statistics. *Am J Epidemiol* 1985; 121:159–167.
2. DeMarais PL, Gertzen J, Weinstein RA. Nosocomial infections in human immunodeficiency virus-infected patients in a long-term-care setting. *Clin Infect Dis* 1997;25:1230–1232.
3. Goetz AM, Squier C, Wagener MM, et al. Nosocomial infections in the human immunodeficiency virus-infected patient: a two-year survey. *Am J Infect Control* 1994;22:334–339.
4. Weber DJ, Becherer PR, Rutala WA, et al. Nosocomial infection rate as a function of human immunodeficiency virus type 1 status in hemophiliacs. *Am J Med* 1991;91:206S–212S.
5. Craven DE, Steger KA, Hirschhorn LR. Nosocomial colonization and infection in persons infected with human immunodeficiency virus. *Infect Control Hosp Epidemiol* 1996;17:304–318.
6. Masur H, Kaplan JE, Holmes KK. Guidelines for preventing opportunistic infections among HIV-infected persons—2002. *Ann Intern Med* 2002;137(5 pt 2):435–473.
7. Palella FJ Jr, Delaney KM, Moorman AC, et al. Declining morbidity and mortality among patients with advanced human immunodeficiency virus infection. HIV Outpatient Study Investigators. *N Engl J Med* 1998;338:853–860.
8. Torres RA, Barr M. Impact of combination therapy for HIV infection on inpatient census. *N Engl J Med* 1997;336:1531–1532.
9. Dybul M, Fauci AS, Bartlett JG, et al. Guidelines for using antiretroviral agents among HIV-infected adults and adolescents. *Ann Intern Med* 2002;137(5 pt 2):381–433.
10. Frank U, Daschner FD, Schulgen G, et al. Incidence and epidemiology of nosocomial infections in patients infected with human immunodeficiency virus. *Clin Infect Dis* 1997;25:318–320.
11. Stroud L, Srivastava P, Culver D, et al. Nosocomial infections in HIV-infected patients: preliminary results from a multicenter surveillance system (1989–1995). *Infect Control Hosp Epidemiol* 1997;18: 479–485.
12. Centers for Disease Control and Prevention. AIDS among persons aged >50 years—United States 1991–1996. *MMWR* 1998;47: 21–27.

13. Fauci AS, Schnittman SM, Poli G, et al. NIH conference. Immunopathogenic mechanisms in human immunodeficiency virus (HIV) infection. *Ann Intern Med* 1991;114:678–693.
14. Feng Y, Broder CC, Kennedy PE, et al. HIV-1 entry cofactor: functional cDNA cloning of a seven-transmembrane, G protein-coupled receptor. *Science* 1996;272:872–877.
15. Perelson AS, Neumann AU, Markowitz M, et al. HIV-1 dynamics in vivo: virion clearance rate, infected cell life-span, and viral generation time. *Science* 1996;271:1582–1586.
16. Mellors JW, Munoz A, Giorgi JV, et al. Plasma viral load and CD4+ lymphocytes as prognostic markers of HIV-1 infection. *Ann Intern Med* 1997;126:946–954.
17. Carpenter CC, Fischl MA, Hammer SM, et al. Antiretroviral therapy for HIV infection in 1997. Updated recommendations of the International AIDS Society-USA panel. *JAMA* 1997;277:1962–1969.
18. O'Brien WA, Hartigan PM, Daar ES, et al. Changes in plasma HIV RNA levels and CD4+ lymphocyte counts predict both response to antiretroviral therapy and therapeutic failure. VA Cooperative Study Group on AIDS. *Ann Intern Med* 1997;126:939–945.
19. Barat LM, Gunn JE, Steger KA, et al. Causes of fever in patients infected with human immunodeficiency virus who were admitted to Boston City Hospital. *Clin Infect Dis* 1996;23:320–328.
20. Afessa B, Green B. Bacterial pneumonia in hospitalized patients with HIV infection: the Pulmonary Complications, ICU Support, and Prognostic Factors of Hospitalized Patients with HIV (PIP) Study. *Chest* 2000;117:1017–1022.
21. Craven DE, Fuller JD, Barber TW, et al. Immunization of adults and children infected with human immunodeficiency virus. II. Use of inactive bacterial and viral vaccines. *Infect Dis Clin Pract* 1992;1: 411–423.
22. Steinhart R, Reingold AL, Taylor F, et al. Invasive Haemophilus influenzae infections in men with HIV infection. *JAMA* 1992;268: 3350–3352.
23. Ho DD, Rota RR, Hirsch MS. Infection of monocyte/macrophages by human T lymphotropic virus type III. *J Clin Invest* 1986;77:1712.
24. Craven DE, Steger KA, La Chapelle R, et al. Factitious HIV infection: the importance of documenting infection. *Ann Intern Med* 1994;121: 763–766.
25. Duncan RA, von Reyn CF, Alliegro GM, et al. Idiopathic CD4+ T-lymphocytopenia—four patients with opportunistic infections and no evidence of HIV infection. *N Engl J Med* 1993;328:393–398.
26. Schacker TW, Hughes JP, Shea T, et al. Biological and virologic characteristics of primary HIV infection. *Ann Intern Med* 1998;128: 613–620.
27. Shelburne SA III, Hamill RJ, Rodriguez-Barradas MC, et al. Immune reconstitution inflammatory syndrome: emergence of a unique syndrome during highly active antiretroviral therapy. *Medicine (Baltimore)* 2002;81:213–227.
28. Jacobson MA. Human immunodeficiency virus-associated immune reconstitution disease. *Am J Med* 2001;110:662–663.
29. Cooney EL. Clinical indicators of immune restoration following highly active antiretroviral therapy. *Clin Infect Dis* 2002;34:224–233.
30. Safdar A, Rubocki RJ, Horvath JA, et al. Fatal immune restoration disease in human immunodeficiency virus type 1—infected patients with progressive multifocal leukoencephalopathy: impact of antiretroviral therapy-associated immune reconstitution.
31. Dieterich DT. Hepatitis C virus and human immunodeficiency virus: clinical issues in coinfection. *Am J Med* 1999;107:79S–84S.
32. Greub G, Ledergerber B, Battegay M, et al. Clinical progression, survival, and immune recovery during antiretroviral therapy in patients with HIV-1 and hepatitis C virus coinfection: the Swiss HIV Cohort Study. *Lancet* 2000;356:1800–1805.
33. Darby SC, Ewart DW, Giangrande PL, et al. Mortality from liver cancer and liver disease in haemophilic men and boys in UK given blood products contaminated with hepatitis C. UK Haemophilia Centre Directors' Organisation. *Lancet* 1997;350:1425–1431.
34. Yee TT, Griffioen A, Sabin CA, et al. The natural history of HCV in a cohort of haemophilic patients infected between 1961 and 1985. *Gut* 2000;47:845–851.
35. Rosenberg PM, Farrell JJ, Abraczinskas DR, et al. Rapidly progressive fibrosing cholestatic hepatitis—hepatitis C virus in HIV coinfection. *Am J Gastroenterol* 2002;97:478–483.
36. Puoti M, Bonacini M, Spinetti A, et al. Liver fibrosis progression is related to CD4 cell depletion in patients coinfected with hepatitis C virus and human immunodeficiency virus. *J Infect Dis* 2001;183: 134–137.
37. De Luca A, Bugarini R, Lepri AC, et al. Coinfection with hepatitis viruses and outcome of initial antiretroviral regimens in previously naive HIV-infected subjects.
38. Sulkowski MS, Moore RD, Mehta SH, et al. Hepatitis C and progression of HIV disease. *JAMA* 2002;288:199–206.
39. John M, Flexman J, French MA. Hepatitis C virus-associated hepatitis following treatment of HIV-infected patients with HIV protease inhibitors: an immune restoration disease? *AIDS* 1998;12:2289–2293.
40. Bica I, McGovern B, Dhar R, et al. Increasing mortality due to end-stage liver disease in patients with human immunodeficiency virus infection. *Clin Infect Dis* 2001;32:492–497.
41. Lindsay MK, Peterson HB, Feng TI, et al. Routine antepartum human immunodeficiency virus infection screening in an inner-city population. *Obstet Gynecol* 1989;74:289–294.
42. Kelen GD, DiGiovanna T, Bisson L, et al. Human immunodeficiency virus infection in emergency department patients. Epidemiology, clinical presentations, and risk to health care workers: the Johns Hopkins experience. *JAMA* 1989;262:516–522.
43. Janssen RS, St Louis ME, Satten GA, et al. HIV infection among patients in U.S. acute care hospitals. Strategies for the counseling and testing of the hospital patients. The Hospital HIV Surveillance Group. *N Engl J Med* 1992;327:445–452.
44. Petrosillo N, Pugliese G, Girardi E, et al. Nosocomial infections in HIV infected patients. Gruppo HIV e Infezioni Ospedaliere. *AIDS* 1999;13:599–605.
45. Padoveze MC, Trabasso P, Branchini ML. Nosocomial infections among HIV-positive and HIV-negative patients in a Brazilian infectious diseases unit. *Am J Infect Control* 2002;30:346–350.
46. Kuehnert MJ, Jarvis WR. Changing epidemiology of nosocomial infections in human immunodeficiency virus-infected patients. *Clin Infect Dis* 1997;25:321–323.
47. Walensky RP, Losina E, Steger-Craven KA, et al. Identifying undiagnosed human immunodeficiency virus: the yield of routine, voluntary inpatient testing. *Arch Intern Med* 2002;162:887–892.
48. Centers for Disease Control and Prevention. Approval of a new rapid test for HIV antibody. *MMWR* 2002;51:1051–1052.
49. Curtis JR. ICU outcomes for patients with HIV infection: a moving target. *Chest* 1998;113:269–270.
50. Casalino E, Mendoza-Sassi G, Wolff M, et al. Predictors of short- and long-term survival in HIV-infected patients admitted to the ICU.
51. Rosenberg AL, Seneff MG, Atiyeh L, et al. The importance of bacterial sepsis in intensive care unit patients with acquired immunodeficiency syndrome: implications for future care in the age of increasing antiretroviral resistance. *Crit Care Med* 2001;29:548–556.
52. Proctor RA. Bacterial sepsis in patients with acquired immunodeficiency syndrome. *Crit Care Med* 2001;29:683–684.
53. Banerjee SN, Emori TG, Culver DH, et al. Secular trends in nosocomial primary bloodstream infections in the United States, 1980–1989. National Nosocomial Infections Surveillance System. *Am J Med* 1991;91:86S–89S.
54. Petrosillo N, Viale P, Nicastri E, et al. Nosocomial bloodstream infections among human immunodeficiency virus-infected patients: incidence and risk factors. *Clin Infect Dis* 2002;34:677–685.
55. Krumholz HM, Sande MA, Lo B. Community-acquired bacteremia in patients with acquired immunodeficiency syndrome: clinical presentation, bacteriology, and outcome. *Am J Med* 1989;86:776–779.
56. Niedt GW, Schinella RA. Acquired immunodeficiency syndrome. Clinicopathologic study of 56 autopsies. *Arch Pathol Lab Med* 1985; 109:727–734.
57. Eisenstein BI. New opportunistic infections—more opportunities. *N Engl J Med* 1990;323:1625–1627.
58. Hirschel B, Francioli P. Progress and problems in the fight against AIDS. *N Engl J Med* 1998;338:906–908.
59. Jacobson MA, Gellermann H, Chambers H. Staphylococcus aureus

bacteremia and recurrent staphylococcal infection in patients with acquired immunodeficiency syndrome and AIDS-related complex. *Am J Med* 1988;85:172–176.
60. Raviglione MC, Battan R, Pablos-Mendez A, et al. Infections associated with Hickman catheters in patients with acquired immunodeficiency syndrome. *Am J Med* 1989;86:780–786.
61. Moore DA, Gazzard BG, Nelson MR. Central venous line infections in AIDS. *J Infect* 1997;34:35–40.
62. Witt DJ, Craven DE, McCabe WR. Bacterial infections in adult patients with the acquired immune deficiency syndrome (AIDS) and AIDS-related complex. *Am J Med* 1987;82:900–906.
63. Whimbey E, Gold JW, Polsky B, et al. Bacteremia and fungemia in patients with the acquired immunodeficiency syndrome. *Ann Intern Med* 1986;104:511–514.
64. Selwyn PA, Alcabes P, Hartel D, et al. Clinical manifestations and predictors of disease progression in drug users with human immunodeficiency virus infection. *N Engl J Med* 1992;327:1697–1703.
65. Weinke T, Schiller R, Fehrenbach FJ, et al. Association between Staphylococcus aureus nasopharyngeal colonization and septicemia in patients infected with the human immunodeficiency virus. *Eur J Clin Microbiol Infect Dis* 1992;11:985–989.
66. Hirschtick RE, Glassroth J, Jordan MC, et al. Bacterial pneumonia in persons infected with the human immunodeficiency virus. Pulmonary Complications of HIV Infection Study Group. *N Engl J Med* 1995; 333:845–851.
67. Centers for Disease Control and Prevention. *Staphylococcus aureus* Resistant to Vancomycin—United States, 2002. *MMWR* 2002;51: 565–567.
68. Yamaguchi E, Chaisson RE. Gram-negative bacteremias in HIV-infected patients. Seventh International Conference on AIDS, Florence, Italy, 1991:539.
69. Kielhofner M, Atmar RL, Hamill RJ, et al. Life-threatening Pseudomonas aeruginosa infections in patients with human immunodeficiency virus infection. *Clin Infect Dis* 1992;14:403–411.
70. Mendelson MH, Gurtman A, Szabo S, et al. Pseudomonas aeruginosa bacteremia in patients with AIDS. *Clin Infect Dis* 1994;18:886–895.
71. Dropulic LK, Leslie JM, Eldred LJ, et al. Clinical manifestations and risk factors of Pseudomonas aeruginosa infection in patients with AIDS. *J Infect Dis* 1995;171:930–937.
72. Fichtenbaum CJ, Woeltje KF, Powderly WG. Serious Pseudomonas aeruginosa infections in patients infected with human immunodeficiency virus: a case-control study. *Clin Infect Dis* 1994;19:417–422.
73. Meynard JL, Barbut F, Guiguet M, et al. Pseudomonas aeruginosa infection in human immunodeficiency virus infected patients. *J Infect* 1999;38:176–181.
74. Horsburgh CR Jr. Mycobacterium avium complex infection in the acquired immunodeficiency syndrome. *N Engl J Med* 1991;324: 1332–1338.
75. du Moulin GC, Stottmeier KD, Pelletier PA, et al. Concentration of Mycobacterium avium by hospital hot water systems. *JAMA* 1988; 260:1599–1601.
76. von Reyn CF, Maslow JN, Barber TW, et al. Persistent colonisation of potable water as a source of Mycobacterium avium infection in AIDS. 1994.
77. Celis R, Torres A, Gatell JM, et al. Nosocomial pneumonia. A multivariate analysis of risk and prognosis. *Chest* 1988;93:318–324.
78. Haley RW, Hooton TM, Culver DH, et al. Nosocomial infections in U.S. hospitals, 1975–1976: estimated frequency by selected characteristics of patients. *Am J Med* 1981;70:947–959.
79. Torres A, Aznar R, Gatell JM, et al. Incidence, risk, and prognosis factors of nosocomial pneumonia in mechanically ventilated patients. *Am Rev Respir Dis* 1990;142:523–528.
80. Chastre J, Fagon JY. Ventilator-associated pneumonia. *Am J Respir Crit Care Med* 2002;165:867–903.
81. Janoff EN, Breiman RF, Daley CL, et al. Pneumococcal disease during HIV infection. Epidemiologic, clinical, and immunologic perspectives. *Ann Intern Med* 1992;117:314–324.
82. Simberkoff MS, El Sadr W, Schiffman G, et al. Streptococcus pneumoniae infections and bacteremia in patients with acquired immune deficiency syndrome, with report of a pneumococcal vaccine failure. *Am Rev Respir Dis* 1984;130:1174–1176.
83. Polsky B, Gold JW, Whimbey E, et al. Bacterial pneumonia in patients with the acquired immunodeficiency syndrome. *Ann Intern Med* 1986;104:38–41.
84. Fleming CA, Craven DE. Smoking and pneumococcal disease. *N Engl J Med* 2000;343:219–220.
85. Casadevall A, Dobroszycki J, Small C, et al. Haemophilus influenzae type b bacteremia in adults with AIDS and at risk for AIDS. *Am J Med* 1992;92:587–590.
86. Feldman C, Kallenbach JM, Miller SD, et al. Community-acquired pneumonia due to penicillin-resistant pneumococci. *N Engl J Med* 1985;313:615–617.
87. Blumberg HM, Rimland D. Nosocomial infection with penicillin-resistant pneumococci in patients with AIDS. *J Infect Dis* 1989;160: 725–726.
88. Smith PF, Stricof RL, Shayegani M, et al. Cluster of Haemophilus influenzae type b infections in adults. *JAMA* 1988;260:1446–1449.
89. Tumbarello M, Tacconelli E, de Gaetano DK, et al. Nosocomial bacterial pneumonia in human immunodeficiency virus infected subjects: incidence, risk factors and outcome. *Eur Respir J* 2001;17: 636–640.
90. Franzetti F, Cernuschi M, Esposito R, et al. Pseudomonas infections in patients with AIDS and AIDS-related complex. *J Intern Med* 1992; 231:437–443.
91. Peruzzi WT, Shapiro BA, Noskin GA, et al. Concurrent bacterial lung infection in patients with AIDS, PCP, and respiratory failure. *Chest* 1992;101:1399–1403.
92. Nichols L, Balogh K, Silverman M. Bacterial infections in the acquired immune deficiency syndrome. Clinicopathologic correlations in a series of autopsy cases. *Am J Clin Pathol* 1989;92:787–790.
93. Haron E, Bodey GP, Luna MA, et al. Has the incidence of Pneumocystis carinii pneumonia in cancer patients increased with the AIDS epidemic? *Lancet* 1988;2:904–905.
94. Chave JP, David S, Wauters JP, et al. Transmission of Pneumocystis carinii from AIDS patients to other immunosuppressed patients: a cluster of Pneumocystis carinii pneumonia in renal transplant recipients. *AIDS* 1991;5:927–932.
95. Singer C, Armstrong D, Rosen PP, et al. Pneumocystis carinii pneumonia: a cluster of eleven cases. *Ann Intern Med* 1975;82:772–777.
96. Chusid MJ, Heyrman KA. An outbreak of Pneumocystis carinii pneumonia at a pediatric hospital. *Pediatrics* 1978;62:1031–1035.
97. Olsson M, Sukura A, Lindberg LA, et al. Detection of Pneumocystis carinii DNA by filtration of air. *Scand J Infect Dis* 1996;28:279–282.
98. Hoover DR, Graham NM, Bacellar H, et al. Epidemiologic patterns of upper respiratory illness and Pneumocystis carinii pneumonia in homosexual men. 1991.
99. Helweg-Larsen J, Tsolaki AG, Miller RF, et al. Clusters of Pneumocystis carinii pneumonia: analysis of person-to-person transmission by genotyping. *Q J Med* 1998;91:813–820.
100. Anderson LJ. Major trends in nosocomial viral infections. *Am J Med* 1991;91:107S–111S.
101. Fuller JD, Craven DE, Steger KA, et al. Influenza vaccination of human immunodeficiency virus (HIV)-infected adults: impact on plasma levels of HIV type 1 RNA and determinants of antibody response. *Clin Infect Dis* 1999;28:541–547.
102. Staprans SI, Hamilton BL, Follansbee SE, et al. Activation of virus replication after vaccination of HIV-1–infected individuals. *J Exp Med* 1995;182:1727–1737.
103. Centers for Disease Control and Prevention. Prevention and treatment of tuberculosis among patients infected with human immunodeficiency virus: principles of therapy and revised recommendations. *MMWR* 1998;47(20):1–53.
104. Barnes PF, Bloch AB, Davidson PT, et al. Tuberculosis in patients with human immunodeficiency virus infection. *N Engl J Med* 1991; 324:1644–1650.
105. Frieden TR, Sterling T, Pablos-Mendez A, et al. The emergence of drug-resistant tuberculosis in New York City. *N Engl J Med* 1993; 328:521–526.
106. Jasmer RM, Hahn JA, Small PM, et al. A molecular epidemiologic

analysis of tuberculosis trends in San Francisco, 1991–1997. *Ann Intern Med* 1999;130:971–978.

107. Small PM, Fujiwara PI. Management of tuberculosis in the United States. *N Engl J Med* 2001;345:189–200.
108. Centers for Disease Control and Prevention. Tuberculosis morbidity—United States, 1997. *MMWR* 1998;47:253–257.
109. Dooley SW, Villarino ME, Lawrence M, et al. Nosocomial transmission of tuberculosis in a hospital unit for HIV-infected patients. *JAMA* 1992;267:2632–2634.
110. Small PM, Hopewell PC, Singh SP, et al. The epidemiology of tuberculosis in San Francisco. A population-based study using conventional and molecular methods. *N Engl J Med* 1994;330:1703–1709.
111. Daley CL, Small PM, Schecter GF, et al. An outbreak of tuberculosis with accelerated progression among persons infected with the human immunodeficiency virus. An analysis using restriction-fragment-length polymorphisms. *N Engl J Med* 1992;326:231–235.
112. Kenyon TA, Ridzon R, Luskin-Hawk R, et al. A nosocomial outbreak of multidrug-resistant tuberculosis. *Ann Intern Med* 1997;127:32–36.
113. Centers for Disease Control and Prevention. Drug susceptible tuberculosis outbreak in a state correctional facility housing HIV-infected inmates: South Carolina, 1999–2000. *MMWR* 2002;49:1041–1044.
114. Valway SE, Sanchez MP, Shinnick TF, et al. An outbreak involving extensive transmission of a virulent strain of Mycobacterium tuberculosis. *N Engl J Med* 1998;338:633–639.
115. Bellamy R, Ruwende C, Corrah T, et al. Variations in the NRAMP1 gene and susceptibility to tuberculosis in West Africans. *N Engl J Med* 1998;338:640–644.
116. Stead WW, Senner JW, Reddick WT, et al. Racial differences in susceptibility to infection by Mycobacterium tuberculosis. *N Engl J Med* 1990;322:422–427.
117. Kallman FJ, Reisner D. Twin studies on the significance of genetic factors in tuberculosis. *Am Rev Tuberc* 1942;47:549–574.
118. Pitchenik AE, Fertel D. Medical management of AIDS patients. Tuberculosis and nontuberculous mycobacterial disease. *Med Clin North Am* 1992;76:121–171.
119. Fischl MA, Uttamchandani RB, Daikos GL, et al. An outbreak of tuberculosis caused by multiple-drug-resistant tubercle bacilli among patients with HIV infection. *Ann Intern Med* 1992;117:177–183.
120. Kramer F, Modilevsky T, Waliany AR, et al. Delayed diagnosis of tuberculosis in patients with human immunodeficiency virus infection. *Am J Med* 1990;89:451–456.
121. Brudney K, Dobkin J. Resurgent tuberculosis in New York City. Human immunodeficiency virus, homelessness, and the decline of tuberculosis control programs. *Am Rev Respir Dis* 1991;144:745–749.
122. Di Perri G, Cruciani M, Danzi MC, et al. Nosocomial epidemic of active tuberculosis among HIV-infected patients. *Lancet* 1989;2:1502–1504.
123. Pierce JR Jr, Sims SL, Holman GH. Transmission of tuberculosis to hospital workers by a patient with AIDS. *Chest* 1992;101:581–582.
124. Pitchenik AE, Rubinson HA. The radiographic appearance of tuberculosis in patients with the acquired immune deficiency syndrome (AIDS) and pre-AIDS. *Am Rev Respir Dis* 1985;131:393–396.
125. Alland D, Kalkut GE, Moss AR, et al. Transmission of tuberculosis in New York City. An analysis by DNA fingerprinting and conventional epidemiologic methods. *N Engl J Med* 1994;330:1710–1716.
126. Centers for Disease Control. Transmission of multidrug-resistant tuberculosis among immunocompromised persons in a correctional system—New York, 1991. *MMWR* 1992;41:509.
127. Dooley SW, Jarvis WR, Martone WJ, et al. Multidrug-resistant tuberculosis. *Ann Intern Med* 1992;117:257–259.
128. Pearson ML, Jereb JA, Frieden TR, et al. Nosocomial transmission of multidrug-resistant Mycobacterium tuberculosis. A risk to patients and health care workers. *Ann Intern Med* 1992;117:191–196.
129. Burman WJ, Gallicano K, Peloquin C. Therapeutic implications of drug interactions in the treatment of human immunodeficiency virus-related tuberculosis. *Clin Infect Dis* 1999;28:419–429.
130. Spradling P, Drociuk D, McLaughlin S, et al. Drug-drug interactions in inmates treated for human immunodeficiency virus and Mycobacterium tuberculosis infection or disease: an institutional tuberculosis outbreak. *Clin Infect Dis* 2002;35:1106–1112.
131. Chien JW, Johnson JL. Paradoxical reactions in HIV and pulmonary TB. *Chest* 1998;114:933–936.
132. DeSimone JA, Pomerantz RJ, Babinchak TJ. Inflammatory reactions in HIV-1–infected persons after initiation of highly active antiretroviral therapy. *Ann Intern Med* 2000;133:447–454.
133. Orlovic D, Smego RA Jr. Paradoxical tuberculous reactions in HIV-infected patients. *Int J Tuberc Lung Dis* 2001;5:370–375.
134. Schluger NW, Perez D, Liu YM. Reconstitution of immune responses to tuberculosis in patients with HIV infection who receive antiretroviral therapy. *Chest* 2002;122:597–602.
135. Jasmer RM, Nahid P, Hopewell PC. Clinical practice. Latent tuberculosis infection. *N Engl J Med* 2002;347:1860–1866.
136. Jasmer RM, Saukkonen JJ, Blumberg HM, et al. Short-course rifampin and pyrazinamide compared with isoniazid for latent tuberculosis infection: a multicenter clinical trial.
137. Beck-Sague C, Dooley SW, Hutton MD, et al. Hospital outbreak of multidrug-resistant Mycobacterium tuberculosis infections. Factors in transmission to staff and HIV-infected patients. *JAMA* 1992;268:1280–1286.
138. Centers for Disease Control. Guidelines for preventing the transmission of tuberculosis in health-care settings, with special focus on HIV-related issues. *MMWR* 1994;43:1–33.
139. Manangan LP, Bennett CL, Tablan N, et al. Nosocomial tuberculosis prevention measures among two groups of US hospitals, 1992 to 1996. *Chest* 2000;117:380–384.
140. Gordin FM, Matts JP, Miller C, et al. A controlled trial of isoniazid in persons with anergy and human immunodeficiency virus infection who are at high risk for tuberculosis. Terry Beirn Community Programs for Clinical Research on AIDS. *N Engl J Med* 1997;337:315–320.
141. Jarvis WR, Hughes JP. Nosocomial gastrointestinal infections. In: Wenzel RP, ed. *Prevention and control of nosocomial infections,* 2nd ed. Baltimore: Williams & Wilkins, 1993:708–740.
142. Zaidi M, Ponce dL, Ortiz RM, et al. Hospital-acquired diarrhea in adults: a prospective case-controlled study in Mexico. *Infect Control Hosp Epidemiol* 1991;12:349–355.
143. Sperber SJ, Schleupner CJ. Salmonellosis during infection with human immunodeficiency virus. *Rev Infect Dis* 1987;9:925–934.
144. Smith PD, Quinn TC, Strober W, et al. NIH conference. Gastrointestinal infections in AIDS. *Ann Intern Med* 1992;116:63–77.
145. Jacobs JL, Gold JW, Murray HW, et al. Salmonella infections in patients with the acquired immunodeficiency syndrome. *Ann Intern Med* 1985;102:186–188.
146. Baskin DH, Lax JD, Barenberg D. Shigella bacteremia in patients with the acquired immune deficiency syndrome. *Am J Gastroenterol* 1987;82:338–341.
147. Perlman DM, Ampel NM, Schifman RB, et al. Persistent Campylobacter jejuni infections in patients infected with the human immunodeficiency virus (HIV). *Ann Intern Med* 1988;108:540–546.
148. Antony MA, Brandt LJ, Klein RS, et al. Infectious diarrhea in patients with AIDS. *Dig Dis Sci* 1988;33:1141–1146.
149. Jacobson MA, Mills J. Serious cytomegalovirus disease in the acquired immunodeficiency syndrome (AIDS). Clinical findings, diagnosis, and treatment. *Ann Intern Med* 1988;108:585–594.
150. Soave R. Cryptosporidiosis and isosporiasis in patients with AIDS. *Infect Dis Clin North Am* 1988;2:485–493.
151. Shadduck JA. Human microsporidiosis and AIDS. *Rev Infect Dis* 1989;11:203–207.
152. Lake-Bakaar G, Quadros E, Beidas S, et al. Gastric secretory failure in patients with the acquired immunodeficiency syndrome (AIDS). *Ann Intern Med* 1988;109:502–504.
153. Simor AE, Bradley SF, Strausbaugh LJ, et al. Clostridium difficile in long-term-care facilities for the elderly. *Infect Control Hosp Epidemiol* 2002;23:696–703.
154. Pulvirenti JJ, Gerding DN, Nathan C, et al. Difference in the incidence of Clostridium difficile among patients infected with human immunodeficiency virus admitted to a public hospital and a private hospital. *Infect Control Hosp Epidemiol* 2002;23:641–647.
155. Barbut F, Meynard JL, Guiguet M, et al. Clostridium difficile-associated diarrhea in HIV-infected patients: epidemiology and risk factors. *J Acquir Immune Defic Syndr Hum Retrovirol* 1997;16:176–181.

156. Tumbarello M, Tacconelli E, Leone F, et al. Clostridium difficile-associated diarrhoea in patients with human immunodeficiency virus infection: a case-control study. *Eur J Gastroenterol Hepatol* 1995;7: 259–263.
157. Steere AC, Hall WJ III, Wells JG, et al. Person-to-person spread of Salmonella typhimurium after a hospital common-source outbreak. *Lancet* 1975;1:319–322.
158. Marrie TJ, Lee SH, Faulkner RS, et al. Rotavirus infection in a geriatric population. *Arch Intern Med* 1982;142:313–316.
159. Jarvis WR, Middleton PJ, Gelfand EW. Significance of viral infections in severe combined immunodeficiency disease. *Pediatr Infect Dis* 1983;2:187–192.
160. Koch KL, Phillips DJ, Aber RC, et al. Cryptosporidiosis in hospital personnel. Evidence for person-to-person transmission. *Ann Intern Med* 1985;102:593–596.
161. Hayes EB, Matte TD, O'Brien TR, et al. Large community outbreak of cryptosporidiosis due to contamination of a filtered public water supply. *N Engl J Med* 1989;320:1372–1376.
162. Carr A, Marriott D, Field A, et al. Treatment of HIV-1–associated microsporidiosis and cryptosporidiosis with combination antiretroviral therapy. *Lancet* 1998;351:256–261.
163. Holmberg SD, Moorman AC, Von Bargen JC, et al. Possible effectiveness of clarithromycin and rifabutin for cryptosporidiosis chemoprophylaxis in HIV disease. HIV Outpatient Study (HOPS) Investigators. *JAMA* 1998;279:384–386.
164. Ravn P, Lundgren JD, Kjaeldgaard P, et al. et al. Nosocomial outbreak of cryptosporidiosis in AIDS patients. *BMJ* 1991;302:277–280.
165. Haley RW, Culver DH, Morgan WM, et al. Identifying patients at high risk of surgical wound infection. A simple multivariate index of patient susceptibility and wound contamination. *Am J Epidemiol* 1985;121:206–215.
166. Schneider PA, Abrams DI, Rayner AA, et al. Immunodeficiency-associated thrombocytopenic purpura (IDTP). Response to splenectomy. *Arch Surg* 1987;122:1175–1178.
167. Wilson SE, Robinson G, Williams RA, et al. Acquired immune deficiency syndrome (AIDS). Indications for abdominal surgery, pathology, and outcome. *Ann Surg* 1989;210:428–433.
168. Whitney TM, Macho JR, Russell TR, et al. Appendicitis in acquired immunodeficiency syndrome. *Am J Surg* 1992;164:467–470.
169. Buehrer JL, Weber DJ, Meyer AA, et al. Wound infection rates after invasive procedures in HIV-1 seropositive versus HIV-1 seronegative hemophiliacs. *Ann Surg* 1990;211:492–498.
170. Guth AA, Hofstetter SR, Pachter HL. Human immunodeficiency virus and the trauma patient: factors influencing postoperative infectious complications. *J Trauma* 1996;41:251–255.
171. Martinez-Gimeno C, Acero-Sanz J, et al. Maxillofacial trauma: influence of HIV infection. *J Craniomaxillofac Surg* 1992;20:297–302.
172. Raviglione MC, Mariuz P, Pablos-Mendez A, et al. High Staphylococcus aureus nasal carriage rate in patients with acquired immunodeficiency syndrome or AIDS-related complex. *Am J Infect Control* 1990; 18:64–69.
173. O'Regan S, Russo P, Lapointe N, et al. AIDS and the urinary tract. *J AIDS* 1990;3:244–251.
174. Kaplan MS, Wechsler M, Benson MC. Urologic manifestations of AIDS. *J AIDS* 1987;30:441–443.
175. Benson MC, Kaplan MS, O'Toole K, et al. A report of cytomegalovirus cystitis and a review of other genitourinary manifestations of the acquired immune deficiency syndrome. *J Urol* 1988;140:153–154.
176. Durand ML, Calderwood SB, Weber DJ, et al. Acute bacterial meningitis in adults. A review of 493 episodes. *N Engl J Med* 1993;328: 21–28.
177. McArthur JC. Neurologic manifestations of AIDS. *Medicine (Baltimore)* 1987;66:407–437.
178. Kales CP, Holzman RS. Listeriosis in patients with HIV infection: clinical manifestations and response to therapy. J *AIDS* 1990;3: 139–143.
179. Mascola L, Lieb L, Chiu J, et al. Listeriosis: an uncommon opportunistic infection in patients with acquired immunodeficiency syndrome. A report of five cases and a review of the literature. *Am J Med* 1988; 84:162–164.
180. Crowe HM, Lichtenberg DA, Craven DE. Nosocomial infection in adult patients with sickle cell anemia. *Infect Control Hosp Epidemiol* 1988;9:405–408.
181. Patterson JE, Madden GM, Krisiunas EP, et al. A nosocomial outbreak of ampicillin-resistant Haemophilus influenzae type b in a geriatric unit. *J Infect Dis* 1988;157:1002–1007.
182. Michelson A, Schuster B, Kamp HD. Paranasal sinusitis associated with nasotracheal and orotracheal long term intubation. *Arch Otolaryngol Head Neck Surg* 1992;118:937–939.
183. Caplan ES, Hoyt NJ. Nosocomial sinusitis. *JAMA* 1982;247: 639–641.
184. Godofsky EW, Zinreich J, Armstrong M, et al. Sinusitis in HIV-infected patients: a clinical and radiographic review. *Am J Med* 1992; 93:163–170.
185. Zurlo JJ, Feuerstein IM, Lebovics R, et al. Sinusitis in HIV-1 infection. *Am J Med* 1992;93:157–162.
186. Hughes WT, Armstrong D, Bodey GP, et al. From the Infectious Diseases Society of America. Guidelines for the use of antimicrobial agents in neutropenic patients with unexplained fever. *J Infect Dis* 1990;161:381–396.
187. Murphy MF, Metcalfe P, Waters AH, et al. Incidence and mechanism of neutropenia and thrombocytopenia in patients with human immunodeficiency virus infection. *Br J Haematol* 1987;66:337–340.
188. Meynard JL, Guiguet M, Arsac S, et al. Frequency and risk factors of infectious complications in neutropenic patients infected with HIV. *AIDS* 1997;11:995–998.
189. Keiser P, Higgs E, Smith J. Neutropenia is associated with bacteremia in patients infected with the human immunodeficiency virus. *Am J Med Sci* 1996;312:118–122.
190. Jacobson MA, Liu RC, Davies D, et al. Human immunodeficiency virus disease-related neutropenia and the risk of hospitalization for bacterial infection. *Arch Intern Med* 1997;157:1825–1831.
191. Moore RD, Keruly JC, Chaisson RE. Neutropenia and bacterial infection in acquired immunodeficiency syndrome. *Arch Intern Med* 1995; 155:1965–1970.
192. Farber BF, Lesser M, Kaplan MH, et al. Clinical significance of neutropenia in patients with human immunodeficiency virus infection. *Infect Control Hosp Epidemiol* 1991;12:429–434.
193. Denning DW, Follansbee SE, Scolaro M, et al. Pulmonary aspergillosis in the acquired immunodeficiency syndrome. *N Engl J Med* 1991; 324:654–662.
194. Pursell KJ, Telzak EE, Armstrong D. Aspergillus species colonization and invasive disease in patients with AIDS. *Clin Infect Dis* 1992;14: 141–148.
195. Till M, Lee N, Soper WD, et al. Typhlitis in patients with HIV-1 infection. *Ann Intern Med* 1992;116:998–1000.
196. Pluda JM, Yarchoan R, Jaffe ES, et al. Development of non-Hodgkin lymphoma in a cohort of patients with severe human immunodeficiency virus (HIV) infection on long-term antiretroviral therapy. *Ann Intern Med* 1990;113:276–282.
197. Krown SE, Myskowski PL, Paredes J. Medical management of AIDS patients. Kaposi's sarcoma. *Med Clin North Am* 1992;76:235–252.
198. Valenti WM, Hall CB, Douglas JR, et al. Nosocomial viral infections. I. Epidemiology and significance. 1980;1:33–37. *Infect Control* 1980; 1:33–37.
199. Morens DM, Bregman DJ, West CM, et al. An outbreak of varicella-zoster virus infection among cancer patients. *Ann Intern Med* 1980; 93:414–419.
200. Cohen PR, Beltrani VP, Grossman ME. Disseminated herpes zoster in patients with human immunodeficiency virus infection. *Am J Med* 1988;84:1076–1080.
201. Jacobson MA, Berger TG, Fikrig S, et al. Acyclovir-resistant varicella zoster virus infection after chronic oral acyclovir therapy in patients with the acquired immunodeficiency syndrome (AIDS). *Ann Intern Med* 1990;112:187–191.
202. Gallant JE, Moore RD, Richman DD, et al. Incidence and natural history of cytomegalovirus disease in patients with advanced human immunodeficiency virus disease treated with zidovudine. The Zidovudine Epidemiology Study Group. *J Infect Dis* 1992;166: 1223–1227.

58

NOSOCOMIAL INFECTIONS IN PATIENTS WITH NEOPLASTIC DISEASES

ADITYA H. GAUR
PATRICIA M. FLYNN

Since the middle of the 20th century, patients with cancer have had an added risk of infection because of the use of immunosuppressive chemotherapy and radiation. In recent years the risk has been enhanced by the use of indwelling central venous catheters (CVCs) (1), more intensive therapy, and the use of bone marrow transplantation. Additionally, patients with neoplastic disease have a more prolonged and repeated contact with the hospital environment, which sometimes involves invasive procedures. Moreover, some patients now admitted with malignancy have an underlying infection with human immunodeficiency virus type 1, imposing a profound effect on the immune system (2). It must be kept in mind that the neoplastic process often has less of an effect on host susceptibility to nosocomial infections than the therapeutic process. One must also appreciate that the main priority is successful anticancer therapy, despite the iatrogenic side effects. Overall, advances in the field of oncology often test the fine balance between more aggressive therapy leading to improved survival and not losing ground because of complications, predominantly infections. Early diagnosis, treatment, containment, and prevention of nosocomial infections are of great importance to the management of neoplastic diseases.

EPIDEMIOLOGY

Cancer patients present the hospital epidemiologist with several special problems. Foremost is the similarity of nosocomial and community-acquired infections (CAIs) in this population. The etiology of an infection in a febrile neutropenic patient acquired at home may be the same as that acquired in the hospital. Many such infections are derived from microorganisms carried as usual flora of the skin and mucous membranes of the alimentary, respiratory, and genitourinary tracts. Under these circumstances, the incubation period cannot be used to determine the relationship of an acute infection to the time of admission to the hospital. Thus, when the cancer patient manifests signs and symptoms of infection while hospitalized, the causative microorganism (e.g., *E. coli, P. aeruginosa, Staphylococcus* species, *Streptococcus* species, *Klebsiella* species, *Candida* species, or *Aspergillus* species) might have been acquired before admission, during a previous hospitalization, or after a current admission to the hospital. The endogenous microbial flora may change after hospitalization. Especially during prolonged hospital courses, microorganisms of the hospital environment may be acquired that will increase the patient's risk for an infectious episode. Despite all this, although immunosuppression and malignancy may lead to some unique types of infections due to opportunistic microorganisms, cancer patients are also susceptible to the same infections encountered in the immunocompetent patient such as respiratory and gastrointestinal viral infections.

The ability to diagnose viral infections with increased sensitivity using polymerase chain reaction (PCR)-based techniques has raised the question about differentiating reactivation of latent viral infections versus a new infection. Latent infections acquired early in life may become activated during immunosuppression and hospitalization. These must be differentiated from acute primary infections caused by the same microorganism that could have been acquired after hospitalization. Notable among these are the herpesvirus infections, including herpes simplex lesions and cytomegalovirus disease. Also, recurrent varicella-zoster virus (VZV) infection in the form of disseminated zoster is sometimes difficult to differentiate from primary varicella. Evidence suggests that some cases of *Pneumocystis carinii* pneumonitis may be acutely acquired infections in the hospital rather than the more usual reactivation of latent infection.

Another problem is difficulty in establishing the etiology of an infectious episode in the immunocompromised cancer patient. Since most infections are due to commensal or opportunistic microorganisms of the normal microbial flora, the isolation of a microorganism by culture may not necessarily prove it to be the cause of the illness. For example, in the febrile neutropenic patient, a microorganism such as *Corynebacterium* species when isolated from a blood culture may be the causative agent or may merely be a skin commensal or contaminant of the culture. Additionally, often the recognition of an infected site is difficult. In the severely neutropenic and anemic patient with cancer, the key signs of infection may be absent because of a lack of inflammatory response. *Staphylococcus aureus* may be introduced nosocomially at the time of a finger stick for a blood count.

Without neutrophils, no infiltration occurs, so swelling and pain of the affected finger may be absent; furthermore, the anemia does not allow the appearance of erythema, so the sole manifestation of the infected finger stick site may be local pain or fever. Meningeal infection in the neutropenic patient occurs without the typical signs of meningeal inflammation such as a stiff neck, and no neutrophils and hypoglycorrhachia will be found in the spinal fluid. Even with fairly extensive bacterial infection in the lung parenchyma, the neutropenic patient may not be able to muster sufficient inflammatory response to create a density recognizable by chest radiograph.

Furthermore, because of the multidisciplinary management, some cancer patients may move through many sites during one hospitalization, such as the operating room, intensive care unit, medical service, physical rehabilitation units, and diagnostic imaging and irradiation departments. Under such circumstances, tracking the source of infection sometimes requires exhaustive epidemiologic investigation.

Finally, standard meaningful definitions of hospital-acquired opportunistic infections are lacking and may vary from one institution to another. When reviewing the literature pertaining to surveillance of nosocomial infections in patients with cancer, one has to be cognizant of the criteria used to define such infections and the denominator used to quantify them; the characteristics of patient populations primarily in terms of risk factors, such as duration of neutropenia; the existing infection control policies, including antimicrobial prophylaxis; and the type of resources available to diagnose infections. In two prospective surveillance studies in adult and pediatric hematology-oncology patients from Bonn, Germany, the authors noted an overall nosocomial infection rate of 11 and 10.8 per 1,000 patient-days, respectively, with roughly 75% of the infections occurring in patients who were neutropenic (3,4). To ensure comparability of surveillance data, these authors recommend that all surveillance studies in the cancer population should include infection rates based on number of patient-days at risk, where "at risk" may be defined as a period of neutropenia.

Thus, the hospital epidemiologist must consider these and other nuances of the compromised host with cancer when searching for nosocomial infections. Molecular techniques to characterize microbes by subcellular and genetic components are evolving as powerful tools for hospital epidemiology. Analysis of chromosomal DNA by pulsed-field gel electrophoresis, ribotyping, and random primer PCR methods permits more precise characterization than more conventional phenotyping techniques.

PATHOGENESIS OF NOSOCOMIAL INFECTIONS IN PATIENTS WITH NEOPLASTIC DISEASE

The primary factor in the pathogenesis of infections in the cancer patient is a defect in host defense. In most patients, the defect is an iatrogenic impairment of the immune system such as suppression of B lymphocytes and antibody production, impairment of T lymphocytes impeding cell-mediated responses, or neutropenia due to intensive chemotherapy or irradiation. However, a breach in the integrity of the skin and mucous membranes is a frequent portal of entry for microbes composing the flora of these sites, especially in the neutropenic patient. A tumor mass may obstruct a vital organ, impair circulation, or invade adjacent tissue, providing a nidus for infection. Because of the extensive use of antibiotics, the normal microbial flora is deranged, and overgrowth of more pathogenic microorganisms occurs. The most frequent single defect predisposing to serious and life-threatening nosocomial infections in cancer patients is neutropenia. Easy access to the absolute neutrophil count plus available data on its predictability for infection make this marker useful in both surveillance and management of cancer patients in hospitals.

The type, dose, and duration of use of anticancer drugs help identify patients at high risk for infection. Not all patients with cancer and not all anticancer drugs are associated with immunosuppression. Anticancer drugs associated with bone marrow suppression leading to neutropenia include cyclophosphamide, chlorambucil, ifosfamide, melphalan, thiotepa, busulfan, procarbazine, nitrosourea compounds, platinum complexes, triazenes, methotrexate, cytarabine, fluorouracil, mercaptopurine, thioguanine, hydroxyurea, dactinomycin, vincristine, vinblastine, and etoposide.

Prednisone, although not a cause of neutropenia, is a potent inhibitor of both humoral and cell-mediated immune responses, especially T-lymphocyte activity. Cyclosporin specifically affects T lymphocytes by decreasing $CD4^+$ lymphocytes and interleukin-2 synthesis. Irradiation and malnutrition cause decreases in T-lymphocyte function.

Some anticancer drugs with little or no effect on the immune response and the neutrophil count are bleomycin, asparaginase, tamoxifen, diethylstilbestrol, testosterone, and megestrol.

Indwelling central catheters and other intravascular access devices, prosthetic devices such as central nervous system shunts and artificial extremities, endotracheal intubation, surgery, and exposure to intensive care unit environments are also important in the pathogenesis of many infections in cancer patients. These are not discussed here because they are covered in Chapters 17, 18, 21, 22, 27, 49, and 67, and because there are no significantly unique features of these infections in the cancer patient.

ETIOLOGIES OF INFECTION

Nosocomial infections in cancer patients can be caused by a variety of infectious microorganisms, but the most common pathogens are bacterial. In previous reports from oncology centers, bacterial microorganisms were isolated in over 75% of nosocomial infections, fungal pathogens in approximately 3% to 10%, and viruses in only 2% (5,6). Although in an oncology intensive care unit fungal infections comprised 22% of nosocomial infections (7), in another study of nosocomial infections in neutropenic patients 19% were due to fungi (8). As mentioned earlier when making comparisons between studies and centers, one has to keep in mind the differences in definitions and in patient and institute characteristics. Polymicrobial infections are not uncommon in this patient population. Robinson et al. (6) noted multiple isolates in one third of their infections. Both multiple bacterial isolates and mixed infections can occur.

Table 58.1 lists most bacteria, fungi, viruses, and protozoa associated with infections in patients with malignancies.

Bacterial Infections

The most important bacterial nosocomial pathogens are *S. aureus, E. coli, P. aeruginosa*, and coagulase-negative staphylococci (5,6) (see Chapters 28, 30, 33, and 34). Together these four microorganisms account for over half of nosocomial bacterial infections in cancer patients.

Gram-Negative Microorganisms

As a family, Enterobacteriaceae are common nosocomial pathogens in cancer patients. *E. coli* and *Klebsiella pneumoniae* predominate (6,9). These microorganisms, along with *Serratia* species (10), *Enterobacter* species (11), and *Citrobacter* species (12), have been isolated in sporadic infections and in epidemics. They are common causes of bacteremia, pneumonia, and urinary tract infections (UTIs). Frequently, patients are already receiving antibiotic therapy when these infections develop (9–12). *P. aeruginosa* is the most notorious pathogen in patients with malignancies. It is associated with nosocomial bacteremia, pneumonia, and urinary tract and wound infection. Although a frequent nosocomial pathogen, it has a special predilection for granulocytopenic hosts. In a review of *P. aeruginosa* infections in cancer patients in the 1990s, Maschmeyer and Braveny (13) note that the proportion of these infections among cases of gram-negative bacteremia over the past two decades has not generally declined with marked local and regional differences in incidence of infections. Infections with *P. aeruginosa* account for approximately 10% of all nosocomial infections in cancer patients (5,6,14). In the hospital environment, *P. aeruginosa* is associated with respiratory equipment, sinks, and fresh fruit and vegetables. Colonization often precedes infection (14,15). The case fatality rate for *P. aeruginosa* infections is reported to be as high as 65% to 70%, which is significantly higher than the rate for other gram-negative bacterial infections (15,16). Newer antimicrobial agents with improved anti-*Pseudomonas* activity may lower the fatality rates (17).

TABLE 58.1. CAUSES OF INFECTIONS IN THE PATIENT WITH CANCER

Bacterial	*Yersinia enterocolitica*
Gram-positive	*Zymononas* species
Bacillus species	Anaerobic coccl and bacilli
Corynebacterium species[a]	*Bacteroides* species
Enterococcus fecalis[a]	*Clostridium* species
Listeria monocytogenes	*Fusobacterium* species
Staphylococcus aureus[a]	*Peptococcus* species
Staphylococcus, coagulase-negative[a]	*Peptostreptococcus* species
Streptococcus pneumoniae[a]	*Propionibacterium* species
Streptococcus pyogenes[a]	*Veillonella* species
Streptococcus, viridans group[a]	Other
Gram-negative	Mycobacteria
Aeromonas species	*Nocardia asteroides*
Acinetobacter species	Nonbacterial
Actinobacillus species	Viral
Alcaligenes species	Adenoviruses[a]
Capnocytophagia species	Cytomegalovirus[a]
Chromobacterium species	Epstein-Barr virus
Citrobacter species	Enteroviruses
Edwardsiella species	Herpesvirus hominis (simplex)[a]
Eikenella species	Influenza viruses
Enterobacter species[a]	Parainfluenza viruses
Erwinia species	Parvovirus
Escherichia coli[a]	Respiratory syncytial virus
Flavobacterium species	Rotavirus[a]
Gardnerella species	Varicella-zoster virus[a]
Hatnia species	Papillomavirus
Haemophilus influenzae[a]	Fungi
Kingella species	*Pseudallescheria boydii*
Klebsiella species[a]	*Alternaria* species
Legionella species	*Aspergillus* species[a]
Moraxella species	*Candida* species[a]
Morganella species	*Coccidiodes immitis*
Neisseria species	*Dreshleria exohilum*
Proteus species[a]	*Fusarium* species
Providencia species	*Geotrichum*
Pseudomonas aeruginosa[a]	*Histoplasma capsulatum*
Pseudomonas, not *aeruginosa*	*Mucor* species
Salmonella species[a]	*Penicillium* species
Serratia marcescens	*Rhizopus* species
Shigella species	Protozoa
Stenotrophomonas maltophilia	*Cryptosporidium* species[a]
	Pneumocystis carinii
	Toxoplasma gondii

[a] Most freauent.

A variety of other gram-negative microorganisms have also been linked with nosocomial infections in cancer patients. The *Legionella* species are fastidious gram-negative bacilli. Approximately 42% of cancer patients with Legionnaire's disease are infected in a hospital setting. Use of steroids and neutropenia appear to have causal roles (18). *Stenotrophomonas maltophilia* (previously *Xanthomonas maltophilia*) has been reported as a cause of bacteremia, UTI, pneumonia, and wound infections in cancer patients. It is most often detected in patients who have received antibiotics and respiratory therapy. The microorganism has been isolated from hospital sinks and respirators. The association between the use of respiratory equipment and isolation of *S. maltophilia* from sputum suggests that the equipment may be a significant reservoir for the microorganism (19).

Gram-Positive Microorganisms

S. aureus was the most frequent bacterial isolate in two surveys of nosocomial pathogens in cancer patients, accounting for 14% to 18% of isolates (5,6). Surgical sites were most often involved. Coagulase-negative staphylococcal infections have increased dramatically over the past decade; these microorganisms are the most common microorganisms isolated from bloodstream infections in some centers (20,21). The rise of these relatively nonpathogenic bacteria has been linked to the use of tunneled CVCs such as the Hickman catheter.

α-Hemolytic streptococci are normal inhabitants of the oropharynx that invade through damaged mucous membranes and cause bacteremia and pneumonia in cancer patients. A syndrome of severe shock and adult respiratory distress syndrome can result. There is a potential causal relationship with cytosine arabinoside administration (22,23).

Clusters of *Corynebacterium jeikeium* bacteremia have been

reported from several cancer centers (24–26). Risk factors include immunosuppression and use of plastic devices such as intravenous catheters. Some evidence suggests that patient-to-patient transmission does not occur (26). The microorganism is resistant to multiple antibiotics, and vancomycin is the suggested therapy.

Anaerobes

Anaerobes are infrequent nosocomial pathogens in the oncology patient and are isolated in less than 5% of infections. Usually, obvious disruption of normal gastrointestinal barriers are apparent when infections do occur (27).

Antibiotic-Resistant Bacteria

Widespread use of antibiotics, both prophylactic and empiric, have resulted in nosocomial infections caused by multiply resistant microorganisms. Methicillin-resistant *S. aureus*, vancomycin-resistant enterococci, and fluoroquinolone-resistant enteric microorganisms have been reported to cause significant problems in an oncology population (28–30). Prudent use of antibiotics and careful surveillance of this population is necessary to detect and control the spread of these pathogens.

Fungal Infections

Candida

Candida albicans is the most common fungal pathogen in cancer patients (see Chapter 39). However, studies have noted increases in the frequency of other *Candida* species, including *C. tropicalis, C. parapsilosis,* and *C. krusei* (31). Within individual cancer centers, a significant species shift has been noted even within the non–*C. albicans* group, such as an increase in *C. parapsilosis* and decrease in *C. tropicalis* (32). Overall, these differences between institutions to some extent are influenced by institutional antifungal prophylaxis guidelines, use of indwelling catheters, as well as types of malignancies treated. Fungemia, pneumonia, UTI, or disseminated disease with involvement of the abdominal viscera may occur. Infections are usually preceded by colonization of the gastrointestinal tract with the offending microorganism, but common-source outbreaks have also been reported. Risk factors include the use of antibiotics, colonization with the microorganism, neutropenia, and the presence of tunneled CVCs.

Aspergillus

Although it is clear that the incidence of invasive aspergillosis has been increasing in patients with cancer, especially those with hematologic malignancies and bone marrow transplant recipients (33), controversy exists regarding the definition of nosocomial versus community-acquired infection. This is in part due to factors such as an unknown incubation period and size of "infectious" inoculum as well as lack of a uniform, reliable methodology for environmental sampling in studies that attempt to trace the source of infection (34). The overall case fatality rate of this disease is very high, with the highest being in bone marrow transplant recipients (35). Sites most often involved include the lungs and paranasal sinuses. Inhalation of conidia is requisite to the development of this infection. Direct inoculation of *Aspergillus* species spores from occlusive materials, such as tape, has also been reported.

Other Fungal Microorganisms

Historically, although *C. albicans* accounts for the majority of infections in compromised patients, recent epidemiological trends indicate a shift toward infections by *Aspergillus* species, non-*albicans Candida* species, as well as previously uncommon hyaline filamentous fungi (such as *Fusarium* species, *Acremonium* species, *Pseudallescheria boydi),* dematiaceous filamentous fungi (such as *Bipolaris* species and *Alternaria* species), and yeast-like pathogens (such as *Trichosporon* species and *Malassezia* species) (36). These emerging pathogens are increasingly encountered as causing life-threatening invasive infections that are often refractory to conventional therapies. Increasing use of antifungal prophylaxis may be linked with the emergence of these microorganisms.

Viral Infections

Overall, viruses account for relatively few nosocomial infections. This number is likely to increase as viral diagnostic technology improves. Known nosocomial pathogens include VZV (37,38), respiratory syncytial virus (RSV) (39), influenza, and rotavirus (40). Hepatitis B and hepatitis C have also been reported from other countries as nosocomial pathogens in children with cancer (41,42).

CLINICAL MANIFESTATIONS

Certain points regarding clinical manifestations of infections in patients with cancer are important to remember. Fever is the most frequent manifestation of nosocomial infection in the cancer patient. When fever occurs, especially in the setting of neutropenia, a diagnostic workup, including a careful history, physical examination, and bacterial and fungal cultures of blood, urine, stool, and any obvious sites of infection such as wounds, should be done before beginning therapy. Bloodstream infections most often present with fever with or without evidence of shock. Catheter-related bacteremias or fungemias may present with chills or rigors after flushing the catheter. If a tunneled CVC is in place, all lumens and ports should be cultured. In addition, if symptoms are present, a chest radiograph, and possibly sinus radiographs, should also be obtained. If no source of infection is identified by the diagnostic workup, the criteria for fever of unknown origin may be met.

Although wound or other cutaneous infections may be diagnosed by the presence of erythema, induration, or purulence at a surgical site, intravenous catheter site, or previously uninvolved area, neutropenic cancer patients often may not be able to mount an inflammatory response, and local infection may be heralded only by pain or fever. This is often the case with perirectal cellulitis, a serious and potentially fatal infection in oncology patients. Rectal pain or pain on defecation should alert clinicians to this possibility. In the absence of neutrophils, extensive bacterial invasion of the meninges may occur without the typical signs of meningeal inflammation, or of the lung without a discernible infiltrate by radiograph, or of the skin without swelling, cellulitis, or formation of pus and abscesses. Alternatively, local or radiographic findings may worsen with the return of neutrophils, often in the presence of improving fever curve and clinical course.

Differentiating an infection from side effects of chemotherapy or radiation can sometimes be very difficult, and not uncommonly empiric treatment for an infection is started while awaiting further information.

SITES OF NOSOCOMIAL INFECTIONS

Bloodstream Infections

Overall, bloodstream infections account for approximately 20% of nosocomial infections in cancer patients (5,6). In two recently published prospective surveillance studies of nosocomial infections in adult and pediatric hematology oncology patients, 43% to 52% of nosocomial infections were bloodstream infections (3,4). The usual definition is the isolation of any pathogen in one or more blood cultures from a patient with clinical symptoms (5,6). Even though microorganisms known to colonize the skin, such as coagulase-negative staphylococci and *Corynebacterium* species (but not *C. jeikeium*), are the most common contaminants of blood cultures, coagulase-negative staphylococcus, especially in the presence of an indwelling catheter, is also a common "true" pathogen.

Currently, gram-positive microorganisms are isolated more often than gram-negative bacteria (8). Before 1960, *S. aureus* was the most common nosocomial pathogen. After adequate antistaphylococcal drugs were introduced, the gram-negative microorganisms gained prominence. More recently, the trend has been toward increasing numbers of gram-positive isolates. Most authors speculate that the increasing use of tunneled CVCs and the concomitant increase in the number of coagulase-negative staphylococcal infections are responsible for this shift (43). The widespread use of second- and third-generation cephalosporins for the empiric treatment of febrile neutropenia has also been speculated to explain this shift. Because these antibiotics have improved gram-negative coverage at the expense of gram-positive coverage, breakthrough nosocomial bacteremias are likely to be of gram-positive origin (44). Fungemia, most often with *Candida* species, is also increasing among oncology patients (45).

Multiple reports note that patients with hematologic malignancies, such as leukemia and lymphoma, are at increased risk of nosocomial bloodstream infections when compared with patients with solid tumors (43,46,47). Mayo and Wenzel (47) noted that leukemics had an infection rate 15 times greater than that of patients with solid tumors. In their study, patients with solid tumors were at no greater risk for bloodstream infections than patients without malignancies.

In addition to different rates of infection, the infecting microorganisms are different for patients with hematologic malignancies compared with those with solid tumors. *E. coli* and *S. aureus* are common pathogens in both groups. Patients with hematologic malignancies have more infections due to *P. aeruginosa* and *K. pneumoniae*, and patients with solid tumors have more infections due to *Bacteroides* species (46). Coagulase-negative staphylococcal infections are also more common in patients with hematologic malignancies (43). Patients who have undergone splenectomy as treatment for malignancy, such as those with Hodgkin's disease, have an increased risk for *Streptococcus pneumoniae* bacteremia (46).

The portal of entry of nosocomial pathogens can often be identified in this population. The most common sites are the respiratory tract, the gastrointestinal tract, and the skin (43,48). Surgical procedures, especially in patients with solid tumors, also provide a common portal of entry (46).

The risk factors for developing nosocomial bloodstream infections include hematologic malignancies, prolonged hospitalization, and bone marrow transplantation (43). Patients with hematologic malignancies are at increased risk because of the intensive cytotoxic chemotherapy, which often renders them pancytopenic for long periods. Mayo and Wenzel (47) noted that over 75% of nosocomial bloodstream infections in leukemic patients occurred when the absolute neutrophil count was below 100 cells/mL. As the intensity of therapy for solid tumor patients increases, so may the rate of nosocomial bloodstream infections.

The prognosis of nosocomial bloodstream infection is related to many factors, including the microorganism causing the sepsis, the source of infection, the absolute neutrophil count, the bone marrow status, and the presence or absence of shock (46). In general, the mortality rate of infections caused by gram-negative microorganisms is greater than that of infections caused by gram-positive microorganisms (43). *P. aeruginosa* and *K. pneumoniae* are often associated with high mortality rates. Bloodstream infections that are polymicrobial or that are associated with pulmonary or intraabdominal infections also carry a high mortality rate (46).

Respiratory Tract Infections

Nosocomial infections of the respiratory tract include pneumonia, sinusitis, pharyngitis, otitis, and rhinitis (see Chapters 22, 23, and 49). These infections account for slightly over 20% of nosocomial infections in cancer patients. Rotstein et al. (5) noted them to be the most common infection at Roswell Park Memorial Institute in 1983 and 1984, accounting for 30% of their reported nosocomial infections.

The most frequently isolated microorganisms include *S. aureus, P. aeruginosa, E. coli,* and *K. pneumoniae* (5,6). Fungal microorganisms, including *Candida* species and *Aspergillus* species, account for a smaller percentage of infections. Frequently, the infecting microorganism is unknown because an invasive procedure would be required to isolate the pathogen. This is common with upper respiratory tract infections such as otitis and sinusitis. Viral infections are also common undiagnosed pathogens of the respiratory tract. Singer et al. (46) reviewed 24 cases of nosocomial pneumonia in cancer patients. Despite invasive diagnostic procedures in 18, there were unclear etiologies in eight, including seven with chronic organizing pneumonia and one with diffuse interstitial pneumonia.

Respiratory tract infections occur most commonly in patients with leukemia/lymphoma and those with solid tumors of the lung and head and neck regions (5,6). Postoperative pneumonias are more often diagnosed in solid tumor patients, because surgical procedures are more often a part of their diagnosis or treatment (5).

Urinary Tract Infections

UTIs have been reported to cause between 17% and 28% of nosocomial infections in this population (5,6) (see Chapter 20). A significant number of UTIs may be asymptomatic, especially in children.

Gram-negative microorganisms, namely *E. coli, K. pneumoniae, P. aeruginosa,* and *Proteus mirabilis,* predominate. The most frequent gram-positive isolates are enterococci. Fungal microorganisms are unusual urinary tract pathogens (5,6).

Patients with cancer are at increased risk for nosocomial UTI when compared with other hospitalized patients (49). Those with underlying diagnoses of prostate, bladder, bone, joint, liver, ovarian, colorectal, or vulvar cancer are the most commonly afflicted (5). As with non-oncology patients, urinary catheterization and manipulation of catheters are often instrumental in the development of nosocomial UTI (49).

Surgical Site Infections

Surgical site infections (SSIs) account for approximately 20% of nosocomial infections in cancer patients (5,6) (see Chapter 21). Identification of infections of surgical sites is usually based on the presence of purulent drainage from the sites. However, special consideration must be given to the neutropenic patient who may manifest infection by serous drainage or erythema and induration alone (6). Patients with solid tumors are most likely to develop SSIs (5,6). This is due to the extensive surgical procedures involved in their diagnosis and treatment. Patients with carcinoma of the vulva or uterus, soft tissue sarcomas, or malignant melanoma are most susceptible. Other high-risk patients include those with gastrointestinal or head and neck malignancies (5,6).

S. aureus is the most common pathogen isolated from SSIs in the cancer patient (5,6). Others frequently noted include *E. coli,* coagulase-negative staphylococci, enterococci, and anaerobes (5,6).

Gastrointestinal Infections

Little information is available about nosocomial gastrointestinal infections in cancer patients (see Chapter 24). The diagnosis should be based on the development of clinical symptoms of diarrhea with or without the isolation of a known pathogen. It is often difficult to distinguish diarrhea associated with gastroenteritis from that caused by chemotherapy-related mucositis. Close communication between the infection control professional and clinical personnel may facilitate this distinction. Potential pathogens include *Salmonella* species, *Shigella* species, rotavirus, other viral agents, and *Clostridium difficile.* In general, surgical patients and those receiving antibiotics are at increased risk of developing *C. difficile*-associated diarrhea (see Chapter 36). These predisposing factors also apply to the oncology patient.

Fever of Unknown Origin

Although not officially recognized by the Centers for Disease Control and Prevention (CDC) as a reportable entity, fever of unknown origin (FUO) is common in the hospitalized cancer patient (3). Despite intensive diagnostic workups and clinical symptoms suggestive of sepsis, pathogens are often not isolated. At St. Jude Children's Research Hospital, FUO accounts for about one third of nosocomial infections in pediatric oncology patients. Rotstein et al. (5) noted that only about 10% of nosocomial infections were classified as FUO in their adult oncology population. Including FUO as a separate, defined clinical entity, Engelhart et al. (3) describe an overall rate of 8.2 per 1,000 days, with two thirds of these episodes occurring during periods of neutropenia. These authors recommend the inclusion of this entity routinely in studies of surveillance of nosocomial infections in patients with cancer.

DIAGNOSIS OF NOSOCOMIAL INFECTIONS IN CANCER PATIENTS

The establishment of a specific etiologic diagnosis in a cancer patient is often difficult because of the commensal nature of the causative microbes and limited capability of the host to respond with recognizable clinical features. Even more difficult is differentiation of nosocomial from CAI. Despite these difficulties in most cancer centers, the specific cause of an infectious episode is established more frequently in the cancer patient than in the noncancer patient. This stems from the urgent need for treatment and more aggressive approaches to diagnosis.

Cultures for Bacteria, Fungi, and Viruses

The most meaningful cultures for bacteria and fungi are those of otherwise sterile body fluids such as blood, spinal fluid, bone marrow, urine, and tissue biopsies. Cultures of specific surface lesions by swab, aspirate, or biopsy require correlation with clinical features, histology, and type of microorganism isolated. Cultures of stool, oropharynx, and normal skin usually provide information only on microbial colonization rather than on the etiology of disease. In certain clinical settings such as a patient with prolonged granulocytopenia with fever unresponsive to antibiotics, the isolation of *Aspergillus* species from the nares or *Candida tropicalis* from the stool or the urine may raise the index of suspicion for invasive fungal disease.

Various techniques are used to diagnose catheter-related infections including paired quantitative CVC and peripheral venous blood cultures and difference in time to detection of blood cultures simultaneously drawn from these two sources (50).

In terms of viral cultures, shell vial spin amplification cultures give a more rapid turnaround time than traditional viral cultures do for detection of cytomegalovirus (CMV) and the more common respiratory viruses including influenza A and B, parainfluenza 1, 2, and 3, RSV, and adenovirus. Respiratory viruses can be significant nosocomial pathogens, and further molecular techniques are sometimes required to differentiate a nosocomial versus a CAI. Although the significance of herpes simplex and VZV isolates is easily discernible because of the typical lesions and illness associated with the overt infections, CMV isolates may be difficult to assess, because the disease patterns associated with this infection are varied, may be nonspecific, and range from asymptomatic latency to life-threatening disease. As mentioned earlier, differentiating a new onset, nosocomial viral infection from reactivation of a latent infection can sometimes be a difficult and fruitless exercise.

For many viruses, viral cultures may eventually be replaced by PCR-based tests. PCR-based assays are currently available or in development for numerous viruses including herpes simplex virus (HSV), CMV, adenovirus, and HHV-6. Although the majority of these tests are done by referral laboratories, centers with a high sample load such as ours are in the process of developing onsite testing facilities. This will facilitate the optimum utilization of this test in terms of turnaround time.

Smears and Stains

Material obtained from infected sites may contain enough of the causative microorganism to permit recognition of the microbe with selective stains and microscopy. Bacterial stains include Gram stain for most bacteria and acid-fast stain for mycobacteria, *Nocardia* species, and *Cryptosporidium* species. Although fungi are usually visualized directly by a Gram stain, a KOH (wet) mount, or a Calcofluor white stain, histopathologically or cytologically, special stains such as the methenamine silver, periodic acid-Schiff, or Papanicolaou stains are used. *P. carinii* can be visualized by a Grocott-Gomori methenamine silver nitrate, Calcofluor white, toluidine blue O, Giemsa, or monoclonal antibody stain. An India ink preparation is made for *Cryptococcus neoformans.* Rapid identification of viruses is based on tests that detect viral antigens such as direct fluorescent-antibody assay or enzyme immunoassay. These tests are currently used to detect respiratory viruses such as RSV, influenza, parainfluenza and adenovirus, HSV, VZV, and gastrointestinal pathogens such as rotavirus.

Tissue Biopsy

Biopsies of various tissues may be obtained for histopathologic examination, for microscopic examination of stained smears, and for culture, including skin biopsy (punch and excisional), lung biopsy (open biopsy and transbronchial), and liver and kidney biopsy (transcutaneous needle biopsy and open biopsy). In experienced hands, transthoracic needle biopsy of chest lesions is a relatively safe and noninvasive tool for the diagnosis of pulmonary fungal disease (51).

Radiography and Imaging

Radiography is most helpful in recognizing pneumonia. Serial chest radiographs are especially helpful in establishing nosocomially acquired pneumonia. Absence of discernible infiltrates does not exclude significant infection of the pulmonary parenchyma in the neutropenic patient. A more sensitive diagnostic test for early diagnosis of chest disease, especially fungal disease, is computed axial tomography (52,53). Even this test has limitations in the setting of a profoundly granulocytopenic host. Computed axial tomography of the liver, spleen, and kidneys is useful in identifying systemic fungal infections. The hypodense distinct lesions are highly suggestive of systemic candidiasis and aspergillosis (54,55).

Newer Technologies

Over the years, molecular techniques are increasingly being used to diagnose nosocomial infections and to investigate the source and spread of infection (39,41,56–58). Techniques being used to investigate outbreaks or in the context of epidemiologic surveillance include DNA-based methods such as plasmid profiling, restriction endonuclease analysis of plasmid and genomic DNA, Southern hybridization analysis using specific DNA probes, and chromosomal DNA profiling using either pulsed-field gel electrophoresis or PCR-based methods (59). Overall, although most of these tools are still in the development phase and have their own limitations, they can be useful supplements to traditional epidemiologic investigations.

Criteria for Nosocomial (Hospital-Acquired) Infections in Cancer Patients

Few studies have provided a perspective of nosocomial infections occurring exclusively in cancer patients (3–6). Due to the epidemiologic nuances mentioned earlier in an immunosuppressed host, the criteria in use for general hospitals such as those used for the CDC's National Nosocomial Infections Surveillance (NNIS) system (60) are not adequate to evaluate nosocomial infections in the immunosuppressed host and require some modifications. Since 1970, an infection surveillance program has been in operation at St. Jude Children's Research Hospital, a 60-bed pediatric oncology center. Criteria were developed to specifically monitor cancer patients. These criteria are outlined here, and results of the surveillance are described to show the pattern of such infections over the past decade, the relationship to several malignancies, and current trends.

General

A. Infections that develop after 48 hours of hospitalization are classified as hospital-acquired infections (HAIs) when the interval between admission and onset of symptoms is greater than the incubation period of the disease and when there is no evidence that the infection was present or incubating at admission. Infection that develops in a patient who was febrile continuously from admission to onset of new symptoms is classified as CAI. Infections that develop in patients who are febrile at admission and become afebrile for 72 or more hours before onset of symptoms are classified as HAI.

B. Infections present on admission and those that become evident during the first 48 hours of hospitalization are classified as CAI unless the infection is directly related to a recent admission.

C. Reactivation of latent infection (e.g., herpes zoster, herpes simplex, *P. carinii* pneumonitis) is classified as CAI.

D. Only the initial infection is counted in patients with multiple infections unless there is anatomic or temporal separation of the infections to suggest different origins.

E. If a new and different microorganism is cultured from a previously infected site, it is counted as HAI only if deterioration in the patient's condition is evident or antibiotics are changed to provide specific coverage of the new pathogen.

Specific

A. *Bacteremia:* One or more positive blood cultures unrelated to an infection present at admission. Propionibacterium, α-hemolytic streptococci, and *Staphylococcus epidermidis* are excluded unless there are two or more positive blood cultures and specific antibiotic therapy is instituted. Postmortem blood cultures are excluded.

B. *Fungemia:* One or more positive blood cultures resulting in antifungal therapy and unrelated to an infection present at admission. Postmortem blood cultures are excluded.

C. *Surgical site infections:* Only infections resulting from procedures performed in the operating room are counted as SSIs (i.e., an infection at a central line site is classified as an SSI only if the line was inserted in the operating room. If the line was inserted at bedside or in the treatment room, the infection is counted as skin and subcutaneous or phlebitis). Any one or more of the following categories qualifies as an SSI:

1. Nonneutropenic patients: purulent drainage with or without culture documentation or antibiotic therapy.
2. Neutropenic patients: <500 neutrophils/mm^3 with
   a. Purulent drainage, or
   b. Erythema and induration with a positive culture and/or antibiotic therapy.
3. Fever ($\geq 38.5°C$) lasting more than 72 hours postoperatively and resulting in antibiotic therapy when the patient was afebrile 2 or more days before surgery.
4. When a patient is returned to surgery because of complications during the postoperative period and evidence of infection is present, it is counted as HAI if there was no evidence of infection during initial surgery.

D. *Skin and subcutaneous:* may be considered procedure-related or procedure-unrelated.

1. Procedure-related: infections resulting from an invasive diagnostic or therapeutic procedure not performed in surgery. Any one or more of the following categories qualifies:
   a. Purulent drainage;
   b. Cellulitis (clinical diagnosis) and antibiotic therapy;
   c. Erythema, tenderness, induration, and fever resulting in antibiotic therapy and/or culture of a microorganism not thought to be a contaminant;
   d. Semiquantitative culture of the catheter tip and/or insertion site section of the catheter resulting in a colony count of at least 15 bacterial colonies in a patient with fever;
   e. Do not include chemical inflammation from drugs known to cause phlebitis or necrosis unless purulent drainage or culture-documented infection is present.
2. Procedure-unrelated: any of the following:
   a. Vesicles of viral origin that become secondarily infected and drain purulent material or when cultures of aspirates from these vesicles reveal a common pathogen (i.e., *S. aureus*).
   b. Purulent dermatitis or decubitus ulcers that drain purulent material or develop cellulitis.
   c. An ulcer in the perineal area that results in antibiotic therapy in a patient who had no signs of ulceration or irritation of the perineum on admission physical examination.

E. *Gastrointestinal:* Clinical signs and symptoms and a positive culture for a known pathogen or diagnostic test for rotavirus, *C. difficile*, or similar microorganism not present on admission. Colonization with a known pathogen (e.g., *Salmonella*) not present on admission stool cultures.

F. *Respiratory*

1. Upper: nose, throat, or ear infection with signs and symptoms at the site involved. Findings such as coryza, streptococcal pharyngitis, otitis media, and mastoiditis qualify. Oral thrush, herpes simplex labialis, and chronic gingivitis are excluded.
2. Lower: any of the following:
   a. Clinical signs and symptoms of lower respiratory tract infection (cough, pleuritic chest pain, purulent sputum, and fever) with or without culture or radiographic documentation.
   b. Radiographic evidence of pneumonia in a patient with fever when atelectasis can be ruled out. There should be no radiographic evidence or signs and symptoms of pneumonia at admission.
   c. Documentation of pneumonia at postmortem examination is included when the patient was admitted without radiographic evidence or signs and symptoms of pneumonia.

G. *Urinary tract*

1. Symptomatic: clinical signs and symptoms (such as fever, dysuria, or frequency) and
   a. A urine culture revealing a colony count exceeding 100,000 colonies of a single microorganism per milliliter on a properly collected and handled specimen. *S. epidermidis* is included in the symptomatic patient, or
   b. Culture of a suprapubic aspirate yielding an isolate not thought to be a contaminant.
2. Asymptomatic
   b. A urine culture colony count exceeding 100,000 of a single microorganism per milliliter plus a negative urine culture at admission obtained while the patient was not on antibiotics, or

b. The recovery of a new and different pathogen in pure culture with a colony count exceeding 100,000 when the patient was admitted with a UTI.
c. *S. epidermidis* is excluded in the asymptomatic patient.

H. *FUO:* All criteria listed below must be met:

1. Fever of at least 38.5°C lasting 24 or more hours.
2. Developing 2 or more days after admission. These 2 or more days must be spent without fever or antibiotic therapy.
3. No evidence of infection at any site on admission.
4. No clinical evidence of infection except fever.
5. No noninfectious cause for the fever can be determined (e.g., sickle cell crisis, aggressive chemotherapy in a patient with a large tumor load, rheumatic fever, systemic lupus erythematosus, rheumatoid arthritis). Postoperative cases with less than 2 days of fever and without antibiotic therapy are included unless a specific infection is identified.

Nosocomial Infections at a Pediatric Cancer Hospital Over One Decade

The aforementioned criteria for identification of nosocomial infections in cancer patients were used to determine the annual infection rates at St. Jude Children's Research Hospital from 1983 through 2001 (Fig. 58.1). During this time, although the mean length of stay in the hospital remained reasonably similar, there seems to be a trend toward a decreasing proportion of nosocomial infections per 1,000 patient-days as well as per number of hospital discharges. It should be pointed out, however, that the intensity of immunosuppressive therapy and the number of cancer patients undergoing bone marrow transplantation tended to increase. It should also be noted that noncontagious patients are kept in private rooms with high-efficiency particulate air (HEPA) filters and unidirectional air flow at portals (positive pressure). No special precautions are given for food, and standard nursing care is provided without protective gowns and masks. Standard universal precautions are practiced unless there are specific indications for transmission-based, airborne, droplet, or contact precautions. Obviously, these data cannot be accurately matched to those of other hospitals unless similar criteria are used for the identification of nosocomial infections, rates are adjusted for severity of illness, and medical practices are comparable. Thus, surveillance data are most valuable to the institution from which they are derived. Seemingly minor institutional practices may be reflected in such data. For example, at St. Jude, cultures of the urine, stool, and throat are routinely taken on admission from all cancer patients. Therefore, the likelihood of identifying true hospital acquisitions of urinary tract and enteric infections is greater than in hospitals wherein routine admission cultures are not done. In some hospitals, this practice would not be prudent. Ideally, each hospital should develop a system that best serves its specific needs for cancer patients.

The nosocomial infection rates by malignancy type, by infection type, and for bone marrow transplant recipients at St. Jude

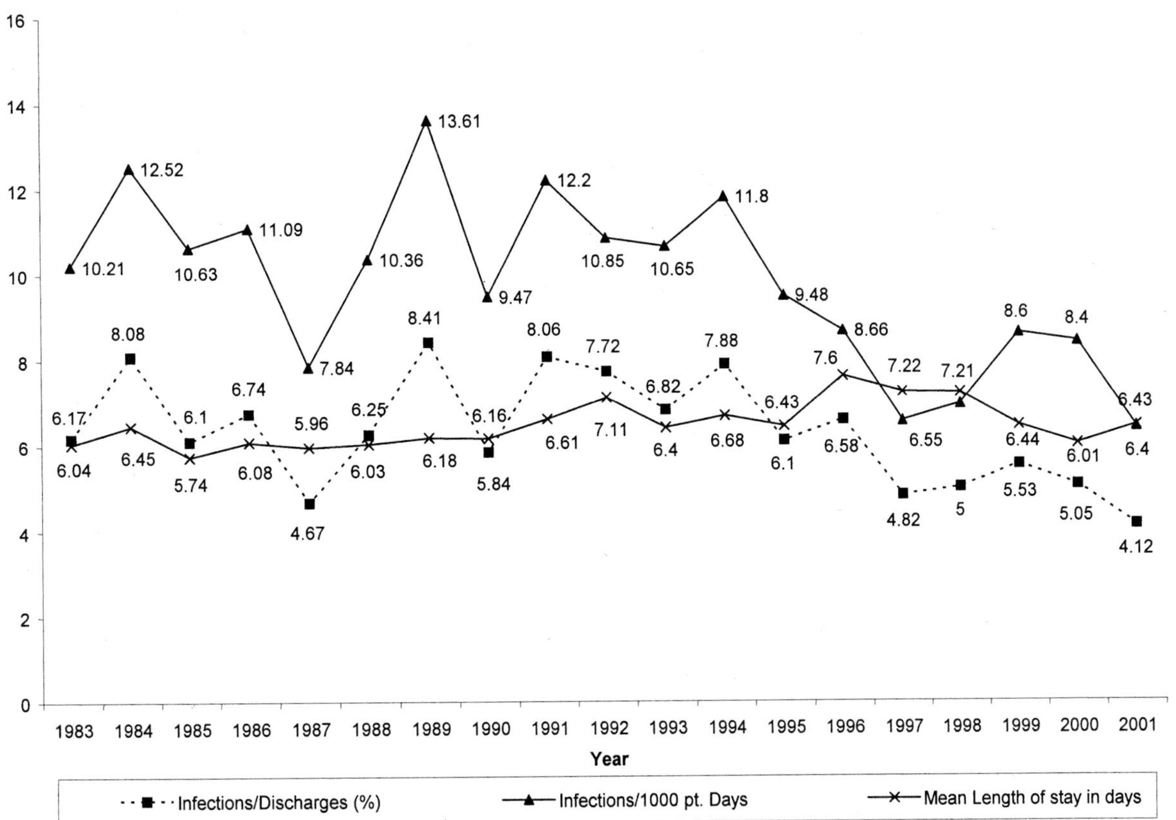

Figure 58.1. Annual nosocomial infection rates at a pediatric oncology center from 1983 to 2001.

during 1997 are summarized in Table 58.2. The rates are based on 2,139 patient discharges and are expressed as number of infections per 1,000 discharges.

It is strikingly obvious that the group at highest risk consists of oncology patients who have undergone bone marrow transplantation. Individuals with acute myelocytic leukemia are at second highest risk for nosocomial infections.

The microbial etiology was identified in 52 of 103 nosocomial infections encountered in 1997 (Table 58.3).

Nosocomial Infections in Adult Neutropenic Cancer Patients

An informative study of nosocomial infections in adults with cancer has been reported by Carlisle et al. (8) from the Albert Einstein Cancer Center in New York. This cancer center at the Montefiore Medical Center, like St. Jude, is a research-oriented 48-bed service. Their study included nosocomial infections in 920 cancer patients admitted over a 3.5-year period who were neutropenic (<1,000/mm^3) for 2 or more consecutive days during hospitalization. Definitions were established to categorize infectious episodes.

The investigators found a high rate of infection in these neutropenic patients, with 46 nosocomial infections per 1,000 neutropenic days. Table 58.4 shows the type of malignancy in relation to the number of days at risk. The sites of infection are shown in Table 58.5 and the causative microorganisms are listed in Table 58.6. Of the 124 bloodstream infections, coagulase-negative staphylococci were found in 42; *E. coli* in 19; streptococci in 19; *Candida* species in 11; *S. aureus* in ten; *Klebsiella* species in ten; and enterococci, *Pseudomonas* species, *Enterobacter* species, *Lactobacillus* species, *Acinetobacter* species, and other bacteria in five or less episodes.

These studies, and earlier studies by Robinson et al. (6), clearly point out the patients within the cancer population at highest risk for nosocomial infections. These are neutropenic patients and patients who have undergone bone marrow transplantation.

TABLE 58.3. ETIOLOGY OF NOSOCOMIAL INFECTIONS IN PEDIATRIC ONCOLOGY PATIENTS IN 1997 (ETIOLOGY IDENTIFIED IN 52 NOSOCOMIAL INFECTIONS)

Etiology	No. of Cases
Bacterial causes (43 cases)	
Bacillus cereus	1
Corynebacterium species	1
Enterococcus	3
Staphylococcus aureus	7
Staphylococcus, coagulase neg.	2
Streptococcus	3
Ochrobactrum anthropi	1
Proteus mirabilis	1
Pseudomonas fluorescens	1
Serratia marcescens	1
Clostridium difficile	1
Escherichia coli	4
Enterobacter species	4
Klebsiella pneumoniae	11
Ureaplasma urealyticum	1
Pseudomonas aeruginosa	2
Fungal causes (10 cases)	
Aspergillus terreus	1
Candida albicans	5
Candida glabrata	1
Candida lusitaniae	1
Candida rugosa	1
Fungi not otherwise specified	1
Viral causes (3 cases)	
Adenovirus	3
Parainfluenza virus	1

Other Unique Nosocomial Infections in Cancer Patients

Perhaps the major serious infection threat to the cancer patient is that caused by the opportunistic fungi, especially candidiasis and aspergillosis. The secular trends in the epidemiology of nosocomial fungal infections in the United States from 1980 to

TABLE 58.2. NOSOCOMIAL INFECTION RATES BY MALIGNANCY TYPE BY INFECTION SITE AND FOR BONE MARROW TRANSPLANT RECIPIENTS DURING 1997 (2, 139 PATIENT DISCHARGES)

	Infections per 1,000 Discharges						
Infection Category	ALL (*n* = 486)	AML (*n* = 221)	ST (*n* = 1,118)	TRNS (*n* = 146)	NHL (*n* = 74)	Other (*n* = 94)	Total (*n* = 2,139)
Bacteremia	1	4	9	2	0	0	16
Surgical site	1	0	4	8	0	0	13
UTI	0	1	3	1	0	0	5
Skin and subcutaneous	2	0	0	0	0	0	2
Respiratory	0	1	9	8	1	0	19
Disseminated fungal	0	1	1	2	0	0	4
Fungemia	2	0	0	2	0	0	4
Gastrointestinal	0	0	0	1	1	0	2
Fever of undetermined etiology	2	4	12	13	1	0	32
Other	3	1	1	1	0	0	6
Total	11	12	39	38	3	0	103

ALL, acute lymphocytic leukemia; AML, acute myelocytic leukemia; ST, solid tumors; TRNS, bone marrow transplant; NHL, non-Hodgkin's lymphoma; UTI, urinary tract infection.

TABLE 58.4. NEUTROPENIC ADULTS WITH CANCER: DAYS AT RISK

Malignancy	Patients (%)	Days at Risk (%)
Hematologic	628 (68)	7,209 (75)
Solid tumor	218 (24)	1,339 (14)
Bone marrow transplant		
Hematologic	26 (3)	456 (5)
Solid tumor	48 (5)	578 (6)

From Carlisle PS, Gucalp R, Wiernik PH, Nosocomial infections in neutropenic cancer patients. *Infect Control Hosp Epidemiol* 1993; 14(6): 320–324, with permission.

TABLE 58.5. SITE-SPECIFIC RATES OF NOSOCOMIAL INFECTIONS BY NUMBER OF NEUTROPENIC PATIENTS (*N* = 920) AND NUMBER OF DAYS AT RISK (*N* = 9,582)

Site	No.	Rate/100 Patients	Rate/1,000 Days at Risk
Overall	444	48.3	46.3
Blood	124	13.5	12.9
Thrush	61	6.6	6.4
Urinary tract	52	5.7	5.4
Respiratory	51	5.5	5.3
Venous access site	43	4.7	4.5
Gastrointestinal tract	32.	3.4	3.3
Skin	31	3.4	3.2
Other	50	5.4	5.2

From Carlisle PS, Gucalp R, Wiernik PH, Nosocomial infections in neutropenic cancer patients. *Infect Control Hosp Epidemiol* 1993; 14(6): 320–324, with permission.

TABLE 58.6. NOSOCOMIAL INFECTIONS IN NEUTROPENIC ADULTS WITH CANCER (*N* = 392)

Microorganisms	No.
Candida	70
Staphylococci, coagulase-negative	67
Escherichia coli	35
Staphylococcus aureus	26
Enterococci	23
Herpes	22
Clostridia	21
Klebsiella	21
Streptococci	21
Pseudomonas	16
Aspergillus	15
Acinetobacter	10
Enterobacter	9
Corynebacterium	8
Citrobacter	3
Proteus	3
Other gram-positive rods	8
Other gram-negative rods	8
Other	6

From Carlisle PS, Gucalp R, Wiernik PH, Nosocomial infections in neutropenic cancer patients. *Infect Control Hosp Epidemiol* 1993; 14(6): 320–324, with permission.

1990 have been described by Beck-Sague and Jarvis (61). During this decade, the NNIS system hospitals reported 30,477 nosocomial fungal infections. During this time, the fungal infection rate increased from 2.0 to 3.8 infections per 1,000 patients discharged. The medical specialty with a high infection rate was oncology, within which rates varied from 8.9 to 10.6 infections per 1,000 discharges. *C. albicans* was the most frequently isolated fungal pathogen (59.7%) followed by other *Candida* species (18.6%). A study of candidemia in cancer patients from November 1992 to October 1994 found that of 249 episodes of candidemia, non-albicans candidemia accounted for 64% (101/159) of episodes in patients with hematologic malignancies and 30% (27/90) of the episodes in patients with solid tumors (62). Although *Aspergillus* causes a much lower rate of infection, it is the mycosis that has been most convincingly associated with the hospital environment. Outbreaks of nosocomial aspergillosis have been reported to be due to hospital construction and renovation activities (63–66). Bone marrow transplant patients are especially susceptible. The source of infection is airborne conidia (spores) of *Aspergillus* species often associated with contaminated air-handling systems. Recent evidence suggests the hospital water distribution system as an additional indoor source for pathogenic fungi (67).

PREVENTION AND CONTROL

Prevention and control of nosocomial infections in patients with neoplastic disease is one of the most important contributors to the overall success of treatment in this patient population. Not only do nosocomial infections add to the morbidity, mortality, and overall cost of care, but, not uncommonly, infectious complications necessitate modifications in dose and scheduling of antineoplastic therapies, potentially compromising the successful treatment of the patient's malignancy. The general principles of infection control that are applied to any hospitalized patient remain the same for patients with neoplastic disease. These include, when indicated, specific transmission-based precautions in addition to standard precautions. Certain additional precautions are taken based on the immunosuppressed state of these patients and their susceptibility to infections by opportunistic pathogens. This is especially true in the very high risk host such as patients who have recently undergone bone marrow transplantation or those with prolonged granulocytopenia. Special precautions to prevent such patients from acquiring infection by filamentous fungi, especially *Aspergillus* species, are extremely important. Certain principles of prevention of nosocomial infections are discussed in the paragraphs that follow, keeping in mind the nuances of a host with a neoplastic disease. Although some preventive measures [e.g., sophisticated air-handling systems, total protected environment (TPE)] are labor intensive, consume a considerable amount of limited healthcare resources, and sometimes lack clear-cut supportive evidence, others (e.g., hand washing, appropriate aseptic technique) are simple, inexpensive, and require very little of the busy healthcare worker's time, and their efficacy is firmly established. Healthcare setups need to individualize their practices based on availability of resources and review of local problems.

Hand Hygiene

Ignaz Philipp Semmelweis, in his classic paper on the prevention of childbed fever in 1861 (68), clearly showed that hand washing is very effective in preventing the spread of nosocomial infection when used assiduously. His insistence, in the 19th century, that students and physicians clean their hands with a chlorine solution before seeing each patient in the clinic represents the first evidence that hand washing with plain soap and water in the setting of heavily contaminated hands may not be enough and the use of an antiseptic agent may be more effective. Since then, the importance of hand antisepsis in prevention of nosocomial infections is well accepted (69,70), and numerous professional societies and committees have published guidelines for appropriate hand hygiene practices. The latest set of guidelines on this subject based on review of existent literature was recently published by the CDC in the *Morbidity and Mortality Weekly Report* (71). The recommendations include use of an alcohol-based hand rub for routinely decontaminating hands in various clinical care situations. Alternatively, the practice of hand washing with antimicrobial soap and water should be continued. Ready access at strategic locations of efficacious hand-hygiene products with low irritancy potential has been emphasized. Use of artificial fingernails or extenders by clinical care providers, especially those taking care of high-risk patients, is discouraged.

It seems clear that the simple act of hand washing greatly reduces the likelihood of transmitting pathogenic microorganisms to hospitalized patients on the hands of healthcare workers. What is also clear is that despite the presence of published guidelines and policies, adherence of healthcare workers to recommended hand-hygiene procedures has been poor, with mean baseline rates of 5% to 81% (71). We recommend that institutions review these guidelines and, based on the resources available, select a hand-hygiene agent or agents and implement a hand-hygiene policy. Periodic monitoring for compliance and focused interventions to improve it, based on the feedback generated, is critical to the success of this intervention (see also Chapter 96).

Infections Associated with Intravascular Devices

Intravascular devices, particularly tunneled CVCs, are used extensively in patients with neoplastic diseases, and infections associated with them result in increased morbidity in the immunocompromised patient. Meticulous attention should be given to establishing effective infection control practices for the insertion and care of these devices. Guidelines for the prevention of intravascular catheter-related infections recommended by a working group including numerous professional organizations were recently published by the CDC (72). These include the use of antimicrobial or antiseptic-impregnated CVCs in adults, recommendations on selection of catheter insertion sites, catheter care, and surveillance for catheter-related infections. Consideration should be given to establishing special intravenous therapy teams to ensure a high level of aseptic technique during catheter insertion and follow-up care. Policies and procedures for infusion therapy should be comprehensive, and persons who perform manipulations of these devices should be thoroughly trained in appropriate infection control techniques (see also Chapters 17 and 18).

Protective Isolation

Although appropriate hand hygiene practices and general principles of antisepsis should be followed with any patient with a neoplastic disease, investigators have explored additional measures to protect certain high-risk patient populations, such as patients with prolonged granulocytopenia or with a recent bone marrow transplant, from acquiring nosocomial infections. These have included elaborate measures for protecting the patient from both extrinsic and intrinsic pathogens, including selective decontamination of the digestive tract, HEPA-filtered air, and food and water low in microbial content. The complexity of such studies makes it difficult to evaluate the effectiveness of simple protective isolation (routine use of gloves, gowns, and masks for all patient contact) as an independent variable. Studies suggest that most bacterial infections in patients with granulocytopenia arise from the patient's own flora, and that colonization by the causative microorganism in nearly half of the infections occurs only after admission to the hospital (73). Contaminated hands of healthcare workers are thought to play a major role in the colonization of these patients. Protective isolation, using only gloves and gowns, has been shown to be effective in reducing infection rates in a pediatric intensive care unit, but patients with immunologic dysfunction were excluded from the study (74). Protective isolation alone has been shown in one study to be of no value in protecting patients with severe granulocytopenia (75). In a randomized clinical trial comparing the role of gown and glove isolation and strict hand washing in the reduction of nosocomial infection in children with solid organ transplantation admitted to a pediatric intensive care unit, Slota et al. (76) found that although the rate of nosocomial infections in both intervention groups was significantly reduced compared to the baseline rate, there was a trend toward a higher reduction in the gown and glove group compared to the hand washing group. Although this study demonstrates the role of gown and glove isolation in certain specific clinical settings and indicates the possibility of some additional benefit of this intervention over simple hand washing, the latter intervention is undeniably relatively inexpensive and simple to implement. Until further studies demonstrating the efficacy and cost-effectiveness of protective isolation in routine care of neoplastic patients in various clinical settings are done, this intervention cannot be uniformly recommended. In the meantime its use as a component of standard infection control procedures such as respiratory or enteric isolation in the setting of documented infections should be continued.

Total Protected Environment (TPE)

Because the causative agents of nosocomial infections in patients with neoplastic diseases include endogenous and a wide variety of exogenous microorganisms, a comprehensive approach to preventing infection and colonization with hospital pathogens has been tried (77,78). This comprehensive approach, total protected environment (TPE), has included the use of protective isolation, selective decontamination of the digestive tract, rigorous antisepsis of the skin and perirectal area, and HEPA-filtered air supplied to the patient in a laminar or turbulent fashion. TPE also includes provision of food and water low in microbial content, sterilization or high-level disinfection of objects before they are taken into the room, and frequent and thorough cleaning and disinfection of room surfaces.

A sterile patient environment cannot be achieved and maintained. Because the patient's endogenous flora and microorganisms in the room and in food and water can only be suppressed, not totally eliminated, a labor-intensive decontamination regimen must be continued throughout the isolation period. TPE is expensive and is beyond the capabilities of many hospitals providing care for patients with neoplastic diseases. Although a reduction in the incidence of infection has been associated with the use of TPE, it must be recognized that since the performance of these studies more than two decades ago, the treatment of infectious complications in neutropenic patients has been improved considerably. Thus, a more relevant question is whether TPE would improve infection-related mortality with the current availability of better treatment options. At this time, a comprehensive approach of TPE is not a standard recommendation for patients with neoplastic disease. Various components of this approach are followed by individual centers, especially those with a bone marrow transplant program.

Air-Handling System

Although provision of clean air is important to any patient, additional measures to eliminate the risk of exposure to filamentous fungi such as *Aspergillus* species, are attempted especially in the high-risk host with prolonged granulocytopenia. Reported outbreaks of nosocomial invasive aspergillosis have been caused by concentration of conidia in hospital ventilation systems (79), contaminated fireproofing materials (80), and air contamination from construction (63–66). One such measure is the use of HEPA filters. The modern HEPA filter, made of superfine spunglass fibers less that 1 mm in diameter, was developed by the Army Chemical Corps and the Naval Research Laboratory in the years immediately after World War II. The maximum allowable penetration of a HEPA filter at any point in the media, frame, or gasket is 0.03% of the challenge concentration of monodispersed thermally generated dioctyl phthalate (DOP) droplets having a count-median diameter of 0.3 ± 0.03 μm.

HEPA-filtered air has been used in many centers as a component of protective isolation to provide ultraclean air to patients during periods of granulocytopenia. In some studies, HEPA-filtered air was delivered to the patient in a unidirectional (formerly called "laminar flow") fashion, and in other studies "life island" units that enclosed the patient's bed in a plastic canopy were used. Unidirectional airflow is not achieved in life island units. A concentration of about 2.12 microorganisms per cubic meter of air can be achieved in life island units and 0.21 microorganisms per cubic meter can be achieved in rooms with unidirectional flow, compared with approximately 106 microorganisms per cubic meter in conventional rooms. Although the efficacy of HEPA filters in preventing aspergillosis seems clear (64,81, 82), the effect on preventing other infections is less certain.

Optimum filtration efficiency using HEPA filters requires considerable effort and resources. HEPA filters should be purchased from a reputable company that scan tests each filter before shipment to ensure that the entire surface of the filter, gasket, and media-frame bonding is free of leaks at or above 0.03% of the challenge concentration of hot DOP. After installation, HEPA filters should be retested by skilled technicians, and leaks at or above 0.01% of the challenge concentration of cold DOP should be repaired. Portable HEPA filtration units have been associated with a decrease in incidence density of aspergillosis cases during a construction-associated outbreak when used in conjunction with other infection control measures (65).

Because new air-handling units sometimes fail to meet design specifications, they should be DOP leak tested before they are placed in operation. We installed a new air handler with HEPA filters as part of a renovation project. DOP leak testing after construction of the unit revealed leaks of greater than 10% between the filter housing and the air handler walls. This represented a 3-log greater penetration of DOP than specified in design criteria and would not have been detected without proper testing. After repairs, no leaks at or above 0.01% were detected.

With proper installation, testing, and maintenance, ultraclean air can be maintained in the patient room. Patients with neoplastic diseases, however, must periodically leave this protected environment for a wide range of diagnostic and therapeutic procedures. Despite the lack of clear-cut data, for a subset of immunocompromised patients identified at high risk for aspergillosis, it is desirable to protect the respiratory tract from opportunistic pathogens during these periods. For this purpose, various masks or respirators may be used. High-efficiency masks have been successfully used in high-risk patients during periods when they are outside their hospital rooms (83). A breakthrough in the manufacture of HEPA-filtered masks is the replacement of delicate fiberglass fibers with durable plastic fibers. This new technology has permitted the production of a durable, lightweight, comfortable mask that readily passes DOP leak tests and should provide the patient with air quality at least as good as that found in HEPA-filtered unidirectional rooms. Another mask in clinical use is the N95 respirator. In the guidelines for Preventing Opportunistic Infections Among Hematopoietic Stem Cell Transplant Recipients published by the CDC, use of the N95 mask (particulate respirator) has been mentioned to prevent mold exposure during transportation near hospital construction or renovation areas since these respirators are regarded as effective against any aerosol (84). For maximal efficacy of any face mask, whether it be the HEPA mask or the N95, proper fit testing and training of the patient is very important. In this regard, unavailability of small masks poses a limitation for their use in infants and small children. In conclusion, although HEPA filters are important, especially to prevent nosocomial aspergillosis in a high-risk host, the correct and optimal installation and use of HEPA filters is relatively complex and expensive.

Other factors related to hospital air handling including appropriate air exchanges and pressurization are equally important in preventing nosocomial airborne infections, especially aspergillosis (85). In a recently published study assessing the ability of hospital air handling systems to filter *Aspergillus*, other fungi, and particles following the implosion of an adjacent building, an encouraging observation was that even standard hospital air handling systems with filtration exceeding minimum American Society of Heating, Refrigeration, and Air Conditioning Engineers (ASHRAE) standards have a significant safety buffer in filtering *Aspergillus* spores (86). HEPA filters likely provide an additional level of safety. Design and maintenance of hospital ventilation systems is discussed in detail in Chapter 89.

In a recent publication, Anaissie et al. (67) submitted evidence to support the theory that hospital water distribution systems may be a potential indoor reservoir of *Aspergillus* species and other molds leading to aerosolization of fungal spores and potential patient exposure. In a high-risk population such as bone marrow transplant patients, these authors recommend the use of sterile (boiled) water for drinking and sterile sponges for bathing. Additionally they recommend cleaning of the floors of the patient shower facilities in order to reduce the air concentration of *Aspergillus* species and other pathogenic airborne molds (87).

Antimicrobial Drugs

The administration of antimicrobial prophylaxis in patients with cancer to prevent both community-acquired and hospital-acquired infections has been most widely studied in neutropenic patients. Initial trials of infection prophylaxis using combinations of nonabsorbable drugs such as aminoglycosides, polymyxins, and vancomycin were followed by studies of orally absorbable agents, primarily trimethoprim-sulfamethoxazole (TMP-SMX) and quinolones. A review of studies of prophylaxis with TMP-SMX by the Infectious Diseases Society of America (IDSA) Fever and Neutropenia Panel found that in most studies there was some benefit in terms of reduced infection rates in the TMP-SMX treated group compared to the placebo group (88). Studies have also shown some benefit of quinolone-based prophylaxis in reducing the rates of infection in neutropenic patients (89,90). Finally with the increase in frequency of fungal infections in patients with neoplastic diseases, especially patients with hematologic malignancy, there has been considerable interest in the role of antifungal prophylaxis. A meta-analysis of studies of the efficacy of antifungal prophylaxis in neutropenic patients observed reductions in use of empirical antifungal therapy, superficial fungal infection, invasive fungal infection, and fungal-infection related mortality (91). Although the benefits of antifungal prophylaxis in terms of infections with *Candida* have been noted, there is no definitive data showing its impact on infections with filamentous fungi.

Despite the data supporting the efficacy of prophylaxis with TMP-SMX, quinolones, fluconazole, and itraconazole in reducing the number of infectious episodes during the neutropenic period, the IDSA Fever and Neutropenia Guidelines Panel remarks "concern about the problem of emerging drug-resistant bacteria and fungi due to extensive antibiotic use, plus the fact that such prophylaxis has not been shown to consistently reduce mortality rates, leads to the recommendation that routine prophylaxis with these drugs in neutropenic patients should be avoided, with the exception of use of TMP-SMX for patients at risk for *P. carinii* pneumonitis" (92).

IMPENDING CHANGES IN NOSOCOMIAL INFECTIONS IN CANCER PATIENTS

Many developments are affecting, or will soon affect, the cancer patient and the pattern of nosocomial infections. Notable are the trends to treat certain patients with fever and neutropenia as outpatients rather than in the hospital and the emergence of antibiotic-resistant bacterial infections. Infection control personnel will need to expand their efforts to match the expansion of the healthcare delivery system and the overall trend to minimize in-hospital treatment of medical conditions. New hospital construction that provides improved physical facilities with better air-handling systems and new approaches to cancer treatment, such as improved bone marrow transplantation and gene therapy, are factors effecting change. In summary, patients with neoplastic diseases, for numerous reasons, are vulnerable to acquiring nosocomial infections. The challenges of diagnosing and managing nosocomial infections in a patient with cancer include difficulties in early diagnosis due to atypical presentation, difficulty in establishing pathogenicity versus mere colonization, problems in sorting out a community versus a hospital source, as well as differentiating a new infection from reactivation of a previous infection. Hospital epidemiologists should continue to reassess the incidence, type, and sources of nosocomial infections for possible changing trends.

REFERENCES

1. Schwarz RE, Groeger JS, Coit DG. Subcutaneously implanted central venous access devices in cancer patients: a prospective analysis. *Cancer* 1997;79(8):1635–1640.
2. Johnson CC, Wilcosky T, Kvale P, et al. Cancer incidence among an HIV-infected cohort. Pulmonary Complications of HIV Infection Study Group. *Am J Epidemiol* 1997;146(6):470–475.
3. Engelhart S, Glasmacher A, Exner M, et al. Surveillance for nosocomial infections and fever of unknown origin among adult hematology-oncology patients. *Infect Control Hosp Epidemiol* 2002;23(5):244–248.
4. Simon A, Fleischhack G, Hasan C, et al. Surveillance for nosocomial and central line-related infections among pediatric hematology-oncology patients. *Infect Control Hosp Epidemiol* 2000;21(9):592–596.
5. Rotstein C, Cummings KM, Nicolaou AL, et al. Nosocomial infection rates at an oncology center. *Infect Control* 1988;9(1):13–19.
6. Robinson GV, Tegtmeier BR, Zaia JA. Brief report: nosocomial infection rates in a cancer treatment center. *Infect Control* 1984;5(6):289–294.
7. Velasco E, Thuler LC, Martins CA, et al. Nosocomial infections in an oncology intensive care unit. *Am J Infect Control* 1997;25(6):458–462.
8. Carlisle PS, Gucalp R, Wiernik PH. Nosocomial infections in neutropenic cancer patients. *Infect Control Hosp Epidemiol* 1993;14(6):320–324.
9. Bodey GP, Elting LS, Rodriquez S, et al. Klebsiella bacteremia. A 10-year review in a cancer institution. *Cancer* 1989;64(11):2368–2376.
10. Saito H, Elting L, Bodey GP, et al. Serratia bacteremia: review of 118 cases. *Rev Infect Dis* 1989;11(6):912–920.
11. Johnson MP, Ramphal R. Beta-lactam-resistant Enterobacter bacteremia in febrile neutropenic patients receiving monotherapy. *J Infect Dis* 1990;162(4):981–983.
12. Samonis G, Anaissie E, Elting L, et al. Review of Citrobacter bacteremia

in cancer patients over a sixteen-year period. *Eur J Clin Microbiol Infect Dis* 1991;10(6):479–485.
13. Maschmeyer G, Braveny I. Review of the incidence and prognosis of Pseudomonas aeruginosa infections in cancer patients in the 1990s. *Eur J Clin Microbiol Infect Dis* 2000;19(12):915–925.
14. Cross A, Allen JR, Burke J, et al. Nosocomial infections due to Pseudomonas aeruginosa: review of recent trends. *Rev Infect Dis* 1983; 5(suppl 5):S837–S845.
15. Schimpff SC, Moody M, Young VM. Relationship of colonization with Pseudomonas aeruginosa to development of Pseudomonas bacteremia in cancer patients. *Antimicrob Agents Chemother* 1970;10: 240–244.
16. Jackson MA, Wong KY, Lampkin B. Pseudomonas aeruginosa septicemia in childhood cancer patients. *Pediatr Infect Dis* 1982;1(4): 239–241.
17. Fergie JE, Shema SJ, Lott L, et al. Pseudomonas aeruginosa bacteremia in immunocompromised children: analysis of factors associated with a poor outcome. *Clin Infect Dis* 1994;18(3):390–394.
18. Nunnink JC, Gallagher JG, Yates JW. Legionnaires' disease in patients with cancer. *Med Pediatr Oncol* 1986;14(2):81–85.
19. Khardori N, Elting L, Wong E, et al. Nosocomial infections due to Xanthomonas maltophilia (Pseudomonas maltophilia) in patients with cancer. *Rev Infect Dis* 1990;12(6):997–1003.
20. Wade JC, Schimpff SC, Newman KA, et al. Staphylococcus epidermidis: an increasing cause of infection in patients with granulocytopenia. *Ann Intern Med* 1982;97(4):503–508.
21. Patrick CC. Coagulase-negative staphylococci: pathogens with increasing clinical significance. *J Pediatr* 1990;116(4):497–507.
22. Cohen J, Donnelly JP, Worsley AM, et al. Septicaemia caused by viridans streptococci in neutropenic patients with leukaemia. *Lancet* 1983; 2(8365–8366):1452–1454.
23. Sotiropoulos SV, Jackson MA, Woods GM, et al. Alpha-streptococcal septicemia in leukemic children treated with continuous or large dosage intermittent cytosine arabinoside. *Pediatr Infect Dis J* 1989;8(11): 755–758.
24. Telander B, Lerner R, Palmblad J, et al. Corynebacterium group JK in a hematological ward: infections, colonization and environmental contamination. *Scand J Infect Dis* 1988;20(1):55–61.
25. Riebel W, Frantz N, Adelstein D, et al. Corynebacterium JK: a cause of nosocomial device-related infection. *Rev Infect Dis* 1986;8(1):42–49.
26. Khabbaz RF, Kaper JB, Moody MR, et al. Molecular epidemiology of group JK Corynebacterium on a cancer ward: lack of evidence for patient-to-patient transmission. *J Infect Dis* 1986;154(1):95–99.
27. Brown EA, Talbot GH, Provencher M, et al. Anaerobic bacteremia in patients with acute leukemia. *Infect Control Hosp Epidemiol* 1989;10(2): 65–69.
28. Kern WV, Andriof E, Oethinger M, et al. Emergence of fluoroquinolone-resistant Escherichia coli at a cancer center. *Antimicrob Agents Chemother* 1994;38(4):681–687.
29. Nourse C, Murphy H, Byrne C, et al. Control of a nosocomial outbreak of vancomycin resistant Enterococcus faecium in a paediatric oncology unit: risk factors for colonisation. *Eur J Pediatr* 1998;157(1):20–27.
30. Rubin LG, Tucci V, Cercenado E, et al. Vancomycin-resistant Enterococcus faecium in hospitalized children. *Infect Control Hosp Epidemiol* 1992;13(12):700–705.
31. Marr KA. The changing spectrum of candidemia in oncology patients: therapeutic implications. *Curr Opin Infect Dis* 2000;13(6):615–620.
32. Safdar A, Perlin DS, Armstrong D. Hematogenous infections due to Candida parapsilosis: changing trends in fungemic patients at a comprehensive cancer center during the last four decades. *Diagn Microbiol Infect Dis* 2002;44(1):11–16.
33. Marr KA, Carter RA, Crippa F, et al. Epidemiology and outcome of mould infections in hematopoietic stem cell transplant recipients. *Clin Infect Dis* 2002;34(7):909–917.
34. Kontoyiannis DP, Bodey GP. Invasive aspergillosis in 2002: an update. *Eur J Clin Microbiol Infect Dis* 2002;21(3):161–172.
35. Lin SJ, Schranz J, Teutsch SM. Aspergillosis case-fatality rate: systematic review of the literature. *Clin Infect Dis* 2001;32(3):358–366.
36. Groll AH, Walsh TJ. Uncommon opportunistic fungi: new nosocomial threats. *Clin Microbiol Infect* 2001;7(suppl 2):8–24.
37. Meyers JD, MacQuarrie MB, Merigan TC, et al. Nosocomial varicella. Part I: outbreak in oncology patients at a children's hospital. *West J Med* 1979;130(3):196–199.
38. Gustafson TL, Lavely GB, Brawner ER Jr, et al. An outbreak of airborne nosocomial varicella. *Pediatrics* 1982;70(4):550–556.
39. Mazzulli T, Peret TC, McGeer A, et al. Molecular characterization of a nosocomial outbreak of human respiratory syncytial virus on an adult leukemia/lymphoma ward. *J Infect Dis* 1999;180(5):1686–1689.
40. Rogers M, Weinstock DM, Eagan J, et al. Rotavirus outbreak on a pediatric oncology floor: possible association with toys. *Am J Infect Control* 2000;28(5):378–380.
41. Widell A, Christensson B, Wiebe T, et al. Epidemiologic and molecular investigation of outbreaks of hepatitis C virus infection on a pediatric oncology service. *Ann Intern Med* 1999;130(2):130–134.
42. Styczynski J, Wysocki M, Koltan S, et al. Epidemiologic aspects and preventive strategy of hepatitis B and C viral infections in children with cancer. *Pediatr Infect Dis J* 2001;20(11):1042–1049.
43. Morrison VA, Peterson BA, Bloomfield CD. Nosocomial septicemia in the cancer patient: the influence of central venous access devices, neutropenia, and type of malignancy. *Med Pediatr Oncol* 1990;18(3): 209–216.
44. Funada H, Machi T, Matsuda T. Bacteremia complicating acute leukemia with special reference to its incidence and changing etiological patterns. *Jpn J Clin Oncol* 1988;18(3):239–248.
45. Wright WL, Wenzel RP. Nosocomial Candida. Epidemiology, transmission, and prevention. *Infect Dis Clin North Am* 1997;11(2): 411–425.
46. Singer C, Kaplan MH, Armstrong D. Bacteremia and fungemia complicating neoplastic disease. A study of 364 cases. *Am J Med* 1977; 62(5):731–742.
47. Mayo JW, Wenzel RP. Rates of hospital-acquired bloodstream infections in patients with specific malignancy. *Cancer* 1982;50(1): 187–190.
48. Kilton LJ, Fossieck BE Jr, Cohen MH, et al. Bacteremia due to gram-positive cocci in patients with neoplastic disease. *Am J Med* 1979;66(4): 596–602.
49. Giongo F, Meroni MR, Busin S. Nosocomial urinary tract infections in neoplastic and non-neoplastic diseases. *Chemioterapia* 1987;6(2 suppl): 503–504.
50. Mermel LA, Farr BM, Sherertz RJ, et al. Guidelines for the management of intravascular catheter-related infections. *Infect Control Hosp Epidemiol* 2001;22(4):222–242.
51. Hoffer FA, Gow K, Flynn PM, et al. Accuracy of percutaneous lung biopsy for invasive pulmonary aspergillosis. *Pediatr Radiol* 2001;31: 144–152.
52. Barnes AJ, Oppenheim BA, Chang J, et al. Early investigation and initiation of therapy for invasive pulmonary aspergillosis in leukaemic and bone marrow transplant patients. *Mycoses* 1999;42(5–6):403–408.
53. Caillot D, Casasnovas O, Bernard A, et al. Improved management of invasive pulmonary aspergillosis in neutropenic patients using early thoracic computed tomographic scan and surgery. *J Clin Oncol* 1997; 15(1):139–147.
54. Bartley DL, Hughes WT, Parvey LS, et al. Computed tomography of hepatic and splenic fungal abscesses in leukemic children. *Pediatr Infect Dis* 1982;1(5):317–321.
55. Flynn PM, Shenep JL, Crawford R, et al. Use of abdominal computed tomography for identifying disseminated fungal infection in pediatric cancer patients. *Clin Infect Dis* 1995;20(4):964–970.
56. Pfaller MA, Herwaldt LA. The clinical microbiology laboratory and infection control: emerging pathogens, antimicrobial resistance, and new technology. *Clin Infect Dis* 1997;25(4):858–870.
57. Peterson LR, Noskin GA. New technology for detecting multidrug-resistant pathogens in the clinical microbiology laboratory. *Emerg Infect Dis* 2001;7(2):306–311.
58. Liu Y, Davin-Regli A, Bosi C, et al. Epidemiological investigation of Pseudomonas aeruginosa nosocomial bacteraemia isolates by PCR-based DNA fingerprinting analysis. *J Med Microbiol* 1996;45(5): 359–365.
59. Pfaller MA. Molecular epidemiology in the care of patients. *Arch Pathol Lab Med* 1999;123(11):1007–1010.

60. Garner JS, Jarvis WR, Emori TG, et al. CDC definitions for nosocomial infections, 1988. *Am J Infect Control* 1988;16(3):128–140.
61. Beck-Sague C, Jarvis WR. Secular trends in the epidemiology of nosocomial fungal infections in the United States, 1980–1990. National Nosocomial Infections Surveillance System. *J Infect Dis* 1993;167(5):1247–1251.
62. Viscoli C, Girmenia C, Marinus A, et al. Candidemia in cancer patients: a prospective, multicenter surveillance study by the Invasive Fungal Infection Group (IFIG) of the European Organization for Research and Treatment of Cancer (EORTC). *Clin Infect Dis* 1999;28(5):1071–1079.
63. Opal SM, Asp AA, Cannady PB Jr, et al. Efficacy of infection control measures during a nosocomial outbreak of disseminated aspergillosis associated with hospital construction. *J Infect Dis* 1986;153(3):634–637.
64. Cornet M, Levy V, Fleury L, et al. Efficacy of prevention by high-efficiency particulate air filtration or laminar airflow against Aspergillus airborne contamination during hospital renovation. *Infect Control Hosp Epidemiol* 1999;20(7):508–513.
65. Loo VG, Bertrand C, Dixon C, et al. Control of construction-associated nosocomial aspergillosis in an antiquated hematology unit. *Infect Control Hosp Epidemiol* 1996;17(6):360–364.
66. Oren I, Haddad N, Finkelstein R, et al. Invasive pulmonary aspergillosis in neutropenic patients during hospital construction: before and after chemoprophylaxis and institution of HEPA filters. *Am J Hematol* 2001;66(4):257–262.
67. Anaissie EJ, Stratton SL, Dignani C, et al. Pathogenic moulds (including Aspergillus spp.) in hospital water distribution systems: A three-year prospective study and clinical implications for patients with hematological malignancies. *Blood* 2003;101(7):2542–2546.
68. Classics in infectious diseases. Childbed fever by Ignaz Philipp Semmelweis. *Rev Infect Dis* 1981;3(4):808–811.
69. Larson E. A causal link between handwashing and risk of infection? Examination of the evidence. *Infect Control* 1988;9(1):28–36.
70. Larson E. Skin hygiene and infection prevention: more of the same or different approaches? *Clin Infect Dis* 1999;29(5):1287–1294.
71. Boyce JM, Pittet D. Guideline for hand hygiene in health-care settings: recommendations of the Healthcare Infection Control Practices Advisory Committee and the HICPAS/SHEA/APIC/IDSA Hand Hygiene Task Force. *MMWR Recomm Rep* 2002;51(RR-16):1–45.
72. O'Grady NP, Alexander M, Dellinger EP, et al. Guidelines for the prevention of intravascular catheter-related infections. Centers for Disease Control and Prevention. *MMWR Recomm Rep* 2002;51(RR-10):1–29.
73. Schimpff SC, Young VM, Greene WH, et al. Origin of infection in acute nonlymphocytic leukemia. Significance of hospital acquisition of potential pathogens. *Ann Intern Med* 1972;77(5):707–714.
74. Klein BS, Perloff WH, Maki DG. Reduction of nosocomial infection during pediatric intensive care by protective isolation. *N Engl J Med* 1989;320(26):1714–1721.
75. Nauseef WM, Maki DG. A study of the value of simple protective isolation in patients with granulocytopenia. *N Engl J Med* 1981;304(8):448–453.
76. Slota M, Green M, Farley A, et al. The role of gown and glove isolation and strict handwashing in the reduction of nosocomial infection in children with solid organ transplantation. *Crit Care Med* 2001;29(2):405–412.
77. Levine AS, Siegel SE, Schreiber AD, et al. Protected environments and prophylactic antibiotics. A prospective controlled study of their utility in the therapy of acute leukemia. *N Engl J Med* 1973;288(10):477–483.
78. Pizzo PA. The value of protective isolation in preventing nosocomial infections in high risk patients. *Am J Med* 1981;70(3):631–637.
79. Lentino JR, Rosenkranz MA, Michaels JA, et al. Nosocomial aspergillosis: a retrospective review of airborne disease secondary to road construction and contaminated air conditioners. *Am J Epidemiol* 1982;116(3):430–437.
80. Aisner J, Schimpff SC, Bennett JE, et al. Aspergillus infections in cancer patients. Association with fireproofing materials in a new hospital. *JAMA* 1976;235(4):411–412.
81. Sherertz RJ, Belani A, Kramer BS, et al. Impact of air filtration on nosocomial Aspergillus infections. Unique risk of bone marrow transplant recipients. *Am J Med* 1987;83(4):709–718.
82. Hahn T, Cummings KM, Michalek AM, et al. Efficacy of high-efficiency particulate air filtration in preventing aspergillosis in immunocompromised patients with hematologic malignancies. *Infect Control Hosp Epidemiol* 2002;23(9):525–531.
83. Raad I, Hanna H, Osting C, et al. Masking of neutropenic patients on transport from hospital rooms is associated with a decrease in nosocomial aspergillosis during construction. *Infect Control Hosp Epidemiol* 2002;23(1):41–43.
84. Guidelines for preventing opportunistic infections among hematopoietic stem cell transplant recipients. *MMWR Recomm Rep* 2000;49(RR-10):1–7.
85. Streifel AJ. In with the good air. *Infect Control Hosp Epidemiol* 2002;23(9):488–490.
86. Srinivasan A, Beck C, Buckley T, et al. The ability of hospital ventilation systems to filter Aspergillus and other fungi following a building implosion. *Infect Control Hosp Epidemiol* 2002;23(9):520–524.
87. Anaissie EJ, Stratton SL, Dignani MC, et al. Cleaning patient shower facilities: a novel approach to reducing patient exposure to aerosolized Aspergillus species and other opportunistic molds. *Clin Infect Dis* 2002;35(8):E86–E88.
88. Hughes WT, Armstrong D, Bodey GP, et al. 1997 guidelines for the use of antimicrobial agents in neutropenic patients with unexplained fever. Infectious Diseases Society of America. *Clin Infect Dis* 1997;25(3):551–573.
89. Engels EA, Lau J, Barza M. Efficacy of quinolone prophylaxis in neutropenic cancer patients: a meta-analysis. *J Clin Oncol* 1998;16(3):1179–1187.
90. Cruciani M, Rampazzo R, Malena M, et al. Prophylaxis with fluoroquinolones for bacterial infections in neutropenic patients: a meta-analysis. *Clin Infect Dis* 1996;23(4):795–805.
91. Bow EJ, Laverdiere M, Lussier N, et al. Antifungal prophylaxis for severely neutropenic chemotherapy recipients: a meta analysis of randomized-controlled clinical trials. *Cancer* 2002;94(12):3230–3246.
92. Hughes WT, Armstrong D, Bodey GP, et al. 2002 guidelines for the use of antimicrobial agents in neutropenic patients with cancer. *Clin Infect Dis* 2002;34(6):730–751.

59

NOSOCOMIAL INFECTIONS IN SOLID ORGAN TRANSPLANT RECIPIENTS

NINA SINGH

Infections remain a significant complication and a leading cause of mortality, particularly within the first year after transplantation. Most infections in transplant recipients are nosocomially acquired and represent either opportunistic infections resulting from iatrogenic immunosuppression or infections resulting from conventional nosocomial pathogens. Within the last decade, the incidence of several opportunistic infections [e.g., cytomegalovirus (CMV) and *Pneumocystis carinii* pneumonia (PCP)] has declined dramatically, largely because of the advent of effective prophylaxis. Instead, nosocomial infections (primarily resulting from bacteria) transmitted from environmental reservoirs or harbored as a result of endogenous colonization in nosocomial settings have emerged as leading infections in organ transplant recipients. In a recent study in liver transplant recipients, 82% of the episodes of fever documented in consecutive patients over a 2-year period were nosocomial, of which 62% were bacterial in origin (1). Fifty-three percent of all infections in heart transplant recipients in another study were nosocomially acquired, and of these 63% were bacterial (2).

Paralleling the trends in nosocomially acquired infections, antimicrobial resistance is increasingly recognized as a problem in the transplant setting. It is noteworthy, however, that the emergence of several of the antibiotic-resistant pathogens was first documented in transplant recipients (3). For example, vancomycin-resistant enterococci (VRE) were initially discovered in liver transplant recipients at several institutions where they eventually became a more widespread problem.

Transplant recipients are uniquely vulnerable to colonization and infection resulting from nosocomial pathogens. Within the same institution, transplant recipients have been shown to have a significantly higher incidence of nosocomial infections than nontransplant patients (4). The predilection of immunocompromised patients to *Legionella* infection is well recognized. However, it is notable that within this subgroup, transplant recipients have the highest risk (5). Among patients undergoing surgical procedures at one institution where legionellosis was documented, renal transplant recipients had an attack rate of 50%, whereas the general hospital population experienced an attack rate of only 0.4% (6). Transplant recipients exposed to tuberculosis during an institutional outbreak were more likely to contract *Mycobacterium tuberculosis* as compared with nontransplant contacts of the source case (7). During a nosocomial outbreak of extended-spectrum β-lactamase–producing *Escherichia coli,* 67% of patients on the liver transplant service, but no other surgical patients on the same floor, were shown to be colonized or infected with the outbreak isolate (8).

This chapter discusses the potential sources, unique risk factors, prevention, and infection control implications for nosocomial infections that may be acquired during or after transplantation.

SOURCES OF NOSOCOMIAL INFECTIONS

Donor-Transmitted Infections

Latent Infections in the Donor

Viral infections latent in the donor have by far the greatest potential for transmission by the transplanted organ and exert a more profound clinical impact in the allograft recipient compared with many other donor-transmitted infections. Thus, serologic screening of the donor for hepatitis B virus (HBV), hepatitis C virus (HCV), CMV, human immunodeficiency virus (HIV), and human T-cell leukemia virus type I (HTLV-I) is routinely recommended (9).

Hepatitis B Virus

The risk of transmission of HBV varies according to the HBV serologic profile of the donor and the recipient and the type of organ transplanted. Allografts from hepatitis B surface antigen (HBsAg)-positive donors can transmit HBV infection not only to recipients who are HBsAg negative but also to the ones who are HBsAg positive. Thus, organ donation from HBsAg-positive donors is recommended only in life-threatening situations, particularly if the recipient has no antibody to hepatitis B surface antigen (anti-HBs). Anti-HBs–positive donors who are negative for HBsAg and antibody to hepatitis B core antigen (anti-HBc) are generally considered unlikely to transmit HBV. HBV DNA, however, may be detectable in these patients by the polymerase chain reaction (PCR). Therefore, the potential for HBV transmission exists for donors with isolated anti-HBs positivity, unless anti-HBs positivity in the donor is the result of HBV vaccination or administration of hepatitis B immunoglobulin (HBIG) (10). Anti-HBc positivity in the absence of HBsAg poses a low but not negligible likelihood of transmission of HBV. The liver may continue to harbor the replicative form of HBV in such donors with the potential of HBV transmission, particularly with the hepatic allograft. Donors with isolated anti-HBc positivity should be considered infectious, although the risk of transmission, especially for the recipients of extrahepatic organs, is low. None of the seven heart transplant recipients, 2.3% (1/42) of the renal, and 50% (3/6) of the liver transplant recipients who received organs from isolated anti-HBc positive donors became infected (11). General consensus is that the organs from anti-HBC positive donors should be used for recipients who are HBsAg positive or who have received HBV vaccine. Transplantation of an anti-HBc positive liver into a nonimmune recipient should be performed only if deemed medically urgent and under a prophylactic regimen of lamivudine with or without HBIG (12).

Hepatitis C Virus

Approximately 5% of all cadaveric organ donors are positive for antibody to HCV (anti-HCV), and 50% of these have detectable HCV viremia by PCR (9). Although anti-HCV–positive donor organs may transmit HCV infection, discarding all HCV-positive organs is not feasible. Transplantation of livers from HCV-positive donors into HCV-positive recipients has not been associated with a decrease in graft or patient survival at 1 to 5 years (13,14). Most transplant centers use HCV-positive donor kidneys only for HCV-positive recipients. The use of anti-HCV–positive organs in anti-HCV–negative recipients may be considered in emergency or life-threatening situations or in selected circumstances, for example, the elderly kidney transplant candidates with limited lifespan or diabetics with end-stage renal disease in whom the gain in quality of life after kidney transplantation might outweigh the risk of HCV, particularly because the long-term outcome of HCV infection in transplant recipients has not been well defined.

Herpesviruses

The donated allograft is a significant and an efficient source of transmission of CMV (15,16). The morbidity from infection is greatest in CMV-seronegative recipients of CMV-positive allografts. Superinfection (i.e., infection with an exogenous strain of CMV in patients with prior evidence of CMV infection) has also been documented. Symptomatic CMV disease occurred more frequently in patients infected with the new CMV strain compared with those with reactivation of the latent virus (17). Donor transmission (documented by molecular typing) has also been demonstrated with other herpesviruses, including herpes simplex virus (HSV), Epstein-Barr virus, and human herpesvirus-6 (HHV-6) (18–21).

Human Immunodeficiency Virus

Donor positivity for HIV by enzyme-linked immunosorbent assay (ELISA) is considered an absolute contraindication to organ donation. Living donors who test negative for HIV antibody may be infectious during the window period between the acquisition of HIV infection and seroconversion. Although HIV p24 antigen may potentially detect HIV infection in such cases, this test is not yet routinely available for organ donors (9). According to the Centers for Disease Control and Prevention's guidelines for HIV screening practices for organ donation, social history suggestive of HIV exposure should be sought in all potential organ donors and may indicate an increased risk of HIV transmission, even in the presence of negative HIV serology (9).

Human T-Cell Leukemia Virus Type I

Although HTLV-I has been documented to be transmitted by blood, the risk of transmission by organ transplantation has not been clearly discerned. Except in life-threatening circumstances, HTLV-I positivity is considered a contraindication to organ donation (9).

Other Pathogens

Transmission of syphilis by organ donation has never been conclusively demonstrated. However, routine serologic screening of all potential donors for syphilis is recommended; recipients of such organs should receive penicillin as prophylaxis post-transplant (22).

Transmission of *M. tuberculosis* to recipients receiving allografts from donors with active tuberculosis has been documented. Transmission of *M. tuberculosis* to two renal transplant recipients from a donor with unrecognized tuberculous meningitis at the time of organ retrieval has been reported (23). Tuberculin-positive donors without clinically overt tuberculosis may also transmit tuberculosis. It is recommended that the recipients of allografts from donors with tuberculin reactivity or a history of tuberculosis receive chemoprophylaxis for tuberculosis after transplantation (24).

Toxoplasma gondii, because of its predilection for latency in muscle tissue, poses a considerable risk for transmission in heart transplant recipients; 50% to 75% of the seronegative recipients of *T. gondii* antibody-positive allografts have developed toxoplasmosis. Because of the paucity of *Toxoplasma* cysts in noncardiac tissue, toxoplasmosis is rarely transmitted by the transplanted organs in renal and liver transplant recipients.

Acquired Infections in the Donor

Life-sustaining measures in critically ill donors may render them susceptible to nosocomially acquired infections with the potential for transmission to the allograft recipients. Two recent studies comprising a large number of patients have shown that donor bacteremia did not portend a higher risk of infectious complications or compromise graft or patient survival (25,26). The most frequent cause of the donor bacteremias in these studies was gram-positive bacteria, of which *Staphylococcus aureus* was the predominant pathogen. Most recipients of organs retrieved from bacteremic donors in the aforementioned studies received antimicrobial therapy. In the study by Lumbreras et al. (25), specific antibiotics were administered to the recipients for 7 to 10 days on receipt of donor blood culture results. In the report by Freeman et al. (26), 91% of the recipients received antibiotics for a mean of 3.8 days. These data suggest that with appropriately administered antibiotic therapy, organs from bacteremic donors can be successfully transplanted without incurring an additional risk for infection or allograft dysfunction in the recipient.

A similar dilemma exists regarding the feasibility of using

organs from donors with bacterial meningitis (27). Lopez-Navidad et al. (27) described the outcome in 16 recipients who had received organs from five patients with bacterial meningitis. The pathogens included *Neisseria meningitidis, Streptococcus pneumoniae,* and *E. coli.* With antibiotic administration ranging from 5 to 10 days, infection caused by the aforementioned bacteria were not documented in any of the recipients. Thus, patients with brain death attributable to bacterial meningitis caused by these bacteria can also be suitable organ donors, if the donor and the recipient receive appropriate antibiotic therapy. An exception, however, is donors with a less commonly encountered bacterial infection, that is, *M. tuberculosis.* Unrecognized active *M. tuberculosis* infection in the donor can be efficiently transmitted to the recipient with deleterious sequelae.

Donor organs colonized with *Candida* or *Aspergillus* may transmit the fungi to lung and heart-lung transplant recipients. Karyotypic analysis of the *Candida albicans* isolates demonstrated identical strains from the donor lung and *C. albicans* isolates causing disseminated infection in a lung transplant recipient (28). Donor organs have also been documented to transmit other fungal infections (e.g., *Cryptococcus neoformans* and *Histoplasma capsulatum*) (29).

Contamination during Organ Procurement

Contamination during harvesting and preservation of the allograft has been reported to occur in 2% to 23% of the kidney allografts. Although some bacteria (e.g., *Staphylococcus epidermidis,* diphtheroid species, and *Propionibacterium acnes*) present little risk of infection to the allograft recipient, more virulent pathogens (e.g., gram-negative rods, particularly *Pseudomonas aeruginosa; S. aureus; Bacteroides* species; and fungi) cultured from the donor or preservation fluid can lead to serious infections (e.g., mycotic aneurysm and anastomotic rupture) in kidney transplant recipients (29).

Blood Products

Although CMV infection has been shown to be transmitted by blood products in organ transplant recipients, the risk is small and has not been shown to correlate with the number of blood products transfused (21). Over a 13 year-period, only 2.6% (3/112) of CMV-seronegative recipients who received CMV-negative renal, heart, lung, or liver allografts were documented to develop transfusion-associated CMV infection (30). Furthermore, transfusion, compared with donor-transmitted CMV infection, has been associated with a lower frequency of symptomatic disease and, therefore, has a less profound clinical impact (31). Although some centers use CMV-seronegative blood products for recipients who are seronegative for CMV, routine testing of blood products for CMV is not recommended.

Since May 1990, all blood products in the United States have been routinely screened for HCV. Consequently, the risk of posttransfusion HCV has declined from 8% to 10% to less than 1% currently.

Environmental Reservoirs and Sources

Environmental sources are significant sites for acquisition of a number of infectious agents, particularly nosocomial pathogens in transplant recipients (Table 59.1). Most cases of *Legionella* in solid organ transplant recipients are nosocomially acquired (32). The source of posttransplant legionellosis in all studies where an environmental link was sought was the hospital's potable water distribution system (5). Restriction fragment length polymorphism patterns documented that the hospital's central hot water supply was the source of legionellosis in a hospital where 14 cases were documented in transplant recipients over an 8-year period (33). Nosocomial legionellosis in heart-lung transplant recipients at one institution was linked to a contaminated ice machine (34).

Outbreaks of invasive aspergillosis in transplant recipients have been linked to construction or demolition activity within or near a hospital; contaminated or poorly maintained ventilation ducts, grids, or air filters; and other dust-generating activities that may aerosolize *Aspergillus* spores. Accommodation of marrow transplant recipients outside of rooms with laminar air flow and high-efficiency particulate air filters during periods of neutropenia have been shown to be a risk factor for invasive aspergil-

TABLE 59.1. MODE OF ACQUISITION OF MAJOR PATHOGENS IN TRANSPLANT RECIPIENTS

Pathogen	Mode of acquisition
Viruses	
Cytomegalovirus	
Seronegative recipient	Donor transmission, rarely transfusions
Seropositive recipient	Reactivation and donor transmission
Herpes simplex virus	Reactivation, rarely donor transmission
Varicella zoster virus	Reactivation, rarely donor transmission
Human herpesvirus-6	Reactivation and donor transmission
Hepatitis C virus	Reactivation, unless donor anti-hepatitis C virus positive
Hepatitis B virus[a]	Rarely donor transmission
Adenovirus	Donor and nosocomial transmission
Respiratory viral infections	Nosocomial and community acquisition
Bacteria	
Staphylococcus aureus	Endogenous nasal colonization, nosocomial transmission
Vancomycin-resistant enterococci	Nosocomial transmission, endogenous gastrointestinal colonization
Pseudomonas aeruginosa	Nosocomial environmental acquisition
Enterobacteriaceae	Endogenous infection, nosocomial transmission Environmental acquisition
Legionella	Environmental acquisition
Mycobacterium tuberculosis	Reactivation, donor transmission, nosocomial transmission
Fungi	
Candida	Endogenous infection (liver transplants), donor transmission (lung transplants)
Aspergillus	Environmental acquisition
Pneumocystis carinii	Reactivation, possibly nosocomial transmission
Cryptococcus neoformans	Unknown
Protozoa	
Toxoplasma gondii	Donor transmission, rarely reactivation

[a]HBsAg-positive donors can transmit hepatitis B virus (HBV) but are not considered acceptable organ donors. Rarely anti-HBs-positive donors (particularly of hepatic allografts) can transmit HBV.

losis (35). A seasonal variation in the incidence of invasive aspergillosis, coinciding with a high outdoor concentration of airborne spores in late summer or fall and a lower concentration in the winter months, has also been observed. The prevailing belief that *Aspergillus* is predominantly an airborne pathogen acquired via inhalation has recently been challenged. It has been proposed that *Fusarium* and *Aspergillus* can be detected in hospital water systems, and aspiration, as opposed to inhalation of *Aspergillus,* may be the mode of acquisition of nosocomial invasive aspergillosis in susceptible hosts (36).

VRE and methicillin-resistant *S. aureus* (MRSA) have become established as endemic pathogens in many institutions and are increasingly recognized as significant microorganisms in transplant recipients. At many centers, VRE, MRSA, or *Clostridium difficile* are currently the most frequent etiologic agents of infections in transplant recipients. Although patient specific variables (e.g., severity of illness, intensity of antimicrobial use, and length of hospital stay) are risk factors for acquisition, environmental contamination and, more importantly, person-to-person transmission are also considered significant factors in the nosocomial spread of these bacteria. Equipment and surfaces in the vicinity of patients colonized and infected with VRE have been shown to become contaminated with VRE; VRE could be recovered for at least 7 days from the surfaces of countertops and after 30 minutes from the stethoscopes (37). Furthermore, epidemiologic studies have documented nosocomial VRE transmission by molecular typing techniques (38). Likewise, pulse-field gel electrophoresis demonstrated that 43% of the MRSA isolates causing invasive infections at a transplant unit shared the same pattern, suggesting nosocomial transmission (39).

C. difficile is currently the most common cause of infectious diarrhea in transplant recipients. Liver transplantation was identified as the most significant independent risk factor for *C. difficile* acquisition in one report (40). Although the precise mode of transmission of *C. difficile* has not been determined, environmental contamination and nosocomial transmission clearly occurs. *C. difficile* was recovered from 9% to 51% of the environmental cultures; objects contaminated with feces (e.g., bed pan, toilet seats, sinks, and scales were most likely to yield *C. difficile*) (41). Positive hand cultures were documented in 59% of the hospital personnel caring for the patients with *C. Difficile,* implicating hands of hospital personnel as a likely mode of transmission (42). Prudent use of antimicrobial agents and measures to curtail nosocomial transmission are key toward effective prevention of infections caused by these pathogens.

TABLE 59.2. RISK FACTORS FOR INFECTION WITH MAJOR NOSOCOMIAL PATHOGENS IN TRANSPLANT RECIPIENTS

Pathogen	Risk factors
Fungi	
Aspergillus	
Lung transplantation	Single lung transplant, CMV infection
Liver transplantation	Poor allograft function, renal failure, particularly a requirement for dialysis, OKT3 use, retransplantation
Heart transplantation	Not determined
Pancreatic transplantation	Not determined
Renal transplantation	Augmented immunosuppression and graft failure requiring hemodialysis
Candida	
Liver transplantation	Prolonged operation time, high transfusion requirement, high serum creatinine, repeat surgeries
Lung transplantation	Donor tracheal colonization
Pancreatic transplantation	Diabetes, exocrine enteric or bladder drainage
Pneumocystis carinii	Augmented immunosuppression, older recipient age, CMV infection
Viruses	
Cytomegalovirus	Donor CMV seropositivity, OKT3 use, allograft rejection, HHV-6 infection
Bacteria	
Vancomycin-resistant *Enterococcus faecium*	Rectal colonization prior to transplant, previous antibiotic use, biliary complications, prolonged hospitalization, surgical reexploration, allograft nonfunction
Methicillin-resistant *Staphylococcus aureus*	Nasal *S. aureus* carriage, prolonged hospitalization, ICU stay
Legionella	Contaminated hospital potable water system, humidifiers, and ice machines
Mycobacterium tuberculosis[a] (risk factors for early-onset tuberculosis)	Nonrenal transplantation, history of prior *M. tuberculosis* (positive tuberculin test or old active tuberculosis on chest radiographs), OKT3 use
Pseudomonas aeruginosa	Donor colonization (lung transplants), cystic fibrosis

CMV, cytomegalovirus; HHV-6, human herpesvirus-6; ICU, intensive care unit.
[a]Early-onset tuberculosis implies infection occurring within 12 months of transplantation.

RISK FACTORS FOR INFECTIONS

Surgical factors, intensity of immunosuppression, and variations in local and systemic host response are among the variables that determine not only the type but the site and severity of infections in different types of organ transplant recipients (Table 59.2).

Liver Transplantation

Liver transplant recipients, by virtue of having hepatic failure and malnutrition before transplantation, represent severely compromised hosts. Many of these patients have concomitant renal failure as a result of hepatorenal syndrome. Renal failure, particularly the requirement for dialysis, was an important predictor of early infections and adversely affected survival after liver transplantation (43,44)

Liver transplant recipients are uniquely susceptible to invasive candidiasis. Most cases originate from endogenous sources; deficient reticuloendothelial function and translocation across the gut mucosa are considered important pathogenetic factors predisposing to invasive candidiasis (45). Vascular and anastomotic complications are also significant risk factors for infectious morbidity in liver transplant recipients. Duct-to-duct biliary anastomosis compared with Roux-en-Y choledochojejunostomy is associated with a lower incidence of infections, because the latter involves the breach of the bowel integrity and sacrificing the sphincter of Oddi, which may promote reflux of bowel contents into the biliary tree (46). Hepatic artery thrombosis may lead to the development of hepatic infarcts with subsequent gangrene and abscess formation. The clinical presentation is usually acute or fulminant, although hepatic artery occlusion may occasionally be occult and present with a clinical picture of unexplained fever and relapsing subacute bacteremia. Hepatic artery thrombosis may also lead to liver abscesses by compromising the biliary vascular supply. Impaired arterial flow to the hepatic allograft preferentially affects the biliary tree because of the biliary tract's almost total reliance on the hepatic arterial blood supply. Hepatic artery thrombosis may thus lead to biliary tract ischemia and biliary leaks, eventually resulting in intrahepatic abscess formation.

The biliary tract may be a source of infection even with an intact vascular supply. Biliary composition is altered during liver transplantation, leading to supersaturation with cholesterol and sludge and stone formation that may predispose to infections (e.g., cholangitis). T-tubes, commonly used to protect duct-to-duct biliary anastomoses, are prone to microbial colonization and form a nidus for the deposition of biliary sludge.

Portal vein thrombosis was shown to be the most significant independent predictor of early bacterial infections after liver transplantation (47). Recurrent viral HCV hepatitis has been documented in nearly 50% of the patients undergoing liver transplantation for end-stage liver disease resulting from HCV. HCV is considered an immunosuppressive and an immunomodulatory virus. Patients with HCV recurrence were significantly more likely to develop late-occurring infections, particularly fungal infections after liver transplantation (48).

Renal Transplantation

Urinary tract and postoperative surgical site infections are two of the most frequent and serious nosocomial infections in renal transplant recipients. Urinary tract infections occur in more than 50% of patients during the first 3 months after transplantation and are the most frequent source of bacteremia during this time. In the absence of antimicrobial prophylaxis, surgical site infections have been reported in up to 20% of patients (49). Organ/space surgical site infections after renal transplantation have been shown to adversely affect graft survival.

Surgical site infections in renal transplant recipients are usually due to staphylococci or gram-negative bacilli (49,50). Staphylococcal infections tended to be associated with incisional surgical site infections and occurred earlier, whereas those due to gram-negative bacilli occurred later; were organ/space surgical site infections; and often led to bacteremia, graft loss, or death. Prolonged urinary catheterization, a surgical site hematoma, a reopened surgical site, and a cadaveric donor graft are risk factors for nosocomial urinary or surgical site infections in renal transplant recipients (51,52). Renal trauma with nephrectomy and graft contamination during transportation may likely account for a higher risk of infection in cadaveric compared with living allograft recipients. Urinary tract infections occurring in the later posttransplant period (beyond 3 months) are usually benign and rarely symptomatic. Antimicrobial prophylaxis has proven highly effective in reducing the rate of urinary tract and surgical site infections in renal transplant recipients. A single perioperative dose of antibiotics led to a reduction in the incidence of surgical site infections from 25% to 2% (53). Prophylaxis with trimethoprim-sulfamethoxazole has been shown to significantly lower the incidence of urinary tract infections, bacteremias, and infections caused by gram-negative bacilli and *S. aureus* when compared with placebo (54).

Heart and Lung Transplantation

Heart and lung transplant recipients are uniquely susceptible to nosocomial bacterial pulmonary infections, particularly in the first month after transplantation. Bacterial pneumonia has been reported in 35% to 48% of the lung and heart-lung transplant recipients (55,56). Impaired mucociliary clearance, loss of cough reflex, postoperative pain with splinting, and donor tracheal colonization are some factors contributing to a high risk of postoperative pneumonia in lung transplant recipients.

Multiply antibiotic-resistant strains of *P. aeruginosa* and *Pseudomonas cepacia* are of particular concern in patients undergoing lung transplantation for cystic fibrosis. One-year mortality was shown to be twofold greater in patients who harbored resistant *Pseudomonas* compared with other patients (57). Indeed, colonization with highly resistant *Pseudomonas* strains is considered a controversial indication for lung transplantation at many centers. Although the infected lung is removed during transplantation, residual colonization of the airway, nasopharynx, and sinuses remains a potential nidus for subsequent infection. Pretransplant bilateral maxillary sinus drainage followed by monthly irrigation with tobramycin led to an improved outcome in cystic fibrosis patients in one study. Some centers use this approach only if clinically significant sinus infection occurs after transplantation (58). An innovative approach using aerosolized colistin and discontinuation of systemic antibiotics led to the emergence of sensitive *Pseudomonas* strains in patients who previously harbored resistant *Pseudomonas* isolates (57). Of 20 cystic fibrosis patients with resistant *Pseudomonas* who received aerosolized colistin, all became colonized with sensitive isolates of *Pseudomonas* within a mean of 45 days. In contrast, only 30% (3/10) of the control candidates who received only systemic antipseudomonal antibiotics became colonized with the sensitive isolates. Five of six patients who received colistin and underwent transplantation continued to harbor sensitive microorganisms after transplantation.

Circulatory support devices (e.g., intraaortic balloon pump and left ventricular assist devices) are required in many potential heart transplant recipients, and their prolonged placement is a major risk factor for bacterial colonization and subsequent nosocomial infections after transplantation. Sternal surgical site infections occur in 5% to 20% of heart and heart-lung transplant recipients; staphylococci, *Enterobacteriaceae,* and *P. aeruginosa* are the most common causative microorganisms. Sternal surgical site infections may directly extend into the mediastinum and predispose to mediastinitis or mycotic aneurysms at the suture sites. Mediastinitis occurs in 2% to 9% of the heart and heart-lung transplant recipients; *S. aureus, P. aeruginosa,* and *C. albicans* have been the most commonly reported microorganisms (59–62). An unusual cause of mediastinitis in transplant recipients is *Mycoplasma hominis* (63).

Pancreatic Transplantation

Surgical site infections, abscesses, or urinary tract infections occur in 7% to 50% of the pancreatic transplant recipients (64–67). Organ/space surgical site infections are a significant cause of graft loss and mortality in these patients. The postoperative infection rates and the causative pathogens depend primarily on the technique used for the drainage of exocrine secretions of the pancreas. Diversion into the small bowel (enteric drainage), free drainage into the peritoneum, drainage into the bladder, and injection of the duct with synthetic polymer are the approaches used for drainage of exocrine secretions. Infection rates are generally the lowest with duct injection and highest with enteric drainage (which facilitates contamination with gastrointestinal bacteria). Infections occurred in 33% (19/57) of the cases who underwent pancreaticojejunostomy, 33% (5/15) in those with free drainage into the peritoneal cavity, and in 3% (1/39) of the cases in which the duct was injected with a synthetic polymer (66). Duct injection, however, is no longer used because of fibrosis that may lead to loss of endocrine function.

Whereas aerobic and anaerobic enteric flora predominate in abscesses associated with enteric drainage, microorganisms in infections in which the viscus has not been opened are usually from the skin flora. *Candida,* however, is a common pathogen in all types of surgical site infections, including those using bladder drainage. A high incidence of *Candida* urinary colonization because of diabetes in these patients along with the nonacidic environment in the bladder created by the exocrine pancreatic secretions facilitate *Candida* colonization.

Small Bowel Transplantation

Unique features predisposing to infections in small bowel transplant recipients are the fact that the contents of the transplanted organ are nonsterile and that these patients require a higher intensity of immunosuppressive therapy to prevent graft rejection (68–72). Virtually all small bowel transplant recipients experience at least one episode of infection; the number of infectious episodes per patient may range from 1 to 11 (median 5) (69). Multivisceral transplant recipients and those undergoing colonic segment transplantation with small bowel transplantation are more likely to develop infections (69). It is noteworthy that small bowel transplant recipients remain susceptible to infections, even in the late posttransplant period (i.e., more than 6 months after transplantation) (69).

Small bowel transplant recipients, particularly CMV-seronegative recipients of seropositive grafts, are uniquely vulnerable to CMV infection and to recurrent episodes of CMV disease (68). CMV disease in recipient-negative donor-positive patients has been shown to adversely affect outcome in these patients. Consequently, some transplant centers do not use CMV-seropositive small bowel grafts for CMV-seronegative recipients (71). Notably, a small bowel graft is involved in 81% to 90% of the patients with CMV disease (68,71).

Bacterial translocation in small bowel transplant recipients predisposes these patients to intraabdominal infections (peritonitis and abscesses). Selective decontamination of the gut after transplantation has been proposed to reduce early postoperative infections in small bowel transplant recipients (70).

TIME OF ONSET

The relative frequency, types of infection, and the specific pathogens encountered after transplantation generally have a predictable time of onset. Thus, infections in transplant recipients must be evaluated in the context of time elapsed since transplantation. These data also have implications relevant for the institution of prophylaxis and the duration of prophylaxis.

Infections During the First 30 Days

Most infections occurring within 30 days of transplantation are a consequence primarily of surgical or technical complications related to transplantation, nosocomial acquisition, and rarely reactivation of latent infections (e.g., herpesviruses) in the recipient. Bacterial infections are by far the most frequently occurring infections during this period; vascular catheter-related infections, nosocomial pneumonia, and surgical site infections are the most common types. Fungal infections likely to be encountered in the first month after transplantation include candidiasis and aspergillosis. Nearly 75% of the cases of invasive candidiasis and aspergillosis in liver transplant recipients occur within the first month and virtually all within 2 months of transplantation (45,73). More recently, however, delayed occurrence of *Aspergillus* infections has been noted; 55% of the cases of invasive aspergillosis in liver transplant recipients occurred after 90 days of transplantation (74). Liver transplant recipients are uniquely susceptible to invasive candidiasis; disruption of the integrity of the bowel and gastrointestinal translocation are the proposed mechanisms. The only significant viral infection occurring within the first 30 days of transplantation is that due to the HSV. However, there is accumulating evidence to suggest that the novel herpesvirus, HHV-6, may also be a pathogen in the early posttransplant period (75). HHV-6 infection characteristically occurs earlier than CMV and may cause fever of unknown origin and idiopathic cytopenia during this period.

Infections Occurring Between 30 and 180 Days

Although nosocomial infections may continue to pose a threat in patients requiring prolonged hospitalization, most infections occurring between 30 and 180 days after transplantation are opportunistic infections related to the effects of immunosuppression. The foremost pathogen in transplant recipients during this time period is CMV; however, infections resulting from *M. tuberculosis, P. carinii, T. Gondii,* and *Nocardia* are also likely to be encountered during this interval. Clinically and histopathologically manifest recurrences of HCV hepatitis usually occurs within 6 months of transplantation. In the absence of immunoprophylaxis for HBV, recurrence of HBV infections in the recipient occur a median of 3 months after transplantation.

Infections Occurring 6 Months or Later

Infectious diseases in the last posttransplant period are typically community-acquired infections similar to those occurring in the general population. However, patients requiring aggressive immunosuppression for recurrent or chronic rejection and those with poorly functioning allografts (e.g., liver transplant recipients with recurrent viral HBV or HCV) continue to be at risk for opportunistic infections. Posttransplant lymphoproliferative disorder, varicella-zoster virus (VZV) infections, cryptococcosis, and infections resulting from dematiaceous fungi typically occur 6 or more months after transplantation.

VIRUSES

Herpesvirus Infections

Cytomegalovirus

CMV has been recognized as one of the most significant pathogens in organ transplant recipients. Depending on the pretransplantation CMV serostatus of the recipient, three distinct epidemiologic patterns of CMV infection exist. Primary infection occurs when a seronegative recipient acquires CMV, either from the transplanted allograft or less commonly from blood products. Reactivation infection results from endogenous reactivation of the latent virus. Superinfection implies acquisition of a new strain of CMV in a patient seropositive for CMV before transplantation. Because 50% to 70% of the general population is seropositive for CMV, most infections in transplant recipients represent reactivation infections. However, the clinical impact of CMV is by far greatest in the context of newly acquired or primary infection. Primary CMV acquisition is associated with a higher rate of CMV infection and symptomatic disease, earlier onset of CMV infection posttransplantation, higher incidence of recurrent episodes of CMV, greater risk of dissemination, and higher mortality (76–78). Symptomatic disease, CMV hepatitis, invasive fungal infections, and death in liver transplantation were more likely to occur when primary infection in the recipient was acquired from the donor organ compared with acquisition from transfusions (31). The time to onset of CMV infection after transplantation is also shorter with donor versus transfusion-associated CMV infection (31). Superinfection, as compared with reactivation infection, is also associated with a higher incidence and severity of symptomatic CMV disease (79).

Risk Factors

CMV serologic status of the recipient and donor is the most significant factor influencing the rate and severity of CMV infection. Eighty percent to 100% of the seronegative recipients of a seropositive donor allograft acquire CMV infection after transplantation. The risk of CMV infection is lowest (<10%) in seronegative recipients of seronegative organ donors. CMV-seropositive recipients have an intermediate risk (40% to 60%) for developing CMV infection. The intensity and type of immunosuppression are also important determinants of the risk of CMV infection (80). Antilymphocyte preparations (e.g., OKT3) are extremely potent reactivators of CMV. Primary immunosuppressive agents (e.g., cyclosporine and tacrolimus), on the other hand, are not efficient reactivators, but, when CMV reactivation occurs, they interfere with the host's ability to limit viral replication (80).

Primary infection with HHV-6, which is considered an immunomodulatory virus, has been proposed to be a risk factor for subsequent CMV invasive disease. Intraoperative hypothermia is a common complication of liver transplant surgery. In a study in liver transplant recipients, intraoperative hypothermia was an independently significant risk factor for early CMV infection and active warming using a convective heating device appeared to curtail this risk (81). Human leukocyte antigen matching and retransplantation have also been shown to be risk factors for CMV infection (77,82).

Pathogenesis

CMV-specific major histocompatibility complex (MHC)-restricted cytotoxic T cells are pivotal in host defense against CMV; clinically significant CMV occurs predominantly among patients without an adequate T-lymphocyte response. Humoral immunity, on the other hand, is an ineffective host defense against CMV, although it may modify (or temper) the severity of infection. Tumor necrosis factor-alpha has been shown to be a powerful promoter of CMV (80,83,84). Any physiologic stimulus for tumor necrosis factor-alpha release (e.g., OKT3, sepsis, and rejection), therefore, has the potential to activate CMV.

CMV is considered an immunosuppressive virus that may facilitate superinfection with opportunistic pathogens (e.g., fungi, gram-negative bacteria, and *P. carinii*) (77,85). Other indirect sequelae of CMV infection include a proposed association with allograft rejection in liver transplant recipients, bronchiolitis obliterans in lung transplant recipients, atherogenesis in heart transplant recipients, and glomerulopathy in renal transplant recipients, although this remains controversial.

Epidemiology and Clinical Features

The overall incidence of CMV infection ranges between 40% and 90% in organ transplant recipients. The highest incidence of CMV infection has been documented in lung or heart-lung transplant recipients (60% to 98%) and the lowest (40% to 50%) in renal transplant recipients. Liver and heart transplant recipients have an intermediate risk of CMV infection (50% to 67%). The frequency of symptomatic disease resulting from CMV ranges from 8% to 15% in renal, 20% to 35% in liver, 27% to 30% in heart, and 55% to 60% in lung transplant recipients. The incidence of CMV infection in small bowel transplant recipients approaches that in lung transplant recipients (68). Small bowel transplant patients also appear to be uniquely susceptible to recurrent episodes of CMV infection (68).

Traditionally, most CMV infections have occurred between 4 and 6 weeks. In patients receiving prolonged antiviral prophylaxis, onset of CMV infection has been noted to be delayed (86–88). A febrile mononucleosis syndrome characterized by fever, arthralgias, myalgias, leukopenia, and atypical lymphocytosis is the most common symptomatic disease caused by CMV, although localized or disseminated tissue invasive disease may also occur. Predilection to involve the transplanted allograft is a peculiar characteristic of CMV. CMV hepatitis occurs most commonly in liver transplant recipients, CMV pneumonitis occurs most commonly in lung transplant recipients, and CMV enteritis occurs most commonly in small bowel transplant recipients. It is proposed that the transplanted allograft may provide a sequestered site for latently infected cells, because MHC mismatches at these sites may prevent the generation of virus-specific cytotoxic T-cell responses (89).

Diagnosis

The diagnosis of CMV infection has traditionally been made by viral isolation, which can take up to 4 weeks. The currently available tests not only allow rapid and reliable diagnosis of CMV infection but also may detect viral shedding at an earlier stage. The shell vial assay for viral cultures uses a monoclonal antibody to detect a 72-kDa immediate early CMV antigen and allows detection of CMV within 16 to 24 hours (90). More recently, a CMV antigenemia assay, with monoclonal antibodies directed against the 63-kDa structural late viral protein, has been developed (91,92). The CMV antigenemia assay is more sensitive and allows earlier detection of CMV than shell vial culture does. Furthermore, results of the antigenemia assay can be quantitated; the number of antigen-positive cells has been shown to correlate with the likelihood of CMV disease and can also be used to monitor response to antiviral therapy. The major drawback of the antigenemia assay is the need for immediate processing of blood samples. Detection of viral DNA by PCR in the leukocyte may be an overly sensitive test for the diagnosis of CMV. Because PCR can detect even minute amounts of viral DNA, it may not differentiate between replicating and latent virus. The precise role of quantitative PCR for the diagnosis of CMV remains to be established. Plasma, as opposed to leukocyte PCR, is specific yet not an excessively sensitive test for the detection of CMV infection (93–95). Its sensitivity is comparable with CMV antigenemia.

Prevention

Matching Donors and Recipients by Serologic Status. Attempts to decrease the morbidity associated with primary donor-acquired CMV infection have included the use of CMV-seropositive donor organs only for seropositive recipients. Although a decrease in graft loss and mortality attributable to CMV was noted in one report (96), others have not shown a significant impact with such an approach. Widespread adoption of this approach, however, is not feasible given the limited organ donor pool.

Prophylaxis. Although several prophylactic strategies have been used for CMV, an optimal approach has not been defined. High-dose acyclovir (800 mg orally four times daily) administered to renal transplant patients for 12 weeks decreased the rate of CMV disease (97). Most subsequent studies in solid organ transplant recipients, including renal transplant patients, showed no benefit of acyclovir in the prevention of CMV disease (98). Ganciclovir, administered intravenously for 2 to 4 weeks, was efficacious against CMV, predominantly in the seropositive patients (99, 100). Ganciclovir for 100 days after transplantation was effective both in seropositive patients and in seronegative recipients of a seropositive allograft; however, the feasibility and cost of administration of ganciclovir for 100 days can be prohibitive (101). A valyl ester of ganciclovir, valganciclovir has significantly improved oral bioavailability as compared with ganciclovir administered orally. Systemic levels equivalent to those achievable with intravenous ganciclovir have been documented with valganciclovir. In high-risk organ transplant recipients, valganciclovir 900 mg once daily had comparable efficacy to oral ganciclovir 1,000 mg three times daily for the prevention of CMV disease (88).

However, the previously mentioned strategies using universal prophylaxis require administration of ganciclovir to all patients, most of whom will not experience CMV infection. With prolonged ganciclovir use, viral resistance remains a potential concern, and it is increasingly documented in transplant recipients (3,102,103).

A preferred approach to the prevention of CMV is to target the patients at highest risk for serious disease resulting from CMV. The success of this approach relies on early identification of CMV infection and on the use of prophylaxis preemptively to prevent asymptomatic infection from progressing to CMV disease. The criterion used to identify high-risk patients may either be a laboratory marker (e.g., viral shedding preceding symptomatic disease) or a clinical event (e.g., institution of OKT3 therapy). Surveillance cultures using a sensitive assay (e.g., CMV antigenemia) offer a significant advantage over the previous culture methods (e.g., shell vial assay) for earlier detection of CMV infection (98,104,105). The preemptive strategy is particularly appealing and perhaps ideal for seropositive patients in whom CMV disease generally is less severe (98). With diligent monitoring, CMV disease can also be prevented in 80% to 100% of the patients with primary CMV infection (106).

Herpes Simplex Virus

HSV infections in transplant recipients present as mucocutaneous lesions resulting from reactivation of the latent virus. However, visceral or disseminated HSV infection can be donor transmitted and may have a fulminant presentation with a grave outcome without antiviral therapy. HSV hepatitis is the most frequently documented site of disseminated HSV infection; its incidence (cases per thousand) is reported to be 2.11 in renal, 2.23 in heart, and 4.81 in liver transplant recipients. In a report comprising 12 cases of HSV hepatitis in solid organ transplant recipients, 33% were due to primary HSV infection believed to be acquired from the donor (107). The median time to onset of HSV hepatitis was 18 days, although it occurred as early as 5 days posttransplantation (107). This characteristic time of onset is in contrast with CMV hepatitis, which usually occurs 30 to 40 days after transplantation. Clinical manifestations of HSV hepatitis include fever, leukocytosis, thrombocytopenia, and marked elevation of hepatocellular liver enzymes. Mortality from primary visceral HSV infection in seronegative recipients was 75%; hypotension, disseminated intravascular coagulation, metabolic acidosis, low platelet count, and high creatinine were significant predictors of mortality (107).

The HSV accounted for 41% of all non-CMV isolates from the respiratory tract in lung transplant recipients; 80% of the isolates were deemed clinically significant and were associated with pneumonitis (108). Another clinical presentation of HSV, predominantly reported in intubated lung and cardiac transplant recipients, is HSV tracheobronchitis that manifested as fever, bronchospasm, leukocytosis, and difficulty weaning. Paradoxically, HSV tracheobronchitis had a more severe presentation and worse outcome in immunocompetent compared with immunosuppressed patients (109). It was proposed that this may be due to a more exuberant local immune response in the immunocompetent patients (109).

Low-dose acyclovir (200 to 400 mg orally three times daily) generally used for 3 to 4 weeks posttransplant is highly effective as prophylaxis for HSV in transplant recipients. At one institution, HSV hepatitis was documented in 12 of 3,536 solid organ transplant recipients before the routine use of acyclovir prophylaxis and in none of the 1,144 patients since the use of acyclovir prophylaxis (107). Longer duration (up to 3 months) of acyclovir is used for lung transplant recipients in some centers (108).

Varicella-Zoster Virus

Up to 70% of the pediatric and 5% of the adult transplant recipients have been reported to be seronegative for VZV (110, 111). Exposure to VZV infection may result in primary varicella in these susceptible patients. Median time to onset of varicella was 2 years after transplantation in one report (110) and 2.4 years in another (112). Visceral dissemination, frequently documented in transplant recipients, is the primary cause of mortality in patients with VZV. Hepatitis, pneumonitis, pancreatitis, gastroenteritis, or meningoencephalitis are the most commonly documented sites of visceral dissemination. Varicella may initially present with acute abdominal pain, and in the absence of skin lesions can defy early recognition. It is notable that up to 16% to 18% of the pediatric transplant recipients may have recurrent varicella infections (112,113).

Varicella-zoster immunoglobulin (VZIG) is recommended for susceptible transplant recipients exposed to varicella. VZIG, however, is not entirely protective; in up to one third of the patients with varicella, lesions have occurred despite VZIG prophylaxis. Some centers use high-dose oral acyclovir for the duration of the incubation period of varicella (i.e., 2 to 3 weeks after exposure of susceptible patients to varicella) (102). Varicella vaccine has been found to be safe and effective in transplant recipients. In 704 pediatric renal transplant recipients who received varicella immunization, 62% had VZV antibodies at 1 year and 42% after 10 years (114). The incidence and severity of varicella was significantly less in the immunized patients (114).

Human Herpesvirus-6

The newest herpesvirus to be considered a pathogen in transplant recipients is HHV-6. HHV-6 is a large double-stranded DNA virus that is antigenically distinct from other human herpesviruses. Its closest phylogenetic relative is CMV; nucleotide sequencing has revealed 66% DNA homology between CMV and HHV-6. On the basis of genomic DNA sequences, cell tropism, and protein expression, two distinct variants of HHV-6, designated as variant A and variant B, have been described (115,116). The two variants differ in virulence; the HHV-6A variant is intrinsically more virulent and neurotropic than the HHV-6B variant (117). Most infections in transplant recipients are due to the HHV-6B variant (117).

Most HHV-6 infections are believe to result from endogenous reactivation of the recipient's latent virus; however, donor transmission has also been documented. Although the precise incidence and clinical sequelae of HHV-6 infection after transplantation remain to be fully elucidated, HHV-6 infection has been reported in 31% to 55% of solid transplant recipients (117). The usual timing of onset is between 2 and 4 weeks posttransplantation. Bone marrow suppression, interstitial pneumonia, encephalopathy, and fever of unknown origin are the most commonly reported clinical manifestations of HHV-6 (117–120). Viral culture remains the gold standard for the diagnosis of HHV-6 infection. A shell vial culture assay (analogous to that for CMV), based on the detection of immediate early antigen of HHV-6 in cell culture, can significantly expedite the time required for detection of HHV-6 compared with the conventional cell culture (117). The role of PCR and antibody titer rises to diagnose active HHV-6 infection has not been fully ascertained. The antiviral susceptibilities of HHV-6 resemble those of CMV (121–123). HHV-6 is sensitive to both ganciclovir and foscarnet and resistant to acyclovir at achievable serum concentrations. The role of prophylaxis for HHV-6 has not yet been fully discerned.

Hepatotropic Viruses

Hepatitis C Virus

End-stage liver disease resulting from HCV has been documented in up to 50% of the patients undergoing liver transplantation in recent years. Up to 95% of the patients with pretransplant HCV infection remain viremic after transplantation, as demonstrated by the presence of HCV RNA in the blood. Clinically and histologically manifest recurrence occurs in 30% to 70% of patients with pretransplant HCV, generally within 1 to 12 months after transplantation (124–126). Progression to cirrhosis has been observed in 15% to 20% of patients 1 to 3 years after initial transplantation. Despite significant morbidity associated with HCV, survival rates in patients with and without HCV recurrence have not been different (126).

The prevalence of HCV positivity in hemodialysis patients ranges between 5% and 54% (127). The number of blood units transfused, the duration of hemodialysis, and the type of dialysis (hemodialysis as opposed to peritoneal dialysis) correlated with a higher incidence of HCV infection in renal transplant candidates (127–129). After transplantation, chronic liver disease has been reported in 10% to 60% of renal transplant recipients and occurred significantly more frequently in patients with HCV compared with those without HCV (128–130). Pretransplant HCV infection, however, does not seem to adversely affect the graft or patient survival after renal transplantation (130,131).

Although most posttransplant HCV infections are due to recurrence of pretransplant HCV, *de novo* infections resulting from acquisition from the donor organ or transfused blood products have been reported. A 35% rate of acquired HCV-RNA infection was reported in 89 liver transplant recipients, most of whom were transplanted before the routine screening of blood products for anti-HCV (124). Routine screening of blood products has led to a significantly lower acquisition rate of HCV (i.e., 2.5% to 4%) (132). HCV has also been transmitted by organs from anti-HCV–positive donors (see the section on sources of nosocomial infections). HCV infection is also considered a significant risk to the personnel involved in the care of HCV-infected transplant patients. The seroprevalence of HCV (7%) in healthcare workers directly involved in the care of liver transplant patients was significantly higher when compared with those not associated with liver transplantation (0.5%) or in volunteer blood donors (0.3%) (133). None of the transplant personnel had hepatitis or a history of transfusion (133). The risk of acquiring HCV after needle stick injuries may be as high as 10%. Serum immunoglobulin is not protective against HCV and is not recommended (also see Chapter 78).

A number of variables are believed to influence the rate and severity of recurrent HCV hepatitis after transplantation, including the level of pretransplant viremia, genotype of the virus, and the intensity of posttransplant immunosuppression (126,134, 135). HCV genotype 1b has been associated with more severe recurrent HCV infection after liver transplantation (126). Corticosteroids have been shown to result in a severalfold increase in the HCV-RNA level. Finally, allograft rejection and steroid-resistant rejection requiring OKT3 can lead to a higher incidence and earlier onset of recurrent HCV hepatitis after liver transplantation (135,136).

Effective prophylaxis against HCV in transplant recipients is not available. It has been shown that polyclonal immunoglobulin preparations against HBsAg administered to liver transplant patients for HBV were also protective against HCV (137). The incidence of HCV viremia in the patients receiving HBIG was significantly lower than in those who did not receive HBIG (54% vs. 94%, $p = .001$). This protective effect may have been due to the presence of anti-HCV in HBIG (137). Prophylaxis with interferon-alpha, administered for 6 months posttransplantation in liver transplant recipients, delayed the occurrence of HCV but decreased neither the incidence nor the severity of recurrent HCV hepatitis (138).

Hepatitis B Virus

The clinical impact of HBV is of greatest importance in the context of liver and renal transplantation. In studies in which long-term immunoprophylaxis was not used, the reinfection rate of the hepatic allograft with HBV was virtually 100% with progression to liver failure and death in as little as 2 to 2.5 years. Anti-HBs immunoprophylaxis has significantly altered the natural history of HBV after liver transplantation. In a large study assessing the outcome in HBsAg-positive patients undergoing liver transplantation, the overall risk of HBV recurrence after 3 years was 67% (139). HBV recurrence was documented in 78% to 90% of patients a mean of 3 months posttransplant in patients who did not receive long-term immunoprophylaxis; recurrence was significantly less (56%) and delayed, occurring a mean of 8 months posttransplant, in patients receiving long-term anti-HBs immunoprophylaxis (139). HBV adversely affects graft and patient survival; survival at 3 years was 54% in patients with HBV recurrence and 83% in those who remained HBsAg negative after transplantation (139).

Several factors influence the recurrence of HBV after transplantation. The risk of recurrence is greater for patients with markers for active replication of HBV before transplantation (e.g., those seropositive for HBeAg or HBV DNA). The risk of HBV recurrence was 83% ±6% in liver transplant recipients seropositive for HBV DNA compared with 58% ±7% in those with neither HBV DNA nor HBeAg at the time of transplantation (139). Fulminant HBV (as opposed to chronic HBV infection) is associated with a lower rate of recurrence. Recurrence was observed in 17% of patients with fulminant HBV compared with 67% in those with chronic HBV cirrhosis (139). Patients with fulminant HBV tend to have lower levels of HBV DNA or replicative HBV. Co-infection with hepatitis delta virus decreases the risk of recurrence in HBV infection after transplantation (139). Delta virus is a naturally occurring inhibitor of HBV replication, and hence HBV DNA levels in delta virus co-infected patients are lower.

Strains of HBV that fail to produce HBeAg because of mutations in the precore region of the HBV genome (also known as precore mutants or HBeAg-deficient mutants) have recently been identified (140). Such patients have high levels of viral DNA in the absence of HBeAg. Patients infected with the precore mutants pretransplant, as opposed to the wild-type virus, have a greater risk of hepatic graft loss resulting from early recurrence (140).

A unique and particularly aggressive syndrome of recurrent HBV infection observed in 12% to 20% of patients with HBV recurrence is fibrosing cholestatic hepatitis, characterized by marked cholestasis and hypoprothrombinemia but only modest increases in serum transaminases (141). Fibrosing cholestatic hepatitis is more likely to occur in patients with pretransplant HBV replication and results in rapid death in almost all cases. A paucity of inflammatory response in this syndrome suggests that the virus may be directly cytopathic.

HBV infection also follows an aggressive clinical course after renal transplantation. Progression of liver disease to cirrhosis and death, however, occurs considerably later than in liver transplantation (i.e., 6 to 8 years after transplantation). Chronic active or persistent hepatitis occurred in 76% of HBsAg-positive patients undergoing renal transplantation compared with 31% in HBsAg-negative patients (142).

The most effective approach to prevent recurrent HBV is the use of combination therapy with lamivudine and HBIG. Prophylaxis with the use of lamivudine monotherapy is not recommended because of the reappearance of HBsAg after liver transplantation in 32% to 50% of the patients. Combination therapy with HBIG and lamivudine prevents HBV recurrence in more than 90% of the patients undergoing liver transplantation for HBV (143,144).

Adefovir dipivoxil and entecavir have been shown to suppress the replication of lamivudine-resistant HBV. In a compassionate-use protocol in 40 patients with lamivudine-resistant HBV awaiting liver transplantation and 127 liver transplant recipients with recurrent HBV resulting from lamivudine-resistant HBV, a two to three log reduction in HBV DNA levels and biochemical improvement was noted (145,146).

Hepatitis G Virus

Hepatitis G virus is a newly identified RNA virus belonging to the family Flaviviridae with an estimated prevalence of 1% to 2% in the volunteer blood donor population in the United States. Sequence analysis suggests that hepatitis G virus and hepatitis GB virus represent independent isolates of the same virus. Hepatitis G virus also bears 26% sequence homology with HCV. Among patients undergoing liver transplantation for end-stage liver disease resulting from HCV, up to 25% may be co-infected with hepatitis G virus. However, hepatitis G virus appears to have minimal clinical impact and influences neither the graft nor patient outcome in liver or renal transplant recipients (147–149). Up to 30% of the patients undergoing liver transplantation for cryptogenic cirrhosis have demonstrated histologic evidence of hepatitis in the absence of any known viruses, including hepatitis G virus (150). It is suspected that as yet unidentified viruses may be the cause of posttransplant hepatitis occurring in the absence of hepatitis A to G viruses (150).

Other Viruses

BK Virus

Within the last decade, BK virus (BKV) has emerged as a significant pathogen in renal transplant recipients. BKV is a polyomavirus that is acquired during childhood. Renal and uroepithelial cells are the main site of latency. Seroprevalence rates in the general population range from 70% to 90%. Nephropathy resulting from BKV has been reported in 1% to 5% of the renal transplant recipients with allograft loss occurring in nearly half of those patients (151). This entity was encountered only rarely before the mid-1990s. Although precise reasons for the recent emergence of BKV as a significant pathogen is unclear, use of novel, more potent immunosuppressive agents (e.g., tacrolimus, mycophenolate mofetil, and sirolimus) is considered to play a role. Donor transmission has been reported; however, most cases of BKV nephropathy occur as a result of reactivation of the latent virus.

The usual time to onset of BKV nephropathy is 28 to 40 weeks posttransplantation. Typical manifestations include a modest rise in creatinine that fails to respond to antirejection therapy. The hallmark of BKV replication are decoy cells, which are urinary epithelial cells bearing ground-glass intranuclear inclusions. Decoy cells, however, lack specificity for the diagnosis. Quantitative BKV viremia, however, has been shown to correlate with BKV nephropathy (152) and may also be used to monitor response to therapy. Specific antiviral therapy for BKV is not available currently. Judicious reduction of immunosuppression has been attempted as a management strategy but may not always be successful. The role of cidofovir for the treatment of BKV nephropathy or that of retransplantation has not been fully defined.

Adenovirus

Adenoviral infections have been documented in up to 10% of the pediatric and 1% to 15% of adult transplant recipients (153–156). Symptomatic disease is more common and generally more severe in pediatric compared with adult patients after transplantation; 60% of the children and 27% of the adult transplant recipients with adenoviral shedding have been shown to have disease resulting from adenovirus (153–155). The precise mode of transmission of adenoviral infections has not been determined, although both donor transmission and nosocomial transmission have been proposed to occur (153–155). In pediatric liver transplant recipients, most severe disease occurred in seronegative children (154), and donor serology was positive in five of six patients evaluated, suggesting that donor transmission is a likely source of infection. Nosocomial acquisition is also a consideration, because several patients with the similar adenovirus strains were found temporally clustered in one report (153).

Hepatitis and pneumonitis are the most common invasive forms of adenoviral disease. Hepatitis in liver transplant recipients, pneumonitis in lung transplant recipients, and hemorrhagic cystitis in renal transplant recipients are the most frequently involved sites of disease. Serotypes 5 and 11 were the most frequent serotypes causing hepatitis and hemorrhagic cystitis, respectively, in transplant recipients. Diagnosis is suggested by the detection of microabscesses with smudgy intranuclear targeted inclusions in histopathologic specimens (157). Immunohistochemistry and culture can be used to confirm adenoviral infection. Although ribavirin has been anecdotally used as therapy (158), an effective prophylaxis for adenoviral infections is currently not available.

Respiratory Viral Infections

The impact of respiratory viral infections [e.g., respiratory syncytial virus (RSV), influenza, and parainfluenza viruses] has not been fully characterized in solid organ transplant recipients. Over a 6-year period, 3.4% of pediatric liver transplant recipients were documented to have RSV infections (159). The median time to diagnosis was 24 days posttransplant. Seventy-six percent of the infections were nosocomially acquired. Early-onset infection and preexisting lung disease portended a more severe disease. Late infections, on the other hand, occurring in the absence of rejection, were usually without untoward sequelae. Of 19 cases of paramyxovirus infection in lung transplant recipients, 9 were due to RSV and 10 due to parainfluenza virus (160). Three cases of parainfluenza type 3 infections in that report occurred within a 3-week period; two of these patients had contact with each other and with hospital personnel during a 1-month period of the infection (160). Influenza can be a serious viral infection in pediatric organ transplant recipients. Of 12 such cases, 5 were exposed to influenza B while hospitalized (161). Annual influenza immunization of pediatric organ transplant recipients, their household contacts, and healthcare workers is recommended (161).

BACTERIAL INFECTIONS

Staphylococci

Staphylococci, particularly *S. aureus,* are increasingly recognized as pathogens in transplant recipients and have emerged as the leading cause of bacterial infections in liver, heart, kidney, and pancreatic transplant recipients at many centers (162–165). This increase largely parallels the more widespread rise in gram-positive infections in the nosocomial setting in recent years. Forty-nine percent of the bacteremias in liver transplant recipients in one report were due to *S. aureus* (163). Although intravascular cannulas, accounting for 54% of all MRSA bacteremias, were the predominant source, wound infections, nosocomial pneumonia, intraabdominal abscess, and peritonitis were also documented as sources of MRSA bacteremia (163). Over one half of the *S. aureus* infections occur in the intensive care unit setting (163). Requirement of invasive procedures, mechanical ventilation, continuous need for intravenous access, and overall debilitated condition of the patients in the intensive care unit provide conditions conducive to the development of nosocomial *S. aureus* infections. *S. aureus* infections generally occur very early after transplantation. In a study in liver transplant recipients, nearly one third of such infections occurred within the first week of transplantation; the median time to onset was 16 days (39). *S. aureus* is also the most frequent cause of endocarditis in organ transplant recipients (166). Notably, 74% of the cases of endocarditis were associated with previous hospital-acquired infection, especially venous access device and wound infections (166).

S. aureus colonization of the anterior nares has recently been shown to be a significant predictor of infections resulting from *S. aureus* in liver transplant patients (39). Overall, nasal carriage was documented in 67% of the patients; infected patients were significantly more likely to be nasal carriers of *S. aureus* compared with the noninfected patients. Pulse-field gel electrophoresis documented that the isolates causing infections matched the isolates from the anterior nares in all cases (39). Furthermore, 43% of infected patients shared the isolates with the same restriction pattern, indicating cross-transmission in the nosocomial setting (39). Eradication of nasal carriage by mupirocin, however, has not been shown to prevent *S. aureus* infections in liver transplant recipients (167). Although 87% of the colonized patients were successfully decolonized, recolonization occurred in 37% (167). Nosocomial transmission leading to exogenous colonization and colonization at non-nasal sites that may be unaffected by nasal administration of mupirocin likely accounted for the failure of mupirocin to decrease *S. aureus* infections (167).

Enterococci

Enterococci, which are normal inhabitants of the gastrointestinal tract, are of greatest relevance in liver transplant recipients. Most enterococcal bacteremias in these patients result from complications related to the biliary tree. Roux-en-Y choledochojejunostomy (which facilitates reflux of enteric bacteria into the biliary tree) and biliary strictures have been shown to be independent risk factors for enterococcal bacteremia after liver transplantation (168).

Vancomycin-resistant *Enterococcus faecium* (VREF) have emerged as nosocomial pathogens of grave concern, particularly after liver transplantation. VREF infections were documented in 10.5% of the liver transplant recipients in one recent study and 16% in another (169,170). Notably, VREF was the most frequently isolated pathogen in infected liver transplant recipients in the latter study. Infections were documented a median of 39 and 42 days after transplantation in two studies (169,170) but considerably earlier (a median of 10 days) in another report (171). Intraabdominal infections were the most frequent site of infection resulting from VREF. VREF fecal carriage before transplantation; previous antibiotic use (including vancomycin); biliary complications; prolonged hospitalization and intensive care unit stay; surgical reexploration; surgical complications during transplantation, including hypotension; and primary nonfunction of the allograft have been identified as significant risk factors for VREF infections (169,170,172). Mortality in the infected patients range between 23% and 50%. Intensive care unit stay before transplantation, hemodialysis, liver failure, and shock have been shown to be independent predictors of mortality in patients with VREF infections (170,172). Not surprisingly, antibiotics have not been effective in reducing mortality; outcome did not differ significantly among patients who received the drugs with activity against the isolate *in vitro* compared with those who received no therapy (169).

VREF colonization once established is often a persistent event; spontaneous conversion to VREF-negative carriage is uncommon. These patients, therefore, remain at risk for invasive infections and a threat for nosocomial transmission. A variety of gut decontamination regimens, including oral bacitracin (173), have been tried; however, none have been shown to be consistently effective. Consequently, infection control practices to prevent nosocomial acquisition and cross-transmission and judicious use of antimicrobial agents, particularly vancomycin, are critically important in curtailing VREF infections.

Mycobacterium tuberculosis

The incidence of tuberculosis in solid organ transplant patients ranges from 0.35% to 5% in the United States and Europe (24,174). However, in highly endemic areas (e.g., India and Pakistan), tuberculosis may develop in 5% to 15% of the transplant patients. The median time to onset after transplantation is 9 months and ranges from 0.5 to 144 months (24,174). Tuberculosis occurs significantly later after transplantation in renal compared with nonrenal transplant recipients. Disseminated disease occurs in nearly one third of the transplant recipients with tuberculosis (24). The gastrointestinal tract is the most frequent extrapulmonary site of tuberculosis in transplant recipients. Other reported extrapulmonary sites of involvement include the skin and osteoarticular tissue, central nervous system, kidneys, and urogenital tract.

Tuberculin reactivity has been documented in 20% of the transplant recipients with tuberculosis, and chest radiographs with evidence of old active tuberculosis were documented in 12% of the patients (24). These patients are more likely to develop tuberculosis earlier after transplantation than those without a history of tuberculin reactivity or abnormal chest radiograph before transplantation. Most tuberculosis infections in transplant recipients represent reactivation of old dormant disease. However, nosocomial acquisition or donor transmission are also well-documented modes of transmission. Tuberculosis has been shown to be transmitted both by living and cadaveric organ donors. Tuberculosis, involving the renal allograft, was documented 35 and 39 days after renal transplantation in two recipients of the same donor who died of hypoglycorrhachic lymphocytic meningitis of unknown etiology; the donor's cerebrospinal fluid culture was positive for *M. tuberculosis* 3 weeks after death (23). One renal allograft recipient of this donor died of disseminated tuberculosis, whereas the second recovered, although rejection secondary to antituberculosis therapy necessitated allograft nephrectomy (23). Two recipients of a single lung transplant from a common donor had the same *M. tuberculosis* isolate as demonstrated by restriction fragment length polymorphism (175). Tuberculosis involving a hepatic allograft was documented in a pediatric transplant recipient who received a living related lateral segment hepatic allograft from the mother (166). Pulmonary tuberculosis was detected concomitantly in the mother who was apparently asymptomatic at the time of donation of the hepatic segmental graft (176).

A nosocomial outbreak involving ten renal transplant patients was documented from one institution; eight of these cases were clustered within a 5-month period (7). The source case was a renal transplant recipient who was exposed to tuberculosis at another hospital. Tuberculosis was not suspected in the source case on admission, thus delaying the isolation precautions. Restriction fragment length polymorphism documented transmission of *M. tuberculosis* from the index case to five renal transplant recipients. The median incubation period for tuberculosis in this outbreak was only 7.5 weeks, and death occurred in five of ten patients a median of 8 weeks after diagnosis (7). It is noteworthy that the exposed transplant recipients were more likely to contract tuberculosis compared with the nontransplant contacts of the source case (7). Overall mortality in organ transplant recipients with tuberculosis is approximately 30% (24). Disseminated compared with localized tuberculosis, prior rejection, and OKT3 receipt were significant predictors of mortality in transplant recipients with tuberculosis.

All transplant recipients should have a tuberculin skin test administered before transplantation. Isoniazid prophylaxis should be considered for the transplant recipients with the characteristics outlined in Table 59.3 regardless of the tuberculin skin test reactivity. A recent study has documented that isoniazid chemoprophylaxis initiated during liver transplant candidacy was safe and effective (177). Such an approach minimizes the exposure to the new allograft to isoniazid and may mitigate potential drug interactions of isoniazid with the immunosuppressive agents. Tuberculin skin test reactivity per se is a controversial indication for prophylaxis in transplant recipients. The rate of tuberculosis among skin-test positive liver transplant candidates and recipients who receive no chemoprophylaxis has been estimated to be 1,585.3 cases per 1,000,000 person-years

TABLE 59.3. INDICATIONS FOR CHEMOPROPHYLAXIS WITH ISONIAZID IN ORGAN TRANSPLANT RECIPIENTS

I. Tuberculin skin reactivity ≥5 mm before transplantation
II. Patients with the following characteristics, regardless of tuberculin skin test reactivity:
    1 Radiographic evidence of old active tuberculosis and no prior prophylaxis
    2. Prior history of inadequately treated tuberculosis
    3. Close contact with an infectious case
    4. Receipt of an allograft from a donor with a history of tuberculosis or tuberculin reactivity
III. Newly infected persons (recent tuberculin skin test converters)

(178). Tuberculosis has been documented in up to 2% of the tuberculin skin-test–negative liver transplant recipients (179). It has been proposed that clinical or radiographic evidence of previous tuberculosis may more reliably identify high-risk patients as compared with the tuberculin skin test result. Optimal management of tuberculin skin test positive or anergic patients, however, remains to be determined.

Legionella

Legionellosis has been reported in 2% to 9% of solid organ transplant recipients with pneumonia; however, at certain institutions, 25% to 38% of the bacterial pneumonias have been due to *Legionella* (5). *Legionella pneumophila* and *Legionella micdadei* are the most common species implicated; however, *Legionella bozemanii, Legionella birminghamensis, Legionella dumoffii,* and *Legionella cincinnatiensis* have also caused infections in transplant recipients.

Inhalation of aerosols containing *Legionella* has been proposed as the mode of transmission for this microorganism. However, aspiration is considered the most likely mode of transmission and *Legionella*-contaminated potable water distribution systems as the predominant source of legionellosis (5). Molecular fingerprinting methods have linked *L. pneumophila* infection in transplant recipients to hospital drinking water (180). Ice machines (34) and ultrasonic humidifiers (181) have also been shown to be the sources of *Legionella* infection after transplantation. Pneumonia is the predominant clinical manifestation of legionellosis, although pericarditis, necrotizing cellulitis, peritonitis, hepatic allograft infection, and hemodialysis fistula infections have also been reported after transplantation (5). Nodular pulmonary densities and cavitation (reported in 50% to 70% of the pulmonary infections in some reports) are characteristic radiographic features but may not be invariably present. *Legionella* are fastidious microorganisms that do not grow on standard bacteriologic media. Selective media containing dyes and antimicrobial agents are needed for optimal growth. Urinary antigen is both sensitive and specific for the detection of *Legionella* and may also be diagnostically useful for detecting *Legionella* in body fluids (e.g., pleural fluids).

It is recommended that hospitals performing large numbers of transplants should routinely culture the hospital water supply for *Legionella,* perhaps once a year (182). If such cultures are positive, specialized *Legionella* laboratory tests, especially culture on selective media and urinary antigen tests, should be made routinely available in the clinical microbiology laboratory. Two disinfection methods for the water supply have emerged as cost effective: superheating the water to 70°C and flushing the distal outlets or the installation of copper-silver ionization units. Hyperchlorination is no longer recommended because of the expense, erratic efficacy, corrosive damage to the piping, and the carcinogenic potential of ingested chlorine. Electric showers have been used when hyperchlorination and superheating and flushing proved inadequate. Unfortunately, this method is unlikely to be effective as a long-term mode of prevention because showering is not the primary mode of transmission.

Nocardiosis

Infections resulting from *Nocardia* species may occur in 2% to 4% of organ transplant recipients; the median time to the onset of nocardiosis after transplantation ranges between 2 and 8 months. Central nervous system involvement occurs in 17% to 38% of these patients. Brain abscesses are usually multiple; meningitis is rare and usually associated with an abscess. An important clue to central nervous system nocardiosis is concomitant skin or subcutaneous lesions from which *Nocardia* species can be readily isolated.

Nocardia is a soil microorganism whose primary portal of entry is the lung. There is evidence to suggest that nosocomial transmission of nocardiosis may occur (183–186). Cases of *Nocardia* infection clustered in time have been reported in renal transplant units. An epidemic strain of *Nocardia* common to the infected patients and environmental dust samples from the unit housing the patients but distinct from environmental isolates elsewhere in the hospital was documented to cause seven infections in a renal transplant and dialysis unit (184). Respiratory isolation of the cases of nocardiosis during outbreaks has been recommended by some (184,185). Trimethoprim-sulfamethoxazole used as prophylaxis for PCP is also effective against nocardiosis.

FUNGAL INFECTIONS

Aspergillus

Invasive aspergillosis remains a devastating fungal infection in all types of transplant recipients. It has, however, unique clinical characteristics and risk factors in different types of solid organ transplant recipients.

Epidemiology

Lung Transplantation

Lung transplant recipients are more likely than other solid organ recipients to develop infection with *Aspergillus* (Table 59.4). Up to 8% of lung transplant recipients develop invasive aspergillosis with an additional 10% demonstrating *Aspergillus* colonization (187–190). Risk factors for *Aspergillus* infection after lung transplantation include CMV infection and single lung transplantation (189,191). Cystic fibrosis is not a risk factor for *Aspergillus* infection posttransplant; isolation of *Aspergillus* species from respiratory secretions of patients with cystic fibrosis pretransplant has not been shown to predict subsequent development of invasive disease (190,192). Most cases of invasive aspergillosis in lung transplant recipients occur within the first 9 months posttransplantation. A unique form of invasive aspergillosis occurring in lung transplant recipients is ulcerative tracheobronchitis.

TABLE 59.4. INCIDENCE OF INVASIVE ASPERGILLOSIS AND MORTALITY IN DIFFERENT TYPES OF SOLID-ORGAN TRANSPLANT RECIPIENTS

Type of transplant	Cumulative incidence of invasive disease (%)	Cumulative incidence of colonization (%)	Crude mortality in patients with invasive aspergillosis (%)
Kidney	0.7	1.7	75
Pancreas	1.3	NA	100
Liver	1.7	0.5	87
Small bowel	3.5	NA	100
Heart	6.2	NA	78
Lung	8.4	10.4	74

NA, data not available.

Liver Transplantation

The incidence of invasive aspergillosis in liver transplant recipients ranges from 1% to 4% (193–197). The infection is most often diagnosed between 2 and 4 weeks after transplantation. A poorly functioning hepatic allograft and renal insufficiency, particularly the requirement for hemodialysis, are considered important risk factors for invasive aspergillosis in liver transplant recipients. Although OKT3 use was shown in early studies to be a risk factor for invasive aspergillosis, a recent large study showed that only 8% of liver transplant recipients with invasive aspergillosis had received OKT3 (195). Approximately 25% of the cases of invasive aspergillosis in liver transplant recipients occur after retransplantation (195). Rarely, the *Aspergillus* infection is confined to the surgical site (producing necrotizing fasciitis) or intraabdominal sites in liver transplant recipients.

Heart Transplantation

Invasive aspergillosis occurs in 1% to 6% of heart transplant recipients (198–201). The median time to development of invasive aspergillosis in these patients is 1 to 2 months. Most infections originate in the lungs, and 20% to 35% disseminate to other organs.

Renal Transplantation

Invasive aspergillosis has been reported in 0.7% to 1% of the patients undergoing renal transplantation (198,202,203). Cases of invasive aspergillosis in renal transplant recipients have usually been pulmonary infections and occasionally disseminated disease. Augmented immunosuppression and graft failure requiring hemodialysis are risk factors for invasive aspergillosis in renal transplant recipients (203).

Diagnosis

Early diagnosis is critically important in reducing the mortality from invasive aspergillosis. *Aspergillus* can be cultured from sputum in only 8% to 34% and from bronchoalveolar lavage fluid in 45% to 62% of patients with invasive pulmonary aspergillosis (204). Respiratory cultures, therefore, may not detect aspergillosis before significant vascular invasion has occurred. Surveillance serologic tests, however, may be potentially more useful. ELISA has been shown to have a sensitivity of 50% to 90% and specificity of 81% to 93% for the diagnosis of invasive aspergillosis (204–206). Furthermore, the antigen detection tests may be positive as long as 28 days before clinical and radiographic signs of invasive aspergillosis become apparent (205). The efficacy of *Aspergillus* antigen detection tests, however, has not been extensively evaluated in solid organ transplant recipients. High-resolution thoracic computed tomography (CT) may be able to raise the index of suspicion for invasive pulmonary aspergillosis soon after the development of symptoms and before culture results are available. Such imaging in neutropenic patients whose fever persisted for more than 2 days despite empiric antibiotic treatment showed findings highly suggestive of invasive pulmonary aspergillosis 5 days earlier than the use of chest roentgenograms (207).

Prevention and Prophylaxis

Outbreaks of aspergillosis have been linked to construction activity within or near a transplant unit and to contaminated or poorly maintained ventilating ducts, grids, and air filters. Outbreaks associated with construction activity in bone marrow transplant recipients have been curtailed by use of laminar air flow units with high-efficiency particulate air filtration. Effective prophylaxis against invasive aspergillosis is currently not available. Although itraconazole is highly active *in vitro* against *Aspergillus,* its efficacy has not yet been demonstrated in clinical trials. Furthermore, the absorption of itraconazole in capsule form can be erratic in transplant recipients. Itraconazole solubilized in cyclodextrin is better absorbed; its efficacy as prophylaxis, however, remains unproven.

Low-dose intravenous amphotericin B (0.1 mg/kg/day) or liposomal intravenous amphotericin B (1 mg/kg/day) have also not been shown to be consistently efficacious. On the contrary, it has been proposed that low-dose amphotericin B may promote the emergence of *Aspergillus* infection (208). Aerosolized amphotericin B prophylaxis administered during the posttransplant hospital stay was shown to reduce the incidence of fungal infections, including aspergillosis in lung, heart-lung, and heart transplant recipients in one report (209). Others have not found it to be effective. Furthermore, the formulation, optimal dosage, and precise mode of delivery of aerosolized amphotericin B preparations has not been determined. Given the lack of availability of effective prophylaxis, preemptive therapy or empiric therapy in selected high-risk patients may be considered as an alternative to prophylaxis.

Candidiasis

With the exception of heart transplant recipients, invasive candidiasis is the most frequently occurring fungal infection in solid organ transplant recipients (45). The incidence of *Candida* infections is highest in liver transplant recipients. Virtually all *Candida* infections are nosocomially acquired, although the source may vary depending on the type of organ transplant recipients. Whereas in liver transplant recipients candidiasis results from endogenous (generally gut) colonization, donor organs are the potential source in heart-lung and lung transplant recipients. Karyotypic analysis has demonstrated *Candida* infection originating in the donor lung as a cause of disseminated disease in a lung transplant recipient (28).

In the earlier studies in liver transplant recipients, 15% to 20% of the patients were documented to have invasive candidiasis (196,210). Intraabdominal infections, with or without subsequent dissemination, are the usual clinical manifestations. Prolonged operation time, retransplantation, greater transfusion requirements, high serum creatinine, and CMV infection were the proposed risk factors for *Candida* infections (Table 59.2). More recently, however, many transplant centers have documented a decline in the incidence of invasive candidiasis, even in the absence of specific antifungal prophylaxis (73,164,211). More conservative immunosuppression but, more importantly, improvement in surgical technique likely accounts for this decline. After pancreatic transplantation, *Candida* infections occur in 15% to 30% of the patients and manifest predominantly as surgical site or bloodstream infections. In heart-lung or lung transplant recipients, the clinical pattern of *Candida* infections may range from tracheobronchitis to systemic invasive disease. Invasive candidiasis in these patients may also result in anastomotic dehiscence, mediastinitis, and mycotic aneurysm. The anastomotic site is particularly vulnerable because of poor blood supply and the presence of suture material. Invasive bronchial infection can then result with breakdown of the anastomosis.

The precise patient population to be targeted, optimal regimen, and duration of antifungal prophylaxis for *Candida* remains controversial. Nystatin-containing selective bowel decontamination regimens have been proposed to lead to a lower incidence of invasive candidiasis in liver transplant recipients (73,211). Its efficacy, however, has never been assessed in a controlled trial. Currently, fluconazole is used for prophylaxis at many liver and pancreatic transplant centers. A randomized trial from Europe compared fluconazole (100 mg once a day) with nystatin (10^6 units every 6 hours) for 28 days after liver transplantation (212). Although the incidence of *Candida* colonization and superficial fungal infections (thrush and cystitis) were decreased, differences in the incidence of invasive candidiasis were not observed in the two groups (212).

Universal use of azole prophylaxis must be undertaken with caution. A major concern with routine azole antifungal prophylaxis is the emergence of azole-resistant *Candida,* a scenario already documented in liver transplant recipients (213). Azole-resistant invasive *Candida glabrata* infection occurred in 4% (4/101) of the liver transplant recipients receiving fluconazole prophylaxis and was the direct cause of death in one patient (213). The routine use of fluconazole is expected to have the potential of selecting fungi innately resistant to fluconazole (e.g., *Aspergillus*). Although this association has not been proved, an unusually high incidence of invasive aspergillosis (8%; 8/101) in liver transplant recipients who routinely received fluconazole prophylaxis prospectively is of concern (213). Finally, the need for fluconazole prophylaxis should be assessed on the basis of the institutional trends in the incidence of invasive candidiasis. Given the low incidence of invasive candidiasis at certain transplant centers, the widespread use of fluconazole prophylaxis for all patients may not be warranted to prevent the infection in 5% of the patients. A more appealing approach might be prophylaxis targeted toward high-risk patients only.

Pneumocystis Carinii

P. carinii has long been classified as a protozoan microorganism on the basis of morphologic features and lack of growth on fungal media. However, gene sequencing of *P. carinii* suggests that the microorganism is indeed a fungus.

Epidemiology

The prevailing assumption has long been that *P. carinii* infection arises from reactivation of endogenous infections acquired in childhood. However, clusters of *P. carinii* infection occurring in transplant recipients have been reported. In one report, all renal transplant recipients affected had attended the same outpatient facility as did patients with advanced HIV infection (214–217). Compared with matched control subjects, PCP cases had more outpatient clinic visits coinciding with visits of HIV-infected patients with *P. carinii* infection (216). Furthermore, *P. carinii* DNA has been demonstrated in more than 50% of the air samples from the hospital rooms of *P. carinii*-infected patients (216). Detection of *P. carinii* DNA was by filtration of air. As molecular epidemiologic techniques become more sophisticated, additional information on such outbreaks may provide more convincing evidence of patient-to-patient transmission of *P. carinii.*

Lung transplant recipients are at greatest risk of developing pulmonary infection with *P. carinii*; in the absence of prophylaxis, PCP may develop in up to 80% of the patients (218). Not all of these patients, however, are symptomatic. Up to 40% of the lung transplant recipients have been shown to have normal chest radiographs, are asymptomatic, and have the microorganism detected on routine posttransplant bronchoscopy. Several factors may account for the high incidence of *P. carinii* infection in lung transplant recipients. First, local defense mechanisms are impaired as a result of lung denervation. Second, it has been hypothesized that an incompatibility exists between the immune effector cells and parenchymal cells in the allograft lung. Infiltrating lymphocytes and mononuclear phagocytes recruited to the infected allograft are derived from the recipient and, therefore, express different MHC antigens than do the donor-derived parenchymal cells (55). Finally, surveillance bronchoscopy may increase the chance of early detection of occult infection. *P. carinii* infection in lung transplant recipients usually occurs in the fourth month after transplantation. Up to 25% of the cases may occur more than a year after transplant; these patients had usually received more intense immunosuppressive therapy.

The incidence of infection with *P. carinii* in patients not receiving PCP prophylaxis is 2% in renal transplant recipients, 5% in heart, and 9% in liver transplant recipients. Most infections occur between 3 and 6 months after transplantation. Between 10% and 20% of the cases occur greater than 6 months posttransplantation, usually in those receiving augmented immunosuppression for rejection (219). Other risk factors for PCP include need for OKT3, CMV infection, and older recipient age. Interestingly, the new immunosuppressive agent mycophenolate mofetil has been shown to have *in vitro* activity against *P. carinii.* In four randomized controlled trials of mycophenolate mofetil use in renal transplant recipients, none of 1,068 patients given mycophenolate mofetil developed *P. carinii* infections compared with 10 of 563 (1.8%) of those randomized not to receive mycophenolate mofetil ($p = .00006$) (220).

Unlike HIV-infected patients, PCP in transplant recipients is rarely diagnosed by examination of an induced sputum sample. Virtually all cases require bronchoalveolar lavage for diagnosis. Co-infection with CMV or bacteria (especially in lung transplant recipients) is common.

Prophylaxis

Prophylaxis with oral trimethoprim-sulfamethoxazole has proven highly efficacious and is recommended for all transplant recipients. Adverse effects of trimethoprim-sulfamethoxazole are relatively uncommon in solid organ transplant recipients. Rash occurs in only 1%. Leukopenia is somewhat more common, occurring in 3% to 20% of patients.

A more controversial issue in prophylaxis of *P. carinii* infection in transplant recipients is the duration of prophylaxis. Many transplant centers (including ours) offer life-long trimethoprim-sulfamethoxazole. Others use it for the first 6 months posttransplantation for heart, renal, and liver transplant recipients and for the first 12 months in lung transplant recipients. The rationale for this approach is that the risk for *P. carinii* infection in stable patients declines substantially 6 months after transplantation. However, cases of PCP have been described several months after discontinuing prophylaxis. At one center, 36% of cases of PCP occurred more than 1 year after transplant and 18% occurred greater than 2 years after transplantation (221). In patients receiving augmented immunosuppression for late-occurring rejection, PCP prophylaxis should be resumed or continued. An additional advantage of trimethoprim-sulfamethoxazole prophylaxis is that it is also effective against other microorganisms such as *Nocardia, Listeria, Toxoplasma,* and *Legionella* in transplant recipients.

Monthly nebulized pentamidine is an alternative prophylaxis in patients intolerant of trimethoprim-sulfamethoxazole. Breakthrough infections, however, have been reported in such patients. Orally administered atovaquone or dapsone would be third-line options. Neither drug has significant interactions with cyclosporine or tacrolimus.

Cryptococcus neoformans

The incidence of *Cryptococcus* in organ transplant recipients ranges from 0.6% to 2.6%. However, there are significant regional variations, with some centers reporting cryptococcosis in up to 5% of the transplant recipients (222). Most cases occur more than 6 months after transplantation; some cases are detected 4 or more years after transplantation. The precise pathogenesis of cryptococcosis is unclear; whether it is a newly acquired or reactivation infection in transplant settings remains unresolved. Given the low incidence of cryptococcosis in transplant recipients and the delayed and often unpredictable time of onset after transplantation, fluconazole prophylaxis is not usually considered necessary in transplant recipients.

Endemic Mycosis (Histoplasmosis, Coccidioidomycosis, and Blastomycosis)

Histoplasmosis has been infrequently reported in transplant recipients. Some 0.3% of renal transplant recipients followed for several years in a nonendemic area of the United States developed histoplasmosis (223). In endemic regions, about 0.5% of renal transplant recipients may develop histoplasmosis (224), although during an outbreak associated with construction activity near a hospital in Indianapolis, the prevalence of disseminated infection rose to 2.1% (224). The median time to onset is 6 to 15 months after transplantation (223,224). In endemic areas, primary infection is thought to be the usual presentation. In contrast, in nonendemic regions, reactivation of latent infection with subsequent hematogenous spread is more likely. Transmission through a cadaveric renal allograft from an infected donor has been described (225). Disseminated disease occurs in more than 75% of the transplant recipients developing histoplasmosis. Culture of *H. capsulatum* remains the gold standard of diagnosis but is often delayed. Serologic tests have proven useful in providing a more rapid diagnosis of histoplasmosis in transplant recipients (224).

Coccidioidomycosis in transplant recipients has been described predominantly from the centers in Arizona and southern California. The risk of overt infection in solid organ transplant recipients in Arizona is about 3% per year, with an overall prevalence of 4.5% for heart transplant recipients (226) and 6.9% for renal transplant recipients (227). In liver transplant recipients in Los Angeles, 0.6% of patients developed overt coccidioidomycosis. The usual time to onset is 2 to 6 months posttransplant (226–228). However, cases have also been reported in the first 4 weeks posttransplantation. Sometimes, this early infection may manifest as fever, a sepsis-like syndrome, and an aggressive pneumonia (228). A subacute presentation occurring several to many months after transplantation, however, is a more common finding. Some patients have disseminated disease with arthritis, meningitis, or skin lesions (229).

Transplant candidates who reside in endemic areas should be screened for coccidioidomycosis before transplantation. Patients at high risk of developing coccidioidomycosis posttransplant include those with detectable titers of coccidioidal antibodies on complement fixation tests, those with radiographic evidence of prior pulmonary infection, and those with a history of active coccidioidomycosis. Prophylactic fluconazole (400 mg/day) should be considered for these patients posttransplant.

Blastomycosis is rarely reported in transplant recipients. A renal transplant recipient has been reported who sustained a needle puncture while working as a veterinarian's assistant and subsequently developed local skin infection and then disseminated disease (230). In this case it was presumed that the infection was transmitted from an infected dog.

Zygomycosis

The incidence of zygomycosis complicating organ transplantation ranges between 0.3% and 5% (231). The usual time to onset is 2 months after transplantation (range, 5 days to 8 years). Most cases are due to *Rhizophus* species, although *Mucor, Absidia,* and *Cunninghamella* have also been reported. Rhinocerebral disease has been observed in 57% of the cases and is the most common clinical presentation. Zygomycosis can be acquired nosocomially; the usual portal of entry is believed to be pulmonary. Adhesive bandages have been incriminated as a source of surgical site infections in transplant recipients.

PROTOZOA

Toxoplasma Gondii

Heart transplantation poses the highest risk for transmission of *T. gondii* because of the parasite's predilection to invade muscular tissue. Fifty percent to 75% of seronegative recipients of seropositive cardiac allografts may develop primary *T. gondii* infection (232). *T. gondii* infections are distinctly unusual in noncardiac transplant recipients.

Most symptomatic infections occur within 6 months of transplantation. Meningoencephalitis, brain abscess, myocarditis, and pneumonitis are the usual clinical manifestations. Demonstration of tachyzoites in tissue sections establishes the diagnosis of acute infection. An immunoperoxidase stain is both sensitive and specific. Tissue cell cultures (e.g., those used for the isolation of viruses) can also detect *T. gondii* in culture within 3 to 6 days (233). Significant changes in antibody titer may not occur in transplant recipients with acute toxoplasmosis. Conversely, a rise in IgM and IgG titers is frequent after heart transplantation without evidence of clinical disease. Prophylaxis with pyrimethamine plus folinic acid for 6 weeks is indicated in seronegative cardiac transplant patients who receive seropositive allografts.

APPROACH TO MAJOR NOSOCOMIAL INFECTIONS IN TRANSPLANT RECIPIENTS

Pulmonary Infiltrates

Pulmonary infiltrates, including those resulting from pneumonitis, remain a serious and frequently encountered complication in transplant recipients. In heart transplant recipients, pulmonary infections have been documented in 28% to 40% of patients (2,162). Fifty-one percent (36/71) of all pulmonary infections in heart transplant recipients in one report were nosocomial in origin; 32% (23/71) were opportunistic and only 17% (12/71) were community-acquired. The latter usually occur in the late posttransplant period (>1 year) (2). Nearly one half of all pneumonias in these patients are bacterial in origin. Prolonged intubation, reintubation, and high-dose corticosteroids were significant risk factors for pneumonia in heart transplant recipients.

The differential diagnosis of pulmonary infiltrates in lung and heart-lung transplant recipients, among other entities, includes acute rejection. Acute rejection may develop in up to 60% of these patients, and most of these episodes occur within the first 3 months. Obliterative bronchitis is a significant late-occurring complication in lung transplant recipients. Rejection and/or infection, particularly resulting from CMV, are proposed to be the leading risk factors.

After liver transplantation, pneumonia occurs in 13% to 34% of patients. Forty-four percent of the liver transplant recipients requiring intensive care unit admission developed pulmonary infiltrates in one study; pulmonary edema (40%), pneumonia (38%), atelectasis (10%), and adult respiratory distress syndrome (8%) were the documented causes (234). Adult respiratory distress syndrome has been reported in 5% to 17% of liver transplant recipients. Large-volume transfusions, liver failure, retransplantation, and sepsis are considered factors predisposing to adult respiratory distress syndrome in these patients (234). Bacteria account for 40% to 67% of all pneumonias in liver transplant recipients. In the earlier reports, viral pneumonitis (CMV or HSV) was documented in 15% to 20% of the pulmonary infections. This incidence, however, has declined to less than 5% in the more recent reports (234). Pneumonias are less common after renal transplantation (occurring in 8% to 16% of the patients) but are nevertheless a significant complication in these patients.

Nosocomial bacterial pneumonitis is the predominant cause of pneumonia in all types of solid organ transplantation; *P. aeruginosa,* Enterobacteriaceae, and *S. aureus* are the bacteria usually implicated. Legionellosis has been reported in 2% to 9% of solid organ transplant recipients with pneumonia (5). Fungal pneumonias in transplant recipients are predominantly due to invasive aspergillosis. Although isolation of *Candida* species from respiratory cultures is common, *Candida* pneumonitis has been documented usually in heart-lung or lung transplant recipients (28). Other less frequent causes of pulmonary infection include cryptococcosis, zygomycosis, coccidioidomycosis, histoplasmosis, and dematiaceous fungi. CMV and to a lesser degree HSV account for most cases of viral pneumonitis. Whereas 5% to 20% of renal, liver, and heart transplant patients develop CMV pneumonitis, the incidence in heart-lung and lung transplant recipients is higher and ranges from 10% to 50%. It is believed that the host immune response is more important for the development of CMV pneumonitis than viral replication is (17). Virus-coded CMV proteins in the lung recognized by host T cells lead to uncontrolled recruitment and accumulation of such cells in the lungs. Pneumonia resulting from RSV generally occurs in pediatric patients and may occur 3 weeks to 2 years after transplantation. Up to 20% to 50% of the cases of RSV are nosocomially acquired. Whereas mortality resulting from RSV in marrow transplant recipients approaches 50%, death resulting from RSV is rare in solid organ transplant recipients. Early identification and isolation of cases, however, is crucial to prevent nosocomial spread.

Given the diversity of likely causes, early and aggressive pursuit of the etiology of pulmonary infection is warranted in all transplant recipients. Although the radiographic appearance of the lesion is never diagnostic, a number of entities may have distinctive or suggestive radiographic characteristics. Nodular pulmonary infiltrates of infectious etiology in liver transplant recipients were most frequently due to *Aspergillus* or *Cryptococcus* in one study (235). However, *S. aureus, Nocardia,* tuberculosis, PCP, CMV, zygomycosis, *Bartonella henselae,* and coccidioidomycosis may present similarly in transplant recipients. Non-infectious causes of pulmonary nodules include metastatic hepatocellular carcinoma, pulmonary calcification, and lymphoproliferative disorders in liver transplant recipients. Pulmonary infarcts, rounded atelectasis, and pulmonary varix in cardiac transplant recipients and acute or chronic rejection in lung transplant patients may have a nodular appearance. Cavitary pneumonia in transplant recipients may be due to *Aspergillus, Cryptococcus, Nocardia, Legionella, M. tuberculosis, Rhodococcus equi,* or other fungi.

CT offers a number of advantages over conventional radiographs, including detection of additional lesions, precise morphology of the lesion, and delineation of mediastinal lymphadenopathy. CTs in patients suspected of having aspergillosis have often revealed lesions that appeared nonspecific or were not visualized on routine x-ray examination. By CT, aspergillosis frequently manifests as nodular lesions, halo signs (nodular opacities with a hazy margin), or an air crescent sign (crescent-shaped area of hyperlucency within a cavitary mass).

Isolation or detection of *Legionella, Nocardia, Cryptococcus, M. tuberculosis,* or *P. carinii* in the sputum or respiratory secretions is diagnostic of pulmonary infection resulting from these pathogens. However, smears and cultures of sputum or respiratory secretions may be diagnostic in fewer than 50% of patients. In a patient with focal air space disease and nondiagnostic noninvasive tests, the choice lies between empiric antibacterial therapy or a diagnostic procedure; we recommend early bronchoscopy with bronchoalveolar lavage. In patients with focal nodular infiltrates, percutaneous needle aspiration is superior to bronchoalveolar lavage with a diagnostic accuracy of 70% to 90%. In patients with diffuse pulmonary infiltrates, bronchoalveolar lavage with or without transbronchial biopsy is the preferred approach. Transbronchial biopsy is particularly valuable for the diagnosis of rejection in lung transplant recipients and for the differentiation of allograft rejection and CMV pneumonitis in these patients. Open lung biopsy should be reserved only for patients with progressive disease refractory to antimicrobial agents in whom bronchoalveolar lavage or percutaneous needle aspiration is nondiagnostic.

Nosocomial Bacteremias

Although the incidence of bacteremia may vary, identifiable portals of entry and defined pathogens exist for most solid organ transplant recipients with bacteremia. The frequency of bacteremia varies from 6% to 10% in kidney, 11% in heart, 11% in pancreatic, and 20% to 25% in liver transplant recipients (165, 236). Ninety-four percent (75/80) of all bacteremias in liver transplant recipients, 56% (15/27) in renal transplant recipients, and 78% (13/18) in heart transplant recipients were nosocomially acquired (236). Pneumonia in heart and heart-lung transplant recipients, urinary tract infections in renal transplant recipients, abdominal and biliary infections in liver transplant recipients, and surgical site and urinary tract infections in pancreatic transplant recipients have been shown to be the most common identifiable sources of bacteremia (165,236). Aerobic gram-negative bacilli constituted 48% of the bacteremic isolates in renal transplant recipients, 49% in liver transplant recipients, and 39% in heart transplant recipients (236). *E. coli, Klebsiella,* and other Enterobacteriaceae were the predominant gram-negative bacteria in renal transplant recipients; *P. aeruginosa* and *Enterobacter* species were predominant in liver transplant recipients; and *P. aeruginosa* and *E. coli* were predominant in heart transplant recipients.

The sources and pathogens causing bacteremias in transplant recipients appear, however, to have undergone a striking evolution in the recent years. Many transplant centers have documented the emergence of gram-positive cocci (enterococci and staphylococci) as foremost pathogens in transplant recipients. In a recent study in liver transplant recipients, intravascular cannulas were by far the most common source, accounting for 39% of all bacteremias (163). Fifty-eight percent of all catheter-associated infections were due to MRSA (163). Within the hospital, intensive care units are the most common site of acquisition of nosocomial bacteremias. Ninety-three percent of the bacteremias in one report were nosocomially acquired, and 52% occurred in the intensive care unit setting (163). Indeed, intensive care unit stay has been shown to be an independent predictor of bacteremic compared with nonbacteremic infections in liver transplant recipients (44). Patients developing bacteremia in the intensive care unit were also more likely to die than those not in the intensive care unit (44); this likely reflected the greater severity of illness of the patients hospitalized in the intensive care unit.

In a study in small bowel transplant recipients, 72% of patients had at least one episode of bloodstream infection (69). Intravascular cannulas accounted for 43% of these infections and were the most frequently identifiable portal of entry. Sixty-two percent of all bloodstream infections were due to gram-positive bacteria (69). In another report, 45% of all bacterial infections and 72% of all bacteremias after small bowel transplantation were due to staphylococci (72).

Most VRE infections originate from an abdominal or biliary source; 38% to 68% of these infections have been associated with bacteremia (170,172). Vancomycin resistance was an independent predicator of mortality in liver transplant recipients with enterococcal bacteremia (170). A noteworthy observation is the predilection of VRE to cause endovascular complications, including mycotic aneurysms and endocarditis (170). Delayed metastatic complications, including endocarditis and osteomyelitis, have also been documented in transplant recipients with MRSA bacteremia. Prophylaxis and infection control measures pertinent to these infections are discussed in the sections on staphylococci and enterococci.

Intraabdominal Infections

Intraabdominal abscesses, peritonitis, and biliary infections are a significant complication after liver transplantation. Intrahepatic abscesses usually occur within 30 days of transplantation; technical problems involving the implanted allograft (e.g., hepatic artery thrombosis, biliary leak, and, rarely, tear of the donor liver) are the primary risk factors. Nearly one half of patients with intrahepatic abscesses may be bacteremic (46). Peritonitis after liver transplantation is typically related to biliary anastomotic leaks or, less frequently, bowel perforation (46). Aerobic enteric gram-negative bacteria, enterococci, anaerobes, and, rarely, *Candida* species are the causal pathogens in most intraabdominal abscesses and peritonitis. An unusual cause of abdominal abscesses in liver transplant recipients is *M. hominis.*

Cholangitis has been documented in 4% to 15% of patients after liver transplantation, with most episodes occurring within 30 days of transplantation. Biliary strictures and biliary leaks are significant predisposing risk factors. Enterococci are characteristically the most common pathogen, whereas anaerobes are encountered rarely. Biliary strictures (e.g., in patients with primary biliary cirrhosis and in those with previous bile duct surgeries) often necessitate Roux-en-Y anastomosis, which is associated with a high rate of intrahepatic and biliary complications. Sterile intraabdominal fluid collections are common after liver transplant surgery. Diagnosis of peritonitis or abscess, thus, requires percutaneous or open drainage and culture. Cultures from abdominal drains often reflect colonization and are not reliable in diagnosing the infection or its etiology.

Central Nervous System Lesions

Although mild neurologic complications may occur in 10% to 47% of organ transplant recipients, 1% to 8% of such patients have major neurologic sequelae or central nervous system lesions. Brain abscesses are among the most serious central nervous system lesions in these patients (237). The frequency of brain abscesses was 0.36% in kidney, 0.63% in liver, and 1.17% in heart and heart-lung transplant recipients (238). Most brain abscesses in solid organ transplant recipients are fungal and represent a nosocomial complication (237,238). Although *Aspergillus* is the most common cause of brain abscesses in organ transplant recipients, less frequently encountered fungal pathogens include *Mucorales, Candida* species, and dematiaceous fungi. Central nervous system lesions resulting from *T. gondii* and *Nocardia* have been reported mainly in heart transplant recipients.

Selby et al. (238) showed that two distinct groups of solid organ transplant recipients existed with regard to timing and susceptibility to brain abscesses. One group, comprised predominantly of liver and renal transplant recipients, developed brain abscesses a median of 24 days posttransplant. Ninety-five percent of these patients were in the intensive care unit and were ventilator dependent; brain abscesses in this setting were exclusively fungal. In the second group, abscesses developed a median of 264 days after transplantation, occurred almost exclusively in heart transplant recipients, and were due to *T. gondii* and *Nocardia.*

Most patients (up to 75%) with fungal brain abscesses have been shown to concurrently have pulmonary lesions resulting from the same fungus (237). A brain biopsy may not be required in such cases.

In the absence of an extraneural focus, brain biopsy should be considered, given the diversity of causal fungal pathogens in such lesions (237).

CONCLUSIONS

Improvement in surgical techniques, the advent of modern immunosuppressive drugs, the availability of rapid and reliable diagnostic modalities, and effective prophylaxis against a number of pathogens have undoubtedly led to a decrease in infectious morbidity and improved outcome in transplant recipients in recent years. Increasing documentation of the emergence of antimicrobial resistance in several key pathogens in transplant recipients, however, is worrisome. Strategies for antimicrobial prophylaxis must comprise approaches that are not only efficacious but minimize the emergence of resistance. Finally, for therapy and prevention to be effective, classic opportunistic infections typically encountered in these patients must be considered and the emerging trends in new infectious agents and the changing epidemiology of these complicating infections must be understood.

REFERENCES

1. Chang FY, Singh N, Gayowski T, et al. Fever in liver transplant recipients: changing spectrum of etiologic agents. *Clin Infect Dis* 1998; 26:59–65.
2. Waser M, Maggiorini M, Luthy A, et al. Infectious complications in 100 consecutive heart transplant recipients. *Eur J Clin Microbiol Infect Dis* 1994;13:12–18.
3. Singh N, Yu VL. Oral ganciclovir usage for cytomegalovirus prophylaxis in organ transplant recipients. Is emergence of resistance imminent? *Dig Dis Sci* 1998;43:1190–1192.
4. Sawyer RG, Crabtree TD, Gleason TG, et al. Impact of solid organ transplantation and immunosuppression on fever, leukocytosis, and physiologic response during bacterial and fungal infections. *Clin Transplantation* 1999;13:260–265.
5. Chow JW, Yu VL. Legionella a major opportunistic pathogen in transplant recipients. *Semin Respir Infect* 1998;13:132–139.
6. Kirby BD, Snyder K, Meyer R, et al. Legionnaires' disease: a report of 65 nosocomial cases and a review of the literature. *Medicine* 1980; 59:188–205.
7. Jereb JA, Burwen DR, Dooley SW, et al. Nosocomial outbreak of tuberculosis in a renal transplant unit: application of a new technique for restriction fragment length polymorphism analysis of *Mycobacterium tuberculosis* isolates. *J Infect Dis* 1993;168:1219–1224.
8. Paterson DL, Muder RR, Squier C, et al. Outbreak of infection with *E. coli* harboring extended spectrum beta-lactamase (ESBL) in a liver transplant unit: could norfloxacin administration to carriers contribute to control? *Clin Infect Dis* 2001;33:126–128.
9. DelMonico FL, Snydman DR. Organ donor screening for infectious diseases. *Transplantation* 1998;65:603–610.
10. Douglas D, Rakela R, Marnish D, et al. Transmission of hepatitis B virus infection from orthotopic donor livers. *Hepatology* 1992;16:49A.
11. Wachs M, Amend W, Ascher N, et al. The risk of transmission of hepatitis B from HBsAg(-), HBcAb(+), HBIgM(-) organ donors. *Transplantation* 1995;59:230.
12. Munoz SJ. Use of hepatitis B core antibody-positive donors for liver transplantation. *Liver Transplantation* 2002;10:S82–S87.
13. Vargas HE, Laskus T, Wang LF, et al. Outcome of liver transplantation in hepatitis C virus-infected patients who received hepatitis C virus-infected grafts. *Gastroenterology* 1999;117:149–153.
14. Torres M, Weppler D, Reddy KR, et al. Use of hepatitis C virus-infected donors for hepatitis C positive OHCT recipients. *Gastroenterology* 1999;117:1253.
15. Ho M, Suwansirikul S, Dowling JN, et al. The transplanted kidney as a source of cytomegalovirus infection. *N Engl J Med* 1975;293: 1109–1112.
16. Betts RF, Freeman RB, Douglas RG, et al. Transmission of cytomegalovirus infection with renal allografts. *Kidney Int* 1975;8:385–392.
17. Grundy JE, Shanley JD, Griffiths PD. Is cytomegalovirus interstitial pneumonitis in transplant recipients an immunopathological condition? *Lancet* 1987;2:996–999.
18. Dummer JS, Armstrong J, Somers J, et al. Transmission of infection with herpes simplex virus by renal transplantation. *J Infect Dis* 1987; 155:202–206.
19. Cen H, Breinig MD, Atchison RW, et al. Epstein-Barr virus transmission via the donor organs in solid organ transplantation: polymerase chain reaction and restriction fragment length polymorphism analysis of IR2, IR3, and IR4. *J Virol* 1991;65:976–980.
20. Ward KN, Gray JJ, Efstathiou S. Primary human herpesvirus 6 infection in a patient following liver transplantation from a seropositive donor. *J Med Virol* 1989;28:69–72.
21. Singh N, Dummer JS, Kusne S, et al. Infections with cytomegalovirus and the herpesviruses in 121 liver transplant recipients: transmission by donated organ and the effect of OKT3 antibodies. *J Infect Dis* 1988;158:124–131.
22. Caballero F, Domingo P, Rabella N, et al. Successful transplantation of organs retrieved from a donor with syphilis. *Transplantation* 1998; 65:598–599.
23. Peters TG, Reiter CG, Boswell RL. Transmission of tuberculosis by kidney transplantation. *Transplantation* 1984;38:514–516.
24. Singh N, Paterson DL. *M. tuberculosis* infection in solid organ transplant recipients: impact and implications for management. *Clin Infect Dis* 1998;27:1266–1277.
25. Lumbreras C, Samz F, Gonazlez A, et al. Clinical significance of donor-unrecognized bacteremia in the outcome of solid-organ transplant recipients. *Clin Infect Dis* 2001;33:722–726.
26. Freeman RB, Giatras I, Falagas ME, et al. Outcome of transplantation of organs procured from bacteremic donors. *Transplantation* 1999; 68:1107–1111.
27. Lopez-Navidad A, Domingo P, Caballero F, et al. Successful transplantation of organs retrieved from donors with bacterial meningitis. *Transplantation* 1997;64:365–368.
28. Kanj SS, Welty-Wolf K, Madden J, et al. Fungal infections in lung and heart-lung transplant recipients: report of 9 cases and review of the literature. *Medicine* 1996;75:142–156.
29. Gottesdiener KM. Transplanted infections: donor-to-host transmission with the allograft. *Ann Intern Med* 1989;110:1001–1016.
30. Preiksaitis JK, Straufman TM. The risk of transfusion-acquired cytomegalovirus (CMV) infection in seronegative solid organ transplant recipients receiving unscreened blood products (1984–1996) (abstract no. 450, p. 191). Seventeenth annual meeting of the American Society of Transplant Physicians, Chicago, 1998.
31. Falagas ME, Snydman DR, Ruthazer R, et al. Primary cytomegalovirus infection in liver transplant recipients: comparison of infections transmitted via donor organs and via transfusions. *Clin Infect Dis* 1996;23:292–297.
32. Ernst A, Gordon FD, Hayek J, et al. Lung abscess complicating *Legionella micdadei* pneumonia in an adult liver transplant recipient. *Transplantation* 1998;65:130–134.
33. Prodinger WM, Bonatti H, Allerberger F, et al. *Legionella* pneumonia in transplant recipients: a cluster of cases of eight years duration. *J Hosp Infect* 1994;26:191–202.
34. Bangsborg JM, Uldum S, Jensen JS, et al. Nosocomial legionellosis in three heart-lung transplant patients: case reports and environmental observations. *Eur J Clin Microbiol Infect Dis* 1995;14:99–104.
35. Wald A, Leisenring W, vanBurik J, et al. Epidemiology of *Aspergillus* infections in a large cohort of patients undergoing bone marrow transplantation. *J Infect Dis* 1997;175:1459–1466.
36. Anaissie E. Invasive aspergillosis: a new look at an old disease. In *Focus on fungal infections.* Orlando, FL, 1998.
37. Noskin GA, Stosor V, Cooper I, et al. Recovery of vancomycin-resistant enterococci on fingertips and environmental surfaces. *Infect Control Hosp Epidemiol* 1995;16:577–581.
38. Morris JG Jr, Shay DK, Hebden JN, et al. Enterococci resistant to multiple antimicrobial agents, including vancomycin: establishment of endeminicity in a university medical center. *Ann Intern Med* 1995; 123:250–259.
39. Chang FY, Singh N, Gayowski T, et al. *Staphylococcus aureus* nasal

colonization and association with infections in liver transplant recipients. *Transplantation* 1998;65:1169–1172.
40. Samore MH, DeGirolami PC, Tlucko A, et al. *Clostridium difficile* colonization and diarrhea at a tertiary care hospital. *Clin Infect Dis* 1994;18:181–187.
41. Kaatz GW, Gitlin SD, Schaberg DR, et al. Acquisition of *Clostridium difficile* from the hospital environment. *Am J Epidemiol* 1998;127: 1289–1294.
42. McFarland LV, Mulligan ME, Kwok RYY, et al. Nosocomial acquisition of *Clostridium difficile* infection. *N Engl J Med* 1998;320: 204–210.
43. Gayowsksi T, Marino IR, Singh N, et al. Orthotopic liver transplantation in high risk patients: risk factors associated with mortality and infectious morbidity. *Transplantation* 1997;65:499–504.
44. Singh N, Gayowski T, Wagener MM, et al. Predictors and outcome of early versus late-onset major bacterial infections in liver transplant recipients receiving tacrolimus (FK506) as primary immunosuppression. *Eur J Clin Micro Infect Dis* 1997;16:821–826.
45. Paya CV. Fungal infections in solid-organ transplantation. *Clin Infect Dis* 1993;16:677–688.
46. Kusne S, Dummer JS, Singh N, et al. Infections after liver transplantation, an analysis of 101 consecutive cases. *Medicine* 1988;67: 132–143.
47. Gayowski T, Marino IR, Doyle HR, et al. A high incidence of native portal vein thrombosis in veterans undergoing liver transplantation. *J Surg Res* 1996;60:333–338.
48. Singh N, Gayowski T, Wagener MM, et al. Increased infections in liver transplant recipients with recurrent hepatitis C virus hepatitis. *Transplantation* 1996;61:402–406.
49. Hoy WE, May AG, Freeman RB. Primary renal transplant wound infections. *N Y State J Med* 1981;81:1469–1473.
50. Lobo PI, Rudolf LE, Kreiger JN. Wound infections in renal transplant recipients—a complication of urinary tract infections during allograft malfunction. *Surgery* 1982;92:491–496.
51. Lapchik MS, Filho AC, Restana JO, et al. Risk factors for nosocomial urinary tract and postoperative wound infections in renal transplant patients: a matched pair case control study. *J Urology* 1992;147: 994–998.
52. Muakkassa WF, Goldman MH, Mendez-Picon G, et al. Wound infections in renal transplant patients. *J Urology* 1983;130:17–19.
53. Tilney NL, Strom TB, Vineyard GC, et al. Factors contributing to the declining mortality rate in renal transplantation. *N Engl J Med* 1978;299:1321–1325.
54. Fox BD, Sollinger HW, Belzer FO, et al. A prospective, randomized double-blind study of trimethoprim-sulfamethoxazole for prophylaxis of infection in renal transplantation: clinical efficacy, absorption, effects on microflora and the cost-benefit of prophylaxis. *Am J Med* 1990;89:255–274.
55. Dauber JH, Paradis IL, Dummer JS. Infectious complications in pulmonary allograft recipients. *Clin Chest Med* 1990;11:291–308.
56. Kramer MR, Marshall SE, Starnes VA, et al. Infectious complications in heart-lung transplantation, analysis of 200 episodes. *Arch Intern Med* 1993;153:2010–2016.
57. Bauldoff GS, Nunley DR, Manzetti JD, et al. Use of aerosolized colistin sodium in cystic fibrosis patients awaiting lung transplantation. *Transplantation* 1997;64:748–752.
58. Lewiston N, King V, Umetsu D, et al. Cystic fibrosis patients who have undergone heart-lung transplantation benefit from maxillary sinus antrostomy and repeated sinus lavage. *Transplant* 1991;23: 1207–1208.
59. Baldwin RT, Radovancevic B, Sweeney MS, et al. Bacterial mediastinitis after heart transplantation. *J Heart Lung Transplant* 1992;11: 545–549.
60. Karwande SV, Renlund DG, Olsen SL, et al. Mediastinitis in heart transplantation. *Ann Thorac Surg* 1992;54:1039–1045.
61. Trento A, Dummer JS, Hardesty RL, et al. Mediastinitis following heart transplant: incidence, treatment and results. *Heart Transplant* 1984;3:336–340.
62. Pearl SN, Weiner MA, Dibbell DG. Sternal infection after cardiac transplantation. Successful salvage utilizing a variety of techniques. *Thorac Cardiovasc Surg* 1982;83:632–634.
63. Steffenson DO, Dummer JS, Granick MS, et al. Sternotomy infections with *Mycoplasma hominis. Ann Intern Med* 1987;106:204–208.
64. Sollinger HW, Ploeg RJ, Eckhoff DE, et al. Two hundred consecutive simultaneous pancreas-kidney transplants with bladder drainage. *Surgery* 1993;114:736–744.
65. Everett JE, Wahoff DC, Statz GKJ, et al. Characterization and impact of wound infection after pancreas transplantation. *Arch Surg* 1994; 129:1310–1317.
66. Hesse UJ, Sutherland DER, Simmons RL, et al. Intra-abdominal infections in pancreas transplant recipients. *Clin Transplantation* 1990;4:287–291.
67. Tesi RJ, Henry ML, Elkhammas EA, et al. Decreased wound complications of combined kidney/pancreas transplants using intraabdominal pancreas graft placement. *Clin Transplantation* 199;4:287–291.
68. Manez R, Kusne S, Green M, et al. Incidence and risk factors associated with the development of cytomegalovirus disease after intestinal transplantation. *Transplantation* 1995;59:1010–1014.
69. Kusne S, Furukawa H, Abu-Elmagd K, et al. Infectious complications after small bowel transplantation in adults: an update. *Transplant Proc* 1996;5:2761–2762.
70. Woodward JE, Mayer D. The unique challenge of small intestinal transplantation. *Br J Hosp Med* 1996;xx:285–290.
71. Reyes J, Bueno J, Kocoshis S, et al. Current status of intestinal transplantation in children. *J Pediatr Surg* 1998;33:243–254.
72. McAlister V, Grant D, Wall W, et al. Immunosuppressive requirements for small bowel/liver transplantation. *Transplant Proc* 1993; 25:1204–1205.
73. Singh N, Gayowski T, Wagener MM, et al. Invasive fungal infections in liver transplant recipients receiving tacrolimus as primary immunosuppressive agent. *Clin Infect Dis* 1997;24:179–184.
74. Singh N, Avery RK, Munoz P, et al. Trends in risk profiles for and mortality associated with invasive aspergillosis among liver transplant recipients. *Clin Infect Dis* 2003;36:46–52.
75. Singh N, Carrigan DR. Human herpesvirus-6 in transplantation: an emerging pathogen. *Ann Intern Med* 1996;124:1065–1071.
76. Hibberd PL, Basgoz N, Fishman J, et al. Primary cytomegalovirus disease is a risk factor for recurrent CMV disease in transplant recipients (abstract H28). Thirty-first Interscience Conference of Antimicrobial Agents and Chemotherapy, 1995, Orlando, FL.
77. Stratta RJ, Shaeffer MS, Markin RS, et al. Cytomegalovirus infection and disease after liver transplantation, an overview. *Diagn Dis Sci* 1992;37:673–688.
78. Hibberd PL, Tolkoff-Rubin NE, Conti D, et al. Preemptive ganciclovir therapy to prevent cytomegalovirus disease in cytomegalovirus antibody-positive renal transplant recipients. A randomized controlled trial. *Ann Intern Med* 1995;123:18–26.
79. Grundy JE, Lui SF, Super M, et al. Symptomatic cytomegalovirus infection in seropositive kidney recipients: reinfection with donor virus rather than reactivation of recipient virus. *Lancet* 1988;2: 132–135.
80. Fietze E, Prosch S, Reinke P, et al. Cytomegalovirus infection in transplant recipients. The role of tumor necrosis factor. *Transplantation* 1994;58:675–680.
81. Paterson DL, Singh N, Stapelfeldt W, et al. Intraoperative hypothermia is an independent risk factor for cytomegalovirus (CMV) infection in liver transplant recipients. *Transplantation* 1999;67: 1151–1155.
82. Manez R, White LT, Linden P, et al. The influence of HLA matching on cytomegalovirus hepatitis and chronic rejection after liver transplantation. *Transplantation* 1993;55:1067–1071.
83. Docke WD, Prosch S, Fietze E, et al. Cytomegalovirus reactivation and tumour necrosis factor. *Lancet* 1994;343:268–269.
84. Haagmans BL, Stals FS, van der Meide PH, et al. Tumor necrosis factor alpha promotes replication and pathogenicity of rat cytomegalovirus. *J Virol* 1994;68:2297–2304.
85. Chatterjee SN, Fiala N, Weiner J. Primary cytomegalovirus and opportunistic infections: incidence in renal transplant recipients. *JAMA* 1978;240:2446–2449.

86. Limaye AP, Corey L, Koelle DM, et al. Emergence of ganciclovir-resistant cytomegalovirus disease among solid organ transplant recipients. *Lancet* 2000;356:645–649.
87. Singh N. Delayed occurrence of cytomegalovirus disease in organ transplant recipients receiving antiviral prophylaxis: are we winning the battle only to lose the war? *Eur J Clin Microbiol Infect* 2002.
88. Paya CV. A randomized, double-blind, double-dummy, active-comparator controlled multi-center study of the efficacy and safety of valganciclovir vs oral ganciclovir for prevention of CMV disease in 372 high-risk (D+/R-) heart, liver and kidney recipients. Forty-second Interscience Conference on Antimicrobial Agents and Chemotherapy, San Diego, September 27–30, 2002.
89. Ho M. Infection and organ transplantation. In: Gelman S, editor. *Anesthesia and organ transplantation.* Philadelphia: WB Saunders, 1987:49–60.
90. Gleaves CA, Smith TF, Shuster EA, et al. Comparison of standard tube and shell vial cell culture techniques for the detection of cytomegalovirus in clinical specimens. *J Clin Microbiol* 1985;21:217–221.
91. The TH, Vander BIJW, VandenBerg AP, et al. Cytomegalovirus antigenemia. *Rev Infect Dis* 1990;12(Suppl):737–744.
92. Gerna G, Zavattoni M, Percivalle E, et al. Rising levels of human cytomegalovirus (HCMV) antigenemia during initial antiviral treatment of solid-organ transplant recipients with primary HCMV infection. *J Clin Microbiol* 1998;36:1113–1116.
93. Patel R, Smith TF, Espy M, et al. A prospective comparison of molecular diagnostic techniques for the early detection of cytomegalovirus in liver transplant recipients. *J Infect Dis* 1995;171:1010–1014.
94. Cunningham R, Harris A, Frankton A, et al. Detection of cytomegalovirus using PCR in serum from renal transplant recipients. *J Clin Pathol* 1995;48:575–577.
95. Schmidt CA, Oettle H, Peng R, et al. Comparison of polymerase chain reaction from plasma and buffy coat with antigen detection and occurrence of immunoglobulin M for the demonstration of cytomegalovirus infection after liver transplantation. *Transplantation* 1995;59:1133–1138.
96. Ackermann JR, LeFor WM, Weinstein S, et al. Four-year experience with exclusive use of cytomegalovirus antibody (CMV-Ab)-negative donors for CMV-Ab-negative kidney recipients. *Transplant Proc* 1988;20(Suppl 1):469–471.
97. Balfour HH, Chace BA, Stepleton JT, et al. A randomized, placebo controlled trial of oral acyclovir for the prevention of cytomegalovirus disease in recipients of renal allografts. *N Engl J Med* 1989;320: 1381–1387.
98. Singh N, Yu VL, Mieles L, et al. High-dose acyclovir compared with short-course preemptive ganciclovir therapy to prevent cytomegalovirus disease in liver transplant recipients, a randomized trial. *Ann Intern Med* 1994;120:375–381.
99. Martin MM, Manez R, Linden P, et al. A prospective randomized trial comparing sequential ganciclovir-high dose acyclovir to high dose acyclovir for prevention of cytomegalovirus disease in adult liver transplant recipients. *Transplantation* 1994;58:779–785.
100. Merigan TC, Renlund DG, Keay S, et al. A controlled trial of ganciclovir to prevent cytomegalovirus disease after heart transplantation. *N Engl J Med* 1993;326:1182–1186.
101. Winston DJ, Wirin D, Shaked A, et al. Randomized comparison of ganciclovir and high-dose acyclovir for long-term cytomegalovirus prophylaxis in liver transplant recipients. *Lancet* 1995;346:69–74.
102. Alain S, Honderlick P, Grenet D, et al. Failure of ganciclovir treatment associated with selection of a ganciclovir resistant cytomegalovirus strain in a lung transplant recipient. *Transplantation* 1997;63: 1533–1536.
103. Rosen HR, Brenner KG, Flora KD, et al. Development of ganciclovir resistance during treatment of primary cytomegalovirus infection after liver transplantation. *Transplantation* 1997;63:476–478.
104. Iberer F, Tscheliessnigg K, Halwache G, et al. Definitions of cytomegalovirus disease after heart transplantation: antigenemia as a marker for antiviral therapy. *Transplant Int* 1996;9:236–242.
105. Verdonck LF, Dekker AW, Rosenberg-Arska M, et al. A risk-adapted approach with a short-course of ganciclovir to prevent cytomegalovirus pneumonia in CMV-seropositive recipients of allogeneic bone marrow transplants. *Clin Infect Dis* 1997;24:901–907.
106. Grossi P, Kusne S, Rinaldo C, et al. Guidance of ganciclovir therapy with pp65 antigenemia in cytomegalovirus-free recipients of livers from seropositive donors. *Transplantation* 1996;61:1659–1660.
107. Kusne S, Schwartz M, Breinig MK, et al. Herpes simplex virus hepatitis after solid organ transplantation in adults. *J Infect Dis* 1991;163: 1001–1007.
108. Holt ND, Gould FKI, Taylor CE, et al. Incidence and significance of noncytomegalovirus viral respiratory infection after adult lung transplantation. *J Heart Lung Transplant* 1997;16:416–419.
109. Schuller D, Spessert C, Fraser VJ, et al. Herpes simplex virus from respiratory tract secretions: epidemiology, clinical characteristics, and outcome in immunocompromised and nonimmunocompromised hosts. *Am J Med* 1993;94:29–34.
110. McGregor RS, Zitelli BJ, Urbach AH, et al. Varicella in pediatric orthotopic liver transplant recipients. *Pediatrics* 1989;83:256–261.
111. Kusne S, Pappo O, Manez R, et al. Varicella zoster virus hepatitis and a suggested management plan for prevention of VZV infection in adult transplant recipients. *Transplantation* 1995;xx:619–621.
112. Feldhoff C, Balfour H, Simmons SR, et al. Varicella in children with renal transplants. *J Pediatr* 1981;98:25–31.
113. Kashtan CE, Cook M, Chavers BM, et al. Outcome of chicken pox in 66 pediatric renal transplant recipients. *J Pediatr* 1997;131:874–877.
114. Broyer M, Tete MJ, Guest G, et al. Varicella and zoster in children after kidney transplantation: long-term results of vaccination. *Pediatrics* 1997;99:35–39.
115. Ablashi D, Agut H, Berneman Z, et al. Human herpesvirus-6 strain groups: a nomenclature. *Arch Virol* 1993;129:363–366.
116. Schirmer EC, Wyatt LS, Yamanishi K, et al. Differentiation between two distinct classes of viruses now classified as human herpesvirus-6. *Proc Natl Acad Sci U S A* 1991;88:5922–5926.
117. Singh N, Gayowski T, Wagener M, et al. Bloodstream infections in liver transplant recipients; changing patterns of microbial origin (abstract). Thirty-sixth Interscience Conference on Antimicrobial Agents and Chemotherapy, New Orleans, 1996.
118. Yoshikawa T, Suga S, Asano Y, et al. A prospective study of human herpesvirus-6 infection in renal transplantation. *Transplantation* 1992;54:879–883.
119. Randhawa PS, Jenkins FJ, Nalesnik MA, et al. Herpesvirus 6 variant A infection after heart transplantation with giant cell transformation in bile ductular and gastroduodenal epithelium. *Am J Surg Pathol* 1997;21:847–853.
120. DesJardin JA, Gibbons L, Cho E, et al. Human herpesvirus 6 reactivation is associated with cytomegalovirus infection and syndromes in kidney transplant recipients at risk for primary cytomegalovirus infection. *J Infect Dis* 1998;178:1783–1786.
121. Agut H, Collandre H, Aubin JT, et al. In vitro sensitivity of human herpesvirus 6 to antiviral drugs. *Res Virol* 1989;140:219–228.
122. Russler SK, Tapper MA, Carrigan DR. Susceptibility of human herpesvirus 6 to acyclovir and ganciclovir [Letter]. *Lancet* 1989;2:382.
123. Streicher HZ, Hung CL, Ablashi DV, et al. In vitro inhibition of human herpesvirus-6 by phosphonoformate. *J Virol Method* 1988;21: 301–304.
124. Wright TL, Donegan E, Hsu HH, et al. Recurrent and acquired hepatitis C viral infection in liver transplant recipients. *Gastroenterology* 1992;103:317–322.
125. Muller H, Otto G, Gosser T, et al. Recurrence of hepatitis C viral infection in liver transplant recipients. *Transplantation* 1992;54: 743–745.
126. Gane EJ, Portman BC, Naumov NV, et al. Long-term outcome of hepatitis C infection after liver transplantation. *N Engl J Med* 1996; 334:815–820.
127. Druwe PM, Michielsen PP, Ramon AM, et al. Hepatitis C and nephrology. *Nephrol Dial Transplant* 1994;9:223–237.
128. Morales JM, Munoz MA, Castellano G, et al. Impact of hepatitis C in long-functioning renal transplants: a clinicopathological followup. *Transplant Proc* 1993;25:1450–1453.
129. Klauser R, Franz M, Traindl O, et al. Hepatitis C antibody in renal transplant patients. *Transplant Proc* 1992;24:286–288.

130. Roth D, Ferrandez JA, Burke GW, et al. Detection of antibody to hepatitis C virus in renal transplant recipients. *Transplantation* 1991; 51:396–400.
131. Stempel CA, Lake J, Kuo G, et al. Hepatitis C—its prevalence in end-stage renal failure patients and clinical course after kidney transplantation. *Transplantation* 1993;55:273–276.
132. Feray C, Gigou M, Samuel D, et al. Natural history of hepatitis C virus (HCV) infection after liver transplantation. *Hepatology* 1992; 16:47A.
133. Goetz A, Ndimbie OK, Wagener MM, et al. Prevalence of hepatitis C infection in health care workers affiliated with a liver transplant center. *Transplantation* 1995;59:990–994.
134. Gayowski T, Singh N, Marino IR, et al. Hepatitis C virus genotypes in liver transplant recipients: impact on posttransplant recurrence, infections, response to interferon-alpha therapy and outcome. *Transplantation* 1997;64:422–426.
135. Sheiner CP, Schwartz ME, Mor E, et al. Severe or multiple rejection episodes are associated with early recurrence of hepatitis C after orthotopic liver transplantation. *Hepatology* 1995;21:30–34.
136. Singh N, Gayowski T, Ndimbie OK, et al. Recurrent hepatitis C virus hepatitis in liver transplant recipients receiving tacrolimus: association with rejection and increased immunosuppression after transplantation. *Surgery* 1996;119:452–456.
137. Feray C, Gigou M, Samuel D, et al. Incidence of hepatitis C in patients receiving different preparations of hepatitis B immunoglobulins after liver transplantation. *Ann Intern Med* 1998;128:810–816.
138. Singh N, Gayowski T, Wannstedt CF, et al. Interferon-alpha as prophylaxis for recurrent viral hepatitis C after liver transplantation. *Transplantation* 1998;75:82–85.
139. Samuel D, Muller R, Alexander G, et al. Liver transplantation in European patients with hepatitis B surface antigen. *N Engl J Med* 1993;329:1842–1847.
140. Angus PW, Locarini SA, McGurghan GW, et al. Hepatitis B virus precore mutant infection is associated with severe recurrent disease after liver transplantation. *Hepatology* 1995;21:14–18.
141. Davies SE, Portmann B, O'Grady JG, et al. Hepatic histological findings after transplantation for chronic hepatitis B virus infection, including a unique pattern of fibrosing cholestatic hepatitis. *Hepatology* 1991;13:150–157.
142. Rao KV, Kasiske BL, Anderson WR. Variability in the morphological spectrum and clinical outcome of chronic liver disease in hepatitis B-positive and B-negative renal transplant recipients. *Transplantation* 1991;51:391–396.
143. Markowitz JS, Martin P, Conrad AJ, et al. Prophylaxis against hepatitis B recurrence following liver transplantation using combination lamivudine and hepatitis B immune globulin. *Hepatology* 1998;28: 585–589.
144. Han S-H, Ofman J, Holt C, et al. An efficacy and cost-effectiveness analysis of combination hepatitis B immune globulin and lamivudine to prevent recurrent hepatitis B after orthotopic liver transplantation compared with hepatitis B immune globulin monotherapy. *Liver Transplant* 2000;6:741–748.
145. Schiff E, Neuhaus P, Tillmann HL, et al. Safety and efficacy of adefovir dipivoxil for the treatment of lamivudine resistant HBV in patients post-liver transplantation. *Hepatology* 2001;34:446A(abst).
146. Shakil AO, Lilly L, Angus P, et al. Entecavir reduces viral load in liver transplant patients who have failed prophylaxis or treatment for hepatitis B. *Hepatology* 2001;34:619A(abst).
147. Cotler SJ, Gretch D, Bronner MP. Hepatitis G virus co-infection does not alter the course of recurrent hepatitis C virus infection in liver transplantation recipients. *Hepatology* 1997;26:432–436.
148. Vargas HE, Laskus T, Radkowski M, et al. Hepatitis G virus coinfection in hepatitis C virus-infected liver transplant recipients. *Transplantation* 1997;64:786–788.
149. Dickson RC, Qian K, Lau JYN. High prevalence of GB virus-C/ hepatitis G virus infection in liver transplant recipients. *Transplantation* 1997;63:1695–1697.
150. Pessoa MG, Terrault NA, Ferrell LD, et al. Hepatitis G virus in patients with cryptogenic liver disease undergoing liver transplantation. *Hepatology* 1997;25:1266–1270.
151. Randhawa PS, Demetris AJ. Nephropathy due to polyomavirus type BK. *N Engl J Med* 2000;342:1361–1362.
152. Hirsch HH, Knowles W, Dickenmann M, et al. Prospective study of polyomavirus type BK replication and nephropathy in renal-transplant recipients. *N Engl J Med* 2002;347:488–496.
153. Michaels MG, Green M, Wald ER, et al. Adenovirus infection in pediatric liver transplant recipients. *J Infect Dis* 1992;165:170–174.
154. Koneru B, Atchison R, Jaffe R, et al. Serologic studies of adenoviral hepatitis following pediatric liver transplantation. *Transplant Proc* 1990;22:1547–1548.
155. Ohori NP, Michaels MG, Jaffe R, et al. Adenovirus pneumonia in lung transplant recipients. *Hum Pathol* 1995;26:1073–1079.
156. McGrath D, Falagas ME, Freeman R, et al. Adenovirus infection in adult orthotopic liver transplant recipients: incidence and clinical significance. *J Infect Dis* 1998;177:459–462.
157. Saad RS, Demetris AJ, Lee RG, et al. Adenovirus hepatitis in the adult allograft liver. *Transplantation* 1997;64:1483–1485.
158. Liles WC, Cushing H, Holt CS, et al. Severe adenoviral nephritis following bone marrow transplantation: successful treatment with intravenous ribavirin. *Transplantation* 1993;12:409–412.
159. Pohl C, Green M, Wald ER, et al. Respiratory syncytial virus infections in pediatric liver transplant recipients. *J Infect Dis* 1992;165: 166–169.
160. Wendt CH, Fox JNK, Hertz MI. Paramyxovirus infection in lung transplant recipients. *J Heart Lung Transplant* 1995;14:479–485.
161. Mauch TJ, Crouch NA, Freese DK, et al. Antibody response of pediatric solid organ transplant recipients to immunization against influenza virus. *J Pediatr* 1995;127:957–960.
162. Miller R, Naftel DC, Bourg RC, et al. Infection after heart transplantation: a multi-institutional study. *J Heart Lung Transplant* 1994;13: 381–393.
163. Singh N, Gayowski T, Wagener MM, et al. Bloodstream infections in liver transplant recipients receiving tacrolimus (FK506): changing pattern of microbial origin. *Clin Transplantation* 1997;11:275–281.
164. Wade JJ, Rolando N, Hallar K, et al. Bacterial and fungal infections after liver transplantation: an analysis of 284 patients. *Hepatology* 1995;21:1328–1366.
165. Lumbreras C, Fernandez I, Velosa J, et al. Infectious complications following pancreatic transplantation: incidence, microbiological, clinical characteristics and outcome. *Clin Infect Dis* 1995;20:514–520.
166. Paterson DL, Dominguez E, Chang FY, et al. Infective endocarditis in solid organ transplant recipients. *Clin Infect Dis* 1998;26:689–694.
167. Paterson DL, Rihs JD, Squier C, et al. Lack of efficacy of mupirocin in the prevention of with *Staphylococcus aureus* in liver liver transplant recipients and candidates. *Transplantation* 2003;75:194–198.
168. Patel R, Badley AD, Larson-Keller J, et al. Relevance and risk factors of enterococcal bacteremia following liver transplantation. *Transplantation* 1996;61:1192–1197.
169. Newell KA, Millis JM, Arnow PM, et al. Incidence and outcome of infection by vancomycin-resistant *Enterococcus* following orthotopic liver transplantation. *Transplantation* 1998;65:439–442.
170. Linden PK, Pasculle AW, Manez R, et al. Differences in outcome for patients with bacteremia due to vancomycin-resistant *Enterococcus faecium* or vancomycin susceptible *E. faecium. Clin Infect Dis* 1996; 22:663–670.
171. Kusne S, Molmenti E, Krystofiak S, et al. Risk factors associated with vancomycin resistant *Enterococcus faecium* (VREF) bacteremia in liver transplant recipients (Abstract J-37). Thirty-seventh Interscience Conference on Antimicrobial Agents and Chemotherapy, Toronto, Canada, 1997.
172. Papanicolaou GA, Myers BR, Meyers J, et al. Nosocomial infections with vancomycin-resistant *Enterococcus faecium in* liver transplant recipients: risk factors for acquisition and mortality. *Clin Infect Dis* 1996;23:760–766.
173. Chia JKS, Nakata M, Park SS, et al. Use of bacitracin therapy for infection due to vancomycin-resistant *Enterococcus faecium. Clin Infect Dis* 1995;21:1520.
174. Aguado JM, Herrero JA, Gavalda J, et al. Clinical presentation and outcome of tuberculosis in kidney, liver, and heart transplant recipients in Spain. *Transplantation* 1997;63:1278–1286.

175. Ridgeway AL, Warner GS, Phillips P, et al. Transmission of mycobacterium tuberculosis to recipients of single lung transplants from the same donor. *Am J Respir Crit Care Med* 1996;153:1166–1168.
176. Kiuchi T, Tanaka K, Inomata Y, et al. Experience of tacrolimus-based immunosuppression in living-related liver transplantation complicated with graft tuberculosis: interaction with rifampicin and side effects. *Transplant Proc* 1996;28:3171–3172.
177. Singh N, Wagener MM, Gayowski T. Safety and efficacy of isoniazid chemoprophylaxis administered during liver transplant candidacy for the prevention of posttransplant tuberculosis. *Transplantation* 2002; 74:892–895.
178. Chaparro SV, Montoya JG, Keeffe EB, et al. Risk of tuberculosis in tuberculin skin test-positive liver transplant patients. *Clin Infect Dis* 1999;29:207–208.
179. Benito N, Sued O, Moreno A, et al. Diagnosis and treatment of latent tuberculosis infection in liver transplant recipients in an endemic area. *Transplantation* 2002;74:1381–1386.
180. Marrie TJ, Johnson WM, Tyler SD, et al. Genomic stability of *Legionella pneumophila* isolates recovered from two cardiac transplant patients with nosocomial Legionnaires' disease. *J Clin Microbiol* 1994; 3085–3087.
181. Phillips SJ, Zeff RH, Gervick D. Legionnaires' disease. *Ann Thorac Surg* 1987;44:564.
182. Singh N, Muder RR, Yu VL, et al. Legionella infection in liver transplant recipients: implications for management. *Transplantation* 1993; 15:1549–1551.
183. Sahathevan M, Harvey FAH, Forbes G, et al. Epidemiology, bacteriology and control of an outbreak of *Nocardia asteroides* infection on a liver transplant unit. *J Hosp Infect* 1991;18:473–480.
184. Stevens DA, Pier AC, Beaman BL, et al. Laboratory evaluation of an outbreak of nocardiosis in immunocompromised hosts. *Am J Med* 1981;71:928–934.
185. Hellyar AG. Experience with *Nocardia asteroides* in renal transplant recipients. *J Hosp Infect* 1988;12:13–18.
186. Baddour LM, Baselski VS, Herr MJ, et al. Nocardiosis in recipients of renal transplants: evidence for nosocomial acquisition. *Am J Infect Control* 1986;14:214–219.
187. Horvath J, Dummer S, Lloyd J, et al. Infection in the transplanted and native lung after single lung transplantation. *Chest* 1993;104: 681–685.
188. Yeldandi V, McCabe MA, Larson R, et al. *Aspergillus* and lung transplantation. *J Heart Lung Transplant* 1995;14:883–890.
189. Westney GE, Kesten S, De Hoyos A, et al. *Aspergillus* infection in single and double lung transplant recipients. *Transplantation* 1996; 61:915–919.
190. Paradowski LJ. Saprophytic fungal infections and lung transplantation—revisited. *J Heart Lung Transplant* 1997;16:524–531.
191. Husni R, Gordon S, Quereshi M, et al. Risk factors for invasive aspergillosis in lung transplant recipients (abstract 33). In program and abstracts of 34th annual meeting of the Infectious Diseases Society of American. New Orleans, 1996.
192. Kanj SS, Tapson V, Davis D, et al. Infections in patients with cystic fibrosis following lung transplantation. *Chest* 1997;112:924–930.
193. Castaldo P, Stratta RJ, Wood RP, et al. Clinical spectrum of fungal infections after orthotopic liver transplantation. *Arch Surg* 1991;126: 149–156.
194. Briegel J, Forst H, Spill B, et al. Risk factors for systemic fungal infections in liver transplant recipients. *Eur J Clin Microbiol Infect Dis* 1995;14:375–382.
195. Singh N, Arnow PM, Bonham A, et al. Invasive aspergillosis in liver transplant recipients in the 1990s. *Transplantation* 1997;64:716–720.
196. Collins LA, Samore MH, Roberts MS, et al. Risk factors for invasive fungal infections complicating orthotopic liver transplantation. *J Infect Dis* 1994;170:644–652.
197. Kusne S, Torre-Cisneros J, Manez R, et al. Factors associated with invasive lung aspergillosis and significance of positive cultures after liver transplantation. *J Infect Dis* 1992;166:1379.
198. Munoz P, Torre J, Bouza E, et al. Invasive aspergillosis in transplant recipients. A large multicentric study. In: Program and abstracts of the 36th Interscience Conference on Antimicrobial Agents and Chemotherapy (New Orleans). Washington DC: American Society for Microbiology, 1996.
199. Faggian G, Livi U, Bortolotti U, et al. Itraconazole therapy for acute invasive pulmonary aspergillosis in heart transplantation. *Transplant Proc* 1989;21:2506–2507.
200. Rabito FJ, Pankey GA. Infections in orthotopic heart transplant patients at the Ochsner Medical Institutions. *Med Clin North Am* 1992; 76:1125–1134.
201. Podzimkova M, Gebauerova M, Malek I, et al. Infectious complications in patients after heart transplantation. *Cor et Vasa* 1993;35: 263–266.
202. Brown RS Jr, Lake JR, Katzman BA, et al. Incidence and significance of *Aspergillus* cultures following liver and kidney transplantation. *Transplantation* 1996;61:666–669.
203. Cofan F, Inigo P, Ricart MJ, et al. Invasive aspergillosis following kidney and kidney-pancreas transplantation. *Nefrologia* 1996;16: 253–260.
204. Paterson DL. Invasive aspergillosis. In: Yu VL, Merrigan T, eds. *Antimicrobial therapy and vaccines.* Baltimore: Williams & Wilkins, 1998.
205. Verweij PE, Dompeling EC, Donnelly JP, et al. Serial monitoring of *Aspergillus* antigen in the early diagnosis of invasive aspergillosis. Preliminary investigations with two examples. *Infection* 1997;25: 86–89.
206. Swanink CMA, Meis JFGM, Rijs AJMM, et al. Specificity of a sandwich enzyme-linked immunosorbent assay for detecting *Aspergillus* galactomannan. *J Clin Microbiol* 1997;35:257–260.
207. Heussel CP, Kauczoe HU, Heussel G, et al. Early detection of pneumonia in febrile neutropenic patients: use of thin-section CT. *Radiology* 1997;169:1347–1353.
208. Singh N, Mieles L, Yu VL, et al. Invasive aspergillosis in liver transplant recipients: association with candidemia, consumption coagulopathy, and failure of prophylaxis with low-dose amphotericin B. *Clin Infect Dis* 1993;17:906–908.
209. Reichenspurner H, Gamberg P, Nitschke M, et al. Significant reduction in the number of fungal infections after lung, heart-lung, and heart transplantation using aerosolized amphotericin B prophylaxis. *Transplant Proc* 1997;29:627–628.
210. Tollemar J, Ericzon BG, Barkhold L, et al. Risk factors for deep candida infections in liver transplant recipients. *Transplant Proc* 1990; 22:1826–1827.
211. Patel R, Portelar D, Bradley AD, et al. *Candida* and non-*Candida* fungal infections after liver transplantation. *Transplantation* 1996;62: 926–934.
212. Lumbreras C, Cuervas-Mons V, Jara P, et al. Randomized trial of fluconazole versus nystatin for the prophylaxis of Candida infection after liver transplantation. *J Infect Dis* 1996;174:583–588.
213. Fortun J, Lopez-San Roman A, Velasco JJ, et al. Susceptibility of *Candida glabrata* strains with reduced susceptibility of azoles in four liver transplant patients with invasive candidiasis. *Eur J Clin Microbiol Infect Dis* 1997;16:314–318.
214. Bensousan T, Garo B, Islam S, et al. Possible transfer of *Pneumocystis carinii* between kidney transplant recipients [Letter]. *Lancet* 1990; 336:1066–1067.
215. Branten AJ, Beckers PJ, Tiggeler RG, et al. *Pneumocystis carinii* pneumonia in renal transplant recipients. *Nephrol Dial Transplant* 1995; 10:1194–1197.
216. Chave JP, David S, Wauters JP, et al. Transmission of *Pneumocystis carinii* from AIDS patients to other immunosuppressed patients: a cluster of *Pneumocystis carinii* pneumonia in renal transplant recipients. *AIDS* 1991;5:927–932.
217. Hennequin C, Page B, Roux P, et al. Outbreak of *Pneumocystis carinii* pneumonia in a renal transplant unit. *Eur J Clin Microbiol Infect Dis* 1995;14:122–126.
218. Gryzan S, Paradis IL, Zeevi A, et al. Unexpectedly high incidence of *Pneumocystis carinii* infection after lung-heart transplantation. Implications for lung defense and allograft survival. *Am Rev Respir Dis* 1988;137:1268–1274.
219. Arend SM, Westendorp RGJ, Kroon FP, et al. Rejection treatment

and cytomegalovirus infection as risk factors for *Pneumocystis carinii* pneumonia in renal transplant recipients. *Clin Infect Dis* 1996;22: 920–925.

220. Paterson D, Singh N. Pulmonary mycoses in solid-organ transplant recipients. In: Sarosi GA, Davies SF, eds. *Fungal infections of the lung.* Baltimore: Lippincott Williams & Wilkins, 2000:239–269.
221. LaRosa S, Gordon S, Kalmadi S, et al. Should prophylaxis for *Pneumocystis carinii* pneumonia (PCP) in solid organ transplant recipients ever be discontinued? (abstract 230) Thirty-fourth annual meeting of the Infectious Diseases Society of America, New Orleans, 1996.
222. Singh N, Gayowski T, Wagener MM, et al. Clinical spectrum of invasive cryptococcosis in liver transplant recipients receiving tacrolimus. *Clin Transplant* 1997;11:66–70.
223. Davies SF, Sarosi GA, Peterson PK. Disseminated histoplasmosis in renal transplant recipients. *Am J Surg* 1979;137:686–691.
224. Wheat LJ, Smith EJ, Sathapatayavongs B, et al. Histoplasmosis in renal allograft recipients. Two large urban outbreaks. *Arch Intern Med* 1983;143:703–707.
225. Wong SY, Allen DM. Transmission of disseminated histoplasmosis via cadaveric renal transplantation: case report. *Clin Infect Dis* 1992; 14:232–234.
226. Hall KA, Sethi GK, Rosado LJ, et al. Coccidioidomycosis and heart transplantation. *J Heart Lung Transplant* 1993;188:491–497.
227. Cohen IM, Galgiani JN, Potter D, et al. Coccidioidomycosis in renal replacement therapy. *Arch Intern Med* 1982;142:489–494.
228. Holt CD, Winston DJ, Kubak B, et al. Coccidioidomycosis in liver transplant patients. *J Infect Dis* 1997;24:216–221.
229. Vartivarian SE, Coudron PE, Markowitz SM. Disseminated coccidioidomycosis. Unusual manifestations in a cardiac transplantation patient. *Am J Med* 1987;83:949–952.
230. Butka BJ, Bennett SR, Johnson AC. Disseminated inoculation blastomycosis in a renal transplant recipient. *Am Rev Respir Dis* 1984;130: 1180–1183.
231. Singh N, Gayowski T, Yu VL. Invasive gastrointestinal zygomycosis in a liver transplant recipient: case report and review of zygomycosis in solid-organ transplant recipients. *Clin Infect Dis* 1995;20:617–620.
232. Luft BJ, Noat Y, Araujo GG, et al. Primary and reactivated *Toxoplasma* infection in patients with cardiac transplants. *Ann Intern Med* 1983; 99:27–33.
233. Shepp DH, Hackman RC, Conley FK, et al. *Toxoplasma gondii* reactivation identified by detection of parasitemia in tissue culture. *Ann Intern Med* 1985;103:218–221.
234. Singh N, Gayowski T, Wagener MM, et al. Pulmonary infiltrates in liver transplant recipients in the intensive care unit. *Transplantation* 1999;67:1138–1144.
235. Paterson DL, Singh N, Gayowski T, et al. Pulmonary nodules in liver transplant recipients. *Medicine* 1998;77:50–58.
236. Wagener MM, Yu VL. Bacteremia in transplant recipients: a prospective study of demographics, etiologic agents, risk factors, and outcomes. *Am J Infect Control* 1992;20:239–247.
237. Bonham CA, Dominguez EA, Fukui MB, et al. Central nervous system lesions in liver transplant recipients: prospective assessment of indications for biopsy and implications for management. *Transplantation* 1998;66:1596–1604.
238. Selby R, Ramirez CB, Singh R, et al. Brain abscess in solid organ transplant recipients receiving cyclosporine-based immunosuppression. *Arch Surg* 1997;132:304–310.

60

INFECTION CONTROL AND PREVENTION IN HEMATOPOIETIC STEM CELL TRANSPLANT PATIENTS

SARA E. COSGROVE
TRISH M. PERL

Bone marrow or hematopoietic stem cell transplantation (HSCT) is a lifesaving therapy for many malignancies and genetic or acquired hematologic syndromes. Worldwide, over 17,000 allogeneic and 30,000 autologous HSCT were performed in 1997 (1). Bone marrow transplantation or HSCT involves the intravenous infusion of hematopoietic stem cells in an attempt to reconstitute the function of the bone marrow. This procedure is used in the treatment of numerous conditions that can be broadly classified into nonmalignant and malignant disorders of marrow function, and malignancies that require high doses of systemic chemotherapeutic agents (2). HSCT is standard therapy for the following nonmalignant conditions: congenital forms of anemia, such as thalassemia, sickle-cell disease, and Diamond-Blackfan anemia; glycogen storage diseases, such as Gaucher's disease; X-linked adrenoleukodystrophy; and diseases that affect immunologic function, such as severe-combined immunodeficiency and Wiskott-Aldrich syndrome. The above indications for HSCT are most common in children, although aplastic anemia is a common nonmalignant indication for HSCT in adults. Although the efficacy of HSCT for nonmalignant disease has not been studied in randomized, clinical trials, in many of these conditions the improved disease-free survival makes HSCT an attractive and at times lifesaving therapy (2).

HSCT is currently employed to treat hematologic malignancies as either a primary treatment, as in acute leukemias, or as a salvage therapy for Hodgkin's disease. Because prolonged marrow aplasia is usually the major dose-limiting toxicity in solid organ tumor chemotherapy, HSCT has been employed to rescue the marrow following chemotherapy. This technique has been used most commonly to treat aggressive or metastatic malignancies such as breast and testicular cancers. In many conditions including acute leukemia, chronic lymphocytic leukemia, Hodgkin's and non-Hodgkin's lymphoma, testicular cancer, and neuroblastoma, HSCT is widely accepted by physicians as standard therapy (2).

The selection of the appropriate HSCT modality depends on the indication for transplant. Treatment of intrinsic bone marrow disorders requires that a nondefective marrow from another individual must be substituted for the diseased one (2). This is known as allogeneic HSCT transplantation. The most serious complication of allogeneic transplantation is graft-versus-host disease (GVHD), which occurs when immunologically competent cells target antigens on the recipient's cells (3,4). The potential immunologic phenomena that accompany foreign cell transplantation are minimized by closely matching the human leukocyte antigen (HLA) of the donor and recipient (2,5).

Recently, some centers have started to perform nonmyeloablative, allogeneic stem cell transplants, which are also known as "minitransplants" or "transplant lite" (6). In these procedures, patients undergo less aggressive chemotherapy or immune-suppressive therapy prior to allogeneic transplant that does not result in complete ablation of the bone marrow (7). The potential advantages of this modality include a decrease in chemotherapy-related toxicities such as mucositis and end-organ toxicity, a theoretic decrease in GVHD, and the ability to treat older or sicker patients. Nonmyeloablative allogeneic stem cell transplants have been used in patients with several disorders including acute leukemias, Hodgkin's and non-Hodgkin's lymphoma, chronic myelogenous leukemia, and multiple myeloma; however, no prospective, randomized, controlled trials have been performed to compare this modality with traditional allogeneic stem cell transplants.

Autologous HSCT transplantation is used to treat conditions in which the patient's own marrow function is normal, such as most solid organ malignancies and lymphomas. Here the recipient serves as his own donor, and bone marrow stem cells are collected prior to treatment for the underlying disease. The most serious complication is relapse of the underlying disease. Thus, the utility of this modality is limited if the bone marrow has been invaded by malignant cells. Techniques to eliminate malignant cells from the recovered marrow, known as purging, have been introduced (2). In addition, although autologous transplantation eliminates the risk of GVHD, the ability to recover sufficient numbers of stem cells to repopulate the marrow limits the ages at which autologous HSCT can be performed.

In the past, bone marrow stem cells were obtained directly from the marrow space by repeated aspiration from the iliac crest. More recently, techniques have been developed to collect stem cells circulating in the peripheral blood. This procedure, peripheral blood stem cell transfer, is more comfortable for the donor and appears to provide more rapid engraftment and, in some studies, higher disease-free survival in the recipient (2). The two terms, *HSCT* and *peripheral blood stem cell transfer,* are used interchangeably in this chapter.

The clinical and physiologic responses and potential complications are similar for patients undergoing HSCT, irrespective of the modality employed. Prior to transplantation, the recipient's own marrow is removed to allow the engraftment of new bone marrow (2). The patients receive a conditioning regimen that usually includes high-dose chemotherapy and total body radiation. This regime purges the patient's existing bone marrow. For example, to clear the bone marrow of diseased cells in a patient with an underlying malignancy, high-dose chemotherapy is directed against the malignancy in question. After the conditioning regimen is completed, the new marrow or graft is infused. At this point, the host is usually granulocytopenic and the peripheral neutrophil count has reached its nadir. The patient remains granulocytopenic and profoundly immunosuppressed until the donated or reinfused stem cells engraft. The time to engraftment depends on a number of factors and usually takes 2 to 3 weeks. Recovery of marrow function is accompanied by a progressive restoration of immunologic competence. In patients undergoing allogeneic HSCT, the process of conditioning and reinfusion of stem cells is similar. However, to minimize the immunologically mediated complications such as GVHD, these patients require additional immunosuppression, such as cyclosporine, corticosteroids, and antithymocyte globulin, or other therapies (2–4,8,9).

The most overwhelming complication of HSCT is profound immunosuppression. Hence, infectious complications are the most common cause of morbidity and mortality among patients undergoing HSCT. Other frequently encountered complications are worthy of mention, because they may alter the recovery of immune function or may be confused with infectious processes. GVHD associated with allogeneic HSCT represents an immunologic response of the graft cells against the host tissues. Some degree of GVHD develops after every allogeneic HSCT and is desirable, because it produces a graft-versus-tumor effect, which results in lower relapse rates (3,4). GVHD occurs in acute or chronic forms and primarily affects the skin, liver, and gastrointestinal tract.

If the transplant is complicated by GVHD, the immune system's recovery is slowed. The graft itself may be depleted of T lymphocytes prior to transplantation to reduce the severity of the subsequent GVHD (2). T-cell depletion increases the risk of a second important complication, that of graft rejection. Graft rejection occurs when residual immunologically active host cells are present because of sensitization from previous blood products and less intensive conditioning regimens. Hence, the primary strategy employed to decrease the risk of rejection has been maximally immunosuppressive conditioning regimens (8). The treatment of GVDH and rejection induces further immunosuppression and decreased antibody and cell-mediated immune responses and may further destroy mucosal surfaces (10). Within the first month following transplantation, patients may experience severe respiratory distress caused by interstitial pneumonia that may be idiopathic in nature and can be associated with diffuse alveolar hemorrhage (11–15). Finally, veno-occlusive disease of the liver can complicate both allogeneic and autologous HSCT (2). This phenomenon, caused by damage to hepatocytes and terminal hepatic venules, may occur in up to 10% to 20% of patients and can mimic a variety of infections (8,16, 17). Veno-occlusive disease usually occurs in the first 30 days after transplantation and is manifested by jaundice, tender hepatomegaly, and ascites, and in severe cases may be associated with progressive hepatic failure and the hepatorenal syndrome. Highly intensive preparatory regimens, grafts from HLA-mismatched donors, and elevated transaminases predispose to veno-occlusive disease (8,16).

PATHOGENESIS AND RISK FACTORS FOR INFECTION

Risk factors for infection among HSCT recipients are multiple but can be classified as endogenous factors, which are those related to the host and the underlying disease, and exogenous factors, which are those related to therapy and the environment. These factors are related, and the contribution of each is difficult to differentiate. The risks of infection and the types of infections vary. Risk can be divided into three periods. The pretransplant period extends from the initiation of the conditioning regimen to the infusion of the transplant. The preengraftment period extends from the infusion of the stem cells to engraftment, heralded by the recovery of the patient's white blood cell count. The postengraftment period can be further divided into the early phase, from engraftment to 100 days posttransplant, and the late phase, from 100 days to approximately 6 months after transplant (10,16). During the pretransplant and pre-engraftment periods, up to 71% of transplant recipients develop documented infections, some of which are fatal (18–20).

Additional risk factors for infection are related to the duration of underlying illness, the type of transplant, presence of renal failure, the degree of histocompatibility mismatch, ABO incompatibility, T-lymphocyte manipulation (depletion), and the presence of viral and fungal infections before the transplant (16,21, 22). Engels et al. (23) found that 55% of patients receiving allogeneic HSCT and 30% of patients with autologous HSCT developed infections during the early phase of HSCT ($p < .01$). Kirk et al. (19) reviewed the early infectious complications in 35 autologous HSCT recipients and found that male gender, total body irradiation, low pretransplant albumin, and mucositis or diarrhea were independent predictors of decreased survival. Age may be an important risk factor for infection, as advancing age considerably increases the risk of GVHD in allogeneic transplantation, and therefore the risk of infection (2,24). In addition, older patients restore their immune systems more slowly.

The role of the patients' underlying illness, hospitalization, and the processes of care are inextricably entangled and each clearly contributes to the patients' risk of developing an infection. In 1969, Johanson et al. (25) published an elegant study that showed that the oropharynx of normal subjects and patients admitted to a psychiatric service were rarely colonized with gram-negative flora. However, 16% of patients with moderate illness and 57% of moribund patients had gram-negative bacilli cultured from the oropharynx. In both groups, the percent of patients colonized with oral gram-negative microorganisms increased proportionally 3 days and 1 week after admission. Not surprisingly, Kramer et al. (26) found that patients with leukemia and lymphoma, with relapsed disease, undergoing chemotherapy, and with granulocytopenia were most likely to develop gram-negative bacteremia and to succumb to infection.

Environment

Among the other sources of potentially colonizing or infecting microorganisms, several hospital sources should be considered. Free-living microorganisms, such as *Pseudomonas* species normally colonize fresh fruits and vegetables and flowers and plants; institutional water sources are potential sources of microorganisms such as *Pseudomonas* species, *Legionella* species, and saprophytic mycobacteria (27–30). Among the most commonly suspected sources of microorganisms and mechanisms of transmission are the fingers and hands of healthcare workers. Schimpff et al. (31) found that 43 of 126 (34%) healthcare workers caring for leukemic patients had gram-negative microorganisms or *Staphylococcus aureus* on their hands (31). Once contaminated, hands may transmit microorganisms to patients. Hands can become contaminated by lotions or by contaminated soaps (32). For example, 12 of 25 (48%) HSCT recipients admitted to a HSCT unit between August and October 1993 became infected or colonized with *Paecilomyces lilacinus* (33). Nine patients (36%) had documented *P. lilacinus* infections. The cause of the outbreak was traced to a contaminated, pharmaceutically prepared skin lotion. Likewise, other agents used in the care of such patients can become contaminated. One dramatic outbreak was reported in which seven of eight patients developed *Pseudomonas aeruginosa* bacteremia serotype 01 (34). Three of five patients without bacteremia were colonized with the outbreak strain. The outbreak strain was also isolated from mouthwash used by the patients, from water, and from two sinks.

The environment including air and water can be a source of infecting microorganisms in these patients particularly for *Aspergillus* species and *Legionella* species. Heating and air conditioning systems can aerosolize the former microorganisms and present a particularly efficient means of spreading *Aspergillus* species. Legionnaires' disease is acquired by inhalation or aspiration of water contaminated by *Legionella* species (35). Aerosols have been generated from cooling towers, air conditioners, and respiratory therapy equipment (36,37). One outbreak of *Stenotrophomonas maltophilia* infections among allogeneic HSCT was linked to a single room on the unit. No source was found, although other outbreaks suggest water may be a source (38, 39). Other epidemiologically important microorganisms that can contaminate hospital water and ice machines include nontuberculous mycobacteria, *P. aeruginosa*, and *Aeromonas hydrophila* (40–42).

In contrast, infections caused by *Aspergillus flavus* and *Aspergillus fumigatus* are related to dispersion of mold via dust. Arnow et al. (43) demonstrated that the mean concentration of *A. fumigatus* and *A. flavus* spores in the air correlated with the incidence of invasive aspergillosis. When the *Aspergillus* concentrations were 0.02 colony-forming units (CFU)/m^3 of air, the incidence of invasive *Aspergillus* infections among high-risk patients was 0.3%. However, when the *Aspergillus* concentrations rose to 1.1 to 2.2 CFU/m^3 of air, the incidence of *Aspergillus* infections among high-risk patients rose to 1.2%. It is not known what concentration is necessary to cause disease, as Rhame et al. (44) reported that 5.4% of HSCT patients developed invasive *Aspergillus* infections when the mean concentration of *A. fumigatus* was 0.9 CFU/m^3 (44). In contrast, Sherertz et al. (45) did not identify cases of invasive aspergillosis when 0.0009 CFU/m^3 of *Aspergillus* was measured in air samples. Thio et al. (46) note that air samples obtained on units that house high-risk patients must be obtained using appropriate high volume samples. We discuss the additional role of these microorganisms below (see Prevention and Control Strategies; see also Chapter 89).

The profound immunosuppression among these patients raises the possibility of acquiring potentially pathogenic microorganisms from sources that are of little concern in other hosts, such as uncooked foods and water. By the time the patient returns home, the immune system has been partially reconstituted, but environmental sources remain a potential problem with sources similar to those found in the hospital setting. The season of the year is a consideration with respect to viral infections. Contact with infected visitors and staff, many of whom may be asymptomatic, is the major risk factor for infection with these viruses.

Pretransplantation Host Risks

The risk of infection during this phase is approximately 12%, with most infections caused by gram-negative bacilli (16). One half of all infectious complications occur in the first 4 to 6 weeks following infusion of bone marrow (18). From the outset, the underlying disease for which the patient is receiving the transplant is likely to be associated with immune function impairment. Chronic lymphocytic leukemia and multiple myeloma are associated with deficient humoral immunity. Hence, these patients frequently have impaired responses to vaccines and immunizations. The patients' overall state of health is often neglected, especially the patients' nutritional status (47). Thus, the patients enter the transplant setting with a predisposition to infection from either their underlying illness or any previous treatments received (16,24).

Furthermore, normal host barriers are frequently compromised in several ways; foremost is the requirement for prolonged central venous access. In addition, urinary catheters may be placed for long periods of time. Medications given to prevent adverse events can alter the normal bacterial flora. For example, cimetidine used to prevent gastritis affects the bacterial flora (48). After treatment with cimetidine, patients had increased bacterial counts and nitrate reducing gram-negative bacteria in the gastric juice. Other investigators have found that chlorhexidine mouthwash may allow gram-negative bacilli to emerge (49). Finally, patients suffer from mucositis induced by the conditioning regimens (50,51). The mucositis creates breaches in the normal mucosal barrier of the oropharynx and gut, thereby allowing bacteria to translocate (52). Up to 50% of patients develop oral mucositis, of which a portion is caused by oral herpes simplex infections (19,23). Schimpff et al. (31) studied 48 patients with acute myelogenous leukemia. Based on serial surveillance cultures and cultures from normally sterile body sites obtained over 2 years, these investigators found that most infections developed from the patients' endogenous flora; 47% of patients became colonized with nosocomially acquired microorganisms. Ultimately, 39/43 (91%) patients who developed bacteremia were colonized with the implicated microorganism prior to developing bloodstream infection (31).

Pre-Engraftment Host Risks

During this early period after HSCT, almost 100% of patients develop a fever higher than 38°C, and 35% to 45% of patients develop infections associated with these fevers (19,20, 23). One group estimated that the overall infection rate during this early period after HSCT was 18 infections per 1,000 patient days (23). The first infection appears a median of 6 days after the transplant (20), although 10% of the infections occurred in the pretransplant period. During this early period, up to 30% of patients develop a bloodstream infection, another 30% develop a catheter-related infection, and 12% develop *Clostridium difficile* diarrhea (20,23). Pneumonia, sinusitis, perirectal abscesses, and diverticulitis occur less frequently (20,23).

HSCT induces profound suppression of the immune system by a variety of mechanisms (2). The agents employed and the intensity of the conditioning regimen produce a profound effect on immune function. For example, the antineoplastic agents used in the conditioning regimens induce lymphocyte and macrophage dysfunction and some, such as cladribine and fludarabine, are potently lymphocytic and induce prolonged $CD4^+$ suppression. Suppression occurs of both the innate and acquired immune systems. Innate immunity is disrupted early in HSCT manifested primarily by the profound neutropenia that occurs in the immediate posttransplant period and that coincides with the period when the patient's natural barriers to infection are most likely to be breached (16). As well as being decreased in numbers, the neutrophils are functionally impaired and display decreased chemotaxis (16). In addition, the risk of developing an infection relates to both the duration and depth of the neutropenia. The risk of infection increases when the absolute neutrophil count (ANC) drops below 1,000 mm^3 and increases sharply when the ANC falls below 500 mm^3 (53). Bodey et al. (53) showed that the risk of serious infections increased from 5 per 100 admissions when the ANC was above 500 cells/mm^3 to 43 infections per 100 admissions when the ANC was below 500 cells/mm^3.

ANCs approaching zero in HSCT patients for the first 2 weeks following transplantation is a common finding (10). Most patients recover white blood cell counts to above 1,000/mm^3 by the 20th to 30th day after transplant (54). The rate of recovery appears to be independent of the quantity of stem cells infused. Even after the neutrophil count recovers and the mucositis resolves, defects in cellular and humoral immunity persist for up to 1 year after transplant (16). Indeed, these immune system abnormalities may persist forever, particularly in the case of allogeneic HSCT requiring continued immunosuppressive drugs (16). Furthermore, defects in neutrophil chemotaxis have been demonstrated among patients with GVHD.

Granulocytopenia allows for otherwise minor localized infections to disseminate. Patients who are neutropenic are at increased risk of developing infections from normal flora of the skin, and urogenital and alimentary tracts (31). Prolonged neutropenia, beyond 2 weeks' duration, however, predisposes to more severe infections, which may in part be due to the selective pressure of antibiotic therapy received earlier in the course of the neutropenia. Later neutropenic infections include those due to highly resistant bacteria, such as *stenotrophomonas maltophilia,* and those due to fungi for which the host is dependent on neutrophil function for their elimination; the most important fungi are *Candida* species and *Aspergillus* species. Recovery from the latter rarely occurs prior to the recovery of the neutrophil count to normal levels.

Postengraftment Host Risks

Several factors influence the degree of immunosuppression experienced after HSCT following recovery of neutrophil function. In allogeneic HSCT the presence of GVHD greatly increases the risk of infection by prolonging the impairment in cellular immunity (55). Ironically the drugs used to treat GVHD produce a similar pattern of immunosuppression. Cyclosporine blocks T-cell activation and corticosteroids block both T- and B-cell function and cause impaired wound healing.

The rates of immune recovery vary, but innate immunity recovers before acquired immunity, accounting in part for the time periods in which different types of infection occur. After resolution of the neutropenia, defects in acquired immunity become apparent as the spectrum of infections switches to include those ordinarily prevented by intact humoral and cellular immunity. Both allogeneic and autologous HSCT are associated with quantitative decreases in lymphocyte counts (56). Furthermore, $CD8^+$ suppressor cell populations recover sooner than the $CD4^+$ helper cells (16). Thus, although the absolute lymphocyte count recovers to normal by the second month posttransplant, cellular immunity remains impaired by an abnormal $CD8^+/CD4^+$ ratio for at least a year after transplantation (56). Complex cellular immune functions, such as the purified protein derivative skin test, can remain absent for over a year after transplantation. In contrast, B-cell functions are reasonably maintained, but antibody production is impaired by defective T-helper cell function. Thus, immunoglobulin G (IgG) levels recover to normal levels within 3 months of transplantation; however, immunoglobulin A (IgA) levels are suppressed for up to a year and responses to vaccination are poor. Furthermore, patients receiving allogeneic HSCT have a high incidence of bloodstream infections even in the absence of neutropenia, and a significant proportion of these episodes are not clearly associated with well-known risk factors such as GVHD or central venous catheters (57).

INCIDENCE AND PREVALENCE OF HEALTHCARE-ASSOCIATED INFECTIONS

The incidence and prevalence of healthcare-associated infections among patients undergoing HSCT has not been well studied. In an early study, 12% of patients hospitalized in an oncology center developed a nosocomial infection (58). The highest incidence of nosocomial infections occurred among patients with acute myelogenous leukemia—30.5 per 1,000 patient days (58). Among patients with acute lymphocytic leukemia, non-Hodgkin's lymphoma, Hodgkin's disease, and breast cancer, the rates reported were 16.7, 13.4, 5.4, and 3.3 per 1,000 patient days, respectively. Carlisle et al. (59) performed prospective surveillance over a 42-month period among neutropenic patients with leukemia and solid organ malignancies, of whom 8% had undergone a HSCT. These authors described 444 infections that were identified among 920 patients during 9,582 days of neutropenia. Overall, 48.3 infections occurred per 100 neutropenic patients (46.3 infections per 1,000 days of risk). The rates of site-specific nosocomial infections per 100 neutropenic patients were 13.5 for bloodstream infections, 5.7 for urinary tract infections, 5.5 for respiratory tract infections, and 3.4 each for skin and gastrointestinal infections. In 88% of infections, pathogens were identified; 35% of pathogens were classified as gram-positive cocci, 27% as gram-negative bacilli, 18% as *Candida* species, 9% as gram-positive bacilli, 6% as viruses, and 4% as *Aspergillus.*

Velasco et al. (60) reported rates of nosocomial infections among patients in an oncology intensive care unit (ICU). They used the National Nosocomial Infections Surveillance (NNIS) system ICU definitions to define infections between 1993 and 1995. Overall, 370 infections were identified among 623 patients and 4,034 patient days. The overall infection rate was 50.0 per 100 patients or 91.7 per 1,000 patient days. Pneumonia was the most common, constituting 28.5% of the nosocomial infections. The urinary tract and bloodstream were the primary sites 25.6% and 24.1% of the time, respectively. Importantly, these authors also reported device-specific rates. The median device specific utilization ratios were 0.63, 0.83, and 0.86 for ventilators, indwelling urinary catheters, and central venous catheters, respectively. This study demonstrated that nosocomial infections correlated significantly with device utilization ($p < .01$), underlying severity of illness ($p < .01$), and average length of ICU stay ($p < .01$). Although the highest device-specific rate was associated with ventilators (41.7/100 ventilator days), the number of catheter days was most strongly correlated with nosocomial infections.

Infections that occur more than 3 months after HSCT have not been well studied. Hoyle and Goldman (61) canvassed 18 of 22 centers performing HSCT in the United Kingdom to determine the prevalence of infections that developed at least 3 months after transplant (61). Six percent of HSCT recipients were readmitted for a serious infection. The most common microorganisms causing serious infections included cytomegalovirus (CMV), *Pneumocystis carinii, Streptococcus pneumoniae, Pseudomonas* species, and *Aspergillus* species. Other groups have shown that 6 months or more after HSCT, recipients remain at an increased risk of *S. pneumoniae* infections and *Pseudomonas* pneumonia (62,63). These studies help us understand the epidemiology of infections among patients who undergo HSCT. However, they only include traditional, inpatient, acute-care settings and do not specifically examine the incidence of nosocomial infections among HSCT recipients. New studies are needed to determine the risk of nosocomial infection among recipients of HSCTs and should bridge the inpatient/outpatient care model that is being adopted by many HSCT centers.

SPECIFIC MICROORGANISMS

Microorganisms are epidemiologically important in this group of patients. We review in detail only those microorganisms that require infection control interventions or have implications for healthcare workers or the environment. Although the risk of developing a blood-borne infection (HIV; hepatitis A, B, C, D, E, G, and H; malaria; Chagas' disease; etc.) is high in this population, we do not cover this subject. An extensive discussion can be found in Chapter 69. Certain infections characteristically occur at different time periods following HSCT (Fig. 60.1). This pattern, however, has been evolving through changes in the management of HSCT patients, such as the use of prophylactic antibiotics and antiviral agents.

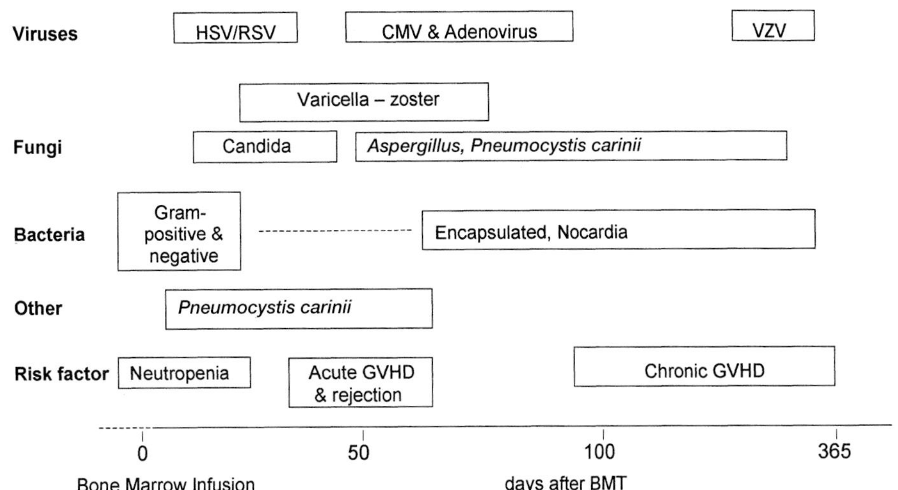

Figure 60.1. Timeline for infectious complications in hematopoietic stem cell transplantation (HSTC) recipients.

Infections in the early posttransplant period are usually due to the host's own flora, colonizing the skin and urogenital and alimentary tracts. The hospital environment, however, alters the profile of microorganisms that colonize individual patients. Owing to the liberal use of broad-spectrum antibiotics in HSCT units, acquisition of highly resistant microorganisms, such as vancomycin-resistant *Enterococcus* (VRE) and *S. maltophilia,* is particularly common. The profound immunosuppression allows these patients to acquire potentially pathogenic microorganisms from sources that are of little concern in other hosts, such as uncooked foods and water. Free-living microorganisms, such as *Pseudomonas* species, normally colonize fresh fruits and vegetables and plants; institutional water sources are potential sources of microorganisms such as *Pseudomonas* species, *Legionella* species, and saprophytic mycobacteria (27). Heating and air conditioning systems can aerosolize the former microorganisms and present a particularly efficient means of spreading microorganisms, such as *Aspergillus* species. Similarly, construction and renovation in and around healthcare institutions have been associated with *Aspergillus* and *Legionella* infections. By the time the patient returns home, the immune system has been partially reconstituted, but environmental sources remain potential problems in ways similar to the hospital setting. During the neutropenic phase immediately following transplantation, pathogens whose removal is dependent on phagocytic function predominate. The earliest of these to occur are infections produced by pyogenic bacteria. It is estimated that 60% of febrile episodes in neutropenic patients are accompanied by bacteremia, but there have been important shifts in the microorganisms responsible for these infections (64). In the 1970s, gram-negative septicemia often caused by *P. aeruginosa, Escherichia coli, Enterobacter cloacae,* and *Klebsiella* species resulted in high mortality of febrile neutropenic patients (65,66). Driven by the extensive use of prophylactic and empiric antibiotic regimens active against gram-negative microorganisms, gram-positive microorganisms have now emerged as the most common pathogens (67). Gram-positive microorganisms now account for 60% of bacteremias in HSCT centers (67,68). Most of these infections are caused by *Staphylococcus epidermidis* and other coagulase-negative staphylococci. Wade et al. (67) found that the incidence of *S. epidermidis* infections increased from 2.0 per 1,000 patient days in 1972 to 14.6 per 1,000 patient days in 1979. More recent prophylactic regimens have led to the emergence of fluoroquinolone resistant gram-negative rods and fungus. Increased use of long-term indwelling venous catheters has also been implicated in the increase in gram-positive infections (67,68). Streptococci, in particular α-hemolytic strains, commonly found in the oral flora have been recovered with increasing frequency owing to the poorer activity of fluoroquinolones against these microorganisms (23). One investigator reported that streptococci cause 71% of bloodstream infections in children undergoing HSCT (69). Likewise, Heimdahl et al. (52) showed that oral microorganisms, particularly α-hemolytic streptococci, caused 24 of 59 infections that occurred in neutropenic patients early after HSCT.

Furthermore, many gram-positive bacteremias, especially those due to *S. epidermidis,* now occur after engraftment (70). Overall, however, the mortality from bacterial infections has decreased with the introduction of aggressive, early therapy directed against gram-negative microorganisms (70). Infections with these microorganisms can still have serious outcomes. In these hosts, Martin et al. (71) found that coagulase-negative staphylococcal bacteremia had an attributable mortality of 13.6%. This elegant study controlled for the severity of underlying disease and was one of the first to highlight the impact of these microorganisms. Investigators have also reported increased mortality in patients with bacteremia due to a viridans species of *Streptococcus* (72). One group studied a cohort of 289 HSCT recipients and noted the mortality associated with gram-positive bacteremia was 27% versus 15% ($p <.02$) in patients with bacteremia caused by other microorganisms (72). Interestingly, gram-positive bacteremia contributed to only five of 52 deaths. One patient with *Streptococcus viridans* bacteremia died from septic shock.

Bacterial Infections

Clostridium difficile

Clostridium difficile is an anaerobic gram-positive rod that produces two toxins, both capable of damaging the mucosa of the colon and leading to pseudomembranous colitis (73). *C. difficile* was first identified as a cause of antibiotic-associated colitis in 1978; it has now become the most common cause of nosocomial diarrhea and inflammatory colitis. *C. difficile* can colonize the gastrointestinal tract, or cause severe diarrhea, pseudomembranous colitis, toxic megacolon, colonic perforation, and even death (73–78). The diagnosis of *C. difficile* disease is discussed in Chapter 36.

Patients who develop *C. difficile*–associated diarrhea have altered intestinal flora related to the use of antibiotics, enemas, and intestinal stimulants (73,79,80). Importantly, broad-spectrum antibiotics commonly used for empiric chemotherapy for neutropenic fevers and prophylaxis against opportunistic infections are associated with *C. difficile* colonization and infections (73, 81–83). In addition, antineoplastic chemotherapeutic agents, especially methotrexate, increase the risk of *C. difficile* infections (84). Gerard et al. (81) recovered *C. difficile* and/or its toxin in 13 of 37 (35%) of hospitalized cancer patients on oral antibiotics and in 15/119 (13%) of other patients ($p <.005$) (81). Up to 30% of patients treated with antibiotics develop diarrhea, and in 20% to 25% of cases of antibiotic-associated diarrhea *C. difficile* is cultured from stool (79,80). The risk of acquisition increases as the patients' length of hospital stay increases, and more than 20% of adults are colonized after a hospitalization of 1 week (73,85). Clabots et al. (86,87) found the rate of acquisition proportionate to the length of hospital stay; 13% of patients hospitalized for 1 to 2 weeks were colonized and 50% of those hospitalized for more than 4 weeks were colonized. In addition, patients who have been recently exposed to a healthcare institution are at increased risk of *C. difficile* colonization and diarrhea (88). *C. difficile* colonization may be a marker for VRE colonization in patients with hematologic malignancies and HSCT (89).

Hence, recipients of HSCT are at high risk of developing *C. difficile* diarrhea. The incidence of acute diarrhea after HSCT is 40% to 50% among adults and up to 83% among children (90,91). Cox et al. (90) found that pathogens accounted for only 13% of the diarrhea, whereas acute GVHD accounted for 48%. No etiology was identified in 39% of diarrheal episodes.

Among patients with infections, the most common infecting microorganisms identified were viruses (12/126 patients—astrovirus and adenovirus) and *C. difficile* (7/126 patients). Other investigators found that microorganisms could be identified in up to 40% of episodes (92). Of the 31 patients where a pathogen was identified, 12 (39%) had adenovirus, 12 (39%) had *C. difficile*, and nine (29%) had rotavirus. More importantly, the mortality rate was 55% among patients with a pathogen isolated and only 13% among those patients who did not develop infectious diarrhea ($p < .0001$). Likewise, Blakey et al. (91) identified the cause of diarrhea in children undergoing HSCT. Enteric pathogens caused diarrhea 52% of the time; 14% of cases of diarrhea were caused by *C. difficile*. Interestingly, other clostridial species including cytotoxin-negative *C. difficile* and *C. innocuum* were excreted in 90% of diarrheal episodes when no enteric pathogen was identified. One study suggests that *C. difficile*–associated diarrhea may be more common among HSCT recipients than previous studies suggest (81,93). Gerard et al. (81) recovered *C. difficile* in 13 of 28 (46%) of cancer patients with diarrhea; seven of 28 (25%) patients were treated for *C. difficile* diarrhea. Yuen et al. (93) prospectively studied HSCT recipients and found that *C. difficile* was the most common microorganism recovered from the diarrheal stools. Among these patients, mortality was no different among patients with and without *C. difficile* isolated from stools.

Nosocomial outbreaks of *C. difficile* have been well documented, including outbreaks in HSCT units (74,75,80, 94–101). Contaminated environmental surfaces are an important and underrecognized reservoir of *C. difficile* spores, and serve as a source of the microorganism from which it can be transmitted to other patients (75,77,102,103). These spores can remain viable on surfaces of inanimate objects for months. *C. difficile* is transmitted directly from patient to patient via the hands of healthcare workers or indirectly through contaminated equipment such as bedpans, urinals, call bells, and contaminated environmental surfaces such as bed rails, floors, and toilet seats (73–75,77,102,103). Outbreak management should include aggressive environmental cleaning and disinfection with a Food and Drug Administration (FDA)-approved or Environmental Protection Agency (EPA)-registered sterilant, use of contact precautions, and minimization of antibiotic use (see also Chapter 36). The use of lyophilized *Saccharomyces boulardii* to reduce diarrhea is not recommended because of the risk of development of fungemia with the microorganism (104).

Legionella Species

Since the first documented legionellosis outbreak in Philadelphia involving American Legion convention delegates in 1976, numerous epidemic and sporadic cases have been reported in the literature (105). The role of *Legionella* as a cause of nosocomial pneumonia is well recognized (106,107). Initially, nosocomial *Legionella* infections were reported in tertiary care centers that housed immunosuppressed patients (105). Outbreaks pointed to HSCT patients as high-risk patients with significant morbidity and mortality of 40% to 50% (105,108–110). Marston et al. (111) found that patients with hematologic malignancies were 22.4 times [95% confidence interval (CI) 19.0–25.9] more likely to die than nonimmunocompromised hosts. These patients are at particular risk of developing a *Legionella* infection because they are neutropenic for long periods of time and have defects in cell-mediated immunity (112). The incidence of healthcare-associated *Legionella* pneumonia among HSCT recipients varies. Several factors contribute to the incidence: (a) the concentration of *Legionella* in the hospital's water supply; (b) the weather and rainfall; (c) the monitoring and treatment strategy for the water supply; and (d) the availability of adequate diagnostic tests (culture, direct fluorescent antigen, and urinary antigen) (108,113–119). Among the 40 *Legionella* species, *Legionella pneumophila* is the most pathogenic, accounting for about 90% of the cases. Furthermore, of more than 14 identified serogroups of *L. pneumophila,* serogroup 1 accounts for more than 80% of the reported cases (111). *L. pneumophila* in the hospital water distribution system has been epidemiologically linked to nosocomially acquired Legionnaires' disease (37,105,109,115, 116,120–123).

Legionnaire's disease is acquired by inhalation of water aerosols or aspiration of water contaminated by *Legionella* (35,124, 125). Aerosols have been generated from cooling towers, air conditioners, humidifiers, evaporative condensers, respiratory therapy equipment, and whirlpool baths (36,37,116,126–136). Other investigators suggest that nasogastric tubes increase the risk of legionellosis presumably by facilitating microaspiration (137,138). The clinical presentation of *Legionella* infection is similar to that in other patients with fever, headache, myalgias, diarrhea, cough, and pneumonia (120). Respiratory insufficiency, sepsis, and multisystem organ failure lead to death (106, 107).

Legionella infection should be considered in any HSCT patient with pneumonia, and appropriate testing for the agent should occur in all cases. Methods for detection of *Legionella* include culture, direct fluorescent antibody testing of bronchoalveolar lavage washings, and urine testing for *L. pneumophila* serogroup 1 antigen. Outbreaks of *L. pneumophila* serogroup 3 and nonpneumophila species in HSCT transplant units emphasize the importance of not relying only on urine testing for diagnosis (123,139).

Surveillance for cases of healthcare-associated *Legionella* should be performed routinely in HSCT patients (104,140). Cases that occur in patients who have been continuously hospitalized for ≥10 days before the onset of illness are considered definite nosocomial cases, and cases that occur 2 to 9 days after admission are considered possible nosocomial cases (104). Appropriate reporting to the hospital epidemiologist or infection control professional (ICP) and the health department should occur in response to a suspected nosocomial case. Hospital epidemiology will initiate an investigation and implement prevention and control measures (see Chapter 35). Additional prevention and control strategies are discussed below (see Prevention and Control Strategies).

Listeria monocytogenes

Listeria monocytogenes is a gram-positive rod that causes serious infections among immunocompromised hosts including those receiving HSCT (141–143). The incidence of listeriosis is 0.39 cases per 100 HSCT (141). Some authors have argued that prophylactic use of antibiotics may prevent these infections, although no studies have been performed. Most commonly the disease presents either as a central nervous system infection or a primary bloodstream infection (141–143). The disease usually presents with fever, headache, and in immunocompromised hosts occasionally nuchal rigidity (26%), vomiting (29%), and diarrhea (19%), or abdominal pain (13%) (143). Depressed consciousness has been reported in up to 42% of patients (143). Recurrent meningitis occurred in two of the patients studied. Mortality, if undiagnosed, can be high. Foods, usually undercooked, containing *Listeria* species are thought to be the source of infection.

Mycobacterium tuberculosis and Nontuberculous Mycobacteria

The frequency of occurrence of *M. tuberculosis* infection in HSCT patients ranges from 0.2% to 5.5% in published studies and is directly related to the incidence of tuberculosis in the general population of the area (144). Most cases reported in the literature are pulmonary infections presenting with fever, cough, and infiltrates on chest radiograph. Other involved sites include the central nervous system, musculoskeletal system, and oral cavity, and these patients may develop multiorgan dissemination (144). Symptom onset is rare during neutropenia, but one quarter of reported cases occur before day 100 (145). The diagnosis of tuberculosis can be challenging, with only a few patients having sputum showing acid-fast bacilli on smear; therefore, therapy should be initiated in suspected cases while culture results are pending. Risk factors for developing tuberculosis included allogeneic transplant [$p < .05$, relative risk (RR) = 23.7], total body irradiation ($p < .05$, RR = 4.9), and chronic GVHD ($p < .05$, RR = 3.6) (146).

Nontuberculous mycobacterial infections have also been described in HSCT patients, with the majority being catheter-related infections caused by rapidly growing mycobacteria such as *Mycobacterium chelonae* and *Mycobacterium fortuitum* (147–149). The diagnosis of respiratory tract disease caused by nontuberculous mycobacteria can be challenging and should be guided by published recommendations (150) (see also Chapters 37 and 38).

Vancomycin-Resistant Enterococcus

Resistance to the glycopeptide antimicrobials vancomycin and teicoplanin in enterococci was first reported in Europe in 1986 and in the United States in 1989. Vancomycin-resistant enterococci (VRE) have become a significant problem in many oncology and HSCT units. The percentage of nosocomial enterococcal isolates that were resistant to vancomycin reported by U.S. ICUs to the NNIS system increased from 0.3% in 1989 to 26.3% in 2000 (151). Jones et al. (152) studied 480 nosocomial enterococcal bloodstream infections from 41 U.S. medical centers and reported that vancomycin resistance occurred in 10% to 20% of all these bloodstream infections.

Risk factors for VRE colonization and infection include host characteristics, hospital factors, and antimicrobial use. Higher severity of illness and the resulting increased length of hospitalization are highly associated with colonization and infection with VRE. A higher incidence of VRE is found in immunocompromised patients such as recipients of an organ or HSCT and patients with neutropenia, hematologic malignancies, renal insufficiency, diabetes, or acquired immune deficiency syndrome (AIDS) (89,153–155). The presence of diabetes, acute renal failure, gastrointestinal procedures, mucositis, and positive *C. difficile* toxin assays has been associated with subsequent development of VRE bacteremia in patients hospitalized on oncology wards (89,156–158). The latter three risk factors suggest that the disruption of the gastrointestinal mucosa of patients colonized with VRE facilitates the translocation of VRE into the bloodstream.

Hospital factors that predict colonization and infection with VRE include location in a high-risk area such as the ICU or oncology unit, length of hospitalization, number of individual contacts with VRE carriers, and overall proportion of patients colonized with VRE on a unit (153,159–161). VRE can be transmitted by person-to-person spread or from the contaminated environment. Most hospital transmission occurs via the contaminated hands of healthcare workers. VRE survives on hands for at least 60 minutes after inoculation and are recovered on the hands in 10% to 43% of workers caring for VRE-colonized patients (162,163). In addition, case-control studies have shown that exposure to a healthcare worker caring for a VRE-infected or -colonized patient increases the risk of acquiring VRE (164). VRE can survive for long periods (up to 7 days) on dry surfaces and is recovered in 7% to 30% of environmental surfaces cultured during outbreaks of VRE (162,165,166). Environmental contamination increases twofold when patients have diarrhea or are colonized in multiple body sites (166,167). VRE outbreaks have been linked to many fomites including contaminated electronic thermometers and ear oxymeters (168,169).

The relationship between antibiotic exposure and colonization and infection with VRE has been extensively studied. The most consistently recognized antimicrobials associated with the acquisition of VRE colonization or infection are vancomycin, extended-spectrum cephalosporins, and antianaerobic agents (160,170–173). Both the total amount of antimicrobials and the therapy are also risk factors for VRE (161). There is a consistent epidemiologic association between previous use of oral vancomycin and subsequent development of VRE colonization, which is likely related to selection pressure in the gastrointestinal tract, leading to the recommendation that oral vancomycin not be used routinely in the therapy of *C. difficile* colitis (161). The relationship between intravenous vancomycin therapy and VRE colonization and infection is more controversial. Although several studies have noted an association between vancomycin and VRE, others have not found an effect (155,167,170–172, 174–179). A meta-analysis from Carmeli et al. (179) showed that the increased risk of VRE acquisition with exposure to vancomycin on crude analysis did not persist in studies that adjusted for length of stay and that used control patients who were VRE negative. Although vancomycin therapy likely does not cause VRE to develop or increase the chance that a patient will acquire VRE, it likely exerts selective pressure in the gastrointestinal tract and increases the burden of preexisting VRE to a detectable level

(161). Consequently, the prudent use of vancomycin in patients at high risk for VRE, particularly HSCT patients, is highly recommended.

Extended spectrum cephalosporins and antianaerobic drugs have also been strongly associated with VRE (155,178,180). Among HSCT patients, Edmond et al. (155) reported that patients who received metronidazole or imipenem were 2.5 times more likely to develop a VRE bloodstream infection. One group was able to reduce the VRE acquisition rate on a leukemia unit by substituting piperacillin-tazobactam for ceftazidime as therapy for febrile neutropenia with no change in vancomycin use (181). The theoretical mechanism of this observation is that extended spectrum penicillins have some activity against enterococci whereas cephalosporins do not, allowing for some reduction of VRE overgrowth in the gastrointestinal tract (161). Although some oncology centers have moved toward the use of extended spectrum penicillins rather than cephalosporins as a means to reduce rates of VRE colonization and infection, further investigation is required in this area.

VRE colonization may persist for up to 1 year (182). Among 253 immunocompromised patients, Lai et al. (183) found 70% of patients were persistent fecal carriers for up to 303 days (median = 41). Of the 49 patients whose later stool cultures no longer grew VRE, four patients became recolonized. Beezhold et al. (184) found that all patients with VRE bloodstream infections were colonized either in the gastrointestinal tract (100%) or on the skin (86%). In fact, VRE colonization may increase the risk of VRE infection by tenfold (185).

The impact of these infections cannot be underestimated in this population. VRE bacteremia is also unequivocally associated with increased mortality in HSCT patients. In a well-designed historical cohort study of 27 leukemic patients with VRE bacteremia, Edmond et al. (160) reported a mortality of 67%, compared to a 30% mortality in closely matched controls without VRE bacteremia. Several studies suggest that VRE infections not only increase hospital length of stay, but also consequently inflate the cost of care to both the hospital and the patient (154,160).

Methicillin-Resistant Staphylococcus aureus (MRSA)

Resistance to methicillin among *S. aureus* was first noted in 1961, the first year that methicillin was available. Since the late 1980s, rates of MRSA in the hospital setting have continued to increase; 55% of nosocomial infections in U.S. ICU patients are due to MRSA, representing a 29% increase in the incidence of MRSA infections over a 4-year period (151). Among HSCT patients, *S. aureus* is a significant pathogen, particularly as a cause of catheter-related bloodstream infection (186). Risk factors for the acquisition of MRSA include previous or prolonged hospitalization, advanced age, recent surgery, enteral feedings, and open skin lesions (187–189). MRSA is transmitted primarily on the hands of healthcare workers; thus, hand hygiene coupled with contact precautions form the backbone of the prevention of transmission of MRSA. One study suggests that the environment and common items in the environment may play a more important role than previously recognized (190). Many centers perform surveillance cultures of the anterior nares at the time of admission and weekly to facilitate the early identification of patients with MRSA. This strategy facilitates the identification and rapid isolation of patients who could be colonized with the microorganism. Given that many of these patients have been previously hospitalized and exposed to antibiotics, we favor such a strategy. Data do not exist at this point to recommend decolonization of this high-risk population, although decolonization strategies have been successful in patients with intravenous catheters (191). Patients with recurrent MRSA infections may benefit from topical nasal treatment with 2% mupirocin calcium ointment. Some investigators recommend the use of chlorhexidine baths with this strategy (192).

Fungal and Mold Infections

A dramatic increase in opportunistic fungal and mold infections has occurred over the last 10 years. *Candida* species is the fourth most frequent isolate recovered from blood cultures in the U.S. (193,194). The Centers for Disease Control and Prevention (CDC) reported an increase in the rate of nosocomial fungal infections from 2.0 to 3.8 per 1,000 discharges (193). Patients housed in oncology units had the second highest rate of nosocomial fungal infections with seven infections per 1,000 discharges (193). In the HSCT population, the increase in invasive fungal infections is largely due to a rise in *Aspergillus* infections (195).

Aspergillus Species

Aspergillus species are thermotolerant fungi that cause significant disease in HSCT recipients. These fungi are ubiquitous, found in soil, water, and decaying material, and produce conidia that are inhaled, leading to colonization and infection in human hosts (196). The most common species causing infection in HSCT patients is *A. fumigatus,* although investigators have observed an increase in non-*fumigatus* species of *Aspergillus* such as *A. niger, A. flavus,* and *A. terreus* over the past few years (197,198). *Aspergillus* species most commonly cause sinusitis and pneumonia, but can disseminate to other organs including the skin and the brain; they are the most common cause of brain abscess in HSCT patients (199–205). Infections occur following a bimodal distribution with an early and a late peak that correlate first with neutropenia and then GVHD and corticosteroid use (206). Baddley et al. (197) reported that the median time to onset of infection at their institution was 102 days, and most infections occurred after post-HSCT day 60. Another group reported that *Aspergillus* is the most common cause of community-acquired pneumonia in allogeneic HSCT patients with GVHD at their institution; 83% of HSCT patients admitted to the hospital for pneumonia were diagnosed with pulmonary aspergillosis (207).

Aspergillus occurs in 4.5% to 28% of HSCT recipients (207). The incidence of this disease is dependent on a number of patient and institutional factors including the conditioning process used during transplantation, type of transplant, the severity of GVHD that develops, corticosteroid use, age and underlying diseases of the patient, the institution's heating and air conditioning system, the presence of construction and renovation, and the season. Wingard et al. (208) found that patients with autologous HSCT developed *Aspergillus* infections while neutropenic and prior to engraftment, whereas allogeneic HSCT patients were significantly more likely to manifest an *Aspergillus* infection after engraftment. The increased incidence of invasive mold infection may also be related to new transplantation modalities such as $CD34^+$-selected autologous peripheral-blood stem cells; further investigations are underway in this area (195). Several authors have shown that acute GVHD and graft rejection increase the risk of aspergillosis (45,208–210). Baddley et al. (197) have suggested that GVHD is a marker for glucocorticosteroid use, which was the only predictor of invasive mold infection in a multivariable analysis of a cohort of 94 adult patients. Prolonged neutropenia has also been shown to increase the risk of aspergillosis (211,212). Finally, many investigators have hypothesized that the widespread and efficacious use of fluconazole for prophylaxis of *Candida* species has contributed to the increase in invasive mold infections that has been noted in the past decade (198,213).

The environment clearly has an impact on whether patients develop disease. Construction and/or renovation and suboptimal maintenance, cleaning, and protection of the environment have been the most important causes of *Aspergillus* infection. Multiple outbreaks reported in the literature have illustrated the risks associated with these activities (Table 60.1) (30,45,46,201, 214–232). Patients housed outside of a high-efficiency particulate air (HEPA) filtered laminar airflow environment are at a tenfold higher risk for developing nosocomial *Aspergillus* infection (45). The use of HEPA filtration with laminar airflow for HSCT recipients can reduce the magnitude of risk for acquiring nosocomial *Aspergillus* infections and is discussed below (see Prevention and Control Strategies).

Diagnosis of *Aspergillus* infection can be challenging. A consensus committee has recently published diagnostic criteria for opportunistic invasive fungal infections to facilitate clinical and epidemiologic research (233). The three categories of disease are proven infection, defined as the recovery of mold from a sterile site or a biopsy specimen showing mold by culture or pathologic examination and a compatible clinical and radiographic presentation; probable infection, defined as recovery of mold from a contiguous, nonsterile site with consistent radiographic and clinical evidence of mold infection; and possible infection, defined as recovery of mold from a nonsterile site or radiographic or clinical evidence of infection (197,233). These definitions are for research and surveillance purposes and should not be used for making clinical decisions. Although tissue biopsy and histologic confirmation of disease is the preferred method of making a clinical diagnosis of *Aspergillus* infection, HSCT patients who have respiratory specimens that grow *Aspergillus* species should be presumed to have invasive disease and should be treated aggressively with an appropriate agent (104,209). Newer diagnostic modalities such as latex agglutination tests, enzyme linked immunosorbent assays, and polymerase chain reaction (PCR) that detect circulating *Aspergillus* antigens have been developed that may allow for earlier detection of invasive disease (234, 235). The purpose of these tests is to provide evidence of invasive aspergillosis prior to detection by chest imaging or clinical symptoms with the intent of initiating treatment earlier.

Infections caused by this microorganism are devastating, with attributable mortality rates ranging from 80% to 95% which have remained relatively constant over the past decade (196–198,236,237). One study of 28 patients who underwent allogeneic HSCT found several factors associated with increased mortality including GVHD status ($p <.0008$) and cumulative prednisone dose the week before the *Aspergillus* infection was diagnosed ($p <.0001$) (210). These authors developed a risk model for mortality and found patients with GVHD who received more than 7 mg/kg of prednisone had a 100% mortality.

Although prophylactic regimens to prevent *Aspergillus* infection have been studied, no approach has been found to be effective in preventing disease. These regimens have included low to moderate dose amphotericin B, aerosolized and intranasal amphotericin B, and lipid formulations of amphotericin B. Consequently, guidelines published by the CDC do not recommend prophylaxis at this time (104). In addition, the guidelines advise against the use of itraconazole capsules as prophylaxis because of poor absorption and kinetics as well as the high frequency of drug interactions with the agent (104).

Candida Species

Twenty-two percent to 25% of HSCT recipients develop *Candida* species infections (18,238–240). *Candida* infections generally occur in the early posttransplant period with a mean time to onset of 2 weeks. The pathogenesis of candidiasis has been proposed to be suppression of normal bacterial flora by antimicrobials, with subsequent overgrowth of yeast in the gastrointestinal tract (241,242). Yeast disseminate via breaks in the mucosal surfaces associated with mucositis or by colonizing long-term intravascular catheters. One study demonstrated that prior use of a Hickman catheter and being colonized at other sites increased the odds of developing candidemia seven- and tenfold, respectively (243).

Risk factors for fungal infection include advanced age, prolonged neutropenia, delayed engraftment, cytotoxic chemotherapy, the use of broad-spectrum antibiotics, the use of steroids, length of hospitalization, presence of GVHD, concomitant CMV disease, and transplantation for acute leukemia (244–246). The intensity of immunosuppression following the initial period of neutropenia provides an additional risk factor for fungal disease. Prospective studies among patients admitted to a medical intensive care unit and an HSCT unit found that risk factors for acquisition of *C. glabrata* included prolonged duration of hospitalization in the unit and prior antimicrobial use (247). Similarly, risk factors for nosocomial acquisition of *C. albicans* include prior antibiotic therapy, length of time spent in the unit, and geographic and temporal links with other patients colonized with these microorganisms (244). Risk factors predicting mortality from *Candida* species include deep fungal infection (RR = 35) and concomitant liver damage due to veno-occlusive disease or GVHD (RR = 7) (248).

The spectrum of fungal disease has changed with widespread use of fluconazole for prophylaxis. Fluconazole (400 mg a day) given from transplant until engraftment has been shown to decrease fungal infections and death from these infections and is now standard practice (249). Prior to the introduction of fluconazole prophylaxis, the mortality attributable to candidemia was 38% (243). *C. albicans* remains the most common

TABLE 60.1. ASPERGILLUS OUTBREAKS AMONG PATIENTS WITH HEMATOLOGIC MALIGNANCY OR (HSCT)

Study	Risk Factors	Site	Cause of Outbreak/Reservoir	No. of Cases	No. of Deaths	Control Measures	Microorganism
Aisner et al. 1976 (215)	Hematologic malignancy Metastatic carcinoma	Pulmonary Sinus	Fireproofing contaminated during construction	8	At least 3	Copper-8-quinonolate	*A. flavus* *A. fumigatus* *A. niger* *Aspergillus* species
Lentino et al. 1982 (216)	Hematologic malignancy Renal transplant recipients	Disseminated	Road construction Window air conditioners	10	6	Not specified	*A. flavus* *A. fumigatus* *A. niger* *Aspergillus* species
Rotstein et al. 1985 (217)	HSCT recipients	Pulmonary Sinus Disseminated	Nebulizer Increased severity of illness	10	10	Not specified	*A. flavus* *A. fumigatus*
Opal et al. 1986 (218)	Hematologic malignancy High-dose corticosteroid therapy Carcinoma	Disseminated	Renovation Construction	11	11	Copper-8-quinonolate to decontaminate work area Airtight barriers HEPA filters in patient rooms Negative pressure in construction area Traffic between construction site and patient areas strictly controlled	*A. flavus* *A. fumigatus* *A. niger* *Aspergillus* species
Allo et al. 1987 (201)	Hematologic malignancy Aplastic anemia	Primary cutaneous *Aspergilius* Disseminated	Contaminated ventilation system in operating room	9	2	Cleaned ventilation system	*A. flavus*
Ruutu et al. 1987 (30)	Hematologic malignancy Bone marrow transplant recipients	Pulmonary Disseminated	Dirty ventilation system	8	6	Cleaned ventilation system Cleaned ventilation ducts and spaces above false ceiling Fittings around HEPA filters resealed Fine filters changed Handles removed from windows Increased speed of ventilation fans	*A. fumigatus*
Perraud et al. 1987 (219)	Hematologic malignancy	Disseminated	Construction/renovation Insulation Blinds	22	18	Not specified	*A. fumigatus*
Sherertz et al. 1987 (45)	HSCT recipients	Disseminated Pulmonary	Not specified	14	Not specified	Laminar airflow HEPA filtration	*A. flavus* *A. fumigatus*
Weems et al. 1987 (220)	Advanced age Renal transplant recipients Hematologic malignancy NICU (colonized cases only)	Disseminated Skin	Major construction with ground site preparation Interior renovation Demolition and modification of HVAC system Excessive dust from: Demolition and contamination of HVAC system Construction traffic	5	At least 4	Windows in patient rooms permanently sealed	*Aspergillus* species *Mucor* species
Barnes et al. 1989 (221)	HSCT recipients	Not specified	Construction	6	6	Laminar airflow	*A. fumigatus*
Hopkins et al. 1989 (222)	Renal transplantation Hematologic malignancy	Pulmonary Disseminated	Construction in central radiology Unfiltered air in construction area	6	2	Renovation completed	*A. fumigatus*
Arnow et al. 1991 (214)	Hematologic malignancy	Pulmonary Disseminated	Inanimate environment	33	Not specified	Filters removed Cleaned gaps Environmental cleaning Inspections of water damage	*A. flavus* *A. fumigatus*

(*continued*)

TABLE 60.1. (*continued*)

Study	Risk Factors	Site	Cause of Outbreak/Reservoir	No. of Cases	No. of Deaths	Control Measures	Microorganism
Flynn et al. 1993 (223)	HSCT recipients Hematologic malignancy Disseminated carcinoma	Pulmonary Disseminated	Renovations two floors below ICU Rerouting of duct work Removal of false ceilings Entry through stairwell/elevator	4 (2) infections (2) colonizations	4	Increased monitoring during outbreak to maintain positive pressure in unit	*A. terreus*
Gerson et al. 1994 (224)	HSCT recipients Hematologic malignancy	Pulmonary Disseminated Sinus Skin	Carpet	13	1	Antimicrobial carpet shampoo Water extraction employed with shampoo	*A. flavus* *A. fumigatus*
Anderson et al. 1996 (225)	Hematologic malignancy Bone marrow transplant recipients	Pulmonary Disseminated	Defective conduit door for trash Contaminated vacuum cleaner	6	At least 1	Vacuum cleaner replaced Duct sealed Itraconazole prophyiaxis	*A. fumigatus* *A. flavus* *A. niger*
Leenders et al. 1996 (226)	Hematologic malignancy	Pulmonary	Not known	5	2	Random amplification of polymorphic DNA analysis Close windows New air handling system maintenance	*A. flavus* *A. fumigatus*
Loo et al. 1996 (227)	Hematologic malignancy Bone marrow transplant recipients	Pulmonary Sinus	Construction	36	17	Portable HEPA filters Copper-8-quinolinolate applied Windows sealed Ceiling tiles replaced Blinds replaced Ventilation system maintained regularly	*A. flavus (8)* *A. fumigatus* *A. niger*
Gaspar et al. 1999 (232)	Hematologic malignancy	Not specified	Construction	11	1	Airtight barriers used to separate construction area from unit Patients moved to another unit	*A. fumigatus*
Lass-Florl et al. 2000 (231)	Hematologic malignancy	Pulmonary Sinus Disseminated	Potted plants on the unit	14	9	Potted plants removed from the unit	*A. terreus*
Thio et al. 2000 (540)	Hematologic malignancy Bone marrow transplant recipients	Disseminated	Construction	29	Not specified	N95 masks wom by patients outside of HEPA filtered areas Floors wet mopped Traffic patterns altered Blinds replaced Outside bricks sealed Pressure adjusted Unit cleaned	*A. flavus*
Oren et al. 2001 (228)	Hematologic malignancy HSCT recipients	Pulmonary	Construction	31/111	8	HEPA filtered unit Amphotericin B IV prophylaxis	*Aspergillus* species
Lai at al. 2001 (230)	Hematologic malignancy Bone marrow transplant recipients	Pulmonary Sinus	Construction	3	2	Unit closed for 2 weeks Air intake duct cleaned Prefilters, filters and HEPA-filtration replaced Carpet replaced with vinyl flooring Unit cleaned Airtight barriers used to separate construction area from unit Amphotericin B IV prophylaxis	*Aspergillus* species *A. flavus* *A. niger* *A. versicolor*
Hahn et al. 2002 (229)	Hematologic malignancy	Pulmonary Sinus	Contaminated wall insulation Construction	10/55	8	HEPA filters placed at intervals in non-BMT wing and at the nursing station Wall insulation decontaminated Floor construction site sealed Itraconazole prophylaxis	*A. flavus*

pathogen isolated in most institutions; however, fluconazole-resistant species, such as *C. glabrata* and *C. krusei,* are a growing problem (193,250). A study of candidemia in Europe evaluated 249 episodes of candidemia in 245 cancer patients and demonstrated an increase in non-*albicans Candida* species; 49% of infections were due to *C. albicans*, but the remaining infections were equally distributed among *C. glabrata* (10%), *C. tropicalis* (11%), *C. parapsilosis* (11%), and other non-*albicans* species (10%) (251). Patients with leukemia and those who had received antifungal prophylaxis were more likely to develop non–*Candida albicans* fungemia. Fluconazole prophylaxis was the single most important risk factor accounting for the increase in *C. krusei* [odds ratio (OR) = 27.07] and *C. glabrata* (OR = 5.08) at one institution (250). The clinical implications of the shift toward non-*albicans* isolates are unclear. One study demonstrated that despite an increase in fluconazole-resistant *C. albicans* and non-*albicans* infections, the attributable mortality rate due to fungemia remained unchanged at 20% since the introduction of fluconazole prophylaxis (246). The authors hypothesize that the decreased mortality may be related to the elimination of more virulent fungal species such as *C. albicans* and *C. tropicalis* during fluconazole therapy.

Nosocomial transmission of *Candida* species has been well documented by molecular typing (252). The major route of transmission is indirect contact between patients by the hands of healthcare workers (244,252,253). In one outbreak of *C. parapsilosis* healthcare workers were implicated, and the outbreak was related to long-term central venous catheters (11,254). The investigators cultured *C. parapsilosis* from the hands of three healthcare workers and found that patients with implantable and semiimplantable central venous catheters were significantly more likely to develop infection (p = .016).

Other Fungal Species

A number of other fungal pathogens, *Trichosporon, Fusarium, Pseudallescheria boydii,* and *Scedosporium prolificans,* are emerging as causes of infection likely due to the increasing intensity of current conditioning regimens, possible selection by extensive use of antifungal agents, and increased awareness of their role as potential pathogens (193,255). These agents, except *Fusarium,* produce spectra of human disease similar to *Aspergillus*. However, the apparent clinical resistance to amphotericin B characterizes these microorganisms (256). All these agents cause infections in patients who are profoundly neutropenic. Although experience is limited, case series report high mortality rates (257). In immunocompromised patients, the mortality rate reaches about 100% despite institution of amphotericin B therapy (258,259).

Fusarium infections in the immunocompromised host disseminate rapidly and produce characteristic skin lesions with central necrosis and an erythematous base that are most often found on the extremities (257,260). *Fusarium* has been reported to cause infection in neutropenic HSCT recipients (261). A recent epidemiologic study showed that *Fusarium* species isolated from the water and from aerosolized water within a hospital were genetically related to isolates from patients infected with *Fusarium* (262). The authors recommend that hospitals with cases of fusariosis consider evaluating the water supply for *Fusarium* species and limiting immunocompromised patients' exposure to tap water.

Trichosporon capitatum has caused septicemia in HSCT patients; in one report, it had been isolated from the stool of three leukemic patients, and all three patients were treated with an azole antifungal compound (263). Lowenthal et al. (264) report a mortality rate of 64% among 42 immunocompromised patients with *Trichosporon cutaneum* infection.

Scedosporium prolificans is a recently recognized agent of bone, soft tissue, and joint infections that occurs with highest frequency in children and young adults and can be fatal in immunocompromised individuals. Pickles et al. (265) reported a hospital-acquired *S. prolificans* infection that did not respond to combinations of surgery, fluconazole, and itraconazole in an immunocompromised patient. The source of these microorganisms is currently debated. Experts argue that the soil, vegetables, and flowers are the source, whereas others provide evidence that contaminated water may be an important reservoir (255). Finally, *Malassezia furfur* and *Malassezia pachydermidis* are lipophilic yeasts that commonly colonize the skin (266). *M. furfur* has usually been described as a cause of catheter-related sepsis in neonates receiving intravenous lipid emulsions in total parenteral nutrition. Barber et al. (266) reported catheter-associated fungemia in seven immunocompromised patients—four adults and three children. Only two of these patients were receiving concurrent intravenous lipid emulsions.

Viral Infections

Viral infections, common among HSCT patients, can be classified as those caused by herpes-family viruses or respiratory viruses.

Respiratory Virus Infection in HSCT Patients

Respiratory virus infections continue to be important problems in HSCT patients. Respiratory syncytial virus (RSV), influenza A and B viruses, parainfluenza virus, picornaviruses, coronavirus, and rhinovirus have been described as agents that affect HSCT patients (267,268). These viruses commonly cause upper respiratory tract infections; however, they often lead to serious lower respiratory tract infections associated with significant morbidity and mortality in the HSCT population. Adenovirus can lead to both respiratory infections and disseminated visceral syndromes (269). Respiratory viruses cause infections in approximately 19% of HSCT patients each season (generally considered to be from November to May in the Northern Hemisphere). Suspicion for respiratory virus infection should be maintained throughout the year, because among viruses, parainfluenza and adenovirus occur year-round. In addition, respiratory viruses are frequent nosocomial pathogens; one group reported that 48% of infections with these agents were acquired within the hospital (267). A study of HSCT patients with respiratory symptoms who had cultures and direct fluorescent antibody examination of nasopharyngeal wash/throat specimens demonstrated that the most common community-acquired respiratory agent was RSV (35%), followed by parainfluenza virus (30%), rhinovirus

(25%), and influenza (11%) (270). Adenovirus was not included in the study because of the difficulty in differentiating new infection from reactivation of latent disease. Patients with radiographic evidence of pneumonia underwent bronchoalveolar lavage; 49% of patients with RSV had pneumonia and 22% of patients with parainfluenza had pneumonia, but pneumonia due to influenza and rhinovirus was uncommon (<10% of patients). In contrast, a more recent study has been reported in which direct immunofluorescence assays were performed on respiratory specimens from 179 patients with HSCT who had 392 episodes of upper respiratory illness (271). Of the 68 (38%) in whom virus was detected, respiratory syncytial virus was detected in 18 patients (26.4%), influenza A or B in 28 (41.2%), and parainfluenza in 7 (10.3%). Fourteen patients (20.6%) had multiple viruses isolated. RSV pneumonia developed in 55.5% of the patients with RSV upper respiratory infections. One of the 15 patients (6.7%) with RSV pneumonia died. Influenza pneumonia was diagnosed in three patients (7.3%). These investigators report a lower mortality than has previously been reported.

Nosocomial transmission has been documented with respiratory viruses, particularly influenza and RSV. Transmission by small particle aerosolization, large droplets, fomites, and contaminated hands is possible; therefore, droplet precautions should be implemented in all patients with upper respiratory tract infection symptoms. Cleaning of the environment is equally important to prevent transmission from contaminated surfaces or fomites. In addition, healthcare workers and family members with these symptoms should not care for or visit patients until symptoms have resolved. Healthcare workers and close contacts of patients should receive an annual influenza vaccination.

Adenovirus

Adenoviruses are nonenveloped, double-stranded DNA viruses 70 to 90 nm in diameter (272). About half of the known serotypes cause human illness (272). In general, type-specific immunity develops after a self-limited, 2-week illness, although latent infection may be established in lymphoid tissue (272). The frequency of acute infection versus reactivation in HSCT patients is unknown. Among HSCT recipients, especially children, the common serotypes that cause disease are 31 in subgroup A; 7, 11, 34, and 35 in subgroup B; 1, 2, 5, and 6 in subgroup C; and 4 in subgroup E (272). One group found that subgroup B serotype 35 was the most prevalent adenovirus strain in their institution, and half of the adult patients infected with this strain had the same serotype recovered from cultures prior to HSCT (273).

Three percent to 20% of HSCT patients develop adenovirus infection, which has many manifestations including upper and lower respiratory tract illness, acute hepatitis, gastrointestinal disease, acute hemorrhagic cystitis, nephritis, conjunctivitis, and central nervous system disease (269,272,274–277). Disseminated adenovirus infection, in which two or more organ systems are involved, also occurs and is associated with a 60% mortality rate (269,277,278). La Rosa et al. (277) examined characteristics of HSCT patients who developed adenovirus infection between 1990 and 1997. The diagnosis was made in 3% of patients and did not have a seasonal variation. Sixty-five percent of cases were diagnosed during the first 100 days posttransplant. Similar numbers of patients had upper respiratory tract illness, enteritis, pneumonia, cystitis, and disseminated disease, and all occurred with similar frequency in patients who underwent allogeneic HSCT compared to autologous HSCT, with the exception of disseminated disease, which was noted only in allogeneic patients. The mortality rate was 26%, with the majority of deaths occurring in patients with pneumonia and disseminated disease. Risk factors for adenovirus infection included receipt of an allogeneic transplant, presence of GVHD, and receipt of concurrent immunosuppressive therapy (277). In addition, others have reported that the incidence of adenovirus is higher in children than adults (279).

The diagnosis of adenovirus infection has traditionally been made by isolation of the virus in culture or by documentation of adenovirus in tissue. PCR is emerging as a promising diagnostic modality that provides a more rapid diagnosis of significant adenovirus infection (280). Unfortunately, there is no established treatment regimen for adenovirus infections; ribavirin and cidofovir have been used for therapy with conflicting results. Because the microorganism can be transmitted from person to person, general infection control practices are important.

Coronavirus

Coronaviruses are a family of single-stranded RNA viruses that cause respiratory disease among humans. Until the 2002–2003 respiratory virus season, two coronavirus strains, OC43 and 229E, were known to cause respiratory disease (281). Patients generally present with mild upper respiratory symptoms, although pneumonia has been described (281,282). Limited data are available about the clinical syndromes among HSCT patients. In a case series of two patients who had received autologous transplants, both developed pneumonia characterized by a dry, nonproductive cough and interstitial infiltrates on radiographs (268). One of the patients survived the infection.

In 2003, severe acute respiratory syndrome was described, which has rejuvenated interest in this virus and the clinical syndromes it causes. Published reports from several cohorts of patients noted a febrile syndrome characterized by cough, myalgias, dyspnea, and occasionally diarrhea with some patients going on to develop respiratory failure. No data have been reported characterizing the spectrum of disease in HSCT patients.

Influenza

Although immunocompromised patients receiving HSCT are considered to be at high risk of acquiring nosocomial influenza, little data are available on resulting pulmonary complications or mortality. Nosocomial outbreaks of influenza often occur during community epidemics and can be explosive among hospitalized high-risk patients. Among HSCT recipients, nosocomial transmission has been documented with the same frequency among neutropenic and nonneutropenic and autologous and allogeneic HSCT recipients (283). Whimbey et al. (283) found that almost one third (29%) of the hospitalized adult HSCT recipients had influenza type A cultured after developing respiratory symptoms. Nosocomial transmission was responsible for 60% of these 68 infections. Seventy-five percent of the cases were complicated by pneumonia and 17% (1/6) of these patients died (see also Chapter 41).

Influenza vaccine should be administered prior to transplantation, because in HSCT patients the response to influenza vaccine is absent for at least 6 months after transplantation (284). Influenza vaccine does not protect patients effectively until 2 years following HSCT. No studies have evaluated the efficacy of chemoprophylaxis or treatment with amantadine, rimantadine, or neuraminidase inhibitors in HSCT patients. Given the morbidity and mortality of this disease in these patients, these agents should be considered for prophylaxis in the event of an influenza exposure or outbreak and for treatment of early influenza as per standard recommendations (285).

Parainfluenza

Parainfluenza virus can cause serious lower respiratory tract disease in both adults and children who undergo HSCT (286). The mortality reported among adult HSCT patients involved in two nosocomial outbreaks of parainfluenza 3 was 33% (287). These outbreaks were caused by introduction of parainfluenza 3 virus strains from a community reservoir into the HSCT population with subsequent person-to-person transmission within the unit (287).

Respiratory Syncytial Virus

Respiratory syncytial virus (RSV) accounts for one third to one half of community-acquired respiratory viral infections among HSCT recipients (267,270). Nosocomial transmission has been well documented, and the risk of nosocomially acquired infection increases during community outbreaks (288). RSV spreads via droplets from respiratory secretions or by contamination of hands or surfaces and subsequent contact with the mucous membranes of the eyes and nose. RSV infection is frequently complicated by pneumonia, and the risk of progression to pneumonia is greater in patients who are pre-engraftment or who had a transplant less than 1 month prior to infection (289). One group of investigators found that 58% (19/33) of the RSV infections in HSCT recipients were complicated by pneumonia, with an associated mortality of 51% (267), and other series have reported mortality rates as high as 80% (289,290). Several observational studies have suggested that aerosolized ribavirin in combination with intravenous immunoglobulin (IVIg) given to patients with RSV involving only the upper respiratory tract may lead to a decrease in the development of pneumonia and subsequent mortality in HSCT patients (291,292). However, no randomized controlled trials have been performed to address the optimal management of RSV infection in HSCT patients (270, 293,294). Prevention of this viral infection like others is the best strategy given the limited therapeutic options and the tremendous morbidity associated with these infections. Comprehensive programs that include surveillance and isolation have been shown to prevent transmission among children (295). A multifaceted infection control strategy is essential in the event of a nosocomial RSV outbreak; prompt identification of cases with active screening, cohorting and isolation of infected patients, screening of staff and visitors for upper respiratory tract symptoms, and staff education have been demonstrated as effective measures in controlling outbreaks on HSCT units (296).

Herpes Viruses Infection in HSCT Patients

Herpes virus infections lead to significant morbidity and mortality in the HSCT population. Although CMV is the most commonly seen herpes virus infection, herpes simplex virus (HSV), varicella-zoster virus (VZV), human herpes virus 6, 7, and 8 (HHV-6, HHV-7, HHV-8), and Epstein-Barr virus (EBV) can all cause disease in HSCT patients. All herpes viruses persist in the host in a latent state; therefore, infection in the HSCT most frequently represents reactivation of latent virus.

Cytomegalovirus

Cytomegalovirus (CMV), a double-stranded DNA herpesvirus, is a major cause of morbidity and mortality among HSCT patients. Asymptomatic infection or symptomatic disease can result from either newly acquired infection from CMV infected bone marrow or blood products or reactivation of previous infection. Risk factors for symptomatic CMV disease in HSCT patients include CMV seropositivity in the HSCT recipient, receipt of CMV seropositive hematopoietic stem cells or blood products by a CMV seronegative recipient, allogeneic HSCT, the development of GVHD, prolonged immunosuppression or lymphopenia following transplantation, and failure of development of a CMV-specific cellular immune response (16, 297–299).

Serious CMV disease most frequently results in interstitial pneumonitis (300). Other manifestations include gastroenteritis, hepatitis, and encephalitis. The overall incidence of developing CMV pneumonia in the first 100 days after transplant is 7% (298). Patients infected with CMV present with nonspecific symptoms such as fever, nonproductive cough, tachypnea, hypoxia, and chest pain (300). CMV is diagnosed usually by identifying CMV in the lower respiratory tract using bronchoalveolar lavage in a patient with signs and symptoms of respiratory disease. Treatment with ganciclovir and IVIg should be started immediately, as delay in initiation of therapy has been associated with increased mortality (301). Despite adequate treatment, mortality from CMV pneumonia remains as high as 20% to 75% (302–305).

A recent review of CMV pneumonia in autologous HSCT recipients at one institution reported that 16 of 795 (2%) autologous HSCT patients developed CMV pneumonitis (306). Patients received HSV prophylaxis with acyclovir from the time of conditioning therapy until engraftment. All patients who developed CMV pneumonia were previously CMV seropositive and all except two had underlying hematologic malignancies. Most cases ($n = 11$) occurred less than 30 days posttransplant, although five cases occurred greater than 100 days posttransplant. Thirty-one percent of patients died. New infection with CMV among CMV-seronegative HSCT patients has dramatically decreased since the use of CMV seronegative or leukocyte-reduced blood products has been implemented. In one study, the rate of exogenous infection was 23% among CMV-seronegative patients getting routine blood products compared to 0% in seronegative patients receiving CMV-seronegative red blood cell and leukocyte-depleted platelets (307). CMV-seronegative blood products are felt to be comparable to filtered leukocyte-reduced blood products with regard to risk of CMV transmission (308). Patients who are seronegative before HSCT should optimally receive hematopoietic stem cells from a seronegative donor. Ljungman et al. (309) showed that patients who were seronegative and had a seronegative donor had a 0% probability of developing CMV disease, whereas seronegative patients with seropositive donors had a 5.4% probability.

Patients who are CMV seropositive at the time of HSCT are at significant risk for developing CMV infection and disease. Historically, 45% to 87% of allogeneic HSCT patients develop CMV infection and 21% to 43% develop disease (300,310). The current standard of care in patients who are seropositive or have received seropositive transplants is to receive prophylactic antiviral therapy or preemptive antiviral therapy after detection of CMV reactivation with diagnostic testing. The rates of CMV disease in HSCT patients are now 5% to 18% (104,299,309). Still, CMV accounts for approximately 15% of the mortality among allogeneic HSCT recipients (311). CMV infection is much less likely to cause serious disease following autologous HSCT (300). The incidence of CMV infection is 45% to 61%; however, only 0.8% to 6.9% of patients develop disease (300). Historically, the majority of CMV infections occur between 30 to 100 days following transplantation, with a median day of onset between the 40th and 50th day (16,300). However, the risk of developing CMV disease later after transplantation appears to be increasing as prophylaxis and preemptive strategies are employed early after HSCT. Nguyen et al. (305) observed that 34 of 541 (6.3%) allogeneic HSCT patients who received ganciclovir prophylaxis until 100 days after the transplant developed CMV pneumonia during the first year after transplant; 74% of episodes occurred after day 100 with a mean occurrence time of 188 days posttransplant. Boeckh et al. (299) studied a cohort of CMV-seropositive allogeneic HSCT patients who received either ganciclovir prophylaxis or ganciclovir therapy, guided by the detection of p65 antigenemia, for 3 months post-HSCT (299). Late CMV disease developed in 26 of 146 (17.8%) patients a median of 169 days after transplant with a range of 96 to 784 days, and the mortality rate was 46%. This trend where CMV infection develops in HSCT cases at longer intervals after the transplant may be related to delayed reconstitution of CMV-specific T-cell immunity in the face of ganciclovir prophylaxis. Patients who are at risk for late CMV infection (allogeneic HSCT patients who have chronic GVHD, steroid use, low CD4 counts, or delay in high avidity anti-CMV antibody, and recipients of matched unrelated or T-cell depleted HSCT) should be screened for evidence of CMV reactivation biweekly (104).

Herpes Simplex Virus

Herpes simplex virus (HSV) infection is an important cause of morbidity in HSCT patients due to the severe mucocutaneous lesions produced by reactivation of latent virus (70). Prior to the routine implementation of prophylaxis, HSV was the most common viral infection seen after HSCT, occurring in up to 80% of seropositive individuals in the first 50 days after HSCT (70,312). Shedding of the virus is most frequent from days 14 through 28 after HSCT (70). In contrast, only 1% of previously seronegative patients excrete the virus. The disease most often involves the oropharynx, but can manifest itself by limited or disseminated cutaneous disease. Less frequently, HSV may produce keratitis, pneumonitis, hepatitis, or encephalitis (70). Importantly, nosocomial transmission of HSV from infected patients to healthcare workers and family members is reported (313,314). Several outbreaks suggest that immunocompromised patients with herpes simplex pneumonia are most likely to transmit the virus (313,314). In one of these studies, molecular typing of strains confirmed that the patients', healthcare workers', and family members' strains were genetically identical (313). An emerging concern is the increasing frequency of HSV strains that are resistant to acyclovir. One study demonstrated that 7% (14/196) of patients undergoing allogeneic HSCT were infected with acyclovir resistant HSV-1; seven cases were also resistant to foscarnet. The major risk factor identified was receipt of a non–geno-identical graft (315) (see Chapter 43).

Human Herpesvirus Types 6 and 7

The scope of disease caused by human herpesvirus types 6 or 7 (HHV-6 or HHV-7) in HSCT patients has yet to be fully elucidated. These viruses are newly recognized; for instance, HHV-6 was first isolated in 1986. Both viruses are frequent causes of febrile infection in children and the etiologic agents of exanthem subitum. Primary infection usually occurs in the first year of life and seroprevalence in adults exceeds 90% (316). Following primary infection, the virus established latency in peripheral blood mononuclear cells as well as salivary glands and neural cells (317). Reactivation of latent virus is felt to be the source of infection in the majority of HSCT patients. Although HHV-6 cannot be cultured from the blood of healthy adults, roughly 40% to 50% of HSCT patients develop HHV-6 viremia 2 to 4 weeks after transplantation (318,319). Patients receiving allogeneic HSCT have been reported to be at higher risk for reactivation of HHV-6 (318). Although most HSCT patients with HHV-6 reactivation are asymptomatic, several studies have demonstrated a correlation between reactivation of HHV-6 and both maculopapular rash and fever following HSCT transplant (318,320–322). Other studies have shown an association between central nervous system symptoms including encephalitis and detection of HHV-6 in cerebrospinal fluid (CSF) (319). Wang et al. (323) examined CSF from 22 allogeneic HSCT patients with central nervous system symptoms and found that 23% (5/22) had detectable HHV-6 DNA and no other potential pathogen identified. In addition, 11 of the 22 patients without detectable HHV-6 had other causes identified that explained central nervous system symptoms. Associations between HHV-6 reactivation in HSCT patients and bone marrow suppression, GVHD, pneumonitis, and CMV disease have also been reported (321,324,325). Nosocomial transmission has not been reported to date. Limited studies have examined HHV-7 infection in these patients. However, in several recent studies it was observed that HHV-7 may act synergistically with CMV infection in transplant recipients (319).

Varicella-Zoster Virus

Varicella-zoster virus (VZV) is the cause of varicella (chicken pox), which represents primary infection, and herpes zoster (shingles), which represents reactivation of latent VZV infection (326). Although varicella is generally a mild disease in children, serious morbidity and mortality are common if infection occurs in immunocompromised patients (327). Among patients developing varicella while receiving chemotherapy for malignancy or immunosuppressive therapy following transplantation, severe disease has been reported in 36% and death in 13% (328,329). In children, 28% not treated with antivirals develop pneumonia (327). The skin lesions may form for up to 2 weeks and crusting may require 3 to 4 weeks (327).

The majority of VZV infections in adults are due to reactivation of latent virus. Although the annual incidence of herpes zoster in normal adults is 0.5%, 13% to 55% of patients undergoing HSCT develop VZV reactivation in the first year after transplant (330). In contrast to HSV infections that usually develop in the first month after HSCT, VZV infections occur a median of 5 months after transplantation (328). Risk factors for reactivation of VZV include chronic GVHD, CD4 lymphocyte count of <200 cells/L, CD8 lymphocyte count of <800 cells/L, and allogeneic transplant (331). Although most patients present with a dermatomal rash, cutaneous dissemination occurs in 6% to 23% of patients, encephalitis occurs in 5% of patients, and visceral involvement is noted in up to 14% of patients (330, 332,333). Visceral involvement most commonly involves the lungs and liver, and abdominal symptoms such as pain, nausea, and vomiting can precede the development of vesicular rash by several days (334). Although antiviral suppression is standard of care for HSV disease, the role of antiviral suppression for the prevention of VZV has not been established in HSCT patients. Although studies have shown that VZV reactivation has been suppressed using oral acyclovir for 6 months after transplant, patients in the studies developed rapid onset of VZV infections after the cessation of therapy (332,335,336). The concerns about development of resistant strains of herpes viruses may outweigh the utility of prophylaxis. Regardless of VZV serologic status, HSCT candidates and recipients should avoid exposure to persons with active VZV infections and to persons who develop a rash after VZV vaccine (104). VZV-seronegative HSCT patients who are exposed to VZV or a vaccinee with a rash and are not immunocompetent should receive VZIG within 96 hours of exposure (104). A recent study by Hata et al. (337) demonstrated that inactivated varicella vaccine given before autologous HSCT and during the first 90 days after significantly reduced the risk of herpes zoster; 33% of unvaccinated patients compared to 13% of vaccinated patients developed zoster. Patients who received the vaccine had earlier development of CD4 T-cell proliferation in response to VZV.

Varicella is extremely contagious, with secondary attack rates of greater than 90% (338,339). The incubation period of varicella ranges from 8 to 21 days, but most patients develop disease between 14 and 16 days after exposure. Patients with varicella become infectious 24 to 48 hours prior to the onset of rash, and viral shedding is prolonged by 2 days in the immunocompromised host (327). Transmission is thought to be due to direct contact with infectious persons. However, based on several outbreaks where patients and/or healthcare workers with no exposure developed varicella, airborne transmission is presumed (340–343). Sawyer et al. (344) used PCR technology to determine whether VZV could be transmitted by aerosol spray. VZV DNA was detected in 64 of 78 (82%) air samples from hospital rooms housing patients with varicella infections and nine of 13 (69%) rooms of patients with herpes zoster. VZV was detected from infected patients' beds for 1 to 6 days following the onset of rash, and on some occasions could be detected outside of the patients' rooms. Interestingly, this study contradicts investigators who suggest fomites are not important in the transmission of VZV (338).

Airborne transmission is suspected to be a primary mechanism of transmission of disease among patients with hematologic malignancy and patients undergoing HSCT (340–343). Leclair et al. (341) described an outbreak of varicella that occurred in a pediatric hospital. Twenty-four of 32 patients hospitalized on an infant ward were exposed and susceptible to varicella. Ultimately 15 (62.5%) patients developed chickenpox after the index case was hospitalized. The patient required mechanical ventilation for varicella pneumonia.

Studies of distribution of air documented increased airflow to those rooms where a higher number of cases occurred. These investigators suggest that increased concentrations of virus and droplets were expelled from the exhaust loop of the ventilator. In a similar instance, Gustafson et al. (343) demonstrated that the risk of children developing varicella was related to how near they came to the index case's room. Eight (11%) exposed children developed varicella. The attack rate was higher for children exposed to the patient early in his disease (8/28; 28.6%). Based on airflow studies, the pressure in all rooms was positive relative to that of the outside corridor. Moreover, 10% of a tracer gas released in the patient's room was measured in corridor air. Furthermore, airborne transmission may occur with herpes zoster that involves more than one dermatome. For instance, an adult patient developed herpes zoster after receiving high-dose steroids, and three nurses developed varicella (342). Two of the three nurses had no contact with the patient (see also Chapter 42).

Other Viruses

Parvovirus

Parvovirus is an uncommon pathogen in the HSCT population, occurring in 1.4% of transplant patients at one institution (345). It has been associated with prolonged anemia and viral shedding in the peritransplant period as well as in patients with chronic GVHD (346–349) (see also Chapter 51).

West Nile Virus

West Nile virus (WNV) is a mosquito-borne flavivirus that is indigenous to Africa, Asia, Australia, and southern Europe

(350). It was first noted in North America in 1999, and the number of yearly cases in the U.S. has continued to increase since that time. It is of concern to caregivers of HSCT patients because of convincing evidence that it can be transmitted by blood transfusion and organ transplantation (351,352). Tests to detect viral nucleic acid within blood products are now available and are being used to assess the blood supply for WNV. In the general population, approximately one in five persons infected with the virus develop a mild febrile illness and only one in 150 develop meningitis or encephalitis (353). However, all of the patients who received organs from a donor who had received blood containing WNV developed clinical WNV; three of the four developed encephalitis and one died, suggesting that the disease is more virulent in immunocompromised hosts (352).

At least two cases of WNV infection are reported in patients who underwent HSCT (354). In both cases the infection was fatal. This population is considered to be at increased risk of infection if they come from areas where WNV is endemic or because they receive blood products. WNV should be suspected in all HSCT patients who have received blood products or have exposure to mosquitoes and present with fevers and neurologic symptoms (355–358). The diverse clinical presentations of WNV neurologic disease include meningoencephalitis, meningitis, flaccid paralysis, ataxia, cranial nerve abnormalities, extrapyramidal signs, myelitis, polyradiculitis, optic neuritis, and seizures. The incubation period is 3 to 14 days, and most patients demonstrate a CSF pleocytosis (353).

Prevention strategies include avoiding exposure to mosquitoes and may include the screening of the blood supply.

Other Pathogens

Other pathogens encountered following HSCT include *P. jiroveci, Nocardia* species, and *Toxoplasma gondii.* All tend to occur later in the posttransplant period, usually between 2 and 6 months, but continued need for immunosuppression and GVHD prolong the period of risk.

Pneumocystis jiroveci

Pneumocystis jiroveci is a fungus that remains an important pathogen among HSCT patients. Prior to the routine use of antimicrobial prophylaxis, *P. jiroveci* pneumonia (PCP) complicated 6.8% to 16% of HSCT and occurred between 40 and 80 days after transplantation (70,359). Since the implementation of prophylaxis, PCP occurs in approximately 2% to 13% of HSCT patients with most cases occurring more than 6 months post-HSCT when prophylaxis is stopped (360,361). Risk factors for PCP include corticosteroid and other immunosuppressant use, relapse, and chronic GVHD, and patients with these risk factors should have prophylaxis continued beyond the standard 6 months. Mortality varies among studies, with rates up to 89% in some reports (362).

Person-to-person transmission of *P. jiroveci* has been proposed based on studies in animal models, geographically and temporally linked clusters of PCP among immunocompromised patients, and rises of *P. jiroveci* antibody titers among persons in contact with patients who have PCP. Vargas et al. (363) reported evidence of nosocomial transmission using a PCR assay. They found that an 8-year-old boy and his contacts (mother, nurse, and physician) had *P. jiroveci* DNA in nasopharyngeal samples. None of the 30 controls having contact less than 5 minutes with the index case had a reactive PCR assay for *P. jiroveci.* Standard precautions are recommended for patients with PCP; however, if evidence of person-to-person spread is suspected or confirmed within a hospital, airborne and contact precautions should be implemented (104).

Nocardia Species

Nocardia species are aerobic actinomycetes that are found in organic matter and soil (364). Nocardial infections are infrequently described in HSCT recipients. Commonly this microorganism produces a focal lung lesion that may cavitate; it frequently disseminates to involve the brain and skin. Disease in this population is commonly associated with a normal white blood cell count (365). Choucino et al. (365) estimate that 0.2% (1 of 554) of autologous HSCT patients and 1.6% (5 of 320) of allogeneic HSCT recipients develop nocardiosis (365). These authors found that the risk of a patient developing nocardial infection was 9.3 times higher among allogeneic HSCT recipients. Among the ten patients studied, these investigators found that all but one had acute or chronic GVHD. Four of the patients had extensive exposure to soil or to organic matter before the nocardial infection developed. Seventy percent of these patients died. Interestingly, three patients developed a nocardial infection despite receiving trimethoprim-sulfamethoxazole (TMP-SMX) prophylaxis. Other investigators also report a high mortality among these patient populations (366–369).

Toxoplasma gondii

Toxoplasma gondii is a protozoan that commonly causes asymptomatic infection in immunocompetent individuals. However, the microorganism can cause life-threatening infection in immunocompromised patients including those undergoing HSCT (370). In these hosts, infection can occur as a new primary infection but most commonly represents reactivation of old disease (95% of cases). Toxoplasmosis most commonly involves the central nervous system, presenting as focal lesions, encephalitis, or rarely, chorioretinitis (370,371). Interstitial pneumonitis and myocarditis also occur in 49% and 17% of cases, respectively (372). In areas of low endemicity, toxoplasmosis occurs in approximately 0.3% of transplants, with higher rates of 2% to 3% seen in France (370,371). Disease most often occurs within the first 6 months after transplant, with a median time to symptom onset of 50 to 64 days (371,372). Risk factors for toxoplasmosis include allogeneic transplant and acute and chronic GVHD; none of the autologous HSCT recipients developed disease in one large series (370).

SITE-SPECIFIC INFECTIONS

Bacteremia and Catheter-Related Infections

Bacteremia or bloodstream infections are reported to be the most common infections in HSCT recipients with an incidence of 38.6% per 100 patients (373). In a longitudinal evaluation 249 episodes of bacteremia occurred over 4 years among 172 patients (373). In this series 81.9% of these infections occurred within 30 days of HSCT, whereas 18% occurred after this time period. The most common microorganisms include coagulase-negative staphylococci and viridans species of *Streptococcus*. These data point to the most common cause of bacteremia, vascular access devices.

Vascular catheters are the most frequently used indwelling devices. Of the approximately 250,000 nosocomial bloodstream infections that occur annually, 30% to 40% occur among patients in hematology-oncology or HSCT units (374,375). Vascular access catheters, frequently implantable catheters, are used in HSCT patients for an extended period of time. However, it is difficult to determine the risk of infection because of variations in the definitions of infection, the time patients are followed, and the types of catheters used. Keung et al. (376) estimated an infection rate of 11.5 per 1,000 catheter-days among 11 HSCT recipients; the rate for bacteremia was 6.7 and the rate for site infection was 4.8. Of the nine catheters removed, eight were removed for infection. In a study of 123 patients who underwent HSCT, 139 double- or triple-lumen catheters were placed and a catheter-related infection occurred in 22 (15.8%); 127 of the 139 catheters were placed percutaneously and remained in place for a mean of 65 ± 55 days (377). Several investigators have noted that HSCT recipients with Hickman catheters are also at risk for catheter-related bloodstream infection, most commonly due to coagulase-negative staphylococcus (298,378). An analysis of 242 HSCT recipients with indwelling Broviac/Hickman catheters who had daily blood cultures drawn showed a catheter-related bloodstream infection rate of 5.28 and an exit site infection rate of 2.59 per 1,000 catheter days. Sixty-five percent of catheter-related infection occurred during neutropenia (186). Although subcutaneous ports are believed to be associated with lower infection rates, no studies have documented this finding in HSCT patients (379).

The CDC has recently developed guidelines for the prevention of catheter-related bloodstream infection, and these should be followed for all HSCT patients with intravascular catheters (375). Recommendations in these guidelines should be followed when long-term catheters are inserted and for their maintenance. Given that many patients are discharged home with indwelling catheters, education regarding prevention of catheter-related infection should be provided to patients and caregivers, including the recommendation that contact with tap water at the catheter site should be avoided (375) (see also Chapters 17, 18, and 19).

Nosocomial Pneumonia

Because of the complications associated with HSCT related to chemotherapy, irradiation, and acute and chronic GVHD, HSCT recipients are susceptible to infections for months after engraftment. Pulmonary complications are seen during the early and late periods after HSCT and are associated with significant morbidity and mortality. The most common early-onset complication is interstitial pneumonitis, occurring in 10% to 40% of patients usually associated with CMV (380,381). Only 20% of pneumonias that occur during the first 100 days after HSCT are caused by bacteria, and these are usually due to gram-negative bacilli (298). Sinopulmonary infections caused by other microorganisms and obstructive airway disease associated with chronic GVHD are among the late-onset problems.

HSCT patients are at a higher risk than general hospital patients for developing nosocomial pneumonia, and 40% to 60% develop adverse pulmonary sequelae (382,383). Pulmonary fungal infections, primarily *Aspergillus* species, may develop in 16% of HSCT patients (196,289,384). Nosocomial pneumonias in immunocompromised hosts can be caused by inhalation of aerosols carrying *Legionella* species or *Aspergillus* species, or as a result of exposure to individuals with RSV or influenza virus. The latter two viruses have emerged as important pathogens in recent years, and outbreaks of nosocomial pneumonia have been documented for both agents (385,386).

Pannuti et al. (196,236) determined the crude and attributable mortality of nosocomial pneumonia in HSCT recipients to be 74.5% and 61.8%, respectively. In this study the most frequent etiologic agents were *Aspergillus* species (36.4%) and CMV (12.7%). Among nonbacterial causes of pneumonia in recipients of allogeneic HSCTs, CMV pneumonia has the highest mortality rate, 91% (13). Diffuse interstitial pneumonia caused by CMV during the postengraftment period occurs in 30% to 40% of the cases (16). Fifty percent of these patients have idiopathic interstitial pneumonia. This entity is equally common in allogeneic and autologous bone marrow transplant recipients.

Sinusitis

Approximately 1.7% of HSCT patients develop sinusitis (387). However, sinusitis is more common among patients with allogeneic than autologous HSCTs (388). Kennedy et al. (387) reported 22 allogeneic, six autologous, and three unrelated donor transplant patients who developed sinusitis among 1,649 patients. The microbiology of sinusitis among HSCT patients depends on many risk factors. Among 41 cultures of the paranasal sinuses obtained from 18 HSCT patients in whom sinusitis developed, the most common microorganisms were gram-negative bacteria (56.7%), gram-positive bacteria (26.7%), and fungi (16.6%) (389). With the increasing use of HSCT and new cytotoxic chemotherapy, patients have become susceptible to sinus disease caused by unusual microorganisms. Invasive fungal sinusitis is becoming increasingly common among HSCT recipients. Fungi, such as *Aspergillus* species, Zygomycetes, and *Curvularia* species, can cause rhinocerebral sinusitis, which is a potentially lethal complication of HSCT-induced neutropenia. Kennedy et al. (387) reported a mortality rate of 62% despite appropriate antifungal therapy and surgical debridement. Sixty-one percent of the patients who died had undergone extensive surgical procedures (see also Chapter 23).

PREVENTION AND CONTROL STRATEGIES

The caveats that make studying infections in HSCT recipients difficult are similar to those in studying prevention. The impact of individual preventive strategies may never be fully understood because (a) large numbers of patients are rarely studied; (b) large numbers of infections are rarely included; (c) multiple antimicrobial agents are administered; (d) interventions such as granulocyte transfusions, granulocyte stimulating factors, and multiple chemotherapeutic regimens are included; (e) the degree and length of neutropenia is not accounted for; (f) the definitions of infections are not similar; (g) the infections are not diagnosed by microbiologic or histologic criteria; and (h) the underlying illnesses are very heterogeneous (390). Nonetheless, healthcare complications must be systematically defined. For example, defining invasive fungal infections or resistant microorganisms are important components of measuring the impact of interventions.

Although we assume that the air, water, and food are safe, in the immunocompromised host these elements may be a source of infection. With the changing paradigm of healthcare, we must pay careful attention to the role played by the home environment, foods, pets, and daily activities in the pathogenesis of complicating infections. Given that the immunosuppression from HSCT lasts much longer than the patient's stay in hospital, many practices should be incorporated into the home environment as well as the hospital setting. Furthermore, as HSCTs are performed in the outpatient setting or as more immunocompromised patients are discharged earlier, prevention strategies should be appropriately incorporated into these environments. Because of the high mortality associated with infection, attention to control and prevention of infections is critical in this high-risk population.

No infection control practice standards for HSCT units exist. Poe et al. (391) sent questionnaires to 91 HSCT programs. These authors found that all programs provided patients with a protective environment. Nonetheless, the type of protective environment varied widely. Overall, 78% of HSCT units had HEPA filtration of ambient air and 18% had sterile laminar air flow rooms. Seventy-seven percent nursed patients in single isolation rooms. Variations also were seen in the type of cover garments worn by staff on entry into patient rooms and by patients on exit from protected environments. Approximately 25% of staff and 14% to 15% of patients used clean or sterile gowns. Most units did not require head or shoe covers. Head covers, shoe covers, and masks were more likely to be required in sterile laminar airflow rooms. Some units required surgical scrubs, whereas others only required standard hand washing. Wide variation also existed in skin, vaginal, and gut decontamination, and mouth care regimens. Finally, approximately 45% of HSCT units reported specific housekeeping practices that were different from those in other units in the hospital.

Despite the limitations of this study and the wide discrepancies in care, guidelines for preventing opportunistic infections among HSCT recipients have been published (104). Additional guidelines outline recommendations for evaluation of the ventilations and plumbing systems, and their maintenance (140). These documents and additional scientific evidence that can be extrapolated from studies in other types of patients can be used to develop an institutional plan. Although some of these guidelines are generally directed to nonimmunocompromised patient populations, they can be applied to HSCT recipients. In addition, the Healthcare Infection Control Practices Advisory Committee (HICPAC) at the CDC has developed several other relevant sets of guidelines, including ones that (a) address prevention and control of VRE (Table 60.2) (392); (b) recommend appropriate hand hygiene methods (393); and (c) provide recommendations to prevent nosocomial pneumonia and that specifically address policies and procedures in HSCT units or their patients (394). The latter guidelines recommend raising the head of the bed to decrease the risk of aspiration, hand hygiene and appropriate mouth care to prevent colonization or cross-contamination by hands of healthcare workers, disinfecting and sterilizing equipment appropriately, and educating patients and hospital staff (394). These guidelines also apply to mechanically ventilated HSCT patients. Importantly, this guideline and the environmental infection control guideline also address the appropriate interventions if an institution has a case of *Aspergillus* or *Legionella* pneumonia.

Beyond the guidelines, several caveats should be further considered in these patients. First, prevention and control of infection in these patients or units where these patients are hospitalized can involve the patients, their caregivers and family members, and their environment. Nosocomial infection may be acquired from infected patients, staff, visitors, or contaminated items in the patients' environment. Although this tenet is true with many patient groups, it particularly applies to HSCT recipients and the units where they are housed. Second, for many diseases, the infection control procedures are multifaceted and include several if not all elements listed below. For example, nosocomial outbreaks or transmission of RSV, influenza, *C. difficile*, and VRE require integrated programs with strict attention to isolation procedures, hand hygiene, and environmental cleaning procedures to control and prevent transmission (Table 60.2). Third, because data are not always available, common sense is critical in developing prevention and control plans. Fourth, although many hospitals complain about the expense associated with such programs, recent studies have shown that these measures may be cost-effective; by decreasing the number of infections in a hospital with a high prevalence of VRE, authors in two studies projected over $100,000 in annual savings (395, 396). Karanfil et al. (295) also projected a savings of $88,000 annually with a comprehensive program to control RSV. Garcia et al. (296) provide another example and reduced the incidence of RSV infections from 4.4 per 1,000 patient days before the interventions were applied to 1.0 per 1,000 patient days after introducing such a program in an HSCT unit.

We discuss the specific elements of programs that can be developed to prevent transmission of epidemiologically important diseases below. Healthcare workers should be educated; feedback should be provided to physicians, providers, and head nurses about infection rates and compliance with policies and procedures; infection control practices (isolation and contact precautions) must be complied with; the environment must be carefully cleaned; and antibiotics must be used judiciously. Furthermore, management always includes strict hand hygiene, limiting exposure to infected persons during the respiratory virus season, screening of patients and healthcare workers, restricting visitors who could be incubating communicable diseases, using appropriate barrier precautions, and furloughing ill healthcare workers. This section reviews infection data so that programs

TABLE 60.2. PREVENTION & CONTROL STRATEGIES FOR SPECIFIC DISEASES

Influenza

For all suspected patients with fever, coryza, cough, and body aches or flu-like symptoms (FLS):
- Active surveillance of all HSCT patients should occur daily in respiratory virus season
- Obtain nasopharyngeal aspirate (or washes) (NPA) specimens for viral culture and antigen detection
- Use strict hand hygiene
- Droplet Precautions
  - Indicated for any patient with bronchiolitis, pneumonia, or FLS
  - Droplet precautions should continue until the culture has been finalized, even in the case of a positive antigen 7 days from the onset of symptoms

Patient placement:
- Private room
- Patient cohorting if private room not available
- Patients should wear surgical masks when outside their rooms

Visitation:
- Visitors who have FLS should not be allowed to visit
- Visitation of children > 12 years should be restricted

Employees:
- Employees who become febrile or have FLS while at home, must stay home
- Employees who become sick while at work must go to the occupational health service and then home
- Employees who have upper respiratory tract symptoms, such as a cough and coryza without fever, should wear surgical masks during patient contact
- Employees must clean hands before and after all patient contact

Prophylaxis:
- Antivirals (amantidine or rimantadine) are the drugs of choice for chemoprophylaxis for Influenza A; use neuraminidase inhibitors (oseltamivir or zanamivir) for influenza B or when strain is unknown in nonimmune persons
- Prophylaxis should be guided by the hospital epidemiologist

Vaccination:
- All personnel, family, and household members should receive the influenza vaccine yearly

Respiratory syncytial virus (RSV)

For all patients suspected with fever, coryza, cough, or FLS:
- Active surveillance of all HSCT patients should occur daily in respiratory virus season
- Obtain nasopharyngeal aspirate (or washes) (NPA) specimens for viral culture and antigen detection
- Use strict hand hygiene
- Droplet/Contact Precautions
  - Indicated for any patient with bronchiolitis, pneumonia, or FLS
  - Droplet/Contact Precautions should continue until the culture has been finalized, even in the case of a positive antigen 7 days from the onset of symptoms

Patient guidelines:
- Use strict hand hygiene
- Private room or patient cohorting
- Droplet/Contact Precautions
- Gloves for contacts
- Gowns and masks for contacts
- Remove all protective attire before leaving the room
- Do not cohort patients with congenital heart disease, chronic lung disease, or immune suppression with patients with RSV

Duration of Droplet Precautions for confirmed cases:
- For patients with immune suppression, including HIV infection, at least 5 days with culture not growing virus and negative antigen
- Precautions may be discontinued only after two consecutive negative RSV antigen tests, obtained 1 week apart

Staff guidelines:
- Healthcare workers with symptoms of viral respiratory infection should be excluded when possible or must wear mask and gloves for all patient contacts
- Minimize contact with patients who have congenital heart disease, chronic lung disease, or immune suppression

Transport guidelines:
- To transport a patient on droplet/contact precautions, place the patient in a clean gown
- No mask is needed on the patient
- Transport person should wear a gown, gloves and mask

Note:
- When gloves are worn, careful attention must be paid to avoid touching other surfaces
- Clean hands after removing gloves

Tuberculosis (TB)

Airborne Precautions:
- Patient with suspected TB or with high-risk exposure based on infection control guidelines

Procedures
- Airborne Precautions rooms should be designated as negative-pressure rooms
- Portable HEPA filter units must be placed in the rooms if they don't have negative pressure
- Healthcare workers entering an airborne precautions room must wear approved respirator (N-95 or PAPR)
- Doors to the patients' rooms must be closed at all times except for entering and exiting
- Time spent in waiting areas must be limited

Patient transportation:
- Notify the accepting unit or diagnostic area
- Wear a surgical mask.

Visitors:
- Visitation to patients on Airborne Precautions should be limited
- Children should not visit patients on airborne precautions.
- During visitations both the patient *and* visitor must wear a surgical mask without exception

Discontinue isolation
- Per hospital protocol

Laboratory:
- Laboratory specimens processed for tuberculosis smear/culture must be performed in the Biosafety level 3 mycobacteriology laboratory
- Susceptibility testing should be performed

Vancomycin-resistant Enterococcus (VRE)

Isolation/precautions approach
- Identification
  - Notify infection control of patients growing VRE-positive isolates
  - Notify the hospital unit
  - Place the patient on Contact Precautions
  - Private room or cohort patients
  - Precautions require:
    - Gown and gloves on entry
    - Precautions to be initiated for outpatients when they are in the exam or treatment rooms
  - Identify readmitted, previously VRE-colonized or -infected patients, and place them on Contact Precautions
  - Discontinue Contact Precautions when approved by infection control
- Hand hygiene
  - Clean hands with an antimicrobial soap (chlorhexidine gluconate) or alcohol-based waterless product after glove removal and before and after patient care

(*continued*)

TABLE 60.2. (*continued*)

- Equipment/supplies
  - Limit supplies brought into the room
  - Dedicate items to VRE colonized/infected patients (e.g., scales, glucometers)
  - Disinfect equipment (e.g., scales, IV pumps) leaving the room with germicide prior to use on another patient
  - Discard dedicated disposable equipment (e.g., thermometers, stethoscopes, and blood pressure cuffs) on patient discharge
  - Transfer the disposable supplies to the next unit caring for the patient
  - Disinfect blood pressure cuffs, stethoscopes and thermometers with approved germicide between patients, in outpatient setting
- Transportation of patient
  - Inpatient area
    - Patient must wear a clean gown prior to leaving the room
    - Wipe the intravenous pump/pole with an approved germicide before leaving the room
    - Wear isolation gown and gloves while transporting patient or patient's equipment
    - Transport patients on equipment easy to clean (i.e., hard, nonporous surfaces)
    - Move disposable supplies (e.g., stethoscopes, blood pressure cuffs) with patients to procedure areas
  - Outpatient areas
    - Communicate the need for precautions to the receiving area
    - Place the contact precautions sticker on the request for services
- Liberties while in isolation
  - Wear a clean gown and clean hands with chlorhexidine gluconate or waterless alcohol-based product prior to leaving the room
  - Use the common areas on the unit (i.e., kitchen, playroom)
- Terminal room cleaning
  - The precaution sign must stay on the door until the room has been disinfected
  - Terminally clean all room surfaces and equipment and launder privacy curtains (around the bed)
  - Clean window curtains if soiled (exception are areas with neutropenic patients; window curtains are removed and cleaned) in the inpatient area
  - Discard disposable supplies
- Operating room (OR)
  - Notify recovery room to allow for appropriate placement of the patient
    - Patient to be placed near a sink and away from other patients in the recovery room
    - Gown and glove during transport
    - Follow standards for routine cleaning between cases in the OR
  - Recovery room/procedures areas/areas without private rooms
    - Gown and glove in patient's immediate environment
    - Attempt to separate the patient and equipment from other patients
  - Stop unnecessary antibiotics
- Antibiotic management: CDC recommends vancomycin restriction
  - Indications for vancomycin
    - Treatment of serious infections due to beta-lactam–resistant gram-positive bacteria
    - Treatment of infections due to gram-positive bacteria in patients with serious beta-lactam allergy
    - *C. difficile*–associated colitis that fails to respond to metronidazole
    - Surgical prophylaxis: AHA guidelines
    - Surgical prophylaxis for implanting prosthetic material or cardiovascular surgery at sites with high rates of methicillin-resistant *S. aureus* (MRSA) or methicillin-resistant *S. epidermidis* (MRSE)
  - Discouraged use of vancomycin
    - Routine surgical prophylaxis
    - Empirical treatment for febrile neutropenic patients (unless strong evidence of infection by gram-positive bacteria)
    - Single positive blood culture for *S. epidermidis*
    - Continued empirical use for presumed infection if cultures fail to confirm need
    - Prophylaxis of lines
    - Selective decontamination
    - Primary treatment of *C. difficile* colitis
    - Topical solutions
  - Inappropriate or excessive use of all antimicrobial agents must be discouraged
  - Third-generation cephalosporins, and antianaerobic agents should be used judiciously
- Surveillance/outbreak control
  - Utilize special infection control measures to control transmission
  - Determine if increased culturing of the environment and/or point prevalence culture surveys are required

can be tailored to the epidemiologic issues in a given hospital and applied to HSCT units. We do not discuss the use of colony-stimulating factors, immunotherapy, and other adjuvant therapies that decrease the duration of neutropenia, dependence on blood products, and length of hospital stay, and hence decrease the risk of infection (397).

Surveillance Activities

Helpful guidelines for appropriate surveillance activities are emerging for institutions that maintain HSCT services (104). They advocate strongly for the development of three types of surveillance—a clinically, a microbiologically, and an environmentally based program to support surveillance functions for epidemiologically important microorganisms and communicable diseases. In addition to routine surveillance, they suggest that infection control programs must have the expertise and resources to respond quickly to outbreaks, clusters, or a case of nosocomial *Legionella* infection (104,140). We have noted many of these recommendations throughout this chapter.

In an era of empiric therapy, diagnosis of infectious etiology is of paramount importance. Clinicians should use and have access to microbiology laboratories with rapid diagnostic capability for influenza, RSV, and *Legionella* (104). Laboratories must have the capability of identifying resistant enterococci and methicillin and vancomycin-resistant *S. aureus* (104). A microbiology laboratory enhances surveillance with diagnostic capabilities for the pathogens and resistance issues that are problems in this population. In addition, clinicians must be encouraged to use diagnostic tests to identify pathogens that are of epidemiologic importance (104,140).

Surveillance activities should target the disease processes and microorganisms that are most problematic in this population at an individual institution and where interventions can take place.

We recommend that, at a minimum, surveillance for healthcare-associated bloodstream infections be done with a focus on those related to catheters and that surveillance be done for nosocomial upper and lower respiratory tract infections with a focus on *Legionella, Aspergillus,* and invasive fungal pathogens, and respiratory viruses, primarily influenza, adenovirus, parainfluenza, and RSV (398). Some groups have advocated that we perform surveillance for fever of unknown origin as this may be the most important clinical entity in neutropenic patients (399). *Legionella* remains a rare but important microorganism that may cause infections in immunocompromised patients; however, clinicians must be taught to order urinary antigen tests and culture and direct fluorescent antibody (DFA) tests on respiratory tract or bronchoalveolar lavage samples (104). Diagnosis of respiratory viruses (nasal washes or nasopharyngeal aspirates for antigens and culture) requires an active surveillance program that implements culturing of all patients with coryza or other upper respiratory tract symptoms during the respiratory virus season. Other surveillance programs that are important to prevent transmission of resistant microorganisms that are microbiologically based include active surveillance programs to identify HSCT colonized with MRSA and VRE. Patients who are not known to be colonized with VRE or MRSA should have weekly perirectal and nares swabs, respectively. If patients have open wounds, we recommend those be cultured for MRSA also. If these programs are run in parallel with the laboratory, selective media can be used to reduce costs. Finally, it is increasingly important to have surveillance in place for some environmental pathogens. Clearly, obtaining air and water samples in the settings of *Aspergillus* or *Legionella* outbreaks or nosocomial cases is recommended; however, there are no guidelines on whether this should be done routinely. Air sampling for fungus or particle counts may help determine if there are breaches in construction projects that could lead to morbidity among these patients. Currently most institutions are approaching environmental surveillance cautiously and are basing it on the epidemiology of the microorganism(s) most often detected in their institution.

Hand Hygiene

General guidelines from HICPAC on hand hygiene and antisepsis should be followed and have recently been revised (393). Since it is well known that microorganisms are transmitted by contaminated hands, appropriate hand hygiene is the cornerstone for controlling the spread of many infectious agents. For example, hand hygiene has been shown to reduce the risk of *C. difficile* transmission (74,75,78,400,401). Furthermore, hand washing with plain soap and water is unreliable and will not remove tenacious microorganisms such as VRE (163). Hence, two primary approaches are used in healthcare settings: hand washing with soaps that have antimicrobial activity, and cleaning with waterless, alcohol-based gels. Hands should be washed with an antiseptic soap containing chlorhexidine gluconate or another antiseptic agent chosen by the institution. Other agents including 0.03% triclosan, hexachlorophene, or chloroxylenol-containing hand-washing soaps have been shown to be effective; however, each has its limitations (393). More recently there has been intense interest in alcohol-based solutions to clean hands because of their efficacy and practicality. A 60% isopropyl alcohol-based solution applied to the hands can reduce VRE isolates on the hands 10,000-fold (163). Recent studies show the superiority of alcohol-based, waterless hand products that have superb activity against resistant microorganisms, skin flora, fungi, and viruses (393).

Proper handwashing and hand cleaning technique should be taught to visitors and healthcare workers. Hand hygiene stations and sinks should be accessible to facilitate their use. We recommend placing alcohol-based products outside of each patient room, in areas where equipment and medications are handled, and in other appropriate areas. Hand hygiene should be practiced before and after each patient contact; after contact with environmental surfaces, equipment, or food; after removal of gloves; and after other activities that may contaminate the hands (393). Following hand hygiene, great care must be exercised to avoid touching the hands on potentially contaminated surfaces, such as doorknobs, bed rails, or countertops (163).

Importantly, the new guidelines specifically recommend that healthcare workers not wear artificial fingernails (393). Nonnative nails, whether artificial, acrylic, or polished (and chipped), can harbor microorganisms that cause infections in all types of patients (402–404). Outbreaks have been associated with healthcare workers wearing artificial nails (405,406). Published data suggest that surgical scrubs, hand washing with soap and water, or application of alcohol-based products do not eliminate these microorganisms (404,407). Because of these data, healthcare workers caring for HSCT patients must not wear artificial or acrylic nails or have polished nails that are chipped (see also Chapter 96).

Blood Product Screening and Prevention of Infection from Extraneous Contamination

As blood products are an important source of several viruses and parasites, screening for agents that cause hepatitis, HIV, and other agents is standard practice in North America. Still, CMV transmission via residual buffy coat cells remains a significant issue in these patients. Among 97 HSCT recipients who were CMV seronegative before transplantation, 57 patients had seronegative marrow donors (307). One of 32 patients who received seronegative products and eight of 25 who received standard blood products developed CMV infection ($p <.007$). However, given the high prevalence of CMV in the general population, it is difficult to procure large amounts of CMV-negative blood for CMV-seronegative patients. In the absence of seronegative products, blood should be depleted of cellular elements. This can be accomplished by several techniques including irradiation or use of specialized filters. Bowden et al. (308) evaluated 502 patients and compared the incidence of CMV infection and disease among those receiving filtered, leukocyte reduced, or CMV seronegative products. No significant differences in the number of infections (1.3% vs. 2.4%; $p = 1.00$) or disease (0% vs. 2.4%, $p = 1.00$) were found among patients who received the seronegative and filtered blood. The probability of developing CMV disease was greater among patients receiving filtered products (2.4% vs. 0% in the seronegative arm, $p = .03$).

Bone marrow for either allogeneic or autologous transplantation is collected from a donor and stored. Infections can occur among recipients of contaminated marrow or blood products (408). Rarely, an infected donor can transmit microorganisms to a patient. More commonly the patient receives contaminated blood products or marrow that was contaminated during processing and storage. Infection caused by viruses (HIV; CMV; HSV; hepatitis A, B, C, and D; adenovirus; EBV; WNV; and rabies), common aerobic bacteria, fungi and yeasts, parasites, and helminths (*Toxoplasma gondii, Trypanosoma cruzi, Plasmodium* species) have been reported (409–423; Guerrero, 1983 #66). To prevent transmission to HSCT recipients, programs now obtain a history and perform a physical examination on the donor (424,425). Donors are asked about high-risk behaviors, previous travel, and signs and symptoms of infection prior to harvesting the marrow, and serum is screened for serologic evidence of disease (54,408,424). Commonly, donors are screened for CMV, EBV, hepatitis B virus (HBV), hepatitis C virus (HCV), *T. gondii,* and other types of dormant infection with dimorphic fungi or *M. tuberculosis.* Finally, some infections, such as HBV, can be prevented by vaccination. In cases where patients cannot be protected using vaccination, novel strategies using passive immunization show promise (426). Daily et al. (426) demonstrated that a HSCT recipient of hepatitis B surface antigen (HBsAg)-positive donor cells was protected with serial injections of hepatitis B immunoglobulin (426). Similar strategies have been used to prevent CMV infection (307).

Bone marrow can be contaminated during harvesting and during the *ex vivo* processing. The amount of contamination that occurs during *in vitro* processing of bone marrow varies between 2.6% and 17% (427–430). Cultured bone marrow from both allogeneic and autologous donors did not grow microorganisms prior to study (428). However, 12/153 (8%) samples grew microorganisms when the marrow was thawed prior to infusion. Gram-negative microorganisms were most commonly isolated including *Pseudomonas* species in 5/12 samples. One patient developed *P. picketti* sepsis following infusion of bone marrow cells. Rowley et al. (427) showed that the risk of contamination of marrow increased as it was manipulated. Finally, Schepers et al. (429) demonstrated a significant decrease in contamination from 5% to 2.6% when appropriate procedures were introduced. Contamination has been traced to heparin and contaminated ficoll separation medium (429,431). To prevent bone marrow contamination, protocols should be established and followed. Centers should use aseptic technique and closed systems to pool stem cells prior to storage (104). Storage requires double bagging to prevent contamination of ports (104). Cultures of the bone marrow should be obtained when it is harvested and when it is defrosted prior to infusion into the recipient.

In addition to marrow contamination, blood products can be a source of infection. Patients can become infected at any time during the transplant procedure when they receive blood or its products (432–436). The risks of infection related to transfused blood and blood products are similar to those from bone marrow. The Red Cross and hospital-based blood banks follow strict guidelines and screening procedures to decrease the risk of transmitting blood-borne pathogens (437) (see also Chapter 69).

Prophylaxis

Antibacterial Prophylaxis

Because of the high mortality of bacterial infections, particularly during the pre-engraftment phase, research has been directed toward the prevention of these infections. Because measures to control bacterial infections have been successful, this may in part contribute to the rise in importance of fungi and viruses as causes of infection in this population. Early broad-spectrum empiric antibiotic therapy may contribute to the bulk of reduction in bacterial infections. Importantly, new guidelines for the use of antimicrobial agents in neutropenic patients have been developed that include a risk assessment, a systematic evaluation of the patient, and a stepwise approach to use of these agents (438). These guidelines provide a measured and thoughtful approach to the use of vancomycin that will help limit resistance (438). From an infection control perspective, the prophylactic use of antibiotics has generated extensive and at times controversial studies that have examined multiple regimens and often include co-interventions, such as a laminar flow room, that make interpretation difficult (Tables 60.3 and 60.4) (9,69, 72,401,439–455).

The rationale for prophylactic administration of antibiotics is based on data that show that the majority of bacterial infections arise during the neutropenic phase from the patient's endogenous flora. Prophylactic antibiotics, therefore, have been used to selectively decontaminate certain body sites. As the gut is the primary reservoir of potentially pathogenic bacteria, attempts at decontamination have focused on this site. The downside of eliminating the resident flora is the potential for selection of other, potentially more resistant, microorganisms. In addition, the benefits of these agents must be balanced against the deleterious effects including toxicity, resistance, fungal overgrowth, and superinfections (452,453,455,456). Although many regimens have been used in the past, this discussion focuses on agents currently in use and on studies focusing on HSCT patients (54,457). These agents appear most useful during periods of neutropenia that last longer than 2 weeks in patients undergoing invasive procedures or with severe mucositis (438, 458).

Investigations in the late 1970s examined the efficacy of nonabsorbable agents for decontamination of the gut (456). Many studies examined a variety of regimens including oral agents such as vancomycin, neomycin, and others, and included other interventions such as protective isolation and low microbial diets (457, 459–461). The overall impact of the agents is difficult to ascertain, given the small size of these studies, but some showed reduction in infection rates. However, the agents were unpalatable and were poorly tolerated by patients (457). Finally, the unexpected consequences include the emergence of resistant microorganisms and infections and superinfections caused by fungi (452,453,455, 456). From animal experiments, investigators discovered that eliminating the anaerobic flora led to increased colonization with resistant microorganisms (456,459). They postulated that anaerobes possess a colonization resistance factor, and therefore that decontamination regimens that did not have substantial anaerobic activity would allow for eliminating pathogenic microorga-

TABLE 60.3. IMPACT OF ORAL ANTIBIOTICS AND GASTROINTESTINAL DECONTAMINATION AMONG PATIENTS WITH HEMATOLOGIC MALIGNANCIES OR UNDERGOING HSCT

Study	*N*	Study Design	Intervention	Effect
Wade et al. 1981 (448)	53 Hematotogic malignancy	Prospective randomized	TMP-SMZ / nystatin (N) vs GENT	Infections: 35 TMP-SMZ / N vs 31 GENT BSI: 5 TMP-SMZ / N vs 8 GENT Deaths: 4 TMP-SMZ / N vs 8 GENT
Pizzo et al. 1983 (445)	150 Hematologic malignancy	Randomized double-blind	TMP-SMZ / erythromycin (E) vs placebo (PL)	Fever: 18.1% TMP-SMZ / E vs 32.2% PL; $p = .009$ Infection: 3.8% TMP-SMZ / E vs 11.9% PL; $p = 0.37$
Wade et al. 1983 (444)	62 Hematologic malignancy	Prospective randomized	TMP-SMZ / Nystatin (N) vs nalidixic acid and nystatin (NL/N), 1–3 days before chemotherapy	Time to infection: 17 days TMP-SMZ / N vs 8 days NL / N; $p = .002$ Duration of granulocytopenia: 23.6 days TMP-SMZ / N vs 13.6 days NL / N; $p = .007$ Deaths: 7 TMP-SMZ / N vs 3 NL/N Gram negative bacilli: greater acquisition in NL / N; $p = .05$
EORTC 1984 (446)	342/545 (evaluable) Hematologic malignancy	Randomized, stratified by diagnosis	TMP-SMZ vs PL	Infection: 64/185 (35%) PL vs 46/177 (26%) TMP-SMZ; $p = .016$ BSI: 32/165 (19%) PL vs 22/177 (12%) TMP-SMZ; $p =$ ns
Dekker et al. 1987 (465)	56 Hematologic malignancy	Randomized	TMP-SMZ + colistin vs ciprofloxacin (C)	C: Decreased colonization with gram-negative bacilli TMP-SMZ: Increased resistant strains
Ferretti et al. 1987 (449)	BMT	Nonrandomized	Chlorhexidine (CH) 0.12%	Decrease in oral soft tissue disease Decrease in oral microorganisms Decrease in *Candida* infections
Karp 1987 (443)	68 Hematologic malignancy	Double-blind, stratified by therapy and diagnosis	Norfloxacin (NF) vs PL at time of chemotherapy, could add oral polymyxin B	Time to fever: 6.3 days NF vs 3.7 days PL; $p = .005$ GNB infections: 4/35 NF vs 13/33 PL No effect on fungi or gram-positive infections No difference in mortality
Attal et al. 1991 (439)	60 BMT	Prospective randomized	Vancomycin (V) vs PL beginning 48 hours before preparative regimen	GP infections: 11/30 PL vs 0/30 V; $p = .002$ BSI: 9/11 PL vs 0 V Deaths: 1 PL vs 0 V V decreased fever and empiric antibiotics
Gluckman et al. 1991 (441)	44 BMT	Prospective randomized	Ofloxacin/amoxicillin (O/A) vs oral vancomycin/tobramycin/ colistin (V/ T/C) 15 days before transplant to 15 days after neutropenia resolved	Resistant bacteria: 5/ 22 O/A vs 2/22 V/T/C Duration of fever: 9.2 days O/A vs 13.7 days V/T/C; $p = .05$
Epstein et al. 1992 (440)	86 Hematologic malignancy	Randomized	Chlorhexidine and nystatin (CH / N) vs chlorthexidine (CH) vs nystatin vs saline	CH decreased oral pathogens No decrease in mucositis
Schmeiser et al. 1993 (442)	101 evaluable BMT	Noncomparative prospective	Ofloxacin	14 patients with proven bacterial infection
EORTC 1994 (541)	551 Hematologic malignancy and BMT	Convenience sample multicenter	Penicillin V (PV) vs placebo and pefloxacin (PL / PF)	Fever: 190/268 (71%) PV vs 213/268 (79%) PL / PF; $p = .083$ BSI: 38/268 (14%) PV vs 58/268 (22%) PL / PF; $p = .03$ Streptococcal BSI: 14/268 (5%) PV vs 27/268 (10%) PL / PF No difference in gram-negative BSI
Lew et al. 1995 (401)	146 Hematologic malignancy and BMT	Double-blind randomized, stratified by diagnosis	TMP-SMZ vs ciprofloxacin (C) with 96 hours of BMT preparation	No difference in fever, duration of neutropenia or incidence of rash BSI: 10 C vs 6 TMP-SMZ *C. difficile* enterocolitis: O C vs 10 TMP-SMZ; $p = .001$ GN infection: O C vs 10 TMP-SMZ
Hidalgo et al. 1997 (468)	40 Hematologic malignancy and BMT	Randomized	Ciprofloxacin (C) vs ciprofloxacin and rifampin (C/R)	Fever: no difference between the two groups C/R did not reduce significantly gram-positive bacteremia C/R higher incidence of drug-related side effects; $p < .05$

(continued)

TABLE 60.3. *(continued)*

Study	N	Study Design	Intervention	Effect
Winston et al. 1998 (452)	209: 166 on Norfloxacin Hematologic malignancy and BMT	Prospective randomized controlled trial; norfloxacin provided to patients nonrandomly	Sulbactam/cefoperoxone (S/C) vs imipenem (I) with or without norfloxacin (NF)	Clinical response 91/103 (88%) S/C vs I 84/104 (81%) 1; $p = 0.17$ 42/166 (25%) on NF developed gram-positive infections vs. 2/37 (5.4%) without prophylactic NF; $p = .007$ Diarrhea 31/103 (30%) S/C vs 1 15/102 (15%); $p = .007$ Superinfections (16%) in both groups
Beelen et al. 1999 (9)	134 Hematologic malignancy and BMT	Prospective randomized clinical trial 5 weeks posttransplant	Ciprofloxacin and metronidazole (C/M) vs ciprofloxacin (C)	Acute GVHD grades II–IV: C/M 22% vs C 54%; $p < .001$ Fecal samples without anaerobic growth: CM 53% vs C 23%; $p < .00001$ Fecal anaerobes in acute GVHD grades II–IV is 100-fold higher than in acute GVHD grades 0–1; $p < .005$
Perea et al. 1999 (453)	31 Solid tumors BMT	Nonrandomized, observational	Ciprofloxacin (C)	Fluoroquinolone-resistant *E. coli* (MIC—8 to 64 mg/L) in 32% of patients Mean number of days of prophylaxis greater in those with resistant strains (8.9 vs 6.4 days) No fluoroquinolone-resistant GNB-BSI
Trenschell et al. 2000 (455)	134 Hematologic malignancy and BMT	Open-label prospective randomized trial	Metronidazole/ciprofloxacin/ fluconazole (M/C/F) vs ciprofloxacin/fluconazole (C/F)	Invasive fungal infections 7/68 (10%) M/C/F vs 11/66 (17%) C/F; $p = .36$ Anaerobic growth in fecal samples: 236/446 (53%) M/C/F vs 96/420 (23%) M/C; $p < .001$ Yeast growth in fecal samples: 334/446 (75%) M/C/F vs 293/475 (62%) M/C; $p < .01$
Prentice et al. 2001 (454)	150 Hematologic malignancy and BMT	Randomized trial	Ciprofloxacin/colistin (C/Col) vs neomycin/colistin (N/Col)	C/Col lower proportion of neutropenic febrile days; $p < .001$ C/Col lower proportion of neutropenic antibiotic days; $p < .001$ Total bacterial isolates 16/64 C/Col vs 44/64 N/Col; $p < .001$ *S. aureus* 0/64 C/Col vs 10/64 N/Col; $p = .001$ Total gram-positive 14/64 C/Col vs 25/64 N/Col; $p = .03$ Total gram-negative 2/64 C/Col vs 16/64 N/Col; $p < .001$

BMT, bone marrow transplant recipients; TMP-SMZ, trimethoprim-sulfamethoxazole; N, nystatin; GENT, gentamicin/nystatin; BSI, bloodstream infection; E, erythromycin; PL, placebo; NL/NY, nalidixic acid/nystatin; C, ciprofloxacin; CH, chlorhexidine; GNB, gram-negative bacilli; NF, norfloxacin; V, vancomycin; O/A, ofloxacin/amoxicillin; V/T/C, vancomycin/tobramycin/colisitin; C/N, chlorhexidine & nystatin; PV, penicillin V; PF, pefloxacin; PL/PF, placebo & pefloxacin; R, rifampin; I, imipenem; S/C, sulbactam/cefoperazone; C/F, ciprofloxacin/fluconazole; M, metronidiazole; C/Col, ciprofloxacin/colistin; N/Col, neomycin/colistin.

nisms without reducing the resistance to colonization by aerobic pathogens (459). Isolation of anaerobic microorganisms may also be associated with higher grades of GVHD (9).

Trimethoprim-sulfamethoxazole (TMP-SMX) has been used to prevent PCP for years, and retrospective data provide information about its utility in preventing bacterial infections (462). In most studies patients receiving TMP-SMX had lower infection rates than patients receiving placebo (438,463). In one large study of adult and pediatric patients who were randomized to placebo or 160/800 mg of TMP-SMX until the neutropenia resolved, those who received TMP-SMX developed fewer infections (26% vs. 39%; $p < .02$) (446). The results are confounded by the use of nonabsorbable antibiotics in some centers. There have been no studies examining the use of TMP-SMX specifically in HSCT recipients, but its use is attractive, as these patients require TMP-SMX for PCP prophylaxis. Unfortunately, drug side effects associated with the higher doses required for gut decontamination, primarily skin manifestations, occurred in approximately 20% of patients (457).

Fluoroquinolones are attractive antimicrobials for use as prophylactic agents; they are well tolerated orally and have limited activity against anaerobes. Studies with these agents show that they are as efficacious as TMP/SMX, if not more so, although they have no activity against *P. carinii* (438). Norfloxacin was the first antibiotic to be compared to TMP-SMX. Four studies showed that the fluoroquinolones reduced gram-negative bacillary infections when compared to TMP-SMX, but two of the studies noted an increase in infections caused by gram-positive bacteria (18,443,464,465). One group documented fewer microbiologically proven infections among patients receiving ciprofloxacin (17% ciprofloxacin vs. 24% norfloxacin) and more patients receiving ciprofloxacin never had a neutropenic fever or required antibiotic therapy (466). Lew et al. (401) randomly assigned 75 patients to receive ciprofloxacin or TMP-SMX and found no difference in infection rates or time to onset of fever. The most recent randomized study reported that patients receiving ciprofloxacin and colistin had a lower proportion of febrile and antibiotic days while neutropenic ($p < .001$; $p < .001$, respectively) (454). Two studies did not show that the addition of rifampin decreased the incidence of febrile episodes (467, 468). One of these studies did not find a decrease in the incidence of gram-positive bacteremia (468).

TABLE 60.4. PREVENTION OF GRAM-POSITIVE INFECTIONS USING ORAL ANTIBIOTICS IN PATIENTS WITH HEMATOLOGIC MALIGNANCIES OR HSCT

Study	*N*	Study Design	Intervention	Effect
De Pauw et al. 1990 (451)	78/89 BMT-evaluable	Nonrandomized	Ciprofloxacin 1 day before BMT	42 episodes BSI 35/42 episodes *S. viridans* BSI
Attal et al. 1991 (439)	60 BMT	Prospective randomized	Vancomyin (V) vs placebo (PL) beginning 48 hours before preparative regimen	GP infections: 11/30 PL vs 0/30 V; *p* = .002 BSI: 9/11 PL vs 0 V Deaths: 1 PL vs 0 V V decreased fever and empiric antibiotics
EORTC 1994 (541)	551 Hematologic maligancy and BMT	Convenience sample multicenter	Penicillin V (PV) vs placebo and pefloxacin (PL/PF)	Fever: 190/268 (71%) PV vs 213/268 (79%) PL/PF; *p* = .083 BSI: 38/268 (14%) PV vs 58/268 (22%) PL/PF; *p* = .03 Streptococcal BSI: 14/268 (5%) PV vs 27/268 (10%) PL/PF No difference in gram-negative BSI
Castagnola et al. 1995 (69)	Not specified BMT (children)	Sequential cohort	PV vs no prophylaxis	Streptococcal BSI: 7/17(41%) PV vs 13/15 (87%) no prophylaxis (*p* significant)
Arns da Cunha et al. 1998 (72)	89 BMT	Sequential cohort	Vancomycin (V) vs penicillin/cefazolin vs no prophylaxis	GP bacteria: 11% V vs 27% penicillin/cefazolin vs 40% no prophylaxis No differences in morbidity
Kern et al. 1994 (450)	131 Hematologic malignancy and BMT	Prospective randomized open label	Roxithromycin (ROX)/ofloxicin (O) vs O	*S. viridans* BSI: 9% (O) vs 0% (ROX/O) *p* = .03 Increased side effects with ROX/O
Gomez-Martin et al. 2000 (467)	130 Solid tumor patients undergoing BMT	Multicenter randomized clinical trial	Ciprofloxacin (C) vs ciprofloxacin/rifampin (C/R)—48 hours before BMT	Reduction overall BSI: 12 C (19%) vs 4 C/R (6.5%); *p* = .05 Decrease in gram-positive BSI: 8 C vs. 2 C/R is not significant; *p* = .05 vs *p* = .09 Increased side effects with C/R (18%) vs 0; *p* = .002
Cordonnier et al. 2002 (458)	513/532 Hematologic maligancy and BMT	Prospective, observation evaluation of consecutive patients at 36 centers	No intervention	*Streptococcus* species risk increased with high-dose cytarabine [OR 2.2; *p* = .04]; antacids [OR 1.6; *p* = 0.4]; nonabsorbable antifungals [OR 4.4 *p* = .02]; *Streptococcus* species infections risk increased with lack of growth factor [OR 2; *p* = .08]; antacids [OR 1.4; *p* = .2]; colimycin [OR 2.6; *p* = .01]; no TMP/SMX [OR 3.3; *p* = .06]; mucositis [OR 1.3; *p* = .14]

BMT, bone marrow transplant recipients; BSI, bloodstream infection; C, ciprofloxacin; V, vancomycin; PL, placebo; PV, penicillin V; PF, pefloxacin; ROX, roxithromycin; O, ofloxacin; T, tobramycin; Tic, ticarcillin; Ceftaz, ceftazidime; Co, colymicin.

The spectrum of microorganisms has shifted with the use of both TMP-SMX and quinolones; gram-positive infections have increased (467). A particularly marked increase in α-hemolytic streptococcal infections was noted in patients receiving ciprofloxacin, which has poor activity against streptococci (23,52, 69). Other risk factors include high-dose cytarabine (OR = 2.2), antacids (OR = 1.6), and nonabsorbable antifungal agents (OR = 4.4) (458). The mortality associated with gram-positive infections is lower than that seen with gram-negative sepsis, and the overall burden of bacterial infections is decreased with prophylaxis (70). Prophylactic strategies to decrease the morbidity associated with these infections have yet to be defined in randomized trials (Tables 60.3 and 60.4). Some centers currently include penicillin V, a first-generation cephalosporin, or vancomycin in their regimen, at least while the patient has mucositis (69,72,439,451). A cohort study among patients suggests that vancomycin may be superior in preventing gram-positive infections, but further trials are needed to confirm this finding (72, 439). To limit exposure to vancomycin, we permit vancomycin to be used for only 7 days after the transplant. This is a procedure not supported by the guidelines (104). Topical decontamination of the oropharynx and skin has also been studied, albeit in a more limited fashion.

Other infections may be prevented by the used of oral antimicrobial agents, although the use of these agents to prevent these diseases has not been specifically tested. Meletis et al. (120) found that oral treatment or decontamination regimens that included fluoroquinolones may prevent Legionnaire's disease. During an outbreak, three of four patients who received nonabsorbable antibiotics developed Legionnaire's disease, and none of the 14 patients who received the quinolone pefloxacin developed *Legionella* infections. These data do not support the use of prophylaxis among HSCT patients on the unit with TMP-SMX or fluoroquinolones in the event of detection of a nosocomial *Legionella* case (104,114,123,469).

Among patients with hematologic malignancies, administration of oral vancomycin, environmental cleaning, and introduction of other measures may prevent colonization with *C. difficile* (83). Lew et al. (401) studied the efficacy and safety of ciprofloxacin and TMP-SMX for the prevention of bacterial infections among patients undergoing HSCT. Ten episodes of *C. difficile* enterocolitis occurred among patients receiving TMP-SMX, whereas no episodes developed in patients receiving ciprofloxacin ($p = .001$). Heizmann et al. (460) examined the effectiveness of gastrointestinal and topical decontamination and isolation in laminar airflow (LAF) units in 20 HSCT patients. *C. difficile* and/or its toxin B were detected in eight patients prior to beginning antimicrobial therapy. No episodes were noted after initiating gastrointestinal and topical decontamination.

Vancomycin flushes, injections, and dwells, or insertion prophylaxis has been used to prevent catheter-related bloodstream infections (470–475). Prophylaxis to prevent infections related to insertion has not been shown efficacious, and centers should follow the recommendations for skin preparation and catheter care described in the national guidelines (375,473,475). Studies examining the impact of vancomycin prophylaxis to prevent line infections report mixed results (470–475). Controversy arises as other components tested including heparin may have impacted the results, and antimicrobial resistance likely develops in this setting.

In summary, prophylaxis is recommended for the prevention of *P. carinii* pneumonia (104,438). There is no consensus on the use of fluoroquinolones or other agents used to prevent infections in neutropenic hosts (104,438). However, the CDC guideline strongly recommends that decisions for prophylaxis be reviewed and discussed with the hospital epidemiologist or infection control practitioner (104). The routine use of vancomycin (or other antimicrobial agents) to prevent central line infections is not recommended (392,438).

Antifungal Chemoprophylaxis

The incidence of fungal infections has increased substantially in the last decade. These infections present insidiously, are difficult to diagnose, and in HSCT may not respond well to antifungal agents. Hence, prevention is an attractive strategy. Most recently, potent antifungal agents with more favorable side-effect profiles have made this approach attractive. Given that *C. albicans* remains the most prevalent fungal infection among patients, most prophylaxis strategies target this microorganism (373). Although other agents have been tried, fluconazole is the antifungal agent used most frequently (249,476–483). There have been two large randomized, placebo-controlled trials of fluconazole prophylaxis among patients (Table 60.5) (249,477–483). Goodman et al. (249) administered 400 mg of fluconazole or placebo daily to 365 HSCT patients when the conditioning regimen started, and discontinued prophylaxis when the neutrophil count was over 1,000/mm^3 for 7 consecutive days or amphotericin B was started. The incidence of superficial and systemic fungal infections [superficial, 8.4% (fluconazole) vs. 33.3% (placebo)] and [systemic, 2.8% (fluconazole) and 15.8% (placebo)] and the mortality attributable to fungal infections, 1 to 179 for patients taking fluconazole vs. 10 to 177 for patients taking placebo, both showed the positive impact of prophylactic fluconazole therapy. Patients (n = 300) randomized to fluconazole in a placebo-controlled trial had significantly lower rates of fungal infections and overall mortality (479). Later studies, including those with prolonged fluconazole administration (up to 75 days after HSCT), have shown a decrease in the subsequent use of parenteral antifungal agents, superficial and invasive fungal infections, and early and late deaths with the use of prophylactic fluconazole (481,482).

A potential problem with the routine use of fluconazole is the selection pressure for infections caused by fluconazole-resistant fungi. The Goodman, Gemio and Slavin groups demonstrated a significant decrease in the number of *C. albicans* infections, but no change in the number of infections due to *C. krusei, Fusarium,* or *Aspergillus* (249,257,479). Wingard et al. (311, 476), however, demonstrated a significant increase in both the rate of *C. krusei* and *C. glabrata* infections and colonization among HSCT patients receiving fluconazole. Despite these findings, several guidelines recommend the routine use of fluconazole (400 mg po qd) (104,438).

Itraconazole is a broad-spectrum triazole that has activity against *Cryptococcus neoformans, Candida* species, and *Aspergillus* species. It can be administered orally and is well tolerated. A randomized, placebo-controlled, double-blind, multicenter trial evaluated the efficacy and safety of itraconazole oral solution among 405 neutropenic patients with hematologic malignancies (480). Proven or suspected deep fungal infection occurred in 24% (48/201) of itraconazole recipients and in 33% (67/204) of placebo recipients ($p = .035$). Candidemia was significantly lower among patients receiving itraconazole as compared to placebo ($p = .01$). No deaths due to candidemia occurred in the itraconazole recipients, compared with four deaths in placebo recipients ($p = .06$).

In another randomized, placebo-controlled trial involving over 200 HSCT patients, those patients receiving placebo developed fungal infections (superficial or systemic) more frequently than those receiving itraconazole (15% vs. 6%; $p = .03$) (483). Among patients with profound and prolonged neutropenia, those receiving placebo used more empirical amphotericin B (61% vs. 22%; $p = .0001$) and developed more systemic fungal infections (19% vs. 6%; $p = .04$). Other studies look promising, although further studies are needed before this can be recommended for routine use (480,484,485).

Low-dose amphotericin B prophylaxis is another prophylactic modality that has also been studied. This agent has an advantage in that it has antifungal activity against *Aspergillus.* The lower dose is used in an attempt to avoid the toxicity of conventional doses of amphotericin B. A number of studies have examined the use of different low-dose protocols in different populations at potential risk with varying results as summarized in Table 60.6 (478,486,487). Rousey et al. (486) administered low-dose amphotericin B to patients starting during the conditioning regimen and demonstrated a statistically significant decrease in both

TABLE 60.5. IMPACT OF ANTIFUNGAL AGENTS AMONG PATIENTS UNDERGOING HSCT

Study	*N* Patient population	Study Design	Intervention	Effect
Wingard et al. 1987 (476)	208 Patients with prolonged neutropenia	Randomized, double-blind, placebo-controlled	Miconazole (MIC) vs placebo (PL)	Fungal sepsis: 1/97 MIC vs 8/11 PL; $p = .03$ Fatal fungal sepsis: 0/1 MIC vs 4/8 PL; $p = .08$
Goodman et al. 1992 (249)	356 BMT recipients	Randomized, double-blind, placebo-controlled	Fluconazole (FLU) vs PL	Fungal infection: Superficial 33.3% PL vs 8.4% FLU; $p = .001$ Systemic 15.8% PL vs 2.8% FLU; $p = .001$ Fewer deaths from acute systemic fungal infection with FLU (1/79) vs PL (10/77); $p = .001$ No differences in overall mortality
O'Donnell et al. 1994 (478)	331 Allogeneic BMT patients	Retrospective	Low-dose amphotericin B (LDAB 5–10 mg/day)	18 systemic mycoses 18 candidemias If treatment was started before high-dose corticosteroids, fungal infections decreased from 30% to 9%; $p = .01$
Riley et al. 1994 (477)	85 BMT recipients	Randomized, double-blind, placebo-controlled	Low-dose amphotericin B (LDAB .1 mg/kg/day) vs placebo (PL)	Fungal infection—systemic: 5/18 (28%) PL vs 0/17 LDAB; $p = .045$ Mean hospitalization: 41.5 days PL (range 22–95) vs 39 days LDAB (range 22–63) Improved survival with LDAB; $p = .08$
Slavin et al. 1995 (479)	300 BMT recipients	Prospective, randomized, double-blind	FLU vs PL for first 75 days after BMT	Fungal infection—proved systemic: 10/52 (19%) FLU vs 26/48 (55%) PL *C. albicans* infection: 0 FLU vs 18 PL ($p = .001$) FLU reduced fungal colonization ($p = .037$)
Menichetti et al. 1999 (480)	405 Hematologic malignancies	Prospective, randomized, double-blind	Itraconazole (IT) vs PL (2.5 mg/kg BID)	Fungal Infections 48/201 (24%) IT vs 67/204 (33%) PL; $p = .035$ Fungemia 1/201 (0.5%) IT vs 8/204 (4%) PL; $p = .001$ *C. albicans* infection: 0 FLU vs 18 PL; $p = .001$ FLU reduced fungal colonization: $p = .037$
Rotstein et al. 1999 (482)	304 Hematologic malignancies or BMT	Prospective, randomized, placebo-controlled	FLU (400 mg/d) vs PL	Use of parenteral antifungal therapy 81/147 (55%) FLU vs 67/133 (50%) PL Invasive fungal infections: 9/141 (6%) FLU vs 32/141 (23%) PL; $p = .0001$ Superficial fungal infections: 10/141 (7%) FLU vs 23/131 (18%) PL; $p = .02$ Reduce colonization: 52/141 (37%) FLU vs 27/141 (19%) PL; $p = .004$ Death: 1/15 (6.7%) FLU vs 6/15 (40%) PL; $p = .04$
Nucci et al. 2000 (483)	219 Patients with hematologic malignancies or having undergone autologous BMT	Prospective, randomized, double-blind, placebo-controlled	IT (100 mg BID) vs PL (100 mg BID)	Overall fungal Infections (deep and superficial): 6/104 (6%) IT vs 16/106 (15%) PL, $p = .03$ Among neutropenic patients, 6% of IT and 19% in PL; $p = .04$ IT reduce fungal infections and colonization
Marr et al. 2000 (481)	300 Blood and HSCT	Prospective follow up of a randomized, double-blind, placebo-controlled trial with 8 years of follow-up	FLU (400 mg/d) vs PL for 75 days after BMT	Survival: 68/152 (45%) FLU vs 41/148 (28%) PL; $p = .0001$ Candidiasis: 4/152 (3%) FLU vs 30/148 (20%) PL; $p < .001$ Early death from *Candida* infections: 1/152 (0.7%) FLU vs 13/148 (9%) PL; $p = .001$ Late death from *Candida* infections: 1/121 (0.8%) FLU vs 8/96(8%) PL; $p = .007$ GVHD: 8/145 (0.6%) FLU vs 20/143 (14%) PL; $p = 0.02$
Boogaerts et al. 2001 (484)	277 Patients with hematologic malignancies, aplastic anemia or having undergone BMT	Open, parallel, randomized, multicenter	IT (100 mg bid) vs amphotericin B/nystatin (AmB/N) (500 mg tid and 2 MU. QID)	Successful prophylaxis in 65% IT vs 53%—AmB/N Deep fungal infections—5% in each group Superficial fungal infections: 3% IT vs 8% PL; $p = .066$ Median time prophylactic failure: IT (37 days) vs AmpB (34 days) Nausea and rash: AmpB + Nystatin No difference in prophylactic efficacy

BMT, bone marrow transplant; LDAB, low-dose amphotericin B; MIC, miconazole; PL, placebo; FLU, fluconazole; IT, itraconazole.

TABLE 60.6. IMPACT OF LOW-DOSE AMPHOTERICIN B AMONG PATIENTS UNDERGOING HSCT

Study	*N*	Study Design	Amphotericin B Dose	Risk Population Studied	Effect
Rousey et al. 1991 (486)	186	Historic cohort study	20 mg/day during conditioning then every other day after BMT	Allogeneic recipients of T-cell–depleted grafts	Incidence of aspergillosis: 3.2% vs 8.9% Greater survival Mortality from *Aspergillus* decreased
Perfect et al. 1992 (487)	188	Randomized placebo-controlled	0.1 mg/kg	Autologous BMT (79% breast cancer)	Fungal infection mortality: ND Overall mortality: infection greater PL (Secondary to multisystem organ failure)
O'Donnell et al. 1994 (478)	331	Retrospective analysis	5–10 mg/d	Patients on steroids for acute GVHD	Fungal infection 29% vs 8%; (p = 0.0004) *Candida* infection 16 vs 3%; (p = 0.0003) *Aspergillus* infection 16 vs 6%; p = 0.36

ND, no difference; BMT, bone marrow transplant; PL, placebo.

overall and *Aspergillus*-specific mortality. When used among patients receiving corticosteroids for acute GVHD, low-dose amphotericin B reduced the risk for fungal infection from 29% to 8% (478). Infectious caused by *Candida* decreased more than those caused by *Aspergillus* (16% to 3% and 16% to 6%, respectively) (478). One investigator found that low-dose amphotericin B prophylaxis did not decrease fungal disease among autologous HSCT patients (487). None of the currently proposed regimens address the issue of late-onset *Aspergillus* infections in allogeneic HSCT patients. Efforts in this group have been limited to attempts at early detection of *Aspergillus* antigen in either blood or urine, but the poor positive and negative predictive values of these tests has prevented their widespread use. Other formulations of amphotericin B have also been studied, including an aerosolized form and a liposomal preparation. Liposomal amphotericin B (AmBisome) was evaluated as prophylaxis during the period of neutropenia, starting when the neutrophil count was less than 500/mm^3.

Ultimately, the selection of an appropriate prophylaxis protocol depends on the epidemiology at a given institution. Daily fluconazole prophylaxis is now recommended (104,438). However, institutions with high rates of fluconazole-resistant *Candida* infections may consider not using fluconazole prophylaxis and instead opt for low-dose amphotericin B. Newer azole agents have not been well studied, and recommendations for their use would be premature. Moreover, ongoing surveillance efforts are necessary to adjust prophylaxis strategies to an evolving microbiologic flora.

Antiviral Chemoprophylaxis

Cytomegalovirus

CMV disease causes significant morbidity and mortality among patients undergoing HSCT, even in the face of antiviral therapy. As such, much effort has been directed toward prevention of CMV disease. Two basic strategies for CMV prevention have been employed: use of antiviral agents in all patients (prophylactic therapy), and screening of at-risk populations for evidence of CMV shedding with early treatment of those patients with evidence of (preemptive therapy). All patients undergoing HSCT should undergo serum testing for anti-CMV antibodies before transplantation (104). In addition, the new HICPAC guidelines strongly recommend that all at risk allogenic HSCT recipients (CMV-seropositive HSCT recipients and CMV-seronegative recipients with a CMV-seropositive donor) should receive either prophylactic or pre-emptive treatment with ganciclovir, with pre-emptive therapy being preferred (104). Various trials have examined the efficacy of several antiviral agents including ganciclovir to prevent CMV infection and disease among HSCT patients (Table 7) (304,88–492).

The data supporting the importance of CMV prevention strategies in all patients for the first 100 days after HSCT is extremely strong (104). Various trials have examined the efficacy of several antiviral agents including ganciclovir to prevent CMV infection among HSCT patients (Table 60.7) (304,488–492). Goodrich et al. (489) evaluated prophylactic ganciclovir compared to placebo among 93 HSCT patients. CMV excretion was significantly decreased in the treatment arm (ganciclovir 3% vs. placebo 45%). While on therapy, one patient receiving ganciclovir developed CMV disease compared to nine patients in the placebo arm. However, there was no difference in mortality at 100 days (ganciclovir 12% vs. placebo 19%) and 180 days (ganciclovir 30% vs. placebo 26%). Three patients receiving ganciclovir developed late-onset CMV disease. Furthermore, neutropenia was significantly more frequent among patients receiving ganciclovir (30% vs. 0%), and these patients were more likely to develop bacterial infection (489). Winston et al. (490) administered ganciclovir (2.5 mg/kg every 8 hours) for 8 days prior to transplantation and again 6 mg/kg weekly from the time neutropenia resolved until 120 days post-HSCT. CMV shedding was significantly decreased (20% vs. 55%) but not CMV disease (10% vs. 24%). Again a significantly greater proportion of ganciclovir-treated patients developed neutropenia (58% vs. 28%), and there was no difference in mortality between the groups (490). These and other studies demonstrate the potential pitfalls of generalized ganciclovir prophylaxis. The high incidence of granulocytopenia potentially exposes a large number of patients who do not have CMV disease to the risk of neutropenic bacterial infections. Furthermore, prophylaxis does not prevent reactivation of CMV later in the patient's course after ganciclovir has been discontinued.

Newer antiviral agents have also been tested. In a large study involving 727 patients in 15 countries, investigators demonstrated valacyclovir was superior to acyclovir (493). In this ran-

TABLE 60.7. RANDOMIZED STUDIES EVALUATING REGIMENS TO PREVENT CYTOMEGALOVIRUS (CMV) DISEASE IN PATIENTS UNDERGOING HSCT

Study	*N*	Study Design	Intervention	Incidence CMV Diseases	Changes in Mortality
Bowden et al. 1986 (307)	97	Randomized trial	Intravenous CMV immunoglobulin and seronegative blood products (CMV-Ig)/neg BP); seronegative blood products alone (neg BP); globulin alone(CMV-Ig); neither (None)	(CMV-Ig)/(neg BP): 5% (neg BP): 13% (CMV-Ig): 24% (None): 40% Seronegative recipients who received negative blood products had less disease (1/32 vs 8/25; $p < .007$)	No mortality reported
Schmidt et al. 1991 (304)	104 BMT	Randomized observation	BAL + cultures and then randomization to ganciclovir (G) vs placebo (PL) in culture positive patients	Disease (pneumonia): 34/40 (85%) CMV positive 12/55 (22%) CMV negative	Culture positive: 5/25 (20%) with ganciclovir 14/20 (70%); RR =0.36; $p = 0.01$
Goodrich et al. 1991 (488)	72	Randomized, double-blind, placebo-controlled	PL vs G	Disease: 15/35 (43%) PL 1/37 (3%) ganciclovir; $p < .00001$	17% placebo vs 3% ganciclovir; $p = 0.04$ 100 days
Goodrich et al. 1993 (489)	93	Placebo-controlled	PL vs G	Infection: 14/31 (45%) placebo 1/33 (3%) ganciclovir Disease: (9/31) 29% placebo (0/31) 0% ganciclovir; $p < .001$	No difference ($p > .05$)
Winston et al. 1993 (490)	95	Placebo-controlled	PL vs G	Infection: 25/45 (56%) placebo 8/40 (20%) ganciclovir; $p < .001$ Disease: 11/45 (24%) placebo 4/40 (10%) ganciclovir; $p = .09$	No difference ($p > .05$)
Einsele et al. 1995 (491)	71	Randomized	Routine culture vs PCR for CMV	Disease: 8/34 (24%) culture 2/37 (5%) PCR; $p = .02$	Mortality 5/34 (15%) culture 0/37 (0%) PCR ($p = 0.02$)
Boeckh et al. 1996 (492)	226	Randomized, double-blind	Screening antigenemia vs ganciclovir	Disease (100 days): 32/226 (14%) antigenemia 6/226 (2.7%) ganciclovir; $p = .002$	No difference ($p > .05$)
Bowden et al. 1995 (542)	502	Prospective, randomized trial	Filtered CMV-negative blood products for CMV-negative BMT recipients	Infection in filtered vs nonfiltered 1.3% vs 2.4%; $p = 1.00$; disease (2.4% vs. 0%; $p = .03$	No mortality reported
Ljungman et al. 2002 (493)	727	Randomized, controlled, double-blind, multicenter trial	Intravenous acyclovir to all patients for 28 days; then oral valacyclovir or acyclovir	Disease; valacyclovir 102 (28%) vs acyclovir 143 (40%); HR 0.59; $p < .0001$	Survival: valacyclovir 76% vs acyclovir 75%
Humar et al. 2001 (543)	118	Randomized, prospective	Posttransplant preemptive screening with bronchoscopy (day 35) then cultures and antigens if signs and symptoms develop or weekly CMV antigenemia	Disease: bronchoscopy 7/58 (12.1%) vs CMV antigenemia 1/60 (1.7%) Presumptive ganciclovir: bronchoscopy 13.8% vs antigenemia 48.3%	No difference
Winston et al. 2003 (544)	168	Randomized	Valacyclovir (oral) vs ganciclovir (intravenous)	Infection: 10/830 (1.2%) valacyclovir vs 16/85 (19%) ganciclovir (HR 1,042; $p = .934$) Disease 2/83 (2%) valacyclovir vs 1/85 (1%) ganciclovir (HR 1,943; $p = .588$)	No mortality reported

ND, no difference; BMT, bone marrow transplant; PL, placebo.

domized, double-blind, placebo-controlled trial, CMV infection or disease developed in 102 (28%) valacyclovir patients, compared with 143 (40%) acyclovir patients (hazard ratio = 0.59; 95% CI, 0.46–0.76; p <.0001). Survival was similar in the two treatment arms (76% and 75% in the valacyclovir and acyclovir groups, respectively). Oral valacyclovir appeared as safe as high-dose oral acyclovir. More recently, Winston et al. (490) demonstrated in a randomized, multicenter trial on CMV-positive HSCT patients that valacyclovir is equally effective to ganciclovir. Patients received either oral valacyclovir, 2 g qid (n = 83), or intravenous ganciclovir, 5 mg/kg q12h for 1 week, then 6 mg/kg once daily for 5 days per week (n = 85), until day 100 after HSCT. CMV infection developed in 12% of the patients who received valacyclovir and in 19% of the patients who received ganciclovir [hazard ratio (HR) = 1.042; 95% CI, 0.391-2.778; p = .934]. CMV disease developed in only two patients who received valacyclovir and in one patient who received ganciclovir (HR = 1.943; 95% CI, 0.176–21.44; p = .588).

The preemptive treatment strategy relies on active surveillance for CMV shedding and initiation of treatment prior to the development of clinical CMV disease. A number of techniques have been employed to detect CMV shedding including shell-vial cultures, detection of pp65 antigen, and detection of CMV-DNA PCR. Shell-vial cultures can take up to 2 days to give a positive result and are therefore less useful in prompt detection of shedding. Detection of CMV pp65 antigen from peripheral white blood cells is currently the most common technique to detect viremia; however, false negative tests can occur if the patient is neutropenic. The highest levels of serum antigen are seen among patients with pneumonitis, gastroenteritis, and viremia. Overall, the positive predictive value for CMV disease in HSCT patients is 53% and the negative predictive value 91%, and the antigen test was positive a median of 10 days before cultures were positive in all pneumonitis patients (492). When compared to prophylactic ganciclovir (5 mg/kg twice a day for 5 days followed by daily ganciclovir until day 100), there was significantly more disease in the CMV antigenemia screening group than in the prophylaxis arm. Only high-grade antigenemia, defined as greater than three positive cells on two slides, was treated with conventional doses of ganciclovir, whereas 40% of patient had low-grade antigenemia. Overall mortality, however, was not affected as the ganciclovir-treated patients had a higher incidence of fungal infections. CMV-DNA PCR can be useful to detect CMV shedding in neutropenic patients; however, positive PCR results do not always correlate with disease. Nonetheless, positive CMV DNA PCR has also been shown to be useful in guiding pre-emptive therapy (491). Even though positive PCR results do not always correlate with disease, one study showed preemptive therapy based on positive CMV DNA PCR reduced the risk of developing CMV-associated and transplant-related mortality from 43.7% to 13% (491). In this study, the PCR was always positive before culture, and although more patients inthe PCR group received ganciclovir, the duration of therapy based on a negative PCR following treatment, was shorter than in the group that depended on culture for CMV detection (491). Currently there is no benefit to routinely administering ganciclovir to HSCT patients who are greater than 100 days posttransplant (104). However, antiviral therapy should be continued after 100 days in HSCT patients in whom virus can be detected.

Controversy still remains regarding the relative merits of both approaches to prevent CMV disease in HSCT patients. Given the potential toxicity of ganciclovir in terms of delayed marrow recovery, better means of defining patients at risk are needed. Currently there is no benefit to routinely administering ganciclovir to HSCT patients who are greater than 100 days post transplant (104). However, antiviral therapy should continue after 100 days in HSCT where virus can be detected.

Other Viruses

Two studies suggest that acyclovir prevents varicella infection (494,495). However, this strategy has not been evaluated among patients undergoing HSCT. Acyclovir may decrease the morbidity associated with VZV infections. Among 40 HSCT patients who were treated with acyclovir for VZV infection, virus was cultured for 2.1 days, and pustules formed, crusted, and healed for a median of 3.5, 8, and 28 days, respectively (496).

Acyclovir should be offered prophylactically to all allogeneic HSCT patients who are HSV seropositive (104). This strategy prevents reactivation of disease. Prophylaxis should be initiated with the conditioning regimen and continued until engraftment occurs or mucositis resolves. Several studies have shown that oral acyclovir prevents the reactivation of oral HSV infections (497, 498). Eighty percent of seropositive patients excrete HSV during the first 50 days after transplantation (70). In contrast, fewer than 1% of seronegative patients excrete virus. Wade et al. (498) gave acyclovir or placebo to 49 HSCT patients for 5 weeks beginning 1 week before transplantation. Five of 24 patients receiving acyclovir developed HSV infection during prophylaxis, compared to 17 of 25 patients receiving placebo (p <.01). The median time to first virus reactivation was significantly longer among patients receiving acyclovir (78 vs. 9 days after transplant, p = .006). Among patients taking a minimum of 40% of their prescribed drug, acyclovir was 96% virologically effective and 100% clinically effective during the period of administration. Preliminary data for valacyclovir prophylaxis suggest that adverse events (hemolytic uremic syndrome and thrombotic thrombocytopenic purpura) should limit its use at this point (104).

Prophylaxis for Other Opportunistic Infections

Prophylaxis with TMP-SMX has been shown to prevent PCP in immunocompromised patients (104,362,438,462). Prophylaxis should be administered from engraftment (or before engraftment if it is delayed) until 6 months for all allogeneic HSCT recipients and for greater than 6 months if patients are receiving immunosuppressive therapy or have chronic GVHD (104). Patients undergoing autologous HSCT should receive prophylaxis if they have underlying hematologic malignancy, receive intense conditioning regimens, or have received fludarabine or 2-CDA (104). Although controversial, prophylaxis with TMP-SMX is not recommended for the prevention of toxoplasmosis in seropositive recipients of allogeneic HSCT (104).

Prophylaxis for Communicable Disease Exposure

Infection control personnel should evaluate HSCT patients who are exposed to communicable diseases based on hospital policy. Personnel need to assess the amount of exposure, how infectious the microorganism is, how it is transmitted, and how immunocompromised the patient is. In several situations additional interventions may be needed. HSCT patients who are not immunocompetent and who are susceptible to varicella and exposed should receive varicella-zoster immunoglobulin (VZIg) within 72 to 96 hours of exposure. Exposure is defined as sharing a room with an infected patient or prolonged face-to-face contact with an infectious person (338). Adults should receive 125 U/10 kg or a maximum of 625 U (338). Acyclovir should be administered preemptively to HSCT patients who are immunocompromised and exposed to VZV infections. Antivirals should be continued for 2 days after the lesions are crusted. Limited data with valacyclovir are available to guide recommendations (104). The varicella vaccine is contraindicated in patients until 24 months after HSCT (104). An inactivated vaccine is being studied currently.

Antiviral agents with activity against influenza, such as amantadine, rimantadine or the newer neuraminidase inhibitors (oseltamivir, zanamivir), are indicated for preemptive therapy (or prophylaxis) during outbreaks and may be administered during influenza season while influenza-like illness is present in the community. Amantadine and rimantadine are preferred for influenza A outbreaks, whereas the neuraminidase inhibitors that have influenza A and B activity should be used for known influenza B outbreaks or in settings where the type of influenza has not been identified. These agents have been used in the setting of influenza in HSCT patients, although little information is available about the efficacy in these patients. Several investigators have used amantadine to protect HSCT patients and found that virus is shed from these patients for 5 to 12 days despite therapy with amantadine (283,499).

Prophylaxis should be administered to patients exposed to *Neisseria meningitidis* infections. Guidelines for prophylaxis of patients exposed to *N. meningitidis* pneumonia should be individualized. One outbreak in the literature describes five oncology patients hospitalized on the same hospital unit, but not in adjacent rooms, who developed *N. meningitidis* colonization or infection (500). The index patient had *N. meningitidis* pneumonia. Based on the extensive transmission associated with this cluster, we believe more liberal standards for prophylaxis are indicated in HSCT patients exposed to patients with *N. meningitidis* pneumonia.

Vaccines for influenza and hepatitis B and the pneumococcal vaccine should be administered to patients undergoing HSCT. These vaccinations are important in preventing infections that occur late after HSCT. The American College of Physicians recommends annual influenza vaccination of immunocompromised individuals and their family members before the winter season. HSCT patients may be vaccinated as soon as 6 months after transplantation. The vaccine has been shown to be efficacious in healthy individuals but may not stimulate an adequate antibody response in individuals receiving chemotherapy. All healthcare workers and staff working on HSCT units should receive an annual influenza vaccination.

Antibiotic Management and Stewardship

Similar to a trend reported in hospitals across the U.S., Ena et al. (501) found that vancomycin use increased 20-fold at one tertiary care center from 1981 to 1991. They also noted that vancomycin use was mostly inappropriate; only one third of vancomycin use was directed against microorganisms resistant to β-lactam antibiotics or used in persons with documented penicillin allergies. Because vancomycin use is a consistent risk factor for colonization and infection with VRE, the CDC developed a set of guidelines that distinguish between appropriate and inappropriate uses of vancomycin (Table 60.2). These guidelines do not support vancomycin use to eradicate MRSA colonization, to treat β-lactam–sensitive microorganisms for convenient dosing, or in response to a single blood culture positive for coagulase-negative staphylococci. The HICPAC guidelines can be modified to best reflect the epidemiology of antibiotic resistance in a geographic area, e.g., the prevalence of MRSA or penicillin-resistant *S. pneumoniae* and the needs in HSCT patients. Nonetheless, efforts to reduce vancomycin use are important. A strict vancomycin-restriction policy can decrease both the overall and the inappropriate use of vancomycin by as much as 50% (170,502). Implementation of modified CDC guidelines resulted in a 40% reduction in vancomycin use in the Johns Hopkins Hospital Oncology Center in Baltimore, Maryland, without any adverse effects on patients.

Antibiotic management including rotation of antibiotics has been proposed as an adjunct to traditional infection control to impact on antimicrobial resistance. Several investigators have proposed antibiotic rotation as a strategy to decrease resistance. Studies have been limited by selection bias, insufficient power, and the failure to control for confounders, including the specific microorganism-drug combination studied, the degree and effectiveness of infection control efforts, the community burden of resistance and the "colonization" pressure, behaviors that may enhance survival of microorganisms, and antimicrobial use outside the hospital. In one study, the authors attempted to decrease the VRE colonization in a hematologic malignancy ward (181). Using a crossover study with 2- to 4-month cycles, empiric use of ceftazidime for neutropenic fevers was associated with a 57% VRE colonization rate. Five infections were reported. In the second phase, piperacillin/tazobactam was used for empiric treatment of neutropenic fevers and the VRE colonization rate decreased to 29%. No infections were identified. In a third cycle patients were treated empirically for neutropenic fevers with ceftazidime alone. The VRE colonization rose to 36%, and three infections were described. A second study on a 20-bed oncology unit evaluated 271 patients over a year (1994–1995) (503). Patients received one of four empiric antibiotic regimens for neutropenic fevers. These regimens were cycled every 4 months with a planned 4-month "washout" period. The regimens included (a) ceftazidime and vancomycin; (b) imipenem; (c) aztreonam and cefazolin; and (d) ciprofloxacin and clindamycin. Forty-two percent completed therapy with the cycle regimen. Almost 80% of the antimicrobial switches were due to persistent fever, 14% were due to breakthrough bacteremia, and 7% related to drug toxicity. There was no impact on enterococcal resistance in the hospital.

Isolation and Barrier Precautions

Isolation and the use of barrier precautions are implemented to prevent patients, fellow patients, or healthcare workers from acquiring communicable diseases or pathogenic microorganisms. Many programs use protective isolation or reverse precautions; however, the data do not support their use among HSCT patients. Most centers now recommend the use of standard precautions (391). Nauseef and Maki (504) compared reverse isolation to standard care and randomized 17 patients (20 episodes) to simple protective isolation (437 days) and 20 patients (23 episodes) to standard care (611 days). No statistically significant differences were observed in the overall incidence of infection, time to onset of first infection, or days with fever. Twenty-seven infections occurred in recipients of standard care (4.4 per 100 days), and 28 infections in isolated patients (6.4 per 100 days). Except for a threefold higher rate of bacteremia among patients in isolation (2.1 vs. 0.7 per 100 days), the profile of infection was similar in the two groups.

We believe that the CDC/HICPAC isolation guidelines for hospitalized patients apply in many respects to HSCT patients (505). The guidelines are formulated using two levels of protection: one is standard and applied to all patients, and the other is based on the potential of disease or microorganism transmission. This new system replaces the previous disease-specific isolation guidelines and has integrated universal precautions and body substance precautions to protect healthcare workers. HSCT units should adopt these isolation and barrier precautions, although some modifications are necessary.

For example, CDC/HICPAC isolation guidelines recommend that VRE-colonized or -infected patients be placed in single rooms, whereas most experts recommend any patient undergoing HSCT be housed in a private room (392). CDC/HICPAC guidelines recommend that healthcare workers wear gloves on entry into the patient's room. We also recommend that gowns be worn upon entering the patient room, irrespective of intent to touch the patient or his/her immediate environment. Gloves and gowns should be discarded before leaving the room. Two studies have shown that gowns and gloves are superior to gloves in preventing transmission of VRE among patients (506, 507). HICPAC guidelines recommend Contact Precautions for all patients infected or colonized with MRSA to prevent transmission of this microorganism (104). Likewise, to prevent transmission of RSV special barriers may be necessary. Gala et al. (508) showed that eye-nose goggles significantly reduced the number of healthcare workers and susceptible infants who developed RSV infection. They noted that 5% of healthcare workers wearing goggles developed RSV infection compared to 34% who did not wear goggles. Likewise, when healthcare workers used these barriers, one child (6%) developed nosocomial RSV infection compared to 43% of children exposed to healthcare workers not wearing goggles. Hence, additional barriers may be required with an extremely vulnerable population. Our experience in the Johns Hopkins Children's Center found that additional barriers reduced RSV transmission among children and we have now expanded the program to all HSCT and leukemia patients (295).

HSCT patients who are infected with varicella should be placed on Airborne and Contact Precautions in a room with negative air pressure (338,505). The CDC recommends that susceptible patients be placed in isolation from 8 to 10 days after exposure to 21 days after exposure or up to 28 days after exposure if VZIg is administered (104,338). Contact Precautions should be continued for 2 days after lesions are crusted. Airborne Precautions are required from 10 to 21 days after the patient was exposed. This isolation must be continued for 28 days after exposure if the patient receives VZIg. Other examples of infectious diseases that require additional isolation include tuberculosis, *N. meningitidis, Yersinia pestis,* MRSA, and scabies, to name a few. Consult the institutional guidelines for disease specific recommendations (see also Chapter 95).

Personal Effects

The role of personal effects in increasing the risk of infection among patients undergoing HSCT is not well studied. Logically, clothes should be clean. Personal effects, toys, and equipment should not make cleaning of the room impossible. In an attempt to improve patient comfort, rooms can become crowded with personal items. These items can collect dust and be difficult to clean. Toys including stuffed animals should be cleaned at least weekly (104). Cleaning procedures are suggested in the HICPAC guidelines (104). Furthermore, it is never clear who should be responsible for cleaning a patient's personal items. One group of investigators cultured teddy bears and found that all had become colonized with bacteria, fungi, or both within a week of hospitalization, and concomitant cultures from patients revealed similar isolates (509). Thus, personal effects should be limited to those that can be disposed of or easily cleaned (104). Water-retaining toys should not be allowed (104,510). Rooms should not become so cluttered with these items that they cannot be cleaned.

Personal Hygiene

Damage to the oral cavity caused by cytotoxic, infectious, and hemorrhagic complications of GVHD is reflected by the severity of the mucositis. The oral cavity is a reservoir for microorganisms. The microorganisms accounting for most oral infections are HSV and *C. albicans* (51). By reducing the number of oral microorganisms through optimal care, the risk of developing a life-threatening systemic infection from an oral source may be reduced. Many HSCT caregivers believe that brushing teeth increases the risk of bacteremia and bleeding. However, problems are more likely to arise when patients are not compliant with good oral hygiene practices (511). Aggressive dental and oral hygiene interventions can ameliorate oral complications prior to transplantation, as elimination of oral infection is paramount for the success of HSCT (104). Daily showers and good perineal care are recommended to optimize skin care (104). Most HSCT teams do not restrict showers, although some have started questioning the role of showers in possible skin erosion and transmission of nosocomial microorganisms to which these patients may be susceptible. In addition to the risk of *Legionella* infections, some authorities suggest water may be a source of fungi (166). Studies are warranted to determine whether showers protect or put at risk hospitalized HSCT patients.

Environmental Controls

Dedicated Equipment

Equipment can be contaminated when exposed to patients, the contaminated hands of healthcare workers, or, rarely, other contaminated equipment (512). Surfaces can remain contaminated with VRE, *C. difficile*, and RSV for long periods of time (75,165,512). Outbreaks have been traced to contaminated equipment (168,169,512). Equipment used for patients with *C. difficile*, SARS, epidemiologically important microorganisms, and VRE should be for their use only (74,75,86,99,162,166). Supplies and equipment should be monitored for dust or potential mold contamination. Sterile dressings and supplies contiguous to the skin should be used for these patients. Similarly, the CDC isolation guidelines recommend cleaning of equipment between patients and, where appropriate, assignment of dedicated equipment to isolated patients to prevent the transmission of nosocomial pathogens (505).

Plants and Fresh Flowers

Plants, fresh flowers, and vases have been shown to harbor bacteria and other microorganisms that are pathogenic for immunocompromised patients. Within 3 days of fresh flowers being placed in water, the water contains up to 1×10^{13} CFU of bacteria per milliliter of water (27). When cultured, *P. aeruginosa, Burkholderia cepacia, P. alcaligenes, A. hydrophila, Acinetobacter* species, *Flavobacterium* species, *E. coli, Klebsiella* species, and *Proteus mirabilis* may be recovered (27). Other authors have found that water cultured from flower vases in hospitals may contain pathogenic fungi as well (28). The microorganism counts increased logarithmically and significantly ($p < .0005$) over time and were not different if distilled or sterile water was substituted for tap water (27). Both Taplin and Mertz (27) and Kates et al. (28) found that water obtained from flower vases contains microorganisms that are highly resistant to antimicrobial agents. Because of these data, most HSCT units do not allow fresh flowers or live plants to be brought in to patients. A recent study found that introducing fresh flowers into the rooms of nonneutropenic, non-HSCT patients did not increase the number of fungi isolated (513). If fresh flowers are allowed, water should be changed every 48 hours and terminal cleaning performed when the patient leaves.

Filtration of Air

Ventilation systems must have certain capacities and should be maintained to protect such high-risk patients (140). HSCT patients, especially allogeneic recipients, should be placed in rooms with greater than 12 air exchanges per hour (104). Airflow should be directed and enter one side of the room and be exhausted from the opposite side. In addition, air pressures should be maintained so that the patient's room is at least 2.5 pascal higher than any adjoining corridors, anterooms, or bathrooms. This requires that rooms be well sealed around windows, electrical outlets, and other sources of air. Based on a large amount of data showing that filtered air decreases the risk of invasive fungal disease, the evidence-based guidelines for preventing opportunistic infections among HSCT recipients recommend several air filtration strategies, such as air filtration with point-of-use HEPA filtration that removes 99.97% of particles greater than 0.3 μm in size (104). Some institutions have built laminar airflow (LAF) rooms, which are more efficient than HEPA filtration alone but are more expensive. We are unaware of any trials that compare HEPA filtration alone to use of LAF. The current guidelines do not recommend LAF. The efficacy of portable machines with HEPA filters is less well studied. Nonetheless, even in rooms or units with HEPA filtration or LAF, the risk of *Aspergillus* infection does not decrease to zero. Patients are still exposed to the ambient air when transported to other areas such as the radiology department. Point-of-use HEPA filters are recommended for allogeneic HSCT and autologous HSCT, especially those with prolonged neutropenia. These recommendations are especially important to implement during periods of construction and renovation. Although we are unaware of data supporting the use, we have patients at Johns Hopkins Hospital wear an N95 mask when they are out of their rooms, outside the hospital, or near construction areas.

Based on extensive epidemiologic data, HSCT patients should be placed in private rooms with specialized air filtration. These recommendations are generated from the experience of multiple investigators. Many investigators have found a significant decrease in *Aspergillus* in air samples and infections among patients with hematologic malignancies and with HSCT (Table 60.8) (44,45,218,221,514). For example, one of these investigators reported 32% (6/19) of the children undergoing HSCTs died of invasive pulmonary aspergillosis during an *Aspergillus* outbreak associated with construction (221). With use of LAF rooms, no more cases of invasive pulmonary aspergillosis occurred (221). More importantly, Passweg et al. (515) compared a group of allogeneic HSCT patients placed in conventional protective isolation (single patient room and any combination of hand washing, gloves, mask, and gown) to a group placed in HEPA-filtered LAF rooms. These investigators found a significantly higher 1-year survival rate and decreased overall risk of transplant-related mortality in the first 100 days posttransplantation in the group treated in HEPA-filtered LAF units compared to those treated by conventional protective isolation.

Other investigators have examined the importance of other interventions in the setting of HEPA filtration or LAF rooms. At least two studies have shown that LAF rooms and gastrointestinal decontamination decrease infection rates and decrease adverse outcomes (516,517). Buckner et al. (516) found that patients in LAF rooms with gastrointestinal tract decontamination had a decreased severity of illness and required fewer granulocyte transfusions (5/46 vs. 22/44; $p < .0001$). Several other investigators advocate use of LAF rooms and sterile diet, gastrointestinal decontamination, and skin cleansing to prevent infections in granulocytopenic patients (515,518–520). However, it is unclear from the currently available literature whether adding sterile diets or skin cleansing to specialized air filtration and antibacterial prophylaxis prevents additional infections (517). To reiterate, HSCT patients, especially allogeneic transplants, should be placed in private rooms with HEPA filtration of air (point of use) with at least 12 air exchanges per hour or an LAF room (104,526). These rooms should be under positive pressure

TABLE 60.8. IMPACT OF DIFFERENT TYPES OF AIR FILTRATION AND THE INCIDENCE OF NOSOCOMIAL ASPERGILLOSIS IN HSCT

Study	Type of Air Filtration	Aspergillus Spore Counts (CFU/m^3)	Incidence of Nosocomial Aspergillosis
Rhame et al. 1984 (44)	Post-HEPA (2 × 4 foot HEPA filter in the room)	2.0 0.8	10/66 (15%) 17/202 (8%)
Rhame et al. 1985 (514)	Post-HEPA (addition of HEPA filter in the corridor)	0.14	4/97 (4%)
Opal et al. 1986 (218)	Portable HEPA filters: Inside rooms Outside rooms	0.8 ± 0.003 1.7 ± 0.2	43 cases/yr 19 cases/yr ($p < .005$)
Sherertz et al. 1987 (45)	Pre-HEPA Post-HEPA (LAF)	0.16–0.40 0.009	11/33 (33%) 0/31 (0%)
Barnes et al. 1989 (221)	Pre-LAF Post-LAF	133 0	6/19 (32%) 0/19 (0%)
Perraud et al. 1992 (545)	Pre-HEPA HEPA	2–24 0–4 ($p < .05$)	Not reported
Loo et al. 1996 (227)	Pre-HEPA HEPA	0–11 0–2 ($p < .05$)	
Mahieu et al. 2000 (546)	HEPA HEPA (during construction)	11 (0–30 CFU/m^3) 397 (17–2,823 CFU/m^3)	Not specified when obtained (6/311 colonized)
Richardson et al. 2000 (547)	Pre-HEPA Portable HEPA filter	0–206 0–15	Not available
Hahn et al. 2002 (229)	Pre-HEPA Post-HEPA		10/55 (18%) 0/36 (0%)
Engelhart et al. 2003 (in press) (548)	Pre-HEPA Portable HEPA filters	8.1 (<0.8–42 CFU/m^3) 5.3 (<0.8–41 CFU/m^3)	0.8/1,000 patient-days in nonfiltered rooms to 0 ($p = 0.33$)

HEPA, high-efficiency particulate air; LAF, laminar airflow.

with respect to the corridors. Although this technology is expensive, the data support improved patient outcomes.

There are no clear guidelines on when or how to monitor the air in a HSCT unit. We follow the CDC guidelines for nosocomial pneumonia and recommend monitoring the air if a case of nosocomial pneumonia caused by *Aspergillus* is identified (104,394). Air should be sampled if additional cases are identified while a source is investigated, with ongoing construction, and prior to opening units to high-risk patients. Air samples should be taken using a high-volume air sampler. Low-volume air samplers are not effective for detection of the low numbers of microorganisms that can be of concern among these patients (46).

The CDC recommends negative pressure rooms with additional special engineering requirements (six to 12 air exchanges per hour and air exhausted to the outside) to prevent transmission of varicella, but other authors suggest negative pressure alone is adequate (338,340). Anderson et al. (340) showed no nosocomial transmission of varicella among 110 susceptible patients who were hospitalized on wards with patients who had varicella. These authors compared this experience to a historical experience in an older hospital without negative pressure rooms. Seven of 41 (17%) susceptible patients hospitalized on the same ward with patients with varicella subsequently developed varicella (see also Chapters 42 and 89).

Construction and Renovation

Construction and renovation projects are common in many hospitals as they strive to update facilities. Construction, whether minor or major, poses special problems for patients undergoing HSCT. Because of their immunosuppression, patients are at risk of developing infections from microorganisms released from construction sites, or from destruction of existing structures and renovation, or from the water supply. Construction, renovation, and maintenance have caused outbreaks of *Aspergillus* infections among patients with altered skin integrity (burns and very premature infants), patients with hematologic malignancies, and those undergoing HSCT (Table 60.9). This association with construction has been based on geographic proximity, temporal relationships, the finding of *Aspergillus* in the environment and supporting molecular typing data, and the control of these infections with appropriate interventions. Despite the lack of direct proof, few people dispute the relationship. Hence any construction or renovation project requires a multidisciplinary team to review the plans for demolition and construction, placement of barriers, and egress and entry to areas (140). All institutions should have a policy for construction and renovation that allows hospital staff to assess the risks any project could pose to patients. Such construction policies should be part of contracts if outside contractors are used for institutionally based projects. Contractors should have back up equipment available and onsite.

The numbers of *Aspergillus* spores in unfiltered ambient air has been measured in several locales and varies from 0.1 to 15 CFU/m^3. The numbers vary with wind, weather conditions, and season (218,521). Streifel et al. (522) showed that the numbers and concentrations of thermotolerant fungi, especially *A. fumigatus*, increase significantly after demolition of a hospital building. The concentration of thermotolerant fungi and *A. fumigatus*

TABLE 60.9. GENERAL RECOMMENDATIONS FOR PREVENTION OF NOSOCOMIAL ASPERGILLOSIS AND OTHER INVASIVE FUNGAL INFECTIONS AMONG HSCT PATIENTS

Category	Specific Element
Ventilation	HEPA filtration or laminar airflow
	Maintain appropriate pressure relationships
	Check window seals, stairwells, vents, ducts
	Maintain >12 air exchanges per hour
Environment	Eliminate carpet and other sources of dust
	Clean rooms (all surfaces) at least daily for dust control
	Avoid dust generating activities (use wet mopping, HEPA vacuuming)
	Eliminate flowers, potted ornamental plants
	Remove wet or damp areas; repair water leaks
	Keep windows closed
	Develop and maintain strict cleaning procedures
	Eliminate areas where water or condensation can collect
	Clean area after any renovation or construction
	Only use toys that can be cleaned and disinfected
	Toys should be routinely cleaned
Personal hygiene	Have patients wear masks (N-95) when out of protected environment
	Consider other protective environments (mobile tents)
	Avoid unprocessed food; certain beans and raw fruits
Construction	Develop policy for construction and renovation with risk levels (see example, Appendix B)
	Seal off construction areas and place under negative pressure; use rigid dust proof barriers; seal doors, etc.
	During outdoor construction seal intake air
	Clean area daily if within the hospital or buildings
	Treat fireproofing with fungicide (copper-8-quinolinolate)
	Assure filters properly sealed in new buildings
	Minimize patient exposure to high-risk activities
	Minimize the traffic through construction area
	Exhaust construction dust
Surveillance	Define disease and find cases of nosocomial infection
	Use large-volume (1,200 L) air samplers to detect *Aspergillus* or fungal spores
	Monitor air and/or environment for *Aspergillus* species if suspected nosocomial infections occur
Cleaning rooms	An oncology patient room must be terminally cleaned (whether occupied or vacant)
	Use thorough cleaning procedures to ensure daily decontamination and cleanliness of the room
	Using approved solutions, remove fingerprints and smudges from light switches, door frames, walls, window sills, and glass; spray the solution on the cleaning cloth or carefully on the wall surface to prevent exposure
Waste removal	Put on gloves, grasp the liner twist and tie closed
	Remove the liner from the basket and replace with a new liner
	Place the waste in a trash cart approved by infection control; wash hands thoroughly again and put on new gloves
Sanitation	Carry all supplies needed into room; make up fresh germicidal solution in the one-gallon pail and in the mop bucket for each room
	Begin sanitizing the room
	Work in a counterclockwise direction around the sanitized surfaces above and below shoulder height
	Move personal belongings temporarily to clean surface areas
	Clean all surfaces including bedside rails, headboard, footboard, and nurse call control (if discharge also clean frame, springs, and wheels); clean ledges, over bed tables, desk tops, telephone (receiver, cord, base, and dial pad), chairs, furniture, door frames and closet bureau outside and top only if room is occupied, and entire unit including top if room is vacated; if the overhead light is surface mounted rather than recessed, wipe with a damp cloth and germicidal solution; clean vents and hard-to-reach areas with a wall mop treated with germicidal solution
	Sanitize the floor by wet mopping with an approved solution; start at the far end of the room and work toward the door; mop around edges of the floor, being careful to remove any dirt from the corners; mop the remainder of the floor, avoid splashing walls and baseboards
	Change mops between each patient room
Restock supplies and inspect room	Wash hands thoroughly again and put on new gloves; replace soap and paper products in restroom and at the sink; if a discharge, make the patient bed according to discharge procedures; area cleaner inspects room to see that all steps have been covered and the room meets approval
	Notify nursing manager or responsible administrator and maintenance of leaks, wet dry wall, or water damage
Cleaning bathroom	Using an approved solution, wipe down surfaces, lower ledges, and pipes of the sink; for more aggressive sink cleaning, use a scouring cleanser to remove soil or stain buildup; clean the mirror with glass cleaner and wipe dry with paper towels; thoroughly clean all ceiling vents, shelves, cabinets, and waste baskets with germicide
	Pay special attention to corners, soap dish, and drain in showers and sinks; sanitize the shower with germicide and a cleaning cloth; wipe the ceramic tile to prevent a soap buildup; check the shower curtain for possible replacement; clean inside toilet bowel with an approved cleanser and clean the outer bowl with an approved germicidal solution, sanitize the inside of the toilet and urinal using a bowl mop saturated with germicide solution; the bowl mop should be worked around, making sure to get into the upper and lower ledges; accidental spills can be cleaned up by flushing with water and wiping the surface dry; the outside surface of the toilet is sanitized by applying germicide on a cleaning cloth and wiping the external surface of the fixture
Administrative	Clean room at least daily
	Terminally clean room on patient discharge or at least every 3 weeks

HEPA, high-efficiency particulate air.

increased by 1.8×10^2 to 10^5 and 3.3×10 to 10^4, respectively, after the building's demolition. Because of these data, construction standards are required for any unit housing HSCT patients (Table 60.9 and Appendix B). These include many elements such as placing appropriate barriers, sealing the barriers, moving high-risk patients away from construction, using negative pressure and HEPA filtration and assuring that the air handling system is functioning properly, and exhausting construction dust appropriately. Because of the risk of transmission of *Aspergillus* or other microorganisms in the air handling systems, construction personnel must work with the institution's engineers to isolate heating and ventilation systems. In addition, airtight barriers have been found to significantly reduce the number of *Aspergillus* spores from 4.2 ± 0.4 spores/m^3 inside the barrier to 1.0 ± 0.3 spores/m^3 outside the barrier (218). Spore counts were also obtained from adjacent hospital units and found to be highest on the floor directly below construction (2.3 ± 1.3 spores/m^3 below the construction site and 1.1 ± 0.6 spores/m^3 in adjacent wards). Implosions require concurrent monitoring to determine whether the air handling system will require manipulation (523). Srinivasan et al. (523) did serial measurements in adjacent buildings and city blocks when a building was imploded near a cancer center. They found that one could easily react to the movement of the debris cloud produced by the implosion, because normal operation of the hospital air handling systems was able to accommodate the modest increase in *Aspergillus,* other fungi, and particles generated by the implosion. In addition, air samples containing *Aspergillus* species were paralleled by particle counts, suggesting these can be used to guide any interventions.

Fireproofing can harbor microorganisms including *Aspergillus.* Copper-8-quinolinolate, a fungicide, is used to decontaminate environmental surfaces. It is highly active against clinically important fungi including *Aspergillus* species and has been used to control several outbreaks (215). It also has the advantage of having persistent antifungal activity and will theoretically prevent fungi or molds from growing if subsequent water damage occurs. Opal et al. (218) cultured a mean of 4.9 ± 1.5 *Aspergillus* spores/m^3 from environmental surfaces in a hospital unit before they were treated with copper-8-quinolinolate. After treating surfaces with this fungicide, a mean of 0.1 ± 0.1 *Aspergillus* spores/m^3 were cultured. Construction traffic patterns should be directed to allow for efficient waste disposal through garbage chutes. If not feasible, construction waste should be removed in covered bins. Floors should be cleaned following the removal of construction waste. Construction personnel should avoid traversing areas where high-risk patients are located. Protective clothing may be appropriate to prevent dissemination of microorganisms into the air. Traffic should be directed away from construction.

Recently, a promising study by Cooper et al. (524) demonstrated what many hospital epidemiologists have known anecdotally. These authors found that the construction measures described above were effective is controlling the amount of ambient *Aspergillus* and *Aspergillus* disease. *Aspergillus* was isolated rarely. The amounts of viable pathogenic fungi were similar between areas under construction and those that were not. There was no difference in the incidence of invasive aspergillosis between 2000 and 2001 (incidence density ratio, 1.2; 95% CI, 0.3 to 4.1).

After construction, one must ensure that the new filters are properly seated. In one hospital, particle counts ranged from 247 to 1,629/m^3 before the new filters were reseated (525). After appropriate installation of the filters, the particle counts decreased to 20 to 35 particles/m^3. We recommend visual inspections to determine whether or not water damage has occurred. Based on the experience of Rhame (526), we further recommend obtaining air samples prior to opening such areas to patients. Finally, other situations warrant evaluation. Gerson et al. (224) reported an outbreak related to carpet tile that was contaminated after a fire. Hence, when damage occurs in a unit due to fire or water, infection control personnel need to inspect the area and consider air and environmental sampling (see also Chapter 88).

Cleaning the Environment

The overall cleanliness of the unit is important. Every hospital should develop a very detailed policy for thorough cleaning of the environment (Table 60.9). Cleaning is required after patients are discharged from a hospital room, or after a patient is seen in the outpatient clinic. If a dedicated clinic room is provided, cleaning at the end of the day may suffice. Many microorganisms can contaminate the environment through contaminated secretions or through transmission on contaminated hands. Because these microorganisms survive in harsh conditions, thorough cleaning is indicated with the appropriate disinfectant. With the exception of hydrogen peroxide (3%), isopropyl alcohol and most disinfectants (sodium hypochlorite, phenolic, and quaternary ammonium compounds) are effective against VRE (527). To prevent transmission of *C. difficile,* phenol-containing disinfectants are recommended for decontamination of inanimate objects and environmental surfaces (75). In an HSCT unit, cleaning and decontamination need to be directed at removing microorganisms that survive in the environment. Accumulation of dust should be prevented. Furthermore, cleaning activities should not generate dust (Table 60.9) (104). Thus, surfaces should be wiped with wet cloths and mops. Special HEPA vacuums are available for areas that have carpeting (104). Anderson et al. (225) noted that airborne *A. fumigatus* rose from 24 CFU/m^3 before vacuuming to 62 CFU/m^3 while the vacuum was being used. A defective disposal conduit door allowed for dispersal of a contaminated aerosol from the ward vacuum cleaner (see also Chapters 77 and 85).

Water and Water Treatment

Water treatment beyond that provided by municipal water systems is primarily aimed at preventing nosocomial *Legionella* infections. Prevention strategies vary by institution and depend on the immunologic status of the patients, the design and construction of the facility, the available resources, and state and local health department regulations (528). Plans to maintain the water systems for healthcare facilities with HSCT patients should be multifaceted, and vary if the response is to a nosocomial *Legionella* case or to colonization (104,112,140). Strategies may include decontamination followed by a maintenance phase. Several caveats must be considered in any plan to treat water and to prevent *Legionella* infections. First, in the initial phase, the effectiveness of a water treatment plan in a hospital water distribution system should be assessed long-term, over 3 to 5 years. Second, most strategies to treat hospital water distribution systems have not been compared to each other. Hence, one is forced to look at the characteristics of the water system in the institution and choose the best engineering and most cost-effective option.

Surveillance for nosocomial *Legionella* in the water is the ultimate test of the efficacy of any water treatment plan. If this approach is taken, a comprehensive plan will provide the most useful information (104,140). Appropriate diagnostic tests must be used to evaluate patients with nosocomial pneumonia and to diagnose *Legionella* infections (104,529). Targeting high-risk patients such as those who have undergone transplantation has been proposed and has the advantage of being cost-efficient (528,530). Goetz and Yu (530) suggest that culturing the water supply and targeting high-risk patients for specialized *Legionella* laboratory tests may help clinicians discover *Legionella* cases in the absence of an outbreak. One strategy requires periodic culturing of the potable water system if more than 30% of cultures of distal outlets (faucets) yield *Legionella* species, or if the system has been decontaminated (531). However, the two HICPAC guidelines that review the benefits of routine environmental sampling found the evidence did not support this practice (104, 140). Documentation of environmental sources of *Legionella* or a case of nosocomial infection should prompt active surveillance, looking for clinical cases and a source of *Legionella*. This approach is based on the theory that in the absence of *Legionella* in water cultures, no cases of nosocomial legionellosis can occur (528). In this case the potable water system, potable water outlets in the patients room, and cooling towers should be cultured by a laboratory with expertise in processing environmental samples. In addition, other potential sources including humidifiers, nebulizers, fountains, irrigation equipment, whirlpools, and ice machines should be investigated. For HSCT we favor the second approach, which includes (a) monitoring the environment (water) serially, (b) obtaining the appropriate diagnostic tests for *Legionella* in patients with nosocomial pneumonia, and (c) investigating the environment when one confirmed or two suspected cases are identified (528,530). Further details of surveillance strategies are outlined in Chapter 35.

If such environmental surveillance cultures yield *Legionella*, the water supply should be decontaminated (see Chapter 35); HSCT patients should be restricted from bathing or showering in *Legionella* contaminated water; water from faucets should not be used in the HSCT area, and sterile water should be used by patients for drinking, brushing teeth, or flushing nasogastric tubes. Disinfection of water supplies can be accomplished by several methods. "Superheat and flush" and hyperchlorination are the two most common measures used for disinfecting the water system (140). Recommendations are found in the 2003 HICPAC guidelines (140). Several recent studies show promising results with novel technologies to treat water that contains *Legionella* and may facilitate compliance with these new guidelines (532–534). At least one of these modalities may remove other potential pathogens from the water supply, although further studies are needed (532). Because some strategies damage water pipes and some chemicals cause untoward health affects, investigators have suggested using several other strategies. For example, Matulonis et al. (112) lowered the chlorine concentration by combining superheating and flushing and ultraviolet irradiation in their strategy. These authors found the incidence of nosocomial *Legionella* pneumonia was 1.5% (3/201) among HSCT patients housed on the unit with treated water, and 22% (33/150) among at-risk patients on regular units. The authors concluded that the multifaceted approach to water treatment reduced the incidence of *Legionella* infections in HSCT patients. Evaluation of decontamination strategies requires an evaluation of the facility, its water system, and the municipal water system (Johns Hopkins evaluation—Appendix C).

Food Preparation and Handling

Careful food preparation is required in all patients but particularly patients undergoing transplantation. Some experts advocate the use of sterile food or low microbial diets (535). With the widespread use of prophylactic antibiotics that remove most pathogenic bacteria from the gastrointestinal tract, low microbial diets are not necessary. However, attention to types of foods and appropriate storage and cooking times is indicated (104). Interest in *Listeria* has increased because of epidemics related to transmission of *Listeria* via contaminated food products (536). Want et al. (536) described an HSCT recipient who developed listeriosis. Chilled cooked foods eaten by a child yielded *L. monocytogenes* on culture, although the strains identified in the food were different from the patient's strain. Formal recommendations have been published that include recommendations for adequately cooking certain foods, although restricted exposure to certain fruits and vegetables and dairy products is advised (104). Other microorganisms that cause food-borne illnesses could also infect these hosts and cause severe illness. Hence, food should be appropriately stored and well cooked.

Visitors

Visitors and family members, although critical to the care of the HSCT patient, can be a source of communicable diseases that can lead to infection. As discussed elsewhere in this section, visitors must wash/clean their hands and follow isolation and barrier precautions. Visitors who are ill with potentially infectious diseases should not be allowed into the institution. Visitors should be screened for diarrhea, vomiting, fever, conjunctivitis, undiagnosed rash, upper respiratory symptoms (cough), recent exposure to people with symptoms consistent with an acute infectious illness, or recently vaccinated with polio, vaccinia, or varicella vaccines. During respiratory virus season, visitors should be screened for respiratory illness and not allowed to visit an HSCT while symptomatic or infectious. Allowing children to visit is very controversial, as they are exposed to many infectious and communicable diseases in school, at play, or in day-care settings. The risks and benefits should be weighed, but additional precautions may be necessary if children are allowed on units. Certainly, more restrictive policies are needed if community or unit-based outbreaks of a communicable disease are in progress. Such strategies have been effectively used to prevent further transmission of influenza, pertussis, SARS, and RSV. All family contacts of patients should have an annual influenza vaccination.

Healthcare Worker Immunization

All healthcare workers should have immunizations required by the institution including measles, mumps, rubella, and evidence of immunity to varicella or of receipt of the varicella vaccine (see Chapters 42, 51, and 80). Tuberculin skin tests should be current. Healthcare workers who work on HSCT units should receive only inactivated polio vaccine. Other vaccines are appropriate, including varicella and influenza. Varicella vaccine can be administered to susceptible healthcare workers working on HSCT units. We believe this is important if susceptible healthcare workers are in contact with susceptible patients, and we require this at our hospitals. If a local, vesicular reaction after the vaccine occurs, the area should be covered (338). Vaccine-associated infections can be spread among household contacts, but no data are available on spread among healthcare workers (537). We have not seen vaccine-associated virus spread nosocomially. More widespread reactions may require the employee to be furloughed (see also Chapter 42).

Most importantly, we feel that all healthcare workers, especially those working with these high-risk patients, should be vaccinated against influenza. Early detection of influenza in healthcare institutions is crucial for preventing nosocomial transmission. Influenza vaccine in healthy, young healthcare workers is 88% efficacious for influenza A and 89% for influenza B (538). In addition, Potter et al. (539) used an elegant study design and demonstrated that vaccinating healthcare workers for influenza reduced influenza-like illness and decreased mortality 47%. Although these studies were not specifically performed among HSCT patients, experts and current guidelines strongly recommend this vaccine (104) (see also Chapters 41 and 80).

CONCLUSION

The prevention and control of nosocomial infections in HSCT recipients and in the units where they are hospitalized is complicated. Prevention and control strategies require a comprehensive understanding of the diseases or the microorganisms and their epidemiology. Interventions are most effective if multidisciplinary. The future challenges will be translating the evidence-based protocols and practices to alternative settings, including rehabilitation and long-term-care institutions and the home. The role of prevention is paramount in these patients. As patients move from a traditional inpatient setting to the outpatient setting, our challenges will include how to define infections, how to find these infections, and how to intervene should an outbreak occur. As antibacterial, antifungal, and antiviral prophylaxis strategies become more sophisticated, new pathogens and increasingly resistant microorganisms or unusual viruses will emerge. Improved diagnostic techniques, rapid molecular typing, and cost-effective surveillance strategies should be developed. The next frontier will be to prevent further antimicrobial resistance from developing and spreading among these patients at risk for infection.

ACKNOWLEDGMENTS

We are grateful to Aneta Gramatikova and Greg Bova, who helped us prepare and edit this chapter, and bring it to fruition, and who developed Appendix C.

APPENDIX A: NOSOCOMIAL INVASIVE FUNGAL INFECTIONS: DEFINITIONS AND CASE CLASSIFICATION FOR HEMATOPOIETIC STEM CELL AND SOLID ORGAN TRANSPLANT, AND HEMATOLOGIC MALIGNANCY PATIENTS, INCLUDING A PROPOSED SURVEILLANCE MECHANISM

Patient Categories

I. Hematopoietic stem cell transplant types
   Allogeneic
   Autologous
II. Leukemia

Definitions

Neutropenia: absolute neutrophil count (ANC) <500 mm^3.

Neutropenia days: duration of neutropenia is calculated as number of days from first ANC <500 mm^3 or first total white blood count (WBC) <1,000 mm^3 to either first ANC/calculated ANC >500 mm^3 for first total WBC in normal range (5,000–10,000 mm^3).

Nosocomial aspergillosis: first occurrence of pulmonary or deep, disseminated aspergillosis in a hospitalized patient during the at-risk periods specified in section IIV below.

Classification Criteria for Nosocomial Invasive Fungal Disease

Definite Case:

Must have consistent clinical picture (febrile, solid organ, bone marrow, lung or heart/lung transplant on broad-spectrum antibiotics) with evidence of invasive aspergillosis by histopathologic examination and (+) culture of aspergillus taken from a sterile site.

Probable Case: Must meet the following criteria:

- Consistent clinical picture with negative histopathologic examination,
- or histopathology not done
- and (+) culture of aspergillus taken from a contiguous, nonsterile site.

Possible Case: Must meet the following criteria:

- Patient with clinical picture and CXR image consistent with aspergillosis
- Negative histopathologic examination or histopathology not done
- No positive culture of aspergillus or positive culture from a non-sterile site
- Treated by clinician with an appropriate antifungal agent at a therapeutic dosage.

Colonized Case:

- Any patient with (+) aspergillus culture and no clinical evidence of fungal infection.

Surveillance Mechanisms

In oncology patients:

Review weekly CT scans and CXRs to look for entries that specify findings consistent with fungal pneumonia or aspergillosis.

Interview weekly ward staff to request names of patients with possible invasive aspergillosis.

Classification of Cases

The case should meet either of the following criteria:

- The infection occurs during the course of the hospitalization in a patient without evidence of pre-existing or incubating aspergillosis upon admission.
- The infection is acquired during hospitalization and becomes evident after hospital discharge.

Definite Nosocomial Case: any case of invasive aspergillosis in which the characteristic symptomatology appears:

- After the second week of admission
- Or within the first week after hospital discharge
- If the last discharge date and current admit date are less than 14 days apart the admissions are considered as one for the purpose of this surveillance

Possible Nosocomial Case: any case of invasive aspergillosis in which the characteristic symptomatology begins:

- During the second week of admission
- Or during the second week after hospital discharge

Numerators and Denominators for Infection Rates

I. *Allogeneic HSCT*
   Numerator: number of allogeneic HSCT patients with aspergillosis.
   At-risk periods: first 100 days after HSCT. If patients have been discharged for 2 weeks, they must be hospitalized again prior to being at risk.
   Denominator: number of patients having allogeneic HSCT.

II. Autologous HSCT
   Numerator: number of autologous HSCT patients with aspergillosis.
   At-risk periods: first 100 days after HSCT. If patients have been discharged for 2 weeks, they must be hospitalized again prior to being at risk.
   Denominator: number of patients having autologous HSCT.

APPENDIX B: EXAMPLE OF A RISK-BASED CONSTRUCTION POLICY

Patient Care Objectives

The intent of this policy is to minimize nosocomial (hospital-acquired) infections in patients that may arise as a result of exposure to microorganisms released into the environment during construction and renovation activities. Controlling dispersal of air- and/or water-borne infectious agents concealed within building components is critical in all of the Johns Hopkins facilities. To this end, all construction and renovation activities shall be defined and managed in such a way that occupants' exposure to dust, moisture, and their accompanying hazards is limited. Controlling construction dust and dirt will further serve to protect staff and visitors, as well as sensitive procedures and equipment, from possible ill effects.

Responsibilities

Facilities Department (FD)

Notify the Hospital Epidemiology and Infection Control (HEIC) Department of planned work to obtain approval prior to start of work (for all new construction or for construction or renovation activities for departments listed in risk groups 3 and 4; see below).

Telecommunication Service (TS), Johns Hopkins Medical Computer Information Services (JHMCIS), Network and Telecommunication Services (NTS)

- Notify HEIC of planned work and obtain approval prior to the start of work in risk groups 3 or 4.
- Follow the approved procedures set up by the FD to minimize the generation of dust.
- Notify appropriate nursing/clinic/department manager of any proposed work and precautionary measures, which will be taken.

- Oversee projects by inspecting barriers, etc. on a routine basis.
- Call Environmental Services to organize any cleanup.

Legal Department (LD)

Include the following language in all construction maintenance, and or renovation contracts: "HEIC shall approve projects involving manipulation of ceiling tiles, performance of dust generating activities, manipulation of HVAC (heating, ventilation, and air conditioning) systems, plumbing, and/or other maintenance repairs prior to the initiation of the project."

Environmental Services (EVS)

- Work with FD to identify areas that need to be damp mopped and clean these areas as scheduled.
- Thoroughly clean new and renovated areas before admitting or readmitting patients.
- Coordinate inspection of final cleaning with HEIC prior to opening/reopening the area.

Nursing Departments (and Other Departments that See Patients)

- Help identify high-risk patients.
- Relocate high-risk patients to unaffected areas before construction/renovation work is initiated.
- Optimally, avoid nonemergent admission/testing/treatment of immunocompromised patients during periods of construction/renovation.

Hospital Infection Control and Epidemiology (HEIC)

- Review procedures that are developed by FD to comply with this policy and submit to HEIC committee for approval.
- Educate managers, medical staff, environmental services personnel, and other staff as needed about risks to immunosuppressed patients exposed to construction dust.
- Determine whether construction poses sufficient increased risk to require/recommend that patients be moved to an area of the hospital/facility where construction is not occurring.
- Review indications for performing environmental cultures with the appropriate departments (health, safety and environment; microbiology laboratory).
- Inspect areas where construction has occurred after final cleaning and approve opening or reopening of the areas.
- Conduct careful environmental investigation, including culture confirmation (as possible), when a cluster of patients with infections potentially related to construction/renovation (aspergillosis, legionellosis, etc.) is identified.

Health, Safety, and Environment (HSE)

- Review air-sampling strategy with HEIC.
- Sample appropriate areas at predetermined time intervals during times of construction/renovation.
- Send all HEIC requested air-samples for culture to the microbiology laboratory for fungal identification (*Aspergillus*) and speciation.

Samples should include selected patient care areas, patient rooms, treatment areas, and predetermined control areas.

Procedures
Construction Guidelines

Facilities Department personnel at Johns Hopkins, who are responsible for managing each construction or renovation project, will:

- Determine the infection control project classification using the matrices (see below). HEIC and the health, safety and environment department may modify, add, or delete guidelines on individual projects in collaboration with the Facilities Department project leader.
- Coordinate the relocation of affected patients and pedestrian traffic routes to areas where there is less potential for exposure to airborne contaminants with the responsible departments.
- Coordinate the preparation of the project area, including the removal of medical supplies, waste, and equipment, prior to the commencement of project activities with the responsible departments.

TABLE A. DEFINITIONS OF CONSTRUCTION ACTIVITY
***Type A*: Inspections and General Upkeep Activities.** Includes but is not limited to: removal of ceiling tiles for visual inspection (limited to 1 tile per 50 square feet); painting (but not sanding); installation of wall covering; electrical trim work; minor plumbing; and activities, which do not generate dust or require cutting into walls or access to ceilings other than for visual inspection.
***Type B*: Small scale, short duration activities, which create minimal dust.** Includes, but is not limited to, installation of telephone and computer cabling, access to chase spaces, cutting into walls or ceiling where dust migration can be controlled.
***Type C*: Any work that generates a moderate to high level of dust.** Includes, but is not limited to, demolition or removal of built-in building components or assemblies, sanding of wall for painting or wall covering, removal of floor covering/wallpaper, ceiling tiles and casework, new wall construction, minor ductwork or electrical work above ceilings, major cabling activities.
***Type D*: Major demolition and construction projects.** Includes, but is not limited to, heavy demolition, removal of a complete ceiling system, and new construction.

Project Classification

Step One

Select *construction activity type from Table A*. (*Construction activity type* is defined by the amount of dust that is generated, the duration of the activity, and the involvement with HVAC systems.) Contact the HEIC Department if any activity is questionable under these guidelines.

Step Two

Select infection control risk group from Table B. (Infection control risk groups are defined are based on project location

TABLE B. DEFINITIONS OF INFECTION CONTROL RISK AREAS/LOCATION

GROUP 0 LOWEST	GROUP 1 LOW	GROUP 2 MEDIUM	GROUP 3 MEDIUM HIGH	GROUP 4 HIGHEST
• Detached buildings	• Office areas • Areas not communi cating with patient care activities	• Patient care & other areas not covered under group 3 or 4 • Laundry • Cafeteria • Dietary • Materials Management • PT/OT/Speech • Admission/Discharge • MRI • Nuclear Medicine • Echocardiography • Laboratories not specified as Group 3 • Public Corridors (through which patients, supplies, and linen pass)	• Emergency Rooms • Radiology • Post-anesthesia Care units (except the Oncology Center) • Labor and Delivery (Nelson 2) • Newborn Nurseries • Newborn Intensive Care unit • Pediatrics (except those listed in group 4) • All Intensive Care Units (except those listed in group 4) • Microbiology lab • Virology lab • Long term/sub-acute units • Pharmacy • Dialysis • Endoscopy • Bronchoscopy areas • Medicine	• Adult and pediatric oncology units including all inpatient units (HSCT, hematologic malignancy services), ICUs and infusion/ outpatient centers • Radiation therapy 2, Chemo infusion 1, clinical area • HIV clinic and inpatient service • Solid organ transplant services • Pharmacy Admixture • Operating Rooms • Post Anesthesia Care Units • C Section Rooms • Sterile Processing • Invasive Radiology • Cardiac Catheterization • Outpatient invasive procedures rooms • Anesthesia and Pump areas

and occupancy.) Contact HEIC Department if any location is questionable under these guidelines. When possible, as in outpatient areas, day-treatment only areas, etc. work should be done after hours since these areas have limited times when patients are seen.

Step Three

Using the construction activity type and the infection control risk group selected from the tables above, use the matrix (Table C) to determine construction classification (class). [Construction classification (class) determines the procedures to be followed during construction and renovation projects.] Contact HEIC Department for "special case" questions.

Step Four

Implement the appropriate infection control construction guideline based on the project classification selected from the construction activity matrix (Table C) in Step Three. (Infection control construction guidelines are procedures to control release(s) of airborne contaminants resulting from construction, demolition, or renovation activities.)

Submittals

Unless previously specified in the construction documents:

- Contractors, or the responsible Johns Hopkins department, will submit report of infection control procedures, including locations and details of barriers, means of creating negative pressure, etc. prior to the start of project for review by health, safety, and environment, HEIC, and facilities departments responsible for managing the project.
- Contractor will submit product data for review as requested.

Execution

Products and Materials

Barrier products that are approved:

- Sheet plastic: fire retardant polyethylene, 6-mil thickness. Dry wall with metal studs.

TABLE C. Construction Activity Matrix

CONSTRUCTION ACTIVITY→ RISK LEVEL ↓	TYPE "A"	TYPE "B"	TYPE "C"	TYPE "D"
Group 0	Class 0	Class 0	Class 0	Class 0
Group 1	Class I	Class II	Class II	Class III/IV
Group 2	Class I	Class II	Class III	Class IV
Group 3	*Class I*	Class III	Class III/IV	Class IV
Group 4	Class III	Class III/IV	Class III/IV	Class IV

TABLE D. INFECTION CONTROL CONSTRUCTION GUIDELINES

CLASS 0	• No infection control measures required.
CLASS I	• Execute work by methods to minimize raising dust from construction operations. • Replace any ceiling tile displaced for visual inspection as soon as possible.
CLASS II	• Provide active means to prevent air-borne dust from dispersing into atmosphere. • Seal unused doors with duct tape. • Contain construction waste before transport in tightly covered containers. • Wet mop and/or vacuum with HEPA filtered vacuum before leaving work area daily. • Place dust-mat at entrance and exit of work area and replace or clean when no longer effective. • Isolate HVAC system in areas where work is being performed. • Wipe casework and horizontal surfaces at completion of project.
CLASS III	• Isolate HVAC system in area where work is being done to prevent contamination of the duct system. • Complete all construction barriers before construction begins. • Maintain negative air pressure within work site utilizing HEPA filtered ventilation units or other methods to maintain negative pressure. Public Safety will monitor air pressure. • Do not remove barriers from work area until complete project is thoroughly cleaned. • Wet mop or vacuum twice per 8-hour period of construction activity or as required in order to minimize tracking. • Remove barrier materials carefully to minimize spreading of dirt and debris associated with construction. Barrier material should be wet wiped, HEPA vacuumed or water misted prior to removal. • Contain construction waste before transport in tightly covered containers. • Place dust-mat at entrance and exit of work area and replace or clean when no longer effective. • Wipe casework and horizontal surfaces at completion of project.
CLASS IV	• Isolate HVAC system in area where work is being done to prevent contamination of duct system. • Complete all construction barriers before construction begins. • Maintain negative air pressure within work site utilizing HEPA filtered ventilation units or other methods to maintain negative pressure. Public Safety will monitor air pressure. • Seal holes, pipes, conduits, and punctures to prevent dust migration. • Construct anteroom and require all personnel to pass through this room. Wet mop or HEPA vacuum the anteroom daily. • During demolition, dust producing work or work in the ceiling, disposable shoes and coveralls are to be worn and removed in the anteroom when leaving work area. • Do not remove barriers from work area until completed project is thoroughly cleaned. • Remove barrier materials carefully to minimize spreading of dirt and debris associated with construction. • Barrier material should be wet wiped, HEPA vacuumed or water misted prior to removal. • Contain construction waste before transport in tightly covered containers. • Place dust-mat at entrance and exit of work area and replace or clean when no longer effective. • Keep work area broom clean and remove debris daily. • Wet mop hard surface areas with disinfectant at completion of project. HEPA vacuum carpeted surfaces at completion of project.

- Solid core, wooden doors in metal frames—painted.
- Portable dust containment system, such as "ZipWall" as manufactured by Zip Wall LLC, Cambridge, MA, or equivalent.

HEPA-filtered ventilation units such as those manufactured by HPA Aire Model PAS 2000 HC or Model PAS 2000 HC or Model PAS 1000HC equipped air filtration units or equivalent. Provide HEPA filter, primary and secondary filters.

Exhaust hoses: heavy duty flexible steel reinforced; ventilator blower hose, WPC such as that manufactured by Federal Hose Mtg. Co. Painsville, OH 44077 or equivalent.

Adhesive walk-off mats: provide minimum size mats of 24 inches × 36 inches such as those manufactured by 3M, St. Paul, MN 55144 or equal.

Disinfectants: Johns Hopkins Hospital approved disinfectant.

Filters: Return and exhaust air ducts shall be covered with 2-inch-thick pleated air filters. Filters to be model #FME-40 as manufactured by Purolator or approved equivalent. Minimum efficiency 25%/35% with minimum of 10 pleats per foot.

Procedures

Isolation

- Construction activities causing disturbances of existing dust, or creating new dust, will be conducted in tight enclosures that cut off flow of particles into adjacent areas.
- Where containment is possible, utilizing building walls and doors (all doors *except construction access doors*) should be closed and sealed with duct tape to prevent dust and debris from escaping.
- Construction, demolition, or reconstruction not capable of containment utilizing, existing building walls and doors, will use one of the following methods of isolation:
- Airtight plastic barriers extending from floor to ceiling decking, or ceiling tiles if not removed. Plastic barrier seams will be sealed with duct tape to prevent dust and debris from escaping.
- Portable dust containment units with polyethylene pulled tight against floor and ceiling.

- Drywall barriers. Seams or joints will be covered or sealed to prevent dust and debris from escaping.

Additional Isolation Requirements

- Seal all penetrations at existing perimeter walls.
- Place isolation barriers at penetration of ceiling envelopes, chases and ceiling spaces to stop movement of air and debris.
- Erect dust barriers at elevator shafts or stairways within the field of construction, allowing for emergency egress.
- Provide anteroom or double entrance openings that allow workers to remove protective clothing or vacuum off existing clothing. Construct anteroom to maintain airflow from clean area through anteroom and into work area.
- Create overlapping flap (minimum of 2 feet wide) at plastic enclosures for personnel access.
- When openings are made into existing ceilings, a portable dust containment or plastic enclosure will be used, sealing off openings, and fitted tightly from ceiling to floor. Any ceiling access panels opened for investigation beyond the sealed areas will be replaced immediately when unattended.
- Direct pedestrian traffic from construction areas away from patient-care areas to limit opening and closing of doors (or other barriers) that may cause dust dispersion, entry of contaminated air, or tracking of dust to patient areas.
- Prevent birds and insects from gaining access to the hospital and hospital air-intact ducts. Exterior openings will remain closed when not in use.

Ventilation

- Negative air pressure will be maintained within the construction area.
- The central HVAC system will be used where possible to help maintain negative air pressure. Contractors will be responsible for blocking off supply ducts and covering return air ducts with 2-inch pleated air filters.
- Where central HVAC systems are not capable of maintaining negative air pressure in the work area, the contractor will provide exhaust fans or HEPA filtered ventilation units to maintain the negative air-pressure within the construction area. Exhaust fans or HEPA filtered ventilation units will run continuously. Contractors are responsible for maintaining equipment and replacement of HEPA and other filters in accordance with the manufacturer's recommendations.
- Construct an anteroom to maintain airflow from clean area through the anteroom and into the work area.

Housekeeping

- Walk-off mats will be used at exits and entrances to the work area. Adhesive walk-off mats should be placed at all doors *exiting* the construction area and carpeted walk-off mats should be placed at all doors *entering* into a construction area.
- Carpeted walk-off dust mats will be vacuumed at least twice per 8-hour shift and at the end of the workday. Any dust tracked outside of the construction area shall be vacuumed or damp-mopped immediately. Vacuum cleaners shall be outfitted with HEPA filters.
- Adhesive walk-off mats should be changed daily, or more frequently as needed, to maintain adhesive surfaces.
- When construction is in an occupied area, the construction area will be vacuumed or damp-mopped at least at the end of each shift. Vacuum cleaners will be outfitted with HEPA filters.

Protective Clothing

- Disposable shoe covers and coveralls are to be worn during demolition.
- Protective clothing will be removed any time the worker leaves the immediate work area.
- Used coveralls and shoe covers will be placed in a sealed plastic bag, prior to removal from the work area, for disposal by the contractor.

Storage of Building Supplies

- Construction materials such as drywall will be stored in clean, dry areas to prevent the growth of bacteria and fungi.
- Ductwork materials will be stored in a clean, dry area to prevent the accumulation of dust in the ductwork prior to installation.

Postconstruction

- The contractor will vacuum and clean all surfaces in the completed construction area, rendering them free of dust prior to the removal of isolation barriers.
- Barrier materials should be removed carefully to minimize spreading of dirt and debris associated with construction. (Barriers should be discarded as construction debris.) Barrier materials should be wet wiped, HEPA vacuumed or water misted prior to removal.
- The contractor will remove all blockages from the air systems.
- The contractor will balance the ventilation system to design specifications (as described in the project manual/agreement.
- Johns Hopkins's facilities department will examine the HVAC equipment and filters for blockage and/or leakage.
- Johns Hopkins's environmental services will perform the final cleaning of newly constructed/renovated areas before allowing patients to enter the areas.

Special Precautions for Water Handling (Plumbing Alterations)

- Exercise caution when handling fluids (e.g., removing plumbing pipes and fixtures) to prevent wetting of building materials and/or contamination of work areas.
- Cap unused domestic water pipe branches at no more than 12 inches from the main line.
- Before an area is turned over for patient occupancy/use, Johns Hopkins's facilities department will test the domestic water for temperature and potability.
- Aerators will not be used on water faucets in patient care/testing/treatment areas.

Supportive Information

BIBLIOGRAPHY

Center for Disease Control and Prevention. Recommendations for prevention of nosocomial pneumonia. *Am J Infect Control* 1994;22:247–292.

APPENDIX C: COMPARISON CHART OF WATER DISINFECTION METHODS IN A HOSPITAL ENVIRONMENT

Item	Disinfection System							Combination Disinfection Systems		
	Super Heating and Flush	Autochlornating/ Inhibitor System	Autochloramine System (Monochloramine)	Chlorine Dioxide	Copper–Silver Ionization System	Ozonation	Ultraviolet	Ultraviolet and Autochlorinating / Inhibitor System	Ultraviolet and Autochloramine System (Monochloramine)	Ultraviolet and Chlorine Dioxide
Used on domestic cold water system	No	Yes	Yes	Yes	Yes	Yes	Yes	Yes	Yes	Yes
Used on domestic hot water system	Yes	Yes	Yes	Yes	Yes	Yes	Yes	Yes	Yes	Yes
Chemical utilized	None	Sodium hypochlorite	Chloramine (chlorine and ammonia)	Chlorine dioxide (sodium chlorite)	Copper and silver (metals)	None	None	Sodium hypochlorite	Chloramine (chlorine and ammonia)	Chlorine dioxide (sodium chlorite)
By-product	None	Trihalomethanes (THMs)	Trihalomethanes (THMs) (far less than chlorine)	Some chemical decomposition in form of chlorite and chlorate	None	Some bromate and formaldehyde	Ozone	Trihalomethanes (THMs)	Trihalomethanes (THMs) (far less than chlorine)	Some chemical decomposition in form of chlorite and chlorate
Effective max. pH	None	7.3 ph	9 pH	10 pH	8 pH	Na	Na	7.8 pH	9 pH	10 pH
Asthetic quality (taste, odor, and clarity)	None	Yes, taste and odor problems	Yes, taste and odor problems	None (below 0.8 ppm); removes most taste and odors problems	Yes, some clarity problems (black water)	Yes, odor problems	None, provided high intensity ozone lamps are not used	Yes, can cause taste and odor problems / only if high-intensity ozone lamps are used	Yes, can cause taste and odor problems / only if high-intensity ozone lamps are used	None (below 0.8 ppm); removes most taste and odors problems, only if high-intensity ozone lamps are used
Impact on equipment and systems	Potential	Potential corrosion problems	Minimal potential corrosion problems	Minimal potential corrosion problems	Minimal potential deposition of copper on steel / localized corrosion	Potential corrosion problems	Potential corrosion problems if high intensity ozone lamps are used	Potential corrosion problems / additional corrosion problems if high-intensity ozone lamps are used	Minimal potential corrosion problems / additional corrosion problems if high-intensity ozone lamps are used	Minimal potential corrosion problems / additional corrosion problems if high-intensity ozone lamps are used
Impact on dialysis equipment	None	None (below 4 ppm)–carbon filters and RO equipment effectively removes chlorine and by-products	Significantly difficult to remove chloramines (monochloramines) and by products at 4 ppm and below; carbon	None (below 0.8 ppm); carbon filters and RO equipment effectively removes chlorine dioxide and by-products	Information currently not available	Information currently not available	None	None (below 4 ppm); carbon filters and RO equipment effectively removes chlorine and by-products	Significantly difficult to remove chloramines (monochloramines) and by-products at 4 ppm and below; carbon	None (below 0.8 ppm); carbon filters and RO equipment effectively removes chlorine dioxide and by-products

(continued)

APPENDIX C: (*continued*)

Item	Disinfection System							Combination Disinfection Systems		
	Super Heating and Flush	Autochlornating/ Inhibitor System	Autochloramine System (Monochloramine)	Chlorine Dioxide	Copper–Silver Ionization System	Ozonation	Ultraviolet	Ultraviolet and Autochlorinating / Inhibitor System	Ultraviolet and Autochloramine System (Monochloramine)	Ultraviolet and Chlorine Dioxide
			filters effective RO membrane not effective; membrane damage possible						filters effective, RO membrane not effective, membrane damage	
Environmental and health effects	Water is at scalding temperature	Produces cabcinogenic THMs.	Produces carcinogenic THMs (less than chlorine).	None; does not produce THMs and can destroy some THMs	Copper is acutely toxic to many aquatic species at levels as low as 50 ppb; system operates between 200–600 ppb copper, 10 to 60 ppb silver	None; bromite identified as an animal carcinogen; effects on humans unknown	None	Produces carcinogenic THMs	Produces carcinogenic THMs (less than chlorine).	None; does not produce THMs and can destroy some THMs
EPA approved primary drinking water disinfectant	No	Yes (below 4 ppm)	Yes (below 4 ppm)	Yes (below 0.8 ppm)	No	No	No	Yes (below 4 ppm)	Yes (below 4 ppm)	Yes (below 0.8 ppm)
Breaks down biofilm (at nominal operating conditions)	Yes	No @ below 50 ppm; minimal above 50 ppm (system operates between 2–3 ppm)	No (system operates at 2–3 ppm)	Yes	Yes/No, depending on ppb	No	No	No @ below 50 ppm; minimal above 50 ppm (system operates between 2–3 ppm)	No (system operates at 2–3 ppm)	Yes
Inhibits biofilm (at nominal operating conditions)	No	Minimal	Minimal	Yes	Yes/No, depending on ppb	No	No	Minimal	Minimal	Yes
Short-term (1–2 days) residual effectiveness against Legionella (disinfection system not operating)	Yes	Yes	Yes, far less effective than chlorine	Yes	Yes	No	No	Yes	Yes (far less effective as chlorine)	Yes

(*continued*)

APPENDIX C: (*continued*)

Item	Disinfection System							Combination Disinfection Systems		
	Super Heating and Flush	Autochlornating/ Inhibitor System	Autochloramine System (Monochloramine)	Chlorine Dioxide	Copper–Silver Ionization System	Ozonation	Ultraviolet	Ultraviolet and Autochlorinating / Inhibitor System	Ultraviolet and Autochloramine System (Monochloramine)	Ultraviolet and Chlorine Dioxide
Long-term (1–2 weeks) residual effectiveness against Legionella (disinfection system not operating)	None	None	Information currently not available	Yes	Yes, for hot water systems only	None	None	None	None	Minimal; some residual protection until biofilm is reestablished; none for bulk water
Flushing required at all fixtures at start up and on periodic bases	Yes	Yes	Yes	Yes	Yes	Yes	Yes	Yes	Yes	Yes
Chlorine shocking of water system required prior to system operating (shocking effects bulk water only—no effect on biofilm)	Na	Yes	Yes	Not required	Not required	Yes	Yes	Yes	Yes	Not required
Estimated for a 800 gpm system (not installed)	Na	$9,000 (approx.)	$9,000 (approx.)	$12,000	$36,000	Not available	$27,000	$36,000 (approx.)	$42,000 (approx.)	$39,000
Estimated installation cost	Na	$5,000 (approx.)	$5,000 (approx.)	$3,000	$5,000	Not available	$10,000	$15,000 (approx.)	$15,000 (approx.)	$13,000
Estimated annual maintenance cost	$12,500 (per event)	$8,000	$8,000	$16,650 @ 1 lb cio_2 or $28,250 @ 2 lbs cio_2	$25,250	Not available	$12,600	$20,600	$20,600	$20,000 @ 1 LB ClO_2 or $32,000 @ 2LBS ClO_2

Opal SM, Asp AA, Cannady PB, et al. Efficacy of infection control measures during a nosocomial outbreak of disseminated aspergillosis-associated with hospital construction. *J Infect Dis* 1986;153:634–637.

Purcell RJ. Controlling Aspergillus contamination in heating ventilation and air-conditioning systems. In: *Plant technology and safety management services: infection control issues in PTSM.* Chicago: Joint Commission of Accreditation of Healthcare Organizations, 1989:23–26.

Developers

Department of Hospital Epidemiology and Infection Control Committee

Facilities Design and Construction Department

Communication and Education

Initial

- This policy will be distributed to all Interdisciplinary Clinical Practice Manual (ICPM) holders and will be available on the Intranet in the ICPM. It will also be located on the HEIC internet site (*www.Hopkins-HEIC.org*).
- An article regarding the new policy will be submitted by HEIC for publication in Hopkins Hot Line.

Ongoing

- HEIC will maintain the ongoing consultative relationship with facilities, environmental services, and health, safety, and environment as needed to provide guidance and education.
- Facilities project managers will educate construction managers (including those of contractors) who will be overseeing construction/renovations. HEIC is available to assist with this education or for consultation as needed.

Key Words

Construction; renovation; building; repairs

REFERENCES

1. Rizzo JD. Physician sees evolving and dynamic role for ABMTR research programs. *ABMTR Newslett* 1998(December);2–10.
2. Armitage JO. Bone marrow transplantation. *N Engl J Med* 1994; 330(12):827–838.
3. Vogelsang GB. Acute and chronic graft-versus-host disease. *Curr Opin Oncol* 1993;5(2):276–281.
4. Vogelsang GB. Graft-versus-host disease: implications from basic immunology for prophylaxis and treatment. *Cancer Treat Res* 1997;77: 87–97.
5. VanBuskirk AM, et al. Transplantation immunology. *JAMA* 1997; 278(22):1993–1999.
6. Djulbegovic B, et al. Nonmyeloablative allogeneic stem-cell transplantation for hematologic malignancies: a systematic review. *Cancer Control* 2003;10(1):17–41.
7. Schouten HC. The role of mini-allotransplants in the treatment of solid tumors. *Ann Oncol* 2002;13(suppl 4):281–286.
8. Rowe JM, et al. Recommended guidelines for the management of autologous and allogeneic bone marrow transplantation. A report from the Eastern Cooperative Oncology Group (ECOG) [see comments]. *Ann Intern Med* 1994;120(2):143–158.
9. Beelen DW, et al. Influence of intestinal bacterial decontamination using metronidazole and ciprofloxacin or ciprofloxacin alone on the development of acute graft-versus-host disease after marrow transplantation in patients with hematologic malignancies: final results and long-term follow-up of an open-label prospective randomized trial. *Blood* 1999;93(10):3267–3275.
10. van der Meer JW, et al. Infections in bone marrow transplant recipients. *Semin Hematol* 1984;21(2):123–140.
11. Cordonnier C, et al. Pulmonary complications occurring after allogeneic bone marrow transplantation. A study of 130 consecutive transplanted patients. *Cancer* 1986;58(5):1047–1054.
12. Weiner RS, et al. Interstitial pneumonitis after bone marrow transplantation. Assessment of risk factors. *Ann Intern Med* 1986;104(2): 168–175.
13. Meyers JD, Flournoy N, Thomas ED. Nonbacterial pneumonia after allogeneic marrow transplantation: a review of ten years' experience. *Rev Infect Dis* 1982;4(6):1119–1132.
14. Pecego R, et al. Interstitial pneumonitis following autologous bone marrow transplantation. *Transplantation* 1986;42(5):515–517.
15. Wingard JR, et al. Interstitial pneumonitis following autologous bone marrow transplantation. *Transplantation* 1988;46(1):61–65.
16. Sable CA, Donowitz GR. Infections in bone marrow transplant recipients. *Clin Infect Dis* 1994;18(3):273–281; quiz 282–284.
17. Dulley FL, et al. Venocclusive disease of the liver after chemoradiotherapy and autologous bone marrow transplantation. *Transplantation* 1987;43(6):870–873.
18. Winston DJ, et al. Infectious complications of human bone marrow transplantation. *Medicine (Baltimore)* 1979;58(1):1–31.
19. Kirk JL Jr, et al. Analysis of early infectious complications after autologous bone marrow transplantation. *Cancer* 1988;62(11):2445–2450.
20. Mossad SB, et al. Early infectious complications in autologous bone marrow transplantation: a review of 219 patients. *Bone Marrow Transplant* 1996;18(2):265–271.
21. Gruss E, et al. [Acute renal failure in the allogeneic transplantation of hemopoietic progenitors. The clinical characteristics in a series of 92 patients]. *Med Clin (Barc)* 1998;111(20):774–775.
22. Benjamin RJ, et al. ABO incompatibility as an adverse risk factor for survival after allogeneic bone marrow transplantation. *Transfusion* 1999;39(2):179–187.
23. Engels EA, et al. Early infection in bone marrow transplantation: quantitative study of clinical factors that affect risk. *Clin Infect Dis* 1999;28(2):256–266.
24. Meyers JD. Infection in bone marrow transplant recipients. *Am J Med* 1986;81(1A):27–38.
25. Johanson WG, Pierce AK, Sanford JP. Changing pharyngeal bacterial flora of hospitalized patients. Emergence of gram-negative bacilli. *N Engl J Med* 1969;281(21):1137–1140.
26. Kramer BS, et al. Role of serial microbiologic surveillance and clinical evaluation in the management of cancer patients with fever and granulocytopenia. *Am J Med* 1982;72(4):561–568.
27. Taplin D, Mertz PM. Flower vases in hospitals as reservoirs of pathogens. *Lancet* 1973(December 8):1279–1281.
28. Kates SG, et al. Indigenous multiresistant bacteria from flowers in hospital and nonhospital environments. *Am J Infect Control* 1991; 19(3):156–161.
29. Ruutu P, et al. Invasive pulmonary aspergillosis: a diagnostic and therapeutic problem. Clinical experience with eight haematologic patients. *Scand J Infect Dis* 1987;19(5):569–575.
30. Ruutu P, et al. An outbreak of invasive aspergillosis in a haematologic unit. *Scand J Infect Dis* 1987;19(3):347–351.
31. Schimpff SC, et al. Origin of infection in acute nonlymphocytic leukemia: significance of hospital acquisition of potential pathogens. *Ann Intern Med* 1972;77:707–714.
32. Morse LJ, Schonbeck LE. Hand lotions—a potential nosocomial hazard. *N Engl J Med* 1968;278(7):376–378.
33. Orth B, et al. Outbreak of invasive mycoses caused by Paecilomyces lilacinus from a contaminated skin lotion. *Ann Intern Med* 1996; 125(10):799–806.
34. Stephenson JR, et al. Gastrointestinal colonization and septicaemia with Pseudomonas aeruginosa due to contaminated thymol mouth-

wash in immunocompromised patients. *J Hosp Infect* 1985;6(4): 369–378.
35. Edelstein PH. Legionnaires' disease. *Clin Infect Dis* 1993;16(6): 741–747.
36. Woo AH, Goetz A, Yu VL. Transmission of Legionella by respiratory equipment and aerosol generating devices. *Chest* 1992;102(5): 1586–1590.
37. Dondero TJ Jr, et al. An outbreak of Legionnaires' disease associated with a contaminated air-conditioning cooling tower. *N Engl J Med* 1980;302(7):365–370.
38. Verweij PE, et al. Nosocomial outbreak of colonization and infection with Stenotrophomonas maltophilia in preterm infants associated with contaminated tap water. *Epidemiol Infect* 1998;120(3):251–256.
39. Labarca JA, et al. Outbreak of Stenotrophomonas maltophilia bacteremia in allogenic bone marrow transplant patients: role of severe neutropenia and mucositis. *Clin Infect Dis* 2000;30(1):195–197.
40. Stine TM, et al. A pseudoepidemic due to atypical mycobacteria in a hospital water supply. *JAMA* 1987;258(6):809–811.
41. Cookson BD, Houang EC, Lee JV. Clustering of aeromonas hydrophila septicaemia. *Lancet* 1981;2(8257):1232.
42. Gebo KA, et al. Pseudo-outbreak of Mycobacterium fortuitum on a human immunodeficiency virus ward: transient respiratory tract colonization from a contaminated ice machine. *Clin Infect Dis* 2002; 35(1):32–38.
43. Arnow PM, et al. Pulmonary aspergillosis during hospital renovation. *Am Rev Respir Dis* 1978;118:549–553.
44. Rhame FS, et al. Extrinsic risk factors for pneumonia in the patient at high risk of infection. *Am J Med* 1984;76(5A):42–52.
45. Sherertz RJ, et al. Impact of air filtration on nosocomial Aspergillus infections. Unique risk of bone marrow transplant recipients. *Am J Med* 1987;83(4):709–718.
46. Thio CL, et al. Refinements of environmental assessment during an outbreak investigation of invasive aspergillosis in a leukemia and bone marrow transplant unit. *Infect Control Hosp Epidemiol* 2000;21(1): 18–23.
47. Henry L. Immunocompromised patients and nutrition. *Prof Nurse* 1997;12(9):655–659.
48. Ruddell WS, et al. Effect of cimetidine on the gastric bacterial flora. *Lancet* 1980;1(8170):672–674.
49. Raybould TP, et al. Emergence of gram-negative bacilli in the mouths of bone marrow transplant recipients using chlorhexidine mouthrinse. *Oncol Nurs Forum* 1994;21(4):691–696.
50. da Fonseca MA. Pediatric bone marrow transplantation: oral complications and recommendations for care. *Pediatr Dent* 1998;20(7): 386–394.
51. Eisen D, Essell J, Broun ER. Oral cavity complications of bone marrow transplantation. *Semin Cutan Med Surg* 1997;16(4):265–272.
52. Heimdahl A, et al. The oral cavity as a port of entry for early infections in patients treated with bone marrow transplantation. *Oral Surg Oral Med Oral Pathol* 1989;68(6):711–716.
53. Bodey GP, et al. Quantitative relationships between circulating leukocytes and infection in patients with acute leukemia. *Ann Intern Med* 1966;64:328–340.
54. Serody JS, Shea TC. Prevention of infections in bone marrow transplant recipients. *Infect Dis Clin North Am* 1997;11(2):459–477.
55. Sable CA, Hayden FG. Orthomyxoviral and paramyxoviral infections in transplant patients. *Infect Dis Clin North Am*, 1995;9(4): 987–1003.
56. Emmanouilides C, Glaspy J. Opportunistic infections in oncologic patients. *Hematol Oncol Clin North Am* 1996;10(4):841–860.
57. Romano V, et al. Bloodstream infections can develop late (after day 100) and/or in the absence of neutropenia in children receiving allogeneic bone marrow transplantation. *Bone Marrow Transplant* 1999; 23(3):271–275.
58. Rotstein C, et al. Nosocomial infection rates at an oncology center. *Infect Control Hosp Epidemiol* 1988;9:13–19.
59. Carlisle PS, Gucalp R, Wiernik PH. Nosocomial infections in neutropenic cancer patients. *Infect Control Hosp Epidemiol* 1993;14(6): 320–324.
60. Velasco E, et al. Nosocomial infections in an oncology intensive care unit. *Am J Infect Control* 1997;25(6):458–462.
61. Hoyle C, Goldman JM. Life-threatening infections occurring more than 3 months after BMT. 18 UK bone marrow transplant teams. *Bone Marrow Transplant* 1994;14(2):247–252.
62. Clark JG, et al. Obstructive lung disease after allogeneic marrow transplantation. Clinical presentation and course. *Ann Intern Med* 1989; 111(5):368–376.
63. Atkinson K, et al. Analysis of late infections in 89 long-term survivors of bone marrow transplantation. *Blood* 1979;53(4):720–731.
64. Flaherty J, et al. Pilot trial of selective decontamination for prevention of bacterial infection in an intensive care unit. *J Infect Dis* 1990; 162(6):1393–1397.
65. Schimpff SC. Empiric antibiotic therapy for granulocytopenic cancer patients. *Am J Med* 1986;80(5C):13–20.
66. Lowder JN, Lazarus HM, Herzig RH. Bacteremias and fungemias in oncologic patients with central venous catheters: changing spectrum of infection. *Arch Intern Med* 1982;142(8):1456–1459.
67. Wade JC, et al. Staphylococcus epidermidis: an increasing cause of infection in patients with granulocytopenia. *Ann Intern Med* 1982; 97:503–508.
68. Pizzo PA, et al. Increasing incidence of gram-positive sepsis in cancer patients. *Med Pediatr Oncol* 1978;5(1):241–244.
69. Castagnola E, et al. Prophylaxis of streptococcal bacteraemia with oral penicillin V in children undergoing bone marrow transplantation. *Support Care Cancer* 1995;3(5):319–321.
70. Walter EA, Bowden RA. Infection in the bone marrow transplant recipient. *Infect Dis Clin North Am* 1995;9(4):823–847.
71. Martin MA, Pfaller MA, Wenzel RP. Coagulase-negative staphylococcal bacteremia: mortality and hospital stay. *Ann Intern Med* 1989; 110:9–16.
72. Arns da Cunha C, et al. Early gram-positive bacteremia in BMT recipients: impact of three different approaches to antimicrobial prophylaxis. *Bone Marrow Transplant* 1998;21(2):173–180.
73. Kelly CP, Pothoulakis C, LaMont JT. Clostridium difficile colitis. *N Engl J Med* 1994;330(4):257–262.
74. McFarland LV, et al. Nosocomial acquisition of Clostridium difficile infection. *N Engl J Med* 1989;320(4):204–210.
75. Gerding DN, et al. Clostridium difficile-associated diarrhea and colitis. *Infect Control Hosp Epidemiol* 1995;16(8):459–477.
76. Heard SR, et al. The epidemiology of Clostridium difficile with use of a typing scheme: nosocomial acquisition and cross-infection among immunocompromised patients. *J Infect Dis* 1986;153(1):159–162.
77. Johnson S, et al. Nosocomial Clostridium difficile colonisation and disease. *Lancet* 1990;336(8707):97–100.
78. Kavan P, et al. Pseudomembraneous clostridium after autologous bone marrow transplantation. *Bone Marrow Transplant* 1998;21(5): 521–523.
79. Bartlett JG. Antibiotic-associated pseudomembranous colitis. *Rev Infect Dis* 1979;1(3):530–539.
80. Zadik PM, Moore AP. Antimicrobial associations of an outbreak of diarrhoea due to Clostridium difficile. *J Hosp Infect* 1998;39(3): 189–193.
81. Gerard M, et al. Incidence and significance of Clostridium difficile in hospitalized cancer patients. *Eur J Clin Microbiol Infect Dis* 1988; 7(2):274–278.
82. Anand A, et al. Epidemiology, clinical manifestations, and outcome of Clostridium difficile-associated diarrhea. *Am J Gastroenterol* 1994; 89(4):519–523.
83. Delmee M, et al. Epidemiology and prevention of Clostridium difficile infections in a leukemia unit. *Eur J Clin Microbiol* 1987;6(6): 623–627.
84. Anand A, Glatt AE. Clostridium difficile infection associated with antineoplastic chemotherapy: a review. *Clin Infect Dis* 1993;17(1): 109–113.
85. Johnson S, Gerding DN. Clostridium difficile–associated diarrhea. *Clin Infect Dis* 1998;26(5):1027–1034; quiz 1035–1036.
86. Clabots CR, et al. Acquisition of Clostridium difficile by hospitalized patients: evidence for colonized new admissions as a source of infection. *J Infect Dis* 1992;166(3):561–567.

87. Johnson S, et al. Treatment of asymptomatic Clostridium difficile carriers (fecal excretors) with vancomycin or metronidazole. A randomized, placebo-controlled trial. *Ann Intern Med* 1992;117(4): 297–302.
88. Samore MH, et al. Clostridium difficile colonization and diarrhea at a tertiary care hospital. *Clin Infect Dis* 1994;18(2):181–187.
89. Roghmann MC, et al. Clostridium difficile infection is a risk factor for bacteremia due to vancomycin-resistant enterococci (VRE) in VRE-colonized patients with acute leukemia. *Clin Infect Dis* 1997;25(5): 1056–1059.
90. Cox GJ, et al. Etiology and outcome of diarrhea after marrow transplantation: a prospective study. *Gastroenterology* 1994;107(5): 1398–1407.
91. Blakey JL, et al. Infectious diarrhea in children undergoing bone-marrow transplantation. *Aust N Z J Med* 1989;19(1):31–36.
92. Yolken RH, et al. Infectious gastroenteritis in bone-marrow-transplant recipients. *N Engl J Med* 1982;306(17):1010–1012.
93. Yuen KY, et al. Clinical significance of alimentary tract microbes in bone marrow transplant recipients. *Diagn Microbiol Infect Dis* 1998; 30(2):75–81.
94. Hanna H, et al. Control of nosocomial Clostridium difficile transmission in bone marrow transplant patients. *Infect Control Hosp Epidemiol* 2000;21(3):226–228.
95. Mayfield JL, et al. Environmental control to reduce transmission of Clostridium difficile. *Clin Infect Dis* 2000;31(4):995–1000.
96. Bartlett JG. Management of Clostridium difficile infection and other antibiotic-associated diarrhoeas. *Eur J Gastroenterol Hepatol* 1996; 8(11):1054–1061.
97. Cartmill TD, et al. Management and control of a large outbreak of diarrhoea due to Clostridium difficile. *J Hosp Infect* 1994;27(1):1–15.
98. Silva J Jr. Clostridium difficile nosocomial infections—still lethal and persistent. *Infect Control Hosp Epidemiol* 1994;15(6):368–370.
99. Jernigan JA, et al. A randomized crossover study of disposable thermometers for prevention of Clostridium difficile and other nosocomial infections. *Infect Control Hosp Epidemiol* 1998;19(7):494–499.
100. Ferroni A, et al. Nosocomial outbreak of Clostridium difficile diarrhea in a pediatric service. *Eur J Clin Microbiol Infect Dis* 1997;16(12): 928–933.
101. Ramos A, et al. [Outbreak of nosocomial diarrhea by Clostridium difficile in a department of internal medicine]. *Enferm Infecc Microbiol Clin* 1998;16(2):66–69.
102. Fekety R, et al. Epidemiology of antibiotic-associated colitis; isolation of Clostridium difficile from the hospital environment. *Am J Med* 1981;70(4):906–908.
103. Savage AM, Alford RH. Nosocomial spread of Clostridium difficile. *Infect Control* 1983;4(1):31–33.
104. Guidelines for preventing opportunistic infections among hematopoietic stem cell transplant recipients. *MMWR Recomm Rep* 2000;49(RR-10):1–125, CE1–7.
105. Stout J, Yu V. Legionellosis. *N Engl J Med* 1997;337(10):682–687.
106. Kirby BD, Harris AA. Nosocomial Legionnaires' disease. *Semin Respir Infect* 1987;2:255–261.
107. Kirby BD, et al. Legionnaires' disease: report of sixty-five nosocomially acquired cases of review of the literature. *Medicine (Baltimore)* 1980;59(3):188–205.
108. Kugler JW, et al. Nosocomial Legionnaires' disease. Occurrence in recipients of bone marrow transplants. *Am J Med* 1983;74(2): 281–288.
109. Kool JL, et al. More than 10 years of unrecognized nosocomial transmission of legionnaires' disease among transplant patients [In Process Citation]. *Infect Control Hosp Epidemiol* 1998;19(12):898–904.
110. Helms CM, et al. Legionnaires' disease associated with a hospital water system: a cluster of 24 nosocomial cases. *Ann Intern Med* 1983; 99(2):172–178.
111. Marston BJ, Lipman HB, Breiman RF. Surveillance for Legionnaires' disease. Risk factors for morbidity and mortality. *Arch Intern Med* 1994;154(21):2417–2422.
112. Matulonis U, Rosenfeld CS, Shadduck RK. Prevention of Legionella infections in a bone marrow transplant unit: multifaceted approach to decontamination of a water system. *Infect Control Hosp Epidemiol* 1993;14(10):571–575.
113. Schwebke JR, Hackman R, Bowden R. Pneumonia due to Legionella micdadei in bone marrow transplant recipients. *Rev Infect Dis* 1990; 12(5):824–828.
114. Benz-Lemoine E, et al. Nosocomial legionnaires' disease in a bone marrow transplant unit. *Bone Marrow Transplant* 1991;7(1):61–63.
115. Stout J, et al. Potable water supply as the hospital reservoir for Pittsburgh pneumonia agent. *Lancet* 1982;1(8270):471–472.
116. Stout J, et al. Ubiquitousness of Legionella pneumophila in the water supply of a hospital with endemic Legionnaires' disease. *N Engl J Med* 1982;306(8):466–468.
117. Marrie TJ, et al. Nosocomial legionnaires' disease: lessons from a four-year prospective study. *Am J Infect Control* 1991;19(2):79–85.
118. Ampel NM, Wing EJ. Legionella infection in transplant patients. *Semin Respir Infect* 1990;5(1):30–37.
119. Muder RR, et al. Nosocomial Legionnaires' disease uncovered in a prospective pneumonia study. *JAMA* 1983;249(23):3184–3188.
120. Meletis J, et al. Legionnaires' disease after bone marrow transplantation. *Bone Marrow Transplant* 1987;2(3):307–313.
121. Patterson WJ, et al. Colonization of transplant unit water supplies with Legionella and protozoa: precautions required to reduce the risk of legionellosis. *J Hosp Infect* 1997;37(1):7–17.
122. Helms CM, et al. Legionnaires' disease associated with a hospital water system. A five-year progress report on continuous hyperchlorination. *JAMA* 1988;259(16):2423–2427.
123. Oren I, et al. Nosocomial outbreak of Legionella pneumophila serogroup 3 pneumonia in a new bone marrow transplant unit: evaluation, treatment and control. *Bone Marrow Transplant* 2002;30(3): 175–179.
124. Yu VL, et al. Lack of evidence for person-to-person transmission of Legionnaires' disease. *J Infect Dis* 1983;147(2):362.
125. Blatt SP, et al. Nosocomial Legionnaires' disease: aspiration as a primary mode of disease acquisition. *Am J Med* 1993;95(1):16–22.
126. Zuravleff JJ, et al. Legionella pneumophila contamination of a hospital humidifier. Demonstration of aerosol transmission and subsequent subclinical infection in exposed guinea pigs. *Am Rev Respir Dis* 1983; 128(4):657–661.
127. Garbe PL, et al. Nosocomial Legionnaires' disease. Epidemiologic demonstration of cooling towers as a source. *JAMA* 1985;254: 521–524.
128. Tobin JO, et al. Legionnaires' disease in a transplant unit: isolation of the causative agent from shower baths. *Lancet* 1980;2(8186): 118–121.
129. Tobin JO, et al. Legionnaires' disease: further evidence to implicate water storage and distribution systems as sources. *Br Med J (Clin Res Ed)* 1981;282(6263):573.
130. Cordes LG, et al. Isolation of Legionella pneumophila from hospital shower heads. *Ann Intern Med* 1981;94(2):195–197.
131. Arnow PM, et al. Nosocomial Legionnaires' disease caused by aerosolized tap water from respiratory devices. *J Infect Dis* 1982;146(4): 460–477.
132. Kaan JA, Simoons-Smit AM, MacLaren DM. Another source of aerosol causing nosocomial Legionnaires' disease. *J Infect* 1985;11(2): 145–148.
133. Gorman GW, et al. Isolation of Pittsburgh pneumonia agent from nebulizers used in respiratory therapy. *Ann Intern Med* 1980;93(4): 572–573.
134. Mastro TD, et al. Nosocomial Legionnaires' disease and use of medication nebulizers. *J Infect Dis* 1991;163(3):667–671.
135. Breiman RF, et al. Role of air sampling in investigation of an outbreak of legionnaires' disease associated with exposure to aerosols from an evaporative condenser. *J Infect Dis* 1990;161(6):1257–1261.
136. O'Mahony MC, et al. The Stafford outbreak of Legionnaires' disease. *Epidemiol Infect* 1990;104(3):361–380.
137. Venezia RA, et al. Nosocomial legionellosis associated with aspiration of nasogastric feedings diluted in tap water. *Infect Control Hosp Epidemiol* 1994;15(8):529–533.
138. Yu VL. Could aspiration be the major mode of transmission for Legionella? *Am J Med* 1993;95(1):13–15.

139. Harrington RD, et al. Legionellosis in a bone marrow transplant center. *Bone Marrow Transplant* 1996;18(2):361–368.
140. Guidelines for environmental infection control in health-care facilities. *MMWR Recomm Rep* 2003;52(RR-10):1–42.
141. Chang J, et al. Listeriosis in bone marrow transplant recipients: incidence, clinical features, and treatment. *Clin Infect Dis* 1995;21(5): 1289–1290.
142. Long SG, Leyland MJ, Milligan DW. Listeria meningitis after bone marrow transplantation. *Bone Marrow Transplant* 1993;12(5): 537–539.
143. Skogberg K, et al. Clinical presentation and outcome of listeriosis in patients with and without immunosuppressive therapy. *Clin Infect Dis* 1992;14(4):815–821.
144. Yuen KY, Woo PC. Tuberculosis in blood and marrow transplant recipients. *Hematol Oncol* 2002;20(2):51–62.
145. Kurzrock R, et al. Mycobacterial pulmonary infections after allogeneic bone marrow transplantation. *Am J Med* 1984;77(1):35–40.
146. Ip MS, et al. Risk factors for pulmonary tuberculosis in bone marrow transplant recipients. *Am J Respir Crit Care Med* 1998;158(4): 1173–1177.
147. Gaviria JM, et al. Nontuberculous mycobacterial infections in hematopoietic stem cell transplant recipients: characteristics of respiratory and catheter-related infections. *Biol Blood Marrow Transplant* 2000; 6(4):361–369.
148. Roy V, Ochs L, Weisdorf D. Late infections following allogeneic bone marrow transplantation: suggested strategies for prophylaxis. *Leuk Lymphoma* 1997;26(1–2):1–15.
149. Roy V, Weisdorf D. Mycobacterial infections following bone marrow transplantation: a 20 year retrospective review. *Bone Marrow Transplant* 1997;19(5):467–470.
150. American Thoracic Society. Diagnostic standards and classification of tuberculosis. *Am Rev Respir Dis* 1990;142(3):725–735.
151. National Nosocomial Infections Surveillance (NNIS) System Report, Data Summary from January 1992–June 2001, issued August 2001. *Am J Infect Control* 2001;29(6):404–421.
152. Jones RN, et al. Nosocomial enterococcal blood stream infections in the SCOPE Program: antimicrobial resistance, species occurrence, molecular testing results, and laboratory testing accuracy. SCOPE Hospital Study Group. *Diagn Microbiol Infect Dis* 1997;29(2): 95–102.
153. Lautenbach E, Bilker WB, Brennan PJ. Enterococcal bacteremia: risk factors for vancomycin resistance and predictors of mortality. *Infect Control Hosp Epidemiol* 1999;20(5):318–323.
154. Linden PK, et al. Differences in outcomes for patients with bacteremia due to vancomycin resistant Enterococcus faecium *or vancomycin-susceptible E. faecium. Clin Infect Dis* 1996;22:663–670.
155. Edmond MB, et al. Vancomycin-resistant Enterococcus faecium bacteremia: risk factors for infection. *Clin Infect Dis* 1995;20:1126–1133.
156. Zaas AK, et al. Risk factors for development of vancomycin-resistant enterococcal bloodstream infection in patients with cancer who are colonized with vancomycin-resistant enterococci. *Clin Infect Dis* 2002;35(10):1139–1146.
157. Kuehnert MJ, et al. Association between mucositis severity and vancomycin-resistant enterococcal bloodstream infection in hospitalized cancer patients. *Infect Control Hosp Epidemiol* 1999;20(10):660–663.
158. Kapur D, et al. Incidence and outcome of vancomycin-resistant enterococcal bacteremia following autologous peripheral blood stem cell transplantation. *Bone Marrow Transplant* 2000;25(2):147–152.
159. Bonten MJ, et al. The role of "colonization pressure" in the spread of vancomycin-resistant enterococci: an important infection control variable. *Arch Intern Med* 1998;158(10):1127–1132.
160. Edmond MB, et al. Vancomycin-resistant enterococcal bacteremia: natural history and attributable mortality. *Clin Infect Dis* 1996;23(6): 1234–1239.
161. Harbarth S, Cosgrove S, Carmeli Y. Effects of antibiotics on nosocomial epidemiology of vancomycin-resistant enterococci. *Antimicrob Agents Chemother* 2002;46(6):1619–1628.
162. Bonilla HF, et al. Colonization with vancomycin-resistant Enterococcus faecium: comparison of a long-term-care unit with an acute-care hospital. *Infect Control Hosp Epidemiol* 1997;18(5):333–339.
163. Wade JJ, Desai N, Casewell MW. Hygienic hand disinfection for the removal of epidemic vancomycin-resistant Enterococcus faecium and gentamicin-resistant Enterobacter cloacae. *J Hosp Infect* 1991;18(3): 211–218.
164. Boyce JM, et al. Outbreak of multidrug-resistant Enterococcus faecium with transferable vanB class vancomycin resistance. *J Clin Microbiol* 1994;32(5):1148–1153.
165. Noskin GA, et al. Recovery of vancomycin-resistant enterococci on fingertips and environmental surfaces [see comments]. *Infect Control Hosp Epidemiol* 1995;16(10):577–581.
166. Weber DJ, Rutala WA. Role of environmental contamination in the transmission of vancomycin-resistant enterococci [editorial; comment]. *Infect Control Hosp Epidemiol* 1997;18(5):306–309.
167. Bonten MJ, et al. Epidemiology of colonisation of patients and environment with vancomycin-resistant enterococci. *Lancet* 1996; 348(9042):1615–1619.
168. Porwancher R, et al. Epidemiological study of hospital-acquired infection with vancomycin-resistant Enterococcus faecium: possible transmission by an electronic ear-probe thermometer. *Infect Control Hosp Epidemiol* 1997;18(11):771–773.
169. Livornese LL Jr, et al. Hospital-acquired infection with vancomycin-resistant Enterococcus faecium transmitted by electronic thermometers [see comments]. *Ann Intern Med* 1992;117(2):112–116.
170. Morris JG, et al. Enterococci resistant to multiple antimicrobial agents, including vancomycin. *Ann Intern Med* 1995;123:250–259.
171. Tornieporth NG, et al. Risk factors associated with vancomycin-resistant Enterococcus faecium infection or colonization in 145 matched case patients and control patients. *Clin Infect Dis* 1996;23(4): 767–772.
172. Montecalvo MA, et al. Outbreak of vancomycin-, ampicillin-, and aminoglycoside-resistant Enterococcus faecium bacteremia in an adult oncology unit. *Antimicrob Agents Chemother* 1994;38(6):1363–1367.
173. Weinstein JW, et al. Resistant enterococci: a prospective study of prevalence, incidence, and factors associated with colonization in a university hospital. *Infect Control Hosp Epidemiol* 1996;17(1):36–41.
174. Boyle JF, et al. Epidemiologic analysis and genotypic characterization of a nosocomial outbreak of vancomycin-resistant enterococci. *J Clin Microbiol* 1993;31(5):1280–1285.
175. Karanfil LV, et al. A cluster of vancomycin-resistant Enterococcus faecium in an intensive care unit [see comments]. *Infect Control Hosp Epidemiol* 1992;13(4):195–200.
176. Handwerger S, et al. Nosocomial outbreak due to Enterococcus faecium highly resistant to vancomycin, penicillin, and gentamicin. *Clin Infect Dis* 1993;16(6):750–755.
177. Cetinkaya Y, Falk PS, Mayhall CG. Effect of gastrointestinal bleeding and oral medications on acquisition of vancomycin-resistant Enterococcus faecium in hospitalized patients. *Clin Infect Dis* 2002;35(8): 935–942.
178. Carmeli Y, Eliopoulos GM, Samore MH. Antecedent treatment with different antibiotic agents as a risk factor for vancomycin-resistant Enterococcus. *Emerg Infect Dis* 2002;8(8):802–807.
179. Carmeli Y, Samore MH, Huskins C. The association between antecedent vancomycin treatment and hospital-acquired vancomycin-resistant enterococci: a meta-analysis. *Arch Intern Med* 1999;159(20): 2461–2468.
180. Pegues DA, et al. Emergence and dissemination of a highly vancomycin-resistant vanA strain of Enterococcus faecium at a large teaching hospital. *J Clin Microbiol* 1997;35(6):1565–1570.
181. Bradley SJ, et al. The control of hyperendemic glycopeptide-resistant Enterococcus species on a haematology unit by changing antibiotic usage. *J Antimicrob Chemother* 1999;43(2):261–266.
182. Montecalvo MA, et al. Natural history of colonization with vancomycin-resistant Enterococcus faecium. *Infect Control Hosp Epidemiol* 1995;16(12):680–685.
183. Lai KK, et al. The epidemiology of fecal carriage of vancomycin-resistant enterococci. *Infect Control Hosp Epidemiol* 1997;18(11): 762–765.
184. Beezhold DW, et al. Skin colonization with vancomycin-resistant enterococci among hospitalized patients with bacteremia. *Clin Infect Dis* 1997;24(4):704–706.

185. Montecalvo MA, et al. A semiquantitative analysis of the fecal flora of patients with vancomycin-resistant enterococci: colonized patients pose an infection control risk. *Clin Infect Dis* 1997;25(4):929–930.
186. Elishoov H, et al. Nosocomial colonization, septicemia, and Hickman/Broviac catheter-related infections in bone marrow transplant recipients. A 5-year prospective study. *Medicine (Baltimore)* 1998; 77(2):83–101.
187. Graffunder EM, Venezia RA. Risk factors associated with nosocomial methicillin-resistant Staphylococcus aureus (MRSA) infection including previous use of antimicrobials. *J Antimicrob Chemother* 2002; 49(6):999–1005.
188. Lucet JC, et al. Prevalence and risk factors for carriage of methicillin-resistant Staphylococcus aureus at admission to the intensive care unit: results of a multicenter study. *Arch Intern Med* 2003;163(2):181–188.
189. Rezende NA, et al. Risk factors for methicillin-resistance among patients with Staphylococcus aureus bacteremia at the time of hospital admission. *Am J Med Sci* 2002;323(3):117–123.
190. Boyce JM, et al. Environmental contamination due to methicillin-resistant Staphylococcus aureus: possible infection control implications. *Infect Control Hosp Epidemiol* 1997;18(9):622–627.
191. Perl TM, Golub JE. New approaches to reduce Staphylococcus aureus nosocomial infection rates: treating S. aureus nasal carriage. *Ann Pharmacother* 1998;32(1):S7–16.
192. Muto CA, et al. SHEA guideline for preventing nosocomial transmission of multidrug-resistant strains of Staphylococcus aureus and enterococcus. *Infect Control Hosp Epidemiol* 2003;24(5):362–386.
193. Fridkin SK, Jarvis WR. Epidemiology of nosocomial fungal infections. *Clin Microbiol Rev* 1996;9(4):499–511.
194. Jarvis WR. Epidemiology of nosocomial fungal infections, with emphasis on Candida species. *Clin Infect Dis* 1995;20(6):1526–1530.
195. Singh N. Trends in the epidemiology of opportunistic fungal infections: predisposing factors and the impact of antimicrobial use practices. *Clin Infect Dis* 2001;33(10):1692–1696.
196. Pannuti C, et al. Nosocomial pneumonia in patients having bone marrow transplant. Attributable mortality and risk factors. *Cancer* 1992;69(11):2653–2662.
197. Baddley JW, et al. Invasive mold infections in allogeneic bone marrow transplant recipients. *Clin Infect Dis* 2001;32(9):1319–1324.
198. Marr KA, Patterson T, Denning D. Aspergillosis. Pathogenesis, clinical manifestations, and therapy. *Infect Dis Clin North Am*, 2002;16(4): 875–894, vi.
199. Schubert MM, et al. Head and neck aspergillosis in patients undergoing bone marrow transplantation. Report of four cases and review of the literature. *Cancer* 1986;57(6):1092–1096.
200. Landoy Z, Rotstein C, Shedd D. Aspergillosis of the nose and paranasal sinuses in neutropenic patients at an oncology center. *Head Neck Surg* 1985;8(2):83–90.
201. Allo MD, et al. Primary cutaneous aspergillosis associated with Hickman intravenous catheters. *N Engl J Med* 1987;317(18):1105–1108.
202. Larkin JA, et al. Primary cutaneous aspergillosis: case report and review of the literature. *Infect Control Hosp Epidemiol* 1996;17(6): 365–366.
203. Johnson AS, et al. Cutaneous infection with Rhizopus oryzae and Aspergillus niger following bone marrow transplantation. *J Hosp Infect* 1993;25(4):293–296.
204. Gerson SL, et al. Invasive pulmonary aspergillosis in adult acute leukemia: clinical clues to its diagnosis. *J Clin Oncol* 1985;3(8):1109–1116.
205. Gerson SL, et al. Discriminant scorecard for diagnosis of invasive pulmonary aspergillosis in patients with acute leukemia. *Am J Med* 1985;79(1):57–64.
206. Wald A, et al. Epidemiology of Aspergillus infections in a large cohort of patients undergoing bone marrow transplantation. *J Infect Dis* 1997;175(6):1459–1466.
207. Alangaden GJ, Wahiduzzaman M, Chandrasekar PH. Aspergillosis: the most common community-acquired pneumonia with gram-negative Bacilli as copathogens in stem cell transplant recipients with graft-versus-host disease. *Clin Infect Dis* 2002;35(6):659–664.
208. Wingard JR, et al. Aspergillus infections in bone marrow transplant recipients. *Bone Marrow Transplant* 1987;2(2):175–181.
209. McWhinney PH, et al. Progress in the diagnosis and management of aspergillosis in bone marrow transplantation: 13 years' experience. *Clin Infect Dis* 1993;17(3):397–404.
210. Ribaud P, et al. Survival and prognostic factors of invasive aspergillosis after allogeneic bone marrow transplantation. *Clin Infect Dis* 1999; 28(2):322–330.
211. Gerson SL, et al. Prolonged granulocytopenia: the major risk factor for invasive pulmonary aspergillosis in patients with acute leukemia. *Ann Intern Med* 1984;100(3):345–351.
212. Weber SF, et al. Interaction of granulocytopenia and construction activity as risk factors for nosocomial invasive filamentous fungal disease in patients with hematologic disorders. *Infect Control Hosp Epidemiol* 1990;11(5):235–242.
213. van Burik JH, et al. The effect of prophylactic fluconazole on the clinical spectrum of fungal diseases in bone marrow transplant recipients with special attention to hepatic candidiasis. An autopsy study of 355 patients. *Medicine (Baltimore)* 1998;77(4):246–254.
214. Arnow PM, et al. Endemic and epidemic aspergillosis associated with in-hospital replication of Aspergillus organisms. *J Infect Dis* 1991; 164(5):998–1002.
215. Aisner J, et al. Aspergillus infections in cancer patients. Association with fireproofing materials in a new hospital. *JAMA* 1976;235(4): 411–412.
216. Lentino JR, et al. Nosocomial aspergillosis: a retrospective review of air\borne disease secondary to road construction and contaminated air conditioners. *Am J Epidemiol* 1982;116(3):430–437.
217. Rotstein C, et al. An outbreak of invasive aspergillosis among allogeneic bone marrow transplants: a case-control study. *Infect Control* 1985;6(9):347–355.
218. Opal SM, et al. Efficacy of infection control measures during a nosocomial outbreak of disseminated aspergillosis associated with hospital construction. *J Infect Dis* 1986;153(3):634–637.
219. Perraud M, et al. Invasive nosocomial pulmonary aspergillosis: risk factors and hospital building works. *Epidemiol Infect* 1987;99(2): 407–412.
220. Weems JJ Jr, et al. Construction activity: an independent risk factor for invasive aspergillosis and zygomycosis in patients with hematologic malignancy. *Infect Control* 1987;8(2):71–75.
221. Barnes RA, Rogers TR. Control of an outbreak of nosocomial aspergillosis by laminar air-flow isolation. *J Hosp Infect* 1989;14(2):89–94.
222. Hopkins CC, Weber DJ, Rubin RH. Invasive aspergillus infection: possible non-ward common source within the hospital environment. *J Hosp Infect* 1989;13(1):19–25.
223. Flynn PM, et al. Aspergillus terreus during hospital renovation [letter]. *Infect Control Hosp Epidemiol* 1993;14(7):363–365.
224. Gerson SL, et al. Aspergillosis due to carpet contamination [letter]. *Infect Control Hosp Epidemiol* 1994;15(4 Pt 1):221–223.
225. Anderson K, et al. Aspergillosis in immunocompromised paediatric patients: associations with building hygiene, design, and indoor air. *Thorax* 1996;51(3):256–261.
226. Leenders A, et al. Molecular epidemiology of apparent outbreak of invasive aspergillosis in a hematology ward. *J Clin Microbiol* 1996; 34(2):345–351.
227. Loo VG, et al. Control of construction-associated nosocomial aspergillosis in an antiquated hematology unit. *Infect Control Hosp Epidemiol* 1996;17(6):360–364.
228. Oren I, et al. Invasive pulmonary aspergillosis in neutropenic patients during hospital construction: before and after chemoprophylaxis and institution of HEPA filters. *Am J Hematol* 2001;66(4):257–262.
229. Hahn T, et al. Efficacy of high-efficiency particulate air filtration in preventing aspergillosis in immunocompromised patients with hematologic malignancies. *Infect Control Hosp Epidemiol* 2002;23(9): 525–531.
230. Lai KK. A cluster of invasive aspergillosis in a bone marrow transplant unit related to construction and the utility of air sampling. *Am J Infect Control* 2001;29(5):333–337.
231. Lass-Florl C, et al. Aspergillus terreus infections in haematological malignancies: molecular epidemiology suggests association with in-hospital plants. *J Hosp Infect* 2000;46(1):31–35.
232. Gaspar C, et al. [Outbreak of invasive pulmonary mycosis in neutro-

penic hematologic patients in relation to remodelling construction work]. *Enferm Infecc Microbiol Clin* 1999;17(3):113–118.
233. Ascioglu S, et al. Defining opportunistic invasive fungal infections in immunocompromised patients with cancer and hematopoietic stem cell transplants: an international consensus. *Clin Infect Dis* 2002; 34(1):7–14.
234. Kami M, et al. Use of real-time PCR on blood samples for diagnosis of invasive aspergillosis. *Clin Infect Dis* 2001;33(9):1504–1512.
235. Buchheidt D, et al. Detection of Aspergillus species in blood and bronchoalveolar lavage samples from immunocompromised patients by means of 2-step polymerase chain reaction: clinical results. *Clin Infect Dis* 2001;33(4):428–435.
236. Pannuti CS, et al. Nosocomial pneumonia in adult patients undergoing bone marrow transplantation: a 9-year study. *J Clin Oncol* 1991; 9(1):77–84.
237. Saugier-Veber P, et al. Epidemiology and diagnosis of invasive pulmonary aspergillosis in bone marrow transplant patients: results of a 5 year retrospective study. *Bone Marrow Transplant* 1993;12(2): 121–124.
238. Morrison VA, Haake RJ, Weisdorf DJ. The spectrum of non-Candida fungal infections following bone marrow transplantation. *Medicine (Baltimore)* 1993;72(2):78–89.
239. Meunier F. Candidiasis. *Eur J Clin Microbiol Infect Dis* 1989;8(5): 438–447.
240. Pirsch JD, Maki DG. Infectious complications in adults with bone marrow transplantation and T-cell depletion of donor marrow. Increased susceptibility to fungal infections. *Ann Intern Med* 1986; 104(5):619–631.
241. McDonald GB, et al. Intestinal and hepatic complications of human bone marrow transplantation. Part I. *Gastroenterology* 1986;90(2): 460–477.
242. McDonald GB, et al. Intestinal and hepatic complications of human bone marrow transplantation. Part II. *Gastroenterology* 1986;90(3): 770–784.
243. Wey SB, et al. Risk factors for hospital-acquired candidemia. A matched case-control study. *Arch Intern Med* 1989;149(10): 2349–2353.
244. Vazquez JA, et al. Nosocomial acquisition of Candida albicans: an epidemiologic study. *J Infect Dis* 1993;168(1):195–201.
245. Goodrich JM, et al. Clinical features and analysis of risk factors for invasive candidal infection after marrow transplantation. *J Infect Dis* 1991;164(4):731–740.
246. Marr KA, et al. Candidemia in allogeneic blood and marrow transplant recipients: evolution of risk factors after the adoption of prophylactic fluconazole. *J Infect Dis* 2000;181(1):309–316.
247. Vazquez JA, et al. Nosocomial Candida glabrata colonization: an epidemiologic study. *J Clin Microbiol* 1998;36(2):421–426.
248. Rossetti F, et al. Fungal liver infection in marrow transplant recipients: prevalence at autopsy, predisposing factors, and clinical features. *Clin Infect Dis* 1995;20(4):801–811.
249. Goodman JL, et al. A controlled trial of fluconazole to prevent fungal infections in patients undergoing bone marrow transplantation. *N Engl J Med* 1992;326(13):845–851.
250. Abi-Said D, et al. The epidemiology of hematogenous candidiasis caused by different Candida species. *Clin Infect Dis* 1997;24(6): 1122–1128.
251. Viscoli C, et al. Candidemia in cancer patients: a prospective, multicenter surveillance study by the Invasive Fungal Infection Group (IFIG) of the European Organization for Research and Treatment of Cancer (EORTC). *Clin Infect Dis* 1999;28(5):1071–1079.
252. Pfaller MA. Nosocomial candidiasis: emerging species, reservoirs, and modes of transmission. *Clin Infect Dis* 1996;22(suppl 2):S89–94.
253. Sanchez V, et al. Nosocomial acquisition of Candida parapsilosis: an epidemiologic study. *Am J Med* 1993;94(6):577–582.
254. Levin AS, et al. Candida parapsilosis fungemia associated with implantable and semi-implantable central venous catheters and the hands of healthcare workers. *Diagn Microbiol Infect Dis* 1998;30(4): 243–249.
255. Rippon JW. The new opportunistic fungal infection: diagnosis, isolation, identification and impact on mycology. Fear of fungi. *Mycopathologia* 1987;99(3):143–146.
256. Goldberg SL, et al. Successful treatment of simultaneous pulmonary Pseudallescheria boydii and Aspergillus terreus infection with oral itraconazole. *Clin Infect Dis* 1993;16(6):803–805.
257. Gamis AS, et al. Disseminated infection with Fusarium in recipients of bone marrow transplants. *Rev Infect Dis* 1991;13(6):1077–1088.
258. Fang CT, et al. Fusarium solani fungemia in a bone marrow transplant recipient. *J Formos Med Assoc* 1997;96(2):129–133.
259. Arrese JE, Pierard-Franchimont C, Pierard GE. Fatal hyalohyphomycosis following Fusarium onychomycosis in an immunocompromised patient. *Am J Dermatopathol* 1996;18(2):196–198.
260. Nucci M, Anaissie E. Cutaneous infection by Fusarium species in healthy and immunocompromised hosts: implications for diagnosis and management. *Clin Infect Dis* 2002;35(8):909–920.
261. Warnock DW. Fungal complications of transplantation: diagnosis, treatment and prevention. *J Antimicrob Chemother* 1995;36(suppl B): 73–90.
262. Anaissie EJ, et al. Fusariosis associated with pathogenic fusarium species colonization of a hospital water system: a new paradigm for the epidemiology of opportunistic mold infections. *Clin Infect Dis* 2001; 33(11):1871–1878.
263. Herbrecht R, et al. Trichosporon capitatum septicemia in immunosuppressed patients. *Pathol Biol* 1990;38:585–588.
264. Lowenthal RM, et al. Invasive Trichosporon cutaneum infection: an increasing problem in immunosuppressed patients. *Bone Marrow Transplant* 1987;2(3):321–327.
265. Pickles RW, et al. Experience with infection by Scedosporium prolificans including apparent cure with fluconazole therapy. *J Infect* 1996; 33(3):193–197.
266. Barber GR, et al. Catheter-related Malassezia furfur fungemia in immunocompromised patients. *Am J Med* 1993;95(4):365–370.
267. Whimbey E, et al. Community respiratory virus infections among hospitalized adult bone marrow transplant recipients. *Clin Infect Dis* 1996;22(5):778–782.
268. Pene F, et al. Coronavirus 229E-related pneumonia in immunocompromised patients. *Clin Infect Dis* 2003;37(7):929–932.
269. Shields AF, et al. Adenovirus infections in patients undergoing bone-marrow transplantation. *N Engl J Med* 1985;312(9):529–533.
270. Bowden R. Respiratory virus infections after bone marrow transplant: the Fred Hutchinson Cancer Research Center experience. *Am J Med* 1997;102(3A):27–30.
271. Machado CM, et al. Low mortality rates related to respiratory virus infections after bone marrow transplantation. *Bone Marrow Transplant* 2003;31(8):695–700.
272. Hierholzer JC. Adenoviruses in the immunocompromised host. *Clin Microbiol Rev* 1992;5(3):262–274.
273. Flomenberg P, et al. Increasing incidence of adenovirus disease in bone marrow transplant recipients. *J Infect Dis* 1994;169(4):775–781.
274. Ambinder RF, et al. Hemorrhagic cystitis associated with adenovirus infection in bone marrow transplantation. *Arch Intern Med* 1986; 146(7):1400–1401.
275. Davis D, Henslee PJ, Markesbery WR. Fatal adenovirus meningoencephalitis in a bone marrow transplant patient. *Ann Neurol* 1988; 23(4):385–389.
276. Carrigan DR. Adenovirus infections in immunocompromised patients. *Am J Med* 1997;102(3A):71–74.
277. La Rosa AM, et al. Adenovirus infections in adult recipients of blood and marrow transplants. *Clin Infect Dis* 2001;32(6):871–876.
278. Munoz FM, Piedra PA, Demmler GJ. Disseminated adenovirus disease in immunocompromised and immunocompetent children. *Clin Infect Dis* 1998;27(5):1194–1200.
279. Baldwin A, et al. Outcome and clinical course of 100 patients with adenovirus infection following bone marrow transplantation. *Bone Marrow Transplant* 2000;26(12):1333–1338.
280. Echavarria M, et al. Prediction of severe disseminated adenovirus infection by serum PCR. *Lancet* 2001;358(9279):384–385.
281. Makela MJ, et al. Viruses and bacteria in the etiology of the common cold. *J Clin Microbiol* 1998;36(2):539–542.
282. Wenzel R, et al. Coronavirus infections in military recruits. Three

year study with coronavirus strains OC43 and 229E. *Am Rev Respir Dis* 1974;109:621–624.
283. Whimbey E, et al. Influenza A virus infections among hospitalized adult bone marrow transplant recipients. *Bone Marrow Transplant* 1994;13(4):437–440.
284. Engelhard D, et al. Antibody response to a two-dose regimen of influenza vaccine in allogeneic T cell-depleted and autologous BMT recipients. *Bone Marrow Transplant* 1993;11(1):1–5.
285. Hayden FG. Prevention and treatment of influenza in immunocompromised patients. *Am J Med* 1997;102(3A):55–60; discussion 75–76.
286. Wendt CH, et al. Parainfluenza virus respiratory infection after bone marrow transplantation. *N Engl J Med* 1992;326(14):921–926.
287. Zambon M, et al. Molecular epidemiology of two consecutive outbreaks of parainfluenza 3 in a bone marrow transplant unit. *J Clin Microbiol* 1998;36(8):2289–2293.
288. Abdallah A, et al. An outbreak of respiratory syncytial virus infection in a bone marrow transplant unit: effect on engraftment and outcome of pneumonia without specific antiviral treatment. *Bone Marrow Transplant* 2003;32(2):195–203.
289. Harrington RD, et al. An outbreak of respiratory syncytial virus in a bone marrow transplant center. *J Infect Dis* 1992;165(6):987–993.
290. Englund JA, et al. Respiratory syncytial virus infection in immunocompromised adults. *Ann Intern Med* 1988;109(3):203–208.
291. Whimbey E, et al. Combination therapy with aerosolized ribavirin and intravenous immunoglobulin for respiratory syncytial virus disease in adult bone marrow transplant recipients. *Bone Marrow Transplant* 1995;16(3):393–399.
292. Ghosh S, et al. Respiratory syncytial virus upper respiratory tract illnesses in adult blood and marrow transplant recipients: combination therapy with aerosolized ribavirin and intravenous immunoglobulin. *Bone Marrow Transplant* 2000;25(7):751–755.
293. Sparrelid E, et al. Ribavirin therapy in bone marrow transplant recipients with viral respiratory tract infections. *Bone Marrow Transplant* 1997;19(9):905–908.
294. Lewinsohn DM, et al. Phase I study of intravenous ribavirin treatment of respiratory syncytial virus pneumonia after marrow transplantation. *Antimicrob Agents Chemother* 1996;40(11):2555–2557.
295. Karanfil LV, et al. Reducing the rate of nosocomially transmitted respiratory syncytial virus [published erratum appears in *Am J Infect Control* 1999;27(3):303]. *Am J Infect Control* 1999;27(2):91–96.
296. Garcia R, et al. Nosocomial respiratory syncytial virus infections: prevention and control in bone marrow transplant patients. *Infect Control Hosp Epidemiol* 1997;18(6):412–416.
297. Hibberd PL, et al. Symptomatic cytomegalovirus disease in the cytomegalovirus antibody seropositive renal transplant recipient treated with OKT3. *Transplantation* 1992;53(1):68–72.
298. Reed EC. Infectious complications during auto-transplantation. *Oncol Clin North Am* 1993;7:771–735.
299. Boeckh M, et al. Late cytomegalovirus disease and mortality in recipients of allogeneic hematopoietic stem cell transplants: importance of viral load and T-cell immunity. *Blood* 2003;101(2):407–414.
300. Zaia JA, Forman SJ. Cytomegalovirus infection in the bone marrow transplant recipient. *Infect Dis Clin North Am* 1995;9(4):879–900.
301. Enright H, et al. Cytomegalovirus pneumonia after bone marrow transplantation. Risk factors and response to therapy. *Transplantation* 1993;55(6):1339–1346.
302. Reed EC, et al. Treatment of cytomegalovirus pneumonia with ganciclovir and intravenous cytomegalovirus immunoglobulin in patients with bone marrow transplants. *Ann Intern Med* 1988;109(10):783–788.
303. Emanuel D, et al. Cytomegalovirus pneumonia after bone marrow transplantation successfully treated with the combination of ganciclovir and high-dose intravenous immune globulin. *Ann Intern Med* 1988;109(10):777–782.
304. Schmidt GM, et al. A randomized, controlled trial of prophylactic ganciclovir for cytomegalovirus pulmonary infection in recipients of allogeneic bone marrow transplants; The City of Hope-Stanford-Syntex CMV Study Group [see comments]. *N Engl J Med* 1991;324(15):1005–1011.
305. Nguyen Q, et al. Late cytomegalovirus pneumonia in adult allogeneic blood and marrow transplant recipients. *Clin Infect Dis* 1999;28(3):618–623.
306. Konoplev S, et al. Cytomegalovirus pneumonia in adult autologous blood and marrow transplant recipients. *Bone Marrow Transplant* 2001;27(8):877–881.
307. Bowden RA, et al. Cytomegalovirus immune globulin and seronegative blood products to prevent primary cytomegalovirus infection after marrow transplantation. *N Engl J Med* 1986;314(16):1006–1010.
308. Bowden RA, et al. A comparison of filtered leukocyte-reduced and cytomegalovirus (CMV) seronegative blood products for the prevention of transfusion-associated CMV infection after marrow transplant [see comments]. *Blood* 1995;86(9):3598–3603.
309. Ljungman P, et al. Results of different strategies for reducing cytomegalovirus-associated mortality in allogeneic stem cell transplant recipients. *Transplantation* 1998;66(10):1330–1334.
310. Winston DJ, Ho WG, Champlin RE. Cytomegalovirus infections after allogeneic bone marrow transplantation. *Rev Infect Dis* 1990; 12(suppl 7):S776–792.
311. Wingard JR, et al. Association of Torulopsis glabrata infections with fluconazole prophylaxis in neutropenic bone marrow transplant patients. *Antimicrob Agents Chemother* 1993;37(9):1847–1849.
312. Bustamante CI, Wade JC. Herpes simplex virus infection in the immunocompromised cancer patient. *J Clin Oncol* 1991;9(10):1903–1915.
313. Perl TM, et al. Transmission of herpes simplex virus type 1 infection in an intensive care unit. *Ann Intern Med* 1992;117(7):584–586.
314. Adams G, et al. Nosocomial herpetic infections in a pediatric intensive care unit. *Am J Epidemiol* 1981;113:126–132.
315. Chen Y, et al. Resistant herpes simplex virus type 1 infection: an emerging concern after allogeneic stem cell transplantation. *Clin Infect Dis* 2000;31(4):927–935.
316. Singh N. Human herpesviruses-6, -7 and -8 in organ transplant recipients. *Clin Microbiol Infect* 2000;6(9):453–459.
317. Caserta MT, Mock DJ, Dewhurst S. Human herpesvirus 6. *Clin Infect Dis* 2001;33(6):829–833.
318. Yoshikawa T, et al. Human herpesvirus 6 viremia in bone marrow transplant recipients: clinical features and risk factors. *J Infect Dis* 2002;185(7):847–853.
319. Yoshikawa T. Human herpesvirus-6 and -7 infections in transplantation. *Pediatr Transplant* 2003;7(1):11–17.
320. Yoshikawa T, et al. Human herpesvirus-6 infection in bone marrow transplantation. *Blood* 1991;78(5):1381–1384.
321. Imbert-Marcille BM, et al. Human herpesvirus 6 infection after autologous or allogeneic stem cell transplantation: a single-center prospective longitudinal study of 92 patients. *Clin Infect Dis* 2000;31(4):881–886.
322. Cone RW, et al. Human herpesvirus 6 infections after bone marrow transplantation: clinical and virologic manifestations. *J Infect Dis* 1999;179(2):311–318.
323. Wang FZ, et al. Human herpesvirus 6 DNA in cerebrospinal fluid specimens from allogeneic bone marrow transplant patients: does it have clinical significance? *Clin Infect Dis* 1999;28(3):562–568.
324. Cone RW, et al. Human herpesvirus 6 in lung tissue from patients with pneumonitis after bone marrow transplantation [see comments]. *N Engl J Med* 1993;329(3):156–161.
325. Drobyski WR, et al. Brief report: fatal encephalitis due to variant B human herpesvirus-6 infection in a bone marrow-transplant recipient. *N Engl J Med* 1994;330(19):1356–1360.
326. Arvin AM. Varicella-zoster virus. *Clin Microbiol Rev* 1996;9(3):361–381.
327. Balfour HH Jr. Varicella zoster virus infections in immunocompromised hosts. A review of the natural history and management. *Am J Med* 1988;85(2A):68–73.
328. Locksley RM, et al. Infection with varicella-zoster virus after marrow transplantation. *J Infect Dis* 1985;152(6):1172–1181.
329. Feldman S, Hughes WT, Daniel CB. Varicella in children with cancer: Seventy-seven cases. *Pediatrics* 1975;56(3):388–397.
330. Arvin AM. Varicella-Zoster virus: pathogenesis, immunity, and clini-

cal management in hematopoietic cell transplant recipients. *Biol Blood Marrow Transplant* 2000;6(3):219–230.
331. Offidani M, et al. A predictive model of varicella-zoster virus infection after autologous peripheral blood progenitor cell transplantation. *Clin Infect Dis* 2001;32(10):1414–1422.
332. Steer CB, et al. Varicella-zoster infection after allogeneic bone marrow transplantation: incidence, risk factors and prevention with low-dose aciclovir and ganciclovir. *Bone Marrow Transplant* 2000;25(6): 657–664.
333. Koc Y, et al. Varicella zoster virus infections following allogeneic bone marrow transplantation: frequency, risk factors, and clinical outcome. *Biol Blood Marrow Transplant* 2000;6(1):44–49.
334. David DS, et al. Visceral varicella-zoster after bone marrow transplantation: report of a case series and review of the literature. *Am J Gastroenterol* 1998;93(5):810–813.
335. Perren TJ, et al. Prevention of herpes zoster in patients by long-term oral acyclovir after allogeneic bone marrow transplantation. *Am J Med* 1988;85(2A):99–101.
336. Ljungman P, et al. Clinical and subclinical reactivations of varicella-zoster virus in immunocompromised patients. *J Infect Dis* 1986; 153(5):840–847.
337. Hata A, et al. Use of an inactivated varicella vaccine in recipients of hematopoietic-cell transplants. *N Engl J Med* 2002;347(1):26–34.
338. Weber DJ, Rutala WA, Hamilton H. Prevention and control of varicella-zoster infections in healthcare facilities. *Infect Control Hosp Epidemiol* 1996;17(10):694–705.
339. Straus SE, et al. NIH conference. Varicella-zoster virus infections. Biology, natural history, treatment, and prevention [published erratum appears in *Ann Intern Med* 1988;109(5):438–439]. *Ann Intern Med* 1988;108(2):221–237.
340. Anderson JD, et al. Lack of nosocomial spread of Varicella in a pediatric hospital with negative pressure ventilated patient rooms. *Infect Control* 1985;6(3):120–121.
341. Leclair JM, et al. Airborne transmission of chickenpox in a hospital. *N Engl J Med* 1980;302(8):450–453.
342. Josephson A, Gombert ME. Airborne transmission of nosocomial varicella from localized zoster. *J Infect Dis* 1988;158(1):238–241.
343. Gustafson TL, et al. An outbreak of airborne nosocomial varicella. *Pediatrics* 1982;70(4):550–556.
344. Sawyer MH, et al. Detection of varicella-zoster virus DNA in air samples from hospital rooms. *J Infect Dis* 1994;169(1):91–94.
345. Gallinella G, et al. Occurrence and clinical role of active parvovirus B19 infection in transplant recipients. *Eur J Clin Microbiol Infect Dis* 1999;18(11):811–813.
346. Weiland HT, et al. Prolonged parvovirus B19 infection with severe anaemia in a bone marrow transplant patient [letter]. *Br J Haematol* 1989;71(2):300.
347. Corbett TJ, et al. Successful treatment of parvovirus B19 infection and red cell aplasia occurring after an allogeneic bone marrow transplant. *Bone Marrow Transplant* 1995;16(5):711–713.
348. Cohen BJ, et al. Chronic anemia due to parvovirus B19 infection in a bone marrow transplant patient after platelet transfusion. *Transfusion* 1997;37(9):947–952.
349. Hsu JW, et al. Parvovirus b19-associated pure red cell aplasia in chronic graft-versus-host disease. *Br J Haematol* 2002;119(1): 280–281.
350. Prowse CV. An ABC for West Nile virus. *Transfus Med* 003;13(1): 1–9.
351. Public health dispatch: investigations of West Nile virus infections in recipients of blood transfusions. *MMWR* 2002;51(43):973–974.
352. Iwamoto M, et al. Transmission of West Nile virus from an organ donor to four transplant recipients. *N Engl J Med* 2003;348(22): 2196–2203.
353. Petersen LR, Marfin AA. West Nile virus: a primer for the clinician. *Ann Intern Med* 2002;137(3):173–179.
354. Hong DS, et al. West Nile encephalitis in 2 hematopoietic stem cell transplant recipients: case series and literature review. *Clin Infect Dis* 2003;37(8):1044–1049.
355. Investigations of West Nile virus infections in recipients of blood transfusions. *MMWR* 2002;51(43):973–974.
356. Update: Investigations of West Nile virus infections in recipients of organ transplantation and blood transfusion—Michigan, 2002. *MMWR* 2002;51(39):879.
357. Update: Investigations of West Nile virus infections in recipients of organ transplantation and blood transfusion. *MMWR* 2002;51(37): 833–836.
358. Investigation of blood transfusion recipients with West Nile virus infections. *MMWR* 2002;51(36):823.
359. Meyers JD, et al. The value of Pneumocystis carinii antibody and antigen detection for diagnosis of Pneumocystis carinii pneumonia after marrow transplantation. *Am Rev Respir Dis* 1979;120(6): 1283–1287.
360. Vasconcelles MJ, et al. Aerosolized pentamidine as Pneumocystis prophylaxis after bone marrow transplantation is inferior to other regimens and is associated with decreased survival and an increased risk of other infections. *Biol Blood Marrow Transplant* 2000;6(1):35–43.
361. Lyytikainen O, et al. Late onset Pneumocystis carinii pneumonia following allogeneic bone marrow transplantation. *Bone Marrow Transplant* 1996;17(6):1057–1059.
362. Tuan IZ, Dennison D, Weisdorf DJ. Pneumocystis carinii pneumonitis following bone marrow transplantation. *Bone Marrow Transplant* 1992;10(3):267–272.
363. Vargas S, et al. Pneumocystis carinii person-to-person transmission from a patient with P carinii pneumonia (PCP) to immunocompetent contact healthcare workers. Infectious Disease Society of America, 37th annual meeting, Denver, November 12–15 1998; abstract 85.
364. McNeil MM, Brown JM. The medically important aerobic actinomycetes: epidemiology and microbiology. *Clin Microbiol Rev* 1994;7(3): 357–417.
365. Choucino C, et al. Nocardial infections in bone marrow transplant recipients. *Clin Infect Dis* 1996;23(5):1012–1019.
366. Hodohara K, et al. Disseminated subcutaneous Nocardia asteroides abscesses in a patient after bone marrow transplantation. *Bone Marrow Transplant* 1993;11(4):341–343.
367. Freites V, et al. Subcutaneous Nocardia asteroides abscess in a bone marrow transplant recipient. *Bone Marrow Transplant* 1995;15(1): 135–136.
368. Chandrasekar PH, Weinmann A, Shearer C. Autopsy-identified infections among bone marrow transplant recipients: a clinico-pathologic study of 56 patients. Bone Marrow Transplantation Team. *Bone Marrow Transplant* 1995;16(5):675–681.
369. Shearer C, Chandrasekar PH. Pulmonary nocardiosis in a patient with a bone marrow transplant. Bone Marrow Transplantation Team. *Bone Marrow Transplant* 1995;15(3):479–481.
370. Slavin MA, et al. Toxoplasma gondii infection in marrow transplant recipients: a 20 year experience. *Bone Marrow Transplant* 1994;13(5): 549–557.
371. Derouin F, et al. Toxoplasmosis in bone marrow-transplant recipients: report of seven cases and review. *Clin Infect Dis* 1992;15(2):267–270.
372. Martino R, et al. Toxoplasmosis after hematopoietic stem cell transplantation. *Clin Infect Dis* 2000;31(5):1188–1195.
373. Ninin E, et al. Longitudinal study of bacterial, viral, and fungal infections in adult recipients of bone marrow transplants. *Clin Infect Dis* 2001;33(1):41–47.
374. Pittet D, et al. Identifying the hospitalized patient at risk for nosocomial bloodstream infection: a population-based study. *Proc Assoc Am Physicians* 1997;109(1):58–67.
375. O'Grady NP, et al. Guidelines for the prevention of intravascular catheter-related infections. Centers for Disease Control and Prevention. *MMWR Recomm Rep* 2002;51(RR-10):1–29.
376. Keung YK, et al. Increased incidence of central venous catheter-related infections in bone marrow transplant patients. *Am J Clin Oncol* 1995; 18(6):469–474.
377. Moosa HH, et al. Complications of indwelling central venous catheters in bone marrow transplant recipients. *Surg Gynecol Obstet* 1991; 172(4):275–279.
378. Petersen FB, et al. Hickman catheter complications in marrow transplant recipients. *JPEN J Parenter Enteral Nutr* 1986;10(1):58–62.
379. Keung YK, et al. Comparative study of infectious complications of

different types of chronic central venous access devices. *Cancer* 1994; 73(11):2832–2837.

380. Giacchino M, et al. [Pulmonary complications after bone marrow transplantation]. *Minerva Pediatr* 1993;45(4):141–150.
381. Slavin MA, Gooley TA, Bowden RA. Prediction of cytomegalovirus pneumonia after marrow transplantation from cellular characteristics and cytomegalovirus culture of bronchoalveolar lavage fluid. *Transplantation* 1994;58(8):915–919.
382. Philit F, et al. [Lung complications of hematopoietic stem cell transplantation]. *Rev Mal Respir* 1996;13(5 suppl):S71–84.
383. Krowka MJ, Rosenow ECD, Hoagland HC. Pulmonary complications of bone marrow transplantation. *Chest* 1985;87(2):237–246.
384. Prodinger WM, et al. Legionella pneumonia in transplant recipients: a cluster of cases of eight years' duration. *J Hosp Infect* 1994;26(3): 191–202.
385. Kapila R, et al. A nosocomial outbreak of influenza A. *Chest* 1977; 71(5):576–579.
386. Eng RHK, et al. Bacteremia and fungemia in patients with acquired immune deficiency syndrome. *Am J Clin Pathol* 1986;86:105–107.
387. Kennedy CA, et al. Impact of surgical treatment on paranasal fungal infections in bone marrow transplant patients. *Otolaryngol Head Neck Surg* 1997;116(6 pt 1):610–616.
388. Savage DG, et al. Paranasal sinusitis following allogeneic bone marrow transplant. *Bone Marrow Transplant* 1997;19(1):55–59.
389. Imamura R, et al. Microbiology of sinusitis in patients undergoing bone marrow transplantation. *Otolaryngol Head Neck Surg* 1999; 120(2):279–282.
390. Young LS. Problems of studying infections in the compromised host. *Rev Infect Dis* 1986;8(suppl 3):S341–349.
391. Poe SS, et al. A national survey of infection prevention practices on bone marrow transplant units. *Oncol Nurs Forum* 1994;21(10): 1687–1694.
392. Recommendations for preventing the spread of vancomycin resistance. Hospital Infection Control Practices Advisory Committee (HICPAC) [published erratum appears in *Infect Control Hosp Epidemiol* 1995;16(9):498]. *Infect Control Hosp Epidemiol* 1995;16(2): 105–113.
393. Boyce JM, Pittet D. Guideline for Hand Hygiene in Health-Care Settings: recommendations of the Healthcare Infection Control Practices Advisory Committee and the HICPAC/SHEA/APIC/IDSA Hand Hygiene Task Force. *Infect Control Hosp Epidemiol* 2002;23(12 suppl):S3–40.
394. Guidelines for prevention of nosocomial pneumonia. Centers for Disease Control and Prevention. *MMWR* 1997;46(RR-1):1–79.
395. Gillis G, Eng-Chong M, Henseleit SE. The financial impact of an outbreak of vancomycin-resistant enterococcus (VRE) colonization in an inpatient/outpatient dialysis program. Abstracts of the 37th ICCAC, September 28–October 1, 1997, Toronto, Ontario, abstract J-86.
396. Montecalvo MA, et al. The cost-benefit of enhanced infection control strategies (EICS) to prevent transmission of vancomycin-resistant enterococci (VRE). Abstracts of the 37th ICCAC, September 28–October 1, 1997, Toronto, Ontario, Abstract J-84.
397. Souetre E, Qing W, Penelaud PF. Economic analysis of the use of recombinant human granulocyte colony stimulating factor in autologous bone marrow transplantation. *Eur J Cancer* 1996;32A(7): 1162–1165.
398. Simon A, et al. Surveillance for nosocomial and central line-related infections among pediatric hematology-oncology patients. *Infect Control Hosp Epidemiol* 2000;21(9):592–596.
399. Engelhart S, et al. Surveillance for nosocomial infections and fever of unknown origin among adult hematology-oncology patients. *Infect Control Hosp Epidemiol* 2002;23(5):244–248.
400. Larson E, et al. Lack of care giver hand contamination with endemic bacterial pathogens in a nursing home. *Am J Infect Control* 1992; 20(1):11–15.
401. Lew MA, et al. Ciprofloxacin versus trimethoprim/sulfamethoxazole for prophylaxis of bacterial infections in bone marrow transplant recipients: a randomized, controlled trial. *J Clin Oncol* 1995;13(1): 239–250.
402. Hedderwick SA, et al. Pathogenic organisms associated with artificial fingernails worn by healthcare workers. *Infect Control Hosp Epidemiol* 2000;21(8):505–509.
403. Wynd CA, Samstag DE, Lapp AM. Bacterial carriage on the fingernails of OR nurses. *AORN J* 1994;60(5):796,799–805.
404. Gross A, Cutright DE, D'Alessandro SM. Effect of surgical scrub on microbial population under the fingernails. *Am J Surg* 1979;138(3): 463–467.
405. Moolenaar RL, et al. A prolonged outbreak of Pseudomonas aeruginosa in a neonatal intensive care unit: did staff fingernails play a role in disease transmission? *Infect Control Hosp Epidemiol* 2000;21(2): 80–85.
406. Parry MF, et al. Candida osteomyelitis and diskitis after spinal surgery: an outbreak that implicates artificial nail use. *Clin Infect Dis* 2001; 32(3):352–357.
407. McNeil SA, et al. Effect of hand cleansing with antimicrobial soap or alcohol-based gel on microbial colonization of artificial fingernails worn by health care workers. *Clin Infect Dis* 2001;32(3):367–372.
408. Gottesdiener KM. Transplanted infections: donor-to-host transmission with the allograft. *Ann Intern Med* 1989;110(12):1001–1016.
409. Hakim M, et al. Toxoplasmosis in cardiac transplantation. *Br Med J (Clin Res Ed)* 1986;292(6528):1108.
410. Tolpin MD, et al. Transfusion transmission of cytomegalovirus confirmed by restriction endonuclease analysis. *J Pediatr* 1985;107(6): 953–956.
411. Curran JW, et al. Acquired immunodeficiency syndrome (AIDS) associated with transfusions. *N Engl J Med* 1984;310(2):69–75.
412. Jaffe HW, et al. Transfusion-associated AIDS: serologic evidence of human T-cell leukemia virus infection of donors. *Science* 1984; 223(4642):1309–1312.
413. Anderson KC, et al. Transfusion-acquired human immunodeficiency virus infection among immunocompromised persons. *Ann Intern Med* 1986;105(4):519–527.
414. Wood CC, et al. Antibody against the human immunodeficiency virus in commercial intravenous gammaglobulin preparations. *Ann Intern Med* 1986;105(4):536–538.
415. Nelson KE, et al. Transmission of retroviruses from seronegative donors by transfusion during cardiac surgery. A multicenter study of HIV-1 and HTLV-I/II infections. *Ann Intern Med* 1992;117(7): 554–559.
416. Lever AM, et al. Non-A, non-B hepatitis occurring in agammaglobulinaemic patients after intravenous immunoglobulin. *Lancet* 1984; 2(8411):1062–1064.
417. Feorino PM, et al. Transfusion-associated acquired immunodeficiency syndrome. Evidence for persistent infection in blood donors. *N Engl J Med* 1985;312(20):1293–1296.
418. Peterman TA, et al. Transfusion-associated acquired immunodeficiency syndrome in the United States. *JAMA* 1985;254(20): 2913–2917.
419. Lutwick LI, et al. The transmission of hepatitis B by renal transplantation. *Clin Nephrol* 1983;19(6):317–319.
420. Villalba R, et al. Acute Chagas' disease in a recipient of a bone marrow transplant in Spain: case report. *Clin Infect Dis* 1992;14(2):594–595.
421. Mourad G, et al. Transmission of Mycobacterium tuberculosis with renal allografts. *Nephron* 1985;41(1):82–85.
422. Peters TG, Reiter CG, Boswell RL. Transmission of tuberculosis by kidney transplantation. *Transplantation* 1984;38(5):514–516.
423. Scowden EB, Schaffner W, Stone WJ. Overwhelming strongyloidiasis: an unappreciated opportunistic infection. *Medicine (Baltimore)* 1978;57(6):527–544.
424. LaRocco MT, Burgert SJ. Infection in the bone marrow transplant recipient and role of the microbiology laboratory in clinical transplantation. *Clin Microbiol Rev* 1997;10(2):277–297.
425. Cisneros JM, Canas E, Pachon J. [Pre-transplant evaluation of the donor and recipient. Recommendations for surveillance and control of infection after transplantation]. *Enferm Infecc Microbiol Clin* 1997; 15(suppl 2):98–103.
426. Daily J, et al. IGIV: a potential role for hepatitis B prophylaxis in the bone marrow peritransplant period. *Bone Marrow Transplant* 1998;21(7):739–742.

427. Rowley SD, et al. Bacterial contamination of bone marrow grafts intended for autologous and allogeneic bone marrow transplantation. Incidence and clinical significance. *Transfusion* 1988;28(2):109–112.
428. Lazarus HM, et al. Contamination during in vitro processing of bone marrow for transplantation: clinical significance. *Bone Marrow Transplant* 1991;7:241–246.
429. Schepers KG, Davis JM, Rowley SD. Incidence of bacterial contamination of bone marrow grafts. *Prog Clin Biol Res* 1992;377:379–384.
430. Farrington M, et al. Bacterial contamination of autologous bone marrow during processing. *J Hosp Infect* 1996;34(3):230–233.
431. Froggatt JWI, et al. Contamination of processed autologous bone marrows from a contaminated lot of density gradient separation medium. *Infect Control Hosp Epidemiol* 1994;15(suppl)(4):22.
432. Buchholz DH, et al. Bacterial proliferation in platelet products stored at room temperature. Transfusion-induced Enterobacter sepsis. *N Engl J Med* 1971;285(8):429–433.
433. Rhame FS, et al. Salmonella septicemia from platelet transfusions. Study of an outbreak traced to a hematogenous carrier of Salmonella cholerae-suis. *Ann Intern Med* 1973;78(5):633–641.
434. Punsalang A, Heal JM, Murphy PJ. Growth of gram-positive and gram-negative bacteria in platelet concentrates. *Transfusion* 1989; 29(7):596–599.
435. Morrow JF, et al. Septic reactions to platelet transfusions. A persistent problem. *JAMA* 1991;266(4):555–558.
436. Murphy S, Gardner FH. Effect of storage temperature on maintenance of platelet viability—deleterious effect of refrigerated storage. *N Engl J Med* 1969;280(20):1094–1098.
437. Tests intended to prevent disease transmission. In: *Standards for blood banks and transfusion services.* Bethesda, MD: American Association of Blood Banks, 1997:19.
438. Hughes WT, et al. 2002 guidelines for the use of antimicrobial agents in neutropenic patients with cancer. *Clin Infect Dis* 2002;34(6): 730–751.
439. Attal M, et al. Prevention of gram-positive infections after bone marrow transplantation by systemic vancomycin: a prospective, randomized trial. *J Clin Oncol* 1991;9(5):865–870.
440. Epstein JB, et al. Efficacy of chlorhexidine and nystatin rinses in prevention of oral complications in leukemia and bone marrow transplantation. *Oral Surg Oral Med Oral Pathol* 1992;73(6):682–689.
441. Gluckman E, et al. Prophylaxis of bacterial infections after bone marrow transplantation. A randomized prospective study comparing oral broad-spectrum nonabsorbable antibiotics (vancomycin-tobramycin-colistin) to absorbable antibiotics (ofloxacin-amoxicillin). *Chemotherapy* 1991;37(suppl 1):33–38.
442. Schmeiser T, et al. Single-drug oral antibacterial prophylaxis with ofloxacin in BMT recipients. *Bone Marrow Transplant* 1993;12(1): 57–63.
443. Karp JE, et al. Oral norfloxacin for prevention of gram-negative bacterial infections in patients with acute leukemia and granulocytopenia. A randomized, double-blind, placebo-controlled trial. *Ann Intern Med* 1987;106(1):1–7.
444. Wade JC, et al. Selective antimicrobial modulation as prophylaxis against infection during granulocytopenia: trimethoprim-sulfamethoxazole vs. nalidixic acid. *J Infect Dis* 1983;147(4):624–634.
445. Pizzo PA, et al. Oral antibiotic prophylaxis in patients with cancer: a double-blind randomized placebo-controlled trial. *J Pediatr* 1983; 102(1):125–133.
446. Trimethoprim-sulfamethoxazole in the prevention of infection in neutropenic patients. EORTC International Antimicrobial Therapy Project Group. *J Infect Dis* 1984;150(3):372–379.
447. Dekker AW, et al. Prevention of infection by trimethoprim-sulfamethoxazole plus amphotericin B in patients with acute nonlymphocytic leukaemia. *Ann Intern Med* 1981;95(5):555–559.
448. Wade JC, et al. A comparison of trimethoprim-sulfamethoxazole plus nystatin with gentamicin plus nystatin in the prevention of infections in acute leukemia. *N Engl J Med* 1981;304(18):1057–1062.
449. Ferretti GA, et al. Chlorhexidine for prophylaxis against oral infections and associated complications in patients receiving bone marrow transplants. *J Am Dent Assoc* 1987;114(4):461–467.
450. Kern WV, et al. A randomized trial of roxithromycin in patients with acute leukemia and bone marrow transplant recipients receiving fluoroquinolone prophylaxis. *Antimicrob Agents Chemother* 1994; 38(3):465–472.
451. De Pauw B, et al. Options and limitations of long-term oral ciprofloxacin as antibacterial prophylaxis in allogeneic bone marrow transplant recipients. *Bone Marrow Transplant* 1990;5:179–182.
452. Winston DJ, et al. Randomized comparison of sulbactam/cefoperazone with imipenem as empirical monotherapy for febrile granulocytopenic patients. *Clin Infect Dis* 1998;26(3):576–583.
453. Perea S, et al. Incidence and clinical impact of fluoroquinolone-resistant Escherichia coli in the faecal flora of cancer patients treated with high dose chemotherapy and ciprofloxacin prophylaxis. *J Antimicrob Chemother* 1999;44(1):117–120.
454. Prentice HG, et al. Oral ciprofloxacin plus colistin: prophylaxis against bacterial infection in neutropenic patients. A strategy for the prevention of emergence of antimicrobial resistance. *Br J Haematol* 2001;115(1):46–52.
455. Trenschel R, et al. Fungal colonization and invasive fungal infections following allogeneic BMT using metronidazole, ciprofloxacin and fluconazole or ciprofloxacin and fluconazole as intestinal decontamination. *Bone Marrow Transplant* 2000;26(9):993–997.
456. Verhoef J, Verhage EA, Visser MR. A decade of experience with selective decontamination of the digestive tract as prophylaxis for infections in patients in the intensive care unit: what have we learned? *Clin Infect Dis* 1993;17(6):1047–1054.
457. Verhoef J. Prevention of infections in the neutropenic patient. *Clin Infect Dis* 1993;17(suppl 2):S359–367.
458. Cordonnier C, et al. Epidemiology and risk factors for gram-positive coccal infections in neutropenia: toward a more targeted antibiotic strategy. *Clin Infect Dis* 2003;36(2):149–158.
459. Bodey GP. Antimicrobial prophylaxis for infection in neutropenic patients. *Curr Clin Top Infect Dis* 1988;9:1–43.
460. Heizmann W, et al. Surveillance cultures and benefit of laminar airflow units in patients undergoing bone marrow transplantation. *Infection* 1987;15(5):337–343.
461. Petersen FB, et al. Laminar air flow isolation and decontamination: a prospective randomized study of the effects of prophylactic systemic antibiotics in bone marrow transplant patients. *Infection* 1986;14(3): 115–121.
462. Hughes WT, et al. Successful chemoprophylaxis for Pneumocystis carinii pneumonitis. *N Engl J Med* 1977;297(26):1419–1426.
463. Hughes WT, et al. 1997 guidelines for the use of antimicrobial agents in neutropenic patients with unexplained fever. Infectious Diseases Society of America. *Clin Infect Dis* 1997;25(3):551–573.
464. Bow EJ, Rayner E, Louie TJ. Comparison of norfloxacin with cotrimoxazole for infection prophylaxis in acute leukemia. The trade-off for reduced gram-negative sepsis. *Am J Med* 1988;84(5):847–854.
465. Dekker AW, Rozenberg-Arska M, Verhoef J. Infection prophylaxis in acute leukemia: a comparison of ciprofloxacin with trimethoprim-sulfamethoxazole and colistin. *Ann Intern Med* 1987;106(1):7–11.
466. Patoia L, et al. Norfloxacin and neutropenia [letter]. *Ann Intern Med* 1987;107(5):788–789.
467. Gomez-Martin C, et al. Rifampin does not improve the efficacy of quinolone antibacterial prophylaxis in neutropenic cancer patients: results of a randomized clinical trial. *J Clin Oncol* 2000;18(10): 2126–2134.
468. Hidalgo M, et al. Lack of ability of ciprofloxacin-rifampin prophylaxis to decrease infection-related morbidity in neutropenic patients given cytotoxic therapy and peripheral blood stem cell transplants. *Antimicrob Agents Chemother* 1997;41(5):1175–1177.
469. Knirsch CA, et al. An outbreak of Legionella micdadei pneumonia in transplant patients: evaluation, molecular epidemiology, and control. *Am J Med* 2000;108(4):290–295.
470. Schwartz C, et al. Prevention of bacteremia attributed to luminal colonization of tunneled central venous catheters with vancomycin-susceptible organisms. *J Clin Oncol* 1990;8(9):1591–1597.
471. Henrickson KJ, et al. Prevention of central venous catheter-related infections and thrombotic events in immunocompromised children by the use of vancomycin/ciprofloxacin/heparin flush solution: a ran-

domized, multicenter, double-blind trial. *J Clin Oncol* 2000;18(6): 1269–1278.
472. Rackoff WR, et al. A randomized, controlled trial of the efficacy of a heparin and vancomycin solution in preventing central venous catheter infections in children. *J Pediatr* 1995;127(1):147–151.
473. Vassilomanolakis M, et al. Central venous catheter-related infections after bone marrow transplantation in patients with malignancies: a prospective study with short-course vancomycin prophylaxis. *Bone Marrow Transplant* 1995;15(1):77–80.
474. Teinturier C, et al. Prevention of gram-positive infections in patients treated with high-dose chemotherapy and bone marrow transplantation: a randomized controlled trial of vancomycin. *Pediatr Hematol Oncol* 1995;12(1):73–77.
475. Ranson MR, et al. Double-blind placebo controlled study of vancomycin prophylaxis for central venous catheter insertion in cancer patients. *J Hosp Infect* 1990;15(1):95–102.
476. Wingard JR, et al. Prevention of fungal sepsis in patients with prolonged neutropenia: a randomized, double-blind, placebo-controlled trial of intravenous miconazole. *Am J Med* 1987;83(6):1103–1110.
477. Riley DK, et al. The prophylactic use of low-dose amphotericin B in bone marrow transplant patients. *Am J Med* 1994;97(6):509–514.
478. O'Donnell MR, et al. Prediction of systemic fungal infection in allogeneic marrow recipients: impact of amphotericin prophylaxis in high-risk patients. *J Clin Oncol* 1994;12(4):827–834.
479. Slavin MA, et al. Efficacy and safety of fluconazole prophylaxis for fungal infections after marrow transplantation—a prospective, randomized, double-blind study. *J Infect Dis* 1995;171(6):1545–1552.
480. Menichetti F, et al. Itraconazole oral solution as prophylaxis for fungal infections in neutropenic patients with hematologic malignancies: a randomized, placebo-controlled, double-blind, multicenter trial. GIMEMA Infection Program. Gruppo Italiano Malattie Ematologiche dell' Adulto. *Clin Infect Dis* 1999;28(2):250–255.
481. Marr KA, et al. Prolonged fluconazole prophylaxis is associated with persistent protection against candidiasis-related death in allogeneic marrow transplant recipients: long-term follow-up of a randomized, placebo-controlled trial. *Blood* 2000;96(6):2055–2061.
482. Rotstein C, et al. Randomized placebo-controlled trial of fluconazole prophylaxis for neutropenic cancer patients: benefit based on purpose and intensity of cytotoxic therapy. The Canadian Fluconazole Prophylaxis Study Group. *Clin Infect Dis* 1999;28(2):331–340.
483. Nucci M, et al. A double-blind, randomized, placebo-controlled trial of itraconazole capsules as antifungal prophylaxis for neutropenic patients. *Clin Infect Dis* 2000;30(2):300–305.
484. Boogaerts M, et al. Itraconazole versus amphotericin B plus nystatin in the prophylaxis of fungal infections in neutropenic cancer patients. *J Antimicrob Chemother* 2001;48(1):97–103.
485. Foot AB, Veys PA, Gibson BE. Itraconazole oral solution as antifungal prophylaxis in children undergoing stem cell transplantation or intensive chemotherapy for haematological disorders. *Bone Marrow Transplant* 1999;24(10):1089–1093.
486. Rousey SR, et al. Low-dose amphotericin B prophylaxis against invasive Aspergillus infections in allogeneic marrow transplantation. *Am J Med* 1991;91(5):484–492.
487. Perfect JR, et al. Prophylactic intravenous amphotericin B in neutropenic autologous bone marrow transplant recipients. *J Infect Dis* 1992; 165(5):891–897.
488. Goodrich JM, et al. Early treatment with ganciclovir to prevent cytomegalovirus disease after allogeneic bone marrow transplantation. *N Engl J Med* 1991;325(23):1601–1607.
489. Goodrich JM, et al. Ganciclovir prophylaxis to prevent cytomegalovirus disease after allogeneic marrow transplant. *Ann Intern Med* 1993; 118(3):173–178.
490. Winston DJ, et al. Ganciclovir prophylaxis of cytomegalovirus infection and disease in allogeneic bone marrow transplant recipients. Results of a placebo-controlled, double-blind trial. *Ann Intern Med* 1993; 118(3):179–184.
491. Einsele H, et al. Polymerase chain reaction monitoring reduces the incidence of cytomegalovirus disease and the duration and side effects of antiviral therapy after bone marrow transplantation. *Blood* 1995; 86(7):2815–2820.
492. Boeckh M, et al. Cytomegalovirus pp65 antigenemia-guided early treatment with ganciclovir versus ganciclovir at engraftment after allogeneic marrow transplantation: a randomized double-blind study. *Blood* 1996;88(10):4063–4071.
493. Ljungman P, et al. Randomized study of valacyclovir as prophylaxis against cytomegalovirus reactivation in recipients of allogeneic bone marrow transplants. *Blood* 2002;99(8):3050–3056.
494. Asano Y, et al. Postexposure prophylaxis of varicella in family contact by oral acyclovir [see comments]. *Pediatrics* 1993;92(2):219–222.
495. Suga S, et al. Effect of oral acyclovir against primary and secondary viraemia in incubation period of varicella [see comments]. *Arch Dis Child* 1993;69(6):639–642; discussion 642–643.
496. Meyers JD, et al. Acyclovir treatment of varicella-zoster virus infection in the compromised host. *Transplantation* 1984;37(6):571–574.
497. Saral R, et al. Acyclovir prophylaxis of herpes-simplex-virus infections. *N Engl J Med* 1981;305(2):63–67.
498. Wade JC, et al. Oral acyclovir for prevention of herpes simplex virus reactivation after marrow transplantation. *Ann Intern Med* 1984; 100(6):823–828.
499. Schepetiuk S, Papanaoum K, Qiao M. Spread of influenza A virus infection in hospitalised patients with cancer [letter]. *Aust N Z J Med* 1998;28(4):475–476.
500. Cohen MS, et al. Possible nosocomial transmission of group Y Neisseria meningitidis among oncology patients. *Ann Intern Med* 1979; 91(1):7–12.
501. Ena J, et al. The epidemiology of intravenous vancomycin usage in a university hospital. A 10-year study [see comments]. *JAMA* 1993; 269(5):598–602.
502. Anglim AM, et al. Effect of a vancomycin restriction policy on ordering practices during an outbreak of vancomycin-resistant Enterococcus faecium. *Arch Intern Med* 1997;157(10):1132–1136.
503. Dominguez EA, et al. A pilot study of antibiotic cycling in a hematology-oncology unit. *Infect Control Hosp Epidemiol* 2000;21(1 suppl): S4–8.
504. Nauseef WM, Maki DG. A study of the value of simple protective isolation in patients with granulocytopenia. *N Engl J Med* 1981; 304(8):448–453.
505. Garner JS. Guideline for isolation precautions in hospitals. The Hospital Infection Control Practices Advisory Committee. *Infect Control Hosp Epidemiol* 1996;17(1):53–80.
506. Srinivasan A, et al. A prospective study to determine whether cover gowns in addition to gloves decrease nosocomial transmission of vancomycin-resistant enterococci in an intensive care unit. *Infect Control Hosp Epidemiol* 2002;23(8):424–428.
507. Puzniak LA, et al. To gown or not to gown: the effect on acquisition of vancomycin-resistant enterococci. *Clin Infect Dis* 2002;35(1):18–25.
508. Gala CL, et al. The use of eye-nose goggles to control nosocomial respiratory syncytial virus infection. *JAMA* 1986;256(19): 2706–2708.
509. Hughes WT, Williams B, Pearson T. The nosocomial colonization of T. Bear. *Infect Control* 1986;7(10):495–500.
510. Buttery JP, et al. Multiresistant Pseudomonas aeruginosa outbreak in a pediatric oncology ward related to bath toys. *Pediatr Infect Dis J* 1998;17(6):509–513.
511. da Fonseca MA, Schubert M, Lloid M. Oral aspects and management of severe graft-vs-host disease in a young patient with beta-thalassemia: case report. *Pediatr Dent* 1998;20(1):57–61.
512. Hall CB, Douglas RG Jr, Geiman JM. Possible transmission by fomites of respiratory syncytial virus. *J Infect Dis* 1980;141(1):98–102.
513. Rupp M, et al. Can fresh flowers and live plants be safely introduced into a bone marrow transplant (BMT) unit? 12th Annual Society of Healthcare Epidemiology of America, 2002;#96.
514. Rhame FS, et al. Endemic Aspergillus airborne spore levels are a major risk for aspergillosis in bone marrow transplant patients. 25th Interscience Conference on Antimicrobial Agents and Chemotherapy, Minneapolis Minnesota, 1985, abstract 147.
515. Passweg JR, et al. Influence of protective isolation on outcome of allogeneic bone marrow transplantation for leukemia. *Bone Marrow Transplant* 1998;21(12):1231–1238.

516. Buckner CD, et al. Protective environment for marrow transplant recipients: a prospective study. *Ann Intern Med* 1978;89(6):893–901.
517. Petersen F, et al. The effects of infection prevention regimens on early infectious complications in marrow transplant patients: a four arm randomized study. *Infection* 1988;16(4):199–208.
518. Schimpff SC, et al. Infection prevention in acute nonlymphocytic leukemia. Laminar air flow room reverse isolation with oral, nonabsorbable antibiotic prophylaxis. *Ann Intern Med* 1975;82(3):351–358.
519. Yates JW, Holland JF. A controlled study of isolation and endogenous microbial suppression in acute myelocytic leukemia patients. *Cancer* 1973;32(6):1490–1498.
520. Bodey GP, et al. Protected environment-prophylactic antibiotic program in the chemotherapy of acute leukemia. *Am J Med Sci* 1971;262(3):138–151.
521. Goodley JM, Clayton YM, Hay RJ. Environmental sampling for aspergilli during building construction on a hospital site. *J Hosp Infect* 1994;26(1):27–35.
522. Streifel AJ, et al. Aspergillus fumigatus and other thermotolerant fungi generated by hospital building demolition. *Appl Environ Microbiol* 1983;46(2):375–378.
523. Srinivasan A, et al. The ability of hospital ventilation systems to filter Aspergillus and other fungi following a building implosion. *Infect Control Hosp Epidemiol* 2002;23(9):520–524.
524. Cooper EE, et al. Influence of building construction work on Aspergillus infection in a hospital setting. *Infect Control Hosp Epidemiol* 2003;24(7):472–476.
525. Rhame FS, Russell AL. Zidovudine after occupational exposure to the human immunodeficiency virus [letter]. *N Engl J Med* 1991;324(4):266–267.
526. Rhame FS. Nosocomial aspergillosis: how much protection for which patients? [editorial]. *Infect Control Hosp Epidemiol* 1989;10(7):296–298.
527. Saurina G, Landman D, Quale JM. Activity of disinfectants against vancomycin-resistant Enterococcus faecium [see comments]. *Infect Control Hosp Epidemiol* 1997;18(5):345–347.
528. Yu V, et al. Legionnella disinfection of water distribution systems: principles, problems, and practice. *Infect Control Hosp Epidemiol* 1993;14:567–570.
529. Ta AC, et al. Comparison of culture methods for monitoring Legionella species in hospital potable water systems and recommendations for standardization of such methods. *J Clin Microbiol* 1995;33(8):2118–2123.
530. Goetz A, Yu VL. Screening for nosocomial legionellosis by culture of the water supply and targeting of high-risk patients for specialized laboratory testing. *Am J Infect Control* 1991;19(2):63–66.
531. Yu VL, et al. Routine culturing for Legionella in the hospital environment may be a good idea: a three-hospital prospective study. *Am J Med Sci* 1987;294(2):97–99.
532. Srinivasan A, et al. A 17-month evaluation of a chlorine dioxide water treatment system to control Legionella species in a hospital water supply. *Infect Control Hosp Epidemiol* 2003;24(8):575–579.
533. Heffelfinger JD, et al. Risk of hospital-acquired legionnaires' disease in cities using monochloramine versus other water disinfectants. *Infect Control Hosp Epidemiol* 2003;24(8):569–574.
534. Stout JE, Yu VL. Experiences of the first 16 hospitals using copper-silver ionization for Legionella control: implications for the evaluation of other disinfection modalities. *Infect Control Hosp Epidemiol* 2003;24(8):563–568.
535. Akers S, Cheney C. The use of sterile and low microbial diets in ultraisolation environments. *J Parenter Enteral Nutr* 1983;7(4):390–397.
536. Want SV, et al. An epidemiological study of listeriosis complicating a bone marrow transplant. *J Hosp Infect* 1993;23(4):299–304.
537. White CJ. Varicella-zoster virus. *Clin Infect Dis* 1997;24:753–763.
538. Wilde JA, et al. Effectiveness of influenza vaccine in health care professionals: a randomized trial. *JAMA* 1999;281(10):908–913.
539. Potter J, et al. Influenza vaccination of health care workers in long-term-care hospitals reduces the mortality of elderly patients [see comments]. *J Infect Dis* 1997;175(1):1–6.
540. Thio CL, et al. Refinements of environmental assessment during an outbreak investigation of invasive aspergillosis in a leukemia and bone marrow transplant unit. *Infect Control Hosp Epidemiol* 2000;21(1):18–23.
541. Reduction of fever and streptococcal bacteremia in granulocytopenic patients with cancer. A trial of oral penicillin V or placebo combined with pefloxacin. International Antimicrobial Therapy Cooperative Group of the European Organization for Research and Treatment of Cancer. *JAMA* 1994;272(15):1183–1189.
542. Bowden RA, et al. A comparison of filtered leukocyte-reduced and cytomegalovirus (CMV) seronegative blood products for the prevention of transfusion-associated CMV infection after marrow transplant. *Blood* 1995;86(9):3598–3603.
543. Humar A, et al. A randomised trial comparing cytomegalovirus antigenemia assay vs screening bronchoscopy for the early detection and prevention of disease in allogeneic bone marrow and peripheral blood stem cell transplant recipients. *Bone Marrow Transplant* 2001;28(5):485–490.
544. Winston DJ, et al. Randomized comparison of oral valacyclovir and intravenous ganciclovir for prevention of cytomegalovirus disease after allogeneic bone marrow transplantation. *Clin Infect Dis* 2003;36(6):749–758.
545. Perraud M, et al. Air filtration and prevention of aspergillary pneumopathies. Preliminary comparative study of two mobile units for bacteriological air purification with recycling. *Nouv Rev Fr Hematol* 1992;34(4):295–299.
546. Mahieu LM, et al. A prospective study on factors influencing aspergillus spore load in the air during renovation works in a neonatal intensive care unit. *J Hosp Infect* 2000;45(3):191–197.
547. Richardson MD, et al. Fungal surveillance of an open haematology ward. *J Hosp Infect* 2000;45(4):288–292.
548. Engelhart S, Hanfland J, Glasmacher A, et al. Impact of portable air filtration units on exposure of haematology-oncology patients to airborne Aspergillus fumigatus spores under field conditions. *J Hosp Infect* 2003;54(4):300–304.

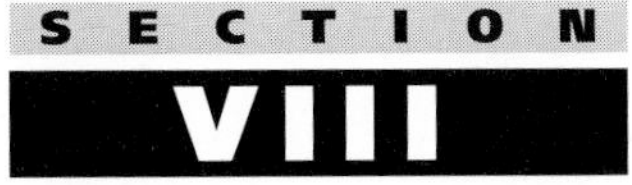

EPIDEMIOLOGY AND PREVENTION OF NOSOCOMIAL INFECTIONS ASSOCIATED WITH DIAGNOSTIC AND THERAPEUTIC PROCEDURES

61

NOSOCOMIAL INFECTIONS ASSOCIATED WITH ANESTHESIA

LOREEN A. HERWALDT
JEAN M. POTTINGER
STACY A. COFFIN
SEBASTIAN SCHULZ-STüBNER

Modern anesthesiology had its origin in the less than honorable pastime of "nitrous oxide capers" and the "ether frolics" of the 1800s (1). William Clark, who participated in those parties, was reportedly the first individual to use ether as an anesthetic, administering it initially during a tooth extraction (2). Soon thereafter, William T. G. Morton, a dentist, administered ether to a patient while John Collins Warren, a professor of surgery at Harvard, removed a tumor from the patient's neck (1). In England, John Snow, who achieved fame for removing the handle of the Broad Street pump and for administering chloroform to Queen Victoria during childbirth, researched many aspects of volatile gas delivery, physiologic effects, and metabolism (3–5). In doing so, Snow elevated anesthesiology from "a rag-and-bottle craft to a specialty based on scientific knowledge" (3).

Unfortunately, Snow did not use his considerable epidemiologic expertise to evaluate whether general anesthesia could be complicated by infections. However, as early as 1873, Skinner (6) raised provocative questions about the infection control practices of anesthesiologists. Since then, numerous anesthesia personnel have investigated whether anesthesia equipment and medications can transmit infections to patients. Various groups have published infection control guidelines for anesthesia practice, including the American Society for Anesthesiology (ASA) (7), the American Association of Nurse Anesthetists (AANA) (8), the Association of Operating Room Nurses (AORN) (9–12), the Centers for Disease Control and Prevention (CDC) (13,14), the Australia and New Zealand College of Anaesthetists (15), the Australian Society of Anaesthetists (16), the Australian Medical Association (17), the New South Wales Health Department (18), the Association of Anaesthetists of Great Britain and Ireland (19), the Department of Health the Netherlands Committee on Infection Prevention (20), and the Societé Francaise d'Anesthesie et de Reanimation (21). Hauer et al. (22) published (in German) a review and critique of hygiene procedures in anesthesia and critical care, and Bimar et al. (23) published their recommendations for infection control in anesthesia. Bowring (24) wrote a short history of infection control in anesthesia. Guidelines and recommendations have proliferated recently. Despite the mass of published material and official guidelines, many important questions remain unanswered.

This chapter reviews and critiques the extant literature on infections associated with anesthesia, particularly the pathogenesis and epidemiology of infections related to general, neuraxial, and intravenous anesthesia; describes outbreaks in which anesthesia personnel served as the reservoirs of infection; discusses practices that put anesthesia personnel at risk for particular occupationally acquired infections; and summarizes measures that can be used to prevent both anesthesia-related and occupationally acquired infections.

INFECTIONS ASSOCIATED WITH GENERAL ANESTHESIA

Pathogenesis

Endotracheal intubation and general anesthesia disrupt the respiratory system's defense mechanisms. The upper airway, which warms, humidifies, and removes large particles from inspired air, is bypassed when an endotracheal tube is inserted. Studies in experimental animals indicate that endotracheal tubes quickly disrupt the ciliated epithelium of the trachea and induce an inflammatory response (25–30). The damaged tracheal epithelium transports mucus poorly.

Drugs used routinely during general anesthesia also debilitate the ciliated epithelium. Opiates directly depress ciliary activity (31), and atropine impairs mucociliary clearance by decreasing bronchial secretions and drying the mucous membranes (32, 33). Dry anesthetic gases damage the ciliated cells and slow mucus flow (34–36). In addition, high concentrations of oxygen cause an inflammatory response in, and sloughing of, the ciliated epithelium (37). Although the extent to which each component of endotracheal intubation, ventilation patterns, and anesthetic drugs and gases damages the respiratory epithelium cannot be determined, data from studies of animals and humans indicate that "the physiologic state of the mucociliary transport system deteriorates under the conditions of intubation, premedication, and [inadequate] humidification used for a routine surgical procedure" (32).

In addition to disrupting the respiratory tract's defenses, the endotracheal tube can transfer bacteria from the patient's pharynx into the trachea (38,39). The endotracheal tube also allows pathogenic microorganisms not present in the patient's preoperative pharyngeal flora to be inoculated directly into the bronchial tree. Redman and Lockey (40) found that none of 46 patients undergoing cardiac operations had coliforms in preoperative cultures of the nose, throat, or larynx. Although most patients were intubated less than 24 hours, cultures of 21 endotracheal tubes yielded gram-negative bacteria, including *Escherichia coli* (17), *Proteus vulgaris* (3), and *Pseudomonas aeruginosa* (1,40). Similarly, Dominquez de Villota et al. (41) found that only one of 28 patients undergoing open-heart operative procedures was colonized preoperatively with a potential pathogen. Immediately after their operations, four patients were colonized with potentially pathogenic microorganisms, including group A β-hemolytic streptococci (one patient), *Pseudomonas stutzeri* (one patient), *Enterococcus faecalis* (one patient), and *Streptococcus pneumoniae* (one patient). After 19 hours, nine patients were colonized by potential pathogens including group A β-hemolytic streptococci (two patients), *P. aeruginosa* (two patients), *Candida albicans* (three patients), *Serratia marcescens* (one patient), and *Klebsiella ozaenae* (one patient) (41). In addition to contaminating the respiratory tract, nasal-tracheal intubation can cause transient bacteremia (42,43).

Epidemiology

Data Suggesting that Anesthesia Equipment Is a Source of Infection

Anesthesia personnel continue to debate whether their equipment transmits pathogenic microorganisms to patients. Numerous authors cite three alleged outbreaks as evidence that contaminated anesthesia machines transmit microorganisms. The initial cluster was reported by Joseph (44), who claimed that "several cases of follicular tonsillitis in all patients administered an anesthetic during a one week period indicated the transfer of microbes from patient to patient by inefficiently sanitized apparatus." However, Joseph provided no additional data to support his claim. Subsequently, Tinne et al. (45) reported an outbreak in which seven cardiothoracic surgery patients, three of whom died, acquired respiratory infections caused by pyocin type 10 *P. aeruginosa. P. aeruginosa* was isolated from numerous sites in the operating room; however, the authors claimed that only those microorganisms taken from the patients, the Ambu rebreathing bag, and a connecting tube of a Bennet ventilator were pyocin type 10. Despite destroying the Ambu bag and treating the ventilator with ethylene oxide after the first two cases were recognized, five additional cases were noted, two of which occurred after the operating unit was extensively decontaminated. Olds et al. (46) reported a cluster of four patients who were colonized or infected with *P. aeruginosa* after cardiac operations. All procedures requiring cardiopulmonary bypass and most other cardiothoracic procedures were performed in one operating room with one anesthesia machine. Before the cluster, anesthesia masks, tubing, rebreathing bags, and connectors were cleaned but not sterilized between cases. *P. aeruginosa* was isolated from the bellows, Y connector, and face mask. One patient was colonized by a strain that was pyocin-typeable, but strains from the index case who had a fatal pneumonia and from one colonized patient were pyocin-nontypeable, as were those from the machine. The authors concluded that the strains were the same and originated from the anesthesia machine because only "7% of *P. aeruginosa* strains are nontypeable" and all of the nontypeable strains displayed the "same duality of phenotype" (46). No further cases occurred after the authors began autoclaving all detachable parts of the anesthesia equipment between cases.

Although the authors of these reports implicated contaminated anesthesia equipment as the source of the infections, their data are less than convincing (44–46). None of the authors conclusively documented the source of the infecting microorganisms. Furthermore, their typing methods evaluated phenotypic, not genotypic, characteristics. Although pyocin typing was state-of-the-art at the time, it does not discriminate between strains as well as modern molecular typing methods do.

Albrecht and Dryden (47) examined postoperative pneumonia rates by retrospectively reviewing the medical records of 220 randomly selected patients. All patients underwent abdominal surgery with general anesthesia and were not infected at the time of the operation. The investigators noted that ten (20%) of the 50 patients who underwent operations before the anesthesia equipment was sterilized and 13 (26%) of the 50 patients who underwent operations when breathing circuits were sterilized but the absorbers were reused acquired postoperative pneumonia. In contrast, only seven (6%) of 120 patients acquired postoperative pneumonia after the anesthesiologists began using sterile breathing circuits and disposable absorbers. The authors claimed that their study provides conclusive evidence that contaminated anesthesia machines transmit bacteria to patients and that these machines should be sterilized between cases. However, the study has several major methodologic flaws that invalidate their results and conclusions. First, they did not clearly define postoperative pneumonia. Second, they did not state whether the persons abstracting the medical records were blinded to the hypothesis being tested. Third, they used historical controls, but they did not substantiate their claim that the "only change was complete cleaning of the breathing circuit between each anesthetic procedure."

Other investigators either obtained cultures from anesthesia equipment after routine use or conducted *in vitro* studies to determine if microorganisms could survive in anesthesia equipment. In general, such experiments identified a wide variety of bacteria contaminating all parts of used anesthesia machines, but the parts of the machine closest to the patient were most heavily contaminated. Joseph (44) isolated primarily saprophytic micrococci and bacilli from breathing circuits and rebreathing bags that were used without being sanitized between cases. The total bacterial counts from the rinse water ranged from 200,000 to 3,400,000 colony-forming units (CFU) for breathing circuits and from 345,000 to 736,000 CFU for rebreathing bags. Stratford et al. (48) obtained cultures from 23 routinely used anesthesia machines. They isolated *Staphylococcus aureus, Staphylococcus albus, E. coli, P. aeruginosa,* viridans streptococci, and *Bacillus* species from reservoir bags, inspiratory tubes, and expiratory tubes with total bacterial counts ranging from as few as ten to as many as 4×10^8 microorganisms. They also noted that the surfaces and knobs of the machines were contaminated with streptococci, *Bacillus* species, *S. aureus,* and *S. albus,* but not with coliforms.

Beck and Zadeh (49) obtained cultures from the four anesthesia machines used in their hospital and found *P. aeruginosa* in the expiratory valve of one machine). Similarly, Dryden (50) found that inspiratory and expiratory valves were frequently contaminated with many different microorganisms. Meeks et al. (51) obtained cultures from anesthesia equipment after use. They grew *Staphylococcus epidermidis* from 73% of face masks, 12% of Y connectors, 6% of breathing circuits, and 6% of rebreathing bags; *S. aureus* from 10% of face masks and 1% of rebreathing tubes; and *Pseudomonas* species from 36% of face masks, 67% of Y connectors, 42% of breathing circuits, and 79% of rebreathing bags. In Livingstone et al.'s (52) study, 13 of 39 (33%) of the rubber masks used to anesthetize tuberculosis patients yielded *Mycobacterium tuberculosis.* Likewise, several investigators who obtained cultures from face masks used to administer nitrous oxide for dental procedures demonstrated that bacteria from a patient's nose and mouth contaminated the apparatus (53–55).

Investigators have also determined that the soda lime canisters in the circuits do not filter bacteria effectively. Using an artificial device, Jenkins and Edgar (56) demonstrated that interposing soda lime did not decrease the number of *S. epidermidis* microorganisms that passed through the canister. Murphy et al. (57) aerosolized eight different bacterial species into a soda lime canister and found that up to 40% of the microorganisms were not retained in the canister. Similarly, Dryden (50) aerosolized *P. aeruginosa* or *Proteus mirabilis* (10^6 CFU/mL) into a canister packed with 450 g of soda lime and used a filter to catch bacteria that passed through the soda lime canister. Cultures of the control filters, which were exposed to aerosolized saline for 90 minutes, were negative, whereas cultures of the test filters were positive after only 2 minutes.

Investigators have noted that the soda lime in the canister is not uniformly bactericidal. Murphy et al. (57) demonstrated that, at room temperature, 1 g of soda lime killed *Klebsiella pneumoniae, C. albicans, S. aureus, P. aeruginosa, S. marcescens, E. coli,* and *S. pneumoniae* within 10 minutes. However, of 1.1×10^5 CFU of *Bacillus subtilis,* 3.1×10^4 CFU survived at 10 minutes, and 1.5×10^3 CFU survived at 30 minutes (57). Dryden (50) demonstrated that 4% sodium hydroxide, Sodasorb extract, and Baralyme extract killed *P. aeruginosa* and *P. mirabilis* within 15 minutes; however, *M. tuberculosis* survived for at least 3 hours in each of the solutions.

Because deliberately contaminating anesthesia machines before use would not be ethical, numerous investigators used laboratory models to simulate the patient–anesthesia machine interaction. To determine whether anesthetic gases could become contaminated when blown through contaminated circuits, Nielsen et al. (58) measured the bacterial content of anesthetic gases before and after passing them through clean and used breathing systems. Gases passed through clean circuits contained 1.2 to 50.2 (median 4.2) CFU of bacteria per 100 L, compared with 3.3 to 129.8 (median 38.5) CFU of bacteria per 100 L for gas passed through used circuits (Mann-Whitney $p < .01$). The authors concluded that anesthetic gases can transfer microorganisms.

Jenkins and Edgar (56) passed oxygen through previously used Y pieces and expiratory limbs of breathing circuits. They recovered *S. aureus* from the oxygen passed through 1 of 11 breathing circuits. Dryden (50) seeded the expiratory valve of a sterile circle absorber with 10^7 CFU of *P. aeruginosa* . He closed the system with a bag at the patient end of the breathing circuit and moved air through the system by manually compressing the breathing bag. Cultures of the inhalation valve obtained 15 minutes into the experiment grew *P. aeruginosa.* Dryden concluded that air moved the bacteria through the circuit.

Rathgeber et al. (59) obtained cultures of used breathing circuits to assess microbiologic contamination. When a filter was used, microorganisms that were isolated from the breathing circuits were not the same microorganisms that were detected in the patients' tracheal aspirates. When no filter was used, the same microorganisms were isolated from the patients' tracheal aspirates and the tubing in 13% of the cases. However, the investigators did not follow these patients to determine if the filters prevented postoperative pneumonia. Therefore, even though they demonstrated that patients' microorganisms can contaminate the breathing circuits and that filters can effectively prevent contamination, they did not show that the filters changed the outcome, i.e., the incidence of postoperative pneumonia.

Investigators from the New South Wales (NSW) Health Department evaluated a cluster of patients who acquired hepatitis C virus (HCV) infection after having operative procedures at a private hospital in Sydney (60). After two persons who had operations on the same day presented to the hospital with acute hepatitis C, NSW health officials tested all patients who had operative procedures during the same session. Three more patients were found to be anti-HCV positive. Surgical personnel were tested and were anti-HCV negative. Patient-to-patient transmission seemed likely, because all five patients were infected with hepatitis C of the same genotype. The investigators noted that the same anesthesia circuit was used without a filter and without decontamination for all 11 patients who had procedures during the implicated session. On the basis of these data, the investigators concluded that the HCV was transmitted through a contaminated anesthesia circuit. They hypothesized that the index case's respiratory secretions containing HCV were introduced into the anesthesia circuit and the virus was transmitted in droplets through minor breaks in the oropharyngeal mucosa of subsequent patients. In response, NSW health officials recommended enforcing an existing guideline that a filter be used in the anesthesia circuit to prevent cross-transmission (18,61).

A number of other agencies, including the AANA (8), the Blood Borne Viruses Advisory Panel of the Association of Anaesthetists of Great Britain and Ireland (19), the Department of Health of the Netherlands Committee on Infection Prevention (20), and the Societé Francaise d'Anesthesie et Reanimation (21) have recommended that an appropriate filter be placed between the patient and the breathing system and that either a new filter or a new breathing circuit should be used for each patient. At present, there is no consensus on whether hydrophobic pleated membrane filters are necessary or whether electrostatic filters are adequate. Most studies of filtration efficiency have indicated that the hydrophobic filters are more efficient (62–64). However, one study of patients undergoing general anesthesia found no difference between hydrophobic filters and electrostatic filters (65). Both filter types significantly decreased the incidence of bacterial contamination in the breathing circuits compared with the level of contamination in endotracheal tubes.

Of note after the guidelines regarding use of filters were published, Heaton et al. (66) conducted a phone survey of hospitals in England to determine whether anaesthetists were following the recommendations. They found that 43 of 55 hospitals routinely used filters in breathing systems. Atkinson et al. (67) conducted a postal survey of 120 hospitals in the United Kingdom, of which 76% replied. Among the respondents, 77.2% of the departments reported that their staff members use a new filter for each patient and 66.3% felt this was a worthwhile practice. However, the respondents felt the primary reason to use filters was to prevent gross contamination of the breathing system but not to prevent transmission of viruses. Only 35.9% of the respondents thought this practice was cost-effective. Daniel and Fowler (68) recently reviewed data in the literature supporting the use of filters in breathing systems.

In summary, the studies reviewed in this section suggest the following:

1. Bacteria can contaminate all parts of anesthesia circuits, but the highest numbers of bacteria contaminate the parts closest to the patient.
2. Some bacteria can be carried by the anesthetic gases from the machine to the patient or vice versa.
3. The soda lime removes bacteria imperfectly, and although it kills many bacterial pathogens, *M. tuberculosis* and *Bacillus* species survive prolonged exposure.
4. Filters decrease contamination of breathing circuits.

Data Suggesting that Anesthesia Equipment Is Not a Source of Infection

In contrast, other anesthesia personnel maintain that anesthesia machines, even when contaminated, do not transmit significant numbers of bacteria. They claim that microorganisms do not survive in the hostile environment of the anesthesia machine. For example, microorganisms are desiccated by the flow of cold, dry anesthetic gases (69). Furthermore, rubber and metal parts of the machine and the highly alkaline condensate at the bottom of the CO_2 absorber inhibit growth of bacteria (70,71).

Stemmermann and Stern (72) asked 14 patients with cavitary tuberculosis to breathe into a basal metabolic rate machine (which is similar to an anesthesia breathing circuit) for 10 minutes and then cough. The investigators did not identify *M. tuberculosis* in smears or cultures of the saline used to wash the masks and tubing. Hence, they concluded that such equipment was unlikely to transmit *M. tuberculosis* from patient to patient.

Du Moulin and Saubermann (70) studied 15 patients anesthetized with sterile machines. Before being anesthetized, two consecutive throat and sputum cultures from each of six patients yielded more than 10 CFU of gram-negative rods, and cultures from nine patients did not yield gram-negative bacteria. Subsequently, the investigators cut the breathing circuits into 14 segments and obtained specimens of the entire surface of each segment. They isolated 1 to 9 CFU per segment, and the microorganisms were randomly distributed along the corrugated tubing. All cultures from machines used on colonized patients were negative. Three cultures from machines used on uncolonized patients were positive; a gram-negative rod was isolated from an expiratory port, and *S. epidermidis* was isolated from a soda lime canister and from a ventilator connection port.

Ping et al. (73) obtained specimens from machines before and after they were used to anesthetize 33 patients who had no symptoms of respiratory disease and 17 patients who had "excessive" lower respiratory tract secretions. Of the 550 cultures obtained from anesthesia equipment immediately before and after use, only five yielded growth. *S. epidermidis* was recovered from one pre- and three postanesthesia cultures obtained from two patients who did not have excessive secretions, and viridans streptococci were recovered from one postanesthesia culture obtained from a patient with excessive secretions.

In a laboratory simulation, Adriani and Rovenstine (74) were unable to grow microorganisms from air blown through soda lime canisters contaminated with large numbers of *E. coli* or *M. tuberculosis* microorganisms. Ziegler and Jacoby (75) used a contaminated machine to ventilate a sterile reservoir bag for 30 minutes. Cultures of the reservoir bag remained negative. Similarly, Pandit et al. (76) were unable to detect microorganisms in the air blown through equipment contaminated with *P. aeruginosa, S. albus,* or *E. faecalis.* After inoculating the expiratory port of a sterile circle system with 10^8 to 10^9 CFU of either *Enterobacter cloacae* or *Flavobacterium* species, du Moulin and Saubermann (70) blew 3 L of nitrous oxide and oxygen per minute through the valve for 3 hours. Every 30 minutes, they obtained samples from the valve and found progressively fewer bacteria in the cultures. They did not recover the indicator microorganisms from other parts of the machine. Ibrahim and Perceval (77) randomly chose 20 used breathing circuits and obtained cultures for bacteria and fungi. In addition, they obtained cultures from ten circuits that had been washed and dried. They also attached ten cleaned circuits to an anesthesia machine, circulated air for 4 hours through the circuits, and then obtained cultures. The investigators claimed that none of the cultures grew significant pathogens. However, *P. aeruginosa, Pseudomonas maltophilia,* and *Pseudomonas alcaligenes* were all grown from some of the circuits after they were used for patients. The investigators also seeded cleaned circuits with viridans streptococci or staphylococcal bacteriophages. They attached these circuits to machines and blew air through them. Air sampling cultures obtained from the distal ends of the tubes were all negative.

Two prospective clinical trials have been cited as evidence that anesthesia machines are not a major source of infections for surgical patients. Garibaldi et al. (78) randomly assigned 257 patients to be anesthetized with disposable corrugated plastic circuits containing bacterial filters (0.22 μm) and 263 patients to be anesthetized with disposable corrugated plastic circuits without filters (78). They were unable to identify a statistically significant difference in postoperative pneumonia rates between the two groups. Their study had 90% power to detect a 50%

difference in pneumonia rates. Feeley et al. (79) found no difference in postoperative pneumonia rates between 138 patients anesthetized with sterile disposable circuits and 155 patients anesthetized using clean reusable circuits. However, their power to detect a 50% difference in rates was only 0.17, $\alpha = 0.05$ (two-tailed chi-square). A 50% difference in pneumonia rates is well beyond what one could expect in a clinical trial. To detect smaller, clinically important differences, one would need to conduct much larger studies. For example, Hess (80) noted that to detect an increase in pneumonia rates from 3% to 5%, 1,500 patients would need to be enrolled to achieve $\alpha = 0.05$, $\beta = 0.20$, and a power of 0.80.

Van Hassel et al. (81) reviewed 9 years of surveillance data. They found lower respiratory tract infections in five of 2,300 (0.2%) patients undergoing operations under regional anesthesia and 31 of 23,500 (0.1%) patients undergoing general anesthesia with tubing that was cleaned only once a day (i.e., was shared by three to seven patients). They changed the soda lime every 3 days and they placed filters at the T pieces only when patients had suspected or overt respiratory tract infections, *M. tuberculosis*, or human immunodeficiency virus (HIV) infection. They concluded that "in our setting, patient factors are most important in the development of postoperative lower respiratory infections and that the role of bacterial filters as a preventive measure is negligible."

In summary, the studies reviewed in this section suggest the following:

1. The environment in the anesthesia machine does not promote survival or growth of bacteria.
2. Some bacteria contaminate the equipment, but anesthetic gases do not move substantial numbers of bacteria toward the patient.
3. Neither filters nor sterile circuits lower pneumonia rates below those seen with clean circuits or with circuits that are changed daily.

Conclusions About the Role of Anesthesia Equipment as a Source of Infection

Despite heated debate, the clinical importance of microorganisms isolated from anesthesia machines and their role in postoperative infections have not been clearly defined. Hogarth (82), after thoroughly reviewing published studies, concluded "there is little evidence to implicate anaesthetic machines and breathing systems as either a source of or vector for bacterial infection of patients undergoing general anaesthesia within the operating theatre." We concur with his assessment. We do not think the outbreaks reported by Joseph (44), Tinne et al. (45), and Olds et al. (46), or the experimental data, provide evidence for transmission of pathogens by anesthesia machines. Furthermore, we do not think Chant et al.'s (60) report provides convincing evidence that contaminated anesthesia circuits transmitted hepatitis C. The latter report did not discuss whether the anesthesia staff complied with critical infection control practices, such as changing gloves between procedures on the same case, changing gloves between cases, and cleaning and disinfecting the anesthesia cart and equipment between cases (83). Moreover, anesthesia circuits have not been implicated in transmission of hepatitis B virus, which is transmitted more readily than is HCV. The report by Chant et al. does suggest that anesthesia and infection control staff must watch for apparent clusters of nosocomial hepatitis C infection and should review the literature frequently to see whether new modes of transmission have been identified for this virus.

Given that the parts of the circuit closest to the patient are most highly contaminated, we agree with the ASA, which recommends that breathing circuits and masks be cleaned and disinfected between cases (7) (see Current Infection Control Guidelines, below). In addition, although filters effectively prevent transfer of bacteria from the patient to the anesthesia machine and from the machine to the patient (84–86), they have not been shown to prevent infections. Thus, we believe that currently available data do not support routine use of filters (7,78, 87) in addition to a clean circuit. Some anesthesiologists insert a filter and a 20-cm swivel connector to the breathing circuit and replace this section after each case. To date this practice has not been evaluated extensively, but it is supported by studies on the efficacy of filters. Patients with active pulmonary tuberculosis who must be given general anesthesia should have a filter in the endotracheal tube or in the expiratory limb of the circuit to reduce the risk of contaminating the anesthesia machine or releasing acid-fast bacteria into the environment (13). The two clinical trials cited above did not identify statistically significant differences in postoperative pneumonia rates between the comparison groups (78,79). However, neither study was designed to detect clinically relevant differences in postoperative pneumonia rates (e.g., 20%). Therefore, clinical trials comparing postoperative pneumonia rates in patients anesthetized with filtered or nonfiltered circuits, with sterile or clean circuits, and sterile or periodically cleaned anesthesia ventilator equipment, are warranted.

INFECTIONS ASSOCIATED WITH NEURAXIAL BLOCKADE

Pathogenesis of Infections Associated with Central Neuraxial Blockade

Microorganisms from exogenous or endogenous sources enter the subarachnoid or epidural space in several ways. Microorganisms from the patient's or anesthesia practitioner's flora can be inoculated directly when the catheter is inserted, as probably occurred in one case reported by North and Brophy (88). In this case, *S. aureus* of the same phage type was isolated from both the epidural abscess and the nose of the anesthesiologist; *S. aureus* with a different phage type was isolated from the patient's nose (88). Several other groups have reported similar cases. Trautmann et al. (89) identified a case of meningitis caused by a *S. aureus* strain that was identical by pulsed-field gel electrophoresis to the *S. aureus* isolate in the anesthesiologist's nose. Schneeberger et al. (90) reported a cluster of meningitis caused by several streptococcal species after subarachnoid neural blockade administered by the same anesthesiologist. The anesthesiologist routinely talked to his patients and did not wear a mask during the procedures. The anesthesiologist complained of recurrent pharyngitis and tonsillitis at the time the first two cases occurred. The investigators concluded that respiratory droplets may have transmitted mouth flora from the anesthesiologist to the patients and, thus, they suggested that all anesthesia personnel wear face masks when performing subarachnoid neural blockade. Assuming that the respiratory tract of anesthesia personnel could be a source of infection, Philips et al. (91) conducted a simulation to assess the efficacy of masks. They seated anesthesia staff in a room with controlled ventilation and asked the volunteers to speak directly at blood agar plates placed 30 cm away. The number of bacteria on the plates was significantly lower when masks were worn.

Microorganisms can also enter the epidural space by hematogenous spread from other body sites, most often skin infections (92), or by migrating along the catheter tract (93,94). A study by Wulf and Striepling (95) suggested that hematogenous spread can occur from infected sites to the epidural space. They performed autopsies on ten patients who had continuous epidural neural blockade for 2 to 21 days after operative procedures. At postmortem examination, seven of nine patients who had both infection and an epidural neural blockade had evidence of epidural infection. The investigators did not find evidence of epidural infection in the nine control patients who had similar underlying infections but did not have an epidural neural blockade. Pinczower and Gyorke (96) reported a case of L1 osteomyelitis caused by *P. aeruginosa* in a 76-year-old man who had a lower respiratory tract infection caused by the same microorganism. Bengtsson et al. (97) reported three cases of spinal space infection in 4 years. The three cases occurred in different hospitals, and three different anesthesiologists did the epidural neural blockades. All three patients had coexisting lower extremity contaminated wounds and two of the three patients were infected with microorganisms that infected their wounds. The investigators concluded that infected lower extremity wounds were a contraindication for epidural anesthesia. Newman (98) did not find any epidural catheter-related infections among over 3,000 patients who had epidural neural blockades for postoperative or posttraumatic analgesia. Thus, Newman did not believe that lower extremity infections were contraindications to epidural anesthesia.

Rarely, contaminated anesthetics are injected into the patient's subarachnoid or epidural space. For example, North and Brophy (88) reported an infection in which *S. aureus* strains with matching phage types were recovered from an abscess and the multidose lidocaine vial. Green and Pathy (99) questioned whether staff can draw up opioids sterilely from ampules, but did not provide evidence to support their concern. They suggested that these drugs be drawn through a filter into a syringe that is then double wrapped and sterilized in ethylene oxide. Raedler et al. (100) obtained cultures of 114 spinal and 20 epidural needles after use for single-injection lumbar anesthesia. Twenty-four cultures (17.9%) grew microorganisms: 15.7% coagulase-negative staphylococci, 1.5% yeasts, and 0.8% each enterococcus, pneumococcus, and micrococcus. However, no infections occurred in the study population. The anesthesiologists who performed these procedures wore "operating room dress," and used sterile gloves and sterile drapes. These authors concluded that it is easy to contaminate the needle and that anesthesiologists need to improve their hygienic measures.

Other investigators evaluated specimens from catheters or syringes. In four studies, 0% to 29% of the catheters were contaminated (101–104) and James et al. (101) found that five of 101 syringes used to inject an anesthetic agent were contaminated. Ross et al. (105) drew up bupivacaine 0.25% into control syringes and into syringes used to induce continuous lumbar epidural neural blockade (test syringe) in 18 obstetric patients). After each dose from the test syringe, cultures were obtained from the contents of both the test and control syringes. Six of 18 test syringes were contaminated with bacteria, compared with one of 18 control syringes. In the five studies cited above, none of the patients acquired infections (101–105). Hence, the authors could not correlate contaminated catheters or syringes with infection.

Yaniv and Potasman (106) reviewed 60 reports of meningitis after subarachnoid or epidural neural blockades or after other "spinal manipulations." Of the 60 infections, 27 (45%) occurred after subarachnoid anesthesia and 4 (6.7%) occurred after epidural anesthesia. Three (5%) of the patients died. Fifty-two of 60 patients had positive cultures, and 43 of those patients were infected with gram-positive microorganisms (33 streptococci and three staphylococci). Only two of the anesthesiologists wore face masks, and most used an iodophor to prepare the skin.

Dawson's (107) review of studies on infections associated with epidural anesthesia indicates that there is no consensus regarding patient risk factors for infectious complications. In addition, the literature includes conflicting reports about the association of the risk of infection with the duration of catheterization and the site of the catheter. Horlocker's (108) review of complications associated with spinal and epidural anesthesia addresses several issues regarding infections after these procedures.

Infections Associated with Epidural Neural Blockade

Epidemiology

Infections rarely complicate short-term epidural neural blockade. Data from two reviews of epidural abscesses suggest that only 1 of 74 infections (1.4%) was related to an epidural catheter (92,109). In 1966, Lund (110) reported no infections in 11,136 epidural blockades. In 1969, Dawkins (111) reviewed more than 350 articles on epidural neural blockade used for operative procedures and for obstetrics. He found no reports of infection after thoracic or lumbar epidural block, but eight (0.2%) of 3,767 sacral epidural blocks were complicated by infection. Dawson (107) recently reviewed the literature and found rates of deep infection ranging from 0% to 0.7% and rates of superficial infection ranging from 1.8% to 12%. Brooks et al. (112) reviewed data from the first 30 months of their pain management service. During this time period, 4,832 procedures were done. Four women (0.08%) who had epidural analgesia for labor and delivery acquired infections. Three infectious were caused by *S. aureus* and one was caused by *S. epidermidis*. Two of the infections were superficial and two were epidural abscesses, one of which was complicated by meningitis.

In a survey of all obstetric units in the U.K., Scott and Hibbard (113) identified one epidural abscess in approximately 506,000 epidural neural blockades given for labor or cesarean section. Palot et al. (114) identified three cases of meningitis in 300,000 patients who had undergone epidural blocks. No infections were identified in three series of obstetric epidural neural blockade that included nearly 12,000 patients (115–117). Together, these studies suggest that three to four serious infections (i.e., epidural abscesses or meningitis) occur per 1 million obstetric epidural neural blocks.

Few studies identified infections associated with epidural neural blockades for operative procedures or for short-term pain relief. Hunt et al. (104) noted one case of localized cellulitis in 102 patients who had catheters in place for fewer than 12 days, and Sethna et al. (118) did not find any infections in approximately 1,200 pediatric surgical patients who had catheters in place for fewer than 8 days. In a retrospective review, Abel et al. (119) did not identify any infections among the 4,392 patients who had epidural catheters placed during operations (mean duration of epidural catheters 2.4 days; range, 0–9 days). Grass et al. (120) reviewed medical records of 5,193 patients who received epidural analgesia for an average of 3.76 days. They did not identify any patients with epidural abscess or meningitis, but one patient had an exit-site infection and two patients had inflammation at the insertion site. McNeely et al. (121) prospectively followed 91 pediatric patients who had epidural catheters in place for 20 to 110 hours, none of whom acquired epidural infection during the study period. Phillips et al. (122) identified three epidural abscesses, all caused by *S. aureus*, among 2,401 patients (0.12%) who had postoperative analgesia over a 5-year period. One of the patients was infected with a methicillin-resistant *S. aureus* (MRSA) strain identical to that infecting another patient on the ward, suggesting person-to-person transmission. The author noted that syringes were used to give the anesthetizing agents to all three patients. They concluded that syringes are easily contaminated and subsequently elected to use 250 mL bags to administer the anesthetizing agents thereafter.

Kost-Byerly et al. (123) evaluated 210 children who had short-term epidural catheters to determine whether caudal catheters were more likely to become infected than lumbar catheters. They did not find any serious systemic infections. Cellulitis occurred in 13% of children with caudal catheters and 3% of those with lumbar catheters. The incidence of cellulitis associated with caudal catheters was not statistically higher for children less than 3 years old (14%) than for those who were older than 3 (9%). Colonization with gram-positive microorganisms did not vary by site, but 16% of the caudal catheters were colonized with gram-negative microorganisms compared with only 3% of the lumbar catheters. Strafford et al. (124) evaluated 1,620 infants, children, and adolescents who had epidural analgesia over a 6-year period. Of these patients, none of the 1,458 patients who had the epidurals for perioperative pain control acquired skin infections or epidural abscesses. On the basis of these data, the authors estimated the incidence of clinical infection to be 0 with a 95% confidence interval (CI) from 0% to 0.03%, or 3/10,000 procedures. One patient of the 162 who had epidural anesthesia to control pain from terminal malignancies had *Candida tropicalis* colonization of a necrotic spinal metastasis.

Holt et al. (125) evaluated epidural catheters inserted by staff in their hospital and in their region. They estimated that 6% of the catheters were colonized, 4.3% were associated with local infections, and 0.7% were associated with meningitis or epidural abscess. In a subsequent letter to the editor, they decreased these estimates to 1.8% for local infections and 0.4% for central nervous system infections, because they felt their original denominator was too small (126). They noted that the median duration of catheterization was 8 days for patients with local infections and 15 days for patients with generalized symptoms (p = .01). They also noted that catheters removed from patients with clinical symptoms were more heavily colonized than those from asymptomatic patients. However, 59 of the 78 catheters that had positive cultures were removed, because the patients were symptomatic, suggesting that this observation was affected by ascertainment bias.

Darchy et al. (127) evaluated 75 patients who had epidural analgesia for ≥48 hours while they were in an intensive care unit (ICU). Nine (12%) patients had local infections, which were defined as discharge at the insertion site and a positive culture, and cultures of catheters from four (1.3%) patients were positive. The authors did not identify any deep infections. They calculated an incidence density rate of 2.7/100 catheter days for local infections and 1.2/100 catheter days for colonized or contaminated catheters. They estimated the upper risk of a spinal space infection to be 4.8% for catheters that remained in place for 4 days.

Epidural catheters inserted for long-term pain control are infected more frequently than those used for short-term pain control. Du Pen et al. (128) followed 350 patients who had long-term epidural catheters and identified 30 superficial (9.3/10,000 catheter-days), eight deep catheter track (2.5/10,000 catheter-days), and 15 epidural space (4.6/10,000 catheter-days) infections. Two of 139 patients (1.4%, or 2.1/10,000 catheter-days) treated by Zenz et al. (129) for pain due to malignancy acquired meningitis. Of 92 cancer patients that Coombs (130) treated with epidural morphine, ten (10.9%) acquired local infections, and two (2.2%) acquired meningitis. Sethna et al. (118) reported one epidural space infection in approximately 150 pediatric patients treated for chronic pain.

Case Reports

Although infections rarely complicate short-term epidural neural blockade, case reports in the literature indicate that such infections do occur and that they can be severe (Table 61.1) (88,95,97,131–164). Of the 45 patients reported, 31 had an epidural or intraspinal abscess. Twenty-six of the 41 infections in which a bacterial pathogen was isolated were caused by *S. aureus,* two infections were caused by *S. epidermidis*, four by *P. aeruginosa*, five by streptococcus species, and one by enterococcus. Three patients died and 23 nearly or fully recovered. See the review by Sarrubi and Vasquez (161) for further information.

TABLE 61.1. INFECTIONS ASSOCIATED WITH EPIDURAL NEURAL BLOCKADE

First Author (Reference)	Year	Indication	Epidural Site	Filter Used	Catheter Duration	Type of Infection	Time from Insertion to Symptoms	Signs and Symptoms	Microorganism	Outcome
Edwards (131)	1943	Vaginal delivery	Caudal	Not specified	Not specified	Epidural abscess, bacteremia	Not specified	Not specified	*S. aureus*	Died 31 days after delivery
Ferguson (132)[a]	1974	Postoperative analgesia	Thoracic	Not specified	2 days	Epidural empyema	4 days	Fever, headache, meningismus	*S. epidermidis*	Sensory impairment, spastic weakness, walks with crutches
							10 days	Urinary retention		
							14 days	Paraparesis		
Saady (133)[a]	1976	Postoperative analgesia	Thoracic	Yes	1.7 days	Epidural abscess	4 days	Fever	*S. aureus*	Sensory impairment, walks with minimal assistance
							8 days	Chills, abdominal pain right upper quadrant		
							9 days	Headache, stiff neck		
							10 days	Urinary retention		
							14 days	Lower extremity paraparesis, no anal tone		
Dougherty (134)	1978	Low back pain	Not specified	Not specified	Epidural injections on three separate occasions by private physician	Meningitis, cellulitis	48 hours after last injection	Fever, headache, photophobia, stiff neck	Gram-positive cocci	Full recovery
North (88)	1979	1. Priapism	Lumbar	No	3 days	Epidural abscess	1 day	Fever	*S. aureus*	Full recovery
							10 days	Stiff neck, dysphagia, back pain, absent ankle jerks		
		2. Fractured ribs, chest injury	Thoracic	Yes	4 days	Epidural abscess	2 days	Fever	*S. aureus*	Sensory impairment
							4 days	Stiff neck, sensory loss T2-T6		
Wenningsted-Torgard (135)	1982	Lower back pain	Lumbar	Not specified	6 days	Skin abscess, spondylitis, bacteremia	10 days	Fever	*S. aureus*	Wedge formation of two vertebral bodies
McDonogh (136)	1984	Fractured ribs	Thoracic	Yes	3.3 days	Epidural abscess	60 hours	Fever	*S. aureus*	Residual left side weakness, uses walking frame, urinary retention
							19 days	Paralysis left leg, weakness right leg, urinary retention, sensory deficit T7-8		

(*continued*)

TABLE 61.1. (*continued*)

First Author (Reference)	Year	Indication	Epidural Site	Filter Used	Catheter Duration	Type of Infection	Time from Insertion to Symptoms	Signs and Symptoms	Microorganism	Outcome
Konig (137)	1985	Knee surgery	Lumbar	Not specified	4 days	Paravertebral and epidural abscesses, osteomyelitis, phlegmonous duritis, myelitis	2 weeks	Pain, lower extremity paraparesis	*S. epidermidis*	Nearly complete recovery
Sollmann (138)	1987	Phantom limb pain	Not specified	Not specified	6 weeks	Large encapsulated "spinal" abscess compressing dura at L4-5	6 weeks	Severe back pain	*P. aeruginosa*	Persistent pain
							5 months	Severe sciatica		
Fine (139)	1988	Neuralgic pain syndrome	Thoracic	Yes	3 days	Site infection, epidural abscess	9 days	Fever, chills, urinary retention	No culture obtained	Sensory impairment
Ready (140)	1989	1. Vaginal delivery	Lumbar	Not specified	50 minutes	Meningitis	24 hours	Headache, stiff neck, fever, back pain, nuchal rigidity	*S. uberis*	Full recovery
		2. Cesarean section	Not specified	Not specified	3 days	Cellulitis	84 hours	Fever	*S. faecalis*	Full recovery
						Meningitis	132 hours	Headache, nuchal rigidity, photophobia, hyperacusis		
Berga (141)	1989	Vaginal delivery	Lumbar	Not specified	Not specified	Meningitis	24 hours	Headache	*S. sanguis*	Full recovery
Chan (142)	1989	Back pain, sciatica	Lumbar	Not specified	One injection by private physician	Epidural abscess	2 days	Fever, chills, rigors	*S. aureus*	Partial recovery, walks with frame
							4 days	Bacteremia		
							6 days	Urinary retention, weakness both legs		
							8 days	Paraplegic, power loss upper extremities		
Goucke (143)	1990	Back pain	Lumbar	Not specified	3 epidural injections	Bacteremia, epidural abscess	23 days after last injection	Back pain, fever, urinary retention	*S. aureus*	Died 7 weeks after laminectomy
Lynch (144)	1990	Intra- and postoperative analgesia	Lumbar	Yes	3 days	Spondylitis	3 days	Fever, chills, headache, back pain	*P. aeruginosa*	9 month recovery, wears lumbar brace, some lumbar pain

(*continued*)

TABLE 61.1. (*continued*)

First Author (Reference)	Year	Indication	Epidural Site	Filter Used	Catheter Duration	Type of Infection	Time from Insertion to Symptoms	Signs and Symptoms	Microorganism	Outcome
Waldmann (145)	1991	Cervical radiculopathy	Cervical	Not specified	3 days	Epidural abscess	3 days	Shaking chills, stiff neck, fever, meningismus	*S. aureus*	Partial use of lower extremities but able to walk
Strong (146)	1991	1. Herpes zoster	Thoracic	Yes	2.5 days 3 days[b]	Epidural abscess	31 days	Pain, headache, stiff neck, fever, right flank pain	*S. aureus*	Full recovery
		2. Reflex sympathetic dystrophy	Cervical	Yes	5 days	Cellulitis	16 days	Cellulitis	Culture negative	Full recovery
					5 days[b]	Epidural abscess	7 weeks	Neck pain radiating to left arm		
Klygis (147)	1991	Vaginal delivery	Not specified	Not specified	Not specified	Epidural abscess	36 hours	Back pain, paresthesias medial thigh and plantar surface of feet, fever	Group G streptococci	Full recovery
Dawson (148)	1991	Postoperative analgesia	Thoracic	Yes	4 days	Epidural abscess	12 days 18 days	Numbness and weakness in leg, urinary incontinence Paraplegia, patulous anus	*S. aureus*	Loss of motor function, requires indwelling urinary catheter, able to take few steps with help
Ferguson (149)	1992	Intra- and postoperative analgesia	Lumbar	Yes	4 days	Cellulitis, epidural infection	7 days	Fever, back pain	*S. aureus*	Not specified
NganKee (150)	1992	Cesarean section	Lumbar	Yes	50 hours	Epidural abscess	5 days	Fever, back pain, rigors, bacteremia, paresthesias, weakness of both legs	*S. aureus*	Full recovery after 8 weeks
Sowter (151)	1992	Intra- and postoperative analgesia	Thoracic	Yes	5 days	Epidural abscess	25 days	Back pain, urinary retention, paresthesias and weakness both legs	*S. aureus*	Paraplegic with indwelling urethral catheter
Shintani (152)	1992	Herpes zoster	Lumbar	Not specified	3 days	Meningitis, epidural abscess	3 days	Headache, nausea, vomiting, fever, somnolence, back pain	Methicillin-resistant *S. aureus*	Full recovery

(*continued*)

TABLE 61.1. (*continued*)

First Author (Reference)	Year	Indication	Epidural Site	Filter Used	Catheter Duration	Type of Infection	Time from Insertion to Symptoms	Signs and Symptoms	Microorganism	Outcome
Nordstrom (153)	1993	Fractured ribs	Thoracic	Yes	6 days	Epidural abscess	19 days	Back pain, numbness both legs, fever, paresis urethral sphincter	*S. aureus*	Incomplete recovery of motor function 4 months after laminectomy
Davis (154)	1993	Vaginal delivery	Lumbar	Not specified	Less than 1 day	Meningitis	40 hours 42 hours	Headache, vomiting Confused, delirium, fever	Group B β-hemolytic Streptococci	Full recovery
Ania (155)	1994	Lumbar pain	Not specified	Not specified	8 days	Meningitis	1 day 3 days	Headache Chills, vomiting	*S. aureus*	Full recovery
Borum (156)	1995	Vaginal delivery	Lumbar	Yes	1 day	Epidural abscess	4 days 6 days	Low back pain, tingling both lower extremities Weakness both lower extremities	*S. aureus*	Full recovery
Liu (157)	1996	Extracorporeal shockwave lithotripsy	Not specified	Not specified	Not specified	Meningitis	2 days	Headache, photophobia	*S. pneumoniae*	Full recovery
Dunn (158)	1996	Intra- and postoperative analgesia	Not specified	Not specified	1 day	Epidural abscess, osteomyelitis	1 day 14 days	Neck and back pain Back pain, nausea, vomiting, pyrexia	*S. aureus*	Mild hip and loin pain 5 months after the operation
Cooper (159)	1996	Chronic back pain	Not specified	Not specified	Injection	Meningitis, cauda equina syndrome	3 days 13 days	Increased back pain, chills, profuse sweating Leg weakness, incontinent of stool	*S. aureus*	Incontinent of stool
Barontini (160)	1996	Transurethral resection of prostate	Lumbar	Not specified	Not specified	Epidural abscess	2 days 4 days	Fever, leg weakness Chills, pain, flaccid paraparesis of leg	No culture obtained	Paraplegia
Pinczower (95)	1996	Postoperative analgesia	Two inter-spaces above the intercristal line	Not specified	4 days	L1 vertebral osteomyelitis	3 weeks	Low back pain	*P. aeruginosa*	Full recovery

(*continued*)

TABLE 61.1. (*continued*)

First Author (Reference)	Year	Indication	Epidural Site	Filter Used	Catheter Duration	Type of Infection	Time from Insertion to Symptoms	Signs and Symptoms	Microorganism	Outcome
Bengtsson (97)	1997	1. Analgesia after a traumatic amputation	L3-4 T12-L1	Yes	1 days[b] 4 days[b]	Meningitis	4 days	High fever, pain and erythema at 2nd insertion site, stiff neck	*P. aeruginosa*	Full recovery
		2. Analgesia for phantom pains after an amputation	Lumbar	Yes	3 days	Soft tissue and interspinal abscess	3 days	High fever, severe headache, erythema *S. aureus* and swelling at insertions site, back pain radiating to right thigh	No culture obtained	Radicular pain in lower back
		3. Analgesia for painful foot ulcers	Lumbar tunneled catheter	Yes	16 days	Psoas abscess at L2-5 tracking to L3-4 intraspinal level	11 days 14 days	High fever Pain radiating from back	*S. aureus*	Full recovery
Sarubbi (161)	1997	1. Analgesia for reflex sympathetic dystrophy	L1-2	Not specified	3 days	Epidural abscess	3 days	High fever, cloudy drainage at catheter exit site	*S. aureus*	Recovered to her baseline
		2. Surgical anesthesia and postoperative analgesia	Not specified	Not specified	2 days	Epidural abscess and meningitis	2 days 5 days	Bilateral leg weakness and double vision Flaccid paralysis, double vision from 3rd nerve palsy, meningismus, sensory level L1	*S. aureus*	Ambulated with a walker at 3 months
Iseki (162)	1998	Analgesia for herpes zoster	11 epidural injections, then: T6-7 T8-9 T7-8		4 days[b] 1 day[b] 6 days[b]	Epidural abscess at T6-7 and inflammation of the perivertebral muscles at T5-7	6 days after the final catheterization	Fever, elevated white blood count and C-reactive protein	Methicillin-resistant *S. aureus*	Full recovery
O'Brien (163)	1999	Analgesia for low back pain	One epidural injection	Not specified	Not applicable	Epidural abscess	3 months	Back pain, bilateral lower extremity pain	*M. fortuitum*	Full recovery

(*continued*)

TABLE 61.1. (*continued*)

First Author (Reference)	Year	Indication	Epidural Site	Filter Used	Catheter Duration	Type of Infection	Time from Insertion to Symptoms	Signs and Symptoms	Microorganism	Outcome
Halkic (164)	2001	Postoperative analgesia	T11-12	Not specified	4 days	Spondylodiscitis at L5-S1	4 days	Lumbar pain radiating to the groin	*Propionibactrium acnes*	Full recovery
Phillips (122)	2002	1. Postoperative analgesia	Thoracic	Not specified	3 days	Epidural abscess	4 days	Low grade fever,	*S. aureus*	Full recovery
							5 days	Higher fever, low back ache, headache, tenderness at insertion site		
		2. Postoperative analgesia	Thoracic	Not specified	3 days	Epidural abscess	3 weeks	Pain at insertion site, weakness in lower extremeties, urinary retention	Methicillin-resistant *S. aureus*	Died of a pulmonary embolus and cardiac arrest

[a] Although discrepancies exist in the two reports, these articles may report the same patient.
[b] Two separate epidural catheters inserted in the same patient.

Infections Associated with Subarachnoid Neural Blockade

Epidemiology

Infections rarely complicate subarachnoid neural blockade, commonly known as spinal anesthesia. Lund (165) reviewed 13 published series accounting for 582,190 subarachnoid neural blockades and found "no prolonged severe neurological sequelae." More recently, Horlocker et al. (166) retrospectively reviewed the medical records of 4,217 patients who had 4,767 subarachnoid neural blockades. They identified two patients who acquired abscesses and did not identify any patients with meningitis. Only four cases of meningitis were reported in eight studies that evaluated approximately 94,000 subarachnoid neural blocks (166–173) (Table 61.2). On the basis of these eight studies, we estimate that the rate of infection is approximately 4.3 per 100,000 subarachnoid neural blockades. Conversely, Kilpatrick and Girgis (174) noted that 17 of 1,429 (1.2%) of patients admitted with meningitis to the Abbassia Fever Hospital in Cairo, Egypt, had recently undergone subarachnoid neural blockade.

Case Reports

Although infections infrequently complicate subarachnoid neural blockade, case reports in the literature indicate that such infections can be serious (Table 61.3) (89,90,93,94,106, 175–187). Of the 26 patients reported, eight had meningitis, four had epidural abscesses, two had soft tissue abscesses, and two had infections of a disc or of a disc space. *S. aureus* caused two and *Pseudomonas* species caused four of the 23 infections in which a bacterial pathogen was identified. Eleven of these infections were caused by streptococcal species. Twenty-one patients recovered fully. Thus, infections associated with subarachnoid neural blockade seem to be somewhat different from those associated with epidural neural blockade in that streptococci were the most common etiologic agents for infections after subarachnoid blockade and patients were more likely to recover fully.

Infections Associated with Combined Epidural and Subarachnoid Neural Blockade

Epidemiology and Case Reports

Anesthesiologists have begun to use both epidural and subarachnoid neural blockade in some patients. Cascio and Heath (188) identified one case of meningitis after about 700 combined epidural and subarachnoid neural blockades. We identified eight case reports of infections (nine infections) after these combined procedures (122,188–194) (Table 61.4). Three of six cases of meningitis were caused by streptococcal species and all three of the epidural abscesses were caused by *S. aureus*. Eight of these patients recovered fully.

TABLE 61.2. MENINGITIS ASSOCIATED WITH SUBARACHNOID NEURAL BLOCKADE

First Author (Reference)	Year	Number of Patients	Number of Infections	Rate of Meningitis
Evans (167)	1945	2,500	0	0
Scarborough (168)	1958	5,000	0	0
Dripps (169)	1954	8,460	0	0
Moore (170)	1966	11,574	0	0
Lund (171)	1968	>21,000	0	0
Sadove (172)	1961	>20,000	3	≈15/100,000
Arner (173)	1952	21,230	1	4.7/100,000
Horlocker (166)	1997	4,217	0	0
Total		>93,981	4	≈4.3/100,000

Infections Associated with Peripheral Nerve Blocks

Epidemiology and Case Reports

Continuous regional anesthetic techniques utilizing peripheral nerve blocks have become more popular in recent years for postoperative pain management especially after orthopedic procedures (195,196). Only a few studies have addressed infectious complications from the indwelling catheters used for these procedures. Bergman et al. (197) identified one patient who had a local *S. aureus* skin infection in the axilla after 48 hours of axillary analgesia among 368 patients (405 axillary catheters). The patient fully recovered with antibiotic treatment. Meier et al. (198) described eight superficial skin infections among 91 patients with continuous interscalene catheters for on average 5 days. Cuvillion et al. (199) obtained cultures of 208 femoral catheters when they were removed after 48 hours. Fifty-four percent of the catheters were colonized with potentially pathogenic bacteria (71% *S. epidermidis*, 10% *Enterococcus* species, and 4% *Klebsiella* species). They also reported three episodes of transient bacteremia, but they did not identify any abscesses or episodes of sepsis (199). None of the groups provided information about the aseptic techniques used for catheter insertion.

To date, guidelines for placement of these catheters have not been published. New complex catheter systems, which require several manipulations during insertion, have been introduced (200). We believe that aseptic technique similar to that recommended for placement of central venous catheters is warranted (201).

Prevention of Infections Associated with Central Neuraxial Blockade

Most reported infections after epidural and subarachnoid neural blockade were caused by bacteria that colonize the skin, respiratory tract, or water. Consequently, we believe anesthesia staff should take precautions to limit contamination from these sources. Most anesthesiologists agree that they should wash their hands with an antimicrobial soap and wear sterile gloves. They also agree that the patient's skin should be prepared with an antimicrobial agent. However, anesthesiologists still debate whether they should wear masks while performing these procedures (202–208). For example, nearly 50% of the anesthesia staff responding to a survey conducted by Panikkar and Yentis (209) reported that they did not wear masks when performing epidural and subarachnoid neural blockade. O'Higgins and Tuckey (210) surveyed 290 anesthesiologists in the U.K., 83% of whom responded. Respondents reported wearing caps (83%), sterile gowns (70%), and masks (66%). Sixty percent reported

TABLE 61.3. INFECTIONS ASSOCIATED WITH SUBARACHNOID NEURAL BLOCKADE

First Author (Reference)	Year	Indication	Type of Infection	Incubation Period	Signs and Symptoms	Microorganism	Outcome	Comments
Corbett (175)	1971	1. Vaginal delivery	Meningitis	36 hours	Fever, headache, stiff neck	*P. aeruginosa*	Full recovery	Three patients infected when a physician rinsed the spinal needle stylet in saline used for consecutive deliveries
		2. Vaginal delivery	Meningitis	3 days	Fever, headache, stiff neck, neck pain, nuchal rigidity	*P. aeruginosa*	Full recovery	
		3. Vaginal delivery	Meningitis	4 days	Fever, headache, nausea	*P. aeruginosa*	Full recovery	
Siegel (176)	1974	Vaginal delivery	Left subgluteal abscess	4 hours	Buttock pain radiating to thigh	*Mimeae*	Full recovery	
				14 days	Severe pain sacroiliac joint			
Loarie (93)	1978	Debride necrotic heel ulcers	Epidural abscess	2 days	Fever, back pain, urinary retention	*S. epidermidis, Bacteroides*	Full recovery	Insulin-dependent diabetic
				15 days	Bilateral lower extremity weakness, absent anal sphincter tone			
Berman (94)	1978	Transurethral evacuation of clot from bladder	Meningitis	1 hour	Shaking chill, fever, back pain, headache, confusion	*Enterococcus*	Not specified	
Beaudoin (177)	1984	Debride and drain infected foot	Epidural abscess	4 days after last subarachnoid neural blockade	Back pain, pain radiating to upper thighs	*Pseudomonas* species	Full recovery	35-year-old insulin-dependent diabetic, received five subarachnoid neural blockades in 10 days
Abdel-Magid (178)	1990	Hemorrhoidectomy	Epidural abscess	15 days	Back pain, leg weakness, urinary retention, fever, bilateral absent ankle reflexes	*Proteus* species	Full recovery	
Roberts (179)	1990	Remove retained placenta	Meningitis	18 hours	Headache, photophobia, fever, chills, positive Kernig's sign, quadriceps weakness	Culture negative	Full recovery	Antibiotics started before the lumbar puncture
Lee (180)	1991	Cesarean section	Meningitis	16 hours	Severe headache	Culture negative	Full recovery	
				22 hours	Nausea, photophobia, decreasing mental status, fever, nuchal rigidity, positive Kernig's sign			
Blackmore (181)	1993	Herniorrhaphy	Meningitis and bacteremia	16 hours	Fever, vomiting, obtundation	*S. mitis*	Full recovery	
Ezri (182)	1994	Hemorrhoidectomy	Meningitis	10 days	Fever	*E. coli*	Full recovery	
				25 days	Malaise, headache, photophobia, dizziness, fever			
Mahendru (183)	1994	Foot amputation	Epidural abscess	3 weeks	Back pain, bilateral lower extremity paresis and weakness	No culture obtained	Died from esophageal carcinoma	Insulin-dependent diabetic
Gebhard (184)	1994	Knee arthroscopy	Discitis	2 months	Back and thigh pain, elevated sedimentation rate	*P. acnes*	Full recovery	

(continued)

TABLE 61.3. (*continued*)

First Author (Reference)	Year	Indication	Type of Infection	Incubation Period	Signs and Symptoms	Microorganism	Outcome	Comments
Newton (185)	1994	Vaginal delivery	Meningitis	12 hours	Headache, photophobia, declining mental status, fever	*S. salivarius*	Full recovery	
Schneeberger (90)	1996	1. Knee arthroscopy	Meningitis	12 hours	Fever, meningeal signs	*S. sanguis*	Full recovery	
		2. Knee arthroscopy	Meningitis	12 hours 2 days	Headache Fever, meningeal signs	*S. mitis*	Full recovery	
		3. Varicose vein stripping	Meningitis	24 hours	Headache, fever, impaired consciousness, meningeal signs	*S. salivarius*	Full recovery	
		4. Varicose vein stripping	Meningitis	12 hours	Headache, fever	*S. cremoris*	Mild-communicating hydrocephalus	Hydrocephalus may have been preexisting
Horlocker (166)	1997	1. Urologic procedure	Disc space infection	1 day 4 months	Low back pain Incapacitating low back pain	*S. aureus*	Full recovery	
		2. Examination under anesthesia	Paraspinal abscess	1 day 11 days	Low back pain Fever	*S. aureus*	Full recovery	
Kaiser (186)	1997	Hysterectomy	Meningitis	12 hours	High fever, severe headache, lumbar pain, lethargy, Glasgow score of 12, nuchal rigidity, positive Kernig's and Brudzinski's signs	*S. salivarius*	Full recovery	
Fernandez (187)	1999	Arthroscopic meniscectomy	Meningitis	18 hours	Severe headache, nausea, vomiting, high fever, nuchal rigidity	*S. mitis*	Full recovery	
Yaniv (106)	2000	Extracorporeal shock wave lithotripsy for ureterolithiasis	Meningitis	12 hours	Fever, severe headache, meningeal signs, elevated white blood cell count	*S. salivarius*	Minor sequealae, mild paresthesia of right thigh	Anesthesiologist wore gown, sterile gloves, face mask
Trautmann (89)	2002	Arthroscopic knee repair	Meningitis	1 day	Fever, nausea, stiff neck	*S. salivarius*	Full recovery	Both patients underwent their operations the same day
		Arthroscopic knee repair	Meningitis	1 day	Headache, nausea, stiff neck	*S. salivarius*	Full recovery	

TABLE 61.4. INFECTIONS ASSOCIATED WITH COMBINED SUBARACHNOID AND EPIDURAL NEURAL BLOCKADE

First Author (Reference)	Year	Indication	Type of Infection	Time of Symptom Onset	Signs and Symptoms	Microorganism	Outcome	Comments
Cascio (188)	1995	Vaginal delivery	Meningitis	16 hours after delivery, ~20 hours after insertion	Fever, headache, chills, photophobia, mild nuchal rigidity	*S. salivarius*	Full recovery	Anesthesiologist wore mask, cap, and sterile gloves, and used povidone-iodine spray for skin antisepsis
Harding (189)	1994	Vaginal delivery	Aseptic meningitis	21 hours after the injection	Severe headache, faint feeling, shortness of breath, urinary retention, aphasia, tingling right side of face, neck stiffness, positive Kernig's sign, low grade fever	No growth	Full recovery	Anesthesiologist scrubbed, wore sterile gown and gloves, and used alcoholic chlorhexidine to prepare the skin
		Vaginal delivery converted to an emergency Cesarean section	Meningitis	3 days after the operation	Headache, fever, vomiting, severe stiff neck, elevated white blood cell count, hypotension, bradycardia	*S. epidermidis*	Full recovery	Alcoholic chlorhexidine used to prepare the skin
Stallard (190)	1994	Analgesia during labor, subsequent Cesarean section	Meningitis	18 hours after the operation	Acute confusion, fever, aphasia, ignored left side, elevated white blood cell count	No growth	Full recovery	Did three procedures to achieve adequate analgesia; anesthesiologist used alcoholic chlorhexidine to prepare the skin and wore mask, gown, and gloves
Aldebert (191)	1996	Vaginal delivery	Meningitis	8 hours after puncture	Headache, nausea, high fever, agitation, nuchal rigidity, positive Babinski sign	Nonhemolytic *Streptococcus*	Full recovery	Anesthesiologist wore mask, gown, cap, and sterile gloves
Dysart (192)	1997	Cesarean section	Epidural abscess	9 days after the operation	Backache, high fever, foot drop, weakness of ankle eversion and inversion, absent ankle jerk reflex, decrease pinprick sensation from L5 to perianal region, elevated erythrocyte sedimentation rate	*S. aureus*	Nearly full recovery; patient had residual numbness in L5 distribution	Anesthesiologist wore a mask, gown, and gloves and used chlorhexidine to prepare the skin
Schroter (193)	1997	Anesthesia for vascular surgery	Epidural abscess	1 day after procedure	Back pain, fever, slight nuchal rigidity, erythema and induration at puncture site and purulent drainage from puncture site, elevated white blood cell count	*S. aureus*	Full recovery	Anesthesiologist wore a mask, surgical hood, sterile gloves, and gown and used povidone-iodine to prepare the skin
Bouhemad (194)	1998	Cesarean section	Meningitis	14 hours after delivery	Fever, severe headache, photophobia, drowsiness, stiff neck, positive Kernig's sign	*S. salivarius*	Full recovery	Anesthesiologist wore gown, gloves, face mask, and cap and used tincture of iodine for skin antisepsis
Phillips (122)	2002	Surgical anesthesia and postoperative analgesia	Epidural abscess L1-2	day 6	Discomfort at the epidural site and severe radicular pain in L2 dermatome, erythema and swelling at site, decreased strength, light touch, and pin prick, and loss of ankle jerk reflex	*S. aureus*	Discharged from hospital 3 months after first operation	Anesthesiologist wore a cap, gown, and sterile gloves and prepared the site with 10% povidone-iodine

scrubbing before cases, 35% washed their hands, and 5% simply put on gloves. Five of the respondents had patients who acquired epidural abscesses. All five anesthesiologists reported wearing caps and four of five used gowns and masks, and four washed their hands before the procedures. Similarly, Sleth's (211) survey found that only 53% of anesthesiologists wore a cap, a mask, and a sterile gown when placing epidural catheters, and only 21% used dressings that allowed staff members to inspect the site continuously. In a letter to the editor, Dolinski and Gerancher (212) quoted data from a study by Philips et al. (91) documenting that surgical masks prevent bacteria from contaminating agar plates placed 30 cm from the mouth and that this effect lasts only for 15 minutes. In addition, they quoted a study by O'Kelly and Marsh (205), the results of which indicate that similar results could be obtained if the subjects didn't talk. Dolinski and Gerancher concluded, "Because it boils down to opinion whether face masks make neuraxis block placement safer, we can neither emphatically recommend the use of face masks nor resolutely recommend they not be worn."

Given the very low rates of infection associated with epidural and subarachnoid neural blockade, we believe it will be very difficult to prove that masks reduce the risk of infection. As noted above, these infections can be very serious, and respiratory bacteria are common etiologic agents. Moreover, anesthesiologists in the United States usually wear masks during operative procedures, even though they are at distance from the operative site. Therefore, it seems prudent they should wear face masks when performing neuraxial blockades. We agree with Wildsmith's (202) recommendation that anesthesia personnel wear masks while performing those procedures. Also, we wonder if the hygienic measures similar to those used for placing central venous catheters should be used for doing these procedures, especially for those in which a catheter will remain in place for hours to days (201). There is evidence that use of full barrier precautions reduces the incidence of catheter-related bloodstream infections (213). Given that the incidence of meningitis and epidural abscess is low, we doubt that the efficacy of full barrier precautions (i.e., the anesthesiologist wears a cap, mask, sterile gloves, and sterile gown and uses a large drape to cover the patient and the patient's bed) can be documented for these procedures. However, these procedures are at least as invasive as placing central venous catheters and the consequences of subsequent infections are at least as bad as those for catheter-associated bloodstream infections.

Dawson et al. (214) evaluated risk factors for infections associated with epidural neural blockade for postoperative pain relief. They found that procedures done between April and August had a sixfold higher risk than those done during other months (95% CI 1.28–28.12, $p = .009$). Procedures for which a syringe was used to administer the anesthetic agent were also at higher risk than those in which a bag was used (the odds ratio for use of a bag was 0.17, 95% CI 0.02–1.34, $p = .05$).

Several investigators have evaluated the agents used to prepare the skin before epidural neural blocks. However there are some methodologic problems with these studies. For example, three of four studies that we reviewed did not report power calculations, and the study conducted by Adam et al. (215), which evaluated 3% povidone-iodine and 1% chlorhexidine in 294 women before deliveries, was not randomized. Kasuda et al. (216) randomly assigned 70 patients to receive either 0.5% chlorhexidine or 10% povidone-iodine. After a median of 49 ± 7 hours, the authors removed the catheters and obtained cultures of the insertion sites and catheter tips. There was no difference in rates of positive cultures. Kinirons et al. (217) (the only investigators who reported a power calculation) cultured catheters removed from 96 children who had epidural catheters for longer than 24 hours. Coagulase-negative staphylococci were the only microorganisms that grew and the colonization rate was lower for the catheters removed from children whose skin was prepared with 0.5% alcoholic chlorhexidine (1/52 catheters, 0.9/100 catheter-days) compared with those removed from children whose skin was prepared with povidone-iodine (5/44 catheters, 5.6/100 catheter-days) (relative risk 0.2, 95% CI 0.1–1.0). They did not identify any epidural space infections. Sato et al. (218) evaluated the efficacy of 0.5% alcoholic chlorhexidine and 10% povidone-iodine in a group of 60 patients who were undergoing back operations under general anesthesia. After prepping and draping the site, the investigators obtained skin biopsies that they evaluated by culture and microscopy. Cultures from skin prepared with the chlorhexidine product were less likely to be positive (5.7%) than were cultures from skin prepared with povidone[iodine (32.4%; $p < .01$). *S. epidermidis, Staphylococcus hyicus,* and *Staphylococcus capitis* grew from skin cultures. However, microscopy of the hair follicles were equally likely to be positive in skin prepared with chlorhexidine (14.3%) and skin prepared with povidone-iodine (11.8%).

Brooks et al. (112) suggested the following precautions for continuous central neuraxial blocks: (a) the anesthesiologist should evaluate whether the infusion should continue if the system becomes disconnected; (b) the exit site should be dressed with a transparent dressing and should be viewed every 8 hours or as necessary; (c) a 0.22-μm 96-hour filter should be included in the infusion system; (d) the tubing, filter, and solution should be changed or the system should be discontinued every 96 hours; and (e) the primary anesthesia and adjuvant bolus dose should be given with a larger syringe that remains attached to the catheter until a continuous analgesia infusion is begun.

Conclusions About the Role of Neuraxial Blockade as a Source of Infection

Infections rarely complicate neuraxial blockades. This fact suggests that the infection control practices used for these procedures are usually adequate. However, because the infections cause substantial morbidity and mortality, anesthesia personnel must maintain strict aseptic technique. In particular for continuous neuraxial blockades, we believe full barrier precautions are warranted (15), that the system should be opened as infrequently as possible, and that chlorhexidine should be considered as the agent for preparing the skin before the procedure. We arrived at these suggestions by extrapolating from data about preventing infections related to central venous catheters. Finally, anesthesia personnel should vigilantly observe their patients after the procedures for signs and symptoms of infection so that infections can be diagnosed and treated immediately. A study by Pegues et al. (219) is relevant to this point. They reviewed medical records from 1980 to 1992 to identify patients who acquired infections associated with short-term epidural catheters, and they followed patients prospectively from January to June 1993. In 1990, they introduced a standardized procedure for inspecting temporary epidural catheters. They identified seven infections during the 12.5-year period, all of which were identified after they introduced the procedures for inspecting catheters. These investigators concluded that the increased incidence may "reflect increased use of epidural catheters for pain management, an improved clinical recognition of these infections, or an ascertainment or misclassification bias associated with retrospective review."

INFECTIONS ASSOCIATED WITH INTRAVENOUS ANESTHESIA

Pathogenesis

Syringes

Bacteria from the hands of healthcare workers can contaminate syringes and their contents. Blogg et al. (220) noted that three of 50 syringes (6%) used repeatedly in an operating room and four of 50 syringes (8%) used repeatedly in an ICU were contaminated with bacteria, including *S. aureus* (two syringes), *E. coli* (two syringes), *S. epidermidis* (three syringes), and viridans streptococci (one syringe) (220). Lessard et al. (221) also obtained cultures from syringes used in their operating rooms and found four contaminated syringes among 100 that were refilled an average of 3.58 times compared with three contaminated syringes among 100 filled only once. Blogg et al. also tested whether bacteria (25×10^6 CFU of *S. marcescens*) on the hands could contaminate syringes when they were refilled. All 15 plastic syringes and 35 of 65 (54%) glass syringes were contaminated after they were refilled twice.

To simulate the common syringe technique, several investigators injected liquid from tuberculin syringes through 26-gauge needles into suspensions of *E. coli* (222–224), *S. aureus* (224), polio virus (225), or ^{3}H-thymide (224). After removing the needles, they examined the syringe contents and found that most were contaminated. Plott et al. (226) took this line of research one step further. They placed 10 mL of sterile water containing 10^6 plaque-forming units of vesicular stomatitis virus into a multidose vial. They then injected 1 mL of sterile water into the vial, withdrew the syringe, changed the needle, drew 1 mL of air into the syringe, injected the air into a second vial, and withdrew 1 mL of water. All of the second vials were contaminated with vesicular stomatitis virus.

Syringes can become contaminated with a patient's blood or with blood-borne pathogens after just one injection into a patient or into an intravenous line. Fleming and Ogilvie (227) found blood in five of 50 syringes (10%) used to inject a vaccine subcutaneously, and Hughes (228) identified red blood cells in 17 of 39 syringes (44%) used to inject saline intramuscularly. Hughes demonstrated that fluid was aspirated from the needle into the syringe when the needle was removed from the syringe. He hypothesized that the syringe used to administer penicillin was contaminated in this manner and subsequently transmitted serum hepatitis to 26 patients. Other investigators confirmed Hughes's hypothesis (222,229). For example, Lutz et al. (222), using an experimental model, calculated that 2×10^{-5} mL of fluid were aspirated into the syringe when they removed the needle. Although minuscule, this volume of blood is 200 to 2,000 times greater than the amount required to transmit hepatitis B virus to chimpanzees (230).

Syringe contents may be contaminated with blood when the syringes are used to administer fluids into intravenous lines. Hein et al. (231) detected visible blood in six and occult blood in eight of 100 injection ports for intravenous tubing. Similarly, Trepanier et al. (232) used Ames Multistix read by a Clinitek 200 module (sensitive to a 1:32,000 dilution) to detect blood in intravenous fluids withdrawn through injection ports. They detected blood in 3.33% (95% CI 2.26–4.73%) of samples withdrawn from the first port and in 0.3% of those withdrawn from the third port (95% CI 0.01–1.84%). When they injected fluids into intravenous tubing through which blood was infusing, 34% (95% CI 24.8–44.1%) of the syringes were contaminated. Using 10-mL syringes, Parlow (233) injected 2-mL aliquots of normal saline into injection ports of intravenous lines used for patients undergoing general anesthesia. After injecting four aliquots per syringe, the investigator removed the needle, filtered the remaining 2 mL of saline, and stained the filter with Papanicolaou's stain. Three of twenty-six samples (11.5%) contained red blood cells.

Investigators at a hospital in Saudi Arabia concluded that malaria was transmitted to 41 patients in a pediatric hospital when a single syringe was used to irrigate numerous patients' heparin locks (234). Nurses reported that they routinely used one syringe to irrigate the heparin locks of three to ten patients. The nurses connected the syringe directly to the catheter hub, and thus did not use needles.

Multidose Vials

Many drugs used by anesthesia personnel are packaged in multidose vials. Ninety-eight percent of anesthesia personnel surveyed by Kempen (235,236) used multidose vials opened by unknown persons, and 75% refilled common syringes from multidose vials and did not subsequently discard the vial. Moreover, a study by Zacher et al. (237) suggests that bacteria contaminating the outside of a multidose vial can be injected into the vial if the vial is not disinfected.

Corley et al. (238) injected at least 1 billion *S. aureus* or *E. coli* microorganisms into vials containing succinylcholine chloride, chloroprocaine, tubocurarine, water for injection, and sodium chloride for injection. After 7 days, 99.6% to 100% of the microorganisms were killed. Of the three anesthetic agents tested, only succinylcholine chloride did not kill all of the bacteria. Highsmith et al. (239) evaluated whether 12 different pathogens persisted in eight drugs commonly packaged in multidose vials. Cultures of procainamide and methohexital were negative at 24 hours. Succinylcholine chloride, regular insulin, potassium chloride, and thiopental killed slowly or allowed limited survival of several microorganisms. If the bacteria were washed in 0.25% peptone broth (i.e., carried some nutrients with them when injected), all 12 microorganisms survived or proliferated in lidocaine. However, if the bacteria were washed in saline, lidocaine supported growth of only *Pseudomonas cepacia*. Bawden et al. (240) inoculated 1 to 100 CFU of *E. coli* or *P. aeruginosa* microorganisms into 30-mL multidose vials of bacteriostatic water with 0.9% benzyl alcohol, 0.9% sodium chloride with 0.9% benzyl alcohol, and 1% lidocaine hydrochloride with 1 mg per milliliter of methylparaben. All cultures were positive at 1 hour, and *E. coli* was recovered from the lidocaine at 16 hours. Longfield et al. (241) inoculated 11 commonly used medications with suspensions of ten bacterial species. When stored at 22°C, atropine and D-tubocurarine were sterile at 4 hours, but lidocaine and heparin still contained viable bacteria at 24 hours. At 4°C, bacteria persisted longer in all medications tested. Plott et al. (226) injected 10^6 plaque-forming units of vesicular stomatitis virus into sterile water, 1% lidocaine, and 1% lidocaine with 1:100,000 epinephrine. All cultures were positive at 1 hour, and cultures of the sterile water and the lidocaine were positive at 1 day. None of the vials contained viable virus at 1 week.

A plethora of culture surveys indicates that the proportion of multidose vials contaminated by bacteria ranges from 0% to 27% (238,240,242–249). In their review of 12 studies published between 1958 and 1983, Longfield et al. (246) noted that all of the studies reporting high rates were done before 1973. On the basis of four studies done after 1973, they estimated that 0.6% of used multidose vials were contaminated with bacteria. Longfield et al. suggested that the differences between the results of earlier and more recent studies might be explained by changes in both the types of drugs packaged in multidose vials and the chemicals used as preservatives. After reviewing 15 papers published between 1958 and 1986, Thompson et al. (250) estimated that 0.5% of used multidose vials become contaminated with bacteria.

Of the studies we evaluated, only one tested used multidose vials for viral contamination. Petty et al. (242) tested 121 used multidose vials for viruses, none of which were positive. Only two studies evaluated used multidose vials for red blood cells. Melnyk et al. (245) evaluated 69 multidose vials; none of the vials were contaminated with bacteria, but one (1.4%) contained red blood cells. Arrington et al. (251) noted that many anesthesia staff members withdrew contents from a medication vial, injected the drug into intravenous tubing, and then used the same needle and syringe to withdraw medication for the next patient. Because they were concerned that this practice could contaminate medication vials, the authors tested vials at the end of the day for the presence of occult blood. The first group consisted of vials reused by staff members who used a single needle and syringe as described above. The second group consisted of vials used by the investigators who placed a new needle on the used syringe to withdraw medication from vials. Eleven of 492 (2.2%) vials in the first group and 1 of 369 (0.3%) in the second group contained occult blood. The authors concluded that their study supported the guidelines of the AANA and CDC that mandate use of a new needle and a new syringe for each patient and each time a vial is entered.

Epidemiology

A number of outbreaks have been caused by contaminated solutions or anesthetic agents (252–270). Of the 18 reports reviewed in Table 61.5, 16 were caused by drugs or solutions that were contaminated by anesthesia or pharmacy personnel, and only one was caused by a drug contaminated by the manufacturer. Eight outbreaks were caused by contaminated propofol (256–258,262,263,265,266). Bennett et al. (270) investigated outbreaks associated with propofol at seven hospitals and found numerous breaks in aseptic technique. For example, anesthesia personnel did not clean vials before opening them and did not wear gloves. They also drew up the drug before the case, transferred syringes containing unused drugs between operating rooms and facilities, and reused syringes. In one hospital, the same strain of *S. aureus* was isolated from the patients and from a lesion on the scalp of the anesthesiologist who prepared the medication. A case-control study implicated exposure to propofol as the risk factor, suggesting that the anesthesiologist contaminated the propofol solution. Kuehnert et al. (263) noted similar faulty technique. Anesthesia personnel often did not wash their hands before preparing the medications, drew up all the propofol doses required for an entire day at one time, and kept the syringes at room temperature throughout the day. In addition, they often used multidose vials that contained large volumes of propofol, and stored the unused doses in the opened vial at room temperature.

Most anesthetic drugs are weak bases dissolved in acidic solutions that inhibit growth of bacteria and fungi (271–273), and most contain a bacteriostatic agent. However, propofol is suspended in a lipid solution that supports bacterial and fungal growth (272–279), and it does not contain a preservative. If anesthesia personnel do not follow aseptic technique when they remove propofol from the glass vial, they can contaminate the solution. The contaminating microorganisms can multiply in propofol while it is infused slowly or while prefilled syringes sit at room temperature. To avoid such problems, the manufacturer recommends that propofol "be drawn into a sterile syringe immediately after the ampoule is opened and administration should commence promptly. Each unit of [propofol] is intended for use in a single patient and the syringe and any unused portion of [propofol] must be discarded at the end of the surgical procedure" (280,281).

Seeberger et al. (282) administer propofol using the following protocol. The anesthesiologist must (a) use only 20-mL ampoules of propofol; (b) use an alcohol-based hand rub before starting the procedure; (c) prepare the syringes, lines, and stopcocks just before the procedure; and (d) discard all unused propofol, and never use propofol from the same ampoule for more than one patient. In addition, an infection control professional conducts continuing education for the anesthesia staff members about good infection control practice and monitors their practice. These investigators reported that between January 1, 1995, and June 30, 1996, they performed 1,407 anesthetic procedures using propofol and 5,026 using thiopentone. Subsequent follow-up revealed that the incidence of catheter-related sepsis of unknown origin was 0.2% for both groups, and the incidence of superficial thrombophlebitis and of fever greater than 38°C of unknown origin was less than 0.1% for both groups. On the basis of these data, they concluded that their precautions were adequate to prevent infections in patients undergoing intravenous anesthesia with propofol.

TABLE 61.5. OUTBREAKS RELATED TO INTRAVENOUS ANESTHESIA

First Author (Reference)	Year	Contaminated Product	Infection	Number of Patients	Microorganism	Comments
Sack (252)	1970	Intravenous solution used for numerous patients	Bacteremia	5	*K. pneumoniae, A. cloacae*	Multiple-dose solution used by same anesthesiologist
Siboni (253) Borghans (254)	1979	Fentanyl	Bacteremia	16	*P. cepacia*	Intrinsic contamination despite methyl- and propyl-p-hydroxybenzoates included as preservatives
Maldonado (255)	1989	Lidocaine multidose vial	Hepatitis	5	Hepatitis B	Vial used for numerous patients by one anesthesiologist
CDC (256) Daily (257)	1990	Propofol infused per pump	Fungemia, endophthalmitis	4	*C. albicans*	Breaks in aseptic technique noted in anesthesia practice
		Propofol infused per pump	Fever, hypertension	2	*M. osloensis*	Same infusion, syringe, and pump used for both patients
CDC (256)	1990	Propofol infused per pump	Bacteremia, surgical site infections	13	*S. aureus*	Same phage type isolated from the patients and the hands of the nurse anesthetist, same infusion used for numerous patients
CDC (256) Villarino (258) CDC (256)	1990 1991 1990	Propofol infused per pump	Fever, surgical site infections	8	*S. aureus*	Same phage type isolated from the patients and from the anesthesiologist's throat
Maki (259)	1991	Fentanyl in predrawn syringes	Bacteremia	3	*P. pickettii*	Narcotic tampering in pharmacy contaminated medication
Froggatt (260)	1991	Common syringe used on numerous patients	Hepatitis	6	Hepatitis B	Medication syringes contaminated by blood from a hepatitis B carrier and used on subsequent patients
Rudnick (261)	1991	Preassembled pressure-monitoring equipment	Bacteremia	9	*P. aeruginosa, E. cloacae, K. pneumoniae*	Pressure monitoring equipment contaminated with floor-washing solution
Veber (262)	1994	Propofol injections	Bacteremia	4	*K. pneumoniae*	Contents of one vial used for four patients over 18 hours
Kuehnert (263)	1997	Propofol injections	Bloodstream infection	5	*S. aureus*	Contents of one vial used on successive patients
Kidd-Ljunggren (264)	1999	Local anesthetic injections	Hepatitis	2	Hepatitis B	A permanent aspiration needle was left in the bottle of local anesthetic; the desired amount was drawn into a syringe; if the patient needed more pain relief, the same syringe was used to obtain the agent; the multidose vial was *not* discarded between patients
Henry (265)	2001	Propofol injections	Bloodstream infection ($n = 5$) Surgical site infection ($n = 2$)	7	*S. marcescens*	One anesthesiologist was associated with all cases but only 14% of the controls; all cases received propofol compared with 24% of controls; no cultures of the environment or the anesthesiologist were positive for the etiologic agent
Massari (266)	2001	Propofol	Hepatitis	4	Hepatitis C	Risk factors for infection included being operated on during the same morning session on the same day as the probable source patient; all five patients were infected with genotype 1b; the only thing all five patients shared was a multidose vial of propofol
Meier (267)	2002	Sedative injections	Hepatitis	>50	Hepatitis C	Nurse anesthetist in a pain clinic used the same needle and syringe to give sedative injections into ports of intravenous lines
Anonymous (268)	2002	Sedative injections	Hepatitis	28	Hepatitis C	Anesthesiologist in an endoscopy clinic obtained sedative from a multidose vial and gave several injections to the same patient with a single needle and syringe; the multidose vial was used for more than one patient; a patient with chronic hepatitis C, genotype 2C, underwent endoscopy at the beginning of the epidemic period
Carbonne (269)	2003	Fentanyl injections	Hepatitis	2	Hepatitis C	A patient had chronic hepatitis C, subtype 1b; repeat doses of fentanyl were obtained from a multidose vial with a used syringe and needle; two patients whose operations followed this patient's operation acquired hepatitis C of the same genotype

Other outbreaks reviewed in Table 61.5 illustrate how various breaks in aseptic technique, including narcotic pilfering (259), use of common syringes (260), and assembling equipment in advance of the procedure (261,263), have led to infections. Although outbreaks associated with contaminated solutions or drugs occur rarely, large numbers of patients can be infected. Most of the reported outbreaks have been related directly to poor aseptic technique, including the unacceptable practices of administering the same solution to more than one patient and entering a multidose vial with a used syringe and needle. Of note, five of the six outbreaks that we added in this revision were outbreaks of viral hepatitis (four hepatitis C, one hepatitis B) (264,266–269). One was related to reuse of syringes (267), and four to misuse of multidose vials (264,266,268,269).

OUTBREAKS ASSOCIATED WITH ANESTHESIA PERSONNEL

Anesthesia personnel have been the reservoir of infection in at least 11 outbreaks (283–294) (Table 61.6). Group A β-hemolytic streptococci disseminated from anesthesia personnel caused five outbreaks of surgical site infections and one outbreak of puerperal sepsis (see Chapters 21 and 55). Anesthesia personnel carried group A β-hemolytic streptococci in the following sites: anus (two outbreaks), anus and throat (one outbreak), throat (one outbreak), and skin lesions (two outbreaks). The source of one outbreak was particularly difficult to identify, because the carrier, an anesthesia technician, was present in the operating room only between cases and not during the operations (290). In two outbreaks of *S. aureus* surgical site infections, the microorganism was disseminated from anesthesiologists with psoriasis. Clearly, the barrier between the anesthesia area and the operative site does not always prevent spread of microorganisms from anesthesia personnel to patients.

Most outbreaks are inadvertent, even if they are related to poor infection control practices. However, outbreaks such as those reported by Maki et al. (259) and Bosch (291,292) demonstrate that on occasion, hospital personnel deliberately put patients at risk. In the outbreak reported by Maki et al., a pharmacy technician replaced stolen fentanyl with nonsterile distilled water. The outbreak described by Bosch is even more frightening. On numerous occasions, an anesthesiologist addicted to morphine and infected with hepatitis C first gave himself morphine and then administered the remaining drug to the patients through the same syringe and needle. He thereby infected at least 171 patients (293). Of note, the two new outbreaks that we added in this edition were both caused by hepatitis C. In each case, the anesthesia provider acquired hepatitis C from a patient and spread the virus to other patients (293,294).

EXPOSURE OF ANESTHESIA PERSONNEL TO PATIENTS' BLOOD AND BODY FLUIDS

Asai et al. (295) screen routinely all patients undergoing elective operations for blood-borne pathogens. Of 6,437 patients screened in a 2-year period, 534 (8.3%) were infected with at least one of these agents. Thus, anesthesiologists frequently care for patients who are infected with these agents.

The proportion of operative procedures in which anesthesia personnel are exposed to blood has varied by study. White and Lynch (296) observed 1,054 blood contacts during 8,502 operative procedures. Anesthesia personnel were exposed to blood in 82 (0.96%) of the cases. The authors noted that fingers, hands, and arms were exposed 70 times, usually when anesthesia personnel inserted intravenous catheters. The face or neck was exposed eight times by blood from the operative field. Legs or feet were exposed four times when blood or bloody irrigation fluid ran off the drapes. In 75 episodes, blood contaminated intact skin, and in two episodes blood contaminated nonintact skin. Five (6%) punctures occurred. Panlilio et al. (297) observed 206 operative procedures and noted that anesthesia staff were exposed to blood in 13 (6.3%). Popejoy and Fry (298) observed blood contact during 190 of 684 operations (28%). Circulating nurses and anesthesia personnel contacted patients' blood more frequently than did surgeons, but surgeons had more frequent percutaneous exposures. The authors noted that "although the anesthesiology staff and circulating nurses reported the greatest number of blood contact events, they were the only individuals who did not consistently wear gloves. Independent observations suggested that they were rarely gloved during the study period."

Several prospective studies indicate that anesthesia personnel are stuck with needles in 0.13% to 0.4% of operative procedures (298–300). During a 3-month period studied by Maz and Lyons (300), a higher proportion of the more experienced anesthesiologists stuck themselves with needles than did the less experienced personnel: four of 15 consultants (27%), two of seven senior registrars (29%), one of six registrars (17%), one of seven senior house officers (14%), and one of seven clinical assistants (14%). Six of the nine needles were contaminated, and only three of the injuries were reported to the proper hospital authorities. In contrast, Jagger et al. (301) observed that residents injured themselves more frequently than did attending physicians in all specialties. Moreover, Heald and Ransohoff (302) estimated the rate of needlestick injuries in anesthesia residents to be 2.5 injuries per resident-year. This rate was lower than that for residents in orthopedics (5.6 injuries per resident-year), general surgery (5.5 injuries per resident-year), and obstetrics and gynecology (4.5 injuries per resident-year) but higher than that for residents in internal medicine (0.75 injuries per resident-year).

Greene et al. (303) studied percutaneous injuries reported by anesthesia personnel from nine hospitals participating in the EPINet surveillance program. All contaminated percutaneous injuries in these personnel resulted from needles, 87% (34 of 39) of which were hollow bore. Seventy-eight percent of these injuries occurred between uses or after use of the device and are therefore considered potentially preventable. In contrast to injuries experienced by anesthesia personnel, fewer than 30% of the injuries to nonanesthesia personnel in the operating rooms were caused by hollow-bore needles. Thus, anesthesia personnel may be less likely to experience percutaneous injuries than are surgeons; however, the needles used by the former usually have hollow bores. In addition, anesthesia personnel use hypodermic needles and large-bore cannula introducers, both of which can carry more blood than suture needles. Thus, the percutaneous

TABLE 61.6. OUTBREAKS RELATED TO ANESTHESIA PERSONNEL

First Author (Reference)	Year	Source	Incubation Period	Infection	Number of Patients	Microorganism	Comments	Time to Recognition	Time to Resolution
Walter (283)	1966	Anesthesiologist	Not specified	Surgical site	10	*S. aureus*	Psoriasis of scalp and extremities, dermatitis on hands; microorganism cultured from nose, throat, hands, and perineum	Not specified	3 years
Payne (284)	1967	Anesthesiologist	2–20 days	Surgical site	33	*S. aureus*	Acute exacerbation of psoriasis resulting in large areas of desquamation	9 days	35 days
Jewett (285)	1968	Anesthesiologist	14–72 hours	Puerperal sepsis	25	Group A β-hemolytic streptococci	Microorganism isolated from hand and shin lesions	6 days	11 days
Schaffner (286)	1969	Anesthesiologist	Not specified	Surgical site	21	Group A β-hemolytic streptococci	Disseminated from an asymptomatic anal carrier	3 weeks	4 months
Gryska (287)	1970	Anesthesiologist	24–48 hours	Surgical site	13	Group A β-hemolytic streptococci	Anal carrier with mild pruritus ani	4 days	30 days
CDC (288)	1976	Anesthesiologist	<48 hours	Surgical site; bacteremia and meningitis	6 1	Group A β-hemolytic streptococci	Asymptomatic throat and anal carrier	Not specified	16 days
Paul (289)	1990	Anesthesiologist	24 hours–16 days	Surgical site	4	Group A β-hemolytic streptococci	Asymptomatic throat carrier	Not specified	30 days
Mastro (290)	1990	Anesthesia technician	6–240 hours	Surgical site	20	Group A β-hemolytic streptococci	Disseminated from a carrier with psoriasis and seborrhea on scalp and ears	23 months	40 months
Bosch (291, 292)	1998, 2000	Anesthesiologist	Not specified	Hepatitis	171	Hepatitis C	Anesthesiologist addicted to morphine and infected with hepatitis C gave himself morphine injections and then gave patients the drug through the same syringe and needle	Not specified	Not specified
Ross (293)	2000	Anesthesia assistant		Hepatitis	5 patients and the anesthesia assistant	Hepatitis C	Index patient may have infected the anesthesia assistant who participated in her operation; 6 weeks later, the anesthesia assistant had acute icterus	Not specified	3 months
Cody (294)	2002	Anesthesiologist	7 weeks	Hepatitis	1	Hepatitis C	Mode of transmission is unclear; anesthesiologist probably acquired hepatitis C from a chronically infected patient	Not specified	Not specified

injuries experienced by anesthesia personnel may be more likely to transmit blood-borne pathogens than are those experienced by surgeons. Jagger et al.'s (301) study confirmed these findings. Most percutaneous injuries observed in this study occurred in the operative site and to nonanesthesia staff; 1.5% of the injuries occurred at the anesthesia cart or machine. However, 16.7% of the injuries sustained by anesthesia personnel were caused by blood-filled, hollow-bore needles.

More recently Greene et al. (304) evaluated contaminated percutaneous injuries (CPIs) among anesthesia personnel at 11 hospitals over a 2-year period. These investigators found that 30% of all CPIs were high-risk exposures, that is, the sharp device was a blood-contaminated hollow-bore needle. Seventy-four percent of these injuries were potentially preventable. They noted that only 26% of CPIs were reported and that reporting rates varied by job category. Student nurse anesthetists reported 64% of their injuries compared with 29% for anesthesia residents, 23% for certified nurse anesthetists, and 19% for staff anesthesiologists. After correcting for under reporting, these investigators calculated a CPI rate of 0.27 CPIs per year per person or 0.42 CPIs per year per full-time equivalent. Patel and Tignor (305) at Yale determined device-specific sharps injury rates. Injuries with hollow-bore needles on Luer-lock syringes occurred at a rate of 1.29/100,000 devices used for anesthesiologists compared with 7.35/100,000 devices used for surgeons. Injuries from intravenous catheters occurred at rates of 1.18/100,000 devices for anesthesiologists and 12.87/100,000 devices for surgeons.

Anesthesia personnel perform numerous procedures during which they may be exposed to patients' blood or body fluids. For example, they insert intravascular catheters, intubate and extubate patients' tracheas, and suction tracheal and oral secretions. Using a questionnaire, Kristensen et al. (306) found that 50% of anesthesiologists had contact with blood during a 1-week period, compared with approximately 40% of orthopedic surgeons and approximately 30% of general surgeons. Furthermore, Kristensen et al. (307) determined that anesthesia personnel contacted patients' blood or body fluids during 36% of common anesthesia procedures (Table 61.7). In a questionnaire survey, Harrison et al. (299) noted that 65 "anaesthetic and related staff" contacted patients' blood or body fluids in 35 of 270 (13%) operations, most frequently while cannulating a vessel.

TABLE 61.7. BLOOD CONTACT DURING ROUTINE ANESTHESIA PROCEDURES (307)

Procedure	Percent Associated with Blood Contact
Injecting a drug intramuscularly	8
Extubating a patient	9
Suctioning the oral cavity, pharynx, or trachea	13
Catheterizing a peripheral vein	18
Doing a lumbar puncture	23
Catheterizing the epidural space	34
Doing an arterial puncture	38
Establishing or discontinuing a blood transfusion	43
Inserting a central venous catheter	87

In addition to contact with visible blood from vessels, the operative site, or contaminated needles, anesthesia personnel are exposed to blood from several less obvious sources. For example, Crisco and DeVane (308) found blood in the mouths of 56 of 168 patients (33%) after tracheal intubation; blood was visible in 12 (7%) and occult in 44 (26%). Thirty-nine patients (23%) had blood on their cheeks, tongue, and posterior soft palate, and for 29 patients (17%) blood was noted on the laryngoscope blade. After tracheal extubation, 58 patients (35%) had overt blood and 59 (35%) had occult blood in their mouths. Blood was found on the distal tip of 113 endotracheal tubes (67%). Similarly, Kristensen et al. (306) noted visible blood on 16 of 29 endotracheal tubes (55%; 95% CI, 36–74%) and occult blood on 6 of 29 endotracheal tubes (21%; 95% CI, 8–40%). Five of 28 suction catheters (18%; 95% CI, 6–37%) were contaminated by visible blood, and 10 (36%; 95% CI, 19–56%) were contaminated by occult blood. Brimacombe et al. (309) determined that cuffed oropharyngeal airways (14%) were more likely than laryngeal mask airways) (LMAs) (3%) to be contaminated with visible blood. Parker and Day (310) found visible blood on 12% of LMAs and 16% of endotracheal tubes after use. However when they tested for occult blood, these investigators found that 76% and 78%, respectively, were contaminated.

In addition, anesthesia personnel may unwittingly contact a patient's blood or body fluids when they touch the anesthetic record (311) or equipment such as the anesthesia machine or touch screens (312). Hall (313) sampled surfaces on "clean" anesthesia machines, carts, and monitors. Of 418 samples, 134 were positive for occult blood and three sites were contaminated with visible blood. (See Current Anesthesia Practice, below, for further studies about this topic.) Perry and Monaghan (314) found visible and occult blood on anesthesia equipment: 35.5% of the tests were positive before the first case of the day, 29.5% were positive after the first case, and 29.5% after the second case. Occult blood was more common than visible blood. They found blood on ventilator controls (25.0%), flowmeter knobs (33.9%), vapor controls (26.8%), electrocardiography cables (64.3%), pulse oximeter probes (19.6%), and blood pressure cuffs (26.8%). Together these studies indicate that anesthesiologists contaminate the environment in which they work with blood, that the equipment is not cleaned adequately, and that anesthesia personnel can unwittingly contact blood during all their activities, not just when they access the vascular system.

INFECTIONS CAUSED BY OCCUPATIONAL EXPOSURE

Hepatitis B Virus

The prevalence of serologic markers for hepatitis B virus (HBV) has ranged from 3.5% to 49% in anesthesia personnel (315–322) compared with only 4.4% to 13.7% (323,324) in the general population. The highest rate of HBV seropositivity, 49%, was noted in an inner city hospital (320), where 27 of 70 anesthesiologists were from areas of the world with a high prevalence of hepatitis B infection and a large proportion of the patients were in high-risk groups. Most point prevalence studies suggest that the proportion of seropositive personnel increases with the duration of anesthesia practice (315–317,319–321). However, in one multicenter point prevalence study, Berry et al. (318) found that hepatitis B seropositivity did not increase with additional years of practice.

Anesthesia personnel were infected with HBV during two outbreaks (325,326). In both outbreaks, the index case was not known to be infected with HBV, routine precautions were taken in the operating room, and the healthcare workers denied touching the patient's blood. Thus, the mode of transmission was not identified.

Hepatitis C Virus

Anesthesia personnel have acquired hepatitis C from patients; some of these staff members subsequently transmitted this virus to patients (see Outbreaks Associated with Anesthesia Personnel, above, and Table 61.6). Bakir et al. (327) described a 33-year-old male Tunisian anesthesiologist who acquired hepatitis C while "training abroad." He was assisting in the care of an accident victim. After the antishock trousers were removed, the anesthesiologist noted a bleeding wound. He instinctively put his bare hand, which had minor cuts, onto the wound. Three months later, he had jaundice, asthenia, hepatitis, and elevated serum transaminases. His hepatitis C serology converted to positive, and he did not respond to treatment with interferon or ribavirin. Greene et al. (304) estimated that the 30-year risk for anesthesiologists acquiring hepatitis C was 0.45% per full-time equivalent (FTE). They estimated that 155 anesthesiologists would acquire hepatitis C over a 30-year period.

Human Immunodeficiency Virus

Although the absolute risk of acquiring HIV infection from occupational exposure has not been determined for anesthesia personnel specifically, one anesthesiologist was infected when he stuck himself with an HIV-contaminated needle (328). Buergler et al. (329) used data in the literature to estimate the risk for anesthesiologists and surgeons of acquiring HIV infection over a 30-year career. They assumed that (a) the risk of needlesticks per year ranges from 0.86 to 2.5 for anesthesiologists and 3.8 to 6.2 for surgeons, (b) the risk of seroconversion from a needlestick ranges from 0.42% to 0.50%, (c) the prevalence of HIV infection in the population would remain constant during the 30-year period and would range from 0.32% to 23.6%, and (d) protective measures would be of no benefit. Using these assumptions, Buergler et al. estimated a cumulative risk for anesthesiologists of 0.05% to 4.5% compared with 0.17% to 13.9% for surgeons. Buergler's estimates have been controversial (330, 331). Subsequently, Greene et al. (304) used different assumptions and estimated the 30-year risk to be only 0.049%, with 17 HIV infections occurring in anesthesiologists during this time period. Regardless of which estimate most closely approximates reality, both estimates suggest that the risk of acquiring HIV infection is measurable. Furthermore, despite the less invasive nature of anesthesia practice, the risk for anesthesiologists overlaps with that of surgeons, and as we noted previously, many exposures among anesthesia personnel are considered high risk because they involved hollow-bore needles that had been in the vascular space.

Herpes Simplex Virus

Herpetic whitlow, infection of the fingers with herpes simplex virus (HSV), occurs rarely in the general population but is a recognized hazard for healthcare workers (see Chapters 43 and 81). Herpes simplex infects the fingers when breaks in the skin are exposed to secretions containing the virus. Serologic surveys indicate that 80% to 90% of the U.S. population has been infected with HSV (332,333). Cross-sectional culture surveys indicate that, at any one time, 2% to 9% of adults and 5% to 8% of children asymptomatically shed HSV in saliva; longitudinal studies suggest that 32% of children and 80% of adults asymptomatically shed HSV in saliva at some points in their lives (334–336). Anesthesia personnel frequently contact patients' oral secretions, and therefore might be at increased risk for acquiring herpetic whitlow (337). Although the frequency of this infection in anesthesia personnel is unknown, individual anesthesiologists and nurse anesthetists have acquired herpetic whitlow from infected patients (338–340).

PREVENTION AND CONTROL OF INFECTION IN THE PRACTICE OF ANESTHESIA

Current Infection Control Guidelines

As noted previously, several agencies, including the ASA (7), the AANA (8), AORN (9–12), CDC (13,14), the Australia and New Zealand College of Anaesthetists (15), the Australian Society of Anaesthetists (16), the New South Wales Health Department (18), and the Association of Anaesthetists of Great Britain and Ireland (19) have published infection control guidelines for the practice of anesthesia (Tables 61.8 through 61.10). In general, the ASA, AANA, and AORN recommend similar procedures. However, the ASA and the AANA recommend substantially different procedures for the care of anesthesia bellows, and they disagree about the need for filters in breathing circuits (Table 61.8). The guidelines published by the ASA are easy to read and are well referenced. They usually state general principles but do not give specific details on how to comply with the guidelines. In contrast, the AANA guidelines are less well organized and are sparsely referenced. However, the AANA gives both general guidelines and specific details on how to comply. The AANA guidelines, but not those produced by the ASA, address such relevant issues as isolation precautions and the HIV-infected anesthesia provider.

Current Anesthesia Practice

Several anesthesiologists have voiced concern about their colleagues' disregard for basic infection control practices. They criticize their colleagues for using common syringes, handling intravenous tubing ports and multidose vials without aseptic technique, recapping needles, failing to maintain separate clean

TABLE 61.8. RECOMMENDATIONS/GUIDELINES FOR INFECTION CONTROL IN ANESTHESIA—EQUIPMENT

Item	ASA (7)	AANA (8)	ANZCA (15)	AORN (9–12)	CDC (14)	Other
Critical: Items that enter or contact an area that is normally sterile. Examples include, but are not limited to, vascular needles, catheters and tubing; syringes; stopcocks; regional block needles and catheters; and urinary catheters.	Use sterile equipment to enter or contact any body area that is normally sterile. Clean reusable items thoroughly and sterilize before reuse. Ensure sterility at the time of use. Follow aseptic techniques when handling and using sterile equipment.	Use sterile items to enter sterile body area or vascular system.		Use sterile items to enter sterile tissue or the vascular system. Clean items thoroughly before disinfection (12).	Sterilize medical devices or patient-care equipment before use. Clean all items thoroughly before sterilizing or disinfecting.	
Semicritical: Items that come in contact with mucous membranes. Examples include, but are not limited to, laryngoscope blades, Magill forceps, endotracheal tube stylets, temperature probes, masks, breathing circuits and connectors, nasal and oral airways, self-inflating resuscitation bags, and esophageal stethoscopes.	Rinse items as soon as possible after use; decontaminate by cleaning, and sterilize or treat with high-level disinfection. Keep endotracheal and endobronchial tubes free from contamination until used.	Sterilize items or treat with high-level disinfection.	Endotracheal tubes, nasal, and pharyngeal airways should be kept sterile until they are used. Reusable face masks must be thoroughly decontaminated and then disinfected before they are reused. Items placed in the upper airway that may cause bleeding, such as laryngoscope blades and temperature probes, must be disinfected before use. The breathing circuit should be sterilized *or* decontaminated and disinfected *or* protected by a new filter. When a filter is used the disposable items between the patient and the filter should be disposed of between each case and the reusable devices should be decontaminated and	Reusable anesthesia equipment that comes in contact with mucous membranes, blood, or body fluid is considered semicritical and should be cleaned and then processed by high-level disinfection, pasteurization, or sterilization between each patient use.	Sterilize or at minimum treat items with high-level disinfection.	Separate used laryngoscope and nondisposable items that are overtly contaminated from clean equipment (372). The part of the breathing circuit between the patient and the filter must either be discarded or cleaned and disinfected after each patient. If a carbon dioxide absorber is also used, the part of the breathing circuit between the absorber and the filter must either be discarded or cleaned and disinfected at the end of each procedure list. If carbon dioxide absorbers are not used, the breathing circuit tubing that conducts the gas to and from the filter must either be discarded or cleaned and disinfected at the end of each procedure or operation list. If a filter is not used, the breathing circuit must either be discarded or cleaned and disinfected after each patient. All anesthetic apparatus that comes in contact with a patient or becomes contaminated with blood or body substances for example airways, endotracheal tubes, laryngoscopes, suckers, forceps, temperature probes, esophageal

(*continued*)

TABLE 61.8. *(continued)*

Item	ASA (7)	AANA (8)	ANZCA (15)	AORN (9–12)	CDC (14)	Other
			disinfected before they are reused.			echo probes, and face masks must be either discarded or cleaned and disinfected after each patient (18).
			Ventilator circuits should be cleaned and disinfected regularly.			A new filter should be placed between the patient and the breathing system *or* a new breathing system should be used for each patient. Expired gas sampling should be done on the breathing system side of the filter. Filters should not be used for pediatric anesthesia; new breathing systems should be used (19).
Noncritical: Items that touch intact skin or do not make contact with the patient.						
1. *Items that touch the patient.* Examples include, but are not limited to, blood pressure cuffs, electrocardiograph cables and electrodes, pulse oximeter and skin temperature sensors, stethoscopes, and head straps.	Clean equipment with a disinfectant at the end of the day and whenever visibly contaminated.	Process equipment with intermediate or low-level disinfection.	Laryngoscope bandles should be decontaminated between uses.	Clean and decontaminate items when contaminated or visibly soiled and at the end of the day.	Wash items with detergent or disinfectant, rinse, and dry.	
2. *Items that do not touch the patient.* Examples include, but are not limited to, exterior surfaces of anesthesia machines, carts, monitors, and tables.	Clean horizontal surfaces of anesthesia machines and carts after each patient.	Clean environmental surfaces with warm water and detergent or with a low- to intermediate-level disinfectant after each patient procedure; terminally disinfect at the end of the day or when contaminated with blood or body fluids.		Clean and decontaminate items when contaminated or visibly soiled and at the end of the day.		

(continued)

TABLE 61.8. (*continued*)

Item	ASA (7)	AANA (8)	ANZCA (15)	AORN (9–12)	CDC (14)	Other
Single-use items	Reuse is not recommended because there are insufficient data on the safety of this practice for anesthesia equipment. Reuse of single-use items shifts the responsibility/liability from the manufacturer to the user. If single-use items are reprocessed, the users must develop a quality assessment program to ensure disinfection/sterilization is adequate and that the function and integrity are not compromised.	Do not reuse, clean, repackage, or resterilize disposable equipment designed for one-time use and labeled as "single-use" items. Hospitals that reprocess and reuse such products, not the manufacturer, are responsible for their safety and effectiveness. Refer to Food and Drug Administration (FDA) guideline. Disposable products that have been opened but not used or manipulated may be resterilized if the manufacturer approves the process.	Items of airway equipment to be placed in direct contact with the respiratory tract and airways labeled by the manufacturer as disposable or for single use only should not be reused.	Single-use items (e.g., suction catheters, breathing circuits, endotracheal tubes, stylets) should be used once and discarded. (a) If a device cannot be cleaned, it cannot be reprocessed and reused; (b) if sterility of a postprocessed device cannot be demonstrated, the device cannot be reprocessed and reused; (c) if the integrity and functionality of a reprocessed device cannot be demonstrated and documented to be as safe for patient care and/or equal to the original device specifications, the device cannot be reprocessed and reused. For further details the reader is referred to the AORN Guidance Statement: Reuse of Single-Use Devices (10)	Do not reprocess items or devices that cannot be cleaned and sterilized or disinfected without altering their physical integrity and function.	FDA compliance policy guide: "The institution or practitioner who reuses a disposable medical device should be able to demonstrate: 1) that the device can be adequately cleaned and sterilized, 2) that the physical characteristics or quality of the device will not be adversely affected, and 3) that the device remains safe and effective for its intended use. Any institution or practitioner who resterilizes and/or reuses a disposable medical device must bear full responsibility for the performance, its safety and effectiveness" (373). (See also Chapter 87.) Medical and Surgical Products Liaison Group and the Association of British Health-Care Industries advise against reuse unless specifically permitted by manufacturers (374). The New South Wales Health Department recommends that medical devices marked "single use only" should not be reused unless (a) testing documents that the devices are not physically or microbiologically less safe than new items; (b) reprocessing is controlled and in accordance with Good Manufacturing Processes defined by the Commonweath Therapeutic Goods Administration; (c) reprocessing must be in accordance with the manufacturer's instructions; (d) standard information is needed for informed patient consent (18).

(*continued*)

TABLE 61.8. (*continued*)

Item	ASA (7)	AANA (8)	ANZCA (15)	AORN (9–12)	CDC (14)	Other
Valves and CO_2 absorber	Clean and disinfect unidirectional valves and CO_2 absorber chambers periodically.	Disassemble, clean, and sterilize CO_2 absorbers and valves prior to reuse. When a patient has a respiratory infection, use disposable devices (e.g., circle system and absorber with bacterial filter, laryngoscope, and airway products) whenever possible.	When a filter is used in the circuit, sterilization of the carbon dioxide absorber before every case is not necessary. The device including the unidirectional valve should be disinfected regularly.	Absorbers and valves should be cleaned when the soda lime is changed according to the manufacturer's written instructions. Particular attention should be paid to the valves. Routine sterilization or high-level disinfection of the internal components of anesthesia machines is considered unnecessary.		
Bellows	Clean and disinfect tubing and bellows at regular intervals, not after each use. Routine sterilization/disinfection of the interior of anesthesia machines is not necessary or feasible.	Sterilize the anesthesia bellows and the bellows base or head after every case unless bacterial filters are used to protect the inspiratory, expiratory, and ventilator limbs of the circuit. When using disposable breathing circuits without bacterial filters, replace the ventilator bellows each time the circuit is replaced and the bellows base or head should be cleaned and sterilized.	Clean and disinfect regularly.	Bellows should be cleaned regularly according to the manufacturer's written instruction. Bellows are thought to represent a low risk for transmission of infection and do not require cleaning and disinfection after each use.		
Filters for breathing circuits	There are insufficient outcome data to support routine use of bacterial filters.	Use breathing circuits with bacterial filters for all cases.			Data do not support using bacterial filters	If used, filters must be discarded after each patient (18).

(*continued*)

TABLE 61.8. *(continued)*

Item	ASA (7)	AANA (8)	ANZCA (15)	AORN (9–12)	CDC (14)	Other
	Use a filter for patients known or suspected to have active tuberculosis.				to prevent nosocomial pulmonary infections (87). Use filter if patient has suspected or confirmed active tuberculosis (13).	At the current state of knowledge, a new bacterial/viral filter should be used for each case. The filter should be placed so as to protect the breathing circuit from possible contamination by the patient (16).
Heated humidifiers		Clean and sterilize humidifiers after each use. Use sterile water.			Sterilize reusable humidifiers or subject them to high-level disinfection after each use (87).	

ASA, American Society of Anesthesiologists; AANA, American Association of Nurse Anesthetists; ANZCA, Australia and New Zealand College of Anaesthetists; AORN, Association of PeriOperative Registered Nurses; CDC, Centers for Disease Control and Prevention.

TABLE 61.9. RECOMMENDATIONS/GUIDELINES REGARDING MEDICATION USE IN ANESTHESIA

Item	ASA (7)	AANA (8)	ANZCA (15)	Other
Preservative-free medications	Use as single-patient, single-dose item. Open at the time of use; discard immediately after use. Swab rubber septum or neck with alcohol before entering. Use sterile needles and syringes to aspirate contents.	Clean the ampule before opening. Use a filtered needle to draw up the medication. Cleanse rubber stoppers before each use.		
Medications drawn up into a syringe	Do not give medications from a syringe to more than one patient. Discard medication drawn into a syringe within 24 hours.	Not addressed.		
Multidose vials	Use aseptic technique. Cleanse rubber stopper. Use sterile needle and syringe each time vial is entered.	Restrict use of multiple dose vials to one patient only unless strict aseptic technique is used. A new sterile syringe and needle should be used each time the vial is penetrated.	Because of the potential for cross-infection, the use of the contents of multiple dose vials and ampules for more than one patient is not recommended except in a dispensing situation where different doses are drawn up before the administration of the first dose to a patient. Likewise, it is recommended that the contents of a single-dose ampule are to be used for one patient only (15).	Single-use ampules or vials of medication must be used for all injections unless alternative systems are set in place to prevent cross-infection (16). A medication may be taken from a multidose vial or ampule only if the medication or solution is not readily available in another form. If any medication is taken from a multidose vial or ampule, a sterile needle and syringe must be used to withdraw the contents. The needle and syringe must be discarded once they have been used. Precautions must be taken to ensure that contaminated material or fluid are not injected into a multidose vial or ampule (18).
Intravenous fluids, tubing, connectors, and disposable pressure transducers	Single-use only.	Single-use only.		
Stopcocks, injection ports, and other portals of access to sterile fluids	Maintain with sterile technique. Keep free of blood and cover with a sterile cap or syringe when not in use. Clean injection ports with appropriate disinfectant before entry.	Use sterile technique for all access ports.		
Use of syringes for more than one patient	Syringes are single-patient-use items. Do not give medications from a syringe to more than one patient. Consider the syringe contaminated after entry into an intravascular line.	Consider syringes and needles as single-use disposable items. Do not reuse needles and syringes. Dispose of all needles and syringes after every use. Once used they are contaminated.		
Noninjectable drugs and ointments and sprays	Discard multidose containers if contaminated or if contamination is suspected. Use unit dose packages whenever possible.	Acknowledge the risk of cross-contamination but do not prescribe practice.		

TABLE 61.10. RECOMMENDATIONS/GUIDELINES TO PROTECT ANESTHESIA PROVIDERS

Item	ASA (7)	AANA (8)	Other
Standard precautions	Use gloves, fluid-resistant mask, face shield, and gown routinely with all patients. Choose barrier commensurate with the expected extent of exposure.	Use standard precautions for all patients. Wear gloves, gowns, mask, and protective eyewear for contact with blood and body fluids. Use transmission-based precautions for patients known to be infected or colonized with epidemiologically important pathogens. See guidelines for specifics.	For the anesthetist's protection protective gloves are worn whenever the hands may contact blood, saliva, or any other body fluid and are to be removed after such a procedure to minimize contamination of the workplace (15). Universal precautions must be adopted for all anaesthetic practice (16). Readers are referred to the Hospital Infection Control Practices Advisory Committee's guideline on isolation precautions that should be released in 2004.
Hand hygiene	Wash hands after touching blood or body fluids whether or not gloves are worn. Wash hands immediately after removing gloves.	Wash hands before and after all contact with patients or specimens, after handling body substances, and after removing gloves.	Frequent hand washing by the anesthetist and the anesthetic technician is a most important infection control measure. Hands should be washed before handling a new patient or equipment to be used on a new patient, after leaving a patient, whenever they become contaminated, and before any invasive procedure (15). Readers are referred to the Hospital Infection Control Practices Advisory Committee's guideline on hand hygiene (375).
Handling needles	Do not recap, bend, break, or remove contaminated needles from syringes by hand. If necessary to recap a needle, use a single-handed technique or a mechanical protection device. Encourage use of needleless systems or shielded needle products. Puncture-resistant containers should be at all work locations.	Do not recap needles or manipulate them in any way. Place used syringes in nearby puncture-resistant containers that are stored upright and labeled as biohazards. Use a mechanical device or one-handed technique if no alternative is available. Alternatives to needles are available for checking sensory awareness.	
Blood exposures	Develop detailed protocol at each facility.	Each facility is obligated to provide postexposure testing, counseling, monitoring, and surveillance.	
Emergency ventilation devices	Mouth pieces, resuscitation bags, and other ventilation devices should be available.	Place equipment needed for emergency resuscitation in areas where the need for resuscitation is probable and predictable. Use ventilation devices rather than mouth-to-mouth resuscitation.	
Personnel with cutaneous lesions	Anesthesiologists should refrain from direct patient contact when they have breaks in the skin or exudative, weeping lesions unless the open area can be protected. Unprotected lesions are a risk to the healthcare worker and the patient.	Not addressed.	Personnel with skin abrasions, cuts or dermatitis must be excluded (16).
Hepatitis B vaccine	Vaccinate all anesthesiologists who do not have documented immunity.	Refers to the OSHA standard. Offer student CRNAs the vaccine at no cost.	Immunization Practices Advisory Committee states that health care workers whose work involves contact with blood should be vaccinated (376). OSHA requires that employers offer the vaccine at no cost to individuals who are exposed to blood (377).
Laser plumes	Hold evacuator nozzles close to the operative field before and 30 seconds after the tissue is vaporized to prevent transmission of viruses.	Not addressed.	

CRNA, Certified Registered Nurse Anesthetist; OSHA, Occupational Safety and Health Administration.

and dirty work spaces, not cleaning and disinfecting equipment after each patient, and not wearing protective barriers (235,236, 312,341–348).

Crow and Green (349) observed 18 surgeons and 10 anesthesiologists during 36 herniorrhaphies to determine whether they complied with 44 "aseptic precautions." Anesthesiologists violated those aseptic precautions nearly twice as often as did the surgeons. During the 36 operations, anesthesiologists were observed to touch the sterile field (two occurrences), have an infection (three occurrences), inadequately separate the operative field from the anesthesia area (three occurrences), wear their masks improperly (seven occurrences), lean over the sterile field (eight occurrences), not wash their hands before the case (24 occurrences), and not cover their hair completely (25 occurrences).

Tait and Tuttle (350) surveyed anesthesiologists to determine how many complied with practices recommended for preventing transmission of infectious agents to patients; 493 of 1149 (43%) completed the survey. Ninety-five percent reported washing their hands after caring for patients they considered to be at high risk for infection, but only 58% washed their hands if they felt the patient was at low risk of infection. Eight-eight percent changed breathing circuits between patients, 99% cleaned laryngoscope blades after each patient, 69% disinfected or sterilized blades, and 60.5% never or rarely disinfected their work surfaces. Forty-seven percent acknowledged that they reused syringes, and 53% said they never reused these devices. el Mikatti et al. (351) did a similar survey in the U.K. They had a better return rate [145 of 213 (68%)] than did Tait and Tuttle. Only 20% of the respondents in the U.K. admitted to ever reusing syringes. However, 49.4% of the anesthesiologists responding to Tait and Tuttle's survey always wore gloves compared with only 14.5% of the respondents to el Mikatti et al.'s survey. The proportion of anesthesiologists who always disinfect the septum of a multidose vial (27.8% U.S., 39.4% U.K.) and who work while sick (upper respiratory tract infection—96% U.S., 94% U.K.; gastrointestinal infection—60.1% U.S., 42.9% U.K.; herpes infection—22% U.S., 32.6% U.K.) was similar in both surveys. Anesthesiologists in both surveys thought their potential to transmit pathogens was low. Both Tait and Tuttle and el Mikatti et al. asked anesthesiologists to describe, using a scale of 0 to 10 (0, no chance of transmission; 10, a significant chance for transmission), the potential for anesthesiologists to transmit pathogens from patient to patient. The median score for anesthesiologists surveyed by Tait and Tuttle was 4.7 compared with only 3 for those surveyed by el Mikatti et al.

Several investigators documented that anesthesia equipment in some institutions is not cleaned and disinfected adequately. Simmons (352) obtained cultures of 20 "clean" handles, all of which grew microorganisms. Although *S. epidermidis, Micrococcus* species, and *Bacillus* species were the most common microorganisms, cultures from 12 of the 20 handles grew group A streptococcus. In addition, one handle each grew *S. aureus*, enterococcus, and *P. aeruginosa* with *Citrobacter*. Phillips and Monaghan (353) tested 65 laryngoscope blades and handles that were "patient-ready" (i.e., had been cleaned and disinfected and were ready to use on the next patient). No visible blood was noted, however, 13 (20%) blades and 26 (40%) of the handles had positive tests for occult blood; blades and handles tested in the afternoon were significantly more likely to be positive compared with those tested in the morning. Morell et al. (354) found similar results; 10.5% of "clean" laryngoscope blades and 50% of "clean" laryngoscope handles were contaminated with occult blood.

Several studies suggest a possible reason that these items are contaminated with blood. Many anesthesia personnel do not routinely clean and disinfect laryngoscope blades, endotracheal tube stylets, and breathing circuits between patients (235,342, 346). Esler et al. (355) did a postal survey of all 289 Royal College tutors in anesthesiology in Great Britain, 239 (82.7%) of whom responded. Of the respondents, 22% autoclaved laryngoscope blades after every use, 19% autoclaved them "often," 41% autoclaved them after high-risk cases, and 18% did not autoclave them. Fifty percent did not dismantle the laryngoscope before cleaning. One third of the respondents did not clean the laryngoscope handle. Forty-nine percent cleaned the handles, 13% autoclaved the handles after high-risk cases, and 5% autoclaved the handle after each case. One third of the respondents said they would not put a randomly selected, ready-to-use laryngoscope from their institutions into their own mouths! Of note, laryngoscope blades are semicritical items and, therefore need to be cleaned and treated at least with high-level disinfection before the next use.

It has been difficult to document that these breaches in infection control practice compromise patients' care. However, Foweraker (356) identified four children in a pediatric cardiology ICU who were infected with *P. aeruginosa.* All four isolates had different phage types. However, the investigators found a laryngoscope blade that had dried secretions around the bulb. *P. aeruginosa* with the same phage type as the strain infecting the one child who died was isolated from the blade. Of note, the staff in this unit did not follow their own cleaning policy. Similarly, Neal et al. (357) reported that eight neonates acquired infections with the same *P. aeruginosa* strain. Dried secretions were found on two neonatal laryngoscopes, and *P. aeruginosa* with the same phage and serotype as the epidemic strain was isolated from cultures of these devices. The laryngoscopes were washed in hot water and detergent and wiped with alcohol. They were then stored loose in a drawer. Nelson et al. (358) reported that *Listeria monocytogenes* possibly was transmitted from one neonate to another by a laryngoscope that was wiped with alcohol and not sterilized as the hospital's policy required. These studies suggest that blood-borne pathogens could be transmitted to patients or to anesthesia personnel via contaminated anesthesia equipment. Laryngoscope blades touch the oral mucosa, and thus, could transmit blood-borne pathogens from patient to patient. Laryngoscope handles and anesthesia carts and machines do not contact patients directly, and thus, may not put patients at risk. However, anesthesia personnel may contaminate their hands when touching these surfaces, putting themselves at risk and putting patients at risk if the staff members do not wash their hands. Further studies are needed to determine whether these items could be a source of infections for individuals (patients or anesthesia staff) or for outbreaks such as that reported by Chant et al. (60).

Anecdotal reports, questionnaires, and studies observing their practice consistently show that many anesthesia personnel do not routinely wear protective equipment to prevent contact with blood and body fluids. Only 16% of anesthesia personnel responding to O'Donnell and Asbury's (359) mail survey stated that they wore gloves for routine daily work. In a similar study, only 9% of anesthesia personnel wore gloves when intubating patients, and 8% wore gloves when inserting peripheral cannulas (299). However, 63% wore gloves to insert arterial lines, and 89% wore gloves to insert central venous catheters (299). Tait and Tuttle (350,360) surveyed anesthesiologists to determine how many complied with guidelines to protect themselves from exposures to blood-borne pathogens. Only 7% of anesthesiologists reported that they wore gowns, and 49.3% reported that they always wore gloves while administering anesthesia. In contrast, only 14.5% of the anesthesiologists responding to el Mikatti et al.'s (351) survey said they always wore gloves. Anesthesiologists who responded to Tait and Tuttle's survey reported that they were more likely to wear gloves if they felt the patient was at high risk for infection with blood-borne pathogens (360). Anesthesiologists who recently entered practice were more likely than their more experienced colleagues to wear gloves for contact with patients felt to be at low risk for infection with a blood-borne pathogen (360). Seventy-eight percent of the respondents reported they had received hepatitis B vaccine (360). Eighty-eight percent sometimes and 10% always recapped needles; nearly 66% used a two-handed technique while recapping. Thirty-two percent of the respondents had sustained injuries with contaminated needles in the preceding 12 months; only 45% reported the incident or sought treatment (360).

In summary, studies consistently indicate that many anesthesia personnel disregard both traditional infection control procedures and those recommended by their own societies. Furthermore, despite the risk of transmitting HBV, HCV, HIV, and other blood-borne diseases, anesthesia personnel continue to use common syringes and procedures that might transmit blood-borne pathogens. In 1990, Kempen and Treiber (347) pointedly stated that "the widespread reeducation of personnel regarding hygiene (universal precautions) due to the AIDS epidemic may have missed anesthetic personnel, as many prevailing anesthetic practices appear quite cavalier regarding nosocomial viral transmission. In 2001, Berry (361) published an editorial in which he commented on a report by Ross et al. (293) in which they described transmission of hepatitis C from a patient to an anesthesia assistant, who then spread this microorganism to other patients. Berry wrote, "The report clearly demonstrates the potential for occupational HCV transmission both from and to patients via tasks performed by anesthesiologists. The disregard of appropriate aseptic techniques and the failure to use standard precautions likely were responsible for the adverse outcomes." Little changed in 11 years!

Preventing Infections in Anesthesia Personnel

Several investigators noted that anesthesia personnel could prevent most of their contact with blood and body fluids by wearing gloves (297–299,301,307). Hence, if anesthesia personnel wore gloves and used other barriers, they could protect themselves against most occupationally acquired infections including HBV, HCV, HIV, and herpetic whitlow. McNamara and Stacey (362) surveyed anesthesia staff at five hospitals in southeast England and found that only 49% knew the published guidelines. Only 29% of the respondents wore gloves routinely. The primary reason anesthesiologists gave for not wearing gloves was that gloves decreased their sense of feel. Some anesthesia staff are concerned that they may increase their risk of injury and that they may contaminate their patients or the environment if they wear gloves while performing procedures. A study by Ben-David and Gaitini (363) suggests that these fears may be unfounded. These investigators observed fewer needlestick injuries and less environmental contamination when personnel wore gloves than when they did not. Although the differences did not reach significance, these data indicate that gloves did not increase the number of injuries or the frequency of contamination.

HBV infection can be prevented by immunizing individuals at high risk and by using appropriate barriers. Hepatitis B vaccine, available in the U.S. since 1982 (364), was accepted slowly by anesthesia personnel. In 1985, only 19% of anesthesia residents surveyed by Berry et al. (318) had been immunized. In 1991, approximately 90% of the anesthesia residents but only 60% of the attending anesthesiologists ($p < .001$) surveyed by Rosenberg et al. (348) had been vaccinated. Two other surveys of anesthesiologists conducted in the late 1980s found vaccination rates of 71% to 74% (299,300).

A case report describes an incident in which respiratory secretions splashed into an anesthesiologist's unprotected eyes during an intubation (365). Subsequently, he acquired bilateral conjunctivitis, fever, myalgia, and pharyngitis. Adenovirus type 14 was isolated from the patient and the anesthesiologist. The authors concluded that face protection would have prevented this exposure, and they recommended that anesthesia personnel wear face protection when intubating patients.

A poignant case report illustrates how performing routine tasks can put anesthesia personnel at risk for HIV infection (328). An anesthesiologist with 20 years of experience inserted a central venous catheter into a patient known to be infected with HIV. After inserting the catheter, the anesthesiologist picked up the 16-gauge needle in his right hand and reached across his left arm to discard it. In the process, he stuck the contaminated needle into his left forearm. Despite beginning azidothymidine (AZT) within 2 hours of the injury, he seroconverted 10 weeks later. In an article (328) and videotape (366) describing the accident, this unfortunate anesthesiologist shared several important lessons. First, the catastrophic procedure was one he had performed hundreds of times. Second, he was working under adverse conditions that forced him to reach across his body with the contaminated needle. Third, and to our mind most important, the accident occurred after he had finished the procedure. He concentrated intently while inserting the line in order to complete the task successfully, but his vigilance dropped while discarding the contaminated needle. Although this is only one case, we conclude that anesthesia personnel should protect themselves by optimizing their work conditions and by concentrating intently during and after procedures, even the most routine.

In summary, numerous studies indicate that anesthesia personnel are frequently exposed to patients' blood and body fluids. The studies also document that anesthesia personnel do not use appropriate barrier precautions. Given that they are frequently exposed to blood but rarely protect themselves, we can only conclude that anesthesia personnel are ignorant of their own risk, deny that they are at risk, or simply are obstinate or cavalier.

CONCLUSION

In 1873, Skinner (6) chastised his colleagues for using their inhalers without cleaning them between patients. He concluded his rebuke as follows:

> It is to be hoped, that the broad hint which I have here given about the repulsiveness and disgusting nature of the practice of permitting more than one patient to breathe through the same instrument, will . . . be acted upon without requiring repetition.

We do not know how Skinner's scathing comments affected his audience. However, another British anesthesiologist published the following editorial in 1964 (367):

> [Anesthesiologists] must be adamant on the question of cleanliness . . . . Only then will they be able to satisfy their colleagues, who will one day surely enquire closely into the part [anesthesiologists] play in hospital cross-infection. This part may well be bigger than is suspected.

Even more recently, Rosenberg (341), an anesthesiologist, bluntly stated:

> The data suggest that anesthesia personnel are aware of their potentially infectious environment but do not implement protective measures for themselves or their patients (341).

One hundred and thirty years after Skinner challenged his colleagues to improve their infection control practices, anesthesia personnel continue to disregard the warnings and guidelines issued by their own colleagues. Why do anesthesia personnel flagrantly disregard basic infection control procedures? What can infection control personnel do to improve compliance? To our knowledge, no published studies have addressed either of these issues. Hence, we offer some of our own untested ideas.

We suggest that anesthesia personnel disregard infection control procedures for several reasons. First, because anesthesia personnel usually do not follow patients throughout the postoperative period, they are unlikely to know which patients develop infections after specific procedures (342). Hence, they are unlikely to associate breaking aseptic technique with patients' infections. Second, anesthesia personnel, like most healthcare workers, learn by watching their mentors. We would argue that the examples set by senior anesthesia personnel might be even more powerful than those in other specialties, because anesthesia trainees work one-on-one with their teachers for prolonged periods. During that time, they watch or perform numerous procedures. Because many anesthesia personnel ignore basic infection control procedures, these bad habits are likely to be transmitted to trainees. McNamara and Stacey (362) suggested that this might be the case when they commented that "all grades are equally at fault. It might be argued that established behaviour is more difficult to change, but it would seem that trainees are learning similar patterns of practice." Third, because anesthesia personnel must do numerous procedures very quickly, they feel that they do not have adequate time to use aseptic technique. Fourth, anesthesiologists work behind a barrier that shields them from the scrutiny of the surgical team. Scrub nurses, or other members of the surgical team, point out breaks in sterile technique that occur in the operative site. However, they are less likely to see errors committed behind the anesthesia barricade. Thus, anesthesiologists rarely get feedback from others regarding their aseptic technique.

What can infection control personnel do to help improve compliance? First, they can educate anesthesia personnel regarding basic infection control procedures, the guidelines published by their own societies, their patients' risk of nosocomial infections, their own risk of occupationally acquired infections, and the Occupational Safety and Health Administration's regulations and fines. Few educational tools specifically address infection control in anesthesia, but the guidelines (7–21) and the videotape (366) mentioned previously are helpful.

Second, infection control personnel should identify a respected anesthesia provider who is interested in infection control issues. Working together, they can more accurately identify the major infection control problems in that particular unit and design practical solutions. Furthermore, proposals designed and presented by an anesthesia provider are more likely to be accepted and used by their colleagues than those imposed by infection control personnel. We have found this collaboration to be very effective at the University of Iowa hospitals and clinics. For example, one of the authors (S. S.-S.), an anesthesiologist, designed an infection control protocol for anesthesiologists. Staff from infection control reviewed and edited the protocol; the chair of anesthesia and the hospital epidemiologist (author L.A.H.) signed the final version. Anesthesia staff members have implemented the protocol, because it was generated internally and was not forced on them by someone who does not understand the contingencies of their practice.

Third, infection control personnel should calculate rates of infections associated with devices inserted by anesthesia personnel and present the data to the anesthesia providers. Although identifying those infections and obtaining the appropriate denominators might be difficult, the data could help anesthesia personnel recognize their own culpability and inspire them to improve their aseptic technique. Such feedback has been shown to reduce infection rates in other settings (368–370). Hajjar and Girard (371) published the results of a study in which they did surveillance for nosocomial infections related to anesthesia. They defined anesthesia-related infections as infections occurring within 72 hours of a general or regional anesthetic procedure. Twenty-five infections met this definition—12 respiratory, nine vascular-catheter associated, two eye, and two mouth—for a rate of 3.4 infections/1,000 patients. These infections could have originated from errors in the operating room, the postanesthesia care unit (PACU), or in the unit to which the patient was transferred after leaving the PACU. Although the origin of these infections is not entirely clear, Hajjar's and Girard's data provide an estimate of the rate and types of infections related to anesthesia practice. We need more studies that address this difficult issue.

Fourth, infection control and anesthesia personnel should

collaborate on studies designed to identify risk factors for infections associated with anesthesia and to assess the mortality, costs, and length of hospital stay attributable to these infections. If we can identify the rates of infection, the human and economic costs, and the risk factors associated with these infections, infection control and anesthesia personnel will be able to design effective preventive measures that will decrease infection rates and improve the quality of patient care.

REFERENCES

1. Key TE. *The history of surgical anesthesia.* New York: Shuman's, 1945: 14–28.
2. Lyman HM. *Artificial anaesthesia and anaesthetics.* New York: William Wood, 1981.
3. Shepard DAE. John Snow and research. *Can J Anaesth* 1989;36: 224–241.
4. Ellis RH. Dr. John Snow. His London residences, and the site for a commemorative London. In: Atkinson RS, Boulton TB, eds. *The history of anaesthesia.* London: Royal Society of Medicine Services, Parthenon, 1989:1–7.
5. Maltby JR, Bamforth BJ. The Wood library-museum's 1858 edition of John Snow's on chloroform and other anesthetics. *Anesth Analg* 1990;71:288–294.
6. Skinner. Anaesthetics and inhalers. *Br Med J* 1873;1:353–354.
7. American Society of Anesthesiologists. The Task Force on Infection Control of the Committee on Occupational Health. *Recommendations for infection control for the practice of anesthesiology,* 2nd ed. Park Ridge, IL: American Society of Anesthesiologists, 1998.
8. American Association of Nurse Anesthetists. *Infection control guide.* Park Ridge, IL: American Association of Nurse Anesthetists, 1997.
9. Anonymous. Recommended practices for cleaning and processing anesthesia equipment. Association of perioperative Registered Nurses. *AORN J* 1999;70:914–917.
10. Anonymous. Reuse of single-use devices. Association of perioperative Registered Nurses. *AORN J* 2001;73:957–962, 964, 966.
11. Anonymous. Recommended practices. Disinfection. Association of Operating Room Nurses. *AORN J* 1992;56:715–720.
12. Association of Operating Room Nurses. Recommended practices. Steam and ethylene oxide (EO) sterilization. Association of Operating Room Nurses. *AORN J* 1992;56:721–730.
13. Centers for Disease Control and Prevention. Guidelines for preventing the transmission of *Mycobacterium tuberculosis* in health-care facilities, 1994. *MMWR* 1994;43:1–132.
14. Centers for Disease Control. CDC guideline for handwashing and hospital environmental control, 1985. Section 2: Cleaning, disinfecting, and sterilizing patient-care equipment. *Infect Control* 1986;7: 236–240.
15. Australia and New Zealand College of Anaesthetists. Policy on infection control in anaesthesia, 1995; updated 2002.
16. Australian Society of Anaesthetists Ltd. ASA position statement. Anaesthesia and HIV and anaesthesia and hepatitis B and C. *http://www.asa.org.au/publications/policies/hiv.htm,* 1994.
17. Australian Medical Association. Position statement. Blood-borne and sexually transmitted viral infections. *http://domino.ama.com.au/AMA-Web,* 1995; amended 2002.
18. New South Wales Health Department. Infection control policy. North Sydney, 1999.
19. Association of Anaesthetists of Great Britain and Ireland. A report received by Council of the Association of Anaesthetists on Blood Borne Viruses and Anaesthesia. Update, 1996.
20. Department of Health of the Netherlands Committee on Infection Prevention. The concept of an individually clean breathing circuit. Department of Health of the Netherlands Committee on Infection Prevention, 1991.
21. Societé Francaise d'Anesthesie et de Reanimation. Recommendations concernant l'hygiene en anesthesia. Societé Francaise d'Anesthesie et de Reanimation, Paris, 1997.
22. Hauer T, Dziekan G, Kruger WA, et al. Sinnvolle und nicht sinnvolle hygienemabnahmen in der anasthesie und auf intensivstationen. *Anaesthesist* 2000;49:96–101.
23. Bimar MC, Hajjar J, Pottecher B. Risque infectieux nosocomial en anesthesia. Recommendations generales. *Ann Fr Anesth Reanim* 1998; 17:392–402.
24. Bowring D. History of infection control in anaesthesia. *Anaesth Intens Care* 1996;24:150–153.
25. Hilding AC, Hilding JA. Tolerance of the respiratory mucous membrane to trauma: surgical swabs and intratracheal tubes. *Ann Otol Rhinol Laryngol* 1962;71:455–479.
26. Way WL, Sooy FA. Histologic changes produced by endotracheal intubation. *Ann Otol Rhinol Laryngol* 1965;74:799–812.
27. Alexopoulos C, Jansson B, Lindholm CE. Mucus transport and surface damage after endotracheal intubation and tracheostomy. An experimental study in pigs. *Acta Anaesth Scand* 1984;28:68–76.
28. Klainer AS, Turndorf H, Wu WH, et al. Surface alterations due to endotracheal intubation. *Am J Med* 1975;58:674–683.
29. Schmidt WA, Schaap RN, Mortensen JD. Immediate mucosal effects of short-term, soft-cuff, endotracheal intubation. *Arch Pathol Lab Med* 1979;103:516–521.
30. Sanada Y, Kojima Y, Fonkalsrud EW. Injury of cilia induced by tracheal tube cuffs. *Surg Gynecol Obstet* 1982;154:648–652.
31. Stoelling RK. *Pharmacology and physiology in anesthetic practice.* Philadelphia: JB Lippincott, 1987.
32. Lichtiger M, Landa JF, Hirsch JA. Velocity of tracheal mucus in anesthetized women undergoing gynecologic surgery. *Anesthesiology* 1975;42:753–756.
33. Annis P, Landa J, Lichtiger M. Effects of atropine on velocity of tracheal mucus in anesthetized patients. *Anesthesiology* 1976;44: 74–77.
34. Burton JDK. Effects of dry anaesthetic gases on the respiratory mucous membrane. *Lancet* 1962;1:235–238.
35. Chalon J, Loew DAY, Malebranche J. Effects of dry anesthetic gases on tracheobronchial ciliated epithelium. *Anesthesiology* 1972;37: 338–343.
36. Forbes AR. Humidification and mucus flow in the intubated trachea. *Br J Anaesth* 1973;45:874–878.
37. Sackner MA, Landa J, Hirsch J, et al. Pulmonary effects of oxygen breathing. 6-hour study in normal men. *Ann Intern Med* 1975;82: 40–43.
38. Nair P, Jani K, Sanderson PJ. Transfer of oropharyngeal bacteria into the trachea during endotracheal intubation. *J Hosp Infect* 1986; 8:96–103.
39. Smith JR, Howland WS. Endotracheal tube as a source of infection. *JAMA* 1959;169:343–345.
40. Redman LR, Lockey E. Colonisation of the upper respiratory tract. *Anaesthesia* 1967;22:220–227.
41. Dominquez de Villota E, Avello F, Granados MA, et al. Early postsurgical bacterial contamination of the airways: a study on 28 open-heart patients. *Acta Anaesth Scand* 1978;22:227–233.
42. Berry FA, Blakenbaker WL, Ball CG. A comparison of bacteremia occurring with nasotracheal and orotracheal intubation. *Anesth Analg* 1973;52:873–876.
43. Berry FA, Yarbrough S, Yarbrough N, et al. Transient bacteremia during dental manipulation in children. *Pediatrics* 1973;51:476–479.
44. Joseph JM. Disease transmission by inefficiently sanitized anesthetizing apparatus. *JAMA* 1952;149:1196–1198.
45. Tinne JE, Gordon AM, Bain WH, et al. Cross-infection by *Pseudomonas aeruginosa* as a hazard of intensive surgery. *Br Med J* 1967;4: 313–315.
46. Olds JW, Kisch AL, Eberle BJ, et al. Pseudomonas aeruginosa respiratory tract infection acquired from a contaminated anesthesia machine. *Am Rev Respir Dis* 1972;105:628–632.
47. Albrecht WH, Dryden GE. Five-year experience with the develop-

ment of an individually clean anesthesia system. *Anesth Analg* 1974; 53:24–28.

48. Stratford BC, Clark RR, Dixson S. The disinfection of anaesthetic apparatus. *Br J Anaesth* 1964;36:471–476.
49. Beck A, Zadeh JA. Infection by anaesthetic apparatus [letter]. *Lancet* 1968;1:533–534.
50. Dryden GE. Risk of contamination from the anesthesia circle absorber: an evaluation. *Anesth Analg* 1969;48:939–943.
51. Meeks CH, Pembleton WE, Hench ME. Sterilization of anesthesia apparatus. *JAMA* 1967;199:276–278.
52. Livingstone H, Heidrick F, Holicky I, et al. Cross-infections from anesthetic face masks. *Surgery* 1941;9:433–435.
53. Hunt LM, Yagiela JA. Bacterial contamination and transmission by nitrous oxide sedation apparatus. *Oral Surg* 1977;44:367–373.
54. Yagiela JA, Hunt LM, Hunt DE. Disinfection of nitrous oxide equipment. *J Am Dent Assoc* 1979;98:191–195.
55. Russell EA, Gross A. Extent of bacterial contamination in nonrebreathing inhalation sedation machine. *Oral Surg* 1979;48:211–213.
56. Jenkins JRE, Edgar WM. Sterilisation of anaesthetic equipment. *Anaesthesia* 1964;19:177–190.
57. Murphy PM, Fitzgeorge RB, Barrett RF. Viability and distribution of bacteria after passage through a circle anaesthetic system. *Br J Anaesth* 1991;66:300–304.
58. Nielsen H, Vasegaard M, Stokke DB. Bacterial contamination of anaesthetic gases. *Br J Anaesth* 1978;50:811–814.
59. Rathgeber J, Kietzmann D, Mergeryan H, et al. Prevention of patient bacterial contamination of anaesthesia-circle-systems: a clinical study of the contamination risk and performance of different heat and moisture exchangers with Electret filter (HMEF). *Eur J Anaesthesiol* 1997; 14:368–373.
60. Chant K, Kociuba K, Crone S, et al. Investigation of possible patient-to-patient transmission of Hepatitis C in a hospital. *NSW Public Health Bull* 1994;5:47–51.
61. Knoblanche GK. Revision of the anaesthetic aspects of an infection control policy following reporting of hepatitis C nosocomial infection. *Anaesth Intensive Care* 1996;24:169–72.
62. Lloyd G, Howells J, Liddle C, et al. Barriers to hepatitis C transmission within breathing systems: efficacy of a pleated hydrophobic filter. *Anaesth Intens Care* 1997;25:235–238.
63. Wilkes AR, Benbough JE, Speight SE, et al. The bacterial and viral filtration performance of breathing system filters. *Anaesthesia* 2000; 55:458–465.
64. Wilkes AR. Measuring the filtration performance of breathing system filters using sodium chloride particles. *Anaesthesia* 2002;57:162–168.
65. Neft MW, Goodman JR, Hlavnicka JP, et al. To reuse your circuit: the HME debate. *AANA J* 1999;67:433–439.
66. Heaton J, Hall AP, Fell D. The use of filters in anaesthetic breathing systems [letter]. *Anaesthesia* 1998;53:407.
67. Atkinson MC, Girgis Y, Broome IJ. Extent and practicalities of filter use in anaesthetic breathing circuits and attitudes towards their use: a postal survey of UK hospitals. *Anaesthesia* 1999;54:37–41.
68. Daniel P, Fowler AJ. Breathing system filter use for infection control and humidification during anesthesia and mechanical ventilation. *Middle East J Anesthesiol* 2001;16:161–184.
69. DeOme KB. The effect of temperature, humidity, and glycol vapor on the viability of air-borne bacteria. *Am J Hyg* 1944;40:239–250.
70. du Moulin GC, Saubermann AJ. The anesthesia machine and circle system are not likely to be sources of contamination. *Anesthesiology* 1977;47:353–358.
71. du Moulin GC, Hedley-Whyte J. Bacterial interactions between anesthesiologists, their patients, and equipment. *Anesthesiology* 1982;57: 37–41.
72. Stemmerman MG, Stern A. Tubercle bacilli in the metabolic apparatus. *Am Rev Tuberc* 1946;53:264–266.
73. Ping FC, Oulton JL, Smith JA, et al. Bacterial filters—are they necessary on anaesthetic machines? *Can Anaesth Soc J* 1979;26:415–419.
74. Adriani J, Rovenstine EA. Experimental studies on carbon dioxide absorbers for anesthesia. *Anesthesiology* 1941;2:1–19.
75. Ziegler C, Jacoby J. Anesthetic equipment as a source of infection. *Curr Res Anesth Analg* 1956;35:451–459.
76. Pandit SK, Mehta S, Agarwal SC. Risk of cross-infection from inhalation anaesthetic equipment. *Br J Anaesth* 1967;39:838–844.
77. Ibrahim JJ, Perceval AK. Contamination of anaesthetic tubing—a real hazard? *Anaesth Intens Care* 1992;20:317–321.
78. Garibaldi RA, Britt MR, Webster C, et al. Failure of bacterial filters to reduce the incidence of pneumonia after inhalation anesthesia. *Anesthesiology* 1981;54:364–368.
79. Feeley TW, Hamilton WK, Xavier B, et al. Sterile anesthesia breathing circuits do not prevent postoperative pulmonary infection. *Anesthesiology* 1981;34:369–372.
80. Hess D. Filters and anesthesia breathing circuits: Can we cut costs without harm? *J Clin Anesth* 1999;11:531–533.
81. van Hassel S, Laveaux M, Leenders M, et al. Bacterial filters in anesthesia: results of 9 years of surveillance. *Infect Control Hosp Epidemiol* 1999;20:58–60.
82. Hogarth I. Anaesthetic machine and breathing system contamination and the efficacy of bacterial/viral filters. *Anaesth Intensive Care* 1996; 24:154–163.
83. Greene ES. Hepatitis C nosocomial infection. *Anaesth Intens Care* 1997;25:86–96.
84. Leijten DTM, Rejger VS, Mouton RP. Bacterial contamination and the effect of filters in anaesthetic circuits in a simulated patient model. *J Hosp Infect* 1992;21:51–60.
85. Berry AJ, Nolte FS. An alternative strategy for infection control of anesthesia breathing circuits: a laboratory assessment of the Pall HEM filter. *Anesth Analg* 1991;72:651–655.
86. Shiotani GM, Nicholes P, Ballinger CM, et al. Prevention of contamination of the circle system and ventilators with a new disposable filter. *Anesth Analg* 1971;50:844–855.
87. Tablan OC, Anderson LJ, Arden NH, et al. Guideline for prevention of nosocomial pneumonia. The Hospital Infection Control Practices Advisory Committee, Centers for Disease Control. *Infect Control Hosp Epidemiol* 1994;15:587–627.
88. North JB, Brophy BP. Epidural abscess: a hazard of spinal epidural anaesthesia. *Aust N Z J Surg* 1979;49:484–485.
89. Trautmann M, Lepper PM, Schmitz FJ. Three cases of bacterial meningitis after spinal and epidural anesthesia. *Eur J Clin Microbiol Infect Dis* 2002;21:43–45.
90. Schneeberger PM, Janssen M, Voss A. Alpha-hemolytic streptococci: a major pathogen of iatrogenic meningitis following lumbar puncture. Case reports and a review of the literature. *Infection* 1996;24:29–33.
91. Philips BJ, Fergusson S, Armstrong P, et al. Surgical face masks are effective in reducing bacterial contamination caused by dispersal from the upper airway. *Br J Anaesth* 1992;69:407–408.
92. Baker AS, Ojemann RG, Swartz MN, et al. Spinal epidural abscess. *N Engl J Med* 1975;293:463–468.
93. Loarie DJ, Fairley HB. Epidural abscess following spinal anesthesia. *Anesth Analg* 1978;57:351–353.
94. Berman RS, Eisele JH. Bacteremia, spinal anesthesia, and development of meningitis. *Anesthesiology* 1978;48:376–377. 95. Wulf H, Striepling E. Postmortem findings after epidural anaesthesia. *Anaesthesia* 1990;45:357–361.
96. Pinczower GR, Gyorke A. Vertebral osteomyelitis as a cause of back pain after epidural anesthesia. *Anesthesiology* 1996;84:215–217.
97. Bengtsson M, Nettelblad H, Sjoberg F. Extradural catheter-related infections in patients with infected cutaneous wounds. *Br J Anaesth* 1997;79:668–670.
98. Newman B. Extradural catheter-related infections in patients with infected cutaneous wounds. *Br J Anaesth* 1998;80:566.
99. Green BGJ, Pathy GV. Ensuring sterility of opioids for spinal administration [letter]. *Anaesthesia* 1999;54:511.
100. Raedler C, Lass-Florl C, Puhringer F, et al. Bacterial contamination of needles used for spinal and epidural anaesthesia. *Br J Anaesth* 1999; 83:657–658.
101. James FM, George RH, Naiem H, et al. Bacteriologic aspects of epidural analgesia. *Anesth Analg* 1976;55:187–190.
102. Shapiro JM, Bond EL, Garman JK. Use of a chlorhexidine dressing to reduce microbial colonization of epidural catheters. *Anesthesiology* 1990;73:625–631.

103. Barreto RS. Bacteriological culture of indwelling epidural catheters. *Anesthesiology* 1962;23:643–646.
104. Hunt JR, Rigor BM, Collins JR. The potential for contamination of continuous epidural catheters. *Anesth Analg* 1977;56:222–225.
105. Ross RM, Burday M, Baker T. Contamination of single dose of bupivacaine vials used repeatedly in the same patient. *Anesth Analg* 1992; 74:S257(abst).
106. Yaniv LG, Potasman I. Iatrogenic meningitis: An increasing role for resistant viridans streptococci? Case report and review of the last 20 years. *Scand J Infect Dis* 2000;32:693–696.
107. Dawson SJ. Epidural catheter infections. *J Hosp Infect* 2001;47:3–8.
108. Horlocker TT. Complications of spinal and epidural anesthesia. *Anesthesiol Clin North Am* 2000;18:461–485.
109. Danner RL, Hartman BJ. Update of spinal epidural abscess: 35 cases and review of the literature. *Rev Infect Dis* 1987;9:265–274.
110. Lund PC. *Peridural analgesia and anesthesia.* Springfield, IL: Charles C Thomas, 1966.
111. Dawkins CJM. An analysis of the complications of extradural and caudal block. *Anaesthesia* 1969;24:554–563.
112. Brooks K, Pasero C, Hubbard L, et al. The risk of infection associated with epidural analgesia. *Infect Control Hosp Epidemiol* 1995;16: 725–726.
113. Scott DB, Hibbard BM. Serious non-fatal complications associated with extradural block in obstetric practice. *Br J Anaesth* 1990;64: 537–541.
114. Palot M, Visseaux H, Botmans C, et al. Epidemiologie des complications de l'analgesie peridurale obstetricale. *Cah Anesthesiol* 1994;42: 229–233.
115. Eisen SM, Rosen N, Winesanker H, et al. The routine use of lumbar epidural anaesthesia in obstetrics: a clinical review of 9,532 cases. *Can Anaesth Soc J* 1960;7:280–289.
116. Holdcroft A, Morgan M. Maternal complications of obstetric epidural analgesia. *Anaesth Intens Care* 1976;4:108–112.
117. Abouleish E, Amortegui AJ, Taylor FH. Are bacterial filters needed in continuous epidural analgesia for obstetrics? *Anesthesiology* 1977; 46:351–354.
118. Sethna NF, Berde CB, Wilder RT, et al. The risk of infection from pediatric epidural analgesia is low. *Anesthesiology* 1992;77(3A): A1158(abst).
119. Abel MD, Horlocker TT, Messick JM, et al. Neurologic complications following placement of 4392 consecutive epidural catheters in anesthetized patients. *Reg Anesth Pain Med* 1998;23(suppl 3):3(abst).
120. Grass JA, Haider N, Group M, et al. Incidence of complications related to epidural catheterization and maintenance for postoperative analgesia. *Reg Anesth Pain Med* 1998;23:108(abst).
121. McNeely JK, Trentadue NC, Rusy LM, et al. Culture of bacteria from lumbar and caudal epidural catheters used for postoperative analgesia in children. *Reg Anesth* 1997;22:428–31.
122. Phillips JMG, Stedeford JC, Hartsilver E, et al. Epidural abscess complicating insertion of epidural catheters. *Br J Anaesth* 2002;89: 778–782.
123. Kost-Byerly S, Tobin JR, Greenberg RS, et al. Bacterial colonization and infection rate of continuous epidural catheters in children. *Anesth Analg* 1998;86:712–716.
124. Stafford MA, Wilder RT, Berde CB. The risk of infection from epidural analgesia in children: a review of 1620 cases. *Anesth Analg* 1995; 80:234–238.
125. Holt HM, Andersen SS, Andersen O, et al. Infections following epidural catheterization. *J Hosp Infect* 1995;30:253–260.
126. Holt HM, Gahrn-Hansen B, Andersen SS, et al. Infections following epidural catheters [letter]. *J Hosp Infect* 1997;35:245.
127. Darchy B, Forceville X, Bavoux E, et al. Clinical and bacteriologic survey of epidural analgesia in patients in the intensive care unit. *Anesthesiology* 1996;85:988–998.
128. Du Pen SL, Peterson DG, Williams A, et al. Infection during chronic epidural catheterization: diagnosis and treatment. *Anesthesiology* 1990; 73:905–909.
129. Zenz M, Piepenbrock S, Tryba M. Epidural opiates: long-term experiences in cancer pain. *Klin Wochenschr* 1985;63:225–229.
130. Coombs DW. Management of chronic pain by epidural and intrathecal opioids: newer drugs and delivery systems. *Int Anesth Clin* 1986; 24:59–74.
131. Edwards WB, Hingson RA. The present status of continuous caudal analgesia in obstetrics. *N Y Acad Med Bull* 1943;19:507–518.
132. Ferguson JF, Kirsch WM. Epidural empyema following thoracic extradural block. Case report. *J Neurosurg* 1974;41:762–764.
133. Saady A. Epidural abscess complicating thoracic epidural analgesia. *Anesthesiology* 1976;44:244–246.
134. Dougherty JH, Fraser RAR. Complications following intraspinal injections of steroids. Report of two cases. *J Neurosurg* 1978;48: 1023–1025.
135. Wenningsted-Torgard K, Heyn J, Willumsen L. Spondylitis following epidural morphine. *Acta Anaesth Scand* 1982;26:649–651.
136. McDonogh AJ, Cranney BS. Delayed presentation of an epidural abscess. *Anaesth Intens Care* 1984;12:364–365.
137. Konig HJ, Schleep J, Krahling KH. Ein fall von querschnitt syndrom nach kontamination eines periduralkatheters. *Reg Anaesth* 1985;8: 60–62.
138. Sollman W-P, Gaab MR, Panning B. Lumbales epidurales hamatom und spinaler abszess nach periduralanaesthesie. *Reg Anaesth* 1987;10: 121–124.
139. Fine PG, Hare BD, Zahniser JC. Epidural abscess following epidural catheterization in a chronic pain patient: a diagnostic dilemma. *Anesthesiology* 1988;69:422–424.
140. Ready LB, Helfer D. Bacterial meningitis in parturients after epidural anesthesia. *Anesthesiology* 1989;71:988–990.
141. Berga S, Trierweiler MW. Bacterial meningitis following epidural anesthesia for vaginal delivery: a case report. *Obstet Gynecol* 1989;74: 437–9.
142. Chan S-T, Leung S. Spinal epidura abscess following steroid injection for sciatica. Illustrated by two case reports. *Spine* 1989;14:106–108.
143. Goucke CR, Graziotti P. Extradural abscess following local anaesthetic and steroid injection for chronic low back pain. *Br J Anaesth* 1990; 65:427–429.
144. Lynch J, Zech D. Spondylitis without epidural abscess formation following short-term use of an epidural catheter. *Acta Anaesthesiol Scand* 1990;34:167–170.
145. Waldman SD. Cervical epidural abscess after cervical epidural nerve block with steroids [letter]. *Anesth Analg* 1991;72:717–718.
146. Strong WE. Epidural abscess associated with epidural catheterization: a rare event? Report of two cases with markedly delayed presentation. *Anesthesiology* 1991;74:943–946.
147. Klygis LM, Reisberg BE. Spinal epidural abscess caused by group G streptococci. *Am J Med* 1991;91:89–90.
148. Dawson P, Rosenfeld JV, Murphy MA, et al. Epidural abscess associated with postoperative epidural analgesia. *Anesth Intens Care* 1991; 19:569–591.
149. Ferguson CC. Infection and the epidural space: a case report. *AANA J* 1992;60:393–396.
150. NganKee WD, Jones MR, Thomas P, et al. Epidural abscess complicating extradural anaesthesia for caesarean section. *Br J Anaesth* 1992; 69:647–652.
151. Sowter MC, Burgess NA, Woodsford PV, et al. Delayed presentation of an extradural abscess complicating thoracic extradural analgesia. *Br J Anaesth* 1992;68:103–105.
152. Shintani S, Tanaka H, Irifune A, et al. Iatrogenic acute spinal epidural abscess with septic meningitis: MR findings. *Clin Neurol Neurosurg* 1992;94:253–255.
153. Nordstrom O, Sandin R. Delayed presentation of an extradural abscess in a patient with alcohol abuse. *Br J Anaesth* 1993;70:368–369.
154. Davis L, Hargreaves C, Robinson PN. Postpartum meningitis. *Anaesthesia* 1993;48:788–789.
155. Ania BJ. *Staphylococus aureus* meningitis after short-term epidural analgesia. *Clin Infect Dis* 1994;18:844–845.
156. Borum SE, McLeskey CH, Williamson JB, et al. Epidural abscess after obstetric epidural analgesia. *Anesthesiology* 1995;82:1523–1526.
157. Liu SS. Pope A. Spinal meningitis masquerading as postdural puncture headache [letter]. *Anesthesiology* 1996;85:1493–1494.
158. Dunn LT, Javed A, Findlay G, et al. Iatrogenic spinal infection following epidural anaesthesia: case report. *Eur Spine J* 1996;5:418–420.

159. Cooper AB, Sharpe MD. Bacterial meningitis and cauda equina syndrome after epidural steroid injections. *Can J Anaesth* 1996;43:471.
160. Barontini F, Conti P, Marello G, et al. Major neurological sequelae of lumbar epidural anesthesia. Report of three cases. *Ital J Neurol Sci* 1996;17:333–339.
161. Sarrubi FA, Vasquez JE. Spinal epidural abscess associated with the use of temporary epidural catheters: report of two cases and review. *Clin Infect Dis* 1997:25:1155–1158.
162. Iseki M, Okuno S, Tanabe Y, et al. Methicillin-resistant Staphylococcus aureus sepsis resulting from infection in paravertebral muscle after continuous epidural infusion for pain control in a patient with herpes zoster. *Anesth Analg* 1998;87:116–118.
163. O'Brien DPK, Rawluk DJR. Iatrogenic *Mycobacterium* infection after an epidural injection. *Spine* 1999;24:1257–1259.
164. Halkic N, Blanc C, Corthesy ME, et al. Lumbar spondylodiscitis after epidural anaesthesia at a distant site [Letter]. *Anaesthesia* 2001;56: 602–603.
165. Lund PC. *Principles and practice of spinal anesthesia.* Springfield, IL: Charles C Thomas, 1971:623.
166. Horlocker TT, McGregor DG, Matsushige DK, et al. A retrospective review of 4767 consecutive spinal anesthetics: central nervous system complications. Perioperative Outcomes Group. *Anesth Analg.* 1997; 84:578–584.
167. Evans FT. Sepsis and asepsis in spinal analgesia. *Proc R Soc Med* 1945; 39:181–185.
168. Scarborough RA. Spinal anesthesia from the surgeon's standpoint. *JAMA* 1958;168:1324–1326.
169. Dripps RD, Vandam LD. Long-term follow-up of patients who received 10,098 spinal anesthetics. *JAMA* 1954;156:1486–1491.
170. Moore DC, Bridenbaugh LD. Spinal (subarachnoid) block. *JAMA* 1966;195:907–912.
171. Lund PC, Cwik JC. Modern trends in spinal anaesthesia. *Can Anaesth Soc J* 1968;15:118–134.
172. Sadove MS, Levin MJ, Rant-Sejdinaj I. Neurological complications of spinal anaesthesia. *Can Anaesth Soc J* 1961;8:405–416.
173. Arner O. Complications following spinal anesthesia. Their significance and a technique to reduce their incidence. *Acta Chir Scand* 1952;104:336–338.
174. Kilpatrick ME, Girgis NI. Meningitis—a complication of spinal anesthesia. *Anesth Analg* 1983;62:513–515.
175. Corbett JJ, Rosenstein BJ. Pseudomonas meningitis related to spinal anesthesia. Report of three cases with a common source. *Neurology* 1971;21:946–950.
176. Siegel RS, Alicandri FP, Jacoby AW. Subgluteal infection following regional anesthesia [letter]. *JAMA* 1974;229:268.
177. Beaudoin MG, Klein L. Epidural abscess following multiple spinal anaesthetics. *Anaesth Intens Care* 1984;12:163–164.
178. Abdel-Magid RA, Kotb HI. Epidural abscess after spinal anesthesia: a favorable outcome. *Neurosurgery* 1990;27:310–311.
179. Roberts SP, Petts HV. Meningitis after obstetric spinal anaesthesia. *Anaesthesia* 1990;45:376–377.
180. Lee JJ, Parry H. Bacterial meningitis following spinal anaesthesia for caesarean section. *Br J Anaesth* 1991;66:383–386.
181. Blackmore TK, Morley HR, Gordon DL. *Streptococcus mitis*-induced bacteremia and meningitis after spinal anesthesia. *Anesthesiology* 1993; 78:592–594.
182. Ezri T, Szmuk P, Guy M. Delayed-onset meningitis after spinal anesthesia [letter]. *Anesth Analg* 1994;79:606–607.
183. Mahendru V. Bacon DR, Lema MJ. Multiple epidural abscesses and spinal anesthesia in a diabetic patient. Case report. *Reg Anesth* 1994; 19:66–68.
184. Gebhard JS, Brugman JL. Percutaneous discectomy for the treatment of bacterial discitis. *Spine* 1994;19:855–857.
185. Newton JA Jr, Lesnik IK, Kennedy CA. *Streptococcus salivarius* meningitis following spinal anesthesia [letter]. *Clin Infect Dis* 1994;18: 840–841.
186. Kaiser E, Suppini A, de Jaureguiberry JP, et al. Meningite aigue a *Streptococcus salivarius* après rachianesthesie. *Ann Fr Anesth Reanim* 1997;16:47–49.
187. Fernandez R, Paz I, Pazos C, et al. Meningitis producida por *Streptococcus mitis* tras anestesia intradural [letter]. *Enferm Infecc Microbiol Clin* 1999;17:150.
188. Cascio M, Heath G. Meningitis following a combined spinal-epidural technique in a labouring term parturient. *Can J Anaesth* 1996;43: 399–402.
189. Harding SA, Collis RE, Morgan BM. Meningitis after combined spinal-extradural anaesthesia in obstetrics. *Br J Anaesth* 1994;73: 545–547.
190. Stallard N, Barry P. Another complication of the combined extradural-subarachnoid technique [letter]. *Br J Anaesth* 1995;75: 370–371.
191. Aldebert S, Sleth JC. Meningite bacterienne après anesthesia rachidienne et peridurale combinee en obstetrique. *Ann Fr Anesth Reanim* 1996;15:687–688.
192. Dysart RH, Balakrishnan V. Conservative management of extradural abscess complicating spinal-extradural anaesthesia for caesarean section. *Br J Anaesth* 1997;78:591–593.
193. Schroter J, Wa Djamba D, Hoffmann V, et al. Epidural abscess after combined spinal-epidural block. *Can J Anaesth* 1997;44:300–304.
194. Bouhemad B, Dounas M, Mercier FJ, et al. Bacterial meningitis following combined spinal-epidural analgesia for labour. *Anaesthesia* 1998;53:290–295.
195. Peng PW, Chan VW. Local and regional block in postoperative pain control. *Surg Clin North Am* 1999;79:345–370.
196. Graf BM, Martin E. [Peripheral nerve block. An overview of new developments in an old technique.] *Anaesthesist* 2001;50:312–322.
197. Bergman BD, Hebl JR, Kent J, et al. Neurologic complications of 405 consecutive continuous axillary catheters. *Anesth Analg* 2003;96: 247–252.
198. Meier G, Bauereis C, Heinrich C. [Interscalene brachial plexus catheter for anesthesia and postoperative pain therapy. Experience with a modified technique.] *Anaesthesist* 1997;46:715–719.
199. Cuvillon P, Ripart J, Lalourcey L, et al. The continuous femoral nerve block catheter for postoperative analgesia: bacterial colonization, infectious rate and adverse effects. *Anesth Analg* 2001;93:1045–1049.
200. Boezaart AP, de Beer JF, du Toit C, et al. A new technique of continuous interscalene nerve block. *Can J Anaesth* 1999;46:275–281.
201. Centers for Disease Control and Prevention. Guidelines for the prevention of intravascular catheter-related infections. *MMWR* 2002; 51(RR-10):1–36.
202. Wildsmith JA. Regional anaesthesia requires attention to detail [letter]. *Br J Anaesth* 1991;67:224–225.
203. Yentis SM. Wearing of face masks for spinal anaesthesia [letter]. *Br J Anaesth* 1992;68:224.
204. Wildsmith JA. Wearing of face masks for spinal anaesthesia [letter]. *Br J Anaesth* 1992;68:224.
205. O'Kelly SW, Marsh D. Face masks and spinal anaesthesia [letter]. *Br J Anaesth* 1993;70:239.
206. Wildsmith JA. Face masks and spinal anaesthesia [letter]. *Br J Anaesth* 1993;70:239.
207. Bromage PR. Postpartum meningitis [letter]. *Anaesthesia* 1994;49: 260.
208. Smedstad KG. Infection after central neuraxial block [editorial]. *Can J Anaesth* 1997;44:235–238.
209. Panikkar KK, Yentis SM. Wearing of masks for obstetric regional anaesthesia. A postal survey. *Anaesthesia* 1996;51:398–400.
210. O'Higgins F, Tuckey JP. Thoracic epidural anaesthesia and analgesia: United Kingdom practice. *Acta Anaesthesiol Scand* 2000;44: 1087–1092.
211. Sleth JC. Evaluation des mesures d'asepsie lors de la realisation d'un catheterisme epidural et perception de son risqué infectieux. Resultats d'une enquete en Languedoc-Roussillon. *Ann Fr Anesth Reanim* 1998; 17:408–414.
212. Dolinski SY, Gerancher JC. Unmasked mischief [letter]. *Anesth Analg* 2001;92:280–281.
213. Raad II, Hohn DC, Gilbreath BJ, et al. Prevention of central venous catheter-related infections by using maximal sterile barrier precautions during insertion. *Infect Control Hosp Epidemiol* 1994;15:231–238.
214. Dawson SJ, Small H, Logan MN, et al. Case control study of epidural

catheter infections in a district general hospital. *Commun Dis Public Health* 2000;3:300–302.

215. Adam MN, Dinulescu T, Mathieu P, et al. Comparaison de l'efficacite de deux antiseptiques dans la prevention de l'infection liee aux catheters periduraux. *Cah Anesthesiol* 1996;44:465–467.
216. Kasuda H, Fukuda H, Togashi H, et al. Skin disinfection before epidural catheterization: comparative study of povidone-iodine versus chlorhexidine ethanol. *Dermatology* 2002;204(suppl 1):42–46.
217. Kinirons B, Mimoz O, Lafendi L, et al. Chlorhexidine versus povidone iodine in preventing colonization of continuous epidural catheters in children. *Anesthesiology* 2001;94:239–244.
218. Sato S, Sakuragi T, Dan K. Human skin flora as a potential source of epidural abscess. *Anesthesiology* 1996;85:1276–1282.
219. Pegues DA, Carr DB, Hopkins CC. Infectious complications associated with temporary epidural catheters. *Clin Infect Dis* 1994;19: 970–972.
220. Blogg CE, Ramsay MAE, Jarvis JD. Infection hazard from syringes. *Br J Anaesth* 1974;46:260–262.
221. Lessard MR, Trepanier CA, Gourdeau M, et al. A microbiological study of the contamination of the syringes used in anaesthesia practice. *Can J Anaesth* 1988;35:567–569.
222. Lutz CT, Bell CE, Wedner HJ, et al. Allergy testing of multiple patients should no longer be performed with a common syringe. *N Engl J Med* 1984;310:1335–1337.
223. Koepke JW, Selner JC. Allergy testing of multiple patients with a common syringe [letter]. *N Engl J Med* 1984;311:1188–1189.
224. Shulan DJ, Weiler JM, Koontz F, et al. Contamination of intradermal skin test syringes. *J Allergy Clin Immunol* 1985;76:226–227.
225. Koepke JW, Reller LB, Masters HA, et al. Viral contamination of intradermal skin test syringes. *Ann Allergy* 1985;55:776–778.
226. Plott RT, Wagner RF, Tyring SK. Iatrogenic contamination of multidose vials in simulated use. A reassessment of current patient injection technique. *Arch Dermatol* 1990;126:1441–1444.
227. Fleming A, Ogilvie AC. Syringe needles and mass inoculation technique. *Br Med J* 1951;1:543–546.
228. Hughes RR. Post-penicillin jaundice. *Br Med J* 1946;2:685–688.
229. Uren R, Commens C, Howman-Giles R. Intradermal injections: a potential health hazard? [letter]. *Med J Aust* 1994;161:226.
230. Barker LF, Maynard JE, Purcell RH, et al. Hepatitis B virus infection in chimpanzees: titration of subtypes. *J Infect Dis* 1975;132:451–458.
231. Hein HAT, Reinhart RD, Wansbrough SR, et al. Recapping needles in anesthesia—is it safe? *Anesthesiology* 1987;67:A161(abst).
232. Trepanier CA, Lessard MR, Brochu JG, et al. Risk of cross-infection related to the multiple use of disposable syringes. *Can J Anaesth* 1990; 37:156–159.
233. Parlow JL. Blood contamination of drug syringes used in anesthesia. *Can J Anaesth* 1989;36:S61–S62(abst).
234. Abulrahi HA, Bohlega EA, Fontaine RE, et al. Plasmodium falciparum malaria transmitted in hospital through heparin locks. *Lancet* 1997;349:23–25.
235. Kempen PM, Learned DW. Anesthesia practice—a vector of infection? *Anesthesiology* 1989;71:A948(abst).
236. Kempen PM. Contamination of syringes [letter]. *Can J Anaesth* 1989; 36:730–731.
237. Zacher AN, Zornow MH, Evans G. Drug contamination from opening glass ampules. *Anesthesiology* 1991;75:893–895.
238. Corley CE, Manos JP, Thomas JD. Multiple dose vials: a source of contamination? *J S C Med Assoc* 1968;64:461–464.
239. Highsmith AK, Greenhood GP, Allen JR. Growth of nosocomial pathogens in multiple-dose parenteral medication vials. *J Clin Microbiol* 1982;15:1024–1028.
240. Bawden JC, Jacobson JA, Jackson JC, et al. Sterility and use patterns of multiple-dose vials. *Am J Hosp Pharm* 1982;39:294–297.
241. Longfield RN, Smith LP, Longfield JN, et al. Multiple-dose vials: persistence of bacterial contaminants and infection control implications. *Infect Control* 1985;6:194–199.
242. Petty WC, Heggers JP, Shelton DF, et al. Viral and bacterial contamination of multiple-dose drug vials kept in anesthesia machines. *Anesthesiology* 1969;30:465–468.
243. Kohan S, Carlin H, Whitehead R. A study of contamination of multiple-dose medication vials. *Hospitals* 1962;36:78,80,82.
244. Rosenzweig AL. Potential health hazards in the multiple-dose vial. *Hospitals* 1964;38:70,72,74.
245. Melnyk PS, Shevchuk YM, Conly JM, et al. Contamination study of multiple-dose vials. *Ann Pharmacother* 1993;27:274–277.
246. Longfield R, Longfield J, Smith LP, et al. Multidose medication vial sterility: an in-use study and a review of the literature. *Infect Control 1984;5:165–169.*
247. Schubert A, Hyams KC, Longfield RN. Sterility of multiple-dose vials after opening. *Anesthesiology* 1985;62:634–636.
248. Young JA, Collette TS, Brehm WF. Sterility of multiple dose vials after repeated use. *Am Surg* 1958;24:811–814.
249. de Silva MI, Hood E, Tisdel E, et al. Multidosage medication vials: a study of sterility, use patterns, and cost-effectiveness. *Am J Infect Control 1986;14:135–138.*
250. Thompson DF, Letassy NA, Gee M, et al. Contamination risks of multidose medication vials: a review. *J Pharm Technol* 1989;5: 249–253.
251. Arrington ME, Gabbert KC, Mazgaj PW, et al. Multidose vial contamination in anesthesia. *AANA J* 1990;58:462–466.
252. Sack RA. Epidemic of gram-negative organism septicemia subsequent to elective operation. *Am J Obstet Gynecol* 1970;107:394–399.
253. Siboni K, Olsen H, Ravn E, et al. Pseudomonas cepacia in 16 nonfatal cases of postoperative bacteremia derived from intrinsic contamination of the anaesthetic fentanyl. *Scand J Infect Dis* 1979;11:39–45.
254. Borghans JGA, Hosli M, Olsen H, et al. *Pseudomonas cepacia* bacteraemia due to intrinsic contamination of an anaesthetic. *Acta Pathol Microbiol Scand* 1979;87:15–20.
255. Maldonado YA, Roesch K, Deresinski SC, et al. Nosocomial hepatitis B outbreak associated with a seronegative health care worker. *Am J Infect Control 1989;17:99(abst).*
256. Centers for Disease Control. Postsurgical infections associated with an extrinsically contaminated intravenous anesthetic agent—California, Illinois, Maine, and Michigan, 1990. *MMWR* 1990;39:426–427,433.
257. Daily MJ, Dickey JB, Packo KH. Endogenous *Candida* endophthalmitis after intravenous anesthesia with propofol. *Arch Ophthalmol* 1991;109:1081–1084.
258. Villarino ME, McNeill MM, Hall WN, et al. Postsurgical infections associated with an extrinsically contaminated intravenous anesthetic agent. Program and Abstracts of the 31st Interscience Conference on Antimicrobial Agents and Chemotherapy, Chicago, September 29–October 2, 1991;156:346.
259. Maki DG, Klein BS, McCormick RD, et al. Nosocomial *Pseudomonas pickettii* bacteremias traced to narcotic tampering. *JAMA* 1991;265: 981–986.
260. Froggatt JW, Dwyer DM, Stephens MA. Hospital outbreak of hepatitis B in patients undergoing electroconvulsive therapy. Program and Abstracts of the 31st Interscience Conference on Antimicrobial Agents and Chemotherapy, Chicago, September 29–October 2, 1991;157: 347.
261. Rudnick JR, Beck-Sague C, Anderson R, et al. Gram-negative bacteremia in open-heart-surgery patients traced to probable tap-water contamination of pressure-monitoring equipment. *Infect Control Hosp Epidemiol* 1996;17:281–285.
262. Veber B, Gachot B, Bedos JP, et al. Severe sepsis after intravenous injection of contaminated propofol [letter]. *Anesthesiology* 1994;80: 712–713.
263. Kuehnert MJ, Webb RM, Jochimsen EM, et al. *Staphylococcus aureus* bloodstream infections among patients undergoing electroconvulsive therapy traced to breaks in infection control and possible extrinsic contamination by propofol. *Anesth Analg* 1997;85:420–425.
264. Kidd-Ljunggren K, Broman E, Ekvall H, et al. Nosocomial transmission of hepatitis B virus infection through multiple-dose vials. *J Hosp Infect* 1999;43:57–62.
265. Henry B, Plante-Jenkins C, Ostrowska K. An outbreak of *Serratia marcescens* associated with the anesthetic agent propofol. *Am J Infect Control 2001;29:312–315.*
266. Massari M, Petrosillo N, Ippolito G, et al. Transmission of hepatitis

C virus in a gynecological surgery setting. *J Clin Microbiol* 2001;39: 2860–2863.
267. Meier B. Reuse of needle at hospital infects 50 with hepatitis C. *New York Times* 2002 Oct 10:
268. Anonymous. Poor injection safety practices are behind spread of nosocomial hepatitis C. *ICP Rep* 2002:84–86.
269. Carbonne A, Thiers V, Germain JM, et al. Patient-to-patient transmission of hepatitis C in a surgery clinic through multi-dose vials (abstract 236). Presented at the 13th annual meeting of the Society for Healthcare Epidemiology of America, April 5–8, 2003, Arlington, Virginia.
270. Bennett SN, McNeil MM, Bland LA, et al. Postoperative infections traced to contamination of an intravenous anesthetic, propofol. *N Engl J Med* 1995;333:147–154.
271. Schmidt RM, Rosenkranz HS. Antimicrobial activity of local anesthetics: lidocaine and procaine. *J Infect Dis* 1970;121:597–607.
272. Berry CB, Gillespie T, Hood J, et al. Growth of micro-organisms in solutions of intravenous anaesthetic agents. *Anaesthesia* 1993;48: 30–32.
273. Sosis M, Braverman B. Growth of *Staphylococcus aureus* in four intravenous anesthetics. *Anesth Analg* 1993;77:766–768.
274. Arduino MJ, Bland LA, McAllister SK, et al. Microbial growth and endotoxin production in the intravenous anesthetic propofol. *Infect Control Hosp Epidemiol* 1991;12:535–539.
275. McLeod GA, Pace N, Inglis MD. Bacterial growth in propofol [letter]. *Br J Anaesth* 1991;67:665–666.
276. Thomas DV. Propofol supports bacterial growth [letter]. *Br J Anaesth* 1991;66:274.
277. Kirk GA, Koontz FP, Chavez AJ. Lidocaine inhibits growth of *Staphylococcus aureus* in propofol. *Anesthesiology* 1992;77:A407(abst).
278. Tessler M, Dascal A, Gioseffini S, et al. Growth curves of *Staphylococcus aureus, Candida albicans,* and *Moraxella osloensis* in propofol and other media. *Can J Anaesth* 1992;39:509–511.
279. Sosis MB, Braverman B, Villaflor E. Propofol, but not thiopental, supports the growth of *Candida albicans. Anesth Analg* 1995;81: 132–134.
280. Patterson JS, Hopkins KJ, Albanese R. Propofol handling techniques [letter]. *Acta Anaesthesiol Scand* 1991;35:370.
281. Patterson JS, Hopkins KJ, Albanese R. Preparation and use of propofol [letter]. *Anaesthesia* 1990;45:1002.
282. Seeberger MD, Staender S, Oertli D, et al. Efficacy of specific aseptic precautions for preventing propofol-related infections: analysis by a quality-assurance programme using the explicit outcome method. *J Hosp Infect* 1998;39:67–70.
283. Walter CW. The infector on the surgical team. *Clin Neurosurg* 1966; 14:361–379.
284. Payne RW. Severe outbreak of surgical sepsis due to *Staphylococcus aureus* of unusual type and origin. *Br Med J* 1967;4:17–20.
285. Jewett JF, Reid DE, Safon LE, et al. Childbed fever—a continuing entity. *JAMA* 1968;206:344–350.
286. Schaffner W, Lefkowitz LB, Goodman JS, et al. Hospital outbreak of infections with group A streptococci traced to an asymptomatic anal carrier. *N Engl J Med* 1969;280:1224–1227.
287. Gryska PF, O'Dea AE. Postoperative streptococcal wound infection. *JAMA* 1970;213:1189–1191.
288. Centers for Disease Control. Hospital outbreak of streptococcal wound infection—Utah. *MMWR* 1976;25:141.
289. Paul SM, Genese C, Spitalny K. Postoperative group A β-hemolytic streptococcus outbreak with the pathogen traced to a member of a healthcare worker's household. *Infect Control Hosp Epidemiol* 1990; 11:643–646.
290. Mastro TD, Farley TA, Elliott JA, et al. An outbreak of surgical-wound infections due to group A streptococcus carried on the scalp. *N Engl J Med* 1990;323:968–972.
291. Bosch X. Hepatitis C outbreak astounds Spain. *Lancet* 1998;351: 1415.
292. Bosch X. Newspaper apportions blame in Spanish hepatitis C scandal. *Lancet* 2000;355:818.
293. Ross RS, Viazov S, Gross T, et al. Transmission of hepatitis C virus from a patient to an anesthesiology assistant to five patients. *N Engl J Med* 2000;343:1851–1854.
294. Cody SH, Nainan OV, Garfein RS, et al. Hepatitis C virus transmission from an anesthesiologist to a patient. *Arch Intern Med* 2002;162: 345–350.
295. Asai T, Matsumoto S, Shingu K. Incidence of blood-borne infectious micro-organisms: would you still not wear gloves? [letter]. *Anaesthesia* 2000;55:591–592.
296. White MC, Lynch P. Blood contact and exposures among operating room personnel: a multicenter study. *Am J Infect Control 1993;21: 243–248.*
297. Panlilio AL, Foy DR, Edwards JR, et al. Blood contacts during surgical procedures. *JAMA* 1991;265:1533–1537.
298. Popejoy SL, Fry DE. Blood contact and exposure in the operating room. *Surg Gynecol Obstet* 1991;172:480–483.
299. Harrison CA, Roger DW, Rosen M. Blood contamination of anaesthetic and related staff. *Anaesthesia* 1990;45:831–833.
300. Maz S, Lyons G. Needlestick injuries in anaesthetists. *Anaesthesia* 1990;45:677–678.
301. Jagger J, Bentley M, Tereskerz P. A study of patterns and prevention of blood exposures in OR personnel. *AORN J* 1998;67:1979–1996.
302. Heald AE, Ransohoff DF. Needlestick injuries among resident physicians. *J Gen Intern Med* 1990;5:389–393.
303. Greene ES, Berry AJ, Arnold WP, et al. Percutaneous injuries in anesthesia personnel. *Anesth Analg* 1996;83:273–278.
304. Greene ES, Berry AJ, Jagger J, et al. Multicenter study of contaminated percutaneous injuries in anesthesia personnel. *Anesthesiology* 1998;89:1362–1372.
305. Patel N, Tignor GH. Device-specific sharps injury and usage rates: an analysis by hospital department. *Am J Infect Control 1997;25:77–84.*
306. Kristensen MS, Wernberg NM, Anker-Moller E. Healthcare workers' risk of contact with body fluids in a hospital: the effect of complying with the universal precautions policy. *Infect Control Hosp Epidemiol* 1992;13:719–724.
307. Kristensen MS, Sloth E, Jensen TKO. Relationship between anesthetic procedure and contact of anesthesia personnel with patient body fluids. *Anesthesiology* 1990;73:619–624.
308. Chrisco JA, DeVane G. A descriptive study of blood in the mouth following routine oral endotracheal intubation. *AANA J* 1992;60: 379–383.
309. Brimacombe JR, Brimacombe JC, Berry AM, et al. A comparison of the laryngeal mask airway and cuffed oropharyngeal airway in anesthetized adult patients. *Anesth Analg* 1998;87:147–152.
310. Parker MRJ, Day CJE. Visible and occult blood contamination of laryngeal mask airways and tracheal tubes used in adult anaesthesia. *Anaesthesia* 2000;55:367–390.
311. Merritt WT, Zuckerberg AL. Contamination of the anesthetic record. *Anesthesiology* 1992;77(3A):A1102(abst).
312. Arkoff H, Ortega RA. Touchscreen technology: potential source of cross-infections [letter]. *Anesth Analg* 1992;75:1073.
313. Hall JR. Blood contamination of anesthesia equipment and monitoring equipment. *Anesth Analg* 1994;78:1136–1139.
314. Perry SM, Monaghan WP. The prevalence of visible and/or occult blood on anesthesia and monitoring equipment. *AANA J* 2001;69: 44–48.
315. Siebke JC, Degre M. Prevalence of viral hepatitis in the staff in Norwegian anaesthesiology units. *Acta Anaesthesiol Scand* 1984;28: 549–553.
316. Malm DN, Mathias RG, Turnbull GW, et al. Prevalence of hepatitis B in anaesthesia personnel. *Can Anaesth Soc J* 1986;33:167–172.
317. Berry AJ, Isaacson IJ, Hunt D, et al. The prevalence of hepatitis B viral markers in anesthesia personnel. *Anesthesiology* 1984;60:6–9.
318. Berry AJ, Isaacson IJ, Kane MA, et al. A multicenter study of the prevalence of hepatitis B viral serologic markers in anesthesia personnel. *Anesth Analg* 1984;63:738–742.
319. Berry AJ, Isaacson IJ, Kane MA, et al. A multicenter study of the epidemiology of hepatitis B in anesthesia residents. *Anesth Analg* 1985; 64:672–676.
320. Fyman PN, Hartung J, Weinberg S, et al. Prevalence of hepatitis B

markers in the anesthesia staff of a large inner-city hospital. *Anesth Analg* 1984;63:433–436.
321. Denes AE, Smith JL, Maynard JE, et al. Hepatitis B infection in physicians. Results of a nationwide seroepidemiologic survey. *JAMA* 1978;239:210–212.
322. Janzen J, Tripatzis I, Wagner U, et al. Epidemiology of hepatitis B surface antigen (HBsAg) and antibody to HBsAg in hospital personnel. *J Infect Dis* 1978;137:261–265.
323. Smith JL, Maynard JE, Berquist KR, et al. Comparative risk of hepatitis B among physicians and dentists. *J Infect Dis* 1976;133:705–706.
324. McQuillan GM, Townsend TR, Fields HA, et al. Seroepidemiology of Hepatitis B virus infection in the United States. *Am J Med* 1989; 87(suppl 3A):5S–10S.
325. Moss ALH. Hospital outbreak of hepatitis B [letter]. *N Z Med J* 1981; 94:65–66.
326. Shanson DC. Hepatitis B outbreak in operating-theatre and intensive care staff [letter]. *Lancet* 1980;2:596.
327. Bakir L, Ayed MB, Chourou O, et al. Hepatitis C virus and professional risk in anesthesia and intensive care: a case report [letter]. *Infect Control Hosp Epidemiol* 1998;19:823.
328. Busby J. Through the valley of many shadows. HIV infected physicians. *Tex Med* 1991;87:36–46.
329. Buergler JM, Kim R, Thisted RA, et al. Risk of human immunodeficiency virus in surgeons, anesthesiologists, and medical students. *Anesth Analg* 1992;75:118–124.
330. Berry AJ. Calculated risk of human immunodeficiency virus infection in anesthesiologists [letter]. *Anesth Analg* 1993;76:912.
331. Green ES. Risk of HIV infection. [letter]. *Anesth Analg* 1993;76:913.
332. Blackwelder WC, Dolin R, Mittal KK, et al. A population study of herpes virus infections and HLA antigens. *Am J Epidemiol* 1982;115: 569–576.
333. Wentworth BB, Alexander ER. Seroepidemiology of infections due to members of the herpesvirus group. *Am J Epidemiol* 1971;94: 496–507.
334. Lindgren KM, Douglas RG, Couch RB. Significance of Herpesvirus hominis in respiratory secretions of man. *N Engl J Med* 1968;278: 517–523.
335. Douglas RG, Couch RB. A prospective study of chronic Herpes simplex virus infection and recurrent Herpes labialis in humans. *J Immunol* 1970;104:289–295.
336. Cesario TC, Poland JD, Wulff H, et al. Six years experience with Herpes simplex virus in a children's home. *Am J Epidemiol* 1969;90: 416–422.
337. Klotz RW. Herpetic whitlow: an occupational hazard. *AANA J* 1990; 58:8–13.
338. DeYoung GG, Harrison AW, Shapley JM. Herpes simplex cross infection in the operating room. *Can Anaesth Soc J* 1968;15:394–396.
339. Louis DS, Silva J. Herpetic whitlow: herpetic infections of the digits. *J Hand Surg* 1979;4:90–93.
340. Orkin FK. Herpetic whitlow—occupational hazard to the anesthesiologist. *Anesthesiology* 1970;33:671–673.
341. Rosenberg AD, Bernstein RL, Ramanathan S, et al. Do anesthesiologists practice proper infection control precautions? *Anesthesiology* 1989;71:A949(abst).
342. Kempen PM. Avoiding nosocomial infection in anaesthesia [letter]. *Can J Anaesth* 1989;36:254–255.
343. Gadalla F, Fong J. Improved infection control in the operating room [letter]. *Anesthesiology* 1990;73:1295.
344. Stevens CK, Wayne S, Downs JB. Anesthesia personnel: HIV knowledge and precautions. *Anesth Analg* 1990;70:S392(abst).
345. Barnette RE, Pietrzak WT, BianRosa JJ. On preventing transmission of viral infections [letter]. *Anesthesiology* 1985;62:845.
346. Greene ES. Quality assurance in infection control. *Anesthesiology* 1990;73:A1061(abst).
347. Kempen PM, Treiber H. Teaching hygienic practices or practicing hygiene as teaching? *Anesth Analg* 1990;70:S199(abst).
348. Rosenberg AD, Bernstein D, Skovron ML, et al. Are anesthesiologists practicing proper infection control precautions? *Anesth Analg* 1991; 72:S228.
349. Crow S, Greene VW. Aseptic transgressions among surgeons and anesthesiologists. *Arch Surg* 1982;117:1012–1016.
350. Tait AR, Tuttle DB. Preventing perioperative transmission of infection: a survey of anesthesiology practice. *Anesth Analg* 1995;80: 764–769.
351. el Mikatti N, Dillon P, Healy TEJ. Hygienic practices of consultant anaesthetists: a survey in the North-West region of the UK. *Anaesthesia* 1999;54:13–18.
352. Simmons SA. Laryngoscope handles: a potential for infection. *AANA J* 2000;68:233–236.
353. Phillips RA, Monaghan WP. Incidence of visible and occult blood on laryngoscope blades and handles. *AANA J* 1997;65:241–246.
354. Morell RC, Ririe D, James RL, et al. A survey of laryngoscope contamination at a university and a community hospital. *Anesthesiology* 1994; 80:960.
355. Esler MD, Baines LC, Wilkinson DJ, et al. Decontamination of laryngoscopes: a survey of national practice. *Anaesthesia* 1999;54:582–598.
356. Foweraker JE. The laryngoscope as a potential source of cross-infection [letter]. *J Hosp Infect* 1995;29:315–316.
357. Neal TJ, Hughes CR, Rothburn MM, et al. The neonatal laryngoscope as a potential source of cross-infection [letter]. *J Hosp Infect* 1995;30:315–317.
358. Nelson KE, Warren D, Tomasi AM, et al. Transmission of neonatal listeriosis in a delivery room. *Am J Dis Child* 1985;139:903–905.
359. O'Donnell NG, Asbury AJ. The occupational hazard of human immunodeficiency virus and hepatitis B infection. I. Perceived risks and preventive measures adopted by anaesthetists: a postal survey. *Anaesthesia* 1992;47:923–928.
360. Tait AR, Tuttle DB. Prevention of occupational transmission of human immunodeficiency virus and hepatitis B virus among anesthesiologists: a survey of anesthesiology practice. *Anesth Analg* 1994;79: 623–628.
361. Berry AJ. Infection control recommendations: their importance to the practice of anesthesiology. *ASA Newslett* 2001;65.
362. McNamara JT, Stacey SG. Poor anaesthetist hygienic practices—a problem across all grades of anesthetist. *Anaesthesia* 1999;54: 718–719.
363. Ben-David B, Gaitini L. The routine wearing of gloves: impact on the frequency of needlestick and percutaneous injury and on surface contamination in the operating room. *Anesth Analg* 1996;83: 623–628.
364. Immunization Practices Advisory Committee. Recommendations of the Immunization Practices Advisory Committee. Update on hepatitis B prevention. *MMWR* 1987;36:353–360, 366.
365. Sidebotham D, Anderson B, Featherstone D, et al. Transfer of adenovirus infection from patient to anaesthetist during emergency tracheal intubation. *Anaesth Intensive Care* 1997;25:83–85.
366. American Society of Anesthesiologists and American Association of Nurse Anesthetists. Infection control in the practice of anesthesia. Produced and distributed in a collaborative effort through an educational grant from Burroughs Wellcome Co.
367. Anonymous. Cross-infection during anaesthesia [editorial]. *Br J Anaesth* 1964;36:465.
368. Nettleman MD, Trilla A, Fredrickson M, et al. Assigning responsibility: using feedback to achieve sustained control of methicillin-resistant *Staphylococcus aureus*. *Am J Med* 1991;91(suppl 3B):228S–232S.
369. Haley RW, Culver DH, White JW, et al. The efficacy of infection surveillance and control programs in preventing nosocomial infections in US hospitals. *Am J Epidemiol* 1985;121:182–205.
370. Cruse PJE, Foord R. The epidemiology of wound infection. A 10-year prospective study of 62,939 wounds. *Surg Clin North Am* 1980; 60:27–40.
371. Hajjar J, Girard R. Surveillance des infections nosomiales liees a l'anesthesie. Etude multicentrique. *Ann Fr Anesth Reanim* 2000;1:47–53.
372. Rosenquist RW, Stock MC. Decontaminating anesthesia and respiratory therapy equipment. *Anesth Clin North Am* 1989;7:951–966.
373. Federal Drug Administration. Compliance policy guide 7124.16. 9/ 24/87. Available from FDA Kansas City Regional Office.
374. Sutcliffe AJ. Can the life of 'single use' breathing systems be extended [editorial]? *Anaesthesia* 1995;50:283–285.

375. Centers for Disease Control and Prevention. Guideline for hand hygiene in health-care settings: recommendations of the healthcare infection control practices advisory committee and the HICPAC/SHEA/APIC/IDSA Hand Hygiene Task Force. *MMWR* 2002;51(RR-16):1.
376. Centers for Disease Control and Prevention. Immunization of health-care workers: Recommendations of the Advisory Committee on Immunization Practices (ACIP) and the Hospital Infection Control Practices Advisory Committee (HICPAC). *MMWR* 1997;46(RR-18):1–41.
377. Department of Labor: Occupational Safety and Health Administration. Occupational exposure to bloodborne pathogens; Final rule, 29 CFR Part 1910. 1030. *Fed Reg* 1991;56:64003–64182.

62

NOSOCOMIAL INFECTIONS ASSOCIATED WITH CARDIAC CATHETERIZATION AND OTHER INVASIVE PROCEDURES IN CARDIOLOGY

MARKUS DETTENKOFER
FRANZ D. DASCHNER

Few prospective studies on nosocomial infections are associated with invasive procedures in cardiology, and most analyses have been done retrospectively. In very few studies were the etiologies, pathogenesis, and epidemiology specifically addressed, primarily because most studies were retrospective. There seem to be, however, no major differences between nosocomial infections associated with invasive devices in cardiology and other foreign body associated infections, which are extensively described in Chapters 17, 18, and 67. Therefore, this chapter mainly describes the incidence rates and types of infections.

INFECTIONS ASSOCIATED WITH CARDIAC CATHETERIZATION

In early publications, bacteremia was reported to occur in 4% to 18% of patients undergoing cardiac catheterization (1,2). However, in these studies, blood for culture was obtained from the intravascular catheter or the vessel from which the catheter was removed. Therefore, it was possible that some of the microorganisms isolated represented contamination of the catheter or the site of insertion. Sande et al. (3) determined the true frequency of bacteremia during and after cardiac catheterization and the true frequency of fever by obtaining 214 blood cultures from 106 patients from a vein in the arm on the side opposite to that of the catheter. All venous samples were sterile; therefore, no bacteremia could be demonstrated during cardiac catheterization.

The mortality and morbidity associated with cardiac catheterization was analyzed over a period of 9 years (1971 to 1979) by Gwost et al. (4). No infection and only two pyrogenic reactions occurred in 1,771 patients. Furthermore, there were only three cases of bacteremia or bacterial endocarditis after 12,367 catheterization procedures reported in a cooperative study (5). Ricci et al. (6) found only five documented infections after review of 7,690 medical records of cardiac catheterizations over a 40-month period.

Between 1980 and 1988, 12,251 arterial punctures for cardiac catheterization, percutaneous transluminal coronary angioplasty (PTCA), or pure diagnostic intraarterial angiography were performed by Würsten et al. (7). The only infectious complications were prolonged healing of a wound in the groin and a severe graft infection necessitating ligation of the common femoral artery.

In a retrospective study from January 1991 to December 1998, Munoz et al. (8) found a bacteremia rate of 0.11% in 22,006 invasive nonsurgical cardiologic procedures (0.24% after PTCA, 0.6% after diagnostic cardiac catheterization, 0.8% after electrophysiologic studies).

The incidence of bacteremia and other infections associated with cardiac catheterization, therefore, seems to be extremely low. Even if synthetic vascular grafts have to be catheterized, the infection rate is very low. Mohr et al. (9) studied 109 percutaneous catheterizations of synthetic vascular grafts in 89 patients to determine the risk of major complications. Ninety-six catheterizations were performed through the inguinal portion of the aortofemoral graft. There were no instances of graft infection, and only one superficial infection developed at a cutaneous puncture site.

Risk of Infection with Reuse of Disposable Cardiac Catheters

In Canada and many European countries the reuse of disposable catheters has been common practice until the end of the last decade. In the United States this practice had been discontinued mainly because of legal concerns, but some centers have started to reuse cardiac catheters involving professional third-party reprocessors (10,11). Several studies have examined the risks of infection with reuse of catheters (see also Chapter 87). Jacobson et al. (12) prospectively studied 341 patients who underwent cardiac catheterization and/or coronary angiography to examine the correlation of adverse effects with the number of times catheters were cleaned and reused. The overall incidence of adverse reactions were hypotension 27%, fever 3%, chills 3%, and all three 0.6%. There were no statistically significant increases in these reactions associated with the reuse of catheters. Bacterial infection did not appear responsible for these reactions, which were thought to be due to angiographic dye. The authors concluded that careful cleaning and reuse of catheters did not obviously increase the risk of infection.

Frank et al. (13) prospectively studied 414 patients who had undergone cardiac catheterization or angiography to determine whether there was an increased risk of bacterial contamination or pyrogenic reactions in patients who received reused cardiac catheters. One hundred sixty-one patients were studied with 426 single-use catheters, 152 with 384 multiple-use catheters that were resterilized once or twice, and 101 patients with 325 multiple-use catheters reprocessed up to ten times. No significant differences between the three groups with respect to fever could be observed. Infectious complications associated with cardiac catheterization or angiography did not occur in any case. It was concluded that careful cleaning, disinfection, and resterilization of intravascular catheters with ethylene oxide (ETO) does not increase the risk of infection. O'Donoghue and Platia (14) surveyed retrospectively 13,395 electrophysiologic studies using 44,950 reused catheters in 12 medical centers. They found one superficial skin infection and eight positive blood cultures. However, blood cultures were only performed when infection was suspected, and no information is given on the denominator. The authors concluded that infections were extremely rare and not significantly different in the catheter reuse group compared with the single-use group and that reuse was safe and cost-effective.

Few studies in the literature provide information on specifically how reuse affects catheter material and function. Zapf et al. (15) presented data concerning mechanical stability of polyethylene catheters (elasticity and maximum tensile strength) when exposed up to 60 times to ETO and concluded that reuse of catheters seems to be possible without loss of mechanical safety. Bentolila et al. (16) studied the effects of reuse on the physical characteristics of five types of angiographic catheters with special emphasis on the possibility that reuse could be associated with blood contamination by loose particles. Samples were taken both from new catheters and from catheters used up to ten times. Routine cleaning and sterilization procedures showed no adverse effect on the maximum tensile strength and elongation at break of catheters. Some biologic debris was occasionally present in reused catheters. However, this appeared to be firmly fixed to the luminal surface and seemed unlikely to be carried into the bloodstream during catheterization. On the other hand, new catheters exhibited a substantially higher loose particle count than catheters that had been properly cleaned and resterilized. It was concluded that properly handled reused angiographic catheters are just as safe for the patient as new catheters. The limit on the number of reuses may depend on the care taken to avoid damage to the luminal surface during cleaning, on aging of the catheter material, and on economic considerations.

One of the main concerns with using resterilized catheters is reactions to endotoxin, which may cause chills, fever, and hypotension. Lee et al. (17) reported reactions in 13% of patients undergoing cardiac catheterization over a 3-month period. New catheters, however, may also contain traces of endotoxin. To establish a baseline for the endotoxin contamination of commercially prepared angiographic catheters, Kundsin and Walter (18) purchased 106 catheters from three manufacturers that were packaged, sterile, and ready for insertion. An additional 25 catheters that were described as unfinished and not sterilized were also obtained from one manufacturer. All catheters contained endotoxin ranging from 6.9 to 55.6 pg per catheter. Twenty-five new sterile catheters were pyrogenic, whereas 106, including the 25 unfinished catheters, were not. The authors also tested 13 catheters that were reprocessed in a cardiac catheterization laboratory. All were found to be pyrogenic, containing as much as 7,800 pg per catheter of endotoxin. Five sequential flushes of each catheter, however, resulted in readily detectable endotoxin activity, indicating a persistent elution of endotoxin from the catheters. Recommendations were then made for processing catheters to eliminate pyrogens.

Buchwalsky et al. (19) recently reported experience in 50,000 interventions, including PTCA, using different reprocessed cardiac catheters. Neither the duration of the intervention nor the catheter-dependent complication rates increased for reused in comparison with single-use catheters.

Avitall et al. (20) investigated, over a period of 1 year, the electrical, mechanical, and physical changes after reuse of 69 catheters used in 336 ablation procedures and concluded that they can be reused an average of five times if careful examination of the ablation tip electrode under appropriate magnification (×30) is performed before each use. The catheters should also be tested for deflection and electrical integrity.

Recommendations for Reprocessing of Cardiac Catheters

In the United States, the Food and Drug Administration (FDA) announced in 2000 that it intended to phase in active enforcement of all its premarket and postmarket requirements for devices to ensure that the cleaning, disinfection, and sterilization of reprocessed single-use devices (SUDs) afforded the same level of safety and effectiveness for patients as new catheters did (*http://www.fda.gov/cdrh/reuse/index.html*). Postmarket requirements such as registration, listing, medical device reporting, medical device tracking, medical device corrections and removals, the quality system regulation, and labeling are also applicable to third-party and hospital reprocessors. This policy led to the comment of a "requiem for reuse of single-use devices in U.S. hospitals" (21). In Germany, the Robert Koch Institute (RKI) recently issued its guideline on reprocessing of medical devices (*http://www.rki.de/GESUND/HYGIENE/ANFORDHYGMED.PDF*). According to this guideline, cardiac catheters are ranked as highly critical medical devices, which require special caution when such devices are reprocessed, and an active external quality control system is required to be in place.

Recommendations Regarding Third-Party Reprocessors of SUDs

The FDA suggests seeking contact with other hospitals to determine their experience with third-party reprocessors and arranging visits to the reprocessors' facilities (*http://www.fda.gov/cdrh/reuse/reuse-faq.html*). In addition, it is recommended to request information regarding FDA inspections, monitoring, and validation.

Recommendations Regarding Cleaning and Sterilizing of Cardiac Catheters

If hospitals decide to reprocess cardiac catheters within their own facilities, the following process is suggested. If these recommendations are followed carefully and are accompanied by strict quality controls, no infectious complications or endotoxic reactions should occur. Resterilization bears the potential for residual chemical contamination with ETO (22). Therefore, residual ETO levels may be substantially reduced by allowing a 14-day waiting period after resterilization or by incorporating a detoxification period immediately after ETO exposure [repeated cycles of steam flushes (23)].

- Flush immediately after use with water or heparinized saline and soak for 20 to 25 minutes.
- Remove and brush the tip and soak in a detergent solution for 30 minutes.
- Push guidewire gently through the catheter lumen to remove any biologic material or debris.
- Hand wash for 5 minutes with detergent solution and rinse intensely with sterile water.
- Blow completely dry with compressed air.
- Inspect carefully for any damage or defect or the presence of organic matter or debris and mark with an indelible marking pen.
- Repackage in sealed envelope and add proper identification.
- Sterilize with ETO.
- Aerate catheters for at least 14 days at room temperature.

INFECTIONS AFTER INTRAAORTIC BALLOON PUMP INSERTION, IMPLANTATION OF A CARDIOVERTER-DEFIBRILLATOR, CORONARY ANGIOPLASTY, STENT IMPLANTATION, LASER THERMAL ANGIOPLASTY, AND PACEMAKER INSERTION

Intraaortic Balloon Pump

Goldberg et al. (24) compared the percutaneous and surgical techniques of intraaortic balloon pump insertion in 101 patients. In the percutaneous group (51 patients), no infection developed, but, in the surgical group, 3 patients developed sepsis with bacteremia (including 1 patient who required vein patch repair of the femoral artery and 1 patient who developed a surgical site infection requiring debridement).

The overall complication rate for 100 consecutive patients treated with the intraaortic balloon pump was 23%, with 5 patients developing surgical site infections and 2 developing septicemia (25). Surgical site problems contributed to the death of one patient. Another patient died with septicemia and an infected aortotomy closure site 4.5 months after the original procedure. An outbreak of *Pseudomonas cepacia* bacteremia associated with a contaminated intraaortic balloon pump was reported by Rutala et al. (26).

Forty-five patients who died after insertion of an intraaortic balloon device were studied at necropsy (27). Thirty-six percent had one or more complications related to the use of the device, one of which was a local surgical site infection not suspected during life. In two other patients in whom the balloon was implanted for septic shock, there was no evidence of seeding of either the balloon catheter or the prosthetic introducer graft.

In a study of 240 consecutive percutaneous intraaortic balloon counterpulsations, Eltchaninoff et al. (28) identified only one case of *Staphylococcus aureus* bloodstream infection and one superficial infection. In the retrospective study by Meco et al. (29), 7 of 116 patients (6%) requiring postoperative intraaortic balloon pump support had infection of the insertion site.

Yang et al. (30) investigated 112 used intraaortic balloons for physical integrity, gas leakage, mechanical performance, surface chemistry and morphology, and physical stability. These intraaortic balloons were all used clinically only once, and the duration of the intraaortic balloons *in vivo* ranged from 6 to 312 hours. Macroscopic examination of the balloons and the outer catheters revealed no obvious change in either shape or color. No discernible abrasions or cracks were observed on the balloons. However, 61% of the balloons were creased and 40% of the central lumens and 21% of the sheaths showed visible bending flaws. Moreover, 65% of the balloons and 38% of the central lumens were contaminated by visible residual organic debris. The authors concluded that the presence of residual organic debris that cannot be eliminated is an indication that such intraaortic balloons should not be reused.

In their prospective study Crystal et al. (31) found an incidence of fever of 47%, true bacteremia of 15%, and sepsis of 12% in 60 patients treated with an intraaortic balloon counterpulsation pump. The authors suggested evaluating the benefit of antibiotic prophylaxis.

Implantable Cardioverter-Defibrillator

The automatic implantable cardioverter-defibrillator (ICD) has been found to be useful in the management of life-threatening ventricular arrhythmias. Marchlinski et al. (32) reported primary infectious complications associated with 6% of cardioverter-defibrillator implantations. In another series by Marchlinski et al. (33) following 26 patients for 13 months, 1 patient developed a superficial incisional surgical site infection 14 days after device implantation and 1 patient acquired a late infection of the generator pocket 3 months after repositioning of a migrated lead and 14 months after initial generator placement. Treatment necessitated removal of both the generator and leads. A partial removal is reserved for patients in whom the risk of complete removal is too high and infection is confined to a part of the ICD (i.e., generator only) (34).

Mela et al. (35) stated that infection is an uncommon (0% to 6.7% reported in the literature) but serious complication after ICD implantation, because complete device removal is often necessary. In their review of 1,700 procedures they found a total of 21 ICD-related infections (1.2%); one fourth of these had systemic signs of infection. Patients with abdominal systems had significantly more infections than patients with pectoral systems (3.2% vs. 0.5%). In a prospective study, Chamis et al. (36) determined the incidence of cardiac device-associated infections among patients with ICD or permanent pacemaker who developed *S. aureus* bacteremia (SAB). In patients with early SAB (<1 year after device placement) they found that 75% of the SAB was related to the device; in patients with late SAB (>1 year) 28.5% were confirmed to be related to the ICD or pacemaker (43% were possible cardiac device infections).

The most common pathogens of infections related to ICD are coagulase-negative staphylococci and *S. aureus* [68% and 23 %, respectively, in the study by Chua et al. (37)].

The decision whether or not to reimplant an ICD after removal of an infected one is controversial. Some authors recommend reimplantation as early as 36 hours after explantation in patients with only local symptoms of infection. The need for reimplantation should be reassessed in every case (37).

With regard to infections, but also to other complications, the single-chamber ICD (SC-ICD) seems to be superior to the dual-chamber ICD (DC-ICD), which may be explainable by the longer operation time and the placement of the second lead of the DC-ICD (infectious complications: 4.1% with the DC-ICD vs. 0% with the SC-ICD) (38).

Percutaneous Transluminal Coronary Angioplasty

No infection was reported during early and long-term follow-up (at least 1 year) of 3,079 patients after coronary angioplasty (39). In a prospective study, 164 PTCAs resulted in one *S. aureus* infection (0.6%) that could be related to the procedure (40).

Malanoski et al. (41) identified a risk of 0.25% for SAB among 1,944 PTCA procedures performed in 25 months at one institution. Cleveland and Gelfand (42) summarized the reported cases of invasive staphylococcal infections associated with PTCA and described three more patients with invasive staphylococcal disease after PTCA of which two patients had received single intravenous antibiotic prophylaxis with 1 g cefazolin. This may very well be explained by the fact that the predominant risk of infection may not have been the procedure itself but more likely the retention of the femoral sheath for more than 24 hours.

McCready et al. (43) noted that septic complications after cardiac catheterization and PTCA are distinctly uncommon, but they described nine cases of septic complications after PTCA resulting in two deaths. Their study suggests that repeated puncture of the same femoral artery and the femoral artery sheath being left in for more than 1 day are risk factors for septic complications (41,43). Cardiac abscess after PTCA have also been described in a patient in whom a problematic and repeated procedure probably led to a direct colonization and subsequent infection of an intimal dissection of the right coronary artery (44).

Siddiqui and Lester (45) described a case of septic arthritis and bilateral endogenous endophthalmitis associated with PTCA. Several cases of septic endarteritis with *S. aureus* after PTCA have been described by different authors (46,47).

In another case report, an epidural abscess occurred in a patient after PTCA. The explanation was that the residual arterial sheath, whose tip was near the aortic bifurcation, was injected with an infected bolus, thus facilitating infection through the lumbar radicular arteries (48). The absence of specific signs may easily cause a delay in recognizing the infection (45,48,49). It has been considered that retention of the sheath for more than 24 hours could be a risk factor for infection. However, prospective studies are not available on this issue (42,50).

Endocarditis following PTCA is such a rare complication that there are merely individual case reports. Wang et al. (51) reported a case of *Candida parapsilosis* endocarditis. Barbetseas et al. (52) reported a case of a patient with infective endocarditis of a prosthetic valve in the aortic position after receiving PTCA. Shibata et al. (53) reported a case of a 73-year-old man who developed infectious endocarditis caused by *S. aureus* after PTCA. A postmortem examination revealed multiple myocardial microabscesses and myocardial infarction resulting from embolic vegetation.

Although infections after PTCA are rare, some have resulted in death (54). Infections may become evident several weeks after the procedure. The longest period between PTCA and the appearance of infectious complications published so far was 1 month (41). Even ultrasonography and computed tomography may fail to reveal vascular infection, and, when there is clinical suspicion of infection, it may be prudent to initiate early surgical exploration (55).

Some authors recommend use of the contralateral inguinal site if PTCA is to follow a recent catheterization (42–44,56,57), whereas others found no correlation between ipsilateral inguinal puncture and infectious complications (40). At present, this question cannot be answered, because none of the cited studies have the statistical power to be able to detect significant differences between contralateral and ipsilateral repuncture.

Risk factors for bacteremia and other infectious complications during cardiac catheterization, mainly during PTCA, are age older than 60 years, congestive heart failure, duration of procedure, number of catheterizations at the same site, difficult vascular access, and an arterial sheath in place for more than 1 day (8,43,58–60).

The most common microorganisms that cause PTCA-related bacteremia are *S. aureus*, coagulase-negative staphylococci, and group B-streptococci (58).

Reuse of Coronary Angioplasty Catheters

One of the pioneer studies on reuse of PTCA catheters was done by Plante et al. (61). In this study two centers were compared; one using new and the other reused catheters. Comparison of the centers led to the conclusion that reuse was associated with a higher rate of adverse clinical events (7.8% vs. 3.8%). This result is in contrast to findings published by Browne et al. (10), who investigated the reuse of PTCA balloon catheters, restored by a process strictly controlled for bioburden and sterility, in patients undergoing PTCA. The study enrolled 107 patients; 106 had a successful laboratory outcome, and 1 required coronary artery bypass graft surgery after failed rescue stenting. The authors concluded that reuse of disposable coronary angioplasty catheters after carefully controlled reprocessing appears to be safe and effective with success rates similar to those of new products and no detectable sacrifice in performance.

Cost-efficacy modeling was then performed by Mak et al. (62) on the basis of Plante et al.'s study using different scenarios. All scenarios included the cost of revascularization resulting from unsuccessful performance of reused catheters. Consequently, the reuse of catheters results in only minimal savings or even a substantial cost increase. However, Mak et al. (63) published a reanalysis of Plante et al.'s results; using logistic regression analysis they demonstrated that adverse effects were not associated with reuse of equipment but rather with other established risk factors of the patient.

Although the prices for new PTCA catheters dropped during the 1990s, the cost for reprocessing has remained stable or may even be rising. A cost-efficiency analysis must, therefore, be based on the individual institution and may well result in a decision to use new catheters (64).

In a small survey with 100 PTCA patients in Cleveland, one third stated that they would refuse the reuse of catheters. Based on the results of their survey, the authors pointed out that a significant minority of patients could make it unacceptable for a hospital to adopt a strategy of balloon catheter reuse. They recommended that at least legal protective measures are adopted, because costs of possible lawsuits could easily neutralize the savings accomplished through reuse (11).

With respect to reuse of PTCA equipment, Krause et al. (65) reviewed the literature, interpreted the current state of knowledge, and presented the main arguments in favor and against reuse. According to the authors, the following conclusions can be drawn:

1. Even assuming that no additional clinical risk is associated with PTCA-catheter reuse, the decision to adopt or reject a reuse policy has to be based on the individual situation at each hospital. Factors to consider include technical and personnel resources of the institution, frequency of PTCA procedures, and the economical and legal environments.
2. The review of the literature shows that authors tend to come to two contradictory conclusions as far as patient safety is concerned. One group of authors claims that PTCA catheters are already being reused in many countries and that there is no evidence for an increased risk. The other group sees a risk in the presence of organic debris in reused catheters, which raises both health and legal issues.

Krause et al. stated that it is unlikely that clinical trials will ever come up with a clear answer to the problem. The best solution to the controversy might be an international committee that develops and updates standard operating procedures for PTCA-catheter reuse, based on the latest scientific evidence and the experience of those countries that already routinely use reprocessed PTCA catheters (65).

Stent Implantation

Gunther et al. (66) described the first case of lethal complications resulting from a myocardial abscess near the stent in the right coronary artery. A second case of fatal outcome resulting from stent infection with *Pseudomonas aeruginosa,* which led to infective mitral endocarditis and saccular aneurysm of the coronary artery, was described by Leroy et al. (67). Studies in a swine model suggest that metallic stents have the potential of becoming infected after bacterial challenge unlike arteries that have undergone angioplasty (68). Seven stent-artery complexes implanted in the iliac arteries of 14 swine were culture positive after an intravenous bacterial challenge with *S. aureus,* whereas only 1 of 14 angioplastied arteries were positive for *S. aureus* (p = .03) (68).

Dieter et al. (69) reported the case of a patient who developed an infected aortic aneurysm after placement of a coronary artery stent. They pointed out that infectious complications have been rare.

Laser Thermal Angioplasty

Laser thermal-assisted balloon angioplasty is used in the treatment of patients with advanced peripheral vascular disease and in high-risk patients who are poor candidates for operative reconstructions. There patients benefited most from minimal-intervention endovascular techniques in which lasers were used as a thermal source or as unguided free energy to recanalize the artery. White et al. (70) followed 28 patients, including 27 who had advanced peripheral vascular disease, for 3 years after laser thermal-assisted balloon angioplasty. Eighteen patients were successfully recanalized, but five amputations were required within 1 month and another six were needed between 8 and 12 months. Early amputations were necessitated by failure of wound healing. Whether this was due to infection, however, was not mentioned in the report.

Diethrich (71) reviewed his experience in treating 1,849 lesions in 894 patients and found no infection. The most common surgical procedures performed were laser angioplasty, patch angioplasty, arterectomy, thrombectomy, femoral-popliteal bypass, and profundoplasty.

If laser-assisted angioplasty, however, is performed in the treatment of prosthetic graft stenosis, the wound infection rate is higher. Diethrich et al. (72) followed 25 symptomatic patients with 28 peripheral prosthetic arterial bypass grafts; 2 patients suffered recurrent thrombosis and 1 developed an inexplicable graft infection 5 months after laser treatment. The latter patient, however, had undergone graft thrombectomy elsewhere 3 months before laser therapy, and the 5-month interval between angioplasty and the identification of the infection would make the laser's role in the etiology doubtful.

Pacemaker Insertion

Insertion in Children

Pacemaker treatment is more complicated in children than in adults, largely because of electrode problems. If infections such as recurrent septicemia occur, the whole system usually has to be removed (73).

Walsh et al. (74) reviewed their 21-year experience with pacemaker implantation in children. Forty-one patients aged 11 days to 19 years at initial pacemaker implantation were followed up to 248 months. Complications included infection in six, and one patient died of a pacemaker-associated infection.

Between 1971 and 1986, 85 pacemakers were implanted at the St. Justine Hospital in Montreal in 57 patients then aged from 1 day to 23 years (mean, 10.3 years). The patients were followed for periods ranging from 15 days to 13.5 years. Only one patient developed a pacemaker-associated infection (75).

Atrial pacing for tachycardia was tested in 23 children and young adults (76). Pacemakers were implanted by the transvenous technique using bipolar leads. Seven patients required reoperations, including five for adapter problems and two for infection.

Nordlander et al. (77) reviewed their clinical experience of pacemaker treatment in children. Pacemaker systems had been implanted in 23 children aged 2 days to 14 years since 1983. Only three local infections developed. They concluded that endocardial pacing is the method of choice even for small children.

Pacemakers can even be implanted in newborns and very small infants. Villain et al. (78) implanted pacemakers in neonates. In eight children, a permanent pacemaker was implanted in the first 2 days of life, and, in six children, the pacemaker was implanted at the age of 2 to 3 months. Only one pacemaker had to be replaced because of infection at 28 months.

Twenty-four children, 15 kg or less in weight, underwent implantation of a permanent pacemaker using the transvenous technique. During a median follow-up period of 3 years and 6 months, two children developed infection (79).

Cohen et al. (80) evaluated possible predictors of pacemaker infections in children. They reported a total of 7.8% infections (30 infections in 385 pacemaker implantations). In a multivariate analysis, trisomy 21 and pacemaker revisions were found as predictors.

Insertion in Adults

Several older publications described infectious complications of pacemakers in adults (81–86). The time from insertion to infection varied from 7 to 31 days, and the only infecting microorganisms were *S. aureus* and *Staphylococcus epidermidis.* Pocket infections usually occurred earlier than septicemia, and the incidence of septicemia was much lower than that of pocket infections. Most recent series have shown infection rates between 0.6% and 2.1% (87,88). In their case report and review of the literature, Voet et al. (89) reported an incidence between 0.3% and 12.6%. This may involve infection of the pocket or the electrodes and may be associated with bacteremia with or without endocarditis. Systemic factors contributing to a higher incidence are diabetes mellitus, thin skin, the use of corticosteroids, age, intravenous catheters, neoplasms, the use of anticoagulants, temporary pacing, dermatologic diseases, and other infectious foci.

One of the most serious infectious complications is pacemaker endocarditis. Arber et al. (90) reported 44 cases and reviewed the literature. Kurup et al. (91) reported the rare case of *Candida tropicalis* pacemaker endocarditis. Between 1980 and 2000, seven of 1,920 patients with pacemaker implantation developed endocarditis in the study by Erdinler et al. (92) The most common pathogen was *S. aureus,* Mezilis et al. (93) described two patients with metastatic pacemaker infections, one caused by *P. aeruginosa* 5 months after implantation and a second by *Streptococcus pneumoniae* 8 years after implantation. Pacemaker infections can also be caused by very rare microorganisms such as *Staphylococcus schleiferi,* a member of the human skin flora (94). A prospective study by Da Costa et al. (95) compared microorganisms isolated at the time of insertion and any infective complication by using ribotyping. Their study supported the hypothesis that pacemaker-related infections are mainly due to local contamination. In general, early infections after implantation tend to be caused by *S. aureus,* whereas late infections are caused by coagulase-negative staphylococci (89).

Several earlier studies on the merits of antibiotic prophylaxis at the time of permanent pacemaker implantation have yielded inconclusive results. A recent meta-analysis of all available randomized trials to evaluate the effectiveness of this measure to reduce infection rates after permanent pacemaker implantation suggests that systemic antibiotic prophylaxis significantly reduces the incidence of potentially serious infective complications. The studies support the use of prophylactic antibiotics at the time of pacemaker insertion to prevent short-term pocket infection, skin erosion, or septicemia (96). The efficacy of antibiotic prophylaxis for late septicemia or endocarditis, however, is unknown.

REFERENCES

1. Kreidberg MB, Chernoff HL. Ineffectiveness of penicillin prophylaxis in cardiac catheterization. *J Pediatr* 1965;66:286–290.
2. Gould L, Lyon AF. Penicillin prophylaxis: cardiac catheterization. *JAMA* 1967;202:662–663.
3. Sande MA, Levinson MD, Lukas DS, et al. Bacteremia associated with cardiac catheterization. *N Engl J Med* 1969;281:1104–1106.
4. Gwost J, Stoebe T, Chesler E, et al. Analysis of the complications of cardiac catheterization over nine years. *Cathet Cardiovasc Diagn* 1982; 8:13–21.
5. Swan HJC. Infections, inflammatory, and allergic complications. *Circulation* 1968;37:49–51.
6. Ricci MA, Trevisani GT, Pilcher DB. Vascular complications of cardiac catheterization [see comments]. *Am J Surg* 1994;167:375–378.
7. Würsten HU, Stricker H, Salzmann C, et al. Periphere Arterienkomplikationen katheterangiographischer Methoden. *Helv Chir Acta* 1990; 57:193–197.
8. Munoz P, Blanco JR, Rodriguez-Creixems M, et al. Bloodstream infections after invasive nonsurgical cardiologic procedures. *Arch Intern Med* 2001;161:2110–2115.
9. Mohr LL, Smith DC, Schaner GJ. Catheterization of synthetic vascular grafts. *J Vasc Surg* 1986;6:854–856.
10. Browne KF, Maldonado R, Telatnik M, et al. Initial experience with reuse of coronary angioplasty catheters in the United States. *J Am Coll Cardiol* 1997;30:1735–1740.
11. Vaitkus PT. Patient acceptance of reused angioplasty equipment. *Am Heart J* 1997;134:127–130.
12. Jacobson JA, Schwartz CE, Marshall HW, et al. Fever, chills, and hypotension following cardiac catheterization with single- and multiple-use disposable catheters. *Cathet Cardiovasc Diagn* 1983;9:39–46.
13. Frank U, Herz L, Daschner FD. Infection risk of cardiac catheterization and arterial angiography with single and multiple use disposable catheters. *Clin Cardiol* 1988;11:785–787.
14. O'Donoghue S, Platia EV. Reuse of pacing catheters: a survey of safety and efficacy. *PACE* 1988;11:1279–1280.
15. Zapf S, Müller K, Haas L. Wiederaufbereitung von Angiographiekathetern. *Rontgen-Blätter* 1987;40:169–172.
16. Bentolila P, Jacob R, Roberge F. Effects of re–use on the physical characteristics of angiographic catheters. *J Med Eng Technol* 1990;14: 254–259.

17. Lee RV, Drabinsky M, Wolfson S, et al. Pyrogen reactions from cardiac catheterization. *Chest* 1973;63:757–761.
18. Kundsin RB, Walter CW. Detection of endotoxin on sterile catheters used for cardiac catheterization. *J Clin Microbiol* 1980;11:209–212.
19. Buchwalsky R, Grove R, Feldkamp E. [25-year experience with reusable heart catheters]. *Z Kardiol* 2001;90:542–549.
20. Avitall B, Khan M, Krum D, et al. Repeated use of ablation catheters: a prospective study. *J Am Coll Cardiol* 1993;2:1367–1372.
21. Favero MS. Requiem for reuse of single-use devices in US hospitals. *Infect Control Hosp Epidemiol* 2001;22:539–541.
22. Aton EA, Murray P, Fraser V, et al. Safety of reusing cardiac electrophysiology catheters. *Am J Cardiol* 1994;74:1173–1175.
23. Ferrell M, Wolf CE, Ellenbogen KA, et al. Ethylene oxide on electrophysiology catheters following resterilization: implications for catheter reuse. *Am J Cardiol* 1997;80:1558–1561.
24. Goldberg M, Rubenfire M, Kantrowitz A, et al. Intraaortic balloon pump insertion: a randomized study comparing percutaneous and surgical techniques. *J Am Coll Cardiol* 1987;9:515–523.
25. McCabe JC, Abel RM, Subramanian VA, et al. Complications of intra-aortic balloon insertion and counterpulsation. *Circulation* 1978;57: 769–773.
26. Rutala WA, Weber DJ, Thomann CA, et al. An outbreak of *Pseudomonas cepacia* bacteremia associated with a contaminated intra-aortic balloon pump. *J Thorac Cardiovasc Surg* 1988;96:157–161.
27. Isner JM, Cohen SR, Virmani R, et al. Complications of the intraaortic balloon counterpulsation device: clinical and morphologic observations in 45 necropsy patients. *Am J Cardiol* 1980;45:260–268.
28. Eltchaninoff H, Dimas AP, Whitlow PL. Complications associated with percutaneous placement and use of intraaortic balloon counterpulsation. *Am J Cardiol* 1993;71:328–332.
29. Meco M, Gramegna G, Yassini A, et al. Mortality and morbidity from intra-aortic balloon pumps. Risk analysis. *J Cardiovasc Surg* 2002;43: 17–23.
30. Yang M, Deng X, Zhang Z, et al. Are intraaortic balloons suitable for reuse? A survey study of 112 used intraaortic balloons. *Artif Organs* 1997;21:121–130.
31. Crystal E, Borer A, Gilad J, et al. Incidence and clinical significance of bacteremia and sepsis among cardiac patients treated with intra-aortic balloon counterpulsation pump. *Am J Cardiol* 2000;86: 1281–1284.
32. Marchlinski FE, Reid PR, Mower MM, et al. Clinical performance of the implantable cardioverter-defibrillator. *PACE* 1984;7:1345–1350.
33. Marchlinski FE, Flores BT, Buxton AE, et al. The automatic implantable cardioverter-defibrillator: efficacy, complications, and device failures. *Ann Intern Med* 1986;104:481–488.
34. Samuels LE, Samuels FL, Kaufman MS, et al. Management of infected implantable cardiac defibrillators. *Ann Thorac Surg* 1997;64: 1702–1706.
35. Mela T, McGovern BA, Garan H, et al. Long-term infection rates associated with the pectoral versus abdominal approach to cardioverter-defibrillator implants. *Am J Cardiol* 2001;88:750–753.
36. Chamis AL, Peterson GE, Cabell CH, et al. *Staphylococcus aureus* bacteremia in patients with permanent pacemakers or implantable cardioverter-defibrillators. *Circulation* 2001;104:1029–1033.
37. Chua JD, Wilkoff BL, Lee I, et al. Diagnosis and management of infections involving implantable electrophysiologic cardiac devices. *Ann Intern Med* 2000;133:604–608.
38. Takahashi T, Bhandari AK, Watanuki M, et al. High incidence of device-related and lead-related complications in the dual-chamber implantable cardioverter defibrillator compared with the single-chamber version. *Circ J* 2002;66:746–750.
39. Cowley MJ, Mullin SM, Kelsey SF, et al. Sex differences in early and long-term results of coronary angioplasty in the NHLBI PTCA Registry. *Circulation* 1985;71:90–97.
40. Shea W, Schwartz RK, Gambino AT, et al. Bacteremia associated with percutaneous transluminal coronary angioplasty. *Cathet Cardiovasc Diagn* 1995;36:5–9.
41. Malanoski GJ, Samore MH, Pefanis A, et al. *Staphylococcus aureus* catheter-associated bacteremia. Minimal effective therapy and unusual infectious complications associated with arterial sheath catheters. *Arch Intern Med* 1995;155:1161–1166.
42. Cleveland KO, Gelfand MS. Invasive staphylococcal infections complicating percutaneous transluminal coronary angioplasty: three cases and review. *Clin Infect Dis* 1995;1:93–96.
43. McCready RA, Siderys H, Pittman JN, et al. Septic complications after cardiac catheterization and percutaneous transluminal coronary angioplasty. *J Vasc Surg* 1991;14:170–174.
44. Timsit JF, Wolff MA, Bedos JP, et al. Cardiac abscess following percutaneous transluminal coronary angioplasty. *Chest* 1993;103:639–641.
45. Siddiqui MA, Lester RM. Septic arthritis and bilateral endogenous endophthalmitis associated with percutaneous transluminal coronary angioplasty. *J Am Geriatr Soc* 1996;44:476–477.
46. Frazee BW, Flaherty JP. Septic endarteritis of the femoral artery following angioplasty. *Rev Infect Dis* 1991;13:620–623.
47. Brummitt CF, Kravitz GR, Granrud GA, et al. Femoral endarteritis due to *Staphylococcus aureus* complicating percutaneous transluminal coronary angioplasty. *Am J Med* 1989;86:822–824.
48. Oriscello RG, Fineman S, Vigario JC, et al. Epidural abscess as a complication of coronary angioplasty: a rare but dangerous complication. *Cathet Cardiovasc Diagn* 1994;33:36–38.
49. Kardaras FG, Kardara DF, Rontogiani DP, et al. Septic endarteritis following percutaneous transluminal coronary angioplasty. *Cathet Cardiovasc Diagn* 1995;34:57–60.
50. Landau C, Lange RA, Hillis LD. Percutaneous transluminal coronary angioplasty. *N Engl J Med* 1994;330:981–993.
51. Wang JH, Liu YC, Le S. *Candida* endocarditis following percutaneous transluminal angioplasty. *Clin Infect Dis* 1998;26:205–206.
52. Barbetseas J, Vyssoulis G, Lambrou S, et al. Embolic stroke after "cured" prosthetic aortic valve endocarditis. *Cardiol Rev* 2002;10: 214–217.
53. Shibata T, Hirai H, Fujii H, et al. Infective endocarditis with myocardial abscesses complicating percutaneous transluminal coronary angioplasty. *J Heart Valve Dis* 2002;11:665–667.
54. Guerin JM, Leibinger F, Mofredj A. Invasive staphylococcal infection complicating coronary angiography without angioplasty. *Clin Infect Dis* 1996;22:886–887.
55. Shea KW, Cunha BA. Invasive staphylococcal infections complicating percutaneous transluminal coronary angioplasty. *Clin Infect Dis* 1996; 22:601.
56. Evans BH, Goldstein EJ. Increased risk of infection after repeat percutaneous transluminal coronary angioplasty. *Am J Infect Control* 1987;15: 125–126.
57. Wiener RS, Ong LS. Local infection after percutaneous transluminal coronary angioplasty: relation to early repuncture of ipsilateral femoral artery. *Cathet Cardiovasc Diagn* 1989;16:180–181.
58. Samore MH, Wessolossky MA, Lewis SM, et al. Frequency, risk factors, and outcome for bacteremia after percutaneous transluminal coronary angioplasty. *Am J Cardiol* 1997;79:873–877.
59. Izumi AK, Samlaska CP, Hew DW, et al. Septic embolization arising from infected pseudoaneurysms following percutaneous transluminal coronary angioplasty: a report of 2 cases and review of the literature. *Cutis* 2000;66:447–452.
60. Ross MJ, Sakoulas G, Manning WJ, et al. *Corynebacterium jeikeium* native valve endocarditis following femoral access for coronary angiography. *Clin Infect Dis* 2001;32:E120–121.
61. Plante S, Strauss BH, Goulet G, et al. Reuse of balloon catheters for coronary angioplasty: a potential cost-saving strategy? *J Am Coll Cardiol* 1994;24:1475–1481.
62. Mak KH, Eisenberg MJ, Eccleston DS, et al. Cost-efficacy modeling of catheter reuse for percutaneous transluminal coronary angioplasty. *J Am Coll Cardiol* 1996;28:106–111.
63. Mak KH, Eisenberg MJ, Plante S, et al. Absence of increased in-hospital complications with reused balloon catheters. *Am J Cardiol* 1996;78: 717–719.
64. van den Brand M. Utilization of coronary angioplasty and cost of angioplasty disposables in 14 western European countries. European Angioplasty Survey Group. *Eur Heart J* 1993;14:391–397.
65. Krause G, Dziekan G, Daschner FD. Reuse of coronary angioplasty balloon catheters: yes or no? *Eur Heart J* 2000;21:185–189.

66. Gunther HU, Strupp G, Volmar J, et al. Coronary stent implantation: infection and abscess with fatal outcome. *Z Kardiol* 1993;82:521–525.
67. Leroy O, Martin E, Prat A, et al. Fatal infection of coronary stent implantation. *Cathet Cardiovasc Diagn* 1996;39:168–170.
68. Hearn AT, James KV, Lohr JM, et al. Endovascular stent infection with delayed bacterial challenge. *Am J Surg* 1997;174:157–159.
69. Dieter RS, Shah P, Pacanowski JP. Aortic arch (pseudo) aneurysm complicating cardiac catheterization. *J Invasive Cardiol* 2001;13: 317–319.
70. White, RA, White GH, Mehringer MC, et al. A clinical trial of laser thermal angioplasty in patients with advanced peripheral vascular disease. *Ann Surg* 1990;212:257–265.
71. Diethrich EB. Laser angioplasty: a critical review based on 1849 clinical procedures. *Angiology* 1990;41:757–767.
72. Diethrich EB, Santiago O, Bahadir I. Laser-assisted angioplasty in the treatment of prosthetic graft stenosis. *Angiology* 1991;42:576–580.
73. DeLeon SY, Bojar R, Koster NK, et al. Recurrent sepsis from retained endocardial electrode in children: successful removal with cardiopulmonary bypass. *PACE* 1984;7:166–168.
74. Walsh CA, McAlister HF, Andrews CA, et al. Pacemaker implantation in children: a 21-year experience. *PACE* 1988;11:1940–1944.
75. Jimenez M, Fournier A, Hery E, et al. Cardiac pacemakers in children. 15 years experience. *Arch Mal Coeurs Vaissaux* 1988;81:665–670.
76. Gillette PC, Zeigler VL, Case CL, et al. Atrial antitachycardia pacing in children and young adults. *Am Heart J* 1991;122:844–849.
77. Nordlander R, Pehrsson SK, Book K, et al. Clinical experience of pacemaker treatment in children. *Scand J Thorac Cardiovasc Surg* 1992; 26:69–72.
78. Villain E, Seletti L, Kachaner J, et al. Artificial cardiac stimulation in the newborn infant with complete congenital atrioventricular block. Study of 16 cases. *Arch Mal Coeurs Vaissaux* 1989;82:739–744.
79. Till JA, Jones S, Rowland E, et al. Endocardial pacing in infants and children 15 kg or less in weight: medium-term follow-up. *PACE* 1990; 13:1385–1392.
80. Cohen MI, Bush DM, Gaynor JW, et al. Pediatric pacemaker infections: twenty years of experience. *J Thorac Cardiovasc Surg* 2002;124: 821–827.
81. Morgan G, Ginks W, Siddons H, et al. Septicemia in patients with an endocardial pacemaker. *Am J Cardiol* 1979;44:221–224.
82. Muers MF, Arnold AG, Sleight P. Prophylactic antibiotics for cardiac pacemaker implantation. *Br Heart J* 1981;46:539–544.
83. Jacobson B, Bluhm G, Julander I, et al. Coagulase-negative staphylococci and cloxacillin prophylaxis in pacemaker surgery. *Acta Pathol Microbiol Immunol Scand [B]* 1983;91:97–99.
84. Harjula A, Järvinen A, Virtanen KS, et al. Pacemaker infections treatment with total or partial pacemaker system removal. *Thorac Cardiovasc Surg* 1985;33:218–220.
85. Bluhm G, Nordlander R, Ransjò U. Antibiotic prophylaxis in pacemaker surgery: a prospective double blind trial with systemic administration of antibiotic versus placebo at implantation of cardiac pacemakers. *PACE* 1986;9:720–726.
86. Smyth EG, Pallister D. Septicaemia in patients with temporary and permanent endocardial pacemakers. *J R Soc Med* 1989;82:396–398.
87. Chauhan A, Grace AA, Newell SA, et al. Early complications after dual chamber versus single chamber pacemaker implantation. *PACE* 1994; 17:2012–2015.
88. Frame R, Brodman RF, Furman S, et al. Surgical removal of infected transvenous pacemaker leads. *PACE* 1993;16:2343–2348.
89. Voet JG, Vandekerckhove YR, Muyldermans LL, et al. Pacemaker lead infection: report of three cases and review of the literature. *Heart* 1999; 81:88–91.
90. Arber N, Pras E, Copperman Y, et al. Pacemaker endocarditis. Report of 44 cases and review of the literature. *Medicine (Baltimore)* 1994;73: 299–305.
91. Kurup A, Janardhan MN, Seng TY. Candida tropicalis pacemaker endocarditis. *J Infect* 2000;41:275–276.
92. Erdinler I, Okmen E, Zor U, et al. Pacemaker related endocarditis: analysis of seven cases. *Jpn Heart J* 2002;43:475–485.
93. Mezilis N, Hough RE, David G, et al. Infections in transvenous cardiac pacemakers: two more cases. *PACE* 1997;20:2992–2994.
94. Célard M, Vandenesch F, Darbas H, et al. Pacemaker infection caused by *Staphylococcus schleiferi,* a member of the human preaxillary flora: four case reports. *Clin Infect Dis* 1997;24:1014–1015.
95. Da Costa A, Lelievre H, Kirkorian G, et al. Role of the preaxillary flora in pacemaker infections: a prospective study. *Circulation* 1998; 97:1791–1795.
96. Da Costa A, Kirkorian G, Cucherat M, et al. Antibiotic prophylaxis for permanent pacemaker implantation. A meta-analysis. *Circulation* 1998;97:1796–1801.

63

INFECTION RISKS OF ENDOSCOPY

JOHN HOLTON

Endoscopic procedures are used worldwide for both diagnostic and therapeutic intervention. Considering the numbers of endoscopies that must be performed annually, the incidence of infection is comparatively low (1,2), although increasing concern has been expressed at cross-contamination during the decontamination process (3). Endoscopic procedures are becoming increasingly complex, particularly in the field of keyhole surgery; however, percutaneous endoscopic surgical procedures have impacted beneficially on the postoperative wound infection rate and by reducing hospital stay have also had an economic benefit. It is therefore important that the potential cross-infectious hazards from the instruments are reduced to a minimum by correct decontamination procedures.

Many endoscopic procedures are carried out with all-metal instruments and they are thus comparatively easy to decontaminate by autoclaving. There are still, however, large numbers of endoscopies performed with instruments that are flexible and heat-sensitive. It is this group of instruments that presents a considerable challenge to effective decontamination, in part because of their complex internal structure, with several very narrow-bore channels and difficult to clean valves and valve seats. An additional factor to be considered is the heavy work load on a clinic and consequently a short turnaround time between patients, thereby potentially making effective decontamination problematic.

Currently there are circumstances that set a particular challenge to the safe decontamination, not only of flexible but also rigid endoscopes, and these circumstances relate to viral and prion contamination of instruments (4). These circumstances take the emphasis for the safe reuse of instruments away from simply killing adherent microorganisms to removal of contaminating "soil" that may contain microbial nucleic acids, hazardous protein, and endotoxin. The availability of the polymerase chain reaction (PCR) has demonstrated that following decontamination procedures (5) it is possible to still detect the presence of microbial nucleic acid and that, although it may not be an infective hazard, it may well be hazardous for the patient by other mechanisms. These considerations have led to a reevaluation of current decontamination procedures by professional organizations and to the circulation of new protocols to deal with contaminated endoscopes (6–12).

To standardize the decontamination procedure for endoscopes, the instruments are now almost universally processed in automated washer/disinfectors. This does not obviate the need for an initial manual cleaning, which is vital to the whole decontamination process, but does ensure that all endoscopes are decontaminated in an identical fashion and frees the endoscopy nurses for other duties in the clinic. There is, however, a downside to the use of automated washer/disinfectors, which relates to recontamination of endoscopes by the machine after the disinfection stage. This is due to the growth of microorganisms within a biofilm present in the tanks and pipes of the washer/disinfector and thus recontamination during the final rinse prior to removal of the instrument from the machine (13). This problem has led to the reporting of pseudo-outbreaks of tuberculosis following bronchoscopy and to actual infection of patients with environmental gram-negative microorganisms. The manufacturers of automated washer/disinfectors have had to redesign the internal architecture of the machines and to otherwise modify them by including a self-disinfection cycle. The problem has also led to the development of systems for the provision of sterile water to the machine from the potable water supplies.

The commonest disinfectant that is used is 2% glutaraldehyde (14–18); however, in the United Kingdom one major manufacturer has withdrawn its product from the market and this has of necessity led to the use of other disinfectants. Glutaraldehyde does have two major disadvantages despite its efficacy as a disinfectant. It is now recognized to be a major cause of occupational allergy, giving rise to both pulmonary and skin hypersensitivity (19,20). Its other main disadvantage is that it acts as a fixative, and with concern expressed over prion proteins and the emphasis placed on soil removal from endoscopes, this characteristic in a disinfectant is unwelcome. The disinfectants that have replaced glutaraldehyde (in the U.K.) are very effective in killing microorganisms but are far more corrosive both to the endoscope and the washer/disinfector.

The area of endoscope decontamination is thus currently in a state of flux, and further developments are anticipated with respect to the processes of decontamination, the nature of disinfectants, and the materials from which endoscopes are manufactured.

TYPES OF ENDOSCOPES

Endoscopes are constructed from a diverse range of materials including plastic, metal, glass, and adhesives. They generally have a complex internal construction with narrow bore channels, external ports, and valves. Many different endoscopes are now produced for a variety of medical interventions, both therapeutic and diagnostic, including bronchoscopy, arthroscopy, laparoscopy, colonoscopy, gastroscopy, and cystoscopy. The endoscopes may be flexible or rigid, the latter usually made entirely of metal and are thus relatively easily decontaminated compared to the flexible endoscopes. They may be used as direct viewing instruments or for the collection of biopsy specimens, as videoendoscopes, or as endoscopes with an ultrasound attachment used for diagnostic purposes.

Endoscopes can be classified as critical instruments—those that penetrate the skin or sterile body cavities—or as semicritical instruments—those that are in contact with mucous membranes. However, this distinction is not clear-cut, as many semicritical instruments may be in contact with pathologic lesions, where the local defenses are breached, or they are used to take specimens, thus breaching local defense mechanisms.

Critical Instruments

These instruments include laparoscopes, cystoscopes, and arthroscopes. Some of these instruments such as the cystoscopes and laparoscopes may be rigid in construction, made out of metal, and are thus autoclavable.

Laparoscopes are used for visualizing the peritoneal cavity, penetrate the skin, and are increasingly used as surgical equipment involved in intraperitoneal operations such as cholecystectomy, hysterectomy, hernia repair, and tubal ligation. Similar instruments may also be used in the thoracic cavity for some surgical procedures.

Arthroscopes are also rigid and autoclavable, and are used for inspecting joint spaces and surgical procedures including meniscectomy. These instruments are also used percutaneously.

Hysteroscopes are used for visualizing the uterus, for removing polyps, for biopsies, and for resection of submucous fibroids.

Cystoscopes are often rigid, although ureteroscopes are flexible. These instruments are used for visualizing the urinary tract, for taking biopsies, removing small tumors and calculi, and dilating stenosed regions of the urinary tract. They may be passed into the renal tract through the urethra or directly into the renal pelvis percutaneously.

Other invasive endoscopes, which may be rigid or flexible, or may or may not have a channel, include angioscopes and ventriculoscopes. In general, the flexible operative endoscopes are heat labile and should be sterilized by ethylene oxide or gas plasma. The rigid ones may be autoclaved.

Semicritical Instruments

These instruments include gastroscopes, duodenoscopes, sigmoidoscopes, proctoscopes, colonoscopes, bronchoscopes, and laryngoscopes. Gastroscopes, duodenoscopes, and colonoscopes are long, flexible instruments, usually with four channels (suction, biopsy, air, and water) and corresponding ports and valves. The suction and biopsy channels are often combined within the insertion tube. Their intricate construction makes them difficult to clean, and the materials from which they are made make them difficult to decontaminate. These instruments are inserted through one of the natural orifices of the body, which has a rich normal flora. Bronchoscopes are thus categorized as semicritical despite the fact they enter a sterile body cavity. These instruments are used both diagnostically and for minor surgical procedures such as polyp removal or diathermy.

Accessories

A wide range of accessories is available for both critical and semicritical endoscopes including forceps, snares, diathermy, bougies, sphincterotomy knives, and lasers. Many of these accessories can be autoclaved, but increasingly manufacturers are supplying single-use disposable accessories. Laser and ultrasonic probes are expensive and not able to be autoclaved.

ETIOLOGY

The commonest microorganisms that cause endoscopy-associated infections or pseudoinfections are opportunistic gram-negative bacteria and mycobacteria that are associated with moisture or biofilms on an endoscopy processing apparatus (21,22). Microorganisms that have frequently been isolated include *Pseudomonas* species (23), *Serratia marcescens, Klebsiella, Escherichia,* and *Salmonella* species (24–31). Bronchoscopy has been associated with contamination or infection caused by *Mycobacterium tuberculosis, Mycobacterium kansasii,* and *Mycobacterium avium* (32–34). Cystoscopy has been associated with infections by *Escherichia, Enterococcus,* and *Proteus* species (35). Percutaneous endoscopy has been associated with skin flora and *Staphylococcus aureus* surgical site infections (36).

Less frequently identified pathogens that may be transmitted by endoscopic procedures include *Helicobacter pylori* (37,38), *Trichosporon asahii* (39), hepatitis B virus (40), and *Strongyloides* (41). Other microorganisms that may be transmitted by endoscopy include *Clostridium difficile, Cryptosporidia,* and enteroviruses.

PATHOGENESIS

Infections are derived either from an external source (exogenous) or from the patient's own microflora (endogenous). Endoscopically transmitted infection reported in the literature has been mainly exogenous, from inadequately decontaminated endoscopes, although endogenous infections have also been reported, particularly in association with urologic or percutaneous procedures.

Exogenous Spread of Infection

There are two main reasons for microorganisms being transmitted to a patient from an endoscope, which are to some extent related. On the one hand, the endoscope may be inadequately decontaminated. On the other hand, microorganisms produce and reside in a biofilm when in a moist environment, such as an endoscope or an endoscope washer/disinfector. Many bacteria secrete a carbohydrate substance, frequently called "slime," which forms the glycocalyx or matrix (the biofilm) within which the microorganisms can survive (42,43). Often biofilms contain complex microbial communities. The dynamics of the biofilm are still poorly understood, but what is certain is that microorganisms within the biofilm are more resistant to biocides than adherent but non–biofilm-associated bacteria or planktonic bacteria (44,45). Additionally, biofilms and the associated bacteria are resistant to hydrodynamic shear forces. Both these characteristics make eradication of microorganisms from endoscopes or endoscope washer/disinfectors difficult and predispose to failure of decontamination processes. The net result is that microorganisms are still present on the endoscope, or the endoscope becomes recontaminated following the decontamination procedure (46,47).

Airborne infection from staff members in the endoscopy room during percutaneous surgical procedures, although possible, is unlikely owing to the small incision produced. During endoscopic surgery the video screen may act as a source of contamination of the surgeons hands, as the electrostatic field generated by the screen facilitates the transfer of microorganisms from the screen to the gloved hands of the surgeon (48).

On the other hand, spread of infection from the patient to the staff is a very real risk during bronchoscopy, particularly when dealing with patients who have tuberculosis. Similar concern has been expressed about staff members acquiring infection with human immunodeficiency virus (HIV) when performing endoscopy on patients who are infected (49). In one study of 427 urologic procedures, contamination of the surgeon's skin or mucous membranes occurred in 32%. Thirty-three percent were endoscopic procedures and in these, contamination of the face or eyes occurred in 46% (50). Although in practice the risks of infection are small, the risks of contamination in some procedures are high, and appropriate physical precautions have been almost universally introduced.

In addition to the transfer of microorganisms to the patient, who may then become colonized, whether or not the patients develop an infection is due to other contributory factors such as their underlying medical condition, the treatment they may be receiving, and whether they already have a focus of infection such as an obstructed bile duct (51).

Endogenous Spread of Infection

Endogenous infection may be due to transfer of microorganisms from one site to another during the insertion or removal of the endoscope. Mouth flora may be transferred to the stomach or to the bronchi during gastroscopy or bronchoscopy. Mouth, stomach, or duodenal flora may be transferred to the biliary or pancreatic system during endoscopic retrograde cholangiopancreatography (ERCP). Intestinal flora may contaminate the oral cavity on removal of a gastroduodenoscope or ERCP. Similarly, skin flora may be introduced into the peritoneal cavity, pleural cavity, or joint; vaginal flora may be introduced into the uterus; fecal, skin, or urethral flora may be introduced into the bladder or kidneys during urological procedures.

INFECTIONS ASSOCIATED WITH ENDOSCOPY

The insertion, manipulation, or removal of the endoscope may be associated with bacteremia, usually with the patient's own microflora but rarely from microorganisms contaminating the endoscope. More usually, pseudoinfections have been reported in the literature, due to contamination of a patient's specimen by a microorganism derived from the endoscope. Percutaneous procedures may be followed by surgical site infections or joint infections, peritonitis, bacteremia, or empyema.

Invasive Endoscopy

Surveys of infective complications following minimally invasive procedures are few, and there is little evidence to show they are due to contaminated endoscopes as opposed to complications of the procedure. Surveys between 1975 and 1980 of, in one case, over 100,000 laparoscopies (52) showed an infection rate of 3% to 4%, with only seven possibly being due to nonsterile equipment. In a second survey of over 10,000 laparoscopies (53), three cases of surgical site infection were reported, none of which were thought to be due to contaminated equipment. In 1991 a prospective study of 1,518 laparoscopic cholecystectomies showed an infection rate of 0.9% to 2.0% (54). In 1999 a retrospective survey of 1,702 laparoscopic cholecystectomies (55) showed an infection rate of 2.3%, with a surgical site infection rate of 0.4%. The commonest infective complication following this procedure is septic complications after spillage of gallstones in the peritoneal cavity (56–58), and not due to a failure of decontamination procedures. In 2002 a Cochrane Review of laparoscopic appendectomy compared to open appendectomy covering 45 studies (59) showed that wound infection following the laparoscopic procedure was half as likely as with the open procedure, but that intraabdominal abscess was three times as likely. It was not suggested that failed decontamination procedures were the cause of any of the infective complications.

Infections following arthroscopy are uncommon, with, in one survey of 12,505 procedures, an infection rate of 0.04% being reported (60). Postprocedure infections do occur, usually with skin flora and usually due to environmental contamination rather that poor decontamination of the arthroscope. In one study, three joint infections occurred in 155 arthroscopies (61), but following alteration of environmental factors, there were no subsequent infections in 222 procedures. In one more recent study, *Candida albicans* infection occurred following arthroscopy. Infectious complications can also follow other laparoscopic orthopedic procedures and in one case lumbar discitis occurred following laparoscopic sacrocolpopexy (62), although there was no indication this was due to failed decontamination.

Cystoscopes were among the first endoscopes to be used, and initially inadequate disinfection was responsible for infection. Many of the cystoscopes can be autoclaved, although flexible heat-sensitive cystoscopes are also used. In the 1950s it was shown that patients were developing infections within a few days of the procedure (63). A number of disinfectants were introduced, and since the use of 2% glutaraldehyde and antibiotic prophylaxis, the postprocedure infection rate is small. In a study of 161 cystoscopies, an infection rate of 7.5% was reported with microorganisms derived from endogenous flora, giving no suggestion that failed decontamination procedures were to blame (64). In a study of 420 patients following flexible cystoscopy, 110 patients donated a postprocedure urine specimen 3 days following the investigation, with 2.7% showing evidence of infection (65). Percutaneous urologic procedures, such as nephrostomy or insertion of ureteral endoprosthesis, in one study had a complication rate of 7%, with 0.87% being due to urinary tract infection. Minor complications of skin inflammation occurred in 5.3%, but in no case was it thought to be due to poor decontamination procedures (66).

Infections are also a complication of cardiovascular cannulation, although there is no suggestion that these infections are due to failed decontamination procedures, as the cannulas are sterile, single-use items. In a retrospective study between 1991 and 1998 of 22,006 procedures, there were 25 cases of bacteremia (0.11%) with 0.24% following percutaneous transluminal coronary angioplasty, 0.06% following cardiac catheterization, and 0.08% following electrophysiologic studies. The majority of the infections were with gram-negative bacteria (67) (see also Chapter 62).

Gastrointestinal Endoscopy

Infections associated with gastrointestinal endoscopy are uncommon, and several surveys dating from the 1970s have shown a rate of less than 1%. In a survey of over 240,000 gastrointestinal endoscopies, only 24 infective complications were reported, including four fatal cases, two of cholangitis and two of pancreatitis (68). In a further study, 116 infective complications were reported, which included bacteremia, hepatitis B, endocarditis, aspiration pneumonia, and Creutzfeldt-Jakob disease (CJD) (14). The microorganisms isolated included enteric gram-negative bacteria such as *Serratia* and *Salmonella*, environmental bacteria such as *Pseudomonas*, and gram-positive bacteria such as *S. aureus*. In a survey in the U.K. of 164,000 endoscopies, the infection rate was 0.74% for ERCP, but of those infected, there was a high mortality rate of 26% (69). Percutaneous endoscopic gastrostomy (PEG) is a procedure for establishing enteral feeding (70). In one study of 166 PEG procedures, the complication rate was 16.3%, with wound infections occurring in 5.4%, including one case of necrotizing fasciitis. Esophagoscopy has been linked to the transmission of *Pseudomonas* with, in some cases, evidence of infection and death following septicemia (71).

Lower respiratory tract infection has also followed endoscopy, again with *Pseudomonas*, which probably relates to aspiration of oral secretions associated with a contaminated endoscope (72).

Following sigmoidoscopy, a 10% prevalence of bacteremia that was detectable over a period of 15 minutes has been reported, although no obvious infective complications were noted (73). Transient bacteremia has also been reported in other studies (74–77).

Procedures involving sclerotherapy with *N*-butyl-2 cyanoacrylate have been shown to have a high rate of bacteremia and peritonitis, ranging from 5% to 53% and 0.5% to 3%, respectively (78,79), and in some cases endocarditis or abscess has occurred following endoscopy (80–82). An alternative approach is the use of a covered needle (Clisco needle) whose tip does not become contaminated during insertion of the endoscope (83). Culture of the tip of covered needles compared to non-covered needles showed a lower contamination rate for the covered needle and by implication this may lower the rate of postprocedure bacteremia. However, endoscopic variceal ligation is replacing sclerotherapy as the method of choice to control bleeding. This procedure has a 3% to 14% risk of bacteremia, with 11/67 patients developing bacteremia and 2/67 developing peritonitis (78).

Salmonella Infections

A microorganism that is easily identified as cross-infection due to a poorly decontaminated endoscope is *Salmonella*, because this microorganism would not normally be found in the environment of an endoscopy room as a contaminant. Cross-infection with *Salmonella* would be likely to cause an infection, even in relatively healthy individuals, in comparison to the environmental opportunist microorganisms commonly linked to failed endoscope decontamination, such as *Klebsiella* and *Pseudomonas*. Most of the cases of transmission of *Salmonella*, and there have been relatively few, date from the 1970s to 1980s, and in all cases disinfectants were used that would be regarded as inappropriate by current standards (29–31). The agents that were used to decontaminate the endoscopes were skin antiseptics—chlorhexidine, cetrimide, povidone-iodine, hexachlorophene, and quaternary ammonium compounds. The majority of reported infections occurred prior to 1983, with only three more cases reported by 1992 and none to the current time. Since the late 1980s, glutaraldehyde and more recently other agents have been used to decontaminate endoscopes, with the effect that there are fewer reported incidents of cross-infection from an endoscope contaminated with enteric gram-negative bacteria.

Endoscopic Retrograde Cholangiopancreatography

Infection following ERCP is more common than with other forms of gastrointestinal endoscopy, particularly when the biliary tree is obstructed. A postal survey of 10,000 endoscopies showed an infection rate of 3%. Most complications were due to pancreatitis, but cholangitis and cases of infected pancreatic pseudocyst also occurred, as did a small number of cases of aspiration pneumonia (84). Exogenous infection leading to septicemia, following the use of a contaminated endoscope for ERCP, has also been reported. The microorganism isolated from the patient's blood, the endoscope, and the water reservoir was *Pseudomonas aeruginosa* (85). In a survey of 690 ERCPs, fever occurred in 12 patients and five of these died of septicemia (86). Microorganisms isolated were *Pseudomonas, Klebsiella, Proteus,* and *Escherichia*. Several other reports have documented infections following ERCP, frequently in association with biliary stasis, and thus likely to be of endogenous origin, but also following the use of inappropriate disinfectants as mentioned previously, or more recently incidents have been reported following recontamination of the endoscope from the endoscope washer/disinfector. In both cases outbreaks due to *Pseudomonas* have been reported (87–90). In one report the post-ERCP infection rate in one hospital increased from 1.6% to 3.6% following the use of a new automated washer/disinfector. The microorganisms causing the bacteremia were *Pseudomonas* and enteric gram-negative bacteria. Seven epidemic strains causing infection were genomically related as shown by macro-restriction DNA analysis and accounted for 55% of the episodes. Effective decontamination of the washer/disinfector led to a reduction in the infection rate to preincident levels (91).

In a report from the United States, *Pseudomonas* was isolated from ten patients following ERCP. Five developed sepsis and one died (92). The same strain (serotype 10) was isolated from the endoscope and persisted in the unit for 9 months. Factors involved in its persistence were probably inadequate decontamination of the endoscope, recontamination from the rinse water of the washer/disinfector, and inadequate drying of the endoscope. *Pseudomonas* has also been implicated in other cases of infection in association with high counts of the microorganism in the biopsy channel and samples of rinse water from the washer disinfector immediately after disinfection with glutaraldehyde (46, 93,94). The mechanism of persistence in this case was lack of circulation of the disinfectant to all areas in the washer/disinfector and the formation of a biofilm containing the microorganism, which acted as a source of recontamination.

Viral Hepatitis Associated with Endoscopy

There is little evidence of viral transmission after endoscopy. Both bronchoscopes and gastroscopes become contaminated with HIV when used on patients with the acquired immune deficiency syndrome (AIDS), yet there is no evidence of transmission following endoscopy. Studies have shown that mechanical cleaning of endoscopes removes even high concentrations of HIV and that glutaraldehyde rapidly inactivates the virus (95). There is a single well-documented case of hepatitis B virus (HBV) transmission between patients (40), but most studies have not been able to document transmission. Of 394 patients followed up after exposure, none showed clinical evidence of infection (96). There have been three reported cases of hepatitis C virus (HCV) transmission, one following ERCP, and two following colonoscopy, and in all cases decontamination was found to have been ineffectively carried out (97). In a study of 19 patients with HCV using molecular techniques to detect the virus, a blood sample taken from the patient was positive prior to the procedure, and 53% of the endoscopes were contaminated with the virus immediately after removal, but after both mechanical cleaning and mechanical cleaning followed by immersion in a disinfection, none were contaminated (98). Thus current decontamination procedures appear to be sufficiently robust to prevent viral transmission following endoscopy.

Bronchoscopy and Infection

A bronchoscope is less complex than a gastrointestinal endoscope, having fewer channels to decontaminate. However, bronchoscopes are used to obtain bronchoalveolar lavage (BAL) specimens in which the pulmonary tree is washed out with saline. There is thus the potential to contaminate the specimen from an inadequately decontaminated endoscope, giving a false clinical impression that the patient is infected. The most frequently reported pseudoinfection is with mycobacterial species, but they have also been reported with *Pseudomonas* found in bronchial washings following bronchoscopy (21). In a study in 1982, 11 of 19 specimens were contaminated with the same serotype 10, which was also isolated from the bronchoscopy channels (99). In another study 82/103 BAL specimens were contaminated by *P. aeruginosa* (100), but again no infections were reported. As with gastrointestinal endoscopy in the 1970s and early 1980s, the disinfectants used were inappropriate. Microorganisms other than *Pseudomonas* have also been linked to outbreaks of pseudoinfections as well as true infective complications. Following bronchoscopy on a patient with *Serratia marcescens* pneumonia, the microorganism was found in the tracheal washings of three other patients (101). Other sources of outbreaks of pseudoinfection have been linked to contaminated sterile water (102) and lens cleaner (103). Finally, *Proteus* species have also been associated with pseudoinfections following bronchoscopy (104).

Gram-negative bacteria are relatively susceptible to disinfectants, compared to the more hardy mycobacteria. Additionally, mycobacteria are also found in water supplies and can grow in biofilm in pipe work. It is therefore not surprising that infections with *M. tuberculosis* and many pseudoinfections with other mycobacterial species have been reported. A retrospective survey of 8,750 bronchoscopies showed that contamination occurred in eight, but there was no evidence of infection (105). *M. tuberculosis* has been isolated from washings of a bronchoscope after it had been decontaminated in povidone-iodine, and transmission was documented from one patient to another in a separate episode. In this case the bronchoscope had also been disinfected in povidone-iodine, and *in vitro* studies showed that this was an ineffective agent for mycobacteria (106). In one month in 1999 five *M. tuberculosis* BAL specimens were reported in one hospital that overall had a low rate of tuberculosis. A retrospective survey for the whole year showed that 19 bronchoscopies had been performed with 10 of 18 BAL specimens positive. Two patients were infected prior to endoscopy and two became infected after the procedure. Six patients had positive specimens but did not develop infection. The majority of the isolates were indistinguishable on restriction fragment length polymorphism analysis. In one of the three endoscopes that was used during this period a small hole was discovered in the sheath, and as leak testing had not been performed regularly, this had allowed a contaminated endoscope to be unwitting used (107).

True infections following bronchoscopy are uncommon. The complication rate of 24,521 bronchoscopic procedures assessed from 192 replies of a questionaire was 0.08% with a mortality of 0.01% (108), with fever in eight patients and pneumonia in two. In a prospective study of 100 bronchoscopies, fever occurred in 16% and lung infiltration in 6% (109). In a prospective study of fever and bacteremia following bronchoscopy in immunocompetent children, of 91 children investigated, 48% developed fever within 24 hours but bacteremia was not detected (110). In those children that developed fever, 40.5% of the BAL specimens had a significant bacterial growth.

There have been numerous reports of pseudoinfections with other mycobacterial species, and on some occasions this has led to inappropriate treatment. In one study *Mycobacterium xenopi* was isolated from 13 clinical specimens, although none had clinical evidence of mycobacterial infection. Five of these patients received antituberculosis therapy (111). An important factor was rinsing bronchoscopes with tap water and gargling with tap water prior to sputum collection. In another study over a period of 37 months, 35% of mycobacterial isolates were *M. xenopi*. Four of the patients had *M. xenopi*–associated disease; the remaining were pseudoinfections. An important risk factor was rinsing bronchoscopes after disinfection in tap water (112). Other mycobacterial species have also been associated with bronchoscopy. A pseudo-outbreak of *Mycobacterium abscessus* occurring in 15 patients was traced to the use of an automated washer/disinfector (13). Pseudo-outbreaks in association with the use of automated washer disinfectors have also been reported with *Mycobacterium chelonae* and *Methylobacterium mesophilicum* (113). Colonization by the microorganisms was linked to bronchoscopy, and the microorganisms were also isolated from the endoscopes, washer disinfectors, and glutaraldehyde taken from the washer/disinfector. Some strains of *Mycobacterium chelonae* are known to be resistant to glutaraldehyde.

Miscellaneous Microorganisms and Sources

Bacillus species have been found in bronchial washing in one hospital, although none of the patients were infected. The source seemed to be the automatic suction valve (114). Fears have been raised that anthrax may be transmitted by endoscopy, although studies of the efficacy of current disinfectants indicate that they would be effective in killing the microorganism (115). An outbreak of *Aeromonas hydrophila* pseudoinfection was reported. The endoscopes were decontaminated with a disinfectant containing a quaternary ammonium compound and glutaraldehyde phenate. The use of 2% glutaraldehyde eradicated the problem (116). *Strongyloides stercoralis* has been transmitted by gastroscopy (41), and also cross-infection with *H. pylori* may occur (37, 38). Fungal infections and pseudoinfections have been reported with *Trichosporon* species (39) and *Aureobasidium* species; the latter was linked to the reuse of plastic stopcocks (117). Finally, in 169 patients following ERCP, 12.7% were positive for *Cryptosporidium* oocytes (118). This is a particular risk for AIDS patients, especially as the microorganism is resistant to most disinfectants. (See Chapter 8 for more information on pseudoinfections.)

CONTROL OF INFECTION

As mentioned, endoscope-associated infection can be either endogenous or exogenous in origin. Endogenous infections may be prevented by appropriate skin preparation or chemoprophylaxis prior to the procedure. Exogenous infections would be prevented by effective decontamination procedures. In this latter category, infections that have followed endoscopy have arisen from the use of inappropriate disinfectants, breakdown in the decontamination process, or recontamination from an automated washer/disinfector.

Several aspects of the prevention of exogenous infection from endoscopes have taken on current importance (119–122). Surveys have shown that there are particular failings in the application of recommended decontamination procedures in many countries (18,123–126). In Britain there is a particular concern that CJD may be transmitted on endoscopes, and this has led to interest in the efficacy of soil removal from endoscopes. Additionally, as current decontamination procedures incorporate the use of automated washer/disinfectors and as there have been pseudoinfections linked to recontamination of an adequately disinfected endoscope from a washer/disinfector, attention has focused on the provision of sterile water for the final rinse of the endoscope. One final current concern in Britain is the removal of 2% glutaraldehyde by one major manufacturer from the marketplace due to problems with sensitization. This has led to the realization that monitoring of staff health is an important issue, as is the assessment of new disinfectants.

Flexible endoscopes are complex, reusable instruments that require unique consideration with respect to decontamination. In addition to the external surface of the endoscope their internal channels are exposed to body fluids and other contaminants. In contrast to rigid endoscopes and some reusable accessories, flexible endoscopes are heat labile and cannot be autoclaved or washed ultrasonically.

The scheme introduced by Spaulding (127) to separate medical devices into critical, semicritical, or noncritical categories depending on their relationship with mucosal surfaces or sterile body cavities does not adequately cover the issues raised by the development of complex, heat-sensitive endoscopes, some of which are introduced into body cavities. This has led to difficulties in sometimes choosing an adequate disinfection regimen and to controversy over the correct regimen for others. According to the Spaulding scheme, arthroscopes and laparoscopes, because they are critical items, should be sterilized. However, mostly these items are decontaminated by high-level disinfection, and the data show that infection following the use of these items is minimal. There is no evidence to suggest that sterilization of these items will reduce the rate of infection, and to do so would involve the use of either ethylene oxide or gas plasma.

Decontamination of Endoscopes

Decontamination is a process that renders the endoscope safe to use on another patient and consists of a mandatory cleaning step followed either by a disinfection or sterilization process. Cleaning removes many of the microorganisms as well as biologic fluids from the surfaces of the endoscope. Thorough cleaning with a detergent (neutral or enzymatic) is one of the main requirements for the effective reprocessing of endoscopes and accessories and is essential to maximize the effectiveness of the subsequent disinfection or sterilization step. Cleaning should comprise an initial mechanical cleaning of the endoscope once removed from the patient, followed by an obligatory clean in an automated washer or washer/disinfector followed by sterilization or high-level disinfection. The cleaning step should include all channels and valves as well as the insertion tube. The channels should be vigorously brushed and the brush sterilized or disposed of (128). The decontamination of reusable accessories was found to be cheaper in one study compared to the use of disposable accessories (129); however, the advantage of using disposable accessories is the lower risk of cross-contamination and the avoidance of the need to track the accessories and record their use in the patient's notes.

Sterilization is defined as the destruction or removal of all viable microorganisms including spores. The Food and Drug Administration (FDA) defines sterilization as a 12-log reduction in the bacterial spore count. The adherence of prions presents a special challenge. In practice, assessment of sterilization in the laboratory requires the killing of spores of *Bacillus subtilis* or *Bacillus stearothermophilus.* According to the Spaulding criteria, cystoscopes, arthroscopes, and laparoscopes should be sterile, but in practice high-level disinfection is frequently used. However, wherever possible, instruments that penetrate a sterile body cavity should be sterilized.

Disinfection is more difficult to define. It implies the removal or destruction of vegetative microorganisms excluding spores; the process reduces the bioload on the endoscope to a safe level, although this may vary with circumstances. In laboratory tests the disinfectant must pass one of the National tests, which usually involves the reduction of a panel of vegetative microorganisms including viruses and mycobacteria by 10^5 in 5 minutes in either clean or dirty conditions, i.e., without or with the addition of an organic soil.

Surface Contamination of Endoscopes

After removal of the endoscope from a patient, it is inevitably contaminated with microorganisms and organic matter. An important consideration is how effectively the decontamination process reduces this contamination. In a study in Italy over a 2-year period, surveillance of contamination of gastroscopes demonstrated that 60.5% were contaminated on the outer surface and the channels were contaminated in 41.3% (130). Similar figures were found for colonoscopes. The microorganisms most frequently isolated were *Pseudomonas* and *Staphylococcus* species. A study investigating the contamination of the air and water channels in endoscopes showed that the air channel in 42 endoscopes and the water channel in only one endoscope was not contaminated (131). There was, however, organic matter present in both channels as determined by amido black staining. This was markedly reduced by effective brushing of the channels. Investigations using sterile, single-use biopsy forceps that had been passed through the channel of an endoscope at different stages of the decontamination cycle showed the effectiveness of the decontamination process (132). The endoscopes were tested prior to use, directly postprocedure, after manual cleaning, and after manual cleaning and exposure to 2% glutaraldehyde, and showed overwhelming contamination with microorganisms immediately after removal from the patient. Microorganisms were present in 25% of cases after manual cleaning and 0% after exposure to glutaraldehyde.

In a further study of the effect of drying on the bioburden of duodenoscopes, endoscopes that had been processed in an automatic washer were sampled through the suction channel at 2, 24, and 48 hours postdisinfection (133). Fifty percent of the endoscopes were contaminated mainly with *Pseudomonas* species and mainly after 48 hours. After an additional drying period was introduced, the contamination fell to 0%, thus emphasizing the importance of drying the endoscope, particularly the channels, prior to storage. Similar results were obtained in a different study (134). In this case the bioburden following removal of the endoscope was 7.0×10^9, which was reduced to 1.3×10^5 by cleaning. Gram-negative bacilli were the most numerous contaminant (*E. coli* and *Bacteroides*) found immediately after removal and *Pseudomonas* after cleaning. In addition to microbial contamination, the endoscopes are also contaminated with organic matter. An investigation of the suction channel from a variety of endoscopes (bronchoscope, duodenoscope, colonoscope) were assessed immediately after removal from the patient and after mechanical cleaning but prior to disinfection or sterilization (135). The highest level of soiling was not unexpectedly found immediately after removal from the patient with high levels of protein, sodium, hemoglobin, bilirubin, carbohydrate, endotoxin, and bacteria. Colonoscopes were the most contaminated. After mechanical cleaning, the levels of most contaminants fell by five- to tenfold with a 3- to 5-log reduction in bacterial contamination. Although cleaning does reduce the level of bioburden and organic contamination, a significant amount still remains.

Transmissible Spongiform Encephalopathies and Endoscopy

Transmissible spongiform encephalopathies (TSE) are a group of neurologic conditions that lead to dementia and are caused by a protein agent called a prion, PrP^{sc}, which is an abnormal variant of a normal cellular protein PrP^{c} (136). Prion proteins are resistant to inactivation by a wide range of sterilization and disinfection processes. The best known of the TSEs is CJD and a modified variant (vCJD) that was first reported in the U.K. in 1996 and that has different clinical and histopathologic appearances. This new-variant CJD is thought to have been transmitted to the human population via food products from beef cattle that were suffering from bovine spongiform encephalopathy (BSE or mad cow disease). Cattle are thought to have contracted BSE by having been fed on processed animal feed. The prion protein of vCJD is found in high concentration in the lymphoreticular system (137) and is thus of particular concern in endoscopy in which biopsies are taken from the small intestine where there is a high concentration of Peyer's patches or ear, nose, and throat (ENT) endoscopy involving the tonsillar tissue (138). The European Society of Gastrointestinal Endoscopy and the U.K. government have issued advice on preventing transmission of vCJD by endoscopy (4,139). The particular concern is the contamination of endoscopes by proteins that are resistant to removal or destruction, because current routine methods of sterilization or high-level disinfection are incapable of inactivating the prion. This places a greater emphasis on the physical cleaning steps prior to sterilization/disinfection and an argument for the use of disposable accessories, particularly biopsy forceps (see also Chapters 47 and 85).

Washer/Disinfectors and Sterile Water

Washer/disinfectors are now recommended as part of the decontamination process rather than a manual wash, as they are more effective and more consistent, and reduce the potential contact with sensitizing agents (140,141). Owing to both the reports of outbreaks of pseudoinfection with gram-negative bacteria and mycobacteria and the importance of removing contaminating organic material from endoscopes, the key role of the washer/disinfector has become an issue. Guidelines have been promulgated on the purchase of washer/disinfectors and the criteria that should be taken into consideration (142). Essentially, the machine must clean, disinfect, and rinse all channels, provide a supply of sterile water for terminal rinsing, contain and filter disinfectant fumes, be equipped with a self-disinfection cycle that irrigates all channels of the washer/disinfector, and finally provide a readout that can be incorporated into the patient's notes.

A controversial issue is the provision of sterile water for the terminal rinsing of endoscopes. In the U.K., HTM 2030 (143) provides precise details on the routine testing of washer/disinfectors to achieve sterile rinse water, even down to the level of allowable endotoxin. However, doubt has been expressed as to its importance, particularly with respect to gastrointestinal endoscopes (144), and concerns have been expressed as to the suitability and practicality of the standards (145). The concern is the ability to actually obtain sterile rinse water, given the difficulty in controlling the formation of biofilm, which makes eradication of the microorganism from the internal channels of the washer disinfector very difficult (146). A study of a new washer/disinfector that was fitted with a water-filtration system to provide a supply of sterile water showed that only 24% of the samples of final rinse water were culture negative over a 6-month period (147). In some cases fungal contamination was found (148). Current methods of trying to obtain sterile water for rinsing include the use of pharmaceutical grade water (which is expensive and impractical), filters, UV light, raised water temperature, and the addition of a biocide.

Decontamination Processes

Items penetrating a sterile body cavity ideally should be sterile, although as discussed above there is some controversy over this. Nevertheless, rigid instruments can be autoclaved. Alternative methods include ethylene oxide, gas plasma, and low temperature steam/formaldehyde or prolonged insertion in a disinfectant. If instruments have been used on a case of CJD, the U.K. recommendations are that they should be incinerated or kept in reserve for future use on a known case of CJD. For operations on known CJD patients, disposable equipment should be used as far as possible. If there is some doubt whether a patient has CJD or not, the instrument or endoscope should be quarantined until a histologic diagnosis is available. Some processes can inactivate the prion protein but can be damaging to instruments, particularly flexible ones. Autoclaving at 134° to 137°C for 18 minutes may be effective in some cases. Immersion in 1 N sodium hydroxide or 20,000 parts per million (ppm) free chlorine or 96% formic acid for 1 hour will inactivate prions (139) but in the routine situation are not practicable (see also Chapter 85).

High-Level Disinfection of Flexible Endoscopes

High-level disinfection of flexible endoscopes involves initial manual cleaning, followed by the use of an automated washer/disinfector that initially mechanically washes the endoscope followed by a period of immersion in a suitable disinfectant. Until recently, 2% glutaraldehyde has been the most commonly used disinfectant. Its advantages are a long in-use life, a broad spectrum of activity, and compatibility with equipment. Its disadvantages are its capacity to cause sensitization in healthcare staff and that it fixes proteins to surfaces. This latter characteristic is unwanted in the light of concerns about prions. Further, some reports have highlighted the emergence of glutaraldehyde-resistance mycobacterial species from the biofilm in washer/disinfectors (149).

Several other agents are now available for high-level disinfection of flexible endoscopes (150,151). Generally, they are more active than glutaraldehyde, providing shorter contact times, but they are also more corrosive to equipment, more expensive, and have a shorter in-use life.

Orthophthalaldehyde

Orthophthalaldehyde (OPA) is a substitute for 2% glutaraldehyde. It has a lower vapor pressure than glutaraldehyde and is thus less likely to cause adverse reactions in healthcare staff, although it does have the same sensitization capacity as glutaraldehyde to exacerbate dermatitis or asthma. It has a similar spectrum of activity to glutaraldehyde, inactivating a broad range of bacteria, viruses, and fungi. It is active against HIV and HBV and is more active than glutaraldehyde against mycobacterial species (152). Its activity against *Cryptosporidia* is, like glutaraldehyde, poor (153). It is similar to glutaraldehyde in its in-use life and in its capacity to fix proteins.

Peracetic Acid

Peracetic acid is available as a liquid disinfectant or as part of a decontamination system incorporating a washer/disinfector (Steris Corporation, Mentor, OH) (154,155). Peracetic acid has a broad spectrum of activity and has greater mycobactericidal activity than glutaraldehyde and is active against glutaraldehyde-resistant mycobacteria (154,156–159). In a comparison with ethylene oxide, peracetic acid was more effective at decontaminating lumina (160), and in a prospective study of contamination in bronchoscopes there was no incidence of cross-contamination in 220 procedures. Additionally, artificial contamination with *Mycobacterium gordonae* was effectively inactivated by peracetic acid (161). It has a shorter in-use life and must be replaced daily. It also is corrosive to flexible endoscopes, and washer/disinfectors have to be modified in order to use the disinfectant.

Chlorine Dioxide

Chlorine dioxide is an effective disinfectant that has a broad spectrum of activity including spores and mycobacteria and some modest activity against cysts of gastrointestinal pathogens such as *Giardia* and *Cryptosporidia* (162–165). It is corrosive and gives off irritant fumes, and some endoscope manufacturers do not recommend that chlorine dioxide be used on their products.

Superoxidized Water

Superoxidized water is the anodal product of the electrolysis of a salt solution. It is vital that the parameters of the electrolysis are adhered to, as an effective agent is only produced by electrolysis of a 0.05% solution of saline at 950 mV. The disinfectant has a broad range of activity (166,167) but is inactivated in the presence or organic matter and adversely affects the polymer coating of some endoscopes. The polymer of endoscopes can be protected with a coating of Optiflex or Scope Protection System (Sterilox Technologies Inc., Mount Olive, NJ). Its active half-life is less than 24 hours and should be used only once and then discarded. The disinfectant could be ideally tailored to be a component of an endoscope/washer disinfector and be continuously produced at the point of use.

Other Agents

Alcohol is an effective antimicrobial against vegetative bacteria including mycobacteria and viruses except for enteroviruses (162,168). Alcohol does not have activity against bacterial spores. Because of the risk of fire, alcohol is not used as a primary disinfectant for endoscopes, but it is useful for flushing the channels as it enhances the drying of the endoscope. Prolonged exposure to alcohol can damage the polymer of the endoscope as well as the lens cement. Other compounds such as iodophors, peroxygen compounds, and quaternary ammonium compounds have been used in the past to decontaminate endoscopes and have been associated with cross-contamination. Newer formulations of some of these agents have been developed, but few data are available on their efficacy, and they are currently not recommended for high-level disinfection of flexible endoscopes.

Gas Plasma Technology

The Sterrad sterilization system (Johnson & Johnson, Irvine, CA) is a low-temperature method that utilizes hydrogen peroxide converted to a plasma, in a vacuum, by MHz electromagnetic radiation. The equipment resembles an autoclave, and like an autoclave a vacuum is drawn prior to injection of hydrogen peroxide. This is then converted to a plasma, and the free radicals kill a wide range of microorganisms including spores and mycobacteria (169–171). For sterilization of endoscopes that have narrow channels, special adaptors are required for the end of each channel, or the channels will not be effectively decontaminated (169). An organic load can also lead to the failure of decontamination (172) (see also Chapters 85 and 86).

CONCLUSION

Infective complications of endoscopy are relatively rare. Few problems of infection occur with operative endoscopes that are sterilized or given high-level disinfection even though they penetrate sterile sites. The majority of infections associated with percutaneous and operative endoscopes relate to endogenous infection. These are principally bacteremia, endocarditis, or abscesses.

Both exogenous and endogenous infections occur in relation to flexible endoscopy, although the incidence is low. Since the advent of totally immersible endoscopes decontaminated with glutaraldehyde and other more potent disinfectants, the incidence of reported cross-infection is low compared to that in the 1970s and early 1980s when nonimmersible endoscopes and inappropriate endoscope disinfectants were more commonly used.

Current concerns in relation to exogenous infection for flexible endoscopy are recontamination of the endoscope from the endoscope washer/disinfector, the provision and value of providing sterile rinse water, and the ability to eradicate biofilm from the washer/disinfector with a total self-disinfection cycle. Another important consideration is the ability to remove organic soil from the endoscope, particularly in relation to contamination by prions and the tracking of instruments to facilitate epidemiologic investigation.

Several agents have been developed and are in use that are more rapidly acting than glutaraldehyde but have a shorter shelf life and are more corrosive. The long-term effects on staff are unknown, reinforcing the need for continual staff monitoring of the long-term health effects. Similarly, long-term follow-up of patients in the community following endoscopy will provide a more accurate quantitation of the burden of postendoscopy infection.

REFERENCES

1. Benjamin SB, Bond JH. Transmission of infection by endoscopy. *Ann Intern Med* 1993;119:440–441.
2. Nelson DB, Barkun AN, Block KP, et al. Technology status evaluation report. Transmission of infection by gastrointestinal endoscopy. *Gastrointest Endosc* 2001;54:824–828.
3. Uttley AHC, Simpson RA. Audit of bronchoscope disinfection: a survey of procedures in England and Wales, and incidence of mycobacterial contamination. *J Hosp Infect* 1994;26:301–308.
4. Axon AT, Beilenhoff U, Bramble MG, et al. Guidelines Committee. European Society of Gastrointestinal Endoscopy (ESGE). Variant Creutzfeldt-Jacob disease (vCJD) and gastrointestinal Endoscopy. *Endoscopy* 2001;33:1070–1080.
5. Deva AK, Vickery K, Zou J, et al. Detection of persistent vegetative bacteria and amplified viral nucleic acid from in-use testing of gastrointestinal endoscopes. *J Hosp Infect* 1998;39:149–157.
6. Anon. Cleaning and disinfection of equipment for gastrointestinal endoscopy. Report of a Working Party for the British Society of Gastrointestinal Endoscopy Committee. *Gut* 1998;42:585–593.
7. Ayliffe G, Minimal Access Therapy Decontamination Working Group. Decontamination of minimally invasive surgical endoscopes and accessories. *J Hosp Infect* 2000;45:263–277.
8. Systchenko R, Marchetti B, Canard JM, et al. Recommendations for the cleaning and disinfection procedures in digestive tract endoscopy. The French Society of Digestive Endoscopy. *Gastroenterol Clin Biol* 2000;24:520–529.
9. Alvarado CJ, Reichelderfer M. APIC guideline for infection prevention and control in flexible endoscopy. Association for Professionals in Infection Control. *Am J Infect Control* 2000;28:138–155.
10. British Thoracic Society Bronchoscopy Guidelines Committee, a Sub-

committee of Standards of Care Committee of British Thoracic Society. British Thoracic Society guidelines on diagnostic flexible bronchoscopy. *Thorax* 2001;56(suppl 1):11–21.

11. Cooke RPD, Feneley RCL, Aycliffe G, et al. Decontamination of urological equipment: interim report of the Working Group of the Standing Committee on Urological Instruments of the British Association of Urological Surgeons. *Br J Urol* 1993;71:5–9.
12. Baker K, McCullagh L. Comparison of actual and recommended ENT endoscope disinfection practices by geographical regions in the United States. *ORL Head Neck Nurs* 1997;15:14–17.
13. Maloney S, Welbel S, Daves B, et al. *Mycobacterium abscessus* pseudoinfection traced to an automated endoscope washer: utility of epidemiologic and laboratory investigation. *J Infect Dis* 1994;169: 1166–1169.
14. Gorse GJ, Messner RL. Infection control practices in gastro-intestinal endoscopy in the United States: a national survey. *Infect Control Hosp Epidemiol* 1991;12:289–296.
15. Rutala WA, Clontz EP, Weber DJ, et al. Disinfection practices for endoscopes and other critical items. *Infect Control Hosp Epidemiol* 1991;12:282–288.
16. Kacmarek RG, Moore RM, McCrohan J, et al. Multistate investigation of the actual disinfection/sterilization of endoscopes in health care facilities. *Am J Med* 1992;92:257–261.
17. Fraise AP, Disinfection in endoscopy. *Lancet* 1995;346:787–788.
18. Ruddy M, Kibbler CC. Endoscopic decontamination: an audit and practical review. *J Hosp Infect* 2002;50:261–268.
19. Burge PS. Occupational risk of glutaraldehyde. *Br Med J* 1989;299: 342.
20. Jachuck SJ, Bound CL, Steel J, et al. Occupational hazard in hospital staff exposed to 2% glutaraldehyde in an endoscopy unit. *J Soc Occup Med* 1989;39:69–71.
21. Kolmos HJ, Lerche A, Kristoffersen K, et al. Pseudo-outbreak of *Pseudomonas aeruginosa* in HIV-infected patients undergoing fiberoptic bronchoscopy. *Scand J Infect Dis* 1994;26:653–657.
22. Wang HC, Liaw YS, Yang PC, et al. A pseudoepidemic of *Mycobacterium chelonae* infection caused by contamination of a fibreoptic bronchoscopy suction channel. *Eur Respir J* 1995;8:1259–1262.
23. Sorin M, Segal-Maurer S, Mariano N, et al. Nosocomial transmission of imipenem-resistant *Pseudomonas aeruginosa* following bronchoscopy associated with improper connection to the Steris System 1 processor. *Infect Control Hosp Epidemiol* 2001;22:409–413.
24. Dean AG. Transmission of *Salmonella typhi* by fiberoptic endoscopy. *Lancet* 1977;2:134.
25. Beecham HJ, Cohen ML, Parkin WE. *Salmonella typhimurium.* Transmission by fiberoptic upper gastrointestinal endoscopy. *JAMA* 1979;241:1013–1015.
26. Hawkey PM, Davies AJ, Viant AC, et al. Contamination of endoscopes by *Salmonella* species. *J Hosp Infect* 1981;2:373–376.
27. Chmel H, Armstrong D. *Salmonella oslo.* A focal outbreak in a hospital. *Am J Med* 1976;60:203–208.
28. Dwyer DM, Klein EG, Istre GR, et al. *Salmonella newport* infections transmitted by fiberoptic colonoscopy. *Gastrointest Endosc* 1987;33: 84–87.
29. Schleisser KH, Rozendaal B, Taal C, et al. Outbreak of *Salmonella agona* infection after upper intestinal fiberoptic endoscopy. *Lancet* 1980;2:1246.
30. O'Connor BH, Bennett JR, Alexander JG, et al. Salmonellosis infection transmitted by fiberoptic endoscopes *Lancet* 1982;2:864–866.
31. Tuffnell PG. *Salmonella* infection transmitted by a gastroscope. *Can J Public Health* 1976;67:141–142.
32. Nelson KE, Larson P, Schraufnagel DE, et al. Transmission of tuberculosis by flexible fiber bronchoscopes. *Annu Rev Respir Dis* 1983; 127:97–100.
33. Michele TM, Cronin WA, Graham NM, et al. Transmission of *Mycobacterium tuberculosis* by a fiberoptic bronchoscope. Identification by DNA fingerprinting. *JAMA* 1997;278:1093–1095.
34. Agerton T, Valway S, Gore B, et al. Transmission of a highly drug resistant strain (strain W1) of *Mycobacterium tuberculosis.* Community outbreak and nosocomial transmission via a contaminated bronchoscope. *JAMA* 1997;278:1073–1077.
35. Lugagne PM, Herve JM, Lebret T, et al. Infection risks of outpatient cystoscopy in men with sterile urine. *Prog Urol* 1997;7:615–617.
36. Mayol J, Garcia-Aguilar J, Ortiz-Oshiro E, et al. Risk of minimal access approach for laparoscopic surgery: multivariate analysis of morbidity related to umbilical trochar insertion. *World J Surg* 1997;21: 529–533.
37. Tytgat GN. Endoscopic transmission of *Helicobacter pylori. Aliment Pharmacol Ther* 1995;9(suppl 2):105–110.
38. Langenberg W, Rauws EA, Oudbier JH, et al. Patient to patient transmission of *Campylobacter pylori* infection by fiberoptic gastroduodenoscopy and biopsy. *J Infect Dis* 1990;161:507–511.
39. Lo Passo C, Pernice I, Celeste A, et al. Transmission of *Trichosporon asahii* oesophagitis by a contaminated endoscope. *Mycoses* 2001;44: 13–21.
40. Birnie GG, Quigley EM, Clements GB, et al. Endoscopic transmission of hepatitis B virus. *Gut* 1983;24:171–174.
41. Mandelstam P, Sugawa C, Silvis SE, et al. Complications associated with oesophagogastroduodenoscopy and with oesophageal dilation. *Gastrointest Endosc* 1976;23:16–19.
42. Dunne WM Jr. Bacterial adhesion: seen any good biofilms lately? *Clin Microbiol Rev* 2002;15:155–166.
43. Gilbert P, Maira-Litran T, McBain AJ, et al. The physiology and collective recalcitrance of microbial biofilm communities. *Adv Microb Physiol* 2002;46:202–256.
44. Russell AD. Antibiotic and biocide resistance in bacteria: introduction. *J Appl Microbiol* 2002;92(suppl):1S–3S.
45. Bardouniotis E, Ceri H, Olson ME. Biofilm formation and biocide susceptibility testing of *Mycobacterium fortuitum* and *Mycobacterium marinum. Curr Microbiol* 2003;46:28–32.
46. Alvarado CJ, Stolz SM, Maki DG. Nosocomial infections from contaminated endoscopes: a flawed automated endoscope washer. An investigation using molecular epidemiology. *Am J Med* 1991;91: 272S–280S.
47. Kressel AB, Kidd F. Pseudo-outbreak of *Mycobacterium chelonae* and *Methylobacterium mesophilicum* caused by contamination of an automated endoscope washer. *Infect Control Hosp Epidemiol* 2001;22: 414–418.
48. Becker R, Kristjanson A, Waller J. Static electricity as a mechanism of bacterial transfer during endoscopic surgery. *Surg Endosc* 1996;10: 397–399.
49. Raufmann JP, Straus EW. Endoscopic procedures in the AIDS patient: risks, precautions, indications and obligations. *Gastroenterol Clin North Am* 1988;17:495–506.
50. McNicholas TA, Jones DJ, Sibley GN. AIDS: the contamination risk in urological surgery. *Br J Urol* 1989;63:565–568.
51. Earnshaw JJ, Clark AW, Thom, BT. Outbreak of *Pseudomonas aeruginosa* following endoscopic retrograde cholangiopancreatography. *J Hosp Infect* 1985;6:95–97.
52. Phillips J, Hulka B, Hulka J, et al. Laparoscopic procedures: the American Association of Gynecologic Laparoscopists Membership survey for 1975. *J Reprod Med* 1977;18:227–232.
53. Loffer FD. Disinfection vs sterilization of gynecological laparoscopic equipment. The experience of the Phoenix Surgicentre. *J Reprod Med* 1980;25:263–266.
54. White JV. Laparoscopic cholecystectomy. The evolution of general surgery. *Ann Intern Med* 1991;115:651–653.
55. McGuckin M, Shea JA, Schwartz JS. Infection and antimicrobial use in laparoscopic cholecystectomy. *Infect Control Hosp Epidemiol* 1999; 20:624–626.
56. Botterill ID, Davides D, Vezakis A, et al. Recurrent septic episodes following gallstone spillage at laparoscopic cholecystectomy. *Surg Endosc* 2001;15:897.
57. DeVincenzo R, Haramati LB, Wolf EL, et al. Gallstone empyema complicating laparoscopic cholecystectomy. *J Thorac Imaging* 2001; 16:174–176.
58. Dashkovsky I, Cozacov JC. Spillage of stones from the gallbladder during laparoscopic cholecystectomy and complication of a retroperitoneal abscess mimicking gluteal abscess in elderly patients. *Surg Endosc* 2002;16:717.
59. Eypasch E, Sauerland S, Lefering R, et al. Laparoscopic versus open

appendectomy: between evidence and common sense. *Dig Surg* 2002; 19:518–522.

60. Johnson LL, Schneider DA, Austin MD, et al. Two percent glutaraldehyde: a disinfectant in arthroscopy and arthroscopic surgery. *J Bone Joint Surg* 1982;64A:237–239.
61. Wind WM, McGrath BE, Mindell ER. Infection following knee arthroscopy. *Arthroscopy* 2001;17:878–883.
62. Kapoor B, Toms A, Hoper P, et al. Infective lumbar discitis following laparoscopic sacrocolpopexy. *J R Coll Surg Edinb* 2002;47:709–710.
63. Miller A, Gillespie WA, Linton KB, et al. Postoperative infection in urology. *Lancet* 1958;2:608–612.
64. Clark KR, Higgs MJ. Urinary infection following out patient flexible cystoscopy. *Br J Urol* 1990;66:503–505.
65. Burke DM, Shackley DC, O'Reilly PH. The community based morbidity of flexible cystoscopy. *Br J Urol* 2002;89:347–349.
66. Kaskarelis IS, Papadaki MG, Malliaraki NE, et al. Complications of percutaneous nephrostomy, percutaneous insertion of ureteral endoprosthesis and replacement procedures. *Cardiovasc Intervent Radiol* 2001;24:224–228.
67. Munoz P, Blanco JR, Rodriguez-Creixems M, et al. Bloodstream infections after invasive nonsurgical cardiologic procedures. *Arch Intern Med* 2001;161:2110–2115.
68. Silva SE, Nebel O, Rogers G, et al. Endoscopic complications. Results of the 1976 American Society for Gastrointestinal Endoscopy Surgery. *JAMA* 1976;235:928–930.
69. Colin-Jones DG, Cocker R, Schiller KFR. Current endoscopic practice in the UK. *Clin Gastroenterol* 1978;7:775–786.
70. Lockett MA, Templeton ML, Byrne TK, et al. Percutaneous endoscopic gastrostomy complications in a tertiary care center. *Am Surg* 2002;68:117–120.
71. Greene WH, Moody M, Hartley R, et al. Oesophagoscopy as a source *of Pseudomonas aeruginosa* sepsis in patients with acute leukaemia: the need for sterilization of endoscopes. *Gastroenterology* 1974;67: 912–919.
72. Noy MF, Harrison L, Holmes GK, et al. The significance of bacterial contamination of fibreoptic endoscopes. *J Hosp Infect* 1980;1:56–61.
73. Le Frock J, Ellis CA, Turchick JB, et al. Transient bacteraemia associated with sigmoidoscopy. *N Engl J Med* 1973;289:467–469.
74. Baltch A, Buhac I Argrawal A, et al. Bacteraemia after upper gastrointestinal endoscopy. *Arch Intern Med* 1977;137:594–597.
75. Mellow MH, Lewis RJ. Endoscopy-related bacteraemia: incidence of positive blood cultures after endoscopy of the upper gastrointestinal tract. *Arch Intern Med* 1976;136:667–669.
76. Norfleet RG, Mulholland DD, Mitchell PD, et al. Does bacteraemia follow colonoscopy? *Gastroenterology* 1976;70:20–21.
77. Norfleet RG, Mitchell PD, Mulholland DD, et al. Does bacteraemia follow upper gastrointestinal endoscopy? *Am J Gastroenterol* 1981;76: 420–422.
78. Lin OS, Wu SS, Chen YY, et al. Bacterial peritonitis after elective endoscopic variceal ligation: a prospective study. *Am J Gastroenterol* 2000;95:214–217.
79. Chen WC, Hou MC, Lin HC, et al. Bacteraemia after endoscopic injection of N-butyl-2-cyanoacrylate for gastric variceal bleeding. *Gastrointest Endosc* 2001;54:214–218.
80. Baskin G. Prospthetic valve endocarditis after endoscopic variceal sclerotherapy: a failure of antibiotic prophylaxis. *Am J Gastroenterol* 1989;84:311–312.
81. Cohen FL, Koerner RS, Taub SJ. Solitary brain abscess following endoscopic injection sclerosis of oesophageal varices. *Gastrointest Endosc* 1985;31:331–333.
82. Dewar TN, Thomson CE, Bass NM. Subdural empyema after endoscopic sclerotherapy. *Am J Med* 1989;87:593–594.
83. Uno Y, Munakata A, Ohtomo Y. Farewell to bacteraemia caused by endoscopic injection-effectiveness of a new injection catheter with a covered tip. *Gastrointest Endosc* 1998;47:523–525.
84. Bilbao MK, Dotter CT, Lee TG, et al. Complications of endoscopic retrograde cholangiopancreatography (ERCP). A study of 10,000 cases. *Gastroenterology* 1976;70:314–320.
85. Doherty DE, Falko JM, Leftkovitz N, et al. *Pseudomonas aeruginosa* sepsis following retrograde cholangiopancreatography (ERCP). *Dig Dis Sci* 1982;27:169–170.
86. Siegman-Igra Y, Spinrad S, Rattan J. Septic complications following endoscopic retrograde cholangiopancreatography (ERCP): the experience in the Tel Aviv Medical Center. *J Hosp Infect* 1988;12:7–12.
87. Earnshaw JJ, Clark AW, Thom BT. Outbreak of *Pseudomonas aeruginosa* following endoscopic retrograde cholangiopancreatography. *J Hosp Infect* 1985;6:95–97.
88. Cryan EMJ, Falkiner FR, Mulvihill TE, et al. *Pseudomonas aeruginosa* cross-infection following endoscopic retrograde cholangiopancreatography. *J Hosp Infect* 1984;5:371–376.
89. Schousboe M, Carter A, Sheppard PS. Endoscopic retrograde cholangiopancreatography: related nosocomial infections. *N Z Med J* 1980; 92:275–277.
90. Elson CO, Hattori K, Blackstone MO. Polymicrobial sepsis following endoscopic retrograde cholangiopancreatography. *Gastroenterology* 1975;69:507–510.
91. Struelens MJ, Rost F, Deplano A, et al. *Pseudomonas aeruginosa* and Enterobacteriaceae bacteraemia after biliary endoscopy: an outbreak investigation using DNA macrorestriction analysis. *Am J Med* 1993; 95:489–498.
92. Allen JL, Allen MO, Olson MM, et al. *Pseudomonas* infection of the biliary system resulting from a contaminated endoscope. *Gastroenterology* 1987;92:759–763.
93. Anon. Nosocomial infection and pseudoinfection from contaminated endoscopes and bronchoscopes—Wisconsin and Missouri. *MMWR* 1991;40:675–678.
94. O'Connor HJ, Babb JR, Ayliff GAJ. *Pseudomonas aeruginosa* infection during endoscopy. *Gastroenterology* 1987;92:1451.
95. Hanson PJ, Jeffries DJ, Collins JV. Viral transmission and fibreoptic endoscopy. *J Hosp Infect* 1991;18(suppl A):136–140.
96. Spach D, Silverstein FE, Stamm WE. Transmission of infection by gastrointestinal endoscopy and bronchoscopy. *Ann Intern Med* 1993; 118:117–128.
97. Ouzan D. Risk of transmission of hepatitis C through endoscopy of the digestive tract. *Presse Med* 1999;28:1091–1094.
98. Deflandre J, Cajot O, Brixko C, et al. Risk of contamination of hepatitis C of endoscopes utilized in gastroenterology hospital service. *Rev Med Liege* 2001;56:696–698.
99. Sammertino MT, Isreal RH, Magnussen CR. *Pseudomonas aeruginosa* contamination of fiberoptic bronchoscopes. *J Hosp Infect* 1982;3: 65–71.
100. Suratt PM, Gruber B, Wellons HA, et al. Absence of clinical pneumonia following bronchoscopy with contaminated and clean bronchofiberscopes. *Chest* 1977;71:52–54.
101. Webb SF, Vall-Spinosa A. Outbreak of *Serratia marcescens* associated with flexible fiberbronchoscope. *Chest* 1975;68:703–708.
102. Siegman-Igra Y, Inbar J, Campus A. An outbreak of pulmonary pseudo-infection by *Serratia marcescens*. *J Hosp Infect* 1985;6: 218–220.
103. Daschner F. Unusual source of contamination of bronchoscopes. *J Hosp Infect* 1982;3:515.
104. Weinstein HJ, Bone RC, Ruth WE. Contamination of a fiberoptic bronchoscope with a *Proteus* species. *Am Rev Respir Dis* 1977;116: 541–543.
105. LeClark P, de Fenoyl O, D'Orbcastel OR, et al. Contamination des fibrescopes bronchiques par les mycobacteries: mythe ou realitie. *Ann Med Interne* 1985;136:482–485.
106. Leers W. Disinfecting endoscopes. How not to transmit *Mycobacterium tuberculosis* by bronchoscopy. *Can Med Assoc J* 1980;123: 275–283.
107. Ramsey AH, Oemig TV, Davis JP, et al. An outbreak of bronchoscopy-related *Mycobacterium tuberculosis* infections due to lack of bronchoscopy leak testing. *Chest* 2002;121:976–981.
108. Credle WF, Smiddy JF, Elliott RC. Complications of fiberoptic bronchoscopy. *Am Rev Respir Dis* 1974;109:67–72.
109. Pereira W, Kovnat DM, Khan MA, et al. Fever and pneumonia after flexible fiberoptic bronchoscopy. *Am Rev Respir Dis* 1975;112:59–64.
110. Picard E, Schwartz S, Goldberg S, et al. A prospective study of fever

and bacteraemia after flexible fiberoptic bronchoscopy in children. *Chest* 2000;117:573–577.

111. Sniadack DH, Ostroff SM, Karlix MA, et al. A nosocomial pseudo-outbreak of *Mycobacterium xenopi* due to a contaminated potable water supply: lessons in prevention. *Infect Control Hosp Epidemiol* 1993;14:636–641.
112. Bennett SN, Peterson DE, Johnson DR, et al. Bronchoscopy-associated *Mycobacterium xenopi* pseudoinfections. *Am J Respir Crit Care Med* 1994;150:245–250.
113. Kressel AB, Kidd F. Pseudo-outbreak of *Mycobacterium chelonae* and *Methylbacterium mesophilicum* caused by contamination of an automated endoscopy washer. *Infect Control Hosp Epidemiol* 2001;22: 414–418.
114. Goldstein B, Abrutyn E. Pseudo-outbreaks of *Bacillus* spores related to fiberoptic bronchoscopy. *J Hosp Infect* 1985;6:194–200.
115. Muscarella LF. Anthrax: is there a risk of cross-infection during endoscopy? *Gastroenterol Nurs* 2002;25:46–48.
116. Esteban J, Gadea I, Fernandez-Roblas R, et al. Pseudo-outbreak of *Aeromonas hydrophila* isolates related to endoscopy. *J Hosp Infect* 1999; 41:313–316.
117. Wilson SJ, Everts RJ, Kirkland KB, et al. A pseudo-outbreak of *Aureobasidium* species lower respiratory tract infections caused by the reuse of a single use stopcock during bronchoscopy. *Infect Control Hosp Epidemiol* 2000;21:470–472.
118. Roberts WG, Green PHR, Ma J, et al. Prevalence of cryptosporidiosis in patients undergoing endoscopy. Evidence for an asymptomatic carrier state. *Am J Med* 1989;87:537–539.
119. Rey JF. Endoscopic disinfection: a worldwide problem. *J Clin Gastroenterol* 1999;28:291–297.
120. Mehta AC, Minai OA. Infection control in the bronchoscopy suite. A review. *Clin Chest Med* 1999;20:19–23.
121. Leung JW. Reprocessing of flexible endoscopes. *J Gastroenterol Hepatol* 2000;15:G73–77.
122. Tandon RK. Disinfection of gastrointestinal endoscopes and accessories. *J Gastroenterol Hepatol* 2000;15:G69–72.
123. Ahuja V, Tandon RK. Survey of gastrointestinal endoscope disinfection and accessory reprocessing practices in the Asia-Pacific region. *J Gastroenterol Hepatol* 2000;15:G78–81.
124. Knieler R. Manual cleaning and disinfection of flexible endoscopes—an approach to evaluating a combined procedure. *J Hosp Infect* 2001;48(suppl A):S84–87.
125. Leiss O, Beilenhoff U, Bader L, et al. Reprocessing of flexible endoscopes and endoscopic accessories- an international comparison of guidelines. *Z Gastroenterol* 2002;40:531–542.
126. Rutala WA, Clontz EP, Weber DJ, et al. Disinfection practices for endoscopes and other semicritical items. *Infect Control Hosp Epidemiol* 1991;12:282–288.
127. Spaulding EH. Chemical disinfection of medical and surgical materials. In: Lawrence CA, Block SS, eds. *Disinfection, sterilization and preservation.* Philadelphia: Lea & Febiger, 1968:517–531.
128. Alfa MJ. Methodology of reprocessing reusable accessories. *Gastrointest Endosc* 2000;10:361–378.
129. Lejeune C, Prost P, Michiels C, et al. Disposable versus reusable biopsy forceps. A prospective cost analysis in the gastrointestinal endoscopy unit of the Dijon University Hospital. *Gastroenterol Clin Biol* 2001;25:669–673.
130. Merighi A, Contato E, Scagliarini R, et al. Quality improvements in gastrointestinal endoscopy: microbiologic surveillance of disinfection. *Gastrointest Endosc* 1996;43:457–462.
131. Ishino Y, Ido K, Koiwai H, et al. Pitfalls in endoscopy reprocessing: brushing of air and water channels is mandatory for high level disinfection. *Gastrointest Endosc* 2001;53:165–168.
132. Kinney TP, Kozarek RA, Raltz S, et al. Contamination of single use biopsy forceps: a prospective in vitro analysis. *Gastrointest Endosc* 2002;56:209–212.
133. Alfa MJ, Sitter DL. In-hospital evaluation of contamination of duodenoscopes: a quantitative assessment of the effect of drying. *J Hosp Infect* 1991;19:89–98.
134. Chu NS, McAlister D, Antonoplos PA. Natural bioburden levels detected on flexible gastrointestinal endoscopes after clinical use and manual cleaning. *Gastrointest Endosc* 1998;48:137–142.
135. Alfa MJ, Degagne P, Olson N. Worst-case soiling levels for patient-used flexible endoscopes before and after cleaning. *Am J Infect Control* 1999;27:392–401.
136. Hansen NJ. Prion diseases (transmissible spongiform encephalopathies):a review. *Endoscopy* 1997;29:584–592.
137. Wadsworth JD, Joiner S, Hill AF, et al. Tissue distribution of protease resistant prion protein in variant Creutzfeldt-Jacob disease using a highly sensitive immunoblotting assay. *Lancet* 2001;358:171–180.
138. Frosh A. Prions and the ENT surgeon. *J Laryngol Otol* 1999;113: 1064–1067.
139. Spencer RC, Ridgway GL, and the vCJD Consensus Group. Sterilization issues in vCJD—towards a consensus. *J Hosp Infect* 2002;51: 168–174.
140. Bradley CR, Babb JR. Endoscope decontamination: automated vs manual. *J Hosp Infect* 1995;30(suppl):537–542.
141. Babb JR, Bradley CR. Endoscope decontamination: where do we go from here? *J Hosp Infect* 1995;30(suppl):543–551.
142. Axon A, Jung M, Kruse A, et al. The European Society of Gastrointestinal Endoscopy (ESGE): check list for the purchase of washer-disinfectors for flexible endoscopes. ESGE Guideline Committee. *Endoscopy* 2000;32:914–919.
143. Anon. Hospital Technical Memorandum 2030. Washer-disinfectors. London: Stationary Office, 1997.
144. Wilcox CM, Waites K, Brookings ES. Use of sterile compared with tap water in gastrointestinal endoscopic procedures. *Am J Infect Control* 1996;24:407–410.
145. Humphreys H, McGrath H, McCormack PA, et al. Quality of final rinse water in washer disinfectors for endoscopes. *J Hosp Infect* 2002; 51:151–152.
146. MacKay WG, Leanord AT, Williams CL. Water, water everywhere nor any a sterile drop to rinse your endoscope. *J Hosp Infect* 2002; 51:256–261.
147. Cooke RP, Whymant-Morris A, Umasankar RS, et al. Bacteria free water for automatic washer-disinfectors: an impossible dream? *J Hosp Infect* 1998;39:63–65.
148. Phillips G, McEwan H, McKay I, et al. Black pigmented fungi in the water pipework supplying endoscope washer disinfectors. *J Hosp Infect* 1999;40:250.
149. Manzoor SE, lambert PA, Griffiths PA, et al. Reduced glutaraldehyde susceptibility in *Mycobacterium chelonae* associated with altered cell wall polysaccharides. *J Antimicrob Chemother* 1999;43:759–765.
150. Rutala WA, Weber DJ. Disinfection of endoscopes: review of new chemical sterilants used for high level disinfection. *Infect Contol Hosp Epidemiol* 1999;20:69–76.
151. Rutala WA, Weber DJ. New disinfection and sterilization methods. *Emerg Infect Dis* 2001;7:348–353.
152. Walsh SE, Maillard JY, Russell AD. Orthophthalaldehyde: a possible alternative to glutaraldehyde for high level disinfection. *J Appl Microbiol* 1999;86:1039–1046.
153. Barbee SL, Weber DJ, Sobsey MD, et al. Inactivation of *Cryptosporidium parvum* oocyst infectivity by disinfection and sterilization processes. *Gastrointest Endosc* 1999;49:605–611.
154. Thamlikitkul V, Trakulsomboon S, Louisirirotchanakul S, et al. Microbial killing activity of peracetic acid. *J Med Assoc Thai* 2001;84: 1375–1382.
155. Duc DL, Ribiollet A, Dode X, et al. Evaluation of the microbiocidal efficacy of Steris System I for digestive endoscopes using Germande and ASTM validation protocols. *J Hosp Infect* 2001;48:135–141.
156. Middleton AM, Chadwick MV, Gaya H. Disinfection of bronchoscopes contaminated in vitro with *Mycobacterium tuberculosis, Mycobacterium avium-intracellulare* and *Mycobacterium chelonae* in sputum using stabilized buffered peracetic acid solution (NuCidex). *J Hosp Infect* 1997;37:137–143.
157. Bradley CR, Babb JR, Ayliffe GA. Evaluation of the Steris System I Peracetic acid endoscope processor. *J Hosp Infect* 1995;29:143–151.

158. Baldry MG. The bactericidal, fungicidal and sporicidal properties of hydrogen peroxide and peracetic acid. *J Appl Bacteriol* 1983;54: 417–423.
159. Stanley PM. Efficacy of peroxygen compounds against glutaraldehyde resistant mycobacteria. *Am J Infect Control* 1999;27:339–343.
160. Alfa MJ, DeGagne P, Olson N, et al. Comparison of liquid chemical sterilization with peracetic acid and ethylene oxide sterilization for long narrow lumens. *Am J Infect Control* 1998;26:469–477.
161. Wallace CG, Agee PM, Demicco DD. Liquid chemical sterilization using peracetic acid. An alternative approach to endoscope reprocessing. *ASAIO J* 1995;41:151–154.
162. Griffiths PA, Babb JR, Fraise AP. Mycobactericidal activity of selected disinfectants using a quantitative suspension test. *J Hosp Infect* 1999; 41:111–121.
163. Coates D. An evaluation of the use of chlorine dioxide (Tristel One Shot) in an automated washer/disinfector (Medivator) fitted with a chlorine dioxide generator for decontamination of flexible endoscopes. *J Hosp Infect* 2001;48:55–65.
164. Winiecka-Krusnell J, Linder E. Cysticidal effect of chlorine dioxide *on Giardia intestinalis* cysts. *Acta Trop* 1998;70:369–72.
165. Korish DG, Mead JR, Madore MS, et al. Effects of ozone, chlorine dioxide, chlorine, and monochloramine on *Cryptosporidium parvum* oocyst viability. *Appl Environ Microbiol* 1990;56:1423–1428.
166. Selkon JB, Babb JR, Morris R. Evaluation of the antimicrobial activity of a new super-oxidised water, Sterilox, for the disinfection of endoscopes. *J Hosp Infect* 1999;41:59–70.
167. Shetty N, Srinivasan S, Holton J, et al. Evaluation of the microbicidal activity of a new disinfectant, Sterilox 2500 against *Clostridium difficile* spores, *Helicobacter pylori*, vancomycin resistant enterococcus species, *Candida albicans* and several mycobacterial species. *J Hosp Infect* 1999;41:101–105.
168. Tyler R, Ayliff GA, Bradley C. Virucidal activity of disinfectants: studies with the polio virus. *J Hosp Infect* 1990;15:339–345.
169. Kyi MS, Holton J, Ridgway GL. Assessment of the efficacy of a low temperature hydrogen peroxide gas plasma sterilization system. *J Hosp Infect* 1995;31:275–284.
170. Rutala WA, Gergen MF, Weber DJ. Comparative evaluation of the sporicidal activity of new low-temperature sterilization technologies: ethylene oxide, 2 plasma sterilization systems and liquid peracetic acid. *Am J Infect Control* 1998;26:393–398.
171. Rutala WA, Gergen MF, Weber DJ. Sporicidal activity of a new low-temperature sterilization technology: the Sterrad 50 sterilizer. *Infect Control Hosp Epidemiol* 1999;20:514–516.
172. Alfa MJ, DeGagne P, Olson N, et al. Comparison of ion plasma, vaporized hydrogen peroxide and 100% ethylene oxide sterilizers to the 12/88 ethylene oxide gas sterilizer. *Infect Control Hosp Epidemiol* 1996;17:92–100.

64

NOSOCOMIAL INFECTIONS ASSOCIATED WITH HEMODIALYSIS

MIRIAM J. ALTER
JEROME I. TOKARS
MATTHEW J. ARDUINO
MARTIN S. FAVERO

Of the patients with end-stage renal disease treated by maintenance hemodialysis in the United States, 91% are on hemodialysis (1). Currently, there are >250,000 chronic hemodialysis patients and >60,000 staff members in approximately 4,000 hemodialysis centers (1). The end-stage renal disease program is administered by the Centers for Medicare and Medicaid Services (CMS, formerly the Healthcare Financing Administration) of the Department of Health and Human Services. It is the only Medicare entitlement that is based on the diagnosis of a medical condition.

Chronic hemodialysis patients are at high risk for infection, because the process of hemodialysis requires vascular access for prolonged periods. In an environment where multiple patients receive dialysis concurrently, repeated opportunities exist for person-to-person transmission of infectious agents, directly or indirectly via contaminated devices, equipment and supplies, environmental surfaces, or hands of personnel. Furthermore, hemodialysis patients are immunosuppressed, which increases their susceptibility to infection, and they require frequent hospitalizations and surgery, which increases their opportunities for exposure to nosocomial infections. This chapter describes the major infectious diseases and several toxic complications due to chemical contamination that can be acquired in the dialysis center setting, the important epidemiologic and environmental microbiologic considerations, and infection control strategies.

BACTERIAL AND CHEMICAL CONTAMINANTS IN HEMODIALYSIS SYSTEMS

A typical hemodialysis system consists of a water supply, a system for mixing water and concentrated dialysis fluid, and a machine to pump the dialysis fluid through the artificial kidney (commonly referred to as the hemodialyzer or dialyzer). The dialyzer is connected to the patient's circulatory system, and blood is pumped through it to accomplish dialysis by means of a membrane to remove waste products from the patient's blood.

Bacterial Contamination of Water

Technical development and clinical use of hemodialysis delivery systems improved dramatically in the late 1960s and early 1970s. However, a number of microbiologic parameters were not accounted for in the design of many hemodialysis machines and their respective water supply systems. There are many situations where certain types of gram-negative water bacteria can persist and actively multiply in aqueous environments associated with hemodialysis equipment. This can result in the production of massive levels of gram-negative bacteria, which can directly or indirectly affect patients by septicemia or endotoxemia.

Gram-negative water bacteria are commonly found in water supplies used for hemodialysis. Under certain circumstances, these microorganisms can persist and multiply in aqueous environments associated with hemodialysis equipment. These bacteria can adhere to surfaces and form biofilms (glycocalyces), which are virtually impossible to eradicate (2–4). Control strategies are designed not to eradicate bacteria but to reduce their concentration to relatively low levels and to prevent their regrowth.

Although certain genera of gram-negative water bacteria (e.g., *Achromobacter, Acinetobacter, Alcaligenes, Aeromonas, Burkholderia, Flavobacterium, Pseudomonas, Ralstonia, Serratia,* and *Xanthomonas*) are most commonly encountered, virtually any bacterium that can grow in water can be a problem in a hemodialysis unit. Several species of nontuberculous mycobacteria may also contaminate water treatment systems, including *Mycobacterium chelonae, M. abscessus, M. fortuitum, M. gordonae, M. mucogenicum* (formerly MCLO), *M. scrofulaceum, M. kansaii, M. avium,* and *M. intracellulare*; these microorganisms do not contain bacterial endotoxin but are comparatively resistant to chemical germicides (5–7).

Gram-negative water bacteria can multiply even in water containing relatively small amounts of organic matter, such as water treated by distillation, softening, deionization, or reverse osmosis, reaching levels of 10^5 to 10^7 colony-forming units (CFU)/mL (8); these levels are not associated with visible turbidity. When treated water is mixed with dialysis concentrate, the resulting dialysis fluid is a balanced salt solution and growth medium almost as rich in nutrients as conventional nutrient broth (8,9). Gram-negative water bacteria growing in dialysis fluids can reach levels of 10^8 to 10^9 CFU/mL, which produce visible turbidity.

Bacterial growth in water used for hemodialysis depends on

the types of water treatment system used, dialysate distribution systems, dialysis machine type, and method of disinfection (5,6, 10) (Table 64.1). Each component is discussed separately below.

Water Supply

Municipal water may be derived from either surface or ground waters, both of which may be contaminated with bacteria and endotoxin (Table 64.1). Endotoxin is particularly likely to be present in surface waters, is not substantially removed by conventional municipal water treatment processes, and may cause pyrogenic reactions (11). Disinfectants such as chlorine and combined chlorine (monochloramine) reduce the numbers of microorganisms but do not eliminate bacteria in municipal water.

Water Treatment Systems

Water used for the production of dialysis fluid must be treated to remove chemical and microbial contaminants. The Association for the Advancement of Medical Instrumentation (AAMI) has published guidelines for the chemical and bacteriologic quality of water used to prepare dialysis fluid (Table 64.2) (12; AAMI, personal communication, July 2003). Some components of the water treatment system may allow amplification of water bacteria. For example, ion exchangers such as water softeners and deionizers do not remove endotoxins or bacteria and provide sites for significant bacterial multiplication (13). Granular activated carbon adsorption media (i.e., carbon filters) are used to remove certain organic chemicals and available chlorine from water, but they also significantly increase the level of water bacteria and do not remove bacterial endotoxins.

A variety of filters are marketed to control bacterial contamination in water and dialysis fluids. Most are inadequate, especially if they are not routinely disinfected or changed frequently. Particulate filters, commonly called prefilters, operate by depth filtration and do not remove bacteria or bacterial endotoxins. These filters can become colonized with gram-negative water bacteria, resulting in higher levels of bacteria and endotoxin in the filter effluent. Absolute filters, including the membrane types, temporarily remove bacteria from passing water. However, some of these filters tend to clog, and gram-negative water bacteria can "grow through" the filter matrix and colonize the downstream surface of the filters within a few days. Further, absolute filters do not reduce levels of endotoxin in the effluent water. These types of filters should be changed regularly in accordance with the manufacturer's directions and disinfected in the same manner and at the same time as the dialysis system.

Ultraviolet irradiation is sometimes used to reduce bacterial contamination in water, but this approach is not recommended (8). Certain populations of gram-negative water bacteria are far more resistant to and may survive ultraviolet radiation. In recirculating dialysis systems, repeated exposures to ultraviolet radiation are used to ensure adequate disinfection; however, this approach allows progressive removal of sensitive microorganisms and multiplication of ultraviolet-resistant microorganisms. In addition, bacterial endotoxins are not affected.

Reverse osmosis is an effective water treatment modality that

TABLE 64.1. FACTORS INFLUENCING MICROBIAL CONTAMINATION IN HEMODIALYSIS SYSTEMS

Factors	Comments
Water supply	
Source of community water	
Groundwater	Contains endotoxin and bacteria
Surface water	Contains high levels of endotoxin and bacteria
Water treatment at dialysis center	Not recommended
None	
Filtration	Particulate filter to protect equipment; does not remove microorganisms
Prefilter	
Absolute filter (depth or membrane)	Removes bacteria but, unless changed frequently or disinfected, bacteria will accumulate and grow through filter; acts as significant reservoir of bacteria and endotoxin
Activated carbon filter	Removes organics and available chlorine or chloramine; significant reservoir of water bacteria and endotoxin
Water treatment devices	
Ion-exchange softener, deionization	Softeners and deionizers are significant reservoirs of bacteria and neither removes endotoxin
Reverse osmosis	Removes bacteria and endotoxin, but must be disinfected; operates at high water pressure
Ultraviolet light	Kills some bacteria, but there is no residual, and ultraviolet-resistant bacteria can develop
Ultrafilter	Removes bacteria and endotoxin; operates on normal line pressure; can be positioned distal to deionizer; must be disinfected
Water and dialysate distribution system	
Distribution pipes	
Size	Oversized diameter and length decrease fluid flow and increase bacteria reservoir for both treated water and centrally prepared dialysate
Construction	Rough joints, dead ends, and unused branches can act as bacterial reservoirs
Elevation	Outlet taps should be located at highest elevation to prevent loss of disinfectant
Storage tanks	Undesirable because they act as reservoir of water bacteria; if present, must be routinely scrubbed and disinfected
Dialysis machines	
Single-pass	Disinfectant should have contact with all parts of machine that are exposed to water or dialysis fluid
Recirculating single-pass, or recirculating (batch)	Recirculating pumps and machine design allow for massive contamination levels if not properly disinfected; overnight chemical germicide treatment recommended

TABLE 64.2. ASSOCIATION FOR THE ADVANCEMENT OF MEDICAL INSTRUMENTATION (AAMI) MICROBIOLOGIC AND ENDOTOXIN STANDARDS FOR DIALYSIS FLUIDS

Type of Hemodialysis Fluid	Maximum Contaminant Level Total Heterotrophs (CFU/mL)	Maximum Contaminant Level Endotoxin (EU/mL)
Water used to prepare dialysate, rinse dialyzers, or prepare dialyzer disinfectant	200	2
Conventional dialysate	2,000/200[a]	No standard/2[b]
Ultrapure dialysate	0.1	0.03
Dialysate for infusion	ND[c]	0.03

[a] 2,000 is the current standard; 200 is the proposed standard.
[b] There is no current standard for endotoxin; 2 is the proposed standard.
[c] Not detectable by routine methods—limit is 1 CFU/1,000 L.
CFU, colony-forming units; EU, endotoxin units.

is used in 97% of U.S. hemodialysis units (14). Reverse osmosis possesses the singular advantage of being able to remove both bacterial endotoxins and bacteria from supply water. However, low numbers of gram-negative and nontuberculous mycobacteria water bacteria can either penetrate this barrier or by other means colonize the downstream portion of the reverse osmosis unit. Consequently, reverse osmosis systems must be disinfected routinely.

We recommend a water treatment system that produces chemically adequate water while avoiding high levels of microbial contamination. The components in the following sequence are well suited for treatment of hard water (15): a set of prefilters, a softener, carbon adsorption tanks (at least two in series are recommended), a particulate filter, a reverse osmosis unit, a deionization unit, and an ultrafilter. As the water passes through these components, it becomes progressively purer chemically, but the level of bacterial contamination increases. Therefore, an ultrafilter is included as the final component to remove bacteria and bacterial endotoxin. The ultrafilter contains membranes similar to those in a reverse osmosis unit but is operated at ordinary water line pressure. Additional source water treatment devices may be added to this system, depending on the chemical quality of the municipal water. If this system is adequately disinfected, the microbial content of water should be well within the recommended guidelines.

Distribution Systems

Water that has passed through the water treatment system (product water) may be distributed to individual dialysis machines where it is combined with dialysate concentrate. Alternately, it may be combined with concentrate in a central location and the resulting dialysis fluid supplied to individual machines. Plastic pipes (usually polyvinyl chloride) are used to distribute water or dialysis fluid to dialysis machines. The use of pipes with a diameter larger than necessary slows the fluid velocity and increases the wetted surface area available for microbial colonization. Increased surface area also results from using pipes that are longer than needed. Gram-negative bacteria in fluids remaining in pipes overnight can multiply rapidly and colonize the wetted surfaces of the pipes, producing bacterial populations and endotoxin in quantities proportional to the volume and surface area. Such colonization results in the formation of a protective biofilm, which is difficult to remove and protects the bacteria from disinfection (16).

Routine disinfection of the water or dialysate distribution system should be performed at least weekly (17). However, the AAMI standards and recommendations, which are consensus documents, do not specify a schedule for disinfection other than suggesting that routine disinfection should be conducted. In many instances, microbiologic monitoring can be used to determine the frequency of disinfection of the water distribution system (18,19).

To prevent disinfectant from draining from pipes by gravity before contact time is adequate, distribution systems should be designed with all outlet taps at equal elevation and at the highest point of the system. Furthermore, the system should be free of rough joints, dead-end pipes, and unused branches and taps. Fluid trapped in such stagnant areas can serve as a reservoir for bacteria that are later inoculated into the distribution system (20).

Storage tanks greatly increase the volume of fluid and surface area of the distribution system. If used, they should be drained frequently, cleaned (including scrubbing of the sides of the tank to remove bacterial biofilm), and disinfected. Also, an ultrafilter distal to the storage tank is recommended.

Hemodialysis Machines

In the 1970s, most dialysis machines were of the recirculating or recirculating single-pass type; their design contributed to relatively high levels of gram-negative bacterial contamination in dialysis fluid. Currently, virtually all centers in the U.S. use single-pass hemodialysis machines. Single-pass machines tend to respond to adequate cleaning and disinfection procedures and, in general, have lower levels of bacterial contamination in their dialysis fluid than do recirculating machines. Levels of contamination in single-pass machines depend primarily on the bacteriologic quality of the incoming water and on the method of machine disinfection (8,21).

A frequent error in disinfecting single-pass systems is introduction of the disinfectant in the same manner and through the same port as the dialysate concentrate. By so doing, the pipes and tubing carrying incoming water or dialysate are not disinfected and may act as a reservoir for bacteria. To ensure adequate disinfection of a single-pass machine, the disinfectant must reach all parts of the system's fluid pathways.

Disinfection of Hemodialysis Systems

Routine disinfection of isolated components of a dialysis system frequently produces inadequate results. Consequently, the total dialysis system (water treatment system, distribution system, and dialysis machine) should be included in the disinfection procedure.

Chlorine-based disinfectants, such as sodium hypochlorite solutions, are convenient and effective in most parts of the dialysis system when used at the manufacturer's recommended concentration. Also, the test for residual available chlorine to confirm adequate rinsing is simple and sensitive. However, because chlorine is corrosive, it is usually rinsed from the system after a short (20- to 30-minute) exposure time. The rinse water invariably contains gram-negative water bacteria that can multiply to significant levels if the system is permitted to stand overnight. Therefore, chlorine disinfectants are best used just before the startup of the dialysis system rather than at the end of the day. In centers dialyzing patients in multiple shifts, it may be reasonable to disinfect with sodium hypochlorite between shifts (this may not be necessary with some single-pass machines if the levels of bacterial contamination are within AAMI limits) and with another disinfectant (formaldehyde, peroxyacetic acid, or glutaraldehyde) at the end of the day.

Aqueous formaldehyde, peroxyacetic acid, or glutaraldehyde solutions produce good disinfection results (22,23). These products are not as corrosive as hypochlorite solutions and can be allowed to remain in the dialysis system for long periods when the system is not operational, thereby preventing regrowth of bacteria. Formaldehyde has good penetrating characteristics but is considered an environmental hazard and potential carcinogen and has irritating qualities that may be objectionable to staff members (24). The Environmental Protection Agency (EPA) has reduced the allowable amount of formaldehyde that can be discharged into the wastewater stream, which has reduced the use of this disinfectant in the dialysis community. Commercial tests (e.g., Formalert, Organon Teknika, Durham, NC) are available and can detect residual formaldehyde in water at concentrations as low as 1 part per million (ppm). Peroxyacetic acid and glutaraldehyde are commercially available and are designed for use with dialysis machines; both are good germicides when used according to the manufacturer's recommendations.

Some dialysis systems use hot-water disinfection for the control of microbial contamination. In this type of system, water heated to greater than 80°C (176°F) is passed through all proportioning, distribution, and patient-monitoring devices at the end of the day. These systems are excellent for controlling bacterial contamination.

Monitoring of Water and Dialysis Fluid

Microbiologic and endotoxin standards for water and dialysis fluids (Table 64.2) (3,12,25–27) were originally based on the results of culture assays performed during epidemiologic investigations and should be used as broad guidelines rather than absolute standards. These standards are in the process of being revised (AAMI, personal communication, July 2003) based on new data on the effects of the microbial quality of hemodialysis fluids on chronic inflammatory response syndrome and anemia management in dialysis patients (28–32).

Water samples should be collected from a source as close as possible to where water enters the dialysate concentrate-proportioning unit. Water samples should be collected at least monthly and repeated when bacteriologic counts exceed 200 CFU/mL and/or endotoxin activity exceeds 2 EU/mL (Table 64.2) (AAMI, personal communication, July 2003) or when changes have been made in the disinfection procedure, the water treatment system, or the water distribution system. Dialysis fluid samples should be collected during or at the termination of dialysis from a source close to where the dialysis fluid either enters or leaves the dialyzer. Dialysis fluid samples should also be collected at least once monthly and repeated when the recommended levels for microbial or endotoxin contamination are exceeded (Table 64.2), when pyrogenic reactions are suspected, or when changes are made in the water treatment system or disinfection protocol. If centers reprocess dialyzers for reuse on the same patient, water used to rinse dialyzers and prepare dialyzer disinfectants also should be assayed at least monthly.

Specimens should be assayed within 30 minutes or refrigerated at 4°C and assayed within 24 hours of collection. Conventional laboratory procedures such as the pour plate, spread plate, or membrane filter technique can be used. Calibrated loops should not be used, because they sample a small volume and are inaccurate. Although standard methods agar, blood agar, and trypticase soy agar were once considered equivalent, it has since been shown that a portion of the gram-negative bacterial flora of bicarbonate dialysis fluid and water has special growth requirements. Microorganisms found in bicarbonate dialysis fluid require a small amount of sodium chloride, and those found in processed water may require a nutrient poor medium. Consequently, to cover both conditions needed, trypticase soy agar is the currently recommended medium; however, one may also use standard plate count, standard methods, or soybean casein digest agars along with commercially available samplers. Blood agar should not be used for this purpose. The assay should be quantitative, not qualitative, and a standard technique for enumeration should be used. Colonies should be counted with the aid of a magnifying device after 48 hours of incubation at 35° to 37°C (3,12,25–27,33). Total viable counts (standard plate counts) are the objective of the assays.

In an outbreak investigation, the assay may need to be both qualitative and quantitative; also, detection of nontuberculous mycobacteria in water may be desirable. In such instances, plates should be incubated for 5 to 14 days.

DIALYSIS-ASSOCIATED PYROGENIC REACTIONS

Gram-negative bacterial contamination of dialysis water or components can cause pyrogenic reactions. Pyrogenic reactions are defined as objective chills (visible rigors) or fever [oral temperature 37.8°C (100°F) or higher] or both in a patient who was afebrile [oral temperature up to 37.0°C (98.6°F)] and who had no signs or symptoms of infection before the dialysis treatment (24). Depending on the type of dialysis system and level of contamination, fever and chills may start 1 to 5 hours after dialysis is initiated. Other symptoms may include hypotension, headache, myalgia, nausea, and vomiting. Pyrogenic reactions can occur with or without bacteremia; because presenting signs and symptoms may not be different in these two instances, blood cultures are necessary.

During the 1990s, an annual average of 20% of the hemodialysis centers in the U.S. reported at least one pyrogenic reaction in the absence of septicemia in patients undergoing dialysis (14). Pyrogenic reactions without bacteremia can result from either the passage of bacterial endotoxin (lipopolysaccharide) in the dialysis fluid across the dialyzer membrane (34,35) or the transmembrane stimulation of cytokine production in the patient's blood by endotoxins in the dialysis fluid (36,37). In other instances, endotoxins can enter the bloodstream directly with fluids that are contaminated with gram-negative bacteria (38, 39). The signs and symptoms of pyrogenic reactions without bacteremia generally abate within a few hours after dialysis has been stopped. If gram-negative bacterial sepsis is associated, fever and chills may persist, and hypotension is more refractory to therapy (11,38).

When a pyrogenic reaction occurs, the following steps are recommended: a careful physical examination to rule out other causes of chills and fever (e.g., pneumonia, vascular access infection, urinary tract infection); blood cultures, other diagnostic tests (e.g., chest radiograph) and cultures as clinically indicated; collection of dialysis fluid from the dialyzer (downstream side) for quantitative and qualitative bacteriologic assays; and recording of the incident in a log or other permanent record. Determining the cause of these episodes is important, because they may be the first indication of a remediable problem.

The higher the level of bacteria and endotoxin in dialysis fluid, the higher the probability they will pass through the dialysis membrane or stimulate cytokine production. In an outbreak of febrile reactions among patients undergoing dialysis, the attack rates were directly proportional to the level of bacterial contamination in the dialysis fluid (8). Prospective studies also demonstrated a lower pyrogenic reaction rate among patients when they underwent dialysis with dialysis fluid that had been filtered and from which most bacteria had been removed compared with patients who underwent dialysis with dialysis fluid that was highly contaminated (mean 19,000 CFU/mL) (40–42).

Among seven outbreaks of bacteremia and pyrogenic reactions not related to dialyzer reuse investigated by the Centers for Disease Control and Prevention (CDC), inadequate disinfection of the water distribution or storage system was implicated in three (Table 64.3). The most recent outbreaks occurred at centers using dialysis machines having a port to dispose of dialyzer priming fluid (waste handling option) (43,44). One-way valves in the waste handling option had not been maintained, checked for competency, or disinfected as recommended, allowing backflow from the drain and contamination of the port.

Hemodialyzer Reuse

Since 1976, the percentage of chronic dialysis centers in the U.S. that reported reuse of disposable hollow-fiber dialyzers has increased steadily (44); the largest increase (139%) occurred during 1976 to 1982, from 18% to 43%, and the highest percentage (82%) was reported in 1997. In 2001, reuse of dialyzers was reported by 76% of centers (CDC, unpublished data).

In 1986, the AAMI's guidelines for reusing hemodialyzers (45) were adopted by the U.S. Public Health Service (USPHS) and later became CMS regulations. In general, dialyzer reuse appears to be safe if performed according to strict and established protocols. Dialyzer reuse has not been associated with transmission of hepatitis B virus (HBV) or hepatitis C virus (HCV) infection but has been associated with pyrogenic reactions (46) (Table 64.3). These adverse events may be the result of the use of incorrect concentrations of chemical germicides or the failure to maintain standards for water quality. Manual reprocessing of dialyzers that does not include a test for membrane integrity, such as the air-pressure leak test, may fail to detect membrane defects and may be a cause of pyrogenic reactions (46).

Some procedures used to reprocess hemodialyzers generally constitute high-level disinfection rather than sterilization (3,47). There are several liquid germicides commonly used for high-level disinfection of dialyzers. Formaldehyde is a chemical solution obtained from chemical supply houses, and is not formulated specifically for dialyzer disinfection. There are chemical germicides specifically formulated for this purpose (e.g., peracetic acid and glutaraldehyde-based products) that are approved by the U.S. Food and Drug Administration (FDA) as sterilants for reprocessing hemodialyzers. In 2001, a peracetic acid formulation was used by 62% of centers that reused dialyzers, formaldehyde by 29%, and glutaraldehyde by 5%; 4% of centers used a heat process (CDC, unpublished data).

In 1983, most centers in the U.S. used 2% aqueous formaldehyde with a contact time of approximately 36 hours for high-level disinfection of disposable dialyzers (48). In 1982, a center using this regimen experienced an outbreak of infections caused by nontuberculous mycobacteria (5). It subsequently was shown that the 2% formaldehyde regimen was not effective against nontuberculous mycobacteria. Rather, a regimen of 4% formaldehyde with a minimum contact time of 24 hours is required to inactivate high numbers of these microorganisms and is recommended as a minimum solution for disinfection of dialyzers (3,46,47). A similar outbreak of systemic mycobacterial infections in five dialysis patients, resulting in two deaths, occurred when high-flux dialyzers were contaminated with mycobacteria during manual reprocessing and were then disinfected with a commercial dialyzer disinfectant prepared at a concentration that did not ensure complete inactivation of mycobacteria (7). These two outbreaks of infection in dialysis patients emphasize the need to use dialyzer disinfectants at concentrations that are effective against the more chemically resistant microorganisms, such as mycobacteria.

Outbreaks of pyrogenic reactions have often resulted from reprocessing dialyzers with water that did not meet AAMI standards (Table 64.3). In most instances, the water used to rinse dialyzers or to prepare dialyzer disinfectants exceeded allowable AAMI microbial or endotoxin standards, because the water distribution system was not disinfected frequently, the disinfectant was improperly prepared, or routine microbiologic assays were improperly performed.

High-Flux Dialysis and Bicarbonate Dialysate

High-flux dialysis uses dialyzer membranes with hydraulic permeabilities five to ten times greater than those of conventional dialyzer membranes. There is concern that bacteria or endotoxin in the dialysate may penetrate these highly permeable high-flux dialyzer membranes.

TABLE 64.3. OUTBREAKS OF DIALYSIS-ASSOCIATED ILLNESSES INVESTIGATED BY THE CENTERS FOR DISEASE CONTROL AND PREVENTION (CDC)

Description (Reference)	Cause(s) of Outbreak	Corrective Measure(s) Recommended
Chemical contamination of dialysate		
Hemolytic anemia in 41 patients (161)	Chloramines in city water not removed completely by carbon filter	Larger carbon filters connected in series; monitor chloramines after each patient shift
Decreased hemoglobin in three pediatric patients (164)	Disinfectant not adequately rinsed from fluid distribution system	Thoroughly rinse germicide from system; use appropriate residual test kit
Severe hypotension in nine patients (165)	Dialysate contaminated with sodium azide from new ultrafilters	Rinse system after modification or installation of new components
Aluminum intoxication in 27 patients (166)	Exhausted deionization tanks unable to remove aluminum from city water	Monitor deionization tanks daily; install reverse osmosis system
Formaldehyde intoxication in five patients; one death (167)	Disinfectant not properly rinsed from fluid distribution system	Eliminate stagnant flow areas; test for residual germicide
Aluminum intoxication in 27 patients; three deaths (160)	Aluminum pump was used to transfer acid concentrate to treatment area	Use components that do not leach harmful substances into dialysis fluids
Fluoride intoxication in eight patients; one death (162)	Excess fluoride in city water; no water treatment by center	Install reverse osmosis system
Fluoride intoxication in nine patients; three deaths (168)	Exhausted deionization tanks discharged a bolus of fluoride	Deionization tanks should be monitored by resistivity meters with audible and visual alarms
Intoxication and death due to volatile organic compounds (CS_2, CH3S, etc) (CDC, unpublished data	Multiple causes: citric acid was used to reduce pH of incoming water to neutral precarbon to aid in adsorption of chlorine; water treatment system not functioning properly	Suspend the use of citric acid for pH control and redesign water treatment system
Bacteremia, fungemia, or pyrogenic reactions not related to dialyzer reuse		
Pyrogenic reactions in 49 patients (11)	Untreated city water contained high levels of endotoxin	Install reverse osmosis system
Pyrogenic reactions in 45 patients (20)	Inadequate disinfection of fluid distribution system	Increase disinfection frequency and germicide contact time
Pyrogenic reactions in 14 patients; two bacteremias; one death (4)	Reverse osmosis water storage tank contaminated with bacteria	Remove or properly disinfect and maintain storage tank
Pyrogenic reactions in six patients; seven bacteremias (169)	Inadequate disinfection of water distribution system and dialysis machines; improper microbial assay procedure	Use correct microbial assay procedure; disinfect water distribution system and dialysis machines according to manufacturer's recommendations
Bacteremia in 35 patients with central vein Catheters (170)	Central vein catheters used as primary access; median duration of infected catheters was 311 days; improper aseptic techniques	Use central vein catheters only when necessary; use appropriate aseptic techniques when inserting and performing catheter care
Three pyrogenic reactions and ten bacteremias in patients treated on machines with a port for disposal of dialyzer priming fluid (WHO) (171)	Incompetent valve allowing backflow from drain to the WHO; bacterial contamination of the WHO	Routine maintenance, disinfection, and check for valve competency of the WHO
Bacteremia in ten patients treated on machines with a port for disposal of dialyzer prime (172)	Incompetent valve allowing backflow from drain to the WHO; bacterial contamination of the WHO	Routine maintenance, disinfection, and check for valve competency of the WHO
Outbreak of pyrogenic reactions and gram-negative bacteremia in 11 patients (four with bacteremia) (17)	Water distribution system and machines were not routinely disinfected or according to manufacturer's instructions; water and dialysate samples were cultured using calibrated loop and blood agar plates—results were always recorded as no growth	Disinfect machines according to manufacturer's instructions; include water distribution system in the weekly disinfection of the RO system
Phialemonium curvatum access infections in four hemodialysis patients, two of these patients died of systemic disease (CDC, unpublished data)	Observations at the facility noted some irregularities in site prep for needle insertion; all affected patients have synthetic grafts; one environmental culture was positive for *P. curvatum* (condensate pan of HVAC serving the dialysis facility)	Review infection control practices, clean and disinfect HVAC system where water accumulates; perform surveillance on all patients
Bacteremia/pyrogenic reactions related to hemodialyzer reuse		
Mycobacterial infections in 27 patients (5)	Inadequate concentration of dialyzer disinfectant	Increase formaldehyde dialyzer disinfectant concentration to 4%
Mycobacterial infection in five high-flux dialysis patients; two deaths (7)	Inadequate concentration of dialyzer disinfectant	Use higher disinfectant concentration and more frequent disinfection of water treatment system

(*continued*)

TABLE 64.3. *(continued)*

Description (Reference)	Cause(s) of Outbreak	Corrective Measure(s) Recommended
Bacteremia and pyrogenic reactions in six patients (173)	Dialyzer disinfectant diluted to improper concentration	Use disinfectant at recommended dilution and verify concentration
Bacteremia in six patients (CDC, unpublished data)	Inadequate concentration of dialyzer disinfectant; water used for reuse did not meet AAMI standards	Use AAMI quality of water; ensure proper germicide concentration in dialyzer
Bacteremia and pyrogenic reactions in six patients (174)	Inadequate mixing of dialyzer disinfectant	Thoroughly mix disinfectant and verify proper concentration
Bacteremia in 33 patients at two dialysis centers (39,175)	Dialyzer disinfectant created holes in dialyzer membrane	Change disinfectant (removed from marketplace by manufacturer)
Bacteremia in six patients; all blood isolates had similar plasmid profiles (176)	Dialyzers contaminated during removal and cleaning of headers with gauze; staff not routinely changing gloves; dialyzers not processed for several hours after disassembly and cleaning	Do not use gauze or similar material to remove clots from header; change gloves frequently; process dialyzers immediately after rinsing and cleaning
Pyrogenic reactions in three high-flux dialysis patients (177)	Dialyzer reprocessed with two disinfectants; water used for reuse did not meet AAMI standards	Do not disinfect dialyzers with multiple germicides; more frequent disinfection of water system
Pyrogenic reactions in 14 high-flux dialysis; one death (178)	Dialyzers rinsed with city water; water for reuse did not meet AAMI standards	Do not rinse or clean dialyzers with city water; disinfect water treatment system more frequently
Pyrogenic reactions in 18 patients (51)	Dialyzers rinsed with city water containing high levels of endotoxin; water used for reuse did not meet AAMI standards	Do not rinse or clean dialyzers with city water; disinfect water treatment system more frequently
Pyrogenic reactions in 22 patients (179)	Water for reuse did not meet AAMI standards; improper microbial assay technique	Use correct microbial assay procedure; disinfect water distribution system
Acute allergic reactions		
Acute allergic reactions in hundreds of patients using reprocessed dialyzers in at least 31 centers (151)	Related to use of ACE inhibitors, and possibly to chemicals used in cleaning dialyzer or inadequate germicide rinse out of dialyzer	No specific recommendations
Transmission of viral agents		
Twenty-six patients seroconverted to HBsAg positive during a 10-month period (180)	Leakage of coil dialyzer membranes and use of recirculating bath dialysis machines	Separation of HBsAg-positive patients and equipment from other patients
Nineteen patients and one staff seroconverted to HBsAg positive during a 14-month period (96)	No specific cause determined; false-positive HBsAg results caused some susceptible patients to be dialyzed with infected patients	Laboratory confirmation of HBsAg-positive results; strict adherence to glove use and use of separate equipment
Twenty-four patients and six staff seroconverted to HBsAg positive during a 10-month period (91)	Staff not wearing gloves; surfaces not properly disinfected; improper handling of needles/sharps resulting in many staff needlesticks	Separation of HBsAg-positive patients and equipment from other patients; proper precautions by staff (e.g., gloves; handling of needles/sharps)
Thirteen patients and one staff seroconverted to HBsAg positive during a 1-month period (95)	Extrinsic contamination of intravenous medication being prepared adjacent to area where blood work was handled	Separate medication preparation area and blood processing for diagnostic tests
Ten patients seroconverted to HBsAg positive in 1 month (181)	Extrinsic contamination of multidose medication vial shared by HBsAg-positive and -susceptible patients	No sharing of supplies, equipment, and medications between patients
Eight patients seroconverted to HBsAg positive during a 5-month period (CDC, unpublished data)	Sporadic screening for HBsAg; HBsAg carriers not separated; major bleeding incident with environmental contamination	Monthly screening of patients for HBsAg; separation of positive patients with dedicated equipment and staff; vaccination of all susceptibles
Seven patients seroconverted to HBsAg-positive during a 3-month period (92)	Same staff caring for HBsAg-positive and -negative patients	Separation of HBsAg-positive patients from other patients; same staff should not care for HBsAg-positive and -negative patients on same shift
Eight patients seroconverted to HBsAg positive during 1 month (148)	Not consistently using pressure transducer filters; same members staff cared for HBsAg-positive and -negative patients on same shift	Use pressure transducer filters and replace after each use; same staff members should not care for HBsAg-positive and -negative patients on same shift
14 patients seroconverted to HBsAg positive during a 6-week period (93)	Failure to review results of admission and monthly HBsAg testing; inconsistent handwashing and use of gloves; adjacent clean and contaminated areas; <20% of patients vaccinated	Proper infection control precautions for dialysis units; routine review of serologic testing; hepatitis B vaccination of all patients

(*continued*)

TABLE 64.3. (continued)

Description (Reference)	Cause(s) of Outbreak	Corrective Measure(s) Recommended
Seven patients seroconverted to HBsAg positive during a 2-month period (93)	Same staff members cared for HBsAg-positive and -negative patients on same shift; common medication and supply carts were moved between stations, and multidose vials were shared; no patients were vaccinated	Dedicated staff for HBsAg-positive patients; no sharing of medication or supplies between any patients; centralized medication and supply areas; hepatitis B vaccination of all patients
Four patients seroconverted to HBsAg positive during a 3-month period (93)	Transmission appeared to occur during hospitalization at an acute care facility	Hepatitis B vaccination of all patients
11 patients seroconverted to HBsAg positive during a 3-month period (93)	Staff, equipment, and supplies were shared between HBsAg-positive and -negative patients; no patients were vaccinated	Dedicated staff for HBsAg-positive patients; no sharing of medication or supplies between patients; hepatitis B vaccination of all patients
Two patients seroconverted to HBsAg positive during a 4-month period (101)	Same staff members cared for HBsAg-positive and -negative patients; no patients were vaccinated	Dedicated staff for HBsAg-positive patients; hepatitis B vaccination of all patients
Thirty-six patients with liver enzyme elevations consistent with non-A, non-B hepatitis (182)	Environmental contamination with blood	Monthly liver enzyme screening; proper precautions (i.e., use of gloves) by staff
Thirty-five patients with liver enzyme elevations consistent with non-A, non-B hepatitis during a 22-month period; 82% of probable cases were anti-HCV positive (183)	Inconsistent use of infection control precautions, especially handwashing and glove use	Strict compliance to aseptic technique and dialysis center precautions
HCV infection developed in 7/41 (17.1%) patients; shift specific attack rates of 29% to 36% (184)	Multidose vials left on top of machine and used by multiple patients; routine cleaning and disinfection of surfaces and equipment between patients not routinely done; arterial line for draining prime waste droped into bucket that was not routinely cleaned between patients	Strict compliance with infection control precautions recommended for all dialysis patients; routine HCV testing
HCV infection developed in 5/75 (6.7%) patients (185)	Sharing of equipment and supplies between chronically infected and susceptible patients; gloves not routinely used; clean and contaminated areas not separated	Strict compliance with infection control precautions recommended for all dialysis patients
HCV infection developed in 3/23 (13%) patients (186)	Supply carts moved between stations and contained both clean supplies and blood-contaminated items; medications prepared in same area used for disposal of used injection equipment	Strict compliance with infection control precautions recommended for all dialysis patients

ACE, angiotensin-converting enzyme; AAMI, Association for the Advancement of Medical Instrumentation; HBsAg, hepatitis B surface antigen; HCV, hepatitis C virus; WHO, waste-handling option.

Another concern is that high-flux dialysis requires the use of bicarbonate rather than acetate dialysate. Acetate dialysate is prepared from a single concentrate with a high salt molarity (4.8 M) that cannot support the growth of most bacteria. Bicarbonate dialysate, however, must be prepared from two concentrates, an acid concentrate with a pH of 2.8 that is not conducive to bacterial growth and a bicarbonate concentrate with a relatively neutral pH and a salt molarity of 1.2 M. Because the bicarbonate concentrate will support rapid bacterial growth (49), its use can increase bacterial and endotoxin concentrations in the dialysate and theoretically may contribute to an increase in pyrogenic reactions, especially when it is used during high-flux dialysis.

Some of this concern appeared justified by the results of surveillance data during the 1990s that showed a significant association between use of high-flux dialysis and reporting of pyrogenic reactions among patients during dialysis (50). However, a prospective study of pyrogenic reactions in patients receiving more than 27,000 conventional, high-efficiency, or high-flux dialysis treatments with a bicarbonate dialysate containing high concentrations of bacteria and endotoxin found no association between pyrogenic reactions and the type of dialysis treatment (51). Although there seem to be conflicting data on the relationship between high-flux dialysis and pyrogenic reactions, centers providing high-flux dialysis should ensure that dialysate meets AAMI microbial standards (Table 64.2).

OTHER BACTERIAL INFECTIONS

The annual mortality rate among hemodialysis patients is 23%, and infections are the second most common cause, accounting for 14% of deaths (1). Septicemia (11.1% of all deaths) is the most common infectious cause of mortality. In studies published from 1997 to 2000 that evaluated rates of bacterial infections in hemodialysis outpatients, bacteremia occurred in 0.63% to 1.7% of patients per month and vascular access infections (with or without bacteremia) in 1.3% to 7.2% of patients per month (52–60). A review of four studies published during 2002 estimated that 1.8% of hemodialysis patients have vascular access associated bacteremia each month, amounting to 50,000 cases nationally per year (61).

Because of the importance of bacterial infections in hemodialysis patients, the CDC initiated an ongoing surveillance project in 1999 (62). All U.S. hemodialysis centers treating outpatients are eligible to enroll. Only bacterial infections associated with hospital admission or intravenous antimicrobial receipt are counted; since infections treated with outpatient oral antimicrobials are excluded, this system likely detects only the more severe infections. During 1999 to 2001, 109 centers reported data. Rates of infection per 100 patient months were 3.2 for all vascular access infections (including access infections both with and without bacteremia), 1.8 for vascular-access associated bacteremia, 1.3 for wound infections not related to the vascular access, 0.8 for pneumonias, and 0.3 for urinary tract infections. Among patients with fistulas or grafts, wounds were the most common site of infection. Among patients with hemodialysis catheters, infections of the vascular access site were most common.

In a study of 27 French hemodialysis centers, 28% of 230 infections in hemodialysis patients involved the vascular access, whereas 25% involved the lung, 23% the urinary tract, 9% the skin and soft tissues, and 15% other or unknown sites (58). Thirty-three percent of infections involved either the vascular access site or were bacteremias of unknown origin, many of which might have been caused by occult access infections. Thus, the vascular access site was the most common site for infection, but accounted for only one third of infections.

Bacterial pathogens causing infection can be either exogenous (i.e., acquired from contaminated dialysis fluids or equipment) or endogenous (i.e., caused by invasion of bacteria present in or on the patient). Exogenous pathogens have caused numerous outbreaks, most of which resulted from inadequate dialyzer reprocessing procedures (e.g., contaminated water or inadequate disinfectant) or inadequate treatment of municipal water for use in dialysis. During 1995 to 1997, four outbreaks were traced to contamination of the waste drain port on one type of dialysis machine (43). Recommendations to prevent such outbreaks are published elsewhere (63).

Contaminated medication vials also are a potential source of bacterial infection for patients. In 1999, an outbreak of *Serratia liquefaciens* bloodstream infections and pyrogenic reactions among hemodialysis patients was traced to contamination of vials of erythropoietin. These vials, which were intended for single use, were contaminated by repeated puncture to obtain additional doses and by pooling of residual medication into a common vial (64).

Vascular Access Infections

Access site infections are particularly important, because they can cause disseminated bacteremia or loss of the vascular access. Local signs of vascular access infection include erythema, warmth, induration, swelling, tenderness, breakdown of skin, loculated fluid, or purulent exudate (53,56,62,65). In the CDC surveillance project, rates of access-associated bacteremia per 100 patient-months were 1.8 overall, and varied by access type: 0.25 for fistulas, 0.53 for grafts, 4.8 for permanent (tunneled, cuffed) catheters, and 8.7 for temporary (nontunneled, noncuffed) catheters (62).

Vascular access infections are caused (in descending order of frequency) by *Staphylococcus aureus* (32–53% of cases), coagulase-negative staphylococci (CNS; 20–32%), gram-negative bacilli (10–18%), nonstaphylococcal gram-positive cocci (including enterococci; 10–12%), and fungi (<1%) (62). The proportion of infections caused by *S. aureus* is higher among patients with fistulas or grafts, and the proportion caused by CNS is higher among patients dialyzed through catheters.

The primary risk factor for access infection is access type, with catheters having the highest risk for infection, grafts intermediate, and native arteriovenous (AV) fistulas the lowest (55, 62,66). Other potential risk factors for vascular access infections include (a) location of the access in the lower extremity; (b) recent access surgery; (c) trauma, hematoma, dermatitis, or scratching over the access site; (d) poor patient hygiene; (e) poor needle insertion technique; (f) older age; (g) diabetes; (h) immunosuppression; and (i) iron overload (53,56,67–69).

Based on the relative risk of both infectious and noninfectious complications, it is recommended that native AV fistulas be used more commonly and hemodialysis catheters less commonly; a goal of no more than 10% of patients maintained with permanent catheter-based hemodialysis treatments is recommended (70). To minimize infectious complications, patients should be referred early for creation of an implanted access, thereby decreasing the time dialyzed through a temporary catheter. Additionally, permanent catheters should be used only in patients for whom implanted access is impossible. During 1995 to 2001, the percentage of patients dialyzed through fistulas increased from 22% to 30%, with most of the increase occurring since 1999 (44; CDC, unpublished data). During the same period, use of grafts decreased from 65% to 44% of patients, and use of catheters increased from 13% to 25%; however, the rate of increase in catheter use appears to be slowing.

Recommendations for preventing vascular access infections have been developed by the National Kidney Foundation (70) and the CDC (71) and recently summarized (72). Selected recommendations for preventing hemodialysis-catheter–associated infection include not using antimicrobial prophylaxis before insertion or during the use of the catheter; not routinely replacing the catheter; using sterile technique (cap, mask, sterile gown, large sterile drapes, and gloves) during catheter insertion; limiting use of noncuffed catheters to 3 to 4 weeks; using the catheter solely for hemodialysis unless there is no alternative; restricting catheter manipulation and dressing changes to trained personnel; replacing catheter-site dressing at each dialysis treatment or if damp, loose, or soiled; disinfecting skin before catheter insertion and dressing changes (a 2% chlorhexidine-based preparation is preferred); and ensuring that catheter-site care is compatible with the catheter material.

In hemodialysis patients, the Infectious Diseases Society of America has recommended treatment with nasal mupirocin in documented *S. aureus* carriers who have a catheter-related bloodstream infection with *S. aureus* and continue to need the hemodialysis catheter (73). Otherwise, the routine use of nasal mupirocin in patients with hemodialysis catheters is not recommended by either the CDC or the National Kidney Foundation (70,71).

Antimicrobial Resistant Bacteria

Hemodialysis patients have been in the forefront of the epidemic of antimicrobial resistance, especially vancomycin resistance. One of the earliest reports of vancomycin-resistant enterococci (VRE) was from a renal unit in London, England, in 1988 (74). The prevalence of VRE stool colonization among dialysis patients has varied from 2.4% at three centers in Indianapolis, Indiana (75), to 9.5% at a university hospital in Baltimore, Maryland (76). In one center with a prevalence of 9%, three patients developed VRE infections in 1 year (77). Among enterococci causing bloodstream infections in hemodialysis patients, 0% to 5% have been reported to be resistant to vancomycin (62,78,79).

Vancomycin resistance in staphylococci has also been reported in dialysis patients. Five of the first six U.S. patients with vancomycin intermediate-resistant *S. aureus* infections identified required dialysis (80). Additionally, the first patient found to be infected with a fully vancomycin-resistant *S. aureus* strain was a chronic hemodialysis patient; vancomycin-resistant *S. aureus* was isolated from a foot wound and temporary catheter exit site (81).

For certain patients, including those infected or colonized with methicillin-resistant *S. aureus* (MRSA) or VRE, contact precautions are used in the inpatient hospital setting. However, contact precautions are not recommended in hemodialysis units for patients infected or colonized with pathogenic bacteria for several reasons. First, although contact transmission of pathogenic bacteria is well documented in hospitals, similar transmission has not been well documented in hemodialysis centers. Transmission might not be apparent in dialysis centers, possibly because it occurs less frequently than in acute-care hospitals or results in undetected colonization rather than overt infection. Also, because dialysis patients are frequently hospitalized, determining whether transmission occurred in the inpatient or outpatient setting is difficult. Second, contamination of the patient's skin, bedclothes, and environmental surfaces with pathogenic bacteria is likely to be more common in hospital settings (where patients spend 24 hours a day) than in outpatient hemodialysis centers (where patients spend approximately 10 hours a week). Third, the routine use of infection control practices recommended for hemodialysis units, which are more stringent than the standard precautions routinely used in hospitals, should prevent transmission by the contact route.

BLOOD-BORNE VIRUSES: VIRAL HEPATITIS AND ACQUIRED IMMUNODEFICIENCY SYNDROME

Recommendations for the control of hepatitis B in hemodialysis centers were first published in 1977 (82), and by 1980 their widespread implementation was associated with a sharp reduction in incidence of HBV infection among both patients and staff members (83). In 1982, hepatitis B vaccination was recommended for all susceptible patients and staff members (84). However, outbreaks of both HBV and HCV infections continue to occur among chronic hemodialysis patients. Other blood-borne pathogens that are potentially transmissible in hemodialysis centers include hepatitis delta virus (HDV) and human immunodeficiency virus (HIV). Hepatitis A and E viruses, which are spread by the fecal-oral route and rarely by blood, have not been associated with hemodialysis.

Hepatitis B Virus

Epidemiology

The incidence and prevalence of HBV infection among chronic hemodialysis patients in the U.S. have dramatically declined, and by 2001 was 0.05% and 0.9%, respectively (85; CDC, unpublished data, 2001). Only 2.9% of all centers reported patients with newly acquired infections; however, 26.5% of centers provided dialysis to one or more chronically infected patients (CDC, unpublished data, 2001).

The chronically infected person is central to the epidemiology of HBV transmission. HBV is transmitted by percutaneous (i.e., puncture through the skin) or permucosal (i.e., direct contact with mucous membranes) exposure to infectious blood or to body fluids that contain blood. All hepatitis B surface antigen (HBsAg)-positive persons are infectious, but those who are also positive for hepatitis B e antigen (HBeAg) circulate HBV at high titers in their blood (10^8 to 10^9 virions/mL) (86,87). With virus titers in blood this high, body fluids containing serum or blood also can contain high levels of HBV and are potentially infectious. Furthermore, HBV at titers of 10^2 to 10^3 virions/mL can be present on environmental surfaces in the absence of any visible blood and still cause transmission (86,88,89).

HBV is relatively stable in the environment and remains viable for at least 7 days on environmental surfaces at room temperature (86,88,89). HBsAg has been detected in dialysis centers on clamps, scissors, dialysis machine control knobs, and doorknobs (90). Thus, blood-contaminated surfaces that are not routinely cleaned and disinfected represent a reservoir for HBV transmission. Dialysis staff members can transfer virus to patients from contaminated surfaces by their hands or gloves or through use of contaminated equipment and supplies.

Most outbreaks of HBV infection among hemodialysis patients (Table 64.3) were caused by cross-contamination to patients via (a) environmental surfaces, supplies (e.g., hemostats, clamps), or equipment that was not routinely disinfected after each use; (b) multiple dose medication vials and intravenous solutions that were not used exclusively for one patient; (c) medications for injection that were prepared in areas adjacent to areas where blood samples were handled; and (d) staff members who simultaneously cared for both HBV-infected and susceptible patients (91–96). Once the factors that promote HBV transmission among hemodialysis patients were identified, recommendations for control were published in 1977 (82). These recommendations included (a) serologic surveillance of patients (and staff members) for HBV infection, including monthly testing of all susceptible patients for HBsAg; (b) isolation of HBsAg-positive patients in a separate room; (c) assignment of staff members to HBsAg-positive patients and not to HBV-susceptible patients during the same shift; (d) assignment of dialysis equipment to HBsAg-positive patients that is not shared by HBV-susceptible patients; (e) assignment of a supply tray to each patient (regardless of serologic status); (f) cleaning and disinfection of nondisposable items (e.g., clamps, scissors) before use on another patient; (g) glove use whenever any patient or hemodialysis equipment is touched and glove changes between each patient (and station); and (h) routine cleaning and disinfection of equipment and environmental surfaces.

The segregation of HBsAg-positive patients and their equipment from HBV-susceptible patients resulted in 70% to 80% reductions in incidence of HBV infection among hemodialysis patients (97–99). The success of isolation practices in preventing transmission of HBV infection is linked to other infection control practices, including routine serologic surveillance and routine cleaning and disinfection. Frequent serologic testing for HBsAg quickly detects patients recently infected with HBV, so isolation procedures can be implemented before cross-contamination can occur. Environmental control by routine cleaning and disinfection procedures reduces the opportunity for cross-contamination, either directly from environmental surfaces or indirectly by hands of personnel.

Despite the current low incidence of HBV infection among hemodialysis patients, outbreaks continue to occur in chronic hemodialysis centers. Investigations of these outbreaks have documented that HBV transmission resulted from failure to use recommended infection control practices, including (a) failure to routinely screen patients for HBsAg or routinely review results of testing to identify infected patients; (b) assignment of staff members to the simultaneous care of infected and susceptible patients; and (c) sharing of supplies, particularly multiple dose medication vials, among patients (93). In addition, few patients had received hepatitis B vaccine. National surveillance data have demonstrated that independent risk factors among chronic hemodialysis patients for acquiring HBV infection include the presence of more than one HBV-infected patient in the hemodialysis center who is not isolated, as well as a <50% hepatitis B vaccination rate among patients (100).

HBV infection among chronic hemodialysis patients also has been associated with hemodialysis provided in the acute-care setting (93,101). Transmission appeared to stem from chronically infected HBV patients who shared staff members, multiple dose medication vials, and other supplies and equipment with susceptible patients. These episodes were recognized when patients returned to their chronic hemodialysis units, and routine HBsAg testing was resumed. Transmission from HBV-infected chronic hemodialysis patients to patients undergoing hemodialysis for acute renal failure has not been documented, possibly because these patients are dialyzed for short durations and have limited exposure. However, such transmission could go unrecognized, because acute renal failure patients are unlikely to be tested for HBV infection.

Other risk factors for acquiring HBV infection include injection drug use, sexual and household exposure to an HBV-infected contact, exposure to multiple sexual partners, male homosexual activity, and perinatal exposure. Dialysis patients should be educated about these other risks and, for those patients chronically infected with HBV, informed that their sexual partners and household contacts should be vaccinated against hepatitis B (102).

Screening and Diagnostic Tests

Several well-defined antigen-antibody systems are associated with HBV infection, including HBsAg and antibody to HBsAg (anti-HBs); hepatitis B core antigen (HBcAg) and antibody to HBcAg (anti-HBc); and HBeAg and antibody to HBeAg (anti-HBe). Serologic assays are commercially available for all of these except HBcAg, because no free HBcAg circulates in blood. One or more of these serologic markers are present during different phases of HBV infection (Table 64.4) (103). HBV infection also can be detected using qualitative or quantitative tests for HBV DNA. These tests are not FDA approved and are most commonly used for patients being managed with antiviral therapy (97,98,104,105).

The presence of HBsAg is indicative of ongoing HBV infection and potential infectiousness. In newly infected persons,

TABLE 64.4. INTERPRETATION OF SEROLOGIC TEST RESULTS FOR HEPATITIS B VIRUS INFECTION

Serologic Markers				
HBsAg	**Total Anti-HBc**	**IgM Anti-HBc**	**Anti-HBs**	**Interpretation**
−	−	−	−	Susceptible, never infected
+	−	−	−	Acute infection early incubation[a]
+	+	+	−	Acute infection
−	+	+	−	Acute resolving infection
−	+	−	+	Past infection, recovered and immune
+	+	−	−	Chronic infection
−	+	−	−	False positive (i.e., susceptible), past infection, or "low-level" chronic infection
−	−	−	+	Immune if titer is ≥ 10 mIU/mL

[a]Transient HBsAg positivity (lasting ≤18 days) might be detected in some patients during vaccination.
HBsAg, hepatitis B surface antigen; anti-HBc, antibody to hepatitis B core antigen; IgM, immunoglobulin M; anti-HBs, antibody to hepatitis B surface antigen.

HBsAg is present in serum 30 to 60 days after exposure to HBV and persists for variable periods. Transient HBsAg positivity (lasting ≤18 days) can be detected in some patients during vaccination (106,107). Anti-HBc develops in all HBV infections, appearing at onset of symptoms or liver test abnormalities in acute HBV infection, rising rapidly to high levels, and persisting for life. Acute or recently acquired infection can be distinguished by presence of the immunoglobulin M (IgM) class of anti-HBc, which persists for approximately 6 months.

In persons who recover from HBV infection, HBsAg is eliminated from the blood, usually in 2 to 3 months, and anti-HBs develops during convalescence. The presence of anti-HBs indicates immunity from HBV infection. After recovery from natural infection, most persons will be positive for both anti-HBs and anti-HBc, whereas only anti-HBs develops in persons who are successfully vaccinated against hepatitis B. Persons who do not recover from HBV infection and become chronically infected remain positive for HBsAg (and anti-HBc), although a small proportion (0.3% per year) eventually clear HBsAg and might develop anti-HBs (108).

In some persons, the only HBV serologic marker detected is anti-HBc (i.e., isolated anti-HBc). Among most asymptomatic persons in the U.S. tested for HBV infection, an average of 2% (range: <0.1% to 6%) test positive for isolated anti-HBc (109); among injecting-drug users, however, the rate is 24% (110). In general, the frequency of isolated anti-HBc is directly related to the frequency of previous HBV infection in the population and can have several explanations. This pattern can occur after HBV infection among persons who have recovered but whose anti-HBs levels have waned or among persons who failed to develop anti-HBs. Persons in the latter category include those who circulate HBsAg at levels not detectable by current commercial assays. However, HBV DNA has been detected in <10% of persons with isolated anti-HBc, and these persons are unlikely to be infectious to others except under unusual circumstances involving direct percutaneous exposure to large quantities of blood (e.g., transfusion) (111). In most persons with isolated anti-HBc, the result appears to be a false positive. Data from several studies have demonstrated that a primary anti-HBs response develops in most of these persons after a three-dose series of hepatitis B vaccine (112,113). No data exist on response to vaccination among hemodialysis patients with this serologic pattern.

A third antigen, HBeAg, can be detected in serum of persons with acute or chronic HBV infection. The presence of HBeAg correlates with viral replication and high levels of virus (i.e., high infectivity). Anti-HBe correlates with the loss of replicating virus and with lower levels of virus. However, all HBsAg-positive persons should be considered potentially infectious, regardless of their HBeAg or anti-HBe status.

Hepatitis C Virus

Epidemiology

Data are limited on current incidence and prevalence of HCV infection among chronic hemodialysis patients. In 2001, 62% of centers reported that they tested patients for antibody to HCV (anti-HCV) (CDC, unpublished data). In the centers that tested, the reported incidence was 0.29% and prevalence was 8.6% [range among end-stage renal disease (ESRD) networks, 5.7% to 11.9%]. Twelve percent of centers reported newly acquired HCV infections among patients. Higher incidence rates have been reported from cohort studies of hemodialysis patients in the U.S. (<1% to 3%) and Europe (3% to 10%) (114–120). Higher prevalences (10% to 36%) also have been reported from studies of patients in individual facilities (114,121).

HCV is most efficiently transmitted by direct percutaneous exposure to infectious blood, and like HBV, the chronically infected person is central to the epidemiology of HCV transmission. Risk factors associated with HCV infection among hemodialysis patients include blood transfusions from unscreened donors and years on dialysis (114,121). The number of years on dialysis is the major risk factor independently associated with higher rates of HCV infection. As the time patients spent on dialysis increased, their prevalence of HCV infection increased from an average of 12% for patients receiving dialysis <5 years to an average of 37% for patients receiving dialysis >5 years (114,121–123).

These studies, as well as investigations of dialysis-associated outbreaks of hepatitis C, indicate that HCV transmission most likely occurs because of inadequate infection control practices. During 1999 to 2000, CDC investigated three outbreaks of HCV infection among patients in chronic hemodialysis centers (CDC, unpublished data, 1999, 2000). In two of the outbreaks, multiple transmissions of HCV occurred during periods of 16 to 24 months (attack rates: 6.6% to 17.5%), and seroconversions were associated with receiving dialysis immediately after a chronically infected patient. Multiple opportunities for cross-contamination among patients were observed, including (a) equipment and supplies that were not disinfected between patient use; (b) use of common medication carts to prepare and distribute medications at patients' stations; (c) sharing of multiple dose medication vials, which were placed at patients' stations on top of hemodialysis machines; (d) contaminated priming buckets that were not routinely changed or cleaned and disinfected between patients; (e) machine surfaces that were not routinely cleaned and disinfected between patients; and (f) blood spills that were not cleaned up promptly. In the third outbreak, multiple new infections clustered at one point in time (attack rate: 27%), suggesting a common exposure event. Multiple opportunities for cross-contamination from chronically infected patients also were observed in this unit. In particular, supply carts were moved from one station to another and contained both clean supplies and blood-contaminated items, including small biohazard containers, sharps disposal boxes, and used Vacutainers containing patients' blood.

Other risk factors for acquiring HCV infection include injection drug use, exposure to an HCV-infected sexual partner or household contact, multiple sexual partners, and perinatal exposure (124,125). The efficiency of transmission in settings involving sexual or household exposure to infected contacts is low, and the magnitude of risk and the circumstances under which these exposures result in transmission are not well defined.

Screening and Diagnostic Tests

FDA-licensed or -approved anti-HCV screening test kits being used in the U.S. comprise three immunoassays: two enzyme immunoassays (EIAs) and one enhanced chemiluminescence immunoassay (CIA) (126). FDA-licensed or -approved supplemental tests include a serologic anti-HCV assay, the strip immunoblot assay (Chiron RIBA HCV 3.0 SIA, Chiron Corp., Emeryville, CA), and nucleic acid tests (NATs) for HCV RNA [including reverse-transcriptase polymerase chain reaction (RT-PCR) amplification and transcription mediated amplification (TMA)].

Anti-HCV testing includes initial screening with an immunoassay. If the screening test is positive, an independent supplemental test with high specificity should be performed to verify the results. Among hemodialysis patients, the proportion of false-positive screening test results averages approximately 15% (126). For this reason, not relying exclusively on anti-HCV screening-test–positive results to determine whether a person has been infected with HCV is critical. Table 64.5 describes the interpretation of HCV testing results both for screening and diagnosis.

For routine HCV testing of hemodialysis patients, the anti-HCV screening immunoassay is recommended, and if positive, supplemental anti-HCV testing using RIBA. RIBA is recommended rather than a NAT because it is a serologic assay and can be performed on the same serum or plasma sample collected for the screening anti-HCV assay. In addition, in certain situations the HCV RNA result can be negative in persons with active HCV infection. As the titer of anti-HCV increases during acute infection, the titer of HCV RNA declines (127). Thus, HCV RNA is not detectable in certain persons during the acute phase of their hepatitis C, but this finding can be transient and chronic infection can develop (128). In addition, intermittent HCV RNA positivity has been observed among persons with chronic HCV infection (129–131). Therefore, the significance of a single negative HCV RNA result is unknown, and the need for further investigation or follow-up is determined by verifying anti-HCV status. In addition, detection of HCV RNA requires that the serum or plasma sample be collected and handled in a manner suitable for NAT and that testing be performed in a laboratory with facilities established for this purpose (test MMWR). Although in rare instances, detection of HCV RNA might be the only evidence of HCV infection, a recent study conducted among almost 3,000 hemodialysis patients in the U.S. found that only 0.07% were HCV RNA positive but anti-HCV negative (CDC, unpublished data).

TABLE 64.5. INTERPRETATION OF TEST RESULTS FOR HEPATITIS C VIRUS INFECTION

Anti-HCV–positive

An anti-HCV–positive result is defined as anti-HCV screening-test–positive and recombinant immunoblot positive (RIBA) or nucleic acid test (NAT) positive; or anti-HCV screening-test–positive, NAT negative, RIBA positive
- An anti-HCV–positive result indicates past or current HCV infection
- An HCV RNA-positive result indicates current (active) infection, but the significance of a single HCV RNA negative result is unknown; it does not differentiate intermittent viremia from resolved infection
- All anti-HCV–positive persons should receive counseling and undergo medical evaluation, including additional testing for the presence of virus and liver disease
- Anti-HCV testing generally does not need to be repeated, once a positive anti-HCV result has been confirmed.

Anti-HCV–negative

An anti-HCV–negative result is defined as anti-HCV screening-test–negative[a]; or anti-HCV screening-test–positive, RIBA negative; or anti-HCV screening-test–positive, NAT negative, RIBA negative
- An anti-HCV–negative person is considered uninfected
- No further evaluation or follow-up for HCV is required, unless recent infection is suspected or other evidence exists to indicate HCV infection (e.g., abnormal liver enzyme levels in immunocompromised persons or persons with no other etiology for their liver disease)

Anti-HCV–indeterminate

An indeterminate anti-HCV result is defined as anti-HCV screening-test–positive, RIBA indeterminate;
- An indeterminate anti-HCV result indicates that the HCV antibody status cannot be determined
- Can indicate a false-positive anti-HCV screening test result, the most likely interpretation in those at low risk for HCV infection; such persons are HCV RNA negative
- Can occur as a transient finding in recently infected persons who are in the process of seroconversion; such persons usually are HCV RNA positive
- Can be a persistent finding in persons chronically infected with HCV; such persons usually are HCV RNA positive

If NAT is not performed, another sample should be collected for repeat anti-HCV testing (≥1 month later)

[a]Interpretation of screening immunoassay test result based on criteria provided by the manufacturer.
From Centers for Disease Control and Prevention. Guidelines for laboratory testing and result reporting of antibody to hepatitis C virus. *MMWR* 2003; 52(RR-3):1–15.

Other Blood-Borne Viruses

Hepatitis Delta Virus

Delta hepatitis is caused by the hepatitis delta virus (HDV), a defective virus that causes infection only in persons with active HBV infection. The prevalence of HDV infection is low in the U.S., with rates of <1% among HBsAg-positive persons in the general population and >10% among HBsAg-positive persons with repeated percutaneous exposures (e.g., injecting-drug users, persons with hemophilia) (132). Areas of the world with high endemic rates of HDV infection include southern Italy, parts of Africa, and the Amazon basin.

Few data exist on the prevalence of HDV infection among chronic hemodialysis patients, and only one transmission of HDV between such patients has been reported in the U.S. (133). In this episode, transmission occurred from a patient who was chronically infected with HBV and HDV to an HBsAg-positive patient after a massive bleeding incident; both patients received dialysis at the same station.

HDV infection occurs either as a co-infection with HBV or as a superinfection in a person with chronic HBV infection. Co-infection usually resolves, but superinfection frequently results in chronic HDV infection and severe disease. High mortality rates are associated with both types of infection. A serologic test that measures total antibody to HDV is commercially available.

Human Immunodeficiency Virus (HIV) Infection

During 1985 to 2001, the percentage of U.S. hemodialysis centers that reported providing chronic hemodialysis for patients with HIV infection increased from 11% to 37%, and the proportion of hemodialysis patients with known HIV infection increased from 0.3% to 1.5% (44; CDC, unpublished data, 2001). HIV is transmitted by blood and other body fluids that contain blood. No patient-to-patient transmission of HIV has been reported in U.S. hemodialysis centers. However, such transmission has been reported in other countries; in one case, HIV transmission was attributed to mixing of reused access needles and inadequate disinfection of equipment (134). HIV infection is usually diagnosed with assays that measure antibody to HIV, and a repeatedly positive EIA test should be confirmed by Western blot or another confirmatory test.

PREVENTING TRANSMISSION OF INFECTIONS AMONG CHRONIC HEMODIALYSIS PATIENTS

Preventing transmission among chronic hemodialysis patients of blood-borne viruses and pathogenic bacteria from both recognized and unrecognized sources of infection requires implementation of a comprehensive infection control program. The components of such a program include infection control practices specifically designed for the hemodialysis setting, including routine serologic testing and immunization, surveillance, and training and education. CDC has published recommendations describing these components in detail (135).

The infection control practices recommended for hemodialysis units (Table 64.6) will reduce opportunities for patient-to-patient transmission of infectious agents, directly or indirectly via contaminated devices, equipment and supplies, environmental surfaces, or hands of personnel. These practices should be carried out routinely for all patients in the chronic hemodialysis setting because of the increased potential for blood contamination during hemodialysis and because many patients are colonized or infected with pathogenic bacteria.

Such practices include additional measures to prevent HBV transmission because of the high titer of HBV and its ability to survive on environmental surfaces (Table 64.6). It is the potential for environmentally mediated transmission of HBV, rather than internal contamination of dialysis machines, that is the focus of infection control strategies for preventing HBV transmission in dialysis centers. For patients at increased risk for transmission of pathogenic bacteria, including antimicrobial-resistant strains, additional precautions also might be necessary in some circumstances. Furthermore, surveillance for infections and other adverse events is required to monitor the effectiveness of infection control practices, as well as training and education of both staff members and patients to ensure that appropriate infection control behaviors and techniques are carried out.

In each chronic hemodialysis unit, policies and practices should be reviewed and updated to ensure that infection control practices recommended for hemodialysis units are implemented and rigorously followed. Intensive efforts must be made to educate new staff members and reeducate existing staff members regarding these practices. Readers should consult the CDC recommendations for details on these practices (135). The following is a summary of selected issues.

Routine Testing

All chronic hemodialysis patients should be routinely tested for HBV and HCV infection, and the results promptly reviewed so that potential episodes of transmission can be identified quickly and patients appropriately managed based on their testing results. Test results (positive and negative) must be communicated to other units or hospitals when patients are transferred for care. Routine testing for HDV or HIV infection for purposes of infection control is not recommended.

Before admission to the hemodialysis unit, the HBV serologic status (i.e., HBsAg, total anti-HBc, and anti-HBs) of all patients should be known. For patients transferred from another unit, test results should be obtained before the patients' transfer. If a patient's HBV serologic status is not known at the time of admission, testing should be completed within 7 days. The hemodialysis unit should ensure that the laboratory performing the testing for anti-HBs can define a 10 mIU/mL concentration to determine protective levels of antibody.

Routine HCV testing should include use of both a screening immunoassay to test for anti-HCV and supplemental or confirmatory testing with an additional, more specific assay. Use of NAT for HCV RNA as the primary test for routine screening is not recommended, because few HCV infections will be identified in anti-HCV negative patients. However, if alanine aminotransferase (ALT) levels are persistently abnormal in anti-HCV negative patients in the absence of another etiology, testing for HCV RNA should be considered. Blood samples collected for NAT should not contain heparin, which interferes with the accurate performance of this assay.

Hepatitis B vaccination is an essential component of prevention in the hemodialysis setting. All susceptible patients and staff should receive hepatitis B vaccine. Susceptible patients who have not yet received hepatitis B vaccine, are in the process of being vaccinated, or have not adequately responded to vaccination should continue to be tested regularly for HBsAg. Detailed recommendations for vaccination and follow-up of hemodialysis patients have been published elsewhere (135).

Management of Infected Patients

Hepatitis B Virus

HBsAg-positive patients should undergo dialysis in a separate room designated only for HBsAg-positive patients. They should use separate machines, equipment, and supplies, and most importantly staff members should not care for both HBsAg-positive and susceptible patients on the same shift or at the same time. Dialyzers should not be reused on HBsAg-positive patients. Because HBV is efficiently transmitted through occupational exposure to blood, reprocessing dialyzers from HBsAg-positive patients might place HBV-susceptible staff members at increased risk for infection.

HBV chronically infected patients (i.e., those who are HBsAg positive, total anti-HBc positive, and IgM anti-HBc negative)

TABLE 64.6. RECOMMENDED INFECTION CONTROL PRACTICES FOR HEMODIALYSIS UNITS:

Infection Control Precautions for All Patients

- Wear disposable gloves when caring for the patient or touching the patient's equipment at the dialysis station; remove gloves and wash hands between each patient or station.
- Items taken into the dialysis station should either be disposed of, dedicated for use only on a single patient, or cleaned and disinfected before taken to a common clean area or used on another patient.
  - Nondisposable items that cannot be cleaned and disinfected (e.g., adhesive tape, clothcovered blood pressure cuffs) should be dedicated for use only on a single patient.
  - Unused medications (including multiple dose vials containing diluents) or supplies (syringes, alcohol swabs, etc.) taken to the patient's station should be used only for that patient and should not be returned to a common clean area or used on other patients.
- When multiple dose medication vials are used (including vials containing diluents), prepare individual patient doses in a clean (centralized) area away from dialysis stations and deliver separately to each patient. Do not carry multiple dose medication vials from station to station.
- Do not use common medication carts to deliver medications to patients. Do not carry medication vials, syringes, alcohol swabs or supplies in pockets. If trays are used to deliver medications to individual patients, they must be cleaned between patients.
- Clean areas should be clearly designated for the preparation, handling, and storage of medications and unused supplies and equipment. Clean areas should be clearly separated from contaminated areas where used supplies and equipment are handled. Do not handle and store medications or clean supplies in the same or an adjacent area to that where used equipment or blood samples are handled.
- Use external venous and arterial pressure transducer filters/protectors for each patient treatment to prevent blood contamination of the dialysis machine's pressure monitor. Change filters/protectors between each patient treatment, and do not reuse them. Internal transducer filters do not need to be changed routinely between patients.
- Clean and disinfect the dialysis station (chairs, beds, tables, machines, etc.) between patients.
  - Give special attention to cleaning control panels on the dialysis machines and other surfaces that are frequently touched and potentially contaminated with patients' blood.
  - Discard all fluid and clean and disinfect all surfaces and containers associated with the prime waste (including buckets attached to the machines).
- For dialyzers and blood tubing that will be reprocessed, cap dialyzer ports and clamp tubing. Place all used dialyzers and tubing in leak-proof containers for transport from station to reprocessing or disposal area.

Schedule for Routine Testing for Hepatitis B Virus (HBV) and Hepatitis C Virus (HCV) Infection

Patient Status	On Admission[a]	Monthly	Semiannual	Annual
All patients	HBsAg, anti-HBc (total), anti-HBs, anti-HCV, ALT			
HBV susceptible, including nonresponders to vaccine		HBsAg		
Anti-HBs positive (≥10 mIU/mL), anti-HBc negative				Anti-HBs
Anti-HBs and anti-HBc positive		No additional HBV testing needed		
Anti-HCV negative		ALT	Anti-HCV	

[a] Results of HBV testing should be known before the patient begins dialysis.
HBsAg Hepatitis B surface antigen; anti-HBc, antibody to hepatitis B core antigen;
anti-HBs, antibody to hepatitis B surface antigen; anti-HCV, antibody to hepatitis C virus;
ALT, alanine aminotransferase.

Hepatitis B Vaccination

- Vaccinate all susceptible patients against hepatitis B.
- Test for anti-HBs 1–2 months after last dose.
  - If anti-HBs is <10 mIU/mL, consider patient susceptible, revaccinate with an additional three doses, and retest for anti-HBs.
  - If anti-HBs is >10 mIU/mL, consider immune, and retest annually.
    - Give booster dose of vaccine if anti-HBs declines to <10 mIU/mL and continue to retest annually.

Management of HBsAg-Positive Patients

- Follow infection control practices for hemodialysis units for all patients.
- Dialyze HBsAg-positive patients in a separate room using separate machines, equipment, instruments, and supplies.
- Staff members caring for HBsAg-positive patients should not care for HBV susceptible patients at the same time (e.g., during the same shift or during patient change-over).

From Centers for Disease Control and Prevention. Recommendations for preventing transmission of infections among chronic hemodialysis patients. *MMWR* 2001;50(RR-5):1–43.

are infectious to others and are at risk for chronic liver disease. They should be counseled regarding preventing transmission to others, their household and sexual partners should receive hepatitis B vaccine, and they should be evaluated (by consultation or referral, if appropriate) for the presence or development of chronic liver disease according to current medical practice guidelines. Persons with chronic liver disease should be vaccinated against hepatitis A, if susceptible.

HBV chronically infected patients do not require any routine follow-up testing for purposes of infection control. However, annual testing for HBsAg is reasonable to detect the small percentage of HBV-infected patients who might lose their HBsAg.

Hepatitis C Virus

HCV transmission within the dialysis environment can be prevented by strict adherence to infection control precautions recommended for all hemodialysis patients (Table 64.6).

Although isolation of HCV-positive patients is not recommended, routine testing for ALT and anti-HCV is important for monitoring the potential for transmission within centers and ensuring that appropriate precautions are being properly and consistently used. Furthermore, HCV-positive patients can participate in dialyzer reuse programs. Unlike HBV, HCV is not transmitted efficiently through occupational exposures. Thus, reprocessing dialyzers from HCV-positive patients should not place staff members at increased risk for infection.

HCV-positive persons should be evaluated (by consultation or referral, if appropriate) for the presence or development of chronic liver disease according to current medical practice guidelines. They also should receive information concerning how they can prevent further harm to their liver and prevent the transmission of HCV to others (136,137). Persons with chronic liver disease should be vaccinated against hepatitis A, if susceptible.

Hepatitis Delta Virus

Because HDV depends on an HBV-infected host for replication, prevention of HBV infection will prevent HDV infection in a person susceptible to HBV. Patients known to be infected with HDV should be isolated from all other dialysis patients, especially those who are HBsAg positive.

Human Immunodeficiency Virus

Infection control precautions recommended for all hemodialysis patients are sufficient to prevent HIV transmission between patients. HIV-infected patients do not have to be isolated from other patients or dialyzed separately on dedicated machines. In addition, they can participate in dialyzer reuse programs. Because HIV is not transmitted efficiently through occupational exposures, reprocessing dialyzers from HIV-positive patients should not place staff members at increased risk for infection.

Bacterial

Contact transmission can be prevented by hand hygiene (138), glove use, and disinfection of environmental surfaces. Infection control precautions recommended for all hemodialysis patients are adequate to prevent transmission for most patients infected or colonized with pathogenic bacteria, including antimicrobial-resistant strains. However, additional precautions should be considered for treatment of patients who might be at increased risk for transmitting pathogenic bacteria. Such patients include those with either an infected skin wound with drainage that is not contained by dressings (the drainage does not have to be culture positive for MRSA or VRE or any specific pathogen) or fecal incontinence or diarrhea uncontrolled with personal hygiene measures. For these patients, consider using the following additional precautions: (a) staff members treating the patient should wear a separate gown over their usual clothing and remove the gown when finished caring for the patient; and (b) dialyze the patient at a station with as few adjacent stations as possible (e.g., at the end or corner of the unit) (135).

Vancomycin is used commonly in dialysis patients, in part because vancomycin can be conveniently administered to patients when they come in for hemodialysis treatments. Prudent antimicrobial use is an important component of the CDC recommendations for preventing the spread of vancomycin resistance (139). This guideline states that vancomycin is *not* indicated for therapy (chosen for dosing convenience) of infections due to β-lactam–sensitive gram-positive microorganisms in patients with renal failure. Depending on the situation, alternative antimicrobials (e.g., cephalosporins) with dosing intervals greater than 48 hours, which would allow postdialytic dosing, could be used. Studies suggest that cefazolin given three times a week in the dialysis unit provides adequate blood levels and could be used to treat many infections in hemodialysis patients (140,141).

Disinfection, Sterilization, and Environmental Hygiene

Good cleaning, disinfection, and sterilization procedures are important components of infection control in the hemodialysis center. The procedures do not differ from those recommended for other healthcare settings (142,143), but the high potential for blood contamination makes the hemodialysis setting unique. Additionally, the need for routine aseptic access of the patients vascular system makes the hemodialysis unit more akin to a surgical suite than to a standard hospital room. Medical items are categorized as critical if they are introduced directly into the bloodstream or normally sterile areas of the body (e.g., needles and catheters); semicritical if they come in contact with intact mucous membranes (e.g., fiberoptic endoscopes); and noncritical if they touch only intact skin (e.g., blood pressure cuffs) (138,142).

Cleaning and housekeeping in the dialysis center have two goals: to remove soil and waste on a regular basis, thereby preventing the accumulation of potentially infectious material, and to maintain an environment that is conducive to good patient care. Crowding of patients and overtaxing of staff members may increase the likelihood of microbial transmission. Adequate cleaning may be difficult if there are multiple wires, tubes, and hoses in a small area. There should be enough space to move completely around each patient's dialysis station without interfering with the neighboring stations. Where space is limited, elimination of unneeded items; orderly arrangement of required items; and removal of excess lengths of tubes, hoses, and wires from the floor can improve accessibility for cleaning. Because of the special requirements for cleaning in the dialysis center, staff should be specially trained in this task.

After each patient treatment, frequently touched environmental surfaces, including external surfaces of the dialysis machine, should be cleaned (with a good detergent) or disinfected (with a detergent germicide). It is the cleaning step that is important for interrupting the cross-contamination transmission routes. Antiseptics, such as formulations with povidone-iodine, hexachlorophene, or chlorhexidine, should not be used, because these are formulated for use on skin and are not designed for use on hard surfaces.

There is no evidence that medical waste is any more infectious than residential waste or has caused disease in the community (144). Wastes from a hemodialysis center that are actually or potentially contaminated with blood should be considered infectious and handled accordingly. Eventually, these items of solid waste should be disposed of properly in an incinerator or sanitary landfill, depending on state or local laws.

Standard protocols for sterilization and disinfection are adequate for processing any items or devices contaminated with blood. Historically there has been a tendency to use "overkill" strategies for instrument sterilization or disinfection and housekeeping protocols. This is not necessary. The floors in a dialysis center are routinely contaminated with blood, but the protocol for floor cleaning is the same as for floors in other health-care settings. Usually, this involves the use of a good detergent-germicide; the formulation can contain a low- or intermediate-level disinfectant.

Blood-borne viruses, such as HBV and HIV, are inactivated by any standard sterilization systems such as standard steam autoclave cycles of 121°C (249.8°F) for 15 minutes, ethylene oxide gas (142), and low-temperature hydrogen peroxide gas plasma (145). Large blood spills should be cleaned to remove visible material, and then the area should receive low- to intermediate-level disinfection following the directions of the germicide manufacturer.

Blood and other specimens, such as peritoneal fluid, from all patients should be handled with care. Peritoneal fluid can contain high levels of HBV and should be handled in the same manner as the patient's blood. Consequently, if the center performs peritoneal dialysis, the same criteria for separating HBsAg-positive patients who are undergoing hemodialysis apply to those undergoing peritoneal dialysis.

HBV has not been grown in tissue cultures, and without a viral assay system, studies on the precise resistance of this virus to various chemical germicides and heat have not been performed. However, the resistance of HBV to heat and chemical germicides may approach that of some other viruses and bacteria but certainly not that of the bacterial endospore or the tubercle bacillus. Further, studies have shown that HBV is not resistant to commonly used high-level and intermediate-level disinfectants (146, 147).

Blood contamination of venous pressure monitors has been implicated in HBV transmission (148). Therefore, venous pressure transducer filters should be used; these filters should not be reused.

In single-pass artificial kidney machines, the internal fluid pathways are not subject to contamination with blood. Although the fluid pathways that exhaust dialysis fluid from the dialyzer may become contaminated with blood in the event of a dialyzer leak, it is unlikely that this blood contamination will reach a subsequent patient. Therefore, disinfection and rinsing procedures should be designed to control contamination with bacterial rather than blood-borne pathogens.

For dialysis machines that use a dialysate recirculating system (such as some ultrafiltration control machines and those that regenerate the dialysate), a blood leak in a dialyzer, especially a massive leak, can result in contamination of a number of surfaces that will contact the dialysis fluid of subsequent patients. However, the procedures that are normally practiced after each use—draining of the dialysis fluid, subsequent rinsing, and disinfection—will reduce the level of contamination to below infectious levels. In addition, an intact dialyzer membrane will not allow passage of bacteria or viruses. Consequently, if a blood leak does occur with either type of dialysis machine, the standard disinfection procedure used for machines in the dialysis center to control bacterial contamination will also prevent transmission of blood-borne pathogens.

NONINFECTIOUS COMPLICATIONS

First-Use and Allergic Reactions

A variety of symptoms attributed to hypersensitivity reactions may occur during dialysis. Symptoms variously reported include increased or decreased blood pressure; dyspnea; cough; conjunctival injection; flushing; urticaria; headache; and pains in the chest, back, and limbs (149). Such symptoms are more common during the first use of a dialyzer and have been termed the "first-use syndrome." These reactions are more common with dialyzers with cuprophan membranes. Some reactions may be associated with residual ethylene oxide in dialyzers. During 1992 and 1993, such reactions were reported by 24% to 27%, respectively, of dialysis centers and were most strongly associated with use of cuprophan and regenerated cellulose membranes (150).

In 1990, several outbreaks of anaphylactoid reactions associated with angiotensin-converting enzyme inhibitors were reported (Table 64.3). Reactions occurred within 10 minutes of initiating dialysis and included nausea, abdominal cramps, burning, flushing, swelling of the face or tongue, angioedema, shortness of breath, and hypotension. One outbreak was linked to reuse of dialyzers (151), but other reports implicated polyacrylonitrile dialyzers in the reactions (152–155). In 1992, the FDA issued a safety alert regarding anaphylactoid reactions in patients on angiotensin-converting enzyme inhibitors, especially those using polyacrylonitrile dialyzers (156).

Dialysis Dementia

Dialysis encephalopathy, or dialysis dementia, is a disorder that affects dialysis patients who for a variety of reasons are subjected to water that has a relatively high content of aluminum, such as community water supplies treated with alum (157, 158). Case definitions of dialysis encephalopathy include three different groups of objective findings:

1. Speech impairment (stuttering, stammering, dysnomia, hypofluency, mutism)
2. Seizure disorder (generalized tonic-clonic, focal, or multifocal seizures)
3. Motor disturbance (myoclonic jerks, motor apraxia, immobility).

The incidence of dialysis dementia reported by hemodialysis centers to the CDC decreased from 0.4% during 1983 to 1985 to 0.1% (129 cases) in 1990, with a case-fatality rate of 21% (159). This decrease may have been related to improvements in water treatment. Specifically, the percent of centers treating water with reverse osmosis, with or without other modalities, increased from 26% in 1980 to 98% in 1996 (14).

To eliminate the possibility of leaching of harmful substances, all components of the water treatment and dialysis fluid preparation and delivery systems should be compatible with all fluid with which they are in contact. In one outbreak, 58 of 85 (68%) dialysis patients at a dialysis center were diagnosed with acute or chronic aluminum intoxication that resulted in three deaths. Investigation revealed that the acidified portion (pH 2.7) of the bicarbonate-based dialysate solution was passed through a pump with an aluminum housing, and aluminum was leached out of the pump and into the dialysate solution in concentrations exceeding 200 ppm and was present in the dialysis fluid (160).

Toxic Reactions

Chemicals in water or as residuals in dialysis fluid can affect dialysis patients. Certain chemicals in water may not be toxic when ingested by humans, but the hemodialysis patient may be exposed directly to 150 L of water per treatment. Two examples will illustrate this problem.

Occasionally, suppliers of community water change their water disinfection patterns by increasing chlorine dosages or by using chloramines. These changes usually occur without the knowledge of the dialysis staff. Chloramines in water used to prepare dialysis fluid must be removed, or the patient will experience acute hemolysis. If the correct water treatment system (activated carbon) is not present or operating in the dialysis center, patients will be exposed to this chemical. In one instance, a dialysis center changed from acetate to bicarbonate dialysate, adding an additional reverse osmosis unit and tanks for preparation and dilution of the dialysate. No changes were made to increase the capacity of the carbon filter, and within a few weeks approximately 100 of the center's dialysis patients were exposed to chloramine-contaminated dialysate when the undersized carbon filters failed. Forty-one patients required transfusion to treat hemolytic anemia caused by the chloramine exposure (161).

Another example of chemical intoxication occurred when a city water treatment plant accidentally fed excessive levels of fluoride into the community water supply, resulting in the death of one dialysis patient and acute illness in several other patients in a hemodialysis center receiving this community water supply. The center's water treatment system was not adequate to remove excessive fluoride from water (162). In both examples, a properly designed water treatment system consisting of adequate carbon filtration for the fluid flow and volume plus the use of reverse osmosis, deionization, and ultrafiltration would have prevented toxic reactions.

There have also been instances in which a disinfectant such as formaldehyde was not sufficiently removed from dialysis systems, and patients were exposed to the chemical. This can be prevented by monitoring the system for complete rinsing using a chemical assay sensitive to the chemical.

In February and March 1996, 101 of 130 patients at a dialysis center in Brazil developed liver disease, visual disturbances, and nausea and vomiting; 50 died (163). The water used to prepare dialysis fluid came from a water reservoir that had a recent algae or cyanobacteria (blue-green algae) bloom. The water received inadequate treatment by the municipal water supplier and the dialysis center. Cyanobacteria are present in bodies of water worldwide. Some species can produce neurotoxins or hepatotoxins that can be fatal to animals that drink water having a heavy growth or bloom of cyanobacteria. During investigation of the Brazil outbreak, a cyanobacterial toxin, Microcystin-LR, was detected in water from the reservoir, treated water at the dialysis center, and case patients' serum and liver tissue. This is the first report of parenteral exposure to cyanobacterial toxins among humans. The outbreak would have been prevented by proper water treatment at the municipal and dialysis center level (163).

A summary of toxic reactions in hemodialysis patients that have been investigated by the CDC is given in Table 64.3.

REFERENCES

1. U.S. Renal Data System. *USRDS 2002 annual data report: atlas of end-stage renal disease in the United States.* Report 15-564. Bethesda, MD: National Institutes of Health, National Institute of Diabetes and Digestive and Kidney Diseases, 2002.
2. Favero MS, Carson LA, Bond WW, et al. Pseudomonas aeruginosa: growth in distilled water from hospitals. *Science* 1971;173(999): 836–838.
3. Favero MS, Bland LA. Microbiologic principles applied to reprocessing hemodialyzers. In: Deane N, Wineman RJ, Bemis JA, editors. *Guide to reprocessing of hemodialyzers.* Boston: Martinus Nijhoff, 1986: 63–73.
4. Favero MS, Petersen NJ, Boyer KM, et al. Microbial contamination of renal dialysis systems and associated health risks. *Trans Am Soc Artif Intern Organs* 1974;20A:175–183.
5. Bolan G, Reingold AL, Carson LA, et al. Infections with Mycobacterium chelonei in patients receiving dialysis and using processed hemodialyzers. *J Infect Dis* 1985;152:1013–1019.
6. Carson LA, Bland LA, Cusick LB, et al. Prevalence of nontuberculous mycobacteria in water supplies of hemodialysis centers. *Appl Environ Microbiol* 1988;54:3122–3125.
7. Lowry P, Beck-Sague CM, Bland L, et al. Mycobacterium chelonae infections among patients receiving high-flux dialysis in a hemodialysis clinic, California. *J Infect Dis* 1990;161:85–90.
8. Favero MS, Petersen NJ, Carson LA, et al. Gram-negative water bacteria in hemodialysis systems. *Health Lab Sci* 1975;12:321–334.
9. Bland LA, Favero MS. *Microbial contamination control strategies for hemodialysis systems.* Oakbrook Terrace, IL: Joint Commission on Accreditation of Healthcare Organizations, Plant, Technology, and Safety Management Series 3, 1989:30–36.
10. Carson LA, Bland LA, Cusick LB, et al. Factors affecting endotoxin levels in fluids associated with hemodialysis procedures. In: Watson SW, Levin J, Novitsky TJ, eds. *Detection of bacterial endotoxins with the Limulus amebocyte lysate test.* New York: Alan R. Liss, 1987: 223–234.
11. Hindman SH, Favero MS, Carson LA, et al. Pyrogenic reactions during haemodialysis caused by extramural endotoxin. *Lancet* 1975;2: 732–734.
12. Association for the Advancement of Medical Instrumentation. American National Standard. Hemodialysis systems. ANSI/AAMI RD5-1992. Arlington, VA: Association for the Advancement of Medical Instrumentation, 1992.
13. Stamm JM, Engelhard WE, Parsons JE. Microbiological study of water-softener resins. *Appl Microbiol* 1969;18:376–386.
14. Tokars JI, Miller ER, Alter MJ, et al. *National surveillance of dialysis-associated diseases in the United States, 1996.* Atlanta, GA: Centers for Disease Control and Prevention, 1998:1–59.
15. Favero MS. Microbiological contaminants. In: *Proceedings of the Association for the Advancement of Medical Instrumentation Technology Assessment Conference: Issues in Hemodialysis.* Arlington, VA: AAMI, 1981:30–33.

16. Anderson RL, Holland BW, Carr JK, et al. Effect of disinfectants on pseudomonads colonized on the interior surface of PVC pipes. *Am J Public Health* 1990;80:17–21.
17. Jackson BM, Beck-Sague CM, Bland LA, et al. Outbreak of pyrogenic reactions and gram-negative bacteremia in a hemodialysis center. *Am J Nephrol* 1994;14(2):85–89.
18. Arduino MJ. Microbiologic quality of water used for hemodialysis. *Contemp Dial Nephrol* 1996;17:17–19.
19. Arduino MJ. What's new in water treatment standards for hemodialysis? *Contemp Dial Nephrol* 1997;18:21–24.
20. Petersen NJ, Boyer KM, Carson LA, et al. Pyrogenic reactions from inadequate disinfection of a dialysis fluid distribution system. *Dialysis Transplant* 1978;7:52,57–60.
21. Favero MS, Carson LA, Bond WW, et al. Factors that influence microbial contamination of fluids associated with hemodialysis machines. *Appl Microbiol* 1974;28:822–830.
22. Petersen NJ, Carson LA, Doto IL, et al. Microbiologic evaluation of a new glutaraldehyde-based disinfectant for hemodialysis systems. *Trans Am Soc Artif Intern Organs* 1982;28:287–290.
23. Townsend TR, Wee SB, Bartlett J. Disinfection of hemodialysis machines. *Dialysis Transplant* 1985;14:274–287.
24. Centers for Disease Control and Prevention. Occupational exposures to formaldehyde in dialysis units. *MMWR* 1986;35(24):399–401.
25. Favero MS, Petersen NJ. Microbiologic guidelines for hemodialysis systems. *Dialysis Transplant* 1977;6:34–36.
26. Bland LA, Favero MS. *Microbiologic and endotoxin considerations in hemodialyzer reprocessing,* vol 3, dialysis 3. Arlington, VA: AAMI Standards and Recommended Practices, 1993:293–300.
27. Association for the Advancement of Medical Instrumentation. American National Standard. Water treatment equipment for hemodialysis applications. ANSI/AAMI RD62–2001. Arlington, VA: Association for the Advancement of Medical Instrumentation, 2001.
28. Baz M, Durand C, Ragon A, et al. Using ultrapure water in hemodialysis delays carpal tunnel syndrome. *Int J Artif Organs* 1991;14(11): 681–685.
29. Lonnemann G. Chronic inflammation in hemodialysis: the role of contaminated dialysate. *Blood Purif* 2000;18(3):214–223.
30. Lonnemann G, Koch KM. Efficacy of ultra-pure dialysate in the therapy and prevention of haemodialysis-associated amyloidosis. *Nephrol Dial Transplant* 2001;16(suppl 4):17–22.
31. Canaud B, Bosc JY, Leray H, et al. Microbiologic purity of dialysate: rationale and technical aspects. *Blood Purif* 2000;18(3):200–213.
32. Schiffl H, Lang SM, Bergner A. Ultrapure dialysate reduces dose of recombinant human erythropoietin. *Nephron* 1999;83(3):278–279.
33. Arduino MJ, Bland LA, Aguero SM, et al. Comparison of microbiologic assay methods for hemodialysis fluids. *J Clin Microbiol* 1991; 29:592–594.
34. Gazenfeldt-Gazit E, Eliahou HE. Endotoxin antibodies in patients on maintenance hemodialysis. *Israel J Med Sci* 1969;5:1032–1036.
35. Laude-Sharpe M, Caroff M, Simard L, et al. Induction of IL-1 during hemodialysis: Transmembrane passage of intact endotoxins (LPS). *Kidney Int* 1990;38:1089–1094.
36. Henderson LW, Koch KM, Dinarello CA, et al. Hemodialysis hypotension: the interleukin hypothesis. *Blood Purif* 1983;1:3–8.
37. Port FK, VanDeKerkhove KM, Kunkel SL, et al. The role of dialysate in the stimulation of interleukin-1 production during clinical hemodialysis. *Am J Kidney Dis* 1987;10:118–122.
38. Kantor RJ, Carson LA, Graham DR, et al. Outbreak of pyrogenic reactions at a dialysis center: association with infusion of heparinized saline solution. *Am J Med* 1983;74:449–456.
39. Murphy J, Parker T, Carson L, et al. Outbreaks of bacteremia in hemodialysis patients associated with alteration of dialyzer membranes following chemical disinfection. *ASAIO J* 1987;16:51(abst).
40. Gordon SM, Oettinger CW, Bland LA, et al. Pyrogenic reactions in patients receiving conventional, high-efficiency, or high-flux hemodialysis treatments with bicarbonate dialysate containing high concentrations of bacteria and endotoxin. *J Am Soc Nephrol* 1992;2: 1436–1444.
41. Pegues DA, Oettinger CW, Bland LA, et al. A prospective study of pyrogenic reactions in hemodialysis patients using bicarbonate dialysis fluids filtered to remove bacteria and endotoxin. *J Am Soc Nephrol* 1992;3:1002–1007.
42. Oliver JC, Bland LA, Oettinger CW, et al. Bacteria and endotoxin removal from bicarbonate dialysis fluids for use in conventional, high-efficiency, and high-flux dialysis. *Artif Organs* 1992;16:141–145.
43. Centers for Disease Control and Prevention. Outbreaks of gram-negative bacterial bloodstream infections traced to probable contamination of hemodialysis machines—Canada, 1995; United States, 1997; and Israel, 1997. *MMWR* 1998;47:55–59.
44. Tokars JI, Frank M, Alter MJ, et al. National surveillance of dialysis-associated diseases in the United States, 2000. *Semin Dial* 2002;15(3): 162–171.
45. Association for the Advancement of Medical Instrumentation. American National Standard. Reuse of hemodialyzers. ANSI/AAMI RD47-1993. Arlington, VA: Association for the Advancement of Medical Instrumentation, 1993.
46. Bland L, Alter M, Favero M, et al. Hemodialyzer reuse: practices in the United States and implication for infection control. *ASAIO J* 1985;31:556–559.
47. Favero MS. Distinguishing between high-level disinfection, reprocessing, and sterilization. Association for the Advancement of Medical Instrumentation, Reuse of Disposables: Implications for quality health care and cost containment. Technology assessment report No. 6. Arlington, VA: Association for the Advancement of Medical Instrumentation, 1983:19–23.
48. Alter MJ, Favero MS, Miller JK, et al. National surveillance of dialysis-associated diseases in the United States, 1988. *ASAIO J* 1990;36: 107–118.
49. Bland LA, Ridgeway MR, Aguero SM, et al. Potential bacteriologic and endotoxin hazards associated with liquid bicarbonate concentrate. *ASAIO J* 1987;33:542–545.
50. Tokars JI, Miller E, Alter MJ, et al. *National Surveillance of Dialysis-Associated Diseases in the United States, 1995.* Atlanta GA: U.S. Department of Health and Human Services, 1998.
51. Gordon S, Tipple M, Bland L, et al. Pyrogenic reactions associated with the reuse of processed hollow-fiber hemodialyzers. *JAMA* 1988; 260:2077–2081.
52. Bloembergen WE, Port FK. Epidemiological perspective on infections in chronic dialysis patients. *Adv Ren Replace Ther* 1996;3(3):201–207.
53. Bonomo RA, Rice D, Whalen C, et al. Risk factors associated with permanent access-site infections in chronic hemodialysis patients. *Infect Control Hosp Epidemiol* 1997;18(11):757–761.
54. Dobkin JF, Miller MH, Steigbigel NH. Septicemia in patients on chronic hemodialysis. *Ann Intern Med* 1978;88(1):28–33.
55. Hoen B, Paul-Dauphin A, Hestin D, et al. EPIBACDIAL: a multicenter prospective study of risk factors for bacteremia in chronic hemodialysis patients. *J Am Soc Nephrol* 1998;9(5):869–876.
56. Kaplowitz LG, Comstock JA, Landwehr DM, et al. A prospective study of infections in hemodialysis patients: patient hygiene and other risk factors for infection. *Infect Control Hosp Epidemiol* 1988;9(12): 534–541.
57. Keane WF, Shapiro FL, Raij L. Incidence and type of infections occurring in 445 chronic hemodialysis patients. *Trans Am Soc Artif Intern Organs* 1977;23:41–47.
58. Kessler M, Hoen B, Mayeux D, et al. Bacteremia in patients on chronic hemodialysis. A multicenter prospective survey. *Nephron* 1993;64(1):95–100.
59. Stevenson KB, Adcox MJ, Mallea MC, et al. Standardized surveillance of hemodialysis vascular access infections: 18-month experience at an outpatient, multifacility hemodialysis center. *Infect Control Hosp Epidemiol* 2000;21(3):200–203.
60. Tokars Light P, Armistead N, et al. Vascular access infections among hemodialysis outpatients. *Am J Kidney Dis* 2001;37:1232–1240.
61. Tokars JI. Bloodstream infections in hemodialysis patients: getting some deserved attention. *Infect Control Hosp Epidemiol* 2002;23(12): 713–715.
62. Tokars JI, Miller ER, Stein G. New national surveillance system for hemodialysis-associated infections: initial results. *Am J Infect Control* 2002;30(5):288–295.
63. Tokars JI, Alter MJ, Arduino MJ. Nosocomial infections in hemodi-

alysis units: strategies for control. In: Jacobsen H, Striker G, Klahr S, eds. *The principles and practice of nephrology.* St. Louis: Mosby, 1995: 337–357.

64. Grohskopf LA, Roth VR, Feikin DR, et al. Serratia liquefaciens bloodstream infections from contamination of epoetin alfa at a hemodialysis center. *N Engl J Med* 2001;344(20):1491–1497.
65. Padberg FT Jr, Lee BC, Curl GR. Hemoaccess site infection. *Surg Gynecol Obstet* 1992;174:103–108.
66. Stevenson KB, Hannah EL, Lowder CA, et al. Epidemiology of hemodialysis vascular access infections from longitudinal infection surveillance data: predicting the impact of NKF-DOQI clinical practice guidelines for vascular access. *Am J Kidney Dis* 2002;39(3):549–555.
67. Besarab A, Bolton WK, Browne JK, et al. The effects of normal as compared with low hematocrit values in patients with cardiac disease who are receiving hemodialysis and epoetin. *N Engl J Med* 1998; 339(9):584–590.
68. Fan PY, Schwab SJ. Vascular access: concepts for the 1990s. *J Am Soc Nephrol* 1992;3(1):1–11.
69. Powe NR, Jaar B, Furth SL, et al. Septicemia in dialysis patients: incidence, risk factors, and prognosis. *Kidney Int* 1999;55(3): 1081–1090.
70. National Kidney Foundation. K/DOQI clinical practice guideline for vascular access, 2000. *Am J Kidney Dis* 2001;37(suppl 1):S137–S181.
71. Centers for Disease Control and Prevention. Guidelines for the prevention of intravascular catheter-related infections. *MMWR* 2002; 51(RR-10):1–29.
72. Berns JS, Tokars JI. Preventing bacterial infections and antimicrobial resistance in dialysis patients. *Am J Kidney Dis* 2002;40(5):886–898.
73. Mermel LA, Farr BM, Sherertz RJ, et al. Guidelines for the management of intravascular catheter-related infections. *Clin Infect Dis* 2001; 32(9):1249–1272.
74. Uttley AH, George RC, Naidoo J, et al. High-level vancomycin-resistant enterococci causing hospital infections. *Epidemiol Infect* 1989;103(1):173–181.
75. Brady JP, Snyder JW, Hasbargen JA. Vancomycin-resistant enterococcus in end-stage renal disease. *Am J Kidney Dis* 1998;32(3): 415–418.
76. Roghmann MC, Fink JC, Polish L, et al. Colonization with vancomycin-resistant enterococci in chronic hemodialysis patients. *Am J Kidney Dis* 1998;32(2):254–257.
77. Fishbane S, Cunha BA, Mittal SK, et al. Vancomycin-resistant enterococci in hemodialysis patients is related to intravenous vancomycin use. *Infect Control Hosp Epidemiol* 1999;20(7):461–462.
78. Dopirak M, Hill C, Oleksiw M, et al. Surveillance of hemodialysis-associated primary bloodstream infections: the experience of ten hospital-based centers. *Infect Control Hosp Epidemiol* 2002;23(12): 721–724.
79. Taylor G, Gravel D, Johnston L, et al. Prospective surveillance for primary bloodstream infections occurring in Canadian hemodialysis units. *Infect Control Hosp Epidemiol* 2002;23(12):716–720.
80. Fridkin SK. Vancomycin-intermediate and -resistant Staphylococcus aureus: what the infectious disease specialist needs to know. *Clin Infect Dis* 2001;32(1):108–115.
81. Chang S, Sievert DM, Hageman JC, et al. Infection with vancomycin-resistant Staphylococcus aureus containing the vanA resistance gene. *N Engl J Med* 2003;348(14):1342–1347.
82. Centers for Disease Control and Prevention. Hepatitis—control measures for hepatitis B in dialysis centers. HEW publication No. [CDC] 78-8358 (Viral Hepatitis Investigations and Control Series). Atlanta: Centers for Disease Control and Prevention, 1977.
83. Alter MJ, Favero MS, Petersen NJ, et al. National surveillance of dialysis-associated hepatitis and other diseases, 1976 and 1980. *Dialysis Transplant* 1983;12:860–865.
84. Centers for Disease Control. Recommendations of the Immunization Practices Advisory Committee (ACIP): inactivated hepatitis B virus vaccine. *MMWR* 1982;31:317–322,327–328.
85. Tokars JI, Miller ER, Alter MJ, et al. National surveillance of dialysis-associated diseases in the United States, 1997. *Semin Dial* 2000;13(2): 75–85.
86. Alter HJ, Seeff LB, Kaplan PM, et al. Type B hepatitis: the infectivity of blood positive for e antigen and DNA polymerase after accidental needlestick exposure. *N Engl J Med* 1976;295(17):909–913.
87. Shikata T, Karasawa T, Abe K, et al. Hepatitis B e antigen and infectivity of hepatitis B virus. *J Infect Dis* 1977;136:571–576.
88. Bond WW, Favero MS, Petersen NJ, et al. Survival of hepatitis B virus after drying and storage for one week. *Lancet* 1981;1:550–551.
89. Favero MS, Bond WW, Petersen NJ, et al. Detection methods for study of the stability of hepatitis B antigen on surfaces. *J Infect Dis* 1974;129(2):210–212.
90. Favero MS, Maynard JE, Petersen NJ, et al. Hepatitis-B antigen on environmental surfaces [letter]. *Lancet* 1973;2:1455.
91. Snydman DR, Bryan JA, Macon EJ, et al. Hemodialysis-associated hepatitis: report of an epidemic with further evidence on mechanisms of transmission. *Am J Epidemiol* 1976;104:563–570.
92. Niu MT, Penberthy LT, Alter MJ, et al. Hemodialysis-associated hepatitis B: report of an outbreak. *Dialysis Transplant* 1989;18: 542–555.
93. Centers for Disease Control and Prevention. Outbreaks of hepatitis B virus infection among hemodialyis patients—California, Nebraska, and Texas, 1994. *MMWR* 1996;45:285–289.
94. Alter MJ, Ahtone J, Maynard JE. Hepatitis B virus transmission associated with a multiple-dose vial in a hemodialysis unit. *Ann Intern Med* 1983;99:330–333.
95. Carl M, Francis DP, Maynard JE. A common-source outbreak of hepatitis B in a hemodialysis unit. *Dialysis Transplant* 1983;12: 222–229.
96. Kantor RJ, Hadler SC, Schreeder MT, et al. Outbreak of hepatitis B in a dialysis unit, complicated by false positive HBsAg test results. *Dialysis Transplant* 1979;8:232–235.
97. Anonymous. Decrease in the incidence of hepatitis in dialysis units associated with prevention programme: public health laboratory survey. *Br Med J* 1974;4:751–754.
98. Najem GR, Louria DB, Thind IS, et al. Control of hepatitis B infection. The role of surveillance and an isolation hemodialysis center. *JAMA* 1981;245:153–157.
99. Alter MJ, Favero MS, Maynard JE. Impact of infection control strategies on the incidence of dialysis-associated hepatitis in the United States. *J Infect Dis* 1986;153:1149–1151.
100. Tokars JI, Alter MJ, Miller E, et al. National surveillance of dialysis associated diseases in the United States, 1994. *ASAIO J* 1997;43: 108–119.
101. Hutin YJ, Goldstein ST, Varma JK, et al. An outbreak of hospital-acquired hepatitis B virus infection among patients receiving chronic hemodialysis. *Infect Control Hosp Epidemiol* 1999;20(11):731–735.
102. Centers for Disease Control and Prevention. Hepatitis B virus: a comprehensive strategy for eliminating transmission in the United States through universal childhood vaccination. Recommendations of the Immunization Practices Advisory Committee (ACIP). *MMWR* 1991; 40(RR-13):1–25.
103. Hoofnagle JH, Di Bisceglie AM. Serologic diagnosis of acute and chronic viral hepatitis. *Semin Liver Dis* 1991;11(2):73–83.
104. Dienstag JL, Schiff ER, Wright TL, et al. Lamivudine as initial treatment for chronic hepatitis B in the United States. *N Engl J Med* 1999; 341(17):1256–1263.
105. Lai C-L, Chien R-N, Leung NWY, et al., and the Asia Hepatitis Lamivudine Study Group. A one-year trial of lamivudine for chronic hepatitis B. *N Engl J Med* 1998;339:61–68.
106. Kloster B, Kramer R, Eastlund T, et al. Hepatitis B surface antigenemia in blood donors following vaccination. *Transfusion* 1995;35(6): 475–477.
107. Lunn ER, Hoggarth BJ, Cook WJ. Prolonged hepatitis B surface antigenemia after vaccination. *Pediatrics* 2000;105(6):E81.
108. McMahon BJ, Alberts SR, Wainwright RB, et al. Hepatitis B-related sequelae. Prospective study in 1400 hepatitis B surface antigen-positive Alaska native carriers. *Arch Intern Med* 1990;150(5):1051–1054.
109. Hadler SC, Murphy BL, Schable CA, et al. Epidemiological analysis of the significance of low-positive test results for antibody to hepatitis B surface and core antigens. *J Clin Microbiol* 1984;19(4):521–525.
110. Levine OS, Vlahov D, Koehler J, et al. Seroepidemiology of hepatitis

B virus in a population of injecting drug users. Association with drug injection patterns. *Am J Epidemiol* 1995;142(3):331–341.

111. Silva AE, McMahon BJ, Parkinson AJ, et al. Hepatitis B virus DNA in persons with isolated antibody to hepatitis B core antigen who subsequently received hepatitis B vaccine. *Clin Infect Dis* 1998;26(4): 895–897.
112. McMahon BJ, Parkinson AJ, Helminiak C, et al. Response to hepatitis B vaccine of persons positive for antibody to hepatitis B core antigen. *Gastroenterology* 1992;103(2):590–594.
113. Lai C-L, Lau JY, Yeoh E-K, et al. Significance of isolated anti-HBc seropositivity by ELISA: implications and the role of radioimmunoassay. *J Med Virol* 1992;36:180–183.
114. Niu MT, Coleman PJ, Alter MJ. Multicenter study of hepatitis C virus infection in chronic hemodialysis patients and hemodialysis center staff members. *Am J Kidney Dis* 1993;22(4):568–573.
115. Fabrizi F, Lunghi G, Guarnori I, et al. Incidence of seroconversion for hepatitis C virus in chronic haemodialysis patients: a prospective study. *Nephrol Dial Transplant* 1994;9(11):1611–1615.
116. Fabrizi F, Martin P, Dixit V, et al. Acquisition of hepatitis C virus in hemodialysis patients: a prospective study by branched DNA signal amplification assay. *Am J Kidney Dis* 1998;31(4):647–654.
117. Pinto dos Santos J, Loureiro A, Cendoroglo N, et al. Impact of dialysis room and reuse strategies on the incidence of hepatitis C virus infection in haemodialysis units. *Nephrol Dial Transplant* 1996;11: 2017–2022.
118. Forns X, Fernandez-Llama P, Pons M, et al. Incidence and risk factors of hepatitis C virus infection in a haemodialysis unit. *Nephrol Dial Transplant* 1997;12(4):736–740.
119. McLaughlin KJ, Cameron SO, Good T, et al. Nosocomial transmission of hepatitis C virus within a British dialysis centre. *Nephrol Dial Transplant* 1997;12(2):304–309.
120. Petrosilla N, Gilli P, Serraino D, et. al. Prevalence of infected patients and understaffing have a role in hepatitis C virus transmission in dialysis. *Am J Kidney Dis* 2001;35(5):1004–1010.
121. Sivapalasingam S, Malak SF, Sullivan JF, et al. High prevalence of hepatitis C infection among patients receiving hemodialysis at an urban dialysis center. *Infect Control Hosp Epidemiol* 2002;23(6): 319–324.
122. Hardy NM, Sandroni S, Danielson S, et al. Antibody to hepatitis C virus increases with time on hemodialysis. *Clin Nephrol* 1992;38(1): 44–48.
123. Selgas R, Martinez-Zapico R, Bajo MA, et al. Prevalence of hepatitis C antibodies (HCV) in a dialysis population at one center. *Perit Dial Int* 1992;12:28–30.
124. Alter MJ. The epidemiology of acute and chronic hepatitis C. *Clin Liver Dis* 1997;1:559–568.
125. Alter MJ. Prevention of spread of hepatitis C. *Hepatology* 2002;36(5 suppl 1):S93–S98.
126. Centers for Disease Control and Prevention. Guidelines for laboratory testing and result reporting of antibody to hepatitis C virus. *MMWR* 2003;52(RR-3):1–15.
127. Busch MP, Kleinman SH, Jackson B, et al. Committee report. Nucleic acid amplification testing of blood donors for transfusion-transmitted infectious diseases: report of the Interorganizational Task Force on Nucleic Acid Amplification Testing of Blood Donors. *Transfusion* 2000;40(2):143–159.
128. Williams IT Gretch D, Fleenor M et al. Hepatitis C virus RNA concentration and chronic hepatitis in a cohort of patients followed after developing acute hepatitis C. In: Margolis HS, Alter MJ, Liang TJ, et al., eds. *Viral hepatitis and liver disease.* Atlanta, GA: International Medical Press, 2002:341–344.
129. Alter MJ, Margolis HS, Krawczynski K, et al. The natural history of community-acquired hepatitis C in the United States. *N Engl J Med* 1992;327:1899–1905.
130. Thomas DL, Astemborski J, Rai RM, et al. The natural history of hepatitis C virus infection: host, viral, and environmental factors. *JAMA* 2000;284(4):450–456.
131. Larghi A, Zuin M, Crosignani A, et al. Outcome of an outbreak of acute hepatitis C among healthy volunteers participating in pharmacokinetics studies. *Hepatology* 2002;36(4 pt 1):993–1000.
132. Hadler SC, Fields HA. Hepatitis delta virus. In: Belshe RB, ed. *Textbook of human virology.* St. Louis, MO: Mosby Year Book, 1991: 749–765.
133. Lettau LA, Alfred HJ, Glew RH, et al. Nosocomial transmission of delta hepatitis. *Ann Intern Med* 1986;104(5):631–635.
134. Velandia M, Fridkin SK, Cardenas V, et al. Transmission of HIV in dialysis centre. *Lancet* 1995;345(8962):1417–1422.
135. Centers for Disease Control and Prevention. Recommendations for preventing transmission of infections among chronic hemodialysis patients. *MMWR* 2001;50(RR-5):1–43.
136. Centers for Disease Control and Prevention. Recommendations for prevention and control of hepatitis C virus (HCV) infection and HCV-related chronic disease. Centers for Disease Control and Prevention. *MMWR Recommend Rep* 1998;47(RR-19):1–39.
137. National Institutes of Health. *Chronic hepatitis C: current disease management.* Washington, DC: National Institute of Diabetes and Digestive and Kidney Diseases, 2000:1–21.
138. Boyce JM, Pittet D. Guideline for Hand Hygiene in Health-Care Settings. Recommendations of the Healthcare Infection Control Practices Advisory Committee and the HIPAC/SHEA/APIC/IDSA Hand Hygiene Task Force. *Am J Infect Control* 2002;30(8):S1–46.
139. Centers for Disease Control and Prevention. Recommendations for preventing the spread of vancomycin resistance. *MMWR* 1995; 44(RR-12):1–13.
140. Fogel MA, Nussbaum PB, Feintzeig ID, et al. Use of cefazolin in chronic hemodialysis patients: a safe and effective alternative to vancomycin. *Am J Kidney Dis* 1998;32(3):401–409.
141. Marx MA, Frye RF, Matzke GR, et al. Cefazolin as empiric therapy in hemodialysis-related infections: efficacy and blood concentrations. *Am J Kidney Dis* 1998;32(3):410–414.
142. Favero MS, Bond WW. Chemical disinfection of medical and surgical materials. In: Block SS, ed. *Disinfection, sterilization and preservation,* 4th ed. Philadelphia: Lea & Febiger, 1991:617–641.
143. Favero MS, Bolyard EA. Microbiologic considerations. Disinfection and sterilization strategies and the potential for airborne transmission of bloodborne pathogens. *Surg Clin North Am* 1995;75(6): 1071–1089.
144. Centers for Disease Control and Prevention. Recommendations for prevention of HIV transmission in health-care settings. *MMWR* 1987; 36:1S-18S.
145. Roberts C, Antonoplos P. Inactivation of human immunodeficiency virus type 1 (HIV-1), hepatitis A virus (HAV), respiratory syncytial virus (RSV), vaccinia virus, herpes simplex virus type 1 (HSV-1), and poliovirus type 2 by hydrogen peroxide gas sterilization. *Am J Infect Control* 1998;26:94–101.
146. Bond WW, Favero MS, Petersen NJ, et al. Inactivation of hepatitis B virus by intermediate-to-high-level disinfectant chemicals. *J Clin Microbiol* 1983;18:535–538.
147. Sattar SA, Tetro J, Springthorpe VS, et al. Preventing the spread of hepatitis B and C viruses: where are germicides relevant? *Am J Infect Control* 2001;29(3):187–197.
148. Centers for Disease Control and Prevention. Outbreak of hepatitis B in a dialysis center. Epidemic Investigation Report EPI 91-17. Atlanta: Centers for Disease Control and Prevention, 1993.
149. Cheung AK. Membrane bioincompatibility. In: Nissenson AR, Fine RN, Gentile DE, eds. *Clinical dialysis.* Norwalk: Appleton & Lange, 1990:69–96.
150. Tokars JI, Alter MJ, Favero MS, et al. National surveillance of dialysis associated diseases in the United States, 1993. *ASAIO J* 1996;42: 219–229.
151. Pegues DA, Beck-Sague CM, Wollen SJ, et al. Anaphylactoid reactions associated with reuse of hollow-fiber hemodialyzers and ACE inhibitors. *Kidney Int* 1992;42:1232–1237.
152. Jadoul M, Struyven J, Stragier A, et al. Angiotensin-converting-enzyme inhibitors and anaphylactic reactions to high-flux membrane dialysis (letter). *Lancet* 1991;337:112.
153. Tielemans C, Madhoun P, Lenaers M, et al. Anaphylactoid reactions during hemodialysis on AN69 membranes in patients receiving ACE inhibitors. *Kidney Int* 1990;38:982–984.
154. van Es A, Henny FC, Lobatto S. Angiotensin-converting-enzyme in-

hibitors and anaphylactoid reactions to high-flux membrane dialysis [letter]. *Lancet* 1991;337:112–113.

155. Verresen L, Waer M, Vanrenterghem Y, et al. Angiotensin-converting-enzyme inhibitors and anaphylactoid reactions to high-flux membrane dialysis. *Lancet* 1990;336:1360–1362.
156. Food and Drug Administration. Severe allergic reactions associated with dialysis and ACE inhibitors. FDA Medical Bulletin, April 22, 1992.
157. Alfrey AC, Mishell JM, Burks J, et al. Syndrome of dyspraxia and multifocal seizures associated with chronic hemodialysis. *Trans Am Soc Artif Intern Organs* 1972;18:257–261.
158. Schreeder MT, Favero MS, Hughes JR, et al. Dialysis encephalopathy and aluminum exposure: an epidemiologic analysis. *J Chron Dis* 1983; 36:581–593.
159. Alter MJ, Favero MS, Miller JK, et al. Reuse of hemodialyzers. Results of nationwide surveillance for adverse effects. *JAMA* 1988;260: 2073–2076.
160. Burwen DR, Olsen SM, Bland LA, et al. Epidemic aluminum intoxication in hemodialysis patients traced to use of an aluminum pump. *Kidney Int* 1995;48:469–474.
161. Tipple MA, Shusterman N, Bland LA, et al. Illness in hemodialysis patients after exposure to chloramine contaminated dialysate. *ASAIO Trans* 1991;37:588–591.
162. Centers for Disease Control. Fluoride intoxication in a dialysis unit-Maryland. *MMWR* 1980;29:134–136.
163. Jochimsen EM, Carmichael WW, An JS, et al. Liver failure and death after exposure to microcystins at a hemodialysis center in Brazil. *N Engl J Med* 1998;338(13):873–878.
164. Gordon S, Bland L, Alexander S, et al. Hemolysis associated with hydrogen peroxide at a pediatric dialysis center. *Am J Nephrol* 1990; 10:123–127.
165. Gordon S, Drachman J, Bland L, et al. Epidemic hypotension in a dialysis center caused by sodium azide. *Kidney Int* 1990;37:110–115.
166. Centers for Disease Control and Prevention. Dialysis dementia from aluminum. Epidemic Investigation Report EPI 81-39. Atlanta: Centers for Disease Control and Prevention, 1982.
167. Centers for Disease Control. Formaldehyde intoxication associated with hemodialysis—California. Epidemic Investigation Report EPI 81-73. Atlanta: Centers for Disease Control, 1984.
168. Arnow PM, Bland LA, Garcia-Houchins S, et al. An outbreak of fatal fluoride intoxication in a long-term hemodialysis unit. *Ann Intern Med* 1994;121:339–344.
169. Centers for Disease Control and Prevention. Pyrogenic reactions and gram-negative bacteremia in patients in a hemodialysis center. Epidemic Investigation Report Epi 91-37. Atlanta: Centers for Disease Control and Prevention, 1991.
170. Centers for Disease Control and Prevention. Bacteremia in hemodialysis patients. Epidemic Investigation Report EPI 92-10. Atlanta: Centers for Disease Control and Prevention, 1992.
171. Jochimsen EM, Frenette C, Delorme M, et al. A cluster of bloodstream infections and pyrogenic reactions among hemodialysis patients traced to dialysis machine waste-handling option units. *Am J Nephrol* 1998;18(6):485–489.
172. Wang S, Levine RB, Carson LA, et al. An outbreak of gram-negative bacteremia in hemodialysis patients traced to hemodialysis machine waste drain ports. *Infect Control Hospital Epidemiol* 1999;20: 746–751.
173. Centers for Disease Control and Prevention. Clusters of bacteremia and pyrogenic reactions in hemodialysis patients—Georgia. Epidemic Investigation Report EPI 86-65. Atlanta: Centers for Disease Control and Prevention, 1987.
174. Beck-Sague CM, Jarvis WR, Bland LA, et al. Outbreak of gram-negative bacteremia and pyrogenic reactions in a hemodialysis center. *Am J Nephrol* 1990;10:397–403.
175. Centers for Disease Control. Bacteremia associated with reuse of disposable hollow-fiber hemodialyzers. *MMWR* 1986;35:417–418.
176. Welbel SF, Schoendorf K, Bland LA, et al. An outbreak of gram-negative bloodstream infections in chronic hemodialysis patients. *Am J Nephrol* 1995;15:1–4.
177. Centers for Disease Control and Prevention. Pyrogenic reactions in patients undergoing high-flux hemodialysis—California. Epidemic Investigation Report EPI 86-80. Atlanta: Centers for Disease Control and Prevention, 1987.
178. Centers for Disease Control and Prevention. Pyrogenic reactions in hemodialysis patients on high-flux hemodialysis—California. Epidemic Investigation Report Epi-87-12. Atlanta: Centers for Disease Control and Prevention, 1987.
179. Rudnick JR, Arduino MJ, Bland LA, et al. An outbreak of pyrogenic reactions in chronic hemodialysis patients associated with hemodialyzer reuse. *Artif Organs* 1995;19:289–294.
180. Snydman DR, Bryan JA, London WT, et al. Transmission of hepatitis B associated with hemodialysis: role of malfunction (blood leaks) in dialysis machines. *J Infect Dis* 1976;134(6):562–570.
181. Alter MJ, Ahtone J, Maynard JE. Hepatitis B virus transmission associated with a multiple-dose vial in a hemodialysis unit. *Ann Intern Med* 1983;99:330–333.
182. Centers for Disease Control and Prevention. Non-A, non-B hepatitis in a dialysis center, Nashville Tennessee. Epidemic Investigation Report EPI-78-96. Phoenix: Centers for Disease Control and Prevention, 1979.
183. Niu MT, Alter MJ, Kristensen C, et al. Outbreak of hemodialysis-associated non-A, non-B hepatitis and correlation with antibody to hepatitis C virus. *Am J Kidney Dis* 1992;19:345–352.
184. Centers for Disease Control and Prevention. Possible ongoing transmission of hepatitis C virus in a hemodialysis unit. Epidemic Investigation Report EPI-99-38. Atlanta: Centers for Disease Control and Prevention, 1999.
185. Centers for Disease Control and Prevention. Transmission of hepatitis C virus among hemodialysis patients. Epidemic Investigation Report Epi-2000. Atlanta: Centers for Disease Control and Prevention, 2000.
186. Centers for Disease Control and Prevention. Transmission of hepatitis C virus in a hemodialysis unit. Epidemic Investigation Report Epi-2000-64. Atlanta: Centers for Disease Control and Prevention, 2000.

65

INFECTIONS ASSOCIATED WITH PERITONEAL DIALYSIS

JEFFREY D. BAND

HISTORICAL PERSPECTIVES

Although peritoneal dialysis has been used to treat acute renal failure for many years, it has only been over the past 20 years that peritoneal dialysis has become a common alternative to hemodialysis for treatment of chronic renal failure. By 1996, more than 32,000 patients in the United States were maintained on chronic peritoneal dialysis (1). Sixteen percent of the United States dialysis population is now undergoing peritoneal dialysis as a form of dialytic therapy.

Two factors have largely contributed to the growth of peritoneal dialysis in the treatment of chronic renal failure. First, the introduction of an implantable, cuffed, indwelling silicone catheter by Tenckhoff and Schecter (2) in 1968 permitted secure and safe access to the peritoneal cavity. Prolonged continuous or intermittent dialysis was now possible. Second, a continuous, portable, and relatively simple dialysis technique was introduced by Popovich et al. (3) in 1976, called continuous ambulatory peritoneal dialysis (CAPD). Modification and simplification of this technique by Oreopoulos et al. (4) in 1978 resulted in fewer interruptions, increased portability, and reduced costs, leading to its popularity and acceptance.

However, peritonitis and, less commonly, catheter exit-site or tunnel infections initially led to cautious growth of this new form of chronic dialytic therapy. Rates of peritonitis as high as two to five episodes per patient-year were reported (5–7). Better patient selection, improved education, and important changes in delivery systems and connectors designed to prevent touch contamination during bag exchanges have significantly reduced rates of peritonitis (8–10). However, the major limitation of chronic peritoneal dialysis is peritonitis and its sequelae. Peritonitis is the most common reason for hospitalization (11), occurring at a rate of one case per 15 patient-months of dialysis (12), and for discontinuation of this form of dialysis (13).

Infections in patients on peritoneal dialysis are largely preventable. Knowledge of the epidemiology and pathogenesis of these infections and sources of infecting microbes is essential to design effective prevention and control strategies.

METHODS OF PERITONEAL DIALYSIS

Peritoneal dialysis may be performed in various settings and with a number of techniques. It involves infusing a dialysis solution composed of balanced salts and various concentrations of glucose into the peritoneal cavity by means of a catheter and achieving ultrafiltration by hyperosmolality; retained metabolites traverse the peritoneum from the bloodstream to the solution.

Acute Peritoneal Dialysis

Acute peritoneal dialysis is generally limited to the patient with newly diagnosed acute renal failure or to other circumstances in which dialysis is anticipated for only a few days. Its origins date back to the 1920s (8). A rigid catheter is inserted into the peritoneal cavity at the bedside after making a small incision, and manual exchanges are performed every 1 to 3 hours as necessary (14). The procedure confers a significant risk of complications, including bowel perforation. Infection is common, especially in cannulations persisting for more than a few days. Some reasons include same location of entry and exit site, lack of an implanted cuff barrier to bacterial migration, migration of the catheter with resultant serosal injury, and the need for frequent exchanges; each poses a risk of contamination.

Chronic Peritoneal Dialysis

Patients with chronic renal failure require maintenance peritoneal dialysis to alleviate symptoms of uremia and correct other metabolic abnormalities. Chronic peritoneal dialysis did not become an acceptable therapeutic alternative to hemodialysis until the mid-1960s, when a semipermanent implantable Silastic catheter was developed by Palmer et al. (15) and modified by Tenckhoff et al. (2,5). Repeated insertions of a peritoneal catheter were no longer necessary to deliver dialysate. The catheter, composed of pliable silicone and usually containing two extraperitoneal Dacron cuffs, is inserted through one incision and tunneled through a subcutaneous tract until the outer end emerges from a new exit site. The Dacron cuffs initiate an inflammatory response in the subcutaneous tissue near the exit site and deep in the abdominal wall, helping to seal the catheter in place, prevent fluid leaks, and limit bacterial migration around the catheter. Chronic peritoneal dialysis can be performed either intermittently or, as is common today, continuously (Fig. 65.1).

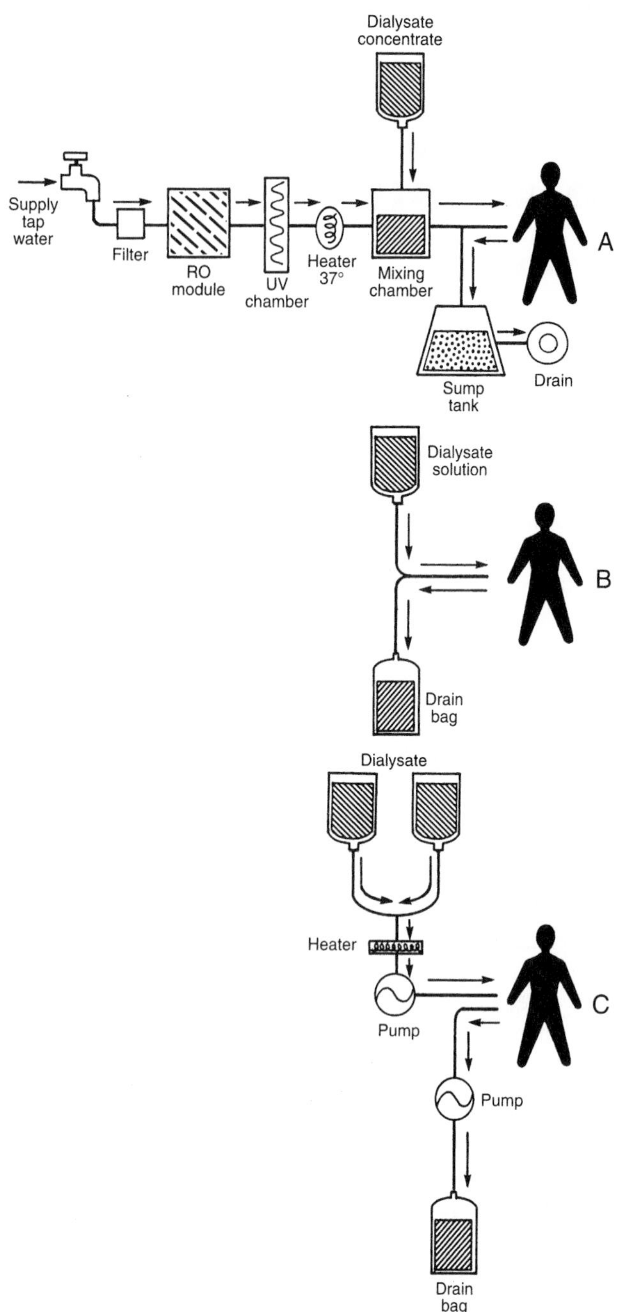

Figure 65.1. Schematic diagrams of peritoneal dialysis systems. **A:** Chronic intermittent peritoneal dialysis (CIPD) by automated machine. **B:** Continuous ambulatory peritoneal dialysis (CAPD). **C:** Continuous cycling peritoneal dialysis (CCPD) by roller pumps.

Chronic Intermittent Peritoneal Dialysis

Chronic intermittent peritoneal dialysis (CIPD) uses prolonged periods in which continuous dialysis is performed, thus permitting at least 48 hours of freedom from dialysis. To perform dialysis, a closed automated dialysis system is used to deliver dialysate to the patient (5–7). To simplify the process and to reduce costs, an automated peritoneal dialysis system was developed that used reverse osmosis (RO) capable of producing sterile pyrogen-free water from tap water, which is then mixed with dialysis concentrate (7). These machines gained widespread popularity in the mid-1970s. Although RO proved to be effective in removing bacterial counts by as much as four logs (16), additional backup systems using heat or ultraviolet (UV) irradiation were added to ensure sterile water. Rates of peritonitis were reduced with these closed systems; however, the machines were found to be quite demanding in terms of maintenance, care, monitoring, and disinfection and may themselves provide a reservoir for pathogens (17). With the meteoric rise of simpler procedures (described later), these machines have largely been replaced.

Continuous Ambulatory Peritoneal Dialysis

CAPD is a form of closed-system continuous dialysis that is machine free. Patients on CAPD manually exchange dialysate, usually four times daily, by using 2 L of dialysate delivered by gravity into the peritoneal cavity. Empty bags, connected to the catheter by extension tubing, collect the effluent, also by gravity, at the end of the dwell time. Fluid from the last exchange of the day dwells overnight in the peritoneal cavity. The technique was pioneered by Popovich et al. (3) in 1976 but initially suffered from high rates of peritonitis and patient inconveniences because of bottled dialysate. Oreopoulos et al. (4) modified the process and replaced the bottled dialysate with plastic dialysate bags, improving convenience, reducing manipulations, and lowering rates of infectious complications. CAPD is, thus, performed without the necessity of machines, is portable, is simple to learn and perform, and has become the procedure of choice for most patients on chronic peritoneal dialysis (10,18–21).

Continuous Cycling Peritoneal Dialysis

A variant of CAPD, continuous cycling peritoneal dialysis (CCPD) combines the principles of continuous automated dialysis during the night with those of prolonged dwell time dialysis during the day by use of a machine cycler allowing for frequent exchanges (22). CCPD has many advantages, including eliminating active dialysis during the day, reducing the number of exchanges, and possibly reducing rates of peritonitis. Disadvantages include cost, machine dependency, and lack of portability. Simpler cyclers will make CCPD an increasingly popular technique.

DEFINITIONS

There are a number of infections associated with peritoneal dialysis. By definition, *peritonitis* signifies inflammation of the peritoneal membranes as a result of infection or other insult. For clinical purposes, the definition proposed by Vas (22), consisting of any two of the following three criteria, is often used to establish a diagnosis of peritonitis: cloudy peritoneal effluent containing more than 100 neutrophils/mm^3, abdominal pain or tenderness, and microorganisms in the peritoneal fluid.

Exit-site infections are usually characterized by the presence of pain, erythema, tenderness, or induration of the catheter site often accompanied by purulent discharge. Infection, when present, is commonly limited to the area between the cutaneous surface (exit site) and the superficial Dacron cuff embedded in the subcutaneous tissue near the skin.

With *tunnel infections,* in which the area between the two Dacron cuffs is commonly referred to as the tunnel (the other cuff is embedded deep in the abdominal wall near the peritoneum), signs of infection include induration, tenderness, or redness of the overlying tissues with or without overt abscess formation.

EPIDEMIOLOGY AND RISK FACTORS ASSOCIATED WITH INFECTION

Regardless of the method of dialysis, infection, especially peritonitis, remains a serious threat to the patient. The incidence of peritonitis associated with an acute dialysis is high, approaching 0.5% to 4% (23). The incidence of peritonitis in patients receiving chronic dialytic therapy varies from center to center and depends on the method of chronic dialysis. However, no study has actually randomized patients with chronic renal failure to receive treatment by the three different methods of chronic dialytic therapy.

Over the years, the incidence of peritonitis associated with CAPD has continued to decrease from early observations of six episodes per patient-year reported in the late 1970s (24,25) to 1.4 episodes or less per patient-year documented by 1988 (26). Further significant reductions have not been achieved since the late 1980s, although some centers have reported rates as low as 0.7 to 0.9 episodes per patient-year (12,27). The initially precipitous drop in infections was largely attributable to enhanced center experience and training (25), substituting plastic dialysis bags for glass bottles, reducing the number of connect-disconnect times (4), incorporating titanium connectors to connect tubing to catheters (28), and developing other methods to reduce touch contamination during bag exchanges (27–29).

Clearly, the risk of developing peritonitis on CAPD increases with time. The period of greatest risk is the first few months of therapy. By the end of 6 months of treatment, the probability of developing at least one episode of peritonitis is 36% (30). This risk increases to 60% by the end of 1 year of treatment, 80% by 2 years, and approaches 90% by 3 years of uninterrupted therapy (26). More than half of all episodes of peritonitis occur in only 25% of all patients on CAPD. Twenty percent of patients develop three or more infections each year, whereas others remain free of infection for 3 or more years (10,31,32).

Several factors place a patient at increased risk for infection, especially peritonitis. These factors have been best studied in patients receiving CAPD. Although age or gender (33) do not appear to be important risk factors [rates may be higher in young children who perform their own therapy as opposed to children who obtain assistance from another family member (34)], underlying disease states may be important. For example, diabetic patients have been found to have higher rates of both peritonitis and exit-site infections (26,35). Lack of compliance with asepsis, lapses in technique, low patient motivation, lack of social support, fewer years of education, and lower socioeconomic status all have been found to be contributing factors to infection (36, 37). The type of catheter design, insertion technique, type of operator, and use of antibiotic prophylaxis at the time of catheter placement do not appreciably influence rates of peritonitis (38). However, data have demonstrated that catheters containing both a superficial and deep Dacron cuff (double-cuffed catheters) were associated with significantly lower rates of peritonitis than single-cuffed catheters (38). Studies have also confirmed that both the type and method of connection used between the dialysis bag and the indwelling peritoneal catheter can influence rates of peritonitis. Patients using connection devices permitting flush before fill systems such as Y-sets (29) or using disconnect systems that sterilize the connection, such as UV radiation (39), had rates of peritonitis significantly lower than those of patients using standard spike connectors (27). Finally, patients who were prescribed intraperitoneal medications and added these medications themselves had higher rates of peritonitis (27).

Intermittent peritoneal dialysis appears to result in lower rates of peritonitis when compared with CAPD. Rates as low as 0.4 to 0.9 episodes per patient-year have been reported (40,41). Perhaps much of this reduction can be attributed to the need for less frequent manipulations. In fact, patients on CIPD perform only 156 to 208 connect-disconnect procedures per year, as opposed to the more than 1,400 required for CAPD. Likewise, patients on CCPD appear to become infected at rates between those described for CIPD and for CAPD (18); these patients perform approximately 700 connect-disconnect procedures annually.

Exit-site or tunnel infections occur more commonly in individuals with concomitant peritonitis. Studies have also demonstrated that nasal carriers of *Staphylococcus aureus* are at increased risk for infection (42–47). Diabetics may also be at increased risk for infection, although this observation may be confounded by the observation of high carriage rates of *S. aureus* in these patients (48). The overall risk of an exit-site or tunnel infection in a patient receiving CAPD approaches 0.2 to 0.7 episodes per patient-year (44,49). Half of patients on CAPD do not develop exit-site infections within 2 years of catheter placement.

Epidemics of peritonitis in patients receiving chronic dialysis have been observed, especially in patients receiving CIPD via machines that use RO to sterilize water that then mixes with a dialysate concentrate (17,50,51). Outbreaks have also occurred as a result of delivering contaminated dialysate to the patient, either directly (52,53) or indirectly by use of water baths to heat the dialysate before infusion (54–56). Contaminated disinfectants used to clean exit sites and tubing ports have also resulted in outbreaks of infection (57).

PATHOGENESIS

Routes of Infection

The four major pathways resulting in peritonitis in patients on dialysis are schematically represented in Fig. 65.2. These include intraluminal transmission of microorganisms (microorganisms gaining entry through the infusion system); periluminal infections (infection of the catheter site with resultant local infection and, at times, spread into the peritoneum); transmural infec-

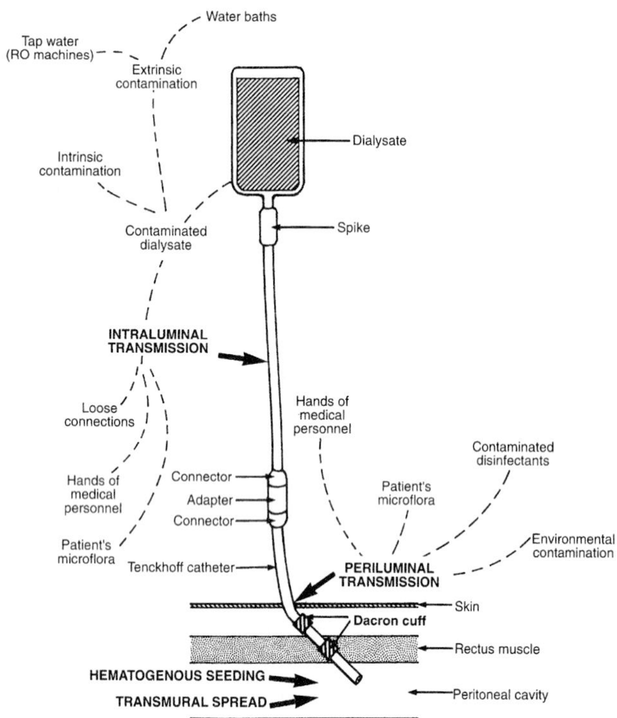

Figure 65.2. Sources of peritonitis and exit-site and tunnel infections in dialysis patients.

tions (peritonitis as a result of intestinal injury, perforation, or transmigration of microorganisms); and hematogenous spread, usually from a site of infection elsewhere. Exit-site or tunnel infections almost always result from a periluminal infection, although peritonitis can cause infection at the deep Dacron cuff of the Silastic catheter with resultant tunnel infection or abscess formation.

Few studies have examined the most common means by which peritonitis develops in patients receiving acute dialytic therapy. Clearly, infection of the catheter site with resultant spread into the peritoneum is a major route of infection. Unlike the situation with chronic dialysis, the cannula is usually inserted directly into the peritoneum after a stab wound is made. A protective tunnel with stabilization by Dacron cuffs is not usually made for short-term acute dialysis. Another important means by which peritonitis may develop in these patients is inadvertent perforation of the bowel during blind catheter placement or as a result of perforation from migration of the rigid catheter during dialysis with injury to the bowel wall. Microorganisms can also be introduced in the lumen during bag or tubing changes.

Contrast this scenario with what is observed in patients on chronic forms of peritoneal dialysis. It appears from inferential and intervention studies that the most important route of infection in these patients is intraluminal. Intraluminal contamination can occur during the numerous connect-disconnect manipulations by means of loose-fitting connectors or malfunctioning clamps, through defects in the plastic tubing or bags, or from the dialysis fluid itself. First, peritonitis occurs at least twice as often as exit-site infections in patients on chronic dialysis (26), suggesting that microorganisms are instilled into the peritoneal cavity. Second, the most common microorganisms causing peritonitis are coagulase-negative staphylococci rather than *S. aureus,* a microorganism found more frequently as a cause of periluminal infections (58). Third, studies have found that a major cause of peritonitis in patients on chronic dialysis is poor technique or observed breaks in technique resulting in intraluminal contamination (59). Fourth, CIPD or CCPD, methods associated with fewer manipulations, have consistently been associated with fewer infections (18,40,41). Finally, incorporating devices or procedures to reduce touch contamination have resulted in fewer infections (27,29).

Contaminated Dialysate

Intrinsic contamination of dialysate has been reported infrequently and may result in infective peritonitis (52) or a sterile peritonitis resulting from delivery of endotoxin (53). In-use or extrinsic contamination may occur during bag exchanges. Fortunately, commercially available dialysate does not support the growth of staphylococci, the most common pathogen responsible for infection, although some gram-negative microorganisms proliferate readily if introduced (60,61). Water-adapted microorganisms such as *Mycobacterium chelonae*-like microorganisms and *Pseudomonas* species have caused outbreaks of peritonitis in patients on CIPD (17,51). Microorganisms such as *M. chelonae*-like organisms not only can live in chlorinated water but also may survive exposure to high concentrations of disinfectants such as formaldehyde (62).

Infection of the catheter site is the second most common cause of peritonitis and the leading cause of exit-site infections in patients on chronic peritoneal dialysis. The implanted catheter never forms a complete sealed junction with the skin; thus, microorganisms are present within the exit site and can result in infection. Although the superficial embedded Dacron cuff is a reasonable barrier, limiting the migration of microorganisms deeper into the abdominal wall or to the peritoneum, its efficacy is clearly not 100% (63). Up to 17% of patients who develop an exit-site infection also have peritonitis (58). *S. aureus* carriers are at high risk for developing an exit-site infection (43–48) as are diabetics (64).

Transmural infections occur as a result of abdominal perforation or injury, inflammation of the serosal surfaces, or transmural migration (65). Rates of peritonitis resulting from intestinal microorganisms are higher in patients with preexisting diverticular disease (66). Infection of the peritoneum or exit site by the hematogenous route is uncommon.

Host Defense Mechanisms

For peritonitis to develop, the patient's host defenses must not be able to contain, destroy, and remove the invading pathogens. Peritoneal fluid normally contains up to 2 million leukocytes/mL, of which more than 80% are mononuclear cells predominately macrophages (67–69). These cells represent the primary cellular barrier against infection (70); patients prone to infection may have fewer macrophages available to combat infection (71). Many microorganisms causing peritonitis require opsonization by heat-stable substances, such as immunoglobulin

G (IgG) and other specific antibodies, or heat-labile components, including complement for efficient removal. Deficiency in IgG or C3 may also predispose patients to infection, as would neutropenia (72).

It is well known that the delivery of dialysate into the peritoneal cavity has a direct adverse effect on host defense mechanisms because of the effects of the low pH and hyperosmolarity of the dialysate. Both acidity and hyperosmolarity reduce the ability of macrophages and polymorphonuclear leukocytes to phagocytize and kill microorganisms (73–75). Also, the presence of extra liters of fluid in the peritoneal cavity during dialysis results in a marked dilutional effect on both cellular and humoral protective factors, resulting in fewer leukocytes per milliliter and a relative opsonic deficiency (72,76).

Obviously, an indwelling peritoneal catheter has adverse effects on the host. A conduit between the outside environment and the peritoneum now exists. The catheter may act as a foreign body, initiating inflammatory changes that predispose to infection, and can serve as a substrate on which colonization may be established. Although Silastic catheters appear to be less thrombogenic than polyurethane catheters (77), all catheters eventually become coated with a fibrin sheath (78). Microorganisms can become embedded in this sheath or in the biofilm produced by many microorganisms, resulting in proliferation with resultant infection. This protective environment may be responsible for the difficulty in eradicating infection by seemingly appropriate antibiotics or for relapses of infection (79).

Finally, patients with end-stage renal failure often have defects in cellular immune functions and are more susceptible to infection in general (80–82).

ETIOLOGIC AGENTS

Causative Microorganisms of Peritonitis

Although numerous microorganisms have been isolated from infected patients on peritoneal dialysis, most of these microorganisms are skin commensals such as coagulase-negative staphylococci (Table 65.1) (22,31,32,44,58,64,83). At least two thirds of all episodes are caused by gram-positive microorganisms; *Staphylococcus epidermidis* is isolated most frequently. The second most common microorganism is *S. aureus,* followed by various streptococcal species. Gram-negative bacteria account for 20% to 30% of all episodes, with *Escherichia coli* and other members of the family Enterobacteriaceae most prevalent. Fewer than 10% of episodes of peritonitis are due to *Pseudomonas aeruginosa* or related microorganisms. Anaerobes are uncommon. When anaerobes are present, the possibility of peritonitis from bowel perforation increases, especially if polymicrobic peritonitis is found.

Peritonitis resulting from fungal microorganisms has been reported to occur in as many as 8% of episodes. The most commonly isolated fungus is *Candida albicans,* followed by other *Candida* species (84,85). Less commonly isolated microorganisms include *Mycobacterium* species and related pathogens. Viral microorganisms and parasites are exceedingly uncommon causes of peritonitis in patients on peritoneal dialysis.

Aseptic peritonitis is a well-described entity. Although the

TABLE 65.1. PREVALENCE OF MICROORGANISMS ISOLATED FROM PATIENTS WITH PERITONITIS AND CATHETER (EXIT-SITE AND TUNNEL) INFECTIONS

Microorganisms	Peritonitis (%)	Catheter infections (%)
Gram-positive aerobic bacteria		
Coagulase-negative staphylococci	40–65	15–20
Staphylococcus aureus	10–25	25–35
Streptococcal species	8–15	2–5
Enterococci	3–7	2–5
Corynebacterium or *Bacillus* species	1–4	2–5
Gram-negative aerobic bacteria		
Escherichia coli	7–12	5–10
Klebsiella species	2–4	2–5
Other Enterobacteriaceae	1–7	1–5
Pseudomonas species	5–9	10–15
Miscellaneous	1–5	1–5
Multiple microorganisms	2–6	25–35
Anaerobes	<5	<1
Fungi	4–8	4–6
Miscellaneous	2–5	3–5

From references 22, 31, 32, 44, 58, 64, 83, with permission.

frequency of culture-negative peritonitis has decreased with improved culture techniques (86), 10% of episodes of peritonitis yield no growth of pathogens on culture. Clearly, some of these episodes represent failure to isolate an infecting microorganism because of the lack of sensitivity of culture techniques (87). Others may be due to a foreign body reaction to the implanted catheter (88), chemical peritonitis (17,89), or delivery of endotoxin into the peritoneum (52).

Causative Microorganisms of Exit-Site or Tunnel Infections

The microbiology of exit-site or tunnel infections differs somewhat from that observed in patients with peritonitis (Table 65.1). Mixed infections, rare in dialysis-associated peritonitis, may be found in up to 30% of these catheter infections (58). The most commonly isolated pathogen is *S. aureus,* accounting for 25% to 35% of all episodes, followed by *S. epidermidis* in 10% to 20% of cases. *Pseudomonas* species are also more frequently recovered from device-related infections than from peritoneal fluid in patients with peritonitis.

Piraino et al. (58) found that 17% of all catheter infections occurred simultaneously with or were followed shortly thereafter by an episode of peritonitis resulting from the same microorganism, supporting the conclusion that exit-site infections can result in peritonitis. Peritonitis and exit-site infections caused by *S. aureus* and *P. aeruginosa* require catheter removal more often than when these same infections are caused by *S. epidermidis.* Others have found high rates of treatment failure when infection was due to fungi (84,85,90). Piraino et al. (58) also found that peritonitis episodes resulting from *S. epidermidis* infrequently had associated exit-site infections, whereas peritonitis caused by *S. aureus* or *Pseudomonas* species were frequently associated with a catheter infection.

Comments on Specific Pathogens

Coagulase-Negative Staphylococci

Eighty percent of coagulase-negative staphylococci belong to the species *S. epidermidis* (91,92); coagulase-negative staphylococci are an important component of the cutaneous flora. Although adherence factors and slime production are thought to be important in pathogenesis of infection, studies have not confirmed this hypothesis. Strains capable of producing slime were not more frequently isolated from episodes of peritonitis (86); in one study, peritonitis-causing strains lacking adherence and slime productivity were more frequently associated with complications (93). Infections resulting from *S. epidermidis* tend to be milder and more responsive to therapy than infections resulting from *S. aureus.*

Staphylococcus aureus

Several studies have found that nasal carriers of *S. aureus* are at higher risk for exit-site infections and peritonitis than noncarriers (42–47,94). Epidemiologic typing has confirmed a high concordance between strains of *S. aureus* isolated from infections and those isolated from the nares (47,94,95). More recently, strains of staphylococci with reduced susceptibilities to glycopeptide antibiotics including vancomycin have been described (96–98), as well as isolates possessing absolute resistance (99,100) (see Chapters 28 and 29).

Enterococci

Although an infrequent cause of initial peritonitis in patients on peritoneal dialysis, enterococci, including vancomycin-resistant strains, have been found in increasing frequency, especially among patients with heavy exposure to antimicrobics. Guidelines for preventing the emergence and spread of vancomycin-resistant enterococci have been published (101) (see Chapter 32).

Enterobacteriaceae

Although the precise origin of these microorganisms as a source of exit-site infections and peritonitis is not known, hand and cutaneous carriage seems more plausible than transmural migration. Ill patients and those with chronic medical problems often are colonized with these microorganisms (102–104). Also, dialysate readily supports the growth of microorganisms such as *E. coli,* as opposed to staphylococcal species; a high index of suspicion for contamination by these microorganisms should be maintained (60,61).

Pseudomonas Species

These microorganisms also colonize the skin of chronically debilitated patients (102–104). Their repeated isolation should also prompt investigation of products, including disinfectants, that might be contaminated (57,105) or exposure to water sources, including pool water or even potable water (106).

Fungi

The source of most yeast is the patient's skin or mucous membranes; less comes from the environment. Established predisposing factors include recently treated bacterial peritonitis, use of broad-spectrum antibiotics, and nosocomial acquisition (85). Infections usually respond poorly to therapy without removal of the peritoneal catheter. Filamentous fungal infections usually arise from environmental contamination. Of these, *Fusarium* species is most common (107).

Mycobacteria

Environmental contamination, especially from water, predisposes to mycobacterial infections resulting from *M. chelonae* and related microorganisms (108). Several outbreaks have been reported in patients receiving intermittent peritoneal dialysis by automated machines (17).

Miscellaneous Microorganisms

Infections resulting from other human flora (e.g., *Haemophilus* species, *Neisseria* species, *Branhamella* species, and *Gardnerella* species) have been reported, as have infections caused by diverse microorganisms, including *Campylobacter* species, *Pasteurella* species, *Listeria* species, and vibrios. Even episodes of peritonitis caused by *Prototheca wickerhamii* have been reported (109).

DIAGNOSTIC CONSIDERATIONS

Clinical Manifestations of Peritonitis and Exit-Site Infections

Most patients who develop peritoneal dialysis-associated peritonitis usually have some complaints of abdominal pain and notice a change in their dialysis effluent from a clear to somewhat cloudy fluid. Onset may be abrupt or relatively indolent depending on the bacterial load and nature of the infecting pathogen. For example, patients who develop peritonitis from *S. aureus* or *P. aeruginosa* have a more aggressive course than patients who have *S. epidermidis* peritonitis (55,58,64,110). Obviously, if peritonitis occurs as a result of bowel perforation, patients usually develop signs of an acute abdomen.

Table 65.2 lists the common manifestations of dialysis-associ-

TABLE 65.2. SYMPTOMS AND SIGNS ASSOCIATED WITH DIALYSIS-ASSOCIATED PERITONITIS

Clinical manifestations	Percentage of patients (range)
Symptoms	
Abdominal pain	73–95
Nausea, vomiting	25–35
Chills	18–23
Diarrhea	6–9
Signs	
Cloudy effluent	86–98
Abdominal tenderness	50–79
Fever (>38°C)	24–34
Drainage problems	10–15

From references 10, 58, 111–113, with permission.

ated peritonitis (10,58,111–113). Of particular importance is the relative infrequency of constitutional manifestations. In general, less than one third of infected patients have fever. However, patients can develop acute illness rapidly (36). Incubation periods range from a few hours to several days.

Exit-site or tunnel infections usually present with pain accompanied by serous or seropurulent drainage. Unless peritonitis is also present, systemic signs or symptoms occur rarely.

Examination of the Peritoneal Fluid

More than 90% of patients with peritonitis have cloudy effluent because of the elevated number of peritoneal leukocytes. Normally, the peritoneal fluid contains less than 60 white blood cells/mm^3; most are mononuclear cells. Infection rapidly results in an increase in the number of white blood cells in the peritoneal fluid and a shift from mononuclear cells to polymorphonuclear leukocytes (67–69,114).

Most patients develop cell counts ranging from a few hundred to several thousand (20,114,115); more than 50% of the cellular component is composed of polymorphonuclear leukocytes (116). Polymorphonuclear leukocyte counts greater than 100/mm^3 in the peritoneal fluid correlate strongly with infection. Occasionally, in some infections, a mononuclear cellular response is found, such as with tuberculous peritonitis. However, most microorganisms associated with dialysis-induced infection result in neutrophilia.

Peritoneal neutrophilia can also be seen in noninfectious inflammatory conditions affecting the peritoneum, including peritonitis caused by chemical irritants or endotoxin, an intraperitoneal bleed, serositis resulting from systemic vasculitis, or primary gastrointestinal disease. Occasionally, peritoneal eosinophilia is observed. Its presence suggests a foreign body (catheter) reaction or an allergy to a catheter component or other product. It is generally a self-limiting process (117).

Gram Staining of Peritoneal Fluid or Drainage from Exit Sites

For cases of suspected peritonitis, preparation of a Gram-stained smear (or other special stains for acid-fast or fungal microorganisms, as appropriate) of the sediment from a centrifuged sample of effluent is important. If the stain is positive, more specific therapy can be instituted, and purely empiric therapy can be avoided. Unfortunately, studies have found a positive Gram stain in only 9% to 35% of cases of peritonitis (118). If purulent drainage is present from an exit-site infection, the Gram stain may prove quite useful in guiding initial therapy.

Culture Methods

Peritoneal dialysate effluent should be cultured as soon as possible in any patient with suspected peritonitis. If this is not feasible, the bag should be stored in a refrigerator and transported to the laboratory within 6 hours.

The optimal method for culturing peritoneal effluent is a matter of considerable controversy. Because the inoculum is usually quite low (20,119), large-volume sampling has resulted in a higher yield. Effluent should generally be concentrated by centrifugation or filtration or inoculated into an enrichment medium (20,22). Use of filters, however, is technically demanding and may result in contamination (120). von Graevenitz and Amsterdam's review (86) of the various microbiologic techniques available is excellent. These authors reviewed studies published before 1987 and found significant problems in comparing various culture methods because of problems in study design and the use of inadequate volumes for direct culturing. They concluded that a minimum of 10 mL of effluent should be cultured, using an enrichment broth with antiphagocytic and lytic properties.

More recently, additional studies have demonstrated that, in addition to concentrating specimens, direct sampling of dialysate into an isolator tube with subsequent inoculation or direct inoculation into semiautomated blood culture systems such as Bactec bottles has been associated with high yields (121–123). An Ad Hoc Advisory Committee on Peritonitis Management (chaired by W.F. Keane, M.D.) recently released a consensus on techniques for sampling and culturing peritoneal dialysis effluent and exit sites (124). Their recommendations are as follows:

1. Peritoneal dialysate effluent should be analyzed as promptly as possible after peritonitis is suspected.
2. An aliquot of 10 to 50 mL should be centrifuged, and the sediment should be examined by Gram stain.
3. Specimens should be cultured by using either concentration methods such as centrifugation (resuspension in nutrient broth or sterile saline with subsequent inoculation of blood and MacConkey agar plates; if a perforated viscus is suspected, anaerobic cultures can also be done; lytic substances such as Triton X can be added to the effluent before centrifugation and may increase the yield of positive cultures) or Millipore filtration. A semiautomated blood culture system for culturing peritoneal dialysis effluents appears to be suitable as well.
4. Using media with antiphagocytic substances and antibiotic binding resins may also result in higher yield.
5. A Calgi swab should be used to culture purulent exudate obtained from an exit site.

COURSE AND PROGNOSIS

Although most patients are not acutely ill, some patients initially develop high-grade toxicity with onset of infection. Blood cultures occasionally are positive. Peritoneal infection also results in impaired ultrafiltration, increased glucose absorption, and tremendous protein losses (125). Infection can result in pulmonary complications resulting from bowel distention with displacement of the diaphragm and pulmonary edema from inadequate volume removal. The inflammatory reaction itself produces a fibrinogen-rich exudate with fibrin clot formation and impaired drainage (40). Repeated episodes can cause scarring with loss of the peritoneal membrane for further ultrafiltration.

Most cases of peritonitis respond promptly to appropriate antimicrobic therapy. However, as discussed previously, certain microorganisms tend to be more difficult to treat or do not respond well to antimicrobial therapy unless the implanted catheter is removed (58 84,85,90). Patients who relapse after seemingly appropriate therapy also usually require catheter removal.

Most exit-site infections can be managed conservatively. However, the presence of a tunnel abscess almost always necessitates removal of the implanted catheter.

PREVENTION AND CONTROL

Despite major advances since the acceptance of chronic peritoneal dialysis as a method of chronic dialytic therapy, infection and catheter-related complications continue to cause significant morbidity. Table 65.3 summarizes important recommendations for prevention.

Prevention largely depends on three factors: proper selection and training of patients, strict adherence to aseptic techniques in all aspects of dialysis, and use of intervention strategies for special at-risk populations.

Patient Selection and Training

Few medical conditions make chronic peritoneal dialysis the method of choice for chronic dialytic therapy. Its ease of performance, ability to be done in the home setting, lower cost when compared with hemodialysis, and, as in the case of CAPD, machine independence have led to greater patient acceptance. Rates of complications are reduced in the highly motivated patient who has received thorough training with continued supervision (36,37,126,127).

Type of Catheter and Insertion Techniques

Although studies have not established that the precise type of catheter inserted has definitely affected rates of infection, Silastic catheters containing both a superficial and a deep Dacron cuff appear to have lower rates of infection when compared with single-cuffed catheters (38). Because silicone can be degraded by iodine or povidone-iodine over time and does not resist biofilm formation (124), newer catheter materials are needed. Bonding of antimicrobic agents to indwelling devices may reduce risks for device-associated infections (128). Studies have not shown definitive advantages for any single method of placement (blind vs. surgical vs. peritoneoscopic insertion) or for placement performed in an operating room suite as opposed to elsewhere; strict attention to asepsis is always important (124). Antimicrobial prophylaxis appears to be warranted immediately before surgical placement of the catheter.

TABLE 65.3. PREVENTION OF INFECTION IN PATIENTS ON CHRONIC PERITONEAL DIALYSIS

Select well-motivated patients and thoroughly instruct them in sterile techniques.
Place the implantable silicone catheter using sterile technique. Double-cuffed catheters may be preferred.
Anchor the catheter site firmly.
Wash hands before all manipulations and avoid touch contamination of tubing connections.
Consider special catheter connectors such as Y-sets using the "flush before fill" concept, patient-assist devices, or connecting devices using ultraviolet sterilization.
Reduce manipulations to a minimum.
Perform daily site care with at least soap and water and inspect site for signs of early infection.
Consider antibiotic prophylaxis only in very limited circumstances (e.g., staphylococcal carriers with frequent exit-site infections).
If using an automated machine using reverse osmosis to "sterilize" tap water, clean and disinfect it regularly.
Treat other sites of infection early to reduce chances of hematogenous or transmural spread to the peritoneum.
Optimize host defenses by good nutrition and care of other medical problems.

Asepsis During Peritoneal Dialysis

Most episodes or peritonitis are due to inadvertent contamination of the dialysis fluid or peritoneal catheter during exchanges (intraluminal contamination). Strict adherence to aseptic practices is essential and can reduce infection rates (59,129). Good hand washing practices using an alcoholic gel rub or antimicrobial soap (130), performing dialysis in a clean and safe environment, and inspecting all supplies for defects before use are important. Numerous connectors and connecting devices have been developed to reduce the possibility of accidental contamination during bag exchanges. These include such items as the titanium adapter (28,131), use of added tubing to permit flush before fill as the Y-connector (29), mechanical patient assist devices (131), connecting devices with in-line bacteriologic filters (119) and devices designed to clean the connections with disinfectants (132,133), UV radiation (39), or heat (134). Studies on the efficacy of these devices have produced contradictory results but definitely show added costs. It does appear that both the UV and Y-connectors have promise; a study of 3,366 CAPD patients who started dialysis at home for the first time between January 1, 1989 and June 30, 1989 demonstrated a relative risk of first peritonitis significantly lower for the Y-set (relative risk 0.6; $p < .01$) and UV set (relative risk 0.75; $p < .01$) when compared with the standard spike connecting set (27). The difference in relative risk between the Y- and UV sets was also statistically significant ($p < .01$). The benefits of the Y-systems on reducing rates of peritonitis was confirmed in another recent study with rates of one episode per 40 months, compared with one episode per 16 months for other systems (135). In Europe, Y-sets containing disinfectants have resulted in fewer episodes of peritonitis when compared with standard connection systems. However, because of fear of accidental chemical peritonitis during use, these modified systems are not popular in the United States. More recently, Y-sets, in which both the dialysis solution and drain bags were preattached, appear to have reduced peritonitis rates further (136).

Systems that permit fewer connections and disconnections have also been associated with reduced rates of peritonitis. Some patients can tolerate three exchanges per day rather than four. Use of the CCPD machine reduces manipulations to twice daily with lower rates of peritonitis (18). Automated intermittent peritoneal dialysis permits even fewer interruptions but may be associated with outbreaks when used at centers or with endemic disease because of problems with disinfection and sterilization (17,40,41,50,51). Formal recommendations for the care of these machines have been published (137).

Site Care and Special Considerations

Daily inspection and care of the exit site is also important, although some controversy exists as to whether such care should include daily showering with soap or additional use of antiseptics on the exit site. One study suggested that rates of exit-site infection can be reduced by using a protective nonocclusive dressing and povidone-iodine cleansing (44); others have not confirmed this observation (124), whereas another small study suggested chlorhexidine to be superior to povidone-iodine (138) for site care. An excellent summary of exit-site practices has recently been updated (139). Infection must be detected and treated early to reduce progression to a tunnel abscess or peritonitis.

S. aureus nasal carriers seem to have benefited from attempts to eliminate carriage by use of various antimicrobic prophylactic agents in some, but not all, studies (42,45). Agents used have included rifampin, trimethoprim-sulfamethoxazole, intranasal bacitracin or mupirocin, or topical mupirocin applied to the exit site (140,141). Recently, a multicenter study involving 267 staphylococcal carriers suggested that monthly application of intranasal mupirocin for 5 days results in a reduction of exit-site infections resulting from *S. aureus* but not to other microorganisms (142). Widespread usage of mupirocin applied topically to the nares or exit site may result in significant development of resistance (143) and may not be cost-effective (144). Unfortunately, more serious infections such as tunnel infections and peritonitis resulting from *S. aureus* were also unaffected by this regimen. However, the epidemiology of infections in staphylococcal carriers is not completely understood, and many chronic carriers do not develop exit-site infections. It might be prudent to restrict such intervention to proven carriers with repeated infections. The device should best be removed after successful renal transplantation (within 4 to 6 weeks after surgery).

Antibiotic Prophylaxis to Reduce Episodes of Peritonitis

Antimicrobial prophylaxis has not resulted in a decrease in early-onset peritonitis after catheter insertion (38) or in a reduction of peritonitis in the long term (145,146). A recent uncontrolled and nonrandomized study suggested that oral prophylaxis with nystatin administered at the time of bacterial peritonitis may reduce subsequent episodes of fungal peritonitis (147).

FUTURE CONSIDERATIONS

Improved catheter materials designed to minimize foreign body reactions, adherence of microorganisms, and biofilm formation; improved techniques of catheter placement and site sealing; and newer delivery systems resulting in fewer episodes of contamination are needed. Enhancing both local and systemic host defense systems may also lead to lower rates of infections in patients on chronic peritoneal dialysis therapy. Trials of a *S. aureus* conjugate vaccine in patients receiving hemodialysis appear promising in preventing systemic infection resulting from *S. aureus* (148) and phase 1 and phase 2 investigations using hyperimmune globulin to *S. aureus* are currently in progress (149).

REFERENCES

1. Renal Data System. USRDS 1997 annual data report. Bethesda, MD: National Institute of Diabetes and Digestive and Kidney Diseases, 1997.
2. Tenckhoff H, Schecter H. A bacteriologically safe peritoneal access device. *Trans Am Soc Artif Int Organs* 1968;14:181–186.
3. Popovich RP, Moncrief JW, Decherd JB, et al. The definition of a novel portable/wearable equilibrium peritoneal dialysis technique. *Am Soc Artif Intern Organs* 1976;5:64(abst).
4. Oreopoulos DG, Robson M, Izalt S, et al. A simple and safe technique for continuous ambulatory peritoneal dialysis. *Trans Am Soc Artif Int Organs* 1978;24:484–487.
5. Tenckhoff H, Blagg CR, Curtis KF, et al. Chronic peritoneal dialysis. *Proc Dial Transplant* 1973;10:363–371.
6. Gutman RA. Automated peritoneal dialysis for home use. *Q J Med* 1978;47:261–280.
7. Tenckhoff H. Meston B, Shilipetar G. A simplified automatic peritoneal dialysis system. *Trans Am Soc Artif Organs* 1972;18:436–439.
8. Boen ST. Overview and history of peritoneal dialysis. *Dial Transplant* 1977;6:12–18.
9. Nolph KD, Cutter SJ, Steinburg SM, et al. Continuous ambulatory peritoneal dialysis in the United States: a three year study. *Kidney Int* 1985;28:198–205.
10. Pollock CA, Ibels LS, Caterson RJ, et al. Continuous ambulatory peritoneal dialysis eight years experience at a single center. *Medicine (Baltimore)* 1989;68:293–308.
11. Lindblad AS, Novak JW, Nolph KD. *Continuous ambulatory peritoneal dialysis in the USA: final report of the National CAPD Registry 1981–1988.* Dordrecht: Kluwer, 1989.
12. Bloembergen WE, Port FK. Epidemiological perspectives on infections in chronic dialysis patients. *Adv Renal Replace Ther* 1996;3: 201–207.
13. Maiorca R, Vonesh EF, Cavilli PL, et al. A multicenter, selection-adjusted comparison of patients and technique survivals on CAPD and hemodialysis. *Perit Dial Int* 1991;11:118–127.
14. Weston RE, Roberts M. Clinical use of stylet-catheter for peritoneal dialysis. *Arch Intern Med* 1965;115:659–662.
15. Palmer RA, Quinton WE, Gray JE. Prolonged peritoneal dialysis for chronic renal failure. *Lancet* 1964;1:700–702.
16. Peterson NJ, Carson LA, Favero JS. Microbiological quality of water in automated peritoneal dialysis systems. *Dial Transplant* 1977;6: 38–40.
17. Band JD, Ward JI, Fraser DW, et al. Peritonitis due to a *Mycobacterium chelonei*-like organism associated with intermittent chronic peritoneal dialysis. *J Infect Dis* 1982;145:9–17.
18. Diaz-Buxo JA, Walker PJ, Farmes CD, et al. Continuous cyclic peritoneal dialysis the Nalli Clinic experience. In: Price JDE, ed. *Peritoneal dialysis. The state of the art.* Princeton, NJ: Communications Media for Education, 1983:23–25.
19. Popovich RP, Moncrief JW, Nolph KD, et al. Continuous ambulatory peritoneal dialysis. *Ann Intern Med* 1978;88:449–456.
20. Rubin J, Rodgers WA, Taylor HM, et al. Peritonitis during continuous ambulatory dialysis. *Ann Intern Med* 1980;92:7–13.
21. Oreopoulos DG. Continuous ambulatory peritoneal dialysis in Canada. *Can Med Assoc J* 1979;120:16–19.
22. Vas SI. Microbiologic aspects of chronic ambulatory peritoneal dialysis. *Kidney Int* 1983;23:328–330.
23. Schoenfield P. Care of the patient on peritoneal dialysis. In: Cogan MG, Schoenfield P, eds. *Introduction to dialysis,* 2nd ed. London: Churchill Livingstone, 1991:236.

24. Popovich RP, Moncrief JE, Nolph JD. Continuous ambulatory peritoneal dialysis (CAPD). *Abstr Am Soc Nephrol* 1977;10:35A.
25. Nolph KD, Sorkin M, Rubin J. Continuous ambulatory peritoneal dialysis: three-year experience at one center. *Ann Intern Med* 1980; 92:609–613.
26. Nolph KD. Current status of CAPD and CCPD. *Dial Transplant* 1988;17:457–460.
27. Port FK, Held PJ, Nolph KD, et al. Risk of peritonitis and technique failure by CAPD connection technique: a national study. *Kidney Int* 1992;42:967–974.
28. Nolph KD. Continuous ambulatory peritoneal dialysis. *Am J Nephrol* 1981;1:1–10.
29. Maiorca R, Contaluppi A, Cancarini GC, et al. Prospective controlled trial of a Y-connector and disinfectant to prevent peritonitis in continuous ambulatory peritoneal dialysis. *Lancet* 1983;2:642–644.
30. Lindblad AS, Novak JW, Nolph KD, et al. The 1987 USA National CAPD Registry Report. *ASAIO Trans* 1988;34:150–156.
31. Swartz RD. Chronic peritoneal dialysis: mechanical and infectious complications. *Nephron* 1987;40:29–37.
32. Williams CC. CAPD in Toronto—an overview. *Perit Dial Bull* 1983; 3:56–58.
33. Renal Data System. NIH CAPD Registry Report from the Data Coordinating Center at the EMMES Corp. Bethesda, MD: National Institute of Digestive and Kidney Diseases, 1987.
34. McClung MR. Peritonitis in children receiving continuous ambulatory peritoneal dialysis. *Pediatr Infect Dis* 1983;2:328–332.
35. Amair P, Khanna R, Leibel B, et al. Continuous ambulatory peritoneal dialysis in diabetics with end-stage renal disease. *N Engl J Med* 1982; 306:625–630.
36. Oreopoulos DG, Williams P, Khanna R, et al. Treatment of peritonitis. *Perit Dial Bull* 1981;1(Suppl):17–19.
37. Rubin J, Ray R, Barnes T, et al. Peritonitis in continuous ambulatory peritoneal dialysis. *Am J Kidney Dis* 1983;2:602–609.
38. Anonymous. Catheter-related factors and peritonitis risk in CAPD patients. *Am J Kidney Dis* 1992;20(Suppl 2):48–54.
39. Popovich RP, Moncrief JW, Sorrels-Akar AJ, et al. The ultraviolet germicidal system: the elimination of distal contamination in CAPD. In: Maher JF, Winchester JF, eds. *Frontiers in peritoneal dialysis.* New York: International Symposium Peritoneal Dialysis, Field and Rich, 1986.
40. Kraus ES, Spector DA. Characteristics and sequelae of peritonitis in diabetics and non diabetics receiving chronic intermittent peritoneal dialysis. *Medicine (Baltimore)* 1983;62:52–57.
41. Diaz-Buxo JA. Does CCPD lower the peritonitis rate? *Contrib Nephrol* 1987;57:191–196.
42. Swartz R, Messana J, Starmann B, et al. Preventing *Staphylococcus aureus* infection during chronic peritoneal dialysis. *J Am Soc Nephrol* 1991;2:1085–1091.
43. Luzar MA, Coles GA, Faller B, et al. Staphylococcus aureus nasal carriage and infection in patients on CAPD. *N Engl J Med* 1990; 322:505–509.
44. Luzar MA, Brown CB, Ball D, et al. Exit site care and exit site infection in continuous ambulatory peritoneal dialysis: results of a randomized multicenter trial. *Perit Dial Int* 1990;10:25–29.
45. Zimmerman SW, Ahrens E, Johnson CA, et al. Randomized controlled trial of prophylactic rifampin for peritoneal dialysis related infections. *Am J Kidney Dis* 1991;18:225–231.
46. Sewell CM, Clarridge J, Lacke C, et al. Staphylococcal nasal carriage and subsequent infection in peritoneal dialysis patients. *JAMA* 1982; 248:1493–1495.
47. Pignatari A, Pfaller M, Hollis R, et al. *Staphylococcus aureus* colonization and infection in patients on chronic ambulatory peritoneal dialysis. *J Clin Microbiol* 1990;28:1898–1902.
48. Tuazon CU, Perez A, Kishaba T, et al. *Staphylococcus aureus* among insulin-injecting diabetic patients. An increased carrier rate. *JAMA* 1975;231:1272.
49. Renal Data System. NIH CAPD Registry. Bethesda, MD: National Institute of Diabetes and Digestive and Kidney Diseases, 1986.
50. Berkelman RL, Godley J, Weber JA, et al. *Pseudomonas cepacia* peritonitis associated with contamination of automated peritoneal dialysis machines. *Ann Intern Med* 1982;96:456–458.
51. Hamory BH, Nevrakias JM, Pearson SK. Peritonitis from automated peritoneal dialysis. *Infect Control* 1984;5:559–561.
52. Karanicolas S, Oreopoulos DG, Izalt S, et al. Epidemic of aseptic peritonitis caused by endotoxin during chronic peritoneal dialysis. *N Engl J Med* 1977;296:1336–1337.
53. Mangram AJ, Archibald LK, Hupert M, et al. Outbreak of sterile peritonitis among continuous cycling peritoneal dialysis patients associated with intrinsically contaminated dialysis fluid. Proceedings of the 37th Interscience Conference on Antimicrobial Agents and Chemotherapy (ICAAC), Abstract J-18, Toronto, Ontario, Canada, September 1997, p. 291.
54. Abrutyn E, Goodhart G, Roos K, et al. *Acinetobacter calcoaceticus* outbreaks associated with peritoneal dialysis. *Am J Epidemiol* 1978; 107:328–335.
55. Kolmos HJ, Anderson KEH. Peritonitis with *Pseudomonas aeruginosa* in hospital patients treated with peritoneal dialysis. *Scand J Infect Dis* 1979;11:207–210.
56. Yuen KY, Seto WH, Ching TY, et al. An outbreak of *Candida tropicalis* peritonitis in patients on intermittent peritoneal dialysis. *J Hosp Infect* 1992;22:65–72.
57. Panlilio AL, Beck-Sague CM, Siegel JD, et al. Infections and pseudo-infections due to povidone-iodine solution contaminated with *Pseudomonas cepacia. Clin Infect Dis* 1992;14:1078–1083.
58. Piraino B, Bernardini J, Sorkin M. A five-year study of the microbiologic results of exit site infections and peritonitis in continuous ambulatory peritoneal dialysis. *Am J Kidney Dis* 1987;10:281–286.
59. Prowant B, Nolph K, Ryan L, et al. Peritonitis in continuous ambulatory peritoneal dialysis: analysis of an 8-year experience. *Nephron* 1986;43:105–109.
60. Verbrugh HA, Keane WF, Conroy WE, et al. Bacterial growth and killing in continuous ambulatory peritoneal dialysis fluids. *J Clin Microbiol* 1984;20:199–203.
61. Sheth NK, Bartell CA, Roth DA. In-vitro study of bacterial growth in continuous ambulatory peritoneal dialysis fluids. *J Clin Microbiol* 1986;23:1096–1098.
62. Hayes PS, McGiboney DL, Band JD, et al. Resistance of *Mycobacterium chelonei*-like organisms to formaldehyde. *Appl Environ Microbiol* 1982;43:722–724.
63. Read RR, Eberwein P, Dasgupta MK, et al. Peritonitis in peritoneal dialysis: bacterial colonization by biofilm spread along the catheter surface. *Kidney Int* 1989;35:614–621.
64. Lane T, Chandran P. Ten-year experience with exit site infections. *Nephron* 1990;55:220–221.
65. Schweinberg FB, Seligman AM, Fine J. Transmural migration of intestinal bacteria. A study based on the use of radioactive *Escherichia coli. N Engl J Med* 1950;242:747–751.
66. Wu G, Khanna R, Vas S, Oreopoulos DG. Is extensive diverticulitis of the colon a contraindication to CAPD? *Perit Dial Bull* 1983;3: 180–183.
67. Haney AF, Muscato JJ, Weinberg JB. Peritoneal fluid cell populations in infertility patients. *Fertil Steril* 1981;35:696–698.
68. Halme J, Becker S, Hammond MG, et al. Pelvic macrophages in normal and infertile women. The role of patent tubes. *Am J Obstet Gynecol* 1982;142:890–895.
69. Parwaresh MR, Radzun HJ, Dommes M. The homogeneity and monocytic origin of human peritoneal macrophages evidenced by comparison of esterase polymorphism. *Am J Pathol* 1981;102: 209–219.
70. Verbrugh HA, Keane WF, Hoidal JR, et al. Peritoneal macrophages and opsonins: antibacterial defense in patients undergoing continuous peritoneal dialysis. *J Infect Dis* 1983;147:1018–1029.
71. Van der Meulen J, Verbrugh HA, Oe PL, et al. Bacterial peritonitis: dirt or defect? In: Maher JF, Winchester JF, eds. *Frontiers in peritoneal dialysis.* New York: International Symposium Peritoneal Dialysis, Field and Rich, 1986.
72. Keane WF, Comty CM, Verbrugh HA, et al. Opsonic deficiency of peritoneal dialysis effluent in continuous ambulatory peritoneal dialysis. *Kidney Int* 1984;25:539–543.

73. Gordon DI, Rice JL, Avery VM. Surface phagocytosis and host defenses in the peritoneal cavity during continuous ambulatory peritoneal dialysis. *Eur J Clin Microbiol Infect Dis* 1990;9:191–197.
74. Duwe AK, Vas SI, Weatherhead JW. Effects of the composition of peritoneal dialysis fluid on chemiluminescence, phagocytosis, and bacterial activity in vitro. *Infect Immun* 1981;33:130–135.
75. Van Bronswijk H, Verbrugh HA, Heezius HC, et al. Dialysis fluid and local host resistance in patients on continuous ambulatory peritoneal dialysis. *Eur J Clin Microbiol Infect Dis* 1988;7:368–373.
76. Twardowski Z, Ksiazek A, Madjan J, et al. Kinetics of continuous ambulatory peritoneal dialysis with few exchanges per day. *Clin Nephrol* 1981;15:119–130.
77. Linder LE, Curelaru I, Gustavsson B, et al. Material thrombogenicity in central venous catheterization: a comparison between soft, antebrachial catheters of silicone elastome and polyurethane. *J Parenter Enteral Nutr* 1984;8:399–342.
78. Marrie TJ, Noble MA, Costerton JW. Examination of the morphology of bacteria adhering to peritoneal dialysis catheters by scanning and transmission electron microscopy. *J Clin Microbiol* 1983;18: 1380–1398.
79. Finkelstein ES, Jekel J, Troidle L, et al. Patterns of infection in patients maintained on long-term peritoneal dialysis therapy with multiple episodes of peritonitis. *Am J Kidney Dis* 2002; 39:1278.
80. Giaccino F, Alloatti S, Guarello F, et al. The influence of peritoneal dialysis on cellular immunity. *Perit Dial Bull* 1982;2:165–168.
81. Montgomerie JZ, Kalmanson GM, Guze LB. Renal failure and infection. *Medicine (Baltimore)* 1968;47:1–32.
82. Peterson PK, Weane WF. Infections in chronic peritoneal dialysis patients. In: Remington JS, Swartz MN, eds. *Current clinical topics in infectious diseases.* New York: McGraw-Hill, 1985:239–260.
83. Bint AJ, Finch RG, Gokal R, et al. Diagnosis and management of peritonitis in continuous ambulatory peritoneal dialysis. Report of a working party of the British Society for Antimicrobial Therapy. *Lancet* 1987;1:845–847.
84. Cheng IKP, Fang GX, Chan TM, et al. Fungal peritonitis complicating peritoneal dialysis: report of 27 cases and review of treatment. *Q J Med New Serv* 1989;71:407–416.
85. Eisenberg ES, Leviton SI, Soeiro R. Fungal peritonitis in patients receiving peritoneal dialysis: experience from 11 patients and review of the literature. *Rev Infect Dis* 1986;8:309–321.
86. von Graevenitz A, Amsterdam D. Microbiological aspects of peritonitis associated with continuous ambulatory peritoneal dialysis. *Clin Microbiol Rev* 1992;5:36–48.
87. Al-Wali W, Baillod R, Hamilton-Miller JMT, et al. Detective work in continuous ambulatory peritoneal dialysis. *J Infect* 1990;20:151–154.
88. Ash S. Chronic peritoneal dialysis catheters: effects of catheter design, materials and location. *Semin Dial* 1990;3:39–46.
89. Picaino B, Bernardini J, Johnston J, et al. Chemical peritonitis due to intraperitoneal vancomycin. *Perit Dial Bull* 1987;7:156–159.
90. Khanna R, McNeely DJ, Oreopoulos DG, Vas SI, et al. Treating fungal infections: fungal peritonitis in CAPD. *BMJ* 1980;280: 1147–1148.
91. Beard-Pegler MA, Gabelish CL, Stubbs E, et al. Prevalence of peritonitis-associated coagulase-negative *Staphylococcus* on the skin of continuous ambulatory peritoneal dialysis patients. *Epidemiol Infect* 1989; 102:365–378.
92. Eisenberg ES, Ambalu SM, Sylagi G, et al. Colonization of skin and development of peritonitis due to coagulase-negative *Staphylococcus* in patients undergoing peritoneal dialysis. *J Infect Dis* 1987;156: 478–482.
93. West TE, Walsche JJ, Krol CP, et al. Staphylococcal peritonitis in patients on continuous ambulatory peritoneal dialysis. *J Clin Microbiol* 1986;23:809–812.
94. Davies SJ, Ogg CS, Cameron JS, et al. *Staphylococcus aureus* nasal carriage, exit site infection, and catheter loss in patients treated with continuous ambulatory peritoneal dialysis (CAPD). *Perit Dial Bull* 1989;9:61–64.
95. Pignatari A, Boyken LD, Herwaldt LA, et al. Application of restriction endonuclease analysis of chromosomal DNA in the study of *Staphylococcus aureus* colonization in continuous ambulatory peritoneal dialysis patients. *Diagn Microbiol Infect Dis* 1992;15:195–199.
96. Smith TL, Pearson ML, Wilcox KR, et al. Emergence of vancomycin resistance in *Staphylococcus aureus. N Engl J Med* 1999;340:493.
97. Hiramatsu K, Hanaki H, Ino T, et al. Methicillin-resistant *Staphylococcus aureus* clinical strain with reduced vancomycin susceptibility. *J Antimicrob Chemother* 1997;40:135–146.
98. Tenover FC, Lancaster MV, Hill BC, et al. Characterization of staphylococci with reduced susceptibilities to vancomycin and other glycopeptides. *J Clin Microbiol* 1998;36:1020–1027.
99. Anonymous. *Staphylococcus aureus* resistant to vancomycin—United States, 2002. *MMWR Morb Mortal Wkly Rep* 2002;51:565.
100. Anonymous. Vancomycin-resistant *Staphylococcus aureus*—Pennsylvania, 2002. *MMWR Morb Mortal Wkly Rep* 2002;51:931.
101. Hospital Infection Control Practices Advisory Committee. Recommendations for preventing the spread of vancomycin resistance. *MMWR Morb Mortal Wkly Rep* 1995;44:1–20.
102. Johanson WG, Pierce AK, Sanford JP, et al. Nosocomial respiratory infections with gram-negative bacilli: the significance of colonization of the respiratory tract. *Ann Intern Med* 1992;77:701.
103. Aly R, Maibach HI, Rahman R, et al. Correlation of human in vivo and in vitro cutaneous antimicrobial factors. *J Infect Dis* 1975;131: 579.
104. Knittle MA, Eitzman DV, Baer H. Role of hand contamination of personnel in the epidemiology of gram-negative nosocomial infections. *J Pediatr* 1975;86:433.
105. Berkelman RL, Lewin S, Allen JR, et al. Pseudobacteremia attributed to contamination of povidone-iodine with *Pseudomonas cepacia. Ann Intern Med* 1981;95:32–36.
106. Gustafson TL, Band JD, Hutcheson RH, et al. *Pseudomonas folliculitis*: an outbreak and review. *Rev Infect Dis* 1983;5:1–8.
107. McNeely DJ, Vas SI, Dombros N, et al. *Fusarium* peritonitis: an uncommon complication of continuous ambulatory peritoneal dialysis. *Perit Dial Bull* 1981;1:94–96.
108. Hakim A, Hisam N, Reuman PD. Environmental mycobacterial peritonitis complicating peritoneal dialysis: three cases and review. *Clin Infect Dis* 1993;16:426–431.
109. Gibb AO, Aggarwal R, Sainson CO. Successful treatment of *Prototheca* peritonitis complicating continuous ambulatory peritoneal dialysis. *J Infect* 1991;22:183–185.
110. Bernardini J, Piraino B, Sorkin M. Analysis of continuous ambulatory peritoneal dialysis-related *Pseudomonas aeruginosa* infections. *Am J Med* 1987;83:829–832.
111. Peterson PK, Matzke G, Keane WF. Current concepts in the management of peritonitis in patients undergoing continuous ambulatory peritoneal dialysis. *Rev Infect Dis* 1987;9:604–612.
112. Valente J, Rappaport W. Continuous ambulatory peritoneal dialysis associated with peritonitis in older patients. *Am J Surg* 1990;159: 579–581.
113. Reddy P, Krol C, Walshe JJ. Characteristics and clinical outcome of CAPD related gram-negative infections. *Kidney Int* 1988;33: 249(abst).
114. Hurley RM, Muogbo D, Wilson GW, et al. Cellular composition of peritoneal effluent: response to peritonitis. *Can Med Assoc J* 1977; 117:1061–1062.
115. Knight KR, Polak A, Crump J, et al. Laboratory diagnosis and oral treatment of CAPD peritonitis. *Lancet* 1982;2:1301–1304.
116. Flanigan MJ, Freeman RM, Lim VS. Cellular response to peritonitis among peritoneal dialysis patients. *Am J Kidney Dis* 1985;6:420–424.
117. Gokal R, Ramos JM, Ward MK, et al. Eosinophilic peritonitis in continuous ambulatory peritoneal dialysis (CAPD). *Clin Nephrol* 1981;15:328–330.
118. Vas SI. Microbiology aspects of peritonitis. *Perit Dial Bull* 1981; 1(Suppl):S11–S14.
119. Spencer RC. Infections in continuous ambulatory peritoneal dialysis. *J Med Microbiol* 1988;27:1–9.
120. Males BM, Walshe JJ, Garringer L, et al. Addi-check filtration, Bactec, and 10-ml culture methods for recovery of microorganisms from dialysis effluent during episodes of dialysis. *J Clin Microbiol* 1986;23: 350–353.

121. Males BN, Walshe JJ, Amsterdam D. Laboratory indices of clinical peritonitis: total leukocyte count, microscopy, and microbiology culture of peritoneal dialysis effluent. *J Clin Microbiol* 1987;25: 2367–2371.
122. Rayner BL, Williams DS, Oliver S. Inoculation of peritoneal dialysis fluid into blood culture bottles improves culture rates. *S Afr Med J* 1993;83:42–43.
123. Woods GL, Washington JA. Comparison of methods for processing dialysate in suspected continuous ambulatory peritoneal dialysis-associated peritonitis. *Diagn Microbiol Infect Dis* 1987;7:155–157.
124. Ad Hoc Advisory Committee on Peritonitis Management. Peritoneal dialysis-related peritonitis treatment recommendations 1993 update and peritoneal catheters and exit site practices: toward optimum peritoneal access. *Perit Dial Intern* 1993;13:14–28.
125. Rubin J, Ray R, Barnes T, et al. Peritoneal abnormalities during infectious episodes of continuous ambulatory peritoneal dialysis. *Nephron* 1981;29:124–127.
126. Fenton SSA. Selection criteria for continuous ambulatory peritoneal dialysis. *Perit Dial Bull* 1982;2:3–7.
127. Corey PN, Steel C. Risk factors associated with time to first infection and time to failure on CAPD. *Perit Dial Bull* 1983;3:S14–S17.
128. Maki DG, Cobb L, Garman JK. An attachable silver-impregnated cuff for prevention of infection with central venous catheters: a prospective randomized multicenter trial. *Am J Med* 1988;85:307.
129. Prowant B, Nolph KD. Five years experience with peritonitis in a CAPD program. *Perit Dial Bull* 1982;2:169–210.
130. Health Care Infection Control Practices Advisory Committee. Guidelines for hand hygiene in health care settings. *MMWR Morb Mortal Wkly Rep* 2002;51(No. RR-16):1.
131. Winchester JF. CAPD systems and solutions. In: Gokal R, ed. *Continuous ambulatory peritoneal dialysis.* London: Churchill Livingstone, 1986:94–109.
132. Gruer LD, Babb JR, Davies JG, et al. Disinfection of hands and tubing of CAPD patients. *J Hosp Infect* 1984;5:305–312.
133. Parsons FM, Ahmed-Jushuf IH, Brownjohn AM, et al. CAPD peritonitis. *Lancet* 1983;1:348–349.
134. Hamilton RW, Disher BA, Dillingham SA, et al. The sterile weld: a new method for connections in continuous ambulatory peritoneal dialysis. *Perit Dial Bull* 1983;3(Suppl 4):8–10.
135. Woodrow G, Turney JH, Brownjohn AM. Technique failure in peritoneal dialysis and its impact on patient survival. *Perit Dial Int* 1997; 17:360–364.
136. Monteon F, Correa-Rotter R, Paniagua R, et al. Prevention of peritonitis with disconnect systems in CAPD: a randomized controlled trial. *Kidney Int* 1998;54:2123.
137. Berkelman RL, Band JD, Petersen NJ. Recommendations for the care of automated peritoneal dialysis machines: can the risk of peritonitis be reduced? *Infect Control* 1984;5:85–87.
138. Jones LL, Tweedy L, Warady BA. The impact of exit site care and catheter design on the incidence of catheter-related infection. *Adv Perit Dial* 1995;11:302–305.
139. Gokal R, Alexander S, Ash S, et al. Peritoneal catheters and exit-site practices toward optimizing peritoneal access: 1998 update. *Perit Dial Int* 1998;18:11.
140. Bernardini J, Piraino B, Holley J, et al. A randomized trial of *Staphylococcus aureus* prophylaxis in peritoneal dialysis patients: mupirocin calcium ointment 2 percent applied to the exit site versus cyclic oral rifampin. *Am J Kidney Dis* 1996;27:695.
141. Vychytil A, Lorenz M, Schneider B, et al. New strategies to prevent *Staphylococcus aureus* infection in peritoneal dialysis patients. *J Am Soc Nephrol* 1998;9:669.
142. Mupiricin Study Group. Nasal mupirocin prevents *Staphylococcus aureus* exit site infection during peritoneal dialysis. *J Am Soc Nephrol* 1996;7:2403–2408.
143. Miller MA, Dascal A, Portnoy J, et al. Development of mupirocin resistance among MRSA after widespread use of nasal mupirocin ointment. *Infect Control Hosp Epidemiol* 1996;17:811.
144. Davey P, Craig AM, Hay C, et al. Cost-effectiveness of prophylactic nasal mupirocin in patients undergoing peritoneal dialysis based on a randomized, placebo-controlled trial. *J Antimicrob Chemother* 1999; 43:105.
145. Low DE, Vas SI, Oreopoulos DG, et al. Randomized clinical trial of prophylactic cephalexin in CAPD. *Lancet* 1980;2:753–754.
146. Churchill DN, Taylor DW, Vas SI, et al. Peritonitis in CAPD patients a randomized clinical trial of trimethoprim-sulfamethoxazole prophylaxis. *Perit Dial Int* 1988;8:125–128.
147. Zaruba K, Peters J, Jungbluth H. Successful prophylaxis for fungal peritonitis in patients on continuous ambulatory peritoneal dialysis: six years experience. *Am J Kidney Dis* 1991;17:43–46.
148. Shinefield H, Black S, Fattom A, et al. Use of a *Staphylococcus aureus* conjugate vaccine in patients receiving hemodialysis. *N Engl J Med* 2002;346:491.
149. Initial safety and pharmacokinetics trial of immune globulin to *S. aureus* capsular polysaccharide (Altistaph^{TM}) in subjects with persistent *S. aureus* bacteremia. Rockville, MD: Nabi Biopharmaceuticals (personal communication).

66

NOSOCOMIAL INFECTIONS ASSOCIATED WITH PHYSICAL THERAPY, INCLUDING HYDROTHERAPY

STEPHEN M. KRALOVIC
CALVIN C. LINNEMANN, JR.

Physical therapists provide a variety of rehabilitative services to patients in hospitals but seldom are implicated as sources of hospital-acquired infections, except for those associated with hydrotherapy. This is surprising from an infection control perspective, because physical therapy provides many opportunities for the transmission of microorganisms between patients. Therapists have direct physical contact with patients, many of whom are severely ill, for mobilization and exercise, and they do not routinely wear gowns and gloves. Therapy is provided either at the bedside or in physical therapy departments. For bedside therapy, the therapist makes rounds from patient to patient and often goes from unit to unit throughout the hospital. For care within departments, patients are transported to a central facility, usually of open design, where many patients are treated at the same time. Hand washing sinks may not be readily available as therapists move between patients. Despite frequent opportunities for cross-infections, either acquired in a central unit or carried from one patient to another during bedside therapy, physical therapists have not been identified as causes of hospital-acquired infections. This may reflect a failure to consider the possibility during outbreak investigations. In contrast to physical therapy in general, hydrotherapy has been shown to be a potential source of infections and is the focus of this chapter. Even in the case of hydrotherapy, proving a role in the transmission of infection has been difficult. The most recent recommendations for infection control practices relative to hydrotherapy demonstrate the lack of strongly supported research findings from which to form guidelines (1).

EPIDEMIOLOGY OF HYDROTHERAPY-RELATED INFECTIONS

Hydrotherapy in the hospital includes immersion tanks, either full-body tanks for debridement of patients with burns and other wounds or extremity tanks; therapeutic whirlpools for cleaning, exercise, or relaxation; and medicinal baths. All of these have been associated with the transmission of infections in the hospital or the community. In the hospital setting, the major concern for infections has been the use of full-body immersion or Hubbard tanks, because these are used for severely ill patients with open wounds who are at high risk for serious infections. The term hydrotherapy is also used to encompass a number of therapeutic modalities under a variety of terms including hydrophysiotherapy, aquatics, swimming pools, pools, physiotherapy pools, whirlpool spas, whirlpool baths, or communal bathing tanks. For purposes of this chapter, we confine the definition of hydrotherapy to individual-use therapeutic modalities; transmission of infection with communal use facilities has been well established.

Epidemics Attributed to Hydrotherapy

Hydrotherapy with immersion tanks has been used in physical therapy for many years, and most large or tertiary care hospitals maintain this equipment in central physical therapy facilities or in burn units. Despite this, only eight epidemic studies involving hydrotherapy have been reported (2–9). Stone and Kolb (2) reported the first epidemic that was attributed to transmission during hydrotherapy in 1971 (Table 66.1). They reported the spread of gentamicin-resistant *Pseudomonas* in a burn unit after the introduction of daily hydrotherapy for all patients with initial burns of less than 10% of total body area or healing wounds with less than 10% full-thickness injury. For 3 years before the use of routine hydrotherapy, gentamicin ointment or cream had been applied to all burn wounds for prophylaxis against *Pseudomonas.* Despite this practice, gentamicin resistance in *Pseudomonas* did not become a problem until hydrotherapy was introduced. The proportion of gentamicin-resistant *Pseudomonas* increased from 2.4% to 37%, with up to 100% of the *Pseudomonas*-contaminated wounds having gentamicin-resistant microorganisms at some time during the patients' hospitalization. When gentamicin prophylaxis was discontinued, gentamicin resistance decreased over a 6-month period. When gentamicin prophylaxis was restarted, gentamicin resistance reappeared. Antibiotics ap-

TABLE 66.1. HOSPITAL OUTBREAKS ATTRIBUTED TO TRANSMISSION DURING HYDROTHERAPY AND EVIDENCE TO SUPPORT AN ASSOCIATION

Microorganism	Clinical service	Site of hydrotherapy	Appearance with introduction or change in hydrotherapy	Environmental surveys	Patient cultures before and after hydrotherapy	Disappearance with modification of hydrotherapy	References
Pseudomonas aeruginosa	Burn unit	Physical therapy dept.	+	+	+	—	Stone and Kolb (2)
Enterobacter cloacae	Burn unit	Burn unit	—	+	—	+[a]	Mayhall, et al. (3)
Pseudomonas aeruginosa	Mainly a gynecologic oncology unit	Physical therapy dept.	+	+	—	+	McGuckin, et al. (4)
Staphylococcus aureus	Hospital-wide	Physiotherapy dept.	—	—	—	—	Rimland (5)
Pseudomonas aeruginosa	Burn unit	Burn unit	—	+	—	+	Tredget, et al. (6)
Pseudomonas aeruginosa	Burn intensive care unit	Burn unit	—	+	—	?	Richard, et al. (7)
Pseudomonas aeruginosa	Burn unit	Burn unit	—	+	—	—	De Vos, et al (8)
Staphylococcus aureus	Burn/plastic surgery unit	Burn unit	—	+	—	+	Embril, et al. (9)

[a] Other control measures were introduced simultaneously with modification of hydrotherapy procedure.

peared to select for resistant *Pseudomonas,* and hydrotherapy facilitated the transmission of these strains between patients.

Environmental cultures showed heavy contamination of the hydrotherapy equipment, including the aerators and agitators, with gentamicin-resistant *Pseudomonas* of the same pyocin type. The cultures remained positive after thorough cleaning. The addition of povidone-iodine resulted in a decrease in the *Pseudomonas* flora but did not eradicate it. Burn wound cultures of patients before and after hydrotherapy showed that 27 of 52 wounds that were not colonized with *Pseudomonas* before hydrotherapy were colonized afterward. Also, *Pseudomonas* was cultured from the hands of 26.7% of the physical therapy workers before they had contact with the patients. Based on the presence or absence of *Pseudomonas* in the cultures from the hydrotherapy tanks or workers' hands, the authors concluded that 11 of the 27 patients may have been colonized from the tank, 9 from the hands of healthcare workers, and 3 from either source. All cultures were negative for the other four patients.

This study, the first to implicate hydrotherapy, still summarizes the current knowledge of the potential role of hydrotherapy in the spread of hospital-acquired infections. Hydrotherapy tanks may be contaminated with bacteria from patients being treated and serve as a reservoir for colonization of other patients. In addition, the therapist's hands, contaminated either from the hydrotherapy equipment or patients, may be a source of transmission to other patients. The addition of a disinfectant to the water suppresses bacterial contamination but does not eradicate it. The most interesting observation was that hydrotherapy did not dramatically increase the colonization of burn wounds with *Pseudomonas.* This suggests a natural limit to the level of *Pseudomonas* colonization of the wounds, but hydrotherapy can facilitate the transmission of a specific microorganism without a marked increase in the level of colonization. These microorganism-specific epidemics would be appreciated only when specific strains are identified by appropriate markers or molecular epidemiologic techniques.

Since this initial report, seven other outbreaks attributed to hydrotherapy in immersion tanks have been reported—four with *Pseudomonas,* two with *Staphylococcus aureus,* and one with *Enterobacter* (3–9) (Table 66.1). The small number of reported outbreaks may reflect the difficulty in distinguishing the role of hydrotherapy from other risk factors in the transmission of infection. In 1979, Mayhall et al. (3) reported an increase of *Enterobacter cloacae* infections in a burn unit with an intensive hydrotherapy program. All patients were debrided and treated with hydrotherapy on admission, and hydrotherapy was repeated twice a day. Liners were used in the tanks with compressed air agitation, but no disinfectants were added to the water. The *E. cloacae* strain was resistant to the topical silver sulfadiazine used for wound care, a situation similar to the gentamicin resistance of the *Pseudomonas* seen in the previous epidemic.

The outbreak began with an increase in *E. cloacae* bacteremias in burn patients that was controlled by improved aseptic technique and hand washing. Despite the decrease in bacteremias, colonization with *E. cloacae* continued over a year and a half. Culture surveys recovered *E. cloacae* in the hydrotherapy area and from the hands of healthcare workers, but antibiogram results for these workers were different from the results obtained from infected patients. The spread of *Enterobacter* in the unit was not controlled until the ratio of staff to patients was increased and changes were made in hydrotherapy procedures. These included the use of a new pair of long disposable gloves and a disposable apron with each patient. It is impossible to determine how much hydrotherapy contributed to the outbreak compared with understaffing, which illustrates the difficulty in establishing the significance of hydrotherapy in transmission of hospital-acquired infections. (For additional information on the epidemiology and prevention of burn wound infections, see Chapter 25.)

A third outbreak attributed to hydrotherapy was reported in 1981 and involved patients on a gynecologic oncology ward (4). During a 2-week period, 11 patients developed *Pseudomonas aeruginosa* wound infections, 10 of whom had received hydrotherapy. Therapy was given as frequently as two to three times a day in unlined tanks without disinfectants added to the water. Between treatments, the tank surfaces were cleaned with a combination of povidone-iodine and sodium hypochlorite, but the solutions were not cycled through the agitators. Sodium hypochlorite cleaning was discontinued after the first infection had occurred. When sodium hypochlorite was reintroduced 2 weeks later, the epidemic stopped. The authors suggested that the infections were spread by hydrotherapy because of inadequate disinfection in the absence of sodium hypochlorite, even though the first case occurred before sodium hypochlorite was stopped. If correct, this would be the only proof that cleaning hydrotherapy tanks with disinfectants decreases infections. The temporal association between the starting and stopping of sodium hypochlorite cleaning and the occurrence of infections suggests a causal relationship, but the authors concede the possibility that the association noted was merely fortuitous. Important information such as the number of patients with open wounds who received hydrotherapy and who were at risk of infection was not determined before or after the changes in sodium hypochlorite use.

A hospital-wide dissemination of methicillin- and tobramycin-resistant *S. aureus* from a physiotherapy department was described by Rimland (5). This retrospective, case-control study implicated the physiotherapy department and the use of the hydrophysiotherapy area ($p = .000067$) on univariate analysis. However, cultures of the environment and of staff in the implicated physiotherapy department were negative, and control measures within the physiotherapy department were not able to prevent further spread of this microorganism once the initial dissemination hospital-wide occurred. No information on how hydrotherapy was performed or techniques of equipment use and cleaning or disinfection was described. Despite this, the study nicely illustrates the open nature of the physical therapy departments to which we referred previously.

Another report of a hospital outbreak associated with hydrotherapy suggested that the best solution to the problem was to discontinue hydrotherapy in the management of burn patients (6). In 1992, Tredget et al. (6) reported an outbreak of *P. aeruginosa* wound infections in a burn unit where daily hydrotherapy was used. The equipment was disinfected after each use with sodium hypochlorite, and the water from the tanks was cultured weekly for bacteria. Three patients were infected, and the *Pseudomonas* cultured from them had the same antibiogram. Restriction fragment length polymorphism analysis and serotyping confirmed that the same microorganism was involved in all three infections. Hydrotherapy was discontinued, and the strain of *Pseudomonas* that infected these three patients disappeared from the unit. *P. aeruginosa* was cultured from the water supply, the hydrotherapy tank, and the hydrotherapy transportation equipment, but the isolates were not typed to determine if these were the epidemic strain. A retrospective study of mortality in the burn unit before and after the discontinuation of hydrotherapy showed a decrease in overall mortality rate from 6.4% to 2.7% and in *Pseudomonas*-related mortality rate from 2.8% to 0%. Although *Pseudomonas*-related mortality decreased, colonization with *Pseudomonas* continued. Colonization occurred later in the hospital course, when patients were more stable and less likely to develop fatal sepsis. They also observed an increase in staphylococcal isolates from wounds after hydrotherapy was stopped.

Even if hydrotherapy was not proven to be the source of the infection in the original three patients, the survey comparing patients with and without hydrotherapy suggested that discontinuation of hydrotherapy does not increase mortality in burn patients and may even have a beneficial effect. However, antibiotic management also changed during this period and may have been responsible for the decrease in mortality. Either way, the authors pointed out that there was no scientific documentation of benefit from hydrotherapy.

An additional outbreak also involved *P. aeruginosa* in a burn unit (7). Hydrotherapy equipment was disinfected with an aldehyde solution. Four patients developed *P. aeruginosa* serotype O:11 bacteremia, and the identical strain was recovered from hydrotherapy equipment, as shown by molecular typing. Changes in hydrotherapy were introduced, but the last infection had occurred 2 months before these modifications, so the association was not clear. It is interesting that a second outbreak with another serotype of *P. aeruginosa* (O:12) occurred at the same time as the O:11 outbreak. The *P. aeruginosa* O:12 was not found in the hydrotherapy equipment and did not disappear when the hydrotherapy was modified. These infections did disappear when anti-*Pseudomonas* antibiotic therapy was improved.

DeVos et al. (8) reported molecular typing analysis of an epidemic of *P. aeruginosa* from a burn department that involved both the intensive care and medical care units. The primary purpose of this study was to demonstrate the usefulness of molecular typing techniques in an epidemiologic investigation. In addition to the patient isolates from the epidemic, the authors typed isolates from environmental cultures from hydrotherapy facilities. A combination of pyoverdine isoelectric focusing, randomly amplified polymorphic DNA polymerase chain reaction (PCR), antibiotic resistance pattern type, and pigment production were the typing methods used. Although the combination of these typing methods indicated a polymicrobial (polyclonal) event, there was a subgroup of isolates (including the environmental hydrotherapy isolates) that constituted a smaller monoclonal epidemic within the larger epidemic. No detailed data regarding hydrotherapy practices or control measures or even an explanation as to the proposed basis for association were provided by the authors.

Finally, an outbreak of methicillin-resistant *S. aureus* (MRSA) was reported involving a combined burn and plastic surgery intensive care unit (9). The isolates from this outbreak were all similar by pulsed-field gel electrophoresis. Hydrotherapy equipment was cultured and yielded growth of the same strain of MRSA as that recovered from patients. The outbreak ceased when the equipment was no longer used. This particular unit did not use immersion hydrotherapy; instead, it used stretcher showering hydrotherapy. Six of the seven cases identified received stretcher hydrotherapy. Despite precautions taken to prevent transmission of disease, the physical limitations of the method precluded application of effective infection control measures. Of 13 environmental cultures taken from the hydrotherapy area, only 2 were positive, 1 from the stretcher frame and 1 from the pistol-grip handheld showerhead. Recovery of MRSA from these two environmental sites represented areas where contact with patients was most likely to occur during the stretcher hydrotherapy procedure.

Another interesting report that did not involve an outbreak investigation was provided by Wisplinghoff et al. (10). A study concerning *Acinetobacter baumannii* colonization and disease was undertaken by the investigators. Although an outbreak investigation was not performed, the authors provided interesting data that hydrotherapy was associated with more serious infectious disease complications. In a retrospective, case-control study, they reviewed risk factors for nosocomial bloodstream infections resulting from *A. baumannii* in adult burn patients. Multivariable logistic regression analysis indicated that use of hydrotherapy was an independent risk factor for *A. baumannii* bacteremia with an odds ratio of 5.5 [95% confidence interval (CI) of 1.11 to 27.76]. Although this study did not describe the form of hydrotherapy used, it reemphasized the potential seriousness of infections that can be associated with water-based treatments of burn patients.

In addition to immersion tanks, infections have been attributed to other water facilities used in the hospital, including whirlpool spas and bathtubs. There is some confusion in terminology, but spas or hot tubs, unlike immersion tanks and bathtubs, are not emptied and disinfected after each patient, and the patients who use them are not as sick as those who are treated in immersion tanks. Infection is prevented by maintaining a bactericidal level of disinfectant in the water at all times and continuous filtration as in swimming pools. Numerous outbreaks of *Pseudomonas* folliculitis and dermatitis and, occasionally, infections resulting from *S. aureus, Legionella pneumophila,* mycobacteria, streptococci, and *Acanthamoeba* have been associated with public or home whirlpools but not with hospital whirlpools. Presumably, this reflects better maintenance in hospitals and use by smaller numbers of people (11). *Pseudomonas* colonizes whirlpools and is suppressed but not eradicated by disinfectants. Any time there is a lapse in quality control, *Pseudomonas* can overgrow and cause disease.

In the past, common bathtubs were often used on hospital wards. Venezia et al. (12) described an outbreak of MRSA in patients with skin disease who used a common bathtub for oatmeal baths. Seven patients developed MRSA bacteremias, and four were shown to be infected by the same strain of MRSA by restriction fragment analysis. These four patients had used the common bathtub. After use of the bathtub was discontinued, transmission of MRSA stopped. This implicates the bathtub as a possible vehicle for transmission of the infections, but the tub was not implicated until after the outbreak, so it was not cultured. Also, the nurse who cared for three patients had psoriasis and was colonized with the same strain of MRSA. She was treated with topical bacitracin, and the MRSA cleared. In retrospect, it was impossible to determine if the nurse was the source of the epidemic rather than the tub or if she was colonized from infected patients.

Burn units have been the reservoir of infection for several large hospital epidemics of MRSA, and environmental surveys during these epidemics recovered MRSA in hydrotherapy facilities (13,14). Crossley et al. (13) noted during an epidemic that MRSA was recovered from hydrotherapy tubs after disinfection with quaternary ammonium compounds. Thompson et al. (14) also found MRSA in their hydrotherapy facilities during an outbreak. With the exception of the findings by Rimland (5), hydrotherapy was not specifically implicated in any MRSA epidemic. This is not surprising, because the major mode of transmission of MRSA is the healthcare worker, and the major reservoir is the colonized patient. Environmental contamination has been considered to have a role in occasional hospital outbreaks of staphylococcal infections, but this has never been proven definitively (15–17).

In addition to common bathtubs, whirlpool baths, which do not have continuous filtration and chlorination as spas do, have been associated with the transmission of *P. aeruginosa* wound infections in nursing homes (18) and severe *P. aeruginosa* infection on a hematologic malignancies unit (19).

Cleaning and Disinfection of Hydrotherapy Equipment

Cleaning and disinfection of immersion tanks between patients should reduce the exposure of patients to potential pathogens. Terminal disinfection after mechanical cleaning might reduce residual bacterial contamination even further. This was evaluated by Turner et al. (20), who did a culture survey in a hydrotherapy facility immediately after patient use, after mechanical scrubbing with a detergent-disinfectant (Vesphene), and after terminal disinfection with a calcium hypochlorite solution (28 g in 1,355 L). During the cleaning process, the turbines were removed, soaked in a germicidal solution, brushed, and then immersed in calcium hypochlorite. The authors found that manual scrubbing with the detergent-disinfectant alone was as effective as scrubbing plus terminal disinfection with calcium hypochlorite in reducing bacterial contamination. The only additional benefit of terminal disinfection was observed in reducing bacterial contamination at the bottom of the tank, which was attributed to the difficulty in cleaning that area.

Because careful cleaning of immersion tanks does not eradicate the *Pseudomonas* flora, disinfectants have been added to the tank water. In the original study Stone and Kolb (2) reported that the addition of povidone-iodine to the water decreased the bacterial load, reducing the percentage of water cultures from filled tanks that were positive for *Pseudomonas* from 15.2% to 3%. They did not indicate if povidone-iodine was added routinely after this observation or if it affected the colonization rate. Smith et al. (21) reported that the addition of sodium hypochlorite to tub water in a concentration of 850 μg/mL decreased bacterial densities on burn wounds less than tenfold. Even the limited effect on bacterial densities was pH dependent and varied by microorganism. Steve et al. (22) evaluated the addition of chlorine in the form of Chloramine-T, with concentrations of 50 to 200 parts per million (ppm) in tank water. At

100 ppm, no bacteria were recovered from the tank water, and, at 150 ppm, the colony counts of cultures from wounds decreased and gram-negative bacteria were reported to be replaced by gram-positive bacteria.

Cardany et al. (23) reported on the addition of sodium hypochlorite to tank water at concentrations of 120, 240, and 780 μg/mL. Their patients were treated in lined hydrotherapy tanks with agitators. When sodium hypochlorite was added, all hydrotherapy water after immersion of patients was sterile. There was also a 10- to 100-fold decrease in bacteria on the burn wounds. The authors reported that patients experienced discomfort on contact with water containing sodium hypochlorite and that agitation of the water produced chlorine vapors, which were irritating to the eyes and noses of personnel.

These studies indicate that the addition of disinfectants such as sodium hypochlorite will decrease the number of bacteria in hydrotherapy water after the treatment of burn patients and should decrease the contamination of hydrotherapy equipment. This should decrease the transmission of infection to other patients using the hydrotherapy equipment, but such an effect has not been demonstrated.

In addition to cleaning, terminal disinfection, and adding disinfectants to the bath water, another technique suggested to reduce contamination in hydrotherapy tanks is the removal of agitators and the use of plastic liners (24,25). The rationale for this is that agitators are very difficult to clean unless removed after each use and soaked in disinfectant, as in the study by Turner et al. (20). The alternative is to remove the agitators and use a new plastic liner for each patient. Air is forced through channels in the liner to provide agitation. However, as Mayhall et al. (3) showed in their study, environmental contamination can occur even when liners are used.

Current Practices in Hydrotherapy Units

There is very little information on current practices in hydrotherapy units, and no universal standards exist. In the United States, the Centers for Disease Control and Prevention (CDC) provided general guidelines for hydrotherapy tanks in 1974 and for public spas and hot tubs in 1985 (26–28). The guidelines for hydrotherapy tanks recommend maintaining a free chlorine residual of 15 mg/L with a pH of 7.2 to 7.6. Tanks should be emptied between each patient use and disinfected. A chlorine solution should be circulated through the agitator of the tank for at least 15 minutes after the last use each day. For public spas and hot tubs, the CDC recommends automatic chemical feeding equipment to maintain 2 to 5 ppm of free residual chlorine or bromine with a pH of 7.2 to 7.8 and a maximum temperature of 104°F. These parameters should be checked hourly. In addition, there should be a filtration system in good working order.

In 1981, McGuckin et al. (29) reported a survey of current practices in hydrotherapy by physical therapy departments in 30 hospitals in the Philadelphia, Pennsylvania, area. Unfortunately, the survey did not distinguish between different types of hydrotherapy equipment but did note wide variations in practices between physical therapy units in the same geographic area. For instance, ten different types of disinfectant solutions were used.

The only comprehensive survey of hydrotherapy practices was reported in 1990 by Thompson et al. (30). This survey was limited to burn care and included 76 hospitals in 39 states. Seventy percent of the burn units used immersion hydrotherapy to some extent. Fifty-seven percent of those had tubs equipped with aerators or agitators, but 70% used tub liners. Thirty-nine percent of the hospitals did not add disinfectants to the tub water. The other hospitals added a hypochlorite (26%), povidone-iodine (14%), chlorhexidine gluconate (13%), Chloramine-T (1%), or a combination of these (7%). Information was not collected on cleaning and terminal disinfection, but 80% of the hospitals monitored the hydrotherapy units with regular microbial cultures. Another survey by Shankowsky et al. (31) confirmed these observations and noted that 18.6% of burn units used showers instead of immersion hydrotherapy.

PREVENTION OF NOSOCOMIAL INFECTIONS IN PHYSICAL THERAPY

The only published recommendations for infection control in physical therapy are those prepared by the Association for Professionals in Infection Control and Epidemiology, and these provide limited guidance because of the lack of information about infection control in physical therapy (32). A comprehensive infection control program for physical therapy must consider facility design and management, personnel practices, and hydrotherapy.

Facilities Design and Management

Physical therapy requires a central facility of open design to provide space for exercise and exercise equipment and for individual treatment tables, with sufficient room for wheelchairs to maneuver and for therapists to move between patients. All mats and tabletops should be covered with impervious materials that can be cleaned frequently with detergents and disinfectants. Cleaning supplies should be readily available to encourage use when needed. The most important design element, from an infection control perspective, is the placement of hand washing sinks and access to alcohol-based hand hygiene products (33). Sinks should be located conveniently for therapists to wash their hands after each patient, without the need to travel long distances. A sink located between every two or three work stations and near open exercise areas and equipment would encourage hand washing. Supplies and equipment should not block access to the sinks. If immersion hydrotherapy is used for burn patients, this should be relegated to a separate facility in or near the burn unit. Hydrotherapy for nonburn patients should be done in the physical therapy facility. Because patient populations using those facilities may differ from other physical therapy patients, it might be advantageous to have the hydrotherapy equipment in a separate room with a separate patient entrance.

Personnel Practices

Patients who are infectious should not be treated in the central facility. Patients with localized wound infections are sometimes treated in physical therapy units, because the wounds can be covered and contained during therapy. However, these patients may have the infecting agent present on other body sites and on clothing. It would seem preferable to provide therapy for such patients in their rooms. Because MRSA infections have become a widespread problem, patients who are colonized but not infected also may be candidates for physical therapy. Nasal colonization in such patients often can be eradicated with topical mupirocin. If not, therapy probably should be done in the patient's room whenever possible. Theoretically, it could be done in a shared facility if the therapists were always careful to wash their hands after patient contact. This has been the practice in some institutions where MRSA colonization has been extensive.

Physical therapists should be thoroughly trained in standard precautions and isolation procedures. A critical aspect of infection control education is to make therapists understand their potential role in transmitting infections as they move from patient to patient in the hospital. Therapists may not be aware of this risk, because they are less likely than other healthcare personnel to continue following patients after the development of nosocomial infections. Hand hygiene should be performed routinely before and after treating all hospitalized patients. Gowns and gloves are particularly important when providing therapy for infected patients because of the direct physical contact with the patient and the patient's clothing. If there is any doubt regarding infection, the therapist should wear gloves and a gown. Annual skin tests for tuberculosis are as important for physical therapists as for other hospital personnel.

Hydrotherapy

The first step is to decide if immersion hydrotherapy is to be used. Tredget et al. (6) suggested that hydrotherapy was not necessary for burn patients and might be harmful. Other approaches are available, such as spraying patients instead of immersing them. If hydrotherapy is to be used for burn patients, the equipment should be easily accessible by or in the burn unit. Although the optimal way to perform immersion hydrotherapy has not been determined by systematic study, experience suggests the following:

1. A written protocol should be developed for hydrotherapy and should include specific instructions for cleaning and disinfection of the tanks.
2. The entire hydrotherapy area including transportation equipment should be considered a potential source of contamination, not just the tub, and should be cleaned appropriately.
3. Personnel should use long gloves (to the elbow or higher) and fluid-impervious gowns to prevent contact with the patient and the bath water.
4. Plastic covers should be placed on stretchers used to immerse the patient in the tub.
5. Disposable plastic liners with channels for agitation with compressed air may avoid the difficulties in cleaning agitators.
6. Faucets should not have stream diverters or aerators. Before filling the tank, the faucet should be flushed with both hot and cold water for at least 60 seconds.
7. After filling the tank, it is reasonable to add a disinfectant to the water.
8. After use, the tub should be drained and mechanically scrubbed with a detergent-disinfectant. Particular attention should be directed to the bottom of the tub and drains.
9. If agitators are used, a germicidal agent such as a chlorine solution (200 to 300 mg/L) should be circulated through the agitator for 15 minutes.
10. After cleaning, the tank should be rinsed with tap water and dried. Between uses, the equipment should be kept dry.
11. There is no demonstrated value for routine environmental cultures of hydrotherapy equipment.

Whirlpool spas, or hot tubs, which have continuous filtration and chlorination should be avoided in the hospital setting because of difficulties in cleaning and maintaining disinfectant levels and the lack of evidence that these are medically necessary or even beneficial. Some obstetric units have experimented with baths, whirlpools, and Jacuzzis (birthing tanks) during labor, which do not have continuous filtration and chlorination, but potential contamination could present significant infection risks (34). Few studies have been conducted regarding potential risk of infection; however, at least one report indicated that a newborn was infected with the same strain of *P. aeruginosa* as was isolated from the birthing tank water (35). (See Chapter 55 on nosocomial infections in obstetric patients.)

Common bathtubs are now used less often in hospitals, and showers are provided in most individual patient rooms. In some settings, such as a burn hospital, bathtubs in individual patient rooms may be appropriate but will require strict adherence to cleaning protocols. Some chronic care facilities may have hydrotherapy pools for exercise, and these should be maintained as in any public swimming facility. This means that the water should be continuously filtered, chlorine residuals maintained at least at 0.4 to 0.6 mg/L, and the pH maintained between 7.2 and 7.6. Patients with infections or those who are fecally incontinent should not use these pools.

CONCLUSIONS

In general, physical therapists should adhere to the same infection control practices as other healthcare workers, including the use of personal protective equipment when there is a potential for contact with blood and body fluids and when caring for patients with infections. Hand washing sinks and alcohol-based hand hygiene products should be readily available in open-design physical therapy facilities. In epidemic investigations, investigators should always consider the possible role of physical therapists in the transmission of infections from patient to patient. Despite decades of use, many questions regarding hydrotherapy remain unanswered. The trend away from the use of immersion hydrotherapy may obviate the need for further investigation, but the facilities currently using hydrotherapy must base decisions on incomplete information. Rigorous cleaning of hydrotherapy equipment between patients and care in avoiding transmission of infectious agents by personnel conducting the hydrotherapy should minimize the risks in most situations.

REFERENCES

1. Centers for Disease Control and Prevention. Guidelines for environmental infection control in healthcare facilities, 2003. Available at *www.cdc.gov/ncidod/hip/enviro/guide.htm* (accessed 1/30/04, last updated 12/3/03).
2. Stone HH, Kolb LD. The evolution and spread of gentamicin-resistant pseudomonads. *J Trauma* 1971;11:586–589.
3. Mayhall CG, Lamb VA, Gayle WE, et al. *Enterobacter cloacae* septicemia in a burn center: epidemiology and control of an outbreak. *J Infect Dis* 1979;139:166–171.
4. McGuckin MB, Thorpe RJ, Abrutyn E. Hydrotherapy: an outbreak of *Pseudomonas aeruginosa* wound infections related to Hubbard tank treatments. *Arch Phys Med Rehabil* 1981;62:283–285.
5. Rimland D. Nosocomial infections with methicillin and tobramycin resistant *Staphylococcus aureus*—implication of physiotherapy in hospital-wide dissemination. *Am J Med Sci* 1985;290:91–97.
6. Tredget E, Shankowsky HA, Joffe AM, et al. Epidemiology of infections with *Pseudomonas aeruginosa* in burn patients: the role of hydrotherapy. *Clin Infect Dis* 1992;15:941–949.
7. Richard P, Le Flock R, Chamoux C, et al. *Pseudomonas aeruginosa* outbreak in a burn unit: role of antimicrobials in the emergence of multiply resistant strains. *J Infect Dis* 1994;170:377–383.
8. De Vos D, Lim A Jr, Pirnay JP, et al. Analysis of *Pseudomonas aeruginosa* isolates by isoelectric focusing of pyoverdine and RAPD-PCR: modern tools for an integrated anti-nosocomial infection strategy in burn wound centres. *Burns* 1997;23:379–386.
9. Embril JM, McLeod JA, Al-Barrak AM, et al. An outbreak of methicillin resistant *Staphylococcus aureus* on a burn unit: potential role of contaminated hydrotherapy equipment. *Burns* 2001;27:681–688.
10. Wisplinghoff H, Perbix W, Seifert H. Risk factors for nosocomial bloodstream infections due to *Acinetobacter baumannii*: a case-control study of adult burn patients. *Clin Infect Dis* 1999;28:59–66.
11. Highsmith AK, McNamara AM. Microbiology of recreational and therapeutic whirlpools. *Toxicity Assess Int J* 1988;3:599–611.
12. Venezia RA, Harris V, Miller C, et al. An outbreak of infections caused by strains of *Staphylococcus aureus* in patients with skin disease using DNA restriction patterns. *Infect Control Hosp Epidemiol* 1992;13:472–476.
13. Crossley K, Landesman B, Zaske D. Investigation of an outbreak of methicillin-resistant *Staphylococcus aureus* resistant to methicillin and aminoglycosides. II. Epidemiologic studies. *J Infect Dis* 1979;139:280–287.
14. Thompson RL, Cabezudo I, Wenzel RP. Epidemiology of nosocomial infections caused by methicillin-resistant *Staphylococcus aureus. Ann Intern Med* 1982;97:309–317.
15. Moore EP, Williams EW. A maternity hospital outbreak of methicillin-resistant *Staphylococcus aureus. J Hosp Infect* 1991;19:5–16.
16. Layton MC, Perez M, Heald P, et al. An outbreak of mupirocin-resistant *Staphylococcus aureus* on a dermatology ward associated with an environmental reservoir. *Infect Control Hosp Epidemiol* 1993;14:369–375.
17. Barg NL. Environmental contamination with *Staphylococcus aureus* and outbreaks: the cause or the effect? *Infect Control Hosp Epidemiol* 1993;14:367–368.
18. Hollyoak V, Allison D, Summers J. *Pseudomonas aeruginosa* wound infections associated with a nursing home's whirlpool bath. *Commun Dis Rep DCR Rev* 1995;5:R100–R102.
19. Berrouane YF, NcNutt L-A, Buschelman BJ, et al. Outbreak of severe *Pseudomonas aeruginosa* infections caused by a contaminated drain in a whirlpool bathtub. *Clin Infect Dis* 2000;31:1331–1337.
20. Turner AG, Higgins MM, Craddock JG. Disinfection of immersion tanks (Hubbard) in a hospital burn unit. *Arch Environ Health* 1974;28:101–104.
21. Smith RF, Blasi D, Dayton SL, et al. Effects of sodium hypochlorite on the microbial flora of burns and normal skin. *J Trauma* 1974;14:938–944.
22. Steve L, Goodhart P, Alexander J. Hydrotherapy burn treatment: use of Chloramine-T against resistant microorganisms. *Arch Phys Med Rehabil* 1979;60:301–303.
23. Cardany CR, Rodeheaver GT, Horowitz JH, et al. Influence of hydrotherapy and antiseptic agents on burn wound bacterial contamination. *J Burn Care Rehabil* 1985;6:230–232.
24. Mansell RE, Orchardt KA. Disinfecting hydrotherapy equipment. *Arch Phys Med Rehabil* 1974;55:318–320.
25. MacMillan BG, Edmonds P, Hummel RP, et al. Epidemiology of *Pseudomonas* in a burn intensive care unit. *J Trauma* 1973;13:627–638.
26. Centers for Disease Control and Prevention. Disinfection of hydrotherapy pools and tanks. U.S. Department of Health and Human Services, Public Health Service. Atlanta, GA: Centers for Diseases Control, 1974.
27. Centers for Disease Control and Prevention. Suggested health and safety guidelines for public spas and hot tubs. U.S. Dept. of Health and Human Services, Public Health Publication 99-960. Atlanta, GA: Centers for Disease Control, 1981 (revised 1985).
28. Garner JS, Favero MS. CDC guidelines for the prevention and control of nosocomial infections. Guidelines for handwashing and hospital environmental control, 1985. *Am J Infect Control* 1986;14:110–126.
29. McGuckin MB, Chung S, Humphrey N, et al. Infection control practices in physical therapy. *Am J Infect Control* 1981;9:18–19.
30. Thompson PD, Bowden ML, McDonald K, et al. A survey of burn hydrotherapy in the United States. *J Burn Care Rehabil* 1990;11:151–155.
31. Shankowsky HA, Callioux LS, Tredget, EE. North American survey of hydrotherapy in modern burn care. *J Burn Care Rehab* 1994;15:143–146.
32. Temple RS. Physical and occupational therapy and rehabilitation medicine In: Pfeiffer JA, ed. *APIC text of infection control and epidemiology.* Washington, DC, APIC, 2000.
33. Boyce JM, Pittet D, et al. Guidelines for hand hygiene in health-care settings. Recommendations of the Healthcare Infection Control Practices Advisory Committee and the HICPAC, SHEA, APIC, IDSA Hand Hygiene Task Force. *MMWR Recomm Rep* 2002;51(RR-16):1–45.
34. Ridgway GL, Tedder RS. Birthing pools and infection control. *Lancet* 1996;347:1051–1052.
35. Hawkins S. Water vs. conventional birth: infection rates compared. *Nursing Times* 1995;91:38–40.

67

INFECTIONS THAT COMPLICATE THE INSERTION OF PROSTHETIC DEVICES

DANIEL P. LEW
DIDIER PITTET
FRANCIS A. WALDVOGEL

The insertion of implants and medical devices has become a common procedure that benefits patients, often in a lifesaving way, who are suffering from a variety of exogenous acquired (trauma, rheumatic fever, hydrocephalus) or degenerative diseases (arthrosis or arthrosclerosis). The number and types of such devices has greatly increased over the past decades. Despite surgical advances and improvements in the materials and design, chronic inflammation and infection continue to be a major complication of their use.

A quantitative estimate of the medical use of foreign devices is complex, because few detailed statistical publications are available. However, as an example, data from various sources indicate that worldwide 3,000,000 central venous cannulas are inserted per year, and more than 500,000 joint arthroplasties and 200,000 pacemaker procedures are performed each year (unpublished information). The number of medical devices is large, because several products are available for each indication from various manufacturers (1) (Table 67.1).

Overall, the problem of infection associated with indwelling devices not only remains important but is also increasing as new devices become available and the number of patients at risk increases. It may be estimated that with the increased longevity of the Western world population, the number of devices will continue to grow.

A fundamental feature of foreign bodies is their exquisite susceptibility to infection. The inoculum of bacteria necessary to induce such postsurgical infections is extremely low when compared with surgery in the absence of a foreign body. In addition, bacteria that are often nonpathogenic and are normally present as skin commensals (i.e., coagulase-negative staphylococci or *Propionibacterium* species) are able to cause infections under these conditions.

The problem of infection associated with indwelling prosthetic devices is, thus, well known and feared by most surgeons. The impact of such infections is profound, because they often result in tissue destruction, serious dysfunction of the prosthetic device, and sometimes systemic dissemination of the pathogen. These infections are difficult to cure with antimicrobial agents and most often necessitate the removal of the device. The incidence of infection associated with medical devices varies with the type of device (Table 67.2). These data are reviewed for each device in later sections of this chapter.

Thus, in few other areas of medical practice has the prevention of infection become so critical and challenging as in surgical procedures associated with the insertion or presence of foreign material. In this chapter, we review the knowledge developed in the area of clinical presentation, diagnosis, and prevention of infection, taking as paradigms the four most often used foreign bodies: orthopedic, vascular devices, cerebrospinal shunts, and breast implants (2–4). The impact of infection associated with intravenous devices is treated in separate chapters (see Chapters 17 and 18).

PATHOPHYSIOLOGY

To understand the pathophysiologic events underlying foreign body infections, it is necessary to characterize three different groups of mechanisms (Fig. 67.1):

1. Foreign surfaces that induce deposition of host proteins
2. Colonizing and invading microorganisms
3. Local function of neutrophils

Experimental work in a large number of laboratories during recent years has been focused on the contribution of each of these elements in the pathogenesis of device-related infection. Some of the major conclusions from these studies are reviewed briefly in the following sections [for a comprehensive textbook in this area see Vaudaux et al. (5)].

Host Proteins Promote Bacterial Adhesion to Foreign Material

Biomaterials implanted in the subcutaneous space are progressively colonized by cellular and fibrillar connective tissue components. This material includes sulfated proteoglycans in addition to collagen and fibronectin. Fibroblasts may contribute by their own protein synthesis machinery to the deposition of extracellular matrix coating the artificial material. When fibrin clots form on the surface of blood-exposed biomaterials, they

TABLE 67.1. MATERIALS COMMONLY USED IN VARIOUS PROSTHETIC IMPLANTS AND MEDICAL DEVICES

Implant or device	Type	Materials
Prosthetic heart valves	Starr-Edwards	Stellite ball, Stellite frame, PET-covered sewing ring
	Björk-Shiley	LTI-carbon disc, Stellite frame, PET-covered sewing ring
	Lillehei-Kaster	LTI-carbon disc. titanium frame, PET-covered sewing ring
	St. Jude Medical	LTI-carbon disc and frame, PET-covered sewing ring
	Omnicarbon	LTI-carbon disc and frame, ULTI-carbon-coated sewing ring
	Hancock, Carpentier-Edwards	Porcine valves, metal frames of different composition
	Xenomedica	PET-covered sewing rings
Left ventricular assist device	Various types	PUR, PET connectors
Total artificial heart	Jarvik-7	PUR, PET cuff-covered PC atrial connectors, PUR drive lines with PET skin buttons, Björk-Shiley valves
Pacemakers	Various types	Titanium, epoxide resin, silicone rubber body package; PUR leads
Vascular grafts	Nontextile, textile (woven, knitted, or velors)	Microporous PTFE, PET, PVA, PAN, nylon, PTFE fiber
Arteriovenous shunts	Scribner subcutaneous	Silicone-rubber-PTFE, PET
Intravascular devices	Short cannulas, long peripheral and central venous catheters, arterial catheters	Steel (needles), FEP, PVC, PET, PE, PUR, PTFE, PP, nylon silicone rubber with PET cuff
	Subclavian hemodialysis catheters	PTFE
Cerebrospinal fluid shunts	Spitz-Holter (VA shunt)	Silicone rubber tube, stainless steel valves, PE silicone rubber shunt PE, silicone rubber
	Other types	
Orthopedic implants	Hip joint prosthesis	Stainless steel, titanium, Co-cr alloys, ceramic femoral components, UHMWPE, polyacetal acetabular cups, PMMA cement
Cranioplastic implants	Skull plate	PMMA titanium
Urologic catheters	Urinary tract catheters, suprapubic catheters	Silicone rubber, latex, silicone-coated latex, silicone rubber
Peritoneal dialysis	Teckhoff-Schechter	Silicone rubber tube with PET cuff
Mammary prostheses	Cronin	Silicone rubber bag filled with silicone gel, PET patches, or covered with PUR
	Arion, simaplast	Silicone rubber bag filled with dextran 70

FEP, fluorinated polyethylene-propylene; LTI, carbon, pyrolytic carbon; PAN, poly(acrylonitrile); PC, polycarbonate; PE, polyethylene; PET, polyethylene terephtalate; PMMA, polymethylmethacrylate; PP, polypropylene; PTFE, polytetrafluoroethylene; PUR, polyurethane; PVA, polyvinylalcohol (Formalinized); PVC, polyvinyl chloride; UHMWPE, ultrahigh molecular weight polyethylene; ULTI, carbon, vapor-deposited carbon.

may also contribute to fibronectin deposition, because fibronectin is known to be covalently cross-linked to fibrin by the action of plasma transglutaminase factor XIII_a (6–9).

The sequence of complex humoral and cellular host responses to biomaterial implants may influence significantly the mode of colonization of the artificial materials by the contaminating microorganisms, in particular staphylococci. Staphylococci possess specific binding sites recognizing a variety of extracellular matrix proteins. Among these, four proteins have received considerable attention over the last few years: fibronectin, fibrinogen, laminin, and thrombospondin (10,11). Adhesion of *Staphylococcus aureus* to biomaterial surfaces coated with extracellular matrix proteins is determined by protein adhesins located on the bacterial cell surface. The fibronectin and fibrinogen binding proteins have been studied in most detail.

TABLE 67.2. FREQUENCY OF FOREIGN BODY INFECTIONS

Device	Infections/prevalence
Prosthetic heart valves	~3.7%
Pacemakers	<1–3%
Vascular grafts	~1.5%
Vascular catheters	0.2–20%
CSF shunts	1.0–27%
Orthopedic implants	
Hip	<2%
Knee	<0.6–11%
CAPD catheters	1.0–6%
Home intravenous therapy (including TPN)	~2%

CAPD, continuous ambulatory peritoneal dialysis; CSF, cerebrospinal fluid; TPN, total parenteral nutrition.

Using a variety of biologic and immunologic assays, variable amounts of fibronectin and fibrinogen deposited on the surface of foreign material were detected. Most adherence-promoting activity to bacteria of inserted biomaterials depends on these surface bound proteins.

The nature of the biomaterial is an important qualitative and quantitative determinant of the deposition of different proteins: The amount of fibronectin deposited onto the surface of inserted central venous catheters is usually low, whereas that of fibrinogen is high. Fibrinogen, however, shows an extensive loss of adherence-promoting activity, which is related to its proteolytic breakdown. Although present in much lower amounts than fibrinogen, intact or fragmented fibronectin actively promotes *S. aureus* adherence onto intravenous catheters.

The pattern is different if the catheters are inserted in arteries instead of veins. Fibrinogen is also present in large amounts but, in this case, is functionally active; the data indicate that fibrinogen is the most important bacterial adherence-promoting protein on arterial catheters. In addition, in devices inserted in arteries, platelets are deposited over the surface and also stimulate

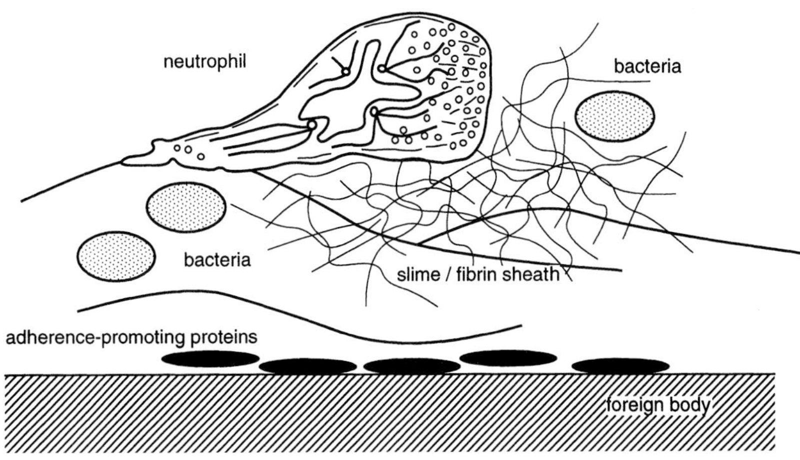

Figure 67.1. Factors contributing to foreign body infections. The key elements involved in the pathogenesis of foreign body infections include host proteins promoting bacterial adhesion to biomaterials, intrinsic properties of colonizing microorganisms that produce amorphous extracellular substance and show markedly reduced susceptibility to antimicrobial killing, and neutrophils whose phagocytic defect impairs their ability to kill bacteria.

S. aureus adherence. It has been shown that thrombospondin, a protein present in the granules of platelets, is the main mediator of this bacteria–cell interaction.

Considerable attention has been given to slime on extracellular material produced by bacteria once they adhere to surfaces. What could be the additional role of slime or extracellular slime substance in these interactions? It is believed that small amounts of *Staphylococcus epidermidis,* which attach to the surface at unique binding sites, can proceed to successfully colonize the surface by producing slime. Slime may stabilize cell-to-cell and cell-to-surface associations, allowing the bacteria to accumulate and divide on the medical device (12). Finally, not much is known about specific binding sites of *S. epidermidis* to extracellular matrix proteins, although the possible presence of an adhesin to fibrinogen has recently been shown for many of these strains (13).

Characteristics of Adherent Bacteria

Recent evidence indicates that fundamental differences exist between bacteria adherent to surfaces and bacteria present in the fluid phase. A variety of microorganisms, in particular coagulase-negative staphylococci, develop an amorphous extracellular substance ("slime" or "exopolymers") after prolonged growth on surfaces. *In vitro* studies demonstrate that microorganisms attached to foreign material and exposed to bactericidal concentrations of antibiotics develop tolerance (i.e., the bacteria become resistant to the lethal effect of the antibiotic). This change in susceptibility has been demonstrated by various approaches. Suspensions of *S. aureus* recovered from the foreign body surface of an experimental animal model (14) showed markedly decreased susceptibilities to *in vitro* killing effects of antistaphylococcal antibiotics compared with the susceptibilities of bacteria of the same strains grown in conventional conditions.

Cell-to-cell signals involved in the bacterial biofilm in *Pseudomonas aeruginosa* may provide a new target to control biofilm formation, but they have not yet been documented for other bacteria.

The use of *in vitro* systems mimicking *in vivo* conditions has also attempted to characterize the development of tolerance. Those studies have shown that the bacteria growing on surfaces, in particular those producing slime, were not killed by bactericidal concentrations of antimicrobial agents. It has been suggested that biofilm-enclosed microorganisms escape antibiotic killing because the extracellular material prevents diffusion and bacterial uptake of antimicrobial agents (Fig. 67.2). Some investigators suggested, however, that the resistance is independent of bacterial slime-producing characteristics. Other factors may be responsible for the decreased susceptibility of attached bacteria (e.g., reduced oxygen tension and pH, nutrient deprivation, or a slow growth rate).

S. aureus small colony variant (SCV) phenotypes are often found in clinical specimens and in foreign body infections. SCV demonstrate slow growth, decreased metabolism, and increased resistance to antibiotics. SCV are able to survive intracellularly and, thus, to escape antibiotics with poor cellular penetration (15,16).

In an *in vitro* system of surface-adherent *S. aureus* growing onto polymethylmethacrylate coverslips coated with pure fibronectin, it was possible to demonstrate a decreased susceptibility to antimicrobial agents within 4 hours after adherence (15). Subpopulations of microorganisms spontaneously released from the surface also showed markedly reduced susceptibilities to antimicrobial killing. In contrast, decreased susceptibility of adherent bacteria to aminoglycosides may be shown to be a specific surface-dependent event, which disappeared on suspension of the bacteria. When adherent, SCV were found to be extremely resistant at concentrations that were effective in controlling adherent non-SCV.

Altered Host Defense in the Vicinity of Foreign Material: A Consequence of Neutrophil Dysfunction

When we investigated neutrophils from animals with experimental foreign body infection, cells recovered from the vicinity of the implant may produce only a weak respiratory burst and had poor bactericidal activity compared with cells collected from the blood of the same animals. This deficiency was due to prior activation of the neutrophils by the foreign material, similar to what occurs during frustrated phagocytosis. This phagocytic

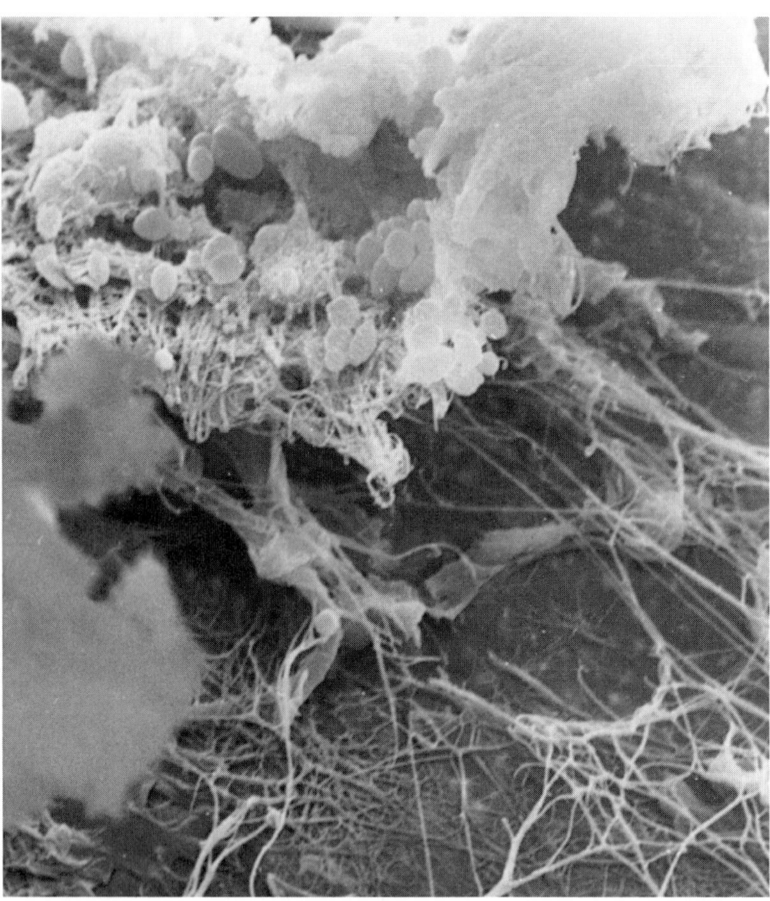

Figure 67.2. Biofilm production in prosthetic infection. Scanning electron micrograph of capsular bone from infected total hip prosthesis. Cocci-shaped bacteria are shown in association with and partly surrounded by extensive biofilm. Amorphous material also includes platelets and destroyed red cells and a fibrinous element. *Staphylococcus epidermidis* was isolated from the specimen. (DP, unpublished data.)

defect may explain the high susceptibility of foreign bodies to infection (17,18).

Another aspect of neutrophil function on foreign surfaces came from studies with a surface phagocytosis assay (19). Whereas bactericidal activity of adherent neutrophils was poor over protein-depleted surfaces, it was increased in the presence of some extracellular matrix proteins such as fibronectin. These proteins are recognized by specific cell surface receptors present in the membrane of neutrophils. Interestingly, fibronectin appeared to enhance both oxygen-dependent and oxygen-independent bactericidal activities of adherent neutrophils.

Additional immunologic components play important roles in the host defenses against infection. Recently, we showed that experimentally enhanced levels of tumor necrosis factor in the area of the foreign body decreases considerably the susceptibility to infection (20).

The extracellular slime substance produced by adherent staphylococci has potent immunomodulatory properties (21). Several neutrophil functions appear to be affected. Chemotactic responsiveness is diminished, and degranulation of specific granule content is increased. Thus, slime appears to interfere with normal surface phagocytosis (Fig. 67.2). Slime also interferes with the blastogenesis of mononuclear cells, decreases the numbers of T and B cells, and inhibits both cytotoxic activity and immunoglobulin production.

In conclusion, the nature of proteins deposited onto the surface of the foreign body and local cytokine levels might explain local defects in cellular host defense, contributing to the persistence of the infection.

INFECTED ORTHOPEDIC PROSTHESES

Joint replacement surgery has become one of the most commonplace prosthetic surgeries over the past decades because of its success in restoring function to disabled arthritic individuals (for review see references 22–25). The initial procedure, total prosthetic hip implantation, was soon followed by total knee replacement, total shoulder replacement, and total elbow replacement. Thus, joint replacement is now a very common operation—more than half a million are carried out each year worldwide. At present, millions of people have implanted prosthetic joints in place.

Infection is, second to loosening, the most common complication of orthopedic implant surgery. For hip surgery, the infection rate should be less than 1.0%, but, for other joints, it may be higher because of proximity to the skin surface and less experience in joint design. An infection rate of 0.5%, when universally attained, is still followed by several thousand new cases of infection each year. Prosthesis removal, which usually is necessary to treat these infections, produces large skeletal defects, shortening of the extremity, and severe functional impairment. Therefore, the patient is facing protracted hospitalization, sizable medical expenses, and, most distressing, renewed disability and occasional death.

Incidence and Risk Factors

Prosthetic joints become infected by two different pathogenetic routes: by introducing microorganisms during the operative procedure and by hematogenous seeding. The postoperative form of infection is the result of wound sepsis contiguous to the prosthesis or operative contamination. During the early postimplantation period when these superficial infections develop, the fascial layers have not healed yet, and the deep periprosthetic tissue is not protected by the usual physical barriers. The freshly implanted biomaterial might also be more susceptible to infection. Any factor or event that delays surgical site healing increases the risk of infection: ischemic necrosis, infected hematomas, surgical site infection (with or without identifiable cellulitis), and suture abscesses are common preceding events for joint sepsis (26–28).

Any bacteremia can induce prosthetic joint infection by hematogenous seeding. In a study of 80 patients with orthopedic prosthesis and *S. aureus* bacteremia, the risk of a prosthesis becoming infected was 34% and 7% for other orthopedic prosthesis. Experimental studies have indicated that although infection of long-standing joint implants by intravenous injection of bacteria is possible, it is easiest to induce the infection in the early postoperative period. Dentogingival infections and manipulations are well-described causes of viridans group streptococcal and anaerobic (peptococci and peptostreptococci) infections of prostheses. Pyogenic skin processes can cause staphylococcal (*S. aureus* and *S. epidermidis*) and streptococcal (groups A, B, C, and G streptococci) infections of joint replacements. Genitourinary and gastrointestinal tract procedures or infections are associated with gram-negative bacillary, enterococcal, and anaerobic infections of prostheses.

Infections have been categorized by the postoperative period in which they occur (Fig. 67.3). By this classification, acute infection (stage 1 infection) is defined as identified within 12 weeks of surgery (up to 40% of total infections); usually associated with low-grade fever; an erythematous, warm, swollen, draining surgical site; and persistent joint pain. In this condition, a distinction may be made between superficial infection (apparently confined to skin or superficial fascia) and deep infection. Subacute infection occurs within 2 years of operation (up to 45% of total infections—stage 2 infection). In this setting, the patient usually develops articular pain after several months of symptom-free ambulation. Late infection (up to 15% of total infections) develops after 2 years of pain-free mobility (stage 3). Many of these late infections are clearly hematogenous in origin. This classification is an artificial categorization and flawed, because a number of factors can influence the timing of symptom appearance; for example, hematogenous infections can produce an acute fulminant presentation resembling early infection despite their late onset.

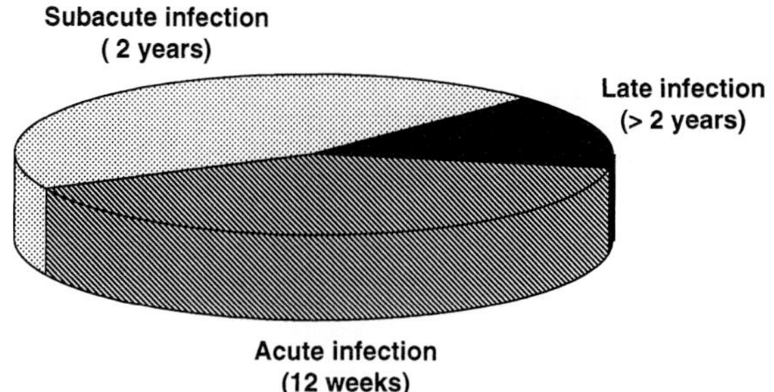

Figure 67.3. Prosthetic device infections. Joint infections complicating prosthetic devices are categorized as follows: acute infections are identified within 12 weeks of surgery, subacute infections occur within 2 years after surgery, and late infections develop more than 2 years after surgery.

Early Infection

The rate of infection after total hip arthroplasty in early surgical series was unacceptably high (29). Wilson et al. reported an infection rate of more than 11% (29), whereas in the early Charnley series (30) the infection rate was 7%. None of these patients were given antibiotic prophylaxis, and standard operating rooms (no air filtration or body exhaust suits) were used. As a result, the source of infection in these early series was thought to be primarily local contamination. This high incidence of sepsis declined after the addition of preventive measures. The introduction of air filtration in addition to prophylactic antibiotics decreased the rate of infection to 0.6% in the later Charnley series (30). Using a similar protocol, Eftekhar et al. reported an infection rate of only 0.5% (29). However, in these series, follow-up was relatively limited. Currently, the rate of infection after total hip arthroplasty is thought to be approximately 1% over the entire lifetime of the prosthesis. This percentage includes operative, perioperative, and late infection.

One of the largest published series comes from the Mayo Clinic where 39,013 total hip or knee prostheses were inserted over 22 years (1969 to 1991) (31). Most patients (>90%) were followed prospectively. The infection rate per 1,000 joint-years was 1.32 for total hip and 2.29 for total knee prostheses. The incidence of prosthetic joint infection fell from 12 and 6 per 1,000 joint-years for total knee and total hip prostheses, respectively, at 0 to 3 months after surgery to less than 2 infections per 1,000 joint-years 24 to 48 months after implantation.

Risk Factors

Conditions favoring total hip arthroplasty infection include a history of postoperative surgical site healing problems, incorrect prophylaxis (32), diabetes (33), and autoimmune diseases. The infection rate for patients with rheumatoid arthritis or systemic lupus erythematosus is twice as high as that of other patients undergoing the same operation but without the underlying disease. In general, the incidence of infection appears to be higher in corticosteroid-dependent patients.

Another risk factor is reintervention. The rate of infection after revision hip surgery is at least twice as high as that after primary total hip arthroplasty. The reason for this increased infection rate is multifactorial. Longer operating times and larger surgical exposures result in the potential for increased direct contamination. In addition, larger exposures required for revision surgery result in increased volumes of devascularized bone and soft tissue and larger dead space, increasing the likelihood for bacterial colonization.

Finally, infection in an artificial joint is a risk factor for developing infection in the same individual bearing another prosthesis. Sixty-eight patients with 159 replacement arthroplasties of more than one major joint inserted between 1975 and 1984 were identified as developing an infection after the first procedure. Subsequent infection in another total joint replacement was documented in ten of these patients. Joint infections were due to the same causative microorganism as the index infection and occurred within the first year after the index infection (34).

Surprisingly, aggressive immunosuppressive therapy does not seem to be an independent risk factor. Local infections complicating large joint replacement in rheumatoid arthritis patients treated with methotrexate versus those not treated with methotrexate were compared in 60 patients who had a total of 92 joint arthroplasties. Treatment in the perioperative period with weekly low-dose pulse methotrexate did not increase the risk of local postoperative infections or poor healing of the surgical site (35).

Late Infection

With the decrease of postoperative infection, late infection is becoming increasingly important, and, in some centers, it may represent 25% to 50% of all cases. The incidence of late infection of total joint prostheses was calculated to be around 0.6%. The microbiology and sources of reported cases of late infections of total joint prostheses of 67 patients reported in the literature have been reviewed (36). The most common pathogen responsible for late prosthetic joint infections was staphylococcus (54%; both *S. aureus* and *S. epidermidis*), even when infections of dental origin were considered. The three most common origins of infection were skin and soft tissue (46%), dental (15%), and urinary tract (13%). *Escherichia coli* was the leading pathogen when the source was the urinary tract (36).

In a recent analysis of a large single-institution series, gram-positive microorganisms accounted for 65% and gram-negative microorganisms for 35% of infections. The most disturbing finding of this study was that *P. aeruginosa* was identified as the infecting microorganism in 12% of all total hip replacement infections. The increasing incidence of gram-negative infection (relative to gram-positive microorganisms) most likely results from improved perioperative technique, with subsequent decreases in the absolute number of early gram-positive infections (29,37).

Epidemiology

Infecting Microorganisms

The data from the Endo-Klinik in Hamburg, Germany (38), indicate that a single pathogen can be identified only in about 70% of cases; the remaining cases are equally divided between polymicrobial and sterile cultures. The pattern of microorganism retrieval from three large series dealing with infected joint replacement is shown in Table 67.3 (31,38a,38b). The predominance of staphylococcal species evenly divided between coagulase-negative staphylococci and *S. aureus* has major implications for surgical prophylaxis (39).

Aerobic streptococci were responsible for a significant number of infections. Gram-negative aerobic bacilli were identified in some series in up to 25% of cases, and anaerobes usually did not account for more than 10% of pathogens. Similar to other prosthetic infections, the full spectrum of microbial agents capable of causing prosthetic joint infections is very large and includes microorganisms ordinarily considered contaminants of cultures, such as corynebacteria, propionibacteria, and *Bacillus* species. Primary infections with fungi (particularly *Candida* species) and mycobacteria have been described rarely.

Risk Factors for Surgical Site Infections

Risk factors for surgical site infections after total knee arthroplasty have been carefully assessed. In a cohort study, stratified analyses identified a preoperative American Society of Anesthesiologists physical status class greater than 3, surgeon X, and early postoperative use of a continuous passive motion device as risk factors associated with surgical site infection after total knee arthroplasty procedures. The authors concluded that surgical technique and the patient's severity of illness were the primary determinants of surgical site infection after total knee

TABLE 67.3. PREDOMINANT MICROORGANISMS ISOLATED IN PROSTHETIC JOINT INFECTION

	Buchholz, et al.[a] (1984) (38a) (%) (n = 869)	Fitzgerald and Jones[b] (1985) (38b) (n = 131) (%)	Mayo Clinic cohort[c] (1969–1991) (31) (n = 1033) (%)
Staphylococcus aureus	32	29	23
Coagulase-negative staphylococci	14	35	25
Other gram-positive microorganisms	12	7	11
Gram-negative aerobes	16	15	11
Anaerobes	9	7	6
Mixed	—	—	14

[a] Single culture only.
[b] Includes polymicrobial infections.
[c] Unknown (sterile *or* not available): 8%.CAPD, continuous ambulatory peritoneal dialysis; CSF, cerebrospinal fluid; TPN, total parenteral nutrition.

arthroplasty. This study demonstrated the complexity of epidemiologic investigation of surgical site infections and the importance of considering patient severity of illness when interpreting surgeon-specific infection rates (28).

Clinical Presentation

Most patients present with a long indolent course characterized by progressively increasing joint pain and the occasional formation of cutaneous draining sinuses and occasionally with fever, soft tissue swelling, or systemic toxicity. In some cases, patients may present with an acute fulminant illness associated with high fever, severe joint pain, local swelling, and erythema. In a large series of infected hip prostheses, the frequencies (in percentages) of these presenting symptoms were as follows: joint pain, 95; fever, 43; periarticular swelling, 38; and wound or cutaneous sinus drainage, 32.

Patients with persistent pain 6 months after total knee arthroplasty must be considered infected until proven otherwise. In a study of 52 patients with knee replacements who had been treated for infection, the workup was evaluated for accuracy in determining infection. Considerable pain was present in 96% of the patients, 77% had swelling of the knee, 27% were febrile, and 27% had active drainage. Pain is, thus, the overriding complaint in patients with such infection (40). The pattern of clinical presentation is determined largely by the nature of the infecting microorganism (i.e., the symptoms may be more prominent in *S. aureus* infections).

Infection must be differentiated from aseptic mechanical problems, which are the most common cause of pain and inflammatory symptoms in these patients (41). The physiopathology of such a reaction is not fully characterized. It is hypothesized that cellular reactions to microparticles derived from biomaterials elicits a detrimental biologic response, which may lead to harmful reactions such as resorption of bone.

Significance of Intraoperative Cultures

The significance of intracapsular cultures in hip replacements has been evaluated in several studies (42,43). In a retrospective study of 1,500 consecutive total hip replacements (44), analysis of cultures taken at the time of operation revealed that positive cultures obtained in primary arthroplasties are not significant.

Evaluation of preoperative cultures before second-stage reimplantation showed that prerevision cultures, grown after discontinuation of antibiotic and before reimplantation, helped to identify the patients in whom the infection might recur. Whether or not therapy should be initiated based on the positivity of intraoperative screening cultures at the time of primary arthroplasty remains unknown.

Significance of Bacterial Growth on Suction Drain Tips

Most postoperative surgical site infections are due to bacterial contamination during surgery (45). However, such contamination is much more frequent than indicated by the rate of postoperative surgical site infection, and, for most wounds, the local defense reactions alone or combined with prophylactic antibiotics are able to eliminate the bacteria. It seems reasonable to assume that if bacteria are detectable in the surgical site in the days after surgery, this is a sign of insufficient bacterial elimination and increased risk of infection.

A study that attempted to investigate further bacterial growth in suction drain fluid and on suction drain tips after clean orthopedic operations was correlated with an increased risk for postoperative surgical site infection. The study included 489 clean orthopedic procedures with implantation of major foreign materials (joint replacements and internal fixations of fractures). Specimens for cultures were taken from the suction drainage system (from the drain fluid, the drain-tube tip, or both). Six superficial and five deep infections were documented after surgery. Only two cultures of drain fluid were positive, and neither of these became infected. Positive drain-tip cultures were seen after 56 operations, and, of these, 5 were followed by infection. Drain tips positive for *S. aureus,* Enterobacteriaceae, or *Streptococcus faecalis* were associated with an increased risk for infection. In contrast, drain-tip cultures growing only coagulase-negative staphylococci, nonhemolytic streptococci, and corynebacteria were not correlated with increased risk for infection.

Several studies have recently evaluated the value of suction drainage fluid culture during clean orthopedic surgery and conclude that systematic culture is not useful for the detection of infection.

Closed suction drainage has become an established routine with the aim of preventing wound hematoma and thereby reducing the risk of infection. However, the benefit of closed suction drainage has never been evaluated in a prospective randomized study. In prospective nonrandomized studies, no advantage was found with closed suction drains. Drainage systems are not without theoretic or experimental risks. In animal experiments, retrograde migration of bacteria along the drain has been observed, increasing the risk of surgical site infection. Furthermore, the presence of a drain as an additional foreign body may weaken the defense reactions and thereby the ability to eliminate contaminating bacteria.

In summary, the previously mentioned data suggest that suction drainage is necessary (46), but early removal of the drains within 24 hours (47) is recommended because drains may harm the host-defense reaction and facilitate infection. Culture of suction fluid during clean orthopedic surgery is not necessary.

Diagnosis

Erythrocyte Sedimentation Rate

Constant joint pain is suggestive of infection, whereas mechanical loosening commonly causes pain only with motion and weight bearing. Persistent elevation of the erythrocyte sedimentation rate (ESR) suggests infection but is neither very sensitive nor very specific (48). The ESR was studied in 79 patients who underwent reoperations for prosthetic hip failures in a study by Thorén (49). Based on postoperative findings, an ESR level of 35 mm was found to represent an acceptable cutoff between infected and noninfected prostheses.

Contrarily, ESR has been one of the more unpredictable tests for identifying subclinical sepsis. Part of the variability in the reported accuracy of ESR relates to the inaccuracy of its measurement. Overall, the average sensitivity in the reviewed series reached 80% with poor specificity, suggesting that ESR is a modestly useful indicator of subclinical infection with a low virulence microorganism. The combined measurement of C-reactive protein levels and ESR seems to be more accurate, but normal values or slight increases were also observed (50). In summary, these parameters are more appropriate for follow-up during therapy than for diagnosis, and both values should be determined preoperatively (45).

Radiology

Plain x-ray films can reveal abnormal lucencies (greater than 2 mm in width) at the bone–cement interface, changes in the position of prosthetic components, cement fractures, periosteal reaction, or motion of components on stress views. The most specific signs for infection are bone resorption and acute or multifocal periostitis (51). In addition, intraarticular injection of dye (arthrography) may reveal abnormal communications between the joint space and multiple defects in the bone–cement interface (22,52). These radiologic abnormalities are found in 50% of septic prostheses. They are related to the duration of infection, because such changes may require 3 to 6 months to become evident. When both distal and proximal components of a prosthetic joint demonstrate radiographic abnormalities, infection is more likely than simple mechanical loosening. However, these x-ray changes are not specific for infection, because they are seen frequently with aseptic processes.

Magnetic resonance (MR) or computed tomography (CT) techniques for evaluating prosthetic joints for infection are of little help. MR images are degraded by metal, usually a component of the prostheses, and CT does not visualize cortical bone accurately.

Radionuclide imaging techniques are clearly preferred and have been extensively used for diagnosing prosthetic joint infection (52). Radioisotopic scans with technetium diphosphonate demonstrate increased uptake in areas of bone with enhanced blood supply or increased metabolic activity. Increased technetium uptake is seen routinely around normal prostheses for 6 months after arthroplasty. After this period, interpretation of a positive scan is controversial. Persistent periprosthetic activity on bone scintigrams has been described even several years after implantation without clinical significance (53). Some authors claim it reflects inflammation and possible loosening but not specifically infection of the implant. Others claim that sequential technetium-gallium bone scanning is also nondiagnostic because of unacceptably low sensitivity and specificity.

Conclusions often state that a normal bone scan excludes the need for surgical intervention to correct loosening or infection as a cause for the patient's pain. Abnormal scans, bone and gallium, do not appear to reliably distinguish between infection and loosening. Strikingly abnormal gallium scans may be associated with "abundant granulation tissue" related to chronic loosening rather than to infection.

The results with indium oxide labeled leukocytes were initially much more appealing (54). When correlated with bone scans, several studies showed sensitivities greater than 88% with similar specificities. However, the difficulties included soft-tissue uptake sometimes not separable from abnormal bone uptake, indium-leukocyte concentration in some arthritides (e.g., rheumatoid arthritis, which may be the underlying disease process that led to the prosthesis), and abnormal indium uptake in the absence of infection. Moreover, indium activity is normally seen in marrow and can be misleading in evaluating infection; the presence of heterotropic bone containing marrow adjacent to the prosthetic joint can confuse the interpretation (54). Finally, indium-leukocyte scans have a decreasing sensitivity for diagnosing infection in bones that are more central than peripheral in location and infections that are more chronic: for chronic hip infection, indium-leukocyte sensitivity is as low as 50%.

Therefore, a normal or negative technetium or indium-labeled leukocyte scan can be considered as strong evidence against the presence of infection (or aseptic loosening), but it is not helpful in establishing a definite diagnosis.

Joint Aspiration

Aspiration of painful total joint replacements has been described as a highly accurate method for identifying infected joints (25,48,55). In 1984, O'Neil and Harris (56) reported the high specificity (98%) of needle aspiration for the diagnosis of infection in 61 total hip arthroplasties; in their series, 12 cases were excluded and judged to be contaminants. Only one infected case was identified, which had not produced any fluid for culture on attempted aspiration. Most contaminants were so judged because the microorganisms were considered to be nonpathogenic skin flora; however, these are now recognized as major participants in the process of subclinical sepsis of orthopedic implants.

Arthrography with hip aspiration was evaluated in a series of 143 patients with hip arthroplasties to determine its effectiveness for diagnosing infection (22). Thirty-three cases of infection were found. On 26 occasions (79%), the causative pathogen was isolated in the joint fluid. In six other cases, infection was revealed from cytologic or arthrographic findings or from both. Hip aspiration arthrography had a sensitivity of 79% for diagnosing the infection and a specificity of 100%. The sensitivity rose to 91% when any one of the following features was observed: leucocytosis of the joint fluid higher than 10,000 elements/mm^3, presence of a fistula or fistulization on arthrography, or isolation of the microorganism in the joint fluid or the rinsing liquid. Arthroscopy biopsy to obtain material for culture and histology is important in chronic arthritis.

Arthrocentesis demonstrates the causative pathogen in 85% to 98% of cases. Fluoroscopic guidance and arthrography are useful in documenting accurate needle placement. When difficulty is encountered in obtaining intraarticular fluid, irrigation with sterile normal saline (without antiseptic preservative additives) can be used to provide the necessary fluid for culture. When initial cultures reveal a relatively avirulent microorganism (*S. epidermidis,* corynebacteria, propionibacteria, and *Bacillus* species), a second aspirate should be considered to confirm the bacteriologic diagnosis and to eliminate the possibility of contamination. Quantitative bacterial cultures by plating are useful in such situations. Growth of significant quantities of microorganisms is very useful information for clinicians. When multiple isolates are present, comparison of genomic DNA from the isolated strains may be useful (57). Operative cultures are definitively diagnostic if the patient has not received antimicrobial therapy for several weeks before the procedure. Multiple specimens of tissue and fluid should be submitted for culture. Because fastidious microorganisms, including anaerobes, may be responsible for prosthetic arthroplasty infections, specimens should be obtained and rapidly cultured on appropriate media.

The sensitivities (in percentages) of different techniques to diagnose infection during operation were as follows: arthrocentesis fluid Gram stain, 0 to 32 (58,59); frozen section histopathology (leukocytic infiltrate in nonosseous periprosthetic tissue), 55 to 84 (58,60); arthrocentesis fluid culture, 85 to 98; and operative culture (osseous and nonosseous periprosthetic tissue), 100 (58).

A controversial study suggested that the incidence of prosthetic joint infections was grossly underestimated by current culture detection methods. Bacteria were observed in 63% of sonicate samples with a monoclonal antibody for *Propionobacterium acnes* and 72% by polymerase chain reaction (PCR) amplification of the IGS RNA gene with universal primers.

The identification of an infected implant before a revision operation is important, because it determines the extent of the surgery required (48). In the presence of infection, cement removal must be complete, and radical excision of infected soft tissue and bone is required. The use of bone grafts is probably contraindicated. Preoperative knowledge of the antibiotic sensitivity of the infecting microorganism will allow the appropriate use of antibiotics both parenterally and in the cement.

Similar to hip prostheses, the workup of an infected total knee arthroplasty should include preoperative aspiration under sterile conditions. Superficial sinus cultures poorly predict the causative pathogen.

Widmer reviewed the estimated likelihood ratio of different tests for diagnosing prosthetic joint infection (60a). The following tests, if positive, rated excellent for diagnosing infection: preoperative aspiration, frozen section from intraoperative samples, and technetium or indium-labeled white blood cell (WBC) scanning. The following tests, if negative, were excellent for absence of infection: indium-labeled IgG scanning and intraoperative culture and a C-reactive protein level less than 1mg/L.

Prevention

Prevention remains the cornerstone infection control procedure for joint replacement. It is efficacious, has few side effects, and is certainly more cost-effective than any other form of therapy. In most centers, general measures are used before surgery; unfortunately, no controlled studies are available regarding the use of these techniques. However, there is little risk to such procedures, and because there is potential benefit they are briefly reviewed here:

- If local skin infection exists, surgical treatment should be delayed until the lesion is healed. If the dentition is poor, cleaning, endodontic procedures (root canals), and extractions should be scheduled before the hip replacement. Urinary tract infection should be treated before operation.
- Many surgeons recommend antimicrobial showers before total hip arthroplasty. Some surgeons suggest a single shower should be taken the night before operation, whereas others use a regimen consisting of showers every 8 hours for 24 to 48 hours before operation.
- Preoperative hair removal may be done using depilatory agents. The advantages of depilatories over shaving is that depilatories do not cause skin breaks. However, many patients are sensitive to these agents, resulting in contact dermatitis that can be associated with higher rates of bacterial colonization. If hair removal is done by shaving, timing is critical. Shaving of the operative site should not be done the night before operation, because it may result in folliculitis and dermatitis in the surgical field. Shaving should be done immediately before operation, just before the patient enters the operating room. Care should also be taken to remove all loose hair from the patient and the patient's gown before the patient enters the surgical theater (see Chapter 21).
- Appropriate care should be taken during skin preparation and draping immediately before the operative procedure. Most operating room protocols include washing of the entire area with an iodophor soap followed by the use of an iodophor paint. Isopropyl alcohol is often used both as a bactericidal agent and as a vehicle to dry the area and increase the adhesion of iodophor-impregnated drapes.

Benefits of Antibiotic Prophylaxis and Ultraclean Air Systems

Animal models have been very useful to assess the utility of various antibiotic regimens in foreign body device-related infections (61–63). Indeed, clinical studies do not allow the separate evaluation of each factor conducive to infection, and experimental studies in this field are limited. The problem can be partly solved by the exclusive study of infection after clean surgery, because in these circumstances, bacteriologic features are well defined; the presence of foreign materials greatly potentiates pathogenic mechanisms, and experimental models are readily available.

Analysis is based on three principles. First, the surgical site must be contaminated, and adherence mechanisms are therefore of paramount importance. Second, most clean surgical sites are found to be contaminated when sampled carefully, and the control of infection is, therefore, more a quantitative than a qualitative problem. Finally, the critical period for the development of infection is short. Antibiotic prophylaxis of 24 hours' duration seems to be effective both clinically and experimentally. As to the timing of initiation of prophylaxis, both experimental studies of foreign body infections (64) and clinical observations indicate that antibiotics should be given within the 2-hour period before surgery.

With these principles as a framework, the effects of antimicrobial agents on microbial factors must be evaluated. The staphylococcal carrier state (whether involving *S. aureus* or coagulase-negative staphylococci) influences the frequency of surgical site infection and can be modified in a positive or negative manner by antibiotics. Bacterial multiplication is influenced by many factors during the first few hours of surgical site infection—a decisive period that offers many therapeutic possibilities. Antibiotic susceptibilities are evidently critical determinants of the efficacy of perioperative antibiotic prophylaxis. Initial resistance and the emergence of resistance by selection or genetic alteration are well-known phenomena, and plasmid transfer among species of staphylococci is a newly observed mechanism of potentially great danger (63).

Norden (65) and Fitzgerald (24) extensively reviewed the literature on antibiotic prophylaxis after total joint replacement (29). Between 1970 and 1980, several studies suggested that antimicrobial prophylaxis reduced the frequency of deep surgical site infection after total joint replacement (66). Hill et al. (67) suggested that prophylaxis with cefazolin significantly reduced the incidence of surgical site infections compared with placebo; however, the site of infection (i.e., prostheses vs. surgical site) was not clearly differentiated. Moreover, when the results were examined according to the type of operating theater used, differences were found to be significant only among patients whose surgery was performed in a conventional theater. When a "hypersterile" theater was used, the rates of infection were the same for the cefazolin-treated and the placebo-treated groups.

Lidwell et al. (68,69) conducted several multicenter studies, including about 8,000 cases, with the major objective of observing the effect of ultraclean operating room air on the infection rate. This investigation demonstrated a clear reduction in the rate of organ/space surgical site infections after surgery in the ultraclean-air operating rooms. The design of the study did not allow for control of the effect of prophylactic antibiotics; however, antibiotic prophylaxis was associated with a lower incidence of infection. The authors suggested that ultraclean air and antibiotic prophylaxis had independent and cumulative effects (70) in preventing surgical site infection but stated that the data were not precise enough to establish this point beyond a doubt and that the study was not set up to examine such a hypothesis.

This area is still controversial. In a prospective study including 7,305 patients, Fitzgerald (24) did not find a statistically significant difference in the infection rate between patients operated on in a conventional operating room and those operated on in a horizontal clean room. Laminar flow is sensitive to the position of operating room equipment and personnel. Salvati et al. (23) showed that the improper positioning of operating room personnel may actually increase the infection rate in a laminar flow room, because it may draw contaminated air onto the field. In addition, laminar air flow is expensive, both in the initial capital expenditure and in operational costs. The question of whether hyperclean air and antibiotic prophylaxis have independent and cumulative effects on the development of surgical site infection remains important, given the cost of hyperclean air systems (71). Table 67.4 summarizes the role of both preventive measures collected from more than 14,000 total hip prosthesis; these data show that both measures are efficient in the prevention of infection and also suggest an independent cumulative effect.

Additional measures being evaluated include total body exhaust suits, special working clothes, and coveralls in the operating room (72). Body exhaust systems also restrict movement by personnel and impair the vision and hearing of the surgeon. Newer models show improvement with regard to movement but still impair the visual field. A cost-benefit analysis study concluded that for departments performing at least 100 total joint replacement procedures per year, a combination of parenteral antibiotic prophylaxis and use of an ultraclean air system is "the most attractive means of prophylaxis from the social point of view." This also appeared to be the most cost-effective system. For departments performing fewer than 100 arthroplasties each year, the authors argued that a combination of parenteral and local antibiotics (the latter delivered in antibiotic-impregnated cement) is the most cost-effective means of reducing infection. In view of the economic costs and the high morbidity associated with infection of prosthetic joints, adherence to these recommendations seems worthwhile until other techniques for the prevention of organ/space surgical site infection are shown to be effective and cost efficient.

Optimal Agents for Prophylaxis

The optimal antimicrobial agent for use in total joint replacement is not clear. Ideally, the agent chosen should be effective in preventing surgical site infection, relatively free of toxicity, and inexpensive. The question of toxicity is important, because agents not anticipated to be toxic may turn out to be so under

TABLE 67.4. ROLE OF ANTIBIOTIC PROPHYLAXIS (AP) AND A CLEAN-AIR ROOM SYSTEM IN PREVENTION OF DEEP INFECTIONS AFTER INSERTION OF TOTAL HIP PROSTHESES

	Regular operating room		Clean-air operating room	
	Without AP	With AP	Without AP	With AP
Number of studies	7	10	3	6
Number of patients	1,880	6,791	2,730	2,754
Number of infections	109	90	18	17
Infection rates				
Range	4.0–11.0%	0.0–3.1%	0.6–1.1%	0.0–1.0%
Average	5.8%	1.3%	0.7%	0.6%
Median	6.5%	1.4%	1.0%	0.75%

From Nelson JP. The operating room environment and its influence on deep wound infections. In: *The hip: proceedings of the Fifth Open Scientific Meeting of the Hip Society*. St. Louis: Mosby, 1977, with permission.

certain conditions. In two Scandinavian studies, for example, the investigators found an unacceptably high incidence of nephrotoxicity, with increases in serum creatinine levels, when dicloxacillin was used prophylactically (73,74). It appears prudent to avoid dicloxacillin as a prophylactic agent in total joint replacement.

Cefazolin has generally been used for prophylaxis in total joint replacement, but there are many reports in the surgical literature that look at newer cephalosporins. Relatively few reported studies have compared various cephalosporins for prophylaxis in total joint replacement. Bryan et al. (75) reported a careful prospective, randomized, double-blind trial comparing cefazolin with cefamandole in total joint replacement. The number of patients studied was relatively small (48 or 49 patients in each group), and the rate of surgical site infection was the same in the two groups. The authors pointed out that given the low incidence of organ/space surgical site infection, a comparative trial large enough to show a true difference between agents is obviously impractical (about 4,800 patients). Despite the lack of other such comparisons, both first-generation (cefazolin) or second-generation cephalosporins (cefamandole and cefuroxime) appear to be appropriate for this indication (65).

Optimal Duration of Prophylaxis

The issue of the optimal duration of antimicrobial prophylaxis has been widely discussed. Pollard et al. (76) indicated that three doses of a cephalosporin for only 12 hours were as effective for prophylaxis as was flucloxacillin given for 14 days. The latter study did not include a control group receiving placebo. However, Hill et al. (77) showed that as few as three doses of antibiotic may constitute effective prophylaxis for this type of surgery. Similarly, Nelson et al. (78) showed that the administration of either nafcillin or cefazolin for 24 hours after surgery was as effective in preventing surgical site infection as the administration of the same antimicrobial agents for 7 days. As stated previously, administration of antibiotics 1 hour before surgery is also an optimal timing (79) with additional doses every 4 hours during the operation (if second-generation cephalosporins are used).

Antibiotic-Containing Cement in Total Joint Replacement

Wahlig et al. (80) noted that patients undergoing total joint replacement of the hip in which gentamicin-containing cement was used had gentamicin in aspirated joint fluid for up to 265 days in one study and in tissue samples for more than 5 years in another study. Concentrations of the drug in surgical site secretions were excellent; levels in serum were acceptably low, never exceeding 3 μg/mL and usually less than 1 μg/mL after 24 hours.

Lynch et al. (81) reported a retrospective review of about 1,500 total joint replacement procedures without prophylactic systemic antibiotics. Plain cement was used in the first 4 years and gentamicin-impregnated cement in the next 4 years. The overall rates of infection for the plain cement and gentamicin cement procedures were 2.2% and 1.3%, respectively; the difference did not reach statistical significance. However, in two subgroups of patients who had undergone previous surgery on the hip, rates of infection were significantly lower for gentamicin-containing cement than for plain cement. The authors concluded that antibiotic-containing cement might be particularly useful for patients undergoing reoperation.

Trippel (82) published a careful review of the entire subject of antibiotic-impregnated cement in total joint replacement. The issues he raised include the following:

1. Many antibiotics appear to be released from the cement in potentially efficacious amounts, but the duration over which these antibiotics continue to be released is less certain. Even for specific combinations of antibiotic and cement, different investigators have derived markedly different data. For example, the period of release of gentamicin from cement has been reported to range from 13 days to 5 years.
2. *In vitro* data suggest that the findings obtained with antibiotic-impregnated cement are highly dependent on experimental conditions. Trippel noted that such conditions are, at best, only rough approximations of the clinical setting.
3. The use of antibiotic-impregnated cement is usually only one of a series of determinant variables in clinical studies. Thus, a lowering of the infection rate is often difficult to attribute to the use of antibiotic-impregnated cement alone.

McQueen et al. (83) performed a well-controlled, prospective, randomized trial including 295 arthroplasties of the hip and knee. The impact of systemic cefuroxime on the development of early infection was compared with that of cefuroxime-impregnated bone cement. The cement group received 1.5 g of cefuroxime in 40 g of cement powder; the parenteral antibiotic group received 1.5 g of cefuroxime intravenously at the induction of anesthesia and two additional doses of 750 mg 6 and 12 hours later. The follow-up period was only 3 months; during that interval, the numbers of infections in the two groups were approximately equal. The observed rate of organ/space surgical site infection was 0.7% in the cement group and 1.3% in the parenteral antibiotic group. The authors demonstrated at least equal efficacy of cefuroxime-impregnated bone cement and parenterally administered cefuroxime in the prevention of early infection in total joint replacement (83). This is probably the best study published regarding the use of antibiotic containing cement.

Espehaug et al. (84) reviewed 10,905 primary cemented total hip replacements in Norway and concluded that systemic antibiotics combined with antibiotic-containing bone cement led to a lower number of infections.

Prophylaxis Against Hematogenous Seeding

Some experimental evidence indicates a high risk of infection of joint implants during bacteremia, especially in the early postoperative period. There is also clear evidence that hematogenous infection of prosthetic joints occurs occasionally secondary to overt infections elsewhere in the body. The skin is the most frequent source of infection followed by the genitourinary tract, the mouth, and the respiratory tract (85). Thus, vigorous treatment of infection elsewhere in the body is required before total joint replacement.

The situation with regard to dental procedures is not clear. Most reported isolates from infected prosthetic joints after dental procedures are microorganisms rarely associated with bacteremia secondary to dental procedures. Only a few reports of oral microorganisms causing late total joint replacement infection after dental work (usually in patients with periodontal disease) are convincing. Careful studies also indicate that the frequency of late prosthetic joint infections associated with dental treatment is low.

A computer simulation model was created by Jacobson et al. (86) to assess the risks and efficacy of no prophylaxis, oral penicillin prophylaxis, and oral cephalexin prophylaxis among dental patients at risk for late prosthetic joint infection. In the framework of the assumptions made by the authors, the analysis suggested a very small risk of infection (29 to 68 cases per 106 dental visits); this risk was lower than that of death from a reaction to an antibiotic. The authors concluded from their model that routine antibiotic prophylaxis for all dental patients with prosthetic joints was not indicated but that prophylaxis might be appropriate in high-risk patients. The clinical profile of high-risk patients remains to be depicted. Obvious periodontal disease is certainly part of the clinical picture (39).

Tsevat et al. (87) used a decision tree to perform a cost-effectiveness analysis and concluded that penicillin prophylaxis was more expensive and less effective than no prophylaxis in this population of patients. Prophylaxis with erythromycin appeared to be the most effective (and the most expensive) alternative. A problem with this study is the estimate by the authors that erythromycin prophylaxis would be 75% effective in preventing joint infection. As they noted in the abstract, "Sensitivity analysis demonstrates that the risk of developing a joint infection is the key parameter in the analysis."

Gillespie (39) analyzed data and assumptions regarding routine antibiotic prophylaxis for dental patients with prosthetic joints and indicated a slight preponderance of evidence in favor of its avoidance. However, in the presence of overt or possible dental sepsis (periodontal disease), prophylaxis was strongly indicated. The reported cases in which dental microorganisms were present in the joint involved patients with proven periodontal disease.

According to the results of the Mayo Clinic cohort study (31), dental procedures constitute a significant risk factor for prosthetic joint infections caused by viridans streptococci compared with infections caused by other pathogens (odds ratio 6.4, 95% confidence interval 2.2 to 18.6). Interestingly, dental procedures were significantly associated only with early and subacute infections.

From the previous discussion, it may be concluded that any patient having an orthopedic implant should be carefully instructed about risks of infection. Patients should be able to carry this information with them continuously; minor infections should be treated aggressively and in particular situations, such as surgery in severe periodontal disease or urologic manipulations in the presence of bacteriuria, antibiotic prophylaxis should be instituted. Prophylaxis is also indicated in patients who have a predisposing condition that increases the risk for infection, such as rheumatoid arthritis or hemophilia. Because no data are available on this specific area, we advise following the recommendations of the American Heart Association regarding the class and dosages of antibiotics to select.

INFECTIONS OF PROSTHETIC HEART VALVES AND VASCULAR GRAFTS

Prosthetic Heart Valve Endocarditis

Incidence and Risk Factors

In three large series reviewed assessing 5,671 recipients of prosthetic heart valves between 1956 to 1982, 220 patients developed prosthetic valve endocarditis (PVE). Actuarial estimates of cumulative risks varied from 1.5% to 4.1% at 12 months and from 3.2% to 5.7% at 60 months (88,89). Each of these studies defined a higher risk period during the initial 6 to 12 months after surgery and a lower risk period thereafter. They also illustrated that prosthetic valves remain vulnerable to infection as long as they are in place.

The effect of specific factors, such as the site of valve implantation and the type of valve implanted (mechanical vs. bioprosthetic valve), on the risk of developing PVE has also been examined. Although no difference has been reported between patients with mitral or aortic prostheses, a difference appears to emerge among mechanical valve recipients as compared with patients with bioprostheses. This difference between type of prosthesis appeared statistically significant in the first months after surgery, whereas the cumulative risk at 5 years was similar for the two valve types.

Calderwood et al. (90) found an enhanced risk for PVE among recipients of multiple prostheses compared with recipients of a single valve. Ivert et al. (91) noted an increased risk of PVE with a longer cardiopulmonary bypass time. These observations suggest that PVE may be associated with more prolonged or complex surgery.

Agnihotri et al. (92) reviewed risk factors in 2,433 patients who underwent valve replacement; endocarditis occurred in 3.7%. Significant risk was observed if prior endocarditis had occurred and even more if *S. aureus* was responsible for preoperative infection. Patients receiving concomitant aortic root replacement were at increased early risk when synthetic material was used.

Pathogenesis Specific to Prosthetic Valve Endocarditis: Early Versus Late Infection

Early infection occurs within 12 months after surgery and represents, for most authors, a nosocomial infection acquired during surgery. Several investigators recovered bacterial species that are commonly associated with early PVE from the operative field and the cardiopulmonary bypass equipment. Postoperative infections resulting from bacteria that are subsequently noted to cause endocarditis have been found in a large percentage of patients with early PVE. Unusual but well-described cases of such nosocomial infection include porcine bioprostheses contaminated by *Mycobacterium chelonae* during production and outbreaks of *Legionella* infection.

The bacteriology of PVE with onset 12 months or more after valve surgery suggests that these infections have been acquired outside the hospital. Incidental infections (e.g., urinary tract infections and furunculosis) and trauma to mucosal surfaces (e.g., genitourinary tract and dental manipulation) may be identified as predisposing events for 50% of patients with late-onset PVE. Microorganisms that enter the blood from the oral cavity and respiratory tract are responsible for late-onset PVE. The recovery of fastidious gram-negative coccobacilli (*Haemophilus* species, *Actinobacillus actinomycetemcomitans, Cardiobacterium hominis, Eikenella corrodens.* and *Kingella* species, so-called HACEK) months and often years after surgery suggests that late-onset PVE is primarily acquired through incidental nonnosocomial infection and bacteremia.

Microbiology

More than 20 years ago, early infections occurring after cardiac surgery were often caused by *S. aureus,* gram-negative bacilli, diphtheroids, and yeasts. The present infrequent role of these microorganisms probably results from multiple factors, including improved surgical techniques and postoperative care that reduced nosocomial infections and improved perioperative antibiotic prophylaxis. Coagulase-negative staphylococci remain the strikingly dominant cause of endocarditis occurring from 2 to 12 months after surgery (Table 67.5).

The microorganisms causing PVE developing more than 12 months after valve implantation become increasingly similar to those associated with native valve endocarditis. During this late postoperative period, the predominant causes of infection are coagulase-negative staphylococci; streptococci; enterococci; *S. aureus;* and fastidious gram-negative coccobacilli, particularly *A. actinomycetemcomitans, C. hominis,* and *Haemophilus* species. A broad range of bacteria have caused sporadic cases of PVE, such as *Corynebacterium* species of the J-K group, *Nocardia asteroides, Bacillus cereus, Listeria monocytogenes, Legionella pneumophila,* and *Legionella dumoffii.*

In the past, fungi have not only accounted for significant numbers of early cases but were also associated with high fatality rates. *Candida* species, followed by *Aspergillus* species, are the two most common fungi causing PVE. Invasive fungi, including *Histoplasma capsulatum, Cryptococcus neoformans,* and *Mucor* species, have caused occasional cases of PVE, as have the so-called saprophytic fungi, *Penicillium chrysogenum, Paecilomyces varioti,* and *Trichosporon cutaneum.* Fungal vegetations formed on prosthetic valves are bulky and may partially occlude the valve orifice or embolize and occlude medium-sized arteries.

TABLE 67.5. PREDOMINANT PATHOGENS OF INFECTIONS ASSOCIATED WITH CARDIAC AND VASCULAR PROSTHESES[a]

Microorganism	Early PVE (≤ 12 mo)	Late PVE (>12 mo)	Vascular prosthesis
Coagulase-negative staphylococci	57%	23%	43%
Staphylococcus aureus	7%	11%	8%
Streptococci (nonenterococcal)	1.5%	27%	5.6%
Enterococci	2.8%	9%	2.8%
Diphtheroids	5.5%	2.3%	—
Gram-negative bacilli	4.2%	2.3%	31%
Fastidious gram-negative coccobacilli	1.5%	16%	—
Fungi	5.5%	2.3%	—
Other (including culture negative)	14%	7%	11%

[a] Results adapted from references 78–82.
PVE, prosthetic valve endocarditis.

Patients with PVE caused by *Legionella* species, mycobacteria, and fungi other than *Candida* species commonly present with negative blood cultures when routine techniques are used. Similarly, in patients with PVE resulting from *Coxiella burnetii* (the etiologic agent for Q fever), blood cultures are negative.

Clinical Features of Prosthetic Valve Endocarditis

The features of PVE are, with the exception of more frequent signs of valve dysfunction and myocardial invasion, similar to those of native valve endocarditis. Most patients present with new murmurs and, particularly, congestive heart failure and cerebrovascular complications. A small proportion of patients present with acute fulminant disease with severe hypotension or septic shock associated with infection resulting from *S. aureus* or *Streptococcus pyogenes.*

Diagnosis

Blood cultures, the primary method by which the cause of PVE is established, are positive in 85% to 95% of patients. Because of the continuous nature of bacteremia in endocarditis, one positive blood culture suggests that multiple cultures will be positive, irrespective of body temperature. The documented persistence of bacteremia over an extended time is a clue to the diagnosis of PVE. Negative blood cultures in patients with PVE are seen most commonly when antibiotics have been administered in the recent past.

Prevention

Patients with PVE continue to experience high mortality rates (30%), and about half of the patients require cardiac surgery as an essential element of therapy. The increased hazard of developing PVE during the initial 6 to 12 months after cardiac surgery associated with operative field and bypass equipment contamination and the persistent occurrence of early postoperative infections suggest that prevention efforts should be focused on the perioperative period.

Placebo-controlled trials demonstrated a significant reduction in surgical site infections when prophylactic antibiotics were administered to patients undergoing cardiac surgery. Similar studies have not yet shown a significant reduction in PVE. Prophylactic antibiotic therapy is, however, well accepted as a routine prescription during cardiac valve replacement surgery. The selection of specific regimens for use in this surgery must consider individual hospital flora (e.g., the prevalence of methicillin-resistant *S. aureus*), the common causes of infection during the 6 to 12 months after surgery, the spectrum of antibiotic activity and the potential toxicities of candidate antibiotics, and the demonstrated efficacy of these agents in properly designed and conducted clinical trials.

In addition, specific regimens must be designed so that antibiotic concentrations exceeding the minimum inhibitory concentrations for the expected pathogens are present in tissues before and throughout the surgical procedure. The failure of prophylaxis may relate to inadequate concentrations in serum at the end of prolonged surgery; thus, the pharmacokinetics and dosing of individual agents must be carefully considered. Based on a literature review, Kaiser (93) recommends using cefazolin (1 g intravenously) preoperatively and every 6 hours thereafter for 48 hours. For patients unable to tolerate β-lactam antibiotics, vancomycin (15 mg/kg intravenously) immediately preoperatively and at 10 mg/kg after the initiation of bypass and every 8 hours postoperatively for 48 hours is recommended. In a study, cefazolin tended to be less effective than cefuroxime and cefamandole in preventing surgical site infections after cardiac surgery.

Vancomycin prophylaxis may also be justified in institutions with a high prevalence of methicillin-resistant *S. aureus* infections. The occurrence of a significant proportion of methicillin-resistant coagulase-negative staphylococcal infections also raises the controversial issue of vancomycin use as the primary prophylactic antimicrobial for prosthetic cardiac surgery.

Patients must also be protected against late-onset PVE. Existing problems likely to give rise to transient bacteremia in the future (e.g., existing dental and gingival disease) should be addressed before an elective valve replacement is performed. Regardless of the time elapsed since cardiac surgery, prosthetic valve recipients should always receive prophylactic antibiotics when undergoing procedures that are associated with bacteremia. The most vigorous prophylaxis regimens recommended in the guidelines of the American Heart Association should be followed whenever possible.

Minor bacterial infections (e.g., furuncles and sinusitis) should be considered a significant threat to a prosthetic valve and treated with antibiotics.

Prognostic Factors

Prognostic factors of overall survival in a series of 122 cases of PVE in the intensive care unit were assessed by Wolff et al. (94). Mortality at 4 months was 34%. In *S. aureus* PVE, the following were predictors of death: prothrombin time less than 30%, concomitant mediastinitis, heart failure, and septic shock. In PVE resulting from other pathogens, prothrombin time less than 30%, renal failure, and heart failure were associated with death.

In conclusion, the prognosis for the satisfactory recovery of patients with PVE has improved significantly over the past decades as a consequence of more effective antimicrobial therapy but particularly as a result of prompt aggressive cardiac surgery in which new techniques for valve replacement and annulus repair have been used. The mean fatality rates for patients with infected cardiac valve prostheses was 54.6% in eight studies summarized in 1982 (95). The overall survival rate for patients with PVE now approaches 80% to 90%. Continued efforts are required to refine the medical and surgical treatment of patients with PVE and, equally important, to prevent PVE (89).

Infections Associated with Vascular Grafts

Artificial conduits represent a major advance in vascular reconstructive surgery, but, from the outset, their use was complicated by the occurrence of graft-related infections. The incidence of such infections has declined over the years because of improvements in surgical technique and materials and, perhaps, because of antimicrobial prophylaxis. Nevertheless, infections of vascular prostheses remain a serious problem, because they are associated with substantial morbidity and mortality (96).

The following discussion focuses exclusively on arterial reconstruction with synthetic grafts.

Incidence

The reported incidence of graft infections ranges from less than 1% to greater than 6%; it varies markedly, however, depending on the anatomic site of the prosthesis. The highest incidence has been observed in grafts crossing the inguinal area.

Pathogenesis and Risk Factors for Infection

Most arterial prosthetic infections are thought to arise from contamination at the time of implantation. The high incidence of graft infections in the groin may be due to the superficial location of the graft that favors cutaneous contamination; surgical site infections occurring at this site may secondarily contaminate the prosthesis.

Richet et al. (97) conducted a prospective multicenter study of 561 vascular surgery patients; 23 (4.1%) developed surgical site infections. Independent risk factors for infection included surgery on lower extremities, delayed surgery, diabetes mellitus, past history of vascular surgery, and short-course antimicrobial prophylaxis.

Microbial Etiology

Staphylococci are the most common microorganisms isolated from vascular prosthetic infections followed by gram-negative bacilli (Table 67.5). Goldstone et al. (96) found that *S. aureus* was the leading pathogen recovered from groin infections occurring within 3.5 months of surgery, whereas coagulase-negative staphylococci predominated among groin infections presenting beyond that interval.

Liekweg and Greenfield (98) reviewed data on 164 well-documented cases of vascular prosthetic infection reported through 1974. *S. aureus* was isolated in fully half of these infections. Other microorganisms isolated, either alone or in mixed infections, were *E. coli,* 13.4%; *Streptococcus* species, 8.5%; *Pseudomonas* species, 6.1%; *Klebsiella* species, 5.4%; *Proteus* species, 4.8%; and coagulase-negative staphylococci, 3.6%. There were also rare isolates of micrococci, enterococci, salmonellae, and anaerobes.

A recent report indicated that the prevalence of MRSA infections in these patients is increasing. Infection of aortic grafts with MRSA appears to be fatal, and lower graft infection is associated with high limb loss (99).

Clinical Presentation

Graft infections may occur within the early postoperative period, but some cases do not become evident until a year or more after surgery. The mean interval between surgery and the recognition of infection in 128 cases reviewed by Liekweg and Greenfield (98) was 27 weeks, but 80% of groin infections became apparent within 5 weeks. Only a few late-onset infections appear to be due to hematogenous spread from other body sites.

Infections of vascular grafts may be quite subtle in their presentation. The appearance of low-grade fever or unexplained laboratory indicators of inflammation (leukocytosis and an elevated ESR) in a patient with a vascular graft should prompt consideration of the possibility of infection. Surgical site purulence, graft thrombosis, or hemorrhage are strongly suggestive of infection.

Approximately one half of all infections present as localized surgical site infections, often with a draining sinus, graft exposure, or both. Such a presentation characterizes infections involving femoropopliteal, iliofemoral, or aortofemoral grafts. Infections may involve only a segment of the prosthesis or may spread extensively along its length.

Infections involving the abdominal aorta may be complicated by the escape of intestinal contents resulting from fistula formation. Such fistulas generally involve the duodenum and communicate with either the paraprosthetic tissues or the prosthesis itself. Manifestations are variable, ranging from low-grade fever to gastrointestinal hemorrhage and acute sepsis, often polymicrobial.

Diagnosis and Complications

Positive blood cultures document the presence of intravascular infection and establish the causative pathogen. A variety of noninvasive and invasive procedures may be helpful. These include CT, nuclear MR, ultrasonography, radionuclide gallium or indium scans, sinograms, needle aspiration, and angiography (89).

A blinded retrospective study was performed recently to determine the sensitivity and specificity of CT in detecting perigraft infection and aortoenteric fistula (100). Comparison of CT findings with operative results revealed that each observer correctly identified as abnormal 33 of 35 cases of perigraft infection either with or without aortoenteric fistula (sensitivity 94%) and that results were falsely positive in three cases (specificity 85%). CT findings ranged from large amounts of perigraft soft tissue and ectopic gas to subtle findings of minimal or no abnormalities; thus, strict criteria must be applied to the interpretation of CTs after aortic surgery (100).

An aortoenteric fistula is among the most challenging problems with which a vascular surgeon is confronted. Secondary fistulas occur in about one third of infected grafts. Unfortunately, the preoperative diagnosis of aortoenteric fistula is established in less than one third of patients, despite the fact that as many as two thirds have suggestive signs or symptoms. Many of these patients are clinically unstable, which often limits the evaluation possible before surgery. Many have signs of an infected aortic graft but no evidence of gastrointestinal blood loss, so suspicion of aortoenteric fistula is not entertained.

Prevention

Potential sites of bacteremic seeding (urinary tract infection, dental abscess, etc.) and local infections of ischemic extremities should be eradicated before placement of a bypass graft. During the operative procedure, strict attention should be given to asepsis and to fastidious surgical technique. Although data are limited, prophylactic antibiotics are believed to be responsible, at least in part, for the decline in infection rates associated with the insertion of vascular prostheses. The use of such prophylaxis is now conventional and is similar to that described in prosthetic cardiac valve insertion.

An attractive alternative approach has been to coat the biomaterial with antibiotics. Type 1 collagen, minimally cross-linked, was used to bind one of three antibiotics (amikacin, chloramphenicol, or rifampin) to coulbe-velour Dacron grafts to develop a prosthesis resistant to infection. The graft bonded with rifampin had inhibitory activity for 1 month with a 50% activity eluted at 5 days, significantly better than the preclotted rifampin graft without collagen bonding. These data suggest that rifampin bonded by collagen can protect a vascular graft against infection with *S. aureus* and *S. epidermidis* for up to 3 weeks after implantation (101).

Because of their vascular location, clearly these prostheses are more exposed to bacteremia and, thus, to hematogenous infection. Data are inadequate to allow a determination of the necessity for antimicrobial prophylaxis in patients with arterial prostheses undergoing dental and surgical procedures. The rationale for such prophylaxis is to prevent the development of an infective arteritis. It is, thus, analogous to the prophylaxis recommended to prevent infective endocarditis in patients with prosthetic heart valves. Paradoxically, the incidence of graft infections induced by bacteremia is quite low. Nevertheless, considering the intravascular location of the prosthesis and the severe implications of such an infection, prophylaxis seems reasonable, particularly during the first 4 months postoperatively when experimental data indicate that the graft is most susceptible to bacteremic seeding. If prophylaxis is elected, the regimens suggested by the American Heart Association are applicable (89).

INFECTIONS OF CENTRAL NERVOUS SYSTEM SHUNTS

Neurosurgeons have increasingly used prosthetic devices within the central nervous system (CNS) for a variety of clinical indications such as hydrocephalus or continuous monitoring of intracranial pressure in posttrauma patients under intensive care.

The reported incidence of infections varies greatly, depending on the nature of the intracerebral device and the period of time the prosthesis is in place, but there is also considerable center-to-center variability in the experience with a single device. The reported incidence of CNS shunt infections has varied between 2% and 31%. Infections appear to be more common in infants and in the elderly (102).

Infections often complicate the external ventricular drainage systems used for intracranial pressure monitoring. Mayhall et al. (103) undertook a prospective epidemiologic study of ventriculostomy-related ventriculitis or meningitis in 172 consecutive neurosurgical patients. The rate of infection was 11%. Independent risk factors for infection included neurosurgical operations, intracranial pressure of 20 mm Hg or more, and ventricular catheterization for more than 5 days. Both intracerebral hemorrhage and irrigation of the intracranial catheter predisposed to the development of infection associated with pressure monitors.

Among children, intraventricular hemorrhage and CNS infections as causes of the hydrocephalus were found to be associated with a higher risk of infection, in particular in young (<6 months) infants (104). Surgical revision for shunt malfunction constitutes an additional risk factor. Retained intracranial catheter fragment or foreign body is a rare condition (105) that may result in recurrent infection (106, 107).

Etiology and Pathogenesis

The leading pathogens responsible for infections of indwelling CNS prostheses are coagulase-negative staphylococci. The second most frequent pathogen is *S. aureus.* A variety of other gram-positive microorganisms, including viridans group streptococci, *S. pyogenes,* enterococci, corynebacteria, and propionibacteria, may be involved. Less frequently, *Haemophilus influenzae* and gram-negative enteric bacteria (e.g., *E. coli, Klebsiella* species, and a variety of others) can cause infections. Infection with gram-negative bacilli is observed more frequently in patients with ventriculoureteral or lumboureteral shunts. *Enterococcus gallinarum* infection was recently reported in a patient with multiple ventriculoperitoneal shunts for multiloculated hydrocephalus resulting from complex meningitis (108).

Most infections are presumed to be due to introduction of the microorganism at the time of surgery or to the contamination of the device by ward personnel during manipulation. The pathogenesis of gram-negative cerebrospinal fluid (CSF) shunt infection is not well understood; bacterial contamination during shunt placement is rather unlikely. Bowel perforation leading to distal colonization of the ventriculoperitoneal shunt with subsequent retrograde migration to the brain is the most common mechanism of infection. Other rare intraabdominal complications include gastric or urinary bladder perforation. Shingadia et al. (107) recently described the case of a 3-year-old boy who experienced ten recurrent episodes of gram-negative ventriculoperitoneal shunt infection with genotypically identical strains over 17 months. Ventriculoscopy revealed the presence of a retained foreign body (either a catheter segment or bone wax) that was successfully removed with no further infection occurring thereafter.

The pathogenesis of CSF shunt infection is mostly characterized by staphylococcal adhesion to the polymeric surface of the catheter. Host proteins (mostly fibrinogen, fibronectin, and vitronectin) are adsorbed to the catheter surface immediately after insertion and promote staphylococcal adhesion to the material. The CSF vitronectin level has been found to be elevated in patients with CSF shunt infection, together with activated complement factor C9 on catheters, suggesting that activation of complement close to the device surface may also contribute to the pathogenesis of infection (109).

Clinical Manifestations

The most common presentation of CNS shunt infection is nonspecific, consisting of fever, nausea, vomiting, malaise, or signs of increased intracranial pressure. The latter suggests obstruction or malfunction of the shunt. In most cases, these symptoms appear within a few weeks to months after insertion. Obvious surgical site infection may also be evident, generally in patients who develop infection in the immediate postoperative period. Classic signs of meningeal irritation were present in more than one third of shunt infections in the study of Schoenbaum et al. (110).

In patients with ventriculoperitoneal shunts, an inflammatory exudate may lead to loculation of CSF, resulting in the formation of a peritoneal cyst. These cysts are often palpable in infants and can be visualized by ultrasonography or CT.

At times, patients infected with microorganisms representative of normal skin flora, such as coagulase-negative staphylococci and *Propionibacterium* species (anaerobic diphtheroids), may pursue an extremely indolent clinical course. Such patients may exhibit only intermittent low-grade fever and malaise with little or no change in spinal fluid cell count, glucose, or protein. Under such circumstances, the physician must be careful to differentiate CNS shunt infections from intercurrent viral or bacterial infections of the upper respiratory, urinary, or gastrointestinal tract.

Infections of intracranial pressure-monitoring devices often occur in patients with altered sensorium. Therefore, fever is the most frequent indicator of the presence of infection. Similar to CNS shunt infections, signs of meningeal irritation are usually not present. Clinical diagnosis is further complicated by the fact that these patients are often critically ill and have many other potential sources of infection, both nosocomial and nonnosocomial.

Diagnosis

CSF obtained by lumbar puncture is often not diagnostic of shunt infection. There is usually only a modest inflammatory reaction in the CSF, with an average of 75 to 100 WBCs/mm^3. CSF protein values range from 15 to 925 mg/dL, and there is only a mild degree of hypoglycorrhachia. Because CSF shunt infections are often indolent, the peripheral WBC count may not be elevated.

The procedure of choice for the definitive diagnosis of shunt infection is aspiration of the shunt reservoir or valve to obtain CSF for examination and culture. Cultures of CSF obtained by this technique are almost always positive. By contrast, CSF cultures obtained by lumbar puncture are often negative. CSF cultures were positive in 20 of 21 and in 34 of 36 specimens obtained by direct aspiration of the shunt in two representative series.

At the time of the initial insertion of a ventricular catheter, tissues damage induces some inflammatory reaction including platelet adhesion to silicone rubber. Serum proteins, in particular immunoglobulins, albumin, fibronectin, vitronectin, and fibrinogen, also adhere to the shunt surface (111). These adsorbed proteins can act as opsonins and stimulate macrophages and monocytes to produce growth factors and other cytokines that potentiate the inflammatory response. Most proteins also facilitate initial bacterial adherence. Obstructed catheters are often associated with acute and chronic inflammatory cell infiltrate, in particular lymphocytes, macrophages, and neutrophils, and multinucleate foreign body giant cells. Eosinophils may be detected in CSF samples. Case reports suggest that hypersensitivity to silicone rubber can occur. Wierbitzky et al. (112) examined eosinophils at the time of shunt obstruction or malfunction in a series of 83 children with regard to possible infection. In more than half of the 32 children with more than 4% of eosinophils in the CSF, bacterial growth was documented; there was a correlation between growth of *S. epidermidis* and the occurrence of CSF eosinophilia ($p < .05$), suggesting that the latter might indicate persistent infection.

Patients with infected ventriculojugular-atrial shunts generally have bacteremia and positive blood cultures. For example, in one series, 13 of 17 patients with infected ventriculojugular-atrial shunts had positive blood cultures. In another series, 95% of patients with infected ventriculojugular-atrial shunts from whom blood specimens were obtained had positive cultures. The ventriculoperitoneal shunt apparatus is not in direct contact with the bloodstream and, as such, patients with ventriculoperitoneal shunt infections almost never have positive blood cultures (113).

Epidemiology

The distribution of bacteria in the operating room environment and its relation to ventricular shunt infections has been studied. After routine skin preparation, bacteria were collected by placing Millipore filters on the patient's prepped skin underneath the drapes, on top of the drapes in the operative field, and/or on the sterile instrument table and left in place for the duration of the operation. In 48 patients, full-thickness skin biopsies taken at the initial incision were cultured in lieu of skin surface cultures. Perioperative CSF cultures and subsequent shunt infections were monitored. Of the 288 environmental (skin and surfaces) cultures, 24 were positive (20 coagulase-negative staphylococci and 4 *S. aureus*). Positive environmental cultures were more likely to occur in a room other than the designated neurosurgical operating room. The occurrence of positive environmental cultures correlated with positive CSF cultures, although the microorganisms were not always the same. Coagulase-negative staphylococci were the most common microorganisms isolated from all sites. It was concluded that bacteria most often associated with shunt infections are airborne in the operating room rather than originating from the patient's skin. Furthermore, they are distributed in the highest concentration near the surgical team. Maintaining a designated operating room in which traffic is limited and requiring operating room personnel to observe strict adherence to covering skin surfaces may help to reduce shunt infection rates (102).

Antimicrobial Prophylaxis

Unfortunately, most studies dealing with antimicrobial prophylaxis are uncontrolled, retrospective, and only include a small number of patients. Thus, these studies have led to controversial results and lack of universal guidelines.

As in other types of infections associated with biomaterials, there has been a marked lowering of the incidence of infections associated with the insertion of indwelling CNS prosthetic devices over the past 25 years, presumably as a result of improvements in technique and materials. Nevertheless, infection remains a significant hazard for patients requiring these devices. Most infections are due to gram-positive cocci, particularly *S. epidermidis,* and occur within the first few weeks to months after implantation.

Both accurate diagnosis and appropriate treatment depend on the isolation and identification of the infecting microorganism. However, well-designed controlled trials studying various management strategies are lacking. Likewise, only a few of the numerous reports of antimicrobial prophylaxis for infection of CNS shunts meet generally agreed on criteria for an acceptable clinical trial (114). At present, the efficacy of such prophylaxis remains to be determined (102,115).

Trends in the results of several placebo-controlled prospective studies reported so far justify the use of antibiotic prophylaxis during implantation and revision of artificial catheters for CSF drainage. Langley et al. (114) conducted a meta-analysis to determine the value of antimicrobial prophylaxis in CSF shunt placement. Using stringent criteria, 12 randomized controlled studies were selected representing 1,359 patients. Only one of these trials achieved statistical significance favoring the use of antimicrobial prophylaxis. Prophylaxis was, however, associated with a significant reduction in subsequent infection in the analysis combining the results of the 12 trials (Mantel-Haenszel weighted risk ratio = 0.52, 95% confidence interval 0.37 to 0.73, $p = .0002$), corresponding with a 48% risk reduction.

Based on these and previous data, antimicrobial prophylaxis is strongly recommended for CSF shunt placement. The administration of a single perioperative dose of an antibiotic targeted at the pathogens that most often infect shunts (i.e., *S. epidermidis* and *S. aureus*) is recommended.

Continuous prophylactic antibiotics are widely used for patients with external ventricular drains (EVDs) despite the lack of evidence for such a practice. Some neurosurgeons recommend the use of periprocedural antibiotics only; others use no antibiotic. Ventriculitis is the most significant complication of EVD, affecting from 0% to 27% of patients (103,116). The risk of infection increases during the first 10 days of EVD placement. Most studies examining ventriculostomy-related infection have used prophylactic antibiotics administered for the entire duration of EVD use. Alleyne et al. (116) recently reported the results of a retrospective cohort study in two groups of patients who received cefuroxime (1.5 g every 8 hours) for the entire duration of EVD, that is, an average of 9.2 days compared with cefuroxime given periprocedural only (maximum of 3 doses). The overall rate of ventriculitis (3.9%) was similar in the two groups. Such a low infection rate may be related to the routine intravenous use of antibiotics initiated before the skin was prepared to ensure optimal tissue level at time of catheter placement, routine skin infection with povidone-iodine (Betadine) solution, careful tunneling of the EVD device for at least 4 cm, and the use of a closed drainage and monitoring system. Because the long-term use of antimicrobials may select for resistant microorganisms, we recommend the use of periprocedural antibiotics only; however, their efficacy alone still must be proven in a prospective, randomized control study. (See also Chapters 27 and 49.)

Epidural Catheters

According to the results of a prospective study of 80 epidural catheters used for postoperative analgesia (117), the pathogenesis of epidural catheter-related infection mimics that of intravenous catheters. The incidence of infection was 11% in this series; insertion site infection resulting from coagulase-negative staphylococci assessed by semiquantitative culture of the catheter occurred in most cases (89%) (see Chapter 61).

INFECTION IN BREAST IMPLANTS

Mammary implants are used in breast augmentation and reconstruction after mastectomy. They may be placed above the muscle and deep to the gland (subglandular) or deep to the muscle (submuscular). Surgical approaches are either inframammary, periareolar, or transaxillary. The implants consist of silicone gel contained within a silicone rubber envelope. An alternative design consists of an outer silicone shell filled with saline, glycerides, or soja oil. The latter two have been recently withdrawn from the market. Polyurethane (PUR)-coated breast prostheses have been developed with the hope of diminishing the incidence of capsular contracture. Temporary or permanent tissue expanders, made of silicone envelopes expandable with saline introduced through a remote filling port, are used in breast reconstruction to stretch out overlying skin and muscle.

Incidence and Risk Factors

Infection after breast implant placement is uncommon. Infections were observed in 2.5% of all operations in a worldwide survey of complications in 10,941 patients who underwent breast augmentation (the incidence was 1.7% for acute postoperative and 0.8% for late infections) (118). More recent large epidemiologic retrospective cohort studies with long-term follow-up found similar infection rates, 2% to 2.5% (119,120).

Risk factors for breast implant-associated infection have not been carefully assessed in prospective studies with long-term follow-up. Almost all studies are retrospective, and case series do not permit the identification of risk factors for infection. Surgical technique and the patient's underlying condition constitute the most important determinants. In particular, breast reconstruction after mastectomy and radiotherapy for cancer are associated with a higher risk for infection and other complications after surgery (119). Excellent surgical technique to prevent formation of hematomata and the occurrence of tissue ischemia is mandatory. In contrast to widespread supposition, the rough-surfaced, textured, or PUR-coated implants do not carry a greater susceptibility to infection than smooth silicone implants do (121).

Nipple piercing may constitute an additional risk factor for breast implant infection (122). It was recently described in a 40-year-old woman who opted to have her right nipple pierced 6 months after bilateral breast augmentation. Two weeks after piercing, she presented with unilateral cellulitis of the nipple areola and surrounding skin and further spread of infection around the right breast implant.

Other possible predisposing factors include skin penetrating accidents, general surgery, dental work, pyoderma, preceding infectious processes, breast trauma, breast massage, and breast skin irritation (121).

Microbiology of the Breast

The human breast is not a sterile anatomic structure; it contains endogenous flora derived from the nipple ducts essentially similar to those found in normal skin. Multiple breast ducts provide a passage from the skin surface to deep within the breast tissue. Coagulase-negative staphylococci were isolated from 53% of specimens in women undergoing breast augmentation or reduction (123); a third of the cultures showed no growth. Microorganisms identified were diphtheroids and lactobacilli (9%), *Bacillus* species (5%), and α-hemolytic streptococci (3%). Anaerobic microorganisms were mostly *P. acnes.* Cultures of material milked from the nipples before breast augmentation grew mainly *S. epidermidis* (16/24, 67%) but also *Bacillus subtilis* (2/24) and diphtheroids (2/24) (124).

Clinical Features

Acute Infection

According to published studies, the incidence of postsurgical implant infections is generally low but correlates with the complexity of the surgical condition. Acute postsurgical infection has been encountered in 0% to 4% (118,121,125–135). Most infections occur during the first month after implantation (121). Because of the lack of a consensus on definitions in the literature, it is difficult to obtain exact estimates of the incidence of infection. Acute infections around breast implants are usually associated with fever, rapidly evolving pain, and marked breast erythema (121,136,137); onset occurs between 6 days and 6 weeks after surgery (median, 10 to 12 days) (138). Ultrasound examination confirms the presence of a fluid collection around the breast implant in most cases. Overall, neither the type of implant nor the surgical procedure appears to have a significant influence on the timing of infection (121).

Although the infection rate rarely exceeds 2% to 3% of patients after augmentation mammoplasty, it is sometimes higher after reconstruction. The probability of infection is up to tenfold higher in women with reconstruction and depends on the degree of preexisting tissue scarring and skin atrophy resulting from cancer surgery and radiation therapy (124–126,138–142). Twenty-four percent to 29% of patients developed implant infections in some series (136,143).

De Cholnoky (118) observed that infections were more common after subcutaneous mastectomy with immediate implant placement than with delayed placement. Infection was less likely to occur in a two-stage procedure in another series (144). In contrast, infection occurred with equal frequency in both the immediate and delayed groups in the series reported by Slavin and Colen in 1990 (145). One hypothesis is that in immediate reconstruction, there is no time for host defense mechanisms to cleanse the tissue of bacteria before the insertion of the prosthesis. With delayed reconstruction, there has been time for bacteria to have been removed from the tissue. The time of implant placement is another important parameter possibly related with an increased risk for infection. Reconstruction, which is performed after mastectomy and axillary node dissection have been performed, may be associated with a higher rate of infection. Furthermore, unlike augmentation surgery, reconstructive surgery is associated with a higher incidence of hematoma and delayed scarring because of the extension of the dissection and secondary skin ischemia. Finally, the use of tissue expanders at the time of immediate reconstruction, especially in the case in which there is to be surgery of the contralateral breast, should be undertaken with caution (136).

In patients with reconstruction and revision, the adhesive bandage of the surgical site dressing may cause a severe contact dermatitis at the surgical site, paving the way for infection of the skin and implant. In this condition, the causative microorganisms included Enterobacteriaceae and *P. aeruginosa* in one series (121).

Toxic shock syndrome after the placement of mammary prostheses is another form of acute infection. In 1983, Barnett et al. (146) reported a 32-year-old woman who had periareolar subglandular placement of double lumen implants and developed sore throat with fever to 39°C, watery diarrhea, myalgias, lethargy, and a rash on the extremities on the fourth postoperative day. On day 7, the rash extended, and the patient developed hypotension and acute respiratory distress syndrome. Although there were no overt signs of infection, both prostheses were removed; purulent material was found around the right prosthesis, which grew *S. aureus.* The patient received broad-spectrum antibiotic coverage and gradually stabilized. Since then, there have been several reports of toxic shock syndrome after breast implant surgery (147,148). In all of the cases, *S. aureus* infection was acquired perioperatively. Median interval between surgery and toxic shock syndrome was 4 days (148). The symptoms may begin in the first 12 to 24 hours after surgery; this is much earlier than the usual surgical site infection. The primary surgical site is rarely impressive, and there is usually neither inflammation nor purulence. The surgical site, when opened, typically harbors a seroma that grows exotoxin toxic shock syndrome toxin-1 (TSST-1) producing *S. aureus.* Early recognition and implant removal is life saving.

An additional case of possible toxic shock syndrome that developed 11 days following elective removal of bilateral breast implants and open capsulectomies has been described (149). The infection most likely resulted from an infected hematoma and possible extracapsular silicone granulomas.

Implant-associated infections caused by nontuberculous mycobacteria have been documented in 15 cases in six states in the United States and were implicated in dozens more. The syndrome of late-developing, massive, odorless, severe effusion with negative routine cultures may suggest requesting special acid-fast cultures and stains. Nontuberculous mycobacteria have been recovered from silastic lens prostheses, porcine valves, and sterile saline. They have a wide distribution including soil, water, hospital and operating room water conduits, and dust. Infections resulting from nontuberculous mycobacteria probably were acquired intraoperatively, with a median time of 28 days after surgery in one series (150). This is, however, a rare event. In a questionnaire to 2,734 plastic surgeons covering 12 months in 1978, the overall rate of infection was 254 in 39,455 breast augmentations (0.64 per 100 operations), and nontuberculous mycobacteria were recovered in only 5 (0.013 per 100 operations).

In a follow-up study (151), the authors reported the clinical and epidemiologic features of 17 cases of periprosthetic nontuberculous mycobacteria (*Myocbacterium fortuitum* and *Mycobacterium chelonae*) infection over 3.5 years. Most cases (n = 11) were reported from four surgical practices in Florida and Texas. In all cases the breast implant was removed. Thirty-seven additional cases associated with augmentation mammaplasty identified between 1979 and 1988 were reported by Wallace et al. (152); 19 of 35 isolates revealed different phenotypes. Rapidly growing nontuberculous mycobacterial surgical site infection occurring after cosmetic surgery and breast implantation in particular are reported regularly (153,154). In most cases, it is difficult to ascertain the source of contamination; a skin marking solution was identified as a possible source in one investigation (155). (See also Chapter 38.)

Late Infection

The knowledge concerning late infections that occur months or years after implantation is mostly anecdotal. In the absence of a mammary implant registry, it proves very difficult to collect comprehensive data. Moreover, because of the length of intervening time, patients with late infection may not be seen by the surgeons who performed the implantation; as participants in a survey, they obviously are not in the position to report such patients (121). Nevertheless, we believe that several useful conclusions can be drawn from our current analysis of the literature.

In view of the numerous women who presently carry mammary implants, the question of late infection and its prevention is of particular importance. Such infections rarely occurred in the survey of 10,941 patients with breast augmentation (0.8%) (118). There were 27 observations with the smooth-surface implants a few months to several years after operation.

Late infection usually results from a secondary bacteremia, an infection at another site, or an invasive procedure. Case reports are illustrative. A patient with breast augmentation developed a sty in one eye 8 months after implantation and noticed the signs of inflammation in one of her breasts 3 days later (121). The implant was removed and found to be infected with *S. epidermidis.* Another patient with augmentation contracted a hemorrhagic cystitis caused by *P. aeruginosa* 2.5 years after implantation that spread within a few days to the implant site (121). A bilateral infection occurred suddenly 1.5 years after insertion of breast prostheses and was presumed to be related to an infected molar tooth (118). Another prosthesis became infected 3 years after insertion, presumably after an axillary hydradenitis (156). Another patient with reconstruction lost her implant because of *S. aureus* infection 7 months after surgery, immediately after a severe bacterial stomatitis (121). Other examples of late breast implant infections include conditions as diverse as *Clostridium perfringens* infection after extensive dental treatment (157); *Klebsiella pneumoniae* infection following breast augmentation combined with abdominoplasty (158); *Enterococcus avium* infection that developed 16 years after implantation (159); infection resulting from *Bacteroides fragilis* occurring 6 weeks after peritonitis resulting from colonic perforation 40 years after augmentation mammaplasty (160); breast implant infection in a human immunodeficiency virus (HIV) patient with disseminated *Mycobacterium avium* complex infection (161); breast implant infection caused by *Pasteurella multocida* in a 47-year-old woman who owned several cats and cared for them closely during the recovery period (162); and other unusual infections resulting from *Brucella* species (163), *Listeria* species (164), *Trichosporon beigelii* (165), or *Candida albicans* (166).

A major conclusion from these reports is that the probability of late implant infection has been shown to be low. Nevertheless, implant carriers should understand that any implant site may act as a trap for bacteria, particularly when bloodstream infections occur. As a consequence, any potentially severe bacterial infection anywhere in the body should be recognized as early as possible and treated with systemic antibiotics promptly and aggressively if one wishes to cut down on these rare late implant infections. Likewise, invasive dental or surgical procedures, especially when performed under septic conditions, should possibly be performed with antibiotic prophylaxis.

The possibility of local bacterial invasion along the milk ducts must be kept in mind. A total of 139 implants from 72 consecutive symptomatic patients were entered into a prospective clinical study (137). The most common local implant symptoms were breast pain (93%), capsular contracture (91%), axillary pain (39%), and upper extremity paresthesia (29%). Almost half (47%) of the implants were culture positive; *P. acnes* was isolated most frequently (57%), followed by *S. epidermidis* (41%) and *E. coli* (1.5%). No fungal infection was identified. The average age of culture-positive implants was 12.2 years. The rate of culture positivity was similar in reconstruction patients as compared with the augmentation group. In the culture-positive group, axillary pain and skin rash were identified at a significantly higher frequency compared with the culture-negative group. There were no significant differences for other local symptoms, including breast pain and capsular contracture. Culture positivity was not significantly associated with systemic symptoms (including fatigue, arthralgias, or fibromyalgia), the number implant surgeries, or implant localization (121).

Low-Grade Infection and Capsular Contracture

Formation of an acellular collagenous sheath around an inert foreign material usually follows the placement of a prosthesis. However, contracture of this scar around a soft deformable implant will lead to a hard spherical mass; this type of envelope is referred to as a capsule. Factors thought to be associated with capsular contracture include infection, hematoma, silicone bleed, and individual predisposition for hypertrophic scarring. Implant filler material (silicone, saline, bilumen), placement (submuscular, subglandular, subcutaneous), and surface texture might also affect the risk of capsular contracture (167).

A current hypothesis for the possible origin of capsular contracture around breast implants is that it may be caused by a low-grade or subclinical infection that can be prevented by antibiotics (168–170). Some studies suggest that the endogenous flora of the breast is most likely responsible for breast infections after surgery and may be associated with fibrous contracture of the breast after subglandular augmentation (118,128–130).

Studies of implant patients have shown that many (20% to 60%) implant pockets are culture positive, most often with *S. epidermidis* (170), which frequently correlates with and may cause capsular contracture (169,170). Cultures performed at the time of surgical capsulotomy were frequently positive, predominantly growing *S. epidermidis* and *P. acnes* (169,171,172). Based on this finding, these authors began to use antibiotics in the implant pocket (169) or in the implants themselves (171) with a decreased incidence of capsular contracture. The possible benefit of local povidone-iodine irrigation at time of implant placement with or without intraprosthetic cephalothin or antibiotic-steroid foam irrigation has been suggested by Burkhardt et al. (171). In a prospective controlled study of 124 patients undergoing breast augmentation an overall 50% reduction in capsule formation was observed in the treatment groups. The practice of breast-pocket irrigation with various antimicrobial solutions, in particular povidone-iodine, is supported by some data and extensive clinical practice among most plastic surgeons (173). The recent and controversial decision in 2000 by the Food and Drug Administration (FDA) in the United States that contact of any breast implant with povidone-iodine is contraindicated (because povidone-iodine may be associated with deflation of saline-filled prostheses in a small proportion of patients) is troublesome and places surgeons who continue to use it at medicolegal risk. Among several antibiotic-containing solutions, only the combination of bacitracin (or vancomycin), cefazolin, and gentamicin proved to be as efficacious *in vitro.* The clinical effectiveness of the procedure and the impact of its use on possible resistance acquisition remain to be tested (173).

However, the source of bacteria may be the skin or breast ducts (124). Ransjö et al. (174) found that the female breast contained bacteria in more than 80% of samples. It was suggested that these bacteria might play a role in the development of capsular contracture. Bacterial isolates were mostly coagulase-negative staphylococci in aerobic and propionibacteria in anaerobic cultures. Experimental studies by Shah et al. (170) in which implant capsules in rabbits were deliberately seeded with *S. epidermidis* demonstrated increased hardness and thickness of the capsule. Intraluminal antibiotics reduced capsule hardness in this rabbit model. Similarly, minocycline and rifampin impregnated, saline-filled silicone implants were less likely to be colonized and cause *S. aureus* infection than unimpregnated implants when inserted subcutaneously in another rabbit model (175). However, the clinical effectiveness and the potential for resistance development need further study before such strategies may be used in human medicine.

Although possible adverse effects of microorganisms have been implicated in symptomatic breast implant patients, the clinical relevance of microbial colonization on implant surfaces removed from symptomatic patients and its possible impact on integrity remain unclear. In a prospective evaluation of 139 implants from 72 symptomatic patients, Ahn et al. (172) found that 47% of implants were culture-positive (mostly *P. acnes,* 56%, and *S. epidermidis,* 41%) and that 47% of the culture-positive implants were intact and 33% ruptured. Culture positivity was not significantly associated with symptoms.

A prospective outcome study was conducted on 100 consecutive patients who requested explantation of their silicone gel breast implants after January 6, 1992 (the moratorium) (176). All patients were extensively evaluated preoperatively and postoperatively. The mean duration of implantation was 12 years. At time of explantation, 25% of the capsules were calcified; 42% were culture-positive. The prevalence of higher grade capsular contracture (classes III to V) was 61%; it was related to implant location, duration *in situ,* and capsular calcification ($p < .05$) but not to capsular colonization or implant integrity. Thus, more research must be conducted to understand the possible relation between bacterial colonization and breast implant capsular contracture.

Prophylactic Antibiotics

The need for prophylaxis in breast surgery is controversial. Although most experts do not recommend prophylaxis routinely for breast procedures, they do recommend prophylaxis in cases of implant placement.

Brand (121) reported the results of a large survey (54,661 implants) of a group of 73 plastic surgeons with long-term experience in mammary augmentation and reconstruction. Most respondents adhered routinely to one or both of the following two prophylactic measures: systemic administration of antibiotic (most commonly a cephalosporin) starting before surgery and continuing for up to 1 week after implantation and irrigation of the surgical pocket and rinsing of the implant before insertion in a solution containing either an antiseptic or an antibiotic (cephalosporin, bacitracin, neosporin, etc). In the absence of a control group, the effectiveness of these measures cannot be ascertained.

Systemic antibiotic prophylaxis at the time of surgery was associated with a significant reduction of the infection rate (0.42% vs. 0.87%) in a large study of 39,455 patients undergoing breast augmentation (132). The prophylactic regimen should be directed against the most likely infecting microorganisms, in particular staphylococci. A single dose, given just before the procedure, provides adequate tissue concentrations throughout the operation. In case of a prolonged procedure or important blood loss, we recommend a second dose. First- or second-generation cephalosporins are the most widely used antibiotics for this indication. In this context, some authors have proposed incorporation of an antibiotic in the expander fluid (177). Cephalothin and gentamicin placed within the lumen of inflatable breast implants *in vitro* have been shown to diffuse outward through the silicone shell. The use of intraluminal cephalothin and gentamicin *in vivo* has significantly reduced the incidence of capsular contracture after both primary breast augmentation and secondary open capsulotomy (168).

Several authors recommend antibiotic prophylaxis be given beforehand when a patient with breast implants is to have any dental procedure. It must be stressed, however, that there is no scientific evidence at the present to support such a recommendation.

CONCLUSIONS: TOWARD PREVENTING MEDICAL DEVICE-ASSOCIATED INFECTIONS

The growing need for and the increasing use of prosthetic materials and implanted medical devices of all kinds have led to technical improvement not only of materials but also of the implantation techniques. Thus, complication rates have decreased over the years, as has the incidence of infections. Surgeons have become more cognizant of the danger of infections associated with foreign bodies, and their prevention has become a major priority for the medical community.

Overall, three major strategies have been developed to prevent these complications: a sterile environment, better operating procedures, and the appropriate use of antibacterial agents. Only the latter lends itself to a well-controlled, randomized, and double-blinded clinical trial. Thus, many improvements in the setting of medical device complications seem to reflect improved medical or surgical practice, without proof based on randomized studies. Thus far, sterile environment and different quality of surgical procedures can hardly be randomized.

The role of antibiotic prophylaxis in preventing implant-associated infections has now been firmly established for a variety of prostheses. Even so, no regimen can be considered as foolproof, and it has to be understood that even the best antibiotic is probably insufficient in the presence of a high bacterial inoculum and/or improper surgical practice. So far, systemic antibiotic prophylaxis has proven efficacy for prosthetic heart valve replacement, orthopedic prosthesis implantation (hip and knee), and insertion of vascular prostheses; in these conditions, systemic antibiotics decrease the risk of early infections. To extrapolate from these results to other procedures, several factors have to be taken into account, which have been demonstrated to be important either in the previously named studies or in experimental models. These encompass, among others, the timing of administration (the foreign material has to be inserted into tissues soaked with the appropriate antibiotic), the dosage and route of administration and pharmacokinetics and tissue penetration (adequate tissue levels of antibiotics probably must be sustained for 6 to 12 hours after the procedure), and the type of infecting microorganism. (By definition, no prophylaxis can take into consideration all likely microorganisms and resistance patterns.) With these simple concepts, new clinical and experimental studies can be conceived for alternative and expanded programs regarding other prosthetic infections.

There is, however, room for many new and imaginative studies in this field. The role of antibiotics incorporated into orthopedic devices, vascular grafts, ventricular shunts, prosthetic heart valves, and, in particular, intravascular catheters must be better defined. Local liberation of stable antibiotic by novel devices must be investigated. Incorporation of other antibacterial substances, such as silver impregnation, bonding of copolymers with antiseptic agents, and quaternary amines containing organosilicons, must be explored further. With the ultimate goal of total sterility, these strategies should find access to clinical use in the near future.

Finally, the materials used for medical devices are presently under intense investigation. Without conceiving new materials—because many of the presently available materials have shown excellent mechanical qualities—their surfaces may be altered to create a more physiologic interface with the host tissue. Changes in surface characteristics such as roughness, surface charge, and adhesive properties for host proteins and/or bacteria, may be another means to decrease infection rates. Finally, masking of adherence—sites of host proteins deposited on foreign surfaces—may prevent initial adherence of the microorganisms, making them easy prey for activated phagocytes. Clearly, this will continue to be an area for high priority not only for the field of infectious diseases but also for biotechnology.

REFERENCES

1. Dankert J, Hogt AH, Feijen J. Biomedical polymers: bacterial adhesion, colonization and infection. *CRC Crit Rev Biocompatib* 1986;2:219–301.
2. Sugarman B, Young EJ. *Infections associated with prosthetic devices.* Boca Raton, FL: CRC Press, 1984:1–285.
3. Young EJ, Sugarman B. Introduction to prosthetic devices and their regulation in the united states. In: Young EJ, Sugarman B, eds. *Infections associated with prosthetic devices.* Boca Raton, FL: CRC Press, 1984:1–10.
4. Bisno AL, Waldvogel FA. *Infections associated with indwelling medical devices,* 2nd ed. Washington, DC: American Society for Microbiology, 1994:1–398.
5. Vaudaux P, Lew DP, Waldvogel FA. Host factors predisposing to foreign body infections. In: Bisno AL, Waldvogel FA, eds. *Infections associated with indwelling medical devices.* Washington, DC: American Society for Microbiology, 1989:3–26.
6. Kudryk BJ, Grossman ZD, McAfee JG, et al. Monoclonal antibodies as probes for fibrin(ogen) proteolysis. In: Chatal JF, ed. *Monoclonal antibodies in immunoscintigraphy.* Boca Raton, FL: CRC Press, 1989:365–398.
7. Francis CW, Marder VJ. A molecular model of plasmic degradation of crosslinked fibrin. *Semin Thromb Hemost* 1982;8:25–35.
8. Doolittle RF. Fibrinogen and fibrin. *Annu Rev Biochem* 1984;53:195–229.
9. Vaudaux P, Pittet D, Haeberli A, et al. Fibronectin is more active than fibrin or fibrinogen in promoting *Staphylococcus aureus* adherence to inserted intravascular catheters. *J Infect Dis* 1993;167:633–641.
10. Brown EJ, Goodwin JL. Fibronectin receptors of phagocytes. Characterization of the arg-gly-asp binding proteins of human monocytes and polymorphonuclear leukocytes. *J Exp Med* 1988;167:777–793.
11. Herrmann M, Vaudaux P, Pittet D, et al. Fibronectin, fibrinogen and laminin act as mediators of adherence of clinical staphylococcal isolates to foreign material. *J Infect Dis* 1988;158:693–701.
12. Christensen GD, Baddour LM, Hasty DL, et al. Microbial and foreign body factors in the pathogenesis of medical device infections. In: Bisno AL, Waldvogel FA, eds. *Infections associated with indwelling medical devices.* Washington, DC: American Society for Microbiology, 1989:27–59.
13. Nilsson M, Frykberg L, Flock J, Pei L, et al. A fibrinogen-binding protein of *Staphylococcus epidermidis. Infect Immun* 1998;66:2666–2673.
14. Chuard C, Lucet EC, Rohner P, et al. Resistance of *Staphylococcus aureus* recovered from infected foreign body in vivo to killing by antimicrobials. *J Infect Dis* 1991;163:1369–1373.
15. Chuard C, Vaudaux PE, Proctor RA, et al. Decreased susceptibility to antibiotic killing of a stable small colony variant of *Staphylococcus aureus* in fluid phase and on fibronectin-coated surfaces. *J Antimicrob Chemother* 1997;39:603–608.
16. Vesga O, Groeschel MC, Otten MF, et al. *Staphylococcus aureus* small colony variants are induced by the endothelial cell intracellular milieu. *J Infect Dis* 1996;173:739–742.
17. Lew DP, Zubler R, Vaudaux P, et al. Decreased heat-labile opsonic activity and complement levels associated with evidence of C3 breakdown products in infected pleural effusions. *J Clin Invest* 1979;63:326–334.
18. Zimmerli W, Lew DP, Waldvogel FA. Pathogenesis of foreign body infection. Evidence for a local granulocyte defect. *J Clin Invest* 1984;73:1191–1200.
19. Herrmann M, Jaconi MEE, Dahlgren C, et al. Neutrophil bactericidal activity against *Staphylococcus aureus* adherent on biological surfaces. *J Clin Invest* 1990;86:942–951.
20. Vaudaux P, Grau GE, Huggler E, et al. Contribution of tumor necrosis factor to host defense against staphylococci in a guinea pig model of foreign body infections. *J Infect Dis* 1992;166:58–64.
21. Peters G, Gray ED, Johnson GM. Immunomodulating properties of extracellular slime substance. In: Bisno AL, Waldvogel FA, eds. *Infections associated with indwelling medical devices.* Washington, DC: American Society for Microbiology, 1989:61–74.
22. Brause BD. Infected orthopedic protheses. In: Bisno AL, Waldvogel FA, eds. *Infections associated with indwelling medical devices.* Washington, DC: American Society for Microbiology, 1989:111–127.
23. Salvati EA, Small RD, Brause BD, et al. Infections associated with orthopedic devices. In: Sugarman B, Young EJ, eds. *Infections associated with prosthetic devices.* Boca Raton, FL: CRC Press, 1984:181–218.
24. Fitzgerald RH Jr. Total hip arthroplasty sepsis—prevention and diagnosis. *Orthop Clin North Am* 1992;23:259–264.
25. Cuckler JM, Star AM, Alavi A, et al. Diagnosis and management of the infected total joint arthroplasty. *Orthop Clin North Am* 1992;22:523–530.
26. Rasul AT Jr, Tsukayama D, Gustilo RB. Effect of time of onset and depth of infection on the outcome of total knee arthroplasty infections. *Clin Orthop* 1991;273:98–104.
27. Sanderson PJ. Infection in orthopaedic implants. *J Hosp Infect* 1991;18(Suppl A):367–375.
28. Gordon SM, Culver DH, Simmons BP, et al. Risk factors for wound infections after total knee arthroplasty. *Am J Epidemiol* 1990;131:905–916.
29. Nasser S. Prevention and treatment of sepsis in total hip replacement surgery. *Orthop Clin North Am* 1992;23:265–277.
30. Charnley J. Postoperative infection after total hip replacement with special reference to air contamination in the operating room. *Clin Orthop* 1972;87:167–187.
31. Steckelberg JM, Osmon DR. Prosthetic joint infections. In: Bisno AL, Waldvogel FA, eds. *Infections associated with indwelling medical devices,* 2nd ed. Washington, DC: American Society for Microbiology, 1994:259–290.
32. Fernandez Arjona M, Gomez-Sancha F, Peinado Ibarra F, et al. Risk infection factors in the total hip replacement. *Eur J Epidemiol* 1997;13:443–446.
33. Espehaug B, Havelin LI, Engesaeter LB, et al. Patient-related risk factors for early revision of total hip replacements. A population register-based case-control study of 674 revised hips. *Acta Orthop Scand* 1997;68:207–215.
34. Murray RP, Bourne MH, Fitzgerald RH Jr. Metachronous infections in patients who have had more than one total joint arthroplasty. *J Bone Joint Surg [Am]* 1991;73A:1469–1474.
35. Perhala RS, Wilke WS, Clough JD, et al. Local infectious complications following large joint replacement in rheumatoid arthritis patients treated with methotrexate versus those not treated with methotrexate [see comments]. *Arthritis Rheum* 1991;34:146–152.
36. Maderazo EG, Judson S, Pasternak H. Late infections of total joint prostheses. A review and recommendations for prevention. *Clin Orthop* 1988;131–142.
37. Schmalzried TP, Amstutz HC, Au M, et al. Etiology of deep sepsis in

total hip arthroplasty: the significance of hematogenous and recurrent infections. *Clin Orthop* 1992;280:200–207.
38. Buchholz HW, Elson RA, Englebrecht E, et al. Management of deep infection of total hip replacement. *J Bone Joint Surg* 1981;63B: 342–353.38a. Buccholz K, von Foerster G. Infection in artificial joint replacement. *Krankenpfl J* 1984;22:4–6.38b. Fitzgerald RH Jr, Jones DR. Hip implant infection. Treatment with resection—arthroplasty and late total hip arthroplasty. *Am J Med* 1985;78:225–228.
39. Gillespie WJ. Infection in total joint replacement. *Infect Dis Clin North Am* 1990;4:465–484.
40. Windsor RE. Management of total knee arthroplasty infection. *Orthop Clin North Am* 1992;22:531–538.
41. Whyte W, Hodgson R, Tinkler J, et al. The isolation of bacteria of low pathogenicity from faulty orthopaedic implants. *J Hosp Infect* 1981;2:219–230.
42. Dupont JA. Significance of operative cultures in total hip arthroplasty. *Clin Orthop* 1986;211:122–127.
43. Lidwell OM, Lowbury EJ, Whyte W, et al. Bacteria isolated from deep joint sepsis after operation for total hip or knee replacement and the sources of the infections with *Staphylococcus aureus. J Hosp Infect* 1983;4:19–29.
44. Tietjen R, Stinchfield FE, Michelsen CB. The significance of intracapsular cultures in total hip operations. *Surg Gynecol Obstet* 1977;144: 699–702.
45. Sorensen AI, Sorensen TS. Bacterial growth on suction drain tips. Prospective study of 489 clean orthopedic operations. *Acta Orthop Scand* 1991;62:451–454.
46. Benoni G, Fredin H. Low- or high-vacuum drains in hip arthroplasty? a randomized study of 73 patients. *Acta Orthop Scand* 1997;68: 133–137.
47. Kim Y, Cho S, Kim R. Drainage versus nondrainage in simultaneous bilateral total knee arthroplasties. *Clin Orthop* 1998;347:188–193.
48. Roberts P, Walters AJ, McMinn DJW. Diagnosing infection in hip replacements. The use of fine-needle aspiration and radiometric culture. *J Bone Joint Surg [Br]* 1992;74B:265–269.
49. Thorén B. Erythrocyte sedimentation rate in infection of total hip replacements. *Orthopedics* 1991;14:495–497.
50. Sanzen L, Sundberg M. Periprosthetic low-grade hip infections. Erythrocyte sedimentation rate and c-reactive protein in 23 cases. *Acta Orthop Scand* 1997;68:461–465.
51. Malghem J, Mosseray A, Vande Berg B, et al. Radiologic aspects of the loosening of cemented hip prostheses: mechanical, septic or granulomatous etiology?. *J Belge Radiol* 1997;80:173–184.
52. Alazraki NP. Diagnosing prosthetic joint infection [editorial; comment]. *J Nucl Med* 1990;31:1955–1957.
53. Palestro CJ, Swyer AJ, Kim CK, et al. Infected knee prosthesis: diagnosis with In-111 leukocyte, Tc-99m sulfur colloid, and Tc-99m MDP imaging. *Radiology* 1991;179:645–648.
54. Palestro CJ, Kim CK, Swyer AJ, et al. Total-hip arthroplasty: periprosthetic indium-111-labeled leukocyte activity and complementary technetium-99m-sulfur colloid imaging in suspected infection [see comments]. *J Nucl Med* 1990;31:1950–1955.
55. Lopitaux R, Levai JP, Raux P, et al. Value of puncture-arthrography in the diagnosis of infection of total hip arthroplasty (in French). *Rev Chir Orthop Reparatrice Appar Mot* 1992;78:34–37.
56. O'Neill DA, Harris WH. Failed total replacement: assessment by plain radiographs, arthrograms, and aspiration of the hip joint. *J Bone Joint Surg* 1984;66A:540–546.
57. Perdreau-Remington F, Rank DR, Lopez FA, et al. Identifying multiple isolates through the comparison of genomic DNAs in a patient with infected hip prosthesis. *West J Med* 1998;168:128–130.
58. Levitsky KA, Hozack WJ, Balderston RA, et al. Evaluation of the painful prosthetic joint. Relative value of bone scan, sedimentation rate, and joint aspiration. *J Arthroplasty* 1991;6:237–244.
59. Chimento GF, Finger S, Barrack RL. Gram stain detection of infection during revision arthroplasty. *J Bone Joint Surg [Br]* 1996;78B: 838–839.
60. Lonner JH, Desai P, Dicesare PE, et al. The reliability of analysis of intraoperative frozen sections for identifying active infection during revision hip or knee arthroplasty. *J Bone Joint Surg [Am]* 1996;78: 1553–1558.
60a. Widmer AF. New developments in diagnosis and treatment of infection in orthopedic implants. *Clin Infect Dis* 2001;33(Suppl 2):594.
61. Zimmerli W, Waldvogel FA, Vaudaux P, et al. Pathogenesis of foreign body infection: description and characteristics of an animal model. *J Infect Dis* 1982;146:487–497.
62. Bouchenaki N, Vaudaux P, Huggler E, et al. Successful single-dose prophylaxis of *Staphylococcus aureus* foreign body infection in guinea pigs by fleroxacin. *Antimicrob Agents Chemother* 1990;34:21–24.
63. Waldvogel FA, Vaudaux P, Pittet D, et al. Perioperative antibiotic prophylaxis of wound and foreign body infections: microbial factors affecting efficacy. *Rev Infect Dis* 1991;13:S782–S789.
64. Tshefu K, Zimmerli W, Waldvogel FA. Short-term administration of rifampin in the prevention or eradication of infection due to foreign bodies. *Rev Infect Dis* 1983;5(Suppl):S474–S480.
65. Norden CW. Antibiotic prophylaxis in orthopedic surgery. *Rev Infect Dis* 1991;13:S842–S846.
66. Hirschmann JV. Antibiotics in the prevention of infection associated with prosthetic devices. In: Sugarman B, Young EJ, eds. *Infections associated with prosthetic devices.* Boca Raton, FL: CRC Press, 1984: 269–278.
67. Hill C, Flamant R, Mazas F, et al. Prophylactic cefazolin versus placebo in total hip replacement. Report of a multicentre double-blind randomised trial. *Lancet* 1981;1:795–796.
68. Lidwell OM, Lowbury EJL, Whyte W, et al. Effect of ultraclean air in operating rooms on deep sepsis in the joint after total hip or knee replacement: a randomized study. *BMJ* 1982;285:10–14.
69. Lidwell OM, Elson RA, Lowbury EJ, et al. Ultraclean air and antibiotics for prevention of postoperative infection. A multicenter study of 8,052 joint replacement operations. *Acta Orthop Scand* 1987;58: 4–13.
70. Klenerman L, Seal D, Sullens K. Combined prophylactic effect of ultraclean air and cefuroxime for reducing infection in prosthetic surgery. *Acta Orthop Belg* 1991;57:19–24.
71. Schutzer SF, Harris WH. Deep-wound infection after total hip replacement under contemporary aseptic conditions. *J Bone Joint Surg [Am]* 1988;70:724–727.
72. Blomgren G, Hoborn J, Nystrom B. Reduction of contamination at total hip replacement by special working clothes. *J Bone Joint Surg [Br]* 1990;72:985–987.
73. Isacson J, Collert S. Renal impairment after high doses of dicloxacillin prophylaxis in joint replacement surgery. *Acta Orthop Scand* 1984; 55:407–410.
74. Hedstrom SA, Hybbinette CH. Nephrotoxicity in isoxazolyl penicillin prophylaxis in hip surgery. *Acta Orthop Scand* 1988;59:114–117.
75. Bryan CS, Morgan SL, Caton RJ, et al. Cefazolin versus cefamandole for prophylaxis during total joint arthroplasty. *Clin Orthop* 1988;228: 117–122.
76. Pollard JP, Hughes SPF, Scott JE, et al. Antibiotic prophylaxis in total hip replacement. *BMJ* 1979;1:707–709.
77. Hill C, Flamant R, Mazas F, et al. Prophylactic cefazolin versus placebo in total hip replacement. Report of a multicentre double-blind randomized trial. *Lancet* 1981;1:795–797.
78. Nelson CL, Green TG, Porter RA, et al. One day versus seven days of preventive antibiotic therapy in orthopedic surgery. *Clin Orthop* 1983;176:258–263.
79. Classen DC, Evans RS, Pestotnik SL, et al. The timing of prophylactic administration of antibiotics and the risk of surgical-wound infection [see comments]. *N Engl J Med* 1992;326:281–286.
80. Wahlig H, Hameister W, Grieben A. Uber die freisetzung von gentamycin aus polymethylmethacryalat. I. Experimentelle untersuchungen in vitro. *Langenbecks Arch Chir* 1972;331:169–192.
81. Lynch M, Esser MP, Shelley P, et al. Deep infection in Charnley low-friction arthroplasty. Comparison of plain and gentamicin-loaded cement. *J Bone Joint Surg* 1987;69A:355–360.
82. Trippel SB. Antibiotic-impregnated cement in total joint arthroplasty. *J Bone Joint Surg* 1986;68A:1297–1302.
83. McQueen MM, Hughes SP, May P, et al. Cefuroxime in total joint

arthroplasty. Intravenous or in bone cement. *J Arthroplasty* 1990;5: 169–172.

84. Espehaug B, Engesaeter LB, Vollset SE, et al. Antibiotic prophylaxis in total hip arthroplasty. Review of 10,905 primary cemented total hip replacements reported to the Norwegian arthroplasty register, 1987 to 1995. *J Bone Joint Surg [Br]* 1997;79:590–595.
85. Deacon JM, Pagliaro AJ, Zelicof SB, et al. Prophylactic use of antibiotics for procedures after total joint replacement. *J Bone Joint Surg [Am]* 1996;78:1755–1770.
86. Jacobson JJ, Schweitzer SO, Kowalski CJ. Chemoprophylaxis of prosthetic joint patients during dental treatment: a decision-utility analysis. *Oral Surg Oral Med Oral Pathol* 1991;72:167–177.
87. Tservat J, Durand-Zaleski I, Pauker SG. Cost-effectiveness of antibiotic prophylaxis for dental procedures in patients with artificial joints. *Am J Public Health* 1989;79:739–743.
88. Harris RL, Wilson WR, Williams TW. Infections associated with prosthetic heart valves. In: Sugarman B, Young EJ, eds. *Infections associated with prosthetic devices.* Boca Raton, FL: CRC Press, 1984: 89–112.
89. Karchmer AW, Bisno AL. Infections of prosthetic heart valves and vascular grafts. In: Bisno AL, Waldvogel FA, eds. *Infections associated with indwelling medical devices.* Washington, DC: American Society for Microbiology, 1989:129–159.
90. Calderwood S, Swinski L, Waternaux C. Risk factors for the development of prosthetic valve endocarditis. *Circulation* 1985;72:31–37.
91. Ivert TSA, Dismukes WE, Cobbs CG, et al. Prosthetic valve endocarditis. *Circulation* 1984;69:223–232.
92. Agnihotri AK, McGiffin DC, Galbraith AJ, et al. The prevalence of infective endocarditis after aortic valve replacement. *J Thorac Cardiovasc Surg* 1995;110:1708–1720.
93. Kaiser AB. Antimicrobial prophylaxis of infections associated with foreign bodies. In: Bisno AL, Waldvogel FA, eds. *Infections associated with indwelling medical devices.* Washington, DC: American Society for Microbiology, 1989:277–287.
94. Wolff M, Witchitz S, Chastang C, et al. Prosthetic valve endocarditis in the ICU. Prognostic factors of overall survival in a series of 122 cases and consequences for treatment decision. *Chest* 1995;108:688–694.
95. Mayer KH, Schoenbaum SC. Evaluation and management of prosthetic valve endocarditis. *Prog Cardiovasc Dis* 1982;25:43–54.
96. Goldstone J, Malone JM, McIntyre KE. Infections associated with prosthetic arterial grafts. In: Sugarman B, Young EJ, eds. *Infections associated with prosthetic devices.* Boca Raton, FL: CRC Press, 1984: 123–141.
97. Richet HM, Chidiac C, Prat A, et al. Analysis of risk factors for surgical wound infections following vascular surgery. *Am J Med* 1991; 91(Suppl 3B):170S–172S.
98. Liekweg WG, Greenfield LJ. Vascular prosthetic infections: collected experience and results of treatment. *Surgery* 1977;81:335–342.
99. Nasima A, Thompson MM, Naylor AR, et al. The impact of MRSA on vascular surgery. *Eur J Vasc Endovasc Surg* 2001;22:211–214.
100. Low RN, Wall SD, Jeffrey RB, et al. Aortoenteric fistula and perigraft infection: evaluation with CT1. *Radiology* 1990;175:157–162.
101. Chervu A, Moore WS, Chvapil M, et al. Efficacy and duration of antistaphylococcal activity comparing three antibiotics bonded to Dacron vascular grafts with a collagen release system. *J Vasc Surg* 1991; 13:897–901.
102. Bisno AL. Infections of central nervous system shunts. In: Bisno AL, Waldvogel FA, eds. *Infections associated with indwelling medical devices.* Washington, DC: American Society for Microbiology, 1989:93–109.
103. Mayhall CG, Archer NH, Lamb VA, et al. Ventriculostomy-related infections. A prospective epidemiologic study. *N Engl J Med* 1984; 310:553–559.
104. Dallacasa P, Dappozo A, Galassi E, et al. Cerebrospinal fluid shunt infections in infants. *Childs Nerv Syst* 1995;11:643–648.
105. Sayers MP. Shunt complications. *Clin Neurosurg* 1975;23:393–400.
106. McKinsey DS, Stanford W, Smith DL. Detection of the source of recurrent *Staphylococcus aureus* bacteremia by ultrafast computerized tomography. *Rev Infect Dis* 1991;13:893–895.
107. Shingadia D, Grant J, Bendet M, et al. Multiple recurrent gram-negative cerebrospinal shunt infections associated with a patient with a retained ventricular foreign body. *Pediatr Neurosurg* 1999;31: 155–158.
108. Kurup A, Tee KWS, Loo LH, et al. Infection of central nervous system by motile enterococcus: first case report. *J Clin Microbiol* 2001; 39:820–822.
109. Lundberg F, Li DQ, Falkenback D, et al. Presence of vitronectin and activated complement factor C9 on ventriculoperitoneal shunts and temporary ventricular drainage catheters. *J Neurosurg* 1999;90: 101–108.
110. Schoenbaum SC, Gardner P, Shillit J. Infections of cerebrospinal fluid shunts: epidemiology, clinical manifestations, and therapy. *J Infect Dis* 1975;131:543–552.
111. Del Bigio MR. Biological reactions to cerebrospinal fluid shunt devices: a review of the cellular pathology. *Neurosurgery* 1998;42: 319–325.
112. Wierbitzky SK, Ahrens N, Becker T, et al. The diagnostic importance of eosinophil granulocytes in the CSF of children with ventricular-peritoneal shunt systems. *Acta Neurol Scand* 1998;97:201–203.
113. Roos KL, Scheld WM. Central nervous system infections. In: Crossley KB, Archer GL, eds. *The staphylococci in human disease.* New York: Churchill Livingstone, 1998:413.
114. Langley JM, LeBlanc JC, Drake J, et al. Efficacy of antimicrobial prophylaxis in placement of cerebrospinal fluid shunts: meta-analysis. *Clin Infect Dis* 1993;17:98–103.
115. Abendschein W. Salvage of infected total hip replacement: use of antibiotic/PMMA spacer. *Orthopedics* 1992;15:228–229.
116. Alleyne CH Jr, Hassan M, Zabramski JM. The efficacy and cost of prophylactic and periprocedural antibiotics in patients with external ventricular drains. *Neurosurgery* 2000;47:1124–1127, discussion 1127–1129.
117. Sanchez-Mora D, Mermel L, Parenteau S, et al. Epidural catheter infection: epidemiology and pathogenesis. Interscience Conference on Antimicrobial Agents and Chemotherapy, New Orleans, October 17–20, 1993.
118. De Cholnoky T. Augmentation mammaplasty. Survey of complications in patients by 265 surgeons. *Plast Reconstr Surg* 1970;45: 573–577.
119. Gabriel SE, Woods JE, O'Fallon WM, et al. Complications leading to surgery after breast implantation. *N Engl J Med* 1997;336:677–682.
120. Kjoller K, Holmich LR, Jacobsen PH, et al. Epidemiological investigation of local complications after cosmetic breast implant surgery in Denmark. *Ann Plast Surg* 2002;48:229–237.
121. Brand KG. Infection of mammary prostheses: a survey and the question of prevention. *Ann Plast Surg* 1993;30:289–295.
122. Javaid M, Shibu M. Breast implant infection following nipple piercing. *Br J Plast Surg* 1999;52:676–677.
123. Thornton JW, Argenta LC, McClatchey KD, et al. Studies on the endogenous flora of the human breast. *Ann Plast Surg* 1988;20:39–42.
124. Courtiss EH, Goldwyn RM, Anastasi GW. The fate of breast implants with infections around them. *Plast Reconstr Surg* 1979;63:812–816.
125. Schatten WE. Reconstruction of the breasts following mastectomy with polyurethane-covered, gel-filled prosthesis. *Ann Plast Surg* 1984; 12:147–156.
126. Hester TR, Nahai F, Bostwick J, et al. A 5 year experience with polyurethane-covered mammary prostheses for treatments of capsular contracture, primary augmentation mammaplasty, and breast reconstruction. *Clin Plast Surg* 1988;12:569–585.
127. Perras C. The prevention and treatment of infection following breast implants. *Plast Reconstr Surg* 1965;35:659.
128. Cronin TD, Greenberg RL. Our experiences with the silastic gel breast prosthesis. *Plast Reconstr Surg* 1970;46:1–7.
129. Cronin TD, Persoff MM, Upton J. Augmentation mammoplasty: complications and etiology. In: Owsley JQJ, Peterson RA, eds. *Symposium on aesthetic surgery of the breast.* St. Louis: Mosby, 1978.
130. Scully SJ. Augmentation mammaplasty without capsular contracture. *Ann Plast Surg* 1981;6:262–270.
131. Mahler D, Hauben DJ. Retromammary versus retropectoral breast augmentation. *Ann Plast Surg* 1982;8:370–374.
132. Clegg HW, Bertagnoll P, Hightower AW, et al. Mammaplasty-associ-

ated mycobacterial infection: a survey of plastic surgeons. *Plast Reconstr Surg* 1983;72:165–172.
133. McGrath MH, Burkhardt BR. The safety and efficacy of breast implants for augmentation mammaplasty. *Plast Reconstr Surg* 1984;74: 550–560.
134. Dolsky RL. Polyurethane-coated implants. *Plast Reconstr Surg* 1985; 76:974–975.
135. Whidden PG. Augmentation mammoplasty. *Transplant Implant Today* 1986;3:43–51.
136. Armstrong RW, Berkowitz RL, Bolding F. Infection following breast reconstruction. *Ann Plast Surg* 1989;23:284–288.
137. Ahn CY, Ko CY, Wagar EA, et al. Microbial evaluation: 139 implants removed from symptomatic patients. *Plast Reconstr Surg* 1995;98: 1225–1229.
138. Jabaley ME, Das SK. Late breast pain following reconstruction with polyurethane-covered implants. *Plast Reconstr Surg* 1986;78: 390–395.
139. Schlenker JD, Bueno RA, Ricketson G, et al. Loss of implants after subcutaneous mastectomy and reconstruction. *Plast Reconstr Surg* 1978;62:853–861.
140. Capozzi A, Pennisi VR. Clinical experience with polyurethane-covered gel filled mammary prostheses. *Plast Reconstr Surg* 1981;68: 512–518.
141. Eyssen JE, Von Werssowetz AL, Middleton GD. Reconstruction of the breast using polyurethane-coated prostheses. *Plast Reconstr Surg* 1984;3:415–419.
142. Slade LC. Subcutaneous mastectomy: acute complications and long-term follow-up. *Plast Reconstr Surg* 1984;73:415–419.
143. Herman D, Wilk A, Meyer C, et al. Notre expérience du risque infectieux dans la chirurgie prothétique mammaire. *Agressologie* 1992; 33:188–190.
144. Worton EW, Siefert LN. Augmentation mammaplasty: a review of fifty consecutive patients. In: Owsley JQJ, Peterson RA, eds. *Symposium on aesthetic surgery of the breast.* St. Louis: Mosby, 1978:341–343.
145. Slavin SA, Colen SR. Sixty consecutive breast reconstructions with the inflatable expander: a critical appraisal. *Plast Reconstr Surg* 1990; 86:910–919.
146. Barnett A, Lavey E, Pearl RM, et al. Toxic shock syndrome from an infected breast prosthesis. *Ann Plast Surg* 1983;10:408–410.
147. Freedman AM, Jackson IT. Infections in breast implants. *Infect Dis Clin North Am* 1989;3:275–287.
148. Holm C, MuhlBauer W. Toxic shock syndrome in plastic surgery patients: case report and review of the literature. *Aesthetic Plast Surg* 1998;22:222–224.
149. Walker LE, Breiner MJ, Goodman CM. Toxic shock syndrome after explantation of breast implants: a case report and review of the literature. *Plast Reconstr Surg* 1997;99:875–879.
150. Hoffman PC, Fraser DW, Robicsek F, et al. Two outbreaks of sternal wound infections due to organisms of the *Mycobacterium fortuitum* complex. *J Infect Dis* 1981;143:533–538.
151. Clegg HW, Bertagnoll P, Hightower HW, et al. Infections due to organisms of *Mycobacterium fortuitum* complex after augmentation mammaplasty: clinical and epidemiological features. *J Infect Dis* 1983; 147:427–433.
152. Wallace RJ, Steele LC, Labidi A, et al. Heterogeneity among isolates of rapidly growing mycobacteria responsible for infections following augmentation mammaplasty despite case clustering in Texas and other southern coastal states. *J Infect Dis* 1989;160:281–288.
153. Heistein JB, Mangino JE, Ruberg RL, et al. A prosthetic breast implant infected with *Mycobacterium fortuitum. Ann Plast Surg* 2000; 44;330–333.
154. Haiavy J. Tobin H. *Mycobacterium fortuitum* infection in prosthetic breast implants. *Plast Reconstr Surg* 2002;109:2124–2128.
155. Safranek TJ, Jarvis WR, Carson LA, et al. *Mycobacterium chelonae* wound infections after plastic surgery employing contaminated gentian violet skin-marking solution. *N Engl J Med* 1987;317:197.
156. Gibney J. The long-term results of tissue expansion for breast reconstruction. *Clin Plast Surg* 1987;14:509–518.
157. Hunger JG, Padilla M. Cooper-Vastola S. Late *Clostridium perfringens* breast implant infection after dental treatment. *Ann Plast Surg* 1996; 36:309–312.
158. Bernardi C, Saccomanno F. Late *Klebsiella pneumoniae* infection following breast augmentation: case report. *Aesthetic Plast Surg* 1998; 22:222–224.
159. Ablaza VJ, LaTrenta GS. Late infection of a breast prosthesis with *Enterococcus avium. Plast Reconstr Surg* 1998;102:227–230.
160. Petit F, Maladry D, Werther JR, et al. Late infection of breast implant, complication of colonic perforation. Review of the literature. Role of preventive treatment. *Ann Chir Plast Esthet* 1998;43:559–562.
161. Eliopoulos DA, Lyle G. *Mycobacterium avium* infection in a patient with the acquired immunodeficiency syndrome and silicone breast implants. *South Med J* 1999;92:80–83.
162. Johnson LB, Busuito MJ, Khatib R. Breast implant infection in a cat owner due to *Pasteurella multocida. J Infect* 2000;41;110–111.
163. Memish ZA, Alazzawi M, Bannatyne R. Unusual complications of breast implants: *Brucella* infection. *Infection* 2001;29:291–292.
164. Gnanadesigan N, Pechter EA, Mascola L. *Listeria* infection of silicone breast implants. *Plast Reconstr Surg* 1994;94:531–533.
165. Reddy BT, Torres HA, Kontoyiannis DP. Breast implant infection caused by *Trichosporon beigelii. Scand J Infect Dis* 2002;343:143–144.
166. Niazi ZB, Salzberg CA, Montecalvo M. *Candida albicans* infection of bilateral polyurethane-coated silicone gel breast implants. *Ann Plast Surg* 1996;37:91–93.
167. Embrey M, Adams EE, Cunningham B, et al. A review of the literature on the etiology of capsular contracture and a pilot study to determine the outcome of capsular contracture interventions. *Aesthetic Plast Surg* 1999;23:197–206.
168. Burkhardt BR, Fried M, Schnur PL, et al. Capsules, infection and intraluminal antibiotics. *Plast Reconstr Surg* 1981;68:43–49.
169. Dubin D. The etiology, pathophysiology, predictability, and early detection of spherical scar contracture of the breast: a detailed explanation and protocol for prevention of spherical scar contracture of the breast. Presented at the Annual Meeting of the American Society for Aesthetic Plastic Surgery, Orlando, FL, 1990.
170. Shah Z, Lehman JA, Tan J. Does infection play a role in breast capsular contracture? *Plast Reconstr Surg* 1981;68:34–38.
171. Burkhardt BR, Dempsey PD, Schnur PL, et al. Capsular contracture: a prospective study of the effect of local antibacterial agents. *Plast Reconstr Surg* 1986;77:919–921.
172. Ahn CY, Ko CY, Wager EA, et al. Microbial evaluation: 139 implants removed from symptomatic patients. *Plast Reconstr Surg* 1996;98: 1225–1229.
173. Adams WP Jr, Conner WC, Barton FE Jr, et al. Optimizing breast-pocket irrigation: the post-Betadine era. *Plast Reconstr Surg* 2001;107: 1596–1601.
174. Rasnjö U, Asplund OA, Gylbert L, et al. Bacteria in the female breast. *Scand J Plast Reconstr Surg* 1985;19:87–89.
175. Darouiche RO, Meader R, Mansouri MD, et al. In vivo efficacy of antimicrobe-impregnated saline-filled silicon implants. *Plast Reconstr Surg* 2002;109:1352–1357.
176. Peter W, Smith D, Fornasier V, et al. An outcome analysis of 100 women after explantation of silicone gel breast implants. *Ann Plast Surg* 1997;39:9–19.
177. Nordström REA. Antibiotics in the tissue expander to decrease the rate of infection. *Plast Reconstr Surg* 1988;81:137–138.

68

NOSOCOMIAL INFECTIONS ASSOCIATED WITH RESPIRATORY THERAPY

KEITH S. KAYE
DAVID J. WEBER
WILLIAM A. RUTALA

The most representative data on the incidence of nosocomial infections has been provided by the Centers for Disease Control and Prevention (CDC) via the National Nosocomial Infections Surveillance (NNIS) system. According to the NNIS system data, nosocomial pneumonia is the second leading cause of hospital-acquired infection, accounting for approximately 15% of all hospital-associated infections and 24% to 27% of all infections acquired in medical intensive care and coronary care units (1–3). The frequency (episodes per 100 hospitalizations) of hospital-acquired pneumonia is 0.2 to 0.94, the lower rates being reported from small private hospitals and the higher rates from large academic hospitals (1,4). The median rates of ventilator-associated nosocomial pneumonia (per 1,000 days ventilated) in intensive care units (ICUs) range from 2.4 (respiratory ICU) to 15.9 (trauma ICU) (5). The frequency of nosocomial pneumonia is reportedly higher in selected patient populations, ranging from 0.66 to 1.47 in the elderly (6,7), 1.7 to 7.2 among newborn ICU patients (4,8), and 2.0 to 21.6 among adult ICU residents (9–14). A point prevalence study of ICUs in 17 Western European countries revealed that 20.6% of all patients had an ICU-acquired infection; pneumonia accounted for 46.9% and lower respiratory tract infections (not pneumonia) accounted for 17.8% of all ICU-acquired infections (15).

Multiple risk factors for nosocomial pneumonia have been identified by univariate analysis: abdominal or thoracic surgery (12,16,17), advanced age (12,17), altered mental status (6,7,13, 17), prior episodes of large-volume aspiration (6,7,10,16,18), H_2 blocker therapy (7,18,19), steroid therapy (18), ICU residence (7,16), nasogastric intubation (6,7,12,16), previous antibiotic use (7,16,20,21), rapidly or ultimately fatal disease (10, 12), trauma (13,14), neurologic disease (14), underlying chronic lung disease (16), and intubation with mechanical ventilation (7,10,13,16). The risk factors for ICU-acquired pneumonia have been reviewed (22,23). Most (7,10,16,18,24) but not all (12) multivariable analyses have shown that mechanical ventilation is a major risk factor for nosocomial pneumonia, with odds ratios ranging from 1.3 to 12.1 (for positive studies). Few investigators have included variables related to type of respiratory care procedures in their multivariable analysis. Joshi et al. (12) found a 2.95-fold increased risk of nosocomial pneumonia associated with recent bronchoscopy in ICU patients.

This chapter focuses on nosocomial infections associated with respiratory therapy. The epidemiology of nosocomial pneumonia in general has been reviewed by several authors since 1990 (25–44) (see Chapter 22). Several reviews have focused on the prevention of nosocomial pneumonia, especially ventilator-associated pneumonia (29,37,39,45,46).

PATHOGENESIS OF NOSOCOMIAL PNEUMONIA AND ROLE OF RESPIRATORY CARE EQUIPMENT

Nosocomial pneumonia may occur by three major routes: (a) aspiration of oropharyngeal flora; (b) inhalation of infectious aerosols; and (c) hematogenous spread from a distant focus of infection. Colonization of the oropharynx and gastrointestinal tract by pathogenic gram-positive and gram-negative bacilli, followed by aspiration in the setting of impaired host defenses, is the major cause of nosocomial pneumonia.

Contaminated respiratory care equipment may lead to nosocomial pneumonia by two routes. First, respiratory care equipment may serve as a reservoir for microorganisms, especially gram-negative bacilli. Fluid-containing devices such as nebulizers and humidifiers may become heavily contaminated by bacteria capable of multiplying in water. Pathogens may then be spread to the patient by hospital personnel or by aerosolization into room air. Second, contaminated equipment may lead to direct airway inoculation of microorganisms if it is directly linked to a ventilatory system or if contaminated medications are instilled by aerosolization. The role of inhalation and respiratory care equipment in nosocomial pneumonia has been reviewed several times in the era of medical/surgical intensive care (13,23,28–34,36,37,41,44,46–53).

Fluid-containing respiratory devices are the major environment-associated reservoirs for nosocomial pneumonia; however, most or all phases of respiratory support have been linked to nosocomial respiratory infections or suggested as potential environmental reservoirs. These include mechanical ventilation bags (MVBs), ventilators, aerosolized medications, bronchoscopy, suction catheters, and respiratory support personnel. Evidence suggests that alterations in infection control practices during the 1960s decreased the number of cases of nosocomial pneumonia from environmental sources (54).

INFECTIONS ASSOCIATED WITH INTUBATION AND MECHANICAL VENTILATION

Pathophysiology of Infection

Intubation for respiratory support increases the patient's risk of nosocomial pneumonia. Nasotracheal or orotracheal intubation predisposes patients to bacterial colonization and nosocomial pneumonia by the following pathophysiologic alterations (52,55,56): (a) it causes sinusitis and trauma to the nasopharynx (nasotracheal tube); (b) it impairs swallowing of secretions; (c) it acts as a reservoir for bacterial proliferation; (d) it increases bacterial adherence and colonization of airways; (e) it requires the presence of a foreign body that traumatizes the oropharyngeal epithelium; (f) it causes ischemia secondary to cuff pressure; (g) it impairs ciliary clearance and cough; (h) it can cause leakage of secretions around the cuff; and (i) it requires suctioning to remove secretions. Mechanical ventilation also exposes the patient to fluid-filled devices, such as in-line nebulizers and humidifiers, which are used to provide humidification or medications.

Incidence of Respiratory Infections

Multiple studies have demonstrated that mechanical ventilation is a major predisposing factor for nosocomial pneumonia (18,24,25,57–80). Direct comparisons of the various studies requires caution because of important differences in study design, including patient population, period of study, criteria for entry into the study, and criteria for diagnosis of pneumonia. However, the following generalizations can be made: between 15% and 40% of patients who undergo mechanical ventilation for more than 48 hours develop nosocomial pneumonia, and the case-fatality rate is exceedingly high.

INFECTIONS ASSOCIATED WITH COMPONENTS OF MECHANICAL VENTILATION

Ventilators

The internal machinery of mechanical ventilators is not considered an important source of bacterial contamination of inhaled air (81). In the 1960s, the use of a high-efficiency bacterial filter interposed between the machinery and the main breathing circuit was advocated to eliminate contaminants from the driving gas and to prevent retrograde contamination of the machine by patients (82,83). The filters were shown, however, to alter the function of the ventilators by impeding high gas flows. Later studies have not shown that a filter placed between the inspiratory phase circuit and the patient prevents infection (84,85).

Placement of a filter or condensate trap on the expiratory limb of the mechanical-ventilator circuit may help prevent cross-contamination of the ventilated patient's immediate environment (86,87), but the importance of such filters in preventing nosocomial pneumonia has not been demonstrated.

Periodic sterilization or high-level disinfection of the internal ventilator machinery is unnecessary; however, ventilator circuits should be sterilized or subjected to high-level disinfection between patient uses. Failure to properly clean and sterilize ventilator circuits between patients has led to outbreaks with *Pseudomonas aeruginosa* (88) and *Acinetobacter calcoaceticus* var. *anitratus* (89). The failure to properly disinfect ventilator temperature probes between patients has led to outbreaks of *Burkholderia cepacia* pneumonia (90,91).

Nebulizer Equipment

Nebulizers have been a significant source of nosocomial pneumonia. Nebulizers with large-volume (greater than 500 mL) reservoirs, including those used in intermittent positive-pressure breathing (IPPB) machines and ultrasonic or spinning-disk room-air "humidifiers," pose the greatest risk of pneumonia to patients, probably because of the total amount of aerosol they generate (29). Other types of nebulizers include small-volume nebulizers for administration of medications, most commonly bronchodilators. Such small-volume nebulizers may be placed in the inspiratory circuit of mechanical ventilators or hand-held.

Nebulizers used in association with mechanical ventilators may be inserted into the inspiratory phase tubing of the mechanical ventilator circuit for the administration of medications or used to provide humidification of air. In-line medication nebulizers may become contaminated by reflux of tubing condensate (92) or use of contaminated solutions (93). Contaminated nebulizers may then lead to nosocomial pneumonia via direct instillation of pathogenic bacteria into the lung. Botman and de Krieger (94) demonstrated that small-volume nebulizers frequently become colonized with pathogenic bacteria, and that nebulizers are associated with an increased risk of respiratory colonization of patients. The risk of pneumonia is related to the production of contaminated bacterial droplets less than 4 μm in diameter (52). Particles larger than 10 μm are trapped in the nasopharynx or trachea, whereas particles smaller than 4 μm may be delivered into the patient's terminal bronchioles and alveoli. Craven et al. (52) emphasized that the risk of pneumonia is related to the size and number of the aerosol particles, the concentration of pathogenic bacteria, and whether aerosol particles are delivered directly into the endotracheal tube or into the oropharynx. The temperature of the reservoir fluid is also critically important, because most nosocomial pathogens cannot survive for long periods in distilled water or saline at temperatures above 50°C. Decreases in the frequency of nebulizer contamination were shown to relate to decreases in the occurrence of necrotizing pneumonia (54).

In addition to the previously mentioned mechanisms of contamination, in-line, fine-particle nebulizers used to humidify air mixed with oxygen from a wall oxygen outlet may become contaminated when ambient air contains bacteria (95,96).

Contaminated nebulizers have been responsible for several

outbreaks. Four cases of *Legionella pneumophila* pneumonia resulted when contaminated tap water was used in jet nebulizers to humidify oxygen administered by face mask (97). Failure to disinfect nebulizers between patients led to an outbreak of *Serratia marcescens* pneumonia (94). Use of contaminated ultrasonic nebulizers in IPPB machines has led to infections with *S. marcescens* (98,99) and *P. aeruginosa* (100).

Mechanical Ventilation with Humidification

Humidification of inspiratory air is an important aspect of ventilator management. Humidification may be achieved by bubble-through humidifiers, which produce minimal aerosols, or wick humidifiers, which produce no aerosols (101,102). Bubble-through humidifiers are usually heated to temperatures that reduce or eliminate bacterial pathogens (102). For these reasons, current humidification practices are not believed to pose a significant risk of pneumonia to ventilated patients (29). However, one study that purposely used contaminated water found that although colony counts in bubble-through humidifiers decreased with time, viable microorganisms remained throughout the study (103). Further, when bubble-through humidifiers were heated, both condensate and effluent gas rapidly became contaminated. Additional studies are required of actual ventilators in use to assess the importance of humidification as a risk factor for nosocomial pneumonia. It is currently recommended that sterile water be used to fill these humidifiers (29) because tap or distilled water may harbor relatively heat-resistant *Legionella* species (104,105).

A potential risk factor for pneumonia in patients using mechanical ventilation with humidification is the condensate that forms in the inspiratory-phase tubing of the ventilator circuit. This condensate forms as a result of the difference in the temperatures of the inspiratory-phase gas and ambient air. Condensate formation is increased if the tubing is unheated compared to the use of heated bubble-through humidifiers. Both the ventilator tubing and condensate rapidly become colonized by gram-negative and gram-positive bacteria during use. The colonizing pathogens originate from the patient, and thus, the highest levels of bacteria are closest to the endotracheal tube, with lower levels near the humidifier reservoir. Craven et al. (106) demonstrated that 33% of inspiratory circuits became colonized by oropharyngeal flora from the patient within 2 hours of use, and 80% were colonized within 24 hours of use. They hypothesized that spillage of this contaminated fluid into the patient's respiratory tract, as might occur during procedures such as patient suctioning or transportation for clinical studies, might lead to nosocomial pneumonia. Contaminated condensate can also serve as a reservoir for respiratory pathogens, which can be transmitted person to person via the hands of medical personnel if staff members fail to wash their hands following ventilator manipulation.

The frequency of ventilator tubing changes and its relationship to the incidence of nosocomial pneumonia has been investigated by several research groups (Table 68.1). In a landmark study, Craven et al. (107) reported that ventilator tubing could be safely changed every 48 hours as opposed to the then-recommended 24-hour changes. Despite this study, which was published in 1982, a 1990 survey of 40 ICUs in England reported that 62% of ICUs continued to change tubing every 24 hours (108). The CDC guideline on nosocomial pneumonia recommends that the breathing circuit be changed no more frequently than 48 hours but states that "the exact maximum time that a circuit can be safely left unchanged on a patient has yet to be

TABLE 68.1. RATES OF VENTILATOR-ASSOCIATED PNEUMONIA AND FREQUENCY FOR CHANGE OF TUBING CIRCUITS FOR MECHANICAL VENTILATION

Reference	Year	Study Design	Humidifier	Circuit	Interval for Circuit Changes (No. of Days)	No. of Patients with Pneumonia	% of Patients with Pneumonia	Incidence (VAP/1,000 Ventilator Days)	*p* Value
Dreyfuss et al. (76)	1991	Randomized	Wick/bubble	Standard	2	35	31	24.6	NS
					None	28	29	28.6	
Boher et al. (109)	1992	Before/after	NA	NA	2	1,172	NA	18	NA
					7	518	NA	13	
Mermel et al. (110)	1994	Randomized	NA	Standard heated wire	2–3	60	7	25	NS
					7	56	2	7	
Hess et al. (111)	1995	Before/after	Bubble	Standard	2	1,708	5.5	9.6	NA
					7	1,715	4.6	8.6	
Kollef et al. (115)	1995	Randomized	Wick	Standard	7	153	29	17.4	NS
					None	147	24	16.4	
Long et al. (112)	1996	Randomized	Wick	Heated wire	2–3	213	13	9	NS
					7	234	11	10	
Kotilainen et al. (113)	1997	Before/after	NA	Heated wire	3	88	9.1	12.9	NS
					7	146	6.2	7.4	
Fink et al. (114)	1998	Before/after	Wick	Standard	2	343	NA	11.3	.0004[a]
					7	137	NA	3.2	
				Heated wire	30	157	NA	6.6	

NA, not available; NS, not statistically significant.
[a] Two-day interval compared with 7-day and 30-day intervals (7-day versus 30-day difference not significant, $p = .27$).

determined" (29). Studies among adult patients demonstrated that changing ventilator circuits at 7 days does not increase the risk of ventilator-associated pneumonia and results in significant cost savings (109–114) (Table 68.1). Additional studies evaluating 30-day or no circuit changes suggest that a further lengthening of the interval for circuit changes is likely to be both safe and cost-effective (76,114,115) (Table 68.1). Limited data are available among neonatal ICU patients. One study reported that changing ventilator circuits at 24- versus 48-hour intervals resulted in reduced circuit colonization (116), whereas another study reported no pneumonias in infants managed with either thrice weekly or once weekly tubing changes (112). The current data indicate that breathing circuits should be changed no more frequently than every 7 days (117), and ventilator circuits probably do not need to be changed on a routine basis, but only when a circuit is contaminated. This practice is likely to be modified when additional data regarding the safety of longer duration of circuit changes become available.

Filling the in-line humidifier with contaminated water has led to an outbreak of *Pseudomonas fluorescens* infections (118). The reuse of inadequately disinfected ventilator circuits has led to outbreaks with *A. calcoaceticus* var. *anitratus* (119,120) and *Pseudomonas* species (121). Reusable ventilator tubing should be thoroughly cleaned and dried after patient use and then sterilized with ethylene oxide gas, subjected to high-level disinfection with a Food and Drug Administration (FDA)-cleared chemical sterilant, or pasteurized (see Chapters 85 and 86). Only sterile water should be used in humidifiers and nebulizers.

Condensate formation can be eliminated by the use of a heat-moisture exchanger (HME) or a hygroscopic condenser humidifier (also known as an "artificial nose") (122,123). The HME eliminates the need for a humidifier by recycling heat and moisture exhaled by the patient. Because a humidifier is not used, no condensate forms in the inspiratory tubing of the ventilator circuit. Thus, bacterial colonization of the tubing is avoided, and the need to routinely change the ventilator tubing is eliminated. Potential problems with HMEs include increased dead space and resistance to breathing, and leakage around the endotracheal tube with drying of sputum and blockage of the tracheobronchial tree (124). Several investigators have reported on the use of an HME (125–133). Prospective studies demonstrate that changing HMEs every 48 to 72 hours rather than every 24 hours did not affect their efficacy or the incidence of nosocomial pneumonia (130,134). In addition, randomized studies found no difference in the infection rates of patients assigned to a hydrophobic HME or a hygroscopic HME (133,134). Multiple randomized trials have compared the rates of ventilator-associated pneumonia in patients in whom an in-line HME was used compared to patients managed with a conventional heated-wire humidifier (127–129,131,132). The rates of pneumonia were lower with use of the HME [range of relative risks (RRs), 0.35 to 0.85]; one study reached statistical significance (132). Use of the HME is both cost-effective and reduces the rate of late-onset, nosocomial ventilator-associated pneumonia (132,135).

Manual Ventilation Bags

Manual ventilation bags are used for urgent ventilation, during routine suctioning of the intubated patient, during transport of the intubated patient, and to ventilate patients during chest physiotherapy. The exterior surface and connecting port of MVBs are routinely contaminated during use. Secretions left in the bag may be aerosolized and/or sprayed into the lower respiratory tract of patients. Further, the exterior surface may serve as a reservoir for pathogens transmitted person to person on the hands of healthcare personnel. Contaminated MVBs have been linked to epidemics of *A. calcoaceticus pneumonia* (120, 136). Thompson et al. (137) demonstrated that, in patients with gram-negative bacteria in their sputum, 71% of the MVB valves and 29% of the air samples taken from the exhalation valve assemblies were culture-positive for the same microorganisms. Weber et al. (138) cultured the interior and exterior surfaces of MVBs used on 14 ICU patients whose respiratory tracts were colonized or infected. Overall, 51 simultaneous cultures of MVB components resulted in the following findings: (a) the MVB exterior surface was culture-positive 100% of the time; (b) the MVB exhalation port was culture-positive 96% of the time; and (c) the MVB interior surfaces were culture-positive only 12% of the time. In three instances (6%), the MVB port became colonized with a pathogen prior to its appearance in the patient's respiratory tract, suggesting that the MVB was the source for the colonizing pathogen.

Contaminated MVBs may serve as a source for nosocomial infection by colonizing the hands of medical personnel who then may cross-transmit such pathogens directly to other patients or to respiratory or other medical equipment, and by introducing pathogens into patients. The following guidelines have been suggested for the prevention of nosocomial respiratory tract infections associated with MVBs (138). First, all medical personnel should wash their hands before and immediately after any contact with patients or potentially contaminated equipment such as MVBs. Second, MVBs should be sterilized or subjected to high-level disinfection between patients. Third, the MVB should be cleaned of visible secretions daily and then disinfected with alcohol. Both the exterior surface and the MVB exhalation valve should be disinfected. The interior surface does not need to be disinfected during routine use. When reprocessed in an appropriate area of the ICU or in central processing, if tenacious sputum cannot be removed from the exhalation port, the port should be disassembled, cleaned, and sterilized or subjected to high-level disinfection.

Prevention of Nosocomial Pneumonia

Several authors have summarized measures that may reduce the incidence of ventilator-associated pneumonia (25,29,36,37, 39,41,44–46,139). These measures include (a) use of aseptic technique for respiratory tract manipulation; (b) proper disinfection and maintenance of respiratory equipment; (c) no routine change of ventilator circuits (change only when visibly soiled or mechanically malfunctioning); (d) hand hygiene (with soap and water or a waterless hand antiseptic) after contact with mucous membranes or contaminated equipment, whether or not gloves are worn; (e) elevation of the head of the bed to 30 to 45 degrees; (f) continuous subglottic suctioning; and (g) noninvasive ventilation to reduce the incidence of mechanical ventilation (140). Additional measures include (a) identification and elimination

TABLE 68.2. RECOMMENDATIONS FOR THE PREVENTION OF NOSOCOMIAL PNEUMONIA INVOLVING RESPIRATORY CARE EQUIPMENT

Prevention Strategy	CDC 1994 (29)	Kollef 1999 (45)	CDC 2002[a]
Decontaminate hands with soap and water or with a waterless antiseptic agent after contact with mucous membranes, respiratory secretions, or objects contaminated with respiratory secretions, whether or not gloves are worn	IA	B	IA
Thoroughly clean all equipment and devices to be sterilized	—	—	IA
Whenever possible, use steam sterilization of high-level disinfection by wet heat pasteurization for reprocessing semicritical equipment or devices	IB	—	IA
When rinsing is necessary after chemical disinfection of semicritical equipment or devices used on the respiratory tract, use sterile or pasteurized water	IB	—	IA
Do not routinely sterilize or disinfect the internal machinery of mechanical ventilators	IA	—	IB
Do not change routinely, on the basis of duration of use, the ventilatory circuit that is in use on an individual patient; change the circuit when it is visibly soiled or mechanically malfunctioning	Change $\geq$ 48 hours, IA	A	IA
Sterilize reusable breathing circuits and bubbling wick humidifiers, or subject them to high-level disinfection between their uses on different patients	IB	—	IB
Periodically drain and discard any condensate that collects in the tubing of a mechanical ventilator, taking precautions not to allow condensate to drain toward the patient	IB	C	IA
Place a filter at the distal end of the expiratory-phase tubing of the breathing circuit to collect condensate	U	—	U
Do not place bacterial filters between the humidifier reservoir and the inspiratory-phase tubing of the breathing circuit of a mechanical ventilator	IB	—	II
Use sterile or pasteurized water to fill bubbling humidifiers	II	—	IB
Preferentially use a closed, continuous-feed humidification system	U	—	U
When cost-effective and unless medically contraindicated, use a heat-moisture exchanger (HME) to prevent pneumonia in a patient receiving mechanical ventilation	U	A	II
Change an HME that is in use on a patient when it malfunctions mechanically or becomes visibly soiled	IB	—	IB
Do not change routinely more frequently than every 48 hours an HME that is in use on a patient	No routine change, IB	—	IB
Daily change of HME	—	A	—
Do not change routinely (in the absence of gross contamination or malfunction) the breathing circuit attached to an HME while it is in use on a patient	IB	—	II
Follow manufacturers' instructions for use and maintenance of wall oxygen humidifiers unless data show that modifying the instructions poses no threat to the patient and is cost-effective	IB	—	IB
Between patients, change the tubing, including any nasal prongs or mask, used to deliver oxygen from a wall outlet	IB	—	IB
Use only sterile or pasteurized fluid for nebulization and dispense the fluid into the nebulizer aseptically	IA	—	IA
Do not routinely sterilize or disinfect the internal machinery of anesthesia equipment	IA	—	IB
Do not routinely sterilize or disinfect the internal machinery of pulmonary-function testing machines between uses on different patients	II	—	II
Unless there is a filter between the mouthpiece and tubing of pulmonary-function testing equipment, sterilize or subject to high-level disinfection or pasteurization reusable mouthpieces and tubing or connectors between uses on different patients	IB	—	IB
Do not use large volume room-air humidifiers that create aerosols unless they can be sterilized or subjected to high-level disinfection at least daily and filled with sterile water	IA	—	IB
Use of either the multiuse closed-system suction catheter or the single-use open-suction catheter	U	—	U
If the closed-system suction is used, change the in-line suction catheter when it malfunctions or becomes visibly soiled	—	—	IB
If the open-system suction is employed, use a sterile single-use catheter	II	—	II
Use only sterile or pasteurized fluid to remove secretions from the suction catheter if the catheter is to be used for reentry into the patient's lower respiratory tract	IB	— —	IB
Remove devices such as endotracheal tubes from patients as the clinical indications are resolved	IB	C	IB
As much as possible, and unless there are medical contraindications, use noninvasive positive-pressure ventilation delivered continuously by facial or nasal mask, instead of performing endotracheal intubation, in patients with hypoxemia or acute respiratory failure	—	C	II
Use an endotracheal tube with a dorsal lumen above the endotracheal cuff to allow drainage (by continuous suctioning) of tracheal secretions that accumulate in the patient's subglottic area	U	A	IB
If there is not a medical contraindication, elevate at an angle of 30 to 45 degrees the head of a patient at high risk of aspiration pneumonia	IB	B	IB
Routine use of "kinetic" beds or continuous lateral rotational therapy for prevention of healthcare-associated pneumonia in critically ill and/or immobilized patients	—	—	U

CDC classification: IA, strongly recommended for all hospitals and strongly supported by well-designed experimental or epidemiologic studies; IB, strongly recommended for all hospitals and viewed as effective by experts in the field and a consensus of HICPAC based on strong rationale and suggestive evidence, even though definitive studies may not have done; II, suggested for implementation in many hospitals—recommendations may be supported by suggestive clinical or epidemiologic studies, a strong theoretical rationale, or definitive studies applicable to some but not all hospitals; U (unresolved issue), practices for which insufficient evidence regarding efficacy exists.

Kollef classification: A, supported by at least two randomized controlled investigations; B, supported by at least one randomized controlled investigation; C, supported by nonrandomized concurrent-cohort investigations, historical-cohort investigations, or case series; D, supported by randomized controlled investigations of other nosocomial infections; U, undetermined or not yet studied in clinical investigations.

[a] The CDC pneumonia guideline was in draft form at the time of preparation of this chart. The recommendations in the final guideline may differ.

CDC, Centers for Disease Control and Prevention; HICPAC, Healthcare Infection Control Practices Advisory Committee.

of environmental reservoirs for pathogens; (b) use of barrier precautions for colonized and infected patients; (c) extubation and removal of nasogastric tubes as soon as clinically possible; (d) avoidance of oversedation and paralytics; (e) discontinuation of bladder catheters as soon as clinically possible; (f) use of proper endotracheal suctioning techniques; (g) maintaining adequate endotracheal cuff pressures; and (h) control of antibiotic use. Table 68.2 summarizes the current CDC guidelines relevant to this chapter for the prevention of nosocomial pneumonia.

Studies evaluating airway management of mechanically ventilated patients have been reviewed (37,53). The following conclusions are justified by the current scientific literature. First, ventilator circuits should be changed no more frequently than every 7 days (76,110,112,114,115). Current studies support the recommendation that routine changes of the ventilatory circuit at any set interval are unnecessary. Second, the type of endotracheal suction system does not appear to influence the rate of ventilator-associated pneumonia, but results from various studies have conflicted. Two trials comparing open and closed suctioning systems showed no significant difference; range of RRs, 0.84 to 0.91 (73,141); but in a later study, use of a closed suctioning system was associated with a significantly decreased risk for ventilator-associated pneumonia (adjusted RR 0.29, $p = .05$) (142). Additional studies are needed to determine the impact of closed suctioning on reduction of risk for ventilator-associated pneumonia. Third, lower rates of ventilator-associated pneumonia and decreased hospital costs may correspond with the avoidance of heated humidifiers and use of HMEs (six trials, one showing a significant difference; range of RRs, 0.34 to 0.90) (53,127–129, 131,132,143). Fourth, the use of endotracheal tubes that allow continuous aspiration of subglottic secretions has been associated with a reduced risk of pneumonia (four trials, two showing a significant difference; range of RRs, 0.22 to 0.61) (38,53, 144–146). Lower rates of pneumonia with use of kinetic versus conventional beds have been demonstrated in several studies, but significant reductions have been demonstrated in only two studies (six trials, two showing a significant difference; range of RRs, 0.22 to 0.78) (147–152). In addition, complicating factors relating to patient discomfort and problems maintaining IV access occurred in several of the studies and may limit the use of kinetic beds. For this reason, routine use of kinetic beds has not been recommended by the CDC. Finally, noninvasive positive pressure ventilation can be used in certain patient populations as an alternative to endotracheal intubation and mechanical ventilation (140,153) and has been shown to significantly decrease the risk for pneumonia in one randomized study (RR, 0.13) (154).

INFECTIONS ASSOCIATED WITH OTHER RESPIRATORY CARE PROCEDURES

Bronchoscopy

Infection Risks

Flexible fiberoptic bronchoscopy is widely used as a diagnostic and therapeutic modality to procure pulmonary specimens for microbial identification via special stains and cultures to obtain specimens for cytologic and histopathologic examination, to aid in intubation, to provide pulmonary toilet, and to remove foreign bodies (155–158). Overall, flexible bronchoscopy has proven to be an invaluable and safe diagnostic procedure. A mail survey of more than 24,000 bronchoscopies by Credle et al. (159) revealed a rate of major complications of 0.08% and only two cases of pneumonia. A later survey by Suratt et al. (160) that included information on approximately 48,000 bronchoscopies did not mention infections complications. A prospective study of 100 patients undergoing flexible bronchoscopy detected temperatures greater than 101°F and/or a new or more extensive pulmonary infiltrate on chest radiography in 16 patients (161). These findings resolved without antimicrobial therapy in all but one patient, and bacteremia was not demonstrated in any patient. However, in a similar study involving 43 consecutive bronchoscopies, Kane et al. (162) reported no instances of postprocedure fever or bacteremia. A survey of 51 European centers that performed a total of 7,446 pediatric bronchoscopies reported the following incidence of fever (not defined): rigid bronchoscopy less than 5% of cases—22 centers, 5% to 10% of cases—four centers, and more than 10% of cases—one center; fiberoptic bronchoscopy less than 5% of cases—30 centers, 5% to 10% of cases—five centers, and more than 10% of cases—three centers (163). The significance of the fever was not analyzed.

Mechanism of Nosocomial Infections

Bronchoscopes routinely become contaminated with a patients' respiratory flora during use. Because many hospitalized patients are colonized with gram-negative bacilli, contamination with these microorganisms is likely. Bronchoscopes may also become contaminated with environmental flora via airborne spread, rinses with nonsterile tap water, contact with contaminated transport cases, or use of nonsterile brushes. The major environmental agents of concern are bacteria that survive in water (e.g., *Pseudomonas,* nontuberculous mycobacteria). Mycobacteria are of particular concern, because they are relatively resistant to disinfectants. In the setting of impaired host defenses, use of contaminated bronchoscopes may lead to colonization or infection of the patient. Use of contaminated scopes may also result in pseudoepidemics in which cultures obtained at the time of bronchoscopy represent colonization of the scope as opposed to colonization or infection of the patient. Although the patient is not infected, such false-positive cultures may have serious consequences, leading to inappropriate therapy of the patient with the risk of drug toxicity and/or an inappropriate diagnosis, which may lead to failure to consider other explanations of the patient's original symptoms and signs (see Chapter 8).

Nosocomial Outbreaks

Nosocomial outbreaks associated with flexible bronchoscopy have been reviewed (50,51,164,165) (Table 68.3). Contaminated equipment has resulted in cross-transmission leading to infection and pseudoepidemics (166–218) (see also Chapter 8).

These outbreaks highlight the critical importance of proper cleaning and disinfection. Problems uncovered by these out-

TABLE 68.3. PSEUDOEPIDEMICS AND INFECTIONS TRANSMITTED BY FLEXIBLE BRONCHOSCOPES

Reference	Year	Microorganism	Isolates	Infections	Deaths	Source of Contamination
Webb and Vall-Spinosa (166)	1975	*Serratia marcescens*	3	3	1	Biopsy channel; disinfection failure
Surratt et al. (167)[a]	1977	*Pseudomonas aeruginosa*	82	—	—	Data not provided
Weinstein et al. (178)[a]	1977	*Proteus* species	8	—	—	Disinfection failure
Hussain (168)	1978	*P. aeruginosa*	1	1	0	Biopsy suction value
Markovitz (169)	1979	*P. pseudomallei*	1	1	0	Data not provided
Steere et al. (170)[a]	1979	*Mycobacterium gordonae*	52	—	—	Contaminated green dye added to cocaine for topical anesthesia
Leers (171)	1980	*M. tuberculosis*	1	0	0	Improper cleaning/disinfection
Schleupner and Hamilton (184)[a]	1980	*Trichosporon cutaneum*, *Penicillium* species	8	—	—	Contaminated cocaine solution used for topical anesthesia
Martone et al. (188)[a]	1981	*B. cepacia*	21	—	—	Contaminated lidocaine and normal saline setups, inadequate disinfectant
Sammartino et al. (182)	1982	*P. aeruginosa*	11	1	0	Inner channel
Dawson et al. (179)	1982	*M. intracellulare*	2	—	—	Plastic tubing; disinfection failure
Nelson et al. (172)	1983	*M. tuberculosis*	2	1	0	Disinfection failure
Pappas et al. (173)	1983	*M. chelonae*	72	2	1	Punctured suction channels
Siegman-Igra et al. (185)[a]	1985	*S. marcescens*	4	—	—	Terminal rinse with tap water
Goldstein and Abrutyn (186)[a]	1985	*Bacillus* species	14	—	—	Automated suction valve
Stine et al. (189)[a]	1987	*M. gordonae*	8	—	—	Terminal tap water rinse?
Prigogine et al. (181)[a]	1988	*M. tuberculosis*	8	—	—	Automatic aspiratory adapter
Wheeler et al. (174)[a]	1989	*M. avium*	2	—	—	Suction valve
Wheeler et al. (174)	1989	*M. tuberculosis*	3	1	0	Suction valve
Hoffmann et al. (175)[a]	1989	*Rhodotorula rubra*	30	—	—	Tub water, cleaning brushes
Jackson et al. (176)[a]	1989	*Sporothrix cyanescens*	4	—	—	Dust created during renovations
Nye et al. (180)[a]	1990	*M. chelonae*	4	—	—	Terminal rinse with contaminated tap water
CDC (190)[a]	1991	*M. chelonae*	14	—	—	Automated washer/disinfector; 10-minute disinfection, terminal tap water rinse
Fitch et al. (191)	1991	*M. chelonae*	21	0	0	Multiple: terminal tap water rinse, automated washer/disinfector
Nicolle et al. (177)	1992	*Blastomyces dermatitidis*	2	—	—	Failure to properly clean scope (microorganism rendered nonviable)
Gubler et al. (192)[a]	1992	*M. chelonae, M. gordonae*	12	—	—	Water tank of automated washer/disinfector
Fraser et al. (193)[a]	1992	*M. chelonae*	14	—	—	Automated cleaner/disinfector
Whitlock et al. (194)[a]	1992	*Rhodotorula rubra*	11	—	—	Suction valve and rubber biopsy valve
Maloney et al. (195)[a]	1994	*M. abscessus*	15	—	—	Automated washer/disinfector
Bennett et al. (196)[a]	1994	*M. xenopi*	13	—	—	Terminal tap water rinse; contaminated hot water tank
Kolmos et al. (197)[a]	1994	*P. aeruginosa*	8	—	—	Suction channels (not cleaned prior to disinfection)
Wang et al. (198)[a]	1995	*M. chelonae*	18	—	—	Suction channels
Hagan et al. (199)[a]	1995	*R. rubra*	11	—	—	Suction channels
Cox et al. (200)[a]	1997	*M. chelonae*	34	—	—	Lidocaine sprayers used on multiple patients
Blanc et al. (201)[a]	1997	*P. aeruginosa*	35	—	—	Automated washer/disinfector
Agerton et al. (202)[a]	1997	*M. tuberculosis (MDR)*	4	2 (disease 1)	—	Improper disinfection, bronchoscopes not fully immersed in disinfectant
Michele et al. (203)	1997	*M. tuberculosis*	1	1	—	Improper disinfection; failure to use enzymatic cleaner, sterilize biopsy forceps, and completely immerse bronchoscope
Mitchell et al. (219)[a]	1997	*Legionella pneumophilia*	3	—	—	Use of contaminated rinse, failure of 70% ethanol flush

(Continued)

TABLE 68.3. Continued

Reference	Year	Microorganism	Isolates	Infections	Deaths	Source of Contamination
Wallace et al. (204)[a]	1998	*M. abscessus*	12	—	—	Automated endoscope reprocessor and manual disinfection
Wallace et al. (204)[a]	1998	*M. abscessus*	30	—	—	Automated endoscope reprocessor
Wallace et al. (204)[a]	1998	*M. fortuitum*	4	—	—	Automated endoscope reprocessor
CDC (220)	1999	*M. tuberculosis*	4	0	—	Automated endoscope reprocessor
CDC (220)[a]	1999	*Mycobacterium avium-intracelluare*	7	—	—	Automated endoscope reprocessor: use of channel adapters provided by bronchoscope manufacturer instead of connector kit provided by automated endoscope reprocessor manufacturer
Strelczyk (205)[a]	1999	Acid-fast bacilli	10	—	—	Automated endoscope reprocessor: inadequate channel connectors provided by bronchoscope manufacturer
Schelenz and French (206)	2000	*Pseudomonas aeruginosa*	—	—	—	Automated endoscope reprocessor
Gillespie et al. (207)[a]	2000	*Mycobacterium chelonae*	2	—	0	Automated endoscope reprocessor
Wilson et al. (208)[a]	2000	*Aureobasidium* species	10	—	—	Reuse of single-use stopcocks
Larson et al. (209)[a]	2001	*M. tuberculosis*	2	—	0	Automated endoscope reprocessor and improper cleaning
Kressel and Kidd (211)[a]	2001	*M. chelonae, Methylobacterium mesophilicum*	20	—	0	Automated endoscope reprocessor
Kramer et al. (210)[a]	2001	*P. aeruginosa*	2	—	0	Automated endoscope reprocessor: contaminated disinfectant due to inadequate concentration
Sorin et al. (212)	2001	*P. aeruginosa*	18	3	1	Automated endoscope reprocessor: inappropriate channel connectors
Ramsey et al. (213)	2002	*M. tuberculosis*	9	3	0	Defective bronchoscope
Srinivasan et al. (214)	2003	*P. aeruginosa*	—	—	—	Defective bronchoscope: loosened biopsy port
Kirschke et al. (221)	2003	*P. aeruginosa*	17	1	—	Defective bronchoscope: loosened biopsy port
Rossetti et al. (216)[a]	2002	*M. gordonae*	16	0	— 0	Automated endoscope reprocessor
Singh et al. (217)[a]	2003	*Trichoporum mucoides*	6	0		Defective bronchoscope
Silva et al. (218)[a]	2003	*P. aeruginosa, S. marcescens*	41	0	0	Inproper rinsing

[a] Pseudoepidemic.
Adapted from Weber, DJ, Rutala, WA. Lessons from outbreaks associated with bronchosocopy. *Infect Control Hosp Epidemiol* 2001;22:403–408.

breaks include failure to properly remove debris from scope channels by brushing (171,177,197), use of inadequate disinfectants (171,172,178,179,196,210), use of contaminated tap water (175,179,192,196,216,219), and failure to dismantle all equipment (168,174,181). Detection of outbreaks (195,196, 202,203,206,211–213,219,220) and determination of the environmental reservoir (195,196,206,211,219) have been aided by molecular typing of outbreak pathogens. Several specific issues in proper cleaning and disinfection of bronchoscopes warrant further elaboration. First, all scope components (e.g., suction valves) must be dismantled and appropriately cleaned and disinfected. Second, terminal rinses to remove residual glutaraldehyde must be done with sterile water. Third, damaged scopes leading to protected foci for microorganisms may lead to cross-transmission despite use of adequate cleaning and disinfectants (173, 213,214,221). Finally, properly cleaned bronchoscopes must be sterilized with ethylene oxide or peracetic acid, or disinfected with an appropriate high-level disinfectant such as 2% glutaraldehyde. Outbreaks have occurred when the disinfectant used was 70% alcohol (178), povidone-iodine (171), alcohol plus povidone-iodine (172), cetrimide plus chlorhexidine (179), or 0.13% glutaraldehyde-phenate (196). Further, the disinfectant must be in contact with all surfaces for the correct exposure time and at the appropriate temperature (173,176,190). Exposure times of less than 20 minutes do not reliably inactivate mycobacteria. Preventing nosocomial transmission of microorganisms by bronchoscopy requires meticulous attention to hand washing and proper cleaning and disinfection of the bronchoscopes. Appropriate care must also be taken by bronchoscopy personnel not to contact pathogens from the patient via airborne transmission (see Chapters 37, 81, and 89).

Guidelines for Disinfection of Bronchoscopes

General guidelines for the disinfection of medical equipment are available (165,222–224) (see Chapter 63). Bronchoscopes should be sterilized or high-level disinfected between patients; however, because of the pressures of time, most scopes are subjected to high-level disinfection. By definition, high-level disinfection may not inactivate bacterial endospores. The microorganisms most resistant to inactivation are bacterial endospores and mycobacteria. Diluted glutaraldehyde preparations (less than 2%) do not reliably inactivate mycobacteria with a 20-minute exposure time (225). Of concern, many hospitals employ either inadequate exposure times or inappropriate disinfectants (226). U.S. guidelines differ from those of the Research Committee of the British Thoracic Society in several important aspects, including special handling for bronchoscopes used on immunocompromised patients and disinfection times (227). Current practice should be based on the more recent U.S. guidelines.

Spirometry

Spirometry is a basic function test that allows the measurement of forced vital capacity and time-related indicators of dynamic pulmonary function (228,229). Data obtained from the forced expiration maneuver can be used to generate flow-volume and volume-time curves. Such measures are widely used in diagnosing pulmonary disorders, evaluating the risks associated with intraabdominal surgery, and assessing the response to bronchodilators. In recent years, much attention has been paid to standardizing spirometry equipment and methods (230–232). Several outbreaks have been linked to the use of contaminated spirometers (233–235). In mechanically ventilated patients, contaminated spirometers have been linked to cross-transmission of *Stenotrophomonas maltophilia* (155,233) and *A. calcoaceticus* var. *anitratus* (234). Hazaleus et al. (235) reported transmission of *Mycobacterium tuberculosis* infection to 1 of 22 patients who underwent pulmonary function testing using a dry-seal spirometer within 12 days of its use for a patient with active pulmonary tuberculosis. Few studies have carefully evaluated the potential of spirometers as vehicles for cross-transmission of microorganisms. Rutala et al. (236) prospectively examined the extent of microbial contamination of two commonly marketed dry-rolling spirometers following use for patients with a heavily colonized or infected respiratory tract. The investigation revealed that the mouthpieces became contaminated with the patients' oral flora and with the associated respiratory pathogen; 14% of tubing samples after patient testing contained the respiratory pathogen. All other equipment samples (e.g., interior surface of the machine) were negative for the respiratory pathogen. These data suggest that changing the mouthpieces and tubing between patients will eliminate the possibility of cross-transmission, and that it is unnecessary to routinely clean the interior surfaces of the machine. Burgos et al. (237) found frequent colonization of the proximal tubing, distal tubing, water, and water-bell of a water-sealed spirometer; however, no transmission of potentially pathogenic microorganisms from equipment to patients or vice versa was demonstrated.

Room Humidifiers

Cool-mist humidifiers have been linked to nosocomial epidemics of sepsis or pneumonia caused by *A. calcoaceticus* var. *anitratus* (238), *A. calcoaceticus* var. *Lwoffi* (239), *P. aeruginosa* (240), and *Legionella pneumophila* (97,241). Experiments using tap water contaminated with *L. pneumophila* have demonstrated that cool-mist humidifiers can readily generate aerosols of *Legionella* that disseminate throughout a two-bed patient room (242). Nonaerosol humidifiers used to humidify wall oxygen may also support the growth of *P. aeruginosa* (243) and have been linked to respiratory infections with this pathogen (244,245).

Inhaled Medication

Direct instillation of aerosolized contaminated medications is a well-established, although unusual, cause of lower respiratory tract infection (50). Both colonization and pneumonia caused by *Klebsiella pneumoniae* resulted from the use of a contaminated stock bottle containing a bronchodilator (246). Contamination of saline vials used in respiratory care equipment has led to multiple outbreaks (98,247–249). Use of contaminated multidose saline vials for IPPB treatments was reported to lead to both pneumonia and sepsis with *S. marcescens* (98). Intrinsic contamination of single-dose vials of tracheal irrigant solution has led to multiple outbreaks of pulmonary colonization with *Ralstonia pickettii* (247,249,250). Following one of these outbreaks, experiments revealed that *R. pickettii* is capable of proliferating in 0.9% sodium chloride solution and that *R. pickettii* is not fully retained by a 0.2-μm cartridge filter (251). Manipulation of disposable saline squeeze vials for use during suctioning frequently leads to contamination of the vial contents with coagulase-negative staphylococci, *Staphylococcus aureus,* streptococci, and enterococci (252). In several cases, the contaminating pathogen was isolated from the nurse's hands, suggesting that contamination occurred during opening of the vial. Despite its frequency, whether such contamination leads to lower respiratory tract infection has not been evaluated.

Of note, symptoms resembling neonatal sepsis have resulted from inadvertent administration of inhaled epinephrine (253).

Aspiration of Contaminated Medications

An outbreak of neonatal listeriosis was traced to bathing of infants with mineral oil from a multidose container that was contaminated by *Listeria monocytogenes* (254). Aspiration of the contaminated oil presumably led to clinical infection and sepsis. Aspiration of commercial charcoal has reportedly led to colonization and, possibly, infection with *Aspergillus niger, Paecilomyces variotti,* and *Penicillium* species (255). The authors noted that commercial charcoal is not a sterile preparation, and its use may lead to colonization in immunocompromised patients.

Ingestion of Contaminated Foods or Medications

Ingestion of contaminated ice led to the development of nosocomial pneumonia due to *Legionella pneumophila* in a long-term ventilated patient (256). Ice machines may serve as the reservoir for nosocomial pathogens, and appropriate management, including periodic cleaning, is indicated (257).

The addition of food dye contaminated with *P. aeruginosa* to nasogastric tube feedings to monitor for possible aspiration led to a cluster of infections in ventilated patients (258). The outbreak was terminated by replacing the multidose bottles with single-use vials.

An investigation of nursing home outbreaks of respiratory infection caused by *Legionella sainthelensi* identified history of a stroke and eating pureed food as risk factors for infection (259). The association of these variables with swallowing disorders suggests that aspiration of contaminated potable water was the cause of *Legionella* infection.

Contaminated mouthwash led to a large pseudo-outbreak of *B. cepacia* from respiratory tract specimens of intubated patients at two hospitals (260,261). Swabbing with the mouthwash was used for routine oral care for all case patients. *B. cepacia* was grown from unopened bottles of the mouthwash, and the pseudo-outbreak ended after use of the mouthwash was discontinued.

Hospital Personnel with Dermatitis

Nosocomial infections have occasionally been linked to colonized or infected respiratory therapists. An epidemic of nosocomial respiratory tract infections due to *A. calcoaceticus* was linked to a respiratory therapist with chronic dermatitis who had persistent hand colonization and who contaminated sterile respiratory care equipment (262). Nosocomial hepatitis B was reported to have been acquired from a therapist with exudative dermatitis during placement of intraarterial catheters (263). Careful hand washing and the use of sterile gloves should minimize transmission of infection during invasive procedures (264). Healthcare workers with weeping or exudative dermatitis should refrain from direct patient care or handling of patient care equipment until the dermatitis has resolved (see also Chapter 99).

Suctioning Apparatus

The collection of body fluids using suction is accomplished by portable pumps or wall vacuum lines. Suction is most commonly used to clear the upper respiratory tract (pharynx and trachea) of secretions in sedated or intubated patients. Suction collection units can lead to nosocomial infections either by producing aerosols containing potential bacterial pathogens or by serving as an environmental reservoir (265). Transmission to patients can occur through contamination of the hands of healthcare personnel during manipulation of the suction unit or through retrograde spread to the patient undergoing suction.

The use of older or improperly designed suction units has resulted in aerosolization of potential microbial pathogens, most commonly aerobic gram-negative bacilli or *S. aureus* (266–268). Contaminated suction units that generate aerosols have led to outbreaks caused by *Klebsiella aerogenes* (269), *P. aeruginosa* (270), and *Salmonella montevideo* (271). Contaminated suction units, along with other environmental reservoirs, have been linked to neonatal infections caused by *P. mirabilis* (272) and *P. aeruginosa* (270,273,274), and to adult infections caused by *K. aerogenes* (269) and *P. aeruginosa* (275–277).

Prevention of nosocomial infections caused by spread of the contaminated secretions contained in suction units requires use of units designed to prevent aerosolization of body fluids or overflow, disinfection between patient uses, disposal of fluids in a non–patient-care area, and hand washing after handling (29).

Tracheal suctioning has occasionally led directly to nosocomial infections. Withdrawal of the suction catheter across the patient's face has reportedly led to serious nosocomial eye infections, most frequently due to *P. aeruginosa* (278). Van Dyke and Spector (279) reported transmission of herpes simplex virus type I from a physician with herpes labialis to an infant during suctioning for meconium aspiration (279). Standard guidelines should be used by hospital personnel performing tracheal suctioning to minimize the risk of nosocomial infection (Table 68.2).

Three studies have compared "open" and "closed" methods for suctioning patients (73,141,142). The first two studies did not detect a difference in the incidence of nosocomial pneumonia. "Closed" suctioning was associated with fewer arrhythmias and less desaturation in one study (141) but with an increased rate of colonization in a second study (73). However, in a more recent study, open suctioning was associated with a 3.5-fold increase in ventilator-associated pneumonia (142). The current data do not favor either mode of suctioning as superior in regard to prevention of pneumonia.

Four studies have compared the incidence of pneumonia in patients when endotracheal tubes that allowed continuous aspiration of subglottic secretions versus standard endotracheal tubes were used (38,144–146). All studies demonstrated that the use of continuous aspiration of subglottic secretions reduced the rate of pneumonia (RRs, 0.22 and 0.61), but only two studies reached statistical significance (144,146). Continuous aspiration of subglottic secretions appears to be an effective method to prevent ventilator-associated pneumonia, and additional, adequately powered studies are warranted.

REFERENCES

1. Horan TC, White JW, Jarvis WR, et al. Nosocomial infection surveillance, 1984. *MMWR CDC Surveill Summ* 1986;35(1):17SS–29SS.
2. Richards MJ, Edwards JR, Culver DH, et al. Nosocomial infections

in coronary care units in the United States. National Nosocomial Infections Surveillance System. *Am J Cardiol* 1998;82(6):789–793.

3. Richards MJ, Edwards JR, Culver DH, et al. Nosocomial infections in medical intensive care units in the United States. National Nosocomial Infections Surveillance System. *Crit Care Med* 1999;27(5): 887–892.
4. Wenzel RP, Osterman CA, Hunting KJ. Hospital-acquired infections. II. Infection rates by site, service and common procedures in a university hospital. *Am J Epidemiol* 1976;104(6):645–651.
5. National Nosocomial Infections Surveillance (NNIS) System Report, data summary from January 1992 to June 2002, issued August 2002. *Am J Infect Control* 2002;30(8):458–475.
6. Harkness GA, Bentley DW, Roghmann KJ. Risk factors for nosocomial pneumonia in the elderly. *Am J Med* 1990;89(4):457–463.
7. Hanson LC, Weber DJ, Rutala WA. Risk factors for nosocomial pneumonia in the elderly. *Am J Med* 1992;92(2):161–166.
8. Hemming VG, Overall JC Jr, Britt MR. Nosocomial infections in a newborn intensive-care unit. Results of forty-one months of surveillance. *N Engl J Med* 1976;294(24):1310–1316.
9. Daschner FD, Frey P, Wolff G, et al. Nosocomial infections in intensive care wards: a multicenter prospective study. *Intensive Care Med* 1982;8(1):5–9.
10. Cunnion K. *Risk factors for nosocomial pneumonia: comparing adult critical care populations.* University of North Carolina School of Public Health, 1991.
11. Stevens RM, Teres D, Skillman JJ, et al. Pneumonia in an intensive care unit. A 30-month experience. *Arch Intern Med* 1974;134(1): 106–111.
12. Joshi N, Localio AR, Hamory BH. A predictive risk index for nosocomial pneumonia in the intensive care unit. *Am J Med* 1992;93(2): 135–142.
13. Chevret S, Hemmer M, Carlet J, et al. Incidence and risk factors of pneumonia acquired in intensive care units. Results from a multicenter prospective study on 996 patients. European Cooperative Group on Nosocomial Pneumonia. *Intensive Care Med* 1993;19(5): 256–264.
14. Kropec A, Schulgen G, Just H, et al. Scoring system for nosocomial pneumonia in ICUs. *Intensive Care Med* 1996;22(11):1155–1161.
15. Vincent JL, Bihari DJ, Suter PM, et al. The prevalence of nosocomial infection in intensive care units in Europe. Results of the European Prevalence of Infection in Intensive Care (EPIC) Study. EPIC International Advisory Committee. *JAMA* 1995;274(8):639–644.
16. Celis R, Torres A, Gatell JM, et al. Nosocomial pneumonia. A multivariate analysis of risk and prognosis. *Chest* 1988;93(2):318–324.
17. Arozullah AM, Khuri SF, Henderson WG, et al. Development and validation of a multifactorial risk index for predicting postoperative pneumonia after major noncardiac surgery. *Ann Intern Med* 2001; 135(10):847–857.
18. Tejada Artigas A, Bello Dronda S, Chacon Valles E, et al. Risk factors for nosocomial pneumonia in critically ill trauma patients. *Crit Care Med* 2001;29(2):304–309.
19. Messori A, Trippoli S, Vaiani M, et al. Bleeding and pneumonia in intensive care patients given ranitidine and sucralfate for prevention of stress ulcer: meta-analysis of randomised controlled trials. *BMJ* 2000;321(7269):1103–1106.
20. Husni RN, Goldstein LS, Arroliga AC, et al. Risk factors for an outbreak of multi-drug-resistant Acinetobacter nosocomial pneumonia among intubated patients. *Chest* 1999;115(5):1378–1382.
21. Hanes SD, Demirkan K, Tolley E, et al. Risk factors for late-onset nosocomial pneumonia caused by Stenotrophomonas maltophilia in critically ill trauma patients. *Clin Infect Dis* 2002;35(3):228–235.
22. Cook DJ, Kollef MH. Risk factors for ICU-acquired pneumonia. *JAMA* 1998;279(20):1605–1606.
23. Fleming CA, Balaguera HU, Craven DE. Risk factors for nosocomial pneumonia. Focus on prophylaxis. *Med Clin North Am* 2001;85(6): 1545–1563.
24. George DL, Falk PS, Wunderink RG, et al. Epidemiology of ventilator-acquired pneumonia based on protected bronchoscopic sampling. *Am J Respir Crit Care Med* 1998;158(6):1839–1847.
25. George DL. Epidemiology of nosocomial ventilator-associated pneumonia. *Infect Control Hosp Epidemiol* 1993;14(3):163–169.
26. Craven DE, Steger KA, Barat LM, et al. Nosocomial pneumonia: epidemiology and infection control. *Intensive Care Med* 1992; 18(suppl 1):S3–9.
27. Inglis TJ. Pulmonary infection in intensive care units. *Br J Anaesth* 1990;65(1):94–106.
28. Craven DE, Steger KA, Barber TW. Preventing nosocomial pneumonia: state of the art and prospective for the 1990s. *Am J Med* 1991; 91:44–53.
29. Tablan OC, Anderson LJ, Arden NH, et al. Guideline for prevention of nosocomial pneumonia. The Hospital Infection Control Practices Advisory Committee, Centers for Disease Control and Prevention. *Infect Control Hosp Epidemiol* 1994;15(9):587–627.
30. Garrard CS, A'Court CD. The diagnosis of pneumonia in the critically ill. *Chest* 1995;108(2 suppl):17S–25S.
31. Craven DE, Steger KA. Epidemiology of nosocomial pneumonia. New perspectives on an old disease. *Chest* 1995;108(2 suppl):1S–16S.
32. Mayhall CG. Nosocomial pneumonia. Diagnosis and prevention. *Infect Dis Clin North Am* 1997;11(2):427–457.
33. Craven DE, Steger KA. Ventilator-associated bacterial pneumonia: challenges in diagnosis, treatment, and prevention. *New Horiz* 1998; 6(2 suppl):S30–45.
34. McEachern R, Campbell GD Jr. Hospital-acquired pneumonia: epidemiology, etiology, and treatment. *Infect Dis Clin North Am* 1998; 12(3):761–779,x.
35. Lynch JP 3rd. Hospital-acquired pneumonia: risk factors, microbiology, and treatment. *Chest* 2001;119(2 suppl):373S–384S.
36. Eggimann P, Pittet D. Infection control in the ICU. *Chest* 2001; 120(6):2059–2093.
37. Engemann J, Kaye KS. Ventilator-associated pneumonia. *Semin Infect Control* 2001;1(4):255–266.
38. Kollef MH, Skubas NJ, Sundt TM. A randomized clinical trial of continuous aspiration of subglottic secretions in cardiac surgery patients. *Chest* 1999;116(5):1339–1346.
39. Koeman M, van der Ven AJ, Ramsay G, et al. Ventilator-associated pneumonia: recent issues on pathogenesis, prevention and diagnosis. *J Hosp Infect* 2001;49(3):155–162.
40. Weber D, Raasch RH, Rutala WA. Healthcare-acquired Pneumonia. *Curr Treat Opt Infect Dis* 2002;4:141–151.
41. Keenan SP, Heyland DK, Jacka MJ, et al. Ventilator-associated pneumonia. Prevention, diagnosis, and therapy. *Crit Care Clin* 2002;18(1): 107–125.
42. Mehta RM, Niederman MS. Nosocomial pneumonia. *Curr Opin Infect Dis* 2002;15(4):387–394.
43. Chastre J, Fagon JY. Ventilator-associated pneumonia. *Am J Respir Crit Care Med* 2002;165(7):867–903.
44. Kollef MH. Epidemiology and risk factors for nosocomial pneumonia. Emphasis on prevention. *Clin Chest Med* 1999;20(3):653–670.
45. Kollef MH. The prevention of ventilator-associated pneumonia. *N Engl J Med* 1999;340(8):627–634.
46. Ferrer R, Artigas A. Clinical review: non-antibiotic strategies for preventing ventilator-associated pneumonia. *Crit Care* 2002;6(1):45–51.
47. Bergogne-Berezin E. Treatment and prevention of nosocomial pneumonia. *Chest* 1995;108(2 suppl):26S–34S.
48. Reinarz JA, Pierce AK, Mays BB, et al. The potential role of inhalation therapy equipment in nosocomial pulmonary infections. *J Clin Invest* 1965;44:831–839.
49. Hovig B. Lower respiratory tract infections associated with respiratory therapy and anaesthesia. *J Hosp Infect* 1981;2:301–305.
50. Rutala WA, Weber DJ. Environmental issues and nosocomial infections. In: Farber BF, ed. *Infection control in intensive care.* New York: Churchill Livingstone, 1987:131–171.
51. Weber DJ, Rutala WA. Environmental issues and nosocomial infections. In: Wenzel RP, ed. *Prevention and control of nosocomial infections,* 3rd ed. Baltimore: Williams & Wilkins, 1997:491–514.
52. Craven DE, Barber TW, Steger KA, et al. Nosocomial pneumonia in the 1990s: update of epidemiology and risk factors. *Semin Respir Infect* 1990;5(3):157–172.
53. Cook D, De Jonghe B, Brochard L, et al. Influence of airway manage-

ment on ventilator-associated pneumonia: evidence from randomized trials. *JAMA* 1998;279(10):781–787.

54. Pierce AK, Sanford JP, Thomas GD, et al. Long-term evaluation of decontamination of inhalation-therapy equipment and the occurrence of necrotizing pneumonia. *N Engl J Med* 1970;282(10):528–531.
55. Levine SA, Niederman MS. The impact of tracheal intubation on host defenses and risks for nosocomial pneumonia. *Clin Chest Med* 1991;12(3):523–543.
56. Koerner RJ. Contribution of endotracheal tubes to the pathogenesis of ventilator-associated pneumonia. *J Hosp Infect* 1997;35(2):83–89.
57. Bryant LR, Trinkle JK, Mobin-Uddin K, et al. Bacterial colonization profile with tracheal intubation and mechanical ventilation. *Arch Surg* 1972;104(5):647–651.
58. Zwillich CW, Pierson DJ, Creagh CE, et al. Complications of assisted ventilation. A prospective study of 354 consecutive episodes. *Am J Med* 1974;57(2):161–170.
59. Lareau SC, Ryan KJ, Diener CF. The relationship between frequency of ventilator circuit changes and infectious hazard. *Am Rev Respir Dis* 1978;118(3):493–496.
60. Cross AS, Roup B. Role of respiratory assistance devices in endemic nosocomial pneumonia. *Am J Med* 1981;70(3):681–685.
61. du Moulin GC, Paterson DG, Hedley-Whyte J, et al. Aspiration of gastric bacteria in antacid-treated patients: a frequent cause of postoperative colonisation of the airway. *Lancet* 1982;1(8266):242–245.
62. Mauritz W, Graninger W, Schindler I, et al. [Pathogenic flora in the gastric juice and bronchial secretion of long-term ventilated intensive-care patients]. *Anaesthesist* 1985;34(4):203–207.
63. Braun SR, Levin AB, Clark KL. Role of corticosteroids in the development of pneumonia in mechanically ventilated head-trauma victims. *Crit Care Med* 1986;14(3):198–201.
64. Craven DE, Kunches LM, Kilinsky V, et al. Risk factors for pneumonia and fatality in patients receiving continuous mechanical ventilation. *Am Rev Respir Dis* 1986;133(5):792–796.
65. Rashkin MC, Davis T. Acute complications of endotracheal intubation. Relationship to reintubation, route, urgency, and duration. *Chest* 1986;89(2):165–167.
66. Ruiz-Santana S, Garcia Jimenez A, Esteban A, et al. ICU pneumonias: a multi-institutional study. *Crit Care Med* 1987;15(10):930–932.
67. Daschner F, Kappstein I, Schuster F, et al. Influence of disposable ("Conchapak") and reusable humidifying systems on the incidence of ventilation pneumonia. *J Hosp Infect* 1988;11(2):161–168.
68. Daschner F, Kappstein I, Engels I, et al. Stress ulcer prophylaxis and ventilation pneumonia: prevention by antibacterial cytoprotective agents? *Infect Control Hosp Epidemiol* 1988;9(2):59–65.
69. Fagon JY, Chastre J, Domart Y, et al. Nosocomial pneumonia in patients receiving continuous mechanical ventilation. Prospective analysis of 52 episodes with use of a protected specimen brush and quantitative culture techniques. *Am Rev Respir Dis* 1989;139(4): 877–884.
70. Jimenez P, Torres A, Rodriguez-Roisin R, et al. Incidence and etiology of pneumonia acquired during mechanical ventilation. *Crit Care Med* 1989;17(9):882–885.
71. Klein BS, Perloff WH, Maki DG. Reduction of nosocomial infection during pediatric intensive care by protective isolation. *N Engl J Med* 1989;320(26):1714–1721.
72. Reusser P, Zimmerli W, Scheidegger D, et al. Role of gastric colonization in nosocomial infections and endotoxemia: a prospective study in neurosurgical patients on mechanical ventilation. *J Infect Dis* 1989; 160(3):414–421.
73. Deppe SA, Kelly JW, Thoi LL, et al. Incidence of colonization, nosocomial pneumonia, and mortality in critically ill patients using a Trach Care closed-suction system versus an open-suction system: prospective, randomized study. *Crit Care Med* 1990;18(12):1389–1393.
74. Jacobs S, Chang RW, Lee B, et al. Continuous enteral feeding: a major cause of pneumonia among ventilated intensive care unit patients. *JPEN J Parenter Enteral Nutr* 1990;14(4):353–356.
75. Torres A, Aznar R, Gatell JM, et al. Incidence, risk, and prognosis factors of nosocomial pneumonia in mechanically ventilated patients. *Am Rev Respir Dis* 1990;142(3):523–528.
76. Dreyfuss D, Djedaini K, Weber P, et al. Prospective study of nosocomial pneumonia and of patient and circuit colonization during mechanical ventilation with circuit changes every 48 hours versus no change. *Am Rev Respir Dis* 1991;143(4 Pt 1):738–743.
77. Jarvis WR, Edwards JR, Culver DH, et al. Nosocomial infection rates in adult and pediatric intensive care units in the United States. National Nosocomial Infections Surveillance System. *Am J Med* 1991; 91(3B):185S–191S.
78. Mosconi P, Langer M, Cigada M, et al. Epidemiology and risk factors of pneumonia in critically ill patients. Intensive Care Unit Group for Infection Control. *Eur J Epidemiol* 1991;7(4):320–327.
79. Kollef MH. Ventilator-associated pneumonia. A multivariate analysis. *JAMA* 1993;270(16):1965–1970.
80. Cook DJ, Walter SD, Cook RJ, et al. Incidence of and risk factors for ventilator-associated pneumonia in critically ill patients. *Ann Intern Med* 1998;129(6):433–440.
81. Holdcroft A, Lumley J, Gaya H. Why disinfect ventilators? *Lancet* 1973;1(7797):240–241.
82. Hellewell J, Jeanes AL, Watkin RR, et al. The Williams bacterial filter. Use in the intensive care unit. *Anaesthesia* 1967;22(3):497–503.
83. Bishop CRW, Williams SR. The use of an absolute filter to sterilize the inspiratory air during intermittent positive pressure respiratory. *Br J Anaesth* 1963;35:32–34.
84. Garibaldi RA, Britt MR, Webster C, et al. Failure of bacterial filters to reduce the incidence of pneumonia after inhalation anesthesia. *Anesthesiology* 1981;54(5):364–368.
85. Feeley TW, Hamilton WK, Xavier B, et al. Sterile anesthesia breathing circuits do not prevent postoperative pulmonary infection. *Anesthesiology* 1981;54(5):369–372.
86. Christopher KL, Saravolatz LD, Bush TL, et al. The potential role of respiratory therapy equipment in cross infection. A study using a canine model for pneumonia. *Am Rev Respir Dis* 1983;128(2): 271–275.
87. Dyer ED, Peterson DE. How far do bacteria travel from the exhalation valve of IPPB equipment? *Anesth Analg* 1972;51(4):516–519.
88. Phillips I, Spencer G. Pseudomonas aeruginosa cross-infection due to contaminated respiratory apparatus. *Lancet* 1965;2(7426): 1325–1327.
89. Vanderbroucke-Grauls C, Kerver AJH, Rommes JH, et al. Endemic *Acinetobacter anitratus* in a surgical intensive care unit: mechanical ventilators as reservoir. *Eur J Clin Microbiol Infect Dis* 1988;7: 485–489.
90. Weems JJ Jr. Nosocomial outbreak of Pseudomonas cepacia associated with contamination of reusable electronic ventilator temperature probes. *Infect Control Hosp Epidemiol* 1993;14(10):583–586.
91. Berthelot P, Grattard F, Mahul P, et al. Ventilator temperature sensors: an unusual source of Pseudomonas cepacia in nosocomial infection. *J Hosp Infect* 1993;25(1):33–43.
92. Craven DE, Lichtenberg DA, Goularte TA, et al. Contaminated medication nebulizers in mechanical ventilator circuits. Source of bacterial aerosols. *Am J Med* 1984;77(5):834–838.
93. Sanders CV Jr, Luby JP, Johanson WG Jr, et al. Serratia marcescens infections from inhalation therapy medications: nosocomial outbreak. *Ann Intern Med* 1970;73(1):15–21.
94. Botman MJ, de Krieger RA. Contamination of small-volume medication nebulizers and its association with oropharyngeal colonization. *J Hosp Infect* 1987;10(2):204–208.
95. Kelsen SG, McGuckin M. The role of airborne bacteria in the contamination of fine particle nebulizers and the development of nosocomial pneumonia. *Ann NY Acad Sci* 1980;353:218–229.
96. Kelsen SG, McGuckin M, Kelsen DP, et al. Airborne contamination of fine-particle nebulizers. *JAMA* 1977;237(21):2311–2314.
97. Arnow PM, Chou T, Weil D, et al. Nosocomial Legionnaires' disease caused by aerosolized tap water from respiratory devices. *J Infect Dis* 1982;146(4):460–467.
98. Cabrera HA. An outbreak of Serratia marcescens, and its control. *Arch Intern Med* 1969;123(6):650–655.
99. Ringrose RE, McKown B, Felton FG, et al. A hospital outbreak of Serratia marcescens associated with ultrasonic nebulizers. *Ann Intern Med* 1968;69(4):719–729.

100. McNamara MJ, Hill MC, Balows A, et al. A study of the bacteriologic patterns of hospital infections. *Ann Intern Med* 1967;66(3):480–488.
101. Rhame FS, Streifel A, McComb C, et al. Bubbling humidifiers produce microaerosols which can carry bacteria. *Infect Control* 1986;7(8): 403–407.
102. Goularte TA, Manning M, Craven DE. Bacterial colonization in humidifying cascade reservoirs after 24 and 48 hours of continuous mechanical ventilation. *Infect Control* 1987;8(5):200–203.
103. Gilmour IJ, Boyle MJ, Streifel A, et al. The effects of circuit and humidifier type on contamination potential during mechanical ventilation: a laboratory study. *Am J Infect Control* 1995;23(2):65–72.
104. Zuravleff JJ, Yu VL, Shonnard JW, et al. Legionella pneumophila contamination of a hospital humidifier. Demonstration of aerosol transmission and subsequent subclinical infection in exposed guinea pigs. *Am Rev Respir Dis* 1983;128(4):657–661.
105. Alary M, Joly JR. Factors contributing to the contamination of hospital water distribution systems by legionellae. *J Infect Dis* 1992;165(3): 565–569.
106. Craven DE, Goularte TA, Make BJ. Contaminated condensate in mechanical ventilator circuits. A risk factor for nosocomial pneumonia? *Am Rev Respir Dis* 1984;129(4):625–628.
107. Craven DE, Connolly MG Jr, Lichtenberg DA, et al. Contamination of mechanical ventilators with tubing changes every 24 or 48 hours. *N Engl J Med* 1982;306(25):1505–1509.
108. Cadwallader HL, Bradley CR, Ayliffe GA. Bacterial contamination and frequency of changing ventilator circuitry. *J Hosp Infect* 1990; 15(1):65–72.
109. Boher M, Lohse S, Glasby C, et al. Impact of 7-day ventilator tubing changes on nosocomial lower respiratory tract infections. *Am J Infect Control* 1992;20:103(abst).
110. Mermel L, Eveloff S, Short K, et al. The risk of pneumonia associated with the use of heated wire versus conventional ventilator circuits—a prospective trial. *Infect Control Hosp Epidemiol* 1994;15(pt 2): 42(abst).
111. Hess D, Burns E, Romagnoli D, et al. Weekly ventilator circuit changes. A strategy to reduce costs without affecting pneumonia rates. *Anesthesiology* 1995;82(4):903–911.
112. Long MN, Wickstrom G, Grimes A, et al. Prospective, randomized study of ventilator-associated pneumonia in patients with one versus three ventilator circuit changes per week. *Infect Control Hosp Epidemiol* 1996;17(1):14–19.
113. Kotilainen HR, Keroack MA. Cost analysis and clinical impact of weekly ventilator circuit changes in patients in intensive care unit. *Am J Infect Control* 1997;25(2):117–120.
114. Fink JB, Krause SA, Barrett L, et al. Extending ventilator circuit change interval beyond 2 days reduces the likelihood of ventilator-associated pneumonia. *Chest* 1998;113(2):405–411.
115. Kollef MH, Shapiro SD, Fraser VJ, et al. Mechanical ventilation with or without 7-day circuit changes. A randomized controlled trial. *Ann Intern Med* 1995;123(3):168–174.
116. Malecka-Griggs B. Microbiological assessment of 24- and 48-h changes and management of semiclosed circuits from ventilators in a neonatal intensive care unit. *J Clin Microbiol* 1986;23(2):322–328.
117. Stamm AM. Ventilator-associated pneumonia and frequency of circuit changes. *Am J Infect Control* 1998;26(1):71–73.
118. Redding PJ, McWalter PW. Pseudomonas fluorescens cross-infection due to contaminated humidifier water. *Br Med J* 1980;281(6235): 275.
119. Cefai C, Richards J, Gould FK, et al. An outbreak of Acinetobacter respiratory tract infection resulting from incomplete disinfection of ventilatory equipment. *J Hosp Infect* 1990;15(2):177–182.
120. Hartstein AI, Rashad AL, Liebler JM, et al. Multiple intensive care unit outbreak of Acinetobacter calcoaceticus subspecies anitratus respiratory infection and colonization associated with contaminated, reusable ventilator circuits and resuscitation bags. *Am J Med* 1988; 85(5):624–631.
121. Im SW, Fung JP, So SY, et al. Unusual dissemination of pseudomonads by ventilators. *Anaesthesia* 1982;37(11):1074–1077.
122. Shelly M, Bethune DW, Latimer RD. A comparison of five heat and moisture exchangers. *Anaesthesia* 1986;41(5):527–532.
123. MacIntyre NR, Anderson HR, Silver RM, et al. Pulmonary function in mechanically-ventilated patients during 24-hour use of a hygroscopic condensor humidifier. *Chest* 1983;84(5):560–564.
124. Branson RD, Davis K Jr, Campbell RS, et al. Humidification in the intensive care unit. Prospective study of a new protocol utilizing heated humidification and a hygroscopic condenser humidifier. *Chest* 1993;104(6):1800–1805.
125. Gallagher J, Strangeways JE, Allt-Graham J. Contamination control in long-term ventilation. A clinical study using a heat- and moisture-exchanging filter. *Anaesthesia* 1987;42(5):476–481.
126. Misset B, Escudier B, Rivara D, et al. Heat and moisture exchanger vs heated humidifier during long-term mechanical ventilation. A prospective randomized study. *Chest* 1991;100(1):160–163.
127. Martin C, Perrin G, Gevaudan MJ, et al. Heat and moisture exchangers and vaporizing humidifiers in the intensive care unit. *Chest* 1990; 97(1):144–149.
128. Roustan JP, Kienlen J, Aubas P, et al. Comparison of hydrophobic heat and moisture exchangers with heated humidifier during prolonged mechanical ventilation. *Intensive Care Med* 1992;18(2): 97–100.
129. Dreyfuss D, Djedaini K, Gros I, et al. Mechanical ventilation with heated humidifiers or heat and moisture exchangers: effects on patient colonization and incidence of nosocomial pneumonia. *Am J Respir Crit Care Med* 1995;151(4):986–992.
130. Djedaini K, Billiard M, Mier L, et al. Changing heat and moisture exchangers every 48 hours rather than 24 hours does not affect their efficacy and the incidence of nosocomial pneumonia. *Am J Respir Crit Care Med* 1995;152(5 pt 1):1562–1569.
131. Hurni JM, Feihl F, Lazor R, et al. Safety of combined heat and moisture exchanger filters in long-term mechanical ventilation. *Chest* 1997;111(3):686–691.
132. Kirton OC, DeHaven B, Morgan J, et al. A prospective, randomized comparison of an in-line heat moisture exchange filter and heated wire humidifiers: rates of ventilator-associated early-onset (community-acquired) or late-onset (hospital-acquired) pneumonia and incidence of endotracheal tube occlusion. *Chest* 1997;112(4):1055–1059.
133. Thomachot L, Viviand X, Arnaud S, et al. Comparing two heat and moisture exchangers, one hydrophobic and one hygroscopic, on humidifying efficacy and the rate of nosocomial pneumonia. *Chest* 1998; 114(5):1383–1389.
134. Davis K Jr, Evans SL, Campbell RS, et al. Prolonged use of heat and moisture exchangers does not affect device efficiency or frequency rate of nosocomial pneumonia. *Crit Care Med* 2000;28(5):1412–1418.
135. Salemi C, Padilla S, Canola T, et al. Heat-and-moisture exchangers used with biweekly circuit tubing changes: effect on costs and pneumonia rates. *Infect Control Hosp Epidemiol* 2000;21(11):737–739.
136. Stone JW, Das BC. Investigation of an outbreak of infection with Acinetobacter calcoaceticus in a special care baby unit. *J Hosp Infect* 1986;7(1):42–48.
137. Thompson AC, Wilder BJ, Powner DJ. Bedside resuscitation bags: a source of bacterial contamination. *Infect Control* 1985;6(6):231–232.
138. Weber DJ, Wilson MB, Rutala WA, et al. Manual ventilation bags as a source for bacterial colonization of intubated patients. *Am Rev Respir Dis* 1990;142(4):892–894.
139. Bonten MJ, Weinstein RA. Infection control in intensive care units and prevention of ventilator-associated pneumonia. *Semin Respir Infect* 2000;15(4):327–335.
140. Girou E, Schortgen F, Delclaux C, et al. Association of noninvasive ventilation with nosocomial infections and survival in critically ill patients. *JAMA* 2000;284(18):2361–2367.
141. Johnson KL, Kearney PA, Johnson SB, et al. Closed versus open endotracheal suctioning: costs and physiologic consequences. *Crit Care Med* 1994;22(4):658–666.
142. Combes P, Fauvage B, Oleyer C. Nosocomial pneumonia in mechanically ventilated patients, a prospective randomised evaluation of the Stericath closed suctioning system. *Intensive Care Med* 2000;26(7): 878–882.
143. Kollef MH, Shapiro SD, Boyd V, et al. A randomized clinical trial comparing an extended-use hygroscopic condenser humidifier with

heated-water humidification in mechanically ventilated patients. *Chest* 1998;113(3):759–767.

144. Mahul P, Auboyer C, Jospe R, et al. Prevention of nosocomial pneumonia in intubated patients: respective role of mechanical subglottic secretions drainage and stress ulcer prophylaxis. *Intensive Care Med* 1992;18(1):20–25.
145. Valles J, Artigas A, Rello J, et al. Continuous aspiration of subglottic secretions in preventing ventilator-associated pneumonia. *Ann Intern Med* 1995;122(3):179–186.
146. Smulders K, van der Hoeven H, Weers-Pothoff I, et al. A randomized clinical trial of intermittent subglottic secretion drainage in patients receiving mechanical ventilation. *Chest* 2002;121(3):858–862.
147. Whiteman K, Nachtmann L, Kramer D, et al. Effects of continuous lateral rotation therapy on pulmonary complications in liver transplant patients. *Am J Crit Care* 1995;4(2):133–139.
148. Summer W, Curry P, Haponik EF, et al. Continuous mechanical turning of intensive care unit patients shortens length of stay in some diagnostic-related groups. *J Crit Care* 1989;4(1):45–53.
149. Gentilello L, Thompson DA, Tonnesen AS, et al. Effect of a rotating bed on the incidence of pulmonary complications in critically ill patients. *Crit Care Med* 1988;16(8):783–786.
150. Fink MP, Helsmoortel CM, Stein KL, et al. The efficacy of an oscillating bed in the prevention of lower respiratory tract infection in critically ill victims of blunt trauma. A prospective study. *Chest* 1990; 97(1):132–137.
151. deBoisblanc BP, Castro M, Everret B, et al. Effect of air-supported, continuous, postural oscillation on the risk of early ICU pneumonia in nontraumatic critical illness. *Chest* 1993;103(5):1543–1547.
152. Kirschenbaum L, Azzi E, Sfeir T, et al. Effect of continuous lateral rotational therapy on the prevalence of ventilator-associated pneumonia in patients requiring long-term ventilatory care. *Crit Care Med* 2002;30(9):1983–1986.
153. Nourdine K, Combes P, Carton MJ, et al. Does noninvasive ventilation reduce the ICU nosocomial infection risk? A prospective clinical survey. *Intensive Care Med* 1999;25(6):567–573.
154. Antonelli M, Conti G, Rocco M, et al. A comparison of noninvasive positive-pressure ventilation and conventional mechanical ventilation in patients with acute respiratory failure. *N Engl J Med* 1998;339(7): 429–435.
155. Jolliet P, Chevrolet JC. Bronchoscopy in the intensive care unit. *Intensive Care Med* 1992;18(3):160–169.
156. Wood RE. Pediatric bronchoscopy. *Chest Surg Clin North Am* 1996; 6(2):237–251.
157. Borchers SD, Beamis JF, Jr. Flexible bronchoscopy. *Chest Surg Clin North Am* 1996;6(2):169–192.
158. Lee A, Wu CL, Feins RH, et al. The use of fiberoptic endoscopy in anesthesia. *Chest Surg Clin North Am* 1996;6:329–347.
159. Credle WF Jr, Smiddy JF, Elliott RC. Complications of fiberoptic bronchoscopy. *Am Rev Respir Dis* 1974;109(1):67–72.
160. Suratt PM, Smiddy JF, Gruber B. Deaths and complications associated with fiberoptic bronchoscopy. *Chest* 1976;69(6):747–751.
161. Pereira W, Kovnat DM, Khan MA, et al. Fever and pneumonia after flexible fiberoptic bronchoscopy. *Am Rev Respir Dis* 1975;112(1): 59–64.
162. Kane RC, Cohen MH, Fossieck BE Jr, et al. Absence of bacteremia after fiberoptic bronchoscopy. *Am Rev Respir Dis* 1975;111(1): 102–104.
163. Barbato A, Magarotto M, Crivellaro M, et al. Use of the paediatric bronchoscope, flexible and rigid, in 51 European centres. *Eur Respir J* 1997;10(8):1761–1766.
164. Spach DH, Silverstein FE, Stamm WE. Transmission of infection by gastrointestinal endoscopy and bronchoscopy. *Ann Intern Med* 1993; 118(2):117–128.
165. Weber DJ, Rutala WA. Lessons from outbreaks associated with bronchoscopy. *Infect Control Hosp Epidemiol* 2001;22(7):403–408.
166. Webb S, Vall-Spinosa, A. Outbreak of Serratia marcescens associated with the flexible fiberbronchoscope. *Chest* 1975;68:703–708.
167. Suratt PM, Gruber B, Wellons HA, et al. Absence of clinical pneumonia following bronchoscopy with contaminated and clean bronchofiberscopes. *Chest* 1977;71(1):52–54.
168. Hussain SA. Fiberoptic bronchoscope-related outbreak of infection with Pseudomonas. *Chest* 1978;74(4):483.
169. Markovitz A. Inoculation by bronchoscopy. *West J Med* 1979;131(6): 550.
170. Steere AC, Corrales J, von Graevenitz A. A cluster of Mycobacterium gordonae isolates from bronchoscopy specimens. *Am Rev Respir Dis* 1979;120(1):214–216.
171. Leers WD. Disinfecting endoscopes: how not to transmit Mycobacterium tuberculosis by bronchoscopy. *Can Med Assoc J* 1980;123(4): 275–280.
172. Nelson KE, Larson PA, Schraufnagel DE, et al. Transmission of tuberculosis by flexible fiberbronchoscopes. *Am Rev Respir Dis* 1983; 127(1):97–100.
173. Pappas SA, Schaaff DM, DiCostanzo MB, et al. Contamination of flexible fiberoptic bronchoscopes. *Am Rev Respir Dis* 1983;127(3): 391–392.
174. Wheeler PW, Lancaster D, Kaiser AB. Bronchopulmonary cross-colonization and infection related to mycobacterial contamination of suction valves of bronchoscopes. *J Infect Dis* 1989;159(5):954–958.
175. Hoffmann KK, Weber DJ, Rutala WA. Pseudoepidemic of Rhodotorula rubra in patients undergoing fiberoptic bronchoscopy. *Infect Control Hosp Epidemiol* 1989;10(11):511–514.
176. Jackson L, Klotz SA, Normand RE. A pseudoepidemic of Sporothrix cyanescens pneumonia occurring during renovation of a bronchoscopy suite. *J Med Vet Mycol* 1990;28(6):455–459.
177. Nicolle LE, McLeod J, Romance L, et al. Pseudo-outbreak of blastomycosis associated with contaminated bronchoscopes. *Infect Control Hosp Epidemiol* 1992;13(6):324.
178. Weinstein HJ, Bone RC, Ruth WE. Contamination of a fiberoptic bronchoscope with Proteus species. *Am Rev Respir Dis* 1977;116(3): 541–543.
179. Dawson DJ, Armstrong JG, Blacklock ZM. Mycobacterial cross-contamination of bronchoscopy specimens. *Am Rev Respir Dis* 1982; 126(6):1095–1097.
180. Nye K, Chadha DK, Hodgkin P, et al. Mycobacterium chelonei isolation from broncho-alveolar lavage fluid and its practical implications. *J Hosp Infect* 1990;16(3):257–261.
181. Prigogine T, Glupczynski Y, Van Molle P, et al. Mycobacterial cross-contamination of bronchoscopy specimens. *J Hosp Infect* 1988;11(1): 93–95.
182. Sammartino MT, Israel RH, Magnussen CR. Pseudomonas aeruginosa contamination of fibreoptic bronchoscopes. *J Hosp Infect* 1982; 3(1):65–71.
183. Weinstein RA, Stamm WE. Pseudoepidemics in hospital. *Lancet* 1977;2(8043):862–864.
184. Schleupner CJ, Hamilton JR. A pseudoepidemic of pulmonary fungal infections related to fiberoptic bronchoscopy. *Infect Control* 1980; 1(1):38–42.
185. Siegman-Igra Y, Inbar G, Campus A. An "outbreak" of pulmonary pseudoinfection by Serratia marcescens. *J Hosp Infect* 1985;6(2): 218–220.
186. Goldstein B, Abrutyn E. Pseudo-outbreak of Bacillus species: related to fibreoptic bronchoscopy. *J Hosp Infect* 1985;6(2):194–200.
187. Richardson AJ, Rothburn MM, Roberts C. Pseudo-outbreak of Bacillus species: related to fibreoptic bronchoscopy. *J Hosp Infect* 1986; 7(2):208–210.
188. Martone WJ, Osterman CA, Fisher KA, et al. Pseudomonas cepacia: implications and control of epidemic nosocomial colonization. *Rev Infect Dis* 1981;3(4):708–715.
189. Stine TM, Harris AA, Levin S, et al. A pseudoepidemic due to atypical mycobacteria in a hospital water supply. *JAMA* 1987;258(6): 809–811.
190. Centers for Disease Control. Nosocomial infection and pseudoinfection from contaminated endoscopes and bronchoscopes- Wisconsin and Missouri. *MMWR CDC Surveill Summ* 1991;40:675–678.
191. Fitch LE, Uttley AH, Honeywell KM, et al. Cross contamination of bronchial washings. *J Hosp Infect* 1991;17(4):322–324.
192. Gubler JG, Salfinger M, von Graevenitz A. Pseudoepidemic of nontuberculous mycobacteria due to a contaminated bronchoscope cleaning

machine. Report of an outbreak and review of the literature. *Chest* 1992;101(5):1245–1249.

193. Fraser VJ, Jones M, Murray PR, et al. Contamination of flexible fiberoptic bronchoscopes with Mycobacterium chelonae linked to an automated bronchoscope disinfection machine. *Am Rev Respir Dis* 1992;145(4 pt 1):853–855.
194. Whitlock WL, Dietrich RA, Steimke EH, et al. Rhodotorula rubra contamination in fiberoptic bronchoscopy. *Chest* 1992;102(5): 1516–1519.
195. Maloney S, Welbel S, Daves B, et al. Mycobacterium abscessus pseudoinfection traced to an automated endoscope washer: utility of epidemiologic and laboratory investigation. *J Infect Dis* 1994;169(5): 1166–1169.
196. Bennett SN, Peterson DE, Johnson DR, et al. Bronchoscopy-associated Mycobacterium xenopi pseudoinfections. *Am J Respir Crit Care Med* 1994;150(1):245–250.
197. Kolmos HJ, Lerche A, Kristoffersen K, et al. Pseudo-outbreak of pseudomonas aeruginosa in HIV-infected patients undergoing fiberoptic bronchoscopy. *Scand J Infect Dis* 1994;26(6):653–657.
198. Wang HC, Liaw YS, Yang PC, et al. A pseudoepidemic of Mycobacterium chelonae infection caused by contamination of a fibreoptic bronchoscope suction channel. *Eur Respir J* 1995;8(8):1259–1262.
199. Hagan ME, Klotz SA, Bartholomew W, et al. A pseudoepidemic of Rhodotorula rubra: a marker for microbial contamination of the bronchoscope. *Infect Control Hosp Epidemiol* 1995;16(12):727–728.
200. Cox R, deBorja K, Bach MC. A pseudo-outbreak of Mycobacterium chelonae infections related to bronchoscopy. *Infect Control Hosp Epidemiol* 1997;18(2):136–137.
201. Blanc DS, Parret T, Janin B, et al. Nosocomial infections and pseudoinfections from contaminated bronchoscopes: two-year follow up using molecular markers. *Infect Control Hosp Epidemiol* 1997;18(2): 134–136.
202. Agerton T, Valway S, Gore B, et al. Transmission of a highly drug-resistant strain (strain W1) of Mycobacterium tuberculosis. Community outbreak and nosocomial transmission via a contaminated bronchoscope. *JAMA* 1997;278(13):1073–1077.
203. Michele TM, Cronin WA, Graham NM, et al. Transmission of Mycobacterium tuberculosis by a fiberoptic bronchoscope. Identification by DNA fingerprinting. *JAMA* 1997;278(13):1093–1095.
204. Wallace RJ Jr, Brown BA, Griffith DE. Nosocomial outbreaks/pseudo-outbreaks caused by nontuberculous mycobacteria. *Annu Rev Microbiol* 1998;52:453–490.
205. Strelczyk K. Pseudo-outbreak of acid-fast bacilli. *Am J Infect Control* 1999;27:18(abst).
206. Schelenz S, French G. An outbreak of multidrug-resistant Pseudomonas aeruginosa infection associated with contamination of bronchoscopes and an endoscope washer-disinfector. *J Hosp Infect* 2000;46(1): 23–30.
207. Gillespie TG, Hogg L, Budge E, et al. Mycobacterium chelonae isolated from rinse water within an endoscope washer-disinfector. *J Hosp Infect* 2000;45(4):332–334.
208. Wilson SJ, Everts RJ, Kirkland KB, et al. A pseudo-outbreak of Aureobasidium species lower respiratory tract infections caused by reuse of single-use stopcocks during bronchoscopy. *Infect Control Hosp Epidemiol* 2000;21(7):470–472.
209. Larson L, Lambert L, Stricof R, et al. *Mycobacterium tuberculosis* contamination and potential exposure from a bronchoscope, Pennsylvania—2000. 11th Annual Scientific Meeting of the Society for Healthcare Epidemiology of America, Toronto, Ontario, Canada, 2001.
210. Kramer M, Krizek L, Gebel J, et al. Bronchoscopic transmission of Pseudomonas aeruginosa due to a contaminated disinfectant solution from an automated dispenser unit. Abstract 118. 11th Annual Scientific Meeting of the Society of Healthcare Epidemiology in America, Toronto, Ontario, Canada, 2001.
211. Kressel AB, Kidd F. Pseudo-outbreak of Mycobacterium chelonae and Methylobacterium mesophilicum caused by contamination of an automated endoscopy washer. *Infect Control Hosp Epidemiol* 2001; 22(7):414–418.
212. Sorin M, Segal-Maurer S, Mariano N, et al. Nosocomial transmission of imipenem-resistant Pseudomonas aeruginosa following bronchoscopy associated with improper connection to the Steris System 1 processor. *Infect Control Hosp Epidemiol* 2001;22(7):409–413.
213. Ramsey AH, Oemig TV, Davis JP, et al. An outbreak of bronchoscopy-related Mycobacterium tuberculosis infections due to lack of bronchoscope leak testing. *Chest* 2002;121(3):976–981.
214. Srinivasan A, Wolfenden LL, Song X, et al. An outbreak of Pseudomonas aeruginosa infections associated with flexible bronchoscopes. *N Engl J Med* 2003;348(3):221–227.
215. Kirschke DL, Jones TF, Craig AS, et al. Pseudomonas aeruginosa and Serratia marcescens contamination associated with a manufacturing defect in bronchoscopes. *N Engl J Med* 2003;348(3):214–220.
216. Rossetti R, Lencioni P, Innocenti F, et al. Pseudoepidemic from Mycobacterium gordonae due to a contaminated automatic bronchoscope washing machine. *Am J Infect Control* 2002;30(3):196–197.
217. Singh N, Belen O, Leger MM, et al. Cluster of Trichosporon mucoides in children associated with a faulty bronchoscope. *Pediatr Infect Dis J* 2003;22(7):609–612.
218. Silva CV, Magalhaes VD, Pereira CR, et al. Pseudo-outbreak of Pseudomonas aeruginosa and Serratia marcescens related to bronchoscopes. *Infect Control Hosp Epidemiol* 2003;24(3):195–197.
219. Mitchell DH, Hicks LJ, Chiew R, et al. Pseudoepidemic of Legionella pneumophila serogroup 6 associated with contaminated bronchoscopes. *J Hosp Infect* 1997;37(1):19–23.
220. Centers for Diseas Control. Bronchoscopy-related infections and pseudoinfections—New York, 1996 and 1998. *MMWR CDC Surveill Summ* 1999(48):557–560.
221. Kirschke D, Jones TF, Craig AS, et al. Pseudomonas aeruginosa associated with a design change in specific models of bronchoscopes, Tennessee, 2001. The 12th Annual Meeting of the Society for Healthcare Epidemiology of America, Salt Lake City, Utah, 2002.
222. Rutala WA. APIC guideline for selection and use of disinfectants. 1994, 1995, and 1996 APIC Guidelines Committee. Association for Professionals in Infection Control and Epidemiology, Inc. *Am J Infect Control* 1996;24(4):313–342.
223. Rutala WA. Disinfection, sterilization and waste disposal. In: Wenzel RP, ed. *Prevention and control of nosocomial infections,* 3rd ed. Baltimore: Williams & Wilkins; 1997:539–593.
224. Rutala WA, Weber DJ, Committee HICPA. Guideline for disinfection and sterilization in health-care facilities. *MMWR (in press).*
225. Rutala WA, Cole EC, Wannamaker NS, et al. Inactivation of Mycobacterium tuberculosis and Mycobacterium bovis by 14 hospital disinfectants. *Am J Med* 1991;91(3B):267S–271S.
226. Rutala WA, Clontz EP, Weber DJ, et al. Disinfection practices for endoscopes and other semicritical items. *Infect Control Hosp Epidemiol* 1991;12(5):282–288.
227. Woodcock A, Campbell I, Collins JV, et al. Bronchoscopy and infection control. *Lancet* 1989;2(8657):270–271.
228. Ruppel GL. Spirometry. *Respir Care Clin North Am* 1997;3(2): 155–181.
229. Anonymous. Peak flow meters and spirometers in general practice. *Drug Ther Bull* 1997;35(7):52–55.
230. The American Thoracic Society. Standardization of spirometry—1987 update. Statement of the American Thoracic Society. *Am Rev Respir Dis* 1987;136(5):1285–1298.
231. Ali BA, Abro YM, Javed NH, et al. Standardization of different spirometers. *Respiration* 1988;53(1):58–63.
232. Glindmeyer HW, Jones RN, Barkman HW, et al. Spirometry: quantitative test criteria and test acceptability. *Am Rev Respir Dis* 1987; 136(2):449–452.
233. Carroll AR, Goularte RA, McGinley KN, et al. An outbreak of *Pseudomonas maltophilia* in intensive care units traced to contaminated respiratory equipment. 12th Annual Association for Practitioners in Infection Control Educational Conference, Cincinnati, Ohio, 1985.
234. Irwin RS, Demers RR, Pratter MR, et al. An outbreak of acinetobacter infection associated with the use of a ventilator spirometer. *Respir Care* 1980;25(2):232–237.
235. Hazaleus RE, Cole J, Berdischewsky M. Tuberculin skin test conversion from exposure to contaminated pulmonary function testing apparatus. *Respir Care* 1981;26(1):53–55.

236. Rutala DR, Rutala WA, Weber DJ, et al. Infection risks associated with spirometry. *Infect Control Hosp Epidemiol* 1991;12(2):89–92.
237. Burgos F, Torres A, Gonzalez J, et al. Bacterial colonization as a potential source of nosocomial respiratory infections in two types of spirometer. *Eur Respir J* 1996;9(12):2612–2617.
238. Smith PW, Massanari RM. Room humidifiers as the source of Acinetobacter infections. *JAMA* 1977;237(8):795–797.
239. Gervich DH, Grout CS. An outbreak of nosocomial Acinetobacter infections from humidifiers. *Am J Infect Control* 1985;13(5):210–215.
240. Grieble HG, Colton FR, Bird TJ, et al. Fine-particle humidifiers. Source of Pseudomonas aeruginosa infections in a respiratory-disease unit. *N Engl J Med* 1970;282(10):531–535.
241. Kaan JA, Simoons-Smit AM, MacLaren DM. Another source of aerosol causing nosocomial Legionnaires' disease. *J Infect* 1985;11(2): 145–148.
242. Woo AH, Yu VL, Goetz A. Potential in-hospital modes of transmission of Legionella pneumophila. Demonstration experiments for dissemination by showers, humidifiers, and rinsing of ventilation bag apparatus. *Am J Med* 1986;80(4):567–573.
243. Ahlgren EW, Chapel JF, Dorn GL. Pseudomonas aeruginosa infection potential of oxygen humidifier devices. *Respir Care* 1977;22(4): 383–385.
244. Goodison RR. Pseudomonas cross-infection due to contaminated humidifier water. *Br Med J* 1980;281(6250):1288.
245. Torres Marti A, Agusti AG, de Celis R, et al. The ethiopathogenic role of oxygen humidifiers connected to intermittent mandatory ventilation valves on nosocomial pneumonias. *Am Rev Respir Dis* 1985; 131(5):803.
246. Mertz JJ, Scharer L, McClement JH. A hospital outbreak of Klebsiella pneumonia from inhalation therapy with contaminated aerosol solutions. *Am Rev Respir Dis* 1967;95(3):454–460.
247. Gardner S, Shulman ST. A nosocomial common source outbreak caused by Pseudomonas pickettii. *Pediatr Infect Dis* 1984;3(5): 420–422.
248. Meltz DJ, Grieco MH. Characteristics of Serratia marcescens pneumonia. *Arch Intern Med* 1973;132(3):359–364.
249. McNeil MM, Solomon SL, Anderson RL, et al. Nosocomial Pseudomonas pickettii colonization associated with a contaminated respiratory therapy solution in a special care nursery. *J Clin Microbiol* 1985;22(6):903–907.
250. Centers for Disease Control. Nosocomial *Ralstonia pickettii* colonization associated with intrinsically contaminated saline solution—Los Angeles, California. *MMWR CDC Surveill Summ* 1998;47:285–286.
251. Anderson RL, Bland LA, Favero MS, et al. Factors associated with Pseudomonas pickettii intrinsic contamination of commercial respiratory therapy solutions marketed as sterile. *Appl Environ Microbiol* 1985;50(6):1343–1348.
252. Rutala WA, Stiegel MM, Sarubbi FA, Jr. A potential infection hazard associated with the use of disposable saline vials. *Infect Control* 1984; 5(4):170–172.
253. Solomon SL, Wallace EM, Ford-Jones EL, et al. Medication errors with inhalant epinephrine mimicking an epidemic of neonatal sepsis. *N Engl J Med* 1984;310(3):166–170.
254. Schuchat A, Lizano C, Broome CV, et al. Outbreak of neonatal listeriosis associated with mineral oil. *Pediatr Infect Dis J* 1991;10(3): 183–189.
255. George DL, McLeod R, Weinstein RA. Contaminated commercial charcoal as a source of fungi in the respiratory tract. *Infect Control Hosp Epidemiol* 1991;12(12):732–734.
256. Graman PS, Quinlan GA, Rank JA. Nosocomial legionellosis traced to a contaminated ice machine. *Infect Control Hosp Epidemiol* 1997; 18(9):637–640.
257. Rutala WA, Weber DJ. Water as a reservoir of nosocomial pathogens. *Infect Control Hosp Epidemiol* 1997;18(9):609–616.
258. File TM Jr, Tan JS, Thomson RB Jr, et al. An outbreak of Pseudomonas aeruginosa ventilator-associated respiratory infections due to contaminated food coloring dye—further evidence of the significance of gastric colonization preceding nosocomial pneumonia. *Infect Control Hosp Epidemiol* 1995;16(7):417–418.
259. Loeb M, Simor AE, Mandell L, et al. Two nursing home outbreaks of respiratory infection with Legionella sainthelensi. *J Am Geriatr Soc* 1999;47(5):547–552.
260. From the Centers for Disease Control and Prevention. Nosocomial Burkholderia cepacia infection and colonization associated with intrinsically contaminated mouthwash—Arizona, 1998. *JAMA* 1999; 281(4):318.
261. Matrician L, Ange G, Burns S, et al. Outbreak of nosocomial Burkholderia cepacia infection and colonization associated with intrinsically contaminated mouthwash. *Infect Control Hosp Epidemiol* 2000; 21(11):739–741.
262. Buxton AE, Anderson RL, Werdegar D, et al. Nosocomial respiratory tract infection and colonization with Acinetobacter calcoaceticus. Epidemiologic characteristics. *Am J Med* 1978;65(3):507–513.
263. Snydman DR, Hindman SH, Wineland MD, et al. Nosocomial viral hepatitis B. A cluster among staff with subsequent transmission to patients. *Ann Intern Med* 1976;85(5):573–577.
264. Occupational Safety and Health Administration, Department of Labor. Occupational exposure to bloodborne pathogens: final rule. Occupational Safety and Health Administration, Department of Labor, 1991:CPR part 1910.1030.
265. Zelechowski GP. Suction collection and its relation to nosocomial infection. *Am J Infect Control* 1980;8(1):22–25.
266. Robertshaw RG. Aerosol production by suction apparatus and methods of containment. *J Hosp Infect* 1982;3(4):379–383.
267. Rees TA. Bacteria in suction machines. *Lancet* 1970;1(7640):240.
268. Ranger I, O'Grady F. Dissemination of micro-organisms by a surgical pump. *Lancet* 1958;2:299–300.
269. Blenkharn JI, Hughes VM. Suction apparatus and hospital infection due to multiply-resistant Klebsiella aerogenes. *J Hosp Infect* 1982;3(2): 173–178.
270. Rubbo SD, Gardner JF, Franklin JC. Source of Pseudomonas aeruginosa infection in premature infants. *J Hyg (Lond)* 1966;64(1): 121–128.
271. Rubenstein A, Fowler, RN. Salmonellosis of the newborn with transmission by delivery room resuscitators. *Am J Public Health* 1955;45: 1109–1114.
272. Becker AH. Infection due to *Proteus mirabilis* in newborn nursery. *Am J Dis Child* 1962;104:355–359.
273. Bassett DC, Thompson SA, Page B. Neonatal infections with Pseudomonas aeruginosa associated with contaminated resuscitation equipment. *Lancet* 1965;1(7389):781–784.
274. Haji TC, Sangam A, Willmot IC, et al. Four-year surveillance of a special care baby unit for Pseudomonas aeruginosa. *J Hosp Infect* 1981; 2(1):77–83.
275. Lowbury EJ, Thom BT, Lilly HA, et al. Sources of infection with Pseudomonas aeruginosa in patients with tracheostomy. *J Med Microbiol* 1970;3(1):39–56.
276. Beck A, Zadeh JA. Infection by anaesthetic apparatus. *Lancet* 1968; 1(7541):533–534.
277. Stiver HG, Clark J, Kennedy J, et al. Pseudomonas sternotomy wound infection and sternal osteomyelitis. Complications after open heart surgery. *JAMA* 1979;241(10):1034–1036.
278. Hilton E, Adams AA, Uliss A, et al. Nosocomial bacterial eye infections in intensive-care units. *Lancet* 1983;1(8337):1318–1320.
279. Van Dyke RB, Spector SA. Transmission of herpes simplex virus type 1 to a newborn infant during endotracheal suctioning for meconium aspiration. *Pediatr Infect Dis* 1984;3(2):153–156.

69

NOSOCOMIAL INFECTIONS ASSOCIATED WITH TRANSFUSION OF BLOOD AND BLOOD PRODUCTS

CHARLES J. SCHLEUPNER

The transfusion of blood and blood products exposes recipient patients to both noninfectious and infectious adverse events (1). Approximately 11 to 12 million units of blood are transfused annually, with an average of 3.5 units per patient and up to five donor sources per transfused patient (2). Most recipients of blood and blood products are unaware of the 1% or greater risk of ill effects associated with transfusion (2). From 1976 through 1985, 355 deaths were reported to the U.S. Food and Drug Administration (FDA) as a result of transfusion, for a mortality risk of 0.001% or 1 in 100,000 patients transfused (2). Infections accounted for 27.3% of these deaths. In contrast, during 1994 only 24 deaths were reported to the FDA related to infusion and only 8% were related to infection (3). The remainder of deaths are related to immunologic reactions or to errors of processing or administration. The nonfatal adverse effects range from minor inconveniences to life-threatening emergencies; they may occur immediately during or within hours of the transfusion or may be delayed for weeks, months, or years. The physician should always consider the risk of such ill occurrences in the decision to transfuse. Although the public desires absolute safety in a product regardless of cost (4,5), physicians can defend a moderate approach to the addition of further testing safeguards resulting from the marked increase of safety of transfused blood in the United States over the last 10 years (6–10). This chapter reviews the potential infections transmitted by blood and blood products (Table 69.1) and their prevention.

NONINFECTIOUS COMPLICATIONS

The noninfectious complications of blood transfusion include acute hemolytic reactions, which may be immunologically or nonimmunologically mediated and account for 53% to 67% of deaths, and nonhemolytic reactions, which are usually febrile or allergic in nature and account for 19% to 25% of deaths resulting from transfusion (1–3). Other nonhemolytic reactions include volume overload, transfusion-related acute lung injury, posttransfusion purpura, hemosiderosis, graft-versus-host disease in severely immunosuppressed hosts, and processing errors (1, 11). Some of these noninfectious complications are obviated by routine measures. They are not life threatening and can be medically managed when they occur. Advanced leukocyte reduction filters during transfusion may be useful to reduce some of these reactions (9,12). Removal of leukocytes before storage may be very important for reduction of transfusion reactions associated with platelets because of the presence of cytokines generated by leukocytes in the plasma phase of stored platelet concentrates (13,14).

INFECTIOUS COMPLICATIONS

It was not until the early twentieth century that transfusion was made feasible for nonterminally ill patients. The new methods included anticoagulation techniques, classification of blood type isoagglutinins (15), and storage of donor blood. Previously, only direct donor-to-recipient transfusions were reluctantly and rarely performed because of the high frequency of often severe complications (16). With the advent of this technology, the infectious complications of blood transfusion became recognized. By World War I, potential donors with malaria, syphilis, and fever were excluded (17). The increased number of transfusions during World War II led to the recognition of posttransfusion hepatitis (PTH) (18). However, even before this description, the American Red Cross Donor Service had deferred all potential blood donors with a history of jaundice within 6 months (19).

The organized collection of blood and blood products for civilian use began in 1947. Hepatitis B virus (HBV) was defined serologically by 1972; its partial control has led to our understanding of other causes of PTH, including hepatitis C virus (HCV), hepatitis delta virus (HDV), hepatitis G virus (HGV), other non-A, non-B hepatitis viral agents, cytomegalovirus (CMV), Epstein-Barr virus (EBV), and, rarely, hepatitis A virus (HAV) (8,10,20–24). The epidemic of human immunodeficiency virus type 1 (HIV-1) infections led to its recognition in the early 1980s as transmissible by blood and blood products (25). Other infectious agents transmitted by blood and blood products include protozoa, filaria, spirochetes, other viruses, and bacteria (1,8–10,20–24).

The remainder of this section reviews each of these pathogens and the prevention of their transmission by blood transfusion

TABLE 69.1. INFECTIOUS COMPLICATIONS OF TRANSFUSION OF BLOOD OR BLOOD PRODUCTS

I. Transfusion-related immunosuppression with secondary infection
   a. Postsurgical patients
   b. Patients with burns affecting more than 10% of body surface area
II. Infections transmitted by transfusion
   a. Hepatitis
      1. HAV
      2. HBV
      3. HCV
      4. HDV
      5. HGV (GBV-C)
      6. Other non-A, non-B agent(s) (TT virus, SEN virus)
      7. CMV
      8. EBV, HHV-8
   b. Other viral infections
      1. HIV-1 and HIV-2
      2. HTLV-I and HTLV-II
      3. Parvovirus B19
      4. Colorado tick fever virus
      5. West Nile virus
      6. Vaccinia virus
   c. Prion of Creutzfeldt-Jakob disease
   d. Protozoal diseases
      1. Malaria
      2. Babesiosis
      3. Trypanosomiasis
      4. Toxoplasmosis
      5. Leishmaniasis
   e. Spirochetal infections
      1. Syphilis
      2. Relapsing fever
      3. Lyme disease (?)
   f. Bacterial infections
      1. Brucellosis
      2. Salmonellosis
      3. Yersinosis
      4. Gram-positive or gram-negative contaminants
   g. Parasitic infestations (loiasis, other filaria)
   h. Rickettsioses

CMV, cytomegalovirus, EBV, Epstein-Barr virus; GBV-A, B, GB virus A and B, respectively; HAV, HBV, HCV, HDV, HGV, hepatitis A, B, C, D, G virus, respectively; HIV-1, HIV-2, human immunodeficiency virus types 1 and 2, respectively; HTLV-I, HTLV-II, human T-cell leukemia virus types I and II, respectively.

after a brief discussion of the recently recognized phenomenon that blood transfusion may cause immunosuppression and thereby predispose the recipient to infections. Table 69.2 summarizes the most recent donor selection criteria of the American Association of Blood Banks (AABB) for the protection of recipients of donor blood (26).

Infections after Noncontaminated Blood Transfusion

Several authors have reviewed the observations that blood transfusions may result in suppression of the recipient's immune defenses, leading to secondary infections (27–30), in addition to an association of transfusion with recurrence of malignancy and increased (renal) allograft survival (12,29,31–33). Using multivariable analysis, Tartter (34) and others (35) have pre-

TABLE 69.2. AMERICAN ASSOCIATION OF BLOOD BANKS CRITERIA FOR PROTECTION OF RECIPIENTS OF DONOR BLOOD (2003)

1. Appearance of good health in donor
   a. Oral temperature of donor ≤37.5°C (99.5°F)
   b. Permanent exclusion for stigmata of injectable drug use or for use of a needle, even once, for nonprescription drug administration
   c. Deferral for alcoholism
   d. Deferral for 12 months after treatment for syphilis or gonorrhea
2. Deferral of donor for 2 weeks after live attenuated bacterial or viral vaccine receipt, except for 4 weeks after rubella or varicella-zoster vaccine and for 1 year after rabies vaccine given for a rabies prone animal bite
3. Donor deferral for 12 months after HBIG
4. Donor deferral if donor was given blood or potentially infected blood products during previous 12 months
5. Permanent donor deferral
   a. If history of hepatitis after age 11 years
   b. If HBsAg (confirmed) or anti-HBc positive (positive at two different donations)
   c. If anti-HCV, HTLV-I/II, or HIV-1/2 seropositive
   d. If in a high-risk group for HIV-1/2 infection
   e. If prior donation led to hepatitis, HTLV-I/II, or HIV-1/2 infection in recipient
   f. A history of babesiosis or Chagas' disease
   g. Donors with a family history of Creutzfeldt-Jakob disease, donor after receipt of human pituitary growth hormone or dura-mater grafts, and donor at risk for variant Creutzfeldt-Jakob disease
6. Donor deferral for 12 months after
   a. Application of a tattoo or unsterile body piercing
   b. Mucous membrane exposure to blood or skin penetration by an instrument contaminated with blood or a body fluid
   c. Sexual exposure to a person with viral hepatitis or confirmed positive test for HBsAg
   d. Sexual contact with a person infected with or at high risk for HIV infection
   e. An ALT determination on one occasion greater than or equal to twice normal or on two occasions abnormal but less than twice normal[a]
   f. Incarceration for >72 hours in a correctional institution
   g. History of syphilis or gonorrhea, reactive screening test for syphilis, or completion of therapy for syphilis or gonorrhea
7. Donor deferral due to malaria (plasma donations excepted)
   a. 3-year deferral for those after recovery from malaria
   b. 3-year deferral for travelers after return from a malaria endemic area if free of symptoms suggestive of malaria
   c. 3-year deferral for immigrants after departure from malaria endemic areas if asymptomatic
   d. 12-month deferral of residents from countries that are malaria free but who have traveled to an area where malaria is endemic (acceptance as donor if symptom free)
8. Donor deferral until 14 days after recovery from suspected or documented West Nile virus (WNV) infection, or until 28 days from onset of illness (suspect or known to be WNV)
9. Donor deferral after smallpox vaccination without complications for 21 days or until scab has fallen off, whichever is longer; donor deferral after smallpox vaccination with complication until 14 days after resolution of complication
10. Donor is provided opportunity in confidence to declare collected blood unsuitable for transfusion by Confidential Unit Exclusion (CUE) bar code sticker or call-back system

ALT, alanine aminotransferase; anti-HBc, antibody to hepatitis B core antigen; HBIG, hepatitis B immune globulin; HBsAg, hepatitis B surface antigen; HCV, hepatitis C virus; HIV-1/2, human immunodeficiency virus types I and II, HTLV-I/II, human T-cell leukemia virus types I and II.
[a] Requirement deleted 6/20/95 but practice continues at some centers.
From American Association of Blood Banks, *Proposed standards for blood banks and transfusion services*, 22nd ed. Bethesda, MD: American Association of Blood Banks, 2003, with permission.

sented data associating blood transfusion with infection after colorectal cancer surgery. Subsequently, reports have made similar associations after surgery for trauma (36–39), Crohn's disease (40), gastrointestinal bleeding (41), open fractures of an extremity (42), and coronary artery bypass surgery (43,44) and with healthcare-associated infections in critical care patients (45). Increased rates of infection after noncontaminated blood transfusion have also been documented in humans with burns affecting more than 10% of their bodies (46); initial studies in an animal burn model indicated similar findings (47,48). However, reports after elective surgery have failed to document such an association (49,50).

The proposed mechanism accounting for these observations is immunosuppression induced by the transfusion; Waymack and Alexander (51) noted a higher incidence of tumor recurrence and reduced survival among oncologic surgery patients who received perioperative blood transfusions. Waymack et al. (52,53) suggested that the mechanism of this immunosuppression may be alteration of macrophage arachidonic acid metabolism. Elevations of prostaglandin E and a decrease of interleukin-2 (IL-2) production have been documented in animal models after allogeneic transfusion (52–54). Lenhard et al. (55) reported decreased lymphocyte antigen responsiveness in transfused patients with chronic renal failure before renal transplantation; Lenhard et al. (56) also documented increased circulating blood monocytes with augmented prostaglandin E production in transfused patients with chronic renal failure. An analogy with the immunosuppression of pregnancy resulting from a blunted IL-2 response and upregulation of interleukin-4 (IL-4) and interleukin-10 (IL-10) has been summarized (31). These altered cytokine kinetics may lead to enhanced Th2 and depressed Th1 responses. Other authors have suggested optional unproven mechanisms for the observed immunomodulation after transfusion, including antigen-induced anergy and immune tolerance, and the effects of transfused cytokines (28,31–33,57). These reported immunologic abnormalities in transfusion recipients have not been linked with potentially transfused agents (e.g., CMV).

Current data suggest that transfusion is a modulator of the immune system. However, considering the problems associated with multivariable analysis of the uncontrolled studies, an independent role for transfusion as an immune suppressant is not yet definitive (28,31–33). However, in one recent prospective randomized trial of postoperative infection (57) and one review, a dose-dependent relationship of transfusion to infection risk and immune suppression has been supported (30).

Several methods are available for avoiding the potential immunosuppressive effects of transfusion linked with surgery and trauma. Improved surgical techniques with attention to hemostasis may avoid much of the need for transfusion. Furthermore, there is minimal scientific justification for the current hemoglobin level (10 g/dL) at which transfusion is said to be indicated (58,59). The decreased blood viscosity associated with reduced hemoglobin concentrations of anemia may increase cardiac output and partially compensate for decreased oxygen delivery to tissues (59,60). Acceptance of reduced indications for transfusion according to hemoglobin concentration and the use of autologous blood for transfusion (self-donated preoperatively or intraoperatively recovered blood) will reduce these immunosuppressive effects of transfusion (59). Other preventive techniques include the use of leukocyte-reduced blood products, such as frozen deglycerolized red blood cells (RBCs) or RBCs after treatment with second-generation micropore or third-generation absorption blood filters, and the use of blood alternatives (e.g., hemoglobin solutions depleted of erythrocyte stroma, chemically modified hemoglobin solutions, and artificial RBCs or neohemocytes) (12,61–66). These leukocyte-depletion techniques also prevent some febrile transfusion reactions (66). The stimulation of the patient's bone marrow with erythropoietin to produce RBCs is another method to avoid transfusion.

The concepts of immunomodulation and increased infection risk after allogeneic blood transfusion have been unified mechanistically through the appreciation of cytokine release by leukocytes during blood storage (14,32,33,35). A number of studies have demonstrated that leukocyte-depletion of transfused RBCs may have favorable effects on infection rates, morbidity, and/or mortality (67–70). These studies further support the role of cytokines derived from leukocytes as a cause of described, although marginally documented, ill effects of transfusion (26). However, leukocyte depletion of RBCs is not universally accepted (71).

Infections after Transfusions Contaminated with Pathogens

Febrile reactions, defined as a temperature rise of 1°C or more, may be associated with 1% to 3% of all RBC transfusions (66). In addition to an infective cause, either ongoing in the recipient or rarely resulting from bacterial contamination of the transfused blood product (see later discussion), fever may also follow a hemolytic transfusion reaction or may be associated with cytokines or antibodies in the transfused blood products or antibodies in the recipient against leukocyte or platelet antigens (14,66). Such febrile reactions may present as acute noncardiogenic pulmonary edema resulting from either reactive lipid products or antileukocyte antibodies or in association with the platelet refractory state (failure of the platelet count to rise after transfusion because of rapid antibody-mediated clearance). These febrile reactions are most commonly seen in multiply transfused alloimmunized recipients, in multiparous female recipients of transfused blood or blood products, or after transfusion of blood or blood products from multiparous female donors. These reactions can be avoided by using leukocyte-depleted blood products (9,14,33,66). Febrile antiplatelet reactions may resolve with leukocyte depletion, but the platelet refractory state is seldom benefited.

Another febrile reaction related to transfusion of immunoincompetent and, rarely, normal hosts occurs 1 to 2 weeks after transfusion with the presentation of fever and erythroderma (72, 73). This transfusion-associated graft-versus-host disease is not infectious and is usually not confused with a febrile transfusion reaction.

The most frequent serious transfusion complication is the transmission of infection, of which hepatitis and, more recently, HIV-1 are the most important. Parenteral transmission of hepatitis was not recognized until 1883 when an outbreak occurred among recipients of a smallpox vaccine of human origin (74).

In 1938 and again in 1942, a yellow fever vaccine stabilized with human serum was reported to have caused jaundice among recipients (75,76); a virus was presumed to have contaminated the human serum. Subsequently, epidemiologic studies and human volunteer experiments defined two forms of viral hepatitis: hepatitis A or infectious hepatitis, believed to be transmitted only orally (short incubation period of 15 to 50 days), and hepatitis B or serum hepatitis, associated with parenteral exposure (long incubation period of 50 to 180 days) (77). Although it was known that both forms of hepatitis could be transmitted parenterally by blood and that hepatitis A could be acquired orally from various body fluids, physicians identified the form of hepatitis by exposure history until 1965 when Blumberg and associates (78,79) serendipitously associated Australia antigen with the surface antigen of hepatitis B. The development of serologic assays for hepatitis B and subsequently hepatitis A opened the door to our evolving understanding of the other agents of PTH (80–82) (Table 69.3).

Hepatitis A

Much of the epidemiologic information contrasting hepatitis A and hepatitis B resulted from human volunteer studies performed in the 1940s (77) and at the Willowbrook State School in New York between 1956 and the late 1960s (83,84). These and other studies defined the differences of incubation periods and antigenicity, the presence of HAV in feces, and the lack of chronic carriage of HAV (77,83–85). HAV was first visualized in stool using immune electron microscopy in 1973 (86); this finding ultimately led to methods for detection of serum antibody to HAV. The periods of viremia, clinical illness, and aspartate aminotransferase elevation have been related (Fig. 69.1); the transience of the immunoglobulin A (IgA) antibody response, followed by a persisting immunoglobulin G (IgG) response, has also been defined by both radioimmunoassays (RIAs) and enzyme immunoassays (EIAs) (87–90). Although IgM antibody usually disappears within 3 to 6 months after infection, it may persist for more than 300 days in 10% to 15% of patients (91). Because of the lack of an HAV carrier state and the brevity of HAV viremia (usually 2 weeks or less, with onset of viremia 7 to 10 days before onset of clinical symptoms, Fig. 69.1), frequent episodes of PTH A are unlikely (9,19,81,82,92,93). With few exceptions, this has been the case (94–100). Usually, PTH A occurs as a sporadic case report after blood donation during the incubation period of the illness (99,100). Unfortunately, several outbreaks have been due to single contaminated units of blood being transfused to multiple infants, resulting in nursery outbreaks with secondary and tertiary cases (95,97,98,100) (see Chapter 45). One recent outbreak occurred among cancer patients treated with IL-2 and lymphokine-activated killer lymphocytes apparently resulting from contaminated serum in the lymphocyte culture medium (99); another outbreak occurred among patients with hemophilia given clotting factor concentrates inadequately treated to inactivate HAV (101). These few reported outbreaks might have been prevented by serologic testing for antibody against HAV; however, the 50% seroprevalence rate for HAV IgG antibody among Americans by age 50, the possible persistence of IgM antibodies for 3 to 6 months after infection despite lack of infectivity, the frequency of symptoms during the viremic phase of the illness (84), and the rarity of fatal illness resulting from HAV are strong arguments against the economic or medical merit of routine testing of donor blood for HAV antibody (9,20,93,102). The estimated current residual risk of acquiring HAV from a unit of transfused blood is 0.0001% (9). The prompt administration of immune serum globulin (ISG) prophylaxis would be appropriate for a recipient of blood found, after transfusion, to contain HAV (20). The elimination of febrile symptomatic patients as blood donors will also generally prevent HAV transmission. Frequent recipients of clotting factor concentrates are candidates for receipt of HAV vaccine (23,101).

Hepatitis B

Blumberg et al.'s classic seroepidemiologic studies of diverse populations led to the discovery of a unique antigen in Australian aborigines and recipients of multiple transfusions, which was called Australia antigen (78,79,103,104). The terminology subsequently evolved from hepatitis-associated antigen to hepatitis B antigen and finally to hepatitis B surface antigen (HBsAg) when it was associated with the surface lipoprotein of HBV (105,106). HBsAg can be found in serum of patients developing acute hepatitis B for 30 to 60 days before illness and may persist for variable periods after clinical recovery (Fig. 69.2). Persistence for longer than 6 months is defined as the chronic carrier state. Antibody against HBsAg (anti-HBs) develops as HBsAg disappears and accounts for long-term immunity (107).

TABLE 69.3. ESTABLISHED POSTTRANSFUSION HEPATITIS VIRUSES

Virus	Virus synonym	Family	Nucleic acid	Incubation period (days)	Chronicity
HAV	Infectious hepatitis	Picorna	RNA	16–50	None
HBV	Serum hepatitis	Hepadna	DNA	50–180	Yes
HCV	Classic non-A, non-B, hepatitis	Flavi	RNA	28–60	Yes
HDV	Delta	Unknown	RNA	21–50	Yes
HGV	Non-A, non-B, non-C hepatitis	Flavi	RNA	ND	Yes
CMV		Herpes	DNA	ND	No[a]
EBV		Herpes	DNA	ND	No[a]

CMV, cytomegalovirus; EBV, Epstein-Barr virus, HAV, HBV, HCV, HDV, HGV, hepatitis A, B, C, D, G, virus, respectively; ND, not defined.
[a] Establishes latent infection in leukocytes.

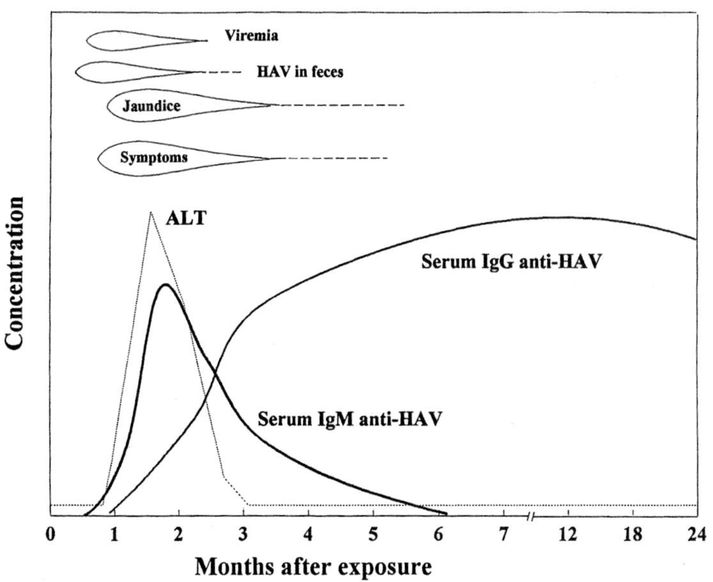

Figure 69.1. The clinical, virologic, and serologic course of acute hepatitis A virus infection. (From Feinstone SM, Gust ID. Hepatitis A virus. In: Mandell GL, Bennett JE, Dolin R, eds. *Principles and practice of infectious diseases,* 5th ed. Philadelphia: Churchill Livingstone, 2000:1920–1940, with permission.)

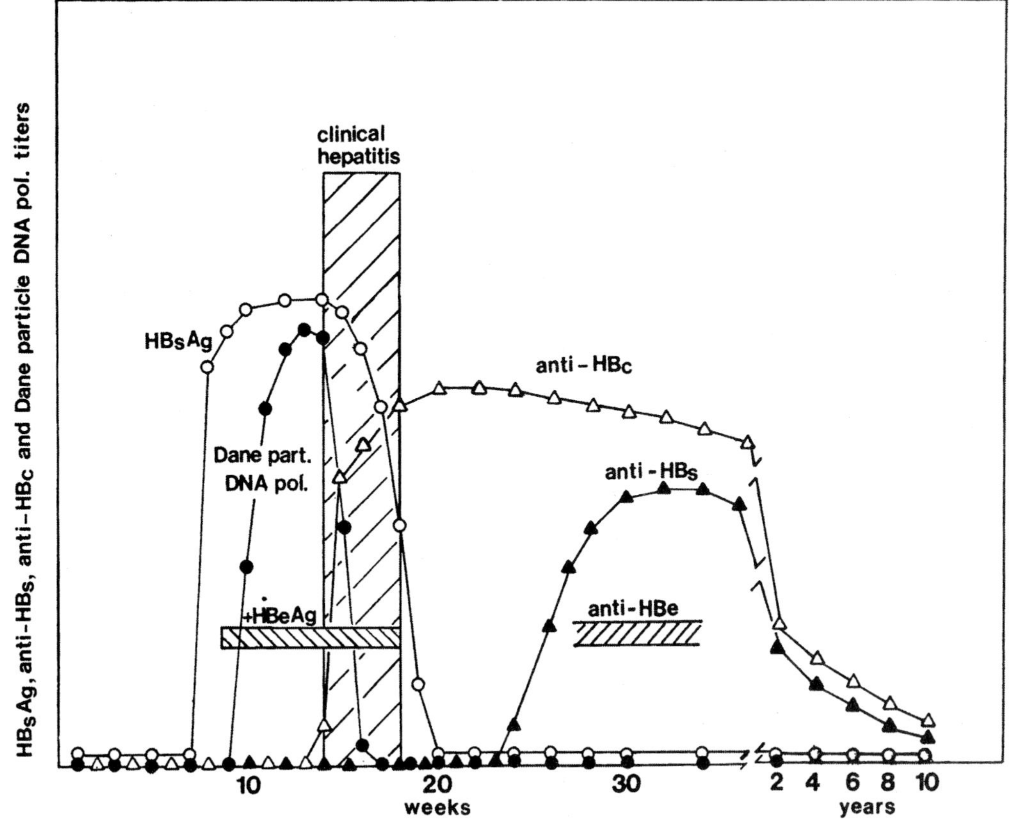

Figure 69.2. The clinical and serologic course of acute hepatitis B infection. (From Robinson WS. Hepatitis B virus and hepatitis D virus. In: Mandell GL, Bennett JE, Dolin R, eds. *Principles and practice of infectious diseases,* 5th ed. Philadelphia: Churchill Livingstone, 2000:1652–1685, with permission.)

Hepatitis B core antigen, reflecting active viral replication, transiently appears in the blood during acute infection, only to be replaced by its antibody (anti-HBc) (108). Anti-HBc appears during acute infection as an IgM antibody and is replaced in up to 80% of patients by a persistent IgG antibody during convalescence (109) (Fig. 69.2).

Hepatitis B e antigen (HBeAg) is a soluble product of HBV infection found transiently in serum during acute hepatitis B and in the serum of patients with chronic hepatitis (110–112) (Fig. 69.2). The presence of HBeAg correlates with the presence of HBV virions in serum. Antibody to HBeAg is more commonly found in chronic asymptomatic carriers of HBsAg (111,112). HBeAg is associated with increased maternal-fetal HBV transmission and transmission via accidental needlestick (113–115).

Transmission of HBV occurs through percutaneous or transmucosal inoculation of HBV in blood or infectious body fluids (primarily semen and breast milk). Inoculation may occur by contaminated needles, during sexual contact, at birth, or during transfusion. Continuous household or institutional contact with an infected person may presumably transmit infection via inapparent exposures.

Acute hepatitis B causes a chronic viral carrier state in 6% to 10% of infected adults and 90% of infected newborns with or without chronic hepatitis (25% of carriers). The most serious sequelae in chronic carriers of HBsAg are cirrhosis and hepatocellular carcinoma. Approximately 750,000 to 1 million chronic HBsAg carriers live in the United States (116). These individuals serve as a potential reservoir within the pool of blood donors. High-risk groups for chronic carriage of HBV are shown in Table 69.4.

Before the development of assays for HBsAg, it was believed that HBV accounted for most cases of PTH. When use of the first-generation immunodiffusion assays for HBsAg was initiated voluntarily on donor blood in 1969 and became mandatory in 1972 (Table 69.5), it was anticipated that PTH would be virtually eliminated. Although there were marked reductions in the frequency of PTH (30% to 55%) and mortality related to transfusion, the problem persisted. Hepatitis B continues to account for at least 10% of cases of PTH (9,116,117). Recently published risk estimates for PTH resulting from HBV are as high as 1 in 63,000 units, with HCV and HBV accounting for 88% of the risk of viral transmission by transfusion (8).

TABLE 69.4. HIGH-RISK GROUPS FOR ACQUIRING HEPATITIS B INFECTION

1. Parenteral drug users
2. Heterosexual men and women and homosexual men with multiple partners
3. Household contacts and sexual partners of chronic HBV carriers
4. Infants born to HBV-infected women
5. Patients and staff in institutions for the developmentally disabled
6. Recipients of plasma-derived products (before current inactivation techniques)
7. Hemodialysis patients
8. Healthcare and public safety workers with frequent exposure to blood
9. Persons born in areas endemic for HBV
10. Alaskan natives
11. Prison inmates

HBV, hepatitis B virus.

The transmission of HBV via transfusion has been reduced to present levels because of the screening of all blood donors for HBsAg with more sensitive assays. Counterimmunoelectrophoresis was introduced in 1972 to 1973, and sensitivity for HBsAg detection was further increased by currently available RIAs, reversed passive hemagglutination, and EIAs (116–121). With the successive introduction of second-generation counterimmunoelectrophoresis and current third-generation tests for HBsAg (Table 69.5), Alter et al. (122–124) documented the parallel reduction of PTH resulting from HBV. This reduction was likely augmented because of current American Red Cross donor selection and deferral procedures and the elimination of paid donors in favor of all-volunteer donors (9,10,116,117, 122–125). HBeAg, associated with parenteral and maternal-fetal HBV transmission, has been found more frequently in paid blood donors (15%) compared with volunteer donors (5%) (126). Further reduction of PTH resulting from HBV may also be due to the fact that asymptomatic HBsAg carriers continue to be removed from the donor pool through repeat donor testing (20,127). Fig. 69.3 presents the current algorithm for screening donor blood for HBV.

The residual frequency of PTH resulting from HBV is apparently due to the fact that HBsAg is circulating at undetectable levels for current screening assays; some of these donor units can be eliminated by screening for anti-HBc (128–133). Such donor unit screening was initiated in 1986 (Table 69.5) as a surrogate test for non-A, non-B PTH but is believed to have contributed further to the reduction of HBV-related PTH. It is estimated that because of the institution of surrogate screens for non-A, non-B PTH [anti-HBc and alanine aminotransferase (ALT), the incidence of HBV-associated PTH has further decreased by up to 84% (134). However, this reduction may also have been affected somewhat at that time by more stringent donor population screening to prevent transfusion-related HIV-1 transmission (116), because the incidence of PTH was already further dropping before the initiation of anti-HBc screening (135). Regardless, the risk of HBV-related PTH has currently dropped at least to 0.002% per transfusion recipient (8,116). However, further reduction may require more sensitive assays, because 4% to 12% of HBV-DNA carriers are seronegative for HBsAg, HBcAb, and other HBV serologic markers (23). HBV mutations may account for these falsely negative serologic tests (8,23).

In addition to the marked reduction of PTH caused by HBV resulting from HBsAg and anti-HBc testing of each donor unit of blood, the recent development of the nucleic acid testing (NAT) for whole blood (to assay for HBV DNA in plasma of donors without HBsAg and with normal ALT) has the potential to decrease the already low rate of PTH resulting from HBV (136,137). It is projected that an additional 81 HBV infected units of blood would be detected annually among the 12 million screened units (8), thereby potentially reducing the risk of HBV transmission by transfusion by 42% to 0.0004% to 0.0009% per unit (8,9,127). One must assess the benefit of such polymerase chain reaction (PCR) assays for HBV DNA versus their cost,

TABLE 69.5. SEROLOGIC TESTS FOR INFECTIOUS AGENTS PERFORMED ON BLOOD AND BLOOD PRODUCTS BEFORE TRANSFUSION

Assay	Target disease	Date initiated
Non-treponemal test[a]	Syphilis	1939–1941
HBsAg (immunodiffusion)	Hepatitis B	July 1972[b]
HBsAg (CIE)	Hepatitis B	1972–1973[b]
HBsAg (RIA or EIA)	Hepatitis B	September 1975[b]
HIV-1 antibody (EIA)	HIV-1 infection	March 1985[b]
HTLV-I antibody (EIA)[c]	HTLV-I infection	December 1988[b]
ALT	Hepatitis B, C, and non-A, non-B, non-C	Summer 1986[b,d]
Anti-HBc	Hepatitis B, C, and non-A, non-B, non-C	Fall 1987[b]
Anti-HCV 1.0 (EIA)	Hepatitis C	May 2, 1990[b]
Anti-HCV 2.0 (EIA)	Hepatitis C	March, 1992[b]
HIV-1/2 antibody (EIA)	HIV-1, HIV-2 infection	June 1, 1992[b]
HIV-1 p24 antigen	HIV-1 infection	March 14, 1996[b]
Anti-HCV 3.0 (EIA)	Hepatitis C	May 1996[e]
HTLV-I/II (EIA)	HTLV-I and HTLV-II	February 15, 1998[b]
NAT for HIV-1, HCV[f]	HIV-1, HCV	April, 1999

ALT, alanine aminotransferase; anti-HBc, antibody to hepatitis B core antigen; anti-HCV, antibody to hepatitis C virus; CIE, counter immunoelectrophoresis; EIA, enzyme immunoassay; HBsAg, hepatitis B surface antigen; HIV-1/2, human immunodeficiency virus types 1 and 2; HTLV-I/II, human T-cell leukemia virus types I and II; RIA, radioimmunoassay.
[a] *Most large centers are now using a treponemal test, an automated MHA-TP.*
[b] *Required by Food and Drug Administration (FDA).*
[c] *With significant HTLV-II cross-reactivity.*
[d] *Requirement deleted June 20, 1995; donation discarded only if ALT ≥2 × normal if ALT test is continued by donor center.*
[e] FDA approved.
[f] NAT, nucleic acid testing; 16 minipool testing.

because the cost-to-benefit ratio is likely to be high (8). Despite not having implemented NAT for HBV, a recent report from hemophilia treatment centers failed to reveal any HBV seroconversions between May 1998 and June 2002 (93).

If it were established within 1 to 2 weeks of receipt that a patient had been administered a unit of HBV-contaminated blood, there are no data that the use of HBV vaccine or hepatitis B immune globulin would be of value. In this unusual situation, one could argue for the use of both preparations, as after parenteral exposure, in an attempt at least to modify the anticipated illness. When it can be anticipated that a person is going to receive multiple future transfusions (e.g., a hemophiliac), HBV vaccine should be administered as early in life as possible. However, the mainstays of prevention of PTH B for most patients are deferral of high-risk donors and serologic testing and NAT of donor units. Given the recommendations of the Immunization Practices Advisory Committee for universal childhood HBV vaccination, the risk of PTH resulting from HBV should become even smaller (138). Without NAT, the risk of transmission of HBV via transfusion has remained stable in the United States (9,10,127). This stability and the lack of an increasing relative risk of HBV transmission probably reflect an effect of universal childhood immunization, in addition to continued refinement of donor deferral criteria and use of antigen and antibody testing.

Delta Hepatitis

Delta agent hepatitis was initially described in 1977 by Rizzetto et al. (139) in Turin, Italy, and was reviewed by Hoofnagle in 1989 (140). Although endemic to southern Italy, this virus has a worldwide but geographically variable distribution, including the Middle East and parts of Africa and South America. In nonendemic areas, such as the United States and Western Europe, the delta virus is found primarily in injectable drug users and multiply transfused patients, including hemophiliacs (141). HDV is a defective RNA virus that replicates only in the presence of HBV with circulating HBsAg (140). It is composed of an inner low-molecular-weight RNA genome associated with the internal delta antigen protein and coated with HBsAg as the surface protein (142).

HDV infection occurs in only two settings: as a simultaneous co-infection with acute HBsAg-positive hepatitis B or as a superinfection superimposed on the chronic HBsAg carrier state (140–142). During co-infection, although the ensuing hepatitis may be severe, biphasic, and protracted with a 2% to 20% mortality rate, most patients recover as hepatitis B resolves and fewer than 5% of patients develop chronic hepatitis (141,143). The mortality rate resulting from co-infection of HDV with HBV contrasts with the less than 1% mortality rate associated with hepatitis B alone (140). Illness associated with HDV is defined by a resurgence of the ALT serum levels after an initial decline, concomitant with the appearance of a transient anti-HDV–IgM response and followed by the development of low titer anti-HDV–IgG (140,143). These antibody responses may be detected by commercially available RIAs and EIAs (144,145).

In contrast to acute co-infection, when HDV infection is superimposed on the chronic HBsAg carrier state, most patients (70%) develop chronic hepatitis with continued presence of HBsAg and HDV in the serum (143). Sixty percent to 70% of patients with chronic delta hepatitis develop cirrhosis, and most

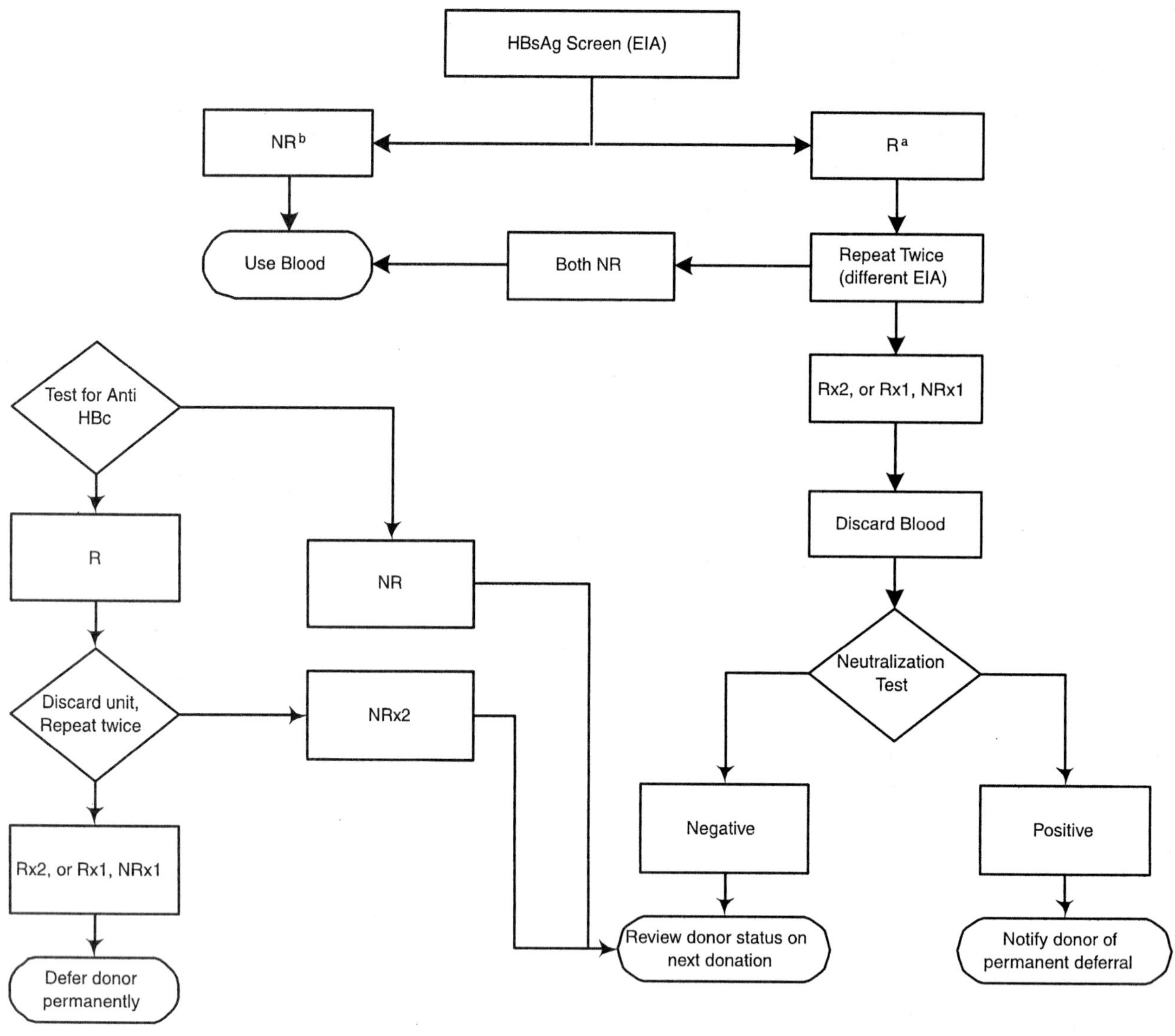

Figure 69.3. Algorithm for screening of donor blood for hepatitis B. R[a], reactive; NR[b], nonreactive.

of these die from liver disease (146). Chronic HDV infection is documented by the persistence of anti-HDV–IgM in high titer (143). HDV antigen may also be detected in the liver.

Because HDV is usually parenterally spread, its frequency in PTH associated with HBV (HBsAg positive) has been evaluated; 3.5% of 262 patients with PTH resulting from HBV were positive for anti-HDV (147). Of these patients, 2.5% of those with self-limited disease were anti-HDV positive, whereas 14.5% of those with fatal hepatitis were infected with HDV. These data raise serious concerns for transfusion recipients; however, screening for HBsAg in each donor unit provides a high degree of protection for HBsAg-negative blood donor recipients (147). HDV antibody screening is not needed. However, the HBsAg-positive prospective transfusion recipient is at some risk, especially if multiply transfused. In addition to the usual HBsAg screen of donor blood, blood-derivative recipients who are HBsAg carriers should be given products from single or minipool plasma sources (147). Furthermore, all donors with ALT elevations should be eliminated as blood sources for HBsAg-positive recipients.

Hepatitis C and Non-A, Non-B Hepatitis

After the introduction of testing of all donor blood for HBsAg, it quickly became apparent that not all PTH was due to HBV (20,81,82). Hepatitis A was also quickly excluded as a potential cause of the residual PTH (81,92), as were CMV and EBV (81,148,149). It was concluded that another virus (or viruses) accounted for most of PTH cases in the United States, initially designated non-A, non-B or type C PTH (150,151). Much of the epidemiologic description of non-A, non-B hepatitis is now applicable to HCV, which caused most cases of non-A, non-B PTH (152–155).

HCV is believed to be the most common cause of nonalcoholic liver disease in the United States. The prevalence of HCV in the U.S. population is 1.8%; 73% of patients with chronic infection have genotype 1, with the remaining predominately genotypes 2 and 3 (156). The risk factors for infection somewhat parallel those of HBV. Among well-defined factors, transfusion (5% to 10%) and injectable drug use (60%) have accounted for most infections; transfusion is a declining risk (8-10,127,153, 156–158). The risk of transfusion-related HCV infection declined between 1981 and 1988 from 17% to 6% before antibody screening. (159). Antibody to HCV is found in up to 85% of injectable drug users (160,161). Other high-risk groups include prisoners, patients with transfusion-dependent bleeding disorders, and hemodialysis patients (158,160–163). Sexual, household, and perinatal transmission and receipt of intravenous immune globulin are less important risks for HCV (158,160, 164–166); sporadic cases without defined exposure have declined (from 40% to 50%) to 5% of new cases (158,159,167). In the contemporary era of home intravenous infusion therapy, risks for HCV infection previously recognized in other sites have emerged in the household setting; a recent report suggests that transmission of HCV from an HCV-infected mother to her hemophiliac child may occur via accidental percutaneous (ungloved) needlestick during venipuncture for clotting factor infusion (168). A family history of liver disease and prior history of blood transfusion, tattooing, sexual promiscuity, injectable drug use, intranasal cocaine use, and male ear piercing have been associated with anti-HCV positivity among blood donors (169, 170).

Approximately 75% of cases of HCV are subclinical, but, when symptomatic, hepatitis C is clinically and biochemically identical to other forms of hepatitis (152,158). Fig. 69.4 depicts the clinical, serologic, and biochemical course of HCV infection. Fifty percent to 85% of patients with hepatitis C develop chronic hepatitis (23,152,171,172). Despite resolution of hepatitis after HCV infection, HCV RNA can often be detected by PCR, indicating HCV persistence in asymptomatic biochemically normal patients (about 30% of chronic carriers) (158,171). Symptoms or serum ALT level do not correlate with disease severity (171,173). Most patients develop chronic active hepatitis with or without cirrhosis (171,172,174,175). Cirrhosis may variably appear in 20% to 50% or more of patients (152,158,175). Chronic hepatitis C has also been linked with hepatocellular carcinoma (158,176–178). Patients seropositive for HCV antibody but with normal ALT values, no HCV RNA in serum, and normal hepatic histology, although uncommon, (up to 15% of those infected) probably have recovered from HCV infection (172).

There are several recent studies assessing the outcome of PTH resulting from HCV. Seeff et al. (179) reported a study of long-term mortality after non-A, non-B PTH in 568 patients matched with two control groups, both of which comprised patients who had been transfused but had normal ALT values after transfusion. After an average of 18 years of follow-up, overall death rates did not differ between patients with PTH and control subjects; there was a small statistically significant increase in deaths resulting from liver disease in the patients with PTH (3.3% vs. 2.0% and 1.1% in the control groups). Tong et al. (180) defined that PTH resulting from HCV evolves into a progressive disease; chronic active hepatitis (23%), cirrhosis (51%), and hepatocellular carcinoma (5.3%) are noteworthy sequelae. The study by Tong et al. was retrospective with a less well-defined population than the prospectively evaluated population reported by Seefe et al. Goedert et al. (181) recently reported 137 hemophiliac patients with end-stage renal disease (ESRD) and HCV infection; ESRD was significantly associated with HIV-1, older age, HBV co-infection, and a low CD4 cell count. A recent study suggests a more benign outcome (45% viral clearance by PCR) in children infected via transfusion (182).

Before the development of the current serologic tests to detect HCV, surrogate markers for non-A, non-B hepatitis were used as screening methods for donor blood. Initially, ALT assays were proposed to help reduce non-A, non-B PTH (183–185). Up to 45% of donor units implicated in transmission of PTH have ALT elevations greater than 60 IU/L (134). Discarding units of blood positive for anti-HBc was subsequently shown to reduce posttransfusion non-A, non-B hepatitis (186,187) (Fig. 69.5). Approximately 53% of blood donors implicated in PTH and

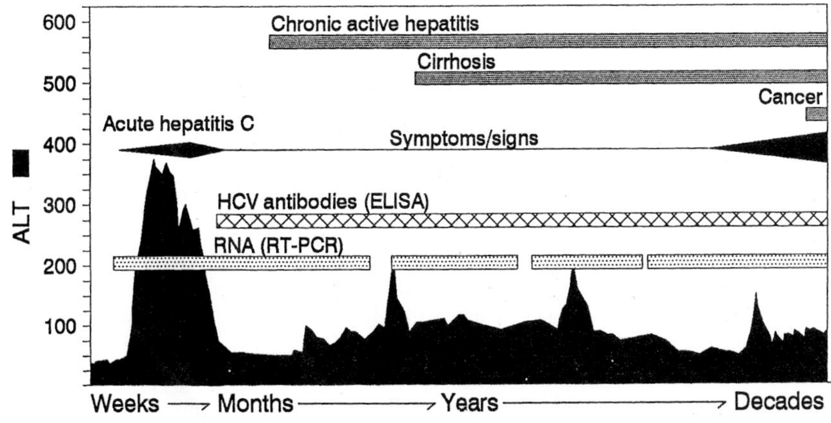

Figure 69.4. The clinical, biochemical, and serologic course of acute hepatitis C infection. (From Thomas DL, Lemon SM. Hepatitis C. In: Mandell GL, Bennett JE, Dolin R, eds. *Principles and practice of infectious diseases,* 5th ed. Philadelphia: Churchill Livingstone, 2000:1736–1760, with permission.)

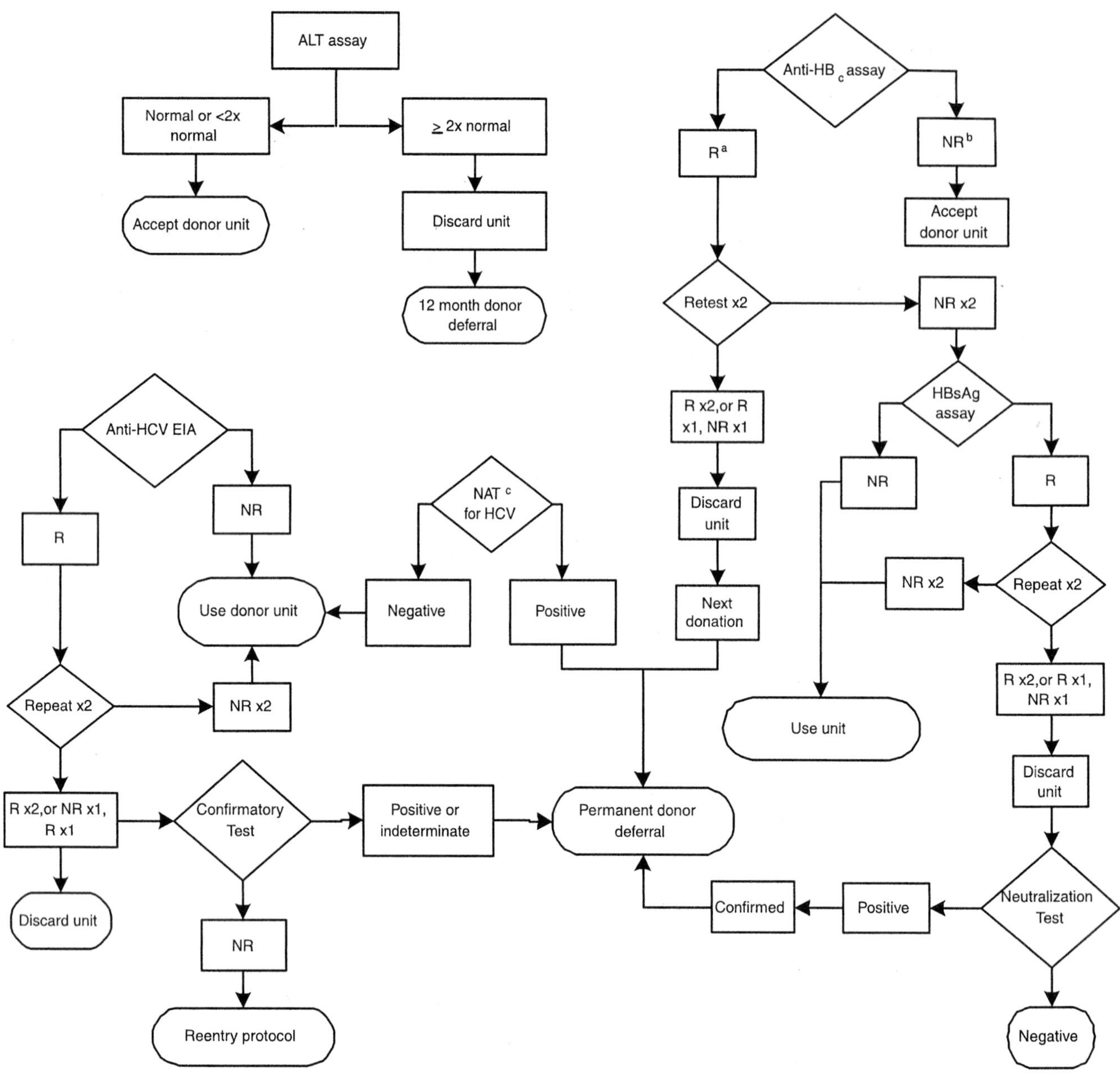

Figure 69.5. Algorithm for screening of donor blood for hepatitis C and hepatitis non-A, non-B, non-C. The requirement for alanine aminotransferase screening was rescinded on June 20, 1995. R[a], reactive; NR[b], nonreactive.

positive for anti-HCV have anti-HBc (134). The use of these assays instituted in 1986 and 1987, respectively (Table 69.5), led to an approximately 30% to 40% reduction of PTH (134). Since 1985, blood transfusion as a source for acquiring HCV has decreased to only 4% of new cases (171).

Contemporary molecular biologic techniques led to the discovery of HCV. Nucleic acid extraction of infectious chimpanzee plasma led to the isolation of viral RNA, its transcription to DNA, and expression after insertion into a phage. Screening of several million DNA sequences for production of proteins that reacted with antibody in the serum of patients with non-A, non-B PTH led to the discovery of a polypeptide (C100-3) that was developed as an antibody-capture RIA for HCV (155). This assay was quickly shown to detect 65% of donor blood capable of transmitting chronic PTH and 17% of acute PTH (188). This commercially available antibody capture RIA was adapted also to an EIA, which has been shown to detect HCV as a cause of PTH (189–191). Initial enthusiasm for this assay dampened because of the delayed seroconversion and, therefore, potential seronegativity of blood donors infected with HCV despite the greater sensitivity of first-generation EIAs compared with RIAs (161,192–195). The sensitivity of the EIA and RIA for preventing non-A, non-B PTH resulting from HCV was variably estimated at 60% to 85% (157,192,196). First-generation assays for anti-HCV became positive up to a year after acute hepatitis C, and up to 20% of patients remained seronegative by these assays (161,190). An explanation for patients with PTH who are seronegative for HCV by first-generation assays might be the presence of another agent of non-A, non-B PTH; more likely, this phenomenon usually reflected the relative insensitivity of these first-generation screening assays (197). Regardless, contrasting the period when only surrogate tests for non-A, non-B PTH were used to the period after 1990 when the first-generation assays were implemented, Donahue et al. (198) demonstrated an 84% reduction of the risk of PTH resulting from HCV among transfused cardiac surgery patients (Table 69.6).

The ability to prevent PTH resulting from HCV was further improved by second-generation EIAs that incorporated detection of antibodies to the core antigen (C22-3 protein) and the C200 antigen, which combines the epitopes included in the c33c and C100-3 proteins (coded by the NS-3 and NS-4 regions of the RNA genome) (23,157). Wang et al. (199) demonstrated 100% sensitivity of a second-generation EIA incorporating these three antigens compared with 83% sensitivity of the first-generation assay; the newer assay also detected anti-HCV 6 weeks earlier than the single-antigen EIA. Using dot-blot assays, several groups demonstrated that antibodies to the c33c or core proteins (C22) consistently appeared before C100-3 from 4 to 13 weeks after transfusion (200,201).

In addition to their sensitivity, another concern with the first-generation anti-HCV EIAs and RIAs was their positive predictive value. A positive EIA or RIA was confirmed by the more specific recombinant immunoblot assay (RIBA) in only 19% to 60% of cases (196,202–205), with only one study showing 100% correlation of the screening EIA with RIBA (192). Newer RIBA and matrix (a semiautomated immunoblot) assays each contain four recombinant antigens (206). In high-risk populations, 70% to 100% of sera repeatedly reactive by second-generation EIAs were determined to be true positives by the RIBA or matrix assays, whereas fewer than 50% of repeatedly reactive second-generation EIAs are true positive in low-risk populations (171,206).

Despite the limitations of first-generation EIAs, on May 2, 1990, an anti-HCV first-generation screening assay became mandatory on all donor blood (Table 69.5). Blood banks began using the second-generation EIA for antibody to HCV on April 6, 1992. Because of the previously discussed suboptimal sensitivity of these assays for HCV infection in a donor unit, the screening of donor blood for ALT level and anti-HBc were considered as important surrogate markers for PTH and were retained as required assays until June 20, 1995 when the requirement for ALT assays was rescinded (Table 69.5 and Fig. 69.5) (23,26, 157,196,202,203,207).

Third-generation EIAs were initially tested in Europe and then approved by the FDA in May 1996 for use by blood donation centers. Similar to the second-generation assays, these third-generation assays incorporate recombinant antigens and include those described previously for the second-generation products in addition to the protein product of the NS-5 region of the genome (RNA polymerase) (23,208,209). These assays detect all genotypes and offer marginal improvement in reducing the seroconversion window (by 12 days) and the potential infectivity of a donor unit (15% reduction of an already low rate) (23,208, 209). All HCV-antibody positive specimens by EIA are confirmed as positive by RIBA; a second-generation RIBA now incorporates the same recombinant antigens as the newer EIAs.

Table 61.6 summarizes the estimates of the frequency of non-A, non-B PTH after each of these assays were implemented on donor blood. The risk of PTH was estimated to be less than 0.5% per patient transfused with the use of the third-generation EIA (23,171,206). In addition to screening for HBsAg and antibody to HIV-1 and the adoption of a totally volunteer blood

TABLE 69.6. RATES OF POSTTRANSFUSION HEPATITIS (PTH) DUE TO NON-A, NON-B AGENTS ACCORDING TO TIMING OF VARIOUS BLOOD DONOR SCREENING PRACTICES BEFORE 1985 THROUGH PRESENT

		Rate of non-A, non-B PTH	
Years	Screening practice	Per patient transfused (%)	Per unit transfused (%)
Pre-1985	Reference period	8–10	—
1985–1987	Donor self-deferral, HIV-1 antibody	4.5	0.45–0.52
1987–1990	Above plus surrogate markers (ALT, anti-HBc)	4.4	0.19–0.36
1990–1992	Above plus first-generation EIA for anti-HCV	1.08	0.03–0.07
1992–1996	Second-generation EIA for anti-HCV	<0.5 (estimate)	0.0001 (Ref. 8)
1996–1999	Third-generation EIA for anti-HCV	Unknown	0.0008 (Ref. 23)
1999–present	Third-generation EIA for anti-HCV, plus NAT for HCV	Unknown	Unknown

ALT, alanine aminotransferase; anti-HBc, antibody to hepatitis B core antigen; anti-HCV, antibody to hepatitis C virus; EIA, enzyme immunoassay; HIV-1, human immunodeficiency virus type 1; NAT, nucleic acid testing.

donor system with donor screening for HIV-1 infection risks, screening for ALT, anti-HBc, and especially anti-HCV have had a major impact on the reduction of PTH, as shown in Table 69.6. Donor questionnaire screening and donor unit serologic screening produced an overall low prevalence of anti-HCV positivity among volunteer blood donors (<0.5%) (161,192,193, 196,202,206). The frequency of anti-HCV positivity has been found to be higher among paid blood donors (10%) compared with volunteer groups (0.36%), correlating with previous observations of the higher frequency of non-A, non-B PTH related to these donor groups (210). Despite this low prevalence in volunteer donors, anti-HCV screening has demonstrated an impact (Table 69.6) because of the frequency of PTH (58–95%) after transfusion of anti-HCV reactive donor units and because of the ability of second- and third-generation EIAs for anti-HCV to detect 90% or more of donor units that transmit HCV (157,161,190,192,194,196,206). The residual risk with the third-generation EIA was related to the possible 12- to 14-week window period after infection with HCV before the appearance of antibody (211).

Because of the added sensitivity of the second- and third-generation EIAs for anti-HCV, a reentry protocol was allowed by the AABB in the past because of the 50% false-positive rate of these EIAs among low-risk volunteer blood donors (206). This reentry protocol is no longer used. With these added screening tools, the risk of PTH has declined to less than 0.5% of transfused patients, a risk comparable with or less than the risk of hepatitis in nontransfused hospitalized patients (153,157,206). Furthermore, 58% to 80% of the patients developing PTH develop persistent ALT elevations and 26% to 85% have chronic hepatitis; 90% of these patients are anti-HCV reactive (134,139, 149,166,170,182). Therefore, with current blood donor unit serologic screening there is the potential not only to reduce PTH resulting from HCV by 90% or more but also to reduce chronic hepatitis resulting from HCV after transfusion by 80% to 90% (188,206). On June 20, 1995, the prior requirement for ALT assays on all donor units was made optional when sensitive second- and now third-generation EIAs for anti-HCV are used. Required ALT testing was made optional because of rejection of many acceptable donors, especially males, because ALT assays are subject to interlaboratory variation and because the risk of PTH in groups receiving blood screened with or without ALT testing was equivalent (207).

The use of NAT has further enhanced the ability to decrease the already low frequency of PTH resulting from defined HCV infection in donor blood (158,212–215). PCR can detect HCV RNA within 59 days of infection (8). With resolution of PTH resulting from HCV, HCV RNA detected by PCR has been shown to clear from blood as antibody levels decrease (201). Before NAT for HCV, the risk of PTH resulting from HCV had been reduced to approximately 0.001% per unit of blood (8,9). The addition of NAT in 1999 has further reduced this risk to 0.00005%, an estimated 72% further risk reduction (8, 9,127,216). Despite NAT, HCV can still be transmitted by anti-HCV- and NAT-negative blood products (217). However, Dodd et al. (127) have documented the very low risk of HCV hepatitis after transfusion; they reported only 74 units of blood from more than 19 million drawn between March 1999 and February 2002 that were HCV antibody negative but HCV-RNA positive, for a rate of one positive unit per 267,700 units. In addition, the Centers for Disease Control and Prevention (CDC) has reported no transfusion-related HCV seroconversions among 11,171 hemophiliac patients between May 1998 and June 2002 (93). These improved safety data reflect an estimated decrement of the window period of infectivity of donor blood for HCV from 82 days with current antibody tests alone to 23 to 36 days by also incorporating NAT (8,218). PTH has become an uncommon event, reflecting the current safety of the blood supply.

Additional potential methods to prevent PTH resulting from HCV await development of a vaccine. Studies evaluating pretransfusion or posttransfusion administration of ISG have demonstrated conflicting results (219–221). The variable efficacy probably reflects inconsistent anti-HCV content of preparations. ISG is not given in this setting (158).

Other unsolved issues regarding non-A, non-B PTH remain. Only 91% of non-A, non-B PTH is associated with anti-HCV reactivity (157,161,190). Although the incubation periods for anti-HCV–positive and anti-HCV–negative PTH are the same (6 to 12 weeks) (197), anti-HCV–positive patients are more seriously ill and have twice the incidence of chronic hepatitis (157,197). Other agents remain yet to be defined to account for the 9% of cases of PTH that are not due to HAV, HBV, or HCV (8–10,127,197,222,223).

Hepatitis G

Similar to the original work with HCV, in 1996 Linnen et al. (224) reported the cloning of HGV from the plasma of two patients, one with non-A, non-B hepatitis and the other asymptomatic with intermittent enzyme elevations. This group reported that HGV was genomically similar to another human virus isolate from a surgeon ill with hepatitis in the 1960s, termed GB virus C. HGV is a member of the Flavivirus family, along with HCV and GB virus C. Using reverse transcriptase PCR technology, 2 of 12 patients with PTH were found positive for HGV RNA by Linnen et al. (224), as were 5 of 38 patients with non-A to non-E community-acquired hepatitis. Four of the latter five patients remained HGV-RNA positive for 2 to 9 years without evidence of chronic hepatitis. In addition, Linnen et al. reported 13 of 779 (1.7%) of volunteer blood donors with normal ALT values positive for HGV RNA, as were 11 of 709 donors (1.5%) with ALT elevations. These authors reported HGV to be globally distributed.

Subsequent studies have confirmed this work and have found HGV in hemodialysis and postoperative patients, presumably transfusion associated (225–227). Several authors have reported on the clinical disease associated with HGV, whether alone or in association with HCV; HGV is at worst a cause of mild acute hepatitis (227,228), but frequently infection with HGV is asymptomatic without evidence of hepatitis (227–229). HGV does not augment disease when accompanying HCV (227–231). HGV was not associated with chronic hepatitis (226,227,229). HGV is also prevalent in injectable drug users and hemophiliacs; HGV can be passed vertically mother-to-child and after heterosexual or homosexual contact with HGV-positive partners (227). Its modes of transmission parallel HCV generally. Tanaka et al. (230) reported HGV responsiveness to interferon-α, but most patients relapsed.

Despite the prevalence of HGV in the volunteer blood donor population (1% to 4%), its role in PTH remains to be determined, because 75% of patients with transfusion-acquired HGV lack biochemical evidence of hepatitis (227,228). Those with hepatitis have only mild elevations asynchronous with their HGV-RNA levels (228). The relevance of HGV (and GB virus C) to PTH remains to be defined with broader seroepidemiologic, biochemical, and clinical studies. Currently there appears to be no reason to test blood donors for HGV (232,233).

Cytomegalovirus

CMV is a member of the herpesvirus family of DNA viruses. Like other members of this group of viruses, latency is the rule after recovery from acute infection. Acquired CMV infection rarely presents as hepatitis (234). Epidemiologically, CMV is acquired by human-to-human contact, congenitally or perinatally from mother to child by contact with cervical secretions, postnatally by an infant via breast milk, and in settings for the care of multiple children (e.g., in neonatal nurseries, in day care centers, and in the family setting) (235) (see Chapter 44). CMV is also transmitted by heterosexual or homosexual contact, by transfusion of donor blood, and by transplantation of donor organs (235).

CMV infections are classified as primary (with seroconversion from negativity to positivity), reactivation of an endogenous infection, or reinfection with a new exogenous strain of CMV (in a seropositive host) (234,235). The latter two forms of infection can be distinguished by using restriction enzyme DNA analysis, but this is not routinely practical (236). Because there are no accurate data on the proportion of reactivation and reinfection for CMV posttransfusion infections, these two forms of infection are called recurrent infections (234,235).

Depending on socioeconomic stratum and age, the seroprevalence of CMV ranges from 25% to 88% (234–240). In studies of CMV infection after transfusion in normal hosts before 1972, the incidence varied from 16% to 67% (234). Most of these infections were asymptomatic. Risk factors for transmission included increasing number of units of blood transfused, use of fresh blood, and use of seropositive blood (234). After 1972, transfusions became less common and involved little or no fresh whole blood, especially in cardiac surgery. Concomitant CMV posttransfusion infections have decreased to 1.2% to 17% (234). In contrast to fresh whole blood, leukocytes containing CMV (monocytes and polymorphonuclear leukocytes) survive storage poorly at 2° to 6°C (234). This observation correlates with the observed reduction of CMV posttransfusion infection rates; studies have shown that 86% of patients infected with CMV after transfusion had received fresh whole blood, compared with 11% of uninfected patients (241,242). Dworkin et al. (243) demonstrated a greater likelihood of isolation of CMV from donor blood during the first 5 days after collection, with infrequent isolation thereafter. In addition to fresh whole blood, granulocyte transfusions have been associated with an especially high risk of CMV infection in compromised hosts (244–246). The difficulty with isolating CMV from donor leukocytes may be a reflection of the small number of leukocytes infected or the need for a posttransfusion host-versus-graft reaction to reactivate the virus (234).

The reduction in overall CMV-related transfusion infections since 1972 also suggests that only a subset of CMV-infected donors (most of whom are seropositive) can transmit infection via donated blood (234,247). This observation is paralleled by the infrequency with which CMV can be isolated from donor blood (234). The receipt of blood from a CMV-seropositive donor significantly correlates with the infrequent residual posttransfusion CMV infections observed since 1972 (248); this has been very well defined in transfused neonates (249). An increased frequency of transmission also correlates with receipt of blood from a donor positive for CMV-IgM antibody (248,250). The pathogenesis of CMV infection after transfusion involves several factors: the volume of blood transfused, activation of leukocytes harboring CMV, and survival of donor cells in the recipient to allow CMV replication (250).

CMV infection can be diagnosed by direct examination of tissues or exfoliated cells for intranuclear inclusions; however, this lacks sensitivity for active infection (251,252). Isolation of CMV in cell culture from blood (leukocytes) is more sensitive and specific for active infection but labor intensive (1 to 4 weeks for positivity). The development of fluorescein-labeled monoclonal antibodies for "immediate-early" and "early" antigen detection permits the diagnosis of CMV infection in cell culture within 24 to 48 hours (253–256). Such antibodies can also be used directly to stain biopsied tissue (253,257,258). CMV DNA probes with hybridization and electron microscopy of tissues and leukocytes are limited to research applications generally and have been reported to have lower sensitivity (234,240). "Nested" PCR has been applied to various body fluids, including cerebrospinal fluid and blood, for the diagnosis of active CMV infection in HIV-1 infected patients (235). This has not been applied to the blood donor setting.

CMV-specific antibodies can be detected by a variety of techniques (complement fixation, indirect hemagglutination, indirect immunofluorescence, anticomplement immunofluorescence, latex agglutination, RIA, and EIA) (234,235). Several of these can be applied to the detection of CMV-IgM antibody, including RIA and EIA (259).

CMV disease most frequently occurs in a seronegative individual after primary infection and usually manifests as mononucleosis; however, posttransfusion CMV infection is usually asymptomatic. Therefore, there is no need to provide CMV-seronegative blood or blood products to immunocompetent recipients (234,250).

The groups at risk for serious posttransfusion CMV infection are seronegative pregnant women, seronegative premature infants, seronegative organ transplant recipients who received an organ from a seronegative donor, seronegative oncology patients receiving chemotherapy, and seronegative patients with HIV-1 infection (235,260,261). Seronegative premature neonates (less than 1,200 g) receiving CMV-seropositive blood are at greater risk for pneumonia, hepatitis, hemolytic anemia, and thrombocytopenia (250,262). Mortality may reach 40%. This subgroup warrants routine receipt of CMV-seronegative blood (see Chapter 44).

Transplant patients developing primary infection (via a transplanted organ or transfusion) develop more serious disease (235, 261). In renal transplantation, the seropositive kidney donor is the major source of CMV (263,264); seronegative transplant recipients receiving kidneys from seronegative donors rarely become infected and have better graft survival than those receiving kidneys from seropositive donors (265–267). It is prudent to provide seronegative recipients of seronegative renal transplants with CMV-seronegative blood (234,250). The same comments apply to heart transplantation (250,268). Better-controlled studies in solid-organ transplant patients are needed, however (250). The data are less clear and less well defined for donor blood in the bone marrow transplantation setting; however, prophylactic granulocyte transfusions, if given during bone marrow transplantation, should be from CMV-seronegative donors if the recipient is seronegative because of the high frequency of symptomatic and fatal infections (244–246,250,269). The use of CMV-seronegative or leukocyte-depleted cellular blood products is warranted in seronegative recipients of bone marrow transplants from CMV-seronegative donors (12,250,260,261,269,270). Such practices have reduced the risk of transfusion-associated CMV infection in this setting (23 to 37%) to 1% to 4%.

Preiksaitis et al. (271) recently documented the low risk of transfusion-related CMV disease in CMV-seronegative children with malignancy because of their low frequency of exposure via transfusion and because of leukocyte depletion of transfused units. In oncology patients, currently available data do not support screening donor blood for CMV (234). Leukocyte-depleted cellular blood products may be indicated in patients with hematologic malignancies who are CMV-seronegative to prevent CMV-associated morbidity (12,261,272). A similar argument can be made for the exceptional HIV-1–infected patient who is seronegative for CMV (250,260,261).

When indicated and necessary, the screening of donor blood for CMV antibodies is problematic because of the high frequency of seropositivity in the population (240,273). At least in the neonatal setting, screening only for evidence of acute or reactivated CMV infection (i.e., CMV IgM) in donor blood will increase the size of the donor pool while reducing posttransfusion disease (234,274). It has been demonstrated that the risk of transmitting CMV is reduced by using leukocyte-depleted blood, either as frozen deglycerolized RBCs or leukocyte-filtered RBCs (12,250,272,275–279). Differential centrifugation of platelet units may also enhance their safety (250). These practices are time consuming and expensive but at times warranted. The use of CMV immune globulin may have some role for preventing CMV-related complications in premature neonates born to CMV-seropositive mothers and in bone marrow transplant recipients, but ganciclovir appears to be more effective in the latter setting and in patients with HIV-1 infection (234,235, 280–282). The effect of the attenuated CMV vaccine in preventing CMV complications of transfusion has been disappointing (235).

Epstein-Barr Virus and Human Herpesvirus 6 and 8

EBV is another member of the herpesvirus family of DNA viruses that is prone to latency in B lymphocytes and pharyngeal epithelial cells. Transfusion-related EBV infection is rare, with only a few recognized cases in the literature despite a 90% seroprevalence among blood donors (261,283–287). Seroconversion after transfusion is usually associated with mild or inapparent clinical illness (284,287). However, Alfieri et al. (288) documented the development of B-cell lymphoproliferative disease in a liver transplant patient after transfusion of EBV-positive donor blood. Because of the seroprevalence of prior infection in the population, screening donor blood is not indicated. Leukocyte-depleted RBCs may prevent transmission from a seropositive donor even during acute infection; leukocyte depletion is prudent in compromised hosts, especially in the transplant setting (261,287–289).

Although no precautions are yet indicated for human herpesvirus-6 (HHV-6) uninfected potential transfusion recipients (60% to 100% of adults are infected), further experience is needed before use of seronegative donor blood can be recommended for seronegative compromised hosts (261,287). HHV-6 has limited recognized pathogenic potential in immunocompromised adults (261).

Human herpesvirus 8 (HHV-8) has been associated with Kaposi's sarcoma, primary-effusion lymphomas, and multicentric Castleman's disease (290). HHV-8 remains latent in peripheral blood mononuclear cells (291). Its seroprevalence is 0% to 3% of volunteer blood donors but from 12% to 36% in homosexual males and injection drug users (290,292). In a study of women who had a history of injection drug use or high-risk sexual behavior, HHV-8 seropositivity was associated with black race; Hispanics; lower level of education; and infection with syphilis, HBV, HCV, and HIV-1 (292). Although there is the potential for transmission by transfusion, the low seroprevalence of HHV-8 in U.S. volunteer blood donors make transmission unlikely. There are no recognized consequences of transfusion-mediated infection at this time (261,290).

Human Immunodeficiency Virus Type 1

Within several years after the epidemic of the acquired immunodeficiency syndrome (AIDS) was recognized, its epidemiology was recognized to include transmission by sexual contact and by sharing blood-contaminated needles (293–295). Avoiding sexual contact and needle sharing with homosexual males, individuals with multiple sexual partners, and individuals using injectable drugs have become confirmed methods for avoiding infection with HIV-1, the cause of AIDS. Initially, the only mechanism for reducing what appeared to be transmission by transfusion was voluntary self-deferral of donors in high-risk groups, including sexual partners of members of the high-risk groups mentioned previously (296). This directive to blood banks for voluntary blood donor deferral was issued on March 4, 1983 (295). The first cases of transfusion-associated AIDS were reported in patients with hemophilia A (297). Subsequent reports included infants and other adults without risk for AIDS other than transfusion (296). The risk of transfusion was subsequently stressed to potential recipients by the recommendation for signed informed consent for nonemergent transfusions, issued on May 8, 1986.

Whole blood, blood cellular components, plasma, and clotting factors were implicated in transmission of HIV-1 (298,299). Immune globulin preparations and hepatitis B vaccine (plasma derived) were noninfectious. Ninety percent to 100% of patients transfused with blood contaminated with HIV-1 became infected (8,300,301). Because blood donors with HIV-1 infection are usually asymptomatic, self-deferral by those in high-risk groups was important, in addition to assaying for antibody. The risk of HIV-1 infection and AIDS was great for hemophiliacs before 1985; coupled with donor deferral and HIV-1 antibody testing, moist heat or solvent detergent treatment of clotting factors has reduced this risk to a very low level for pooled plasma products (302–306).

After the isolation of HIV-1 in 1983 to 1984 (307–310), serologic tests for detection of antibodies to HIV-1 in patients with AIDS were described (311–313). The assay techniques for these antibodies were quickly developed by private industry as an EIA, and blood centers within the United States initiated donor screening in March 1985 (314). The blood supply was thereby rendered safer (315). Despite the lack of specificity of an initially positive EIA, this screening EIA soon was also used as a diagnostic test, coupled with a confirmatory Western blot (WB).

Because of this evolving diagnostic function of the EIA, the CDC and American Red Cross established alternate test sites in April 1985 for anonymous testing to prevent high-risk individuals from using blood donor sites for diagnostic purposes (316). Individuals recommended for testing gradually evolved to include, in addition to the high-risk groups mentioned previously, pregnant women at high risk for HIV-1 infection, attendees of sexually transmissible diseases clinics and drug abuse clinics, and recipients of transfusions between 1978 and 1985. During this time, the definition of high-risk behavior warranting HIV-1 antibody testing and deferral from donating blood was expanded to include a single homosexual encounter since 1977, sexual contact with a prostitute, and residence in sub-Saharan Africa (because of HIV-2 risk). These attempts at high-risk donor self-deferral were effective except among injectable drug users (317, 318). This broadened definition of high-risk individuals was promulgated because of the window period after infection before antibody to HIV-1 can be detected (see later discussion).

In June 1986, notification was mandated for recipients of units of blood or blood products transfused before March 1985 that were subsequently determined to be seropositive for HIV-1. This "lookback program" allowed earlier medical evaluation, management, and observation of the natural history of HIV-1 infection in patients with well-defined dates of exposure.

With the use of the EIA, WB, and an antigen-capture EIA (313,319,320) the serology of HIV-1 infection was defined (Fig. 69.6). HIV-1 is composed of several structural (glyco) proteins that elicit antibodies (313). The core protein of 24,000 molecular weight (p24) correlates with active viral replication, appears early after infection, and coincides generally with plasma HIV-1 RNA levels (Fig. 69.6); its disappearance correlates with development of anti-p24. The envelope glycoprotein of 160,000 molecular weight (gp 160) is composed of a transmembrane subunit (gp 41) and an attachment subunit (gp 120); the host makes an antibody to each of these components. Internal polymerase gene products include the reverse transcriptase protein (p66, p51) and an endonuclease (p31); antibodies are made against both of these gene products. The first-generation EIA detected antibody to any of these proteins, because an impure virus lysate was used; however, the WB (and a radioimmunoprecipitation assay) allow differentiation of antibodies to each antigen (313). Other confirmatory antibody assays used to demonstrate infection with HIV-1 are available, but further testing of blood beyond antibody assays necessitates tests for HIV-1 detection [p24 antigen capture EIA, viral culture, or NAT (proviral DNA or viral RNA)] (313).

Because a lysate of human cells infected with HIV-1 was used as the antigen source for the first-generation EIA, antibodies to human cell antigens (and not viral antigens) in human serum caused false positivity of the EIA and resulted in its lack of specificity despite sensitivity; although the WB assay for antibodies used the same lysate, the viral (glyco) proteins were separated from each other and from contaminating human cell antigens electrophoretically, thereby allowing differentiation of antibodies and greater specificity (316).

The sequence available for testing for HIV-1 in donor units is depicted in Fig. 69.7. The criteria for a positive WB have been debated but were defined by the CDC as the presence of antibody to p24 and antibody to either gp 41 or gp 120/160 (321). Using this sequence of testing (Fig. 69.7), estimates of the frequency of transfusion of donor blood infected with HIV-1 ranged from 3 to 26 per 1 million transfusions with early

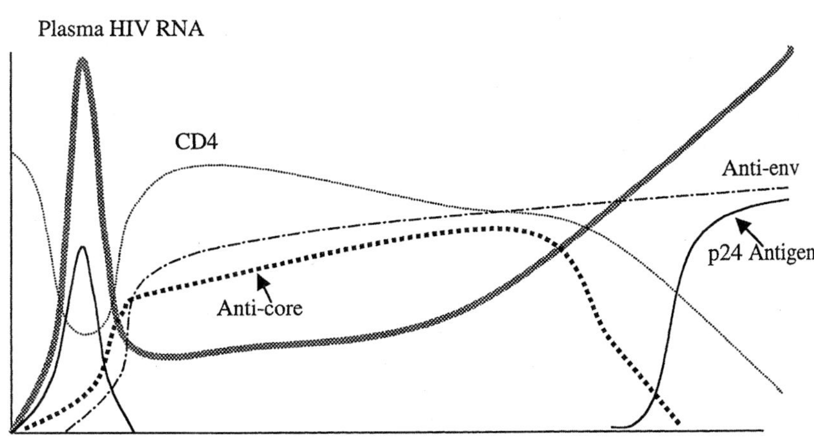

Figure 69.6. Chronology of human immunodeficiency virus type 1 infection defined by presence of core (p24) antigen and antibodies to core protein and envelope (gp 41) glycoprotein. (From Demeter LM, Reichman RC. Detection of human immunodeficiency virus infection. In: Mandell GL, Bennett JE, Dolin R, eds. *Principles and practice of infectious diseases,* 5th ed. Philadelphia: Churchill Livingstone, 2000:1369–1374, with permission.)

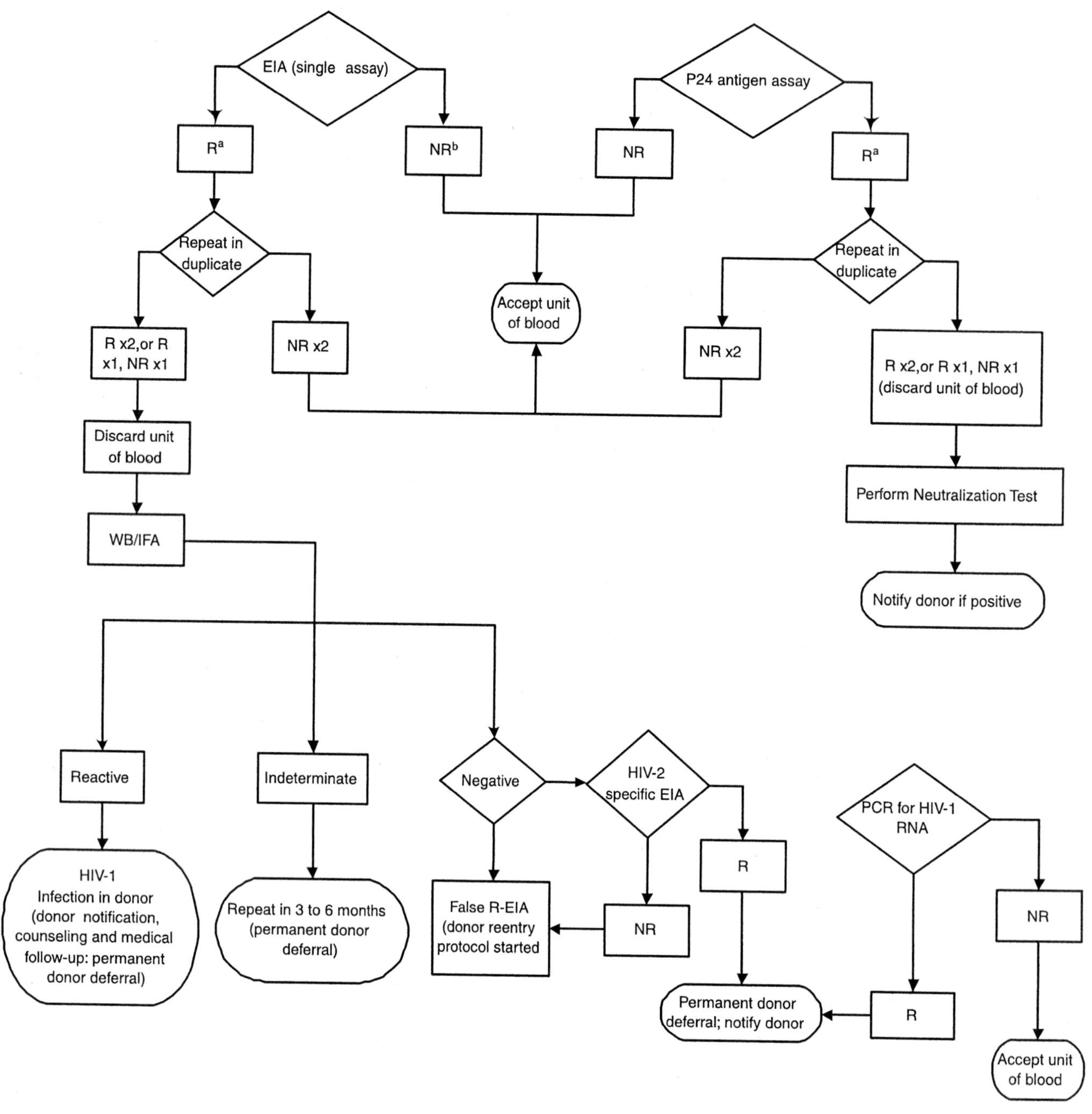

Figure 69.7. Algorithm for screening donor blood for human immunodeficiency virus type 1 and type 2 infections. R[a], reactive; NR[b], nonreactive.

EIAs (322–326). The most recent estimate using contemporary antibody assays approximates the lower frequency of 1 in 493,000 donor units (.0002%) (8). The entire antibody testing sequence even with first-generation EIA and WB had a positive predictive value of 81% to 100% with a 99% to 100% specificity (327). Follow-up evaluations of blood donors with indeterminate WB patterns (Fig. 69.7)—the presence of one or more antibodies but not enough to meet the definition of positive—have shown that these donors or recipients of their blood never develop serologic evidence of infection (328–332) (361).

Because of the window period with EIAs for HIV-1 antibody (between infection of a patient and seroconversion), rare transmission of HIV-1 could occur by transfusion (8,333,334). The window period was estimated at 42 to 45 days with the HIV-1 viral lysate EIAs and at 22 to 25 days with the contemporary HIV-1 recombinant protein supplemented EIAs (second- and third-generation EIAs) (8,23,335,336). This window period may be further reduced to 6 to 16 days by assaying for p24 antigen or HIV-1 DNA in leukocytes by PCR (8,23,336,337). Detection of HIV-1 RNA by PCR may reduce the window period after infection to 11 to 13 days (8,23,336). Proposals to initiate p24 antigen testing on all blood and plasma donor units were not supported in the scientific community because of minimal estimated benefit (five to ten infected donor units detected per year in the United States) (23,336–339). Despite this, in August 1995, the FDA recommended p24 antigen detection assays on all donor units (340). The first p24 test was licensed in March 1996, at which time antigen screening of donor blood ensued (23) (Table 69.5). The algorithm for such testing is incorporated into Fig. 69.7.

In an attempt to make the blood supply additionally safe, in April 1999 NAT for HIV-1 was initiated on all donor blood in the United States (341). PCR for both HIV-1 and HCV have been combined and applied to minipools of plasma from 16 donated units of blood for cost efficiency (342–344); when positive by the combined assay, individual units that were part of the plasma minipool then undergo NAT for HIV-1 and HCV. It is estimated that the window period (preseroconversion) is also shortened by PCR for HIV-1 by 14 to 15 days (the window for HCV is also shortened by 26 days) (218).

As a result of the current blood donor unit testing algorithm, including the third-generation EIA, P24 antigen capture EIA, and PCR for RNA, the risk of receiving a unit of blood transmitting HIV-1 is estimated to be 0.00004% to 0.0005% (or 1 per 200,000 to 2,000,000 units transfused (9,93,127). Despite such sensitivity of the testing algorithm and very low risk, transmission of HIV-1 from an infected unit to two recipients has been reported in Singapore (345).

The rarity of HIV-1 infection in seronegative blood donors has been confirmed by the use of HIV-1 culture and the PCR to detect HIV-1 infection in donor blood (9,93,346). In addition to all blood donors being screened for HIV-1 infection, all organ, tissue, and semen donors undergo self-deferral for high risk and are screened for antibody to HIV-1 (305); transmission has occurred in this setting (347). The estimate of the prevalence of HIV-1 infection among blood donors in the United States with antibody screening alone was 7.7 to 13 per 100,000 donors (or 0.00077% to 0.013%) (348,349). The estimated risk of a transfusion recipient being given an HIV-1–positive unit of blood with antibody screening had ranged between 1 in 40,000 and 1 in 150,000 (350); however, more recent estimates place this risk much lower, as described previously (9,93,127,349). Because 40% of HIV-1–seropositive individuals also have anti-HBc, screening for this surrogate marker of HCV and for prior HBV infection has also contributed somewhat to the risk reduction for HIV-1 transmission when antibody tests alone were used as screening (134). The continued value of the anti-HBc assay in this regard has recently been questioned (351). Screening donated blood for syphilis also possibly contributed to further risk reduction for HIV-1.

As evidence for this continued risk reduction for receipt of a unit of blood capable of transmitting HIV-1, Dodd et al. (127) reported that from March 1999 through February 2002 more than 19 million units of blood were tested by NAT; five of these units were seronegative for HIV-1 but positive for HIV-1 RNA, for a rate of 1 per 3,962,000 units. These safety data reflect an estimated decrement of the window period of infectivity of donor blood for HIV-1 from 22 days with current antibody tests alone to 8 to 11 days by also incorporating NAT (9,218). This rate is very close to that projected by Schreiber et al. (8) and in keeping with the fact that the risk of receiving a HIV-1 infected unit of blood today is so low that it is more easily estimated than measured (8,127). Other transfusion risks now deserve more attention for their potential clinical benefit than further efforts at risk reduction for HIV-1.

In addition to self-deferral for those in high-risk groups and antibody screening, other attempts have been made to enhance the safety of blood for HIV-1 infection. Leukocyte filtration may reduce but not eliminate the infectivity of donor blood (352). Experimental studies of photoinactivation of HIV-1 in whole blood have been reported (306,353). Immune globulin preparations are already safe because of Cohn fractionation, and clotting factor and plasma products have been made safe by the application of heat treatment with steam vapor and solvent-detergent treatment (299,301,306). Additional chemical treatments of clotting factors have been suggested, in addition to the possible future use of monoclonal antibodies to inactivate HIV-1 (301). Synthetic production of clotting factors by genetic engineering and the use of artificial blood may also become available (see later discussion).

Human Immunodeficiency Virus Type 2

HIV-2 is a retrovirus currently endemic in West Africa. It is similar to HIV-1 and produces a similar illness; it has been reported in immigrants to the United States (354–356). Despite the low prevalence of HIV-2 infection in the United States, screening of donor blood for antibodies to HIV-2 began in June 1992 using a combined HIV-1 and HIV-2 recombinant viral protein antigen preparation as an EIA (357). The testing algorithm for HIV-2, if the combined HIV-1 and HIV-2 EIA is positive but assays for HIV-1 are negative, follows that outlined in Fig. 69.7 for HIV-1. If the serum specimen is repeatedly reactive by the combined HIV-1 and HIV-2 EIA, a WB for HIV-1 is performed; if this is negative or indeterminate, an HIV-2–specific EIA is performed, followed by an HIV-2–specific WB (357). The first two cases of HIV-2 infection among blood donors have been reported (358), but this is a rare event.

Human T-Cell Leukemia Virus Types I and II

Human T-cell leukemia virus type I (HTLV-I) is a chronic latent retrovirus infection epidemiologically linked to the islands of southwestern Japan and the Caribbean, where 20% of adults and 2% to 5% of blacks are seropositive (354–356). This virus is also endemic in the southeastern United States. HTLV-I infection is rare overall in the United States population, occurring in 9 to 80 of 100,000 blood donors (348,356,359–361). In Italy, this infection has been found serologically in 290 of every 100,000 donors; this higher rate of infection is believed to reflect frequent infection among persons using injectable drugs in Italy (362). Transmission occurs from mother to child; by sexual contact; by contaminated needles; and by transfusion of whole blood, packed cells, and platelets (354,355). Although not totally safe, blood derivatives such as coagulation factors seem to be free of transmission risk because of the intraleukocytic location of the virus (354,355). From 30% to 63% of recipients of cellular blood products, 40% of platelet recipients, and 28% of recipients of RBC units from infected donors become infected; cell-free products may pose no risk (360,363–365). Storage of units of RBCs for more than 14 days may eliminate the risk of transmission of HTLV-I and HTLV-II from an infected donor (364). Antibodies have become detectable by 3 to 6 weeks after transfusion with units seropositive for anti-HTLV-I; IgM antibodies, detected early, became undetectable within a few months. Although the risk of transmission of HTLV-I infection by transfusion had been estimated at 0.024% per unit before HTLV-I EIA screening (326,365), more recent estimates of this risk suggest that the rate may be as low as 0.00015% to 0.002% (8, 366). The combined HTLV-I and HTLV-II viral lysate and recombinant antigen EIAs have resulted in this lowered risk.

Infection with HTLV-I has been linked with the development of human T-cell leukemia, which may be either a smoldering or fulminant leukemia, associated with hypercalcemia, hepatosplenomegaly, lymphadenopathy, and skin lesions (355). Circulating lymphocytes with indented nuclei are suggestive of the disease. After a latency of up to 20 years, the risk of developing this leukemia after HTLV-I infection is estimated at 1 in 80 (355). HTLV-I infection has also been linked with tropical spastic paraparesis (367).

HTLV-II is not linked definitively with any particular disease process but has been associated with atypical hairy cell leukemia and a chronic neurodegenerative disease (354,365,368,369). Transmission of HTLV-II is epidemiologically linked with transfusion but primarily with injectable drug use in the United States (348,370–372). Murphy et al. (361) have associated HTLV-II transmission, focused on the West Coast, with injectable drug use and secondary sexual transmission; seroprevalence among blood donors from 1991 to 1995 was 0.0223% (361).

Because of the 84% homology of the p24 core antigens of HTLV-I and HTLV-II, the EIA for HTLV-I may detect infection with HTLV-II (366,371). Although the incidence of HTLV-II infection in the United States is low, in some areas HTLV-II is at least as common as HTLV-I (361,364). A specific HTLV-II screening test for donor blood is currently not performed; a combined HTLV-I and HTLV-II EIA serves this function (365,371).

Serologic methods used to document HTLV-I and HTLV-II infection include EIA, immunofluorescence, WB, and radioimmunoprecipitation assay (355,365,371). The EIA and WB are similar to those performed for HIV-1, with similar gene products. The first-generation EIAs used HTLV-I viral lysates or recombinant gene products as antigens for antibody detection (365); these assays had a high degree of cross-reactivity for HTLV-II but failed to detect 9% to 45% of HTLV-II–positive blood specimens (359,365,371). They were also prone to some false positivity for HTLV-I; however, recent surveys suggest a specificity of 98% and sensitivity of 96% to 99% for HTLV-I–infected donor units (371). There was no cross-reactivity of HTLV-I–positive specimens in the HIV-1 EIA (355); however, 70% to 78% of HIV-1 EIA positive, WB indeterminate specimens reacted in the HTLV-I EIA (355). On November 29, 1988, the FDA issued the initial directive for anti-HTLV-I testing of all blood donated for cellular products (but not for plasma). The algorithm for testing follows that for HIV-1 (Fig. 69.7).

Second-generation EIAs for HTLV-I and HTLV-II have combined the viral lysate or recombinant gene antigens with a recombinant transmembrane envelope antigen (rgp21e) that cross-reacts between HTLV-I and HTLV-II (365,373). Although this assay remains incompletely sensitive for HTLV-II, its specificity and sensitivity for HTLV-I antibodies was much improved (365). Newer third-generation EIAs for HTLV-I and HTLV-II were introduced, combining both HTLV-I and HTLV-II recombinant antigens or viral lysates; these assays are variably more sensitive than second-generation assays (365). In 1998, the combined HTLV-I and HTLV-II viral lysate or recombinant antigen EIA was instituted by blood centers (Table 69.5).

For repeatedly reactive anti-HTLV-I and HTLV-II EIA donor units, specimens are initially tested with a WB that can differentiate infection with HTLV-I or HTLV-II (365). However, the WB is indeterminate in 38% to 75% of anti-HTLV-I and anti-HTLV-II reactive donor units (365). Most of these indeterminate specimens are PCR negative, implying a high WB false positivity resulting from indeterminate reactions. A recently developed RIBA is more specific, resolving 66% of WB indeterminate reactions (365). Therefore, the RIBA may be a more sensitive and specific confirmatory assay for HTLV-I and HTLV-II than WB, because it can detect antibodies to the viral envelope glycoprotein; WB is more sensitive for antibodies to core proteins, which are the frequent cause of false positivity (362). However, other surveys report improved HTLV-I and HTLV-II WB specificity (>97%), but there are also continued problems with its sensitivity (<65%) (371).

DNA PCR has been used to confirm HTLV-I and HTLV-II infection in lymphocytes of seropositive donors. Of patients with a positive HTLV-I and HTLV-II EIA, DNA PCR confirms infection with HTLV-II in 42% to 52% (347,359). By DNA PCR, up to 15% of persons with a positive EIA may be uninfected with either virus (359).

HTLV-I or HTLV-II infection has been found in 0.014% to 0.021% of all blood donors in the United States (359). After institution of screening of all donor blood by the HTLV-I EIA, this rate dropped for HTLV-I and HTLV-II to about 0.0014% (359,366). The risk of HTLV-II is about three times higher in first-time blood donors compared with HTLV-I (10). There is considerable geographic variation in seroprevalence. Generally, higher seropositivity rates for blood donors for HTLV-II are seen on the West Coast (359,361). Rates are highest among African Americans, Hispanics, and Asians; among injectable drug users or their sexual contacts; among persons born in the Caribbean or Japan; and among persons with a history of blood transfusion. In addition to serologic screening, self-deferral of these high-risk groups (as for HIV-1) is an important adjunct to the prevention of HTLV-I and HTLV-II transmission by transfusion. The risk of transmitting HTLV-I or HTLV-II is estimated at 1 in 641,000 units (8), but may range from 1 in

250,000 to 2,000,000 units (9). In addition, the overall risk for HTLV-II infection in blood donors is declining (127).

The use of leukocyte filtration is unwarranted to prevent the rare instance of possible transmission of HTLV-I or HTLV-II from a seronegative donor (12). A lookback program has been mandated, but, because of the long latency of HTLV-I infection and the infrequency of symptomatic disease, its value is in question except for long-term epidemiology.

TT Virus and Sen Virus

TT virus (TTV) is named for the initials of the patient in whom it was initially defined in 1997; this patient had hepatitis, thereby linking TTV possibly to non-A, non-B, non-C, non-D, non-E hepatitis (374,375). TTV is a circular, single-stranded DNA virus with up to 16 genotypes, which was initially thought to be another agent of PTH (374). TTV is present in 7.5% to 10% of volunteer blood donors in the United States but has a much greater seroprevalence in less well-developed areas of the globe, varying from 14% to 86% of populations (374). TTV is epidemiologically linked to multiply transfused patients and injectable drug users but probably also has a common fecal-oral route of spread (374). Although TTV is transmitted by transfusion and found in higher titer in liver than in serum, it is not associated with hepatitis or other liver disease, despite its apparent replication there (374,376–379). Given these data, there is no reason to assess prospective donor units for the presence of TTV at this time.

SEN virus (SENV) was isolated from an injectable drug user and reported in 2000 (380). SENV is a circular, single-stranded DNA virus with eight strains (A through H) that is related to TTV and has a seroprevalence in blood donors of 1.8% to 13%. Up to 70% of multiply transfused patients are seropositive (380, 381). SENV-H is most common in the United States and up to 20% to 76% of patients with HCV are SENV seropositive (381); however, the presence of SENV does not affect the severity of HCV or the response to therapy for HCV, despite long-term persistence of SENV. Without a relationship to hepatitis or other disease, there is no reason to test donor units for SENV presently.

West Nile Virus

West Nile virus (WNV) is an Old World Flavivirus, previously endemic in Africa, Asia, the Middle East, and southern Europe (382). Since its initial recognition in 1937 in an ill woman in the West Nile region of Uganda, there have been infrequent human outbreaks; notable exceptions have been an Israeli nursing home outbreak in 1957 and outbreaks in Romania (1996), Russia (1999), and Israel (1999 and 2000) (382, 383). In late summer 1999, eight patients with encephalitis were initially recognized as a WNV outbreak in New York City; this led to the recognition of 59 patients hospitalized for WNV infection (384). In subsequent years WNV has spread via its mosquito vector and/or its migratory bird definitive hosts (crows, ravens, blue jays) to at least 44 of 48 continental United States (385). Humans and horses are dead-end hosts after the bite of an infected mosquito (382). In the United States there were 3,389 human cases during 2002 with 201 deaths. Four of every five patients are asymptomatic, and only one in 10 infected patients seek medical attention (382). One in 150 infected patients develops meningoencephalitis or a polio-like syndrome (382,386).

Because of the presence of mild illness after infection, especially in young adults (the likely blood donor population), and because of an incubation period of 3 to 14 days (382,383), the potential for transfusion transmission associated with viremia exists. During the WNV epidemic of 2002, at least 6 patients developed confirmed WNV infection via transfusions with an additional 27 suspected occurrences (387). During the epidemic in New York City in 1999, the risk that a blood donor would have WNV in the blood was estimated at 2 per 10,000 donors (388). Because of these risks, the FDA released its "Final Guidance" for assessing donor suitability and blood product safety regarding possible WNV infection in the donor on October 25, 2002 (Table 69.2) (389). Techniques for antibody detection and NAT for WNV are under rapid development. The potential for WNV transmission via transfusion in future years hopefully will be greatly decreased.

Colorado Tick Fever Virus, Parvovirus, and Vaccinia Virus

Other potential viral causes of posttransfusion infection include Colorado tick fever virus and parvovirus B19. The rarity of reports of transmission by transfusion and the usual association of illness in the potential blood donor with Colorado tick fever virus infection argue for no additional donor precautions at this time (287,390,391).

However, questions continue to be raised about the need for studies to define the risk of B19 transfusion-related infection, to improve detection techniques, and to refine inactivation techniques (392). These concerns are raised because of continued but infrequently recognized episodes of transfusion-related infection (393–396) and one reported episode of B19 transmission by intravenous immune globulin (397). Although fresh frozen plasma and albumin are safe, 10% of clotting factor concentrates are contaminated because of incomplete inactivation by dry heat, wet heat, or solvent/detergent treatments (392,398–400). Plasma pools usually have detectable B19 DNA (401). The frequency of B19 DNA is stated to be one in 20,000 to 50,000 donors (401). However, this frequency among Pittsburgh blood donors was reported to be 0.1% during June and July, the peak of the B19 season (402); 2 of 11 recipients of B19 DNA positive blood developed clinically apparent infection. However, clinically consequential B19 posttransfusion infection is uncommon (400,401). Accordingly, the FDA proposed that any screening process for plasma pools only be capable of detecting B19 in pools with less than 10^4 genome copies per milliliter (401).

Vaccinia virus is a double-stranded DNA virus, related to cowpox virus, which has been used to immunize humans against smallpox (caused by variola virus). Use of this vaccine on a routine basis had ceased in 1971 to 1972, and in 1977 the last case of smallpox was documented in Somalia (403). Because of the terrorist threat to use biologic weapons, on December 13, 2002 a presidential decision was made to initiate a smallpox vaccination campaign for individuals likely to encounter the first patients after a bioterrorist exposure. During a secondary phase additional healthcare workers, emergency personnel, policemen, and fireman on a voluntary basis were to receive the vaccine.

After percutaneous inoculation, vaccinia virus multiplies locally causing in succession a papule, vesicle, and pustule, which ruptures, crusts, and heals with scab formation. Investigations using the New York City Board of Health strain of vaccinia have documented viremia during disseminated vaccinia infection (404,405); there are reports from 1930 and 1953 of isolation of vaccinia virus from blood 3 to 10 days after vaccination (406). Accordingly, because of the potential for vaccinia viremia in a recent recipient of smallpox vaccine, the FDA has issued a "Final Guidance" in December 2002 recommending blood donor deferral for 21 days after vaccine receipt or until the scab has separated if there are no complications to vaccination; this and deferral if complications develop are summarized in Table 69.2 (406).

Prion Disease

Creutzfeldt-Jakob disease (CJD) is suspected to be transmitted by a proteinaceous infectious particle (prion). After a 4- to 25-year latency, CJD has been recognized as acquired by corneal and dura mater transplants from infected donors, through use of human pituitary-derived growth hormone, and through reuse of electroencephalographic electrodes. A group in the United Kingdom has reported the transmission of bovine spongiform encephalopathy (BSE) to sheep via transfusion of whole blood from a sheep with incubating BSE (407,408). There are no data in humans to support transfusion of blood or blood products as a mechanism for transmission of CJD. More than 100 recipients of blood from patients who later developed CJD are being followed, some for more than 27 years; none has developed CJD during follow-up (409). There is a greater concern for transmission of variant CJD by blood products (409); it is postulated that variant CJD might be transmitted more efficiently with a shorter incubation period. Surveillance and lookback studies are underway (410). Despite the inadequacy of present plasma product treatments for prion inactivation, no cases of CJD nor its variant have been detected in frequent recipients of plasma products (409).

In 1987, the FDA required permanent deferral of potential blood donors treated with human pituitary-derived growth hormone; on August 8, 1995, permanent donor deferral was also required for recipients of dura mater grafts and for donors with a family history of CJD (23). The twenty-second edition of the AABB guidelines also apply permanent deferral status to anyone at risk for variant CJD (26) (Table 69.2). Notification is also required for physicians who cared for patients who previously received blood products from such donors.

Malaria

Transfusion-related malaria is the most common transfusion-induced parasitic infection worldwide, especially in the tropics, but it is rare in the United States (411). The average annual rate has remained 0.25 cases per million units of blood collected through 1987 or about three cases per year (410,411). Mungai et al. (412) reported 93 cases of transfusion-transmitted Malaria between 1963 and 1999 in the United States; 35% were due to *Plasmodium falciparum* and 27% each were due to *Plasmodium vivax* and *Plasmodium malariae* (412). Approximately 62% of these cases could have been prevented by appropriate application of donor guidelines. Since its eradication from the United States in the 1940s, *P. malariae* had been the most common form of malaria associated with transfusion in nonendemic areas because of its persistence; however, *P. falciparum* and *P. vivax* are now becoming more important because of immigration and air travel associated with tourism (411,412). This is also the experience in Canada (413). In the last decade most infected donors were immigrants (412).

Malaria has been transmitted by transfusion of whole blood, fresh plasma, and platelets (410,411). The incubation period after transfusion is from 1 to 4 weeks. Diagnosis in the transfused patient often is delayed because of lack of a history of travel to an endemic area. Increased morbidity and occasional mortality result. Malaria has also been transmitted by renal transplantation (411). Nosocomial transmission by needlestick and a multidose vial have been described (411). The current guidelines recommended by the AABB (Table 69.2) should enhance prevention of this transfusion-related illness. The risk of transfusion of a unit of blood in the United States from a donor with malaria is estimated at one for every 3 to 4 million units (306).

Direct smear of donated blood for parasites is insensitive for detection (412). Serologic screening with indirect fluorescent antibody or indirect hemagglutination is one of the most sensitive methods available for diagnosing plasmodial infection, but its disadvantages as a screening test include cost, seronegativity during early parasitemia, and exclusion of immune donors after adequate treatment (411,414,415). Detection of circulating antigens and nucleic acids (e.g., by PCR) are very sensitive techniques that may become useful (416). A combination of antigen and antibody detection can enhance sensitivity for plasmodial infection to 88% (415). Smith et al. (417) reported a technique to prevent transfusion-related infection by photoinactivation of plasmodia in blood using a photosensitizing dye.

Babesiosis

Babesia microti is a zoonotic protozoal parasite transmitted to humans in nature by a tick bite and occasionally by transfusion (418–420). Babesiosis is second only to malaria as a reported transfusion-transmitted protozoal infection (419). The protozoan parasitizes RBCs. Most infections in endemic areas (primarily the Northeast, California, northern Midwest, and Northwest) are asymptomatic or subclinical unless in a splenectomized host, when infection may be fatal (418). Serosurveys of blood donors in the Northeast have shown seropositivity rates of 3.7% without a clinical history consistent with infection, and parasitemia occurs in 50% or more of seropositive patients (306,421). Because of the subclinical nature of acute infection, presumably with parasitemia, the possibility of transfusion-related illness is expected, especially during May through September, when the primary vector, the nymphal tick, feeds. The estimated annual incidence of transfusion-associated babesiosis is less than one case per million units transfused (419).

Transmission by packed RBCs, frozen-thawed blood, and platelets (because of free parasites in plasma) from asymptomatic donors has been well documented (410,420,422–425). The parasite may survive for up to 35 days at 4°C liquid storage (426). The incubation period in posttransfusion babesiosis is 6 to 9 weeks, which is longer than for tick-borne disease (1 to 3 weeks). The longer incubation period after transfusion is surprising, because up to 30% of RBCs may be parasitized in the infected normal host (427). Clinical disease in transfusion recipients is unusual, however (419).

Prevention of transfusion-related disease relies on recognizing acute illness in a potential blood donor, deferring individuals from highly endemic areas from donating blood during May through September, avoiding donors with fever within the 2 months before donation, and eliminating potential donors with a history of tick bite (418,419). A history of babesiosis is cause for permanent donor deferral (26) (Table 69.2). Serologic screens using indirect fluorescent antibody are not practical and are insensitive early in disease (418,419). PCR is not yet available. Inactivation techniques applied to donor blood with promising results have included gamma irradiation, combined psoralens with ultraviolet light, and photosensitization with pheophorbide (419). As deer herds increase in endemic areas, transmission by tick bite will increase, thereby enhancing the likelihood of an infected blood donor. Physicians must remain aware of babesiosis as a potential transfusion-related illness in an endemic area.

Trypanosomiasis

African trypanosomiasis (or sleeping sickness) is rarely transmitted by transfusion, because infected patients are usually symptomatic when parasitemic and thereby unsuitable blood donors; unusual asymptomatic parasitemic patients have accounted for rare transfusion-related disease (410).

In contrast, blood transfusion is the second most common means for transmission of American trypanosomiasis, or Chagas' disease, in the endemic countries of Central or South America (428). *Trypanosoma cruzi,* the etiologic agent, is usually transmitted by various species of hematophagous triatomine insects (or reduviid bugs). Both mammals and humans are infected. The signs and symptoms of acute infection are so mild that they are unnoticed by the host or at least not attributed to *T. cruzi.* Untreated, such hosts remain infected for life, and parasitemia may be detected years after infection in up to 50% of patients (306,410). Up to 20% to 40% of infected patients may develop cardiac or gastrointestinal symptoms after years or decades.

In Central and South America, 18 to 20 million people may be infected, and Chagas' disease is the most common transfusion-transmitted infection (306,428,429). Because of recent immigration to the United States from these areas (because of social unrest), especially from Mexico, it is estimated that 100,000 persons in the United States are infected with *T. cruzi* (430). The seroprevalence of *T. cruzi* in the U.S. blood donor population ranges from 0.01% to 0.2% (431). The potential for infection of the United States blood supply has been recognized, but concerns have been heightened by several reports of acute symptomatic infection in immunocompromised hosts (410, 432–434). Whole blood, packed RBCs, and platelets have a higher risk of infection than plasma; the parasite can survive storage at 4°C for 18 to 21 days and can survive freezing (426). Transmission by renal transplantation has also been documented (410). Although the likelihood of transmission by blood from an infected donor may range from 13% to 49%, most posttransfusion infections are asymptomatic in immunocompetent hosts (428,435). Those reports of more serious illness typical for compromised hosts raise concern about more widespread transfusion-related infection. Seropositivity rates in Los Angeles County have been reported to be 2.4% to 4% (436,437). A report of questionnaire results of blood donors in 18 California donor centers identified risk factors for Chagas' disease in 1 of every 340 donors (living in endemic area for more than 1 year, living in dwellings with mud walls or thatched roofs, transfusion in endemic area, or history of Chagas' disease) (437). With an up to 4% serologic positivity rate in a similar population, an infection rate of 1 in 8,500 donors can be estimated in this donor population (437). Other serosurveys demonstrated infection in populations in Texas and New Mexico (437). A Southwest Region American Red Cross serosurvey demonstrated 3 reactive units among 100,089 tested (431).

Prevention in the United States is problematic. Detection of parasitemia is unlikely during chronic infection. Serologic testing with complement fixation, indirect hemagglutination, EIA, and the direct agglutination or recombinant immunoassays, used in areas of high endemicity, is impractical in the United States because of low infection rates of blood donors and the low specificity of these tests; all require confirmation with a second, different assay (414,428,438). As suggested by the AABB, it is more practical to defer donors with a history of Chagas' disease or exposure by prior travel or residence in endemic countries (428). A transfusion history in an area endemic for Chagas' disease should also be included as a deferral criterion (437). Heightened awareness by health professionals about the potential transmission of *T. cruzi* by blood transfusion is also warranted, especially where Latin American immigrants have concentrated, such as Los Angeles, Chicago, New York City, Washington DC, Miami, and possibly Texas and New Mexico (414,426,428,431,437). If the possibility of transfusion-related Chagas' disease increases in certain cities because of immigration, serologic screening or treatment of donor blood with gentian violet or crystal violet may become indicated (428). Both inactivating dyes are used in Latin America with good results.

Toxoplasmosis

Toxoplasmosis is a common infection of mammals and humans usually acquired orally or congenitally and possibly by aerosol. The etiologic microorganism *Toxoplasma gondii* may survive at 4°C for up to 50 days (426). Transmission by a transplanted organ (heart, kidney, bone marrow) has been documented (410). Because asymptomatic prolonged parasitemia is uncommon, transmission by transfused blood is possible but has been documented only rarely (439,440). For this reason and the lack of adequately sensitive and specific assays, routine screening of blood donors is unwarranted and not feasible (306). Prevention of transmission by donor serologic screening or by use of prophylactic pyrimethamine in the transplant recipient has been described (411,414).

Leishmaniasis

Leishmania species have worldwide distribution in humans and mammals; the microorganism is transmitted by sandflies (or by *Phlebotomus* species in India). *Leishmania* microorganisms parasitize leukocytes and the organs containing tissue monocytes/macrophages; when found in blood, they are within leukocytes. Transfusion-induced infection is rare, with only a few reported cases (410,426). None has occurred in the United States (414,426). In endemic areas there is the potential for transfusion transmission. Among 21 EIA-positive asymptomatic volunteer blood donors in Rio de Janeiro, 5 were positive by NAT for DNA of *Leishmania donovani* (441).

In the United States, the immigrant or traveler with infection would most likely be deferred because of signs of acute or chronic infection. No preventive measures are usually warranted except those outlined in Table 69.2 (306). However, military operations in the Middle East during 1991 resulted in a few cases of viscerotropic *Leishmania tropica* infection among returning military personnel. For this reason, the AABB, with the military, recommended deferral of military and civilian blood donors until January 1, 1993, if they had recently been in this area. However, donors of plasma for further processing were not and need not be deferred.

Syphilis

Treponema pallidum is usually transmitted sexually or congenitally; less commonly, infection occurs by kissing, direct inoculation or, in the past, by transfusion (442,443). Infection with *T. pallidum* induces a disseminated vasculitis with spirochetemia and secondary cutaneous, cardiovascular, neurologic, and other organ system effects. Transmission via transfused blood was recognized as early as 1915 (442,443). Most infectious donors were in the primary or secondary stages of disease. However, many transfusion-related cases were probably unrecognized. Transfusion-related syphilis has not been recognized since 1966 (444). The reasons for the lack of transfusion-transmitted syphilis include (1) serologic screening of all donor blood, (2) the low incidence of syphilis in blood donors, (3) an all volunteer blood donor pool, (4) deferral of high-risk individuals, (5) the impact of refrigeration on spirochete survival, and (6) the frequent administration of antibiotics to transfusion recipients (445).

Although *T. pallidum* can survive in stored blood at 4°C for up to 4 days, its survival at clinically relevant concentrations may be only 2 days. During storage of blood at 4°C that was highly contaminated experimentally with *T. Pallidum,* blood remained infectious for up to 5 days (446). Platelets, which are stored at 22°C, may also transmit syphilis (446).

Today, donated blood is routinely screened for syphilis in the United States, usually with the Venereal Disease Research Laboratory (VDRL) assay, rapid plasma reagin, or, most recently, the automated microhemagglutination-*T. pallidum*; the VDRL and rapid plasma reagin are nontreponemal tests that have lower sensitivity and specificity than treponemal tests (442, 445). It is argued that donor blood should continued to be screened for syphilis for multiple reasons: (1) the incidence of syphilis is increasing; (2) there is an increasing demand for fresh blood components, obviating the inactivation of *T. pallidum* with storage for 72 hours at 4°C; (3) screening identifies donors at high risk for other sexually transmissible diseases (e.g., HIV-1 infection) (447); (4) the cost of screening is low; (5) screening remains legally required by the FDA, despite a decision by the AABB in 1985 to drop its requirement for syphilis screening; and (6) screening identifies patients in need of therapy (442, 445,448). Other preventive measures for deferring donors who might be infected with *T. pallidum* are defined in Table 69.2.

Despite these arguments for continued screening, a strong case has been defined by Schmidt (443) to discontinue such screenings. A recent publication adds support to this opinion; Orton et al. (449) reported that between 1998 and 1999, among 169 sera that were FTA-ABS positive, none was positive for *T. pallidum* DNA and/or RNA. Therefore, even among units of blood screened as seropositive for *T. pallidum,* none is likely to be infectious. Policy evolution in this regard awaits further study, as outlined by Orton (445), given the desire for a zero-risk blood supply.

Lyme Disease

Lyme disease is a tick-borne borreliosis caused by *Borrelia burgdorferi.* Like syphilis, Lyme disease results from vasculitis with associated spirochetemia. Its serologic diagnosis has become more reliable but remains somewhat cumbersome serologically to differentiate active versus treated disease (450). Although knowledge of the pathogenesis of Lyme disease supports the potential of transmission by transfusion, no case has yet been reported (418,451). The microorganism has been shown to survive in stored blood experimentally for up to 60 days at 4°C, in fresh frozen plasma at less than 18°C for 45 days, and in platelet concentrates for 6 days at 20° to 24°C (451–453). At this time, serologic screening of donor blood is not needed nor are additional historical questions for the donor (306). Noteworthy is a report documenting the lack of seroconversion among nine recipients of antibody-positive donor blood (454). In addition, Perdrizet et. al. (424) have reported a renal transplant patient who acquired babesiosis from a unit of blood donated by a patient who also developed Lyme disease 2 days after blood donation; the transfusion recipient remained free of Lyme disease (424).

Relapsing Fever

Relapsing fever is another form of borreliosis transmitted by a louse or tick; the former serves as a vector from human to human, whereas the latter serves as a vector from the mammalian reservoir to humans. *Borrelia recurrentis* and the *Borrelia* species of the tick-borne form of the disease can apparently survive in citrated blood, because there are rare case reports of infection by transfusion (455,456). These are unusual events, and no donor-related preventive screening is appropriate at this time.

Bacterial Infections

Transfusion reactions resulting from bacterial contamination are usually due to one of two sources: contamination during collection and processing or a bacteremia undetected in the donor at the time of collection (9,306,457–462). It is difficult to distinguish these two potential mechanisms in a given circumstance. However, most contaminants of units of RBCs have been gram-negative microorganisms with low pathogenicity, including *Serratia* and *Pseudomonas* species, suggesting processing contamination. The relatively few gram-positive isolates are most likely skin flora that contaminated the blood at the time of collection. One recent epidemic of *Serratia marcescens* bacteremia was traced to contamination of blood collection bags during manufacture (463). A recommendation was made for production of blood packs with sterile exterior surfaces.

One report documented that during such events, adverse reactions developed in 38 of 76 patients during transfusion, including fever (80%), chills (53%), hypotension (37%), and nausea with vomiting (26%) (457). There was a 35% mortality rate overall. In the remainder of the patients, reactions developed from 15 minutes to 17 days after the transfusion (457,458).

A subset of the gram-negative rods contaminating transfused RBCs or blood products in reviews (457–462) and other reports (464–472) most likely reflected disease in the donor. The report of two thalassemic patients with transfusion-acquired brucellosis and a more recent report reflect the potential for chronic asymptomatic *Brucella* species bacteremia with acquisition by transfusion (464,472).

Most striking, however, are reports of *Yersinia enterocolitica* acquired via transfused RBCs (458,460,461,465–471). *Yersinia* species account for up to 80% of episodes of sepsis syndromes secondary to transfusions with RBCs from a donor infected with a bacterium (460). Up to 60% of donor recipients may die with this syndrome (460,461). This scenario reflects the recognized potential for this microorganism to persist in the intestinal mucosa and lymphoid tissue after acute illness resolves, from whence it may stimulate the immune system and create reactive immunologic sequelae and occult bacteremia (473). Furthermore, storage conditions for RBCs are almost ideal for supporting growth (460). This microorganism can grow at 4°C in blood and survives intracellularly in leukocytes; in addition, during storage, some hemolysis occurs, releasing hemoglobulin and iron; the latter is a growth factor for the microorganism. After an initial drop in bacterial counts following blood collection (obviating any value to culture at the time of collection), bacterial counts surge within leukocytes during storage (470). This has prompted recommendations for decreased storage times from 42 to 25 days, among others (461,470). This microorganism also becomes resistant to complement-mediated lysis at temperatures below 20°C, especially when plasma has been removed (474). Prestorage leukodepletion of RBC units after initial storage at 20°C for 3 to 8 hours does reduce but not totally eliminate the risk of transfusion of *Yersinia* (and coagulase-negative staphylococci) contaminated units of blood (461,475,476).

Bartonella bacilliformis, a gram-negative bacillus, is an intraerythrocytic parasite endemic to the highlands of the western Andes in Peru, Ecuador, and Colombia, where it is transmitted by sandflies. Bacteremia is detected in 5% of apparently healthy persons in these areas. Transfusion-related infection might occur if a carrier immigrated to the United States (426).

Platelet units, especially random donor pools compared with single-donor apheresis products, are a particular problem with regard to potential bacterial contamination, because they are stored at room temperature for up to 5 days before use (23, 459,462,477). The incidence of a serious transfusion-associated sepsis episode is 1 in 50,000 for platelets, tenfold higher than for RBCs (462). Among transfusion-related fatalities reported to the FDA between 1986 and 1991, platelet transfusions accounted for 21 of 29 bacterially mediated deaths (23). The eight remaining deaths were due to transfused RBC units. It is estimated that up to 10% of platelet pools used for transfusion are contaminated with bacteria (478), but bacterial contamination has been documented by culture in 0.06% to 0.28% of pooled platelet concentrate transfusions and in 0.005% to 0.03% of single-donor apheresis platelet transfusions (23). Most contaminants are skin flora such as *Bacillus* species and coagulase-negative staphylococci, but gram-negative microorganisms may also play a role (458,459,479,480). The use of pH and glucose measurements on stored platelet concentrates to detect bacterial contamination immediately before transfusion have been variably successful (481,482). Automated microbiologic culturing of platelet concentrates is a promising technique for reduction of the risk with random donor pools (483,484). Blajchman and Goldman (462) have discussed these and other prevention techniques.

Given the potential problem of bacterial contamination of blood and blood products with its associated morbidity and mortality, suggested revisions for handling of donor blood have been made. Platelet storage time is limited to 5 days. Efforts for the prevention of contamination during collection and processing need reemphasis (457–459,462). Physicians should be aware of the potential for bacterial contamination of transfused products and, therefore, culture the unit being transfused and the recipient's blood when such a reaction is suspected (457–459). Staining the residual blood in the bag might give a more immediate answer as to the cause. The CDC has suggested testing RBCs stored for 25 days or more for bacteria or endotoxin before administration (468). This could be accomplished with microscopy using various stains, with culture, with nucleic acid hybridization or PCR, and with a limulus lysate assay for endotoxin (459–462). None of these tests is really practical nor sufficiently sensitive. Such reactions to bacterial contaminants in transfused products are probably more common than reporting would reflect (457,462). Regarding the use of platelet transfusions in thrombocytopenic patients, recent data suggest that the reduced platelet threshold should be lowered to 10,000/mm^3 before transfusion (485–488). A reduction of the number of platelet-related episodes of sepsis and mortality may thereby be achieved.

Parasitic Infestations

Several tissue nematodes pose a remote potential transfusion hazard because of chronic asymptomatic microfilaremia; these include the microfilariae *Brugia malayi, Loa loa, Wuchereria bancrofti, Mansonella ozzardi,* and *M. perstans* (411,414,426). Transfused microfilaria are unable to complete their life cycle after intravenous inoculation; they are cleared rapidly in the recipient or may persist in the circulation for up to 2 years, usually without associated symptoms or only a mild febrile reaction (414). The unlikelihood of such contamination of donor blood in the United States and the good outcome argue against a need to screen donors or donated blood (414).

Rickettsioses

The rickettsia produce illness after insect vector inoculation (except for *Coxiella burnetii*) by producing a vasculitis. With microorganism replication in endothelial cells and the organs with tissue monocyte/macrophages, rickettsemia occurs during the incubation period and during acute illness. There are two remote reports of rickettsioses being transmitted by blood taken from donors during the incubation period of their illness; one was associated with Q fever in the recipient (489) and the other was associated with Rocky Mountain spotted fever (490). *Ehrlichia chaffeensis* has survived experimental inoculation into refrigerated, stored RBCs for 11 days (418). *Ehrlichia phagocytophilia* has been transmitted by blood transfusion in sheep and isolated from refrigerated stored blood from naturally infected patients for up to 2 weeks (418). Eastlund et al. (491) reported a case of human granulocytic ehrlichiosis in a 75-year-old man after RBC transfusion. None of these rare occurrences with rickettsia warrants donor screening other than that outlined in Table 69.2 (418).

OTHER MECHANISMS FOR REDUCING TRANSFUSION RISKS

Additional attempts to reduce the risk of infection after transfusion have proceeded along several avenues other than serologic screening; these include physical or chemical treatment of blood or blood products for sterilization, the use of directed and autologous (instead of allogeneic) blood transfusion, and the development of blood substitutes.

Factor VIII and IX concentrates are produced as lyophilized products after Cohn ethanol fractionation of plasma pools. These products unfortunately contained infectious hepatitis viruses and HIV-1 before 1984 when dry heat treatment of the lyophilized powder at 60°C for 24 hours was begun. However, although HIV-1 was inactivated, HBV and HCV remained viable. Subsequently adopted procedures, such as pressurized steam treatment of wetted lyophilized concentrates, pasteurization (liquid factor VIII and IX are heated at 60°C for 10 hours), and purification of these factors with monoclonal antibody affinity columns have succeeded in rendering these products safe (1,492, 493). The shortcoming of these procedures is reduction of factor yield. Therefore, more promising methods using virucidal solvents or detergents are now used; also, further purified factor concentrates (by anionic exchange chromatography) to reduce alloantigen contaminants that might stimulate the immune system in an HIV-1–infected patient (thereby augmenting viral replication) are used (306,494). Virus inactivation in fresh-frozen plasma has been accomplished by treatment with methylene blue, solvents and detergents, radiation, and heating (493,495, 496).

Plasma protein fractions and albumin are also products of Cohn ethanol fractionation of plasma pools. After separation from plasma, they are subjected to pasteurization at 60°C for 10 hours; all infectious viral particles are inactivated along with clotting factors (1).

In addition to photoinactivation of malaria parasites in blood as a physicochemical means of rendering blood noninfectious (see previous discussion), several authors have reported chemical inactivation of HIV-1 in whole blood and plasma with aluminum phthalocyanine derivatives that left erythrocytes intact (353,497,498). Such chemical sterilization of blood may offer hope for an even safer blood supply in the future. A variety of other photochemical inactivation procedures for virus and bacterial pathogens, including psoralens (S-59), have been recently investigated for cellular blood products (306,499–501).

During the last decade, there has been a decline in the collection of homologous volunteer donor blood (9,502). Fortunately, this has not compromised the national blood supply, because it was offset by autologous donations and a decline in the use of transfused blood and blood products (9). All of these occurrences relate to the concern about transfusion-associated HIV-1 infection. After the definition of HIV-1 epidemiology, there was initial interest in the use of directed donations by friends, family, or another selected person for an individual recipient (503). The disadvantages of such a policy were emphasized by many advisory bodies. These problems included the following: (1) a valid medical history is more uncertain when obtained from a solicited donor known to the recipient than from a volunteer donor; (2) the anonymity of the donor is not preserved, leading to potential legal liability; (3) such nonvoluntary donors have a higher risk of transmitting PTH (503,504); (4) such directed donors create an apparent double standard of transfusion medicine that may be, ironically, less safe; and (5) there are logistic problems with such a program (503). Fortunately, such programs have been phased out after a patient education program (505).

Autologous blood donation (ABD) is perhaps the safest form of transfusion therapy, because it avoids isoimmunization and eliminates the risk of transmission of infectious agents except for contaminating bacteria (506–508). Autologous transfusion can be one of four types: (1) remote preoperative storage; (2) immediate preoperative phlebotomy with acute normovolemic hemodilution; (3) intraoperative recovery; and (4) postoperative recovery (from drainage tubes and reinfusion). Remote preoperative donation and storage is the most commonly practiced type (507–510). By 1992, 8.3% of all blood donated was for this purpose (507). Up to 70% of patients can have their total transfusion needs satisfied by this technique (510). However, although decreasing exposure to allogeneic blood, preoperative autologous donation may lead to increased transfusion of such donors (511). Unfortunately, up to half of autologous units are discarded; they are not used for allogeneic transfusion and the practice is, therefore, wasteful (507,508). Unexpectedly, the safety of autologous donor units is less (12 times the rate of reactions to allogeneic units) and their use has declined since the early 1990s (9,507,508).

Immediate preoperative phlebotomy is a similar second option (9,507,508). Potential problems related to such a practice are multiple. The safety of immediate preoperative autologous donations with normovolemic hemodilution has been raised, because patients are generally older with cardiovascular disease (510). Curiously, severe donor reactions have been infrequent and use of allogeneic units is reduced with this practice (507, 508).

Overall, the need and extent of serologic testing for autologous donor units has been questioned; it seems prudent not to exempt such donor units and to discard them if they are found to be infected to protect healthcare workers and a potential accidental recipient other than the donor (510). The potential autologous donor can be prohibited if the presence of an infectious agent precludes making donor units safe for handling. There are other logistical problems with such a program, and a residual risk of transfusion reactions exists (hemolysis, sepsis from bacterial contaminants, and pulmonary edema) (507).

Two other forms of autologous transfusions, intraoperative and postoperative salvage of blood followed by autologous transfusion, have become safer because of methodologic improvements (507,508,512). Concerns remain about such transfusions in patients with infection (506,507,513); the presence of malignancy is generally a contraindication to autologous transfusion after intraoperative salvage (506,507). Bacterial contamination, metabolic complications, and air embolism after use of perioperatively salvaged blood are recognized risks (508,512). The success of perioperative prophylactic antibiotics has been reported recently (514). There is also a question as to whether or not perioperative RBC salvage actually reduces allogeneic transfusion requirements (507).

More recent concerns about ABD relate to its cost effectiveness (515–520). Table 69.7 defines the approximate costs to blood donation centers for marketing a unit of homologous RBCs; total costs approximate $195 per unit but costs may vary by region. Blood donation centers at times sell units of RBCs for less than their cost by offsetting expenses through profits on other blood products. In contrast, a unit after ABD costs approximately 50% more because of the labor-intensive donation process and costs of processing and storage (520). In addition, 9% to 10% of ABD units are used, because they are available only for elective procedures. Few centers allow crossover of ABD units to the homologous donor pool of blood for safety reasons (507,516); therefore, most if not all ABD units are discarded. Despite low rates of use, there are associated higher transfusion rates than for allogeneic blood for the population served (criteria are not as stringently applied by surgeons) and thereby costs of administration accrue (511). ABD has been judged not to be cost effective for total hip and knee replacement (516) and for coronary artery bypass surgery and transurethral prostate resection (517,519). These findings have probably contributed to the reported decline of ABD (9). Despite large cost disadvantages, some knowledgeable physicians still present an argument for continuing ABD because of the fewer noninfectious complications and the recipient's peace of mind (521); however, Medicare and some private insurers will not cover ABD (507,521, 522).

TABLE 69.7. ESTIMATED COST PER UNIT OF DONOR BLOOD OBTAINED AT BLOOD DONATION CENTERS, 2003

Item	Amount ($)	Percent of cost
Donor recruitment	10	5
Collection personnel[a]	50	26
Product management[b]	6	3
Product processing[c]	4	2
Product testing[d]	40	20
Overhead	85	44
Total	195	100

[a]RN, LPN, phlebotomist.
[b]Distribution costs.
[c]Centrifugation, etc.
[d]Venereal Disease Research Laboratory (VDRL) assay; hepatitis B surface antigen (HBsAg); antibody for hepatitis B core antigen (anti-HBc); and antibodies for hepatitis C virus (HCV), human immunodeficiency virus types 1 and 2 (HIV 1/2), and human T-cell leukemia virus types I and II (HTLV-I/II); nucleic acid testing (NAT) for HIV-I and HCV.

The development of safe and effective blood substitutes has been disappointing despite the reduction of infection risk (507). Perfluorocarbons have been ineffective for oxygen delivery and are toxic to leukocytes (1,507,508). RBC stroma-free hemoglobin solutions are used only in emergency situations because of their short half-life after transfusion (1,523). Hemoglobin encapsulated in liposomes has a longer half-life, but there is concern about compromise of the organs with tissue monocytes/macrophages where it is cleared (1). Preoperative use of recombinant erythropoietin has resulted in reduced need for allogeneic transfusions (508).

Approximately 12 million units of blood are transfused annually in the United States at an average cost of $219 (or more) to the patient (502,520). Of this cost, approximately 37% is attributed to acquisition charges from blood donation centers, 13% to handling by the hospital blood bank, 43% to laboratory tests for crossmatching, and 7% to blood administration charges (520). In addition to these costs, about 2 to 3 of 10,000 recipients (2 per 100,000 units transfused) suffer a serious or fatal infectious complication of transfusion, perhaps necessitating a more prolonged hospitalization or additional laboratory charges (9,524). Because much of the present cost of a unit of transfused blood is related to screening for transmissible diseases (up to 20% of blood donation center charges) (Table 69.7), any further reduction of infection risk is least expensively accomplished through prudent use of transfusions according to suggested guidelines (9,59,508). Furthermore, it is estimated that 13% to 50% of transfusions are unneeded (59). Some recent studies have documented the lack of benefit of overzealous transfusion thresholds. In intensive care patients, the use of a threshold of less than 7.0 g of hemoglobin was associated with a lower 30-day mortality compared with a 10-g threshold (525). The exception to this policy appears to be patients older than 55 years and those with cardiac disease (526,527). However, in the patient group with cardiac disease undergoing interventions, unnecessary transfusions have led to additional costs and potential morbidity (525). The case for a moderate position has been summarized by Valeri et al. (528).

A review of the management of a severely anemic patient

who refused transfusion (a Jehovah's Witness) provides perspective for the management of many patients (529). At this time, there is no functional substitute for blood when it is required. Clinicians must continue to strive to make a very low infection risk product even safer while practicing cost-effective medicine by reducing reliance on overused blood products. Furthermore, given the results of the SHOT initiative indicating that most transfusion-related morbidity and mortality in Great Britain today is related to noninfectious complications of transfusion, one should give considerable attention in the United States to quality improvement initiatives to improve further the safety of blood products (530).

REFERENCES

1. Boral LI, Henry JB. Transfusion medicine. In: Henry JB, ed. *Clinical diagnosis and management by laboratory methods,/i> 18th ed. Philadelphia: WB Saunders, 1991:930–975.*
2. Sazama K. Reports of 355 transfusion-associated deaths: 1976 through 1985. *Transfusion* 1990;30:583–590.
3. Linden JV, Tourault MA. Decrease in frequency of transfusion fatalities. *Transfusion* 1997;37:243–244.
4. Schmidt PJ. Introducing new tests before transfusion. Who shall decide? *Arch Pathol Lab Med* 1994;118:454–456.
5. Hanson M. Blood donor screening—factors influencing decision making. *Arch Pathol Lab Med* 1994;118:457–461.
6. Dodd RY. The Risk of transfusion-transmitted infection. *N Engl J Med* 1992;327:419–421.
7. Sloand EM, Pitt E, Klein HG. Safety of the blood supply. *JAMA* 1995;274:1368–1373.
8. Schreiber GB, Busch MP, Kleinman SH, et al. The risk of transfusion-transmitted viral infections. *N Engl J Med* 1996;334:1685–1690.
9. Goodnough LT, Brecher ME, Kanter MH, et al. Transfusion medicine (first of two parts). *N Engl J Med* 1999;340:438–447.
10. Glynn SA, Kleinman SH, Schrieber GB, et al. Trends in incidence and prevalence of major transfusion-transmissible viral infections in US blood donors, 1991–1996. *JAMA* 2000;284:229–235.
11. Silliman CC, Paterson AJ, Dickey WO, et al. The association of biologically active lipids with the development if transfusion-related acute lung injury: a retrospective study. *Transfusion* 1997;37:719–726.
12. Lane TA. Leukocyte reduction of cellular blood components—effectiveness, benefits, quality control, and costs. *Arch Pathol Lab Med* 1994;118:392–404.
13. Heddle NM, Klama L, Singer J, et al. The role of the plasma from platelet concentrations in transfusion reactions. *N Engl J Med* 1994;331:625–628.
14. Brand A. Passenger leukocytes, cytokines, and transfusion reactions. *N Engl J Med* 1994;331:670–671.
15. Landsteiner K. Zur Kenntnis der antifermentativen, lytisichen and agglutinierenden Wirkungen des Blutserums in der Lymphe. *Zentrbl Bakteriol Mikrobiol Hyg [A]* 1900;27:357–360.
16. Oberman HA. The evolution of blood transfusion. *Univ Mich Med Center J* 1967;33:68–74.
17. Tabor E. *Infectious complications of blood transfusion.* New York: Academic Press, 1982.
18. Beeson PB. Jaundice occurring one to four months after transfusion of blood or plasma. *JAMA* 1943;121:1332–1334.
19. Kendrick DB. Blood program in World War II. Washington, DC: Office of the Surgeon General, Department of the Army, 1964: 674–675, 778–780.
20. Conrad ME. Disease transmissible by blood transfusion: viral hepatitis and other infectious disorders. *Semin Hematol* 1981;18:122–146.
21. Bayer WL, Tegtmeier GE, Barbara JAJ. The significance of non-A, non-B hepatitis, cytomegalovirus and the acquired immune deficiency syndrome in transfusion practice. *Clin Hematol* 1984;13:253–269.
22. Bove JR. Transfusion-transmitted diseases other than AIDS and hepatitis. *Yale J Biol Med* 1990;63:347–351.
23. Menitove JE. Transfusion-transmitted infections: update. *Semin Hematol* 1996;33:290–301.
24. Dodd, RY. Epidemiology of transfusion-transmitted diseases. In: Anderson KC and Ness PM, eds. *Scientific basis of transfusion medicine: implications for clinical practice,* 2nd ed. Philadelphia: WB Saunders, 2000:455–471.
25. Curran JW, Lawrence DN, Jaffe H, et al. Acquired immune deficiency syndrome (AIDS) associated with transfusions. *N Engl J Med* 1984;310:69–75.
26. American Association of Blood Banks. *Proposed standards for blood banks and transfusion services* 22nd ed. Bethesda, MD: American Association of Blood Banks, 2003.
27. Tartter PI. Blood transfusion and postoperative infections. *Transfusion* 1989;29:456–459.
28. Triulzi DJ, Blumberg N, Heal JM. Association of transfusion with postoperative bacterial infection. *Crit Rev Clin Lab Sci* 1990;28:95–107.
29. Waymack JP. Sequelae of blood transfusions. *Infect Med* 1991;8:7–15.
30. Blumberg N. Allogenic transfusion and infection: economic and clinical implications. *Semin Hematol* 1997;34:34–40.
31. Blumberg N, Heal JM. The transfusion immunomodulation theory: the Th1/Th2 paradigm and an analogy with pregnancy as a unifying mechanism. *Semin Hematol* 1996;33:329–340.
32. Blajchman MA. Immunomodulatory effects of allogeneic blood transfusions: clinical manifestations and mechanisms. *Vox Sanguinis* 1998;74(Suppl 2):315–319.
33. Vamvakas EC, Blajchman MA. Deleterious clinical effects of transfusion-associated immunomodulation: fact or fiction? *Blood* 2001;97:1180–1195.
34. Tartter PI. Blood transfusion and infectious complications after colorectal cancer surgery. *Br J Surg* 1988;75:789–792.
35. Jensen LS, Kissmeyer-Nielson P, Wolff B, et al. Randomised comparison of leucocyte-depleted versus buffy-coat-poor blood transfusion and complications after colorectal surgery. *Lancet* 1996;348:841–845.
36. Dellinger EP, Oreskovich MR, Wertz MJ, et al. Risk of infection after laparotomy for penetrating abdominal injury. *Arch Surg* 1984;119:20–27.
37. Nichols RL, Smith JW, Klein DB, et al. Risk of infection after penetrating abdominal trauma. *N Engl J Med* 1984;311:1065–1070.
38. Dawes LG, Aprahamian C, Condon RE, et al. Risk of infection after colon injury. *Surgery* 1986;100:796–803.
39. Claridge JA, Sawyer RG, Schulman AM, et al. Blood transfusions correlate with infections in trauma patients in a dose-dependent manner. *Am Surg* 2002;68:566–572.
40. Tartter PI, Driefuss RM, Malon AM, et al. Relationship of postoperative septic complications and blood transfusions in patients with Crohn's disease. *Am J Surg* 1988;155:43–48.
41. Christou NV, Meakins JL, Gotto D, et al. Influence of GI bleeding on host defense and susceptibility to infection. *Surg Forum* 1979;30:46–47.
42. Dellinger EP, Miller SD, Wertz MJ, et al. Risk of infection after open fracture of the arm or leg. Presented at the International Symposium on the Biology of Transfusion Induced Immunosuppression, Snowbird, UT, January, 1988.
43. Miholic J, Hudec M, Domanig E, et al. Risk factors for severe bacterial infections after valve replacement and aortocoronary bypass operations: analysis of 246 cases by logistic regression. *Ann Thorac Surg* 1985;40:224–228.
44. Ottino G, DePaulis R, Pansini S, et al. Major sternal wound infection after open-heart surgery: a multivariate analysis of risk factors in 2,579 consecutive operative procedures. *Ann Thorac Surg* 1987;44:173–179.
45. Taylor RW, Manganaro LM, O'Brien JO, et al. Impact of allogenic packed red blood cell transfusion on nosocomial infection rates in the critically ill patient. *Crit Care Med* 2002;30:2249–2254.
46. Graves TA, Cioffi WG, Mason AD Jr, et al. Relationship of transfusion and infection in a burn population. *J Trauma* 1989;29:948–954.

47. Waymack JP, Robb E, Alexander JW. Effect of transfusion of immune function in a traumatized animal model. *Arch Surg* 1987;122: 935–939.
48. Waymack JP, Warden GD, Miskell P, et al. Effect of varying number and volume of transfusions on mortality rate after septic challenge in an animal model. II. Effect on mortality rate after septic challenge. *World J Surg* 1987;11:387–391.
49. Sauaia A, Alexander W, Moore EE. Autologous blood transfusion does not reduce postoperative infection rates in elective surgery. *Am J Surg* 1999;178:549–555.
50. Vamvakas EC, Carven JH. Length of storage of transfused red cells and postoperative morbidity in patients undergoing coronary artery bypass graft surgery. *Transfusion* 2000;40:101–109.
51. Waymack JP, Alexander JW. Blood transfusion as an immunomodulator: a review. *Comp Immunol Microbiol Infect Dis* 1986;9:177–183.
52. Waymack JP, Gallon L, Barcelli U, et al. Effect of blood transfusions on immune function. III. Alterations in macrophage arachidonic acid metabolism. *Arch Surg* 1987;122:56–60.
53. Waymack JP, Balakrishnan K, McNeal N, et al. Effect of blood transfusions on macrophage-lymphocyte interaction in an animal model. *Ann Surg* 1986;204:681–685.
54. Stephan RN, Kisala JM, Dean RE, et al. Effect of blood transfusion on antigen presentation and on interleukin-2 generation. *Arch Surg* 1988;123:235–240.
55. Lenhard V, Maassen G, Grossewild H, et al. Effect of blood transfusions on immunoregulatory mononuclear cells in prospective transplant recipients. *Transplant Proc* 1983;15:1011–1015.
56. Lenhard V, Gesma D, Opelz G. Transfusion-induced release of prostaglandin E and its role in the activation of T-suppressor cells. *Transplant Proc* 1985;17:2380–2382.
57. Houbiers JG, van de Velde CJ, van de Watering LM, et al. Transfusion of red cells is associated with increased incidence of bacterial infection after colorectal surgery: a prospective study. *Transfusion* 1997;37:126–134.
58. Kowalyshyn TJ, Prager D, Young J. A review of the present status of preoperative hemoglobin requirements. *Anesth Analg* 1972;51:75–79.
59. Welch HG, Meehan KR, Goodnough LT. Prudent strategies for elective red blood cell transfusion. *Ann Intern Med* 1992;116:393–402.
60. Horstman BH, Gleser M, Wolfe D, et al. Effects of hemoglobin reduction on VO2 max and related hemodynamics in exercising dogs. *J Appl Physiol* 1974;37:97–102.
61. Albert ED, Scholz S, Meixner U, et al. B-matching of pretransplant blood transfusion is associated with poor graft survival. *Transplant Proc* 1981;13:175–177.
62. DeVenuto F, Friedman HI, Neville JR, et al. Appraisal of hemoglobin solution as a blood substitute. *Surg Gynecol Obstet* 1979;149: 417–436.
63. Palani CK, De Woskin R, Moss GS. Scope and limitations of stroma free hemoglobin solution as an oxygen-carrying blood substitute. *Surg Clin North Am* 1975;55:3–10.
64. DeVenuto F, Zegna A. Preparation and evaluation of pyridoxalated-polymerized human hemoglobin. *J Surg Res* 1983;34:205–212.
65. Hunt CA, Burnette RR, MacGregor RD, et al. Synthesis and evaluation of a prototypal artificial red cell. *Science* 1985;230:1165–1168.
66. Lane TA, Anderson KC, Goodnough LT, et al. Leukocyte reduction in blood component therapy. *Ann Intern Med* 1992;117:151–162.
67. van de Watering LMG, Hermans J, Houbiers JGA, et al. Beneficial effects of leukocyte depletion of transfused blood on postoperative complications in patients undergoing cardiac surgery. A randomized clinical trial. *Circulation* 1998;97:562–568.
68. Tarter PI, Mohandas K, Azar P, et al. Randomized trial comparing packed red cell blood transfusion with and without leukocyte depletion for gastrointestinal surgery. *Am J Surg* 1998;176:462–466.
69. Fransen E, Maessen J, Dentener M, et al. Impact of blood transfusion on inflammatory mediator release in patients undergoing cardiac surgery. *Chest* 1999;116:1233–1239.
70. Rios JA, Korones DN, Heal JM, et al. WBC-reduced blood transfusions and clinical outcome in children with acute lymphoid leukemia. *Transfusion* 2001;41:873–877.
71. Thurer RL, Luban NLC, AuBuchon JP, et al. Universal WBC reduction. *Transfusion* 2000;40:751–752.
72. Anderson KC, Weinstein HJ. Transfusion associated graft-versus-host disease. *N Engl J Med* 1990;323:315–321.
73. Capon SM, Depond WD, Tyan DB, et al. Transfusion associated graft-versus-host disease in an immunocompetent patient. *Ann Intern Med* 1991;114:1025–1026.
74. Lurman. Eine icterusepidemie. *Berlin Klin Wschr* 1885;22:20–27.
75. Findlay GM, MacCallum FO. Hepatitis and jaundice associated with immunization against certain virus diseases. *Proc R Soc Med* 1938; 31:799–805.
76. Minutes, Meeting of Subcommittee of Blood Substitutes, Division of Medical Sciences, National Research Council, May 12, 1942, October 20, 1942, and February 24, 1943.
77. MacCallum FO. Scientific discussion (infective hepatitis). *Lancet* 1947;2:435–436.
78. Blumberg BS, Alter HJ, Visnich S. A new antigen in leukemia sera. *JAMA* 1965;191:541–546.
79. Blumberg BS, Gerstley BJS, Hungerford DA, et al. A serum antigen (Australia antigen) in Down's syndrome, leukemia, and hepatitis. *Ann Intern Med* 1967;66:924–931.
80. Ginsberg AL, Conrad ME, Bancroft WH, et al. Prevention of epidemic HAA-positive hepatitis with gamma globulin: use of a simple radioimmune assay to detect HAA. *N Engl J Med* 1972;286:562–566.
81. Feinstone SM, Kapikian AZ, Purcell RH, et al. Transfusion-associated hepatitis not due to viral hepatitis type A or B. *N Engl J Med* 1975; 292:767–770.
82. Knodell RG, Conrad ME, Deinstag JL, et al. Etiological spectrum of post-transfusion hepatitis. *Gastroenterology* 1975;69:1278–1285.
83. Krugman S, Ward R, Giles JP. The natural history of infectious hepatitis. *Am J Med* 1962;32:717–728.
84. Krugman S, Giles JP, Hammond J. Infectious hepatitis: evidence for two distinctive clinical, epidemiological, and immunological types. *JAMA* 1967;200:365–373.
85. Krugman S, Giles JP. Viral hepatitis: new light on an old disease. *JAMA* 1970;212:1019–1029.
86. Feinstone SM, Kapikian AZ, Purcell RH. Hepatitis A: detection by immune election microscopy of a viruslike antigen associated with acute illness. *Science* 1973;182:1026–1028.
87. Bradley DW, Fields HA, McCaustland KA, et al. Serodiagnosis of viral hepatitis A by a modified competitive binding radioimmunoassay for immunoglobulin M anti-hepatitis A virus. *J Clin Microbiol* 1979; 9:120–127.
88. Locarnini SA, Coulepis AG, Stratton AM, et al. A solid-phase enzyme-linked immunosorbent assay for detection of hepatitis A specific immunoglobulin M. *J Clin Microbiol* 1979;9:459–465.
89. Flehmig B, Ranke M, Berthold H, et al. A solid-phase radioimmunoassay for detection of IgM antibodies to hepatitis A virus. *J Infect Dis* 1979;140:169–175.
90. Stafford SES, Needleman SB, Decker RH. Radioimmunoassay for detection of antibody to hepatitis A virus. *J Clin Pathol* 1980;74: 25–31.
91. Kao HW, Ashcavai M, Redeker AG. The persistence of hepatitis A IgM antibody after acute clinical hepatitis A. *Hepatology* 1984;4: 933–936.
92. Hollinger FB, Khan NC, Oefinger PE, et al. Posttransfusion hepatitis type A. *JAMA* 1983;250:2313–2317.
93. Centers for Disease Control and Prevention. Blood safety monitoring among persons with bleeding disorders—United States, May 1998–June 2002. *MMWR Morb Mortal Wkly Rep* 2003:51; 1152–1154.
94. Goodman RA. Nosocomial hepatitis A. *Ann Intern Med* 1985;103: 452–454.
95. Noble RC, Kane MA, Reeves SA, et al. Posttransfusion hepatitis A in a neonatal intensive care unit. *JAMA* 1984;252:2711–2715.
96. Sherertz RJ, Russell BA, Reuman PD. Transmission of hepatitis A by transfusion of blood products. *Arch Intern Med* 1984;144: 1579–1580.
97. Azimi PH, Roberto RR, Guralnik J, et al. Transfusion acquired hepa-

titis A in a premature infant with secondary nosocomial spread in an intensive care nursery. *Am J Dis Child* 1986;140:23–27.
98. Giacoia GP, Kasprisin DO. Transfusion-acquired hepatitis A. *South Med J* 1989;82:1357–1360.
99. Weisfuse IB, Graham DJ, Will M, et al. An outbreak of hepatitis-A among cancer patients treated with interleukin-2 and lymphokine-activated killer cells. *J Infect Dis* 1990;161:647–652.
100. Lee KK, Vargo LR, Le CT, et al. Transfusion-acquired hepatitis A outbreak from fresh frozen plasma in a neonatal intensive care unit. *Pediatr Infect Dis J* 1992;11:122–123.
101. Centers for Disease Control and Prevention. Hepatitis A among persons with hemophilia who received clotting factor concentrate—United States, September–December 1995. *MMWR Mortal Morb Wkly Rep* 1996;45:29–32.
102. Lemon SA. Type A viral hepatitis. New developments in an old disease. *N Engl J Med* 1985;313:1059–1067.
103. Prince AM. An antigen detected in the blood during the incubation period of serum hepatitis. *Proc Natl Acad Sci U S A* 1968;60:814–821.
104. Giles JP, McCollum RW, Berndston LW Jr, et al. Viral hepatitis-relation of Australia/SH antigen to the Willowbrook MS-2 strain. *N Engl J Med* 1969;281:119–121.
105. Almeida JD, Rubenstein D, Stott J. New antigen antibody system in Australia-antigen positive hepatitis. *Lancet* 1971;2:1125–1127.
106. Deinstag JL, Alaama A, Mosley JW, et al. Etiology of sporadic hepatitis B surface antigen negative hepatitis. *Ann Intern Med* 1977;87:1–6.
107. Holland PV, Alter HJ. The clinical significance of hepatitis B virus antigens and antibodies. *Med Clin North Am* 1975;59:849–855.
108. Hoofnagle JH, Gerety RJ, Barker LF. Antibody to hepatitis B core antigen. *Am J Med Sci* 1975;270:179–187.
109. Chau KH, Hargie MP, Decker RH, et al. Serodiagnosis of recent hepatitis B infection by IgM class anti-HBc. *Hepatology* 1983;3: 142–149.
110. Tabor E, Russell RP, Gerety RJ. Hepatitis B surface antigen (and e antigen) in pleural effusion: a case report. *Gastroenterology* 1977;73: 1157–1159.
111. Chadwick RG, Thomas HC, Sherlock S. e Antigen in agammaglobulinemia. *Lancet* 1978;1:616–617.
112. Magnius LO, Lindholm A, Lundin P. A new antigen antibody system. Clinical significance in long-term carriers of hepatitis B surface antigen. *JAMA* 1975;231:356–359.
113. Alter HJ, Seeff LB, Kaplan PM, et al. Type B hepatitis: the infectivity of blood positive for e antigen and DNA polymerase after accidental needlestick exposure. *N Engl J Med* 1976;295:909–913.
114. Okada K, Kamiyama I, Inomata M, et al. e Antigen and anti e in the serum of asymptomatic carrier mothers as indicators of positive and negative transmission of hepatitis B virus to their infants. *N Engl J Med* 1976;294:746–749.
115. Takahashi K, Imai M, Tsuda F, et al. Association of Dane particles with e antigen in the serum of asymptomatic carriers of hepatitis B surface antigen. *J Immunol* 1976;117:102–105.
116. Centers for Disease Control and Prevention. Public Health Service inter-agency guidelines for screening donors of blood, plasma, organs, tissues, and semen for evidence of hepatitis B and hepatitis C. *MMWR Mortal Morb Wkly Rep* 1991;40:1–17.
117. Aach RD, Kahn RA. Posttransfusion hepatitis: current perspectives. *Ann Intern Med* 1980;92:939–946.
118. Hollinger FB, Werch J, Melnick JL. A prospective study indicating that double-antibody radioimmunoassay reduces the incidence of posttransfusion hepatitis B. *N Engl J Med* 1974;290:1104–1109.
119. Polesky HF, Hanson MR. Comparison of viral hepatitis marker test methods based in AABB-CAP survey data. *Am J Clin Pathol* 1981; 26(Suppl):521–524.
120. Schable CA, Maynard JE. Serodiagnosis of acute hepatitis B virus infection by a modified competitive binding radioimmunoassay. *J Clin Microbiol* 1982;16:973–975.
121. Ratnam S, Tobin AM. Comparative evaluation of commercial enzyme immunoassay kits for detection of hepatitis B seromarkers. *J Clin Microbiol* 1987;25:432–433.
122. Alter HJ, Holland PV, Purcell RH, et al. Posttransfusion hepatitis after exclusion of commercial and hepatitis B antigen positive donors. *Ann Intern Med* 1972;77:691–699.
123. Alter HJ, Purcell RH, Holland PV, et al. Clinical and serological analysis of transfusion-associated hepatitis. *Lancet* 1975;2:838–841.
124. Alter HJ. How frequent is posttransfusion hepatitis after the introduction of third generation donor screening for hepatitis B? What is its probable nature? An international forum. *Vox Sang* 1977;32: 346–363.
125. Koretz RL, Gitnick GL. Prevention of posttransfusion hepatitis: role of sensitive hepatitis B antigen screening, tests source of blood and volume of transfusion. *Am J Med* 1975;59:754–760.
126. Tabor E, Goldfield M, Black HC, et al. Hepatitis B e antigen in volunteer and paid blood donors. *Transfusion* 1980;20:192–198.
127. Dodd RY, Notari EP, Stramer SL. Current prevalence and incidence of infectious disease markers and estimated window-period risk in the American Red Cross blood donor population. *Transfusion* 2002;42: 975–979.
128. Hoofnagle JH, Seeff LB, Bales Z, et al. Type B hepatitis after transfusion with blood containing antibody to hepatitis B core antigen. *N Engl J Med* 1978;298:1379–1383.
129. Lander JJ, Gitnick GL, Gelb LH, et al. Anticore antibody screening of transfused blood. *Vox Sang* 1978;34:77–80.
130. Katchaki JN, Siem TH, Brouwer R, et al. Detection and significance of anti-HBc in the blood bank: preliminary results of a controlled prospective study. *J Virol Meth* 1980;2:119–125.
131. Stevens CE, Aach RD, Hollinger FB, et al. Hepatitis B virus antibody in blood donors and the occurrences of non-A, non-B hepatitis in transfusion recipients: an analysis of the transfusion-transmitted viruses study. *Ann Intern Med* 1984;101:733–738.
132. Koziol DE, Holland PV, Alling DW, et al. Antibody to hepatitis B core antigen as a paradoxical marker for non-A, non-B hepatitis agents in donated blood. *Ann Intern Med* 1986;104:488–495.
133. Larsen J, Hetland G, Skaug K. Posttransfusion hepatitis B transmitted by blood from a hepatitis B surface antigen-negative hepatitis B virus carrier. *Transfusion* 1990;30:431–432.
134. Dodd RY, Popovsky MA. Antibodies to hepatitis B core antigen and the infectivity of the blood supply. *Transfusion* 1991;31:443–449.
135. Alter MJ, Hadler SC, Margolis HS, et al. The changing epidemiology of hepatitis B in the United States. Need for alternative vaccination strategies. *JAMA* 1990;263:1218–1222.
136. Sun CF, Pao CC, Wu SY, et al. Screening for hepatitis B virus in healthy blood donors by molecular DNA hybridization analysis. *J Clin Microbiol* 1988;26:1848–1852.
137. Wang JT, Wang TH, Sheu JC, et al. Detection of hepatitis B virus DNA by polymerase chain reaction in plasma of volunteer blood donors negative for hepatitis B surface antigen. *J Infect Dis* 1991;163: 397–399.
138. Centers for Disease Control and Prevention. Hepatitis B virus: a comprehensive strategy for eliminating transmission in the United States through universal childhood vaccination. *MMWR Mortal Morb Wkly Rep* 1991;40:1–25.
139. Rizzetto M, Canese MG, Arico S, et al. Immunofluorescence detection of new antigen-antibody system (delta/anti-delta) associated to hepatitis B virus in liver and serum of HBsAg carriers. *Gut* 1977;18: 997–1003.
140. Hoofnagle JH. Type D (delta) hepatitis. *JAMA* 1989;261: 1321–1325.
141. Rizzetto M, Gerin JL, Purcell RH, et al. *Hepatitis delta virus and its infection.* New York: Alan R. Liss, 1987.
142. Rizzetto M. The delta agent. *Hepatology* 1983;3:729–737.
143. Farci P, Gerin JL, Aragona M, et al. Diagnostic and prognostic significance of the IgM antibody to the hepatitis delta virus. *JAMA* 1986; 255:1443–1446.
144. Crivelli O, Rizzetto M, Lavarini C, et al. Enzyme-linked immunosorbent assay for detection of antibody to the hepatitis B surface antigen-associated delta antigen. *J Clin Microbiol* 1981;14:173–177.
145. Puig J, Fields HA. Development of an enzyme immunoassay using recombinant expressed antigen to detect hepatitis delta virus antibodies. *J Clin Microbiol* 1989;27:2222–2225.
146. Rizzetto M, Verme G, Recchia S, et al. Chronic HBsAg hepatitis

with intrahepatic expression of delta antigen. An active and progressive disease unresponsive to immunosuppressive treatment. *Ann Intern Med* 1983;98:437–441.

147. Rosina F, Saracco G, Rizzetto M. Risk of posttransfusion infection with the hepatitis delta virus. *N Engl J Med* 1985;312:1488–1491.
148. Prince AM, Grady GF, Hazzi C, et al. Long-incubation posttransfusion hepatitis without serological evidence of exposure to hepatitis B virus. *Lancet* 1974;2:241–246.
149. Dienstag JL, Feinstone SM, Purcell RH, et al. Non-A non-B posttransfusion hepatitis. *Lancet* 1977;1:560–562.
150. Mosely JW, Redeker AG, Feinstone SM, et al. Multiple hepatitis viruses in multiple attacks of acute viral Hepatitis. *N Engl J Med* 1977;296:75–78.
151. Shimizu YK, Feinstone SM, Purcell RH, et al. Non-A, non-B hepatitis: ultrastructural evidence for two agents in experimentally infected chimpanzees. *Science* 1979;205:197–200.
152. Dienstag JL. Non-A, non-B hepatitis I. Recognition epidemiology, and clinical features. *Gastroenterology* 1983;85:439–462.
153. Czaja AJ, Davis GL. Hepatitis non-A, non-B: manifestations and implications of acute and chronic disease. *Mayo Clin Proc* 1982;57: 639–652.
154. Choo QL, Kuo G, Weiner Al, et al. Isolation of a cDNA clone derived from a blood-borne non-A, non-B hepatitis genome. *Science* 1989; 244:359–362.
155. Kuo G, Choo QL, Alter GL, et al. An assay for circulating antibodies to a major etiologic virus of human non-A, non-B hepatitis. *Science* 1989;244:362–364.
156. Alter MJ, Kruszon-Moran D, Nainan OV, et al. The prevalence of hepatitis C virus infection in the United States, 1988 through 1994. *N Engl J Med* 1999;341;556–562.
157. Aach RD, Stevens CE, Hollinger FB, et al. Hepatitis C virus infection in post-transfusion hepatitis. *N Engl J Med* 1991;325:1326–1328.
158. Gross JB Jr. Clinician's guide to hepatitis C. *Mayo Clin Proc* 1998; 73:355–361.
159. Gill P. Transfusion-associated hepatitis C: reducing the risk. *Transfusion Med Rev* 1993;7:104–111.
160. Alter MJ, Hadler SC, Judson FN, et al. Risk factors for acute non-A, non-B hepatitis in the United States and association with hepatitis C virus infection. *JAMA* 1990;264:2231–2235.
161. Esteban JI, Viladomiu L, Gonzalez A, et al. Hepatitis C virus antibodies among risk groups in Spain. *Lancet* 1989;2:294–297.
162. Zeldis JB, Depner TA, Kuramoto IK, et al. The prevalence of hepatitis C virus antibodies among hemodialysis patients. *Ann Intern Med* 1990;112:958–960.
163. Rumi MG, Colombo M, Gringeri A, et al. High prevalence of antibody to hepatitis C virus in multitransfused hemophiliacs with normal transaminase levels. *Ann Intern Med* 1990;112:379–380.
164. Alter MJ, Sampliner RE. Hepatitis C: and miles to go before we sleep. *N Engl J Med* 1989;321:1538–1540.
165. Bjoro K, Froland SS, Yun Z, et al. Hepatitis C infection in patients with primary hypogammaglobulinemia after treatment with contaminated immune globulin. *N Engl J Med* 1994;331:1607–1611.
166. Schiff RI. Transmission of viral infections through intravenous immune globulin. *N Engl J Med* 1994;331:1649–1650.
167. Francis DP, Hadler SC, Prendergast TJ, et al. Occurrence of hepatitis A, B and non-A, non-B in the United States: CDC Sentinel County Hepatitis Study I. *Am J Med* 1984;76:69–74.
168. Centers for Disease Control and Prevention. Transmission of hepatitis C virus infection associated with home infusion therapy for hemophilia. *MMWR Mortal Morb Wkly Rep* 1997;46:597–599.
169. Esteban JI, Lopez-Talavera JC, Genesca J, et al. High rate of infectivity and liver disease in blood donors with antibodies to hepatitis C virus. *Ann Intern Med* 1991;115:443–449.
170. Conry-Cantilena C, VanRaden M, Gibble J, et al. Routes of infection, viremia, and liver disease in blood donors found to have hepatitis C virus infection. *N Engl J Med* 1996;334:1691–1696.
171. Alter MJ, Margolis HS, Krawczynski K, et al. The natural history of community-acquired hepatitis C in the United States. *N Engl J Med* 1992;327:1899–1905.
172. Shakil AO, Conry-Cantilena C, Alter HJ, et al. Volunteer blood donors with antibody to hepatitis C virus: clinical, biochemical, virologic, and histologic features. *Ann Intern Med* 1995;123:330–337.
173. Bodenheimer HC, Lefkowitch J, Lindsay K, et al. Histological and clinical correlationsin chronic hepatitis C. *Hepatology* 1990;12:844.
174. Schoeman MN, Liddle C, Bilous M, et al. Chronic non-A, non-B hepatitis: lack of correlation between biochemical and morphological activity, and effects of immunosuppressive therapy on disease progression. *Aust N Z J Med* 1990;20:56–62.
175. Davis GL, Balart LA, Schiff ER, et al. Treatment of chronic hepatitis C with recombinant interferon alfa: a multicenter randomized, controlled trial. *N Engl J Med* 1989;321:1501–1506.
176. Colombo M, Kuo G, Choo QI, et al. Prevalence of antibodies to hepatitis C virus in Italian patients with hepatocellular carcinoma. *Lancet* 1989;2:1006–1008.
177. Bruix J, Barrera JM, Calvet X, et al. Prevalence of antibodies to hepatitis C virus in Spanish patients with hepatocellular carcinoma and hepatic cirrhosis. *Lancet* 1989;2:1004–1006.
178. Yu MC, Tong MJ, Coursaget P, et al. Prevalence of hepatitis B and C viral markers in black and white patients with hepatocellular carcinoma in the United States. *J Natl Cancer Inst* 1990;82:1038–1041.
179. Seeff LB, Buskell-Bales Z, Wright EC, et al. Long-term mortality after transfusion-associated non-A, non-B hepatitis. *N Engl J Med* 1992;327:1906–1911.
180. Tong MJ, El-Farra NS, Reikes AR, et al. Clinical outcomes after transfusion-associated hepatitis C. *N Engl J Med* 1995;332: 1463–1466.
181. Goedert JJ, Eyster ME, Lederman MM, et al. End-stage liver disease in persons with hemophilia and transfusion-associated infections. *Blood* 2002;100:1584–1589.
182. Vogt M, Lang T, Frosner G, et al. Prevalence and clinical outcome of hepatitis C infection in children who underwent cardiac surgery before the implementation of blood-donor screening. *N Engl J Med* 1999;341:866–870.
183. Aach RD, Szmuness W, Mosley JW, et al. Serum alanine aminotransferase of donors in relation to the risk of non-A, non-B hepatitis in recipients. *N Engl J Med* 1981;304:989–994.
184. Alter HJ, Purcell RH, Holland PV, et al. Donor transaminase and recipient hepatitis: impact on blood transfusion services. *JAMA* 1981; 246:630–634.
185. Friedman LS, Dienstag JL, Watkins E, et al. Evaluation of blood donors with elevated serum alanine aminotransferase levels. *Ann Intern Med* 1987;107:137–144.
186. Stevens CE, Aach RD, Hollinger FB, et al. Hepatitis B virus antibody in blood donors and the occurrence of non-A, non-B hepatitis in transfusion recipients. *Ann Intern Med* 1984;101:733–738.
187. Koziol DE, Holland PV, Alling DW, et al. Antibody to hepatitis B core antigen as a paradoxical marker for non-A, non-B hepatitis agents in donated blood. *Ann Intern Med* 1986;104:488–495.
188. Miyamura T, Saito I, Ketayama T, et al. Detection of antibody against antigen expressed by molecularly cloned hepatitis C virus cDNA: application to diagnosis and blood screening for posttransfusion hepatitis. *Proc Natl Acad Sci U S A* 1990;87:983–987.
189. Sansonno D, Dammacco F. Antibodies to hepatitis C virus in non-A, non-B post-transfusion and cryptogenetic chronic liver disease. *Lancet* 1989;2:798–799.
190. Alter HJ, Purcell RH, Shih JW, et al. Detection of antibody to hepatitis C virus in prospectively followed transfusion recipients with acute and chronic non-A, non-B hepatitis. *N Engl J Med* 1989;321: 1494–1500.
191. Wang JT, Wang TH, Lin JT, et al. Hepatitis C virus in a prospective study of posttransfusion non-A, non-B hepatitis in Taiwan. *J Med Virol* 1990;32:83–86.
192. Esteban JI, Gonzalez A, Hernandez JM, et al. Evaluation of antibodies to hepatitis C virus in a study of transfusion-associated hepatitis. *N Engl J Med* 1990;323:1107–1112.
193. Stevens CE, Taylor PE, Pindyck J, et al. Epidemiology of hepatitis C virus. *JAMA* 1990;263:49–53.
194. Tremolada F, Casarin C, Tagger A, et al. Antibody to hepatitis C virus in post-transfusion hepatitis. *Ann Intern Med* 1991;114:277–281.
195. Taliani G, DeBac C, Maiozzi S, et al. HCV transmission by fresh

packed red cells from anti-HCV negative donors. *Lancet* 1991;338: 62.

196. Barrera JM, Bruguera M, Ercilla MG, et al. Incidence of non-A, non-B hepatitis after screening blood donors for antibodies to hepatitis C virus and surrogate markers. *Ann Intern Med* 1991;115:596–600.
197. Alter HJ. Descartes before the horse: I clone, therefore I am: the hepatitis C virus in current perspective. *Ann Intern Med* 1991;115: 644–649.
198. Donahue JG, Munoz A, Ness PM, et al. The declining risk of post-transfusion hepatitis C virus infection. *N Engl J Med* 1992;327: 369–373.
199. Wang JT, Wang TH, Lin JT, et al. Improved serodiagnosis of post-transfusion hepatitis C virus infection by a second-generation immunoassay based on multiple recombinant antigens. *Vox Sang* 1992;62: 21–24.
200. Vallari DS, Jett BW, Alter HJ, et al. Serological markers of posttransfusion hepatitis C viral infection. *J Clin Microbiol* 1992;30:552–556.
201. Lelie PN, Cuypers TM, Reesink HW, et al. Patterns of serological markers in transfusion transmitted hepatitis C virus infection using second-generation HCV assays. *J Med Virol* 1992;37:203–209.
202. Menitove JE, Richards WA, Destree M, et al. Early US experience with anti-HCV kit in blood donors. *Lancet* 1990;336:244–245.
203. Alberti A, Chemello L, Cavalletto D, et al. Antibody to hepatitis C virus and liver disease in volunteer blood donors. *Ann Intern Med* 1991;114:1010–1012.
204. Skidmore S. Recombinant immunoblot assay for hepatitis C antibody. *Lancet* 1990;335:1346.
205. Weiner AJ, Truett MA, Rosenblatt J, et al. HCV testing in low-risk population [Letter]. *Lancet* 1990;336:695.
206. Alter MJ. Review of serologic testing for hepatitis C virus infection and risk of post-transfusion hepatitis C. *Arch Pathol Lab Med* 1994; 118:342–345.
207. NIH Consensus Development Panel on Infectious Disease Testing for Blood Transfusions. Infectious disease testing for blood transfusions. *JAMA* 1995;274:1374–1379.
208. Barrera JM, Francis B, Ercilla G, et al. Improved detection of anti-HCV in post-transfusion hepatitis by a third-generation ELISA. *Vox Sang* 1995;68:15–18.
209. Vrielink H, Zaauer HL, Reesink HW, et al. Comparison of two anti-hepatitis C virus enzyme-linked immunosorbent assays. *Transfusion* 1995;35:601–604.
210. Dawson GJ, Lesniewski RR, Stewart JL, et al. Detection of antibodies to hepatitis C virus in US blood donors. *J Clin Microbiol* 1991;29: 551–556.
211. Farci P, Alter HJ, Wong D, et al. A long-term study of hepatitis C virus replication in non-A, non-B hepatitis. *N Engl J Med* 1991;325: 98–104.
212. Weiner AJ, Kuo G, Bradley DW, et al. Detection of hepatitis C viral sequences in non-A, non-B hepatitis. *Lancet* 1990;335:1–3.
213. Zanetti AR, Tanzi E, Zehender G, et al. Hepatitis C virus RNA in symptomless donors implicated in post-transfusion non-A, non-B hepatitis. *Lancet* 1990;336:448.
214. Farci R, Wang D, Alter HJ, et al. Detection of HCV sequences by PCR in hepatitis C virus infection: relationship to antibody response and clinical outcome. *Hepatology* 1990;12:904.
215. Tedeschi V, Seeff LB. Diagnostic tests for hepatitis C: where are we now? *Ann Intern Med* 1995;123:383–385.
216. Gresens CJ, Holland PV. The disappearance of transfusion-transmitted hepatitis C virus infections in the United States. *Clin Liver Dis* 2001;5:1105–1113.
217. Schuttler CG, Caspari G, Jursch CA, et al. Hepatitis C virus transmission by a blood donation negative in nucleic acid amplification tests for viral RNA. *Lancet* 2000;355:41–42.
218. Kolk DP, Dockter J, Linnen J, et al. Significant closure of the human immunodeficiency virus type 1 and hepatitis C virus preseroconversion detection windows with a transcription-mediated-amplification-driven assay. *J Clin Microbiol* 2002;40:1761–1766.
219. Knodell RG, Ginsberg AL, Conrad ME, et al. Efficacy of prophylactic gamma-globulin in preventing non-A, non-B post-transfusion hepatitis. *Lancet* 1976;1:557–561.
220. Seeff LB, Zimmerman HJ, Wright EC, et al. Liver physiology and disease. A randomized, double-blind controlled trial of the efficacy of immune serum globulin for the prevention of post-transfusion hepatitis. *Gastroenterology* 1977;72:111–121.
221. Sanchez-Quijano A, Lissen E, Diaz-Torres MA, et al. Prevention of post-transfusion, non-A, non-B hepatitis by non-specific immunoglobulin in heart surgery patients. *Lancet* 1988;1:1245–1249.
222. Tabor E. The three viruses of non-A, non-B hepatitis. *Lancet* 1985; 1:743.
223. Dodd RY. Hepatitis C, other types of non-B parenteral hepatitis and blood transfusion. *Dev Biol Stand (Basel)* 1993;81:35–40.
224. Linnen J, Wages J Jr, Zhang-Keck Z-Y, et al. Molecular cloning and disease association of hepatitis G virus: a transfusion-transmissible agent. *Science* 1996;271:505–508.
225. Masuko K, Mitsui T, Iwano K, et al. Infection with hepatitis GB virus C in patients on maintenance hemodialysis. *N Engl J Med* 1996; 334:1485–1490.
226. Wang J-T, Tsai F-C, Lee C-Z, et al. A prospective study of transfusion-transmitted GB virus C infection: similar frequency but different clinical presentation compared with hepatitis C virus. *Blood* 1996; 88:1881–1886.
227. Kleinman S. Hepatitis G virus biology, epidemiology, and clinical manifestations: implications for blood safety. *Transfusion Med Rev* 2001;15:201–212.
228. Alter HJ, Nakatsuji Y, Melpolder J, et al. The incidence of transfusion-associated hepatitis G virus infection and its relation to liver disease. *N Engl J Med* 1997;336:747–754.
229. Alter MJ, Gallagher M, Morris TT, et al. Acute non-A-E hepatitis in the United States and the role of hepatitis G virus infection. *N Engl J Med* 1997;336:741–746.
230. Tanaka E, Alter HJ, Nakatsuji Y, et al. Effect of hepatitis G virus infection on chronic hepatitis C. *Ann Intern Med* 1996;125:740–743.
231. Tan D, Matsumoto A, Conry-Cantilena C, et al. Analysis of hepatitis G virus (HGV) RNA, antibody to HGV envelope protein, and risk factors for blood donors coinfected with HGV and hepatitis C virus. *J. Infect Dis* 1999;179:1055–1061.
232. Alter HJ. G-pers creepers, where'd you get those papers? A reassessment of the literature on the hepatitis G virus. *Transfusion* 1997;37: 569–572.
233. Mushahwar IK. Recently discovered blood-borne viruses: are they hepatitis viruses or merely endosymbionts? *J Med Virol* 2000;62: 399–404.
234. Tegtmeier GE. Cytomegalovirus infection as a complication of blood transfusion. *Semin Liver Dis* 1986;6:82–95.
235. Crumpacker CS. Cytomegalovirus. In: Mandell GL, Bennett JE, Dolin R, eds. *Principles and practice of infectious diseases,* 5th ed. New York: Churchill Livingstone, 2000:1586–1599.
236. Huang ES, Huong SM, Tegtmeier GE, et al. Cytomegalovirus: genetic variation of viral genomes. *Ann N Y Acad Sci* 1990;354: 332–346.
237. Glazer JP, Friedman HM, Grossman RA, et al. Live cytomegalovirus vaccination of renal transplant candidates: a preliminary trial. *Ann Intern Med* 1979;91:676–683.
238. Dworsky M, Yow M, Stagno S, et al. Cytomegalovirus infection of breast milk and transmission in infancy. *Pediatrics* 1983;72:295–299.
239. Krech U. Complement-fixing antibodies against cytomegalovirus in different parts of the world. *Bull WHO* 1973;49:103–106.
240. Zhang LJ, Hanff P, Rutherford C, et al. Detection of human cytomegalovirus DNA, RNA, and antibody in normal donor blood. *J Infect Dis* 1995;171:1002–1006.
241. Wilhelm JA, Matter L, Schopfer K. Risk of CMV transmission to non-immunocompromised patients from seropositive blood donors. *Experientia* 1985;41:550(abst).
242. Wilhelm JA, Matter L, Schopfer K. The risk of transmitting cytomegalovirus to patients receiving blood transfusions. *J Infect Dis* 1986;154: 169–171.
243. Dworkin RJ, Drew WL, Miner RC, et al. Survival of cytomegalovirus in viremic blood under blood bank storage conditions. *J Infect Dis* 1990;161:1310–1311.
244. Winston DJ, Ho WG, Howell CL, et al. Cytomegalovirus infections

associated with leukocyte transfusions. *Ann Intern Med* 1980;93: 671–675.
245. Hersman J, Meyers JD, Thomas ED, et al. The effect of granulocyte transfusions on the incidence of cytomegalovirus infection after allogeneic marrow transplantation. *Ann Intern Med* 1982;96:149–152.
246. Nichols WG, Price T, Boeckh M. Cytomegalovirus infections in cancer patients receiving granulocyte transfusions. *Blood* 2002;99: 3483–3484.
247. Preiksaitis JK, Grument FC, Smith WK, et al. Transfusion-acquired cytomegalovirus infection in cardiac surgery patients. *J Med Virol* 1985;15:283–290.
248. Beneke JS, Tegtmeier GE, Alter HJ, et al. Relation of titers of antibodies to CMV in blood donors to the transmission of cytomegalovirus infection. *J Infect Dis* 1984;150:883–888.
249. Monif GRG, Daicoff GI, Flory FL. Blood as a potential vehicle for the cytomegaloviruses. *Am J Obstet Gynecol* 1976;126:445–448.
250. Preiksaitis JK. Indications for the use of cytomegalovirus-seronegative blood products. *Transfusion Med Rev* 1991;5:1–17.
251. Smith TF, Holley KE, Keys TF, et al. Cytomegalovirus studies of autopsy tissue. I. Virus isolation. *Am J Clin Pathol* 1975;63:854–858.
252. Macasaet FF, Holley KE, Smith TF, et al. Cytomegalovirus studies of autopsy tissue. II. Incidence of inclusion bodies and related pathologic data. *Am J Clin Pathol* 1975;63:859–865.
253. Griffiths PD, Panjwani DD, Stirk PR, et al. Rapid diagnosis of cytomegalovirus infection in immunocompromised patients by detection of early antigen fluorescent foci. *Lancet* 1984;2:1242–1245.
254. Gleaves CA, Smith TF, Shuster EA, et al. Rapid detection of cytomegalovirus in MRC-5 cells inoculated with urine specimens by using low speed centrifugation and monoclonal antibody to an early antigen. *J Clin Microbiol* 1984;19:917–919.
255. Gleaves CA, Smith TF, Shuster EA, et al. Comparison of standard tube and shell vial culture techniques for the detection of cytomegalovirus in clinical specimens. *J Clin Microbiol* 1985;21:217–221.
256. Alpert G, Mazeron MC, Colimon R, et al. Rapid detection of human cytomegalovirus in the urine of humans. *J Infect Dis* 1985;152: 631–633.
257. Goldstein LC, McDougall J, Hackman R, et al. Monoclonal antibodies to cytomegalovirus: rapid identification of clinical isolates and preliminary use in diagnosis of cytomegalovirus pneumonia. *Infect Immun* 1982;38:273–281.
258. Volpi A, Whitley RJ, Ceballos R, et al. Rapid diagnosis of pneumonia due to cytomegalovirus with specific monoclonal antibodies. *J Infect Dis* 1983;147:1119–1120.
259. Griffiths PD. Diagnostic techniques for cytomegalovirus infection. *Clin Haematol* 1984;13:631–644.
260. Pamphilon DH, Rider JR, Barbara JAJ, et al. Prevention of transfusion-transmitted cytomegalovirus infection. *Transfusion Med* 1999;9: 115–123.
261. Kühn JE. Transfusion-associated infections with cytomegalovirus and other human herpesviruses. *Infuse Ther Transfus Med* 2000;27: 138–143.
262. Yeager AS, Grumet FC, Hafleigh EB, et al. Prevention of transfusion-acquired cytomegalovirus infections in newborn infants. *J Pediatr* 1981;98:281–287.
263. Betts RF, Freeman RB, Douglas RG Jr, et al. Transmission of cytomegalovirus infection with renal allograft. *Kidney Int* 1975;8: 387–394.
264. Ho M, Suwansirikul S, Dowling JN, et al. The transplanted kidney as a source of cytomegalovirus infection. *N Engl J Med* 1975;293: 1109–1112.
265. Betts RF, Freeman RB, Douglas RG Jr, et al. Clinical manifestations of renal allograft derived primary cytomegalovirus infection. *Am J Dis Child* 1977;131:759–763.
266. Thomas F, Lee HM, Wolf JS, et al. Monitoring and modulation of immune reactivity in human transplant recipients. *Surgery* 1976;79: 408–413.
267. Chou S, Kim DY, Norman DJ. Transmission of cytomegalovirus by pretransplant leukocyte transfusions in renal transplant candidates. *J Infect Dis* 1987;155:565–567.
268. Preiksaitis JK, Rosno S, Grument C, et al. Infections due to herpesviruses in cardiac transplant recipients: role of the donor heart and immunosuppressive therapy. *J Infect Dis* 1983;14:974–981.
269. Bowden RA, Slichter SJ, Sayers MH, et al. Use of leukocyte-depleted platelets and cytomegalovirus seronegative red blood cells for prevention of primary cytomegalovirus infection after marrow transplant. *Blood* 1991;78:246–250.
270. Miller WJ, McCullough J, Balfour HH Jr, et al. Prevention of cytomegalovirus infection after bone marrow transplantation: a randomized trial of blood product screening. *Bone Marrow Transplant* 1991; 7:227–234.
271. Preiksaitis JK, Desai S, Vaudry W, et al. Transfusion- and community-acquired cytomegalovirus infection in children with malignant disease: a prospective study. *Transfusion* 1997;37:941–946.
272. deGraan-Hentzen YCE, Gratama JW, Mudde GC, et al. Prevention of primary cytomegalovirus infection in patients with hematologic malignancies by intensive white cell depletion of blood products. *Transfusion* 1989;29:757–760.
273. Dodd RY, Nath N, Pielech M, et al. Prevalence of infection by four hepatotropic viruses in a voluntary donor population. *Transfusion* 1981;22:422(abst).
274. Lamberson HV Jr, McMillan JA, Weiner LB, et al. Prevention of transfusion-associated cytomegalovirus (CMV) infection in neonates by screening blood donors for IgM to CMV. *J Infect Dis* 1988;157: 820–823.
275. Lang DJ, Ebert PA, Rodgers BM, et al. Reduction of postperfusion cytomegalovirus infections after the use of leukocyte-depleted blood. *Transfusion* 1977;17:391–395.
276. Tolkoff-Rubin NE, Rubin RH, Keller EE, et al. Cytomegalovirus infection in dialysis patients and personnel. *Ann Intern Med* 1978; 89:625–628.
277. Brady MT, Milam JD, Anderson DC, et al. Use of deglycerolized red blood cells to prevent posttransfusion infection with cytomegalovirus in neonates. *J Infect Dis* 1984;150:334–339.
278. Taylor BJ, Jacobs RF, Baker RL, et al. Frozen deglycerolized blood prevents transfusion-acquired cytomegalovirus infections in neonates. *Pediatr Infect Dis* 1986;5:188–191.
279. Gilbert GL, Hayes K, Hudson IL, et al. Prevention of transfusion-acquired cytomegalovirus infection in infants by blood filtration to remove leukocytes. *Lancet* 1989;1:1228–1231.
280. Winston DJ, Ho WG, Lin CH, et al. Intravenous immune globulin for prevention of cytomegalovirus infection and interstitial pneumonia after bone marrow transplantation. *Ann Intern Med* 1987;106: 12–18.
281. Schmidt GM, Horak DA, Niland JC, et al. A randomized, controlled trial of prophylactic ganciclovir for cytomegalovirus pulmonary infection in recipients of allogeneic bone marrow transplants. *N Engl J Med* 1991;324:1005–1011.
282. Snydman DR, Werner BG, Meissner HC, et al. Use of cytomegalovirus immunoglobulin in multiply transfused premature neonates. *Pediatr Infect Dis J* 1995;14:34–40.
283. Gerber P, Walsh JH, Rosenblum EN, et al. Association of EB-virus infection with the post-perfusion syndrome. *Lancet* 1969;1:593–596.
284. Henle W, Henle G, Scriba M, et al. Antibody responses to the Epstein-Barr virus and cytomegaloviruses after open-heart and other surgery. *N Engl J Med* 1970;282:1068–1074.
285. Turner AR, MacDonald RN, Cooper BA. Transmission of infectious mononucleosis by transfusion of pre-illness plasma. *Ann Intern Med* 1972;77:751–753.
286. Solem JH, Jorganson W. Accidentally transmitted infectious mononucleosis. *Acta Med Scand* 1969;186:433.
287. Sayers MH. Transfusion-transmitted viral infections other than hepatitis and human immunodeficiency virus infection-cytomegalovirus, Epstein-Barr virus, human herpesvirus-6, and human parvovirus B19. *Arch Pathol Lab Med* 1994;118:346–349.
288. Alfieri C, Tanner J, Carpentier L, et al. Epstein-Barr virus transmission from a blood donor to an organ transplant recipient with recovery of the same virus strain from the recipient's blood and oropharynx. *Blood* 1996;87:812–817.
289. Jacobs RF. Frozen deglycerolized blood and transmission of Epstein-Barr virus. *J Infect Dis* 1986;153:800.

290. Strauss SE. Human herpesvirus type 8 (Kaposi's sarcoma-associated herpesvirus). In: Mandell GL, Bennett JE, Dolin R, eds. *Principles and practices of infectious diseases,* 5th ed. New York: Churchill Livingston, 2000:1618–1621.
291. Blackbourn DJ, Ambroziak J, Lennette E, et al. Infectious human herpesvirus 8 in a healthy North American blood donor. *Lancet* 1997; 349:609–611.
292. Cannon MJ, Dollard SC, Smith DK, et al. Blood-borne and sexual transmission of human herpesvirus 8 in women with or at risk for human immunodeficiency virus infection. *N Engl J Med* 2001;344: 637–643.
293. Centers for Disease Control and Prevention. *Pneumocystis pneumonia*—Los Angeles. *MMWR Mortal Morb Wkly Rep* 1981;30: 250–252.
294. Centers for Disease Control and Prevention. Kaposi's sarcoma and *Pneumocystis* pneumonia among homosexual men—New York City and California. *MMWR Mortal Morb Wkly Rep* 1981;30:305–308.
295. Centers for Disease Control and Prevention. Prevention of acquired immunodeficiency syndrome (AIDS): report of inter-agency recommendations. *MMWR Mortal Morb Wkly Rep* 1983;32:101–103.
296. Sandler SG, Katz AJ. Impact of AIDS on blood services in the United States. *Vox Sang* 1984;46:1–7.
297. Centers for Disease Control and Prevention. *Pneumocystis carinii* pneumonia among persons with hemophilia A. *MMWR Mortal Morb Wkly Rep* 1982;31:365–367.
298. Curran JW, Lawrence DN, Jaffe H, et al. Acquired immune deficiency syndrome (AIDS) associated with transfusions. *N Engl J Med* 1984; 310:69–75.
299. Evatt BL, Ramsey RB, Lawrence DN, et al. The acquired immune deficiency syndrome (AIDS) in patients with hemophilia. *Ann Intern Med* 1984;100:499–504.
300. Ward JW, Bush TJ, Perkins HA, et al. The natural history of transfusion-associated infection with human immunodeficiency virus. *N Engl J Med* 1989;321:947–952.
301. Donegan E, Stuart M, Niland JC, et al. Infection with human immunodeficiency virus type 1 (HIV-1) among recipients of antibody-positive blood donations. *Ann Intern Med* 1990;113:733–739.
302. Schimpf K, Brackmann HH, Kreuz W, et al. Absence of anti-human immunodeficiency virus types 1 and 2 seroconversion after the treatment of hemophilia A or Von Willebrand's disease with pasteurized factor VIII concentrate. *N Engl J Med* 1989;321:1148–1152.
303. Remis RS, O Shaughnessy MV, Tsoukas C, et al. HIV transmission to patients with hemophilia by heat-treated, donor-screened factor concentrate. *Can Med Assoc J* 1990;142:1247–1254.
304. Epstein JS, Fricke WA. Current safety of clotting factor concentrates. *Arch Pathol Lab Med* 1990;114:335–340.
305. Centers for Disease Control and Prevention. Safety of therapeutic products used for hemophilia patients. *MMWR Mortal Morb Wkly Rep* 1988;37:441–444, 449–450.
306. Snyder EL, Dodd RY. Reducing the risk of blood transfusion. *Hematology* 2001;433–442.
307. Barre-Sinoussi F, Chermann JC, Rey F, et al. Isolation of a T-lymphotropic retrovirus from a patient at risk for acquired immune deficiency syndrome (AIDS). *Science* 1983;220:868–871.
308. Popovic M, Sarngadharan MG, Read E, et al. Detection, isolation, and continuous production of cytopathic retroviruses (HTLV-III) from patients with AIDS and pre-AIDS. *Science* 1984;224:497–500.
309. Gallo RC, Salahuddin SZ, Popovic M, et al. Frequent detection and isolation of cytopathic retroviruses (HTLV-III) from patients with AIDS and at risk for AIDS. *Science* 1984;224:500–503.
310. Levy JA, Hoffman AD, Kramer SM, et al. Isolation of lymphocytopathic retroviruses from San Francisco patients with AIDS. *Science* 1984;225:840–843.
311. Sarngadharan MG, Popovic M, Bruch L, et al. Antibodies reactive with human T-lymphotropic retroviruses (HTLV-III) in serum of patients with AIDS. *Science* 1984;224:506–508.
312. Brun-Vezinet F, Rouzioux C, Barre-Sinoussi F, et al. Detection of IgG antibodies to lymphadenopathy-associated virus in patients with AIDS or lymphadenopathy syndrome. *Lancet* 1984;1:1253–1256.
313. Demeter LM, Reichman RC. Detection of human immunodeficiency virus infection. In: Mandell GE, Bennett JE, Dolin R, eds. *Principles and practices of infectious diseases,* 5th ed. New York: Churchill Livingstone, 2000:1369–1374.
314. Centers for Disease Control and Prevention. Provisional Public Health Service inter-agency recommendations for screening donated blood and plasma for antibody to the virus causing acquired immunodeficiency syndrome. *MMWR Mortal Morb Wkly Rep* 1985;34:1–5.
315. Schorr JB, Berkowitz A, Cumming PD, et al. Prevalence of HTLV-III antibody in American blood donors. *N Engl J Med* 1985;313: 384–385.
316. Centers for Disease Control and Prevention. Human T-lymphotropic virus type III/lymphadenopathy-associated virus antibody testing at alternate sites. *MMWR Mortal Morb Wkly Rep* 1986;35:284–287.
317. Ness PM, Douglas D, Koziol D, et al. Decreasing seroprevalence of human immunodeficiency virus type 1 in a regional blood donor population. *Transfusion* 1990;30:201–206.
318. Nelson KE, Vlahov D, Margolick J, et al. Blood and plasma donations among a cohort of intravenous drug users. *JAMA* 1990;263: 2194–2197.
319. Goudsmit J, DeWolf F, Paul DA, et al. Expression of human immunodeficiency virus antigen (HIV-Ag) in serum and cerebrospinal fluid during acute and chronic infection. *Lancet* 1986;2:177–180.
320. Goudsmit J, Lange JMA, Paul DA, et al. Antigenemia and antibody titers to core and envelope antigens in AIDS, AIDS-related complex, and subclinical human immunodeficiency virus infection. *J Infect Dis* 1987;155:558–560.
321. Centers for Disease Control and Prevention. Interpretation and use of the Western blot assay for serodiagnosis of human immunodeficiency virus type 1 infections. *MMWR Mortal Morb Wkly Rep* 1989; 38(Suppl 7):1–7.
322. Ward JW, Holmberg SD, Allen JR, et al. Transmission of human immunodeficiency virus (HIV) by blood transfusion screened as negative for HIV antibody. *N Engl J Med* 1988;318:473–478.
323. Bove JR. Transfusion-associated hepatitis and AIDS. *N Engl J Med* 1987;317:242–244.
324. Menitove JE. The decreasing risk of transfusion-associated AIDS. *N Engl J Med* 1989;321:966–968.
325. Cumming PD, Wallace EL, Schorr JB, et al. Exposure of patients to human immunodeficiency virus through the transfusion of blood components that test antibody-negative. *N Engl J Med* 1989;321: 941–946.
326. Cohen ND, Munoz A, Reitz BA, et al. Transmission of retroviruses by transfusion of screened blood in patients undergoing cardiac surgery. *N Engl J Med* 1989;320:1172–1176.
327. MacDonald KL, Jackson JB, Bowman RJ, et al. Performance characteristics of serologic tests for human immunodeficiency virus type 1 (HIV-1) antibody among Minnesota blood donors. *Ann Intern Med* 1989;110:617–621.
328. van der Poel CL, Lelie PN, Reesink HW, et al. Blood donors with indeterminate anti-p24^{gag} reactivity in HIV-1 Western blot: absence of infectivity to transfused patients and in virus culture. *Vox Sang* 1989;56:162–167.
329. Leitman SF, Klein HG, Melpolder JJ, et al. Clinical implications of positive tests for antibodies to human immunodeficiency virus type 1 in asymptomatic blood donors. *N Engl J Med* 1989;321:917–924.
330. Jackson JB, MacDonald KL, Caldwell J, et al. Absence of HIV infection in blood donors with indeterminate western blot tests for antibody to HIV-1. *N Engl J Med* 1990;322:217–222.
331. Dock NL, Kleinman SH, Rayfield MA, et al. Status of human immunodeficiency virus infection in individuals with persistently indeterminate Western blot patterns: prospective studies in a low prevalence population. *Arch Intern Med* 1991;151:525–530.
332. Jackson JB, Hanson MR, Johnson GM, et al. Long-term follow-up of blood donors with indeterminate human immunodeficiency virus type 1 results on Western blot. *Transfusion* 1995;35:98–102.
333. Centers for Disease Control and Prevention. Transfusion-associated human T-lymphotropic virus type III/lymphadenopathy-associated virus infection from a seronegative donor Colorado. *MMWR Mortal Morb Wkly Rep* 1986;35:389–391.
334. Centers for Disease Control and Prevention. Persistent lack of detecta-

ble HIV-1 antibody in a person with HIV infection—Utah, 1995. *MMWR Mortal Morb Wkly Rep* 1996;45:181–185.
335. Petersen LR, Satten GA, Dodd R, et al. Duration of time from onset of human immunodeficiency virus type 1 infectiousness to development of detectable antibody. *Transfusion* 1994;34:283–289.
336. Busch MP, Lee LLL, Satten GA, et al. Time course of detection of viral and serologic markers preceding human immunodeficiency virus type 1 seroconversion: implications for screening of blood and tissue donors. *Transfusion* 1995;35:91–97.
337. Alter HJ, Epstein JS, Swenson SG, et al. Prevalence of human immunodeficiency virus type 1 p24 antigen in U.S. blood donors an assessment of the efficacy of testing in donor screening. *N Engl J Med* 1990;323:1312–1317.
338. LePont F, Costagliola D, Rouzioux C, et al. How much would the safety of blood transfusion be improved by including p24 antigen in the battery of tests? *Transfusion* 1995;35:542–547.
339. Busch MP, Alter HJ. Will human immunodeficiency virus p24 antigen screening increase the safety of the blood supply and, if so, at what cost? *Transfusion* 1995;35:536–539.
340. Centers for Disease Control and Prevention. U.S. Public Health Service guidelines for testing and counseling blood and plasma donors for human immunodeficiency virus type 1 antigen. *MMWR Mortal Morb Wkly Rep* 1996;45:1–9.
341. Stramer SL, Caglioti S, Strong DM. NAT of the United States and Canadian blood supply. *Transfusion* 2000;40:1165–1168.
342. AuBuchon JP, Birkmeyer JD, Busch MP. Cost-effectiveness of expanded human immunodeficiency virus-testing protocols for donated blood. *Transfusion* 1997;37:45–51.
343. Yerly S, Pedrocchi M, Perrin L. The use polymerase chain reaction in plasma pools for the concomitant detection of hepatitis C virus and HIV type 1 RNA. *Transfusion* 1998;38:908–914.
344. Kemper M, Witt D, Madsen T, et al. The effects of dilution on the outcome of pooled plasma testing with HIV type 1 (HIV-1) RNA genome amplification as compared to the outcome of individual-unit testing with other HIV-1 markers. *Transfusion* 1998;38:469–472.
345. Ling AE, Robbins KE, Brown TM, et al. Failure of routine HIV-1 tests in a case involving transmission with preseroconversion blood components during the infectious window period. *JAMA* 2000;284: 210–214.
346. Busch MP, Eble BE, Khayam-Bashi H, et al. Evaluation of screened blood donations for human immunodeficiency virus type 1 infection by culture and DNA amplification of pooled cells. *N Engl J Med* 1991;325:1–5.
347. Centers for Disease Control and Prevention. Human immunodeficiency virus infection transmitted from an organ donor screened for HIV antibody—North Carolina. *MMWR Mortal Morb Wkly Rep* 1987;36:306–308.
348. Lee HH, Swanson P, Rosenblatt JD, et al. Relative prevalence and risk factors of HTLV-I and HTLV-II infection in U.S. blood donors. *Lancet* 1991;337:1435–1439.
349. Lackritz EM, Satten GA, Aberle-Grasse J, et al. Estimated risk of transmission of the human immunodeficiency virus by screened blood in the United States. *N Engl J Med* 1995;333:1721–1725.
350. Heymann SJ, Brewer TF, Feinberg HV, et al. How safe is safe enough? New infections and the U.S. blood supply. *Ann Intern Med* 1992; 117:612–614.
351. Korelitz JJ, Busch MP, Kleinman SH, et al. Relationship between antibody to hepatitis B core antigen and retroviral infections in blood from volunteer donors. *Transfusion* 1996;36:232–237.
352. Rawal BD, Busch MP, Endow R, et al. Reduction of human immunodeficiency virus-infected cells from donor blood by leukocyte filtration. *Transfusion* 1989;29:460–462.
353. Matthews JL, Sogandares-Bernal F, Judy MM, et al. Preliminary studies of photoinactivation of human immunodeficiency virus in blood. *Transfusion* 1991;31:636–641.
354. Kloser PC, Mangia AJ, Leonard J, et al. HIV-2-associated AIDS in the United States. *Arch Intern Med* 1989;149:1875–1877.
355. Larson CJ, Taswell HF. Human T-cell leukemia virus type I (HTLV-I) and blood transfusion. *Mayo Clin Proc* 1988;63:869–875.
356. Williams AE, Fang CT, Slamon DJ, et al. Seroprevalence and epidemiological correlates of HTLV-I infection in U.S. blood donors (erratum in *Science* 1989;244:757). *Science* 1988;240:643–646.
357. Centers for Disease Control and Prevention. Testing for antibodies to human immunodeficiency virus type-2 in the United States. *MMWR Mortal Morb Wkly Rep* 1992;41:1–9.
358. Centers for Disease Control and Prevention. Update: HIV-2 infection among blood and plasma donors—United States, June 1992–June 1995. *MMWR Mortal Morb Wkly Rep* 1995;44:603–606.
359. Centers for Disease Control and Prevention. Human T-lymphotropic virus type I screening in volunteer blood donors—United States, 1989. *MMWR Mortal Morb Wkly Rep* 1990;39:915, 921–924.
360. Centers for Disease Control and Prevention and the U.S.P.H.S. Working Group. Guidelines for counseling persons infected with human T-lymphotropic virus type I (HTLV-1) and type II (HTLV-II). *Ann Intern Med* 1993;118:448–454.
361. Murphy EL, Watanabe K, Nass CC, et al. Evidence among blood donors for a 30-year-old epidemic of human T lymphotropic virus type II infection in the United States. *J Infect Dis* 1999;180: 1777–1783.
362. deStasio G, Canavaggio M, Rizzi L, et al. Screening for anti human T-lymphotropic virus antibody in blood donors and polytransfused patients in Apulia (Italy). *Vox Sang* 1990;59:167–171.
363. Okochi K, Sato H, Hinuma Y. A retrospective study on transmission of adult T-cell leukemia virus by blood transfusion: seroconversion in recipients. *Vox Sang* 1984;46:245–253.
364. Kleinman S, Swanson P, Allain JP, Lee H. Transfusion transmission of human T-lymphotropic virus types I and II: serologic and polymerase chain reaction results in recipients identified through look-back investigations. *Transfusion* 1993;31:14–18.
365. Vrielink H, Zaaijer HL, Reesink HW. The clinical relevance of HTLV type I and II in transfusion medicine. *Transfusion Med Rev* 1997;11: 173–179.
366. Nelson KE, Donahue JG, Munoz A, et al. Transmission of retroviruses from seronegative donors by transfusion during cardiac surgery. *Ann Intern Med* 1992;117:554–559.
367. Roman GC. The neuroepidemiology of tropical spastic paraparesis. *Ann Neurol* 1988;23(Suppl):S113–S120.
368. Kalyanaraman VS, Sacngadharan MG, Robert-Guroff M, et al. A new subtype of human T-cell leukemia virus (HTLV-II) associated with a T-cell variant of hairy cell leukemia. *Science* 1982;218:571–573.
369. Hjelle B, Appenzeller O, Mills R, et al. Chronic neurodegenerative disease associated with HTLV-II infection. *Lancet* 1992;339: 645–646.
370. Tedder RS, Shanson DC, Jeffries DJ, et al. Low prevalence in the U.K. of HTLV-I and HTLV-II infection in subjects with AIDS with extended lymphadenopathy and at risk of AIDS. *Lancet* 1984;2: 125–128.
371. Centers for Disease Control and Prevention. Update: serologic testing for human T-lymphotropic virus type I, United States, 1989 and 1990. *MMWR Mortal Morb Wkly Rep* 1992;41:259–262.
372. Donegan E, Busch MP, Galleshaw JA, et al. Transfusion of blood components from a donor with human T-lymphotropic virus type II (HTLV-II) infection. *Ann Intern Med* 1990;113:555–556.
373. Zhang X, Constantine NT, Bansal J, et al. Evaluation of a new generation synthetic peptide combination assay for detection of antibodies to HIV-1, HIV-2, HTLV-I, and HTLV-II simultaneously. *J Med Virol* 1992;38:49–53.
374. Bendinelli M, Pistello M, Maggi F, et al. Molecular properties, biology, and clinical implications of TT virus, a recently identified widespread infectious agent of humans. *Clin Microbiol Rev* 2001;14: 98–113.
375. Desai SM, Muerhoff AS, Leary TP, et al. Prevalence of TT virus in US blood donors and populations at risk for acquiring parenterally transmitted viruses. *J Infect Dis* 1999;179:1242–1244.
376. Matsumoto A, Yeo AET, Shih JWK, et al. Transfusion-associated TT virus infection and its relationship to liver disease. *Hepatology* 1999; 30:283–288.
377. Bowden S, Locarnini S. TT virus: an agent of transfusion-associated hepatitis or yellow herring? *J Gastroenterol Hepatol* 1999;14:299–300.
378. Kobayashi M, Chayama K, Arase Y, et al. Prevalence of TT virus

before and after blood transfusion in patients with chronic liver disease treated surgically for hepatocellular carcinoma. J. *Gastroenterol Hepatol* 1999;14:358–363.

379. Lefrère, JJ, Roudot-Thoraval F, Lefrère F, et al. Natural history of the TT virus infection through follow-up of TTV DNA-positive multiple-transfused patients. *Blood* 2000;95:347–351.
380. Umemura T, Yeo AET, Sottini A, et al. SEN virus infection and its relationship to transfusion-associated hepatitis. *Hepatology* 2001;33: 1303–1311.
381. Kao JH, Chen W, Chen PJ, et al. SEN virus infection in patients with chronic hepatitis C: preferential coinfection with hepatitis C genotype 2a and no effect on response to therapy with interferon plus ribavirin. *J Infect Dis* 2003;187:307–310.
382. Petersen LR, Marfin AA. West Nile virus: a primer for the clinician. *Ann Intern Med* 2002;137:173–179.
383. Petersen LR, Roehrig JT. West Nile virus: a reemerging global pathogen. *Emerg Infect Dis* 2001;7:611–614.
384. Nash D, Mostashari F, Fine A, et al. The outbreak of West Nile virus infection in the New York City area in 1999. *N Engl J Med* 2001; 344:1807–1814.
385. Centers for Disease Control and Prevention. Provisional surveillance summary of the West Nile virus epidemic–United States, January—November 2002. *MMWR* 2002;51:1129–1133.
386. Centers for Disease Control and Prevention. Acute flaccid paralysis syndrome associated with West Nile virus infection–Mississippi and Louisiana, July—August 2002. *MMWR* 2002;51:825–828.
387. Centers for Disease Control and Prevention. Public health dispatch: investigations of West Nile virus infections in recipients of blood transfusion. *MMWR* 2002;51:973–974.
388. Biggerstaff BJ, Petersen LR. Estimated risk of West Nile virus transmission through blood transfusion during an epidemic in Queens, New York City. *Transfusion* 2002;42:1019–1026.
389. Food and Drug Administration. Recommendations for the assessment of donor suitability and blood and blood product safety in cases of known or suspected West Nile virus infections. *Final guidance,* issued May 1, 2003.
390. Hughes LE, Casper EA, Clifford CM. Persistence of Colorado tick fever virus in red blood cells. *Am J Trop Med Hyg* 1974;23:530–532.
391. Centers for Disease Control and Prevention. Transmission of Colorado tick fever virus by blood transfusion—Montana. *MMWR Mortal Morb Wkly Rep* 1975;24:422–427.
392. Mosley JW. Should measures be taken to reduce the risk of human parvovirus (B19) infection by transfusion of blood components and clotting factor concentrates? *Transfusion* 1994;34:744–746.
393. Mortimer PP, Luban NLC, Kelleher JF, et al. Transmission of serum parvovirus-like virus by clotting factor concentrates. *Lancet* 1983;2: 482–484.
394. Lefrère JJ, Mariotti M, Thauvin M. B19 parvovirus DNA in solvent/detergent-treated anti-haemophilia concentrates. *Lancet* 1994;343: 211–212.
395. Zanella A, Rossi F, Cesana C, et al. Transfusion-transmitted human parvovirus B19 infection in a thalassemic patient. *Transfusion* 1995; 35:769–772.
396. Cohen BJ, Beard S, Knowles WA, et al. Chronic anemia due to parvovirus B19 infection in a bone marrow transplant patient after platelet transfusion. *Transfusion* 1997;37:947–952.
397. Hayakawa F, Imada K, Towatari M, et al. Life-threatening human parvovirus B19 infection transmitted by intravenous immune globulin. *Br J Hematol* 2002;118:1187–1189.
398. Lefrère JJ, Mariotti M, De La Croix I, et al. Albumin batches and B19 parvovirus DNA. *Transfusion* 1995;35:389–391.
399. McOmish F, Yap PL, Jordan A, et al. Detection of parvovirus B19 in donated blood: a model system for screening by polymerase chain reaction. *J Clin Microbiol* 1993;31:323–328.
400. Azzi A, Morfini M, Mannucci PM. The transfusion-associated transmission of parvovirus B19. *Transfusion Med Rev* 1999;13:194–204.
401. Brown KE, Young NS, Alving BM, et al. Parvovirus B19: implications for transfusion medicine. Summary of a workshop. *Transfusion* 2001; 41:130–135.
402. Jordan J, Tiangco B, Kiss J, et al. Human parvovirus B19: prevalence of viral DNA in volunteer blood donors and clinical outcomes of transfusion recipients. *Vox Sang* 1998;75:97–102.
403. Henderson DA, Inglesby TV, Bartlett JG, et al. Smallpox as a biological weapon. Medical and Public Health Management. *JAMA* 1999; 281:2127–2137.
404. Blattner RJ, Norman JO, Heys FM, et al. Antibody response to cutaneous inoculation with vaccinia virus: viremia and viruria in vaccinated children. *J Pediatr* 1964;64:839–852.
405. Kempe CH. Studies on smallpox and complications of smallpox vaccination. *Pediatrics* 1960;26:176–189.
406. Food and Drug Administration. Final guidance: recommendations for deferral of donors and quarantine and retrieval of blood and blood products in recent recipients of smallpox vaccine (vaccinia virus) and certain contacts of smallpox vaccine recipients. December, 2002.
407. Houston F, Foster JD, Chong A, et al. Transmission of BSE by blood transfusion in sheep. *Lancet* 2002;356:999–1000.
408. Huner N, Foster J, Chong A, et al. Transmission of prion diseases by blood transfusion. *J Gen Virol* 2002;83:2897–2905.
409. Hoots WK, Abrams C, Tankersley D. The impact of Creutzfeldt-Jakob disease and variant Creutzfeldt-Jakob disease on plasma safety. *Transfusion Med Rev* 2001;15(Suppl 1):45–59.
410. Guerrero IC, Weniger BC, Schultz MG. Transfusion malaria in the United States, 1972–1981. *Ann Intern Med* 1983;99:221–226.
411. Lettau LA. Nosocomial transmission and infection control aspects of parasitic and ectoparasitic diseases. Part II. Blood and tissue parasites. *Infect Control Hosp Epidemiol* 1991;12:111–121.
412. Mungai M, Tegtmeier G, Chamberland M, et al. Transfusion-transmitted malaria in the United States from 1963 through 1999. *N Engl J Med* 2001;344:1973–1978.
413. Slinger R, Giulivi A, Bodie-Colllins M, et al. Transfusion-transmitted malaria in Canada. *CMAJ* 2001;164:377–379.
414. Shulman IA. Parasitic infections and their impact on blood donor selection and testing. *Arch Pathol Lab Med* 1994;118:366–370.
415. Silvie O, Thellier M, Rosenheim M, et al. Potential value of *Plasmodium falciparum*-associated antigen and antibody detection for screening of blood donors to prevent transfusion-transmitted malaria. *Transfusion* 2002;42:357-362.
416. Bruce-Chwatt LJ. From Laveran's discovery to DNA probes: new trends in diagnosis of malaria. *Lancet* 1987;2:1509–1511.
417. Smith OM, Traul DL, McOlash L, et al. Evaluation of merocyanine–540-sensitized photoirradiation as a method for purging malarially infected red cells from blood. *J Infect Dis* 1991;163:1312–1317.
418. McQuiston JH, Childs JE, Chamberland ME, et al. Transmission of tick-bourne agents of disease by blood transfusion: a review of known and potential risks in the United States. *Transfusion* 2002;40: 274–284.
419. Pantanowitz L, Telford SR III, Cannon ME. The impact of babesiosis on transfusion medicine. *Transfusion Med Rev* 2002:16:131–143.
420. Mintz ED, Anderson JF, Cable RG, et al. Transfusion-transmitted babesiosis: a case report from a new endemic area. *Transfusion* 1991; 31:365–368.
421. Popovsky MA, Lindberg LE, Syrek AL, et al. Prevalence of *Babesia* antibody in a selected blood donor population. *Transfusion* 1988;28: 59–61.
422. Herwaldt BL, Kjemtrup AM, Conrad PA, et al. Transfusion-transmitted babesiosis in Washington state: first reported case caused by a WA1-type parasite. *J Infect Dis* 1997;175:1259–1262.
423. Dobroszycki J, Herwaldt BL, Boctor F, et al. A cluster of transfusion-associated babesiosis cases traced to a single asymptomatic donor. *JAMA* 1999;281:927–930.
424. Perdrizet GA, Olson NH, Krause PJ, et al. Babesiosis in a renal transplant recipient acquired through blood transfusion. *Transplantation* 2000;70:205–208.
425. Kain KC, Jassoum SB, Fong IW, et al. Transfusion-transmitted babesiosis in Ontario: first reported case in Canada. *Can Med Assoc J* 2001; 164:1721–1723.
426. Shulman IA, Appleman MD. Transmission of parasitic and bacterial infections through blood transfusion within the U.S. *Crit Rev Clin Lab Sci* 1991;28:447–459.

427. Iacopino V, Earnhart T. Life-threatening babesiosis in a woman from Wisconsin. *Arch Intern Med* 1990;150:1527–1528.
428. Schmunis GA. Trypanosoma, the etiologic agent of Chagas' disease: status in the blood supply in endemic and nonendemic countries. *Transfusion* 1991;31:547–557.
429. Schmunis GA, Zicker F, Pinheiro F, et al. Risk for transfusion-transmitted infectious diseases in Central and South America. *Emerg Infect Dis* 1998;1:5–11.
430. Skolnick A. Does influx from endemic areas mean more Chagas' disease [news]? *JAMA* 1989;262:1433.
431. Leiby DA, Fucci MH, Stumpf RJ. *Trypanosoma cruzi* in a low-to moderate-risk blood donor population: seroprevalence and possible congenital transmission. *Transfusion* 1999;39:310–315.
432. Grant IH, Gold JWM, Wittner M, et al. Transfusion-associated acute Chagas' disease acquired in the United States. *Ann Intern Med* 1989; 111:849–851.
433. Nickerson P, Orr P, Schroeder ML, et al. Transfusion-associated *Trypanosoma cruzi* infection in a non-endemic area. *Ann Intern Med* 1989; 111:851–853.
434. Cimo PL, Luper WE, Scouros MA. Transfusion-associated Chagas' disease in Texas: report of a case. *Tex Med* 1993;89:48–50.
435. Kirchhoff LV. Is *Trypanosoma cruzi* a new threat to our blood supply? *Ann Intern Med* 1989;111:773–775.
436. Kerndt PR, Waskin HA, Kirchhoff LV, et al. Prevalence of antibody to *Trypanosoma cruzi* among blood donors in Los Angeles, California. *Transfusion* 1991;31:814–818.
437. Galel SA, Kirchhoff LV. Risk factors for *Trypanosoma cruzi* infection in California blood donors. *Transfusion* 1996;36:227–231.
438. Oelemann WMR, Vanderborght BOM, Verissimo Da Costa GC, et al. A recombinant peptide antigen line immunoassay optimized for the confirmation of Chagas' disease. *Transfusion* 1999;39:711–717.
439. Siegel SE, Lund MN, Gelderman AH, et al. Transmission of toxoplasmosis by leukocyte transfusion. *Blood* 1971;37:388–394.
440. Miller MJ, Aronson WJ, Remington JS. Late parasitemia in asymptomatic acquired toxoplasmosis. *Ann Intern Med* 1969;71:139–145.
441. Otero AC, da Silva VO, Luz KG, et al. Occurrence of *Leishmania donovani* DNA in donated blood from seroreactive Brazilian blood donors. *Am J Trop Med Hyg* 2000;62:128–131.
442. DeSchryver A, Meheus A. Syphilis and blood transfusion: a global perspective. *Transfusion* 1990;30:844–847.
443. Schmidt PJ. Syphilis, a disease of direct transfusion. *Transfusion* 2001; 41:1069–1071.
444. Chambers RW, Foley HT, Schmidt PJ. Transmission of syphilis by fresh blood components. *Transfusion* 1969;9:32–34.
445. Orton S. Syphilis and blood donors: what we know, what we do not know, and what we need to know. *Transfusion Med Rev* 2001;15: 282–292.
446. Van der Sluis, JJ, ten Kate FJW, Vuzevski VD, et al. Transfusion syphilis, survival of *Treponema pallidum* in stored donor blood. I. Dose dependence of experimentally determined survival times. *Vox Sang* 1985;49:390–399.
447. Ramsey G, Soltis F, Bowman R, et al. Syphilis serology in blood donors: a possible surrogate marker for human immunodeficiency virus risk. *Vox Sang* 1991;60:165–168.
448. Greenwalt TJ, Rios JA. To test or not to test for syphilis: a global problem. *Transfusion* 2001;41:976.
449. Orton SL, Liu H, Dodd RY, et al. Prevalence of circulating Treponema pallidum DNA and RNA in blood donors with confirmed-positive syphilis tests. *Transfusion* 2002;42:94–99.
450. Steere AC. *Borrelia burgdorferi* (Lyme disease, Lyme borreliosis). In: Mandell GL, Bennett JE, Dolin R, eds. *Principles and practice of infectious diseases,* 5th ed. Philadelphia: Churchill Livingstone, 2000: 2504–2518.
451. Aoki SK, Holland PV. Lyme disease another transfusion risk? *Transfusion* 1989;29:646–650.
452. Badon SJ, Fister RD, Cable RG. Survival of *Borrelia burgdorferi* in blood products. *Transfusion* 1989;29:581–583.
453. Nadelman RB, Sherer C, Mack L, et al. Survival of *Borrelia burgdorferi* in human blood stored under blood banking conditions. *Transfusion* 1990;30:298–301.
454. Bohme M, Schwenecke S, Fuchs E, et al. Screening of blood donors and recipients for *Borrelia burgdorferi* antibodies: no evidence of *B. burgdorferi* infection transmitted by transfusion. *Infusionsther Transfusionsmed* 1992;19:204–207.
455. Wang CW, Lee CU. Malaria and relapsing fever after blood transfusion including the report of a case of congenital transmission of relapsing fever. *Chin Med J* 1936;50:241–248.
456. Hira PR, Husein SF. Some transfusion-induced parasitic infections in Zambia. *J Hyg Epidemiol Microbiol Immunol* 1979;23:436–444.
457. Morduchowicz G, Pitlik SD, Huminer D, et al. Transfusion reactions due to bacterial contamination of blood and blood products. *Rev Infect Dis* 1991;13:307–314.
458. Sazama K. Bacteria in blood for transfusion. *Arch Pathol Lab Med* 1994;118:350–365.
459. Wagner SJ, Friedman LI, Dodd RY. Transfusion-associated bacterial sepsis. *Clin Microbiol Rev* 1994;7:290–302.
460. Klein HG, Dodd RY, Ness PM, et al. Current status of microbial contamination of blood components: summary of a conference. *Transfusion* 1997;37:95–101.
461. Readin FC, Brecher ME. Transfusion-related bacterial sepsis. *Curr Opin Hematol* 2001;8:380–386.
462. Blajchman MA, Goldman M. Bacterial contamination of platelet concentrates: incidence, significance, and prevention. *Semin Hematol* 2001;38(Suppl 11):20–26.
463. Heltberg O, Skov F, Gerner-Smidt P, et al. Nosocomial epidemic of *Serratia marcescens* septicemia ascribed to contaminated blood transfusion bags. *Transfusion* 1993;33:221–227.
464. Economidou J, Kalafatas P, Vatopoulou T, et al. Brucellosis in two thalassemic patients infected by blood transfusion from the same donor. *Acta Haemat* 1976;55:244–249.
465. Jacobs J, Jamaer D, Vandeven J, et al. *Yersinia enterocolitica* in donor blood: a case report and review. *J Clin Microbiol* 1989;27:1119–1121.
466. Aber RC. Transfusion-associated Yersinia. *Transfusion* 1990;30: 193–195.
467. Wilkinson TJ, Colls BM, Chambers ST, et al. Blood transfusion acquired *Yersinia enterocolitica* sepsis: two cases. *N Z Med J* 1991;104: 121–122.
468. Centers for Disease Control and Prevention. *Yersinia enterocolitica* bacteremia and endotoxin shock associated with red blood cell transfusions—U.S., 1991. *JAMA* 1991;265:2174–2175.
469. Centers for Disease Control and Prevention. Red blood cell transfusions contaminated with *Yersinia enterocolitica*—United States, 1991–1996, and initiation of a national study to detect bacteria-associated transfusion reactions. *MMWR Mortal Morb Wkly Rep* 1997; 46:553–555.
470. Theakston EP, Morris AJ, Streat SJ, et al. Transfusion transmitted *Yersinia enterocolitica* infection in New Zealand. *Aust N Z J Med* 1997; 27:62–67.
471. Blei F, Puder DR. *Yersinia enterocolitica* bacteremia in a chronically transfused patient with sick cell anemia case report and review of the literature. *Am J Pediatr Hematol Oncol* 1993;15:430–434.
472. Doganay M, Aygen B, Esel D. Brucellosis due to blood transfusion. *J Hosp Infect* 2001;49:151–152.
473. Hoogkamp-Korstanje JAA, deKoning J, Hesseman J. Persistence of *Yersinia enterocolitica* in man. *Infection* 1988;16:81–85.
474. Gibb AP, Martin KM, Davidson GA, et al. Modeling the growth of *Yersinia enterocolitica* in donated blood. *Transfusion* 1994;34: 304–310.
475. Siblini L, Lafeuillade B, Ros A, et al. Reduction of *Yersinia enterocolitica* load in deliberately inoculated blood: the effects of blood prestorage temperature and WBC filtration. *Transfusion* 2002;42: 422–427.
476. Ali A, Lyn P, Bordossy L, et al. Reduction by in-line leukocyte filtration of bacterial contaminants is more effective after an 8 hour hold at 22c than at 4c. *Transfusion* 1997;37(Suppl):12S.
477. Ness P, Braine H, King K, et al. Single-donor platelets reduce the risk of septic platelet transfusion reactions. *Transfusion* 2001;41:857–861.
478. Goldman M, Blajchman MA. Blood product-associated bacterial sepsis. *Transfusion Med Rev* 1991;5:73–83.

479. Centers for Disease Control and Prevention. Bacterial contamination of platelet pools—Ohio, 1991. *MMWR Mortal Morb Wkly Rep* 1992; 41:36–37.
480. Leiby DA, Kerr KL, Campos JM, et al. A retrospective analysis of microbial contaminants in outdated random-donor platelets from multiple sites. *Transfusion* 1997;37:259–263.
481. Wagner SJ, Robinette D. Evaluation of swirling, pH, and glucose tests for the detection of bacterial contamination in platelet concentrates. *Transfusion* 1996;36:989–993.
482. Burstain JM, Brecher ME, Workman K, et al. Rapid identification of bacterially contaminated platelets using reagent strips: glucose and pH analysis as markers of bacterial metabolism. *Transfusion* 1997;37: 255–258.
483. Wagner SJ, Robinette D. Evaluation of an automated microbiologic blood culture device for detection of bacteria in platelet components. *Transfusion* 1998;38:674–679.
484. Brecher ME, Means N, Jere CS, et al. Evaluation of an automated culture system for detecting bacterial contamination of platelets: an analysis with 15 contaminating organisms. *Transfusion* 2001;41: 477–482.
485. Rebulla P, Finazzi G, Marangoni F, et al. The threshold for prophylactic platelet transfusions in adults with acute myeloid leukemia. *N Engl J Med* 1997;337:1870–1875.
486. Kruskall MS. The perils of platelet transfusions. *N Engl J Med* 1997; 337:1914–1915.
487. Wandt H, Frank M, Ehninger G, et al. Safety and cost effectiveness of a 10 x 10^9/L trigger for prophylactic platelet transfusions compared with the traditional 20 x 10^9/L trigger: a prospective comparative trial in 105 patients with acute myeloid leukemia. *Blood* 1998;91: 3601–3606.
488. Schiffer CA, Anderson KC, Bennett CL, et al. Platelet transfusion for patients with cancer: clinical practice guidelines of the American Society of Clinical Oncology. *J Clin Oncol* 2001;19:1519–1538.
489. Centers for Disease Control and Prevention. Q fever. *MMWR Mortal Morb Wkly Rep* 1976;47:86–87.
490. Wells GM, Woodward TE, Fiset P, et al. Rocky Mountain spotted fever caused by blood transfusion. *JAMA* 1978;239:2763–2765.
491. Eastlund T, Persing D, Mathiesen D, et al. Human granulocytic ehrlichiosis after red cell transfusion. *Transfusion* 1999;39(Suppl): 117S.
492. Mannucci PM, Morfini M, Gatti L, et al. No hepatitis after treatment with a modified factor IX concentrate in previously untreated hemophiliacs. *Ann Intern Med* 1985;103:226–227.
493. Rodell MB, Bergman GE. Safety of monoclonal antibody purified factor VIII. *Lancet* 1990;336:188.
494. Mannucci PM, Schimpf K, Brettler DB, et al. Low risk for hepatitis C in hemophiliacs given a high-purity, pasteurized factor VIII concentrate. *Ann Intern Med* 1990;113:27–32.
495. Solheim BG, Rollag H, Svennevig JL, et al. Viral safety of solvent/detergent-treated plasma. *Transfusion* 2000;40:84–90.
496. Biesert L, Suhartono H. Solvent/detergent treatment of human plasma—a very robust method for virus inactivation. Validated virus safety of OCTAPLAS. *Vox Sang* 1998;71(Suppl 1):207–212.
497. Wieding JU, Hellstern P, Kohler M. Inactivation of viruses in fresh-frozen plasma. *Ann Hematol* 1993;67:259–266.
498. Horowitz B, Williams B, Rywkin S, et al. Inactivation of viruses in blood with aluminum phthalocyanine derivatives. *Transfusion* 1991; 31:102–108.
499. Lin L, Cook DN, Wiesehahn GP, et al. Photochemical inactivation of viruses and bacteria in platelet concentrates by use of a novel psoralen and long-wavelength ultraviolet light. *Transfusion* 1997;37: 423–435.
500. Wagner SJ, Skripchenko A, Robinette D, et al. Preservation of red cell properties after virucidal phototreatment with dimethylmethylene blue. *Transfusion* 1998;38:729–737.
501. Corash L. New technologies for the inactivation of infectious pathogens in cellular blood components and the development of platelet substitutes. *Baillières Clin Haematol* 2000;13:549–563.
502. Surgenor DM, Wallace EL, Hao SHS, et al. Collection and transfusion of blood in the United States, 1982–1988. *N Engl J Med* 1990; 322:1646–1651.
503. Kruskall MS, Umlas J. Acquired immunodeficiency syndrome and directed blood donations. A dilemma for American medicine. *Arch Surg* 1988;123:23–25.
504. Morad Z, Suleiman AB, Kong CT. Hepatitis in renal transplant recipients with and without donor-specific blood transfusion. *Transplant Proc* 1989;21:1825–1826.
505. Liver H, Lachman M, Badon S. The impact of a patient education program on directed donations. *Transfusion* 1991;31:518–520.
506. Popovsky MA, Devine PA, Taswell HF. Intraoperative autologous transfusion. *Mayo Clin Proc* 1985;60:125–134.
507. Goodnough LT, Brecher ME, Kanter MH, et al. Transfusion medicine (second of two parts). Blood conservation. *N Engl J Med* 1999; 340:525–533.
508. Spahn DR, Casutt M. Eliminating blood transfusion. *Anesthesiology* 2000;93:242–255.
509. Thomas MJG, Desmond MJ, Gillon J. Consensus conference on autologous transfusion. General background paper. *Transfusion* 1996; 36:628–632.
510. Thomas MJG, Gillon J, Desmond MJ. Consensus conference on autologous transfusion. Preoperative autologous donation. *Transfusion* 1996;36:633–639.
511. Forgie MA, Wells PS, Laupacis A, et al. Preoperative autologous donation decreases allogeneic transfusion but increases exposure to all red blood cell transfusion. *Arch Intern Med* 1998;158:610–616.
512. Desmond MJ, Thomas MJG, Gillon J, et al. Consensus conference on autologous transfusion. Perioperative red cell salvage. *Transfusion* 1996;36:644–651.
513. Boudreaux JP, Bornside GH, Cohn I. Emergency autotransfusion: partial cleansing of bacteria-laden blood by cell washing. *J Trauma* 1983;23:31–35.
514. Wollinsky KH, Oethinger M, Büchele M, et al. Autotransfusion bacterial contamination during hip arthroplasty and efficacy of cefuroxime prophylaxis. *Acta Orthop Scand* 1997;68:225–230.
515. Renner SW, Howanitz PJ, Bachner P. Preoperative autologous blood donation in 612 hospitals. A College of American Pathologists Q-probes study of quality issues in transfusion practice. *Arch Pathol Lab Med* 1992;116:613–619.
516. Birkmeyer JD, Goodnough LT, AuBuchon JP, et al. The cost-effectiveness of preoperative autologous blood donation for total hip and knee replacement. *Transfusion* 1993;33:544–551.
517. Birkmeyer JD, AuBuchon JP, Littenberg B, et al. Cost-effectiveness of preoperative autologous donation in coronary artery bypass grafting. *Ann Thorac Surg* 1994;57:161–169.
518. Kruskall MS, Yomtovian R, Dzik WH, et al. On improving the cost-effectiveness of autologous blood transfusion practices. *Transfusion* 1994;34:259–264.
519. Etchason J, Petz L, Keeler E, et al. The cost effectiveness of preoperative autologous blood donations. *N Engl J Med* 1995;332:719–724.
520. Forbes JM, Anderson MD, Anderson GF, et al. Blood transfusion costs: a multicenter study. *Transfusion* 1991;31:318–323.
521. Rutherford CJ, Kaplan HS. Autologous blood donation: can we bank on it? *N Engl J Med* 1995;332:740–742.
522. Yomtovian R, Kruskall MS, Barber JP. Autologous-blood transfusion: the reimbursement dilemma. *J Bone Joint Surg [Am]* 1992;74A: 1265–1272.
523. Palani CK, DeWoskin R, Moss GS. Scope and limitations of stroma-free hemoglobin solution as an oxygen-carrying blood substitute. *Surg Clin North Am* 1975;55:3–10.
524. Dodd RY. The risk of transfusion-transmitted infection. *N Engl J Med* 1992;327:419–421.
525. Moscucci M, Ricciardi M, Eagle KA, et al. Frequency, predictors, and appropriateness of blood transfusion after percutaneous coronary interventions. *Am J Cardiol* 1998;81:702–707.
526. Hebert PC, Wells G, Blajchman MA, et al. A multicenter, randomized, controlled clinical trial of transfusion requirements in critical care. *N Engl J Med* 1999;340:409–417.

527. Wu WC, Rathore SS, Wang Y, et al. Blood transfusion in elderly patients with acute myocardial infarction. *N Engl J Med* 2001;345: 1230–1236.
528. Valeri CR, Crowley JP, Loscalzo J. The red cell transfusion trigger: has a sin of commission now become a sin of omission? *Transfusion* 1998;38:602–610.
529. Mann MC, Votto J, Kambe J, et al. Management of the severely anemic patient who refuses transfusion: lessons learned during the care of a Jehovah's Witness. *Ann Intern Med* 1992;117:1042–1048.
530. Williamson LM, Lowe S, Love EM, et al. Serious hazards of transfusion (SHOT) initiative: analysis of the first two annual reports. *BMJ* 1999;319:16–19.

70

NOSOCOMIAL INFECTIONS ASSOCIATED WITH PROCEDURES PERFORMED IN RADIOLOGY

BRUCE S. RIBNER

The radiology department has traditionally been considered a low-risk environment for nosocomial infections. However, major advances in the field of radiology over the past few decades, with the introduction of isotope scanning, ultrasound, computed tomography, magnetic resonance imaging, and the development of interventional radiology, have increased the potential for the transmission of infectious pathogens to both patients and healthcare workers. Unfortunately, an appreciation for the occurrence of nosocomial infections associated with these radiologic procedures has not kept pace with this technology (1). Few radiology texts address nosocomial infections associated with radiologic procedures. In addition, most invasive radiologic procedures introduced over the past few decades have not been prospectively analyzed for measures that could decrease the occurrence of nosocomial infections resulting from them. This is due, in part, to the rather limited time during which the radiologist interacts with the patient, and the resulting difficulty in achieving the long-term follow-up required to identify nosocomial infections.

This chapter summarizes the infectious complications associated with radiologic procedures and the infection control practices that might decrease the occurrence of these infections. As conclusive data regarding the prevention of nosocomial infections are lacking for many of these procedures, reliance is placed largely on related procedures performed in other specialties of medicine in which interventions that reduce the nosocomial transmission of infectious pathogens have been identified.

INFECTION CONTROL POLICY

The radiology suite experiences a steady stream of a wide variety of patients each day. Patients referred from the ambulatory care and emergency areas are intermixed with inpatients requiring diagnostic procedures. All of these patients can contaminate the environment of the radiology service with infectious pathogens. Chin supports and chest racks used in obtaining chest radiographs (2), radiography tables (2), radiographic film markers (3), barium enema equipment (4), x-ray tubes (5), and x-ray film and developing solutions (6) may all become contaminated with multiple microorganisms from patients. In addition, the ease with which *Clostridium difficile* contaminates the environment of the patient colonized with this microorganism (7) makes it likely that contamination of the radiology area with *C. difficile* occurs as well. This environmental contamination may result in the subsequent spread of pathogenic microorganisms from these objects to other patients. In addition to fomite transmission, potential pathogens may be spread to patients visiting the radiology area via the airborne route. Hopkins et al. (8) traced an outbreak of invasive aspergillosis in their hospital to construction activity in the radiology suite. Patients visiting the radiology suite for diagnostic procedures were infected when there was inadequate containment of aspergillus spores generated during renovation. Similarly, investigations of hospital outbreaks of multidrug-resistant tuberculosis have revealed that most cases were acquired within the facilities via the airborne route. A major factor in most of these outbreaks was a delay in initiating the isolation of patients infected with pulmonary tuberculosis (9). Many of these patients had made multiple visits to the radiology department with no precautions taken to prevent the transmission of respiratory pathogens, making it likely that some transmission occurred within the radiology department.

Given the large numbers of both diagnosed and undiagnosed infected patients presenting to the radiology department, and the potential for these patients to contaminate both objects and the air with pathogenic microorganisms, the foundation of any program for the prevention of nosocomial infections in the radiology department must begin by establishing good infection control policies. Among other issues, these policies must address the effective disinfection of environmental surfaces likely to act as fomites. The cleaning of these surfaces must be performed with an Environmental Protection Agency (EPA)-registered germicide (see Chapter 85) between all patients, with more rigorous cleaning protocols at periodic intervals (see Chapter 77). A material that can be either discarded or easily disinfected between patients should cover surfaces that may be difficult to disinfect, such as switches and control panels. Policies should ensure that all disposable items are discarded after a single patient use, as such items are not designed for reprocessing and reuse on multiple patients. Attention must also be given to the appropriate cleaning and disinfection of all reusable equipment, with the level of disinfection determined by the intended use of the item (see Chapter 85). Items that enter tissues or vascular spaces require sterilization. Items that contact mucous membranes or nonintact skin require high-level disinfection. Items that contact intact skin require only low-level disinfection.

The radiology department must also establish good communication with the clinical areas referring patients to the department so as to identify patients who may require transmission-based precautions. Patients on transmission-based precautions must have those precautions continued in the radiology department. When possible, patients on transmission-based precautions should undergo their procedures late in the day when traffic in the department is light and more attention can be given to environmental cleaning. These patients should also spend the minimum time possible in the radiology department so as to limit the potential exposure of susceptible patients and staff.

Due to concern about the nosocomial transmission of tuberculosis in the radiology suite (see Chapter 37), the Centers for Disease Control and Prevention (CDC) has published specific recommendations for precautions to be followed in radiology departments (9). Patients with known or suspected tuberculosis should wear a properly fitted surgical mask when in the department. When possible, an area in the department should be specially ventilated for Airborne Precautions. This requires a net negative air pressure in relation to surrounding areas, sufficient air changes to remove droplet nuclei between patients, and either direct exhausting of all air to the outside (preferred) or filtration of air through high-efficiency particulate air (HEPA) filters before it is recirculated. In facilities with a high incidence of tuberculosis, ventilation in waiting areas should also be designed and maintained to reduce the risk of tuberculosis transmission. This should include provisions for direct exhausting of all air to the outside (preferred) or HEPA filtration of all air before it is recirculated. A goal of 10 to 12 air changes per hour for such waiting areas has been established (10,11).

STANDARD PRECAUTIONS

The infection control measures discussed above protect employees and patients from the transmission of most potential pathogens. However, attention to the transmission of blood-borne pathogens in the workplace increased in the 1980s. Hepatitis B virus (HBV) and the human immunodeficiency virus (HIV) are the blood-borne pathogens that have attracted the most attention from healthcare workers and regulatory agencies (12).

Personnel working in radiology departments historically have not been considered a group at high risk for infection with blood-borne pathogens (12–14). However, radiology personnel are increasingly performing procedures that can result in exposure to blood and other potentially infectious materials (materials epidemiologically linked with the transmission of blood-borne pathogens) (15). Because a high percentage of patients infected with HBV (16) or HIV (17) are unidentified during their encounter with the healthcare system, it is essential that all patients be approached as though they are infected with blood-borne pathogens. This concept of using Universal Precautions (see Chapter 95) for blood and other potentially infectious materials of all patients was first suggested by the CDC in 1987 (18). These precautions were subsequently mandated by the Occupational Safety and Health Administration for all healthcare workers (12). In 1996, the CDC recommended replacement of universal precautions with standard precautions, a change aimed at focusing more attention on pathogens that are not primarily blood-borne (19). Reports have detailed how these precautions can be applied to the radiology department (15,19–22). In general, these recommendations mirror those for other areas of the hospital in which similar procedures are performed (Table 70.1).

TABLE 70.1. STANDARD PRECAUTIONS AS APPLIED TO RADIOLOGY

- Wash hands promptly and thoroughly after patient contact or contact with blood, body fluids, excretions, or secretions.
- All personnel who could be exposed to blood or other potentially infectious material must receive training on these risks and on ways to minimize these risks.
- Employees must be offered hepatitis B immunization free of charge within 10 days of being assigned to tasks that pose a risk of exposure to blood or other potentially infectious materials.
- Disposable sharps, such as needles and scalpels, must be discarded immediately after use into puncture-resistant containers located as close as practical to the point of use. Sharps should not be recapped, bent, or otherwise manipulated before being discarded.
- All personnel who are present at procedures that could involve contact with blood, body fluids, secretions, excretions, mucous membranes, or nonintact skin of patients must use appropriate barrier precautions. This may involve use of gloves, gowns, masks, goggles, or face shields, depending on the degree of potential exposure. Interventional radiologists may need to consider the length of the procedure when establishing gloving policies. Hansen et al. (22) found that 23% of the gloves worn for more than 2 hours during interventional radiology procedures were perforated by the end of the procedure. Few of these perforations were noted by the wearer. Similar data from other studies could support double-glove policies or the routine changing of gloves during prolonged interventional procedures.

SPECIFIC PROCEDURES

Radiographic Studies of the Gastrointestinal Tract

The spread of enteric pathogens during radiologic procedures of the gastrointestinal tract has been a matter of concern for a number of years. Meyers (4) and Steinbach et al. (23) demonstrated retrograde contamination of the apparatus used for administering barium during the performance of barium enemas. This equipment became heavily contaminated with fecal contents by the end of the procedure. Hervey (24) reported an outbreak of typhoid fever traced to an apparatus that resembles the equipment used to administer barium during a barium enema. In his investigation, as in those by Meyers and by Steinbach et al., it was noted that fecal contents could contaminate the apparatus and its tubing via retrograde flow during the procedure. Although the apparatus was cleaned between patients, sufficient microorganisms remained in the apparatus to infect patients on whom it was subsequently used. Similarly,

Meyers and Richards (25) were able to demonstrate that six of seven patients who underwent barium enemas after contamination of the bag contents with poliovirus became infected with the polio virus as documented by rises in serum neutralization antibodies to the virus. In a related report, 36 cases of amebiasis were traced to a contaminated colonic irrigation machine in an outpatient chiropractic clinic (26). Although the irrigation equipment was cleaned after each patient use, cultures of the machine immediately after cleaning revealed heavy contamination with fecal coliforms. The ease with which *C. difficile* contaminates the environment of colonized and infected patients (7) makes it likely that this bacterium is also present where gastrointestinal procedures are performed.

Given this potential for the transmission of enteric pathogens, all equipment used in barium enema procedures either must be subjected to high-level disinfection or must be disposable. In fact, disposable kits have replaced reusable equipment in most facilities (27,28).

Several investigators have documented bacteremia associated with radiologic studies of the gastrointestinal tract. In two large studies, 11% (29) and 23% (30) of patients undergoing barium enemas had bacteremia. In both reports, the bacteremia could be detected within 1 minute of the start of the procedure. This bacteremia was transient and could be documented only for 30 minutes. Radiologic findings and colonic pathology did not influence the likelihood of the occurrence of bacteremia. Bacteremia was most likely to occur during the maximal distention of the colon. In evaluating the patients in these studies, no adverse effects of the bacteremia could be documented. However, one episode of *Clostridium perfringens* sepsis has been reported in a patient with acute leukemia who underwent a barium enema (31). Although the transient bacteremia associated with the barium enema is unlikely to adversely affect most patients, bacterial endocarditis after a barium enema has been reported in one patient (32). This has, in turn, raised the question of antibiotic prophylaxis for the prevention of infective endocarditis (33,34). However, barium enemas have not been found to be a risk factor in studies evaluating the epidemiology of bacterial endocarditis. Although a definitive answer is probably not possible, the current consensus is to avoid the use of prophylactic antibiotics for patients undergoing barium enemas.

Ultrasound Procedures in Radiology

Ultrasonography has become an increasingly popular mode of evaluating a wide range of tissues. It is estimated that the average ultrasound machine may be used on as many as 30 patients a day, giving this equipment the potential to serve as an important fomite for the transmission of pathogens between patients (35). Although many of these procedures restrict the ultrasound probe to contact with intact skin, probes are also being utilized for procedures in which they come into contact with mucous membranes and normally sterile tissues, occasionally in the operating room. Several studies have documented heavy contamination of the ultrasound probe, especially after contact with a mucous membrane (35–37).

The standard manufacturer's recommendation for disinfection of the ultrasound probe is to soak the probe in a dilute sodium hypochlorite solution or an EPA-registered germicide for the time specified by the germicide's manufacturer, frequently 20 minutes. Unfortunately, the multiple procedures scheduled for these probes frequently preclude such long soak times. In addition, the probes may be damaged by total immersion in these solutions due to leakage around the seals or deterioration of the acoustic lens or rubber seals (35,38). In practice, routine cleaning of the probe followed by low-level disinfection with an alcohol wipe seems appropriate when procedures involve contact only with intact skin. For procedures where the probe comes into contact with mucous membranes or nonintact skin, thorough cleaning followed by high-level disinfection with an EPA-registered germicide is recommended (39,40). Because of the difficulty in achieving high-level disinfection, it is recommended that a new sheath, such as a condom, cover probes that will be in contact with mucous membranes or sterile tissues for each such procedure (39,40).

Endoscopic Procedures in Radiology

Other subspecialists such as gastroenterologists, pulmonologists, and surgeons perform endoscopic procedures much more frequently than they are performed by radiologists. Often, endoscopy is not performed in the radiology suite but rather in patient care areas, in the operating room, or in other dedicated areas such as laboratories within the hospital or ambulatory center. To the extent that endoscopy is performed in areas outside of radiology, general infection control policies similar to those recommended for the radiology suite need to be implemented.

Endoscopic procedures of the pulmonary tract (41,42), upper gastrointestinal tract (32,42–44), lower gastrointestinal tract (32,42), and biliary tract (42,45) have all been associated with nosocomial bacteremia and infections. *Salmonella* species and *Pseudomonas aeruginosa* are the most common pathogens isolated in infections after gastrointestinal endoscopy, whereas *Mycobacterium tuberculosis*, atypical mycobacteria, and *P. aeruginosa* are the most common isolates in infections after bronchoscopy (42). In general, *P. aeruginosa* and atypical mycobacteria tend to come from environmental contamination of the equipment, whereas *Salmonella* and *M. tuberculosis* originate in patients previously studied with the endoscopes.

Risk factors for nosocomial infections after endoscopy tend to fall into two categories. The major patient risk factor that increases the likelihood of bacteremia and infection following endoscopic gastrointestinal procedures is the inability to establish adequate drainage of the biliary tract after endoscopic retrograde cholangiopancreatography (ERCP) (33,45–47). This finding has led several authors to recommend that prophylactic antibiotics be administered to patients undergoing ERCP in whom adequate drainage cannot be established after the procedure. However, data are lacking to define the appropriate timing and the agents to be used (45–47).

As in the case of the barium enema, the question of antibiotic prophylaxis for the prevention of infective endocarditis after ERCP has been raised (32,33,47). The current consensus is to use prophylactic antibiotics in patients at moderate or high risk of endocarditis who are undergoing ERCP when biliary obstruction exists (33,47). Such increased-risk patients would include those with prosthetic heart valves, a previous history of bacterial endocarditis, congenital heart disease, acquired valvular dysfunction, hypertrophic cardiomyopathy, mitral prolapse with regurgitation or thickened leaflets, surgically constructed systemic-pulmonary shunts or conduits, and patients with synthetic vascular grafts for the first year after placement of the graft. Antibiotic prophylaxis in these patients should include parenteral agents directed against enterococci, most typically parenteral ampicillin or vancomycin together with gentamicin. As infections other than endocarditis after ERCP are rarely due to the enterococcus, this still leaves unresolved the issue of additional prophylaxis against other pathogens when adequate drainage cannot be established.

Failure to adequately disinfect the endoscope and associated equipment appears to be another major risk factor for bacteremia and sepsis associated with endoscopic procedures. Contaminated water bottles (48), inappropriate disinfectants (41), scope designs that make adequate disinfection of the endoscope difficult (49), and inadequate quality control over cleaning procedures for the endoscopes (50) have all contributed to nosocomial infections. (For a detailed discussion on cleaning and disinfection of endoscopes, see Chapter 63).

Myelography

Myelography is associated with an extremely low rate of nosocomial infections. Given the anatomic location of these infections, however, they can be catastrophic. Seventeen cases of meningitis after myelography have been reported (51–53). Oropharyngeal streptococci have caused most of these infections. The presumed source of these bacteria has been the oropharynx of the individual performing the procedure. This has been attributed to the fact that those performing the myelography frequently do not wear masks. The low incidence of this infectious complication has impeded the implementation of more stringent infection control measures (53). Nonetheless, the wearing of masks would appear to be a logical low-cost precaution for the prevention of this potentially lethal infection.

Vascular Radiology

Vascular radiology covers a wide range of procedures performed both by radiologists and cardiologists. As such, these procedures may be carried out both in the radiology suite and in designated catheterization laboratories outside of the radiology suite (see Chapter 62).

Simple angiography procedures generally have a very low rate of infectious complications. Although endocarditis after coronary angiography has been reported (54), prospective studies have found low rates of bacteremia and infectious intravascular complications associated with angiography. Sande et al. (55) found that none of 106 patients undergoing cardiac catheterization had detectable bacteremia or postprocedural intravascular infections. Shawker et al. (56) were able to detect bacteremia in 4 of 100 patients undergoing angiography of various vessels. Three of the four episodes were caused by inadequate sterilization of the catheter before the procedure. None of these patients developed any infectious sequelae. Infections at the insertion site of the catheter also appear to be quite infrequent. Laslett and Sabin (57) found no evidence of insertion site infection in 504 percutaneous left-sided heart catheterizations. Leaman and Zelis (58) were able to collect data on 107,203 cardiac catheterization procedures through a survey of 250 facilities. Only 0.06% of catheterizations performed by percutaneous insertion were reported to lead to insertion site infections. Catheterizations performed by cutdown had an insertion site infection rate of 0.62%. Although low, this was ten times the rate of site infection that occurred after percutaneous insertions.

In formulating infection control standards for simple angiography, it is generally agreed that the preparation of the insertion site should involve the same disinfection techniques as are used for other intravascular devices. Individuals performing the procedure should wash their hands with an antiseptic-containing hand washing agent before donning sterile gloves. Strict attention must be given to proper cleaning and sterilization of guidewires and catheters that are reused. For angiography performed via the percutaneous insertion technique, it would appear that the remaining elements of the environment might be less critical in preventing insertion site infections. Laslett and Sabin (57) and Leaman and Zelis (58) could demonstrate no benefit from the use of caps and masks by personnel performing the angiography in preventing site infections. Unfortunately, they did not address the issue of gowns for personnel involved in performing the procedure. Given the potential for inadvertent contact of the catheter with the body or arms of the personnel directly involved in the procedure, gowns for these individuals would seem appropriate, although there is no documentation that they are necessary. Leaman and Zelis's observations indicate that gowns do not appear to be necessary for ancillary personnel and observers.

The tenfold increase in insertion site infections associated with angiography performed via the cutdown approach would argue for avoiding this technique whenever possible. When the cutdown approach was required, Leaman and Zelis (58) found that the use of masks, caps, and gowns for all personnel and observers significantly decreased the rate of site infections. They also demonstrated a significant correlation between the number of cutdown procedures performed by a laboratory per year and the rate of insertion site infections. Laboratories performing more than 150 cutdown procedures per year had an insertion site infection rate of 0.49%. In contrast, laboratories performing fewer than 150 such procedures per year had an insertion site infection rate nearly three times greater (1.43%). This difference was statistically significant. This observation would argue for the importance of the learning curve in preventing nosocomial site infections associated with angiography.

Standard precautions require the consideration of attire not only to protect the patient from infection but also to protect the healthcare worker from exposure to blood and other potentially infectious materials. Thus, although the wearing of masks, caps, and gowns by personnel may not have been documented to prevent nosocomial infections in patients undergoing percutaneous angiography, the potential for blood exposure during these procedures requires the use of this attire to protect the healthcare worker from exposures (see Chapter 95). In addition, eye protection, such as goggles or face shields, is essential.

Interventional vascular radiology has moved substantially beyond simple angiography. Angioplasty, arthrectomy, the placement of intravascular stents, and embolotherapy are procedures that were introduced into the modern radiology suite and catheterization laboratory during the 1980s. Most of these procedures have been associated with low rates of nosocomial infection. Gardiner et al. (59) recorded no infectious complications in 453 transluminal angioplasties. However, Frazee and Flaherty (60) were able to identify ten patients with septic endarteritis of the femoral artery after percutaneous transluminal coronary angioplasty. Zollikofer et al. (61) noted no nosocomial infections after the placement of intravascular arterial stents in 21 vessels, but Gordon et al. (62) documented an episode of renal artery arteritis after placement of a renal artery stent and were able to find reports of four other cases of iliac artery arteritis after stent placement. Both Frazee and Flaherty and Gordon et al. found that reuse of an indwelling catheter or sheath left in a groin for more than 24 hours, repeated procedures, local hematoma formation, and increased procedure time increased the risk of arteritis.

Percutaneous transcatheter embolization is the intravascular deposition of particulate, liquid, or mechanical agents or an autologous blood clot to produce vessel occlusion (63). This procedure has been associated with a high number of postprocedural infections in certain settings. Whereas Higashida et al. (64) detected no infectious complications after the balloon embolization of 215 intracranial neurovascular aneurysms, Hemingway (65) recorded seven deaths from sepsis among 410 embolization procedures involving a variety of arteries. All seven patients who died had embolization of hepatic lesions. Although the patients who died were all extremely ill at the time of the procedure, it is of note that all deaths occurred among the early cases performed by their group. A decrease in sepsis as a complication of embolization was observed as the group gained experience with the procedure and as prophylactic antibiotics were introduced into their protocol. Embolization of the spleen has also been associated with a high rate of infectious complications. Initial reports cited the almost universal occurrence of splenic abscesses and sepsis after splenic embolization (66,67). After modification of this procedure, with a change to partial rather than total splenic embolization, the introduction of strict sterile technique, and the introduction of antibiotic prophylaxis, Spigos et al. (68) were able to perform splenic embolization on 13 patients without any postprocedural infectious complications. Since these modifications were introduced together, it is impossible to evaluate the efficacy of each intervention separately. Although not explicitly stated, the improvement in patient outcome occurred, as noted in Hemingway's series, as the author gained experience with the procedure.

Infection control guidelines in these newer forms of interventional vascular radiology should parallel those used for standard angiography. Strict attention to the disinfection of the insertion site and careful hand washing with an antiseptic-containing agent before donning sterile gloves are important. In angioplasty, arthrectomy, stent placement, and embolization of intracranial vessels, infectious risks appear to be small. However, adherence to Standard Precautions requires the use of masks, gowns, gloves, and goggles or face shields. The Society of Cardiovascular and Interventional Radiology has developed quality improvement guidelines for percutaneous transcatheter embolization (63). Antibiotic prophylaxis is recommended for embolization of the spleen and for other body sites where bacterial contamination is likely, such as the colon, open trauma, and liver. In the embolization of hepatic and splenic vessels, the potential for severe infectious complications appears to be great. Pending more detailed studies, strict attention to sterile technique, the use of prophylactic antibiotics, and performance of the procedure by those with the most experience would seem to offer the greatest benefit in preventing nosocomial infections.

Nonvascular Interventional Radiology

Nonvascular interventional radiology has evolved since the 1970s to include percutaneous biopsies, diagnostic and therapeutic aspiration of fluid, treatment of strictures, and removal of stones. Of these, the image-guided percutaneous biopsy has become the most frequently performed interventional radiologic procedure (69). Infections after such biopsies are uncommon. The Society of Cardiovascular and Interventional Radiology has set a performance standard for infectious complications of 1% for all biopsies and 3% for prostate biopsies (70).

The ability to drain visceral abscesses and collections of fluid, often in lieu of a surgical procedure, has become an increasingly important radiologic intervention. As might be expected, these drainage procedures are associated with a higher rate of infectious complications than are percutaneous biopsies. The Society of Cardiovascular and Interventional Radiology has set a threshold of 4% for septic shock and 10% for bacteremia associated with all abscess and fluid drainage procedures (71). vanSonnenberg et al. (72) summarized the outcomes of 250 percutaneous abscess and fluid drainage procedures. Two patients experienced sepsis with hypotension, and five others had bacteremia with fever after the procedure. One patient had secondary infection of a noninfected lymphocele after percutaneous drainage. An additional six patients were noted to have infections at the catheter insertion site. Again, as in other interventional radiologic procedures, the authors emphasized that most infectious complications occurred early in the group's experience with the technique. It is also worth noting that although the infectious complication rate approached 6%, it was lower than the rate observed in an equivalent population undergoing surgical procedures to drain fluid collections (73).

Percutaneous transhepatic drainage of the biliary tract for acute relief of obstruction is an extension of the percutaneous drainage procedure. Drainage in most such patients is either palliative, when the obstruction is secondary to malignancy, or a preoperative measure to decrease the degree of patient illness when obstruction is secondary to cholelithiasis, stricture, or malignancy (74–77). Most of these patients have evidence of cholangitis with multiple bacterial pathogens before the procedure, often with bacteremia. Given the degree of preexisting illness in many of these patients, it is not surprising that some series have reported high rates of infectious complications. Thus, Hamlin et al. (75) noted sepsis in 1% of the patients undergoing percutaneous transhepatic drainage; Kadir et al. (74) and Joseph et al. (77) noted sepsis in 27% and 33%, respectively, of the patients on whom they performed this procedure. Joseph et al. were able to decrease this rate by 50% through the administration of prophylactic antibiotics. Again, the surgical literature suggests that equivalent patients undergoing surgical decompression would experience sepsis over 50% of the time (74).

Related procedures performed increasingly on the biliary tract include transhepatic cholangiography, placement of endoprostheses through a blocked duct, balloon dilation of strictures, and removal of stones. In general, the infectious complications associated with these procedures occur at approximately the same rate as those associated with percutaneous transhepatic drainage (69,78,79).

Percutaneous genitourinary procedures are most commonly performed to relieve obstruction secondary to neoplasms, stones, or strictures (69). These procedures have fewer infectious complications than do the analogous procedures performed on the biliary tract. Yoder et al. (80) reported that five of 65 patients undergoing nephrostomy placement for pyonephrosis had septic complications, but none died. Similarly, Stables et al. (81) summarized the results of nephrostomy placement in 516 patients. Ten (2%) developed nosocomial infections, most commonly pyelonephritis or the exacerbation of pyonephrosis. There were no deaths as compared with a 6% mortality rate in equivalent patients undergoing surgical drainage procedures. Cochran et al. (82) retrospectively reviewed 56 percutaneous nephrostomy procedures. Existence of struvite stones, abnormal urinalysis (not defined by authors), and positive urine cultures (criteria not given by authors) were believed to increase the likelihood of sepsis. Patients with one or more of these risk factors (the high-risk group) had a 50% chance of developing sepsis after percutaneous nephrostomy, as compared with a 14% likelihood of developing sepsis if none of these risk factors (low-risk group) were present. Antibiotic administration did not alter the rate of infection in the low-risk group but decreased the occurrence of sepsis by 80% in the high-risk group.

Although there are few prospective data evaluating interventions for the prevention of nosocomial infections after nonvascular interventional radiology (78), a consensus appears to have emerged as to which infection control measures may help to reduce the rate of infectious complications associated with these procedures. With the exception of the percutaneous biopsy, these procedures are associated with a high rate of infectious complications with substantial morbidity and mortality. It is generally accepted that these procedures must be performed in an environment approaching that used for the equivalent surgical procedures. Strict adherence to sterile technique with the creation of a sterile field appears to be appropriate (73). All personnel involved in the procedure should wear caps, masks, gowns, and gloves. The simplest procedure required to establish drainage and decompression should be performed with a minimum of manipulation and distention during the initial procedure (73, 81,83). Although prophylactic antibiotics have clearly been found to reduce the risk of nosocomial infections in a few studies, their exact role has not been determined (78). Antibiotic prophylaxis is unlikely to be of benefit in percutaneous biopsy procedures given the low rate of infectious complications associated with these procedures. Transhepatic and genitourinary procedures are followed by much higher rates of infectious complications, many of which will likely benefit from prophylactic antibiotics. Other drainage procedures are associated with much lower rates of infection. Further research is required to determine which, if any, of these procedures will benefit from prophylactic antibiotics. If prophylactic antibiotics are used, they should be administered no sooner than 1 hour before commencing the procedure. For most procedures, prophylactic antibiotics should not be continued after the procedure. However, for certain percutaneous drainage procedures, continuing antibiotics for 24 to 48 hours after the procedure may be appropriate (78). Specific agents to be used depend on the body site involved and local susceptibility patterns.

As with vascular interventional procedures, experience is important; rates of nosocomial infections are reduced as groups gain experience (72). As in vascular interventional radiology, all personnel must observe standard precautions.

Radiolabeled Imaging Studies

Radiolabeled imaging studies appear to be associated with a low rate of infectious complications. Proper attention to technique, as is required in all intravascular access procedures, is essential. In addition, because materials are removed from the patient, processed in another area, and then reinjected into the patient, strict protocols must be developed to prevent the contamination of the material to be reinjected. A reminder of the care required in dealing with these materials is provided by the report of three patients who received intravenous injections of blood or other materials from patients infected with HIV while undergoing nuclear medicine procedures (84). All three episodes occurred as a result of preventable administration errors. At the time of the report, two of three patients had developed infection with HIV. As a result of these errors, the CDC published recommendations to be followed when nuclear medicine procedures are performed (84). These are summarized in Table 70.2

TABLE 70.2. RECOMMENDED POLICIES FOR INSTITUTIONS OR CLINICS IN WHICH NUCLEAR MEDICINE PROCEDURES ARE PERFORMED

- All healthcare providers should receive training on infection control procedures.
- Written infection control policies and procedures for nuclear medicine should be promulgated and disseminated. These should include procedures to follow in the event of a potential emergency, such as an administration error.
- All doses and syringes should be checked for identification and radioassayed before injection.
- All syringes should be labeled with appropriate identifying information, including the patient's name and the pharmaceutical. A unique identification number should also be used.
- Consideration should be given to the implementation of a system when administering biologic products that requires that two persons cross-check all labeling of product to be injected, the prescription, and patient identification.
- Contaminated and used syringes should be disposed of safely and appropriately.
- An administration error should be immediately reported to supervisory personnel. Patients involved should be managed according to policies established for blood exposures.

From Centers for Disease Control. Patient exposures to HIV during nuclear medicine procedures. *MMWR* 1992;41:575–579, with permission.

Oral Radiology

The dental profession has a long tradition of concern for infection control issues (see Chapter 54). Dentists were one of the first groups identified as being at high risk .for occupational HBV infection (85). In addition, dental personnel have been recognized as being potentially exposed to a wide variety of other pathogens, including *M. tuberculosis*, staphylococci, streptococci, cytomegalovirus, herpes simplex virus, HIV, and viral respiratory pathogens (86). The documented transmission of HBV (87), staphylococci, streptococci (5), and other infectious pathogens (86) to patients has further reinforced interest in infection control in dentistry. Further, dentistry remains one of only two professions in which transmission of HIV from a healthcare worker to patients has been documented (88).

Although many procedures within dentistry can lead to the transmission of infectious pathogens, dental radiology has been clearly associated with contamination of the office environment and transmission of microorganisms between patients. The radiographic equipment, dental chair, headrest, adjacent horizontal surfaces (89), radiographic film, film developer, and darkroom (6) may all become contaminated with oropharyngeal pathogens during the course of oral radiology. These pathogens, in turn, may be transmitted to healthcare workers or patients. Design features frequently contribute to this potential for the transmission of microorganisms. The control panel for radiology equipment in the dental operatory is frequently not designed for effective disinfection (89), and it is difficult to aseptically remove the film from a film packet contaminated with oral secretions (6).

In response to these concerns regarding the potential for spread of infectious pathogens between patients and between patients and healthcare workers in dentistry, the CDC (86) and several dental organizations (90,91) have published infection control guidelines for dental radiology (Table 70.3).

TABLE 70.3. INFECTION CONTROL GUIDELINES FOR DENTAL RADIOLOGY

- All patients should be treated as potentially infectious.
- Gloves should be worn during all radiographic procedures and while handling contaminated film packets, supplies, and equipment. Gloves should also be worn during cleanup procedures.
- The exposure switch and cone should be covered with paper backed by an impervious material, aluminum foil, or clear plastic wrap. These should be changed between patients. If covering is not possible, the switch and cone must be disinfected between patients.
- Operators should avoid touching environmental surfaces with contaminated gloves.
- Film packets and supplies should be obtained before seating the patient.
- All materials and instruments used during patient care should be kept on work surfaces that are covered. If this is not possible, work surfaces should be disinfected with an EPA-registered and ADA-accepted disinfectant between patients.
- Nondisposable instruments such as intraoral film holders, beam-aligning devices, and panoramic bite blocks should be sterilized between patients.
- All darkroom surfaces that are contaminated by film packets must be disinfected regularly.
- Contaminated film packets should be wiped dry and carried to the darkroom in a disposable container.
- Gloves should be worn while handling contaminated film packets. The films should be dropped onto a disposable towel without touching the films. Contaminated packets and gloves should be discarded before film processing.
- The use of daylight loaders is discouraged, because they are easily contaminated.

EPA, Environmental Protection Agency; ADA, American Dental Association.

REFERENCES

1. Joffre F, Otal P, d'Othee BJ. Plea for a surgical conscience in the interventional radiology suite. *Cardiovasc Intervent Radiol* 1998;21:445–447.
2. Meyers PH. Contamination of patient-contact surfaces in radiology departments. *JAMA* 1969;209:772.
3. Hodges A. Radiographic markers: friend or fomite. *Radiol Technol* 2001;73:183–185.
4. Meyers PH. Contamination of barium enema apparatus during its use. *JAMA* 1960;173:1589–1590.
5. White SC, Glaze S. Interpatient microbiological cross-contamination after dental radiographic examination. *J Am Dent Assoc* 1978;96:801–804.
6. Bachman CE, White JM, Goodis HE, et al. Bacterial adherence and contamination during radiographic processing. *Oral Surg Oral Med Oral Pathol* 1990;70:669–673.
7. McFarland LV, Mulligan ME, Kwok RYY, et al. Nosocomial acquisition of Clostridium difficile infection. *N Engl J Med* 1989;320:204–210.
8. Hopkins CC, Weber DJ, Rubin RH. Invasive aspergillus infection: possible non-ward common source within the hospital environment. *J Hosp Infect* 1989;13:19–25.
9. Centers for Disease Control. Nosocomial transmission of multidrug-resistant tuberculosis among HIV-infected persons. *MMWR* 1991;40:585–591.
10. Centers for Disease Control. Guidelines for preventing the transmission of Mycobacterium tuberculosis in health-care facilities, 1994. *MMWR* 1994;43(RR-13):1–132.
11. Lindberg PR. *Improving hospital ventilation systems for tuberculosis infection control.* 1993 Plant, Technology and Safety Management Series, Number 1. Oakbrook Terrace, IL: Joint Commission on Accreditation of Healthcare Organizations, 1993.
12. Occupational Safety and Health Administration. Occupational exposure to bloodborne pathogens: final rule. December 6, 1991;56(235) 29 CFR Part 1910.1030;64175–64182.
13. West DJ. The risk of hepatitis B infection among health professionals in the United States: a review. *Am J Med Sci* 1984;287:26–33.
14. Centers for Disease Control. Surveillance for occupationally acquired HIV infection United States, 1981–1992. *MMWR* 1992;41:823–825.
15. Heller RM, Horev G, Kirchner SG, et al. AIDS awareness in the conduct of radiologic procedures: guidelines to safe practice. *Radiology* 1988;166:563–567.
16. Kane MA, Hadler SC, Margolis HS, et al. Routine prenatal screening for hepatitis B surface antigen. *JAMA* 1988;259:408–409.
17. Baker JL, Kelen GD, Sivertson KT, et al. Unsuspected human immunodeficiency virus in critically ill emergency patients. *JAMA* 1987;257:2609–2611.
18. Centers for Disease Control. Recommendations for prevention of HIV transmission in health-care settings. *MMWR* 1987;36(suppl 2S):3S–18S.
19. Garner JS. Guideline for isolation precautions in hospitals. *Infect Control Hosp Epidemiol* 1996;17:53–80.
20. Wall SD, Olcott EW, Gerberding JL. AIDS risk and risk reduction in the radiology department. *AJR* 1991;157:911–917.
21. Sniffen JM. Infection Control. In: Kandarpa K, Aruny JE, eds. *Handbook of interventional radiologic procedures,* 2nd ed. Boston: Little, Brown, 1996:362–364.
22. Hansen ME, McIntire DD, Miller GL. Occult glove perforations: fre-

quency during interventional radiology procedures. *AJR* 1992;159:131–135.
23. Steinbach HL, Rousseau R, McCormack KR, et al. Transmission of enteric pathogens by barium enema. *JAMA* 1960;174:1207–1208.
24. Hervey CR. A series of typhoid fever cases infected per rectum. *Am J Public Health* 1929;19:166–171.
25. Meyers PF, Richards M. Transmission of polio virus vaccine by contaminated barium enema with resultant antibody rise. *AJR* 1964;91:864–865.
26. Istre GR, Kreiss K, Hopkins RS, et al. An outbreak of amebiasis spread by colonic irrigation at a chiropractic clinic. *N Engl J Med* 1982;307:339–342.
27. Pochaczevsky R, Sherman RS, Meyers PH. A disposable kit for barium enemas. *Radiology* 1961;77:831–833.
28. Dreyfuss JR, Robbins LL, Murphy JT. Disposable, plastic unit for barium-enema examination. *Radiology* 1961;77:834–835.
29. Le Frock JL, Ellis CA, Klainer AS, et al. Transient bacteremia associated with barium enema. *Arch Intern Med* 1975;135:835–837.
30. Butt J, Hentges D, Pelican G, et al. Bacteremia during barium enema study. *AJR* 1978;130:715–718.
31. Richman LS, Short WF, Cooper WM. Barium enema septicemia. Occurrence in a patient with leukemia. *JAMA* 1973;226:62–63.
32. Ward RL. Endocarditis complicating ulcerative colitis. *Gastroenterology* 1977;73:1189–1190.
33. Shorvon PJ, Eykyn SJ, Cotton PB. Gastrointestinal instrumentation, bacteraemia, and endocarditis. *Gut* 1983;24:1078–1093.
34. Dajani AS, Taubert KA, Wilson W, et al. Prevention of bacterial endocarditis. Recommendations by the American Heart Association. *JAMA* 1997;277:1794–1801.
35. Fowler C, McCracken D. US probes: risk of cross infection and ways to reduce it—comparison of cleaning methods. *Radiology* 1999;213:299–300.
36. Spencer P, Spencer RC. Ultrasound scanning of post-operative wounds: the risks of cross infection. *Clin Radiol* 1988;39:245–246.
37. Muradali D, Gold WL, Phillips A, et al. Can ultrasound probes and coupling gel be a source of nosocomial infection in patients undergoing sonography? An in vivo and in vitro study. *AJR* 1995;164:1521–1524.
38. Karadeniz YM, Kilic D, Altan SK, et al. Evaluation of the role of ultrasound machines as a source of nosocomial and cross-infection. *Invest Radiol* 2001;36:554–558.
39. Rutala WA. APIC guideline for selection and use of disinfectants. *Am J Infect Control* 1996;24:313–342.
40. American Institute of Ultrasound in Medicine: Ultrasound Practice Committee Report for Cleaning and Preparing Endocavitary Ultrasound Transducers Between Patients. American Institute of Ultrasound in Medicine, October 1995, modified June 11, 1999. (Posted on the AIUM Web site.)
41. Wheeler PW, Lancaster D, Kaiser AB. Bronchopulmonary cross-colonization and infection related to mycobacterial contamination of suction valves of bronchoscopes. *J Infect Dis* 1989;159:954–958.
42. Spach DH, Silverstein FE, Stamm WE. Transmission of infection by gastrointestinal endoscopy and bronchoscopy. *Ann Intern Med* 1993;118:117–128.
43. Pritchard TM, Foust RT, Cantey JR, et al. Prosthetic valve endocarditis due to *Cardiobacterium hominis* occurring after upper gastrointestinal endoscopy. *Am J Med* 1991;90:516–518.
44. Bianco JA, Pepe MS, Higano C, et al. Prevalence of clinically relevant bacteremia after upper gastrointestinal endoscopy in bone marrow transplant recipients. *Am J Med* 1990;89:134–136.
45. Cotton PB, Lehman G, Vennes J, et al. Endoscopic sphincterotomy complications and their management: an attempt at consensus. *Gastrointest Endosc* 1991;37:383–393.
46. Motte S, Deviere J, Dumonceau JM, et al. Risk factors for septicemia following endoscopic biliary stenting. *Gastroenterology* 1991;101:1374–1381.
47. Anonymous. Antibiotic prophylaxis for gastrointestinal endoscopy. American Society for Gastrointestinal Endoscopy. *Gastrointest Endosc* 1995;42:630–635.
48. Bass DH, Oliver S, Bornman PC. *Pseudomonas* septicaemia after endoscopic retrograde cholangiopancreatography an unresolved problem. *S Afr Med J* 1990;77:509–511.
49. Favero MS. Strategies for disinfection and sterilization of endoscopes: the gap between basic principles and actual practice. *Infect Control Hosp Epidemiol* 1991;12:279–281.
50. Kaczmarek RG, Moore RM, McCrohan J, et al. Multi-state investigation of the actual disinfection/sterilization of endoscopes in health care facilities. *Am J Med* 1992;92:257–261.
51. Schelkun SR, Wagner KF, Blanks JA, et al. Bacterial meningitis following Pantopaque myelography. A case report and review of the literature. *Orthopedics* 1985;8:73–76.
52. de Jong J, Barrs ACM. Lumbar myelography followed by meningitis. *Infect Control Hosp Epidemiol* 1992;13:74–75.
53. Watanakunakorn C, Stahl C. *Streptococcus salivarius* meningitis following myelography. *Infect Control Hosp Epidemiol* 1992;13:454.
54. Winchell P. Infectious endocarditis as a result of contamination during cardiac catheterization. *N Engl J Med* 1953;248:245–246.
55. Sande MA, Levinson ME, Lukas DS, et al. Bacteremia associated with cardiac catheterization. *N Engl J Med* 1969;281:1104–1106.
56. Shawker TH, Kluge RM, Ayella RJ. Bacteremia associated with angiography. *JAMA* 1974;229:1090–1092.
57. Laslett LJ, Sabin A. Wearing of caps and masks not necessary during cardiac catheterization. *Cathet Cardiovasc Diagn* 1989;17:158–160.
58. Leaman DM, Zelis RF. What is the appropriate dress code for the cardiac catheterization laboratory? *Cathet Cardiovasc Diagn* 1983;9:33–38.
59. Gardiner GA, Meyerovitz MF, Stokes KR, et al. Complications of transluminal angioplasty. *Radiology* 1986;159:201–208.
60. Frazee BW, Flaherty JP. Septic endarteritis of the femoral artery following angioplasty. *Rev Infect Dis* 1991;13:620–623.
61. Zollikofer CL, Antonucci F, Stuckmann G. Intravascular stents in the treatment of arterial occlusive disease. In: Kadir S, ed. *Current practice of interventional radiology.* Philadelphia: BC Decker, 1991.
62. Gordon GI, Vogelzang RL, Curry RH, et al. Endovascular infection after renal artery stent placement. *J Vasc Intervent Radiol* 1996;7:669–672.
63. Drooz AT, Lewis CA, Allen TE, et al. Quality improvement guidelines for percutaneous transcatheter embolization. *J Vasc Intervent Radiol* 1997;8:889–895.
64. Higashida RT, Halbach VV, Dowd CF, et al. Intracranial aneurysms: interventional neurovascular treatment with detachable balloons results in 215 cases. *Radiology* 1991;178:663–670.
65. Hemingway AP. Complications of embolotherapy. In: Kadir S, ed. *Current practice of interventional radiology.* Philadelphia: BC Decker, 1991.
66. Goldstein Hm, Wallace S, Anderson JH, et al. Transcatheter occlusion of abdominal tumors. *Radiology* 1976;120:539–545.
67. Castaneda-Zuniga WR, Hammerschmidt DE, Sanchez R, et al. Nonsurgical splenectomy. *AJR* 1977;129:805–811.
68. Spigos DG, Jonasson O, Mozes M, et al. Partial splenic embolization in the treatment of hypersplenism. *AJR* 1979;132:777–782.
69. Mueller PR, vanSonnenberg E. Interventional radiology in the chest and abdomen. *N Engl J Med* 1990;322:1364–1374.
70. Cardella JF, Bakal CW, Bertino RE, et al. Quality improvement guidelines for image-guided percutaneous biopsy in adults. *J Vasc Intervent Radiol* 1996;7:943–946.
71. Bakal CW, Sacks D, Burke DR, et al. Quality improvement guidelines for adult percutaneous abscess and fluid drainage. *J Vasc Intervent Radiol* 1995;6:68–70.
72. vanSonnenberg E, Mueller PR, Ferrucci JT. Percutaneous drainage of 250 abdominal abscesses and fluid collections. *Radiology* 1984;151:337–341.
73. Hunter DW, Simmons RL, Hulbert JC. Antibiotics for radiologic interventional procedures. *Radiology* 1988;166:572–573.
74. Kadir S, Baassiri A, Barth KH, et al. Percutaneous biliary drainage in the management of biliary sepsis. *AJR* 1982;138:25–29.
75. Hamlin JA, Friedman M, Stein MG, et al. Percutaneous biliary drainage: complications of 118 consecutive catheterizations. *Radiology* 1986;158:199–202.

76. Lois JF, Gomes AS, Grace PA, et al. Risks of percutaneous transhepatic drainage in patients with cholangitis. *AJR* 1987;148:367–371.
77. Joseph PK, Bizer LS, Sprayregen SS, et al. Percutaneous transhepatic biliary drainage. *JAMA* 1986;255:2763–2767.
78. Spies JB, Rosen RJ, Lebowitz AS. Antibiotic prophylaxis in vascular and interventional radiology: a rational approach. *Radiology* 1988;166:381–387.
79. Clark CD, Picus D, Dunagan WC. Bloodstream infections after interventional procedures in the biliary tract. *Radiology* 1994;191:495–499.
80. Yoder IC, Pfister RC, Lindfors KK, et al. Pyonephrosis: imaging and intervention. *AJR* 1983;141:735–740.
81. Stables DP, Ginsberg NJ, Johnson ML. Percutaneous nephrostomy: a series and review of the literature. *AJR* 1978;130:75–82.
82. Cochran ST, Barbaric ZL, Lee JJ, et al. Percutaneous nephrostomy tube placement. *Radiology* 1991;179:843–847.
83. van Waes PF, Simoons-Smit IM. Use of antibiotics in interventional radiologic procedures: an important lesson still to be learned. *Radiology* 1988;166:570–571.
84. Centers for Disease Control. Patient exposures to HIV during nuclear medicine procedures. *MMWR* 1992;41:575–579.
85. Smith JL, Maynard JE, Berquist KR, et al. Comparative risk of hepatitis B among physicians and dentists. *J Infect Dis* 1976;133:705–706.
86. Centers for Disease Control. Recommended infection-control practices for dentistry. *MMWR* 1993;42(RR-8):1–12.
87. Ahtone J, Goodman RA. Hepatitis B and dental personnel: transmission to patients and prevention issues. *J Am Dent Assoc* 1983;106:219–222.
88. Centers for Disease Control. Update: investigations of patients who have been treated by HIV-infected health-care workers. *MMWR* 1992;41:344–346.
89. Infection control in dental radiology. In: Cottone JA, Terezhalmy GT, Molinari JA, eds. *Practical infection control in dentistry.* Philadelphia: Lea & Febiger, 1991.
90. American Academy of Oral and Maxillofacial Radiology. Infection control guidelines for dental radiographic procedures. *Oral Surg Oral Med Oral Pathol* 1992;73:48–49.
91. Council on Dental Materials, Instruments, and Equipment; Council on Dental Practice; Council on Dental Therapeutics. Infection control recommendations for the dental office and the dental laboratory. *J Am Dent Assoc* 1988;116:241–248.

71

INFECTIONS ASSOCIATED WITH HYPERBARIC OXYGEN THERAPY AND HYPERBARIC CHAMBERS, AND RESEARCH IN ALTITUDE CHAMBERS AND SATURATION DIVING

JON T. MADER
JUE WANG

The ability to explain the spread of an infection to a patient or group of patients and to apply the principles of infection control to prevent further spread are the skills most characteristic of the hospital epidemiologist. Knowledge of what happens in a given area of a hospital or in various outpatient settings is crucial to understanding outbreaks of nosocomial infection.

This chapter discusses hyperbaric and hypobaric chambers and saturation diving. The physical settings for patients treated in hyperbaric chambers, for healthy subjects exposed to hypobaric altitude chambers and for divers exposed to pressurized chambers for saturation diving, are described. With this knowledge, infection control experts will be in a better position to assess the likelihood of transmission of infections under such conditions. This chapter also discusses infection control procedures, isolation precautions, and possible scenarios for nosocomial transmission of infection.

HYPERBARIC OXYGEN THERAPY

Hyperbaric oxygen (HBO) therapy is defined as the treatment of a patient who is entirely enclosed within a pressure vessel and is breathing 100% oxygen at a pressure greater than that at sea level [1 atmosphere absolute (ATA)] (1). For routine treatments, the pressure is usually 2.0 to 2.8 ATA, which is equivalent to 33 to 60 feet of seawater. However, there are certain diving complications such as air embolism and decompression sickness where pressures up to 6.0 ATA (165 feet of seawater) are used as part of the treatment. The list of indications for such treatments is fairly varied and includes both infectious and noninfectious diseases and diving accidents (Table 71.1). Approval of these indications is based on the report of the Hyperbaric Oxygen Therapy Committee (1) of the Undersea and Hyperbaric Medical Society, which continually reviews evidence of efficacy for each indication.

It is important to note that all discussions in this chapter relate to systemic HBO therapy. Topical oxygen therapy has been shown to be of no benefit (2) because oxygen is not significantly absorbed through the skin.

Hyperbaric treatments can be given in either an outpatient or an inpatient setting, and there are many freestanding hyperbaric units not affiliated with hospitals. In the hospital setting, even critically ill patients can receive HBO treatments. In the multiplace chambers of many hospitals, patients can receive the same level of intensive care and monitoring that they would ordinarily receive in an intensive care unit. In a few centers, surgical procedures can be performed during HBO treatments (3).

The rationale for use of HBO in each clinical setting is fairly specific and is based on well-documented HBO mechanisms of activity. In bacterial infections, HBO has a direct or indirect effect on aerobic and anaerobic microorganisms. HBO increases the oxygen tension in infected tissue, including bone. HBO does not have a direct effect on aerobic microorganisms. In fact, hyperbaric conditions induce aerobic microorganisms to produce increased concentrations of superoxide dismutase, an oxygen radical detoxifying enzyme. However, hyperbaric oxygenation does increase the oxygen tension in infected tissue, thereby promoting the oxygen-dependent intracellular killing mechanisms of the polymorphonuclear leukocyte and to a lesser extent the macrophage. Thus, HBO provides the necessary substrate (oxygen) for the killing of aerobic and anaerobic microorganisms by the polymorphonuclear leukocyte (4,5). HBO also has a direct effect on strictly anaerobic microorganisms through the production of toxic radicals. The toxic oxygen radicals have a direct cidal effect on *Peptococcus* species, *Peptostreptococcus* species, and *Fusobacterium* species. For clostridial myonecrosis, oxygen levels above 250 mm Hg can inhibit the production of α-toxin (6) that causes systemic toxicity. However, to actually kill the oxygen-tolerant *Clostridium* species, Po_2 levels in excess of 1,200 mm Hg must be achieved. *Bacteroides* species are also oxygen tolerant.

HBO provides adequate oxygen for fibroblast activity, leading to angiogenesis and wound healing in hypoxic tissues. HBO

TABLE 71.1. APPROVED INDICATIONS FOR USE OF HYPERBARIC OXYGEN THERAPY

Air or gas embolism
Carbon monoxide poisoning and smoke inhalation, carbon monoxide poisoning complicated by cyanide poisoning
Clostridial myonecrosis (gas gangrene)
Crush injury, compartment syndrome, and other acute traumatic ischemias
Decompression sickness
Enhancement of healing in selected problem wounds, including nonhealing wounds in the diabetic; wounds failing to generate granulation tissue; arterial insufficiency ulcers; and others
Exceptional blood loss anemia
Necrotizing soft tissue infections, including necrotizing fasciitis, Fournier's gangrene, and mixed aerobic/anaerobic necrotizing cellulitis
Chronic refractory osteomyelitis
Radiation tissue damage (osteoradionecrosis and soft tissue radionecrosis)
Threatened soft tissue flaps and grafts
Thermal burns
Adjunctive hyperbaric oxygen in intracranial abscess

From Camporesi EM, ed. *Hyperbaric oxygen therapy: a committee report.* Bethesda, MD: Undersea and Hyperbaric Medical Society, 1996, with permission.

treatments can oxygenate wounds that are otherwise too hypoxic to heal, such as diabetic foot wounds. A Po_2 of less than 30 mm Hg is not conducive to collagen production by the fibroblast, neutrophilic killing of microorganisms, or angiogenesis (the budding of capillary endothelial cells to generate capillaries within a newly formed collagen connective tissue framework). The partial pressure of oxygen in ischemic, traumatized, or infected tissues is often less than 30 mm Hg. HBO can increase the oxygen level significantly, thus promoting wound healing (7). In chronic refractory osteomyelitis, a hypoxic state exists in bone, impairing osteoclast and osteoblast activity. HBO facilitates correction of bone hypoxia, thereby allowing resorption of micronecrotic foci of bone and facilitating bone healing (8).

HBO is used to treat carbon monoxide intoxication, failing flaps, air embolism, and decompression sickness. HBO has been shown to decrease the local inflammatory response in damaged tissue. Zamboni et al. (9) showed that HBO significantly reduced neutrophil endothelial adherence in damaged venules. Thom et al. (10) demonstrated that HBO inhibited β_2-integrin–dependent adherence to damaged endothelium. Polymorphonuclear leukocytes, which do not adhere to damaged endothelium, do not release toxic oxygen radicals into the adjacent tissue. Toxic oxygen radicals and their subsequent interactions in the tissues may lead to an intense inflammatory response.

HBO has also been shown to facilitate entry of antibiotics into bacterial cells when antibiotic transport is oxygen dependent (11). Also, some antibiotics have been shown to have a decreased efficacy in an anaerobic environment. These antibiotics include aminoglycosides, vancomycin, and the quinolones. Additive effects of HBO and antibiotics have been observed for tobramycin, trimethoprim-sulfamethoxazole, and nitrofurantoin. Known mechanisms in other clinical settings have been fully reviewed (12,13).

Types of Chambers

Two types of hyperbaric chambers currently are in use. The monoplace chamber, which is used to treat one patient at a time, is pressurized with 100% oxygen. It is usually made of acrylic materials. The multiplace chamber usually holds two or more patients with tenders (e.g., nurses, respiratory technicians, and hyperbaric technicians) to care for the patients. These are usually metal chambers and are pressurized with room air. Patients breathe 100% oxygen, either through tight-fitting face masks such as the Scott mask or through more comfortable plastic hoods such as the Sealong or Duke hood. The hoods are either taped tightly around the patient's shoulders or placed over the head with a rubber diaphragm to retain gasses. There are intake and outflow tubes from the hoods. An intubated patient can receive oxygen directly through the endotracheal tube. Oxygen lines enter the chamber through penetrators from an oxygen source, which may be either the central hospital oxygen system or separate oxygen tanks. In-line filters are placed between the oxygen source and chamber supply to trap particulate material.

Potential for Infection Transmission

Potential for patient infection by a transmissible pathogen during a hyperbaric chamber treatment is about the same as it is for the classic nosocomial routes that are described throughout this volume (14). Patients treated in outpatient HBO chamber centers are also at risk of acquiring the usual types of contagious diseases reported for outpatient clinic settings (15).

Respiratory Route

A number of respiratory infections are transmitted by the airborne route, by droplet nuclei containing bacteria or viral particles, or by large respiratory droplets dispersed over short distances. Theoretically, some infections could be transmitted from a patient or tender to another patient when treatments take place in a multiplace chamber. However, no study has documented that this occurs more frequently inside the chamber than would occur outside the chamber.

Infections that can be transmitted from the respiratory tract by droplet nuclei or by larger respiratory droplets include pulmonary tuberculosis; *Haemophilus influenzae* epiglottitis, meningitis, or pneumonia; *Neisseria meningitidis* pneumonia, meningitis, or bacteremia; *Bordetella pertussis* (whooping cough); measles; mumps; rubella; respiratory syncytial virus infection; and varicella-zoster virus infections. A patient with herpes zoster may shed the virus from skin lesions and transmit the virus to a nonimmune individual through the airborne route. After such an exposure, the individual would develop chickenpox (16,17). Prudence would dictate that patients or tenders with the infection should avoid being in a chamber with other patients or tenders who are known to be nonimmune or whose immune status is unknown.

During a standard treatment, which lasts about 2 hours, each patient is breathing oxygen from a separate supply line for approximately 75% of the time. Because each patient has his or her own air source, there is a lower probability of contracting airborne infections from contagious patients than if they were sharing the air at sea level with a contagious patient, although there are no data to confirm this.

Mullins et al. (18) found that hospital air often contains the fungus *Aspergillus fumigatus* and other *Aspergillus* species. Infection with *A. fumigatus* has been reported in immunocompromised patients who inhaled spores from sources in the environment (19,20). Routine changing of hospital ventilation system filters is indicated to prevent heavy contamination with *Aspergillus* species (21). Although no infections have been reported secondary to contamination of hyperbaric chamber filters, there is no reason to doubt that such an event could occur, leading to invasive fungal pulmonary infections. Thus, hyperbaric personnel should clean and change chamber air filters routinely. If any patient receiving HBO treatments acquires such an infection, an epidemiologic investigation should include culture of chamber filters.

There is circumstantial evidence that nosocomial pneumonia can be caused by aerosolization of *Legionella pneumophila* with cooling towers and evaporative condensers as the modes of dissemination (22); however, this has been questioned (23). Inhalation of aerosolized tap water by humidifiers has been linked to hospital-acquired Legionnaire's disease (24) (see Chapter 35). A prospective study in which *Legionella* species infection was shown to be the most common cause of nosocomial pneumonia in a population of oncologic head and neck surgery patients (25) seems to support this concept. Such patients also tend to aspirate as a result of oral surgery. Thus, patients with head and neck cancers could develop nosocomial pneumonia during hyperbaric treatment, either by aspiration or by the airborne route (including legionellosis). Head and neck cancer patients, particularly if they have received radiotherapy to the head and neck area, are frequently treated with HBO for wound-healing problems, osteoradionecrosis of the mandible, and for neck flap problems.

The human immunodeficiency virus is not transmitted by the respiratory route. Therefore, universal precautions, without any special modifications, are effective in preventing the transmission of blood-borne infections during hyperbaric therapy.

Contact Transmission

Many patients treated with HBO have open wounds. These are often open actively draining wounds in diabetics that may be infected with *Staphylococcus* species. Other conditions treated with HBO include clostridial myonecrosis, mixed aerobic/anaerobic necrotizing fasciitis, and necrotizing fasciitis caused by *Streptococcus pyogenes.*

One of the questions HBO staff members ask at a multiplace chamber installation is, Can patient X be treated with patients Y and Z? Alternatively, the question is, Can patients A and B be treated together by only one nurse, or are two nurses necessary?

Patients are always treated while their wounds are dressed, even if their wound is draining. The wounds do not need to be exposed to oxygen, because the hyperoxygenation occurs through the circulatory route. This reduces the risk of contamination from secretions from open wounds. Only dressings that have drainage soaking through the dressing or that became contaminated before or while being applied can spread infection (26,27). It is recommended that the nurse/tender wear gloves while caring for such a patient. If the nurse/tender needs to tend to another patient with an open wound, intravenous line, or catheter, or if a manipulation is needed at another body site during the same treatment, gloves should be changed between patients or sites, as has been recommended elsewhere (28). Alternatively, for patients with actively draining wounds, assigning nurses on a one-to-one basis might be advantageous. Particular attention should be paid to preventing transmission of infection by fomites.

It is of the utmost importance to prevent the patient-to-patient spread of microorganisms such as methicillin-resistant *Staphylococcus aureus* and other multiply resistant *Staphylococcus* species, multiply-resistant *Pseudomonas aeruginosa*, and other gram-negative rods. The burn patient population provides reservoirs for these microorganisms. Many patients treated with HBO for nonhealing wounds are often simultaneously receiving whirlpool treatments and hydrotherapy in Hubbard tanks. Outbreaks of *P. aeruginosa* wound infections related to Hubbard tank treatments, but unrelated to HBO, have been reported when sodium hypochlorite as a tank disinfectant was discontinued; the outbreaks resolved when this disinfectant was reinstituted (29).

Infections that spread by the fecal-oral route cause infectious gastroenteritis and may be acquired in the hospital or during HBO therapy. *Salmonella* species, *Shigella* species, enterotoxigenic *Escherichia coli, Campylobacter jejuni*, and *Yersinia enterocolitica* have all been implicated in hospital outbreaks, particularly in newborn infants. Hepatitis A and other viral agents are also transmitted through the fecal-oral route. *Clostridium difficile* colitis is usually associated with overgrowth of the microorganism during antibiotic therapy. The microorganism is highly communicable, and cross-contamination occurs in patients of all ages. Once the environment becomes contaminated, the spores may remain viable on surfaces for up to 5 months. Thus, the chamber and its environmental surfaces should be carefully cleaned with hypochlorite solution after each treatment of a patient with this infection and at regular intervals (30). Such patients should be treated alone or should not share tenders in a multiplace chamber. (For additional details on control of *C. difficile* infections, see Chapter 36.)

HBO is often used in the treatment of clostridial myonecrosis (gas gangrene). The causative agent for clostridial myonecrosis is often *Clostridium perfringens*. The initiation of the disease is often from the direct inoculation of the appropriate clostridial species in an area within a wound with decreased oxidation/reduction potential (31).

Necrotizing soft tissue infections are also treated with HBO. Necrotizing soft tissue infections are also known as Fournier's gangrene, anaerobic cellulitis, necrotizing fasciitis, and Meleney's synergistic gangrene, among others. The pathogenesis of the disease usually involves the compromise of mucocutaneous barriers that can occur in infected decubitus and diabetic ulcers. Many patients treated with HBO have decubitus and diabetic ulcers. It is not inconceivable that patients with these types of wounds could contract the bacteria that cause necrotizing soft tissue infections at hyperbaric facilities if proper precautions are not taken (31).

Additional Infection Control Measures

An important infection control measure in HBO therapy is cleaning face masks and hoods used for delivery of oxygen between uses to prevent overgrowth of surface bacteria that could aerosolize on reuse. Each patient is usually assigned a personally labeled hood or mask for the duration of his or her therapy. The hood or mask is cleaned after HBO treatment with quaternary ammonium compounds as recommended by the manufacturer. Quaternary ammonium compounds are low-level disinfectants that can disinfect items, which will come in contact with the skin. All hoods, neck seals, and tubing should be properly discarded after the patient has completed his or her prescribed course of treatments.

Storage of water for long periods for use in suppression of fire in the potentially higher oxygen environment of a hyperbaric chamber theoretically could lead to overgrowth of a number of microorganisms. The only risk of contaminating patients with these microorganisms would be from the use of the water. Use of bactericidal solutions might reduce the risk significantly, although troublesome microorganisms, such as nontuberculous mycobacteria, may persist (32).

Surface areas should undergo standard cleaning with a combined bactericidal, virucidal, and tuberculocidal detergent. Chamber personnel should keep a sharps receptacle for easy disposal of needles in the chamber to decrease the risk of needle sticks.

If an environmental reservoir is suspected in an outbreak of nosocomial infections, microbiologic sampling may be indicated during the investigation; however, microbiologic surveillance of the environment in an HBO chamber is not routinely warranted. Culturing of environmental surfaces during an investigation should be based on clues from the epidemiologic data and should be done using a written protocol that specifies the surfaces to be sampled.

There are clearly no data and no rationale to justify empty-chamber pressurization as a means to kill bacteria and sterilize the chamber because the direct antibacterial effect of HBO would be limited to anaerobes that are usually not the bacteria that cause nosocomial infections; the antibacterial effect on aerobes is mediated by the host response, which is absent in an empty chamber.

Surveillance is more important than environmental cultures. Acquisition of any nosocomial infection by any HBO patient should be reported directly to an infection control professional or committee at the institution. This would also include outpatients, because 20% to 70% of postoperative surgical site infections do not become apparent until after discharge (33). Reporting the information could make it possible to identify and control a common-source outbreak that might affect other patients in the hospital. It should be remembered that patients treated in medical HBO chambers come from a variety of specialty and subspecialty services from all patient settings and occasionally from other hospitals. Thus, a common source might not be easily discerned.

ALTITUDE (HYPOBARIC) CHAMBERS

Background

Classically, medicine has considered patients with abnormal physiology or illnesses in a normal environment. With the inception of aviation and space operations, aerospace medicine has emerged to deal with flight crew members and their normal adaptive physiology in the abnormal environment of flight.

Altitude chambers, also known as hypobaric chambers, simulate exposure to altitudes from 2,500 feet above sea level [13.5 pounds per square inch absolute (PSIA) = 700 mm Hg] to 25,000 feet (5.5 PSIA = 282 mm Hg). High-altitude chambers can simulate the pressure environment up to 100,000 feet and even to the vacuum of space (34).

Unlike hyperbaric facilities, which are routinely used therapeutically, altitude chambers are not used to directly treat medical conditions. Their primary role is in physiologic training and research involving healthy individuals. Numerous governmental agencies, military bases, universities, and other organizations provide instruction to military and civilian pilots in high-altitude physiology and recognition of individual responses to hypoxia. Additionally, altitude chambers are regularly used in the training of spaceflight crews.

In a typical session, ambient pressure is reduced to simulate the reduced pressure at high altitude. Now chamber occupants must breathe from an enriched oxygen source via face mask to compensate for the reduced atmospheric pressure. The physiologic effects of early hypoxia may then be demonstrated by brief oxygen mask removal under careful supervision.

Physiologic Training

In an actual or simulated high-altitude environment, there are altered physiologic demands on the body. Decreased available oxygen, lowered barometric pressure, temperature extremes, confused sensory input, and acceleration are some of the typical stresses experienced during flight. Pilots must not only possess excellent psychomotor skills and be free of infirmity or disability (35), they must also be familiar and experienced with the high-altitude environment, changes in ambient pressure during normal ascent and descent, rapid decompression during emergencies, and their own individual, often insidious, reactions to the onset of hypoxia. Altitude chamber experience teaches physiologic self-awareness. It is an essential part of military aviation training and is highly recommended for civilian pilots. For most, it is their first familiarization with the potential hazards of the high-altitude flight environment.

In the United States, federal aviation regulations require high-altitude physiology training for cockpit and cabin crews operating above 25,000 feet. For pilots who fly aircraft with service ceilings above 18,000 feet, the National Transportation Safety Board has also recommended physiology training. The Federal Aviation Administration (FAA) offers evidence that civilian pilots who fly at altitudes of 10,000 feet during the day and 5,000 feet at night would benefit from physiologic training. Since 1965, the Civil Aeromedical Institute of the FAA in Oklahoma City, Oklahoma, has instructed over 15,000 students in high-altitude physiology with altitude chamber training flights. Typical training sessions simulate flight to 25,000 feet, accompanied by a 3- to 5-second decompression from 8,000 to 18,000 feet (36).

Research

Altitude chambers have been widely used to study both human and animal physiology. A number of investigations have studied aspects of altitude-induced hypoxia in normal subjects, such as the effects of drugs on performance, the prevention of altitude-induced decompression illness, or the effects of hypoxia on contact lenses. Short-term hypoxic exposures in hypobaric chambers over several hours are useful in studying acute mountain sickness (37). As a medical assessment tool, hypobaric facilities are sometimes used for diagnostic evaluation of a medically restricted aircrew to assess susceptibility to altitude-induced decompression illness. Astronaut training uses altitude chambers to prepare crew members for extravehicular activity and to evaluate pressure suit controls and reliability. Yet other research involves developing crew survival systems using positive pressure breathing technology capable of life support during recovery from extreme altitudes.

Infections in Altitude Chambers

Like hyperbaric chambers, altitude chambers used in training or research expose individuals to a closed controlled environment. In any such environment, there is potential for transmission of an infectious agent between individuals. One study of a submarine crew implicates a closed ventilation system in airborne transmission of tuberculosis (38). Yet relatively less study of infectious diseases susceptibility and transmission in humans has been made in altitude chambers compared with hyperbaric facilities. Although generally only healthy individuals are exposed to the modified hypobaric environment, infection control and prevention are nonetheless important to safe operation of altitude chambers.

Animal studies have for decades illustrated that exposure to reduced barometric pressure and/or hypoxia may affect host susceptibility to infectious diseases (39–42). Both animal and human studies have indicated several possible mechanisms by which hypoxia may result in immunosuppression, including blunted cell-mediated immune responses and increased cortisol release (43). The potential for a hypoxia-induced increase in susceptibility to viral, bacterial, or fungal diseases may be present in altitude chamber activities. Similar infection control measures, as those discussed for hyperbaric chambers, should be regularly used with particular attention to the cleaning of oxygen face masks.

Implications for Spaceflight

Carefully evaluating the risk of infections in the closed environments of environmental chambers may have implications for spaceflight. The hazard of infectious diseases among the crew members in long-duration manned spaceflight is related to the unique conditions of spacecraft environment. Confinement in a small, enclosed volume, with special problems of waste disposal and personal hygiene and microgravity present special features that favor transmission of microorganisms. Alterations in microbial flora related to space radiation-induced genetic variants may lead to increased virulence of commensal flora. To prevent the development and transmission of infectious diseases in spaceflight, the effects of spaceflight on microorganism function, particularly infectivity and pathogenicity, and on the human immune system must be understood.

Previous investigations have reported that spaceflight may produce a stimulating effect on microbial metabolism. The studies performed on Shuttle Missions STS-63 and STS-69 have shown that liquid suspension bacterial cultures of both *E. coli* and *B. subtilis* grow to higher cell concentrations in spaceflight than on earth (44). Lapchine et al. (45) published the results of two experiments performed in 1982 and 1985 (Cytos 2 during the French-Soviet Mission and "Antibio" in the Biorack program of the European Space Agency). The results showed a modification in the structure of the cell wall of *S. aureus* under electron microscopy and an increase of antibiotic resistance in bacteria during growth in flight. These changes in morphology and physiology may significantly alter the pathogenicity of microorganisms in the space environment.

Accumulating evidence suggests that the human immunity may be altered in astronauts exposed to the conditions of long-term spaceflight. Among the parameters affected are leukocyte blastogenesis, natural killer (NK) cell activity, leukocyte subset distribution, cytokine production (including interferons and interleukins), and macrophage maturation and activity (46,47). Alterations in leukocyte subset distribution have also been reported after flight of humans and animals in space (48). These changes start to occur after only a few days in spaceflight, and some changes continue throughout long-term spaceflight. Although no major nonphysiologic health problems have been reported during or following spaceflight, diseases resulting from immunosuppression could occur on long-duration missions and could include bacterial, fungal, and viral infections in addition to an increased incidence of neoplasia.

As longer duration missions with larger crews are planned, new issues and questions related to infections in closed environments will arise. Microorganisms from many sources will lead to general contamination of the space environment. The primary source of microorganisms in spaceflight is the crew members themselves. Healthy individuals carry large amounts of bacteria on their skin, and in their respiratory and gastrointestinal tracts. Animal and plant payloads may also serve as another source of microorganisms in the spaceflight environment. Reducing the risk to the crew from microorganisms requires monitoring both the spacecraft environment and the flight crews. Comprehensive monitoring and evaluation of crew members, payloads, and supplies need to conducted before and after flight.

In the weeks and days before launch, spaceflight crew members undergo careful medical evaluation, including detailed physical and laboratory examinations. During the Apollo program, a comprehensive program of preflight isolation and epidemiologic surveillance was implemented, known as the Flight Crew Health Stabilization Program (FCHSP). This program provided immunizations and strict infection control preventive measures to minimize crew member exposure to infectious agents. It also enabled prompt diagnosis and treatment of any disease in crew members and their families. No infectious diseases occurred in crew members before, during, or after flight when the FCHSP was in effect (49) (Table 71.2).

Current space shuttle operations address infection control in a variety of ways. Any preflight illness or infection in a crew member results in a flight postponement. Crew members are also quarantined before flight, with restricted visits during the week before launch. After flight, exposed cabin surfaces are wiped with isopropyl alcohol to reduce bacterial buildup. No significant positive culture results have been obtained from either air or surface samples inside the orbiter, either before or after flight. Although fluid shifts associated with microgravity exposure during flight may predispose crew members to nasal congestion and upper respiratory infections during flight, there are no data to indicate that an infectious disease or pathogen is any more transmissible during spaceflight.

During current shuttle missions, a normobaric [14.7 pounds per square inch (psi)] and normoxic (O_2 21% or 3.1 psi) cabin environment is generally maintained. However, preparing for extravehicular activity (EVA) and minimizing the risk of decompression sickness (DCS) requires equilibrating at a lower tissue nitrogen concentration. Thus, for a period up to 24 hours before EVA, on-board cabin pressure is reduced to 10.2 psi at 27% O_2. EVA is then conducted in a 4.3 psi pressure suit at 95% O_2. The effects of repeated EVA exposure to this normoxic but hypobaric environment with regard to infection needs to be more clearly elucidated. Other lines of research may someday explore the potential radioprotective role of mild hypoxia during a long-duration mission (50).

TABLE 71.2. ILLNESS OCCURRENCE IN SPACE CREWS BEFORE THE FLIGHT CREW HEALTH STABILIZATION PROGRAM[a]

Illness	Number Involved	Phase
Bends	2	In flight
Upper respiratory disease	8	Preflight
Viral gastrointestinal infection	3	Preflight
Eye or skin irritation (fiberglass)	3	In flight
Skin infection	2	In flight
Trauma	1	Landing
Urinary tract infection	1	In flight
Contact dermatitis	2	In flight
Arrhythmia	2	In flight
Arrhythmia	2	Postflight
Laceration	1	Preflight
Serous otitis	1	In flight
Eye and finger injury	1	In flight
Sty	1	In flight
Boil	1	In flight
Back strain	1	Postflight
Rash	1	In flight
Fatigue work–rest cycles	3	In flight
Toxic pneumonia	3	Reentry

[a] Does not include isolated premature ventricular beats or premature atrial beats or motion sickness.
From Dehart RL. *Fundamentals of aerospace medicine*. Philadelphia: WB Saunders, 1981, with permission.

Space medicine is still in its infancy. With greater experience in low earth orbit, with larger crews, and with longer missions, we can look to longitudinal studies to establish a relative or direct measurement of infection transmission risks associated with spaceflight. As the number and duration of flights increase, unique medical and physiologic problems will require innovative solutions (51).

SATURATION DIVING

Humans have participated in undersea operations for centuries. The growing realization of the potential of the ocean environment as a virtually untapped wealth of resources has led to an unprecedented interest in developing techniques for employment of people at increasing depths and for longer periods of time. Industrial and military operational needs have set the pace for exploitation of the sea, with further stimulation from scientific salvage efforts. The past half century has witnessed tremendous progress in people's ability to live in an environment that is essentially hostile to human existence. Recent advances in offshore oil resources exploration and production, undersea mining, and salvage and search and rescue techniques depend on the effort to extend people's ability to live and work under water—the development of saturation diving.

Saturation diving is used extensively for maintenance and inspection of offshore sub-sea oil production systems. The saturation period includes compression, bottom time (working period), and decompression. A typical saturation period is between 12 and 24 days, during which the divers live in pressurized chambers on board a diving vessel in an atmosphere of pressurized helium and oxygen. When working, the divers dress in a protective diving suit, in which heated sea water is continuously flushed on to the diver's skin to maintain thermal balance. The ambient absolute pressure is dependent on the working depth (normally 50 to 200 m) and the partial pressure of oxygen is dependent on the phase of the dive. The ambient temperature in the chambers varies with working depth, but is often around 28° to 30°C. The relative humidity is generally high and may reach 80% to 90%. During recompression, occupational saturation divers live in a closed, high-humidity environment with close physical contact. Cutaneous infections are frequent health complications during saturation diving (52,53). *P. aeruginosa* is frequently recognized as the causative agent of otitis externa and cutaneous infections (54). Saturation divers are particularly prone to cutaneous infections as they are routinely confined to warm, moist living conditions for prolong periods. Also, seawater has a rich variety of microorganisms that are capable of causing infections. The potential effects of saturation diving on human immunity are also a concern. Saturation diving has been shown to induce lymphocyte subset changes, including a decrease in the CD4/CD8 ratio, a decrease in the fraction of CD4 T cells, and an increase in NK cells (55,56). It has also been postulated that the decreased resistance to skin and other infections that are encountered in deep sea divers may be due to a decreased functional killing capacity of neutrophilic granulocytes (57).

Recently, Wang et al. (58) reported a molecular epidemiology investigation of an outbreak of methicillin-resistant *S. aureus* (MRSA) cutaneous infection, which involved all six members of a diving team during a 45-day saturation dive. The cutaneous infections involved different body sites including the nose, external ear canal, neck, back, and extremities. These infections did not respond to multiple courses of oral antibiotics or topical application of antibiotic ointment. This is the first report of spread of MRSA within a group of healthy divers in a saturation diving chamber. In this study, all MRSA isolates shared the same antibiotic sensitivity pattern, suggesting a common source. Molecular typing by pulsed-field gel electrophoresis (PFGE) confirmed that all MRSA isolates belonged to the same clone. The MRSA strain that caused the outbreak was most likely introduced by a colonized or infected diver. Direct or indirect contact was the likely mode of transmission of MRSA to the other divers.

Nasal carriage of *S. aureus* appears to play a key role in the epidemiology and pathogenesis of infection. The nasal colonization rate in the general diver population is unknown. In our study of six divers, MRSA nasal carriage was found in three out of the six divers. PFGE demonstrated that the *S. aureus* isolates obtained from the anterior nares of three divers and from the cutaneous infections of five divers were all the same strain.

We recommend implementation of a program for prevention of *S. aureus* outbreaks in saturation diving facilities including (a) identification of early cutaneous infections by pre-diving physical examinations; (b) good hygiene and Universal Precautions during the course of saturation diving; (c) judicious use of antibiotics, including topical agents, to reduce selection of resistant microorganisms; (d) obtaining cultures from lesions to guide antibiotic therapy; (e) eradication of MRSA nasal carriage by topical application of mupirocin; and (f) thorough environmental cleaning (including chamber and diving equipment) after each saturation dive.

CONCLUSION

The enclosed environments of hyperbaric and altitude chambers and pressurized chambers for saturation diving can potentiate the spread of transmissible pathogens. It is crucial to understand the importance of infection control procedures and to ensure their implementation, whether the people inside these chambers are patients and tenders, spaceflight trainees and crew members, or saturation divers. Only through surveillance will infections associated with such environments be recognized and prevented. Further research on the epidemiology and prevention and control of infections acquired in such chambers is needed.

REFERENCES

1. Camporesi EM, ed. *Hyperbaric oxygen therapy: a committee report.* Bethesda, MD: Undersea and Hyperbaric Medical Society, 1996.
2. Leslie CA, Sapico FL, Guiunas VJ, et al. Randomized controlled trial of topical hyperbaric oxygen for treatment of diabetic foot ulcers. *Diabetes Care* 1988;11:111–115.
3. Bakker DJ. *The use of hyperbaric oxygen in the treatment of certain infectious diseases especially gas gangrene and acute dermal gangrene.* Wageningen, the Netherlands: Drukkerij Veenman B.V., 1984.
4. Beaman L, Beamen BL. The role of oxygen and its derivatives in microbial pathogenesis and host defense. *Annu Rev Microbiol* 1984;38: 27–48.
5. Park MK, Myers RAM, Marzella L. Oxygen tensions and infections: modulation of microbial growth, activity of antibiotics, and immunologic responses. *Clin Infect Dis* 1992;14:720–740.
6. Van Unnik AJM. Inhibition of toxin production in *Clostridium perfringens* in vitro by hyperbaric oxygen. *Antonie Van Leeuwenhoek* 1965; 31:181–186.
7. Sheffield PJ. Tissue oxygen measurements. In: Davis JD, Hunt TK, eds. *Problem wounds: the role of oxygen.* New York: Elsevier, 1988.
8. Mader JT, Adams KR, Wallace WR, et al. Hyperbaric oxygen as adjunctive therapy for osteomyelitis. *Infect Dis Clin North Am* 1990;4: 433–440.
9. Zamboni WA, Roth AC, Russell RC, et al. Morphologic analysis of the microcirculation during reperfusion of ischemic skeletal muscle and the effect of hyperbaric oxygen. *Plast Reconstr Surg* 1993;91: 1110–1123.
10. Thom SR, Mendiguren I, Hardy K, et al. Inhibition of human neutrophil beta2-integrin-dependent adherence by hyperbaric O2. *Am J Physiol* 1997;272:C770–C777.
11. Mader JT, Adams KR, Couch LA, et al. Population of tobramycin by hyperbaric oxygen in experimental pseudomonas aeruginosa osteomyelitis (abstract 1331). In: *Programs and Abstracts of the 27th Interscience Conference on Antimicrobial Agents and Chemotherapy.* Washington DC: American Society for Microbiology, 1987:328.
12. Parks MK, Muhvich KH, Myers RA, et al. Effects of hyperbaric oxygen in infectious diseases: basic mechanisms. In: Kindwasll EP, ed. *Hyperbaric medicine practice.* Flagstaff, AZ: Best Publishing, 1994:141–164.
13. Wang J, Li F, Calhoun JH, et al. The roles and effectiveness of adjunctive hyperbaric oxygen therapy in the management of musculoskeletal disorders. *J Postgrad Med* 2002;48:226–231.
14. Jacoby I. How to prevent chamber disease transmission. *Pressure* 1991; 20:1–10.
15. Goodman RA, Solomon SL. Transmission of infectious diseases in outpatient health care settings. *JAMA* 1991;265:2377–2381.
16. Weber DJ, Rutala WA, Parham C. Impact and costs of varicella prevention in a university hospital. *Am J Public Health* 1988;78:19–23.
17. Josesphson A, Gombert ME. Airborne transmission of nosocomial varicella from localized zoster. *J Infect Dis* 1988;158:238–241.
18. Mullins J, Harvey R, Seaton A. Sources and incidence of airborne *Aspergillus fumigatus. Clin Allergy* 1976;6:209–217.
19. Aisner J, Schimpff SC, Bennett JE, et al. *Aspergillus* infection in cancer patients: association with fireproofing materials in a new hospital. *JAMA* 1976;235:411.
20. Lentino JR, Rosenkranz MA, Michaels JA, et al. Nosocomial aspergillosis: a retrospective review of airborne disease secondary to road construction and contaminated air conditioners. *Am J Epidemiol* 1982; 116:430.
21. Arnow PM, Saidgh M, Costas C, et al. Endemic and epidemic Aspergillosis associated with in-hospital replication of *Aspergillus* organisms. *J Infect Dis* 1991;164:998–1002.
22. Kaufmann A, McDade J, Patton C, et al. Pontiac fever: isolation of the etiologic agent (*Legionella pneumophila*) and demonstration of its mode of transmission. *Am J Epidemiol* 1981;114:337–347.
23. Muder R, Yu VL, Woo A, et al. Mode of transmission of *L. pneumophila*: a critical review. *Arch Intern Med* 1986;146:1607–1612.
24. Arnow P, Chou T, Weil D, et al. Nosocomial Legionnaire's disease caused by aerosolized tap water from respiratory devices. *J Infect Dis* 1982;146:460–467.
25. Johnson JT, Yu VL, Best M, et al. Nosocomial legionellosis uncovered in surgical patients with head and neck cancer: implications for epidemiologic reservoir and mode of transmission. *Lancet* 1985;2:298–300.
26. Mead JH, Lupton GP, Dillavou CL, et al. Cutaneous *Rhizopus* infection: occurrence as a postoperative complication associated with an elasticized adhesive dressing. *JAMA* 1979;242:272–274.
27. Pearson RD, Valenti WM, Steigbigel RT. *Clostridium perfringens* wound infection associated with elastic bandages. *JAMA* 1980;244: 1128–1130.
28. Patterson JE, Vecchio J, Pantelick EL, et al. Association of contami-

nated gloves with transmission of *Acinetobacter calcoaceticus* var. *anitratus* in an intensive care unit. *Am J Med* 1991;91:479–483.
29. McGuckin MB, Thorpe RJ, Abrutyn E. Hydrotherapy: an outbreak of *Pseudomonas aeruginosa* wound infections related to Hubbard tank treatments. *Arch Phys Med Rehabil* 1981;62:283–285.
30. Kaatz GW, Gitlin SD, Schaberg DR, et al. Acquisition of *Clostridium difficile* from the hospital environment. *Am J Epidemiol* 1988;127:1289–1294.
31. Brown RB, Sands M. Infectious disease indications for hyperbaric oxygen therapy. *Comp Ther* 1995;21:663–667.
32. Carson LA, Petersen NJ, Favero MS, et al. Growth characteristics of atypical mycobacteria in water and their comparative resistance to disinfectants. *Appl Environ Microbiol* 1978;36:839–846.
33. Holtz TH, Wenzel RP. Postdischarge surveillance for nosocomial wound infection: a brief review and commentary. *Am J Infect Control* 1992;20:206–213.
34. Hitchcock FA. Paul Bert and the beginnings of aviation medicine. *Aerospace Med* 1971;42:1101.
35. Guyton AC. *Textbook of medical physiology,* 6th ed. Philadelphia: WB Saunders, 1981.
36. Shaw RV II. *Training of civilian aircrews in altitude chambers. Federal Aviation Administration, Federal Air Surgeon's Medical Bulletin.* Oklahoma City: Civil Aeromedical Institute, 1992:92–94.
37. Savourey G, Guinet A, Besnard Y, et al. Are the laboratory and field conditions observations of acute mountain sickness related? *Aviat Space Environ Med* 1997;68:895–899.
38. Suzuki S, Nakabayashi K, Ohkouchi H, et al. Tuberculosis in the crew of a submarine. *Jpn J Thorac Dis* 1997;35:61–66.
39. Schmidt JP. Resistance to infectious disease versus exposure to hypobaric pressure and hypoxic, normoxic or hyperoxic atmospheres. *Fed Proc* 1969;3:1099–1103.
40. Schmidt JP, Barrington JD, Pindak FF. Hematologic changes associated with viral infection and hypobaric hypoxic. *Aerospace Med* 1970;41:602–607.
41. Giron DJ, Pindak FE, Schmidt JP. Effect of hypobaric hypoxia on MM virus infection. *Aerospace Med* 1970;41:854–855.
42. Stunkard JA, Schmidt JP, Cordaro JT. Resistance to bacterial infection in a hypobaric normoxic environment. *Aerospace Med* 1970;41:873–875.
43. Meehan RT. Immune suppression at high altitude. *Ann Emerg Med* 1987;16:974–979.
44. Kacena MA, Manfredi B, Todd P. Effects of space flight and mixing on bacterial growth in low volume cultures. *Microgravity Sci Technol* 1999;12:74–77.
45. Lapchine L, Moatti N, Gasset G, et al. Antibiotic activity in space. *Drugs Exp Clin Res* 1986;12:933–938.
46. Levin DS, Greenleaf JE. Immunosuppression during spaceflight deconditioning. *Aviat Space Environ Med* 1998;69:172–177.
47. Sonnenfeld G. Immune responses in space flight. *Int J Sports Med* 1998;19:S195–204.
48. Taylor GR, Konstantinova IV, Sonnenfeld G, et al. Changes in the immune system during and after spaceflight. *Adv Space Biol Med* 1997;6:1–32.
49. Nicogossian A, Parker J. *Space physiology and medicine.* NASA SP-447. Washington, DC: Government Printing Office, 1983.
50. Nicogossian A, Huntoon CL, Pool SL. *Space physiology and medicine,* 3rd ed. Philadelphia: Lea & Febinger, 1994:112–113.
51. Dietlein LF, Johnston RS. U.S. manned space flight: the first twenty years. A biological status report. *Acta Astronautica* 1981;8:893–906.
52. Schane W. Prevention of skin problems in saturation diving. *Undersea Biomed Res* 1991;18:205–207.
53. Alcock SR. Acute otitis externa in divers working in the North Sea: a microbiological survey of seven saturation dives. *J Hyg (Lond)* 1977;78:395–409.
54. Ahlen C, Mandal LH, Iversen OJ. Identification of infectious Pseudomonas aeruginosa strains in an occupational saturation diving environment. *Occup Environ Med* 1998;55:480–484.
55. Matsuo H, Shinomiya N, Suzuki S. Hyperbaric stress during saturation diving induces lymphocyte subset changes and heat shock protein expression. *Undersea Hyperb Med* 2000;27:37–41.
56. Shinomiya N, Suzuki S, Hashimoto A, et al. Effects of deep saturation diving on the lymphocyte subsets of healthy divers. *Undersea Hyperb Med* 1994;21:277–286.
57. Benestad HB, Hersleth IB, Hardersen H, et al. Functional capacity of neutrophil granulocytes in deep-sea divers. *Scand J Clin Lab Invest* 1990;50:9–18.
58. Wang J, Corson K, Mader JT. Diver's nose: the source of MRSA outbreak in a saturation diving chamber? (abstract). In: *Programs and Abstracts of the Oxygen 2002.* La Jolla, CA: Undersea & Hyperbaric Medical Society, 2002.

72

INFECTION CONTROL IN GENE THERAPY

DAVID J. WEBER
MARTIN E. EVANS
WILLIAM A. RUTALA

The last two decades has seen a dramatic increase in the number of gene therapy protocols being conducted in the United States and around the world. The first gene therapy protocol in the U.S. was initiated in 1990 for treatment of severe combined immunodeficiency (1). As of 2002, 636 gene therapy protocols had been initiated worldwide, which had enrolled 3,496 patients (Table 72.1) (2). The proliferation of clinical gene therapy trials reflects our developing understanding of the genetic basis of many diseases and rapid advances in molecular biology including the ability to produce vectors capable of transferring genetic material into somatic cells. However, the need for careful assessment of the potential benefits and risks of all gene therapy trials has been highlighted by the death of a patient during a gene therapy trial (3) and the development of leukemia in two other patients who underwent retrovirus-mediated gene transfer to correct X-linked severe combined immunodeficiency syndrome (4,5).

This chapter provides an overview of gene therapy technology and regulatory requirements for research in the U.S., and discusses the infection control aspects of clinical trials using gene transfer. Readers interested in gene therapy are referred elsewhere for reviews of the general methods and vectors used in gene therapy (6–15), the history of gene therapy (16), the ethics of gene therapy (17–24), regulatory aspects of gene therapy (25, 26), and liability issues (27). Reviews have covered the use of gene therapy in the following medical conditions: autoimmune diseases (28–30), cancer (31–34), human immunodeficiency virus (HIV) infection (35,36), genetic diseases (37–39), and disorders of the nervous system (40).

Recommendations for infection control of gene therapy have been discussed in an editorial (41), consensus conference (42), and an excellent review (43).

BACKGROUND

Gene therapy is a term that can be applied to any clinical therapeutic procedure in which genes are intentionally introduced into human somatic cells (8). Prior to considering gene therapy, several requirements must be fulfilled. First, the gene(s) in question must be identified, and the nature of the defect characterized. Genetic diseases can be defined by the aberrant, specific gene expression that differs from the disease-free state. This variance may be due to a gene product that is absent or deficient [e.g., the cystic fibrosis transmembrane regulator (CFTR) protein] (44,45), one that is abnormally present (e.g., Epstein-Barr virus nuclear antigen-1 in Hodgkin's disease) (46), or abnormal regulation or expression of normal cellular products (i.e., downregulation of human leukocyte antigens by adenovirus). Second, it is important to understand which tissues express the defect, and how accessible they are to manipulation. For example, while hemophilia B is caused by inadequate production of factor IX by the liver, factor IX does not require precise metabolic regulation, and even small amounts of production of factor IX by any cell line could prevent disease manifestations. Thus, hemophilia B is potentially amenable to *ex vivo* manipulation of hematopoietic cells or fibroblasts (47). The key technologies that have facilitated the utilization of gene therapy include new methods by which cellular genes could be isolated (cloned), manipulated (engineered), and transferred into human cells. To obtain a therapeutic effect, there are basically three options for somatic gene therapy: (a) replacement of defective or missing genes for the treatment of inherited diseases, (b) augmentation of normal gene function or introduction of additional genetic information that interferes with proliferative diseases, and (c) blocking disease triggering or supporting genes like oncogenes on the deoxyribonucleic acid (DNA) or ribonucleic acid (RNA) level (Table 72.2). In brief, these three options could be thought of as gene replacement, gene addition, and gene correction (14).

Human gene therapy is currently limited to manipulations affecting somatic, differentiated cells. Germline gene therapy, where reproductive cells are treated for the correction of a genetic disease being transferred to the patient's descendants, is not likely to become acceptable as a feasible strategy in the foreseeable future. Due to the potential risks and unpredictable results, germline gene therapy has never been authorized in humans.

There are two main approaches to gene therapy: *in vivo,* in which genes are delivered directly to target cells in the body,

TABLE 72.1. APPROVED GENE THERAPY PROTOCOLS THROUGH 2002

Trial Division	Subdivision	Protocols, Number (% of Trials within Subdivision)	Patients, Number (% of Trials within Subdivision)
Country of origin	United States	505 (79.4%)	2,088 (60.4%)
	Other	131 (20.6%)	1,409 (39.6%)
Clinical phase	I	420 (66%)	1,804 (51.6%)
	I/II	134 (21.1%)	914 (26.1%)
	II	73 (11.5%)	507 (14.5%)
	III	5 (0.8%)	Not available
Diseases addressed	Cancer	403 (63.4%)	2,392 (68.4%)
	Monogenic diseases	78 (12.3%	309 (8.8%)
	Infectious diseases	41 (6.4%)	408 (11.7%)
	Vascular diseases	51 (8.0%)	86 (2.5%)
	Other diseases	12 (1.9%)	21 (0.6%)
	Gene marking	49 (7.7%)	274 (7.8%)
Sources of target cells	Autologous	358 (58.2%)	2,758 (78.9%)
	Allogeneic	36 (5.7%)	246 (7.0%)
	Autologous and allogeneic	4 (0.6%)	166 (4.9%)
	Syngeneic	7 (1.1%)	61 (1.7%)
	Allogeneic and syngeneic	1 (0.2%)	8 (0.2%)
	Xenogeneic	3 (0.5%)	30 (0.9%)
	Not specified	213 (33.7%)	225 (6.4%)
Vector	Retrovirus	217 (34.1%)	1,755 (50.2%)
	Adenovirus	171 (26.9%)	644 (18.4%)
	Lipofection	77 (12.1%)	619 (17.7%)
	Naked/plasmid DNA	70 (11.0%)	123 (3.5%)
	Pox virus	39 (6.1%)	88 (2.5%)
	Adeno-associated virus	15 (2.4%)	36 (1.0%)
	RNA transfer	6 (0.9%)	30 (0.9%)
	Herpes simplex virus	5 (0.8%)	21 (0.6%)
	Others	11 (1.7%)	35 (1.0%)
	Not stated	25 (3.9%)	143 (4.1%)
Route of administration	Intratumor	152 (23.9%)	1,217 (34.8%)
	Intravenous	115 (18.1%)	320 (9.2%)
	Subcutaneous	64 (10.1%)	562 (16.1%)
	Bone marrow transplantation	45 (7.1%)	276 (7.9%)
	Intramuscular	49 (7.7%)	343 (9.8%)
	Intraperitoneal	22 (3.5%)	107 (3.1%)
	Intranasal	20 (3.1%)	162 (4.6%)
	Other	108 (17%)	269 (7.7%)
	Multiple routes	21 (3.3%)	90 (2.6%)
	Not specified	40 (6.3%)	148 (4.2%)

Adapted from ref. 2.

TABLE 72.2. STRATEGIES FOR USE OF GENE TRANSFER

Strategy	Method	Example
Supplementation	Transfer a functional gene into cells that have a defective gene	Cure severe immunodeficiency by replacing a defective adenosine deaminase gene with the normal gene by means of a retroviral vector
Immunotherapy	Deliver a gene that will elicit an immune response when the gene product is expressed	Infect with vaccinia containing prostate-specific antigen gene
Cancer therapy	Deliver a therapeutic gene into cancer cells	Infect cancer cells with adenovirus containing the gene for necrosis factor
Chemoprotection	Transfer a gene for drug resistance into normal cells to protect them from chemotherapy	Transfer a multidrug resistance gene into normal bone marrow cells; transplant the cells and administer chemotherapy to kill unprotected tumor cells
Ablative therapy	Deliver a gene that will allow activation of a prodrug leading to cell death	Insert the herpes simplex virus thymidine kinase gene into tumor cells and administer ganciclovir
Antiviral therapy	Deliver a gene into infected cells that interferes with viral replication	Transfer the gene for hairpin ribozyme, which cleaves HIV-1 RNA, into HIV-infected cells
Marking	Insert a gene into cells to identify them when the gene is expressed	Infect harvested bone marrow cells with a retrovirus containing neomycin phosphotransferase gene; after transplantation, look for cells producing the enzyme as evidence for engraftment

Adapted from Evans ME, Lesnaw JA. *Clin Infect Dis* 2002;35:597–605.

and *ex vivo,* in which target cells are genetically manipulated outside the body and then reimplanted (8). To carry out gene therapy, the exogenous gene is transferred in an expression cassette, including the promoter, which regulates expression of the new gene, often in the form of a complement DNA (cDNA), and stop signals to terminate translation (6). The exogenous or therapeutic gene can be isolated from the genome of a human, another animal, a plant, a bacterium, or a virus, and may code for any type of protein (6). Depending on the choice of the regulatory element, which controls the expression of the therapeutic gene, gene expression can be high or low level, specific to certain cell types, or even continuously variable, and can respond to local environmental factors such as the partial pressure of oxygen or the concentration of a drug (6).

The expression cassette is transferred to target cells using a vector. The most commonly used vector systems include retroviruses, lentiviruses, adenovirus, adeno-associated virus, poxviruses such as vaccinia, and herpes simplex virus (Table 72.3). Each delivers the expression cassette via distinct mechanisms and each has unique advantages and disadvantages (Table 72.4). Although viral vectors have been most commonly used, nonviral vector systems are of increasing scientific interest. Nonviral vector systems include plasmid-liposome complexes, newer kinds of vectors that sheath DNA in nonlipid coats, and naked DNA (7, 48–50).

To date, the many obstacles to successful gene therapy have not been overcome. The ideal gene delivery vehicle would efficiently and specifically transfer the gene to target cells, and subsequently obtain high, regulatable, and durable levels of gene expression (7). In addition, an ideal vector should not evoke an immune response (unless designed to do so), should be nontoxic to the recipient and easily purified in high concentration, and there should be no risk of recombination or replication (unless desired). Current obstacles to successful gene therapy include low efficiency of gene transfer to the target cell, inadequate regulation of the therapeutic gene in the transduced cell, and maintaining long-term, stable gene expression at an appropriate level.

TABLE 72.3. VECTORS USED FOR GENE THERAPY

Vector	Genome Size, kbp	Gene(s) Deleted or Inserted	Packaging Cell Line
Murine retroviruses	7–11	*gag, pol,* and *env*	HEK 293
Lentiviruses	7–11	All except *gag, pol,* and *rev*; additional deletions in long terminal repeats to produce self-inactivating vectors	HEK 293
Adenoviruses	36–38	E1a, E2, E3, E4, or all genes leaving signal sequences	HEK 293
Adeno-associated viruses	4.7	*cap* and *rep*	HEK 293 with plasmid bearing adenovirus helper functions
Vaccinia	130–380	No deletions; therapeutic gene inserted into silent regions of the genome or into nonessential genes (e.g., the thymidine kinase gene)	Not applicable
Herpesviruses	120–240	Immediate-early genes	
Plasmids and viruslike particles		Not applicable	Not applicable

Adapted from Evans ME, Lesnaw JA. *Clin Infect Dis* 2002;35:597–605.

COMMONLY USED VECTORS

Retroviruses

Retroviruses (e.g., murine leukemia virus) are the most popular vectors for gene transfer. Lentiviruses (e.g., HIV) may also be used in a similar fashion. When murine leukemia virus or other retroviral vectors are used for gene therapy, the genes required for retrovirus replication, such as *gag, pol,* and/or *env,* are deleted and the therapeutic gene inserted in their place (51–55). As a result of these deletions the vector is unable to replicate. Lentiviruses are increasingly used, because they overcome some of the limitations of the murine leukemia virus vectors. Multiple gene deletions in the lentivirus vectors make it extremely unlikely that the vector could be reactivated. In addition, the vectors are engineered to be replication incompetent by deleting sequences in the terminal signal (i.e., long terminal repeats) that are essential for gene expression. These vectors are resistant to complement and can be infused directly into the circulation, where they infect quiescent or dividing cells expressing CD4 on their surface (56).

Retroviruses are advantageous, because they elicit little immune response and because they integrate into the host genome. They offer the potential for stable long-term gene expression. A major concern is that oncoviruses may induce insertional mutations and transform target cells into cancer cells.

Adenoviruses

Adenoviruses are icosahedral, large, nonenveloped, double-stranded DNA viruses. Because of several advantages (Table 72.4), adenoviral vectors are widely used (57–59). There are four adenovirus gene regions, designated E1 through E4, that encode proteins necessary for viral replication. Early gene therapy trials utilized vectors that were constructed by deleting portions of E1 and inserting the transgene. Although the goal of this method was to develop a replication incompetent vector, it was subsequently demonstrated that cytokines (e.g., interleukin-6) could supply the function of the E1 region and permit low-level vector replication. In addition, E1-deleted adenovirus could replicate in the presence of co-infection with other DNA viruses, such as papillomavirus or cytomegalovirus. For this reason, modern vectors have deletions in additional regions of E2, E3, and/or E4. Growth of adenovirus vectors in the HEK 293 packaging cell line has led to recombination between the vector and viral gene sequences present in the packaging cell line with the genera-

TABLE 72.4. ADVANTAGES, DISADVANTAGES AND INFECTION CONTROL CONCERNS BY VECTOR

Vector	Advantages	Disadvantages	Infection Control Concerns
Murine retroviruses	Little immune response; potential for stable integration into host chromosome; amphotropic viruses for a wide variety of tissues	Inefficient *ex vivo* transfer; genes insert randomly and therefore have risk of insertional mutagenesis; inactivated by complement; only infect actively dividing cells; size of transgene limited	Minimal hazard when they are incubated with host cells *ex vivo*; secondary infections via accidental inoculation unlikely
Lentiviruses	Little immune response; potential for stable integration into host chromosome (life-long gene expression); can be administered *in vivo* because they are complement resistant	Insertional mutagenesis; limited to CD4+ cells unless pseudotyped with vesicular stomatitis or Ebola virus surface glycoprotein	Secondary infections via accidental inoculation possible
Adenoviruses	High titers can be grown; not integrated into host genome; large capacity for transgenes; infect dividing and non-dividing cells; very stable virus; can be administered *in vivo*	Systemic infection possible; elicits an immune response that may limit repeated use; genes may function transiently	Stable in the environment; potential transmission via contaminated fomites, close personal contact, or droplets; relatively resistant to some disinfectants
Adeno-associated viruses	Integrates into host chromosome; infects dividing and non-dividing cells, can be administered *in vivo*; does not elicit an immune response; requires helper virus for expression	Small capacity for transgenes; risk of insertional mutagenesis; association with male infertility; problems with expansion of production capacity	Prudent to use same precautions as for adenovirus
Vaccinia	Can accommodate a large transgenes; can be lypholized; does not integrate into host chromosome	Replication-competent vector with many adverse reactions; immune response may limit usefulness	Infection can be transmitted via contact or droplet routes; may cause severe disease in immunocompromised contacts or contacts with underlying skin disorders; vaccinators should receive vaccinia vaccine
Herpesviruses	Produced at high levels; targets non-dividing nerve cells; can accommodate large transgene; latency	Latency	If cutaneous infection present transmission may occur via direct contact
Alphaviruses	Produced at high levels; broad host range high RNA replication rate in cytoplasm, extreme transgene expression levels	Short-term expression mode, strong cytotoxic effects on host cells	Adverse reactions following accidental inoculation possible
Plasmids and viruslike particles	Safe; gene expression can be regulated	Low gene transfer efficiency; unstable in most body tissues	None

Adapted from Evans ME, Lesnaw JA. *Clin Infect Dis* 2002;35:597–605.

tion of replication-competent adenovirus. The use of alternative cell lines may minimize this problem (60).

Adeno-Associated Viruses

Adeno-associated virus is a single-stranded DNA virus. The virus is usually found as a provirus integrated into chromosome 19 of the host cell genome, where it remains inert until helper viruses supply the missing proteins or genes needed for replication. Helper viruses include herpesviruses, adenoviruses, or vaccinia virus. Replication-defective vectors can be constructed by removing all internal viral coding sequences of the wild-type strain and inserting the transgene. The use of adeno-associated viral vectors and their advantages and disadvantages are reviewed elsewhere (61–63).

Poxviruses

Vaccinia virus, the vaccine agent used in the eradication of smallpox, is being used as a gene therapy vector. Unlike other vectors it has not been engineered to be replication incompetent. Instead, transgenes are inserted into silent regions of the vaccinia genome.

Herpesviruses

Herpes simplex is an enveloped double-stranded DNA virus that infects sensory neural cells where it remains in a latent state. Replication incompetent virus can be produced by mutations in the required immediate-early genes. Transgenes can be inserted into these replication incompetent vectors. The use of herpes virus vectors is reviewed elsewhere (64,65).

Alphaviruses

Replication-deficient vectors have been engineered for several alphaviruses such as Semliki Forest virus, Sindbis virus, and Venezuelan equine encephalitis (66,67). The recombinant particles from these vectors are generated by cotransfection of alphavirus replicon and helper virus RNA, which therefore, upon infection of host cells, leads to one round of RNA replication, but no further production of virus progeny (67). These vectors are attractive because of the potential for high-titer production, broad host range, and large transgene expression capacity.

INFECTION CONTROL

Key aspects of infection control include protection of researchers and healthcare workers administering gene therapy vector and caring for subjects of gene therapy research, environmental and equipment disinfection, and laboratory safety. Institutional guidelines should be based on the vector used.

Protection of Healthcare Workers

Currently, there are no National Institutes of Health (NIH), Food and Drug Administration (FDA), or Centers for Disease Control and Prevention (CDC) infection control guidelines for minimizing the hazards to healthcare personnel caring for patients on gene therapy protocols or for preventing person-to-person transmission of gene therapy vectors. NIH requires persons submitting gene therapy protocols to describe the hazards of the proposed therapy to persons other than the patients being treated (68). Specifically, the investigator must answer the following questions:

1. On what basis are potential public health benefits or hazards postulated?
2. Is there a significant possibility that the added DNA will spread from the patient to other persons or the environment?
3. What precautions will be taken against such spread (e.g., patient sharing a room, healthcare workers, or family members)?
4. What measures will be undertaken to mitigate the risks, if any, to public health?
5. In light of possible risks to offspring, including vertical transmission, will birth control measures be recommended to patients? Are such concerns applicable to healthcare personnel?

However, NIH guidelines do not discuss how to assess the level of risk, what level of risk is acceptable, or measures to minimize such risks.

The goal of the infection control policies should be to minimize the risk of transmission of the gene vector to healthcare providers and visitors. For protocols that involve removal of the target cell with *ex vivo* alteration followed by reinfusion, environmental controls should be adequate to prevent hazardous exposure of healthcare personnel. For protocols that involve administration of vectors that could result in potentially transmittable diseases (e.g., vaccinia, adenovirus), use of appropriate personnel protective equipment as recommended in the CDC's isolation guidelines (69) should be sufficient to protect healthcare workers (Table 72.5). Special precautions may be advised for use of certain vectors. For example, persons administering vaccinia-based products should be screened and if no contraindications are present, immunized with vaccinia.

For directly administered gene vectors, prevention should focus on the known modes of transmission of the vector. Standard Precautions, as described by the CDC, should form the basis for rational infection control measures. At our current stage of knowledge, the use of Contact and Droplet Precautions (gloving and masking before entering the room) for vectors transmitted by the contact or droplet routes appears warranted. For vectors infused directly into the patient, Standard Precautions should be adequate.

All gene therapy protocols should include guidance on the management of healthcare workers accidentally exposed to a gene therapy vector.

Disinfection

Proper disinfection of work areas, instruments, and spills is critical to prevent person-to-person transmission of pathogens

TABLE 72.5. RECOMMENDED BIOSAFETY LEVELS FOR PHARMACY AND TRANSMISSION PRECAUTIONS USED FOR PATIENTS UNDERGOING GENE THERAPY

Vector	Recommended Biosafety level	Intravenous	Intramuscular or Intratumoral	Aerosol	Intradermal
Murine retroviruses	2	S	NA	NA	NA
Lentiviruses	3	S	NA	NA	NA
Adenoviruses					
At $\leq 10^{13}$ pfu/dose	2	S	S	C, D	NA
At $>10^{13}$ pfu/dose	2	D, C	D, C	A, D, C	NA
Adeno-associated viruses	1	S	S	C, D	NA
Vaccinia	2	NA	NA	NA	S
Herpesviruses	2	S	S	NA	NA
Alphaviruses	2 or 3 (depends on specific virus)	S	S	NA	NA
Plasmids and viruslike particles	1	S	S	S	NA

A, Airborne Precautions; C, Contact Precautions; D, Droplet Precautions; NA, not applicable; S, Standard Precautions; pfu, plaque-forming units
Adapted from Evans ME, Lesnaw JA. *Clin Infect Dis* 2002;35:597–605.

via contaminated hands. The environmental stability and susceptibility of microorganisms varies. Among gene therapy vectors adenoviruses are likely to be the most environmentally stable. Healthcare-associated outbreaks have been reported with both poxviruses and adenoviruses. Although most transmission is likely via droplet transmission, contaminated fomites have also played an important role. CDC guidelines for the disinfection of environmental surfaces and equipment should be scrupulously followed (70,71). In general, an Environmental Protection Agency (EPA)-registered hospital disinfectant should be used for cleaning environmental surfaces. A 1:10 diluted preparation of household bleach (sodium hypochlorite) would be effective against all currently used vectors. Infection control personnel should consult with the manufacturer of the gene therapy vector for their recommendations on the most effective surface disinfectant. EPA approved high-level disinfectants would be adequate for semicritical patient equipment. However, care must be taken [appropriate use of personal protective equipment (PPE)] during the cleaning steps to protect healthcare workers from accidental infection. When possible, initial decontamination following by cleaning and then high-level disinfection should be undertaken.

Laboratory Safety

Gene therapy vectors may represent a laboratory hazard during their construction. The U.S. Public Health Service has provided an excellent guideline for assuring the safe handling of microbes (72). Strict adherence to this guideline is recommended for all microbiologic and biomedical laboratories (Table 72.5). The key principle of biosafety ensconced in the guideline is "containment," a collection of engineering controls designed to allow the safe handling of infectious materials in the laboratory environment. *Primary containment,* the protection of personnel and the immediate laboratory environment from exposure to infectious agents, is provided by good microbiologic techniques and the use of appropriate safety equipment (e.g., biologic safety cabinets, enclosed containers). Preexposure immunization may be available and recommended (e.g., vaccinia vaccine for personnel working with this agent as gene therapy vector). *Secondary containment,* the protection of the environment external to the laboratory from exposure to infectious material, is provided by a combination of facility design and operational practices (e.g., specialized ventilation systems to ensure directional air flow, controlled access zone).

The U.S. Public Health Guideline groups all microbes into four categories depending on several factors including pathogen virulence, modes of transmission, and availability of vaccine and treatment. The pathogen group then defines four levels of recommended biosafety (BSL-1 to BSL-4) that require increasingly elaborate primary and secondary containment:

- BSL-1 practices, safety equipment, and facility design and construction are appropriate for undergraduate and secondary educational training and teaching laboratories, for other laboratories in which work is done with defined and characterized strains of viable microorganisms not known to consistently cause disease in healthy adult humans (e.g., adeno-associated virus).
- BSL-2 practices, safety equipment, and facility design and construction are applicable to clinical, diagnostic, teaching, research, or production facilities in which work is done with the broad spectrum of indigenous moderate-risk agents that are present in the community and associated human disease of varying severity (e.g., murine retroviruses, adenovirus). Primary hazards to personnel working with these agents relate to accidental percutaneous or mucous membrane exposures, or ingestion of contaminated materials.
- BSL-3 practices, safety equipment, and facility design and construction are applicable to clinical, diagnostic, teaching, research, or production facilities in which work is done with indigenous or exotic agents with a potential for respiratory transmission, and which may cause serious and potentially lethal infection (e.g., lentiviruses). Primary hazards to personnel working with these agents relate to autoinoculation, ingestion, and exposure to infectious aerosols.
- BSL-4 practices, safety equipment, and facility design and construction are applicable for work with dangerous and exotic agents that pose a high individual risk of life-threatening disease, which may be transmitted via the aerosol route and for which there is no available vaccine or therapy (e.g., no current gene therapy vectors fall into this class). The primary hazards to personnel working with BSL-4 agents are respiratory exposure to infectious aerosols and exposure of mucous membranes or nonintact skin to infectious droplets, and autoinoculation.

Management of Research Subjects

It would be ideal to either use or engineer live vectors that have a self-limited life span. In this case, research volunteers should be maintained on precautions until proven vector-free. Informed consent should include agreeing to isolation requirements. Prior agreement with state or local health departments can be sought to allow the use of a limited, legally enforced quarantine for patients who seek to leave the hospital and who may endanger the community. Quarantine measures should be individually reviewed by a biosafety committee whenever instituted. Should volunteers exposed to live vectors decide to leave containment prior to the end of their quarantine period, they should be contacted by appropriate county or state health department personnel.

Retrovirus

Murine retroviral gene transfer is usually performed *ex vivo* in a laboratory under carefully controlled conditions. Since there is no evidence that wild-type murine retroviruses cause human disease, these vectors probably do not represent a risk even if directly inoculated into the bloodstream. Newer murine-based vectors that have been engineered to be complement resistant and lentiviral vectors are theoretically capable of causing human disease. However, replication competent lentivirus vectors have not been reported and hence infection, although theoretically possible, is highly unlikely.

Standard precautions as used to prevent HIV transmission should be effective in preventing transmission of retroviral vectors. Whenever possible, needleless devices should be used to minimize the likelihood of accidental percutaneous injury. There is no need to isolate patients, use dedicated equipment, restrict visitors, use special precautions for waste disposal, or require special handling of linens or eating utensils.

Adenoviruses

In persons with normal host defenses adenoviruses cause minor illnesses such as conjunctivitis, respiratory tract disease, and gastroenteritis. In persons with abnormal host defenses adenoviruses may cause serious illnesses including pneumonia, gastrointestinal hemorrhage, cystitis, and hepatic necrosis. The mortality rate has been reported to be as high as 60% among stem-cell transplant patients and as high as 20% among renal or liver transplant patients with adenoviral infections. Currently there is no effective prophylactic vaccine or therapy.

Initially the use of adenoviral vectors generated two concerns: first, that the vector might recombine with wild-type virus and become replication competent; and second, that replication competent adenovirus reactivants in the treatment inoculum might be shed by patients who had undergone gene therapy, leading to transmission of infection to healthcare workers, visitors, family members, or other patients. For this reason, elaborate infection control measures were initially employed. However, published trials in which inocula of $\leq 10^{13}$ virus particles were used have not demonstrated either shedding or significant numbers of replication competent recombinants. It is still not known if therapy with higher titers of virus would present a hazard.

Because of concerns that complementation by wild-type adenoviruses could lead to the development of replication competent virus, it may be prudent to screen prospective gene therapy patients and healthcare workers for clinical signs of adenovirus infection. Subjects with possible active infection should be deferred from entering the trial; healthcare workers with possible infection should be reassigned to care for other patients. Pharmacy staff preparing adenoviral vectors should work in a level-2 biosafety cabinet and wear appropriate PPE (gloves, gowns). The vector should be transferred in a container clearly marked with a biohazard label. Air in syringes or tubing should be expressed in the pharmacy, not at the bedside.

Adenoviruses are extremely hardy and can survive on surfaces for an extended period of time. Surface disinfection should be performed after the subject has left his/her room. Only disposable equipment should be used, or equipment should be disinfected following patient use. Because of the theoretical risk of aerosol transmission if high-titer vector is provided, it would be reasonable to manage such patients on Droplet Precautions.

Adeno-Associated Virus

Only limited data are available on the frequency of vector shedding or reactivant shedding. Theoretically, adeno-associated virus vectors could be transmitted by the respiratory or fecal-oral route as is adenovirus. In absence of specific guidelines, it seems reasonable to use the same guidelines for adeno-associated viral vectors as are recommended for adenoviral vectors.

Poxviruses

Vaccinia is administered most commonly by intradermal scarification or intradermal injection. The virus is likely to be shed from the immunization site until the lesion completely scabs and heals over. Administration of vaccinia vectors should be done using aseptic technique (gloves) in a private room. Because vaccinia vectors are not designed to be replication defective, the risk of cross-infection with this vector is greater than for other gene therapy vectors. The risk of contact transmission can be minimized by keeping the vaccination site covered with a semipermeable or gauze dressing. An occlusive dressing should not be used. Contaminated dressings should be managed and disposed of as regulated medical waste. All personnel working with vaccinia vectors should be screened and, unless contraindicated, provided with vaccinia immunization. Personnel with a contraindication to vaccinia immunization should be prohibited from manipulating vaccinia vectors. Vaccinia vaccine should be provided only with informed consent. Vaccinated healthcare personnel should be managed as recommended by the CDC during the postvaccination period.

Vaccinated subjects may be managed using Standard Precautions. If they develop generalized vaccinia, progressive vaccinia, or eczema vaccinatum, they should be placed on Contact and Airborne Precautions. There are no special recommendations for the handling of eating utensils. Potentially contaminated clothes and bed linens should be managed appropriately during transport and either washed with hot water followed by drying or washed with bleach.

Herpesviruses

Only limited information is available on the shedding of herpes simplex virus (HSV) vectors. Transmission is possible with direct contact with lesions. However, the use of standard precautions should prevent transmission. Although, HSV can survive on fomites for up to 4 hours, fomite-mediated transmission has not been reported.

REGULATION

The institutions with major regulatory responsibility over human gene therapy are the NIH and the FDA, which have overlapping jurisdiction in the U.S. Within the NIH, the Office of Recombinant DNA Activities (ORDA) is responsible for reviewing and coordinating all activities related to the NIH Guidelines for Research Involving Recombinant DNA Molecules (68). The Recombinant DNA Advisory Committee (RAC) is a public advisory committee that advises the NIH director concerning recombinant DNA research. Within the FDA, gene therapy oversight falls within the Center for Biologics Evaluation and Research (CBER).

Experiments involving the deliberate transfer of recombinant DNA or DNA- or RNA-derived recombinant DNA into human subjects (human gene transfer) cannot be initiated without simultaneous submission to both NIH/ORDA and FDA of such information on the proposed experiment as is prescribed by those agencies. Investigational new drug (IND) applications shall be submitted to the FDA in the format described in 21 CFR, Chapter 1, Subchapter D, Part 312, Subpart B, Section 23, IND Content and Format. Gene therapy regulations were last updated by NIH in April 2002 (68) and by the FDA in March 1998 (73). Investigators should adhere to the most recent regulations, which can be found on the NIH *(www.nih.gov/od/orda/guidelines.htm)* and FDA *(www.fda.gov/cber/guidelines.htm)* Web sites.

Because the field is evolving so rapidly, regulation of these biologics is handled on a case-by-case basis but follows a common set of principles (68)

PRODUCT PREPARATION AND MONITORING

Key regulatory and safety aspects of product preparation include (a) an adequate rationale for efficacy of therapy; (b) vector source materials, which should be characterized and documented thoroughly, and viral vectors or plasmids, which should be generated from cloned and characterized constructs and subjected to confirmatory identity tests; (c) a detailed understanding and description of the procedure for selection of the final gene construct, method of transfer of the gene construct into the host cell, and selection and characterization of the recombinant host cell clone including vector copy number and physical state of the final vector construct inside the host cell (i.e., integrated or extra chromosomal); (d) a master viral bank, which should be created when a virus, with or without a therapeutic gene, is used as a seed in the manufacture of a therapeutic vector; and (e) demonstration of lot-to-lot reproducibility.

Additional important factors in the preparation of material for human gene therapy include the following: (a) sterility of the final product must be maintained (e.g., freedom from bacteria, fungi, *Mycoplasma,* and adventitious viruses); (b) in the case of replication defective or replication-selective vectors, master viral banks should be demonstrated to be free of replication-competent viruses, which may arise as a result of contamination or recombination during the generation of the master viral bank; (c) products made by cells and required for therapeutic activity should be shown to be biologically active, and this activity must be quantitated and shown adequate to produce the desired effect *in vivo*; (d) for genetically altered *in vitro* cells, evidence should be available as to whether cells survive and continue to function *in vivo*; and (e) for directly administered vectors, a highly sensitive assay should be available for detecting infection with the vector. In addition to being highly sensitive, the assay should also be specific for detection of the genetically altered vector.

This last point has been a concern since the inception of the RAC in 1974 and is a critical issue in infection control. There are many viral-like sequences endogenous in mammalian genomes, and the possibility exists that a vector could recombine with endogenous sequences or with a coincident superinfecting virus. Consequently, vectors have been designed that would require multiple recombination events, each one unlikely to produce a replication-competent virus (74). There has been a report of a replication-competent retrovirus found in the production of a vector to be used in a human protocol but not yet implemented in subjects (75).

DEVELOPING AN INFECTION CONTROL POLICY

Infection control recommendations are based on the microbiology and epidemiology of the vector used in the gene therapy protocol. Infection control policies should be altered after scientific studies provide data to liberalize or alter the recommendations. Unfortunately, there are only limited data on which to base our current recommendation, because data on transmissibility of vectors (e.g., shedding) and production of replication competent vectors has often been considered proprietary. The development of infection control guidelines, should gene therapy enter general medical use, will be imprecise, because data on which to base recommendations is limited by the small size of current trials, multitude of vectors in current use, highly selected patient populations, and handling of vectors by highly skilled researchers. Further the limited number and small size of trials makes it impossible to assess the possibility of rare adverse events.

The issues to be assessed in developing infection control policies are described in Table 72.6. In general, patients should be placed on isolation precautions based on the vector, mode of transmission, and risk of transmission. All patients should be managed using Standard Precautions. Other CDC precaution categories should be used as previously described. Measures should be in place to prevent sharps injuries.

Gene therapy vectors should be managed in the laboratory using NIH biosafety guidelines. Research personnel should be trained in the proper use of PPE. Vectors should be disposed of as regulated medical waste. Surface decontamination should be performed using EPA registered hospital disinfectants unless the vector requires other agents to ensure inactivation. In general, the pharmacy should adhere to similar safety guidelines such as preparing vectors for administration in an appropriate biosafety cabinet and use of appropriate PPE.

TABLE 72.6. COMPONENTS OF AN INFECTION CONTROL POLICY REGARDING GENE THERAPY

- Basis of infection control policy
  - Vector employed
  - Method of vector administration
  - Ability of vector to cause disease in the patient
  - Mode of transmission of the vector (i.e., contact, droplet, airborne)
  - Infectivity (i.e., transmissibility)
  - Ability of vector to cause disease in healthcare personnel
  - Potential for development of replication competent vector
  - Environmental stability (i.e., survival)
  - Susceptibility to disinfectants
- Hospital care issues
  - Isolation precautions
  - Visitor guidelines
  - Restrictions on patient travel outside hospital room
  - Disinfection: surface, equipment
  - Restrictions on healthcare personnel allowed to care for patient
  - Laboratory risks: via percutaneous injury, via aerosolization
  - Monitoring: research subject, medical staff, environment, visitors

The infection control policy should also address the screening and potential exclusion of personnel (e.g., workers with potential adenovirus infection), need for immunizations (e.g., vaccinia immunization), and management of personnel with accidental exposure to the vector (e.g., sharps injury).

CONCLUSION

Gene therapy is at the cutting edge of science. Appropriate infection control practices will need to be based on technologic advancements within the field of gene therapy, scientific assessment of the adequacy of current containment practices, and ongoing evaluation of risks to study volunteers and healthcare personnel.

REFERENCES

1. Blaese RM, Culver KW, Miller DA, et al. T lymphocyte-directed gene therapy for ADA-SCID: initial trial results after 4 years. *Science* 1995; 270:475–480.
2. *Wiley Journal of Gene Medicine* web site *http://www.wiley.co.uk/genetherapy/clinical/*.
3. Thompson L. Human gene therapy. Harsh lesions, high hopes. *FDA Consumer* 2000;34:19–24.
4. Hacein-Bey-Abina S, Von Kalle C, Schmidt M, et al. LMO2-associated clonal T cell proliferation in two patients after gene therapy for SCID-XI. *Science* 2003;302:415–419.
5. Kohn DB, Sadelain M, Gloriso JC. Occurrence of leukaemia following gene therapy of X-linked SCID. *Nature Rev Cancer* 2003;3:477–488.
6. Feuerbach FJ, Crystal RG. Progress in human gene therapy. *Kidney Int* 1996;49:1791–1794.
7. Friedmann T. Overcoming the obstacles to gene therapy. *Sci Am* 1997; 276:96–101.
8. Russell SJ. Science, medicine and the future. Gene therapy. *Br Med J* 1997;315:1289–1292.
9. Gorecki DC, MacDermot KD. Gene therapy: panacea or placebo? I. Strategies and limitations of gene therapy. *Arch Immunol Ther Exp (Warsz)* 1997;45:367–374.
10. Gorecki DC, MacDermot KD. Gene therapy: panacea or placebo? II. Main applications of gene therapy. *Arch Immunol Ther Exp (Warsz)* 1997;45:375–381.
11. Sandhu JS, Keating A, Hozumi N. Human gene therapy. *Crit Rev Biotechnol* 1997;17:307–326.
12. Anderson WF. Human gene therapy. *Nature* 1998;392(suppl):25–30.
13. Duque MDPM, Sanchez-Preito R, Lieonart M, et al. Perspectives in gene therapy. *Histol Histopathol* 1998;13:231–242.
14. Kmiec EB. Gene therapy. *Am Sci* 1999;87:240–247.
15. Balicki D, Beuthler E. Gene therapy of human disease. *Medicine* 2002; 81:69–86.
16. Friedmann T. The road toward human gene therapy—a 25-year perspective. *Ann Med* 1997;29:575–577.
17. Fletcher JC. Evolution of ethical debate about human gene therapy. *Hum Gene Ther* 1990;1:55–68.
18. Juengst ET. The NIH points to consider and the limits of human gene therapy. *Hum Gene Ther* 1990;1:425–433.
19. Fletcher JC, Richter G. Human fetal gene therapy: moral and ethical questions. *Hum Gene Ther* 1996;7:1605–1614.
20. Hillman AL, Brenner MK, Caplan AL, et al. Gene therapy: socioeconomic and ethical issues. *Hum Gene Ther* 1996;7:1139–1144.
21. Bayertz K. Ethical aspects of gene therapy and molecular genetic diagnosis. *Cytokines Mol Ther* 1996;2:207–211.
22. King NMP. Rewriting the points to consider: the ethical impact of guidance document language. *Hum Gene Ther* 1999;10:133–139.
23. Dettweiler U, Simon P. Points to consider for ethics committees in human gene therapy trials. *Bioethics* 2001;15:491–500
24. Smith L, Byers JF. Gene therapy is the post-Gelsinger era. *JONA's Healthcare Law Ethics Regul* 2002;4:104–110.
25. Cohen-Haguenauer O. Gene therapy: regulatory issues and international approaches to regulation. *Curr Opin Biotech* 1997;8:361–369.
26. Cornetta K, Smith FO. Regulatory issues for clinical gene therapy trials. *Hum Gene Ther* 2002;13:1143–1149.
27. Palmer JG. Human gene therapy: suggestions for avoiding liability. *Ann NY Acad Sci* 1994;716:294–305.
28. Trucco M, Robbins PD, Thomson AW, et al. Gene therapy strategies to prevent autoimmune disorders. *Curr Gene Ther* 2002;1:341–354.
29. Tarner IH, Fathman CG. The potential for gene therapy in the treatment of autoimmune disease. *Clin Immunol* 2002;104:204–216.
30. Robbins PD, Evans CH, Chernajovky Y. Gene therapy for arthritis. *Gene Ther* 2003;10:902–911.
31. Vile RG, Russell SJ, Lemoine NR. Cancer gene therapy: hard lessons and new courses. *Gene Ther* 2000;7:2–8.
32. Arceci RJ, Cripe TP. Emerging cancer-targeted therapies. *Pediatr Clin North Am* 2002;49:1339–1368.
33. Parney IF, Chang LJ. Cancer immunogene therapy: a review. *J Biomed Sci* 2003;10:37–43.
34. Douglas JT. Cancer gene therapy. *Technol Cancer Res Treat* 2003;2: 51–64.
35. Amado RG, Mitsuyasu RT, Zack JA. Gene therapy for the treatment of AIDS: animal models and human clinical experience. *Frontiers Biosci* 1999;4:D468–475.
36. Statham S, Morgan RA. Gene therapy: clinical trials for HIV. *Curr Opinion Mol Ther* 1999;1:430–436.
37. Desnick RJ, Schuchman EH. Gene therapy for genetic diseases. *Acta Paediatr Jpn* 1998;40:191–203.
38. Knoell DL, Tiu IM. Human gene therapy for hereditary diseases: a review of trials. *Am J Health Sys Pharm* 1998;55:899–904.
39. Howe S, Thrasher AJ. Gene therapy for inherited immunodeficiencies. *Curr Hematol Rep* 2003;2:328–334.
40. Ho DY, Sapolsky RM. Gene therapy for the nervous system. *Sci Am* 1997;276:116–120.
41. Weber DJ, Rutala WA. Gene therapy: a new challenge for infection control. *Infect Control Hosp Epidemiol* 1999;20:530–532.
42. Evans ME, Jordan CT, Chang SM, et al. Clinical infection control in gene therapy: a multidisciplinary conference. *Infect Control Hosp Epidemiol* 2000;21:659–673.
43. Evans ME, Lesnaw JA. Infection control for gene therapy: a busy physician's primer. *Clin Infect Dis* 2002;35:597–605.
44. Zeitlin PL. Therapies directed at the basic defect in cystic fibrosis. *Clin Chest Med* 1998;19:515–525.
45. Griesenbach U, Ferrari S, Geddes DM, et al. Gene therapy progress and prospects: cystic fibrosis. *Gene Ther* 2002;9:1344–1350.
46. Jarrett RF. Epstein-Barr virus and Hodgkin's disease. *Epstein-Barr Virus Rep* 1998;5:77–85.
47. Monahan PE, White GC. Hemophilia gene therapy: update. *Curr Opinion Hematol* 2002;9:430–436.
48. Wivel NA, Wilson JM. Methods of gene delivery. *Hematol Oncol Clin North Am* 1998;12:483–501.
49. Felgner PL. Nonviral strategies for gene therapy. *Sci Am* 1997;276: 102–106.
50. Rolland AP. From genes to gene medicines: recent advances in nonviral gene therapy. *Crit Rev Ther Drug Carrier Syst* 1998;15:143–198.
51. Takeuchi Y, Pizzato M. Retrovirus vectors. *Adv Exp Med Biol* 2000; 465:23–35.
52. Kim SH, Kim S, Robbins PD. Retroviral vectors. *Adv Virus Res* 2000; 55:545–563.
53. Weber E, Anderson WF, Kasahara N. Recent advances in retrovirus vector-mediated gene therapy: teaching an old vector new tricks. *Curr Opinion Mol Ther* 2001;3:439–453.
54. Hansen AC, Pedersen FS. Safety features of retroviral vectors. *Curr Opinion Mol Ther* 2002;4:324–333.
55. Brenner S, Malech HL. Current developments in the design of onco-retrovirus and lentivirus vector systems for hematopoietic cell gene therapy. *Biochim Biophys Acta* 2003;1640:1–24.
56. Zufferey R. Production of lentiviral vectors. *Curr Topics Microbiol Immunol* 2002;261:107–121.

57. Breyer B, Jiang W, Cheng H, et al. Adenoviral vector-mediated gene transfer for human gene therapy. *Curr Gene Ther* 2001;1:149–162.
58. Vorburger SA, Hunt KK. Adenoviral gene therapy. *Oncologist* 2002; 7:46–59.
59. Bauerschmitz GJ, Baker SD, Hemminki A. Adenoviral gene therapy for cancer: from vectors to targeted and replication competent agents. *Int J Oncol* 2002;21:1161–1174.
60. Fallaux FJ, Bout A, van der Velde I, et al. New helper cells and matched early region 1–deleted adenovirus vectors prevent generation of replication-competent adenoviruses. *Hum Gene Ther* 1998;9:1909–1917.
61. Lai CM, Lai YK, Rakoczy PE. Adenovirus and adeno-associated virus vectors. *DNA Cell Biol* 2002;21:895–913.
62. Wright JF, Qu G, Tang C, et al. Recombinant adeno-associated virus: formulation challenges and strategies for a gene therapy vector. *Curr Opinion Drug Discovery Dev* 2003;6:174–178.
63. Lehtonen E, Tenenbaum L. Adeno-associated viral vectors. *Int Rev Neurobiol* 2003;55:65–98.
64. Lilley CE, Branston RH, Coffin RS. Herpes simplex virus vectors for the nervous system. *Curr Gene Ther* 2001;1:339–358.
65. Burton EA, Fink DJ, Glorioso JC. Gene delivery using herpes simplex virus vectors. *DNA Cell Biol* 2002;21:915–936.
66. Lundstrom K. Alphavirus vectors for gene therapy applications. *Curr Gene Ther* 2001;1:19–29.
67. Lundstrom K. Latest development in viral vectors for gene therapy. *Trends Biotech* 2003;21:117–122.
68. National Institutes For Health. Guidelines for research involving recombinant DNA molecules (NIH guidelines), April 2002. *www.nih.-gov/od/orda/guidelines.htm.*
69. Gardner JS, Hospital Infection Control Practices Advisory Committee. Guideline for isolation precautions in hospitals. *Infect Control Hosp Epidemiol* 17:53–80, 1996.
70. Rutala WA, Weber DJ. Guideline for disinfection in health-care facilities. *MMWR (in press).*
71. Centers for Disease Control and Prevention. Guidelines for environmental infection control in health-care facilities. *MMWR* 2002;52(RR-10):1–44.
72. U.S. Department of Health and Human Services. *Biosafety in Microbiology and Biomedical Laboratories,* 4th ed. Washington, DC: U.S. Government Printing Office, 1999.
73. Center for Biologics Evaluation and Research, Food and Drug Administration. Guidance for human somatic cell therapy and gene therapy, March 1998. *Hum Gene Ther* 1998;9:1513–1524 (also *www.fda.gov/cber/guidelines.html*).
74. Anderson WF, McGarrity GJ, Moen RC. Report to the NIH recombinant DNA Advisory Committee on murine replication-competent retrovirus (RCR) assays (February 17, 1993). *Hum Gene Ther* 1993;4: 311–321.
75. Department of Health and Human Services, Recombinant DNA Advisory Committee, National Institutes of Health. Regulatory issues. *Hum Gene Ther* 1998;9:911–932.

73

INFECTION IN XENOTRANSPLANTATION—A MODEL FOR DETECTION OF UNKNOWN PATHOGENS

JAY A. FISHMAN

XENOTRANSPLANTATION: THE BACKGROUND

Over 80,000 people are awaiting human organs for transplantation in the United States, with at least an equal number in other countries. However, despite efforts to promote donation, 17 people in the U.S. die each day while on the waiting lists due to the lack of available organs. In 1907, the father of modern transplantation biology, Alexis Carrel, suggested that the future of transplantation for the treatment of organ failure was "heterotransplantation" now termed *xenotransplantation.* Xenotransplantation, the transplantation of cells, tissues, or vascularized organs from nonhuman species into human recipients, has reemerged as a potential solution to the growing shortage of human organ and tissue donors. Xenografts may serve as either permanent replacements or as a bridge to the availability of human-derived organs. In addition to vascularized grafts or tissues (e.g., pancreatic islets), bone marrow transplantation across species' lines may provide novel therapies for hematopoietic and metabolic diseases and AIDS, or serve as a mechanism for inducing chimerism and tolerance to transplanted solid xenografts (1,2).

A series of clinical xenotransplants have been performed including grafts of blood vessels, skin, and heart valves, fetal pancreatic islet cells and neural tissue from swine, and hearts and livers from nonhuman primates. None of these transplants has resulted in prolonged graft survival and none has been associated with unusual infections. The majority of such grafts have been lost to immunologic rejection (both humoral and cellular), molecular incompatibilities (e.g., clotting and complement activation), or infection due to what are considered common pathogens of organ transplant recipients. Genetic modifications of donor swine to prolong graft survival have included the insertion of human complement regulatory proteins and deletion in swine of the genes encoding the Gal, α-1,3-gal sugars, the main target of hyperacute humoral graft rejection. These recent advances have enhanced the likelihood that xenografts may survive to clinical utility. However, the intensity of immune suppression needed to maintain graft function in animal models suggests that infection and malignancy will remain significant barriers to xenotransplantation even as the immune barriers are being breached.

Although significant immunologic hurdles remain to the broad clinical application of xenotransplantation, public attention has focused largely on the ethical issues raised by interspecies transplantation and on the possible spread of infection from nonhuman species to human xenograft recipients and into the community at large. This risk of infection was considered in terms of the risk of the spread of common pathogens of the donor species, generally considered to be primates or swine, to humans via infection of the xenograft tissue. However, experience with immunocompromised patients including those with solid organ and hematopoietic transplants, with AIDS, or undergoing chemotherapy, has suggested that novel pathogens, possibly those not normally associated with human disease, may emerge in these "sentinel chickens" for infection (3–7). This risk has been termed "xenosis" or "xenozoonosis." This theoretical concern has gained some substance with the isolation of a novel porcine endogenous retrovirus (PERV) and the demonstration that this family of viruses is capable of infecting human cells *in vitro.* The description of other potential pathogens has further increased the level of concern. Conversely, xenotransplantation may provide a unique benefit when compared with human allografts. Xenografts may be resistant to infection by common human pathogens (e.g., HIV, hepatitis B and C, cytomegalovirus) and provide a novel approach to replacement of tissues damaged by persistent infection. Xenografts may also provide a vehicle for the transmission of genetic therapies.

Limited clinical trials of porcine xenotransplantation have been initiated without adverse infectious complications. A central problem remains the detection of potential human pathogens derived from other species and the assessment of the level of risk for xenosis. Information in this area has evolved rapidly due to ongoing studies of large animal models using immunosuppressive regimens comparable to those anticipated for use in clinical trials. In developing strategies for clinical xenotransplantation, the risk for xenosis must be assessed and minimized, and balanced against the potential benefits to transplant recipients (4).

BARRIERS TO SUCCESSFUL CLINICAL XENOTRANSPLANTATION

The main hurdles to successful xenotransplantation have been immunologic. The primary barrier to xenotransplantation has been hyperacute rejection (HAR) (1,12–14). HAR is the effect of preformed ("natural") antibodies present in humans and other New World primates against a ubiquitous Gal, α-1,3-gal epitope on (porcine) vascular endothelia. With HAR, the binding of antibody with complement deposition results in the death of the vascularized xenograft within minutes after implantation. Evolving antigraft humoral and cellular immunity and rejection contribute further to graft injury (15–19). Strategies to prevent hyperacute rejection have included depletion of antibody to the Gal, α-1,3-gal epitope and genetic engineering of swine to express human complement regulatory proteins on porcine xenografts so as to decrease complement deposition and tissue injury. It is of interest that some of these complement regulatory proteins also serve as cellular receptors for human pathogens (e.g., measles) to which swine are not naturally susceptible (20). Recently, genetic engineering of a number of heterozygous "knockout" swine has been reported without the gene for α-1,3-galactosyltransferase (GGTA1) and unable to produce the sugar molecule targeted by HAR (21). Homozygous knockout pigs have been born recently with preclinical studies getting underway. The effect of these manipulations is not yet known. It is notable that the natural antibodies may provide an immunologic defense against human infection by retroviruses, parasites and other common microorganisms that carry the Gal, α-1,3-gal epitope. Thus, depletion of such antibodies may pose a risk to the host. "Tolerance induction" (antigen specific immunologic unresponsiveness) and a variety of immunosuppressive regimens are under study to prevent chronic, cellular rejection. The impact of such manipulations (e.g., does the tolerant host also become tolerant of latent infections carried by the tissues?) remains to be determined.

THE CONCEPT OF XENOSIS AND RISK

Transplantation poses a unique epidemiologic hazard due to the efficiency of the transmission of pathogens, particularly viruses, with the cells of viable grafts (8). Most infections after transplantation that are not related to technical complications or nosocomial colonization, are due to exposures to community-acquired pathogens (e.g., influenza) or to reactivation of latent infection (e.g., cytomegalovirus, *Toxoplasma gondii*) from the host or the allograft in the setting of immune suppression. Infection in the immunocompromised host is often due to microorganisms of little native virulence in the immunologically normal host. The terms *xenosis, direct zoonosis,* and *xenozoonosis* imply that non–human-derived infection has developed after the natural barriers to infection, including skin and mucosal surfaces, have been bypassed by implantation of a xenograft (9).

Whether microorganisms transplanted into a host replicate or cause disease depends on the nature of the microorganisms, the efficacy of the host's inflammatory and immune responses, and the availability of the appropriate substrate for infection (cells with appropriate receptors, tissues with needed nutrients, oxygen, pH, etc.). Should the microorganism adapt (e.g., mutation, acquisition of novel nucleic acids) so as to survive within the human host, predictions based on the "normal" nature of the microorganism will become invalid. In xenotransplantation, predictions about infectious risks are based largely on extrapolation from experience in allotransplantation and on data related to specific pathogens identified in preclinical models. Novel human pathogens, however, may remain unrecognized until infection develops in the xenograft recipient. Few of these factors can be evaluated with certainty prior to performing xenograft implantation in humans or, possibly, in related primate species.

TABLE 73.1. NONRECOGNITION OF INFECTION ASSOCIATED WITH XENOGRAFT TRANSPLANTATION

High background rate of opportunistic infection in compromised hosts
Previously unknown or unrecognized pathogens
New syndromes or altered clinical manifestations in the transplant recipient
Low incidence or scattered or sporadic cases
Masked symptoms due to co-infection with other opportunistic pathogens
Absence of specific diagnostic tests for animal-derived microorganisms
Common syndromes (respiratory, liver, gastrointestinal)
Latency or carrier (colonization) state without clinical manifestations

A number of factors may increase the risk of infection in xenotransplantation: (a) the xenograft serves as a reservoir from which donor microorganisms are introduced and replicate without the need of a "vector" to achieve disease transmission; (b) novel clinical syndromes may be unrecognized, given the high background rate of infection and diminished signs of inflammation in the immunocompromised transplant recipient (Table 73.1); (c) microbiologic assays for microorganisms from nonhuman species may not exist; (d) donor-derived microorganisms may be nonpathogens in the native host species but may cause disease in a new host ("xenotropic microorganisms"), or may acquire new characteristics (genetic recombination or mutation) (10,11); and (e) donor–recipient incompatibility of the major transplantation antigens required for cellular immune function [i.e., major histocompatibility complex (MHC) antigens] may reduce the efficacy of the host's immune response to infection within the xenograft.

IDENTIFYING POTENTIAL HUMAN PATHOGENS

Although there are many microorganisms from other species that infect humans, some are likely to pose a particular threat to the immunocompromised human host (Table 73.2). Without confirmation in animal models or in humans, such predictions are merely educated guesses based on experience with comparable microorganisms in immunocompromised humans. Specific microorganisms may increase in virulence with passage in a new host (evolutionary adaptation) or may cause no disease in their native species while causing disease in xenograft recipients (12). To reduce this risk as much as possible, exclusion criteria (Table 73.3) have been generated for microorganisms likely to cause

TABLE 73.2. CATEGORIES OF POTENTIAL PATHOGENS RESULTING FROM XENOTRANSPLANTATION

Traditional zoonosis: well-characterized clinical syndromes of humans (e.g., *Toxoplasma gondii*); specific diagnostic assays generally available

Species-specific: microorganisms incapable of causing infection outside the xenograft (e.g., porcine cytomegalovirus); some tests available, few standardized assays available for humans

Potential pathogens: microorganisms of broad "host range," which may spread beyond the xenograft (e.g., adenovirus); few specific diagnostic assays available

Unknown pathogens: microorganisms not known to be human pathogens and for which clinical syndromes and microbiologic assays are not available

- New virulence characteristics within a host; i.e., xenotropic microorganisms
- Viral recombinants resulting from intentional genetic modification of donor diseases resulting from multiple simultaneous infections (e.g., lymphosis of cattle due to *Babesia* and viral co-infection)

disease in xenograft recipients. From these criteria, lists of microorganisms have been generated to guide the breeding of source animals for xenotransplantation (Table 73.4). Such lists, although inexact in the absence of clinical experience, serve a variety of purposes in the progress of xenotransplantation: (a) microorganisms thought to pose an unacceptable risk to the recipient can be bred out of a donor herd prospectively (designated pathogen-free, DPF); (b) microbiologic assays for these microorganisms can be developed for clinical use; (c) studies in preclinical xenograft models may clarify the biology of these microorganisms; and (d) prophylactic strategies can be developed for microorganisms not "removed" from donors.

Microorganism exclusion lists vary with the donor species and the use intended for the xenograft. Thus, pancreatic islets may pose different risks for infection and/or require different immune suppression than whole, vascularized pancreases; neural cells placed in the brain may provide a risk different from that posed by a xenografted liver or heart. Such lists of designated pathogens (e.g., for swine, Table 73.5) provide a basis for microbiologic screening of source animals and/or of cells and tissues intended for xenotransplantation.

Such microbiologic standards must be "dynamic"—rigorously tested and subject to revision based on experimental and clinical data. Standards for testing must also reflect the evolution of testing strategies [e.g., quantitative assays or reverse-transcriptase polymerase chain reaction (RT-PCR)] and adjusted for

TABLE 73.3. SCREENING XENOGRAFT SOURCE ANIMALS: MICROBIOLOGIC EXCLUSION CRITERIA

Known pathogens of humans (e.g., rabies, *Mycobacterium tuberculosis*)

Known pathogens of immunocompromised human hosts (e.g., *Toxoplasma gondii, Strongyloides* species)

Similar to pathogens of transplant recipients (e.g., porcine cytomegalovirus adenovirus)

Antibiotic-resistant microorganisms (bacteria, viruses)

Viruses at high risk for recombination (e.g., parvovirus, rotavirus)

Organ-specific exclusion list (e.g., *Mycoplasma* species in lung donors)

TABLE 73.4. MICROBIAL AGENTS OF SWINE KNOWN TO CAUSE INFECTION IN HUMANS

Bacteria:
Actinobacillus species
Actinomyces pyogenes
Bacillus anthracis
Brucella suis
Campylobacter coli
Campylobacter jejuni
Chlamydia psittaci
Clostridium perfringens
Clostridium septicum
Clostridium tetani
Erysipelothrix rhusiopathiae
Haemophilius species
Listeria monocytogenes
Mycobacterium avium complex
Mycobacterium bovis
Mycobacterium tuberculosis
Pasteurella multocida
Pseudomonas aeruginosa
Pseudomonas pseudomallei
Salmonella cholerasuis
Salmonella enteriditis
Salmonella typhimurium
Shigella species
Staphylococcus aureus
Streptococcus group E
Streptococcus pneumoniae
Streptococcus suis
Yersinia enterocolitica
Yersinia pseutotuberculosis

Fungi:
Aspergillus species
Candida albicans
Coccidioides immitis
Cryptococcus neoformans
Histoplasma capsulatum
Microsporum nanum (ringworm)
Nocardia asteroides
Petriellidium boydii
Pneumocystis carinii
Prototheca (algae)
Zygomycetes (*Mucor, Rhizopus, Absida*)

Parasites (protozoa/helminths):
Ascaris suum
Cryptosporidium species
Gnathostoma spinigerum
Isospora species
Paragonimus westermani
Sarcocystis suihominis
Spirometra species
Schistosoma japonicum
Toxoplasma gondii
Trichinella spiralis

Viruses:
Encephalomyocarditis virus
Foot and mouth disease Virus
Parainfluenza virus-1
Rabies
Swine influenza (H_1N_1, H_3N_2)

TABLE 73.5. "DESIGNATED-PATHOGEN-FREE" MINIATURE SWINE

For xenotransplantation, examples of microorganisms to exclude:

Bacteria:
Brucella suis
Leptospira
Listeria monocytogenes
Mycobacterium bovis
Mycobacterium tuberculosis
Mycobacterium avium-intracellulare complex
Mycoplasma hyopneumoniae (lung transplant)
Salmonella
- *typhi*
- *typhimurium*
- *cholerasuis*

Shigella species

Streptococus suis

Fungi:
Candida species (lesions)
Histoplasma capsulatum
Aspergillus species (colonized or lesions)
Cryptococcus neoformans

Parasites:
Ascaris suum
Cryptosporidium parvum
Strongyloides ransomi
Toxoplasma gondii
Trichinella spiralis, Neospora
Isospora species

Echinococcus species

Viruses:
Porcine hepatitis E
Encephalomyocarditis virus
- Influenza virus (porcine and human)
- Porcine cytomegalovirus
- Porcine γ = herpesvirus (PGHV or PLHV)
- Porcine reproductive and respiratory Syndrome virus
- Porcine circovirus
- Porcine parvovirus; rotavirus
- Rabies virus
- Pseudorabies virus
- Nipah (Hendra-like) and Menangle virus

differences in the use of specific tissues, immunosuppressive regimens, and the geographic region in which tissues are procured.

SOURCE SPECIES

Swine is the source species for organs most often considered for use in humans. Although nonhuman primates are closer immunologically ("concordant species"), ethical issues, the risk of transmission of viruses known to be infectious for humans, poor size matches, and the expense and difficulty in breeding have excluded this option (22–25). Potential infectious risks associated with the use of nonhuman primates as organ donors for humans have led the U.S. Food and Drug Administration (FDA) to preclude the use of these species as organ donors for humans. Swine, although immunologically dissimilar from humans ("discordant species"), are easier and less costly to breed, can be good size matches for humans, and may be genetically engineered to express or suppress specific genes relevant to transplantation. The best-studied swine include those genetically engineered to express human complement regulatory proteins (h-DAF) and the National Institutes of Health (NIH) miniature swine. The latter herds have some advantages for possible human use including genetic homogeneity (including of histocompatibility antigens), the ability to control microbial flora in the closed herd, the capacity to establish genetic knockouts or to introduce transgenes, and extensive investigation for studies of immunologic tolerance (1,2). Both fetal and adult tissues have been studied. Other species have not been investigated as xenografts sources for human use to any great extent.

POTENTIAL PATHOGENS FROM SWINE: BREEDING

Swine have been developed for studies of transplantation immunology and are being developed commercially as potential organ donors for humans. Infections in these animals following bone marrow and solid organ transplantation have been studied. Historically, routine prophylaxis using broad-spectrum antimicrobial agents in swine has resulted in the selection and dissemination of highly antimicrobial-resistant bacteria and colonization with yeasts. Infections related to surgical sites and intravenous catheters were due to gram-negative bacteria including *Klebsiella pneumoniae* and *Pseudomonas aeruginosa* with resistance to multiple antibiotics. Subsequently, animals entering the facility became colonized with resistant microorganisms within 7 days following arrival. In addition, common colonizing bacteria of swine causing bacteremic infections included *Enterococcus faecalis, Staphylococcus aureus, Streptococcus suis, Actinomyces pyogenes, Pasteurella multocida,* and *Candida albicans.* With antimicrobial restrictions both in the facility and in the farms rearing these animals, routine isolation of antibiotic-resistant bacteria from mouth, nares, and rectum disappeared (4,6,24). Thus, antimicrobial use must be restricted in the rearing of potential xenograft donors.

Zoonotic infections of humans with swine-derived pathogens have been observed in meat handlers, in farmers, and in individuals ingesting undercooked pork products. Ingestion has resulted in many bacterial and parasitic infections, including those due to *Salmonella* species, *Cholera suis, Brucella,* and *Trichinella spiralis* species. Significant infections in butchers and farmers have included rabies, anthrax, brucellosis, *Cholera* species, *Campylobacter* and *Cryptosporidia* gastroenteritides, toxoplasmosis, leptospirosis, listeriosis, erysipeloid, salmonellosis, and yersiniosis. Infections due to *S. suis* are considered an occupational hazard for European meat handlers. No excess mortality due to infection has been described in these workers. Of the common pathogens derived from swine, swine influenza (general H1N1 or H3N2 subtypes) has had the greatest impact, causing the human influenza pandemic of 1918–1919 and multiple subsequent outbreaks. Up to 20% of slaughterhouse workers and 25% of swine have serologic evidence of exposure to these agents. Recombinant strains of influenza (H1N2) have been observed in swine populations in which H1N1 strains are endemic, and co-infection from humans with other strains (H3N2) occurs. There is no evidence of increased virulence of these "new" strains. However, such populations of swine may serve as a reservoir for human infection.

Most clinical laboratories lack microbiologic assays adequate for the complete speciation of many common pathogens derived from swine including a variety of aerobic streptococci, *Haemophilus, Campylobacter,* and *Pasteurella* species. In our animals, clinical isolates have been characterized by veterinary laboratories, often using assays not approved for human use. *S. suis,* in particular, causes severe metastatic infection in humans including bacterial meningoencephalitis. Serologic tests to measure human antibodies against porcine-specific microorganisms or porcine serologies against human-specific pathogens are not available for studies of epidemiology. Further, serologic assays are often of limited use in immunocompromised individuals who may fail to develop antibody responses rapidly enough for use in clinical diagnosis. As a result, new microbial pathogens from swine will require the development of new microbiologic assays for clinical use. These tests must include both culture systems and assays for microorganism-specific proteins and nucleic acids.

Exposures to products derived from pigs and other nonhuman species have had no demonstrable adverse effects on individuals or the general population. Screening of cesarean-derived porcine fetal tissues intended for human xenotransplantation has been reported for pancreatic islet cells implanted into the kidney capsule or portal vein. These investigators have focused on the reduction or elimination of common pathogens of swine in tissue preparation. Bjoersdorff et al. (26,27) used a serologic and microbiologic screening program for preparations of islet-like cell clusters. Antibodies were found in donor swine to *Leptospira interrogans* and *Aspergillus fumigatus.* Bacterial cultures were rarely (4%) positive from the endometrium or amniotic fluid, and negative from the transplanted cell preparations. Viral, fungal, and parasitic evaluations were also negative. When transplanted into humans, no infections were reported. Transplantation of porcine fetal brain cells for the treatment of refractory Parkinson's disease and intractable seizures with minimal immune suppression have been achieved without infectious complications to date. Transplantation into the central nervous system may be less subject to immune rejection or cellular inflammation than other tissues. The impact of this location on the activation of infection cannot be predicted.

Xenotransplantation from swine to nonhuman primates and rodents has achieved only limited survival (3 to 8 weeks). This represents a relatively limited period of observation for the emergence of latent infection. "Archiving" of tissue and serum samples from donor animals and recipients will be essential in the tracking of any unsuspected or novel pathogen in clinical trials.

The need for herd isolation and continuous surveillance of animals intended for organ derivation places a significant burden on the developers of animals for human organ donation. Meticulous record keeping of all breeding conditions and archived specimens of animal tissues and sera must be maintained to allow prospective and retrospective evaluation of infectious hazards from each animal and/or herd. Barrier (isolation) facilities for isolated herds of animals appear essential. However, it is likely that the manner in which the level of safety created by the exclusion criteria or lists of microorganisms is achieved need not be uniform as long as the transplanted tissues do not pose a microbiologic hazard to the recipient. For example, the need to develop pathogen-free herds of animals may be reduced if the absence of potential pathogens can be demonstrated, or such microorganisms removed, during processing. Thus, cellular transplants (e.g., bone marrow, microencapsulated tissues) pose a different set of opportunities and challenges than do vascularized organ grafts. The goal, therefore, is not to establish the use of a single technology for animal husbandry but to achieve the microbiologic end point of optimal safety. Achievement of microbiologic standards must be monitored through the routine screening of sentinel animals from the donor herds. In addition, food sources must be carefully selected to avoid the introduction of microorganisms and prions. The development of breeding technology includes a variety of facilities for the isolation of herds from other animals (including rodents) and arthropod vectors. The development and use of such facilities must be documented so as to comply with regulatory authorities and to ensure optimal animal welfare standards. Health screening must not be limited to infectious diseases risks. Inbreeding may increase the incidence of congenital malformations or of inborn errors of metabolism, which must be identified and excluded from source animals.

Primate-Derived Pathogens

Perhaps the best-characterized accidental human exposure to animal-derived virus was the contamination of the Salk polio vaccine virus and adenovirus vaccines with simian virus 40 (SV40). SV40 was secreted by the rhesus monkey cells used to grow the vaccine strains of virus. SV40 was undetected, because the virus causes no cytopathic effect in the monkey cell lines used for vaccine production ("xenotropic"). SV40, an oncogenic agent in monkeys, was ingested or injected into over one million individuals without adverse effects on morbidity or mortality, including leukemia or other forms of carcinoma by 10 years following exposure (in 1960). Careful analysis is complicated by the presence of cross-reacting antigens for serologic testing and by the relatively short follow-up period. More recent data suggest a possibly increased frequency of SV40 DNA sequence in some mesotheliomas. Increasing numbers of infections due to other polyomaviruses (JC and BK) have been described in immunocompromised individuals. Human infections due to nonhuman primate viruses have been well documented in regard to Marburg virus from African green monkey kidneys used for vaccine production, herpes B virus, and SIV.

Few data are available regarding the activation of infection following primate to human xenotransplantation (22,25). Infections including *Aspergillus* fungemia and bacterial peritonitis following an anastomotic leak have complicated the recoveries of immunosuppressed recipients of livers from nonhuman primates. Patients have not developed serologic evidence of infection due to B-virus or other unsuspected pathogens, but further studies of the recipients (nucleic acid hybridization or polymerase chain reaction amplification) for such pathogens are needed.

Given the potential hazard of exposure to primate-derived infections, the FDA states that xenotransplants from nonhuman primates would expose "recipients, their close contacts, and the public at large . . . to significant infectious disease risk" (Guidance for Industry, FDA, March 1999). In particular, a large group of viruses capable of replicating in human cells have been identified in most nonhuman primate species.

NOVEL VIRUSES IN XENOTRANSPLANTATION

After transplantation, cell-associated viruses are a common form of infection in recipients. The most common infections are those due to herpesviruses [cytomegalovirus (CMV), human herpesviruses (HHV) 6, 7, and 8, Epstein-Barr virus (EBV), herpes simplex], community acquired respiratory viruses (influenza, respiratory syncytial virus), hepatitis viruses, polyomaviruses, and papillomaviruses. In the transplant recipient, viral infection has been associated with (a) viral syndromes (fever, neutropenia, lymphadenopathy) and tissue injury (retinitis, hepatitis) or allograft and xenograft injuries (e.g., nephritis, carditis, pneumonitis); (b) increased rate of graft rejection via upregulation of cell surface antigens and a proinflammatory cytokine milieu; (c) systemic immune suppression that predisposes to other opportunistic infections (e.g., *Pneumocystis carinii, Aspergillus species,* or *Nocardia asteroides*); and (d) contribution to the development of malignancy (e.g., anogenital and squamous carcinoma with papillomavirus, lymphoma with EBV).

The ability of unknown pathogens to replicate and adapt to the human host following transplantation is unknown. Altered tissue tropism, mutation, or recombination with host or donor nucleic acids has been described in animal models. Xenotropic viruses or defective viruses are also well known. Many of the conditions associated with viral activation (e.g., immune suppression, graft-versus-host disease, graft rejection, viral coinfection, cytotoxic therapy) will be present in the xenograft recipient.

In our studies of pig-to-primate xenotransplantation, immune suppression increases the replication of PERV, porcine cytomegalovirus (PCMV), and porcine lymphotropic herpesvirus (PLHV), and possibly others (30–38).

Endogenous Retroviruses

A unique concern in xenotransplantation is the risk of retroviral infection. Exogenous human retroviral infections (HTLV-1, HTLV-2, and HIV) have been transmitted with tissues during organ transplantation and associated with active infection. The course of accidentally transmitted infection due to HIV-1 is accelerated in transplant recipients, manifesting disease (AIDS) within 6 months (28,29). Concerns about retroviral transmission in xenotransplantation relate to the potential for "silent" transmission, i.e., manifestations of retroviral infection may be clinically inapparent. The activation of latent virus and the development of clinical manifestations, if any, may be delayed for over a decade and may not occur during the life span of the recipient. Further, the manifestations of retroviral infection may be clinically inapparent: altered gene regulation, oncogenesis, or recombination.

Endogenous γ-retroviruses, which are infectious for human cells *in vitro,* have been described in many mammalian species including baboons (BaEV), cats (RD114), and mice (murine ERV). Three closely related, replication competent C-type porcine endogenous retroviruses (PERV A, B, C) have been identified, which appear to have closest phylogenetic relatedness to the gibbon-ape leukemia virus (GALV) and the Koala retrovirus (KoRV) (33,34,39). These strains carry distinct *env* genes and belong to different receptor interference groups. The *env* region is responsible for host range determination—receptor binding by the virus to target cells and variation in antigenicity. Production of PERV is assayed using either quantitative DNA PCR or RT-PCR methods. Proviral DNA is found in the germ lines and expressed by porcine cell lines and in the cells and tissues of normal swine (34). PERV has been detected in all strains of swine tested with significant variability in the amount of virus produced and the copy number of possible full-length proviral sequences (range 8 to 50).

PERV A and B infect many human cell lines and primary cell cultures (32,33,39–42). PERV that is infectious for human cells *in vitro* appears to contain a recombinant *env* gene consisting of portions of PERV A and PERV C. The role of such recombinants *in vivo* is unknown. Thus, swine with incomplete genomic provirus (i.e., PERV A without a complete *env* gene) might be able to generate infectious virus in the presence of infectious PERV C. In species with endogenous viruses (mice) pseudotyping of virus (packaging in host viral envelope) occurs, which complicates analysis of studies of pig tissues in murine hosts.

No evidence of infection has been demonstrated of human cells *in vivo* and no disease due to this family of viruses has been described in swine or humans to date (33,41,43–46). In studies of individuals with transient exposure to pig tissues (by splenic perfusion, skin grafts for burns), there may be some persistence of porcine cells or nucleic acids in circulation without evidence of PERV infection of human cells *in vivo.* Some data suggest that primary cell lines of primates (baboons, gorilla, and macaques) can be infected by PERV A, B, and possibly C, which enhances the value of preclinical studies in primates.

Open reading frames (ORFs) of additional B, C, and D type retroviruses exist in the porcine genome. Most are small ORFs (300 base pairs) of unknown significance (42).

PERV messenger RNAs (mRNAs) are expressed spontaneously in all pig tissues under consideration for xenotransplantation in all types of swine tested to date. There is significant variation between tissues in the sizes and amounts of some of the PERV mRNA transcripts, consistent with *in vivo* recombination or processing in different tissues.

Viral expression is amplified by stimulation of swine peripheral blood lymphocytes *in vitro* and by immune suppression *in vivo.*

Herpesviruses

Activation of latent α-, β-, and γ-herpesvirus infections is one of the most important problems in transplantation (8). The herpesviruses are activated during periods of intensified immune suppression or immune dysfunction and by immune reactivity to grafts (rejection) (47–50). Comparable viruses exist in mice, primates, and swine. The replication of PCMV is enhanced in a pig-to-primate model of xenotransplantation (30,36). PCMV infection has been associated with tissue-invasive infection in porcine xenografts in baboon hosts and appears to participate in the induction of endothelial injury and consumptive coagulopathy (CC) in some animals. It is unclear whether the syndrome of CC in animal models is due to endothelial activation by viral infection (and secretion of tissue factor), immune injury (antibodies or cells), or other unidentified factors. PCMV does not appear to cause invasive disease in baboon recipients of porcine xenografts based on molecular and histologic evaluations (30). However, intensive immune suppression used in studies of xenotransplantation may result in a significant risk of reactivation of latent PCMV. Of note, early weaning of swine appears to reduce the incidence of CMV infection and improve the survivals in pig-to-baboon xenotransplantation of porcine kidneys and hearts. Recent data suggest that porcine CMV may have reduced susceptibility to ganciclovir, foscarnet, and cidofovir *in vitro.*

A porcine γ-herpesvirus (PLHV) has been described in association with a syndrome of lymphoid proliferation in swine undergoing experimental allogeneic hematopoietic stem cell transplantation and with characteristics similar to posttransplantation lymphoproliferative disease (PTLD) (37,38,51,52). Based on sequence analysis, this virus is indistinguishable from porcine lymphotropic herpesvirus-1 (PLHV-1) and has some genetic homology with known sequences of lymphocryptovirus (EBV) and the rhadinoviruses (HHV-8). The role of this virus in the pathogenesis of porcine PTLD is under investigation. In allogeneic transplantation models, the risk of PTLD in swine is related to the overall intensity of immune suppression, the MHC disparity between donor and host, the degree of T-cell depletion, and the PLHV activation that precedes B-cell proliferation.

Other Potential Pathogens

A variety of novel pathogens have been described in swine. The role of such microorganisms *in vivo* in the context of immune suppression remains to be established. These include porcine circovirus (PCV) types 1 and 2 (with PCV-2 causing a wasting syndrome particularly in concert with parvovirus infection), porcine reproductive and respiratory syndrome virus, porcine encephalomyocarditis virus, influenza viruses, African swine fever virus, hepatitis E–like virus, pseudorabies virus, and polyomaviruses of swine. The interactions of such potential pathogens, the possibility of pseudotyping of viruses, and the role of herpesviruses in enhancing infection remain to be clarified.

ROUTINE MONITORING FOR XENOGENEIC INFECTION

In xenograft recipients the risks of infection and rejection necessitate lifelong monitoring. In addition to the recipients, some individuals are potentially at heightened risk for infection derived from either the donor animals or from the recipient. This would include first-degree relatives or sexual contacts of recipients and xenograft donor animal handlers, and these individuals need to be considered for inclusion in any monitoring scheme. Individuals should be monitored at fixed intervals and for periods of increased risk of infection including during symptomatic infections and periods of increased immune suppression.

The tests to be performed are of four types: (a) cultures to identify and isolate microorganisms for further study; (b) nucleic acid (DNA or mRNA) detection; (c) microorganism-specific antigen detection tests (e.g., enzyme-linked immunosorbent assay, ELISA), particularly for the detection of microorganisms not easily isolated by available culture techniques; and (d) serologic testing for epidemiologic evaluation of exposures to novel microorganisms. The frequency of routine testing for the recipient might be weekly for 3 months, alternate weeks for 3 months, monthly for 6 months, and quarterly thereafter, consistent with a common schedule for posttransplantation clinical care. Following periods of fever or of clinical infection (see below), monitoring would be increased to weekly for 1 to 2 months and then revert to the previous level of surveillance. Samples should be stored on relatives, intimate contacts, and animal handlers every 6 months, with more frequent monitoring (monthly) if the animals or recipients developed signs of infection or were determined to be infected with a xenograft-derived pathogen.

Testing should include archiving of specimens for future study; routine bacterial, fungal, and viral cultures on cells of human and donor origin; PCR for PERV mRNA and DNA using both sera and leukocytes; control assays for porcine chimerism; and cocultivation of peripheral blood leukocytes with human and donor cell lines. The U.S. Public Health Service is intimately involved in the procurement, storage, and testing of samples for retroviral infection resulting from exposure to pig-derived tissues.

Optimal assays for PERV have not been defined; RT-PCR may be more informative regarding viral infection, and standard (DNA) PCR is subject to more artifact from donor cellular contamination. Each assay must be standardized and certified as to reliability. Each positive assay for PERV must be confirmed in independent assays before informing the physician and patient and acting upon the possibility of xenogeneic infection.

PARADIGM FOR THE MANAGEMENT OF PATIENTS WITH SIGNS OF INFECTION

Organ transplant recipients frequently manifest signs of infection. Infection, graft rejection, posttransplantation lymphoproliferative disorder, and other etiologies of organ dysfunction may be indistinguishable on clinical grounds. In xenograft recipients, these signs may be manifestations of common, community-acquired infections or latent infections reactivated in the recipient. However, the risk that these symptoms are the result of infection, possibly xenosis, will require an organized management strategy. The key features of such a scheme are not dissimilar to the approach taken for allograft recipients:

- Full microbiologic evaluation prior to the initiation of antimicrobial therapy
- Radiologic studies often accompanied by invasive diagnostic testing (needle or surgical biopsies)
- Early empiric antimicrobial therapy directed at the most likely pathogens
- Hospital admission and isolation from other patients until the nature of the process is further defined; special precautions (e.g., respiratory, secretions, neutropenia) dictated by the patients' clinical presentation
- Universal precautions for all patients

Available data will dictate special testing to be performed on archived specimens and at the breeding colony. In the event of the recognition of a novel recombinant microorganism or severe infectious illness without explanation, strict isolation with high-efficiency particulate air (HEPA) filtration will be required.

BENEFITS OF XENOTRANSPLANTATION

Concerns regarding potential infectious risks of xenotransplantation have generally overwhelmed discussions about the potential benefits of this technology in terms of the transmission of infection to graft recipients. However, some of the major infectious hazards of allotransplantation can be addressed via elective xenotransplantation should this become practical for broad clinical application. Some of the unique benefits of xenotransplantation are derived from the following:

- Careful microbiologic screening of the animals used for xenotransplantation (as compared with the relatively limited screening of human sera and tissues prior to use in allotransplantation).
- The potential resistance of the xenogeneic tissues to infection by human pathogens including HIV (1 and 2), HTLV, hepatitis viruses, and herpes viruses (including human CMV). For example, porcine cytomegalovirus does not appear to infect baboon tissues *in vivo* (30). This "species specificity" may reflect the absence of receptors or of cellular "machinery" necessary for viral replication in human cells (53).
- Limited duration of exogenous immune suppression is a component of many proposed xenotransplantation protocols, which include immunologic tolerance induction. If these are applied clinically, the risk of common opportunistic infections will be reduced.

- Reduced duration of hospitalization for donor and recipients. At present, cadaver donor organs are derived from hospitalized patients potentially infected with nosocomial pathogens. Similarly, transplant recipients often have prolonged in-hospital waiting times for allografts. During this time, they become colonized with nosocomial microorganisms and may develop infection related to intravenous and urinary catheters or respiratory and cardiac assist devices.
- Patients can receive their transplants at the time of greatest clinical need.

INFECTIOUS RISKS, SURVEILLANCE, AND THE SEARCH FOR NOVEL PATHOGENS

The assessment of infectious risks associated with clinical xenotransplantation is central to the acceptance of this technology by the community and to optimal care for these patients. Thus, it is important to investigate potential pathogens in both preclinical models and in xenograft recipients. Some progress has been made in defining the risks due to known pathogens. The cloning of PERV and the identification of other viruses has allowed the development of assays for these agents. However, the greatest risk of transmission of infection in xenotransplantation may be due to unknown microorganisms, microorganisms that cause asymptomatic or delayed infection, and for which, by definition, microbiologic assays do not exist. Some of these should be identifiable in preclinical models, although others may appear only in clinical trials. Keys to the identification of potential human pathogens include (a) prospective studies to identify new or unsuspected infectious agents, and (b) a commitment to share clinical and preclinical data that suggest the presence of unusual infectious events in xenotransplantation. Without a commitment to sharing epidemiologic data, the occasional infectious event or novel syndrome is likely to remain unrecognized—below the epidemiologic "radar screen."

Efforts have been made to define some of the administrative hurdles to optimizing safety in clinical xenotransplantation (see the "Consultation on Xenotransplantation Surveillance" sponsored by the OECD, World Health Organization, and Health Canada, *http://www.oecd.org*). These emphasize the need for

- shared definitions for xenogeneic infectious diseases events (case definition, laboratory assays, and specific microorganisms);
- facilitation of reporting of "health events" in xenotransplantation trials and linkage to source animal data;
- international cooperation in reporting, recording, and response to adverse events associated with xenotransplantation (database development);
- agreement on the nature of the investigation to be undertaken in the setting of infection in xenotransplantation;
- archiving of clinical samples for epidemiologic studies and for basic research; and
- recognition that unknown microorganisms may cause disease in immunocompromised individuals.

These programmatic components will allow clinical investigators, public health officials, and the public to recognize and assess the occurrence of novel infections of all types, not just those related to xenotransplantation. A number of national and international databanks already exist for the detection of unusual clusters of infectious events (e.g., outbreaks of Hantavirus, *Salmonella,* Ebola). The coordination of such systems on an international basis will enhance the safety of xenotransplantation as this technology approaches clinical application.

NEW TECHNOLOGIES

Epidemics of novel pathogens (AIDS, Hantavirus, BK polyomavirus in renal transplantation) and outbreaks of known pathogens (Norwalk-like viruses on cruise ships, Leishmaniasis, Ebola) suggest that gaps exist in the tools available for prospective epidemiologic surveillance. Similarly, recent episodes of bioterrorism (*Anthrax* bacillus) suggest a need for broader microbial surveillance and improved reporting techniques. Newer molecular techniques are beginning to be applied in xenotransplantation to address the question, What new pathogens are present that might pose a risk to immunosuppressed human recipients? The goal is to detect new nucleic acid or protein markers specific for unknown pathogens. This strategy is the same used to detect the "unculturable" microorganisms responsible for non-A, non-B hepatitis (hepatitis C) and Whipple's disease. Use of broad-range hybridization probes or PCR primers, molecular differential display, genetic subtraction libraries, and microarray technologies can be linked to data from the human genome project and advances in proteomics to detect novel pathogens in human hosts after accidental exposure (epidemiology), intentional infection (bioterrorism), or unknown exposure (xenotransplantation).

In bioterrorist attacks, as in all of medicine, those hosts who are immunologically least capable of fighting off infection have the greatest morbidity after exposure. Thus, influenza and anthrax have disproportionate mortality in the elderly, those with comorbid conditions (heart, lung liver, and kidney disease), and in those with underlying immune deficiencies (organ transplant recipients, cancer patients, patients treated with corticosteroids). As a result, immunocompromised hosts, including those undergoing allo- and xenotransplantation, will serve as the best sentinel population for novel surveillance strategies. In this manner, new pathogens may be uncovered before they have a significant impact on human health. The cost of such screening will be more modest (DNA extractions, sequencing, comparison with databases) than many "anti-bioterrorist" strategies currently under development. The coupling of the search for known pathogens with a prospective search for unknown microorganisms would provide a new vision of the growing spectrum of human disease.

ACKNOWLEDGMENTS

These studies were supported by Public Health Services grant NIH-NIAID PO1-AI45897.

REFERENCES

1. Sachs DH. Mixed chimerism as an approach to transplantation tolerance. *Clin Immunol* 2000;95(1 pt 2):S63–68.
2. Sachs DH. The pig as a potential xenograft donor. *Vet Immunol Immunopathol* 1994;43:185–191.
3. Michaels MG, Simmons RL. Xenotransplant-associated zoonoses. Strategies for prevention. *Transplantation* 1994;57(1):1–7.
4. Fishman JA. Xenosis and xenotransplantation: addressing the infectious risks posed by an emerging technology. *Kidney Int Suppl* 1997;58: S41–45.
5. Bach FH, et al. Uncertainty in xenotransplantation: individual benefit versus collective risk. *Nature Med* 1998;4(2):141–144.
6. Fishman JA. The risk of infection in xenotransplantation. Introduction. *Ann NY Acad Sci* 1998;862:45–51.
7. Fishman JA. Infection in xenotransplantation: a clinical approach. *Transplant Proc* 1999;31(6):2225–2227.
8. Fishman JA, Rubin RH. Infection in organ-transplant recipients. *N Engl J Med* 1998;338(24):1741–1751.
9. Fishman JA. Miniature swine as organ donors for man: strategies for the prevention of xenotransplant-associated infections. *Xenotransplantation* 1994;1:47–57.
10. Isfort R, et al. Retrovirus insertion into herpesvirus in vitro and in vivo. *Proc Natl Acad Sci USA* 1992;89:991–995.
11. Javier RT, Sedarati F, Stevens JG. Two avirulent herpes simplex viruses generate lethal recombinants in vivo. *Science* 1986;234:746–748.
12. Buhler L, et al. Pig kidney transplantation in baboons: anti-Gal(alpha)1-3Gal IgM alone is associated with acute humoral xenograft rejection and disseminated intravascular coagulation. *Transplantation* 2001; 72(11):1743–1752.
13. Alwayn IP, et al. The problem of anti-pig antibodies in pig-to-primate xenografting: current and novel methods of depletion and/or suppression of production of anti-pig antibodies. *Xenotransplantation* 1999; 6(3):157–168.
14. Yamada K, et al. Mechanisms of tolerance induction and prevention of cardiac allograft vasculopathy in miniature swine: the effect of augmentation of donor antigen load. *J Thorac Cardiovasc Surg* 2000;119(4 pt 1):709–719.
15. Platt JL, Saadi S. The role of complement in transplantation. *Mol Immunol* 1999;36(13–14):965–971.
16. Platt JL. The immunological barriers to xenotransplantation. *Crit Rev Immunol* 1996;16(4):331–358.
17. Bach FH, et al. Modification of vascular responses in xenotransplantation: inflammation and apoptosis. *Nature Med* 1997;3(9):944–948.
18. Ferran C, et al. Xenotransplantation: progress toward clinical development. *Adv Nephrol* 1997;27:391–420.
19. Platt JL. Prospects for xenotransplantation. *Pediatr Transplant* 1999; 3(3):193–200.
20. Rosengard AM, et al. Tissue expression of human complement inhibitor, decay-accelerating factor, in transgenic pigs. A potential approach for preventing xenograft rejection. *Transplantation* 1995;59(9): 1325–1333.
21. Lai L, et al. Production of alpha-1,3-galactosyltransferase knockout pigs by nuclear transfer cloning. *Science* 2002;295(5557):1089–1092.
22. Michaels MG, et al. Distinguishing baboon cytomegalovirus from human cytomegalovirus: importance for xenotransplantation. *J Infect Dis* 1997;176(6):1476–1483.
23. Michaels M. Xenozoonoses and the xenotransplant recipient. *Ann NY Acad Sci* 1998;862:100–104.
24. Fishman JA. Infection and xenotransplantation. Developing strategies to minimize risk. *Ann NY Acad Sci* 1998;862:52–66.
25. Michaels MG, et al. Detection of infectious baboon cytomegalovirus after baboon-to-human liver xenotransplantation. *J Virol* 2001;75(6): 2825–2828.
26. Bjoersdorff A, et al. Microbiologic screening as a preparatory step for clinical xenografting of porcine fetal islet-like cell clusters. *Transplant Proc* 1992;24(2):674–676.
27. Groth CG, et al. Transplantation of porcine fetal islet-like cell clusters into eight diabetic patients. *Transplant Proc* 1993;25(1 pt 2):970.
28. Bowden RA, et al. Progression of human immunodeficiency virus type-1 infection after allogeneic marrow transplantation. *Am J Med* 1990; 88(5N):49N–52N.
29. Schwarz A, et al. The effect of cyclosporine on the progression of human immunodeficiency virus type 1 infection transmitted by transplantation—data on four cases and review of the literature. *Transplantation* 1993;55(1):95–103.
30. Mueller NJ, et al. Activation of cytomegalovirus in pig-to-primate organ xenotransplantation. *J Virol* 2002;76(10):4734–4740.
31. Stoye JP, et al. Endogenous retroviruses: a potential problem for xenotransplantation? *Ann NY Acad Sci* 1998;862:67–74.
32. Patience C, Takeuchi Y, Weiss RA. Infection of human cells by an endogenous retrovirus of pigs. *Nature Med* 1997;3(3):282–286.
33. Le Tissier P, et al. Two sets of human-tropic pig retrovirus. *Nature* 1997;389(6652):681–682.
34. Akiyoshi DE, et al. Identification of a full-length cDNA for an endogenous retrovirus of miniature swine. *J Virol* 1998;72(5):4503–4507.
35. Qari SH, et al. Susceptibility of the porcine endogenous retrovirus to reverse transcriptase and protease inhibitors. *J Virol* 2001;75(2): 1048–1053.
36. Fryer JF, et al. Quantitation of porcine cytomegalovirus in pig tissues by PCR. *J Clin Microbiol* 2001;39(3):1155–1156.
37. Goltz M, et al. Sequence analysis of the genome of porcine lymphotropic herpesvirus 1 and gene expression during posttransplant lymphoproliferative disease of pigs. *Virology* 2002;294(2):383–393.
38. Huang CA, et al. Posttransplantation lymphoproliferative disease in miniature swine after allogeneic hematopoietic cell transplantation: similarity to human PTLD and association with a porcine gammaherpesvirus. *Blood* 2001;97(5):1467–1473.
39. Takeuchi Y, et al. Host range and interference studies of three classes of pig endogenous retrovirus. *J Virol* 1998;72(12):9986–9991.
40. Blusch JH, et al. Infection of nonhuman primate cells by pig endogenous retrovirus. *J Virol* 2000;74(16):7687–7690.
41. Martin U, et al. Productive infection of primary human endothelial cells by pig endogenous retrovirus (PERV). *Xenotransplantation* 2000; 7(2):138–142.
42. Patience C, et al. Multiple groups of novel retroviral genomes in pigs and related species. *J Virol* 2001;75(6):2771–2775.
43. Patience C, et al. No evidence of pig DNA or retroviral infection in patients with short-term extracorporeal connection to pig kidneys. *Lancet* 1998;352(9129):699–701.
44. Heneine W, et al. No evidence of infection with porcine endogenous retrovirus in recipients of porcine islet-cell xenografts. *Lancet* 1998; 352(9129):695–699.
45. Paradis K, et al. Search for cross-species transmission of porcine endogenous retrovirus in patients treated with living pig tissue. The XEN 111 Study Group. *Science* 1999;285(5431):1236–1241.
46. Cunningham DA, et al. Analysis of patients treated with living pig tissue for evidence of infection by porcine endogenous retroviruses. *Trends Cardiovasc Med* 2001;11(5):190–196.
47. Hirsch MS. Immunological activation of oncogenic viruses: interrelationship of immunostimulation and immunosuppression. *Johns Hopkins Med J Suppl* 1974;3:177–185.
48. Hirsch MS. Immunological activation of endogenous oncogenic viruses. *Ann NY Acad Sci* 1976;276:529–535.
49. Olding LB, Jensen FC, Oldstone MB. Pathogenesis of cytomegalovirus infection. I. Activation of virus from bone marrow-derived lymphocytes by in vitro allogenic reaction. *J Exp Med* 1975;141(3):561–572.
50. Olding LB, Kingsbury DT, Oldstone MB. Pathogenesis of cytomegalovirus infection. Distribution of viral products, immune complexes and autoimmunity during latent murine infection. *J Gen Virol* 1976;33(2): 267–280.
51. Ulrich S, Goltz M, Ehlers B. Characterization of the DNA polymerase loci of the novel porcine lymphotropic herpesviruses 1 and 2 in domestic and feral pigs. *J Gen Virol* 1999;80(pt 12):3199–3205.
52. Ehlers B, Ulrich S, Goltz M. Detection of two novel porcine herpesviruses with high similarity to gammaherpesviruses. *J Gen Virol* 1999; 80(pt 4):971–978.
53. Michaels MG, et al. Lack of susceptibility of baboons to infection with hepatitis B virus. *Transplantation* 1996;61(3):350–351.

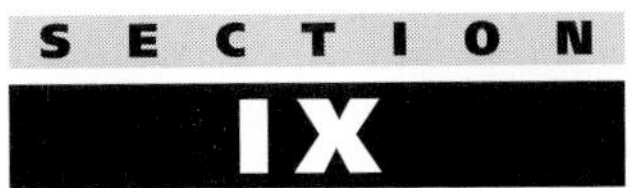

EPIDEMIOLOGY AND PREVENTION OF NOSOCOMIAL INFECTIONS RELATED TO HOSPITAL SUPPORT SERVICES

74

CENTRAL STERILE SUPPLY

LYNNE M. SEHULSTER
JANET K. SCHULTZ

The central sterile supply (CSS), or sterile processing department, is a specialized service area of virtually all hospitals and an increasing number of nonhospital healthcare settings (e.g., ambulatory surgical centers). This service area is responsible for collecting and receiving reusable patient care items, instruments, and devices used during the provision of healthcare and for decontaminating, processing, packaging, sterilizing, storing, and dispensing these items to all parts of the healthcare facility. CSS may also manage the distribution of sterile, single-use, disposable patient-care items. Reliable sterilization of surgical instruments, textiles, utensils, and innumerable other items essential to medical care is one of the oldest and most basic measures for the prevention of healthcare-associated infection, dating back to the studies of Pasteur and Koch over a century ago (1). The delivery of sterile products for use in patient care, however, depends not only on the efficacy of the sterilization process itself but also on a well-designed facility, good infection control practices, effective quality control, and other aspects of device processing and handling before, during, and after sterilization (2). These other considerations include appropriate strategies to facilitate instrument decontamination and cleaning and a thorough understanding of the sterilization process and the factors that affect its success or failure. Furthermore, technology, employee education, safety, and productivity are important considerations for operation of an efficient CSS (3). The CSS should have in place policies and procedures governing all aspects of activity within the unit. Key elements in these documents include, but are not limited to (a) engineering and facilities management requirements, (b) infection control, (c) quality assurance and process management, (d) occupational safety and health, (e) training, (f) traffic control, and (g) oversight of instrument reprocessing located elsewhere in the facility.

GENERAL CENTRAL STERILE SUPPLY AREA DESIGN AND ENVIRONMENT

Central sterile supply is divided generally into distinct areas based on their specific function (4). These task-based areas include (a) the receiving, cleaning, and decontamination area; (b) the decasing or breakout area; (c) the personnel support area; (d) the preparation and packaging area; (e) the textile assembly area (pack room); (f) sterilization area(s); (g) the sterile storage area; (h) equipment and cart holding area; (i) the equipment storage area; (j) the administrative area; and (k) the housekeeping equipment storage area (5). These areas should be partitioned into separate units whenever possible; this is especially true for the cleaning and decontamination area, which has special ventilation requirements (i.e., negative air pressure and vented to the outside) compared to the other CSS areas. The design of a CSS department takes into account the flow of the work load and the type of materials distribution system. Distribution may be accomplished by automation (e.g., vertical or horizontal conveyor, pneumatic tube systems), powered delivery carts, or manual pickup and delivery. Handwashing facilities should be conveniently located throughout all areas within CSS (4,5). CSS departments may or may not serve as materials management units for the facility. If this function is assigned to CSS, the decasing/breakout area is used to accommodate the unpacking and distribution of manufactured clean supplies (5). The personnel support area provides space for toilet, shower, and locker facilities for employees. The textile assembly area is where clean textiles are inspected, folded, repaired as needed, and assembled into wrapped packs (5). This function may or may not be duplicated by the facility's laundry.

Adequate humidity, ventilation, and temperature control are important for (a) prevention of environmental contamination of reprocessed items, (b) provision of appropriate storage of sterile goods, and (c) maintenance of a safe workplace. Temperatures in CSS areas vary, but most center on 75°F (24°C). The exception is for the cleaning/decontamination area, where temperatures are in the range of 60° to 68°F (15.6° to 20°C) (5). This provides an adequate comfort range for the workers who must wear substantial protective attire throughout the day. Humidity levels in CSS should be set in the range of 35% to 60% (4,5). The ventilation system should be designed so that air flows from clean areas into relatively soiled areas and is exhausted to the outside or, if recirculated, passed through an appropriate bank of filters [e.g., a high-efficiency particulate air (HEPA) filter] for return to the system (4–6). Four- to ten air changes per hour (ACH) are specified for CSS ventilation, with a minimum of six to ten ACH in the cleaning/decontamination area and a minimum of ten ACH in the area where the sterilizer equipment is located (4,5). The areas under negative pressure (i.e., cleaning/decontamination, sterilizer loading area, and restrooms/housekeeping) are vented directly to the outside, whereas air from the other areas of CSS can be recirculated. The availability and configuration of systems that provide steam, hot and cold water (or water of a temperature specified by reprocessing equipment manufacturers), distilled or demineralized water, compressed air, nitrogen, vacuum sources, electrical power, air exhaust, and drainage of sewage are important to consider when installing equipment (3,5). The electrical system in the unit should allow for the safe and efficient operation of equipment. Availability of a source of uninterrupted power is recommended in the event of an emergency (5).

Moist heat sterilization methods (i.e., saturated steam under pressure) remain the primary choice for terminal reprocessing of heat-stable instruments and devices. The quality of the steam is critical to the efficient operation of these sterilizers, and there should be sufficient steam capacity engineered into the system to accommodate this demand. Hospital boiler systems may not be capable of providing steam of sufficient quality; self-contained packaged steam generators are another option. Steam delivered to the steam sterilizers should be saturated steam with a steam quality between 97% and 100% (5). The purity of the steam should meet or exceed International Standards Organization (ISO) recommendations for limits on heavy metals, conductivity, pH, appearance, hardness, chlorine, phosphate, and evaporate residue (5,7).

INSTRUMENT AND DEVICE REPROCESSING: PREVENTION AND CONTROL OF HEALTHCARE-ASSOCIATED ADVERSE OUTCOMES

Effective sterilization of items depends not only on reliable operation of the gas, steam, or low-temperature sterilizers, but also on correct methods of cleaning, packaging, arrangement of items in the sterilizer, and storage of these items.

Cleaning and Decontamination

The essential first step to any terminal reprocessing strategy for reusable medical instruments and devices is the reduction of bioburden. Debris such as blood, mucus, oil, or other foreign matter interferes with the sterilization process by acting as a barrier to the sterilizing agent (8–10). Additionally, cleaning and decontamination of used instruments renders those instruments safe for CSS staff to handle during further reprocessing (11). Retained debris can also affect the functionality of a device at the point of use, resulting in additional patient-safety concerns (12).

Cleaning is defined as the removal of all adherent visible soil from the surfaces, crevices, joints, and lumina of instruments. Decontamination is the physical or chemical process that renders a potentially contaminated, inanimate [illegible] safe for further handling (10,12–15). The techniques for instrument cleaning and decontamination are hand scrubbing, ultrasonic cleaning, and processing with a washer-sterilizer or washer-decontaminator (12).

Manual Cleaning

Manual cleaning of instruments at the sink is still done and may be necessary for powered equipment and some extremely delicate items or to apply direct water pressure to contaminated lumina. Cleaning agents commonly used in manual cleaning contain surfactants, and some mechanical cleaning action (i.e., scrubbing, brushing) is needed for the effective removal of organic matter. During the cleaning and decontamination process, personnel must wear appropriate protective apparel (e.g., fluid-impervious gown or apron with full sleeves, latex or vinyl gloves that resist puncture or tearing during the process, face shield or surgical mask and goggles, a hair covering, and impervious shoe covers). Such items provide the worker with protection from wetness and exposure to body fluids and tissues (16). Splatter or aerosols generated during hand scrubbing should be kept to a minimum through appropriate cleaning techniques (e.g., keeping brushes under water during scrubbing) (10).

Whenever possible, hand scrubbing should be avoided, because it increases the worker's contact with contaminated surfaces and involves the added danger of handling sharp and pointed objects, thereby increasing the risk of sustaining percutaneous injuries (PIs). Sharp instruments should not be cleaned by hand when they can be effectively washed in a machine. Furthermore, contaminated, reusable sharps must not be stored or reprocessed such that the worker would have to reach into a container to retrieve the item (17). Alternatives that can help prevent these injuries include using forceps retrieval, or a perforated tray so that the devices can be cleaned *in situ.*

Ultrasonic Cleaning

Ultrasonic cleaning is a method that reduces the need for hand scrubbing. The ultrasonic washer cleans by cavitation, a process whereby sound waves produce vigorous microscopic implosions of tiny vapor bubbles on the surface of objects immersed in the cleaning chamber. This agitation causes a vacuum-scrubbing action, pulling out fine debris particles from manually inaccessible surfaces (e.g., box-lock joints and serrations). Items should be rinsed to remove gross soil before being placed in the ultrasonic washer. When grossly soiled items are placed into the ultrasonic washer, the process is less effective, because the debris absorbs the sound waves. The water needs to be changed more frequently as well. Ultrasonic technology produces aerosols that reflect the fluid contents of the chamber; operation of the ultrasonic cleaner unit without a chamber cover allows these aerosols to escape. Because of this, the ultrasonic washer should be located in the decontamination area of the CSS. The potential hazards to personnel from aerosolization of such contaminated fluids should be considered when planning CSS worker safety programs. Exposure to such fluids should be prevented by use of engineering controls, changes in work practices, or use of personal protective equipment. The unit's chamber should be disinfected, rinsed, and dried at the end of the day. The manufacturer's directions should be followed for optimal results (14,15, 17–19).

Automated Reprocessing Systems

Washer-sterilizers use one of two methods to wash chamber contents. The first is a flooding technique, in which the chamber partially fills with water to which detergent has been added and then is agitated by blowing steam into the chamber through the water. These units generally operate at 270°F (132°C). This is an inefficient cleaning method that should not be relied on when there are lumened or complex devices in the load. The second method is generally used in larger, tunnel-type units. In these, rotating spray arms create water jets that clean by impingement. In this second category, most machines reach a temperature of 285°F (141°C) (14).

Washer-decontaminator or washer-disinfector machines easily remove excessive amounts of debris from instruments by using spraying water aimed to cover all parts of the load. The numerous water jets allow excellent cleaning even if instruments are grossly soiled. The agitation of the water is such that it cleans instruments thoroughly without tossing them about, thereby reducing the risk of damage to delicate items. The operating water temperature is generally around 140°F (60°C), below the level at which protein rapidly coagulates, making removal easier than at higher temperatures (12,18). Appropriate soap and disinfectant should be used in accordance with the manufacturer's instructions (14).

The use of automated cleaning/decontaminating systems offers some advantages over manual cleaning. The process is controllable and minimizes worker contact with contaminated items (11,20). Automation can enhance the quality assurance for the cleaning portion of the overall instrument reprocessing strategy. A wide variety of mechanical washer/cleaners from a number of manufacturers is available, and new technology continues to be developed. New innovations that increase worker safety and protection are especially in demand (21).

The cleaning and terminal reprocessing of flexible fiberoptic and video endoscopes and bronchoscopes are often performed by specially trained technicians in the care units where these instruments are used. Effective reprocessing of these instruments begins the moment they are removed from the patient (22). All surfaces of the endoscope or bronchoscope should be kept moist until cleaning and further reprocessing can be performed. Automated endoscope reprocessing systems (AERs) for washing and disinfection are being used increasingly for the reprocessing of these instruments primarily for the effectiveness of the process, but also because of space limitations in the care unit. One critical point to remember is that all AERs on the market today require that the endoscope or bronchoscope be manually rinsed so that gross soil is removed before placing the instrument in the AER. Some units also require the use of special connection devices that may be specific to a type or model of instrument (23). Use of appropriate connectors helps to ensure that the liquid chemical sterilant or high-level disinfectant can effectively reach the interior surfaces of the instrument's channels (24). It is important that these automated systems are cleaned and maintained regularly in accordance with the manufacturer's instructions to prevent the colonization of the equipment with bacteria (e.g., *Pseudomonas aeruginosa,* or nontuberculous mycobacteria). Outbreaks of healthcare-associated infections and episodes of pseudoinfections related to endoscopy and bronchoscopy have been attributed to contaminated washer-disinfectors through molecular epidemiology and strain identification techniques (23, 25–27). Bacteria, particularly those microorganisms commonly found in tap water (e.g., *Pseudomonas* species), can become resident in poorly maintained equipment through the formation of biofilms that may help protect the bacteria from inactivation with liquid chemical germicides (27–32). This phenomenon has led some to explore ways to enhance quality assurance of the process in the interest of patient safety. A recent issue of debate is the sampling of the AER rinse water to help verify that in-line bacteriologic filters are performing according to specifications (31). This position, however, is not widely embraced by the endoscopy community at present (33).

Other Considerations

Instruments should be kept moist prior to cleaning. Dried-on debris is more difficult to remove. Disinfection or sterilization cannot be accomplished if gross contamination is present on the instruments at the time when the final reprocessing steps are initiated (8,12,13,15,34). Instruments should be covered with a wet cloth and then contained for transport to CSS. Soaking instruments in water or other fluid during transport is discouraged because of the risk of spills and the danger of injury to workers in lifting heavy basins or containers. Once in the CSS area, instruments contaminated with organic matter may be immersed in an enzyme detergent solution to enhance manual or mechanical cleaning effectiveness. Enzyme soaks keep debris suspended in solution, preventing its deposition and drying onto the surface of instruments. When employing this method, care should be taken to use the appropriate use-dilution, water temperature, and soak times as provided by the specific manufacturer of the enzyme detergent. Additionally, workers may get a false sense of security about the safety of handling the instruments immersed in a presoaking solution. These instruments are not yet safe to handle without personal protective equipment.

The use of an appropriate detergent avoids damage to instruments, prolongs their use-life, and prevents the creation of crevices in which debris can collect (17,35). One inadvertent result of the implementation of standard precautions has been the increasing use of disinfectant/detergent agents for presoaking or manually cleaning medical instruments. Agents that contain chlorinated compounds (e.g., bleach) or that are highly acidic or alkaline can damage the surface layer of stainless steel instruments, resulting in corrosion and weakening. It is important to use only those detergent and disinfectant products specifically labeled for instrument cleaning. Hard surface disinfectant/detergents registered by the U.S. Environmental Protection Agency (EPA) are generally intended for cleaning and disinfecting large environmental surfaces (e.g., floors, walls, and table tops) and are not appropriate for use on instruments.

No single approach to decontamination and cleaning is effective for all instruments and degrees of contamination. Risks and benefits are associated with each method, and it is the responsibility of the healthcare facility to use all available information to determine the best methods for its CSS.

Packaging

Materials used for hospital instrument wrapping and packaging should provide a cost-effective means of containment to maintain the sterility of the contents (5,36). An intact wrapper impervious to extraneous microbes, moisture, dust, and soil, and strong enough to resist punctures and tears during normal handling, theoretically should protect properly sterilized material indefinitely. However, such materials may also impede the passage of steam, ethylene oxide (EO), or the sterilants in low-temperature sterilizing systems, thus interfering with the sterilization process. Therefore, compromises from this ideal must be made for items processed in healthcare facilities because of the limited choices available for terminal sterilization. Additionally, wrapping materials should (a) provide a seal of proven integrity, (b) be resistant to delamination when the pack is opened, (c) be free of pinholes, (d) allow suitable printing or labeling, (e) minimize the generation of nonviable particles, (f) provide evidence of tampering, and (g) produce minimal or no lint if fabric is used (37–39).

Packaging materials should be compatible with the sterilization process. When the steam sterilization process is used, the materials should allow adequate air removal, steam penetration, and drying. When gas sterilization is used, materials should allow adequate penetration and release of the gaseous sterilant and moisture. Packaging materials should also be inexpensive, impervious to bacteria, sealable before sterilization, and flexible enough to permit swift wrapping and unwrapping (36,40,41). Materials should be evaluated and selected according to their performance properties rather than according to whether they are woven, nonwoven, reusable, or disposable (42). Manufacturers of sterilizer equipment should provide the user with some indication of which packaging materials are suitable for their units.

Muslin (i.e., 140 thread count, 100% cotton fabric) was the standard for many years in packaging for healthcare facilities. That product is no longer available for purchase as a wrapper. However, many improved reusable and single-use materials are available in the marketplace. The product must be cleared by the Food and Drug Administration (FDA) for use as a sterilization wrapper. In addition, consideration should be given to requiring that the material pass the American Society for Testing and Materials (ASTM) standard test method for resistance of protective clothing materials to synthetic blood (43). Patching of reusable fabrics is acceptable as long as the patches are applied with adhesive and not sewn in place. The critical factor is the amount of nonoccluded surface left after patching and folding (44).

Policies and procedures for in-house packaging should be written, reviewed annually, and readily available within the institution (36–49).

Sterilization Process

General Principles

The first thing that must be considered before subjecting a cleaned, reusable device or patient-care item to a sterilizing process is whether or not the materials are compatible with the process. Saturated steam sterilization is the most commonly available processing method in healthcare facilities and should be used whenever the device or instrument can tolerate this process, both because of the inherent reliability and robustness of the process and its low cost relative to other methods. Heat-sensitive materials are being incorporated increasingly into modern medical devices and patient-care items. A number of modern, low-temperature sterilizing systems provide alternatives for the sterilization of heat-sensitive materials. Some materials may be incompatible with some of these newer processes, and such interactions may physically degrade the item, destroy its material, or leave toxic residuals on or in the treated item (49,50).

It is important to remember, however, that all sterilizing systems have inherent limitations and that no single system can be used effectively for all instruments and devices (51). A common problem with any sterilizing system is the ability of the sterilizing agent (e.g., steam, gas, gas plasma) to diffuse throughout the chamber and the load, so that the agent makes contact with all interior and exterior surfaces of the items undergoing sterilization. In steam autoclaves, trapped air, either in the chamber or within an instrument or container, can prevent effective penetration of the steam to all surfaces in the load. Instrument design (i.e., long, narrow lumina) can pose significant challenges both for effectiveness of the cleaning procedures and sterilant diffusion. Load configuration and density must be carefully controlled to allow air removal, sterilant penetration, and drying in steam sterilization cycles. This is especially critical if the sterilizer relies on gravity displacement to remove air. For sterilizers that have mechanisms to assist in air removal (e.g., pulsing steam or vacuum conditioning phases), the configuration and density issues are not as great, but drying may still be a problem if the sterilizer is overloaded. The performance of low-temperature systems, including EO and gas plasma, is particularly affected by the presence of residual organic matter, salt, and moisture (52).

All articles to be sterilized should be arranged so that all surfaces are directly exposed to the sterilizing agent for the prescribed time and at the prescribed temperature. All hinged instruments should be open and/or unlocked. Reliable sterilization depends on both the sterilant's contact with all surfaces of the item and the duration of that contact. All articles should be aligned on sterilization carriers or in the sterilizer so as not to interfere with air removal and introduction of sterilant. Instrument sets should be placed in perforated wire mesh bottom trays or in instrument container systems (5,19). They should not be tilted on edge, as this results in the concentration of metal mass at the bottom of the tray. This arrangement interferes with drying (12). Wrapped trays should not be stacked, as instrument damage can result. Rigid reusable sterilization container systems may be horizontally stacked if the container design permits adequate penetration of the sterilant. The container manufacturer's written instructions on this point should be followed.

When items are nested in one package, they should be separated by absorbent towels or other moisture-absorbent material. This enhances the passage of steam to all surfaces during sterilization and facilitates drying by preventing the pooling of condensate. Nested items should be positioned in the same direction so that (a) air pockets are not created, (b) condensate can drain out, and (c) sterilant can circulate freely (53).

Performance records for all sterilizers should be maintained for each cycle, including load contents and retained for the period indicated by the individual healthcare facility and/or the state's statute of limitations. Records for implantable devices should allow for tracking from the sterilizer to the point of use.

These records may be used as documentation for product recall and quality assurance (5,19,54). All packages should have internal and external chemical indicators appropriate for the sterilizing system used (i.e., steam or low-temperature systems using EO or gas plasma).

Methods to Monitor the Sterilization Process

Monitoring the sterilization process is an important quality-assessment procedure for infection control in CSS. The three forms of monitoring are (a) physical monitoring (observing and recording the parameters of sterilizer functioning, such as time, temperature, pressure, or gas concentration); (b) chemical monitoring (color- or physical-change indicators that detect exposure to sterilizing agents or conditions); and (c) biologic monitoring (spore testing, the most important check on sterilizer function).

Physical data are usually the first indications of the adequacy of a sterilization process. For steam sterilizers that use a vacuum assist to remove air at the beginning of the cycle, a Bowie-Dick type test should be run daily to ensure that this system is working properly. For each sterilization cycle, the mechanical readings should be checked on the printout at the conclusion of the cycle. Sterilizers without such printouts (either in digital or chart form) are not appropriate for acute care facilities and should be phased out of use in office-based settings as soon as economically feasible. Any deviation from the expected normal readings of the various parameters (e.g., time or temperature) should alert the operator to potential problems.

Chemical indicators are devices to provide information relative to the achievement of one or several of the conditions necessary to destroy microorganisms by a sterilization process. Thus, when used in a sterilization process, chemical indicators can indicate that a device has been exposed to a sterilization process (throughput or process indicator), or may provide more detailed information on the exposure conditions endured by the device. They can be useful for (a) monitoring product flow, to make sure that unprocessed product is not mistaken for that which has been sterilized; (b) ensuring the use of proper packing, and sterilizer load configurations; and (c) ensuring the proper functioning of the processing equipment (5,55). Chemical indicators are intended for use in conjunction with other process monitoring systems. The American Association for Medical Instrumentation (AAMI) and the ISO have designated six classes of chemical indicators, five of which are commercially available (56–58). These classes are (a) throughput indicators, or external indicators; (b) air removal indicators (Bowie-Dick type tests) (59); (c) steam penetration indicators (available in Europe but not in the U.S.); (d) multiparametric indicators, or integrators that respond to two or more critical parameters of the sterilization process; and (e) class 5 indicators that correlate to the performance of a biologic indicator within a specific range of sterilization conditions (56,58). The sixth classification is that of an emulator, and no such product is commercially available in the U.S.

In addition, there are indicators that rely on an enzyme reaction. One such product contains only the enzyme itself and is regarded by the FDA as a chemical indicator (either class 4 or 5, depending on data submitted to the FDA). Another type relies on the reaction of an enzyme that is actually in the spore coat of a microorganism known to be resistant to the method of sterilization (see below). This second type can be used either as an early readout indicator when only the enzyme reaction is used, or as a typical biologic indicator if the spores are actually incubated in the growth media.

In the early 20th century, microbiologists and clinicians began to seek further assurances of sterility of reprocessed items beyond monitoring the physical variables, and suspensions of bacterial spores came into use as a biologic means of monitoring steam sterilization. The earliest culture control used was garden soil to which had been added a number of sporulating cultures of known resistant laboratory strains. In the late 1950s, commercially manufactured biologic indicators (BIs) began to be used in U.S. hospitals (1,60). These consisted of standardized preparations of *Geobacillus stearothermophilus* (formerly known as *Bacillus stearothermophilus*) spores with defined heat-kill characteristics.

BIs are defined in the AAMI standard as a calibration of microorganisms in or on a carrier put up in a package that maintains the integrity of the inoculated carrier, is convenient to the user, and serves to demonstrate whether the conditions were adequate to achieve sterilization (5,55). BIs are standardized bacterial spore populations known to be resistant to the particular sterilant and physical methods of sterilization to be monitored. Thus, no single BI can be used reliably to monitor all of the various physical methods of sterilization. There are three basic types of BIs: (a) paper strips inoculated with bacterial spores; (b) self-contained BIs, in which the spores are enclosed in a carrier; and (c) enzyme-based BIs (61). Of these, only the enzyme-based BIs are capable of providing rapid readout of results, generally in a matter of hours, as opposed to the 48 hours incubation required for determining growth.

At present, the Joint Commission on Accreditation of Healthcare Organizations (JCAHO), AAMI, and the Association of Perioperative Registered Nurses (AORN) recommend using *G. stearothermophilus* spores for steam sterilizers and peracetic acid-based systems, and *Bacillus atrophaeus* (formerly known as *Bacillus subtilis* var. *niger*) spores for EO sterilizers, hydrogen peroxide gas plasma sterilizers, and dry heat ovens (62, 63). The Centers for Disease Control and Prevention (CDC) concurs with the use of gram-positive bacterial spores for BIs (9,64). Manufacturers of low-temperature sterilizer equipment should provide the user with information on the proper selection of an indicator system for use with their equipment. All hospital steam autoclaves should be monitored at least weekly with BIs, although many healthcare facilities are monitoring their equipment daily. The JCAHO, AORN, and AAMI also recommend monitoring every load sterilized by EO. Each load containing implantable objects should be monitored with a spore test. The JCAHO, AORN, and CDC further recommend that sterilizer loads containing implantables or intravascular devices should not be released until the spore test has been reported as negative. It is recognized, however, that in an emergency situation it may not be possible to quarantine implantable items for 48 hours, especially if the assay of the indicator is dependent on growth of survivors. Rapid BIs (e.g., enzyme-based BIs) may alleviate this situation. The enzyme-based BI measures a spore-specific enzyme, α-D-glucosidase, which is inactivated proportionally with the inactivation of the spore population. The assay of this enzyme-based indicator can be accomplished in a matter of minutes, and it has been shown that this BI is equivalent in sensitivity to the more conventional BIs (65). The availability of this type of BI may encourage more healthcare facilities to incorporate this quality assurance process into their services. A questionnaire survey of U.S. hospitals in the late 1980s showed that 30% of 120 hospitals used a spore test with all loads containing implants. Few hospitals using spore tests quarantined the items until results were available (66). The AAMI has recently endorsed the routine release of all steam-sterilized loads, including implantables, based on the results of the enzyme readout only for the enzyme/spore combination BI (63).

The BI pack should be placed in the area of the sterilizer that will present the most challenge to all sterilization parameters. For steam sterilizers, the BI should be placed at the front on the bottom and near the door in a routinely loaded sterilizer. For EO sterilization, the BI should be in the center of the load. Each manufacturer of a sterilizer should provide instructions on test pack placement for that sterilizer, since these may differ based on design and cycle considerations.

BIs are designed such that the inoculum size should reflect the expected degree of contamination plus a margin of safety. Currently, commercially available BIs fall in the range of 10^4 to 10^6 spores for *G. stearothermophilus* and center at 10^6 spores for *B. atrophaeus*. Additionally, the resistance of these cultivated spores is generally higher than that found in native species of the same type. Because the BIs have 10^4 to 10^6 spores per unit (which is far in excess of the expected bioburden remaining on thoroughly cleaned instruments and patient care items), and the resistance is considered to be greater than the microorganisms on the healthcare items undergoing sterilization, the probability of nonsterility of the items in the load is considered to be less than 1 in 1,000,000 after a 12-log reduction of the BI (67). This provides for a sterility assurance level of 10^{-6}.

Since their development, commercial BIs have shown significant variability (68,69). Despite appeal for standardized BI methodology, problems with sporadically false-positive BIs continue to occur (70,71). There are several factors that may influence the occurrence of a false-positive BI, many of which relate to human error. Use of a self-contained BI can minimize handling and the inadvertent introduction of contamination. BIs used with some of the new low-temperature systems are generally not self-contained and require open transfer for assay. The extra handling may produce false positive BIs more often (72).

A single positive test does not necessarily indicate sterilizer failure. If available, a presumptive identification of the growing microorganism should be performed. This can be done by Gram stain and microscopic examination to ascertain that the microorganism is of the *Bacillus* species (i.e., gram-positive rods). While this is occurring, equipment failure should be ruled out. Immediate service should be requested to detect any sterilizer malfunction. If a sterilizer malfunction is identified, the equipment should be taken out of service and all items processed in that load should be recalled, cleaned, and reprocessed (9). Once a sterilizer is repaired, it is necessary to challenge the unit to confirm proper operation. This approach is also used when it becomes necessary to switch steam sterilizers over to an auxiliary supply of steam. The unit should be operated until two consecutive runs return negative BI results before the unit is returned fully to service. Ordinarily, this will mean that steam sterilizers may be down for several hours after repair, whereas EO sterilizers, peracetic acid, and gas plasma units may be off-line for at least 7 days (72). It is important to recognize that the use of a BI does not guarantee sterility but rather provides an additional mechanism for monitoring the sterilizer cycle beyond the graphic temperature-pressure record and chemical indicators. A negative BI test offers further assurance that the sterilizer variables and exposure time were what was intended. It can be inferred that there is a very high probability that all viable microorganisms remaining on the cleaned items contained in the load were killed (1,73–75).

Storage

The sterile storage area should be adjacent to the sterilizing area, preferably in a separate, enclosed, limited-access, and well-ventilated area to provide protection against dust, moisture, and temperature and humidity extremes (5,6). The maintenance of optimal environmental conditions in the storage area minimizes the potential for contamination of sterile supplies. There should be a minimum of six to ten total ACH, and the relative humidity should be maintained in the range of 35% to 50% (4,5). The area should also be free of insects and other vermin that seek the warmth of reprocessed packages for habitat.

Sterile materials should be stored at least 8 to 10 inches from the floor, at least 18 inches from the ceiling, and at least 2 inches from outside walls. The items should be positioned so that packaging is not crushed, bent, compressed, or punctured, all of which will compromise the sterility of the contents. The contents of any sterilized package should be considered contaminated if the packaging is damaged. All wrapped sterilized packages should be handled and stored in a manner that minimizes stress and pressure (45). Storage of supplies on floors, windowsills, and areas other than designated shelving counters or carts should be avoided (5,54). Open shelves, cupboards, or drawers are acceptable, but articles stored in drawers may need special protection against physical damage (48). Some hospitals have utilized movable shelves to maximize storage capacity when space is limited (76).

Every package that has been sterilized within the facility should be imprinted or labeled with a load control number that indicates the sterilizer used, the cycle or load number, the date of sterilization, and an expiration date. The term *shelf life*, as used with respect to a sterilized product, is defined as the period during which sterility can be maintained. Shelf-life considerations create more misconceptions, confusion, and misleading information than any other facet of the preparation and use of sterilized products (37–40,43). There are reports in the technical literature describing the length of time sterile goods can be stored and still be considered sterile, with safe storage times reported to range from as short as 1 week to indefinitely (9,40). To add to the confusion, some reports discuss neither the wrapping material used nor conditions for storage in relation to the safe storage periods (45,77). Some studies suggested that safe storage times ranged from 2 days to 9 months depending on the wrapper/storage combination. The problem related to most studies is that the conclusions became a standard for all hospitals regardless of the barrier properties of the wrappers used or the hospital's control over the environmental factors that really affect shelf life. No trend toward increased probability of contamination over time was observed for any pack type studied. The studies were not ready to call any storage time safe or unsafe. They observed, however, that storage periods up to 50 weeks did not increase the probability of contamination regardless of the wrapping material used (nonbarrier woven, barrier nonwoven, or polypropylene peel pouches), storage location, or dust cover use (9, 37,38,53).

Loss of sterility of package contents is considered event related, not time related, and depends in part on the type of packaging used (78). Event-related factors include (a) frequency and method of handling; (b) storage area conditions such as location, space, open/closed shelving, temperature, humidity; and (c) the presence of dust, insects, flooding, and vermin (36). Sterility of package contents is considered compromised if packages become wet or are dropped on the floor, or if the packaging is torn, punctured, or otherwise comes apart.

Shelf life and expiration dating policies must be decided by each individual healthcare facility. Because of the differences in both packaging materials used and facilities for storage, it is impossible to recommend shelf times that would be universally applicable for sterile items.

Inventory control means that the correct quantity and quality of supplies is readily available to meet demands. A stock rotation policy and procedure should be developed for all areas of the facility in which sterile supplies are stored. Supplies should be placed on shelves so that expiration dates are readily visible. Correct stock rotation minimizes waste by reducing the number of sterile items that will have to be reprocessed or discarded. This approach helps to ensure that devices that may no longer be sterile are not inadvertently used (36).

Distribution of Sterile Goods

Packs transported to operating rooms and other areas within the healthcare facility should be provided with an additional outer dust-protection cover that can be removed before the pack is taken into the clean zone. This can be applied either to the individual packages or to the total cart. The transporting vehicle should be reserved for CSS use (5,36).

Maintenance

Preventive maintenance of all sterilizers should be performed according to individual policy on a scheduled basis by qualified personnel, using the sterilizer manufacturer's service manual as a reference (19). Sterilizers should be inspected and cleaned daily or at intervals recommended by the manufacturer to prevent the accumulation of residue that may transfer to packaging in the chamber. The time-temperature charting devices and temperature-pressure gauges should be calibrated after any repair affecting sterilizer performance and at least every 6 months or at the interval recommended by the sterilizer manufacturer (5,19).

HEALTHCARE-ASSOCIATED INFECTIONS AND OTHER ADVERSE OUTCOMES LINKED TO CENTRAL STERILE SUPPLY PROCESSES AND MATERIALS

Infections, injuries, and other adverse outcomes associated with CSS processes or materials can be divided into two groups: those affecting patients and the quality of their medical care, and occupational hazards and risks for the CSS work force.

Adverse Outcomes for Patients

The margin for allowable error implicit in modern sterilization procedures is sufficiently large for those based on physical methods of microbial inactivation, such that there is minimal risk that items in a load will fail to achieve sterility in the event of a potential sterilizer malfunction, especially if the microbial bioburden on reprocessed items has been reduced before sterilization by proper cleaning. As a consequence, healthcare-associated infection, particularly bacterial infection, traced to mechanical failure of sterilization equipment has been infrequent (1) (see Chapter 86).

Several aspects of the instrument reprocessing strategy, however, can be associated with adverse outcomes for patients if recommended practices are not followed. In 1961, three cases of surgical site infection caused by *Clostridium perfringens* were reported as a result of inadequate cleaning of instruments and sterilizer failure (79). Transmission from the index case to the other patients was linked to residual contamination on the surgical instruments. Another episode traced to sterilizer failure in a hospital resulted in six cases of *P. aeruginosa* meningitis or intraabdominal abscesses (80). Possible failure of flash sterilization processing of implantable neurosurgical devices was epidemiologically implicated in this outbreak. Bacteremias and fungemias have been associated with improperly sterilized pressure transducer domes (81). Improperly sterilized surgical equipment was linked to an outbreak of postsurgical nasal cellulitis in which *Mycobacterium chelonae* was recovered from patients undergoing surgical rhinoplasty (82). Improper packing of surgical linens/drapes prior to autoclaving was associated with an outbreak of polymicrobial ventriculitis in a surgical intensive care unit (83). Tight packaging of the linens prevented the sterilant from penetrating throughout the pack. Additionally, the hospital failed to run routine process indicators (i.e., Bowie-Dick testing, BIs). Another episode resulting in transmission of nontuberculous mycobacteria (NTM) was linked to deficiencies in disinfection or sterilization practices in the operating room (OR) and major defects in the autoclave located in the OR (84). Inadequate sterilization and rinsing surgical instruments with tap water, coupled with minimal training in instrument reprocessing strategies, were implicated in an outbreak of *M. chelonae* abscesses after liposuction in a physician's office-based practice (85). These latter two outbreaks illustrate the problems that may occur with instrument reprocessing activities that are based elsewhere in the healthcare facility. Lack of experience with proper instrument reprocessing and attendant quality assurance can be problematic, especially if the workers and the processes in these areas do not have any oversight from infection control or CSS personnel.

Proper maintenance of the equipment in CSS is very important in the prevention of healthcare-associated adverse outcomes for patients. One outbreak of diffuse lamellar keratitis (DLK) was attributed to endotoxin exposure from sterilized instruments (86). Biofilms of gram-negative bacteria built up in the sterilizer's water reservoir, presumably diminishing the quality of the steam and thereby resulting in the transfer of endotoxin to the instruments. Biofilm control measures were implemented and a significant reduction in the development of DLK was observed.

Materials compatibility with sterilants has emerged in the forefront with the development of new options for sterilization. Therefore, it is important to review fully the advantages and limitations of new sterilization technologies so that it is clearly understood which items and materials can be safely reprocessed. An outbreak of corneal decompensation among patients receiving elective intraocular surgery was associated with residual copper and zinc in lumened, copper, and brass surgical instruments sterilized with the Plazlyte system (AbTox, Mundelein, IL), a sterilizer that is no longer marketed in the U.S. (87). The contact of the instruments' metals with the sterilant in this system produced toxic by-products that resulted in ocular damage, with some of the cases experiencing irreversible conditions.

Reuse of Single-Use Medical Devices and Patient Care Items

Over the past 10 years or so, there has been a growing interest in reuse of instruments and items clearly labeled as single-use only. Many of these devices appear to sustain little obvious wear and tear after their one-time use on the patient, and it is tempting to consider cleaning and reprocessing these devices.

However, there are a number of factors that should be considered when evaluating whether or not a single-use device can be reused safely (e.g., difficulties in cleaning, presence of long narrow lumina, chemical coatings, integrity and compatibility of materials, and continued performance of the instrument according to specifications) (88). The medical literature is mixed on this issue. Some *in vitro* studies lend support to the practice of reusing these items (89–91), whereas others point to definite problems encountered with cleaning and with materials integrity or compatibility (92–97). There is potential for injury, infection, or other adverse outcome to occur. In a Brazilian hospital, several patients undergoing cardiac catheterization with reprocessed catheters experienced pyrogenic reactions. The catheters were sterilized by EO after being cleaned several times at CSS. Analysis of the water used to reprocess catheters revealed elevated endotoxin levels; endotoxin was also detected in the reprocessed catheters (98).

Most of the reprocessing of single-use medical devices in the U.S. is now being done by commercial companies commonly known as "third-party reprocessors." These companies receive used, contaminated items from healthcare facilities. They then decontaminate, clean, inspect/test, package, and sterilize the devices. These reprocessed items are then returned to the healthcare facility for use. The FDA has now promulgated regulations governing the reuse of single-use devices as is presently occurring in U.S. hospitals (99–104). Although there are little available data on specific incidents of harm caused to patients because of the reuse of these devices, the government has concluded that the potential risks are such that reprocessing entities should be regulated in the same way as original medical device manufacturers. The FDA now considers hospitals that reprocess devices labeled for single use as manufacturers as well. The regulations do not apply to office-based practices, independent ambulatory surgery centers, or clinics at this time. Additionally, the regulations exclude devices that are reprocessed after being opened but not used. However, the FDA has begun fact-finding on this latter topic and may move forward with regulations (103).

Reprocessors must comply with all of the pre- and post-market regulations governing medical device manufacturing, including the need for pre-market clearance if required for that specific device, registration and listing as a manufacturer, mandatory reporting of adverse events, medical device tracking (if required for a specific device), corrections and removals, labeling, and compliance with the Quality System Regulation (105). The FDA maintains a very helpful Web site on reuse issues and regulation (104). A thorough discussion of this issue and the attendant regulations is found in Chapter 87.

Contract, Off-Site Reprocessing Services

Healthcare facilities are under constant demand to reduce expenditures wherever possible while not compromising the quality of patient care. This discussion often comes up when it is time to replace outdated and old equipment (106). Some healthcare facilities have opted to out-source their reusable instrument reprocessing service to a contractor, based largely on economic assessment. Many off-site contractors provide the instruments, devices, linens, and other durable goods in addition to the reprocessing service. This means that the healthcare facility can reduce its instrument inventory and largely eliminate an in-house service that has potential occupational risks for injury and infection. The disadvantages to utilizing such a service include the possible elimination of the facility infrastructure that would normally support instrument reprocessing, and the lack of "favorite" instruments from the physician/surgeon's perspective (unless arrangements to retain these instruments are built into the contract) (107). Healthcare facilities are often expected to remove gross soil from the instruments before the contractor comes for instrument pickup. Contractors then fully clean and reprocess the instruments accordingly, and transport them back to the facility in a manner that prevents the reprocessed instruments from becoming contaminated prior to use. The frequency of pickup and delivery is dictated by the work volume of the facility. The company should provide CSS staff with full documentation of its operation, including the details of quality assurance and infection control. CSS staff should be confident that all aspects of the terminal reprocessing services provided by an outsourcer would be equal to or better than those provided in-house. Contract services also provide backup instrument reprocessing services on an as-needed basis, such as during emergency shutdown of a hospital's CSS or during construction and renovation of CSS areas (107).

Occupational Risks for Healthcare Workers in Central Sterile Supply

Occupationally Acquired Infections

Central sterile supply workers encounter blood, tissues, body substances, and fluids contaminated with these proteinaceous materials on a daily basis. According to standard precautions, the blood from all patients should be considered infectious, and used instruments and items should be considered potentially infective and handled with extraordinary care (108). There is a recognized risk of exposure to blood-borne pathogens [i.e., human immunodeficiency virus (HIV-1), hepatitis B virus (HBV), and hepatitis C virus (HCV)] for CSS personnel during the reprocessing of reusable medical devices. Inherent in the manual cleaning/decontamination process is power spraying, splashing, and the potential for puncture wounds. CSS workers, therefore, are considered appropriate candidates for hepatitis B vaccination and should be offered the vaccine accordingly (16, 109,110).

CSS personnel performing decontamination should wear protective apparel, including an impervious gown and shoe covers, heavy gloves, and eye goggles or face shields. Although proper technique when handling patient-care items is extremely important, minimizing the amount of contact with these items may be a more practical approach for reducing the risk of exposure to potentially infectious fluids (111,112). Automated equipment, such as washer-decontaminators, washer-sterilizers, and ultrasonic cleaners, aids in reducing manual processing. However, these machines may produce a spray from the fluids contained within, and this should be considered when one is planning programs for protection of workers (see also Chapters 78 and 79).

Even though properly attired with personal protective equipment, healthcare workers in CSS are still at risk for injuries and infections by puncturing themselves with sharp, contaminated instruments. Disposable sharps need to be discarded in an approved sharps container at the point of use. Reusable instruments should be placed in a puncture-resistant container for safe transport to the decontamination area (112). Percutaneous injuries (PIs), including needle sticks, have been reported by CSS personnel (108,111). In a CDC surveillance study, occupational PIs sustained at CSS represented less than 1% of the PIs in the institutions and were either associated with improperly disposed needles or occurred during the cleaning/handling of sharp instruments (S. Campbell, CDC, personal communication, 1998). It is not clear, however, if such exposure episodes among CSS workers have resulted in notable transmission of blood-borne infection. CDC surveillance of healthcare personnel with HIV/AIDS as of December 2001 does not identify CSS workers as a separate occupational category, and there are only four possible cases listed for "Other Health-Care Occupation" (113).

Nevertheless, CSS workers should be trained on the importance of promptly reporting occupational exposures to blood and body fluids (16). In a survey conducted in the mid-1990s to assess the level and reasons of underreporting of PIs sustained by healthcare workers, 9% of workers in CSS recalled at least one PI in the preceding 12 months; 50% of the injuries were not reported to the hospital surveillance system, because the healthcare worker believed that the injury was associated with a low risk of infection (S. Campbell, CDC, personal communication, 1998).

Risks Associated with Ethylene Oxide Sterilization

Ethylene oxide (EO) has been produced commercially and used as a sterilizing agent for many years and is mutagenic for several microorganisms. Its use, however, is being phased out in healthcare settings because of environmental concerns relating to emissions and inherent health risks for both CSS workers and patients who come in contact with EO vapors and surface residuals, respectively. EO has produced tumors (114) and teratogenic effects and maternal toxicity (115) when injected into mice. Some evidence of carcinogenicity of EO has been found in humans (116). Study of spontaneous abortions in hospital staff suggested that exposure to EO in hospitals may carry a risk of spontaneous abortion among CSS staff (117).

To use EO in the safest possible manner, three guidelines need to be followed: (a) provide safe devices that are sterile, unaltered, and with no undesirable residues; (b) protect workers from chronic EO exposure; and (c) take steps to prevent hazardous episodes of leaks, fires, or explosions (118).

Aeration of Instruments, Devices, and Items After Ethylene Oxide Sterilization

Excessive levels of residual EO or EO by-products (ethylene glycol, ethylene chlorohydrin) on medical devices are harmful. Ethylene oxide and ethylene chlorohydrin can be removed from items after sterilization. Therefore, it is imperative that all instruments and devices subjected to EO sterilization are fully aerated to eliminate EO residuals prior to handling and use. Items (e.g., prosthetic devices, instruments, or catheters) improperly aerated can cause serious chemical burns or tissue irritation (117–120). Ethylene glycol is not removed by aeration. Therefore, precautions such as making certain that no liquid exists in the load, selection of a quality gas source, and routine maintenance of the sterilizer are needed to prevent its formation.

Aeration of EO-reprocessed instruments and patient care items at ambient conditions in an open, unrestricted area is unacceptable, because it would unnecessarily expose workers to EO. For safety purposes, aeration should be accomplished by using in-chamber aeration within the sterilizer if the unit is so designed, or by using properly designed mechanical aeration cabinets that accurately control airflow and temperature and that are exhausted to the outside (118,120). Adequate aeration time must be allowed after sterilization so that residual EO can be reduced to a level safe for both personnel and patients. Length of aeration depends on many variables, including (a) composition, form, density, and weight of the sterilized item; (b) product packing, loading, and mass; (c) type of EO sterilization system used; (d) temperature of the aeration chamber; (e) number of filtered air changes per hour, and air flow characteristics; and (f) intended use of the item (external application or implantable device) (19,118,119). Polyvinylchloride is one of the most challenging materials from which EO residue must be eliminated. No standard times for aeration can be reliably given without consulting the device, sterilizer, and packaging manufacturers. Items can require as short as a few hours or as long as several days in an aeration cabinet to reduce EO to safe levels.

In 1978, the FDA proposed limits on the amount of residual EO (30 μg/kg/day for 30 days) that can remain on sterilized medical devices for human patients. These limits were based on histologic and hematologic studies in rodents and dogs (120). The FDA has raised the allowable residual limit of EO to 250 parts per million (ppm) on devices subjected to EO sterilization, with the exception of those devices used in donor and patient blood collection (product codes 81GKT and 81KSR) (121). More recently, the ISO and AAMI have adopted a philosophy that the limit should depend on the intended use of the device and the length of contact with human tissue so that the dose to tissue is considered, not just the amount retained in the device (121–125).

Preventing Occupational Exposure to Ethylene Oxide

Each worker must be informed of the possible health effects of exposure to EO. This information must include an explanation of the requirements of the Occupational Safety and Health Administration (OSHA) standard on occupational exposure to EO and must identify the areas and tasks in which there is potential exposure to EO emissions (126).

OSHA published a final ruling on EO in 1984 that reduced the permissible worker 8-hour time-weighted exposure level of EO from 50 ppm of air to 1 ppm of air. In 1988, OSHA amended its existing standard by adopting an excursion limit for EO of 5 ppm of air averaged over a 15-minute sampling period (49,126). Workers who are exposed to EO emissions at or above the action level (0.5 ppm) for at least 30 days per year, even if an approved respirator is used, must have medical examinations at least annually.

Restrictions on EO use have included the amount permitted to exit the sterilizers to the atmosphere. These restrictions have been imposed by individual states and air pollution control boards (127). These restrictions not only ensure that occupational exposure to EO is minimized but also prevent the passive exposure of patients, other hospital workers, visitors, and individuals in or near the healthcare facility. All EO sterilizers and aerators must be directly vented out of the workplace to the outside atmosphere (4). The vent line must not terminate within 25 feet (7.6 m) of any building air intake. A greater distance may be needed in some situations, depending on the direction of prevailing winds and the location of buildings (122,127).

Desirable EO sterilizer safety features include, but are not limited to (a) purge of the system at the end of cycle, (b) door-locking and sealing mechanisms, (c) audible alarm at the end of the EO cycle, (d) automatic door controls, and (d) audible and/or visual alarms for system failures. Scrubbers that convert EO to less toxic ethylene glycol have been used successfully to control EO emissions (118,122).

CSS personnel should ask instrument and device manufacturers for written instructions on the proper sterilization and aeration times for their products when EO is the recommended sterilant for successful reprocessing. CSS personnel also have to develop, implement, and enforce aeration policies and procedures. Aeration recommendations should be carried out in an uninterrupted cycle to prevent unnecessary operator exposure to EO due to opening the aerator door. Policies regarding early removal of devices that have not been completely aerated must be established through the hospital's infection control committee, legal counsel, and/or risk management committee (119) (see also Chapter 86).

CONCLUSION

Central sterile supply is an example of the person–machine interface that is so visible in the delivery of healthcare. Sterility assurance depends on the performance of both employees and equipment. Several processes have been developed to replace EO (e.g., ozone, hydrogen peroxide plasma, hydrogen peroxide liquid). Because of the constant changes in this field, it is crucial that professionals involved with CSS have a solid scientific understanding of the basic principles of cleaning, decontamination, disinfection and sterilization, and current clinical practices (128).

REFERENCES

1. Maki DG, Hassemer CA. Flash sterilization: carefully measured haste. *Infect Control* 1987;18:307–310.
2. Pugliese G, Hubbard C. Central services, linens and laundry. In: Bennett JV, Brachman PS, eds. *Hospital infections*, 4th ed. Philadelphia: Lippincott-Raven, 1998:325–332.
3. Drake A. Reflections on renovation in central service. *J Health Mater Manage* 1990;8:24–25.
4. American Institute of Architects and U.S. Department of Health and Human Services. *Guidelines for design and construction of hospitals and health-care facilities*. Washington, DC: American Institute of Architects Press, 2001.
5. Association for the Advancement of Medical Instrumentation. *Steam sterilization and sterility assurance in health care facilities*. ANSI/AAMI ST46:2002. Arlington, VA: AAMI, 2002.
6. U.S. Department of Health, Education, and Welfare. *Minimum requirements of construction and equipment for hospital and medical facilities*. DHEW Publication No. (HRA) 79-14500. Hyattsville, MD: Bureau of Health Facilities Financing, Compliance, and Conversion, 1982.
7. International Organization for Standardization. *Sterilization for health care products—requirements for validation and routine control of moist heat sterilization in health care facilities*. ISO 13683. Geneva, Switzerland: ISO, 1996.
8. Greene VW. Microbiological contamination control in hospitals. Part 6—roles of central service and the laundry. *JAHA* 1970;44:99–103.
9. Garner JS, Favero MS. CDC Guideline for handwashing and hospital environmental control, 1985. *Infect Control* 1986;7:231–240.
10. Association for the Advancement of Medical Instrumentation. *Safe handling of biological decontamination of reusable medical devices in health care facilities and nonclinical settings*. ANSI/AAMI ST35-2003. Arlington, VA: AAMI, 2003.
11. Miles RS. What standards should we use for the disinfection of large equipment? *J Hosp Infect* 1991;18(suppl A):264–273.
12. Schultz JK. Decontamination recommended practices. In: Reichert M, Young J, eds. *Sterilization technology for the health care facility*, 2nd ed. Gaithersburg, MD: Aspen, 1997.
13. Harrison SK, Evans WJ Jr, LeBlanc DA, et al. Cleaning and decontaminating of medical instruments. *J Health Mater Manage* 1990;8: 36–42.
14. Ryan P. Concepts of cleaning technologies and processes. *J Health Mater Manage* 1987;5:20–27.

15. Graham GS. Decontamination: a microbiologist's perspective. *J Health Mater Manage* 1988;6:36–41.
16. U.S. Department of Labor, Occupational Safety and Health Administration. Occupational exposure to bloodborne pathogens. Final rule. 29 CFR Part 1910.1030. *Fed Reg* 1991;56:64175–64182.
17. Miller CH, Palenik CJ. Sterilization, disinfection and asepsis in dentistry. In: Block SS, ed. *Disinfection, sterilization and preservation,* 5th ed. Philadelphia: Lippincott Williams & Wilkins, 2001:1049–1068.
18. Crow S. Washer decontamination: an evaluation. *Infect Control Hosp Epidemiol* 1990;10:220–221.
19. Association of periOperative Registered Nurses. Sterilization in the perioperative practice setting. *In: AORN standards and recommended practices.* Denver: Association of periOperative Registered Nurses (AORN), 2003:237–366.
20. Jette LP, Lambert NG. Evaluation of two hot water washer disinfectors for medical instruments. *Infect Control Hosp Epidemiol* 1988; 9:194–199.
21. Drake A, Ayers L. Validation of the microbial safety of instruments/utensils following automated thermal disinfection. Proceeding of the 18th Annual Conference and International Meeting of Association for Practitioners of Infection Control, Nashville, TN, 1991.
22. Society of Gastroenterology Nurses and Associates. *Standards of infection control in reprocessing flexible gastrointestinal endoscopes.* Chicago: SGNA, 2000. At: *http://www.sgna.org/resources/guideline3.cfm.*
23. Alvarado CJ, Stolz SM, Maki DG. Nosocomial infections from contaminated endoscopes: a flawed automated endoscope washer. an investigation using molecular epidemiology. *Am J Med* 1991;3B: 275S–280S.
24. FDA and CDC Public Health Advisory. Infection from endoscopes inadequately reprocessed by automated endoscope reprocessing systems. September 10, 1999. At: *http://www.fda.gov/cdrh/safety/endoreprocess.pdf.*
25. Blanc DS, Parret T, Janin B, et al. Nosocomial infections and pseudoinfections from contaminated bronchoscopes: two-year follow-up using molecular markers. *Infect Control Hosp Epidemiol* 1997;18: 134–136.
26. Allen JI, O'Connor AM, Olson MM, et al. *Pseudomonas* infection of the biliary system resulting from use of a contaminated endoscope. *Gastroenterology* 1987;92:759–763.
27. Gubler JGH, Salfinger M, von Graevenitz A. Pseudoepidemic of nontuberculous mycobacteria due to a contaminated bronchoscope cleaning machine. Report of an outbreak and review of the literature. *Chest* 1992;101:1245–1249.
28. Fraser VJ, Jones M, Murray PR, et al. Contamination of flexible fiberoptic bronchoscopes with *Mycobacterium chelonae* linked to an automated bronchoscope disinfection machine. *Am Rev Respir Dis* 1992;145:853–855.
29. Maloney S, Welbel S, Daves B, et al. *Mycobacterium abscessus* pseudoinfection traced to an automated endoscope washer: utility of epidemiologic and laboratory investigation. *J Infect Dis* 1994;169: 1166–1169.
30. Merighi A, Contato E, Scagliarini R, et al. Quality improvement in gastrointestinal endoscopy: microbiologic surveillance of disinfection. *Gastrointest Endosc* 1996;43:457–462.
31. Muscarella LF. Application of environmental sampling to flexible endoscope reprocessing: the importance of monitoring the rinse water. *Infect Control Hosp Epidemiol* 2002;23:285–289.
32. Mitchell DH, Hicks LJ, Chiew R, et al. Pseudoepidemic of *Legionella pneumophila* serogroup 6 associated with contaminated bronchoscopes. *J Hosp Infect* 1997;37:19–23.
33. Nelson DB, Jarvis WR, Rutala WA, et al. Multi-society guideline for reprocessing flexible gastrointestinal endoscopes. *Infect Control Hosp Epidemiol* 2003;24:532–537.
34. Cooke EM. HIV and decontamination procedures. *Br Med J* 1989; 299:72–73.
35. Morgan DR, Lamont TJ, Dawson JD, et al. Decontamination of instruments and control of cross infection in general practice. *Br Med J* 1990;300:1379–1380.
36. Association of periOperative Registered Nurses. Recommended practices for selection and use of packaging systems. In: *AORN standards, practices and guidelines.* Denver: Association of periOperative Registered Nurses (AORN), 2003.
37. Mayworm D. Sterile shelf life and expiration dating. *J Hosp Supply Proc Distr* 1984;2:32–35.
38. Klapes NA, Greene VW, Langhols AC, et al. Effect of long-term storage on sterile status of devices in surgical packs. *Infect Control* 1987;8:289–293.
39. Fiuke C. CSR wrapping and packaging. *J Health Mater Manage* 1989; 7:77–80.
40. Mallison GF, Standard PG. Safe storage times for sterile packs. *Mater Manage Central Serv* 1974;48:77–80.
41. Alder VG, Alder FI. Preserving the sterility of surgical dressings wrapped in paper and other materials. *J Clin Pathol* 1961;14:76–79.
42. Belkin NL. Central service guidelines present challenges for in-house packaging. *Hospitals JCAH* 1978;52:146–148.
43. American Society for Testing and Materials (ASTM). *Guidelines for protective apparel.* ASTM, 1993:11.
44. Association for the Advancement of Medical Instrumentation. *Processing of reusable surgical textiles for use in health care facilities.* ANSI/AAMI ST65:2000. Arlington, VA: AAMI, 2000.
45. Standard PG, Mackel DC, Mallison GF. Microbial penetration of muslin and paper-wrapped packs stored on open shelves and in closed cabinets. *Appl Microbiol* 1971;22:432–437.
46. Fallon RJ. Wrapping of sterilized articles. *Lancet* 1963;2:785.
47. Speers R, Shooter RA. The use of double-wrapped packs to reduce contamination of the sterile contents during extraction. *Lancet* 1966; 2:469–470.
48. Allen SM, Crowley N, Cunliffe AC, et al. Central sterile supply. *Lancet* 1965;2:1343.
49. Cyr WH, Glasser ZR. Limits for residues of ETO on sterilized medical devices: considerations of carcinogenic risks. Proceedings and Abstracts of ASM International Symposium on Chemical Germicides, Atlanta, 1990.
50. U.S. Food and Drug Administration. FDA safety alert: warning regarding the use of the Abtox Plazlyte sterilization system. Rockville, MD: U.S. Department of Health and Human Services, Food and Drug Administration, April 13, 1998.
51. Rutala WA, Weber DJ. Clinical effectiveness of low-temperature sterilization technologies. *Infect Control Hosp Epidemiol* 1998;19: 798–804.
52. Alfa MJ, Olson N, Degagne P, et al. New low temperature sterilization technologies: microbiocidal activity and clinical efficacy. In: Rutala, WA, ed. *Disinfection, sterilization, and antisepsis in health care.* Washington, DC, Champlain, NY: Association for Professionals in Infection Control and Epidemiology, and Polysciences, 1998:67–78.
53. Greene VW, Borlaug GM, Nelson E. Effects of patching on sterilization of surgical textiles. *AORN J* 1981;33:1249–1261.
54. Joslyn LJ. Sterilization by heat. In: Block SS, ed. *Disinfection, sterilization and preservation,* 5th ed. Philadelphia: Lippincott Williams & Wilkins, 2001:695–728.
55. Berube R, Oxborrow GS, Gaustad JW. Sterility testing: validation of sterilization processes and sporicide testing. In: Block SS, ed. *Disinfection, sterilization and preservation,* 5th ed. Philadelphia: Lippincott Williams & Wilkins, 2001:1047–1057.
56. Association for the Advancement of Medical Instrumentation. *Sterilization of health care products—chemical indicators—part 1: general requirements.* ANSI/AAMI ST60-1996. Arlington, VA: AAMI, 1996, American National Standard.
57. Association for the Advancement of Medical Instrumentation. *Chemical indicators—guidance for selection, use, and interpretation of results.* AAMI TIR 25-1999. Arlington, VA: AAMI, 1999.
58. International Organization for Standardization. *Sterilization of health care products: chemical indicators. Part 1, general requirements.* Geneva, Switzerland: ISO, 1995.
59. Association for the Advancement of Medical Instrumentation. *Sterilization of health care products—chemical indicators. Part 2: class 2 indicators for air removal test sheets and packs.* Arlington, VA: AAMI, 1999.
60. Kereluk K, Gammon R, Lloyd RS. Microbiological aspects of sterilization. II. microbial resistance. *Appl Microbiol* 1970;19:153–156.
61. Favero MS. Developing indicators for monitoring sterilization. In:

Rutala, WA, ed. *Disinfection, sterilization, and antisepsis in health care.* Washington, DC, Champlain, NY: Association for Professionals in Infection Control and Epidemiology, and Polysciences, 1998: 119–132.

62. Joint Commission on Accreditation of Health Care Organizations. *Accreditation manual for hospitals.* Chicago: JCAHO, 2001.
63. Association for Advancement of Medical Instrumentation. *Sterilization of health care products—biological indicators—part 1: general.* ANSI/AAMI ST59-1999. Arlington, VA: AAMI, 1999, American National Standard.
64. Centers for Disease Control and Prevention. Guidelines for infection control in dental health-care settings, 2003. *MMWR* 2003;52 (RR-17): 1–61.
65. Rutala WA, Gergen MF, Weber DJ. Evaluation of a rapid readout biological indicator for flash sterilization with three biological indicators and three chemical indicators. *Infect Control Hosp Epidemiol* 1993; 14:390–394.
66. Gurevich I, Yannelli B, Cunha BA. Survey of techniques used for sterilization of facial implants. *Am J Infect Control* 1989;17:35–38.
67. Kotilainen HR, Gantz NM. An evaluation of three biological indicator systems in flash sterilization. *Infect Control* 1987;8:311–316.
68. Lee C, Montville TJ, Sinskey AJ. Comparison of the efficacy of steam sterilization indicators. *Appl Environ Microbiol* 1979;37:1113–1117.
69. Perkins RE, Bodman HA, Kundsin RB, et al. Monitoring steam sterilization of surgical instruments: a dilemma. *Appl Environ Microbiol* 1981;42:383–384.
70. Everly BJ, Lattimer JM, Matsen JM, et al. False positive spore strip sterility tests with steam sterilization. *Am J Infect Control* 1983;11: 71–73.
71. Maki DM, Alvarado C, Davis JP. False positive results of spore tests in ETO sterilizers, Wisconsin. *MMWR* 1981;30:239–240.
72. Sandrick K. Positive action. *Materials Management* 1998;7:16–21.
73. Reich R, Morien LL. Influence of environmental storage relative humidity on BI resistance, viability, and moisture content. *Appl Environ Microbiol* 1982;43:609–614.
74. Birnbaum D, Ayers H, Carlson LD. Failure of sterilization process indicators. *Infect Control* 1987;8:491–492.
75. Tornello JD. Flash sterilization: evaluating biological indicators. *AORN J* 1986;43:1289–1294.
76. McFaddin C, Earnhardt K. Sterile supply storage—finding a place for everything. *AORN J* 1999;70:686–688.
77. Standard PG, Mallison GF, Mackel DC. Microbial penetration through three types of double wrappers for sterile packs. *Appl Microbiol* 1973;26:59–62.
78. Hunstiger CA, Greene VW. Maintaining sterile integrity of hospital produced packs. *J Sterile Serv Manage* 1987:21–24.
79. Eichoff TC. An outbreak of surgical wound infections due to *Clostridium perfringens. Surg Gynecol Obstet* 1962;114:102–108.
80. Ho JL, Highsmith AK, Wong ES, et al. Common source *Pseudomonas aeruginosa* infection in neurosurgery. Proceedings and Abstracts of the Annual Meeting of the American Society for Microbiology, Dallas, TX, 1981.
81. Beck-Sague CM, Jarvis WR. Epidemic bloodstream infections associated with pressure transducers: a persistent problem. *Infect Control Hosp Epidemiol* 1989;10:54–59.
82. Soto LE, Bobadilla M, Villalobos Y, et al. Post-surgical nasal cellulitis outbreak due to *Mycobacterium chelonae. J Hosp Infect* 1991;19: 99–106.
83. Esel D, Doganay M, Bozdemir N, et al. Polymicrobial ventriculitis and evaluation of an outbreak in a surgical intensive care unit due to inadequate sterilization. *J Hosp Infect* 2002;50:170–174.
84. Chadha R, Grover M, Sjarma A, et al. An outbreak of post-surgical wound infections due to *Mycobacterium abscessus. Pediatr Surg Int* 1998;13:406–410.
85. Meyers H, Brown-Elliott BA, Moore D, et al. An outbreak of *Mycobacterium chelonae* infection following liposuction. *Clin Infect Dis* 2002;34:1500–1507.
86. Holland SP, Mathias RG, Morck DW, et al. Diffuse lamellar keratitis related to endotoxins release from sterilizer reservoir biofilms. *Ophthalmology* 2000;107:1227–1233.
87. Duffy RE, Brown SE, Caldwell KL, et al. An epidemic of corneal destruction caused by plasma gas sterilization. The Toxic Cell Destruction Syndrome Investigative Team. *Arch Ophthalmol* 2000;118: 1167–1176.
88. Cogdill CP, Quaglia L. How safe and effective is reuse of single-use only medical devices? *Biomed Instrumentation Technol* 1998;32: 434–435.
89. Avitall B, Khan M, Krum D, et al. Repeated use of ablation catheters: a prospective study. *J Am Coll Cardiol* 1993;22:1367–1372.
90. Shaw JP, Eisenberg MJ, Azoulay A, et al. Reuse of catheters for percutaneous transluminal coronary angioplasty: effects on procedure time and clinical outcomes. *Catheter Cardiovasc Interv* 1999;48:54–60.
91. Roach SK, Kozarek RA, Raltz SL, et al. *In vitro* evaluation of integrity and sterilization of single-use argon beam plasma coagulation probes. *Am J Gastroenterol* 1999;94:139–143.
92. Chan AC, Ip M, Koehler A, et al. Is it safe to reuse disposable laparoscopic trocars? An *in vitro* testing. *Surg Endosc* 2000;14:1042–1044.
93. Luijt DS, Schirm J, Savelkoul PH, et al. Risk of infection by reprocessed and resterilized virus-contaminated catheters; an *in-vitro* study. *Eur Heart J* 2001;22:378–384.
94. Heeg P, Roth K, Reichl R, et al. Decontaminated single-use devices: an oxymoron that may be placing patients at risk for cross-contamination. *Infect Control Hosp Epidemiol* 2001;22:542–549.
95. Brown SA, Merritt K, Woods TP, et al. Effects of different disinfection and sterilization methods on tensile strength of materials used for single-use devices. *Biomed Instrum Technol* 2002;36:23–27.
96. Alfa MJ, Nemes R. Inadequacy of manual cleaning for reprocessing single-use, triple-lumen sphinctertomes: simulated-use testing comparing manual with automated cleaning methods. *Am J Infect Control* 2003;31:193–207.
97. Chaufour X, Deva AK, Vickery K, et al. Evaluation of disinfection and sterilization of reusable angioscopes with the duck hepatitis B model. *J Vasc Surg* 1999;30:277–282.
98. Duffy R, Couto B, Starling C, et al. Improving water quality can reduce pyrogenic reactions associated with cardiac catheter reuse. *Infect Control Hosp Epidemiol* 2003;24:955–960.
99. U.S. Food and Drug Administration. Enforcement priorities for single-use devices reprocessed by third parties and hospitals. August 14, 2000. *Fed Reg* 2000;65:49583–49585. Also available at: *http://www.fda.gov/cdrh/reuse/reuse-documents.html#8.*
100. U.S. Food and Drug Administration. Labeling recommendations for single-use devices reprocessed by third parties and hospitals: final guidance for industry and FDA. July 30, 2001. At: *http://www.fda.gov/cdrh/comp/guidance/1392.pdf.*
101. U.S. Food and Drug Administration. Medical device user fee and modernization act of 2002; validation data in premarket notification submissions (510(k)s) for reprocessed single-use medical devices. Guidance for industry and FDA staff. At: *http://www.fda.gov/cdrh/ode/guidance/1216.pdf.*
102. U.S. Government Accounting Office. GAO report: single-use medical devices: little available evidence of harm from reuse, but oversight warranted. June 20, 2000. GAO/HEHS-00–123.
103. U.S. Food and Drug Administration. Determining hospital procedures for opened-but-unused, single-use medical devices: Request for comments and information. *Fed Reg* 2002;67:55269–55270.
104. U.S. Food and Drug Administration. Reuse of single-use devices information. At: *http://www.fda.gov/cdrh/reuse/.*
105. U.S. Food and Drug Administration. 21 CFR, Parts 801 and 820: Labeling: quality systems regulations. Washington, DC: Government Printing Office, 1998:14–38,143–156.
106. Giarraputo D. In-house versus off-site sterilization. *Hosp Materiel Manage Q* 1990;12:49–55.
107. Morganstern KH. Contract processing and sterilization. *J Health Mater Manage* 1991;16,19–20,22,24.
108. Centers for Diseases Control. Recommendations for prevention of HIV transmission in health-care settings. *MMWR* 1987;36(suppl S): 2S–17S.
109. Centers for Disease Control and Prevention. Immunization of health-care workers: recommendations of the Advisory Committee on Immunization Practices (ACIP) and the Hospital Infection Control Prac-

tices Advisory Committee (HICPAC). *MMWR* 1997;46(RR-18): 1–42.

110. Centers for Disease Control and Prevention. Updated U.S. Public Health Service guidelines for the management of occupational exposures to HBV, HCV, and HIV and recommendations for postexposure prophylaxis. *MMWR* 2001;50(RR-11):1–42.
111. Haiduven DJ, DeMaio TM, Stevens DA. A five year study of needlestick injuries significant reduction associated with communication, education, and convenient placement of sharps containers. *Infect Control Hosp Epidemiol* 1992;13:265–271.
112. Kennedy PB, Gualteney JM. Brief report: the detection of blood on gloved hands of CSS personnel and cleaned instruments used for procedures on patient units. *Infect Control Hosp Epidemiol* 1988;9: 117–118.
113. Centers for Disease Control and Prevention. Issues in healthcare settings. Surveillance of healthcare personnel with HIV/AIDS, as of December 2001. At: *http://www.cdc.gov/ncidod/hip/BLOOD/hivpersonnel.htm.*
114. Dunkelberg H. On the oncogenic activity of ETO and propylene oxide in mice. *Br J Cancer* 1979;30:588–589.
115. La Borde J, Kimmel C. The teratogenicity of ETO administered intravenously to mice. *Toxicol Appl Pharmacol* 1980;56:16–22.
116. Hogsted C, Rohlen O, Berndtsson BS, et al. A cohort study of mortality and cancer incidence in ETO production workers. *Br J Industr Med* 1979;36:276–280.
117. Hemminki KK, Mutanen P, Saloniemi I, et al. Spontaneous abortions in hospital staff in sterilizing instruments with chemical agents. *Br Med J* 1982;284:1461–1463.
118. Joslyn LJ. Gaseous chemical sterilization. In: Block SS, ed. *Disinfection, sterilization and preservation,* 5th ed. Philadelphia: Lippincott Williams & Wilkins, 2001:580–595.
119. American Society for Hospital Service Personnel, American Hospital Association. *Ethylene oxide for use in hospitals. A manual for health care personnel,* 3rd ed. Chicago: American Hospital Association, 1998: 95–99.
120. U.S. Food and Drug Administration. Ethylene oxide, ethylene chlorohydrin, and ethylene glycol: proposed maximum residue limits and maximum levels of exposure. *Fed Reg* 1978;43:27474–27483.
121. U.S. Food and Drug Administration. Guidance for ANSI/AAMI/ISO 10993-7; 1995. Biological evaluation of medical devices, Part 7: ETO sterilization residuals (revised 8/20/98).
122. Association for the Advancement of Medical Instrumentation. *Ethylene oxide sterilization in health care facilities: safety and effectiveness.* ANSI/AAMI ST41-1999. Arlington, VA: AAMI, 1999.
123. Association for the Advancement of Medical Instrumentation. *Biological evaluation of medical devices, Part 7: ethylene oxide residuals.* ANSI/AAMI/ISO 10993–7: 1995/revised 2001. Arlington, VA: AAMI, 2001.
124. Association for the Advancement of Medical Instrumentation. *Guidance for ANSI/AAMI/ISO 10993-7:1995.* AAMI TIR 19:1998. Arlington, VA: AAMI, 1998.
125. Association for the Advancement of Medical Instrumentation. *Amendment 1 to AAMI TIR 19-1998.* AAMI TIR 19: 1998/A1:1999. Arlington, VA: AAMI, 1999.
126. U.S. Department of Labor, Occupational, Safety and Health Administration. 29 CFR 1910.1047 Subpart Z. Occupational exposure to ethylene oxide, final standard. *Fed Reg* 1988;53:11413–11438.
127. U.S. Environmental Protection Agency. Assessment of ethylene oxide as a potentially toxic air pollutant: Notice. *Fed Reg* 1985;50: 40285–40289.
128. Young JH, Whitbourne J. New sterilization technologies. In: Reichert M, Young JH, eds. *Sterilization technology.* Gaithersburg, MD: Aspen, 1993:265–270.

75

PHARMACY SERVICE

CYRUS C. HOPKINS

The hospital pharmacist and the pharmacy service are essential elements of any infection control program. The formal statement of the American Society of Health-System Pharmacists (ASHP) describes three major roles of pharmacists in infection control: reducing the transmission of infection, promoting the rational use of antimicrobial agents, and educating patients, health professionals, and the public (1). The latter two roles are self-evident, and provide a valuable overlap and indeed synergy with the work of infection control professionals. There is one element of the role of the pharmacy, however, that is unique: the preparation and distribution of medications and other sterile materials. This role is the subject of this chapter.

PHARMACY-PROVIDED MATERIALS AS A SOURCE OF CONTAMINATION

Epidemiologic Overview

The distribution of any contaminated product could produce the epidemic pattern of a common-source outbreak. However, in the case of contaminated sterile products, this is often obscured by the scope of the epidemic, in particular by the time and space over which it may occur. The simplest common-source outbreak (caused by, for example, a shared meal) results from a single exposure in time and place. The epidemic curve reflects a well-defined, circumscribed population at risk, and the incubation period of the agent. In the case of contaminated medications, however, the exposure occurs over a period of time in the form of many single-case exposures, involving populations that can range from a few patients in a single unit to hundreds in many countries. Further confusion in analysis results from secondary cross-infection. In the analysis of these infections, exposure is more often measured as colonization or a positive culture, rather than as a clinical infection. On the other hand, the discovery of a contaminated product in use requires clinical and epidemiologic interpretation: it may be meaningless, it may be associated with a common-source epidemic, or it may be a part of a complex epidemic pattern with aspects of both common-source and person-to-person transmission with successive users.

The original source of the contamination, and the vehicles involved as inanimate vectors, will determine the scope and nature of the epidemic. The hospital pharmacy is but one step in a complex chain of processes that lead from manufacture to use. Contamination of a sterile product may occur before arrival in the hospital pharmacy; during the course of dispensing, repackaging, or compounding in the pharmacy; or after it leaves the pharmacy, usually at the point of use. Corresponding to each of these, there may arise three distinct types of epidemics, which will be discussed separately.

The first type, contamination occurring in a manufactured product outside the hospital, is often described as "intrinsic." It is important to point out, however, that contamination of a presumably sterile product is now rarely an issue of a manufacturing pharmacy's providing contaminated materials. Manufacturing pharmacies operate under strict supervision, and almost always have strict internal quality standards. However, perhaps in response to a number of external factors, more and more hospitals, 20% in a recent survey (2), have out-sourced the compounding of some medications. These medications would be considered "intrinsic," though the epidemiology and etiology are quite different.

Contamination during preparation or compounding within the pharmacy is also rarely an issue now. Particularly in the early literature, a number of outbreaks were described as pharmacy based, but some situations were poorly defined. These reports often described defective techniques that are no longer used in pharmacy practice. The modern pharmacy operates under strict guidelines of quality with appropriate quality-control measures, and is infrequently the source of infectious materials.

On the other hand, contamination of a product released or distributed by the pharmacy as a sterile product and subsequently contaminated in use is far more likely. Examples of this type continue to appear, and may involve both inpatient and outpatient sources of care. Regardless of the source, incidents of contamination at first may seem to implicate products coming from the pharmacy, whether the pharmacy is the distributor or the source. Therefore, pharmacy data and personnel may be involved in the analysis and control of these outbreaks.

The major differences between the epidemic patterns of these three sites of contamination involve differences of scale in time and in space.

Prepharmacy Contamination

Items contaminated in manufacturing (intrinsic contamination) are likely to be distributed over wide geographic areas and used over long periods of time. The outbreaks associated with these products, therefore, are disseminated widely in time and in space. Thus, the epidemic is detectable over wide areas (even nationally) and in many institutions. A delay in using these products may initially obscure the common-source nature of the outbreak, and investigation on a national scale is often required. Occasionally, a carefully focused surveillance system and an alert observer can recognize these outbreaks even on a very local scale, particularly if it involves a very unusual microorganism in an unusual site. The nationwide epidemic of contaminated intravenous fluids in 1970 to 1971, for example, lasted for months (3) but was also suspected in one hospital within a month. A small hospital in Coeur d'Alene, Idaho, suspected it with its second case! (4). More recently, this same recognition of a highly unusual microorganism in unusual sites allowed recognition of a multistate transmission of contaminated injectable steroids after only five cases of infection occurred, since these were infections of the central nervous system (CNS) and joints with *Exophiala*, an unusual fungal microorganism, in generally immunocompetent hosts (5). Earlier, on an international scale, contamination of two lots of fentanyl with *Pseudomonas cepacia* resulted in only 16 cases of bacteremia in 2 months, but nine were in Denmark and seven were in Holland (6,7).

An extraordinary array of products have been contaminated in the course of commercial manufacture, from antiseptic solutions (8) to single-dose vials of saline (9). Many involve disinfectant solutions, which seem to be disproportionately represented (10,11), in which sterilization of the end product was often inadequate. Even nonsterile items, when heavily contaminated, can create infection if inadvertently placed in the wrong site (12) or when used in a highly susceptible patient, such as a neonate (13). In many instances, the specific defect in production is not described in the literature. For those that are, however, it is worth noting that many defects partly resulted from processes that are no longer recommended, such as failure to sterilize the final product (14). Indeed, the vast majority of described outbreaks of manufacturer-related contamination occurred some years ago, though they are still being described in other countries (15,16). One interesting feature of industrial contamination is that in some circumstances the same problem may return, thus causing return of the epidemic (17).

Although this reduction in contaminations may be partly due to earlier detection, it is also likely that much of it is the result of improved practices in manufacturing. The contributions of prior studies in hospital epidemiology in effecting these changes are significant, and continuing vigilance in hospital epidemiology, as well as in the pharmaceutical industry, will continue to be important in identifying new hazards. Continuing meticulous observation of quality standards by the industry should make manufacturer-related contamination a rare problem, and its potential for causing significant infection is still further reduced by good infection control practices that define or restrict the duration of use of medications, materials, or intravenous fluid systems used on nursing units in the hospital.

The more widespread use of out-sourcing of compounding, however, has introduced a new source of contamination of the intrinsically contaminated materials, though the source will appear the same to the hospital epidemiologist. One outbreak associated with out-sourced compounding has been described (5), but this case report may suggest serious underreporting of the problem, as a number of other similar situations are appearing in the literature (18).

In a recognized outbreak, just as in any hazard notification, the pharmacy, as the agent distributing the materials, is obliged to locate any unused portions of an affected lot or medication and must have a mechanism for its removal from patient care areas. The remaining portion of the affected lot must be either returned or tested as part of an ongoing epidemic investigation. Whenever possible, other recipients of potentially contaminated materials should be identified and followed, although this requires information about distribution that often is insufficient or unavailable. Distribution of prepackaged contaminated materials cannot be prevented by any reasonable, or recommended, quality control strategies of the pharmacy services of the hospital; routine sterility testing of reliably produced sterile products is not appropriate. Under extraordinary epidemic conditions, of course, such sampling may be an important part of the investigation.

Contamination in the Pharmacy

The pharmacy service is directly responsible for the prevention of contamination of sterile products within the pharmacy. Outbreaks in which the source was adequately evaluated and specifically related to pharmacy services are uncommonly reported in the medical literature. When the details are known, the analysis demonstrates that several steps in the complex process can be the source of contamination. The microorganism often reflects the source, as in any clinical epidemiologic investigation.

The well-documented outbreaks that involve contamination of a sterile product in the process of preparation fall into two types. The first involves a contaminated solution used in the formulation of a product. In one case, a phosphate buffer used in the formulation of amphotericin B became contaminated and resulted in meningitis and bacteremia with *Enterobacter agglomerans, Pseudomonas fluorescens,* and *Pseudomonas aeruginosa* in a single patient (19). In a second case, seven bacteremias were epidemiologically related to a contaminated potassium-chloride additive, though this was not microbiologically documented (20). The persistent use of multiple-use sterile solutions in pharmacy preparation was discouraged as early as 1973 (21), though similar reused or stock solutions continue to be found in other sites of preparation (22,23).

The second type of contamination involves a piece of equipment, often a container, pump, syringe, or tubing, that is repeatedly used in the formulation or preparation of sterile fluids (24–26). In one case this outbreak was identified by bacteriologic monitoring that discovered *Enterobacter cloacae* in sampled aliquots and was related to a pressure canister used in preparation of the solution (24). *Candida* outbreaks were traced back to a contaminated vacuum system in a pharmacy used to prepare parenteral solutions (25,26).

Many or all of the practices identified as responsible for these outbreaks would now generally be eliminated under current recommendations for pharmacy practice. The recommendations concerning the appropriate practices and subsequent end-product sterility testing programs might be expected to identify, and thus prevent, many of these situations. Certainly, the reuse of open stock solutions, the continuing use of contaminated equipment, and the absence of final sterilization should generally not occur. Two components of control are thus identified: quality control in the process, and final sampling of the end product. These are discussed below. Both are available for products prepared in a pharmacy; neither is likely to be available for products prepared at the site of use.

Given standard practices of pharmacy services, well-described outbreaks demonstrated to have been pharmacy-centered are now very rare in the United States.

Increased concern about out-sourcing practices have also led to guidelines for the hospital pharmacist to oversee these services, since the ultimate responsibility for the provision of these products still rests with the hospital pharmacy (27).

Contamination at Site of Use

Contamination of products subsequent to release to the work site as sterile products is now much more common than prepharmacy or pharmacy contamination. These cases involve a defect in use, usually at the site of care, that resulted in contamination of a product originally distributed as sterile. The specific service doing the admixture or contaminating the product is often not clearly defined. When described, these cases often include the repeated use of bottles of stock solutions, or using solutions that were topped-off by adding additional solutions to fluid in the base of a container. Some of this contamination was done in formulation or preparation areas that may or may not have been connected to the pharmacy, while many were done in the care unit itself.

With good practices (especially nursing), this mode of contamination should also be very uncommon. Such contamination is likely to be confined to localized areas within a single institution, often a single ward or office. In some situations, multiple units sharing a common product could all be affected [e.g., the use of contaminated ventilation nebulizers in several intensive care units (ICUs)] (28). The presence of several cases, particularly if caused by an unusual microorganism or if occurring at an unusual site, may lead to the conclusion that an item prepared in the pharmacy is responsible. However, careful epidemiologic investigation, assuming adequate reporting and identification of similar infections in other parts of the hospital, can exclude contamination of the same pharmacy product in other areas and suggest in-use contamination of the product. Such outbreaks have included a variety of materials, from intravenously administered flush solutions (29) to multiply used medications from a multidose vial (MDV) (30), especially ophthalmic solutions (31). The agents involved also vary widely with the item and the nature of contamination. Repeated use of the same product or device over a short period may allow more unusual microorganisms to be transferred by these routes. For example, from a patient source, hepatitis B can contaminate a heparin-saline flush solution (30). Some of the cross-contamination can be reduced by appropriate policy requirements such as the prohibition against reusing syringes or reentering an MDV. A recent dramatic example of such practices outside of the hospital resulted in a large outbreak of *Serratia liquefaciens* bloodstream infections originating in a hemodialysis center (32).

The role of MDVs in outbreaks, however, often remains unclear. Although MDVs seem a logical source of risk, and can, in rare instances, cause common source outbreaks, they are infrequently involved and can only rarely be shown to be contaminated (33). Indeed, purposeful contamination of such units is infrequently sustained under conditions of use, as most microorganisms will not survive in these solutions, particularly when they contain a bacteriostatic preservative (34,35). But contamination can be demonstrated by simulated use (36). Therefore, single-dose vials are strongly recommended.

It is important to note that many of the earlier epidemics resulting from contamination of medications or solutions prepared on the ward were also the result of practices that are no longer recommended. Indeed, it is now widely agreed that such preparation should be done in the pharmacy under careful quality monitoring (37). Some personnel in patient care areas try to improvise or develop their own on-site methods of formulation or mixing. They should bear in mind examples of earlier outbreaks caused by these practices. The variety of means of contamination is apparently endless; nefarious substitution of syringes of stolen fentanyl with unsterile water to support illicit drug use sets a new low (38). Virtually, any product can become contaminated with repeated use, provided it will support the growth of a contaminating microorganism. These products can then cause outbreaks in selected units either directly, as with contaminated nebulizers causing lower respiratory tract infection (39), or by creating colonization in a fluid or tissue that later serves as a reservoir for subsequent infections, as in colonization of the pharynx by contaminated mouthwash solution (40). Even surface solutions used in nonsterile sites can become contaminated and serve as a source of outbreaks with resistant microorganisms (41). Even saline can do so, either as a direct contaminant (17) or as the source of a pseudoepidemic (42). A striking demonstration of the varieties of extrinsic contamination is found in recent experience with propofol, an oil-based anesthetic agent that though itself sterile, has been responsible for several outbreaks of bloodstream infections. Seven such outbreaks, with at least five different microorganisms, were described in the initial report (43).

Understanding the extent of the cross-infection or the mode of contamination of the product may still require a careful analytic investigation. Although the pharmacy may not be ultimately implicated in these epidemics, their staffs and data are often involved in the investigation. Pharmacists will also appropriately participate in deciding on the recommended specifications of use of some of these products (especially, for example, the duration of use of MDVs).

ETIOLOGY

The microorganisms identified in pharmacy-centered outbreaks related to contaminated pharmacologic products are heterogeneous and vary with the contaminated product that serves as the source. Generally, this favors microorganisms capable of survival and growth in a liquid medium. Hence, the predilection toward relatively few species of aerobic gram-negative bacilli when found in liquid media such as intravenous fluids (44) or the preferential growth and isolation of fungi and yeasts in hyperalimentation solutions (45).

In some fluids, the use of germicidal preservatives may further limit the microorganisms capable of growing in these solutions to very few, more hardy, and relatively more resistant microorganisms such as *Xanthomonas* and *Pseudomonas* species (46). Contamination of commercially prepared solutions, therefore, is less representative of the flora found in clinical specimens. The same is true of pharmacy-based sources, though there may be added opportunity for contamination by *Candida* species or skin flora from the pharmacist.

In contrast, contamination in use can also be caused by a wide variety of other microorganisms potentially found in the patient's environment or on the hands of healthcare workers. Many of the associations of disseminated disease with pharmacy-prepared solutions either are supported by the ability to grow in these solutions (47) or may be cases of contamination in use, often from the patient's skin (48). Some of this contamination is via skin flora from handling by those preparing or using the product, and some is from contamination of equipment or fluid by a patient who earlier received the same product. In such a case, contamination of intravenous sites (48), injection sites (49), or even epidural sites (50) can result in outbreaks of unusual microorganisms, like *Mycobacterium chelonae* or *Malassezia furfur* (48,49). Almost any solution can be responsible for the spread of resistant microorganisms. Contamination of sterile items for multiple use probably occurs more often than we recognize. Some primary bacteremias or infected wounds or injection sites could presumably result from this mechanism, but without multiple cases that can be linked epidemiologically or without evidence of contamination, there is no way to relate these cases to the pharmacy. Except when fluid contamination in the presence of unusual gram-negative bacilli is highly suspected, these outbreaks are likely to remain undetected.

Colonization Versus Disease

Solutions released by the pharmacy can occasionally be shown to be contaminated but not related to adverse patient events. Most forms of contamination of nonsterile solutions pose little or no risk, except perhaps in a highly susceptible host. Enteral feeding solutions, for example, can be shown to have high levels of bacterial contamination, particularly when tested in use (51). However, unless contaminated by enteric pathogens or toxin-producing pathogens, this contamination, even at high levels, is not likely to be directly clinically significant. Still, even high levels of contamination with microorganisms that are not enteric pathogens may indirectly cause disease. Heavily colonized enteral feedings have been associated with a higher incidence of pneumonia or bacteremia with the same microorganism (52), though the mechanism is unclear. Certainly, such contamination, if detected after preparation, may serve as an indicator of lapses in technique of preparation that need to be identified, but if they are detected only after a period of use in a contaminated site, they may be less significant. On the other hand, a recent outbreak demonstrated the hazard of enteral feedings containing a dye contaminated with *Burkholderia cepacia* (53). This dye had been added for the purpose of detecting aspiration, and the direct contribution to disease was as likely to have been aspiration as contamination.

Detection by Cultures

Routine culturing of products prepared by the pharmacy is an inefficient and unreliable means of detecting contaminated materials, particularly since these sampling systems should ordinarily find a very low frequency of contamination. End-product culturing of processed or repackaged materials may still be a useful way to allow early discovery of lapses in technique, thereby indirectly preventing epidemic disease in patients. Accordingly, strategies for culturing the end product remain part of the standard recommended procedure.

The identification of contaminated solutions obtained by a program of quality inspection should be distinguished from pseudoepidemics, which have also been described in relation to pharmacy-prepared solutions. Many of these are caused by multiply used items contaminated in use. When manufactured or pharmacy-processed germicidal solutions (54,55) are contaminated, they generally cause clusters of positive cultures resulting from technical contamination that occurs while clinical specimens are obtained or handled for diagnostic evaluation.

QUALITY ASSURANCE

Since hospital pharmacy services and the infection control community are both increasingly aware of the potential risks of the types of contamination described above, increasing attention has been given to the safe preparation of pharmacy products. Two components of the recommended quality assurance programs are described in this section.

Preparation of Sterile Products

Over the years, a number of recommendations applicable to preparation and compounding of sterile products have been made. Through the 1990s, the most widely used by far, according to a survey, had been the recommendations of the National Coordinating Committee on Large Volume Parenterals (NCCLVP) of the American Society of Hospital Pharmacists (56), which cover a wide variety of issues concerning intravenous therapy. Supporting recommendations are regularly updated in the *United States Pharmacopoeia* (57). In addition, in separate documents, the Food and Drug Administration (FDA) requires adherence to current good manufacturing practices for manufacturing pharmacies. Guidelines of the Centers for Disease Control and Prevention (CDC) and the Joint Commission for Accreditation of Healthcare Organizations (JCAHO) are more general.

More recently, in an attempt to bring these guidelines into currently accepted practice, the American Society of Hospital Pharmacists issued a set of guidelines for each of these areas. These guidelines reflect and build on the prior work and recommendations and are supported by both experiential and experimental data (37). The final report of these recommendations largely supplants the prior recommendations, and is likely to provide the standard of practice for these services. Therefore, it is worth describing in more detail, though for implementation the document itself must be carefully studied.

These recommendations describe increasingly stringent criteria for preparation of materials, presenting three levels of risk. The identification of which processes belong in which risk level remains somewhat arbitrary and, within generally described guidelines is left up to the professional judgment of the pharmacist. The general guidelines emphasize differences in the interval between preparation and use (depending on how the products are stored) or in the source of the materials. Even the most basic class (risk level 1) requires written policies that address, in some (specified) detail, a number of features, including education and training, competency testing, storage and handling, facilities and equipment, dress and conduct, process validation, preparation technique, labeling, and documentation.

The infection control principles enumerated in these recommendations will be familiar to most infection control professionals (ICPs). It is instructive to recognize that many areas are analogous to clinical settings. For example, the segregation of a clean (or aseptic) area, with traffic control, is a familiar concept to ICPs; the recommendation of a requirement for reassessment and documentation of competency for sterile product preparation will particularly interest those concerned with supervision and quality assurance. The end-product testing and evaluation of a risk level 1 preparation does not include microbiologic documentation or sampling.

Risk level 2 defines a more rigid set of controls, especially including some environmental monitoring of the area in which these products are prepared, and the description of each method includes limits of acceptability. For preparation of materials in this class, a more rigidly defined clean room with positive pressure is specified. Environmental and end-product testing techniques are specified; some techniques are described below. Sampling of the surfaces of the site used to prepare the materials is specified here but is only recommended at this risk level.

Risk level 3 presents the highest risk, since it includes materials prepared from unsterile components, and therefore has still more stringent specifications. These include means of monitoring the physical environment of the aseptic preparation area and environmental microbiologic sampling. These items require a process of terminal sterilization. The techniques of sterilization are specifically described, including the size of the filter (generally 0.22 μm), followed by integrity testing. If other techniques of sterilization are used, the method must not alter the pharmaceutical properties of the product.

Stratification of Risk

Under any circumstance, some contamination may inadvertently occur, sometimes the result of an imperfect technique. Any contamination may be significant under some conditions if at a sufficiently high level, or with certain microorganisms, or occurring frequently enough as to raise concern about the sterility of the manufacturing or handling process as a whole. Accordingly, specific sampling methods have been proposed for continuing use in pharmacy quality monitoring. Among the many items prepared in hospital pharmacies, different items reflect different degrees of risk.

1. Nonsterile compounded items, though not intended to be sterile, should have an acceptable microbial level. Accordingly, the United States Pharmacopeia National Formulary (USP-NF) specifies certain acceptable levels of microbial contamination of nonsterile products that should not be exceeded (57), though routine culturing of these items is not recommended.
2. Total parenteral nutrition solutions have often been implicated as causes of, or at least risk factors for, bacteremia or fungemia. Much of the evidence is based on circumstantial observations that growth of the agent can be maintained, often preferentially, in the solution (45). On some occasions, a specific defect in the formulation of the product in the pharmacy has been identified as the cause (26). Often, this analysis is confounded by a high prevalence of the microorganisms in the environment of the patient, which allows contamination of a specimen or a device at the bedside. This can occur either via an external route or, potentially, by allowing transient fungemia or bacteremia to colonize a catheter tip.

   Nevertheless, since some of these outbreaks can be related to the process of preparation, meticulous care should be used in preparation of these solutions, and periodic sampling of the prepared product is desirable. Testing techniques may often need to be modified for specific preparations, particularly those containing lipids (58,59).
3. Sterile products or solutions, especially in risk level 3, must be released only with a program of end-product testing. For these programs, a formal sampling plan should be specifically described, including careful consideration of the sampling methods, the responsibility for handling the samples, and the designation of responsibility for reviewing, reporting, and acting on the results.

   Ophthalmic solutions, because of their demonstrated potential for contamination and infection, often have separate recommendations from the pharmaceutical community (60). These solutions can be responsible for outbreaks of disease. In the vast majority of these cases, the contamination occurs in use rather than in pharmacy preparation. Both the frequency of contamination in use and the frequent occurrence of subsequent cross-infection may relate, in part, to the need to have the delivery system (or dropper) so close to the conjunctiva that contact is very likely and cross-infection by direct contact more probable.

Assessment of Progress

Since 1990, the ASHP has been vigorously advocating and educating its members about quality assurance activities. Earlier surveys of members pointed out several areas of concern (56); later surveys have demonstrated improvement, particularly in orientation and training. It is worth noting that at the time of the 1995 survey, only 6.2% of members were out-sourcing compounding of sterile materials (61), although in 2002 it may be as high as 20% (2). Recent position statements and other educational and review activities of the ASHP society show vigorous support for the programs outlined above.

FORMULARY AND ANTIBIOTIC CONTROL

By virtue of its control over hospital formularies and of the distribution of medications within the hospital, the hospital pharmacy is often in a position to contribute significantly to defining and directing the appropriate use of antibiotics. Hospital pharmacists are committed to this goal, working in conjunction with other members of the healthcare teams (1). Contributions to this end can occur either at a system-wide level or in individual case management. There are two objectives: (a) to prevent the emergence of resistance by limiting the use of antibiotics of excessively broad spectrum or by narrowing the spectrum for a specific case, and (b) to limit cost, either system-wide or case by case, by the selection of the most cost-effective alternatives (62,63). The means to these ends have been varied and reflect quite different institutional philosophies and uses of resources, but the most obvious process is the elimination of some alternatives from the hospital formulary altogether (64). This decision generally can be best made by a structured review of new drugs, compared with other available alternatives, by a physician's committee working with the pharmacy staff. The alternatives can be evaluated with respect to both clinical and fiscal issues and can be effectively supported on both grounds (65). Effective institution of such a process generally needs to be associated with a vigorous countermarketing or other educational program (66,67), and is likely to work only with the visible participation and support of clinical leaders and role models, particularly from the infectious diseases community.

Also, the clinician user can be prompted to select one drug or combination over another either by a direct prompt or reminder for those with computer order-entry systems (68–70) or by recommending programs, guidelines, or pathways for clinical situations, particularly in teaching settings. In some situations, the reporting of only some of the antibiotic sensitivity results from particular isolates may direct clinicians to pick antibiotics from those presented as sensitive, and require further inquiry and effort to ascertain susceptibility results to other agents. Providing cost data to the clinicians may also reduce costs. Furthermore, in many institutions, the need to obtain approval for the use of certain antibiotics or for the use of certain antibiotics in higher-than-recommended doses may effectively control antibiotic use, but it requires the continuous availability of the approvers to discuss their guidelines. Approvers can be either pharmacists or infectious diseases physicians.

Some antibiotic courses have recommended durations that can be defined by predetermined stop-orders, which require active intervention by the clinician in order to override. This practice is particularly effective for perioperative prophylactic antibiotics, for which a strong clinical consensus can be developed in support of a limited course. Finally computer entry of orders allows more precise definition of duration and specific dose administration, which can often be adjusted for other parameters, such as weight and renal function. Such merging of computer databases will also allow identification of adverse events of a number of kinds, from adverse drug reactions to nosocomial infections (71).

Pharmacy oversight, required by the JCAHO mandate to review the appropriateness of use of medications provided, can sometimes be used to review patterns of use.

PHARMACY RECORDS AND REVIEW

In addition to case-by-case review of the use of antibiotics, pharmacy records and information systems can sometimes be helpful in several other activities relevant to infection control activities, depending heavily on the information system. System-wide analysis of antibiotic utilization, distribution, and cost can at least help to identify developing trends for which further information might be useful, though there are no generally acceptable benchmark levels of use for comparison. Such data can often be projected in conjunction with data on emerging patterns of resistance to support teaching efforts aimed at reducing the use of particular antibiotics (72).

Pharmacy records may occasionally be useful in other epidemic investigations as when an agent is thought (or shown) to be contaminated, and some inquiry is required as to the possible involvement or infection of other patients.

Pharmacy records can also provide one source for screening for nosocomial infection in a surveillance system (73) by identifying patients begun on antibiotics in the hospital, though established definitions are necessary to find possible cases for further screening. Identifying antibiotic use alone cannot be used as a predictive risk factor for subsequent infection, but an integrated system incorporating other data can be used (71,74).

CONCLUSION

Increasingly careful attention to the quality and sterility processing of pharmaceutical materials has made epidemics originating from either hospital pharmacies or manufactured products exceedingly rare in the United States, but out-sourcing of compounding has become an area of concern. Constant vigilance in quality assurance techniques by pharmacists and manufacturers and continuing awareness on the part of infection control professionals should maintain this favorable situation. Both disciplines can work cooperatively on the appropriate use of antimicrobials.

REFERENCES

1. American Society of Health-System Pharmacists. ASHP statement on the pharmacist's role in infection control. *Am J Health-Syst Pharm* 1998;55:1724–1726.
2. Pedersen CA, Schneider PJ, Scheckelhoff DJ. ASHP national survey of pharmacy practice in hospital settings: dispensing and administration—2002. *Am J Health-Syst Pharm* 2003;60:50–68.
3. Maki DG, Rhame FS, Mackel DC, et al. Nationwide epidemic of septicemia caused by contaminated intravenous products. 1. Epidemiologic and clinical features. *Am J Med* 1976;60:471–485.
4. West R. Personal communication.
5. Centers for Disease Control and Prevention. Exophiala infection from

contaminated injectable steroids prepared by a compounding pharmacy—United States, July–November 2002. *MMWR* 2002;51: 1109–1112.

6. Siboni K, Olsen H, Ravin E, et al. *Pseudomonas cepacia* in 16 nonfatal cases of postoperative bacteremia derived from intrinsic contamination of the anaesthetic fentanyl. *Scand J Infect Dis* 1979;11:39–45.
7. Borghans JGA, Hosli MC, Olsen H, et al. *Pseudomonas cepacia* bacteremia due to intrinsic contamination of an anaesthetic. *Acta Pathol Microbiol Scand [B]* 1979;87:15–20.
8. Panlilio AL, Beck-Sague CM, Siegel JD, et al. Infections and pseudoinfections due to povidone-iodine solution contaminated with *Pseudomonas cepacia. Clin Infect Dis* 1992;14:1078–1083.
9. Gardner S, Shulman ST. A nosocomial common source outbreak caused by *Pseudomonas pickettii. Pediatr Infect Dis* 1984;3:420–422.
10. Malizia WF, Gangardosa EJ, Goley AF. Medical intelligence. Benzalkonium chloride as a source of infection. *N Engl J Med* 1960;263: 800–802.
11. Dixon RE, Kaslow RA, Mackel DC, et al. Aqueous quaternary ammonium antiseptics and disinfectants. *JAMA* 1976;236:2415–2417.
12. George DL, McLeod R, Weinstein RA. Contaminated commercial charcoal as a source of fungi in the respiratory tract. *Infect Control Hosp Epidemiol* 1991;12:732–734.
13. Matsaniotis NS, Syriopoulou VP, Theodoridou MC, et al. *Enterobacter* sepsis in infants and children due to contaminated intravenous fluids. *Infect Control* 1984;5:471–477.
14. Martone WM, Osterman CA, Fisher KA, et al. *Pseudomonas cepacia:* implications and control of epidemic nosocomial colonization. *Rev Infect Dis* 1981;3:708–715.
15. Fernandez C, Wilhemi I, Andradas E, et al. Nosocomial outbreak of *Burkholderia pickettii* infection due to a manufactured intravenous product used in three hospitals. *Clin Infect Dis* 1996;22(6):1092–1095.
16. Garrett DO, McDonald LC, Wanderley A, et al. An outbreak of neonatal deaths in Brazil associated with contaminated intravenous fluids. *J Infect Dis* 2002;186:81–86.
17. Labarca JA, Trick WE, Peterson CL, et al. A multistate nosocomial outbreak of Ralstonia pickettii colonization associated with and intrinsically contaminated respiratory care solution. *Clin Infect Dis* 1999;29: 1281–1286.
18. Young D. Outsourced compounding can be problematic: community pharmacies linked to contaminated injectables (news). *Am Soc Health-Syst Pharm* 2002;59:2261–2264.
19. Sarubbi FA, Wilson MB, Lee M, et al. Nosocomial meningitis and bacteremia due to contaminated amphotericin B. *JAMA* 1978;239: 416–418.
20. Edwards KE, Allen JR, Miller MJ, et al. *Enterobacter aerogenes* primary bacteremia in pediatric patients. *Pediatrics* 1978;62:304–306.
21. Farrand RJ, Williams A. Evaluation of single-use packs of hospital disinfectants. *Lancet* 1973;1:591–593.
22. McGuckin MB, Thorpe RJ, Koch KM, et al. An outbreak of *Achromobacter xylosoxidans* related to diagnostic tracer procedures. *Am J Epidemiol* 1982;115:785–793.
23. Safranek TJ, Jarvis WR, Carson LA, et al. *Mycobacterium chelonae* wound infections after plastic surgery employing contaminated gentian violet skin-marking solution. *N Engl J Med* 1987;317:197–201.
24. Talbot GH, Miller DE, Doorley M, et al. *Enterobacter cloacae*–contaminated cardioplegia solution: discovery and eradication of a pharmacy reservoir. *Am J Infect Control* 1984;12:239–244.
25. Plouffe JF, Brown DG, Silva J Jr, et al. Nosocomial outbreak of *Candida parapsilosis* fungemia related to intravenous infusions. *Arch Intern Med* 1977;137:1686–1689.
26. Solomon SL, Khabbaz RF, Parker RH, et al. An outbreak of *Candida parapsilosis* bloodstream infections in patients receiving parenteral nutrition. *J Infect Dis* 1984;149:98–101.
27. American Society of Health-System Pharmacists. ASHP Guidelines on outsourcing pharmaceutical services. *Am J Health-Syst Pharm* 1998;55: 1611–1617.
28. Sanders CV, Luby JA, Johanson WG, et al. *Serratia marcescens* infections from inhalation therapy medications: nosocomial outbreak. *Ann Intern Med* 1970;73:15–21.
29. Van Laer F, Raes D, Vandamme P, et al. An outbreak of *Burkholderia cepacia* with septicemia on a cardiology ward. *Infect Control Hosp Epidemol* 1998;19(2):112–113.
30. Oren I, Hershow RC, Ben-Porath E, et al. A common-source outbreak of fulminant hepatitis B in a hospital. *Ann Intern Med* 1989;110: 691–698.
31. D Angelo LJ, Hierholzer JC, Holman RC, et al. Epidemic keratoconjunctivitis caused by adenovirus type 8: epidemiologic and laboratory aspects of a large outbreak. *Am J Epidemiol* 1981;113:44–49.
32. Grohskopf LA, Roth VR, Feikin DR, et al. Serratia liquefaciens bloodstream infections from contamination of epoetin alfa at a hemodialysis center. *N Engl J Med* 2001;344:1491–1497.
33. Nakashima AK, Highsmith AK, Martone WJ. Survival of *Serratia marcescens* in benzalkonium chloride and in multiple-dose medication vials: relationship to epidemic septic arthritis. *J Clin Microbiol* 1987;25: 1019–1021.
34. Plott RT, Wagner RF, Tyring SK. Iatrogenic contamination of multidose vials in simulated use. A reassessment of current patient injection technique. *Arch Dermatol* 1990;126:1441–1444.
35. de Silva MI, Hood E, Tisdel E, et al. Multidosage medication vials: a study of sterility, use patterns, and cost-effectiveness. *Infect Control* 1986;14:135–138.
36. Bawden JC, Jacobson JA, Jackson JC, et al. Sterility and use patterns of multiple dose vials. *Am J Hosp Pharm* 1982;39:294–297.
37. American Society of Health-System Pharmacists. ASHP guidelines on quality assurance for pharmacy-prepared sterile products. *Am J Health-Syst Pharm* 2000;57:1150–1169.
38. Maki DG, Klein BS, McCormick RD, et al. Nosocomial *Pseudomonas pickettii* bacteremia traced to narcotic tampering. A case for selective drug screening of health care personnel. *JAMA* 1991;265:981–986.
39. Hamill RJ, Houston ED, Georghiou PR, et al. An outbreak of *Burholderia* (formerly *Pseudomonas*) *cepacia* respiratory tract colonization and infection associated with nebulized albuterol therapy. *Ann Intern Med* 1995;122:762–766.
40. Bosic C, Davin-Regli A, Chanel R, et al. A *Serratia marcesean* nosocomial outbreak due to contamination of nexitidine solution. *J Hosp Infect* 1996;33:217–224.
41. Gaillot O, Maruejouls C, Abachin E, et al. Nosocomial outbreak of *Klebsiella pneumoniae* producing SHV-5 extended-spectrum beta-lactamase, originating from a contaminated ultrasonography coupling gel. *J Clin Microbiol* 1998;36(5):1357–1360.
42. Granowitz EV, Keenholtz SL. A pseudoepidemic of *Alcaligenes xylosoxidans* attributable to contaminated saline. *Am J Infect Control* 1998; 26(2):146–148.
43. Bennett SN, McNeil MM, Bland LA, et al. Postoperative infections traced to contamination of an intravenous anesthetic, propofol. *N Engl J Med* 1995;333(3):147–154.
44. Maki DG, Martin WT. Nationwide epidemic of septicemia caused by contaminated infusion products. IV. Growth of microbial pathogens in fluids for intravenous infusion. *J Infect Dis* 1975;131:267–272.
45. Goldmann DA, Martin WT, Worthington JW. Growth of bacteria and fungi in total parenteral nutrition solutions. *Am J Surg* 1973;126: 314–318.
46. Corbett JJ, Rosenstein BJ. *Pseudomonas meningitis* related to spinal anesthesia. Report of three cases with a common source of infection. *Neurology* 1971;21:946–950.
47. Mertz JJ, Scharer L, McClement JH. A hospital outbreak of *Klebsiella* pneumonia from inhalation therapy with contaminated aerosol solutions. *Am Rev Respir Dis* 1967;95:454–460.
48. Garcia CR, Johnston BL, Corvi G, et al. Intravenous catheter-associated *Malassezia furfur* fungemia. *Am J Med* 1987;83:790–792.
49. Gremillion DH, Mursch SB, Lerner CJ. Injection site abscesses caused by *Mycobacterium chelonei. Infect Control* 1983;4:25–28.
50. Birnbach DJ, Stern DJ, Murray O, et al. Povidone-iodine and skin disinfection before initiation of epidural anesthesia. *Anesthesiology* 1998;88:668–672.
51. Ole S, Kamiya A, Hironagak, et al. Microbial contamination of enteral feeding solution and its prevention. *Am J Infect Control* 1992;20: 202–205.
52. Thurn J, Crossley K, Gergts A, et al. Enteral hyperalimentation as a source of nosocomial infection. *J Hosp Infect* 1990;15:203–217.

53. Gravel D, Sample ML, Ramotr K, et al. outbreak of Burkholderia cepacia in the adult intensive care unit traced to contaminated indigo-carmine dye. *Infect Control Hosp Epidemiol* 2002;23:103–106.
54. Schleupner CJ, Hamilton JR. A pseudoepidemic of pulmonary fungal infections related to fiberoptic bronchoscopy. *Infect Control* 1980;1: 38–42.
55. Berkelman RL, Lewin S, Allen JR, et al. Pseudobacteremia attributed to contamination of povidone-iodine with *Pseudomonas cepacia. Ann Intern Med* 1980;95:32–36.
56. Crawford SY, Narducci WA, Augustine SC. National survey of quality assurance activities for pharmacy-prepared sterile products in hospitals. *Am J Hosp Pharm* 1991;48:2398–2413.
57. *The United States pharmacopeia,* 26th rev., and the national formulary, 21st ed. Rockville, MD: United States Pharmacopeial Convention, 2003.
58. Murray PR, Sandrock MJ. Sterility testing of a total nutrient admixture with a biphasic blood-culture system. *Am J Hosp Pharm* 1991;48: 2419–2421.
59. Levchuk JW, Nolly RJ, Lander N. Method for testing the sterility of total nutrient admixtures. *Am J Hosp Pharm* 1988;45:1311–1321.
60. American Society of Hospital Pharmacists ASHP technical assistance bulletin on pharmacy-prepared ophthalmic products. *Am J Hosp Pharm* 1993;50:1462–1463.
61. Santell J, Kamalich RF. National survey of quality assurance activities for pharmacy-prepared sterile products in hospitals and home infusion facilities—1995. *Am J Health-Syst Pharm,* 1996.53(21): 2591–2605.
62. Coleman RW, Rodondi LC, Kaubisch S, et al. Cost-effectiveness of prospective and continuous parenteral antibiotic control: experience at the Palo Alto Veterans Affairs Medical Center from 1987 to 1989. *Am J Med* 1991;90:439–444.
63. Hawkins VA, Powell MF. Justification for a pediatric satellite pharmacy at a tertiary-care institution. *Am J Hosp Pharm* 1992;49:2192–2197.
64. Garlbaldi RA, Burke J. Practice forum: surveillance and control of antibiotic use in the hospital. *Am J Infect Control* 1991;19:164–170.
65. Hess DA, Mahoney CD, Johnson, et al. Integration of clinical and administrative strategies to reduce expenditures for antimicrobial agents. *Am J Hosp Pharm* 1990;47:585–591.
66. Avorn J, Soumerai SB. Special article: improving drug-therapy decisions through educational outreach. A randomized controlled trial of academically based detailing. *N Engl J Med* 1983;308:1457–1463.
67. Manning PR, Lee PV, Clintworth WA, et al. Changing prescribing practices through individual continuing education. *JAMA* 1986;253: 230–231.
68. Snyder LL, Clyne KE, Wagner JC. Antibiotic sensitivity and the prescribing information sheet: assisting the prescribing physician. *Am J Infect Control* 1990;18:399–404.
69. Avorn J, Soumerai SB, Taylor W, et al. Reduction of incorrect antibiotic dosing through a structured educational order form. *Arch Intern Med* 1988;143:1720–1724.
70. Larsen RA, Evans RS, Burke JP, et al. Improved perioperative antibiotic use and reduced surgical wound infections through use of computer decision analysis. *Infect Control Hosp Epidemiol* 1989;10:316–320.
71. Bates, DW, Evans RS, Murff H, et al. Detecting adverse events using information technology. *J Am Med Inform Assoc* 2003;10:115–128.
72. Burke JP, Classen DC, Pestotnik SL, et al. The HELP system and its application to infection control. *J Hosp Infect* 1991;18:424–431.
73. Evans RS, Burke JP, Classen DC, et al. Computerized identification of patients at high risk for hospital-acquired infection. *Am J Infect Control* 1992;20:4–10.
74. Hirschhorn LR, Currier JS, Platt R. Electronic surveillance of antibiotic exposure and coded discharge diagnoses as indicators of postoperative infection and other quality assurance measures. *Infect Control Hosp Epidemiol* 1993;14:21–28.

76

VOLUNTEER SERVICES

KATHY B. MILLER

Volunteer workers have a long history of service in U.S. healthcare facilities. They provide important adjunct services to patients and families in practically every hospital in the United States, regardless of size. However, there are no reports of nosocomial infections associated with exposures to volunteers, and a review of the medical literature has produced no citations specifically dealing with the infection risks or preventive measures necessary to protect both patients and volunteers from communicable disease transmission.

In some facilities, no distinction is made between volunteers and employees. The Centers for Disease Control and Prevention refer to healthcare workers as all the paid and unpaid persons working in healthcare settings who have the potential for occupational exposure (1,2). Volunteers are often managed under the employee health program for routine testing and immunizations. In the current economic healthcare environment, a pragmatic approach to managing the infection risks is recommended. By identifying the types of volunteer services provided and conducting a risk assessment to evaluate the risk of disease transmission likely to occur from volunteer-patient contact, an effective cost-efficient infection control program can be established.

TYPES OF VOLUNTEER SERVICES

Volunteers provide a wide variety of services throughout hospitals and medical centers. They are usually identified with activities such as greeting and escorting patients and families, working in gift shops, running errands, filling water pitchers, and delivering mail and flowers. However, volunteers may also assist in outpatient clinics, laboratories, radiology departments, day care centers, long-term care facilities, and food service areas. The type of volunteer-patient contact and the categories of disease transmission likely to occur must be evaluated. Based on information reported by Diekema and Doebbeling (3), Table 76.1 lists modes of transmission for diseases that potentially can be transmitted between patients and volunteers and individuals at high risk of developing complications. The type of facility or area in which the volunteer will be working must also be assessed. In long-term care facilities, for example, measles and hepatitis B cause less concern and receive less consideration than tuberculosis and influenza (4).

Because the most common volunteer services involve only casual contact, such as providing patient information and assistance and escort and transport services, volunteers would appear to be at greatest risk of developing diseases transmitted by the airborne route, either by droplet nuclei or small-particle aerosols. These include infections resulting from varicella zoster virus (chickenpox), rubella, rubeola, *Mycobacterium tuberculosis,* and influenza. Individuals who work on pediatric, oncology, transplant, and infectious diseases units or services are especially at risk. Conversely, patients may be at risk for developing infections from exposure to volunteers with diseases transmitted by the airborne route. Volunteers who have direct patient contact, especially with the pediatric population, or contact with blood or body fluids, as in a laboratory setting, are also at risk of contracting diseases spread by the fecal-oral (i.e., *Salmonella, Shigella,* and rotavirus) and blood-borne [i.e., hepatitis B, human immunodeficiency virus (HIV)] routes.

Based on previous experience and data summarized and reported by Sherertz and Hampton (5) and Decker and Schaffner (6) on the risk of transmission between patients and hospital personnel, Table 76.2 lists diseases that may be transmitted between patients and volunteers. Efforts to minimize the risk of transmission should be directed toward the higher risk diseases.

RECOMMENDATIONS

Guidelines for the protection of both patients and volunteers from communicable diseases should be established by each facility. These guidelines should be administered by the facility's employee health program, if such a program exists, or the contract occupational health service.

Preplacement examinations should be offered to all new volunteers and should include at least the following (3,5):

A. Health history
   1. Past or current communicable diseases and medical conditions
      a. Chickenpox (varicella-zoster virus)
      b. Tuberculosis
      c. Hepatitis (viral)
      d. Any other infectious diseases as indicated by past exposure history (i.e., skin eruptions, bacterial or viral gastroenteritis)
      e. Any immunocompromising disorders or therapies (i.e., leukemia, lymphoma, systemic lupus erythema-

TABLE 76.1. COMMUNICABLE DISEASES, MODES OF TRANSMISSION, AND INDIVIDUALS AT HIGH RISK

Disease	Mode of Transmission	Individuals at High Risk
VZV	Droplet nuclei Direct contact with respiratory secretions and vesicular fluid	Pregnant women Seronegative immunocompromised hosts Neonates
Rubella	Respiratory droplets	Pregnant women
Tuberculosis	Droplet nuclei	—
Conjunctivitis (adenovirus)	Respiratory droplets Direct contact with contaminated inanimate reservoirs Fecal-oral (in children)	— —
Rubeola	Droplet nuclei	Pregnant women Immunocompromised hosts
Influenza	Respiratory droplets	>65 years of age; <14 years of age Immunocompromised hosts
Mumps	Respiratory droplets	Postpubertal men Pregnant women
Pertussis	Respiratory droplets	
RSV	Direct contact with infected secretions and fomites	Neonates, young children (<2 years of age)
Rotavirus	Fecal-oral	Neonates, young children (<5 years of age)
Group A streptococcus	Respiratory droplets	—
Hepatitis A	Fecal-oral Blood transfusion	Neonates, children
Hepatitis B	Direct contact with blood, body fluids (percutaneous, mucous membrane, or nonintact skin exposure)	Healthcare workers
Hepatitis C	Percutaneous exposure	Healthcare workers
HSV	Direct contact with open lesions, body fluids	Infants, immunocompromised hosts
Salmonella/*Shigella*	Fecal-oral	
CMV	Direct contact with body fluids, blood transfusion	Pregnant women Immunocompromised hosts
HIV	Direct contact with blood, body fluids (percutaneous, mucous membrane, or nonintact skin exposure)	—
Parvovirus B19	Respiratory droplets	Pregnant women
Pneumococcal pneumonia	Respiratory droplets	>65 years of age Immunocompromised hosts Underlying cardiac, liver, renal, or pulmonary disease
Haemophilus influenzae	Respiratory droplets	>65 years of age Immunocompromised hosts
Meningococcal meningitis	Respiratory droplets Direct contact with respiratory secretions or laboratory cultures	Underlying pulmonary disease or alcoholism —

CMV, cytomegalovirus; HIV, human immunodeficiency virus; HSV, herpes simplex virus; RSV, respiratory syncytial virus; VZV, varicella-zoster virus.

tosus, diabetes mellitus, rheumatoid arthritis, cytotoxic therapy, corticosteroid therapy, HIV infection)

2. Immunization status
   a. Rubella
   b. Rubeola
   c. Mumps
   d. Varicella
   e. Diphtheria
   f. Pertussis
   g. Tetanus
   h. Tuberculosis
   i. Hepatitis A and hepatitis B
   j. Pneumococcus (for volunteers >65 years of age or those with underlying immunocompromising conditions or cardiac, liver, renal, or pulmonary disease)
   k. *Haemophilus influenzae* (for volunteers >65 years of age or those with underlying immunocompromising conditions or pulmonary disease)

B. Skin testing with purified protein derivative (PPD) for tuberculosis including those with a history of Bacille Calmette-Guérin (BCG) vaccination. If the first skin test is negative, the skin test should be repeated at an interval of at least 7 days, and the results of the second test (negative or positive) recorded in the volunteer's health record (1). Two-step skin testing is used to detect persons infected with *M. tuberculosis* in the remote past whose skin test has become negative (see Chapter 37). Testing of PPD-negative volunteers should be repeated at regular intervals as determined by a risk assessment performed by the employee health or infection control services. Volunteer workers who have a documented history of a positive PPD or completion of therapy for active disease or prophylaxis should be excluded from testing unless they develop signs or symptoms suspicious for tuberculosis (1). HIV-infected volunteers should be informed of the potential for exposure to tuberculosis in the healthcare facility, especially when working with

TABLE 76.2. RISK OF INFECTION TRANSMISSION BETWEEN PATIENTS AND VOLUNTEERS

	Risk of Transmission	
Disease	Patient to Volunteer	Volunteer to Patient
Chickenpox/varicella	High	High
Rubella	High	High
Tuberculosis	High	High
Conjunctivitis (viral)	High	High
Rubeola	High	Low
Influenza	Intermediate	Intermediate
Mumps	Intermediate	Intermediate
Pertussis	Intermediate	Intermediate
RSV	Intermediate	Intermediate
Rotavirus	Intermediate	Intermediate
Group A streptococcus	Intermediate	Intermediate
Hepatitis A	Low	Low
Hepatitis B	Low	Low
Hepatitis C	Low	Low
HSV	Low	Low
Salmonella/Shigella	Low	Low
CMV	Low	Low
HIV	Low	Low
Parvovirus B19	Low	Low
Pneumococcus	Low	Low
Haemophilus influenzae	Low	Low
Neisseria meningitidis	Low	Low

CMV, cytomegalovirus; HSV, herpes simplex virus; HIV, human immunodeficiency virus; RSV, respiratory syncytial virus.

high-risk patient populations (i.e., acquired immunodeficiency syndrome, pulmonary disease) (7).

C. Laboratory tests, depending on the institution's immunization strategy
   1. Rubeola titers on volunteers born during or after 1957 who do not have documentation of appropriate vaccination (i.e., two doses of live measles virus vaccine) or physician-diagnosed measles (2)
   2. Rubella titers on volunteers born during or after 1957 who do not have documentation of appropriate vaccination (i.e., at least one dose of live rubella virus vaccine); rubella titers on all women who could become pregnant and who do not have documentation of prior rubella vaccination or laboratory evidence of past infection (2)
   3. Varicella titers on all volunteers without a definite history for chickenpox. Individuals with a reliable history of chickenpox can be considered to have immunity (8, 9).
   4. Routine serologic screening for hepatitis B is no longer recommended. Screening is not necessary for potential vaccine recipients, and vaccination is not hazardous to individuals who are chronic carriers or who are already immune (3).

D. Vaccinations
   1. Measles, mumps, and rubella—if during the preplacement examination it is determined that a volunteer does not have immunity to rubeola, rubella, or mumps by vaccination, laboratory evidence, or physician diagnosis, vaccination is recommended. This includes unvaccinated individuals born before 1957 who do not have a history of physician diagnosis or laboratory evidence of measles immunity or a positive serologic test indicating immunity to rubella. Rubella vaccination or laboratory evidence of immunity is especially important for female volunteers of childbearing age who could become pregnant. According to the Centers for Disease Control and Prevention, all medical or nonmedical, paid or volunteer personnel who work in healthcare facilities should be immune to rubeola and rubella. In addition, immunity to mumps is highly desirable. Serologic testing is not necessary before immunization unless it is considered to be cost-effective by the healthcare facility. The measles-mumps-rubella trivalent vaccine should be considered whenever any of its component vaccines is indicated. However, a monovalent or bivalent vaccine can be used if the recipient has documented evidence of immunity to one or two components (2). The healthcare facility may want to consider mandatory vaccination for volunteers who lack immunity and work in high-risk areas (i.e., pediatrics, obstetrics and gynecology).
   2. Varicella—unless contraindicated, varicella virus vaccine is recommended for all susceptible nonpregnant hospital personnel who lack a definite history or laboratory evidence of immunity (8,10).

      Female volunteers of childbearing age who will be working in high-risk areas must be informed of risks and procedures to follow on notification of pregnancy. Pregnant volunteers without documented immunity to measles, mumps, or rubella by immunization or serology should not be allowed to work with patients suspected of having or known to have these diseases. Pregnant volunteers with an uncertain or negative history for chickenpox who have not been vaccinated with the varicella virus vaccine should not be permitted to work with patients with suspected or known chickenpox or herpes zoster unless they have a positive serologic test indicating prior infection with the varicella-zoster virus. Pregnant volunteers who have received the varicella vaccine in the past should be tested for varicella antibody to ensure protective levels of antibody before they are exposed to patients with chickenpox or herpes zoster.
   3. Hepatitis B—hepatitis B vaccine should be made available to anyone who may be exposed to blood or body fluids, including volunteers working in clinical laboratories and handling specimens who are at risk of percutaneous, mucous membrane, or nonintact skin exposures (11,12). Recipients must be encouraged to complete the entire series of injections. Vaccine acceptance and completion rates are less than 50% for most healthcare worker groups (13).
   4. Influenza—influenza vaccine should be made available to employees before the beginning of the influenza season each year, usually between October and mid-November. Typically, influenza occurs on a seasonal basis between December and April. Vaccination of healthcare workers has been shown to be effective in reducing the impact of influenza in healthcare settings (14–16).

5. Hepatitis A—hepatitis A vaccine may be beneficial for volunteers who have exposure to fecal excretions or work in high-risk areas (i.e., pediatrics, food service departments) (3).
6. Pneumococcal and *H. influenzae* vaccines—volunteers who are older than 65 years or immunocompromised may benefit from these vaccines (3, 6).

Volunteer workers who are exposed to patients or personnel with communicable illnesses or who have significant exposure to blood or body fluids should be evaluated by the employee health or infection control services. Individuals requiring postexposure prophylaxis and/or testing should be evaluated, treated, and followed up according to established guidelines for occupational exposure. Depending on the disease and type of exposure, susceptible volunteers may need to be excluded from patient contact until they have passed through the incubation period for the specific disease (see Chapters 51 and 99). Volunteers with fever, cough, colored or bloody sputum, exudative skin lesions, rash, nausea, vomiting, diarrhea, conjunctivitis, night sweats, jaundice, fatigue, or unexplained weight loss should be evaluated by the employee health service or their private physician and excluded from work until the illness or skin infection has resolved.

CONCLUSIONS

Although there are no published guidelines for the protection of volunteer workers, it is the responsibility of every facility to protect patients, employees, and volunteers from communicable diseases acquired by contact with infected individuals. Volunteers should be included and addressed in each facility's preventive medicine policy.

Volunteers should be evaluated according to the type of services that they will be performing and the areas in which they will be working. A risk assessment should be performed to identify any exposure-prone activities. An education program should be provided to all volunteer workers to include proper hand washing, basic concepts of disease transmission, factors affecting their own immune status, potential for occupational exposure, use of standard precautions, benefits of vaccination programs, signs and symptoms of communicable diseases, and importance of reporting significant symptoms to the employee health or infection control services and remaining at home until illness has resolved (1, 4,17).

REFERENCES

1. Centers for Disease Control and Prevention. Guidelines for preventing the transmission of *Mycobacterium tuberculosis* in health care facilities. *MMWR Morb Mortal Wkly Rep* 1994;43:1–132.
2. Centers for Disease Control and Prevention. Measles, mumps, and rubella—vaccine use and strategies for elimination of measles, rubella, congenital rubella syndrome and control of mumps: recommendations of the advisory committee on immunization practices (ACIP). *MMWR Morb Mortal Wkly Rep* 1998;47:1–57.
3. Diekema DJ, Doebbeling BN. Employee health and infection control. *Infect Control Hosp Epidemiol* 1995;16:292–301.
4. Smith PW, Rusnak PG. Infection prevention and control in the long-term care facility. *Am J Infect Control* 1997;25:488–512.
5. Sherertz RJ, Hampton AL. Infection control aspects of hospital employee health. In: Wenzel RP, ed. *Prevention and control of nosocomial infections.* Baltimore: Williams & Wilkins, 1993.
6. Decker MD, Schaffner W. Nosocomial diseases of health care workers spread by the airborne or contact routes (other than tuberculosis). In: Mayhall CG, ed. *Hospital epidemiology and infection control.* Baltimore: Williams & Wilkins, 1996.
7. Centers for Disease Control and Prevention. USPHS/IDSA guidelines for the prevention of opportunistic infections in persons infected with human immunodeficiency virus: a summary. *MMWR Morb Mortal Wkly Rep* 1995;44:1–34.
8. Lyznicki JM, Bezman RJ, Genel M. Immunization of healthcare workers with varicella vaccine. *Infect Control Hosp Epidemiol* 1998;19: 348–353.
9. Weber DJ, Rutala WA, Hamilton H. Prevention and control of varicella-zoster infections in healthcare facilities. *Infect Control Hosp Epidemiol* 1996;17:694–705.
10. Centers for Disease Control and Prevention. Prevention of varicella: recommendations of the advisory committee on immunization practices (ACIP). *MMWR Morb Mortal Wkly Rep* 1996;45:1–36.
11. Centers for Disease Control and Prevention. Protection against viral hepatitis: recommendations of the advisory committee on immunization practices (ACIP). *MMWR Morb Mortal Wkly Rep* 1990;39:1–26.
12. Cardo DM, Bell DM. Bloodborne pathogen transmission in health care workers. *Infect Dis Clin North Am* 1997;11:331–346.
13. Corser WD. Occupational exposure of health care workers to bloodborne pathogens. *AAOHN J* 1998;46:246–252.
14. Centers for Disease Control and Prevention. Prevention and control of influenza: recommendations of the advisory committee on immunization practices (ACIP). *MMWR Morb Mortal Wkly Rep* 1998;47: 1–26.
15. Centers for Disease Control and Prevention. Guidelines for prevention of nosocomial pneumonia. *MMWR Morb Mortal Wkly Rep* 1997;46: 1–79.
16. Evans ME, Hall KL, Berry SE. Influenza control in acute care hospitals. *Am J Infect Control* 1997;25:357–362.
17. Adal KA, Flowers RH, Anglim AM, et al. Prevention of nosocomial influenza. *Infect Control Hosp Epidemiol* 1996;17:641–648.

77

ENVIRONMENTAL SERVICES

DONALD VESLEY
ANDREW J. STREIFEL

ENVIRONMENTAL RESERVOIRS AND THE EPIDEMIOLOGIC CHAIN

The relationship between the physical environment of healthcare facilities and infection control has long been debated. Continuing advances in medical technology and pharmacology have given physicians many options for preventing nosocomial infections unrelated to the physical environment. Restrictive and time-consuming barriers and procedures such as laminar-flow rooms with attendant aseptic technique have generally been in disfavor relative to the pharmacologic approach to preserving immune competence. At the same time, passive environmental controls such as filtration and pressurization systems to provide spore-free environments continue to be used in increasingly sophisticated ways. Legitimate questions remain as to the extent to which environmental reservoirs contribute to nosocomial infections. An argument can legitimately be made that cleanliness needs no further epidemiologic justification and that all hospitalized patients are entitled to a clean and odor-free environment. However, legitimate questions can also be raised as to allocation of resources to environmental controls that have no epidemiologic basis. An example is the extent to which chemical germicides should be used on environmental surfaces as opposed to nongermicidal cleaning methods that appear to yield equivalent microbiologic reductions (1).

One reason for continued disagreement over the importance of environmental reservoirs is failure to consider historical perspective and thus the starting point for measuring significance. People have rightly come to expect a high level of sanitation in medical facilities, a level that has already achieved a major reduction in infection incidence, and are now dealing with a very different set of infection determinants focusing largely on patient susceptibility factors. The writings of Florence Nightingale based on her experiences in the Crimean War in the 1850s reveal the striking contrasts of the two centuries (2). She devoted whole chapters to pure air, pure water, efficient drainage, cleanliness, and light, which she considered the cornerstones of good health and prevention of mortality. In her detailed journals, she documented survival data in the hospital where she cared for British soldiers of the Crimean War. She documented dramatic changes in mortality from February 1855 (420/1,000) to September 1855 (22/1,000), which she attributed to "nursing care and sanitary measures" (3). Her changes included such basics as scrub brushes, laundry tubs, and clean dressings for wounds, all replacing abominably filthy conditions associated with the pest houses of the time. Thus, the question that should be addressed today is not whether the environment is important—it obviously is—but how best to use available infection control practices most cost effectively to protect patients and healthcare workers from infectious hazards. In this chapter, we review a variety of environmental reservoirs relative to evidence linking these reservoirs to disease and distinguish between linkage to disease and evidence of lower contamination levels (which may or may not be worthwhile) regardless of disease linkage. In this chapter we emphasize two developments, which we consider most significant in this ongoing attempt to define the role of the physical environment in nosocomial infections. First, as antibiotic resistance problems mount and higher percentages of infections become more difficult to treat one has little choice but to fall back on environmental cleanliness as a cornerstone preventive component of infection control. The second development is the continuing refinement of DNA fingerprinting technology, which more and more enables identification of specific sources of infection and determination of relatedness of infection clusters. We cite a number of examples and predict that this technology will eventually shed further light on the importance of environmental controls.

LITERATURE REVIEW

Association of Reservoirs with Nosocomial Infections

Although the literature is replete with accounts of microbial contamination in a great variety of hospital settings, most of these articles describe contamination levels, not infection levels, and prescriptions for reducing these contamination levels do not necessarily translate into reduced incidence of nosocomial infection. Even when specific correlation to infection rates is suggested, the evidence is often tenuous, and direct association to an environmental source is difficult to prove. One area where investigators seem to be convinced that environmental sources contribute to infection is that of *Aspergillus* infections in severely immunocompromised patients. Humphries et al. (4) attributed two invasive *Aspergillus* infections in an intensive therapy unit to spores accumulating in fibrous insulation material above a perforated metal ceiling. Arnow et al. (5) similarly attributed an increase in *Aspergillus* incidence to growth of microorganisms on filters and claimed that improved environmental maintenance and filter removal were associated with a fourfold reduction in aspergillosis incidence over a 2-year period. Table 77.1 lists environmental sources of fungi in the hospital (5–18).

Air

The controversy over the role of airborne microbes as a source of surgical site infections has gone on for many decades. In theory, a surgical site exposing sterile tissue is susceptible to invading microorganisms from many sources. Certainly, rigid aseptic techniques and the need to sterilize any item entering a surgical site has long been accepted practice. Similarly, the need for filtration and high dilution rates of operating room air has also been accepted. However, proof of airborne infection of surgical sites has been hard to come by, and demonstrated effectiveness of specific controls as a means of reducing infection incidence has similarly been hard to prove. Walter et al. (19) claimed to have demonstrated a specific airborne surgical infection, and Hart (20) published the results of a 29-year study claiming significant benefit of ultraviolet installations for limiting surgical site infection. Other investigators, however, have failed to confirm these conclusions. In particular, Ayliffe and Beard (21) and Howe and Marston (22), while confirming that good filtration and dilution could reduce airborne contamination levels, could find no association of such reductions with infection prevention. In a general review of indoor microbial aerosols, Spendlove and Fannin (23) made the point that little is known about the true significance of these aerosols relative to human health and that continued research is needed. The sources of mold are many in the biologic world and the indoor environment can be controlled when emphasis is on filtration, air exchanges, and pressure management (24). It becomes imperative to control sources close to the patients at risk to opportunistic microbes such as *Aspergillus fumigatus.* (See also Chapter 89.)

TABLE 77.1. ENVIRONMENTAL FUNGAL SOURCES IN HOSPITALS

Source	Reference	Patient infection claim
Ventilation system	Fox (6)	Surgical wounds
Fireproofing material	Aisner (7)	Yes
Blankets	Noble (8)	No
Air conditioner	Lentino (9) Wadowsky (10)	Yes
Insulation	Arnow (5), Fox (6)	Yes
Construction projects	Krasinski (11)	Yes
Demolition	Streifel (12)	No
Track dirt (1976)	Arnow (13)	Yes
Road construction	Lentino (9)	Yes
Plants	Staib (14)	No
Pigeons	Kyriakides (15)	Yes
Food	Falken (16)	Colonization
Housekeeping	Rhame (17)	No
Moldy wood (1981)	Streifel (18)	No

Water Reservoirs

The literature is replete with reports of improperly disinfected medical devices that are implicated in nosocomial infections, particularly devices such as respiratory therapy equipment that are associated with water reservoirs of one kind or another (25) or devices that have hard-to-clean channels such as fiberoptic endoscopes (26). Similarly, a number of environmental water reservoirs have quite clearly been associated with infection involving aerosolization from these sources. Examples include faucet aerators associated with *Pseudomonas* infections (27) and shower heads associated with legionellosis (28,29) (see Chapter 35). Weber et al. (30) recently confirmed by pulsed-field gel electrophoresis that faucet aerators were contaminated with identical strains of *Stenotrophomonas maltophilia* found to colonize a cluster of patients in a surgical intensive care unit. They attributed the problem to low-level contamination of potable water subsequently amplified in the faucet aerators. Jonas et al. (31) compared three methods of DNA typing to compare environmental and patient isolates of *Legionella pneumophila.* Although all three methods detected one prominent genotype, amplified fragment length polymorphism (AFLP) had better interassay reproducibility and concordance than either macrorestriction analysis (MRA) or arbitrarily primed polymerase chain reaction (AP-PCR). MRA was also cited as an important tool for epidemiologic investigation of nosocomial infections by Luck et al. (32) who used that technique to match *Legionella* isolates from four patients with identical strains isolated from the hot water supply of the hospital. Legionellosis is a disease important in the lexicon of nosocomial infections for which an environmental reservoir has clearly been identified (warm water reservoirs in buildings) and for which specific preventive environmental protocols are recommended and generally accepted. Edelstein (33) reviewed some of these recommendations. They include hyperchlorination (6 to 20 mg/L) followed by long-term continuous chlorination at 1 to 2 mg/L or intermittent elevation of water temperature to 60°C to 70°C with or without chlorination. An additional example of aerosolization from a water reservoir was reported by Grieble et al. (34). They associated a rise in gram-negative septicemias with aerosolization from a waste hydropulping system that had been installed in a new Veterans Administration hospital. They also suggested that closing down the system halted the outbreak.

Hydrotherapy pools and tanks are another water reservoir wherein the combination of organic debris from infected patients and elevated water temperature clearly support growth of microorganisms; not surprisingly, several investigators have associated these tanks with infections. Examples include McGuckin et al. (35) reporting on an outbreak of *Pseudomonas aeruginosa* wound infection and Mayhall et al. (36) describing a bacteremia outbreak of *Enterobacter cloacae* (see Chapter 66). Rutala and Weber (37) reviewed the subject of water reservoirs of nosocomial pathogens. They listed more than a dozen such reservoirs identified in hospitals, including potable water, sinks, faucet aerators, showers, ice and ice machines, eyewash stations, dental-unit water systems, dialysis water, water baths, ice baths, tub immersion, toilets, and flower vases. All these sources have been specifically shown to harbor nosocomial pathogens, and regardless of the uncertain epidemiologic significance of such reservoirs, prudent control measures are available to limit microbial growth and such measures should be used. The authors also pointed out the growing importance of molecular epidemiology for typing pathogens in these reservoirs. DNA fingerprinting by pulsed-field gel electrophoresis is an example of a technique that can be used to match clinical and environmental strains. That technique was used by Buttery et al. (38) to link a *P. aeruginosa* outbreak to water-retaining bath toys in a toy box. Finally, Verweig et al. (39) used random arbitrary polymorphic DNA (RAPD) PCR analysis to link an infant death from *S. maltophilia* infection to contaminated tap water. They concluded that preterm infants should not be washed using tap water. Water has been implicated as a potential reservoir for filamentous fungi (40,41), and it is logical that spores could become entrapped in water and distributed to susceptible patients. This contamination was not associated with growth in water but at the interface of water and air (42). Although eliminating all of these microbes seems easy to do with high-efficiency particulate air (HEPA) quality filters, it would seem more efficient to provide sterile water for drinking. The potential sources in municipal water include soil, expansion tanks, evaporative pans, or potential biofilm within the water distribution system.

Infant Formula

As early as 1990, Clark et al. (43) used plasmid analysis, chromosomal restriction endonuclease analysis, ribotyping, and multilocus enzyme electrophoresis to match isolates of *Enterobacter sakazakii* from patients with isolates from infant formula, strongly implicating the formula as the source of those infections.

Environmental Surfaces

Environmental surfaces have long been something of an enigma for healthcare facilities. Although no one disputes the desirability of keeping these facilities clean or that esthetic considerations alone justify the cost of routine housekeeping, it is more difficult to justify the routine use of costly disinfectants on hospital floors and furnishings. No one has seriously proposed that such products in themselves can prevent nosocomial infections. It was demonstrated in the 1960s by Vesley and Michaelsen (44) and by Finegold et al. (45) that detergents (or even hot tap water) without chemical disinfectants can achieve microbial reduction equivalent to that of disinfectants. It has also been demonstrated by Vesley et al. (1) that dry cleaning with a chemically treated mop before wet cleaning accounts for most of the microbial load reduction on floor surfaces in hospitals. Dharan et al. (46) compared germicidal treatments to detergent only cleaning of floors and furniture in a 4-month trial in Switzerland. They concluded that microbial levels could be reduced but failed to observe any change in nosocomial infection rates in more than 1,000 patients. Maki et al. (47) performed an elaborate study of microbes on floors, walls, and other surfaces of an old hospital; then, before occupancy, they performed the same study in a new hospital that was replacing it. They reported no change in infection rates in the new hospital despite an absence of the surface pathogens immediately on occupancy. The old surface contamination patterns were reestablished in 6 to 12 months, leading the authors to conclude that the environment was contaminated by the patients rather than the other way around. Similarly, Danforth et al. (48) compared infection rates over a 3-month period on eight acute care nursing units that had been cleaned with either a disinfectant or a detergent. The rates were not significantly different (8.0 per 100 discharges in the units cleaned with disinfectant vs. 7.1 per 100 discharges in the units cleaned with a detergent).

The emergence of vancomycin-resistant enterococci (VRE) as a major nosocomial pathogen in the 1990s has rekindled some of the arguments about the importance of environmental surfaces. Weber and Rutala (49) reviewed this subject and hypothesize that "there is sufficient evidence to state that inanimate surfaces likely play a role in the transmission of VRE." They support this view by citing the survival of VRE on environmental surfaces for hours and claim that such contaminants can colonize hands. They also call into question the adequacy of current terminal cleaning practices for eliminating VRE from environmental surfaces. The seriousness of the VRE problem and recent confirmation of the first vancomycin-resistant *Staphylococcus aureus* certainly warrants close surveillance of the role of the environment. However, it remains difficult to determine whether such environmental surfaces play a role in initiating infection or, as others have claimed, merely reflect the presence of a source patient contaminating his or her surroundings.

A relationship was established by Alberti et al. (50) between the environmental contamination of a hematology-oncology ward and the incidence of invasive nosocomial aspergillosis. The conclusions of such evaluations indicate the importance of environmental control of contamination. In other words the hospital environment should be kept clean for the sake of infection control.

Soiled Linen

Soiled linen is another source of contaminants that has drawn some attention in hospitals. Again, the need for clean bedding is not at issue. Clearly, every patient is entitled to freshly laundered bedding as a matter of routine practice. However, the manipulation of soiled bedding is recognized as a major contributor to airborne contamination, and the question becomes "Does aerosolization contribute to nosocomial infection?" For example, Michaelsen and Vesley (51) reported a significant increase in air contamination even on the upper stories of a hospital when soiled linen was pulled from a basement chute closet, but the importance of such an observation relative to infection transmission has not been established. Colbeck (52) claimed a reduced incidence of skin boils after disinfection of blankets, but the evidence was purely circumstantial.

Construction Projects

One correlation of an environmental source relative to patient colonization that has been documented fairly consistently is that of building construction projects and fungal infection. Arnow et al. (13), Sarubbi et al. (53), and Krasinski et al. (11) have all demonstrated recovery of *Aspergillus* from patients, which they traced to specific construction activities. Streifel et al. (12) reported that careful control measures during a building demolition project successfully prevented patient fungal colonization despite an enormous increase in fungal air contamination resulting from demolition. In a related finding, Streifel et al. (18) associated airborne *Penicillium* spores with leaking pipes in a rotting wood cabinet in a medication room (Fig. 77.1). Thus, special precautions to contain contaminants during ongoing remodeling and new construction projects would appear to be one environmental control situation that is justifiable for infection prevention reasons. Carter and Barr (54) reviewed construction-related nosocomial infection outbreaks, citing particularly *Aspergillus* and *Legionella* as often construction related. They make specific recommendations for environmental control during construction including barriers, signs, traffic control, and ventilation suggestions.

Little information is available for specific management of barriers for respective construction projects. Choosing an appropriate barrier for type of job is dependent on length of project or type of disruption. Barriers can be either long-term or short-term. Consideration for the length of a project in a critical space is important for project management. Risk factors that take into account the nature of the healthcare area being remodeled and what is being disrupted should be included in decision making. Streifel (24) provided an example of barrier differences in microbial counts when a bathroom was dismantled using a substantial barrier and portable HEPA filtration. Also, Rautiala et al. (55) provided comparison methods for three types of barriers in controlling microbes during renovation. The study showed that the methods used were effective at preventing movement of microbes to adjacent spaces but did not minimize the exposure to workers in the construction zone. Such efforts demonstrate the effectiveness of barriers when they have negative pressure or airflow from clean areas to dirty areas. The levels of pressurization to achieve such control have not been recommended. Levels at or greater than 2.5 pascal (Pa) would be acceptable for protected environments. Alevantis et al. (56) found that a pressure differential of 8 Pa prevented the migration of environmental tobacco smoke. Smoke serves as a good surrogate, so that the barriers where critical control is necessary should be designated as smoke barriers, which is common in healthcare construction because of interim life safety code requirements (57).

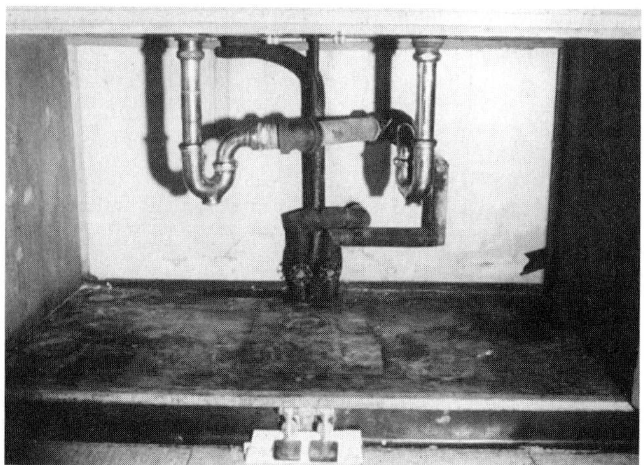

Figure 77.1. Mold accumulation in wooden cabinet under hand wash sink.

Control of internal sources of mold during maintenance and renovation are a challenge, but external construction control is contingent on protecting the external shell of the building from penetration by excavation aerosols. This can be complicated if the building requiring protection is a high rise. The lower portion of a high rise building has a natural tendency to pull air into the building to satisfy heat rising through the structure. Occupants using close proximity areas for smoking or normal pedestrian traffic may create an opening in the building to enhance the movement of excavation aerosol into the protected clinical structure. Control of entrances to a critical building is essential to protect the building from external projects.

Regardless of the project, a risk assessment is necessary to recognize the status of the clinical areas affected and the type of project impact on those areas. For example, if the windows are to be replaced on a hospital building, efforts to ensure pressure control on the internal connections are critical, and an airlock (ante) egress room may be necessary to ensure air pressure control. Likewise, if work is scheduled on a roof, efforts to protect that roof surface from puncture is critical for water damage control. Water damage control is essential for ensuring minimal mold growth inside of a building. If water damage occurs because of leaks, broken piping, or heavy rainfall, mold growth on modern building material such as gypsum board will occur if drying does not occur within 72 hours. Unprotected elevator shafts have resulted in multistory mold contamination occurring in a university hospital that required removal of the elevator shaft fire-rated gypsum board. A specification in the construction documents stated that the gypsum board was to be installed and protected from weather conditions required that the moldy board be removed at the contractor's expense. This is still cheaper than the litigation potential if the moldy board was left in place while the hospital initiated a program for bone marrow transplantation and a patient developed a mold infection. Under such circumstances, the knowledge that the elevator shafts were moldy and not removed would be suspected as the source of infection and subjected to major problems. Contract specifications for a construction project should be provided in the bid documents to ensure basic consideration for clean to dirty airflow, construction traffic, roof protection, water damage management, and assurance that the spaces to be occupied by immune-compromised patients such as bone marrow transplant units have definable protective parameters such as pressure differential, air changes per hour, and filtration (58). The "Guidelines for Environmental Infection Control" (*MMWR Morb Mortal Wkly Rep*June 6, 2003) will certainly add to the coordination of construction management in healthcare facilities as part of the justification involved with the infection control risk assessment. (See also Chapter 88.)

Food Sources

Another potential environmental source for introduction of opportunistic microorganisms into hospitals is on raw food products. Shooter et al. (59) isolated *P. aeruginosa* from salads and other cold foods in London area hospitals and then showed that some patients apparently acquired similar strains. Kominos et al. (60) reported on the introduction of *P. aeruginosa* into a hospital via raw vegetables such as carrots, celery, and tomatoes but presented no evidence of direct association with nosocomial infection. Sanborn (61), on the other hand, claimed that an outbreak caused by *Salmonella chester* was traced to contamination of a cutting board by a raw turkey, and Levine et al. (62) similarly implied that equipment contaminated by egg products was at least partially to blame for numerous cases of salmonellosis reported from nursing homes. Thus, careful attention to the basics of food sanitation can certainly be justified as an infection control practice.

Plants and Flowers

Cut flowers, and particularly the vase water in which they are displayed, have been well established as a source of opportunistic pathogens. Taplin and Merz (63) detected gentamicin-resistant gram-negative rods in 23 of 75 vases tested in a burn unit and associated the removal of these flowers with a decrease in wound colonization. Schoroth and Cho (64) and Rosenzweig (65) also detected gram-negative microorganisms on flowers or in flower water but did not implicate these microorganisms in patient infection. Potted plants have been reported by Staib et al. (14), Burge et al. (66), and Smith et al. (67) as potential sources of aerosolized fungal spores, but none of these authors presented evidence of epidemiologic significance for their findings.

Solid Waste

In recent years, most of the attention related to hospital solid wastes has focused on infectious waste issues, particularly on treatment and disposal of these wastes after they leave the hospital (see Chapter 100). A 1997 report indicated that three active cases of tuberculosis and 13 additional conversions resulted from clogged filters in a shredder at a commercial infectious waste treatment facility in Washington (68). The lesson is that decontamination must precede shredding to prevent such incidents from occurring. The effect of such wastes within the hospital has received very little attention in recent years, undoubtedly because of the lack of evidence linking such wastes to nosocomial infections. An elaborate survey of hospital waste handling and its contribution to microbial contamination of air and surfaces was described by Bond and Michaelsen (69). They concluded that contamination emanating from solid wastes was relatively insignificant and was greatly overshadowed by contamination levels resulting from the handling of soiled laundry. The quantitative and qualitative aspects of that study were detailed by Greene et al. (70,71).

DISCUSSION AND RECOMMENDATIONS

The role of the environment in nosocomial infections has been studied and debated for many years. Looking objectively at the evidence, it seems that much of the confusion relates to semantics rather than to scientific differences of opinion. Identification of reservoirs, issues of survival and infectivity of microorganisms, the relative importance of immune suppression, the role of autogenous versus exogenous sources, and the identification of transmission paths and portals of entry are now well understood. The previous sections have identified specific reports wherein environmental reservoirs have been cited (with varying degrees of evidence) as the source of cases or outbreaks of nosocomial illness, of colonization without illness, or, even more frequently, simply as reservoirs or hiding places for opportunistic microorganisms without epidemiologic association of any kind. Depending on the definition of environment and particularly of the interface between people, instruments, and equipment and the traditional air, water, or surfaces (floors, walls, and furniture), all of which can conceivably be lumped together as environment, one can conclude a greater or lesser role for environmental transmission. For example, everyone agrees on the importance of hand washing in preventing nosocomial infection, but is hand washing an environmental issue (involving products and methods) or is it simply a personal practice issue?

In a 1981 review, McGowan (72) suggested that the interest in the role of environmental factors in nosocomial infections is that they appear more amenable to control than do other facets of the problem. He argued against the routine monitoring of such environments as being of limited value, a position now shared by almost all practitioners in this field, and argued for selective monitoring only for clearly defined objectives, such as to support epidemiologic investigations or to monitor sterilization processes. Rhame (17) reviewed the role of the inanimate environment in nosocomial infections and differentiated types of evidence related to environmental involvement. He made the point that many reports merely indicate that a particular microorganism was cultured from a particular fomite with or without proliferation, the implication being that the environment becomes contaminated from infected or colonized patients not the other way around. He correctly downplayed these reports relative to the fewer case-control or prospective epidemiologic studies.

Thus, it is not possible to generalize meaningfully about environmental transmission. Instead, specific items and areas of the institutional environment must be considered separate entities, and environmental manipulation must be consistent with efficient operation and productive infection control practice. For example, there is sufficient evidence for the potential of hot water reservoirs to harbor *Legionella* microorganisms and to transmit those microorganisms to patients to warrant environmental intervention to prevent that problem. Conversely, there is insufficient evidence linking floor contamination to disease transmission to justify the use of expensive disinfectants for routine cleaning. Instead, esthetic cleanliness based on effective soil removal and odor control is clearly justifiable as the expectation of all patients.

Recommendations for Environmental Control

One is left with having to design, construct, and maintain a complex physical environment for the care of increasingly susceptible hospital patients. Although one may quibble over the epidemiologic significance of this environment, we believe that current knowledge should enable clinicians to proceed with this task in a sensible, science-based, and cost-effective manner, confident that they are enhancing infection control practice and doing their duty for the patients that they are charged with protecting. In the following section, we propose some of these approaches without apology. "Guidelines for Environmental Infection Control" (*MMWR Morb Mortal Wkly Rep* June 6, 2003) is followed as part of the environment of care especially as it relates to Joint Commission on Accreditation of Healthcare Organizations (JCAHO) accreditation and funding stipulations promulgated by Medicare funding. Such "carrot sticks" will certainly help to define the cost-effective measures necessary to maintain a healthcare facility as a safe environment of care.

General Considerations

A modern healthcare facility should be designed for efficient traffic flow, with particular attention to separation of dirty and clean areas. Among the clean areas, operating rooms and bone marrow transplantation facilities should be considered at the cleanest end of the spectrum. Unnecessary traffic should be effectively excluded from any critical care area. Air handling systems should be designed flexibly to allow higher volume air circulation in critical areas. Higher air volumes are needed to accommodate varying temperature and humidity conditions but should never be allowed to compromise contamination control airflow patterns. Air should move generally from cleaner to dirtier locations. Air intakes should be well separated from dirty air discharges and located away from loading docks subject to diesel fumes (see Chapter 89).

Maintenance of Ventilation Systems

Duct and fan systems should be subject to routine maintenance and cleaning practices, including regular filter changes. It is important to remove dust and lint accumulations periodically. However, protocols should be developed to ensure that such maintenance does not release accumulated buildup of lint or other debris that could aerosolize opportunistic fungal spores. Fig. 77.2 presents an example of heavy lint buildup on a bathroom exhaust grill. Particular attention must also be paid to avoiding high moisture conditions with resultant mold growth in ducts or on insulating materials (Fig. 77.3).

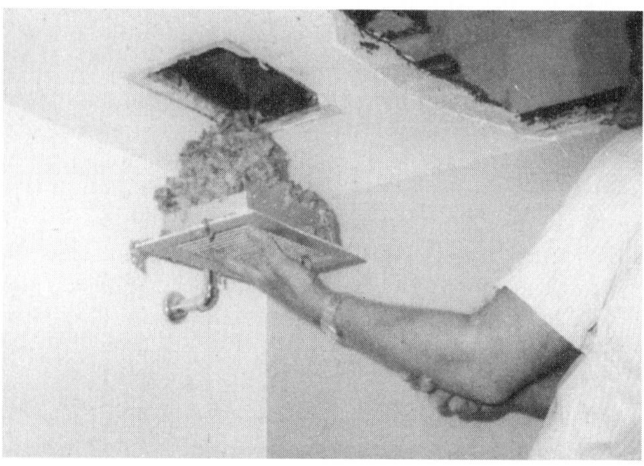

Figure 77.2. Bathroom exhaust debris.

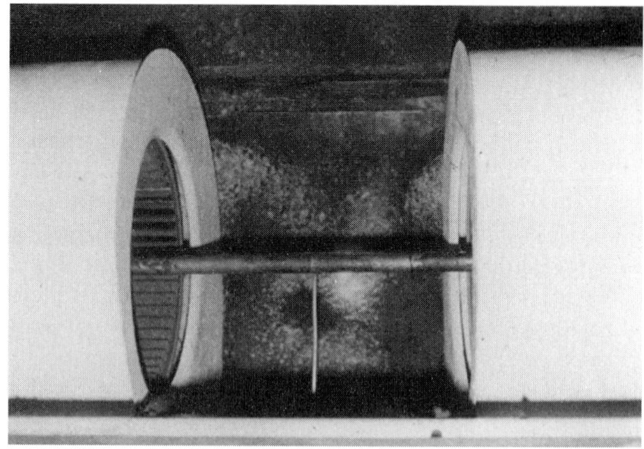

Figure 77.3. Fan coil with mold on wet insulation.

Control During Construction Projects

The large number of ongoing renovation projects in healthcare facilities requires particular attention to detail to avoid outbursts of airborne fungi or bacteria. Written procedures should be in place to ensure consistency of these efforts, particularly as they pertain to the most critical areas of the facility. Erection of physical barriers to isolate renovation projects may often be necessary. Ventilation systems may need to be shut down temporarily or airflow may need to be rerouted to protect sensitive areas. Control over elevators to facilitate removal of debris or supply of building materials, without mingling with patients and staff members, may be necessary. Finally, traffic flow patterns for construction personnel vis-à-vis patients and healthcare workers should be defined and monitored. Table 77.2 lists some of the considerations for external project planning. Water damage management, external and internal, can poten-

TABLE 77.2. EXTERNAL CONSTRUCTION PLANNING

Pest management
Building seal
Windows and doors
Employee access
Ventilation assurance for protected hospital areas
Filtration integrity
Appropriate airflow
Air changes per hour
Pressurization
Water damage plan
Roof protection
Water damage-resistant gypsum board
Emergent response for water damage
Outage planning
Ventilation
Plumbing
Electricity

tially be an important factor for preventing mold colonization of a building. Prolonged wetting of modern building materials such as gypsum board and ceiling tiles can establish significant mold reservoirs in a building that could be problematic later. Bid specification should address such incidents with a plan for delegating responsibility for drying or removal of the materials before mold contaminates the internal clinical areas of a healthcare facility.

General Housekeeping

Housekeeping protocols should take into account the need for continuous surveillance over potential buildup of moisture conditions and subsequent fungal proliferation. Dust suppression practices should be emphasized, and cleaning of vents and air conditioners should be routine. Any use of vacuum cleaners should incorporate exhaust filters. Specific spill cleanup procedures should be in place with clear designation of responsibility for such cleanups. Attention should also be paid to ongoing availability of all supplies needed for emergency spill cleanup. Types of chemical disinfectants should be carefully chosen and should follow Centers for Disease Control and Prevention guidelines. Frequently, nongermicidal cleaning products are sufficient at lower cost than sanitizers or disinfectants and have the added benefit of a lower probability of causing chemical sensitivity problems (see Chapter 85).

Maintenance of Water Reservoirs

Specific measures for ensuring the absence of water contaminants such as *Legionella* have been discussed. Control of temperature, periodic superheating, maintenance of chlorine residuals, routine cleaning of storage tanks and other reservoirs, and avoidance of dead-ends or other promoters of stagnation are all important features of preventive maintenance of water reservoirs (see Chapter 35). In special systems, such as renal dialysis units, ultraviolet light and/or bacterial filters may be appropriate to ensure consistent control (see Chapter 64).

CONCLUSIONS

Since this chapter was first drafted about 5 years ago, hundreds of additional articles have been published detailing contamination problems in healthcare facilities. In this revision, we have attempted to update the original chapter to reflect any significant new information. The looming threat of antibiotic resistance overcoming pharmacologic innovation clouds the future but brings us again to emphasize basics of microbial contamination control. Although medical practice, facilities, and equipment for patient care have become more sophisticated and automated, the basic premise of the original chapter has not changed: controlling and minimizing levels of conventional and opportunistic microbial pathogens in healthcare environments is an integral and important aspect of nosocomial infection control.

REFERENCES

1. Vesley D, Klapes NA, Benzoe K, et al. Microbiological evaluation of wet and dry floor sanitization systems in hospital patient rooms. *Appl Environ Microbiol* 1987;53:1042–1045.
2. Nightingale F. *Notes on nursing: what it is and is not,* 2nd ed. New York: Harrison and Sons, 1860.
3. Clemons B. Florence Nightingale. *Score* 1981;6:23–27.
4. Humphries H, Johnson EM, Warnock DW, et al. An outbreak of aspergillosis in a general ITU. *J Hosp Infect* 1991;18:167–177.
5. Arnow PM, Sadigh M, Costas C, et al. Endemic and epidemic aspergillosis associated with in-hospital replication of *Aspergillus* organisms. *J Infect Dis* 1991;1964:998–1002.
6. Fox BC, Chamberlin L, Kulich P, et al. Heavy contamination of operating room air by *Penicillium* species: identification of the source and attempts at decontamination. *Am J Infect Control* 1990;18:300–306.
7. Aisner J, Schimpff SC, Bennett JE, et al. *Aspergillus* infections in cancer patients: association with fireproofing materials in a new hospital. *JAMA* 1976;235:411–412.
8. Noble WC, Clayton YM. Fungi in the air of hospital wards. *J Gen Microbiol* 1963;32:397–402.
9. Lentino JR, Rosenkranz MA, Michaels JA, et al. Nosocomial aspergillosis: a retrospective review of airborne disease secondary to road construction and contaminated air conditioners. *Am J Epidemiol* 1982; 116:430–437.
10. Wadowsky RM, Benner SM. Distribution of the genus *Aspergillus* in hospital room air conditioners. *Infect Control* 1987;8:516–518.
11. Krasinski K, Holzman RS, Hanna B, et al. Nosocomial fungal infection during hospital renovation. *Infect Control* 1985;6:278–282.
12. Streifel AJ, Lauer JL, Vesley D, et al. *Aspergillus fumigatus* and other thermotolerant fungi generated by hospital building demolition. *Appl Microbiol* 1983;46:375–378.
13. Arnow PM, Anderson RL, Mainous PD, et al. Pulmonary aspergillosis during building renovation. *Am Rev Respir Dis* 1978;118:49–53.
14. Staib F, Tompak B, Thiel D, et al. *Aspergillus fumigatus* and *Aspergillus niger* in two potted ornamental plants, cactus *(Peiphyllum truncatum)* and clivia *(Clivia miniata)*. Biological and epidemiological aspects. *Mycopathologia* 1978;66:27–30.
15. Kyriakides GK, Zinneman HH, Hall WH, et al. Immunologic monitoring and aspergillosis in renal transplant patients. *Am J Surg* 1976; 13:246–252.
16. Falken MC, Streifel AJ, Marx SS, et al. Food does not appear to be a source of fungal disease in marrow transplant recipients (abstract). American Society for Microbiology 86th annual meeting, Washington DC, March 1986.
17. Rhame FS. The inanimate environment. In: Bennet JV, Brachman PS, eds. *Hospital infections,* 3rd ed. Boston: Little, Brown and Company, 1992.
18. Streifel AJ, Stevens PP, Rhame RS. In-hospital source of airborne penicillium species spores. *J Clin Microbiol* 1987;25:1–4.
19. Walter CW, Kundsin RB, Brubaker MM. The incidence of airborne wound infection during operation. *JAMA* 1963;186:122–127.
20. Hart D. Bacterial ultraviolet radiation in the operating room. Twenty-nine year study for the control of infections. *JAMA* 1960;172: 1019–1028.
21. Ayliffe GAJ, Beard MA. A system of air recirculation and antibacterial surface treatment in a surgical ward. *J Clin Pathol* 1962;15:242–246.
22. Howe CW, Marston AT. A study on sources of post-operative staph infection. *Surg Gynecol Obstet* 1962;115:266–275.
23. Spendlove CJ, Fannin KF. Source, significance, and control of indoor microbial aerosols: human health aspects. *Public Health Rep* 1983;98: 227–244.
24. Streifel AJ. Aspergillosis and construction. In: Kundsin RB, ed. *Architectural design and indoor microbial pollution.* New York: Oxford University Press, 1988.
25. Reinarz JA, Pierce AK, Mays BB, et al. The potential role of inhalation therapy equipment in nosocomial pulmonary infection. *J Clin Invest* 1965;44:831–839.
26. Earnshaw JJ, Clark AW, Thom BT. Outbreak of *Pseudomonas aerugi-*

nosa following endoscope retrograde cholangiopancreatography. *J Hosp Infect* 1985;6:95–97.
27. Wilson MG, Nelson RC, Phillips LH, et al. New source of *Pseudomonas aeruginosa* in a nursery. *JAMA* 1961;1756:1146–1148.
28. Bollin GE, Plouffe JF, Para MF, et al. Aerosols containing *Legionella pneumophila* generated by shower heads and hot-water faucets. *Appl Environ Microbiol* 1985;50:1128–1131.
29. Dennis PJ, Wright AE, Rutter DA, et al. *Legionella pneumophila* in aerosols from shower baths. *J Hyg* 1984;93:349–353.
30. Weber, DJ, Rutala WA, Blanchett CN, et al. Faucet aerators: a source of patient colonization with *Stenotropomonas maltophilia. Am J Infect Control* 1999;27:59–63.
31. Jonas D, Meyer HG, Matthes P, et al. Comparative evaluation of three different genotyping methods for investigation of nosocomial outbreaks of Legionnaires' disease in hospitals. *J Clin Microbiol* 2000;38: 2284–2291.
32. Luck PC, Kohler J, Maiwald M, et al. DNA polymorphisms in strains of *Legionella pneumophila* serogroups 3 and 4 detected by macrorestriction analysis and their use for epidemiological investigation of nosocomial legionellosis. *Appl Environ Microbiol* 1995;61:2000–2003.
33. Edelstein PH. Environmental aspects of *Legionella. ASM News* 1985; 51:460–467.
34. Grieble HG, Bird TJ, Nidea HM, et al. Chute hydropulping waste disposal system: a reservoir of enteric bacilli and *Pseudomonas* in a modern hospital. *J Infect Dis* 1974;130:602–607.
35. McGuckin MB, Thorpe RJ, Arbrutyn E. An outbreak of *Pseudomonas aeruginosa* wound infections related to Hubbard tank treatments. *Arch Phys Med Rehab* 1981;62:283–287.
36. Mayhall CG, Lamb VA, Gayle WE Jr, et al. *Enterobacter cloacae* septicemia in a burn center: epidemiology and control of an outbreak. *J Infect Dis* 1979;139:166–171.
37. Rutala WA, Weber DJ. Water as a reservoir of environmental pathogens. *Infect Control Hosp Epidemiol* 1997;18:609–616.
38. Buttery JP, Alabaster SJ, Heine RG, et al. Multiresistant *Pseudomonas aeruginosa* outbreak in a pediatric oncology ward related to bath toys. *Pediatr Infect Dis J* 1998;17:509–513.
39. Verwieg, PE, Meis JF, Christmann V, et al. Nosocomial outbreak of colonization and infection with *Stenotrophomonas maltophilia* in preterm infants associated with contaminated tapwater. *Epidemiol Infect* 1998;120:251–256.
40. Warris A, Gaustad J, Eis GF, et al. Recovery of filamentous fungi from water in a paediatric bone marrow transplantation unit. *J Hosp Infect* 2001;47:143–148.
41. Anaissie E, Kuchar R, Rex J, et al. Fusariosis associated with pathogenic *Fusarium* species colonization of a hospital water system: a new paradigm for epidemiology of opportunistic mold infections. *Clin Infect Dis* 2001;33:1871–8.
42. Fridkin S, Kremer F, Bland L, et al. *Acremonium kiliense* endophthalmitis that occurred after cataract extraction in an ambulatory surgical center and was traced to an environmental reservoir. *Clin Infect Dis* 1996;22:222–227.
43. Clark NC, Hill HC, O'Hara CM, et al. Epidemiologic typing of *Enterobacter sakazakii* in two neonatal nosocomial outbreaks. *Diagn Microbiol Infect Dis* 1990;13:467–472.
44. Vesley D, Michaelsen GS. Application of a surface sampling technic to the evaluation of bacteriological effectiveness of certain hospital housekeeping procedures. *Health Lab Sci* 1964;1:107–113.
45. Finegold SM, Sweeney EE, Gaylor DW, et al. Hospital floor decontamination: controlled blind studies in evaluation of germicides. *Antimicrob Agents Chemother* 1963:250–258
46. Dharan S, Mououga P, Copin P, et al. Routine disinfection of patients' environmental surfaces. Myth or reality? *J Hosp Infect* 1999;42: 113–117.
47. Maki DG, Alvarado CJ, Hassemer CA, et al. Relation of the inanimate hospital environment to endemic nosocomial infections. *N Engl J Med* 1982;307:1562–1566.
48. Danfoth D, Nicolle LE, Hume K, et al. Nosocomial infections on nursing units with floors cleaned with a disinfectant compared with detergent. *J Hosp Infect* 1987;10:229–235.
49. Weber DJ, Rutala WA. Role of environmental contamination in the transmission of vancomycin-resistant enterococci. *Infect Control Hosp Epidemiol* 1997;18:306–309.
50. Alberti C, Bouakline A, Ribaud P, et al. Relationship between environmental fungal contamination and the incidence of invasive aspergillosis in haematology patients. *J Hosp Infect* 2001;48:198–206.
51. Michaelsen GS, Vesley D. Dissemination of airborne microorganisms in an institutional environment. In: *Proceedings of a Symposium on Surface Contamination, Oak Ridge, TN, June 1964.* Oxford and New York: Pergamon Press, 1964.
52. Colbeck JC. The hospital environment: its place in the hospital staphylococcus infection problem. *Am J Public Health* 1960;50:468–473.
53. Sarubbi FA, Kopf HB, Milson MB, et al. Increased recovery of *Aspergillus flavus* from respiratory specimens during hospital construction. *Am Rev Respir Dis* 1982;125:33–38.
54. Carter CD, Barr BA. Infection control issues in construction and renovation. *Infection Control Hosp Epidemiol* 1997;18:587–596.
55. Rautiala S, Reopenen T, Nevalainen A, et al. Control of exposure to airborne viable microorganisms during remediation of moldy buildings: report of three case studies. *J Am Ind Hyg Assoc* 1998;59:455–460.
56. Alevantis LE, Liu K-S, Hayward SB, et al. Effectiveness of ventilation in 23 designated smoking areas in California office buildings. Proceedings of IAQ-94 ASHRAE, Atlanta, GA, 1995.
57. Code for Safety to Life From Fire in Buildings and Structures. National Fire Protection Association Rule 101, 1994. Reference code 1008.5.2 WFPA.1 Batterymarch Park, Quincey, MA.
58. Streifel AJ, Marshal JW. *Parameters for ventilation controlled environments in hospitals. Design construction and operation of healthy buildings.* Atlanta, GA: ASHRAE Press, 1997:305–309.
59. Shooter RA, Cooke EM, Gaya H, et al. Food and medicaments as possible sources of hospital strains of *Pseudomonas aeruginosa. Lancet* 1969;1:1227–1229.
60. Kominos SD, Copeland CE, Grosiak B, et al. Introduction of *Pseudomonas aeruginosa* into hospitals via vegetables. *Appl Microbiol* 1972;24: 567–570.
61. Sanborn WR. The relationship of surface contamination to the transmission of disease. *Am J Public Health* 1963;53:1278–1283.
62. Levine WC, Smart JR, Archer DL, et al. Foodborne disease outbreaks in nursing homes, 1975 through 1987. *JAMA* 1991;266:2105–2109.
63. Taplin D, Merz PM. Flower vases in hospitals as reservoirs of pathogens. *Lancet* 1973;2:1279–1281.
64. Schoroth MN, Cho JJ. No evidence that *Pseudomonas* on chrysanthemums harms patients. *Lancet* 1973;2:906–907.
65. Rosenzweig AL. Contaminated flower vases. *Lancet* 1973;2:568–569.
66. Burge HA, Solomon WR, Muilenberg ML. Evaluation of indoor plantings as allergen exposure sources. *J Allergy Clin Immunol* 1982;70: 101–108.
67. Smith V, Streifel A, Rhame FS, et al. Potted plant fungal spore shedding. Proceedings of the American Society of Microbiologists Annual Meeting, Miami Beach, FL, 1988.
68. Waste workers stricken with TB; health officials probe operation. *Occupational Health and Safety Letter* 1997;Dec 22:200.
69. Bond RG, Michaelsen GS. Bacterial contamination from hospital solid wastes. Final report under grant no. EF-00007-04. Bethesda, MD: Institute of Allergy and Infectious Disease, National Institutes of Health, 1964.
70. Greene VW, Vesley D, Bond RG, et al. Microbiological contamination of hospital air. I. Quantitative studies. *Appl Microbiol* 1962;10: 561–567.
71. Greene VW, Vesley D, Bond RG, et al. Microbiological contamination of hospital air. II. Qualitative studies. *Appl Microbiol* 1962;10: 568–571.
72. McGowan JE. Environmental factors in nosocomial infection a selective focus. *Rev Infect Dis* 1981;3:760–769.

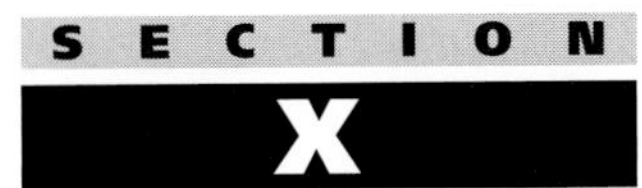

EPIDEMIOLOGY AND PREVENTION OF NOSOCOMIAL INFECTIONS IN HEALTHCARE WORKERS

78

NOSOCOMIAL VIRAL HEPATITIS IN HEALTHCARE WORKERS

SUSAN E. BEEKMANN
DAVID K. HENDERSON

Viral hepatitis was first recognized as an occupational hazard for healthcare workers nearly half a century ago when a blood bank worker acquired viral hepatitis after sustaining multiple needlesticks (1). Since then, we have witnessed an explosion of knowledge in the fields of both basic virology and hospital epidemiology. Five primarily hepatotropic viruses (hepatitis A–E, see Chapter 45) have been identified and characterized, their modes of occupational transmission have been determined, and strategies for prevention have been developed. This chapter addresses the nosocomial epidemiologies of these five agents and does not specifically address the several additional agents that currently contribute to the viral hepatitis alphabet, including the agent called hepatitis French (origin) virus (HFV) (hepatitis F) (2); the bloodborne GB agents [GB virus A (GBV-A), GB virus B (GBV-B), and GB virus C (GBV-C) (3,4)], which rarely cause hepatitis; and hepatitis G virus (HGV), a common, easily transmitted bloodborne agent that is closely related to GBV-C and causes clinically mild, if any, hepatitis (5–8), and may not, in fact, be hepatotropic (9). Until these non–A–E hepatitis viruses and other putative hepatitis agents (10–12) are formally recognized as hepatitis viruses and have their respective epidemiologies delineated, general infection control practices for protecting healthcare workers from enterically transmitted or parenterally transmitted agents, as appropriate, are indicated. This chapter focuses on the etiology of occupationally acquired viral hepatitis, the epidemiology of these viruses in the hospital setting, and the specific prevention and control strategies for each of the five hepatotropic agents identified above.

ETIOLOGY AND EPIDEMIOLOGY

The risk of occupational transmission of each of the hepatitis viruses differs according to the infective body substance, the modes of transmission, the occupations and work responsibilities of healthcare workers, the varying prevalences of infection in the patient population, healthcare workers' immune statuses, and the workers' compliance with infection control procedures. An overview of the five major hepatitis viruses, risks for occupational transmission in the healthcare setting, modes of occupational transmission, relevant prevention strategies, and currently imprecise or unanswered questions are presented in Table 78.1. Factors affecting the risks for occupational transmission for each virus are as follows:

Hepatitis A Virus

Although healthcare workers are generally not considered to be at substantially increased risk for acquiring hepatitis A virus (HAV) infection (13–17), occupational transmission of this virus has been well documented and occurs, albeit rarely, under unusual circumstances. Most HAV transmission in healthcare settings occurs from index patients who are asymptomatic, from those in whom the infection is otherwise unsuspected and/or undiagnosed, from patients who are in the prodromal phase of the infection when viral shedding in the stool is maximal, in instances in which infection control procedures are less than optimal, and in settings in which patients are incontinent of feces (18–33). Occupational HAV transmission occurs primarily via the fecal-oral route, following direct or indirect contact with the index patient's fecal material and is generally only recognized when a cluster of cases occurs. Although healthcare workers can acquire HAV from contaminated food or drink (34–36), occupational infection usually occurs following direct contact with infectious patients. Neonatal intensive care units may provide a unique setting for nosocomial/occupational transmission, because several reported outbreaks, some with widespread secondary transmission, have occurred in this setting (20,22,23,28,31, 37,38). Outbreaks in neonatal intensive care units have most frequently followed the rare occurrence of transfusion-acquired infection of a neonate. Unless staff members practice strict hand washing and environmental cleaning, neonatal and pediatric intensive care settings may provide optimal opportunities for fecal contamination of healthcare workers' hands and environmental surfaces. HAV can survive on workers' hands and this aspect of HAV epidemiology may contribute to the indirect spread of the virus to other patients and staff members (39).

Although occupational HAV infection occurs rarely in U.S. healthcare workers, seroepidemiologic studies in other countries suggest that selected healthcare workers may be at increased risk for occupational infection. One study proposed that HAV is an occupational hazard in Germany, ranking third, with respect

TABLE 78.1. MAJOR HEPATITIS VIRUSES AND OCCUPATIONAL TRANSMISSION TO HEALTHCARE WORKERS

Feature	Hepatitis A (HAV)	Hepatitis B (HBV)	Hepatitis C (HCV)	Hepatitis D (HDV)	Hepatitis E (HEV)
Occupational transmission problem	Rare	Common	Infrequent	Uncommon	Rare
Major mode of occupational transmission	Fecal/oral	Blood	Blood	Blood	Fecal/oral
Isolation precautions for patient	Standard Precautions	Standard Precautions	Standard Precautions	Standard Precautions	Standard Precautions
Prophylaxis for occupational exposure	Ig	Hepatitis B vaccine and HBIg	None	Hepatitis B vaccine and HBIg for persons without HBV infection; none available for HBV carriers	None available
Controversy/ alternative approaches/ unresolved issues	Adjunctive HAV immunization for individuals at risk	Additional booster dose of HBV vaccine for healthcare workers who fail to maintain protective antibody levels	No postexposure prophylaxis, but some advocate either preemptive therapy or watchful waiting (see text)	None	None

Ig, immunoglobulin; HBIg, hepatitis B immunoglobulin.

to morbidity statistics, among infectious occupational diseases, based on frequency of compensation (40). Compared to the general population, medical occupational groups with the highest anti-HAV seroprevalences, in decreasing order, included medical charwomen, food handlers, pediatric nurses, other nurses, and physicians. Another study in Belgium found that healthcare workers in a pediatric hospital had a higher seroprevalence of anti-HAV than workers in general hospitals (41), and a study in France reported a higher seroprevalence among nursing staff when compared to nonmedical employees (42).

Various studies have investigated risk factors for occupational infection with HAV. Factors that facilitate fecal-oral spread enhance transmission. Fecal material from most normal HAV-infected patients is usually easily contained and presents a limited risk to staff members who practice good hand washing and rigorously follow infection control procedures. Conversely, patients who are incontinent of feces and those who have diarrhea present a much higher risk. Factors associated with occupational infection include an index case with diarrhea or incontinent of feces (19,21,22,24–27,29,30,32); an index case hospitalized during the prodromal period of maximal virus fecal excretion (18,19, 21,24–30,43); adult patients who have poor hygiene (43); and less-than-optimal adherence to recommended infection control procedures, including lack of adherence to standard and/or enteric precautions (29,33,38,43). One study identified four additional activities that may have enhanced fecal-oral spread in the occupational setting: sharing food with patients or their families, drinking coffee, sharing cigarettes, and eating in the nurses' office on an intensive care unit (30). Another study identified risk factors for transmission to staff during an outbreak in a neonatal intensive care unit, including caring for an infant with HAV infection, drinking beverages in the unit, and not wearing gloves when taping an intravenous line (31). This study also documented prolonged viral excretion in infected neonates; some infected infants excreted virus for 4 to 5 months after infection. This prolonged period of viral excretion in neonates and infants may also contribute to the risk for nosocomial transmission. Other studies in neonatal intensive care units found that risk of occupational infection was greater among staff members who did not routinely wash their hands after treating an infected infant (38) and among staff members who cared for the index (i.e., infected) case for longer periods of time (28). Another outbreak investigation in a burn treatment center implicated eating on the hospital ward as the single most important risk factor for HAV infection among staff members (44). Vomitus, bile-stained emesis, or bile-contaminated nasogastric suction material may also serve as a reservoir for HAV transmission (21, 25,29,45), since there is evidence that HAV is excreted in bile (46). One study that involved an index patient who had neither diarrhea nor fecal incontinence identified intensive handling of infectious bile, rather than contact with feces, as the most likely mode of transmission (45). Other likely factors contributing to this outbreak included inadequate terminal cleaning of equipment, food consumption in the unit, and inadequate hand washing practices (45).

Because most patients are hospitalized for hepatitis A only after they become jaundiced (and at a time when viral excretion is often substantially reduced from peak excretion during the prodromal stage of infection), these patients are generally considered less infectious. Although fecal excretion of HAV may persist longer in children than in adults, quantitative determinations may be important to determine the risk of exposure to infected pediatric patients (47).

Reported attack rates for occupationally acquired HAV have varied, ranging from a low of 2% of exposed susceptible staff members (29), to 10% (21), 12% (24), 4% to 16% (23), 3% to 30% (28), and 21% to 50% (25). Reasons for the wide variability in attack rates may include varying definitions of occupational exposure to the index case, varying levels of infectivity of source patients, varying intensity of exposures, and the effectiveness and timing of prophylactic immunoglobulin administration.

Hepatitis B Virus

Historically, the highest risk for occupationally acquired hepatitis among healthcare workers has been associated with exposure to hepatitis B virus (HBV); in fact, before the advent of the hepatitis B vaccine, HBV infection was the major occupational risk to healthcare workers (48). In the 1980s, the annual incidence of HBV infection among healthcare workers in the U.S. was staggering. The Centers for Disease Control and Prevention (CDC) estimated that in the mid-1980s approximately 12,000 HBV infections occurred annually in healthcare workers who had frequent occupational exposure to blood or other potentially infectious materials, with an annual rate of infection between 4.89 and 6.63 per 1,000 exposed susceptible workers (49). Of these 12,000 occupationally infected workers each year, CDC scientists estimated that 3,000 developed symptomatic clinical illnesses, more than 600 were hospitalized, and more than 250 of these healthcare workers died. The CDC estimated that between 600 and 1,200 of these healthcare workers became chronic hepatitis B carriers. Since the HBV vaccine was developed and aggressive hepatitis B vaccination of healthcare workers in the U.S. has been promoted, HBV infections among healthcare providers has decreased dramatically to an estimated 400 annually by 1995 (50).

Numerous studies have documented that healthcare workers exposed to blood are at high risk for acquiring HBV infection. In one of the earliest studies, Williams et al. (51) investigated a large epidemic of hepatitis B infections among hospital personnel and found that clinical hepatitis attack rates and HBV antibody prevalence rates correlated with occupational exposure to blood from patients being treated with hemodialysis. Transmission was thought to occur by both accidental parenteral and so-called inapparent parenteral routes of inoculation of contaminated blood. Pattison et al. (52) studied workers in a large community hospital between 1972 and 1974 and found a significant association between frequency of blood contact and prevalence of HBV, but no association between frequency of patient contact and HBV prevalence. The first nationwide, cross-sectional seroepidemiologic survey of occupationally acquired HBV infection among physicians was conducted by Denes et al. (53) in 1975–1976. They found that infection rates were higher among those practicing in urban settings, that the risk for infection increased with the number of years in practice, and that infection rates were highest among pathologists and surgeons. Dienstag and Ryan (54) studied workers at a large urban hospital and found that the prevalence of HBV serologic markers increased as a function of contact with blood, years in a healthcare occupation, and age, but not as a function of contact with patients, years of education, previous needlestick, transfusion, or globulin injection. The highest seroprevalences were found among emergency room nurses, pathology staff members, blood bank staff members, laboratory technicians, intravenous teams, and surgical house officers. Similar high-risk occupations (emergency room, medical and surgical intensive care units, and dentistry and oral surgery) were identified by Jovanovich et al. (55) in a study conducted in an urban hospital.

Snydman et al. (56) conducted a multiinstitutional seroepidemiologic survey of hospital employees in 1980 and 1981 and found that the duration of employment for laboratory workers, surgical staff members, and medical staff members was associated with increased risk for having HBV markers. In this latter study, the highest gradient of risk in these occupations occurred during the first 5 years of employment. Another large multiinstitutional study of nearly 5,700 hospital employees conducted by Hadler et al. (57) controlled for nonoccupational risk factors and confirmed the earlier findings of Dienstag and Ryan that occupational blood exposure, but not patient contact, was associated with risk for prior HBV infection. Hadler et al. also found that the frequency of needle accidents during daily work was directly related to HBV seroprevalence. The occupational group with the highest HBV infection rate was clinical laboratory and blood bank technicians, who routinely handled large numbers of blood specimens. In general, these and similar studies in the pre–HBV-vaccine era may be summarized by noting that healthcare workers who have occupational exposure to blood had a prevalence of HBV markers several times both that of workers who did not have blood exposure as well as that of the general population. This prevalence of HBV infection increased with increasing years of occupational exposure. HBV infection was related to the degree and frequency of blood exposure and not to the degree of patient contact.

West (58) reviewed studies evaluating the risk for HBV infection in healthcare providers and found the risk to be approximately four times elevated when compared to the risk for infection in the at-large adult population. In West's review, physicians and dentists were found to be five to ten times more likely to experience hepatitis B infection, and surgeons, dialysis personnel, personnel providing care for developmentally disabled individuals, and clinical laboratorians to be at tenfold or higher risks for HBV infection (58).

The risk of occupational exposure to HBV depends on several other factors besides occupation and frequency of occupational exposures. The prevalence of HBV infection in the patient population also influences the risk for occupational exposure. Because HBV prevalence is generally higher in urban settings, workers in urban hospitals have been found to be at higher risk for HBV infection (53) than are workers in rural hospitals (59). Renal dialysis patients (see Chapter 64) who require frequent blood transfusions and have suppressed immune responses have long been known to be at high risk, both for acquiring HBV infection as well as for developing chronic HBV infections. For this reason, the staff caring for dialysis patients is at increased risk for occupational HBV infection (58,60,61). Workers in hospitals serving large numbers of other patient population groups at risk for HBV infection, such as intravenous drug users, homosexual men, prison inmates, the developmentally disabled, or immigrants from highly endemic areas, are also at higher risk for occupational exposure and infection with HBV (62). Patients who are asymptomatic HBV carriers are the primary reservoir for HBV infection in the healthcare setting. Broad-scale testing to identify infected patients is neither practical nor cost-effective.

In one study, testing patients who reported a history of hepatitis would have detected fewer than 20% of HBV-infected patients (63).

The infectivity of the source material also influences the risk of acquiring HBV infection. Although hepatitis B surface antigen (HBsAg) has been detected in nearly all body fluids, blood is considered the most infectious and is probably responsible for most occupationally acquired infections. The infectivity of blood is generally correlated with the presence of HBV DNA polymerase or hepatitis B early antigen (HBeAg) in the blood. The risk for HBV infection after a percutaneous (needlestick) exposure to blood from an HBV-infected individual has been estimated to range from 19% to 37% if the donor blood is HBeAg-positive (64,65). In the dental setting, saliva, particularly bloody saliva, is also considered to represent a substantial infectious risk.

The type of exposure to blood or other potentially infectious materials also influences the risk of acquiring infection. Percutaneous exposures, such as needlesticks or injuries with contaminated sharp instruments, are associated with the highest risks for occupational infection. Very small inocula of HBsAg-positive blood may produce infection, since the blood of acute or chronic HBV carriers may contain as many as 10^{13} virus particles of HBV per milliliter of blood (48). Infectivity studies in chimpanzees have demonstrated that serum positive for HBeAg is infectious in dilutions up to 10^{-8} (66). Despite the fact that percutaneous exposures are the most efficient route of infection, the CDC estimates that fewer than 20% of HBV-infected healthcare workers recall an injury/exposure of this type (67). Thus, other, so-called inapparent parenteral, exposures account for a substantial fraction of occupational HBV infections. Preexisting cuts, dermatitis, other skin lesions, or mucous membranes may provide portals of entry for HBV infection. Blood-contaminated inanimate objects or environmental surfaces also have been implicated in occupational transmission in certain settings. In one study, sustaining paper cuts while handling laboratory computer cards in a hospital clinical laboratory was associated with an outbreak of HBV infection (68). Before strict infection prevention measures were implemented in hemodialysis centers, environmental contamination with blood that subsequently resulted in contaminated workers' hands was hypothesized to facilitate HBV transmission (69,70). Contamination of mucous membranes of the eye or mouth, which may occur with accidental splashes or pipetting accidents, also may result in HBV transmission (71).

More recent seroprevalence studies in healthcare workers have documented the importance of hepatitis B vaccine in preventing infections. Thomas et al. (72) studied 943 healthcare personnel in an inner city hospital. Their multivariable analysis identified only one risk factor—absence of HBV vaccination—to be independently associated with HBV infection in this population of healthcare workers. Similarly, Panlilio et al. (73) studied 770 surgeons for markers of HBV infection and found two risk factors—not receiving hepatitis B vaccine and practicing surgery for at least 10 years—for HBV infection. Another study in 114 operating room personnel in Pakistan also documented that nonvaccinated workers were more likely to be infected with HBV (121). Supplementing these seroprevalence studies, Lanphear et al. (74) investigated the incidence of clinical HBV infection in hospital workers and found a dramatic decrease associated with increased immunity due to vaccination.

Hepatitis C Virus

Our current understanding of the role of hepatitis C virus (HCV) in occupationally acquired infections is less clear than for HAV and HBV and is complicated by the evolving understanding of the pathogenesis and immunopathogenesis of exposure and infection with this flavivirus (see Chapter 45).

Since the parenteral mode of transmission of HCV has been clearly established as a primary route of infection for transfusion recipients and intravenous substance users, by analogy to HBV, occupational transmission of HCV in the healthcare setting—including transmission from patients to staff, from patient to patient, and from infected providers to their patients—is likely to be linked to apparent and inapparent parenteral exposure to blood. To date, exposure to blood remains the primary vehicle for occupationally acquired HCV infection, as is evidenced by the overwhelming majority of the cases of occupational infection that have been described in the literature (75–91). HCV also has been transmitted by a punch (92). HCV RNA has been detected in saliva (93–95), and two cases suggest that transmission of HCV occurred following human bites (96, 97). Abe et al. (98) also provided experimental documentation of HCV transmission by saliva. When present in saliva, HCV titers are lower than in blood. The potential infectivity of saliva may have important implications for patient-to-provider transmission, primarily in the dental healthcare setting. HCV RNA also has been detected in a variety of other body fluids from infected patients, including menstrual fluid (99), semen (95, 100,101), urine (95), spinal fluid (102), and ascites (95). The relevance of these latter body substances to the transmission of HCV is unclear. In summary, blood is the body substance that presents the most risk for HCV transmission in the healthcare setting. Despite the fact that transmission of HCV resulting from exposures to body fluids other than blood has not yet been documented, presumably because viral titers in these fluids are substantially lower than in blood, other body substances may present measurable risks for occupational infection, particularly if the healthcare worker is exposed by the parenteral route and/or receives a large inoculum.

Parenteral exposures represent the primary mode of occupationally acquired infection, as is evidenced by the overwhelming majority of the cases of occupational infection that have been described in the literature (79–91). However, two cases of HCV infection have been documented following mucosal exposures to blood (103,104). Extensive HCV environmental contamination of instruments and surfaces in hemodialysis (105–109) and dental surgery settings (110) can occur, and such HCV environmental contamination has been suggested to play a role in transmission of HCV. However, to our knowledge, transmission of a specific HCV strain through environmental contamination has not yet been documented. Transmission resulting from environmental contamination should be an extremely uncommon occurrence if proper sterilization and disinfection procedures are practiced and if current standards of infection control are followed.

Numerous cases of nosocomial transmission from patient to patient (often as a result of cross-contamination from an index case, for example, in hemodialysis, from the use of multidose vials for sequential patients, reuse of spring-loaded finger-stick devices, and contamination of endoscopes and other devices for invasive procedures) have been reported in the literature. A detailed discussion of this topic is beyond the scope of this chapter (see Chapter 45).

Recognizing the epidemiologic similarities between HCV and HBV, several investigators attempted to assess the risk of occupational infection by testing healthcare workers for the serologic prevalence of HCV antibodies, when serologic tests for HCV became available. Interpretation of these studies must take into account both the limitations of the serologic assays (111) and the inadequacy of assessing only the humoral immune response as a measure of exposure and HCV infection (112). Many of the published studies employed the first-generation anti-HCV test that detects an antibody directed against a nonstructural HCV protein, anti-c100-3, and that has low sensitivity and specificity for diagnosing HCV infection when compared with second- and third-generation tests. Even later generation anti-HCV antibody tests still may not detect 100% of infected persons, and tests designed to detect circulating HCV RNA may be necessary to identify some infected individuals. In addition, the anti-HCV tests have a high rate of false positivity in populations with a low prevalence of infection, and supplemental tests for specificity are necessary. The recombinant immunoblot assay (RIBA) or another supplemental HCV neutralization assay should be used to verify repeatedly reactive enzyme immunoassays. Even HCV RNA detection assays are problematic. These tests are subject to false-positive and false-negative results following improper collection, handling, or storage of test samples, and their interpretation is not conclusive: a single negative test may not indicate lack of infection but may be due to fluctuating RNA levels (113), and a single positive test should be repeated to exclude the high likelihood of contamination and a falsely positive assay. In summary, the evolving diagnostic technology has complicated comparisons of HCV seroprevalence and incidence among the various published studies.

Keeping these limitations in mind, Table 78.2 summarizes published studies of anti-HCV seroprevalence among many diverse types of healthcare workers (72,73,114–160).

In addition to the substantial variation in study design, the differences in healthcare worker populations studied, and the differences in the technologies used for detection, other considerations further complicate comparing and interpreting these studies. HCV seroprevalence varies geographically, so similar occupational groups from different locations cannot be compared directly, and local comparison groups are needed for determining if particular healthcare worker groups are at increased risk. Because blood donor seroprevalence data are readily available, blood donors were often used for comparison in these prevalence studies. However, blood donors are not a good comparison group, because they are preselected to avoid a history of hepatitis as well as a history of risk factors for bloodborne infections (161). Most of these studies were not designed to investigate risk factors for HCV seroprevalence, or had too few HCV seropositive subjects to do so. Those studies that did identify risk factors for HCV infection found associations with increasing age (125,146), years in healthcare occupations (127, 142,146), a history of blood transfusions (124,146), and a history of prior needlestick injuries (124,135). In aggregate, given the limitations of the study designs, testing methodology, and selection bias, these studies suggest that healthcare workers' risk of HCV infection is only minimally higher than that of volunteer blood donors, and appears to be approximately tenfold lower than the occupational/nosocomial risks posed by HBV in the healthcare setting.

Table 78.3 summarizes the results of HCV incidence studies conducted in various populations of healthcare workers who had sustained occupational exposures to HCV (83,87,131,133,139, 141,146,162–179). Although most of studies employed anti-HCV antibody testing as the primary detection system for HCV infection, nine of the studies used polymerase chain reaction (PCR) technology to attempt to detect HCV RNA as a marker for infection among individuals who had sustained parenteral exposures to blood from patients known to harbor HCV infection (87,131,164,171,173–175,177,179).

Several factors contribute to the wide variance in the transmission rates (0–22.2%) observed in these studies: different study designs and testing methods, widely differing sample sizes, variable populations of workers followed, different types of exposures, different infectivity of source patients, and potential geographic variability. Recognizing these limitations and acknowledging that the studies are not directly comparable, the pooled infection rate following percutaneous exposures was 1.9%. The risk for infection following other types of exposures has been less intensively studied, but, to date, no infections have been identified in the longitudinal studies following either mucous membrane or other less commonly occurring exposures. Monitoring for infection by measuring HCV RNA may be a more reliable marker for HCV viremia and infectivity (165,180–182), but even when PCR monitoring is combined with antibody testing, the risk for infection may still be underestimated, because neither of these technologies identifies individuals who mount only a brisk cellular response and quickly clear the infection (112). Noting all of these limitations, if one pools the data from the nine studies that used RNA PCR testing, the calculated transmission rate for percutaneous injuries is somewhat higher (3.6%) than is found in the studies assessing incidence by anti-HCV antibody tests alone.

At least four cohort studies of hospital workers initially negative for anti-HCV have attempted to measure incidence of HCV infection. In the first study, samples collected from 960 dental staff during 1979–1981 were retrospectively tested for anti-HCV and two were found to seroconvert, for an incidence of 0.15 per 100 person years of follow-up (122). In the second, in a cohort of hospital staff in Cincinnati followed from 1980 to 1989, six cases of occupationally acquired non-A, non-B hepatitis occurred, for an incidence of 21 cases per 100,000 healthcare workers per year (139). Four of the six cases were confirmed to be HCV infection. This incidence was approximately three times higher than that of non-healthcare workers. The third study followed 765 hospital workers in Italy who were screened for HCV in 1986 and retested in 1992 (143). One worker became infected, for an annual incidence of HCV infection of 0.02%.

TABLE 78.2. SEROPREVALENCE STUDIES OF ANTI–HEPATITIS C VIRUS (HCV) AMONG HEALTHCARE WORKERS

Study Location and Population (Reference)	HCV Assay[a]	Number Tested	% Anti-HCV Seroprevalence	Comparison Group, Number Tested (% Seroprevalance);
Italy, hospital workers (114)	Not specified	945	4.8	Blood donors, 3,575 (1.1) Factory workers, 576 (10.0)
India, healthcare workers (115)	Not specified	90	0	
England, hospital workers (116)	EIA-1	100	0	
Austria, hospital workers (117)	EIA-1	294	2.0	Voluntary blood donors, number not specified (0.7)
Germany, healthcare workers (118)	EIA-1	217	2.8	Blood donors, 500 (0.4)
Germany, hospital workers (119)	EIA-1	738	1.1	
Italy, healthcare workers (120)	EIA-1	1,008	4.1	Blood donors, 3,572 (0.95)
Pakistan, operating room personnel (121)	EIA-1	114	4.4	Blood donors, number not specified (0.7)
United States, dental personnel (122)	EIA-1, RIBA-1	960	1.0	
New York, hemodialysis workers (123)	EIA-1, RIBA	51	2.0	
California, hospital workers (124)	EIA-1, SN	1,677	1.4	
New York, surgeons (73)	EIA-1, SN	770	0.9	
United States and Canada, orthopedic surgeons (125)	EIA-1, SN	3,262	0.8	
New York, healthcare workers (126)	EIA-1, RIBA	158	1.3	
New York, dentists (127)	EIA-1, RIBA	456	1.8	Non-healthcare worker controls matched by graduate education level, 723 (0.1)
Connecticut, healthcare workers (128)	EIA-1, RIBA-2	243	1.6	
Japan, hospital workers (129)	EIA-1, RIBA	1,097	2.5	Blood donors, 526 (1.1)
Japan, acupuncturists (129)	EIA-1, RIBA	183	5.5	Blood donors, 710 (3.2)
United States, hemodialysis workers (130)	EIA-1, SN	142	1.4	
Italy, hospital workers (131)	EIA-1, RIBA	1,347	0.7	Volunteer blood donors, number not specified (0.9)
Maryland, hospital workers (72)	EIA-1 or EIA-2, RIBA	943	0.7	Blood donors, 104,239 (0.4)
Wales, dental surgeons (132)	EIA-2	94	0	Blood donors, number not specified (0.3)
Italy, hospital workers (133)	EIA-2, SN	635	0.6	
Japan, hemodialysis workers (134)	EIA-2	152	8.6	Blood donors, 919 (1.5)
Italy, healthcare workers (135)	EIA-2, SN	407	1.2	General population, 253 (0.8)
Germany, hospital workers (136)	EIA-2, RIBA-2	1,033	0.6	Volunteer blood donors, 2,113 (0.24)
Taiwan, dentists (137)	EIA-2, PCR	461	0.7	Volunteer blood donors, number not specified (0.95 by EIA-1)
South Africa, nurses (138)	EIA-2, SN	212	0	Volunteer blood donors, 35,685 (0.3)
Ohio, clinical and laboratory based healthcare workers (227)	EIA-2, RIBA-2	861	2.0	Volunteer blood donors, 20,304 (0.5)
California, healthcare workers (140)	EIA-1, EIA-2, RIBA-2	851	1.4	
London, healthcare workers (141)	EIA-2, RIBA-2	1,053	0.3	Blood donors, number not specified (0.3)
Belgium, hemodialysis nurses (142)	EIA-2, RIBA-2	120	4.1	Blood donors, number not specified (0.6)
Italy, healthcare workers (143)	EIA-2, RIBA	937	0.9	Voluntary blood donors, 1,136 (0.5), pregnant women, 657 (0.8)
Sweden, healthcare workers (144)	EIA-2, SN	880	0.7	Blood donors, number not specified (0.6)
France, hospital employees (145)	EIA-2, RIBA-2	430	0.9	Office workers, 180 (1.7)
Italy, healthcare workers (146)	EIA-2, RIBA-2	3,073	2.2	Blood donors, 11,000 (0–1.7%)
Italy, psychiatric hospital workers (147)	EIA-2, RIBA-2	145	1.4	
England, hospital workers (148)	EIA-2, EIA-3	1,949	0.2	Blood donors, 1,350 (0.1)
Belgium, hospital workers (149)	EIA-3, RIBA-3	2,031	1.5	
Italy, hospital workers (150)	RIBA-2	472	2.5	
Japan, hospital workers (151)	EIA-2	1,638	2.8	
U.K., dental workers (152)	EIA-3, EIA-3, PCR	167	1.2	
Hungary, hospital workers (153)	EIA-2, EIA-3, RIBA-2	409	2.4	
Lebanon, hospital workers (154)	EIA-3, EIA-3, PCR	502	0.4	Blood donors, 600 (0.4)
Mexico, medical residents (155)	EIA-3, RIBA-2	89	1.1	
India, hospital workers (156)	EIA-3, RIBA-3	200	0	
Switzerland, dental workers (157)	EIA-3, EIA-3 RIBA-3, PCR	1,056	0.09	
Syria, healthcare workers (158)	EIA-3	189	3.0	
Italy, hospital workers (159)	EIA-3	4,517	1.97	
Libya, hospital workers (160)	EIA-3	459	2.0	

[a]EIA, enzyme immunoassay; RIBA, recombinant immunoblot assay; SN, supplemental neutralization; PCR, polymerase chain reaction.

TABLE 78.3. LONGITUDINAL STUDIES ASSESSING OCCUPATIONAL RISK FOR HEPATITIS C VIRUS (HCV) INFECTION FOLLOWING PARENTERAL OCCUPATIONAL EXPOSURES TO BLOOD FROM PATIENTS INFECTED WITH HEPATITIS C

First Author (Reference)	Year	Location	Parenteral HCV Exposures	HCV Infections	% HCV Infected	Testing Methodology	Comments
Kiyosawa[a] (162)	1991	Japan	110	3[a]	2.7[a]	EIA-1, RIBA-1	
Francavilla (133)	1992	Italy	30	0	0	EIA-2	
Hernandez (163)	1992	Spain	81	0	0	EIA-2, RIBA	
Marranconi (83)	1992	Italy	117	3	2.6	EIA, RIBA	
Mitsui (164)	1992	Japan	68	7	10.3	EIA-2, PCR	
Stellini (131)	1993	Italy	30	0	0	EIA-1, RIBA-1, PCR	
Sodeyama (165)	1993	Japan	62	3	4.8	EIA-2	
Lanphear (139)	1994	U.S.	50	3	6	EIA-2, SN	
Perez-Trallero (166)	1994	Spain	53	1	1.9	EIA-2, EIA-3	
Petrosillo (167)	1994	Italy	61	0	0	EIA-2, RIBA-2	Dialysis settings
Ippolito (168)	1994	Italy	123[b]	2[b]	1.6	EIA-2, RIBA-2	HIV co-infected sources
Zuckerman (141)	1994	U.K.	24	0	0	EIA-2, RIBA-2	
Puro[b] (146)	1995	Italy	97	1[b]	1.0	EIA-2, RIBA-2	
Puro[b] (169)	1995	Italy	436	4[b]	0.9	EIA-2, RIBA-2	
Puro[b] (170)	1995	Italy	61	0	0	EIA-2, RIBA-2	HIV uninfected sources
Arai (171)	1996	Japan	56	3	5.4	RIA-1, PHA-2, PCR	
Mizuno (87)	1997	Japan	37	2	5.4	EIA-2, PCR, sequencing	
Serra (172)	1998	Spain	443	3	0.7	EIA-2, EIA-3	
Takagi (173)	1998	Japan	251	4	1.6	EIA-1, EIA-2, PCR	
Veeder (174)	1998	U.S.	9	2	22.2	EIA, PCR	
Hamid (175)	1999	Pakistan	53	2	3.8	EIA-2, PCR	
Hasan (176)	1999	Kuwait	24	0	0	EIA-2, RIBA	
Baldo (177)	2002	Italy	68	0	0	EIA-3, RIBA-2, PCR	
Regez (178)	2002	Netherlands	23	0	0	EIA-3, RIBA-2	
Wang (179)	2002	Taiwan, ROC	14	1	7.1	EIA-3, RIBA-2, PCR	
Total (see text)			2,381	44	1.8		

[a] Some patients may overlap with ref. 165.
[b] Some patients may be counted more than once from these studies reported by the same set of investigators.
EIA-1, first-generation enzyme immunoassay; EIA-2, second-generation immunoassay; EIA-3, third-generation immunoassay; RIBA-1, first-generation recombinant immunoblot assay; RIBA-2, second-generation recombinant immunoblot assay; PCR, polymerase chain assay; RIA, radioimmunoassay; PHA, passive hemagglutination; SN, supplemental neutralization.
Modified from Henderson DK. Managing occupational risks for hepatitis C transmission in the healthcare setting. *Clin Microbiol Rev* 2003; 16:(3): 546–568.

The fourth cohort study, conducted in San Francisco, observed a single seroconversion between 1984 and 1992, and found an incidence density rate of 0.08 per 100 person-years (140). For perspective, this study also measured an incidence density rate of 3.05 per 100 person-years for HBV among nonvaccinated susceptible workers and 0.055 for HIV. A population-based surveillance system for acute viral hepatitis in Italy found that in 1991 healthcare workers were 2.95 times as likely to acquire acute hepatitis C compared to the general population, and in 1994 they were 1.72 times as likely (183).

The findings of a low seroprevalence of HCV infection among healthcare workers and the moderate risk of documented transmission by needlestick injury suggest that the occupational risk of HCV infection exists and is intermediate between the 0.3% per percutaneous exposure risk for occupational HIV exposure (184) and the 19% to 37% risk for parenteral exposure to an "e" antigen positive, HBV-infected source (64,65). The most probable reason for the lower risk is that titers of HCV circulating in blood are relatively low (probably 2 to 3 logs lower than HBV titers, as noted above) (66,183), so that transmission by small inocula such as needlesticks or other injuries in the occupational setting is less efficient than is the case for HBV. However, because most HCV infections are persistent, the prevalence of HCV infection in some patient populations actually may be higher than for hepatitis B (185), providing a larger pool of potential sources for occupational infection. Because of the wide variability in HCV prevalence by geographic region and patient populations, occupational risk will necessarily vary by these conditions.

As noted above, recent studies of the immunopathogenesis of HCV infection suggest that none of the techniques that have been applied in the longitudinal studies of risk for occupational HCV infection may provide a true denominator of healthcare workers sustaining occupational HCV infections. Anecdotal case reports document HCV antigen circulation in individuals who never made anti-HCV antibody, despite the development of productive HCV infection (186). Additionally, some investigators have suggested that both antibody tests and tests for circulating HCV nucleic acid underestimate the true denominator of exposures, further suggesting that the most sensitive measure of past exposure may well be assessment of specific cellular immunity directed against HCV (112). As noted above, none of the longitudinal studies of healthcare workers measured cellular immune responses.

Further cohort incidence studies and exposure follow-up studies, with larger numbers of workers, employing both HCV

RNA testing and sensitive measures of cellular immune responses directed against HCV will be needed to define more precisely the occupational risk of HCV infection.

Hepatitis D Virus

Hepatitis D virus (HDV), formerly called the delta agent, is a defective virus that needs HBV as a helper virus (see Chapter 45). Thus, HDV may infect healthcare workers either as a co-infection with HBV (i.e., a simultaneous exposure) or as a superinfection when healthcare workers already have HBV infection. The extent of HDV infection in healthcare workers has not been determined, because HDV antibody testing is not routinely performed (187). Even if HDV antibody screening were routine, the prevalence would be difficult to determine, because infection may elicit only a transient and low-titered response (188). Nevertheless, there is anecdotal evidence for occupational HDV transmission in a hemodialysis nurse (189), and documented evidence for transmission to a surgeon following a deep needlestick injury (190).

Because of its dependence on HBV, the epidemiology and mode of transmission of HDV are similar to those of hepatitis B. Worldwide, approximately 5% of HBsAg carriers are infected with HDV (191). However, not all HBV-infected individuals have the same risk for HDV infection, because geographic and risk group distribution vary substantially. Patient populations that include HBV-infected persons from HDV-endemic areas, such as southern Italy, the Amazon basin, the Middle East, and certain Pacific islands, are more likely to be co-infected with HDV, and therefore present a greater risk to healthcare workers. Among risk groups for HBV infection, HBV-infected hemophiliacs, intravenous drug abusers, and hemodialysis patients are more likely to be co-infected with HDV than are homosexual men.

Hepatitis E Virus

The etiologic agent of the syndrome of enterically transmitted non-A, non-B hepatitis prevalent in India, Pakistan, Nepal, southwestern China, central Asia, the former Soviet Union, and parts of Africa and Mexico is now recognized to be the hepatitis E virus (HEV) (see Chapter 45). HEV is not prevalent in the U.S., although the disease has been imported from endemic areas by immigrants or travelers (192–196). However, although still very rare, the first cases acquired within the U.S. have been reported (197), and a new strain, called HEV US-1, has been identified as the cause in one instance (198,199). Caution is required when interpreting results from seroprevalence studies; results of assays for antibody to HEV vary widely and are highly discrepant among populations in non–HEV-endemic areas (200–202) (see Chapter 45).

HEV, as is the case for HAV, is transmitted by the fecal-oral route. In the epidemic setting, fecal contamination of water is the most common vehicle for transmission (203). Although person-to-person transmission can occur, infection in household contacts is uncommon (204), suggesting that this mode of transmission is relatively inefficient. Some recent studies have suggested that there may be a reservoir for HEV infection in animals (205). Medical staff members in refugee camps have become infected (206). However, the exact mode of transmission in this report is unknown, and the fact that sanitation conditions in refugee camps differ significantly from those in most healthcare settings must be recognized. As with HAV, a period of viremia occurs during the prodromal phase of illness, before virus is shed in the feces, so bloodborne transmission is also possible (207). Presumptive transmission of HEV to a doctor and two nurses has been reported following exposure to amniotic fluid, blood, and stool from a patient with acute hepatitis E acquired following travel to India (208). Until more information becomes available, the risk for occupational acquisition of HEV by healthcare workers in most settings should be considered real, but rare, occurring only under distinctly unusual circumstances in the U.S.

Some recent evidence suggests that hepatitis E may have a zoonotic reservoir, with pigs and possibly rats serving as reservoirs for human infection (205,209). Critical information about hepatitis E and its etiology, epidemiology, and prevention was developed within 20 years; serologic tests have been developed, and a candidate vaccine is being evaluated in clinical trials (phase III clinical trials).

PATHOGENESIS

Other than the clear association of needles, scalpels, and other medical "sharps" with the bloodborne hepatitis syndromes, the pathogenesis of these syndromes in the healthcare setting is not substantially different from the pathogenesis in the community. Chapter 45 thoroughly discusses the pathogenesis of these syndromes.

CLINICAL MANIFESTATIONS

Similarly, the clinical manifestations of the viral hepatitis infections arising as a result of occupational exposures in healthcare workers are generally similar to those in other adults (see Chapter 45). An exception may exist for occupationally acquired HCV. One follow-up study suggested that when hepatitis C develops following occupational exposure, the disease tends to be mild and transient (164) in contrast to transfusion-acquired hepatitis C, which tends to become persistent and chronic. Another study of community-acquired HCV infection, however, found that the frequency of development of chronic hepatitis is similar regardless of how the HCV infection is initially contracted but that severe chronic disease in the form of chronic active hepatitis is more common following transfusion-acquired infection (perhaps because of an inoculum effect) (210). Further studies are needed to confirm these preliminary observations.

DIAGNOSIS

The diagnosis of hepatitis infections in healthcare workers who have sustained occupational exposures is no different from diagnosis in a patient presenting with a hepatitis syndrome (see

Chapter 45). One diagnosis-related issue that is worthy of some emphasis (especially when the source patient is known) is that of determining the hepatitis infection status of the source patient. When the source patient is identifiable and his/her hepatitis infection status is not known, documenting the source patient's infection status will facilitate both risk assessment and the healthcare worker's postexposure management and follow-up and, in the event that the source patient is found to be infected with the same virus, will likely solidify the healthcare worker's compensation claim. As is done with postexposure testing of source patients for human immunodeficiency virus (HIV) infection, we feel strongly that such testing should be done with the informed consent of the source patient. State laws vary regarding the need for informed consent for testing. In occupational exposure settings, some states permit testing of available serum without consent. Hospitals and infection control committees should construct (and follow) policies that are consonant with their state and local laws. A major controversy currently exists concerning the use of periodic monitoring by RNA PCR of healthcare workers who have sustained occupational exposures to a source patient's blood for the so-called preemptive therapy or watchful waiting strategies (211) (discussed in more detail below).

PREVENTION AND CONTROL

As the hepatitis viruses differ in their modes of transmission and mechanisms of immunity, so will their methods of prevention and control. Components of a multidimensional prevention program include (a) education and training of staff members; (b) administrative controls (identification and isolation of infectious patients); (c) engineering controls [e.g., adequate hand washing facilities, proper selection and use of sharps disposal containers (212) and safety equipment such as protective needle-safety devices]; (d) safe work practices and appropriate use of protective barrier equipment to minimize occupational exposures [practicing Standard (Universal) Precautions with all patients]; and (e) employee immunization and postexposure management through occupational health services. Prevention of HAV and HEV infection focuses primarily on interrupting fecal-oral transmission, whereas HBV, HCV, and HDV are bloodborne pathogens requiring different precautions and strategies. Education and training of staff members regarding the methods of infection control and specific prevention strategies is the most important and fundamental component of prevention. When accidental exposures occur, appropriate postexposure prophylaxis, if available, should be administered. Postexposure prophylaxis strategies vary for each virus; currently HAV and HBV are the only hepatitis viruses for which there are vaccines for preexposure prevention and immune globulins for postexposure prevention.

Hepatitis A Virus

To prevent occupational transmission of HAV, healthcare workers should practice good basic infection control techniques, particularly strict hand washing, with all patients. Because virus is shed in the feces in the highest concentrations during the incubation period and early in the prodromal period (when hepatitis A infection may not be suspected), identifying and isolating infectious patients may not be possible. In the neonatal or pediatric hospital setting in particular, HAV infections are usually asymptomatic and unsuspected. Hospitalized patients known to have had a recent exposure to known or suspected hepatitis A should undergo serologic studies, should receive appropriate immunoprophylaxis, and should be isolated appropriately. When a patient is known or suspected to have hepatitis A or has unspecified hepatitis consistent with a viral etiology, the CDC traditionally recommended enteric precautions through the first week after onset of jaundice (213). The CDC's current guidelines recommend standard precautions for most patients with hepatitis A, but Contact Precautions for patients who are diapered or incontinent (214). Contact Precautions should be maintained for duration of hospitalization for infants and children less than 3 years old, for 2 weeks after onset of symptoms in children 3–14 years old, and until 1 week after onset of symptoms for others. Standard Precautions dictate that gloves should be worn when handling all feces or feces-contaminated articles from all patients. Gloves should be worn routinely for contact with patients who have diarrhea or are incontinent of feces. To minimize inapparent contact with fecal material, healthcare workers should wash their hands after even minimal patient contact, and environmental contamination must be minimized by cleaning and disinfection procedures.

In the event of occupational exposure to HAV, postexposure prophylaxis with immunoglobulin (Ig) is recommended (62, 215,216). Immunization with the hepatitis A vaccine is another reasonable postexposure immunoprophylaxis strategy, with or without the passive administration of Ig. As a practical matter, however, Ig is seldom used during the primary outbreak, because the index case is often not diagnosed until after the first cluster of infections has occurred. In the healthcare setting, Ig is more commonly employed to prevent secondary transmission. When administered before exposure or during the incubation period, Ig protects against clinical illness (i.e., Ig may not prevent infection but minimizes the clinical signs and symptoms of infection). Protective effects are greatest when administered early in the incubation period, and Ig should be given no later than 2 weeks after exposure. Serologic screening of exposed workers for anti-HAV is not recommended, because screening is more costly than administering Ig and would unnecessarily delay Ig administration, compromising its efficacy. For postexposure prophylaxis, a single intramuscular dose of 0.02 mL/kg of standard lot Ig is recommended. Because the risk of occupational transmission in healthcare workers is so low, Ig is not recommended for preexposure prophylaxis.

Inactivated hepatitis A vaccines have been marketed for more than 5 years (217) and the CDC's Advisory Committee on Immunization Practices (ACIP) has issued recommendations concerning their use (215,216). Because healthcare workers in general are not at high risk for HAV infection, preexposure use of the vaccine in healthcare workers has not been recommended by the ACIP. However, selected workers, such as those in laboratories or primate animal facilities who work with HAV, should be vaccinated. For outbreaks occurring in hospitals or institutions for developmentally challenged patients, the CDC still recommends aggressive use of Ig, as there are no data concerning the role of hepatitis A vaccine in these settings, though some investigators (particularly those from outside the U.S. in settings in which the risk for transmission may be higher) have recommended it (33). Because the vaccine should be administered at least 2 weeks prior to exposure to HAV, Ig is still recommended for postexposure prophylaxis. In one of the authors' institution, however, the occupational medical service occasionally makes exceptions to the CDC's general recommendations. If the exposed healthcare worker is likely to have additional future exposures to HAV and both immediate and long-term protection is desired, both the vaccine and Ig may be administered. Vaccine should be administered with a different syringe at a different site from the Ig; the ultimate antibody titer obtained is likely to be lower than when the vaccine is given alone. Both hepatitis A vaccines currently available in the U.S. require two doses, the second administered 6 months after the first (VAQTA) or 6 to 12 months after the first (HAVRIX). Vaccine protection has been shown to persist for at least 6 years (218), is likely to last for at least 10 years, and possibly for as long as 50 years (219, 220).

One study has examined the cost-effectiveness of vaccinating medical students for hepatitis A and concluded that, although the cost per year of life saved was similar to that of many other medical interventions, in order to be cost-saving, the incidence of hepatitis A infection would have to be at least ten times higher than the present rate (221). One selected set of healthcare workers who should be considered for hepatitis A vaccination is individuals identified as harboring chronic HCV infection. A recent study documented the substantial risk of fulminant hepatitis and death among persons with chronic hepatitis C who acquired HAV infection (222), and universal vaccination of all HCV-infected individuals has been proposed (223).

Fortunately, unlike HBV, HCV, and HDV infections, HAV does not result in a chronic infection state requiring difficult management decisions and long-term work restriction. Healthcare workers with hepatitis A infection should be restricted from patient contact and food handling until 7 days after onset of jaundice (224).

Hepatitis B Virus

Of all the hepatitis syndromes, prevention efforts in the healthcare setting have focused most aggressively on occupational HBV infection. Results of these efforts are encouraging, but there are still opportunities for improvement. The CDC estimates that the incidence of HBV in healthcare workers declined from 17,000 per year in 1983 to approximately 400 annual infections in 1995 (50). This decline is generally attributed to the introduction of the hepatitis B vaccine in 1982, the institution of universal blood and body fluid precautions in 1987, and the issuance of the Occupational Safety and Health Administration's (OSHA) bloodborne pathogens standard in 1991 (50, 74,225–227). The use of postexposure prophylaxis, and, to a much lesser extent, patient screening to identify those infected with HBV for special precautions also may have contributed to decreased infections.

Because the source patients for most occupationally acquired HBV infections are never identified, all patients should be assumed to be infectious. This concept is the cornerstone of Universal/Standard Precautions and was originally developed in 1987 to address concerns about the transmission of HIV (see Chapter 79). All healthcare workers who have potential occupational exposure to blood or other potentially infectious materials must receive training in the various aspects of Universal/Standard Precautions: administrative and engineering controls, appropriate work practices, and use of protective barrier equipment to minimize occupational exposures. Such training is required both by the OSHA final rule on bloodborne pathogens (67) and by federal law. Engineering controls include the provision of hand washing facilities and equipment designed to minimize percutaneous injuries (e.g., impervious needle disposal units and self-blunting, shielded, or needleless devices). Work practices include appropriate hand washing, safe handling of needles and other sharp devices, and avoiding risky behaviors such as oral pipetting, recapping needles, and improper handling or disposal of needles and other sharp instruments. Employees must also know how and when to use appropriate protective barrier equipment, such as gloves, gowns, masks, and eye protection, to prevent occupational exposure to blood or other infectious substances. Employee training should also include safe disposal of infectious wastes, housekeeping practices to prevent environmental contamination, and first-aid procedures and injury reporting procedures to follow in the event of an occupational exposure. A summary of specific methods to reduce exposure to blood and other body fluids in the higher-risk operating room setting has also been published (228).

Hepatitis B Vaccine

Healthcare institutions are also required by the OSHA final rule to provide hepatitis B vaccine free of charge to all at-risk employees; workers who refuse the vaccine are required to sign a declination. Despite the fact that the vaccine provides the best available means of protection from hepatitis B, it has, unfortunately, been underutilized. The original hepatitis B vaccine licensed for use in the U.S. in 1981 was derived from human plasma, and, the vaccine's proven safety and efficacy notwithstanding, vaccination programs were plagued with unfounded safety concerns about possible contamination with other bloodborne pathogens. Currently the two U.S.-licensed vaccines are marketed, and both are genetically engineered by inserting the gene for HBsAg into the yeast *Saccharomyces cerevisiae* and harvesting the HBsAg particles produced in culture. The recommended dose and schedule for immunizing healthcare workers is 1.0 mL, injected into the deltoid muscle, at 0, 1, and 4 to 6 months. An adequate antibody response is generally considered to be at least 10 milli–International Units (mIU)/mL0, which is approximately equivalent to 10 sample ratio units (SRU) by radioimmunoassay (RIA) or a positive test result by enzyme immunoassay (EIA) (62).

Several factors affect the immunogenicity of the vaccine. Care must be taken to prevent freezing the vaccine during shipping and storage, or vaccine potency will be reduced. The vaccine manufacturer's recommended schedule should be followed. Satisfactory protection is obtained if the vaccine doses are administered at longer intervals, but optimal protection does not occur until the third dose. The response may be suboptimal if the vaccine is administered by gluteal injection, rather than being injected into the deltoid muscle. However, age of the recipient is probably the most important determinant of vaccine response. Vaccine response ranges from 90% to 95% among young adults to only 50% to 70% in vaccinees over 60 years of age (229, 230). Persons with immunosuppressive illnesses, such as renal failure and HIV infection, and persons with chronic diseases, such as diabetes and chronic liver disease, also have diminished vaccine responses. Smokers have been found to have decreased immune responses compared to nonsmokers (229,231–233), and obesity is also associated with diminished response (229, 233,234). Unlicensed, reduced vaccine dosages and intradermal routes of injection have been studied extensively, but the OSHA final rule stipulates that vaccine must be provided to healthcare workers according to current recommendations of the U.S. Public Health Service (USPHS) (224).

Prevaccination antibody testing of potential vaccine recipients for evidence of existing immunity is not necessary, but may be sensible if the prevalence of prior infection in the population to be immunized is greater than 10%. The decision to implement a screening program should be based on an institution-specific cost-benefit analysis considering the HBV seroprevalence rate among employees, the cost of serologic screening to the institution, and the costs of vaccination (62). The issue of postvaccination anti-HBs testing has been more controversial. The recent decline in the occupational HBV transmission rate has been proposed as one argument against routine testing (235). Although postvaccination assessment of antibody response was not recommended routinely in the past, testing was advisable for persons 50 years of age or older, those who were vaccinated with unlicensed dosages or routes of administration, those with immunosuppressive conditions or chronic diseases, and those whose subsequent management depended on knowing their immune status (such as dialysis staff members) (62,229). In one of the authors' institution, postvaccination testing is offered to anyone who desires it. The CDC's ACIP and Healthcare Infection Control Practices Advisory Committee (HICPAC) now recommend that postvaccination testing be performed 1 to 2 months after the third dose for healthcare workers who have contact with patients or blood and are at ongoing risk for injuries with sharp instruments or needlesticks (224). Other researchers have proffered what they believe to be a more cost-effective strategy of not performing postvaccination antibody testing, but instead providing postexposure testing and prophylaxis (236). Unfortunately, in our view, this approach has significant limitations. Workers who have inapparent or unreported occupational exposures would not benefit from this alternate strategy, nor would nonresponders be identified and counseled accordingly.

Workers who do not respond adequately to the primary series (nonresponders) may respond to additional vaccine doses. Nonresponders should be revaccinated with a second, three-dose series or be evaluated to determine if they are positive for HBsAg (224). Revaccinated workers should be retested after completion of the second vaccine series. Nonresponders who are HBsAg-negative should also be counseled that they are susceptible to HBV infection, they should practice scrupulous universal precautions, and they need hepatitis B immunoglobulin (HBIg) for postexposure prophylaxis (see below). The CDC further recommends that workers in chronic dialysis centers who do not respond to the vaccine should be tested for HBsAg and anti-HBs semiannually (237). Alternate vaccine formulations appear promising and may be effective in immunizing some nonresponders to current vaccines (238).

The USPHS does not currently recommend either booster doses for workers who initially respond to the vaccine but whose antibody levels decline over time or periodic serologic testing to monitor anti-HBs levels (224). Studies of duration of vaccine-induced immunity in healthy young adults have shown that between 28% and 50% of those who responded to vaccination lost adequate levels of antibody by 5 years, and 30% to 60% had no or low antibody levels by 8 years (229). However, data suggest that, in the rare instances in which HBV infection occurs in adult vaccine responders, the infection is transient and does not result in clinical illness. Other studies have shown that there is excellent persistence of immunologic memory for up to 10 to 11 years following vaccination (50,239,240). Some institutions do offer booster doses of vaccine to healthcare workers who have previously responded to hepatitis B vaccination, who remain in at-risk professions, and whose anti-HBs antibody titers have dropped into the negative range (Table 78.4).

Another consideration is emphasizing the importance of vaccination of healthcare workers during orientation, training, and/or before occupational exposures can occur. This approach has two advantages: it may increase vaccine acceptance, and it will prevent infection in trainees who are unskilled and at increased risk of accidental injuries while learning techniques. Studies to determine vaccine coverage among healthcare workers have reported variable results. One study of randomly selected hospitals conducted in 1992 found that only 51% of eligible (and therefore presumably at-risk) employees were vaccinated with three doses of vaccine (226). A large study of American and Canadian orthopedic surgeons found that the prevalence of vaccination decreased steadily with age, from 90% of 20- to 29-year-old surgeons to only 35% of those 60 years old or older (125). Only 55% of hospital-based surgeons in a multicenter survey reported receiving all three doses of vaccine (73). Another national study determined that only 66.5% of eligible employees had received three doses of the vaccine, although coverage was somewhat higher (75%) in workers with frequent exposure to potentially infectious body fluids (50). Hospitals with increased vaccination coverage often provided incentives, used employee performance measures (e.g., supervisors were notified if an employee refused vaccination, sanctions were imposed for refusing vaccination, or vaccination was required as a condition of employment), sent reminder notices when vaccine doses were due, and used a computerized tracking system. Clearly, we are making progress, but efforts are still needed to improve vaccine acceptance among healthcare workers. Although there is no precedent for federal law requiring workers to receive a vaccine, mandatory immunization of susceptible healthcare workers has been proposed as the best strategy to further prevent occupational and nosocomial hepatitis B infection. Many healthcare institutions and medical schools have adopted this strategy.

TABLE 78.4. GUIDELINES FOR MANAGEMENT OF HEPATITIS EXPOSURES TO BLOOD AND OTHER POTENTIALLY INFECTIOUS MATERIALS AT THE NATIONAL INSTITUTES OF HEALTH (NIH) CLINICAL CENTER

Laboratory Results Obtained on Source (Donor) Patient[a]	Exposed HCWs' HB Vaccine Status	Exposed HCWs' Laboratory Studies Ordered[b]	Exposed HCWs' Laboratory Results	HCW Treatment[c] and Follow-Up
HBsAg+ or unknown, possibly HBsAg+	Unvaccinated	HBsAg, anti-HBs, ALT/AST	Anti-HBs+	None
			Anti-HBs−	HBIg, begin HB vaccine series.[d] Obtain HBsAg, anti-HBs, anti-HBc, ALT/AST in 3 and 6 months.
	Vaccinated, known nonresponder (anti-HBs−)	HBsAg, anti-HBs, ALT/AST	HBsAg+ and anti-HBs−	None
			HBsAg− and anti-HBs−	HBIg and either: initiate revaccination as soon as possible or 2nd HBIg dose in 1 month. Obtain HBsAg, anti-HBs, anti-HBc, ALT/AST in 3 and 6 months.
	Vaccinated, undocumented anti-HBs response	HBsAg, anti-HBs, ALT/AST	Anti-HBs+	None
			Anti-HBs−	HBIG and initiate revaccination as soon as possible. Obtain HBsAg, anti-HBs, anti-HBc, ALT/AST in 3 and 6 months.
	Vaccinated, known responder (anti-HBs+)	Anti-HBs	Anti-HBs+	None
			Anti-HBs−	HB vaccine booster dose.
HCV PCR +, anti-HCV + or unknown, possible anti-HCV+		Anti-HCV, ALT/AST; PCR for HCV RNA	Anti-HCV+	None. If unvaccinated, begin HB vaccine series. Refer for follow-up.
			Anti-HCV−	If unvaccinated, begin HB vaccine series. Obtain anti-HCV, ALT/AST at 3 and 6 months. Repeat HCV PCR at q2 week intervals for 6 months. If positive, follow closely for resolution of infection (see text). After 4 months of positivity, refer for consideration of IFN-α treatment.[e] Obtain anti-HAV. If anti-HAV neg., begin HA vaccine series.
AST/ALT abnormal, anti-HCV−, NANB suspected, or unknown, possible NANB		Anti-HCV, ALT/AST	ALT/AST abnormal, NANB suspected	None. If unvaccinated, begin HB vaccine series.
			ALT/AST abnormal or normal, NANB not suspected	None. If unvaccinated, begin HB vaccine series. Obtain anti-HCV, ALT/AST at 3 and 6 months.

HCW, healthcare worker; HBsAg, hepatitis B surface antigen; anti-HBs, antibody to hepatitis B surface antigen; anti-HBc, antibody to hepatitis B core antigen; ALT, alanine aminotransferase; AST, aspartate aminotransferase; anti-HCV, antibody to hepatitis C virus; HBIg, hepatitis B immune serum globulin, 0.06 mL/kg IM, as soon as possible (value beyond 7 days unknown); HB vaccine, hepatitis B vaccine; anti-HBs+, ≥10 sample ratio units (SRU) by radioimmunoassay (RIA) or positive by enzyme immunoassay (EIA); anti-HAV, antibody to hepatitis A virus; HA vaccine, hepatitis A vaccine; NANB, non-A, non-B, non-C hepatitis; IFN, interferon.

[a] If the source of the exposure is known, obtain written, informed consent and order HBsAg, anti-HCV, and AST/ALT.

[b] If resources permit, obtain informed consent and freeze an aliquot of serum for future reference.

[c] Unless HCW is known to be positive for HBsAg or has adequate levels of anti-HBs, postexposure treatment should always include counseling and initiation of HB vaccine series (if unvaccinated or if HB vaccine series is incomplete), or administration of booster doses if indicated.

[d] Alternatively, if the employee refuses vaccine, administer HBIG as soon as possible and repeat in 1 month.

[e] Not a current United States Public Health Service (USPHS) recommendation.

Courtesy of Dr. James M. Schmitt, Occupational Medical Service, National Institutes of Health (modified).

MANAGEMENT OF EMPLOYEES SUSTAINING OCCUPATIONAL EXPOSURES

The CDC recommends (224,241), and the OSHA final bloodborne standard requires, that postexposure prophylaxis be provided to employees experiencing adverse exposures to hepatitis B. Healthcare institutions should have established protocols for providing immediate appropriate first aid for injuries and exposures, mechanisms for reporting employee injuries/exposures, and protocols to manage these exposures (242) (see Chapter 79). Table 78.4 summarizes the management of employees following exposures to blood or other potentially infectious materials as practiced at the Clinical Center, National Institutes of Health (NIH) (243). Although the complete protocol also includes other bloodborne pathogens, such as HIV and human T-cell lymphotropic virus, only the hepatitides are discussed here (see Chapter 79). Management of exposures includes assessing the type, source, and circumstances of the exposure incident; evaluating the source (donor) patient for clinical, epidemiologic, and laboratory evidence of hepatitis; and evaluating the hepatitis

B vaccination history and hepatitis infection/immunity status of the exposed healthcare worker. Prophylactic treatment must be provided to susceptible healthcare workers as soon as possible following accidental occupational percutaneous or mucosal exposures to HBsAg-positive blood. A regimen combining HBIg and hepatitis B vaccine provides both short- and long-term protection and is the treatment of choice. At the Clinical Center, we often already know not only the vaccination status and HBV immunity status of the exposed healthcare worker but also the hepatitis status of many of the patients participating in research protocols. In many hospitals, this information will not be readily available, and employee treatment may have to be initiated pending laboratory test results. The most recent CDC recommendations (241) for prophylaxis should be followed. As soon as possible following the exposure, the vaccination status and immunity status of the exposed worker should be reviewed. If the exposed worker has not been vaccinated or has not completed vaccination, the vaccine series should be started and a single dose of HBIg (0.06 mL/kg) should be given as soon as possible, preferably within 24 hours of exposure. The vaccine should be administered in the deltoid at a separate site and can be given simultaneously with HBIg or within 7 days of exposure. If the exposed worker has already been vaccinated for hepatitis B and is known to have detectable antibody (anti-HBs ≥10 mIU/mL), no treatment is indicated. If the exposed worker has already been vaccinated and is known to be a nonresponder (anti-HBs <10 mIU/mL), either administration of a single dose of HBIg and initiation of revaccination are indicated, or a dose of HBIg should be given as soon as possible followed by a second dose 1 month later. If the exposed worker has been vaccinated but the employee's anti-HBs response status is unknown, the worker should be tested for antibody; if adequate, no treatment is indicated; if <10 mIU/mL, a single dose of HBIg and a vaccine booster dose should be given. CDC recommendations (224,241) should be consulted for prophylaxis of healthcare workers when the source is HBsAg-negative, not tested for HBsAg, or the status is unknown.

The occupational medical service (employee health service) plays an especially important role in the management of employees who have sustained occupational exposures to bloodborne pathogens. Counseling exposed employees is a crucial component of postexposure management. Counseling these employees is complex, labor-intensive, and often time-consuming and emotionally draining (244). The counselor should collect the epidemiologic details relevant to the exposure (i.e., how and why the exposure took place). In addition, the counselor should (a) provide the exposed healthcare worker with estimates (based on the literature) of the risk of infection associated with exposures of the type sustained by the worker; (b) discuss in detail the therapeutic postexposure management options (e.g., HBIg, vaccine), and the short- and long-term side effects associated with these options; (c) discuss the plan for follow-up (and the importance of compliance with that plan); (d) discuss precautions that may be useful to avoid transmission to others should the injury result in infection; (e) provide emotional support for the exposed worker; (f) respond to any questions related to the exposure; and (g) encourage the exposed employee to call or return with additional questions (244).

MANAGEMENT OF EMPLOYEES WHO ARE CHRONIC CARRIERS OF HEPATITIS B

The risk of HBV being transmitted from an infected healthcare provider to a patient is virtually nonexistent in the setting of routine patient care contact. A small but nonetheless real risk for provider-to-patient HBV transmission does exist for invasive patient contact (i.e., situations accompanied by some risk for the patient to be exposed to the blood of the healthcare provider). Personnel who are HBeAg-positive HBV carriers present a slightly higher level of risk to their patients. Through 1994, investigators at the CDC identified 42 instances of provider-to-patient HBV transmission (infecting over 375 patients) (245), and instances continue to occur. When the HBeAg status of the infected workers responsible for provider-to-patient transmission has been determined, nearly all have been e-antigen positive, with rare exceptions: four surgeons all of whom harbored a virus that was a precore mutant (i.e., one genetically unable to express HBeAg but still capable of assembling infectious virions) (246) and another case also involving a surgeon (247). With the exception of providers who have been shown to transmit infection to patients, historically no restrictions had been placed on healthcare workers who were chronically infected with HBV (248–250). Although contrary to previously issued guidelines and recommendations, new guidelines were issued by the CDC in July 1991 recommending that healthcare workers who perform exposure-prone invasive procedures be aware of their HBV infection statuses; those who are found to be HBeAg-positive should not perform such procedures unless they have sought the counsel of an expert review panel and been advised under what circumstances (if any) they would be allowed to perform these procedures (250). Further, these guidelines note that HBeAg-positive healthcare workers should inform prospective patients about their (i.e., the provider's) infection status (250). Congress subsequently mandated that states must implement the CDC guidelines or certify state guidelines as equivalent as a condition for continued federal public health funding. Consequently, local or state public health officials should be contacted to determine the regulations or recommendations applicable in a given area. In August 1993, the United Kingdom health departments issued revised guidelines requiring vaccination of all nonimmune healthcare workers who perform procedures "in which injury to the worker could result in blood contaminating the patient's open tissues." They further require postvaccination testing to document response to the vaccine and practice restrictions for surgeons who are found on postvaccine testing to be HBeAg carriers (251). Because of the recently published incidents of HBeAg-negative surgeons transmitting hepatitis B infection, others are proposing HBV DNA quantitation testing of HBeAg-negative workers to determine infectivity and permission to perform high-risk procedures (252,253). Preliminary investigations in HBeAg-negative hepatitis B carriers in Britain suggest that 38% of HBeAg-negative carriers may be potentially infectious if the presence of DNA by genome amplification were the criterion used to define infectivity, and 20% would be considered infectious if presence of the precore mutant were the criterion used (254).

A thorough discussion of the problems raised by excluding

practitioners infected with bloodborne pathogens is beyond the scope of this chapter. These complex management issues have been addressed in detail elsewhere (255–260). The Society for Healthcare Epidemiology of America (SHEA) has issued detailed recommendations regarding the management of healthcare workers infected with bloodborne pathogens (260). SHEA recommends that HBeAg-positive workers routinely should double glove and should not perform activities that have been identified epidemiologically as associated with a risk for provider-to-patient HBV transmission despite the use of appropriate infection control procedures (e.g., vaginal hysterectomy, major pelvic surgery, and cardiac surgery). SHEA further recommends that HBV-infected healthcare workers should not be required to disclose their infection status to any patient, except for situations in which a patient has clearly been exposed to the worker's blood or other potentially infectious body fluid.

Two clusters of HBV infection from HBeAg-positive surgeons have occurred, despite increased attention to infection control measures. Four patients acquired clinical hepatitis B infection from an orthopedic surgeon (261), and 19 patients of a thoracic surgery resident became infected (262). No specific events or breaks in technique were identified in either cluster that could have led to the transmissions, although the surgical resident did not wear double gloves. In further investigations, the CDC had the resident perform laboratory simulations of tying surgical knots for an hour, which resulted in paper-cut–like skin lesions on the index fingers, and HBsAg and HBV DNA were detected in rinsings from his gloves. These lesions, combined with serous exudates and glove failure, could theoretically have caused HBV contamination of the patients' surgical wounds.

The management of practitioners who are chronically infected with bloodborne pathogens is complex for a variety of reasons. Because of the extremely limited data available, no single approach to this complex issue addresses all the relevant issues. Further, individuals who hold quite disparate positions with respect to the patients' right to know and the providers' right to privacy and medical confidentiality likely will have polar views of any individual approach to managing infected providers. Historically, science has provided the foundation for sentient public health policy. In many respects, the hepatitis B–infected practitioner has been "additional baggage" on the bandwagon of public sentiment being driven by societal anxiety about iatrogenic HIV transmission (255). Nonetheless, as additional data accumulate, the argument for considering the management of providers infected with each of the bloodborne viral infections on the evidence that relates specifically to that infection becomes increasingly more compelling.

Hepatitis C Virus

Unfortunately, unlike hepatitis B, there are no passive or active immunization products to prevent HCV infection. Prevention relies primarily on healthcare workers practicing universal precautions (see discussion in Hepatitis B Virus, above, and Chapter 79); universal precautions have also been shown to decrease transmission to patients in a high-risk setting (263).

MANAGEMENT OF EMPLOYEES SUSTAINING OCCUPATIONAL EXPOSURES TO HCV

The issue of postexposure prevention of HCV infection remains controversial. Testing for antibodies to HCV in source patients and in the exposed healthcare worker is subject to the limitations of serologic testing discussed previously. The HCV antibodies identified in the currently available antibody assays are not neutralizing for HCV and are not protective, due to substantial HCV strain variability that permits multiple infections (122,264,265). Therefore, anti-HCV identified in the "baseline" serum of an exposed employee does not indicate immunity. Conversely, HCV antibodies present in the source patient are not necessarily markers for infectivity of the source patient (although the source should be assumed to be infectious); such antibodies do not distinguish among acute, chronic, or resolved infection. Even third-generation anti-HCV testing will still not detect 5% to 10% of persons with HCV infection (113). HCV RNA testing by the PCR method is probably the best currently available test to identify source patients who are HCV-infected and infectious. As noted above, even the PCR methodology is fraught with complexity.

Current U.S. Public Health Service Guidelines

The CDC, in collaboration with HICPAC, has issued recommendations for follow-up of healthcare workers following occupational exposure to HCV (266,267). These recommendations emphasize that institutions should have policies and procedures for follow-up of personnel who sustain percutaneous or permucosal exposure to anti-HCV–positive blood. Such policies should include, at a minimum, (a) for the source, baseline testing for anti-HCV; (b) for the exposed worker, baseline and follow-up (e.g., 6-month) testing for anti-HCV and alanine aminotransferase activity; (c) confirmation by supplemental anti-HCV testing of all anti-HCV results reported as repeatedly reactive by EIA; (d) recommending against immediate postexposure prophylaxis with Ig or antiviral agents (e.g., interferon); and (e) education of workers about the risk for and prevention of bloodborne infections, including hepatitis C, in occupational settings, with the information routinely updated to ensure accuracy.

Several other potential interventions have been proposed for managing occupational exposures to HCV, including immunoprophylaxis with Ig, preemptive therapy of acute infection with immunomodulators, so-called watchful waiting with immunomodulators (211), and postexposure chemoprophylaxis (or chemoprophylaxis plus immunoprophylaxis with immunomodulators). Each of these approaches is worthy of additional consideration.

Immunoprophylaxis with Immunoglobulin

The issue of postexposure immunoprophylaxis with Ig also has been controversial, because no data demonstrate the efficacy of Ig in this setting. Data from earlier trials of Ig to prevent posttransfusion non-A, non-B hepatitis demonstrated mixed results (268–270). Although the CDC recommendations (62) once stated that "it may be reasonable to administer Ig (0.06 mL/kg) as soon as possible after exposure," more recent data have led the HICPAC to no longer endorse this practice (266, 271). In fact, neither of the authors' institutions offers postexposure treatment with Ig for occupational exposures to HCV. Although plasma pools for fractionation to derive Ig in the U.S. once included antibodies for HCV (272), currently the U.S. and other countries screen plasma donors and exclude HCV-positive donors; thus, Ig products no longer contain antibodies to HCV and therefore offer no theoretical benefit (267,273). Postexposure studies in experimentally infected chimpanzees have demonstrated that neither anti-HCV–negative intravenous Ig nor specially prepared hepatitis C Ig (containing significant titers of anti-HCV antibody) prevents HCV infection (274).

Postexposure Immunoprophylaxis with Immunomodulators

Immediate postexposure, short-duration interferon treatment has been attempted, but was not successful in preventing infection (86). For several theoretical reasons (delineated in detail in ref. 211), and in spite of inferences in the literature suggesting its efficacy, no current rationale supports the use of immunomodulating substances in the immediate postexposure setting. As noted above, one could actually mount reasonable arguments as to why immunomodulators should not be administered in the very early phase of infection.

Postexposure Antiviral Chemoprophylaxis

Agent(s) with clearly defined antiviral activity against HCV (as compared with immunomodulatory activities) have yet to be made available in the healthcare market. Some agents that are designed to have specific anti-HCV activity are in the drug-development process. In the absence of data demonstrating both the relative safety (i.e., since the transmission risk is, at most, 2% to 3%, then 97% to 98% of those given the agent would not need the treatment) as well as efficacy of anti-HCV agents, no recommendation can be made about their potential use in the postexposure setting. Should some of these compounds be demonstrated to have specific antiviral activity against HCV (and to be reasonably safe), they could become candidates for postexposure chemoprophylaxis for occupational exposure to HCV (211).

Preemptive Treatment of Acute HCV Infection vs. Watchful Waiting and Treatment of Established HCV Infection (211)

Another proposed postexposure management strategy, first suggested by Schiff et al. (122) in 1990, involves weekly monitoring of exposed persons for HCV RNA and initiating interferon treatment when infection is either first detected, preemptive treatment, or when it appears that the infection may become chronic (275). The practicality of such an approach notwithstanding, definitive data are not yet available to document the efficacy of this approach, though many institutions in the U.S. are adopting this approach or some modification of it (276).

Perhaps one of the most compelling arguments for the use of one of the PCR monitoring strategies is the remarkable experience published over the past few years describing the treatment of patients who have the acute hepatitis C syndrome (277–283). These studies have shown cure/resolution rates among patients who received treatment for their acute infections that are much higher than one would expect, based on the experience treating patients who have chronic HCV infection (284–286). In one of the studies of the therapy of acute hepatitis C, HCV RNA was undetectable and alanine aminotransferase levels were entirely normal in 43 of the 44 patients who were studied (282). This 98% cure rate dwarfs any previously published study of the treatment of HCV infection.

Comparing the treatment of patients with the acute hepatitis C syndrome with those who are chronically infected may not be entirely appropriate. Immunologic responses to HCV infection are complex, and individuals who develop acute hepatitis at the time of infection may represent a population of individuals who are capable of mounting more aggressive immunologic responses to the infection. Other studies of therapy of acute hepatitis C have produced similar, but not quite so striking, successes (279,287,288).

Despite the fact that all of the studies describing the treatment of early or acute HCV infection have substantial limitations (discussed in detail in refs. 211 and 275), the outcomes associated with the therapy of the acute hepatitis C syndrome almost uniformly suggest that treatment of acute HCV infection is advantageous. The recently published NIH Consensus Conference on Hepatitis C concluded that patients identified with acute hepatitis C should received therapy with immunomodulators (283).

Following this approach, an institution's occupational medicine staff monitors healthcare workers who have sustained occupational exposures (at approximately 2-week intervals following an occupational exposure to HCV) using HCV RNA-PCR. In some institutions, if infection is definitively identified (as demonstrated by repeatedly positive HCV RNA detection from the serum of the exposed worker), interferon therapy is initiated. Regimens selected have varied. Jaeckel et al. (282) used a regimen of 5 million units of interferon alpha-2b subcutaneously daily for 4 weeks and then the same dose administered three times per week for an additional 20 weeks.

Others have suggested watchful waiting, also using PCR monitoring. Following this strategy, the institution's occupational medicine staff would also monitor the exposed healthcare worker at 2-week intervals by HCV PCR, and then closely follow individuals who become HCV PCR positive to see if chronic infection develops. One approach has been to recommend interferon treatment only for those who remain HCV-RNA-PCR positive and have elevated alanine aminotransferase levels 2 to 4 months into the course of their infections (211,275,283). This approach allows a substantial fraction of individuals to resolve their infections spontaneously and would not put individuals who spontaneously recover at risk for the substantial toxicity associated with therapy with interferon (275). Both these approaches have merit and both have at least anecdotal support in the literature. The preemptive therapy approach has been used successfully in several instances (88,171,173,179,289), and unsuccessfully in others (86). The case report describing failure of a postexposure interferon intervention provides indirect support for the watchful waiting strategy. In this case the exposed individual received postexposure prophylaxis with interferon-α, 5 million units per day intramuscularly for 4 days, beginning on the day of exposure (86). One month later, he developed elevated aminotransferase levels and was positive for HCV RNA by PCR; 11 weeks later, his anti-HCV antibody test was positive, and 6 months after the exposure his liver biopsy demonstrated chronic persistent hepatitis. The patient subsequently was treated with a 6-month course of interferon-α and was apparently cured (86).

The CDC has not made formal recommendations concerning the use of either of these latter two strategies; however, as noted above, a substantial number of hospitals in the U.S. have adopted these strategies for managing occupational HCV exposures (276). Both the preemptive therapy and watchful waiting models represent entirely reasonable approaches to the management of occupational HCV exposure based on the currently available information. Monitoring for HCV by PCR, monitoring alanine aminotransferase levels, and making management decisions based on these data and the individual's clinical status represents perhaps the most reasonable approach to postexposure management, in our view and seems, in our opinion, to represent a substantially improved strategy over the current USPHS recommendation to monitor anti-HCV antibody at 3 months and 6 months following exposure (241,290). The watchful waiting strategy is the approach currently in use at the Clinical Center at the NIH.

MANAGEMENT OF EMPLOYEES WHO ARE CHRONICALLY INFECTED WITH HEPATITIS C

The transmission of HCV from healthcare provider to patient has been reported uncommonly, albeit with some increased frequency in the past 3 years. As is the case for HBV carriers, individuals chronically infected with HCV are unlikely to transmit infection during routine patient contact. The risk for provider-to-patient HCV transmission during invasive patient contact (in which the patient may be exposed to the blood of the healthcare provider) is very small and, because of the lower titers of virus present in the circulation, is likely to be even lower than the risk for HBV transmission. Several cases of iatrogenic HCV transmission have been reported in the past few years, primarily in Europe, and specifically in the United Kingdom (291–301).

The first published instance of provider-to-patient transmission was detected in a posttransfusion hepatitis study conducted in Spain (292) when patients were found to have become infected with HCV despite the fact that all blood donors tested negative for anti-HCV and HCV RNA (although an instance in which HCV transmission was suspected but not proven had been described from the U.K. a year earlier) (291). In the Spanish study, patients had undergone heart valve replacements performed by the same surgeon, who was subsequently found to be anti-HCV–positive, to have high titers of HCV RNA, and to have elevated liver function tests. The surgeon and five patients had infections with HCV genotype 3 I (a rare genotype in Spain); genotype comparison of the sequences and phylogenetic-tree analysis indicated a common epidemiologic origin for these viral strains. The surgeon reported sustaining percutaneous injuries frequently, most of which occurred while tying the wires during closure of the sternum, and many injuries were not noticed until after completion of the procedure. He also reported infrequent percutaneous injuries with sharp objects and needles; after such an injury he would remove the instrument from the field and change gloves. The surgeon did not recall an instance of bleeding into a patient's wound, and he had no history of dermatitis. Although the precise mode of transmission remains unknown, these findings suggest that transmission was associated with percutaneous injuries.

The analysis of the case from the U.K. cited above as initially described in 1995 (291) was ultimately published in 1999 (302). In this investigation, one of 278 potentially exposed patients developed HCV infection with a strain identical to their surgeon's strain (302). A third case of hepatitis C transmission from a gynecologic surgeon to his patients was reported from the U.K. in 1999 (295); however, the complete details of the large look-back investigation are not yet available. More than 4,500 former and current patients of the HCV-infected gynecologic surgeon were contacted and eight were found to have HCV strains identical to the surgeon's (298,303). An additional case of provider-to-patient transmission occurred in a child who acquired infection through probable percutaneous exposure to his mother's HCV-infected blood during infusion of clotting-factor concentrate (304). Sequence analysis indicated the mother's and child's HCV strains were identical. While attempting infusions, the mother did not wear gloves and recalled instances of pricking her finger with the needle (drawing a visible quantity of blood), but she could not recall if she continued to use the same needle for the infusion.

Ross et al. (305) evaluated 207 of the 229 surgical patients of an HCV-infected orthopedic surgeon in Germany and found three of the 207 to be HCV infected (as determined by a positive HCV-antibody test). One of the three was infected with an HCV isolate that was virtually identical to the surgeon's. The patient had undergone a total hip arthroplasty with trochanteric osteotomy. These same investigators also evaluated patients of a German gynecologic surgeon who was found to be HCV infected. The gynecologist transmitted HCV infection to a single patient on whom he had performed a cesarean section (301). None of the surgeon's nearly 3,000 patients were found to have acquired infection (301). In the single case of healthcare provider–to-patient transmission of HCV reported to date from the U.S., Cody et al. (299) documented HCV transmission from an anesthesiologist who had acute HCV infection to a patient for whom the physician had provided anesthesia care during the patient's thoracic surgical operation. None of an additional 348 patients for whom this physician had provided anesthesia services were found to be infected.

Two additional look-back studies are underway in the U.K. involving 2,650 patients of two HCV-infected providers (300, 303). Four infections have been linked to the two providers (three in the first study and only one in the second) (300,303).

A major outbreak of provider-to-patient HCV transmission

was reported in Spain, where an HCV-infected anesthetist, a morphine addict, infected over 200 postoperative patients by giving himself part of the syringe contents of postoperative opioid analgesia first, and then giving the remainder to the patients using the same syringe (293,296).

In summary, only these few instances of iatrogenic HCV transmission have been documented to date (and only one of these occurred in the U.S.). The fact that the number of cases in Europe has increased substantially over the past several years is a matter of substantial concern. Nonetheless, iatrogenic transmission appears to be an extremely rare event, occurring only during unusual invasive circumstances from providers who have high titers of HCV RNA. There are currently no USPHS recommendations suggesting restriction of U.S. healthcare workers with HCV infection; in fact, existing guidelines suggest these practitioners need not be restricted (267,306). Based on the U.S. experience to date, practice restrictions are probably unnecessary, unless transmission has been documented. Each infected provider should be evaluated individually. Conversely, because of the number of iatrogenic cases of HCV infection recently detected in the U.K., the U.K. government has recently recommended practice restrictions for HCV-infected providers (307). If the U.K. experience is ultimately borne out in the U.S., current policies may need revision.

Hepatitis D Virus

Prevention of HDV in healthcare workers is best accomplished by preventing primary HBV infection. Although preliminary immunization studies in animals show some promise in limiting HDV infection (308), no agents are currently available for active or passive immunization of healthcare workers who are already infected with HBV against HDV. This situation is worrisome, because workers who are already infected with HBV are at risk of developing severe acute illness and chronic liver disease should they acquire HDV superinfection (188). This possibility provides an additional compelling reason for healthcare workers to become vaccinated against HBV. Preliminary experimental studies of treatment of chronic HDV infection with interferon-α indicate that HDV replication may be inhibited, but this response may be transient. In one study, treatment for a year with high doses of interferon alpha-2a resulted in improvement in about half of treated patients, but relapse was still common (309). Further long-term studies are needed to clarify the role of interferon-α in the therapy of HDV infection (310). Currently, the only preventive measure available for those infected with HBV is scrupulous adherence to universal precautions to minimize occupational exposures to blood.

Hepatitis E Virus

HEV transmission to healthcare workers in most developed countries is extremely rare. The diagnosis of HEV infection should be considered in travelers who have diarrhea and hepatitis and are returning from endemic areas. Precautions similar to those for preventing nosocomial acquisition of HAV should be adequate to prevent fecal-oral transmission. Workers in settings in which HEV may be present, such as refugee camps, should be especially careful to practice meticulous hand washing after patient contact and before eating and smoking (206). Unlike HAV, no agents are currently available for immunization or passive immunoprophylaxis following exposure to HEV. An experimental vaccine has been successful in monkeys (311), and a recombinant vaccine is currently in phase III clinical trials (205,209). Ig manufactured in nonendemic areas is likely not to be protective because of a lack of antibody to HEV (312), and the efficacy of Ig from endemic areas is unknown. There is conflicting evidence that IgG anti-HEV protects against hepatitis E and HEV infection in monkeys and humans. Earlier studies suggested that protective antibodies exist (311,313), but a later study demonstrated that passive immunization with HEV antibodies was not protective (314). No HEV-specific Ig is currently available for protection from HEV.

REFERENCES

1. Leibowitz S, Greenwald L, Cohen I, et al. Serum hepatitis in a blood bank worker. *JAMA* 1949;140:1331–1333.
2. Deka N, Sharma M, Mukerjee R. Isolation of the novel agent from human stool samples that is associated with sporadic non-A, non-B hepatitis. *J Virol* 1994;68:7810–7815.
3. Leary T, Muerhoff A, Simons J, et al. Sequence and genomic organization of GBV-C: a novel member of the Flaviviridae associated with human non–A-E hepatitis. *J Med Virol* 1996;48:60–67.
4. Simons J, Pilot-Matias T, Leary T, et al. Identification of two flavivirus-like genomes in the GB hepatitis agent. *Proc Natl Acad Sci USA* 1995;92:3401–3405.
5. Alter M, Gallagher M, Morris T, et al. Acute non-A–E hepatitis in the United States and the role of hepatitis G virus infection. *N Engl J Med* 1997;336:741–746.
6. Alter HJ, Nakatsuji Y, Melpolder J, et al. The incidence of transfusion-associated hepatitis G virus infection and its relation to liver disease. *N Engl J Med* 1997;336(11):747–754.
7. Heuft H, Berg T, Schreier E, et al. Epidemiological and clinical aspects of hepatitis G virus infection in blood donors and immunocompromised recipients of HGV-contaminated blood. *Vox Sang* 1998;74:161–167.
8. Linnen J, Wages J Jr, Zhang-Keck ZY, et al. Molecular cloning and disease association of hepatitis G virus: a transfusion-transmissible agent. *Science* 1996;271(5248):505–508.
9. Pessoa M, Terrault N, Detmer J, et al. Quantitation of hepatitis G and C viruses in the liver: evidence that hepatitis G virus is not hepatotropic. *Hepatology* 1998;27:877–880.
10. Arankalle V, Chadha M, Tsarev S, et al. Seroepidemiology of water-borne hepatitis in India and evidence for a third enterically-transmitted hepatitis agent. *Proc Natl Acad Sci USA* 1994;91:3428–3432.
11. Miyake Y, Sugiyama K, Goto K, et al. Using polymerase chain reaction to detect the etiological virus of serologically non-A, non-B, non-C fulminant hepatitis in Japanese children. *Acta Paediatr Jpn* 1998;40:102–104.
12. Okamoto H, Nishizawa T, Kato N, et al. Molecular cloning and characterization of a novel DNA virus (TTV) associated with post-transfusion hepatitis of unknown etiology. *Hepatol Res* 1998;10:1–16.
13. Gibas A, Blewett DR, Schoenfeld DA, et al. Prevalence and incidence of viral hepatitis in health workers in the prehepatitis B vaccination era. *Am J Epidemiol* 1992;136:603–610.
14. Francis DP. Occurrence of hepatitis A, B, and non-A/non-B in the United States. *Am J Med* 1984;76:69–74.
15. Kashiwagi S, Hayashi J, Ikematsu H, et al. Prevalence of immunologic markers of hepatitis A and B infection in hospital personnel in Miyazaki Prefecture, Japan. *Am J Epidemiol* 1985;122:960–969.
16. Maynard JE. Viral hepatitis as an occupational hazard in the health care profession. In: Vyas GN, Cohen SN, Schmid R, eds. *Viral hepati-*

tis: etiology, epidemiology, pathogenesis and prevention. Philadelphia: Franklin Institute, 1978:321–331.

17. Szmuness W, Dienstag JL, Purcell RH, et al. Hepatitis type A and hemodialysis: a seroepidemiologic study in 15 U.S. centers. *Ann Intern Med* 1977;87:8–12.
18. Center for Disease Control. Outbreak of viral hepatitis in the staff of a pediatric ward—California. *MMWR* 1977;26:77–78.
19. Orenstein WA, Wu E, Wilkins J, et al. Hospital-acquired hepatitis A: report of an outbreak. *Pediatrics* 1981;67:494–497.
20. Seeberg S, Brandberg Å, Hermodsson S, et al. Hospital outbreak of hepatitis A secondary to blood exchange in a baby. *Lancet* 1981;1: 1155–1156.
21. Goodman RA, Carder CC, Allen JR, et al. Nosocomial hepatitis A transmission by an adult patient with diarrhea. *Am J Med* 1982;73: 220–226.
22. Klein BS, Michaels JA, Rytel MW, et al. Nosocomial hepatitis A: a multinursery outbreak in Wisconsin. *JAMA* 1984;252:2716–2721.
23. Noble RC, Kane MA, Reeves SA, et al. Posttransfusion hepatitis A in a neonatal intensive care unit. *JAMA* 1984;252:2711–2715.
24. Krober MS, Bass JW, Brown JD, et al. Hospital outbreak of hepatitis A: risk factors for spread. *Pediatr Infect Dis J* 1984;3:296–299.
25. Reed CM, Gustafson TL, Siegel J, et al. Nosocomial transmission of hepatitis A from a hospital-acquired case. *Pediatr Infect Dis J* 1984; 3:300–303.
26. Edgar WM, Campbell AD. Nosocomial infection with hepatitis A. *J Infect* 1985;10:43–47.
27. Skidmore SJ, Gully PR, Middleton JD, et al. An outbreak of hepatitis A on a hospital ward. *J Med Virol* 1985;17:175–177.
28. Azimi PH, Roberto RR, Guralnik J, et al. Transfusion-acquired hepatitis A in a premature infant with secondary nosocomial spread in an intensive care nursery. *Am J Dis Child* 1986;140:23–27.
29. Baptiste R, Koziol DE, Henderson DK. Nosocomial transmission of hepatitis A in an adult population. *Infect Control* 1987;8:364–370.
30. Drusin LM, Sohmer M, Groshen SL, et al. Nosocomial hepatitis A infection in a paediatric intensive care unit. *Arch Dis Child* 1987;62: 690–695.
31. Rosenblum LS, Villarino ME, Nainan OV, et al. Hepatitis A outbreak in a neonatal intensive care unit: risk factors for transmission and evidence of prolonged viral excretion among preterm infants. *J Infect Dis* 1991;164:476–482.
32. Earl A, O'Keete J, Huston M, et al. A nosocomial outbreak of hepatitis A among nursing staff on a medical unit. *Am J Infect Control* 1991; 19:116.
33. Petrosillo N, Raffaele B, Martini L, et al. A nosocomial and occupational cluster of hepatitis A virus infection in a pediatric ward. *Infect Control Hosp Epidemiol* 2002;23(6):343–345.
34. Earl A, Larson R, Seweryn S, et al. Hepatitis A outbreak among students and employees of a university medical center. *Am J Infect Control* 1994;22:124.
35. Eisenstein AB, Aach RD, Jacobsohn W, et al. An epidemic of infectious hepatitis in a general hospital: possible transmission by contaminated orange juice. *JAMA* 1963;185:171–174.
36. Meyers JD, Romm FJ, Tihen WS, et al. Food-borne hepatitis A in a general hospital: epidemiologic study of an outbreak attributed to sandwiches. *JAMA* 1975;231:1049–1053.
37. Lee KK, Vargo LR, Lê CT, et al. Transfusion-acquired hepatitis A outbreak from fresh frozen plasma in a neonatal intensive care unit. *Pediatr Infect Dis J* 1992;11:122–123.
38. Watson JC, Fleming DW, Borella AJ, et al. Vertical transmission of hepatitis A resulting in an outbreak in a neonatal intensive care unit. *J Infect Dis* 1993;167(567–571).
39. Mbithi JN, Springthorpe S, Boulet JR, et al. Survival of hepatitis A virus on human hands and its transfer on contact with animate and inanimate surfaces. *J Clin Microbiol* 1992;30:757–763.
40. Hofmann F, Wehrle G, Berthold H, et al. Hepatitis A as an occupational hazard. *Vaccine* 1992;10(suppl):S82–S84.
41. Van Damme P, Cramm M, Van der Auwera J-C, et al. Hepatitis A vaccination for health care workers. *BMJ* 1993;306:1615.
42. Germanaud J. Hepatitis A and health care personnel. *Arch Intern Med* 1994;154:820–822.
43. Jensenius M, Ringertz SH, Berild D, et al. Prolonged nosocomial outbreak of hepatitis A arising from an alcoholic with pneumonia. *Scand J Infect Dis* 1998;30(2):119–123.
44. Doebbeling B, Li N, Wenzel R. An outbreak of hepatitis A among health care workers: risk factors for transmission. *Am J Public Health* 1993;83:1679–1684.
45. Hanna J, Loewenthal M, Negel P, et al. An outbreak of hepatitis A in an intensive care unit. *Anaesth Intens Care* 1996;24:440–444.
46. Bradley DW, Hollinger B, Hornbeck CL, et al. Isolation and characterization of hepatitis A virus. *Am J Clin Pathol* 1976;65:876–889.
47. Tassopoulos NC, Papaevangelou GJ, Ticehurst JR, et al. Fecal excretion of Greek strains of hepatitis A virus in patients with hepatitis A and in experimentally infected chimpanzees. *J Infect Dis* 1986;154: 231–237.
48. Hadler SC. Hepatitis B virus infection and health care workers. *Vaccine* 1990;8:S24–28.
49. Department of Labor, Department of Health and Human Services. Joint advisory notice: protection against occupational exposure to hepatitis B virus (HBV) and human immunodeficiency virus (HIV). *Fed Reg* 1987;52::41818–41824.
50. Mahoney FJ, Stewart K, Hu H, et al. Progress toward the elimination of hepatitis B virus transmission among health care workers in the United States. *Arch Intern Med* 1997;147:2601–2605.
51. Williams SV, Huff JC, Feinglass EJ, et al. Epidemic viral hepatitis, type B, in hospital personnel. *Am J Med* 1974;57:904–911.
52. Pattison CP, Maynard JE, Berquist KR, et al. Epidemiology of hepatitis B in hospital personnel. *Am J Epidemiol* 1975;101:59–64.
53. Denes AE, Smith JL, Maynard JE, et al. Hepatitis B infection in physicians: results of a nationwide seroepidemiologic survey. *JAMA* 1978;239(3):210–212.
54. Dienstag JL, Ryan DM. Occupational exposure to hepatitis B virus in hospital personnel: infection or immunization. *Am J Epidemiol* 1982;115:26–39.
55. Jovanovich JF, Saravolatz LD, Arking LM. The risk of hepatitis B among select employee groups in an urban hospital. *JAMA* 1983;250: 1893–1894.
56. Snydman DR, Muñoz A, Werner BG, et al. A multivariate analysis of risk factors for hepatitis B virus infection among hospital employees screened for vaccination. *Am J Epidemiol* 1984;120:684–693.
57. Hadler SC, Doto IL, Maynard JE, et al. Occupational risk of hepatitis B infection in hospital workers. *Infect Control* 1985;6:24–31.
58. West DJ. The risk of hepatitis B infection among health professionals in the United States: a review. *Am J Med Sci* 1984;287(2):26–33.
59. Harris JR, Finger RF, Kobayashi JM, et al. The low risk of hepatitis B in rural hospitals: results of a seroepidemiologic survey. *JAMA* 1984; 252:3270–3272.
60. Chalmers TC. Hemodialysis-associated hepatitis. *JAMA* 1973;225: 412–414.
61. Snydman DR, Bregman D, Bryan JA. Hemodialysis-associated hepatitis in the United States, 1974. *J Infect Dis* 1977;135:687–691.
62. Centers for Disease Control. Protection against viral hepatitis: Recommendations of the Immunization Practices Advisory Committee (ACIP). *MMWR* 1990;39:1–26.
63. Mosley JW. Measures to prevent intrahospital transmission of HBV. In: Szmuness W, Alter HJ, Maynard JE, eds. *Viral hepatitis.* Philadelphia: Franklin Institute, 1982:547–562.
64. Seefe LB, Wright EC, Zimmerman HJ, et al. Type B hepatitis after needlestick exposure: prevention with hepatitis B immune globulin: final report of the Veterans' Administration Cooperative Study. *Ann Intern Med* 1978;88:285–293.
65. Werner BJ, Grady GF. Accidental hepatitis-B-surface- antigen-positive inoculations: use of "e" antigen to estimate infectivity. *Ann Intern Med* 1982;97:367–369.
66. Tabor E, Purcell RH, Gerety RJ. Primate animal models and titered inocula for the study of human hepatitis A, hepatitis B, and non-A, non-B hepatitis. *J Med Primatol* 1983;12:305–318.
67. Department of Labor OSHA. Occupational exposure to bloodborne pathogens; final rule. *Fed Reg* 1991;56:64175–64182.
68. Pattison CP, Boyer KM, Maynard JE, et al. Epidemic hepatitis in a

clinical laboratory: possible association with computer card handling. *JAMA* 1974;230:854–857.

69. Alter MJ, Favero MS, Maynard JE. Impact of infection control strategies on the incidence of dialysis-associated hepatitis in the United States. *J Infect Dis* 1986;153:1149–1151.
70. Snydman DR, Bryan JA, Macon EJ, et al. Hemodialysis-associated hepatitis: report of an epidemic with further evidence on mechanisms of transmission. *Am J Epidemiol* 1976;104:563–570.
71. Francis DP, Maynard JE. The transmission and outcome of hepatitis A, B, and non-A, non-B: a review. *Epidemiol Rev* 1979;1:17–31.
72. Thomas DL, Factor SH, Kelen GD, et al. Viral hepatitis in health care personnel at The Johns Hopkins Hospital. The seroprevalence of, and risk factors for, hepatitis B virus and hepatitis C virus infection. *Arch Intern Med* 1993;153(14):1705–1712.
73. Panlilio AL, Shapiro CN, Schable CA, et al. Serosurvey of human immunodeficiency virus, hepatitis B virus, and hepatitis C virus infection among hospital-based surgeons. Serosurvey Study Group. *J Am Coll Surg* 1995;180(1):16–24.
74. Lanphear BP, Linnemann CC, Cannon CG, et al. Decline of clinical hepatitis B in workers at a general hospital: relation to increasing vaccine-induced immunity. *Clin Infect Dis* 1993;16:10–14.
75. Center for Disease Control. Non-A, non-B hepatitis infection transmitted via a needle—Washington. *MMWR* 1979;28:157–158.
76. Ahtone J, Francis D, Bradley D, et al. Non-A, non-B hepatitis in a nurse after percutaneous needle exposure. *Lancet* 1980;1:1142.
77. Henderson DK, Saah AJ, Zak BJ, et al. Risk of nosocomial infection with human T-cell lymphotropic virus type III/lymphadenopathy-associated virus in a large cohort of intensively exposed health care workers. *Ann Intern Med* 1986;104(5):644–647.
78. Mayo-Smith MF. Type non-A, non-B and type B hepatitis transmitted by a single needlestick. *Am J Infect Control* 1987;15:266–267.
79. Schlipkoter U, Roggendorf M, Cholmakow K, et al. Transmission of hepatitis C virus (HCV) from a haemodialysis patient to a medical staff member. *Scand J Infect Dis* 1990;22(6):757–758.
80. Vaqlia A, Nicolin R, Puro V, et al. Needlestick hepatitis C virus seroconversion in a surgeon. *Lancet* 1990;336(8726):1315–1316.
81. Cariani E, Zonaro A, Primi D, et al. Detection of HCV RNA and antibodies to HCV after needlestick injury. *Lancet* 1991;337:850.
82. Seefe LB. Hepatitis C from a needlestick injury. *Ann Intern Med* 1991;115(5):411.
83. Marranconi F, Mecenero V, Pellizzer GP, et al. HCV infection after accidental needlestick injury in health-care workers. *Infection* 1992; 20(2):111.
84. Tsude K, Fujiyama S, Sato S, et al. Two cases of accidental transmission of hepatitis C to medical staff. *Hepatogastroenterology* 1992;39(1): 73–75.
85. Suzuki K, Mizokami M, Lau J, et al. Confirmation of hepatitis C virus transmission through needlestick accidents by molecular evolutionary analysis. *J Infect Dis* 1994;170(6):1575–1578.
86. Nakano Y, Kiyosawa K, Sodeyama T, et al. Acute hepatitis C transmitted by needlestick accident despite short duration interferon treatment. *J Gastroenterol Hepatol* 1995;10(5):609–611.
87. Mizuno Y, Suzuki K, Mori M, et al. Study of needlestick accidents and hepatitis C virus infection in healthcare workers by molecular evolutionary analysis. *J Hosp Infect* 1997;35:149–154.
88. Noguchi S, Sata M, Suzuki H, et al. Early therapy with interferon for acute hepatitis C acquired through a needlestick. *Clin Infect Dis* 1997;24(5):992–994.
89. Ridzon R, Gallagher K, Ciesielski C, et al. Simultaneous transmission of human immunodeficiency virus and hepatitis C virus from a needle-stick injury. *N Engl J Med* 1997;336(13):919–922.
90. Norder H, Bergstrom A, Uhnoo I, et al. Confirmation of nosocomial transmission of hepatitis C virus by phylogenetic analysis of the NS5-B region. *J Clin Microbiol* 1998;36(10):3066–3069.
91. Sulkowski MS, Ray SC, Thomas DL. Needlestick transmission of hepatitis C. *JAMA* 2002;287(18):2406–2413.
92. Abel S, Cesaire R, Cales-Quist D, et al. Occupational transmission of human immunodeficiency virus and hepatitis C virus after a punch. *Clin Infect Dis* 2000;31(6):1494–1495.
93. Wang J-T, Wang T-H, Lin J-T, et al. Hepatitis C virus RNA in saliva of patients with post-transfusion hepatitis C infection. *Lancet* 1991;337:48.
94. Young KC, Chang TT, Liou TC, et al. Detection of hepatitis C virus RNA in peripheral blood mononuclear cells and in saliva. *J Med Virol* 1993;41(1):55–60.
95. Liou TC, Chang TT, Young KC, et al. Detection of HCV RNA in saliva, urine, seminal fluid, and ascites. *J Med Virol* 1992;37(3): 197–202.
96. Dusheiko GM, Smith M, Scheuer PJ. Hepatitis C virus transmitted by human bite. *Lancet* 1990;336:503–504.
97. Figueiredo J, Borges A, Martinez R, et al. Transmission of hepatitis C virus but not human immunodeficiency virus type 1 by a human bite. *Clin Infect Dis* 1994;19:546–547.
98. Abe K, Kurata T, Shikata T, et al. Experimental transmission of non-A, non-B hepatitis by saliva. *J Infect Dis* 1987;155:1078–1079.
99. Silverman AL, Puccio JE, Kulesza GW, et al. HCV RNA is present in the menstrual blood of women with chronic hepatitis C infection. *Am J Gastroenterol* 1994;89(8):1201–1202.
100. Fiore RJ, Potenza D, Monno L, et al. Detection of HCV RNA in serum and seminal fluid from HIV-1 co-infected intravenous drug addicts. *J Med Virol* 1995;46(4):364–367.
101. Leruez-Ville M, Kunstmann JM, De Almeida M, et al. Detection of hepatitis C virus in the semen of infected men. *Lancet* 2000; 356(9223):42–43.
102. Laskus T, Radkowski M, Bednarska A, et al. Detection and analysis of hepatitis C virus sequences in cerebrospinal fluid. *J Virol* 2002; 76(19):10064–10068.
103. Sartori M, La TG, Agiletta M, et al. Transmission of hepatitis C via blood splash into conjunctiva. *Scand J Infect Dis* 1993;25(2): 270–271.
104. Rosen H. Acquisition of hepatitis C by a conjunctival splash. *Am J Infect Control* 1997;25:242–247.
105. Allander T, Medin C, Jacobson SH, et al. Transmission of hepatitis C virus by transfer of an infected individual to a new dialysis unit. *Nephron* 1996;73(1):110.
106. Le Pogam S, Le Chapois D, Christen R, et al. Hepatitis C in a hemodialysis unit: molecular evidence for nosocomial transmission. *J Clin Microbiol* 1998;36(10):3040–3043.
107. Wreghitt TG. Blood-borne virus infections in dialysis units—a review. *Rev Med Virol* 1999;9(2):101–109.
108. Abacioglu YH, Bacaksiz F, Bahar IH, et al. Molecular evidence of nosocomial transmission of hepatitis C virus in a haemodialysis unit. *Eur J Clin Microbiol Infect Dis* 2000;19(3):182–186.
109. Delarocque-Astagneau E, Baffoy N, Thiers V, et al. Outbreak of hepatitis C virus infection in a hemodialysis unit: potential transmission by the hemodialysis machine? *Infect Control Hosp Epidemiol* 2002; 23(6):328–334.
110. Piazza M, Borgia G, Picciotto L, et al. Detection of hepatitis C virus-RNA by polymerase chain reaction in dental surgeries. *J Med Virol* 1995;45:40–42.
111. De Medina M, Schiff E. Hepatitis C: diagnostic assays. *Semin Liver Dis* 1995;15:33–40.
112. Takaki A, Wiese M, Maertens G, et al. Cellular immune responses persist and humoral responses decrease two decades after recovery from a single-source outbreak of hepatitis C. *Nat Med* 2000;6(5): 578–582.
113. Alter MJ, Mast EE, Moyer LA, et al. Hepatitis C. *Infect Dis Clin North Am* 1998;12(1):13–26.
114. De Luca M, Ascione A, Vacca C, et al. Are health-care workers really at risk of HCV infection? *Lancet* 1992;339:1364–1365.
115. Amarapurkar D. Prevalence of hepatitis C antibodies in health-care workers. *Lancet* 1994;344:339.
116. Mortimer PP, Cohen BJ, Litton PA, et al. Hepatitis C virus antibody. *Lancet* 1989;2:798.
117. Hofmann H, Kunz C. Low risk of health care workers for infection with hepatitis C virus. *Infection* 1990;18(5):286–288.
118. Polywka S, Laufs R. Hepatitis C virus antibodies among different groups at risk and patients with suspected non-A, non-B hepatitis. *Infection* 1991;19:81–84.

119. Abb J. Prevalence of hepatitis C virus antibodies in hospital personnel. *Int J Med Microbiol* 1991;274:543–547.
120. Libanore M, Bicocchi R, Ghinelli F, et al. Prevalence of antibodies to hepatitis C virus in Italian health care workers. *Infection* 1992;20:50.
121. Mujeeb S, Khatri Y, Khanani R. Frequency of parenteral exposure and seroprevalence of HBV, HCV, and HIV among operating room personnel. *J Hosp Infect* 1997;38:133–137.
122. Schiff E, de Medina M, Hill M, et al. Prevalence of anti-HCV in the VA dental environment form 1979–1981. *Hepatology* 1990;12:849(abst).
123. Forseter G, Wormser G, Adler S, et al. Hepatitis C in the health care setting. II. Seroprevalence among hemodialysis staff and patients in suburban New York City. *Am J Infect Control* 1993;21(1):5–8.
124. Polish L, Tong M, Co R, et al. Risk factors for hepatitis C virus infection among health care personnel in a community hospital. *Am J Infect Control* 1993;21:196–200.
125. Shapiro C, Tokars J, Chamberland M, The American Academy of Orthopaedic Surgeons Serosurvey Study Committee. Use of the hepatitis-B vaccine and infection with hepatitis B and C among orthopaedic surgeons. *J Bone Joint Surg* 1996;78A:1791–1800.
126. Wormser GP, Forseter G, Joline C, et al. Hepatitis C infection in the health care setting. I. Low risk from parenteral exposure to blood of human immunodeficiency virus-infected patients. *Am J Infect Control* 1991;19(5):237–242.
127. Klein RS, Freeman K, Taylor PE, et al. Occupational risk for hepatitis C virus infection among New York City dentists. *Lancet* 1991;338:1539–1542.
128. Cooper BW, Krusell A, Tilton RC, et al. Seroprevalence of antibodies to hepatitis C virus in high-risk hospital personnel. *Infect Control Hosp Epidemiol* 1992;13:82–85.
129. Nakashima K, Kashiwagi S, Hayashi J, et al. Low prevalence of hepatitis C virus infection among hospital staff and acupuncturists in Kyushu, Japan. *J Infect* 1993;26:17–25.
130. Niu M, Coleman P, Alter M. Multicenter study of hepatitis C virus infection in chronic hemodialysis patients and hemodialysis center staff members. *Am J Kidney Dis* 1993;22:568–573.
131. Stellini R, Calzini A, Gussago A, et al. Low prevalence of anti-HCV antibodies in hospital workers. *Eur J Epidemiol* 1993;9:674–675.
132. Herbert AM, Walker DM, Davies KJ, et al. Occupationally acquired hepatitis C virus infection. *Lancet* 1992;339(8788):305.
133. Francavilla E, Rinaldi R, Cattelan AM, et al. Low prevalence of antibodies to hepatitis C virus in hospital employees. *Infection* 1992;20(5):295.
134. Fujiyama S, Kawano S, Sato S, et al. Prevalence of hepatitis C virus antibodies in hemodialysis patients and dialysis staff. *Hepatogastroenterol* 1992;39:161–165.
135. Campello C, Majori S, Poli A, et al. Prevalence of HCV antibodies in health-care workers from northern Italy. *Infection* 1992;20:224–226.
136. Jochen AB. Occupationally acquired hepatitis C virus infection. *Lancet* 1992;339(8788):304.
137. Kuo MY-P, Hahn L-J, Hong C-Y, et al. Low prevalence of hepatitis C virus infection among dentists in Taiwan. *J Med Virol* 1993;40:10–13.
138. Soni P, Tait D, Kenoyer D, et al. Hepatitis C virus antibodies among risk groups in a South African area endemic for hepatitis B virus. *J Med Virol* 1993;40:65–68.
139. Lanphear BP, Linnemann CC, Cannon CG, et al. Hepatitis C virus infection in healthcare workers: risk of exposure and infection. *Infect Control Hosp Epidemiol* 1994;15(12):745–750.
140. Gerberding JL. Incidence and prevalence of human immunodeficiency virus, hepatitis B virus, hepatitis C virus, and cytomegalovirus among health care personnel at risk for blood exposure: final report from a longitudinal study. *J Infect Dis* 1994;170:1410–1417.
141. Zuckerman J, Clewley G, Griffiths P, et al. Prevalence of hepatitis C antibodies in clinical health-care workers. *Lancet* 1994;343(8913):1618–1620.
142. Jadoul M, Akrout M, Cornu C, et al. Prevalence of hepatitis C antibodies in health-care workers. *Lancet* 1994;344:339.
143. Di Nardo V, Bonaventura M, Chiaretti B, et al. Low risk of HCV infection in health care workers. *Infection* 1994;22:115.
144. Struve J, Aronsson B, Frenning B, et al. Prevalence of antibodies against hepatitis C virus infection among health care workers in Stockholm. *Scand J Gastroenterol* 1994;29:360–362.
145. Germanaud J, Barthez J-P, Causse X. The occupational risk of hepatitis C infection among hospital employees. *Am J Public Health* 1994;84:122.
146. Puro V, Petrosillo N, Ippolito G, et al. Occupational hepatitis C virus infection in Italian health care workers. *Am J Public Health* 1995;85:1272–1275.
147. Di Nardo V, Petrosillo N, Ippolito G, et al. Prevalence and incidence of hepatitis B virus, hepatitis C virus and human immunodeficiency virus among personnel and patients of a psychiatric hospital. *Eur J Epidemiol* 1995;11:239–242.
148. Neal K, Dornan J, Irving W. Prevalence of hepatitis C antibodies among healthcare workers of two teaching hospitals. Who is at risk? *BMJ* 1997;314:179–180.
149. De Brouwer C, Lecomte A. HCV antibodies in clinical health-care workers. *Lancet* 1994;344:962.
150. De Mercato R, Guarnaccia D, Ciannella G, et al. Hepatitis C virus among health care workers. *Minerva Med* 1996;87(11):501–504.
151. Miyajima I, Sata M, Murashima S, et al. Prevalence of hepatitis C antibodies in health care personnel. *Kansenshogaku Zasshi* 1997;71(2):103–107.
152. Lodi G, Porter SR, Teo CG, et al. Prevalence of HCV infection in health care workers of a UK dental hospital. *Br Dent J* 1997;183(9):329–332.
153. Mihaly I, Lukacs A, Telegdy L, et al. Screening for hepatitis C of hospital personnel at the Szent Laszlo Hospital of Budapest. *Orv Hetil* 1996;137(50):2791–2794.
154. Irani-Hakime N, Aoun J, Khoury S, et al. Seroprevalence of hepatitis C infection among health care personnel in Beirut, Lebanon. *Am J Infect Control* 2001;29(1):20–23.
155. Villasis-Keever MA, Pena LA, Miranda-Novales G, et al. Prevalence of serological markers against measles, rubella, varicella, hepatitis B, hepatitis C, and human immunodeficiency virus among medical residents in Mexico. *Prev Med* 2001;32(5):424–428.
156. Ganju SA, Goel A. Prevalence of HBV and HCV infection among health care workers (HCWs). *J Commun Dis* 2000;32(3):228–230.
157. Weber C, Collet S, Fried R, et al. Low prevalence of hepatitis C virus antibody among Swiss dental health care workers. *J Hepatol* 2001;34(6):963–964.
158. Othman BM, Monem FS. Prevalence of hepatitis C virus antibodies among health care workers in Damascus, Syria. *Saudi Med J* 2001;22(7):603–605.
159. Sulotto F, Coggiola M, Meliga F, et al. Degree of hepatitis C infection risk in the health care setting. *Med Lav* 2002;93(1):34–42.
160. Daw MA, Elkaber MA, Drah AM, et al. Prevalence of Hepatitis C virus antibodies among different populations of relative and attributable risk. *Saudi Med J* 2002;23(11):1356–1360.
161. Shapiro CN. Occupational risk of infection with hepatitis B and hepatitis C virus. *Surg Clin North Am* 1995;75(6):1047–1056.
162. Kiyosawa K, Sodeyama T, Tanaka E, et al. Hepatitis C in hospital employees with needlestick injuries. *Ann Intern Med* 1991;115(5):367–369.
163. Hernandez ME, Bruguera M, Puyuelo T, et al. Risk of needle-stick injuries in the transmission of hepatitis C virus in hospital personnel. *J Hepatol* 1992;16(1–2):56–58.
164. Mitsui T, Iwano K, Masuko K, et al. Hepatitis C virus infection in medical personnel after needlestick accident. *Hepatology* 1992;16(5):1109–1114.
165. Sodeyama T, Kiyosawa K, Urushihara A, et al. Detection of hepatitis C virus markers and hepatitis C genomic-RNA after needlestick accidents. *Arch Intern Med* 1993;153(13):1565–1572.
166. Perez-Trallero E, Cilla G, Saenz JR. Occupational transmission of HCV. *Lancet* 1994;344(8921):548.
167. Petrosillo N, Puro V, Ippolito G, the Italian study group on blood-borne occupational risk in dialysis. Prevalence of hepatitis C antibodies in health-care workers. *Lancet* 1994;344:339–340.

168. Ippolito G, Puro V, De Carli G. Risk of Occupational HIV infection after needlestick. Paper presented at 10th International Conference on AIDS, August 7–12, 1994, Yokohama, Japan.
169. Puro V, Petrosillo N, Ippolito G. Risk of hepatitis C seroconversion after occupational exposures in health care workers. Italian Study Group on Occupational Risk of HIV and Other Bloodborne Infections. *Am J Infect Control* 1995;23(5):273–277.
170. Puro V, Petrosillo N, Ippolito G, et al. Hepatitis C virus infection in healthcare workers. *Infect Control Hosp Epidemiol* 1995;16:324–325.
171. Arai Y, Noda K, Enomoto N, et al. A prospective study of hepatitis C virus infection after needlestick accidents. *Liver* 1996;16(5):331–334.
172. Serra C, Torres M, Campins M. Occupational risk of hepatitis C virus infection after accidental exposure. Catalonia Group for the Study of the Occupational Risk of HCV Infection at Hospitals. *Med Clin (Barc)* 1998;111(17):645–649.
173. Takagi H, Uehara M, Kakizaki S, et al. Accidental transmission of HCV and treatment with interferon. *J Gastroenterol Hepatol* 1998; 13(3):238–243.
174. Veeder A, Stellrecht K, Steinmann A, et al. Hepatitis C infection in health care workers following percutaneous exposures to HCV positive sources (abstract). Paper presented at the eighth annual meeting of the Society for Healthcare Epidemiology of America, 1998, Orlando, Florida.
175. Hamid SS, Farooqui B, Rizvi Q, et al. Risk of transmission and features of hepatitis C after needlestick injuries. *Infect Control Hosp Epidemiol* 1999;20(1):63–64.
176. Hasan F, Askar H, Al Khalidi J, et al. Lack of transmission of hepatitis C virus following needlestick accidents. *Hepatogastroenterology* 1999; 46(27):1678–1681.
177. Baldo V, Floreani A, Dal Vecchio L, et al. Occupational risk of bloodborne viruses in healthcare workers: a 5-year surveillance program. *Infect Control Hosp Epidemiol* 2002;23(6):325–327.
178. Regez RM, Rietra PJ, van der Linden CT, et al. Reducing the risk of blood-transmitted infections of HIV, hepatitis B or C virus in a teaching hospital in Amsterdam—evaluation of a protocol for needlestick accidents among hospital staff during the period 1997–2001. *Ned Tijdschr Geneeskd* 2002;146(13):617–621.
179. Wang TY, Kuo HT, Chen LC, et al. Use of polymerase chain reaction for early detection and management of hepatitis C virus infection after needlestick injury. *Ann Clin Lab Sci* 2002;32(2):137–141.
180. Farci P, London WT, Wong DC, et al. The natural history of infection with hepatitis C virus (HCV) in chimpanzees: comparison of serologic responses measured with first- and second-generation assays and relationship to HCV viremia. *J Infect Dis* 1992;165:1006–1011.
181. Farci P, Alter HJ, Wong D, et al. A long-term study of hepatitis C virus replication in non-A, non-B hepatitis. *N Engl J Med* 1991;325: 98–104.
182. Cristiano K, Di Bisceglie A, Hoofnagle JH, et al. Hepatitis C viral RNA in serum of patients with chronic non-A, non-B hepatitis: detection by the polymerase chain reaction using multiple primer sets. *Hepatology* 1991;14:51–55.
183. Stroffolini T, Marzolini A, Palumbo F, et al. Incidence of non-A, non-B and HCV positive hepatitis in healthcare workers in Italy. *J Hosp Infect* 1996;33(2):131–137.
184. Henderson DK, Gerberding JL. Healthcare worker issues, including occupational and nonoccupational postexposure management. In: Dolin RMH, Saag MS, eds. *AIDS therapy,* 2nd ed. New York: Churchill Livingstone, 2003:327–346.
185. Kelen GD, Green GB, Purcell RH, et al. Hepatitis B and hepatitis C in emergency department patients. *N Engl J Med* 1992;326: 1399–1404.
186. Morand P, Dutertre N, Minazzi H, et al. Lack of seroconversion in a health care worker after polymerase chain reaction-documented acute hepatitis C resulting from a needlestick injury. *Clin Infect Dis* 2001; 33(5):727–729.
187. Lettau LA. The A, B, C, D, and E of viral hepatitis: spelling out the risks for healthcare workers. *Infect Control Hosp Epidemiol* 1992;13: 77–81.
188. Rizzetto M. The delta agent. *Hepatology* 1983;3:729–737.
189. Marinucci G, Valeri L, Di Giacomo C, et al. Spread of delta in a group of haemodialysis carriers of HBsAg. In: Verme G, Bonino F, Rizzetto M, eds. *Viral hepatitis and delta infection.* New York: Alan R. Liss, 1983:151–154.
190. Lettau LA, Alfred HJ, Glew RH, et al. Nosocomial transmission of delta hepatitis. *Ann Intern Med* 1986;104:631–635.
191. Rizzetto M. Hepatitis delta virus: biology and infection. In: Shikata T, Purcell RH, Uchida T, eds. *Viral hepatitis C, D and E.* Amsterdam: Elsevier, 1991:327–333.
192. De Cock KM, Bradley DW, Sandford NL, et al. Epidemic non-A, non-B hepatitis in patients from Pakistan. *Ann Intern Med* 1987;106: 227–230.
193. Dawson GJ, Mushahwar IK, Chau KH, et al. Detection of long-lasting antibody to hepatitis E virus in a US traveller to Pakistan. *Lancet* 1992;340:426–427.
194. Bader T, Krawczynski K, Polish L, et al. Hepatitis E in a U.S. traveler to Mexico. *N Engl J Med* 1991;325:1659.
195. Centers for Disease Control and Prevention. Hepatitis E among U.S. travelers, 1989–1992. *MMWR* 1993;42:1–4.
196. Smalley D, Brewer S, Dawson G, et al. Hepatitis E virus infection in an immigrant to the United States. *South Med J* 1996;89:994–996.
197. Munoz S, Bradley D, Martin P, et al. Hepatitis E virus found in patients with apparent fulminant non-A, non-B hepatitis. *Hepatology* 1992;16:76A.
198. Kwo P, Schlauder G, Carpenter H, et al. Acute hepatitis E by a new isolate acquired in the United States. *Mayo Clin Proc* 1997;72: 1133–1136.
199. Schlauder G, Dawson G, Erker J, et al. The sequence an phylogenetic analysis of a novel hepatitis E virus isolated from a patient with acute hepatitis reported in the United States. *J Gen Virol* 1998;79:447–456.
200. Mast E, Alter M, Holland P, et al. Evaluation of assays for antibody to hepatitis E virus by a serum panel. *Hepatology* 1998;27:857–861.
201. Thomas D, Yarbough P, Vlahov D, et al. Seroreactivity to hepatitis E virus in areas where the disease is not endemic. *J Clin Microbiol* 1997;35:1244–1247.
202. Ghabrah T, Tsarev S, Yarbough P, et al. Comparison of tests for antibody to hepatitis E virus. *J Med Virol* 1998;55:134–137.
203. Clayson E, Vaughn D, Innis B, et al. Association of hepatitis E virus with an outbreak of hepatitis at a military training camp in Nepal. *J Med Virol* 1998;54:178–182.
204. Purcell RH, Ticehurst JR. Enterically transmitted non-A, non-B hepatitis: epidemiology and clinical characteristics. In: Zuckerman AJ, ed. *Viral hepatitis and liver disease.* New York: Alan R. Liss, 1988: 131–137.
205. Worm HC, van der Poel WH, Brandstatter G. Hepatitis E: an overview. *Microbes Infect* 2002;4(6):657–666.
206. Centers for Disease Control. Enterically transmitted non-A, non-B hepatitis—East Africa. *MMWR* 1987;36:241–244.
207. Chauhan A, Jameel S, Dilawari JB, et al. Hepatitis E virus transmission to a volunteer. *Lancet* 1993;341:149–150.
208. Robson SC, Adams S, Brink N, et al. Hospital outbreak of hepatitis E. *Lancet* 1992;339:1424–1425.
209. Hyams KC. New perspectives on hepatitis E. *Curr Gastroenterol Rep* 2002;4(4):302–307.
210. Alter MJ, Margolis HS, Krawczynski K, et al. The natural history of community-acquired hepatitis C in the United States. *N Engl J Med* 1992;327:1899–1905.
211. Henderson DK. Managing occupational risks for hepatitis C transmission in the healthcare setting. *Clin Microbiol Rev* 2003;16(3): 546–568.
212. National Institute for Occupational Safety and Health. *Selecting, evaluating, and using sharps disposal container.* Washington, DC: U.S. Department of Health and Human Services, January 1998.
213. Garner J, Simmons B. Guideline for isolation precautions in hospitals. *Infect Control* 1983;4(suppl):245–325.
214. Garner JS. Guideline for isolation precautions in hospitals. The Hospital Infection Control Practices Advisory Committee. *Infect Control Hosp Epidemiol* 1996;17(1):53–80.
215. Centers for Disease Control and Prevention. Prevention of hepatitis A through active or passive immunization: recommendations of the Advisory Committee on Immunization Practices (ACIP). *MMWR* 1996;45(RR-15):1–30.

216. Centers for Disease Control and Prevention. Prevention of hepatitis A through active or passive immunization: Recommendations of the Advisory Committee on Immunization Practices (ACIP). *MMWR Recomm Rep* 1999;48(RR-12):1–37.
217. Lemon S, Thomas D. Vaccines to prevent viral hepatitis. *N Engl J Med* 1997;336:196–204.
218. Werzberger A, Kuter B, Nalin D. Six years' follow-up after hepatitis A vaccination. *N Engl J Med* 1998;338:1160.
219. Wiedermann G, Kundi M, Ambrosch F, et al. Inactivated hepatitis A vaccine: long-term antibody persistence. *Vaccine* 1997;15:612–615.
220. Koff R. Hepatitis A. *Lancet* 1998;351:1643–1649.
221. Smith S, Weber S, Wiblin T, et al. Cost-effectiveness of hepatitis A vaccination in healthcare workers. *Infect Control Hosp Epidemiol* 1997; 18:688–691.
222. Vento S, Garofano T, Renzini C, et al. Fulminant hepatitis associated with hepatitis A virus superinfection in patients with chronic hepatitis C. *N Engl J Med* 1998;338:286–290.
223. Berenguer M, Wright T. Are HCV-infected individuals candidates for hepatitis A vaccine? *Lancet* 1998;351:924–925.
224. Centers for Disease Control and Prevention. Immunization of health-care workers: recommendations of the Advisory Committee on Immunization Practices (ACIP) and the Hospital Infection Control Practices Advisory Committee (HIC-PAC). *MMWR* 1997;46(RR-18): 1–42.
225. Alter MJ, Hadler SC, Margolis HS, et al. The changing epidemiology of hepatitis B in the United States. Need for alternative vaccination strategies. *JAMA* 1990;263:1218–1222.
226. Agerton T, Mahoney F, Polish L, et al. Impact of the bloodborne pathogens standard on vaccination of healthcare workers with hepatitis B vaccine. *Infect Control Hosp Epidemiol* 1995;16:287–291.
227. Lanphear BP. Trends and patterns in the transmission of bloodborne pathogens to health care workers. *Epidemiol Rev* 1994;16(2): 437–450.
228. Howard RJ, Fry DE, Davis JM, et al. Hepatitis C virus infection in healthcare workers. Surgical Infection Society. *J Am Coll Surg* 1997; 184(5):540–552.
229. Hadler SC, Margolis HS. Hepatitis B immunization: vaccine types, efficacy, and indications for immunization. *Curr Clin Top Infect Dis* 1992;12:282–308.
230. Havlichek D, Rosenman K, Simms M, et al. Age-related hepatitis B seroconversion rates in health care workers. *Am J Infect Control* 1997; 25:418–420.
231. Coleman PJ, Shaw FE, Serovich J, et al. Intradermal hepatitis B vaccination in a large hospital employee population. *Vaccine* 1991;9: 723–727.
232. Shaw FE, Guess HA, Roets JM, et al. Effect of anatomic injection site, age and smoking on the immune response to hepatitis B vaccination. *Vaccine* 1989;7:425–430.
233. Roome AJ, Walsh SJ, Cartter ML, et al. Hepatitis B vaccine responsiveness in Connecticut public safety personnel. *JAMA* 1993;270(24): 2931–2934.
234. Wood RC, MacDonald KL, White KE, et al. Risk factors for lack of detectable antibody following hepatitis B vaccination of Minnesota health care workers. *JAMA* 1993;270(24):2935–2939.
235. Rhame FS. Reduced development of anti-HBs in vaccinated health care workers. *Infect Dis Alert* 1993;12:79–80.
236. Alimonos K, Nafziger A, Murray J, et al. Prediction of response to hepatitis B vaccine in health care workers: whose titers of antibody to hepatitis B surface antigen should be determined after a three-dose series, and what are the implications in terms of cost-effectiveness? *Clin Infect Dis* 1998;26:566–571.
237. Department of Health and Human Services. Draft guideline for infection control in health care personnel, 1997; notice. *Fed Reg* 1997; 62(173):47275–47327.
238. Zuckerman J, Sabin C, Craig F, et al. Immune response to a new hepatitis B vaccine in healthcare workers who had not responded to standard vaccine: randomised double blind dose-response study. *BMJ* 1997;314:329–333.
239. Wainwright RB, Bulkow LR, Parkinson AJ, et al. Protection provided by hepatitis B vaccine in a Yupik Eskimo population—results of a 10-year study. *J Infect Dis* 1997;175(3):674–677.
240. Bulkow L, Wainwright R, McMahon B, et al. Increases in levels of antibody to hepatitis B surface antigen in an immunized population. *Clin Infect Dis* 1998;26:933–937.
241. Centers for Disease Control and Prevention. Updated U.S. Public Health Service Guidelines for the Management of Occupational Exposures to HBV, HCV, and HIV and Recommendations for Postexposure Prophylaxis. *MMWR* 2001;50(RR-11):1–52.
242. Gerberding JL, Henderson DK. Management of occupational exposures to bloodborne pathogens: hepatitis B virus, hepatitis C virus, and human immunodeficiency virus. *Clin Infect Dis* 1992;14:1179–1185.
243. Henderson DK. Human immunodeficiency virus in the health-care setting, Chapter 285. In: Mandell G, Dolin R, Bennett J, eds. *Principles and practice of infectious diseases,* 4th ed. New York: Churchill-Livingstone, 1995:2632–2656.
244. Fahey BJ, Beekmann SE, Schmitt JM, et al. Managing occupational exposures to HIV-1 in the healthcare workplace. *Infect Control Hosp Epidemiol* 1993;14(7):405–412.
245. Bell D, Shapiro CN, Chamberland ME, et al. Preventing bloodborne pathogen transmission from health-care workers to patients: the CDC perspective. *Surg Clin North Amer* 1995;75:1189–1203.
246. The Incident Investigation Teams and Others. Transmission of hepatitis B to patients from four infected surgeons without hepatitis B e antigen. *N Engl J Med* 1997;336:178–184.
247. Halle M. Patients want ban on operations by doctors with hepatitis B. *BMJ* 1996;313:576.
248. Alter HJ, Chalmers TC, Freeman BM, et al. Health-care workers positive for hepatitis B surface antigen. Are their contacts at risk? *N Engl J Med* 1975;292(9):454–457.
249. Alter HJ, Chalmers TC. The HBsAg positive health worker revisited. *Hepatology* 1981;1:467–470.
250. Centers for Disease Control. Recommendations for preventing transmission of human immunodeficiency virus and hepatitis B virus to patients during exposure-prone invasive procedures. *MMWR* 1991; 40(RR-8):1–9.
251. UK Department of Health, UK Advisory Group on Hepatitis. *Protecting health care workers and patients from hepatitis B.* Heywood Lancashire, England: UK Department of Health, 1993.
252. Poole C. Hepatitis B and health-care workers. *Lancet* 1997;350:218.
253. Noone P, Symington I, Carman W. Hepatitis B and health-care workers. *Lancet* 1997;350:219.
254. Boxall E, Ballard A. Fifth of e antigen negative carriers of hepatitis B virus should not perform exposure prone procedures. *BMJ* 1997; 314:144.
255. Henderson DK. The HIV- or HBV-infected healthcare provider and society's perception of risk: science, nonscience, and nonsense. *Ann Allergy* 1992;68:197–199.
256. Weber DJ, Hoffmann KK, Rutala WA. Management of the healthcare worker infected with human immunodeficiency virus: lessons from nosocomial transmission of hepatitis B virus. *Infect Control Hosp Epidemiol* 1991;12:625–630.
257. Henderson DK. Management of health-care workers who are infected with the human immunodeficiency virus or other bloodborne pathogens. In: DeVita V, Hellman S, Rosenberg S, eds. *AIDS—etiology, diagnosis, treatment, and prevention,* 3rd ed. Philadelphia: Lippincott, 1993.
258. Henderson DK. Human immunodeficiency virus infection in patients and providers. In: Wenzel R, ed. *Prevention and control of nosocomial infections,* 2nd ed. Baltimore, MD: Williams & Wilkins, 1992:42–57.
259. Rhodes RS, Telford GL, Hierholzer WJ Jr, et al. Bloodborne pathogen transmission from healthcare worker to patients. Legal issues and provider perspectives. *Surg Clin North Am* 1995;75(6):1205–1217.
260. Henderson DK, The AIDS/Tuberculosis Subcommittee of the Society for Healthcare Epidemiology of America. Management of healthcare workers infected with hepatitis B virus, hepatitis C virus, human immunodeficiency virus, or other bloodborne pathogens. AIDS/TB Committee of the Society for Healthcare Epidemiology of America. *Infect Control Hosp Epidemiol* 1997;18(5):349–363.

261. Johnston B, Langille D, LeBlanc J, et al. Transmission of hepatitis B related to orthopedic surgery (Abstract). *Infect Control Hosp Epidemiol* 1994;15:352.
262. Harpaz R, Von Seidlein L, Averhoff FM, et al. Transmission of hepatitis B virus to multiple patients from a surgeon without evidence of inadequate infection control. *N Engl J Med* 1996;334(9):549–554.
263. Jadoul M, Coarnu C, van Ypersele de Strihou C, Universitaires Cliniques St-Luc (UCL) Collaborative Group. Universal precautions prevent hepatitis C virus transmission: a 54 month follow-up of the Belgian multicenter study. *Kidney Int* 1998;53:1022–1025.
264. Farci P, Alter H, Govindarajan S, et al. Lack of protective immunity against reinfection with hepatitis C virus. *Science* 1992;258:135–140.
265. Farci P, Alter H, Wong D, et al. Prevention of hepatitis C virus infection in chimpanzees after antibody-mediated *in vitro* neutralization. *Proc Natl Acad Sci USA* 1994;91:7792–7796.
266. Centers for Disease Control and Prevention. Recommendations for follow-up of health-care workers after occupational exposure to hepatitis C virus. *MMWR* 1997;46(26):603–606.
267. Centers for Disease Control and Prevention. Risk of acquiring hepatitis C for health care workers and recommendations for prophylaxis and follow-up after occupational exposure. *Hepatitis surveillance report no. 56.* Atlanta, GA: U.S. Department of Health and Human Services, 1995:3–6.
268. Knodell RG, Conrad ME, Ginsberg AL, et al. Efficacy of prophylactic gamma-globulin in preventing non-A, non-B post-transfusion hepatitis. *Lancet* 1976;1:557–561.
269. Seeff LB, Zimmerman HJ, Wright EC, et al. A randomized, double blind controlled trial of the efficacy of immune serum globulin for the prevention of post-transfusion hepatitis. *Gastroenterology* 1977; 72:111–121.
270. Sanchez-Quijano A, Pineda JA, Lissen E, et al. Prevention of post-transfusion non-A, non-B hepatitis by non-specific immunoglobulin in heart surgery patients. *Lancet* 1988;1:1245–1249.
271. Pugliese G. Data lacking for postexposure prophylaxis with immune serum globulin following HCV exposure. *Infect Control Hosp Epidemiol* 1994;15:212.
272. Finlayson JS, Tankersley DL. Anti-HCV screening and plasma fractionation: the case against. *Lancet* 1990;335:1274–1275.
273. Miller MA, Orenstein P, Amihod B. Administration of immune serum globulin following exposure to hepatitis C virus. *Clin Infect Dis* 1993;16(2):335.
274. Krawczynski K, Alter M, Tankersley D, et al. Effect of immune globulin on the prevention of experimental hepatitis C virus infection. *J Infect Dis* 1996;173:822–828.
275. Hoofnagle JH. Therapy for acute hepatitis C. *N Engl J Med* 2001; 345(20):1495–1497.
276. Alvarado-Ramy F, Alter MJ, Bower W, et al. Management of occupational exposures to hepatitis C virus: current practice and controversies. *Infect Control Hosp Epidemiol* 2001;22(1):53–55.
277. Cammà C, Almasio P, Craxì A. Interferon as treatment for acute hepatitis C. A meta-analysis. *Dig Dis Sci* 1996;41:1248–1255.
278. Calleri G, Colombatto P, Gozzelino M, et al. Natural beta interferon in acute type-C hepatitis patients: a randomized controlled trial. *Ital J Gastroenterol Hepatol* 1998;30(2):181–184.
279. Vogel W. Treatment of acute hepatitis C virus infection. *J Hepatol* 1999;31(suppl 1):189–192.
280. Jaeckel E, Manns MP. The course and therapy of acute hepatitis C viral infection. Is a prevention of its becoming chronic possible? *Z Gastroenterol* 2000;38(5):387–395.
281. Hoey J, Wooltorton E. Early treatment of acute hepatitis C infection may lead to cure. *Can Med Assoc J* 2001;165(11):1527.
282. Jaeckel E, Cornberg M, Wedemeyer H, et al. Treatment of acute hepatitis C with interferon alfa-2b. *N Engl J Med* 2001;345(20): 1452–1457.
283. Alberti A, Boccato S, Vario A, et al. Therapy of acute hepatitis C. *Hepatology* 2002;36(5 suppl):S195–200.
284. Liang TJ, Rehermann B, Seeff LB, et al. Pathogenesis, natural history, treatment, and prevention of hepatitis C. *Ann Intern Med* 2000; 132(4):296–305.
285. Bonkovsky HL, Mehta S. Hepatitis C: a review and update. *Dis Mon* 2001;47(12):610–647.
286. Di Bisceglie AM, Hoofnagle JH. Optimal therapy of hepatitis C. *Hepatology* 2002;36(5):S121–S127.
287. Pimstone NR, Powell JS, Kotfila R, et al. High dose (780 MIU/52 weeks) interferon monotherapy is highly effective treatment for acute hepatitis C. *Gastroenterology* 2000;118(5):960A.
288. Vogel W, Graziadei I, Umlauft F, et al. High-dose interferon-alpha2b treatment prevents chronicity in acute hepatitis C: a pilot study. *Dig Dis Sci* 1996;41(12 suppl):81S–85S.
289. Oketani M, Higashi T, Yamasaki N, et al. Complete response to twice-a-day interferon-beta with standard interferon-alpha therapy in acute hepatitis C after a needle-stick. *J Clin Gastroenterol* 1999;28(1): 49–51.
290. Centers for Disease Control and Prevention. Recommendations for prevention and control of hepatitis C virus (HCV) infection and HCV-related chronic disease. Centers for Disease Control and Prevention. *MMWR Recomm Rep* 1998;47(RR-19):1–39.
291. Public Health Laboratory Service. Hepatitis C Transmission from health care worker to patient. *PHLS Commun Dis Rep* 1995;5(26): 121.
292. Esteban JI, Gomez J, Martell M, et al. Transmission of hepatitis C virus by a cardiac surgeon. *N Engl J Med* 1996;334(9):555–560.
293. Bosch X. Hepatitis C outbreak astounds Spain. *Lancet* 1998;351: 1415.
294. Brown P. Surgeon infects patient with hepatitis C. *BMJ* 1999; 319(7219):1219.
295. Public Health Laboratory Service. Transmission of hepatitis C virus from surgeon to patient prompts lookback. *Commun Dis Rep CDR Wkly* 1999;9(44):387.
296. Bosch X. Newspaper apportions blame in Spanish hepatitis C scandal. *Lancet* 2000;355(9206):818.
297. Public Health Laboratory Service. Hepatitis C lookback exercise. *Commun Dis Rep CDR Wkly* 2000;10(23):203, 206.
298. Public Health Laboratory Service. Two hepatitis C lookback exercises—national and in London. *Commun Dis Rep CDR Wkly* 2000; 10(14):125,128.
299. Cody SH, Nainan OV, Garfein RS, et al. Hepatitis C virus transmission from an anesthesiologist to a patient. *Arch Intern Med* 2002; 162(3):345–350.
300. Public Health Laboratory Service. Hepatitis C lookback in two Trusts in the south of England. *Public Health Lab Serv* [Commun Dis Rep CDR Wkly CDR Wkly (Electronic)]. October 31, 2002. Available at *http://www.phls.org.uk/publications/cdr/PDFfiles/2001/cdr2101.pdf.*
301. Ross RS, Viazov S, Thormahlen M, et al. Risk of hepatitis C virus transmission from an infected gynecologist to patients: results of a 7-year retrospective investigation. *Arch Intern Med* 2002;162(7): 805–810.
302. Duckworth GJ, Heptonstall J, Aitken C. Transmission of hepatitis C virus from a surgeon to a patient. The Incident Control Team. *Commun Dis Public Health* 1999;2(3):188–192.
303. Pugliese G, Favero MS. Healthcare worker-to-patient transmission of HCV in the UK. *Infect Control Hosp Epidemiol* 2000;21(9):619.
304. Centers for Disease Control and Prevention. Transmission of hepatitis C virus infection associated with home infusion therapy for hemophilia. *MMWR* 1997;46:597–599.
305. Ross RS, Viazov S, Roggendorf M. Phylogenetic analysis indicates transmission of hepatitis C virus from an infected orthopedic surgeon to a patient. *J Med Virol* 2002;66(4):461–467.
306. Alter MJ. Prevention of spread of hepatitis C. *Hepatology* 2002;36(5 suppl 1):S93–98.
307. Public Health Laboratory Service. New guidance on hepatitis C infected health care workers. *Public Health Lab Serv* [Commun Dis Rep CDR Wkly CDR Wkly (Electronic)]. August 22, 2002. Available at *http://www.phls.org.uk/publications/cdr/archive02/News/news3402.html#hepC.*
308. Karayiannis P, Saldanha J, Jackson A, et al. Partial control of hepatitis delta virus superinfection by immunisation of woodchucks (*Marmota monax*) with hepatitis delta antigen expressed by a recombinant vaccinia or baculovirus. *J Med Virol* 1993;41:210–214.

309. Farci P, Mandas A, Coiana A, et al. Treatment of chronic hepatitis D with interferon alfa-2a. *N Engl J Med* 1994;330:88–94.
310. Karayiannis P, Saldanha J, Monjardino J, et al. Prevention and treatment of hepatitis delta virus infection. *Prog Clin Biol Res* 1991;364: 377–383.
311. Tsarev SA, Tsareva TX, Emerson SU, et al. Successful passive and active immunization of cynomolgus monkeys against hepatitis E. *Proc Natl Acad Sci USA* 1994;91:10198–10202.
312. Purcell R. Enterically transmitted non-A, non-B hepatitis. *Prog Liver Dis* 1990;9:497–504.
313. Bryan JP, Tsarev SA, Iqbal M, et al. Epidemic hepatitis E in Pakistan: patterns of serologic response and evidence that antibody to hepatitis E virus protects against disease. *J Infect Dis* 1994;170:517–521.
314. Chauhan A, Dilawari J, Sharma R, et al. Role of long-persisting human hepatitis E virus antibodies in protection. *Vaccine* 1998;16: 755–756.

79

NOSOCOMIAL HUMAN IMMUNODEFICIENCY VIRUS INFECTION IN HEALTHCARE WORKERS

SUSAN E. BEEKMANN
DAVID K. HENDERSON

By December 2001, human immunodeficiency virus type 1 (HIV-1) infection had resulted in more than 816,000 cases of the acquired immunodeficiency syndrome (AIDS) in the United States, almost 468,000 of whom have died (1). Established risk factors for infection include both homosexual and heterosexual sexual contact, perinatal exposure, and parenteral exposure. Parenteral exposure includes such specific risks as sharing needles during intravenous drug use and receiving blood, blood products, or tissues that are contaminated by HIV. Healthcare workers, in addition to these traditional risk behaviors, are at occupational risk for acquiring HIV infection following parenteral or mucous membrane exposure to blood or blood-containing body fluids from HIV-infected patients.

Exposure to contaminated body fluids from HIV-infected patients and the potential for acquiring occupational HIV infection are issues that usually result in substantial healthcare worker anxiety. Even though the risk for occupational infection with hepatitis B virus (see Chapter 78) in the healthcare environment has been documented since 1949 (2) and is associated with significantly more morbidity and mortality in the healthcare setting than is HIV, a clear focus on defining and minimizing healthcare workplace risks was not developed until the HIV epidemic was well underway (3,4). Since the early 1980s, the subject of occupationally acquired HIV infection has received extensive media coverage, both in the lay press and in scientific forums. This chapter discusses these occupational risks in the context of available scientific knowledge, to provide a somewhat broader perspective regarding the risks for HIV transmission in society.

ETIOLOGY

HIV-1 is the only retrovirus that has been associated with serious occupational morbidity and mortality. Several cases of simian immunodeficiency virus (SIV) seroconversion have been reported (5,6), but this virus has not yet been shown to cause disease in humans, and the SIV-seropositive laboratory workers remain well. Because several other human retroviruses have routes of transmission similar to those of HIV-1 [e.g., HIV-2, human T-cell lymphotrophic virus I (HTLV-I) (7), and HTLV-II], occupational transmission of these viruses may someday be detected, although no reports of occupational infection with these other agents have been published. Nonetheless, risks of transmission associated with other retroviruses are likely to be extremely low, and current guidelines for prevention of transmission of HIV-1 are thought to be adequate to prevent transmission of all bloodborne viruses, including other retroviruses.

PATHOGENESIS

HIV derives a major survival advantage from its ability to target the immune system by infecting $CD4^+$ T cells and by inducing a specific cytokine milieu. The wide range of immunologic abnormalities in HIV-infected patients results primarily from the impairment of T-cell–mediated immunity. Observations that substantial viral replication occurs in lymphatic tissue during the period of clinical latency (8), whereas only low levels of virus are detected in peripheral lymphocytes (9), reinforce the insidious nature of the immunopathogenic effects of this virus. Several factors (i.e., postulated cofactors) have been suggested to enhance viral replication, often via lymphocyte activation. Inoculum size and certain inherent properties of the virus (e.g., syncytium-inducing viral phenotype) appear to confer greater overall HIV pathogenicity and may shorten the time to development of symptomatic HIV infection. The addition of HIV protease inhibitors to the armamentarium of antiretroviral drugs has dramatically improved the prognosis for HIV-infected persons (10–12). Combination antiretroviral therapy has been clearly linked with reductions in morbidity and mortality, with the most dramatic reductions coinciding with increases in the use of protease inhibitors (13). Despite these therapeutic advances, reservoirs of HIV-1 have been identified that represent major impediments to eradication, including latent $CD4^+$ T cells, macrophages, and dendritic cells (14,15).

Evidence has accumulated that infection of Langerhans cells, which are dendritic cells of the epidermis, plays a pivotal role in early transmucosal and transepidermal transmission (16). HIV infection of these Langerhans cells is regulated by surface expression of CD4 and HIV co-receptors, specifically CCR5. Langerhans cells, which represent only 2% to 3% of all epidermal cells, become infected within 24 hours of exposure, and within an additional 24 to 48 hours this cell population has migrated from epithelial tissue to lymphoid tissue (17,18). Within 5 days, HIV is detectable in peripheral blood in the SIV model. In addition, a molecule called DC-SIGN functions as an attachment factor and mediates capture of HIV by dendritic cells without infection of these cells (16). HIV captured by dendritic cells maintains infectivity for 25 days *in vitro* in the absence of replication within dendritic cells, whereas free virus rapidly loses its infectious potential. Langerhans cells are the major epidermal cell type that is involved in transmission of HIV to lymphoid tissue (19). Thus, ability to block infection of dendritic cells by HIV may importantly impact occupational transmission of HIV. Additionally, since systemic HIV infection is not thought to occur immediately following exposure, a brief window of opportunity may allow modification of viral replication in the initial target cells or lymph nodes with postexposure antiretroviral treatment.

Once occupational transmission of HIV has occurred, the pathogenesis of infection is not thought to be different from that following other modes of transmission (see Chapter 57). As occurs with other HIV transmission modalities, some healthcare workers who have acquired occupational HIV infection have progressed quite rapidly to AIDS, whereas others remain asymptomatic after many years of infection.

DIAGNOSIS AND CLINICAL MANIFESTATIONS

The clinical and laboratory manifestations of HIV infection are generally no different for healthcare workers who acquire occupational infections than they are for persons infected through other routes. Findings that may be useful in establishing the diagnosis of HIV infection of healthcare workers are discussed in detail in this section.

HIV-specific antibodies usually appear from 6 weeks to 4 months following exposure. An analysis of 51 seroconversions in healthcare workers determined that the estimated median interval from exposure to seroconversion was 46 days, with a mean interval of 65 days (20). Serodiagnosis consists of screening enzyme-linked immunosorbent assays (ELISAs) followed by a diagnostic Western blot when the ELISA is positive. On evaluation using the Western blot technique, antibodies to the group-specific antigen/core (GAG) proteins (i.e., p18, p24, and/or p55) may be the first to appear, but antibodies to the envelope (ENV) (e.g., gp120, gp160, gp41) and polymerase (POL) gene products (e.g., p31) develop thereafter, confirming the serodiagnosis of HIV infection. Rapid HIV antibody testing with high sensitivity and specificity (99.6% and 100%, respectively) and 20-minute turnaround time is now widely available (OraSure Technologies, Bethlehem, PA). Rapid testing may facilitate source patient testing and decrease the length of time healthcare workers take postexposure prophylaxis, pending the source patient HIV test result.

Delayed seroconversion has been suggested following sexual exposures (21,22), and the relatively low-inoculum exposures sustained by healthcare workers could result in latent HIV infection and delayed seroconversion. Postexposure prophylaxis does not appear to prolong time to development of HIV antibodies (23). Ninety-five percent of healthcare workers seroconverting after occupational HIV exposure have done so within 6 months of the exposure (23) when routine testing has been performed.

According to the Centers for Disease Control and Prevention (CDC), two cases of delayed seroconversion occurring in healthcare workers have been reported (23). These healthcare workers had both tested seronegative for HIV at least 6 months following exposure, but were seropositive within 12 months after the exposure. One of these delayed seroconversions was associated with concomitant exposure to hepatitis C virus, and this individual developed co-infection with hepatitis C that was rapidly fatal (24). CDC models indicate that the upper 95th percentile of the distribution of time between exposure and seroconversion is 190 days, and that 5% of healthcare workers are estimated to seroconvert in more than 6 months following exposure (25). Acute retroviral syndrome (26–28) associated with primary HIV infection has been a relatively common finding among healthcare workers in whom documented occupational HIV infection has occurred. This syndrome usually occurs 4 to 6 weeks after the occupational exposure. The CDC reported that 81% of healthcare workers experienced a syndrome compatible with primary HIV infection a median of 25 days after exposure (20). This clinical syndrome has been described as resembling acute infectious mononucleosis; fever, rash, malaise, myalgias/arthralgias, headaches, night sweats, pharyngitis, and lymphadenopathy have been documented (26–28). Laboratory abnormalities have also been described, including reduced total lymphocyte count, elevated sedimentation rate, and elevated transaminases and alkaline phosphatase levels.

Core (p24) antigenemia may be detected coincident with the onset of symptoms and usually resolves within several weeks to months as antibodies to p24 are produced and become detectable in the peripheral circulation (29). Several investigators have also detected the presence of virus by culture and/or by polymerase chain reaction (PCR) in cerebrospinal fluid, peripheral blood mononuclear cells (PBMCs), and plasma before the development of an antibody response in persons with nonoccupational exposures (27,30–32). Plasma HIV RNA levels are highest immediately after acquisition and then rapidly decrease (33). These direct virus assays [including HIV p24 antigen enzyme immunoassay (EIA), PCR for HIV RNA, and the branched-chain DNA assay] consistently detect infections 1 to 2 weeks earlier than the most sensitive antibodies, but they still do not become positive until weeks or months postexposure and they may revert to negative following antibody seroconversion (25). Interestingly, no association between plasma HIV RNA levels at the time of seroconversion and subsequent rate of $CD4^+$ cell loss or AIDS progression has been detected (33). The use of PCR to detect circulating viral RNA will likely supplant the use of the p24 antigen test, although the p24 assay turnaround time is much shorter than for the PCR assay in some centers.

Although direct virus assays have been used as ancillary tests in the diagnosis of occupational HIV infection, these tests should not routinely be used to detect infection in exposed healthcare workers (25). These tests may be helpful in defined adjunctive circumstances, such as when the ELISA is positive but the Western blot is indeterminate, or when symptoms are consistent with the acute retroviral syndrome but serologic testing remains negative for more than several weeks. A negative direct virus assay should never be the basis for excluding infection. Although ultrasensitive direct virus assays are available (quantitation of HIV-1 RNA down to 50 copies/mL), the risk for false-positive results increases accordingly.

Symptoms consistent with the acute retroviral syndrome signal that HIV antibodies will appear, usually within 1 to 10 weeks (27) if infection has indeed occurred. Healthcare workers who sustain occupational exposures should be educated about the symptoms of the seroconversion illness and should be instructed to seek urgent attention in the employee health clinic if these symptoms appear. In most occupational seroconversions, HIV seropositivity has not been documented as part of the routine serologic follow-up but has been detected after the healthcare worker seeks medical attention for an illness consistent with seroconversion. Nonetheless, the CDC recommends HIV antibody testing at 6 weeks, 3 months, and 6 months following the occupational exposure (34). The National Institutes of Health (NIH) Clinical Center Occupational Medical Service also elects to check HIV antibody status at 12 months following exposure, although this is not routinely recommended by the CDC because of the rarity of delayed seroconversion events (34). Because of the anecdotal experience with delayed HIV seroconversion occurring following concomitant exposures to HIV and hepatitis C virus (HCV), most authorities would recommend extending follow-up to 12 months following simultaneous exposures to hepatitis C and HIV.

EPIDEMIOLOGY

Occupational injuries and exposures to blood and body fluids continue to be commonplace in virtually every healthcare setting. Healthcare workers who sustain these injuries and exposures often react immediately with anxiety, fear, and concern over their risk for acquiring HIV. Framing the issue of HIV transmission risk is quite complex. Nonetheless, more than a decade of dealing with HIV infection in the healthcare workplace has led to a fairly extensive database characterizing these occupational risks.

Perception of risk is clearly affected by the news media and publicity regarding recent cases of occupational infection. The sensationalism that has traditionally accompanied HIV-related issues in the media has artificially inflated perceptions of occupational risk. We frequently find that both the lay public and, particularly, healthcare workers believe that large numbers of occupational HIV infections have been documented. Depending on the definition of occupational infection chosen for the analysis, one can arrive at quite disparate assessments of the number of occupational HIV infections documented in the U.S. (35).

REPORTS OF OCCUPATIONAL INFECTIONS

A wide variety of sources have provided information about HIV infection in healthcare workers (35). Several general types of case reports have appeared in the literature, ranging from healthcare workers in whom HIV seroconversions have been documented following an occupational exposure, to healthcare workers who are found to be seropositive but in whom the seropositivity cannot be linked to a discrete injury or exposure.

Documented seroconversions are generally defined as cases in which a healthcare worker sustains an injury with a device contaminated with blood from an HIV-seropositive or indeterminate source; the healthcare worker is documented to be HIV-seronegative at the time of the exposure, and then the healthcare worker develops serologic evidence of HIV infection within the ensuing 6 months. Documented seroconversions are the source of the most detailed and reliable epidemiologic information about occupational infections and are, in fact, the standard against which other types of information about occupational HIV infection can be measured. Through June 30, 2001, 57 cases of occupational seroconversions had been documented either in the medical literature or in individual case reports to the CDC that meet the criteria established for this category of occupational infection (1). Of the 57 infected healthcare workers, 48 had percutaneous injuries, five had mucocutaneous exposures, two had both percutaneous and mucous membrane exposures, and two had unknown routes of exposure.

In addition to these documented seroconversions, a number of additional cases of HIV infection have been categorized by the CDC as possible occupational infections. All of the individuals placed in this category have worked in a healthcare setting some time since 1978, and all deny behavioral or transfusion risks for HIV infection. Each of the healthcare workers in this category retrospectively reported a "source unknown" exposure or an occupational exposure to blood, body fluids, or laboratory solutions containing HIV, but these individuals either did not report their exposures or were not tested for HIV at baseline or shortly after the exposure event (to demonstrate that the individuals were not already infected when the exposure occurred). Some fraction of the 137 healthcare workers in this broad category as of June 30, 2001, undoubtedly acquired occupational infection from the incriminated exposure; nonetheless, these cases are less clear, because the seroconversion events were not documented (1). The possible occupational infection category exhibits different demographics from the set of individuals who have documented occupational infections, and likely includes individuals who have confounding community-based risk for infection (35).

Nonetheless, when both categories are combined, the total number of documented and/or possible occupational HIV infections in the U.S. through June 30, 2001, is 194. Ippolito et al. (36) reported 94 documented and 170 possible cases worldwide through September 1997. Since the overwhelming majority of these cases have been reported as anecdotes, these data provide only limited insight into the magnitude of risk for occupational infection (i.e., based on these data, one can state only that healthcare workers are at risk for occupational HIV infection). Some conclusions can be drawn, however, from the cases of documented seroconversions regarding the epidemiology of occupational infection. For example, by examining cases of documented seroconversion for circumstances of occupational exposure, one can gain substantial insight into the types of exposures likely to result in transmission of HIV. Even these relatively small databases provide evidence that the risk associated with mucocutaneous exposures appears to be lower than the risk associated with percutaneous injuries.

DATA DESCRIBING THE MAGNITUDE OF RISK OF HIV TRANSMISSION IN THE HEALTHCARE SETTING

Longitudinal cohort studies of healthcare workers involved in the day-to-day care of HIV-infected patients and in the handling and processing of specimens from such patients provide the best available data regarding the magnitude of risk for transmission in the healthcare setting. A number of prospective studies have followed healthcare workers who have sustained documented exposure to blood or blood-containing body fluids from HIV-infected patients. In all of these studies, healthcare workers undergo baseline and follow-up HIV serologic testing (at a minimum) any time a healthcare worker sustains a percutaneous exposure to blood from an HIV-infected patient. The average risk of HIV infection following percutaneous exposure to HIV-infected blood has remained at approximately 0.3% [95% confidence interval (CI) = 0.2% to 0.5%] for a number of years.

Similarly, other prospective studies are currently examining the risk associated with mucous membrane exposures to blood or body fluids from HIV-infected patients. Although mucous membrane exposures that resulted in HIV transmission have been reported anecdotally (36,37), no seroconversions have occurred following the mucous membrane exposures that were prospectively collected from enrollees in these longitudinal studies.

FACTORS THAT MIGHT MODIFY THE RISK OF TRANSMISSION

Although these data are reasonably specific, and confidence intervals around the calculated risks of transmission are narrow, we still lack sufficient information to predict which injuries will result in transmission of infection. Many of the percutaneous injuries that have been associated with documented seroconversions have been quite deep or extensive or have involved injection of a volume of blood into the healthcare worker, whereas other percutaneous injuries associated with transmission have been relatively minor. Mucous membrane or nonintact skin exposures that resulted in transmission have almost uniformly been quite extensive (e.g., the contact with blood has been for a prolonged period (>15 minutes) or has involved large areas of skin surface). Occasionally, injuries that one might intuitively think would have a higher than average risk for infection have not resulted in infection. For example, a healthcare worker at the NIH Clinical Center sustained a severe injury with a bone marrow aspiration needle that had been used on a patient with end-stage HIV disease; the needle actually penetrated through the palm and was visible from the dorsum of the worker's hand. This exposure did not transmit HIV infection. The epidemiologic factors contributing to the risk for occupational infection have been explored using the case-control method (38).

Thirty-three cases of occupational HIV seroconversion following percutaneous exposures to HIV-infected blood and 665 controls who did not seroconvert were studied by Cardo et al. (38) at the CDC. Multivariable logistic regression identified several risk factors associated with HIV transmission after percutaneous exposure: deep injury [odds ratio (OR) 15, 95% CI 6.0–41], visible blood on device (OR 6.2, 95% CI 2.2–21), procedure involving needle in artery or vein (OR 4.3, 95% CI 1.7–12), terminal illness in source patient (OR 5.6, 95% CI 2.0–16), and postexposure use of zidovudine (OR 0.19, 95% CI 0.06–0.52). Increased risk was associated with factors that are indirect measures of the inoculum size (i.e., the quantity of blood transferred in the exposure) or higher viral burden (i.e., source patient in the terminal stage of AIDS). Thus, although the average risk of HIV transmission following a percutaneous exposure is 0.3%, the risk of transmission following exposures involving large quantities of blood or high viral titers may be substantially higher than the average risk. Corroborating evidence for the factors identified by the case-control study were supplied by a laboratory study that demonstrated that more blood is transferred by deeper injuries and hollow-bore needles (39). Mast and Gerberding (40) also determined that glove use reduced the transferred blood volume by nearly 50% in their laboratory model.

Despite our inability to predict with precision which exposures result in transmission of HIV infection, the documented seroconversions have provided us with specific information about which body fluids have resulted in transmission. Of the 57 documented seroconversions, 49 exposures were to HIV-infected blood, one to visibly bloody pleural fluid, four to an unspecified fluid, and three to a concentrated viral preparations in a laboratory (34). Thus, blood appears to be the major clinical risk associated with transmission. A case report documented transmission of HIV to a laboratory technician from Germany who sustained an accidental splash of serum from an infected patient to his eye (41). Transmission in this case was likely facilitated by failure to wash the eye and by the technician's concomitant conjunctivitis related to a contact lens present in his eye at the time of exposure. Blood, visibly bloody body fluid, and now serum clearly remain the primary risk for transmission of HIV (36).

The type of needle or sharp object involved in the injury also appears to affect the risk of transmission. To date, to our knowledge, no cases of occupational infection have been definitively linked to an exposure resulting from a solid (i.e., suture) needle. Transmission has been associated with several types of hollow-bore needles (including injection needles and intravenous catheters) and other sharp objects (including contaminated broken glass, scalpels, and an orthopedic pin) (36).

Finally, certain source patient variables, and, perhaps, even several factors relating to the recipient healthcare worker's status, likely affect transmission. Source patients with terminal HIV disease were found to be associated with higher risks of HIV transmission in the case-control study discussed previously (38).

Although data regarding specific measurement of HIV viral burden were not available to the CDC researchers, the increased risk of HIV transmission from source patients who are in the late-stage of HIV infection likely is a surrogate marker for RNA plasma levels as measured by RNA PCR or the branched-chain DNA assay. Some also have postulated that the recipient healthcare worker's histocompatibility with the source patient [i.e., human leukocyte antigen (HLA) type, etc.] or, any concurrent viral illnesses such as Epstein-Barr virus, cytomegalovirus infection, or infection with human herpesvirus-6 that results in increased CD4 expression, or the presence of chronic inflammation at or around the skin entry site, might also influence the risk of transmission. Despite this educated speculation, the numbers of cases of documented seroconversions with these data available are too few to permit adequate characterization of these risks.

COMPARISON OF THE RISK OF HIV TRANSMISSION TO THE RISK OF TRANSMISSION OF OTHER BLOODBORNE PATHOGENS

When addressing the risk of acquiring occupational HIV infection, healthcare workers must be able to place that risk into the broader perspective of risk associated with other bloodborne pathogens such as hepatitis B and hepatitis C (see Chapter 78). Hepatitis B has long been recognized as a significant cause of healthcare worker morbidity and mortality; healthcare worker risks associated with hepatitis C have only been documented and partially characterized in the past several years (42,43).

The CDC estimated in 1987 that 12,000 cases of hepatitis B infection per year occurred among healthcare workers in the U.S. and that 500 healthcare workers were hospitalized each year because of the complications of occupationally acquired hepatitis B (44). Additionally, prior to the full-scale implementation of hepatitis B immunization, approximately 200 workers died each year from occupational hepatitis B or its complications (45). More recently, Mahoney et al. (46) found that the calculated number of hepatitis B virus infections among healthcare workers declined from 17,000 in 1983 to 400 in 1995. This dramatic decline was associated with implementation of universal precautions policies, with licensure of recombinant-DNA hepatitis B vaccines, and the OSHA Bloodborne Pathogens Standard.

The risk associated with hepatitis C appears to be lower than the risk associated with hepatitis B; healthcare workers with frequent blood contact account for 1% to 2% of reported cases of hepatitis C infection (47), and seroprevalence studies indicate that healthcare workers' risk of hepatitis C infection is only slightly higher than that of volunteer blood donors. Several small prospective studies have measured the risk of transmission after percutaneous exposure and the average risk was 1.9% (see Chapter 78) (48) with a range from approximately 0% (in six studies, summarized in ref. 42) to 22% (49), depending on the size of the population studied and the assays used to test source patients and employees, among other important variables. Lower rates of transmission have been associated with the use of the (much less sensitive) first-generation hepatitis C serologic test and with an interesting geographic distribution (see Chapter 78).

The morbidity and mortality associated with occupational exposure and infection with hepatitis B far outstrips the impact of HIV on healthcare occupations. For comparison, through June 2001, a cumulative total of 26 U.S. healthcare workers are known to have developed AIDS following occupational exposure and infection (34). Despite the dramatic decline in the incidence of hepatitis B infections among healthcare workers in the U.S. (46), thousands of healthcare workers have died from the complications of occupationally acquired hepatitis B. Because acceptance of the hepatitis B vaccine is not uniform and because 6% to 10% of healthcare workers do not respond to immunization, the number of occupational infections with HBV will likely continue to eclipse those associated with HIV. The impact of HCV in the healthcare setting is just beginning to be appreciated. Whereas the average infection rate following occupational exposure is only 1.9%, traditional teaching suggests that as many as 85% of the healthcare workers who acquire occupational infection develop chronic infection and that approximately two thirds of those who become chronically infected develop persistently elevated liver enzymes and are at increased risk for liver failure, cirrhosis, and hepatocellular carcinoma.

PREVENTION AND CONTROL

Indirect evidence demonstrates that zidovudine postexposure prophylaxis may reduce the risk of HIV transmission (38,50); however, because of the toxicity and inconvenience of the agents administered as postexposure prophylaxis, the attention of the healthcare community should be focused first on preventing occupational exposures as a means of preventing transmission of HIV. The U.S federal government has issued regulations that have just this intent. In 1991, the Occupational Safety and Health Administration (OSHA) issued regulations (51) that were designed to ensure employer compliance with full implementation of universal precautions (52). This Bloodborne Pathogen Standard also mandates that employers offer hepatitis B immunization to healthcare workers at risk for occupational exposure at no cost to the employee.

Primary Prevention of Exposures in the Healthcare Workplace

In the time that has elapsed since the initial cluster of cases of *Pneumocystis carinii* pneumonia was identified in Los Angeles in the summer of 1981 (53), the CDC has issued a series of guidelines with the goal of preventing transmission of HIV infection to healthcare providers (3,34,44,52,54–64). The concept of universal precautions, or use of blood and body-fluid precautions for the care of all patients, was first proposed by the CDC in 1985 (3) and again in 1986 (58). The August 1987 guidelines (frequently referred to as the universal precautions guidelines) consolidated and updated all previous CDC recommendations concerning the prevention of occupational infection with HIV (52).

The 1987 universal precautions guidelines (summarized in

Table 79.1) strongly emphasized the need for every healthcare worker to consider all patients as potentially infected with HIV or other bloodborne pathogens and to adhere to infection-control precautions for minimizing the risk of exposure to blood and body fluids from all patients. These guidelines have been updated by the Healthcare Infection Control Practices Advisory Committee (HICPAC) (65). Universal Precautions and body substance isolation (66) are now amalgamated into a single set of guidelines called Standard Precautions (65).

Although the use of Universal Precautions, now called Standard Precautions (see Chapter 95), has been advocated as a means to prevent occupational exposures to blood and other body fluids, neither the efficacy nor the cost-effectiveness of these admittedly labor-intensive and costly (67) precautions has been demonstrated definitively. Furthermore, Standard Precautions, with its emphasis on barrier precautions, may not prevent percutaneous injuries, which are the major risk associated with occupational infections, although appropriate handling and disposal of needles and other sharp objects is an integral component of these guidelines.

TABLE 79.1. SUMMARY OF UNIVERSAL PRECAUTIONS: RECOMMENDATIONS FOR PREVENTION OF HIV TRANSMISSION IN HEALTHCARE SETTINGS

Universal blood and body fluid precautions should be consistently used for all patients since only serologic testing reliably identifies all patients infected with HIV or other bloodborne pathogens.

Universal Precautions apply to blood and bloody body fluids, semen and vaginal secretions, tissues, cerebrospinal fluid, synovial fluid, pleural fluid, peritoneal fluid, pericardial fluid, and amniotic fluid.

Appropriate barrier precautions should routinely be followed to prevent skin and mucous membrane exposure when contact with blood or other body fluids of any patient is anticipated.

Gloves are required for touching blood and body fluids, mucous membranes, or nonintact skin of all patients; for handling items soiled with blood or body fluids; and for performing vascular access procedures.

Masks and protective eyewear or face shields are required when droplets of blood or other body fluids might be generated that could contact mucous membranes (eyes, nose, mouth).

Gowns are required when splashes of fluids might be generated.

Hand washing is required after contamination with blood or other body fluids and immediately after gloves are removed.

Precautions should be taken to prevent sharps injuries during procedures, during cleaning of instruments, and during disposal of used needles.

Needles should never be recapped, purposely bent or broken, or removed from disposable syringes.

Disposable syringes and needles, scalpels, and other sharps should be placed in puncture-resistant containers for disposal; these containers should be placed as close as practical to the area where sharps are being used.

Mouthpieces, resuscitation bags, or other ventilation devices should be available where their use can be readily anticipated.

Healthcare workers who have exudative lesions or weeping dermatitis should refrain from all direct patient care.

Pregnant healthcare workers should be especially familiar with and should strictly adhere to the concepts of Universal Precautions.

HIV, human immunodeficiency virus.
From Centers for Disease Control. Recommendations for prevention of HIV transmission in health-care settings. *MMWR* 1987; 36(suppl 2S): 1S–19S; and Centers for Disease Control. Update: universal precautions for prevention of transmission of human immunodeficiency virus, hepatitis B virus, and other bloodborne pathogens in health-care settings. *MMWR* 1988; 37: 377–382, 387–388.

Studies of the efficacy of standard precautions have produced inconsistent results. At least one study has concluded that universal precautions training was associated with increased incidence of injuries (68), whereas others have reported stable exposure rates (69). Some studies have shown decreases in recapping or needle-disposal device-related injuries, but stable (or slightly increased) overall injury rates (70–74). The studies indicating that implementation of Universal Precautions did not decrease overall injury rates almost uniformly indicate poor healthcare worker compliance with Universal Precautions or fail to assess compliance in any way. Several other groups have reported trends toward fewer needlestick injuries in association with Universal Precautions (67,75). Investigators at the NIH Clinical Center reported that implementation of Universal Precautions was associated with a significant decrease in both cutaneous (76) and reported parenteral exposures to blood (77). A review of published percutaneous injury rates per 100 employees found that more recent injury rates (following implementation of the Bloodborne Pathogens Standard in 1992; see below) are lower than those based on pre-1992 data (78). To the extent that these precautions are actually followed, they will very likely reduce occupational exposures to bloodborne pathogens. Ensuring compliance, however, is a challenging matter. Despite these controversies, Universal/Standard Precautions have been widely implemented and are now mandated by the OSHA (51).

This mandate was published by the Department of Labor as the "Occupational Exposure to Bloodborne Pathogens; Final Rule" in the *Federal Register* in December 1991 (the details of this final rule are summarized in Table 79.2) (51). Employers, including hospitals and virtually any setting in which exposure to blood might occur, are now required to have in place an exposure control plan that mandated implementation of Universal Precautions by 1992. In addition, a series of other requirements have been imposed, including extensive documentation and record-keeping regarding compliance with these regulations. Other requirements relate to engineering and work practice controls, use of appropriate personal protective equipment, detailed housekeeping standards, and requirements for biohazard labeling. Free hepatitis B immunization is now required for all employees with any potential for exposure; healthcare workers who decline vaccination must sign an "informed refusal," the content of which is specified in the final rule. Finally, the OSHA has established an obligatory federal standard of practice for employers when an employee is involved in an exposure incident; current recommendations of the U.S. Public Health Service (USPHS) must be implemented following an exposure incident.

Certain portions of the final rule were impatiently awaited by occupational medicine and hospital epidemiology personnel, in particular the requirement to document compliance with the hepatitis B vaccination. Although the rates of occupational hepatitis B have decreased dramatically with the OSHA final rule and use of Universal Precautions (46), absolute protection can only be assured with evidence of serologic immunity. Prior to publication of the OSHA final rule, the CDC estimated that only 30% to 40% of healthcare workers had been vaccinated (79,80). In 1995, Agerton et al. (81) concluded that the OSHA final rule resulted in a greater awareness by healthcare workers of their risk for hepatitis B and an increase in the number of workers receiving the vaccine; nonetheless, only 51% of eligible workers had completed a vaccination series. Other portions of the final rule, such as the exposure determination requirement, in which employers must list all job classifications in which some employees have occupational exposure to blood, and then list every task and procedure performed by the employees in those job classifications, are remarkably onerous and have undoubtedly greatly increased the workload of hospital epidemiology personnel with, in our opinion, little likely benefit to the employee.

MANAGEMENT OF OCCUPATIONAL EXPOSURES

Healthcare institutions have ethical and now legal responsibilities to develop and implement protocols for managing healthcare workers who are occupationally exposed to bloodborne pathogens. However, given the major gaps in the available scientific data regarding these issues, the optimal management of employees sustaining exposures remains elusive. Thus, this issue, which is particularly difficult for the healthcare workers who sustain the exposures, is likely to remain as problematic for hospital administrators, hospital legal staff members, hospital epidemiologists, infection control professionals, hospital infection control committees, and healthcare employees, who often are responsible for development and implementation of policies and procedures designed to manage exposed employees.

In addition to the routine difficulties inherent in any occupational exposure, HIV-related exposures present the additional concern of secondary transmission of HIV to significant others. Healthcare workers who sustain occupational HIV exposures often react with profound anxiety and experience severe emotional and psychological stress. Managing these exposures is complex, labor-intensive, and often emotionally draining for the physician/counselor in the occupational health service (82).

Postexposure management of occupational exposures should be routinely taught and reinforced during hospital epidemiology and occupational health interactions with healthcare workers (e.g., during orientation of new employees and during initial and recurring Standard Precautions training). Institutions should not defer disseminating this information until after an exposure; all healthcare workers should be aware of the appropriate procedures to follow irrespective of whether an exposure has occurred. The process of immediate postexposure management should consist of three basic steps: administration of immediate first aid at the work site, informing one's supervisor of the event if the supervisor is immediately available, and immediately reporting to the occupational medical service (or through another institutionally established reporting mechanism). We encourage our employees to report all exposures for two reasons: first, proper treatment (e.g., first aid and—when appropriate or desirable—postexposure chemoprophylaxis) can be administered, and second, reporting allows documentation of work-related exposures and facilitates workers' compensation claims when such claims are appropriate.

Although no data address the efficacy of immediate application of first aid in preventing transmission of occupational bloodborne infections, most authorities recommend administration of first aid immediately following an exposure as a logical action (34,83). Given a lack of data with which to make a scientific recommendation regarding first aid, selection of agents for decontamination (e.g., soap and water, chlorhexidine, iodophors, peroxide) should depend, in part, on which agents are most readily available. Although following an established institutional regimen seems an entirely reasonable approach, occupational medicine staff should explain that no study documents the efficacy of these first-aid interventions in preventing occupational infection with bloodborne pathogens. In fact, an anecdotal report documents occupational infection with HIV despite the immediate application of first aid, including thoroughly rinsing the injury site (a cut from glass contaminated with blood from an AIDS patient) with undiluted bleach (84). At the NIH Clinical Center, our routinely recommended procedure is immediately to scrub the site of the injury or cutaneous exposure with a povidone-iodine solution and to attempt to "milk" the site of a transcutaneous exposure to express blood. Clinical Center guidelines also recommend that mucous membrane exposures affecting the mouth or nose be rinsed thoroughly with water or saline; exposures affecting the eyes should be rinsed thoroughly with water, saline, or sterile irrigants (82,85).

Once the site has been decontaminated, the healthcare worker should inform his or her supervisor about the exposure (if the supervisor is in the immediate vicinity or can be reached within a minute or two) so that the supervisor can provide coverage while the employee is away from the area. The healthcare worker should then report immediately to the institution's employee health service. Reporting of exposures is essential both to ensure adequate care for the injured employee and to assist the institution in making necessary policy and procedural changes to minimize risks of injury to other employees. To facilitate reporting, a mechanism should be defined and widely publicized and must be capable of being activated at any time of the day. A number of institutions have implemented 24-hour-a-day hotlines staffed by expert clinicians who can coordinate both exposure reporting and employee management. Clinicians who provide first-line response to employees exposed to patients known or suspected to be HIV-infected should be prepared to provide state-of-the-art medical management of occupational exposures but also must be prepared for and capable of dealing with the extreme anxiety and occasional hysteria associated with these exposures.

Education and counseling are important components of the management of occupational exposures to bloodborne pathogens. Employees sustaining exposures to blood or body fluids from patients known or suspected to be HIV-infected need counseling regarding (a) the epidemiology, routes of transmission, and transmissibility of HIV; (b) the risk for occupational transmission of HIV following such an injury; (c) the importance of notifying the occupational health service of any acute febrile illness; and (d) techniques effective in minimizing the risk for transmission of HIV to sexual partners (82).

Management of employees sustaining exposures to blood or body fluids from patients whose HIV status is unknown is confounded by the problems associated with testing the source patients. Each institution should develop a policy for the management of exposures when the source patient is either unable or refuses to consent to these tests that is consonant with state and/or local laws. Many states have laws that either permit testing of source patients in certain circumstances even if consent is refused or legally require informed consent for testing.

For institutions to achieve and maintain roles as healthcare worker advocates, the medical confidentiality and privacy of healthcare workers who sustain occupational exposures and/or infections must be preserved. Each employee who sustains an occupational exposure must be apprised fully of the procedures used for ensuring confidentiality and reassured that records will not be released without his or her consent. To maintain privacy, laboratory samples should never be submitted with identifiers that can be traced to an individual. Additionally, access to records of occupational exposures should be strictly controlled. We recommend that records of HIV, hepatitis B, and hepatitis C testing of employees be maintained separately from routine employee health records. Indeed, the OSHA requires that the employer obtain a copy of the evaluating healthcare professional's written opinion only, which must include a statement that the employee has been informed of the results of the evaluation and told about any medical conditions resulting from exposure that may require further evaluation and treatment. All other medical findings or diagnoses must be kept confidential and not included in the written report provided to the employer (51) (Table 79.2).

TABLE 79.2. REQUIREMENTS OF THE OCCUPATIONAL SAFETY AND HEALTH ADMINISTRATION'S BLOODBORNE PATHOGENS STANDARD

Hospitals and other healthcare employers are required to:

Develop an exposure control plan that identifies employees with occupational risk of exposure to blood or body fluid.

Train all employees annually on occupational risks and methods to reduce risk of exposure.

Maintain records of employee training for 3 years and of medical evaluations for the duration of employment plus 30 years.

Use warning labels and signs to identify biohazards; red bags or containers are allowed to substitute for the label in many cases.

Implement engineering and work practice controls for worker protection, including specific requirements for:
- Hand washing
- Safe handling and disposal of sharps
- Employee conduct in areas of potential exposure
- Management, storage, and shipping of specimens

Provide personal protective clothing and equipment:
- Employees must be trained how and when to use equipment.
- Cleaning, laundering, repair, and replacement are the employer's responsibility.

Maintain detailed housekeeping standards, including requirements for special handling and bagging of "contaminated" laundry.

Provide voluntary hepatitis B vaccine at no cost to employees:
- Prevaccination screening cannot be required.
- Employees declining vaccination must sign an "Informed Refusal," the content of which is specified.

Provide medical evaluation after exposure incidents:
- Ensure testing of the source patient when consent is obtained.
- Provide postexposure prophylaxis as recommended by the U.S. Public Health Service.

Institute additional precautions for HIV and HBV research and production facilities, where applicable.

HIV, human immunodeficiency virus; HBV, hepatitis B virus.
From Code of Federal Regulations 29 CFR 1910.100.

SECONDARY PREVENTION OF HIV TRANSMISSION—POSTEXPOSURE ANTIRETROVIRAL PROPHYLAXIS FOLLOWING OCCUPATIONAL EXPOSURES

Ideally, primary prevention of occupational HIV infection would obviate the need for postexposure prophylaxis. Unfortunately, neither implementation of Standard Precautions nor use of safer devices will prevent all injuries. Postexposure antiretroviral chemoprophylaxis has become the standard of care following at-risk injuries and exposures (34,50,86,87). Currently, the USPHS recommends that postexposure prophylaxis should be available as soon as possible following exposure (34), and the OSHA final rule mandates employer compliance with USPHS recommendations (51). Basic recommendations for postexposure prophylaxis now include a two-drug regimen using two nucleoside analogs (zidovudine plus lamivudine, lamivudine plus stavudine, or stavudine plus didanosine) for 4 weeks (34). An expanded regimen incorporating a third drug, usually a protease inhibitor, is recommended for exposures that are associated with an increased risk for transmission. In instances in which resistance to antiretroviral agents incorporated in the basic regimen is anticipated, the CDC has recommended using a combination of three agents to which the source patient's HIV isolate has not been exposed.

Whereas definitive evidence of the efficacy of chemoprophylaxis is still lacking, these recommendations for postexposure prophylaxis were based on several pieces of evidence (50,88). The retrospective case-control study results discussed previously in this chapter were initially presented in 1994 (89) and then in final form in 1997 (38). This study documented an association between use of zidovudine postexposure prophylaxis and an 80% reduction in risk for HIV seroconversion (90). This association was surprising and initially greeted with skepticism (88), particularly since a retrospective case-control study design is not optimal for assessing the efficacy of postexposure prophylaxis. Nonetheless, the association held true even with the addition of cases from the United Kingdom, France, and Italy. Although the magnitude of the protective effect may be altered with the future addition of more cases, the conclusion drawn from these data is that "chemoprophylaxis may well be worthwhile after occupational exposure and may be a reasonable option after any type of exposure to HIV" (88). With a risk for infection of 0.2%, the sample-size requirements for a placebo-controlled trial are formidable. For example, assuming that a candidate agent is 80% effective and assuming a power of 80%, 17,110 healthcare workers would be needed for a double-blinded placebo-controlled trial to demonstrate significance at the .05 level. Thus, definitive proof of the efficacy of postexposure prophylaxis, apart from the retrospective case control study, is unlikely to ever be established.

Zidovudine has also been shown to decrease the risk of mother–infant transmission of HIV (91). Only approximately 30% of the decrease in risk of vertical transmission following use of zidovudine prophylaxis was found to be attributable to a reduction in maternal viral burden, which suggests that newborns benefit from a substantial chemoprophylactic effect, effective preemptive therapy for HIV infection, or both (92). Abbreviated zidovudine regimens have also been shown to be effective in decreasing the ratio of prenatal HIV transmission (93–95). Strikingly, in some of these studies, antiviral efficacy was demonstrated in instances in which only the infant received therapy (i.e., true postexposure prophylaxis) (94,96). In addition, postexposure prophylaxis has been shown to prevent or ameliorate retroviral infection in some animal studies (97). Taken together, these pieces of evidence provide the foundation for the current USPHS recommendations (34).

Animal studies have provided insight, to both the safety as well as the efficacy of postexposure chemoprophylaxis regimens. Not surprisingly, given the fact that these agents are active at the level of nucleic acids, long-term studies of the chronic administration of antiretroviral agents to animals have identified some toxicities (98–100).

Studies evaluating the efficacy of antiretroviral agents in preventing retroviral infections in animal models provide some of the best available evidence that these agents might, in fact, be of value in preventing occupational HIV infection. Whereas the results of the first such studies were relatively discouraging (101–113), more recent studies have clearly demonstrated that antiretrovirals can prevent infection when the drugs are administered at, or shortly following, infection. Most of the initial studies demonstrated some drug effect (i.e., treated animals fare slightly better than controls, but all animals became infected) (101–113). Beginning in 1992 (114), studies in mouse and macaque models have demonstrated effective chemoprophylaxis (114–119). Three sets of studies warrant special mention. The early studies of Ruprecht et al. (120,121) using the Rauscher murine leukemia virus (RMLV) model demonstrated as early as 1990 that either zidovudine or zidovudine plus interferon-α could prevent RMLV viremia. Subsequent studies with this model demonstrated chemoprophylactic efficacy of zidovudine (117). Böttiger et al. (116) studied a new agent BEA-005 (also known as 2,3′-dideoxy-3′-hydroxymethyl cytidine) in a macaque model and showed that all BEA-005–treated animals that had been injected intravenously or exposed intrarectally to either HIV-2 or SIV were protected, irrespective of the viral agent or the route of inoculation. Tsai et al. (118) administered a new nucleotide analog agent, (R)-9-[2-phosphonylmethoxypropyl] adenine [PMPA, now Food and Drug Administration (FDA)-approved as Tenofovir DF], to several sets of macaques that had been infected intravenously with SIV. One set of animals was given PMPA at the time of infection, one set was given PMPA 4 hours after infection, and a third set was given the agent 24 hours after infection. All of the untreated control animals became infected, and none of the animals in any of the treatment groups developed any sign of SIV infection.

These animal models have also been used to evaluate factors that might modulate the efficacy of postexposure chemoprophylaxis. In the RMLV model the efficacy of antiretroviral prophylaxis is directly dependent on both the size of the viral inoculum administered and the presence of intact cellular immune mechanisms in the animals studied (117). In the macaque model, Tsai et al. (122) demonstrated the importance of both timely administration of chemoprophylaxis and extended therapy. In their model, all of the animals that were treated for a total of 28 days remained uninfected, whereas only half the animals treated for 10 days were uninfected; none of the macaques treated for only 3 days were protected. Tsai et al. also demonstrated that delay of treatment was detrimental in the model. None of the animals that received postexposure chemoprophylaxis within 24 hours of intravenous infection developed productive SIV infection, whereas only 50% of the animals treated at 48 hours after infection and 25% of animals treated at 72 hours after infection were protected from SIV infection.

The evidence provided by these animal studies is invaluable. The data clearly demonstrate that antiretroviral agents can prevent retroviral infections in these models. They do not, however, guarantee that the same can be said for prevention of HIV infection in humans.

Failure of zidovudine following occupational injuries to healthcare workers has been documented in at least 22 instances (34,123). Fourteen of the 23 source persons were known to have been treated with antiretroviral therapy prior to the exposure. Antiretroviral resistance testing of source patient virus was performed in eight instances, and in four the virus was found to have reduced sensitivity to drug(s) used for postexposure prophylaxis. Six additional cases of zidovudine failure following larger or direct intravenous inocula have occurred: two seroconversions occurred after direct intravenous inoculation of HIV-infected blood during nuclear medicine procedures (124,125), another occurred after a deep stab injury inflicted on a prison guard (126), the fourth case occurred following suicidal self-inoculation of blood (127), and the fifth seroconversion occurred after transfusion of an entire unit of contaminated blood (98). An additional case of suicidal self-inoculation was reported in which the exposed individual did not become infected after postexposure prophylaxis with zidovudine, lamivudine, indinavir, ritonavir, and nevirapine. The authors suggest that the absence of infection was related to the small size of viral inoculum (2 mL blood with viral load <50 copies/mL), administration of postexposure prophylaxis, and development of an HIV-specific T-cell response (128). Interestingly, genotypic resistance did not correlate with a lack of protection in the ACTG 076 study of zidovudine administration to attempt to prevent vertical transmission of HIV. Nonetheless, exposure to a strain of HIV with reduced sensitivity to zidovudine may influence the likelihood of failure of postexposure chemoprophylaxis. Other hypothesized reasons for the failure of zidovudine postexposure prophylaxis include a high viral titer or large inoculum exposure, time factors including delayed initiation or premature discontinuation of postexposure prophylaxis, host factors including cellular immune responsiveness, and the source patient's virus including the presence of syncytia-forming strains (129). Although anecdotal reports of failure provide useful insight into both injury circumstances and specific issues regarding administration of zidovudine, these reports indicate only that the efficacy of zidovudine chemoprophylaxis is not 100%, and they do not, in themselves, prove lack of efficacy.

Delayed seroconversion following zidovudine prophylaxis has been a theoretical concern, since some of the animal data indicate that administration of zidovudine may merely delay viremia (102). A review of zidovudine prophylaxis failure published in 1997 determined that ten of 11 healthcare workers experienced an acute retroviral illness between 13 and 75 days (median 22 days) following the exposure, and all had seroconverted by 6 months following the exposure (129). These data are consistent with seroconversion data from healthcare workers who had not received postexposure prophylaxis.

The role of zidovudine-resistant strains of HIV in the failure of zidovudine chemoprophylaxis is unclear. Many reports of transmission of zidovudine-resistant isolates have been published (130,131), and studies show a prevalence of zidovudine resistance mutations in viral sequences from newly infected individuals of 5% to 10% (132,133). Studies on blood collected from a nationally representative sample of more than 1,900 HIV-infected patients in 1999 found that 78% of patients who had a measurable viral load had resistance to at least one antiretroviral drug (134). Extrapolating the results to all HIV-infected patients receiving care in the U.S., more than half are estimated to be infected with drug-resistant virus. The highest level of resistance (70%) was associated with nucleoside reverse-transcriptase inhibitors; the prevalence of drug resistance was significantly higher among those who had more advanced HIV disease. Additionally, at least one report suggests that zidovudine resistance-associated mutations present at the time of seroconversion may persist for at least 3 years in the absence of treatment (135–137). Little et al. (138) reported in 2002 that the frequency of high-level resistance to one or more antiretroviral drugs increased from 3.4% (1995–1998) to 12.4% (1999–2000) among 202 subjects in ten North American cities. Thus, the source patient's treatment history should be taken into account when determining the appropriate antiretroviral drugs for postexposure prophylaxis. However, as noted above, the relative importance of genotypic resistance to zidovudine to the chemoprophylaxis setting is not clear. Maternal zidovudine-resistant virus was predictive of transmission to the infant in one study, independent of viral load, in mothers with moderately advanced HIV disease, many of whom had been treated with zidovudine before pregnancy (139). Nonetheless, data regarding perinatal transmission suggest that perinatal HIV transmission may be established by a relatively restricted number of virus particles and that drug-resistant forms may be less able to establish infection than the wild-type virus (140,141). To further support this notion, several groups have found that virus with three-class multidrug resistance is infrequently transmitted, which may reflect the poor replication capacity of these extensively mutated viruses (132, 133,142,143).

Combination regimens, particularly those using three or more drugs, have been proven superior to monotherapy or double nucleoside therapy in HIV-infected patients (11,12,144, 145). Current guidelines define highly active antiretroviral therapy (HAART) as the cornerstone of care for HIV-infected patients. HAART typically involves three or more drugs that inhibit the replication of HIV by various mechanisms (146). There are no data to address the efficacy of other antiretroviral agents added to the basic single-drug regimen for postexposure prophylaxis. Theoretically, a combination of drugs with activity at different stages of viral replication could offer an additive preventive effect, particularly for occupational exposures with increased risks of transmission.

Currently, the routine use of three drugs for all occupational HIV exposures is not recommended (34). The USPHS has concluded that the use of a highly potent regimen (i.e., three drugs) can be justified for exposures that pose an increased risk for transmission, but that the additional potential toxicity may not be justified for lower risk exposures (34). The basic two-drug regimen is recommended for less severe exposures (e.g., solid needle and superficial injury) and HIV-infected sources with asymptomatic HIV infection or known low viral load (<1,500 RNA copies/mL). If the injury is more severe (e.g., large-bore hollow needle, deep puncture, visible blood on device, or needle used in patient's artery or vein) or the HIV-infected source has symptomatic HIV infection, AIDS, acute seroconversion, or known high viral load, then the expanded three-drug regimen is recommended. The two-drug basic regimens currently recommended by the USPHS include zidovudine plus lamivudine, lamivudine plus stavudine, or didanosine plus stavudine (Table 79.3). Zidovudine plus lamivudine may be the preferred choice in areas where zidovudine and lamivudine resistance has not become a widespread problem, as it is available in a combination formula (Combivir, GlaxoSmithKline, Research Triangle Park, NC) and includes the agent for which the most postexposure prophylaxis data are available. The addition of a protease inhibitor as a third drug for postexposure prophylaxis following high-risk exposures is based on the demonstrated efficacy of these agents in reducing viral burden, as well as their interference at a different site of viral replication (i.e., after viral integration has occurred) than for nucleoside analog reverse-transcriptase inhibitors. However, protease inhibitors have potentially serious drug interactions when used concomitantly with other medications. These agents also have serious side effects when used as an agent for combination postexposure prophylaxis, including nephrolithiasis, hepatitis, and pancytopenia (34). Nonetheless, an analysis determined that triple-drug combination therapy following moderate-to-high risk occupational exposures is cost-effective for society (147). If combination postexposure prophylaxis is minimally more effective than zidovudine alone, then the added expense of including other drugs in the drug regimen is clearly justified.

Tenofovir, (R)-9-[2-phosphonylmethoxypropyl] adenine (PMPA), is a recently FDA-approved nucleotide analog with documented efficacy in animal models (118,122) and a good safety profile. It is also available in a once-daily (one tablet) formulation for ease of use and, it is hoped, improved adherence. Tenofovir likely represents at least one reasonable addition to the list of agents that might be selected as part of a postexposure chemoprophylaxis regimen when the CDC releases updated recommendations in 2004.

A significant number of healthcare workers begin postexposure prophylaxis with two or more drugs after exposure to a source patient of unknown serostatus (148). Postexposure prophylaxis continues until the ELISA result is available, which may take up to 5 days. CDC HIV Postexposure Prophylaxis Registry data indicate that a healthcare worker taking only a few days of prophylaxis pending the source patient HIV test result is as likely as a healthcare worker taking the full 28-day course of prophylaxis to experience toxicity, since the median time to onset of symptoms was 3 to 4 days (148). Use of a rapid HIV screening test (see Diagnosis and Clinical Manifestations, above) will likely prevent the need for any medication and thus should decrease

TABLE 79.3. SUMMARY OF POSTEXPOSURE PROPHYLAXIS OPTIONS FOR HEALTHCARE WORKERS EXPOSED TO HIV

Basic Regimen		Expanded Regimen
Two nucleoside analogs		Two nucleoside analogs plus One additional drug
	Indications	
Occupational HIV exposures categorized as "less severe" (e.g., solid needle, superficial injury); source with asymptomatic infection or low viral load		Occupational HIV exposures categorized as "more severe" (e.g., deep puncture, visible blood on device); source with symptomatic infection or high viral load, or known drug resistance
	Antiretroviral Agents	
Choice of one regimen	Zidovudine + lamivudine Lamivudine + stavudine Stavudine + didanosine	*Choice of one regimen*
	Indinavir Nelfinavir Efavirenz Abacavir	*Choice of one*

HIV, human immunodeficiency virus.

healthcare worker anxiety as well as drug toxicity, and decrease costs for the institution (149,150).

Reasonable toxicity data are now available for zidovudine postexposure prophylaxis. At the NIH and San Francisco General Hospital, a multicenter collaborative study has been completed regarding the safety and toxicity of zidovudine administered to healthcare workers following occupational exposure (151). The zidovudine regimen used in this study consisted of 1,200 mg/day on days 1 to 3, followed by 1,000 mg/day on days 4 to 28. These investigators reported a mean decrease in hemoglobin values from 13.9 g/dL at baseline to 13.2 g/dL at 4 weeks for 105 healthcare workers who took zidovudine for at least 22 days. The maximum decrease in absolute neutrophil count was 1,200/mm^3 at week 4 following exposure. In this study, hematologic toxicities correlated neither with body weight nor with reported subjective toxicities. No nonhematologic objective toxicity was reported (151). Symptoms of drug intolerance (nausea, fatigue, headache) occurred in a substantial number of subjects (152). Forty-nine percent of 674 subjects experienced at least one adverse effect (most commonly nausea) in one study (153); other investigators reported that subjective toxicities were experienced by 69% of 155 healthcare workers who took zidovudine for at least 1 week (151). Despite the symptoms experienced by a majority of healthcare workers, laboratory evidence of significant objective toxicity was rare.

The Italian Registry of Antiretroviral Postexposure Prophylaxis observed hemoglobin values in the 9.5- to 11-g/dL range in 3% of healthcare workers and a neutrophil count of less than 1,000 cells/mm^3 in two healthcare workers (153). These same authors observed a transient increase of serum alanine aminotransferase to three times the upper limit of normal in seven healthcare workers. Prophylaxis was continued in each of these cases and all laboratory values returned to baseline within 1 to 2 weeks after a completed course of prophylaxis (153).

An increasing body of evidence documents the toxicity of antiretrovirals other than zidovudine in uninfected healthcare workers and in patients with early (or primary) HIV infection. A recent study examined the effects of HAART on patients with primary HIV infection (154). Commonly reported side effects for protease inhibitors include nausea, diarrhea, headache, mild liver function test abnormality, hyperglycemia, and nephrolithiasis (34,155). A multicenter collaborative study for occupational exposures examined the safety and adherence with combination postexposure prophylaxis regimens (156). Thirty-six of 54 healthcare workers took two drugs (zidovudine plus lamivudine), 16 took three drugs (zidovudine plus lamivudine plus indinavir), and two workers took didanosine plus stavudine. Twenty-eight percent discontinued prophylaxis early because of symptoms. Liver function abnormalities developed in two individuals, and prophylaxis was discontinued in both cases. The first individual was also receiving isoniazid prophylaxis. The second individual was exposed concomitantly to hepatitis C virus and HIV. This latter exposure resulted in acute hepatitis C infection; HIV was first diagnosed 12 months after the exposure (156). Additional toxicity data are provided by a report of ten healthcare workers receiving a three-drug combination regimen (86). All ten workers had some side effects, including gastrointestinal disturbance, fatigue, headache, and confusion. Three workers stopped postexposure prophylaxis early because of symptomatology. Wang et al. (148) reported on the postexposure prophylaxis (PEP) experiences of healthcare workers enrolled in the HIV PEP Registry; 308 of 492 (63%) enrolled healthcare workers took at least three antiretroviral agents; 340 of 449 (76%) healthcare workers with 6 weeks of follow-up reported some symptoms while on postexposure prophylaxis: nausea (57%), fatigue or malaise (38%), headache (18%), vomiting (16%), diarrhea (14%), and myalgias or arthralgias (6%). Median time to onset of each of the five most frequent symptoms was 3 to 4 days. Only 37 (8%) workers with 6 weeks of follow-up were reported to have laboratory abnormalities, most of which were unremarkable. Similar proportions of workers who took two drugs as compared with three drugs completed regimens as prescribed. However, significantly

TABLE 79.4. SUMMARY OF LABORATORY TESTING FOR HEALTHCARE WORKERS RECEIVING POSTEXPOSURE PROPHYLAXIS

	HIV Antibody	CBC with Differential[a]	Chemistry Panel[b]	Urine Pregnancy Test for Females
Baseline	X	X	X	X
2 weeks		X	X	
4 weeks		X	X	
6 weeks	X	[c]	[c]	
3 months	X			
6 months	X			
12 months	X			
Suspected acute retrovira syndrome	IX	X	X	
Suspected drug toxicity		X	X	

[a] CBC with differential should consist of a basic hematology panel with white blood cell differential and platelet count.
[b] Chemistry panel should consist of routine electrolytes, glucose, creatinine, serum glutamic-oxaloacetic transaminase (SGOT)(AST), serum glutamic-pyruvic transaminase (SGPT)(ALT), alkaline phosphatase, bilirubin, amylase.
[c] Only if previous results indicate toxicity.

more healthcare workers taking three drug regimens reported adverse events. Another recent report of healthcare worker post-exposure prophylaxis experience indicated that 10/46 (22%) stopped treatment secondary to adverse events or symptoms (157).

The immediate management of an occupational exposure should include the administration of first aid and rinsing and/or decontaminating of the exposure site as soon as is reasonably possible (i.e., as soon as patient and healthcare worker safety permits). At the NIH Clinical Center we recommend the following management approach for healthcare workers who have sustained occupational exposures to HIV (82,83): Wounds should be washed with soap and water, then irrigated with sterile saline, a disinfectant or other suitable solution. Healthcare workers who have sustained a mucosal exposure involving the mouth and nose should flush the exposed area extensively with water or sterile irrigants. For exposures involving the eyes, the involved area(s) should be irrigated with clean water, saline, or sterile fluids designed as ocular irrigants. All exposures should be reported immediately to the employee's supervisor and to the institution's occupational medical service. Each institution should work aggressively to develop mechanisms that facilitate both the reporting of exposures as well as the provision of follow-up care. The mechanisms should be widely publicized in the institution. Where feasible, institutions should offer access to consultants who are expert about the pathogenesis of HIV infection, the risk for occupational HIV infection, and the safety, efficacy, and known toxicities associated with the administration of antiretroviral agents. All institutional occupational medical systems must protect the confidentiality and medical privacy of the exposed worker. For healthcare workers who sustain documented occupational exposures to HIV, we advocate serologic studies at or as near to the exposure event as is possible (to document baseline seronegativity), with follow-up studies at 6 weeks, 3 months, 6 months, and 1 year following exposure. All exposed workers should be offered the opportunity to take postexposure antiretroviral chemoprophylaxis (described above). Once the baseline serology, hematology, and chemistry studies are drawn, healthcare workers who elect chemoprophylaxis should be followed for signs of drug toxicity while on therapy. Studies that we routinely order for healthcare workers electing postexposure chemoprophylaxis are detailed in Table 79.4. Additionally, supplementary studies, including PCR or branched-chain DNA assays, are ordered if the healthcare worker develops symptoms suggestive of the seroconversion illness.

MANAGEMENT OF THE HIV-INFECTED HEALTHCARE WORKER

In July 1990, the CDC published a report of possible iatrogenic transmission of HIV to a patient during an invasive dental procedure (158) followed 6 months later by another report documenting identification of four additional patients apparently infected with HIV by the same dentist in Florida (159). Two years later, a sixth patient was also identified as having been infected with the same strain of HIV as that from the dentist (160). These events, as well as the drama surrounding the tragic stories of the infected patients of the dentist who have chosen to make their plights public, alarmed the public and prompted calls for practice restrictions for HIV-infected healthcare workers.

Assessment of Risk for Transmission of HIV from Healthcare Worker to Patient

Discovery of the cluster of patients infected by the Florida dentist highlighted the need for additional data on the risk of HIV transmission from an HIV-infected provider to patients. These anecdotal cases of transmission, similar to the cases of transmission from patient to healthcare worker, indicate that provider-to-patient transmission is possible but do not quantify the level of risk associated with infected providers. Scrutiny of the procedures that were performed by the dentist on the infected patients also provides little useful information, because some of the patients had no more than what would be considered routine (i.e., noninvasive) dental work.

A second instance of transmission from provider to patient has been reported from France (161). An orthopedic surgeon most likely was infected with HIV in May 1983. The diagnosis of HIV seropositivity and AIDS was made simultaneously in March 1994. A total of 968 patients were serologically tested for HIV out of 3,004 who had undergone at least one invasive procedure by the surgeon. One patient, who had undergone two very lengthy hip procedures in 1992 and 1993, was determined to have seroconverted. Although no specific exposure incidents were recognized during the procedures, the patient was seronegative before the operation performed by the surgeon, and had a particularly prolonged duration of exposure to risk (the initial procedure lasted more than 10 hours). The surgeon's viral load could have been elevated at the time of the operation on this patient, and phylogenetic analysis indicated a close relationship between the patient's and the surgeon's viruses. The French National Public Health Network believes the case for transmission, based on the epidemiologic investigation and confirmed by viral sequencing, to be highly probable.

Another possible case of transmission, in this instance nurse to patient, again from France, was reported in 2000 (162). Phylogenetic analysis strongly suggests an HIV-infected nurse as the source of infection, although the authors do not provide any epidemiologic information as to the possible route of infection. The nurse was also co-infected with HCV, and both HIV and HCV were diagnosed 3 weeks after she provided care for the patient and transmission likely occurred. At the time of diagnosis, the source nurse had an HIV viral load of 1.8×10^5 copies/mL, her $CD4^+$ cell count was 94 per mm^3, and she was diagnosed with advanced hepatic cirrhosis with a blood clotting disorder (163). Hepatitis C was not transmitted to the patient. Investigators suggest that the nurse's high viral load associated with severe blood clotting disorders may have enhanced the risk of HIV transmission, although the nurse reported no percutaneous blood injury. A look-back study reported testing 2,310 of 7,580 patients (30%), and no additional cases of HIV infection were identified (163).

Based on our knowledge of routes of transmission from patients to providers, the primary risk for transmission of HIV is through exposure of the patient's bloodstream to blood from an infected provider (164). Based on this assumption, most authorities have concluded that routine patient-care activities pose no measurable risk for transmission (61,165). The CDC recommends that, if universal/standard precautions and the correct infection control procedures are followed, infected healthcare workers should not be restricted from performance of routine patient-care activities including drawing blood or starting intravenous lines. To transmit infection, a sharp object would first have to be contaminated with the provider's blood and then would have to recontact the patient's tissues. Whereas a number of studies have described the risk for surgeons sustaining exposures during surgical procedures (166–169), none of these studies attempted to assess the recontact risk. Two direct observational studies have attempted to address the patient's risk for exposure to a provider's blood during a surgical procedure (170, 171). In the first study, investigators from the CDC estimated that a surgical sharp object that had potentially injured a resident or attending surgeon had approximately a one in three chance of recontacting the tissues of the patient. This estimate was based on 28 recontacts following 88 observed injuries in surgeons; other authorities, including surgeons with years of operative experience, feel that this estimate of 32% may substantially overestimate the actual recontact risk. In the second preliminary study addressing potential for recontact injuries, occupational injuries during surgery were categorized as "definite" and "possible" (171). These investigators found that three of nine "definite" provider injuries recontacted the patient, whereas two of seven "possible" injuries recontacted the patient.

The CDC then used the estimated recontact risk to calculate a risk for provider-to-patient infection (172). This calculated risk for HIV infection associated with a patient undergoing a single invasive procedure performed by an HIV-infected surgeon was estimated to be between 1 in 42,000 and 1 in 420,000 procedures, and the similar risk for hepatitis B infection was estimated to be approximately 1 in 420 to 1 in 4,200 procedures. This risk assessment has several limitations, including its reliance on a single, as yet unconfirmed, estimate of recontact risk. Additionally, data regarding magnitude of transmission risk from patient to provider were used to estimate the reverse risk from provider to patient. Most provider injuries result from hollow-bore needles; yet, to our knowledge, no cases of patient-to-provider transmission have yet been documented following an exposure to a contaminated surgical needle. Conversely, most patient exposures are likely to arise from surgical needles; the inocula associated with these injuries are likely to be smaller than those associated with hollow-bore needles. Therefore, the risk of transmission of 0.2% to 0.3% based on patient-to-provider exposure and transmission data may overestimate the actual risk associated with a typical patient exposure. Finally, these risk estimates do not consider the provider's experience and skill level. Clearly, the risk for adverse exposures and, therefore, the even lower risk of patient exposure vary substantially among providers. For example, a surgeon with 15 years of experience may be substantially less likely to injure himself or herself than is a novice surgeon performing the identical procedure.

Other than the CDC estimate cited above, several additional estimates of the risk for provider-to-patient transmission of HIV have been published (172–175). These estimates range from one infection per 21 million hours of surgery (174) to one infection per 130,000 procedures (175).

An important issue that is not considered in any of the current risk assessment models is the potential infectivity of the medical practitioner. For example, iatrogenic transmission of hepatitis B has occurred almost exclusively from providers who were carriers of HBeAg. One exception to this rule is the reports of iatrogenic transmission of hepatitis B precore mutants that may be deficient in assembling the e antigen (176). Hepatitis B e antigenemia is a surrogate marker for viral burden. Individuals with circulating e antigen have high-grade HBV viremia. Based on these data, the CDC has issued formal recommendations about the management of HBeAg-positive providers who perform invasive procedures (61). Despite the wide availability of HIV viral load testing, either by reverse-transcriptase PCR (RT-PCR) technology or using a branched-chain DNA assay, current recommendations for HIV-infected practitioners do not take viral burden into account, rather addressing all HIV-infected practitioners, irrespective of the stage of HIV disease. As we learn more about the relative risk associated with varying viral burdens, these guidelines should probably be revisited.

LOOK-BACK NOTIFICATIONS FOR PATIENTS OF INFECTED PROVIDERS

A series of retrospective "look-back" studies have provided additional, albeit indirect, information about the risk of HIV transmission from provider to patient. In all of these studies, patients have been offered HIV testing retrospectively after a healthcare provider has been determined to be HIV-infected. According to the CDC, 51 HIV-seropositive healthcare workers had prompted HIV antibody testing of 22,171 patients by January 1, 1995 (172). To date, no additional iatrogenic infections have been documented in these studies. In fact, no HIV-infected patients have been identified for 37 of these infected healthcare workers; one or more HIV-infected patients were identified for 14 healthcare workers (the number of HIV-infected patients per healthcare worker ranged from 1 to 41). Of the 113 infected patients identified in these look-back studies, investigations have been completed for 110 patients. Twenty-eight were known to have been previously infected, 62 had established risk factors other than care by an HIV-infected provider, 15 had other potential chances for exposure (e.g., exchange of sex for drugs or money and/or multiple sex partners), and five had no risk identified. Genetic sequencing of the virus in the case of the infected Florida dentist indicated that six of the nine HIV-infected patients in the practice were infected with HIV strains that were closely related to those of the dentist (177,178).

A series of well-publicized look-back studies has been published from around the U.S. (179–189), which may have left the impression that look-back studies are now a standard of care whenever an HIV-infected healthcare worker who has performed invasive procedures in his or her practice is publicly identified. Indeed, many of these studies were the response of an institution or public health agency to a public outcry precipitated by discovery of an infected provider. Epidemiologists and other professionals responsible for follow-up of an infected provider must bear in mind that the risk of transmission associated with patient contact and even most, if not all, invasive procedures is negligible, and many experts argue that these studies are of extremely limited utility. The CDC has concluded that the risk for transmission of HIV from a healthcare worker to a patient is very small, and that retrospective patient notification need not be routine (172).

According to guidelines published by the Society for Healthcare Epidemiology of America, look-back notification should be considered in the following circumstances: (a) after a proven case of transmission of HIV, hepatitis B, or any other bloodborne pathogen to an index case; and (b) following a serious breach in infection control practices during invasive procedures performed by an infected healthcare worker (165). Look-back studies should not be undertaken for HIV-infected healthcare workers who do not perform invasive procedures. Two of the published look-back studies also detailed the costs incurred. Danila et al. (181) estimated that the costs associated with a study of an HIV-infected family physician totaled approximately $130,000, which was one third of the entire annual Minnesota Department of Health budget for statewide AIDS and HIV surveillance. A second look-back study estimated that the total costs incurred by initial patient notification and testing were $158,500 (189). Given the current efforts to control spiraling healthcare costs, look-back notifications in general may be an inappropriate use of diminishing resources.

Draft guidelines recently made available by the U.K. National Health Service (NHS) (*www.doh.gov.uk/aids*) advise that it is no longer necessary to notify every patient who has undergone an exposure-prone procedure by an infected healthcare worker because of the low risk of transmission and the anxiety caused to patients and the wider public. The NHS defines three categories of exposure-prone procedures; only for category 3 procedures where fingertips are out of sight for a significant part of the procedure and in which there is a distinct risk of injury (e.g., hysterectomies, cesarean sections, open cardiac surgery procedures) is patient notification necessary. HIV-infected healthcare workers, however, are prohibited from performing any exposure-prone procedure, including local anesthetic injections in dentistry and removal of hemorrhoids.

POLICY ISSUES

In summary, only three instances (eight patients infected through three healthcare workers) of iatrogenic HIV transmission have been documented to date. Additionally, the published risk estimates, even with their inherent limitations, support the conclusion that the risk of HIV transmission from provider to patient is extremely small, perhaps negligible, even during invasive procedures. Clearly, we all face, and accept, risks of a much higher magnitude each day. Indeed, 10 to 20 persons die from penicillin-related anaphylaxis per million first doses administered, and 250 persons per million die from car accidents per year (for those driving 10,000 miles per year) as compared with the risk of 1 to 24 seroconversions per million invasive procedures by an infected provider (190). Despite widespread acceptance of risks associated with driving a car and taking penicillin, the public continues to demand zero risk for provider-to-patient transmission of HIV. Although zero risk sounds inherently attractive, attainment is impossible. Even HIV-testing every provider annually (or more frequently) would miss some cases, especially incident cases in the so-called window of infectivity, and would result in unnecessary restrictions on those who test falsely positive. Additionally, the costs associated with minimizing this minuscule risk would be extraordinary (191–194). Developing sound public health policy for managing infected providers remains difficult, if not impossible, when anxiety and hysteria shape public perceptions of risk.

Another traditional concern of the medical establishment is that of *primum non nocere* (first, do no harm). This concept is reinforced from each provider's first days as a student in a healthcare profession, yet we all recognize that doing no harm is impossible. The realistic goal is to minimize the harm that we do while keeping risks in appropriate perspective. Other risks, including such issues as the competence levels of practicing providers and provider substance abuse, undoubtedly result in a much higher level of patient morbidity and mortality than the risk associated with competent HIV-infected providers. Thus, to reduce patient risk, one could certainly marshal a cogent argument for implementing routine drug and alcohol testing and mandatory competence reviews of healthcare professionals rather than implementing mandatory HIV-testing programs.

A final issue of concern relates to disability law and the concept of *significant risk*, which was adopted in the *School Board v. Arline* case (195), in which the U.S. Supreme Court determined that a disabled teacher who had chronic tuberculosis could not be discharged from her job, because she was disabled as a result of her condition and did not present a significant risk for transmission of tuberculosis. This concept has been reaffirmed twice, in the Civil Rights Restoration Act of 1988 (Public Law 100-259, 134, Congressional Record H.587-8) and, more recently, in the Americans with Disabilities Act of 1990 (Public

Law 101-336, 104 Stat. 327) (see Chapter 104). Mandating practice restrictions in order to reduce a risk that is lower than other accepted risks would essentially undermine current disability law by legally redefining the concept of significant risk (196).

Despite the Americans with Disabilities Act, the courts have, with few exceptions, upheld restrictions of HIV-infected healthcare workers from practice (197). Despite the legal standard that the employer bears the burden of proving that the practice poses a significant risk of harm, in reality the courts have shifted the burden to healthcare workers to show they pose virtually no risk. The CDC guidelines recommend use of an expert review panel to determine the ranges of acceptable practice, but the courts have twice upheld employer restrictions despite expert review panel advice that the healthcare worker should continue to practice (198,199).

Thus the issues surrounding the management of providers infected with bloodborne pathogens are exceedingly complex. As more knowledge is gained about the risks for iatrogenic spread of hepatitis B, hepatitis C, and HIV, management strategies may become more straightforward. The constellation of problems associated with the management of HIV-infected healthcare workers will undoubtedly continue to haunt the medical profession for years to come. Obtaining data to aid decisions about the most appropriate management of infected providers will be extraordinarily difficult given existing societal perceptions and the magnitude of risk associated with infected providers. Nonetheless, as a discipline, the hospital epidemiology community must assume leadership through educational efforts and by placing these risks into appropriate perspective with other risks, whether occupational, iatrogenic, or societal. Finally, based on our current understanding of the magnitude of risk for provider-to-patient transmission of bloodborne pathogens, we feel that prevention efforts should be focused on strategies to prevent occupational exposures to blood and body fluids. We believe the limited research capital available should be used to develop (a) devices and procedures that minimize risks of injury, (b) interventions that influence improvements in practitioners' workplace practices, (c) better approaches to educate healthcare workers and patients about risk and risk perception, and (d) sensible strategies to manage these risks.

REFERENCES

1. Centers for Disease Control and Prevention. Surveillance of health care workers with HIV/AIDS. December 6, 2001. Available at: *http://www.cdc.gov/hiv/stats/hasr1201/tabl17.htm.*
2. Leibowitz S, Greenwald L, Cohen I, et al. Serum hepatitis in a blood bank worker. *JAMA* 1949;140:1331–1333.
3. Centers for Disease Control. Summary and recommendations for preventing transmission of infection with human T-lymphotropic virus type III/lymphadenopathy–associated virus in the workplace. *MMWR* 1985;34:681–686,691–685.
4. Centers for Disease Control. Recommendations for protection against viral hepatitis. *MMWR* 1985;34(22):313–324,329–335.
5. Centers for Disease Control. Seroconversion to simian immunodeficiency virus in two laboratory workers. *MMWR* 1992;41(36):678–681.
6. Centers for Disease Control. Anonymous survey for simian immunodeficiency virus (SIV) seropositivity in SIV-laboratory researchers—United States, 1992. *MMWR* 1992;41(43):814–815.
7. Advisory Committee on Infection within Hospitals. *Management of HTLV-III/LAV infection in the hospital.* Chicago: American Hospital Association, 1986.
8. Pantaleo G, Graziosi C, Demarest J, et al. HIV infection is active and progressive in lymphoid tissue during the clinically latent stage of disease. *Nature* 1993;362:355–358.
9. Piatak M, Saag MS, Yang LC, et al. High levels of HIV-1 in plasma during all stages of infection determined by competitive PCR. *Science* 1993;259:1749–1754.
10. Louie JK, Hsu LC, Osmond DH, et al. Trends in causes of death among persons with acquired immunodeficiency syndrome in the era of highly active antiretroviral therapy, San Francisco, 1994–1998. *J Infect Dis* 2002;186(7):1023–1027.
11. Hammer SM, Squires KE, Hughes MD, et al. A controlled trial of two nucleoside analogues plus indinavir in persons with human immunodeficiency virus infection and CD4 cell counts of 200 per cubic millimeter or less. *N Engl J Med* 1997;337:725–733.
12. Gulick RM, Mellors JW, Havlir D, et al. Treatment with indinavir, zidovudine, and lamivudine in adults with human immunodeficiency virus infection and prior antiretroviral therapy. *N Engl J Med* 1997; 337:734–739.
13. Palella FJ Jr, Delaney KM, Moorman AC, et al. Declining morbidity and mortality among patients with advanced human immunodeficiency virus infection. HIV Outpatient Study Investigators. *N Engl J Med* 1998;338(13):853–860.
14. Finzi D, Hermankova M, Pierson T, et al. Identification of a reservoir for HIV-1 in patients on highly active antiretroviral therapy. *Science* 1997;278:1295–1300.
15. Schrager LK, D'Souza MP. Cellular and anatomical reservoirs of HIV-1 in patients receiving potent antiretroviral combination therapy. *JAMA* 1998;280(1):67–71.
16. Piguet V, Blauvelt A. Essential roles for dendritic cells in the pathogenesis and potential treatment of HIV disease. *J Invest Dermatol* 2002; 119(2):365–369.
17. Hu J, Gardner MB, Miller CJ. Simian immunodeficiency virus rapidly penetrates the cervicovaginal mucosa after intravaginal inoculation and infects intraepithelial dendritic cells. *J Virol* 2000;74(13): 6087–6095.
18. Spira AI, Marx PA, Patterson BK, et al. Cellular targets of infection and route of viral dissemination after an intravaginal inoculation of simian immunodeficiency virus into rhesus macaques. *J Exp Med* 1996;183(1):215–225.
19. Blauvelt A, Glushakova S, Margolis LB. HIV-infected human Langerhans cells transmit infection to human lymphoid tissue *ex vivo. AIDS* 2000;14(6):647–651.
20. Centers for Disease Control and Prevention. Public Health Service guidelines for the management of health-care worker exposures to HIV and recommendations for postexposure prophylaxis. *MMWR* 1998;47(RR-7):1–33.
21. Ranki A, Krohn M, Allain J-P, et al. Long latency period precedes overt seroconversion in sexually transmitted human-immunodeficiency virus infection. *Lancet* 1987;2:589–593.
22. Wolinsky SM, Rinaldo CR, Kwok S, et al. Human immunodeficiency virus type 1 (HIV-1) infection a median of 18 months before a diagnostic western blot: evidence from a cohort of homosexual men. *Ann Intern Med* 1989;111(12):961–972.
23. Ciesielski CA, Metler RP. Duration of time between exposure and seroconversion in healthcare workers with occupationally acquired infection with human immunodeficiency virus. *Am J Med* 1997; 102(5B):115–116.
24. Ridzon R, Gallagher K, Ciesielski C, et al. Simultaneous transmission of human immunodeficiency virus and hepatitis C virus from a needle-stick injury. *N Engl J Med* 1997;336(13):919–922.
25. Busch MP, Sattem GA. Time course of viremia and antibody seroconversion following human immunodeficiency virus exposure. *Am J Med* 1997;102(suppl 5B):117–124.
26. Fox R, Eldred LJ, Fuchs EJ, et al. Clinical manifestations of acute infection with human immunodeficiency virus in a cohort of gay men. *AIDS* 1987;1(1):35–38.
27. Ho DD, Sarngadharan MG, Resnick L, et al. Primary human T-

lymphotropic virus type III infection. *Ann Intern Med* 1985;103(6 pt 1):880–883.
28. Kessler HA, Blaauw B, Spear J, et al. Diagnosis of human immunodeficiency virus infection in seronegative homosexuals presenting with an acute viral syndrome. *JAMA* 1987;258:1196–1199.
29. Gaines H, Sonnerborg A, Czajkowski J, et al. Antibody response in primary human immunodeficiency virus infection. *Lancet* 1987:1249–1253.
30. Albert J, Gaines H, Sonnerborg A, et al. Isolation of human immunodeficiency virus (HIV) from plasma during primary HIV infection. *J Med Virol* 1987;23(1):67–73.
31. Daar ES, Moudgil T, Meyer RD, et al. Transient high levels of viremia in patients with primary human immunodeficiency virus type 1 infection. *N Engl J Med* 1991;324(14):961–964.
32. Stramer SL, Heller JS, Coombs RW, et al. Markers of HIV infection prior to IgG antibody seropositivity. *JAMA* 1989;262:64–69.
33. Schacker TW, Hughes JP, Shea T, et al. Biological and virologic characteristics of primary HIV infection. *Ann Intern Med* 1998;128(8):613–620.
34. Centers for Disease Control and Prevention. Updated U.S. Public Health Service guidelines for the management of occupational exposures to HBV, HCV, and HIV and recommendations for postexposure prophylaxis. *MMWR* 2001;50(RR-11):1–52.
35. Beekmann SE, Fahey BJ, Gerberding JL, et al. Risky business: using necessarily imprecise casualty counts to estimate occupational risks for HIV-1 infection. *Infect Control Hosp Epidemiol* 1990;11:371–379.
36. Ippolito G, Puro V, Heptonstall J, et al. Occupational human immunodeficiency virus infection in health care workers: worldwide cases through September 1997. *Clin Infect Dis* 1999;28(2):365–383.
37. Beltrami EM, Williams IT, Shapiro CN, et al. Risk and management of blood-borne infections in health care workers. *Clin Microbiol Rev* 2000;13(3):385–407.
38. Cardo DM, Culver DH, Ciesielski CA, et al. A case-control study of HIV seroconversion in health care workers after percutaneous exposure. *N Engl J Med* 1997;337(21):1485–1490.
39. Mast ST, Woolwine JD, Gerberding JL. Efficacy of gloves in reducing blood volumes transferred during simulated needlestick injury. *J Infect Dis* 1993;168:1589–1592.
40. Mast S, Gerberding JL. Factors predicting infectivity following needlestick exposure to HIV: an in vitro model. *Clin Res* 1991;39:58A.
41. Eberle J, Habermann J, Gurtler LG. HIV-1 infection transmitted by serum droplets into the eye: a case report. *AIDS* 2000;14(2):206–207.
42. Henderson DK. Managing occupational risks for hepatitis C transmission in the healthcare setting. *Clin Microbiol Rev* 2003;16:546–568.
43. Beekmann SE, Henderson DK. Health care workers and hepatitis: Risk for infection and management of exposures. *Infect Dis Clin Pract* 1992;1(6):424–428.
44. Centers for Disease Control. Protection against viral hepatitis: recommendations of the Immunization Practices Advisory Committee (ACIP). *MMWR* 1990;39:1–26.
45. Department of Labor, Department of Health and Human Services. Joint advisory notice: protection against occupational exposure to hepatitis B virus (HBV) and human immunodeficiency virus (HIV). *Fed Reg* 1987;52:41818–41824.
46. Mahoney FJ, Stewart K, Hu H, et al. Progress toward the elimination of hepatitis B virus transmission among health care workers in the United States. *Arch Intern Med* 1997;147:2601–2605.
47. Alter MJ. Epidemiology of hepatitis C in the west. *Semin Liver Dis* 1995;15:5–14.
48. Alter MJ, Mast EE, Moyer LA, et al. Hepatitis C. *Infect Dis Clin North Am* 1998;12(1):13–26.
49. Veeder A, Stellrecht K, Steinmann A, et al. Hepatitis C infection in health care workers following percutaneous exposures to HCV positive sources (abstract). Paper presented at the eighth annual meeting of the Society for Healthcare Epidemiology of America, 1998, Orlando, Florida.
50. Henderson DK. HIV postexposure prophylaxis in the 21st century. *Emerg Infect Dis* 2001;7(2):254–258.
51. Department of Labor OSHA. Occupational exposure to bloodborne pathogens; final rule. *Fed Reg* 1991;56:64175–64182.
52. Centers for Disease Control. Recommendations for prevention of HIV transmission in health-care settings. *MMWR* 1987;36(suppl 2S):1S–19S.
53. Centers for Disease Control. *Pneumocystis* Pneumonia. *MMWR* 1981;30:250–252.
54. Centers for Disease Control. Acquired immune deficiency syndrome: precautions for clinical and laboratory staffs. *MMWR* 1982;31:577–580.
55. Centers for Disease Control. Acquired immunodeficiency syndrome (AIDS): precautions for health-care workers and allied professionals. *MMWR* 1983;32:450–451.
56. Centers for Disease Control. Recommended infection-control practices for dentistry. *MMWR* 1985;35:237–242.
57. Centers for Disease Control. Recommendations for preventing possible transmission of human T-lymphotropic virus type III/lymphadenopathy-associated virus from tears. *MMWR* 1985;34:533–534.
58. Centers for Disease Control. Recommendations for preventing transmission of infection with human T-lymphotropic virus type III/lymphadenopathy-associated virus during invasive procedures. *MMWR* 1986;35:221–223.
59. Centers for Disease Control. Update: universal precautions for prevention of transmission of human immunodeficiency virus, hepatitis B virus, and other bloodborne pathogens in health-care settings. *MMWR* 1988;37::377–382;387–388.
60. Centers for Disease Control. *Guidelines for prevention of transmission of human immunodeficiency virus and hepatitis B virus to health-care and public-safety workers—a response to PL 100–607. The Health Omnibus Programs Extension Act, 1988.* Washington, DC: Department of Health and Human Services, 1989.
61. Centers for Disease Control. Recommendations for preventing transmission of human immunodeficiency virus and hepatitis B virus to patients during exposure-prone invasive procedures. *MMWR* 1991;40(RR-8):1–9.
62. Centers for Disease Control and Prevention. Recommended infection control practices for dentistry. *MMWR* 1993;42(RR-8):1–12.
63. Centers for Disease Control and Prevention. Recommendations for follow-up of health-care workers after occupational exposure to hepatitis C virus. *MMWR* 1997;46(26):603–606.
64. Centers for Disease Control and Prevention. Public Health Service Task Force recommendations for the use of antiretroviral drugs in pregnant women infected with HIV-1 for maternal health and for reducing perinatal HIV-1 transmission in the United States. Centers for Disease Control and Prevention [published errata appear in *MMWR* 1998;47(14):287 and 199824;47(15):315]. *MMWR* 1998;47(RR-2):1–30.
65. Garner JS. Guideline for isolation precautions in hospitals. The Hospital Infection Control Practices Advisory Committee. *Infect Control Hosp Epidemiol* 1996;17(1):53–80.
66. Lynch P, Jackson MM, Cummings MJ, et al. Rethinking the role of isolation practices in the prevention of nosocomial infection. *Ann Intern Med* 1986;107:243–246.
67. Doebbeling BN, Wenzel RP. The direct costs of universal precautions in a teaching hospital. *JAMA* 1990;264:2083–2087.
68. McCormick RD, Meisch MG, Ircink FG, et al. Epidemiology of hospital sharps injuries: a 14-year prospective study in the pre-AIDS and AIDS eras. *Am J Med* 1991;91(suppl 3B):301S-307S.
69. Edmond M, Khakoo R, McTaggart B, et al. Effect of bedside needle disposal units on needle recapping frequency and needlestick injury. *Infect Control Hosp Epidemiol* 1988;9:114–116.
70. Krasinski K, LaCouture R, Holzman RS. Effect of changing needle disposal systems on needle puncture injuries. *Infect Control* 1987;8:59–62.
71. Linnemann CC, Cannon C, DeRonde M, et al. Effect of educational programs, rigid sharps containers, and universal precautions on reported needlestick injuries in healthcare workers. *Infect Control Hosp Epidemiol* 1991;12:214–219.
72. Ribner BS, Ribner BS. An effective educational program to reduce

the frequency of needle recapping. *Infect Control Hosp Epidemiol* 1990; 11:635–638.

73. Saghafi L, Raselli P, Francillon C, et al. Exposure to blood during various procedures: results of two surveys before and after the implementation of universal precautions. *Am J Infect Control* 1992;20(2): 53–57.
74. Sellick JA, Hazamy PA, Mylotte JM. Influence of an educational program and mechanical opening needle disposal boxes on occupational needlestick injuries. *Infect Control Hosp Epidemiol* 1991;12: 725–731.
75. Wong ES, Stotka JL, Chinchilli VM, et al. Are universal precautions effective in reducing the number of occupational exposures among health care workers? A prospective study of physicians on a medical service. *JAMA* 1991;265:1123–1128.
76. Fahey BJ, Meehan PE, Henderson DK. The risk of HIV-1 transmission in health care workers. *Infect Med* 1988;5:224–237.
77. Beekmann SE, Vlahov D, Koziol DE, et al. Implementation of universal precautions was temporally associated with a sustained, progressive decrease in percutaneous exposures to blood or body fluids. *Clin Infect Dis* 1994;18(4):562–569.
78. Beekmann SE, Vaughn TE, McCoy KD, et al. Hospital bloodborne pathogens programs: program characteristics and blood and body fluid exposure rates. *Infect Control Hosp Epidemiol* 2001;22(2):73–82.
79. Centers for Disease Control and Prevention. Protection against viral hepatitis. Recommendations of the Immunization Practices Advisory Committee (ACIP). *MMWR* 1990;39(RR-2):1–26.
80. Hadler SC. Hepatitis B virus infection and health care workers. *Vaccine* 1990;8:S24–28.
81. Agerton T, Mahoney F, Polish L, et al. Impact of the bloodborne pathogens standard on vaccination of healthcare workers with hepatitis B vaccine. *Infect Control Hosp Epidemiol* 1995;16:287–291.
82. Fahey BJ, Beekmann SE, Schmitt JM, et al. Managing occupational exposures to HIV-1 in the healthcare workplace. *Infect Control Hosp Epidemiol* 1993;14(7):405–412.
83. Gerberding JL, Henderson DK. Management of occupational exposures to bloodborne pathogens: hepatitis B virus, hepatitis C virus, and human immunodeficiency virus. *Clin Infect Dis* 1992;14:1179–1185.
84. Henderson DK, Fahey BJ, Willy ME, et al. Risk for occupational transmission of human immunodeficiency virus type 1 (HIV-1) associated with clinical exposures: a prospective evaluation. *Ann Intern Med* 1990;113:740–746.
85. Jaffe HA, Schmitt JM. AIDS in the workplace. In: Rom W, ed. *Environmental and occupational medicine,* 2nd ed. Boston: Little, Brown, 1992:685–713.
86. Sepkowitz KA, Rivera P, Louther J, et al. Postexposure prophylaxis for human immunodeficiency virus: frequency of initiation and completion of newly recommended regimen. *Infect Control Hosp Epidemiol* 1998;19:506–508.
87. Sistrom MG, Coyner BJ, Gwaltney JM, et al. Frequency of percutaneous injuries requiring postexposure prophylaxis for occupational exposure to human immunodeficiency virus. *Infect Control Hosp Epidemiol* 1998;19:504–506.
88. Henderson DK. Postexposure treatment of HIV—taking some risks for safety's sake. *N Engl J Med* 1997;337(21):1542–1543.
89. Cardo D, Srivastava P, Ciesielski C, et al. Case-control study of HIV seroconversion in health care workers after percutaneous exposure to HIV-infected blood (Abstract I236). Paper presented at the 34th Interscience Conference on Antimicrobial Agents and Chemotherapy, 1994, Orlando, FL.
90. Centers for Disease Control and Prevention. Case-control study of HIV seroconversion in health-care workers after percutaneous exposure to HIV-infected blood—France, United Kingdom, and United States, January 1988–August 1994. *MMWR* 1995;44(50):929–933.
91. Connor EM, Sperling RS, Gelber R, et al. Reduction of maternal-infant transmission of human immunodeficiency virus type 1 with zidovudine treatment. Pediatric AIDS Clinical Trials Group Protocol 076 Study Group. *N Engl J Med* 1994;331(18):1173–1180.
92. Sperling RS, Shapiro DE, Coombs RW, et al. Maternal viral load, zidovudine treatment, and the risk of transmission of human immunodeficiency virus type 1 from mother to infant. Pediatric AIDS Clinical Trials Group Protocol 076 Study Group. *N Engl J Med* 1996; 335(22):1621–1629.
93. Shaffer N, Chuachoowong R, Mock PA, et al. Short-course zidovudine for perinatal HIV-1 transmission in Bangkok, Thailand: a randomised controlled trial. Bangkok Collaborative Perinatal HIV Transmission Study Group. *Lancet* 1999;353(9155):773–780.
94. Wade NA, Birkhead GS, Warren BL, et al. Abbreviated regimens of zidovudine prophylaxis and perinatal transmission of the human immunodeficiency virus. *N Engl J Med* 1998;339(20):1409–1414.
95. Wiktor SZ, Ekpini E, Karon JM, et al. Short-course oral zidovudine for prevention of mother-to-child transmission of HIV-1 in Abidjan, Cote d'Ivoire: a randomised trial. *Lancet* 1999;353(9155):781–785.
96. Bulterys M, Orloff S, Abrams E, et al. Impact of zidovudine post-perinatal exposure prophylaxis on vertical HIV-1 transmission: a prospective cohort study in four US cities (abstract 15). Paper presented at the Global Strategies for the Prevention of HIV Transmission from Mothers to Infants, September 1–6 1999, Toronto, Ontario, Canada.
97. Black RJ. Animal studies of prophylaxis. *Am J Med* 1997;102(suppl 5B):39–44.
98. Centers for Disease Control. Public Health Service statement on management of occupational exposure to human immunodeficiency virus, including considerations regarding zidovudine postexposure use. *MMWR* 1990;39(RR):1– 14.
99. Lewis W, Dalakas MC. Mitochondrial toxicity of antiviral drugs. *Nat Med* 1995;1(5):417–422.
100. Luster MI, Rosenthal GJ, Cao W, et al. Experimental studies of the hematologic and immune system toxicity of nucleoside derivatives used against HIV infection. *Int J Immunopharmacol* 1991;1(99): 99–107.
101. Fazely F, Haseltine WA, Rodger RF, et al. Postexposure chemoprophylaxis with ZDV or ZDV combined with interferon-alpha: failure after inoculating rhesus monkeys with a high dose of SIV. *J Acquir Immune Defic Syndr* 1991;4(11):1093–1097.
102. Gerberding JL, Marx P, Gould R, et al. Simian model of retrovirus chemoprophylaxis with constant infusion zidovudine plus or minus interferon alpha (abstract). Paper presented at the 31st Interscience Conference on Antimicrobial Agents and Chemotherapy, 1991, Washington, DC.
103. Hayes KA, Lafrado LJ, Erickson JG, et al. Prophylactic ZDV therapy prevents early viremia and lymphocyte decline but not primary infection in feline immunodeficiency virus-inoculated cats. *J AIDS* 1993; 6(2):127–134.
104. Hayes KA, Wilkinson JG, Frick R, et al. Early suppression of viremia by ZDV does not alter the spread of feline immunodeficiency virus infection in cats. *J AIDS Hum Retrovirol* 1995;9(2):114–122.
105. Lundgren B, Bottiger D, Ljungdahl-Stahle E, et al. Antiviral effects of 3′-fluorothymidine and 3′-azidothymidine in cynomolgus monkeys infected with simian immunodeficiency virus. *J AIDS* 1991;4: 489–498.
106. Martin LN, Murphey CM, Soike KF, et al. Effects of initiation of 3′-azido,3′-deoxythymidine (zidovudine) treatment at different times after infection of rhesus monkeys with simian immunodeficiency virus. *J Infect Dis* 1993;168(4):825–835.
107. Mathes L, Polas P, Hayes K, et al. Pre- and postexposure chemoprophylaxis: evidence that 3′-azido-3′-deoxythymidine inhibits feline leukemia virus disease by a drug-induced vaccine response. *Antimicrob Agents Chemother* 1992;36:2715–2721.
108. McClure HM, Anderson DC, Fultz P, et al. Prophylactic effects of AZT following exposure of macaques to an acutely lethal variant of SIV (SIV/SMM/PBj-14) (abstract). Paper presented at the 5th International Conference on AIDS, 1989, Ottawa, Canada.
109. McCune JM, Namikawa R, Shih CC, et al. Suppression of HIV infection in AZT-treated SCID-hu mice. *Science* 1990;247(4942): 564–566.
110. Morrey JD, Okleberry KM, Sidwell RW. Early-initiated zidovudine therapy prevents disease but not low levels of persistent retrovirus in mice. *J AIDS* 1991;4:506–512.
111. Ruprecht RM, O'Brien LG, Rossoni LD, et al. Suppression of mouse viraemia and retroviral disease by 3′-azido-3′deoxythymidine. *Nature* 1986;323:467–469.

112. Shih CC, Kaneshima H, Rabin L, et al. Postexposure prophylaxis with zidovudine suppresses human immunodeficiency virus type 1 infection in SCID-hu mice in a time-dependent manner. *J Infect Dis* 1991;163(3):625–627.
113. Tavares L, Roneker C, Johnston K, et al. 3′-Azido-3′deoxythymidine in feline leukemia virus-infected cats: a model for therapy and prophylaxis of AIDS. *Cancer Res* 1987;47:3190–3194.
114. Van Rompay KK, Marthas ML, Ramos RA, et al. Simian immunodeficiency virus (SIV) infection of infant rhesus macaques as a model to test antiretroviral drug prophylaxis and therapy: oral 3′-azido-3′-deoxythymidine prevents SIV infection. *Antimicrob Agents Chemother* 1992;36(11):2381–2386.
115. Böttiger D, Putkonen P, Oberg B. Prevention of HIV-2 and SIV infections in cynomolgus macaques by prophylactic treatment with 3′-fluorothymidine. *AIDS Res Hum Retroviruses* 1992;8(7):1235–1238.
116. Böttiger D, Johansson NG, Samuelsson B, et al. Prevention of simian immunodeficiency virus, SIVsm, or HIV-2 infection in cynomolgus monkeys by pre- and postexposure administration of BEA-005. *AIDS* 1997;11(2):157–162.
117. Ruprecht RM, Bronson R. Chemoprevention of retroviral infection: success is determined by virus inoculum strength and cellular immunity. *DNA Cell Biol* 1994;13(1):59–66.
118. Tsai CC, Follis KE, Sabo A, et al. Prevention of SIV infection in macaques by (R)-9-(2-phosphonylmethoxypropyl)adenine. *Science* 1995;270(5239):1197–1199.
119. Putkonen P, Makitalo B, Bottiger D, et al. Protection of human immunodeficiency virus type 2–exposed seronegative macaques from mucosal simian immunodeficiency virus transmission. *J Virol* 1997; 71(7):4981–4984.
120. Ruprecht RM, Bernard LD, Gama Sosa MA, et al. Murine models for evaluating antiretroviral therapy. *Cancer Res* 1990;50(17 suppl): 5618S–5627S.
121. Ruprecht RM, Mullaney S, Bernard LD, et al. Vaccination with a live retrovirus: the nature of the protective immune response. *Proc Natl Acad Sci USA* 1990;87(14):5558–5562.
122. Tsai CC, Emau P, Follis KE, et al. Effectiveness of postinoculation (R)-9-(2-phosphonylmethoxypropyl) adenine treatment for prevention of persistent simian immunodeficiency virus SIVmne infection depends critically on timing of initiation and duration of treatment. *J Virol* 1998;72(5):4265–4273.
123. Hawkins DA, Asboe D, Barlow K, et al. Seroconversion to HIV-1 following a needlestick injury despite combination post-exposure prophylaxis. *J Infect* 2001;43(1):12–15.
124. Centers for Disease Control. Patient exposures to HIV during nuclear medicine procedures. *MMWR* 1992;41:575–578.
125. Lange JMA, Boucher CAB, Hollak CEM, et al. Failure of zidovudine prophylaxis after accidental exposure to HIV-1. *N Engl J Med* 1990; 322:1375–1377.
126. Jones PD. HIV transmission by stabbing despite zidovudine prophylaxis. *Lancet* 1991;338:884.
127. Durand E, LeJeunne C, Hugues FC. Failure of prophylactic zidovudine after suicidal self-inoculation of HIV-infected blood. *N Engl J Med* 1991;324:1062.
128. Aberle JH, Schmied B, Vetter N, et al. Absence of human immunodeficiency virus infection after intentional injection of infected blood. *Clin Infect Dis* 2002;35:26–28.
129. Jochimsen EM, Luo CC, Beltrami JF, et al. Investigations of possible failures of postexposure prophylaxis following occupational exposures to human immunodeficiency virus. *Arch Intern Med* 1999;159(19): 2361–2363.
130. Erice A, Mayers DL, Strike DG, et al. Brief report: Primary infection with zidovudine-resistant human immunodeficiency virus type 1. *N Engl J Med* 1993;328(16):1163–1165.
131. Wainberg MA, Friedland G. Public health implications of antiretroviral therapy and HIV drug resistance. *JAMA* 1998;279(24): 1977–1983.
132. Yerly S, Kaiser L, Race E, et al. Transmission of antiretroviral-drug-resistant HIV-1 variants. *Lancet* 1999;354(9180):729–733.
133. Little SJ, Daar ES, D'Aquila RT, et al. Reduced antiretroviral drug susceptibility among patients with primary HIV infection. *JAMA* 1999;282(12):1142–1149.
134. Stephenson J. Sobering levels of drug-resistant HIV found. *Jama* 2002;287(6):704–705.
135. Quigg M, Rebus S, France AJ, et al. Mutations associated with zidovudine resistance in HIV-1 among recent seroconverters. *AIDS* 1997; 11:835–836.
136. Montaner JSG, Singer J, Schechter MT, et al. Clinical correlates of *in vitro* resistance to zidovudine. Results of the multicentre Canadian AZT trial. *AIDS* 1993;7:189–196.
137. Japour AJ, et al. Prevalence and clinical significance of zidovudine resistance mutations in human immunodeficiency virus isolated from patients after long-term zidovudine treatment. *J Infect Dis* 1995;171: 1172–1179.
138. Little SJ, Holte S, Routy JP, et al. Antiretroviral-drug resistance among patients recently infected with HIV. *N Engl J Med* 2002; 347(6):385–394.
139. Welles SL, Pitt J, Colgrove R, et al. HIV-1 genotypic zidovudine drug resistance and the risk of maternal-infant transmission in the women and infants transmission study. The Women and Infants Transmission Study Group. *AIDS* 2000;14(3):23–271.
140. Colgrove R, Pitt J, Chung PH, et al. Selective vertical transmission of HIV-1 zidovudine resistance mutations. Paper presented at the 5th Conference on Retroviruses and Opportunistic Infections, 1998, Chicago, IL.
141. Colgrove R, Pitt J, Chung PH, et al. Selective vertical transmission of HIV-1 antiretroviral resistance mutations. *AIDS* 1998;12(17): 2281–2288.
142. Yerly S, Vora S, Rizzardi P, et al. Acute HIV infection: impact on the spread of HIV and transmission of drug resistance. *AIDS* 2001; 15(17):2287–2292.
143. Grant RM, Hecht FM, Warmerdam M, et al. Time trends in primary HIV-1 drug resistance among recently infected persons. *JAMA* 2002; 288(2):181–188.
144. Lafeuillade A, Poggi C, Tamalet C, et al. Effects of a combination of zidovudine, didanosine, and lamivudine on primary human immunodeficiency virus type 1 infection. *J Infect Dis* 1997;175:1051–1055.
145. Manion DJ, Hirsch MS. Combination chemotherapy for human immunodeficiency virus-1. *Am J Med* 1997;102(suppl 5B):76–80.
146. HIV/AIDS Treatment Information Service. Guidelines for the use of antiretroviral agents in HIV-infected adults and adolescents. November 10, 2003. *www.aidsinfo.gov/guideline*
147. Pinkerton SD, Holtgrave DR, Pinkerton HJ. Cost-effectiveness of chemoprophylaxis after occupational exposure to HIV. *Arch Intern Med* 1997;157(17):1972–1980.
148. Wang SA, Panlilio AL, Doi PA, et al. Experience of healthcare workers taking postexposure prophylaxis. *Infect Control Hosp Epidemiol* 2000; 21:780–785.
149. Kallenborn JC, Price TG, Carrico R, et al. Emergency department management of occupational exposures: cost analysis of rapid HIV test. *Infect Control Hosp Epidemiol* 2001;22:289–293.
150. Greub G, Maziero A, Burgisser P, et al. Spare post-exposure prophylaxis with round-the-clock HIV testing of the source patient. *AIDS* 2001;15(18):2451–2452.
151. Fahrner R, Beekmann S, Koziol D, et al. Safety of zidovudine administered as post-exposure chemoprophylaxis to healthcare workers sustaining HIV-related occupational exposures. 34th Interscience Conference on Antimicrobial Agents and Chemotherapy, 1994, Orlando, FL.
152. Beekmann SE, Fahrner R, Henderson DK, et al. Zidovudine safety and tolerance among uninfected healthcare workers: a brief update. *Am J Med* 1997;102(5B):63–64.
153. Ippolito G, Puro V, The Italian Registry of Antiretroviral Prophylaxis. Zidovudine toxicity in uninfected healthcare workers. *Am J Med* 1997;102(5B):58–62.
154. Berrey MM, Schacker T, Collier AC, et al. Treatment of primary human immunodeficiency virus type 1 infection with potent antiretroviral therapy reduces frequency of rapid progression to aids. *J Infect Dis* 2001;183(10):1466–1475.
155. Lee LM, Henderson DK. Tolerability of postexposure antiretroviral

prophylaxis for occupational exposures to HIV. *Drug Saf* 2001;24(8): 587–597.

156. Fahrner R, Beekmann SE, Nelson L, et al. Combination post-exposure prophylaxis (PEP): a prospective study of HIV-exposed health care workers (HCW). Paper presented at the 12th International Conference on AIDS, July 1998, Geneva.
157. Garb JR. One-year study of occupational human immunodeficiency virus postexposure prophylaxis. *J Occup Environ Med* 2002;44(3): 265–270.
158. Centers for Disease Control. Possible transmission of human immunodeficiency virus to a patient during an invasive dental procedure. *MMWR* 1990;39(29):489–493.
159. Centers for Disease Control. Update: Transmission of HIV infection during an invasive dental procedure—Florida. *MMWR* 1991;40(2): 21–33.
160. Hillis DM, Huelsenbeck JP. Support for dental HIV transmission. *Nature* 1994;369:24–25.
161. Lot F, Seguier JC, Fegueux S, et al. Probable transmission of HIV from an orthopedic surgeon to a patient in France. *Ann Intern Med* 1999;130(1):1–6.
162. Goujon CP, Schneider VM, Grofti J, et al. Phylogenetic analyses indicate an atypical nurse-to-patient transmission of human immunodeficiency virus type 1. *J Virol* 2000;74(6):2525–2532.
163. Astagneau P, Lot F, Bouvet E, et al. Lookback investigation of patients potentially exposed to HIV type 1 after a nurse-to-patient transmission. *Am J Infect Control* 2002;30(4):242–245.
164. Beekmann SE, Doebbeling BN. Frontiers of occupational health. New vaccines, new prophylactic regimens, and management of the HIV-infected worker. *Infect Dis Clin North Am* 1997;11(2):313–329.
165. Henderson DK, The AIDS/Tuberculosis Subcommittee of the Society for Healthcare Epidemiology of America. Management of healthcare workers infected with hepatitis B virus, hepatitis C virus, human immunodeficiency virus, or other bloodborne pathogens. AIDS/TB Committee of the Society for Healthcare Epidemiology of America. *Infect Control Hosp Epidemiol* 1997;18(5):349–363.
166. Gerberding JL, Littell C, Tarkington A, et al. Risk of exposure of surgical personnel to patients' blood during surgery at San Francisco General Hospital. *N Engl J Med* 1990;322(25):1788–1793.
167. Lowenfels AB, Wormser GP. Frequency of puncture injuries in surgeons and estimated risk of HIV infection. *Arch Surg* 1989;124: 1284–1286.
168. Panlilio AL, Foy DR, Edwards JR, et al. Blood contacts during surgical procedures. *JAMA* 1991;265:1533–1537.
169. Popejoy SL, Fry DE. Blood contact and exposure in the operating room. *Surg Gynecol Obstet* 1991;172(6):480–483.
170. Tokars JI, Bell DM, Culver DH, et al. Percutaneous injuries during surgical procedures. *JAMA* 1992;267(21):2899–2904.
171. Gerberding JL, Ramiro N, Perlman J, et al. Intraoperative blood exposures at San Francisco General Hospital: provider injuries and patient recontacts. Paper presented at the 31st annual meeting of the Infectious Diseases Society of America, 1993, New Orleans.
172. Robert LM, Chamberland ME, Cleveland JL, et al. Investigations of patients of health care workers infected with HIV: the Centers for Disease Control and Prevention database. *Ann Intern Med* 1995; 122(9):653–657.
173. Rhame FS. The HIV-infected surgeon. *JAMA* 1990;264:507–508.
174. Lowenfels AB, Wormser G. Risk of transmission of HIV from surgeon to patient. *N Engl J Med* 1991;325:888–889.
175. Gostin L. HIV-infected physicians and the practice of seriously invasive procedures. *Hastings Center Rep* 1989;19(1):32–39.
176. Public Health Laboratory Service Communicable Disease Surveillance Centre Incident Investigation Teams and others. Transmission of hepatitis B to patients from four infected surgeons without hepatitis B e antigen. *N Engl J Med* 1997;336(3):178–184.
177. Ciesielski C, Marianos D, Ou C-Y, et al. Transmission of human immunodeficiency virus in a dental practice. *Ann Intern Med* 1992; 116(10):798–805.
178. Ou CY, Ciesielski CA, Myers G, et al. Molecular epidemiology of HIV transmission in a dental practice. *Science* 1992;256(5060): 1165–1171.
179. Armstrong FP, Miner JC, Wolfe WH. Investigation of a health care worker with symptomatic human immunodeficiency virus infection: an epidemiological approach. *Milit Med* 1987;152:414–418.
180. Comer RW, Myers DR, Steadman CD, et al. Management considerations for an HIV-positive dental student. *J Dent Educ* 1991;55: 187–191.
181. Danila RN, MacDonald KL, Rhame FS, et al. A look-back investigation of patients of an HIV-infected physician. Public health implications. *N Engl J Med* 1991;325(20):1406–1411.
182. Dickinson GM, Morhart RE, Klimas NG, et al. Absence of HIV transmission from an infected dentist to his patients. An epidemiologic and DNA sequence analysis. *JAMA* 1993;269(14):1802–1806.
183. Mishu B, Schaffner W, Horan JM, et al. A surgeon with AIDS: lack of evidence of transmission to patients. *JAMA* 1990;264:467–470.
184. Porter JD, Cruickshank JG, Gentle PH, et al. Management of patients treated by surgeon with HIV infection. *Lancet* 1990;335:113–114.
185. Rogers AS, Froggatt JW, Townsend T, et al. Investigation of potential HIV transmission to the patients of an HIV-infected surgeon. *JAMA* 1993;269(14):1795–1801.
186. Sacks JJ. AIDS in a surgeon. *N Engl J Med* 1985;313:1017–1018.
187. Sacks JJ. More on AIDS in a surgeon. *N Engl J Med* 1986;314:1190.
188. Staver S. AIDS "look-back" dilemma: should patients be told about infected doctors? *Am Med News* 1991(June 10):38.
189. von Reyn CF, Gilbert TT, Shaw FE Jr, et al. Absence of HIV transmission from an infected orthopedic surgeon: a 13-year look-back study. *JAMA* 1993;269(14):1807–1811.
190. Henderson DK. Human immunodeficiency virus infection in patients and providers. In: Wenzel R, ed. *Prevention and control of nosocomial infections,* 2nd ed. Baltimore: Williams & Wilkins, 1992:42–57.
191. Russo G, LaCroix S. A second look at the cost of mandatory human immunodeficiency virus and hepatitis B virus testing for health-care workers performing invasive procedures. *Infect Control Hosp Epidemiol* 1992;13(2):107–110.
192. Gerberding JL. Expected costs of implementing a mandatory human immunodeficiency virus and hepatitis B virus testing and restriction program for health-care workers performing invasive procedures. *Infect Control Hosp Epidemiol* 1991;12:443–447.
193. Owens DK, Nease RJ. Occupational exposure to human immunodeficiency virus and hepatitis B virus: a comparative analysis of risk. *Am J Med* 1992;92(5):503–512.
194. Phillips KA, Lowe RA, Kahn JG, et al. The cost-effectiveness of HIV testing of physicians and dentists in the United States. *JAMA* 1994; 271(11):851–858.
195. *School Board v. Arline.* 480 U.S. 273, 1987.
196. Feldblum C. Disability anti-discrimination laws and HIV testing of health-care providers. *Courts Health Sci Law* 1991;2:136–142.
197. Gostin LO. A proposed national policy on health care workers living with HIV/AIDS and other blood-borne pathogens. *JAMA* 2000; 284(15):1965–1970.
198. *Doe v. University of Maryland Medical System Corporation.* 50 F3d 1261, 1264, 4th circuit, 1995.
199. *Doe v. Washington University.* 780 F Supp 628, ED Mo, 1991.

80

VACCINATION OF HEALTHCARE WORKERS

MICHAEL D. DECKER
DAVID J. WEBER
WILLIAM A. SCHAFFNER

It has been said that sanitation and vaccination have made the two greatest contributions to the health of mankind. This importance is mirrored within healthcare institutions. For healthcare workers (HCWs) and for their patients, sanitation (better known within hospitals as hygiene or infection control) may be the first line of defense against infectious agents, but HCW vaccination is an essential second line of defense to prevent spread of infection from patients to HCWs, among HCWs, and from HCWs to patients.

Accordingly, ensuring the immunity of HCWs to infection or disease caused by relevant infectious agents is an essential component of any healthcare institution's occupational health program, to accomplish two fundamental legal and moral duties: protection of the workers from the risks of the workplace, and protection of the patients from the risks posed by infectious HCWs.

High rates of immunity among HCWs are required if patients are to be protected from infection spread by HCWs, as even a single infected HCW can expose many patients. Unfortunately, it has proven impossible to attain the necessary high vaccination rates through purely voluntary programs. Screening has repeatedly shown substantial proportions of hospital staff to be susceptible to vaccine-preventable diseases, in the absence of a policy requiring immunity. For example, numerous studies of hospital workers in the early 1990s showed that 5% to 10% were susceptible to measles, despite national recommendations regarding measles immunity (1–5). Indeed, the last major outbreaks of measles in the United States were predominantly fueled by spread within healthcare institutions. As cohorts born after the disappearance of epidemic measles enter the workforce, the proportion susceptible will increase unless immunity is confirmed and vaccinations provided to the susceptible. For example, a recent study reported that 9% of adult healthcare workers hired at a cancer hospital between 1998 and 1999 were seronegative for measles antibody, compared with 4% of those of the same age hired between 1983 and 1988 (6).

The problem of continued HCW susceptibility to vaccine-preventable diseases is not, of course, limited to measles. Even following adoption by the Occupational Safety and Health Administration (OSHA) of the Bloodborne Hazard Standard, with its requirement to offer hepatitis B vaccine to all exposed workers, substantial numbers of HCWs remain susceptible (particularly physicians, who typically are not employees and thus not subject to the standard). Similarly, surveys of HCWs have reported low rates of acceptance of influenza immunization. Selected studies of hepatitis B and influenza vaccine coverage rates are shown in Table 80.1 (7–20).

Many institutions (and some jurisdictions) have adopted policies requiring the demonstration of immunity to selected diseases as a condition of service in various capacities or units. Although the proportion of institutions with such policies continues to increase, as recently as 1995 a survey of children's hospitals showed the following frequency of policies requiring measles, mumps, rubella, and varicella vaccination: medical students, 47% to 74%; resident physicians, 70% to 91%; hospital-based physicians, 40% to 55%; and private or community-based physicians, only 15% to 26% (21).

Although one might argue that it is the worker's right to decline vaccination and accept the risk of infection, no one would argue that the worker has a right to infect patients. Accordingly, we consider "informed refusal" of vaccination to be permissible only for infections that are not expected to place the patient at jeopardy. (For employees, hepatitis B has been placed in this category as a matter of law by the Bloodborne Hazards Standard, despite numerous outbreaks of healthcare provider-to-patient transmission of hepatitis B; but physicians typically are not employees, and vaccination can be made a condition of surgical or other privileges, even if not a condition of employment). For those vaccine-preventable infections among HCWs that place patients at risk, we urge the adoption of policies that make demonstrated immunity (or valid medical waiver) a condition of employment (or privileges) in positions that would place the patient at risk in the event of HCW infection.

ORGANIZATION OF THE IMMUNITY (VACCINATION) PROGRAM

As alluded to above, it is important that the occupational health team understand that they need to operate an immunity

TABLE 80.1. HEPATITIS B AND INFLUENZA VACCINE COVERAGE OF HEALTHCARE WORKERS: SELECTED STUDIES

Vaccine	First Author	Year(s)	Study Location	Healthcare Workers Evaluated	Immunization Rate
Hepatitis B	Shapiro (8)	1991	3,411 orthopedic surgeons	Orthopedics	65%
	Panlilio (14)	1991–92	21 hospitals	General surgery, orthopedics, gynecology	55%
	Agerton (13)	1992	150 hospitals, United States	All staff	51%
	Cleveland (9)	1992	U.S. dentists	Dentists	85%
	Gyawali (15)	1994	London teaching hospital	Staff with blood exposure	78%
	Mahoney (16)	1994–95	200 U.S. hospitals	Staff eligible for hepatitis B vaccine	66.5%
Influenza	Weingarten (7)	1986–87	Los Angeles hospital	House staff and nurses	3.5%
	McArthur (11)	1991	1,270 extended-care facilities, Canada	All staff	>75% in only 3.7% of facilities
	Nichol (12)	1993–94	Minneapolis hospital	Physicians and nurses	61.2%
	Zadeh (17)	1995–98	Nursing homes, nine U.S. states	All staff	46%
	Cui (18)	1996–98	43 nursing homes, Hawaii	All staff	38%
	Russell (19)	1998	136 nursing homes, Alberta, Canada	All staff	29.9%
	Stevenson (20)	1999	Nursing homes, Canada	All staff	35%

program, not simply a vaccination program. The goal is to identify the susceptibilities of the workers to relevant infections and to take such steps (typically, vaccination) as may be appropriate to ensure their continued immunity.

The services provided by the institution, and the characteristics of the patient populations served, need to be considered in determining these policies. Some infections (e.g., rubella and varicella) are much more likely to be associated with serious complications in adult HCWs, and at the same time some infections that are common and often minor among HCWs can be life-threatening to patients with underlying chronic illnesses (e.g., influenza), immunosuppression (e.g., vaccinia), etc. The presence of special programs or populations (e.g., transplant units) will further alter the nature and scope of the vaccination and immunity policies. With these considerations in mind, the institution must decide which of the infections with potential for spread to, or through, HCWs, warrant monitoring of HCW immunity; which warrant offering of immunization to the susceptible (with the option to decline); and which warrant mandatory immunization (or demonstrated immunity).

The institution has no obligation under the Occupational Safety and Health Act with respect to workers (e.g., volunteers, medical or other students, contract workers, etc.) who are not employees. Unfortunately, because microbes are unaware of this legal nuance, patient protection requires that the institution's vaccination and immunity policy apply to all workers, irrespective of their employment status, including workers with direct patient care responsibilities (e.g., nurses, respiratory technicians, physical therapists, physicians, students), workers without direct patient care responsibilities (e.g., environmental service workers, security), contract or service workers, and emergency medical personnel.

All HCWs new to a healthcare facility should receive a prompt review (within 10 working days) of their immunity with respect to vaccine-preventable diseases. Immunity is most commonly demonstrated by documentation of immunization; for those persons believed to be immune on the basis of natural infection, serologic documentation or verified physician diagnosis should be required. Unless immune, the HCW should be appropriately immunized. As a general rule, serologic screening for immunity before immunization is neither necessary nor cost-effective. However, healthcare facilities might find certain screening programs to be cost-effective, given the cost of the screening test, the cost of the vaccine, and the prevalence of immunity in the local HCW population. In addition, facilities might wish to permit screening at the worker's request (either at the institution's or the worker's expense).

The institution may also wish to make available to HCWs vaccinations that are not necessary for the protection of patients but that are indicated for other reasons. For example, the establishment and maintenance of immunity to diphtheria and tetanus toxins is universally recommended, and ensuring the timely provision of tetanus and diphtheria toxoid (Td) boosters through the employee health service will eliminate concerns about tetanus prophylaxis in the event of (possibly unreported) occupational injury.

When vaccines are provided, appropriate information should be recorded in the employee's medical record (Table 80.2). Signed informed consent (or refusal, if appropriate) specific to each vaccine should be obtained before immunization. Vaccine information statements (22) must be provided for vaccines covered by the National Childhood Vaccine Injury Act (including measles, mumps, rubella, polio, diphtheria, tetanus, pertussis, hepatitis A, hepatitis B, *Haemophilus influenzae* type b, meningococcal, pneumococcal, and varicella vaccines; influenza vaccine is expected to be added to this list in 2004. Vaccine information statements are also available for yellow fever and smallpox vaccines. Any adverse events occurring after immunization should be reported to the Vaccine Adverse Events Reporting System (23).

TABLE 80.2. DATA TO RECORD WHEN PROVIDING VACCINES TO HEALTHCARE WORKERS

Employee name
Employee identification number
Date of birth
Signed informed consent (or refusal, if relevant)
Date of immunization (or refusal)
Vaccine provided (or declined)
Name of vaccine manufacturer
Lot number of vaccine
Site of immunization
Route of immunization
Date of next scheduled dose or booster (if applicable)
Adverse events (if any)
Name, title, and address of person providing vaccine

The immunization status of all HCWs should be recorded in their employee medical record. A mechanism should be established to track immune status, including the need for and timing of repeat immunization, with effective recall and enforcement provisions.

VACCINES RECOMMENDED FOR HEALTHCARE WORKERS: GENERAL GUIDELINES

Recommendations regarding the vaccination of HCWs have been issued by the Centers for Disease Control and Prevention (CDC) and its advisory bodies (24–26), the American College of Physicians (ACP) (27), the American Academy of Pediatrics (28), and others (29–36). Many of these recommendations are updated periodically (see Table 80.3 for on-line sources of information).

TABLE 80.3. ON-LINE SOURCES FOR CURRENT VACCINE INFORMATION AND VACCINATION RECOMMENDATIONS

General Information Concerning Vaccines And Vaccine-Preventable Diseases
- CDC's National Immunization Program: *http://www.cdc.gov/nip/default.htm*
- Allied Vaccine Group: *http://www.vaccine.org/*
- American Academy of Pediatrics Childhood Immunization Support Program: *http://www.cispimmunize.org/index.html*
- American College of Physicians Adult Immunization Initiative: *http://www.acponline.org/aii/?hp*
- The Immunization Action Coalition: *http://www.immunize.org/*

Recommendations
- Recommendations of the ACIP: *http://www.cdc.gov/nip/publications/acip-list.htm*

Vaccine manufacturers (package inserts, etc.)
- Aventis Pasteur: *https:www.vaccineshoppe.com/* (login not required for package inserts and other information)
- GlaxoSmithKline Vaccines: *http://gskvaccines.com/* (login not required for package inserts and other information)
- Merck & Co., Inc: *http://www.merckvaccines.com/vaccineInfo_frmst.html*
- Wyeth Vaccines: *http://www.vaccineworld.com/wv_home.asp*

ACIP, Advisory Committee on Immunization Practices; CDC, Centers for Disease Control and Prevention.

All HCWs should be immune to mumps, measles, rubella, and varicella, and all HCWs with potential exposure to blood or body fluids should be immune to hepatitis B (Table 80.4). Influenza vaccine should be offered to all HCWs yearly (and strongly encouraged, if not mandated). In special circumstances, HCWs or laboratory personnel should be offered immunization with other vaccines, including Bacille Calmette-Guérin (BCG), hepatitis A, quadrivalent meningococcal, inactivated poliomyelitis, rabies, typhoid, and vaccinia (Table 80.5).

HCWs who are immunocompromised, pregnant, or have certain underlying chronic diseases can pose special considerations in the provision of immunizations (Table 80.6) (37–51). Some routinely recommended vaccines (especially live virus vaccines such as measles, mumps, rubella, varicella, and BCG) may be contraindicated, and some vaccines not routinely recommended for HCWs may be indicated (e.g., pneumococcal, meningococcal, and *H. influenzae* type b vaccines). In addition, for some indicated vaccines, higher antigen doses or postimmunization serologic evaluation may be indicated (e.g., hepatitis B vaccine in people with renal failure). When an otherwise mandatory vaccine is contraindicated for a given HCW, the worker should be individually evaluated for the possibility of altering his or her assignment to reduce risk to patients or to the HCW.

Immunization of pregnant HCWs raises a number of issues. For some live-attenuated and all inactivated or toxoid vaccines, the risks from immunization during pregnancy are largely theoretical (26,27). For such vaccines, the benefit of immunization outweighs the potential risks for adverse reactions, especially when the risk of exposure is high, infection would pose a special risk to the mother or fetus, and the vaccine is unlikely to cause harm. Furthermore, newer information continues to confirm the safety of vaccines given inadvertently during pregnancy. Female HCWs should have been immunized against measles, mumps, rubella, varicella, tetanus, diphtheria, and hepatitis B as adolescents (26). However, as this may not have occurred (or immunity may not have been produced), it is especially important that all HCWs be screened for rubella immunity (by serology as history is often unreliable), because of the consequences of infection for the developing fetus. Because of the theoretical risks, live attenuated viral vaccines (mumps, measles, rubella, and varicella) should be deferred for pregnant women.

Pregnant HCWs may receive combined tetanus and diphtheria toxoid (Td) (26,52). Women who are in their second or third trimester (>14 weeks pregnant) during respiratory virus season should receive influenza immunization (26,53). If otherwise indicated, susceptible pregnant women may receive hepatitis A, hepatitis B, inactivated influenza, meningococcal, pneumococcal, rabies, typhoid Vi polysaccharide, and inactivated poliomyelitis vaccines (formulations containing trace or no thimerosal are preferable, when available) (26). Breast-feeding does not adversely affect the response to immunization and is not a contraindication for any of the currently recommended vaccines. The indications for using immune globulins in pregnant women are the same as those for women who are not pregnant.

Before the administration of any vaccine, the HCW should be evaluated for the presence of any condition that is listed as a vaccine contraindication or precaution (54). If such a condition is present, the risks and benefits of vaccination need to be care-

TABLE 80.4. VACCINES STRONGLY RECOMMENDED FOR ALL PERSONS WHO PROVIDE HEALTHCARE TO PATIENTS OR WHO WORK IN INSTITUTIONS THAT PROVIDE HEALTHCARE

Vaccine	Recommendation	Schedule (Adults)	Major Contraindications	Special Considerations
Measles	All HCWs (including those born before 1957) who cannot document either receipt of two doses of live vaccine on or after their first birthday or laboratory evidence of immunity should receive at least one dose of vaccine; MMR is preferred unless immunity to mumps and rubella are documented	0.5 mL SC, second dose at least 1 mo later	Pregnancy; hypersensitivity to gelatin, neomycin, or eggs; immunocompromised state[a]; recent receipt of immunoglobulin	Persons vaccinated during 1963–7 with a killed measles vaccine alone, killed vaccine followed by live vaccine, or with a vaccine of unknown type should be revaccinated with two doses of live measles virus vaccine
Mumps	Vaccinate unless born before 1957 or physician-diagnosed disease, laboratory evidence of immunity, or prior receipt of vaccine is documented; MMR preferred unless contraindicated	0.5 mL SC, no booster	Pregnancy; hypersensitivity to gelatin, neomycin, or eggs; immunocompromised state[a]; recent receipt of immunoglobulin	MMR is preferred unless contraindicated or immunity to measles and rubella are documented
Rubella	Vaccinate unless male born before 1957,[b] or documentation of physician-diagnosed disease, laboratory evidence of immunity, or prior receipt of vaccine	0.5 mL SC, no booster	Pregnancy; hypersensitivity to gelatin or neomycin; immunocompromised state[a]; recent receipt of immunoglobulin	MMR is preferred unless contraindicated or immunity to measles and mumps are documented
Varicella	Consider vaccinating (see Special Considerations) unless physician-diagnosed disease, laboratory evidence of immunity, or prior receipt of vaccine is documented; acceptability of a personal history of disease (not physician-diagnosed) depends on nature of patient population (risk profile)	0.5 mL SC, second dose 4–8 wk later if ≥13 yr of age	Pregnancy; hypersensitivity to gelatin or neomycin; immunocompromised state[a]; recent receipt of immunoglobulin; avoid salicylate use for 6 weeks after vaccination	Susceptibles can be identified by serotesting all HCWs, only those with a negative or uncertain history of chickenpox, or by simply immunizing all those with a negative or uncertain history
Hepatitis B	All HCWs at risk for exposure to blood or body fluids; vaccinate unless laboratory evidence of immunity or prior receipt of three doses of vaccine with an appropriate schedule is documented	1.0 mL IM (deltoid) at 0, 1, 6 mo; booster doses not necessary	Hypersensitivity to common baker's yeast	Prevaccination serologic screening is not necessary. HCWs who have contact with patients or blood should be tested 1–2 months after vaccination to determine response (see text)
Influenza	All HCWs who have contact with patients at high risk for influenza or its complications; HCWs who work in chronic care facilities; schedule and Contraindications shown are for trivalent inactivated vaccine (see Special Considerations)	0.5 mL IM yearly	Hypersensitivity to eggs (or thimerosal, for formulations containing thimerosal), no evidence exists of risk to mother or fetus when the vaccine is administered to a pregnant woman	Trivalent inactivated vaccine is preferred over live attenuated intranasal vaccine for immunization of HCWs, due to the theoretical risk of spread to immunosuppressed and other at-risk patients

Adapted from Immunization of health-care workers: recommendations of the Advisory Committee on Immunization Practices (ACIP) and the Hospital Infection Control Practices Advisory Committee (HICPAC). *MMWR* 1997;46(RR-18):1–42.
IM, intramuscularly; MMR, measles, mumps, and rubella vaccine; SC, subcutaneously
Note: The package insert and ACIP recommendations should be consulted for specific guidance regarding indications, storage, administration, precautions, and contraindications.
[a] Persons immunocompromised because of immune deficiency diseases, human immunodeficiency virus infection, leukemia, lymphoma or generalized malignancy, or immunosuppressed as a result of therapy with corticosteroids (i.e., ≥2 mg/kg body weight or 20 mg/day of prednisone for ≥2 weeks), alkylating drugs, antimetabolites, or radiation). Also see Table 80.6.
[b] Many authorities would also vaccinate males born before 1957 unless immunity is demonstrated.

fully weighed by the healthcare provider and the employee. The most common contraindication is a history of an anaphylactic reaction to a previous dose of the vaccine or to a vaccine component. Factors that are not contraindications to immunization include the following: breast-feeding or household contact with a pregnant woman (exception: vaccinia); reaction to a previous vaccination consisting only of mild-to-moderate local tenderness, swelling, or both, or fever less than 40.5°C; mild acute illness with or without low-grade fever; current antimicrobial therapy (except for oral typhoid vaccine) or convalescence from a recent illness; personal history of allergies (except a history of an anaphylactic reaction to a vaccine component); and family history of allergies, adverse reactions to vaccination, or seizures (27).

TABLE 80.5. VACCINES THAT MAY BE INDICATED FOR HEALTHCARE WORKERS (HCWS) OR LABORATORY PERSONNEL

Vaccine	Recommendation	Schedule	Major Contraindications	Special Considerations
BCG (for tuberculosis prevention)	ndicated only for HCWs in localities where (1) multidrug-resistant tuberculosis is prevalent; (2) a strong likelihood of infection exists; and (3) full implementation of infection control precautions has been inadequate in controlling the spread of infection	One percutaneous dose of 0.3 mL; no booster recommendation	Immunocompromised state[a] or pregnancy	BCG vaccination of U.S. HCWs is discouraged as it would interfere with subsequent PPD screening programs and can result in complications
Hepatitis A	Not routinely indicated for HCWs; persons who work with HAV-infected primates or with HAV in a research laboratory setting should be vaccinated	Two doses IM either 6–12 mo apart (*Vaqta*) or 6 mo apart (*Havrix*)	History of anaphylaxis to a previous dose; hypersensitivity to 2-phenoxyethanol, formalin, or (*Havrix* only) neomycin	
Meningococcal polysaccharide (serogroups A, C, Y, W135)	Not routinely indicated for HCWs except personnel with laboratory or industrial exposure to *N. meningitidis* aerosols; may be useful during an outbreak due to a type included in the vaccine	0.5 mL IM; consider booster dose within 3–5 yrs if exposure continues	Sensitivity to thimerosal (used in multi-dose presentation only)	A conjugate quadrivalent vaccine (A, C, Y, W-135) is expected to become available soon and should provide superior and more durable immunogenicity
Pertussis	Not currently recommended, but see Special Considerations; once adult acellular formulations are licensed in the U.S., they likely will be recommended for outbreak control, for persons having prolonged close contact with infants not yet fully immunized, and perhaps routinely (as TdaP) in place of Td	0.5 mL IM; booster schedule not yet determined, but likely will be similar to Td	Hypersensitivity to any component of the vaccine	Adolescent-adult formulations of acellular pertussis vaccines are licensed in Canada, Europe, and elsewhere, and likely will be licensed in the U.S. in the next few years
Poliomyelitis	All persons should be immune; immune status should be confirmed for HCWs in close contact with people who may be excreting wild virus and laboratory personnel handling specimens that may contain wild virus	Unimmunized adults: two doses of IPV given SC 4–8 wk apart, followed by a third dose at 6–12 months	Hypersensitivity to 2-phenoxyethanol, formaldehyde, neomycin, streptomycin or polymyxin B	Use only IPV; OPV can, rarely, result in paralysis of recipients or their contacts (OPV is not available in the U.S.)
Rabies	Not routinely indicated for HCWs except personnel working with rabies virus or infected animals in diagnostic or research activities	Preexposure: 1.0 mL IM on days 0, 7, and 21 or 28; follow standard guidelines for postexposure prophylaxis	*Imovax*: none; *RabAvert*: hypersensitivity to bovine gelatin, chicken protein, neomycin, chlortetracycline, or amphotericin B	Postexposure prophylaxis boosters may be required despite primary immunization
Typhoid	Not routinely indicated for HCWs except laboratory personnel who frequently work with *Salmonella typhi*	One 0.5 mL dose IM (Vi polysaccharide vaccine); booster doses of 0.5 mL every 2 yr; *or* four oral doses (Ty21a) on alternate days; as per manufacturer revaccinate with the entire four-dose series every 5 yr	History of severe local reaction or anaphylaxis to a previous dose of vaccine; Ty21a should not be administered to immunosuppressed[a] persons or to persons receiving antimicrobials	Do not use the killed whole-cell vaccine; the Vi polysaccharide vaccine (*Typhim VI*) may be preferable because Ty21a (*Vivotif*) is a live attenuated product that poses a theoretical risk of transmission to patients by recently immunized HCWs
Vaccinia	Not routinely indicated for HCWs except personnel who directly handle cultures or animals contaminated with recombinant vaccinia or Orthopox viruses (monkeypox, cowpox) that infect humans, or as part of pre-event vaccination program (see Special Considerations)	One dose administered with a bifurcated needle; boosters every 10 yr	Pregnancy; breast-feeding; history of eczema in worker or close family contacts; other acute, chronic, or exfoliative skin conditions; immunosuppression in vaccine recipient or household contact; hypersensitivity to polymyxin B, streptomycin, tetracycline, neomycin, glycerin, or phenol	Vaccine is available only from CDC Drug Services; a bioterrorism-related pre-event vaccination program was conducted among HCWs in 2002 and early 2003 but subsequently became inactive

Adapted from Immunization of health-care workers: recommendations of the Advisory Committee on Immunization Practices (ACIP) and the Hospital Infection Control Practices Advisory Committee (HICPAC). *MMWR* 1997;46(RR-18):1–42.

BCG, Bacille Calmette-Guérin; HDCV, human diploid cell vaccine; IM, intramuscularly; IPV, inactivated poliovirus vaccine; OPV, oral poliovirus vaccine; PCEC, purified chick embryo cell culture rabies vaccine; PPD, purified protein derivative (tuberculin); SC, subcutaneously.

Notes: 1. Excluded are vaccines not currently available in the U.S. for civilian use (e.g., anthrax, plague).

2. This table only considers indications related to occupational exposures of HCWs; these and other (e.g., Td, pneumococcal, etc.) vaccines may be indicated for persons, whether HCWs or not, who meet certain exposure or risk criteria.

3. The package insert and ACIP recommendations should be consulted for specific guidance regarding indications, storage, administration, precautions, and contraindications.

[a] Persons immunocompromised because of immune deficiency diseases, human immunodeficiency virus infection, leukemia, lymphoma or generalized malignancy, or immunosuppressed as a result of therapy with corticosteroids (i.e., $\geq$2 mg/kg body weight or 20 mg/day of prednisone for $\geq$2 weeks), alkylating drugs, antimetabolites, or radiation).

TABLE 80.6. RECOMMENDATIONS CONCERNING IMMUNIZATION OF HEALTHCARE WORKERS WITH SPECIAL CONDITIONS

Vaccine	Pregnancy	HIV Infection	Severe Immunosuppression[a]	Asplenia	Renal Failure	Diabetes	Alcoholism and Alcoholic Cirrhosis
BCG	C	C	C	UI	UI	UI	UI
Hepatitis A	UI	UI	UI	UI	UI	UI	R[b]
Hepatitis B	R	R	R	R	R	R	R
Influenza, inactivated	R[c]	R	R	R	R	R	R
Influenza, live attenuated[d]	C	C	C	C	C	C	C
Measles, mumps, rubella	C	R[e]	C	R[b]	R	R	R
Meningococcus	UI	UI	UI	R	UI	UI	UI
Poliovirus, inactivated[f,g]	UI	UI	UI	UI	UI	UI	UI
Pneumococcus	UI	R[b]	R[b]	R[b]	R[b]	R[b]	R[b]
Rabies	UI	UI	UI	UI	UI	UI	UI
Tetanus/diphtheria[f]	R[b]	R[b]	R[b]	R[b]	R[b]	R[b]	R[b]
Typhoid, Vi polysaccharide	UI	UI	UI	UI	UI	UI	UI
Typhoid, Ty21a[d]	UI	C	C	UI	UI	UI	UI
Varicella	C	C	C	R	R	R	R
Vaccinia	C	C	C	UI	UI	UI	UI

Adapted from Adapted from Immunization of health-care workers: recommendations of the Advisory Committee on Immunization Practices (ACIP) and the Hospital Infection Control Practices Advisory Committee (HICPAC). *MMWR* 1997;46(RR-18):1–42.
BCG, bacille Calmette-Guérin; HIV, human immunodeficiency virus; IPV, inactivated poliovirus vaccine; MMR, measles-mumps-rubella vaccine; R, recommended; C, contraindicated; UI, use if indicated.
Note: The package insert and ACIP recommendations should be consulted for specific guidance regarding indications, precautions, and contraindications.
[a] Severe immunosuppression can be the result of congenital immunodeficiency; HIV infection, leukemia, lymphoma, generalized malignancy, or therapy with alkylating agents, antimetabolites, radiation, or large amounts of corticosteroids.
[b] Recommendation is based on the person having the indicated underlying condition, not their status as HCW.
[c] Recommended for women who will be in the second or third trimester of pregnancy during the influenza season.
[d] Because of the theoretical risk of transmission to patients of the live attenuated agent contained in this vaccine, use of the alternative inactivated vaccine is preferred.
[e] Generally contraindicated in persons with HIV infection; recommended for children (no official recommendation for serosusceptible adults) with $CD4^+$ >200/μL; consider reimmunization if initial immunization was given when $CD4^+ \geq 200$ μL and if $CD4^+$ increases to ≥200 μL due to highly active antiretroviral therapy.
[f] All persons, whether HCW or not, should be immune unless specifically contraindicated.
[g] Immunization with IPV is recommended for unvaccinated healthcare workers who have close contact with persons who may be excreting wild poliovirus. Healthcare workers who have a primary series of OPV or IPV who are directly involved with the provision of care to patients who may be excreting poliovirus may receive another dose of IPV. Except in the context of mass immunization to control circulating wild polio, use only IPV; OPV can, rarely, result in paralysis of recipients or their contacts (OPV is not available in the U.S.).

USE OF VACCINES FOR POSTEXPOSURE PROPHYLAXIS OR OUTBREAK CONTROL

Those who have had to respond to the spread within their institution of a vaccine-preventable illness understand quite clearly how preferable it is to have previously vaccinated their HCWs. The virtual impossibility of identifying and immunizing susceptible HCWs sufficiently rapidly during an outbreak of measles, mumps, rubella, or varicella to avoid spread to another generation of susceptible HCWs or patients offers a powerful inducement for policies requiring immunity before assignment to duty. Moreover, these vaccines are not known to provide protection when given to a susceptible person following exposure. In contrast, tetanus toxoid (Td toxoids preferred) (55), hepatitis B vaccine (56), vaccinia (45), and rabies vaccine (41) are effective when given promptly following exposure, and hepatitis A vaccine may provide at least partial protection (57). Varicella vaccine may provide protection if given within 72 hours of exposure, but it should not be relied on to prevent further transmission by exposed HCWs because of incomplete efficacy (58). Immunization of HCWs with hepatitis A, meningococcal, or acellular pertussis vaccine may be indicated to control an institutional or community outbreak. In the event of widespread influenza activity, additional supplies of influenza vaccine may be difficult to obtain, adding further importance to a robust annual influenza vaccination program. Outbreaks of measles or polio are now highly unlikely (except, perhaps, in distinct communities that reject vaccination), but either would trigger large-scale immunization drives. Finally, passive vaccination with immunoglobulin is useful for postexposure prophylaxis for hepatitis A, hepatitis B, measles, rabies, tetanus, varicella, and vaccinia.

GUIDELINES FOR THE USE OF SELECTED VACCINES

The following subsections provide additional information regarding the vaccine-preventable diseases for which immunization of HCWs is recommended, either universally (Table 80.4) or in special circumstances (Table 80.5). For each vaccine, administration schedules and contraindications are summarized in these tables, and recommendations concerning immunization of healthcare workers with special conditions are provided in Table 80.6. Management of the vaccine-preventable diseases themselves and management of exposures to those diseases (other than postexposure vaccination) are covered in detail in other chapters, to which readers will be referred.

Hepatitis A Vaccine

Background

Hepatitis A virus (HAV) is highly endemic in the U.S., with 13,397 cases (4.91 cases per 100,000) reported to the CDC in 1999 (59), a figure that probably represents less than 10% of actual infections. The incidence of HAV varies by race (among U.S. residents highest in Native Americans and Native Alaskans), location (in the U.S. higher west of the Mississippi River), and age. Globally, incidence and median age of onset are closely related to socioeconomic and developmental status, with higher rates and lower median ages of onset in less-developed countries. In the U.S., schoolchildren 5 to 14 years of age have the highest reported incidence. However, infection in infants and young children often is asymptomatic, so the age distribution of reported cases may not be representative of the underlying age distribution of infection. Sources of infection include household or sexual contact with a person with HAV (22% to 26% of reported cases), with a child or employee in a day-care center (14% to 16%), or with an international traveler (4% to 6%) (60). The majority of cases are sporadic, with no identified source. Food- or water-borne outbreaks classically account for only 2% to 3% of cases, but are becoming more common with globalization of the U.S. food supply.

Hepatitis A results in substantial morbidity with significant costs caused by medical care and lost work time. Approximately 11% to 22% of people who develop hepatitis A require hospitalization (46). In the U.S., an estimated 100 deaths per year are attributable to acute hepatitis A (there is no chronic infection).

Nosocomial Outbreaks

Although several cohort studies have failed to demonstrate HCWs to be at increased risk for hepatitis A compared with control populations (61–64), some European researchers have reported that HCWs had higher than expected rates of seropositivity to hepatitis A (65,66). A number of nosocomial outbreaks of HAV have been reported (67–83). These reports suggest a common set of circumstances: a source patient who was not jaundiced, in whom hepatitis was not suspected, and who had fecal incontinence or diarrhea. Risk factors for HAV transmission to personnel include activities that increase the risk of fecal-oral contamination, including caring for a person with unrecognized HAV infection (67–76); sharing food, beverages, or cigarettes with patients, their families, or the staff (70,76–78); nail biting; handling bile without proper precautions (76); and not washing hands or wearing gloves when providing care to an infected patient (73,74,76,78) (see also Chapters 45 and 81).

Vaccination

Although current recommendations do not support routine immunization of U.S. HCWs except in areas where hepatitis A is highly endemic (24), cost-benefit analyses have suggested that the cost of hepatitis A vaccination in HCWs, per life-year saved, was similar to that of other standard medical interventions (84). As with other special use vaccines, HCWs should be encouraged to review with their local medical provider their own risks and benefits for hepatitis A vaccine.

Hepatitis B Vaccine

Background

Exposure to blood-borne pathogens via parenteral or mucosal contact can expose HCWs to the risk of acquiring numerous infections, foremost among these (in terms of risk, prevalence, and aggregate burden) being hepatitis B. Seroprevalence surveys conducted prior to the availability of hepatitis B virus (HBV) vaccine showed HCWs to be at threefold to fivefold higher risk of HBV infection than the general U.S. population (85–88), with the risk of infection proportionate to the extent and duration of blood contact. The use of HBV vaccine among HCWs, coupled with the institution of universal (now standard) precautions and other preventive measures such as needleless devices, has markedly reduced that risk. Mahoney et al. (16) reported that HBV infection among HCWs declined from 17,000 in 1983 to 400 in 1995. This 95% decline in incidence observed among HCWs was 1.5-fold greater than the reduction in incidence in the general U.S. population during the same time period.

Nosocomial Exposures

HCWs are at risk of hepatitis B acquisition for several reasons. First, HCWs have high rates of exposure to blood (89). For example, a 1988 survey of New York City surgeons found that 86% had at least one puncture injury in the preceding year (90). A survey of U.S. and Canadian orthopedic surgeons in 1991 found that 87.4% had a blood–skin contact and 39.2% a percutaneous blood contact in the previous month (91). Second, the virus can persist in the environment, being able to survive drying and storage at 25°C and 42% relative humidity for 1 week (92). Third, HBV is highly transmissible; the titer of infectious particles is extraordinarily high in the blood of actively infected persons. Consequently, rates of disease transmission after a percutaneous injury with a contaminated sharp range from 6% to 30% (93–95). HBV infection also can be acquired via mucosal exposure, exposure to nonintact skin, or ocular exposure (60), and has been transmitted to patients by a worker with severe exudative dermatitis while obtaining arterial blood gases (96). Fourth, a substantial number of patients have inapparent infections; for example, a study of consecutive blood samples submitted to the chemistry laboratory of an urban hospital in 1987 revealed that only 28% of hepatitis B surface antigen (HBsAg)-positive specimens were labeled with a biohazard label as required (97). Finally, many HCWs remain unimmunized.

Many outbreaks of healthcare provider–to-patient transmission of hepatitis B have been described (98–102). Transmission typically occurs during an invasive procedures, with the most important risk factors being e-antigen positivity of the HCW, degree of invasiveness of the procedure, the infected HCW not wearing gloves, or injury (often inapparent) to the infected HCW (see also Chapters 45, 78, and 81).

Vaccination

OSHA has mandated since 1991 that all healthcare employees be offered hepatitis B immunization. Employees may refuse immunization but must sign a declination form. Employees who decline hepatitis B vaccine cite a desire to avoid medications, the perception that they are at low risk for occupationally acquired HBV infection, and concern about side effects (103). Availability of educational materials directed at these issues may be helpful in minimizing refusals.

Protective serum titers of anti-HBsAg ($\geq$10 mIU/mL) develop in 90% of healthy adults who receive three intramuscular (IM) doses of hepatitis B vaccine (104–106). Independent risk factors for failure to seroconvert following HBV vaccine include smoking, female gender, higher body mass index, and older age (107). The two currently available hepatitis B vaccines, Recombivax HB and Engerix-B, are equally immunogenic and are interchangeable; either can be used (in its recommended dose) to complete an immunization series begun with the other (104). Immunogenicity is not reduced when hepatitis B vaccine is given with other vaccines. Pregnancy is not a contraindication to hepatitis B vaccine. All injections should be provided in the deltoid because gluteal injection can result in poor immunogenicity.

The usual vaccination schedule consists of three doses administered at 0, 1, and 6 months. A schedule of 0, 1, and 2 months or 0, 1, and 4 months should be considered for unimmunized HCWs at high risk of HBV (e.g., hemodialysis workers, cardiac surgeons), with a fourth dose given at 12 months to ensure long-term protection (108,109). All HCWs should have an anti-HBsAg titer obtained 1 to 2 months after the third immunization (110). HCWs with postimmunization titers <10 mIU/mL should receive up to three additional IM doses of hepatitis B vaccine; serum antibody can be checked 1 to 2 months after each dose, with vaccination terminated if immunity is achieved. (Laboratories using test kits that simply report "positive" or "negative" must consult the product literature or manufacturer to determine the minimum antibody level able to return a positive result.) If protection is not achieved following the third additional (sixth total) dose, the HCW should be considered a nonresponder. Following a subsequent exposure, the HCW should be tested for the presence of HBsAg and given hepatitis B immune globulin as indicated for postexposure prophylaxis.

Symptomatic hepatitis B is rare in immunized people who developed protective levels of antibody, even though there is eventual loss of detectable antibody in up to 50% of those people 5 to 10 years after immunization. For this reason, there is currently no recommendation for periodic boosting of HCWs who have responded to hepatitis B vaccine (58,111). Nonetheless, many institutions provide postexposure serologic testing of exposed HCWs and offer a booster dose of vaccine for those with antibody levels <10 mIU/mL, not because of medical need but in consideration of the anxieties of the exposed worker.

Influenza Vaccine

Background

Influenza is characterized by the abrupt onset of fever, myalgia, sore throat, and nonproductive cough. During influenza epidemics, the hospitalization rate for the elderly and for persons with underlying health problems (especially cardiopulmonary) may increase twofold to fivefold compared with nonepidemic periods (112). Of the 23 influenza seasons between 1972 and 1992, 19 were associated with excess mortality, nine with more than 20,000 influenza-associated excess deaths, and four with more than 40,000 excess deaths (113,114).

Influenza is a single-stranded RNA virus that occurs in three basic antigen types (A, B, and C) based on nuclear material. Type A infects humans and other animals (especially fowl, other birds, and pigs) and is antigenically characterized by two surface proteins, hemagglutinin (associated with cell attachment), and neuraminidase (associated with cell penetration). In recent years, most influenza A human disease has been caused by viruses expressing hemagglutinin types H1, H2, or H3 and neuraminidase types N1 or N2. Infection with a strain expressing a given hemagglutinin and neuraminidase reduces the likelihood and severity of subsequent infection by strains expressing those types, but confers little or no protection against viruses expressing other types. Influenza A hemagglutinins and neuraminidases of given types undergo continual antigenic modification (antigenic drift, due to point mutations) that can reduce, sometimes markedly, the protection conferred by infection with an earlier strain of the same subtype, leading to epidemics. At unpredictable intervals, an influenza A strain undergoes a genetic shift (probably due to recombination events within an avian or porcine host that is simultaneously infected with a human and an animal strain) and produces a new subtype, to which there is no protection from infection with previous strains, leading to pandemics. In the past 125 years, there have been four pandemics, due to H3N2 in 1889, H1N1 in 1919 (the "Spanish flu"), H2N2 in 1957 (the "Asian flu"), and H3N2 in 1968 (the "Hong Kong flu"). In recent years, both H1N1 and H3N2 have circulated (114). In addition, there have been isolated instances of human infection due to human–animal recombinant influenza A viruses (e.g., the Hong Kong chicken-market outbreak of H5 virus or the Netherlands H6 cases), but (perhaps due to aggressive containment efforts, or perhaps due to inherent characteristics) none have spread widely.

Influenza B infects only humans, predominantly children, and typically causes milder illness than does influenza A. Influenza B is genetically more stable than influenza A.

The composition of each year's influenza vaccine is determined about 6 months before influenza season each year (to allow time for manufacture), based on recommendations by the World Health Organization (WHO) and national advisory groups that monitor strains circulating worldwide. Unfortunately, new strains sometimes arise too late to be included in that year's vaccine.

Influenza virus appears to spread from person to person by small particle aerosol transmission. Although aerosol transmission is well established, nosocomial transmission via fomites and contaminated hands remains possible. Influenza virus is shed for up to 5 days after onset of illness by adults and up to 7 days by children.

Nosocomial Exposures

Nosocomial acquisition of influenza is common (115–136), typically in association with community outbreaks; HCWs acquire infection from patients or in the community, and then spread infection to other HCWs and patients, endangering patients and disrupting the provision of care (115–119,137). Influenza infection among staff is common during the winter season and results in substantial absenteeism. Attack rates of 25% to 80% are often observed among both patients and staff during outbreaks. Similarly, nosocomial outbreaks within extended-care facilities (e.g., for the elderly) can result in substantial morbidity and mortality (137–155).

The nosocomial spread of influenza cannot be prevented with measures instituted only when influenza is known to circulate, because identification of all patients with influenza is unlikely to be accomplished (119) and community indicators of influenza activity (e.g., visits to acute ambulatory care centers for upper respiratory illness) cannot be relied on to provide warning of influenza among hospitalized patients (117).

On the other hand, high influenza immunization rates among HCWs has been shown to result in a decrease in the attack rate of influenza among patients (156,157). For example, patients in facilities with more than 60% of the staff immunized experienced less influenza-related mortality and illness compared with patients in facilities without immunized staff (156).

For all these reasons, routine annual influenza immunization of HCWs is essential and has been recommended for many years. Recommendations for prevention and control of nosocomial influenza have been published and are summarized in Table 80.7 (120,121,158–164) (see also Chapters 41 and 81).

Vaccination

Influenza vaccine is suitable for any person without specific contraindication who wishes to reduce his or her risk of influenza disease; a randomized, controlled trial in a general working population has demonstrated that providing influenza vaccine is cost-effective (165). Vaccination is strongly recommended for all persons aged 6 months or older who are at increased risk for complications of influenza because of age or underlying medical condition. Those at increased risk for influenza-related complications include all persons aged 6 through 23 months; all persons aged 50 years or older; residents of extended-care facilities or long-term-care facilities that house people of any age who have chronic medical conditions; adults and children who have required regular medical follow-up or hospitalization during the previous year because of chronic metabolic diseases (including diabetes mellitus), renal dysfunction, hemoglobinopathies, or immunosuppression; persons aged 6 months to 18 years who are receiving long-term aspirin therapy and therefore may be at risk for developing Reye syndrome after influenza; and women who will be in the second or third trimester of pregnancy during the influenza season (53).

TABLE 80.7. CDC RECOMMENDATIONS FOR THE PREVENTION AND CONTROL OF NOSOCOMIAL INFLUENZA

Prevention

1. Educate personnel about the epidemiology, modes of transmission, and means of preventing the spread of influenza
2. Establish mechanism(s) by which hospital personnel are promptly alerted of an increase in influenza activity in the local community
3. Arrange for laboratory tests to be available to clinicians, for use when clinically indicated, to confirm the diagnosis of influenza and other acute viral respiratory diseases promptly, especially during November through April
4. Offer vaccine to outpatients and inpatients at high risk of complications from influenza, beginning in September and continuing until influenza activity has begun to decline
5. Vaccinate HCWs before the influenza season each year, preferably between mid-October and mid-November
6. Isolate patients with known or suspected influenza in a private room, preferably under negative pressure
7. Institute masking of individuals who enter the room of a patient with influenza
8. Evaluate HCWs with febrile upper respiratory illnesses and consider removal from duties that involve direct patient care (use more stringent guidelines for staff working in high-risk areas, such as intensive care units, nurseries, or with severely immunocompromised patients)
9. During community or hospital outbreaks, restrict hospital visitors who have a febrile respiratory illness

Control of nosocomial influenza outbreaks

1. Early in the outbreak, obtain a nasopharyngeal swab or nasal-wash specimen from patients with recent onset of symptoms suggestive of influenza for virus culture or antigen detection
2. Administer current influenza vaccine to unvaccinated patients and staff
3. Administer antiviral prophylaxis to all uninfected patients in an involved unit for whom it is not contraindicated
4. Administer antiviral prophylaxis to all unvaccinated staff members for whom it is not contraindicated and who are in the involved unit or taking care of high-risk patients
5. If the cause of the outbreak is confirmed to be influenza and vaccine has been administered only recently to susceptible patients and personnel, continue antiviral prophylaxis until 2 weeks after the vaccination
6. To the extent possible, do not allow contact between those at high risk of complications from influenza and patients or staff who are taking antiviral treatment for an acute respiratory illnesses; prevent contact during and for 2 days after the latter discontinue treatment; a failure to isolate patients treated with amantadine or rimantadine may result in the dissemination of drug-resistant strains

Adapted from Tablan OC, Anderson LJ, Arden NH, et al. Guideline for prevention of nosocomial pneumonia. *Infect Control Hosp Epidemiol* 1994;15:587–27.
CDC, Centers for Disease Control and Prevention; HCW, healthcare worker.

Most pertinently, influenza vaccine is recommended for HCWs, because they can transmit influenza virus to people at high risk, and moreover are needed for patient care during influenza outbreaks. Indeed, mandatory influenza immunization of HCWs is being considered by at least one leading healthcare institution. The CDC specifically recommends immunization for the following HCWs: physicians, nurses, and other personnel in both hospital and outpatient care settings; employees of nursing homes and long-term-care facilities who have contact with patients or residents; and providers of home care to people at high risk (e.g., visiting nurses and volunteer workers) (53). Unfortunately, despite these recommendations, many HCWs choose not to take influenza vaccine (165–167). Reasons offered by HCWs who decline influenza immunization have included desire to avoid medications, inconvenient vaccine administration, concern about side effects, belief that influenza can be caused by the vaccine, and belief that the vaccine is ineffective (7,12,103). Institution-wide influenza immunization programs that are highly publicized, bring the program to the worker, take advantage of social or peer pressure, and reward participation have shown the greatest success. Institutions should consider introducing innovative methods of taking vaccine to workers, such as provision by mobile carts on hospital wards, offering vaccine to house staff and students in clinics and conferences, etc. (158).

Measles-Mumps-Rubella Vaccine

Background

The widespread use of Measles-Mumps-Rubella (MMR) vaccine in the U.S., coupled with the hemisphere-wide measles eradication program, has led to record-low incidences of measles, mumps, and rubella. In 2002, there were reported only 34 cases of measles (of which 18 were imported), 270 cases of mumps, 18 cases of rubella, and one congenital rubella syndrome (168).

All three diseases are transmitted by the droplet route; measles, perhaps the most contagious disease known, also is transmitted by the airborne route. All three infections are contagious prior to development of clinically recognizable illness. Moreover, a history of prior disease does not reliably predict prior infection and immunity, and consequently, many unimmunized HCWs may falsely believe themselves immune.

Measles is highly dangerous; during the last major U.S. outbreak, one of every 500 infected persons died. Rubella is less serious, but is of special concern because of its ability to cause congenital abnormalities in the fetuses of up to 90% of women with confirmed infection in the first trimester of pregnancy. Mumps is typically a mild illness in children, but meningoencephalitis, oophoritis, pancreatitis, and nephritis can occur, especially in adults, and epididymo-orchitis occurs in 20% to 40% of postpubertal men and may eventuate in testicular atrophy. Orchitis has been reported among male HCWs who developed mumps as a result of hospital exposure (169).

Nosocomial Exposures

Nosocomial measles is well documented in the literature (170–202) and has played an important role in the propagation of community outbreaks (170–172). Measles was acquired in a medical setting by 1.1% of all cases between 1980 and 1984 (173) and 3.5% of all cases between 1985 and 1989 (174), representing up to 53% of the cases in certain outbreaks (171, 175–180). Spread of measles has also occurred in outpatient settings, including emergency departments and physician offices, with transmission occurring even 75 minutes after the departure of the index case (176,181–186). People who visited an emergency department have been shown to have a 4.9-fold (187) to 5.2-fold (172) higher risk of developing measles one incubation period later compared with those who did not have such visits. Nosocomial outbreaks have led to hospitalization of infected staff (188), severe complications in infected patients (189), and occasionally death of patients (170,188). The cost of controlling a single outbreak has ranged from $28,000 to more than $100,000 (170,188).

Nosocomial outbreaks of mumps have been reported infrequently (169,203–207), but transmission from patient to patient (203–205) and from patient to healthcare provider (169, 204–206) has been reported. In one case, it was suggested that an asymptomatically infected hospital nurse introduced mumps into a children's hospital (203). During the 1986–1987 Tennessee mumps epidemic, six HCWs in three different hospitals developed mumps after nosocomial exposure (204). Nosocomial rubella also is well documented in the literature (208–225). Sources of rubella infection have included both people with acute infection and infants with congenital rubella (208–210). Hospital-acquired infection of pregnant staff members has led to the termination of pregnancy (210,212).

Absence of a mandatory program requiring MMR immunity results in a subpopulation of susceptible HCWs capable of propagating epidemics. Although these diseases presently are rare, they are not eradicated, and they are so communicable—especially measles—that rapid nosocomial spread will inevitably occur following each index case, unless exceptionally high vaccination rates are maintained (see also Chapters 51 and 81).

Vaccination

All HCWs should be immune to mumps, measles, and rubella. Immunity may be demonstrated by meeting one of the following: (a) birth before 1957, for rubella (except women with childbearing potential) and mumps, but not measles (24); outbreak investigations have revealed that 4.0% to 9.0% of people born before 1957 were susceptible to measles (195,226,227); (b) laboratory evidence of immunity (people with indeterminate levels should be considered susceptible); (c) physician-diagnosed disease (measles or mumps, but not rubella); or (d) evidence of appropriate immunizations (228). Hospitals that do not implement this recommendation should assess the immunity of HCWs born before 1957, in the same manner as for younger HCWs, during a community or institutional outbreak of measles. Rubella vaccine is recommended for all female HCWs with childbearing potential (24) or, alternatively, for all persons regardless of gender (28) who do not have evidence of rubella immunity, including people born before 1957.

About 95% of subjects respond to a first dose of measles vaccine. However, measles is so contagious that it can propagate in a population that is 95% immune. Because nearly 95% of initial nonresponders will respond to a second dose, two doses of measles vaccine (MMR is preferred) are recommended to reduce the pool of susceptibles. Revaccination with MMR may also be indicated for mumps control, because studies have shown that mumps can occur in a highly vaccinated population (229).

Meningococcal Vaccine

Background

Neisseria meningitidis is responsible for 2,500 to 3,000 cases of invasive meningococcal disease annually in the U.S., the majority of these in persons 23 to 64 years of age (230,231). This relatively uncommon disease is notorious for its high rates of morbidity and mortality, and its ability to maim or kill a healthy person overnight. Even with the best medical care, fatality rates are 9% to 12% (up to 40% for meningococcal sepsis), and 11% to 19% of survivors of meningococcal disease experience serious sequelae such as hearing loss, neurologic disability, or amputation (231).

There are five serogroups of *N. meningitidis* that are important in human disease (based on the capsular polysaccharide and denoted A, B, C, Y, and W-135). Humans are the only natural reservoir for *N. meningitidis*. The microorganism colonizes the nasopharynx, and is carried by 5% to 10% of the population at any given point in time; carriage can give rise to type-specific antibody. Transmission is by droplet or nasopharyngeal secretions. Disease arises from invasion of capsule-producing strains in persons lacking specific anticapsular antibody.

In the U.S., nearly all cases of invasive meningococcal disease are sporadic, but certain populations (including military recruits, college freshmen living in dormitories, and persons with terminal complement deficiencies or asplenia) are at elevated risk of invasive meningococcal disease, and small epidemics occur regularly. Household or other close contacts are at 200 to 1,000 times the risk of developing meningococcal disease as is the general public (232), and secondary attack rates in households average 2% to 5% (233)

Effective vaccines exist for four of the five common serogroups (all but B). In the U.S., a quadrivalent polysaccharide vaccine is currently available, and a quadrivalent conjugate vaccine is expected to be licensed in 2004 or 2005. Bivalent, trivalent, and quadrivalent polysaccharide vaccines and monocomponent (type C) conjugate vaccines are available in various other countries.

Nosocomial Exposures

Although person-to-person transmission of *N. meningitidis* appears to require relatively prolonged close contact (233,234), the existence of epidemics, the elevated secondary attack rates in households, the known elevated risk of disease among social clusters (military recruits, college freshmen, concertgoers, bar patrons, etc.) (231), and especially the fearsome consequences of invasive meningococcal disease give rise to substantial anxiety among HCWs caring for patients diagnosed with the disease. And indeed, nosocomial (233,235–238) and laboratory-based (239) transmission have occurred, but sufficiently uncommonly that vaccination is not routinely recommended for HCWs (235) (see also Chapters 47 and 81).

Vaccination

Vaccination is currently recommended for research, industrial, and clinical laboratory personnel who are exposed routinely to *N. meningitidis* in solutions that may be aerosolized (230). In addition, institutions might elect to immunize selected staff members who have heightened likelihood of (or anxiety concerning) caring for patients with invasive meningococcal disease. As we went to press, Offit and Peter (240) noted, "Although [universal administration of] the meningococcal vaccine may be an inefficient use of public health resources, the decision to receive the vaccine could save lives and prevent the devastating consequences of meningococcal infection . . . . Policies and practices should be established to inform parents and patients about the availability of vaccines that can prevent diseases such as invasive meningococcal infections." In addition, once the quadrivalent conjugate vaccine is licensed, it is likely that official recommendations will be revisited.

Pertussis Vaccine

Background

In the U.S., the reported annual incidence of pertussis has declined from a high of 260,000 cases prior to routine vaccination to a low of some 1,300 cases in 1977 (241). Subsequently, however, pertussis has progressively increased, with 9,771 cases reported in 2002 (168). Most of this increase has occurred among infants younger than 6 months (too young to be fully immunized) and adolescents and adults (due to waning vaccine-induced immunity) (242). Because the classic whoop often is not seen with adult pertussis, the disease is commonly misdiagnosed (e.g., as bronchitis). However, studies using sophisticated diagnostic methods have demonstrated that *Bordetella pertussis* is a common cause of prolonged cough illness in adults (243–245). Deville et al. (246) followed HCWs for 5 years and found that 90% of subjects had serologic evidence of new infection during that period; 55% had evidence of two infections, 17% had evidence of three infections, and 4% had evidence of four infections.

Nosocomial Exposures

Many nosocomial pertussis outbreaks have been reported (247–257). Although the source case most commonly was an infected patient in whom pertussis was unrecognized (247–249), infected HCWs (250,251) and visitors (252) have also served as sources. Secondarily infected HCWs, in turn, serve as the source for additional cases in the institution (250,251,253,258) or their own households (248,250) (see also Chapter 81).

Vaccination

Pertussis immunization classically has ceased around age 6 years, because adverse reactions to whole-cell vaccine among older persons have not been tolerable. However, effective acellular pertussis vaccines have been developed that are highly effective but little more reactogenic than a standard tetanus-diphtheria booster (259–265). Adolescent-adult formulations of such vaccines have been licensed in Canada, Europe, and elsewhere and are expected to be licensed in the U.S. within a few years (266).

Once licensed, it is likely that adult acellular pertussis vaccine, combined with diphtheria and tetanus toxoids, will be recommended for some or all HCWs in lieu of the usual diphtheria-tetanus booster. Meanwhile, in the event of a nosocomial outbreak, consideration could be given to administration of half doses of pediatric diphtheria-tetanus-acellular pertussis (DTaP) vaccine (with informed consent) as part of an outbreak control program (254,255,266).

Typhoid Vaccine

Background

Typhoid fever now is relatively rare in the U.S., with fewer than 500 cases reported annually. The disease remains common, however, in areas of the world where fecal contamination of food or drinking water occur. The majority of cases in Western countries occur among travelers to other countries (267).

Nosocomial Exposures

Although *Salmonella* is a common cause of nosocomial infectious diarrhea, such cases in the U.S. usually involve the animal serotypes (268–273) rather than *Salmonella typhi* (274–282). Transmission to HCWs other than laboratorians working with *S. typhi* is distinctly uncommon (see also Chapter 81).

Vaccination

Two modern vaccines exist, a live-attenuated oral vaccine (not recommended for HCWs, due to the theoretical risk of spread to patients) and a killed parenteral vaccine based on the capsular polysaccharide. A conjugate version of the latter vaccine has been developed but is not yet licensed. Vaccination is recommended for microbiology laboratorians who work frequently with *S. typhi.*

Vaccinia (Smallpox Vaccine)

Background

Smallpox, one of the greatest killers of mankind, was eradicated as a natural disease in 1977 (283). Unfortunately, it is now known that the Soviet Union weaponized smallpox during the 1980s, stockpiling enormous quantities of the virus whose present whereabouts are not known with certainty (284). The consequent fear that smallpox might be used as a bioterror agent spurred efforts by the U.S. and other governments to reestablish stockpiles of smallpox vaccine (vaccinia). In addition, in 2002–2003 the U.S. promulgated a pre-event vaccination program designed to ensure the availability of immunized cadres that could respond to a smallpox release (285). However, due primarily to concerns about vaccine adverse events (283) but also, perhaps, to doubts as to the likelihood of such an event, vaccine uptake among HCWs was so low that the program was functionally suspended in 2003.

Nosocomial Exposures

Prior to the eradication of natural smallpox, the threat of nosocomial spread of infection was averted through universal vaccination. Subsequently, until the issue of bioterror protection arose, the only indication for the (somewhat hazardous) vaccination of HCWs was to prevent the potentially more hazardous consequences of inadvertent infection with vaccinia among laboratory and HCWs occupationally exposed to vaccinia, recombinant vaccinia viruses, and other orthopoxviruses that can infect humans (286) (see Chapters 81, 111, and 112).

Vaccination

In the U.S., vaccinia is available only through the public health authorities. As of publication time, vaccination against smallpox was recommended by the CDC only for laboratorians (or, presumably, other HCWs) who work with orthopoxviruses (for this indication, contact CDC) and for public health and healthcare response team members (for this indication, contact your state or local health department).

Varicella Vaccine

Background

Varicella-zoster virus (VZV) is the causative agent of varicella (chickenpox). Following acute infection, the virus remains latent in the trigeminal and dorsal root ganglia for life, and from there may erupt on occasion to cause herpes zoster (shingles) (287). Although varicella is generally a mild disease in children, it is often more serious in adults, and substantial morbidity and mortality are common if infection occurs in neonates, pregnant women, or the immunocompromised (287). VZV is most commonly transmitted from person to person by the droplet route, but true airborne transmission may also occur. The secondary attack rate of varicella among susceptible people in the household setting has ranged from 61% to 87% (288–290). Herpes zoster is also infectious, although analysis of households suggests that the risk of transmission is lower than that for varicella.

Varicella disease appears to have declined sharply in the U.S. following incorporation of the varicella vaccine into the childhood vaccination schedule (291). Paradoxically, this heightens the importance of an institutional varicella immunity program, as those who escaped infection in childhood [in the prevaccine era, at least 5% of persons aged 20 to 29 (292)] and were left susceptible are likely to remain so, absent vaccination.

Nosocomial Exposures

Control of varicella is important in healthcare facilities because varicella and zoster are highly contagious, with many reported nosocomial outbreaks (290,293–313); infection in adults frequently results in complications, including hospitalization (294,314,315); infection in pregnant women may lead to both maternal (287) and fetal (316–318) complications; and immunosuppressed persons, who make up a progressively larger proportion of hospital inpatients, are at high risk of complications (294,319–326).

Studies conducted prior to widespread varicella vaccination have indicated that a report of prior varicella by an HCW is predictive of immunity as measured by serology (327). However, as exposure opportunities are reduced by childhood immunization programs, the proportion of such reports that are false positive must inevitably rise, and active screening will increasingly be necessary. A history of prior household exposure to VZV is not predictive of immunity (328). Among HCWs with a negative or uncertain history of VZV infection, serosusceptibility has ranged from 4% to 47% (293,296,297,330–334). Overall, a median of 3% of HCWs are susceptible to varicella (296–298, 329,330,332–334), absent an institutional immunization program, and 2% to 16% of susceptible staff will develop clinical varicella after nosocomial exposure to VZV (293,294,296) (see Chapters 42 and 81).

Vaccination

Due to its high communicability and potential for serious consequences, the appearance of active varicella infection within a healthcare institution is an infection control emergency. In the absence of assurance of HCW immunity, the management of such VZV exposure incidents is burdensome and expensive. Accordingly, many institutions (particularly those with pediatric, obstetric, transplant, chemotherapy, or similar programs) have elected to require demonstrated immunity among HCWs working with such patients. Decision and cost-effectiveness analysis methods have been used to demonstrate that immunization of HCWs susceptible to varicella is cost-effective for healthcare facilities (335–338).

We recommend that HCWs be screened for VZV immunity at the time of initial employment (or, for current employees, at time of next tuberculosis or similar screening). HCWs with a reliable history of VZV infection may be considered immune; all others should undergo serologic testing and, if negative, be considered for immunization with two doses of vaccine at least 4 weeks apart. Postimmunization serology is not recommended.

There appears to be virtually no risk of transmission of the vaccine virus from healthy people who do not develop a rash postimmunization. HCWs who develop an injection site rash may continue to work with nonimmunocompromised patients, provided that the lesions are covered. HCWs with a generalized rash should be furloughed until the rash is resolved. In the authors' experience, this has been approximately 5 days. The rash should not automatically be assumed to be due to vaccine, especially if exposure to a case of chickenpox has occurred in the preceding 3 weeks.

CONCLUSION

All HCWs should be immune to measles, mumps, rubella, and varicella. All those with the potential for exposure to blood or potentially contaminated body fluids should be immune to hepatitis B. Absent specific contraindication, those who are susceptible should be offered the appropriate vaccines; prevaccination serologic testing is not medically required but may be offered at the institution's discretion.

In addition, all HCWs should be immunized annually against influenza. HCWs also should receive tetanus-diphtheria and pneumococcal vaccines as recommended for the general public. Hepatitis A vaccine may be indicated based on local or regional epidemiology. Once licensed, adult acellular pertussis vaccine should be administered to all HCWs having prolonged close contact with infants not yet fully immunized, and should be considered for routine use in lieu of Td. Finally, selected HCWs may be candidates for other available vaccines, including meningococcus, polio, plague, rabies, typhoid, and vaccinia.

REFERENCES

1. Schwarcz S, McCaw B, Fukushima P. Prevalence of measles susceptibility in hospital staff. Evidence to support expanding the recommendations of the Immunization Practices Advisory Committee. *Arch Intern Med* 1992;152:1481–1483.
2. Wright LJ, Carlquist JF. Measles immunity in employees of a multihospital healthcare provider. *Infect Control Hosp Epidemiol* 1994;15:8–11.
3. Huang KG, Spence MR, Deforest A, et al. Measles immunization in HCWs. *Infect Control Hosp Epidemiol* 1994;15:4.
4. Stover BH, Adams G, Kuebler CA, et al. Measles-mumps-rubella immunization of susceptible hospital employees during a community measles outbreak: cost-effectiveness and protective efficacy. *Infect Control Hosp Epidemiol* 1994;15:18–21.
5. Willey ME, Koziol DE, Fleisher T, et al. Measles immunity in a population of healthcare workers. *Infect Control Hosp Epidemiol* 1994;15:12–17.
6. Seo SK, Malak SF, Lim S, et al. Prevalence of measles antibody among young adult healthcare workers in a cancer hospital: 1980s versus 1998–1999. *Infect Control Hosp Epidemiol* 2002;23:276–278.
7. Weingarten S, Riedinger M, Bolton LB, et al. Barriers to influenza vaccine acceptance. *Am J Infect Control* 1989;17:202–207.
8. Shapiro CN, Tokars JI, Chamberland ME. Use of the hepatitis-B vaccine and infection with hepatitis B and C among orthopedic surgeons. *J Bone Joint Surg* 1996;78:1791–1800.
9. Cleveland JL. Hepatitis B vaccination and infection among U.S. dentists, 1983–1993. *J Am Dent Assoc* 1996;127:1385–1390.
10. McArthur MA, Simor AE, Campbell B, et al. Influenza and pneumococcal vaccination and tuberculin skin testing programs in long-term care facilities: where do we stand? *Infect Control Hosp Epidemiol* 1995;16:18–24.
11. McArthur MA, Simor AE, Campbell B, et al. Influenza vaccination in long-term-care facilities: structuring programs for success. *Infect Control Hosp Epidemiol* 1999;20:499–503.
12. Nichol KL, Hauge M. Influenza vaccination of healthcare workers. *Infect Control Hosp Epidemiol* 1997;18:189–194.
13. Agerton TB, Mahoney FJ, Polish LB, et al. Impact of the bloodborne pathogens standard on vaccination of healthcare workers with hepatitis B vaccine. *Infect Control Hosp Epidemiol* 1995;16:287–291.
14. Panlilio AL, Shapiro CN, Schable CA, et al. Serosurvey of human immunodeficiency virus, hepatitis B virus, and hepatitis C virus infection among hospital-based surgeons. *J Am Coll Surg* 1995;180:16–24.
15. Gyawali P, Rice PS, Tilzey AJ. Exposure to blood borne viruses and the hepatitis B vaccination status among healthcare workers in inner London. *Occup Environ Med* 1998;55:570–572.
16. Mahoney FJ, Stewart K, Hu H, et al. Progress toward the elimination of hepatitis B virus transmission among health care workers in the United States. *Arch Intern Med* 1997;157:2601–2605.
17. Zadeh MM, Bridges CB, Thompson WW, et al. Influenza outbreak detection and control measures in nursing homes in the United States. *J Am Geriatr Soc* 2000;48:1310–1315.
18. Cui XW, Nagao MM, Effler PV. Influenza and pneumococcal vaccination coverage levels among Hawaii statewide long-term-care facilities. *Infect Control Hosp Epidemiol* 2001;22:519–521.
19. Russell ML. Influenza vaccination in Alberta long-term care facilities. *Can Med Assoc J* 2001;164:1423–1427.
20. Stevenson CG, McArthur MA, Naus M, et al. Prevention of influenza and pneumococcal pneumonia in Canadian long-term care facilities: how are we doing? *Can Med Assoc J* 2001;164:1413–1419.

21. Lane NE, Paul RI, Bratcher DF, et al. A survey of policies at children's hospitals regarding immunity of healthcare workers: Are physicians protected? *Infect Control Hosp Epidemiol* 1997;18:400–404.
22. *http://www.cdc.gov/nip/publications/VIS/default.htm.*
23. Vaccine Adverse Event Report System (VAERS). *http://www.fda.gov/cber/vaers/vaers.htm.*
24. Bolyard EA, Tablan OC, Williams WW, et al., and the Hospital Infection Control Practices Advisory Committee. Guideline for infection control in healthcare personnel. *Infect Control Hosp Epidemiol* 1998;19:407–463.
25. Immunization of health-care workers: recommendations of the Advisory Committee on Immunization Practices (ACIP) and the Hospital Infection Control Practices Advisory Committee (HICPAC). *MMWR* 1997;46(RR-18):1–42.
26. General recommendations on immunization: recommendations of the Advisory Committee on Immunization Practices (ACIP) and the American Academy of Family Physicians. *MMWR* 2002;51(RR-2): 1.
27. ACP Task Force on Adult Immunization and Infectious Disease Society of America. *Guide for adult immunization,* 3rd ed. Philadelphia: American College of Physicians, 1994.
28. Committee on Infectious Diseases, American Academy of Pediatrics. *Red book: 2003 report of the Committee on Infectious Diseases,* 26th ed. Elk Grove Village, IL: American Academy of Pediatrics, 2003.
29. Krause PJ, Gross PA, Barrett TL, et al. Quality standard for assurance of measles immunity among healthcare workers. *Infect Control Hosp Epidemiol* 1994;15:193–199.
30. Beekmann SE, Doebbeling BN. Frontiers of occupational health: new vaccines, new prophylactic regimens, and management of the HIV-infected worker. *Infect Dis Clin North Am* 1997;11:313–329.
31. Weber DJ, Rutala WA. Selection and use of vaccines for healthcare workers. *Infect Control Hosp Epidemiol* 1997;18:682–687.
32. Kessler ER. Vaccine-preventable diseases in health care. *Occup Med* 1997;12:731–739.
33. Poland GA, Haiduven DJ. Immunization in the health-care worker. In: *APIC text of infection control and epidemiology.* Association for Professionals in Infection Control and Epidemiology, 2000: 80.1–80.32.
34. Poland GA, Schaffner W, Publiese G, eds. *Immunizing healthcare workers: a practical approach.* Thorofare, NJ: SLACK.
35. Zimmermann RK, Ball JA. Adult vaccinations. *Prim Care* 2001;25: 763–790.
36. DeCastro MG, Denys GA, Fauerbach LL, et al. APIC position paper: immunization. *Am J Infect Control* 1999;27:52–53.
37. Poliomyelitis prevention in the United States: introduction of a sequential vaccination schedule of inactivated poliovirus vaccine followed by oral poliovirus vaccine: recommendations of the Advisory Committee on Immunization Practices (ACIP). *MMWR* 1997; 46(RR-3):1–25.
38. Control and prevention of meningococcal disease: recommendations of the Advisory Committee on Immunization Practices (ACIP). *MMWR* 1997;46(RR-5):1–11.
39. Control and prevention of serogroup C meningococcal disease: evaluation and management of suspected outbreaks: recommendations of the Advisory Committee on Immunization Practices (ACIP). *MMWR* 1997;46(RR-5):13–21.
40. The role of BCG vaccine in the prevention and control of tuberculosis in the United States: a joint statement by the Advisory Committee for the Elimination of Tuberculosis and the Advisory Committee on Immunization Practices. *MMWR* 1996;45(RR-4):1–18.
41. Rabies prevention—United States, 1991: recommendations of the Immunization Practices Advisory Committee (ACIP). *MMWR* 1991; 40(RR-3):1–19.
42. Prevention of plague: recommendations of the Advisory Committee on Immunization Practices (ACIP). *MMWR* 1996;45(RR-14):1–15.
43. Typhoid immunization: recommendations of the Immunization Practices Advisory Committee (ACIP). *MMWR* 1990;39(RR-10):1–5.
44. Typhoid immunization: recommendations of the Immunization Practices Advisory Committee (ACIP). *MMWR* 1994;43(RR-14):1–7.
45. Vaccinia (smallpox) vaccine: recommendations of the Immunization Practices Advisory Committee (ACIP). *MMWR* 1991;40(RR-14): 1–10.
46. Prevention of hepatitis A though active or passive immunization: recommendations of the Advisory Committee on Immunization Practices (ACIP). *MMWR* 1999;48(RR-12):1–37.
47. Use of anthrax vaccine in the United States: recommendations of the Advisory Committee on Immunization Practices (ACIP). *MMWR* 2001;49(RR-15).
48. Recommendations of the Advisory Committee on Immunization Practices (ACIP): use of vaccines and immune globulin in persons with altered immunocompetence. *MMWR* 1993;42(RR-4):1–18.
49. Loutan L. Vaccination of the immunocompromised patient. *Biologicals* 1997;25:231–236.
50. Pirofski L-A, Casadevall A. Use of licensed vaccines for active immunization of the immunocompromised host. *Clin Microbiol Rev* 1998; 11:1–26.
51. Weber DJ, Weigle K, Rutala WA. Immunization of workers with altered host defenses. In: Poland GA, Schaffner W, Publiese G (eds). *Immunizing healthcare workers: a practical approach.* Thorofare, NJ: SLACK.
52. Faix RG. Immunization during pregnancy. *Clin Obstet Gynecol* 2002; 45:42–58.
53. Centers for Disease Control and Prevention. Prevention and control of influenza: recommendations of the Advisory Committee on Immunization Practices (ACIP). *MMWR* 2003;52(RR-8):1–34.
54. Update: Vaccine side effects, adverse reactions, contraindications, and precautions: recommendations of the Advisory Committee on Immunization Practices (ACIP). *MMWR* 1996;45(RR-12):1–35.
55. Diphtheria, tetanus, and pertussis: recommendations of the Immunization Practices Advisory Committee (ACIP). *MMWR* 1991;40(RR-10):1–28.
56. Hepatitis B virus: a comprehensive strategy for eliminating transmission in the United States through universal childhood vaccination: recommendations of the Immunization Practices Advisory Committee (ACIP). *MMWR* 1991;40(RR-13):1–25.
57. Andre F, Van Damme P, Safary A, et al. Inactivated hepatitis A vaccine: immunogenicity, efficacy, safety and review of official recommendations for use. *Expert Rev Vaccines* 2002;1(1):9–23.
58. Prevention of varicella: updated recommendations of the Advisory Committee on Immunization Practices (ACIP). *MMWR* 1999; 49(RR-6):1–5.
59. Summary of notifiable diseases, United States. *MMWR* 2002;49(52): 1–100.
60. Kew MC. Possible transmission of serum (Australia-antigen-positive) hepatitis via the conjunctiva. *Infect Immun* 1973;7:823–824.
61. Kashiwagi S, Hayashi J, Ikematsu H, et al. Prevalence of immunologic markers of hepatitis A and B infection in hospital personnel in Miyazaki Prefecture, Japan. *Am J Epidemiol* 1985;122:964–969.
62. Gibas A, Blewett DR, Schoenfield DA, et al. Prevalence and incidence of viral hepatitis in healthcare workers in the prehepatitis B vaccination era. *Am J Epidemiol* 1992;136:1791–1800.
63. Abb J. Prevalence of hepatitis A virus antibodies in hospital personnel. *Gesundheitswesen* 1994;56:377–379.
64. Papaevangelou GJ, Roumeliotou-Karayannis AJ, Contoyannis PC. The risk of hepatitis A and B virus infections from patients under care without isolation precaution. *J Med Virol* 1981;7:143–148.
65. Germanaud J. Hepatitis A and health care personnel [letter]. *Arch Intern Med* 1994;154:820.
66. Van Damme P, Cramm M, Van der Auwera J-C, et al. Hepatitis A vaccination for healthcare workers. *BMJ* 1993;306:1615.
67. Goodman RA, Carder CC, Allen JR, et al. Nosocomial hepatitis A transmission by an adult patient with diarrhea. *Am J Med* 1982;73: 220–226.
68. Krober MS, Bass JW, Brown JD, et al. Hospital outbreak of hepatitis A: risk factors for spread. *Pediatr Infect Dis J* 1984;3:296–299.
69. Klein BS, Michaels JA, Rytel MW, et al. Nosocomial hepatitis A: a multinursery outbreak in Wisconsin. *JAMA* 1984;252:2716–2721.
70. Reed CM, Gustafson TL, Siegel J, et al. Nosocomial transmission of hepatitis A from a hospital-acquired case. *Pediatr Infect Dis J* 1984; 3:300–303.

71. Skidmore SJ, Gully PR, Middleton JD, et al. An outbreak of hepatitis A on a hospital ward. *J Med Virol* 1985;17:175–177.
72. Baptiste R, Koziol DE, Henderson DK. Nosocomial transmission of hepatitis A in an adult population. *Infect Control* 1987;8:364–370.
73. Watson JC, Flemming DC, Borella AJ, et al. Vertical transmission of hepatitis A resulting in an outbreak in a neonatal intensive care unit. *J Infect Dis* 1993;167:567–571.
74. Doebbeling BN, Li N, Wenzel RP. An outbreak of hepatitis A among healthcare workers: risk factors for transmission. *Am J Public Health* 1993;83:1679–1684.
75. Burkholder BT, Coronado VG, Brown J, et al. Nosocomial transmission of hepatitis A in a pediatric hospital traced to an anti-hepatitis A virus-negative patient with immunodeficiency. *Pediatr Infect Dis J* 1995;14:261–266.
76. Hanna JN, Loewenthal MR, Negel P, et al. An outbreak of hepatitis A in an intensive care unit. *Anaesth Intensive Care* 1996;24:440–444.
77. Drusin LM, Sohmer M, Groshen SL, et al. Nosocomial hepatitis A infection in a pediatric intensive care unit. *Arch Dis Child* 1987;62: 690–695.
78. Rosenblum LS, Villarino ME, Nainan OV, et al. Hepatitis A outbreak in a neonatal intensive care unit: risk factors for transmission and evidence of prolonged viral excretion among preterm infants. *J Infect Dis* 1991;164:476–482.
79. Eisenstein AB, Aach RD, Jacobson W, et al. An epidemic of infectious hepatitis in a general hospital: probable transmission by contaminated orange juice. *JAMA* 1993;185:171–184.
80. Meyers JD, Romm FJ, Tihen WS, et al. Food-borne hepatitis A in a general hospital: epidemiologic study of an outbreak attributed to sandwiches. *JAMA* 1975;231:1049–1053.
81. Azimi PH, Roberto RR, Guralnik J, et al. Transfusion-acquired hepatitis A in a premature infant with secondary nosocomial spread in an intensive care nursery. *Am J Dis Child* 1986;140:23–27.
82. Lee KK, Vargo LR, Le CT, et al. Transfusion-acquired hepatitis A outbreak from fresh frozen plasma in a neonatal intensive care unit. *Pediatr Infect Dis J* 1992;11:122–123.
83. Jensenius M, Ringertz SH, Bell H, et al. Prolonged nosocomial outbreak of hepatitis A arising from an alcoholic with pneumonia. *Scand J Infect Dis* 1998;30:119–123.
84. Smith S, Weber S, Wiblin T, et al. Cost-effectiveness of hepatitis A vaccination in healthcare workers. *Infect Control Hosp Epidemiol* 1997; 18:688–691.
85. Segal HE, Llewellyn CH, Irwin G, et al. Hepatitis B antigen and antibody in the U.S. Army: prevalence in healthcare personnel. *Am J Public Health* 1976;66:67–671.
86. Denes AE, Smith JL, Maynard JE, et al. Hepatitis B infection in physicians: results of a nationwide seroepidemiologic survey. *JAMA* 1978;239:210–212.
87. Dienstag JL, Ryan DM. Occupational exposure to hepatitis B virus in hospital personnel: infection or immunization? *Am J Epidemiol* 1982;115:26–39.
88. Hadler SC, Doto IL, Maynard JE, et al. Occupational risk of hepatitis B infection in hospital workers. *Infect Control* 1985;6:24–31.
89. Beltrami EM, Williams IT, Shapiro CN, et al. Risks and management of blood-borne infections in health care workers. *Clin Microbiol Rev* 2000;13:385–407.
90. Lowenfels AB, Wormser GP, Jain R. Frequency of puncture injuries in surgeons and estimated risk of HIV infection. *Arch Surg* 1989; 124:1284–1286.
91. Tokars JI, Chamberland ME, Schable CA, et al. A survey of occupational blood contact and HIV infection among orthopedic surgeons. *JAMA* 1992;268:489–494.
92. Bond WW, Favero MS, Peterson NJ, et al. Survival of hepatitis B virus after drying and storage for one week. *Lancet* 1981;1:550–551.
93. Grady GF, Lee VA, Prince AM, et al. Hepatitis B immune globulin for accidental exposures among medical personnel: final report of a multicenter controlled trial. *J Infect Dis* 1978;138:625–638.
94. Seeff LM, Wright EC, Zimmerman HJ, et al. Type B hepatitis after needle-stick exposure: prevention with hepatitis B immune globulin. *Ann Intern Med* 1978;88:285–293.
95. Werner BG, Grady GF. Accidental hepatitis-B-surface-antigen-positive inoculations. *Ann Intern Med* 1982;97:367–369.
96. Snydman DR, Hindman SH, Wineland MD, et al. Nosocomial viral hepatitis B: a cluster among staff with subsequent transmission to patients. *Ann Intern Med* 1976;85:573–577.
97. Handsfield HH, Cummings MJ, Swenson PD. Prevalence of antibody to human immunodeficiency virus and hepatitis B surface antigen in blood samples submitted to a hospital laboratory: implications for handling specimens. *JAMA* 1987;258:3395–3397.
98. Weber DJ, Hoffmann KK, Rutala WA. Management of the healthcare worker infected with human immunodeficiency virus: lessons from nosocomial transmission of hepatitis B virus. *Infect Control Hosp Epidemiol* 1991;12:625–630.
99. Bell DM, Shapiro CN, Ciesielski CA, et al. Preventing bloodborne pathogen transmission from health-care workers to patients. *Surg Clin North Am* 1995;75:1189–1203.
100. Harpaz R, Von Seidlein L, Averhoff FM, et al. Transmission of hepatitis B virus to multiple patients from a surgeon without evidence of inadequate infection control. *N Engl J Med* 1996;334:549–554.
101. Incident Investigation Team and Others. Transmission of hepatitis B to patients from four infected surgeons without hepatitis B "e" antigen. *N Engl J Med* 1997;336:178–184.
102. Chiarella LA, Cardo DM, Panlilio A, et al. Risks and prevention of bloodborne virus transmission from infected healthcare providers. *Semin Infect Control* 2001;1:61–72.
103. Christian MA. Influenza and hepatitis B vaccine acceptance: a survey of healthcare workers. *Am J Infect Control* 1991;19:177–184.
104. Lemon SM, Thomas DL. Vaccines to prevent viral hepatitis. *N Engl J Med* 1997;336:196–204.
105. Koff RS. Hepatitis vaccines. *Infect Dis Clin North Am* 19xx;15:83–95.
106. Mahoney FJ. Update on diagnosis, management, and prevention of hepatitis B virus infection. *Clin Microbiol Rev* 1999;12:351–356.
107. Wood RC, MacDonald KL, White KE, et al. Risk factors for lack of detectable antibody following hepatitis B vaccination on Minnesota health care workers. *JAMA* 1993;270:2935–2939.
108. Jilg W, Schmidt M, Deinhardt F. Vaccination against hepatitis B: comparison of three different vaccination schedules. *J Infect Dis* 1989; 160:766–769.
109. Hadler SC, de Monzon A, Lugo DR, et al. Effect of timing of hepatitis B vaccine doses on response to vaccine Yucca Indians. *Vaccine* 1989; 7:106–110.
110. Hadler SC, Francis DP, Maynard JE, et al. Long-term immunogenicity and efficacy of hepatitis B vaccine in homosexual men. *N Engl J Med* 1986;315:209–214.
111. Cardo DM, Bell DM. Bloodborne pathogen transmission in healthcare workers. *Infect Dis Clin North Am* 1997;11:331–346.
112. Barker WH. Excess pneumonia and influenza associated hospitalizations during influenza epidemics in the United States, 1970–78. *Am J Public Health* 1986;76:761–765.
113. Influenza surveillance—United States, 1992–93 and 1993–94. *MMWR* 1997;46(SS-1):1–12.
114. Anonymous. Influenza. In: Atkinson W, Wolfe C, eds. *Epidemiology and prevention of vaccine-preventable diseases,* 7th ed. Atlanta: Centers for Disease Control and Prevention and the Public Health Foundation, 2002:190–204.
115. Balkovic ES, Goodman RA, Rose FB, et al. Nosocomial influenza A (H1N1) infection. *Am J Med Tech* 1980;46:318–320.
116. Van Voris LP, Belshe RB, Shaffer JL. Nosocomial influenza B virus infection in the elderly. *Ann Intern Med* 1982;96:153–158.
117. Hammond GW, Cheang M. Absenteeism among hospital staff during an influenza epidemic: implications for immunoprophylaxis. *Can Med Assoc J* 1984;131:449–452.
118. Suspected nosocomial influenza cases in an intensive care unit. *MMWR* 1988;37:3–4,9.
119. Pachucki CT, Pappas SAW, Fuller GF, et al. Influenza A among hospital personnel and patients. *Ann Intern Med* 1989;149:77–80.
120. Evert RJ, Hanger HJC, Jennings LC, et al. Outbreaks of influenza A among elderly hospital inpatients. *N Z Med J* 1996;109:272–274.
121. Evans ME, Hall KL, Berry SE. Influenza control in acute care hospitals. *Am J Infect Control* 1997;25:357–362.

122. Meibalane R, Sedmak GV, Sasidharan P, et al. Outbreak of influenza in a neonatal intensive care unit. *J Pediatr* 1977;91:974–976.
123. Kapila R, Lintz DI, Tecson FT, et al. A nosocomial outbreak of influenza A. *Chest* 1977;71:576–579.
124. Rivera M, Gonzalez N. An influenza outbreak in a hospital. *Am J Nurs* 1982;82:1836–1838.
125. Bean B, Rhame FS, Hughes RS, et al. Influenza B: hospital activity during a community outbreak. *Diagn Microbiol Infect Dis* 1983;1: 177–183.
126. Weingarten S, Friedlander M, Rascon D, et al. Influenza surveillance in an acute-care hospital. *Arch Intern Med* 1988;148:113–116.
127. Grayston JT, Diwan VK, Cooney M, et al. Community- and hospital-acquired pneumonia associated with Chlamydia TWAR infection demonstrated serologically. *Arch Intern Med* 1989;149:169–173.
128. Serwint JR, Miller RM. Why diagnose influenza infections in hospitalized pediatric patients? *Pediatr Infect Dis J* 1993;12:200–204.
129. Whimbey E, Elting LS, Couch RB, et al. Influenza A virus infections among hospitalized adult bone marrow transplant recipients. *Bone Marrow Transplant* 1994;13:437–440.
130. Scheputiuk S, Papanaoum K, Quao M. Spread of influenza A virus infection in hospitalized patients with cancer. *Aust N Z J Med* 1998; 28:475–476.
131. Munoz FM, Campbell JR, Atman RL, et al. Influenza A virus outbreak in a neonatal intensive care unit. *Pediatr Infect Dis J* 1999;18: 811–815.
132. Cunney RJ, Bialachowski A, Thornley D, et al. An outbreak of influenza A in a neonatal intensive care unit. *Infect Control Hosp Epidemiol* 2000;21:449–454.
133. Weinstock DM, Eagan J, Malak SA, et al. Control of influenza on a bone marrow transplant unit. *Infect Control Hosp Epidemiol* 2000; 21:730–732.
134. Barlow G, Nathwani D. Nosocomial influenza infection. *Lancet* 2000; 355:1187.
135. Malavaud S, Malavaud B, Sanders K, et al. Nosocomial influenza virus A (H3N2) infection in a solid organ transplant department. *Transplantation* 2001;72:5325–537.
136. Sagrera X, Ginovart G, Raspall F, et al. Outbreaks of influenza A virus infection in neonatal intensive care units. *Pediatr Infect Dis J* 2002;21:196–200.
137. Serie C, Barme M, Hannoun C, et al. Effects of vaccination on an influenza epidemic in a geriatric hospital. *Dev Biol Stand* 1977;39: 317–321.
138. Hall WN, Goodman RA, Noble GR, et al. An outbreak of influenza B in an elderly population. *J Infect Dis* 1981;144:297–302.
139. Goodman RA, Orenstein WA, Munro TF, et al. Impact of influenza A in a nursing home. *JAMA* 1982;247:1451–1453.
140. Arroyo JC, Postic B, Brown A, et al. Influenza A/Philippines/2/82 outbreak in a nursing home: limitations of influenza vaccination in the aged. *Am J Infect Control* 1984;12:329–334.
141. Christie RW, Marquis LL. Immunization roulette: influenza occurrence in five nursing homes. *Am J Infect Control* 1985;13:174–177.
142. Horman JT, Stetler HC, Israel E, et al. An outbreak of influenza A in a nursing home. *Am J Public Health* 1986;76:501–504.
143. Patriarca PA, Weber JA, Parker RA, et al. Risk factors for outbreaks of influenza in nursing homes. *Am J Epidemiol* 1986;124:114–119.
144. Strassburg MA, Greenland S, Sorvillo FJ, et al. Influenza in the elderly: report of an outbreak and a review of vaccine effectiveness reports. *Vaccine* 1986;4:38–44.
145. Arden NH, Patriarca PA, Fasano MB, et al. The role of vaccination and amantadine prophylaxis in controlling an outbreak of influenza A (H3N2) in a nursing home. *Arch Intern Med* 1988;148:865–868.
146. Gross PA, Rodstein M, LaMontage JR, et al. Epidemiology of acute respiratory illness during an influenza outbreak in a nursing home. *Arch Intern Med* 1988;148:559–561.
147. Mast EE, Harmon MW, Gravenstein S, et al. Emergence and possible transmission of amantadine-resistant viruses during nursing home outbreaks of influenza A (H3N2). *Am J Epidemiol* 1991;134: 988–997.
148. Control of influenza A outbreaks in nursing homes: Amantadine as an adjunct to vaccine—Washington, 1989–90. *MMWR* 1991;40: 842–845.
149. Outbreak of influenza A in a nursing home—New York, December 1991–January 1992. *MMWR* 1992;41:129–131.
150. Degelau J, Somani SK, Cooper SL, et al. Amantadine-resistant influenza A in a nursing facility. *Arch Intern Med* 1992;152:390–392.
151. Taylor JL, Dwyer DM, Coffman T, et al. Nursing home outbreak of influenza A (H3N2): evaluation of vaccine efficacy and influenza case definition. *Infect Control Hosp Epidemiol* 1992;13:93–97.
152. Morens DM, Rash VM. Lessons from a nursing home outbreak of influenza A. *Infect Control Hosp Epidemiol* 1995;16:275–280.
153. Issacs S, Dickenson C, Brimmer G. Outbreak of influenza A in an Ontario nursing home—January 1997. *Canada Comm Dis Rep* 1997; 23:105–108.
154. Bowles SK, Kennie N, Ruston L, et al. Influenza outbreak in a long-term care facility: considerations for pharmacy. *Am J Health-System Pharm* 1999;56:2303–2307.
155. Atkinson WL, Arden NH, Patriarca PA, et al. Amantadine prophylaxis during an institutional outbreak of type A (H1N1) influenza. *Arch Intern Med* 1986;146:1751–1756.
156. Potter J, Stott DJ, Roberts MA, et al. Influenza vaccination of health care workers in long-term-care hospitals reduces the mortality of elderly patients. *J Infect Dis* 1997;175:1–6.
157. Carman WF, Elder AG, Wallace LA, et al. Effects of influenza vaccination on health-care workers on mortality of elderly people in long-term care: a randomized controlled trial. *Lancet* 2000;355:93–97.
158. Adal KA, Flowers RH, Anglim AM, et al. Prevention of nosocomial influenza. *Infect Control Hosp Epidemiol* 1996;17:641–648.
159. Fedson DS. Prevention and control of influenza in institutional settings. *Hosp Pract* 1989;24:87–96.
160. Graman PS, Hall CB. Nosocomial viral infections. *Semin Respir Infect* 1989;4:253–260.
161. Graman PS, Hall CB. Epidemiology and control of nosocomial viral infections. *Infect Dis Clin North Am* 1989;3:815–841.
162. Gravenstein S, Miller BA, Drinka P. Prevention and control of influenza A outbreaks in long-term care facilities. *Infect Control Hosp Epidemiol* 1992;13:49–54.
163. Tablan OC, Anderson LJ, Arden NH, et al. Guideline for prevention of nosocomial pneumonia. *Infect Control Hosp Epidemiol* 1994;15: 587–627.
164. Gomolin IH, Leib HB, Arden NH, et al. Control of influenza outbreaks in the nursing home: guidelines for diagnosis and management. *J Am Geriatr Soc* 1995;43:71–74.
165. Nichol KL, Lind A, Margolis KL, et al. The effectiveness of vaccination against influenza in healthy, working adults. *N Engl J Med* 1995; 333:889–893.
166. Ohrt CK, McKinney WP. Achieving compliance with influenza immunization of medical house staff and students: a randomized controlled study. *JAMA* 1992;267:1377–1380.
167. Nafziger DA, Herwaldt LA. Attitudes of internal medicine residents regarding influenza vaccination. *Infect Control Hosp Epidemiol* 1994; 15:32–35.
168. Centers for Disease Control and Prevention. Final 2002 reports of notifiable diseases. *MMWR* 2003;52:741–749.
169. Faoagali JL. An assessment of the need for vaccination amongst junior medical staff. *N Z Med J* 1976;84:147–150.
170. Raad II, Sherertz RJ, Rains CS, et al. The importance of nosocomial transmission of measles in the propagation of a community outbreak. *Infect Control Hosp Epidemiol* 1989;10:161–166.
171. Measles—Washington. *MMWR* 1990;39:473–476.
172. Farizo KM, Stehr-Green PA, Simpson DM, et al. Pediatric emergency room visits: a risk factor for acquiring measles. *Pediatrics* 1991;87: 74–79.
173. Davis RM, Orenstein WA, Frank JA, et al. Transmission of measles in medical settings: 1980 through 1984. *JAMA* 1986;255:1295–1298.
174. Atkinson WL, Markowitz LE, Adams NC, et al. Transmission of measles in medical settings—United States, 1985–1989. *Am J Med* 1991;91(suppl 3B):320S–324S.
175. Measles among children of migrant workers—Florida. *MMWR* 1983; 32:471–472,477–478.

176. Measles—Hawaii. *MMWR* 1984;33:702,707–711.
177. Measles—Puerto Rico. *MMWR* 1985;34:169–172.
178. Istre GR, McKee PA, West GR, et al. Measles spread in medical settings: an important focus of disease transmission. *Pediatrics* 1987; 79:356–358.
179. Measles—Dade County, Florida. *MMWR* 1987;36:45–48.
180. McGrath D, Swanson R, Weems S, et al. Analysis of a measles outbreak in Kent County, Michigan in 1990. *Pediatr Infect Dis J* 1992; 11:385–389.
181. Imported measles with subsequent airborne transmission in a pediatrician's office—Michigan. *MMWR* 1983;32:401–403.
182. Remington PL, Hall WN, Davis IH, et al. Airborne transmission of measles in a physician's office. *JAMA* 1985;253:1574–1577.
183. Bloch AB, Orenstein WA, Ewing WM, et al. Measles outbreak in a pediatric practice: airborne transmission in an office setting. *Pediatrics* 1985;75:676–683.
184. Measles transmitted in a medical office building—New Mexico. *MMWR* 1987;36:25–27.
185. Ward J, El-Saadi O. Measles in the waiting room: a cautionary tale. *Aust Fam Physician* 1999;28:1103.
186. Blake KV, Nguyen OTK, Capon AG. Nosocomial transmission of measles in western Sydney. *Med J Aust* 2001;175:442.
187. Miranda AC, Falcao JM, Dias JA, et al. Measles transmission in health facilities during outbreaks. *Int J Epidemiol* 1994;23:843–848.
188. Rivera ME, Mason WH, Ross LA, et al. Nosocomial measles infection in a pediatric hospital during a community-wide epidemic. *J Pediatr* 1991;119:183–186.
189. Freebeck PC, Clark S, Fahey PJ. Hypoxemic respiratory failure complicating nosocomial measles in a healthy host. *Chest* 1992;02: 625–626.
190. Measles—Texas. *MMWR* 1981;30:209–211.
191. Measles in medical settings—United States. *MMWR* 1981;30: 125–126.
192. Anonymous. Measles nearly eliminated, but still poses a nosocomial risk. *Hosp Infect Control* 1982;9:133–136.
193. Interstate transmission of measles in a gypsy population—Washington, Idaho, Montana, California. *MMWR* 1983;32:659–662.
194. Dales LG, Kizer KW. Measles transmission in medical facilities. *West J Med* 1985;142:415–416.
195. Watkins NM, Smith RP Jr, St. Germain DL, et al. Measles (rubeola) infection in a hospital setting. *Am J Infect Control* 1987;15:201–206.
196. Sienko DG, Friedman C, McGee HB, et al. A measles outbreak at university medical settings involving healthcare providers. *Am J Public Health* 1987;77:1222–1224.
197. Measles—Los Angeles County, California. *MMWR* 1989;38: 49–52,57.
198. Markowitz LE, Preblud SR, Orenstein WA, et al. Patterns of transmission in measles outbreaks in the United States, 1985–1986. *N Engl J Med* 1989;320:75–81.
199. de Swart RL, Wertheim-van Dillen PME, van Binnendijk RS, et al. Measles in a Dutch hospital introduced by a immunocompromised infant from Indonesia infected with a new virus genotype. *Lancet* 2000;355:201–202.
200. Mendelson GMS, Roth CE, Wreghitt TG, et al. Nosocomial transmission of measles to healthcare workers. Time for a national screening and immunization policy for NHS staff? *J Hosp Infect.*
201. Biellik RJ, Clements CJ. Strategies for minimizing nosocomial measles transmission. *Bull WHO* 1997;75:367–375.
202. Measles—New Hampshire. *MMWR* 1984;33:549–554,559.
203. Brunell PA, Brickman A, O'Hare D, et al. Ineffectiveness of isolation of patients as a method of preventing the spread of mumps. *N Engl J Med* 1968;279:1357–1361.
204. Wharton M, Cochi SL, Hutcheson RH, et al. Mumps transmission in hospitals. *Arch Intern Med* 1990;150:47–49.
205. Fischer PR, Brunetti C, Welch V, et al. Nosocomial mumps: report of an outbreak and its control. *Am J Infect Control* 1996;24:13–18.
206. Glick D. An isolated case of mumps in a geriatric population. *J Am Geriatr Soc* 1970;18:642–644.
207. Sparling D. Transmission of mumps. *N Engl J Med* 1969;280:276.
208. Schiff GM, Dine MS. Transmission of rubella from newborns. *Am J Dis Child* 1965;110:447–451.
209. Nosocomial rubella infection—North Dakota, Alabama, Ohio. *MMWR* 1981;29:629–631.
210. Sheridan E, Aitken C, Jeffries D, et al. Congenital rubella syndrome: a risk for immigrant populations. *Lancet* 2002;359:674–675.
211. Polk BF, White JA, DeGirolami PC, et al. An outbreak of rubella among hospital personnel. *N Engl J Med* 1980;303:541–545.
212. Heseltine PNR, Ripper M, Wohlford P. Nosocomial rubella—consequences of an outbreak and efficacy of a mandatory immunization program. *Infect Control* 1985;6:371–374.
213. Giles JW, Smith IM. The study of a rubella outbreak. *J Iowa Med Soc* 1972;62:238–341.
214. Carne S, Dewhurst CJ, Hurley R. Rubella epidemic in a maternity unit. *BMJ* 1973;1:444–446.
215. Baba K, Yabuuchi H, Okuni H, et al. Rubella epidemic in an institution: protective value of live rubella vaccine and serological behavior of vaccinated, revaccinated and naturally immune groups. *Biken J* 1978;21:25–31.
216. Exposure of patients to rubella by medical personnel—California. *MMWR* 1978;27:123.
217. Rubella in hospital personnel and patients—Colorado. *MMWR* 1979; 28:325–327.
218. McLaughlin MC, Gold LH. The New York rubella incident: a case for changing hospital policy regarding rubella testing and immunization. *Am J Public Health* 1979;69:287–289.
219. Gladstone JL, Millian SJ. Rubella exposure in an obstetric clinic. *Obstet Gynecol* 1981;57:182–186.
220. Strassburg MA, Imagawa DT, Fannin SL, et al. Rubella outbreak among hospital employees. *Obstet Gynecol* 1981;57:283–288.
221. Rubella in hospitals—California. *MMWR* 1983;32:37–39.
222. Strassburg MA, Stephenson TG, Habel LA, et al. Rubella in hospital employees. *Infect Control* 1984;5:123–126.
223. Storch GA, Gruber C, Benz B, et al. A rubella outbreak among dental students: Description of the outbreak and analysis of control measures. *Infect Control* 1985;6:150–156.
224. Jacobson JT. Rubella: one hospital's experience. *Am J Infect Control* 1987;15:136–137.
225. Poland GA, Nichol KL. Medical students as sources of rubella and measles outbreaks. *Arch Intern Med* 1990;150:44–46.
226. Braunstein H, Thomas S, Ito R. Immunity to measles in a large population of varying age. *Am J Dis Child* 1990;144:296–298.
227. Smith E, Wong VK. Measles susceptibility of hospital personnel. *Arch Intern Med* 1993;153:1011.
228. Bertin ML. Communicable diseases: infection, prevention for nurses at work and home. *Nurs Clin North Am* 1999;34:509–526.
229. Hersh BS, Fine PE, Kent WK, et al. Mumps outbreaks in a highly vaccinated population. *J Pediatr* 1991;119:187–193.
230. Centers for Disease Control and Prevention. Prevention and control of meningococcal disease, and meningococcal disease and college students: recommendations of the Advisory Committee on Immunization Practices (ACIP). *MMWR* 2000;49:1–20.
231. Rosenstein NE, Perkins BA, Stephens DA, et al. Meningococcal disease. *N Engl J Med* 2001;344:1378–88.
232. Shapiro ED. Prophylaxis for contacts of patients with meningococcal or *Haemophilus influenzae* type B disease. *Pediatr Infect Dis* 1982;1: 132–138.
233. Artenstein MS, Ellis RE. The risk of exposure to a patient with meningococcal meningitis. *Milit Med* 1968;133:474–477
234. Fallon RJ. Hospital-acquired meningococcaemia. *J Hosp Infect* 1992; 20:121–132.
235. Centers for Disease Control. Nosocomial meningococcemia—Wisconsin. *MMWR* 1978;27:358–363.
236. Cohen MS, Steere AC, Baltimore R, et al. Possible nosocomial transmission of group Y Neisseria meningitidis among oncology patients. *Ann Intern Med* 1979;91:7–12.
237. Rose HD, Lenz IE, Sheth NK. Meningococcal pneumonia: a source of nosocomial infection. *Arch Intern Med* 1981;141:575–577.
238. Riewerts-Eriksen NH, Espersen F, Laursen L, et al. Nosocomial outbreak of group C meningococcal disease. *BMJ* 1989;298:568–569.

239. Centers for Disease Control. Laboratory-acquired meningococcemia—California and Massachusetts. *MMWR* 1991;40:46–47,55.
240. Offit PA, Peter G. The meningococcal vaccine—public policy and individual choices. *N Engl J Med* 2003;349(24):2353–2356.
241. Centers for Disease Control and Prevention. Pertussis vaccination: use of acellular pertussis vaccines among infants and children: recommendations of the Advisory Committee on Immunization Practices. *MMWR* 1997;46(RR-7):1–25.
242. Guris D, Strebel PM, Bardenheier B, et al. Changing epidemiology of pertussis in the United States: increasing reported incidence among adolescents and adults, 1990–1996. *Clin Infect Dis* 1999;28: 1230–1237.
243. Mink C, Cherry JD, Christenson P, et al. A search for Bordetella pertussis infection in university students. *Clin Infect Dis* 1992;14: 464–471.
244. Rosenthal S, Strebel P, Cassiday P, et al. Pertussis infection among adults during the 1993 outbreak in Chicago. *J Infect Dis* 1995;171: 1650–1652.
245. Wright SW, Edwards KM, Decker MD, et al. Pertussis infection in adults with persistent cough. *JAMA* 1995;13:1044–1046.
246. Deville JG, Cherry JD, Christenson PD, et al. Frequency of unrecognized Bordetella pertussis infections in adults. *Clin Infect Dis* 1995; 21:639–642.
247. Kurt TL, Yeager AS, Guenette S, et al. Spread of pertussis by hospital staff. *JAMA* 1972;221:264–267.
248. Linneman CC, Ramundo N, Perlstein PH, et al. Use of pertussis vaccine in an epidemic involving hospital staff. *Lancet* 1975;2: 540–543.
249. Addiss DG, Davis JP, Meade BD, et al. A pertussis outbreak in a Wisconsin nursing home. *J Infect Dis* 1991;164:704–710.
250. Steketee RW, Wassilak SGF, Adkins WN, et al. Evidence for a high attack rate and efficacy of erythromycin prophylaxis in a pertussis outbreak in a facility for the developmentally disabled. *J Infect Dis* 1988;157:434–440.
251. Tanaka Y, Fujinaga K, Goto A, et al. Outbreak of pertussis in a residential facility for handicapped people. *Dev Biol Stand* 1991;73: 329–332.
252. Valenti WM, Pincus PH, Messner MK. Nosocomial pertussis: possible spread by a hospital visitor. *Am J Dis Child* 1980;134:520–521.
253. Fisher MC, Long SS, McGowan KL, et al. Outbreak of pertussis in a residential facility for handicapped people. *J Pediatr* 1989;114: 934–939.
254. Shefer A, Dales L, Nelson M, et al. Use and safety of acellular pertussis vaccine among adult hospital staff during an outbreak of pertussis. *J Infect Dis* 1995;171:1053–1056.
255. Christie CDC, Glover AM, Willke MJ, et al. Containment of pertussis in the regional pediatric hospital during the greater Cincinnati epidemic of 1993. *Infect Control Hosp Epidemiol* 1995;16:556–563.
256. Wright SW, Edwards KM, Decker MD, et al. Pertussis seroprevalence in emergency department staff. *Ann Emerg Med* 1994;24:413–417.
257. Wright SW, Decker MD, Edwards KM. Incidence of pertussis infection in healthcare workers. *Infect Control Hosp Epidemiol* 1999;20: 120–123.
258. Weber DJ, Rutala WA. Management of healthcare workers exposed to pertussis. *Infect Control Hosp Epidemiol* 1994;15:411–415.
259. Edwards KM, Decker MD, Graham BS, et al. Adult immunization with acellular pertussis vaccine. *JAMA* 1993;269:53–56.
260. Keitel WA, Muenz LR, Decker MD, et al. A randomized clinical trial of acellular pertussis vaccines in healthy adults: dose-response comparisons of 5 vaccines and implications for booster immunization. *J Infect Dis* 1999;180:397–403.
261. Halperin SA, Smith B, Russell M, et al. An adult formulation of a five-component acellular pertussis vaccine combined with diphtheria and tetanus toxoids is safe and immunogenic in adolescents and adults. *Vaccine* 2000;18:1312–1319.
262. Rothstein EP, Pennridge Pediatric Associates, Anderson EL, et al. An acellular pertussis vaccine in healthy adults: safety and immunogenicity. *Vaccine* 1999;17:2999–3006.
263. van der Wielen M, van Damme P, Joosens E, et al. A randomized controlled trial with a diphtheria-tetanus-acellular pertussis (dTpa) vaccine in adults. *Vaccine* 2000;18:2075–2082.
264. Minh NNT, He Q, Edelman K, et al. Immune responses to pertussis antigens eight years after booster immunization with acellular vaccines in adults. *Vaccine* 2000;18:1971–1974.
265. Turnbull FM, Heath TC, Jalaludin BB, et al. A randomized trial of two acellular pertussis vaccines (dTpa and pa) and a licensed diphtheria-tetanus vaccine (Td) in adults. *Vaccine* 2001;19:628–636.
266. Edwards KM, Decker MD. Pertussis Vaccine. In: Plotkin S, Orenstein WA, eds. *Vaccines,* 4th ed. Philadelphia: WB Saunders, 2004: 471–528.
267. Centers for Disease Control and Prevention. Typhoid immunization—recommendations of the Advisory Committee on Immunization Practices (ACIP). *MMWR* 1994;43(RR-14):1–7
268. Baine WB, Gangarosa EJ, Bennett JV, et al. Institutional salmonellosis. *J Infect Dis* 1973;128:357–359.
269. Centers for Disease Control. Salmonellosis—Baltimore, Maryland. *MMWR* 1970;19:314.
270. Steere AC, Craven PJ, Hall WJI, et al. Person-to-person spread of *Salmonella typhimurium* after a hospital common-source outbreak. *Lancet* 1975;1:319–322.
271. Lintz D, Kapila R, Pilgrim E, et al. Nosocomial *Salmonella* epidemic. *Arch Intern Med* 1976;136:968–973.
272. Mendis NM, De La Motte PU, Gunatillaka PD, et al. Protracted infection with Salmonella bareilly in a maternity hospital. *J Trop Med Hyg* 1976;79:142–150.
273. Standaert SM, Hutcheson RH, Schaffner W. Nosocomial transmission of salmonella gastroenteritis to laundry workers in a nursing home. *Infect Control Hosp Epidemiol* 1994;15:22–26.
274. Tissot Guerraz F, Reverdy ME, Cetre JC, et al. A case of nosocomial typhoid in a pediatric ward. *Arch Fr Pediatr* 1990;47(7):543.
275. Dean AG. Transmission of *Salmonella typhi* by fiberoptic endoscopy. *Lancet* 1977;2(8029):134.
276. Zejdl J, Kavanova R, Cech M. Nosocomial epidemic of typhoid fever in 2 hospital wards of the North Bohemian region. *Cesk Epidemiol Mikrobiol Imunol* 1968;17(5):313–318.
277. Maudgal DP, Shafi MS, Northfield TC. Duodenal intubation as a source of typhoid fever. *Dig Dis Sci* 1982;27:549–552.
278. Blaser MJ, Feldman RA. Acquisition of typhoid fever from proficiency-testing specimens. *N Engl J Med* 1980;303(25):1481.
279. Blaser MJ, Lofgren JP. Fatal salmonellosis originating in a clinical microbiology laboratory. *J Clin Microbiol* 1981;13(5):855–858.
280. Blaser MJ, Hickman FW, Farmer JJ 3rd, et al. *Salmonella typhi*: the laboratory as a reservoir of infection. *J Infect Dis* 1980;142(6): 934–938.
281. Walia I, Narayan JP. Epidemic typhoid among nurses. *Nurs J India* 1986;77(10):255–256,278.
282. DuPont HL. Nosocomial salmonellosis and shigellosis [editorial]. *Infect Control Hosp Epidemiol* 1991;12:707–709.
283. Centers for Disease Control and Prevention. Vaccinia (smallpox) vaccine: recommendations of the Advisory Committee on Immunization Practices (ACIP). *MMWR* 2001;50(RR-10):1–25
284. Alibek K, Handelman S. *Biohazard: the chilling true story of the largest covert biological weapons program in the world—told from inside by the man who ran it.* New York: Random House, 1999.
285. Centers for Disease Control and Prevention. Recommendations for using smallpox vaccine in a pre-event vaccination program: supplemental recommendations of the Advisory Committee on Immunization Practices (ACIP) and the Healthcare Infection Control Practices Advisory Committee (HICPAC). *MMWR* 2003;52(RR-7):1–16.
286. Centers for Disease Control and Prevention. Vaccinia (smallpox) vaccine: recommendations of the Advisory Committee on Immunization Practices (ACIP). *MMWR* 1991;40(RR-14):1–11
287. Gershon AA, Takahashi M, Seward J. Varicella vaccine. In: Plotkin S, Orenstein WA, eds. *Vaccines,* 4th ed. Philadelphia: WB Saunders, 2004:783–823.
288. Simpson REH. Infectiousness of communicable diseases in the household (measles, chickenpox, and mumps). *Lancet* 1952;2:549–554.
289. Ross AH. Modification of chickenpox in family contacts by administration of gamma globulin. *N Engl J Med* 1962;267:369–376.

290. Josephson A, Karanfil L, Gombert ME. Strategies for the management of varicella-susceptible healthcare workers after a known exposure. *Infect Control Hosp Epidemiol* 1990;11:309–313.
291. Seward JF, Watson BM, Peterson CL, et al. Varicella disease after introduction of varicella vaccine in the United States, 1995–2000. *JAMA* 2002;287:606–611.
292. Kilgore PE, Kruszon-Moran D, Seward JF, et al. Varicella in Americans from NHANES III: implications for control through routine immunization. *J Med Virol* 2003;70(suppl 1):S111–118.
293. Weber DJ, Rutala WA, Parham C. Impact and costs of varicella prevention in a University Hospital. *Am J Public Health* 1988;78:19–23.
294. Miller E, Marshall R, Vurdien J. Epidemiology, outcome and control of varicella-zoster infection. *Rev Med Microbiol* 1993;4:222–230.
295. Hyams PJ, Stuewe MCS, Heitzer V. Herpes zoster causing varicella (chickenpox) in hospital employees: cost of a casual attitude. *Am J Infect Control* 1984;12:2–5.
296. Krasinski K, Holzman RS, LaCouture R, et al. Hospital experience with varicella-zoster virus. *Infect Control* 1986;7:312–316.
297. Stover BH, Cost KM, Hamm C, et al. Varicella exposure in a neonatal intensive care unit: case report and control measures. *Am J Infect Control* 1988;16:167–172.
298. Gustafson TL, Shehab Z, Brunell PA. Outbreak of varicella in a newborn intensive care nursery. *Am J Dis Child* 1984;138:548–550.
299. Evans P. An epidemic of chickenpox. *Lancet* 1940;2:339–340.
300. McKendrick GDW, Emond RTD. Investigation of cross-infection in isolation wards of different designs. *J Hyg Camb* 1976;76:23–31.
301. Morens DM, Bregman DJ, West CM, et al. An outbreak of varicella-zoster virus infection among cancer patients. *Ann Intern Med* 1980; 93:414–419.
302. Leclair JM, Zaia JA, Levin MJ, et al. Airborne transmission of chickenpox in a hospital. *N Engl J Med* 1980;302:450–453.
303. Scheifele D, Bonner M. Airborne transmission of chickenpox [letter]. *N Engl J Med* 1980;303:281–282.
304. Asano Y, Iwayama S, Miyata T, et al. Spread of varicella in hospitalized children having no direct contact with an indicator zoster case and its prevention by a live vaccine. *Biken J* 1980;23:157–161.
305. Faizallah R, Green HT, Krasner N, et al. Outbreak of chickenpox from a patient with immunosuppressed herpes zoster in hospital. *BMJ* 1982;285:1022–1023.
306. Gustafson TL, Lavely GB, Brawner ER, et al. An outbreak of airborne nosocomial varicella. *Pediatrics* 1982;70:550–556.
307. Tsujino G, Sako M, Takahashi M. Varicella infection in a children's hospital: prevention by vaccine and an episode of airborne transmission. *Biken J* 1984;27:129–132.
308. Anderson JD, Bonner M, Schiefele DW, et al. Lack of nosocomial spread of varicella in a pediatric hospital with negative pressure ventilated patient rooms. *Infect Control* 1985;6:120–121.
309. Josephson A, Gombert M. Airborne transmission of nosocomial varicella from localized zoster. *J Infect Dis* 1988;158:238–241.
310. Morgan-Capner P, Wilson M, Wright J, et al. Varicella and zoster in hospitals. *Lancet* 1990;335:1460.
311. Friedman CA, Temple DM, Robbins KK, et al. Outbreak and control of varicella in a neonatal intensive care unit. *Pediatr Infect Dis J* 1994; 13:152–153.
312. Faoagali JL, Darcy D. Chickenpox outbreak among the staff of a large, urban adult hospital: costs of monitoring and control. *Am J Infect Control* 1995;23:247–250.
313. Kavaliotis J, Loukou I, Trachana M, et al. Outbreak of varicella in a pediatric oncology unit. *Med Pediatr Oncol* 1998;31:166–169.
314. Wharton M. The epidemiology of varicella-zoster virus infection. *Infect Dis Clin North Am* 1996;10:571–581.
315. Choo PW, Donahue JG, Manson JE, et al. The epidemiology of varicella and its complications. *J Infect Dis* 1995;172:706–712.
316. Gershon AA. Varicella-zoster virus: prospects for control. *Adv Pediatr Infect Dis* 1995;10:93–124.
317. Birthistle K, Carrington D. Fetal varicella syndrome—a reappraisal of the literature. *J Infect* 1998;36(suppl 1):25–29.
318. Sauerbrei A, Wutzler P. The congenital varicella syndrome. *J Perinatol* 2000;20:548–554.
319. Feldman S, Hughes WT, Daniel CB. Varicella in children with cancer: seventy-seven cases. *Pediatrics* 1975;56:388–397.
320. Feldhoff CM, Balfour HH, Simmons RL, et al. Varicella in children with renal transplants. *J Pediatr* 1981;98:25–31.
321. Locksley RM, Flournoy N, Sullivan KM, et al. Infection with varicella-zoster virus after marrow transplantation. *J Infect Dis* 1985;152: 1172–1181.
322. Meyers JD, MacQuarrie MB, Merigan TC, et al. Nosocomial varicella: Part 1. Outbreak in oncology patients at a children's hospital. *West J Med* 1979;130:196–199.
323. Morgan ER, Smalley LA. Varicella in immunocompromised children. *Am J Dis Child* 1983;137:883–885.
324. Whitley R, Hilty M, Haynes R, et al. Vidarabine therapy of varicella in immunosuppressed patients. *J Pediatr* 1982;101:125–131.
325. Feldman S, Lott L. Varicella in children with cancer: impact of antiviral therapy and prophylaxis. *Pediatrics* 1987;80:255–262.
326. McGregor RS, Zitelli BJ, Urback AH, et al. Varicella in pediatric orthotopic liver transplant recipients. *Pediatrics* 1989;83:256–261.
327. Gallagher J, Quaid B, Cryan B. Susceptibility to varicella zoster virus infection in health care workers. *Occup Med* 1996;46:289–292.
328. Myers MG, Rasley DA, Hierholzer WJ. Hospital infection control for varicella virus infections. *Periatrics* 1982;70:199–202.
329. Steele RW, Coleman MA, Fiser M, et al. Varicella-zoster in hospital personnel: skin test reactivity to monitor susceptibility. *Pediatrics* 1982;70:604–608.
330. Alter SJ, Hammond JA, McVey CJ, et al. Susceptibility to varicella-zoster virus among adults at high risk for exposure. *Infect Control* 1986;7:448–451.
331. Haiduven-Griffiths D, Fecko H. Varicella in hospital personnel: a challenge for the infection control practitioner. *Am J Infect Control* 1987;15:207–211.
332. McKinney WP, Horowitz MM, Battiola RJ. Susceptibility of hospital-based healthcare personnel to varicella-zoster virus infections. *Am J Infect Control* 1989;17:26–30.
333. Shehab ZM, Brunell PA. Susceptibility of hospital personnel to varicella-zoster virus. *J Infect Dis* 1984;150:786.
334. Haiduven DJ, Hench CP, Stevens DA. Postexposure varicella management of nonimmmune personnel: an alternative approach. *Infect Control Hosp Epidemiol* 1994;15:329–334.
335. Nettleman MD, Schmid M. Cost-effectiveness of varicella vaccination in hospital employees [abstract 70]. Program and Abstracts of the Sixth Annual Meeting of SHEA, Washington, DC, 1996.
336. Hamilton HA. A cost minimization analysis of varicella vaccine in healthcare workers. Thesis. Chapel Hill, NC: Department of Epidemiology, University of North Carolina School of Public Health, 1996.
337. Gray AM, Fenn P, Weinberg J, et al. An economic analysis of varicella vaccination for health care workers. *Epidemiol Infect* 1997;119: 209–220.
338. Tennenberg AM, Brassared JF, Lieu JV, et al. Varicella vaccination for healthcare workers at a university hospital: an analysis of costs and benefits. *Infect Control Hosp Epidemiol* 1997;18:405–411.

81

NOSOCOMIAL DISEASES OF HEALTHCARE WORKERS SPREAD BY THE AIRBORNE OR CONTACT ROUTES (OTHER THAN TUBERCULOSIS)

MICHAEL D. DECKER
WILLIAM SCHAFFNER

By virtue of their profession, healthcare workers are at greater risk of acquiring certain illnesses than are non–healthcare workers. This chapter discusses diseases spread by the contact or airborne routes for which healthcare workers are at elevated risk or that pose a particular problem for infection control and employee health staff. Notwithstanding the occasional nosocomial report, diseases that occur in the healthcare setting incidentally (e.g., food-borne illness arising in the hospital's cafeteria) are not considered. Similarly, only those diseases to which the immunologically normal healthcare worker is susceptible are covered.

Issues posed by the viral hepatitides and the human immunodeficiency virus (HIV) are covered in Chapters 78 and 79 respectively; tuberculosis is discussed in Chapter 37; infections of particular pertinence to laboratory workers are discussed in Chapter 82; infections pertinent to prehospital and posthospital healthcare workers are reviewed in Chapters 83 and 84; and issues consequent to bioterrorism are found in Chapters 109 to 112. This chapter enumerates the remaining nosocomial airborne and contact-spread diseases for which healthcare workers are at elevated risk, reviews their epidemiology and prevention in healthcare institutions, and discusses some of the special challenges they pose for the infection control team. Pathogenesis, diagnosis, and therapy of these diseases are not addressed in detail, because they are discussed in other chapters of this text and elsewhere.

METHODS OF SPREAD

As Brachman (1) and others have pointed out, contact and airborne spread represent two ends of a spectrum. The spectrum begins with direct physical contact, as seen with herpes simplex or syphilis. Such person-to-person spread includes most fecal-oral transmission. Disease may be transmitted by indirect contact, in which the victim encounters an intermediate object that previously was in contact with the source; such a circumstance could arise, for example, through careless handling of contaminated equipment or used dressings. Disease can be spread via respiratory droplets expelled by a cough or sneeze; the cloud of expelled particles can impact persons or other objects within several feet, but the droplets do not travel farther before they settle to the ground. Finally, if respiratory droplets are sufficiently small, their moisture entirely evaporates while airborne, leaving any contained infectious particles suspended in the air. These droplet nuclei can be transported in the air over substantial distances. Under appropriate circumstances, other tiny particles (e.g., desquamated skin squames, fungal spores) may also be spread afar on the wind. Many diseases are spread by more than one of these routes. Additional pathways for the spread of disease include the blood-borne, common-source, and vector-borne routes. The diseases of transcendent importance spread by the blood-borne route are hepatitis B and C (Chapter 78) and HIV infection (Chapter 79). In the United States, healthcare workers generally are not at elevated risk of common-source or vector-borne diseases because of their occupation.

Humans long have pondered the origins of disease, and through the ages, the issue of airborne contagion has been raised many times. The Greek physician Galen stated, "When many sicken and die at once, we must look to a single common cause, the air we breathe" (2). Hamlet bemoaned "this foul and pestilent canopy, the air," but 1500 years after Galen, Sydenham said it was not the air itself, but "pestilential particles" carried by the air that conveyed disease (2). Despite these prophetic speculations, Galen was responsible for establishing the dominance of the theory that deranged humors were responsible for disease, a belief to which Sydenham subscribed and which persisted until overthrown by the discoveries of the anatomists, pathologists, and microbiologists of the nineteenth century.

The discoveries of Louis Pasteur and others refocused attention on the possible spread of disease through the air to such an extent that Tyndall was moved to write "the floating dust of the air . . . mingled with it the special germs which produce the epidemic, being thus enabled to sow pestilence and death over nations and continents" (3). But soon, belief in the airborne spread of disease ebbed again because of the elucidation of the causes and modes of transmission of fecal-oral diseases, such as cholera; vector-borne diseases, such as malaria; and the venereal diseases, such as syphilis. These discoveries had so reduced the attraction of the concept of airborne spread that by 1910, Chapin (4) stated in his *Sources and Modes of Infection,* "Bacteriology teaches that former ideas in regard to the manner in which diseases may be airborne are entirely erroneous; that most diseases are not likely to be dust-borne, and they are spray-borne only for 2 or 3 feet."

There opinion lay for 20 years, not overturned even by the great influenza pandemic until Wells (5) articulated the concept of droplet nuclei, infectious particles that can remain suspended in the air for many hours after the droplet itself has evaporated and that can be carried a considerable distance on air currents. Wells promptly proceeded to test his theory by placing ultraviolet lights in selected classrooms of two schools (6). In a subsequent measles epidemic, the attack rate was dramatically higher in the control classes. Riley later collaborated with Wells to demonstrate the airborne transmission of tuberculosis (7,8). Similar experiments, coupled with more sophisticated epidemiologic observations of outbreaks, have established the importance of the airborne route of spread for many diseases.

VIRAL INFECTIONS

Common Respiratory Viruses

Few healthcare workers would rank the common respiratory viruses first on a list of the diseases to which their work exposes them, but we would speculate that these illnesses cause more disruption and lost productivity than all the others we discuss combined.

Influenza

The prototype of these illnesses is influenza. Influenza epidemics occur with distressing frequency within healthcare institutions, with predictable consequences; increased absenteeism or reduced efficiency of staff members and increased mortality, morbidity, and length of stay among the patients. Indeed, immunization of healthcare workers results in significantly reduced morbidity (43% reduction in influenzalike illness) and mortality (44% reduction) among geriatric patients in long-term care facilities (9).

The capacity of influenza for explosive spread was demonstrated by an outbreak among 53 persons stranded aboard a grounded airliner for 3 hours: within 3 days, 72% of the passengers were ill with influenza A. When the "Asian" influenza A pandemic of 1957 reached the Oklahoma City Veterans' Hospital, 19 (39%) of 49 patients on the neurologic ward were affected, three of whom died; all but one of the physicians on the ward were "incapacitated" (10). During the same epidemic, eight (62%) of 13 unvaccinated staff members studied at the New York Hospital developed influenza, as compared to 7 (35%) of 20 vaccinated staff (11). Influenza A/Bangkok (H3N2) produced illness in one third of patients and staff members on affected wards at a Chicago hospital (12). The same strain of influenza caused a 70% increase in absenteeism during a 2-week period among employees of a Winnipeg, Canada, hospital, which incurred excess sick-leave costs of $24,500 (1980 Canadian dollars) (13). Reports of nosocomial outbreaks of influenza B appear to be less common than reports of influenza A. This finding may merely reflect the greater prevalence of influenza A in recent years, although one report of hospital surveillance during an influenza B epidemic found no clusters of disease despite 25 cases detected by culture (14).

Influenza is spread via infected nasopharyngeal secretions. Attempts in 1918 to transmit the pandemic strain failed because of improper technique; it was not until 1937 that Smorodintseff and associates demonstrated experimental transmission by droplets (15). Spread is believed predominantly to involve respiratory droplets, as well as direct person-to-person spread through contact with infected secretions. Airborne spread is plausible but not as well documented as with such diseases as tuberculosis and varicella. The airliner outbreak was marked by mingling of the occupants, a vigorously coughing source patient, and a nonfunctioning ventilation system, and thus, it may have been entirely caused by droplet spread.

Given the opportunities for exposure to influenza during a community outbreak, the only realistic approach to prevention among healthcare workers is through immunization. Unfortunately, achieving high immunization rates among healthcare workers has proven difficult (16–18). Hospital-wide influenza immunization programs that are highly publicized, bring the program to the worker, take advantage of social or peer pressure, and reward participation may find greater success. In an established outbreak, cohort isolation may help prevent spread to other patients (19) but likely would be of little benefit to the work force, given the ubiquitous opportunities for exposure during an outbreak. Amantadine and rimantadine as well as the neuraminidase inhibitors zanamivir and oseltamivir can protect from influenza A, should a worker at high risk of complications escape the immunization program. Infected employees should not work in order to prevent spread to other personnel and, particularly, to patients. Infected healthcare workers may also expose persons with a high risk of complications in their houses, yet another reason for them to be immunized (20). (For more information on influenza, see Chapter 41.)

Parainfluenza

Parainfluenza infections are most problematic among infants and young children, and spread on pediatric wards is well documented. These outbreaks often involve the staff (21,22); an outbreak investigated at the Children's Hospital National Medical Center was shown to affect six of 17 neonates along with 18 of 52 nursing personnel (22). Although the disease is relatively mild among older children and healthy adults, it can be a problem in long-term-care facilities, affecting both patients and staff, with patient deaths reported (23). Of the various strains of parainfluenza virus, type 3 appears to be implicated more often in nosocomial outbreaks. The spread of parainfluenza often is indolent (24), and the virus appears to be relatively hardy; droplets may contaminate environmental surfaces with virus that survives for many hours (25).

Spread of parainfluenza virus is by direct contact and by large droplets, which may create the potential for indirect contact spread. Airborne spread is plausible but has not been demonstrated. Immunity is not durable and reinfection occurs throughout life. Thus far, efforts to develop vaccines have not been fruitful. Thus, protection of the healthcare worker rests on identification and isolation of cases with use of contact and, perhaps, droplet precautions. (Note: All references to specific forms of isolation precautions, such as standard or Droplet Precautions, refer to the isolation strategies described by the Hospital Infection Control Practices Advisory Committee of the United States Public Health Service (26) (see also Chapter 48).

Respiratory Syncytial Virus

Respiratory syncytial virus (RSV) is the most important respiratory pathogen of infants and young children, in whom it is the predominant cause of bronchiolitis and pneumonia (27,28). Community-based outbreaks occur every winter and spring, and essentially the entire population has serologic evidence of infection by age 3 years. Immunity is short-lived and reinfection can occur annually. Thus, RSV spreads readily to healthcare workers. The disease is mild in previously infected adults, who may be asymptomatic or experience symptoms of the common cold (29). Despite their mild illness, however, infected healthcare workers can serve as a source of infection for pediatric (30,31) and other (23,32–35) patients in whom infection may be dangerous.

Hall et al. (30) studied nosocomial RSV during a community outbreak and found that 45% of infants hospitalized 1 week or more acquired infection as did 10 of 24 staff members. Indeed, in the absence of effective barrier precautions, 30% to 60% of healthcare workers caring for RSV-infected children acquired infection (36,37).

RSV infection appears to be acquired through inoculation of the eyes or nose by direct and indirect contact with infectious respiratory secretions (29,37). Use by caregivers of eye-nose goggles markedly reduces spread of the disease (36,38), probably by preventing self-inoculation via contaminated hands; others have shown similar benefit through use of gloves and gowns (39) or gloves, gowns, and masks (40). To curtail both direct and indirect contact spread, use of Standard and Contact Precautions is appropriate. As is so often the case, scrupulous hand washing is the key to prevention of infection (see also Chapter 48).

Adenovirus

The adenoviruses are responsible for a variety of syndromes: typical upper respiratory infections (e.g., cough, coryza, pharyngitis), particularly of children; febrile acute respiratory disease of military recruits; epidemic keratoconjunctivitis; pharyngoconjunctival fever; and, uncommonly, pneumonia (41). Spread can be explosive, particularly in closed groups, such as military recruits or shipyard workers.

A number of outbreaks of epidemic keratoconjunctivitis have been documented in healthcare facilities. Most often, these outbreaks involve spread to patients exposed to contaminated ophthalmologic equipment or solutions or to a caregiver's unwashed hands (42–48). Healthcare workers have acquired conjunctivitis not only through care of patients with conjunctivitis but also through care of patients with other adenovirus infections such as pneumonia (49) when appropriate isolation precautions were not observed (see also Chapter 26).

Although less common, outbreaks of respiratory disease resulting from adenovirus are more serious. A 1980 outbreak at Children's Hospital in San Diego, California, involved six patients (of whom four died) as well as 300 (78%) of 383 employees, of whom 15% developed conjunctivitis, 28% diarrhea, and 72% upper respiratory symptoms (50). The outbreak was terminated by strict isolation, cohorting, furlough of ill employees, and closure to new admissions. A smaller but similar outbreak in a neonatal intensive care nursery resulted in two patient deaths and infection of nine patients and ten staff members (51). An outbreak in a pediatric long-term-care facility resulted in 11 deaths and 28 cases (46% attack rate) among patients; 22% of staff members (23 of 106) acquired illness (52). An outbreak in another pediatric long-term-care facility following infection in one infant spread to involve two staff members and 10 (30%) of 33 patients, of whom two died (53).

Although respiratory illness is rarely serious among adults, it may be more severe among residents of long-term-care facilities (23, 54). The infection can be fatal among the immunocompromised (55).

Good evidence supports the spread of adenovirus by direct contact, indirect contact, droplets, and (predominantly among children) the fecal-oral route. Airborne spread is plausible, but we are not aware of a nosocomial outbreak that cannot be explained by contact or droplet spread. Airborne spread does not appear to be necessary to explain epidemics among military recruits, given their prolonged close contact and the opportunity for droplet spread. Contact Precautions should be used for patients with adenovirus conjunctivitis; Droplet Precautions should be added for those with adenovirus respiratory infection. Environmental decontamination can be difficult, because the adenovirus is unusually hardy; alcohol and chlorhexidine are not reliable agents for disinfection. A variety of vaccines have been used with success in the military, but none is available for civilian use (see also Chapter 48).

Rhinovirus and Coronavirus

The rhinoviruses and coronaviruses cause the common cold—coryza, with variable cough, and pharyngitis. More than 100 serotypes of rhinovirus are known (virtually ensuring the opportunity each year to encounter a virus to which one is not yet immune), as well as an as-yet-undetermined number of coronaviruses. Although the rhinoviruses and the usual coronaviruses are virologically distinct, they are clinically and epidemiologically similar enough to be considered together. Widespread community outbreaks caused by these viruses occur every winter, with low-level spread throughout the year. As every parent knows, incidence rates are highest among young children and decline with increasing age among adults (apart from a higher incidence among adults with young children). Schools and homes are the major foci of dissemination (56). Given the ubiquitous opportunities for exposure and the usually benign outcome, healthcare workers may not view the common cold as a target for infection control. Transmission does occur between patients and caregivers, however, with outcomes that are burdensome for caregivers and potentially serious for selected patients, such as the immunocompromised, the very young (28), or the elderly (57). For example, Valenti et al. (31) investigated an outbreak of viral respiratory disease in a neonatal intensive care unit (NICU) and determined that one half of the cases were caused by RSV and one half were caused by rhinovirus; respiratory illnesses were similarly serious in the two groups of infants (31). The investigation showed that the infants acquired their infections from their caregivers, 31% of whom had been ill in the preceding week. Unlike other viral respiratory infections, rhinovirus infections do not appear to be significantly more dangerous among the healthy elderly (23), although lower respiratory tract involvement has been seen (58), and can have severe consequences among those with chronic pulmonary disease (57).

During infection, rhinovirus is present in high titer in nasal secretions but only in low titer, if at all, in oral or pharyngeal secretions (56). Volunteer studies have shown that infection is acquired readily via the nose or conjunctiva but poorly via the oral route. Although the virus is relatively hardy and can survive drying on environmental surfaces for several hours, the overwhelmingly most important route of spread is nose to hand to nose or eye. Prevention of spread of infection to or from workers is best accomplished through use of standard precautions, with particular attention to hand washing. Workers should be encouraged to stay home at times of profuse catarrh.

SARS (Severe Acute Respiratory Syndrome) Coronavirus

Severe acute respiratory syndrome (SARS) is a new disease that began in southern China late in 2002 and spread rapidly to Hong Kong, Singapore, Taiwan, Vietnam, and Canada (59). Few cases were documented in the United States. A new coronavirus was quickly established as its cause. Although definitive information concerning the nuances of transmission still is lacking, it is clear that droplet and close contact spread occur, sometimes with astounding efficiency from so-called super-spreaders. Aided by a large, distinctive, and malfunctioning sewage system transmission from virus excreted in feces may have occurred in a high-rise housing complex in Hong Kong. The role of conventional fecal-oral transmission and the role of environmental contamination remain uncertain.

Nosocomial transmission to healthcare workers (with some fatal results) was a prominent feature in virtually every country experiencing the disease (59–64). The United States was spared almost all nosocomial spread. This may have been the happy consequence of intensive education by the Centers for Disease Control and Prevention (CDC), the good fortune of not having a super-spreader enter the country, or other unknown factors.

Much of the nosocomial spread of SARS was attributed to inconsistent observance of strict Airborne Precautions and inconstant use of personal protective equipment, particularly during aerosol-generating activities. Droplet Precautions have been shown to be effective in reducing transmission risk. If SARS recurs, the fastidious use of isolation and personal protective equipment will be critical to avoiding spread of the virus to healthcare professionals (see also Chapter 113).

Enteric Viruses

Coxsackievirus, Echovirus, Poliovirus, and Miscellaneous Enteroviruses

The enteroviruses cause a variety of syndromes, including aseptic meningitis, encephalitis, poliomyelitis, herpangina, epidemic myalgia, upper and lower respiratory disease, hand-foot-mouth disease, conjunctivitis, pericarditis, and myocarditis (65). In the United States, enterovirus infections occur almost exclusively between May and November, peaking in the summer months (66). Many enterovirus infections are associated with exanthems. These viruses are so common, and their manifestations so varied, that recognition of transmission or identification of the causative agent often occurs only when a distinctive outbreak occurs.

Enterovirus infections are common in children, for whom they are generally mild. Infections are more likely to be serious among infants and adults, who experience a greater frequency of cardiac or neurologic involvement (65). For example, an outbreak of echovirus 30 in a day-care center came to attention when 13 parents developed aseptic meningitis (67). Similarly, in an outbreak of coxsackievirus B5 infection in a newborn nursery, illness was sporadic and mild among full-term infants but more prevalent and severe among premature infants; two nurses developed severe pleurodynia and fever (68). A New Zealand hospital experienced a dual outbreak involving echovirus 11 and coxsackievirus B3 (69). Eleven infants and 12 staff members developed meningitis; about one-half the infections were nosocomial. Modlin (70) reviewed 16 nursery outbreaks of echovirus and found hospital personnel to be involved in nine cases. In a unique outbreak of hand-foot-mouth disease in Utah, 17 (13%) of 136 operating suite personnel—but no patients—developed clinical disease resulting from contact spread following illness in an index surgical technician (71).

All enteroviruses reside in the gastrointestinal tract, and thus most spread is by direct contact involving the fecal-oral route. Many of these viruses, however, can be recovered from the oropharynx during illness, and some are much more readily isolated from throat or conjunctiva than stool and have been experimentally transmitted by coughing (65). Thus, Standard Precautions should be supplemented by Contact Precautions or droplet precautions whenever the specific clinical syndrome suggests a risk of spread by those routes. As always, hand washing is likely the most important single preventive strategy.

Poliovirus infection has been eradicated from the Western Hemisphere (72). Until worldwide eradication is achieved, occasional imported cases may be seen in the United States. However, the risk of spread will remain confined to sects that shun immunization unless immunization efforts wane in this country. The use of live attenuated oral poliovirus vaccine (OPV) has been abandoned in the United States. The risk of vaccine-associated disease was once seen at a rate of about one case per 2.6 million doses (73). In countries were OPV is still used, a risk of vaccine-associated paralytic disease exists in contacts of OPV recipients, raising a theoretical concern of infection in a healthcare worker, although we find no evidence that such an event has ever occurred. In addition, transmission should be prevented by standard precautions. Thus, verification of primary poliovirus immunization of healthcare workers is recommended only for (a) those working with poliovirus in the laboratory; (b) those who might care for, or handle specimens from, a patient excreting wild poliovirus; or (c) in the event of an outbreak (see also Chapters 24 and 50).

Rotavirus, the Norovirus, and Related Viruses

Rotavirus is the principal etiologic agent of infantile diarrhea and is responsible for up to one half of all episodes of acute diarrheal disease in infants and young children. The Norwalk-like viruses, a growing group of similar yet genetically diverse members of the Caliciviridae, consist of Norovirus (formerly, Norwalk virus) and a host of other small (27 nm, as compared to 70 nm for rotavirus) round-structured viruses (SRSVs) such as the Snow Mountain, Hawaii, and Marin County agents (74). These agents appear to be responsible for two thirds of all non-bacterial gastroenteritis (75). An additional but much smaller proportion of viral gastroenteritis is attributable to the astroviruses, other caliciviruses, and minireoviruses. The coronaviruses [especially including the toroviruses (76)], adenoviruses, enteroviruses, and parvoviruses, discussed elsewhere in this chapter, can also cause gastroenteritis.

Several nosocomial outbreaks of rotavirus have been documented in neonatal or pediatric units, usually initiated by admission of children involved in a community outbreak (77–84). Although each of these outbreaks involved substantial nosocomial spread of infection to hospitalized infants and children, no healthcare workers were reported to acquire illness. Several rotavirus outbreaks among geriatric populations have also been reported (85–88). In contrast to the experience with pediatric outbreaks, infection and illness occurred among staff members in each of these geriatric outbreaks. Another outbreak, involving somewhat less-elderly patients on a cardiology ward, also involved the staff (89), as did an outbreak on an obstetrics unit (90). Whether this difference in likelihood of illness among staff members reflects random chance, differing host adaptation of viral strains, or systematic differences in infection control practices is unclear.

Rotavirus is spread by the fecal-oral route, principally via the hands of healthcare workers. The virus is highly stable, but environmental contamination does not appear to be an important pathway of transmission in an outbreak. Similarly, despite occasional isolation of the virus from pharyngeal secretions, airborne spread does not appear likely. Standard Precautions should be sufficient, supplemented by Contact Precautions for diapered or incontinent patients. Of interest, quaternary ammonium disinfectants appear to be ineffective against rotavirus; bleach or phenolics should be used if rotavirus environmental contamination is a concern (91). (For additional information on enteric viruses, see Chapters 24 and 50.)

Noroviruses and other SRSVs cause explosive outbreaks of gastroenteritis in the home, school, and community settings, particularly in the winter and spring. The gastroenteritis is marked by sudden onset of vomiting and diarrhea. Rates of secondary spread are high, and disease often involves school-aged children, parents and caregivers, and some young children. Of 90 outbreaks reported to the CDC from January 1996 to June 1997, 43% involved nursing homes and hospitals (92). In a Tennessee outbreak, 55% of patients and 61% of the nursing staff in a long-term-care hospital became ill in a 10-day period (93); an outbreak in a similar facility in Los Angeles involved 55% of residents and 25% of staff members (94). Although attack rates have been higher among patients than staff in most outbreaks, this outcome is not always the case. In a recent North Carolina outbreak, 31% of staff and 11% of patients were ill (95). A 3-week outbreak at a 600-bed Toronto, Canada, hospital involved 27% of the 2,379-person staff, as well as 10% of their household contacts (96). The outbreak appeared to be centered in the emergency room, where 69% of the staff and 33% of visitors acquired illness; an extensive investigation suggested spread of infection by the airborne route. Investigation of a cruise-ship outbreak the following year similarly suggested a role for airborne or droplet spread (97). Investigators of several subsequent outbreaks have concluded that airborne or droplet transmission occurred (94,98–102), although some commentators remain skeptical (74,103). Caul (101) has pointed out that, based on electron micrographic studies, each ounce of vomitus contains 30 million viral particles; only 10 to 100 are required to cause infection. Projectile vomiting associated with Norovirus gastroenteritis may aerosolize infectious droplets. This view is supported by data such as those of Chadwick and McCann (99), who found that staff members exposed to nearby vomiting had a fourfold elevated risk of illness; nearby vomiting and close patient contact remained as the only significant independent predictors in a multiple logistic regression.

The appropriate choice of isolation precautions for Norovirus and related gastroenteritis is somewhat contentious; Standard Precautions may not be sufficient. Although unproven, the plausibility of Droplet spread and the epidemiologic evidence supporting that route of transmission appear to be sufficient to warrant droplet precautions when confronted by forceful vomiting caused by Norovirus-like agents. The evidence that environmental contamination plays a role in disease transmission is insufficient to recommend Contact Precautions, although, as is recommended for rotavirus, Contact Precautions should be considered in the event of fecal incontinence or other gross soiling. Nosocomial outbreaks may require cohorting and furloughing of involved staff members until they are well; most affected institutions have employed elaborate environmental decontamination, the need for which is unproven, but perhaps prudent (see also Chapters 24 and 50).

Hepatitis A

The hepatitis A virus causes an acute, self-limited infection whose clinical manifestations vary with age. Children typically experience mild or no illness; adults commonly develop malaise, nausea, vomiting, and icterus. Fulminant hepatitis and death are rare (0.1–0.5%) (104). The disease is clinically indistinguishable from several other viral hepatitides, and serologic diagnosis is required.

Nosocomial transmission is thought to be unusual. Most nosocomial outbreaks arise following admission of a patient not suspected to have hepatitis A, who either has subclinical infection, is in the prodrome, or is serologically false-negative because of immune deficiency (105), emphasizing the need to follow standard precautions for all patients. For example, three physicians caring for a 21-month-old girl with unsuspected anicteric hepatitis A became infected and ill; another developed subclinical infection (106). Of 58 susceptible workers exposed to a patient who had vomiting, diarrhea, and fecal incontinence during the 8 days preceding jaundice, six (10.3%) acquired infection (107). An outbreak in one NICU affected 13 infants, 22 nurses, eight other staff, and four household contacts (108); an outbreak in another NICU involved four infants and ten staff members. Investigations of such outbreaks have repeatedly identified two sets of behaviors as risk factors for worker infection: (a) a failure to wash hands, wear gloves, or both (107–109); and (b) eating, drinking, or smoking in the patient care unit (108,110,111).

Hepatitis A is transmitted almost exclusively by the fecal-oral route. A brief viremic phase occurs, during which blood-borne transmission is possible; airborne transmission has been alleged in at least one report (112) but is unlikely. The virus is present in high concentrations in the stool, and Standard Precautions should be supplemented with Contact Precautions in the case of fecal incontinence (including diapered infants).

Excellent vaccines have been developed and licensed. Although considered indicated among U.S. healthcare personnel only for susceptibles in areas where hepatitis A is highly endemic (113), cost-benefit analyses have suggested that the cost of hepatitis A vaccination in healthcare workers, per life-year saved, was similar to that of other standard medical interventions (114) (see Chapter 45).

Herpes Viruses

Infections caused by the herpes viruses are among the most common diseases of humans. The herpes viruses are not cleared following primary infection but, rather, reside permanently in target tissue. The viruses remain capable of reactivation, which might result in clinical disease on a regular basis (herpes simplex), occasionally (varicella-zoster virus), or only in the face of immune compromise [cytomegalovirus (CMV)]. The herpes viruses have been incriminated as risk factors for several neoplasms, and those that are lymphotropic alter immune function during active infection.

Herpes Simplex Virus

Herpes simplex virus (HSV) infection is common. In the United States, by age 45, 70% to 80% of the population has acquired antibody to HSV-1, the strain associated with oral lesions; 15% to 20% of whites and 40% to 60% of blacks have antibody to HSV-2, the strain associated with genital lesions. Infection with either strain is lifelong; following primary infection, the virus travels along sensory nerves and becomes latent within sensory ganglia. In a recurrence, the virus reactivates, travels peripherally from the ganglia along the nerves, and reestablishes cutaneous infection (115). Of importance to the healthcare worker, active virus can also be demonstrated in oral or genital secretions when no cutaneous or mucosal lesion is evident.

Although herpes virus can cause a variety of clinical syndromes, only one is routinely of pertinence to the healthcare worker: whitlow, a term derived from the middle-English whit flaw, or a flaw in the quick of the nail. Both HSV-1 and HSV-2 can cause whitlow; prior oral or genital infection does not necessarily protect one from acquiring a new infection of the finger (116). Workers with frequent exposure to oral secretions, such as dental workers, respiratory care personnel, and anesthesia staff members, are at greatest risk (117–120). Oral transmission can occur during mouth-to-mouth resuscitation (121), and at least one outbreak has been reported involving transmission between nurses and patients in a pediatric intensive care unit (ICU) with further household spread (122).

Under most circumstances, compliance with standard precautions should ensure protection from infection with HSV. Workers should glove (both hands) before contact with any oral secretions, including before airway suctioning. Contact Precautions should be considered when dealing with neonatal, disseminated, or severe primary herpes infection (see Chapter 43). Workers with whitlow should be restricted from contact with patients or their environment, and restriction from contact with high-risk patients may be appropriate for workers with orofacial herpes lesions.

Varicella-Zoster Virus

The varicella-zoster virus (VZV) is the etiologic agent of chickenpox; reactivation of the latent virus in previously infected persons produces the disease known as herpes zoster (shingles). Chickenpox is common among children, in whom the disease is generally mild; severity of illness increases with age of the subject. Despite repeated epidemics in schools, a small proportion of adults escape childhood infection and remain susceptible. Nearly all healthcare workers (98–100%) with a clinical history of chickenpox are immune as measured by serology (123), but 4% to 47% (median, 15%) of those with a negative or uncertain history of prior chickenpox are susceptible (123). In one study, the rate of susceptibility was higher among those less than 35 (7.5%) than those more than 35 years of age (0%) (124). Primary infection in susceptible adults can (but usually does not) cause serious disease, including varicella pneumonitis, which can be fatal. Two groups are at special risk from primary varicella infections: the immunocompromised, among whom the mortality rate may approach 20%; and newborns whose mothers develop primary infection from 5 days before to 2 days after giving birth. The combination of absent transplacental antibody and massive exposure places these infants at high risk, and the mortality rate can approach 30% (125).

Countless nosocomial outbreaks of VZV infection have been reported; indeed, it would be surprising to learn of a hospital caring for pediatric patients that has been spared. The high communicability of VZV, the routine presence in the hospital of immunocompromised patients at risk of serious or fatal disease if infected, and the presence of a core of susceptible healthcare workers make the management of VZV exposure one of the most challenging tasks of the infection control worker. This task is complicated by the fact that VZV is one of the few agents of nosocomial infection capable of true airborne spread (126–134). Airborne spread of VZV can arise from patients (or personnel) with primary infection (133), from patients with disseminated zoster (128–130), or rarely from patients with localized zoster (132). Of course, the infection can be transmitted by contact as well as through the air.

Management of VZV exposure incidents is burdensome and expensive. In a 1-year period at their hospital, Krasinski et al. (135) recorded 95 VZV infections (93 inpatients, two staff members), resulting in six exposure incidents involving 156 patients and 353 staff members. Fifty-one patients and 101 staff members denied prior VZV infection, but serology confirmed five and 11, respectively, to be susceptible. Three secondary infections occurred, six courses of varicella-zoster immune globulin (VZIG) were administered, and 13 staff members were furloughed, at a cost of 356 hours of infection control staff time and $41,500. Similarly, Weber et al. (136) documented exposures in 121 patients and more than 300 staff members in a single year, of whom 11 and 49, respectively, were serosusceptible; costs of managing these exposures totaled $55,934. Given the frequency of VZV exposure incidents and the burden they impose, it is not surprising that the appropriate management of exposure events has been much debated (137–148).

For hospitals providing care to immunocompromised pediatric patients, a comprehensive approach is recommended; certain elements may not be required in institutions lacking pediatric or immunodeficient patients. With the licensure of a safe and effective varicella vaccine, immunization of susceptible employees is now the cornerstone of the varicella control program and is cost effective (123,149,150). Susceptible employees can be identified by serotesting all employees, serotesting only those with a negative or uncertain history of chickenpox, or by forgoing serotesting and simply immunizing all those with a negative or uncertain history; the choice of strategy will depend on the institution's assessment of the relative costs of vaccine and serology, the rate of seronegativity in its employees, and the risk it is willing to accept of missing the detection and vaccination of a susceptible person (113,123,151).

Immunization of staff does not address all concerns. Although seroconversion is not ensured following vaccination, postvaccination serology is not helpful and is not recommended (113). In addition, vaccinees can develop a mild generalized rash, and may pose a risk of infection to susceptible patients. The institution should develop policies concerning management of vaccinated employees who develop a rash illness or who are subsequently exposed to varicella. Employees with chickenpox, as well as immunosuppressed employees with zoster, must be excluded; otherwise, healthy employees with covered zoster lesions may work, except with high-risk patients.

When an exposure event occurs, unvaccinated susceptible employees with exposure (i.e., those who have provided care without the required precautions) are furloughed from the 8th to the 21st days following exposure (113). Only employees known to be immune are assigned to care for patients with active VZV infection. Contact Precautions are used for all patients with VZV infection, and Airborne Precautions are added for those with primary varicella or disseminated zoster. Finally, exposed susceptible patients are discharged as soon as possible; if not discharged by the 8th day following exposure, they are placed in isolation through the 21st day or until discharged. VZIG is considered for exposed susceptible persons with impaired immune responses, including pregnant females (see Chapters 42, 51, and 99).

Epstein-Barr Virus

The Epstein-Barr virus (EBV) is the principal causative agent of infectious mononucleosis and has been implicated as a cause of Burkitt's lymphoma and nasopharyngeal carcinoma. From 30% to 95% of children have antibodies to EBV by age 6; the proportion is higher in less-developed countries. After children, young adults are the most commonly infected group, in whom infection is more likely to be symptomatic (152).

Transmission appears to require exchange of saliva and otherwise does not occur even with prolonged close contact. Few reports suggest nosocomial spread. Ginsburg et al. (153) reported an outbreak of infectious mononucleosis at an outpatient clinic in which five (17%) of 29 staff members developed clinical disease with serologic confirmation of recent EBV infection. The only possible route of transmission identified by the authors was the communal use of poorly washed coffee cups. One additional report noted the development of mononucleosis, reported to be serologically confirmed, in five (17%) of 29 laboratory workers; three had been involved in performing mononucleosis tests on serum specimens.

EBV is apparently transmitted rarely, if ever, to healthcare workers, and no supplement to Standard Precautions is indicated in the care of patients infected with EBV.

Cytomegalovirus

Nearly everyone acquires cytomegalovirus (CMV) infection at some point in life; age at first infection follows a pattern similar to that previously described for EBV, with larger proportions of children infected earlier in life in less-developed countries. Infection is most often asymptomatic or associated with nonspecific symptoms, but in less than 1% of cases may cause mononucleosis, hepatitis, or respiratory, gastrointestinal, or neurologic disease. As with the other herpes viruses, CMV infection is lifelong, and subsequent immunocompromise permits the virus to reactivate and cause respiratory, gastrointestinal, ophthalmologic, or other disease. In addition, CMV is one of the five classic teratogenic infections; primary or subclinical recurrent maternal infection during pregnancy can cause transplacental infection and neurologic damage to the fetus. Most fetal infections result from recurrent, rather than primary, maternal infection; the risk of fetal infection is about 1% for pregnant women with CMV antibody (154).

Concern regarding fetal CMV infection has stimulated substantial anxiety among healthcare workers, although to our knowledge, no nosocomial outbreak of CMV has ever been reported. Numerous studies of seroprevalence and seroconversion rates have been performed among nurses and other staff members who care for young children (155–170); although some studies found some elevation in risk (often not reaching statistical significance), none concluded that healthcare workers incurred a material additional risk as compared to the risk associated with routine home and community life. In recent years, anxiety concerning CMV appears to have subsided. This reaction may reflect reassurance by the cited data and by the adoption of universal precautions—or perhaps distraction by a new concern, HIV. CMV is excreted in urine and saliva, as well as stool, tears, breast milk, semen, and cervical secretions (154). Droplet or airborne spread does not appear to occur, even during mechanical ventilation (171). Adherence to Standard Precautions is adequate to protect the worker (see Chapter 44).

Human Herpesviruses 6–8

Human herpesvirus 6 (HHV-6) has been identified as the causative agent of *roseola infantum* (also known as exanthem subitum and sixth disease). Roseola, the last of the classic exanthems of childhood to be differentiated, occurs commonly in children between the ages of 6 months, after waning of maternal antibody, and 4 years, by which age almost all children are seropositive (172). Within this age range, HHV-6 is a common cause of febrile illness, accounting for 20% of emergency room visits by infants 6 to 12 months old (173). Reactivation during the year or two following primary infection was found in 16% of subjects (173), and the occurrence of occasional outbreaks (174) suggests that reinfection of children is possible. Primary infection of adults is rare, because most acquire immunity in childhood, but when it occurs, it can produce lymphadenopathy, hepatitis, or a mononucleosis-like syndrome (175). Serious or fatal HHV-6 reactivation has been demonstrated in recipients of bone marrow and, to a lesser extent, liver transplants. However, no evidence of transmission to healthcare workers exists as yet; thus, no infection control measures beyond standard precautions are needed. Serologic studies show that infection with human herpesvirus 7 is widespread in childhood. The virus may be another cause of *roseola infantum*; otherwise, its clinical significance is uncertain. Human herpesvirus 8 seems to resemble EBV in its ability to transform lymphocytes, and appears to be important in the cause of Kaposi's sarcoma (176) and has produced bone marrow failure in patients with kidney transplants (177). Standard precautions are indicated.

Herpesvirus Simiae

Herpesvirus simiae, also known as simian herpesvirus B, is enzootic in rhesus, cynomolgus, and other macaque monkeys in whom it behaves much as HSV-1 does in humans. The disease can be transmitted to humans by the bite of a monkey; of 23 patients known to have symptomatic infections prior to 1987, 18 died of encephalitis. Only one known instance of spread from human to human has been reported, but it is noteworthy for occurring in the course of providing nursing care: the wife of a monkey handler repeatedly applied cortisone cream both to her husband's wound and to her own excoriated dermatitis; he died, but she received acyclovir and her disease did not progress (178). Standard precautions appear to be sufficient to prevent transmission to the healthcare worker (179).

Other Major Childhood Viruses

Measles

Measles, perhaps the most contagious disease extant, is an acute exanthematous infection caused by the rubeola virus (180). It has been known since ancient times and was ranked first among the exanthems by the 19th-century nosologists (181). Illness begins with cough, coryza, and fever; an enanthem (Koplik's spots) and a maculopapular exanthem follow. Measles is the most dangerous of the common exanthematous diseases of childhood. Even in healthy children, the disease can progress to pneumonia or, less commonly, encephalitis; bacterial pneumonia can also complicate the course. Chronic complications include subacute sclerosing panencephalitis. Measles infection is more serious in adults and in immunocompromised individuals. A safe, effective live attenuated vaccine exists, and its widespread use has reduced the incidence of measles in the United States, previously as high as 500,000 cases per year, nearly to zero.

The exceptional communicability of measles permitted continued epidemics in past years, despite relatively high immunization levels. Measles outbreaks typically involve one or both of two groups: (a) infants too young to be immunized and young children who escaped immunization, and (b) young adults (including healthcare workers) with primary vaccine failure (about 2% to 5% of vaccinees). These problems have been addressed with substantial success by vigorous immunization campaigns and by implementing a two-dose immunization schedule, which gives a second opportunity to immunize those who failed to seroconvert when first vaccinated (182). History makes it clear, however, that any slippage in immunization rates will lead to a resurgence of measles consequent to importations from areas of the world where active transmission continues.

Reports of measles infections among healthcare workers caused by nosocomial outbreaks are frequent (183–193), and the frequency of such events climbed during the 1980s. For the 5-year period 1980–1984, 241 cases of measles (1.1% of all cases from 1980 to 1984) were acquired in healthcare settings; of the 241 cases, 24% were among staff members (184). In the next 5-year period, 1,209 medical-setting cases were identified (3.5% of all cases during the period); 28% of the infections occurred in staff members (189). Most of these cases represented a failure to immunize, not a failure of vaccine; only 20% of staff members for whom immunization status was known were documented to have received even one dose of vaccine. From 1985 through 1991, 2,997 measles cases were acquired in medical facilities, representing 4% of the total in that period (194). As measles has been brought under greater control, the mean age of patients has shifted upward (27% of cases from 1993 to 1995 were in persons older than 20 years of age), and the proportion of cases acquired in medical settings increased (to 14% for the period 1992–1995) (195).

Nosocomial measles is a serious matter, involving substantial risk to patients and staff. During 1988, Children's Hospital in Los Angeles admitted 37 patients with measles (188). Six cases were unsuspected, exposing 107 patients and 24 staff members. Twelve patients and seven employees developed measles; one patient died, and two workers were hospitalized with pneumonia. Eight hundred workers required vaccination, and 211 workdays were lost. Others have recounted the disruption and expense associated with these outbreaks (190,196,197). In addition to jeopardizing healthcare workers and inpatients, nosocomial outbreaks can play an important role in propagating measles in the community (187,188,198,199).

Like varicella, measles is spread readily by the airborne route. In 1937, Wells placed ultraviolet lights in selected classrooms of two schools (6). In a subsequent measles epidemic, the attack rate was dramatically higher in the control classrooms, indicating causation of measles by an airborne agent susceptible to inactivation by ultraviolet light. Analyses of other outbreaks have confirmed the potential for airborne spread (186,200,201), and Airborne Precautions should be used for patients known or suspected to have measles. Isolation strategies, however, clearly do not eliminate the risk of nosocomial measles; healthcare workers must be immune. Authorities now are willing to categorize as immune all persons born before 1957 (182,194–195, 202–205). From 1985 through 1991, 29% of healthcare workers reported with measles were born before 1957. Numerous serosurveys support the view that persons in this older group are less likely to be susceptible than younger persons (206–212). Thus, because of the virtual absence of measles in the United States today, the 1957 demarcation is practical.

Immunization program costs can be minimized by devising program strategies that optimize the balance between obtaining preimmunization serology (to immunize only the susceptible) and immunizing without serology (a less expensive alternative if most will need immunization) (206,212–214). The ideal measles prevention program would require that regardless of age, every worker with patient contact show documentation of receipt of two doses of measles vaccine after the first birthday, at least 1 month apart, or serologic evidence of immunity (a documented physician diagnosis of natural measles infection might also be accepted). Immunization would be required, as necessary, to satisfy this standard. However, substantial practical difficulties are encountered with this approach. Many workers properly immunized in childhood cannot document that fact and, thus, would require either serologic screening or two immunizations. If serologic screening is pursued, rubella immunity also should be assayed; more workers are susceptible to rubella than to measles (204), and primary vaccine failure could have occurred with either antigen. Finally, a program incorporating serologic screening incurs substantial overhead associated with tracking of results and recall of employees.

The Advisory Committee on Immunization Practices (ACIP) recommended in December 1997 that all healthcare workers born after 1956 be required to show proof of immunity or receipt of two doses of vaccine; those born before 1957 should be considered for one dose of vaccine without proof of immunity (215). A simpler alternative approach is to give one injection of combined measles-mumps-rubella (MMR) vaccine to every employee who cannot document immunity or adequate prior immunization. Although this approach is not as comprehensive as the ideal program, the shortfall in immunization coverage would be limited to those persons who were susceptible to measles prior to this immunization, who failed to respond to this immunization, and who would have responded to a second injection given a month later. Data from Willy et al. (211) suggest that this strategy would leave 0.7% more of the work force susceptible (or equivocal) than would the ideal program (6.1% initially susceptible, 14.1% nonresponders to first vaccination, 81.8% responders to second vaccination). In comparison, programs that do not immunize persons born before 1957 leave 1.6% (211) to 6.4% (207) of employees susceptible; those that immunize only new hires can be expected to have substantial numbers of susceptible employees for many years.

Regardless of program strategy, MMR vaccine should be used rather than monovalent measles vaccine. As discussed later, the consequences of nosocomial rubella can be disastrous, and many healthcare workers remain susceptible to mumps. No ill effects ensue from immunizing those already immune, and persons not yet immune require immunization. Individuals responsible for employee immunization programs will find helpful the previously cited program analyses (206,212–214), the analysis of vaccine response by Willy et al. (211), and the detailed recommendations published in a 1994 consensus paper (205) (see Chapter 51).

Rubella

Rubella (German measles) is another of the common exanthematous infections of childhood. Categorized as "third disease" when it was clinically differentiated from measles and scarlet fever 100 years ago, rubella is less contagious than measles and substantially less dangerous (except to the fetus). Postnatally acquired infection is commonly mild, and complications are rare apart from arthritis or arthralgia, which can affect up to one third of women (children and men are relatively spared). The arthritis may take several months to resolve and rarely may become chronic (216).

The importance of rubella derives from its potential for devastating damage to the fetus. Depending on fetal age, infection may result in fetal death, heart defects, deafness, cataracts or glaucoma, retardation, and a host of other congenital maladies. The risk of fetal damage declines with maturity, from a high of 60% during the first 2 months of pregnancy. Once a susceptible woman is exposed, no intervention is likely to alter subsequent events favorably. Prevention of congenital rubella syndrome depends on establishing prior immunity.

Several nosocomial rubella outbreaks have involved staff members and patients (217–228); Hispanic patients and staff are apparently particularly susceptible. Such outbreaks can have substantial consequences. For example, a nosocomial outbreak in Boston involved 47 healthcare workers, one of whom terminated her early pregnancy (219); rubella in an obstetrics clinic nurse exposed 151 obstetrics patients and 44 employees (220); an obstetrician and two other staff members of a prenatal clinic developed rubella, exposing 56 susceptible pregnant women and infecting 2 (224); 15 cases of rubella among staff members of an obstetrics service led to exposure of 231 pregnant women, of whom 25% were susceptible (223). The national immunization program has substantially curtailed circulation of wild rubella virus, and such outbreaks have become rare. At the same time, however, the reduced circulation of wild virus has reduced the opportunity for women who escaped childhood immunization to acquire natural immunity prior to entering the childbearing years. The potential for rubella outbreaks among hospital personnel clearly remains should a case be introduced; serosurveys indicate that 4% to 6% of new hires are susceptible (229,230), and 19% of practicing obstetricians surveyed in 1994 had neither been immunized nor been demonstrated to be immune by serology (231).

Persons infected with rubella are infectious from 10 days before until 5 days after rash onset. Rubella is believed to be spread by respiratory droplets; airborne spread is plausible but has not been demonstrated. Droplet Precautions are recommended for management of patients with rubella, but as with measles, infections can be expected among employees despite isolation precautions unless the employees are immune.

A safe, effective live attenuated virus vaccine was introduced in 1969. Although the vaccine can cause a febrile illness as well as transient arthritis, these effects are less common, milder, and shorter-lived than with natural infection. Congenital rubella syndrome has not been demonstrated following vaccination, but the vaccine virus can cross the placenta; therefore, the vaccine should not be given to women who might be pregnant or become pregnant within 3 months. As discussed with respect to measles, employee health programs likely will find it more cost-effective to immunize with MMR all those who cannot document prior immunization than to perform serology for both measles and rubella (194). Either approach, however, is less expensive than managing the consequences of an outbreak such as those previously described (219,227) (see Chapter 51).

Mumps

Mumps is an acute viral infection that, in unimmunized populations, occurs predominantly among school-aged children. Illness begins with nonspecific symptoms of a viral syndrome, followed by acute nonsuppurative parotitis that may be unilateral or bilateral. The swelling may be painful and accompanied by fever, but it resolves within a week. Other glands may be affected; epididymo-orchitis occurs in 20% to 40% of postpubertal men and may eventuate in testicular atrophy. Rarer manifestations include meningoencephalitis, oophoritis, pancreatitis, and nephritis (232). A safe and effective live attenuated virus vaccine has been available since 1967. However, use of mumps vaccine was not required in many jurisdictions until relatively recently, and a substantial population escaped immunization (202,233). Mumps is much less contagious than measles, varicella, or rubella, and many adults remain susceptible. Outbreaks of mumps have occurred in healthcare facilities with transmission from patient to worker (234–236) and from healthcare worker to patient (237). Mumps is spread by droplets and by contact with saliva, which is infectious for up to 9 days prior to the parotitis. Thus, although droplet precautions are appropriate, they are unlikely to be implemented before transmission has occurred; prevention of nosocomial transmission requires immunization. A policy of immunizing with MMR all persons who cannot document adequate prior immunization would obviate the need to perform yet another serology (see Chapter 51).

Parvovirus

The parvoviruses cause infections marked by bone marrow suppression and reductions in blood cell counts in a number of species. Parvovirus B19 is the cause of (a) erythema infectiosum, the fifth of the classic exanthems of childhood; (b) transient aplastic crisis in patients with chronic anemias; and (c) fetal infections, leading to hydrops or abortion. Erythema infectiosum is a generally mild illness marked by a "slapped cheek" facial rash and variable, often lacy, extremity rash. Arthritis and arthralgia may occur, most often in adults (238).

Outbreaks in schools and the community are common. Patients with erythema infectiosum are no longer infectious by the time the rash appears, but patients with transient aplastic crisis or immunodeficiency are viremic while ill. Nosocomial outbreaks with spread to healthcare workers have been described (239–241), but the risk to healthcare workers is low (242), particularly as compared to school or day-care employees (243,244), who are more commonly in contact with children incubating erythema infectiosum. Indeed, apparent nosocomial outbreaks may merely reflect transmission outside the hospital during a communitywide outbreak (245). Parvovirus is believed to be spread by direct contact, blood, and respiratory droplets; true airborne spread has not been demonstrated, and the possible role of fomites is undefined. Standard Precautions are sufficient for care of uncomplicated erythema infectiosum but should be supplemented by droplet precautions for patients with transient aplastic crisis or other parvovirus syndromes (see Chapter 51).

Rare and Exotic Viruses

In this section we briefly consider a number of viral infections that rarely, if ever, are encountered in U.S. hospitals. Some are relatively benign but might be capable of spread to healthcare workers. Others have frightening reputations that are undeserved, because they have no demonstrated potential for spread to healthcare workers. A few have earned their formidable reputations and require caution, particularly including some of the hemorrhagic fever viruses.

Hemorrhagic Fever Viruses

The viruses known to cause hemorrhagic fever (HF) in humans differ in their structure and genetics but share the ability to cause a generalized illness that can be severe, marked by involvement of visceral organs (e.g., hepatitis, nephritis, carditis) and by thrombocytopenia or other coagulation defects that lead to disseminated intravascular coagulation or other bleeding diatheses. Humans likely are not the primary hosts for any of these viruses, with the possible exception of dengue. The two most important routes of exposure are insect bites (yellow fever, dengue, Rift Valley fever, Crimean-Congo HF, Kyasanur Forest disease, and Omsk HF) and exposure to infectious rodent urine either directly or, more often, via contaminated airborne dust (Lassa fever, Argentine HF, Bolivian HF, and Hantaan and related HFs); the natural route of exposure is not known for Marburg and Ebola HFs (246–250). Laboratory-acquired infections have been reported for Hantaan HF (251) and Kyasanur Forest disease (252), but person-to-person transmission is not known to occur with yellow fever, dengue, Argentine HF, Bolivian HF, Rift Valley fever, Hantaan HF, Kyasanur Forest disease, or Omsk HF, and these diseases are not discussed further here (the hantavirus group is discussed in the next section).

Lassa Fever

Of the four HFs with known potential for nosocomial spread, the best known is Lassa fever. The disease was first recognized following infection of three nurses at a missionary hospital in Nigeria, of whom two died (253). The next year, an outbreak in the same community led to the death of a missionary physician who became infected through a cut received while performing an autopsy on a presumed Lassa fever patient (254). Two years later, an outbreak in a Liberian missionary hospital led to illness in three patients and seven staff members; one nurse and all three patients died, for a case fatality rate of 36% (255). However, subsequent studies have shown that the disease is endemic in West Africa, with infection rates of 10% to 20%, and that 90% to 95% of these infections are mild or inapparent (256). Thus, the extraordinary precautions recommended and implemented by the CDC with the first case imported to the United States (257) were significantly relaxed in later recommendations (258–260), because it became apparent that attention to barrier precautions prevented nosocomial infections (259–261).

Outcome of Lassa fever is correlated with the degree and persistence of viremia; exceptionally high titers of virus can be found in blood. Prevention of nosocomial transmission must focus on avoidance of inoculation or aerosolization of blood. Primary human infection arises from inhalation of dust or aerosols contaminated with infected rodent urine. Person-to-person transmission of Lassa fever has occurred both in the household and the hospital setting, but initial fears of droplet or airborne transmission have not been substantiated. Because spread by direct contact is a possibility, it is appropriate to supplement Standard Precautions with Contact Precautions (see Chapters 47 and 111).

Marburg Virus

In 1967, several hundred African green monkeys imported from Uganda for medical research arrived in Marburg, Germany. Subsequently, 25 researchers working with monkey kidneys or tissue cultures became ill with a viral HF; seven died, as did 13 of the monkeys (246,250). Six close contacts of the researchers also acquired illness; none died. The causative agent was determined to be a unique filamentous virus (filovirus). The virus has been identified in only a few subsequent sporadic cases of infection in Africa, several of which involved person-to-person transmission to medical staff members (262,263). The natural reservoir and routes of transmission remain unknown (264). The disease is clearly transmissible by the respiratory route from laboratory specimens, but person-to-person infection appears to require close contact. Pending further data, use of Contact Precautions and careful attention to Standard Precautions (especially with respect to blood) appears appropriate. Tissue and laboratory specimens should be handled with caution and processed so as to ensure containment (see Chapters 47 and 111).

Ebola Virus

Two simultaneous outbreaks of viral HF in neighboring regions of Sudan and Zaire in 1976 heralded the existence of yet another African HF virus (265). Of the identified cases in Sudan and Zaire, 55% and 88%, respectively, died, reflecting substantial differences in the two viral subtypes (250). The outbreaks were accompanied by nosocomial and household spread, but investigation of the only other known human outbreak, 2 years later, showed that person-to-person transmission required blood exchange or close personal contact (266).

The Ebola virus is similar to the Marburg virus, joining it as the only other member of the filovirus family. As with Marburg virus, the natural reservoir of Ebola virus remains unidentified. Monkeys are susceptible and experience a high mortality rate (267), which suggests that they are not among the natural hosts. The discovery of Ebola virus epidemics among medical research monkeys held in U.S. and Philippine primate centers caused considerable alarm and prompted strict new screening and quarantine regulations (268,269). This Reston subtype of Ebola virus was highly virulent for monkeys, but it produced only subclinical infection among the exposed humans (270).

More than 25 years had passed since the last recognized outbreak of human disease caused by Ebola virus when a large new outbreak involving the Zaire subtype began in early 1995 in Kikwit, Zaire. As in previous outbreaks, provision of medical care without use of standard infection control precautions led to an explosive nosocomial outbreak, with many worker and patient deaths at Kikwit General Hospital; job-specific attack rates ranged from 31% for physicians to 10% for nurses to 4% for other workers (271). Another outbreak now is underway along the remote northern border between Gabon and Congo (272).

Disease is spread by contact with infected blood or tissues; parenteral exposure is particularly lethal. Although epidemiologic and pathologic evidence suggest that aerosol spread is possible, (270), the importance of this route is uncertain. Standard Precautions should be supplemented with comprehensive contact Precautions; Droplet Precautions are not known to be necessary but their use, particularly when dealing with the highly lethal Zaire subtype, should depend on the clinical circumstances (see Chapters 47 and 111).

Both Ebola and Marburg virus can persist in tissues for several months following acute infection, emphasizing the need for careful handling. As with Lassa and Marburg viruses, it is recommended to supplement Standard with full Contact Precautions.

Crimean-Congo Hemorrhagic Fever

The fourth of the HFs shown to spread from person to person, Crimean-Congo HF, was first described among Russian troops in Crimea in 1944. Found in the Balkans, Siberia, China, the Middle East, and Africa, the virus is normally transmitted by ticks but can be spread by close contact, and several nosocomial outbreaks have occurred (246,248,273–275). Nosocomial transmission can be prevented by attention to barrier precautions (274); Contact Precautions should also be used (see Chapters 47 and 111).

Other arenaviruses have been associated with sporadic secondary transmission (276). For example, Sabiá virus has infected at least two laboratory workers (277); although transmission to healthcare workers as a consequence of clinical duties has not been reported, enhanced infection control precautions have been proposed for care of such patients (277).

Hantavirus Group

Hantaan and related viruses are the etiologic agents of the HF with renal syndrome seen in Korea (Korean HF), China, Siberia, and southeastern Europe. Spread is through inhalation of dust or aerosols contaminated with infected rodent urine or, rarely, a rodent bite; person-to-person transmission is unknown. In June 1993, a previously unrecognized syndrome consisting of nonspecific viral symptoms progressing rapidly to respiratory failure, interstitial pulmonary edema, and death was described among residents of the southwestern United States (278). Investigation showed the causative agent to be a previously unrecognized hantavirus (now named the Sin Nombre virus). Although the syndrome is new, the reservoir (the deer mouse) and route of transmission appear to be typical of the hantavirus family (279). The deer mouse resides in much of the United States, and cases of hantavirus pulmonary syndrome have been described in various locales (280,281). Little evidence supports nosocomial spread, and Standard Precautions should be sufficient.

Human Papillomavirus

A large number of papillomaviruses produce various forms of warts and other epithelial tumors. Spread is believed to be by close contact and would be prevented by Standard Precautions. However, one interesting report showed the presence of intact papillomavirus deoxyribonucleic acid (DNA) in the vapor produced by laser treatment of warts and other verrucae (282). Whether human infection at any site could arise from such an exposure is speculative, but prudence suggests ensuring proper exhaust of the vapor.

Pox Viruses

Smallpox, a colossus of death, no longer strides the earth but lies imprisoned under heavy guard in Russia and Atlanta, awaiting final destruction (283). Only as smallpox neared defeat by the milkmaid's friend, vaccinia, did smallpox reveal beyond doubt its ability to attack not only those nearby, via contact, but also distant victims through the air; to prove its prowess, it claimed as its final victim a photographer infected in her office by air wafted from a nearby research laboratory (284,285).

Vaccinia too, its task completed, had largely disappeared, although vaccination continued for laboratorians working with orthopox and vaccinia viruses (286). After the terrorist attacks of September 11, 2001, smallpox bioterrorism preparedness activities included a program of vaccinating public health workers and some hospital workers. This program is further discussed in Chapter 80.

Vaccinia can be passed from person to person by contact with the active vaccinial lesion, but no viremia is present in the normal host (287), and respiratory spread does not occur; contact precautions are sufficient. The theoretical possibility of airborne spread exists with the progressive vaccinia that can occur in the immunocompromised, although it has not been demonstrated; should such a case be encountered (or smallpox be unleashed once again), Airborne Precautions would be indicated.

The large genome of vaccinia makes it attractive as a carrier of inserted genetic material, the hybrid then being used to infect a patient and thereby accomplishing gene therapy. This process raises numerous infection control issues, which are discussed in detail elsewhere (288; and see Chapter 72); vaccination of clinical staff working with patients given vaccinial recombinants may be appropriate.

Monkeypox produces a disease that is similar in appearance to smallpox but is not readily transmitted from person to person (287). During the summer of 2003 an outbreak of monkeypox occurred in the United States among persons who had purchased imported exotic pets (Gambian giant rats among them) and prairie dogs that had become cross-infected at the animal distribution facility (289). No transmission to healthcare providers was detected. CDC's ACIP suggested that vaccinia vaccine (smallpox vaccine) might be a useful preventive measure among potentially exposed healthcare workers. Not much, if any, vaccine was used for that purpose. Molluscum contagiosum and orf require close contact for transmission (290); Standard Precautions are sufficient.

Rabies and the Other Encephalitis Viruses

Vector-borne encephalitis viruses include (a) eastern, western, and Venezuelan equine encephalitis virus; (b) St. Louis and tick-borne encephalitis viruses; (c) the California encephalitis virus group (including La Crosse and Jamestown Canyon viruses); (d) Powassan, Louping Ill, and Negishi viruses as well as West Nile virus. Most strains are spread by mosquitoes, some by ticks; primary host species include horses, birds, deer, rodents, and pigs. None of the viruses are transmitted from person to person, although some have infected laboratory workers exposed to aerosols (247,248,292).

West Nile virus arrived in the United States in 1999, causing an outbreak of meningoencephalitis among largely elderly residents of New York City (291). Over succeeding mosquito transmission seasons it has spread stepwise across the entire United States. Although the vast majority of human infections are acquired from mosquito bites, transplacental transmission to a fetus, transmission via breast milk, and acquisition from an infected organ donor as well as from transfused blood have been documented. No special risk to healthcare workers has been shown.

Lymphocytic choriomeningitis (LCM) virus, related to the Lassa fever virus, shares its characteristic of being spread by exposure to infectious rodent urine; rodent bites have also been implicated. Unlike Lassa virus, LCM virus is not known to spread from person to person. Several outbreaks of LCM have affected medical center staff, but all have been attributable to contact or presence in the same room with rodents being used in research (249,293–296).

Rabies, one of the most feared diseases, is a viral zoonosis transmitted to humans through the bite of an infected mammal. Rabies is the most uniformly fatal infection known; survival is nearly unprecedented once symptoms begin. Consequently, anxiety among healthcare workers is intense once a patient has been diagnosed with rabies, and scores or even hundreds of healthcare workers are commonly administered rabies prophylaxis following diagnosis of a patient. Although rabies virus can be isolated from a variety of human tissues and fluids, including saliva (297), a well-documented instance of person-to-person transmission of rabies has never occurred, apart from corneal transplantation (297,298). One report describes two possible cases in Ethiopia of human-to-human transmission (both involving saliva: one bite and one kiss), but these cases were not laboratory-confirmed (299).

No evidence supports droplet, airborne, or environmental transmission from human sources for any of these agents; therefore, Standard Precautions are sufficient. Healthcare workers involved with a rabies case do not need prophylaxis unless mucous membranes or nonintact skin were exposed to potentially infectious body fluids (298). Preexposure immunization is indicated for those working with rabies virus or likely to come into contact with potentially rabid animals (see Chapter 47).

Prions

Prions are poorly understood, small, protein-containing particles that can be detected in the brain in certain pathologic states and appear to be responsible for a number of slowly progressive neurodegenerative diseases. These transmissible spongiform encephalopathies include Creutzfeldt-Jakob disease (CJD), kuru, Gerstmann-Sträussler-Scheinker disease, and fatal familial insomnia in humans, and scrapie, bovine spongiform encephalopathy (mad cow disease), transmissible mink encephalopathy, and related diseases in animals. Purified prion material derived from the aforementioned diseases can induce the disease in a healthy host when injected (or, in the case of kuru, when ingested). No one has been able to demonstrate nucleic acids in prions, and their reproduction might involve an alteration in a protein normally encoded by the host (300).

Person-to-person spread of CJD has occurred in connection with corneal transplants (301), dural grafts (302), contaminated neurosurgical instruments (303), and cadaver-derived growth hormone (304) or gonadotropin (305). Kuru is acquired by ingestion of infected human brain, and new-variant CJD is a rare sequela to ingestion of beef products from cattle with mad cow disease (306). The evidence strongly indicates that CJD and related diseases do not spread by the airborne or contact routes, and Standard Precautions are sufficient when caring for patients with these diseases. However, prions are extremely resistant to inactivation and retain infectivity even in formalin-fixed tissue. Patient specimens and contaminated equipment (e.g., needles, surgical instruments) must be handled with particular care, and detailed recommendations have been offered for their decontamination (307) (see Chapters 47 and 85).

CHLAMYDIAL, RICKETTSIAL, AND MYCOPLASMAL INFECTIONS

Chlamydiae

Like the viruses, members of the order Chlamydiae are obligate intracellular parasites. Three species have been identified: *Chlamydia trachomatis,* the cause of trachoma and lymphogranuloma venereum; *Chlamydia psittaci,* the agent of psittacosis; and *Chlamydia pneumoniae,* previously called the TWAR agent, which causes an atypical pneumonia. (The first two recognized isolates were identified at the University of Washington and were obtained from a Taiwanese child in 1965 and a student with acute upper respiratory infection in 1983). Humans are the natural hosts of *C. trachomatis* and *C. pneumoniae,* whereas *C. psittaci* is a pathogen of animals, particularly psittacine birds (parrots), and infects humans only secondarily. *C. trachomatis* is spread by contact with infected secretions, and Standard Precautions are sufficient to protect healthcare workers.

C. psittaci is spread through the air, but it is uncertain whether person-to-person transmission occurs. Several nosocomial outbreaks have been described in the literature that were attributed at the time to psittacosis (308–310), but they either antedated the recognition of *C. pneumoniae* (to which bird owners are as susceptible as anyone else) and might well have been caused by the latter agent (311), or rested on serologic results that were less than fully conclusive (312,313) (see Chapter 47). *C. pneumoniae* has been implicated in outbreaks of pneumonia in various closed communities such as classrooms and military barracks; nosocomial outbreaks appear to be very rare. In at least one outbreak, serologic data support the impression of nosocomial spread of chlamydial pneumonia, but whether the species was accurately identified is unclear (310).

Although droplet spread of chlamydial pneumonia cannot be excluded, current evidence does not appear to justify imposition of Droplet Precautions; Standard Precautions should suffice (26).

Rickettsiae

The rickettsiae are also obligate intracellular parasites. Those of the genus *Rickettsia* all have nonhuman mammalian reservoirs, are transmitted to humans by insect vectors, and survive only briefly outside a host. The lone member of the genus *Coxiella* behaves quite differently. *C. burnetii,* the etiologic agent of Q fever, is a gram-negative coccobacillus that can sporulate and thereby survive outside the host for extended periods (314). Q fever (so named because its cause was a query) is a zoonosis of ungulates (e.g., sheep and cattle) that can cause an acute and chronic febrile illness in humans. Humans are highly susceptible; a single microorganism can cause disease. Outbreaks of Q fever have occurred not only among those who work with ungulates but also those nearby. Included among the latter group have been a number of healthcare workers exposed to sheep used in research at their medical centers (315–320). Laboratory workers are also at risk (321); indeed, the first recognized case of Q fever in the U.S. was acquired occupationally by a National Institutes of Health physician (322). However, despite the fact that *C. burnetii* can be isolated from human milk, placenta, and blood, no evidence indicates transmission to healthcare workers during normal clinical duties, and Standard Precautions are sufficient.

Mycoplasmas

The members of the *Mycoplasma* and closely related *Ureaplasma* species are the smallest free-living microorganisms known. Because they have fastidious growth requirements, they are difficult to culture on artificial media and are found in nature only in close relation with their hosts. Of the numerous mycoplasmas isolated from humans and potentially involved in human disease, only one has been associated with outbreaks among healthcare workers: *Mycoplasma pneumoniae,* a prominent cause of the atypical pneumonia syndrome.

M. pneumoniae infections occur sporadically or as outbreaks in closed populations such as families, schools, and military barracks (323). Younger persons are more susceptible and tend to have milder disease. Outbreaks among staff members have been described in healthcare institutions in Finland, Ohio, Texas, and New York (324,325). Transmission is believed to be by respiratory droplets, and Droplet Precautions should be followed.

BACTERIAL INFECTIONS

Bacterial Enteric Infections

Salmonellae

The salmonellae are aerobic gram-negative bacilli that inhabit the intestinal tracts of humans and animals. Some strains are specific to humans or other species, whereas others have a broad host range. Salmonellae routinely cause gastroenteritis but can induce a wide variety of diseases in humans. *Salmonella typhi,* the causative agent of typhoid fever, produces the most serious illness in humans but many of the animal salmonellae can produce serious or fatal disease, particularly in the elderly (326).

Salmonella is a common cause of nosocomial infectious diarrhea, particularly in newborn and pediatric units, which account for 50% of reported nosocomial cases (327). Between 1963 and 1972, 28% of reported *Salmonella* outbreaks in the United States occurred in healthcare institutions (328); case-fatality ratios were less than 1% in most hospital units but rose to 3% in pediatric units, 7% in nurseries, and 9% in nursing homes.

Nosocomial outbreaks often involve healthcare workers (329–332), who occasionally become chronic carriers. One unusual nosocomial outbreak involved spread of *Salmonella* infection from patients to nursing home laundry workers who handled soiled sheets without use of gloves or other barrier precautions and who routinely ate in the laundry room (333).

Salmonella is spread by the fecal-oral route and, notwithstanding the rare report suggesting alternative routes of spread (334), Standard Precautions are sufficient to protect the worker. In addition, soiled laundry must be handled in accord with established recommendations, and food should not be consumed in work areas (see Chapters 24 and 50). Two excellent typhoid vaccines, one oral, one parenteral (as well as an older parenteral vaccine that should no longer be used) are now available, and immunization is indicated for laboratorians working with *S. typhi.*

Shigella

Shigella species are the principal etiologic agents of bacillary dysentery; *S. dysenteriae* causes the most severe disease, whereas *S. sonnei* has been the most common isolate in recent years. Shigellosis is easily transmitted, because the infective dose is 100 microorganisms or fewer. The disease is marked by abdominal cramping and watery diarrhea that becomes bloody or mucoid, usually accompanied by fever. Illness typically lasts 1 week but can be prolonged (327,335). Nosocomial outbreaks of *Shigella* are much less common than are *Salmonella* outbreaks but can be a particular problem in long-term-care and custodial institutions for children and for the elderly (336–340). In each of the cited outbreaks, staff members acquired infection from patients and often facilitated the spread of infection.

Shigella species are transmitted solely by the fecal-oral route, and Standard Precautions normally are sufficient to protect the worker. Because of the low infective dose, Contact Precautions should be used when managing diapered or incontinent patients.

Cholera

Vibrio cholerae causes cholera, a toxin-mediated profuse watery diarrhea that can cause prostration in the first hour and death from dehydration in the second. Cholera, described in ancient Greek and Sanskrit texts, circled the globe in six successive epidemic waves during the 19th and early 20th centuries. Epidemic cholera returned in 1991 in South America, establishing a new endemic focus (341).

Spread of cholera is by the fecal-oral route. On rare occasions, humans may become carriers. Nosocomial transmission to patients has occurred (342,343), but little evidence indicates transmission to healthcare workers. As with other highly transmissible gastroenteritides, Standard Precautions should be supplemented with Contact Precautions when caring for diapered infants or fecally incontinent patients (see Chapters 24 and 50).

Other Bacterial Agents of Diarrhea

Clostridium difficile secretes a toxin that causes pseudomembranous colitis. Risk of the disease is substantially elevated in patients whose normal bowel flora have been depleted by treatment with antibiotics, particularly broad-spectrum cephalosporins (344). *C. difficile* is an important nosocomial pathogen spread by direct and indirect contact (345,346), and standard precautions should be supplemented with contact precautions. Healthcare workers might acquire the microorganism occupationally, but normally would not be expected to manifest illness. However, full-blown pseudomembranous colitis has been reported in staff members who were taking a bowel-active antibiotic during a nosocomial outbreak of disease (347,348) (see Chapter 36).

Escherichia coli is the most common of the aerobic enteric bacteria that colonize the normal intestinal tract. There are numerous strains, some of which can be important causes of enteric disease. Enteroinvasive *E. coli* microorganisms behave like *Shigella* and cause dysentery; enterotoxigenic strains cause a cholera-like illness; the enterohemorrhagic *E. coli* O157:H7, often associated with undercooked ground beef, causes bloody diarrhea. All strains are spread by the fecal-oral route and require Contact Precautions only when managing diapered or incontinent patients. Similar precautions are recommended for the bacterial diarrheas not discussed here.

Bacterial Diseases Spread by the Respiratory Route

Diphtheria

Diphtheria, described by Hippocrates, has been a fearsome disease; an epidemic in New England in the early 18th century killed one third of all children, and in the early 1920s diphtheria was the leading cause of death of Canadian children aged 2 to 14 years (349). Epidemics occurred at approximately 25-year intervals until modern times; the disease has nearly been eradicated through use of diphtheria toxoid vaccines. The causative microorganism is *Corynebacterium diphtheriae,* a gram-positive bacillus for which humans are the only known reservoir. The microorganism colonizes the respiratory tract or skin wounds, where it may be asymptomatic or produce mild inflammation. The microorganism does not invade, but if it is infected by the toxin-encoding bacteriophage, it can liberate a toxin that interferes with ribosomal protein synthesis, causing local accumulation of killed cells and inflammatory residue (the pseudomembrane), myocarditis, neuropathies, and nephritis. Skin carriage can be common in certain groups; for example, 86% of diphtheria cases among urban alcoholics in Seattle, Washington, were cutaneous (350). Spread of the microorganism to others occurs more readily from those with skin carriage than from those with pharyngeal carriage (351).

Adequate antibody to the toxin largely protects from the serious consequences of infection but does not eradicate carriage of the microorganism. Because introduction of toxigenic strains into the community can result in disease if immunization levels are inadequate, it is pertinent that 22% to 62% of U.S. adults under 40 years of age and 41% to 84% of persons 60 years and older lack protective levels of diphtheria antitoxin (352). The possible consequences of widespread adult susceptibility to diphtheria were illustrated in Russia and other former Soviet states, which experienced a massive outbreak of diphtheria in the 1990s following decreased childhood immunization programs, resulting in 140,000 cases and 4,000 deaths (353). Although diphtheria has become rare in the U.S. and Western Europe, outbreaks involving patients and staff members have occurred in healthcare institutions (354,355). Serotesting during one hospital outbreak found 37% of staff members to be susceptible. Diphtheria is spread both by respiratory droplets and by direct contact. Droplet Precautions are appropriate for cases with respiratory tract disease, and Contact Precautions should be implemented for those with cutaneous diphtheria. Employee health programs should ensure that employees have been immunized within the past 10 years with tetanus and diphtheria toxoids (Td) adsorbed, for adult use (352).

Pertussis

Guillaime Baillou described an outbreak in Paris of a disease he called "quinta" in 1578; in 1679, Thomas Sydenham renamed the disease pertussis, meaning violent cough. The disease is highly contagious and spreads via respiratory droplets. When *Bordetella pertussis* microorganisms enter the respiratory tract, they attach via their fimbriae to cilia, causing ciliary stasis, cell death, and shedding of respiratory mucosal cells. Because they do not invade, they largely escape cellular host defenses, continuing to produce local damage and, through their toxins, systemic disease, until the host finally is able to clear the microorganisms. The onset is insidious, seeming like a typical cold or upper respiratory infection with little fever. Within a week or so, a cough appears that progresses within another week or two to paroxysms. In a paroxysm, the patient may produce up to a dozen short coughs with no intervening inspiration; cyanosis and vomiting often occur. Finally, after perhaps expelling some thick mucus from the bronchial tree, a desperate inspiration through a narrowed glottis produces the characteristic whoop. This phase continues for up to 4 weeks and then gradually subsides; nonparoxysmal cough may persist for as long as 6 months. Pertussis is one of the most contagious of the infectious diseases, and is a significant health problem worldwide, with more than 60 million cases and 500,000 to 600,000 deaths annually (356).

Pertussis can be an important cause of respiratory disease in adults (357–364), who experience a less severe syndrome marked by a debilitating cough that persists for many months. One quarter to one fifth of adults with persistent cough have laboratory evidence of recent pertussis infection (365,366). Several hospital outbreaks have been reported in which staff members became infected by symptomatic patients and subsequently spread disease to other patients and adult contacts (367–373), and studies have demonstrated both the prevalence and incidence of pertussis among healthcare workers (374–376). Unfortunately, adverse reactions to conventional whole-cell pertussis vaccine are common and severe among adults; for example, significant local reactions were noted in as many as 97% of adult recipients of whole-cell pertussis vaccine in one hospital outbreak (368). Because standard pertussis vaccine is not given beyond age 6, antibody wanes with age, and adolescents and adults become increasingly susceptible to pertussis. In turn, they act as a reservoir of disease able to expose and infect infants not yet immunized (376–378). These factors are thought to be important in the current epidemic of pertussis: there were 7,796 cases of pertussis reported in 1996, the highest total in nearly 30 years (379, 380).

Acellular pertussis (aP) vaccines have been developed that are licensed for use in children and that appear to be safe and immunogenic in adults (381–385). If they become licensed for adult use, as is likely within a few years, employee health programs should utilize tetanus-diphtheria acellular pertussis (TdaP) rather than Td for booster immunizations. Meanwhile, in the event of a nosocomial outbreak, consideration can be given to the provision (with informed consent) of a half-dose of pediatric TdaP vaccine to at-risk workers (386–388).

Droplet Precautions should be used when managing known or suspected pertussis infection. Erythromycin or its more recent derivatives (e.g., azithromycin) can be used for prophylaxis of exposed healthcare workers and others (373), but may fail (389); work restrictions are appropriate for symptomatic employees (341,390).

Streptococcus

Streptococcus pyogenes (group A *Streptococcus*) is one of the most common and dangerous bacterial pathogens. Group A streptococci colonize the throats of 15% to 20% of schoolchildren; anal, vaginal, scalp, and other cutaneous carriage also occurs. The microorganism commonly causes acute pharyngitis and cutaneous infections, including erysipelas, and was the most common cause of puerperal sepsis in the days before Semmelweis. The group A streptococcus can cause fatal deep infections, including pneumonia, sepsis, myositis, and necrotizing fasciitis, and it can cause nonsuppurative sequelae, including rheumatic fever and nephritis (391).

Streptococcal toxins are responsible for streptococcal toxic shock syndrome and for scarlet fever (second disease, the only classic exanthematous disease of childhood caused by a bacterium). Most reported nosocomial outbreaks of group A streptococcal disease have involved transmission from healthcare workers to patients, resulting in wound (392) or skin and soft tissue (393) infections. Healthcare workers can acquire colonization or infection of the pharynx or of the skin (particularly at wound sites). During a recent 3-year period, the CDC received reports of ten nosocomial clusters of invasive group A streptococcal infection involving spread to healthcare workers, resulting in toxic shock, pneumonia, cellulitis, lymphangitis, and pharyngitis (394–396).

Group A streptococcus is spread readily by contact, by respiratory droplets, and by contaminated common sources such as food and drink (396). Reports have also apparently documented the airborne spread of group A streptococci (15), but such events are probably rare. Contact precautions should be used for persons with purulent wound infections (including burns), unless the infections are minor and well contained by bandages. Droplet precautions should be implemented for management of patients with group A streptococcal respiratory tract infection, including pharyngitis, pneumonia, or scarlet fever (which is most commonly associated with pharyngeal infection). Standard Precautions, including careful hand washing, remain essential (see Chapters 21 and 31), and should be supplemented with Contact Precautions when dealing with major infected skin wounds and with Droplet Precautions when dealing with pharyngitis, pneumonia, or scarlet fever in infants and young children (26). Infected workers with draining lesions should be excluded and treated, as should asymptomatic carriers who have been epidemiologically implicated in transmission (113,397,398).

Pneumococcus

Streptococcus pneumoniae is a major cause of bacterial pneumonia, sinusitis, otitis, and meningitis, and can cause a host of other serious infections. Previously uniformly susceptible to penicillin, pneumococci increasingly manifest reduced susceptibility or resistance to penicillin, erythromycin, and even third-generation cephalosporins (399–401). Unlike group A streptococci, pneumococci elaborate few toxins; their ability to cause disease resides in their capacity to reproduce in host tissues and to stimulate a vigorous inflammatory response.

The pneumococcus colonizes the nasopharynx in 5% to 10% of adults and 20% to 40% of children (402). Infection is seasonal, increasing in the winter months, and more likely at the extremes of age. Outbreaks of pneumococcal disease usually occur in circumstances of prolonged close contact (403–408) and are uncommon but not unprecedented in hospitals (408); several nursing home outbreaks have been documented (409–413). Spread is by respiratory droplet but, as noted, usually requires prolonged close contact. In most cases, Standard Precautions will be sufficient, but Droplet Precautions are recommended when the infecting pneumococcus is resistant to antibiotics.

Healthcare workers are not a group recommended to receive the present polysaccharide polyvalent pneumococcal vaccine. Conjugate pneumococcal vaccines, which link the capsular polysaccharide to a carrier protein and thereby stimulate the T-cell–dependent arm of the immune system, are used routinely in young children (413).

Meningococcus

Neisseria meningitidis has a fearsome reputation as the causative agent of epidemic cerebrospinal fever and, indeed, is capable of producing rapidly fatal sepsis or meningitis. However, the microorganism is not nearly as communicable as fables (and television) portray. Epidemics of meningococcal disease occur throughout the world, and transmission undoubtedly occurs with prolonged close contact (414,415). Household or other close contacts are at 200 to 1,000 times the risk of developing meningococcal disease as is the general public (416); secondary attack rates in households average 2% to 5% (414). However, although nosocomial (414,417–420) and laboratory-based (421) transmission have occurred, such transmission is distinctly unusual and appears to be more likely to occur with meningococcal pneumonia (417–419) than with meningitis or sepsis (414).

Transmission is by respiratory droplets, and Droplet Precautions are appropriate for patients with invasive meningococcal disease, particularly pneumonia, until 24 hours after institution of effective therapy. Chemoprophylaxis should be offered to workers having prolonged close contact or contact with respiratory secretions without appropriate barrier protection and might consist of orally administered ofloxacin (or equivalent), 400 mg once, or rifampin, 600 mg twice daily for 2 days. Healthcare workers are not a group recommended to receive the present polysaccharide meningococcal vaccine. However, future combination vaccines incorporating conjugate pneumococcal and meningococcal antigens will probably become available, and such vaccines may become recommended for healthcare workers (see Chapter 47).

Haemophilus influenzae

Haemophilus influenzae is a gram-negative bacillus indigenous to humans, commonly carried in the pharynx and, less often, the conjunctivae and genital tract. In past years, *H. influenzae* type b (Hib) was the most common cause of meningitis among children between 1 month and 2 years of age. However, following licensure of the conjugate Hib vaccines (422), invasive Hib disease among children has virtually disappeared (423). Pneumonia caused by *H. influenzae* occurs among adults but tends to be restricted to those with lung disease, alcoholism, or other compromise. Nosocomial outbreaks of type b and nontypable *H. influenzae* have been reported (424–428), but spread to healthcare workers appears to be unlikely. Use of Droplet Precautions for patients with invasive *H. influenzae* infections is recommended to prevent spread of the microorganism to other patients, particularly unimmunized children, the elderly, and the immunocompromised.

Plague

> The hand of the Lord was against the city with a very great destruction: and he smote the men of the city, both small and great, and they had emerods in their secret parts.1st Samuel 5:9

Yersinia pestis, the causative microorganism of plague, is a gram-negative bacillus that is zoonotic among rodents. Although some of the pestilences described in First Samuel and other books of the Bible may have been the disease we now know as plague, the first epidemic ascribed with confidence to that disease was the Great Epidemic of Justinian, which took the lives of 25% of the population of the Roman Empire in 542 A.D. (429). Two more great epidemics swept the world in the 14th (the "Black Death") and late 19th (the "Bombay Plague") centuries. In modern times, plague persists in endemic foci in the western U.S., Southeast Asia, east Africa, and South America. In the U.S., 362 cases of human plague were reported from 1944 to 1993. The disease is slowly becoming more widespread and, in the last decade, has been reported from Texas, Oklahoma, and every contiguous state in or west of the Rockies. As suburban development has extended, the household has become the most common site of exposure, and domestic cats allowed to roam in endemic areas have become important sources of transmission to cat owners and veterinarians (430).

There are three distinct forms of plague. Bubonic plague is characterized by markedly swollen and tender inguinal, axillary, or other lymph nodes (buboes), and is typically spread by the bite of a flea (or similar pest). Bubonic plague commonly eventuates in sepsis. However, septicemia can occur directly, without development of a bubo, and is called septicemic plague. Finally, pulmonary involvement permits direct human-to-human spread of the disease, causing pneumonic plague. In the absence of prompt antibiotic therapy, fatality rates for bubonic, septicemic, and pneumonic plague are 70%, 100%, and 100%, respectively; even with antibiotics, 33% of patients with septicemic plague die, three times the rate of those with bubonic plague (431). The outbreak of pneumonic plague in India in late 1994 served as a reminder that the disease remains dangerous; of 276 persons hospitalized in the first 3 weeks of the outbreak with a diagnosis of plague, 56 (20%) died (432).

Pneumonic plague is spread by respiratory droplets. Because any case of plague may progress to pulmonic involvement, all patients with plague should be placed on Droplet Precautions until the patient has received an effective antibiotic for 24 to 48 hours (433); persons known to have respiratory tract disease should remain on Droplet Precautions for at least 72 hours following initiation of effective therapy. Care should be taken with laboratory specimens not to create aerosols, but otherwise they may be handled normally (see Chapter 47).

Brucellosis

Brucellosis is a zoonosis due to any of several species of *Brucella.* Like typhoid fever, brucellosis is an enteric fever characterized by fever (undulant if untreated), malaise, headache, and possibly, lymphadenopathy, visceromegaly, and depression; most organ systems can become involved. Nearly all cases occur in persons with close contact with infected animals. Airborne transmission in the laboratory (434,435) is a potential problem if proper safeguards are not followed (see Chapter 82), and transmission to nurses and physicians caring for infected patients has occurred (435) but is rare. Standard Precautions are sufficient to prevent transmission during clinical care.

Legionellosis

Nosocomial outbreaks of legionellosis (either pneumonia or Pontiac fever) attributable to environmental sources have been reported on multiple occasions, as detailed in Chapter 35. Although the exposure of staff members to these environmental sources is often similar to that of patients, overt disease is rare among staff members even when common among patients, reflecting the relationship between pulmonary or other compromise and development of clinical disease. Nonetheless, serologic surveys of hospital staff members support the hypothesis that subclinical or mild disease occurs among healthy staff members in an outbreak resulting from an environmental source (436–438). Despite suggestions in the early literature (436), no good evidence supports person-to-person spread of *Legionella* infection, and cautious prior CDC recommendations for "secretion" precautions (439) have been withdrawn; Standard Precautions suffice (26).

Bacterial Diseases Spread by Contact

Staphylococcus aureus

Staphylococcus aureus is a gram-positive microorganism that intermittently colonizes normal human skin and, particularly, the nares. The microorganism is hardy and survives well on environmental surfaces. Healthy mucous membranes and skin are adept at preventing invasion by *S. aureus,* but a break allows invasion that can lead to serious local, metastatic, or systemic infection. The increasing prominence of methicillin-resistant *S. aureus* (MRSA) has heightened concern among clinicians, infection control workers, and other staff members.

Colonization with *S. aureus* becomes more likely as exposure and opportunities increase (440). Colonization of healthcare workers with MRSA is likely in direct proportion to its prevalence in their environment (441,442), except when contact precautions are followed (443). In turn, the likelihood that healthy workers will acquire staphylococcal infection of minor wounds, or that staphylococci will invade through minor wounds to cause serious illness, increases with their prevalence of carriage (440, 444–446).

Spread of staphylococci is almost exclusively by direct and indirect contact, notwithstanding demonstration of the possibility of airborne spread (447,448). Prevention of spread depends on scrupulous attention to Standard Precautions supplemented by Contact Precautions when environmental contamination is likely (e.g., staphylococcal scalded skin syndrome; exfoliative dermatitis; furunculosis, especially in children; infected burns, especially if large) or when dealing with MRSA (see Chapters 28 and 29).

Vancomycin-Resistant Enterococcus

Infection control workers who once had MRSA nightmares now dream about vancomycin-resistant *Enterococcus* (VRE). Indeed, VRE is a legitimate source of anxiety (see Chapter 32), and it can be transmitted readily from patient to patient on the hands of healthcare workers, but it poses no personal threat to the workers themselves.

Syphilis

Treponema pallidum, the causative agent of syphilis, is a spirochete for which humans are the only known natural host. The microorganism causes a complex and chronic infection that begins with the primary skin or mucosal lesion (chancre), progresses to secondary dissemination throughout the body, and then becomes latent. Ten to 30 years later, 10% to 20% of patients with untreated disease will progress to tertiary disease with cardiovascular, neurologic, gummatous, or other complications (449).

T. pallidum is a fragile microorganism that survives poorly apart from the body. Transmission is by contact with the chancre, mucous patches, condylomata lata, nasal discharge of babies congenitally infected, or other moist sources in primary and secondary stages of the disease. Prior to the routine use of gloves, primary infection of the hands of physicians and other healthcare workers was occasionally recognized (450), but such events are now exceedingly rare (451,452). Standard Precautions are sufficient to prevent transmission.

Gonorrhea

Neisseria gonorrhoeae, the causative agent of gonorrhea, is a gram-negative diplococcus that primarily infects columnar or cuboidal epithelium. Consequently, the major risk of nosocomial transmission to healthcare workers involves conjunctivitis, usually due to inoculation of the eye by a contaminated finger. Although pharyngeal infection occurs, subsequent respiratory transmission does not appear to be a concern. The skin lesions of disseminated gonococcal infection rarely contain viable microorganisms (451).

Unwitting transmission to a healthcare worker is most likely in association with unrecognized disease in patients admitted for other reasons. A particular concern is gonococcal ophthalmia neonatorum, which may occur despite prophylaxis and may remain unrecognized for days. Once again, Standard Precautions are sufficient to prevent transmission (see Chapter 26).

FUNGAL INFECTIONS

With rare exceptions, fungi are not transmitted from person to person, and healthy workers are not at risk of acquiring fungal infection from patients. Of the deep fungal infections, histoplasmosis, blastomycosis, and coccidioidomycosis have caused outbreaks among healthy persons, but workers in healthcare institutions are no more likely to be involved in such outbreaks than workers in other kinds of facilities in the same geographic area.

Symptomatic infection with *Cryptococcus, Aspergillus,* or *Mucorales* rarely or never occurs in normal hosts, and in any event, the microorganisms are abundant in nature. However, *Coccidioides* (and perhaps others of the dimorphic fungi) can germinate and grow in the filamentous form if patient drainage is left undisturbed for several days in bandages and casts; once aerial structures have developed, they are capable of releasing infectious spores (453). Otherwise healthy workers can become sensitized to *Aspergillus* antigens and experience allergic bronchopulmonary aspergillosis when exposed to air from, for example, contaminated humidifiers (one possible cause of "sick building syndrome"), but healthcare workers are not at particularly elevated risk of such exposures.

Sporotrichosis, chromomycosis, or mycetoma could be transmitted by means of a contaminated sharps injury, but neither airborne nor contact spread is plausible. *Candida* is a normal human commensal that can cause opportunistic illness (e.g., thrush, vaginal candidiasis) in otherwise healthy persons, but such infections are usually endogenous. Person-to-person transmission occurs on rare occasions (e.g., newborn thrush, balanitis), but the usual circumstances are not applicable to healthcare workers.

The fungal infections most readily transmitted from person to healthy person are the dermatophytoses, as we are repeatedly reminded by the advertisements for athlete's foot tonics. Although rare, nosocomial outbreaks of ringworm and other dermatophyte infections have occurred and involved staff members (454,455). Standard Precautions should be sufficient to prevent spread of fungal infections to the healthy worker.

PROTOZOAL AND PARASITIC INFECTIONS

Amebiasis, giardiasis, cryptosporidiosis, isosporosis, microsporidiosis, enterobiasis, hymenolepiasis, strongyloidiasis, and many of the other diseases caused by intestinal protozoa and helminths are transmitted by the fecal-oral route and, thus, could be transmitted by contact between a patient and an unwary worker. Proper attention to standard precautions and hand washing will prevent such infections. Certain of the blood and tissue parasites are well known to be transmitted to healthcare workers by needlestick (especially malaria, but leishmania, trypanosomiasis, or babesiosis could be transmitted similarly), through laboratory accidents (especially toxoplasmosis), or through other blood-to-blood exposures (456), but otherwise, person-to-person transmission does not occur (457). Transmission of trichomoniasis from patient to patient by contaminated fomites is possible, but the requisite genital contact should not occur among staff.

Pneumocystis carinii is a protozoan (or perhaps fungus) that appears to be ubiquitous, because 70% to 80% of children have antibodies by age 4 years (458). Transmission appears to be by air, and several nosocomial outbreaks have been reported (458, 459). Nonetheless, immunocompetent workers are not at risk (nor are most immunocompromised workers, because they already carry the microorganism, but such workers should avoid exposure). Standard Precautions are sufficient for all these infections.

The parasites with demonstrated ability to cause nosocomial outbreaks involving staff and patients are the ectoparasites. Nosocomial transfer of pediculosis (head, body, or pubic lice) is possible, but unlikely, because sharing of clothing or bedding (or direct pubic contact) is generally required for transmission (460). In contrast, numerous nosocomial outbreaks of scabies have occurred (460–464), and such outbreaks can be widespread and persistent. *Sarcoptes scabiei,* the itch mite, burrows into the skin and lays eggs; sensitization to mite antigens leads to intense pruritus. Disease is transmitted by direct or indirect contact. Infestation in the normal host involves one to two dozen mites; immunocompromised hosts [e.g., those with alcoholism, Down syndrome, leprosy, or acquired immune deficiency syndrome (AIDS)] can develop "Norwegian" or crusted scabies marked by proliferation of thousands of mites, resulting in hyperkeratotic and crusted skin. Such persons are highly contagious. Management of a nosocomial outbreak is difficult and stressful (461–469). If infestation is widespread, all potentially involved persons must be treated simultaneously (within 24 to 48 hours) on two occasions 1 week apart, and all routes of indirect contact (laundry, shared lockers, etc.) must be identified and managed. Fortunately, the mite survives only 48 hours outside the body, permitting decontamination of fomites by storage. Prevention largely depends on a high index of suspicion regarding dermatitis, particularly in immunocompromised patients. Those patients known or suspected to have scabies should be managed with Contact Precautions until properly treated.

Several nosocomial outbreaks of infestations caused by pigeon mites have been reported. The disease can mimic scabies, but unlike the itch mite, the pigeon mite can survive for months between meals (460). Workers or, more often, patients can become infested, usually through proximity to ducts, air conditioners, or cracks that lead to pigeon roosts.

Myiasis is seen not uncommonly as a presenting condition in inner-city emergency rooms and can occur as a nosocomial infestation of wounds or mucus membranes. However, transmission to workers is not possible (see Chapter 46).

NONINFECTIOUS DISEASES

Some diseases are spread to healthcare workers by air or by contact but are not infectious. These diseases fall into two principal categories: allergic and toxic.

Diseases Caused by Allergic Reactions

Serious allergic reactions to latex are increasingly being recognized among patients and staff (465–480). An estimated 7% of surgeons and 35% of spina bifida patients have immunoglobulin E (IgE) antibodies to latex. Numerous allergic reactions have been reported, many severe, and several healthcare workers have had to leave practice. For highly sensitized workers, direct contact with latex is not required; anaphylaxis has been induced when someone nearby changed gloves (471). Early signs of sensitization to latex should prompt an immediate switch to vinyl or other gloves before such extreme sensitization occurs. (See Chapter 99).

Hypersensitivity pneumonitis can occur in response to numerous fungi and likely to bacterial components as well (481); such reactions may be important in certain cases of "sick building syndrome." Numerous outbreaks of infection attributed to airborne or droplet dispersal of bacteria by humidifiers and air handling systems have occurred among patients who are susceptible because of intubation, presence of wounds, indwelling devices, and so on (448,482–485). Infection of healthy staff by such routes is not known to occur, but the potential for hypersensitivity pneumonitis exists. Prevention depends on proper attention to maintenance and sterile precautions.

Finally, workers highly sensitized to certain drugs can be at risk from exposure to those drugs; for example, the simple flushing of a syringe containing penicillin might adversely affect a worker with high-level penicillin allergy. Employees of pharmaceutical manufacturers have had allergic reactions to drug dusts, but fortunately, modern-day hospital pharmacists do not use mortar and pestle nearly as often as their predecessors.

Diseases Caused by Toxic Exposures

Healthcare workers are exposed to a remarkable variety of chemicals that are known to be toxic by the contact or respiratory routes; ethylene oxide, glutaraldehyde, formaldehyde, xylene, chemotherapeutic agents, pentamidine, ribavirin, and anesthetic gases are among the substances with known toxic potential, most of which are subject to regulation by the Occupational Safety and Health Administration (OSHA). Depending on the substance, workers must be provided with appropriate training and personal protection, material safety data sheets must be provided, warning labels must be displayed, environmental and personal exposure levels must be monitored, and proper disposal must be ensured. Because many of these toxic substances are pertinent to infection control, the infection control worker should be familiar with the staff and operations of the industrial safety program of the institution.

ORGANIZATIONAL ISSUES

Special Populations

Specific policies should be developed to address certain sensitive issues: (a) healthcare workers infected with HIV (see Chapter 79); (b) workers with chronic infectious hepatitis (see Chapter 78); (c) workers with immune compromise, of whatever cause (see Chapters 57–60 and 79); and (d) pregnant employees. Pregnant employees often object to providing care to patients with selected infections out of fear that doing so will pose a risk to the fetus. This concern is almost never justified, and pregnant employees should not be routinely excluded from care of any

TABLE 81.1. SUMMARY OF ADVISORY COMMITTEE ON IMMUNIZATION. PRACTICES (ACIP) RECOMMENDATIONS ON IMMUNIZATION OF HEALTHCARE WORKERS WITH SPECIAL CONDITIONS (MODIFIED FROM ACIP RECOMMENDATIONS).

Vaccine	Diabetes	Pregnancy	HIV Infection	Alcoholic Cirrhosis	Severe Immunosuppression[a]	Alcoholism Asplenia	Renal Failure
BCG	UI	C	C	UI	UI	UI	UI
Hepatitis A	UI	UI	UI	UI	UI	UI	R[b]
Hepatitis B	R	R	R	R	R	R	R
Influenza	R[c]	R	R	R	R	R	R
Measles, mumps, rubella	C	R§	C	R	R	R	R
Meningococcus	UI	UI	UI	R[d]	UI	UI	UI
Polio, IPV[e]	UI	UI	UI	UI	UI	UI	UI
Polio, OPV[e]	UI	C	C	UI	UI	UI	UI
Pneumococcus†	UI	R	R	R	R	R	R
Rabies	UI	UI	UI	UI	UI	UI	UI
Tetanus/diphtheria†	R	R	R	R	R	R	R
Typhoid, inactivated & Vi	UI	UI	UI	UI	UI	UI	UI
Typhoid, Ty21a	UI	C	C	UI	UI	UI	UI
Varicella	C	C	C	R	R	R	R
Vaccinia	UI	C	C	UI	UI	UI	UI

BCG, bacille Calmette-Guérin; C, contraindicated; IPV, poliovirus vaccine inactivated; OPC, poliovirus vaccine live oral; R, recommended; UI,use if indicated.
[a] Severe immunosuppression can be the result of congenital immunodeficiency, leukemia, lymphoma, generalized malignancy or therapy with alkylating agents, antimetabolites, radiation, or large amounts of corticosteroids.
[b] Recommendation is based on the person's underlying condition rather than occupation.
[c] Women who will be in the second or third trimester of pregnancy during influenza season.
[d] Contraindicated in persons with human immunodeficiency virus infection and severe immunosuppression; see text.
[e] Vaccination is recommended for unvaccinated healthcare workers who have close contact with patients who may be excreting wild polioviruses. Primary vaccination with IPV is recommended because the risk for vaccine-associated paralysis after administration of OPV is higher among adults than among children. Healthcare workers who have had a primary series of OPV or IPV who are directly involved with the provision of care to patients who may be excreting poliovirus may receive another dose of either IPV or OPV. Any suspected case of poliomyelitis should be investigated immediately. If evidence suggests transmission of wild poliovirus, control measures to contain further transmission should be instituted immediately, including an OPV vaccination campaign.
From Bolyard EA, Tablan OC, Williams WW, et al., and the Hospital Infection Control Practices Advisory Committee. Guideline for infection control in healthcare personnel, 1998. *Infect Control Hosp Epidemiol* 1998;19:407–463.

particular patients (110). On the other hand, women who are or might become pregnant should be counseled concerning the importance of complying with established precautions, particularly when dealing with patients infected with agents having known potential for complicating pregnancy (110,486). Vaccination recommendations for special populations of healthcare workers are summarized in Table 81.1.

Vaccination Program

Organization of the employee health service is detailed in Chapter 99, and we will not duplicate that material here except to stress the importance of a comprehensive and well-documented vaccination program. The employee health service should maintain a vaccination registry that documents all vaccinations ever received by all employees; the value of these data in the event of an exposure event or outbreak is enormous. In addition, the institution should, in its own self-interest, ensure up-to-date vaccination (or documented immunity) of all employees with respect to diphtheria, tetanus, hepatitis B, measles, mumps, rubella, varicella, and influenza. Other vaccines may be indicated for certain employees (e.g., laboratory researchers or those working in special units), and if indicated should be provided at no cost, such as vaccinia, rabies, hepatitis A, polio, and typhoid (see also Chapter 80).

SUGGESTED READINGS

The topics of this chapter have been the subject of several recent comprehensive reviews or guidelines (26,110,486–488), which may provide additional information.

REFERENCES

1. Brachman PS. Epidemiology of nosocomial infections. In: Bennett JV, Brachman PS, eds. *Hospital infections,* 3rd ed. Boston/Toronto/London: Little, Brown, 1992:3–20.
2. Winslow CEA. *Conquest of epidemic diseases.* Princeton, NJ: Princeton University Press, 1943.
3. Riley RL. Historical background. *Ann NY Acad Sci* 1980;353:3–9.
4. Chapin CV. *Sources and modes of infection.* New York: John Wiley, 1910.
5. Wells WF. On air-borne infection. Study II. Droplets and droplet nuclei. *Am J Hyg* 1934;20:611–618.
6. Wells WF, Wells MW, Wilder TS. The environmental control of epidemic contagion. I. An epidemiologic study of radiant disinfection of air in day schools. *Am J Hyg* 1942;35:97–121.
7. Riley RL, Mills CC, Nyka W, et al. Aerial dissemination of pulmonary tuberculosis: a two-year study of contagion in a tuberculosis ward. *Am J Hyg* 1959;70:185–196.
8. Riley RL, Mills CC, O'Grady F, et al. Infectiousness of air from a tuberculosis ward. Ultraviolet irradiation of infected air: comparative infectiousness of different patients. *Am Rev Respir Dis* 1962;84: 511–525.
9. Potter J, Stott DJ, Roberts MA, et al. Influenza vaccination of health

care workers in long-term-care hospitals reduces the mortality of elderly patients. *J Infect Dis* 1997;175:1–6.

10. Muchmore HG, Felton FG, Scott LV. A confirmed hospital epidemic of Asian Influenza. *J Okla State Med Assoc* 1960;53:142–145.
11. Blumenfeld HL, Kilborne ED, Louria DB, et al. Studies on influenza in the pandemic of 1957–1958. I. An epidemiologic, clinical, and serologic investigation of an intrahospital epidemic, with a note on vaccination efficacy. *J Clin Invest* 1959;38:199–212.
12. Centers for Disease Control. Influenza A in a hospital—Illinois. *MMWR* 1981;30:79–80,85.
13. Hammond GW, Cheang M. Absenteeism among hospital staff during an influenza epidemic: implications for immunoprophylaxis. *Can Med Assoc J* 1984;131:449–452.
14. Bean B, Rhame FS, Hughes RS, et al. Influenza B: hospital activity during a community epidemic. *Diagn Microbiol Infect Dis* 1983;1: 177–183.
15. Robertson OH. Air-borne infection. *Science* 1943;97:495–502.
16. Adal KA, Flowers RH, Anglim AM, et al. Prevention of nosocomial influenza. *Infect Control Hosp Epidemiol* 1996;17:641–648.
17. Nichol KL, Hauge M. Influenza vaccination of healthcare workers. *Infect Control Hosp Epidemiol* 1997;18:189–194.
18. Harbarth S, Siegrist C-A, Schira J-C, et al. Influenza immunization: improving compliance of healthcare workers. *Infect Control Hosp Epidemiol* 1998;19:337–342.
19. Valenti WM, Menegus MA. Nosocomial viral infections: IV. Guidelines for cohort isolation, the communicable disease survey, collection and transport of specimens for virus isolation, and considerations for the future. *Infect Control* 1981;2:236–245.
20. Ong AKY, Srimanunthipol J, Frankel RI. Influenza vaccination status of healthcare workers and the extent of their domestic contact with individuals at high risk for influenza-related complications. *Infect Control Hosp Epidemiol* 2000;21:735–737.
21. Moisiuk SE, Robson D, Klass L, et al. Outbreak of parainfluenza virus type 3 in an intermediate care neonatal nursery. *Pediatr Infect Dis J* 1998;17:49–53.
22. Singh-Naz N, Willy M, Riggs N. Outbreak of parainfluenza virus type 3 in a neonatal nursery. *Pediatr Infect Dis J* 1990;9:31–33.
23. Falsey AR. Noninfluenza respiratory virus infection in long-term care facilities. *Infect Control Hosp Epidemiol* 1991;12:602–608.
24. Hall CB. Hospital-acquired pneumonia in children: the role of respiratory viruses. *Semin Respir Infect* 1987;2:48–56.
25. Brady MT, Evans J, Cuartas J. Survival and disinfection of parainfluenza viruses on environmental surfaces. *Am J Infect Control* 1990;18: 18–23.
26. Garner JS, Hospital Infection Control Practices Advisory Committee. Guideline for isolation precautions in hospitals. *Infect Control Hosp Epidemiol* 1996;17:53–80.
27. Chanock RM, Kim HW, Vargosko AJ, et al. Respiratory syncytial virus I. Virus recovery and other observations during 1960 outbreak of bronchiolitis, pneumonia, and minor respiratory diseases in children. *JAMA* 1961;176:647–652.
28. Hall CB. Nosocomial viral respiratory infections: perennial weeds on pediatric wards. *Am J Med* 1981;70:670–676.
29. Chanock RM, McIntosh K, Murphy BR, et al. Respiratory syncytial virus. In: Evans AS, ed. *Viral infections of humans: epidemiology and control,* 3rd ed. New York and London: Plenum, 1991:525–544.
30. Hall CB, Douglas RGJ, Geiman JM, et al. Nosocomial respiratory syncytial virus infections. *N Engl J Med* 1975;293:1343–1346.
31. Valenti WM, Clarke TA, Hall CB, et al. Concurrent outbreaks of rhinovirus and respiratory syncytial virus in an intensive care nursery: epidemiology and associated risk factors. *J Pediatr* 1982;100: 722–726.
32. Guidry GG, Black-Payne CA, Payne DK, et al. Respiratory syncytial virus infection among intubated adults in a university medical intensive care unit. *Chest* 1991;100:1377–1384.
33. Takimoto CH, Cram DL, Root RK. Respiratory syncytial virus infections on an adult medical ward [see comments]. *Arch Intern Med* 1991;151:706–708.
34. Englund JA, Anderson LJ, Rhame FS. Nosocomial transmission of respiratory syncytial virus in immunocompromised adults. *J Clin Microbiol* 1991;29:115–119.
35. Harrington RD, Hooton TM, Hackman RC, et al. An outbreak of respiratory syncytial virus in a bone marrow transplant center. *J Infect Dis* 1992;165:987–993.
36. Agah R, Cherry JD, Garakian AJ, et al. Respiratory syncytial virus (RSV) infection rate in personnel caring for children with RSV infections. Routine isolation procedure vs routine procedure supplemented by use of masks and goggles. *Am J Dis Child* 1987;141:695–697.
37. Hall CB. Respiratory syncytial virus: its transmission in the hospital environment. *Yale J Biol Med* 1982;55:219–223.
38. Gala CL, Hall CB, Schnabel KC, et al. The use of eye-nose goggles to control nosocomial respiratory syncytial virus infection. *JAMA* 1986;256:2706–2708.
39. Leclair JM, Freeman J, Sullivan BF, et al. Prevention of nosocomial respiratory syncytial virus infections through compliance with glove and gown isolation precautions. *N Engl J Med* 1987;317:329–334.
40. Snydman DR, Greer C, Meissner HC, et al. Prevention of nosocomial transmission of respiratory syncytial virus in a newborn nursery. *Infect Control Hosp Epidemiol* 1988;9:105–108.
41. Monto AS. Acute respiratory infections. In: Last JM, Wallace RB, eds. *Maxcy-Rosenau-Last public health and preventive medicine,* 13th ed. Norwalk, CT: Appleton & Lange, 1992:125–130.
42. Dawson C, Darrell R. Infections due to adenovirus type 8 in the United States. I. An outbreak of epidemic keratoconjunctivitis originating in a physician's office. *N Engl J Med* 1963;268:1031–1034.
43. Laibson PR, Ortolan G, Duprt-Strachan S. Community and hospital outbreak of epidemic keratoconjunctivitis. *Arch Ophthalmol* 1968;80: 467–473.
44. Wegman DH, Guinee VF, Millian SJ. Epidemic keratoconjunctivitis. *Am J Public Health* 1970;60:1230–1237.
45. Keenlyside RA, Hierholzer JC, D'Angelo LJ. Keratoconjunctivitis associated with adenovirus type 37: an extended outbreak in an ophthalmologist's office. *J Infect Dis* 1983;147:191–198.
46. Warren D, Nelson KE, Farrar JA, et al. A large outbreak of epidemic keratoconjunctivitis: problems in controlling nosocomial spread. *J Infect Dis* 1989;160:938–943.
47. Takeuchi R, Nomura Y, Kojima M, et al. A nosocomial outbreak of epidemic keratoconjunctivitis due to adenovirus type 37. *Microbiol Immunol* 1990;34:749–754.
48. Rosenbach KA, Nadiminti V, Vincent AL, et al. An outbreak of adenoviral keratoconjunctivitis. *Infect Med* 2002;19:436–438.
49. Levandowski RA, Rubenis M. Nosocomial conjunctivitis caused by adenovirus type 4. *J Infect Dis* 1981;143:28–31.
50. Straube RC, Thompson MA, Van Dyke RB, et al. Adenovirus type 7b in a children's hospital. *J Infect Dis* 1983;147:814–819.
51. Finn A, Anday E, Talbot GH. An epidemic of adenovirus 7a infection in a neonatal nursery: course, morbidity, and management. *Infect Control Hosp Epidemiol* 1988;9:398–404.
52. Porter JD, Teter M, Traister V, et al. Outbreak of adenoviral infections in a long-term pediatric facility, New Jersey, 1986/87. *J Hosp Infect* 1991;18:201–210.
53. Singh-Naz N, Brown M, Ganeshanathan M. Nosocomial adenovirus infection: molecular epidemiology of an outbreak. *Pediatr Infect Dis J* 1993;12:922–925.
54. Uemura T, Kawashitam T, Ostuka Y, et al. A recent outbreak of adenovirus type 7 infection in a chronic inpatient facility for the severely handicapped. *Infect Control Hosp Epidemiol* 2000;21: 559–560.
55. Brummitt CF, Cherrington JM, Katzenstein DA, et al. Nosocomial adenovirus infections: molecular epidemiology of an outbreak due to adenovirus 3a. *J Infect Dis* 1988;158:423–432.
56. Gwaltney JM Jr. Rhinoviruses. In: Evans AS, ed. *Viral infections of humans: epidemiology and control,* 3rd ed. New York and London: Plenum, 1991:593–616.
57. Wald TG, Shult P, Krause P, et al. A rhinovirus outbreak among residents of a long-term care facility. *Ann Intern Med* 1995;123: 588–593.
58. Nicholson KG, Baker DJ, Gaquhar A, et al. Acute upper respiratory

tract viral illness and influenza immunization in homes for the elderly. *Epidemiol Infect* 1990;105:609–618.

59. Peiris JSM, Yuen KY, Osterhaus ADME, et al. The severe acute respiratory syndrome. *N Engl J Med* 2003;349:2431–2441.
60. Avendano M, Derkach P, Swan S. Clinical course and management of SARS in health care workers in Toronto: a case series. *Can Med Assoc J* 2003;168:1649–1660.
61. Varia, M, Wilson S, Sarwal S, et al. Investigation of a Nosocomial outbreak of severe acute respiratory syndrome (SARS) in Toronto, Canada. *Can Med Assoc J* 2003;169:285–292.
62. Scales DC, Green K, Chan AK, et al. Illness in intensive care staff after brief exposure to severe acute respiratory syndrome. *Emerging Infect Dis* 2003;9:1205–1210.
63. Ho AS, Sung JJY, Chan-Yeung M. An outbreak of severe acute respiratory syndrome among hospital workers in a community hospital in Hong Kong. *Ann Intern Med* 2003;139:564–567.
64. Seto WH, Tsang D, Yung RWH, et al. Effectiveness of precautions against droplets and contact in prevention of Nosocomial transmission of severe acute respiratory syndrome (SARS). *Lancet* 2003;361: 1519–1520.
65. Melnick JL. Enteroviruses. In: Evans AS, ed. *Viral infections of humans: epidemiology and control,* 3rd ed. New York and London: Plenum, 1991:191–263.
66. Moore M. From the Centers for Disease Control: Enteroviral disease in the United States, 1970–1979. *J Infect Dis* 1982;146:103–108.
67. Helfand RF, Khan AS, Pallansch MA, et al. Echovirus 30 infection and aseptic meningitis in parents of children attending a child care center. *J Infect Dis* 1994;169:1133–1137.
68. Brightman VJ, Scott TF, Westphal M, et al. An outbreak of coxsackie B-5 virus infection in a newborn nursery. *J Pediatr* 1966;69:179–192.
69. Reiss-Levy E, Baker A, Don N, et al. Two concurrent epidemics of enteroviral meningitis in an obstetric neonatal unit. *Aust NZ J Med* 1986;16:365–372.
70. Modlin JF. Perinatal echovirus infection: insights from a literature review of 61 cases of serious infection and 16 outbreaks in nurseries. *Rev Infect Dis* 1986;8:918–926.
71. Johnston JM, Burke JP. Nosocomial outbreak of hand-foot-and-mouth disease among operating suite personnel. *Infect Control* 1986; 7:172–176.
72. Centers for Disease Control. Certification of poliomyelitis eradication—the Americas, 1994. *MMWR* 1994;43:720–722.
73. Nkowane BM, Wassilak SG, Orenstein WA, et al. Vaccine-associated paralytic poliomyelitis. United States: 1973 through 1984. *JAMA* 1987;257:1335–1340.
74. Kapikian AZ, Chanock RM. Viral gastroenteritis. In: Evans AS, ed. *Viral infections of humans: epidemiology and control,* 3rd ed. New York and London: Plenum, 1991:293–340.
75. Kaplan JE, Gary GW, Baron RC, et al. Epidemiology of Norwalk gastroenteritis and the role of Norwalk virus in outbreaks of acute nonbacterial gastroenteritis. *Ann Intern Med* 1982;96:756–761.
76. Jamieson FB, Wang EEL, Bain C, et al. Human torovirus: a new nosocomial gastrointestinal pathogen. *J Infect Dis* 1998;178: 1263–1269.
77. Chapin M, Yatabe J, Cherry JD. An outbreak of rotavirus gastroenteritis on a pediatric unit. *Am J Infect Control* 1983;11:88–91.
78. Noone C, Banatvala JE. Hospital acquired rotaviral gastroenteritis in a general paediatric unit. *J Hosp Infect* 1983;4:297–299.
79. Srinivasan G, Azarcon E, Muldoon MR, et al. Rotavirus infection in normal nursery: epidemic and surveillance. *Infect Control* 1984;5: 478–481.
80. Dennehy PH, Peter G. Risk factors associated with nosocomial rotavirus infection. *Am J Dis Child* 1985;139:935–939.
81. Cone R, Mohan K, Thouless M, et al. Nosocomial transmission of rotavirus infection. *Pediatr Infect Dis J* 1988;7:103–109.
82. Ringenbergs ML, Davidson GP, Spence J, et al. Prospective study of nosocomial rotavirus infection in a paediatric hospital. *Aust Pediatr J* 1989;25:156–160.
83. Raad II, Sherertz RJ, Russell BA, et al. Uncontrolled nosocomial rotavirus transmission during a community outbreak. *Am J Infect Control* 1990;19:24–28.
84. Gaggero A, Avendano LF, Fernandez J, et al. Nosocomial transmission of rotavirus from patients admitted with diarrhea. *J Clin Microbiol* 1992;30:3294–3297.
85. Marrie TJ, Lee SHS, Faulkner RS, et al. Rotavirus infection in a geriatric population. *Arch Intern Med* 1982;142:313–316.
86. Cubitt WD, Holzel H. An outbreak of rotavirus infection in a long-stay ward of a geriatric hospital. *J Clin Pathol* 1980;33:306–308.
87. Abbas AMA, Denton MD. An outbreak of rotavirus infection in a geriatric hospital. *J Hosp Infect* 1987;9:76–80.
88. Lewis DC, Lightfoot NF, Cubitt WD, et al. Outbreaks of astrovirus type 1 and rotavirus gastroenteritis in a geriatric in-patient population. *J Hosp Infect* 1989;14:9–14.
89. Holzel H, Cubitt DW, McSwiggan DA, et al. An outbreak of rotavirus infection among adults in a cardiology ward. *J Infect* 1980;2:33–37.
90. Hildreth C, Thomas M, Ridgway GL. Rotavirus infection in an obstetric unit. *Br Med J* 1981;282:231.
91. Sattar SA, Hacobsen H, Rahman H, et al. Interruption of rotavirus spread through chemical disinfection. *Infect Control Hosp Epidemiol* 1994;15:751–756.
92. Fankhauser RL, Noel JS, Monroe SS, et al. Molecular epidemiology of "Norwalk-like viruses" in outbreaks of gastroenteritis in the United States. *J Infect Dis* 1998;178:1571–1578.
93. Gustafson TL, Kobylik B, Hutcheson RH, et al. Protective effect of anticholinergic drugs and psyllium in a nosocomial outbreak of Norwalk gastroenteritis. *J Hosp Infect* 1983;4:367–374.
94. Gellert GA, Waterman SH, Ewert D, et al. An outbreak of acute gastroenteritis caused by a small round structured virus in a geriatric convalescent facility. *Infect Control Hosp Epidemiol* 1990;11:459–464.
95. Caceres VM, Kim DK, Bresee JS, et al. A viral gastroenteritis outbreak associated with person-to-person spread among hospital staff. *Infect Control Hosp Epidemiol* 1998;19:162–167.
96. Sawyer LA, Murphy JJ, Kaplan JE, et al. 25- to 30-nm virus particle associated with a hospital outbreak of acute gastroenteritis with evidence for airborne transmission. *Am J Epidemiol* 1988;127: 1261–1271.
97. Ho MS, Glass RI, Monroe SS, et al. Viral gastroenteritis aboard a cruise ship. *Lancet* 1989;2:961–965.
98. Chadwick PR, Walker M, Rees AE. Airborne transmission of a small round structured virus [letter—see comments]. *Lancet* 1994;343:171.
99. Chadwick PR, McCann R. Transmission of a small round structured virus by vomiting during a hospital outbreak of gastroenteritis. *J Hosp Infect* 1994;26:251–259.
100. Chadwick P. Airborne transmission of a small round structured virus [letter—reply]. *Lancet* 1994;343:609.
101. Caul EO. Small round structured viruses: airborne transmission and hospital control. *Lancet* 1994;343:1240–1242.
102. Sloan DSG. Role of small round viruses and small round structured viruses [letter—comment]. *Lancet* 1994;344:128.
103. Noah ND. Airborne transmission of a small round structured virus [letter—comment]. *Lancet* 1994;343:608–609.
104. Hadler SC, Margolis HS. Viral hepatitis. In: Evans AS, ed. *Viral infections of humans: epidemiology and control,* 3rd ed. New York and London: Plenum, 1991:351–391.
105. Burkholder BT, Coronado CG, Brown J, et al. Nosocomial transmission of hepatitis A in a pediatric hospital traced to an anti-hepatitis A virus-negative patient with immunodeficiency. *Pediatr Infect Dis J* 1995;14:261–266.
106. Orenstein WA, Wu E, Wilkins J, et al. Hospital-acquired hepatitis A: report of an outbreak. *Pediatrics* 1981;67:494–497.
107. Goodman RA, Carder CC, Allen JR, et al. Nosocomial hepatitis A transmission by an adult patient with diarrhea. *Am J Med* 1982;73: 220–226.
108. Rosenblum LS, Villarino ME, Nainan OV, et al. Hepatitis A outbreak in a neonatal intensive care unit: risk factors for transmission and evidence of prolonged viral excretion among preterm infants. *J Infect Dis* 1991;164:476–482.
109. Watson JC, Fleming DW, Borella AJ, et al. Vertical transmission of hepatitis A resulting in an outbreak in a neonatal intensive care unit. *J Infect Dis* 1993;167:567–571.
110. Drusin LM, Sohmer M, Groshen SL, et al. Nosocomial hepatitis A

infection in a paediatric intensive care unit. *Arch Dis Child* 1987;62: 690–695.

111. Doebbeling BN, Li N, Wenzel RP. An outbreak of hepatitis A among health care workers: risk factors for transmission. *Am J Public Health* 1993;83:1679–1684.
112. Aach RD, Evans J, Losee J. An epidemic of infectious hepatitis possibly due to airborne transmission. *Am J Epidemiol* 1968;87:99–109.
113. Bolyard EA, Tablan OC, Williams WW, et al., and the Hospital Infection Control Practices Advisory Committee. Guideline for infection control in healthcare personnel, 1998. *Infect Control Hosp Epidemiol* 1998;19:407–463.
114. Smith S, Weber S, Wiblin T, et al. Cost-effectiveness of hepatitis A vaccination in healthcare workers. *Infect Control Hosp Epidemiol* 1997; 18:688–691.
115. Corey L. Herpes simplex virus. In: Mandell GL, Douglas RG Jr, Dolin R, eds. *Principles and practice of infectious diseases,* 5th ed. New York: Churchill Livingstone, 2000:1564–1580.
116. Blank H, Haines HG. Experimental human reinfection with herpes simplex virus. *J Invest Dermatol* 1973;61:223–225.
117. Dunbar C. Herpetic whitlow: an occupational hazard for nursing personnel. *Heart Lung* 1978;7:645–646.
118. Greaves WL, Kaiser AB, Alford RH, et al. The problem of herpetic whitlow among hospital personnel. *Infect Control* 1980;1:381–385.
119. Klotz RW. Herpetic whitlow: an occupational hazard. *AANA J* 1990; 58:8–13.
120. Avitzur Y, Amir J. Herpetic whitlow infection in a general pediatrician—an occupational hazard. *Infection* 2002;30:234–236.
121. Hendricks AA, Shapiro EP. Primary herpes simplex infection following mouth-to-mouth resuscitation. *JAMA* 1980;243:257–258.
122. Adams G, Stover BH, Keenlyside RA, et al. Nosocomial herpetic infections in a pediatric intensive care unit. *Am J Epidemiol* 1981; 113:126–132.
123. Weber DJ, Rutala WA, Hamilton H. Prevention and control of varicella-zoster infections in healthcare facilities. *Infect Control Hosp Epidemiol* 1996;17:694–705.
124. McKinney WP, Horowitz MM, Battiola RJ. Susceptibility of hospital-based health care personnel to varicella-zoster virus infections. *Am J Infect Control* 1989;17:26–30.
125. Whitley RJ. Varicella-zoster virus. In: Mandell GL, Douglas RG Jr, Dolin R, eds. *Principles and practice of infectious diseases,* 5th ed. New York: Churchill Livingstone, 2000:1580–1586.
126. Greene D, Barenberg LH, Greenberg B. Effect of irradiation of the air in a ward on the incidence of infections of the respiratory tract. *Am J Dis Child* 1941;61:273–275.
127. Habel K. Mumps and chickenpox as air-borne diseases. *Am J Med* 1945;209:75–78.
128. Asano Y, Iwayama S, Miyata T, et al. Spread of varicella in hospitalized children having no direct contact with an indicator zoster case and its prevention by a live vaccine. *Biken J* 1980;23:157–161.
129. Leclair JM, Zaia JA, Levin MJ, et al. Airborne transmission of chickenpox in a hospital. *N Engl J Med* 1980;302:450–453.
130. Gustafson TL, Lavely GB, Brawner ERJ, et al. An outbreak of airborne nosocomial varicella. *Pediatrics* 1982;70:550–556.
131. Tsujino G, Sako M, Takahashi M. Varicella infection in a children's hospital: prevention by vaccine and an episode of airborne transmission. *Biken J* 1984;27:129–132.
132. Josephson A, Gombert ME. Airborne transmission of nosocomial varicella from localized zoster. *J Infect Dis* 1988;158:238–241.
133. Menkhaus NA, Lanphear B, Linnemann CC. Airborne transmission of varicella-zoster virus in hospitals [letter—comment]. *Lancet* 1990; 336:1315.
134. Sawyer MH, Chamberlin CJ, Wu YN, et al. Detection of varicella-zoster virus DNA in air samples from hospital rooms. *J Infect Dis* 1994;169:91–94.
135. Krasinski K, Holzman RS, LaCouture R, et al. Hospital experience with varicella-zoster virus. *Infect Control* 1986;7:312–316.
136. Weber DJ, Rutala WA, Parham C. Impact and costs of varicella prevention in a university hospital. *Am J Public Health* 1988;78:19–23.
137. Riley RL. Airborne transmission of chickenpox [letter]. *N Engl J Med* 1980;303:281.
138. Scheifele D, Bonner M. Airborne transmission of chickenpox [letter]. *N Engl J Med* 1980;303:281–282.
139. Leclair JM, Zaia JA, Levin MH, et al. Airborne transmission of chickenpox [letter]. *N Engl J Med* 1980;303:282.
140. Anderson JD, Bonner M, Scheifele DW, et al. Lack of nosocomial spread of Varicella in a pediatric hospital with negative pressure ventilated patient rooms. *Infect Control* 1985;6:120–121.
141. Preblud SR. Nosocomial varicella: worth preventing, but how? *Am J Public Health* 1988;78:13–15.
142. Stover BH, Cost KM, Hamm C, et al. Varicella exposure in a neonatal intensive care unit: case report and control measures. *Am J Infect Control* 1988;16:167–172.
143. Haiduven-Griffiths D, Fecko H. Varicella in hospital personnel: a challenge for the infection control practitioner. *Am J Infect Control* 1987;15:207–211.
144. Lipton SV, Brunell PA. Management of varicella exposure in a neonatal intensive care unit. *JAMA* 1989;261:1782–1784.
145. Josephson A, Karanfil L, Gombert ME. Strategies for the management of varicella-susceptible healthcare workers after a known exposure. *Infect Control Hosp Epidemiol* 1990;11:309–313.
146. Morgan-Capner P, Wilson M, Wright J, et al. Varicella and zoster in hospitals. *Lancet* 1990;335:1460.
147. Sutherland S, Honeywell K, Lee S, et al. Varicella and zoster in hospitals. *Lancet* 1990;335:1460–1461.
148. Haiduven DJ, Hench CP, Stevens DA. Postexposure varicella management of nonimmune personnel: an alternative approach. *Infect Control Hosp Epidemiol* 1994;15:329–334.
149. Tennenberg AM, Brassard JE, Van Lieu J, et al. Varicella vaccination for healthcare workers at a university hospital: an analysis of costs and benefits. *Infect Control Hosp Epidemiol* 1997;18:405–411.
150. Nettleman MD, Schmid M. Controlling varicella in the healthcare setting: the cost effectiveness of using varicella vaccine in healthcare workers. *Infect Control Hosp Epidemiol* 1997;18:504–508.
151. Lyzinicki JM, Bezman RJ, Genel M. Report of the council on scientific affairs, American Medical Association: immunization of healthcare workers with varicella vaccine. *Infect Control Hosp Epidemiol* 1998;19:348–353.
152. Evans AS, Niederman JC. Epstein-Barr virus. In: Evans AS, ed. *Viral infections of humans: epidemiology and control,* 3rd ed. New York and London: Plenum, 1991:265–292.
153. Ginsburg CM, Henle G, Henle W. An outbreak of infectious mononucleosis among the personnel of an outpatient clinic. *Am J Epidemiol* 1976;104:571–575.
154. Gold E, Nankervis GA. Cytomegalovirus. In: Evans AS, ed *Viral infections of humans: epidemiology and control,* 3rd ed. New York and London: Plenum, 1991:169–190.
155. Young AB, Reid D, Grist NR. Is cytomegalovirus a serious hazard to female hospital staff? *Lancet* 1983;1:975–976.
156. Dworsky ME, Welch K, Cassady G, et al. Occupational risk for primary cytomegalovirus infection among pediatric health-care workers. *N Engl J Med* 1983;309:950–953.
157. Lipscomb JA, Linnermann CC Jr, Hurst PF, et al. Prevalence of cytomegalovirus antibody in nursing personnel. *Infect Control* 1984; 5:513–518.
158. Hatherley LI. Is primary cytomegalovirus infection an occupational hazard for obstetric nurses? A serological study. *Infect Control* 1986; 7:452–455.
159. Friedman HM, Lewis MR, Nemerofsky DM, et al. Acquisition of cytomegalovirus infection among female employees at a pediatric hospital. *Pediatr Infect Dis* 1984;3:233–235.
160. Onorato IM, Martone WJ, Stansfield SK. Epidemiology of cytomegaloviral infections: recommendations for prevention and control. *Rev Infect Dis* 1985;7:479–497.
161. Brady MT. Cytomegalovirus infections: occupational risk for health professionals. *Am J Infect Control* 1986;14:197–203.
162. Adler SP. Nosocomial transmission of cytomegalovirus. *Pediatr Infect Dis* 1986;5:239–245.
163. Balfour CL, Balfour HH Jr. Cytomegalovirus is not an occupational risk for nurses in renal transplant and neonatal units. Results of a prospective surveillance study. *JAMA* 1986;256:1909–1914.

164. Plotkin SA. Cytomegalovirus in hospitals. *Pediatr Infect Dis J* 1986; 5:177–178.
165. Brady MT, Demmler GJ, Anderson DC. Cytomegalovirus infection in pediatric house officers: susceptibility to and rate of primary infection. *Infect Control* 1987;8:329–332.
166. Blackman JA, Murph JR, Bale JF Jr. Risk of cytomegalovirus infection among educators and health care personnel serving disabled children. *Pediatr Infect Dis J* 1987;6:725–729.
167. Pomeroy C, Englund JA. Cytomegalovirus: epidemiology and infection control. *Am J Infect Control* 1987;15:107–119.
168. Flowers RH, Torner JC, Farr BM. Primary cytomegalovirus infection in pediatric nurses: a meta-analysis. *Infect Control Hosp Epidemiol* 1988;9:491–496.
169. Balcarek KB, Bagley R, Cloud GA, et al. Cytomegalovirus infection among employees of a children's hospital. No evidence for increased risk associated with patient care. *JAMA* 1990;263:840–844.
170. Tookey P, Peckham CS. Does cytomegalovirus present an occupational risk? [editorial]. *Arch Dis Child* 1991;66:1009–1010.
171. Faix RG. Lack of aerosol dispersal of cytomegalovirus during mechanical ventilation. *Pediatr Infect Dis J* 1989;8:330–332.
172. Committee on Infectious Diseases. *2000 Red Book: Report of the Committee on Infectious Diseases,* 25th ed. Elk Grove Village, IL: American Academy of Pediatrics, 2000.
173. Hall CB, Long CE, Schnabel KC, et al. Human herpesvirus-6 infection in children. A prospective study of complications and reactivation. *N Engl J Med* 1994;331:432–438.
174. Okuno T, Mukai T, Baba K, et al. Outbreak of exanthem subitum in an orphanage. *J Pediatr* 1991;119:759–761.
175. Kimberlin DW. Human herpesviruses 6 and 7: identification of newly recognized viral pathogens and their association with human disease. *Pediatr Infect Dis J* 1998;17:59–68.
176. Levy JA. Three new human herpesviruses (HHV 6, 7, and 8). *Lancet* 1997;349:558–562.
177. Luppi M, Barozzi P, Schulz TF, et al. Bone marrow failure associated with human herpes virus 8 infection after transplantation. *N Engl J Med* 2000; 343: 1378–1385.
178. Centers for Disease Control. B-virus infection in humans—Pensacola, Florida. *MMWR* 1987;36:289–290,295–296.
179. Cohen JI, Davenport DS, Stewart JA, et al. Recommendations for prevention of and therapy for exposure to B virus (*Cercopithecine herpesvirus 1*). *Clin Infect Dis* 2002;35:1191–1203.
180. Gershon AA. Measles virus (rubeola). In: Mandell GL, Douglas RG Jr, Bennett JE, eds. *Principles and practice of infectious diseases,* 3rd ed. New York: Churchill Livingstone, 2000;1801–1809.
181. Shapiro L. The numbered diseases: first through sixth. *JAMA* 1965; 194:680–686.
182. Centers for Disease Control. Measles prevention: recommendations of the Immunization Practices Advisory Committee (ACIP). *MMWR* 1989;38(S-9):1–18.
183. Centers for Disease Control. Measles in medical settings—United States. *MMWR* 1981;30:125–126.
184. Davis RM, Orenstein WA, Frank JAJ, et al. Transmission of measles in medical settings: 1980 through 1984. *JAMA* 1986;255: 1295–1298.
185. Watkins NM, Smith RPJ, St. Germain DL, et al. Measles (rubeola) infection in a hospital setting. *Am J Infect Control* 1987;15:201–206.
186. Sienko DG, Friedman C, McGee HB, et al. A measles outbreak at university medical settings involving health care providers. *Am J Public Health* 1987;77:1222–1224.
187. Raad II, Sherertz RJ, Rains CS, et al. The importance of nosocomial transmission of measles in the propagation of a community outbreak. *Infect Control Hosp Epidemiol* 1989;10:161–166.
188. Rivera ME, Mason WH, Ross LA, et al. Nosocomial measles infection in a pediatric hospital during a community-wide epidemic. *J Pediatr* 1991;119:183–186.
189. Atkinson WL, Markowitz LE, Adams NC, et al. Transmission of measles in medical settings—United States, 1985–1989. *Am J Med* 1991;91:320S–324S.
190. Rank EL, Brettman L, Katz-Pollack H, et al. Chronology of a hospital-wide measles outbreak: lessons learned and shared from an extraordinary week in late March 1989. *Am J Infect Control* 1992;20:315–318.
191. Gurevich I. Varicella zoster and herpes simplex virus infections. *Heart Lung* 1992;21:85–91.
192. Enguidanos R, Mascola L, Frederick P. A survey of hospital infection control policies and employee measles cases during Los Angeles County's measles epidemic, 1987 to 1989. *Am J Infect Control* 1992;20: 301–304.
193. Ammari LK, Bell LM, Hodinka RL. Secondary measles vaccine failure in healthcare workers exposed to infected patients. *Infect Control Hosp Epidemiol* 1993;14:81–86.
194. Atkinson WL. Measles and healthcare workers. *Infect Control Hosp Epidemiol* 1994;15:5–7.
195. Steingart KR, Thomas AR, Dykewicz CA, et al. Transmission of measles virus in healthcare settings during a communitywide outbreak. *Infect Control Hosp Epidemiol* 1999;20:115–119.
196. Gurevich I, Barzarga RA, Cunha BA. Measles: lessons from an outbreak. *Am J Infect Control* 1992;20:319–325.
197. Eagan J. Measles: an infection control nightmare. *RN* 1991;54:26–29.
198. Farizo KM, Stehr-Green PA, Simpson DM, et al. Pediatric emergency room visits: a risk factor for acquiring measles. *Pediatrics* 1991;87: 74–79.
199. McGrath D, Swanson R, Weems S, et al. Analysis of a measles outbreak in Kent County, Michigan in 1990. *Pediatr Infect Dis J* 1992; 11:385–389.
200. Riley EC, Murphy G, Riley RL. Airborne spread of measles in a suburban elementary school. *Am J Epidemiol* 1978;107:421–432.
201. Centers for Disease Control. Imported measles with subsequent airborne transmission in a pediatrician's office—Michigan. *MMWR* 1983;32:401–402.
202. Decker MD, Schaffner W. Immunization of hospital personnel and other health care workers. *Infect Dis Clin North Am* 1990;4:211–221.
203. Murray DL. Vaccine-preventable diseases and medical personnel. Ensure the immunity of all! [editorial—comment]. *Arch Intern Med* 1990;150:25–26.
204. Weber DJ, Rutala WA, Orenstein WA. Prevention of mumps, measles, and rubella among hospital personnel. *J Pediatr* 1991;119: 322–326.
205. Krause PJ, Gross PA, Barrett TL, et al. Quality standard for assurance of measles immunity among health care workers. *Infect Control Hosp Epidemiol* 1994;15:193–199.
206. Subbarao EK, Amin S, Kumar ML. Prevaccination serologic screening for measles in health care workers [see comments]. *J Infect Dis* 1991; 163:876–878.
207. Houck P, Scott-Johnson G, Krebs L. Measles immunity among community hospital employees. *Infect Control Hosp Epidemiol* 1991;12: 663–668.
208. Schwarcz S, McCaw B, Fukushima P. Prevalence of measles susceptibility in hospital staff. Evidence to support expanding the recommendations of the Immunization Practices Advisory Committee [see comments]. *Arch Intern Med* 1992;152:1481–1483.
209. Kim M, LaPointe J, Liu FJG. Epidemiology of measles immunity in a population of healthcare workers. *Infect Control Hosp Epidemiol* 1992;13:399–402.
210. Wright LJ, Carlquist JF. Measles immunity in employees of a multihospital healthcare provider [see comments]. *Infect Control Hosp Epidemiol* 1994;15:8–11.
211. Willy ME, Koziol DE, Fleisher T, et al. Measles immunity in a population of healthcare workers. *Infect Control Hosp Epidemiol* 1994;15: 12–17.
212. Stover BH, Adams G, Kuebler CA, et al. Measles-mumps-rubella immunization of susceptible hospital employees during a community measles outbreak: cost-effectiveness and protective efficacy [see comments]. *Infect Control Hosp Epidemiol* 1994;15:18–21.
213. Huang KG, Spence MR, Deforest A, et al. Measles immunization in HCWs [letter]. *Infect Control Hosp Epidemiol* 1994;15:4.
214. Sellick JA Jr, Longbine D, Schifeling R, et al. Screening hospital employees for measles immunity is more cost effective than blind immunization. *Ann Intern Med* 1992;116:982–984.
215. Centers for Disease Control and Prevention. Immunization of

healthcare workers: recommendations of the Advisory Committee on Immunization Practices (ACIP) and the Hospital Infection Control Practices Advisory Committee (HICPAC). *MMWR* 1997;46(RR-18): 1–42.

216. Gershon AA. Rubella (German measles). In: Mandell GL, Douglas RG Jr, Dolin R, eds. *Principles and practice of infectious diseases,* 5th ed. New York: Churchill Livingstone, 2000;1708–1714.
217. Baba K, Yabuuchi H, Okuni H, et al. Rubella epidemic in an institution: protective value of live rubella vaccine and serological behavior of vaccinated, revaccinated and naturally immune groups. *Biken J* 1978;21:25–31.
218. McLaughlin MC, Gold LH. The New York rubella incident: a case for changing hospital policy regarding rubella testing and immunization. *Am J Public Health* 1979;69:287–289.
219. Polk BF, White JA, DeGirolami PC, et al. An outbreak of rubella among hospital personnel. *N Engl J Med* 1980;303:541–545.
220. Gladstone JL, Millian SJ. Rubella exposure in an obstetric clinic. *Obstet Gynecol* 1981;57:182–186.
221. Evans ME, Schaffner W. Rubella immunization of hospital personnel: a debate. *Infect Control* 1981;2:387–390.
222. Centers for Disease Control. Nosocomial rubella infection—North Dakota, Alabama, Ohio. *MMWR* 1981;29:630–631.
223. Strassburg MA, Imagawa DT, Fannin SL, et al. Rubella outbreak among hospital employees. *Obstet Gynecol* 1981;57:283–288.
224. Fliegel PE, Weinstein WM. Rubella outbreak in a prenatal clinic: management and prevention. *Am J Infect Control* 1982;10:29–33.
225. Centers for Disease Control. Rubella in hospitals—California. *MMWR* 1983;32:37–39.
226. Strassburg MA, Stephenson TG, Habel LA, et al. Rubella in hospital employees. *Infect Control* 1984;5:123–126.
227. Storch GA, Gruber C, Benz B, et al. A rubella outbreak among dental students: description of the outbreak and analysis of control measures. *Infect Control* 1985;6:150–156.
228. Heseltine PN, Ripper M, Wohlford P. Nosocomial rubella—consequences of an outbreak and efficacy of a mandatory immunization program. *Infect Control* 1985;6:371–374.
229. Fraser V, Spitznagel E, Medoff G, et al. Results of a rubella screening program for hospital employees: a five-year review (1986–1990). *Am J Epidemiol* 1993;138:756–764.
230. Ferson MJ, Robertson PW, Whybin LR. Cost effectiveness of prevaccination screening of health care workers for immunity to measles, rubella and mumps. *Med J Aust* 1994;160:478–482.
231. Schoenhoff DD, Lane TW, Hansen CJ. Primary prevention and rubella immunity: overlooked issues in the outpatient obstetric setting. *Infect Control Hosp Epidemiol* 1997;18:633–636.
232. Baum SG, Litman N. Mumps virus. In: Mandell GL, Douglas RG Jr, Dolin R, eds. Principles and practice of infectious diseases, 3rd ed. New York: Churchill Livingstone, 2000:1776–1781.
233. Wharton M, Cochi SL, Hutcheson RH, et al. A large outbreak of mumps in the post-vaccine era. *J Infect Dis* 1988;158:1253–1260.
234. Glick D. An isolated case of mumps in a geriatric population. *J Am Geriatr Soc* 1970;18:642–644.
235. Faoagali JL. An assessment of the need for vaccination amongst junior medical staff. *NZ Med J* 1976;84:147–150.
236. Wharton M, Cochi SL, Hutcheson RH, et al. Mumps transmission in hospitals [see comments]. *Arch Intern Med* 1990;150:47–49.
237. Sparling D. Transmission of mumps [Letter]. *N Engl J Med* 1969; 280:276.
238. Centers for Disease Control. Risks associated with human parvovirus B19 infection. *MMWR* 1989;38:81–88,93–97.
239. Bell LM, Naides SJ, Stoffman P, et al. Human parvovirus B19 infection among hospital staff members after contact with infected patients [see comments]. *N Engl J Med* 1989;321:485–491.
240. Pillay D, Patou G, Hurt S, et al. Parvovirus B19 outbreak in a children's ward. *Lancet* 1992;339:107–109.
241. Shishiba T, Matsunaga Y. An outbreak of erythema infectiosum among hospital staff members including a patient with pleural fluid and pericardial effusion. *J Am Acad Dermatol* 1993;29:265–267.
242. Ray SM, Erdman DD, Berschling JD, et al. Nosocomial exposure to parvovirus B19: low risk of transmission to healthcare workers. *Infect Control Hosp Epidemiol* 1997;18:109–114.
243. Gillespie SM, Cartter ML, Asch S, et al. Occupational risk of human parvovirus B19 infection for school and day-care personnel during an outbreak of erythema infectiosum [see comments]. *JAMA* 1990; 263:2061–2065.
244. Adler SP, Manganello AM, Koch WC, et al. Risk of human parvovirus B19 infections among school and hospital employees during endemic periods. *J Infect Dis* 1993;168:361–368.
245. Dowell SF, Torok TJ, Thorp JA, et al. Parvovirus B19 infection in hospital workers: community or hospital acquisition? *J Infect Dis* 1995;172:1076–1079.
246. LeDuc JW. Epidemiology of hemorrhagic fever viruses. *Rev Infect Dis* 1989;11(suppl 4):S730–S735.
247. Tsai TF. Flavivirus (yellow fever, dengue, dengue hemorrhagic fever, Japanese encephalitis, St. Louis encephalitis, tick-borne encephalitis) In: Mandell GL, Douglas RG Jr, Dolin R, eds. *Principles and practice of infectious diseases,* 5th ed. New York: Churchill Livingstone, 2000: 1714–1736.
248. Peters CJ. California encephalitis hantavirus pulmonary syndrome and bunyavirid hemorrhagic fevers. In: Mandell GL, Douglas RG Jr, Dolin R, eds. *Principles and practice of infectious diseases,* 5th ed. New York: Churchill Livingstone, 2000:1849–1855.
249. Peters CJ. Lymphocytic choriomeningitis virus, Lassa virus, the South American hemorrhagic fevers. In: Mandell GL, Douglas RG Jr, Dolin R, eds. *Principles and practice of infectious diseases,* 5th ed. New York: Churchill Livingstone,2000:1855–1862.
250. Peters CJ. Marburg and Ebola virus hemorrhagic fevers. In: Mandell GL, Douglas RG Jr, Dolin R, eds. *Principles and practice of infectious diseases,* 5th ed. New York: Churchill Livingstone, 2000:1821–1823.
251. Desmyter J, LeDuc JW, Johnson KM, et al. Laboratory rat associated outbreak of haemorrhagic fever with renal syndrome due to Hantaan-like virus in Belgium. *Lancet* 1983;2:1445–1448.
252. Banerjee K, Gupta NP, Goverdhan MK. Viral infections in laboratory personnel. *Ind J Med Res* 1979;69:363–373.
253. Frame JD, Baldwin JM, Gocke DJ, et al. Lassa fever, a new virus disease of man from West Africa. I. Clinical description and pathological findings. *Am J Trop Med Hyg* 1970;19:670–676.
254. White HA. Lassa fever. A study of 23 hospital cases. *Trans R Soc Trop Med Hyg* 1972;66:390–401.
255. Monath TP, Mertens PE, Patton R, et al. A hospital epidemic of Lassa fever in Zorzor, Liberia, March–April 1972. *Am J Trop Med Hyg* 1973;22:773–779.
256. Frame JD, Casals J, Dennis EA. Lassa virus antibodies in hospital personnel in western Liberia. *Trans R Soc Trop Med Hyg* 1979;73: 219–224.
257. Zweighaft RM, Fraser DW, Hattwick MA, et al. Lassa fever: response to an imported case. *N Engl J Med* 1977;297:803–807.
258. Holmes GP, McCormick JB, Trock SC, et al. Lassa fever in the United States: investigation of a case and new guidelines for management. *N Engl J Med* 1990;323:1120–1142.
259. Centers for Disease Control. Management of patients with suspected viral hemorrhagic fever. *MMWR* 1988;37(S-3):1–16.
260. Johnson KM, Monath TP. Imported Lassa fever—reexamining the algorithms [editorial]. *N Engl J Med* 1990;323:1139–1141.
261. Helmick CG, Webb PA, Scribner CL, et al. No evidence for increased risk of Lassa fever infection in hospital staff. *Lancet* 1986;2: 1202–1205.
262. Gear JS, Cassel GA, Gear AJ, et al. Outbreak of Marburg virus disease in Johannesburg. *Br Med J* 1975;4:489–493.
263. Smith DH, Johnson BK, Isaacson M, et al. Marburg-virus disease in Kenya. *Lancet* 1982;1:816–820.
264. Conrad JL, Isaacson M, Smith EB, et al. Epidemiologic investigation of Marburg virus disease, Southern Africa, 1975. *Am J Trop Med Hyg* 1978;27:1210–1215.
265. Bowen ET, Lloyd G, Harris WJ, et al. Viral haemorrhagic fever in southern Sudan and northern Zaire. Preliminary studies on the aetiological agent. *Lancet* 1977;1:571–573.
266. Baron RC, McCormick JB, Zubeir OA. Ebola virus disease in south-

ern Sudan: hospital dissemination and intrafamilial spread. *Bull WHO* 1983;61:997–1003.
267. Hayes CG, Burans JP, Ksiazek TG, et al. Outbreak of fatal illness among captive macaques in the Philippines caused by an Ebola-related filovirus. *Am J Trop Med Hyg* 1992;46:664–671.
268. Centers for Disease Control. Ebola virus infection in imported primates—Virginia, 1989. *MMWR* 1989;38:831–832, 837–838.
269. Centers for Disease Control. Update: Ebola-related filovirus infection in nonhuman primates and interim guidelines for handling nonhuman primates during transit and quarantine. *MMWR* 1990;39: 22–24,29–30.
270. Preston R. *The hot zone.* New York: Random House, 1994.
271. Tomori O, Bertolli J, Rollin PE, et al. Serologic survey among hospital and health center workers during the Ebola hemorrhagic fever outbreak in Kikwit, Democratic Republic of the Congo, 1995. *J Infect Dis* 1999;179(suppl 1):S98–101.
272. Thacker PD. An Ebola epidemic simmers in Africa. *JAMA* 2003; 290: 317–319.
273. Burney MI, Ghafoor A, Saleen M, et al. Nosocomial outbreak of viral hemorrhagic fever caused by Crimean Hemorrhagic fever-Congo virus in Pakistan, January 1976. *Am J Trop Med Hyg* 1980;29:941–947.
274. Suleiman MN, Muscat-Baron JM, Harries JR, et al. Congo/Crimean haemorrhagic fever in Dubai. An outbreak at the Rashid Hospital. *Lancet* 1980;2:939–941.
275. van Eeden PJ, Joubert JR, van de Wal BW, et al. A nosocomial outbreak of Crimean-Congo haemorrhagic fever at Tygerberg Hospital. Part I. Clinical features. *S Afr Med J* 1985;68:711–717.
276. Peters CJ, Jahrling PB, Khan AS. Patients infected with high-hazard viruses: scientific basis for infection control. *Arch Virol* 1996; 11(suppl):141–168.
277. Armstrong LR, Dembry L-M, Rainey PM, et al. Management of a Sabiá virus-infected patient in a US hospital. *Infect Control Hosp* 1999; 20:176–182.
278. Centers for Disease Control. Update: outbreak of hantavirus infection—southwestern United States, 1993. *MMWR* 1993;42:441–443.
279. Centers for Disease Control. Update: hantavirus disease—southwestern United States, 1993. *MMWR* 1993;42:570–572.
280. Centers for Disease Control. Hantavirus pulmonary syndrome—United States, 1993 (published erratum appears in *MMWR* 1994;43(7):127). *MMWR* 1994;43:45–48.
281. Centers for Disease Control. Hantavirus pulmonary syndrome—Northeastern United States, 1994. *MMWR* 1994;43: 548–556.
282. Garden JM, O'Banion MK, Shelnitz LS, et al. Papillomavirus in the vapor of carbon dioxide laser-treated verrucae. *JAMA* 1988;259: 1199–1202.
283. Dumbell K. What should be done about smallpox virus? *Lancet* 1987; 2:957–958.
284. Wehrle PF, Posch J, Richter KH, et al. An airborne outbreak of smallpox in a German hospital and its significance with respect to other recent outbreaks in Europe. *Bull WHO* 1970;43:669–679.
285. Hawkes N. Science in Europe: smallpox death in Britain challenges presumption of laboratory safety. *Science* 1979;203:855–856.
286. Mackett M. Vaccinia virus recombinants: potential vaccines. *Acta Trop (Basel)* 1987;445(suppl 12):94–97.
287. Neff JM. Variola (smallpox) and monkeypox viruses. In: Mandell GL, Douglas RG Jr, Dolin R, eds. *Principles and practice of infectious diseases,* 5th ed. New York: Churchill Livingstone, 2000:1555–1556.
288. Evans ME, Lesnaw JA. Infection control in gene therapy. *Infect Control Hosp Epidemiol* 1999;20:568–576.
289. Centers for Disease Control and Prevention. Update: multistate outbreak of monkeypox-Illinois, Indiana, Kansas, Missouri, Ohio and Wisconsin, 2003. *MMWR* 2003;52:561–564.
290. Neff JM. Parapox viruses and molluscum contagiosum and tanapox viruses. In: Mandell GL, Douglas RG Jr, Dolin R, eds. *Principles and practice of infectious diseases,* 5th ed. New York: Churchill Livingstone, 2000:1556–1557.
291. Petersen LR, Marfin AA, Gubler DJ. West Nile virus. *JAMA* 2003; 290:524–528.
292. Markoff L. Alphaviruses In: Mandell GL, Douglas RG Jr, Dolin R, eds. *Principles and practice of infectious diseases,* 5th ed. New York: Churchill Livingstone, 2000:1703–1708.
293. Baum SG, Lewis AMJ, Rowe WP, et al. Epidemic nonmeningitic lymphocytic-choriomeningitis-virus infection: an outbreak in a population of laboratory personnel. *N Engl J Med* 1966;274:934–936.
294. Hinman AR, Fraser DW, Douglas RG, et al. Outbreak of lymphocytic choriomeningitis virus infections in medical center personnel. *Am J Epidemiol* 1975;101:103–110.
295. Bowen GS, Calisher CH, Winkler WG, et al. Laboratory studies of a lymphocytic choriomeningitis virus outbreak in man and laboratory animals. *Am J Epidemiol* 1975;102:233–240.
296. Dykewicz CA, Dato VM, Fisher-Hoch SP, et al. Lymphocytic choriomeningitis outbreak associated with nude mice in a research institute [published erratum appears in *JAMA* 1992;268(7):874]. *JAMA* 1992; 267:1349–1353.
297. Anderson LJ, Williams LPJ, Layde JB, et al. Nosocomial rabies: investigation of contacts of human rabies cases associated with a corneal transplant. *Am J Public Health* 1984;74:370–372.
298. Centers for Disease Control and Prevention. Human rabies prevention—United States, 1999: recommendations of the Advisory Committee on Immunization Practices (ACIP). *MMWR* 1999;48(No RR-1):1–19.
299. Fekadu M, Edeshaw T, Wondimagegnehu A, et al. Possible human-to-human transmission of rabies in Ethiopia. *Ethiop Med J* 1996;34: 123–127.
300. Tyler KL. Prions and diseases of the central nervous system (transmissible neurodegenerative diseases). In: Mandell GL, Bennett JE, Dolin R, eds. *Mandell, Douglas and Bennett's principles and practice of infectious diseases,* 5th ed. New York: Churchill Livingstone, 2000: 1971–1985.
301. Duffy P, Wolf J, Collins G, et al. Letter: possible person-to-person transmission of Creutzfeldt-Jakob disease. *N Engl J Med* 1974;290: 692–693.
302. Miyashita K, Inuzuka T, Kondo H, et al. Creutzfeldt-Jakob disease in a patient with a cadaveric dural graft. *Neurology* 1991;41:940–941.
303. Will RG, Matthews WB. Evidence for case-to-case transmission of Creutzfeldt-Jakob disease. *J Neurol Neurosurg Psychiatry* 1982;45: 235–238.
304. Brown P, Gajdusek DC, Gibbs CJ Jr, et al. Potential epidemic of Creutzfeldt-Jakob disease from human growth hormone therapy. *N Engl J Med* 1985;313:728–731.
305. Dumble LJ, Klein RD. Creutzfeldt-Jakob legacy for Australian women treated with human pituitary gonadotropins [letter]. *Lancet* 1992; 340:847–848.
306. Johnson RT, Gibbs CJ Jr. Creutzfeldt-Jakob disease and related transmissible spongiform encephalopathies. *N Engl J Med* 1998;339: 1994–2004.
307. Dormont D. How to limit the spread of Creutzfeldt-Jakob disease. *Infect Control Hosp Epidemiol* 1996;17:521–528.
308. Fisher HR, Helsby RJ. Three cases of psittacosis with two deaths. *Br Med J* 1931;1:887–888.
309. Olson BJ, Treuting WL. An epidemic of a severe pneumonitis in the bayou region of Louisiana. *Public Health Rep* 1944;59:1299–1311.
310. Broholm KA, Bottiger M, Jernelius H, et al. Ornithosis as a nosocomial infection. *Scand J Infect Dis* 1977;9:263–267.
311. Pether JVS, Wang S, Grayston JT. Chlamydia pneumoniae, strain TWAR, as the cause of an outbreak in a boys' school previously called psittacosis. *Epidemiol Infect* 1989;103:395–400.
312. Huches C, Maharg P, Rosario P, et al. Possible nosocomial transmission of psittacosis. *Infect Control Hosp Epidemiol* 1997;18:165–168.
313. Schaffner W. Birds of a feather—do they flock together? *Infect Control Hosp Epidemiol* 1997;18:162–164.
314. Marrie TJ. Coxiella burnetii (Q fever). In: Mandell GL, Bennett JE, Dolin R, eds. *Mandell, Douglas and Bennett's principles and practice of infectious diseases,* 5th ed. New York: Churchill Livingstone, 2000: 2043–2050.
315. Hornibrook JW, Nelson KR. An institutional outbreak of pneumonitis. I. Epidemiological and clinical studies. *Public Health Rep* 1940; 55:1936–1944.

316. Dyer RE, Topping NH, Bengtson IA. Isolation and identification of causative agent. *Public Health Rep* 1940;55:1945–1954.
317. Schachter J, Sung M, Meyer KF. Potential danger of Q fever in a university hospital environment. *J Infect Dis* 1971;123:301–304.
318. Meiklejohn G, Reimer LG, Graves PS, et al. Cryptic epidemic of Q fever in a medical school. *J Infect Dis* 1981;144:107–113.
319. Simor AE, Brunton JL, Salit IE, et al. Q fever: hazard from sheep used in research. *Can Med Assoc J* 1984;130:1013–1016.
320. Graham CJ, Yamauchi T, Rountree P. Q fever in animal laboratory workers: an outbreak and its investigation. *Am J Infect Control* 1989; 17:345–348.
321. Johnson JEI, Kadull PJ. Laboratory acquired Q fever. A report of fifty cases. *Am J Med* 1966;41:391–403.
322. Bayer RA. Q fever as an occupational illness at the National Institutes of Health. *Public Health Rep* 1982;97:58–60.
323. Baum SG. Mycoplasma pneumoniae and atypical pneumonia. In: Mandell GL, Bennett JE, Dolan R, eds. *Mandell, Douglas and Bennett's principles and practice of infectious diseases,* 5th ed. New York: Churchill Livingstone, 2000:2018–2027.
324. Kleemola M, Jokinen C. Outbreak of Mycoplasma pneumoniae infection among hospital personnel studied by a nucleic acid hybridization test. *J Hosp Infect* 1992;21:213–221.
325. Centers for Disease Control. Outbreaks of Mycoplasma pneumoniae respiratory infection—Ohio, Texas, and New York, 1993. *MMWR* 1993;42:931,937–939.
326. Miller SI, Pegues DA. Salmonella species, including Salmonella typhi. In: Mandell GL, Bennett JE, Dolin R, eds. *Mandell, Douglas and Bennett's principles and practice of infectious diseases,* 5th ed. New York: Churchill Livingstone, 2000:2344–2363.
327. DuPont HL. Nosocomial salmonellosis and shigellosis [editorial]. *Infect Control Hosp Epidemiol* 1991;12:707–709.
328. Baine WB, Gangarosa EJ, Bennett JV, et al. Institutional salmonellosis. *J Infect Dis* 1973;128:357–359.
329. Centers for Disease Control. Salmonellosis—Baltimore, Maryland. *MMWR* 1970;19:314.
330. Steere AC, Craven PJ, Hall WJI, et al. Person-to-person spread of *Salmonella typhimurium* after a hospital common-source outbreak. *Lancet* 1975;1:319–322.
331. Lintz D, Kapila R, Pilgrim E, et al. Nosocomial *Salmonella* epidemic. *Arch Intern Med* 1976;136:968–973.
332. Mendis NM, De La Motte PU, Gunatillaka PD, et al. Protracted infection with *Salmonella bareilly* in a maternity hospital. *J Trop Med Hyg* 1976;79:142–150.
333. Standaert SM, Hutcheson RH, Schaffner W. Nosocomial transmission of salmonella gastroenteritis to laundry workers in a nursing home. *Infect Control Hosp Epidemiol* 1994;15:22–26.
334. Bate J, James U. *Salmonella typhimurium* infection dust-borne in a children's ward. *Lancet* 1958;2:713–715.
335. DuPont HL. Shigella species (bacillary dysentery). In: Mandell GL, Bennett JE, Dolin R, eds. *Mandell, Douglas and Bennett's principles and practice of infectious diseases,* 5th ed. New York: Churchill Livingstone, 2000:2363–2369.
336. Weissman JB, Hutcheson RH. Shigellosis transmitted by nurses. *South Med J* 1976;69:1341–1346.
337. Laboratory Centers for Disease Control. Outbreak of *Shigella flexneri* in a nursing home—Alberta. *Can Dis Week Rep* 1988;14:99–101.
338. Horan MA, Gulati RS, Fox RA, et al. Outbreak of *Shigella sonnei* dysentery on a geriatric assessment ward. *J Hosp Infect* 1984;5: 210–212.
339. Bachrach SJ. Successful treatment of an institutional outbreak of shigellosis. *Clin Pediatr* 1981;20:127–131.
340. Hunter PR, Hutchings PG. Outbreak of *Shigella sonnei* dysentery on a long stay psychogeriatric ward. *J Hosp Infect* 1987;10:73–76.
341. Seas C, Gotuzzo E. Vibrio cholerae In: Mandell GL, Bennett JE, Dolin R, eds. *Mandell, Douglas and Bennett's principles and practice of infectious diseases,* 5th ed. New York: Churchill Livingstone, 2000: 2266–2272.
342. Mhalu FS, Mtango FD, Msengi AE. Hospital outbreaks of cholera transmitted through close person-to-person contact. *Lancet* 1984;2: 82–84.
343. Ryder RW, Rahman ASMM, Alim ARMA, et al. An outbreak of nosocomial cholera in a rural Bangladesh hospital. *J Hosp Infect* 1986; 8:275–282.
344. Nelson DE, Auerbach SB, Baltch AL, et al. Epidemic *Clostridium difficile*–associated diarrhea: role of second- and third-generation cephalosporins. *Infect Control Hosp Epidemiol* 1994;15:88–94.
345. McFarland LV, Mulligan ME, Kwok RYY, et al. Nosocomial acquisition of *Clostridium difficile* infection. *N Engl J Med* 1989;320: 204–210.
346. Samore M, Killgore G, Johnson S, et al. Multicenter typing comparison of sporadic and outbreak *Clostridium difficile* isolates from geographically diverse hospitals. *J Infect Dis* 1997;176:1233–1238.
347. Delmee M. *Clostridium difficile* infection in health-care workers. *Lancet* 1989;2:1095.
348. Johnson S, Samore MH, Mathis SD, et al. Clostridium difficile diarrhea in health care workers. In: *Program and abstracts of the 9th Annual Scientific Meeting of the Society for Healthcare Epidemiology of America,* April 18–20, San Francisco, abstract 31.
349. MacGregor RR. *Corynebacterium diphtheriae.* In: Mandell GL, Bennett JE, Dolin R, eds. *Mandell, Douglas and Bennett's principles and practice of infectious diseases,* 5th ed. New York: Churchill Livingstone, 2000:2190–2198.
350. Harnisch JP, Tronca E, Nolan CM, et al. Diphtheria among alcoholic urban adults: a decade of experience in Seattle. *Ann Intern Med* 1989; 111:71–82.
351. Larsson P, Brinkhoff B, Larsson L. *Corynebacterium diphtheriae* in the environment of carriers and patients. *J Hosp Infect* 1987;10:282–286.
352. Centers for Disease Control. Update on adult immunization. Recommendations of the Immunization Practices Advisory committee (ACIP). *MMWR* 1991;40(RR-12):1–94.
353. Vitek CR, Wharton M. Diphtheria in the former Soviet Union: reemergence of a pandemic disease. *Emerg Infect Dis* 1998;4:539–550.
354. Gray RD, James SM. Occult diphtheria infection in a hospital for the mentally subnormal. *Lancet* 1973;1:1105–1106.
355. Anderson GS, Penfold JB. An outbreak of diphtheria in a hospital for the mentally subnormal. *J Clin Pathol* 1973;26:606–615.
356. Muller AS, Leeuwenberg J, Pratt DS. Pertussis: epidemiology and control. *Bull WHO* 1986;64:321–331.
357. Linnemann CC Jr, Nasenbeny J. Pertussis in the adult. *Annu Rev Med* 1977;28:179–185.
358. Morse SI. Pertussis in adults. *Ann Intern Med* 1968;68:953–954.
359. Robertson PW, Goldberg H, Jarvie BH, et al. Bordetella pertussis infection: a cause of persistent cough in adults. *Med J Aust* 1987;146: 522–525.
360. Cherry JD, Baraff LJ, Hewlett E. The past, present, and future of pertussis. The role of adults in epidemiology and future control [see comments]. *West J Med* 1989;150:319–328.
361. Mortimer EA Jr. Pertussis and its prevention: a family affair [comment]. *J Infect Dis* 1990;161:473–479.
362. Aoyama T, Takeuchi Y, Goto A, et al. Pertussis in adults. *Am J Dis Child* 1992;146:163–166.
363. Hewlett EL. Pertussis in adults: significance for disease transmission and immunisation policy [editorial]. *J Med Microbiol* 1992;36: 141–142.
364. Cromer BA, Goydos J, Hackell J, et al. Unrecognized pertussis infection in adolescents. *Am J Dis Child* 1993;147:575–577.
365. Mink CM, Cherry JD, Christenson P, et al. A search for *Bordetella pertussis* infection in university students. *Clin Infect Dis* 1992;14: 464–471.
366. Wright SW, Edwards KM, Decker MD, et al. Pertussis infection in adults with persistent cough. *JAMA* 1995;273:1044–1046.
367. Kurt TL, Yeager AS, Guenette S, et al. Spread of pertussis by hospital staff. *JAMA* 1972;221:264–267.
368. Linnemann CC Jr, Ramundo N, Perlstein PH, et al. Use of pertussis vaccine in an epidemic involving hospital staff. *Lancet* 1975;2: 540–543.
369. Valenti WM, Pincus PH, Messner MK. Nosocomial pertussis: possible spread by a hospital visitor. *Am J Dis Child* 1980;134:520–521.
370. Broome CV, Preblud SR, Bruner B, et al. Epidemiology of pertussis, Atlanta, 1977. *J Pediatr* 1981;98:362–367.

371. Addiss DG, Davis JP, Meade BD, et al. A pertussis outbreak in a Wisconsin nursing home. *J Infect Dis* 1991;164:704–710.
372. Herwaldt LA. Pertussis in adults. What physicians need to know. *Arch Intern Med* 1991;151:1510–1512.
373. Weber DJ, Rutala WA. Management of healthcare workers exposed to pertussis. *Infect Control Hosp Epidemiol* 1994;15:411–415.
374. Wright SW, Edwards KM, Decker MD, et al. Pertussis seroprevalence in emergency department staff. *Ann Emerg Med* 1994;24:413–417.
375. Wright SW, Decker MD, Edwards KM. Incidence of pertussis infection in healthcare workers. *Infect Control Hosp Epidemiol* 1999;20: 120–123.
376. Nelson JD. The changing epidemiology of pertussis in young infants. The role of adults as reservoirs of infection. *Am J Dis Child* 1978; 132:371–373.
377. Weber DJ, Rutala WA. Management of healthcare workers exposed to pertussis. *Infect Control Hosp Epidemiol* 1994;15:411–415.
378. Farizo KM, Cochi SL, Zell ER, et al. Epidemiological features of pertussis in the United States, 1980–1989. *Clin Infect Dis* 1992;14: 708–719.
379. Centers for Disease Control. Resurgence of pertussis—United States, 1993. *MMWR* 1993;42:952–953,959–960.
380. Centers for Disease Control. Quarterly immunization table. *MMWR* 1998;47:67.
381. Edwards KM, Decker MD, Graham BS, et al. Adult immunization with acellular pertussis vaccine. *JAMA* 1993;269:53–56.
382. Herwaldt LA. Pertussis and pertussis vaccines in adults [editorial—comment]. *JAMA* 1993;269:93–94.
383. Keitel WA, Muenz LM, Decker MD, et al. A randomized clinical trial of acellular pertussis vaccines in healthy adults: dose-response comparisons of five vaccines and implications for booster immunization. *J Infect Dis* 1999; 180: 397–403.
384. Rothstein EP, Anderson EL, Decker MD, et al. An acellular pertussis vaccine in healthy adults; safety and immunogenicity. *Vaccine* 1999; 17: 2999–3006.
385. Christie CDC, Garrison KMK, Kiely L, et al. A trial of acellular pertussis vaccine hospital workers during the Cincinnati pertussis epidemic of 1993. *Clin Infect Dis* 2001;33:997–1003.
386. Shefer A, Dales L, Nelson M, et al. Use and safety of acellular pertussis vaccine among adult hospital staff during an outbreak of pertussis. *J Infect Dis* 1995;171:1053–1056.
387. Edwards KM, Decker MD, Pertussis vaccine. In: Plotkin SK, Orenstein WA, eds. *Vaccines,* 4th ed. Philadelphia: Saunders, 2004: 471–528.
388. Christie CDC, Glover AM, Willke MJ, et al. Containment of pertussis in the regional pediatric hospital during the greater Cincinnati epidemic of 1993. *Infect Control Hosp Epidemiol* 1995;16:556–563.
389. Halsey NA, Welling MA, Lehman RM. Nosocomial pertussis: a failure of erythromycin treatment and prophylaxis. *Am J Dis Child* 1980; 134:521–522.
390. Haiduven DJ, Hench CP, Simpkins SM, et al. Standardized management of patients and employees exposed to pertussis. *Infect Control Hosp Epidemiol* 1998;19:861–864.
391. Bisno AL, Stevens DL. Streptococcus pyogenes (including streptococcal toxic shock syndrome and necrotizing fasciitis). In: Mandell GL, Bennett JE, Dolin R, eds. *Mandell, Douglas and Bennett's principles and practice of infectious diseases.* 5th ed. New York: Churchill Livingstone, 2000:2101–2117.
392. Schaffner W, Lefkowitz LB, Goodman JS, et al. Hospital outbreak of infections with group A streptococci traced to an asymptomatic anal carrier. *N Engl J Med* 1969;280:1224–1225.
393. Ramage L, Green K, Pyskir D, et al. An outbreak of fatal nosocomial infections due to group A streptococcus on a medical ward. *Infect Control Hosp Epidemiol* 1996;17:429–431.
394. Schwartz B, Elliott JA, Butler JC, et al. Clusters of invasive group A streptococcal infections in family, hospital, and nursing home settings. *Clin Infect Dis* 1992;15:277–284.
395. Kakis A, Gibbs L, Eguia J, et al. An outbreak of group A streptococcal infection among health care workers. *Clin Infect Dis* 2002; 35: 1353–1359.
396. Decker MD, Lavely GB, Hutcheson RH Jr, et al. Food-borne streptococcal pharyngitis in a hospital pediatrics clinic. *JAMA* 1985;253: 679–681.
397. Weber DJ, Rutala WA. Management of healthcare workers with pharyngitis or suspected streptococcal infections. *Infect Control Hosp Epidemiol* 1996;17:753–761.
398. The prevention of invasive Group A streptococcal infections workshop participants. Prevention of invasive Group A streptococcal disease among household contacts of case patients and among post partum and post surgical patients; recommendations from the Centers for Disease Control and Prevention. *Clin Infect Dis* 2002;35:950–959.
399. Decker MD, Gregory DW, Boldt J, et al. The detection of penicillin-resistant pneumococci. The compliance of hospital laboratories with recommended methods. *Am J Clin Pathol* 1985;84:357–360.
400. Centers for Disease Control. Prevalence of penicillin-resistant *Streptococcus pneumoniae*—Connecticut, 1992–1993. *MMWR* 1994;43: 216–217,223.
401. Centers for Disease Control. Drug-resistant *Streptococcus pneumoniae*—Kentucky and Tennessee, 1993. *MMWR* 1994;43:23–26,31.
402. Musher DM. *Streptococcus pneumoniae.* In: Mandell GL, Bennett JE, Dolin R, eds. *Mandell, Douglas and Bennett's principles and practice of infectious diseases,* 5th ed. New York: Churchill Livingstone, 2000: 2128–2128.
403. DeMaria A Jr, Browne K, Berk SL, et al. An outbreak of type 1 pneumococcal pneumonia in a men's shelter. *JAMA* 1980;244: 1446–1449.
404. Mercat A, Nguyen J, Dautzenberg B. An outbreak of pneumococcal pneumonia in two men's shelters. *Chest* 1991;99:147–151.
405. Cherian T, Steinhoff MC, Harrison LH, et al. A cluster of invasive pneumococcal disease in young children in child care. *JAMA* 1994; 271:695–697.
406. Hoge CW, Reichler MR, Dominguez EA, et al. An epidemic of pneumococcal disease in an overcrowded, inadequately ventilated jail. *N Engl J Med* 1994;331:643–648.
407. Crum NF, Wallace MR, Lamb CR, et al. Halting a pneumococcal pneumonia outbreak among United States Marine Corps trainees. *Am J Prevent Med* 2003;25:107–111.
408. Cartmill TD, Panigrahi H. Hospital outbreak of multiresistant *Streptococcus pneumoniae* [letter—see comments]. *J Hosp Infect* 1992;20: 130–132.
409. McNeely DF, Lyons J, Conte S, et al. A cluster of drug-resistant *Streptococcus pneumoniae* among nursing home patients. *Infect Control Hosp Epidemiol* 1998;19:476–477.
410. Sheppard DC, Bartlett KA, Lampiris HW. *Streptococcus pneumoniae* transmission in chronic-care facilities: description of an outbreak and review of management strategies. *Infect Control Hosp Epidemiol* 1998; 19:851–853.
411. Nuorti JP, Butler JC, Crutcher JM, et al. An outbreak of multidrug-resistant pneumococcal pneumonia and bacteremia among unvaccinated nursing home residents. *N Engl J Med* 1998;338:1861–1868.
412. Gleich S, Morad Y, Echague R, et al. Streptococcus pneumoniae serotype 4 outbreak in a home for the aged: report and review of recent outbreaks. *Infect Control Hosp Epidemiol* 2000;21:711–717.
413. Black S, Shinefield H, Fireman B, et al. Efficacy, safety and immunogenicity of heptavalent pneumococcal conjugate vaccine in children. *Pediatr Infect Dis J* 2000;19:187–195.
414. Artenstein MS, Ellis RE. The risk of exposure to a patient with meningococcal meningitis. *Milit Med* 1968;133:474–477.
415. Fallon RJ. Hospital-acquired meningococcaemia. *J Hosp Infect* 1992; 20:121–132.
416. Shapiro ED. Prophylaxis for contacts of patients with meningococcal or *Haemophilus influenzae* type B disease. *Pediatr Infect Dis* 1982;1: 132–138.
417. Centers for Disease Control. Nosocomial meningococcemia—Wisconsin. *MMWR* 1978;27:358–363.
418. Cohen MS, Steere AC, Baltimore R, et al. Possible nosocomial transmission of group Y *Neisseria meningitidis* among oncology patients. *Ann Intern Med* 1979;91:7–12.
419. Rose HD, Lenz IE, Sheth NK. Meningococcal pneumonia: a source of nosocomial infection. *Arch Intern Med* 1981;141:575–577.

420. Riewerts-Eriksen NH, Espersen F, Laursen L, et al. Nosocomial outbreak of group C meningococcal disease. *BMJ* 1989;298:568–569.
421. Centers for Disease Control. Laboratory-acquired meningococcemia—California and Massachusetts. *MMWR* 1991;40:46–47,55.
422. Decker MD, Edwards KM, Bradley R, et al. Comparative trial in infants of four conjugate *Haemophilus influenzae* type B vaccines [see comments]. *J Pediatr* 1992;120:184–189.
423. Centers for Disease Control. Progress toward elimination of *Haemophilus influenzae* type B disease among infants and children—United States, 1987–1993. *MMWR* 1994;43:144–148.
424. Patterson JE, Madden GM, Krsiiunas EP, et al. A nosocomial outbreak of ampicillin-resistant *Haemophilus influenzae* type B in a geriatric unit. *J Infect Dis* 1988;157:1002–1007.
425. Bachrach S. An outbreak of *Haemophilus influenzae* type B bacteraemia in an intermediate care hospital for children. *J Hosp Infect* 1988; 11:121–126.
426. Hekker TA, van der Schee AC, Kempers J, et al. A nosocomial outbreak of amoxicillin-resistant non-typable *Haemophilus influenzae* in a respiratory ward [see comments]. *J Hosp Infect* 1991;19:25–31.
427. Howard AJ, Owens D, Musser JM. Cross-infection due to *Haemophilus influenzae* type B in adults [Letter—see comments]. *J Hosp Infect* 1991;19:70–72.
428. McGechie PB. Nosocomial bacteraemia in hospital staff caused by *Haemophilus influenzae* type B [letter—comment]. *J Hosp Infect* 1992; 21:159–160.
429. O'Neill YV. Diseases of the Middle Ages. In: Kiple KF, ed. *The Cambridge world history of human disease.* Cambridge, UK: Cambridge University Press, 1993:270–279.
430. Centers for Disease Control. Human plague—United States, 1993–1994. *MMWR* 1994;43:242–246.
431. Butler T. Yersinia species (including plague). In: Mandell GL, Bennett JE, Dolin R, eds. *Mandell, Douglas and Bennett's principles and practice of infectious diseases,* 5th ed. New York: Churchill Livingstone, 2000; 2406–2414.
432. 4 plague deaths bring India's total to 56 in 3 weeks. *Orlando Sentinel* 1994;A-16.
433. White ME, Gordon D, Poland JD, et al. Recommendations for the control of *Yersinia pestis* infections. *Infect Control* 1980;1:326–329.
434. Olle-Goig JE, Canela-Soler J. An outbreak of *Brucella melitensis* infection by airborne transmission among laboratory workers. *Am J Public Health* 1987;77:335–338.
435. Kiel FW, Khan MY. Brucellosis among hospital employees in Saudi Arabia. *Infect Control Hosp Epidemiol* 1993;14:268–272.
436. Saravolatz L, Arking L, Wentworth B, et al. Prevalence of antibody to the Legionnaires' disease bacterium in hospital employees. *Ann Intern Med* 1979;90:601–603.
437. Marrie TJ, George J, Macdonald S, et al. Are health care workers at risk for infection during an outbreak of nosocomial Legionnaires' disease? *Am J Infect Control* 1986;14:209–213.
438. O'Mahony MC, Stanwell-Smith RE, Tillett HE, et al. The Stafford outbreak of Legionnaires' disease. *Epidemiol Infect* 1990;104: 361–380.
439. Jarvis WR. Recommended precautions for patients with Legionnaires' disease. *Infect Control* 1982;3:401–402.
440. Decker MD, Lybarger JA, Vaughn WK, et al. An outbreak of staphylococcal skin infections among river rafting guides. *Am J Epidemiol* 1986;124:969–976.
441. Cookson B, Peters B, Webster M, et al. Staff carriage of epidemic methicillin-resistant *Staphylococcus aureus* [see comments]. *J Clin Microbiol* 1989;27:1471–1476.
442. Opal SM, Mayer KH, Stenberg MJ, et al. Frequent acquisition of multiple strains of methicillin-resistant *Staphylococcus aureus* by healthcare workers in an endemic hospital environment. *Infect Control Hosp Epidemiol* 1990;11:479–485.
443. Jernigan JA, Titus MG, Gröschel DHM, et al. Effectiveness of contact isolation during a hospital outbreak of methicillin-resistant *Staphylococcus aureus. Am J Epidemiol* 1996;143:496–504.
444. Sheagren JN. *Staphylococcus aureus.* The persistent pathogen (first of two parts). *N Engl J Med* 1984;310:1368–1373.
445. Chow JW, Yu VL. *Staphylococcus aureus* nasal carriage in hemodialysis patients. Its role in infection and approaches to prophylaxis. *Arch Intern Med* 1989;149:1258–1262.
446. Boyce JM. Methicillin-resistant *Staphylococcus aureus* in hospitals and long-term care facilities: microbiology, epidemiology, and preventive measures. *Infect Control Hosp Epidemiol* 1992;13:725–737.
447. Mortimer EA Jr, Wolinsky E, Gonzaga AJ, et al. Role of airborne transmission in staphylococcal infections. *Br Med J* 1966;1:319–322.
448. Gundermann KO. Spread of microorganisms by air-conditioning systems—especially in hospitals. *Ann NY Acad Sci* 1980;353:209–217.
449. Lossick JG, Kraus SJ, Syphilis. In: Evans AS, ed. *Bacterial infections of humans: epidemiology and control,* 2nd ed. New York and London: Plenum, 1991:675–695.
450. Whitney CM. The physician's danger in treating patients who have syphilis. *Am J Syph* 1928;12:1–12.
451. Rein MF. Nosocomial sexually transmitted diseases. *Infect Control* 1984;5:117–122.
452. Normand R, Klotz SA, Tudor S. Annual syphilis serology testing in hospital employees: is it beneficial? *Am J Infect Control* 1988;16: 30–33.
453. Eckmann BH, Schaefer GL, Huppert M. Bedside interhuman transmission of coccidioidomycosis via growth on fomites: an epidemic involving six persons. *Am Rev Respir Dis* 1964;89:175–185.
454. Arnow PM, Sadigh M, Costas C, et al. Endemic and epidemic aspergillosis associated with in-hospital replication of *Aspergillus microorganisms. J Infect Dis* 1991;164:998–1002.
455. Lewis SM, Lewis BG. Nosocomial transmission of *Trychophyton tonsurans tinea corporis* in a rehabilitation hospital. *Infect Control Hosp Epidemiol* 1997;18:322–325.
456. Chen K-T, Chen C-J, Chang P-Y, et al. A nosocomial outbreak of malaria associated with contaminated catheters and contrast medium of a computed tomographic scanner. *Infect Control Hosp Epidemiol* 1999;20:22–25.
457. Lettau LA. Nosocomial transmission and infection control aspects of parasitic and ectoparasitic diseases. Part I. Introduction/enteric parasites. *Infect Control Hosp Epidemiol* 1991;12:59–65.
458. Lettau LA. Nosocomial transmission and infection control aspects of parasitic and ectoparasitic diseases. Part II. Blood and tissue parasites. *Infect Control Hosp Epidemiol* 1991;12:111–121.
459. Chave J-P, David S, Wauters J-P, et al. Transmission of *Pneumocystis carinii* from AIDS patients to other immunosuppressed patients: a cluster of *Pneumocystis carinii pneumonia* in renal transplant recipients. *AIDS* 1991;5:927–932.
460. Lettau LA. Nosocomial transmission and infection control aspects of parasitic and ectoparasitic diseases. Part III. Ectoparasites/summary and conclusions. *Infect Control Hosp Epidemiol* 1991;12:179–185.
461. Degelau J. Scabies in long-term care facilities. *Infect Control Hosp Epidemiol* 1992;13:421–425.
462. Pasternak J, Richtmann R, Ganme APP, et al. Scabies epidemic: price and prejudice. *Infect Control Hosp Epidemiol* 1994;15:540–542.
463. Yonkosky D, Ladia L, Gackenheimer L, et al. Scabies in nursing homes: an eradication program with permethrin 5% cream. *J Am Acad Dermatol* 1990;23:1133–1136.
464. Clark J, Friesen DL, Williams WA. Management of an outbreak of Norwegian scabies. *Am J Infect Control* 1992;20:217–220.
465. Gonzalez E. Latex hypersensitivity: a new and unexpected problem. *Hosp Pract* 1992;27:137–140, 145–148.
466. Obasanjo OO, Wu P, Conlon M, et al. An outbreak of scabies in a teaching hospital: lessons learned. *Infect Control Hosp Epidemiol* 2001; 22:13–18.
467. Zafar AB, Beidas SO, Sylvester LK. Control of transmission of Norwegian scabies. *Infect Control Hosp Epidemiol* 2002;23:278–279.
468. DeShazo RD, Williams DF, Moak ES. Fire ant attacks on residents in health care facilities: a report of two cases. *Ann Intern Med* 1999; 131:424–429.
469. Sussman GL. Latex allergy: its importance in clinical practice. *Allergy Proc* 1992;13:67–69.
470. Bubak ME, Reed CE, Fransway AF, et al. Allergic reactions to latex among health-care workers [see comments]. *Mayo Clin Proc* 1992; 67:1075–1079.
471. Baur X, Ammon J, Chen Z, et al. Health risk in hospitals through

airborne allergens for patients presensitised to latex. *Lancet* 1993;342: 1148–1149.

472. Decter BM, Gorra J. Allergic reactions to latex [letter—comment]. *Mayo Clin Proc* 1993;68:202.
473. Akasawa A, Matsumoto K, Saito H, et al. Incidence of latex allergy in atopic children and hospital workers in Japan. *Int Arch Allergy Immunol* 1993;101:177–181.
474. deShazo RD. Latex-induced anaphylaxis [editorial—comment]. *South Med J* 1993;86:977–978.
475. Hitchens JT. Latex gloves: friend or foe? *AANA J* 1993;61:379–381.
476. Yassin MS, Lierl MB, Fischer TJ, et al. Latex allergy in hospital employees. *Ann Allergy* 1994;72:245–249.
477. Markey J. Latex allergy: implications for healthcare personnel and infusion therapy patients. *J Intraven Nurs* 1994;17:35–39.
478. Reis JG. Latex sensitivity. Controlling health care workers', patients' risks. *AORN J* 1994;59:615–617,620–621.
479. Mendyka BE, Clochesy JM, Workman ML. Latex hypersensitivity: an iatrogenic and occupational risk. *Am J Crit Care* 1994;3:198–201.
480. Salkie ML. Allergens in the workplace. *Clin Biochem* 1994;27:81–85.
481. Burrell R. Microbiological agents as health risks in indoor air. *Environ Health Perspect* 1991;95:29–34.
482. Grieble HG, Colton FR, Bird TJ, et al. Fine particle humidifiers: source of *Pseudomonas aeruginosa* infections in a respiratory-disease unit. *N Engl J Med* 1970;282:531–534.
483. Pierce AK, Sanford JP. Bacterial contamination of aerosols. *Arch Intern Med* 1973;131:156–159.
484. Smith PW, Massanari RM. Room humidifiers as the source of *Acinetobacter* infections. *JAMA* 1977;237:795–797.
485. Allen KD, Green HT. Hospital outbreak of multi-resistant *Acinetobacter anitratus:* an airborne mode of spread? *J Hosp Infect* 1987;9: 110–119.
486. Mirza A, Wyatt M, Begue RE. Infection control practices and the pregnant health care worker. *Pediatr Infect Dis J* 1999;18:18–22.
487. Sepkowitz KA. Occupationally acquired infections in health care workers. Part I. *Ann Intern Med* 1996;125:826–834.
488. Sepkowitz KA. Occupationally acquired infections in health care workers. Part II. *Ann Intern Med* 1996;125:917–928.

82

NOSOCOMIAL INFECTIONS IN DIAGNOSTIC LABORATORIES

DAVID L. SEWELL

Advances in medical and surgical interventions, world travel, global climate changes, and threats of bioterrorism are rapidly changing healthcare and pose a challenge in controlling occupationally acquired infections (1–4). Historically, workers in diagnostic laboratories have always been at higher risk for infection from exposure to infectious materials (5). Today, the laboratory worker is faced with increased exposure to infectious material from the recognition of new infectious agents, potential use of bioterrorism agents, increasing antimicrobial resistance, and introduction of new diagnostic techniques and instrumentation. In addition, improper handling of biologic wastes or episodes of laboratory-acquired infection (LAI) could lead to the spread of microorganisms outside the laboratory, although this occurrence has been rare. Thus, implementation and adherence to effective prevention and control measures should be important to all who work in the laboratory environment (6). Interestingly, laboratory workers must be constantly reminded of these hazards, because they often minimize the risk either through constant daily exposure or risk-taking behavior (7). This chapter considers microorganisms likely to cause infections in hospital laboratory workers, usual modes by which these microorganisms are transmitted in the laboratory, and appropriate control measures for preventing such incidents.

OCCURRENCE OF LABORATORY-ACQUIRED INFECTION

The risk of LAI has been recognized since the end of the nineteenth century but the true incidence is unknown, even today, because of the lack of adequate reporting systems. In the world literature, LAIs are usually reported as individual cases or compiled through laboratory surveys. Often, accurate documentation of the LAI is lacking in these reports. The most extensive surveys in the United States were conducted by Sulkin and Pike from 1949 to 1970 (8–10). More recent surveys reviewed LAIs in Utah (11) and in public health laboratories (12). Based on these limited data, Wilson and Reller (13) estimated that the annual incidence of LAIs in the United States was between 1 and 5 per 1,000 employees. More systematic surveys of LAIs have occurred in the United Kingdom from 1970 to 1995 (14–16). The most recent retrospective survey for occupationally acquired infections in 397 laboratories (1994 to 1995) in the United Kingdom found an overall incidence rate of 16.2 per 100,000 person-years compared with 82.7 infections per 100,000 person-years for a similar survey conducted in 1988 to 1989, suggesting that control measures may be reducing the incidence of infections (16). Because of the lack of adequate modern data on LAIs, control measures are proposed and implemented on the basis of old data (11), experience with one infectious agent applied to others, the epidemiology of relevant microorganisms from nonlaboratory settings, and hazard analysis (17). Although laboratory workers will always be at risk for infection, adherence to safety measures will significantly reduce the risk.

The previous data document the occupational risk associated with handling patient specimens and microbiologic cultures. By contrast, few reports document the spread of laboratory pathogens from the laboratory to other hospital areas or to the community (18). Thus, the risk of infection to laboratory workers is greatest from specimens originating in the community or hospitalized patients, and the danger of diagnostic laboratory microorganisms affecting the community is small.

Mode of Transmission and Etiology

In laboratories, the factors that influence occupationally acquired infections are related to host susceptibility and behavior, the virulence and availability of the pathogen, and the work environment (5). The most common types of exposure that cause infections include inhalation of aerosols generated by accidents and work practices; percutaneous inoculation through accidents with needles, blades, and broken glassware; ingestion; and contamination of mucous membranes and skin (5,19). Often the specific exposure incident is not easily identifiable other than working with infectious material in a diagnostic laboratory environment. In the past, *Brucella* species, *Mycobacterium tuberculosis, Coxiella burnetii,* hepatitis B virus (HBV), *Francisella tularensis,* and *Salmonella* species caused most of the LAIs (9). During the 1980s, laboratory workers were most frequently infected with *M. tuberculosis, Salmonella* species, *Shigella* species, HBV, and hepatitis C virus (HCV) (11,12,14,15). In the 1990s, biosafety measures have emphasized the reduction of infection from blood-borne pathogens in all healthcare workers (HCWs).

The risk of acquiring a blood-borne infection is influenced by the prevalence of infection in patients, the amount of blood involved, the type of exposure, the concentration of pathogen in the blood or body fluid, and the availability of postexposure prophylaxis (6,20). In addition to infections from human immunodeficiency virus (HIV), HBV, and HCV, blood-borne transmission of at least 20 different agents has been reported (21). However, non–blood-borne infections from enteric pathogens, *Brucella* species, and *Neisseria meningitidis* continue to cause LAIs (17,22–24). A list of selected microorganisms that may cause laboratory infections is illustrated in Table 82.1. A more complete compilation can be found in selected publications (6, 17,25–27). The following is a categorization of these microorganisms by their likely mode of spread within the laboratory environment.

Blood-borne Viruses

The blood-borne viruses (HIV, HBV, HCV) pose the infection risk of greatest concern to hospital workers (6,20,28). As of June 30, 2001, the Centers for Disease Control and Prevention (CDC) had received reports of 57 HCWs in the United States who are documented as having seroconverted to HIV and 137 other reports classified as possible occupational transmission *(http://www.cdc.gov/hiv/pubs/facts/hcwsurv.htm).* These individuals include 19 laboratory workers (16 of who were clinical laboratory workers). Forty-eight of the 57 documented exposures were percutaneous exposures, 5 were mucocutaneous, 2 were both, and 2 were an unknown route of exposure. Forty-nine HCWs were exposed to HIV-infected blood, 3 to concentrated virus, 1 to visibly bloody fluid, and 4 to unspecified fluid. Twenty-six of these individuals developed acquired immunodeficiency syndrome (AIDS). It is estimated that the individual HCW experiences approximately 30 needlestick injuries per 100 beds per year (29) and that laboratory workers experience more mucocutaneous exposures (30).

The risk of infection from HIV, HBV, and HCV following occupational exposure to infected blood is related to the concentration of the virus in blood. HBV can be present in concentrations of 10^8 to 10^9 infectious particles/mL blood, and the concentrations of HIV and HCV are 10^0 to 10^4 and 10^2 to 10^3 particles/mL blood, respectively (6,20). The risk of infection following a percutaneous exposure is approximately 18% (6% to 30%) for HBV, 1.8% (0% to 7%) for HCV, and 0.3% (0% to 0.9%) for HIV. Following the mandatory requirement that employers provide HBV vaccination at no cost to their employees, the incidence of HBV infections in HCWs decreased 95% from 1983 to 1995 (31). The prevalence of HCV infection among HCWs (1% to 2%) appears no greater than the rate observed in the general population (6,20). Although the blood-borne viruses are found in many different body fluids and tissues, the transmission of HCV, HIV, and HBV is most often associated with blood or visibly bloody body fluids.

Airborne Mycobacteria and Bacteria

The transmission of *M. tuberculosis* and *Mycobacterium bovis* in healthcare facilities and clinical laboratories is a recognized risk (32). Since 1953 the tuberculosis case rate has declined tenfold from 53 cases per 100,000 to 5.6 per 100,000 in 2001 and decreased 40% from 1992 when the case rate most recently peaked in the United States *(http://www.cdc.gov/nchstp/tb/surv/surv2001/default.htm).* The presence of tubercle bacilli in specimens other than respiratory secretions (e.g., gastric aspirates, cerebrospinal fluid (CSF), urine, exudates, and tissue) may result in nosocomial transmission to HCWs and autopsy personnel (33). In addition, infection may result from direct parenteral inoculation by laboratory workers (34). However, the greatest risk to laboratory personnel is from exposure to aerosols generated during handling of liquid specimens, preparation of frozen sections, and performing autopsies (6). Other bacteria that may be transmitted by airborne droplets or aerosols include *Corynebacterium diphtheriae; N. meningitidis; Bordetella pertussis; Streptococcus pyogenes;* and the potential agents of bioterrorism, *Bacil-*

TABLE 82.1. SELECTED MICROORGANISMS INVOLVED IN LABORATORY INFECTION EPISODES REPORTED IN MEDICAL JOURNALS DURING THE PERIOD 1994–2002 BY MICROORGANISM GROUP

Group and Microorganism	Type of Laboratory	Year of Publication	References
Bacteria			
Brucellosis	Diagnostic, Research	2000, 2001	22, 24
Toxigenic E. coli	Diagnostic	1996, 1998	46, 49
N. meningitidis	Diagnostic	2001	23
Shigellosis	Diagnostic	1997	43
Tuberculosis	Diagnostic, Anatomic	1998, 2001	33, 34
Viruses			
Human immunodeficiency virus	Anatomic	1997	76
Sabia virus	Research	1995	55
West Nile virus	Diagnostic	2002	56
Parasites			
Leishmaniasis	Diagnostic	1997	87
Rickettsiae			
Scrub typhus	Research	2001	42
Fungi			
Penicillium marneffei	Diagnostic	1994	39

lus anthracis, Yersinia pestis, Brucella species, *F. tularensis,* and *Burkholderia pseudomallei* (6,25,35–38). Brucellosis is a commonly reported LAI in research and animal laboratories but also occurs in clinical laboratories (22,24). The agent of whooping cough, *B. pertussis,* has caused at least 12 LAIs in the past 20 years (5). *N. meningitidis* is an infrequent cause of LAIs but has been associated with fatal outcomes and should be handled in a manner that minimizes risk for exposure to aerosols or droplets (23). Worldwide, 16 probable cases of LAIs have occurred from 1986 to the present with six probable cases occurring in the United States from 1996 to 2001. The source isolates were recovered from blood or CSF in five of the six cases and probably CSF or middle ear fluid in the sixth case. In 15 of the 16 worldwide cases, common laboratory procedures were not performed in a biologic safety cabinet and may have contributed to the exposure incidents.

Airborne Fungi

Laboratory-acquired fungal infections have been reported infrequently after 1980. Generally, fungal infections are acquired from the inhalation of the conidia of *Coccidioides immitis, Histoplasma capsulatum,* or *Blastomyces dermatitidis* and in one report *Penicillium marneffei* (5,17,19,39). Occasionally, cutaneous infections occur following accidental inoculation (40,41). Coccidioidomycosis and histoplasmosis are the most likely fungal infections to be transmitted in the laboratory (17). Arthroconidia from laboratory cultures of *C. immitis* easily become airborne, whereas spherules from tissue are much less likely to be aerosolized. Laboratory-acquired histoplasmosis also results primarily from handling laboratory cultures. The infective conidia are small and likely to become airborne, resist drying, and can cause infection after small inocula are inhaled. Pulmonary infection resulting from *B. dermatitidis* has followed inhalation of the conidia by laboratory workers, but this is much less frequent than cases of coccidioidomycosis or histoplasmosis.

Airborne Viruses, Chlamydia, and Rickettsiae

Most LAIs from *C. burnetii* arise from aerosols generated in animal research laboratories although there are a few reports of parenteral and mucous membrane transmissions (5,19,25). LAIs from *Rickettsia typhi, Rickettsia coronii,* and*Orientia tsutsugamushi* have also been reported (5,42). Before 1960, psittacosis was "among the most commonly reported laboratory-associated infections" (25), but only sporadic cases have been reported in the past 20 years (5). Psittacosis case-fatality rates are high compared with those of infections resulting from other agents. The microorganism *Chlamydia psittaci* may be present in tissues, feces, nasal secretions, and blood specimens. Few infections occur from exposure to *Chlamydia trachomatis* and generally result from mucous membrane exposure. Respiratory viral infections acquired in the laboratory are probably underreported, because it is difficult to document occupational acquisition. These viruses can be aerosolized by manipulation of specimens or cultures. Most laboratory-acquired viral infections, other than infections from the blood-borne viruses, occur in animal research laboratories following exposure to aerosols or contamination of skin and mucous membranes (5).

Contact-acquired Enteric Bacteria, Viruses, and Parasites

Infections from the enteric bacterial pathogens, *Salmonella* species and *Shigella* species, are commonly reported LAIs and are probably underreported (5,11,16,25,43). Infections generally occur from handling laboratory specimens and microbiologic cultures or occasionally from ingestion of intentionally contaminated food (44). *Salmonella typhi* causes the most serious infection (45). Gastroenteritis resulting from *Vibrio* species, *Campylobacter* species, enterotoxigenic *Escherichia coli,* and hepatitis A (HAV) and hepatitis E (HEV) viruses is infrequently reported (5,46–49). The shedding of HAV and probably HEV is diminished by the time a patient is symptomatic, decreasing the risk of transmission in the healthcare facility (4).

Parasitic diseases are receiving increasing attention because of world travel and increased susceptibility in immunocompromised individuals (50). Laboratory-acquired malaria, leishmaniasis, trypanosomiasis, and toxoplasmosis infections have all been reported. The two most frequently reported infections from accidental exposure are from *Trypanosoma cruzi* and *Toxoplasma gondii.* The rate of occurrence of laboratory accidents during work with *T. gondii* is reported to be one accident per 9,300 hours of exposure (51) or 1 infection per 24 person-years (50). The infection rate for working with *T. cruzi* is calculated to be 1 infection per 46 person-years. These infections ranged from asymptomatic to fatal in one case for each microorganism. Herwaldt (50) also reported on *Plasmodium* species (34 cases) and *Leishmania* species (12 cases) infections. Most of the infections associated with blood and tissue protozoa occurred from parenteral exposure but other routes included skin and mucous membrane exposure and ingestion. Only 21 cases of LAIs with intestinal protozoans have been reported and involved *Cryptosporidium parvum, Isospora belli,* and *Giardia lamblia.* Fewer reports have involved the helminths, including *Schistosoma* species, *Strongyloides* species, and *Ancylostoma* species. The most probable route of infection was ingestion of contaminated material although a few cases were associated with aerosols or skin penetration.

Contact-associated Bacteria and Fungi

S. pyogenes, Staphylococcus aureus, Neisseria gonorrhoeae, and *N. meningitidis* all have caused laboratory infection in association with parenteral inoculation or droplet exposure of mucous membranes from laboratory cultures of the microorganism or from clinical specimens. A few LAIs resulting from *Cryptococcus neoformans, B. dermatitidis,* and *Sporothrix schenckii* have occurred in which the proposed mode of spread was direct contact, splash, or percutaneous inoculation.

Bacteria, Fungi, Spirochetes, Viruses, and Rickettsia with Multiple Modes of Transmission

Many microorganisms, including the potential agents of bioterrorism, are transmitted by multiple exposure routes such as aerosols, contamination of skin and mucous membranes, ingestion, and percutaneous inoculation. Brucellosis is highly infectious and often causes multiple infections in research or laboratory workers following an accident (22,24). Infections often occur when laboratory workers do not recognize the pathogen and neglect to take necessary safety precautions (52). The practice of "sniffing" plates for characteristic odors associated with a specific bacterium should be curtailed (5). In addition to aerosol transmission, laboratory-acquired brucellosis has occurred from direct skin contact with cultures or with other infectious material, percutaneous inoculation, and spray onto mucous membranes. These same transmission routes are important for *B. anthracis,* the agent of anthrax; *F. tularensis,* the cause of tularemia; *C. diphtheriae,* the agent of diphtheria, and *Y. pestis,* the agent of plague. All of these bacteria should be handled with biosafety level (BSL) 2 and 3 safety precautions (37). *B. pseudomallei,* the microorganism responsible for melioidosis, is cited as a rare cause of LAIs but has been associated with a fatal outcome (53). Direct contact with microbiologic cultures or specimens, ingestion, autoinoculation, and exposure to infectious aerosols and droplets all have been implicated in transmission of *B. pseudomallei.* Fortunately, the agent of Q fever, *C. burnetii,*is rare in the United States, so the risk for diagnostic laboratory-acquired Q-fever infection in this country is minor compared with that in many other parts of the world. The microorganism is present in blood, urine, feces, milk, and tissue specimens and resists drying. Airborne spread is the most likely route for laboratory transmission, but parenteral inoculation occurs as well. An extremely small inoculum can produce disease.

Leptospira interrogans, the cause of leptospirosis, can be present in urine, blood, and tissues of infected patients. Ingestion, accidental parenteral inoculation, and contact of skin or mucous membranes with cultures or infected specimens all have led to laboratory worker infection. Likewise, syphilis has been an LAI and its agent, *Treponema pallidum,* can be present not only in blood but also in cutaneous, mucous membrane, and other lesions. Laboratory spread of this microorganism follows from parenteral inoculation, contact of mucous membranes or broken skin with infectious clinical materials, and possibly infectious aerosols. Most laboratory-acquired viral infections occur in animal research facilities and include numerous agents (5). Arenavirus (54), Sabia virus (55), West Nile virus (56), and other viruses causing hemorrhagic disease have caused laboratory infections. Lymphocytic choriomeningitis virus infections in laboratory workers occur in diagnostic facilities when cell cultures become contaminated with the virus, leading to possible aerosolization or skin or mucous membrane contamination. Specimens suspected of harboring the agent of smallpox, variola major, should not be cultured but rather shipped directly to CDC or a state health laboratory (37,38). Accidental parenteral inoculations are likely sources for laboratory-acquired rickettsial infections, but several infections with typhus have been associated with aerosols or infected airborne particles, and cases of Rocky Mountain spotted fever probably have occurred by this route as well (19,42). Because most diagnostic clinical laboratories do not perform cultures for rickettsia, these infections are more likely to be a risk in research laboratories.

RESERVOIRS AND MODES OF SPREAD

As detailed previously, a variety of modes of transmission have been noted in cases of LAIs and include inhalation, ingestion, inoculation, and contamination of skin and mucous membranes (6,17,19,25).

Perhaps the most likely mode of transmission is due to accidental inoculation of skin or soft tissue with needles or other sharps such as scalpels and broken glass from specimen containers. Nearly all pathogenic microorganisms can produce infection by this route, which is the most frequent route of transmission for blood-borne pathogens such as HIV or the hepatitis viruses (6). Hopefully, the accidental percutaneous inoculation of infectious material by laboratory personnel will decrease with the increased use of plastic collection tubes, needleless systems, and engineered safety devices (6,57,58). Needles should not be used in the laboratory unless there is no other alternative.

Although the intact skin is an excellent barrier to penetration by microorganisms, it does contain minor cuts and abrasions that serve as portals of entry. Contamination of mucous membranes by splashes and sprays of infectious material can lead to the laboratory transmission of HIV and other pathogenic agents to laboratory workers (5,6,25,27). In animal research facilities, bites and scratches from infected animals present a risk for transmission of an agent.

As on patient care wards, transmission by hand to skin and mucous membrane of the mouth, eye, and nose can cause an infection (59). Ingestion may occur following mouth pipetting, transfer of microorganisms on contaminated fingers or pencils, accidental splashes, or consumption of food and beverages in the laboratory. The laboratory environment is contaminated during the workday from routine specimen processing and the other work practices that produce aerosols or splatters and results in the contamination of hands (25,27,60). This stresses the importance of avoiding poor personal hygiene practices, such as applying cosmetics and adjusting contact lenses in the laboratory. Cases associated with contamination of food, drink, or tobacco products also have declined, because attention has been paid to eliminating eating, drinking, and smoking in the laboratory. Indirect contact with microorganisms can occur when environmental objects (e.g., specimen containers, test requisitions, instruments) or surfaces become contaminated with microorganisms. Accidents or spills also can lead to contamination of the workbench or other equipment, which may lead to contamination by hand contact.

Airborne spread is one mode of transmission of great concern in the laboratory (6,37, 61). Many laboratory procedures generate aerosols, droplets, or droplet nuclei that can be associated with direct transmission of infection through inhalation by the laboratory worker. Droplet nuclei (<5 μm in diameter) tend to remain suspended in air and move throughout the room or to build on air currents and reach the alveoli of the lungs when inhaled (62,63). Relevant procedures that generate aerosols include use of bacteriology loops for transferring cultures and flaming them afterward; pipetting (especially with fixed automatic pipettes); using syringes and needles; opening tubes and bottles; using centrifuges and blenders; performing autopsies; harvesting viral cultures; lyophilizing; and breaking culture plates, bottles, and tubes. These work practices also produce droplets that contaminate counters or floor surfaces, permitting transmission from these surfaces to hands. Microorganisms in blood droplets can survive for several days after drying on work surfaces or instruments (64).

GUIDELINES FOR PREVENTION

Laboratory safety is demanded by the standards of the Occupational Safety and Health Administration (OSHA), which are driven by the premise that the employer must provide a safe workplace (20,28,65–68). Compliance with current OSHA standards is subject to assessment by the agency's inspectors; thus, these regulations are perhaps of greatest importance to clinical diagnostic laboratories. Other groups, such as the CDC (69,70), the National Institutes of Health (25), the College of American Pathologists (CAP), and the National Coordinating Committee for Laboratory Standards (6) all provide guidelines or regulations for laboratory safety. OSHA, the National Institute for Occupational Safety and Health (NIOSH), the CAP, and the Joint Commission on Accreditation of Healthcare Organizations include safety among their checklists for laboratory inspectors. State and local licensing inspections and federal inspections for participation in Medicare also focus on safety issues.

Guidelines for laboratory safety from these groups cover exposures to chemical agents, fire, and other aspects, but the highlight of each is the prevention of laboratory infection. The following discussion is guided by these various regulations and guidelines and centers on the clinical diagnostic laboratory. The prevention of infection in autopsy, surgical pathology, and research and referral laboratories follows the same general plan considered here, but its implementation varies dramatically in each site according to the work done and the microorganisms involved (6).

Each laboratory must assess its specific risk from handling infectious material and design an exposure control plan to minimize these potential risks. Safety practices, usually containment measures, are designed to reduce or eliminate the exposure of laboratory workers to infectious material (6,25). These practices vary with the pathogenicity and infectious dose of the agent, the routes of transmission, the work performed, and the availability of treatment or prophylaxis (25,71,72). The CDC/National Institutes of Health guidelines (25) recommend four levels of biosafety (Table 82.2), and each successive level suggests increased occupational risk and more stringent containment practices. These classifications are similar to those adopted by the World Health Organization (WHO) based on increasing level of risk to the individual and community and availability of effective treatment and prevention (73). The clinical diagnostic laboratory typically encounters microorganisms as shown in Table 82.2; thus, further discussion focuses on elements in BSLs 2 and 3. Laboratories that use, receive, or store select agents must address, in addition to BSL 2 to 4 safety practices, security and reporting issues (74). Additional safety practices are necessary for work in research and anatomic laboratories (6,75–77).

OSHA regulations for prevention of infection emphasize engineering controls, work practices modification, and personal

TABLE 82.2. BIOSAFETY LEVEL OF MICROORGANISMS ENCOUNTERED IN THE LABORATORY AND SELECTED MICROORGANISMS REPRESENTATIVE OF THE LEVEL

Level	Description	Examples	Examples Likely to be Encountered in Diagnostic Clinical Laboratories
1	Microorganisms not known to cause disease in healthy adult humans	*Bacillus subtilis*	None
2	Moderate-risk microorganisms present in the community and associated with human disease of varying severity	Hepatitis B virus, *Salmonella* species, *Toxoplasma*	Most microorganisms present, other than those listed below (this level is also appropriate for human specimens where the presence of an infectious agent is unknown)
Mod. Level 2	Microorganisms requiring selected precautions more stringent than level 2 but not to the extent of level 3 (consult reference below for additional measures recommended)	*B. anthracis,* West Nile virus	*Ascaris, B. pertussis, C. botulinum. Y. pestis* Creutzfeldt-Jakob agent, *Fasciola, Legionella pneumophila, Schistosoma, Taenia solium, Toxoplasma*
3	Agents with a potential for respiratory transmission and that may cause serious and potentially lethal infection	*Coxiella burnetii*, B virus, *Rickettsia* species, St. Louis encephalitis virus, Venezuelan equine virus, yellow fever virus, lymphocytic choriomeningitis virus, rabies virus, vesicular stomatitis virus	*Brucella* species, *Chlamydia* species, *C. immitis, F. tularensis, H. capsulatum, M. tuberculosis, S. schenckii*
4	Dangerous agents that pose a high individual risk of life-threatening disease, which may be transmitted by aerosol route and for which there is no available vaccine or therapy	Junin virus, Lassa virus, Marburg virus, smallpox virus	None

From Ref. 25, 37, and 56.

protection by immunization and protective equipment (67,68). Guidelines for the clinical diagnostic laboratory can be placed in these same general categories and compared for BSLs 2 and 3 (Tables 82.3 to 82.5). Most guidelines are common to both BSLs 2 and 3 (Table 82.3), whereas some are unique to level 2 (Table 82.4), and others are specific to level 3 protection (Table 82.5). Many of these elements are pertinent to other hospital areas and to laboratories; such policies are discussed in detail in other chapters and are reviewed only briefly here. Several elements of infection prevention are more relevant to the laboratory than to other areas, and these are discussed at greater length in the following sections.

TABLE 82.3. CONTROL MEASURES FOR PREVENTION OF LABORATORY-ASSOCIATED NOSOCOMIAL INFECTIONS THAT ARE COMMON TO BIOSAFETY LEVELS 2 AND 3[a]

A. Engineering controls
1. Only needle-locking syringes or disposable syringe-needle units are used for injection or aspiration of infectious materials
2. Needles and syringes or other sharps are used only when there is no alternative, such as for parenteral injection, phlebotomy, or aspiration of fluid from diaphragm bottles
3. Syringes that resheath the needle, needleless systems, and other safe devices are used when possible
4. Plasticware is substituted for glassware whenever possible
5. Used disposable needles are carefully placed in conveniently located puncture-resistant containers. Nondisposable sharps are placed in a hard-walled container for transport to a processing area for decontamination, preferably by autoclaving
6. Cultures, tissues, and specimens of body fluids are placed in containers that prevent leakage during collection, transport, handling, processing, storage, or shipping
7. Materials with high concentrations or large volumes of infectious agents may be centrifuged in the open laboratory only if sealed rotor heads or centrifuge safety cups are used and if these rotors or safety cups are opened only in a biologic safety cabinet
8. An eyewash facility is readily available
9. Rugs are not used, because proper decontamination following a spill is difficult
10. Bench tops are impervious to water and resistant to acids, alkali, organic solvents, and moderate heat
11. Laboratory furniture is sturdy, and spaces between benches, cabinets, and equipment are accessible for cleaning
12. Open windows are fitted with fly screens
13. A method for decontamination of infectious or regulated laboratory wastes is available (e.g., autoclave, chemical disinfection, incinerator)

B. Work practice modification
1. Hands are washed after handling infectious material, after removing gloves, and before leaving the laboratory
2. Food is stored outside the work area in cabinets or refrigerators designated for this purpose only
3. Mouth pipetting is prohibited; mechanical pipetting devices are used
4. All procedures are performed carefully to minimize splashes or aerosols
5. Work surfaces are decontaminated at least once a day and after any spill of viable material
6. All cultures, stocks, and other regulated wastes are decontaminated before disposal by an approved decontamination method such as autoclaving
7. Materials to be decontaminated outside of the immediate laboratory are placed in a durable, leak-proof container and closed for transport
8. Materials to be decontaminated off-site from the laboratory are packaged in accordance with applicable local, state, and federal regulations before removal from the facility
9. An insect and rodent control program is in effect
10. A biosafety manual is prepared or adopted
11. Personnel are advised of special hazards and are required to read and follow instructions on practices and procedures
12. Personnel receive appropriate training on potential hazards associated with the work involved, the necessary precautions to prevent exposures, and exposure evaluation procedures. Annual updates, or additional training as necessary for procedural or policy changes, are provided
13. A high degree of precaution always is taken with any contaminated sharp items, including needles and syringes, slides, pipettes, capillary tubes, and scalpels
14. Used disposable needles are not bent, sheared, broken, recapped, removed from disposable syringes, or otherwise manipulated by hand before disposal; they are placed in appropriate containers (see above)
15. Broken glassware is not handled directly by hand but is removed by mechanical means (e.g., brush, dustpan, tongs, forceps)
16. Containers of contaminated needles, sharps, and broken glass are decontaminated before disposal according to local regulations
17. Laboratory equipment and work surfaces are decontaminated with an appropriate disinfectant routinely, after work with infectious materials is finished, and especially after contamination by infectious material (e.g., spills, splashes)
18. Contaminated equipment is decontaminated before it is sent for repair or maintenance or packaged for transport
19. Spills and accidents resulting in overt exposures to infectious materials are reported immediately to the laboratory director

C. Personal protection
1. Personnel receive appropriate immunizations or tests (e.g., tuberculin skin test) for the agents potentially handled or potentially present
2. Medical evaluation, surveillance, and treatment are provided as appropriate, and written records are maintained following any exposure to infectious agents
3. Persons who wear contact lenses in laboratories should also wear goggles or a face shield
4. Protective laboratory coats, smocks, gowns, or uniforms designated for laboratory use are worn while in the laboratory
5. Protective clothing is removed and left in the laboratory before leaving for non-laboratory areas and is either disposed of in the laboratory or laundered by the institution, never taken home by personnel
6. Gloves are worn when hands might contact infectious materials, contaminated surfaces, or equipment. They are disposed of when contaminated, removed when work with infectious materials is complete, and are not worn outside the laboratory
7. Disposable gloves are not washed or reused

[a] As defined by the Centers for Disease Control and Prevention with the National Institutes of Health (25) and the Occupational Safety and Health Administration (67).

TABLE 82.4. REQUIREMENTS FOR BIOSAFETY LEVEL 2 THAT DIFFER FROM THOSE FOR BIOSAFETY LEVEL 3[a]

A. Engineering controls
 1. Properly maintained biologic safety cabinets, preferably class II or other appropriate personal protective equipment or physical containment devices are used for procedures that could create infectious aerosols or splashes. These may include centrifuging, grinding, blending, vigorous shaking or mixing, sonic disruption, opening containers of infectious materials whose internal pressures are different from ambient pressure, and harvesting infected tissues
 2. Each laboratory contains a sink for hand washing

B. Work practice modification
 1. Access to the laboratory is limited or restricted when work with infectious agents is in progress
 2. Eating, drinking, smoking, handling contact lenses, and applying cosmetics are not permitted in the "work area" (laboratory for level 3)
 3. Only persons who have been advised of the potential hazard(s) and meet specific entry requirements (e.g., immunization) enter the laboratory
 4. When the infectious agents in use in the laboratory require special provisions for entry (e.g., immunization), a hazard warning sign incorporating the universal biohazard symbol is posted on the access door to the laboratory work area. The sign identifies the agent, lists names and telephone numbers of responsible persons, and indicates the special requirements for entering the laboratory

C. Personal protection
 1. Face protection (e.g., masks, goggles, faceshield) is used for anticipated splashes or sprays of infectious materials when the microorganisms must be manipulated outside the biologic safety cabinet
 2. When appropriate, considering the agents handled, baseline serum specimens for personnel are collected and stored. Additional serum specimens may be collected periodically, depending on the agents handled or the function of the facility.

[a] As defined by the Centers for Disease Control and Prevention with the National Institutes of Health (25) and the Occupational Safety and Health Administration (67).

Engineering Controls

Airflow handling is an essential element in several clinical care areas of a hospital where microorganisms likely to be spread by airborne transmission are encountered, especially *M. tuberculosis* and certain fungi (68). In the laboratory, however, the potential for encountering BSL 3 microorganisms that can be spread by air is so much greater that certain standards and guidelines beyond those for the rest of the institution are mandatory (61,78). Aerosolization can result from use of blenders, both low- and high-speed centrifuges, and automatic pipettes. Loops used for inoculation of microbiologic cultures can lead to aerosolization if not flamed properly. Other standard and seemingly innocuous laboratory procedures such as pipetting, accidentally dropping infected liquids on a counter, and inoculating a tube with a syringe all can generate aerosols. If one adds to this the presence in clinical specimens of microorganisms prone to spread by the airborne route (e.g., *M. tuberculosis, H. capsulatum, C. immitis,* and certain viruses), the need for control of aerosols becomes crucial. Thus, building design that ensures inward directional airflow into the laboratory from corridors and hallways and similar engineering for direct exhaust of the air without recirculation are crucial for laboratories handling airborne pathogens. For BSL 3 laboratories, airflow is monitored to ensure that the ventilation system does not fail (61,69). Air ventilation in the autopsy room is also critical and the room should be under negative pressure, provide 12 air exchanges per hour, and be exhausted directly to the outside (6).

Biologic safety cabinets (BSCs) are designed to contain the highly infectious agents that are transmitted by an airborne route through infectious splashes or aerosols generated by microbiologic procedures (6,61,79). There are three types of BSCs (Class I, II, and III), but most routine clinical laboratories use Type II BSCs that provide protection to the user and prevent external contamination of the materials inside the cabinet. An effective containment system for handling BSL 2 and 3 agents requires that the BSC is properly maintained, that the BSC be certified annually or whenever the cabinet is moved, and that well-trained employees use good microbiologic technique (6). The characteristics of each type of cabinet and procedures for their correct use have been reviewed and extensively described elsewhere (6, 61,68).

Other engineering controls for decreasing the risk associated with handling infectious material include safety engineered devices and instruments, sharps containers, safety containers for centrifuges, plastic containers and collection devices for specimens, mechanical pipettes and diluters, bench tops impervious to liquids, and personal protection equipment. These controls are discussed in depth in other publications (6,26).

Work Practice Modification

Laboratory workers cannot identify specimens that contain infectious agents and, therefore, must practice standard precautions, which is the concept that all patients and all laboratory specimens are potentially infectious and capable of transmitting infection (6,70,80). These guidelines represent the first level of protection for the laboratory worker from a wide variety of pathogens. Hand washing is a fundamental procedure to reduce duration of exposure and transmission of an infectious agent within the healthcare facility, including the laboratory. Adequate hand washing should occur before leaving the laboratory, after removing gloves, and after obvious hand contamination by using traditional soap and water or an alcohol-based gel (81). Some work practices promote the transfer of microorganisms from surfaces to hands to mucous membranes and are universally prohibited in the laboratory. These prohibited practices include eating or storing food, drinking, applying cosmetics or contact lens, smoking, chewing gum, and mouth pipetting. Workers with skin lesions or dermatitis on the hands or wrists should not handle potentially infectious materials without adequate protection (82).

Personnel who collect and transport specimens should be adequately trained. Whether transported by hand or pneumatic tube, specimens should be placed in a leak-proof primary container. This primary container is placed in a leak-proof secondary container that is usually a sealable plastic bag. Secondary containers and specimen storage areas should be labeled with a biohazard label to alert individuals to the potential infectious haz-

TABLE 82.5. REQUIREMENTS FOR BIOSAFETY LEVEL 3 THAT DIFFER FROM THOSE FOR BIOSAFETY LEVEL 2[a]

A. Engineering controls
1. The laboratory is separated from areas with unrestricted traffic flow. Passage through two sets of self-closing doors is the basic requirement for entry. A clothes change room (shower optional) may be included in the passageway
2. A ducted exhaust air ventilation system is provided. This system creates directional airflow that draws air from clean areas into the laboratory toward contaminated areas. The air is not recirculated to any other area of the building. It is discharged to the outside with filtration and other treatment optional. The outside exhaust must be dispersed away from occupied areas and air intakes
3. The high-efficiency particulate air (HEPA)-filtered exhaust air from class II or class III biologic safety cabinets is discharged directly to the outside or through the building exhaust system (for class II cabinets, exhaust air can be recirculated if the cabinet is tested and certified at least every 12 months). Discharged air to the building exhaust system is connected in a manner that avoids any interference with air balance of the cabinets or building exhaust system
4. Properly maintained biologic safety cabinets are used (class II or III, as appropriate)
5. Continuous flow centrifuges or other equipment that may produce aerosols are contained in devices that exhaust air through HEPA filters before discharge into the laboratory
6. Outside of a biologic safety cabinet, appropriate combinations of personal protective equipment are used (special protective clothing, masks, gloves, face protection, or respirators) in combination with physical containment devices (e.g., centrifuge safety cups, sealed centrifuge rotors) for manipulation of cultures or other materials that may be a source of infectious aerosols
7. Laboratory doors are kept closed when testing or experiments are in progress
8. Each laboratory contains a sink for hand washing. The sink is foot, elbow, or automatically operated and is near the laboratory exit door
9. The interior surfaces of walls, floors, and ceilings are water-resistant so they can be easily cleaned. Penetrations in these surfaces are sealed or capable of being sealed to facilitate decontamination
10. Windows in the laboratory are closed and sealed

B. Work practice modification
1. Eating, drinking, smoking, handling contact lenses, and applying cosmetics are not permitted in the laboratory ("work area" for level 2)
2. Persons who are at increased risk of infection or to whom infection may be unusually hazardous are not allowed in the laboratory. Access is restricted to persons whose presence is required for program or support purposes
3. Only persons who have been advised of the potential hazard(s), meet specific entry requirements (e.g., immunization), and comply with all entry and exit procedures enter the laboratory
4. When infectious materials are in the laboratory, a hazard warning sign incorporating the universal biohazard symbol is posted on all laboratory and animal room access doors. The sign identifies the agent, lists names and telephone numbers of responsible persons, and indicates any specific requirements for entering the laboratory, such as the need for immunizations, respirators, or other personal protective measures
5. The laboratory director ensures that, before working with microorganisms at biosafety level 3, all personnel demonstrate proficiency in standard microbiologic practices and techniques and in the practices and operations specific to the laboratory facility. This might include prior experience in handling human pathogens or cell cultures or a specific training program
6. All manipulations involving infectious materials are conducted in biologic safety cabinets or other physical containment devices within the containment module. No work in open vessels is conducted on the open bench
7. All potentially contaminated waste materials (e.g., gloves, laboratory coats) from laboratories are decontaminated before disposal or reuse
8. Spills of infectious materials are decontaminated, contained, and cleaned up by appropriate professional staff members or others properly trained and equipped to work with concentrated infectious material
9. Animals and plants not related to the work being conducted are not permitted in the laboratory

C. Personal protection
1. Outside of a biologic safety cabinet, appropriate combinations of personal protective equipment are used (special protective clothing, masks, gloves, face protection, or respirators) in combination with physical containment devices (e.g., centrifuge safety cups, sealed centrifuge rotors) for manipulation of cultures or other materials that may be a source of infectious aerosols
2. Face protection (goggles and mask or face shield) is worn for manipulations of infectious materials outside the biologic safety cabinet
3. Protective laboratory clothing such as solid-front or wrap-around gowns, scrub suits, or coveralls must be worn in, and not worn outside, the laboratory
4. Reusable laboratory clothing is to be decontaminated before being laundered
5. Baseline serum specimens for personnel are collected and stored for all laboratory and other at-risk personnel. Additional serum specimens may be collected periodically, depending on the agents handled or the function of the facility

[a] As defined by the Centers for Disease Control and Prevention with the National Institutes of Health (25) and the Occupational Safety and Health Administration (67).

ard. Needles should be removed before transporting a syringe to the laboratory.

Specimen processing in microbiology requires special steps to prevent infection and should be performed in a BSC. For example, when entering a blood culture bottle with a needle and syringe, the vial should never be held in the worker's hand and the bottle should be placed behind a splashguard or in a BSC. Similarly, unfixed slides should always be handled as if they contained infectious materials (6). Special steps are needed for dealing with the potential hazards associated with the use of diagnostic instruments (6).

Prompt decontamination of spills is particularly important in the laboratory. Most laboratory spills involve blood, other body fluids, or microbiologic media that often contain high concentrations of protein. Because many disinfectants are less active in the presence of these proteins, the bulk of the spilled liquid must be adsorbed before disinfection (6,82). For large spills of microbiologic cultures, the spill is flooded with an appropriate disinfectant and left to stand for 20 minutes before clean-up (6). Phenolic disinfectants are not recommended for use on contaminated medical devices that come in contact with laboratory workers but may be used on laboratory instruments, floors, and countertops. Also, instrument parts made in part or wholly of aluminum are corroded by sodium hypochlorite, so other disinfectants are preferred for disinfection of laboratory instruments containing these parts.

Surveillance of accidents and exposures is a key feature of infection control in all hospital areas but is especially important in the laboratory. The essential components of postexposure management include incident reporting, wound management, evaluation of the transmission risk, and consideration of postexposure prophylaxis (6,20,28). The incident is reported to the supervisor, no matter how trivial the injury or exposure may be and includes the date and time of exposure, the details of the accident, information on the source person, and medical evaluation of the injured employee. The immediate reporting of the incident establishes a time relationship, in the event that an infection develops, and permits preventive measures to be implemented. OSHA regulations require that the facility's exposure control plan includes hepatitis B vaccination at no cost to the employee, postexposure evaluation and follow-up, communication of potential hazards to employees, and appropriate records and reporting (6,20,28,57,58). (See Chapters 78, 79, and 99.)

Follow-up for the individual is vital; equally important is the periodic and regular analysis of the incidents that occur in a given laboratory. Laboratory, occupational health, and infection control personnel should cooperate in the compilation and analysis of incident report data to search for common patterns, to eliminate identified risk factors, and to modify laboratory procedures to minimize occurrence of these incidents (64). Procedures for medical follow-up of exposure to blood-borne pathogens are dealt with elsewhere.

Surface cleaning of the laboratory bench or other surfaces must be meticulous, because these surfaces are likely to be contaminated with potential pathogens (60). Many surfaces (countertops, floors, equipment, centrifuges, etc.) become contaminated by microorganisms during routine processing of clinical specimens and cultures. These surfaces should be carefully disinfected at the completion of work and after accidental spills to prevent contamination of laboratory employees and visiting medical personnel who may unknowingly carry the agent to other parts of the facility or the community (60). All unnecessary material should be removed from these surfaces to facilitate proper cleaning and disinfection.

Waste disposal and handling of biologic materials at the end of processing are especially important topics for the laboratory, because of the volume of the materials involved and because the processing of the specimens often involves amplification of the potential pathogen (83). The laboratory is a major generator of biohazardous waste and should segregate the material into designated categories such as routine, chemical, and biohazardous waste for proper decontamination and disposal. Fortunately, the same procedures used in other parts of the facility apply to laboratory waste. (See Chapter 100.)

The shipment of infectious material is regulated by national and international rules and regulations promulgated by the U.S. Department of Transportation, International Airline Transport Association, and the WHO and are beyond the scope of this chapter (73,84,85).

Personal Protection

Immunization

Laboratory workers must be encouraged to participate in the same immunization program that is offered throughout the institution (6,86). This includes, at a minimum, provision of HBV immunization at no cost to the employee. The laboratory worker may be at greater risk of exposure to body fluids containing one of the hepatitis viruses, so it might be worth the special effort to emphasize immunization to laboratory employees. Immunizing trainees against HBV is particularly important, because the risk of infection often is high during training.

Bacillus Calmette-Guérin (BCG) vaccine is made from an attenuated strain of *M. bovis.* It is not routinely offered to hospital workers in the United States, because a positive tuberculin skin test when the vaccine is effective is thought to be a hindrance to surveillance for natural tuberculous infection and because adverse effects are associated with immunization (e.g., abscess at the injection site). However, it may be considered for laboratory employees who process large volumes of specimens containing *M. tuberculosis.* Other possible vaccines for laboratory workers include meningococcal polysaccharide vaccine, rabies vaccine, polio vaccine, and typhoid vaccine. Primary prevention in the laboratory should focus on biosafety practices, but these vaccines are a consideration for personnel who work with these agents on a frequent and regular basis. At this time, smallpox vaccination is recommended only for those individuals in the laboratory who directly handle cultures of the smallpox virus.

Personal Protective Equipment

Gloves, masks, and gowns are used throughout a hospital to protect workers from contact with blood and other potentially infectious materials. The laboratory is no exception to this practice, because all specimens handled in the laboratory are considered potentially infectious. Laboratory workers must be trained in the appropriate use, limitations, and disposal of personal protective equipment. In general only powder-free latex or other nonlatex gloves should be used in the laboratory as part of the standard precaution guidelines. Puncture-resistant gloves should be available in the autopsy suite or when handling scalpels and other sharps. In addition to protective clothing, laboratory workers should wear face shields or work behind splashguards when removing stoppers or withdrawing samples from specimen tubes (6). When extensive soaking by potentially infectious material is a possibility, waterproof coats, gowns, or aprons should be worn. Respiratory protection in the form of NIOSH-approved masks (e.g., N95 particulate respirator) is recommended when working with *M. tuberculosis* or other similar BSL 3 microorganisms (6,25). Shoes should cover the feet to protect the skin from spills or dropped sharps. All personal protective equipment, including laboratory coats, gowns, or other protective covers, should not be worn outside the laboratory area.

ACKNOWLEDGMENT

This chapter contains information presented in Chapter 74 by John E. McGowan Jr. in the second edition of this book.

REFERENCES

1. Peterson LR, Brossette SE. Hunting health care-associated infections from the clinical microbiology laboratory: passive, active, and virtual surveillance. *J Clin Microbiol* 2002;40:1–4.
2. Kiska DL. Global climate change: an infectious disease perspective. *Clin Microbiol Newslett* 2000;22:81–86.
3. Weinstein RA. Nosocomial infection update. *Emerg Infect Dis* 1998; 416–420.
4. Aitken C, Jeffries DJ. Nosocomial spread of viral disease. *Clin Microbiol Rev* 2001;14:528–546.
5. Harding AL, Byers KB. Epidemiology of laboratory-associated infections. In: Fleming DO, Hunt DL eds. *Biological safety: principles and practices,*, 3rd ed. Washington, DC: American Society for Microbiology, 2000:35–54.
6. NCCLS. *Protection of laboratory workers from occupationally acquired infections; approved standard.* M29-A2. Wayne, PA: NCCLS, 2001,
7. Straton CW. Occupationally acquired infections: a timely reminder. *Infect Control Hosp Epidemiol* 2001;22:8–9.
8. Pike RM. Laboratory-associated infections. Summary and analysis of 3921 cases. *Health Lab Sci* 1976;13:105–114.
9. Pike RM. Laboratory-associated infections: incidence, fatalities, causes and prevention. *Annu Rev Microbiol* 1979;33:41–66.
10. Sulkin SE, Pike RM. Viral infections contracted in the laboratory. *N Engl J Med* 1949;241:205–213.
11. Jacobson JT, Orlob RB, Clayton JL. Infections acquired in clinical laboratories in Utah. *J Clin Microbiol* 1985;21:486–489.
12. Vesley D, Hartmann HM. Laboratory-acquired infections and injuries in clinical laboratories: a 1986 survey. *Am J Public Health* 1988;78: 1213–1215.
13. Wilson ML, Reller LB. Clinical laboratory-acquired infections. In: Bennett JV, Brachman PS, eds. *Hospital infections,* 4th ed. Philadelphia: Lippincott-Raven, 1998:343–355.
14. Grist NR, Emslie JA. Association of Clinical Pathologists' surveys of infection in British clinical laboratories, 1970–1989. *J Clin Pathol* 1994;47:391–394.
15. Grist NR, Emslie JA. Infections in British clinical laboratories, 1986–7. *J Clin Pathol* 1989;42:677–681.
16. Walker D, Campbell D. A survey of infections in United Kingdom laboratories, 1994–1995. *J Clin Pathol* 1999;52:415–418.
17. Sewell DL. Laboratory-associated infections and biosafety. *Clin Microbiol Rev* 1995;8:389–405.
18. Reuben B, Band JD, Wong P, et al. Person-to-person transmission of *Brucella melitensis. Lancet* 1991;337:14–15.
19. Voss A. Prevention and control of laboratory-acquired infections. In: Murray PR, Baron EJ, Pfaller MA, et al., eds. *Manual of clinical microbiology,* 7th ed. Washington, DC: American Society for Microbiology, 1999:165–173.
20. Beltrami EM, Williams IT, Shapiro CN, et al. Risk and management of blood-borne infections in health care workers. *Clin Microbiol Rev* 2000;13:385–407.
21. Collins CH, Kennedy DA. Microbiological hazards of occupational needlestick and 'sharps' injuries. *J Appl Bacteriol* 1987;62:385–402.
22. Fiori PL, Mastrandrea S, Rappelli P, et al. *Brucella abortus* infection acquired in microbiology laboratories. *J Clin Microbiol* 2000;38: 2005–2006.
23. Centers for Disease Control and Prevention. Laboratory-acquired meningococcal disease-United States, 2000. *MMWR Morb Mortal Wkly Rep* 2000;51:141–144.
24. Memish ZA, Mah MW. Brucellosis in laboratory workers at a Saudi Arabian hospital. *Am J Infect Control* 2001;29:48–52.
25. Centers for Disease Control and Prevention, National Institutes of Health. *Biosafety in microbiological and biomedical laboratories,* 4th ed. Washington, DC: U.S. Government Printing Office (HHS Publ. No. CDC 93-8395), 1999.
26. Fleming DO, Hunt DL, eds. *Biological safety: principles and practices,* 3rd ed. Washington, DC: American Society for Microbiology, 2000.
27. Collins CH. *Laboratory-acquired infections: history, incidence, causes, and prevention.* Oxford, United Kingdom: Butterworth-Heinemann Ltd, 1993.
28. Centers for Disease Control and Prevention. Updated U.S. public health service guidelines for the management of occupational exposures to HBV, HCV, and HIV and recommendations for postexposure prophylaxis. *MMWR Morb Mortal Wkly Rep* 2001;50:1–42.
29. National Institute for Occupational Safety and Health. NIOSH alert: preventing needlestick injuries in health care settings. NIOSH publication 2001-108. 1999; November 1-24. NIOSH-Publications Dissemination Cincinnati, OH.
30. Lymer UB, Schutz AA, Isaksson B. A descriptive study of blood exposure incidents among healthcare workers in a university hospital in Sweden. *J Hosp Infect* 1997;35:223–235.
31. Mahoney FJ, Steward H, Hu H, et al. Progress toward elimination of hepatitis B virus transmission among health care workers in the United States. *Arch Intern Med* 1997;157:2601–2605.
32. Kao AS, Ashford DA, McNeil MM, et al. Descriptive profile of tuberculin skin testing programs and laboratory-acquired tuberculosis infections in public health laboratories. *J Clin Microbiol* 1997;35: 1847–1851.
33. D'Agata EMC, Wise S, Stewart A, et al. Nosocomial transmission of *Mycobacterium tuberculosis* from an extrapulmonary site. *Infect Control Hosp Epidemiol* 2001;22:10–12.
34. Genee D, Siegret HH. Tuberculosis of the thumb following a needlestick injury. *Clin Infect Dis* 1998;26:210–211.
35. Coggin JH Jr. Bacterial pathogens. In: Fleming DO, Hunt DL eds, *Biological safety: principles and practices,* 3rd ed. Washington, DC: American Society for Microbiology, 2000:65–88.
36. Kakis A, Gibbs L, Eguia J, et al. An outbreak of group A streptococcal infection among health care workers. *Clin Infect Dis* 2002;35: 1353–1359.
37. Gilchrist MJR, McKinney WP, Miller JM, et al. Cumitech 33. In Snyder JW, coordinating ed. *Laboratory safety, management, and diagnosis of biological agents associated with bioterrorism.* Washington, DC: American Society for Microbiology, 2000.
38. Miller JM. Agents of bioterrorism: preparing for bioterrorism at the community health care level. *Infect Dis Clinics North Am* 2001;15: 1127–1156.
39. Hilmarsdottir I, Coutellier A, Elbaz J, et al. A French case of laboratory-acquired disseminated *Penicillium marneffei* infection in a patient with AIDS. *Clin Infect Dis* 1994;19:357–358.
40. Cooper CR, Dixon DM, Salkin IF. Laboratory-acquired sporotrichosis. *J Med Vet Mycol* 1992;30:169–171.
41. Larson DM, Eckman MR, Alber CL, et al. Primary cutaneous (inoculation) blastomycosis: an occupational hazard to pathologists. Am J Clin Pathol 1983;79:253–255.
42. Oh M, Kim N, Huh M, et al. Scrub typhus pneumonitis acquired through the respiratory tract in a laboratory worker. *Infection* 2001; 29:54–56.
43. Mermel LA, Josephson SL, Dempsey J, et al. Outbreak of *Shigella sonnei* in a clinical microbiology laboratory. *J Clin Microbiol* 1997;35: 3163–3165.
44. Kolavic SA, Kimura A, Simons SL, et al. An outbreak of *Shigella dysenteriae* type 2 among laboratory workers due to intentional food contamination. *JAMA* 1997;278:396–398.
45. Ashdown LR, Cassidy J. Successive *Salmonella give* and *Salmonella typhi* infections, laboratory-acquired. *Pathology* 1991;23:233–234.
46. Rao GG, Saunders BP, Masterton RG. Laboratory acquired verotoxin producing *Escherichia coli* (VTEC) infection. *J Hosp Infect* 1996;33: 228–230.

47. Burnens AP, Zbinden R, Kaempf L, et al. A case of laboratory acquired with *Escherichia coli* O157:H7. *Zbl Bakt* 1993;279:512–517.
48. Penner JL, Hennessy JN, Mills SD, et al. Application of serotyping and chromosomal restriction endonuclease digest analysis in investigating a laboratory-acquired case of *Campylobacter jejuni*. *J Clin Microbiol* 1983; 18:1427–1428.
49. Coia JE. Nosocomial and laboratory-acquired infection with *Escherichia coli* O157. *J Hosp Infect* 1998;40:107–113.
50. Herwaldt BL. Laboratory-acquired parasitic infections from accidental exposures. *Clin Microbiol Rev* 2001;14:659–688.
51. Parker SL, Holliman RE. Toxoplasmosis and laboratory workers: a case-control assessment of risk.*Med Lab Sci* 1992;49:103–106.
52. Batchelor BI, Brindle RJ, Gilks GF, et al. Biochemical mis-identification of *Brucella melitensis* and subsequent laboratory-acquired infections. *J Hosp Infect* 1992;22:159–162.
53. Ashdown LR. Melioidosis and safety in the clinical laboratory. *J Hosp Infect* 1992;21:301–306.
54. Vasconcelos PF, Travassos da Rosa RA, Rodrigues SG, et al. Laboratory-acquired human infection with SP H 114202 virus (Arenavirus: Arenaviridae family): clinical and laboratory aspects. *Rev Inst Med Trop Sao Paulo* 1993;35:521–525.
55. Barry M, Russi M, Armstrong L, et al. Brief report: treatment of a laboratory-acquired Sabia virus infection. *N Engl J Med* 1995;333: 294–296.
56. Centers for Disease Control and Prevention. Laboratory-acquired West Nile virus infections-United States, 2002. *MMWR Morb Mortal Wkly Rep* 2002;51:1133–1135.
57. Occupational Safety and Health Administration. Occupational exposure to bloodborne pathogens: needlestick and sharps injuries; final rule. *Federal Register* 2001;66:5317–5325.
58. NCCLS. Implementing a needlestick and sharps injury prevention program in the clinical laboratory; a report. Standard X3-R. Wayne, PA: NCCLS, 2002.
59. Bolyard EA, Tablan OC, Williams WW, et al. Guideline for infection control in healthcare personnel, 1998. *Infect Control Hosp Epidemiol* 1998;19:407–463.
60. Collins SM, Hacek DM, Degan LA, et al. Contamination of the clinical microbiology laboratory with vancomycin-resistant enterococci and multidrug-resistant Enterobacteriaceae: implications for hospital and laboratory workers. *J Clin Microbiol* 2001;39:3772–3774.
61. Richmond JY, Knudsen RC, Good RC. Biosafety in the clinical mycobacteriology laboratory. *Clin Lab Med* 1996;16:527–550.
62. Cole EC, Cook CE. Characterization of infectious aerosols in health care facilities: an aid to effective engineering controls and preventive strategies. *Am J Infect Control* 1998;26:453–464.
63. Gilchrist MJR, Fleming DO. Biosafety precautions for *Mycobacterium tuberculosis* and other airborne pathogens. In: Fleming DO, Hunt DL eds. *Biological safety: principles and practices,* 3rd ed. Washington, DC: American Society for Microbiology, 2000:209–219.
64. Groschel DHM, Strain BA. Laboratory safety in clinical microbiology. In: Balows Hausler WJ Jr, Herrmann KL, Isenberg HD, et al., eds. *Manual of clinical microbiology,* 5th ed. Washington, DC: American Society for Microbiology, 1991:49–58.
65. Occupational Safety and Health Administration. Enforcement procedures for the occupational exposure to bloodborne pathogens. CPL 2-2.69 2001.
66. Occupational Safety and Health Administration. Occupational exposure to bloodborne pathogens: request for information. *Federal Register* 1998;63:48250–48252. OSHA, Washington, DC.
67. Occupational Safety and Health Administration. Occupational exposure to bloodborne pathogens: final rule. *Federal Register* 1991;56: 64003–64182.
68. Occupational Safety and Health Administration. Occupational exposure to tuberculosis: proposed rule. *Federal Register* 1997;62:52149–54309.
69. Centers for Disease Control and Prevention. Guidelines for preventing the transmission of *Mycobacterium tuberculosis* in health-care facilities. *MMWR Morb Mortal Wkly Rep* 1994;43:1–128.
70. Garner JS, Hospital Infection Control Practices Advisory Committee. Guideline for isolation precautions in hospitals. *Infect Control Hosp Epidemiol* 1996;17:53–80.
71. Fleming DO. Risk assessment of biological hazards. In: Fleming DO, Hunt DL eds, *Biological safety: principles and practices,* 3rd ed. Washington, DC: American Society for Microbiology, 2000:57–64.
72. Knudsen RC. Risk assessment for biological agents in the laboratory. In: Richmond JY, ed. *Rational basis for biocontainment: proceedings of the Fifth National Symposium on Biosafety.* Mundelein, IL: American Biological Safety Association, 1998.
73. World Health Organization. *Laboratory biosafety manual,* 2nd ed. Geneva: WHO, 1993.
74. Centers for Disease Control and Prevention. Laboratory security and emergency response guidance for laboratories working with select agents. *MMWR Morb Mortal Wkly Rep* 2002;51:1–6.
75. Cipriano M. *Cumitech 36, Biosafety considerations for large-scale production of microorganisms.* Washington, DC: American Society for Microbiology, 2002.
76. Johnson MD, Schaffner W, Atkinson J, et al. Autopsy risk and acquisition of human immunodeficiency virus infection: a case report and reappraisal. *Arch Pathol Lab Med* 1997;121:64–66.
77. McCaskie AW, Calder SJ, Roberts M, et al. Sectioning fresh human bone: the reduction of aerosol and physical hazards. *Br J Biomed Sci* 1997;54:88–90.
78. Crane JT, Richmond JY. Design of biomedical laboratory facilities. In: Fleming DO, Hunt DL eds, *Biological safety: principles and practices,* 3rd ed. Washington, DC: American Society for Microbiology, 2000: 283–311.
79. Stuart DG. Primary barriers: biological safety cabinets, fume hoods, and glove boxes. In: Fleming DO, Hunt DL eds, *Biological safety: principles and practices,* 3rd ed. Washington, DC: American Society for Microbiology, 2000:313–330.
80. Henderson DK. Raising the bar: the need for standardizing the use of "standard precautions" as a primary intervention to prevent occupational exposures to bloodborne pathogens. *Infect Control Hosp Epidemiol* 2001;22:70–72.
81. Centers for Disease Control and Prevention. Guideline for hand hygiene in health-care settings. *MMWR Morb Mortal Wkly Rep* 2002;51: 1–47.
82. Hunt DL. Standard (universal) precautions for human specimens. In: Fleming DO, Hunt DL eds. *Biological safety: principles and practices,* 3rd ed. Washington, DC: American Society for Microbiology, 2000: 355–367.
83. Zaki AN, Campbell JR. Infectious waste management and laboratory design criteria. *Am Indust Hyg Assoc J* 1997;58:800–808.
84. U.S. Department of Transportation, Research and Special Programs Administration. Hazardous materials: revision to standards for infectious substances and genetically modified organisms; final rule. *Federal Register* 2002;67:53117–53144.
85. International Air Transport Association. Dangerous goods regulations, 41st ed. 2000, 57–88. IATA, Montreal, Quebec Canada.
86. Sepkowitz KA. Occupationally acquired infections in health care workers, part I. *Ann Intern Med* 1996;125:826–834.
87. Knobloch J, Demar M. Accidental *Leishmania mexicana* infection in an immunocompromised laboratory technician. *Trop Med Int Health* 1997;2:1152–1155.

83

PREVENTION OF OCCUPATIONALLY ACQUIRED INFECTIONS IN PREHOSPITAL HEALTHCARE WORKERS

JAMES M. MELIUS

Prehospital healthcare workers include an estimated 250,000 healthcare workers (1). Many work for modern well-equipped emergency medical systems in major metropolitan areas. Others volunteer their time for local rescue companies with very limited resources, often in rural areas. Some are full-time professional healthcare workers dedicated to a career in emergency medical services, whereas others may only provide voluntary services for a few hours per month or may only occasionally have to provide emergency medical care as part of their full-time jobs as firefighters or police officers.

Working in the prehospital environment is in many ways similar to providing care in hospitals and other healthcare facilities. Prehospital healthcare workers encounter a variety of seriously ill patients with many types of illness, and, like other healthcare workers, emergency medical workers face an increased risk of acquiring a number of different infectious diseases as a result of their work. The increasing risk of a bioterroism incident expands the number of conditions that must be considered.

Prehospital healthcare workers usually spend only a short time with each patient. This limited contact undoubtedly lowers their risk of acquiring a patient-related infection. However, a number of other factors may increase this risk.

In responding to traffic accidents or entering the homes of their patients, these workers provide medical care in many different settings over which they have little control. In most situations, they do not have complete information on the patient's medical condition. This lack of control of their work environment and incomplete diagnostic information have significant implications in preventing the transmission of infectious diseases from the patients to these workers.

Another important difference from many other healthcare workers is the variety of types of organizations that employ these workers and the lack of programs within those organizations for providing infection control services. In some cases, the organizations may lack the resources or commitment for the operation of good infection control programs. Although infection control programs for prehospital workers have improved in recent years in response to the need for better infection control, there are still large disparities among different organizations.

This chapter provides an overview of the infectious diseases risks faced by prehospital healthcare workers and of the methods useful for their prevention. These preventive steps are quite similar to those used in other healthcare settings. Therefore, this chapter emphasizes preventive approaches especially important to prehospital healthcare workers rather than reiterating infection control procedures described elsewhere in this book. Finally, the chapter briefly discusses approaches for organizing better preventive programs for these workers.

PREHOSPITAL HEALTHCARE

Prehospital healthcare workers include many thousands of healthcare workers in many organizational settings. Some work full time as emergency medical care workers for private or public providers. Others spend most of their time conducting other tasks (e.g., fire fighting) but must occasionally provide emergency medical care. Others volunteer their services, spending a few to many hours every week with volunteer rescue squads (usually in rural areas).

These workers also differ in their medical training. Some have years of specialized training for their careers and frequent updating of their medical training. Others have only very limited emergency care training and little continued training because of their other job requirements.

The common tasks performed by these workers include the provision of emergency medical care outside the hospital (or healthcare facility) setting and the transport of these patients to healthcare facilities. The types of patient being cared for obviously varies among different prehospital care providers. Some mainly transport patients who are not critically ill, whereas others mainly respond to trauma incidents. Geographic location and many other factors obviously affect the potential exposure of these workers to people with communicable diseases.

The workplace for prehospital healthcare providers can be viewed as including four settings: (1) the accident scene or other place where initial care for the patient is provided, (2) the transport vehicle, (3) the healthcare facility receiving area (usually emergency room), and (4) the facility in which the responder is stationed (e.g., hospital, fire house). From the perspective of infection control, the third setting is not discussed in this chapter. However, it should be noted that emergency medical providers may be at some risk for acquiring infections even after arrival at the healthcare facility.

The site of the initial care (e.g., patient's residence, accident scene) is probably the most problematic of the four locations. In contrast to most other healthcare workers, the emergency medical responder usually has little information about the patient's condition when initially providing medical care at the scene. Thus, the responder is usually not aware of whether the patient has a communicable disease. Collection of some diagnostic information is obviously a critical aspect of providing initial emergency care, but information about a specific infectious disease often will not be obtained. Often, a specific infectious disease will not be diagnosed until after the patient has been hospitalized.

In providing care, the responder usually must rely on verbal information from the patient or family that may not fully reflect the patient's medical condition. In some cases, the patient may be unconscious and otherwise unable to provide any information, and knowledgeable family members may not be present. In the absence of specific diagnostic information, the responder must depend on his or her initial physical assessment of the patient, perhaps with additional knowledge such as the likelihood of the patient having an infectious disease because of the geographic location (i.e., how common is the disease in that area).

The responder not only lacks diagnostic information but must provide emergency medical care at the site. In many cases, this care must be provided at the patient's residence. The responders may have a very limited work area and poor lighting, making certain procedures, such as starting intravenous lines, difficult. In addition, the patient may be combative or otherwise difficult to manage, further increasing the risk of this type of procedure. For airborne communicable diseases, there may be increased risk of exposure, because the responder must work in a residential environment in which the patient has been staying. This area may lack adequate ventilation and may have contaminated surfaces.

An accident or trauma scene may pose additional dangers. In addition to the limited space, poor lighting, and other problems, the trauma scene may have broken glass and other sharp objects that could contribute to the spread of blood-borne pathogens. In some cases, the responder may have to spend a long period stabilizing the patient until the patient can be extricated from a motor vehicle. Taking proper infection control precautions in a confined space with a seriously injured patient may be quite difficult.

Another aspect of providing emergency care at the scene that is obvious but is especially important is that all protective equipment that is needed at the scene must be carried by the responders. If they do not bring the necessary equipment with them, the equipment must either be retrieved from their transport vehicle or from their station or not used at all. Anticipating what will be needed and then providing ready access to that equipment can be quite challenging (2). The availability of equipment may be particularly problematic for responders who most often fulfill other duties (e.g., law enforcement or fire fighting) but are also expected to provide emergency medical care.

The situation in transport vehicles is somewhat better. The patient is usually stable enough to be transported. Better medical and monitoring equipment is also available. However, this setting also has a number of problems. First, patients often must be rapidly transported to the hospital and may often be in very critical condition. Medical care and procedures such as starting intravenous lines must be conducted very quickly. Most transport vehicles have very little room, further compounding this problem. Transport also may cause problems because of the movement of the vehicle during transport. This is obviously a problem while trying to perform procedures during transport (e.g., insertion of intravenous lines). Another potential problem is that most emergency transport vehicles are poorly ventilated. Most ventilation either comes from opening windows or from the vehicle's heating or cooling systems, which often simply recirculate most of the air in the vehicle (3).

Another site where emergency medical responders work is their station. In some cases, this may be a hospital. In others, it may be a fire house or similar structure. Some responders may even work from their homes (e.g., rural volunteer units). This location is most important in terms of infection control in that responders must often return to that site to clean their equipment. Proper equipment and practices for this setting are obviously important.

OCCUPATIONALLY ACQUIRED INFECTIONS

Prehospital healthcare workers share many of the risks of occupationally acquired infections with healthcare workers in other settings. Although most of their contacts with infectious patients are relatively brief, the lack of information about the patient's conditions and difficult environmental conditions may increase their risk relative to the more controlled hospital environment.

There is relatively little documentation of the actual risk of occupationally acquired infections among emergency medical providers. Hepatitis B has probably received the most attention (4). However, other infections have occasionally been reported. For example, there is a case report of toxic shock syndrome in a firefighter from a *Streptococcus pyogenes* infection acquired from cardiopulmonary resuscitation of an infected child (5).

The best documentation of the infectious diseases risk for prehospital healthcare workers comes from a survey of the emergency medical service in Portland, Oregon (6). Using verbal and written exposure reports and other sources, the author documented 256 reported infectious disease exposure incidents over a 2-year period (1988 to 1989). The incidence of reported exposures was 4.4 per 1,000 emergency medical service calls. Of these, approximately 24% involved respiratory exposure and 47% involved exposure of intact skin. Approximately 29% involved the exposure of nonintact skin or mucous membranes to blood or other body fluids or needlesticks. Fourteen incidents involving either needlesticks or exposure of nonintact skin or mucous membranes to blood or other body fluids were reported over the 2-year period. Although difficult to generalize to other emergency medical settings, these data do provide some sense of the scope of infectious diseases exposures for prehospital healthcare workers.

A survey of emergency medical service workers serving three inner city emergency departments focused only on occupational blood contact (7). Based on 62 self-reported blood contact incidents while transporting 2,472 patients, the study estimated that each worker had 12.3 blood contacts per year, including 0.2 annual percutaneous exposures. Bleeding patients were the main source of the exposures.

Another survey of paramedics in Florida conducted in 1987 found 110 reported needlestick injuries based on 300 returned questionnaires from a mail survey of 500 paramedics in that state (8). More than one third were reported to have occurred while workers were recapping needles.

Some earlier surveys of prehospital healthcare workers for hepatitis B markers provides some indication of these workers risk for that disease. A study of 59 Seattle, Washington, paramedics found that 25% had evidence of antibody to hepatitis B surface or core antigen (9). A similar survey of 338 Houston, Texas, paramedics found the prevalence of hepatitis antibodies to be approximately 26%, whereas a survey of Boston, Massachusetts, paramedics and emergency medical technicians found the prevalence to be approximately 28% (10,11). A recent review article summarizes much of the available literature on hepatitis B risk for public safety workers (4)

There is little documentation of the prevalence or incidence of other occupationally acquired infections in prehospital healthcare workers. Based on the type of work, one would expect them to be potentially at risk for the same types of infections as other healthcare workers (especially emergency room workers) (see Chapters 78,79, and 81). However, the incidence of particular infections is difficult to estimate.

ATTITUDES

A number of studies have discussed attitudes and precautionary behaviors among prehospital healthcare providers regarding the implementation of precautions for blood-borne infections. These studies have shown that these providers have been very concerned about the risk of acquiring human immunodeficiency virus (HIV) infection from their work (12–14). Many preferred not to treat HIV-infected patients. However, few reported actually refusing to provide treatment. Inadequate training was a major concern among providers in one survey. Cost of hepatitis B immunization was another concern in a study of paramedics in Florida (8).

Legal Requirements

Requirements for qualifications and training for prehospital healthcare workers vary from state to state. Most states do not have specific regulations regarding infection control practices and training, although many receive some training in this area and may be held to some general standard of practice. However, in the last few years, the federal government has gotten more involved in regulating infection control practices through occupational safety and health regulation, specifically in the area of blood-borne infections (1). Although the scope of this regulation (see Chapters 79 and 104) clearly covers prehospital healthcare workers, legal coverage of the standard varies. Many states do not provide occupational safety and health regulation or enforcement for public employees. The federal Occupational Safety and Health Administration (OSHA) does not cover public employees if the state does not provide such coverage. Coverage for volunteer rescue squads or fire departments also varies from state to state. More recently, OSHA has issued enforcement guidelines for protecting healthcare workers from the risk of tuberculosis. A more comprehensive standard has been proposed and is currently under review.

One very troublesome issue for prehospital healthcare providers has been the issue of notification of providers after they have transported and cared for patients with infectious diseases. Although confidentiality protection for HIV-infected patients has contributed to this difficulty, other factors are also important. The infected patient may not be diagnosed for some time after admission. Most often, the prehospital care provider is not employed by the healthcare facility in which the patient is diagnosed, and infection control staff members in that facility may not be aware of the potential exposure of the prehospital care provider. Difficulties in communication and patient confidentiality further complicate this situation.

A number of states have passed laws requiring that healthcare facilities notify prehospital healthcare providers if they have transported a patient with an infectious disease that could be transmitted to the provider (15). The scope and requirements of these laws vary from state to state. The Ryan White Act passed by Congress in 1990 mandated the development of a notification system for all prehospital care providers. For potentially fatal infections spread by airborne routes, healthcare facilities were required to notify the prehospital care provider if a patient whom he or she had transported was diagnosed with such an infection. For blood-borne infections, prehospital healthcare providers were allowed to inquire about a patient's diagnosis through a designated liaison if the prehospital healthcare provider was significantly exposed (e.g., needlestick) while transporting the patient. The law included a mechanism for review of the significance of the exposure and for protecting the confidentiality of the patient. The Department of Health and Human Services has now implemented this portion of the legislation. This requirement has helped to improve communication between prehospital care providers and hospitals regarding these issues.

PROGRAMS

Although infection control activities for prehospital healthcare workers are essentially the same as for other healthcare workers, some issues should be emphasized.

First, emergency medical providers are often unaware of the patient's diagnosis when arriving at the site of care or during transport to a healthcare facility. Therefore, standard protocols for the application of infection control procedures are especially important. Standard adherence to universal precautions for all patient care activities is an obvious example. Another approach would be to initiate certain precautions for specific types of patients triggered by their symptoms or by knowledge of the presence of specific infectious diseases in their service area. Assuming that all infectious patients can be individually identified at the scene is not good practice. Any selective protocols need to be simple and easy to apply.

Second, proper protective equipment must be available for use at the scene. This includes equipment such as masks and gloves needed during patient care and equipment for disposal. Requiring used needles to be brought back to the station for disposal increases the risk for these providers (8). Use of self-capping intravenous catheters for prehospital emergency care workers has been shown to result in a marked decrease in reported needlestick injuries (16,17). A recent study among 477 active EMS workers in Arizona on the use of a spring-loaded automatic retracting lancet device reduced the rate of needlestick injuries from 16 per 954 person-years to 2 per 477 person-years (17). The responsible parties need to ensure that necessary equipment is available. Proper equipment for cleaning used equipment in the station is also important. Cleaning such equipment in an area used for food preparation (e.g., responder's home or in a fire house) is not good practice. Proper procedures for medical waste disposal also need to be followed (see Chapter 100).

Third, proper infection control practices need to be adapted to the situation when the responder may have other job duties such as law enforcement or fire fighting. If the responder may arrive at the scene equipped for one type of duty but then must act as an emergency medical responder, proper equipment needed for infection control must still be provided (2).

Adequate training is extremely important. The application of standard practices throughout the provider organization is critical, because the providers usually will not base their use of precautions on prior knowledge of whether the patient has an infection. All staff members need to be appropriately trained and familiar with the infection control practices for the organization.

The threat of a bioterrorism attack will pose additional challenges to the development and delivery of infection control programs for prehospital workers. Currently, these and other medical care organizations are in the process of implementing the nation's new smallpox vaccination program—a very complex and difficult task for many prehospital responder organizations (18). The bioterrorism threat will require additional training and other resources. Meeting this challenge will also place more emphasis on the need for improved administration of the infection control programs for these organizations and on the necessity for better and more rapid communication with public health authorities.

ORGANIZATION OF SERVICES

Perhaps the most difficult issue with the implementation of infection control programs for prehospital care providers is the organization of these services given the different types of organizations in which these responders work (19,20). Other than hospital-based responders, the organization and provision of the necessary training and medical services needed for a good infection control program must be implemented by the provider organization. The following suggestions apply mainly to other types of organizations (e.g., fire departments, rescue squads).

First, given the growing importance and complexity of good infection control programs for these workers, one person in each organization must be made fully responsible for this program. Implementation of program elements can be delegated to others in the organization, but there needs to be a single position responsible for the overall program. This responsibility includes training, procurement and placement of proper equipment, and medical follow-up. This person must seek input from all parts of the organization to ensure that the infection control program is being properly implemented. Joint labor–management health and safety committees are one means for obtaining this input.

Second, there needs to be some liaison with a medical provider capable of providing the medical care and advice needed for the infection control program. This could be the infection control staff at the major hospital serviced by the responder. It could also be the emergency medical department providing emergency medical training or consultation for the responder organization. This medical liaison is critical for two functions. First, they can assist with infection control training and provide consultation on specific issues. Second, they can provide the medical consultation needed for issues related to immunization, surveillance programs, and incident follow-up. Although both are important, the latter best illustrates the need for such a medical liaison. Prompt follow-up medical care is critical after an incident such as a needlestick injury. Attempting to arrange such follow-up without any planning or preparation puts a great burden on the person at risk. It is far better to have developed a comprehensive medical program as part of the overall infection control program.

Many prehospital care providers have limited finances and are already strained by the requirements of providing good medical service. Additional training and immunizations may add to the financial strains, but such assistance is critical to the development and operation of a good infection control program.

CONCLUSIONS

Although there are few data on the extent of occupationally acquired infections among prehospital healthcare workers, their risk appears to be similar to that of other emergency care workers. The development of good infection control programs for these workers is hampered by the nature of the work and the diversity of organizations providing such care. However, sound infection control programs for these workers have been developed and should be beneficial.

REFERENCES

1. Occupational Safety and Health Administration, U.S. Department of Labor. Occupational exposure to bloodborne pathogens; final rule. *Federal Register* 1991;56:64004–64182.
2. Shell H. The Phoenix fanny pack. An infection protection accessory for all occasions. *J Emerg Med Serv* 1998;20(4):68–73.

3. National Institute for Occupational Safety and Health. Health hazard evaluation report. HETA95-0031-2601 University of Medicine and Dentistry of New Jersey. National Institute for Occupational Safety and Health, Cincinnati, OH 1996.
4. Rischitelli G, Harris J, McCauley L, et al. The risk of acquiring hepatitis B or C among public safety workers: a systematic review. *Am J Prev Med* 2001; 20(4):299–306.
5. Valenzuela TD, Hooton TM, Kaplan EL, et al. Transmission of toxic strep syndrome from an infected child to a firefighter during CPR. *Ann Emerg Med* 1991;20:90–92.
6. Reed E, Daya MR, Jui J, et al. Occupational infectious disease exposures in EMS personnel. *J Emerg Med* 1993;11:9–16.
7. Marcus R, Srivastava PU, Bell DM, et al. Occupational blood contact among prehospital providers. *Ann Emerg Med* 1995;25:776–779.
8. Klontz KC, Gunn RA, Caldwell JS. Needlestick injuries and hepatitis B immunizations in Florida paramedics: a statewide survey. *Ann Emerg Med* 1991;20:1310–1313.
9. Valenzuela TD, Hook EW, Copass MK, et al. Occupational exposure to hepatitis B in paramedics. *Arch Intern Med* 1985;145:1976–1977.10 Pepe PE, Hollinger FB, Troisi CL, et al. Viral hepatitis risk in urban emergency medical services personnel. *Ann Emerg Med* 1986;15: 454–457.
11. Kunches LM, Craven DE, Werner BG, et al. Hepatitis B exposure in emergency medical personnel. Prevalence of serological markers and need for immunization. *Am J Med* 1983;75:269–272.
12. Eastham JN, Thompson ME, Ryan PA. Treatment and career attitudes of prehospital care providers associated with potential exposure to HIV/ AIDS. *Am J Emerg Med* 1991;9:122–126.
13. Smyser MS, Bryce J, Joseph JG. AIDS-related knowledge, attitudes, and precautionary behaviors among emergency medical personnel. *Public Health Rep* 1990;105:496–504.
14. Thompson ME, Eastham JN. Prehospital providers AIDS knowledge and attitudes. *Md Med J* 1989;38:1027–1032.
15. Steele LJ. When universal precautions fail. Communicable disease notification laws for emergency responders. *J Legal Med* 1990;11:451–480.
16. O'Connor RE, Krall SP, Megaregel RE, et al. Reducing the rate of paramedic needlesticks in emergency medical services: the role of self-capping intravenous catheters. *Acad Emerg Med* 1996;3:668–674.
17. Peate WF. Preventing needlesticks in emergency medical system workers. *J Occup Environ Med* 2001;43(6):554–557.
18. Centers for Disease Control and Prevention. Guidelines for smallpox vaccination for state and local health departments. LDL, Atlanta, GA. December 2002.
19. National Fire Protection Association 1581. Standard on fire department infection control program. National Fire Protection Association. Quincy, MA, 1991.
20. International Association of Fire Fighters. Infectious diseases and the fire and emergency services. International Association of Fire Fighters. Washington, DC, 1992.

84

PREVENTION OF OCCUPATIONALLY ACQUIRED INFECTIONS IN POSTHOSPITAL HEALTHCARE WORKERS

CHARLES W. STRATTON IV

Infectious diseases can be transmitted from one human to another by a number of different mechanisms. Some of these mechanisms such as aerosolized respiratory droplets pose a direct threat to persons nearby, whereas others involve direct contact or exposure to biologic specimens from infected patients. Healthcare workers, consequently, are known to be at risk for contracting an infection from patients or patient specimens (1–6). Such risks for occupationally acquired infections in healthcare workers have long been appreciated, as is evident by the protective clothing once worn during the plague epidemic of the fourteenth century (Fig. 84.1). The evolving severe acute respiratory syndrome (SARS) epidemic (7), the threat of bioterrorism (8), and the ongoing acquired immunodeficiency syndrome (AIDS) epidemic (9) has focused considerable attention on occupationally acquired infections. Such attention has resulted in Centers for Disease Control and Prevention (CDC) infection control guidelines for SARS (10), Public Health Service (PHS) regulations for select agents and toxins (11), and Occupational Safety and Health Administration (OSHA) regulations for blood-borne pathogens (12). The reemergence of tuberculosis (13,14) similarly has resulted in CDC guidelines (15) and federally mandated regulations (16).

Several important references related to reducing the risk of occupationally acquired infections in healthcare workers are readily available. The National Committee for Clinical Laboratory Standards (NCCLS) offers Document M29-A2, "Protection of Laboratory Workers from Occupationally Acquired Infections" (17). The CDC also offers guidelines for infection control in hospital personnel (18). These guidelines include recommendations for nonpatient healthcare personnel, management of exposures, prevention of transmission of infections in microbiology and biomedical laboratories, and prevention of latex barrier hypersensitivity reactions.

More persons in the United States today are employed in the healthcare sector than in any other industry (19). Historically, most of these workers have been employed in the hospital setting. Thus, occupationally acquired infections in healthcare workers have received the greatest attention for workers in the hospital setting. Hospitals have developed comprehensive infection control programs and occupational health services that address the prevention of occupationally acquired infections. However, as we enter the twenty-first century, the horizons of infection control are expanding (20) because of the recognition that the risk of infections transmitted from patients to healthcare workers is not limited to hospital workers but extends to out-of-hospital healthcare workers (21). Today, healthcare is delivered in outpatient, transitional care, long-term care, rehabilitative care, home care, and private office settings (22). The out-of-hospital setting is receiving increasing attention, and infection control requirements and activities have been established (23, 24). Chapter 83 covers the prehospital healthcare worker, whereas this chapter covers the prevention of occupationally acquired infections in posthospital healthcare workers.

EXAMPLES OF POSTHOSPITAL HEALTHCARE WORKERS AND THEIR RISK FOR OCCUPATIONALLY ACQUIRED INFECTIONS

The definition of posthospital healthcare workers continues to evolve (22). Outpatient healthcare workers and medical personnel at reference laboratories, for example, can be either prehospital or posthospital healthcare workers. Following are examples of common categories of posthospital healthcare workers and their risk for occupationally acquired infections.

Pathologists and Medical Technologists

Although pathologists and medical technologists generally work in the hospital setting, they may be involved in either hospital care or posthospital care. For example, pathologists and medical technologists who are involved in surgical pathology, cytology, and clinical laboratories are usually involved in hospital care, whereas pathologists and morgue personnel involved in autopsies could be considered posthospital healthcare workers. Moreover, some pathologists and medical technologists work in reference laboratories that are not associated with a hospital. As nonhospital-associated freestanding operations, these reference

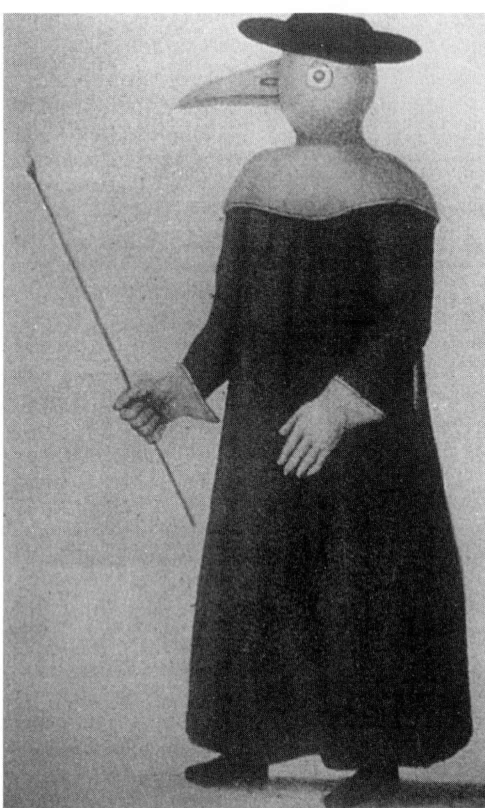

Figure 84.1. Protective garb worn by healthcare workers in the Middle Ages to protect themselves against plague.

laboratories most often do not have the assistance of hospital infection control professionals and, hence, may fall short in providing protective measures appropriate to the infectious risks. The use of such freestanding reference laboratories for testing of specimens from hospitalized patients and for testing of specimens from patients in the prehospital and posthospital setting is increasing. This, in turn, has resulted in potential infectious risks for personnel involved in the packaging, handling, and transport of medical specimens. Accordingly, the PHS and NCCLS have developed regulations and guidelines for proper procedures for the handling and transport of diagnostic specimens and etiologic agents (11,25). Moreover, NCCLS, the CDC, and the National Institutes of Health (NIH) address biosafety issues in microbiology and biomedical laboratories (17, 26). All pathologists and medical technologists have unique risks for occupationally acquired infections because of contact with patient specimens. The risk for pathologists and medical technologists involved in clinical laboratories is covered in Chapter 82. The risks for pathologists who perform autopsies (17,27) are addressed in this chapter. Biosafety considerations for autopsies are important topics that often are not addressed by hospital infection control committees.

Home Healthcare Workers

Cost containment has shifted a great deal of medical care from the hospital setting to the outpatient setting. Although the home setting is considered to have fewer infection risks, studies have not confirmed this (28). Clearly some patients receiving home healthcare have infections and, thus, pose a risk for home healthcare workers (29). These patients are often elderly and may have unrecognized tuberculosis (30). AIDS patients are another group of patients commonly cared for in a domiciliary setting (31). Such infection risks in the home healthcare setting are only beginning to be studied. Research is needed to delineate such risks and to identify ways to minimize or prevent these infections from being transmitted to home healthcare workers. This topic is discussed in Chapter 107.

Residential Long-Term Healthcare Workers

The number of persons entering assisted living facilities and nursing homes for residential long-term care is substantial and is increasing. Many of these nursing home, residential care, and assisted-living patients enter such facilities directly from the hospital. The need for residential long-term care facilities to provide comprehensive infection control programs is well recognized (32). A number of infectious diseases problems are common to long-term care facilities and often are unappreciated (33). Atypical presentation of infections is generally acknowledged and may lead to delays in diagnosis and treatment of infections such as tuberculosis. The physical plant of many long-term care facilities is often a factor; many residents live in confined settings with few private rooms, and rooms appropriate for isolation often are not available. Finally, many long-term care facilities experience rapid turnover of personnel, and residential long-term care workers frequently have less training than those in the hospital setting. Long-term care facilities need a well-developed infection control program that in part identifies and minimizes the risk of occupationally acquired infections. Such programs can be developed best with the assistance of the hospital-based infection control professional (34). (See Chapter 106.)

Outpatient Healthcare Workers

The delivery of healthcare continues to shift from the hospital setting to the outpatient setting (22). For example, an increasing number of surgical procedures are done on an outpatient basis, and postoperative complications are now seen by emergency departments (35). Thus, many outpatient healthcare workers can be considered posthospital workers and share the risks of posthospital healthcare workers. The Joint Commission on Accreditation of Healthcare Organizations (JCAHO) is actively reviewing infection control programs for outpatient services that are affiliated with hospitals.

Rehabilitation Facility Workers

Another shift in providing healthcare has been the establishment of rehabilitation facilities. Follow-up care of many illnesses is now carried out in these facilities, and nosocomial infections are common (36). Healthcare workers in these facilities have similar risks to hospital workers, yet these rehabilitation facilities may not be associated with a hospital and have access to infection control professionals and policies. Surveillance and infection control measures, nonetheless, are needed.

Dialysis Facility Workers

Freestanding dialysis facilities have become very common. Clearly, the risk for many blood-borne pathogens in such facilities is high (37). These centers may not have access to infection control professionals and policies; however, surveillance and infection control measures clearly are needed.

Healthcare Laundry Workers

Freestanding healthcare laundries serving multiple hospitals have been established in many cities. The risk for these workers is high for certain infections, including blood-borne pathogens because of the presence of sharp objects such as needles (38). Workers in these laundries also are at risk for scabies. Laundries may not have access to infection control professionals and policies.

Funeral Home Workers

The risk for exposure to infectious agents during autopsies is becoming better known and has resulted in guidelines for performing autopsies to minimize this risk (17,27,39). In particular, guidelines designed to minimize the risk of human immunodeficiency virus (HIV) infection have been developed (40,41). Funeral home workers can be considered posthospital healthcare workers and share some of the same risks as a pathologist performing an autopsy (42). A study of funeral practitioners has noted a low rate of occupational exposures and a high rate of hepatitis B vaccination in comparison with prior studies, which suggests both improved education for and compliance with the recommendations for preventing transmission of blood-borne pathogens in the workplace (43). Such efforts should be continued.

Trash Haulers and Landfill Operators

The potential for exposure to infectious diseases in trash haulers and landfill operators is a very important issue (44,45). Although minimal (46,47), the risk is real and should be controlled. The proper disposal of medical waste is a key factor in controlling this risk; NCCLS Document GP5-A "Clinical Laboratory Waste Management: Approved Guideline" addresses this topic (48), and federal law now requires compliance (49). (See Chapter 100.)

EPIDEMIOLOGY OF OCCUPATIONALLY ACQUIRED INFECTIONS

Although quite a few pathogens can be transmitted to a worker in the healthcare setting, there are relatively few mechanisms by which such transmission can occur. The most common and important mechanisms of transmission are exposure to aerosols, exposure to blood or body fluids via direct contact or inoculation, and hand-to-mouth transmission. These are reviewed in some detail.

Exposure to Aerosols

The transmission of *Mycobacterium tuberculosis* occurs mainly by inhalation of droplet nuclei (50). There is also evidence that in some cases the coronavirus responsible for SARS has been spread by droplet nuclei (7). These droplets are airborne particles and must be less than 5 μm in size to reach the alveolar spaces. Droplet nuclei can be produced when persons with pulmonary or laryngeal infections speak, sneeze, cough, or sing. If these persons are in a healthcare setting such as a nursing home, and the diagnosis of tuberculosis or SARS is unknown, they become a risk to healthcare workers. Healthcare workers in laboratories are also at risk for airborne pathogens, because there are certain manipulations with patient samples that may produce an aerosol. An important example of such a manipulation is dropping of fluids containing microbial suspensions (e.g., urine containing *M. tuberculosis* microorganisms because of renal tuberculosis) onto a hard surface, producing an aerosol. Working with *Neisseria meningitidis* cultures are also considered a risk, and microbiology technologists should be immunized against this pathogen.

The risk of aerosolized *M. tuberculosis* from patients with unsuspected tuberculosis to posthospital healthcare workers such as home healthcare, nursing home, and clinic healthcare workers has become quite clear with the resurgence of tuberculosis in the United States. This risk increases in settings such as outpatient clinics where many sick people congregate in waiting and treatment rooms or halls and is also increased in communities where the incidence of HIV and/or tuberculosis is high. Outbreaks of tuberculosis among healthcare workers have occurred (51–53); some have involved multidrug-resistant *M. tuberculosis* (52,53). This risk can best be appreciated by considering the tuberculosis skin test conversion rates among healthcare workers that have ranged from 0.11% to 10% (54,55). This risk increases considerably in healthcare workers who are exposed to persons from countries where tuberculosis is endemic, to HIV patients, and to patients known to have tuberculosis; the skin test conversion rates in such settings have ranged from 18% to 55% (56,57). Transmission of tuberculosis to healthcare workers can be a major problem requiring prevention and control (57). This problem is covered in great detail in Chapter 37.

A less well-appreciated, but equally important, risk for posthospital healthcare workers such as pathologists and funeral home workers is the risk for aerosolized transmission of infectious agents when working with deceased patients (58). In addition to the risk of dropping body fluids containing microbial suspensions, a number of other procedures associated with autopsies produce an aerosol. For example, the Rokitansky method, in which the abdominal and thoracic organs are eviscerated as a unit, continues to be commonly used at autopsy. However, this method involves blunt blind dissection in both cavities, which is cumbersome and creates unnecessary aerosols. The NCCLS now recommends removing organs singly (the Virchow technique) to avoid the more hazardous aerosolization risk associated with complete evisceration by the Rokitansky method

(17). The NCCLS also recommends that organs not be photographed until they have been fixed in formalin to decrease the risk of aerosolized microorganisms. Unfortunately, this does not provide complete protection against aerosolized *M. tuberculosis* because this pathogen survives fixation in formalin, although the fixation does decrease the number of mycobacteria and thus lessens the degree of infectivity (59). The need to saw the calvarium is perhaps the most problematic autopsy procedure, because it unavoidably creates an aerosol. Aerosolization can be minimized by doing this procedure inside a plastic bag or plastic head frame, using a hand saw (difficult to do), or having a vacuum attached to the oscillating saw.

Another important risk factor for aerosolization during an autopsy is the use of side-arm faucet water aspirators to remove pleural or peritoneal fluids from these body cavities, because these aspirating devices produce an infectious aerosol. Side-arm faucet water suction devices should not be used in autopsy suites or in funeral homes. Instead, they should be replaced by surgical-type vacuum reservoirs that are attached to the hospital vacuum lines that have appropriate traps, filters, and regulators (60).

Air flow in the autopsy suites (but not funeral homes) has been addressed by the American Society of Heating, Refrigerating, and Air Conditioning Engineers and by the CDC (15). Adequate air flow is an important means of minimizing the risk of aerosolized pathogens. Both groups recommend that autopsy suites have at least 12 total air exchanges per hour and that autopsy room air be exhausted directly to the outside. In addition, the College of American Pathologists recommends that autopsies on high-risk patients be done only in rooms with good ventilation (60,61).

It is important to have a clear understanding of what constitutes good ventilation. There are three important engineering factors that allow good ventilation/control of air within a room. First, negative pressure in the room should be maintained with respect to surrounding areas. This means that air should move from an area of low infectivity (i.e., outside the room) to an area of higher infectivity (i.e., inside the room). Second, the number of air changes in the room should be increased, which can substantially decrease the risk of the transmission of aerosolized pathogens by dilution and removal of these pathogens. Good ventilation also dictates that within-room mixing of air (i.e., ventilation efficiency) is adequate. This is usually accomplished by placing air supply outlets in the ceiling and exhaust inlets near the floor. This provides a downward movement of clean air, which travels through the breathing zone to the floor area for exhaust. Third, there should be adequate exhaust to the outside. Because the air in a high-risk room such as the autopsy suite is likely to be contaminated with infectious droplet nuclei, it should not be recirculated within the room or within the building. Instead, this potentially contaminated air should be exhausted to the outside, away from intake vents, people, and animals. An episode in a medical examiner's office in Syracuse, New York, (53) illustrates this point. Two workers in the Onondaga County medical examiner's office were infected by *M. tuberculosis* after they were exposed during autopsies on cadavers of prison inmates who had been infected with *M. tuberculosis* before death. In addition to the two workers who contracted clinical manifestations of tuberculosis, the tuberculin skin tests of 30% of the staff in the medical examiner's office converted to positive; this included a secretary whose desk was right under the ventilation system that circulated air from the morgue. The examiner's office responded to this episode by installing a new ventilation system, adding ultraviolet treatment of the air in the morgue, and initiating a respiratory protection program for personnel who worked in the morgue. Chapter 89 provides additional information on the design and maintenance of ventilation systems and prevention of airborne infections.

If adequate ventilation is not possible, healthcare workers who have any possibility of being exposed to aerosolized infectious particles should participate in a respiratory protection program. This is accomplished by wearing particulate respirators. A standard surgical mask is not a particulate respirator because lack of a tight face seal allows particles between 1 and 3 μm to be inhaled. Disposable particulate respirators are available. There are two types: the dust/mist filter, which excludes particles of 2 μm, and the fume filter, which excludes particles 0.6 to 1.0 μm. The CDC has published guidelines for the use of particulate respirators that include training, fit testing, care, and maintenance (15); OSHA requires that a fume filter be used in particulate respirators (16).

Exposure to Blood or Body Fluids via Direct Contact or Inoculation

It is well appreciated today that exposure to blood or body fluids via direct contact or inoculation can result in the transmission of a number of pathogens, of which the best known examples are hepatitis B virus (HBV) and HIV. The risk of HIV has increased the awareness of this problem. Numerous incidents of exposure of healthcare workers to HIV-infected blood have been evaluated in multiple prospective studies. These studies have identified HIV infections, usually involving individuals who had been punctured with needles; seroconversions are rare in staff members with intact skin. The rate of infection with HIV in healthcare workers after exposure to HIV-infected blood is approximately 0.3% (62). It is instructive to review seroconversions in healthcare workers analyzed by the CDC (62), including six from prospective studies. Of the 34 individuals with seroconversion, 12 were nurses, 11 were laboratory workers, 4 were physicians, and the other 7 were from other occupational groups. All underwent HIV seroconversion within 1 year of exposure, which had been mucocutaneous contact or percutaneous inoculation with blood or fluids containing HIV. Of the 28 percutaneous inoculations, 14 occurred while drawing venous blood and 2 occurred while drawing arterial blood; 5 of these were associated with carrying out intravenous infusions. Of the remaining injuries, two had occurred while injecting laboratory specimens, one while holding a specimen vial and two while manipulating a transvenous pacemaker. The remaining injuries were a result of other or unknown causes. Most of these percutaneous inoculations occurred after unexpected movement by a patient, a co-worker, or equipment (seven exposures); inadequate needle disposal (nine exposures); and recapping of needles (seven exposures). Thirteen of these 28 occurred through the workers' gloved hands. Of the five mucocutaneous exposures that resulted in seroconversion, one involved pressure hemostasis with an ungloved hand, three occurred during accidents involving blood spillage, and one involved an individual who was sprayed with concentrated virus. The CDC has concluded that the most frequent cause of occupational transmission of HIV or HBV is injury by a needle contaminated with the virus (62). However, other mechanisms such as virus-contaminated body fluids being splashed on mucosal membranes and, to a lesser degree, skin clearly are important. Finally, but most importantly, postexposure prophylaxis with antiretroviral therapy with zidovudine (ZDV) has been found to be associated with a greater than 80% reduction in the risk of occupational infection (63). Prophylaxis clearly is important (64,65). For this reason, the PHS recommends that ZDV, lamivudine, and sometimes a protease inhibitor such as indinavir should be given prophylactically within 1 to 2 hours of a high-risk exposure to HIV (65). (See Chapter 79.)

PREVENTION

Prevention of Exposure to Blood and Body Fluids

Strategies are needed to reduce the occupational exposure to infectious agents by inoculation and/or direct contact. These are summarized in Table 84.1. Chapters 45, 78, and 79 cover nosocomial infections in healthcare workers caused by infectious agents acquired by exposure to blood and body fluids or by direct contact with other infectious substances. Specific risks associated with autopsies and appropriate preventive measures are discussed further in this chapter.

TABLE 84.1. STRATEGIES FOR RISK REDUCTION FROM OCCUPATIONAL EXPOSURE TO INFECTIOUS AGENTS BY INOCULATION OR DIRECT CONTACT

Strategy	Comment
Improved education/training on the safe handling and disposal of needles	This is an approach that will most rapidly reduce risks
Modifications of work-practice habits involving the way devices are used	The proper education/training should lead to such changes in habit
Improvements in personal protective-equipment to include design, comfort, and availability and use and aimed at providing a better barrier between the blood/body fluids of a patient and the healthcare worker	Although this is a slower process than education, it can be done in a short period; education and training on the use of personal protective equipment obviously is needed to ensure its proper use
Engineering controls that are designed to eliminate the problem	Examples are needle-free devices for intravenous access and devices that cover a needle after use; these are the least-rapid strategies to implement
Administrative controls and policies to ensure the implementation of such controls	Examples are postexposure management procedures and vaccination against hepatitis B virus; these, like education and training, can be implemented quite rapidly

Autopsy protocols (17,27,39–41,59-61,66) should include measures to prevent or minimize exposure of the prosector and his or her assistant to potentially contaminated tissues and body fluids by direct contact or via inoculation. These measures should also prevent other areas of the autopsy suite from becoming contaminated so that bystanders, housekeeping personnel, and others will not be exposed to contaminated tissue and fluids. In short, autopsy precautions should be directed at the prevention of needlesticks, accidental cuts, and splash or direct contamination of mucous membranes or skin in any person who for any reason enters the autopsy suite. A rational approach to the safe conduct of autopsies includes (17,27,39) performance of autopsies by experienced and well-trained personnel, use of appropriate safety-oriented devices, a safe work environment, appropriate work practices, appropriate vaccination against vaccine-preventable diseases such as hepatitis B, and Universal Precautions. These are discussed in greater detail.

Experienced and Well-Trained Personnel

It is logical to assume that the risk of accidental injury is greatest among the inexperienced. This has been confirmed by a study wherein a laceration injury occurred in 1 of every 11 autopsies conducted by pathology residents. In contrast, one such injury occurred for every 53 autopsies performed by staff pathologists (67). In addition, there should not be time constraints (self-imposed or otherwise) that could lead to hurried carelessness. For this reason, many pathology departments do not routinely conduct autopsies after 4 p.m.

There must be a sufficient number of experienced and well-trained personnel. Most autopsies are done with two persons, the prosector and his or her assistant. A logical recommendation is to have a third person (17,27). This third person functions as a circulator and does not directly participate in the autopsy procedure. Thus, the prosector and his or her assistant are "dirty," whereas the circulator remains clean, avoiding direct contact with contaminated tissues and body fluids. The circulator's tasks include the following:

1. Preparation of the 0.5% sodium hypochlorite solution from commercial bleach solution by diluting the latter 1:10. This solution is used to swab surfaces and/or to soak instruments.
2. Preparation of plastic biohazard bags for bagging soiled linens from the stretcher and for the gowns and scrub suits, which are deposited in plastic bags after the autopsy has been finished. Other plastic bags are prepared for waste such as gloves, masks, and foot covers, which will be incinerated. All bags must be labeled with a biohazard tag as per OSHA regulations (12) and with the disposition (incineration or laundering). Many medical centers now have colored bags to indicate the disposition (e.g., red for incineration, orange for laundering).
3. Assistance in the collection of all specimens by bringing clean containers to the table in which specimens may be placed. Also, the propane gas cylinder can be lit for the searing spatula. The circulator should do all paperwork such as laboratory requisitions. The circulator also ensures that specimen con-

tainers are washed clean and wiped with 0.5% sodium hypochlorite solution, the caps and covers are tightly fastened, the containers are labeled with biohazard tags and the deceased's name and hospital number, and the containers are placed in waterproof bags for transportation to the various laboratories for further processing and studies. Finally, the circulator attaches the accompanying laboratory requisitions to the proper specimens.
4. Assistance in providing any instruments or other supplies to the prosector.
5. Recording the organ weights and other descriptive notes, often using dictating equipment.
6. Adjusting the lamp and microphone over the autopsy table.
7. Communication with physicians, nursing supervisors, funeral directors, and other relevant personnel so that the telephone receiver does not get contaminated by the prosector.
8. Handling of containers in which tissues for fixation are to be placed to avoid contamination of the outer surface of the container.
9. Wiping up any drops of blood or body fluids that may fall on the floor around the autopsy table. Gloves should be worn. Paper towels and 0.5% sodium hypochlorite solution are used. This minimizes any soiling of the autopsy floor.

Use of Appropriate Safety Devices

Safety devices for the routine autopsy have become an important aspect of Universal Precautions and are well documented and described (12,17). Particularly important in the autopsy suite are personal protective items. Eyes should be protected by goggles or face shields. Eye glasses are often worn instead of goggles or face shields but provide only minimal protection for the eyes. Goggles under which eye glasses can be worn are available. Surgical caps and masks should be worn for the performance of the autopsy. The mask is particularly important for the prevention of tuberculosis. These masks should not be the standard surgical mask but instead a disposable particulate respirator. OSHA, of course, requires a fume filter that excludes particles 0.6 to 1.0 μm in size. A number of pathologists use and are very pleased with powered respirators. Scrub suits should be worn. These should have long sleeves with either attached or separately provided water-repellent sleeves. The scrub suit must not be worn outside of the autopsy suite. Surgical gowns have been recommended (17). These should be waterproof disposable gowns with disposable forearm guards. A waterproof apron must be worn. Protective shoes should be worn. These are not to leave the autopsy suite. Waterproof shoe coverings should be worn over these shoes; these should be disposable. Two pairs of gloves are recommended because latex loses its integrity after a period of use (68). Frequent changing of the outer pair is recommended. Many prosectors now use a fine-mesh metallic glove or a Kevlar "fish" glove. The latter was developed for workers cleaning fish and is very flexible and not clumsy. These Kevlar gloves can be purchased more cheaply from a sporting goods store than from a laboratory safety catalog. If such gloves are not worn routinely, they should be worn for high-risk procedures such as removing the pelvic organs or cutting the ribs. Ribs should not be cut through the bony portion but instead should be incised medial to the costochondral junction. Uncalcified cartilage, unlike bone cuts with spicules, will not scratch or puncture the skin if there is unexpected contact. A safe yet practical approach to gloving is a pair of tight-fitting latex surgical gloves underneath Kevlar gloves, with a larger pair worn on top of the Kevlar gloves. The outer pair should be changed frequently.

Other safety devices concern the use of instruments and their design. There should be only one blade in the dissection field at any given time. Blades with rounded ends are available. Changing blades should not be attempted with forceps and clamps, because these contribute to flying blades. When an oscillating (Stryker) saw is used, a vacuum device can be attached to minimize aerosols. Alternatively, a damp towel can be held over the saw by a second person or a clear plastic bag can be used to contain the entire procedure. Many prosectors now recommend that the cranium be opened with a hand saw, although this is exceedingly difficult. Blunt needles are available for aspirating body fluids.

Safe Work Environment

It is the responsibility of each medical center to provide an adequately equipped and safe morgue facility. Of utmost importance is proper ventilation. Good lighting is important. A shower should be available in both the men's and women's locker rooms. All surfaces should be of a material that is easy to clean (e.g., stainless steel); contaminated surfaces should be promptly cleansed and treated with an appropriate disinfectant. Floors and walls are best painted with enough coats of epoxy paint to seal such materials as cinder blocks, bricks, tile, and concrete. The floors should have drains connected with appropriate traps and filters to the hospital drainage system. High-pressure hose sprays should be avoided during the autopsy cleanup procedure. Similarly, side-arm faucet water aspirators that use the Bernoulli principle to create an inexpensive suction device should be avoided, because these may create an infectious aerosol. Instead, surgical-type vacuum reservoirs that are properly connected to the hospital system should be available.

Appropriate Work Practices

Work practices and attitudes regarding the transmission of infectious diseases during the autopsy are evolving and are being shaped by new scientific evidence. For example, Bankowski et al. (69) described the postmortem recovery of human immunodeficiency virus type 1 (HIV-1) from the plasma and mononuclear cells of patients with AIDS. Recovery of infectious HIV-1 from 51% of blood samples of deceased AIDS victims should prompt pathologists and morticians to reevaluate policies regarding universal precautions and the handling of known HIV-1–infected cadavers. Of particular interest in this comprehensive evaluation is the authors noting that time from death until specimen acquisition was the only factor significantly associated with recovery of HIV-1. No HIV-1 was recovered from cadavers sampled more than 21 to 25 hours after death. Thus, delaying an autopsy for 24 hours may markedly decrease the potential HIV-1 infectivity. However, it is clear that the risks are not entirely eliminated by postponement of the autopsy. Infectious HIV has been recovered from tissue, bone, and blood after a postmortem interval of 6 days and from an unfixed spleen specimen stored at 20°C for 14 days after death (70). Unfortunately, a 24-hour delay in the autopsy would not be well received by funeral directors and embalmers who already have identified significant delays in obtaining autopsied cases from hospitals (71).

Hepatitis B Vaccination

Healthcare workers with occupationally acquired HBV infection have died from this infection (72). Despite all the concern about autopsies in the AIDS era, among the greatest risks to pathologists continues to be viral hepatitis (73), both hepatitis B and hepatitis C. The prevalence of anti-hepatitis B antibody in pathologists is 27%, exceeded only by surgeons at 28% (74). The risk of acquiring HBV infection from occupational exposure depends on the nature and frequency of exposure to blood or to body fluids containing blood (75). The risk of infection is at least 30% after a percutaneous exposure to blood from a hepatitis B e antigen-seropositive source (76). Unlike HIV-1, hepatitis B vaccination is readily available, and all pathologists who are seronegative for hepatitis B should be vaccinated. Vaccination for hepatitis B has been shown to effectively prevent nosocomial hepatitis B (77,78), and the CDC now recommends such vaccination (79). (See Chapter 78.)

Universal Precautions

The concept of Universal Precautions is quite simple. This concept recognizes that medical history and examination cannot reliably identify all patients with blood-borne pathogens; therefore, blood and body fluid precautions should be used *consistently* for *all* patient specimens. This approach is recommended by the CDC and is referred to as "universal blood and body fluid precautions." All patient tissues, blood, and body fluids should be considered potentially infectious. This concept is further discussed in Chapters 78 and 79.

The concept of Universal Precautions is extremely important to undertakers and mortuary workers (42,58). Although all deceased patients known to have a contagious disease should have the body bag marked with a biohazard or blood precautions tag to warn funeral directors and other mortuary personnel, not all cases of transmissible infectious diseases are identified at the time of death. The greatest risk for mortuary workers is the injection and distribution of embalming fluid, which displaces the natural body fluids. This procedure carries the risk of needlestick injuries, direct contact with displaced body fluids, and aerosolization of displaced body fluids. Therefore, mortuary workers should follow the same precautions as outlined for the autopsy.

After the introduction of Universal Precautions in 1986, with reaffirmation by the CDC in subsequent publications (80,81), a modified approach (82) was published in 1988. The difference between these two proposals is that, initially, all body fluids were treated as if they were equally infectious; the modified approach excluded certain body fluids unless they were contaminated with blood. Subsequent experience has revealed that compliance with universal precautions is not ideal, with perceived risk and appropriate education as important factors in compliance (83–86). Nonetheless, these guidelines remain prudent today and are summarized in Table 84.2.

It is important to realize that these guidelines are only for blood-borne infections and do not address transmission of aerosolized infectious pathogens. It was initially estimated that the cost of universal precautions would be between $1 and $10 per patient admitted to hospitals in the United States (87). Subsequent data (88) found that the cost of implementing the CDC Universal Precautions in a university hospital were closer to the $10 per patient estimate. Finally, it should also be realized that no data confirm the efficacy of these guidelines. Nonetheless, they are sensible if they are followed correctly.

Prevention of Diseases Transmitted by Hand-to-Mouth Contact

Although airborne transmission and direct contact and inoculation of infectious pathogens are the most common risks for occupationally acquired infections in posthospital healthcare workers, hand-to-mouth transmission is nevertheless an important mechanism in the pathogenesis of these infections. Basically, the mechanism consists of a healthcare worker contaminating his or her hand(s) with an infectious agent from a patient and then transferring this pathogen to his or her mouth. As might be anticipated, most of these infections involve pathogens that cause diarrheal illnesses, although viral hepatitis is another infection that can be transmitted by hand-to-mouth contact (i.e., fecal-oral contamination).

Fecal-oral contamination occurs, because many patients have poor personal hygiene and soil the environment, after which poor hand washing practices by healthcare workers result in transmission of the diarrheal illness to themselves.

Outbreaks of diarrhea in long-term care facilities appear to be a common problem (33,89). The risk for nursing home workers and posthospital healthcare workers can be appreciated by reviewing a number of illustrative reports. Maryland has reported

TABLE 84.2. MODIFIED RECOMMENDATIONS FOR UNIVERSAL PRECAUTIONS

Following the precautions with:
- Amniotic fluid
- Blood and other body fluids containing visible blood
- Cerebrospinal fluid
- Pericardial fluid
- Peritoneal fluid
- Pleural fluid
- Semen
- Synovial fluid
- Tissues
- Vaginal secretions

It is not necessary to follow the precautions with the following body fluids unless they are contaminated with blood:
- Feces
- Nasal secretions
- Sputum
- Sweat
- Tears
- Urine
- Vomitus

numerous outbreaks of gastroenteritis in nursing homes with most outbreaks caused by Norwalk-like viruses (90). During an average outbreak, almost one third of residents and one fifth of staff members are infected. Others have reported similar findings (91). The CDC has reported that Norwalk-like viruses are a common cause of outbreaks of acute gastroenteritis on cruise ships and nursing homes (92). One nursing home report (93) described an outbreak of *Giardia lamblia* that originated with an infected meal and then progressed by fecal-oral contamination and eventually affected 35 residents and 38 employees of the facility. Other bacterial pathogens have caused serious gastroenteritis outbreaks in the nursing home setting. For example, *Escherichia coli* 0157:H7 caused a period of enteritis exceeding 18 days in 33% of nursing home residents and 13% of staff members (94). Finally, HIV-infected patients are recognized as commonly having diarrhea caused by enteric viruses (95). Clearly, the problem of fecal-oral transmission in posthospital healthcare workers is important.

Healthcare workers who are at risk for outbreaks spread by fecal-oral contamination must practice good hand washing techniques themselves and reinforce the importance of hand washing for everyone within the facility, including healthcare workers, competent patients and residents, and visiting friends and family members. In addition, supplies of soap, towels, and gloves must be adequate throughout the facility. If hand washing is difficult to do, the substitution of a waterless alcohol hand rub is recommended (96). The use of gloves must include changing gloves before going from one patient to another and washing hands each time a pair of gloves is removed. This is because many pathogens can stick to the latex gloves after contamination, and adherence persists despite washing the gloves with soap, chlorhexidine, or isopropyl alcohol (97).

Finally, although the concept of interrupting or preventing outbreaks of infections with hand washing began with Semmelweis in 1847 (98) and is still considered necessary, the actual role of hand washing remains somewhat controversial even today (99). Moreover, compliance with hand washing recommendations has been poor (100,101), leading to the use of alcoholic preparations that require no water (97,102). The subject of hand washing and hand disinfection is extensively covered in Chapter 96. Hand washing is vital to interrupt the fecal-oral route of transmission of infection (103,104).

KEY INFECTIOUS PATHOGENS OF CONCERN FOR POSTHOSPITAL HEALTHCARE WORKERS

A diverse group of specific pathogens are involved in nosocomial infections. These are discussed in detail in Section V of this book. Management and work-ups of healthcare workers exposed to nosocomial pathogens and to other infectious pathogens is important, and guidelines for this have been published (105,106). Some infectious pathogens are of minimal risk for occupationally acquired infections in posthospital healthcare workers (e.g., coagulase-negative staphylococci). On the other hand, a number of infectious pathogens may or may not be associated with nosocomial infections per se but are of particular concern to posthospital healthcare workers such as prosectors and morticians. Examples of these pathogens include HIV-1, rabies virus, and the human transmissible spongiform encephalopathies agent. These and other agents of particular concern to posthospital healthcare workers are briefly discussed in this section.

Human Immunodeficiency Virus

HIV-1, as already mentioned, is responsible for altering the approach to prevention of occupational exposure to infectious agents in the healthcare workplace (107). Mechanisms for transmission of HIV-1 to posthospital healthcare workers include direct contact (e.g., splashing mucosal surfaces) and inoculation. To date, there is no evidence for airborne transmission or fecal-oral transmission. Obviously, the posthospital healthcare workers at risk include all those involved with blood and body fluids of premortem or postmortem AIDS victims and the trash haulers and landfill operators who may be exposed to improperly disposed needles. The key to prevention of HIV-1 infections in these persons is to prevent exposure. A number of these preventive measures were discussed previously in this chapter.

Additional measures include decontaminating any spills of blood or body fluids in the work area with 5% sodium hypochlorite. All instruments used for AIDS patient care should be soaked in disinfectant for 30 minutes before routine washing. HIV-1 is inactivated by a wide range of disinfectants (108,109), including 50% ethanol, 3% hydrogen peroxide, phenolic compounds (e.g., Lysol), iodophor compounds (e.g., Betadine), and sodium hypochlorite (household bleach) in a freshly prepared 1:10 dilution in water (final concentration 0.5%). Because of their corrosive action, soaking instruments in bleach solutions should be limited to 30 minutes. Instruments using electronic devices that are an integral part of the equipment are more difficult to disinfect. Fortunately, studies have shown that HIV-1 is reliably eliminated by routine disinfection for such electronic instruments (110). In addition, there are now guidelines for disinfection practices for semicritical items (111). (See Chapter 74.)

Disposable needles must be used and disposed of properly. These needles should not be purposely bent, clipped, recapped, or otherwise manipulated by hand. A puncture-resistant container for sharp instruments should be within easy reach and must be used. Needles and syringes should be dropped into this container after use. Additional guidelines for the selection and use of needles and syringes by hospital personnel are provided in Chapter 97.

The risk for acquiring HIV-1 infection from an occupational exposure has been studied extensively in numerous prospective studies. These studies consistently have documented a comparatively low rate of infection per percutaneous exposure. When results of these studies are combined, the magnitude of risk for HIV-1 infection appears to be 0.32% per exposure (112). This means that, in general, one might expect between three and four occupational infections for every 1,000 parenteral exposures to blood from HIV-1–infected patients. The risk may be higher or lower, depending on the severity of injury. For example, if a large volume of blood is injected via a needlestick injury, the risk is considered higher than with a low volume. The risk for

HIV-1 infection after a mucous membrane exposure is believed to be lower but is not zero.

A retrospective case control study (62) to identify risk factors for HIV seroconversion among healthcare workers after a percutaneous exposure to HIV-infected blood found that workers were more likely to become infected if they were exposed to a larger amount of blood (i.e., presence of visible blood on the device before injury, needle had been placed directly into the patient's vein or artery, or deep injury). Increased rates of transmission were also noted from terminally ill patients with AIDS that has been attributed to an increased titer of HIV in the blood of these patients.

If a posthospital healthcare worker is exposed to HIV-1, a number of issues must be addressed (112–114). The first is immediate and aggressive first aid. This may not eliminate the risk for HIV-1 infection after exposure but is probably of some help in reducing the healthcare worker's postinjury emotional and psychologic stress. Current recommendations for first-aid measures after exposure to HIV-1 include vigorous scrubbing of parenteral injury sites for 10 minutes with 10% povidone-iodine solution. Milking the wound site to promote bleeding is encouraged. Exposure of mucous membranes to HIV-1 should be followed by irrigation of these membranes with normal saline for 15 minutes. Immediately after completion of these first-aid measures, the employee should report the occupational exposure formally to appropriate persons. These include the responsible supervisor and medical personnel (e.g., occupational medical service, if available; emergency room if not). The safety officer and quality assurance personnel, if applicable, may be informed as well. The healthcare worker should be advised, however, that discussing the exposure widely with coworkers may prove to be a problem if the exposure does result in infection.

When appropriate medical personnel are notified, they should evaluate the injury, review and repeat first-aid measures, and initiate medical and psychologic therapy. The postinjury evaluation should include he route of exposure, the source (i.e., specific blood or body fluid involved), the likely volume of inoculum, the condition of the source patient (i.e., the stage of HIV-1 infection and history of any antiretroviral therapy), the amount of time (if any) between the removal of a needle (or other sharp instrument) and the penetration of the exposed worker, the extent of injury, the type and promptness of first-aid measures, and the health status and anxiety level of the injured healthcare worker. The worker's hepatitis B and hepatitis C infection status should be determined, because occupational hepatitis is also a potential problem (115,116). Postexposure management for occupational exposure to hepatitis B and C virus are discussed in each respective section.

All parenteral injuries should be treated equally with identical initial postinjury triage and management for all reported injuries. Such identical triage and initial management tactics allow for the potential lack of a precise occupational exposure history from an anxious healthcare worker, serve to reassure the injured worker, and place the institution in a clear position of healthcare worker advocacy.

Because of the common and often extreme emotional reaction of exposed healthcare workers, initial guidance about relative risk may not be comprehended at the initial encounter and should be reviewed again at later counseling sessions. It is important that several such counseling sessions are scheduled soon after the exposure. Counseling should include relevant estimates of the risk for infection associated with the type of exposure experienced by the healthcare worker. Most exposed workers find the relatively low 1/360 to 1/500 risk associated with parenteral exposure to HIV-1 to be somewhat reassuring. However, the counselor must explain that these figures represent an average risk and that the worker's specific injury may be associated with a higher or lower risk for infection. Counseling initially should address the rationale for considering antiretroviral prophylaxis. This must be done quickly, because prophylaxis should be initiated as soon as possible after the exposure. Counseling must include a plan for follow-up to include such measures as serologic testing and additional counseling. In addition, counseling should include the possibility that the exposure may result in infection, and precautions that may avoid transmission to others should be discussed. Finally, counseling should provide emotional support for the worker and should address all questions related to the exposure. This support may need to include other members of the worker's family. It is useful to provide a standard written summary for the counseling and advice provided so that lack of retention of the information because of the emotional state of the worker does not cause a problem.

A major issue with occupational exposure to HIV-1 has been whether or not to offer chemoprophylaxis. Part of the reason for this problem was that initially it was unknown whether ZVD could prevent HIV infection if it was administered before and/or during exposure. An animal study used infant rhesus macaques to investigate the efficacy of ZVD prophylaxis in preventing simian immunodeficiency virus (SIV) infection after a low dose of SIV (117). In this study, ZVD prophylaxis given 2 hours before the SIV dose effectively prevented infection. Clinical experience with ZVD prophylaxis (62) has revealed that such prophylaxis is useful. Currently, postexposure prophylaxis with multiple antiretroviral agents is recommended (63–65,112). This postexposure prophylaxis should be initiated within the first 2 hours but could be instituted as late as 1 to 2 weeks after HIV exposure in high-risk exposures. ZVD should be considered for all regimens because of sufficient data to support its use in this setting. In addition, lamivudine should be added to ZDV therapy for increased antiretroviral activity and activity against ZVD-resistant strains. Finally, a protease inhibitor such as indinavir should be added for high-risk exposure or if ZVD-resistant strains are likely. The latest CDC guidelines for prophylaxis should be obtained and reviewed; these are constantly being updated.

Most medical centers offer antiretroviral postexposure chemoprophylaxis to healthcare workers who sustain parenteral or mucous membrane occupational exposures to HIV-1, provided these institutions are able to provide emergency evaluation, treatment, and consultation 24 hours a day, 7 days a week. (See Chapter 79.) Clearly, it is much more difficult to offer such therapy to many posthospital healthcare workers. Such workers may want to participate, if possible, in an ongoing program at a local medical center.

Counseling is an extremely important aspect of postexposure care of the employee yet can be extremely difficult to provide to most posthospital healthcare workers. Such counseling can be complex, labor intensive, and time consuming. Because guidelines for counseling have been established (114) and are used at many medical centers, such centers may be able to provide this kind of counseling to posthospital healthcare workers on a contractual basis. Appropriate follow-up is needed and can also be supplied by the counseling service. For a more thorough review of this topic, see Chapter 79.

Hepatitis B Virus

HBV is the etiologic agent causing a form of acute hepatitis that characteristically has a long incubation period (40 to 120 days) after the initial contact with the infectious virion (118). This form of hepatitis was first recognized in 1833 after administration of smallpox vaccine that contained human lymphatic fluids. It was not until the 1940s and 1950s that the percutaneous transfer of material containing human serum was appreciated as an important route of transmission (119). Unfortunately, the appreciation of this route resulted in the name "serum jaundice" or "serum hepatitis" as opposed to the shorter incubation variety [i.e., that caused by hepatitis A virus (HAV)], which was called "infectious hepatitis." Although the name serum jaundice accurately describes the first recognized route, it implies that this is the only route. That is not the case with HBV, because it has become clear in recent years that HBV is most commonly spread by routes that do not involve direct percutaneous transfer (120). Examples of these routes include sexual contact, transmission from mothers to their newborn infants, and contact with saliva (120,121).

HBV is a well-recognized occupational hazard in the healthcare worker (72,122). As with HIV, the major routes involving healthcare workers are percutaneous transfer and exposure of mucosal tissues and open sores to blood or body fluids containing the virus. As already mentioned, the prevalence of HBV antibody in physicians such as pathologists and surgeons approaches 30% (72). Overall, healthcare workers who frequently encounter blood or blood products have an intermediate risk for HBV infections; approximately 1% to 2% of these workers are hepatitis B surface antigen (HBsAg)-positive, whereas 15% to 30% of workers have other markers, such as anti-HBs and antibody to hepatitis B core antigen (anti-HBc).

For healthcare workers, the most effective way to deal with the threat of hepatitis B is by preexposure immunization with hepatitis B vaccine (123). There are two types of vaccines available from Merck, Sharp, and Dohme; the first, a plasma-derived vaccine (Heptavax-B), was licensed in 1981; the second, a recombinant vaccine (Recombivax-HB), was licensed in 1986. Subsequently, a second recombinant vaccine (Engerix-B, SmithKline Beecham) was licensed. Prospective, double-blind, placebo-controlled trials have shown greater than 90% protection (124). Those few individuals who later became infected with HBV have been among the vaccine recipients who failed to convert. The presence of anti-HBs antibody in the serum of healthcare workers after a course of three vaccinations with hepatitis B vaccine can be detected by serologic testing, and the occasional failure of vaccination can be identified. Healthcare workers who do not respond to or do not complete the primary vaccination series should be revaccinated with a second three-dose vaccine series or evaluated to determine whether they are HBsAg seropositive (79). Revaccinated healthcare workers should be tested for anti-HBs at the completion of the second series. Vaccine-induced antibodies decline gradually with time, and as many as 60% of those who initially respond to vaccination will lose detectable anti-HBs by 8 years (77).

Healthcare workers should be vaccinated against hepatitis B not only to protect their own health but also to prevent spread of hepatitis B infection to patients (125) or their families if healthcare workers become infected. Despite the availability of vaccines for over a decade, with vaccination available for free in many cases, and the cogent reasons for such vaccination, there are still healthcare workers involved in posthospital care who have not been vaccinated. The worry of possible transmission of AIDS in the plasma-derived vaccine has been shown to be groundless (126). The ability of the HBV vaccine to protect healthcare workers is clearly documented (77,78). There is no reason whatsoever for healthcare workers not to receive vaccination against HBV, and all should do so (79).

For those workers who are not vaccinated and who are potentially exposed by accidental needlestick injury, mucosal splash with body fluids, or other such incident, a plan similar to that outlined for HIV is useful. In addition, postexposure prophylaxis of hepatitis B with hepatitis B vaccine and hepatitis B immune globulin is useful and should be undertaken (127). For additional details, see Chapters 50 and 78.

Other Types of Viral Hepatitis

The ability to serologically diagnose acute viral hepatitis caused by infection with HAV or HBV has led to the recognition of other viral hepatitis agents that are predominantly transmitted either by the percutaneous (blood) or the fecal-oral routes. These agents are grouped as non-A, non-B hepatitis agents. The first of these described was the hepatitis delta virus (HDV), which is made up of a single-stranded RNA (1,700 nucleotides) surrounded by a protein coat (128). This protein coat is encoded by the delta virus genome and has an outer membranous protein envelope consisting of HBsAg encoded by the HBV. This HBsAg-containing envelope allows the delta virus to attach to hepatic cells. The delta virus is then infectious, provided that the new host has an active hepatitis B infection, because the delta virus co-infects with and requires the function of active HBV for its replication. The delta virus can infect a person simultaneously along with hepatitis B or superinfect a person who is already infected with hepatitis B. The duration of infection caused by the HDV, of course, is determined by the duration of and cannot outlast the hepatitis B infection. HDV thus also should be screened for in any situations involving potential transmission of hepatitis B infection.

The molecular cloning of a parenterally transmitted virus, referred to as hepatitis C virus (HCV), has been described (129) and is the recognized cause of most non-A, non-B hepatitis in the developed world. Because of its blood-borne route of transmission and its prevalence, this type of hepatitis is of concern to healthcare workers and is discussed separately.

A second form of non-A, non-B hepatitis is epidemiologically distinct, is transmitted by the fecal-oral route, and causes large epidemics in third-world countries. Additional work (130) suggests that a single virus is responsible for most of this form of hepatitis seen worldwide. This virus is hepatitis E virus and, like HAV, is of somewhat less concern to the healthcare worker, because this virus is transmitted only by the fecal-oral route.

Hepatitis C

HCV is of particular concern to healthcare workers, because its routes of transmission are similar to those of hepatitis B and because of the potential long-term untoward effects. In fact, one of the most disturbing features of HCV to healthcare workers exposed to this agent is the fact that this viral infection of the liver has a propensity to progress to chronic hepatitis with biochemical evidence of chronic hepatitis (131). In addition, long-term follow-up studies have shown that 20% to 25% of patients ultimately develop cirrhosis of the liver. HCV is currently considered one of the major causes of cirrhosis in the United States and ranks as one of the most common reasons for liver transplantation in adults. Multiple reports have shown that healthcare workers are at risk for HCV infection (132–136).

Although HCV to date has not been cultured, the development of an assay to detect antibody against a recombinant polypeptide of HCV has allowed investigators to pursue the epidemiologic study of this infection. Confirmatory HCV testing has become commercially available and includes the Abbott MATRIX-HCV immunoblot assay and the Ortho-Chiron recombinant immunoblot assay. However, the interpretation of these anti-HCV assay results is limited by several factors, including lack of detection in approximately 5% of infected patients; inability to distinguish between acute, chronic, and past infections; prolonged interval between the onset of acute illness with HCV and seroconversion; and false-positive rates as high as 50% in areas with low prevalence of HCV infection (137).

Despite these remarkable advances, the epidemiology of this infection in healthcare workers is not yet totally clear. What is now known is that transmission of HCV by blood products has been unequivocally demonstrated. Hepatitis C is, in fact, the most common cause of posttransfusion hepatitis. Transmission of HCV by organ transplantation has also been documented (138). In addition, this form of hepatitis has been shown to have sexual, vertical, and intrafamilial spread.

Several case reports have demonstrated transmission of HCV infection from anti-HCV–seropositive patients to healthcare workers as a result of accidental needlestick injury or lacerations with sharp instruments (129,136). The rate of anti-HCV seroconversion averaged 1.8%, whereas studies using HCV detection by polymerase chain reaction (PCR) assay revealed a 10% rate of transmission (130,131,136).

High-risk source patients for HCV infection clearly would include parenteral drug abusers, hemophilia patients, dialysis patients, multiply transfused patients, and patients with unexplained acute or chronic liver disease or enzyme elevation. Recommendations for follow-up of healthcare workers after occupational exposure to HCV now exist (139,140), and regulations for the prevention of occupationally acquired HCV have been established (12). Unfortunately, effective postexposure prophylaxis for HCV has not yet been determined. However, combination therapy of chronic hepatitis C with peginterferon-alpha-2a and oral ribavirin now appears to be a valuable first-line treatment option (141). This combination may in time prove useful for postexposure prophylaxis for HCV. In the meantime, medical centers should use the same general approach for HCV as that used for HIV and HBV. This approach should also be applied to posthospital healthcare workers. Readers wishing more information are referred to Chapters 50 and 78.

Mycobacterium tuberculosis

After a steady decline in the incidence of tuberculosis from the mid-1950s to the mid-1980s, tuberculosis has again become a major health problem in the United States because of an increasing incidence and a similar increase in the numbers of multidrug-resistant strains (13,14,142–146). The reasons for this resurgence are complex and include the AIDS epidemic, increasing numbers of homeless persons, increased migration from countries with a high prevalence of tuberculosis, increased crowding in housing among the poor, increased numbers of residents in long-term care facilities, decreased compliance in tuberculosis therapeutic regimens, atypical tuberculosis in AIDS patients, delayed recognition of tuberculosis, delayed recognition of multidrug-resistant isolates, and inadequate hospital facilities for treating patients with tuberculosis (50-53,147–153). The risk of acquiring tuberculosis by healthcare workers has increased (54-57,154–161). The nosocomial transmission of tuberculosis has even been reported from patients with draining lesions (158,159). Posthospital healthcare workers, like all others, are at greater risk for tuberculosis, as shown by outbreaks in nursing homes (33) and autopsy suites (53,58).

Measures to prevent the spread of tuberculosis in posthospital healthcare workers are identical to those used to prevent the spread in hospitals and include infection control measures for source control and engineering controls (15,16,162–164). Infection control measures should be standardized based on guidelines from the CDC (15) and documented in an appropriate procedure manual. Such control measures include rapidly identifying and isolating patients with presumptive tuberculosis, having patients cover their mouths when coughing, using masks, and initiating antituberculosis therapy as soon as the diagnosis is established. Engineering controls include rapid air exchange, negative pressure ventilation with air exhausted to the outside, high-efficiency particulate air (HEPA) filters, and ultraviolet lighting.

Many nosocomial outbreaks of tuberculosis have been related to lack of adherence to proper infection control measures for tuberculosis and/or to inadequate functioning of isolation rooms (151–157). If hospitals have such problems, facilities in which posthospital healthcare workers are employed, such as nursing homes or patient homes, can hardly be expected to have adequate isolation rooms.

Although establishing and maintaining effective isolation rooms is necessary for preventing transmission of tuberculosis, such rooms alone do not offer sufficient protection for healthcare workers who take care of patients. This is because such persons who are physically close to patients with active tuberculosis will be exposed to infectious aerosols before ventilation can reduce the aerosol concentration significantly. Thus, healthcare workers who care for patients should wear appropriate respirators. The definition of an appropriate respirator currently is debated. The CDC defines an appropriate respirator as a "particulate respirator," which is the same as what the National Institute for Occupational Safety and Health (NIOSH) calls a "disposable dust/mist-filter respirator" (15). This type of respirator excludes particles 2 μm in diameter. NIOSH instead recommends a fume filter that uses HEPA-filter media and excludes particles 0.6 to 1 μm in size (16,162). Finally, all types of air-purifying respirators allow some inward leakage of droplet nuclei around the face seal. Particulate respirators permit 10% to 20% leakage, whereas a powered air-purifying respirator with qualitative or quantitative fit testing as recommended by NIOSH (162) for high-risk medical procedures such as bronchoscopy permit far less leakage (2%).

The CDC has released guidelines for preventing tuberculosis transmission in healthcare facilities (15), and these should help clarify many of these issues. In addition, OSHA has issued guidelines (16) for enforcement of tuberculosis protection requirements as delineated in 29 CFR 1910. Key elements of these tuberculosis protection requirements include the following:

1. Healthcare workers who enter rooms occupied by patients with suspected or known infectious tuberculosis or who perform high-risk procedures (e.g., bronchoscopy) on such individuals must use NIOSH-approved fume (HEPA) respirators. In addition, a complete respiratory protection program, including qualitative (irritant fume) or quantitative fit testing of respirators, must be in place.
2. Records of employee exposure to tuberculosis, of tuberculosis skin testing, and of medical evaluations and treatment for tuberculosis are subject to OSHA record-keeping rules. Any positive tuberculosis skin test in an employee (other than preemployment) would be presumed to be occupational and should be recorded on the OSHA 200 log as would any clinical infection with tuberculosis.
3. Medical management of any clinical manifestations of tuberculosis, including positive skin tests, is the responsibility of the employer. In addition, employers are expected to establish tuberculin skin testing programs for the early identification of personnel with tuberculous infection. Finally, like the bloodborne pathogen standard, employers will be expected to have yearly training/educational programs for tuberculosis.

This clarification of OSHA regulations (16,164) is an important step. Employers of healthcare workers, including posthospital healthcare workers, have access to additional information on control of tuberculosis (165–167), including the use of screening methods (168) and vaccination (169). Readers wishing additional information on tuberculosis should read Chapter 37, whereas Chapter 89 addresses the design and maintenance of hospital ventilation systems.

Methicillin-resistant *Staphylococcus aureus*

Infections caused by *S. aureus* continue to be an important clinical problem (170). The emergence of antimicrobial resistance has been a consistent characteristic of this pathogen, with resistance generally following the widespread use of a particular antimicrobial agent (171). This was seen for penicillin in the 1940s, erythromycin in the 1950s, methicillin in the 1960s, ciprofloxacin in the 1980s, and vancomycin in the twenty-first century. Methicillin-resistant *S. aureus* (MRSA) was first seen in the 1960s (172); although the term *methicillin resistance* is somewhat misleading, because these isolates are resistant to many other antimicrobial agents such as aminoglycosides, clindamycin, and ciprofloxacin (171). This multidrug resistance makes therapy and/or eradication very difficult. Moreover, resistance has raised the level of concern in healthcare workers who frequently deal with nosocomial staphylococcal infections and worry that they may become colonized and subsequently become infected themselves or transmit this pathogen to their patients or family. Since the 1960s, MRSA has spread worldwide (173) and today is commonly found in hospitals, in long-term care facilities, and in the community (174–176). The recent report of vancomycin-resistant *S. aureus* containing the *vanA* resistance gene (177) is very worrisome because vancomycin resistance in MRSA strains will make therapy of staphylococcal infections more difficult.

Colonization of healthcare workers by MRSA is common (178,179). Although the carriage on the hands may only be transient, *S. aureus* (both susceptible strains and MRSA) adheres well to human nasal epithelial cells (180). Thus, healthcare workers may develop nasal colonization with MRSA, which may then be a significant risk factor for infection by spread of the colonizing strain (181–183). Because of universal precautions, many healthcare workers now routinely wear gloves when taking care of patients. Unfortunately, some wear one pair of gloves while taking care of several patients. Hand washing sometimes is done between patients without removing the gloves. Staphylococci adhere well to gloves, and washing while wearing gloves facilitates transfer of *S. aureus* through the glove to the hand (184). Obviously, hands should be washed between patients with an antimicrobial soap (185) after gloves are removed. Finally, the transfer of MRSA from inanimate objects to the hands of healthcare workers may be a real problem, as suggested by a number of reports (186,187).

Although this possible mechanism remains controversial (188), there are clearly instances wherein inanimate objects can harbor staphylococci or perhaps other pathogens. Perhaps wearing gloves facilitates the transfer of the staphylococci from the inanimate object to the hands of a healthcare worker and, if improper hand washing techniques are used, from the hands of a healthcare worker to a patient. Bedrails are now thought to be an important factor in such transmission and may deposit microorganisms on the clothing of healthcare workers as they lean on these rails while caring for a patient. The use of gowns and gloves for routine care of patients with known colonization by multidrug-resistant microorganisms has been recommended.

Healthcare workers have noted the increase in nosocomial infections caused by MRSA and are concerned that they may become colonized or infected. Such concern about infection is valid because a number of reports have documented these kinds of infections in healthcare personnel (189–192). The frequency of nasal carriage among healthcare workers ranges from 20% to

90%, but fewer than 10% of healthy nasal carriers disperse the microorganisms into the air (193). However, nasal carriers with upper respiratory symptoms can disseminate the microorganisms into the air more effectively. It should be somewhat comforting for healthcare workers to understand that they alone can prevent such colonization and infection with MRSA by proper hand washing techniques. These techniques are covered in detail in Chapter 96. Additional information on *S. aureus* and on MRSA is found in Chapters 28 and 29.

Group A Streptococcus

Group A streptococcus (*Streptococcus pyogenes*) is one of the most common and ubiquitous of human pathogens and causes an impressive variety of infections. These include acute pharyngitis, impetigo, sinusitis, otitis, peritonsillar and retropharyngeal abscess, pneumonia, scarlet fever, toxic shock syndrome, erysipelas, cellulitis, lymphangitis, puerperal sepsis, vaginitis, myositis, gangrene, necrotizing fasciitis, septic arthritis, suppurative thrombophlebitis, bacteremia, endocarditis, and osteomyelitis. This pathogen is also known for its association with two nonsuppurative sequelae, acute rheumatic fever and acute glomerulonephritis, which are related to specific immune responses by the host. It is no wonder that healthcare workers are concerned about this microorganism.

Although *S. pyogenes* is not generally viewed as a nosocomial pathogen, outbreaks have been described in hospitals and nursing homes (194–197). Thus, healthcare workers are at risk for this infection. Because *S. pyogenes* is such a ubiquitous pathogen, it is difficult to determine if a healthcare worker has a group A streptococcal infection resulting from work-related acquisition. However, certain streptococcal infections in healthcare workers or others are more easily delineated as having been caused by a single source. One report describes the nosocomial transmission of *S. pyogenes* from a single source patient to 24 healthcare workers (198). Another report describes foodborne streptococcal pharyngitis, which has been reported in a hospital pediatric clinic after a potluck luncheon (199). Healthcare workers with pharyngitis or other types of suspected streptococcal infections are at risk for spreading this pathogen (200). It is for this reason that restriction from patient care activities and food handling is indicated for healthcare workers with group A streptococcal infections until 24 hours after they have received appropriate antimicrobial therapy. Unfortunately, asymptomatic carriage of *S. pyogenes* by healthcare workers also can result in nosocomial outbreaks (201,202).

S. pyogenes is spread by respiratory secretions. This mechanism of transmission is facilitated by the ability of these streptococci to adhere to human epithelial cells (203) via lipoteichoic acid (204), which is present at the streptococcal cell wall and adheres to surface fibronectin on the surface of oral epithelial-cell membranes (205). Heavily encapsulated strains of *S. pyogenes* seem to be more readily transmitted from person to person than those with minimal hyaluronate capsules (206). This may be due to initial attachment of the capsule to mucus. Once attached to human oral mucosal tissue, the group A streptococci may simply become colonizers of this tissue or may cause invasive streptococcal infections. Throat cultures of approximately 20% of persons with pharyngitis are positive for *S. pyogenes.* Unfortunately, if a control group without pharyngitis is also cultured for *S. pyogenes,* the cultures of 20% of this group are also positive (207). It can be very difficult to differentiate active streptococcal pharyngitis from the carrier state in a symptomatic person (208). The antistreptolysin O titer and other similar antibody titers such as antihyaluronidase and antideoxyribonuclease (DNase) B are useful, because these antibody titers become elevated with active infection. These are obtained as a single serologic test referred to as the "streptozyme test."

In addition to causing acute pharyngitis, group A streptococci are also recognized for their propensity to cause skin infections. This is not unexpected when the pathogenesis of these skin infections is understood (209,210). Fibronectin, the attachment site on mucosal epithelial cells, is also found in other tissues such as blood vessels, in which it stabilizes cell-to-cell and cell-to-substrate attachments to endothelial cells (211). Damage to blood vessels and their endothelial lining such as caused by an abrasion or any other such skin surface wound will expose the fibronectin in the endothelial lining and offer an attachment site for *S. pyogenes.* With 20% of the population carrying group A streptococci in their nasopharynx, it is no wonder that occasional injuries to the skin become infected by this pathogen.

S. pyogenes remains susceptible to β-lactam agents and is relatively easy to treat. If it were not for the sequelae of acute rheumatic fever and acute glomerulonephritis, these infections would not cause as much concern. Concern by healthcare workers has increased recently, because acute rheumatic fever, after declining for many years (212), has reemerged and remains a problem (213,214). This reemergence has been associated with a concomitant increase in the rate of isolation of very mucoid well-recognized rheumatogenic serotypes (e.g., types 1, 3, 5, 6, and 18).

The sequelae of both acute rheumatic fever and acute glomerulonephritis are now thought to be related to a host immune response to M protein. This protein is a filamentous molecule consisting of two protein chains in a coiled configuration extending about 60 nm above the surface of the streptococcus (215). The M protein is antigenic and can be studied using serologic methodology. The M serotype appears to be one marker of rheumatogenicity, and those M serotypes most strongly associated with acute rheumatic fever and postpharyngeal and postpyodermal acute glomerulonephritis appear to be distinct (216). Indeed, purification of M protein combined with genetic analysis demonstrated distinct structural differences between the M proteins of streptococci associated with acute rheumatic fever and those known to cause acute glomerulonephritis (217). Of clinical interest is the fact that the acute rheumatogenic sequelae can be prevented by timely treatment of the streptococcal infection, whereas the glomerulonephritic sequelae are not influenced by antimicrobial therapy.

From the viewpoint of prevention of streptococcal infection and sequelae in posthospital healthcare workers, it does not make sense to be overly concerned about a pathogen that can be isolated from 20% of the population in general. However, it would seem prudent to exercise some precautions when taking care of a patient with known group A streptococcal infection. Precautions taken for wound infections with a multiresistant pathogen such as MRSA (to include gloves and gown) would appear appropriate. This is because group A streptococci have been transmitted from infected patients to healthcare workers who have had contact with infectious secretions (218), and these infected workers have subsequently acquired a variety of group A streptococcal illnesses. Equally important is the fact that healthcare workers who have become carriers of group A streptococcus have been linked to sporadic outbreaks of streptococcal infections (201, 219–221). See Chapter 31 for additional information on group A streptococci.

Rabies Virus

The name *rabies* comes from Latin and means "rage" or "madness." Rabies has been the object of human fear ever since the disease was first recognized in antiquity (222–224). Cases of human rabies have increased in the United States in the past decade; many of these are bat-associated cryptic cases (225). Thus, concerns about the possible transmission of rabies to healthcare workers is not at all surprising. This concern most often involves hospitalized patients with suspected or proven rabies (226) and hospital healthcare workers. When patients with rabies die, similar concerns are voiced by prosectors and funeral home employees. Moreover, these posthospital healthcare workers may deal with a death by unknown causes in which the etiologic role of rabies is not recognized until long after the autopsy has been completed (225).

These concerns, although not supported by actual case reports in which healthcare workers have become infected by rabies after direct exposure to an infected patient, are based on some data that clearly allow for the possibility of such transmission. Indeed, rabies virus has been detected in human tracheal secretions, saliva, nasal swabs, and human tissue (227), and airborne transmission in a laboratory worker has been described (228). The virus has never been detected in blood, urine, or feces.

As with any potentially transmissible infection, it is useful for the healthcare worker to understand the pathogenesis of rabies (229). The rabies virus is present in high titers in infected animals saliva and is introduced during a bite to the muscle tissue of another animal. The virus may attach to and enter peripheral nerve cells immediately if a large inoculum is introduced by the bite such that the virus comes into direct contact with these nerves. Otherwise, the inoculated rabies virus attaches to the plasma membrane of human cells via a glycoprotein present in spike-like projections in the outer layer (230). A proposed binding site on human cells is the nicotinic acetylcholine receptor (231). Usually, the rabies virus is amplified by replication in skeletal-muscle cells near the site of inoculation until the concentration of virus is high enough to reach and attach to unmyelinated sensory and motor terminals (232). Once attached to the nerve cells, rabies virus readily enters the cell and then is able to travel through nerve cells, from one to the next via the endplates, until it reaches the central nervous system (229). Once the virus has entered the nerve cells, it is sequestered from the immune system, and immunization from then on will be ineffective. Once the rabies virus reaches the spinal cord via retrograde axoplasmic flow at 8 to 20 μm/day, the first symptoms of the infection—pain or paresthesia at the wound site—may occur (233). This is followed by rapidly progressive encephalitis as the virus first disseminates through the central nervous system. The virus next spreads throughout the body along the peripheral nerves. On arrival via peripheral nerves to the salivary glands, the rabies virus is shed in the saliva.

It is also useful to review the epidemiology of rabies (224, 225). Human rabies is uncommon in the United States, primarily because of canine rabies-control programs; dogs account for less than 5% of the cases in animals. Moreover, ready access to improved human rabies biologicals (human rabies immune globulin and rabies vaccine) has been responsible, in part, for preventing rabies in those persons who come in contact with potentially rabid animals such as bats (bat rabies is enzootic in the United States, with cases reported from all of the 48 contiguous states), raccoons (predominant in the southeast and the northeast), foxes (predominant in upper New York State and upper Vermont and in parts of Arizona and Texas), skunks (predominant in California and the south-central and north-central states), and coyotes (predominant in the Texas panhandle).

Of particular interest to infection control professionals is that in a study of 14 patients with rabies treated in U.S. hospitals, 576 contacts of the patients received postexposure prophylaxis (234). Seventy percent of those who received postexposure prophylaxis were medical personnel, most of whom were nurses and respiratory therapists, who would have the greatest contact with saliva. Another example is that of an 11-year-old girl in New York State who died of unknown meningoencephalitis and was later found to have died of rabies when routine histopathologic slides of brain tissue were reviewed approximately 2 to 3 weeks after death. When the diagnosis was made, rabies postexposure prophylaxis was administered to 55 persons, including 8 family members, 3 friends, 35 healthcare workers, 5 members of the autopsy team, 3 transport personnel, and 1 mortician (235). Thus, 9 of 55 were posthospital healthcare workers.

It becomes clear that a rapid antemortem diagnosis of rabies is important. The importance of early suspicion of rabies is not that the course or prognosis of rabies can be altered but that measures to reduce the number of persons potentially exposed to the rabies virus during patient care can be reduced, and those persons who are candidates for postexposure prophylaxis can be more easily identified. Rabies should be considered in the differential diagnosis of any acute progressive encephalitis of unknown etiology. Other clinical manifestations suggestive of rabies include paresthesia at an injury site, hydrophobia (patients withdraw when offered a drink and have difficulty swallowing oral secretions; strep throat is often blamed for these symptoms), and copious salivation. Once rabies is considered in the differential diagnosis, it is possible to make an antemortem diagnosis of human rabies by sending cerebrospinal fluid (CSF), serum, saliva, and a biopsy of nuchal skin or of brain tissue to the state laboratory or CDC. Tests for antibodies in the CSF and serum, PCR and/or cultures for rabies virus in the CSF and saliva, and fluorescent antibody tests for tissue inclusion bodies can be diagnostic.

Appropriate infection control measures are also indicated whenever a patient is suspected of being infected with rabies (236). Wearing gloves, gowns, masks, and goggles is indicated for healthcare workers caring for possible rabies patients or for posthospital healthcare workers participating in an autopsy, involved in transportation of the patient, or involved as a mortician. In addition, respiratory precautions (as done with active pulmonary tuberculosis) should be followed, because transmission of rabies through inhalation of virus has been reported (228). Finally, inoculation of some body fluids (such as saliva or tracheal secretions but not blood) could transmit rabies and should be avoided, whenever possible, with preventive measures such as those used for AIDS patients.

Preexposure and postexposure rabies prophylaxis for healthcare workers has not been satisfactorily delineated to date, and decisions regarding postexposure prophylaxis should be made on a case-by-case basis after discussion with public health authorities (79,237). The lack of such guidelines for who should or should not receive prophylaxis most often results in overuse of this preventive measure because of the high level of anxiety associated with rabies (234). Fortunately, guidelines for preexposure and postexposure rabies prophylaxis have been published (79,237).

When rabies prophylaxis has been decided on as a preventive measure, there are clear guidelines as to how to do this (79,237). The initial step in prevention of rabies in healthcare workers is to provide local wound treatment if the exposure involved a wound (e.g., a leak of respiratory or salivary fluid through a latex glove to an open wound). This treatment is similar to that used for HIV exposure via an open cut or wound and consists of immediate and thorough washing with soap and water or other antiseptic preparation for hand washing. Human rabies immune globulin and rabies vaccine should be used for exposures that do not involve bites and bites and cuts if the risk is high (e.g., a confirmed case and a respiratory therapist who cared for this patient). Ideally, treatment with both should be initiated for high-risk healthcare personnel. For low-risk persons, treatment can be delayed for up to 48 hours, pending the results of laboratory tests. The usual interval between exposure and prophylactic treatment for rabies in the United States is 5 days (234), which suggests that delays do not seriously compromise successful prophylaxis. Remember, however, that the pathogenesis involves a race between the immunoglobulins and attachment and penetration of the rabies virus to nerve cells. Thus, it would be predicted that longer delays and/or higher inoculum would occasionally result in prophylaxis failures, which have been reported (235, 236).

Prophylaxis consists of both the human rabies immune globulin and the vaccine. The human rabies immune globulin should be given in a dose of 20 IU/kg, with one half of this dose injected into the wound area and one half given intramuscularly in the gluteal area (79,237). Two rabies vaccines are currently available: human diploid-cell rabies vaccine (HDCV: Imovax Rabies) and rabies vaccine absorbed (RVA), which are considered equivalent in terms of safety and efficacy. There are two approved schedules for rabies prophylaxis in the United States. The first is a postexposure schedule in which 1.0 mL of HDCV or RVA is given intramuscularly in the deltoid area on days 0, 3, 7, 14, and 28. The preexposure schedule is most often given to persons such as veterinarians and other animal handlers and consists of 1.0 mL of HDCV or RVA intramuscularly in the deltoid area on days 0, 7, and 21 or 28 or 0.1 mL of HDCV intradermally in the skin over the deltoid area on days 0, 7, and 21 or 28. Boosters may be needed if there is continuing risk. Although vaccination is quite effective, it is not 100% effective (238,239). (See also Chapter 47.)

Transmissible Spongiform Encephalopathies Agent

The transmissible spongiform encephalopathies are degenerative diseases of the central nervous system caused by prions (240). They may be sporadic, infectious, or inherited in origin and are believed to be caused by abnormally configured host-encoded prion proteins that accumulate in the central nervous system. Human prion diseases include Creutzfeldt-Jakob disease and a variant of Creutzfeldt-Jakob disease that is caused by a prion strain indistinguishable from bovine spongiform encephalopathy in cattle (241,242). Although quite rare, Creutzfeldt-Jakob disease has been described as a risk for healthcare workers (243, 244). Because this progressive and relentless neurologic disease has a 100% mortality rate, it is not surprising that healthcare workers are aware of this rare disease and are concerned about the risk for transmission.

Creutzfeldt-Jakob disease is one of four recognized forms of spongiform encephalopathies in humans. The other three are kuru, Gerstmann-Sträussler Scheinker syndrome, and fatal familial insomnia syndrome. There are also animal forms of spongiform encephalopathies, such as scrapie in sheep and goats and bovine spongiform encephalopathy in cattle and dairy cows. The bovine spongiform encephalopathy has been termed "mad cow disease" by the lay press. These spongiform encephalopathies appear to be caused by novel infectious pathogens called prions (240). Prion means *pro*teinaceous *in*fectious particles, which are small particles in brain tissue that produce a neuropathic spongiform change. Infected brains demonstrate an amyloid protein that can transmit an identical spongiform disease to experimentally inoculated animals (245). Because prions resist inactivation by procedures and agents that modify nucleic acids and appear to consist only of an amyloid protein (246), they are now considered an abnormal derivative of normal protein that results in infectious amyloidosis. Thus, it appears that an abnormal protein seed molecule is able to serve as a template for the alteration of other normal precursor protein molecules that are being produced in the cell. The precursor protein of these various spongiform encephalopathies is a membrane-anchored glycoprotein that is found in most organs and cell types, including neurons. The exact biologic role of the protein is unknown. Mutation of the coding gene for this precursor protein has been associated with inherited spongiform encephalopathies. This precursor protein coded by the mutated gene then acts as a template to normal precursor protein and alters these proteins such that they aggregate as insoluble amyloid fibrils. The mutation of this gene can be transmitted to offspring, and about 10% of cases of Creutzfeldt-Jakob disease have been recognized as familial. Familial prion disease causing Creutzfeldt-Jakob disease appears to be an autosomal dominant disorder, like Huntington's disease. When the mutated gene is introduced in genetic material of transgenic mice, spontaneous central nervous system degeneration occurs and is characterized by clinical signs indistinguishable from experimental murine scrapie. Moreover, neuropathy consisting of spongiform morphology and astrocytic gliosis is identical in both. The genetic disease caused by this mutation can become contagious if the altered protein itself is transmitted from an infected host to a normal host. This has been seen in experimental animal inoculation and with iatrogenic inoculation of humans by contaminated neurosurgical instruments, corneal and dura mater grafts, and pituitary hormone extracts. This abnormal protein then acts as a seed molecule to produce template-induced polymerization of normal proteins in the newly infected host.

From an infection control standpoint, the risk of transmission of Creutzfeldt-Jakob disease in healthcare personnel is limited to inoculation with infected central nervous system material (247, 248). Clearly, patients known or suspected of having Creutzfeldt-Jakob disease become a potential problem in this regard if neurosurgical or autopsy procedures are performed. The precautions taken to prevent the transmission of HIV would be similar, the goal being to reduce the chance of inoculation injury. The World Health Organization (WHO) has developed infection control guidelines for transmissible spongiform encephalopathies (249). Moreover, a detailed description of precautions has been developed by the American Neurological Association and is available for those who wish more details (250). Finally, comprehensive recommendations for disinfection and sterilization of medical devices contaminated by the Creutzfeldt-Jakob agent have been published (251). (See also Chapter 47.)

REFERENCES

1. Sepkowitz KA. Occupationally acquired infections in health care workers. Part 1. *Ann Intern Med* 1996;125:826–834.
2. Sepkowitz KA. Occupationally acquired infections in health care workers. Part 2. *Ann Intern Med* 1996;125:917–928.
3. Swinker M. Occupational infections in health care workers: prevention and intervention. *Am Fam Physician* 1997;56:2291–2300, 2303–2306.
4. Lipscomb J, Rosenstock L. Healthcare workers: protecting those who protect our health. *Infect Control Hosp Epidemiol* 1997;18:397–399.
5. Chong CY, Goldman DA, Huskins WC. Prevention of occupationally acquired infections among health-care workers. *Pediatr Rev* 1998;19: 219-230.
6. Sharbaugh RJ. The risk of occupational exposure and infection with infectious disease. *Nurs Clin North Am* 1999;34:493–508.
7. Li TS, Buckley TA, Yap FH, et al. Severe acute respiratory syndrome (SARS): infection control. *Lancet* 2003;361:1386.
8. Bozeman WP, Dilbero D, Schauben JL. Biologic and chemical weapons of mass destruction. *Emerg Med Clin North Am* 2002;20: 975–993.
9. Petrosillo N, Puro V, De Carli G, et al. Risks faced by laboratory workers in the AIDS era. *J Biol Regul Homeost Agents* 2001;15: 243–248.
10. Centers for Disease Control and Prevention. Updated interim domestic infection control guidance in the health care and community setting for patients with suspected SARS, March 18, 2003. Available at *http://www.cdc.gov/ncidod/sars/infectioncontrol.htm* (accessed).
11. Public Health Service. 42 CFR Part 73, Possession, use, and transfer of select agents and toxins; Interim Final Rule, *Federal Register* 2002; 240:76886.
12. US Department of Labor, Occupational Safety and Health Administration. 29 CFR Part 1910.1030, Blood-borne pathogens; Final Rule. *Federal Register* 2001;66:5352.
13. Tiruviluamala P, Reichman LB. Tuberculosis. *Ann Rev Public Health* 2002;23:403–426.
14. Navin TR, McNabb SJ, Crawford JT. The continued threat of tuberculosis. *Emerg Infect Dis* 2002;8:1187.
15. Centers for Disease Control and Prevention. Guidelines for preventing the transmission of *Mycobacterium tuberculosis* in health care facilities. *MMWR Mortal Morb Wkly Rep* 1994;43:1–132.
16. US Department of Labor, Occupational Safety and Health Administration. 29 CFR Part 1910. Occupational exposure to tuberculosis; Proposed Rule. *Federal Register* 1997;62:54159.
17. National Committee for Clinical Laboratory Standards. *Protection of laboratory workers from occupationally acquired infections,* 2nd ed. Approved guideline. NCCLS document M29-A2. Villanova, PA: NCCLS, 2001.
18. Bolyard EA, Tablan OC, Williams WW, et al. Guideline for infection control in healthcare personnel, 1998. *Infect Control Hosp Epidemiol* 1998;19:407–463.
19. Udasin IG. Health care workers. *Prim Care* 2000;27:1079–102.
20. Wade BH. Outpatient/out of hospital care issues. In: Wenzel RP, ed. *Prevention and control of nosocomial infections,* 3rd ed. Philadelphia: Williams & Wilkins, 1997:243–259.
21. Stratton CW. The expanding horizons of infection control. *Infect Control Hosp Epidemiol* 1995;16:192–193.
22. Jarvis WR. Infection control and changing health-care delivery systems. *Emerg Infect Dis* 2001;7:170–173.
23. Willy ME. The epidemiology and control of communicable diseases (in the outpatient setting). *Lippincotts Prim Care Pract* 1999;3:82–92.
24. Friedman C, Barnette M, Busk AS, et al. Requirements for infrastructure and essential activities of infection control and epidemiology in out-of-hospital settings: a Consensus Panel report. *Am J Infect Control* 1999;27:418–430.
25. National Committee for Clinical Laboratory Standards. *Procedures for the handling and transport of domestic specimens and etiologic agents,* 3rd ed. Approved standard. NCCLS document H5-A3. Villanova, PA: NCCLS, 1994.
26. Centers for Diseases Control and Prevention, National Institutes for Health. *Biosafety in microbiology and biomedical laboratories,* 4th ed. Atlanta, GA: U.S. Department of Health and Human Services, Public Health Service, 1999.
27. Nolte KB, Taylor DG, Richmond JY. Biosafety considerations for autopsy. *Am J Forensic Med Pathol* 2002;23:107–122.
28. Rhinehart E. Infection control in home care. *Emerg Infect Dis* 2001; 7:208–211.
29. White MC. Infections and infection risks in home care settings. *Infect Control Hosp Epidemiol* 1992;13:535–539.
30. Garvey CM. Tuberculosis management in the home setting. *Caring* 1994;13:12–13.
31. Yeargin P, Johnson C. Home care for patients with AIDS. Professional and personal perspectives. *Adv Nurse Pract* 2001;9:61, 63–64.
32. Nicolle LE. Preventing infections in non-hospital settings: long-term care. *Emerg Infect Dis* 2001;7:205–207.
33. Strausbaugh LJ, Sukumar SR, Joseph CL. Infectious disease outbreaks in nursing homes: an unappreciated hazard for frail elderly persons. *Clin Infect Dis* 2003;36:870–876.
34. Satterfield N. Infection control in long-term care facilities: the hospital-based practitioner's role. *Infect Control Hosp Epidemiol* 1993;14: 40–47.
35. Hatlestad D. Surgery: not just for hospitals anymore. Part 2: EMS response to postoperative complications. *Emerg Med Serv* 2002;31: 81–84, 86.
36. Golloit F, Astagneau P, Cassou B, et al. Nosocomial infections in geriatric long-term-care and rehabilitation facilities: exploration in the development of a risk index for epidemiological surveillance. *Infect Control Hosp Epidemiol* 2001;22:746–753.
37. Zuckerman M. Surveillance and control of blood-borne virus infections in haemodialysis units. *J Hosp Infect* 2002;50:1–5.
38. Perry PA. Dirty and dangerous. Sharps hazards lurk in hospital laundries. *Health Facil Manage* 2001;14:33–35.
39. Orenstein JM. Guidelines for high risk or potentially high risk autopsy cases. *Pathologist* 1984;38:33–34.
40. Maas AE. AIDS autopsy precautions. *Pathologist* 1985;39:20–21.
41. Reichert CM. New safety considerations for the acquired immuno-

deficiency syndrome autopsy. *Arch Pathol Lab Med* 1992;116: 1109–1110.
42. Bakhshi SS. Code of practice for funeral workers: managing infection risk and body bagging. *Commun Dis Public Health* 2001;4:283–287.
43. Gershon RMM, Vlahov D, Farzadegan H, et al. Occupational risk of human immunodeficiency virus, hepatitis B virus, and hepatitis C virus among funeral service practitioners in Maryland. *Infect Control Hosp Epidemiol* 1995;16:194–197.
44. Rutala WA, Mayhall CG. Medical waste. *Infect Control Hosp Epidemiol* 1992;13:38–48.
45. Hageman JP. Handling, storage, treatment, and disposal of mixed wastes at medical facilities and academic institutions. *Health Phys* 2002;82(Suppl 5):S66–S76.
46. Carson EK. The hazards of medical waste. *Imprint* 1994;41:81–83.
47. Keene JH. Medical waste: a minimal hazard. *Infect Control Hosp Epidemiol* 1991;12:682–685.
48. National Committee for Clinical Laboratory Standards. *Clinical laboratory waste management: approved guideline.* NCCLS document GP5-A. Villanova, PA: NCCLS, 1993.
49. Research and Special Programs Administration (RSPA), DOT. Hazardous materials: revision to standards for infectious substances. Final Rule. *Federal Register* 2002;67:53117.
50. Nardell EA. Dodging droplet nuclei: reducing the probability of nosocomial tuberculosis transmission in the AIDS era. *Am Rev Respir Dis* 1990;142:501–503.
51. Couldwell DL, Dore GJ, Harkness JL, et al. Nosocomial outbreak of tuberculosis in an outpatient HIV treatment room. *AIDS* 1996; 10:521–525.
52. Cleveland JL, Kent J, Gooch BF, et al. Multidrug-resistant *Mycobacterium tuberculosis* in an HIV dental clinic. *Infect Control Hosp Epidemiol* 1995;16:7–11.
53. Ussery XT, Bierman JA, Valway S, et al. Transmission of multidrug-resistant *Mycobacterium tuberculosis* among persons exposed in a medical examiner's office, New York. *Infect Control Hosp Epidemiol* 1995; 16:160–165.
54. McKenna MT, Hutton MD, Cauthen G, et al. The association between occupation and tuberculosis: a population based survey. *Am J Respir Crit Care Med* 1996;154:587–589.
55. Larsen NM, Biddle CL, Sotir MJ, et al. Risk of tuberculin skin test conversion among health care workers: occupational versus community exposure and infection. *Clin Infect Dis* 2002;35:796–801.
56. Menzies D, Fanning A, Yuan L, et al. Tuberculosis among health care workers. *N Engl J Med* 1995;332:92–98.
57. Wenger PN, Otten J, Breeden A, et al. Control of nosocomial transmission of multidrug-resistant *Mycobacterium tuberculosis* among healthcare workers and HIV-infected patients. *Lancet* 1995;345: 235–240.
58. Sterling TR, Pope DS, Bishai WR, et al. Transmission of *Mycobacterium tuberculosis* from a cadaver to an embalmer. *N Engl J Med* 2000; 342:246–248.
59. Demiryurek D, Bayramoglu A, Ustacelebi S. Infective agents in fixed human cadavers: a brief review and suggested guidelines. *Anat Rec (New Anat)* 2002;269:194–197.
60. *Safety precautions for the high-risk autopsy.* VCR educational tape from the College of American Pathologists.
61. Geller SA, Gerber MA. Guidelines for high risk autopsy cases. In: Hutchins GM, ed. *Autopsy performance and reporting.* Skokie, IL: College of American Pathologists, 1990:67–75.
62. Cardo DM, Culver DH, Ciesielski C, et al. A case-controlled study of HIV seroconversion in health care workers after percutaneous exposure. *N Engl J Med* 1997;337:1485–1490.
63. Henderson DK. Postexposure treatment of HIV—taking some risks for safety's sake. *N Engl J Med* 1997;337:1542–1543.
64. Gerberding JL. Prophylaxis for occupational exposure to HIV. *Ann Intern Med* 1996;125:497–501.
65. Centers for Disease Control and Prevention. Update: provisional public health service recommendations for chemoprophylaxis after occupational exposure to HIV. *MMWR Mortal Morb Wkly Rep* 1996;45: 468–472.
66. Geller SA. The autopsy in acquired immunodeficiency syndrome: how and why. *Arch Pathol Lab Med* 1991;115:610–613.
67. O'Brian DS. Patterns of occupational hand injury in pathology: the interaction of blades, needles, and the dissectors digits. *Arch Pathol Lab Med* 1991;115:610–613.
68. Richardson JM, Redford LK, Morton H, et al. Protective garb [Letter]. *N Engl J Med* 1988;318:1333.
69. Bankowski MJ, Landay AL, Staes B, et al. Postmortem recovery of human immunodeficiency virus type 1 from plasma and mononuclear cells: implications for occupational exposure. *Arch Pathol Lab Med* 1992;116:1124–1127.
70. Nyberg M, Suni J, Haltia M. Isolation of human immunodeficiency virus (HIV) at autopsy one to six days postmortem. *Am J Clin Pathol* 1990;94:422–425.
71. Heckerling PS, Williams MJ. Attitudes of funeral directors and embalmers toward autopsy. *Arch Pathol Lab Med* 1992;116:1147–1151.
72. Shapiro CN. Occupational risk of infection with hepatitis B and hepatitis C virus. *Surg Clin North Am* 1995;75:1047–1056.
73. Maynard JE. Nosocomial viral hepatitis. *Am J Med* 1981;70:439–444.
74. Denes AE, Smith JL, Maynard JE, et al. Hepatitis B infection in physicians. Results of a nationwide seroepidemiologic survey. *JAMA* 1978;239:210–212.
75. Hadler SC, Doto IL, Maynard JE, et al. Occupational risk of hepatitis B infection in hospital workers. *Infect Control* 1985;6:24–31.
76. Shapiro CN. Tokars JI, Chamberland ME. American Academy of Orthopaedic Surgeons Serosurvey Study Committee. Use of the hepatitis B vaccine and infection with hepatitis B and C among orthopaedic surgeons. *J Bone Joint Surg Am* 1996;78A:1791–1800.
77. Hadler SC, Margolis HS. Hepatitis B immunization vaccine types, efficacy, and indication for immunization. *Curr Clin Top Infect Dis* 1992;12:282–308.
78. Minnesota Department of Health. Reduced development of anti-HBS in vaccinated health care workers. *Dis Control Newslett* 1992;20: 77–84.
79. Centers for Disease Control and Prevention. Immunization of healthcare workers: recommendations of the Advisory Committee on Immunization Practices (ACIP) and the Hospital Infection Control Practices Advisory Committee (HICPAC). *MMWR Mortal Morb Wkly Rep* 1997;46:1–42.
80. Update: human immunodeficiency virus infections in health care workers exposed to blood of infected patients. *MMWR Mortal Morb Wkly Rep* 1987;36:286–289.
81. Recommendation for prevention of HIV transmission in health-care settings. *MMWR Mortal Morb Wkly Rep* 1987;36(Suppl 2):1S–18S.
82. Universal precautions for prevention of transmission of human immunodeficiency virus, hepatitis B virus, and other bloodborne pathogens in health-care settings. *MMWR Mortal Morb Wkly Rep* 1988;37: 377–382, 387–388.
83. Gershon RRM, Vlahov D, Felknor SA, et al. Compliance with universal precautions among health care workers at three regional hospitals. *Am J Infect Control* 1995;23:225–236.
84. Jeffe DB, Mutha S, L Ecuyer PB, et al. Healthcare workers attitudes and compliance with Universal Precautions: gender, occupation, and specialty differences. *Infect Control Hosp Epidemiol* 1997;18:710–712.
85. Nelsing S, Nielsen TL, Nielsen JO. Noncompliance with universal precautions and the associated risk of mucocutaneous blood exposure among Danish physicians. *Infect Control Hosp Epidemiol* 1997;18: 692–698.
86. McCoy KD, Beekmann SE, Ferguson KJ, et al. Monitoring adherence to standard precautions. *Am J Infect Control* 2001;29:24–31.
87. Wenzel RP. Interaction of man and microbe: implications of the AIDS epidemic for hospital epidemiology. *Am J Infect Control* 1988; 16:214–220.
88. Doebbeling BN, Wenzel RP. The direct costs of universal precautions in a teaching hospital. *JAMA* 1990;264:2083–2087.
89. Bennett RG. Diarrhea among residents of long-term care facilities. *Infect Control Hosp Epidemiol* 1993;14:397–404.
90. Green KY, Belliot G, Taylor JL, et al. A predominant role for Norwalk-like viruses as agents of epidemic gastroenteritis in Maryland nursing homes for the elderly. *J Infect Dis* 2001;185:133–146.

91. Reid JA, Breckon D, Hunter PR. Infection of staff during an outbreak of viral gastroenteritis in an elderly person's home. *J Hosp Infect* 1990; 16:81–85.
92. Centers for Disease Control. Rorovirus activity—United States, 2002. *MMWR Morb Mortal Wkly Rep* 2003;52:41–45.
93. White KE, Hedberg CW, Edmonson LM, et al. An outbreak of giardiasis in a nursing home with evidence for multiple modes of transmission. *J Infect Dis* 1989;160:298–304.
94. Carter AO, Borczyk AA, Carlson JAK, et al. A severe outbreak of *Escherichia coli* 0157:H7 associated hemorrhagic colitis in a nursing home. *N Engl J Med* 1987;317:1496–1500.
95. Grohmann GS, Glass RI, Pereira HG, et al. Enteric viruses and diarrhea in HIV-infected patients. *N Engl J Med* 1993;329:14–57.
96. Widmer AF. Replace hand washing with use of a waterless alcohol hand rub? *Clin Infect Dis* 2000;31:136–142.
97. Doebbeling BN, Pfaller MA, Houston AK, et al. Removal of nosocomial pathogens from the contaminated glove. Implications for glove reuse and handwashing. *Ann Intern Med* 1988;109:394–398.
98. Lesky E. *The Vienna Medical School of the 19th century.* Baltimore: Johns Hopkins University, 1976:124–186.
99. Perceval A. Wash hands, disinfect hand, or don't touch? Which, when, and why? *Infect Control Hosp Epidemiol* 1993;14:273–275.
100. Albert RK, Condie F. Handwashing patterns in medical intensive care units. *N Engl J Med* 1981;304:1465–1466.
101. Graham M. Frequency and duration of handwashing in an intensive care unit. *Am J Infect Control* 1990;18:77–81.
102. Voss A, Widmer AF. No time for handwashing? Handwashing versus alcoholic rub: can we afford 100% compliance. *Infect Control Hosp Epidemiol* 1997;18:205–208.
103. Black RE, Dykes AC, Anderson K, et al. Handwashing to prevent diarrhea in day-care centers. *Am J Epidemiol* 1981;113:445–451.
104. Kahn MV. Interruption of shigellosis by handwashing. *Trans R Soc Trop Med Hyg* 1982;76:164–168.
105. Schmid MM, Miller ED. Managing exposures to infections. In: Wenzel RP, ed. *Prevention and control of nosocomial infections,* 3rd ed. Baltimore: Williams & Wilkins, 1997:437–460.
106. Herwaldt LA, Pottinger JM, Carter CD, et al. Exposure workups. *Infect Control Hosp Epidemiol* 1997;18:850–871.
107. Jaffe HA, Schmitt J. AIDS in the workplace. In: Rom WN, ed. *Environmental and occupational medicine,* 2nd ed. Boston: Little, Brown and Company, 1992:685–713.
108. Martin LS, McDougal JS, Loskoski SL. Disinfection and inactivation of the human T-lymphotrophic virus type III/lymphadenopathy associated virus. *J Infect Dis* 1986;162:400–403.
109. Rutala WA. APIC guideline for selection and use of disinfectants. *Am J Infect Control* 1996;24:313–324.
110. Hanson PJV, Gor D, Jeffries DJ, et al. Elimination of high titer HIV from fiberoptic endoscopes. *Gut* 1990;31:657—–659.
111. Rutala WA, Clontz EP, Weber DJ, et al. Disinfection practices for endoscopes and other semi-critical items. *Infect Control Hosp Epidemiol* 1991;12:282–296.
112. Chiarello LA, Gerberding JL. Human immunodeficiency virus in health care settings. In: Mandell GL, Bennett JE, Dolin R, eds. *Principles and practice of infectious diseases,* 5th ed. New York: Churchill Livingstone, 2000:3052–3066.
113. Fahey BJ, Beekmann SE, Schmitt JM, et al. Managing occupational exposures to HIV-1 in the healthcare workplace. *Infect Control Hosp Epidemiol* 1993;14:405–412.
114. Gerberding JL, Henderson KD. Management of occupational exposure to bloodborne pathogens: hepatitis B virus, hepatitis C virus, and human immunodeficiency virus. *Clin Infect Dis* 1992;14:1179–1185.
115. Perrillo RP, Regenstein FG, Roodman ST. Chronic hepatitis B in asymptomatic homosexual men with antibody to the human immunodeficiency virus. *Ann Intern Med* 1986;105:382–383.
116. Hayashi PH, Flynn N, McCurdy SA, et al. Prevalence of hepatitis C virus antibodies among patients infected with human immunodeficiency virus. *J Med Virol* 1991;3:177–180.
117. Van Rompay KKA, Marthas ML, Ramos RA, et al. Simian immunodeficiency virus (SIV) infection of infant rhesus macaques as a model to test antiretroviral drug prophylaxis and therapy: oral 3′-azido-3′-deoxythymidine prevents SIV infection. *Antimicrob Agents Chemother* 1992;36:2381–2386.
118. Seeger C, Mason WS. Hepatitis B virus biology. *Microbiol Mol Biol Rev* 2000;64:51–68.
119. Paul RJ, Havens WP, Sabin AB, et al. Transmission experiments in serum jaundice and infectious hepatitis. *JAMA* 1945;128:911–915.
120. Hersh T, Melnick JL, Goyal RK, et al. Nonparenteral transmission of viral hepatitis type B (Australian antigen-associated serum hepatitis). *N Engl J Med* 1971;285:1363–1364.
121. Alter JH, Purcell RH, Gerin JL. Transmission of hepatitis B to chimpanzees by hepatitis B surface antigen-positive saliva and semen. *Infect Immun* 1977;16:928–933.
122. Maynard JE. Viral hepatitis as an occupational hazard in the health care professional. In: Vyas GN, Cohen SN, Schmid R, eds. *Viral hepatitis: a contemporary assessment of etiology, epidemiology, pathogenesis, and prevention.* Philadelphia: Franklin Institute, 1978:321–331.
123. Kreider SD, Lang WR. Hepatitis B vaccine. *N Engl J Med* 1984;310: 466–467.
124. McLean AA, Buynak EB, Kuter BJ, et al. Clinical experience with hepatitis vaccine. In: *Proceedings of the symposium on hepatitis B: the virus, the disease, the vaccine.* New York: Plenum Press, 1984.
125. Syndmen DR, Hinman SH, Wineland MD. Nosocomial viral hepatitis B: a cluster among staff with subsequent transmission to patients. *Ann Intern Med* 1976;85:523–525.
126. Stevens CE. No increased incidence of AIDS in recipients of hepatitis B vaccine. *N Engl J Med* 1983;308:1163–1164.
127. Center for Disease Control. Post-exposure prophylaxis of hepatitis B. *Ann Intern Med* 1984;101:351–354.
128. Columbo M, Cambieri R, Rumi M, et al. Long-term delta superinfection in hepatitis B surface antigen carriers and its relationship to the course of chronic hepatitis. *Gastroenterology* 1983;85:235–239.
129. Alter MJ, Hadler SC, Judson FN, et al. Risk factors for acute non-A, non-B hepatitis in the United States and association with hepatitis C virus infection. *JAMA* 1990;264:2231–2235.
130. Reyes GR, Purdy MA, Kim JP, et al. Isolation of a cDNA from the virus responsible for enterically transmitted non-A, non-B hepatitis. *Science* 1990;247:1335–1339.
131. Farci P, Alter HJ, Wong D, et al. A long-term study of hepatitis C virus replication in non-A, non-B hepatitis. *N Engl J Med* 1991;325: 98–104.
132. Herbert AM, Walker DM, Kavies KJ, et al. Occupationally acquired hepatitis C virus infection. *Lancet* 1992;339:305.
133. Zuckerman J, Clewley G, Griffiths P, et al. Prevalence of hepatitis C antibodies in clinical health-care workers. *Lancet* 1994;343: 1618–1620.
134. Petrosilla M, Puro V, Ipolito G, and the Italian Study Group on Bloodborne Occupational Risk in Dialysis. Prevalence of hepatitis C antibodies in health-care workers. *Lancet* 1994;344:339–340.
135. Lanphear BP, Linneman CC, Cannon CG, et al. Hepatitis C virus in health care workers: risk of exposure and infection. *Infect Control Hosp Epidemiol* 1994;15:745–750.
136. Mitsui T, Iwano K, Masuko K, et al. Hepatitis C virus infection in medical personnel after needlestick accident. *Hepatology* 1992;16: 1109–1114.
137. Alter MJ. The detection, transmission, and outcome of hepatitis C virus infection. *Infect Agents Dis* 1993;2:155–166.
138. Pereira BJ, Milford EL, Kirkman RL, et al. Transmission of hepatitis C virus by organ transplantation. *N Engl J Med* 1991;325:454–460.
139. Centers for Disease Control and Prevention. Recommendations for prevention and control of hepatitis C virus (HCV) infection and HCV-related chronic disease. *MMWR Mortal Morb Wkly Rep* 1998; 47:1–39.
140. Alvardo-Ramy F, Alter MJ, Bower W, et al. Management of occupational exposures to hepatitis C virus: current practice and controversies. *Infect Control Hosp Epidemiol* 2001;22:53–55.
141. Keating GM, Curran MP. Peginterferon-alpha-2a (40kD) plus ribavirin: a review of its use in the management of chronic hepatitis C. *Drugs* 2003;63:701–730.
142. Fatkenheur G, Taelman H, Lepage P, et al. The return of tuberculosis. *Diag Microbiol Infect Dis* 1999;34:139–146.

143. Snider DE Jr, Roper WLE. The new tuberculosis. *N Engl J Med* 1992; 326:703–705.
144. Pearson ML, Jereb JA, Frieden TR, et al. Nosocomial transmission of multidrug resistant *Mycobacterium tuberculosis. Ann Intern Med* 1992;117:191–196.
145. Jarvis WR. Nosocomial transmission of multidrug-resistant *Mycobacterium tuberculosis. Am J Infect Control* 1995;23:146–151.
146. Bloch AB, Rieder HL, Kelly GD, et al. The epidemiology of tuberculosis in the United States. *Clin Chest Med* 1989;10:297–312.
147. Addington WW. Patient compliance: the most serious remaining problem in the control of tuberculosis in the United States. *Chest* 1979;76:741–743.
148. Barnes PF, Bloch AB, Davidson PT, et al. Tuberculosis in patients with human immunodeficiency virus infection. *N Engl J Med* 1991; 324:1644–1650.
149. Beck-Sague CM, Dooley SW, Hutton MD, et al. Hospital outbreak of multidrug-resistant *Mycobacterium tuberculosis* infections: factors in transmission to staff and HIV-infected patients. *JAMA* 1992;268: 1280–1286.
150. Zara S, Blumberg HM, Beck-Sague C, Hass WH, et al. Nosocomial transmission of *Mycobacterium tuberculosis*: role of health care workers in outbreak propagation. *J Infect Dis* 1995;172:1542–1549.
151. Dooley SW, Villarino ME, Lawrence M, et al. Nosocomial transmission of tuberculosis in a hospital unit for HIV-infected patients. *JAMA* 1992;267:2632–2635.
152. Nicas M, Sprinson JE, Royce SE, et al. Isolation rooms for tuberculosis control. *Infect Control Hosp Epidemiol* 1993;14:619––622.
153. Catanzara A. Nosocomial tuberculosis. *Am Rev Respir Dis* 1982;125: 559–562.
154. Beck-Sague C, Dooley SW, Hutton MD, et al. Hospital outbreak of multidrug-resistant *Mycobacterium tuberculosis* infections: factors in transmission to staff and HIV-infected patients. *JAMA* 1992;268: 1280–1286.
155. Haley CE, McDonald RC, Rossi L, et al. Tuberculosis epidemic among hospital personnel. *Infect Control Hosp Epidemiol* 1989;10: 204–210.
156. DiPerri G, Cadeo G, Costelli F, et al. Transmission of HIV-associated tuberculosis to health care workers. *Infect Control Hosp Epidemiol* 1993;14:67–72.
157. Sepkowitz KA. Tuberculosis and the health care worker: a historical perspective. *Ann Intern Med* 1994;120:71–79.
158. Frampton MW. An outbreak of tuberculosis among hospital personnel caring for a patient with a skin ulcer. *Ann Intern Med* 1992;117: 312–313.
159. Hutton MD, Steao WW, Cauthento M, et al. Nosocomial transmission of tuberculosis associated with a draining tuberculous abscess. *J Infect Dis* 1990;161:286–295.
160. Jereb JA, Klevens M, Privett TD, et al. Tuberculosis in health care workers at a hospital with an outbreak of multidrug-resistant *Mycobacterium tuberculosis. Arch Interm Med* 1995;155:854–859.
161. Rattner SL, Fleischer JA, Davidson BL. Tuberculin positivity and patient contact in healthcare workers in the urban United States. *Infect Control Hosp Epidemiol* 1996;17:369–371.
162. Riley RL, Nardell EA. Controlling transmission of tuberculosis in health care facilities: ventilation, filtration, and ultraviolet air disinfection. In: *Plant, technology and safety management series, controlling occupational exposures to tuberculosis.* Oakbridge Terrace, IL: Joint Commission on Accreditation of Healthcare Organizations, 1993.
163. National Institute for Occupational Safety and Health. *NIOSH recommended guidelines for personal respiratory protection of workers in healthcare facilities potentially exposed to tuberculosis.* Atlanta, GA: National Institute for Occupational Safety and Health, 1992.
164. Kelley D. Rules to live by. Official guidelines on preventing the spread of TB. U.S. Department of Labor/OSHA. *J Emerg Med Serv* 1999; 24:S14.
165. Stroud LA, Tokars JI, Grieco MN, et al. Evaluation of infection control measures in preventing the nosocomial transmission of multidrug-resistant *Mycobacterium tuberculosis* in a New York City hospital. *Infect Control Hosp Epidemiol* 1995;16:141–147.
166. Pugiliese G, Tapper ML. Tuberculosis control in health care. *Infect Control Hosp Epidemiol* 1996;17:369–371.
167. Maloney SA, Pearson ML, Gordon MT, et al. Efficacy of control measures in preventing nosocomial transmission of multidrug-resistant tuberculosis to patients and health care workers. *Ann Intern Med* 1995;122:90–95.
168. Centers for Disease Control and Prevention. Screening for tuberculosis infection in high-risk populations: recommendations of the Advisory Council for the Elimination of Tuberculosis. *MMWR Mortal Morb Wkly Rep* 1995;44:19–34.
169. Brewer T, Colditz G. Bacille Calmette-Guerin vaccination for prevention of tuberculosis in health care workers. *Clin Infect Dis* 1995;20: 136–142.
170. Lowy FD. *Staphylococcus aureus* infections. *N Engl J Med* 1998;339: 520–530.
171. Smith TL, Jarvis WR. Antimicrobial resistance in *Staphylococcus aureus. Microbes Infect* 1999;1:795–805.
172. Barber M. Methicillin-resistant staphylococci. *J Clin Pathol* 1961;14: 385–393.
173. Ayliffe GA. The progressive intercontinental spread of methicillin-resistant *Staphylococcus aureus. Clin Infect Dis* 1997;24(Suppl 1): S74–S79.
174. Edmond MB, Wallace SE, McClish DK, et al. Nosocomial blood stream infections in United States hospitals: a three-year analysis. *Clin Infect Dis* 1999;29:239–244.
175. Crossley K. Long-term care facilities as sources of antibiotic-resistant nosocomial pathogens. *Curr Opin Infect Dis* 2001;14:455–459.
176. Herold BC, Immergluck LC, Maranan MC, et al. Community-acquired methicillin-resistant *Staphylococcus aureus* in children with no identified predisposing risk. *JAMA* 1998;279:593–598.
177. Chang S, Sievert DM, Hageman JC, et al. Infection with vancomycin-resistant *Staphylococcus aureus* containing the vanA resistance gene. *N Engl J Med* 2003;348:1342–1347.
178. Cookson B, Peters B, Webster M, et al. Staff carriage of epidemic methicillin-resistant *Staphylococcus aureus. J Clin Microbiol* 1989;27: 1471–1476.
179. Opal SM, Mayer KH, Stenberg, MJ, et al. Frequent acquisition of multiple strains of methicillin-resistant *Staphylococcus aureus* by health care workers in an epidemic hospital environment. *Infect Control Hosp Epidemiol* 1990;11:479–485.
180. Ward TT. Comparison of *in-vitro* adherence of methicillin-sensitive and methicillin-resistant *Staphylococcus aureus* to human nasal epithelial cells. *J Infect Dis* 1992;166:400–404.
181. Chou JW, Yu VL. *Staphylococcus aureus* nasal carriage in hemodialysis patients: its role in infection and approaches to prophylaxis. *Arch Intern Med* 1989;149:1258–1262.
182. Reboli AC, John JF, Platt CG, et al. Methicillin resistant *Staphylococcus aureus* outbreak in a Veterans Affairs Medical Center: importance of carriage of the organism by hospital personnel. *Infect Control Hosp Epidemiol* 1990;11:291–296.
183. Boyce JM, Opal SM, Byone-Potter G, et al. Spread of methicillin-resistant *Staphylococcus aureus* in a hospital after exposure to a health care worker with chronic sinusitis. *Clin Infect Dis* 1993;17:496–504.
184. Doebbling BN, Pfaller MA, Houston AK, et al. Removal of nosocomial pathogens from the contaminated glove. Implications for glove reuse and handwashing. *Ann Intern Med* 1988;109:394–398.
185. Onesko KM, Wienke EC. The analysis of the impact of a mild, low-iodine, lotion soap on the reduction of nosocomial methicillin-resistant *Staphylococcus aureus*: a new opportunity for surveillance by objectives. *Infect Control* 1987;8:284–288.
186. Ndawula EM, Brown L. Mattresses as reservoirs of epidemic methicillin-resistant *Staphylococcus aureus* [Letter]. *Lancet* 1991;337:488.
187. Layton MC, Perez M, Heald P, et al. An outbreak of mupirocin- and methicillin-resistant *Staphylococcus aureus* on a dermatology ward associated with an environmental reservoir. *Infect Control Hosp Epidemiol* 1993;14:369–375.
188. Barg NL. Environmental contamination with *Staphylococcus aureus* and outbreaks: the cause or the effect? *Infect Control Hosp Epidemiol* 1993;14:367–368.
189. Simmons BP, Munn C, Gelfand M. Toxic shock in a hospital em-

ployee due to methicillin-resistant *Staphylococcus aureus* [Letter]. *Infect Control Hosp Epidemiol* 1986;7:350.

190. Brennen C, Muder RR. Conjunctivitis associated with methicillin-resistant *Staphylococcus aureus* in a long-term facility. *Am J Med* 1990; 88:14–17.
191. Muder RR, Brennen C, Wagener MM, et al. Methicillin-resistant staphylococcal colonization and infection in a long-term care facility. *Ann Intern Med* 1991;114:107–112.
192. Muder RR, Brennen C, Goetz AM. Infection with methicillin-resistant *Staphylococcus aureus* among hospital employees. *Infect Control Hosp Epidemiol* 1993;14:576–578.
193. Sheretz RJ, Reagan DR, Hampton KD, et al. A cloud adult: the *Staphylococcus aureus*-virus interaction revisited. *Ann Intern Med* 1996; 124:539–547.
194. Reid RI, Briggs RS, Seal DV, et al. Virulent *Streptococcus pyogenes*: outbreak and spread within a geriatric unit. *J Infect Dis* 1983;6: 219–225.
195. Ruben FL, Norden CW, Heisler B, et al. An outbreak of *Streptococcus pyogenes* infections in a nursing home. *Ann Intern Med* 1984;101: 494–496.
196. Schwartz B, Elliot JA, Butler JC, et al. Clusters of invasive group A streptococcal infections in family, hospital, and nursing home settings. *Clin Infect Dis* 1992;15:277–284.
197. Ramage L, Green K, Pyskir D, et al. An outbreak of fatal nosocomial infections due to group A streptococcus on a medical ward. *Infect Control Hosp Epidemiol* 1996;17:429–431.
198. Kakis A, Gibbs L, Eguia J, et al. An outbreak of group A streptococcal infection among health care workers. *Clin Infect Dis* 2002;35: 1353–1359.
199. Decker MD, Lavely GB, Hutcheson RH Jr, et al. Food-borne streptococcal pharyngitis in a hospital pediatrics clinic. *JAMA* 1986;253: 679–681.
200. Weber DJ, Rutala WA, Denny FW Jr. Management of healthcare workers with pharyngitis or suspected streptococcal infections. *Infect Control Hosp Epidemiol* 1996;17:753–761.
201. Kolmos HJ, Svendsen RN, Nielsen SV. The surgical team as a source of postoperative wound infections caused by *Streptococcus pyogenes. J Hosp Infect* 1997;35:207–214.
202. Centers for Disease Control and Prevention. Nosocomial group A streptococcal infections associated with asymptomatic heath-care workers—Maryland and California, 1997. *MMWR Morb Mortal Wkly Rep* 1999;48:163–166.
203. Beachey EH, Simpson WA, Ofek I, et al. Attachment of *Streptococcus pyogenes* to mammalian cells. *Rev Infect Dis* 1983;5(Suppl 4): S670–S677.
204. Beachey EH, Ofek I. Epithelial cell binding of group A streptococci by lipoteichoic acid on fimbriae denuded of M protein. *J Exp Med* 1976;143:759–771.
205. Simpson WA, Courtney HS, Ofek I. Interactions of fibronectin with streptococci: the role of fibronectin as a receptor for *Streptococcus pyogenes. Rev Infect Dis* 1987;9(Suppl 4):S351–S359.
206. Kass EH, Seastone CV. The role of the mucoid polysaccharide (hyaluronic acid) in the virulence of group A hemolytic streptococci. *J Exp Med* 1944;79:319–330.
207. Stromberg A, Schwan A, Cars O. Throat carrier rates of beta-hemolytic streptococci among health adults and children. *Scand J Infect Dis* 1988;20:411–417.
208. Kaplan EL, Top FH Jr, Dudding BA, et al. Diagnosis of streptococcal pharyngitis: differentiation of active infection from the carrier state in the symptomatic child. *J Infect Dis* 1971;123:490–501.
209. Peter G, Smith AL. Group A streptococcal infections of the skin and pharynx. *N Engl J Med* 1977;297:311–317.
210. Smyth EG, Weinbren MJ. Severe group A streptococcal infection. *Lancet* 1988;2:454–455.
211. Hekman CA, Luskotoff DJ. Fibrinolytic pathways and the endothelium. *Semin Thromb Hemost* 1987;13:514–527.
212. Gordis L. The virtual disappearance of rheumatic fever in the United States: lessons in the rise and fall of disease. *Circulation* 1985;72: 1155–1162.
213. Bisno AL. The resurgence of acute rheumatic fever in the United States. *Annu Rev Med* 1990;41:319–329.
214. Stollerman GH. Rheumatic fever in the 21st century. *Clin Infect Dis* 2001;33:806–813.
215. Fischetti VA, Jones KF, Hollingshead SK, et al. Structure, function, and genetics of streptococcal M protein. *Rev Infect Dis* 1988;10(Suppl 2):S356–S359.
216. Berrios X, Quesney F, Morales A, et al. Acute rheumatic fever and poststreptococcal glomerulonephritis in an open population: comparative studies of epidemiology and bacteriology. *J Lab Clin Med* 1986; 108:535–542.
217. Khandke KM, Fairwell T, Manjula BN. Difference in the structural features of streptococcal M proteins from nephritogenic and rheumatogenic serotypes. *J Exp Med* 1987;166:151–162.
218. Valenzuela TD, Hooton TM, Kaplan EL, et al. Transmission of toxic strep syndrome from an infected child to a firefighter during CPR. *Ann Emerg Med* 1991;20:90–92.
219. Richman DD, Breton SJ, Goldmann DA. Scarlet fever and group A streptococcal surgical wound infection traced to an anal carrier. *J Pediatr* 1977;90:387–390.
220. Mastro TD, Farley TA, Elliot JA, et al. An outbreak of surgical-wound infections due to group A streptococcus carried on the scalp. *N Engl J Med* 1990;323:968–972.
221. Viglionese A, Nottebart VF, Bodman HA, et al. Recurrent group A streptococcal carriage in a health care worker associated with widely separated nosocomial outbreaks. *Am J Med* 1991;91(Suppl 3B): S329–S333.
222. Steele JH, Fernandez PJ. History of rabies and global aspects. In: Baer GM, ed. *The natural history of rabies,* 2nd ed. Boca Raton, FL: CRC Press, 1991:1–24.
223. Fishbein DB, Robinson LE. Current concepts: rabies. *N Engl J Med* 1997;329:1632–1638.
224. Ruppercht CE, Hanlon CA, Hemachudha T. Rabies re-examined. *Lancet Infect Dis* 2002;2:327–343.
225. Messenger SL, Smith JS, Ruppecht CE. Emerging epidemiology of bat-associated cryptic cases of rabies in humans in the United States. *Clin Infect Dis* 2002;35:738–747.
226. Helmick CG, Tauxe RV, Vernon AA. Is there risk to contacts of patients with rabies? *Rev Infect Dis* 1987;9:511–518.
227. Warrell DA, Warrell MJ. Human rabies and its prevention: an overview. *Rev Infect Dis* 1988;10:S726–S731.
228. Winkler WG, Fashinell TR, Leffingwell L, et al. Airborne rabies transmission in a laboratory worker. *JAMA* 1973;226:1219–1221.
229. Tsiang H. Pathophysiology of rabies virus infection of the nervous system.*Adv Virus Res* 1993;42:375–412.
230. Wunner WH, Larson JK, Dietzschold B, et al. The molecular biology of rabies viruses. *Rev Infect Dis* 1988;10(Suppl 4):S771–S784.
231. Lentz TL, Burrage TG, Smith AL, et al. Is the acetylcholine receptor a rabies virus receptor? *Science* 1982;215:182–184.
232. Murphy FA, Bauer SP. Early street rabies virus infection in striated muscle and later progression to the central nervous system. *Intervirology* 1974;3:256–268.
233. Wilson JM, Hettiarachchi J, Wijesuriya LM. Presenting features and diagnosis of rabies. *Lancet* 1975;2:1139–1140.
234. Helmick CG. The epidemiology of human rabies postexposure prophylaxis, 1980–1981. *JAMA* 1983;250:1990–1996.
235. Centers for Disease Control and Prevention. Human rabies—New York, 1993. *MMWR Morbid Mortal Wkly Rep* 1993;42:799, 806.
236. Weber DJ, Rutala WA. Risks and prevention of nosocomial transmission of rare zoonotic diseases. *Clin Infect Dis* 2001;32:446–456.
237. Centers for Disease Control and Prevention. Human rabies prevention—United States, 1999: recommendations of the Immunization Practices Advisory Committee (ACIP). *MMWR Mortal Morb Wkly Rep* 1999;48:1–21.
238. Rabies vaccine failures. *Lancet* 1988;1:917–918.
239. Shill M, Baynes RD, Miller SD. Fatal rabies encephalitis despite appropriate post-exposure prophylaxis: a case report. *N Engl J Med* 1987; 316:1257–1258.

240. Prusiner SB. Prions. *Proc Natl Acad Sci U S A* 1998;95:13363–13383.
241. Andrews NJ, Farrington CP, Ward HJ, et al. Deaths from variant Creutzfeldt-Jakob disease in the UK. *Lancet* 2003;361:751–752.
242. Centers for Disease Control and Prevention. Probable variant Creutzfeldt-Jakob disease in a U.S. resident—Florida, 2002. *MMWR Morb Mortal Wkly Rep* 2002;51:927–929.
243. Brown P, Gibbs CJ Jr, Gajdusek DC, et al. Transmission of Creutzfeldt-Jacob disease from formalin-fixed, paraffin-embedded human brain tissue [Letter]. *N Engl J Med* 1986;315:1614–1615.
244. Miller DC. Creutzfeldt-Jacob disease in histopathology technicians [Letter]. *N Engl J Med* 1988;318:853–854.
245. Manuelidis EE, Angelo JN, Gorgacz EJ, et al. Experimental Creutzfeldt-Jakob disease transmitted via the eye with infected cornea. *N Engl J Med* 1977;296:1334–1336.
246. Hetz C, Soto C. Protein misfolding and disease: the case of prion disorders. *Cell Mol Life Sci* 2003;60:133–143.
247. Weissmann C, Enari M, Klohn P-C, et al. Transmission of prions. *J Infect Dis* 2002;186(Suppl 2):S157–S165.
248. Weber DJ, Rutala WA. Managing the risk of nosocomial transmission of prion diseases. *Curr Opin Infect Dis* 2002;15:421–425.
249. World Health Organization. WHO infectious control guidelines for transmissible spongiform encephalopathies. Report of a WHO consultation, Geneva, Switzerland, 23-26 March 1999. Available at *http://www.who.int/csr/resources/publications/bse/WHO_CDS_CSR_APH_2000_3/en/*.
250. Committee on Health Care Issues, American Neurological Association. Precautions in handling tissues, fluids, and other contaminated materials from patients with documented or suspected Creutzfeldt disease. *Ann Neurol* 1986;19:75–77.
251. Rutala WA, Weber DJ. Creutzfeldt-Jakob diseases: recommendations for disinfection and sterilization. *Clin Infect Dis* 2001;32: 1348–1356.

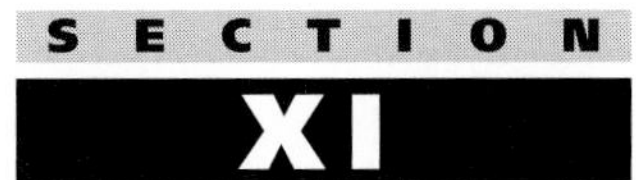

DISINFECTIONS AND STERILIZATION

85

SELECTION AND USE OF DISINFECTANTS IN HEALTHCARE

WILLIAM A. RUTALA
DAVID J. WEBER

Each year in the United States there are approximately 27,000,000 surgical procedures and an even larger number of invasive medical procedures (1). For example, there are at least 10 million gastrointestinal endoscopies per year (2). Each of these procedures involves contact by a medical device or surgical instrument with a patient's sterile tissue or mucous membranes. A major risk of all such procedures is the introduction of infection. Failure to properly disinfect or sterilize equipment carries not only the risk associated with breach of the host barriers but the additional risk of person-to-person transmission (e.g., hepatitis B virus) and transmission of environmental pathogens (e.g., *Pseudomonas aeruginosa*).

Achieving disinfection and sterilization through the use of disinfectants and sterilization practices is essential for ensuring that medical and surgical instruments do not transmit infectious pathogens to patients. Since it is unnecessary to sterilize all patient-care items, healthcare policies must identify whether cleaning, disinfection, or sterilization is indicated based primarily on the items' intended use.

Multiple studies in many countries have documented lack of compliance with established guidelines for disinfection and sterilization (3–6). Failure to comply with scientifically based guidelines has led to numerous outbreaks (6–10). This chapter presents a pragmatic approach to the judicious selection and proper use of disinfection processes, based on well-designed studies assessing the efficacy (via laboratory investigations) and effectiveness (via clinical studies) of disinfection procedures.

DEFINITION OF TERMS

Sterilization is the complete elimination or destruction of all forms of microbial life and is accomplished in healthcare facilities by either physical or chemical processes. Steam under pressure, dry heat, ethylene oxide (ETO) gas, hydrogen peroxide gas plasma, and liquid chemicals are the principal sterilizing agents used in healthcare facilities. Sterilization is intended to convey an absolute meaning, not a relative one. Unfortunately, some health professionals as well as the technical and commercial literature refer to "disinfection" as "sterilization" and items as "partially sterile." When chemicals are used for the purposes of destroying all forms of microbiologic life, including fungal and bacterial spores, they may be called chemical sterilants. These same germicides used for shorter exposure periods may also be part of the disinfection process (i.e., high-level disinfection).

Disinfection describes a process that eliminates many or all pathogenic microorganisms on inanimate objects with the exception of bacterial spores. Disinfection is usually accomplished by the use of liquid chemicals or wet pasteurization in healthcare settings. The efficacy of disinfection is affected by a number of factors, each of which may nullify or limit the efficacy of the process. Some of the factors that affect both disinfection and sterilization efficacy are the prior cleaning of the object; the organic and inorganic load present; the type and level of microbial contamination; the concentration of and exposure time to the germicide; the nature of the object (e.g., crevices, hinges, and lumina); the presence of biofilms; the temperature and pH of the disinfection process; and, in some cases, the relative humidity of the sterilization process (e.g., ETO).

By definition, then, disinfection differs from sterilization by its lack of sporicidal property, but this is an oversimplification. A few disinfectants kill spores with prolonged exposure times (3 to 12 hours) and are called chemical sterilants. At similar concentrations but with shorter exposure periods (e.g., 20 minutes for 2% glutaraldehyde), these same disinfectants kill all microorganisms with the exception of large numbers of bacterial spores and are called high-level disinfectants. Low-level disinfectants may kill most vegetative bacteria, some fungi, and some viruses in a practical period of time (≤10 minutes), whereas intermediate-level disinfectants may be cidal for mycobacteria, vegetative bacteria, most viruses, and most fungi, but do not necessarily kill bacterial spores. The germicides differ markedly among themselves primarily in their antimicrobial spectrum and rapidity of action. Table 85.1 lists the methods of sterilization and disinfection. Table 85.2 lists the characteristics desired in an ideal disinfectant.

Cleaning, on the other hand, is the removal of visible soil (e.g., organic and inorganic material) from objects and surfaces, and it normally is accomplished by manual or mechanical means using water with detergents or enzymatic products. Thorough cleaning is essential before high-level disinfection and sterilization since inorganic and organic materials that remain on the

TABLE 85.1. METHODS OF STERILIZATION AND DISINFECTION

	Sterilization		Disinfection		
	Critical items (will enter tissue or vascular system or blood will flow through them)		High-level (semicritical items; [except dental] will come in contact with mucous membrane or nonintact skin)	Intermediate-level (some semicritical items[1] and noncritical items)	Low-level (noncritical items; will come in contact with intact skin)
Object	Procedure	Exposure Time	Procedure (exposure time 12–30 min at ≥20°C)[2,3]	Procedure (exposure time ≤10 min)	Procedure (exposure time ≤10 min)
Smooth, hard Surface[1,4]	A	MR	D	J[5]	K
	B	MR	E	K	L
	C	MR	F	M	M
	D	10 h	H	N	N
	F	6 h	I[6]		O
	G	12 m			
	H	3–8 h			
Rubber tubing and catheters[3,4]	A	MR	D		
	B	MR	E		
	C	MR	F		
	D	10 h	H		
	F	6 h	I[6]		
	G	12 m			
	H	3–8 h			
Polyethylene tubing and catheters[3,4,7]	A	MR	D		
	B	MR	E		
	C	MR	F		
	D	10 h	H		
	F	6 h	I[6]		
	G	12 m			
	H	3–8 h			
Lensed instruments[4]	A	MR	D		
	B	MR	E		
	C	MR	F		
	D	10 h	H		
	F	6 h			
	G	12 m			
	H	3–8 h			
Thermometers (oral and rectal)[8]				K[8]	
Hinged instruments[4]	A	MR	D		
	B	MR	E		
	C	MR	F		
	D	10 h	H		
	F	6 h	I[6]		
	G	12 m			
	H	3–8 h			

Modified from 13,15,16,391

A, Heat sterilization, including steam or hot air (see manufacturer's recommendations, steam sterilization processing time from 3–30 minutes, see Table 10)
B, Ethylene oxide gas (see manufacturer's recommendations, generally 1–6 hours processing time plus aeration time of 8–12 hours at 50–60°C)
C, Hydrogen peroxide gas plasma (see manufacturer's recommendations, processing time between 45–72 minutes; endoscopes or medical devices with lumens >40 cm or a diameter <3 mm cannot be processed at this time in the United States)
D, Glutaraldehyde-based formulations (≥2% glutaraldehyde, caution should be exercised with all glutaraldehyde formulations when further in-use dilution is anticipated); glutaraldehyde (0.95%) and 1.64% phenol/phenate. One glutaraldehyde-based product has a 5 minute exposure time at 35°C.
E, Ortho-phthalaldehyde 0.55%
F, Hydrogen peroxide 7.5% (will corrode copper, zinc, and brass)
G, Peracetic acid, concentration variable but ≥.2% is sporicidal. Peracetic acid immersion system operates at 50–56°C.
H, Hydrogen peroxide (7.35%) and 0.23% peracetic acid; hydrogen peroxide 1% and peracetic acid 0.08% (will corrode metal instruments)
I, Wet pasteurization at 70°C for 30 minutes with detergent cleaning
J, Sodium hypochlorite (5.25–6.15% household bleach diluted 1 : 50 provides >1000 ppm available chlorine; will corrode metal instruments)
K, Ethyl or isopropyl alcohol (70–90%)
L, Sodium hypochlorite (5.25–6.15% household bleach diluted 1 : 500 provides >100 ppm available chlorine)
M, Phenolic germicidal detergent solution (follow product label for use-dilution)
N, Iodophor germicidal detergent solution (follow product label for use-dilution)
O, Quaternary ammonium germicidal detergent solution (follow product label for use-dilution)
MR, Manufacturer's recommendations.
NA, Not applicable

[1] See text for discussion of hydrotherapy.
[2] The longer the exposure to a disinfectant, the more likely it is that all microorganisms will be eliminated. Ten-minute exposure is not adequate to disinfect many objects, especially those that are difficult to clean, because they have narrow channels or other areas that can harbor organic material and bacteria. Twenty-minute exposure at 20°C is the minimum time needed to reliably kill *M. tuberculosis* and nontuberculous mycobacteria with a 2% glutaraldehyde. With the exception of >2% glutaraldehydes, follow the FDA-cleared high-level disinfection claim. Some high-level disinfectants have a reduced exposure time (e.g., ortho-phthalaldehyde at 12 minutes at 20°C), because of their rapid activity against mycobacteria or reduced exposure time due to increased mycobactericidal activity at elevated temperature (2.5% glutaraldehyde at 5 minutes at 35°C).
[3] Tubing must be completely filled for disinfection and liquid chemical sterilization; care must be taken to avoid entrapment of air bubbles during immersion.
[4] Material compatibility should be investigated when appropriate.
[5] Used in laboratory where cultures or concentrated preparations or microorganisms have spilled. This solution may corrode some surfaces.
[6] Pasteurization (washer-disinfector) or respiratory therapy or anesthesia equipment is a recognized alternative to high-level disinfection. Some data challenge the efficacy of some pasteurization units.
[7] Thermostability should be investigated when appropriate.
[8] Do not mix rectal and oral thermometers at any stage of handling or processing.

TABLE 85.2. PROPERTIES OF AN IDEAL DISINFECTANT

1. Broad spectrum: should have a wide antimicrobial spectrum
2. Fast acting: should produce a rapid kill
3. Not affected by environmental factors: should be active in the presence of organic matter (e.g., blood, sputum, feces) and compatible with soaps, detergents, and other chemicals encountered in use
4. Nontoxic: should not be harmful to the user or patient
5. Surface compatibility: should not corrode instruments and metallic surfaces and should not cause the deterioration of cloth, rubber, plastics, and other materials
6. Residual effect on treated surfaces: should leave an antimicrobial film on the treated surface
7. Easy to use with clear label directions
8. Odorless: should have a pleasant odor or no odor to facilitate its routine use
9. Economical: should not be prohibitively high in cost
10. Solubility: should be soluble in water
11. Stability: should be stable in concentrate and use-dilution
12. Cleaner: should have good cleaning properties
13. Environmentally friendly: should not damage the environment on disposal

Modified from 193.

surfaces of instruments interfere with the effectiveness of these processes. Decontamination is a procedure that removes pathogenic microorganisms from objects so they are safe to handle, use, or discard.

The suffix *-cide* or *-cidal* indicates a killing action. For example, a germicide is an agent that can kill microorganisms, particularly pathogenic microorganisms (germs). The term *germicide* includes both antiseptics and disinfectants. Antiseptics are germicides applied to living tissue and skin, whereas disinfectants are antimicrobials applied only to inanimate objects. In general, antiseptics are used only on the skin and not for surface disinfection, and disinfectants are not used for skin antisepsis, because they may cause injury to skin and other tissues. Other words with the suffix *-cide* (e.g., virucide, fungicide, bactericide, sporicide, and tuberculocide) can kill the type of microorganism identified by the prefix. For example, a bactericide is an agent that kills bacteria (11–16).

A RATIONAL APPROACH TO DISINFECTION AND STERILIZATION

Over 30 years ago, Earle H. Spaulding (12) devised a rational approach to disinfection and sterilization of patient-care items or equipment. This classification scheme is so clear and logical that it has been retained, refined, and successfully used by infection control professionals and others when planning methods for disinfection or sterilization (11,13,15,17,18). Spaulding believed that the nature of disinfection could be understood more readily if instruments and items for patient care were divided into three categories based on the degree of risk of infection involved in the use of the items. The three categories he described were critical, semicritical, and noncritical. This terminology is employed by the 1985 Centers for Disease Control and Prevention (CDC) in several of its guidelines: for handwashing and hospital environmental control (19), for the prevention of transmission of human immunodeficiency virus (HIV) and hepatitis B virus (HBV) to healthcare and public-safety workers (20), and for environmental infection control and prevention in healthcare facilities (21).

Critical Items

Critical items are so called because of the high risk of infection if such an item is contaminated with any microorganism, including bacterial spores. Thus, it is critical that objects that enter sterile tissue or the vascular system be sterile, because any microbial contamination could result in disease transmission. This category includes surgical instruments, cardiac and urinary catheters, implants, and ultrasound probes used in sterile body cavities. Most of the items in this category should be purchased as sterile or be sterilized by steam sterilization if possible. If heat-sensitive, the object may be treated with ETO, hydrogen peroxide gas plasma, or by liquid chemical sterilants if other methods are unsuitable. Table 85.1 lists several germicides categorized as chemical sterilants. These include ≤2.4% glutaraldehyde-based formulations, 0.95% glutaraldehyde with 1.64% phenol/phenate, 7.5% stabilized hydrogen peroxide, 7.35% hydrogen peroxide with 0.23% peracetic acid, 0.2% peracetic acid, and 0.08% peracetic acid with 1.0% hydrogen peroxide. Liquid chemical sterilants can be relied on to produce sterility only if cleaning, to eliminate organic and inorganic material, precedes treatment and if proper guidelines as to concentration, contact time, temperature, and pH are met.

Semicritical Items

Semicritical items are those that come in contact with mucous membranes or nonintact skin. Respiratory therapy and anesthesia equipment, some endoscopes, laryngoscope blades, esophageal manometry probes, rectal manometry catheters, and diaphragm fitting rings are included in this category. These medical devices should be free of all microorganisms, although small numbers of bacterial spores may be present. Intact mucous membranes, such as those of the lungs or the gastrointestinal tract, generally are resistant to infection by common bacterial spores but susceptible to other microorganisms such as bacteria, mycobacteria, and viruses. Semicritical items minimally require high-level disinfection using chemical disinfectants. Glutaraldehyde, hydrogen peroxide, ortho-phthalaldehyde (OPA), and peracetic acid with hydrogen peroxide are cleared by the Food and Drug Administration (FDA) and are dependable high-level disinfectants provided the factors influencing germicidal procedures are met (Table 85.1). When a disinfectant is selected for use with certain patient-care items, the chemical compatibility after extended use with the items to be disinfected also must be considered.

Although the complete elimination of all microorganisms in/on an instrument with the exception of small numbers of bacterial spores is the traditional definition of high-level disinfection, the FDA requires a more defined end point. For example, the FDA accepts a 6-$\log_{10}$ reduction of microorganisms (i.e., specific strains of mycobacteria), with the exception of small numbers of bacterial spores, as proof of high-level disinfection. This is noteworthy, as complete elimination of microorganisms (e.g., *Mycobacterium chelonae*) on a contaminated instrument occurs with a starting inoculum of $\leq 10^6$ colony-forming units (CFU) but may not occur if the starting inoculum is $>10^6$ CFU. However, cleaning followed by high-level disinfection should eliminate sufficient pathogens to prevent transmission of infection (22,23).

Laparoscopes and arthroscopes entering sterile tissue ideally should be sterilized between patients. However, they sometimes undergo only high-level disinfection between patients in the U.S. (24–26). As with flexible endoscopes, these devices may be difficult to clean or to do high-level disinfection/sterilization due to their intricate device design (e.g., long narrow lumina, hinges). Meticulous cleaning must precede any high-level disinfection/sterilization process. Although sterilization is preferred, there are no published outbreaks resulting following high-level disinfection of these scopes when properly cleaned and high-level disinfected. Newer models of these instruments can withstand steam sterilization that for critical items would be preferable to high-level disinfection.

Semicritical items should be rinsed with sterile water after high-level disinfection to prevent their contamination with microorganisms that may be present in tap water, such as nontuberculous mycobacteria (10,27,28), *Legionella* (29–31), or gram-negative bacilli such as *Pseudomonas* (15,17,32–34). In circumstances where rinsing with sterile water rinse is not feasible, a tap water or filtered water (0.2μm filter) rinse should be followed by an alcohol rinse and forced air drying (24,34,35). Forced-air drying markedly reduces bacterial contamination of stored endoscopes, most likely by removing the wet environment favorable for bacterial growth (35). After rinsing, items should be dried and stored (e.g., packaged) in a manner that protects them from recontamination.

Some items that may come in contact with nonintact skin for a brief period of time (i.e., hydrotherapy tanks, bed side rails) are usually considered noncritical surfaces and are disinfected with intermediate-level disinfectants (e.g., phenolic, iodophor, alcohol, chlorine) (21). Since hydrotherapy tanks have been associated with spread of infection, some facilities have chosen to disinfect them with recommended levels of chlorine (21,36).

In the past it was recommended that mouthpieces and spirometry tubing be high-level disinfected (e.g., glutaraldehyde), but it was unnecessary to clean the interior surfaces of the spirometers (37). This was based on a study that showed that mouthpieces and spirometry tubing become contaminated with microorganisms, but there was no bacterial contamination of the surfaces inside the spirometers. More recently, filters have been used to prevent contamination of this equipment distal to the filter; such filters and the proximal mouthpiece should be changed between patients.

Noncritical Items

Noncritical items are those that come in contact with intact skin but not mucous membranes. Intact skin acts as an effective barrier to most microorganisms; therefore, the sterility of items coming in contact with intact skin is "not critical." Examples of noncritical items are bedpans, blood pressure cuffs, crutches, bed rails, linens, some food utensils, bedside tables, patient furniture, and floors. In contrast to critical and some semicritical items, most noncritical reusable items may be decontaminated where they are used and do not need to be transported to a central processing area. There is virtually no risk of transmitting infectious agents to patients via noncritical items (33) when they are used as noncritical items and do not contact nonintact skin and/or mucous membranes. However, these items (e.g., bedside tables, bed rails) could potentially contribute to secondary transmission by contaminating hands of healthcare workers or by contact with medical equipment that will subsequently come in contact with patients (11,38–42). Table 85.1 lists several low-level disinfectants that may be used for noncritical items. The exposure time listed in Table 85.1 is less than or equal to 10 minutes. Most Environmental Protection Agency (EPA)-registered disinfectants have a 10-minute label claim. However, multiple investigators have demonstrated the effectiveness of these disinfectants against vegetative bacteria [e.g., *Listeria, Escherichia coli, Salmonella*, vancomycin-resistant enterococci (VRE), methicillin-resistant *Staphylococcus aureus* (MRSA)], yeasts (e.g., *Candida*), mycobacteria (e.g., *Mycobacterium tuberculosis*), and viruses (e.g., poliovirus) at exposure time of 30 to 60 seconds (39–57). These products should be used in accordance with the manufacturers' recommendations (e.g., use-dilution, shelf-life, storage, material compatibility, safe use and disposal) but often are not; one study showed that only 14% of sampled disinfectants had the correct concentration (58).

Mops and reusable cleaning cloths are regularly used to achieve low-level disinfection. However, they are commonly not kept adequately cleaned and disinfected, and if the water-disinfectant mixture is not changed regularly (e.g., after every three to four rooms, no longer than 60-minute intervals), the mopping procedure may actually spread heavy microbial contamination throughout the healthcare facility (59). In one study, standard laundering provided acceptable decontamination of heavily contaminated mop heads but chemical disinfection with a phenolic was less effective (59). The frequent laundering of mops (e.g., daily), therefore, is recommended.

Changes in Disinfection and Sterilization Since 1981

The table contained in the CDC Guideline for Environmental Control prepared in 1981 as a guide to the appropriate selection and use of disinfectants has undergone several important changes (Table 85.1) (13). First, formaldehyde-alcohol has been deleted as a recommended chemical sterilant or high-level disinfectant, because it is irritating and toxic and not commonly used. Second, several new chemical sterilants have been added, including hydrogen peroxide, peracetic acid (51,60,61), and peracetic acid and hydrogen peroxide in combination. Third, 3% phenolics and iodophors have been deleted as high-level disinfectants because of their unproven efficacy against bacterial spores, *M. tuberculosis*, and/or some fungi (48,62). Fourth, isopropyl alcohol and ethyl alcohol have been excluded as high-level disinfectants (13) because of their inability to inactivate bacterial spores and because of the inability of isopropyl alcohol to inactivate hydrophilic viruses (e.g., poliovirus, Coxsackie virus) (63). Fifth, a 1:16 dilution of 2.0% glutaraldehyde–7.05% phenol–1.20% sodium phenate (which contained 0.125% glutaraldehyde, 0.440% phenol, and 0.075% sodium phenate when diluted) has been deleted as a high-level disinfectant, because this product was removed from the marketplace in December 1991 because of a lack of bactericidal activity in the presence of organic matter; a lack of fungicidal, tuberculocidal, and sporicidal activity; and reduced virucidal activity (43,48,49,62, 64–70). Sixth, the exposure time required to achieve high-level disinfection has been changed from 10 to 30 minutes to 12 minutes or more depending on the scientific literature and the FDA-cleared label claim (23,48,60,67,71–75). Of note, one glutaraldehyde product has an FDA-cleared label claim of 5 minutes when used at 35°C (76).

Several new subjects have been added to the guideline: an expanded section on disinfection and sterilization of Creutzfeldt-Jakob disease (CJD) agent; inactivation of bioterrorists agents; decontamination of bone; surface disinfection; microbial contamination of disinfectants; air disinfection; and disinfection in the hemodialysis unit.

DISINFECTION OF HEALTHCARE EQUIPMENT

Concerns with Implementing the Spaulding Scheme

One problem with implementing the Spaulding scheme is that of oversimplification. For example, it does not consider problems with reprocessing of complicated medical equipment that often is heat-sensitive or problems of inactivating certain types of infectious agents (e.g., prions such as CJD agent). Thus, in some situations it is still difficult to choose a method of disinfection, even after considering the categories of risk to patients. This is especially true for a few medical devices (e.g., arthroscopes, laparoscopes) in the critical category, because there is controversy about whether they should be sterilized or high-level disinfected (24,77). Heat-stable scopes (e.g., many rigid scopes) should be steam sterilized. Some of these items cannot be steam sterilized, because they are heat-sensitive; further, sterilization by using ETO may be too time-consuming for routine use between patients (new technologies, such as hydrogen peroxide gas plasma and peracetic acid reprocessor, provide faster cycle times). However, evidence that sterilization of these items improves patient care by reducing the infection risk is lacking (25, 78–82). Many newer models of these instruments can withstand steam sterilization, which for critical items is the preferred method.

Another problem with implementing the Spaulding scheme is how an instrument in the semicritical category (e.g., endoscopes) should be processed that would be used with a critical instrument that would have contact with sterile body tissues. For example, is an endoscope used for upper gastrointestinal tract investigation still a semicritical item when it is used with sterile biopsy forceps or when it is used in a patient who is bleeding heavily from esophageal varices? Provided that high-level disinfection is achieved, and all microorganisms with the exception of bacterial spores have been removed from the endoscope, then the device should not represent an infection risk and should remain in the semicritical category (83–85). There are no reports of infection with spore-forming bacteria from appropriately high-level disinfected endoscopes.

An additional problem with the implementation of the Spaulding system is that the optimal contact time to achieve high-level disinfection has not been defined or varies among professional organizations, resulting in different strategies for disinfecting different types of semicritical items (e.g., endoscopes, applanation tonometers, endocavitary transducers, cryosurgical instruments, and diaphragm fitting rings). The impact of this variability is discussed below. Until simpler and effective alternatives are identified for device disinfection in clinical settings, it would be prudent to follow the recommendations in this chapter and in the guidelines of the CDC (17,20,86–88).

Reprocessing of Endoscopes

Physicians use endoscopes to diagnose and treat numerous medical disorders. Although endoscopes represent a valuable diagnostic and therapeutic tool in modern medicine and the incidence of infection associated with use has been reported as very low (about 1 in 1.8 million procedures) (89), more healthcare-associated outbreaks have been linked to contaminated endoscopes than to any other medical device (6–8). To prevent the spread of healthcare-associated infections, all heat-sensitive endoscopes (e.g., gastrointestinal endoscopes, bronchoscopes, nasopharyngoscopes) must be properly cleaned and at a minimum subjected to high-level disinfection following each use. High-level disinfection can be expected to destroy all microorganisms, although when high numbers of bacterial spores are present, a few spores may survive.

Flexible endoscopes, by virtue of the types of body cavities they enter, acquire high levels of microbial contamination (bioburden) during each use (90). For example, the bioburden found on flexible gastrointestinal endoscopes following use has ranged from 10^5 to 10^{10} CFU/mL, with the highest levels being found in the suction channels (90–93). The average load on bronchoscopes before cleaning was 6.4×10^4 CFU/mL. Cleaning reduces the level of microbial contamination by 4 to 6 $\log_{10}$ (74). Using HIV-contaminated endoscopes, several investigators have shown that cleaning completely eliminates the microbial contamination on the scopes (94,95). Similarly, other investigators found that ETO sterilization or high-level disinfection (soaking in 2% glutaraldehyde for 20 minutes) were effective only when the device was first properly cleaned (96).

High-level disinfectants cleared for marketing by the FDA include formulations with ≥2.4% glutaraldehyde, 0.55% OPA, 0.95% glutaraldehyde with 1.64% phenol/phenate, 7.35% hydrogen peroxide with 0.23% peracetic acid, 1.0% hydrogen peroxide with 0.08% peracetic acid, and 7.5% hydrogen peroxide (76). Although all of these products have excellent antimicrobial activity, certain products based on oxidizing chemicals [e.g., 7.5% hydrogen peroxide and 1.0% hydrogen peroxide with 0.08% peracetic acid (the latter is no longer marketed)] have limited use, because they may cause cosmetic and functional damage to endoscopes (60). Two newer formulations (0.95% glutaraldehyde with 1.64% phenol/phenate, and 7.35% hydrogen peroxide with 0.23% peracetic acid) have been FDA-cleared but data regarding antimicrobial activity or materials compatibility have not yet been published in the scientific literature. ETO sterilization of flexible endoscopes is infrequent, because it requires a lengthy processing and aeration time (e.g., 12 hours) and is a potential hazard to staff and patients. The two products that are most commonly used for reprocessing endoscopes in the U.S. are glutaraldehyde and an automated, liquid chemical sterilization process that uses peracetic acid (97). The American Society of Gastrointestinal Endoscopy (ASGE) recommends glutaraldehyde solutions that do not contain surfactants, because the soapy residues of surfactants are difficult to remove during rinsing (2). OPA has begun to replace glutaraldehyde in many healthcare facilities as it possesses several potential advantages over glutaraldehyde: it causes no known irritation to the eyes and nasal passages, it does not require activation or exposure monitoring, and it has a 12-minute high-level disinfection claim in the U.S. (60). Disinfectants that are not FDA cleared and should not be used for reprocessing endoscopes include iodophors, chlorine solutions, alcohols, quaternary ammonium compounds, and phenolics. These solutions may still be in use outside the U.S., but their use should be strongly discouraged because of lack of proven efficacy against all microorganisms or materials incompatibility.

The FDA cleared a package label for 2.4% glutaraldehyde that requires a 45-minute immersion at 25°C to achieve high-level disinfection (i.e., 100% kill of *M. tuberculosis*). However, available data suggest that *M. tuberculosis* levels can be reduced by at least 8 $\log_{10}$ with cleaning (4 $\log_{10}$) (74,92,93,98) followed by chemical disinfection for 20 minutes at 20°C (4 to 6 $\log_{10}$) (74,84,99). Based on these data, the Association for Professionals in Infection Control (APIC) (100), the Society of Gastroenterology Nurses and Associates (SGNA) (34,101) and ASGE (2) recommend that equipment be immersed in 2% glutaraldehyde at 20°C for at least 20 minutes for high-level disinfection (2,18, 50,74,85,99,102–106). In the absence of independently validated data regarding alternative exposure times of high-level disinfectants, the manufacturers' recommendations to achieve high-level disinfection should be followed. Currently, such data are available only for 2% glutaraldehyde solutions.

Flexible endoscopes are particularly difficult to disinfect (107) and easy to damage because of their intricate design and delicate materials (108). Meticulous cleaning must precede any sterilization or high-level disinfection of these instruments. Failure to perform good cleaning may result in a sterilization or disinfection failure and outbreaks of infection may occur. Several studies have demonstrated the importance of cleaning in experimental studies with the duck HBV (96,109), HIV (110), and *Helicobacter pylori* (111).

Examining healthcare-associated infections related only to endoscopes through July 1992, Spach et al. (6) found that 281 infections were transmitted by gastrointestinal endoscopy and 96 were transmitted by bronchoscopy. The clinical spectrum ranged from asymptomatic colonization to death. *Salmonella* species and *P. aeruginosa* repeatedly were identified as causative agents of infections transmitted by gastrointestinal endoscopy, and *M. tuberculosis* (TB), atypical mycobacteria, and *P. aeruginosa* were the most common causes of infections transmitted by bronchoscopy. Major reasons for transmission were inadequate cleaning, improper selection of a disinfecting agent, failure to follow recommended cleaning and disinfection procedures (6, 8,33), and flaws in endoscope design (112,113) or automated endoscope reprocessors (7). Failure to follow established guidelines has continued to lead to infections associated with gastrointestinal endoscopes (8) and bronchoscopes (7). Potential device-associated problems should be reported to the FDA's Center for Devices and Radiologic Health. One multistate investigation found that 23.9% of the bacterial cultures from the internal channels of 71 gastrointestinal endoscopes grew ≥100,000 colonies of bacteria after completion of all disinfection/sterilization procedures and before use on the next patient (114).

Automated endoscope reprocessors (AERs) offer several advantages compared to manual reprocessing: they automate and standardize several important reprocessing steps (115–117), reduce the likelihood that an essential reprocessing step will be skipped, and reduce personnel exposure to high-level disinfectants or chemical sterilants. Failure of AERs has been linked to outbreaks of infections (118) or colonization (7,119), and the AER water filtration system may not be able to reliably provide bacteria-free rinse water (120,121). It is critical that correct connectors between the AER and the device are established to ensure complete flow of disinfectants and rinse water (7,122). In addition, some endoscopes such as the duodenoscopes [e.g., endoscopic retrograde cholangiopancreatography (ERCP)] contain features (e.g., elevator-wire channel) that require a flushing pressure that is not achieved by most AERs and must be reprocessed manually using a 2- to 5-mL syringe. New duodenoscopes equipped with a wider elevator-channel that AERs can reliably reprocess may be available in the future (117). Outbreaks involving removable endoscope parts (123,124) such as suction valves and endoscopic accessories designed to be inserted through flexible endoscopes such as biopsy forceps emphasize the importance of cleaning to remove all foreign matter before high-level disinfection or sterilization (125). Some types of valves are now available as single-use, disposable products (e.g., bronchoscope valves) or steam sterilizable products (e.g., gastrointestinal endoscope valves).

There is a need for further development and redesign of AERs (7,126) and endoscopes (108,127) so that they do not represent a potential source of infectious agents. Endoscopes employing disposable components (e.g., protective barrier devices or sheaths) can provide an alternative to conventional liquid chemical high-level disinfection/sterilization (128). Another new technology is a swallowable camera-in-a-capsule that travels through the digestive tract and transmits color pictures of the small intestine to a receiver that is worn outside the body. At present, this capsule will not replace colonoscopy.

Recommendations for the cleaning and disinfection of endoscopic equipment have been published and should be strictly followed (2,34,100,101,129–132). Unfortunately, audits have shown that personnel do not adhere to guidelines on reprocessing (133–135) and outbreaks of infection continue to occur (136–138). To ensure that reprocessing personnel are properly trained, there should be initial and annual competency testing for each individual who reprocesses endoscopic instruments (34, 139).

In general, endoscope disinfection or sterilization with a liquid chemical sterilant involves five steps after leak testing: (a) clean—mechanically clean internal and external surfaces, including brushing internal channels and flushing each internal channel with water and a detergent or enzymatic cleaners (leak testing is recommended for endoscopes before immersion); (b) disinfect—immerse endoscope in high-level disinfectant (or chemical sterilant) and perfuse (eliminates air pockets and ensures contact of the germicide with the internal channels) disinfectant into all accessible channels such as the suction/biopsy channel and air/water channel and expose for a time recommended for specific products; (c) rinse—rinse the endoscope and all channels with sterile water or filtered water (commonly used with AERs); if this is not feasible, use tap water; (d) dry—rinse the insertion tube and inner channels with alcohol and dry with forced air after disinfection and before storage; and (e) store the endoscope in a way that prevents recontamination and promotes drying (e.g., hung vertically).

One study demonstrated that reprocessed endoscopes (e.g., air/water channel, suction/biopsy channel) were generally negative [100% after 24 hours; 90% after 7 days (1 CFU of coagulase-negative staphylococci in one channel)] for bacterial growth when stored by hanging in a vertical position in a ventilated cabinet (140). Because tap water may contain low levels of microorganisms, some have suggested that only sterile water, which may be prohibitively expensive (141), or AER filtered water be used. The suggestion to use only sterile water or filtered water is not consistent with published guidelines that allow tap water with an alcohol rinse and forced air-drying (2,34,100) or the scientific literature (35,84). In addition, there has been no evidence of disease transmission when tap water followed by an alcohol rinse and forced air-drying has been used. AERs produce filtered water via passage through a bacterial filter (e.g., 0.2μm). Filtered rinse water was identified as a source of bacterial contamination in a recent study that cultured the accessory and suction channels of endoscopes and the internal chambers of AERs between 1996 and 2001 and reported 8.7% of samples collected between 1996 and 1998 had bacterial growth with 54% being *Pseudomonas* species (142). Following the introduction of a system of hot water flushing of the piping (60°C for 60 minutes daily), the frequency of positive cultures fell to approximately 2% with only rare isolation of >10 CFU/mL.

In addition to these practices, a protocol should be developed that ensures that the user knows whether an endoscope has been appropriately cleaned and disinfected (e.g., using a room or cabinet for processed endoscopes only) or has not been reprocessed. Confusion can result when users leave endoscopes on movable carts, and it is unclear whether the endoscope has been processed or not. Although one guideline has recommended that an endoscope (e.g., a duodenoscope) should be reprocessed immediately before its use (131), other guidelines do not require this activity (2,34), and with the exception of the Association of periOperative Registered Nurses (AORN), professional organizations do not recommend that reprocessing be repeated so long as the original processing is done correctly.

As part of a quality assurance program, healthcare facility personnel may consider random bacterial surveillance cultures of processed endoscopes to ensure high-level disinfection or sterilization (7,143,144). Reprocessed endoscopes should be free of microbial pathogens except for small numbers of relatively avirulent microbes that represent exogenous environmental contamination (e.g., coagulase-negative staphylococci, *Bacillus* species, diphtheroids). It has also been suggested that the final rinse water used during endoscope reprocessing be microbiologically cultured at least monthly (145). The microbiologic standard that should be met has not been set. However, neither the routine culture of reprocessed endoscopes nor the final rinse water has been validated by correlating viable counts on an endoscope to infection following an endoscopic procedure. If culturing of reprocessed endoscopes were done, sampling the endoscope would assess water quality as well as other important steps (e.g., disinfectant effectiveness, exposure time, cleaning) in the reprocessing procedure. A number of methods for sampling endoscopes and water have been described (21,140,142,144,146, 147).

The carrying case used to transport clean and reprocessed endoscopes outside of the healthcare environment should not be used to store an endoscope or to transport the instrument within the healthcare facility. A contaminated endoscope should never be placed in the carrying case as the case can also become contaminated. When the endoscope is removed from the case and properly reprocessed and put back in the case, the endoscope can become recontaminated by the case. If the carrying case becomes contaminated, it should be discarded (Olympus America, written communication, June 2002).

Infection control professionals should ensure that institutional policies are consistent with national guidelines, and conduct infection control rounds periodically (e.g., at least annually) in areas where endoscopes are reprocessed to make certain there is compliance with policy. Breaches in policy should be documented and corrective action instituted. In incidents in which endoscopes were not exposed to a high-level disinfection process, all patients were assessed for possible acquisition of HIV, HBV, and hepatitis C virus (HCV). This highlights the importance of rigorous infection control (148,149).

Laparoscopes, Arthroscopes, and Cystoscopes

Although high-level disinfection appears to be the minimum standard for processing laparoscopes, arthroscopes, and cystoscopes between patients (24,77,150,151), there continues to be debate about this practice (80,81,152). However, neither side in the high-level disinfection versus sterilization debate has sufficient data on which to support its conclusions. Proponents of high-level disinfection refer to membership surveys (25) or institutional experiences (78) involving over 117,000 and 10,000 laparoscopic procedures, respectively, that cite a low risk of infection (<0.3%) when high-level disinfection is used for gynecologic laparoscopic equipment. Only one infection in the membership survey was linked to spores. In addition, studies conducted by Corson et al. (153,154) demonstrated growth of common skin microorganisms (e.g., *Staphylococcus epidermidis*, diphtheroids) from the umbilical area even after skin preparation with povidone-iodine and ethyl alcohol. Similar microorganisms were recovered in some instances from the pelvic serosal surfaces or from the laparoscopic telescopes, suggesting that the microorganisms probably were carried from the skin into the peritoneal cavity. Proponents of sterilization focus on the possibility of transmitting infection by spore-forming microorganisms. Researchers have proposed several reasons why sterility was not necessary for all laparoscopic equipment: only a limited number of microorganisms (usually ≤ 10) are introduced into the peritoneal cavity during laparoscopy; minimal damage is done to inner abdominal structures with little devitalized tissue; the peritoneal cavity tolerates small numbers of spore-forming bacteria; equipment is simple to clean and disinfect; surgical sterility is relative; the natural bioburden on rigid lumened devices is low (155); and no evidence that high-level disinfection, instead of sterilization, increases the infection risk (78,80,81). With the advent of laparoscopic cholecystectomy, there is justifiable concern with high-level disinfection as the degree of tissue damage and bacterial contamination is greater than with laparoscopic procedures in gynecology. Failure to completely dissemble, clean, and high-level disinfect the parts of a laparoscope has led to patient infections (156). Data from one study suggested that disassembly, cleaning, and proper assembly of laparoscopic equipment used in gynecologic procedures before steam sterilization presents no risk of infection (157).

As with laparoscopes and other equipment that enter sterile body sites, arthroscopes ideally should be sterilized before used. Older studies demonstrated that these instruments were commonly (57%) only high-level disinfected in the U.S. (24,77). A more recent survey, although with a response rate of only 5%, reported that high-level disinfection was used in 31% of the healthcare facilities and sterilization in the remainder (26). Presumably this is because the incidence of infection is low and the few infections are probably unrelated to the use of high-level disinfection rather than sterilization. In a retrospective study of 12,505 arthroscopic procedures, Johnston et al. (79) found an infection rate of 0.04% (five infections) when arthroscopes were soaked in 2% glutaraldehyde for 15 to 20 minutes. Four infections were caused by *S. aureus,* whereas the other was an anaerobic streptococcal infection. Since these microorganisms are very susceptible to high-level disinfectants such as 2% glutaraldehyde, the origin of these infections was likely the patient's skin. There are two case reports of *Clostridium perfringens* arthritis when the arthroscope was disinfected with glutaraldehyde for an exposure time that is not effective against spores (158,159).

Although only limited data are available, there is no evidence to demonstrate that high-level disinfection of arthroscopes, laparoscopes, or cystoscopes poses an infection risk to the patient. For example, a prospective study compared the reprocessing of arthroscopes and laparoscopes (per 1,000 procedures) with ETO sterilization to high-level disinfection with glutaraldehyde and found no statistically significant difference in infection risk between the two methods (i.e., ETO, 7.5/1,000 procedures; glutaraldehyde, 2.5/1,000 procedures) (80). The debate about high-level disinfection versus sterilization of laparoscopes and arthroscopes will go unsettled until there are published well-designed, randomized clinical trials. In the meantime, the recommendations of this chapter and the APIC and CDC guidelines should be followed (15,17,88). That is, laparoscopes, arthroscopes, cystoscopes, and other scopes that enter normally sterile tissue should be subjected to a sterilization procedure before each use; if this is not feasible, they should receive at least high-level disinfection.

Tonometers, Diaphragm Fitting Rings, Cryosurgical Instruments, and Endocavitary Probes

Disinfection strategies for other semicritical items (e.g., applanation tonometers, rectal/vaginal probes, cryosurgical instruments, and diaphragm fitting rings) are highly variable. For example, one study revealed that no uniform technique was in use for disinfection of applanation tonometers, with disinfectant contact times varying from <15 seconds to 20 minutes (24). In view of the potential for transmission of viruses [e.g., herpes simplex virus (HSV), adenovirus 8, or HIV] (160) by tonometer tips, the CDC recommends (86) that the tonometer tips be wiped clean and disinfected for 5 to 10 minutes with either 3% hydrogen peroxide, 5,000 parts per million (ppm) chlorine, 70% ethyl alcohol, or 70% isopropyl alcohol. Structural damage to Schiøtz tonometers has been observed with a 1:10 sodium hypochlorite (5,000 ppm chlorine) and 3% hydrogen peroxide (161). After disinfection, the tonometer should be thoroughly rinsed in tap water and air dried before use. Although these disinfectants and exposure times should kill pathogens that can infect the eyes, there are no studies that provide direct support (162, 163). The guidelines of the American Academy of Ophthalmology for preventing infections in ophthalmology focus on only one potential pathogen, HIV (164). Because a short and simple decontamination procedure is desirable in the clinical setting, swabbing the tonometer tip with a 70% isopropyl alcohol wipe is sometimes practiced (163). Preliminary reports suggest that wiping the tonometer tip with an alcohol swab and then allowing the alcohol to evaporate may be an effective means of eliminating HSV, HIV, and adenovirus (163,165,166). However, since these studies involved only a few replicates and were conducted in a controlled laboratory setting, further studies are needed before this technique can be recommended. In addition, two reports have found that disinfection of pneumotonometer tips between uses with a 70% isopropyl alcohol wipe contributed to outbreaks of epidemic keratoconjunctivitis caused by adenovirus type 8 (167,168).

There are also limited studies that evaluated disinfection techniques for other items that contact mucous membranes, such as diaphragm fitting rings, cryosurgical probes, transesophageal echocardiography probes (169), or vaginal/rectal probes used in sonographic scanning. Lettau et al. (87) of the CDC supported the recommendation of a diaphragm-fitting ring manufacturer that involved using a soap-and-water wash followed by a 15-minute immersion in 70% alcohol. This disinfection method should be adequate to inactivate HIV, HBV, and HSV even though alcohols are not classified as high-level disinfectants, because their activity against picornaviruses is somewhat limited (63). There are no data on the inactivation of human papillomavirus by alcohol or other disinfectants, because *in vitro* replication of complete virions has not been achieved. Thus, although alcohol for 15 minutes should kill pathogens of relevance in gynecology, there are no clinical studies that provide direct support for this practice.

Vaginal probes are used in sonographic scanning. A vaginal probe and all endocavitary probes without a probe cover are semicritical devices as they have direct contact with mucous membranes (e.g., vagina, rectum, pharynx). Although one could argue that the use of the probe cover changes the category, this chapter proposes that a new condom/probe cover should be used to cover the probe for each patient, and since condoms/probe covers may fail (169–172), high-level disinfection of the probe also should be performed. The relevance of this recommendation is reinforced with the findings that sterile transvaginal ultrasound probe covers have a very high rate of perforations even before use (0%, 25%, and 65% perforations from three suppliers) (172). After oocyte retrieval use, Hignett and Claman (172) found a very high rate of perforations in used endovaginal probe covers from two suppliers (75% and 81%), whereas Amis et al. (173) and Milki and Fisch (170) demonstrated a lower rate of perforations after use of condoms (0.9% and 2.0%, respectively). Rooks et al. (174) found that condoms were superior to commercially available probe covers for covering the ultrasound probe (1.7% for condoms versus 8.3% leakage for probe covers). These studies underscore the need for routine probe disinfection between examinations.

Although most ultrasound manufacturers recommend the use of 2% glutaraldehyde for high-level disinfection of contaminated transvaginal transducers, the use of this agent has been questioned (175), because it may shorten the life of the transducer and may have toxic effects on the gametes and embryos (176). An alternative procedure for disinfecting the vaginal transducer has been offered by Garland and de Crespigny (177). It involves the mechanical removal of the gel from the transducer, cleaning the transducer in soap and water, wiping the transducer with 70% alcohol or soaking it for 2 minutes in 500 ppm chlorine, and rinsing with tap water and air drying. The effectiveness of this and other methods (173) has not been validated in either rigorous laboratory experiments or clinical use. High-level disinfection with a product that is not toxic to staff, patients, probes, and retrieved cells (e.g., hydrogen peroxide) should be used until such time as the effectiveness of alternative procedures against microbes of importance at the cavitary site is scientifically demonstrated. Other probes such as rectal, cryosurgical, and transesophageal probes/devices should also be subjected to high-level disinfection between patients.

Ultrasound probes may also be used during surgical procedures and have contact with sterile body sites. These probes may be covered with a sterile sheath to reduce the level of contamination on the probe and reduce the risk of infection. However, since the sheath does not provide complete protection of the probe, the probes should be sterilized between each patient use as with other critical items.

Some cryosurgical probes are not fully immersible. When reprocessing these probes, the tip of the probe should be immersed in a high-level disinfectant for the appropriate time (e.g., 20 minutes exposure with 2% glutaraldehyde) and any other portion of the probe that could have mucous membrane contact could be disinfected by immersion or wrapping with a cloth soaked in a high-level disinfectant to allow the recommended contact time. After disinfection, the probe should be rinsed with tap water and dried before use. Healthcare facilities that use nonimmersible probes should replace them as soon as possible with fully immersible probes.

As with other high-level disinfection procedures, proper cleaning of probes is necessary to ensure the success of the subsequent disinfection (178). Muradali et al. (179) demonstrated a reduction of vegetative bacteria inoculated on vaginal ultrasound probes when the probes were cleaned with a towel. No information is available on either the level of contamination of such probes by potential viral pathogens such as HBV and human papilloma virus (HPV) or their removal by cleaning (such as with a towel). Because these pathogens may be present in vaginal and rectal secretions and contaminate probes during use, high-level disinfection of the probes after such use is recommended.

Dental Instruments

Scientific articles and increased publicity about the potential for transmitting infectious agents in dentistry have focused attention on dental instruments as possible agents for pathogen transmission (180,181). The American Dental Association recommends that surgical and other instruments that normally penetrate soft tissue or bone (e.g., forceps, scalpels, bone chisels, scalers, and surgical burs) be classified as critical devices that should be sterilized after each use or discarded. The recommendations for dental instruments are somewhat unique in that instruments that are not intended to penetrate oral soft tissues or bone (e.g., amalgam condensers, and air/water syringes) but may come in contact with oral tissues are classified as semicritical but are recommended to be sterilized after each use (182). This is consistent with recommendations from CDC and FDA (183, 184). Handpieces that cannot be heat sterilized should be retrofitted to attain heat tolerance. Handpieces that cannot be retrofitted and thus are not able to be heat sterilized should not be used (184). Chemical disinfection is not recommended for critical or semicritical dental instruments. Methods of sterilization that may be used for critical or semicritical dental instruments and materials that are heat-stable include steam under pressure (autoclave), chemical (formaldehyde) vapor, and dry heat (e.g., 320°F for 2 hours). The steam sterilizer is the method most commonly used by dental professionals (185). All three sterilization procedures can be damaging to some dental instruments, including steam-sterilized handpieces (186).

Several studies have demonstrated variability among dental practices while trying to meet these recommendations (187, 188). For example, 68% of respondents believed they were sterilizing their instruments but did not use appropriate chemical sterilants or exposure times, and 49% of respondents did not challenge autoclaves with biologic indicators (187). Other investigators using biologic indicators have found a high portion (15–65%) of positive spore tests after assessing the efficacy of sterilizers used in dental offices. In one study of Minnesota dental offices, operator error, rather than mechanical malfunction (189), caused 87% of sterilization failures. Common factors in the improper use of sterilizers include chamber overload, low temperature setting, inadequate exposure time, failure to preheat the sterilizer, and interruption of the cycle.

Mail-return sterilization monitoring services use spore strips to test sterilizers in dental clinics, but delay caused by mailing to the test laboratory could potentially cause false-negative results. Studies revealed, however, that the poststerilization time and temperature after a 7-day delay had no influence on the test results (190). Miller and Sheldrake (191) also found that delays (7 days at 27°C and 37°C, 3-day mail delay) did not cause any predictable pattern of inaccurate spore tests (191).

Uncovered operatory dental surfaces (e.g., countertops, chair switches, and light handles) should be disinfected between patients. This can be accomplished using products that are registered with the EPA as "hospital disinfectants." There are several chemical classes (e.g., phenolics) that can be used for this purpose (182,192,193). If waterproof surface covers are used to reduce contamination of surfaces and are carefully removed and replaced between patients, the protected surfaces do not need to be disinfected between patients (unless visibly contaminated) but should be disinfected at the end of each working day.

Decontamination of Bone

Bone is the second most frequently transplanted tissue in humans, after blood (194). The risk of infections transmissible by allografts (e.g., bones, tendons, and ligaments) depends on the technique applied for procurement, preservation, and bacteriologic control, and on the prevalence of infectious carriers. HIV (195) and *Clostridium sordelli* (196) have been transmitted by bone transplantation. Despite the infection control measures employed to select the donors, the risk of infectious agents associated with the tissue obtained for transplantation cannot be ignored, and a safe, dependable method of secondary sterilization without damaging the tissue or recipient is essential. Two sterilization methods (gamma irradiation and ETO) that would inactivate spores have been associated with problems (e.g., weakened tissue, increased toxicity) that limit their use in processing of tissues for transplantation.

Recently, a system to sterilize musculoskeletal tissues (e.g., bones, tendons) for use in bone grafting was developed using various chemical solutions to remove endogenous materials (e.g., blood, and bone marrow) and inactivate infectious agents. This vacuum-pressure cleaning system uses detergent, hydrogen peroxide, and alcohol in two cycles. Preliminary studies have shown it is effective in eliminating *B. stearothermophilus* spores (197).

Although not often mentioned, instances have occurred in which a graft has been dropped on the operating room floor. To determine the amount of microbial contamination that occurs when the graft is dropped, surplus bone specimens from 50 procedures were dropped and submitted for culture. No positive cultures were obtained (198). Another study evaluated the most effective method for disinfecting contaminated human bone-tendon allografts (i.e., beef muscle, cadaveric human bone-tendon allografts, and Achilles tendon-calcaneus allografts) (199). A 2% and 4% chlorhexidine irrigation solution and 4% chlorhexidine/triple antibiotic bath completely disinfected the test tissues after an exposure time of 10 to 12 minutes.

Disinfection of HBV-, HCV-, HIV- or Tuberculosis-Contaminated Devices

Should we sterilize or high-level disinfect semicritical medical devices contaminated with blood from patients infected with HBV, HCV, or HIV or with respiratory secretions from patients with pulmonary tuberculosis? The CDC recommendation for high-level disinfection is appropriate, because experiments have demonstrated the effectiveness of high-level disinfectants to inactivate these and other pathogens that may contaminate semicritical devices (54,55,64,72,95,106,110,200–215). Nonetheless, some healthcare facilities have modified their disinfection procedures when endoscopes are used with a patient known or suspected to be infected with HBV, HIV, or *M. tuberculosis* (24, 216). This is inconsistent with the concept of standard precautions that presumes that all patients are potentially infected with bloodborne pathogens (207). Several studies have highlighted the inability to distinguish HBV- or HIV-infected patients from noninfected patients on clinical grounds (217–219). It also is likely that mycobacterial infection will not be clinically apparent in many patients. In most instances, hospitals that altered their disinfection procedure used ETO sterilization on the endoscopic instruments, because they believed this practice reduced the risk of infection (24,216). ETO is not routinely used for endoscope sterilization because of the lengthy processing time. Endoscopes and other semicritical devices should be managed the same way whether or not the patient is known to be infected with HBV, HCV, HIV, or *M. tuberculosis*.

An evaluation of a manual disinfection procedure to eliminate HCV from experimentally contaminated endoscopes provided some evidence that cleaning and 2% glutaraldehyde for 20 minutes should prevent transmission (215). Using experimentally contaminated hysteroscopes, Sartor etal. (105) detected HCV by polymerase chain reaction (PCR) in one (3%) of 34 samples following cleaning with a detergent, but no samples were positive following treatment with a 2% glutaraldehyde solution for 20 minutes. Rey et al. (103) demonstrated complete elimination of HCV (as detected by PCR) from endoscopes used on chronically infected patients following cleaning and disinfection for 3 to 5 minutes in glutaraldehyde. Similarly, Chanzy et al. (215) used PCR to demonstrate complete elimination of HCV following standard disinfection of experimentally contaminated endoscopes. The inhibitory activity of a phenolic and a chlorine compound on HCV showed that the phenolic inhibited the binding and replication of HCV but the chlorine was ineffective, probably due to its low concentration and its neutralization in the presence of organic matter (220).

Disinfection in the Hemodialysis Unit

Hemodialysis systems include hemodialysis machines, water supply, water treatment systems, and the distribution system. During hemodialysis, patients have acquired bloodborne viruses and pathogenic bacteria (221–223). Cleaning and disinfection are important components of infection control in a hemodialysis center. Disinfectants used to reprocess hemodialyzers, hemodialysis machines, and water treatments systems are now regulated by the FDA as a class II medical device, subject to 510[k] clearance.

Disinfection on noncritical surfaces (e.g., dialysis bed or chair, countertops, external surfaces of dialysis machines, and equipment—scissors, hemostats, clamps, blood pressure cuffs, stethoscopes) should be done with low-level disinfectants unless the item is visibly contaminated with blood, in which case a tuberculocidal agent (or a disinfectant with specific label claims for HBV and HIV) should be used (222,224). This procedure accomplishes two goals: it removes soil on a regular basis, and maintains an environment that is consistent with good patient care. Disinfection of hemodialyzers is accomplished with peracetic acid, formaldehyde, glutaraldehyde, heat and citric acid, and chlorine-containing compounds. Disinfection of hemodialysis systems is normally accomplished by chlorine-based disinfectants (e.g., sodium hypochlorite), aqueous formaldehyde, heat pasteurization, ozone, or peracetic acid. All products must be used according to the manufacturers' recommendations. Some dialysis systems use hot-water disinfection for the control of microbial contamination.

Since about 80% of U.S. chronic hemodialysis centers reprocess (i.e., reuse) dialyzers for the same patient, high-level disinfection is also common in dialysis centers. Three disinfectants were commonly used in a 2000 survey: a peracetic acid formulation was used by 59% of centers that reused dialyzers, formaldehyde by 31%, and glutaraldehyde by 5%. A heat process (221,222, 225) was used by 4%. Detailed infection control recommendations, to include disinfection and sterilization and the use of dedicated machines for hepatitis B surface antigen (HBsAg)-positive patients, in the hemodialysis setting may be found in two reviews (221,222).

Inactivation of *Clostridium difficile*

The source of healthcare-associated acquisition of *C. difficile* in nonepidemic settings has not been determined. The environment and carriage on the hands of healthcare personnel have been considered as possible sources of infection. Carpeted rooms occupied by a patient with *C. difficile* are more heavily contaminated with *C. difficile* than noncarpeted rooms (226). Since *C. difficile* may display increased levels of spore production when exposed to non–chlorine-based cleaning agents and the spores are more resistant than vegetative cells to commonly used surface disinfectants (227), some investigators have recommended the use of dilute solutions of hypochlorite (1,600 ppm available chlorine) for routine environmental disinfection of rooms of patients with *C. difficile*–associated diarrhea or colitis (228) or in units with high *C. difficile* rates (229). Mayfield et al. (229) showed a marked reduction in *C. difficile*–associated diarrhea rates in the bone marrow transplant unit (from 8.6 to 3.3 cases per 1,000 patient-days) during the period of bleach disinfection (1:10 dilution) of environmental surfaces compared to cleaning with a quaternary ammonium compound. Thus, use of a diluted hypochlorite should be considered in units with high *C. difficile* rates. However, studies have shown that asymptomatic patients constitute an important reservoir within the healthcare facility and that person-to-person transmission is the principal means of transmission between patients. Thus, handwashing, barrier precautions, and meticulous environmental cleaning with a low-level disinfectant (e.g., germicidal detergent) should be effective in preventing the spread of the microorganism (230).

Contaminated medical devices such as colonoscopes could serve as vehicles for the transmission of *C. difficile* spores. For this reason, investigators have studied commonly used disinfectants and exposure times to assess whether current practices may be placing patients at risk. Data demonstrate that 2% glutaraldehyde reliably kills *C. difficile* spores using exposure times of 5 to 20 minutes (70,231,232).

Inactivation of Creutzfeldt-Jakob Disease Agent

Creutzfeldt-Jakob disease (CJD) is a degenerative neurologic disorder of humans with an incidence in the U.S. of approximately 1 case/million population/year (233,234). CJD is thought to be caused by a proteinaceous infectious agent or prion. CJD is related to other human transmissible spongiform encephalopathies (TSEs) that include kuru (zero incidence, now eradicated), Gertsmann-Sträussler-Scheinker (GSS) syndrome (1/billion), and fatal familial insomnia syndrome (FFI) (<1/billion). Prion diseases do not elicit an immune response, result in a noninflammatory pathologic process confined to the central nervous system, have an incubation period of years, and usually are fatal within 1 year of diagnosis.

Recently, a new variant form of CJD (vCJD) has been recognized that is acquired from cattle with bovine spongiform encephalopathy (BSE, or "mad-cow" disease). As of November 4, 2002, a total of 138 vCJD cases have been reported worldwide, 128 in the United Kingdom, six in France, and one each in Italy, Ireland, Canada, and the U.S. (235). Each of the latter three cases had resided in the U.K. during the U.K. outbreak of BSE (L Schonberger, written communication, 2002). Compared with CJD patients, vCJD patients are younger (29 vs. 65 years of age), have a longer duration of illness (14 vs. 4.5 months), and present with sensory and psychiatric symptoms that are uncommon with CJD.

The agents of CJD and other TSEs exhibit an unusual resistance to conventional chemical and physical decontamination methods. Since the CJD agent is not readily inactivated by conventional disinfection and sterilization procedures and because of the invariably fatal outcome of CJD, the procedures for disinfection and sterilization of the CJD prion have been both cautious and controversial for many years.

CJD occurs as both a sporadic and familial disease. Less than 1% of CJD episodes have resulted from healthcare-associated transmission; the majority result from use of contaminated tissues or grafts. Iatrogenic CJD has been described in humans in three circumstances: after use of contaminated medical equipment on patients undergoing invasive procedures (two confirmed cases); after patients received extracted pituitary hormones (>130 cases); and after patients received an implant of contaminated grafts from humans (cornea, three cases; dura mater, >110 cases) (236,237). All known instances of iatrogenic CJD have resulted from exposure to infectious brain, pituitary, or eye tissue. Tissue infectivity studies in experimental animals have determined the infectiousness of different body tissues

(Table 85.3) (238,239). Transmission via stereotactic electrodes is the only convincing example of transmission via a medical device. The electrodes had been implanted in a patient with known CJD and then cleaned with benzene and "sterilized" with 70% alcohol and formaldehyde vapor. Two years later, these electrodes were retrieved and implanted into a chimpanzee in which the disease developed (240). The method used to sterilize these electrodes would not currently be considered an adequate method for sterilizing medical devices. The infrequent transmission of CJD via contaminated medical devices probably reflects the inefficiency of transmission unless dealing with neural tissue and the effectiveness of conventional cleaning and current disinfection and sterilization procedures (241). Retrospective studies suggest four other episodes may have resulted from use of contaminated instruments in neurosurgical operations (242,243). An index CJD case was identified in one case and in this case the surgical instruments were cleaned with soap and water followed by exposure to dry heat for an unspecified time and temperature (243). All six cases of CJD associated with neurosurgical instruments occurred in Europe between 1953 and 1976 and details of the reprocessing methods for the instruments are incomplete (L. M. Sehulster, written communication, 2000). There are no known episodes of CJD attributable to the reuse of devices contaminated with blood or via transfusion of blood products. The risk of occupational transmission of CJD to a healthcare worker is remote. Healthcare workers should use standard precautions when caring for patients with CJD.

To minimize the possibility of use of neurosurgical instruments that have been potentially contaminated during procedures performed on patients in whom CJD is later diagnosed, healthcare facilities should consider using the sterilization guidelines outlined below for neurosurgical instruments used during brain biopsy done on patients in whom a specific lesion has not been demonstrated (e.g., by magnetic resonance imaging or computed tomography scans). Alternatively, neurosurgical instruments used in such patients could be disposable (241) or instruments quarantined until the pathology of the brain biopsy is reviewed and CJD excluded.

The inactivation of prions by disinfectant and sterilization processes has been studied by several investigators, but these studies do not reflect the reprocessing procedures in a clinical setting. First, these studies have not incorporated a cleaning procedure that normally reduces microbial contamination by 4 $\log_{10}$ (15) and reduces protein contamination (244–246). Second, the prion studies have been done with tissue homogenates, and the protective effect of tissue may explain, in part, why the CJD agent is difficult to inactivate (247). Brain homogenates have been shown to confer thermal stability to small subpopulations of the scrapie agent and some viruses. Third, results of inactivation studies of prions have been inconsistent due to the use of differing methodologies, which may have varied by prion strain, prion concentration, test tissue (intact brain tissue, brain homogenates, partially purified preparations), test animals, duration of follow-up of inoculated animals, exposure container, method of calculating log-reductions in infectivity, concentration of the disinfectant at the beginning and end of an experiment, cycle parameters of the sterilizer, and exposure conditions. Despite these limitations, there is some consistency in the results (241, 248). To provide scientifically based recommendations, research in which actual medical instruments are contaminated with prions (including vCJD) followed by cleaning and either conventional sterilization or disinfection, or special prion reprocessing, should be undertaken.

Based on the disinfection studies many, but not all, disinfection processes fail to inactivate clinically significant numbers of prions (Table 85.4) (249–263). There are four chemicals that reduce the prion titer by $>3 \log_{10}$ in 1 hour: chlorine, a phenolic (based on ortho-phenylphenol, p-tertiary-amylphenol and ortho-benzyl-para-chlorophenol) at >0.9%, guanidine thiocyanante, and sodium hydroxide. Of these four chemical compounds, chlorine has provided the most consistent prion inacti-

TABLE 85.3. COMPARATIVE FREQUENCY OF INFECTIVITY IN ORGANS/TISSUE/BODY FLUIDS OF HUMANS WITH TRANSMISSIBLE SPONGIFORM ENCEPHALOPATHIES

Infectious Risks[1]	Tissue
High	Brain (including dura mater), spinal cord, eyes
Low	Cerebrospinal fluid, liver, lymph node, kidney, lung, spleen, placenta
None	Peripheral nerve, intestine, bone marrow, whole blood, leukocytes, serum, thyroid gland, adrenal gland, heart, skeletal muscle, adipose tissue, gingiva, prostate, testis, tears, nasal mucus, saliva, sputum, urine, feces, semen, vaginal secretions, milk

Modified from 236, 241, 706.
[1] Infectious risks: high=transmission to inoculated animals > 50%; low=transmission to inoculated animals ≥10–20% (except for lung tissue, for which transmission is 50%); none=transmission to inoculated animals 0% (several tissues in this category had few tested specimens).

TABLE 85.4. EFFICACY OF CHEMICAL DISINFECTANTS IN INACTIVATING PRIONS

Ineffective chemical disinfectants ($\leq$3-$\log_{10}$ reduction in 1 hour)	Effective chemical disinfectants ($>$3-$\log_{10}$ reduction in 1 hour)
Alcohol 50%	Chlorine >1,000 ppm
Ammonia 1.0M	Guanidine thiocyanate
Chlorine dioxide 50 ppm	Guanidine thiocyanate
Formaldehyde 3.7%	A phenolic disinfectant (see CJD text) >0.9%
Glutaraldehyde 5%	
Hydrochloric acid 1.0 N	
Hydrogen peroxide 3%	
Iodine 2%	
Peracetic acid	
Phenol/phenolics 0.6%	
Potassium permanganate 0.1–0.8%	
Sodium deoxycholate 5%	
Sodium dodecyl sulfate 0.5–5%	
Tego (dodecyl-di[aminoethyl]-glycine) 5%	
Triton X-100 1%	
Urea 4–8 M	

Modified from 241, 707.

vation results (241). However, the corrosive nature of chlorine makes it unsuitable for semicritical devices such as endoscopes.

Prions also exhibit an unusual resistance to conventional physical decontamination methods (Table 85.5). Although there is some disagreement on the ideal time and temperature cycle for autoclaving, the recommendation for 134°C for ≥18 minutes (prevacuum) and 132°C for 60 minutes (gravity displacement) are based on the scientific literature (251–253,255,259,262, 264,265). Some investigators also have found that combining sodium hydroxide (e.g., 0.09 N for 2 hours) with steam sterilization for 1 hour at 121°C results in complete loss of infectivity (255,265). However, the combination of sodium hydroxide and steam sterilization may be deleterious to surgical instruments (248), sterilizers, as well as sterilizer operators who could be breathing vaporized chemicals unless engineering controls or use of personal protective equipment (PPE) prevents exposure.

The disinfection and sterilization recommendations for CJD in this chapter are based on the belief that infection control measures should be predicated on epidemiologic evidence linking specific body tissues or fluids to transmission of CJD, infectivity assays demonstrating that body tissues or fluids are contaminated with infectious prions, cleaning data using biologic indicators and proteins (74,244,245), inactivation data of prions, the risk of disease transmission with the use of the instrument or device, and a review of other recommendations (11, 266,267; L. M. Sehulster, written communication, 2000). Other CJD recommendations have been based primarily on inactivation studies (15,248,268). Thus, the three parameters integrated into disinfection and sterilization processing are the risk of the patient's having a prion disease, the comparative infectivity of different body tissues, and the intended use of the medical device (11,266,267; L. M. Sehulster, written communication, 2000). High-risk patients include those with known prion disease; rapidly progressive dementia consistent with possible prion disease; familial history of CJD, GSS, FFI; patients known to carry a mutation in the *PrP* gene involved in familial TSEs; a history of dura mater transplants; or a known history of cadaver-derived pituitary hormone injection. High-risk tissues include brain, spinal cord, and eye. All other tissues are considered low or no risk (Table 85.3). Critical devices are defined as devices that enter sterile tissue or the vascular system (e.g., implants). Semicritical devices are defined as devices that contact nonintact skin or mucous membranes (e.g., endoscopes). The AORN recommended practices for reprocessing surgical instruments exposed to CJD are consistent with the following recommendations (241,269).

TABLE 85.5. EFFICACY OF STERILIZATION PROCESSES IN INACTIVATING PRIONS

Ineffective sterilization processes (≤3-$\log_{10}$ reduction in 1 hour)	Effective sterilization processes (>3-$\log_{10}$ reduction in 1 hour)
Autoclaving at conventional exposure conditions (121°C for 15 minutes)	Autoclaving at 134°C for 18 minutes (prevacuum sterilizer)
Dry heat	Autoclaving 121–132°C for 1 hr (gravity displacement sterilizer)
Ethylene oxide	0.09N or 0.9N NaOH for 2 hours plus 121°C for 1 hour (gravity displacement sterilizer)
Formaldehyde	
Boiling	
Ultraviolet light	

Modified from 241,707.

Recommendations for disinfection and sterilization of prion-contaminated medical devices are as follows. For high-risk tissues, high-risk patients, and critical or semicritical medical devices, clean the device and sterilize preferably using a combination of sodium hydroxide and autoclaving as recommended by the World Health Organization (WHO) (236) [e.g., immerse in 1 N NaOH (1 N NaOH is a solution of 40 g NaOH in 1 L of water) for 1 hour; remove and rinse in water, then transfer to an open pan and autoclave (121°C gravity displacement or 134°C porous or prevacuum sterilizer) for 1 hour; or immerse instruments in 1 N NaOH for 1 hour and heat in a gravity displacement sterilizer at 121°C for 30 minutes; clean; and subject to routine sterilization], or by autoclaving at 134°C for 18 minutes in a prevacuum sterilizer, or 132°C for 1 hour in a gravity displacement sterilizer. The temperature should not exceed 134°C since under certain conditions the effectiveness of autoclaving actually declines as the temperature is increased (e.g., 136°C, 138°C) (264). The combined use of autoclaving in sodium hydroxide has raised concerns of possible damage to autoclaves (T. K. Moore, written communication, October 2002), and hazards to operators due to the caustic vapors. This risk can be minimized by the use of polypropylene containment pans and lids designed for condensation to collect and drip back into the pan (270). Hot NaOH is more caustic than NaOH at room temperature, so even greater care should be taken to avoid exposure to it when hot (D. Asher, written communication, November 2002). Instruments should be kept wet or damp until they are decontaminated and they should be decontaminated as soon as possible after use. Dried films of tissue are more resistant to prion inactivation by steam sterilization compared to tissues that were kept moist. This may relate to the rapid heating that occurs in the film of dried material compared to the bulk of the sample, and the rapid fixation of the prion protein in the dried film (259). It also appears that prions in the dried portions of the brain macerates are less efficiently inactivated than undisturbed tissue. Prion-contaminated medical devices that are impossible or difficult to clean should be discarded. Flash sterilization should not be used for reprocessing. To minimize environmental contamination, noncritical environmental surfaces should be covered with plastic-backed paper and when contaminated with high-risk tissues the paper should be properly discarded. Environmental surfaces (noncritical) contaminated with high-risk tissues (e.g., laboratory surfaces) should be cleaned and then spot decontaminated with a 1:10 dilution of hypochlorite solutions.

For added safety, one could consider reprocessing critical or semicritical devices contaminated with low-risk tissues from high-risk patients with special prion reprocessing. Although low risk tissue has been found to transmit CJD at a low frequency (Table 85.3), this has been demonstrated only when low-risk tissue is inoculated into the brain of a susceptible animal. However, in humans, medical instruments contaminated with low-risk tissue would be unlikely to transmit infection following conventional cleaning and sterilization since the instruments would not be used in the central nervous system. Environmental surfaces contaminated with low-risk tissues require only standard (i.e., blood-contaminated) disinfection (11,241,266). Since noncritical surfaces are not involved in disease transmission, the normal exposure time (≤10 minutes) is recommended.

Most of the data that form the basis of these recommendations have been generated from studies of the prions responsible for sporadic CJD or animal TSE diseases (e.g., scrapie). Limited data are available on which to base recommendations for the prevention of vCJD. To date, there have been no reports of human-to-human transmission of vCJD by blood or tissue. Unlike sporadic CJD, patients with vCJD have prions detectable in the lymphoid tissue. Furthermore, prion proteins may be detectable before the onset of clinical illness. This has raised concern about the possible human-to-human transmission of vCJD by medical instruments contaminated with such tissues. On the basis of these concerns, the use of prion disinfection and sterilization guidelines (or single-use instruments) has been proposed in the U.K. for instruments used in dental procedures (271), eye procedures (272), or tonsillar surgery (273) on patients at high risk of sporadic CJD or vCJD. Following complications (death in one patient and increased bleeding) associated with the use of single-use instruments in tonsillar surgery, it is now advised in the U.K. that given the balance of risk, surgeons can return to using reusable surgical equipment. If epidemiologic and infectivity data show that these tissues represent a transmission risk, then CJD sterilization precautions (or use of disposable equipment) could be extended to equipment used for these procedures (274). In addition, chronic wasting disease in deer and elk have been spreading in the midwestern U.S. Transmission of chronic wasting disease to humans has not been described.

OSHA Bloodborne Pathogen Standard

In December 1991, the Occupational Safety and Health Administration (OSHA) promulgated a standard entitled "Occupational Exposure to Bloodborne Pathogens" to eliminate or minimize occupational exposure to bloodborne pathogens (275). One component of this requirement is that all equipment and environmental and working surfaces be cleaned and decontaminated with an appropriate disinfectant after contact with blood or other potentially infectious materials. Although the OSHA standard does not specify the type of disinfectant or procedure, the OSHA compliance document (276) suggests that a germicide must be tuberculocidal to kill the HBV. Thus, it suggests that a tuberculocidal agent should be used to clean blood spills on noncritical surfaces. To follow the OSHA compliance document, a tuberculocidal disinfectant (e.g., phenolic, chlorine) would be needed to clean a blood spill. This caused concern among housekeeping managers who tried to identify disinfectant detergents claiming to be tuberculocidal on the assumption that such products would be effective in eliminating transmission of HBV. This directive could be problematic on a practical level for three reasons. First, nontuberculocidal disinfectants such as quaternary ammonium compounds inactivate the HBV (208). Second, noncritical surfaces are rarely, if ever, involved in disease transmission (33). Third, the exposure times that manufacturers use to achieve their label claims are not employed in healthcare settings to disinfect noncritical surfaces. For example, to make a label claim against HBV, HIV, or *M. tuberculosis,* a manufacturer must demonstrate inactivation of these microorganisms when exposed to a disinfectant for 10 minutes. This cannot be practically achieved for disinfection of environmental surfaces in a healthcare setting. The EPA will allow a label of a shorter exposure time when supported by test data. Multiple scientific papers have demonstrated significant microbial reduction with exposure times of less than 10 minutes (39–49,51–57). For this reason and since exposure times of 10 minutes or greater are not feasible for disinfection of environmental surfaces in healthcare settings, most healthcare facilities apply the disinfectant and allow it to dry (~1 minute). However, contact times should be at least 30 seconds to achieve significant microbial inactivation.

In February 1997, OSHA amended its policy and stated that EPA-registered disinfectants that are labeled as effective against HIV and HBV would be considered as appropriate disinfectants "provided such surfaces have not become contaminated with agent(s) or volumes of or concentrations of agent(s) for which higher level disinfection is recommended." When bloodborne pathogens other than HBV or HIV are of concern, OSHA continues to require the use of EPA-registered tuberculocidal disinfectants or hypochlorite solution (diluted 1:10 or 1:100 with water) (207,277). Recent studies demonstrate that, in the presence of large blood spills, a 1:10 final dilution of hypochlorite solution should be initially used to inactivate bloodborne viruses (56,214) to minimize risk of disease to the healthcare worker from percutaneous injury during the cleanup process.

Emerging Pathogens (*Cryptosporidium, H. pylori, E. coli* O157:H7, Rotavirus, Human Papilloma Virus, Norwalk Virus)

Emerging pathogens are of growing concern to the general public and infection control professionals. Relevant pathogens include *Cryptosporidium parvum, H. pylori, E. coli* O157:H7, HIV, HCV, rotavirus, multidrug-resistant *M. tuberculosis,* and nontuberculosis mycobacteria (e.g., *M. chelonae*). The susceptibility of each of these pathogens to chemical disinfectants/sterilants has been studied. With the exceptions discussed below, all of these emerging pathogens are susceptible to currently available chemical disinfectants/sterilants (278).

Cryptosporidium is resistant to chlorine at concentrations used in potable water. *C. parvum* is not completely inactivated by most disinfectants used in healthcare including ethyl alcohol (279), glutaraldehyde (279,280), 5.25% hypochlorite (279), peracetic acid (279), OPA (279), phenol (279,280), povidone-iodine (279,280), and quaternary ammonium compounds (279). The only chemical disinfectants/sterilants able to inactivate greater than 3 $\log_{10}$ of *C. parvum* were 6% and 7.5% hydrogen peroxide (279). Sterilization methods will fully inactivate *C. parvum,* including steam (279), ethylene oxide (279,281), and hydrogen peroxide gas plasma (279). Although most disinfectants are ineffective against *C. parvum,* current cleaning and disinfection practices appear satisfactory to prevent healthcare-associated transmission. For example, endoscopes are unlikely to represent an important vehicle for the transmission of *C.*

parvum because the results of bacterial studies indicate mechanical cleaning will remove approximately 10^4 microorganisms and drying rapidly results in loss of *C. parvum* viability (e.g., 30 minutes, 2.9 $\log_{10}$ decrease, and 60 minutes, 3.8 $\log_{10}$ decrease) (279).

Chlorine at ~1 ppm has been found capable of eliminating approximately 4 $\log_{10}$ of *E. coli* O157:H7 within 1 minute in a suspension test (57). Electrolyzed oxidizing water at 23°C was effective in 10 minutes in producing a 5-$\log_{10}$ decrease in *E. coli* O157:H7 inoculated onto kitchen cutting boards (282). The following disinfectants eliminated >5 $\log_{10}$ of *E. coli* O157:H7 within 30 seconds: a quaternary ammonium compound, a phenolic, a hypochlorite (1:10 dilution of 5.25% bleach), and ethanol (46). Disinfectants including chlorine compounds are able to reduce *E. coli* O157:H7 experimentally inoculated onto alfalfa seeds or sprouts (283,284) or beef carcass surfaces (285).

Only limited data are available on the susceptibility of *H. pylori* to disinfectants. Using a suspension test, Akamatsu et al. (53) assessed the effectiveness of a variety of disinfectants against nine strains of *H. pylori.* Ethanol (80%) and glutaraldehyde (0.5%) killed all strains within 15 seconds; chlorhexidine gluconate (0.05%, 1.0%), benzalkonium chloride (0.025%, 0.1%), alkyldiaminoethylglycine hydrochloride (0.1%), povidone-iodine (0.1%), and sodium hypochlorite (150 ppm) killed all strains within 30 seconds. Both ethanol (80%) and glutaraldehyde (0.5%) retained similar bactericidal activity in the presence of organic matter, whereas the other disinfectants showed reduced bactericidal activity. In particular, the bactericidal activity of povidone-iodine (0.1%) and sodium hypochlorite (150 ppm) was markedly decreased in the presence of dried yeast solution with killing times increased to 5 to 10 minutes and 5 to 30 minutes, respectively.

Immersion of biopsy forceps in formalin before obtaining a specimen does not affect the ability to culture *H. pylori* from the biopsy specimen (286). The following methods have been demonstrated to be ineffective for eliminating *H. pylori* from endoscopes: cleaning with soap and water (104,287), immersion in 70% ethanol for 3 minutes (288), instillation of 70% ethanol (111), instillation of 30 mL of 83% methanol (287), and instillation of 0.2% Hyamine solution (289). The differing results with regard to the efficacy of ethyl alcohol are unexplained. Cleaning followed by use of 2% alkaline glutaraldehyde (or automated peracetic acid) has been demonstrated by culture to be effective in eliminating *H. pylori* (104,287,290). Epidemiologic investigations of patients who had undergone endoscopy with endoscopes mechanically washed and disinfected with 2.0% to 2.3% glutaraldehyde have revealed no evidence of person-to-person transmission of *H. pylori* (111,291). Disinfection of experimentally contaminated endoscopes using 2% glutaraldehyde (10-, 20-, and 45-minute exposure times) or the peracetic acid system (with and without active peracetic acid) has been demonstrated to be effective in eliminating *H. pylori* (104). *H. pylori* DNA has been detected by PCR in fluid flushed from endoscope channels following cleaning and disinfection with 2% glutaraldehyde (292). The clinical significance of this finding is unclear. *In vitro* experiments have demonstrated a >3.5-$\log_{10}$ reduction in *H. pylori* after exposure to 0.5 mg/L of free chlorine for 80 seconds (293).

An outbreak of healthcare-associated rotavirus gastroenteritis on a pediatric unit has been reported (294). Person-to-person transmission via the hands of healthcare workers was the proposed mechanism. Prolonged survival of rotavirus on environmental surfaces (90 minutes to more than 10 days at room temperature) and hands (>4 hours) has been demonstrated. Rotavirus suspended in feces can survive for a longer period of time (295,296). Vectors for this infection have included air, hands, fomites, water, and food (296). Products with demonstrated efficacy (>3 $\log_{10}$ reduction in virus) against rotavirus within 1 minute include 95% ethanol, 70% isopropanol, some phenolics, 2% glutaraldehyde, 0.35% peracetic acid, and some quaternary ammonium compounds (52,297–299). In a human challenge study, a disinfectant spray (0.1% ortho-phenylphenol and 79% ethanol), sodium hypochlorite (800 ppm free chlorine), and a phenol-based product (14.7% phenol diluted 1:256 in tap water) when sprayed onto contaminated stainless steel disks, were effective in interrupting the transfer of a human rotavirus from stainless steel disk to fingerpads of volunteers after an exposure time of 3 to 10 minutes. A quaternary ammonium product (7.05% quaternary ammonium compound diluted 1:128 in tap water) and tap water allowed transfer of virus (45).

There are no data on the inactivation of human papillomavirus by alcohol or other disinfectants because *in vitro* replication of complete virions has not been achieved. Similarly, little is known about the inactivation of Norwalk virus and Norwalk virus–like particles (members of the family Caliciviridae and important causes of gastroenteritis in humans), as they cannot be grown in tissue culture. Inactivation studies with a closely related cultivable virus (i.e., feline calicivirus) have shown the effectiveness of chlorine, glutaraldehyde, and iodine-based products, whereas the quaternary ammonium compound, detergent, and ethanol failed to inactivate the virus completely (300).

Inactivation of Bioterrorism Agents

Regarding the potential for biologic terrorism (301,302), the CDC has categorized several agents as "high priority" because they can be easily disseminated or transmitted person to person, cause high mortality, and are likely to cause public panic and social disruption (303). These agents include *Bacillus anthracis* (anthrax), *Yersinia pestis* (plague), variola major (smallpox), *Clostridium botulinum* toxin (botulism), *Francisella tularensis* (tularemia), filoviruses (Ebola hemorrhagic fever, Marburg hemorrhagic fever); and arenaviruses [Lassa (Lassa fever), Junin (Argentine hemorrhagic fever)], and related viruses (303).

Sterilization and disinfection have a role regarding the potential agents of bioterrorism. First, the susceptibility of these agents to germicides *in vitro* is similar to other related pathogens. For example, variola is similar to vaccinia (63) and *B. anthracis* is similar to *B. atrophaeus* (formerly *B. subtilis)* (304). Thus, one can extrapolate from the larger database available on the susceptibility of genetically similar microorganisms. Second, many of the potential bioterrorist agents are stable enough in the environment that contaminated environmental surfaces or fomites could lead to transmission of agents such as *B. anthracis, F. tularensis,* variola major, *C. botulinum* toxin, and *C. burnetti* (305). Third, data suggest that current disinfection and sterilization practices are appropriate for the management of patient care equipment and environmental surfaces when potentially contaminated patients are evaluated in or admitted to a healthcare facility following exposure to a bioterrorist agent. For example, sodium hypochlorite may be used for surface disinfection (*http://www.epa.gov/pesticides/factsheets/bleachfactsheet.htm*). In instances where the healthcare facility is the site of a bioterrorist attack, environmental decontamination may require special decontamination procedures (e.g., chlorine dioxide gas for anthrax spores; *http://www.epa.gov/pesticides/factsheets/chlorinedioxidefactsheet.htm*). Use of disinfectants for decontamination following a bioterrorist attack requires crises exemption from the EPA (*http://www.epa.-gov/opprd001/section18/*). Of only theoretical concern is the possibility that a bioterrorism agent could be engineered to be less susceptibility to disinfection and sterilization processes.

Toxicologic, Environmental, and Occupational Concerns

Health hazards associated with the use of germicides in healthcare vary from mucous membrane irritation to death, with the latter involving accidental injection by mentally disturbed patients (306). Although variations exist in the degree of toxicity ([Hess, 1991 #9210]; 307,308), all disinfectants should be used with the proper safety precautions (309) and for the intended purpose only.

The key factors associated with assessing the health risk of a chemical exposure include the duration, intensity (i.e., how much chemical is involved), and route (e.g., skin, mucous membranes, and inhalation) of the exposure. Toxicity may be acute or chronic. Acute toxicity usually results from an accidental spill of a chemical substance. The exposure of personnel is sudden and often produces an emergency situation. Chronic toxicity results from repeated exposure to low levels of the chemical over a prolonged period. The responsibility for informing workers of the chemical hazards in the workplace and implementing control measures rests with the employer. The OSHA Hazard Communication Standard (Code of Federal Regulations 29 CFR 1910.1200, 1915.99, 1917.28, 1918.90, 1926.59, and 1928.21) requires manufacturers and importers of hazardous chemicals to develop Material Safety Data Sheets (MSDSs) for each chemical or mixture of chemicals. Employers must have MSDSs readily available to employees who work with the products and thus may be exposed.

Exposure limits have been published for many chemicals used in healthcare to aid in providing a safe environment and are discussed in each section of this chapter as relevant. Only the exposure limits published by OSHA carry the legal force of regulations. OSHA publishes a limit as a time weighted average (TWA), that is, the average concentration for a normal 8-hour workday and a 40-hour workweek to which nearly all workers may be repeatedly exposed to a chemical without adverse health effects. For example, the permissible exposure limit (PEL) for ethylene oxide is 1.0 ppm, 8-hour TWA. The National Institute for Occupational Safety and Health (NIOSH) develops recommended exposure limits (RELs). RELs are recommended by NIOSH as being protective of worker health and safety over a working lifetime. This limit is frequently expressed as a 40-hour TWA exposure for up to 10 hours per day during a 40-hour workweek. These exposure limits are designed for inhalation exposures. Irritant and allergic affects may occur below the exposure limits, and skin contact may result in dermal effects or systemic absorption apart from inhalation. The current RELs can be accessed via the NIOSH Web page (*www.cdc.gov/niosh*). Guidelines on exposure limits are also provided by the American Conference of Governmental Industrial Hygienists (ACGIH) (310). Additionally, information about workplace exposures and methods to reduce them (e.g., work practices, engineering controls, PPE) is available on the OSHA (*www.osha.gov*) and the NIOSH Web sites.

Some states have excluded the disposal of certain chemical germicides (e.g., glutaraldehyde, formaldehyde, and some phenols) or limited certain concentrations via the sewer system. These rules are intended to minimize environmental harm. If healthcare facilities exceed the maximum allowable concentration for a chemical (e.g., $\geq$5.0 mg/L), they have three options. First, they can switch to alternative products. For example, they can change from glutaraldehyde to another disinfectant for high-level disinfection or from phenolics to quaternary ammonium compounds for low-level disinfection. Second, they can collect the disinfectant and dispose of it as a hazardous chemical. Third, they can use a commercially available small-scale treatment method (e.g., neutralize glutaraldehyde with glycine).

The safe disposal of regulated chemicals is important throughout the medical community. In the case of disposal of large volumes of spent solutions, users may decide to neutralize the microbicidal activity prior to disposal (e.g., glutaraldehyde). This can be accomplished by reaction with chemicals such as sodium bisulfite (311,312) or glycine (313).

European authors have suggested that disinfection by heat rather than chemicals should be used for instruments and ventilation therapy equipment. The concerns for chemical disinfection include the toxic side effects for the patient caused by chemical residues on the instrument or object, occupational exposure to toxic chemicals, and the danger of recontamination by rinsing the disinfectant with microbially contaminated tap water (314).

Disinfection in Ambulatory Care, Home Care, and the Home

With the advent of managed healthcare, increasing numbers of patients are now being cared for in ambulatory care and in home settings. Many of these patients have communicable diseases, immunocompromising conditions, or invasive devices. Therefore, adequate disinfection in these settings is necessary to provide a safe patient environment. Since the ambulatory care setting (i.e., outpatient facilities) provides the same infection risk as the hospital, the Spaulding classification scheme described above should be followed (Table 85.1) (15).

The home environment should be a much safer setting than hospitals or ambulatory care. Epidemics should not be a problem and cross-infection should be rare. Among the products recommended for home disinfection of reusable objects are bleach, alcohol, and hydrogen peroxide. It has been recommended by APIC that reusable objects (e.g., tracheostomy tubes) that touch mucous membranes be disinfected by immersion in 70% isopropyl alcohol for 5 minutes, or 3% hydrogen peroxide for 30 minutes. Additionally, a 1:50 dilution of 5.25% to 6.15% sodium hypochlorite (household bleach) (3 minutes) should be effective (315,316). Noncritical items (e.g., blood pressure cuffs, crutches) can be cleaned with a detergent. Blood spills should be handled as per OSHA regulations as described above. In general, sterilization of critical items is not practical in homes but theoretically could be accomplished by chemical sterilants or boiling. Single-use disposable items can be used or reusable items sterilized in a hospital (317,318).

Some environmental groups advocate "environmentally safe" products as alternatives to commercial germicides in the home-care setting. These alternatives (e.g., ammonia, baking soda, vinegar, Borax, liquid detergent) are not registered with the EPA and should not be used for disinfecting, because they are ineffective against *S. aureus*. Borax, baking soda, and detergents are also ineffective against *Salmonella typhi* and *E. coli*; however, undiluted vinegar and ammonia are effective against *S. typhi* and *E. coli* (46,319,320). Common commercial disinfectants designed for home use have also been found effective against selected antibiotic-resistant bacteria (46).

Public concerns have been raised that the use of antimicrobials in the home may promote the development of antibiotic-resistant bacteria (321,322). This issue is unresolved and needs to be considered further via scientific and clinical investigations. Although the public health benefits resulting from the use of disinfectants in the home environment are unknown, it is known that many sites in the home kitchen and bathroom are microbially contaminated (323), and the use of hypochlorites results in a marked reduction of bacteria (324). It is also known from laboratory studies that many commercially prepared household disinfectants are effective against common pathogens (46) and can interrupt surface-to-human transmission of pathogens (41). The "targeted hygiene concept," which means identifying situations and areas (e.g., food preparation surfaces and bathroom) where there is a risk of transmission of pathogens, may be a reasonable way to identify when disinfection may be appropriate (325).

Susceptibility of Antibiotic-Resistant Bacteria to Disinfectants

As with antibiotics, reduced susceptibility (or acquired resistance) of bacteria to disinfectants can arise by either chromosomal gene mutation or the acquisition of genetic material in the form of plasmids or transposons (326–331). When there is a change in bacterial susceptibility that renders an antibiotic ineffective against an infection previously treatable by that antibiotic, the bacteria are referred to as "resistant." In contrast, reduced susceptibility to disinfectants does not correlate with failure of the disinfectant, because concentrations used in disinfection still greatly exceed the cidal level. Thus, the word *resistance* when applied to these changes is incorrect and the preferred term is *reduced susceptibility* or *increased tolerance* (329,332).

MRSA and VRE are recognized as important healthcare-associated agents. It has been known for years that some antiseptics and disinfectants are, on the basis of minimum inhibitory concentrations (MICs), somewhat less inhibitory to *S. aureus* strains that contain a plasmid-carrying gene encoding resistance to the antibiotic gentamicin (329). For example, Townsend et al. (333) found that gentamicin resistance also encodes reduced susceptibility to propamidine, quaternary ammonium compounds, and ethidium bromide, and Brumfitt et al. (334) found MRSA strains less susceptible than methicillin-sensitive *S. aureus* (MSSA) strains to chlorhexidine, propamidine, and the quaternary ammonium compound cetrimide. Al-Masaudi et al. (335) found the MRSA and MSSA strains to be equally sensitive to phenols and chlorhexidine, but MRSA strains were slightly more tolerant to quaternary ammonium compounds. Studies have established the involvement of two gene families [*qac*CD (now referred to as *smr*) and *qac*AB] in providing protection against agents that are components of disinfectant formulations such as quaternary ammonium compounds. Tennent et al. (336) propose that staphylococci evade destruction because the protein specified by the *qac*A determinant is a cytoplasmic-membrane–associated protein involved in an efflux system that actively reduces intracellular accumulation of toxicants such as quaternary ammonium compounds to intracellular targets.

Other studies demonstrated that plasmid-mediated formaldehyde tolerance is transferable from *Serratia marcescens* to *E. coli* (337) and plasmid-mediated quaternary ammonium tolerance is transferable from *S. aureus* to *E. coli* (338). Tolerance to mercury and silver is also plasmid borne (326,328–331).

Since the concentrations of disinfectants used in practice are much higher than the MICs observed, even for the more tolerant strains, the clinical relevance of these observations is questionable. Several studies have found antibiotic-resistant hospital strains of common healthcare-associated pathogens (i.e., *Enterococcus, P. aeruginosa, Klebsiella pneumoniae, E. coli S. aureus,* and *S. epidermidis*) to be equally susceptible to disinfectants as antibiotic-sensitive strains (46,339–341). The susceptibility of glycopeptide-intermediate *S. aureus* was similar to vancomycin-susceptible MRSA (342). Based on these data, routine disinfection and housekeeping protocols do not need to be altered because of antibiotic resistance provided the disinfection method is effective (343,344). A study that evaluated the efficacy of selected cleaning methods (e.g., QUAT-sprayed cloth, and QUAT-immersed cloth) for eliminating VRE found that currently used disinfection processes are likely highly effective in eliminating VRE. However, surface disinfection must involve contact with all contaminated surfaces (343).

Lastly, does the use of antiseptics or disinfectants facilitate the development of disinfectant-tolerant microorganisms? Based on current evidence and reviews (321,322,331,332,345), the development of enhanced tolerance to disinfectants in response to disinfectant exposure can occur. However, it is not important in clinical terms since the level of tolerance is low and unlikely to compromise the effectiveness of disinfectants where much higher concentrations are used (332).

The issue of whether low-level tolerance to germicides selects for antibiotic-resistant strains is unsettled but may depend on the mechanism by which tolerance is attained. For example, changes in the permeability barrier or efflux mechanisms may affect susceptibility to antibiotics and germicides, but specific changes to a target site may not. Some researchers have suggested that the use of disinfectants or antiseptics (e.g., triclosan) could facilitate the development of antibiotic-resistant microorganisms

(321,322,346). Although there is evidence in laboratory studies of low-level resistance to triclosan, the concentrations of triclosan in these studies were low (generally <1 μg/mL) and dissimilar from the higher levels used in antimicrobial products (2,000–20,000 μg/mL) (347,348). Thus, researchers can create laboratory-derived mutants that demonstrate reduced susceptibility to antiseptics or disinfectants. In some experiments, such bacteria have demonstrated reduced susceptibility to certain antibiotics (322). There is no evidence that using antiseptics/disinfectants selects for antibiotic-resistant microorganisms in nature or that mutants survive in nature (349). In addition, there are fundamental differences between the action of antibiotics and disinfectants. Antibiotics are selectively toxic and generally have a single target site in bacteria, thereby inhibiting a specific biosynthetic process. Germicides generally are considered to be nonspecific antimicrobials because of a multiplicity of toxic effect mechanisms or target sites and are broader spectrum in the types of microorganisms against which they are effective (329,332).

The rotational use of disinfectants in some environments (e.g., pharmacy production units) has been recommended and practiced in an attempt to prevent the development of resistant microbes (350,351). Currently, there are rare case reports about appropriately used disinfectants that have resulted in a clinical problem arising from the selection or development of nonsusceptible microorganisms (352).

Surface Disinfection: Should We Do It?

The effective use of disinfectants constitutes an important factor in preventing healthcare-associated infections. Surfaces are considered noncritical items as they come in contact with intact skin. Use of noncritical items or contact with noncritical surfaces carries little risk of transmitting a pathogen to patients or staff. Thus, the routine use of germicidal chemicals to disinfect hospital floors and other noncritical items is controversial (353,354). In 1991, Favero and Bond (355) provided an expansion of the Spaulding scheme by dividing the noncritical environmental surfaces into housekeeping surfaces and medical equipment surfaces. The classes of disinfectants used on housekeeping and medical equipment surfaces may be similar. However, the frequency of decontaminating may vary (see manufacturers' recommendations). Medical equipment surfaces (e.g., blood pressure cuffs, stethoscopes, hemodialysis machines, and x-ray machines) may become contaminated with infectious agents and may contribute to the spread of healthcare-associated infections (224). For this reason, noncritical medical equipment surfaces should be disinfected with an EPA-registered low- or intermediate-level disinfectant. Use of a disinfectant provides antimicrobial activity that is likely to be achieved with minimal additional cost or work.

Environmental surfaces (e.g., bedside table) also may potentially contribute to cross-transmission by hand contamination of healthcare personnel due to contact with contaminated surfaces, medical equipment, or patients (44,356). A recent paper reviews the epidemiologic and microbiologic data regarding the use of disinfectants on noncritical surfaces (357).

Table 85.6 lists seven reasons for using a disinfectant on noncritical surfaces. Five of these are particularly noteworthy and support the use of a germicidal detergent. First, hospital floors become contaminated with microorganisms by settling of airborne bacteria; by contact with shoes, wheels, and other objects; and occasionally by spills. The removal of microbes is a component in the control of healthcare-associated infections. In an investigation on the cleaning of hospital floors, the use of soap and water (90% reduction) was less effective in reducing the numbers of bacteria than was a phenolic disinfectant (94–99.9% reduction) (358). However, a few hours after floor disinfection the bacterial count was nearly back to the pretreatment level. Second, detergents become contaminated and result in seeding the patient's environment with bacteria. Investigators have shown that mop water becomes increasingly dirty during cleaning, and mop water becomes contaminated if soap and water is used rather than a disinfectant. For example, Ayliffe et al. (359) found that bacterial contamination in soap and water without a disinfectant increased from 10 to 34,000 CFU/mL after cleaning a ward, whereas the contamination in a disinfectant solution did not change (20 CFU/mL). Dharan et al. (360) also found that the use of detergents on floors and patient room furniture increased the bacterial contamination in the patients' environmental surfaces after cleaning (average increase = 103.6 CFU/24 cm^2) (360). In addition, Engelhart et al. (361) recently described a *P. aeruginosa* outbreak in a hematology-oncology unit associated with contamination of the surface cleaning equipment when nongermicidal cleaning solutions instead of disinfectants

TABLE 85.6. EPIDEMIOLOGIC EVIDENCE ASSOCIATED WITH THE USE OF SURFACE DISINFECTANTS OR DETERGENTS ON NONCRITICAL SURFACES

Justification for Use of Disinfectants for Noncritical Surfaces
Surfaces may contribute to transmission of epidemiologically important microbes (e.g., vancomycin-resistant *Enterococcus*, methicillin-resistant *S. aureus*, viruses)
Disinfectants are needed for surfaces contaminated by blood and other potentially infective material
Disinfectants are more effective than detergents in reducing microbial load on floors
Detergents become contaminated and result in seeding the patient's environment with bacteria
Disinfection of noncritical equipment and surfaces is recommended for patients on isolation precautions by the Centers for Disease Control and Prevention.
Advantage of using a single product for decontamination of noncritical surfaces, both floors and equipment
Some newer disinfectants have persistent antimicrobial activity
Justification for Using a Detergent on Floors
Noncritical surfaces contribute minimally to endemic healthcare-associated infections
No difference in healthcare-associated infection rates when floors are cleaned with detergent versus disinfectant
No environmental impact (aquatic or terrestrial) issues with disposal
No occupational health exposure issues
Lower costs
Use of antiseptics/disinfectants selects for antibiotic-resistant bacteria (?)
More aesthetically pleasing floor

Modified from 357.

were used for decontamination of the patients' environment. Third, the CDC recommends in its isolation guideline that noncritical equipment contaminated with blood, body fluids, secretions, or excretions be cleaned and disinfected after use. The same guideline recommends that, in addition to cleaning, disinfection of the bedside equipment and environmental surfaces (e.g., bed rails, bedside tables, carts, commodes, doorknobs, and faucet handles) is indicated for certain pathogens, especially enterococci, which can survive in the inanimate environment for prolonged periods (362). Fourth, OSHA requires that surfaces contaminated with blood and other potentially infectious materials (e.g., amniotic, pleural fluid) be disinfected. Fifth, using a single product throughout the facility may simplify both training and appropriate practice.

There also are reasons for using a detergent alone on floors since noncritical surfaces contribute minimally to endemic healthcare-associated infections (363), and no differences have been found in healthcare-associated infection rates when floors are cleaned with detergent versus disinfectant (360,364,365). However, these studies have been small, of short duration, and suffer from low statistical power since the outcome, healthcare-associated infections, is one of low frequency. The low rate of infections makes it difficult statistically to demonstrate the efficacy of an intervention. Since housekeeping surfaces are associated with the lowest risk of disease transmission, some researchers have suggested that either detergents or a disinfectant/detergent could be used (355). Although there are no data that demonstrate a reduction in healthcare-associated infection rates with the use of surface disinfection of floors, there are data that demonstrate a reduction in microbial load associated with the use of disinfectants. Given this information and that environmental surfaces (e.g., bedside table, bed rails) in close proximity to the patient and in outpatient settings (366) have been demonstrated to become contaminated with epidemiologically important microbes such as VRE and MRSA (40,366–368) and these microorganisms survive on various hospital surfaces (369,370), some have suggested that these surfaces should be disinfected on a regularly scheduled basis (357). Spot decontamination on fabrics that remain in hospitals or clinic rooms while patients move in and out (e.g., privacy curtains) also should be considered. One study demonstrated the effectiveness of spraying the fabric with 3% hydrogen peroxide (371). Future studies should evaluate the level of contamination on noncritical environmental surfaces as a function of high and low hand contact and whether some surfaces (e.g., bed rails) near the patient with high contact frequencies require more frequent disinfection. Regardless of whether a detergent or disinfectant is used on surfaces in a healthcare facility, cleaning should be undertaken on a routine basis and when environmental surfaces are dirty or soiled in order to provide an aesthetically pleasing environment and to prevent potentially contaminated objects from serving as a source for healthcare-associated infections (372). The value of designing surfaces (e.g., hexyl-polyvinylpyridine) that kill bacteria on contact (373) or have sustained antimicrobial activity (374) should be further evaluated.

Heavy microbial contamination of wet mops and cleaning cloths and the potential for spread of such contamination have been recognized by several investigators (59,375). They have shown that wiping hard surfaces with contaminated cloths may result in contamination of hands, equipment, and other surfaces (59,376). Data have been published that can be used to formulate effective policies for decontamination and maintenance of reusable cleaning cloths. For example, heat was the most reliable treatment of cleaning cloths as a detergent washing followed by drying at 80°C for 2 hours produced elimination of contamination. Alternatively, immersing the cloth in hypochlorite (4,000 ppm) for 2 minutes produced no detectable survivors in 10 of 13 cloths (377). If reusable cleaning cloths or mops are used, decontamination should occur regularly to prevent surface contamination during cleaning with subsequent transfer of microorganisms from these surfaces to patients or equipment via the hands of healthcare workers.

Air Disinfection

The use of a disinfectant spray-fog technique for antimicrobial control of hospital rooms has been used. This technique of spraying of disinfectants is an unsatisfactory method of decontaminating air and surfaces and is not recommended for general infection control in routine patient-care areas (362). Disinfectant fogging is rarely, if ever, used in U.S. healthcare facilities for air and surface disinfection in patient-care areas. Methods (e.g., filtration, ultraviolet germicidal irradiation, chlorine dioxide) to reduce air contamination in the healthcare setting are discussed in another guideline (21).

Microbial Contamination of Disinfectants

Contaminated disinfectants and antiseptics have been occasional vehicles of healthcare infections and pseudoepidemics for more than 50 years. A summary of the published reports describing contaminated disinfectants and antiseptic solutions leading to healthcare-associated infections has been published (378). Since this summary, additional reports have been published (379–381). When examining the reports of disinfectants found contaminated with microorganisms, there are several noteworthy observations. Perhaps most importantly, high-level disinfectants/liquid chemical sterilants have not been associated with outbreaks due to intrinsic or extrinsic contamination. Another feature of these outbreaks has been that members of the genus *Pseudomonas* (e.g., *P. aeruginosa*) are the most frequent isolates from contaminated disinfectants, being the agents recovered from 80% of the contaminated products. Their ability to remain viable or grow in use-dilutions of disinfectants is unparalleled. This survival advantage for *Pseudomonas* is presumably due to their nutritional versatility, their unique outer membrane that constitutes an effective barrier to the passage of germicides, and/or their efflux systems. Although the concentrated solutions of the disinfectants have not been demonstrated to be contaminated at the point of manufacture, Newman et al. (382) found that an undiluted phenolic may be contaminated by a *Pseudomonas* species during use. In most of the reports that describe illness associated with contaminated disinfectants, the product was used to disinfect patient-care equipment such as cystoscopes, cardiac catheters, and thermometers. The germicides used as disinfectants that were reported contaminated include chlorhexidine, quaternary ammonium compounds, phenolics, and pine oil.

The following control measures should be instituted to reduce the frequency of bacterial growth in disinfectants and the threat of serious healthcare-associated infections from the use of such contaminated products (378). First, some disinfectants should not be diluted and those that are must be prepared correctly to achieve the manufacturer's recommended use-dilution. Second, we must learn from the literature what inappropriate activities result in extrinsic contamination (i.e., at the point of use) of germicides and prevent their recurrence. Common sources of extrinsic contamination of germicides in the reviewed literature are the water to make working dilutions, contaminated containers, and general contamination of the hospital areas where the germicides are prepared and/or used. Third, stock solutions of germicides must be stored as indicated on the product label. Currently, the EPA verifies manufacturers' efficacy claims against microorganisms. These measures should provide assurance that products that meet the EPA registration requirements are capable of achieving a certain level of antimicrobial activity when used as directed.

FACTORS AFFECTING THE EFFICACY OF DISINFECTION AND STERILIZATION

The activity of germicides against microorganisms depends on a number of factors, some of which are intrinsic qualities of the microorganism, whereas others depend on the chemical and external physical environment. An awareness of these factors should lead to a better utilization of disinfection and sterilization processes; thus they will be briefly reviewed. More extensive consideration of these and other factors may be found elsewhere (11,12,14,383,384).

Number and Location of Microorganisms

All other conditions remaining constant, the larger the number of microbes present, the longer it takes for a germicide to destroy all of them. This relationship was illustrated by Spaulding when he employed identical test conditions and demonstrated that it took 30 minutes to kill 10 *B. atrophaeus* (formerly *Bacillus subtilis*) spores but 3 hours to kill 100,000 *B. atrophaeus* spores. This reinforces the need for scrupulous cleaning of medical instruments before disinfection and sterilization. By reducing the number of microorganisms that must be inactivated, one correspondingly shortens the exposure time required to kill the entire microbial load. Researchers have also shown that aggregated or clumped cells are more difficult to inactivate than monodispersed cells (385).

The location of microorganisms also must be considered when assessing factors affecting the efficacy of germicides. Medical instruments with multiple pieces must be disassembled, and equipment such as endoscopes that have crevices, joints, and channels are more difficult to disinfect than flat-surface equipment, because it is more difficult to penetrate all parts of the equipment with a disinfectant. Only surfaces in direct contact with the germicide will be disinfected, so there must be no air pockets, and the equipment must be completely immersed for the entire exposure period. Manufacturers should be encouraged to produce equipment that is engineered so cleaning and disinfection may be accomplished with ease.

Innate Resistance of Microorganisms

Microorganisms vary greatly in their resistance to chemical germicides and sterilization processes (Fig. 85.1) (327). Intrinsic resistance mechanisms in microorganisms to disinfectants varies. For example, spores are resistant to disinfectants, because the spore coat and cortex act as a barrier, mycobacteria have a waxy cell wall that prevents disinfectant entry, and gram-negative bacteria possess an outer membrane that acts as a barrier to the uptake of disinfectants (326,328–330). Implicit in all disinfection strategies is the consideration that the most resistant microbial subpopulation controls the sterilization or disinfection time. That is, to destroy the most resistant types of microorganisms-bacterial spores, the user needs to employ exposure times and a concentration of germicide needed to achieve complete destruction. With the exception of prions, bacterial spores possess the highest innate resistance to chemical germicides, followed by coccidia (e.g., *Cryptosporidium*), mycobacteria (e.g., *M. tuberculosis*), nonlipid or small viruses (e.g., poliovirus, and coxsackievirus), fungi (e.g., *Aspergillus* and *Candida*), vegetative bacteria (e.g., *Staphylococcus* and *Pseudomonas*), and lipid or medium-size viruses (e.g., herpes and HIV). The germicidal resistance exhibited by the gram-positive and gram-negative bacteria is similar with some exceptions (e.g., *P. aeruginosa,* which shows greater resistance to some disinfectants) (352,386,387). *P. aeruginosa* has also been shown to be significantly more resistant to a variety of disinfectants in its naturally occurring state as compared to cells subcultured on laboratory media (386). *Rickettsiae, Chlamydiae,* and mycoplasma cannot be placed in this scale of relative resistance, because information on the efficacy of germicides against these agents is limited (388). Since these microorganisms contain lipid and are similar in structure and composition to other bacteria, it might be predicted that they would be inactivated by the same germicides that destroy lipid viruses and vegetative bacteria. A known exception to this supposition is *Coxiella burnetti,* which has demonstrated resistance to disinfectants (389).

Concentration and Potency of Disinfectants

With other variables constant, and with one exception (i.e., iodophors), the more concentrated the disinfectant, the greater its efficacy and the shorter the time necessary to achieve microbial kill. Generally not recognized, however, is that all disinfectants are not similarly affected by concentration adjustments. For example, quaternary ammonium compounds and phenol have a concentration exponent of 1 and 6, respectively; thus halving the concentration of a quaternary ammonium compound requires a doubling of its disinfecting time, but halving the concentration of a phenol solution requires a 64-fold (i.e., 26) increase in its disinfecting time (348,390).

It is also important to consider the length of the disinfection time, which is dependent on the potency of the germicide. This

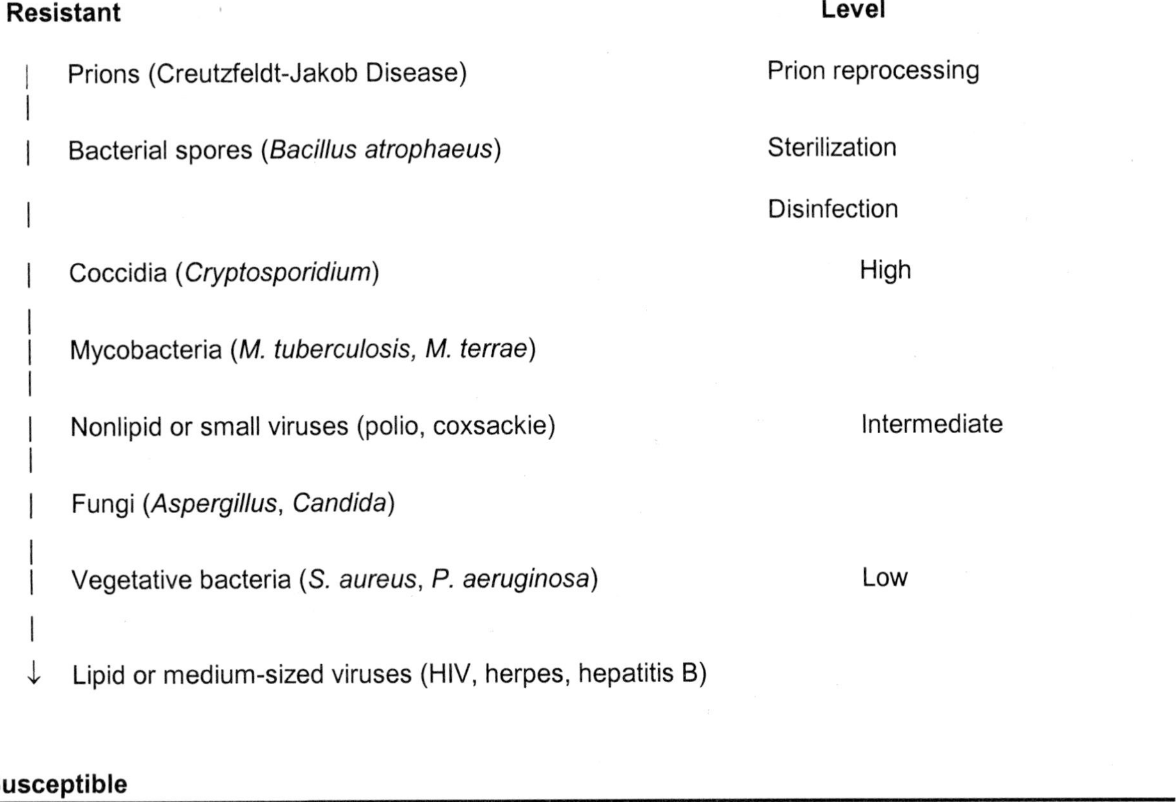

Figure 85.1. Decreasing order of resistance of microorganisms to disinfection and sterilization and the level of disinfection or sterilization. Modified from 11, 329.

was illustrated by Spaulding, who demonstrated using the mucin-loop test that 70% isopropyl alcohol destroyed 10^4 *M. tuberculosis* in 5 minutes, whereas a simultaneous test with 3% phenolic required 2 to 3 hours to achieve the same level of microbial kill (12).

Physical and Chemical Factors

Several physical and chemical factors—temperature, pH, relative humidity, and water hardness—also influence disinfectant procedures. For example, the activity of most disinfectants increases as the temperature increases but there are exceptions. Further, too great an increase in temperature causes the disinfectant to degrade, weakens its germicidal activity, and may produce a potential health hazard.

An increase in pH improves the antimicrobial activity of some disinfectants (e.g., glutaraldehyde, quaternary ammonium compounds) but decreases the antimicrobial activity of others (phenols, hypochlorites, and iodine). The pH influences the antimicrobial activity by altering the disinfectant molecule or the cell surface.

Relative humidity is the single most important factor influencing the activity of gaseous disinfectants/sterilants such as ETO, chlorine dioxide, and formaldehyde.

Water hardness (i.e., high concentration of divalent cations) reduces the rate of kill of certain disinfectants. This occurs because divalent cations (e.g., magnesium and calcium) in the hard water interact with the disinfectant to form insoluble precipitates (11,391).

Organic and Inorganic Matter

Organic matter in the form of serum, blood, pus, fecal, or lubricant material may interfere with the antimicrobial activity of disinfectants in at least two ways. Most commonly the interference occurs by a chemical reaction between the germicide and the organic matter, resulting in a complex that is less germicidal or nongermicidal, leaving less of the active germicide available for attacking microorganisms. Chlorine and iodine disinfectants, in particular, are prone to such interaction. Alternatively, organic material may protect microorganisms from attack by acting as a physical barrier (392).

The effects of inorganic contaminants on the sterilization process were studied in the 1950s and 1960s (393,394). These studies and more recent studies show the protection of microorganisms to all sterilization processes due to occlusion in salt crystals (244,395). This further emphasizes the importance of meticulous cleaning of medical devices before any sterilization or disinfection procedure since both organic and inorganic soils are easily removed by washing (244).

Duration of Exposure

Items must be exposed to the appropriate germicide for the minimum contact time specified on the products labeling unless scientific studies demonstrate an alternative time is effective. All lumina and channels of endoscopic instruments must come in contact with the disinfectant. Air pockets interfere with the disinfection process and items that float on the disinfectant will not be disinfected. The disinfectant must be introduced reliably into the internal channels of the device. The exact times for disinfecting medical items are somewhat elusive because of the effect of the aforementioned factors on disinfection efficacy. Contact times that have proved reliable are presented in Table 85.1, but, in general, the longer contact times are more effective than shorter ones.

Biofilms

Microorganisms may be protected from disinfectants due to the production of thick masses of cells (396) and extracellular materials or biofilms (397–403). Biofilms are microbial masses attached to surfaces that are immersed in liquids. Once these masses are formed, microbes may be resistant to the disinfectants by multiple mechanisms including higher resistance of older biofilms, genotypic variation of the bacteria, microbial production of neutralizing enzymes, and physiologic gradients within the biofilm (e.g., pH). Although new decontamination methods are being investigated for removal of biofilms, chlorine remains the most efficient product (404). Investigators have hypothesized that the glycocalyx-like cellular masses on the interior walls of polyvinyl chloride pipe would protect embedded microorganisms from some disinfectants and serve as a reservoir for continuous contamination (397,398,405). Biofilms have been found in whirlpools (406), dental unit waterlines (407), and numerous medical devices (e.g., contact lenses, pacemakers, hemodialysis systems, urinary catheters, central venous catheters, endoscopes) (402,404,408). Their presence may have serious implications for immunocompromised patients and patients with indwelling medical devices. Enzymes can be used for the degradation of biofilms (409), but no products are registered by the EPA or FDA for this purpose.

CHEMICAL DISINFECTANTS

Alcohol

Overview

In the healthcare setting, "alcohol" refers to two water-soluble chemical compounds whose germicidal characteristics are generally underrated: ethyl alcohol and isopropyl alcohol (410). These alcohols are rapidly bactericidal rather than bacteriostatic against vegetative forms of bacteria; they also are tuberculocidal, fungicidal, and virucidal but do not destroy bacterial spores. Their cidal activity drops sharply when diluted below 50% concentration, and the optimum bactericidal concentration is in the range of 60% to 90% solutions in water (volume/volume) (411, 412).

Mode of Action

The most feasible explanation for the antimicrobial action of alcohol is denaturation of proteins. This is supported by the observation that absolute ethyl alcohol, a dehydrating agent, is less bactericidal than mixtures of alcohol and water, because proteins are denatured more quickly in the presence of water (412,413). Protein denaturation also is consistent with the observations by Sykes (414) that alcohol destroys the dehydrogenases of *E. coli,* and Dagley et al. (415) that ethyl alcohol increases the lag phase of *Enterobacter aerogenes* and this could be reversed by the addition of certain amino acids. The latter authors concluded that the bacteriostatic action was due to the inhibition of the production of metabolites essential for rapid cell division.

Microbicidal Activity

Methyl alcohol (methanol) has the weakest bactericidal action of the alcohols and thus is seldom used in healthcare (416). The bactericidal activity of various concentrations of ethyl alcohol (ethanol) was examined by Morton (411) against a variety of microorganisms in exposure periods ranging from 10 seconds to 1 hour. *P. aeruginosa* was killed in 10 seconds by all concentrations of ethanol from 30% to 100% (v/v), whereas *S. marcescens, E. coli,* and *Salmonella typhosa* were killed in 10 seconds by all concentrations of ethanol from 40% to 100%. The gram-positive microorganisms *S. aureus* and *Streptococcus pyogenes* were slightly more resistant, being killed in 10 seconds by ethyl alcohol concentrations from 60% to 95%. Coulthard and Sykes (417) found isopropyl alcohol (isopropanol) slightly more bactericidal than ethyl alcohol for *E. coli* and *S. aureus.*

Ethyl alcohol, at concentrations of 60% to 80%, is a potent virucidal agent inactivating all of the lipophilic viruses (e.g., herpes, vaccinia, influenza virus) and many hydrophilic viruses [e.g., adeno-, entero-, rhino-, and rotaviruses but not hepatitis A virus (51)]. Isopropyl alcohol is not active against the nonlipid enteroviruses but is fully active against the lipid viruses (63). Studies also have demonstrated the ability of ethyl and isopropyl alcohol to inactivate HBV (203,204) and the herpes virus (418), and ethyl alcohol to inactivate HIV (206), rotavirus, echovirus, and astrovirus (419).

In testing the effect of ethyl alcohol against *M. tuberculosis,* Smith (420) noted that 95% ethanol killed the tubercle bacilli in sputum or water suspension within 15 seconds. In 1964, Spaulding stated that alcohols were the germicide of choice for tuberculocidal activity and they should be the standard by which all other tuberculocides were compared. For example, he compared the tuberculocidal activity of iodophor (450 ppm), a substituted phenol (3%), and isopropanol (70%/volume) using the mucin-loop test (10^6 *M. tuberculosis* per loop) and determined that the contact times needed for complete destruction were 120 to 180 minutes, 45 to 60 minutes, and 5 minutes, respectively. The mucin-loop test is a severe test developed for the purpose of producing long survival times. Thus, these figures should not be extrapolated to the exposure times that are needed when these germicides are being used on medical or surgical material (410).

Ethyl alcohol (70%) was the most effective concentration for killing the tissue phase of *Cryptococcus neoformans, Blastomyces dermatitidis, Coccidioides immitis,* and *Histoplasma capsulatum* and the culture phases of the latter three microorganisms aerosolized onto various surfaces. The culture phase was more resistant to the action of ethyl alcohol and required about 20 minutes to disinfect the contaminated surface, compared to <1 minute for the tissue phase (421,422).

Isopropyl alcohol (20%) has been shown to be effective in killing the cysts of *Acanthamoeba culbertsoni* (423) as have chlorhexidine, hydrogen peroxide, and thimerosal (424).

Uses

Alcohols are not recommended for sterilizing medical and surgical materials principally because of their lack of sporicidal action and their inability to penetrate protein-rich materials. Fatal postoperative wound infections with *Clostridium* have occurred when alcohols were used to sterilize surgical instruments contaminated with bacterial spores (425). Alcohols have been used effectively to disinfect oral and rectal thermometers (426, 427), hospital pagers (428), scissors (429), stethoscopes (430), and fiberoptic endoscopes (431,432). Alcohol towelettes have been used for years to disinfect small surfaces such as rubber stoppers of multiple-dose medication vials or vaccine bottles. Furthermore, alcohol is occasionally used to disinfect external surfaces of equipment [e.g., stethoscopes, ventilators, manual ventilation bags (433)], CPR manikins (434), ultrasound instruments (435), or medication preparation areas. Two studies demonstrated the effectiveness of 70% isopropyl alcohol to disinfect reusable transducer heads in a controlled environment (436, 437). In contrast, Beck-Sague and Jarvis (438) described three bloodstream infection outbreaks when alcohol was used to disinfect transducer heads in an intensive care setting.

The documented shortcomings of alcohols on equipment are that they damage the shellac mountings of lensed instruments, tend to swell and harden rubber and certain plastic tubing after prolonged and repeated use, bleach rubber and plastic tiles (410), and damage tonometer tips (deterioration of the glue) after the equivalent of one working year of routine use (439). Lingel and Coffey (440) also found that tonometer biprisms soaked in alcohol for 4 days developed rough front surfaces that could potentially cause corneal damage. This appeared to be caused by a weakening of the cementing substances used to fabricate the biprisms. Corneal opacification has been reported when tonometer tips were swabbed with alcohol immediately before intraocular pressure measurements were taken (441). Alcohols are flammable and consequently must be stored in a cool, well-ventilated area. They also evaporate rapidly, and this makes extended exposure time difficult to achieve unless the items are immersed.

Chlorine and Chlorine Compounds

Overview

Hypochlorites are the most widely used of the chlorine disinfectants and are available in a liquid (e.g., sodium hypochlorite) or solid (e.g., calcium hypochlorite) form. The most prevalent chlorine products in the U.S. are aqueous solutions of 5.25% to 6.15% sodium hypochlorite, which usually are called household bleach. They have a broad spectrum of antimicrobial activity, do not leave toxic residues, are unaffected by water hardness, are inexpensive and fast acting (316), remove dried or fixed microorganisms and biofilms from surfaces (245), and have a low incidence of serious toxicity (442–444). Sodium hypochlorite at the concentration used in domestic bleach (5.25–6.15%) may produce ocular irritation or oropharygeal, esophageal, and gastric burns (307,445–449). Other disadvantages of hypochlorites include corrosiveness to metals in high concentrations (>500 ppm), inactivation by organic matter, discoloring or "bleaching" of fabrics, release of toxic chlorine gas when mixed with ammonia or acid (e.g., household cleaning agents) (450–452), and relative instability (315). The microbicidal activity of chlorine largely is attributed to undissociated hypochlorous acid (HOCl). The dissociation of HOCl to the less microbicidal form (hypochlorite ion OCl^-) is dependent on pH. The disinfecting efficacy of chlorine decreases with an increase in pH that parallels the conversion of undissociated HOCl to hypochlorite ion (453,454). A potential hazard is the production of the carcinogen bis-chloromethyl ether when hypochlorite solutions come into contact with formaldehyde (455) and the production of the animal carcinogen trihalomethane when hot water is hyperchlorinated (456). The EPA has decided after reviewing environmental fate and ecologic data that the currently registered uses of hypochlorites will not result in unreasonable adverse effects to the environment (457).

Alternative compounds that release chlorine and are used in the healthcare setting include demand-release chlorine dioxide, sodium dichloroisocyanurate, and chloramine T. The advantage of these compounds over the hypochlorites is that they retain chlorine longer and so exert a more prolonged bactericidal effect. Sodium dichloroisocyanurate tablets are stable, and the microbicidal activity of solutions prepared from sodium dichloroisocyanurate tablets may be greater than that of sodium hypochlorite solutions containing the same total available chlorine for two reasons. First, with sodium dichloroisocyanurate only 50% of the total available chlorine present is free (HOCl and OCl^-), whereas the remainder is combined (mono- or dichloroisocyanurate), and as free available chlorine is used up the latter is released to restore the equilibrium. Second, solutions of sodium dichloroisocyanurate are acidic whereas sodium hypochlorite solutions are alkaline and the more microbicidal type of chlorine (HOCl) is believed to predominate (458–461). Disinfectants based on chlorine dioxide are prepared fresh as required by mixing the two components [base solution (citric acid with preservatives and corrosion inhibitors) and the activator solution (sodium chlorite)]. *In vitro* suspension tests showed that solutions containing about 140 ppm chlorine dioxide achieved a reduction factor exceeding 10^6 of *S. aureus* in 1 minute and of *B. atrophaeus* spores in 2.5 minutes in the presence of 3 g/L bovine albumin. The potential for damaging equipment requires consideration as long-term use can result in damage to the outer plastic coat of the insertion tube (462).

Mode of Action

The exact mechanism by which free chlorine destroys microorganisms has not been elucidated. Inactivation by chlorine may result from a number of factors: oxidation of sulfhydral enzymes and amino acids; ring chlorination of amino acids; loss of intracellular contents; decreased uptake of nutrients; inhibition of protein synthesis; decreased oxygen uptake; oxidation of respiratory components; decreased adenosine triphosphate production; breaks in DNA; and depressed DNA synthesis (332,454). The actual microbicidal mechanism of chlorine may involve a combination of these factors or the effect of chlorine on critical sites (332).

Microbicidal Activity

Low concentrations of free available chlorine (e.g., HOCl, OCl^-, and elemental chlorine—Cl_2) have a biocidal effect on mycoplasma (25 ppm) and vegetative bacteria (<5 ppm) in seconds in the absence of an organic load (388,454). Higher concentrations (1,000 ppm) of chlorine are required to kill *M. tuberculosis* using the Association of Official Analytical Chemists (AOAC) tuberculocidal test (64). A concentration of 100 ppm will kill ≥99.9% of *B. atrophaeus* spores within 5 minutes (463, 464) and destroy mycotic agents in <1 hour (454). Klein and DeForest (63) reported that 25 different viruses were inactivated in 10 minutes with 200 ppm available chlorine. Several studies have demonstrated the effectiveness of diluted sodium hypochlorite and other disinfectants to inactivate HIV (54). Chlorine (500 ppm) showed inhibition of *Candida* after 30 seconds of exposure (47). Experiments using the AOAC use-dilution method have shown that 100 ppm of free chlorine will kill 10^6 to 10^7 *S. aureus, Salmonella choleraesuis,* and *P. aeruginosa* in <10 minutes (315). Since household bleach contains from 5.25% to 6.15% sodium hypochlorite, or 52,500 to 61,500 ppm available chlorine, a 1:1,000 dilution provides about 53 to 62 ppm available chlorine and a 1:10 dilution of household bleach provides about 5,250 to 6,150 ppm.

Some data are available for chlorine dioxide that support manufacturers' bactericidal, fungicidal, sporicidal, tuberculocidal, and virucidal label claims (465–468). A chlorine dioxide generator has been shown effective for decontamination of flexible endoscopes (462). Chlorine dioxide can be produced by mixing solutions such as a solution of chlorine with a solution of sodium chlorite (454). In 1986 a chlorine dioxide product was voluntarily removed from the market when its use was found to cause cellulose-based dialyzer membranes to leak, which allowed bacteria to migrate from the dialysis fluid side of the dialyzer to the blood side (469).

Sodium dichloroisocyanurate at 2,500 ppm available chlorine has been found to be effective against bacteria in the presence of up to 20% plasma compared to 10% plasma for sodium hypochlorite at 2,500 ppm (470).

Uses

Hypochlorites are widely used in healthcare facilities in a variety of settings (316). Inorganic chlorine solution is used for disinfecting tonometer heads (162) and for spot disinfection of counter tops and floors. A 1:10 to 1:100 dilution of 5.25% to 6.15% sodium hypochlorite (i.e., household bleach) (20,207, 471,472) or an EPA-registered tuberculocidal disinfectant (15) has been recommended for decontaminating blood spills. For small spills of blood (i.e., drops of blood) on noncritical surfaces, the area can be disinfected with a 1:100 dilution of 5.25% to 6.15% sodium hypochlorite or an EPA-registered tuberculocidal disinfectant. Since hypochlorites and other germicides are substantially inactivated in the presence of blood (56,470,473,474), large spills of blood require that the surface be cleaned before an EPA-registered disinfectant or a 1:10 (final concentration) solution of household bleach is applied. If there is a possibility of a sharps injury, there should be an initial decontamination (60,307), followed by cleaning and terminal disinfection (1:10 final concentration) (56). Extreme care should always be employed to prevent percutaneous injury. At least 500 ppm available chlorine for 10 minutes is recommended for decontamination of CPR training manikins (475). Full-strength bleach is recommended for self-disinfection of needles and syringes used for illicit drug use when needle exchange programs are not available. The difference in the recommended concentrations of bleach reflects the difficulty of cleaning the interior of needles and syringes and the use of needles and syringes for parenteral injection (476). Clinicians should not alter their use of chlorine on environmental surfaces based on testing methodologies that do not simulate actual disinfection practices (477,478). Other uses in healthcare include as an irrigating agent in endodontic treatment (479) and for disinfecting manikins, laundry, dental appliances, hydrotherapy tanks (21,36), regulated medical waste before disposal (316), and the water distribution system in hemodialysis centers and hemodialysis machines (221).

Chlorine has long been favored as the preferred disinfectant in water treatment. Hyperchlorination of a *Legionella*-contaminated hospital water system (21) resulted in a dramatic decrease (30% to 1.5%) in the isolation of *L. pneumophila* from water outlets and a cessation of healthcare-associated Legionnaires' disease in the affected unit (456,480). Chloramine T (481) and hypochlorites (36) have been used in disinfecting hydrotherapy equipment.

Hypochlorite solutions in tap water at a pH >8 stored at room temperature (23°C) in closed, opaque plastic containers may lose up to 40% to 50% of their free available chlorine level over a period of 1 month. Thus, if a user wished to have a solution containing 500 ppm of available chlorine at day 30, a solution containing 1,000 ppm of chlorine should be prepared at time 0. There is no decomposition of sodium hypochlorite solution after 30 days when stored in a closed brown bottle (315).

The use of powders, composed of a mixture of a chlorine-releasing agent with highly absorbent resin, for disinfecting body fluid spills has been evaluated by laboratory tests and hospital ward trials. The inclusion of acrylic resin particles in formulations markedly increases the volume of fluid that can be soaked up as the resin can absorb 200 to 300 times its own weight of fluid, depending on the fluid consistency. When experimental formulations containing 1%, 5%, and 10% available chlorine were evaluated by a standardized surface test, those containing 10% demonstrated bactericidal activity. One problem with chlorine-releasing granules is that chlorine fumes can be generated when they are applied to urine (482).

Formaldehyde

Overview

Formaldehyde is used as a disinfectant and sterilant both in the liquid and gaseous states. The liquid form is considered briefly here, and a review of the gaseous form may be found elsewhere (483). Formaldehyde is sold and used principally as a water-based solution called formalin, which is 37% formaldehyde by weight. The aqueous solution is a bactericide, tuberculocide, fungicide, virucide, and sporicide (63,73,484–486). OSHA indicated that formaldehyde should be handled in the workplace as a potential carcinogen and set an employee exposure standard for formaldehyde that limits an 8-hour TWA exposure to a concentration of 0.75 parts formaldehyde per million parts of air (0.75 ppm) (487,488). The standard includes a second permissible exposure limit in the form of a short-term exposure limit (STEL) of 2 ppm that is the maximum exposure allowed during a 15-minute period (489). Ingestion of formaldehyde can be fatal, and long-term exposure to low levels in the air or on the skin can cause asthma-like respiratory problems and skin irritation such as dermatitis and itching. For these reasons, employees should have limited direct contact with formaldehyde, and these considerations limit its role in sterilization and disinfection processes. Key provisions of the OSHA standard that protects workers from exposure to formaldehyde can be found in Title 29 of CFR 1910.1048 (and equivalent regulations in states with OSHA-approved state plans) (490).

Mode of Action

Formaldehyde inactivates microorganisms by alkylating the amino and sulfhydral groups of proteins and ring nitrogen atoms of purine bases (355).

Microbicidal Activity

A wide range of microorganisms are destroyed by varying concentrations of aqueous formaldehyde solutions. Klein and DeForest (63) demonstrated inactivation of poliovirus in 10 minutes required an 8% concentration of formalin, but all other viruses tested were inactivated with 2% formalin. Four percent formaldehyde is a tuberculocidal agent, inactivating 10^4 *M. tuberculosis* in 2 minutes (73), and 2.5% formaldehyde inactivated about 10^7 *S. typhi* in 10 minutes in the presence of organic matter (485). Rubbo et al. (73) demonstrated that the sporicidal action of formaldehyde was slower than that of glutaraldehyde when they performed comparative tests with 4% aqueous formaldehyde and 2% glutaraldehyde against the spores of *B. anthracis*. The formaldehyde solution required a contact time of 2 hours to achieve an inactivation factor of 10^4, whereas glutaraldehyde required only 15 minutes.

Uses

Although formaldehyde-alcohol is a chemical sterilant and formaldehyde is a high-level disinfectant, the healthcare uses of formaldehyde are limited by its irritating fumes and the pungent odor that is apparent at very low levels (<1 ppm). For these reasons and others, such as it is also a suspected human carcinogen that is linked to nasal cancer and lung cancer (491), this germicide is excluded from Table 85.1. When it is employed there is generally limited direct employee exposure; however, excessive exposures to formaldehyde have been documented for employees of renal transplant units (487,492) and students in a gross anatomy laboratory (493). Formaldehyde is used in the healthcare setting to prepare viral vaccines (e.g., poliovirus, influenza), as an embalming agent, to preserve anatomic specimens, and, in the past, for sterilizing surgical instruments, especially when mixed with ethanol. A 1997 survey found that formaldehyde was used for reprocessing hemodialyzers by 34% of the hemodialysis centers in the U.S., a 60% decrease from 1983 (494,495). If used at room temperature, a concentration of 4% with a minimum exposure time of 24 hours is required to disinfect disposable hemodialyzers that are reused on the same patient (496,497). Aqueous formaldehyde solutions (1–2%) also have been used to disinfect the internal fluid pathways of dialysis machines (497). To minimize a potential health hazard to dialysis patients, the dialysis equipment must be thoroughly rinsed and tested for residual formaldehyde before use.

Paraformaldehyde, a solid polymer of formaldehyde, may be vaporized by heat for the gaseous decontamination of laminar flow biologic safety cabinets when maintenance work or filter changes require access to the sealed portion of the cabinet.

Glutaraldehyde

Overview

Glutaraldehyde is a saturated dialdehyde that has gained wide acceptance as a high-level disinfectant and chemical sterilant (97). Aqueous solutions of glutaraldehyde are acidic and generally in this state are not sporicidal. Only when the solution is "activated" (made alkaline) by use of alkalinating agents to pH 7.5 to 8.5 does the solution become sporicidal. Once activated, these solutions have a shelf life of minimally 14 days because of the polymerization of the glutaraldehyde molecules at alkaline pH levels. This polymerization blocks the active sites (aldehyde groups) of the glutaraldehyde molecules that are responsible for its biocidal activity.

Novel glutaraldehyde formulations (e.g., glutaraldehyde-phenol-sodium phenate, potentiated acid glutaraldehyde, stabilized alkaline glutaraldehyde) produced in the past 30 years have overcome the problem of rapid loss of activity (e.g., a use life of 28 to 30 days) while generally maintaining excellent microbicidal activity (498–502). However, it should be recognized that antimicrobial activity is dependent not only on age but also on use conditions such as dilution and organic stress. Manufacturers' literature for these preparations suggests that the neutral or alkaline glutaraldehydes possess superior microbicidal and anticorrosion properties when compared to acid glutaraldehydes, and a few published reports substantiate these claims (464,503,504). However, two studies found no difference in the microbicidal activity of alkaline and acid glutaraldehydes (64,505). The use of glutaraldehyde-based solutions in healthcare facilities is widespread because of their advantages: excellent biocidal properties;

activity in the presence of organic matter (20% bovine serum); and noncorrosive action to endoscopic equipment, thermometers, rubber, or plastic equipment. The advantages, disadvantages, and characteristics of glutaraldehyde are listed in Tables 85.7 and 85.8.

Mode of Action

The biocidal activity of glutaraldehyde is a consequence of its alkylation of sulfhydral, hydroxyl, carboxy, and amino groups of microorganisms, which alters RNA, DNA, and protein synthesis. Scott and Gorman (506,507) provide an extensive review of the mechanism of action of glutaraldehydes.

Microbicidal Activity

The *in vitro* inactivation of microorganisms by glutaraldehydes has been extensively investigated and reviewed (506,507). Several investigators showed that ≥2% aqueous solutions of glutaraldehyde, buffered to pH 7.5 to 8.5 with sodium bicarbonate, were effective in killing vegetative bacteria in less than 2 minutes; *M. tuberculosis,* fungi, and viruses in less than 10 minutes; and spores of *Bacillus* and *Clostridium* species in 3 hours (464,506–511). Spores of *C. difficile* are more rapidly killed by 2% glutaraldehyde than are spores of other species of *Clostridium* and *Bacillus* (70,231,232). There have been reports of microorganisms with significant resistance to glutaraldehyde, including some mycobacteria (*M. chelonae, M. avium-intracellulare, M. xenopi*) (512–514), *Methylobacterium mesophilicum* (515), *Trichosporon,* fungal ascospores (e.g., *Microascus cinereus, Cheatomium globosum*), and *Cryptosporidium* (279,516). *M. chelonae* persisted in a 0.2% glutaraldehyde solution used to store porcine prosthetic heart valves (517).

Collins and Montalbine (503) reported that 2% alkaline glutaraldehyde solution inactivated 10^5 *M. tuberculosis* cells present on the surface of penicylinders within 5 minutes at 18°C. However, subsequent studies conducted by Rubbo et al. (73) questioned the mycobactericidal prowess of glutaraldehydes. They showed that 2% alkaline glutaraldehyde has slow action (20 to >30 minutes) against *M. tuberculosis* and compares unfavorably with alcohols, formaldehydes, iodine, and phenol. Collins (518) demonstrated that suspensions of *Mycobacterium avium, M. intracellulare,* and *M. gordonae* were more resistant to inactivation by a 2% alkaline glutaraldehyde (estimated time to complete inactivation, 60 minutes) than were virulent *M. tuberculosis* (estimated time to complete inactivation, 25 minutes). Collins (75) also showed that the rate of kill was directly proportional to the temperature and that sterility of a standardized suspension of *M. tuberculosis* could not be achieved within 10 minutes. A recently FDA-cleared chemical sterilant containing 2.5% glutaraldehyde uses increased temperature (35°C) to reduce the time required to achieve high-level disinfection (5 minutes) (76), but its use

TABLE 85.7. COMPARISON OF THE CHARACTERISTICS OF SELECTED CHEMICALS USED PRIMARILY AS HIGH-LEVEL DISINFECTANTS

	HP (7.5%)	PA (0.2%)	Glut (≥2.0%)	OPA (0.55%)	HP/PA (7.35%/.23%)
HLD Claim	30 m @ 20°C	NA	20–90 m @ 20°–25°C	12 m @ 20°C	15 m @ 20°C
Sterilization Claim	6 h @ 20°	12 m @ 50–56°C	10 h @ 20°–25°C	None	3 h @ 20°C
Activation	No	No	Yes (alkaline glut)	No	No
Reuse life[1]	21d	Single use	14–30 d (acid glut-1 yr)	14d	14d
Shelf Life Stability[2]	2 y	6 mo	2 y	2 y	2 y
Disposal Restrictions	None	None	Local[3]	Local[3]	None
Materials Compatibility	Good	Good	Excellent	Excellent	No data
Monitor MEC[4]	Yes (6%)	No	Yes (1.5% or higher)	Yes (0.3% OPA)	No
Safety	Serious eye damage (safety glasses)	Serious eye and skin damage (conc soln)[5]	Respiratory	Eye irritant, stains skin	Eye damage
Processing	Manual or automated	Automated	Manual or automated	Manual or automated	Manual
Organic material resistance	Yes	Yes	Yes	Yes	Yes
OSHA exposure limit	1 ppm TWA	PA-none	0.05 ppm Ceiling	None	HP-1 ppm TWA
Sterilant Cost[6]	$24.99/gal	$4.95/container	$13.00/gal	$35.00/gal	$32.00/gal
Cost profile (per cycle)[7]	$0.40 (manual), $1.59 (automated)	$4.95 (automated)	$0.31 (manual), $1.24 (automated)	$0.83 (manual)	$0.76 (manual)

Modified from 60.
Abbreviations: HLD=high-level disinfectant; HP=hydrogen peroxide; PA=peracetic acid; glut=glutaraldehyde; PA/HP=peracetic acid and hydrogen peroxide; OPA=ortho-phthalaldehyde (FDA cleared as a high-level disinfectant, included for comparison to other chemical agents used for high-level disinfection); m=minutes; h=hours; NA=not applicable; TWA=time-weighted average for a conventional 8-hour workday.
[1] number of days a product can be reused as determined by re-use protocol
[2] time a product can remain in storage (unused)
[3] no U.S. EPA regulations, but some states and local authorities have additional restrictions
[4] MEC=minimum effective concentration, the lowest concentration of active ingredients at which the product is still effective
[5] Conc soln=concentrated solution
[6] figure includes only the cost of the processing solution (suggested list price to healthcare facilities in August 2001)
[7] per cycle cost profile assumes maximum use life (e.g., 21 days for hydrogen peroxide, 14 days for glutaraldehyde), 3 reprocessing cycles per day, 1-gallon basin for manual processing, and 4-gallon tank for automated processing

TABLE 85.8. SUMMARY OF ADVANTAGES AND DISADVANTAGES OF CHEMICAL AGENTS USED AS CHEMICAL STERILANTS[1] OR AS HIGH-LEVEL DISINFECTANTS

Sterilization Method	Advantages	Disadvantages
Peracetic Acid/Hydrogen Peroxide	• No activation required • Odor or irritation not significant	• Materials compatibility concerns (lead, brass, copper, zinc) both cosmetic and functional • Limited clinical experience • Potential for eye and skin damage
Glutaraldehyde	• Numerous use studies published • Relatively inexpensive • Excellent materials compatibility	• Respiratory irritation from glutaraldehyde vapor • Pungent and irritating odor • Relatively slow mycobactericidal activity • Coagulates blood and fixes tissue to surfaces • Allergic contact dermatitis
Hydrogen Peroxide	• No activation required • May enhance removal of organic matter and microorganisms • No disposal issues • No odor or irritation issues • Does not coagulate blood or fix tissues to surfaces • Inactivates *Cryptosporidium* • Use studies published	• Material compatibility concerns (brass, zinc, copper, and nickel/silver plating) both cosmetic and functional • Serious eye damage with contact
Ortho-phthalaldehyde	• Fast acting high-level disinfectant • No activation required • Odor not significant • Excellent materials compatibility claimed • Does not coagulate blood or fix tissues to surfaces claimed	• Stains skin, mucous membranes, clothing, and environmental surfaces • Limited clinical experience • More expensive than glutaraldehyde • Eye irritation with contact • Slow sporicidal activity
Peracetic Acid	• Rapid sterilization cycle time (30–45 minutes) • Low temperature (50–55°C) liquid immersion sterilization • Environmental friendly by-products (acetic acid, O_2, H_2O) • Fully automated • Single-use system eliminates need for concentration testing • Standardized cycle • May enhance removal of organic material and endotoxin • No adverse health effects to operators under normal operating conditions • Compatible with many materials and instruments • Does not coagulate blood or fix tissues to surfaces • Sterilant flows through scope facilitating salt, protein, and microbe removal • Rapidly sporicidal • Provides procedure standardization (constant dilution, perfusion of channel, temperatures, exposure)	• Potential material incompatibility (e.g., aluminum anodized coating becomes dull) • Used for immersible instruments only • Biological indicator may not be suitable for routine monitoring • One scope or a small number of instruments can be processed in a cycle • More expensive (endoscope repairs, operating costs, purchase costs) than high-level disinfection • Serious eye and skin damage (concentrated solution) with contact • Point-of-use system, no sterile storage

Modified from 60.

[1] All products effective in presence of organic soil, relatively easy to use, and have a broad spectrum of antimicrobial activity (bacteria, fungi, viruses, bacterial spores, and mycobacteria). The above characteristics are documented in the literature; contact the manufacturer of the instrument and sterilant for additional information. All products listed above are FDA-cleared as chemical sterilants except OPA, which is an FDA-cleared high-level disinfectant.

is limited to automatic endoscope reprocessors equipped with a heater. In another study employing membrane filters for measurement of mycobactericidal activity of 2% alkaline glutaraldehyde, Collins (72) demonstrated that complete inactivation was achieved within 20 minutes at 20°C when the test inoculum was 10^6 *M. tuberculosis* per membrane. Several investigators have demonstrated that glutaraldehyde solutions inactivate 2.4 to >5.0 $\log_{10}$ of *M. tuberculosis* in 10 minutes (including multidrug-resistant *M. tuberculosis*) and 4.0 to 6.4 $\log_{10}$ of *M. tuberculosis* in 20 minutes (48,50,64,67,71,72,75,518). On the basis of these data and other studies, 20 minutes at room temperature is the minimum exposure time needed to reliably kill *Mycobacteria* and other vegetative bacteria with a ≥2% glutaraldehyde (2,15,18,23,50,74,85,99,102–106).

Dilution of glutaraldehyde during use commonly occurs, and studies show a glutaraldehyde concentration decline after a few days of use in an automatic endoscope washer (519,520). This occurs because instruments are not thoroughly dried and water is carried in with the instrument, which increases the solution's volume and dilutes its effective concentration (521). This emphasizes the need to ensure that semicritical equipment is disinfected with an acceptable concentration of glutaraldehyde. Data suggest that 1.0% to 1.5% glutaraldehyde is the minimum effective concentration for >2% glutaraldehyde solutions when used as a high-level disinfectant (67,503,504,520). Chemical test strips or liquid chemical monitors (521,522) are available for determining whether an effective concentration of glutaraldehyde is present despite repeated use and dilution. The frequency of testing should be based on how frequently the solutions are used (e.g., used daily, test daily; used weekly, test before use; used 30 times per day, test each tenth use), but the strips should not be used to extend the use life beyond the expiration date. Data suggest the chemicals in the test strip deteriorate with time (523) and a manufacturer's expiration date should be placed on the bottles. The bottle of test strips should be dated when opened and used for the period of time indicated on the bottle (e.g., 120 days). The results of test strip monitoring should be documented. The glutaraldehyde test kits have been preliminarily evaluated for accuracy and range (523), but the reliability has been questioned (524). The concentration should be considered unacceptable or unsafe when the test indicates a dilution below the product's minimum effective concentration (MEC) (generally to 1.0% to 1.5% glutaraldehyde or lower) by the indicator not changing color.

A 2.0% glutaraldehyde–7.05% phenol–1.20% sodium phenate product that contained 0.125% glutaraldehyde–0.44% phenol–0.075% sodium phenate when diluted 1:16 was not recommended as a high-level disinfectant because of its lack of bactericidal activity in the presence of organic matter and its lack of tuberculocidal, fungicidal, virucidal, and sporicidal activity (43,48,49,62,64–70,525). In December 1991, the EPA issued an order to stop the sale of all batches of this product based on efficacy data that showed that this product is not effective against spores and possibly other microorganisms or inanimate objects as claimed on the label (526). A new diluted glutaraldehyde containing 0.95% glutaraldehyde with 1.64% phenol/phenate has been cleared by the FDA as a high-level disinfectant. The other glutaraldehyde sterilants cleared by the FDA as of January 2002 contain 2.4% to 3.4% glutaraldehyde and are used undiluted (76).

Uses

Glutaraldehyde is used most commonly as a high-level disinfectant for medical equipment such as endoscopes (60,97,432), spirometry tubing, dialyzers (527), transducers, anesthesia and respiratory therapy equipment (528), hemodialysis proportioning and dialysate delivery systems (495,529), and reuse of laparoscopic disposable plastic trocars (530). Glutaraldehyde is noncorrosive to metal and does not damage lensed instruments, rubber, or plastics. Glutaraldehyde should not be used for cleaning noncritical surfaces as it is too toxic and expensive.

Colitis believed due to glutaraldehyde exposure from residual disinfecting solution in the endoscope solution channels has been reported and is preventable by careful endoscope rinsing (307,531–541). One study found that residual glutaraldehyde levels were higher and more variable after manual disinfection (<0.2–159.5 mg/L) than after automatic disinfection (0.2–6.3 mg/L) (542). Similarly, keratopathy and corneal decompensation were caused by ophthalmic instruments that were inadequately rinsed after soaking in 2% glutaraldehyde (543,544).

Healthcare workers can become exposed to elevated levels of glutaraldehyde vapor when equipment is processed in poorly ventilated rooms, when spills occur, during activation or changeover of glutaraldehyde solutions (545), or when there are open immersion baths. Acute or chronic exposure may result in skin irritation or dermatitis, mucous membrane irritation (eye, nose, mouth), or pulmonary symptoms (307,546–550). Epistaxis, allergic contact dermatitis, asthma, and rhinitis also have been reported in healthcare workers exposed to glutaraldehyde (547, 551–558).

Glutaraldehyde exposure should be monitored to ensure a safe work environment. Testing can be done by four techniques: a silica gel tube/gas chromatography with a flame ionization detector, dinitrophenylhydrazine (DNPH)-impregnated filter cassette/high-performance liquid chromatography (HPLC) with an ultraviolet (UV) detector, a passive badge/HPLC, or a handheld glutaraldehyde air monitor (559). The silica gel tube and the DNPH-impregnated cassette are suitable for monitoring the 0.05-ppm ceiling limit. The passive badge, with a 0.02-ppm limit of detection, is considered marginal at the ACGIH ceiling level. The ceiling level is thought to be too close to the glutaraldehyde meter's 0.03-ppm limit of detection to provide confidence in the readings (559). ACGIH does not require a specific monitoring schedule for glutaraldehyde; however, a monitoring schedule is needed to ensure that the level is less than the ceiling limit. For example, monitoring should be done initially to determine glutaraldehyde levels, after procedural or equipment changes, and in response to worker complaints (560). In the absence of an OSHA PEL or NIOSH REL, if the glutaraldehyde level is higher than the ACGIH ceiling limit of 0.05 ppm, it would be prudent to take corrective action and repeat monitoring (560).

Engineering and work practice controls that may be used to combat these problems include ducted exhaust hoods, air systems that provide 7 to 15 air exchanges per hour, ductless fume hoods with absorbents for the glutaraldehyde vapor, tight-fitting lids on immersion baths, personal protection (e.g., nitrile or butyl rubber gloves but not natural latex gloves; goggles) to minimize skin or mucous membrane contact, and automated endoscope processors (7,561). If engineering controls fail to maintain levels below the ACGIH, institutions may consider the use of respirators [e.g., a half-face respirator with organic vapor cartridge (551) or a type C supplied air respirator with a full face piece operated in a positive pressure mode (562)]. In general, engineering controls are preferred over work practice and administrative controls, as they do not require the active participation of the healthcare worker. Even though enforcement of the OSHA ceiling limit was suspended in 1993 by the U.S. Court of Appeals (490), it is prudent to limit employee exposure to 0.05 ppm (per ACGIH) since at this level glutaraldehyde is irritating to the eyes, throat, and nose (307,490,550,563). If glutaraldehyde disposal via the sanitary sewer system is restricted, sodium bisulfate can be used to neutralize the glutaraldehyde and make it safe for disposal.

Hydrogen Peroxide

Overview

The literature contains several accounts of the properties, germicidal effectiveness, and potential uses for stabilized hydrogen peroxide in the healthcare setting. Published reports ascribe good germicidal activity to hydrogen peroxide and attest to its bactericidal, virucidal, sporicidal, and fungicidal properties (564–566). The advantages, disadvantages, and characteristics of hydrogen peroxide are listed in Tables 85.7 and 85.8.

Mode of Action

Hydrogen peroxide works by the production of destructive hydroxyl free radicals that can attack membrane lipids, DNA, and other essential cell components. Catalase, produced by aerobic and facultative anaerobes that possess cytochrome systems, may protect cells from metabolically produced hydrogen peroxide by degrading hydrogen peroxide to water and oxygen. This defense is overwhelmed by the concentrations used for disinfection (564,565).

Microbicidal Activity

Hydrogen peroxide is active against a wide range of microorganisms, including bacteria, yeasts, fungi, viruses, and spores (69,565). Schaeffer et al. (567) demonstrated the bactericidal effectiveness and stability of hydrogen peroxide in urine against a variety of healthcare-associated pathogens. They showed that microorganisms with high cellular catalase activity (e.g., *S. aureus, S. marcescens,* and *Proteus mirabilis*) required 30 to 60 minutes of exposure to 0.6% hydrogen peroxide for a 10^8 reduction in cell counts, whereas microorganisms with lower catalase activity (e.g., *E. coli, Streptococcus* species, and *Pseudomonas* species) required only 15 minutes exposure. Wardle and Renninger (568) investigated 3%, 10%, and 15% hydrogen peroxide for reducing spacecraft bacterial populations and got a complete kill of 10^6 spores (i.e., *Bacillus* species) with a 10% concentration and a 60-minute exposure time. A 3% concentration for 150 minutes killed 10^6 spores in six of seven exposure trials (568). Sagripanti and Bonifacino (569,570) found that a 10% hydrogen peroxide solution resulted in a 10^3 decrease in *B. atrophaeus* spores and a 10^5 or greater decrease when tested against 13 other pathogens in 30 minutes at 20°C. A 3.0% hydrogen peroxide solution was ineffective against VRE after 3- and 10-minute exposure times (571) and caused only a 2-$\log_{10}$ reduction in the number of *Acanthamoeba* cysts in approximately 2 hours (572). A 7% stabilized hydrogen peroxide proved to be sporicidal (6 hours exposure time), mycobactericidal (20 minutes), and fungicidal (5 minutes) at full strength, and virucidal (5 minutes) and bactericidal (3 minutes) at a 1:16 dilution when using a quantitative carrier test (566). The 7% solution of hydrogen peroxide, tested after 14 days of stress (in the form of germ-loaded carriers and respiratory therapy equipment), was found to be sporicidal (>7 $\log_{10}$ reduction in 6 hours), mycobactericidal (>6.5 $\log_{10}$ reduction in 25 minutes), fungicidal (>5 $\log_{10}$ reduction in 20 minutes), bactericidal (>6 $\log_{10}$ reduction in 5 minutes), and virucidal (5 $\log_{10}$ reduction in 5 minutes) (573). Synergistic sporicidal effects were observed when spores were exposed to a combination of hydrogen peroxide (5.9% to 23.6%) and peracetic acid (574). The antiviral activity of hydrogen peroxide against rhinovirus was demonstrated in studies by Mentel and Schmidt (575). The time required for inactivating three serotypes of rhinovirus using a 3% hydrogen peroxide solution was 6 to 8 minutes; this time increased with decreasing concentrations (18–20 minutes at 1.5%, 50–60 minutes at 0.75%).

Concentrations of hydrogen peroxide from 6% to 25% have promise as chemical sterilants. The product marketed as a sterilant is a premixed, ready-to-use chemical that contains 7.5% hydrogen peroxide and 0.85% phosphoric acid (to maintain a low pH) (60). The mycobactericidal activity of 7.5% hydrogen peroxide has been corroborated by Sattar (576), who showed the inactivation of >10^5 multidrug resistant *M. tuberculosis* after a 10-minute exposure (576). Thirty minutes were required for >99.9% inactivation of polio and hepatitis A viruses (577). Mbithi et al. (51) showed that 3% and 6% hydrogen peroxide were unable to inactivate the hepatitis A virus in 1 minute using a carrier test. The effectiveness of 7.5% hydrogen peroxide at 10 minutes was compared to 2% alkaline glutaraldehyde at 20 minutes in manual disinfection of endoscopes; no significant difference in germicidal activity was observed (578). There also were no complaints received from the nursing or medical staff in terms of odor or toxicity. In one study, 6% hydrogen peroxide (unused product was 7.5%) was more effective in the high-level disinfection of flexible endoscopes than was the 2% glutaraldehyde solution (579). A new, rapid-acting 13.4% hydrogen peroxide formulation (currently not FDA-cleared) has demonstrated sporicidal, mycobactericidal, fungicidal, and virucidal efficacy. Manufacturer's data demonstrate that this solution sterilizes in 30 minutes and provides high-level disinfection in 5 minutes (580). This product has not been used long enough to evaluate material compatibility to endoscopes and other semicritical devices, and further assessment by instrument manufacturers should be done.

Under normal conditions, hydrogen peroxide is extremely stable when properly stored (e.g., in dark containers). The decomposition or loss of potency in small containers is less than 2% per year at ambient temperatures (581).

Uses

Commercially available 3% hydrogen peroxide is a stable and effective disinfectant when used on inanimate surfaces. It has been used in concentrations from 3% to 6% for the disinfection of soft contact lenses (e.g., 3% for 2 to 3 hours) (564,582,583), tonometer biprisms (440), ventilators (584), fabrics (371), and endoscopes (579). Hydrogen peroxide was effective in spot-disinfecting fabrics in patients' rooms (371). Corneal damage from a hydrogen peroxide–soaked tonometer tip that was not properly rinsed has been reported (585). Hydrogen peroxide also has been instilled into urinary drainage bags in an attempt to eliminate the bag as a source of bladder bacteriuria and environmental contamination (586). Although the instillation of hydrogen peroxide into the bag reduced microbial contamination of the bag, this procedure did not reduce the incidence of catheter-associated bacteriuria (586).

A chemical irritation resembling pseudomembranous colitis, which was caused by either 3% hydrogen peroxide or a 2% glutaraldehyde, has been reported (532). An epidemic of pseudomembrane-like enteritis and colitis in seven patients in a gastrointestinal endoscopy unit also has been associated with inadequate rinsing of 3% hydrogen peroxide from the endoscope (587).

As with other chemical sterilants, dilution of the hydrogen peroxide must be monitored by regularly testing the minimum effective concentration (i.e., 7.5% to 6.0%). Compatibility testing by Olympus America of the 7.5% hydrogen peroxide found both cosmetic changes (e.g., discoloration of black anodized metal finishes) (60) and functional changes with the tested endoscopes (Olympus, written communication, October 15, 1999).

Iodophors

Overview

Iodine solutions or tinctures have long been used by health professionals, primarily as antiseptics on skin or tissue. Iodophors, on the other hand, have been used both as antiseptics and disinfectants. An iodophor is a combination of iodine and a solubilizing agent or carrier; the resulting complex provides a sustained-release reservoir of iodine and releases small amounts of free iodine in aqueous solution. The best-known and most widely used iodophor is povidone-iodine, a compound of polyvinylpyrrolidone with iodine. This product and other iodophors retain the germicidal efficacy of iodine but unlike iodine are generally nonstaining and are relatively free of toxicity and irritancy (588,589).

Several reports that documented intrinsic microbial contamination of antiseptic formulations of povidone-iodine and poloxamer-iodine (590–592) caused a reappraisal of the chemistry and use of iodophors (593). It was found that "free" iodine (I_2) contributes to the bactericidal activity of iodophors, and dilutions of iodophors demonstrate more rapid bactericidal action than does a full-strength povidone-iodine solution. The reason for the observation that dilution increases bactericidal activity is unclear but it has been suggested that dilution of povidone-iodine results in weakening of the iodine linkage to the carrier polymer with an accompanying increase of free iodine in solution (591). Therefore, iodophors must be diluted according to the manufacturers' directions to achieve antimicrobial activity.

Mode of Action

Iodine is able to penetrate the cell wall of microorganisms quickly and it is thought that the lethal effects result from a disruption of protein and nucleic acid structure and synthesis.

Microbicidal Activity

Published reports on the *in vitro* antimicrobial efficacy of iodophors demonstrate that iodophors are bactericidal, mycobactericidal, and virucidal but may require prolonged contact times to kill certain fungi and bacterial spores (12,62–64,297, 594–597). Berkelman et al. (594) found that three brands of povidone-iodine solution demonstrated more rapid kill (seconds to minutes) of *S. aureus* and *M. chelonae* at a 1:100 dilution than did the stock solution. Klein and DeForest (63) demonstrated the virucidal activity of 75 to 150 ppm available iodine against seven viruses. Other investigators have questioned the efficacy of iodophors against poliovirus in the presence of organic matter (596) and rotavirus SA-11 in distilled or tap water (297). Manufacturers' data demonstrate that commercial iodophors are not sporicidal, but they are tuberculocidal, fungicidal, virucidal, and bactericidal at their recommended use-dilution.

Uses

Besides their use as an antiseptic, iodophors have been used for the disinfection of blood culture bottles and medical equipment such as hydrotherapy tanks, thermometers, and, in the past, endoscopes. Antiseptic iodophors are not suitable for use as hard-surface disinfectants because of concentration differences. Iodophors formulated as antiseptics contain less free iodine than those formulated as disinfectants (355). Iodine or iodine-based antiseptics should not be used on silicone catheters as the silicone tubing may be adversely affected (598).

Ortho-phthalaldehyde (OPA)

Overview

OPA is a high-level disinfectant that received FDA clearance in October 1999. It contains 0.55% 1,2-benzenedicarboxaldehyde or OPA. OPA solution is a clear, pale-blue liquid with a pH of 7.5. The advantages, disadvantages, and characteristics of OPA are listed in Tables 85.7 and 85.8.

Mode of Action

Preliminary studies on the mode of action of OPA suggest that both OPA and glutaraldehyde interact with amino acids, proteins, and microorganisms. However, OPA is a less potent cross-linking agent. This is compensated for by the lipophilic aromatic nature of OPA that is likely to assist its uptake through the outer layers of mycobacteria and gram-negative bacteria (599,600). OPA appears to kill spores by blocking the spore germination process (601).

Microbicidal Activity

Studies have demonstrated excellent microbicidal activity in *in vitro* studies (60,91,279,374,602–611). For example, Gregory et al. (603) demonstrated that OPA has superior mycobactericidal activity (5-$\log_{10}$ reduction in 5 minutes) compared to glutaraldehyde. The mean times required to produce a 6-$\log_{10}$ reduction for *M. bovis* using 0.21% OPA was 6 minutes compared to 32 minutes using 1.5% glutaraldehyde. OPA showed good activity against the mycobacteria tested, including the glutaraldehyde-resistant strains, but 0.5% OPA was not sporicidal with 270 minutes of exposure. Increasing the pH from its unadjusted level (about 6.5) to pH 8 improved the sporicidal activity of OPA (604). Chan-Myers and Roberts (607) showed that the level of biocidal activity was directly related to the temperature. A greater than 5-$\log_{10}$ reduction of *B. atrophaeus* spores was observed in 3 hours at 35°C as compared to 24 hours at 20°C. Also, with an exposure time at or below 5 minutes, a decrease in biocidal activity was observed with increasing serum concentration. However, there was no difference in efficacy when the exposure time was 10 minutes or longer. Walsh et al. (604) also found OPA effective (>5-$\log_{10}$ reduction) against a wide range of microorganisms, including glutaraldehyde-resistant mycobacteria and *B. atrophaeus* spores.

Uses

OPA has several potential advantages compared to glutaraldehyde. It has excellent stability over a wide pH range (pH 3–9), is not a known irritant to the eyes and nasal passages, does not require exposure monitoring, has a barely perceptible odor, and requires no activation. OPA, like glutaraldehyde, has excellent material compatibility. A potential disadvantage of OPA is that it stains proteins gray (including unprotected skin) and thus must be handled with caution (60). However, skin staining would indicate improper handling that requires additional training or PPE (gloves, eye and mouth protection, fluid-resistant gowns). PPE should be worn when handling contaminated instruments, equipment, and chemicals (374). In addition, equipment must be thoroughly rinsed to prevent discoloration of a patient's skin or mucous membranes.

Since OPA was only recently cleared for use as a high-level disinfectant, only limited clinical studies are available. In a clinical-use study, exposure of 100 endoscopes for 5 minutes to OPA resulted in a >5-$\log_{10}$ reduction in bacterial load. Further, OPA was effective over a 14-day usage cycle (91). Manufacturer's data show that OPA lasts longer in an automatic endoscope reprocessor before reaching its MEC limit (MEC after 82 cycles) compared to glutaraldehyde (MEC after 40 cycles) (374). Disposal must be done in accordance with local and state regulations. If OPA disposal via the sanitary sewer system is restricted, glycine (25 g/gallon) can be used to neutralize the OPA and make it safe for disposal.

The high-level disinfectant label claims for OPA solution at 20°C vary worldwide, e.g., 5 minutes in Europe, Asia, and Latin America; 10 minutes in Canada and Australia; and 12 minutes in the U.S. These label claims are different worldwide because of differences in the test methodology and requirements for licensure.

Peracetic Acid

Overview

Peracetic, or peroxyacetic, acid is characterized by a very rapid action against all microorganisms. Special advantages of peracetic acid are that it lacks harmful decomposition products (i.e., acetic acid, water, oxygen, hydrogen peroxide), it enhances removal of organic material (612), and leaves no residue. It remains effective in the presence of organic matter and is sporicidal even at low temperatures. Peracetic acid can corrode copper, brass, bronze, plain steel, and galvanized iron, but these effects can be reduced by additives and pH modifications. It is considered unstable, particularly when diluted; for example, a 1% solution loses half its strength through hydrolysis in 6 days, whereas 40% peracetic acid loses 1% to 2% of its active ingredients per month (565). The advantages, disadvantages, and characteristics of peracetic acid are listed in Tables 85.7 and 85.8.

Mode of Action

Little is known about the mechanism of action of peracetic acid, but it is thought to function similarly to other oxidizing agents; that is, it denatures proteins, disrupts the cell wall permeability, and oxidizes sulfhydral and sulfur bonds in proteins, enzymes, and other metabolites (565).

Microbicidal Activity

Peracetic acid inactivates gram-positive and gram-negative bacteria, fungi, and yeasts in ≤5 minutes at <100 ppm. In the presence of organic matter, 200 to 500 ppm is required. For viruses, the dosage range is wide (12–2,250 ppm), with poliovirus inactivated in yeast extract in 15 minutes with 1,500 to 2,250 ppm. One study showed that 3.5% peracetic acid was ineffective against the hepatitis A virus after 1-minute exposure using a carrier test (51). With bacterial spores, 500 to 10,000 ppm (0.05% to 1%) inactivates spores in 15 seconds to 30 minutes using a spore suspension test (565,569,613,614).

Uses

An automated machine using peracetic acid to chemically sterilize medical (e.g., endoscopes, arthroscopes), surgical, and dental instruments is used in the U.S. (615–617). As previously noted, dental handpieces should be steam sterilized. The sterilant, 35% peracetic acid, is diluted to 0.2% with filtered water at a temperature of 50°C. Simulated-use trials have demonstrated excellent microbicidal activity (99,617–621), and three clinical trials have demonstrated both excellent microbial killing and no clinical failures leading to infection (81,622,623). The high efficacy of the system was demonstrated by Alfa et al. (621), who compared the efficacies of the system with that of ETO. Only the peracetic acid system was able to kill 6 $\log_{10}$ of *M. chelonae, Enterococcus faecalis,* and *B. atrophaeus* spores with both an organic and inorganic challenge. An investigation by Fuselier and Mason (81) compared the costs, performance, and maintenance of urologic endoscopic equipment processed by high-level disinfection (with glutaraldehyde) with those of the peracetic acid system and reported no clinical differences between the two systems. However, the use of this system led to increased costs when compared to high-level disinfection, including costs for processing ($6.11 vs. $0.45 per cycle), purchasing and training ($24,845 vs. $16), installation ($5,800 vs. $0), and endoscope repairs ($6,037 vs. $445) (81). Further, three clusters of infection using the peracetic acid automated endoscope reprocessor were linked to inadequately processed bronchoscopes when inappropriate channel connectors were used with the system (624).

These clusters highlight the importance of training, proper model-specific endoscope connector systems, and quality control procedures to ensure compliance with endoscope manufacturer's recommendations and professional organization guidelines. An alternative high-level disinfectant available in the U.K. contains 0.35% peracetic acid. Although this product is rapidly effective against a broad range of microorganisms (625–627), it tarnishes the metal of endoscopes and is unstable, resulting in only a 24-hour use life (627).

Peracetic Acid and Hydrogen Peroxide

Overview

Two chemical sterilants are available that contain peracetic acid plus hydrogen peroxide [0.08% peracetic acid plus 1.0% hydrogen peroxide (no longer marketed), 0.23% peracetic acid plus 7.35% hydrogen peroxide]. The advantages, disadvantages, and characteristics of peracetic acid and hydrogen peroxide are listed in Tables 85.7 and 85.8.

Microbicidal Activity

The bactericidal properties of peracetic acid and hydrogen peroxide have been demonstrated (628). Manufacturer's data demonstrated that this inactivated all microorganisms with the combination of peracetic acid and hydrogen peroxide with the exception of bacterial spores within 20 minutes. The 0.08% peracetic acid plus 1.0% hydrogen peroxide product was effective in inactivating a glutaraldehyde-resistant mycobacterium (629).

Uses

The combination of peracetic acid and hydrogen peroxide has been used for disinfecting hemodialyzers (630). The percentage of dialysis centers using a peracetic acid–hydrogen peroxide–based disinfectant for reprocessing dialyzers increased from 5% in 1983 to 56% in 1997 (495). Olympus America (written communication, April 15, 1998) does not endorse the use of 0.08% peracetic acid plus 1.0% hydrogen peroxide on any Olympus endoscope due to cosmetic and functional damage, and will not assume liability for chemical damage as a result of the use of this product. This product is not currently available. A newer chemical sterilant with 0.23% peracetic acid and 7.35% hydrogen peroxide has been cleared by the FDA, and its characteristics, advantages, and disadvantages are shown in Tables 85.7 and 85.8. Olympus America (written communication, September 13, 2000) tested the 7.35% hydrogen peroxide and 0.23% peracetic acid product and concluded it was not compatible with its flexible gastrointestinal endoscopes based on immersion studies where the test insertion tubes had failed due to swelling and loosening of the black polymer layer of the tube.

Phenolics

Overview

Phenol has occupied a prominent place in the field of hospital disinfection since its initial use as a germicide by Lister in his pioneering work on antiseptic surgery. In the past 30 years, however, work has been concentrated on the numerous phenol derivatives or phenolics and their antimicrobial properties. Phenol derivatives originate when a functional group (e.g., alkyl, phenyl, benzyl, halogen) replaces one of the hydrogen atoms on the aromatic ring. Two phenol derivatives commonly found as constituents of hospital disinfectants are ortho-phenylphenol and ortho-benzyl-para-chlorophenol. The antimicrobial properties of these compounds and many other phenol derivatives are much improved over those of the parent chemical. Phenolics are absorbed by porous materials and the residual disinfectant may cause tissue irritation. In 1970 Kahn (631) reported that depigmentation of the skin is caused by phenolic germicidal detergents containing para-tertiary butylphenol and para-tertiary amylphenol.

Mode of Action

Phenol, in high concentrations, acts as a gross protoplasmic poison, penetrating and disrupting the cell wall and precipitating the cell proteins. Low concentrations of phenol and higher molecular-weight phenol derivatives cause bacterial death by the inactivation of essential enzyme systems and leakage of essential metabolites from the cell wall (632).

Microbicidal Activity

Published reports on the antimicrobial efficacy of commonly used phenolics showed that they were bactericidal, fungicidal, virucidal, and tuberculocidal (12,54,62,64,206,387,486, 632–638). One study demonstrated little or no virucidal effect of a phenolic against coxsackie B4, echovirus 11, and poliovirus 1 (636). Similarly, Klein and DeForest (63) observed that 12% ortho-phenylphenol failed to inactivate any of the three hydrophilic viruses after a 10-minute exposure time, although 5% phenol was lethal for these viruses. A 0.5% dilution of a phenolic (2.8% ortho-phenylphenol and 2.7% ortho-benzyl-para-chlorophenol) inactivated HIV (206), and a 2% solution of a phenolic (15% ortho-phenylphenol and 6.3% para-tertiary-amylphenol) inactivated all but one of 11 fungi tested (62).

Manufacturers' data using the standardized AOAC methods demonstrate that commercial phenolics are not sporicidal but are tuberculocidal, fungicidal, virucidal, and bactericidal at their recommended use-dilution. Attempts to substantiate the bactericidal label claims of phenolics using the AOAC use-dilution method have failed on occasion (387,637). However, these same studies have shown extreme variability of test results among laboratories testing identical products.

Uses

Many phenolic germicides are EPA-registered as disinfectants for use on environmental surfaces (e.g., bedside tables, bed rails, laboratory surfaces) and noncritical medical devices. Phenolics are not FDA-cleared as high-level disinfectants for use with semicritical items but could be used to preclean or decontaminate critical and semicritical devices prior to terminal sterilization or high-level disinfection.

The use of phenolics in nurseries has been questioned because of the occurrence of hyperbilirubinemia in infants placed in bassinets where phenolic detergents were used (639). In addition, Doan et al. (640) demonstrated bilirubin level increases in phenolic-exposed infants compared to nonphenolic-exposed infants when the phenolic was prepared according to the manufacturers' recommended dilution. If phenolics are used to clean nursery floors, they must be diluted according to the recommendation on the product label. Phenolics (and other disinfectants) should not be used to clean infant bassinets and incubators while occupied. If phenolics are used to terminally clean infant bassinets and incubators, the surfaces should be rinsed thoroughly with water and dried before the infant bassinets and incubators are reused (15).

Quaternary Ammonium Compounds

Overview

The quaternary ammonium compounds are widely used as disinfectants. There have been some reports of healthcare-associated infections associated with contaminated quaternary ammonium compounds used to disinfect patient-care supplies or equipment such as cystoscopes or cardiac catheters (641,642). The quaternary ammonium compounds are good cleaning agents, but high water hardness (643) and materials such as cotton and gauze pads may make them less microbicidal because of insoluble precipitates and because cotton and gauze pads absorb the active ingredients. As with several other disinfectants (e.g., phenolics, iodophors) gram-negative bacteria have been found to survive or grow in them (378). Chemically, the quaternaries are organically substituted ammonium compounds in which the nitrogen atom has a valence of 5, four of the substituent radicals (R1–R4) are alkyl or heterocyclic radicals of a given size or chain length, and the fifth (X-) is a halide, sulfate, or similar radical (644). Each compound exhibits its own antimicrobial characteristics, hence the search for one compound with outstanding antimicrobial properties. Some of the chemical names of quaternary ammonium compounds used in healthcare are alkyl dimethyl benzyl ammonium chloride, alkyl didecyl dimethyl ammonium chloride, and dialkyl dimethyl ammonium chloride. The newer quaternary ammonium compounds (i.e., fourth generation), referred to as twin-chain or dialkyl quaternaries (e.g., didecyl dimethyl ammonium bromide and dioctyl dimethyl ammonium bromide), purportedly remain active in hard water and are tolerant of anionic residues (645).

A few case reports have documented occupational asthma as a result of exposure to benzalkonium chloride (646).

Mode of Action

The bactericidal action of the quaternaries has been attributed to the inactivation of energy-producing enzymes, denaturation of essential cell proteins, and disruption of the cell membrane (645). Evidence in support of these and other possibilities is provided by Sykes (644) and Petrocci (647).

Microbicidal Activity

Results from manufacturers' data sheets and from published scientific literature indicate that the quaternary ammonium compounds sold as hospital disinfectants are generally fungicidal, bactericidal, and virucidal against lipophilic (enveloped) viruses; they are not sporicidal and generally not tuberculocidal or virucidal against hydrophilic (nonenveloped) viruses (12,47–49, 51,52,54,62,64,300,647–649). Best et al. (48) and Rutala et al. (64) demonstrated the poor mycobactericidal activities of quaternary ammonium compounds. Attempts to reproduce the manufacturers' bactericidal and tuberculocidal claims using the AOAC tests with a limited number of quaternary ammonium compounds have failed on occasion (64,387,637). Studies have shown, however, extreme variability of test results among laboratories testing identical products (387,637).

Uses

The quaternary ammonium compounds are commonly used in ordinary environmental sanitation of noncritical surfaces such as floors, furniture, and walls. EPA-registered quaternary ammonium compounds are appropriate to use when disinfecting medical equipment that comes into contact with intact skin (e.g., blood pressure cuffs).

Miscellaneous Inactivating Agents

Other Germicides

Several compounds have antimicrobial activity but for various reasons have not been incorporated into our armamentarium of healthcare disinfectants. These include mercurials, sodium hydroxide, β-propiolactone, chlorhexidine gluconate, cetrimide-chlorhexidine, glycols (triethylene and propylene), and the Tego disinfectants. A detailed examination of these agents is presented in two authoritative references (14,384).

A peroxygen-containing formulation had marked bactericidal action when used as a 1% weight/volume solution and virucidal activity at 3% (43) but did not have mycobactericidal activity at concentrations of 2.3% and 4% and exposure times ranging between 30 and 120 minutes (650). It also required 20 hours to kill *B. atrophaeus* spores (651). A powder-based peroxygen compound for disinfecting contaminated spill was strongly and rapidly bactericidal (652).

Metals such as silver, iron, and copper could be used for the disinfection of water, reusable medical devices, or incorporated into medical devices (e.g., intravascular catheters) (653–658). Preliminary data suggest they are effective against a wide variety of microorganisms.

Nanoemulsions, composed of detergents and lipids in water, have been shown in preliminary studies to have activity against vegetative bacteria, enveloped viruses, *Bacillus* spores, and *Candida*. This product represents a potential agent for use as a topical biocidal agent (659–661).

"Superoxidized Water"

Reports have examined the microbicidal activity of a new disinfectant, "superoxidized water." The concept of electrolyzing saline to create a disinfectant or antiseptics is appealing as the basic materials of saline and electricity are cheap and the end product (i.e., water) is not damaging to the environment. The main products of this water are hypochlorous acid at a concentration of about 144 mg/L and chlorine. As with any germicide, the antimicrobial activity of superoxidized water is strongly affected by the concentration of the active ingredient (available free chlorine) (662). The disinfectant is generated at the point of use by passing a saline solution over coated titanium electrodes at 9 amps. The product generated has a pH of 5.0 to 6.5 and an oxidation-reduction potential (redox) of >950 mV. Although "superoxidized water" is intended to be generated fresh at the point of use, when tested under clean conditions the disinfectant is effective within 5 minutes when 48 hours old (663). Unfortunately, the equipment required to produce the product may be expensive as parameters such as pH, current, and redox potential must be closely monitored. The solution has been shown to be nontoxic to biologic tissues. Although the solution is claimed by the manufacturer in the U.K. to be noncorrosive and nondamaging to endoscopes and processing equipment, one flexible endoscope manufacturer (Olympus Key-Med, U.K.) has voided the warranty on the endoscopes if superoxidized water is used to disinfect them (664).

The antimicrobial activity of this new, recently FDA-cleared (FDA correspondence, September 18, 2002) high-level disinfectant has been tested against bacteria, mycobacteria, viruses, fungi, and spores (663,665,666). Data have shown that freshly generated superoxidized water is rapidly effective (<2 minutes) in achieving a 5-$\log_{10}$ reduction of pathogenic microorganisms (e.g., *M. tuberculosis, M. chelonae,* poliovirus, HIV, MRSA, *E. coli, Candida albicans, Enterococcus faecalis, P. aeruginosa*) in the absence of organic loading. However, the biocidal activity of this disinfectant was substantially reduced in the presence of organic material (5% horse serum) (663,666). No bacteria or viruses were detected on artificially contaminated endoscopes after 5 minutes exposure to superoxidized water (667). Additional studies are needed to determine if this solution may be used as an alternative to other disinfectants or antiseptics for handwashing, skin antisepsis, room cleaning, or equipment disinfection (e.g., endoscopes, dialyzers) (374,665,668).

Metals as Microbicides

Comprehensive reviews of antisepsis (669), disinfection (391), and antiinfective chemotherapy (670) barely mention the antimicrobial activity of heavy metals (657,658). Nevertheless, it has been known since antiquity that some heavy metals possess antiinfective activity. Heavy metals such as silver have been used for prophylaxis of conjunctivitis of the newborn, topical therapy for burn wounds, and bonding to indwelling catheters, and the use of heavy metals as antiseptics or disinfectants is also being reexplored.

Clinical uses of other heavy metals include the use of copper-8-quinolinolate as a fungicide against *Aspergillus,* copper-silver ionization for *Legionella* disinfection (671–673), the use of organic mercurials as an antiseptic (e.g., mercurochrome) and preservative/disinfectant (e.g., thimerosal—currently being removed from vaccines) in pharmaceuticals and cosmetics (658).

Ultraviolet (UV) Radiation

UV has a wavelength range between 328 and 210 nm (3, 280 and 2,100 Å). Its maximum bactericidal effect occurs at 240 to 280 nm. Mercury vapor lamps emit more than 90% of their radiation at 253.7 nm, which is near the maximum microbicidal activity (674). Inactivation of microorganisms is due to destruction of nucleic acid via induction of thymine dimers. UV has been employed in the disinfection of drinking water, air (674), titanium implants (675), and contact lenses (676). Studies have shown that bacteria and viruses are more easily killed by UV light than are bacterial spores (674). UV has several potential applications. but unfortunately its germicidal effectiveness and use is influenced by the following factors: organic matter; wavelength; type of suspension; temperature; type of microorganism; and UV intensity, which is affected by distance and dirty tubes (677). The application of UV in the healthcare environment (i.e., operating rooms, isolation rooms, and biologic safety cabinets) is limited to the destruction of airborne microorganisms or inactivation of microorganisms located on surfaces. The effect of UV radiation on postoperative wound infections has been investigated by means of a double-blind, randomized study in five university medical centers. After following 14,854 patients over a 2-year period, the investigators reported the overall wound infection rate to be unaffected by UV, although there was a significant reduction (3.8% to 2.9%) in postoperative infection in the "refined clean" surgical procedures (678). No data support the use of UV lamps in isolation rooms, and this practice has caused at least one epidemic of UV-induced skin erythema and keratoconjunctivitis in hospital patients and visitors (679).

Pasteurization

Pasteurization is not a sterilization process; its purpose is to destroy all pathogenic microorganisms with the exception of bacterial spores. The time-temperature relation for hot-water pasteurization is generally >70°C (158°F) for 30 minutes. The water temperature should be monitored as part of a quality assurance program (680). Pasteurization of respiratory therapy (681, 682) and anesthesia equipment (683) is a recognized alternative to chemical disinfection. The efficacy of this process has been tested using an inoculum that the authors believed might simulate contamination by an infected patient. Using a large inoculum (10^7) of *P. aeruginosa* or *A. calcoaceticus* in sets of respiratory tubing before processing, Gurevich et al. (681) demonstrated that machine-assisted chemical processing was more efficient than machine-assisted pasteurization with a disinfection failure rate of 6% and 83%, respectively. Other investigators found hot water disinfection to be effective (inactivation factor >5 $\log_{10}$) for the disinfection of reusable anesthesia or respiratory therapy equipment (682,683).

Flushing and Washer Disinfectors

Flushing and washer disinfectors are automated and closed equipment that clean and disinfect objects from bedpans and washbowls to surgical instruments and anesthesia tubes. Items such as bedpans and urinals can be cleaned and disinfected in flushing disinfectors. They have a short cycle of a few minutes. They clean by flushing with warm water, possibly with a detergent, and then disinfect by flushing the items with hot water at approximately 90°C for 1 minute, or with steam. Since this machine empties, cleans, and disinfects, manual cleaning is eliminated, fewer disposable items are needed, and less chemical germicides are used. A microbiologic evaluation of one washer/disinfector demonstrated that suspensions of *Enterococcus faecalis* or poliovirus were completely inactivated (684). Other studies have shown that strains of *Enterococcus faecium* are able to survive the British standard for heat disinfection of bedpans (80°C for 1 minute). The significance of this finding with reference to the potential for enterococci to survive and disseminate in the healthcare environment is debatable (685–687). These machines are available and used in many European countries.

Surgical instruments and anesthesia equipment, which are more difficult to clean, are run in washer disinfectors with a longer cycle of some 20 to 30 minutes with the use of a detergent. These machines also disinfect by hot water at approximately 90°C (688).

Registration and Neutralization of Germicides

Any discussion of germicidal efficacy would be incomplete without commenting on the evaluation and registration of germicides to assure that they meet manufacturers' label claims. Chemical germicides formulated as disinfectants or chemical sterilants in the U.S. are registered and regulated in interstate commerce by the Antimicrobial Division, Office of Pesticides Program, EPA. The authority for this activity was mandated by the Federal Insecticide, Fungicide, and Rodenticide Act (FIFRA) of 1947. In the past, the EPA required manufacturers of chemical germicides formulated as sanitizers, disinfectants, or chemical sterilants to test formulations by using accepted methods for microbicidal activity, stability, and toxicity to animals and humans. In June 1993, the FDA and EPA issued a memorandum of understanding that divided responsibility for review and surveillance of chemical germicides between the two agencies. Under the agreement, the FDA regulates chemical sterilants used on critical and semicritical devices, and the EPA regulates disinfectants used on noncritical surfaces (689). In 1996, Congress passed the Food Quality Protection Act (FQPA), which amended FIFRA in regard to several products regulated by both the EPA and FDA. One provision of FQPA is that regulation of liquid chemical sterilants used on critical and semicritical medical devices (EPA continues to register nonmedical chemical sterilants) was removed from the jurisdiction of EPA and now rests solely with the FDA (690). The FDA and EPA have considered the impact of FQPA, and the FDA has published its final guidance document on production submissions and labeling, January 2000.

The methods that EPA has used for registration are standardized by the AOAC; however, a survey of the scientific literature indicates numerous deficiencies associated with these tests (51, 67,71,396,636,637,691–696) that cause them to be neither accurate nor reproducible (387,637). As part of their regulatory authority, the EPA and FDA support the development and validation of methods for assessing disinfection claims (697,698). For example, the EPA has supported the work of Sattar and Springthorpe (611), who have developed a two-tier quantitative carrier test that can be used to assess sporicidal, mycobactericidal, bactericidal, fungicidal, virucidal, and protozoacidal activity of chemical germicides. The EPA is accepting label claims against HBV using the duck hepatitis B model to quantify disinfectant activity (109,699). The EPA also may do the same for HCV using the bovine viral diarrhea virus as a surrogate. Antiseptics are considered to be antimicrobial drugs used on living tissue and thus are regulated by the FDA under the Food, Drug, and Cosmetic Act. The FDA regulates liquid chemical sterilants/high-level disinfectants intended to process critical and semicritical devices. The FDA has published recommendations on the types of test methods that manufactures should submit to the FDA for 510[k] clearance for such agents.

For nearly 30 years, the EPA also performed intramural pre- and postregistration efficacy testing of some chemical disinfectants, but in 1982 this was stopped, reportedly for budgetary reasons. Thus, manufacturers presently do not need to have microbiologic activity claims verified by the EPA or an independent testing laboratory when registering a disinfectant or chemical sterilant (700). This occurred at a time when the frequency of contaminated germicides and infections secondary to their use had increased (378). Investigations that demonstrated that interlaboratory reproducibility of test results was poor and manufacturers' label claims were not verifiable (387,637) and symposia sponsored by the American Society for Microbiology (696) heightened awareness of these problems and reconfirmed the need to improve the AOAC methods and reinstate a microbiologic activity verification program. A General Accounting Office report, "Disinfectants: EPA Lacks Assurance They Work" (701), seemed to provide the necessary impetus for EPA to initiate some corrective measures, which include cooperative agreements to improve the AOAC methods and independent verification testing for all products labeled as sporicidal and disinfectants labeled as tuberculocidal. These measures will eventually improve the aforementioned problems if interest and funds are sustained. A list of products registered with the EPA and labeled for use as sterilants, tuberculocides, or against HIV and/or HBV is available through the EPA's Web site: *http://www.epa/oppad001/chemregindex.htm*. Organizations (e.g., Organization for Economic Cooperation and Development) are working to achieve harmonization of germicide testing and registration requirements.

One of the difficulties associated with the evaluation of the bactericidal activity of disinfectants is preventing bacteriostasis due to disinfectant residues that are carried over into the subculture media. Likewise, small amounts of disinfectants on environmental surfaces may make it difficult to get an accurate bacterial count when performing microbiologic sampling of the healthcare environment as part of an epidemiologic or research investigation. One of the ways these problems may be overcome is by employing neutralizers that inactivate residual disinfectants (702–704). Two commonly used neutralizing media for chemical disinfectants are Letheen Media and D/E Neutralizing Media. The former contains lecithin to neutralize quaternaries and polysorbate 80 (Tween 80) to neutralize phenolics, hexachlorophene, formalin, and, with lecithin, ethanol. The D/E Neutralizing media neutralize a broad spectrum of antiseptic and disinfectant chemicals, including quaternary ammonium compounds, phenols, iodine and chlorine compounds, mercurials, formaldehyde, and glutaraldehyde (705). A review of neutralizers used in germicide testing has been published (703).

CONCLUSION

When properly used, disinfectants can ensure the safe use of invasive and noninvasive medical devices. However, current disinfection guidelines must be strictly followed.

REFERENCES

1. Mangram AJ, Horan TC, Pearson ML, et al. Guideline for prevention of surgical site infection, 1999. Hospital Infection Control Practices Advisory Committee. *Infect Control Hosp Epidemiol* 1999;20:250–278.
2. American Society for Gastrointestinal Endoscopy. Position statement: reprocessing of flexible gastrointestinal endoscopes. *Gastrointest Endosc* 1996;43:541–546.
3. Uttley AH, Simpson RA. Audit of bronchoscope disinfection: a survey of procedures in England and Wales and incidents of mycobacterial contamination. *J Hosp Infect* 1994;26:301–308.
4. Zaidi M, Angulo M, Sifuentes-Osornio J. Disinfection and sterilization practices in Mexico. *J Hosp Infect* 1995;31:25–32.
5. McCarthy GM, Koval JJ, John MA, et al. Infection control practices across Canada: do dentists follow the recommendations? *J Can Dent Assoc* 1999;65:506–511.
6. Spach DH, Silverstein FE, Stamm WE. Transmission of infection by gastrointestinal endoscopy and bronchoscopy. *Ann Intern Med* 1993;118:117–128.
7. Weber DJ, Rutala WA. Lessons from outbreaks associated with bronchoscopy. *Infect Control Hosp Epidemiol* 2001;22:403–408.
8. Weber DJ, Rutala WA, DiMarino AJ Jr. The prevention of infection following gastrointestinal endoscopy: the importance of prophylaxis and reprocessing. In: DiMarino AJ Jr, Benjamin SB, eds. *Gastrointestinal diseases: an endoscopic approach.* Thorofare, NJ: Slack, 2002:87–106.
9. Meyers H, Brown-Elliott BA, Moore D, et al. An outbreak of *Mycobacterium chelonae* infection following liposuction. *Clin Infect Dis* 2002;34:1500–1507.
10. Lowry PW, Jarvis WR, Oberle AD, et al. *Mycobacterium chelonae* causing otitis media in an ear-nose-and-throat practice. *N Engl J Med* 1988;319:978–982.
11. Favero MS, Bond WW. Chemical disinfection of medical and surgical materials. In: Block SS, ed. *Disinfection, sterilization, and preservation.* Philadelphia: Lippincott Williams & Wilkins, 2001:881–917.
12. Spaulding EH. Chemical disinfection of medical and surgical materials. In: Lawrence C, Block SS, eds. *Disinfection, sterilization, and preservation.* Philadelphia: Lea & Febiger, 1968:517–531.
13. Simmons BP. CDC guidelines for the prevention and control of nosocomial infections. Guideline for hospital environmental control. *Am J Infect Control* 1983;11:97–120.
14. Block SS. *Disinfection, sterilization, and preservation.* Philadelphia: Lippincott Williams & Wilkins, 2001.
15. Rutala WA, 1994, 1995, and 1996 APIC Guidelines Committee. APIC guideline for selection and use of disinfectants. Association for Professionals in Infection Control and Epidemiology. *Am J Infect Control* 1996;24:313–342.
16. Rutala WA. Disinfection, sterilization and waste disposal. In: Wenzel RP, ed. *Prevention and control of nosocomial infections.* Baltimore: Williams and Wilkins, 1997:539–593.
17. Garner JS, Favero MS. CDC Guideline for handwashing and hospital environmental control, 1985. *Infect Control* 1986;7:231–243.
18. Rutala WA. APIC guideline for selection and use of disinfectants. *Am J Infect Control* 1990;18:99–117.
19. Garner JS, Favero MS. CDC guidelines for the prevention and control of nosocomial infections. Guideline for handwashing and hospital environmental control, 1985. Supersedes guideline for hospital environmental control published in 1981. *Am J Infect Control* 1986;14:110–129.
20. Centers for Disease Control. Guidelines for prevention of transmission of human immunodeficiency virus and hepatitis B virus to health-care and public-safety workers. *MMWR* 1989;38:1–37.
21. Centers for Disease Control. Draft guideline for environmental infection control in healthcare facilities, 2001.
22. Foliente RLKB, Aprecio RM, Bains HJ, et al. Efficacy of high-level disinfectants for reprocessing gastrointestinal endoscopes in simulated-use testing. *Gastrointest Endosc* 2001;53:456–462.
23. Kovacs BJ, Chen YK, Kettering JD, et al. High-level disinfection of gastrointestinal endoscopes: are current guidelines adequate? *Am J Gastroenterol* 1999;94:1546–1550.
24. Rutala WA, Clontz EP, Weber DJ, et al. Disinfection practices for endoscopes and other semicritical items. *Infect Control Hosp Epidemiol* 1991;12:282–288.
25. Phillips J, Hulka B, Hulka J, et al. Laparoscopic procedures: the American Association of Gynecologic Laparoscopists' Membership Survey for 1975. *J Reprod Med* 1977;18:227–232.
26. Muscarella LF. Current instrument reprocessing practices: results of a national survey. *Gastrointest Nurs* 2001;24:253–260.
27. Wright EP, Collins CH, Yates MD. *Mycobacterium xenopi* and *Mycobacterium kansasii* in a hospital water supply. *J Hosp Infect* 1985;6:175–178.
28. Wallace RJ Jr, Brown BA, Driffith DE. Nosocomial outbreaks/pseudo-outbreaks caused by nontuberculous mycobacteria. *Annu Rev Microbiol* 1998;52:453–490.
29. Mitchell DH, Hicks LJ, Chiew R, et al. Pseudoepidemic of *Legionella pneumophila* serogroup 6 associated with contaminated bronchoscopes. *J Hosp Infect* 1997;37:19–23.
30. Meenhorst PL, Reingold AL, Groothuis DG, et al. Water-related nosocomial pneumonia caused by *Legionella pneumophila*serogroups 1 and 10. *J Infect Dis* 1985;152:356–364.
31. Atlas RM. *Legionella*: from environmental habitats to disease pathology, detection and control. *Environ Microbiol* 1999;1:283–293.
32. Rutala WA, Weber DJ. Water as a reservoir of nosocomial pathogens. *Infect Control Hosp Epidemiol* 1997;18:609–616.
33. Weber DJ, Rutala WA. Environmental issues and nosocomial infections. In: Wenzel RP, ed. *Prevention and control of nosocomial infections.* Baltimore: Williams and Wilkins, 1997:491–514.
34. Society of Gastroenterology Nurses and Associates. Standards for infection control and reprocessing of flexible gastrointestinal endoscopes. *Gastroenterol Nurs* 2000;23:172–179.
35. Gerding DN, Peterson LR, Vennes JA. Cleaning and disinfection of fiberoptic endoscopes: evaluation of glutaraldehyde exposure time and forced-air drying. *Gastroenterology* 1982;83:613–618.
36. Turner AG, Higgins MM, Craddock JG. Disinfection of immersion tanks (Hubbard) in a hospital burn unit. *Arch Environ Health* 1974;28:101–104.
37. Rutala DR, Rutala WA, Weber DJ, et al. Infection risks associated with spirometry. *Infect Control Hosp Epidemiol* 1991;12:89–92.
38. Ray AJ, Hoyen CK, Taub TF, et al. Nosocomial transmission of vancomycin-resistant enterococci from surfaces. *JAMA* 2002;287:1400–1401.
39. Sattar SA, Lloyd-Evans N, Springthorpe VS, et al. Institutional outbreaks of rotavirus diarrhoea: potential role of fomites and environmental surfaces as vehicles for virus transmission. *J Hyg (Lond)* 1986;96:277–289.
40. Weber DJ, Rutala WA. Role of environmental contamination in the transmission of vancomycin-resistant enterococci. *Infect Control Hosp Epidemiol* 1997;18:306–309.
41. Ward RL, Bernstein DI, Knowlton DR, et al. Prevention of surface-

to-human transmission of rotaviruses by treatment with disinfectant spray. *J Clin Microbiol* 1991;29:1991–1996.
42. Sattar SA, Jacobsen H, Springthorpe VS, et al. Chemical disinfection to interrupt transfer of rhinovirus type 14 from environmental surfaces to hands. *Appl Environ Microbiol* 1993;59:1579–1585.
43. Tyler R, Ayliffe GA, Bradley C. Virucidal activity of disinfectants: studies with the poliovirus. *J Hosp Infect* 1990;15:339–345.
44. Gwaltney JM Jr, Hendley JO. Transmission of experimental rhinovirus infection by contaminated surfaces. *Am J Epidemiol* 1982;116: 828–833.
45. Sattar SA, Jacobsen H, Rahman H, et al. Interruption of rotavirus spread through chemical disinfection. *Infect Control Hosp Epidemiol* 1994;15:751–756.
46. Rutala WA, Barbee SL, Aguiar NC, et al. Antimicrobial activity of home disinfectants and natural products against potential human pathogens. *Infect Control Hosp Epidemiol* 2000;21:33–38.
47. Silverman J, Vazquez JA, Sobel JD, et al. Comparative in vitro activity of antiseptics and disinfectants versus clinical isolates of *Candida* species. *Infect Control Hosp Epidemiol* 1999;20:676–684.
48. Best M, Sattar SA, Springthorpe VS, et al. Efficacies of selected disinfectants against *Mycobacterium tuberculosis*. *J Clin Microbiol* 1990;28: 2234–2239.
49. Best M, Kennedy ME, Coates F. Efficacy of a variety of disinfectants against *Listeria*spp. *Appl Environ Microbiol* 1990;56:377–380.
50. Best M, Springthorpe VS, Sattar SA. Feasibility of a combined carrier test for disinfectants: studies with a mixture of five types of microorganisms. *Am J Infect Control* 1994;22:152–162.
51. Mbithi JN, Springthorpe VS, Sattar SA. Chemical disinfection of hepatitis A virus on environmental surfaces. *Appl Environ Microbiol* 1990;56:3601–3604.
52. Springthorpe VS, Grenier JL, Lloyd-Evans N, et al. Chemical disinfection of human rotaviruses: efficacy of commercially-available products in suspension tests. *J Hyg (Lond)* 1986;97:139–161.
53. Akamatsu T, Tabata K, Hironga M, et al. Transmission of *Helicobacter pylori* infection via flexible fiberoptic endoscopy. *Am J Infect Control* 1996;24:396–401.
54. Sattar SA, Springthorpe VS. Survival and disinfectant inactivation of the human immunodeficiency virus: a critical review. *Rev Infect Dis* 1991;13:430–447.
55. Resnick L, Veren K, Salahuddin SZ, et al. Stability and inactivation of HTLV-III/LAV under clinical and laboratory environments. *JAMA* 1986;255:1887–1891.
56. Weber DJ, Barbee SL, Sobsey MD, et al. The effect of blood on the antiviral activity of sodium hypochlorite, a phenolic, and a quaternary ammonium compound. *Infect Control Hosp Epidemiol* 1999;20: 821–827.
57. Rice EW, Clark RM, Johnson CH. Chlorine inactivation of *Escherichia coli* O157:H7. *Emerg Infect Dis* 1999;5:461–463.
58. Pentella MA, Fisher T, Chandler S, et al. Are disinfectants accurately prepared for use in hospital patient care areas? *Infect Control Hosp Epidemiol* 2000;21:103.
59. Westwood JC, Mitchell MA, Legace S. Hospital sanitation: the massive bacterial contamination of the wet mop. *Appl Microbiol* 1971; 21:693–697.
60. Rutala WA, Weber DJ. Disinfection of endoscopes: review of new chemical sterilants used for high-level disinfection. *Infect Control Hosp Epidemiol* 1999;20:69–76.
61. Russell AD. Bacterial spores and chemical sporicidal agents. *Clin Microbiol Rev* 1990;3:99–119.
62. Terleckyj B, Axler DA. Quantitative neutralization assay of fungicidal activity of disinfectants. *Antimicrob Agents Chemother* 1987;31: 794–798.
63. Klein M, DeForest A. The inactivation of viruses by germicides. *Chem Specialists Manuf Assoc Proc* 1963;49:116–118.
64. Rutala WA, Cole EC, Wannamaker NS, et al. Inactivation of *Mycobacterium tuberculosis* and *Mycobacterium bovis* by 14 hospital disinfectants. *Am J Med* 1991;91:267S–271S.
65. Robison RA, Bodily HL, Robinson DF, et al. A suspension method to determine reuse life of chemical disinfectants during clinical use. *Appl Environ Microbiol* 1988;54:158–164.
66. Isenberg HD, Giugliano ER, France K, et al. Evaluation of three disinfectants after in-use stress. *J Hosp Infect* 1988;11:278–285.
67. Cole EC, Rutala WA, Nessen L, et al. Effect of methodology, dilution, and exposure time on the tuberculocidal activity of glutaraldehyde-based disinfectants. *Appl Environ Microbiol* 1990;56:1813–1817.
68. Power EG, Russell AD. Sporicidal action of alkaline glutaraldehyde: factors influencing activity and a comparison with other aldehydes. *J Appl Bacteriol* 1990;69:261–268.
69. Rutala WA, Gergen MF, Weber DJ. Sporicidal activity of chemical sterilants used in hospitals. *Infect Control Hosp Epidemiol* 1993;14: 713–718.
70. Rutala WA, Gergen MF, Weber DJ. Inactivation of *Clostridium difficile* spores by disinfectants. *Infect Control Hosp Epidemiol* 1993;14: 36–39.
71. Ascenzi JM, Ezzell RJ, Wendt TM. A more accurate method for measurement of tuberculocidal activity of disinfectants. *Appl Environ Microbiol* 1987;53:2189–2192.
72. Collins FM. Use of membrane filters for measurement of mycobactericidal activity of alkaline glutaraldehyde solution. *Appl Environ Microbiol* 1987;53:737–739.
73. Rubbo SD, Gardner JF, Webb RL. Biocidal activities of glutaraldehyde and related compounds. *J Appl Bacteriol* 1967;30:78–87.
74. Rutala WA, Weber DJ. FDA labeling requirements for disinfection of endoscopes: a counterpoint. *Infect Control Hosp Epidemiol* 1995; 16:231–235.
75. Collins FM. Kinetics of the tuberculocidal response by alkaline glutaraldehyde in solution and on an inert surface. *J Appl Bacteriol* 1986; 61:87–93.
76. Food and Drug Administration. Sterilants and high level disinfectants cleared by FDA in a 510(k) as of January 30, 2002 with general claims for processing reusable medical and dental devices, *htpp://www.fda.-gov/cdrh/ode/germlab.html.*, 2001.
77. Crow S, Metcalf RW, Beck WC, et al. Disinfection or sterilization? Four views on arthroscopes. *AORN J* 1983;37:854–9, 862–868.
78. Loffer FD. Disinfection vs. sterilization of gynecologic laparoscopy equipment. The experience of the Phoenix Surgicenter. *J Reprod Med* 1980;25:263–266.
79. Johnson LL, Shneider DA, Austin MD, et al. Two per cent glutaraldehyde: a disinfectant in arthroscopy and arthroscopic surgery. *J Bone Joint Surg* 1982;64:237–239.
80. Burns S, Edwards M, Jennings J, et al. Impact of variation in reprocessing invasive fiberoptic scopes on patient outcomes. *Infect Control Hosp Epidemiol* 1996;17(suppl):P42.
81. Fuselier HA Jr, Mason C. Liquid sterilization versus high level disinfection in the urologic office. *Urology* 1997;50:337–340.
82. Muscarella LF. High-level disinfection or "sterilization" of endoscopes? *Infect Control Hosp Epidemiol* 1996;17:183–187.
83. Miles RS. What standards should we use for the disinfection of large equipment? *J Hosp Infect* 1991;18:264–273.
84. Lee RM, Kozarek RA, Sumida SE, et al. Risk of contamination of sterile biopsy forceps in disinfected endoscopes. *Gastrointest Endosc* 1998;47:377–381.
85. Kinney TP, Kozarek RA, Raltz S, et al. Contamination of single-use biopsy forceps: A prospective in vitro analysis. *Gastrointest Endosc* 2002;56:209–212.
86. Centers for Disease Control. Recommendations for preventing possible transmission of human T-lymphotropic virus type III/lymphadenopathy-associated virus from tears. *MMWR* 1985;34:533–534.
87. Lettau LA, Bond WW, McDougal JS. Hepatitis and diaphragm fitting. *JAMA* 1985;254:752.
88. Rutala WA, Weber DJ, Committee HICPA. Guideline for disinfection and sterilization in healthcare facilities. *Am J Infect Control (in press).*
89. Schembre DB. Infectious complications associated with gastrointestinal endoscopy. *Gastrointest Endosc Clin North Am* 2000;10:215–232.
90. Chu NS, Favero M. The microbial flora of the gastrointestinal tract and the cleaning of flexible endoscopes. *Gastrointest Endosc Clin North Am* 2000;10:233–244.
91. Alfa MJ, Sitter DL. In-hospital evaluation of orthophthalaldehyde as

a high level disinfectant for flexible endoscopes. *J Hosp Infect* 1994;26:15–26.

92. Vesley D, Melson J, Stanley P. Microbial bioburden in endoscope reprocessing and an in-use evaluation of the high-level disinfection capabilities of Cidex PA. *Gastroenterol Nurs* 1999;22:63–68.
93. Chu NS, McAlister D, Antonoplos PA. Natural bioburden levels detected on flexible gastrointestinal endoscopes after clinical use and manual cleaning. *Gastrointest Endosc* 1998;48:137–142.
94. Hanson PJ, Gor D, Clarke JR, et al. Contamination of endoscopes used in AIDS patients. *Lancet* 1989;2:86–88.
95. Hanson PJ, Gor D, Clarke JR, et al. Recovery of the human immunodeficiency virus from fibreoptic bronchoscopes. *Thorax* 1991;46:410–412.
96. Chaufour X, Deva AK, Vickery K, et al. Evaluation of disinfection and sterilization of reusable angioscopes with the duck hepatitis B model. *J Vasc Surg* 1999;30:277–282.
97. Cheung RJ, Ortiz D, DiMarino AJ Jr. GI endoscopic reprocessing practices in the United States. *Gastrointest Endosc* 1999;50:362–368.
98. Urayama S, Kozarek RA, Sumida S, et al. Mycobacteria and glutaraldehyde: is high-level disinfection of endoscopes possible? *Gastrointest Endosc* 1996;43:451–456.
99. Jackson J, Leggett JE, Wilson DA, et al. *Mycobacterium gordonae* in fiberoptic bronchoscopes. *Am J Infect Control* 1996;24:19–23.
100. Alvarado CJ, Reichelderfer M. APIC guideline for infection prevention and control in flexible endoscopy. Association for Professionals in Infection Control. *Am J Infect Control* 2000;28:138–155.
101. Society of Gastroenterology Nurses and Associates. Guideline for the use of high-level disinfectants and sterilants for reprocessing of flexible gastrointestinal endoscopes. *Gastroenterol Nurs* 2000;23:180–187.
102. Martin MA, Reichelderfer M, 1991, and 1993 APIC Guidelines Committee. APIC guidelines for infection prevention and control in flexible endoscopy. *Am J Infect Control* 1994;22:19–38.
103. Rey JF, Halfon P, Feryn JM, et al. Risk of transmission of hepatitis C virus by digestive endoscopy. *Gastroenterol Clin Biol* 1995;19:346–349.
104. Cronmiller JR, Nelson DK, Jackson DK, et al. Efficacy of conventional endoscopic disinfection and sterilization methods against *Helicobacter pylori* contamination. *Helicobacter* 1999;4:198–203.
105. Sartor C, Charrel RN, de Lamballerie X, et al. Evaluation of a disinfection procedure for hysteroscopes contaminated by hepatitis C virus. *Infect Control Hosp Epidemiol* 1999;20:434–436.
106. Hanson PJ, Chadwick MV, Gaya H, et al. A study of glutaraldehyde disinfection of fibreoptic bronchoscopes experimentally contaminated with *Mycobacterium tuberculosis*. *J Hosp Infect* 1992;22:137–142.
107. Merighi A, Contato E, Scagliarini R, et al. Quality improvement in gastrointestinal endoscopy: microbiologic surveillance of disinfection. *Gastrointest Endosc* 1996;43:457–462.
108. Bond WW. Endoscope reprocessing: Problems and solutions. In: Rutala WA, ed. *Disinfection, sterilization, and antisepsis in healthcare.* Champlain, NY: Polyscience Publications, 1998:151–163.
109. Deva AK, Vickery K, Zou J, et al. Establishment of an in-use testing method for evaluating disinfection of surgical instruments using the duck hepatitis B model. *J Hosp Infect* 1996;33:119–130.
110. Hanson PJ, Gor D, Jeffries DJ, et al. Elimination of high titre HIV from fibreoptic endoscopes. *Gut* 1990;31:657–659.
111. Wu MS, Wang JT, Yang JC, et al. Effective reduction of *Helicobacter pylori* infection after upper gastrointestinal endoscopy by mechanical washing of the endoscope. *Hepatogastroenterology* 1996;43:1660–1664.
112. Kirschke DL, Jones TF, Craig AS, et al. *Pseudomonas aeruginosa* and *Serratia marcescens* contamination associated with a manufacturing defect in bronchoscopes. *N Engl J Med* 2003;348:214–220.
113. Srinivasan A, Wolfenden LL, Song X, et al. An outbreak of *Pseudomonas aeruginosa* infections associated with flexible bronchoscopes. *N Engl J Med* 2003;348:221–227.
114. Kaczmarek RG, Moore RM Jr, McCrohan J, et al. Multi-state investigation of the actual disinfection/sterilization of endoscopes in health care facilities. *Am J Med* 1992;92:257–261.
115. Bradley CR, Babb JR. Endoscope decontamination: automated vs. manual. *J Hosp Infect* 1995;30:537–542.
116. Muscarella LF. Advantages and limitations of automatic flexible endoscope reprocessors. *Am J Infect Control* 1996;24:304–309.
117. Muscarella LF. Automatic flexible endoscope reprocessors. *Gastrointest Endosc Clin North Am* 2000;10:245–257.
118. Alvarado CJ, Stolz SM, Maki DG. Nosocomial infections from contaminated endoscopes: a flawed automated endoscope washer. An investigation using molecular epidemiology. *Am J Med* 1991;91:272S–280S.
119. Fraser VJ, Jones M, Murray PR, et al. Contamination of flexible fiberoptic bronchoscopes with *Mycobacterium chelonae* linked to an automated bronchoscope disinfection machine. *Am Rev Respir Dis* 1992;145:853–855.
120. Cooke RP, Whymant-Morris A, Umasankar RS, et al. Bacteria-free water for automatic washer-disinfectors: an impossible dream? *J Hosp Infect* 1998;39:63–65.
121. Muscarella LF. Deja Vu . . . All over again? The importance of instrument drying. *Infect Control Hosp Epidemiol* 2000;21:628–689.
122. Rutala WA, Weber DJ. Importance of lumen flow in liquid chemical sterilization. *Am J Infect Control* 1999;20:458–459.
123. Dwyer DM, Klein EG, Istre GR, et al. *Salmonella newport* infections transmitted by fiberoptic colonoscopy. *Gastrointest Endosc* 1987;33:84–87.
124. Wheeler PW, Lancaster D, Kaiser AB. Bronchopulmonary cross-colonization and infection related to mycobacterial contamination of suction valves of bronchoscopes. *J Infect Dis* 1989;159:954–958.
125. Bond WW. Virus transmission via fiberoptic endoscope: recommended disinfection. *JAMA* 1987;257:843–844.
126. Lynch DA, Porter C, Murphy L, et al. Evaluation of four commercial automatic endoscope washing machines. *Endoscopy* 1992;24:766–770.
127. Bond WW. Disinfection and endoscopy: microbial considerations. *J Gastroenterol Hepatol* 1991;6:31–36.
128. Nelson D. Newer technologies for endoscope disinfection: electrolyzed acid water and disposable-component endoscope systems. *Gastrointest Endosc Clin North Am* 2000;10:319–328.
129. Kruse A, Rey JF. Guidelines on cleaning and disinfection in GI endoscopy. Update 1999. The European Society of Gastrointestinal Endoscopy. *Endoscopy* 2000;32:77–80.
130. British Thoracic Society. British Thoracic Society guidelines on diagnostic flexible bronchoscopy. *Thorax* 2001;56:1–21.
131. Association of Operating Room Nurses. *Recommended practices for use and care of endoscopes. 2000 standards, recommended practices, and guidelines.* Denver, CO: AORN, 2000:243–247.
132. British Society of Gastroenterology. Cleaning and disinfection of equipment for gastrointestinal endoscopy. Report of a working party of the British Society of Gastroenterology Endoscope Committee. *Gut* 1998;42:585–593.
133. Jackson FW, Ball MD. Correction of deficiencies in flexible fiberoptic sigmoidoscope cleaning and disinfection technique in family practice and internal medicine offices. *Arch Fam Med* 1997;6:578–582.
134. Orsi GB, Filocamo A, Di Stefano L, et al. Italian National Survey of Digestive Endoscopy Disinfection Procedures. *Endoscopy* 1997;29:732–738; quiz 739–740.
135. Honeybourne D, Neumann CS. An audit of bronchoscopy practice in the United Kingdom: a survey of adherence to national guidelines. *Thorax* 1997;52:709–713.
136. Michele TM, Cronin WA, Graham NM, et al. Transmission of *Mycobacterium tuberculosis* by a fiberoptic bronchoscope. Identification by DNA fingerprinting. *JAMA* 1997;278:1093–1095.
137. Bronowicki JP, Venard V, Botte C, et al. Patient-to-patient transmission of hepatitis C virus during colonoscopy. *N Engl J Med* 1997;337:237–240.
138. Agerton T, Valway S, Gore B, et al. Transmission of a highly drug-resistant strain (strain W1) of *Mycobacterium tuberculosis*. Community outbreak and nosocomial transmission via a contaminated bronchoscope. *JAMA* 1997;278:1073–1077.
139. Food and Drug Administration, Centers for Disease Control and Prevention. FDA and CDC public health advisory: infections from endoscopes inadequately reprocessed by an automated endoscope re-

processing system, Food and Drug Administration, Rockville, MD, 1999.
140. Riley R, Beanland C, Bos H. Establishing the shelf life of flexible colonoscopes. *Gastroenterol Nurs* 2002;25:114–119.
141. Humphreys H, McGrath H, McCormick PA, et al. Quality of final rinse water used in washer-disinfectors for endoscopes. *J Hosp Infect* 2002;51:151–153.
142. Pang J, Perry P, Ross A, et al. Bacteria-free rinse water for endoscope disinfection. *Gastrointest Endosc* 2002;56:402–406.
143. Leung J, Vallero R, Wilson R. Surveillance cultures to monitor quality of gastrointestinal endoscope reprocessing. *Am J Gastroenterol* 2003; 98.
144. Moses FM, Lee J. Surveillance cultures to monitor quality of gastrointestinal endoscope reprocessing. *Am J Gastroenterol* 2003;98:77–81.
145. Muscarella LF. Application of environmental sampling to flexible endoscope reprocessing: the importance of monitoring the rinse water. *Infect Control Hosp Epidemiol* 2002;23:285–289.
146. Bond WW, Hedrick ER. Microbiological culturing of environmental and medical-device surfaces. In: Isenberg HD, Gilchrist MJR, eds. *Clinical microbiology procedures handbook, section 11, epidemiologic and infection control microbiology.* Washington, DC: American Society for Microbiology, 1992:11.10.1–11.10.9.
147. Murray PR, Baron EJ, Pfaller MA, et al., eds. *Manual of clinical microbiology.* Washington, DC: American Society for Microbiology Press, 1999.
148. Murphy C. Inactivated glutaraldehyde: Lessons for infection control. *Am J Infect Control* 1998;26:159–160.
149. Carsauw H, Debacker N. Recall of patients after use of inactive batch of Cidex disinfection solution in Belgian hospitals, Fifth International Conference of the Hospital Infection Society, Edinburgh, September 15–18, 2002.
150. Ad hoc Committee on Infection Control in the Handling of Endoscopic Equipment. Guidelines for preparation of laparoscopic instrumentation. *AORN J* 1980;32:65–66,70,74,76.
151. Taylor EW, Mehtar S, Cowan RE, et al. Endoscopy: disinfectants and health. Report of a meeting held at the Royal College of Surgeons of England, February 1993. *J Hosp Infect* 1994;28:5–14.
152. Hulka JF, Wisler MG, Bruch C. A discussion: laparoscopic instrument sterilization. *Med Instrum* 1977;11:122–123.
153. Corson SL, Block S, Mintz C, et al. Sterilization of laparoscopes. Is soaking sufficient? *J Reprod Med* 1979;23:49–56.
154. Corson SL, Dole M, Kraus R, et al. Studies in sterilization of the laparoscope: II. *J Reprod Med* 1979;23:57–59.
155. Chan-Myers H, McAlister D, Antonoplos P. Natural bioburden levels detected on rigid lumened medical devices before and after cleaning. *Am J Infect Control* 1997;25:471–476.
156. Rodrigues C, Mehta AC, Jha U, et al. Nosocomial *Mycobacterium chelonae* infection in laparoscopic surgery. *Infect Control Hosp Epidemiol* 2001;22:474–475.
157. Marshburn PB, Rutala WA, Wannamaker NS, et al. Gas and steam sterilization of assembled versus disassembled laparoscopic equipment. Microbiologic studies. *J Reprod Med* 1991;36:483–487.
158. Bernhang AM. Clostridium pyoarthrosis following arthroscopy. *Arthroscopy* 1987;3:56–58.
159. D'Angelo GL, Ogilvie-Harris DJ. Septic arthritis following arthroscopy, with cost/benefit analysis of antibiotic prophylaxis. *Arthroscopy* 1988;4:10–14.
160. Weber DJ, Rutala WA. Nosocomial ocular infections. In: Mayhall CG, ed. *Infection control and hospital epidemiology.* Philadelphia: Lippincott Williams & Wilkins, 1999:287–299.
161. Chronister CL. Structural damage to Schiotz tonometers after disinfection with solutions. *Optom Vis Sci* 1997;74:164–166.
162. Nagington J, Sutehall GM, Whipp P. Tonometer disinfection and viruses. *Br J Ophthalmol* 1983;67:674–676.
163. Craven ER, Butler SL, McCulley JP, et al. Applanation tonometer tip sterilization for adenovirus type 8. *Ophthalmology* 1987;94: 1538–1540.
164. American Academy of Ophthalmology. Updated recommendations for ophthalmic practice in relation to the human immunodeficiency virus. American Academy of Ophthalmology, San Francisco, CA, 1988.
165. Pepose JS, Linette G, Lee SF, et al. Disinfection of Goldmann tonometers against human immunodeficiency virus type 1. *Arch Ophthalmol* 1989;107:983–985.
166. Ventura LM, Dix RD. Viability of herpes simplex virus type 1 on the applanation tonometer. *Am J Ophthalmol* 1987;103:48–52.
167. Koo D, Bouvier B, Wesley M, et al. Epidemic keratoconjunctivitis in a university medical center ophthalmology clinic; need for re-evaluation of the design and disinfection of instruments. *Infect Control Hosp Epidemiol* 1989;10:547–552.
168. Jernigan JA, Lowry BS, Hayden FG, et al. Adenovirus type 8 epidemic keratoconjunctivitis in an eye clinic: risk factors and control. *J Infect Dis* 1993;167:1307–1313.
169. Fritz S, Hust MH, Ochs C, et al. Use of a latex cover sheath for transesophageal echocardiography (TEE) instead of regular disinfection of the echoscope? *Clin Cardiol* 1993;16:737–740.
170. Milki AA, Fisch JD. Vaginal ultrasound probe cover leakage: implications for patient care. *Fertil Steril* 1998;69:409–411.
171. Storment JM, Monga M, Blanco JD. Ineffectiveness of latex condoms in preventing contamination of the transvaginal ultrasound transducer head. *South Med J* 1997;90:206–208.
172. Hignett M, Claman P. High rates of perforation are found in endovaginal ultrasound probe covers before and after oocyte retrieval for *in vitro* fertilization-embryo transfer. *J Assist Reprod Genet* 1995;12: 606–609.
173. Amis S, Ruddy M, Kibbler CC, et al. Assessment of condoms as probe covers for transvaginal sonography. *J Clin Ultrasound* 2000;28: 295–298.
174. Rooks VJ, Yancey MK, Elg SA, et al. Comparison of probe sheaths for endovaginal sonography. *Obstet Gynecol* 1996;87:27–29.
175. Odwin CS, Fleischer AC, Kepple DM, et al. Probe covers and disinfectants for transvaginal transducers. *J Diagn Med Sonog* 1990;6: 130–135.
176. Benson WG. Exposure to glutaraldehyde. *J Soc Occup Med* 1984;34: 63–64.
177. Garland SM, de Crespigny L. Prevention of infection in obstetrical and gynaecological ultrasound practice. *Aust N Z J Obstet Gynaecol* 1996;36:392–395.
178. Fowler C, McCracken D. US probes: risk of cross infection and ways to reduce it—comparison of cleaning methods. *Radiology* 1999;213: 299–300.
179. Muradali D, Gold WL, Phillips A, et al. Can ultrasound probes and coupling gel be a source of nosocomial infection in patients undergoing sonography? An in vivo and in vitro study. *AJR* 1995;164: 1521–1524.
180. Lewis DL, Arens M, Appleton SS, et al. Cross-contamination potential with dental equipment. *Lancet* 1992;340:1252–1254.
181. Lewis DL, Boe RK. Cross-infection risks associated with current procedures for using high-speed dental handpieces. *J Clin Microbiol* 1992; 30:401–406.
182. American Dental Association. Infection control recommendations for the dental office and the dental laboratory. *J Am Dent Assoc* 1996; 127:672–680.
183. Centers for Disease Control. Recommended Infection-Control Practices for Dentistry, 1993. *MMWR* 1993;41:1–12.
184. Department of Health and Human Services. Food and Drug Administration. Dental handpiece sterilization, Food and Drug Administration, Rockville, MD, 1992.
185. Silverstone SE, Hill DE. Evaluation of sterilization of dental handpieces by heating in synthetic compressor lubricant. *Gen Dent* 1999; 47:158–160.
186. Goodman HS, Carpenter RD, Cox MR. Sterilization of dental instruments and devices: an update. *Am J Infect Control* 1994;22:90–94.
187. Gurevich I, Dubin R, Cunha BA. Dental instrument and device sterilization and disinfection practices. *J Hosp Infect* 1996;32:295–304.
188. Smith A, Dickson M, Aitken J, et al. Contaminated dental instruments. *J Hosp Infect* 2002;51:233–235.
189. Hastreiter RJ, Molinari JA, Falken MC, et al. Effectiveness of dental

office instrument sterilization procedures. *J Am Dent Assoc* 1991;122: 51–56.

190. Andres MT, Tejerina JM, Fierro JF. Reliability of biologic indicators in a mail-return sterilization-monitoring service: a review of 3 years. *Quintessence Int* 1995;26:865–870.
191. Miller CH, Sheldrake MA. The ability of biological indicators to detect sterilization failures. *Am J Dent* 1994;7:95–97.
192. Miller CH. Cleaning, sterilization and disinfection: basics of microbial killing for infection control. *J Am Dent Assoc* 1993;124:48–56.
193. Molinari JA, Gleason MJ, Cottone JA, et al. Comparison of dental surface disinfectants. *Gen Dent* 1987;35:171–175.
194. Angermann P, Jepsen OB. Procurement, banking and decontamination of bone and collagenous tissue allografts: guidelines for infection control. *J Hosp Infect* 1991;17:159–169.
195. Centers for Disease Control. Transmission of HIV through bone transplantation: Case report and public health recommendations. *JAMA* 1988;260:2487–2488.
196. Centers for Disease Control. Update: Allograft-associated bacterial infections—United States, 2002. *MMWR* 2002;51:207–210.
197. Bianchi J, Buskirk D, Kao Kopf P, et al. Batch processed allograft bone versus single donor processing for antimicrobial capacity, 25th annual meeting, American Association of Tissue Banks, Washington, DC, August 25–29, 2001.
198. Presnal BP, Kimbrough EE. What to do about a dropped bone graft. *Clin Orthop Rel Res* 1993;296:310–311.
199. Burd T, Conroy BP, Meyer SC, et al. The effects of chlorhexidine irrigation solution on contaminated bone-tendon allografts. *Am J Sports Med* 2000;28:241–244.
200. Sarin PS, Scheer DI, Kross RD. Inactivation of human T-cell lymphotropic retrovirus (HTLV-III) by LD. *N Engl J Med* 1985;313:1416.
201. Sarin PS, Scheer DI, Kross RD. Inactivation of human T-cell lymphotropic retrovirus. *Environ Microbiol* 1990;56:1423–1428.
202. Ascenzi JM. Standardization of tuberculocidal testing of disinfectants. *J Hosp Infect* 1991;18:256–263.
203. Bond WW, Favero MS, Petersen NJ, et al. Inactivation of hepatitis B virus by intermediate-to-high-level disinfectant chemicals. *J Clin Microbiol* 1983;18:535–538.
204. Kobayashi H, Tsuzuki M. The effect of disinfectants and heat on hepatitis B virus. *J Hosp Infect* 1984;5:93–94.
205. Spire B, Barre-Sinoussi F, Montagnier L, et al. Inactivation of lymphadenopathy associated virus by chemical disinfectants. *Lancet* 1984; 2:899–901.
206. Martin LS, McDougal JS, Loskoski SL. Disinfection and inactivation of the human T lymphotropic virus type III/Lymphadenopathy-associated virus. *J Infect Dis* 1985;152:400–403.
207. Centers for Disease Control. Recommendations for prevention of HIV transmission in health-care settings. *MMWR* 1987;36:S3–S18.
208. Prince DL, Prince HN, Thraenhart O, et al. Methodological approaches to disinfection of human hepatitis B virus. *J Clin Microbiol* 1993;31:3296–3304.
209. Prince DL, Prince RN, Prince HN. Inactivation of human immunodeficiency virus type 1 and herpes simplex virus type 2 by commercial hospital disinfectants. *Chem Times Trends* 1990;13:13–16.
210. Sattar SA, Springthorpe VS, Conway B, et al. Inactivation of the human immunodeficiency virus: an update. *Rev Med Microbiol* 1994; 5:139–150.
211. Kaplan JC, Crawford DC, Durno AG, et al. Inactivation of human immunodeficiency virus by Betadine. *Infect Control* 1987;8:412–414.
212. Hanson PJ, Gor D, Jeffries DJ, et al. Chemical inactivation of HIV on surfaces. *Br Med J* 1989;298:862–864.
213. Hanson PJ, Jeffries DJ, Collins JV. Viral transmission and fibreoptic endoscopy. *J Hosp Infect* 1991;18:136–140.
214. Payan C, Cottin J, Lemarie C, et al. Inactivation of hepatitis B virus in plasma by hospital in-use chemical disinfectants assessed by a modified HepG2 cell culture. *J Hosp Infect* 2001;47:282–287.
215. Chanzy B, Duc-Bin DL, Rousset B, et al. Effectiveness of a manual disinfection procedure in eliminating hepatitis C virus from experimentally contaminated endoscopes. *Gastrointest Endosc* 1999;50: 147–151.
216. Reynolds CD, Rhinehart E, Dreyer P, et al. Variability in reprocessing policies and procedures for flexible fiberoptic endoscopes in Massachusetts hospitals. *Am J Infect Control* 1992;20:283–290.
217. Handsfield HH, Cummings MJ, Swenson PD. Prevalence of antibody to human immunodeficiency virus and hepatitis B surface antigen in blood samples submitted to a hospital laboratory. Implications for handling specimens. *JAMA* 1987;258:3395–3397.
218. Baker JL, Kelen GD, Sivertson KT, et al. Unsuspected human immunodeficiency virus in critically ill emergency patients. *JAMA* 1987; 257:2609–2611.
219. Kelen GD, Fritz S, Qaqish B, et al. Unrecognized human immunodeficiency virus infection in emergency department patients. *N Engl J Med* 1988;318:1645–1650.
220. Agolini G, Russo A, Clementi M. Effect of phenolic and chlorine disinfectants on hepatitis C virus binding and infectivity. *Am J Infect Control* 1999;27:236–239.
221. Favero MJ, Tokars JI, Arduino MJ, et al. Nosocomial infections associated with hemodialysis. In: Mayhall CG, ed. *Infection control and hospital epidemiology.* Philadelphia: Lippincott Williams & Wilkins, 1999:897–917.
222. Centers for Disease Control. Recommendations for preventing transmission of infections among chronic hemodialysis patients. *MMWR* 2001;50:1–43.
223. Velandia M, Fridkin SK, Cardenas V, et al. Transmission of HIV in dialysis centre. *Lancet* 1995;345:1417–1422.
224. Guinto CH, Bottone EJ, Raffalli JT, et al. Evaluation of dedicated stethoscopes as a potential source of nosocomial pathogens. *Am J Infect Control* 2002;30:499–502.
225. Tokars JI, Frank M, Alter MJ, et al. National Surveillance of Dialysis-Associated Diseases in the United States, 2000. *Semin Dialysis* 2002; 15:162–171.
226. Skoutelis AT, Westenfelder GO, Beckerdite M, et al. Hospital carpeting and epidemiology of *Clostridium difficile. Am J Infect Control* 1994;22:212–217.
227. Wilcox MH, Fawley WN. Hospital disinfectants and spore formation by *Clostridium difficile. Lancet* 2000;356:1324.
228. Kaatz GW, Gitlin SD, Schaberg DR, et al. Acquisition of *Clostridium difficile* from the hospital environment. *Am J Epidemiol* 1988;127: 1289–1294.
229. Mayfield JL, Leet T, Miller J, et al. Environmental control to reduce transmission of *Clostridium difficile. Clin Infect Dis* 2000;31: 995–1000.
230. McFarland LV, Mulligan ME, Kwok RY, et al. Nosocomial acquisition of *Clostridium difficile* infection. *N Engl J Med* 1989;320: 204–210.
231. Hughes CE, Gebhard RL, Peterson LR, et al. Efficacy of routine fiberoptic endoscope cleaning and disinfection for killing *Clostridium difficile. Gastrointest Endosc* 1986;32:7–9.
232. Dyas A, Das BC. The activity of glutaraldehyde against *Clostridium difficile. J Hosp Infect* 1985;6:41–45.
233. Centers for Disease Control. Surveillance for Creutzfeldt-Jakob disease—United States. *MMWR* 1996;45:665–668.
234. Johnson RT, Gibbs CJ Jr. Creutzfeldt-Jakob disease and related transmissible spongiform encephalopathies. *N Engl J Med* 1998;339: 1994–2004.
235. Centers for Disease Control. Probable variant Creutzfeldt-Jakob diseases in a U.S. resident-Florida, 2002. *MMWR* 2002;51:927–929.
236. World Health Organization. WHO infection control guidelines for transmissible spongiform encephalopathies, *http://www.who/cds/csr/aph/2000.3.*
237. Brown P, Preece M, Brandel JP, et al. Iatrogenic Creutzfeldt-Jakob disease at the millennium. *Neurology* 2000;55:1075–1081.
238. Brown P. Environmental causes of human spongiform encephalopathy. In: Baker H, Ridley RM, eds. *Methods in molecular medicine: prion diseases.* Totowa, NJ: Humana Press, 1996:139–154.
239. Brown P, Gibbs CJ, Rodgers-Johnson P, et al. Human spongiform encephalopathy: the National Institutes of Health series of 300 cases of experimentally transmitted disease. *Ann Neurol* 1994;35:513–529.
240. Bernoulli C, Siegfried J, Baumgartner G, et al. Danger of accidental person-to-person transmission of Creutzfeldt-Jakob Disease by surgery. *Lancet* 1977;1(8009):478–479.

241. Rutala WA, Weber DJ. Creutzfeldt-Jakob disease: recommendations for disinfection and sterilization. *Clin Infect Dis* 2001;32:1348–1356.
242. Nevin S, McMenemey WH, Behrman S, et al. Subacute spongiform encephalopathy-A subacute form of encephalopathy attributable to vascular dysfunction (spongiform cerebral athrophy). *Brain* 1960;83: 519–569.
243. Foncin J-F, Gaches J, Cathala F, et al. Transmission iatrogene interhumaine possible de maladie de Creutzfeldt-Jakob avec atteinte des grains du cervelet. *Rev Neurol (Paris)* 1980;136:280.
244. Jacobs P. Cleaning: Principles, methods and benefits. In: Rutala WA, ed. *Disinfection, sterilization, and antisepsis in healthcare.* Champlain, NY: Polyscience Publications, 1998:165–181.
245. Merritt K, Hitchins VM, Brown SA. Safety and cleaning of medical materials and devices. *J Biomed Mater Res* 2000;53:131–136.
246. Alfa MJ, Jackson M. A new hydrogen peroxide-based medical-device detergent with germicidal properties: Comparison with enzymatic cleaners. *Am J Infect Control* 2001;29:168–177.
247. Rohwer RG. Virus like sensitivity of the scrapie agent to heat inactivation. *Science* 1984;223:600–602.
248. Steelman VM. Activity of sterilization processes and disinfectants against prions (Creutzfeldt-Jakob disease agent). In: Rutala WA, ed. *Disinfection, sterilization, and antisepsis in healthcare.* Champlain, NY: Polyscience Publications, 1998:255–271.
249. Brown P, Gibbs CJ Jr, Amyx HL, et al. Chemical disinfection of Creutzfeldt-Jakob disease virus. *N Engl J Med* 1982;306:1279–1282.
250. Brown P, Rohwer RG, Green EM, et al. Effect of chemicals, heat, and histopathologic processing on high-infectivity hamster-adapted scrapie virus. *J Infect Dis* 1982;145:683–687.
251. Kimberlin RH, Walker CA, Millson GC, et al. Disinfection studies with two strains of mouse-passaged scrapie agent. Guidelines for Creutzfeldt-Jakob and related agents. *J Neurol Sci* 1983;59:355–369.
252. Taguchi F, Tamai Y, Uchida A, et al. Proposal for a procedure for complete inactivation of the Creutzfeldt-Jakob disease agent. *Arch Virol* 1991;119:297–301.
253. Taylor DM, Fraser H, McConnell I, et al. Decontamination studies with the agents of bovine spongiform encephalopathy and scrapie. *Arch Virol* 1994;139:313–326.
254. Manuelidis L. Decontamination of Creutzfeldt-Jakob disease and other transmissible agents. *J Neurovirol* 1997;3:62–65.
255. Ernst DR, Race RE. Comparative analysis of scrapie agent inactivation methods. *J Virol Methods* 1993;41:193–201.
256. Dickinson AG, Taylor DM. Resistance of scrapie agent to decontamination. *N Engl J Med* 1978;299:1413–1414.
257. Hartley EG. Action of disinfectants on experimental mouse scrapie. *Nature* 1967;213:1135.
258. Zobeley E, Flechsig E, Cozzio A, et al. Infectivity of scrapie prions bound to a stainless steel surface. *Mol Med* 1999;5:240–243.
259. Taylor DM. Inactivation of transmissible degenerative encephalopathy agents: a review. *Vet J* 2000;159:10–17.
260. Tateishi J, Tashima T, Kitamoto T. Practical methods for chemical inactivation of Creutzfeldt-Jakob disease pathogen. *Microbiol Immunol* 1991;35:163–166.
261. Taylor DM. Resistance of the ME7 scrapie agent to peracetic acid. *Vet Microbiol* 1991;27:19–24.
262. Brown P, Rohwer RG, Gajdusek DC. Newer data on the inactivation of scrapie virus or Creutzfeldt-Jakob disease virus in brain tissue. *J Infect Dis* 1986;153:1145–1148.
263. Flechsig E, Hegyi I, Enari M, et al. Transmission of scrapie by steel-surface-bound prions. *Mol Med* 2001;7:679–684.
264. Taylor DM. Inactivation of prions by physical and chemical means. *J Hosp Infect* 1999;43(suppl):S69–S76.
265. Taylor DM, Fernie K, McConnell I. Inactivation of the 22A strain of scrapie agent by autoclaving in sodium hydroxide. *Vet Microbiol* 1997;58:87–91.
266. Favero MS. Current issues in hospital hygiene and sterilization technology. *J Infect Control* (Asia Pacific Edition) 1998;1:8–10.
267. Favero MS. Current status of sterilisation technology. *Zentr Steril* 1998;6:159–165.
268. Committee on Health Care Issues ANA. Precautions in handling tissues, fluids, and other contaminated materials from patients with documented or suspected Creutzfeldt-Jakob disease. *Ann Neurol* 1986;19:75–77.
269. Association for peri-Operative Registered Nurses. Recommended practices for cleaning and caring for surgical instruments and powered equipment. *AORN J* 2002;75:727–741.
270. Brown SAMK. Use of containment pans and lids for autoclaving caustic solutions. *Am J Infect Control* 2002 *(in press).*
271. Bagg J, Sweeney CP, Roy KM, et al. Cross infection control measures and treatment of patients at risk of Creutzfeldt-Jakob disease in UK general dental practice. *Br Dent J* 2001;191:87–90.
272. Tullo A, Buckley R, M P. CJD and the eye. *Eye* 2000;14:259–260.
273. Kirkpatrick WNA, Waterhouse N. Pharyngoplasty and the risk of variant CJD transmission. *Br J Plast Surg* 2001;54:552–561.
274. Weber DJ, Rutala WA. Managing the risk of nosocomial transmission of prion diseases. *Curr Opinion Infect Dis* 2002;15:421–425.
275. Occupational Safety and Health Administration. Occupational exposure to bloodborne pathogens; final rule. *Fed Reg* 1991;56: 64003–64182.
276. Occupational Safety and Health Administration. OSHA instruction CPL 2–2.44C. Office of Health Compliance Assistance, Washington, DC, 1992.
277. Occupational Safety and Health Administration. OSHA Memorandum from Stephen Mallinger. EPA-Registered disinfectants for HIV/HBV, Washington, DC, 1997.
278. Rutala WA, Weber DJ. Infection control: the role of disinfection and sterilization. *J Hosp Infect* 1999;43:S43–55.
279. Barbee SL, Weber DJ, Sobsey MD, et al. Inactivation of *Cryptosporidium parvum* oocyst infectivity by disinfection and sterilization processes. *Gastrointest Endosc* 1999;49:605–611.
280. Wilson JA, Margolin AB. The efficacy of three common hospital liquid germicides to inactivate *Cryptosporidium parvum* oocysts. *J Hosp Infect* 1999;42:231–237.
281. Fayer R, Graczyk TK, Cranfield MR, et al. Gaseous disinfection of *Cryptosporidium parvum* oocysts. *Appl Environ Microbiol* 1996;62: 3908–3909.
282. Venkitanarayanan KS, Ezeike GO, Hung YC, et al. Inactivation of *Escherichia coli* O157:H7 and *Listeria monocytogenes* on plastic kitchen cutting boards by electrolyzed oxidizing water. *J Food Prot* 1999;62: 857–860.
283. Taormina PJ, Beuchat LR. Behavior of enterohemorrhagic *Escherichia coli* O157:H7 on alfalfa sprouts during the sprouting process as influenced by treatments with various chemicals. *J Food Prot* 1999;62: 850–856.
284. Taormina PJ, Beuchat LR. Comparison of chemical treatments to eliminate enterohemorrhagic *Escherichia coli* O157:H7 on alfalfa seeds. *J Food Prot* 1999;62:318–324.
285. Castillo A, Lucia LM, Kemp GK, et al. Reduction of *Escherichia coli* O157:H7 and *Salmonella typhimurium* on beef carcass surfaces using acidified sodium chlorite. *J Food Prot* 1999;62:580–584.
286. Graham DY, Osato MS. Disinfection of biopsy forceps and culture of *Helicobacter pylori* from gastric mucosal biopsies. *Am J Gastroenterol* 1999;94:1422–1423.
287. Kaneko H, Mitsuma T, Kotera H, et al. Are routine cleaning methods sufficient to remove *Helicobacter pylori* from endoscopic equipment? *Endoscopy* 1993;25:435.
288. Langenberg W, Rauws EA, Oudbier JH, et al. Patient-to-patient transmission of *Campylobacter pylori* infection by fiberoptic gastroduodenoscopy and biopsy. *J Infect Dis* 1990;161:507–511.
289. Miyaji H, Kohli Y, Azuma T, et al. Endoscopic cross-infection with *Helicobacter pylori. Lancet* 1995;345:464.
290. Fantry GT, Zheng QX, James SP. Conventional cleaning and disinfection techniques eliminate the risk of endoscopic transmission of *Helicobacter pylori. Am J Gastroenterol* 1995;90:227–232.
291. Shimada T, Terano A, Ota S, et al. Risk of iatrogenic transmission of *Helicobacter pylori* by gastroscopes. *Lancet* 1996;347:1342–1343.
292. Roosendaal R, Kuipers EJ, van den Brule AJ, et al. Detection of *Helicobacter pylori* DNA by PCR in gastrointestinal equipment. *Lancet* 1993;341:900.
293. Johnson CH, Rice EW, Reasoner DJ. Inactivation of *Helicobacter pylori* by chlorination. *Appl Environ Microbiol* 1997;63:4969–4970.

294. Chapin M, Yatabe J, Cherry JD. An outbreak of rotavirus gastroenteritis on a pediatric unit. *Am J Infect Control* 1983;11:88–91.
295. Keswick BH, Pickering LK, DuPont HL, et al. Survival and detection of rotaviruses on environmental surfaces in day care centers. *Appl Environ Microbiol* 1983;46:813–816.
296. Ansari SA, Spingthorpe S, Sattar SA. Survival and vehicular spread of human rotaviruses: possible relation to seasonality of outbreaks. *Rev Infect Dis* 1991;13:448–461.
297. Sattar SA, Raphael RA, Lochnan H, et al. Rotavirus inactivation by chemical disinfectants and antiseptics used in hospitals. *Can J Microbiol* 1983;29:1464–1469.
298. Lloyd-Evans N, Springthorpe VS, Sattar SA. Chemical disinfection of human rotavirus-contaminated inanimate surfaces. *J Hyg (Lond)* 1986;97:163–173.
299. Tan JA, Schnagl RD. Inactivation of a rotavirus by disinfectants. *Med J Aust* 1981;1:19–23.
300. Doultree JC, Druce JD, Birch CJ, et al. Inactivation of feline calicivirus, a Norwalk virus surrogate. *J Hosp Infect* 1999;41:51–57.
301. Leggiadro RJ. The threat of biological terrorism: a public health and infection control reality. *Infect Control Hosp Epidemiol* 2000;21: 53–56.
302. Henderson DA. The looming threat of bioterrorism. *Science* 1999; 283:1279–1282.
303. Centers for Disease Control. Biological and chemical terrorism: strategic plan for preparedness and response. *MMWR* 2000;49(RR-4): 1–14.
304. Brazis AR, Leslie JE, PW K, et al. The inactivation of spores of *Bacillus globigii* and *Bacillus anthracis* by free available chlorine. *Appl Microbiol* 1958;6:338–342.
305. Weber DJ, Rutala WA. Risks and prevention of nosocomial transmission of rare zoonotic diseases. *Clin Infect Dis* 2001;32:446–456.
306. Chataigner D, Garnier R, Sans S, et al. [Acute accidental poisoning with hospital disinfectant. 45 cases of which 13 with fatal outcome]. *Presse Med* 1991;20:741–743.
307. Weber DJ, Rutala WA. Occupational risks associated with the use of selected disinfectants and sterilants. In: Rutala WA, ed. *Disinfection, sterilization, and antisepsis in healthcare.* Champlain, NY: Polyscience Publications, 1998:211–226.
308. Cokendolpher JC, Haukos JF. *The practical application of disinfection and sterilization in health care facilities.* Chicago: American Hospital Association, 1996.
309. Oie S, Kamiya A. Assessment of and intervention for the misuse of aldehyde disinfectants in Japan. *Infect Control Hosp Epidemiol* 2002; 23:98–99.
310. American Conference of Governmental Industrial Hygienists (ACGIH). *Threshold limit values for chemical substances and physical agents and biological exposure indices.* Cincinnati: ACGIH, 2001.
311. Jordan SLP, Russo MR, Blessing RL, et al. Glutaraldehyde safety: inactivation and disposal. Abstract. *Am J Infect Control* 1997;25: 154–155.
312. Jordan SL. The correct use of glutaraldehyde in the healthcare environment. *Gastroenterol Nurs* 1995;18:143–145.
313. Cheung HY, Brown MR. Evaluation of glycine as an inactivator of glutaraldehyde. *J Pharm Pharmacol* 1982;34:211–214.
314. Daschner F. The hospital and pollution: role of the hospital epidemiologist in protecting the environment. In: Wenzel RP, ed. *Prevention and control of nosocomial infections.* Baltimore: Williams & Wilkins, 1997:595–605.
315. Rutala WA, Cole EC, Thomann CA, et al. Stability and bactericidal activity of chlorine solutions. *Infect Control Hosp Epidemiol* 1998;19: 323–327.
316. Rutala WA, Weber DJ. Uses of inorganic hypochlorite (bleach) in health-care facilities. *Clin Microbiol Rev* 1997;10:597–610.
317. Rutala WA, Weber DJ. Principles of disinfecting patient-care items. In: Rutala WA, ed. *Disinfection, sterilization, and antisepsis in healthcare.* Champlain, NY: Polyscience Publications, 1998:133–149.
318. Luebbert P. Home care. In: Pfeiffer JA, ed. *APIC text of infection control and epidemiology,* vol 1. Washington, DC: Association for Professionals in Infection control and epidemiology, 2000:44–47.
319. Parnes CA. Efficacy of sodium hypochlorite bleach and "alternative" products in preventing transfer of bacteria to and from inanimate surfaces. *Environ Health* 1997;59:14–20.
320. Karapinar M, Gonul SA. Effects of sodium bicarbonate, vinegar, acetic and citric acids on growth and survival of *Yersinia enterocolitica. Int J Food Microbiol* 1992;16:343–347.
321. McMurry LM, Oethinger M, Levy SB. Triclosan targets lipid synthesis. *Nature* 1998;394:531–532.
322. Moken MC, McMurry LM, Levy SB. Selection of multiple-antibiotic-resistant (mar) mutants of *Escherichia coli* by using the disinfectant pine oil: roles of the *mar* and *acr*AB loci. *Antimicrob Agents Chemother* 1997;41:2770–2772.
323. Scott E, Bloomfield SF, Barlow CG. An investigation of microbial contamination in the home. *J Hyg (Lond)* 1982;89:279–293.
324. Rusin P, Orosz-Coughlin P, Gerba C. Reduction of faecal coliform, coliform and heterotrophic plate count bacteria in the household kitchen and bathroom by disinfection with hypochlorite cleaners. *J Appl Microbiol* 1998;85:819–828.
325. International Scientific Forum on Home Hygiene. *www.ifh-homehygiene.org.*
326. Russell AD, Russell NJ. Biocides: activity, action and resistance. In: Hunter PA, Darby GK, Russell NJ, eds. *Fifty years of antimicrobials: past perspectives and future trends.* England: Cambridge University Press, 1995:327–365.
327. Russell AD. Bacterial resistance to disinfectants: Present knowledge and future problems. *J Hosp Infect* 1998;43:S57–S68.
328. Russell AD. Plasmids and bacterial resistance to biocides. *J Appl Microbiol* 1997;83:155–165.
329. Russell AD. Bacterial resistance to disinfectants: present knowledge and future problems. *J Hosp Infect* 1998;43:S57–68.
330. Russell AD. Principles of antimicrobial activity and resistance. In: Block SS, ed. *Disinfection, sterilization, and preservation.* Philadelphia: Lippincott Williams & Wilkins, 2001:31–55.
331. McDonnell G, Russell AD. Antiseptics and disinfectants: activity, action, and resistance. *Clin Microbiol Rev* 1999;12:147–179.
332. Gerba CP, Rusin P. Relationship between the use of antiseptics/disinfectants and the development of antimicrobial resistance. In: Rutala WA, ed. *Disinfection, sterilization and antisepsis: principles and practices in healthcare facilities.* Washington, DC: Association for Professional in Infection Control and Epidemiology, 2001:187–194.
333. Townsend DE, Ashdown N, Greed LC, et al. Transposition of gentamicin resistance to staphylococcal plasmids encoding resistance to cationic agents. *J Antimicrob Chemother* 1984;14:115–124.
334. Brumfitt W, Dixson S, Hamilton-Miller JM. Resistance to antiseptics in methicillin and gentamicin resistant *Staphylococcus aureus. Lancet* 1985;1:1442–1443.
335. Al-Masaudi SB, Day MJ, Russell AD. Sensitivity of methicillin-resistant *Staphylococcus aureus* strains to some antibiotics, antiseptics and disinfectants. *J Appl Bacteriol* 1988;65:329–337.
336. Tennent JM, Lyon BR, Midgley M, et al. Physical and biochemical characterization of the qacA gene encoding antiseptic and disinfectant resistance in *Staphylococcus aureus. J Gen Microbiol* 1989;135:1–10.
337. Kaulfers PM, Laufs R. [Transmissible formaldehyde resistance in *Serratia marcescens*]. *Zentralbl Bakteriol Mikrobiol Hyg [B]* 1985;181: 309–319.
338. Tennent JM, Lyon BR, Gillespie MT, et al. Cloning and expression of *Staphylococcus aureus*plasmid-mediated quaternary ammonium resistance in *Escherichia coli. Antimicrob Agents Chemother* 1985;27: 79–83.
339. Rutala WA, Stiegel MM, Sarubbi FA, et al. Susceptibility of antibiotic-susceptible and antibiotic-resistant hospital bacteria to disinfectants. *Infect Control Hosp Epidemiol* 1997;18:417–421.
340. Anderson RL, Carr JH, Bond WW, et al. Susceptibility of vancomycin-resistant enterococci to environmental disinfectants. *Infect Control Hosp Epidemiol* 1997;18:195–199.
341. Sakagami Y, Kajimura K. Bactericidal activities of disinfectants against vancomycin-resistant enterococci. *J Hosp Infect* 2002;50:140–144.
342. Sehulster LM, Anderson RL. Susceptibility of glycopeptide-intermediate resistant *Staphylococcus aureus* (GISA) to surface disinfectants, hand washing chemicals, and a skin antiseptic. Abstract Y-3. 98th

General Meeting of American Society for Microbiology, May, 1998: 547.
343. Rutala WA, Weber DJ, Gergen MF. Studies on the disinfection of VRE-contaminated surfaces. *Infect Control Hosp Epidemiol* 2000;21: 548.
344. Byers KE, Durbin LJ, Simonton BM, et al. Disinfection of hospital rooms contaminated with vancomycin-resistant *Enterococcus faecium. Infect Control Hosp Epidemiol* 1998;19:261–264.
345. Russell AD, Suller MT, Maillard JY. Do antiseptics and disinfectants select for antibiotic resistance? *J Med Microbiol* 1999;48:613–615.
346. Levy SB. The challenge of antibiotic resistance. *Sci Am* 1998;278: 46–53.
347. Jones RD, Jampani HB, Newman JL, et al. Triclosan: a review of effectiveness and safety in health care settings. *Am J Infect Control* 2000;28:184–196.
348. Russell AD, McDonnell G. Concentration: a major factor in studying biocidal action. *J Hosp Infect* 2000;44:1–3.
349. Russell AD, Maillard JY. Reaction and response-relationship between antibiotic resistance and resistance to antiseptics and disinfectants. *Am J Infect Control* 2000;28:204–206.
350. Murtough SM, Hiom SJ, Palmer M, et al. Biocide rotation in the healthcare setting: is there a case for policy implementation? *J Hosp Infect* 2001;48:1–6.
351. Murtough SM, Hiom SJ, Palmer M, et al. A survey of rotational use of biocides in hospital pharmacy aseptic units. *J Hosp Infect* 2002;50: 228–231.
352. Gebel J, Sonntag H-G, Werner H-P, et al. The higher disinfectant resistance of nosocomial isolates of *Klebsiella oxytoca*: how reliable are indicator organisms in disinfectant testing? *J Hosp Infect* 2002;50: 309–311.
353. Ruden H, Daschner F. Should we routinely disinfect floors? *J Hosp Infect* 2002;51:309.
354. Rutala WA, DJ W. Should we routinely disinfect floors? Reply to Professor F. Daschner. *J Hosp Infect* 2002;51:309–311.
355. Favero MS, Bond WW. Chemical disinfection of medical and surgical materials. In: Block SS, ed. *Disinfection, sterilization, and preservation.* Philadelphia: Lea & Febiger, 1991:617–641.
356. Rheinbaben FV, Schunemann S, Grob T, et al. Transmission of viruses via contact in a household setting: experiments using bacteriophage OX174 as a model virus. *J Hosp Infect* 2000;46:61–66.
357. Rutala WA, Weber DJ. Surface disinfection: should we do it? *J Hosp Infect* 2001;48(suppl A):S64–S68.
358. Ayliffe GAJ, Collins DM, Lowbury EJL. Cleaning and disinfection of hospital floors. *Br Med J* 1966;2:442–445.
359. Ayliffe GA, Collins BJ, Lowbury EJ, et al. Ward floors and other surfaces as reservoirs of hospital infection. *J Hyg (Lond)* 1967;65: 515–536.
360. Dharan S, Mourouga P, Copin P, et al. Routine disinfection of patients' environmental surfaces. Myth or reality? *J Hosp Infect* 1999; 42:113–117.
361. Engelhart SKL, Glasmacher A, Fischnaller E, et al. *Pseudomonas aeruginosa* outbreak in a haematology-oncology unit associated with contaminated surface cleaning equipment. *J Hosp Infect* 2002;52:93–98.
362. Garner JS. Guideline for isolation precautions in hospitals. The Hospital Infection Control Practices Advisory Committee. *Infect Control Hosp Epidemiol* 1996;17:53–80.
363. Maki DG, Alvarado CJ, Hassemer CA, et al. Relation of the inanimate hospital environment to endemic nosocomial infection. *N Engl J Med* 1982;307:1562–1566.
364. Daschner F, Rabbenstein G, Langmaack H. [Surface decontamination in the control of hospital infections: comparison of different methods (author's transl)]. *Dtsch Med Wochenschr* 1980;105:325–329.
365. Danforth D, Nicolle LE, Hume K, et al. Nosocomial infections on nursing units with floors cleaned with a disinfectant compared with detergent. *J Hosp Infect* 1987;10:229–235.
366. Smith TL, Iwen PC, Olson SB, et al. Environmental contamination with vancomycin-resistant enterococci in an outpatient setting. *Infect Control Hosp Epidemiol* 1998;19:515–518.
367. Boyce JM, Potter-Bynoe G, Chenevert C, et al. Environmental contamination due to methicillin-resistant *Staphylococcus aureus*: possible infection control implications. *Infect Control Hosp Epidemiol* 1997; 18:622–627.
368. Bonten MJM, Hayden MJ, Nathan C, et al. Epidemiology of colonisation of patients and environment with vancomycin-resistant enterococci. *Lancet* 1996;348:1615–1619.
369. Neely AN, Maley MP. Survival of enterococci and staphylococci on hospital fabrics and plastic. *J Clin Microbiol* 2000;38:724–726.
370. Wendt C, Wiensenthal B, Dietz E, et al. Survival of enterococci on dry surfaces. *J Clin Microbiol* 1998;36:3734–3736.
371. Neely AN, Maley MP. The 1999 Lindberg award. 3% hydrogen peroxide for the gram-positive disinfection of fabrics. *J Burn Care Rehabil* 1999;20:471–477.
372. Griffith CJ, Cooper RA, Gilmore J, et al. An evaluation of hospital cleaning regimes and standards. *J Hosp Infect* 2000;45:19–28.
373. Tiller JC, Liao CJ, Lewis K, et al. Designing surfaces that kill bacteria on contact. *Proc Natl Acad Sci USA* 2001;98:5981–5985.
374. Rutala WA, Weber DJ. New disinfection and sterilization methods. *Emerg Infect Dis* 2001;7:348–353.
375. Whitby JL, Rampling A. *Pseudomonas aeruginosa* contamination in domestic and hospital environments. *Lancet* 1972;1:15–17.
376. Scott E, Bloomfield SF. The survival and transfer of microbial contamination via cloths, hand and utensils. *J Appl Bacteriol* 1990;68: 271–278.
377. Scott E, Bloomfield SF. Investigations of the effectiveness of detergent washing, drying and chemical disinfection on contamination of cleaning cloths. *J Appl Bacteriol* 1990;68:279–283.
378. Rutala WA, Cole EC. Antiseptics and disinfectants—safe and effective? *Infect Control* 1984;5:215–218.
379. Oie S, Huang Y, Kamiya A, et al. Efficacy of disinfectants against biofilm cells of methicillin-resistant *Staphylococcus aureus. Microbios* 1996;85:223–230.
380. Sartor C, Jacomo V, Duvivier C, et al. Nosocomial *Serratia marcescens* infections associated with extrinsic contamination of a liquid nonmedicated soap. *Infect Control Hosp Epidemiol* 2000;21:196–199.
381. Reiss I, Borkhardt A, Fussle R, et al. Disinfectant contaminated with *Klebsiella oxytoca* as a source of sepsis in babies. *Lancet* 2000;356:310.
382. Newman KA, Tenney JH, Oken HA, et al. Persistent isolation of an unusual *Pseudomonas* species from a phenolic disinfectant system. *Infect Control* 1984;5:219–222.
383. Bean HS. Types and characteristics of disinfectants. *J Appl Bacteriol* 1967;30:6–16.
384. Russell AD, Hugo WB, Ayliffe GAJ. *Principles and practice of disinfection, preservation and sterilization.* Oxford, England: Blackwell Scientific, 1999.
385. Gillis RJ, Schmidt WC. Scanning electron microscopy of spores on inoculated product surfaces. *MD* 1983:46–49.
386. Favero MS, Petersen NJ, Carson LA, et al. Gram-negative water bacteria in hemodialysis systems. *Health Lab Sci* 1975;12:321–334.
387. Rutala WA, Cole EC. Ineffectiveness of hospital disinfectants against bacteria: a collaborative study. *Infect Control* 1987;8:501–506.
388. Lee DH, Miles RJ, Perry BF. The mycoplasmacidal properties of sodium hypochlorite. *J Hyg (Lond)* 1985;95:243–253.
389. Scott GH, Williams JC. Susceptibility of *Coxiella burnetii* to chemical disinfectants. *Ann NY Acad Sci* 1990;590:291–296.
390. Russell AD. Factors influencing the efficacy of antimicrobial agents. In: Russell AD, Hugo WB, Ayliffe GAJ, eds. *Principles and practice of disinfection, preservation and sterilization.* Oxford: Blackwell Science, 1999:95–123.
391. Rutala WA. Selection and use of disinfectants in healthcare. In: Mayhall CG, ed. *Infection control and hospital epidemiology.* Philadelphia: Lippincott Williams & Wilkins, 1999:1161–1187.
392. Lewis DL, Arens M. Resistance of microorganisms to disinfection in dental and medical devices. *Nat Med* 1995;1:956–958.
393. Abbott CF, Cockton J, Jones W. Resistance of crystalline substances to gas sterilization. *J Pharm Pharmacol* 1956;8:709–720.
394. Doyle JE, Ernst RR. Resistance of *Bacillus subtilis* var. *niger* spores occluded in water-insoluble crystals to three sterilization agents. *Appl Microbiol* 1967;15:726–730.
395. Gorham RA, Jacobs P, Roberts CG. Laboratory artifacts due to pro-

tein and salt crystals on the inactivation of *Bacillus stearothermophilus. J Hosp Infect* 1998;40:abstract P.9.2.2.

396. Cole EC, Rutala WA, Carson JL, et al. *Pseudomonas* pellicle in disinfectant testing: electron microscopy, pellicle removal, and effect on test results. *Appl Environ Microbiol* 1989;55:511–513.
397. Anderson RL, Holland BW, Carr JK, et al. Effect of disinfectants on pseudomonads colonized on the interior surface of PVC pipes. *Am J Public Health* 1990;80:17–21.
398. Anderson RL, Vess RW, Carr JH, et al. Investigations of intrinsic *Pseudomonas cepacia* contamination in commercially manufactured povidone-iodine. *Infect Control Hosp Epidemiol* 1991;12:297–302.
399. LeChevallier MW, Cawthon CD, Lee RG. Inactivation of biofilm bacteria. *Appl Environ Microbiol* 1988;54:2492–2499.
400. LeChevallier MW, Cawthon CD, Lee RG. Factors promoting survival of bacteria in chlorinated water supplies. *Appl Environ Microbiol* 1988; 54:649–654.
401. Costerton JS, Steward PS, Greenberg EP. Bacterial biofilms: a common cause of persistent infections. *Science* 1999;284:1318–1322.
402. Donlan RM, Costerton JW. Biofilms: Survival mechanisms of clinically relevant mirocorganisms. *Clin Microbiol Rev* 2002;15:167–193.
403. Dunne WM. Bacterial adhesion: Seen any good biofilms lately? *Clin Microbiol Rev* 2002;15:155–166.
404. Marion-Ferey K, Pasmore M, Stoodley P, et al. Biofilm removal from silicone tubing: an assessment of the efficacy of dialysis machine decontamination procedures using an in vitro model. *J Hosp Infect* 2003; 53:64–71.
405. Brown ML, Aldrich HC, Gauthier JJ. Relationship between glycocalyx and povidone-iodine resistance in *Pseudomonas aeruginosa* (ATCC 27853) biofilms. *Appl Environ Microbiol* 1995;61:187–193.
406. Price D, Ahearn DG. Incidence and persistence of *Pseudomonas aeruginosa* in whirlpools. *J Clin Microbiol* 1988;26:1650–1654.
407. Anonymous. Dental Unit Waterlines: Approaching the Year 2000. ADA Council on Scientific Affairs. *J Am Dent Assoc* 1999;130: 1653–1664.
408. Donlan RM. Biofilms: a source of infection? In: Rutala WA, ed. *Disinfection, sterilization and antisepsis: principles and practices in healthcare facilities.* Washington, DC: Association for Professional in Infection Control and Epidemiology, 2001:219–226.
409. Johansen C, Falholt P, Gram L. Enzymatic removal and disinfection of bacterial biofilms. *Appl Environ Microbiol* 1997;63:3724–3728.
410. Spaulding EH. Alcohol as a surgical disinfectant. *AORN J* 1964;2: 67–71.
411. Morton HE. The relationship of concentration and germicidal efficiency of ethyl alcohol. *Ann NY Acad Sci* 1950;53:191–196.
412. Ali Y, Dolan MJ, Fendler EJ, et al. Alcohols. In: Block SS, ed. *Disinfection, sterilization, and preservation.* Philadelphia: Lippincott Williams & Wilkins, 2001:229–254.
413. Morton HE. Alcohols. In: Block SS, ed. *Disinfection, sterilization, and preservation.* Philadelphia: Lea & Febiger, 1983:225–239.
414. Sykes G. The influence of germicides on the dehydrogenases of *Bact. coli.* Part I. The succinic acid dehydrogenase of *Bact. coli. J Hyg (Camb)* 1939;39:463–469.
415. Dagley S, Dawes EA, Morrison GA. Inhibition of growth of *Aerobacter aerogenes*: the mode of action of phenols, alcohols, acetone and ethyl acetate. *J Bacteriol* 1950;60:369–378.
416. Tilley FW, Schaffer JM. Relation between the chemical constitution and germicidal activity of the monohydric alcohols and phenols. *J Bacteriol* 1926;12:303–309.
417. Coulthard CE, Sykes G. The germicidal effect of alcohol with special reference to its action on bacterial spores. *Pharmaceut J* 1936;137: 79–81.
418. Tyler R, Ayliffe GA. A surface test for virucidal activity of disinfectants: preliminary study with herpes virus. *J Hosp Infect* 1987;9: 22–29.
419. Kurtz JB, Lee TW, Parsons AJ. The action of alcohols on rotavirus, astrovirus and enterovirus. *J Hosp Infect* 1980;1:321–325.
420. Smith CR. Alcohol as a disinfectant against the tubercle bacillus. *Public Health Rep* 1947;62:1285–1295.
421. Kruse RH, Green TD, Chambers RC, et al. Disinfection of aerosolized pathogenic fungi on laboratory surfaces. 1. Tissue phase. *Appl Microbiol* 1963;11:436–445.
422. Kruse RH, Green TD, Chambers RC, et al. Disinfection of aerosolized pathogenic fungi on laboratory surfaces. II. Culture phase. *Appl Microbiol* 1964;12:155–160.
423. Connor CG, Hopkins SL, Salisbury RD. Effectivity of contact lens disinfection systems against *Acanthamoeba culbertsoni. Optom Vis Sci* 1991;68:138–141.
424. Turner NA, Russell AD, Furr JR, et al. *Acanthamoeba*spp., antimicrobial agents and contact lenses. *Sci Prog* 1999;82:1–8.
425. Nye RN, Mallory TB. A note on the fallacy of using alcohol for the sterilization of surgical instruments. *Boston Med Surg J* 1923;189: 561–563.
426. Frobisher M, Sommermeyer L, Blackwell MJ. Studies on disinfection of clinical thermometers. I. Oral thermometers. *Appl Microbiol* 1973; 1:187–194.
427. Sommermeyer L, Frobisher M. Laboratory studies on disinfection of rectal thermometers. *Nurs Res* 1973;2:85–89.
428. Singh D, Kaur H, Gardner WG, et al. Bacterial contamination of hospital pagers. *Infect Control Hosp Epidemiol* 2002;23:274–276.
429. Embil JM, Zhanel GG, Plourde J, et al. Scissors: a potential source of nosocomial infection. *Infect Control Hosp Epidemiol* 2002;23: 147–151.
430. Zachary KC, Bayne PS, Morrison VJ, et al. Contamination of gowns, gloves, and stethoscopes with vancomycin-resistant enterococci. *Infect Control Hosp Epidemiol* 2001;22:560–564.
431. Babb JR, Bradley CR, Deverill CE, et al. Recent advances in the cleaning and disinfection of fibrescopes. *J Hosp Infect* 1981;2: 329–340.
432. Garcia de Cabo A, Martinez Larriba PL, Checa Pinilla J, et al. A new method of disinfection of the flexible fibrebronchoscope. *Thorax* 1978;33:270–272.
433. Weber DJ, Wilson MB, Rutala WA, et al. Manual ventilation bags as a source for bacterial colonization of intubated patients. *Am Rev Respir Dis* 1990;142:892–894.
434. Cavagnolo RZ. Inactivation of herpesvirus on CPR manikins utilizing a currently recommended disinfecting procedure. *Infect Control* 1985; 6:456–458.
435. Ohara T, Itoh Y, Itoh K. Ultrasound instruments as possible vectors of staphylococcal infection. *J Hosp Infect* 1998;40:73–77.
436. Talbot GH, Skros M, Provencher M. 70% alcohol disinfection of transducer heads: experimental trials. *Infect Control* 1985;6:237–239.
437. Platt R, Lehr JL, Marino S, et al. Safe and cost-effective cleaning of pressure-monitoring transducers. *Infect Control Hosp Epidemiol* 1988; 9:409–416.
438. Beck-Sague CM, Jarvis WR. Epidemic bloodstream infections associated with pressure transducers: a persistent problem. *Infect Control Hosp Epidemiol* 1989;10:54–59.
439. Chronister CL, Russo P. Effects of disinfecting solutions on tonometer tips. *Optom Vis Sci* 1990;67:818–821.
440. Lingel NJ, Coffey B. Effects of disinfecting solutions recommended by the Centers for Disease Control on Goldmann tonometer biprisms. *J Am Optom Assoc* 1992;63:43–48.
441. Soukiasian SH, Asdourian GK, Weiss JS, et al. A complication from alcohol-swabbed tonometer tips. *Am J Ophthalmol* 1988;105: 424–425.
442. Jakobsson SW, Rajs J, Jonsson JA, et al. Poisoning with sodium hypochlorite solution. Report of a fatal case, supplemented with an experimental and clinico-epidemiological study. *Am J Forensic Med Pathol* 1991;12:320–327.
443. Heidemann SM, Goetting MG. Treatment of acute hypoxemic respiratory failure caused by chlorine exposure. *Pediatr Emerg Care* 1991; 7:87–88.
444. Hoy RH. Accidental systemic exposure to sodium hypochlorite (Clorox) during hemodialysis. *Am J Hosp Pharm* 1981;38: 1512–1514.
445. Landau GD, Saunders WH. The effect of chlorine bleach on the esophagus. *Arch Otolaryngol* 1964;80:174–176.
446. French RJ, Tabb HG, Rutledge LJ. Esophageal stenosis produced

by ingestion of bleach: report of two cases. *South Med J* 1970;63: 1140–1144.
447. Ward MJ, Routledge PA. Hypernatraemia and hyperchloraemic acidosis after bleach ingestion. *Hum Toxicol* 1988;7:37–38.
448. Ingram TA. Response of the human eye to accidental exposure to sodium hypochlorite. *J Endodont* 1990;16:235–238.
449. Haag JR, Gieser RG. Effects of swimming pool water on the cornea. *JAMA* 1983;249:2507–2508.
450. Mrvos R, Dean BS, Krenzelok EP. Home exposures to chlorine/chloramine gas: review of 216 cases. *South Med J* 1993;86:654–657.
451. Reisz GR, Gammon RS. Toxic pneumonitis from mixing household cleaners. *Chest* 1986;89:49–52.
452. Gapany-Gapanavicius M, Yellin A, Almog S, et al. Pneumomediastinum. A complication of chlorine exposure from mixing household cleaning agents. *JAMA* 1982;248:349–350.
453. Hoffman PN, Death JE, Coates D. The stability of sodium hypochlorite solutions. In: Collins CH, Allwood MC, Bloomfield SF, Fox A, eds. *Disinfectants: their use and evaluation of effectiveness.* London: Academic Press, 1981:77–83.
454. Dychdala GR. Chlorine and chlorine compounds. In: Block SS, ed. *Disinfection, sterilization, and preservation.* Philadelphia: Lippincott Williams & Wilkins, 2001:135–157.
455. Gamble MR. Hazard: formaldehyde and hypochlorites. *Lab Anim* 1977;11:61.
456. Helms C, Massanari R, Wenzel R, et al. Control of epidemic nosocomial legionellosis: a 5 year progress report on continuous hyperchlorination of a water distribution system. Abstracts of 27th Interscience Conference of Antimicrobial Agents and Chemotherapy, 1987:349: 158.
457. Environmental Protection Agency. R.E.D. facts sodium and calcium hypochlorite salts, 1991.
458. Coates D. Comparison of sodium hypochlorite and sodium dichloroisocyanurate disinfectants: neutralization by serum. *J Hosp Infect* 1988; 11:60–67.
459. Coates D. A comparison of sodium hypochlorite and sodium dichloroisocyanurate products. *J Hosp Infect* 1985;6:31–40.
460. Coates D, Wilson M. Use of sodium dichloroisocyanurate granules for spills of body fluids. *J Hosp Infect* 1989;13:241–251.
461. Bloomfield SF, Uso EE. The antibacterial properties of sodium hypochlorite and sodium dichloroisocyanurate as hospital disinfectants. *J Hosp Infect* 1985;6:20–30.
462. Coates D. An evaluation of the use of chlorine dioxide (Tristel One-Shot) in an automated washer/disinfector (Medivator) fitted with a chlorine dioxide generator for decontamination of flexible endoscopes. *J Hosp Infect* 2001;48:55–65.
463. Williams ND, Russell AD. The effects of some halogen-containing compounds on *Bacillus subtilis* endospores. *J Appl Bacteriol* 1991;70: 427–436.
464. Babb JR, Bradley CR, Ayliffe GAJ. Sporicidal activity of glutaraldehydes and hypochlorites and other factors influencing their selection for the treatment of medical equipment. *J Hosp Infect* 1980;1:63–75.
465. Brown DG, Skylis TP, Fekety FR. Comparison of chemical sterilant/disinfectant solutions against spores of *Clostridium difficile.* Abstracts of the American Society for Microbiology, 1983:Q39,267.
466. Grant D, Venneman M, Burns RM. Mycobactericidal activity of Alcide an experimental liquid sterilant. Abstracts of the Annual Meeting of the American Society of Microbiology, 1982:Q101,226.
467. Korich DG, Mead JR, Madore MS, et al. Effects of ozone, chlorine dioxide, chlorine, and monochloramine on *Cryptosporidium parvum* oocyst viability. *Appl Environ Microbiol* 1990;56:1423–1428.
468. Griffiths PA, Babb JR, Fraise AP. Mycobactericidal activity of selected disinfectants using a quantitative suspension test. *J Hosp Infect* 1999; 41:111–121.
469. Centers for Disease Control. Bacteremia associated with reuse of disposable hollow-fiber hemodialyzers. *MMWR* 1986;35:417–418.
470. Bloomfield SF, Miller EA. A comparison of hypochlorite and phenolic disinfectants for disinfection of clean and soiled surfaces and blood spillages. *J Hosp Infect* 1989;13:231–239.
471. Centers for Disease Control. Acquired immune deficiency syndrome (AIDS): precautions for clinical and laboratory staffs. *MMWR* 1982; 31:577–580.
472. Garner JS, Simmons BP. Guideline for isolation precautions in hospitals. *Infect Control* 1983;4:245–325.
473. Van Bueren J, Simpson RA, Salman H, et al. Inactivation of HIV-1 by chemical disinfectants: sodium hypochlorite. *Epidemiol Infect* 1995;115:567–579.
474. Coates D. Disinfection of spills of body fluids: how effective is a level of 10,000 ppm available chlorine? *J Hosp Infect* 1991;18:319–322.
475. Anonymous. Recommendations for decontaminating manikins used in cardiopulmonary resuscitation training, 1983 update. *Infect Control* 1984;5:399–401.
476. Centers for Disease Control. Use of bleach for disinfection of drug injection equipment. *MMWR* 1993;42:418–419.
477. Shapshak P, McCoy CB, Rivers JE, et al. Inactivation of human immunodeficiency virus-1 at short time intervals using undiluted bleach. *J AIDS* 1993;6:218–219.
478. Shapshak P, McCoy CB, Shah SM, et al. Preliminary laboratory studies of inactivation of HIV-1 in needles and syringes containing infected blood using undiluted household bleach. *J AIDS* 1994;7: 754–759.
479. Brystrom A, Sundqvist G. Bacteriologic evaluation of the effect of 0.5 percent sodium hypochlorite in endodontic therapy. *Oral Surg Oral Med Oral Pathol* 1983;55:307–312.
480. Helms CM, Massanari RM, Zeitler R, et al. Legionnaires' disease associated with a hospital water system: a cluster of 24 nosocomial cases. *Ann Intern Med* 1983;99:172–178.
481. Steve L, Goodhart P, Alexander J. Hydrotherapy burn treatment: use of chloramine-T against resistant microorganisms. *Arch Phys Med Rehabil* 1979;60:301–303.
482. Coates D, Wilson M. Powders, composed of chlorine-releasing agent acrylic resin mixtures or based on peroxygen compounds, for spills of body fluids. *J Hosp Infect* 1992;21:241–252.
483. Tulis JJ. Formaldehyde as a gas. In: Phillips GB, Miller WS, eds. *Industrial sterilization.* Durham: Duke University Press, 1972: 209–238.
484. Emmons CW. Fungicidal action of some common dsinfectants on two dermatophytes. *Arch Dermatol Syphil* 1933;28:15–21.
485. McCulloch EC, Costigan S. A comparison of the efficiency of phenol, liquor cresolis, formaldehyde, sodium hypochlorite and sodium hydroxide against *Eberthella typhi* at various temperatures. *J Infect Dis* 1936;59:281–284.
486. Sagripanti JL, Eklund CA, Trost PA, et al. Comparative sensitivity of 13 species of pathogenic bacteria to seven chemical germicides. *Am J Infect Control* 1997;25:335–339.
487. NIOSH. Formaldehyde: evidence of carcinogenicity. NIOSH Current Intelligence Bulletin 34. DHEW (NIOSH) Publication No. 81-111, 1981.
488. Occupational Safety and Health Administration. OSHA amends formaldehyde standard. *Occupational Safety and Health News* 1991:1.
489. Occupational Safety and Health Administration. OSHA Fact Sheet: Formaldehyde. U.S. Department of Labor, 2002.
490. Occupational Safety and Health Administration. Air Contaminants Final Rule. *Fed Reg* 1993;58:35338–5351.
491. Occupational Safety and Health Administration. OSHA Fact Sheet: Formaldehyde. U.S. Department of Labor, 2002.
492. Centers for Disease Control. Occupational exposures to formaldehyde in dialysis units. *MMWR* 1986;35:399–401.
493. Centers for Disease Control. Formaldehyde exposures in a gross anatomy laboratory—Colorado. *MMWR* 1983;52:698–700.
494. Tokars JI, Miller ER, Alter MJ, et al. National surveillance of dialysis associated diseases in the United States, 1995. *ASAIO J* 1998;44: 98–107.
495. Tokars JI, Miller ER, Alter MJ, et al. National surveillance of dialysis-associated diseases in the United States, 1997. *Semin Dialysis* 2000; 13:75–85.
496. Favero MS, Alter MJ, Tokars JI, et al. Dialysis-associated disease and their control. In: Bennett JV, Brachman PS, eds. *Hospital infections.* Boston: Little, Brown, 1998:357–380.
497. Bland LA, Favero MS. Microbial contamination control strategies for

hemodialysis system. Plant, Technology & Safety Management Series: infection control issues in PTSM 1990, Oakbrook Terrace, Illinois.
498. Boucher RM. Potentiated acid 1,5 pentanedial solution—a new chemical sterilizing and disinfecting agent. *Am J Hosp Pharm* 1974; 31:546–557.
499. Miner NA, McDowell JW, Willcockson GW, et al. Antimicrobial and other properties of a new stabilized alkaline glutaraldehyde disinfectant/sterilizer. *Am J Hosp Pharm* 1977;34:376–382.
500. Pepper RE. Comparison of the activities and stabilities of alkaline glutaraldehyde sterilizing solutions. *Infect Control* 1980;1:90–92.
501. Leach ED. A new synergized glutaraldehyde-phenate sterilizing solution and concentrated disinfectant. *Infect Control* 1981;2:26–30.
502. Miner NA, Ross C. Clinical evaluation of ColdSpor, a glutaraldehyde-phenolic disinfectant. *Respir Care* 1991;36:104–109.
503. Collins FM, Montalbine V. Mycobactericidal activity of glutaraldehyde solutions. *J Clin Microbiol* 1976;4:408–412.
504. Masferrer R, Marquez R. Comparison of two activated glutaraldehyde solutions: Cidex Solution and Sonacide. *Respir Care* 1977;22: 257–262.
505. Jette LP, Ringuette L, Ishak M, et al. Evaluation of three glutaraldehyde-based disinfectants used in endoscopy. *J Hosp Infect* 1995;30: 295–303.
506. Scott EM, Gorman SP. Glutaraldehyde. In: Block SS, ed. *Disinfection, sterilization, and preservation.* Philadelphia: Lippincott Williams & Wilkins, 2001:361–381.
507. Scott EM, Gorman SP. Glutaraldehyde. In: Block SS, ed. *Disinfection, sterilization, and preservation.* Philadelphia: Lea & Febiger, 1991: 596–616.
508. Stonehill AA, Krop S, Borick PM. Buffered glutaraldehyde—a new chemical sterilizing solution. *Am J Hosp Pharm* 1963;20:458–465.
509. Borick PM, Dondershine FH, Chandler VL. Alkalinized glutaraldehyde, a new antimicrobial agent. *J Pharm Sci* 1964;53:1273–1275.
510. Russell AD. Glutaraldehyde: current status and uses. *Infect Control Hosp Epidemiol* 1994;15:724–733.
511. Hanson PJ, Bennett J, Jeffries DJ, et al. Enteroviruses, endoscopy and infection control: an applied study. *J Hosp Infect* 1994;27:61–67.
512. van Klingeren B, Pullen W. Glutaraldehyde resistant mycobacteria from endoscope washers. *J Hosp Infect* 1993;25:147–149.
513. Griffiths PA, Babb JR, Bradley CR, et al. Glutaraldehyde-resistant *Mycobacterium chelonae* from endoscope washer disinfectors. *J Appl Microbiol* 1997;82:519–526.
514. Dauendorffer JN, Laurain C, Weber M, et al. Evaluation of the bactericidal efficiency of a 2% alkaline glutaraldehyde solution on *Mycobacterium xenopi. J Hosp Infect* 2000;46:73–76.
515. Webster E, Ribner B, Streed LL, et al. Microbial contamination of activated 2% glutaraldehyde used in high-level disinfection of endoscopes (abstract). *Am J Infect Control* 1996;24:153.
516. Casemore DP, Blewett DA, Wright SE. Cleaning and disinfection of equipment for gastrointestinal flexible endoscopy: interim recommendations of a Working Party of the British Society of Gastroenterology. *Gut* 1989;30:1156–1157.
517. Laskowski LF, Marr JJ, Spernoga JF, et al. Fastidious mycobacteria grown from porcine prosthetic-heart-valve cultures. *N Engl J Med* 1977;297:101–102.
518. Collins FM. Bactericidal activity of alkaline glutaraldehyde solution against a number of atypical mycobacterial species. *J Appl Bacteriol* 1986;61:247–251.
519. Leong D, Dorsey G, Klapp M. Dilution of glutaraldehyde by automatic endoscope machine washers: the need for a quality control program. Abstracts of the 14th Annual Educational Conference of Association for Practitioners in Infection Control, 1987:108:130.
520. Mbithi JN, Springthorpe VS, Sattar SA, et al. Bactericidal, virucidal, and mycobactericidal activities of reused alkaline glutaraldehyde in an endoscopy unit. *J Clin Microbiol* 1993;31:2988–2995.
521. Kleier DJ, Averbach RE. Glutaraldehyde nonbiologic monitors. *Infect Control Hosp Epidemiol* 1990;11:439–441.
522. Kleier DJ, Tucker JE, Averbach RE. Clinical evaluation of glutaraldehyde nonbiologic monitors. *Quintessence Int* 1989;20:271–277.
523. Overton D, Burgess JO, Beck B, et al. Glutaraldehyde test kits: evaluation for accuracy and range. *Gen Dent* 1989;37:126,128.
524. Cooke RPD, Goddard SV, Chatterley R, et al. Monitoring glutaraldehyde dilution in automated washer/disinfectors. *J Hosp Infect* 2001; 48:242–246.
525. Ayliffe GA, Babb JR, Bradley CR. Disinfection of endoscopes. *J Hosp Infect* 1986;7:296–299.
526. Centers for Disease Control. Federal regulatory action against sporicidin cold sterilizing solution. *MMWR* 1991;40:880–881.
527. Husni L, Kale E, Climer C, et al. Evaluation of a new disinfectant for dialyzer reuse. *Am J Kidney Dis* 1989;14:110–118.
528. Townsend TR, Wee SB, Koblin B. An efficacy evaluation of a synergized glutaraldehyde-phenate solution in disinfecting respiratory therapy equipment contaminated during patient use. *Infect Control* 1982; 3:240–244.
529. Petersen NJ, Carson LA, Doto IL, et al. Microbiologic evaluation of a new glutaraldehyde-based disinfectant for hemodialysis systems. *Trans Am Soc Artif Intern Organs* 1982;28:287–290.
530. Gundogdu H, Ocal K, Caglikulekci M, et al. High-level disinfection with 2% alkalinized glutaraldehyde solution for reuse of laparoscopic disposable plastic trocars. *J Laparoendosc Adv Surg Tech [A]* 1998;8: 47–52.
531. Castelli M, Qizilbash A, Seaton T. Post-colonoscopy proctitis. *Am J Gastroenterol* 1986;81:887.
532. Jonas G, Mahoney A, Murray J, et al. Chemical colitis due to endoscope cleaning solutions: a mimic of pseudomembranous colitis. *Gastroenterology* 1988;95:1403–1408.
533. Levine DS. Proctitis following colonoscopy. *Gastrointest Endosc* 1988; 34:269–272.
534. Riney S, Grimes M, Khalife K, et al. Diarrhea associated with disinfection of sigmoidoscopes. *Am J Infect Control* 1991;19:109(abst).
535. Durante L, Zulty JC, Israel E, et al. Investigation of an outbreak of bloody diarrhea: association with endoscopic cleaning solution and demonstration of lesions in an animal model. *Am J Med* 1992;92: 476–480.
536. Burtin P, Ruget O, Petit R, et al. Glutaraldehyde-induced proctitis after endorectal ultrasound examination: a higher risk of incidence than expected? *Gastrointest Endosc* 1993;39:859–860.
537. Babb RR, Paaso BT. Glutaraldehyde proctitis. *West J Med* 1995;163: 477–478.
538. Ryan CK, Potter GD. Disinfectant colitis. Rinse as well as you wash. *J Clin Gastroenterol* 1995;21:6–9.
539. Rozen P, Somjen GJ, Baratz M, et al. Endoscope-induced colitis: description, probable cause by glutaraldehyde, and prevention. *Gastrointest Endosc* 1994;40:547–553.
540. West AB, Kuan SF, Bennick M, et al. Glutaraldehyde colitis following endoscopy: clinical and pathological features and investigation of an outbreak. *Gastroenterology* 1995;108:1250–1255.
541. Dolce P, Gourdeau M, April N, et al. Outbreak of glutaraldehyde-induced proctocolitis. *Am J Infect Control* 1995;23:34–39.
542. Farina A, Fievet MH, Plassart F, et al. Residual glutaraldehyde levels in fiberoptic endoscopes: measurement and implications for patient toxicity. *J Hosp Infect* 1999;43:293–297.
543. Dailey JR, Parnes RE, Aminlari A. Glutaraldehyde keratopathy. *Am J Ophthalmol* 1993;115:256–258.
544. Courtright P, Lewallen S, Holland SP, et al. Corneal decompensation after cataract surgery. An outbreak investigation in Asia. *Ophthalmology* 1995;102:1461–1465.
545. Leinster P, Baum JM, Baxter PJ. An assessment of exposure to glutaraldehyde in hospitals: typical exposure levels and recommended control measures. *Br J Ind Med* 1993;50:107–111.
546. Beauchamp RO, St. Clair MB, Fennell TR, et al. A critical review of the toxicology of glutaraldehyde. *Crit Rev Toxicol* 1992;22:143–174.
547. Corrado OJ, Osman J, Davies RJ. Asthma and rhinitis after exposure to glutaraldehyde in endoscopy units. *Hum Toxicol* 1986;5:325–328.
548. Norback D. Skin and respiratory symptoms from exposure to alkaline glutaraldehyde in medical services. *Scand J Work Environ Health* 1988; 14:366–371.
549. Mwaniki DL, Guthua SW. Occupational exposure to glutaraldehyde in tropical climates. *Lancet* 1992;340:1476–1477.
550. Centers for Disease Control. Symptoms of irritation associated with exposure to glutaraldehyde. *MMWR* 1987;36:190–191.

551. Wiggins P, McCurdy SA, Zeidenberg W. Epistaxis due to glutaraldehyde exposure. *J Occup Med* 1989;31:854–856.
552. Di Prima T, De Pasquale R, Nigro M. Contact dermatitis from glutaraldehyde. *Contact Derm* 1988;19:219–220.
553. Fowler JF Jr. Allergic contact dermatitis from glutaraldehyde exposure. *J Occup Med* 1989;31:852–853.
554. Fisher AA. Allergic contact dermatitis of the hands from Sporicidin (glutaraldehyde-phenate) used to disinfect endoscopes. *Cutis* 1990; 45:227–228.
555. Nethercott JR, Holness DL, Page E. Occupational contact dermatitis due to glutaraldehyde in health care workers. *Contact Derm* 1988;18: 193–196.
556. Gannon PF, Bright P, Campbell M, et al. Occupational asthma due to glutaraldehyde and formaldehyde in endoscopy and x ray departments. *Thorax* 1995;50:156–159.
557. Chan-Yeung M, McMurren T, Catonio-Begley F, et al. Occupational asthma in a technologist exposed to glutaraldehyde. *J Allergy Clin Immunol* 1993;91:974–978.
558. Schnuch A, Uter W, Geier J, et al. Contact allergies in healthcare workers. Results from the IVDK. *Acta Derm Venereol* 1998;78: 358–363.
559. Wellons SL, Trawick EG, Stowers MF, et al. Laboratory and hospital evaluation of four personal monitoring methods for glutaraldehyde in ambient air. *Am Ind Hyg Assoc J* 1998;59:96–103.
560. Newman MA, Kachuba JB. Glutaraldehyde: a potential health risk to nurses. *Gastroenterol Nurs* 1992;14:296–300, discussion 300–301.
561. Association for the Advancement of Medical Instrumentation. *Safe use and handling of glutaraldehyde-based products in healthcare facilities.* Arlington, VA: AAMI, 1995.
562. Anonymous. Material Safety Data Sheet. *Glutaraldehyde.* New York: Occupational Health Services, 1992.
563. Rutala WA, Hamory BH. Expanding role of hospital epidemiology: employee health—chemical exposure in the health care setting. *Infect Control Hosp Epidemiol* 1989;10:261–266.
564. Turner FJ. Hydrogen peroxide and other oxidant disinfectants. In: Block SS, ed. *Disinfection, sterilization, and preservation.* Philadelphia: Lea & Febiger, 1983:240–250.
565. Block SS. Peroxygen compounds. In: Block SS, ed. *Disinfection, sterilization, and preservation.* Philadelphia: Lippincott Williams & Wilkins, 2001:185–204.
566. Sattar SA, Springthorpe VS, Rochon M. A product based on accelerated and stabilized hydrogen peroxide: evidence for broad-spectrum germicidal activity. *Can J Infect Control* 1998;Winter:123–130.
567. Schaeffer AJ, Jones JM, Amundsen SK. Bacterial effect of hydrogen peroxide on urinary tract pathogens. *Appl Environ Microbiol* 1980; 40:337–340.
568. Wardle MD, Renninger GM. Bactericidal effect of hydrogen peroxide on spacecraft isolates. *Appl Microbiol* 1975;30:710–711.
569. Sagripanti JL, Bonifacino A. Comparative sporicidal effect of liquid chemical germicides on three medical devices contaminated with spores of *Bacillus subtilis. Am J Infect Control* 1996;24:364–371.
570. Sagripanti JL, Bonifacino A. Effects of salt and serum on the sporicidal activity of liquid disinfectants. *J AOAC Int* 1997;80:1198–1207.
571. Saurina G, Landman D, Quale JM. Activity of disinfectants against vancomycin-resistant *Enterococcus faecium. Infect Control Hosp Epidemiol* 1997;18:345–347.
572. Kilvington S. Moist-heat disinfection of *Acanthamoeba* cysts. *Rev Infect Dis* 1991;13:S418.
573. Sattar SA, Adegbunrin O, Ramirez J. Combined application of simulated reuse and quantitative carrier test to assess high-level disinfection: Experiments with an accelerated hydrogen peroxide-based formulation. *Am J Infect Control* 2002;30:449–457.
574. Leaper S. Influence of temperature on the synergistic sporicidal effect of peracetic acid plus hydrogen peroxide in *Bacillus subtilis*SA22(NCA 72–52). *Food Microbiol* 1984;1:199–203.
575. Mentel R, Schmidt J. Investigations on rhinovirus inactivation by hydrogen peroxide. *Acta Virol* 1973;17:351–354.
576. Sattar SA. Effect of liquid chemical germicides on mycobacteria including multi-drug resistant isolates of *Mycobacteria tuberculosis.* Abstracts of the 37th Interscience Conference on Antimicrobial Agents of Chemotherapy; September 28–October 1, 1997, Toronto, Ontario, Canada, 1977:E166.
577. *Sporox sterilant and high-level disinfectant technical report.* Montvale, NJ: Reckitt & Colman, 1997:1–12.
578. Sattar SA, Taylor YE, Paquette M, et al. In-hospital evaluation of 7.5% hydrogen peroxide as a disinfectant for flexible endoscopes. *Can J Infect Control* 1996;11:51–54.
579. Vesley D, Norlien KG, Nelson B, et al. Significant factors in the disinfection and sterilization of flexible endoscopes. *Am J Infect Control* 1992;20:291–300.
580. Hobson DW, Seal LA. Evaluation of a novel, rapid-acting, sterilizing solution at room temperature. *Am J Infect Control* 2000;28:370–375.
581. Anonymous. Hydrogen peroxide, ACS reagent. Vol. 2001: Sigma Product Information Sheet, *http://www.sigma.sial.com/sigma/proddata/h0904.htm.*
582. Silvany RE, Dougherty JM, McCulley JP, et al. The effect of currently available contact lens disinfection systems on *Acanthamoeba castellanii* and *Acanthamoeba polyphaga. Ophthalmology* 1990;97:286–290.
583. Moore MB. *Acanthamoeba keratitis* and contact lens wear: the patient is at fault. *Cornea* 1990;9:S33–35; discussion S39–40.
584. Judd PA, Tomlin PJ, Whitby JL, et al. Disinfection of ventilators by ultrasonic nebulisation. *Lancet* 1968;2:1019–1020.
585. Levenson JE. Corneal damage from improperly cleaned tonometer tips. *Arch Ophthalmol* 1989;107:1117.
586. Thompson RL, Haley CE, Searcy MA, et al. Catheter-associated bacteriuria. Failure to reduce attack rates using periodic instillations of a disinfectant into urinary drainage systems. *JAMA* 1984;251:747–751.
587. Bilotta JJ, Waye JD. Hydrogen peroxide enteritis: the "snow white" sign. *Gastrointest Endosc* 1989;35:428–430.
588. Gottardi W. Iodine and iodine compounds. In: Block SS, ed. *Disinfection, sterilization, and preservation.* Philadelphia: Lea & Febiger, 1991: 152–166.
589. Gottardi W. Iodine and iodine compounds. In: Block SS, ed. *Disinfection, sterilization, and preservation.* Philadelphia: Lippincott Williams & Wilkins, 2001:159–184.
590. Craven DE, Moody B, Connolly MG, et al. Pseudobacteremia caused by povidone-iodine solution contaminated with *Pseudomonas cepacia. N Engl J Med* 1981;305:621–623.
591. Berkelman RL, Lewin S, Allen JR, et al. Pseudobacteremia attributed to contamination of povidone-iodine with *Pseudomonas cepacia. Ann Intern Med* 1981;95:32–36.
592. Parrott PL, Terry PM, Whitworth EN, et al. *Pseudomonas aeruginosa* peritonitis associated with contaminated poloxamer-iodine solution. *Lancet* 1982;2:683–685.
593. Favero MS. Iodine—champagne in a tin cup. *Infect Control* 1982;3: 30–32.
594. Berkelman RL, Holland BW, Anderson RL. Increased bactericidal activity of dilute preparations of povidone-iodine solutions. *J Clin Microbiol* 1982;15:635–639.
595. Chang SL. Modern concept of disinfection. *J Sanit Eng Div Proc Am Soc Civ Eng* 1971:689–705.
596. Wallbank AM, Drulak M, Poffenroth L, et al. Wescodyne: lack of activity against poliovirus in the presence of organic matter. *Health Lab Sci* 1978;15:133–137.
597. Carson JA, Favero MS. Comparative resistance of nontuberculous mycobacteria to iodophor germicides. Abstracts of the Annual Meeting of the American Society for Microbiology, 1984:Q101:221.
598. Medcom. Medcom Frequently Asked Questions. *www.medcompnet.-com/faq/faq/html,* 2000.
599. Simons C, Walsh SE, Maillard JY, et al. A note: ortho-phthalaldehyde: proposed mechanism of action of a new antimicrobial agent. *Lett Appl Microbiol* 2000;31:299–302.
600. Walsh SE, Maillard JY, Simons C, et al. Studies on the mechanisms of the antibacterial action of ortho-phthalaldehyde. *J Appl Microbiol* 1999;87:702–710.
601. Cabrera-Martinez RM, Setlow B, Setlow P. Studies on the mechanisms of the sporicidal action of ortho-phthalaldehyde. *J Appl Microbiol* 2002;92:675–680.
602. Gordon MD, Ezzell RJ, Bruckner NI, et al. Enhancement of myco-

bactericidal activity of glutaraldehyde with a,B-unsaturated and aromatic aldehydes. *J Indust Microbiol* 1994;13:77–82.

603. Gregory AW, Schaalje GB, Smart JD, et al. The mycobactericidal efficacy of ortho-phthalaldehyde and the comparative resistances of *Mycobacterium bovis, Mycobacterium terrae,* and *Mycobacterium chelonae. Infect Control Hosp Epidemiol* 1999;20:324–330.
604. Walsh SE, Maillard JY, Russell AD. Ortho-phthalaldehyde: a possible alternative to glutaraldehyde for high level disinfection. *J Appl Microbiol* 1999;86:1039–1046.
605. Roberts CG, Chan Myers H. Mycobactericidal activity of dilute ortho-phthalaldehyde solutions. In: Abstracts in Environmental and General Applied Microbiology, Q-265, ASM 98th General Meeting, Atlanta, Georgia, 1998:464–465.
606. Chan-Myers H. Sporicidal activity of ortho-phthalaldehyde as a function of temperature. *Infect Control Hosp Epidemiol* 2000;21:101(abst).
607. Chan-Myers H, Roberts C. Effect of temperature and organic soil concentration on biocidal activity of ortho-phthalaldehyde solution (abstract). 2000 Education Meeting of the Association for Professional in Infection Control and Epidemiology, Minneapolis, MN, 2000:31.
608. Bruckner NI, Gordon MD, Howell RG. Odorless aromatic dialdehyde disinfecting and sterilizing composition. US Patent 4,851,449. July, 1989.
609. McDonnell G, Pretzer D. New and developing chemical antimicrobials. In: Block SS, ed. *Disinfection, sterilization, and preservation.* Philadelphia: Lippincott Williams & Wilkins, 2001:431–443.
610. Fraud S, Maillard J-Y, Russell AD. Comparison of the mycobactericidal activity of ortho-phthalaldehyde, glutaraldehyde, and other dialdehydes by a quantitative suspension test. *J Hosp Infect* 2001;48: 214–221.
611. Sattar SA, Springthorpe VS. New methods for efficacy testing of disinfectants and antiseptics. In: Rutala WA, ed. *Disinfection, sterilization and antisepsis: principles and practices in healthcare facilities.* Washington, DC: Association for Professional in Infection Control and Epidemiology, 2001:174–186.
612. Tucker RC, Lestini BJ, Marchant RE. Surface analysis of clinically used expanded PTFE endoscopic tubing treated by the STERIS PROCESS. *ASAIO J* 1996;42:306–313.
613. Lensing HH, Oei HL. Investigations on the sporicidal and fungicidal activity of disinfectants. *Zentralbl Bakteriol Mikrobiol Hyg [B]* 1985; 181:487–495.
614. Sagripanti JL, Bonifacino A. Comparative sporicidal effects of liquid chemical agents. *Appl Environ Microbiol* 1996;62:545–551.
615. Crow S. Peracetic acid sterilization: a timely development for a busy healthcare industry. *Infect Control Hosp Epidemiol* 1992;13:111–113.
616. Malchesky PS. Medical applications of peracetic acid. In: Block SS, ed. *Disinfection, sterilization, and preservation.* Philadelphia: Lippincott Williams & Wilkins, 2001:979–996.
617. Mannion PT. The use of peracetic acid for the reprocessing of flexible endoscopes and rigid cystoscopes and laparoscopes. *J Hosp Infect* 1995; 29:313–315.
618. Bradley CR, Babb JR, Ayliffe GA. Evaluation of the Steris System 1 Peracetic Acid Endoscope Processor. *J Hosp Infect* 1995;29:143–151.
619. Duc DL, Ribiollet A, Dode X, et al. Evaluation of the microbicidal efficacy of Steris System I for digestive endoscopes using GERMANDE and ASTM validation protocols. *J Hosp Infect* 2001;48: 135–141.
620. Alfa MJ, Olson N, Degagne P, et al. New low temperature sterilization technologies: microbicidal activity and clinical efficacy. In: Rutala WA, ed. *Disinfection, sterilization, and antisepsis in healthcare.* Champlain, NY: Polyscience Publications, 1998:67–78.
621. Alfa MJ, DeGagne P, Olson N, et al. Comparison of liquid chemical sterilization with peracetic acid and ethylene oxide sterilization for long narrow lumens. *Am J Infect Control* 1998;26:469–477.
622. Seballos RJ, Walsh AL, Mehta AC. Clinical evaluation of a liquid chemical sterilization system for flexible bronchoscopes. *J Bronch* 1995;2:192–199.
623. Wallace CG, Agee PM, Demicco DD. Liquid chemical sterilization using peracetic acid. An alternative approach to endoscope processing. *ASAIO J* 1995;41:151–154.
624. Centers for Disease Control and Prevention. Bronchoscopy-related infections and pseudoinfections—New York, 1996 and 1998. *MMWR* 1999;48:557–560.
625. Babb JR, Bradley CR. Endoscope decontamination: where do we go from here? *J Hosp Infect* 1995;30:543–551.
626. Middleton AM, Chadwick MV, Gaya H. Disinfection of bronchoscopes, contaminated in vitro with *Mycobacterium tuberculosis, Mycobacterium avium-intracellulare* and *Mycobacterium chelonae* in sputum, using stabilized, buffered peracetic acid solution ("Nu-Cidex"). *J Hosp Infect* 1997;37:137–143.
627. Holton J, Shetty N. In-use stability of Nu-Cidex. *J Hosp Infect* 1997; 35:245–248.
628. Alasri A, Roques C, Michel G, et al. Bactericidal properties of peracetic acid and hydrogen peroxide, alone and in combination, and chlorine and formaldehyde against bacterial water strains. *Can J Microbiol* 1992;38:635–642.
629. Stanley P. Destruction of a glutaraldehyde-resistant mycobacterium by a per-oxygen disinfectant. *Am J Infect Control* 1998;26:185(abst).
630. Fleming SJ, Foreman K, Shanley K, et al. Dialyser reprocessing with Renalin. *Am J Nephrol* 1991;11:27–31.
631. Kahn G. Depigmentation caused by phenolic detergent germicides. *Arch Dermatol* 1970;102:177–187.
632. Prindle RF. Phenolic compounds. In: Block SS, ed. *Disinfection, sterilization, and preservation.* Philadelphia: Lea & Febiger, 1983: 197–224.
633. Hegna IK. A comparative investigation of the bactericidal and fungicidal effects of three phenolic disinfectants. *J Appl Bacteriol* 1977;43: 177–181.
634. Hegna IK. An examination of the effect of three phenolic disinfectants on *Mycobacterium tuberculosis. J Appl Bacteriol* 1977;43:183–187.
635. Bergan T, Lystad A. Antitubercular action of disinfectants. *J Appl Bacteriol* 1971;34:751–756.
636. Narang HK, Codd AA. Action of commonly used disinfectants against enteroviruses. *J Hosp Infect* 1983;4:209–212.
637. Cole EC, Rutala WA, Samsa GP. Disinfectant testing using a modified use-dilution method: collaborative study. *J Assoc Off Anal Chem* 1988;71:1187–1194.
638. Goddard PA, McCue KA. Phenolic compounds. In: Block SS, ed. *Disinfection, sterilization, and preservation.* Philadelphia: Lippincott Williams & Wilkins, 2001:255–281.
639. Wysowski DK, Flynt JW Jr, Goldfield M, et al. Epidemic neonatal hyperbilirubinemia and use of a phenolic disinfectant detergent. *Pediatrics* 1978;61:165–170.
640. Doan HM, Keith L, Shennan AT. Phenol and neonatal jaundice. *Pediatrics* 1979;64:324–325.
641. Shickman MD, Guze LB, Pearce ML. Bacteremia following cardiac catheterization. *N Engl J Med* 1959;260:1164–1166.
642. Ehrenkranz NJ, Bolyard EA, Wiener M, et al. Antibiotic-sensitive *Serratia marcescens* infections complicating cardiopulmonary operations: contaminated disinfectant as a reservoir. *Lancet* 1980;2: 1289–1292.
643. Shere L. Some comparisons of the disinfecting properties of hypochlorites and quaternary ammonium compounds. *Milk Plant Monthly* 1948(March):66–69.
644. Sykes G. *Disinfection and sterilization.* London: E & FN Spon Ltd, 1965.
645. Merianos JJ. Surface-active agents. In: Block SS, ed. *Disinfection, sterilization, and preservation.* Philadelphia: Lippincott Williams & Wilkins, 2001:283–320.
646. Purohit A, Kopferschmitt-Kubler MC, Moreau C, et al. Quaternary ammonium compounds and occupational asthma. *Int Arch Occup Environ Health* 2000;73:423–427.
647. Petrocci AN. Surface active agents: quaternary ammonium compounds. In: Block SS, ed. *Disinfection, sterilization, and preservation.* Philadelphia: Lea & Febiger, 1983:309–329.
648. Smith CR, Nishihara H, Golden F, et al. The bactericidal effect of surface-active agents on tubercle bacilli. *Public Health Rep* 1950;48: 1588–1600.
649. Sattar SA, Springthorpe VS, Karim Y, et al. Chemical disinfection of non-porous inanimate surfaces experimentally contaminated with four human pathogenic viruses. *Epidemiol Infect* 1989;102:493–505.

650. Broadley SJ, Furr JR, Jenkins PA, et al. Antimycobacterial activity of 'Virkon'. *J Hosp Infect* 1993;23:189–197.
651. Angelillo IF, Bianco A, Nobile CG, et al. Evaluation of the efficacy of glutaraldehyde and peroxygen for disinfection of dental instruments. *Lett Appl Microbiol* 1998;27:292–296.
652. Coates D. Disinfectants and spills of body fluids. *Nurs RSA* 1992;7: 25–27.
653. Landeen LK, Yahya MT, Gerba CP. Efficacy of copper and silver ions and reduced levels of free chlorine in inactivation of *Legionella pneumophila. Appl Environ Microbiol* 1989;55:3045–3050.
654. Pyle BH, Broadaway SC, McFeters GA. Efficacy of copper and silver ions with iodine in the inactivation of *Pseudomonas cepacia. J Appl Bacteriol* 1992;72:71–79.
655. Yahya MT, Landeen LK, Messina MC, et al. Disinfection of bacteria in water systems by using electrolytically generated copper:silver and reduced levels of free chlorine. *Can J Microbiol* 1990;36:109–116.
656. Liu Z, Stout JE, Tedesco L, et al. Controlled evaluation of copper-silver ionization in eradicating *Legionella pneumophila* from a hospital water distribution system. *J Infect Dis* 1994;169:919–922.
657. Weber DJ, Rutala WA. Use of metals and microbicides in the prevention of nosocomial infections. In: Rutala W, ed. *Disinfection, sterilization, and antisepsis in healthcare.* Champlain, NY: Polyscience Publications, 1995:271–285.
658. Weber DJ, Rutala WA. Use of metals as microbicides in preventing infections in healthcare. In: Block SS, ed. *Disinfection, sterilization, and preservation.* Philadelphia: Lippincott Williams & Wilkins, 2001: 415–430.
659. Hamouda T, Hayes MM, Cao ZH, et al. A novel surfactant nanoemulsion with broad-spectrum sporicidal activity against *Bacillus* species. *J Infect Dis* 1999;180:1939–1949.
660. Hamouda T, Myc A, Donovan B, et al. A novel surfactant nanoemulsion with a unique non-irritant topical antimicrobial activity against bacteria, enveloped viruses and fungi. *Microbiol Res* 2001;156:1–7.
661. Hamouda T, Baker JR Jr. Antimicrobial mechanism of action of surfactant lipid preparations in enteric Gram-negative bacilli. *J Appl Microbiol* 2000;89:397–403.
662. Sampson MNMA. Not all super-oxidized waters are the same. *J Hosp Infect* 2002;52:227–228.
663. Selkon JB, Babb JR, Morris R. Evaluation of the antimicrobial activity of a new super-oxidized water, Sterilox®, for the disinfection of endoscopes. *J Hosp Infect* 1999;41:59–70.
664. Fraise AP. Choosing disinfectants. *J Hosp Infect* 1999;43:255–264.
665. Tanaka H, Hirakata Y, Kaku M, et al. Antimicrobial activity of superoxidized water. *J Hosp Infect* 1996;34:43–49.
666. Shetty N, Srinivasan S, Holton J, et al. Evaluation of microbicidal activity of a new disinfectant: Sterilox® 2500 against *Clostridium difficile* spores, *Helicobacter pylori*, vancomycin resistant *Enterococcus* species, *Candida albicans* and several *Mycobacterium* species. *J Hosp Infect* 1999;41:101–105.
667. Tsuji S, Kawano S, Oshita M, et al. Endoscope disinfection using acidic electrolytic water. *Endoscopy* 1999;31:528–535.
668. Tanaka N, Fujisawa T, Daimon T, et al. The use of electrolyzed solutions for the cleaning and disinfecting of dialyzers. *Artif Organs* 2000;24:921–928.
669. Rotter ML. Handwashing, hand disinfection, and skin disinfection. In: Wenzel RP, ed. *Prevention and control of nosocomial infections.* Baltimore: Williams & Wilkins, 1997:691–709.
670. Mandel GL, Bennett JE, Dolin R. *Principles and practices of infectious diseases.* New York: Livingstone, 2000.
671. Goetz A, Yu VL. Copper-silver ionization: cautious optimism for *Legionella* disinfection and implications for environmental culturing. *Am J Infect Control* 1997;25:449–451.
672. Miuetzner S, Schwille RC, Farley A, et al. Efficacy of thermal treatment and copper-silver ionization for controlling *Legionella pneumophila* in high-volume hot water plumbing systems in hospitals. *Am J Infect Control* 1997;25:452–457.
673. Stout JE, Lin YS, Goetz AM, et al. Controlling *Legionella* in hospital water systems: experience with the superheat-and-flush method and copper-silver ionization. *Infect Control Hosp Epidemiol* 1998;19: 911–914.
674. Russell AD. Ultraviolet radiation. In: Russell AD, Hugo WB, Ayliffe GAJ, eds. *Principles and practices of disinfection, preservation and sterilization.* Oxford: Blackwell Science, 1999:688–702.
675. Singh S, Schaaf NG. Dynamic sterilization of titanium implants with ultraviolet light. *Int J Oral Maxillofac Implants* 1989;4: 139–146.
676. Dolman PJ, Dobrogowski MJ. Contact lens disinfection by ultraviolet light. *Am J Ophthalmol* 1989;108:665–669.
677. Shechmeister IL. Sterilization by ultraviolet irradiation. In: Block SS, ed. *Disinfection, sterilization, and preservation.* Philadelphia: Lea & Febiger, 1991:553–565.
678. National Research Council. Postoperative wound infections—the influence of ultraviolet irradiation of the operating room and of various other factors. *Ann Surg* 1964;160:1–125.
679. Sensakovic JW, Smith LG. Nosocomial ultraviolet keratoconjunctivitis. *Infect Control* 1982;3:475–476.
680. Cefai C, Richards J, Gould FK, et al. An outbreak of respiratory tract infection resulting from incomplete disinfection of ventilatory equipment. *J Hosp Infect* 1990;15:177–182.
681. Gurevich I, Tafuro P, Ristuccia P, et al. Disinfection of respirator tubing: a comparison of chemical versus hot water machine-assisted processing. *J Hosp Infect* 1983;4:199–208.
682. Rutala WA, Weber DJ, Gergen MF, et al. Efficacy of a washer-pasteurizer for disinfection of respiratory-care equipment. *Infect Control Hosp Epidemiol* 2000;21:333–336.
683. Jette LP, Lambert NG. Evaluation of two hot water washer disinfectors for medical instruments. *Infect Control Hosp Epidemiol* 1988; 9:194–199.
684. Dempsey KM, Chiew RF, McKenzie JA, et al. Evaluation of the cleaning and disinfection efficacy of the DEKO-190; award-based automated washer/disinfector. *J Hosp Infect* 2000;46:50–54.
685. Kearns AM, Freeman R, Lightfoot NF. Nosocomial enterococci: resistance to heat and sodium hypochlorite. *J Hosp Infect* 1995;30: 193–199.
686. Bradley CR, Fraise AP. Heat and chemical resistance of enterococci. *J Hosp Infect* 1996;34:191–196.
687. Chadwick PR, Oppenheim BA. Vancomycin-resistant enterococci and bedpan washer machines. *Lancet* 1994;344:685.
688. Nystrom B. New technology for sterilization and disinfection. *Am J Med* 1991;91:264S–266S.
689. Anonymous. Memorandum of understanding between the Food and Drug Administration, Public Health Service, and the Environmental Protection Agency. 1993.
690. Ulatowski TA. Current activities concerning the premarket evaluation of infection control devices at the Food and Drug Administration. In: Rutala WA, ed. *Disinfection, sterilization, and antisepsis in healthcare.* Champlain, NY: Polyscience Publications, 1998:1–7.
691. Cole EC, Rutala WA. Bacterial numbers on penicylinders used in disinfectant testing: use of 24 hour adjusted broth cultures. *J Assoc Off Anal Chem* 1988;71:9–11.
692. Cole EC, Rutala WA, Alfano EM. Comparison of stainless steel penicylinders used in disinfectant testing. *J Assoc Off Anal Chem* 1988; 71:288–289.
693. Cole EC, Rutala WA, Carson JL. Evaluation of penicylinders used in disinfectant testing: bacterial attachment and surface texture. *J Assoc Off Anal Chem* 1987;70:903–906.
694. Cole EC, Rutala WA, Samsa GP. Standardization of bacterial numbers of penicylinders used in disinfectant testing: interlaboratory study. *J Assoc Off Anal Chem* 1987;70:635–637.
695. Alfano EM, Cole EC, Rutala WA. Quantitative evaluation of bacteria washed from stainless steel penicylinders during AOAC use-dilution method. *J Assoc Off Anal Chem* 1988;71:868–871.
696. Favero MS, Groschel DHM. *Chemical germicides in the health care field: current status and evaluation of efficacy and research needs.* Washington, DC: American Society for Microbiology, 1987.
697. Sattar SA. Microbicidal testing of germicides: an update. In: Rutala WA, ed. *Disinfection, sterilization, and antisepsis in healthcare.* Champlain, NY: Polyscience Publications, 1998:227–240.
698. Best M. *Development of a combined carrier test for disinfectant efficacy.* Ottawa, Canada: University of Ottawa, 1994.

699. Sanders FT. Environmental protection agency's role in the regulation of antimicrobial pesticides in the United States. In: Rutala WA, ed. *Disinfection, sterilization and antisepsis: principles and practices in healthcare facilities.* Washington, DC: Association for Professional in Infection Control and Epidemiology, 2001:28–40.
700. Groschel DHM. Caveat emptor: do your disinfectants work? *Infect Control* 1983;4:144.
701. United States General Accounting Office. Disinfectants: EPA lacks assurance they work, 1990.
702. Johnston MD, Lambert RJW, Hanlon GW, et al. A rapid method for assessing the suitability of quenching agents for individual biocides as well as combinations. *J Appl Microbiol* 2002;92:784–789.
703. Russell AD. Neutralization procedures in the evaluation of bactericidal activity. In: Collins CH, Allwood MC, Bloomfield SF, Fox A, eds. *Disinfectants: their use and evaluation of effectiveness.* London: Academic Press, 1981:45–59.
704. Russell AD, Ahonkhai I, Rogers DT. Microbiological applications of the inactivation of antibiotics and other antimicrobial agents. *J Appl Bacteriol* 1979;46:207–245.
705. Engley FB Jr, Dey BP. A universal neutralizing medium for antimicrobial chemicals. *Chem Specialists Manuf Assoc Proc* 1970:100–106.
706. Geertsma RE, van Asten JAAM. Sterilization of prions: Requirements, complications, implications. *Zentr Steril* 1995;3:385–394.
707. Rutala WA, Weber DJ. Management of equipment contaminated with Creutzfeldt-Jakob disease. In: Rutala WA, ed. *Disinfection, sterilization and antisepsis: principles and practices in healthcare facilities.* Washington, DC: Association for Professionals in Infection Control and Epidemiology, 2001:167–172.

86

STERILIZATION AND PASTEURIZATION

JOHN H. KEENE

Although chemicals have been used empirically for centuries to preserve foods, sterilization methods for medical equipment and devices are a relatively recent development. The recognition and acceptance of germs as a causative agent of disease led, in the mid- to late 1800s, to the realization that removal of germs from surgical instruments and other hospital equipment would protect patients from life-threatening infections. Pasteur's laboratory experiments led him to discover the dust on his laboratory instruments and that passing them through a flame before use prevented contamination of his experiments (1). The use of heat as a sterilizing agent was not readily accepted, but as the positive results became known, more emphasis was placed on sterilization processes in the medical field.

Sterilization has become a prerequisite for certain procedures and devices, and a whole industry has been developed to provide new, better, and more cost-effective ways of ensuring sterilization of medical equipment and devices. It is important to understand the terminology and technology of sterilization and to recognize the importance of following appropriate procedures to achieve sterilization. In addition, it is important to understand the need for and methodology of validating and documenting sterilization procedures. Failure to implement the appropriate sterilization process leads to contamination of critical instrumentation, infection of patients, and potential loss of life.

In many cases, the destruction of common pathogens is sufficient for a particular process. However, it is important to remember that any microorganism in the wrong place at the right time is a potential pathogen. Because the current patient population is at particular risk for infection due to immune incompetence (patients infected with the human immunodeficiency virus, transplant patients, cancer chemotherapy patients, and elderly patients), sterilization verification becomes even more important.

In addition to their concern for proper sterilization processes and protection of patients, healthcare administrators must also be concerned with the health and safety of their personnel and the potential for environmental contamination. Sterilization processes designed to destroy microorganisms carry with them the potential to harm the personnel who must perform the processes and the potential to result in environmental damage. Appropriate mechanisms for minimizing personnel exposure and environmental release must be developed and incorporated in the operation of the healthcare facility.

DEFINITIONS

Disinfection is a process that results in the destruction of infectious agents on inanimate objects but does not necessarily destroy all bacterial spores. The process may be a result of treatment with chemicals or physical agents. Although the term *disinfection* is often used synonymously with *sterilization,* it is not the same, and the two processes should be considered separately. Disinfection is the subject of Chapter 85 and is not further considered here.

Sterilization, on the other hand, is defined as a process that results in the destruction or elimination of all forms of life, including bacterial spores. The term is most often used in the context of destroying microorganisms. Sterilization is an absolute in that a material, when sterile, cannot be contaminated with any form of viable microorganism. However, the term has been used to denote the filter treatment of fluids that removes bacteria, fungi, and spores but not viruses. Therefore, one must understand the limitations of the sterilization process before accepting the product as truly sterile.

The verification of sterility would necessarily depend on the ability of personnel to demonstrate the destruction of all living microorganisms. Such verification would suppose that we have knowledge of all living microorganisms and can demonstrate their existence. Because this is virtually impossible and totally impractical, the efficacy of sterilization processes is most often demonstrated through the use of known highly resistant microorganisms as indicators, and the verification of sterility becomes a matter of probability. The assurance of the completion of the sterilization process is different for differing operations and is measured by the percentage of reduction, or log reduction (D value), in initial counts of biologic indicators that is accomplished by the process.

Pasteurization is historically defined as the heating of materials to temperatures of around 60°C for 30 minutes to destroy pathogens that may be present, although other time/temperature relationships have also been used. The process of pasteurization is also used for the reduction of infectious agents in liquids and has been tried in the processing of various devices, particularly anesthesia equipment and various types of scopes. It should be noted that this is not sterilization and should not be used for devices when there is a critical need for a sterilized product.

Filtration is another mechanism for treatment of air and fluids to reduce microbial contamination. Although filtration is often referred to as a sterilization process, it is possible for viral particles and bacteria to pass through many filters. Properly chosen and controlled, however, this process can be used to ensure that fluids and air are free from bacterial, mold, and particulate contamination.

CRITERIA OF STERILIZATION

Several criteria of sterilization as an absolute process should be recognized:

1. Thermal death time: the time required to kill all spores at a specified temperature;
2. D value: the time required to reduce the microbial population by 90% or 1 log;
3. F value: the time in minutes required to kill all the spores in suspension when at a temperature of 121°C or 250°F.

The D and F values can be used to evaluate various methods of sterilization.

PRINCIPLES OF STERILIZATION

The kinetics of inactivation and principles of thermal destruction of microorganisms are beyond the scope of this chapter; interested readers are referred to the excellent treatises of Wickamanayake and Sproul (2) and Pflug and Holcomb (3).

The efficacy of various sterilization processes depends on a number of factors. Each factor that must be considered in choosing a particular process and determining the efficacy of that process is discussed below.

Natural Resistance

Sterilization depends on the inactivation of microbial life processes faster than the microorganism can replace or repair the destroyed cell material. Death curves for microorganisms are generally accepted to be logarithmic, and variations from log death curves are considered to be due to variations in the nature of the microorganisms in question (4). Some antimicrobial agents (chemical disinfectants and antibiotics) react with crucial enzymes or interfere with enzyme systems within the cell. Cells that are not killed by the initial insult often are genetically different from those that are killed and have altered enzymes or enzyme systems that allow for survival. These microorganisms then multiply and become the resistant population. Sterilization processes do not lead to resistant populations because, by definition, all microorganisms are killed by the process.

However, even in regard to sterilization processes, genetics do play a significant role in protection of microorganisms. For example, bacterial spores are significantly more resistant to various sterilization processes than are vegetative cells. The natural resistance of spores is primarily due to the chemical composition of the spore coat and differs for different genera and species.

The requirements for sterilization differ for different microorganisms according to the genetic makeup of the microorganism. Some microorganisms grow well at temperatures normally used for pasteurization and must be treated at higher temperatures. Some microorganisms can rapidly repair radiation damage; thus, the level and duration of radiation treatment must be increased to ensure inactivation. Some microorganisms can find their way through filter materials, and the final use of the filtrate must be considered. This is not to imply that sterilization cannot be accomplished, but only to point out that the process must be carefully determined and scrupulously monitored to ensure the desired result.

Microbial Load and Extraneous Organic Materials

The final outcome of the sterilization process depends on the numbers of microorganisms initially present in the material to be sterilized, and the values that define the process all depend on the initial number of microorganisms. Therefore, the higher the number of microorganisms in or on the materials to be treated, the longer or more concentrated the treatment must be to achieve sterilization.

In addition to the effect of bioburden on the final outcome of the sterilization process, extraneous organic materials also contribute to the efficacy of the process. As with microorganisms, excess organic material increases the duration of, and changes the requirements for, the sterilization process. Organic material serves to protect the microorganisms from the effects of the specific process and may cause process failure.

Sterilization processes have been developed to ensure successful sterilization. Because, in a practical sense, sterilization is a statistical phenomenon, we must assume that a given process will result in complete kill of any microorganisms present, and our assumption must be based on the monitoring data obtained from that process.

GENERAL REQUIREMENTS FOR STERILIZATION PROCESSES

As in disinfection processes, a number of factors, aside from the natural resistance of spores and other microorganisms, affect the efficacy of any sterilization process. These factors include time, temperature, relative humidity (RH), pH, and standardization of loads.

Time

All sterilization processes require time for completion. The time required primarily depends on the process (e.g., wet heat, dry heat, gas, radiation). In addition, the time depends on the presence or absence of organic material and bioburden. The time required for adequate processing is determined by the use of indicator microorganisms that are known to be particularly resistant to the process being used. The sterilization process is defined in terms of time required to kill all spores present or to reduce the number of microorganisms present by 90%. Because microbial death curves tend to be exponential, extrapolations can ensure that appropriate times are used to allow for destruction of the microorganisms that might be present.

Temperature

Microorganisms generally have an optimal growth temperature above which they do not grow well or they die. Therefore, increasing the temperature of a sterilization process above the optimal growth temperature for the microorganism in question would increase the efficacy of a process.

Relative Humidity

The role of RH has been studied with regard to both heat sterilization processes and chemical (gas) processes. RH is defined as the ratio of the actual water vapor pressure in a system to the saturated water vapor pressure of the system at the same temperature. This term describes the water conditions in the atmosphere and as such inherently describes the water condition of the microbial cell or spore. Water activity is the relative water availability in a cell or spore and depends on the RH. There is an inverse relationship of cell resistance to water activity. It appears that, in most instances, the more water available to the vegetative cells or spores, the faster the heat inactivation process. Any sterilization process should account for the RH (5).

pH

As with disinfectant activity, the pH of the suspending medium appears to play a role in the sensitivity of microorganisms and spores to heat inactivation. A number of studies have demonstrated that a lowered pH may result in decreased resistance to heat treatment for bacterial species and spores, but the opposite is true for yeasts (3). It is postulated that pH changes alter the degree of dissociation of materials in solution, resulting in a shift of the oxidation reduction potential, thus affecting the survival of microorganisms.

Load Standardization

For all contained sterilization processes, it is important that loads be standardized to ensure a uniform process. Loads can vary in a number of ways, including the number of packs, the volume of the packs, the size of the packs, and the contents of the packs. Failure to standardize loads (i.e., instrument packs, linens, routine loads) adds another variable to the process. Theoretically, if a sterilization container/process [e.g., autoclave, ethylene oxide (ETO) unit] is tested and validated with a given load, any change in that load could result in a failure of the process. However, as a practical matter, the parameters of sterilization are chosen to ensure overkill, and failure of the process is most often due to actual equipment failure or to failure of personnel to monitor or to adequately follow the instructions for performing the process.

HEAT STERILIZATION PROCESSES

Since the beginning of recorded time, heat in one form or another has been used to cleanse and purify. In the medical field, hot air ovens, which require extended process times to be effective, have been used to sterilize materials and equipment that must be kept dry. On the other hand, moist heat (steam sterilization) processes have been found to be a more rapid and effective method of sterilization for those materials with which they are compatible.

Steam Sterilization

Steam sterilization is the most common of all the sterilization procedures used in the healthcare facility, because steam under pressure has been found to effectively destroy even the most resistant bacterial spores during a brief exposure. Steam sterilization is universally used except where heat and moisture damage may occur to the material being sterilized.

Various types of steam sterilization equipment (autoclaves) have been developed and used with success over the years. It has been demonstrated that moisture is a necessary part of the steam sterilization process, because without moisture the process reverts to a dry heat process and requires longer exposure times. The major design features of steam sterilization equipment involve the mechanisms for removal of air from the load, thus ensuring complete mixing of the steam and elimination of cold spots in the autoclave. These mechanisms include gravity displacement, mass flow dilution, pressure pulsing, high vacuum, and pressure pulsing with gravity displacement. All these methods have been developed to help remove air from the system and from the materials to be sterilized to optimize efficiency and efficacy. Each method has its own deficiencies because of the physics and thermodynamics of steam, air, and water mixtures. The pressure pulsing gravity displacement system has been found to be most useful for general use, because it reduces the thermal lag on heating of the load to the desired exposure temperature.

Factors that can affect the efficacy of the steam sterilizer include the air tightness of the sterilizer, atmospheric pressure, quality of steam, and characteristics of the load. In autoclaves that use the vacuum process, air from outside the vessel may be brought in through leaks in the system. This may result in a failure of the system because of uneven heating and spot dry conditions. Autoclaves operated at or below atmospheric pressure are inherently subject to air leaks, and continued vigilance with regard to maintenance of equipment is necessary to minimize potential problems. Joslyn (4) has described a new mechanism whereby sterilization is performed using a pulse method in which the steam pulses are performed at pressures above atmospheric pressure. This process should eliminate problems associated with air leaks because it is performed completely under positive pressure conditions.

The quality of the steam introduced into the sterilizer is also important in ensuring appropriate operation of the device. The quality of steam is defined by the weight of dry steam in a mixture of dry saturated steam and water in the system. Ideally, 100% saturated steam is required for proper operation of steam sterilizing equipment. Most equipment is designed with a steam separator and baffle that removes the water from the steam and directs the pure saturated steam to the chamber at the required velocity.

An appropriately designed autoclave operates efficiently regardless of the quality of the steam delivered to the equipment except when the separator or baffle malfunctions. Decreased steam quality (i.e., increased water content) may result in saturation of the materials such as dressings, wrappings, or linens. Excessive moisture then reduces the diffusion of steam throughout the load and, specifically, throughout the moisture laden packs. This may result in trapped air in the pack and increased time requirements for sterilization. In addition, grossly wet materials do not dry easily when the sterilization cycle is completed, and wet packs easily become contaminated.

Rutala et al. (6) showed that the type of container in which bags of waste were treated in a gravity displacement steam sterilizer had a significant effect on the sterilization time. These workers found that stainless steel containers allowed for optimal heat transfer and decreased the time required to sterilize the waste.

Although steam sterilization is the most common sterilization process used in the healthcare facility and personnel are most familiar with the process, the maintenance and operation of the equipment must still be closely monitored. The process is extremely complex and can be affected by a number of variables. Personnel responsible for steam sterilization in a healthcare facility should be familiar with all requirements for proper operation of the process. An excellent reference on the subject is found in the Association for the Advancement of Medical Instrumentation's recommended practice (7). Failure to understand the steam sterilization process, the equipment operation, or the validation process could lead to sterilization failure and contamination of critical medical supplies.

Flash Sterilization

The process of flash sterilization is often used for treatment of items that have become contaminated in the operating suite and will be needed again in a short time. As mentioned in the section on steam sterilization, sterilization requires removal of air and replacement of that air with saturated steam. Materials to be flash sterilized may inherently trap air in the system (e.g., porous linen, lumens of instruments), and varying conditions are necessary with these types of materials to ensure appropriate treatment. Flash sterilization for nonporous items is accomplished by heating to 270°F (132°C) for 3 minutes, or 10 minutes for porous materials, in a gravity displacement steam sterilizer. The actual sterilization cycle is the time required to heat up, treat, and cool down the sterilizer and therefore can take as long as 5 to 7 minutes for the 3-minute cycle and 12 to 18 minutes for the 10-minute cycle (8).

This process undoubtedly results in the destruction of most vegetative cells and viruses provided they are not protected by excess organic matter and the bioburden is low. Experimental evidence in the laboratory also indicates that the times and temperatures are sufficient to inactivate spores of *Bacillus stearothermophilus.* However, spore testing with commercial self-contained biologic indicators is often misleading (9). In addition, when this process is used, there is rarely time, before the use of the sterilized item, to allow for incubation of biologic indicators. Because of difficulties in verifying the validation process, Garner and Favero (10) have recommended against the use of flash sterilization for implantable items.

The cleanliness of the instruments to be sterilized, the condition of the autoclave, failure to document loads, and autoclave parameters all may affect the outcome of the process. It is important to recognize the shortcomings of flash sterilization and to use this process sparingly if protection of patients from wound contamination is to be ensured.

Dry Heat Sterilization

Dry heat (hot air ovens) has been used for many years as a method for sterilizing glassware, instruments, and other critical supplies that, for various reasons, could not be sterilized by steam sterilization procedures. Although wet heat sterilization is defined as sterilization at an RH of 1% or 100%, the parameters of dry heat treatment are not so easily determined. Dry heat sterilization takes place at an RH of between 0% and greater than 99%. The conditions for effective dry heat sterilization depend on the amount of water in the materials to be sterilized and in the environment of the dry heat sterilizer. At any given temperature, the lower the RH, the longer the time required for sterilization in a dry heat process. An understanding of this phenomenon explains the conflicting requirements established by various regulatory agencies in different countries with regard to the parameters of dry heat sterilization. Generally, in the United States, the requirement for dry heat treatment of containers for pharmaceutical products is 170°C for 2 hours. The American process includes a significant protection factor if one assumes that the British Pharmacopeia requirement of 150°C for 1 hour is also efficacious (11).

Dry heat sterilization advantages include low corrosiveness and deep penetration. However, the heating process is slow, and long sterilizing times are required. Materials may also be damaged by exposure to high temperatures for long periods.

Although a number of testing procedures have been developed to demonstrate the dry heat inactivation of microbial cells and spores, none of these is readily acceptable as a routine mechanism for deciding the exact time and temperature to be used for the process in the hospital. A description of these tests is beyond the scope of this chapter. It should be sufficient to recognize that the process recommended in the *U.S. Pharmacopeia* includes an appropriate protection factor and therefore should be a safe procedure when necessary.

GAS STERILIZATION

Since before the time of Hippocrates and the proclamation of the belief that infections were caused by miasmas and bad vapors, humans have sought a means of combating infectious diseases through the use of gaseous agents. The use of incense and frankincense was associated with concepts of purification of the air. Spices were placed in foods in the hope that their strong odors would prevent spoilage. In more recent times, the aerosolization of carbolic acid in operating rooms by Joseph

Lister, the use of sulfur dioxide and chlorine for terminal disinfection of a sick room, and the introduction of the use of formaldehyde for the same purpose did much to stimulate research on methods and mechanisms of gas sterilization. During the early part of this century, it was discovered that the terminal gas sterilization of sick rooms with formaldehyde was not as important as previously thought, and the emphasis on gas sterilization in the medical field declined.

With the advent of modern medical science and its plastics, electronics, disposables, and other heat-labile components, a new interest has developed in gaseous sterilization procedures for the medical field. Several gaseous agents have been used successfully to sterilize medical devices, instruments, and equipment. However, these agents can be toxic to people as well as the microorganism they are designed to destroy, and caution is needed to ensure appropriate protection of personnel and patients from exposure to many of these gaseous sterilants.

Ethylene Oxide

Phillips and Kaye (12), in a series of reports, reviewed the early literature concerning the use of ETO as a bactericidal agent. They proposed an alkylation reaction as the mechanism of action of this material and established the basic conditions under which ETO was most effective as a sterilizing agent. This was the beginning of a new era in the field of medical device sterilization. The development of ETO sterilization methods and procedures, pioneered by Phillips and Kaye and continued by numerous other investigators, has led to the widespread use of disposable equipment and supplies in the hospital industry. This trend has done much to decrease the possibility of cross-contamination and has aided in the battle against hospital-acquired infections. It has, however, also led to the discovery of the toxic effects of ETO, and the safety procedures for the use of this material must be carefully considered to avoid personnel, patient, and environmental exposure.

ETO is a colorless gas that is highly reactive with many different types of chemicals. ETO gas is highly flammable and explosive. However, mixture of the gas with carbon dioxide (13) or other gaseous carriers (fluorocarbons) (14) significantly reduces the fire hazards associated with the pure substance and allows its use, in special vessels, for sterilization. Mixtures of ETO in fluorocarbons appear to be more advantageous for use in hospitals, but information on the potential environmental hazards of these compounds has limited their use (15–17).

As was mentioned above, ETO mixtures have been used in sterilization processes. With the concern over fluorocarbons, processes have been developed using vacuum vessels in which a series of evacuations and backfills with nitrogen are used to ensure that the oxygen level remaining is insufficient to support combustion when pure ETO is added. The equipment used for the sterilization process is complex and has been developed to ensure appropriate mixing and control of the factors required (e.g., temperature, RH, ETO concentration) to achieve sterilization (18).

Formaldehyde

Formaldehyde has been shown, under appropriate conditions of temperature and humidity, to be both sporicidal and bactericidal. Although the use of formaldehyde in the decontamination of sick rooms in hospitals was considered helpful in the early part of this century, further study of the practice indicated that such a drastic method was not necessary to ensure cleanliness of rooms occupied by contagious persons. However, formaldehyde is still used as a fumigant for rooms and buildings in which massive contamination has occurred, such as mold growth in water-damaged buildings and in the terminal decontamination of high-containment biologic laboratories. It is the sterilizing gas of choice for decontamination of biologic safety cabinets and high-efficiency particulate air (HEPA) filter units.

Formaldehyde is generated by heating either paraformaldehyde or formalin to release the gaseous formaldehyde, and the activity of the formaldehyde depends on its condensation on contaminated surfaces. A procedure for microbiologic decontamination using paraformaldehyde has been published by the National Sanitation Foundation International (19).

Formaldehyde has also been demonstrated to be toxic to humans and has been classified as a potential carcinogen. The Occupational Safety and Health Administration (OSHA) has thus developed a standard regarding potential personnel exposure (20). Anyone using this material would be wise to review current federal and state regulations that might apply to both personnel exposure and environmental release.

Low-Temperature Steam Formaldehyde Process

Although pure formaldehyde has not been found to be particularly useful for medical device sterilization in the United States, European investigators have demonstrated that a combination of low-temperature steam and formaldehyde (LTSF) can be used. This process was first described by Alder et al. (21) in England. It was initially designed for the processing of cystoscopes and similar devices. Since that time, equipment has been developed that provides the necessary controlled conditions for sterilization of a wide variety of medical devices. Kanemitsu et al. (22) evaluated an LTSF sterilizer and concluded that this methodology was particularly useful because of its excellent efficacy, short handling time, and safety. However, these authors warned that the size of the load in the sterilizer affected its efficacy and that small loads were preferable to larger ones for processing.

The process involves the injection of dry formaldehyde gas into the treatment vessel followed by injection of steam to ensure an internal temperature of about 73°C and a holding time of 2 hours. The process is completed, and the residual formaldehyde is removed by further steam flushes and an introduction of sterile filtered air (23). As with ETO sterilization, the potential for residual formaldehyde on the surface of sterilized devices is a major concern. Nystrom (24) reported that studies in Sweden have shown that residual formaldehyde can consistently be kept under 5 mg/cm^3. Nystrom also stated that the occupational exposure resulting from the operation of this process is well below the threshold limit value of 0.6 mg/m^3 mandated by Swedish occupational health regulations.

Proponents of the process point to the facts that treated equipment needs less aeration than ETO does and that the increased temperature of operation increases the probability of sterilization success. In the U.S., however, this process has not been well accepted, probably because a reliable commercial process has not been validated, and there is considerable concern regarding the toxic and allergenic nature of formaldehyde.

Alternatives to Ethylene Oxide Sterilization

Concern over the hazards associated with the use of ETO have prompted many investigators to evaluate alternative methods for sterilizing heat-labile devices and instruments, including vapor phase hydrogen peroxide (VPHP) and various gas plasma technologies. Although not yet in widespread use, these technologies are beginning to be evaluated by healthcare facilities as safer more environmentally friendly alternatives to ETO processes.

Vapor Phase Hydrogen Peroxide

Liquid hydrogen peroxide (H_2O_2) has long been known for its ability to sterilize and its relative safety. Graham and Rickloff (25) reported on the development of a process using gaseous H_2O_2 at low concentrations and ambient temperatures to sterilize equipment and devices. It appears that sterilization can be achieved with this material with relatively short contact times. One of the major concerns of using relatively powerful oxidants for sterilizing medical devices has been the potential for damage to the devices. The short contact times required for the vapor phase H_2O_2 process appear to allow for reduced potential damage to devices because of possible oxidation.

Vapor phase H_2O_2 technology seems to have considerable potential in its use to replace ETO for the sterilization of heat-labile materials. Johnson et al. (26) and Klapes and Vesley (27) reported that VPHP generators have shown sporicidal activity and that, in their studies, the process shows promise as an effective and safe alternative method of sterilization. However, much work is still to be done with regard to such factors as compatibility studies and efficacy. In addition, the penetrability of H_2O_2 vapor through cellulosics is limited by absorption, which further limits the type of packaging available for this process. Nonetheless, VPHP sterilization is a promising alternative to more toxic and potentially environmentally hazardous methods of sterilization.

Plasma Gas Sterilization

Other alternatives to ETO sterilization have been developed and are currently available for use in healthcare facilities for the processing of heat-sensitive devices. These low-temperature plasma technologies include the Plaslyte (AbTox, Mundelein, IL) system that uses gaseous peracetic acid and the Sterrad (Advanced Sterilization Products, Irvine, CA) system that uses low-temperature H_2O_2 gas plasma (LT-HPGP). The ion plasma sterilization processes operate at relatively low temperatures by exposing peracetic acid or H_2O_2 to either strong electric or magnetic fields. Such exposure results in the formation of an ion plasma that contains reactive radicals that are known to be reactive with almost all molecules essential for metabolism and reproduction of living cells (e.g., DNA, RNA, proteins, etc.).

These technologies have stimulated interest in healthcare facility personnel, because they have short turnaround times compared with ETO sterilizers and are both more environmentally friendly and safer to use. Rutala and Weber (28) summarized the disadvantages of these methodologies. The authors stated that the use of the peracetic acid plasma method was limited to stainless steel surgical instruments (excluding lumen devices and hinged instruments). In addition, no liquids or materials that might be harmed by vacuum could be treated. The LT-HPGP process was limited by U.S. Food and Drug Administration (FDA) restrictions on treatment, by this method, of endoscopes and other medical devices with lumina longer than 12 inches or having a lumen diameter less than one-quarter inch (6 mm). Cellulose, linens, and liquids also cannot be processed in this device. Finally, the LT-HPGP process requires special packaging of devices and a special tray for processing.

A number of studies have demonstrated the efficacy of the LT-HPGP against viruses and parasites in the laboratory (29, 30). The efficacy of both processes in the treatment of medical devices was evaluated by comparison with the ETO 12/88 process by Alfa et al. (31). These authors concluded that the margin of safety for the methods tested was less than that of the 12/88 method and were concerned that even the 12/88 method failed to kill microorganisms in narrow lumen devices when salt or serum was present. They emphasized the need for scrupulous cleaning of the lumen of medical devices before treatment to ensure sterilization. Such research emphasizes the need for strict adherence to cleaning protocols before treatment of devices and provides valuable insight into a number of problems that can be associated with any alternative sterilization techniques. Bar et al. (32), concerned about reports of mycobacterial contamination of bronchoscopes, studied the use of LT-HPGP for the sterilization of these devices. Their results indicated that bronchoscopes washed and disinfected by conventional "washer/disinfector" as well as "intensive washing" (washing followed by glutaraldehyde treatment) still showed the presence of mycobacterium DNA, by nucleic acid amplification technique. Those scopes sterilized by the LT-HPGP were all negative by this test methodology. The authors concluded that LT-HPGP sterilization would be recommended if the nucleic acid amplification technique was to be used for the diagnostic procedure to verify sterility of the treated bronchoscopes.

Feldman and Hui (33) studied the compatibility of LT-HPGP sterilization with various medical devices and materials. The authors reported that in their studies of over 600 individual resterilizable devices from more than 125 manufacturers, approximately 95% of the devices could be safely sterilized by this process. They listed various materials that could be considered for LT-HPGP processing, including stainless steel (300 series), aluminum (600 series), titanium, glass, silica ceramic, and a number of plastics and elastomers. They also studied numerous adhesives and provided a listing of the adhesives that proved to be most compatible with the process.

Although these alternative methods have been developed in response to the patient, occupational, and environmental safety hazards associated with the use of ETO sterilizers, they may not themselves be without potential hazard. A recent report of several cases of corneal endothelial decompensation resulting from surgery with instruments sterilized in the peracetic acid plasma system has raised questions about the possible interaction of the sterilizing agents with the brass-containing parts of the instruments, resulting in release of metal compounds that can cause corneal decompensation. Studies are currently underway to verify the connection between the sterilization process and the injuries (34). Ikarashi et al. (35) also reported on the cytotoxicity of various medical materials exposed to a VPHP sterilization process, thus emphasizing the requirement for further investigation regarding the need for aeration to remove cytotoxic residuals from materials treated by the alternative techniques.

IONIZING RADIATION

Although ionizing radiation is not commonly used in the hospital for the sterilization of equipment and medical devices, it is an important process in the manufacture and packaging of devices used in the healthcare facility. Many of the devices that are supplied sterile to the hospital, such as plastic hypodermic syringes and catheters, are formulated to be sterilized by gamma radiation and may be damaged or may not properly function when sterilized in any other manner. These items are considered to be single-use items and are not to be resterilized once they have been opened and contaminated, unless the manufacturer guarantees the safety of the device after resterilization (see Chapter 87). Radiation causes little or no damage to the materials treated and leaves no residual radioactivity. Radiation of drugs, pharmaceuticals, and tissues for transplantation has also been successful.

Although there are a number of proposals for explaining the radiation inactivation of microorganisms, the effect of radiation appears to be a result of damage to DNA. Resistance to radiation treatment appears to depend on the microorganism's ability to repair the DNA damage (36,37). As with other sterilization processes, it has been generally accepted that bacterial spores are the most resistant microorganisms, and that demonstration of the killing of spores is an appropriate demonstration of the efficacy of the radiation sterilization process. It appears that although bacterial spores are the most resistant and gram-negative rods appear to be the least resistant to radiation damage, a number of inherently radiation-resistant microorganisms do exist and could be present in or on items to be sterilized. Members of the genus *Deinococcus* appear to be extremely resistant to radiation (38). In addition, other microorganisms (specific *Moraxella, Arthrobacter, Acinetobacter,* and *Pseudomonas* species) have been shown to exhibit enhanced resistance to radiation damage.

Procedures for ensuring the sterility of irradiated products have been proposed by the Association for the Advancement of Medical Instrumentation (39). These procedures are based on the known bioburden of the product, dose of irradiation, and good manufacturing procedures as required by the FDA.

FILTRATION

Although filtration is an important process in the preparation of a variety of liquid products used in the healthcare facility, in general it cannot be considered a mechanism for sterilization. Strict interpretation of the term *sterilization* implies killing or removal of all forms of life. Filters in use for the sterilization of such items as intravenous additives, drugs, and vaccines are, for the most part, bacterial filters. They do not, nor are they designed to, remove viruses. On the other hand, the materials that are treated by filtration are not expected to have live virus in them. Still, the fact that this process is designed for removal of bacteria must be considered.

Processing of fluids in the healthcare setting is discussed by Eudailey (40). Procedures for ensuring the quality of filtered materials, with particular reference to hospital pharmacy prepared intravenous fluids and hyperalimentation fluids, are presented in a number of articles on the subject (41–44).

The type of filter to be used for a particular operation depends on the operation and the requirements for the final product. Different types of filters are used for specific processes. The filter media range from deep filters of various materials (e.g., fiberglass, cotton, resins, porcelain, diatomaceous earth) to membrane filters of cellulose and other polymers. Depth filters have the advantage of being able to handle large amounts of contaminants throughout their thickness and can often retain particles smaller than their normal size rating because of adsorption of the particles on the filter. These filters, however, have some disadvantages. They tend to allow media migration in that the filter media may be released and travel through the filter and in fact may contaminate the product. There may also be a release of microorganisms as material passes through the filter during long process times. The filters may also retain significant amounts of fluid product, which can be a problem if the product is particularly valuable. Membrane filters, on the other hand, do not suffer from the problems of media migration or potential release of filtered microorganisms. They are efficient, and there is no retention of fluid product. The major disadvantage of the membrane filter is the fact that it tends to get clogged by excess dirt in the system.

It should be noted that filtration is also important in the removal of microorganisms and particulates from gases and air. The filtration capacity of such filters primarily depends on impaction, diffusion, and electrostatic charge. Particles traveling in an air stream tend to stay in that stream. Filtration is accomplished when the particles in the air stream have an impact on the surface of the filter fibers. The higher the air velocity, the greater the surface area of the filter, and the smaller the diameter of the fibers, the higher the probability of impaction. Diffusion also plays a part in the filtration process. Low-velocity air flow favors diffusion of the particulates to the filter surface, and very small (low-mass) particles tend to diffuse in the depths of the filter and are intercepted by the filter. HEPA filters have an efficiency of at least 99.97% at 0.3μm. These filters, by design, are more efficient for particle sizes above and below 0.3 μm.

Laminar-flow HEPA filtration units have been suggested for operating rooms, isolation rooms, and laboratories. It should be noted that at the point of release from the filters, the air is sterile, but as with any other sterilization process, the air quickly becomes contaminated from contact with unsterile materials. The use of these units should be tempered with an understanding of their limitations and the potential for recontamination of the air. It should also be noted that the filters used to remove infectious agents from the air are considered to be contaminated with those infectious agents. Personnel charged with maintenance, testing, and removal of the filters should be appropriately cautioned with regard to the hazards involved with these procedures.

PASTEURIZATION

Pasteurization is a process of inactivation of the vegetative cells of pathogenic bacteria and of viruses by heating at relatively low temperatures. The process has found widespread use in the food industry since its development by Louis Pasteur. The actual time/temperature conditions for pasteurization vary with the type of material being treated and the personnel performing the process. Historically, pasteurization for milk involves heating to approximately 60°C for 30 minutes or to 70°C for 15 to 20 seconds. Anesthesia equipment has been pasteurized by using an exposure to hot water at 75°C for 10 minutes (45). Treatment of plasma fractions at 60°C for 6 hours has been used for inactivation of viruses in the production of blood products (46). All these processes use the principle of heat inactivation of vegetative cells and viruses to ensure appropriate kill times.

The major disadvantages of pasteurization in the treatment of critical materials is the lack of standardization of the equipment and difficulty of validation. Because this is not a sterilization process, extreme care must be taken to ensure that the process is performed so that agents considered to be particularly important are inactivated.

VALIDATION

Major research studies on sterilization indicate that there is more to be learned with regard to sterilization processes (2,3). Research in the laboratory has been directed at the mechanisms of action of various sterilization processes, and the results have been conflicting, because there is so much variation in the conditions of the studies. Although much has been learned, the information gained is not always directly applicable to the real-world process in that microorganisms are not the same and conditions with regard to composition of loads, organic load, and bioburden are constantly changing. Therefore, any validation process must consider the variability inherent in the process and demonstrate overkill if sterilization is to be ensured.

Historically, the spores of bacteria have been thought to be the most resistant microorganisms with regard to heat, radiation, and chemicals. It has been natural to assume that processes that result in inactivation of these spores would provide a significant margin of safety to ensure sterility of the products treated by these processes. Spore suspension testing requires specific laboratory procedures and considerable incubation time. Alternative chemical indicators have been developed and compared with spore tests with good results (47), but spore testing continues to be the standard.

Although indicators are an important part of quality assurance of sterilization processes, the validation of the process and documentation of the actual operating parameters of the process are of paramount importance. It should be noted that spore and chemical indicators testing can only be as good as the placement of the spore suspensions or indicators. Failure to place the indicators in appropriate places in the load leads to false-negative results (i.e., apparent sterility when the items are not really sterilized). All sterilization processes should be thoroughly evaluated before being put into service and at regular intervals. Autoclaves should be mapped with thermocouples to determine potential cold spots. Filter systems should be tested for leakage. Gas sterilization units should be appropriately validated for such factors as gas concentration, temperature, and RH.

The sterility assurance level for a particular sterilization process is not routinely determined in the healthcare facility, because personnel lack expertise in the procedures. Young (48) has discussed cycle times and safety factors for steam and ETO sterilization cycles to be used in hospitals. Validation of healthcare facility sterilization equipment is primarily performed by the manufacturer of the equipment. To ensure appropriate sterilization processes, healthcare facility personnel must ensure that all manufacturer recommendations are met. The daily operation of the sterilizing processes must be documented by personnel performing the process. This documentation should be reviewed for each operation, and any malfunction should be noted and appropriate action taken to ensure that the product either has been properly treated or is returned for reprocessing.

In light of the advent of new medical devices, intricately designed with heat-sensitive parts and narrow lumina, the mechanisms for appropriate sterilization become a matter of concern for patient safety. In a provocative editorial, Rutala and Weber (28) questioned whether or not, because of the development of low-temperature sterilization technologies, there is a need to redefine sterilization. Current FDA requirements stipulate that a sterilizer's microbicidal performance must be tested under specified simulated use conditions, which include that the test articles must be inoculated with 10^6 colony-forming units (CFU)/unit of the most resistant test microorganism prepared with inorganic and organic test loads. The inocula must be placed in various locations on the test articles, including those least favorable to penetration and contact with the sterilant (49). Rutala and Weber, however, argue that these requirements may be too restrictive and that the requirements for efficacy should include the demonstration by instrument/device manufacturers that cleaning followed by a sterilization process can inactivate a clinically relevant inoculum of highly resistant microorganisms in the presence of an organic load in the most inaccessible location in the device. They note that the responsibility for defining the efficacy of new sterilization technologies should be met by the FDA, the device manufacturer, or the sterilizer manufacturer.

It seems logical that medical device manufacturers should take the lead in the evaluation of new sterilization processes for their own devices and that they should recommend the safest, most environmentally friendly, and cost-effective technologies available. Healthcare personnel must be aware of the problems associated with new and existing technologies and ensure that whatever process is used, it will be safe and effective.

MATERIALS DEGRADATION

New methodologies always bring with them new benefits as well as new potential hazards. New sterilization technologies are no exception. The benefits of new technologies must be reviewed and verified so that decisions can be made regarding the efficacy of medical devices as related to the sterilization process. Nuutinen et al. (50) studied the effect of various sterilization processes on the physical and mechanical properties of self-reinforced bioabsorbable fibers made out of polylactide (PLLA). The intrinsic viscosity, crystallinity, and mechanical properties (modulus of elasticity, yield strength, and ultimate tensile strength) were tested before and immediately after each sterilization treatment, as well as up to 30 weeks *in vitro*. Compared with unsterilized fibers, the intrinsic viscosity was markedly decreased after radiation sterilization (gamma and electron beam), and the loss in mechanical properties was accelerated during *in vitro* degradation. Plasma and ethylene oxide (one and two cycles) did not markedly alter the properties of the samples after sterilization or during *in vitro* degradation. The authors concluded that their data are important for determining the effect of various sterilization processes on the physical and mechanical properties of polylactide-based materials and can be used to predict how fast degradation of the mechanical properties of the self-reinforced PLLA will occur. They can also be used to tailor the degradation kinetics to optimize implant design.

With the advent of new medical devices that are heat sensitive, the search for a safe, effective sterilization methodology that is compatible with the device materials has accelerated. Although the use of various oxidizing agents, coupled with ionization procedures (as in LT-HPGP), or VPHP generators have become more popular and are replacing the more toxic ETO processes, there are potential problems with the integrity of the materials treated by these processes. Hopper et al. (51) postulated that conventional polyethylene liners cross-linked by sterilization with gamma radiation in air had better *in vivo* wear performance than non–cross-linked liners sterilized with gas plasma. The polyethylene liners that had been sterilized with gamma radiation in air had a significantly lower wear rate than did the gas-plasma–sterilized liners. The authors concluded that *in vivo* wear of conventional polyethylene liners that had been sterilized with gamma radiation in air was, on average, 50% less than that of non–cross-linked liners sterilized with gas plasma. In a comprehensive study of the safety of plasma-based sterilization, Lerouge et al. (52) used both the Sterrad and Plazlyte processes to evaluate the induction of surface modifications on polymeric medical devices. They observed surface oxidation and wettability changes on all surfaces sterilized by these techniques. The type and severity of the modification varied with the sterilizer and the type of polymer sterilized. It should be noted that these observed changes have not been shown to be particularly detrimental to patients, but further studies need to be performed to ensure the safety of this technology.

NOSOCOMIAL INFECTIONS

Sterilization and disinfection processes for medical devices and equipment have been developed specifically to prevent infections due to contamination of these materials. Obviously, if a material has been sterilized and is kept from being contaminated before use, there is no chance of infection in a patient exposed to it. Failure to appropriately perform or monitor the sterilization process or unvalidated changes in equipment or product, however, may result in an unsterilized product.

Bryce et al. (53) reported on an outbreak of *Bacillus cereus* in intensive care unit patients on respirators. The infections were traced to ventilator circuitry that had been pasteurized. The infections were due to the presence of a spore-forming microorganism, and the method for treatment of the equipment was not sufficient to kill the spores of the offending microorganism. A similar outbreak involving *Flavobacterium meningosepticum* was reported by Pokrywka et al. (54). In this outbreak, it was discovered that the pasteurization units were operating at suboptimal temperatures, thus allowing survival of the microorganisms.

Kaczmarek et al. (55) studied disinfection/sterilization practices for endoscopes in healthcare facilities and reported that the disinfection/sterilization procedures are not always optimal and that variation occurred even within hospitals. Pattison et al. (46) reported on an outbreak of hepatitis B associated with transfusion of commercially prepared plasma protein fraction that had undergone pasteurization in the preparation process. Nineteen of 31 patients receiving the plasma fraction had developed illness compatible with hepatitis B. The plasma had been subjected to treatment at 60°C for 10 hours, but the authors suggest that the process was inadequate to destroy the hepatitis B virus.

Although the study of Kaczmarek et al. concentrated on disinfection procedures and a number of outbreaks of nosocomial infection have been traced to inadequately disinfected materials and devices, few cases of nosocomial infection have been traced specifically to failure of sterilization processes. The notable exceptions are the outbreaks of nosocomial sepsis that have been traced to commercial intravenous fluids. Duma et al. (56) reported an outbreak of septicemias specifically related to intravenous infusions in 1971. Goldmann et al. (57) reported a nationwide outbreak of *Enterobacter* and *Erwinia* (*Enterobacter agglomerans*) infections traceable to commercial intravenous fluids that occurred in 1971. Goldmann et al. suggested that appropriate surveillance data were available before the dates of the outbreak and were sufficient to predict that there was a problem and that proper analysis of the data could have prevented the outbreak. In 1981, a second outbreak of nosocomial *Enterobacter* infections was traced to contaminated commercial intravenous fluids (58). During this outbreak, the contamination was shown to be present in the screw caps of bottles. The contamination was apparently protected from coming in contact with steam during the sterilization cycle by the design of the cap and thus was not subject to appropriate sterilizing conditions. These outbreaks point to the need for constant attention to detail with regard to ensuring the effectiveness of sterilization cycles and to review of surveillance data with particular regard to infections with exotic microorganisms associated with apparently sterile devices and fluids.

HEALTH AND SAFETY

Sterilization processes are designed, by definition, to eliminate all forms of life. As a result, these processes are inherently hazardous to those personnel involved with them. It is imperative that personnel understand the hazards of the process that they are required to perform. They must be trained in the use of appropriate personal protective equipment and understand and be able to carry out emergency procedures that would minimize personnel exposure to the sterilization process. Table 86.1 shows some of the potential hazards associated with major sterilization processes and includes reference to the OSHA standards that specifically apply. It is obvious that the hazards of sterilization processes involve both potential physical hazards such as heat and radiation and potential exposures to chemically hazardous materials such as the sterilant gases and their carriers. The administrative and supervisory personnel of each facility must recognize the hazards associated with the processes being performed in that facility, must develop appropriate safety procedures to protect the personnel involved, and must ensure that those procedures are being followed.

Ethylene Oxide Safety

A number of reports have demonstrated the dangers of ETO to both patients and personnel. Both human and animal studies suggest that ETO is a potential occupational carcinogen, causing leukemia and other cancers. ETO has also been linked to reproductive damage, including spontaneous abortions, cytogenetic damage, neurologic effects ranging from nausea and dizziness to peripheral paralysis, and tissue irritation (59).

OSHA has issued a standard (60) that sets a limit on worker exposure to ETO averaged over an 8-hour day. The standard was amended in 1988 to further reduce the health risk associated with ETO by requiring control of short-term exposures as well.

The key provisions of the ETO standard include a limit on workplace exposure of one part ETO per million parts air (1 ppm) averaged over an 8-hour day, and an excursion limit of 5 ppm averaged over a sampling period of 15 minutes. Employee rotation is prohibited as a means of compliance with the excursion limit.

TABLE 86.1. POTENTIAL OCCUPATIONAL HAZARDS ASSOCIATED WITH MAJOR STERILIZATION PROCESSES

Sterilization Process	Potential Hazards	OSHA Standards (29 CFR)
Steam (including flash sterilization)	Heat Super heated water	
Dry heat ovens	Heat	
Gas		
ETO	Toxic, carcinogenic, possible teratogen, dermatologic problems	1910:1047 (1910.134)a
Formaldehyde	Toxic, probable human carcinogen, irritant, dermatologic problems	1910:1048 (1910:134)a
Radiation	Exposure to radiation source	1910:96
Filters		
HEPA	Infectious agents trapped in filter	

OSHA, Occupational Safety and Health Administration; ETO, ethylene oxide; HEPA, high-efficiency particulate air.

Where the excursion limit is exceeded, employers must do the following:

1. Use engineering controls and work practices to reduce exposure. These controls and practices may be supplemented by the use of respirators where necessary.
2. Establish and implement a written compliance program to achieve the excursion limit.
3. Establish exposure monitoring and training programs for employees subjected to ETO exposure above the excursion limit.
4. Identify as a regulated area any location in which airborne concentrations of ETO are expected to exceed the excursion limit.
5. Place warning labels on containers capable of releasing ETO to the extent that an employee's exposure would foreseeably exceed the excursion limit.

Respirators can be used to control exposure only until feasible engineering and work practice controls are being implemented; during maintenance, repair, and other operations for which engineering controls are not feasible; in work situations wherein feasible engineering and work practice controls do not reduce exposures below the permissible exposure limit; and in emergencies.

OSHA has set an action level of 0.5 ppm. If the 8-hour time-weighted airborne concentration of ETO is at or exceeds the action level, employers must begin periodic exposure monitoring and medical surveillance. Employers who demonstrate that worker exposures are below the action level need not comply with most provisions of the standard.

If employers have not monitored worker exposures within the past year, they must do so for each job classification in a work area during each shift; representative sampling is permitted under certain circumstances. The frequency of subsequent monitoring depends on the results of the initial sampling. All monitoring may be observed by workers and their designated representatives.

A comprehensive medical surveillance program must be conducted by or under the supervision of a licensed physician. Workers must receive a medical examination before assignment to an area in which exposure is at or above the prescribed level, annually if they are exposed at this level for 30 days or more during the year, upon request if they develop symptoms suggesting overexposure or want medical advice concerning the effects of ETO exposure on their ability to produce a healthy child, and when they end employment in an area of exposure.

Other requirements include identification of excessive exposure areas, communication of hazard to affected employees, and OSHA record keeping.

Patient Safety

Because of the potential toxicity and resultant hazard to patients, it is important for persons using ETO for sterilization of medical devices to ensure adequate aeration for treated materials. The aeration process reduces ETO residues in and on the devices to a level that will not cause problems for patients or personnel exposed to the treated materials.

Formaldehyde Safety

Studies indicate that formaldehyde is a potential human carcinogen (20). Airborne concentrations above 0.1 ppm can cause irritation of the eyes, nose, and throat. The severity of irritation increases as concentrations increase; at 100 ppm, exposure to formaldehyde is immediately dangerous to life and health. Dermal contact causes various skin reactions, including sensitization, which might force sensitized persons to find other work.

To protect workers exposed to formaldehyde, the OSHA formaldehyde standard (61) applies to formaldehyde gas, its solutions, paraformaldehyde, and a variety of other materials that serve as sources of the substance. In addition to setting permissible exposure levels and exposure monitoring and training, the standard requires medical surveillance and medical removal of sensitized personnel, record keeping, regulation of potentially hazardous areas, hazard communication, and emergency procedures. Employers are to ensure primary reliance on engineering and work practices to control exposure. Selection and maintenance of appropriate personal protective equipment by employers is also required. If respirators are necessary, compliance with the OSHA respiratory protection standard is required. In addition, training is required at least annually for all employees exposed to formaldehyde concentrations of 0.1 ppm or greater.

The permissible exposure limit for formaldehyde in all workplaces covered by the OSHA Act is 0.75 ppm measured as an 8-hour time-weighted average. The standard includes a 2 ppm short-term exposure limit (STEL) (i.e., maximum exposure allowed during a 15-minute period). The action level is 0.5 ppm measured over 8 hours.

As with the ETO standard, the formaldehyde standard requires that the employer conduct initial monitoring to identify all employees who are exposed to formaldehyde at or above the action level or STEL and to accurately determine the exposure of each employee so identified. If the exposure level is maintained below the STEL and the action level, employers may discontinue exposure monitoring until such time as there is a change that could affect exposure levels. The employer must also monitor employee exposure promptly upon receiving reports of formaldehyde-related signs and symptoms.

A medical removal protection provision is included in the standard for employees suffering significant adverse effects from formaldehyde exposure. This provision requires that such employees are removed to jobs with less exposure until their condition improves, or for a period of 6 months, or until a physician determines that they will not be able to return to any workplace with formaldehyde exposure.

Occupational Safety and Health Administration Hazard Communication

The hazard communication standard (62) requires identification and appropriate labeling of all hazardous chemicals in the workplace. This standard also requires appropriate training and medical monitoring of personnel. In addition to the general requirements of the hazard communication standard, other standards for specific hazardous chemicals also require certain labeling.

The formaldehyde standard specifically delineates requirements for labeling of formaldehyde, including mixtures and solutions composed of 0.1% or greater formaldehyde and for materials capable of releasing formaldehyde in excess of 0.1 ppm. Hazard labeling, including a warning that formaldehyde presents a potential cancer hazard, is required where formaldehyde levels, under reasonably foreseeable conditions of use, could exceed 0.5 ppm. The ETO standard also has provisions for labeling containers that might release substantial quantities of ETO in excess of the excursion limits set by the standard.

Environmental Safety

In addition to the potential for personnel exposure, environmental concerns must be addressed. This is particularly true for the release of agents such as ETO and formaldehyde. The carrier for ETO may also be a potential environmental hazard, because the chlorinated and fluorinated hydrocarbons that have historically been used as a carrier to minimize the explosiveness of the ETO have been banned. These agents can be toxic in the environment and are regulated by either federal or state regulations concerned with toxic releases to air and water. It is important to realize that such environmental regulations are constantly being evaluated and revised by the regulatory sector, and specific references to such regulations in any textbook would undoubtedly be dated. It should be sufficient to warn that administrative and supervisory personnel must evaluate the release of these materials from the facility with regard to specific applicable regulations.

REFERENCES

1. Block SS. Historical review. In: Block SS, ed. *Disinfection, sterilization, and preservation.* Philadelphia: Lea & Febiger, 1991:1–17.
2. Wickamanayake GB, Sproul OJ. Kinetics of the inactivation of microorganisms. In: Block SS, ed. *Disinfection, sterilization, and preservation.* Philadelphia: Lea & Febiger, 1991:72–84.
3. Pflug IJ, Holcomb RG. Principles of thermal inactivation of microorganisms. In: Block SS, ed. *Disinfection, sterilization, and preservation.* Philadelphia: Lea & Febiger, 1991:85–131.
4. Joslyn LJ. Sterilization by heat. In: Block SS, ed. *Disinfection, sterilization, and preservation.* Philadelphia: Lea & Febiger, 1991:495–526.
5. Pflug IJ. The role of water in heat sterilization. *Pharmaceut Manufact* 1984;August:16–17.
6. Rutala WA, Stiegel M, Sarubbi F Jr. Decontamination of laboratory microbiological waste by steam sterilization. *Appl Environ Microbiol* 1982;43:1311–1316.
7. Association for the Advancement of Medical Instrumentation. *Good hospital practice: steam sterilization and sterility assurance. Recommended practice.* Arlington, VA: AAMI, 1988.
8. Howard WJ. The controversy of flash sterilization. *Today's OR Nurse* 1991;January:24–27.
9. Reich R, Fitzpatrick B. Flash sterilization. *J Hosp Suppl Process Distrib* 1985;May/June:60–63.
10. Garner J, Favero M. CDC Guidelines for the prevention and control of nosocomial infections guideline for handwashing and hospital environmental control. *Am J Infect Control* 1986;14:110–129.
11. Bruch CW. Dry-heat sterilization for planetary-impacting spacecraft.

Proceedings of the National Conference on Spacecraft Sterilization Technology, NASA SP-108, 1996.

12. Phillips CR, Kaye S. Sterilizing action of gaseous ethylene oxide. I. Review. *Am J Hyg* 1949;50:270–279.
13. Coward H, Jones G. Limits of flammability of gases and vapor. Bureau of Mines Bulletin No. 503, 1952.
14. Kaye S. Non-inflammable ethylene oxide sterilant. U.S. Patent No. 2,891,838, 1959.
15. Environmental Protection Agency. U.S. EPA assessment of ethylene oxide as a potentially toxic air pollutant. October 2, 1985. *Fed Reg* 1985;50:40286.
16. Environmental Protection Agency. U.S. EPA protection of stratospheric ozone. August 12, 1986. *Fed Reg* 1986;53:30566.
17. Environmental Protection Agency. Protection of stratospheric ozone. April 3, 1989. *Fed Reg* 1989;54:13502.
18. Parisi A, Young W. Sterilization with ethylene oxide and other gases. In: Block SS, ed. *Disinfection, sterilization, and preservation.* Philadelphia: Lea & Febiger, 1991:580–595.
19. National Sanitation Foundation. Class II (laminar flow) biohazard cabinetry, NSF 49 1992. NSF International Standard, 1992.
20. U.S. Dept. of Labor. OSHA formaldehyde standard. 29 CFR 1910: 1048.
21. Alder V, Brown A, Gillespie W. Disinfection of heat sensitive material by low temperature steam and formaldehyde. *J Clin Pathol* 1966;19: 83–89.
22. Kanemitsu K, Kunishima H, Imasaka T, et al. Evaluation of a low-temperature steam and formaldehyde sterilizer. J Hosp Infect. 2003; 55(1):47–52.
23. Ayliffe GAJ. The use of ethylene oxide and low temperature steam/ formaldehyde in hospitals. *Infection* 1989;17:109–110.
24. Nystrom B. New technology for sterilization and disinfection. *Am J Med* 1991;91(suppl 3B):264S–266S.
25. Graham GS, Rickloff J. The feasibility of terminally sterilizing heat sensitive products with hydrogen peroxide gas. Presented at the fall meeting of the Parenteral Drug Association, San Francisco, CA, November, 1992.
26. Johnson J, Arnold J, Nail S, et al. Vaporized hydrogen peroxide sterilization of freeze dryers. *J Parenter Sci Technol* 1992;46:215–225.
27. Klapes NA, Vesley D. Vapor phase hydrogen peroxide as a surface decontaminant and sterilant. *Appl Environ Microbiol* 1992;56: 503–506.
28. Rutala W, and Weber D. Low-temperature sterilization technologies: do we need to redefine sterilization? *Infect Control Hosp Epidemiol* 1996; 17:87–91.
29. Vassal S, Favennec L, Ballet J, et al. Hydrogen peroxide gas plasma sterilization is effective against *Cryptosporidium parvum* oocysts. *Am J Infect Control* 1998;26:136–138.
30. Roberts C, Antonoplos P. Inactivation of human immunodeficiency virus type 1, hepatitis a virus, respiratory syncytial virus, vaccinia virus, herpes simplex virus type 1, and poliovirus type 2 by hydrogen peroxide gas plasma sterilization. *Am J Infect Control* 1998;26:94–101.
31. Alfa M, DeGagne P, Olson N, et al. Comparison of ion plasma, vaporized hydrogen peroxide, and 100% ethylene oxide sterilizers to the 12/ 88 ethylene oxide gas sterilizer. *Infect Control Hosp Epidemiol* 1996; 17:92–100.
32. Bar W, Marquez de Bar G, Naumann A, et al. Contamination of bronchoscopes with Mycobacterium tuberculosis and successful sterilization by low-temperature hydrogen peroxide plasma sterilization. *Am J Infect Control* 2001:29(5):306–311.
33. Feldman L, Hui H. Compatibility of medical devices and materials with low-temperature hydrogen peroxide gas plasma. *Med Device Diagn Ind* December 1997.
34. Anonymous. Corneal decompensation after intraocular ophthalmic surgery—Missouri, 1998. *MMWR* 1998;47:306–309.
35. Ikarashi Y, Tsuchiya T, Nakamura A. Cytotoxicity of medical materials sterilized with vapour-phase hydrogen peroxide. *Biomaterials* 1995;16: 177–183.
36. Davies R, Sinskey A, Botstein D. Deoxyribonucleic acid repair in a highly resistant *Salmonella typhimurium. J Bacteriol* 1973;114: 357–366.
37. Town C, Smith K, Kaplan H. Production and repair of radiochemical damage in *Escherichia coli* deoxyribonucleic acid, its modification by culture conditions and relation to survival. *J Bacteriol* 1971;105:127.
38. Brooks BW. Red pigmented micrococci: a basis for taxonomy. *Int J System Bacteriol* 1980;30:627.
39. Association for the Advancement of Medical Instrumentation. *Process control guidelines for radiation sterilization of medical devices.* Arlington, VA: AAMI, 1981.
40. Eudailey W. Membrane filters and membrane-filtration processes for healthcare. *Am J Hosp Pharm* 1983;40:1921–1923.
41. Crawford S, Narducci W, Augustine S. National survey of quality assurance activities for pharmacy-prepared sterile products in hospitals. *Am J Hosp Pharm* 1991;48:2398–2413.
42. National Coordinating Committee on Large Volume Parenterals. Recommendations to pharmacists for solving problems with large volume parenterals. *Am J Hosp Pharm* 1976;33:231–236.
43. Levchuk J, Nolly R, Lander N. Method for testing the sterility of total nutrient admixtures. *Am J Hosp Pharm* 1988;45:1311–1321.
44. Akers M, Wright G, Carlson K. Sterility testing of antimicrobial-containing injectable solutions prepared in the pharmacy. *Am J Hosp Pharm* 1991;48:2414–2418.
45. Craig DB, Cowan S, Forsyth W, et al. Disinfection of anaesthesia equipment by a mechanized pasteurization method. *Can Anaesth Soc J* 1975;22:219–223.
46. Pattison CP, Klein C, Leger R, et al. An outbreak of type B hepatitis associated with transfusion of plasma protein fraction. *Am J Epidemiol* 1976;103:399–407.
47. Hirsch A, Manne S. Bioequivalent chemical steam sterilization indicators. *Med Instrum* 1984;18:272–275.
48. Young JH. Comparison of in-hospital and industrial sterilization of medical devices. *J Health Care Mater Mgmt* 1986;4:29–34.
49. Food and Drug Administration, Division of General and Restorative Devices. Guidance on premarket notification [510(K)] submissions for sterilizers intended for use in health care facilities. Washington, DC: FDA, March 1993.
50. Nuutinen JP, Clerc C, Virta T, et al. Effect of gamma, ethylene oxide, electron beam, and plasma sterilization on the behaviour of SR-PLLA fibres in vitro. *J Biomater Sci Polym Ed.* 2002;13(12):1325–36.
51. Hopper RH Jr, Young AM, Orishimo KF, et al. Effect of terminal sterilization with gas plasma or gamma radiation on wear of polyethylene liners. *J Bone Joint Surg* 2003;85A(3):464–468.
52. Lerouge S, Tabrizian M, Wertheimer M, et al. Safety of plasma-based sterilization: Surface modifications of polymeric medical devices induced by Sterrad and Plazlyte processes. *Bio-Med Mat Eng* 2002:12: 3–13.
53. Bryce E, Smith J, Tweeddale M, et al. Dissemination of *Bacillus cereus* in an intensive care unit. *Infect Control Hosp Epidemiol* 1993;14: 459–462.
54. Pokrywka M, Viazanko K, Medvick J, et al. A *Flavobacterium meningosepticum* outbreak among intensive care patients. *Am J Infect Control* 1993;21:139–145.
55. Kaczmarek RG, Moore R, McCrohan J, et al. Multi-state investigation of the actual disinfection/sterilization of endoscopes in health care facilities. *Am J Med* 1991;92:257–261.
56. Duma R, Warner J, Dalton H. Septicemia from intravenous infusions. *N Engl J Med* 1971;284:257–260.
57. Goldmann D, Dixon R, Fulkerson C, et al. The role of nationwide nosocomial infection surveillance in detecting epidemic bacteremia due to contaminated intravenous fluids. *Am J Epidemiol* 1978;108: 207–213.
58. Matsaniotis N, Syriopoulou V, Theodoridou M, et al. Enterobacter sepsis in infants and children due to contaminated intravenous fluids. *Infect Control* 1984;5:471–477.
59. Keene JH. The mutagenicity, toxicity, and potential carcinogenicity of ethylene oxide. MPH thesis. Chapel Hill, NC: University of North Carolina, School Of Public Health, 1980:35.
60. U.S. Dept. of Labor. OSHA ethylene oxide standard. 29 CFR 1910: 1047.
61. U.S. Dept. of Labor. OSHA formaldehyde standard. 29 CFR 1910.1048
62. U.S. Dept. of Labor. OSHA hazard communication standard. 29 CFR 1910:1200.

87

REUSE OF MEDICAL DEVICES LABELED FOR SINGLE-USE

VELVL W. GREENE

It is difficult for those who have no personal experience with the purchase, processing, and distribution of medical devices in hospitals to appreciate the magnitude and diversity of this enterprise. These are the "tools of the trade," tens of thousands of different products, many of which contact or penetrate some part of some patient some time and whose aggregate cost is in the multibillion dollar range. Superficial attempts to classify the medical device world into neat and precise categories usually oversimplify the picture and understate its complexity. Still, one traditional classification has served hospital workers well for nearly a century, their identification as either *reusables* or *disposables.*

1. Reusable devices, also called *durables,* are usually fabricated from metal, glass, rubber, or woven textiles. They are purchased from an original equipment manufacturer (OEM) in "factory release" condition and before use on a patient are inspected, cleaned, wrapped, and sterilized in the hospital's central supply service (CSS). After use on a patient, they are again cleaned, inspected, packaged, and sterilized. Although the initial unit cost might be high, the ultimate cost is considerably reduced after repeated cycles of use and in-house reprocessing.
2. Disposable devices are traditionally constructed from inexpensive, heat-sensitive materials such as plastics. They are purchased from an OEM, factory-sterilized and packaged, ready-for-use. The original cost is usually low enough so that recycling does not make economic sense. They are intended to be used just once and then discarded. If they are designed for direct patient care, they are usually labeled "for single-use only."

After decades of separate but equal coexistence in the hospital, the distinctions between reusables and disposables started to blur. By the middle 1970s, for various economic reasons hospitals were replacing more and more of their traditional durable and reusable devices with the less expensive disposables. At the same time, there was a revolution in medical technology. Almost daily advances and innovations in diagnosis and treatment and the wholesale adoption of these new techniques created an urgent demand for the instruments and devices that enabled the techniques to be performed. The disposable medical device industry happily responded to this need by fabricating many of these relatively complicated and sophisticated devices, using the same kind of nondurable raw materials found in their simpler, traditional disposables. They were considerably more expensive than the latter but for a variety of reasons they were still labeled for single-use only. In the hospital world of the 1970s, discarding anything that could be used again was not acceptable. Moreover, by this time in history, hospitals had significantly improved their sterilizing competence. (See Chapters 74 and 86.) Recycling was an ecologic and economic virtue. All the incentives for recycling disposable medical devices were in place.

It soon became a common practice. The same common sense that justified discarding urine collection bags, after a single use, rebelled against discarding, after only one use, expensive sphincterotomes that "have a lot of life left in them." Then like now, the hospital world was under constant pressure to cut costs of a "runaway" healthcare system.

Parenthetically, during the same period of the late 1970s, some hospitals were experiencing some strange infections (see Chapter 47). They were advised to discard perfectly good reusables that had been used on patients exposed to or suffering from the so-called slow viruses (today known as prions), which were surprisingly refractory to the conventional sterilizing treatments of steam, EO, and strong germicides. Thus, disposables were reused and reusables were discarded.

A new nomenclature was in order and it evolved. The colloquial term disposable, once descriptive and appropriate (this chapter, in previous editions of the text, was actually titled "Reuse of Disposable Devices"), is considered today somewhat archaic and even pejorative. The new term, adopted by the Center of Devices and Radiological Health (CDRH) of the Food and Drug Administration (FDA) is single-use devices (SUDs) or "medical devices labeled for single-use." To avoid ambiguity (and the subtle inference that if a device is called disposable it probably is) the terminology in the rest of the chapter conforms to that used by the agency.

What defines a SUD or distinguishes it from a reusable? It certainly is not purchase cost or technical complexity. The FDA implies it is the presence or absence of the OEM's label warning against reuse. The hospital uses a more pragmatic definition: if the device, after use, can be returned to a satisfactory state of sterility and function, it can be reused. However, the most important single feature that should distinguish SUDs from reusable devices is the intent of the OEM (or arguably, lack of intent). Quite simply, if the OEM intends for the device to be reused, it will be specifically designed for that purpose and fabricated from the appropriate durable materials. If, on the other hand, it is intended to be used once and then discarded, this intent will significantly influence the device design and material selection.

Two terms, *safe* and *functional,* lie at the heart of the SUD reuse controversy. Clinicians all agree that any device that poses a demonstrable risk of infection or malfunction should have no place in the care of humans. Thus, the first and basic question is whether SUDs, recycled after use, are as safe to use and as functionally reliable as the original SUD purchased from the OEM who fabricated it in a facility that was approved by CDRH and that met their rigorous quality assurance (QA) standards. Another point of interest is whether the original SUD is equivalent to the traditional reusable device it is replacing—the one routinely recycled through the CSS. In addition, it would also be interesting to compare the safety and reliability of recycled SUDs to recycled reusables. Only then can one debate disagreements about economic incentives, legal ramifications, ethical issues, and bureaucratic oversight. Finally, one can raise the question about where the reprocessing should be done—in the hospital, in a facility controlled by the OEM, or by so-called third-party reprocessors.

The FDA might have preempted all debate. The agency has recently reexamined its regulatory policy and decided to extend the existing SUD manufacturing regulations, which in the past applied only to OEMs, to hospitals and any third parties who reprocess SUDs. There are those who think that this means the end of SUD reuse. Others worry about burgeoning bureaucracy and intrusion of federal government regulators into hospital practice.

This chapter reviews some of the more reliable published studies dealing with the risks of reusing SUDs. To provide some perspective, it describes the historical evolution of device processing in hospitals. It reviews the aims and strategies of the recent FDA action. Finally, it discusses some of the nonmedical issues that still fuel the reuse controversy whether or not the FDA actually implements its new regulations and whether or not they succeed in solving the reuse problem.

A brief explanation might be in order for essentially ignoring two types of devices commonly included in discussions of SUD reuse: endoscopes and hemodialyzers. They are routinely recycled in hospitals and are relatively difficult to clean and sterilize. Moreover, the former may sometimes have attachments labeled for single-use only. However, the endoscope is basically a durable device sold to the hospital with full intention and knowledge that it will be reused many times and reprocessed either in the hospital or in a commercial facility. The dialyzer was once labeled as a SUD, but today the manufacturer is obligated by the FDA to provide instructions for reprocessing and reusing.

HISTORICAL INSIGHTS

Medical Devices and Nosocomial Infections

Not too long ago humans lived in a world of epidemiologic naivety. The common fomite phobia that prevailed in the Western world since the discovery of bacteria was also shared by hospitals. From the time of Lister until the 1960s, any medical device—durables or single-use—would be among the first suspects in a case of nosocomial infection. If doorknobs, kitchen cutlery, and pencil erasers were considered serious vehicles for disease agent transmission, what was one to think about devices that came into intimate contact with a patient's skin, mucous membranes, blood, and deep tissue? Actually, the suspicions were not groundless, particularly if the devices had previously been used on patients with overt infections or who might have been carriers. Equally as important, hospital sterilizing facilities and skills had not achieved the level expected today. Packaging was primitive, gravity steam autoclaves frequently failed, poststerilization recontamination was not uncommon, and the parameters and protocols of modern QA were still being perfected.

Perhaps the first documented case of a nosocomial infection, attributed to a contaminated medical device, was described by Semmelweis (1) more than a century ago. During a postmortem examination of a woman who died from puerperal fever, a student assistant accidentally pricked the finger of the pathology instructor, Jakob Kolletschka, with the dissection knife. Kolletschka, who was Semmelweis's friend and teacher, developed a sore at the puncture site, was hospitalized within a week, and died shortly thereafter with the generalized inflammatory symptoms of puerperal fever.

Medicine did not yet know much about microbes or infectious diseases, but Semmelweis intuitively recognized the reservoir of infection (cadaver), the path of transmission (knife), and the portal of entry (puncture wound) for "the cadaverous particles [that] caused his death." Students of medical history know that this reasoning, although originally rejected, really anticipated many of the modern concepts about antisepsis, asepsis, disinfection, and surgical sterility. For the purpose of this chapter, however, it is cited only to show that nosocomial infections attributed to medical devices long predate the practice of reusing disposables. They even predate the germ theory.

After Louis Pasteur, Joseph Lister, and their contemporaries established the etiologic connection between microbes and infectious diseases, the medical world began to focus its attention on the disinfection of devices and materials used in surgery (2). Metal instruments, sponges, and sutures made from silk and catgut were soaked in corrosive and potent chemicals like carbolic acid, sublimate of mercury, and formalin. The number of device-related infections were reduced, but both patients and practitioners experienced irritation and tissue toxicity caused by the disinfectants.

The invention of the steam autoclave, about 1890, was the major breakthrough that essentially solved both problems associated with medical and surgical devices—the risk of infections and chemical toxicity. Most of these devices and materials, at least the critical ones that would contact the very susceptible interior tissues of the body or would be used for parenteral and vascular injections, were made from glass, metal, rubber, cotton, or wool. They could be cleaned and wrapped and then sterilized by steam. After removal from the autoclave, they would remain wrapped and sterile and unexposed to any contaminating sources until opened by the physician just before use.

Evolution of Hospital In-house Sterilization

Thus began the remarkable hospital cottage industry known as the central sterilization department (CSD), central sterile supply, supply processing and distribution (SPD), or any of the dozens of other terms used to describe the same generic task. For nearly a century, these enterprises have been recycling used devices and instruments, originally only from surgery and then from all over the hospital, for safe and efficient reuse.

The steam autoclave, the mainstay of the CSS for nearly a century, was joined in the 1970s by EO sterilizers—the gas autoclave. The combination of both systems permitted the hospital to sterilize nearly anything it wanted to, including heat-sensitive materials such as plastics, electronics, optical systems, batteries, and motors—all of which would have been destroyed by the moisture, heat, and pressure of the steam autoclave. In recent years, more sophisticated sterilization systems, including vapor phase hydrogen peroxide and plasma gas, have been introduced to treat heat-labile devices and instruments in the hospital (see Chapter 86).

Considering the epidemiologic potential, remarkably few nosocomial infections can be attributed to medical devices sterilized in the modern hospital CSS. This is ample empirical evidence that the sterilizers in use today are reliable and that the hospital reprocessing system works. The used devices are decontaminated, cleaned, and inspected by personnel specially trained for the task. The packs containing the devices to be sterilized are assembled, wrapped, and positioned in the autoclaves according to rigorous protocols. Vacuum pumps remove any air that would prevent penetration of the sterilizing gas. Chemical indicators sensitive to heat or EO are placed in every pack to verify that the contents are actually exposed to the desired sterilizing conditions. The steam and gas autoclaves used for sterilizing are designed for overkill margins of safety to reduce the probability of survival of viable bacterial spores (that are orders of magnitude more resistant than any normal nosocomial pathogen) to less than 1/1,000,000 per pack. The autoclaves are challenged at least once per week with biologic indicators (dried spore suspensions) that monitor their continuing functional reliability. Furthermore, the sterilized packs are stored under strictly controlled environmental conditions until opened and used. (3)

In addition to the risk of transmitting infections, users of medical devices face additional problems. Even durable devices wear out and break down; sharps become dull, springs lose their tension, metal rusts. Repeated cleaning and sterilizing cycles accelerated the deterioration. QA programs can be implemented to reduce the number of impaired devices from entering the system, but much depends on the frequency and sophistication of the inspection. Good QA costs money and most middle-sized and small hospitals cannot afford sophisticated QA. However, they can afford the consequences of failure even less. For such institutions, a ready-to-use device whose sterility and function was warranted by an OEM would always be welcome, particularly if it was cheap enough to be discarded after use.

SINGLE-USE DEVICES AND THEIR REUSE

Hospital Supply Industry and the Plastics Revolution

Even during the very early years of in-house sterilization and recycling, hospitals recognized that certain devices and materials, such as surgical dressings, gauze bandages, and catgut sutures, were difficult to reuse. The practice was uneconomical, or inefficient, or, in the case of Listerian dressings—cloth plastered with pitch, paraffin, and carbolic acid—simply too messy. The manufacture of these items was, consequently, relegated to an embryonic hospital supply industry, and the concept of the prepackaged, presterilized disposable, today known as a SUD, was born (4).

These two sterilizing enterprises—the hospital's recycling program for reusables and industry's production of SUDs—enjoyed a somewhat symbiotic relationship for close to 50 years until the end of World War II when the plastics revolution swept the country. It was quickly evident that many items recycled by the hospital (e.g., gloves, tubing, syringes, bedpans, dishes, bottles, and linens) formerly made from durable metal, glass, rubber, and woven textiles could now be made much cheaper from the abundant variety of new plastics and synthetic compounds that were being developed and introduced at an unprecedented rate, and these devices were truly disposable. They were fabricated from heat-sensitive materials that would disintegrate in the hospital's steam autoclave, which was the only sterilizing system universally available until the early 1970s. No one wanted to reuse these things anyway; economically, it was not worth the effort. By the middle 1970s, as many as possible of the hospitals' reusable devices, those traditionally recycled in the CSS, were gradually being replaced by presterilized SUDs.

Ironically, during these plastics years, the greatest concerns hospitals had about the prepackaged factory-sterilized SUDs were their sterility! With typical professional arrogance, they assumed that only doctors and nurses could properly sterilize medical devices. The sterility concern was resolved after 1976, when the Medical Device Amendments became part of the Food, Drug, and Cosmetics Act. Today, the shoe is on the other foot, and questions are legitimately raised as to whether the in-house hospital sterility standards are as good as those of industry (5).

Biotechnology and Medical Devices

When the incentives for purchasing SUDs were entirely economic and the SUDs were mostly cheaper replacements for simple items like bedpans and gloves, the only real concerns dealt with inventory management, the space available for storage, and the potential environmental impact of disposing of megatons of refuse (6).

The dimensions of the SUD problem changed again during the technology revolution mentioned previously. Hospitals began purchasing an amazing variety of complex gadgetry based on electronic circuitry, membrane technology, expensive optics, and miniaturized components. Today, it is estimated that more than two thirds of the tens of thousands of sterile devices used daily in American hospitals are SUDs. They include the original cheap disposable items and modern arthroscopy instruments, laparoscopic dissectors, and endotracheal tubes. Furthermore, the standards of sterility and reliability they must meet are regulated by federal law.

Quality Assurance in the SUD Industry

The labeling of SUDs for single-use only is, in part, a consequence of the strict testing and manufacturing requirements imposed before the device can be released for sale. The manufacturer must be able to demonstrate both theoretically and empirically to the CDRH that the sterilizing process used is adequate to destroy all resistant contaminants that would be found on the original device and that the probability of contamination on the final product is actually less than one microbe on a million devices. The construction, organization, and sanitary conditions of the manufacturing facilities are regulated by guidelines known as good manufacturing practices (GMPs), and all of this is subject to inspection. Because the manufacturer cannot control any of these manufacturing standards anywhere except in his or her own factory, and one presumes that QA and GMPs are relevant to the safety and effectiveness of the finished device, the manufacturer is protecting himself or herself from liability, as well as protecting the consumer from harm, by warning the world that the product is guaranteed only for the first use.

Often overlooked but essential to the understanding of this problem is the well-known fact that cleaning and sterilizing sophisticated medical devices are not always routine procedures, simply accomplished by passing them through a washer followed by an autoclave. The devices must be designed and fabricated with cleaning and sterilizing in mind; concomitantly the recycling process should be designed with the device and its idiosyncrasies in mind (3). Otherwise, the process might fail. The cleaning and sterilizing agents used might not pass through narrow apertures or gain access to all of the critical surfaces or the interior of long narrow lumens, or the chemicals used might corrode or weaken these surfaces. The manufacturers of reusable devices not only design them to be compatible with repeated processing in the hospital's CSS and select fabrication material that can stand up to multiple cycles of use and reprocessing they also provide detailed protocols and instructions to CSS personnel about how to render a used device once again safe and functional. Quite different circumstances prevail in the SUD industry. Here the OEM designs the device to be cleaned, tested, packaged, and sterilized by personnel under his or her supervision and in his or her own facility.

Incentives for Reuse

It would be reasonable to imagine that the single-use warning label would convince the hospital's management not to recycle a SUD and many hospitals have heeded the warning. Cost-saving imperatives are compelling, however, particularly if the hospital's management is convinced that the enterprise is technically feasible. Most hospitals that are big enough to gain economically from reuse of SUDs have also invested considerable capital in modern sterilizing equipment. They are also the ones that would suffer most from legal and economic sanctions imposed by the community relative to hospital wastes. Moreover, as Mayhall (7) pointed out nearly two decades ago, there are several good reasons for in-house sterilization of SUDs, other than economics. For example, a hospital might want to recycle used SUDs when the delivery of new SUDs has been interrupted, when a package has been opened or damaged and the sterile status of the unused SUD is unknown, or when an unused and presterilized SUD is being incorporated into a new pack that will be sterilized as a unit.. A hospital will simply ignore the OEM's warning when the Puritan streak, so deeply ingrained in American hospitals, convinces the hospital that discarding a device is wasteful, expensive, and probably sinful. The attitude of many healthcare professionals was summarized in a succinct declaration at the Association for the Advancement of Medical Instrumentation (AAMI) 1983 conference: "We had not regarded woven catheters as disposable devices. The fact that they are *declared disposable* means next to nothing" (8).

Magnitude of the Reuse Practice

No one knows who was the first to resterilize and use again a medical device labeled for single-use only and exactly when it was done. Several lines of evidence point to specialists who were working with expensive SUDs during the early 1970s. At the National Workshop on Reuse of Consumables in Hemodialysis in 1982 and at the AAMI Technology Assessment Conference on the Reuse of Disposables in 1983, the issue came out of the closet and some brave pioneers, particularly in the fields of hemodialysis and cardiac angiography, described their own empirical success with recycling. This should not be surprising. Modern medicine is the home of innovation and "stretching the envelope." What is surprising is the speed with which SUD reuse swept through the hospital world and its acceptance as a routine, even unquestionable practice.

At the 1984 Georgetown University Conference, an informal survey of 204 respondents revealed that 82% were aware of the reuse of one or more types of SUDs in their own institutions. Only 6% stated that their facilities either had a policy prohibiting reuse or did not reuse SUDs; 12% were either unaware of reuse in their institution or did not answer the question (9). At this conference, the FDA cited surveys that showed that in 14% of hospitals were reusing at least selected SUDs in 1976 and that this number increased to 90% by 1982 (10). Also at this conference, the Centers for Disease Control and Prevention (CDC) described the growth of the common practice of reusing hemodialyzers in dialysis centers. During the period 1976 to 1980, 17% to 18% of the centers were reusing. In 1982, this proportion increased to 43%, and it was anticipated that this would rise to 60% by 1983. In the early 1980s, 52% of patients undergoing dialysis in centers reimbursed by the Health Care Financing Administration were in reuse programs (11).

In the Georgetown informal survey, the most common SUDs reused were hemodialyzers (46% of respondents), cardiovascular catheters and guidewires (31%), respiratory therapy breathing circuits (18%), biopsy needles (17%), cautery devices (16%), anesthesia breathing circuits (14%), and endotracheal tubes (10%). Of the respondents, 5% to 10% indicated that they reused suture staple removers, syringes, orthopedic appliances, suction canisters, tracheal tubes, and Bovie cords. These were followed by a list of 31 devices, the reuse of which was reported by less than 5% of the respondents (9).

Reuse in Canadian Hospitals

A survey of 1,238 Canadian hospitals (1,065 responded) in 1986 is probably the most reliable and certainly the most comprehensive report on the prevalence of SUD reuse during those years. It revealed that, among the larger hospitals (more than 200 beds), 86% regularly and 6% occasionally reused single-use medical devices; only 8% never reused. Among the smaller hospitals, 50% never reused, 38% said they reused regularly, and 12% said they did so only occasionally or during emergencies. Interestingly, only 38% of hospitals that regularly reused had written procedures for reuse, and only 32% indicated a mechanism for determining the number of times a device was reused. Cost-analysis studies to demonstrate the economic justification for reuse had been undertaken by only 29% of regular reusers (12).

The Canadian survey, surprisingly, does not even mention hemodialyzers and ranks the frequency of reuse reporting among the 377 hospitals that regularly reuse SUDs as follows: Bain circuits, 67% to 70%; nebulizers-humidifiers, 61% to 71%; endotracheal tubes, 13% to 19%; other breathing circuits, 47% to 58%; transducer domes, 7% to 8%; cardiac catheters, 7% to 20%; and arterial catheter needles, 0% to 8%.

Current Reuse Prevalence

The data cited previously reflect the situation in the 1980s. By the year 2000, a number of reliable surveys suggested that only 20% to 30% of American hospitals were reusing SUDs and that one third of those hospitals relied on a third-party reprocessing company to do the job. The Government Accounting Office (GAO) report (13) that summarized these surveys also provided the most comprehensive and certainly the most objective evaluation of the SUD reuse issue known to me.

The most recent update on reuse prevalence is derived from an FDA telephone survey of all hospitals in the country (except military and Veterans Administration institutions) carried out between December 2001 and February 2002 (14) The response rate was nearly 80% and verified that 24% reuse SUDs. The most common devices reused were sequential compression device (SCD) sleeves (15.8%), followed by "drill bits, saws, blades, or burrs" (7.3%), "biopsy forceps, snares" (6.2%), "endoscopic/laparoscopic scissors, graspers, dissectors, or clamps" (6.1%), and electrophysiology (EP) catheters (3.9%). Nearly half of all hospitals with more than 250 beds reuse SUDs, compared with only 12.3% of hospitals with less than 50 beds. This probably reflected the new FDA regulations that were looming on the hospitals' horizons; most reusers (84%) used the services of third-party reprocessors. The majority of the remaining in-house reprocessors (60% of the 15.4%) were small hospitals with less than 100 beds.

MEDICAL RISKS ASSOCIATED WITH REUSE OF SINGLE-USE DEVICES

The recycling of SUDs poses two kinds of problems: medical risks that may result in physical and physiologic harm and nonmedical problems that derive from the economics, possible liability, and ethics of the practice.

Among the potential medical risks, Phillips (15) included the following:

1. Infection risk: the medical device in question may become contaminated during the first use or during the reprocessing procedure. If for any reason the hospital's CSD is incapable of properly resterilizing the device (see Chapter 86), it becomes a potential infection hazard to any patient on whom it will be reused.
2. Pyrogens: medical devices may become contaminated with gram-negative bacteria during patient use or subsequent rinsing in contaminated water. Sterilization destroys the viable microorganisms, but the residual lipopolysaccharide or endotoxins may remain. These chemicals can cause febrile reactions in patients even if the reused device is sterile (see Chapters 62 and 64).
3. Toxic residues: the recycling process involves decontaminating, cleaning, and sterilizing with a variety of germicides, detergents, and toxic gases. If these chemical residuals are not completely removed, they can irritate and harm the tissues of the patient on whom they are reused.
4. Bioincompatibility: devices that have been implanted in a patient or that have had significant contact with the patient's body tissues and fluids may become coated with some of his or her unique cells and biochemicals. If the device is reused on another patient without scrupulous cleaning and removal of those biochemicals, they might generate foreign-tissue reactions and lead to immunologic rejection of the device.
5. Functional reliability: as devices are used over and over again, it might be expected that they will gradually lose the original functional reliability that they had when new. The electronic, mechanical, optical, and physical properties of any device usually deteriorate with age and repeated use. How can a hospital determine the number of times a device can be safely reused without experimenting and placing patients at risk?
6. Physical integrity and sterile barriers. What is the effect of repeated use, cleaning, and sterilizing on such properties as tensile strength of a device, burst pressure, leak pressure, surface finish, dimensional tolerances, and membrane integrity? Do the materials used to construct medical devices suffer from fatigue? How many times can they be reused safely before failure?

All of the risks, catalogued previously, are consistent with theory and have happened in practice. However, they apply to all devices, reusables and previously used SUDs, which are really the subjects of concern in this chapter. In theory, used SUDs pose even greater risks because of several extenuating circumstances that have already been alluded to previously, such as the questionable ability of the average hospital CSS to conduct technically demanding QA tests of safety and function, the common use of nondurable raw materials for SUD fabrication, the inability of CSS cleaning and sterilizing practices to process a SUD that has not been designed or constructed to be compatible with the CSS system, and the unwillingness of the SUD manufacturers to provide instructions for reprocessing a given device.

No matter how compelling the theory, what is the evidence

that SUD reuse poses a real risk for real patients? There are three potential sources for this kind of information: hospital and medical record surveys, anecdotal reports, and systematic epidemiologic studies.

DOCUMENTING REUSE PROBLEMS

Two studies from the early 1980s (16,17) are characteristic of the time and the type of information then available. In one 326-bed hospital there were 623 instrument failures in 22 months. Seventy percent of these were associated with SUDs. No mention was made whether these were new or reused devices. In a 452-bed university-affiliated hospital there were 224 incidents of equipment failure in 36 months. The majority involved SUDs being used for the first time. The stated policy of this hospital was not to reuse. Thirty-six of the 224 incidents involved invasive procedures.

Perhaps the most comprehensive and certainly the most recent survey was reported by the FDA (18), based on their medical device report (MDR) system. The CDRH is supposed to receive "event reports" about inadvertent outcomes (e.g., injuries) in the field that can be attributed to medical devices, but they concede that the MDR system does not enable accurate assessment of failure rates. Their most recent evaluation is based on the 3 years from 1996 to 1999. Of 300,000 reports submitted, 219 involved hemodialyzers (which are strictly speaking, not really SUDs), and 245 other adverse events could possibly be attributed to reuse of 70 different SUDs.

In truth, the general impression shared about the risks of reusing SUDs is derived not from MDRs but from historical anecdotes reports of isolated events that occurred 20 or 30 years ago. These events actually happened and were sufficiently newsworthy to receive wide publicity or sufficiently egregious to result in generous damage awards after litigation. However, there is rarely sufficient information from anecdotal reports to compare relative risks (RR) of infections, endotoxic reactions, or equipment failure associated with reused SUDs vis-à-vis unused SUDs vis-à-vis classical reusable devices. Some of these reports are cited as evidence that the concerns described previously are not just theoretical and that reprocessing and reuse of disposable devices do (or did) involve some health risks.

Perhaps the most notorious incident involving a reused product was the Mosely case—a legal action in which a doctor and a hospital were held liable for $970,000 in damages after a cardiac catheter broke and became lodged in a patient's thigh. This was actually a reusable device labeled by the manufacturer for a maximum of three uses. However, it had been reused at least 19 times and had been recalled by the manufacturer 9 years before the incident. When the manufacturer's representative contacted the hospital after the recall, he was informed that none of the items remained in use. However, a search revealed that 53 of the dated catheters were in stock; they were used regularly although some had not even been sterilized (19).

A more recent and relevant case of structural weakening because of SUD reuse was described by Fishman (20). An aluminum stylet, the manufacturer of which had cautioned against reuse, broke off in the esophagus of a 72-year-old patient during intubation and ultimately perforated her duodenum. Apparently, the cleaning and sterilizing procedure caused the stylet to lose its malleability, and the metallic structure was sufficiently compromised to permit breakage.

Butler and Worthley (21) reported several adverse outcomes associated with the reuse of flow-directed balloon-tipped catheters and demonstrated that devices resterilized with EO were less rigid and had an increased incidence of balloon rupture compared with new devices. The greatest incidence of rupture occurred during the third use, and they recommended that the instrument be recleaned and resterilized for only one extra use; beyond this limit, both function and structure were significantly compromised. Repeated EO sterilization can also weaken the structural integrity of single-use (polyvinylchloride) esophageal stethoscopes. Bryson et al. (22) described how one of these devices, which had been cleaned and resterilized "for economy," fragmented during a routine thoracotomy and had to be removed in several pieces in the recovery room.

Resterilization with EO caused structural damage to a thin (0.003 in.) polycarbonate membrane in the single-use dome of a blood pressure transducer. As the number of sterilizations increased, the probability of a defect also increased. The minute cracks that resulted, cracks that could not be detected by routine CSD monitoring, seriously compromised the sterile integrity of the device. In a 1976 outbreak, 25 patients developed primary bacteremia with *Serratia marcescens,* and four died during the 4.5-month period when single-use domes were being reused on blood pressure transducers (23).

In fairness, it should be reported that contaminated reusable pressure transducers were also implicated in a number of other nosocomial infections episodes during the 1970s (24,25). The outbreaks involved *S. marcescens, Pseudomonas* species, *Enterobacter* species, *Candida* species, and hepatitis B virus and were responsible for several fatalities. In these cases, however, improper cleaning and sterilization of the devices were blamed not compromise of sterile membrane barriers. When appropriate sterilization and disinfection practices were introduced, the outbreaks were brought under control.

In contrast to the cardiac catheter experiences described previously, the infection risk associated with the reuse of single-use plastic insulin syringes seems negligible. Reports from California (26), Virginia (27), Ireland (28), Scotland (29), and Australia (30) all agree that the practice combines both cost benefits and safety. Nearly all of this reuse involves a given patient reusing the same syringe, and the insulin for injection is formulated with antibacterial agents that suppress growth of contaminants. However, these findings cannot be extrapolated to the hospital, where cross-infection via inadequately sterilized devices is much more probable.

Other reports of infections associated with the reuse of SUDs incriminated hemodialyzers and blood lancets. The lancet incident occurred in a private physician's office in which 18 cases of hepatitis B could be traced to a nurse's reuse of single-use blood lancets for hemoglobin testing (31). One wonders how much money that nurse actually saved.

Reprocessed hemodialyzers identified as SUDs have not only been incriminated as sources of infection but also have been reported as the sources of pyrogenic reactions (32). The infection problem is being solved by more comprehensive high-level disinfection protocols, but the pyrogen control is much more complex. This finding has serious implications because of the prevalence of reuse of these devices and the general acceptance that, if the hemodialyzer's reuse is restricted to the same patient, the procedure is actually beneficial. The dialyzer situation is thoroughly reviewed in Chapter 64.

Endotoxic reactions were also observed following reuse of cardiac catheters (33,34) (see Chapter 62). Again the problem was not so much intrinsic to reuse as it was to inadequacy of the reprocessing system. Jacobson et al. (35) conducted a carefully controlled trial of patients studied with both single-use and reused catheters. They concluded that if the catheters were carefully cleaned and reused, there was no statistical difference in infection rates or endotoxic reactions between new and reused devices.

Most of the anecdotal events reported previously occurred 2 decades ago, when recycling protocols for used SUDs were still in early stages of development. It should not come as a surprise that infections and pyrogenic reactions occurred. Over the years, however, hospitals learned from their mistakes and perfected more suitable recycling processes for various SUDs just as they did previously for durable devices. It may not be fair to assume that the problems described previously are still current. What is the risk situation now?

Systematic studies of SUD-reuse problems do exist and some are very well designed and executed. Their most common drawback, usually beyond control of the investigators, is inadequate sample size, lack of suitable controls, and the inability to "blind" the clinician who is doing the procedure and evaluating the outcome. These faults seriously limit the generalization of their findings to other hospitals or devices. Some studies may be flawed by commercial bias. Not surprisingly, those sponsored by SUD suppliers suggest that reuse results in considerable numbers of QA failures. In contrast, hospitals and physicians who practice SUD reuse and who have a financial incentive to do so point to impressive track records with no adverse iatrogenic events. It is quite possible that both are right. Much depends on what one is looking for and how hard (and long) one looks. Several recent reports are cited as examples.

Jacob and Bentolila (36) described an extensive and comprehensive study of contaminated angioplastic catheters conducted at two hospitals in Quebec. They challenged the hospitals' sterilizing systems (EO) with a variety of catheters, various bioloads inside and outside the lumens, and heavy loads of liquid and dried blood occluding the microbial contamination. They concluded that the risk of infection is not significantly higher with reused catheters than with new ones. They also verified that their presterilizing cleaning technique with pyrogen-free water and judicious choice of cleaning chemicals solved the pyrogen and toxic residual problem. Mechanical tests on several types of SUDs revealed that they did not become more fragile after multiple use but emphasized that this aspect of safety must be established de novo for every new type of catheter that is purchased.

Kazorek and his colleagues (37–39) conducted several prospective studies on the reuse of sphincterotomes and biopsy forceps sold as SUDs. They ascertained the sterilizability of the devices after artificial challenges with contaminants and after use in the clinical setting and the number of times that the devices could be reused before a critical malfunction would occur. Most important, they carried out a cost analysis of comparing reusable, disposable, and reprocessed disposable devices. Although some of their clinical trials enrolled too few patients to reach broad generalized conclusions, there is no doubt that these workers could successfully practice modern gastroenterology with reused SUDs and save significant sums of money for their hospital.

A randomized, double-blind, controlled clinical trial was conducted in Kuwait by Zubaid et al. (40) to compare the safety (clinical success) and efficacy (angiographic success) of reused versus new coronary angioplasty balloon catheters. There were no significant differences in incidence of balloon failure in the two groups, the angiographic success rate was similar, and the number of catheters used per lesion, amount of contrast, and procedural and fluoroscopy time were similar. After 30 days, the incidence of major adverse cardiac events was similar and the incidence of fever no different.

In contrast to the studies that demonstrated feasibility of reuse, Heeg et al. (41) in Germany concluded that none of the SUDs they studied (biopsy forceps and papillotomes) were effectively cleaned, disinfected, or sterilized. Moreover, there was some material damage to the structure of the fragile devices. The scanning electron micrographs of the residual contamination on the SUDs after reprocessing dramatically demonstrated the inadequacy of the cleaning process. In all fairness, however, it should be emphasized that these investigators were also unable to sterilize reusable biopsy forceps, papillotomes, and a stone retrieval basket that had been included as controls. Is it possible that the bottom line of this study—sponsored by a leading SUD manufacturer—is the self-serving conclusion not to reprocess anything—neither SUDs nor reusables?

A significant contribution to the debate was made by Chaufer et al. (42) in Australia who evaluated the transmission of live viruses via reusable angioscopes. Thirteen of these devices became contaminated with duck hepatitis B virus (DHBV)-containing blood after examining an infected duck. After a variety of cleaning, disinfection (glutaraldehyde), and sterilizing (EO) treatments (and combinations of these), the angioscopes were reused to examine healthy ducks. All 38 control (no treatment) birds became infected. No disease was transmitted by devices properly cleaned and sterilized. However, if the instruments were inadequately cleaned, DBHV survived despite disinfection or sterilization. Perhaps the *a fortieri* argument may be made that if it is so difficult to render reusable devices safe and effective (devices designed for recycling and backed by decades of empirical success), the probability of succeeding with recycled SUDs is considerably diminished.

This point is reinforced by an *in vitro* study recently published by Luijt et al. (43). They deliberately contaminated disposable catheters with an RNA virus (echovirus-11) and a DNA virus (adenovirus-2), reprocessed them by cleaning and sterilizing with glutaraldehyde, and simulated their reuse. After performing polymerase chain reaction (PCR) and cell culture assays they concluded that, even after vigorous cleaning and sterilization, virus was still present in the device and that catheters labeled for single-use only should not be reprocessed.

Plante et al. (44) stirred the crucible of controversy somewhat with a 1994 study that challenged the official premise of the Ministry of Health of their own province (36), namely that reuse of coronary catheters is safe, effective, and economically justified. These investigators conducted a prospective observational study of 693 patients undergoing coronary angioplasty in two hospitals, one of which reused single-use catheters and the other one did not. Reuse involved more devices per procedure (2.4 vs. 1.5), had a higher incidence of initial balloon failure (10.2 vs. 3.3), prolonged procedure time (81 vs. 68 minutes), and required an increased volume of contrast medium (201 vs. 165 ml). Reuse was also associated with a higher rate of adverse clinical events (7.8% vs. 3.8%). There was no significant difference in the very low incidence of fever in either group (3/320 vs. 1/373) and in no case did the fever appear to be related to the catheterization procedure. To be fair, they reported that the hospital that reused the SUDs saved $110,000 CDN during the 10-month course of the study.

It is quite common when faced with research results that contradict one's own position—in this case, the argument that SUD reuse is safe, effective, and economical—to reanalyze the opponent's contradictory data, preferably with a sophisticated statistical technique that might discover serious flaws. Two years after it appeared, a reanalysis of Plante's paper was published by Mak et al. (45) in an equally distinguished journal. The latter made several justifiable criticisms and his new calculations dampened the difference in outcomes between the patients treated with only new SUDs and those in whom SUDs were reused. However, he could not counter the observation that reused catheters failed more frequently than new ones, required more frequent replacement, and significantly lengthened duration of the procedure.

The bottom line regarding nosocomial infection risks associated with reusing SUDs is that they exist and may not be dismissed as trivial. However, there is no compelling evidence, certainly not from recent studies and not from consideration of the prevalence of the practice, that these risks are significantly higher than those experienced with new SUDs or traditional reusables. The other problems cited by Phillips (15), namely pyrogens, toxic residues, bioincompatiblity, functional reliability, and physical integrity really require further and more systematic study before reaching rational conclusions about risks of SUD reuse. The overwhelming impression conveyed by the most reliable sources is that the harder one looks the more one finds and much depends on who is looking. A scanning electron microscope reveals residuals that could be missed by ordinary light microscopes. Tests that measure compression strength, leak rates, resonant frequency, and other equally arcane criteria that are used by QA engineers to judge function and integrity might reject devices as unsuitable even if the physician claims that "they work fine." The duration of an angioplastic procedure probably depends as much (or more) on the patient and the physician as it does on the number of times that the catheter has been recycled. In the past, hospitals have focused much of their attention on the cleaning, sterilizing, and infection problems of used SUDs and largely ignored structural and functional QA. It may very well be the case that the latter should play a greater role in deciding whether to continue reuse practice or, at the very least, in making device-by-device decisions. The only answers currently available are track records of empirical success. Moreover, without a fuller and more comprehensive record of all device-related events, one cannot tell whether the damage resulted from reuse per se (as would be suggested by theory), whether the process used to recycle them was inadequate and correctable, or whether the process was simply not carried out properly. The track record suggests that many items labeled as SUDs can actually be recycled several times safely.

Nonmedical Problems Associated with Reuse of Disposables

Even if the technical and medical issues are in order, certain economic, legal, and moral ramifications of SUD reuse suggest strongly that the practice should be severely curtailed or at least more deeply reexamined. This is not be the appropriate medium for a thorough analysis of these issues, but a brief review of some of the questions that have been raised should illustrate the point.

Power and Politics

The debate about reusing SUDs goes beyond the ivory towers of academia and the drab cubicles of bureaucracy. It reflects a serious struggle between several powerful forces—the hospital world, healthcare professionals, the device supply industry, government regulators, and others—with some very significant stakes in contention: turf control, money, the health of the public, hospital traditions, and employment of the working poor. The numbers and diversity of groups whose members stand to lose or gain—sometimes their very livelihood—depending on decisions reached about reusing or discarding SUDs is impressive [e.g., see the Web site maintained by the Association for Advancement of Medical Instrumentation (AAMI)] (46). Each side tries to present those data and arguments that paint it in the best possible light and tries to obfuscate the opposition. Under these circumstances, scientific truth and objectivity is sometimes difficult to ascertain

Economics

The original justification for reusing SUDs—saving money—has been challenged from the very beginning (47–49). These authorities point out that most hospitals involved in SUD reuse do not carry out proper cost-accounting studies that would validate such savings and that those few who do studies overlook a number of direct and indirect costs involved. For example, they do not factor into the equation the extra time required to do a procedure with reprocessed SUDs that may be functional but not quite as flexible or manageable as new unused devices (44) or the number of recycled devices that would be rejected by the practitioner during the procedure. They ask about the point in the reuse sequence at which savings move from "negligible" to "significant": Do we reuse a SUD to save $100 or $10 but do not think it worthwhile to save $5? How many times? Until it fails or when it reaches the 50% point in its "life expectancy" cycle? Who decides?

Critics of reuse claim that hospitals do not even factor into their economic incentive calculations the potential legal costs that will be faced if a patient dies or is injured by a SUD used contrary to manufacturers' warnings. Others emphasize the costs of establishing a proper QA program to minimize such events; they point out that if a hospital had to spend money on QA, the savings realized from reuse of disposables would soon evaporate. This is apparently what will happen when the new FDA policy transfers SUD reprocessing from the hospital to a commercial, outside facility.

Some of the most biting criticism of SUD reuse deals with the question, "Who really benefits economically?" Is the patient examined with a cardiac catheter, previously used 20 times, charged less than the patient who was number 10 in line? Is it fair to charge them the same? And if we do, is it the average cost of a reused SUD, or the prorated cost after each reuse, or the original price of the brand new one? Does the hospital pocket the savings? Or the insurance company? Or Medicare? Do we even tell the insurance carrier that we are using reprocessed SUDs and charging as if they were new?

Legal Considerations

Liability questions associated with SUD reuse are as intriguing and frustrating as those of economics. The point is that there is no specific law against reuse that would expose the reuser to criminal charges. However, there are more than a million attorneys in the United States, most of whom earn their livelihood from litigation and a large number of these from litigation in the fields of medical malpractice, product liability, and personal injury. There is remarkably little statute law on the books dealing with the reuse issue, and there is a dearth of case law on the subject. Until the FDA's initiative in 2000 to treat reprocessing of SUDs as a manufacturing activity that came under its jurisdiction (see later) there was a confusing hodgepodge of directives, guidelines, regulations, advisories, licensing criteria, and codes emanating from governmental agencies, professional associations, and conference proceedings that related to safety and effectiveness of reused devices. The jungle is always ecologically ripe for an explosion of litigation. Good reviews of the liability issues relative to SUD reuse can be found in the 1983 AAMI report (50) and the 1984 Georgetown conference proceedings (51); a brief but more recent summary was published in the 1992 Emergency Care Research Institute (ECRI) newsletter (19) already cited. It should also be noted that he new FDA initiative does not ban reuse in the hospital. The hospital may still be caught in the "litigation net" along with the third-party reprocessor if some undesirable event occurs and plaintiff's attorney demonstrates that reuse, in that particular case, of a device labeled for single-use only was a negligent act.

Ethical Concerns

The ethical arguments against the reuse of SUDs are even more compelling than the economic uncertainties and the fears of litigation presented previously. If by reusing SUDs, the hospital is exposing itself to unnecessary legal liability and associated costs of litigation, the practice has little, if any, moral justification and requires very little further analysis. Win or lose, the litigation will certainly raise the costs of medical care, and the practice has a negligible, even questionable, benefit to the patient or the hospital.

However, the moral issues go much deeper. How do we reconcile patient autonomy and justice in a situation in which one patient gets a brand new device and the next gets a device for which the manufacturer denies responsibility? How do we frame the informed consent questions? Who will be first and who last? How did the hospital originally determine the limits of reuse before it started the practice? Or was this a kind of empirical clinical trial on human beings without their informed consent and without permission from the institutional review board? The questions about charging for SUDs have been mentioned previously; they might sound flippant and insignificant in view of the huge costs of medical care, but there are some basic issues of honesty and potential fraud involved.

The fundamental ethical question in SUD reuse, as in most other biomedical issues, must deal with the beneficence of any practice versus all of the other values, such as justice, autonomy, and risk of harm (52). Here the answer seems clear. Except for the case of previously used dialyzers (with which some benefits to the patient are clinically discernible along with some risks), a patient treated or diagnosed with a reused SUD is no better off and is theoretically at higher risk than a patient exposed to the prepackaged, presterilized, and previously unused device. If there are other benefits, such as monetary savings for the patient, this might become a question of informed consent. If the patient will be deprived of treatment or care because the only device available has been previously used and reprocessed, this is also a matter of informed consent. However, the bottom line is benefit to the patient, and, until the advocates of reuse can demonstrate this with data, the practice should be avoided.

THE NEW FDA APPROACH TO THE ISSUE OF SUD REUSE

The Medical Device Amendments of 1976 require the FDA to see that devices that enter the market are safe and effective and to ensure that they remain that way. The position of the FDA then, a position which has not really changed today, is that their regulatory authority relates to manufacture of medical devices rather than to their use (10). Thus, when some medical practitioners started to recycle their more expensive and sophisticated SUDs in the 1970s to save money, the FDA did not exert any regulatory efforts to outlaw the practice, although they were aware of its rapidly rising prevalence and the early reports of associated casualties (23). They issued guidelines in 1981, addressed to the institutions and practitioners who "reprocess and reuse disposable medical devices," instructing them to be able to demonstrate "(1) that the device can be adequately cleaned and sterilized, (2) that the physical characteristics or quality of the device will not be adversely affected, and (3) that the device remains safe and effective. Also, the user must bear full responsibility for reuse." Sixteen years after these positions were presented at the Georgetown Conference (10) the FDA completely reversed its approach to SUD reuse.

The current director of CDRH read a statement (18) before

a Senate committee in June, 2000, in which he stated that the FDA "has re-examined its policy on this issue" and reached a "decision to treat all reprocessors of SUDs, whether third-party firms or hospitals, in a similar manner," namely as manufacturers of medical devices and subject to the same licensing, inspection, regulation, and noncompliance penalties as commercial OEMs. In other words, the FDA, which is constrained from simply banning SUD reuse because that is essentially a medical practice option, is redefining some aspects of the SUD-reprocessing operation to accomplish the same end.

A used SUD would now be considered "raw material." The cleaning, testing, packaging, and sterilizing steps that are daily done to recycle reusable devices in every CSS in the country, would be considered a manufacturing process when recycling SUDs. The hospital in which this was done would now be recognized as an OEM, which would ironically be required to label the reprocessed used devices for single-use only! Because of this, the hospital would have to adhere to all of the premarketing requirements incumbent on all OEMs of medical devices and go through the technical and bureaucratic steps of validating their procedures and QA standards through the CDRH. The details, deadlines, fines for noncompliance, and updates of FDA new approach can be accessed on the Internet (53).

In previous editions, the chapter on SUD reuse ended with a plea to hospitals to " . . . do what they do best—provide medical and surgical and rehabilitative care to patients—and let industry do what it does best—supply safe and effective devices to the hospital and practitioner." The new FDA policy seems to reinforce this advice. Certainly the decreased prevalence of SUD recycling, cited earlier, demonstrates that the practice in American hospitals has dropped significantly in the last few years. However, if the new directives just remove the in-house phase of reprocessing, transfer it to a third-party, and continue to allow devices to be used over and over again contrary to the advice of the original manufacturer, the legal and ethical issues have not been resolved. It should be emphasized once again that, if a medical device is not designed for reuse, it should not be reused or it should not be reused until the patient is aware of what is taking place and consents to it.

Actually, those with the most experience in the field believe that this is not only the end of SUD reprocessing in the American hospital but also that it is the end of SUD reuse, period! In a brilliant essay Favero (54) suggested that hospitals do not want to become nor will they be able to afford the cost of becoming OEMs. Furthermore, the third-party reprocessors have also been redefined as OEMs and will have to dance the same dance as the real OEM with respect to manufacturing practices, premarket approval, inspections, QA validations, ad infinitum. In turn, the extra costs that OEM status will entail and which they will have to pass on to their hospital customers will reduce any financial advantage that used SUDs used to have over brand-new ones.

Perhaps this is what FDA wanted in the first place—to terminate SUD reuse without banning it. If so, it is an ingenious ploy. Why they changed their mind after nearly 3 decades of basic inaction except for guidelines and platitudes is another subject for historians to elucidate, particularly because they did it just when the hospitals were getting so proficient at recycling. One of the more noteworthy quotations from the Senate hearing stated "Despite a lack of clear data that directly link injuries to reuse, FDA has concluded that the practice of reprocessing SUDs merits increased regulatory oversight" (18).

Will the next FDA policy reexamination lead it to extend its oversight to the world of reusable devices? Will Dr. Favero's next requiem be offered for the venerable hospital institution known as the CSS?

CONCLUSIONS

Analysis of the historical, epidemiologic, and regulatory literature pertaining to the reuse in hospitals of medical devices labeled for single-use only or SUDs leads to the following conclusions:

1. Compared with previously unused devices, reused SUDs should in theory pose increased risks of infection; a higher incidence of febrile reactions from pyrogenic residuals; irritation from toxic residues deposited by cleaning and sterilizing chemicals; immunologic reactions to foreign tissue residues on previously implanted devices; a higher incidence of electronic, mechanical, optical, and physical malfunctions; and diminished physical integrity of the device and integral sterile barriers.
2. In clinical practice, however, empirical evidence from institutions that have been reusing SUDs for decades does not support the premise that the practice demonstrably endangers their patients' life and health.
3. Systematic and controlled prospective studies in this field provide contradictory results. Many of the studies are flawed by inadequate sample numbers to provide the statistical power that would demonstrate safety. Investigator bias and commercial bias permeate the literature. The field is in need of some good systematic studies using large numbers of experimental animals.
4. The economic, legal, and ethical aspects of SUD reuse are not the same as those of reprocessing. Even a hospital that delegates the latter to a third-party processor is obligated to obtain informed consent from patients before using them, to make sure that the allocation of new and reused devices is fair, and to return the savings—if any—to the patient.
5. The reuse debate may quickly become (or already has become) moot because of the recent FDA initiative to classify both hospitals and third-party reprocessors of SUDs as device manufacturers who must conform to all of the restrictions and testing standards previously demanded only from commercial manufacturers. This initiative not only removes the economic incentive for reuse but also actually adds a regulatory disincentive. In effect, both SUD reprocessing and reuse will fade from the scene and might disappear.

REFERENCES

1. Semmelweis IF. *The etiology, concept, and prophylaxis of childbed fever—1860.* Madison: University of Wisconsin Press, 1983. Carter KC, translator and editor.
2. Richardson RG. *Surgery: old and new frontiers.* New York: Scribner, 1968:75–81.

3. Perkins JJ. *Principles and methods of Sterilization in health sciences,* 2nd ed. Springfield, IL: Charles Thomas Publishers, 1969.
4. Kilmer FB. Modern surgical dressings. *Am J Pharm* 1897:69:24–39.
5. Bruch CW. *Inhospital versus industrial sterility assurance: is there a double standard? Inhospital sterility assurance-current perspectives.* Technology Assessment Report 4-82. Arlington, VA: AAMI, 1982:19–22.
6. Brown RM, ed. *Use and disposal of single use items in health care facilities.* Ann Arbor, MI: National Sanitation Foundation, 1968.
7. Mayhall CG. Types of disposable medical devices reused in hospitals. *Infect Control* 1986;7:491–494.
8. Sones M. *Position of the Society for Cardiac Angiography. Reuse of disposables.* Technology Assessment Report 6-83. Arlington, VA: AAMI, 1983:92.
9. Institute for Health Policy Analysis. *Reuse of disposable medical devices in the 1980s.* Washington, DC: Georgetown University Medical Center, 1984.
10. Villforth JC. Position of the US Food and Drug Administration. In: *Reuse of disposable medical devices in the 1980s.* Washington, DC: Georgetown University Medical Center, 1984:91–94.
11. Favero M. Position of the Centers for Disease Control. In: *Reuse of disposable medical devices in the 1980s.* Washington, DC: Georgetown University Medical Center, 1984:98–101.
12. Campbell BA, Wells GA, Palmer WN, et al. Reuse of disposable medical devices in Canadian hospitals. *Am J Infect Control* 1987;15: 196–200.
13. General Accounting Office (GAO). Single-use medical devices: little available evidence of harm from reuse but oversight warranted. Letter Report, 06/20/2000, GAO/HEHS-00-123. Available at *http://www.aami.org/reuse/.*
14. Food and Drug Administration. Survey on the reuse and reprocessing of single-use devices (SUDs) in US hospitals—executive summary. Updated 10/16/02. Available at *http://www.fda.gov/cdrh/Reuse/survey-execsum.html.*
15. Phillips GB. *Reuse of products labeled for single use only. Inhospital sterility assurance-current perspectives.* Technology Assessment Report 4-82. Arlington, VA: AAMI, 1982:52–54.
16. Beck WC, Geffert JP, Comella LH. Lessons learned from the Hospital Experience Reporting System. *Med Instrum* 1983;17: 343–346.
17. Bancroft M, Bushnell LS. *Hospital experience reporting system.* Final report, Food and Drug Administration Contract 223-80-5090, 26 Mar 1984. Silver Spring, MD: Center for Devices and Radiological Health.
18. Feigal DW. Statement before the Senate Committee on Health, Education, Labor and Pensions June 27, 2000. Available at *http://www.fda.gov/ola/2000/suds2.html.*
19. ECRI. *Reusing disposable products. Operating room risk management.* Plymouth Meeting, PA: ECRI, October, 1992.
20. Fishman RL. Reuse of a disposable stylet with life threatening complications. *Anesth Analg* 1991;72:266–267.
21. Butler L, Worthley LIG. Reuse of flow-directed balloon-tipped catheters. *BMJ* 1982;284:207. 22. Bryson TK, Saidman LJ, Nelson W. A potential hazard connected with the resterilization and reuse of disposable equipment. *Anesthesiology* 1979;50:370.
23. Sterilization and disinfection of hospital supplies. *MMWR Morb Mortal Wkly Rep* 1977;26:266.
24. Weinstein RA, Stamm WE, Kramer L, et al. Pressure monitoring devices-overlooked source of nosocomial infections. *JAMA* 1976;236: 936–938.
25. Donowitz LG, Marsik FJ, Hoyt JW, et al. *Serratia marcescens* bacteremia from contaminated pressure transducers. *JAMA* 1979;242: 1749–1751.
26. Crouch M, Jones A, Kleinbeck E, et al. Reuse of disposable syringe-needle units in the diabetic patient. *Diabetes Care* 1979;2:418–420.
27. Hodge RH, Krongaard L, Sande MA, et al. Multiple use of disposable insulin syringe-needle units. *JAMA* 1980;244:266–267.
28. Collins BJ, Richardson SG, Spence BK, et al. Safety of reusing disposable plastic insulin syringes. *Lancet* 1983;1:559–560.
29. Strathclyde Diabetic Group. Disposable or non-disposable syringes and needles for diabetics? *BMJ* 1983;286:369–370.
30. Stepanas TV, Turley H, Tuohy E. Reuse of disposable insulin syringes. *Med J Aust* 1982;1:311–313.
31. Phillips GB. *The reuse of single use medical devices: issues and impacts.* Washington, DC: Health Industry Manufacturers Association, 1984.
32. Gordon SM, Tipple M, Bland LA, et al. Pyrogen reactions associated with the reuse of disposable hollow-fibre hemodialyzers. *JAMA* 1988; 260:2077–2081.
33. Endotoxic reactions associated with the reuse of cardiac catheters—Massachusetts. *MMWR Morb Mortal Wkly Rep* 1979;28:25–27.
34. Kundsin RB, Walter CW. Detection of endotoxin on sterile catheters used for cardiac catheterization. *J Clin Microbiol* 1980;1:209–212.
35. Jacobson JA, Schwartz CE, Marshall HW, et al. Fever, chills, and hypotension following cardiac catheterization with single- and multiple-use disposable catheters. *Cathet Cardiovasc Diagn* 1982;9:39–46.
36. Jacob R, Bentolila P. The reuse of single-use catheters. Report submitted to the Ministre de la Sante et des Services sociaux du Quebec by the Conseil d'evaluation des technologies de la sante. Conseil d'evaluation: Montreal, Canada 1993.
37. Kozarek RA, Raltz SL, Merriam LD, et al. Disposable versus reusable biopsy forceps: a prospective evaluation of costs. *Gastrointest Endosc* 1996;43:10–13.
38. Kozarek RA, Raltz SL, Ball TJ, et al. Reuse of disposable sphincterotomes for diagnostic and therapeutic ERCP: a one-year prospective study. *Gastrointest Endosc* 1999;49:39–42.
39. Lee RM, Vido F, Kozarek RA, et al. In vitro and in vivo evaluation of a reusable double-channel sphincterotome. *Gastrointest Endosc* 1999; 49:477–482.
40. Zubaid M, Thomas CS, Salman H, et al. A randomized study of the safety and efficacy of reused angioplasty balloon catheters. *Indian Heart J* 2001;53:167–171.
41. Heeg P, Roth K, Reichl R, et al. Decontaminated single-use devices: an oxymoron that may be placing patients at risk for cross contamination. *Infect Control Hosp Epidemiol* 2001;22:542–549.
42. Chaufour X, Deva AK, Vickery K, et al. Evaluation of disinfection and sterilization of reusable angioscopes with the duck hepatitis B model. *J Vasc Surg* 1999;30:277–282.
43. Luijt DS, Schirm J, Savelkoul PH, et al. Risk of infection by reprocessed and resterilized virus-contaminated catheters; an in vitro study. *Eur Heart J* 2001;22:378–384.
44. Plante S, Strauss BH, Goulet G, et al. Reuse of balloon catheters for coronary angioplasty: a potential cost-saving strategy? *J Am Coll Cardiol* 1994;24:1475–481.
45. Mak KH et al. Absence of increased in-hospital complications with reused balloon catheters *Am J Cardiol* 1996;78:717–719.
46. AAMI resources on reuse of single-use devices. Updated 01-31-02. Available at *http://www.aami.org/reuse.*
47. Romeo AA. The economics of reuse. In: *Reuse of disposable medical devices in the 1980s.* Washington, DC: Georgetown University Medical Center, 1984:43–49.
48. Duffie ER. Concerns of the medical device industry. In: *Reuse of disposable medical devices in the 1980s.* Washington, DC: Georgetown University Medical Center, 1984:107–112.
49. Jarvis AE. *Reuse and product development, production, quality assurance, and cost. Reuse of disposables.* Technology Assessment Report 6-83. Arlington, VA: AAMI, 1983:62–64.
50. Salman SL. *Reuse and insurance coverage. Reuse of disposables.* Technology Assessment Report 6-83. Arlington, VA: AAMI, 1983:41–43.
51. Novak N. Legal concerns surrounding the reuse of disposable medical devices. In: *Reuse of disposable medical devices in the 1980s.* Washington, DC: Georgetown University Medical Center, 1984:56–72.
52. Beauchamp TL. *Moral problems in the reuse of disposable medical devices in the 1980s.* Washington, DC: Georgetown University Medical Center, 1984:50–55.
53. Reuse of single-use devices: Key Government documents. Available at *http://www.fda.gov/cdrh/reuse/index.html.*
54. Favero MS. Requiem for reuse of single-use devices in US hospitals. *Infect Control Hosp Epidemiol* 2001;22:539–541.

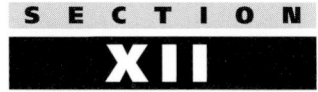

PREVENTION OF INFECTIONS ACQUIRED BY PATIENTS IN HEALTHCARE FACILITIES RELATED TO CONSTRUCTION, RENOVATION, DEMOLITION, AND VENTILATION SYSTEMS

88

PREVENTION OF INFECTIONS RELATED TO CONSTRUCTION, RENOVATION, AND DEMOLITION

JUDENE BARTLEY

PATIENT SAFETY, HEALING ENVIRONMENTS AND INFECTIOUS RISKS

Patient Safety Initiatives

The Institute of Medicine's (IOM) first report on patient safety in 1999 seized the nation's attention, focusing on the importance of the healthcare environment's effect on patient outcomes (1). The Agency for Healthcare Research and Quality (AHRQ) was charged with developing a plan to reduce adverse outcomes and improve the safety of workers and patients. This focus on medical safety continues to develop in healthcare organizations across the United States (2). Care delivery processes occur in physical structures intended to be healing environments, enhancing patient's health outcomes. Coincident with the emphasis on patient safety, accreditation agencies such as the Joint Commission on Accreditation of Healthcare Organizations (JCAHO) also encourages facilities to ensure that the environment of care (EOC) in facilities does not serve as a reservoir for pathogens. Implicit in this emphasis on the EOC is preventive maintenance for critical utility systems that deliver ventilation and water to patient care areas.

Microbial Hazards Associated with Construction and Renovation

The physical environment in a healthcare facility may pose risks to occupants (e.g., patients, personnel and visitors), if enhancements to the environment are carried out without a basic understanding of the potential for creating hazards and the associated morbidity and/or mortality. Physical hazards, infectious risks among them, may occur as the result of well-intentioned designs that may have unexpected consequences. For example, hospital epidemiologists need to balance proposals for a water feature such as a water wall, with potential risks of disease from water-borne opportunistic infectious agents such as *Legionella* species. A clearer picture of infectious hazards associated with care delivery environments has emerged over the past decades. Healthcare epidemiologists and other infection control professionals (ICPs) are increasingly recognizing that such risks may occur during construction, renovation, or preventive maintenance or from damage following natural or manmade disasters. New knowledge gained from disease outbreaks and successful interventions can be incorporated by architectural and engineering communities to improve designs, resulting in truly healing environments. It is essential that architects, engineers, healthcare epidemiologists, infectious disease specialists, infection control (IC) personnel, safety specialists, and others balance planning for construction and renovation with a thorough knowledge of infectious hazards, preventive techniques, and effective interventions to ensure the safest and most patient friendly environment. Rubin et al. (3) analyzed reports in the literature describing associations between the EOC and occurrence of infectious diseases. Of the reports in this review, almost all were observational and the few randomized controlled trials that were conducted had small sample sizes and lacked statistical power thereby precluding definitive conclusions. Therefore, most knowledge from studies of the role of the EOC on healthcare-associated infections (HAIs) is derived from investigation of clusters of disease. This evidence suggests that an overall cause-effect relationship does exist between healthcare environmental factors and therapeutic outcomes, but it is evident that there is a great need for more research. These experiences do provide information on mitigating risks and designing the EOC to prevent disease transmission.

Airborne Microorganisms

Most studies that have associated disease transmission with construction or renovation have involved improper ventilation design or maintenance that allowed exposure of highly immunocompromised populations such as bone marrow transplant patients to opportunistic pathogens (e.g., *Aspergillus* species). Airborne infectious agents (e.g., *Mycobacterium tuberculosis*) affect the health of patients and healthcare personnel (HCP). Insights gained from infectious diseases outbreak investigations have been used to mitigate risks of nosocomial exposure during construction or renovation. Interventions that were frequently associated with decreased infection rates or that terminated outbreaks have been steadily incorporated as standard design requirements by guideline-setting agencies (4,5). Selected examples of risk mitigation or prevention are summarized in this section to underscore the importance of specific design issues such as controlling dissemination of particulates and airborne pathogens during demolition and ensuring that the design of heating, ventilation, and air conditioning (HVAC) systems meet the needs for general and special patient care areas [e.g., operating rooms (ORs), interventional cardiology units, and airborne infection isolation rooms (AIIRs)]. Sources of airborne contaminants and infectious agents are closely related with water- and moisture-related conditions. Representative outbreaks are also discussed considering primarily the major mode of infectious agent transmission.

Construction and Airborne Sources

Air quality management during construction is key to preventing transmission of opportunistic microorganisms to susceptible patients, most notably highly immunosuppressed patients. Key publications of outbreaks related to *Aspergillus* species and related fungi received increased attention in the 1970s and are summarized elsewhere (6,7) (see Chapter 60). Transmission of airborne infectious agents may originate from patient reservoirs (Chapter 37), from laboratories and autopsy rooms (Chapters 82 and 84), and from dust and soil introduced into the facilities during construction (8,9). The relationship between facility HVAC and airborne nosocomial infections is discussed elsewhere in this text (Chapter 89). Numerous studies have confirmed the process by which construction activity brings outdoor contaminants into a building normally "protected" by multiple systems. Key findings from investigations describing airborne microbial contamination associated with construction between 1976 to 2002 are summarized in Table 88.1 (10–61).

Soil and dust become vehicles for particulates, which carry microorganisms, leading to infection and disease in specific populations. This process has been described in several excellent studies (23,24,62,63). Dust particles from excavation (aside from irritation from fumes and chemicals) become the vehicle for introducing opportunistic microorganisms into the air handling systems or HVAC (33,64).

External Demolition and Implosions. Excavation has been cited as the major problem with external demolition and implosions (65). Recent reports regarding the impact of large-scale demolition (e.g., implosion) have provided important new information about whole-building HVAC and air pressurization. Facility-associated cases of aspergillosis have been related to depressurization, drawing contaminants into a facility adjacent to another building that was imploded (54,66,67) (see Chapter 89). Intrusion of contaminants during nearby building implosions producing larger than normal burdens of dust and contaminants has been measured; proper planning can reduce the risk from this increased burden (68,69). Preemptive measures include cancelling elective surgery for patients at high risk, sealing windows and doors, additional filtering, and maintaining positive air pressure for special areas. A fire in a nearby building may also have resulted in transmission of *Aspergillus* species through open windows by imbedding spores in carpeting (36).

Indoor Environment. *Aspergillus* species and *Rhizopus* are among the most important fungi introduced during construction and are characterized by an ability to grow in an indoor environment under favorable temperature and moisture conditions (13,14,24). Other fungi that gain access through building penetrations include *Penicillium* species, *Cladosporium* species, and similar airborne contaminants (33,63,70).

Air Handlers. Many publications have addressed the importance of appropriate air handling during construction to reduce the risk of transmission of airborne pathogens such as *Aspergillus* species to susceptible patients. Appropriate air handling includes zonal use of high-efficiency particulate air (HEPA) filters, provision of negative air pressure (39,45,71,72), dedicated exhaust, and physical isolation of the construction area from patient care areas (24,32,40). Numerous patient outbreaks of bacterial and fungal infections associated with aerosols from contaminated ventilation ducts, grills, damaged barriers (e.g., bird screens, ventilation fans), and vacuum cleaners reinforce the importance of maintaining an intact air handling system (11,43,50).

Room Design and Location. Room design must consider location of supply air and exhaust vents, critical determinants in transmitting airborne contaminants (33,41). Negative air pressure in pediatric oncology units, for example, was shown to reduce the spread of varicella-zoster virus (VZV) among workers and patients (16). Lower bloodstream infection and mortality rates were reported for burn patients in enclosed intensive care unit (ICU) beds than for patients in open wards (73). Multiple outbreaks related to *M. tuberculosis* were terminated with properly designed and improved maintenance of negative air pressure (isolation) rooms (74).

The Surgical Suite Environment. The OR environment has been studied extensively in an attempt to reduce infectious risks in patients undergoing orthopedic joint replacement. The literature on reductions in surgical site infection (SSI) rates, primarily found in total joint arthroplasty, is reviewed elsewhere (75–77). The focus for this chapter relates to contamination of the OR during construction and renovation from airborne fungi and other pathogens (27,28,31,78–85). A summary of the general issues and interventions to mitigate these problems have been reported elsewhere (8,9,28,82,86) (see Chapter 89). Multiple interventions in ORs have led to steady reductions in infectious outcomes for surgical patients. As a result, current standards include increased outside air and total air exchanges per hour, improved air filtration efficiency, proper humidification, and filter location in air handlers serving ORs (15,31,42). Major studies by Lidwell (87,88) focused on the use of ultraclean (laminar airflow) HEPA-filtered air in clean orthopedic surgical procedures. These studies, together with other multisite studies (80, 89), led to a better understanding of the independent contribution of ultraclean air in reducing clean SSIs; its effect is comparable to the use of preoperative prophylactic antibiotics. Accordingly, laminar airflow HEPA filtration may be considered for specific high-risk populations to reduce SSIs. However, definitive evidence on efficacy of elaborate laminar airflow in prevention of SSIs is lacking.

Water-Borne Microorganisms

Contaminated water can be a source of water-borne pathogens. Those at greatest risk are immunocompromised patients,

TABLE 88.1. AIRBORNE MICROBIAL CONTAMINATION ASSOCIATED WITH CONSTRUCTION—SELECTED STUDIES BY YEAR AND MICROORGANISM

Year	Author	Microorganism	Population/location	Epidemiologic factors	Remedial measures or preventive measures
1976	Aisner, et al. (10)	*Aspergillus flavus, Aspergillus fumigatus, Aspergillus niger, Aspergillus* species	Hematology, solid tumor	False ceilings; moisture fireproofing materials	Solid, sealed ceiling
1976	Kyriakides, et al. (11)	*A. fumigatus*	Renal transplant	Ventilation contaminated with bird droppings	Replaced bird screen; repair malfunctioning exhaust fan
1978	Arnow, et al. (12)	*A. fumigatus*	Hematology	Building materials, wet	Replace water damaged materials
1982	Lentino, et al. (13)	*A. flavus, A. fumigatus, A. niger, Aspergillus* species	Hematology, renal transplant	Contaminated window AC units; road construction	Removal of window AC units (suggested)
1982	Sarubbi, et al. (14)	*A. flavus*	Medical-surgical	Construction dust; improperly functioning air handler	Repair of defective air handler
1984	deSilva and Rissing (15)	Bacteria, multiple	Cardiac surgery	Ineffective operating room air handler; unacceptable SSI	Changes to air handler to increase AC/H; improved filter efficiency, constant temp/RH, increased positive pressure
1985	Anderson, et al. (16)	Varicella zoster	Pediatrics	Isolation rooms without negative pressure	Negative pressure, no anterooms; no cases of nosocomial transmission
1985	Krasinski, et al. (17)	*Penicillium, Zygomycetes, Aspergillus* species	Newborn	Improperly functioning air handler	Barriers/negative pressure in construction area
1986	Opal, et al. (18)	*A. flavus, A. fumigatus, A. niger, Aspergillus* species	Hematology, medical ICU	Construction/renovation activity; ineffective barriers and air handler	Physical sealed barriers; portable HEPA filter machines; Air handler treated with copper 8 quinolinolate
1987	Allo, et al. (19)	*A. flavus*	Hematology, operating room (OR)	Contaminated OR ventilation system	Cleaned ventilation system
1987	Ruutu, et al. (20)	*A. fumigatus*	Hematology, bone marrow transplant (BMT)	Contaminated OR ventilation system	Cleaned ventilation system including ducts; filters changed, HEPA filter framing sealed
1987	Perraud, et al. (21)	*A. fumigatus*	Hematology	False ceilings; acoustic insulation	Barriers; evacuate high-risk patients during renovation
1987	Sherertz, et al. (22)	*A. flavus, A. fumigatus*	BMT	Efficiency of laminar air flow; HEPA filtration	Horizontal LAF HEPA filtration improved outcome
1987	Streifel, et al. (23)	*Penicillium* species	BMT	Moisture; rotted wood cabinets released spores into room air	Replace with nonporous surfaces around sink
1987	Weems, et al. (24)	*Aspergillus* species, *Rhizopus, Mucorales* species	Hematology, renal transplant, BMT	Construction/demolition activity; excessive dust; improperly functioning air handler; open windows	Construction plans: HVAC; permanently sealed barriers against infiltration from windows
1989	Barnes and Rogers (25)	*A. fumigatus*	BMT	Construction	Laminar air flow units
1989	Hopkins, et al. (26)	*A. fumigatus*	Renal transplant, hematology	Construction in centrally located radiology suite	Preventive measures in areas where patients are treated outside of room
1990	Mehta (27)	*A. fumigatus, Aspergillus* species	Open heart surgery, OR	Ineffective air handler; proximity of contamination to air intake; lack of preventive maintenance	Pigeons' nest adjacent to air intake removed; change of prefilters; use of HEPA filtration
1990	Fox, et al. (28)	*Penicillium* species, *Cladosporium* species, *Aspergillus* species	OR	Ventilation duct lined with contaminated fiberglass insulation	Decontamination of air handler ductwork; filter replacement
1990	Jackson, et al. (29)	*Sporothrix cyanescens*	Bronchoscopy suite	Renovation of suite; pseudoepidemics from dust	Appropriate barriers and negative pressure
1991	Arnow (30)	*A. flavus, A. fumigatus*	Hematology	Improperly sealed air filters	Filters removed and cleaned; addressed water damage
1991	Everett and Kipp (31)	Bacteria, multiple	Surgical patient	Inefficient OR ventilation system	Changes in number of OR air changes; temperature
1991	Humphreys, et al. (32)	*A. fumigatus, Aspergillus* species	ICU	Perforated ceiling; fibrous insulation	Solid ceiling; proper insulation
1992	Abzug, et al. (33)	*Mucorales, Zygomycetes*	Pediatric, leukemia	Air intakes proximity to heliport	Modifications to helipad design and HEPA filters
1992	Hruszkewycz, et al. (34)	*Penicillium* species, *Aspergillus* species	Laboratory pseudooutbreak	Improper airflow during renovation near lab; false ceiling in work area	Sealed ceilings; proper use of lab hoods; appropriate air flow controls
1993	Flynn, et al. (35)	*A. terreus*	ICU, BMT, hematology	Renovation adjacent to ICU affecting ventilation duct; false ceiling removal	Adjusted pressure relationships between ICU and renovation area, including stairwell, elevators
1994	Gerson, et al. (36)	*A. flavus, A. fumigatus*	BMT, leukemia	Open window; fire contaminated carpet	Modifications of carpet cleaning/extraction procedures

(continued)

TABLE 88.1. *(continued)*

Year	Author	Microorganism	Population/location	Epidemiologic factors	Remedial measures or preventive measures
1994	Iwen, et al. (37)	*Aspergillus* species, Mixed fungi	BMT unit, hematology	Improper air flow; suspected infiltration from windows	Sealed windows and balanced air flow; replaced HEPA filters
1995	Stroud, et al. (38)	Multidrug resistant *M. tuberculosis*	AIDS patients	Improper air changes and pressure relationships for isolation rooms	Adjusted ventilation according to CDC guideline for prevention of transmission of MTB
1995	Alvarez, et al. (39)	*Scedosporium prolificans*	Hematology unit	Internal renovation; ventilation system	Moved patients to another floor level
1996	Bryce, et al. (40)	*A. fumigatus, A. niger, A. terreus*	Med surg ICU, burn unit patients	Renovation in central supply area, contaminated supplies used in ICU, burn patients	Sealed off construction area with temporary vents; cleaning of supplies (external surfaces)
1996	Cotterill, et al. (41)	Methicillin-resistant *Stapylococcus aureus*	ICU	Open window; improper air intake/exhaust	Windows closed; redesigned bed placement
1996	Fridkin, et al. (42)	*Acremonium kiliense*	Ambulatory surgery	Poorly designed air handler; contaminated humidifier	Redesign; changed HEPA filters; proper maintenance of pressure relationships
1996	Anderson, et al. (43)	*A. flavus, A. fumigatus, A. niger*	BMT, pediatric oncology unit	Improper air flow from clinical waste disposal area; contaminated vacuum	Sealing of disposal room and ducts; use of HEPA-filter vacuum cleaners
1996	Leenders, et al. (44)	*A. flavus, A. fumigatus*	Hematology	Environmental source not identified	Windows closed; new air handler
1996	Loo, et al. (45)	*A. flavus, A. fumigatus, A. niger*	BMT, hematology unit	Construction; demolition; perforated ceiling tiles	Solid ceiling; HEPA machines; use of Copper 8 quinolinolate
1996	Philpot-Howard (46)	*Aspergillus* species and other filamentous fungi	Hematology patients	Construction; ventilation parameters	Preventive maintenance of air supply; use of barrier
1996	Pittet, et al. (47)	*Aspergillus* species	COPD	Insufficient air filter replacement	Monitor filter function; replaced filters
1997	Dearborn, et al. (48)	*Stachybotrys atra*	Infants	Water damage; suspect release of airborne toxin (residences)	Decontamination with diluted bleach
1998	Tabbara, et al. (49)	*A. fumigatus*	Cataract, OR ocular surgery	Hospital construction	Proper maintenance of physical structure
1998	Kumari, et al. (50)	Methicillin-resistant *S. aureus*	Orthopedic patients	Ventilation grills	Air handler cleaned; maintained proper pressure relationships
1999	Cornet, et al. (51)	*Aspergillus* species	Hematology	Renovation and dust production	Use of portable HEPA filters versus LAFR HEPA
1999	Garrett, et al. (52)	*Aspergillus* species	Rheumatology patients	Construction not sealed off; improper pressure relationships and air changes	Adjusted ventilation according to CDC guidelines (TB)
1999	Laurel, et al. (53)	*A. niger*	Laboratory pseudooutbreak	Construction; installation of ventilation duct adjacent to biological safety cabinet (BSC)	Cleaning, pre-filter; HEPA filter changes; construction protocols for laboratory
2000	Thio, et al. (54)	*A. flavus*	BMT, hematology	Pressure relationship of units to whole hospital; negative pressure	HEPA; readjust pressure relationships to ensure hospital as a whole slightly positive
2001	Burwen, et al. (55)	*A. flavus*	Hematology-oncology	Distance from renovation; construction activity	Screen and use HEPA filtered air; applicable CDC guidelines
2001	Lai (56)	*A. niger, Aspergillus* species	BMT, patient wards	Construction adjacent to BMT unit	BMT site tightly sealed; high-risk patients to avoid site during construction
2001	Oren, et al. (57)	*A. flavus, Aspergillus* species	Leukemia, BMT patients	Construction; natural ventilation	Ward with air filtration using HEPA filters
2001	Pegues, et al. (58)	*Aspergillus* species	Heart-lung transplant	Renovation; dust production	Removal of carpeting; replacement of ceiling tiles
2002	Hahn, et al. (59)	*A. flavus, A. niger*	Hematology-oncology	Contaminated insulation in affected unit and nurses station	Installation of HEPA filters
2002	Kistemann, et al. (60)	*Aspergillus* species	COPD and corticosteroids	Reconstruction; pigeon droppings; water damage from leakage	Clean up of area; maintenance/precautions to reduce exposure of high-risk patients to the environment
2002	Raad, et al. (61)	*A. fumigatus, A. flavus A. terreus, Aspergillus* species	Hematology	Construction dust outside of protected BMT area	High-risk patients wear high efficiency masks during transport outside room during construction

AC, air conditioning; AC/H, ; AIDS, acquired immunodeficiency syndrome; CDC, Centers for Disease Control and Prevention; COPD, chronic obstructure pulmonary disease; HEPA, high-efficiency particulate air; HVAC, heating, ventilation, and air conditioning; ICU, intensive care unit; SSI, surgical site infection; TB, tuberculosis.

and many outbreak investigations have identified potable water systems and storage tanks, shower heads, and ice machines as sources of water-borne pathogens (90–93). Table 88.2 summarizes findings from investigations of clusters of infection caused by water-borne pathogens (92,94–111). *Legionella* species, for example, have been implicated in patient infections acquired through inhalation of aerosols spread from contaminated storage tanks, shower heads, and equipment that used tap water, such as water baths, and/or entire water systems (103,112–116). A review of nosocomial water-borne infections excluding those caused by *Legionella* species revealed 43 outbreaks with associated deaths of almost 1,400 per year and called for provision of sterile rather than potable water for high-risk patients during hospitalization (117). Maintenance of drinking water quality depends on good design and preventive maintenance and surveillance for nosocomial infections that includes a high index of suspicion for infectious agents associated with moisture and water distribution systems. One study assessed the risk of bacterial pathogens in drinking water in an attempt to determine if dose-response relationships could be developed, and whether or not potable water poses a public health hazard (118). The results included a ranking of water-associated microorganisms from

TABLE 88.2. WATER-ASSOCIATED CONTAMINATION ASSOCIATED WITH CONSTRUCTION—SELECTED STUDIES BY YEAR AND MICROORGANISM

Year	Author	Microorganism	Population/location	Epidemiologic factors	Remedial measures or preventive measures
1981	Cordes, et al. (94)	*Legionella pneumophila* serogroup 6	Hospital patient rooms	Contaminated water supply; shower heads	Decontamination of shower heads
1981	Crane, et al. (92)	*P. paucimobilis*	Intensive care unit (ICU)	Contaminated tap water	Thermal decontamination of water system; revised procedures for use of tap water for equipment
1986	Panwalker and Funse (95)	*Mycobacterium gordonae*	Hospital	Contaminated ice machines	Disinfection; preventive maintenance
1991	Burns, et al. (96)	*Mycobacterium fortuitum*	Alcoholism rehabilitation unit	Ward showers; tap supply	Disconnected and disinfected showers
1993	Hlady, et al. (97)	*Legionella pneumophila* serogroup 1	Hotel	Decorative water fountain	Proper heat and maintenance
1993	Sniadeck, et al. (98)	*Mycobacterium xenopi*	Hospital rooms	Water supply (pseudooutbreak)	Maintain temperature greater than 120°F (49°C; preferably 54°C)
1994	Prodinger, et al. (99)	*Legionella pneumophila* serogroup 1	Renal allograft	Water distribution system	Replaced central water supply with individual electric water heaters in each room
1995	Bangsborg, et al. (100)	*Legionella pneumophila* serogroups 1 and 6	Heart-lung transplant	ICU kitchen ice machine	Disinfection of machine; preventive maintenance
1997	Graman, et al. (101)	*Legionella pneumophila* serogroup 6	Ventilator patients	Ice machine	Replace supply line and treatment of water system
1997	Patterson, et al. (102)	*Legionella pneumophila, Legionella bozemanii, Legionella gormanii*	General hospital	Water storage and distribution systems	Maintain hot water above 58°C
1998	Kool, et al. (103)	*Legionella pneumophila, Legionella* species	Transplant center	Water system	Hyperchlorination
1999	Biurrun, et al. (104)	*Legionella pneumophila* serogroup 6	General hospital	Water distribution system	Copper-silver ionization and continuous chlorination system
1999	Weber, et al. (105)	*Stentotrophomonas maltophilia*	Surgical ICU	Potable water aerators	Removal or routine disinfection
2000	Kappstein, et al. (106)	*Acinetobacter junii*	Pediatric oncology	Contaminated aerators	Remove, use aerators with radially/vertically arranged lamellae (not mesh)
2000	Knirsch, et al. (107)	*Legionella micdadei*	Solid organ transplant	Hot water sources	Treat hot water supply
2000	Stout, et al. (108)	*Legionella pneumophila* serogroup 1	LTC residents	Water distribution system	Install copper-silver ionization system
2000	Borau, et al. (109)	*Legionella pneumophila* serogroup 6	ICU patients	Hot water system	Elevate hot water temperature
2002	Grove, et al. (110)	*Legionella longbeachae*	ICU patients	Cooling tower; pigeon's nest 1–2 cm from vent; demolition	Removal of nest; PM cooling towers
2002	Darelid, et al. (111)	*Legionella pneumophila* serogroup 1	General hospital	Water distribution system	Maintain water temperature 55°C

studies reported primarily from medical centers. Although the purpose of the study was not directly related to construction, the review does confirm the expected frequency of opportunistic microorganisms causing serious infections associated with water. These opportunistic microorganisms are of concern because of their potential for direct or indirect transmission from taps and sinks or through inhalation of aerosols generated from construction activities. Even contaminated condensation from window air conditioning units when combined with other work practices can lead to invasive infections such as *Acinetobacter* species bloodstream infections in high-risk pediatric populations (119).

Moisture and Fungi

Excessive moisture around pipes and insulation, condensation in drain pans, and flooding from broken pipes can lead to extensive environmental fungal contamination. Such contamination has been associated, for example, with water-soaked cabinets in medication rooms (23,62). Static water systems can provide a reservoir of microorganisms in the healthcare environment by supporting their growth. Nonsterile water used for invasive patient-related procedures can result in direct or indirect transmission of microorganisms to patients (92,98,120). A recent report of fungal endophthalmitis from *Acremonium kiliense* following cataract surgery in an ambulatory surgery setting demonstrated the process by which contaminated humidifier water functioned as a reservoir for an infectious agent eventually spreading through the airborne route by way of the ventilation system (42). Typically nosocomial transmission of fungi is airborne; however, there is emerging evidence that potable water in health facilities may also be a significant reservoir, suggesting that prompt disinfection of high water-use areas such as showers is an important measure to prevent exposure to fungal pathogens (121).

Legionella Species

Annually there are estimates of between 8,000 to 18,000 hospitalizations for legionellosis (122). However, reported hospital outbreaks predominate in the literature because of the fatal effects on susceptible patient populations; they have helped characterize *Legionella* and identify key risk factors from affected individuals (123–126). Although each reported outbreak of legionellosis improved the epidemiologic profile of this pathogen, endemic, sporadic cases (representing most of the observed cases) still evade full understanding. The mode of transmission implicates not only cooling towers, potable water reservoirs, and distribution systems (124,125,127,128) but also water-related equipment (e.g., medication nebulizers) (129) and potable water used for nasogastric feeding (93).

Legionella species from nearby environmental water sources enter hospital water systems, multiply in cooling towers and evaporative condensers, and/or contaminate the potable water system. Because infection develops after inhaling airborne water droplets containing *Legionella* species, any opportunity for contaminated water to aerosolize is of concern during construction and renovation. Major construction has been associated with numerous nosocomial outbreaks or clusters (112). Potential mechanisms include release of this microorganism from vibration or significant changes in water pressure. These disturbances loosen corrosion and disturb biofilms thereby releasing *Legionella* species in water system pipes. Excavation permits the microorganism to be released from the soil; the microorganisms eventually enter cooling towers, air intakes, or water systems, leading to direct inhalation from water sources (130). Summaries of outbreaks have been described in the Centers for Disease Control and Prevention (CDC) guidelines and other government and private recommendations for detection and treatment (130–135).

CHANGES IN HEALTHCARE DELIVERY AND IMPACT ON CONSTRUCTION TRENDS

Construction Costs

Annual construction and design surveys in the United States indicate a continued major expenditure on healthcare construction and renovation. Changes in patient acuity, aging, and reduced capitol funds have affected construction expenditures in a number of ways. Recent trends show dollars are spent primarily on inpatient specialty beds (e.g., cardiac and cancer) along with increasing demands for assisted-living and skilled nursing centers. Construction for hospitals, nursing homes, and outpatient facilities in 2001 totaled 3,362 projects, at a cost of $15.7 billion (136). However, 76% of the projects involved either expansion or renovation at a cost of $8.7 billion—more than half of total construction expenditures. The increasing age of U.S. healthcare facilities generates a constant need for repair and remediation work (cabling, room additions). These processes increase risks of environmental contamination, affecting air and water quality. Natural disasters (e.g., flooding) add additional opportunities for contaminating healthcare delivery sites. New concerns for protecting buildings from airborne contaminants from intentional release of biologic agents or unintended manmade disasters have focused additional attention to the building envelope, ventilation management, and the isolation room capacity (137, 138).

Costs of Healthcare-Associated Disease

Outbreak investigations documenting health outcomes resulting from contamination are associated with multiple healthcare settings but focus primarily on hospitals. Although the actual percentage of HAIs directly related to construction is unknown, one can consider costs in terms of one significant airborne infectious agent, *Aspergillus* species. *Aspergillus* can be either community-acquired or nosocomial, but it is difficult to always distinguish between them. The total cost impact is enormous. For example, in considering aspergillosis alone for 1 year (1996), costs were estimated at $633.1 million. Although the number of aspergillosis-related hospitalizations are a small percentage of the total hospitalizations (10,190 hospitalizations; 1, 970 deaths), the average length of stay (LOS) attributable to treating this disease is 17.3 days, costing an average $62,426 [95% confidence interval (CI) $52,670 to $72,181] based on 176,272 hospital days (95% CI 147,163 to 206,275 days) (139).

The case fatality rate for aspergillosis averages 58%, but for bone marrow transplant recipients it reaches 86.7% (140) (see Chapter 60). A better assessment of risks and their mitigation can enable architects to design and plan for patient-friendly and safer facilities.

DESIGNING FOR DISEASE PREVENTION AND HEALTH PROMOTION

Healthcare Study Design

This section focuses on design and construction of healthcare environments that plan to reduce risks of adverse outcomes learned from past experience and that emphasize infection prevention and control during new construction and renovation (external and internal). Suggestions and recommendations to prevent and control infectious risks are based on published investigations occurring most frequently in hospitals; these recommendations may need tailoring for other healthcare delivery sites. Design professionals are increasingly interested in identifying individual variables that affect patient outcomes and worker productivity, forming a growing science around the relationship between the built environment and quality of care (141). The *built* or physical environment is defined as any aspect of the environment that is constructed by design experts such as architects or designers. More attention is being given to designing facilities that are cost-effective, efficient, and functional for staff while cultivating a caring, healing environment for patients.

Collaborative efforts between the Picker Institute and the Center for Health Design resulted in initiatives to analyze and improve patient outcomes (142,143). Focus groups identified properties that were important for healing and well-being of patients in acute, ambulatory, or long-term care settings. Participants identified the need for an environment that enables a connection to staff, is conducive to well-being, is convenient and accessible, allows confidentiality and privacy, cares for the family, is considerate of impairments, provides connection to the outside world, and provides safety and security. It is noteworthy that participants identified physical conditions *only* in terms of comfort (temperature, lighting, and cleanliness) but not in terms of illnesses (e.g., *M. tuberculosis* associated with ventilation structures). Although numerous studies have reinforced the importance of a safe physical environment, patient perceptions have a powerful—but not always measurable—impact on patient outcomes (142,143).

Current and Future Design and Materials

Because of the paucity of scientific evidence, ICPs must rely on fundamental principles such as the epidemiology of infectious diseases to determine what interventions are most likely to be effective in preventing infection. Evidence from prevention of HAIs through use of antimicrobial-impregnated medical devices is leading to incorporation of antimicrobial surface or polymer treatments to minimize environmental reservoirs of potential pathogens (144,145). Other architectural and utility system features under study include ventilation systems that provide 100% exhaust, design of microbial-resistant building materials (e.g., glass mat faced gypsum board), use of ultraviolet germicidal irradiation to prevent biofouling of air handling units, and design features that minimize buildup of biofilms in potable water systems (146). Of the published studies with better research designs there were findings that environmental features can correlate with health outcomes; therefore, improvement in outcomes may be possible through design interventions that are guided by sound scientific inquiry. However, studies that contain data about the effect of the environment are surprisingly scarce. The need for broadened research is striking; many factors have never been investigated. Many studies have significant flaws that render conclusions suspect or cast doubt on the ability to generalize the findings to other populations. Future research should be more carefully designed to ensure that groups of patients being compared under various conditions do not differ in other ways, thus preventing skewed results. Current efforts include designing the safest possible hospitals in the broadest sense of safety (147–149) and considering IC issues in design (145, 150).

A number of engineering studies directed at determining ideal ventilation for patient rooms (151) or AAIRs (152) have provided a foundation for design recommendations (153). Additional studies of areas needing special ventilation such as the OR suite have and will continue to drive changes in specific parameters for consensus guidelines. Interestingly, a computer modeling study of efficacy of OR HVAC design found that increasing the number of air changes per hour was not as important as air velocity, and unidirectional airflow at the surgical site was more important than location (high or low) of exhaust ducts (154).

Floor covering materials such as carpeting have been studied extensively, and, although it is colonized with a variety of pathogens (e.g., *Clostridium difficile*), no direct link to patient infections has been found (36,155,156). Accordingly, carpet in patient care areas should be chosen with respect to aesthetics and cleanability and not because of risk to patients. Current interest in surfaces and treatment or incorporation of antimicrobial products into the surface matrix to inhibit microbial growth are available commercially. However, most efficacy studies involve *in vitro* investigations; more research is needed to determine if such measures can prevent HAIs (157).

REGULATORY AND ACCREDITATION AGENCIES' GUIDELINES AND STANDARDS THAT IMPACT CONSTRUCTION

Agencies with Impact on Design and Physical Environment

Standards and guidelines issued or enforced by the following agencies have had major impact on the physical structure of healthcare settings. There are many agencies and professional associations that have a direct impact or provide resources to plan, design, and better construct facilities; some of note include the following:

1. American Institute of Architects/Academy of Architecture for Health and the Facilities Guideline Institute (AIA/AAH/

FGI): "2001 Guidelines for Design and Construction of Hospitals and Healthcare Facilities"—minimum standards for most states (4)
2. Centers for Medicare and Medicaid Services (CMS), formerly Health Care Finance Administration (HCFA): "Hospital Conditions of Participation (COP)"—for Medicare and Medicaid (158)
3. JCAHO: "Comprehensive Accreditation Manual for Hospitals: The Official Handbook" (159)
4. CDC/Healthcare Infection Control Practices Advisory Committee (HICPAC): "Guidelines for Environmental Infection Control for Healthcare Facilities" (160) and numerous other guidelines (5,161–164)
5. Other agencies
   - Occupational Safety and Health Administration (OSHA): tuberculosis, construction, bloodborne pathogens, and legionellosis (133,165,166)
   - National Institute of Occupational Safety and Health (NIOSH): HVAC, sharps containers, and air sampling (167–169)
   - State and local standards (170)
6. Professional organizations with resources and/or standards
   - Association for Professionals in Infection Control and Epidemiology (APIC): state-of-the-art report (SOAR); infection control risk assessment (ICRA) (8,9,171)
   - American Society of Healthcare Engineering (ASHE): contractor certificate program including ICRA; monographs
   - American Society of Heating, Refrigerating and Air-conditioning (ASHRAE): basic design research; design handbooks

Relationship between AIA/FGI Guidelines and Regulations

Changes related to facility design aimed at reducing infectious risks are evident in many of the revised standards. For example, the 2001 AIA/FGI guidelines (minimum standards) added explicit requirements for design consideration termed an ICRA. CMS requirements are consistent with the AIA/FGI guidelines, although CMS uses additional physical plant standards to enforce the COP and the Life Safety Code (LSC), currently the 2000 LSC. In addition to CMS, more than 40 states adopted the AIA/FGI guidelines as minimum design standards or adapted them with state-specific regulations governing physical plant and safety issues, transforming guidelines to regulatory status. Facilities accredited by JCAHO must consider the EOC standards that became effective January 1, 2001, because these impact utility management standards for all facilities. In 2002, JCAHO added specific standards for design and construction that reflect the 2001 AIA/FGI guidelines requirement for a risk assessment that state, "When planning demolition, construction, or renovation work, the hospital conducts a proactive risk assessment using risk criteria to identify hazards that may potentially compromise patient care in occupied areas of the hospital's buildings. The scope and nature of the activities should determine the extent of risk assessment required. The risk criteria should address the impact demolition, renovation, or new construction activities have on air quality requirements, IC, utility requirements, noise, vibration, and emergency procedures. As required, the hospital selects and implements proper controls to reduce risk and minimize impact of these activities" (159). The CDC guideline for environmental IC supports many key guidelines and recommendations and provides strength-ranked recommendations based on peer-reviewed scientific evidence (160).

AIA/FGI: Key Design Agency

The AIA/FGI with assistance from the U.S. Department of Health and Human Services publishes minimum guidelines that have been wholly adopted by most states and the Indian Health Service; the remaining states accept them with some modifications. Chapters address outpatient care sites, nursing homes, hospice, assisted living, and rehabilitation settings in addition to the basic hospital guidelines. Although the 1996 to 1997 *Guidelines for Design and Construction of Hospitals and Health Care Facilities* required an ICRA, the impact was narrowly confined to determining numbers of AIIRs (172). The AIA/FGI 2001 guidelines expanded ICRA based on the facility's patient or resident population and programs (4).

INFECTION CONTROL RISK ASSESSMENT—DESIGN AND CONSTRUCTION ASPECTS

Concept—The Infection Control Risk Assessment

Infection Control Risk Assessment—Construction Projects

The AIA/FGI guidelines recognize that renovation and new construction in existing facilities can create conditions that may be hazardous to occupants. The 1996 to 1997 edition of the guidelines required construction and major renovation assessments during project planning related to specific risks. The current 2001 guidelines lend stronger weight to IC input at the *initial stages* of planning and design of a project by requiring documentation of an ICRA (4). The ICRA is considered a process requiring documentation of *continued involvement* of IC throughout specific projects. ICRA is a determination of the potential risk of transmission of various agents, particularly biologic, in the facility but expands far beyond determining optimal numbers of isolation rooms or location of hand washing stations. Instead, ICRA supports design of the EOC toward systems that prevent transmission of infection and ensures a safe environment for patients, personnel, and visitors. For example, an important component of ICRA is determining locations and installation of dedicated exhaust when cleaning and disinfection of medical equipment is anticipated. Furthermore, preliminary evidence suggests that ICUs with a central nursing station surrounded by private rooms permits easy visualization and response to rapid changes in patient status (150). Such architectural arrangements, although not directly related to preventing disease transmission, enhance spatial separation of patients and facilitate communication thereby improving safety for patients and personnel.

The 2001 guidelines state that "the ICRA shall be conducted by a panel with expertise in IC, risk management, facility design, construction, ventilation, safety, and epidemiology. The panel *shall provide documentation* of the risk assessment during planning, design, and construction. The ICRA shall only address building areas anticipated to be affected by construction. The design professional shall incorporate the specific, construction-related requirements of the ICRA in the contract documents. The contract documents shall require the constructor to implement these specific requirements during construction" (4). The specific elements to be addressed include the following:

1. Impact of disruption on patients and employees
2. Patient placement or relocation
3. Placement of effective barriers to protect susceptible patients from airborne contaminants such as *Aspergillus* species
4. Air handling needs in surgical services, airborne infection isolation and protective environment (PE) rooms, laboratories, local exhaust systems for hazardous agents, and other special areas
5. Determination of additional numbers of airborne infection isolation or PE rooms
6. Consideration of the domestic water system to limit *Legionella* species and other water-borne opportunistic pathogens

ICRA and Long-Range Planning and Design

Although the ICRA as described by the guidelines is basic, it is equally important to step back and consider the long-range planning that goes into the overall master facility plan and the critical need for early and continuous input from IC. Although the language of the ICRA clearly calls for input during planning, it is applied most frequently to specific projects. APIC published a strategy in 2000 for assessing healthcare facilities for infectious risks during construction in the APIC SOAR on construction and renovation and recommended an ICRA similar to that later required by AIA/FGI guidelines and in the draft CDC environmental IC guidelines. However, the tactics begin with developing a *construction and renovation policy (CRP), a multidisciplinary team, and a process to implement the policy* (9).

Once a system is in place providing for oversight, the application of the guidelines fit into each specific project. The guidelines require documentation of an ICRA for each *specific* project; they are not retrospective and apply only to new construction or major renovation. However, the approaches may be applied to smaller repair or preventive maintenance projects as appropriate. Thus, development of a broad-based CRP is an efficient and effective method to address basic principles that affect all projects, using the CRP as reference point for the facility. Recommended resources for a CRP include the AIA/FGI guidelines, the CDC environmental IC guidelines, the APIC SOAR, and Canadian guidelines for *Aspergillus* and *Legionella.*

Infection Control Risk Assessment—Overview for Planning and Design

Teams

Multidisciplinary planning committees vary according to the size, although all resources agree that an assessment panel must include professionals with expertise in IC, risk management, facility design, construction, ventilation, safety, and epidemiology. The panel is most effective if it includes an administrator and major stakeholders such as environmental services and the patient care manager most affected by the construction or renovation. If a CRP is developed and approved, it becomes the basis of the ICRA for major or minor processes. A key first step is identification of a multidisciplinary planning group involving design professionals, engineers, risk and safety, IC and epidemiology, the IC committee (or committee charged with development and review of the IC policy), and administrators representing special program needs.

Construction and Renovation Policy

A comprehensive CRP requiring IC input is the fundamental strategy that ensures timely notification of the ICP (or person with IC responsibilities) for early program planning. Once established, the ICP should be made aware of planned projects as a matter of routine. This in turn ensures that an IC evaluation of the project will be provided from concept to completion as now required by the ICRA. The evaluation should include design of the EOC, construction preparation and demolition, intraconstruction operations and maintenance, project completion with postconstruction cleanup, and monitoring. The ICRA documentation process fits future projects from small to complex (8, 171).

Construction and Renovation Policy Elements

The policy should address overall planning, designing, and monitoring processes, anticipating that future projects will vary in degree of complexity. It should ensure that input is required in all phases (i.e., structural design and specific practices to protect occupants during the preconstruction, intraconstruction, and postconstruction phases).

Basic issues include the authority and responsibility for establishing internal and subcontractor coordination of each stage of the project. The policy should be submitted for approval by the facility's board of trustees and reviewed and approved periodically (e.g., annually). Specific elements that should be included in the policy include the authority and responsibility for establishing internal and subcontractor coordination of (a) construction preparation and demolition, (b) intraconstruction operations and maintenance, (c) project completion and postconstruction cleanup, and (d) monitoring.

A comprehensive policy is the basis of *individual project* ICRAs. The CRP should also anticipate remediation responses in the event of major disruptions. Elements include the following:

- Authority and communication lines to determine if or how patient unit closure will occur
- Planning for air handling and water systems and plumbing as appropriate
- Expectations for contractor accountability in the event of breaches in IC practices and related written agreements
- Patient area risk assessment—location or admission criteria

- Criteria for emergency work interruptions (stop and start processes)
- Education: for whom and by whom
- Occupational health expectations for subcontractors before start, as needed
- Traffic patterns for patients, HCP, and visitors
- Transport and approval for disposal of waste materials
- Emergency preparedness plans for major utility failures with IC implications, including location and responsibilities
- Commissioning—what testing will be done to determine that delivered projects meet the owner's expectations
- Monitoring processes

Integration of the CRP and ICRA

Once approved, a CRP becomes the 'driver' to ensure appropriate and continuous input from IC into (a) the structural design processes to identify appropriate and timely IC practices and (b) involvement in specific projects during each construction phase, focusing on patient and worker protection from construction activity.

Infection Control Risk Assessment—Design

Population Assessment

Long-range planning for major new construction projects begins with assessments of the organization's patient population to identify the type and structure needed by defined programs. For example, an elderly population requires different support structure than an organ transplant unit. Reviewing communicable disease reports to local public health agencies and historical summaries of HAI may suggest the need for increased numbers of private rooms for AIIRs. There are major differences across the United States for the types and prevalence of disease requiring ventilation controls, which affect the need for AIIRs or PEs.

Budget Issues

Healthcare epidemiology and infection control (HEIC) staff participation is critical in the initial planning and approval meetings during the programming or design phase. Issues frequently addressed include budget, space constraints including storage and equipment cleaning areas, air handling units, hand washing facilities, appropriate finishes, specific products with infectious implications, and applicable regulations. HEIC staff should be prepared to support their position and recommendations with published citations whenever feasible, especially when a recommendation is not budget neutral (8,9,64,86). HEIC staff frequently work with consultants during the planning phase of specific projects, including architectural and construction companies in a "partnering" process. Consulting an environmental expert might also be necessary if the size and complexity of construction provides considerable risk to highly susceptible patients because of location, prolonged time of construction, work conducted over continuous shifts, and likelihood of air handlers sustaining frequent interruptions. These variables increase risks to patients and personnel and may require environmental testing. If appropriate, budgets for environmental consultants and anticipated testing or environmental monitoring must be considered at the earliest stage of planning. Major design components that must be addressed include design to support IC practice and design and number and type of isolation rooms (i.e., AIIR or PE).

Special Environments—AIIR and PE

New Construction or Renovation

AIA/FGI guidelines outline the design characteristics for AIIR, including no minimum requirement for anterooms. Anterooms may be useful for supplies and accommodating personal protection equipment but are not needed to maintain negative air pressure of the room with respect to the adjacent corridor. The guidelines do not support dual-purpose positive and negative ventilation (i.e., rooms "switched" from negative to positive air pressure) because of concerns over reliability and maintenance of intended pressurization relationships. AIIR in new construction or renovation require a negative airflow of at least 12 air exchanges/hour (ACH). Although audible alarms may be used to monitor AIIR, current guidelines for new construction require permanently installed *visual* mechanisms to constantly monitor the direction of airflow (4). AIIRs also require self-closing doors and tight sealing of the room. If the air cannot be exhausted directly to the outside, it must be filtered through HEPA filters before it is recirculated to the facility's HVAC system.

PEs are not required by the guidelines because they are dependent on the program of the organization. However, the guidelines appendix provides suggestions for PE design (4). These designs are consistent with CDC guidelines regarding tuberculosis and pneumonia (5,161). Planning for a population needing PE should consider the one condition that requires an anteroom to achieve proper airflow (i.e., a highly immunosuppressed patient who is infected with an airborne infectious agent like VZV requires positive pressure in the room to protect from other airborne infectious agents like *Aspergillus* and also requires removal of the air to ensure protection of caregivers from VZV). The guidelines offer two designs to accomplish the pressure relationships, both requiring an anteroom.

Ventilation and Mechanical Systems and Basic Infrastructure

Long-range planning requires attention to key systems such as HVAC, including recommended ventilation and filtration specifications and mechanical systems involving water supply and plumbing. Key parameters for HVAC include filtration efficiency, air exchanges, pressurization relationships, humidity, and temperature. Recommended ranges for each of these are outlined in detail in the guidelines and elsewhere in this text (4) (see Chapter 89).

Rooms and Storage Supporting Infection Control Practice

The guidelines require specific areas such as utility rooms (soiled and clean), instrument processing, holding, and workrooms. Storage of movable and modular equipment is critical from both a life safety and cleanliness viewpoint. The public perception of clutter is frequently associated with contamination and is seen as an IC problem. Stretchers, wheelchairs, intravenous (IV) poles, and other large patient care equipment are generally shared among units. Adequate space is needed to store, remove, clean, and maintain the items in an orderly fashion and reduce damage to surfaces and must be located away from normal traffic (4). In addition CMS and state-based enforcement agencies emphasize clear, unobstructed corridors in healthcare facilities.

Design and Surfaces

Ideally, surfaces are designed to include cleanability; problems can be avoided if surfaces near plumbing fixtures are smooth, nonporous, and water resistant. Operating and delivery rooms and isolation and sterile processing areas also need smooth finishes that are free of fissures or open joints and crevices that retain or permit passage of dirt particles (4,170,173). Planning may include consideration of light fixtures that have flat surfaces for ease in wiping clean. Window ledges are dust-collecting horizontal spaces that can be eliminated with a minimum width of nonporous material. Seamless, sealed floors are required to be clean not waxed and having rounded corners and edges aids in reducing the accumulation of debris from traffic, fluids, and dirt. Noncloth furniture resists absorption of moisture and stains, making cleaning more effective and efficient. Stainless steel surfaces, in particular, are both resilient and easily sanitized. Selection of surface materials, therefore, must balance use life, cleanability, cost, and maintenance.

Selection of Building Materials

The construction materials vary for flooring (identify precise location of carpet or vinyl); walls; headwall components; windows; doors; countertops; plumbing fixtures (i.e., sinks, faucets, handles, etc.); lighting; electrical outlets; furnishings (e.g., bed, chairs, bedside tables); and computers, equipment, and supplies storage areas. Choices should consider selection of latex-free construction materials for all items, sizes, dimensions, colors, finishes, securement, and seams. Counter space required for various activities should have countertops that are seamless, nonporous, and durable against multiple germicidal cleanings.

IC aspects associated with construction materials must be included along with those of local fire marshal requirements and state and local mandated codes and standards. General IC considerations include nonporous surfaces that are easily cleaned with Environmental Protection Agency (EPA) registered germicides. They should also consider hands-free, foot pedal, or sensor-activated faucets; lids; handles; dispensers; and controls to the extent feasible. HEIC staff should evaluate materials that withstand harsh chemical contact without corrosion, staining, or disruption of function and durability. Modifications that reduce soil and debris reservoirs include seamless design, rounded corners, sealed seams, wall bumpers, handrails, and electronic door openers. Counter space required for various activities should have countertops that are seamless, nonporous, and durable against multiple germicidal cleanings. Drawers and containers for storage should be constructed from seamless, molded materials with rounded corners to prevent cracks, crevices, or folded edges that attract soil and are difficult to clean (150,174).

Furnishings, Fixtures, and Equipment

Furniture

Modular furniture not easily moved should be installed on raised platforms or suspended in some manner to achieve a minimum 6-in. to 12-in. clearance from the floor to allow pull out for cleaning or to allow cleaning underneath. Attention must be paid to storage units with electrical or computer connections. Upholstered furniture should be managed like carpeting (including disposal) in the event of major soaking and contamination as a result of floods, leaks, or sewage. If furniture is affected by only steam moisture, it can be dried. Hardwood with intact laminate can be cleaned and disinfected with dilute bleach. Laminated furniture that has exposed particle board beneath the surface or other furniture composed of pressed wood or chipboard supports fungal contamination and growth when wet and should be discarded if it becomes soaked (9,64).

Hand Washing Stations and Hand Cleaning Agent Dispenser Placement

Design and placement of hand washing stations becomes more critical with the additional consideration of waterless alcohol-based hand rubs and has an impact in the event of plumbing disruptions or lack of preventive maintenance.

Number and Design. The guidelines for new construction recommend the minimum number of hand washing facilities for hospital patient rooms as one in the toilet room and one in the patient room outside of the privacy curtain to ensure that HCP can carry out standard precautions. Having a sink in a patient or resident room and in the toilet room supports essential IC practices. IC plays a critical role in recommending proper placement of hand wash facilities. In addition, IC support for a sink standard of minimum dimensions may prevent installation of small "cup" sinks that challenge proper hand washing (170). The guidelines describe permissible types of controls for hand washing facilities in various areas.

Placement. Improper placement can add to the environmental reservoir of contaminants. Sinks must be convenient and accessible, but nearby surfaces should also be nonporous to resist fungal growth (64,170). One source recommends a minimum distance of 15 ft from all inpatient beds or bassinets and 25 ft from outpatient chairs, stretcher, and treatment areas to ensure access (170). Hand washing facilities should also be situated to avoid splashing (suggesting at least 36 in. from patients or clean supplies) or equipped with a splash guard to avoid splash contamination (170). CDC hand hygiene guidelines (175) make a strong recommendation for addition of waterless alcohol-based hand antiseptic agents as part of a facility's overall hand hygiene program. Dispenser location has emerged as one of the critical issues to address for this class of products. For example the CDC guideline recommends that these not be placed near the hand washing stations to reduce confusion between them and antimicrobial soap used with water. Since the publication of these guidelines, there has been an increase in the adoption of waterless alcohol-based hand antiseptics by U.S. healthcare facilities. Theoretical concern of flammability of this class of hand hygiene agents has prompted fire safety officials in several states to restrict location of dispensers to patient care rooms or suites and prohibit them in exit or egress corridors (176). Perceptions that waterless hand hygiene products will supplant the need for hand washing stations also are unfounded. Both traditional washing with soap and water and the waterless products are needed, and the ICRA process should ensure adequate provision for new construction and renovation.

Cabinets. Areas beneath sinks should not be considered storage areas because of proximity to sanitary sewer connections and risk of leaks or water damage. Clean or sterile patient items should be not be placed beneath sanitary sewer pipe connections or stored with soiled items; cleaning materials are the only items acceptable to be stored under sinks, from a regulatory aspect (170). Facilities may develop design standards excluding storage space beneath sinks, thus preventing misuse and need for cleaning. As noted earlier, cabinet construction materials need to be nonporous to resist fungal growth.

Aerators. Aerated sink faucets located near patients, particularly in ICUs, may be a risk because of their ability to enhance growth of water-borne microorganisms. The faucet aerator has been identified as a reservoir and possible source of infection within the hospital. Rutala (177) noted that the most convincing evidence for the role of faucet aerators is provided by Fierer et al. In this study, premature infants became infected with *Pseudomonas aeruginosa* from delivery room resuscitation equipment contaminated by a faucet aerator. Rutala concluded that the degree of importance of aerators as reservoirs for nosocomial pathogens remains unknown. Because *Legionella* species grow well in the sediment formed in aerators, Freije et al. (135) recommend aerator removal. Proper sink design and dimensions can reduce splashing and risks of general contamination, while eliminating concerns for aerators completely.

Flush Sinks and Hoppers

Clinical sinks are frequently located in soiled utility rooms for disposal of body fluids and liquids but warrant similar considerations for moisture and contamination. Clinical or "flushing rim" sinks remove contaminated fluids in a manner similar to toilets and are not intended as utility or instrument cleaning sinks. Splashguards are valuable but inclusion may depend on sink design and use. If staff members are not routinely required to use face protectors, a splashguard should be required.

Whirlpool and Spa-like Bathing Facilities

Various types of bathing facilities are now available for mothers in birthing rooms and as additional amenity for some patient care rooms. Recommendations for cleaning have been compared with hydrotherapy tanks and equipment cleaning procedures (9). However, plumbing for a traditional whirlpool bath circulates water through piping and jets that are inaccessible to mechanical cleaning. Potential risks for cross-transmission of contaminants is, therefore, possible, especially if used during labor given the likelihood of introducing blood or other body fluids, which can be trapped in the pipe system. Pipeless whirlpool baths are commercially available, and cleanability using an *in vitro* testing protocol has been verified by the National Sanitation Foundation (Sanijet Corp., Coppell, TX; *www.sanijet.com*). Controlled trials comparing traditional to pipeless whirlpool baths are lacking, and the evidence demonstrating disease transmission from these systems is anecdotal. Communication with state regulators, cleaning and disinfecting the tub and jets with specific spa-cleaning products, and proper draining and flushing sequences are essential when considering installation (9).

Eyewash Stations

OSHA directs proper use and placement of eyewash stations with distance determined by the pH of the involved chemicals. Source water in stationary eyewash stations may stand unused in the incoming pipes at room temperature for long periods, providing a reservoir for potential pathogens (177). After a report of *Acanthamoeba* in eyewash stations, OSHA issued a bulletin recommending cleaning and disinfection methods. The schedule follows the American National Standards Institute Z358-1981 recommendations for flushing the system 3 minutes each week (120).

Dispenser Placement—Sharps Containers

Location of disposal containers should consider ease of visibility to avoid overfilling and should be within easy horizontal reach of the user. Systems should have secure locking and enable easy replacement. When containers are fixed to a wall, the vertical height should allow the worker to view the opening or access the container. NIOSH recommendations suggest ergonomic considerations for installation heights or creative approaches for specialty areas (168). Sufficient temporary storage space for filled containers must be in design planning (166). If a mobile cart mechanism is used, construction materials for the carts and containers must be fluid resistant, have appropriate biohazard signage, be puncture proof, and have a secure closure (166). Sharps containers and needle boxes are currently wall mounted in close proximity to the point of use; the containers are usually replaced when two-thirds full (168). Location, placement on the wall, and so forth must consider use such as residents' needs for medication, the main medication preparation area, and treatment rooms. Although this may be addressed in furnishings, it is appropriate to consider it with waste management. CMS also addresses proper storage and containment of waste in dumpsters and the management of the loading dock (e.g., free of debris and covered receptacles) (158).

Ice Machines

Ice availability for human consumption and medical nursing treatment may be located in the nutritional area or a clean room. Because contamination frequently occurs with ice because of inadequate machine maintenance or contamination during collection and handling of ice, an ice delivery method should be designed to minimize contamination. When icemaking equipment is accessible to patients or visitors it should be self-dispensing to avoid touch contamination. The ICP should ensure that the ice machine is designed to deliver ice without permitting the receptacle and human hands from coming in contact with the dispensing port. The drainage tray should permit routine cleaning and disinfection and eliminate any standing water source. Direct access and storage bins with ice scoops should be avoided (178). If a wall collection and removal system is planned, then construction materials and mechanisms would need to address IC aspects of containment and confinement with risk-reduction cleaning capabilities.

ICRA for Construction and Renovation Projects—Process

Overview

A good CRP supports long-range planning as discussed previously and provides guidance for individual construction projects, large or small. An ICRA for a specific construction project ensures appropriate planning for major new construction that also involves excavation and/or demolition or basic steps for simpler renovation projects. The ICRA team reviews the plan with considerable attention to detail by making inquiries to clarify understanding before a sign-off is completed. HEIC staff assess the plans, paying particular attention to the specific requirements cited for the building improvement. HEIC staff should focus on both the general and specific design aspects that influence and/or impact desired IC practices. If IC input does not occur in the beginning phase, there may be problems later with the infrastructure systems, such as air, water, traffic, and disruptions that impact on residents. For example, air quality may be compromised because of infrequent filter changes, leading to aerosolized fungi released from dust during the demolition phase (8,9) (see Chapter 89). Water may become contaminated with microbes when numerous dead-end pipe junctions contain stagnant water or when old piping is disrupted in replacement phases. Problems also occur when chlorine and/or temperature interventions to control *Legionella* are not maintained. A recent report documents that plumbing in even newly constructed nursing homes was readily colonized with *Legionella* (108).

Patients

The ICRA team assesses the inherent susceptibility of the patient (e.g., degree of immunosuppression as in a bone marrow transplant patient) and the risk associated with the degree of invasiveness for procedures (e.g., patient undergoing surgery). The degree of dust and moisture is also assessed according to the size of the project, the length of time of the project, and the frequency of shift. After the assessment is made, a determination of the impact on the populations and the impact on areas adjacent to the construction site is made. Fig. 88.1 describes one widely used process using a matrix that matches levels of patient risk with levels of anticipated construction dust.

The risk score determines needed interventions based on the following:

- Construction activity—project complexity in terms of dust generation and duration of activity
- Patients—assessment of the population at risk and location in terms of invasive procedures

The matrix grid format immediately leads to identifying the following:

- Number and types of necessary controls and IC interventions
- Signatures of all parties, thus providing accountability for the mutually agreed on plan (9,171)

The process is made efficient by incorporating the precautions that can be determined using a decision-support matrix and a checklist in the form of a permit with signatures. Submission of an IC permit is an additional step and a useful method that is designed to assess the complexity of the project as a matrix of risk groups (patients and environment) (Fig. 88.1). The precautions, internal and/or external, include determining appropriate protection of occupants from demolition, ventilation and water management following planned or unplanned power outages, movement of debris, traffic flow, cleanup, and acceptance of the final renovation from the constructor. Whether or not this matrix method is used, there are key issues that should still occur:

- Routine submission of scheduled project lists from facility management to IC, enabling IC to be proactively aware of projects and to anticipate IC needs
- Submission of an "IC permit" or "project approval signature block" before the beginning of projects, beyond required project lists (9,171). Formats may range from simple checklists to questionnaires designed to assist staff members in assessing risks and identifying prevention strategies

Worker and Contractor Expectations

Contracting companies receiving the documentation that describes steps to take to protect patients must also consider management of contractor employees for security and IC purposes. Requirements for contract workers must be spelled out in project manual specifications documents. Expectations include control methods such as badges (pictures), point of entrance or access to the construction site, or entrance to the hospital. Check-in and checkout procedures, specific areas for donning and removing protective garb, and eating and toilet facilities should be identified well before the project begins. Health requirements and educational issues vary by project but should be included in principle as items that must be determined by mutual agreement between the owner (healthcare organization) and the construction company or companies.

Obtaining the cooperation of contractors is key to ensure that the hired work crew observes appropriate behavior when entering a hospital site. Provision of training and education by ICPs and healthcare professionals to contractors and subcontractors is the first step in creating a stronger sense of partnership. Training should include information on hygiene, traffic patterns, availability of protective wear (e.g., shoe covers and cover gowns), and other dust containment recommendations. Tendering documents should include all expected necessary containment recommendations. These recommendations may include that dust on clothing and boots be removed before entering the healthcare facility; that entrance to high-risk patient and staff

Infection Control Risk Assessment Matrix Of Precautions For Construction and Renovation

Step One:

Using the following table, *identify* the Type of Construction Project Activity (Type A-D)

TYPE A	**Inspection and Non-Invasive Activities** Includes, but is not limited to: ▪ removal of ceiling tiles for visual inspection limited to 1 tile per 50 square feet ▪ painting (but not sanding) ▪ wallcovering, electrical trim work, minor plumbing, and activities which do not generate dust or require cutting of walls or access to ceilings other than for visual inspection
TYPE B	**Small scale, short duration activities which create minimal dust** Includes, but is not limited to: ▪ installation of telephone and computer cabling ▪ access to chase spaces ▪ cutting of walls or ceiling where dust migration can be controlled
TYPE C	**Work that generates a moderate to high level of dust or requires demolition or removal of any fixed building components or assemblies** Includes, but is not limited to: ▪ sanding of walls for painting or wall covering ▪ removal of floorcoverings, ceiling tiles and casework ▪ new wall construction ▪ minor duct work or electrical work above ceilings ▪ major cabling activities ▪ any activity which cannot be completed within a single workshift
TYPE D	**Major demolition and construction projects** Includes, but is not limited to: ▪ activities which require consecutive work shifts ▪ requires heavy demolition or removal of a complete cabling system ▪ new construction

Step 1 ______________________________

Figure 88.1. Infection Control Risk Assessment Matrix of Precautions for Construction and Renovation and Infection Control Construction Permit. (Forms modified and provided courtesy of J Bartley, ECSI Inc, Beverly Hills, MI 2002. Steps 1 to 3 adapted with permission from Kennedy V, Barnard B, St Luke's Episcopal Hospital, Houston TX; and Fine C, CA; Steps 4 to 14 adapted with permission from Fairview University Medical Center, Minneapolis MN.)

Step Two:

Using the following table, *identify* the Patient Risk Groups that will be affected.
If more than one risk group will be affected, select the higher risk group:

Low Risk	Medium Risk	High Risk	Highest Risk
▪ Office areas	▪ Cardiology ▪ Echocardiography ▪ Endoscopy ▪ Nuclear Medicine ▪ Physical Therapy ▪ Radiology/MRI ▪ Respiratory Therapy	▪ CCU ▪ Emergency Room ▪ Labor & Delivery ▪ Laboratories (specimen) ▪ Newborn Nursery ▪ Outpatient Surgery ▪ Pediatrics ▪ Pharmacy ▪ Post Anesthesia Care Unit ▪ Surgical Units	▪ Any area caring for immunocompromised patients ▪ Burn Unit ▪ Cardiac Cath Lab ▪ Central Sterile Supply ▪ Intensive Care Units ▪ Medical Unit ▪ Negative pressure isolation rooms ▪ Oncology ▪ Operating rooms including C-section rooms

Step 2____

Step Three: **Match the** following on the matrix below:

Construction Project Activity (Type *A, B, C, D*) from Step One, with the ...
Patient Risk Group (*Low, Medium, High, Highest*) to find the ...

Class of Precautions (*I, II, III or IV*) or level of infection control activities required.
Class I-IV or Coded Precautions are delineated on the following page.

Class of Precautions: Construction Project by Patient Risk

Construction Project Activity

Patient Risk Group	TYPE A	TYPE B	TYPE C	TYPE D
LOW Risk Group	I	II	II	III/IV
MEDIUM Risk Group	I	II	III	IV
HIGH Risk Group	I	II	III/IV	IV
HIGHEST Risk Group	II	III/IV	III/IV	IV

Note: Infection Control permit/approval will be required before construction begins when the Construction Project Activity and Class of Precautions indicate that **Class III** or **Class IV** control procedures are necessary.

Step 3____

Description of Required Infection Control Precautions by Class

	During Construction Project	Upon Completion of Project
CLASS I	1. Execute work by methods to minimize raising dust from construction operations 2. Immediately replace any ceiling tiles displaced for visual inspection	1. Clean work area upon completion of task
CLASS II	1. Provide active means to prevent airborne dust from dispersing into atmosphere 2. Water mist work surfaces to control dust 3. Seal unused doors with duct tape 4. Block off and seal air vents 5. Place dust mat at entrance and exit of work area 6. Remove or isolate HVAC system in areas where work is being performed	1. Wipe work surfaces with disinfectant 2. Contain construction waste before transport in tightly covered containers 3. Wet mop and/or vacuum with HEPA filtered vacuum before leaving work area 4. Remove isolation of HVAC system in areas where work is being performed
CLASS III	1. Remove or isolate HVAC system in area where work is being done to prevent contamination of duct system 2. Complete all critical barriers (i.e. sheetrock, plywood, plastic) to seal area from non-work area or implement control cube method (cart with plastic covering and sealed connection to work site with HEPA vacuum for vacuuming prior to exit) before construction begins 3. Maintain negative air pressure within work site utilizing HEPA equipped air filtration units 4. Contain construction waste before transport in tightly covered containers 5. Cover transport receptacles or carts, tape covering unless solid lid	1. Do not remove barriers from work area until completed project is inspected by the owner's Safety Department and Infection Control Department and thoroughly cleaned by the owner's Environmental Services Department 2. Remove barrier materials carefully to minimize spreading of dirt and debris associated with construction 3. Vacuum work area with HEPA filtered vacuums 4. Wet mop area with disinfectant 5. Remove isolation of HVAC system in areas where work is being performed
CLASS IV	1. Remove or isolate HVAC system in area where work is being done to prevent contamination of duct system 2. Complete all critical barriers (i.e. sheetrock, plywood, plastic) to seal area from non work area or implement control cube method (cart with plastic covering and sealed connection to work site with HEPA vacuum for vacuuming prior to exit) before construction begins 3. Maintain negative air pressure within work site utilizing HEPA equipped air filtration units 4. Seal holes, pipes, conduits, and punctures appropriately 5. Construct anteroom and require all personnel to pass through this room so they can be vacuumed using a HEPA vacuum cleaner before leaving work site or they can wear cloth or paper coveralls that are removed each time they leave the work site 6. All personnel entering work site are required to wear shoe covers. Shoe covers must be changed each time the worker exits the work area 7. Do not remove barriers from work area until completed project is inspected by the owner's Safety Department and Infection Control Department and thoroughly cleaned by the owner's Environmental Services Department	1. Remove barrier material carefully to minimize spreading of dirt and debris associated with construction 2. Contain construction waste before transport in tightly covered containers 3. Cover transport receptacles or carts tape covering unless solid lid 4. Vacuum work area with HEPA filtered vacuums 5. Wet mop area with disinfectant 6. Remove isolation of HVAC system in areas where work is being performed

Step 4. Identify the areas surrounding the project area, assessing potential impact

Unit Below	Unit Above	Lateral	Lateral	Behind	Front
Risk Group	Risk Group	Risk Group	Risk Group	Risk Group	Risk Group

Step 5. Identify specific site of activity eg, patient rooms, medication room, etc.

____

Step 6. Identify issues related to: ventilation, plumbing, electrical in terms of the occurrence of probable outages.

____

Step 7. Identify containment measures, using prior assessment. What types of barriers? (Eg, solids wall barriers); Will HEPA filtration be required?

____

(Note: Renovation/construction area shall be isolated from the occupied areas during construction and shall be negative with respect to surrounding areas)

Step 8. Consider potential risk of water damage. Is there a risk due to compromising structural integrity? (eg, wall, ceiling, roof)

Step 9. Work hours: Can or will the work be done during non-patient care hours?

Step 10. Do the plans allow for adequate number of isolation/negative airflow rooms?

Step 11. Do the plans allow for the required number & type of handwashing sinks?

Step 12. Does the infection control staff agree with the minimum number of sinks for this project? (Verify against AIA/FGI Guidelines for types and area)

Step 13. Does the infection control staff agree with the plans relative to clean and soiled utility rooms?

Step 14. Plan to discuss the following containment issues with the project team. (Eg, traffic flow, housekeeping, debris removal [how and when]),

____

____

____

Appendix

Identify and communicate the responsibility for project monitoring that includes infection control concerns and risks. ICRA may be modified throughout the project; revisions must be communicated to the Project Manager.

Infection Control Construction Permit

	Permit No:
Location of Construction:	Project Start Date:
Project Coordinator:	Estimated Duration:
Contractor Performing Work:	Permit Expiration Date:
Supervisor:	Telephone:

YES	NO	CONSTRUCTION PROJECT ACTIVITY	YES	NO	PATIENT RISK GROUP
		TYPE A: Inspection, non-invasive activity			GROUP 1: Low Risk
		TYPE B: Small scale, short duration activities which create minimal dust			GROUP 2: Medium Risk
		TYPE C: Activity generates moderate to high levels of dust, requires greater than 1 work shift for completion			GROUP 3: Medium/High Risk
		TYPE D: Major demolition and construction activities Requiring consecutive work shifts			GROUP 4: Highest Risk

CLASS I	1. Execute work by methods to minimize raising dust from construction operations. 2. Immediately replace any ceiling tile displaced for visual inspection.	3. Minor Demolition for Remodeling
CLASS II	1. Provides active means to prevent air-borne dust from dispersing into atmosphere 2. Water mist work surfaces to control dust while cutting. 3. Seal unused doors with duct tape. 4. Block off and seal air vents. 5. Wipe surfaces with disinfectant.	6. Contain construction waste before transport in tightly covered containers. 7. Wet mop and/or vacuum with HEPA filtered vacuum before leaving work area. 8. Place dust mat at entrance and exit of work area. 9. Remove or isolate HVAC system in areas where work is being performed.
CLASS III **Date** **Initial**	1. Obtain infection control permit before construction begins. 2. Isolate HVAC system in area where work is being done to prevent contamination of the duct system. 3. Complete all critical barriers or implement control cube method before construction begins. 4. Maintain negative air pressure within work site utilizing HEPA equipped air filtration units. 5. Do not remove barriers from work area until complete project is thoroughly cleaned by Env. Services Dept.	6. Vacuum work area with HEPA filtered vacuums. 7. Wet mop with disinfectant 8. Remove barrier materials carefully to minimize spreading of dirt and debris associated with construction. 9. Contain construction waste before transport in tightly covered containers. 10. Cover transport receptacles or carts. Tape covering. 11. Remove or isolate HVAC system in areas where work is being performed/
Class IV **Date** **Initial**	1. Obtain infection control permit before construction begins. 2. Isolate HVAC system in area where work is being done to prevent contamination of duct system. 3. Complete all critical barriers or implement control cube method before construction begins. 4. Maintain negative air pressure within work site utilizing HEPA equipped air filtration units. 5. Seal holes, pipes, conduits, and punctures appropriately. 6. Construct anteroom and require all personnel to pass through this room so they can be vacuumed using a HEPA vacuum cleaner before leaving work site or they can wear cloth or paper coveralls that are removed each time they leave the work site.	7. All personnel entering work site are required to wear shoe covers 8. Do not remove barriers from work area until completed project is thoroughly cleaned by the Environmental Service Dept. 9. Vacuum work area with HEPA filtered vacuums. 10. Wet mop with disinfectant. 11. Remove barrier materials carefully to minimize spreading of dirt and debris associated with construction. 12. Contain construction waste before transport in tightly covered containers. 13. Cover transport receptacles or carts. Tape covering. 14. Remove or isolate HVAC system in areas where work is being done.

Additional Requirements:	
______ Date/Initials:	______ Exceptions/Additions to this permit Date/ Initials: are noted by attached memoranda
Permit Request By:	Permit Authorized By:
Date:	Date:

traffic areas be avoided; that cover gowns and booties be made available for workers; and that workers be provided with portable toilets for their use only and with potable water to wash, preferably outside of occupied healthcare facility grounds. These precautions help limit the amount of dust that is introduced into the healthcare facility. A partnership with contractors helps ensure greater respect for IC concerns among construction workers and raise the level of IC awareness regarding the different phases of the project, particularly high dust-generating activities (e.g., demolition of a targeted building) (67). Select aspects that should be in place for contractors and subcontractors include the following:

1. Proof of liability and worker's compensation insurance
2. Training on owner (facility) safety and IC policies and any other federal, state, and local authority having jurisdictional requirements
3. Identification of hazardous chemicals planned for use and material safety data sheets (MSDS) provided to owner
4. Spill response plans outlined for hazardous chemicals
5. Personal protective equipment (PPE) available and notice of anticipated generation of hazardous waste
6. Location and access to owner emergency care services
7. Assessment and documentation of interim life safety measures (ILSM)
8. Evacuation and fire safety response plans confirmed
9. Plans for worksite dust containment reinforced and attention to wall or floor penetrations

PRECONSTRUCTION

Project Management ICRA Team Sets the Stage

Worker Risk Assessment and Education

Health, Training, and Education

Health risk evaluations for potential exposures depend on the type of construction planned. Facility staff overseeing or working with outside contractors should assist in determining potential environmental risks for facility workers or contractors. Policies should include provisions for training and by whom (facility or contractor). Training must be appropriate to the task (e.g., staff entering air systems for preventive maintenance, such as changing filters, should be alerted to the potential for airborne dust containing spores of microorganisms and arrange to first turn off fans and don a mask). Staff members working in sanitary or septic sewage systems, drainage pipes, and so forth should be alerted to the risks of moisture and fungal contamination (8,9, 82,161,163,177). Agreements should be developed appropriate to the project regarding provisions for pertinent health protection, vaccinations, tuberculosis assessment and purified protein derivative (PPD) skin testing, or related education before workers begin construction. Requirements vary with degree of environmental risk and proximity to the patient population.

As agreements are completed, they should provide evidence that workers have received appropriate health protection as noted previously and should include the following information:

- Facility exposure control plan(s) for IC, hazardous chemicals, and life safety
- How to seek help and report exposures (e.g., first-aid location and initial steps to report exposures)
- Use of particulate respirators or other PPE
- Risk prevention for unexpected safety issues, such as noxious fumes, asbestos, and so forth (9,161–164) (see Chapter 89)
- The facility should be satisfied that provisions have been made for effective IC education designed to address facility-specific needs related to potential infectious risk exposures as described previously (9,160–164)

Preparation for Demolition and Construction

The project teams provide ongoing planning and monitoring during area preparation and throughout the demolition, construction, cleanup, preparation for return to service, and final project review (4, 8,159). Before construction begins, the focus of preparations should be on isolation of the construction or renovation area. Some sources categorize projects in terms of minor or major risk based on the level of needed barriers; checklists are developed accordingly (9,64).

External Excavation Precautions

External excavation is ideally conducted during off-hours so that air handlers can be adjusted; the goal is to protect the intake as much as possible. Small projects require similar planning and vary by degree, but preparation still requires early communication with facility management. Specific educational needs (e.g., OSHA), regulations, and health issues for patients and workers need to be addressed. A final customized checklist should be appended to the CRP (9).

Inspection of the Worksite

Daily inspections should be made, particularly at the start of a project. Recording inspections and observations is recommended. The inspection should look at major areas, including the following:

- Dust containment barriers at the source are appropriate
- The frequency in wetting excavated soil or demolished building, truck, and equipment path is adequate
- Doors, windows, and other ports of entry located near the project are sealed or barred from use
- Construction worker behavior, such as removing dust and observing good hygiene before entering into health care grounds, is acceptable
- Waste is kept to a minimum

It is recommended that an inspection worksheet or checklist be created, with daily inspections and observations recorded and copies given to the designated individuals who can correct the situation when necessary. The worksheet should include key precautions to observe and a follow-up segment. These worksheets act as a means of communication, and, if a problem arises, they become evidence that due diligence was exercised by ICPs and other healthcare professionals (67).

Internal Issues

Type and Extent of Construction

Project complexity varies with time, numbers of workers, whether contractors work continuous shifts, scope and degree of activity (high or low dust generation), and proximity to patients with varying degrees of risk for infection.

Internal Renovations

Internal projects require much additional planning, compared to external construction. Patient areas or units that cannot be closed or that are adjacent to a major renovation require special planning (e.g., OR additions adjacent to an active surgical suite). These situations may justify environmental monitoring beyond visual inspection to detect increased airborne contamination and to plan interventions (5,8,9,18,24,82,160).

General Issues

Patient Location during Construction

There should be no flow-through traffic in the area, meaning routing patterns for staff traffic and visitor access traffic must be planned and designated, and signage must be posted for ease in compliance. Adherence to existing codes and standards for the size of corridors and doorways remains in effect. Visitors or residents investigating progress during construction may place themselves and construction workers at risk. This requires considerable monitoring by staff to ensure a safe environment surrounding the renovation and/or construction.

Risk Factors

Managing infectious risks during construction means collaboration among all personnel. These risks include dust and debris compromising the environment, airborne microbes carried to immunocompromised residents, an unbalanced ventilation system affecting air quality, water contamination, accumulated and multiple waste reservoirs, ineffective dustproof barriers, to name a few. Depending on the location of the construction and the proximity to resident care areas, residents may have to be relocated to a safer unit. Meticulous maintenance of physical barriers and infrastructure systems (i.e., air, water, etc.) are required as risk reduction efforts. Airborne debris of particulate matter may carry microbes that contaminate the air and are especially hazardous to residents who may inhale the debris and develop respiratory infections and/or complications. Control of airflow patterns (e.g., clean to dirty); interruption of utility, building, and equipment services; and communication requirements should be specified in the project bid proposal to ensure construction specification compliance.

Environmental Control and Containment

Containment

Isolating the construction site by physical dust control partitions requires floor to deck (solid compartment separation between floors above dropped ceiling) walls made of airtight fire-rated barriers, usually consisting of drywall or plywood with caulked seams or heavy duty plastic with sealed seams and gasketed door frames. Site access points are controlled entries for those authorized to enter. These egress paths are located where minimal debris can be transferred from the construction side to the cleaner areas of the facility. Personnel authorized for entry are commonly identified by badge and protective gear, such as hard hats. Emphasis is placed on dust control, which is a constant challenge during the project; diligent cleaning efforts are critical. Dust collection mats with adhesive surface can also assist with minimizing migration of dust and debris carried by construction personnel. These mats typically have several layers that can be removed as needed when the exposed surface becomes loaded with dust. Daily cleaning by gathering gross debris for disposal is necessary before damp mopping the area as a dust control mechanism. Containment is further practiced when a debris exit path is marked and a delivery point of materials and supplies is designated.

Containment also includes HVAC systems. Measures such as sealing of grills or vents against construction debris; frequent changing of filters within the ventilation ducts; ensuring that the window seals are leak proof and airtight; and, if chutes are used to remove demolition materials, monitoring for negative pressure and ensuring that the chutes are closed when nonoperational or during duct cleaning are all important aspects to address.

During construction, unintentional water contamination of porous, acoustical ceiling tiles and/or fireproofing and filter materials may occur. Prompt removal of damaged, moisture-laden materials reduces the potential for fungal spore release (9,160, 173).

Dust and Debris Control—Barrier Systems. The area should be isolated, as the project requires. Small, short duration projects generating minimal dust may use fire-rated plastic sheeting but should be sealed at full ceiling height with at least 2-foot overlapping flaps for access to entry. Any project that produces moderate to high levels of dust requires rigid, dust-proof, and fire-rated barrier walls (e.g., drywall) with caulked seams for a tight seal. Large, dusty projects need an entry vestibule for clothing changes and tool storage. The entry area should have gasketed door frames; tight seals should be maintained at the full perimeter of walls and wall penetrations. An interim plastic dust barrier may be required to protect the area while the rigid impervious barrier is being constructed. Cleaning is required at completion of the barrier construction; plans should also describe a terminal barrier removal process that minimizes dust dispersal (9,64).

Ventilation.

Air System Flow. It should be determined whether the construction area uses fresh (outside) or recirculated air; filters should be added or return vents covered as needed with filter material or plastic. Air must flow from clean to dirty areas (4,8,9) (see Chapter 89).

Negative Air Pressure. The air within the construction area must be negative with respect to surrounding areas and with no disruption of air systems of adjacent areas. Constant negative pressure within the zone should be monitored with an alarmed device, which must be maintained and monitored by construction personnel. Exhaust from construction air should be directed outside or exhaust vents in the construction area should be sealed to prevent recirculation if possible. If the exhaust must tie into a recirculated air system, a prefilter and high-efficiency filter (95%) should be used before exhaust to prevent contamination of the ducts. Fans should be turned off before opening ductwork, and necessary interruptions (e.g., fire drills) should be planned for to minimize risk (4,9,64). Portable HEPA filtration devices can also aid in capture of particulates that might be aerosolized during demolition of drywall, removal of flooring materials, and so forth. Such devices can also facilitate creation of negative pressure by adding a flexible duct from the exhaust pathway of the portable device directly outside, if feasible. Other variables to address include the following:

- The status of sealed penetrations and intact ceilings should be verified in adjacent areas.
- Air exchange rates and pressure relationships: It should be verified that the facility can maintain proper rates in critical areas near construction activity, ensure air is not being recirculated without filtration from the construction area elsewhere, and provide accountability for and frequency of testing air pressures throughout the project (8,9,64).
- Vibration or disturbances: Drilling and other sources of vibration have potential to dislodge dust collected above suspended or false ceilings; vibrations loosen corrosion within water pipes as well. Plans should require vacuuming of affected areas and flushing debris from water systems before reoccupancy (8,24, 115,135).
- Specification of temperature and humidity ranges: Determine limits as appropriate (4,9,86,158).
- Monitoring: Consideration must include risks of malfunction or complete loss of utilities. Both visual cues and particulate air monitoring may be used. The type and frequency of monitoring, evaluation of results, and follow-up action by designated parties are essential to planning (8,9,64).

Traffic Control

Control

The safety approach to traffic control is signage that identifies construction areas and restricts entry to authorized construction personnel who have appropriate protective equipment. The IC perspective is to divert nonessential traffic (e.g., patients, HCP, or visitors) from the site, thereby reducing risk of exposure to or dissemination of airborne pathogens carried by dust. If intersection of patient care areas and construction is unavoidable, the route should be designed to minimize risks of exposure to infectious agents even if they have donned personal protective attire (masks). Visitors are guided to the most direct but safest route to visit residents. Because visitors are potential reservoirs of infectious agents transmissible to susceptible residents, they should be assessed for symptoms of communicable infectious diseases whether construction projects are in progress or not. Designated entry and exit procedures must be defined. Egress paths should be free of debris, designated elevators should be used during scheduled times, and only authorized personnel should be allowed to enter the construction zone. Signage should direct pedestrian traffic away from the construction area and materials (8,9,24,64).

Debris Management: Windows, Chutes

Debris. Used materials should be removed in carts with tightly fitted covers, using designated traffic routes. Medical waste containers (sharps or other medical regulated waste) should be removed by the facility before start of the project. Efforts should be made to minimize use of elevators with transport during the lowest period of activity. Debris should be removed daily and at times specified by agreements. If chutes are used to direct debris outside, HEPA-filtered negative air machines should be used, and the chute opening should be sealed when not in use. Filters should be bagged and sealed before being transported out of the construction area (8,9,24,64).

Exterior Windows. Windows should be sealed to minimize infiltration from excavation debris.

Patient Equipment—Contamination of Patient Rooms, Supplies, and Equipment

Worksite Garb

Contractor personnel clothing should be free of loose soil and debris before leaving the construction area. If protective apparel is not worn, a HEPA-filtered vacuum should be used to remove dust from clothing before leaving the barricade. PPE (e.g., face shields, gloves, respirators) is worn as appropriate. Contractors entering invasive procedure areas should be provided with disposable jump suits and head and shoe coverings. Protective clothing should be removed before exiting the work area. Tools and equipment should be damp wiped before entry and exit from the work areas (8,9,64).

Barriers

Areas around construction should be monitored to maintain protection of in-use patient care areas as described. Patient doors adjacent to construction area should be kept closed, with appropriate traffic control (8,9).

Storage

Sites should be designated for new and damaged construction materials (9).

Contractor Cleaning

The construction zone should be maintained in a clean manner by contractors and swept or HEPA-vacuumed daily or more frequently as needed to minimize dust. Adjacent areas should be damp mopped daily or more frequently as needed. Walk-off mats may minimize tracking of heavy dirt and dust from construction areas (8,9).

Facility Cleaning

Contracts should clearly specify responsibilities and expectations for routine and terminal cleaning before opening the newly renovated or construction zone (8,9).

Site Cleanliness

Monitoring the area proximal to the barriers surrounding the project site is usually delegated to the housekeeping and support service. Frequent cleaning is basic to maintaining dust control. Project site cleaning is an ongoing activity that should be viewed as a critical success factor in reducing risk. A question may be raised concerning the need for air testing of particulate matter to determine site cleanliness. A more productive approach is a preventive one, that is, establish routine cleaning frequencies at the same rate that a facility might institute *if* air testing demonstrated that dust levels were high.

The IC and safety aspects of maintaining a clean work area include reduced clutter and fall hazards, diminished exposure to airborne debris that may cause infectious or allergic responses, and enhanced visibility to perform the work at hand. CMS is also concerned with providing an environment that is free from hazards (e.g., wet floors not identified with signage or blocked access) (158). Similar concerns arise throughout construction or renovation projects and require vigilance on everyone's part to maintain safety and control dust.

Standard housekeeping IC practices are followed. Housekeeping equipment should be designated for this area. Fresh germicidal solutions are used and changed often. Chemically treated dust cloths and mop heads should not be shaken and are laundered daily. Vacuum and suction machines are equipped with high-efficiency filters and changed frequently for maximum benefit in controlling airborne dispersal of dust and microorganisms. Frequency of filter changes is workload dependent and based on filter efficiency and performance effectiveness.

INTRACONSTRUCTION PHASE AND THE ROLE OF A HOSPITAL EPIDEMIOLOGY AND INFECTION CONTROL PROGRAM

Communication

Once renovation or construction has begun, the ICP should be available to provide maintenance and operational input. Frequency of input or meetings depends on the scope of the project. Specific concerns must be customized in each project and include IC practices, education, and monitoring. The ICP is vital in educating and supporting "users or owners" to manage their area under construction (e.g., educating staff members on how to monitor their own performance as much as possible). In more complex projects, the ICP may assist directly or make provisions for items already outlined. A number of areas involving specific ICP involvement are discussed later.

Environmental Rounds

An efficient method to integrate key IC and life safety issues is the use of rounds, using simple checklists based on the items addressed previously (171). ICPs can advise or participate in rounds, which should be scheduled as often as necessary and include a variety of observable "indicators" such as barriers (doors, signage), air handling (windows closed), project area (debris, cleaning), traffic control, and dress code. It may be necessary on occasion to schedule rounds after normal hours or on weekends if that is when construction or renovation is scheduled (8,9,64).

Environmental Monitoring Activities during Construction

There are currently no recommendations for routine environmental culturing during construction. Enhanced targeted patient surveillance (e.g., respiratory illnesses consistent with aspergillosis or legionellosis) near construction areas should be part of the ICRA. Other control measures previously discussed must be continuously monitored. However, when an outbreak associated with construction is suspected or identified, water or air sampling may be indicated. It is vitally important to establish a hypothesis with clear and measurable goals. Culturing or sampling procedures should be defined before initiation (e.g., asbestos, fungal, or particulates). Sampling procedures relative to the suspected agent(s) and sources should be used. The investigator must be cognizant of the many pitfalls associated with the interpretation of environmental data. Therefore, as part of the investigation planning, it is important to establish parameters for interpreting collected data.

Outcome or Process Measures

Projects may be approached as performance improvement initiatives using outcome measures (e.g., SSI rates) or process measures (measuring compliance) using visual observations, airborne particulate monitors, satisfaction surveys, and so forth (9, 18,160).

Impact on Special Areas

Patients requiring AIIRs need close monitoring to ensure that negative-pressure relationships are maintained, particularly when there is potential for disruption of pressure relationships (8,9,32,179). Intake areas such as emergency departments need planning to triage potentially infectious patients (4,5,160). If highly susceptible patients cannot be relocated, indicators should be identified to trigger planned intervention (8,9,18,24,64). Immunosuppressed populations in bone marrow transplantation units or protected environments, ICUs, and so forth require special planning. The goal is to minimize patient exposure to major construction activity; therefore, nonemergency admissions should be avoided during periods of major excavation. If delaying admissions is not an option, patients should be located in areas as remote as possible from construction activity (8,9).

Patient Location and Transport

Healthcare providers should plan patient care activities to minimize exposure to construction sites. At least one study found that critically ill, ventilator-dependent patients transported from the ICU for diagnostic or therapeutic procedures was an independent risk factor for development of ventilator-associated pneumonia (9). To decrease exposure for patients during construction activities the following should be considered:

- Provide treatment in the patient's room
- Transport via an alternate route
- Schedule transport or procedures during periods with minimal construction activity
- Minimize waiting and procedure times near construction zones
- Mask patient or provide other barriers (e.g., covering open wounds) based on patient's clinical status

Emergent Issues—Interruption of Utility Services

Utility services may be interrupted during any type of construction. Infectious agents may contaminate air-handling units, medical vacuum, and water systems after planned or unplanned power disruptions. HEIC can provide input into emergency preparedness to reduce the potential risks of contamination. Response plans should include assessment of the population at risk and cleanup should focus on steps to prevent, detect, and reduce risk from infectious hazards. For example, as power is reestablished after an interruption, dampers and fans of air handling units resume operation. Dust and particulate matter released during this process may transmit allergenic or infectious agents such as *Aspergillus* species to patients and staff (8,9,17,24,64, 135). Therefore, IC policies for areas in which invasive procedures are performed should require sufficient time to clear the air of potential contaminants before resuming the room(s) use. Ventilation time should be based on the number of air changes per hour required by the area. The NIOSH chart for removal efficiency of airborne contaminants may provide guidance, but its use should be tempered by its assumptions (5,160). In the event of major contamination of patient care areas, plans should specify responsibilities for these decisions and for intensified cleaning, environmental surveillance of airborne infectious agents, and restriction of water use until testing or flushing determines safe use.

POSTCONSTRUCTION

Postconstruction and Cleanup

Project Checklists

Check-off lists of expected practices identified at the beginning of the project should be reviewed for items agreed on before the area is returned to full service or patient occupancy. A useful tool during review is the contractor's "punchlist" to ensure that missed details have been addressed (e.g., installations of soap dispensers or designated types of hand washing and sink controls) (8,9,171).

Owner Preinspections before Move-in

Suggested check points for inspections include validating air systems by verifying air balances and pressures, checking electrical current of wall outlets, testing suction capability of wall units, assessing oxygen and gas delivery ports for ease in delivery and control accuracy, checking illumination sources, flushing water systems, rechecking that sinks are in place and functioning properly, determining if aerators are absent, testing whether soap and towel dispensers are full and functional and whether sharps containers properly placed.

Postconstruction Agreements

Cleanup agreements (e.g., cleaning, air balancing, filter changes, flushing of water systems, etc.) and other utility service checks and cleaning must be established in the early planning phase as discussed previously. These include the following at minimum:

- Contractor cleaning to include area clearance, cleaning, and decontamination and wipedown
- Cleaning after removal of partitions around construction area, minimizing dust production
- Facility-based routine and terminal cleaning before returning area to service
- Provision of time frames for facility review (e.g., 2 weeks) after completion of the project to ensure that all issues were addressed properly
- Systematic review of outcomes in the facility's designated review process, whether by contract or committee structure. Items may range from sealed cabling and electrical penetrations and ceiling tile replacements to the completed punchlist
- Cleaning and replacement of filters and other equipment if affected by major or minor disruptions or conditions that could have contaminated the air or water supply (9,23,62–64)

Steps before Occupancy

Checklists specific to the project should be developed for a walk-through just before occupancy. Core IC issues for inclusion are listed later as applicable. The designated team should do the following:

- Check that sinks are properly located and functioning
- Verify that sinks in critical patient care areas have properly functioning fixtures
- Check for the presence or absence of aerators in these fixtures according to facility policy
- Test whether soap and towel dispensers are filled and functioning
- Check whether surfaces in procedure and service areas are appropriate for use (e.g., smooth, nonporous, water-resistant)
- Verify that air balancing has been completed according to specifications
- Test whether air flows into negative-pressure rooms or out of positive-pressure rooms

In conclusion, the role of HEIC in construction and renovation remains a challenging and exciting one and is the ultimate demonstration of its multidisciplinary nature. Interaction and integration of efforts with other disciplines is consistent with the underlying foundation of HEIC—disease prevention for patients, HCP, and visitors.

REFERENCES

1. Kohn LT, Corrigan JM, Donaldson MS eds. *To err is human: building a safer health system.* Washington, DC: Institute of Medicine National Academy Press, 1999, pp 1–223.
2. Anonymous. Quality Interagency Coordination Task Force, doing what counts for patient safety: federal actions to reduce medical errors and their impact. Report of the Quality Interagency Coordination task force (QUIC) to the president. Washington DC: Agency for Healthcare Quality and Research, 2000. Available at *http://www.quic.gov/report/toc.htm* (accessed 1/24/04).
3. Rubin HR, Owens AJ, Golden G. *Status report (1998): an investigation to determine whether the built environment affects patients' medical outcomes.* Martinez, CA: The Center for Health Design, Inc., 1998:1–80.
4. American Institute of Architects Academy of Architecture for Health, Facilities Guideline Institute. *2001 Guidelines for design and construction of hospitals and healthcare facilities.* Washington, DC: The American Institute of Architects Press, 2001.
5. Centers for Disease Control and Prevention. Guidelines for preventing the transmission of *Mycobacterium tuberculosis* in health-care facilities, 1994. *MMWR Morb Mortal Wkly Rep* 1994;RR-13:1–132.
6. American Thoracic Society Workshop. Achieving healthy indoor air: report of the American Lung Association and American Thoracic Society Workshop 1995. Nov 16–19, Santa Fe, NM. *Am J Respir Crit Care Med* 1997;156:S33–S64.
7. Rhame FS. Prevention of nosocomial aspergillosis. *J Hosp Infect* 1991; 18(Suppl A):466–472.
8. Bartley JM. Construction and renovation. In: Pfeiffer J, ed. *APIC text of infection control and epidemiology.* Washington, DC: Association for Professionals in Infection Control and Epidemiology, 2000: 72.1–72.11.
9. Bartley JM. APIC State-of-the-art-report: the role of infection control during construction in health care facilities. *Am J Infect Control* 2000; 28:156–169.
10. Aisner J, Schimpff SC, Bennett JE, et al. *Aspergillus* infections in cancer patients: association with fireproofing materials in a new hospital. *JAMA* 1976;235:411–412.
11. Kyriakides GK, Zinneman HH, Hall WH, et al. Immunologic monitoring and aspergillosis in renal transplant patients. *Am J Surg* 1976; 131:246–252.
12. Arnow PM, Anderson RI, Mainous PD, et al. Pulmonary aspergillosis during hospital renovation. *Am Rev Resp Dis* 1978;118:49–53.
13. Lentino JR, Rosenkranz MA, Michaels JA, et al. Nosocomial aspergillosis: a retrospective review of airborne disease secondary to road construction and contaminated air conditioners. *Am J Epidemiol* 1982; 116:430–437.
14. Sarubbi FS, Kopf MB, Wilson MB, et al. Increased recovery of *Aspergillus flavus* from respiratory specimens during hospital construction. *Am Rev Resp Dis* 1982;125:33–38.
15. deSilva MI, Rissing JP. Postoperative wound infection following cardiac surgery: significance of contaminated cases performed in the preceding 48 hours. *Infect Control* 1984;5:371–377.
16. Anderson JD, Bonner M, Scheifle DW, et al. Lack of nosocomial spread of varicella in a pediatric hospital with negative pressure ventilated patient rooms. *Infect Control* 1985;6:120–121.
17. Krasinski K, Holzman RS, Hanna B, et al. Nosocomial fungal infection during hospital renovation. *Infect Control* 1985;6:278–282.
18. Opal SM, Asp AA, Cannady PB Jr, et al. Efficacy of infection control measures during a nosocomial outbreak of aspergillosis associated with hospital construction. *J Infect Dis* 1986;153:634–637.
19. Allo MD, Miller J, Townsend T, et al. Primary cutaneous aspergillosis associated with Hickman intravenous catheters. *N Engl J Med* 1987; 317:1105–1108.
20. Ruutu P, Valtonen V, Elonen E, et al. Invasive pulmonary aspergillosis: a diagnostic and therapeutic problem. Clinical experience with eight haematologic patients. *Scand J Infect Dis* 1987;19:569–575.
21. Perraud M, Piens MA, Nicoloyannis N, et al. Invasive nosocomial pulmonary aspergillosis: risk factors and hospital building works. *Epidemiol Infect* 1987; 99:407–412.
22. Sherertz RJ, Belani A, Kramer BS, et al. Impact of air filtration on nosocomial *Aspergillus* infections. Unique risk of bone marrow transplant recipients. *Am J Med* 1987;83:709–718.
23. Streifel AJ, Steven PP, Rhame FS. In-hospital source of airborne *Penicillium* species. J Clin Microbiol 1987;25(Suppl 2):1–4.
24. Weems JJ, Davis BJ, Tablan OC, et al. Construction activity: an independent risk factor for invasive aspergillosis and zygomycosis in patients with hematologic malignancy. *Infect Control* 1987;8:71–75.
25. Barnes RA, Rogers TR. Control of an outbreak of nosocomial aspergillosis by laminar air-flow isolation. *J Hosp Infect* 1989;14:89–94.
26. Hopkins CC, Weber DJ, Rubin RH. Invasive aspergillus infection: possible non-ward common source within the hospital environment. *J Hosp Infect* 1989;13:19–25.
27. Mehta G. *Aspergillus* endocarditis after open-heart surgery an epidemiological investigation. *J Hosp Infect* 1990;15:245–253.
28. Fox BC, Chamberlin L, Kulich P, et al. Heavy contamination of operating room air by *Penicillium* species: identification of the source and attempts at decontamination. *Am J Infect Control* 1990;18: 300–306.
29. Jackson L, Klotz SA, Normand RE. A pseudoepidemic of *Sporothrix cyanescens* pneumonia occurring during renovation of a bronchoscopy suite. *J Med Vet Mycol* 1990;28:455–459.
30. Arnow PM, Sadigh MC, Weil D, et al. Endemic and epidemic aspergillosis associated with in-hospital replication of *Aspergillus* organisms. *J Infect Dis* 1991;164:998–1002.
31. Everett WD, Kipp H. Epidemiologic observations of operating room infections resulting from variations in ventilation and temperature. *Am J Infect Control* 1991;19:277–282.
32. Humphreys H, Johnson EM, Warnock DW, et al. An outbreak of aspergillosis in a general ITU. *J Hosp Infect* 1991;18:167–177.
33. Abzug MJ, Gardner S, Glode MP, et al. Heliport-associated nosocomial mucormycoses. *Infect Control Hosp Epidemiol* 1992;13:325–326.
34. Hruszkewycz V, Ruben B, Hypes CM, et al. A cluster of pseudofungemia associated with hospital renovation adjacent to the microbiology laboratory. *Infect Control Hosp Epidemiol* 1992;13:147–150.
35. Flynn PM, Williams BG, Hethrington SV, et al. *Aspergillus terreus* during hospital renovation [Letter]. *Infect Control Hosp Epidemiol* 1993;14:363–365.
36. Gerson SL, Parker P, Jacobs MR, et al. Aspergillosis due to carpet contamination [Letter]. *Infect Control Hosp Epidemiol* 1994;15: 221–223.
37. Iwen PC, Davis JC, Reed EC, et al. Airborne fungal spore monitoring in a protective environment during hospital construction and correlation with an outbreak of invasive aspergillosis. *Infect Control Hosp Epidemiol* 1994;15:303–306.
38. Stroud LA, Tokars JI, Grieco MH, et al. Evaluation of infection control measures in preventing the nosocomial transmission of multidrug resistant *Mycobacterium tuberculosis. Infect Control Hosp Epidemiol* 1995;16:141–147.
39. Alvarez M, Lopez P, Raon C, et al. Nosocomial outbreak caused by *Scedosporium prolificans (inflatum)*: four fatal cases in leukemic patients. *J Clin Microbiol* 1995;33:3290–3295.
40. Bryce EA. Walker M, Scharf S, et al. An outbreak of cutaneous aspergillosis in a tertiary-care hosp. *Infect Control Hosp Epidemiol* 1996; 17:170–172.
41. Cotterill S, Evans R, Fraise AP. An unusual source for an outbreak of methicillin-resistant *Staphylococcus aureus* on an intensive therapy unit. *J Hosp Infect* 1996;32:207–216.
42. Fridkin SK, Kremer FB, Bland LA, et al. *Acremonium kiliense* endophthalmitis that occurred after cataract extraction in an ambulatory surgical center and as traced to an environmental reservoir. *Clin Infect Dis* 1996;22:222–227.
43. Anderson K, Morris G, Kennedy H, et al. Aspergillosis in immunocompromised paediatric patients: associations with building hygiene, design and indoor air. *Thorax* 1996;51:256–261.
44. Leenders A, van Belkum A, Janssen S, et al. Molecular epidemiology of apparent outbreak of invasive aspergillosis in a hematology ward. *J Clin Microbiol* 1996;34:345–351.
45. Loo VG, Bertrand C, Dixon C, et al. Control of construction-associated nosocomial Aspergillosis in an antiquated hematology unit. *Infect Control Hosp Epidemiol* 1996;17:360–364.

46. Philpot-Howard J. Prevention of fungal infections in hematology patients. *Infect Control Hosp Epidemiol* 1996;17:545–551.
47. Pittet D, Huguenin T, Dharan S, et al. Unusual case of lethal pulmonary aspergillosis in patients with chronic obstructive pulmonary disease. *Am J Respir Crit Care Med* 1996;154:541–544.
48. Dearborn DG, Infeld MD, Smith PG, et al. Update: pulmonary hemorrhage/hemosiderosis among infants. *MMWR Morb Mortal Wkly Rep* 1997;46:33–35.
49. Tabbara KF, al Jabarti AL. Hospital construction-associated outbreak of ocular aspergillosis after cataract surgery. *Ophthalmology* 1998;105: 522–526.
50. Kumari DN, Haji TC, Keer V, et al. Ventilation grilles as a potential source of methicillin-resistant *Staphylococcus aureus* causing an outbreak in an orthopedic ward at district general hospital. *J Hosp Infect* 1998;39:127–133.
51. Cornet M, Levy V, Fleury L, et al. Efficacy of prevention by high-efficiency particulate air filtration or laminar airflow against *Aspergillus* airborne contamination during hospital renovation. *Infect Control Hosp Epidemiol* 1999;20:508–513.
52. Garrett DO, Jochimsen E, Jarvis WR. Invasive *Aspergillus* spp. infections in rheumatology patients. *J Rheumatol* 1999;26:146–149.
53. Laurel VL, Meier PA, Astorga A, et al. Pseudoepidemic of *Aspergillus niger* infections traced to specimen contamination in the microbiology laboratory. *J Clin Microbiol* 1999;37:1612–1616.
54. Thio CL, Smith D, Merz WG, et al. Refinements of environmental assessment during outbreak investigation of invasive aspergillosis in a leukemia and bone marrow transplant unit. *Infect Control Hosp Epidemiol* 2000;21:18–23.
55. Burwen DR, Lasker BA, Rao N, et al. Invasive aspergillosis outbreak on a hematology-oncology ward. *Infect Control Hosp Epidemiol* 2001; 22:45–48.
56. Lai KK. A cluster of invasive aspergillosis in a bone marrow transplant unit related to construction and the utility of air sampling. *Am J Infect Control* 2001;29:333–337.
57. Oren I, Haddad N, Finkelstein R, et al. Invasive pulmonary aspergillosis in neutropenic patients during hospital construction: before and after chemoprophylaxis and institution of FEPA filters. *Am J Hematol* 2001;66:257–262.
58. Pegues CF, Daar ES, Murthy AR. The epidemiology of invasive pulmonary aspergillosis at a large teaching hospital. *Infect Control Hosp Epidemiol* 2001;22:370–374.
59. Hahn T, Cummings M, Michalek AM, et al. Efficacy of high-efficiency particulate air filtration in preventing aspergillosis in immunocompromised patients with hematologic malignancies. *Infect Control Hosp Epidemiol* 2002;23:525–531.
60. Kistemann T, Huneburg H, Exner M, et al. Role of increased environmental *Aspergillus* exposure for patients with chronic obstructive pulmonary disease (COPD) treated with corticosteroids in an intensive care unit. *Int J Hyg Environ Health* 2002;204:347–351.
61. Raad I, Hanna H, Osting C, et al. Masking of neutropenic patients on transport from hospital rooms is associated with a decrease in nosocomial aspergillosis during construction. *Infect Control Hosp Epidemiol* 2002;23:41–43.
62. Streifel AJ, Lauer JL, Vesley D, et al. *Aspergillus fumigatus* and other thermotolerant fungi generated by hospital building demolition. *Appl Environ Microbiol* 1983;46:375–378.
63. Streifel AJ. Aspergillosis and construction. In: Kundsin RB, ed. *Architectural design and indoor microbial pollution.* New York: Oxford University Press, 1988:198–217.
64. University of Minnesota Extension Service, University of Minnesota Building Research Consortium, IAQ Project, Department of Environmental Health and Safety. Health Care Construction and IAQ. Minneapolis, MN, Sept.16–17, 2002. Components available at *http://www.dehs.umn.edu/iaq* (accessed 1/24/04).
65. Dewhurst AG, Cooper MJ, Khan SM, et al. Invasive aspergillosis in immunocompromised patients: potential hazard of building work. *BMJ* 1990;301:802–804.
66. Streifel AJ. In with the good air. *Infect Control Hosp Epidemiol* 2002; 23:488–490.
67. Cheng SM, Streifel AJ. Infection control considerations during construction activities: land excavation and demolition. *Am J Infect Control* 2001;29:321–328.
68. Srinivasan A, Beck C, Buckley T, et al. The ability of hospital ventilation systems to filter *Aspergillus* and other fungi following a building implosion. *Infect Control Hosp Epidemiol* 2002;23:520–524.
69. Bouza E, Pelaez T, Perez-Molina J, et al. Demolition of a hospital building by controlled explosion: the impact on filamentous fungal load in internal and external air. *J Hosp Infect* 2002;52:234–242.
70. Bernstein RS, Sorenson WG, Garabrant D, et al. Exposures to respirable, airborne *Penicillium* from a contaminated ventilation system: environmental and epidemiological aspects. *Am Ind Hyg Assoc J* 1983; 44:161–169(abst).
71. Opal SM, Asp AA, Cannady PB Jr, et al. Efficacy of infection control measures during a nosocomial outbreak of aspergillosis associated with hospital construction. *J Infect Dis* 1996;153:634–637.
72. Pinker S. ORs closed after *Aspergillus* discovered at Royal Vic. *CMAJ* 2001;164:1333.
73. Shirani KZ, McManus AT, Vaughn GM, et al. Effects of environment on infection in burn patients. *Arch Surg* 1986;121:31–36.
74. Jarvis WR. Nosocomial transmission of multi-drug resistant *M. tuberculosis. Am J Infect Control* 1995;23:147–151.
75. Love CB Gordon SL. Total hip replacement. Current bibliographies in medicine (CBM) 94–95. Jan 1991–April 1994. *NIH Infection* 1994: 35–39. Available at *http://www.nlm.nih.gov/pubs/cbm/hip-repl.html* (accessed 1/24/04).
76. Bohn WW, McKinsey DS, Dystra M, et al. The effect of a portable HEPA-filtered body exhaust system on airborne microbial contamination of a conventional operating room. *Infect Control Hosp Epidemiol* 1996;17:419–422.
77. Shaw JA, Bordner MA, Hamory BH. Efficacy of the Steri-Shield filtered exhaust helmet in limiting bacterial counts in the operating room during total joint arthroplasty. *J Arthroplasty* 1996;11:469–473.
78. Ayliffe GA. Role of the operating suite in surgical wound infection. *Rev Inf Dis* 1991;13(Suppl 10):S800–S804.
79. Lidwell OM. Ultraviolet radiation and the control of airborne contamination in the operating room. *J Hosp Infect* 1994;28:245–248.
80. Pittet D, Ducel G. Infectious risk factors related to operating rooms. *Infect Control Hosp Epidemiol* 1994;15:456–572.
81. Hambraeus A. Aerobiology in the operating room—review. *J Hosp Infect* 1988;11(Suppl A):68–76.
82. Haberstich N. Prevention of infection during major construction and renovation in the surgery department of a large hospital. *Am J Infect Control* 1987;15:36A–38A.
83. Howorth F. Prevention of airborne infection during surgery. *Lancet* 1985;8425:386–388.
84. Fitzgerald RH Jr. Microbiologic environment of the conventional operating room. *Arch Surg* 1979;14:772–775.
85. Nelson CL. Environmental bacteriology in the unidirectional (horizontal) operating room. *Arch Surg* 1979;114:778–782.
86. Bartley JM. Environmental control: operating room air quality. *Todays OR Nurse* 1993;15(5):11–18.
87. Lidwell OM, Lowbury EJ, Whyte W, et al. Infection and sepsis after operations for total hip or knee-joint replacement: influence of ultraclean air, prophylactic antibiotics and other factors. *J Hyg (Lond)* 1984;93:505–529.
88. Lidwell OM, Lowbury EJ, Whyte W, et al. Extended follow-up of patients suspected of having joint sepsis after total joint replacement. *J Hyg (Lond)* 1985;95:655–664.
89. Salvati, EA, Robinson RP, Zeno SM, et al. Infection rates after 3175 total hips and total knee replacements performed with and without a horizontal uni-directional filtered air-flow system. *J Bone Joint Surg [Br]* 1982;64-A:535–535.
90. Claesson BEB, Claesson UL-E. An outbreak of endometritis in a maternity unit caused by spread of group A streptococci from a showerhead. *J Hosp Infect* 1995;6:304–311.
91. Ravn P, Lundgren JD, Kjaeldgaard P, et al. Nosocomial outbreak of cryptosporidiosis in AIDS patients. *BMJ* 1991;302:277–280.
92. Crane LR, Tagle LC, Palutke W. Outbreak of *Pseudomonas paucimobilis* in an intensive care facility. *JAMA* 1981;246:985–987.
93. Venezia RA, Agresta MD, Hanley EM, et al. Nosocomial legionellosis

associated with aspiration of nasogastric feedings diluted in tap water. *Infect Control Hosp Epidemiol* 1994;15:529–533.

94. Cordes LG, Wiesenthal AM, Gorman GW, et al. Isolation of *Legionella pneumophila* from hospital shower heads. *Ann Intern Med* 1981; 94:195–197.
95. Panwalker AP, Fuhse E. Nosocomial *Mycobacterium gordonae*: pseudoinfection from contaminated ice machines. *Am J Infect Control* 1986;7:67–70.
96. Burns DN, Wallace RJ Jr, Schultz ME, et al. Nosocomial outbreak of respiratory tract colonization with *Mycobacterium fortuitum*: demonstration of the usefulness of pulse-field gel electrophoresis in an epidemiologic investigation. *Am Rev Respir Dis* 1991;144:1153–1159.
97. Hlady WG, Mullen RC, Mintz CS, et al. Outbreak of Legionnaires' disease linked to a decorative fountain by molecular epidemiology. *Am J Epidemiol* 1993;138:555–562.
98. Sniadeck DH, Ostroff SM, Karlix MA, et al. Nosocomial pseudo-outbreak of *Mycobacterium xenopi* due to contaminated potable water supply: lessons in prevention. *Infect Control Hosp Epidemiol* 1993;14: 637–641.
99. Prodinger WM, Bonatti H, Allerberger F, et al. *Legionella* pneumonia in transplant recipients: a cluster of cases of eight years' duration. *J Hosp Infect* 1994;26:191–202.
100. Bangsborg JM, Uldum S, Jensen JS, et al. Nosocomial legionellosis in three heart-lung transplant patients: case reports and environmental observations. *Eur J Clin Microbiol Infect Dis* 1995;14:99–104.
101. Graman PS, Quinlan GA, Rank JA. Nosocomial legionellosis traced to a contaminated ice machine. *Infect Control Hosp Epidemiol* 1997; 18:637–640.
102. Patterson WJ, Hay J, Seal DV, et al. Colonization of transplant unit water supplies with *Legionella* and protozoa: precautions required to reduce the risk of legionellosis. *J Hosp Infect* 1997 ;37:7–17.
103. Kool JL, Fiore AE, Kioski CM, et al. More than 10 years of unrecognized nosocomial transmission of Legionnaires disease among transplant patients. *Infect Control Hosp Epidemiol* 1998;19:898–894.
104. Biurrun A, Calballero L, Pelaz C, et al. Treatment of a *Legionella pneumophila*-colonized water distribution system using copper-silver ionization and continuous chlorination. *Infect Control Hosp Epidemiol* 1999;20:426–428.
105. Weber DJ, Rutala WA, Blanchet CN, et al. Faucet aerators: a source of patient colonization with *Stenotrophomonas maltophilia. Am J Infect Control* 1999;27:59–63.
106. Kappstein I, Grundmann H, Hauer T, et al. Aerators as a reservoir of *Acinetobacter junii*: an outbreak of bacteraemia in paediatric oncology patients. *J Hosp Infect* 2000;44:27–30.
107. Knirsch CA, Jakob K, Schoonmaker D, et al. An outbreak of *Legionella micdadei* pneumonia in transplant patients: evaluation, molecular epidemiology, and control. *Am J Med* 2000;108:290–295.
108. Stout JE, Brennen C, Muder RR. Legionnaires disease in a newly constructed long-term care facility. *J Am Geriatr Soc* 2000;48: 1589–1592.
109. Borau J, Czap RT, Strellrecht KA, et al. Long-term control of *Legionella* species in potable water after a nosocomial legionellosis outbreak in an intensive care unit. *Infect Control Hosp Epidemiol* 2000;21: 602–603.
110. Grove DI, Lawson PJ, Burgess JS, et al. An outbreak of *Legionella longbeachae* infection in an intensive care unit. *J Hosp Infect* 2002;5: 250–258.
111. Darelid J, Lofgren S, Malmvall BE. Control of nosocomial Legionnaires disease by keeping the circulating hot water temperature above 55 degrees C: experience from a 10-year surveillance programme in a district general hospital. *J Hosp Infect* 2002;50:213–219.
112. Mermel LA, Josephson SL, Giorgio CH, et al. Association of Legionnaires' disease with construction: contamination of potable water? *Infect Control Hosp Epidemiol* 1995;16:76–81.
113. Kool JL, Bergmire-Sweat D, Butler JC, et al. Hospital characteristics associated with colonization of water systems by Legionella and risk of nosocomial Legionnaires disease: a cohort study of 15 hospitals. *Infect Control Hosp Epidemiol* 1999;21:434–435.
114. Struelens MJ, Maes N, Rost F, et al. Genotypic and phenotypic methods for the investigation of a nosocomial *Legionella pneumophila* outbreak and efficacy of control measures. *J Infect Dis* 1992;166:22–30.
115. Yu VL, Zeming L, Stout J, et al. *Legionella* disinfection of water distribution systems: principles, problems and practice. *Infect Control Hosp Epidemiol* 1993;14:567–570.
116. Pegues DA, Carson LA, Anderson RL, et al. Outbreak of *Pseudomonas cepacia*bacteremia in oncology patients. *Clin Infect Dis* 1993;16: 407–411.
117. Anaissie EJ, Penzak SR, Dignani MC. The hospital water supply as a source of nosocomial infections. A plea for action. *Arch Intern Med* 2002; 162:1483–1492.
118. Rusin PA, Rose JB, Haas CN, et al. Risk assessment of opportunistic bacterial pathogens in drinking water. *Rev Environ Contam Toxicol* 1997;152:57–83.
119. McDonald LC, Walker M, Carson L, et al. Outbreak of *Acinetobacter* spp. bloodstream infections in a nursery associated with contaminated aerosols and air conditioners. *Pediatr Infect Dis J* 1998;17:716–722.
120. Miles J. Potentially hazardous amoebae found in eyewash stations. Hazard Information bulletin. United States Dept. of Labor and Occupational Safety and Health Administration. Dec. 1986. Bulletin 19861223. Available at *http://www.osha.gov/dts/hib/hib__data/hib19861223.html* (accessed 1/24/04).
121. Anaissie EJ, Stratton SL, Dignani MC, et al. Pathogenic *Aspergillus* species recovered from a hospital water system: a 3-year prospective study. *Clin Infect Dis* 2002;34:780–789.
122. Marston BJ, Plouffe JF, Tile TM, et al. Incidence of community-acquired pneumonia requiring hospitalization—results of a population-based active surveillance study in Ohio. *Arch Intern Med* 1997; 157:1709–1718.
123. Cohen ML, Broome CV, Paris AL, et al. Fatal nosocomial Legionnaires' disease: clinical and epidemiologic characteristics. *Ann Intern Med* 1979;90:611–613.
124. Haley CE, Cohen ML, Halter J, et al. Nosocomial Legionnaires' disease: a continuing common-source epidemic at Wadsworth Medical Center. *Ann Intern Med* 1979;90:583–586(abst).
125. Dondero TJ Jr, Rendtorff RC, Mallison GF, et al. An outbreak of Legionnaires' disease associated with a contaminated air-conditioning cooling tower. *N Engl J Med* 1980;302:365–370.
126. Hanrahan JP, Morse DL, Scharf VB, et al. A community hospital outbreak of legionellosis. *Am J Epidemiol* 1987;25:639–649.
127. Marrie TJ, MacDonald S, Clarke K, et al. Nosocomial Legionnaires' disease: lessons from a four year prospective study. *Am J Infect Control* 1991;19:79–85.
128. Marrie TJ, Haldane D, MacDonald S, et al. Control of endemic nosocomial Legionnaires' disease by using sterile potable water for high risk patients. *Epidemiol Infect* 1991;107:591–605.
129. Mastro TD, Fields BS, Breiman RF, et al. Nosocomial Legionnaires' disease and use of medication nebulizers. *J Infect Dis* 1991;163: 667–671.
130. Fields BS, Benson RF, Besser RE. Legionella and Legionnaires' disease: 25 years of investigation. *Clin Microbiol Rev* 2002;15:506–26.
131. Centers for Disease Control and Prevention. Respiratory infection—Pennsylvania. *MMWR Morb Mortal Wkly Rep* 1997;46;3: 49–56.
132. Tablan OC, Anderson LJ, Arden NH, et al. and the Hospital Infection Control Advisory Committee. Guidelines for prevention of nosocomial pneumonia. *Am J Infect Control* 1994;22:247–292.
133. Occupational Safety and Health Administration. Legionnaires' disease. In: OSHA technical manual section II: 7:1-46. Available at *http://www.osha.gov/dts/osta/otm/otm__iii/otm__iii__7.html* (accessed 1/24/04).
134. American Society of Heating, Refrigerating and Air-Conditioning Engineers. ASHRAE Standards Committee. 2000 Guideline: minimizing the risk of legionellosis associated with building water systems. 12-2000. Atlanta, GA: American Society of Heating Refrigerating and Air-Conditioning Engineers, 2000.
135. Freije MA, Barbaree JM. *Legionellae control in health care facilities: a guide for minimizing risk.* Indianapolis, IN: HC Information Resources Inc., 1996.
136. Moon S. Building the brand. *Modern Health* 2000;32(3):37–51.

137. National Institute for Occupational Safety and Health, Department of Health and Human Services. Protecting building environments from airborne chemical, biological, or radiological attacks. Publication no. 2002-139 Cincinnati, OH: NIOSH, HHS, 2002. Available at *http://www.cdc.gov/niosh/bldvent/2002-139.html* (accessed 1/24/04).
138. U.S. Army Edgewood Chemical Biological Center (ECBC) and the Protective Design Center (PDC) of the U.S. Army Corps of Engineers. Protecting buildings and their occupants from airborne hazards. Draft report TI 853-01 October 2001. Headquarters U.S. Army Corps of Engineers Engineering and Construction Division Directorate of Military Programs Washington, DC 20314-1000.
139. Dasbach EJ, Davies GM, Teutsch SM. Burden of aspergillosis-related hospitalizations in the United States. *Clin Infect Dis* 2000;31: 1524–1528.
140. Lin S-J, Schranz J, Teutsch SM. Aspergillosis case-fatality rate: systematic review of the literature. *Clin Infect Dis* 2001;32:358–66.
141. Lundstrom T, Pugliese G, Bartley J, et al. Organizational and environmental factors that affect worker health and safety and patient outcomes. *Am J Infect Control* 2002;30:93–106.
142. Gerteis M. Conference overview: through the patient's eyes—improvement strategies that work. *Jt Comm J Qual Improv* 1999;25: 335–342.
143. Fowler E, MacRae S, Stern A, et al. The built environment as a component of quality care: understanding and including the patient's perspective. *Jt Comm J Qual Improv* 1999;25:352–362.
144. Neely AC, Maley MP. Survival of enterococci and staphylococci on hospital fabrics and plastic. *J Clin Microbiol* 2000;38:724–726.
145. Noskin GA, Peterson LR. Engineering infection control through facility design. *Emerg Infect Dis* 2001;7:354–357.
146. Kool JL, Carpenter JC, Fields BS. Effect of monochloramine disinfection of municipal drinking water on risk of nosocomial Legionnaires' disease. *Lancet* 1999;353:272–277.
147. Bilchik GS. New vistas. Evidence-based design projects look into the links between a facility's environment and its care. *Health Facil Manage* 2002;15(8):19–24.
148. Martin C. Putting patients first: integrating hospital design and care. *Lancet* 2000;356:518.
149. Reiling J. Designing a safe hospital. Publication 1 Series Symposium Partnership Symposium, Oct 16–19, 2002 Washington, DC. In: Carlson School of Management, University Minnesota.
150. Bartley J, Bjerke NB. Infection control considerations in critical care unit design and construction: a systematic risk assessment. *Crit Care Nurs Q* 2001;24(3):43–58.
151. Memarzadeh F, Manning A. Thermal comfort, uniformity and ventilation effectiveness in patient rooms: performance assessment using ventilation indices. *ASHRAE Trans* 2000;106:748–761.
152. Memarzadeh F, Jiang J. A methodology for minimizing risk from airborne organisms in hospital isolation room. *ASHRAE Trans* 2000; 106:731–737.
153. Ninomura PE, Bartley J. New ventilation guidelines for health-care facilities. *ASHRAE J* 2001;43:29–33.
154. Memarzadeh F, Manning AP. Comparison of operating room ventilation systems in the protection of the surgical site. *ASHRAE Trans* 2002;108:3–15.
155. Anderson RL, Mackel DC, Stoler BS, et al. Carpeting in hospitals: an epidemiological evaluation. *J Clin Microbiol* 1982;15:408–415.
156. Skoutelis AT, Westenfelder GO, Beckerdite M, et al., Hospital carpeting and epidemiology of *Clostridium difficile. Am J Infect Control* 1994;22:212–217.
157. Environmental Protection Agency (EPA). Consumer articles treated with pesticides. U.S. EPA, 04/28/1998. Available at *http://www.epa.gov/pesticides/factsheets/treatart.htm* (accessed 1/24/04).
158. Centers for Medicare and Medicaid Services. Hospital conditions of participation. Code of Federal Regulations, 42(3):474–496. 42CFR482 2002. Baltimore: Department of Health and Human Services, 2002.
159. Joint Commission on Accreditation of Healthcare Organizations. *Comprehensive accreditation manual for hospitals: the official handbook.* CAH00SJ. Oakbrook Terrace, IL: JCAHO Press, 2003.
160. Centers for Disease Control and Prevention (CDC) and Health-care Infection Control Practices Advisory Committee (HICPAC). Guideline for environmental infection control for health-care facilities. Available at: http://www.cdc.gov/ncidod/hip/enviro/guide.htm (accessed 1/24/04).
161. Centers for Disease Control and Prevention. CDC guidelines for prevention of nosocomial pneumonia. *MMWR Morb Mortal Wkly Rep* 1997;46:RR1:1–79.
162. Garner J. Hospital Infection Control Practices Advisory Committee. Guideline for isolation precautions in hospitals. *Am J Infect Control* 1996;24:24–52.
163. Bolyard EA, Tablan OC, Williams WW, et al. Guideline for infection control in health care personnel, 1998. *Am J Infect Control* 1998;26: 289–354.
164. Centers for Disease Control and Prevention (CDC). Guidelines for preventing opportunistic infections among hematopoietic stem cell transplant recipients. *MMWR Morb Mortal Wkly Rep* 2000;49(RR-10):1–125.
165. Occupational Safety and Health Administration (OSHA), US Department of Labor, 29 CFR 1926.50 and 51. Occupational Safety and Health Administration safety and health regulations for construction. Occupational health and environmental controls: 1979; 1993.
166. Occupational Safety and Health Administration (OSHA).Occupational exposure to bloodborne pathogens: final rule. 29 C.F.R, §1910.1030. *Federal Register* 1991:56:64175–64182.
167. National Institute for Occupational Safety and Health (NIOSH). Building air quality. A guide for building owners and facility managers. Publication 91-114. Cincinnati OH: NIOSH, HHS, 1991. Available at *http://www.cdc.niosh/bldvent/2002-139.html* (accessed 1/24/04).
168. National Institute for Occupational Safety and Health. Selecting, evaluating and using sharps disposal containers. Publication 97-111. Cincinnati, OH: NIOSH, HHS, 1997. Available at *http://www.cdc.niosh/sharps1.html* (accessed).
169. Jensen PA, Schafer MP. Sampling and characterization of bioaerosols. NIOSH manual of analytical methods; revised 6/99. Available at *http://www.cdc.gov/niosh/nmam/pdfs/chapter-j.pdf* (accessed).
170. Michigan Department of Consumer and Industry Services (MDCIS). *Minimum design standards for health care facilities in Michigan.* Lansing: MDCIS Press, 1998. Available at *http://www.michigan.gov/documents/cis_bhs_fhs_standards_health_care_facilities_37364_7.pdf* (accessed 1/24/04).
171. Bartley JM, ed. Association for Professionals in Infection Control and Epidemiology (APIC). *APIC infection control tool kit series, construction and renovation,* 2nd ed. Washington, DC: Association for Professionals in Infection Control and Epidemiology Press, 2002.
172. American Institute of Architects Academy of Architecture for Health. *1996–7 Guidelines for design and construction of hospital and health care facilities.* Washington, DC: American Institute of Architects Press, 1996.
173. Bartley JM. Water issues in healthcare. In: Pfeiffer J, ed. *APIC text of infection control and epidemiology.* Washington, DC: Association for Professionals in Infection Control and Epidemiology Press, 2000: 78.1–78.6.
174. Barber JM. Key considerations in emergency and trauma unit design. *Crit Care Nurs Q* 1991;14(1):71–82.
175. Boyce JM, Pittet D. Guidelines for hand hygiene in health-care settings. *Am J Infect Control* 2002;30(8):S1–46.
176. Office of Fire Safety, MDCIS. Policy 2-25. Alcohol based waterless hand sanitizing cleaner. Oct. 10,2002. Available at *http://www.michigan.gov/cis0,1607, 7-154-10575-55727--,00.html* (accessed 1/24/04).
177. Rutala WA. Water as a reservoir of nosocomial pathogens. *Infect Control Hosp Epidemiol* 1997;18:609–616.
178. Manangan LP, Anderson RL, Arduino MJ, et al. Sanitary care and maintenance of ice-storage chests and making machines in healthcare facilities. *Am J Infect Control* 1998;26:111–112.
179. Pavelchak N, DePersis RP, London M, et al. Identification of factors that disrupt negative air pressurization of respiratory isolation rooms. *Infect Control Hosp Epidemiol* 2000;21:191–195.

89

DESIGN AND MAINTENANCE OF HOSPITAL VENTILATION SYSTEMS AND THE PREVENTION OF AIRBORNE NOSOCOMIAL INFECTIONS

ANDREW J. STREIFEL

A building ventilation system is expected to supply air at a comfortable temperature and humidity level (1,2). In the hospital setting, heating, ventilation, and air conditioning (HVAC) systems must often provide specially conditioned air to protect the health of patients and staff. Certain patients are particularly vulnerable to infection from airborne pathogens (3). Others, such as tuberculosis patients, are potential sources of airborne infection, which may put those around them at risk. To design a proper hospital ventilation system, one must be familiar with both the physical and biologic characteristics of airborne agents causing nosocomial infections. Knowledge of ventilation strategies and equipment used to reduce the potential for airborne transmission of disease requires understanding of airborne particle management for contamination control (4).

The science of aerobiology began with Louis Pasteur's discoveries in the middle nineteenth century. By this time, investigators had made great strides in characterizing airborne flora and fauna and in developing methods for accurate quantitative sampling of these populations. During the 1930s, William Wells published on the infectious capacity of droplets and droplet nuclei. He also studied the air-sterilizing properties of ultraviolet (UV) light. By the 1960s, investigators were reporting on the airborne transmission of a variety of infections, including tuberculosis, influenza, smallpox, and measles. From particle science and fluid dynamics has evolved the study of bioaerosols, which quantitatively describes the generation and dispersal mechanisms that dictate the behavior of airborne microorganisms (5). By applying an understanding of these biologic and physical principles, the hospital can provide a ventilation system that can help protect against the spread of nosocomial or occupationally acquired infection.

BIOAEROSOLS AND INFECTION

For an object to remain airborne, it must be small enough so that the viscosity of the air impedes its fall in response to gravity. Lewis Stokes (6) developed an equation that predicts the falling velocity of a particle as a function of its diameter. Stokes's law for determining the sedimentation velocity (V_s) of particles from 1 to 100 μm in diameter is as follows:

$$V_s = \frac{2}{9}\frac{\sigma - \rho}{\mu}\rho^2$$

where σ is the density of the particle, *g* is the acceleration of gravity, ρ is the density of the medium, *r* is the radius of the particle, and μ is the viscosity of the medium.

Gregory (6) published a table of experimentally observed falling velocities for a number of microorganisms. It can be readily observed that many particles ranging in size from 1 to 5 μm have falling velocities in still air on the order of 1 yard an hour. Many spores, such as those of *Aspergillus fumigatus,* have roughened surfaces that tend to further enhance their buoyancy. Such particles can stay airborne almost indefinitely and can ride on air currents for thousands of miles from their point of origin (Fig. 89.1).

It is important to realize that, if such small particles were entrained in a patient's respiratory airstream, they are of the size most likely to elude the cilial and mucosal defenses of the upper respiratory tract and to deposit in the alveoli of the deep lung (Fig. 89.2). Since the early 1970s, investigators have enhanced the understanding of the respiratory fate of small particles as a function of their Stokes diameter.

Quantitative information about particles is as reliable as the measuring instrumentation. By knowing the airborne spore concentration in a given air body and the tidal volume of the lung, one can estimate the probability of inhaling a certain quantity of pathogenic material. Riley and Nardell (7) used the concept of infectious dose in the form of quanta to predict the probability of infection from the release of infectious particles. Using ventilation, one can achieve protection, to a degree, before reaching a point of diminishing returns (8) for infection control, especially for agents such as *Mycobacterium tuberculosis.*

Reliable assessment of biologic risks from airborne pathogens is difficult because of the variables that are intrinsic to living systems. Two *Aspergillus* spores or influenza virus particles may have widely differing potentials for causing infection, depending on such factors as viability of the spores or particles and the

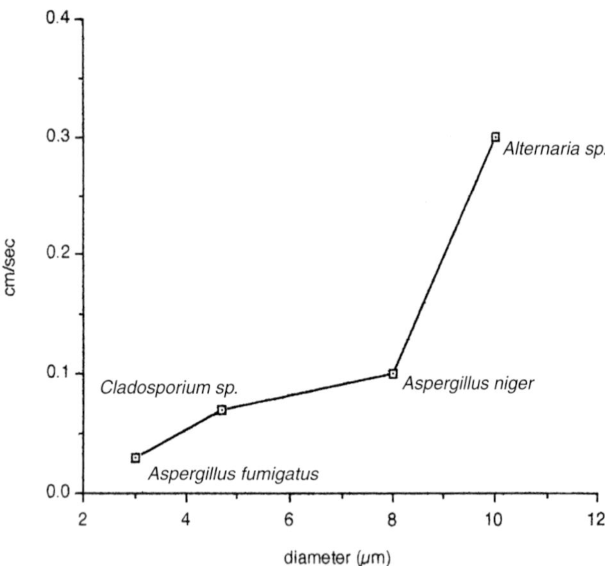

Figure 89.1. Observed terminal velocities of fall of spores and pollen related to diameter. Falling velocity of selected spores in centimeters per second. (From Gregory PH. *The microbiology of the atmosphere,* 2nd ed. New York: John Wiley & Sons, 1973:21, with permission.)

health status of the person inhaling them. To determine control strategies for such agents, it is first necessary to estimate what constitutes an infective dose and then to determine what sort of ventilation control system will reduce concentrations of the suspected pathogen to a safe or noninfective level (9).

GENERAL VENTILATION PRINCIPLES

Although air is a gaseous mixture containing nitrogen, oxygen, carbon dioxide, and a number of trace elements, it behaves in accordance with the principles of fluid dynamics. In descriptions of ventilation systems, air is treated as though it were a liquid flowing through the system. Air moves in response to

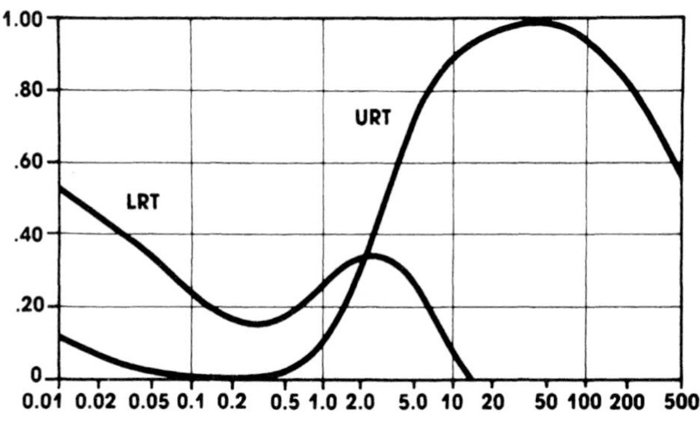

Figure 89.2. Upper and lower respiratory tract (URT and LRT) deposition of idealized spherical particles as a function of diameter. (From Rhame FS, Mazzarella M, Streifel AJ, et al. Evaluation of commercial air filters for fungal spore removal efficiency. Third International Conference on Nosocomial Infections, Atlanta, 1990, with permission.)

pressure. For liquids, the most common source of pressure is gravity. For gases, the most common source of pressure is temperature. The global system of air movement is powered by the rays of the sun. In a building HVAC system, pressure is provided by fans that push or pull air through the building. The most basic rule of airflow in a duct system is that air in must equal air out (10). For any two points in a closed duct, $A_1V_1 = A_2V_2$, where A_1 is the cross-sectional area (measured in square feet) and V_1 is the air velocity (in feet per minute). A_1V_1 gives the airflow in cubic feet per minute (cfm). This equation indicates that if the ducts contract (reducing A), air speed, V, must increase proportionally to maintain the same cubic feet per minute flow rate.

The basic rule of air pressure is $TP = VP - SP$, where TP is the total pressure in the system, VP is the velocity pressure, and SP is the static pressure. Velocity pressure is measured in the direction of airflow and is directly proportional to V, the speed of the moving air. Velocity pressure is always positive. Static pressure is the pressure a body of air exerts on its container, and it can be measured in all directions. Static pressure may be either positive or negative. It is pressure that tends to either burst (positive pressure) or collapse (negative pressure) the duct. If a body of air increases in speed, the velocity pressure increases whereas the static pressure drops.

TP, the total pressure, may be either positive or negative and is the sum of the static and velocity pressure. As a body of air moves through a duct system in response to pressure generated by a fan, the total pressure in the system decreases because of frictional losses between the moving air body and the walls of its container, the duct system. This concept is illustrated by a third equation, $TP_1 = TP_2 - H_L$, which tells that, for a body of air moving from point 1 to point 2, the total pressures at the two points differ by the frictional losses (H_L) caused by the intervening run of duct.

These three rules provide the conceptual framework within which ventilation systems are designed. In a simple recirculating model, the fan creates sufficient positive pressure to force air through the supply duct work and sufficient negative pressure to draw the air out of the rooms into the return duct work and back to the fan, completing the circuit. The pressure generated by the fan must be sufficient to overcome the energy losses created by friction between the moving air and the duct system through which it travels. The duct work blows air into the various rooms through supply openings. The air circulates in the room and then moves toward return openings that draw air back into the return duct system with negative pressure (suction).

The supply and return openings in the room illustrate an important difference between positive and negative pressure ventilation. An individual with healthy lungs can easily blow out a candle at arm's length. The same healthy lungs could not generate enough negative pressure, or suction, to cause the flame to even flicker (11). The supply duct is comparable with blowing out the candle, whereas the exhaust is attempting to suck it out. We refer to the strong directional flow of positively pressured supply air as "throw," whereas the negatively pressured exhaust duct has a "capture velocity" (Fig. 89.3). The control of such a ventilation system is facilitated by a sealed room. A seal on the room allows air to enter and escape only through the ducted

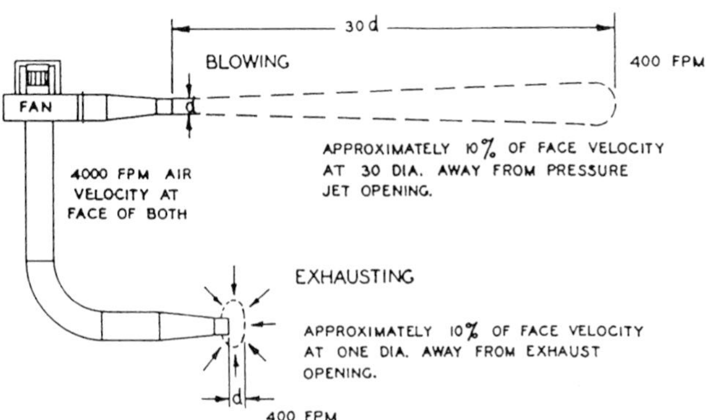

Figure 89.3. Basic difference between flow and pressure openings.

openings. Such measures help to maintain consistent control of the ventilation (12).

HOSPITAL VENTILATION SYSTEMS

In designing a HVAC system for any occupied building, one must properly size ducts and fans to provide the proper air pressures and duct velocities to meet the ventilation requirements of the entire building. Properly sized heating and cooling equipment and noise reduction enter into the total calculations, as does some sort of filtration or air cleaning system. As air recirculates in a building, it builds up an increasing load of gaseous contaminants that are not readily removed by filtration. It is necessary to exhaust a certain percentage of this stale air and replace it with fresh outdoor air to ensure occupant health and comfort (13). A wide variety of systems have been used to meet these criteria. I consider a few of the more common types with an eye toward the needs of the hospital environment.

Central Air Conditioning System

This system brings in fresh outdoor air and mixes it with recirculated air. This air mixture is filtered and conditioned for temperature and humidity according to institutional requirements and then distributed to all building locations. This system is favored for its low cost and simplicity. In a large hospital, the major drawback of centrally conditioned air is the difficulty in adapting it to the specific requirements of local areas, which may have differing heating and cooling needs. This is a particular problem in cold climates in which rooms along the exterior shell require warmer air than rooms in the central core. Large central supply ducts, which reduce noise by slowing airflow, require large amounts of space. Efforts to create local or zone conditions with additional equipment, such as extra heating and cooling coils or booster fans, rapidly increase costs and are often only partially effective.

Dual Duct System

This system has a central system that separately produces two air streams, one hot and the other cold, which are then parallel-ducted throughout the building. Each room is provided with a mixing box in which the two air streams are blended. This allows individual thermostats and volume controls for each room. Although more expensive and difficult to install, this system can provide a number of microclimates without much add-on equipment. The principal drawbacks are the degree of care required in installing the system and the sound baffling required to reduce the noise created by faster airflows within the smaller duct work. Other variations in the air-handling system may be unique to a regional climate condition that design engineers have considered in the ventilation specifications. This may be a factor for the considerations for humidification or dehumidification.

The control of water in the air-handling system is paramount for controlling potential allergens and pathogens associated with growth of microorganisms on fibrous insulation (14,15). The air-handling system variation can depend considerably on design for the climate. All designs require careful maintenance and operational considerations for infection control. For example, a local fan coil system has often been used in hospital areas requiring supplemental cooling. Such climate control is often provided with local systems that recirculate ambient air and provide dehumidification and cooling. Such systems, although engineered for temperature control, do not accommodate air purification control. The drain pans, if not properly maintained, become reservoirs for local fungal contamination (16). Air conditioners may also be reservoirs for fungal growth or accumulation (17, 18). Such systems should be discouraged for areas in which immunocompromised patients are hospitalized. Recent outbreak investigations have demonstrated prolific growth on cold ducted systems either on filters or associated with mixing boxes.

Filtration

Hospital HVAC systems are often required to perform additional tasks related to the prevention of nosocomial infections. By appropriate use of air-filtration technology, a hospital air-handling system can deliver air that is virtually particle free to areas where such a level of protection is needed. The problem presented by such a rigorous filtration system is the energy cost involved. Most filters scrub the air by trapping particles in dense pleated media. Dense filters impede the flow of air and cause a loss of system pressure. To maintain effective air velocities in the duct work, a more powerful fan must be installed to overcome this pressure drop across the filter.

Filters are rated by their percentage of efficiency. A number of different test methods are used to rate air filters (19,20). Most common are the dioctyl phthalate (DOP) and dust spot tests. The DOP test challenges an air filter with an aerosol 0.3 μm in diameter. A light-scattering instrument downstream measures the penetration of the filter by these particles. A filter that can arrest 99.97% of the DOP particles is referred to as a high-efficiency particulate air (HEPA) filter. This method actually counts particles as a measurement of efficiency.

The dust spot test is used to rate less rigorous filters. This test uses atmospheric air or a defined dust as the challenge. Air upstream and downstream from the tested filter is drawn through filter paper. The samples are then compared for opacity using a photometer. Although not quantitative in evaluating particle reduction, this test measures the ability of a filter to reduce the dirt load of an air stream. Kuehn (21) and Rhame et al. (22) have shown that dust spot methods can measure high-efficiency removal of particles.

The most effective hospital filtration system has been evaluated for air cleaning. Outdoor air is initially filtered through 20% to 40% efficient media, mixed with recirculating air, and sent through a 90% dust spot efficient filter. These 90% filters have been demonstrated to provide nearly 100% efficiency in removing particles 1 to 5 mm in diameter with a lower pressure drop than when the 99.97% HEPA filters are used. Modern filters designed with larger surface areas can provide high filter efficiency while maintaining relatively low pressure drops compared with previous versions of the HEPA filter. Distributing such clean air throughout the system provides an additional layer of safety to all occupants at risk for airborne pathogens. Then, where required, rooms or zones can be HEPA-filtered for a higher degree of protection. Modern filtration technology is creating low-pressure drop filters resulting from fiber electrostatic qualities and increased surface area of the filter. Although reduced resistance pressure while maintaining high-filter efficiency is beneficial for cost savings, careful consideration for proven long-term efficiency is necessary to prevent problems (23). High-efficiency filter innovation certainly helps provide sufficient air volume to assist in maintaining essential air quality parameters in hospitals, which often become deficient in air volume delivery and exhaust as the building ages. Such systems reduce risks created by opening and shutting doors and from transporting vulnerable patients for procedures that cannot be performed in specially protected areas. Filtration continues to dominate priorities for air quality (24,25) in prevention of aspergillosis. The combination of appropriate ventilation parameters (filtration, air exchanges, and pressure) helps in the control of the many sources of opportunistic filamentous fungal infections plaguing the immunocompromised host (26).

AREAS REQUIRING SPECIAL VENTILATION

Certain areas in the hospital have special ventilation systems as described in the HVAC handbook (1) and American Institute of Architects guidelines for hospital construction (2). Air systems have been designed to meet these specific needs, most commonly operating rooms, positive-pressure protective environments, negative-pressure isolation units, and local air control flow life islands (Table 89.1). Each of these situations has specific ventilation requirements related to prevention of nosocomial infection or occupational exposure to airborne infectious diseases or medicated aerosols or gases. All operate on the underlying principle that clean air should move from less contaminated to more contaminated areas (clean to dirty airflow). To more clearly illustrate the principles involved, I discuss a specific patient, pathogen, or procedure for each type of situation.

Protective Environments

Operating Room

Surgery is by nature a process requiring invasive procedures that expose host tissues to the outside environment, creating the potential for exposure to external agents, such as bacteria and fungi. Therefore, in the operating room, the surgical site and instrument table should be considered the cleanest area, and infection control efforts should be directed toward providing protection through appropriate ventilation control.

Surgical site infection is a well-documented surgical complication (27). Aseptic technique and prophylactic antibiotics provide the first line of defense, but it has been shown that removing bacteria and fungi from operating room air helps to minimize infection (28,29). Microorganisms shed by humans are the most common airborne agents in a correctly designed operating room with appropriate air filtration (30). Large volumes of air filtered through high-efficiency filters should be provided from panels in the operating room ceiling over the surgical site. The downward force of air from the ceiling supply diffuser provides a focused ventilated area around the surgical site that is constantly washed by a high-volume flow of clean air. Such airflow moves particles away from the operating table toward the air returns at the margins of the room. It is important that this displacement airflow of filtered air is delivered in such a manner that infectious particles shed by the operating team are swept away toward the return ducts and not trapped and recirculated within the vicinity of the procedure. The more objects that interrupt the airflow pattern, the greater the turbulence. Special clean room laminar flow ventilation with HEPA filtration has been used in orthopedic cases to prevent the consequences of surgical site infections. A vertical flow system designed to provide a downward flow of air over the surgical site actually increases the air exchanges in the cleanest zone (31). Air delivery from a horizontal direction does not provide an extra benefit, because personnel and equipment in the way of the directed airflow cause turbulence and potential trajectory of problematic particles toward the surgical site. Vertical flow is preferred over horizontal airflow for space management and infection control considerations (32). Memarzadeh and Manning (33) performed computational fluid dynamic studies which reinforced the empirical findings of Lidwell (32) that a vertical flow with velocity from 30 to 35 linear feet per minute (lfpm) (0.15 to 0.18 m/second) could be achieved at the surgical site. If air supply can provide a laminar flow regimen albeit at a lower velocity than official definition of laminar flow of 90 lfpm (0.45 m/second), control of the shed particles over of the surgical site is realistic.

Pressure management in the protective operating room environment is designated by a positive airflow out of the cleanest area of the operating room suites. This designation does not give guidance for what is necessary to provide that pressurization. Murray et al. (12) have suggested that a differential air volume (supply versus exhaust or return) exceeding 10% to 15% provides the required airflow. This concept works best in a high volume environment like an operating room or in bone marrow transplant rooms, which require higher airflow volumes. Such suggestions have not been validated. Consistent management of pressure is a problem when windows are operable or doors are left open. Using an anteroom or door closure is an essential component for room pressure management. Operating rooms have multiple doors, and, if any of those doors are open, the pressure differential is eliminated until the door is closed. Proce-

TABLE 89.1. SUMMARY OF SPECIAL-VENTILATION HOSPITAL AREAS

	Infectious Disease Isolation Room	Compromised Host Ventilation	Operating Room
Air pressure	Negative	Positive	Positive
Room air changes	≥6 renovation ≥12 new construction	>12	15 or 25
Sealed	Yes	Yes	Yes
Directed airflow	Clean-to-dirty (employee clean)	Clean-to-dirty (patient clean)	Displacement flow in surgical site critical
Filtration supply	90% (dust-spot ASHRAE 52–76)	99.97%[c]	90%
Recalculation	No	Yes	Yes

ASHRAE, American Society for Heating, Refrigerating, and Air Conditioning Engineers.
[a] Minimized infiltration for ventilation control.
[b] Clean-to-dirty (negative) to infectious patient (positive) away from compromised patient.
[c] Fungal filter at point of use—high-efficiency particulate air (HEPA) 99.97% @ 0.3-μm particles.

dural practice for operating rooms should include closed doors, except for egress, while the surgical site is open.

Investigations have shown value in properly clothing the operating room team for maximum contamination control. The surgical team is a potential reservoir of infection. The average person sheds approximately 10^7 particles of sloughed skin per day (34,35). During an hour-long surgical procedure, each individual in the operating theater may shed 10^6 particles. Each one of these particles may be carrying bacteria that can infect a surgical site. However, in the properly ventilated operating room, such shedding should not pose an infectious risk to patients. For operative procedures involving insertion of a prosthetic device and for which ultraclean air may be desired, shedding can be greatly reduced by providing surgical personnel with negatively pressurized evacuated gowns.

Opportunistic environmental microbes such as *Clostridium perfringens* or *Aspergillus* spores should be minimized in an operating room setting. These soil microorganisms are readily filtered from incoming air if filters are installed and maintained properly. Such microorganisms would be expected in air supply systems that have leaks or tears in the filters. A lack of maintenance also is a problem, because it allows a reservoir of microbial growth in the air-delivery system. Such inadequate maintenance or installation must be avoided in the critical surgical areas.

Shed microbes from human attendants must be controlled with the directed airflow and barrier protection. Tunevall and Jorbeck (36) raised the issue that masks do not affect the presence of microbes in a surgical setting. The range of microbial recovery from air sampling suggests that the use of barriers prevents the inadvertent shedding of microbes from exposed areas such as the mouth or hair. Barriers have also been shown to prevent contamination of drapes and the surgical site. With aseptic technique and appropriate ventilation, the exposed skin from both the patient and attendants becomes an important source for microbial exposure in the surgical setting (37). Unclean floors from track dirt and accumulated debris could become an internal source for *C. perfringens* or other soil microorganisms (38) if disturbed. Human source microbes can be controlled with aseptic technique (39) and barrier protection (40). A forced air ventilation system enhances the cleanliness of the critical surgery area. The ventilation system is essential for protecting the surgical site using particle displacement dynamics of properly directed purified air movement.

The patient is also a potential source for infecting the personnel in the operating room setting. The generation of aerosols during the use of cautery and lasers is a matter of concern. Information on the transmission of infectious agents by these procedures is minimal; however, scavenging devices are being used to minimize the presence of obnoxious odors or aerosols in the operating room setting. For example, such local exhaust and filtration systems can be used to capture problematic aerosols generated during the removal of extrapulmonary tuberculosis lesions.

Positive-pressure Room (Protective Environments)

Oncology and Solid Organ Transplant Patient

Modern medical technology has provided methods for transplanting immunologically dissimilar tissue between donor and recipient. The immunosuppressive treatment necessary to prevent rejection of the transplanted organ or tissue puts the host at risk for opportunistic infections. Environmental pathogens causing legionellosis or aspergillosis are common (3,41,42) and must be controlled in a critical hospital setting. These environmental microorganisms pose little threat to the healthy individual protected by normal humoral and cellular immune defenses.

A. fumigatus is a common soil fungus. Its spores range in diameter from 2 to 3.5 μm and are commonly recovered from outdoor air samples. This airborne fungus is cosmopolitan and is commonly recovered when using a volumetric air sampler. This thermotolerant fungus poses a particular risk as a nosocomial pathogen because of its ability to reach the alveoli in the lung and its ability to thrive at 37°C. On inhalation by the granulocytopenic patient, these spores can cause a form of pneumonia that is difficult to diagnose and treat. Peterson et al. (43) noted that 17 of 19 patients with aspergillosis died in a series of 60 patients. Opportunistic filamentous fungal infections seem to be less responsive to conventional antibiotic therapy. Providing spore-free air through filtration and ventilation and local activity control is the best method for preventing infections transmitted by fungal spores (44). Because some patients remain immunocompromised for up to several months, it is also necessary to minimize airborne environmental contamination by microbes in the environment of convalescent transplantation and oncology patients.

The basic ventilation approach in such facilities is to provide positive-pressure ventilation wherein the amount of HEPA-filtered supply air exceeds the amount of air exhausted by at least 10%. The offset should be about 125 cfm between the supply and exhaust/return to provide a substantial difference for ensuring consistent pressure differential in the special ventilation rooms. This difference should be able to establish a pressure differential greater than 0.01 inches water gauge (2.5 Pa). By delivering air at a rate of between six and ten air changes per hour, depending on heating and cooling requirements, and by using supply and return air that ensures thorough mixing, the room can be kept relatively spore-free (45). Supply air diffusers should be located in the ceiling and positioned to throw air down far enough into the room to ensure particle displacement and mixing. In the protected ventilation environment, the filtered air should flow from the vulnerable patient toward the corridor. Such clean to dirty airflow provides air movement that should prevent inhalation of common airborne fungal spores by the patient.

Bone Marrow Transplantation Unit

Simple positive pressure ventilation may not provide sufficient protection for the extremely vulnerable patient. Patients requiring bone marrow transplants are often housed in laminar air flow (LAF) rooms (41). Such rooms are designed with one entire wall of HEPA filters. Fans blow air through these filters at high velocity [about 100 to 150 lfpm (46,47)] and out through high-capacity return ducts located on the opposite wall. Although the term laminar flow is not an accurate description of the fluid dynamics of the airflow under such conditions, the effect is that smoke particles injected into the LAF air stream are swept straight across the room, parallel to the floor, and out through the return. It is as though a piston of clean air is being pushed across the room, driving any contaminants out through the return ducts. To enhance patient protection, all caregivers should work downstream from the patient so as not to impede the protective airflow across the bed. Such rooms provide more than 100 air changes per hour. The high velocity of the airflow can create uncomfortable drafts and excess noise. Housing patients in such an environment is an extreme measure and can be problematic during long periods of convalescence. Because of high cost and limited availability, these LAF systems are difficult to provide for all immunosuppressed patients. Therefore, less drastic ventilation control procedures are often recommended (48,49) (Table 89.2).

TABLE 89.2. COMPONENTS OF A PROTECTED ENVIRONMENT

Sealed room (windows and utility connections)
Increased room air changes (>12)
Highly filtered air (>95% efficient @ 0.3-μm particles)
Positive pressure rooms (>10% or >125 cfm) supply over exhaust/return air volume)
Directed airflow (airflow from the "clean" patient to the "dirty" patient)
Leakage total for room at <0.5 ft^2
Procedural practice modification
Self-closing doors

The problem most frequently associated with contaminated hospital air is construction activity (50). Control of aerosol generation, airflow, filtration, barrier penetration, and traffic requires careful monitoring and supervision to maintain specially ventilated areas. Air filtration and increased room air changes help to prevent infection in areas adjacent to construction activity (51,52). Patients must be continuously confined in such rooms to be totally protected. Items brought into such areas can also be contaminated (53) with fungi from outdoors. The ventilation procedural practices in the patient's room and construction and maintenance practices must be carefully controlled throughout critical care facilities (54). (See Chapter 88.)

Airborne Infectious Disease Control

Negative-Pressure Isolation: Airborne Infection Isolation (AII) Room

Hospitals often house patients who have infectious diseases spread by the airborne route in negative-pressure isolation rooms to prevent escape of pathogens from the room to surrounding areas (Table 89.3). Patients harboring *M. tuberculosis* can pose an occupational risk to the caregiver (see Chapter 37). With the development of antibiotic-resistant *M. tuberculosis,* infections may be difficult to treat and may be fatal in immunocompromised healthcare workers. During contagious stages of the disease, patients can create infectious aerosols by coughing, speaking, singing, or sneezing. The infectious droplets can dry in air to form droplet nuclei 1 to 5 μ in size and float for long periods, increasing the probability of inhalation. A single inhaled tubercle bacillus may be able to produce an infection. Although tuberculosis patients must be isolated to minimize the risk of transmission of infection, the other infectious diseases spread by the airborne route also require isolation using special ventilation (9, 55).

In designing ventilation for isolation rooms, the area of the infected patient should be considered dirty (Fig. 89.4). The current strategy is to provide negative pressure to ventilate the room with exhaust exceeding supply by about more than 10% or by more than 125 cfm difference. It must be noted that the relatively low differential for air volume requires significant sealing of the room to prevent leakage. The room air should be exhausted to the outside or if returned for reuse should be filtered through a HEPA filter. This prevents air contaminated by the patient from escaping into the rest of the hospital and reduces the concentration of airborne tubercle bacilli within the room.

The room exchange rate has been studied with respect to particle removal (9); a point of diminishing returns is reached at about 12 to 15 room air exchanges per hour. The retrofit of older space to the higher air exchanges is difficult and not practi-

TABLE 89.3. INFECTIOUS DISEASES REQUIRING SPECIAL VENTILATION

Herpes Zoster, disseminated
Tuberculosis, pulmonary or laryngeal
Varicella (chickenpox)

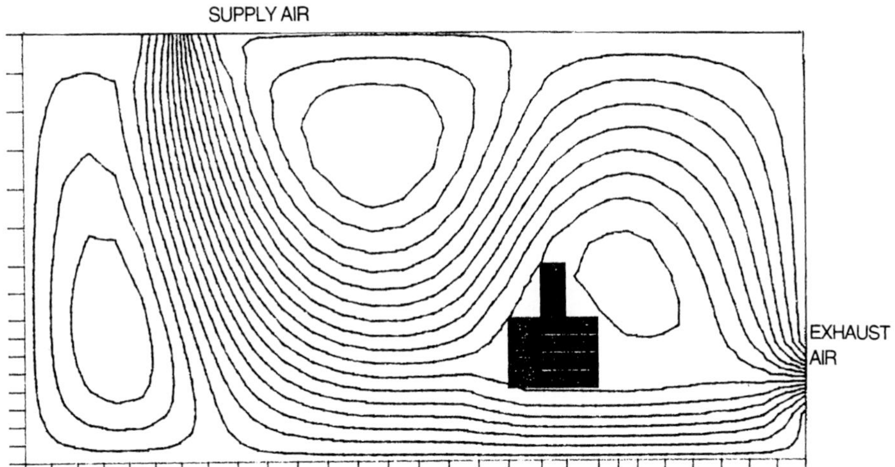

Figure 89.4. Computer simulation of airflow pattern in a patient room that can be used to visualize air patterns in special ventilation rooms. In this example, airflow from the supply air covers the healthcare worker area, passing the "dirty" patient before exhausting.

cal unless new design and construction are planned. To maintain relative pressures, one must ensure that the ventilation in place is working. The control of the airflow depends on the anticipation of exhaust systems deterioration from accumulation of dirt and lint on fan blades and turning vanes. Cleaning the air pathway and exhaust fans helps to ensure consistent pressure relationships.

Installing effective negative-pressure ventilation is more challenging than installing positive-pressure ventilation. The negative-pressure system is easily compromised by air infiltration, and extra attention must be paid to sealing all ducts, doors, walls, and windows of the room. Even if the system is well sealed, it is more difficult to create directional airflow using suction. The clean (employee area) to dirty (patient area) airflow pattern should also be incorporated into isolation room design. The effectiveness of such design features, although intuitive and associated with clean room ventilation methods, must still be verified. There are difficulties in applying exhaust ventilation to clear a room of low concentrations of infectious particles. One study reported that when the concentration of microorganisms is low, a 14-fold increase in fresh air ventilation only reduces concentrations by 10% (8).

Clearly, additional measures are required to make the room of the infectious patient safe. Source control measures, such as surgical masks for patients, local exhaust ventilation near the patient's head, and a respiratory protection plan for employees, are necessary for a comprehensive plan. UV light fixtures mounted high on the walls of the room have been shown to reduce the concentration of airborne bacteria. Riley et al. (56) demonstrated that a 30-watt UV light reduced airborne bacteria at a rate equivalent to 20 air changes per hour of mechanical ventilation. It must be remembered that when using UV light or portable filters to enhance ventilation for particle removal, the devices do increase equivalent room air changes for airborne infectious diseases control but do not satisfy fresh air requirements (13).

Maintenance Considerations

Design of sophisticated hospital ventilation systems must include ongoing routine maintenance as part of the budget for the project (14). Ventilation systems rapidly fail if not carefully installed, monitored, and repaired as needed. Deferred maintenance is a common problem in many hospital systems. In addition, sophisticated ventilation systems have failed to perform as specified because of inadequate installation. Failure to provide the designed supply of air in special ventilation areas by installing a fan with insufficient delivery capability will create ventilation deficiencies. Likewise, a void in the caulk around a window in a positive pressure room can allow windblown spores to enter the patient's room, bypassing the filtration system and exposing the patient. Improperly installed humidification or cooling systems can allow moisture buildup, creating ideal growth conditions in the air-handling system for potentially lethal mold. Poorly designed gaskets and mounting apparatus can allow dirty air to bypass the HEPA filters and contaminate clean areas. The failure to maintain the system may cause the air balance to change because of increased accumulation of lint and dust on filters; this may decrease the exhaust ventilation. Such changes could alter the negative air balance and cause the room to become positively pressurized (Table 89.4).

When designing a high-performance air-handling system, it is vitally important that all components are easily accessible for routine inspection and maintenance. Filter change-out must be performed according to safe maintenance practice (54). Filter efficiency actually increases during use as trapped particles increase the density of the filter media. At the end of a filter's useful life, it is so loaded with particles that it begins to impede system airflow. Monitoring devices such as manometers or gauges should be installed to measure the pressure drop across filters, and when the indicator exceeds manufacturer's specifications, the filter should be changed. Often, these measuring devices are not operable because of neglected maintenance (57). It is difficult to remove and replace the filter without dislodging

TABLE 89.4. VENTILATION HAZARDS

Problem	Consequences	Possible Solutions
Water-damaged building materials (14)	Water leaks can soak wood, wallboard, insulation, wall coverings, ceiling tiles, and carpeting. All can provide microbial habitat when wet. This is especially true for fungi growing on gypsum board.	1. Incorporate fungi static compounds in building materials in areas at risk for moisture problems 2. Replace water-damaged materials 3. Test for moisture and dry in less than 72 hr
Filter bypasses (46)	Rigorous air filtration requires air flow resistance. Air stream will elude filtration if openings are present because of filter damage or poor fit.	1. Use pressure gauges to ensure that filter is performing at proper static pressure 2. Make ease of installation and maintenance criteria for filter selection. 3. Properly train maintenance personnel in HVAC issues 4. Design system with filters downstream from fans 5. Avoid water on filters or insulation
Improper fan setting (57)	Air must be delivered at design volume to maintain pressure balances. Airflow in special vent rooms reverses.	1. Routinely monitor air flow and pressure balances throughout critical parts of HVAC system
Ductwork disconnections (58)	Dislodged or leaky supply duct runs can spill into or leaky returns may draw from hidden areas. Pressure balance will be interrupted, and infectious material may be disturbed and entrained into hospital air supply.	1. Design a ductwork system that is easy to access, maintain, and repair 2. Train maintenance personnel to regularly monitor air flow volumes and pressure balances throughout the system 3. Test critical areas for appropriate airflow
Air flow impedance (11)	Debris, structural failure, or improperly adjusted dampers can block duct work and prevent designed air flow.	1. Design and budget for a duct system that is easy to inspect, maintain, and repair 2. Alert contractors to use caution when working around HVAC system during the construction phase 3. Regularly clean exhaust grills 4. Provide monitoring for special ventilation areas
Open windows (9,18)	Open windows can alter fan induced pressure balances and allow dirty-to-clean air flow.	1. Use sealed windows 2. Design HVAC system to deliver sufficient outdoor dilution ventilation 3. Monitor CO_2 levels in all occupied areas to ensure adequate fresh air supply 4. Sign windows where fire code prohibits sealing
Dirty window air conditioners (17,18)	Dirt, moisture, and bird droppings can contaminate window air conditioners, which can then introduce infectious material into hospital room.	1. Design such devices out of new construction 2. Where they must be used, make sure that they are routinely inspected and cleaned
Inadequate filtration (55)	Infectious particles pass through filter into vulnerable patient areas. Specify appropriate filters during new construction design phase.	1. Specify appropriate filters during new construction design phase 2. Make sure that HVAC fans are sized to overcome pressure demands of filter system 3. Inspect and test filters for proper installation
Maintenance disruptions (53)	Fan shut-offs, dislodged filter cake contaminates downstream air supply and drain pans, compromises airflow in special ventilation areas.	1. Be sure to budget for rigorous maintenance schedule when designing a facility 2. Design system for easy maintenance 3. Ensure good communication between engineering and maintenance personnel 4.Institute an ongoing training program for all involved staff members
Duct contamination (14,15)	Debris is released during maintenance or cleaning.	1. Provide point-of-use filtration in the critical areas 2. Design air handling system with insulation on the exterior of the ducts 3. No fibrous sound attenuators 4. Decontaminate or encapsulate contamination
Depressurized hospital building (61)	Infiltration of unfiltered air into the building during construction caused aspergillosis in oncology patients	1. Ensure building pressure by over supply air volume by rebalancing or upgrading building ventilation 2. Add doors and weather-stripping to prevent air movement during periods of air imbalance 3. Difficult issue with high-rise buildings

Useful equipment: Moisture Meter Model Tramex Moisture Encounter Professional Equipment Item #M253, $~300,00, 1–800 334–9291; Digital pressure gauge, Energy Conservatory, Minneapolis, MN, ~$800.00, 612–827–1117; Copper-8-quinolinolate, Micropel SWR, Microban Systems Inc. Bradock, PA. 412.351.8686.

CO_2, carbon dioxide, HVAC, heating, ventilation, and air conditioning.

trapped contaminants and sending them downstream. The point-of-use filter (placed at the end of the duct just above the diffuser) in the bone marrow transplantation unit minimizes this effect by preventing more than 95% of the released particles from reaching the patient care area (58).

Fans, cooling coils, and condensate pans must be readily accessible for cleaning and repairs. Studies and reports indicate that failure to design hospital HVAC systems with provisions for routine maintenance access can result in untoward clinical consequences (14). Training of personnel in the principles and importance of ventilation is essential. Often, maintenance personnel shut down critical fan systems without notifying persons in the affected areas. Such shut downs are a real threat because of the lack of ventilation control during those times. Fan systems must be routinely maintained, and shut downs must be carefully planned. Likewise, plans for emergency outages must also include provisions for backup motors or redundant systems. For example, contingencies for failure of the ventilation system in a bone marrow transplantation unit should include changes of procedural practice during the absence of ventilation control. For example, on the patient care unit, should the routine cleaning and patient visitation be temporarily suspended during fan outages? If malfunction is persistent, should supplemental ventilation be provided with portable systems? Such scenarios should also be considered for the ventilation for infectious disease isolation in anticipation of planned or unplanned outages. Finally, it is crucial that funds for ongoing maintenance and training are included in the hospital budget.

Provisions must be made for additional patient protection during construction and remodeling projects (57,58). When wall cavities are opened, large quantities of spores might be released from water-damaged areas hidden from view (59). Protective air environments must be secured from penetration by dust and debris generated during remodeling projects. During a large construction project at a Midwestern hospital, the infection control team purchased an optical particle counter to monitor the operating theaters and ensure that the ventilation system was controlling the air quality during construction (60). Microbiologic air monitoring can also be used, but baseline data must first be generated along with construction monitoring during the project. Results are often hard to interpret, and time spent would be lost to the more important aspect of monitoring the compliance to construction specifications related to infection control during construction. On the other hand, commissioning of ventilation systems by air sampling would ensure that specifications for filter installation and operation have been met.

Verification of Ventilation Parameters for Special Ventilation Rooms

Infection control airflow design specifications should also be verified (61). The parameters important for verification are associated with pressurization, room air exchanges, and filtration. Nicas et al. (62) and Rice et al. (63) showed considerable variation of airflow when special ventilation rooms were tested. Rice et al. reported large pressure variation for positively pressurized rooms primarily because of maintenance manipulation of dampers or fan belts. Negatively pressurized rooms had much lower pressure differentials and were considered more stable, but the airflow direction changed from negative to positive more frequently. The fluctuation from negative to positive was probably due in part to a low pressure differential at or about 0.25 Pa (250 Pa per 1.0 inch water gauge). Recently, Streifel and Marshall (64) clarified parameters that could be measured before occupancy of special ventilation areas. Table 89.5 is a listing of the parameters and notably the pressure measurements are listed. The pressure performance must be considered as a range because of constant variation of outdoor conditions, elevator movement, and doors being used.

Testing and proving that airflow is appropriate, air exchanges are sufficient, and filtration is appropriate permit mechanical ventilation to be ruled out as a source for acquisition of *Aspergillus.* Other considerations can, therefore, be explored.

Air Sampling Methods

The nonviable airborne particle can be detected with the use of a particle counter, optical or laser, that allows real-time air quality analysis. It is important to differentiate particle sizes. The most useful devices for measuring particle sizes are those that determine particle size diameters greater than 0.5 μm, 1.0 μm, and 5.0 μm per cubic foot. The particles at greater than 0.5 μm are used for assessing a clean room, and Military Standard 209 (e) is used to classify clean rooms with particles per cubic foot less than a certain number. The classification is based on increments of 10, and a HEPA filtered (99.97% efficient at 0.3-μm diameter particles) operating room or bone marrow transplant environment with no people should be capable of class 1,000 clean room status or better. The definition of a class 1,000 clean room is that there are less than 1,000 particles per cubic foot greater than 0.5 μm in diameter. Such information is especially useful for ensuring filtration integrity or infiltration in a critical environment before the areas are occupied. These devices are useful for determining the cleanest areas. The class of the room designation can be a useful guideline but should not have such a specification for an absolute number that cannot be exceeded.

The viable airborne particle analysis is more complex, because laboratory expertise is necessary. The selection of media, incuba-

TABLE 89.5. RECOMMENDED MEASUREMENTS FOR SPECIAL VENTILATION ROOMS

	Protective	Airborne Infection
Pressure differentials	>2.5 Pa(0.01 in. w.g.[a])	>0.25 Pa(0.001 in. w.g.)
Air exchanges per hour	>12	>12
Filtration	99.97% @ 0.3 μ DOP[b]	90% (dust spot)
Room airflow direction	Out	In
Clean to dirty airflow in room	Patient clean	Patient dirty
Ideal pressure differential	>8 Pa	>2.5 Pa

[a] Water gauge.
[b] Dioctyl phalate.

tion temperature, and skill for identification of environmental microbes are factors that must be considered if an environmental sampling program is initiated. The purpose for sampling should include determination of what the sampling is expected to evaluate. For example, an air-sampling search for human-shed microbes such as *M. tuberculosis* or staphylococcal species should not be considered because of the difficulty in culturing the slow growing *M. tuberculosis* and because staphylococcal species are frequently shed from humans. Aerosols generated by a medical device such as a drill may be instructive for air sample evaluations but certainly are not routine in any setting. Air sampling from a practical point of view should be considered only for evaluation of the presence of airborne fungi.

Evaluation of the air for airborne fungi yields information that may be helpful in preventing infection or determining the source of airborne opportunistic environmental fungi. Sampling for airborne fungi should be used for determining the levels in areas where patients are at risk for infections from these opportunistic fungi. The media used for sampling a hospital environment should be capable of isolating clinically relevant microorganisms. Because the fungi are capable of growth on a variety of media, clinical media such as Sabouraud or inhibitory mold agar provides direct morphologic identification from the recovered isolates. Some environmental media, although excellent for total recovery, may require extensive subculturing for identification (Table 89.6).

The presence of fungi capable of growth at body temperature is of particular concern. The difference between fungi that grow at room temperature (25°C) and body temperature (37°C) are generally greater than one order of magnitude except in highly filtered environments (Table 89.6). The most common in hospital exposure occurs from improperly filtered incoming air or from internal sources that were disrupted because of construction or maintenance. Air sampling will not prevent infections during construction. Air sampling can provide information that should inform infection control professionals that the air quality is good enough for safe patient care, because control measures are in place. It is difficult to detect the short-term high-dose exposures that occur because of environmental disruption.

There are a variety of samplers capable of viable particle air sampling that include volumetric samplers and slit or sieve impactors. It is important that a volume of air is sampled. Settle plates depend on gravity, but single spores are less than 5.0 μm in diameter and are buoyant aerodynamic particles. Clumps of particles settle, but perhaps the most problematic particles are those that are capable of entering the lungs. These respirable particles are less than 5.0 μm in diameter. Collecting the particles in sufficient quantity is essential to detect low concentrations of spores causing nosocomial infection. Arnow et al. (14) reported infection rates of about 1.2% with *Aspergillus flavus* and *A. fumigatus* at 2.2 and 1.1 colony-forming units (CFU)/m^3, respectively. Rhame et al. (65) reported a 5.4% infection rate with *A. fumigatus* at 0.9 CFU/m^3. A major problem with most samplers used in hospitals is low sample volume capability. Most samplers are designed to sample dirty environments. Samplers that sample 1 cfm may fail to detect spores at levels less than 1.0 CFU/m^3. Hospital air samples should be at least 35 cubic feet or 1.0 m^3 to detect low levels of spores. Disadvantages of many samplers include low-volume sampling, drying of media with long sampling times, difficult manipulation of culture plates, and difficult calibration. A slit to agar sampler with a timer up to 60 minutes may be the best choice of sampler dependent on the type of timer, noise levels, and portability.

TABLE 89.6. MEDIA AND INCUBATION TEMPERATURES FOR CULTURING AIR SAMPLES

Appropriate selection of growth media helps to expedite identification
- Sabouraud, Czapek, inhibitory mold agar, etc.

Incubation temperature
- At 25°C, greater numbers of airborne fungi will grow; lower temperatures help to distinguish infiltration or filtration deficiencies
- At 35°C, the temperature selects for pathogen recovery; *Aspergillus fumigatus* and *Aspergillus flavus* are thermotolerant

Interpretation of Data

Timing for detecting airborne fungal levels is important for interpretation of results. For example, activity evaluation with an air sampler may reveal high concentrations of airborne fungi during renovation activity of a water-damaged bathroom. The best use of air sampling is before occupancy to determine proper filter installation and room pressurization. The purpose of such sampling is to establish rank order for the cleanest areas. The best filtration should demonstrate the lowest particle or viable airborne fungal counts. Such numbers are best demonstrated as baseline before occupancy. Subsequent sampling should take into account people and conditions such as incorrect airflow in a protective environment. Exposure to high levels of an airborne infectious agent over a short time is probably the greatest risk to the host. The ability to capture such events is difficult. The sampling of the environment should be to determine if the ventilation systems work according to specification. Therefore, the areas with the best filtration, pressurization, and air exchanges should have the lowest airborne fungal counts. This should also be true for nonviable airborne particles detected with a particle counter.

If pathogens (*A. fumigatus, A. flavus,* or other opportunists capable of growth at body temperature) are recovered from protected environments, consideration should be taken for single-plate hits versus multiple-plate hits from pathogenic fungi. Random isolate recoveries may be represented by a single colony on a plate. Greater than two colonies, for example, *A. fumigatus,* may represent a point source within the patient care environment. Repeat sampling under such circumstances should determine if it was a passing phenomenon (Table 89.7).

Interpretation of the results from air sampling requires a comparison of sample locations. If sampling is requested, the cleanest environment (i.e., operating rooms or bone marrow transplant unit) should have the lowest numbers of microorganisms recovered. The basic comparison should be from clean to cleanest in CFU/m^3. For better results, such comparisons should be done with culture media incubated at room temperature. Room temperature incubation at about 25°C is more sensitive for fungal recovery. The comparison samples for detecting filtration integrity or potential infiltration should also be incubated at room

TABLE 89.7. INTERPRETATION OF AIR SAMPLE DATA

- Rank order determination
  - Clean to cleanest with the lowest counts in the areas with proper ventilation control (pressure, air exchanges, and filtration)
  - Lowest counts in the areas with best filtration.
  - Comparison data necessary (outdoor vs. lobby vs. patient care area)
- Indoor-to-outdoor ratio
  - I/O <1 normal
  - I/O >1 potential problems.
  - Consider outdoor conditions and comparison data colony types
- Qualitative information
  - Pathogen recovery with results >1 CFU pathogen per plate a potential indoor source
  - Comparison to determine homogenous versus heterogeneous population
- Temperature selectivity
  - Pathogens grow at temps >35°C
  - Total fungi more sensitive to I/O at 25°C

CFU, colony-forming unit.

temperature. Qualitative analysis, however, of airborne pathogens such as *A. fumigatus* is better at close to body temperature (>35°C), because the other mesophilic fungi are inhibited, allowing the pathogens to be more easily detected. The pathogens are easily obscured when the samples are incubated at room temperature. Also, the rank order comparison is difficult at the higher temperature, because the differences in levels in highly filtered areas are not very great. For example, the difference in recovery from media incubated at room temperature for samples taken from the nurses' station in the bone marrow transplant unit versus those taken from HEPA-filtered rooms might be 55 and 4 CFU/m^3, whereas the same samples incubated at 35°C might yield 10 and 4 CFU/m^3, respectively. The samples incubated at room temperature are intended to demonstrate ventilation deficiencies, whereas the samples incubated at body temperature should be able to detect pathogens. Pathogen content should be less than 1.0 CFU/m^3 with repeat sampling. Invariably *A. fumigatus* shows up as a single isolate with few, if any, other microorganisms on the sample plate. A combination of factors that demonstrate the cleanest environment with the lowest pathogen counts are important for data interpretation. The value of comparisons with outside recoveries is that levels of *A. fumigatus* are often higher outside the hospital than inside, for example, 9.0 versus 1.0 CFU per sample. When adjusted for CFU/m^3, outside samples have much higher levels than inside, allowing an indoor-to-outdoor ratio of less than 1. However, if the inside levels are higher than outside levels (except during snow cover or after rain), then an internal source may be suspect. The recovery of two or more colonies of a pathogen from media incubated at 35°C may indicate an internal point source (66).

CONCLUSIONS

It is important that infection control, environmental, engineering, and maintenance personnel actively monitor the proper operation of the HVAC system. Smoke tubes can be used to demonstrate airflow movement in special ventilation areas. However, new instruments are capable of measuring very low pressures and should be incorporated into the quality measures necessary for a safe environment of care. All maintenance, surveillance, repair, and construction activities should be coordinated in such a manner as to ensure that precautions to protect the health and well-being of all patients and staff are implemented. Use of pressure (airflow direction), room air changes per hour, and filtration verification specifications are essential for effectively maintaining protective and airborne infection isolation environments.

Protection from Bioaerosols

Concern for the protection of buildings is imminent especially because terrorism is part of the current state of affairs in the world order. Planning to provide an upgrade of building systems for protection certainly is being considered as part of the National Bioterrorism Hospital Preparedness Program. Hospitals should consider such planning; however, certain preparedness for fire protection and common sense planning for natural microbial agents (pathogenic *Aspergillus* species) will certainly help to prepare healthcare buildings for such events. Previous sections of this chapter consider the ventilation requirements for airborne infection isolation. For rooms, the described ventilation parameters will help maintain individual room control of microbial agents spread by the airborne route. The concern for the emergency room waiting areas and sections of the hospital needing to house potentially infectious patients is a challenge. Current fire code requirements for smoke control will aid in the development of a strategic plan for isolating a ward. Hospitals are segmented into smoke control zones, which are smoke compartments. These zones have ventilation dampers and fire stopped walls that will evacuate smoke if fires are detected in that zone. Engineering concepts are being explored to use the smoke control dampers and exhaust systems to help isolate the areas with infectious agents. The criteria for isolation would not be as extreme as the smoke management requirements, but the mechanism should already be in place for establishing the depressurized zone for an AII patient care unit. These concepts will help to establish such areas without the excess cost for configuring an area that may never be required. NIOSH has published a listing of building preparation tasks, if implemented, would help to protect from naturally occurring airborne infectious agents:

http://www.cdc.gov/niosh/bldvent/2002-139.html
http://www.cdc.gov/niosh/docs/2003-136.pdf

It is vitally important to focus on what works, especially on what works consistently. To provide the best possible hospital air quality, state-of-the-art technology is needed. It is equally important, however, to emphasize effective communication and common-sense procedures that will account for the human element, permit the system to function as designed, and meet the goal of providing the best in healthcare. Too many facilities are focused on air sampling for preventive measurements of air quality. Efforts must be taken to ensure ventilation proficiency with the ventilation parameters that will help to control the airborne infectious agents that are potentially pathogenic to humans.

REFERENCES

1. Chapter 7 health care facilities. In: *ASHRAE handbook—HVAC applications.* Atlanta: American Society for Heating, Refrigerating and Air-Conditioning, 1999.
2. Department of Health and Human Services and American Institute of Architects Committee on Health Care Facilities. *Guidelines for construction and equipment of hospital and medical facilities, 1992–93.* Washington DC: American Institute of Architects Press, 2001.
3. Rubin R. The compromised host as sentinel chicken. *N Engl J Med* 1987;317:1151–1153.
4. Ottney TC. Particle management for HVAC system. *ASHRAE J* 1993; 35:26–34.
5. Wolf HW, Skaliy P, Hall LB. Sampling microbiological aerosols. Monograph No. 60. Washington DC: U.S. Department of Health, Education and Welfare, 1959.
6. Gregory PH. *The microbiology of the atmosphere,* 2nd ed. New York: John Wiley & Sons, 1973.
7. Riley R, Nardell E. Clearing the air: the theory and application of ultraviolet air disinfection. *Am Rev Respir Dis* 1989;139:1286–1294.
8. Nardell E, et al. Airborne infection: theoretical limits of protection achievable by building ventilation. *Am Rev Respir Dis* 1991;144: 302–306.
9. Hermans RD, Streifel AJ. Ventilation design. In: Bierbaum PJ, Lippman M, eds. *Workshop on engineering controls for preventing airborne infections in workers in health care and related facilities.* Cincinnati, OH: NIOSH and CDC, 1993.
10. Bond RG, Michelson G, DeRoos R, eds. *Environmental health and safety in health care facilities.* New York: Macmillan, 1993.11. *Industrial ventilation: a manual of recommended practice,* 20th ed. Cincinnati, OH: American Conference of Government Industrial Hygienists, 1988.
12. Murray W, Streifel AJ, O'Dell T, et al. Ventilation for protection of immune compromised patients. *ASHRAE Trans* 1988;94:1185–1191.
13. Ventilation for acceptable indoor air quality. In: *ASHRAE standard.* Atlanta: American Society for Heating, Refrigerating and Air-Conditioning, 1999.
14. Arnow PM, et al. Endemic and epidemic aspergillosis associated with in-hospital replication of *Aspergillus* organisms. *J Infect Dis* 1991;164: 998–1002.
15. Morey R, Williams C. Porous insulation in buildings: a potential source of microorganisms. Proceedings Indoor Air '90 5th International Conference, Toronto, 1990:1–6.
16. Kundsin R, ed. *Architectural design and indoor microbial pollution. Ventilation and disease.* New York: Oxford University Press, 1988.
17. Wadowsky R, Benner S. Distribution of the genus *Aspergillus* in hospital room air conditioners. *Infect Control* 1987;8:516–518.
18. Lentino J, et al. Nosocomial aspergillosis: a retrospective review of airborne disease secondary to road construction and contaminated air conditioners. *Am J Epidemiol* 1982;116:430–437.
19. Method of testing air-cleaning devices used in general ventilation for removing particulate matter. In: 1992 b. *ASHRAE Standard.52.2* Atlanta: American Society of Heating, Refrigerating, and Air-Conditioning Engineers, 1992.
20. Wright M. *Procedures test filtration properties of filters, in clean rooms.* Tulsa, OK: Penn Well Publishing, 1989:30–33.
21. Kuehn TK. *Matching filtration to health requirements.* Minneapolis: University of Minnesota, 1993.
22. Rhame FS, Mazzarella M, Streifel AJ, et al. Evaluation of commercial air filters for fungal spore removal efficiency. Third International Conference on Nosocomial Infections, Atlanta, 1990.
23. Raynor PC, Chae SJ. Dust loading on electrostatically charged filters in a standard test & real HVAC system. *Filtration Separation* 2003; 40:35–39.
24. Hahn T, Cummings M, et al. Efficacy of high efficiency particulate air filtration in preventing aspergillosis in immunocompromised patients with hematologic malignancies. *ICHE* 2002;23:525–531.
25. Cornet M, Levy V, et al. Efficacy of prevention by high efficiency particulate air filtration or laminar airflow against *Aspergillus* airborne contamination during hospital renovation. *ICHE* 1999;20:508–513.
26. Streifel A. Editorial: in with the good air. ICHE 2002;23:488–490.
27. Walter C. The surgeons responsibility for asepsis. *Med Instrum* 1978; 12:149–157.
28. Drake C, et al. Environmental air and airborne infections. *Ann Surg* 1977;185:219–223.
29. Fitzgerald R. Microbiologic environment of the conventional operating room. *Arch Surg* 1979;114:772–775.
30. Hambraeus A, Bengtsson S, Laurell G. Bacterial contamination in a modern operating suite. *J Hyg (Camb)* 1977;79:121–131.
31. Woods JE, et al. Ventilation requirements in hospital operating rooms part 1: control of airborne particles. *ASHRAE Trans* 1986;92:455–459.
32. Lidwell O, et al. Ultraclean air and antibiotics for prevention of postoperative infection. *Acta Orthop Scand* 1987;58:4–13.
33. Memarzadeh F, Manning A. Comparison of operating room ventilation systems in the protection of the surgical site. *ASHRAE Trans* 2002; 108:3–15.
34. Blomgren G, Hoborn J, Nystrom B. Reduction of contamination at total hip replacement by special working clothes. *J Bone Joint Surg [Br]* 1990;6:985–987.
35. Humphreys H, et al. The effect of surgical theatre head-gear on air bacterial counts. *J Hosp Infect* 1991;19:175–180.
36. Tunevall TG, Jorbeck H. Influence of wearing masks on the density of airborne bacteria in the vicinity of the surgical wound. *Eur J Surg* 1992;158:263–266.
37. Whyte W, et al. The relative importance of the routes and sources of wound contamination during general surgery. II. Airborne. *J Hosp Infect* 1992;22:41–44.
38. Clark RP, et al. Ventilation conditions and air-borne bacteria and particles in operating theatres: proposed safe economies. *J Hyg (Camb)* 1985; 95:325–335.
39. Ritter M, et al. The effect that time, touch and environment have upon bacterial contamination of instruments during surgery. *Ann Surg* 1976; 184:642–644.
40. Jalovaara P, Puranen J. Air bacterial and particle counts in total hip replacement operations using non-woven and cotton gowns and drapes. *J Hosp Infect* 1989;14:333–338.
41. Pursell KJ. Invasive pulmonary aspergillosis complicating neoplastic disease. *Semin Respir Infect* 1992;7:96–103.
42. Bodey GP. The emergence of fungi as major hospital pathogens. *J Hosp Infect* 1988;11(Suppl A):411–426.
43. Petersen PK, McGlave P, Ramsay NK, et al. A prospective study of infectious diseases following bone marrow transplantation: emergence of *Aspergillus* and cytomegalovirus as the major causes of mortality. *Infect Control* 1983;4:81–89.
44. Rhame F. Prevention of nosocomial aspergillosis. *J Hosp Infect* 1991; 18(Suppl A):466–472.
45. Streifel AJ, Rhame FS. Hospital air filamentous fungal spore and particle counts in a specially designed hospital. 6th International Conference on Indoor Air Quality and Climate, Helsinki, 1993.
46. Solberg C, et al. Laminar airflow protection in bone marrow transplantation. *Am Soc Microbiol* 1971;21:209–216.
47. Sherertz RJ, et al. Impact of air filtration on nosocomial *Aspergillus* infections. *Am J Med* 1987;83:709–718.
48. Nauseef W, Maki D. A study of the value of simple protective isolation in patients with granulocytopenia. *N Engl J Med* 1981;304:448–453.
49. Rhame F. Nosocomial aspergillosis: how much protection for which patients? *Infect Control Hosp Epidemiol* 1989;10:296–298.
50. Walsh T, Dixon D. Nosocomial aspergillosis: environmental microbiology, hospital epidemiology, diagnosis and treatment. *Eur J Epidemiol* 1989;5:131–142.
51. Sarubbi FA, et al. Increased recovery of *Aspergillus flavus* from respiratory specimens during hospital construction. *Am Rev Respir Dis* 1982; 25:33–38.

52. Rhame F. Endemic nosocomial filamentous fungal disease: a proposed structure for conceptualizing and studying the environmental hazard. *Infect Control* 1986;7:124–125.
53. Staib F, et al. Occurrence of aspergillus fumigatus in West Berlin contribution to the epidemiology of aspergillosis. *Zentralbl Bakteriol Mikrobiol Hyg A* 1978;241:337–357.
54. USEPA, Office of Air and Radiation and USDHHS, NIOSH, 1991. Building air quality: a guide for building owners and facilities managers. Washington DC: USEPA. EPA/400/1091/033.
55. Rousseau C. HVAC system provisions to minimize the spread of tuberculosis bacteria. *ASHRAE Trans* 1993;99:2–4.
56. Riley R, Knight M, Middlebrook G. Ultraviolet susceptibility of BCG and virulent tubercle bacilli. *Am Rev Respir Dis* 1976;113: 413–418.
57. Streifel AJ. Maintenance and engineering. In: Pfeiffer J, ed. *APIC text of infection control and epidemiology.* Washington DC Association of Professionals in Infection Control and Epidemiology, 2000: 76.1–76.8
58. Streifel AJ, Vesley D, Rhames FS. Occurrence of transient high levels of airborne fungal spores. Proceedings of the 6th Conference on Indoor Air Quality and Climate, Toronto, 1990.
59. Opal S, et al. Efficacy of infection control measures during a nosocomial outbreak of disseminated aspergillosis associated with hospital construction. *J Infect Dis* 1986;153:634–637.
60. Streifel A. Aspergillosis and construction. In: Kundsin R, ed. *Architectural design and indoor microbial pollution.* New York: Oxford University Press, 1988.
61. Spendglove WH, Fannin K. Source, significance, and control of indoor microbial aerosols: human and health aspects. *Public Health Rep* 1983; 98:229–244.
62. Nicas M, Sprinson JE, Royce SE, et al. Isolation rooms for tuberculosis control. *Infect Control Hosp Epidemiol* 1993;14:619–622.
63. Rice N, Streifel AJ, Vesley D. An evaluation of hospital special ventilation room pressures. *ICHE* 2001;22:19–23.
64. Streifel AJ, Marshall JW. Parameters for ventilation controlled environments in hospitals. In: *Design, construction, and operation of healthy buildings.* IAQ/1997. Atlanta: American Society for Heating, Refrigerating and Air-Conditioning Press, 1998.
65. Rhame FS, Streifel AJ, Kersey JH, et al. Extrinsic risk factors for pneumonia in the patient at high risk of infection. *Am J Med* 1984;76: 42–52.
66. Streifel AJ. Air cultures for fungi. In: Isenberg HD, ed. *Clinical microbiology procedures handbook.* Washington DC: American Society for Microbiology Press, 2003:13.9.1–13.9.7.

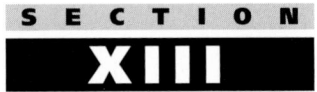

SECTION XIII

ANTIMICROBIAL AGENTS IN HOSPITAL EPIDEMIOLOGY AND INFECTION CONTROL

90

MECHANISMS OF BACTERIAL RESISTANCE TO ANTIMICROBIAL AGENTS

LOUIS B. RICE

The vast majority of antimicrobial agents employed in clinical settings are either natural products or chemical derivatives of natural products. The producers of these agents in nature are generally the microbes themselves, and their development appears to represent an attempt to acquire a selective advantage in mixed microbial environments. Since the production of antibiotics has been occurring in the microbial environment for (presumably) eons, it stands to reason that mechanisms to avoid their lethal action have been developed as well, either by species that produce the antibiotics or those that must share limited space and resources with those that do. In many instances, therefore, our discovery and growing use of antibiotics has led not to the development of resistance genes in bacteria, but merely to the natural selection of intrinsically resistant species or the efficient scavenging of preexisting resistance genes by normally susceptible human pathogens. The emergence of *Lactobacillus* species during therapy with vancomycin and of *Stenotrophomonas maltophilia* during therapy with imipenem are examples of selection of intrinsically resistant species. Other phenotypes of resistance reflect more the ease with which susceptible bacteria can mutate either structural or regulatory genes intrinsic to their species in a manner that results in decreased antibiotic susceptibility. Examples of this type of resistance include extended-spectrum cephalosporin resistance in *Enterobacter* species, fluoroquinolone resistance in many different species of bacteria, or the emerging resistance to linezolid in enterococci. Resistance to some antibiotics, in some species, is not readily achievable by mutation, and thus must be acquired from other sources. This so-called acquired resistance accurately characterizes many different resistance phenotypes, including ampicillin-resistance in *Escherichia coli,* penicillin-resistance in staphylococci, and vancomycin resistance in enterococci and more recently in *Staphylococcus aureus.* Finally, when antimicrobial agents are developed specifically to avoid the lethal action of acquired resistance genes, mutations within the acquired genes themselves can lead to resistance to the newer agents. The emergence of resistance to extended-spectrum cephalosporins in *Klebsiella pneumoniae* and *E. coli* represent this sort of amplified resistance.

Antimicrobial agents are effective, because they target metabolic pathways or enzymes that are specific to bacteria and not to the host. A variety of mechanisms have been shown to result in bacterial resistance. Among these mechanisms are alterations in the antibiotic target such that binding or inhibition of function is decreased to the point of clinical irrelevance, decreased permeability that results in the inability of the agent to reach its target at a critical concentration, efflux of the agent from the cell, and destruction or modification of the antibiotic.

The expression of resistance and virulence by bacteria is often linked, but sometimes in unpredictable ways. Selection of rifampin or streptomycin-resistant mutants in the laboratory is often associated with a decrease in the virulence of the strains when tested in animal models (1). It is presumed that the point mutations in the targets (RNA polymerase in the case of rifampin, the ribosome in the case of streptomycin) lead to subtle but not fatal decreases in function in these resistant strains, conferring a competitive survival disadvantage relative to wild-type strains. Interestingly, continued passage in animals in the absence of antibiotic selective pressure does not always result in reversion to the susceptible genotype. Instead, compensatory mutations frequently occur that mitigate the deleterious affects of the primary mutation, restoring virulence while maintaining resistance (1). Acquired resistance and virulence determinants may also coalesce in environments that favor them, such as the modern hospital. Recent reports suggest that ampicillin- and vancomycin-resistant *Enterococcus faecium* strains isolated in United States hospitals are enriched in potential virulence determinants esp (enterococcal surface protein) and hyaluronidase (2,3). This combination of resistance and virulence may help explain the remarkable increase in importance of *E. faecium* as a nosocomial pathogen over the past decade (4,5).

ANTIMICROBIAL RESISTANCE TRANSFER

Although the primary concern of the hospital epidemiologist is the prevention of spread of bacterial strains among hospitalized patients, it is worthwhile to consider mechanisms by which resistance genes themselves can spread among bacterial strains. A full discussion of the mechanisms of resistance transfer is beyond the scope of this chapter. Nevertheless, a few basic concepts should be understood.

Antimicrobial resistance determinants are commonly incorporated into extrachromosomal, independently replicating elements known as plasmids. Plasmids vary greatly in size (3 to >200 kb) and in the number of incorporated resistance determinants. In addition to genes responsible for replication and for antibiotic resistance, many plasmids also possess genes that stimulate their transfer between strains within a given genus, and occasionally between strains of different (although usually closely related) genera. Large, transferable plasmids have been implicated in the spread of ceftazidime resistance among strains of Enterobacteriaceae, particularly in intensive and chronic care settings (6,7). Many of these plasmids also possess genes encoding resistance to a range of non–β-lactam antimicrobial agents, resulting in the elimination of several antibacterial options with a single transfer event (6,7). Transferable plasmids have also been identified in gram-positive genera, perhaps best characterized by the pheromone-responsive plasmids found in strains of *Enterococcus faecalis* (8). The widespread emergence of high-level gentamicin resistance in enterococci (see below), resulting from the production of a modifying enzyme most commonly encoded on plasmids, is a testament to the efficiency of plasmids in disseminating resistance determinants in this genus (9,10). Enterococci are also known to possess "broad host range" plasmids. These plasmids transfer at a lower efficiency than do the pheromone-responsive plasmids, but have the advantage of being able to transfer to and replicate within a wide variety of species. Recent evidence implicates broad host-range plasmids in the exchange of important resistance genes between enterococci and staphylococci, including β-lactamase production and high-level vancomycin resistance (11–13).

Plasmids need not encode their own transfer genes in order to spread between strains. Nonconjugative plasmids may be mobilized for transfer by conjugative plasmids. In addition, the presence of insertion sequences (small regions of DNA capable of independent movement between replicons) has been shown to facilitate the co-integration of conjugative and nonconjugative plasmids, resulting in a larger, conjugative element (14). Appropriately sized plasmids may also be spread by transduction, resulting from the aberrant incorporation of plasmid rather than bacteriophage DNA into the phage head.

In addition to plasmids, antimicrobial resistance determinants frequently are incorporated into mobile elements known as transposons. Transposons may be rather simple elements whose mobility results from the presence of insertion sequences flanking an antimicrobial resistance determinant (composite transposons), an arrangement in which mobility is due entirely to functions encoded by the insertion sequences (15). Alternatively, transposons may be complex structures incorporating several genes. Tn*21* is a Tn*3*-family transposon that has been found to contain a genetic locus (*tnpI*) that serves as a "hot spot" for the integration of a variety of antimicrobial resistance genes (16). Consequently, several Tn*21*-like transposons conferring resistance to a number of different antimicrobial agents, in varying combinations, have been described (17). These loci, referred to as integrons, appear to be important mechanisms for the dissemination of antimicrobial resistance genes in many gram-negative bacilli (18,19). Recent data indicate that integrons may be critical vehicles of microbial genetic evolution, and have only recently been employed by bacteria for purposes of stockpiling resistance determinants (20). Another Tn*3*-family transposon, Tn*1546* (21), confers resistance to vancomycin and teicoplanin in enterococci and more recently in *S. aureus.* It encodes nine genes involved in the regulation of transposition and the expression of glycopeptide resistance.

In general, transposons participate in the transfer of antimicrobial resistance determinants by virtue of their ability to move between bacterial chromosome and transferable plasmid. Exceptions to this rule are the conjugative transposons of gram-positive bacteria, which can transfer between strains without the necessity of a plasmid intermediate (22). These transposons possess their own genes responsible for transfer between microorganisms. In general, conjugative transposons encode resistance to tetracycline via the *tetM* gene, although some have been found to encode resistance to multiple antimicrobial agents (22). In addition to the transfer of the elements themselves, some investigators have found that the presence of conjugative transposons stimulates the transfer of unrelated chromosomal genes, raising the possibility that these elements could be involved in the transfer of a range of unrelated resistance determinants (11,23). A transposon in the Tn*916* family has been described that encodes VanB-type vancomycin resistance in *E. faecium* (24). Conjugative transposons may also transfer determinants for antibacterial activity as well as antibiotic resistance. Several lactococcal conjugative elements encoding determinants for production of the antibacterial peptide nisin have been described (25).

Other mobile elements involved in the spread of antimicrobial resistance are the insertion sequences (IS elements). These elements do not encode antimicrobial resistance themselves but may aid in the spread of resistance determinants via the formation of composite transposons or by serving as areas of homologous recombination between plasmid and chromosome. Insertion of IS elements may also result in the activation of poorly expressed genes via the presence of promoter sequences within the end of the mobile element (15). Evidence indicates that the expression of imipenem resistance in some strains of *Bacteroides fragilis* is due to the insertion of IS elements upstream of an unexpressed chromosomal gene encoding a carbapenemase (26).

Our ability to thwart the spread of resistance determinants between bacterial strains in the natural environment is, at present, poor. Factors affecting transfer between strains are poorly understood, but in some cases may involve exposure to antimicrobial agents themselves. Transfer of conjugative transposons, for example, has been shown to be increased *in vitro* and *in vivo* after exposure of the donor strain to tetracycline (27,28). It is therefore reasonable to presume that environmental pressure from the overuse of antimicrobial agents plays some role in the spread of these determinants. In addition, the commingling of many different strains of bacteria in the human gastrointestinal tract resulting from hospital and antibiotic exposure as well as from inattention to appropriate infection control techniques probably play roles in the spread of resistant strains. In some cases, institution of infection control measures (such as barrier precautions for infected and colonized patients) has been shown to abort serious outbreaks of resistant microorganisms (29,30). In others, decreasing use of an antibiotic has been associated with a reduction in the prevalence of resistant strains in an institution (31). As such, judicious use of antimicrobial agents and proper attention to infection control recommendations are likely to be our best weapons to combat the spread of resistant bacteria for the foreseeable future.

β-LACTAMS

Mechanism of Action

Targets of β-lactam antibiotics are a series of enzymes involved in the last step of peptidoglycan (cell wall) synthesis. This step involves a cross-linking reaction carried out by transpeptidases in which the terminal D-alanine of the pentapeptide stem of the peptidoglycan is cleaved. The energy resulting from this cleavage is used to form a peptide bond between the fourth residue of the pentapeptide (also D-alanine) and the cross-bridge, which is itself linked to the e-amino of diaminopimelic acid (in gram-negative microorganisms) or lysine (in gram-positive microorganisms) (Fig. 90.1). This cross-link is absolutely required for structural integrity of the bacterial cell wall. β-Lactam antibiotics, such as penicillin, are structural analogs of the pentapeptide terminal D-alanyl:D-alanine (Fig. 90.2) target covalently bound by the transpeptidases. The fact that these transpeptidases also bind penicillin (and other β-lactams) covalently has resulted in referral to them as penicillin-binding proteins (PBPs).

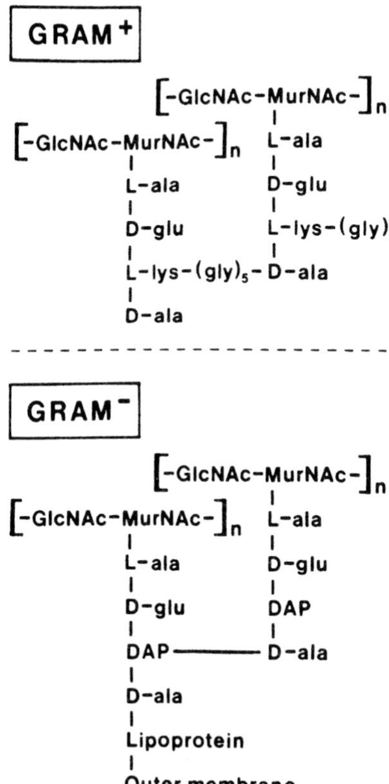

Figure 90.1. Structure of murein in bacteria. The gram-positive pentaglycine cross-link is shown. (From Schaechter M, et al., eds. *Mechanisms of microbial diseases,* 2nd ed. Baltimore: Williams & Wilkins, 1993.)

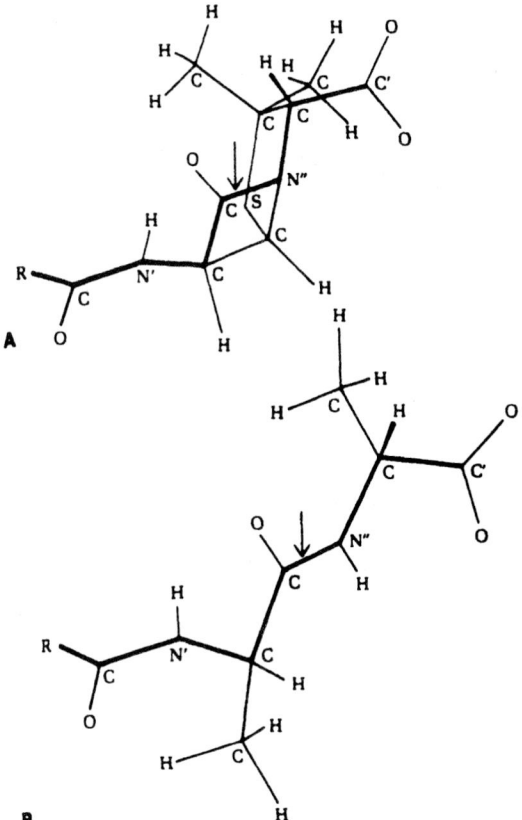

Figure 90.2. Stereochemical models comparing penicillin **(A)** and the D-alanyl-D-alanine terminus of the peptidoglycan **(B)**. *Arrows* indicate the position of the CO–N bond in the β-lactam ring of penicillin and of the CO–N bond in the D-alanyl-D-alanine. (Adapted from Volk WA, et al., eds. *Essentials of medical microbiology.* Philadelphia: JB Lipp3incott, 1991.)

Mechanisms of β-Lactam Resistance

Target Resistance

The binding affinity of β-lactams for their targets, the PBPs, varies with the β-lactam and the PBP. Enterococci, for example, are intrinsically resistant to the cephalosporins, because these β-lactams do not bind the enterococcal PBPs with high affinity (32). Within the genus *Enterococcus, E. faecium* tend to be more resistant to penicillins, because many strains express a low-affinity PBP (PBP5) that carries out cell wall synthesis at penicillin concentrations that inhibit the other PBPs (33).

Many cases of PBP-mediated β-lactam resistance result from the intrinsic characteristics of the PBPs of a given strain. PBP-mediated resistance may also be acquired. Resistance resulting from mutation can be readily demonstrated in the laboratory (34). Resistance to oxacillin in clinical *S. aureus* strains has been attributed to point mutations in PBP genes (34). In species that are naturally transformable (that can absorb naked DNA from the environment), formation of mosaic PBP genes is common. Cloning and sequencing of *Streptococcus pneumoniae* or *Neisseria gonorrhoeae* genes encoding abnormal, low-affinity PBPs responsible for penicillin resistance has shown significant sections of these genes to be of foreign origin. In *S. pneumoniae,* the origin appears to have been from oral streptococci (35); in *N. gonorrhoeae,* from oral commensal neisserial species (36,37). The evolution of mosaic genes most likely occurred via DNA transformation followed by homologous recombination across areas of PBP sequence homology between the native and foreign DNA. Entire low-affinity PBPs can also be acquired by normally susceptible bacteria. Methicillin-resistant *S. aureus* (MRSA) has most commonly acquired low affinity PBP2a, encoded by the *mecA* gene. Recent work suggests that the *mec* region is located within a larger mobile element (designated SCC*mec*) and that this region varies in size depending on how much extra DNA it contains (38). Nosocomial strains (which are resistant to several unrelated classes of antimicrobial agents) contain a larger SCC*mec*, reflecting insertion of additional DNA, some of which encodes additional antimicrobial resistance. In contrast, the recently described MRSA arising in the community (which is generally susceptible to a range of other antimicrobial agents) contains a relatively small SCC*mec* that encodes only resistance to methicillin (39). Recent data suggest that the *mec* region may have been acquired from coagulase-negative staphylococcal species (40).

The expression of resistance encoded by mosaic or acquired PBPs is often dependent on very specific conditions. Several staphylococcal genes, called *fem* (factors essential for methicillin resistance) or *aux* factors, have been identified, the inactivation of which results in reversion to susceptible phenotype despite expression of PBP2a (41). In most cases these *fem* genes encode enzymes responsible for the synthesis of peptidoglycan precursors. The failure to express resistance when these genes are deleted suggests that the PBP2a is very specific in the substrates it will tolerate. Similar supportive genes have been described in *S. pneumoniae* strains that encode mosaic PBP genes (42).

Enterococci are intrinsically resistant to some β-lactams, especially the cephalosporins, at high levels. Resistance is related to the low affinity of these compounds for the enterococcal PBPs (33,43). Strains resistant to even higher levels of the penicillins, in the absence of production of β-lactamase, have been described with increasing frequency (4,44). These strains include several species, but *E. faecium* is most commonly reported from clinical laboratories. Most of these high-level resistant strains possess one or more point mutations in *pbp5* that are thought to lower the affinity for penicillin and other β-lactams (45). It is not clear at present whether the point mutations alone account for all of the penicillin resistance in these strains (46). Enterococcal strains expressing high levels of resistance to β-lactams through low-affinity PBPs are also more resistant to β-lactam–aminoglycoside synergy, even in the absence of high levels of aminoglycoside resistance (47). Single-agent β-lactam therapy is precluded for such strains, leaving the glycopeptides as the antibiotic class of choice. The continued spread of glycopeptide resistance in penicillin-resistant enterococci (see below) is a persistent problem at many large centers (4).

β-Lactamase–Mediated Resistance

A more important and frequent mechanism of bacterial resistance to β-lactam antibiotics, especially in gram-negative bacteria, is the production of β-lactamases, enzymes that hydrolyze the β-lactam ring (Fig. 90.3). The reactive β-lactam ring is required for formation of a covalent bond between the antibiotic and its PBP target. Destruction of this ring results in loss of antimicrobial activity. The β-lactamases form a broad family of enzymes, and along with the PBPs, are classified as serine D, D-peptidases (48). The homologies between many β-lactamases and PBP have led to the suggestion that β-lactamases have evolved from penicillin-binding proteins.

Two classification schemes for the β-lactamases are widely used. The first is based on primary structure and has been proposed by Ambler et al. (49) (Table 90.1). In this scheme, the enzymes of staphylococci, the common plasmid-mediated enzymes of the gram-negative microorganisms and all their variants, one of the enzymes of *Bacillus*, and others are lumped into a single class, class A. A consensus sequence for this class has been proposed (50). The other scheme (Bush-Jacoby-Medeiros classification) relies on the substrate specificity of the enzymes (51) (Table 90.2). There are many more classes and subclasses in this scheme, since single point mutations in the gene encoding an enzyme may result in substantial changes in substrate specificity.

Staphylococcal β-lactamase production became widespread

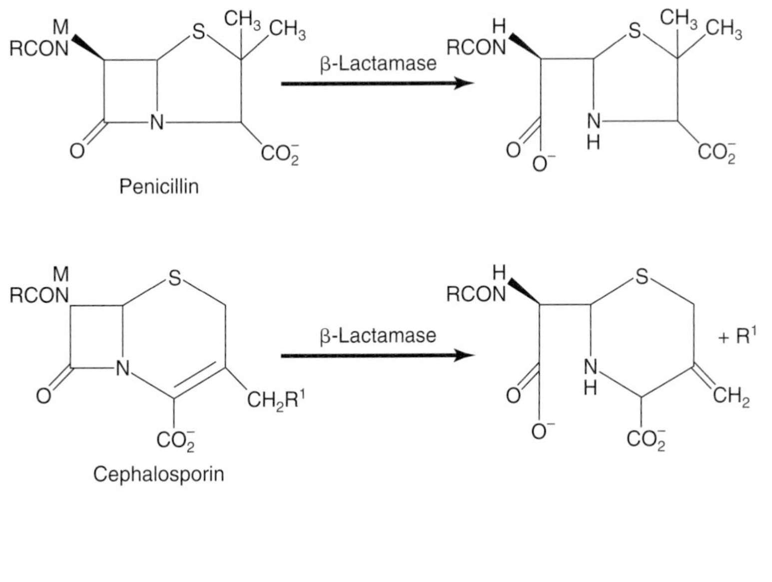

Figure 90.3. Reactions catalyzed by β-lactamase on penicillin and on cephalosporin. (From Neu HC. Contribution of β-lactamases to bacterial resistance and mechanisms to inhibit β-lactamase. *Am J Med* 1985;79(suppl 5B):2–12.)

TABLE 90.1. MOLECULAR CLASSIFICATION OF β-LACTAMASES

Class	Examples
A	TEM, SHV (gram-negative microorganisms), PC1 (*Staphylococcus aureus*)
B	Metallo-β-lactamases
C	*AmpC* gene
D	OXAT-4

From Ambler R.P. The structure of β-lactamases. *Philos Trans R Soc Lond [B]* 1980;289:321–331, with permission.

within a few years of the clinical introduction of penicillin (52, 53). By the mid-1940s, β-lactamase–producing *S. aureus* strains were widespread within hospitals, necessitating the introduction of vancomycin and semisynthetic penicillins such as methicillin, nafcillin, and oxacillin. Although the subsequent decades have not seen significant evolution of the staphylococcal genes resulting in hydrolysis of the semisynthetic penicillins or new cephalosporins, it has been shown that the most common variant of staphylococcal β-lactamase, immunologic type A, is more efficient at hydrolyzing older cephalosporins such as cefazolin, a fact that may be related to failures of antibiotic prophylaxis in some cases (54). The commonly used semisynthetic penicillins are highly effective in treatment of infections due to methicillin-susceptible, β-lactamase–producing staphylococci, as are combinations of β-lactams and β-lactamase inhibitors. The importance of β-lactamase production in gram-positive bacteria remains essentially restricted to staphylococci. Among other gram-positive pathogens, only enterococci have been shown to express β-lactamase (the same β-lactamase as expressed by staphylococci), but reports of such isolates remain quite rare and their clinical importance appears to be minimal.

The epidemiology of β-lactamase–mediated resistance in gram-negative bacilli is far more complex than in gram-positive. Hundreds of different β-lactamases have been described in gram-negative bacteria over the past two decades. The most problematic and prevalent of these enzymes are those that confer resistance to expanded spectrum cephalosporins. Many of these extended-spectrum β-lactamases (ESBLs) are progeny of more narrow spectrum enzymes that fall, like the staphylococcal β-lactamase, into Ambler class A. The most common enzymes of this class among clinical isolates are related to the widely prevalent TEM-1 and SHV-1 enzymes (51). TEM-1 is widely prevalent as the cause of ampicillin resistance in *E. coli, Haemophilus influenzae,* and in some cases *N. gonorrhoeae,* whereas SHV-1 is the chromosomal β-lactamase found in most *K. pneumoniae* strains. TEM-1 and SHV-1 are broad-spectrum β-lactamases that hydrolyze the penicillins (ampicillin, mezlocillin, and piperacillin) with greater efficiency than the cephalosporins (55). Genes encoding ESBLs are most commonly found on transferable plasmids with resistance determinants to numerous other antimicrobial classes. Since the early 1980s, we have observed the emergence of *K. pneumoniae* and *E. coli,* and occasionally other Enterobacteriaceae, producing mutant forms of TEM-1 or SHV-1 capable of hydrolyzing the oxyiminocephalosporins (ceftazidime, cefotaxime, ceftriaxone), aztreonam (a monobactam), and others (55). Although TEM-related enzymes predominated in early ESBL outbreaks, more recent surveys suggest a predominance of SHV-related ESBLs. Moreover, an increasingly greater variety of non–TEM- or SHV-related enzymes continue to be described (56). Strains elaborating ESBLs, most commonly *Klebsiella,* have been responsible for several outbreaks of infection and colonization in Europe and the U.S. More recently, several different ESBLs have been described in *Proteus mirabilis,* especially in Europe (57). Outbreaks have been ascribed to clonal dissemination, plasmid dissemination, or both (31,58,59). The expanded activity of ESBLs results from single or sometimes multiple point mutations in the genes that result in critical amino acid substitutions (55). These point mutations are often found in association with cellular characteristics that serve to enhance the phenotypic expression of resistance, such as location downstream of strong promoters (leading to increased β-lactamase quantity) and reductions in the expression of outer membrane proteins (porins that serve as conduits for entry of antibiotics into the periplasmic space). These enhancing mechanisms may be important predisposing factors for the emergence of ESBLs in the clinical setting, since they would be expected to increase expression of resistance at the single cell level, thereby promoting the survival of initial point mutants in the setting of heavy antibiotic exposure. At least one case study supports the concept of predisposing porin reductions promoting emergence of an ESBL (60).

Mutations to extend the spectrum of TEM-1 or SHV-1 and

TABLE 90.2. CLASSIFICATION OF β-LACTAMASES ACCORDING TO FUNCTION

Group	Description	Examples	Molecular Class
1	Cephalosporin hydrolyzing enzymes not inhibited by clavulanic acid	*AmpC*	C
2a	Penicillin hydrolyzing enzymes inhibited by clavulanic acid	*B. licheniformis* 749	A
2be	Broad-spectrum enzymes inhibited by clavulanic acid	TEM	A
2b	Extended-spectrum enzymes inhibited by clavulanic acid	TEM 3–26	A
2c	Carbenicillin hydrolyzing enzymes inhibited by clavulanic acid	PSE-1.3.4	A
2d	Cloxacillin hydrolyzing enzymes inhibited by clavulanic acid	OXA-1–11	D
2e	Cephalosporin hydrolyzing enzymes inhibited by clavulanic acid	*B. fragilis* G42	A
3	Metallo-β-lactamases	*S. maltophilia* GN12873	B
4	Penicillin hydrolyzing enzymes not inhibited by clavulanic acid	*B. fragilis* G237	?

From Bush K, Jacoby GA, Medeicos AA. A Functional Classification Scheme for β-lactamases and its molecular structure. *Antimicrob Agents Chemoth* 1998; 39:1216.

allow hydrolysis of extended-spectrum cephalosporins commonly yield increased susceptibility to inhibition by β-lactamase inhibitors. In the clinical setting, however, the production of multiple enzymes and/or overproduction of individual enzymes often confers *in vitro* resistance to β-lactam/β-lactamase inhibitor combinations in ESBL producers. The relative scarcity of ESBL producers has made controlled studies of the efficacy of different therapies impractical, but carbapenems have been most effective in animal studies of infections with ESBL producers as well as case reports and small series. The most clinical experience has been with imipenem (58,61).

Resistance to extended-spectrum cephalosporins may also be conferred by expression of regulatory mutants of Bush-Jacoby-Medeiros group 1 (Ambler's class C) β-lactamases. These enzymes are broadly active cephalosporinases (which also hydrolyze penicillins) and resistant to clinically achievable concentrations of β-lactam/β-lactamase inhibitor combinations (51). They are encoded by the *ampC* gene, a chromosomal gene widely disseminated among Enterobacteriaceae and *Pseudomonas aeruginosa.* In some species, such as *E. coli, ampC* is poorly expressed and not under regulatory control due to the absence of the *ampR* gene. The product of the *ampR* gene interacts with different cell wall breakdown products in a manner that results in AmpR becoming either a suppressor or an activator of *ampC* transcription (62–64). Under normal circumstances, cells with inducible AmpC β-lactamases employ *AmpD* (a cellular amidase encoded by *ampD*) to reduce intracellular quantities of cellular breakdown product anhydro-muramyl-tripeptide, which results in an excess of uridine diphosphate (UDP)-muramyl-pentapeptide. UDP-muramyl-pentapeptide interaction with AmpR maintains AmpR as a repressor of *ampC* transcription. When exposed to certain antibiotics that favor production of anhydro-muramyl-tripeptide (such as cefoxitin, clavulanic acid, and imipenem), the ability of AmpD to convert this substrate is overwhelmed, and interaction between anhydro-muramyl-tripeptide and AmpR converts AmpR into an activator of *ampC* transcription (induction). *ampR* is present and *ampC* is under regulatory control in *Enterobacter* species, *Serratia marcescens, Citrobacter freundii,* and *P. aeruginosa,* among others (64–66). Imipenem is an efficient inducer of *ampC* expression, but it is a poor substrate for the *ampC* β-lactamase. It therefore remains active even in the presence of induced β-lactamase (as long as a concomitant mutation decreasing the entry of imipenem into the periplasmic space is not present—see below). Newer cephalosporins such as ceftazidime, ceftriaxone, and others are efficiently hydrolyzed by the AmpC, but are poor inducers and therefore appear active *in vitro* against bacteria expressing inducible AmpC.

Unfortunately, the newer oxyiminocephalosporins (e.g., ceftazidime, cefotaxime, ceftriaxone) are very good selectors of mutants that express high levels of the *ampC* β-lactamase constitutively. Their ability to select constitutive mutants results from their status as weak inducers. Constitutive AmpC production commonly results from null mutations in *ampD,* with subsequent intracellular accumulation of anhydro-muramyl-tripeptide and constitutive activation of *ampC* expression (62). Thus, from among a population of microorganisms, the small number (1 in 10^{6-7}) of preexisting cells with mutations *ampD* are selected for growth by the presence of antibiotic with potent activity against strains in which *ampC* expression is repressed. Once constitutive expression occurs, the strains are essentially resistant to all β-lactams except for carbapenems and cefepime (66). Cefepime's major advantage in this regard appears to be its status as a zwitterion, allowing it to achieve high periplasmic concentrations by rapid passage through the outer membrane. Caution should be exercised in using cefepime to treat deregulated *ampC* mutants of *Enterobacter* species, however, since reports of the emergence of cefepime resistance (associated with a reduction in an outer membrane protein) in these strains during therapy have been published (67).

Although many β-lactams can select for constitutive *ampC* mutants *in vitro,* third-generation cephalosporins are the primary offenders in the clinical setting (68,69). In a study of *Enterobacter* bacteremia by Chow et al. (68), the major class of antibiotics associated with selection of resistance was the newer cephalosporins as opposed (especially) to the newer penicillins. Concomitant use of aminoglycosides did not prevent the emergence of this resistance. In this study, resistance developed in 19% of all patients treated with newer cephalosporins. Therapeutic failure occurred in about half of those patients. For all patients infected with a multiply resistant strain, the mortality rate was significantly increased. Infection with a multiply resistant strain was closely associated with prior use of a new cephalosporin. These data argue for limiting the use of extended-spectrum cephalosporins to forestall the emergence of Enterobacteriaceae resistant to multiple β-lactam antibiotics.

Although *ampC* is chromosomally encoded and generally not transferable, plasmid-encoded versions of these enzymes have been observed in several species of Enterobacteriaceae, including *E. coli* and *K. pneumoniae,* among others (56). These strains express high levels of the AmpC enzyme constitutively and have resistance profiles identical to multiply β-lactam–resistant *Enterobacter* species and *P. aeruginosa.* The most prevalent of these enzymes is CMY-2, derived from the *Citrobacter* AmpC enzyme (70). Plasmid-encoded AmpC enzymes have been found in *E. coli, Salmonella,* and other gram-negative species (56). Currently available β-lactamase inhibitors are poorly active against these enzymes. Thus, the carbapenems are the only therapeutically reliable β-lactams. It is noteworthy, however, that one such enzyme, designated ACT-1, was identified in a porin-deficient strain of *K. pneumoniae*, where it conferred resistance to imipenem and was associated with failures of this antibiotic in clinical settings (71).

Resistance to β-lactam/β-lactamase inhibitor combinations can result from several different mechanisms, all of which involve the production of β-lactamase. As noted above, expression of an AmpC enzyme confers resistance to both cephalosporins and β-lactam/β-lactamase inhibitor combinations. Resistance to inhibitor combinations alone can be conferred by increased production of a normally susceptible enzyme (i.e., TEM-1), permeability defects, or a combination of both mechanisms (72). Specific inhibitor-resistant enzymes can also result from mutation of TEM-1 or SHV-1, similar to extending the cephalosporin spectrum of these β-lactamases (73). Although mutations that extend the spectrum against cephalosporins and those that confer resistance to inhibitors are not strictly incompatible, the extent of resistance conferred against one class of compounds is usually mitigated by the concomitant presence of mutations conferring resistance to the other class (74). These data indicate that the active site of class A enzymes is limited in its flexibility, and that mutations that extend the natural spectrum come at a cost in enzyme efficiency. Human pathogenic bacteria seem to have figured this out by themselves, however, since resistance to both extended-spectrum cephalosporins and β-lactam/β-lactamase inhibitor combinations is quite common in the clinical setting. This phenotype can be conferred by production of AmpC enzymes, by the increased production of an ESBL, or by the expression of more than one enzyme (one an ESBL, the other a more common enzyme such as SHV-1) (75,76).

Although the carbapenems remain the most stable β-lactams to hydrolysis, there are specific enzymes that are efficient at hydrolyzing these compounds. *S. maltophilia* is an intrinsically carbapenem-resistant species that can emerge as an important pathogen in clinical settings (77). It owes its resistance to synthesis of an inducible, zinc-dependent carbapenemase encoded on the chromosome. Several cation (usually zinc)-dependent β-lactamases (generally classified as IMP or VIM enzymes) capable of hydrolyzing carbapenems have been described in several species (78). A French study showed that approximately 1% to 2% of examined *B. fragilis* isolates carried a carbapenemase gene, although the gene was expressed in about only half of these (79). Examination of the strains in which expression occurred revealed an IS element upstream of the carbapenemase gene (80). It is thought that a promoter on the IS element is required for carbapenemase expression (80). Chromosomally encoded class A carbapenemases have been described in scattered isolates of *Enterobacter* and *Serratia* (81), with plasmid-encoded variants described in *K. pneumoniae* and *P. aeruginosa,* but these remain very rare. In *Acinetobacter baumannii,* carbapenem resistance has been associated with expression of class D enzymes (OXA type), but the exact contribution of these enzymes to clinical resistance in *Acinetobacter* remains in question (82).

β-Lactamase Expression Combined with Membrane Changes

It is known that a combination of a permeability deficit plus expression of a β-lactamase with poor hydrolytic activity against carbapenems can lead to clinically important levels of carbapenem resistance. The most well known example of this occurs in *P. aeruginosa.* In this species, a single outer membrane protein (OMP) functioning as a porin, OMP D2, encoded by the *oprD2* gene, is required for transport of imipenem, as well as positively charged amino acids such as lysine (83,84). At the same time, imipenem is an efficient inducer of expression of the AmpC (class Ia) β-lactamase of *P. aeruginosa* and other microorganisms (65). Strains that decrease expression of OMP D2 in their outer membranes are resistant to imipenem. It has been shown (Table 90.3) that OMP-mediated resistance requires expression of the AmpC β-lactamase, even though it is an inefficient hydrolyzer of imipenem (84). Since imipenem is an excellent inducer of β-lactamase expression, it is likely that a combination of the two phenomena results in clinical resistance. This same combination of mechanisms has been shown to lead to carbapenem resistance in *Enterobacter* species and *Proteus rettgeri* (85–87). Mutants

TABLE 90.3. SUSCEPTIBILITY OF MUTANTS OF PSEUDOMONAS AERUGINOSA M2297 TO CARBAPENEMS IN RELATION TO THEIR EXPRESSION OF CHROMOSOMAL β-LACTAMASE AND D2 PORIN

		MIC (μg/mL)[b] of	
Class I β-Lactamase[a]	**D2 porin**	**Imipenem**	**Ceftazidime**
→Inducible ↓	+	1	1
→Derepressed ↓	+	1	32
Basal	+	0.12	1
→Inducible	−	16	1
→Derepressed ↓	−	16	32
Basal	−	0.5	1

MIC, minimal inhibitory concentration.
[a] The arrows show the sequence of mutant derivation. The amount of β-lactamase produced by the inducible microorganisms depended on the presence and concentration of inducers. Derepressed mutants made the enzyme copiously regardless of induction, and basal mutants had only a trace level.
[b] Note that β-lactamase–inducible or derepressed microorganisms were less susceptible to imipenem than were the basal mutants. This protection gave clinical resistance (MIC ≥ 8 μg/mL) only when D2 porin was absent. Moreover, loss of the β-lactamase from the D2 porin–deficient microorganisms caused almost full restoration of imipenem suscaptibility, confirming that resistance required both the enzyme and the impermeability. Ceftazidime, which is a labile weak inducer of the class I enzyme and which cannot traverse the pores formed by D2 porin, retained equal activity against β-lactamase–inducible and basal microorganisms irrespective of their D2 porin expression. However, its activity was lost against the derepressed mutants.
From Livermore DM. Carbapenemases: the next generation of β-lactamases. *ASM News* 1993; 59 : 129–135, with permission.

resistant to carbapenems have been described both in *E. cloacae* and *E. aerogenes,* although these mutants are more easily obtained (in the laboratory) in the latter species (85). Clinical isolates of carbapenem-resistant *K. pneumoniae* expressing a plasmid-mediated AmpC β-lactamase combined with loss of expression of two nonspecific porins have been reported (71).

An emerging area of interest is the impact of efflux pump expression on resistance to β-lactam antibiotics. This phenomenon has been most carefully explored in *P. aeruginosa.* Several classes of efflux pumps have been described in gram-negative bacteria. A full description of the different pump classes is beyond the scope of this chapter. The reader is referred for more detailed information to several excellent reviews (88–90). To understand how these pumps can work in concert to promote resistance to β-lactams and other antimicrobial agents, it is worth considering the case of *P. aeruginosa* and its efflux pumps that fall into the resistance-nodulation-cell division (RND) class. RND pumps are generally tripartite systems composed of a cytoplasmic membrane portion, an outer membrane portion, and a portion that connects the two across the periplasmic space (88). These pumps serve to extrude material from the cytoplasm into the surrounding media, but also appear to be able to efflux material (particularly β-lactam antibiotics) from the periplasm as well. Four RND efflux pumps have been characterized in *P. aeruginosa*—MexAB-OprM, MexCD-OprJ, MexEF-OprN, and MexXY-OprM (Table 90.4) (91,92)— and there are undoubtedly several more. These pumps all have broad substrate specificity. MexAB-OprM is constitutively expressed, whereas MexCD-

TABLE 90.4. RESISTANCE-NODULATION CELL (RND) PUMPS CHARACTERIZED IN *PSEUDOMONAS AERUGINOSA* AND THEIR SUBSTRATE SPECIFICITIES

RND Pump	Substrates
MexAB-OprM	Q, M, T, L, C, novobiocin, β-lactams except imipenem, aminoglycosides under low ionic strength conditions
MexCD-OprJ	Q, M, T, L, C, novobiocin, penicillins except carbenicillin and sulbenicillin, cephems except ceftazidime, flomoxef, meropenem
Mex EF-OprN	Chloramphenicol, quinolones, trimethoprim, carbapenems
MexXY-OprM	Q, M, T, L, C, aminoglycosides, penicillins except carbenicillin and sulbenicillin, cephems except cefsulodin and ceftazidime, meropenem

Q,M,T,L,C, quinolones, macrolides, tetracyclines, lincomycin, chloramphenicol.

OprJ is repressed in most wild-type strains and MexEF-OprN is variably expressed. MexXY-OprM is expressed at low levels, if at all, during normal laboratory growth. MexAB-OprM pumps out a wide variety of β-lactam antibiotics, but cefepime and cefpirome are poor substrates for this pump. Imipenem is not a substrate for any of the pumps. MexCD-OprJ also has broad substrate specificities, but is limited in its ability to pump β-lactams. In contrast to MexAB-OprM, cefepime is a good substrate for this pump (92). There is in general an inverse correlation between expression of MexAB-OprM and MexCD-OprJ, suggesting some form of control over the total quantity of efflux pumps expressed in a cell at a given time (91). However, the levels of expression observed for MexCD-OprJ in strains devoid of MexAB-OprM do not confer resistance to any antibiotics. Overexpression of MexCD-OprJ is required for resistance. MexEF-OprN may efflux meropenem efficiently, but not imipenem. However, expression of the normally repressed MexEF-OprN is associated with decreased expression of outer membrane protein OprD, the porin associated with imipenem entry into the periplasmic space, reductions in which (in association with AmpC expression—see above) are associated with imipenem resistance. Hence, increased expression of MexAB-OprM and derepression MexEF-OprN are associated with almost universal β-lactam resistance, except for modest susceptibility to cefepime. One outbreak of *P. aeruginosa* strains expressing this combination of pumps involved 67 patients and required cefepime-amikacin combinations for successful treatment (93).

Thus, a wide variety of mechanisms lead to β-lactam resistance. At least some of these mechanisms could spread by plasmids and transposable elements. The β-lactam class of antibiotics, representing our least toxic and most potent agents, may no longer offer the therapeutic potential it once did. In my view, a replacement for this class will not be available this decade.

CYCLIC GLYCOPEPTIDES

The cyclic glycopeptides include vancomycin, teicoplanin (not available for clinical use in the U.S.), as well as a number of compounds such as avoparcin, ristocetin, actaplanin, and others that have not been used in human infections (94). These antibiotics are highly active against gram-positive bacteria. Teicoplanin is more active against enterococci, whereas vancomycin tends to be more active against the staphylococci. Molecular weights of cyclic glycopeptides range from 1,200 to 2,000 d. They all have a central-core heptapeptide, of which three amino acids are highly conserved. Some of these amino acids are crucial to the mode of action of this class. Other important glycopeptide components include the chlorine substituents and the sugars (94).

Gram-positive bacteria, most commonly enterococci, expressing resistance to the cyclic glycopeptides have now been described throughout the world, and are causes of significant morbidity and mortality in hospitalized patients, particularly in the U.S. (95,96). The overwhelming majority of vancomycin-resistant enterococci (VRE) are *E. faecium* that also express resistance to ampicillin, the other major antimicrobial agent used to treat enterococcal infections (4). They are also frequently resistant to fluoroquinolones, macrolides, penicillins, and to high levels of aminoglycosides (97), rendering most therapies inactive. In the past few years, three new agents (quinupristin-dalfopristin, linezolid, daptomycin) have been introduced to treat VRE infections, but neither of these agents is immune to the problem of resistance.

The cyclic glycopeptides bind to acyl-D-alanyl:D-alanine at the terminus of the pentapeptide of the peptidoglycan precursor (94). This binding occurs as the precursor is exiting from the cell membrane to the cell wall, at which point the precursor is added on to the growing peptidoglycan by transglycosylase. Glycopeptides prevent cleavage of the terminal D-ala that is required for establishing the peptide cross-link between adjacent peptide chains. Glycopeptide binding of D-Ala:D-Ala is also thought to cause a "steric" inhibition of transglycosylation, because the bulky antibiotic prevents the transglycosylase from interacting with the peptidoglycan. Virtually all bacteria synthesize peptidoglycan terminating in D-Ala:D-Ala. However, since the currently available glycopeptides are larger than the exclusion limits of the porin proteins of gram-negative outer membranes, only gram-positive species are susceptible to clinically achievable concentrations of this class of antibiotics.

Enterococcal vancomycin resistance has been attributed to six different genetic clusters (VanA–E, G) (98–101). A seventh gene cluster conferring vancomycin resistance (VanF) has been described in the biopesticide *Paenobacillus popillae,* but has not been found elsewhere (102). The vancomycin resistance operons can be broadly separated into two groups: those that synthesize peptidoglycan precursors terminating in D-lactate (*vanA, B, D,* hereafter referred to as the lactate operons) and those that synthesize precursors terminating in D-serine (*vanC, E, G,* hereafter referred to as the serine operons). The lactate operons (specifically *vanA* and *vanB*) have spread widely throughout the world and are the predominant operons conferring acquired glycopeptide resistance. They are focused primarily in *E. faecium.* The serine operons are either intrinsic to some minor species of *enterococci VanC* in *Enterococcus casseliflavus, Enterococcus flavescens,* and *Enterococcus gallinarum* or have been described in only very rare isolates of *E. faecalis* (*vanE* and *G*). *vanA* and *vanB* have been described in transposable elements (21,24) and are generally transferable to enterococcal recipients *in vitro,* whereas neither *vanD* nor the serine operons have been shown to be transferable. Structural comparisons of the six different operons are shown in Figure 90.4.

Three functions of the different operons are essential to confer resistance to glycopeptides. First, the resistant substrate must be synthesized (Fig. 90.5). The *vanH* genes of the lactate operons encode a dehydrogenase that converts cellular pyruvate to D-lactate, whereas the *vanT* genes of the serine operons convert cellular L-serine to D-serine (hatched genes in Fig. 90.4). The second critical function is ligating the resistant substrate to D-alanine, forming the depsipeptide that is linked to precursor UDP-muramyl-tripeptide to form the pentapeptide precursor. The ligase genes carry the designation specific to the different operons, *vanA, B, C, D, E,* or *G* (in black in Fig. 90.4). The third essential function is depletion of the cellular pool of normal D-Ala–D-Ala dipeptide, ensuring that the precursors produced are almost exclusively of the resistant variety. In the lactate operons, the *vanX* gene encodes a dipeptidase that efficiently cleaves D-Ala–D-Ala, thereby ensuring incorporation of D-Ala–D-Lac into the pentapeptide precursors. The *vanY* gene of the lactate operons encodes a carboxypeptidase that cleaves the terminal D-Ala from normal pentapeptide precursor, depriving it of the bond breaking that provides the energy to make the peptide cross-link. The *vanY* gene is not essential for resistance, but serves to amplify the level of resistance when it is expressed. The *vanC* operon encodes an enzyme with both dipeptidase and carboxypeptidase activity ($vanXY_C$). A homologous gene is also found in the *VanE* serine operon. The *vanG* operon, however, contains two open reading frames with *vanY* homology ($vanY_{G1}$, $vanY_{G2}$). It has been hypothesized that one or both of these enzymes may also possess dipeptidase activity (101). The *vanA* operon contains a seventh gene, *vanZ,* that results in increased levels of teicoplanin resistance by an unknown mechanism (103). The *vanB* operon contains a seventh gene, designated *vanW,* whose function is unknown at present (104), but which is not required for resistance.

In all of the operons, expression of resistance is conferred by two-component regulatory systems encoded by the *vanS* and *vanR* genes (gray in Fig. 90.4) that are stimulated by the presence of one or more glycopeptides in the milieu (104,105). *vanR* regulates the transcription of the polycistronic message that encodes the three proteins essential for vancomycin resistance. Depending on its phosphorylation state, *vanR* can serve as either a repressor or activator of transcription. The phosphorylation state of *vanR* is determined by *vanS,* the transmembrane sensor component of the two-component system. *vanA* strains are resistant to both vancomycin and teicoplanin, because the presence of both antibiotics induces expression of the *vanA* operon. *vanB* strains remain susceptible to teicoplanin because the operon is not induced by the presence of teicoplanin. Teicoplanin is not a viable therapeutic alternative, however, since mutations resulting in either constitutive expression of the operon or sensitivity of $vanS_B$ to induction by teicoplanin are frequent enough to lead to the emergence of resistance on therapy (106).

Because the *van* operons can serve as the sole source for depsipeptide used in the formation of cell wall precursors, there occasionally have been observed strains that are dependent on vancomycin for survival (107). These strains generally possess mutations that lead to nonfunctional cellular ligase genes (108). Under normal circumstances, bacterial cells that have undergone null mutations in their ligase genes would not survive. However, if these strains possess one of the two primary vancomycin-resistant operons, they can survive as long as vancomycin is present in the environment. These strains have been dubbed "vancomycin-dependent enterococci." They depend on the presence of vancomycin as long as the Van genes are expressed inducibly in the presence of the antibiotic. They provide interesting insight into

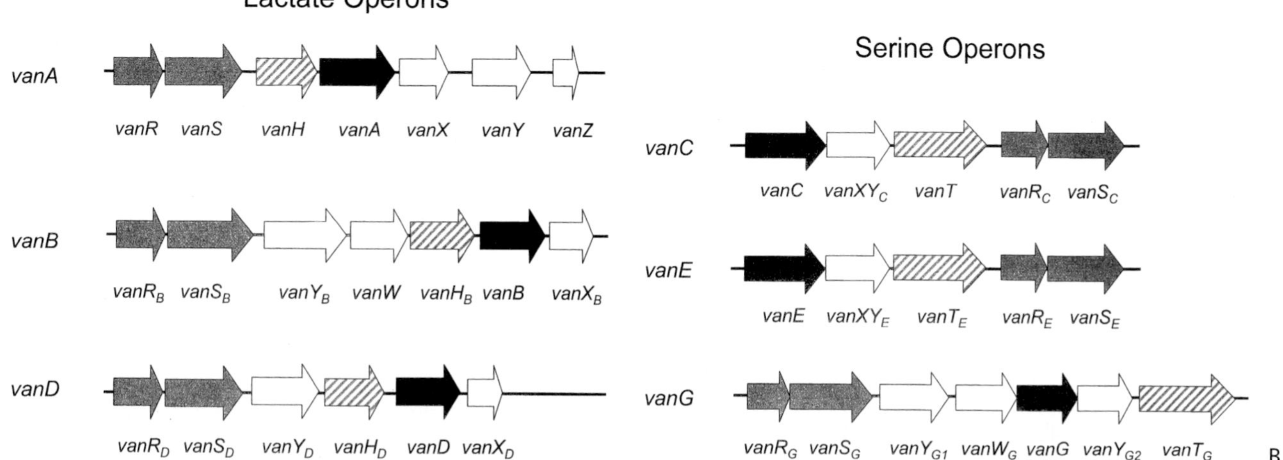

Figure 90.4. **A:**Depiction of lactate vancomycin resistance operons. Individual gene designations are found under the *arrows* representing the extent and direction of transcription of the open reading frames. *Gray* represents regulatory genes. The *hatched markings* represent the dehydrogenase genes, the *black* the ligase genes. (See text for specific functions of the different proteins.) **B:** Depiction of lactate vancomycin resistance operons. Individual gene designations are found under the *arrows* representing the extent and direction of transcription of the open reading frames. *Gray* represents regulatory genes. The *hatched markings* represent the serine racemase genes, the *black* the ligase genes. (See text for specific functions of the different proteins.)

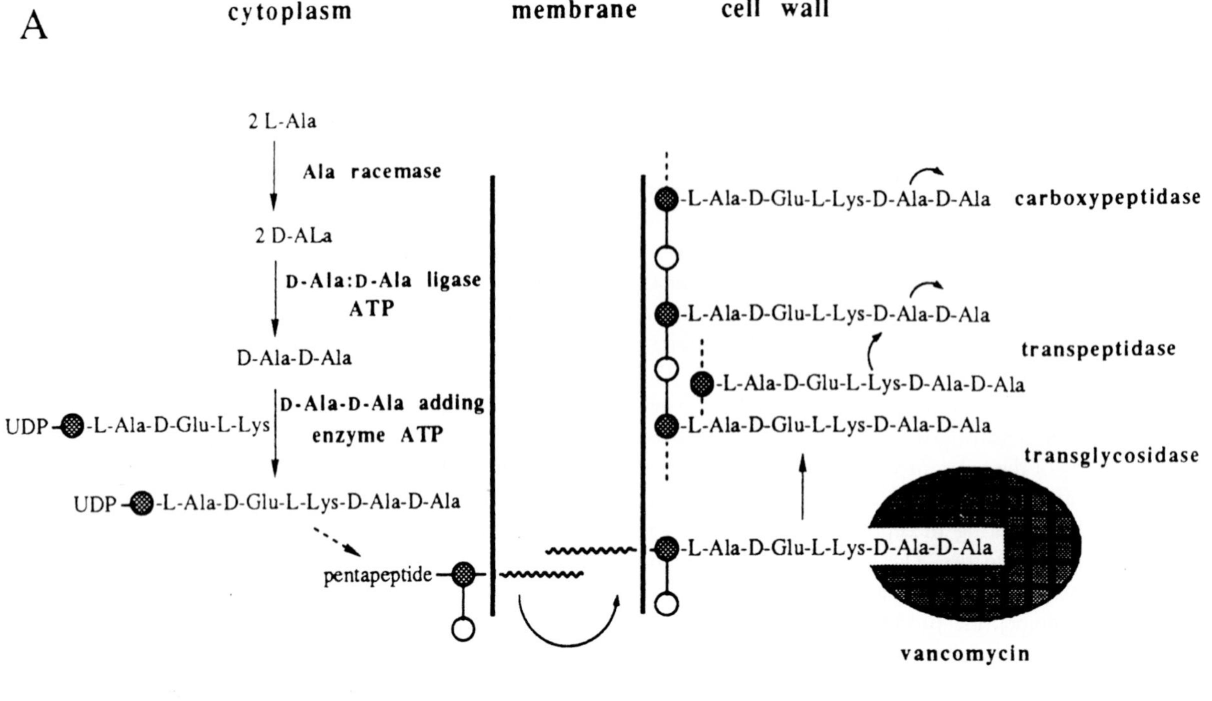

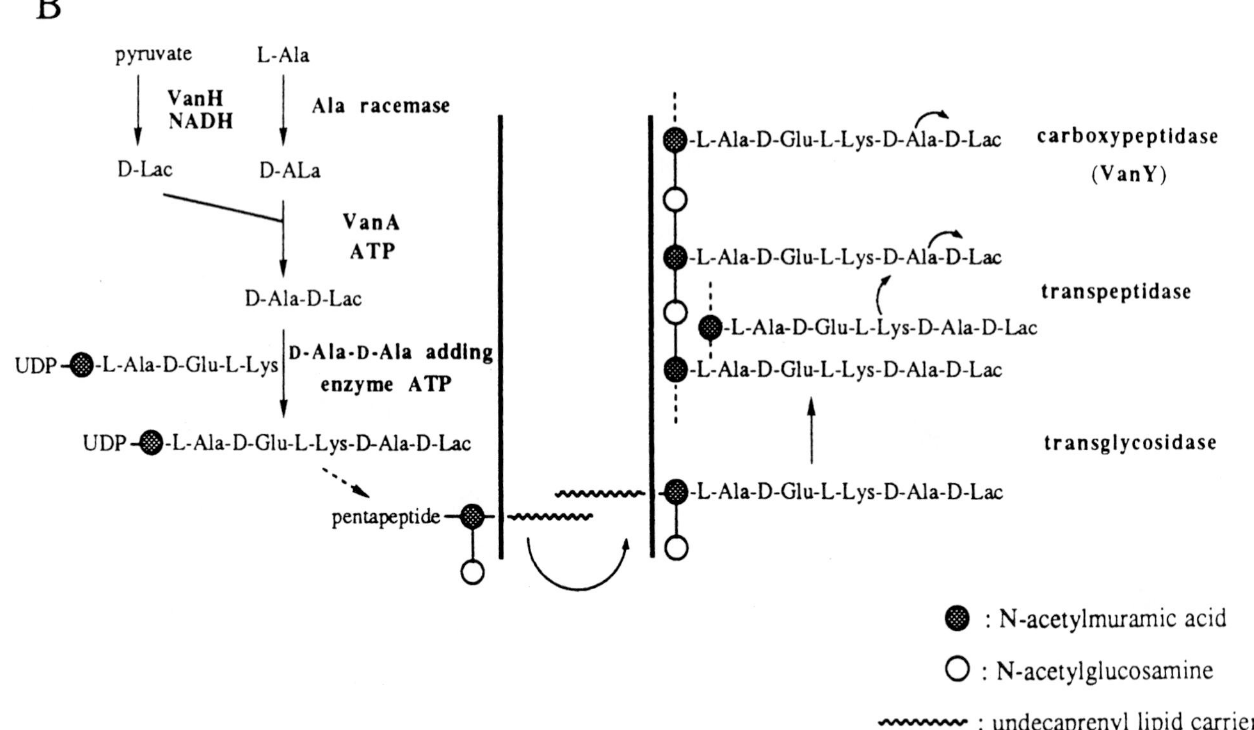

Figure 90.5. Schematic representation of peptidoglycan biosynthesis in glycopeptide-susceptible **(A)** and glycopeptide-resistant **(B)** cells. (From Arthur M, Courvalin P. Genetics and mechanisms of glycopeptide resistance in enterococci. *Antimicrob Agents Chemother* 1993;37:1563–1571.)

the mechanisms of vancomycin resistance but are of little consequence clinically except in terms of detection where growth in the absence of the antibiotic might not be observed. A variant of the *vanD* operon has recently been described that lacks $vanX_D$ and $vanY_D$ activity, but synthesizes lactated precursors exclusively because of constitutive expression in the setting of a null mutation in the normal cellular ligase gene (108).

Both *vanA* and *vanB* operons have been shown to be mobile. The *vanA* operon is characteristically encoded by a ca. 10-kb Tn*3*-family transposon designated Tn*1546* (21). This transposon has been found on plasmids, and it is presumed that the transfer of conjugative plasmids explains most of the genetic variability observed in *vanA* clinical isolates. *vanB* is characteristically encoded in the bacterial chromosome, although rare reports of plasmid-mediated *vanB*-type resistance have been published (109,110). Transfer of *vanB*-type resistance to enterococcal recipients *in vitro* has been observed, and is usually accompanied by the acquisition of large segments of chromosomal DNA (111). Two transposons or transposon-like *vanB* elements have been described. Tn*1547* is composite transposon whose mobility is conferred by flanking copies of IS*256*-related IS elements (112). Tn*5382* (and its likely identical relative Tn*1549*) is a 33-kb transposon with similarities to the conjugative transposons seen frequently in many species of gram-positive cocci (24). The contribution of these various transposons to the genetic variability observed in *vanB*-type enterococci is probably substantial.

Soon after the discovery of the vancomycin resistance operons in enterococci, *in vitro* studies suggested that the *vanA* operon could be transferred and expressed in *S. aureus.* Despite this observation, nearly 15 years passed before the first reports, in 2002, of two clinical *S. aureus* isolates expressing vancomycin resistance (12,13) (in Michigan and Pennsylvania). In both cases, the *vanA* operon has been identified in *S. aureus.* In one instance the vancomycin-resistant *S. aureus* was isolated from a wound also contaminated with *vanA*-expressing *E. faecalis.* Tn*1546* was identified in both strains, although on different plasmids. Fortunately, neither intra- nor interhospital spread of either of these microorganisms has been documented. Nevertheless, their discovery has grave implications for our ability to use vancomycin for the treatment of staphylococcal infections into the future.

Mutational resistance to vancomycin in *S. aureus* has been sporadically reported over the past few years. In virtually all cases, these isolates have been isolated from patients (generally dialysis patients) who have been treated with long-term vancomycin therapy. Resistance is associated with enlargement of the staphylococcal cell wall, and the cell wall itself contains large numbers of unlinked precursors, which can potentially serve as targets for vancomycin binding (113,114). It has been postulated that resistance results from vancomycin being sequestered within the enlarged cell wall (soaked up like a sponge), preventing achievement of adequate concentrations of vancomycin at the cell membrane, where precursors are added to the growing peptidoglycan. It is likely that this mechanism of resistance is favored only in the setting of persistent and significant vancomycin exposure, since spread to other patients has not been documented and reversion to normal (susceptible) phenotype commonly occurs when *in vitro* selection by vancomycin is removed. Animal data does suggest, however, that despite marginal minimum inhibitory concentrations (MICs) (ca. 8–16 μg/mL), this type of resistance will result in vancomycin treatment failure (115).

Staphylococcal strains with decreased susceptibility to teicoplanin have also been described. Mutational resistance to teicoplanin is very common among *S. hemolyticus* and *S. epidermidis* and, with release of teicoplanin for therapy in Europe, has been described in *S. aureus* as well (116,117). Some evidence suggests that PBPs may be involved in the expression of resistance, although the exact mechanism in these strains is still unknown (118). It is possible to select mutants of *S. hemolyticus* and *S. aureus* resistant to vancomycin, but only after multiple steps (119,120). Resistant mutants arising during vancomycin therapy of *S. hemolyticus* infections in the presence of plastic catheters has been reported in humans (117), but these mutants tend to be unstable. The emergence of normally saprophytic microorganisms intrinsically resistant to the glycopeptides (including lactobacilli, leuconostocs, pediococci, and others) as important pathogens has been reviewed (121). These strains predominantly infect immunocompromised patients. The mechanism of glycopeptide resistance is identical to that described for enterococci. They synthesize a peptidoglycan precursor terminating in D-Ala–D-Lac normally (122). For the most part, these microorganisms remain susceptible to the penicillins.

AMINOGLYCOSIDES

Structure and Mechanism of Action

The aminoglycosides are made of three amino sugars in glycosidic linkage (Fig. 90.6). As such, they are polycationic compounds. They are divided into two classes: the streptidine class, of which streptomycin is the only member in clinical use, and the 2-deoxystreptamine class, which includes all other clinically used aminoglycosides. Uptake of aminoglycosides into bacterial cells is via active transport through the cytoplasmic membrane. The intracellular target of all aminoglycosides is the 30S subunit of the ribosome. For streptomycin, only a single ribosomal-binding site exists, whereas for the others, multiple binding sites are available. In gram-negative microorganisms, aminoglycoside uptake probably occurs via a two-stage process in which the cationic antibiotic displaces magnesium ions linking lipid A subunits. This displacement results in disruption of the outer membrane and diffusion of the antibiotic into the periplasmic space. It seems likely that, in addition to its activity at the ribosome, disruption of the cytoplasmic membrane also plays a role in the activity of these agents. Binding to the 30S ribosomal subunit results in extensive translational misreading and synthesis of abnormal proteins, many of which integrate into the membrane, resulting in further disintegration. It is the sum of these effects that is thought to lead to the bactericidal activity of the aminoglycosides.

Mechanisms of Resistance

Simple mutation of genes encoding ribosomal proteins can result in streptomycin resistance, since only a single binding site

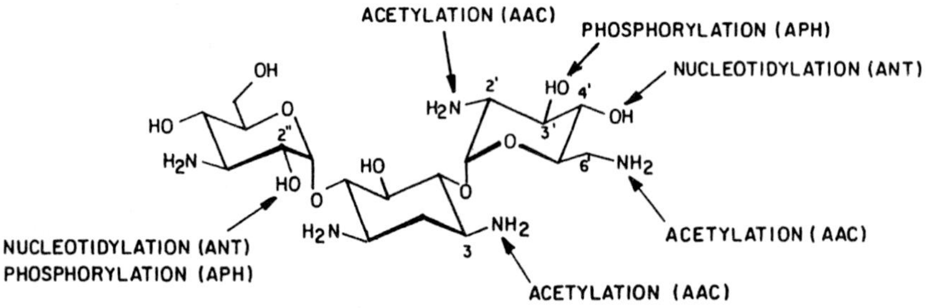

Figure 90.6. Prototypic aminoglycoside showing sites available for modification and modifications that have been shown to occur.

exists for this antibiotic. Ribosomally resistant mutants have been described clinically, primarily in enterococci and mycobacteria. These mutants remain susceptible to the other aminoglycosides. Mutants with altered membrane transport (the so-called small colony-formers) can also be resistant to aminoglycosides. These cells have altered membrane proton motive force and are unable to transport aminoglycosides across the cytoplasmic membrane. Such mutants are less virulent than their wild-type parents (123).

The primary mechanism of bacterial resistance to aminoglycosides is enzymatic modification of the antibiotic (124) (Fig. 90.6). Such chemical modifications prevent binding of the aminoglycoside to the ribosome and may also decrease transport. Three major classes of modifying enzymes have been described that depend on the particular modification involved: phosphorylases, adenyl transferases, and acetyl transferases (Table 90.5). Resistance to all aminoglycosides is achievable by a combination of different enzymes.

The emergence of enzyme-mediated resistance to aminoglycosides in enterococci is a significant clinical problem. Because of their intrinsic tolerance to the bactericidal activity of all cell wall–active agents, effective treatment of serious enterococcal infections requires the synergistically bactericidal combination of a cell wall–active agent and an aminoglycoside. Since the most common genes encoding aminoglycoside resistance in enterococci were derived from the staphylococci, these two genera will be discussed together. Gentamicin resistance in strains of *S. aureus* and *S. epidermidis* first appeared in the U.S. and elsewhere in the mid-1970s (125). In 1979, the first case of high-level resistance to gentamicin, which results in resistance to synergistic bactericidal activity in enterococci, was reported (126). Resistance to aminoglycosides has spread widely in both genera since the first reports.

High-level resistance to gentamicin in both staphylococci and enterococci results from modification of the antibiotic by enzymatic mechanisms. Resistance is most commonly encoded by the *aacA-aphD* resistance gene, the product of which is a 6′-acetyltransferase-2″phosphotransferase (6′-AAC-2″-APH) bifunctional enzyme, a fusion protein that possesses both of the above enzymatic activities (127). The 6′-AAC component of the bifunctional enzyme confers resistance to amikacin, kanamycin, and tobramycin, whereas the 2″-APH component is primarily responsible for resistance to gentamicin and netilmicin. All strains that possess this gene are resistant to all of the above-mentioned aminoglycosides. Streptomycin, which is inactivated by a separate enzyme, is the single clinically available aminoglycoside not inactivated by the bifunctional enzyme. The nucleotide sequences of the genes responsible for the production of the bifunctional enzyme are identical in *S. aureus* and *E. faecalis,* and probably in *E. faecium, S. epidermidis,* and *S. agalactiae* as well (127–129). These genes are often integrated into conjugative plasmids in both staphylococci and enterococci. In addition, the bifunctional enzyme gene has been found integrated into transposons in *S. aureus* (Tn*4001*), *S. epidermidis* (Tn*4031*), and *E. faecalis* (Tn*5281*) (130–132). Nucleotide sequence analysis of the region adjacent to the enterococcal gene and structural analysis of the enterococcal transposable element reveal extensive similarities with Tn*4001* from *S. aureus.* Two additional genes that confer resistance to aminoglycosides in enterococci have been described in the past decade (133). Unlike the bifunctional enzyme, these phosphotransferases do not confer resistance to a wide range of aminoglycosides. In addition, they may confer only relatively low levels of resistance (256 μg/mL) when tested by standard techniques, and therefore may be missed in screening assays designed to detect the more common enzymes. Despite these lower levels of resistance, they do confer a resistance to cell wall–active agent-aminoglycoside synergism, so they may prove to be important for the treatment of endocarditis. The overall prevalence of these enzymes is relatively low at present but it bears watching, and physicians are well advised to consider the possibility that such an enzyme is present when treating serious enterococcal infections.

TABLE 90.5. AMINOGLYCOSIDE-MODIFYING ENZYMES

Acetyltransferases	Phosphotransferases	Adenyltransferases
AAC(1)	APH(2″)-I	ANT(2″)-I
AAC(2′)-I	APH(3′)-I	ANT(3″)-I
AAC(3)-I	APH(3′)-III	ANT(4′)-I
AAC(3)-II	APH(3′)-IV	ANT(4′)-II
AAC(3)-III	APH(3′)-V	ANT(6)-I
AAC(3)-IV	APH(#′)-VI	ANT(9)-I
AAC(3)-VI	APH(3′)-VII	
AAC(3)-VII	APH(3″)-I	
AAC(3′)-VIII	APH(6)-I	
AAC(3)-IX	APH(4)-I	
AAC(3)-X	APH(7″)	
AAC(6′)-I	APH(9)	
AAC(6′)-II		
AAC(6′)-APH(2″)		
AAC(6)-III		
AAC(6)-IV		

From Rather PN. Origins of aminoglycoside modifying enzymes. *Drug Resist Updates* 1998;1:285–291, with permission.

High-level gentamicin resistance in enterococcal isolates has spread rapidly in some hospitals, with one center reporting 55% of nosocomial enterococcal isolates resistant to gentamicin (10). Gentamicin-resistant enterococci appear to be transmitted in the hospital setting on the hands of caregivers. Measures undertaken to limit such transmission have proven effective in containing outbreaks of infection and colonization with these microorganisms (134). A growing body of evidence suggests that serious infection with these strains is associated with a worse prognosis than is associated with infections caused by susceptible isolates (135–137). Episodes of failure (resulting in death or requiring surgical intervention for cure) in the treatment of enterococcal endocarditis caused by gentamicin-resistant strains have been reported (137,138). Fortunately, most enterococcal infections can be successfully treated with a single agent. For more serious infections, it is essential to test all enterococcal isolates for high-level resistance to both gentamicin and streptomycin. Depending on the center, anywhere from 0% to 45% of enterococcal strains exhibiting high-level gentamicin resistance are reported to remain susceptible to streptomycin (136,139). Combinations of cell wall–active agents and streptomycin should be effective in the treatment of strains exhibiting high-level gentamicin resistance but lacking high-level resistance to streptomycin, and vice versa (138,140). At present, there is no reliable bactericidal combination of antibiotics against strains exhibiting high-level resistance to both gentamicin and streptomycin.

In gram-negative microorganisms, aminoglycoside-modifying enzymes are the most important mechanisms of resistance. In general, genes encoding such enzymes are carried on plasmids or transposons and are expressed constitutively. However, in the case of *S. marcescens* and *Providencia stuartii,* aminoglycoside acetyltransferases are normally encoded by chromosomal genes but are not well expressed (141,142). It appears that, in these species, the chromosomally encoded acetyltransferases represent intrinsic housekeeping genes that are responsible for acetylating peptidoglycan (143). Aminoglycosides bear structural resemblance to peptidoglycan, and are acetylated as well. Normally these enzymes are produced in amounts sufficient to acetylate peptidoglycan, but not to result in resistance. Mutants that express these enzymes at high levels can be easily selected, and probably account for many of the aminoglycoside-resistant strains of these species.

Gram-negative bacteria also employ efflux pumps to assist with aminoglycoside resistance. In *P. aeruginosa,* the MexXY-OprM system is most commonly implicated in aminoglycoside efflux (144), but more recent data also implicated MexAB-OprM and an analog of the *E. coli* small multidrug resistance (SMR)-type pump *emrE* ($emrE_{Pae}$) (145). The MexAB-OprM pump effluxes aminoglycosides *in vitro,* but only when tested in low ionic strength media. An RND pump has also been recently implicated in aminoglycoside resistance in *Acinetobacter baumannii* (146). The area of efflux pump-mediated resistance is only beginning to be explored, and there will no doubt be significant discoveries made in this area over the next decade.

Although many clinicians retreat from aminoglycoside use in the therapy for gram-negative infections, there are accumulating data that, at least for a subset of patients, the combination of aminoglycoside with β-lactams is superior to either agent alone, or even to other combinations (68,147). Furthermore, it is unlikely that this beneficial effect is due to the suppression of emerging β-lactam–resistant mutants (68). In addition, the popularization of once-daily aminoglycoside therapy may lead to more aminoglycoside use in the future. Thus, aminoglycoside resistance in gram-negative species may ultimately be more important than is currently thought.

RESISTANCE TO THE FLUOROQUINOLONES

Structure and Mechanism of Action

The quinolone class of antibiotics can be historically traced to nalidixic acid. These antibiotics are potent inhibitors of cellular topoisomerases, enzymes required for winding and unwinding supercoiled, double-stranded DNA (148). Quinolone antibiotics act by inhibiting DNA synthesis. Their targets are two type 2 topoisomerases, DNA gyrase and topoisomerase IV. These two enzymes both exist as tetramers composed of different subunits (GyrA and GyrB of DNA gyrase; ParC and ParE of topoisomerase IV). DNA gyrase maintains negative supercoiling of DNA, whereas topoisomerase IV separates interlocked DNA strands formed during replication, facilitating segregation into daughter cells. Fluoroquinolones bind to the topoisomerase-DNA complexes and disrupt cellular processes involving DNA (replication fork, transcription of RNA, DNA helicase) (149–151). The end result is cellular death by unclear mechanisms.

Fluoroquinolone affinity for the two targets varies with the compound, explaining to some extent differing potencies. The enzyme for which a particular fluoroquinolone has the greatest affinity is referred to as the primary target (152–154). It is generally but not universally true that DNA gyrase is the primary target of fluoroquinolones in gram-negative bacteria, whereas topoisomerase IV is the primary target in gram-positive bacteria.

Alterations in Target Enzymes

The most common mechanism of fluoroquinolone resistance is point mutations of the topoisomerase genes resulting in structural alterations in the topoisomerase enzymes. In *gyrA* and *parC,* resistance-associated mutations are often localized to a region in the enzyme that contains the active site tyrosine covalently linked to the broken DNA strand. This 130 base pair (bp) region of *gyrA* has been referred to as the quinolone-resistance-determining region (QRDR) (155). X-ray crystallographic studies of a fragment of the *gyrA* enzyme suggest that QRDR mutations are clustered in three dimensions, supporting the hypothesis that this region constitutes a part of the quinolone binding site (156). Frequent sites for resistance-associated mutations are serine 83 and aspartate 87 of DNA gyrase and serine 79 and aspartate 83 of *parC* (157).

The level of resistance conferred by a point mutation in the primary target enzyme depends on the change of enzyme affinity created by the mutation and the affinity of the specific fluoroquinolone for the secondary target. As such, fluoroquinolones exhibiting strong affinity for both target enzymes may be less likely to promote the emergence of resistant strains in the clinical setting, since the activity against the secondary target may be enough to inhibit the bacterium even in the presence of primary target mutation. Consistent with this hypothesis, fluoroquinolone-species combinations for which single mutations result in significantly higher MICs (such as ciprofloxacin and *S. aureus* or *P. aeruginosa*) have readily selected out resistant mutants in the clinical setting (158).

Most highly resistant strains exhibit more than one mutation in both the *gyrA* and *parC* enzymes. It is noteworthy in this context that fluoroquinolone resistance conferred by enzyme mutations is to some degree a class resistance in which the activity of all fluoroquinolones is impacted. Thus, although single point mutations conferring resistance to one fluoroquinolone may not yield MICs conferring clinically significant levels of resistance for another, the MICs for the all fluoroquinolone will inevitably be increased. These preexisting mutations may then serve as the template to select additional mutations that result in more broad-spectrum fluoroquinolone resistance. Some experts suggest that this phenomenon should prompt clinicians always to use the most potent fluoroquinolone when treating infections, to prevent the emergence of resistance. Some degree of skepticism about such recommendations is warranted, since potency varies with the microorganism (moxifloxacin may be more potent against *S. pneumoniae* than ciprofloxacin, but the reverse is true for *P. aeruginosa*) and fluoroquinolone concentrations achievable in many areas of the body (such as the gastrointestinal tract) may not approximate those needed to prevent the emergence of resistance. Such recommendations, therefore, should be tested in controlled clinical trials before they are widely adopted.

Mutations in *gyrB* and *parE* are less common than in *gyrA* and *parC* and cluster in the midportion of the subunit (159). The true impact of these mutations on expression of resistance remains to be determined.

Resistance Due to Decreased Intracellular Accumulation

Fluoroquinolones penetrate the outer membrane of gram-negative bacteria through porins, and so the absence of specific porins may theoretically impact the susceptibility. However, diffusion through outer and cytoplasmic membranes is generally sufficient to retain activity against strains solely lacking porins (160). More important in reducing intracellular accumulation of fluoroquinolones is the expression of multidrug resistance pumps (157). All of the pumps described above for *P. aeruginosa* have been shown to efflux fluoroquinolone antimicrobial agents (91,92). By themselves, pumps generally confer only a low level of resistance to fluoroquinolones. However, their expression may amplify the level of resistance conferred by point mutations within the topoisomerase genes. By so doing, they may increase the risk that a given fluoroquinolone will select out resistant mutants through single point mutations.

A transferable, plasmid-mediated form of resistance to fluoroquinolones has been described in a strain of *K. pneumoniae* (161). The gene conferring this resistance has been designated *qnr,* and its mechanism discerned to be protection of the DNA gyrase from interaction with the fluoroquinolone (162). The extent to which *qnr*-like genes will become prevalent in the population remains unknown, but recent data suggest that at present its prevalence in the U.S. is very low (163).

Resistance to Newer Antimicrobial Agents

The emergence and spread of multiresistant enterococci in the past decade, accompanied by the inexorable increase in the prevalence of MRSA, has amplified the importance of finding new agents with clinically important activity against resistant gram-positive cocci. Two such agents have been licensed in the past 5 years. Quinupristin-dalfopristin is a combination of two pristinamycins (one of the streptogramin A class, the other a streptogramin B) that have synergistic activity against *E. faecium* (although they are ineffective against *E. faecalis*) and *S. aureus.* The overall use of this combination has been limited by considerations of cost and toxicities, and by the need to administer through a central venous catheter. Despite its limited use, two forms of resistance have already been noted in *E. faecium.* The first is a low-level resistance whose mechanism remains to be fully defined, but which may involve activation of an efflux pump. Data from a recent clinical study reported that 21% of *E. faecium* isolated exhibited such low-level resistance (95). This type of resistance has not been shown to be transferable, and its impact on therapy remains to be determined. High-level resistance to these mixtures can result from resistance to streptogramin A alone and was first described in staphylococci conferred by genes encoding streptogramin A acetyltransferases [*vat*(A), *vat*(B), and *vat*(C)] or adenosine triphosphate (ATP)-binding efflux genes [*vga*(A), *vga*(B)]. Two acetyltransferase genes have now been described that confer resistance to quinupristin-dalfopristin in *E. faecium—vat*(D) [previously *sat*(A)] and *vat*(E) [previously *sat*(G)]. In most cases, these resistance genes are found along with an *erm* resistance gene (164), suggesting that resistance to both streptogramin A and B may be necessary to confer clinically significant levels of resistance to quinupristin-dalfopristin in *E. faecium.* These genes have been found on transferable plasmids, suggesting that the potential for spread is significant.

Linezolid is the first licensed member of the oxazolidone class of antibiotics. It is active against most multiresistant gram-positive cocci including multiresistant enterococci and *S. aureus.* Linezolid acts by binding to the conglomeration of ribosomes, messenger RNB (mRNA), and transfer RNA (tRNA) known as the initiation complex, thereby inhibiting protein synthesis. Resistance to linezolid has been associated with point mutations in the 23S ribosomal RNA subunit (165). The most common mutation found in resistant isolates has been a G→U change at position 2576 (*E. coli* numbering scheme). The degree of resistance seen in enterococci is related to the percentage of ribosomal RNA (rRNA) genes that have this mutation (166). This type of resistance has not been transferable in any of the cases examined to date. However, the known transferability of enterococci themselves within the healthcare setting creates concern that these strains could become prevalent. One outbreak of such strains in a liver transplant unit has already been reported (167).

CONCLUSION

Despite our best efforts, the elusive promise of the "perfect" antibiotic has not been realized. Experience with the use of antibiotics in the clinical setting has taught us that resistance often emerges soon after the clinical introduction of any antibiotic, and in some cases these resistance determinants spread rapidly once they are present in human pathogens. Resistance may be promoted by the excessive and injudicious use of antimicrobial agents, as well as by poor infection control practices employed in the hospital, day-care centers, and the home. Guidelines for the prevention of resistance in hospitals have been issued jointly by the Society for Healthcare Epidemiology of America and the Infectious Diseases Society of America (168). The guidelines suggest a number of strategies including some aimed at testing the hypotheses and proposals contained within the document. We hope that these suggestions will be implemented so that optimal programs based on data can be introduced.

Since it is our behavior and practices that have amplified the problem of resistance, it stands to reason that altering these behavior patterns may contribute to its control or eradication. A detailed understanding of the mechanisms by which resistance emerges within and spreads among bacterial species is an essential component of any strategy to control antimicrobial resistance in the hospital setting. Intelligent, mechanism-based strategies employing an appropriate mix of infection and antibiotic control offer the best hope for controlling the spread of resistance as well as for the conservation of important and increasingly scarce economic resources.

REFERENCES

1. Bjorkman J, Nagaev I, Berg OG, et al. Effects of environment on compensatory mutations to ameliorate costs of antibiotic resistance. *Science* 2000;287:1479–1482.
2. Willems RJ, Homan W, Top J, et al. Variant esp gene as a marker of a distinct genetic lineage of vancomycin-resistant Enterococcus faecium spreading in hospitals. *Lancet* 2001;357:853–855.
3. Rice LB, Carias L, Rudin S, et al. A potential virulence gene, *hyl*$_{Efm}$, predominates in *Enterococcus faecium* of clinical origin. *J Infect Dis* 2003;187:508–512.
4. Sahm DF, Marsilio MK, Piazza G. Antimicrobial resistance in key bloodstream bacterial isolates: electronic surveillance with the Surveillance Network Database—USA. *Clin Infect Dis* 1999;29:259–263.
5. Murdoch DR, Mirrett S, Harrell LJ, et al. Sequential emergence of antibiotic resistance in enterococcal bloodstream isolates over 25 years. *Antimicrob Agents Chemother* 2002;46:3676–3678.
6. Chanal CM, Sirot DL, Labia R, et al. Comparative study of a novel plasmid-mediated β-lactamase, CAZ-2, and the CTX-1 and CAZ-1 enzymes conferring resistance to broad-spectrum cephalosporins. *Antimicrob Agents Chemother* 1988;32:1660–1665.
7. Rice LB, Willey SH, Papanicolaou GA, et al. Outbreak of ceftazidime resistance caused by extended-spectrum β-lactamases at a Massachusetts chronic care facility. *Antimicrob Agents Chemother* 1990;34: 2193–2199.
8. Dunny GM, Leonard BAB, Hedberg PJ. Pheromone-inducible conjugation in *Enterococcus faecalis*: interbacterial and host-parasite chemical communication. *J Bacteriol* 1995;177:871–876.
9. Murray BE. The life and times of the enterococcus. *Clin Microbiol Rev* 1990;3:46–65.
10. Zervos MJ, Kaufman CA, Therasse PM, et al. Nosocomial infection by gentamicin-resistant *Streptococcus faecalis* : an epidemiologic study. *Ann Intern Med* 1987;106:687–691.
11. Rice LB, Carias LL. Transfer of Tn*5385*, a composite, multiresistance element from *Enterococcus faecalis. J Bacteriol* 1998;180:714–721.
12. Vancomycin-resistant Staphylococcus aureus—Pennsylvania, 2002. *MMWR* 2002;51:902.
13. Clark N, Jevitt L, Kellum M, et al. High-level vancomycin resistance in a clinical isolate of Staphylococcus aureus. Presented at 42nd Interscience Conference on antimicrobial agents and chemotherapy, San Diego, CA, 2002.
14. Heaton MP, Discotto LF, Pucci MJ, et al. Mobilization of vancomycin resistance by transposon-mediated fusion of a VanA plasmid with an Enterococcus faecium sex pheromone-response plasmid. *Gene* 1996;171:9–17.
15. Galas DJ, Chandler M. Bacterial insertion sequences. In: Berg DE, Howe MM, eds. *Mobile DNA.* Washington, DC: American Society for Microbiology, 1989:109–162.
16. Mercier J, Lachapelle J, Couture F, et al. Structural and functional characterization of *tnpI*, a recombinase locus in Tn*21* and related β-lactamase transposons. *J Bacteriol* 1990;172:3745–3757.
17. Partridge SR, Brown HJ, Stokes HW, et al. Transposons Tn1696 and Tn21 and their integrons In4 and In2 have independent origins. *Antimicrob Agents Chemother* 2001;45:1263–1270.
18. Bennett PM. Integrons and gene cassettes: a genetic construction kit for bacteria. *J Antimicrob Chemother* 1999;43:1–4.
19. White PA, McIver CJ, Rawlinson WD. Integrons and gene cassettes in the Enterobacteriaceae. *Antimicrob Agents Chemother* 2001;45: 2658–2661.
20. Rowe-Magnus DA, Guerout AM, Ploncard P, et al. The evolutionary history of chromosomal super-integrons provides an ancestry for multiresistant integrons. *Proc Natl Acad Sci USA* 2001;98:652–657.
21. Arthur M, Molinas C, Depardieu F, et al. Characterization of Tn1546, a Tn3-related transposon conferring glycopeptide resistance by synthesis of depsipeptide peptidoglycan precursors in Enterococcus faecium BM4147. *J Bacteriol* 1993;175:117–127.
22. Clewell DB, Flannagan SE, Jaworski DD. Unconstrained bacterial promiscuity: the Tn*916*-Tn*1545* family of conjugative transposons. *Trends Microbiol* 1995;3:229–236.
23. Torres OR, Korman RZ, Zahler SA, et al. The conjugative transposon Tn*925*: enhancement of conjugal transfer by tetracycline in *Enterococcus faecalis* and mobilization of chromosomal genes in both *Bacillus subtilis* and *E. faecalis. Mol Genl Genet* 1991;225:395–400.
24. Carias LL, Rudin SD, Donskey CJ, et al. Genetic linkage and cotransfer of a novel, *vanB*-containing transposon (Tn*5382*) and a low-affinity penicillin-binding protein 5 gene in a clinical vancomycin-resistant *Enterococcus faecium* isolate. *J Bacteriol* 1998;180: 4426–4434.
25. Rauch PJH, Beerthuyzen MM, De Vos WM. Distribution and evolution of nisin-sucrose elements in *Lactococcus lactis. Appl Environ Microbiol* 1994;60:1798–1804.
26. Podglajen I, Breuil J, Rohaut A, et al. Multiple mobile promoter regions for the rare carbapenem resistance gene of Bacteroides fragilis. *J Bacteriol* 2001;183:3531–3555.
27. Rice LB, Marshall SH, Carias LL. Tn*5381*, a conjugative transposon identifiable as a circular form in *Enterococcus faecalis. J Bacteriol* 1992; 174:7308–7315.
28. Doucet-Populaire F, Trieu-Cuot P, Dosbaa I, et al. Inducible transfer of conjugative transposon Tn*1545* from *Enterococcus faecalis* to *Listeria monocytogenes* in the digestive tracts of gnotobiotic mice. *Antimicrob Agents Chemother* 1991;35:185–187.
29. Boyce JM, Opal SM, Chow JW, et al. Outbreak of multidrug-resistant *Enterococcus faecium* with transferable *vanB* class vancomycin resistance. *J Clin Microbiol* 1994;32:1148–1153.
30. Boyce JM, Mermel LA, Zervos MJ, et al. Controlling vancomycin-resistant enterococci. *Infect Control Hosp Epidemiol* 1995;16: 634–637.
31. Rice LB, Eckstein EC, DeVente J, 1996. Ceftazidime-resistant *Klebsiella pneumoniae* isolates recovered at the Cleveland Department of Veterans Affairs Medical Center. *Clin Infect Dis* 1996;23:118–124.
32. Williamson R, Calderwood SB, Moellering RCJ, et al. Studies on the mechanism of intrinsic resistance to β-lactam antibiotic in group D streptococci. *J Gen Microbiol* 1983;129:813–822.

33. Williamson R, LaBouguenec C, Gutmann L, et al. One or two low affinity penicillin-binding proteins may be responsible for the range of susceptibility of *Enterococcus faecium* to penicillin. *J Gen Microbiol* 1985;131:1933–1940.
34. Tomasz A, Drugeon HB, de Lencestre HM, et al. New mechanism for methicillin resistance in *Staphylococcus aureus*: clinical isolates that lack the PBP2a gene and contain normal penicillin-binding proteins with modified penicillin-binding capacity. *Antimicrob Agents Chemother* 1989;33:1869–1874.
35. Dowson CG, Hutchison A, Brannigan JA, et al. Horizontal transfer of penicillin-binding protein genes in penicillin-resistant clinical isolates of *Streptococcus pneumoniae. Proc Natl Acad Sci USA* 1989;86: 8842–8846.
36. Spratt BG. Hybrid penicillin-binding proteins in penicillin-resistant strains of *Neisseria gonorrhoeae. Nature (Lond)* 1988;332:173–176.
37. Spratt BG, Zhang Q-Y, Jones DM, et al. Recruitment of a penicillin-binding protein gene from *Neisseria flavescens* during the emergence of penicillin resistance in *Neisseria meningitidis. Proc Natl Acad Sci USA* 1989;86:8988–8992.
38. Ito T, Katayama Y, Asada K, et al. Structural comparison of three types of staphylococcal cassette chromosome mec integrated in the chromosome in methicillin-resistant Staphylococcus aureus. *Antimicrob Agents Chemother* 2001;45:1323–1336.
39. Hiramatsu K, Cui L, Kuroda M, et al. The emergence and evolution of methicillin-resistant Staphylococcus aureus. *Trends Microbiol* 2001; 9:486–493.
40. Wu SW, de Lencastre H, Tomasz A. Recruitment of the mecA gene homologue of Staphylococcus sciuri into a resistance determinant and expression of the resistant phenotype in Staphylococcus aureus. *J Bacteriol* 2001;183:2417–2424.
41. Chambers HF. Methicillin resistance in staphylococci: molecular and biochemical basis and clinical implications. *Clin Microbiol Rev* 1997; 10:781–791.
42. Filipe SR, Pinho MG, Tomasz A. Characterization of the murMN operon involved in the synthesis of branched peptidoglycan peptides in Streptococcus pneumoniae. *J Biol Chem* 2000;275:27768–27774.
43. Williamson R, Al-Obeid S, Shlaes JH, et al. Inducible resistance to vancomycin in *Enterococcus faecium* D366. *J Infect Dis* 1989;159: 1095–1104.
44. Grayson ML, Eliopoulos GM, Wennersten CB, et al. Increasing resistance to β-lactam antibiotics among clinical isolates of *Enterococcus faecium*: a 22-year review at one institution. *Antimicrob Agents Chemother* 1991;35:2180–2184.
45. Rybkine T, Mainardi J-L, Sougakoff W, et al. Penicillin-binding protein 5 sequence alterations in clinical isolates of *Enterococcus faecium* with different levels of β-lactam resistance. *J Infect Dis* 1998;178: 159–163.
46. Rice LB, Carias LL, Hutton-Thomas R, et al. Penicillin-binding protein 5 and expression of ampicillin resistance in Enterococcus faecium. *Antimicrob Agents Chemother* 2001;45:1480–1486.
47. Torres C, Tenorio C, Lantero M, et al. High-level penicillin resistance and penicillin-gentamicin synergy in *Enterococcus faecium. Antimicrob Agents Chemother* 1993;37:2427–2431.
48. Joris B, Ghuysen JM, Dive G, et al. The active site serine penicillin-recognizing enzymes as members of the *Streptomyces* R61 D-D peptidase family. *Biochem J* 1988;250:313–324.
49. Ambler RP. The structure of β-lactamases. *Philos Trans R Soc Lond [B]* 1980;289:321–331.
50. Ambler RP, Coulson AFW, Frère JM, et al. A standard numbering scheme for the class A β-lactamases. *Biochem J* 1991;276:269–272.
51. Bush K, Jacoby GA, Medeiros AA. A functional classification scheme for β-lactamases and its correlation with molecular structure. *Antimicrob Agents Chemother* 1995;39:1211–1233.
52. Barber M, Rozwadowska-Dowsenko M. Infection by penicillin-resistant staphylococci. *Lancet* 1948;2:641–644.
53. Lacey RW. Antibiotic resistance plasmids of *Staphylococcus aureus* and their clinical importance. *Bacteriol Rev* 1975;39:1–32.
54. McMurray LW, Kernodle DS, Barg NL. Characterization of a widespread strain of methicillin-susceptible *Staphylococcus aureus* associated with nosocomial infections. *J Infect Dis* 1990;162:759–762.
55. Jacoby GA, Medeiros AA. More extended-spectrum β-lactamases. *Antimicrob Agents Chemother* 1991;35:1697–1704.
56. Bradford PA. Extended-spectrum beta-lactamases in the 21st century: characterization, epidemiology, and detection of this important resistance threat. *Clin Microbiol Rev* 2001;14:933–951.
57. Bonnet R, De Champs C, Sirot D, et al. Diversity of TEM mutants in Proteus mirabilis. *Antimicrob Agents Chemother* 1999;43:2671–2677.
58. Meyer KS, Urban C, Eagan JA, et al. Nosocomial outbreak of *Klebsiella* infection resistant to late-generation cephalosporins. *Ann Intern Med* 1993;119:353–358.
59. Peña C, Pujol M, Ardanuy C, et al. Epidemiology and successful control of a large outbreak due to *Klebsiella pneumoniae* producing extended-spectrum β-lactamases. *Antimicrob Agents Chemother* 1998; 42:53–58.
60. Rasheed JK, Jay C, Metchock B, et al. Evolution of extended-spectrum β-lactam resistance (SHV-8) in a strain of *Escherichia coli* during multiple episodes of bacteremia. *Antimicrob Agents Chemother* 1997; 41:647–653.
61. Schiappa DA, Hayden MK, Matushek MG, et al. Ceftazidime-resistant *Klebsiella pneumoniae* and *Escherichia coli* bloodstream infection: a case-control and molecular epidemiologic investigation. *J Infect Dis* 1996;174:529–536.
62. Jacobs C, Frere J-M, Normark S. Cytosolic intermediates for cell wall biosynthesis and degradation control inducible β-lactam resistance in gram-negative bacteria. *Cell* 1997;88:823–832.
63. Jacobs C, Huang LJ, Bartowsky E, et al. Bacterial cell wall recycling provides cytosolic muropeptides as effectors for beta-lactamase induction. *Eur Mol Biol Org J* 1994;13:4684–4694.
64. Jacobs C, Joris B, Jamin M, et al. AmpD, essential for both β-lactamase regulation and cell wall recycling, is a novel cytosolic *N*-acetylmuramyl-L-alanine amidase. *Mol Microbiol* 1995;15:553–559.
65. Sanders WEJ, Sanders CC. Inducible β-lactamases: clinical and epidemiologic implications for use of newer cephalosporins. *Rev Infect Dis* 1988;10:830–838.
66. Sanders CC. Cefepime: the next generation? *Clin Infect Dis* 1993;17: 369–379.
67. Limaye AP, Gautom RK, Black D, et al. Rapid emergence of resistance to cefepime during treatment. *Clin Infect Dis* 1997;25:339–340.
68. Chow JW, Fine MJ, Shlaes DM, et al. *Enterobacter* bacteremia: clinical features and emergence of antibiotic resistance during therapy. *Ann Intern Med* 1991;115:585–590.
69. Kaye KS, Cosgrove S, Harris A, et al. Risk factors for emergence of resistance to broad-spectrum cephalosporins among Enterobacter spp. *Antimicrob Agents Chemother* 2001;45:2628–2630.
70. Hoyen CM, Hujer AM, Hujer KM, et al. A clinical strain of Escherichia coli possessing CMY-2 plasmid-mediated amp C beta-lactamase: an emerging concern in pediatrics? *Microb Drug Resist* 2002; 8:329–333.
71. Bradford PA, Urban C, Mariano N, et al. Imipenem resistance in *Klebsiella pneumoniae* is associated with the combination of ACT-1, a plasmid-mediated AmpC beta-lactamase, and the loss of an outer membrane protein. *Antimicrob Agents Chemother* 1997;41:563–569.
72. Sanders CC, Iaconis JP, Bodey GP, et al. Resistance to ticarcillin-potassium clavulanate among clinical isolates of the Family *Enterobacteriaceae*: role of PSE-1 β-lactamase and high levels of TEM-1 and SHV-1 and problems with false susceptibility in disk diffusion tests. *Antimicrob Agents Chemother* 2001;32:1365–1369.
73. Bonomo RA, Rice LB. Inhibitor resistant class A beta-lactamases. *Front Biosci* 1999;4:e34–41.
74. Randegger CC, Hachler H. Amino acid substitutions causing inhibitor resistance in TEM beta-lactamases compromise the extended-spectrum phenotype in SHV extended-spectrum beta-lactamases. *J Antimicrob Chemother* 2001;47:547–554.
75. Rice LB, Carias LL, Bonomo RA, et al. Molecular genetics of resistance to both ceftazidime and β-lactam-β-lactamase inhibitor combinations in *Klebsiella pneumoniae* and in vivo response to β-lactam therapy. *J Infect Dis* 1996;173:151–158.
76. Jett BD, Ritchie DJ, Reichley R, et al. In vitro activities of various β-lactam antimicrobial agents against clinical isolates of *Escherichia*

coli and *Klebsiella spp.* resistant to oxyimino cephalosporins. *Antimicrob Agents Chemother* 1995;39:1187–1190.

77. Payne DJ. Metallo-β-lactamases a new therapeutic challenge. *J Med Microbiol* 1993;39:93–99.
78. Nordmann P, Poirel L. Emerging carbapenemases in gram-negative aerobes. *Clin Microbiol Infect* 2002;8:321–331.
79. Podglajen I, Breuil J, Bordon F, et al. A silent carbapenemase gene in strains of *Bacteroides fragilis* can be expressed after a one step mutation. *FEMS Microbiol Lett* 1992;70:21–29.
80. Podglajen I, Breuil J, Collatz E. Insertion of a novel DNA sequence, IS*1186*, immediately upstream of the silent carbapenemase gene *cfiA*, promotes expression of carbapenem resistance in clinical isolates of *Bacteroides fragilis*. *Mol Microbiol* 1994;12:105–114.
81. Rasmussen BA, Bush K. Carbapenem-hydrolyzing beta-lactamases [see comments]. *Antimicrob Agents Chemother* 1997;41:223–232.
82. Naas T, Nordmann P. OXA-type beta-lactamases. *Curr Pharm Des* 1999;5:865–879.
83. Trias J, Nikaido H. Outer membrane protein D2 catalyzes facilitated diffusion of penems and carnbapenems through the outer membrane of *Pseudomonas aeruginosa*. *Antimicrob Agents Chemother* 1990;34: 52–57.
84. Livermore DM. Interplay of impermeability and chromosomal β-lactamase activity in imipenem-resistant *Pseudomonas aeruginosa*. *Antimicrob Agents Chemother* 1992;36:2046–2048.
85. Chow JW, Shlaes DM. Imipenem resistance associated with the loss of a 40 kDa outer membrane protein in *Enterobacter aerogenes*. *J Antimicrob Chemother* 1991;28:499–504.
86. Lee EH, Nicolas MH, Kitzis MD, et al. Association of two resistance mechanisms in a clinical isolate of Enterobacter cloacae with high-level resistance to imipenem. *Antimicrob Agents Chemother* 1991;35: 1093–1098.
87. Raimondi A, Traverso A, Nikaido H. Imipenem- and meropenem-resistant mutants of *Enterobacter cloacae* and *Proteus rettgeri* lack-porins. *Antimicrob Agents Chemother* 1991;35:1174–1180.
88. Nikaido H. Multiple antibiotic resistance and efflux. *Curr Opin Microbiol* 1998;1:516–523.
89. Poole K. Multidrug resistance in Gram-negative bacteria. *Curr Opin Microbiol* 2001;4:500–508.
90. Van Bambeke F, Balzi E, Tulkens PM. Antibiotic efflux pumps. *Biochem Pharmacol* 2000;60:457–470.
91. Li XZ, Barre N, Poole K. Influence of the MexA-MexB-oprM multidrug efflux system on expression of the MexC-MexD-oprJ and MexE-MexF-oprN multidrug efflux systems in Pseudomonas aeruginosa. *J Antimicrob Chemother* 2000;46:885–893.
92. Masuda N, Sakagawa E, Ohya S, et al. Substrate specificities of MexAB-OprM, MexCD-OprJ, and MexXY-oprM efflux pumps in Pseudomonas aeruginosa. *Antimicrob Agents Chemother* 2000;44: 3322–3327.
93. Dubois V, Arpin C, Melon M, et al. Nosocomial outbreak due to a multiresistant strain of Pseudomonas aeruginosa P12: efficacy of cefepime-amikacin therapy and analysis of beta-lactam resistance. *J Clin Microbiol* 2001;39:2072–2078.
94. Barna JCJ, Williams DH. The structure and mode of action of glycopeptide antibiotics of the vancomycin group. *Annu Rev Microbiol* 1984;39:339–357.
95. Vergis EN, Hayden MK, Chow JW, et al. Determinants of vancomycin resistance and mortality rates in enterococcal bacteremia. A prospective multicenter study. *Ann Intern Med* 2001;135:484–492.
96. Lodise TP, McKinnon PS, Tam VH, et al. Clinical outcomes for patients with bacteremia caused by vancomycin-resistant enterococcus in a level 1 trauma center. *Clin Infect Dis* 2002;34:922–929.
97. Eliopoulos GM, Wennersten CB, Gold HS, et al. Characterization of vancomycin-resistant *Enterococcus faecium* isolates from the United States and their susceptibility in vitro to dalfopristin-quinupristin. *Antimicrob Agents Chemother* 1998;42:1088–1092.
98. Arthur M, Reynolds P, Courvalin P. Glycopeptide resistance in enterococci. *Trends Microbiol* 1996;4:401–407.
99. Perichon B, Reynolds P, Courvalin P. VanD-type glycopeptide-resistant *Enterococcus faecium* BM4339. *Antimicrob Agents Chemother* 1997;41:2016–2018.
100. Fines M, Perichon B, Reynolds P, et al. VanE, a new type of acquired glycopeptide resistance in Enterococcus faecalis BM4405. *Antimicrob Agents Chemother* 1999;43:2161–2164.
101. McKessar SJ, Berry AM, Bell JM, et al. Genetic characterization of *vanG*, a novel vancomycin resistance locus in *Enterococcus faecalis*. *Antimicrob Agents Chemother* 2000;44:3224–3228.
102. Patel R, Piper K, Cockerill FR 3rd, et al. The biopesticide Paenibacillus popilliae has a vancomycin resistance gene cluster homologous to the enterococcal VanA vancomycin resistance gene cluster. *Antimicrob Agents Chemother* 2000;44:705–709.
103. Arthur M, Depardieu F, Molinas C, et al. The *vanZ* gene of Tn*1546* from *Enterococcus faecium* BM4147 confers resistance to teicoplanin. *Gene* 1995;154:87–92.
104. Evers S, Courvalin R. Regulation of VanB-type vancomycin resistance gene expression by the vanSB-VanRB two component regulatory system in *Enterococcus faecalis* V583. *J Bacteriol* 1996;178:1302–1309.
105. Arthur M, Depardieu F, Gerbaud G, et al. The VanS sensor negatively controls VanR-mediated transcriptional activation of glycopeptide resistance genes of Tn1546 and related elements in the absence of induction. *J Bacteriol* 1997;179:97–106.
106. Baptista M, Depardieu F, Reynolds P, et al. Mutations leading to increased levels of resistance to glycopeptide antibiotics in VanB-type enterococci. *Mol Microbiol* 1997;25:93–105.
107. Green M, Shlaes JH, Barbadora K, et al. Bacteremia due to vancomycin-dependent *Enterococcus faecium*. *Clin Infect Dis* 1995;20: 712–714.
108. Depardieu F, Reynolds PE, Courvalin P. VanD-type vancomycin-resistant Enterococcus faecium 10/96A. *Antimicrob Agents Chemother* 2003;47:7–18.
109. Woodford N, Jones BL, Baccus Z, et al. Linkage of vancomycin and high-level gentamicin resistance genes on the same plasmid in a clinical isolate of *Enterococcus faecalis*. *J Antimicrob Chemother* 1995;35: 179–184.
110. Rice LB, Carias LL, Donskey CJ, et al. Transferable, plasmid-mediated VanB-type glycopeptide resistance in *Enterococcus faecium*. *Antimicrob Agents Chemother* 1998;42:963–964.
111. Hayden MK, Picken RN, Sahm DF. Heterogeneous expression of glycopeptide resistance in enterococci associated with transfer of *vanB*. *Antimicrob Agents Chemother* 1997;41:872–874.
112. Quintiliani R Jr, Courvalin P. Characterization of Tn*1547*, a composite transposon flanked by the IS*16* and IS*256*-like elements, that confers vancomycin resistance in *Enterococcus faecium* BM4281. *Gene* 1996;172:1–8.
113. Hiramatsu K. Vancomycin resistance in staphylococci. *Drug Resist Updates* 1998;1:135–150.
114. Sieradzki K, Roberts RB, Haber SW, et al. The development of vancomycin resistance in a patient with methicillin-resistant Staphylococcus aureus infection [see comments]. *N Engl J Med* 1999;340:517–523.
115. Climo MW, Patron RL, Archer GL. Combinations of vancomycin and β-lactams are synergistic against staphylococci with reduced susceptibilities to vancomycin. *Antimicrob Agents Chemother* 1999;43: 1747–1753.
116. Kaatz GW, Seo SM, Dorman NJ, et al. Emergence of teicoplanin resistance during therapy of *Staphylococcus aureus* endocarditis. *J Infect Dis* 1990;162:103–108.
117. Schwalbe RS, Stapleton JT, Gilligan PH. Emergence of vancomycin resistance in coagulase negative staphylococci. *N Engl J Med* 1987; 316:927–931.
118. Shlaes DM, Shlaes JH, Vincent S, et al. Teicoplanin-resistant *Staphylococcus aureus* expresses a novel membrane protein and increases expression of penicillin-binding protein 2 complex. *Antimicrob Agents Chemother* 1993;37:2432–2437.
119. Sieradzki K, Tomasz A. Inhibition of cell wall turnover and autolysis by vancomycin in a highly vancomycin-resistant mutant of *Staphylococcus aureus*. *J Bacteriol* 1997;179:2557–2566.
120. Moreira B, Boyle-Vavra S, de Jonge BLM, et al. Increased production of penicillin-binding protein 2, increased detection of other penicillin-binding proteins, and decreased coagulase activity associated with glycopeptide resistance in *Staphylococcus aureus*. *Antimicrob Agents Chemother* 1997;41:1788–1793.

121. Ruoff KL, Kuritzkes DR, Wolfson JS, et al. Vancomycin-resistant gram-positive bacteria isolated from human sources. *J Clin Microbiol* 1988;26:2064–2068.
122. Billot-Klein D, Gutmann L, Sablé S, et al. Modification of peptidoglycan precursors is a common feature of the low-level vancomycin-resistant VANB-type Enterococcus D366 and of the naturally glycopeptide-resistant species *Lactobacillus casei, Pediococcus pentosaceus, Leuconostoc mesenteroides* and *Enterococcus gallinarum. J Bacteriol* 1994;176:2398–2405.
123. Damper PD, Epstein W. Role of the membrane potential in bacterial resistance to aminoglycoside antibiotics. *Antimicrob Agents Chemother* 1981;20:803–808.
124. Shaw KJ, Rather PN, Hare RS, et al. Molecular genetics of aminoglycoside resistance genes and familial relationships of the aminoglycoside-modifying enzymes. *Microbiol Rev* 1993;57:138–163.
125. McGowan JE, Terry PM, Huang TSR, et al. Nosocomial infections with gentamicin-resistant *Staphylococcus aureus*: plasmid analysis as an epidemiologic tool. *J Infect Dis* 1979;140:864–872.
126. Horodniceanu T, Bougueleret L, El-Solh N, et al. High-level plasmid-borne resistance in *Streptococcus faecalis* subsp. *zymogenes. Antimicrob Agents Chemother* 1979;16:686–689.
127. Ferretti JJ, Gilmore KS, Courvalin P. Nucleotide sequence of the gene specifying the bifunctional 6′-aminoglycoside acetyltransferase-2″ aminoglycoside phosphotransferase enzyme in *Streptococcus faecalis* and identification and cloning of the gene regions specifying the two activities. *J Bacteriol* 1986;167:631–638.
128. Lyon BR, May JW, Skurray RA. Tn*4001*: a gentamicin and kanamycin resistance transposon in *Staphylococcus aureus. Mol Genl Genet* 1984;193:554–556.
129. Kaufhold A, Podbielski A, Horaud T, et al. Identical genes confer high-level resistance to gentamicin upon *Enterococcus faecalis, Enterococcus faecium*, and *Streptococcus agalactiae. Antimicrob Agents Chemother* 1992;36:1215–1218.
130. Hodel-Christian SL, Murray BE. Characterization of the gentamicin resistance transposon Tn*5281* from *Enterococcus faecalis* and comparison to staphylococcal transposons Tn*4001* and Tn*4031*. *Antimicrob Agents Chemother* 1991;35:1147–1152.
131. Byrne ME, Gillespie MT, Skurray RA. Molecular analysis of a gentamicin resistance transposonlike element on plasmids isolated from North American *Staphylococcus aureus* strains. *Antimicrob Agents Chemother* 1990;34:2106–2113.
132. Thomas WD, Archer GL. Mobility of gentamicin resistance genes from staphylococci isolated in the United States: identification of Tn*4031*, a gentamicin resistance transposon from *Staphylococcus epidermidis. Antimicrob Agents Chemother* 1989;33:1335–1341.
133. Chow JW. Aminoglycoside resistance in enterococci. *Clin Infect Dis* 2000;31:586–589.
134. Rhinehart E, Smith NE, Wennersten C, et al. Rapid dissemination of β-lactamase-producing, aminoglycoside-resistant *Enterococcus faecalis* among patients and staff on an infant-toddler surgical ward. *N Engl J Med* 1990;323:1814–1818.
135. Wells VD, Wong ES, Murray BE, et al. Infections due to beta-lactamase-producing, high-level gentamicin resistant *Enterococcus faecalis. Ann Intern Med* 1992;116:285–292.
136. Huycke MM, Spiegel CA, Gilmore MS. Bacteremia caused by hemolytic, high-level gentamicin-resistant *Enterococcus faecalis. Antimicrob Agents Chemother* 1991;35:1626–1634.
137. Noskin GA, Till M, Patterson BK, et al. High-level gentamicin resistance in *Enterococcus faecalis* bacteremia. *J Infect Dis* 1991;164: 212–215.
138. Rice LB, Calderwood SB, Eliopoulos GM, et al. Enterococcal endocarditis: a comparison of native and prosthetic valve disease. *Rev Infect Dis* 1991;13:1–7.
139. Markowitz SM, Wells VD, Williams DS, et al. Antimicrobial susceptibility and molecular epidemiology of β-lactamase-producing, aminoglycoside-resistant isolates of *Enterococcus faecalis. Antimicrob Agents Chemother* 1991;35:1075–1080.
140. Wurtz R, Sahm D, Flaherty J. Gentamicin-resistant, streptomycin susceptible *Enterococcus (Streptococcus) faecalis* bacteremia. *J Infect Dis* 1991;163:1393–1394.
141. Rather PN, Orosz E, Shaw KJ, et al. Characterization and transcriptional regulation of the 2′-*N*-acetyltransferase gene from *Providencia stuartii. J Bacteriol* 1993;175:6492–6498.
142. Shaw KJ, Rather P, Sabatelli F, et al. Characterization of the chromosomal *aac(6′)-Ic* gene from *Serratia marcescens. Antimicrob Agents Chemother* 1992;36:1447–1455.
143. Clarke AJ, Francis D, Keenleyside WJ. The prevalence of gentamicin 2′-*N*-acetyltransferase in the *Proteae* and its role in the *O*-acetylation of peptidoglycan. *FEMS Microbiol Lett* 1996;145:201–207.
144. Aires JR, Kohler T, Nikaido H, et al. Involvement of an active efflux system in the natural resistance of Pseudomonas aeruginosa to aminoglycosides. *Antimicrob Agents Chemother* 1999;43:2624–2628.
145. Li XZ, Poole K, Nikaido H. Contributions of MexAB-OprM and an EmrE homolog to intrinsic resistance of Pseudomonas aeruginosa to aminoglycosides and dyes. *Antimicrob Agents Chemother* 2003;47: 27–33.
146. Magnet S, Courvalin P, Lambert T. Resistance-nodulation-cell division-type efflux pump involved in aminoglycoside resistance in Acinetobacter baumannii strain BM4454. *Antimicrob Agents Chemother* 2001;45:3375–3380.
147. Korvick JA, Bryan CS, Farber B, et al. Prospective observational study of *Klebsiella* bacteremia in 230 patients: outcome for antibiotic combinations versus monotherapy. *Antimicrob Agents Chemother* 1992;36: 2639–2644.
148. Hooper DC, Wolfson JS. Mode of action of the quinolone antimicrobial agents: review of recent information. *Rev Infect Dis* 1989;11(suppl 5):S902–S911.
149. Hiasa H, Yousef DO, Marians KJ. DNA strand cleavage is required for replication fork arrest by a frozen topoisomerase-quinolone-DNA ternary complex. *J Biol Chem* 1996;271:26424–26429.
150. Willmott CJ, Critchlow SE, Eperon IC, et al. The complex of DNA gyrase and quinolone drugs with DNA forms a barrier to transcription by RNA polymerase. *J Mol Biol* 1994;242:351–363.
151. Shea ME, Hiasa H. Interactions between DNA helicases and frozen topoisomerase IV—quinolone-DNA ternary complexes. *J Biol Chem* 1999;274:22747–22754.
152. Blanche F, Cameron B, Bernard FX, et al. Differential behaviors of Staphylococcus aureus and Escherichia coli type II DNA topoisomerases. *Antimicrob Agents Chemother* 1996;40:2714–2720.
153. Pan XS, Fisher LM. Streptococcus pneumoniae DNA gyrase and topoisomerase IV: overexpression, purification, and differential inhibition by fluoroquinolones. *Antimicrob Agents Chemother* 1999;43: 1129–1136.
154. Alovero FL, Pan XS, Morris JE, et al. Engineering the specificity of antibacterial fluoroquinolones: benzenesulfonamide modifications at C-7 of ciprofloxacin change its primary target in Streptococcus pneumoniae from topoisomerase IV to gyrase. *Antimicrob Agents Chemother* 2000;44:320–325.
155. Yoshida H, Bogaki M, Nakamura M, et al. Quinolone resistance-determining region in the DNA gyrase *gyrA* gene of *Escherichia coli. Antimicrob Agents Chemother* 1990;34:1271–1272.
156. Morais Cabral JH, Jackson AP, Smith CV, et al. Crystal structure of the breakage-reunion domain of DNA gyrase. *Nature* 1997;388: 903–906.
157. Piddock LJ. Mechanisms of fluoroquinolone resistance: an update 1994–1998. *Drugs* 1999;58:11–18.
158. Coronado VG, Edwards JR, Culver DH, et al. Ciprofloxacin resistance among nosocomial Pseudomonas aeruginosa and Staphylococcus aureus in the United States. National Nosocomial Infections Surveillance (NNIS) System. *Infect Control Hosp Epidemiol* 1995;16: 71–75.
159. Hooper DC. Emerging mechanisms of fluoroquinolone resistance. *Emerg Infect Dis* 2001;7:337–341.
160. Nikaido H, Thanassi DG. Penetration of lipophilic agents with multiple protonation sites into bacterial cells: tetracyclines and fluoroquinolones as examples. *Antimicrob Agents Chemother* 1993;37:1393–1399.
161. Martinez-Martinez L, Pascual A, Jacoby GA. Quinolone resistance from a transferable plasmid. *Lancet* 1998;351(9105):797–799.
162. Tran JH, Jacoby GA. Mechanism of plasmid-mediated quinolone resistance. *Proc Natl Acad Sci USA* 2002;99:5638–5642.

163. Jacoby GA, Chow N, Waites KB. Prevalence of plasmid-mediated quinolone resistance. *Antimicrob Agents Chemother* 2003;47: 559–562.
164. Soltani M, Beighton D, Philpott-Howard J, et al. Mechanisms of resistance to quinupristin-dalfopristin among isolates of Enterococcus faecium from animals, raw meat, and hospital patients in Western Europe. *Antimicrob Agents Chemother* 2000;44:433–436.
165. Prystowsky J, Siddiqui F, Chosay J, et al. Resistance to linezolid: characterization of mutations in rRNA and comparison of their occurrences in vancomycin-resistant enterococci. *Antimicrob Agents Chemother* 2001;45:2154–2156.
166. Marshall SH, Donskey CJ, Hutton-Thomas R, et al. Gene dosage and linezolid resistance in Enterococcus faecium and Enterococcus faecalis. *Antimicrob Agents Chemother* 2002;46:3334–3336.
167. Herrero IA, Issa NC, Patel R. Nosocomial spread of linezolid-resistant, vancomycin-resistant Enterococcus faecium. *N Engl J Med* 2002; 346:867–869.
168. Shlaes DM, Gerding DN, John JF Jr, et al. Society for Healthcare Epidemiology of America and Infectious Diseases Society of America Joint Committee on the Prevention of Antimicrobial Resistance: guidelines for the prevention of antimicrobial resistance in hospitals. *Clin Infect Dis* 1997;25:584–599.

91

ANTIMICROBIAL RESISTANCE IN HOSPITAL FLORA AND NOSOCOMIAL INFECTIONS

G. L. FRENCH

Nosocomial infections may be caused by community microorganisms brought into the hospital by patients or others, or by hospital microorganisms that are infecting or colonizing patients or staff members or contaminating the inanimate environment. To be successful as hospital pathogens, nosocomial bacteria must be able to establish themselves and survive in the hospital environment, colonize the mucosa and skin of patients and staff members, survive on various surfaces during patient-to-patient transmission, and resist antibiotic and sometimes antiseptic therapy (1). Inherent multiple antibiotic resistance, and the ability to acquire additional genetic resistance factors in the face of increasing use of antibiotics, is important for survival. Numerous reports show that microorganisms causing hospital infection and colonizing patients and staff members are more antibiotic-resistant than those in the community. For example, human fecal bacteria are more resistant in hospital populations than such bacteria outside. Acquired antibiotic resistance was rare in *Escherichia coli* isolated from the feces of animals and humans in remote areas of the world before the introduction of antibiotics (2,3), and in London in the 1960s antibiotic resistance was uncommon in fecal microorganisms but increased in patients after they were admitted to the hospital (4). Similarly, fecal microorganisms in hospital sewage were found to be more antibiotic-resistant than those from domestic sewage (5), and antibiotic resistance and multiple resistance increased in sewage microorganisms in outflow from a new hospital in Hong Kong soon after it opened but did not change in microorganisms in sewage from a nearby town (6).

The assessment of antibiotic resistance in hospital bacterial isolates has been hampered by a lack of agreement on how resistance rates should be measured. Artificially high rates may be produced by counting multiple isolates of the same resistant microorganism from the same patient or from different patients during outbreaks. However, it has now been shown that results from the first isolate only of a bacterial species per patient give acceptable antimicrobial susceptibility rates that can be used for comparative purposes (7–9). National resistance rates are often extrapolated from surveillance data derived from a few hospitals in a few centers, with little attention to the use of appropriate denominators. Despite these reservations, we believe resistance is increasing, but the exact levels of resistance in different places and the rate of increase are unclear.

The situation is further complicated by the high rates of hospital-acquired infection and antimicrobial resistance in intensive care units (ICUs). Indeed, laboratory-based resistance rates for all microorganisms in the ICU are the same as rates based on epidemiologic surveillance of hospital-acquired infections only (10). Archibald et al. (11) demonstrated that there was a significant stepwise decrease in the percentage of resistant microorganisms isolated from patients in the ICU, from non-ICU inpatients, and from outpatients. They concluded that resources allocated to control antimicrobial resistance therefore should be concentrated on the hospital and particularly on the ICU. A number of surveillance systems studying hospital-acquired infection and antimicrobial resistance have been set up, including the U.S. Intensive Care Antimicrobial Resistance Epidemiology (ICARE) Project (10) and the European Prevalence of Infection in Intensive Care (EPIC) Study (12). In January 1999, the hospital-wide component was eliminated from the National Nosocomial Infections Surveillance (NNIS) system, because case finding was costly and inaccurate, and rates were unhelpful for national comparison, because they were not risk-adjusted. Perhaps as a reflection of this, the pooled NNIS antimicrobial resistance rates for various nosocomial pathogens for the decade of 1992–2002 show little difference between ICU and non-ICU patients (Table 91.1). The experience of many clinicians supports the view of Archibald et al. (11) that rates are higher in ICU.

Table 91.2 shows results from the NNIS system comparing resistance rates in U.S. ICUs for various pathogens isolated in 1994–1998 and 1999 (13). It can be seen that during this period there was a dramatic increase in resistance rates for several important nosocomial pathogens. In particular there was a 47% increase in vancomycin resistance in enterococci, a 43% increase in methicillin resistance in *Staphylococcus aureus,* and an increase in resistance in *Pseudomonas aeruginosa* of 35% and 49% to imipenem and quinolones, respectively.

TABLE 91.1. POOLED MEANS OF THE DISTRIBUTION OF ANTIMICROBIAL RESISTANCE RATES (%), BY ALL ICUs COMBINED AND NON-ICU INPATIENT AREAS, JANUARY 1998 TO JUNE 2002

Pathogen	ICUs	Non-ICUs
MRSA	51.3	41.4
Methicillin-resistant CNS	75.7	64.0
Vancomycin-resistant *Enterococcus* spp.	12.8	12.0
Ciprofloxacin/ofloxacin-resistant *Pseudomonas aeruginosa*	36.3	27.0
Levofloxacin-resistant *P. aeruginosa*	37.8	28.9
Imipenem-resistant *P. aeruginosa*	19.6	12.7
Ceftazidime-resistant *P. aeruginosa*	13.9	8.3
Piperacillin-resistant *P. aeruginosa*	17.5	11.5
Cef3-resistant *Enterobacter* spp.	26.3	19.8
Carbapenem-resistant *Enterobacter* spp.	0.8	1.1
Cef3-resistant *Klebsiella pneumoniae*	6.1	5.7
Cef3-resistant *Escherichia coli*	1.2	1.1
Quinolone-resistant *E. coli*	5.8	5.3
Penicillin-resistant pneumococci	20.6	19.2
Cefotaxime/ceftriaxone-resistant pneumococci	8.2	8.1

MRSA, Methicillin-resistant *Staphylococcus aureus;* CNS, coagulase-negative staphylococci; Cef3, ceftazidime, cefotaxime, or ceftriaxone; Quinolone, ciprofloxacin, ofloxacin, or levofloxacin; Carbapenem, imipenem or meropenem.
From National Nosocomial Infections Surveillance (NNIS) System Report, data summary from January 1992 to June 2002, issued August 2002. *Am J Infect Control* 2002;30:458–475.

Until recently, typing methods for nosocomial bacteria were usually clumsy, imprecise, or, for many species, unavailable. However, the introduction of genome analysis has provided relatively simple and greatly improved methods for elucidating the epidemiology of most microorganisms of hospital infection (14–16). Similarly, the epidemiology of antibiotic resistance was previously based on phenotypic descriptions. Now that we have a better understanding of the molecular basis of resistance and genetic probes for resistance determinants are more widely available, the molecular epidemiology of resistance genes is becoming clearer (17).

TABLE 91.2. MEAN RESISTANCE RATES IN SELECTED PATHOGENS ASSOCIATED WITH NOSOCOMIAL INFECTIONS IN ICU PATIENTS, JANUARY–MAY 1999 COMPARED WITH THE FIVE YEARS 1994–1998

Antimicrobial/Pathogen	Increase in Resistance (%)
Vancomycin/enterococci	47
Methicillin/*Staphylococcus aureus*	43
Methicillin/coagulase-negative staphylococci	2
3rd cephalosporin/*E. coli*	23
3rd cephalosporin/*K. pneumoniae*	−1
Imipenem/*P. aeruginosa*	35
Quinolone/*P. aeruginosa*	49
3rd cephalosporin/*P. aeruginosa*	<1
3rd cephalosporin/*Enterobacter* spp.	3

3rd, third generation.
From National Nosocomial Infections Surveillance (NNIS) System Report, Data Summary from January 1990–May 1999, Issued June 1999. *Am J Infect Control* 1999;27:520–532.

EMERGENCE OF ANTIBIOTIC RESISTANCE IN NOSOCOMIAL PATHOGENS

Antibiotic Use and Antibiotic Resistance

Hospital patients often have compromised host defenses due to treatment or underlying disease, and therefore are at risk of acquiring infection with both virulent and opportunistic pathogens. Since antibiotic use is concentrated in hospitals, both types of pathogen are more likely to survive and proliferate in the hospital environment and colonize patients if they are resistant to common antimicrobials. Furthermore, infection with resistant microorganisms often fails to respond to initial empirical therapy, increasing the time during which cross-infection may occur. Antimicrobial resistance is thus one of the factors that favor the development of hospital infection, and at any given time the common nosocomial pathogens are often resistant to the antibiotics in current use. The tendency for antibiotic use to promote the emergence of resistant pathogens is called "antibiotic pressure."

The relationship between antibiotic use and antibiotic resistance, and the problems of proving a cause-and-effect relationship, have been well reviewed by McGowan (18). Despite methodologic difficulties, there are many reports of resistance rising during increased antibiotic use and falling after a reduction in use (18). Nevertheless, as McGowan points out, antibiotic pressure is not the only reason why nosocomial pathogens appear increasingly antibiotic-resistant.

Publication Bias

Unusual antimicrobial resistance is a simple and readily available epidemiologic marker for hospital infection. The appearance of urinary tract infection caused by cephalosporin- and aminoglycoside-resistant *Klebsiella pneumoniae,* for example, will be vigorously pursued by the infection control team and perhaps reported in the literature, whereas a similar outbreak with a sensitive strain may go unnoticed and unreported. The tendency of authors to report, and editors to accept, accounts of infection caused by multiply resistant rather than sensitive microorganisms is an example of publication bias (18). Thus, although nosocomial pathogens are usually multiply antibiotic-resistant, this characteristic is sometimes overemphasized.

Opportunistic Infection and Antibiotic Resistance

With advances in medical care, many highly compromised patients are being successfully treated by intensive medical care but remain vulnerable to nosocomial infection. Immunocompromised patients are susceptible to opportunistic pathogens of low virulence, and those undergoing intensive therapy may become infected by free-living bacteria that survive in the hospital environment and are transmitted to patients via equipment such as ventilators and urinary and vascular catheters. These opportunists are often inherently resistant to common antibiotics, probably because they are adapted to live in soil and water, where they are exposed to naturally occurring antimicrobial substances. They are also relatively resistant to disinfectants and can be selected by changing patterns of disinfectant use. These microorganisms include *Pseudomonas, Acinetobacter,* and *Enterobacter* species, which would have become increasing causes of hospital infection even without antibiotic pressure. The coagulase-negative staphylococci, which colonize human skin and are often antibiotic-resistant, rarely, if ever, cause infection in healthy individuals but have become major causes of nosocomial bloodstream infection, because they can adhere to prosthetic implants and vascular catheters. All these inherently resistant microorganisms also tend to acquire further antibiotic resistances in hospitals, encouraged by antibiotic pressure. The emergence of gram-positive nosocomial pathogens, such as the enterococci, is probably directly related to their inherent resistance to the cephalosporins, aminoglycosides, and quinolones during a period of increasing use of these drugs for the treatment of gram-negative infections.

Environmental Contamination and Antibiotic Resistance

Many gram-negative opportunistic pathogens are free-living, nonfastidious in their nutritional requirements, and capable of multiplying at a wide range of temperatures. They can survive and proliferate in wet environmental sites such as hospital water systems (19–24), and sink drains (25–27), and may sometimes spread from these reservoirs to cause infections in patients. These water microorganisms include a number of nonfermenting bacteria, such as *Pseudomonas, Acinetobacter,* and *Flavobacterium* species, which are inherently antibiotic-resistant and can accumulate acquired resistance factors. *Pseudomonas fluorescens* can grow at 48°C and has caused several outbreaks of bacteremia following contamination of refrigerated blood transfusion packs (28). Resistant *Enterobacteriaceae* and gram-positive microorganisms are also sometimes isolated from these environmental sites; for example, *Enterobacter cloacae* has been isolated from ice machines (21) and coagulase-negative staphylococci causing prosthetic valve endocarditis from ice-water baths used during thermodilution cardiac output studies (29). Similarly, outbreaks of disinfectant- and antibiotic-resistant pseudomonads have been reported, associated with contamination of the internal plumbing of endoscope washer-disinfectors (30,31).

Multiresistant gram-negative bacteria such as *Pseudomonas, Burkholderia, Stenotrophomonas, Ralstonia, Acinetobacter, Enterobacter, Klebsiella, Citrobacter, Serratia,* and *Flavobacterium* species may also contaminate and survive in supposedly sterile solutions or clean-water reservoirs associated with hospital equipment. Outbreaks of antibiotic-resistant infection may thus occur when there are failures of sterilization of injectable solutions or breakdowns in the maintenance, decontamination, and disinfection of equipment. For example, a *Pseudomonas* species established itself in the distilled water supply of a hospital pharmacy and contaminated sterilized infusion fluids when the distilled water was used to cool autoclaved bottles (19). Compared with other Enterobacteriaceae, *Enterobacter* species have a special ability to survive and multiply in 5% dextrose solutions (32) and have caused a number of outbreaks of bacteremia following infusion of contaminated fluids (33,34).

Outbreaks due to many different multiresistant gram-negative bacteria have been associated with contaminated hospital equipment such as arterial pressure monitoring systems (35,36), endoscopes (37), suction apparatus, humidifiers, nebulizers, ventilators, and breast pumps (38,39). Similarly, resistant microorganisms such as *Klebsiella, Serratia,* and *Enterobacter* species may contaminate and survive in cold hospital food or enteral feeds given to compromised patients (40,41). Free-living, multiply resistant, gram-negative microorganisms tend to be relatively resistant to disinfectants and bacteriostatic agents. Thus, contamination of disinfectants and multiple-use medications may lead to outbreaks of antibiotic-resistant infection. *P. aeruginosa,* for example, is so resistant to the quaternary ammonium compounds that cetrimide is used in a *Pseudomonas*-selective culture medium! Many strains of methicillin-resistant *S. aureus* (MRSA) and methicillin-resistant *Staphylococcus epidermidis* acquire genes for resistance to disinfectants such as cetrimide and chlorhexidine disinfectants, which may facilitate the spread of these microorganisms in hospitals (42,43).

McGowan (44) has emphasized, however, that the environment is rarely the reservoir for endemic hospital infection and only occasionally acts as the source for individual outbreaks. Furthermore, environmental sites may become contaminated from infected or colonized patients rather than the other way around. Routine surveillance cultures of the hospital environment, therefore, are unjustified, and environmental cultures made during outbreaks should be interpreted with care (44,45).

MECHANISMS AND GENETICS OF ANTIBIOTIC RESISTANCE

Some microorganisms are inherently resistant to common antimicrobials. For example, *K. pneumoniae* is resistant to ampicillin; *Enterobacter* species to ampicillin and many cephalosporins; enterococci to cephalosporins and quinolones; and *P. aeruginosa* to ampicillin, some cephalosporins, and other groups. Some *Pseudomonas* species are inherently resistant to nearly all of the agents active against gram-negative bacteria, the JK coryneforms are resistant to most drugs used for gram-positive infection, and fungi such as *Candida albicans* are inherently resistant to all antibacterial antibiotics. Antibiotic therapy tends to suppress sensitive environmental and commensal bacteria and encourage their replacement with resistant microorganisms. Initially, the more resistant members of generally sensitive species proliferate, and then the inherently resistant genera take over. Highly compromised patients who receive multiple courses of antibiotics commonly become colonized by increasingly resistant microorganisms, often suffering sequential infections with *Klebsiella, P. aeruginosa,* enterococci, and, finally, *Candida.*

Naturally sensitive bacteria may acquire antibiotic resistance caused by a number of mechanisms (46,47). The most common is probably the production of drug-destroying enzymes. This is the typical mechanism by which microorganisms such as *S. aureus* and *E. coli* and other gram-negative bacteria acquire resistance to ampicillin, aminoglycosides, and chloramphenicol. There may be alterations in the permeability of the cell wall, preventing antibiotics from reaching their target sites (or there may be increased antibiotic efflux, resulting in the same effect).

This is the common mechanism of tetracycline resistance and is one of the ways in which microorganisms such as *P. aeruginosa* may acquire resistance to several aminoglycosides simultaneously. Alterations in target sites prevent antibiotics from binding at their sites of action. Changes in the affinities of penicillin-binding proteins result in methicillin resistance in staphylococci, penicillin resistance in pneumococci, and ampicillin resistance in enterococci. Alterations in ribosomal-binding sites may produce acquired resistance to rifampin, fusidic acid, and the macrolides, and alteration of DNA gyrase is the common mechanism of quinolone resistance. Alterations (or substitutions) of enzymes in metabolic pathways are responsible for resistance to sulfonamides and trimethoprim that block bacterial folate metabolism.

Acquired resistance mechanisms may be encoded on the bacterial chromosome or on plasmids, which are independently replicating molecules of extrachromosomal DNA. Resistance may emerge by mutation, which occurs relatively frequently in rapidly multiplying bacteria, or, more commonly, by acquisition of resistance plasmids from other bacteria. The spread of resistance among bacteria by plasmid transfer is sometimes called "infectious resistance." The transmission of DNA between bacteria may occur by bacteriophage transduction (as in the transmission of penicillinase-mediated penicillin-resistance in *S. aureus*), conjugation (the common mechanism of transfer between gram-negative species), or transformation. Transformation was previously regarded as a relatively unimportant mechanism of resistance transfer in clinical bacteria, but there is increasing evidence for its importance in the emergence of resistance in gram-positive microorganisms. Although the host range of many plasmids is restricted, and gram-positive and gram-negative microorganisms tend not to share resistance genes, plasmids can be exchanged between different bacterial species; for example, most ampicillin resistance in *Haemophilus influenzae* is mediated by a β-lactamase that probably originated from *E. coli.*

Resistance genes may be encoded on a variety of transferable elements, including transposons and integrons that can insert into both chromosomes and plasmids. The combination of multiple insertion elements may create large multiple resistance gene packages (48). Integrons encoding multiple antimicrobial resistances are now widespread in Enterobacteriaceae in both hospitals and the community (49,50). There is continuous horizontal transfer of these resistance genes between and within species, and acquisition of multiple resistance favors the proliferation of certain cross-infecting microorganisms in hospitals (51).

The spread of resistance plasmids or transposons among several different bacterial strains or species may produce an epidemic of resistance in commensal and environmental bacteria during an outbreak of hospital infection in patients (52–54). *Klebsiella* and *Serratia* species are particularly good at acquiring and disseminating a variety of resistance plasmids (55–58). Opportunistic pathogens such as these, which can readily acquire new resistances in the face of changing therapy, have become the dominant causes of hospital infection.

THE CHANGING PATTERN OF HOSPITAL INFECTION

The use of antibiotics encourages the development of more resistant bacteria in patient commensal flora and in the hospital environment (4,59–62), leading to antibiotic-resistant hospital-acquired infection. After effective therapy is introduced for one group of such infections, there is a tendency for another group of resistant microorganisms to emerge.

A change in pattern of serious hospital infection after the introduction of antibiotics was first noted by Finland and his colleagues (63). Between 1935 and 1957, antibiotic-sensitive gram-positive pathogens were replaced by penicillin-resistant *S. aureus* and multiresistant gram-negative bacteria such as *E. coli, Klebsiella,* and *Proteus* species. As discussed previously, these gram-negative opportunists emerged not only because they are inherently resistant to common antimicrobials and disinfectants, but also because many of them are free-living microorganisms that can survive in wet sites in the hospital environment (22, 25–27,64,65).

Once the emergence of resistant opportunistic pathogens had been recognized, new, more effective drugs were developed for therapy. The worldwide problem of the multiresistant "hospital staphylococcus" in the 1960s diminished after the introduction of methicillin, oxacillin, and cloxacillin (66,67), and outbreaks of gentamicin-resistant *Klebsiella* and other gram-negative microorganisms seen in the 1970s waned in the 1980s with the use of newer aminoglycosides and cephalosporins.

Since the 1980s, however, the pattern has changed again with a dramatic increase in multiply resistant gram-positive nosocomial infection (1,68). Methicillin-resistant *S. aureus,* resistant to all β-lactams and to many other previously effective agents, has emerged as a worldwide cause of large hospital outbreaks associated with serious morbidity and mortality (66,67,69,70). Coagulase-negative staphylococci are increasingly common hospital pathogens (71), partly because they, too, are often resistant to methicillin and other agents, but also because many strains produce an extracellular slime (72–74) that enables them to colonize intravascular and other plastic prostheses. Finally, many antibiotics used for gram-negative nosocomial infections, including ampicillin, the aminoglycosides, cephalosporins, and quinolones, are ineffective against coryneform bacteria and enterococci, and therefore these species have also emerged as important causes of hospital infection (75).

This is a continuing dynamic situation. Resistant gram-positive bacteria remain a major feature of hospital infection, mainly because of widespread endemic MRSA. However, resistant gram-negative bacteria continue as important nosocomial pathogens, usually causing epidemics or sporadic endogenous infection. Thus the picture now is of hospital infection being dominated by multiply drug resistant (MDR) pathogens of multiple species and gram-reaction.

Since fungi such as *Candida* and *Aspergillus* species are resistant to virtually all antibacterials; multiple courses of therapy in highly compromised patients may result in colonization and infection with these microorganisms. However, because fungi have always been inherently resistant to antibiotics, and serious invasive infection usually occurs only in patients with deficiencies of cell-mediated immunity, changes in antibiotic use have probably had little effect on the incidence of such infections, which account for only a few percent of all nosocomial episodes (71).

Multiresistant aerobic gram-positive bacteria were responsible for 39% of all nosocomial infections analyzed by the U.S. NNIS system between January 1990 and March 1996 (76). Aerobic gram-negative bacteria caused 42% of infections during the same period. *S. aureus* was the commonest isolate of all, followed by *E. coli,* coagulase-negative staphylococci, and *Enterococcus* species. Coagulase-negative staphylococci were the most common microorganisms isolated from blood and enterococci the second most common from urine (after *E. coli*). Gram-positive bacteria were also frequently isolated from ICU patients studied between January 1986 and April 1997 (77), where they were found in 50% of positive blood cultures and 39% of infected wounds.

MULTIRESISTANT PROBLEM MICROORGANISMS

Gram-Negative Bacteria

Escherichia coli

Escherichia coli is the commonest cause of hospital-acquired gram-negative urinary tract infection and septicemia (71). The species is naturally susceptible to ampicillin, but now about 50% to 60% of both hospital and community isolates are resistant (78), usually by the production of β-lactamases, enzymes that bind and destroy β-lactam antibiotics. The most common type of β-lactamase in *E. coli* is TEM-1, accounting for about 80% of such resistance (79–81). TEM-1 is encoded on transferable plasmids and has disseminated throughout the world since its discovery in 1965 (82). Some strains of Enterobacteriaceae, including *E. coli,* produce TEM-2, a similar enzyme that differs from TEM-1 only in a single amino acid. Although ampicillin is now unreliable for the treatment of *E. coli* infection, other drugs usually remain effective, including the cephalosporins, quinolones, and aminoglycosides. *E. coli* can also be treated by the combination of a β-lactam with a β-lactamase inhibitor, such as amoxicillin/clavulanic acid (co-amoxiclav) and ampicillin/sulbactam. The β-lactamase inhibitors prevent the action of TEM-1 or TEM-2 and restore the activity of the β-lactams. This combination is now threatened, because some *E. coli* strains can produce excessive amounts of TEM-1 that swamp the effect of the β-lactamase inhibitor (83,84) or are resistant to it (81).

Mutations in TEM-1 and TEM-2 have resulted in new "extended-spectrum" β-lactamases (ESBLs) that can break down newer cephalosporins and thus render *E. coli* resistant to them. These ESBLs are named TEM-3, TEM-4, etc., and more than 100 of them have been reported (46,85). They are often plasmid-borne and associated with other multiple resistances such as aminoglycoside resistance. However, *E. coli* is not a very epidemic microorganism in hospitals, and hospital outbreaks are more common with ESBL-producing strains of *K. pneumoniae* (see below). Nevertheless, cephalosporin resistance is increasing in hospital isolates of *E. coli,* and in the U.S. NNIS system, resistance to newer cephalosporins in ICU isolates of *E. coli* increased 23% between 1994–1998 and 1999 (Table 91.2) (13).

E. coli can acquire other resistances, including plasmid-borne aminoglycoside resistance and, increasingly, mutational quinolone resistance, but their frequencies vary considerably in different parts of the world (86–88). In the European Antimicrobial Resistance Surveillance System (EARSS) study from 2001, resistance to gentamicin was less than 5% in most European countries but was more than 10% in Israel, Bulgaria, and Malta. In ten of the 20 countries surveilled by EARSS, ciprofloxacin resistance was more than 8%, and ranged between 0% (Estonia) and 21% (Israel) (87).

E. coli is relatively fastidious in its nutritional requirements and does not survive well in the environment. For these reasons, most nosocomial *E. coli* infections are endogenous, arising from commensal bowel flora (89), and they are relatively easy to treat. However, a few outbreaks of hospital and community infection with multiresistant strains have been reported (90,91).

Klebsiella, Enterobacter, and *Serratia* Species

Klebsiella, Enterobacter, and *Serratia* species are common opportunistic pathogens that have similar epidemiologies and clinical presentations. They are all inherently resistant to ampicillin, and *Enterobacter* species and *Serratia* species are resistant to first-generation cephalosporins (78). These enterobacteria have a great facility for acquiring and disseminating resistance plasmids (54,58,92,93), especially among themselves, and *Enterobacter* species may develop chromosomal resistance to newer cephalosporins (94,95). To a greater or lesser extent, they colonize human bowel and patient skin and may spread from person to person on staff members' hands. They may then go on to colonize the urinary and respiratory tracts of patients treated with β-lactams and may produce bacteremia in the immunocompromised host. They are relatively free-living and can also survive and multiply in nutritionally poor wet environments at room temperatures. Because of this, they may contaminate food, enteral feeds, and infusion fluids, leading to widespread common-source outbreaks.

Klebsiella Species

K. pneumoniae is naturally resistant to ampicillin, usually by the production of SHV-1, a β-lactamase similar to TEM-1 and TEM-2, which may be encoded on either the chromosome or, less commonly, on a transferable plasmid (96). Because of this natural resistance, *K. pneumoniae* often replaces commensal *E. coli* in patients treated with ampicillin or similar drugs. The carriage rate in normals is low but increases in hospitalized patients, especially during prolonged hospitalization or antibiotic therapy (97,98). The microorganism can colonize the bowel, the bladder, the upper respiratory tract, and the skin and, in compromised patients, may go on to produce invasive urinary and respiratory tract infection and septicemia. Most colonized patients are asymptomatic, but they may act as sources of cross-infection for others; the outbreak strain is usually transferred on staff members' hands (99,100,101). In addition, *K. pneumoniae* readily acquires other transferable resistances and disseminates them to other strains of *Klebsiella* or other species of Enterobacteriaceae (40,53,54). *K. pneumoniae* (and *Enterobacter* species) appear to have a greater ability than *E. coli* and other Enterobacteriaceae to colonize the skin of patients and to survive on both skin and dry surfaces (89,92,97,98,101). On dry surfaces, about 10% of *E. coli* but only 1% of *Klebsiella* lose plasmid-mediated gentamicin resistance (89). All these factors contribute to the success of *Klebsiella* species as opportunistic hospital pathogens.

During the 1970s, there were frequent reports of hospital outbreaks of gentamicin-resistant *K. pneumoniae,* sometimes associated with significant mortality when highly compromised patients were involved (102–105). The microorganisms often spread between hospitals and into the community. They became endemic in some hospitals and were sometimes associated with the simultaneous appearance of multiple resistances in other strains of *Klebsiella* and in other species of Enterobacteriaceae (55,106,107). In these cases, *K. pneumoniae* appeared to be acting as an engine of resistance dissemination, especially resistance to aminoglycosides (40,92).

Once the epidemiology of resistant *Klebsiella* infection was understood, and following the introduction of newer cephalosporins, these outbreaks became much less common. However, strains of *K. pneumoniae* (and also *Klebsiella ozaenae*) have appeared that are resistant to third-generation cephalosporins and can spread to produce hospital outbreaks (85,108–111). This type of resistance is mediated by the production of ESBLs that can break down some of the newer cephalosporins. These β-lactamases are the result of small mutations in the genes encoding TEM-1, TEM-2, or SHV-1 (46,85), although other families of enzymes may be involved (46,80). They are encoded on plasmids that can transfer to other species, and they are often associated with other multiple resistances, including resistance to aminoglycosides (112). Although ESBL-producing strains are usually susceptible to β-lactam–β-lactamase-inhibitor combinations such as amoxicillin plus clavulanate and ampicillin plus sulbactam, nosocomial isolates may be resistant by hyperproduction of the ESBL (113,114). These multiresistant strains may also acquire resistance to quinolones by mutation. Thus, recent isolates are often resistant to all the common β-lactams, aminoglycosides, and quinolones, and reliably susceptible only to the carbapenems.

Outbreaks with these new multiresistant *Klebsiella* species seem to have an epidemiology similar to that of the gentamicin-resistant *Klebsiella* outbreaks of the 1970s. They can cause large hospital outbreaks, sometimes with dissemination between hospitals (115), and the outbreak strains can pass aminoglycoside and cephalosporin resistances to other bacterial species (116). Initially these new multiply-resistant Klebsiellas were seen sporadically in Europe (108–110), but much larger outbreaks have been reported from many countries around the world (113, 117–127). These microorganisms are also causing sporadic infections with increasing frequency: in a survey of 35 European ICUs, ESBL producers accounted for 23% of 966 sequential *Klebsiella* isolates (128).

Klebsiella oxytoca has been shown by DNA hybridization to be a distinct species of *Klebsiella* and may even belong in a different genus (129). It is a less common cause of human infection than *K. pneumoniae* but has emerged as an important nosocomial opportunist that also can produce and disseminate resistance to aminoglycosides and the newer β-lactam antibiotics (80, 107,130–132). The epidemiologies and clinical presentations of these two species are similar.

Enterobacter Species

There are now 11 named species of *Enterobacter,* including microorganisms previously allocated to the genera *Aerobacter* and *Erwinia.* The most frequent species isolated from clinical material is *Enterobacter cloacae,* which is much more common than the next most frequent species, *Enterobacter aerogenes* (34,36). In the United States, *Enterobacter* species have replaced *Klebsiella* species as the third most common cause of gram-negative nosocomial infection after *E. coli* and *P. aeruginosa* (47,94,133). This is probably due to the selection of resistant mutants by the increasing clinical use of cephalosporins. *Enterobacter* species are inherently resistant to first-generation cephalosporins and can develop chromosomally mediated resistance to second- and third-generation cephalosporins (133–135), sometimes during the treatment of individual patients (136). *Enterobacter* species possess an inducible chromosomally encoded class I β-lactamase that is normally suppressed by a repressor gene and is produced in large amounts only after exposure to certain β-lactams. Full resistance to second- and third-generation cephalosporins results when stably derepressed mutants appear that express the class I β-lactamase constitutively. These mutants are selected by cephalosporin therapy and produce the β-lactamase continuously.

Enterobacter species have a similar ability to that of *Klebsiella* species to survive on skin and dry surfaces (89), but *Enterobacter* species are more able to survive in nutritionally poor fluids such as 5% dextrose and have often caused outbreaks associated with contaminated intravenous solutions (32–34). Although *Enterobacter* species are well recognized as nosocomial pathogens, they appear to cause hospital outbreaks less frequently than *Klebsiella* species or *Serratia* species. Several studies have shown that the emergence of multiresistant *Enterobacter* species is related to use of second- and third-generation cephalosporins, especially as prophylaxis (61,133).

Serratia Species

These are small aerobic gram-negative bacilli whose normal habitat is soil and water, but they are sometimes found as mucosal commensals of humans. There are several species, of which the most common in clinical material is *Serratia marcescens* followed by *Serratia liquefaciens,* previously known as *Enterobacter liquefaciens.* They are inherently resistant to cephalosporins and polymyxins and readily acquire resistance factors to ampicillin and aminoglycosides, but they are usually susceptible to cotrimoxazole (137). Multiresistant *Serratia* species have become more common, but the degree of resistance varies in different areas (137–140). They produce typical opportunistic infections, having a similar epidemiology and clinical presentation to *Klebsiella* and *Enterobacter* species, although *Serratia* species are the least common of the three. Most clinical isolates represent colonizations, but bacteremia sometimes occurs.

Pseudomonas and *Pseudomonas*-Like Species

These are nonfermenting, aerobic, gram-negative bacteria that are widely distributed in nature, are nonfastidious in their nutritional requirements, and can survive and multiply in many wet environmental sites, often at ambient or low temperatures. They also readily colonize mucous membranes of compromised patients who have been treated with multiple courses of antibiotics. Although they have little pathogenicity for normal individuals, they are resistant to many common antimicrobials and disinfectants and flourish as environmental opportunistic pathogens in intensive care and similar units. Since these microorganisms survive in many types of liquid media, they are sometimes the cause of "pseudobacteremia"; that is, they may be isolated from blood culture bottles following ward or laboratory contamination rather than patient infection (141). Colonized patients may later go on to develop invasive disease, but the mere isolation of a pseudomonad from a clinical specimen does not necessarily indicate infection, and individual patients should be assessed clinically before treatment decisions are made. Although many species of *Pseudomonas* and *Pseudomonas*-like microorganisms have been isolated from clinical material, the ones that cause most problems of antibiotic-resistant nosocomial infection are *P. aeruginosa, Stenotrophomonas* (formerly *Xanthomonas* or *Pseudomonas*) *maltophilia, Burkholderia* (formerly *Pseudomonas*) *cepacia,* and *Ralstonia* (formerly *Pseudomonas or Burkholderia*) *pickettii. Achromobacter xylosoxidans* is a nonfermenting gram-negative bacillus that behaves like *Pseudomonas* and causes similar hospital infections.

Pseudomonas aeruginosa

This is the most common pseudomonad isolated from clinical specimens and the most frequent species causing invasive infection. It accounts for about 10% of all hospital-acquired infection and is about the third most common cause of hospital-acquired gram-negative bacteremia after *E. coli* and *K. pneumoniae* (71). It is a normal commensal of humans, colonizing skin, nose, throat, and stool in a widely varying number (0–40%) of healthy subjects (97). Hospitalized patients have a higher rate of colonization of these sites, which increases with length of stay (59,61, 142). Colonization is encouraged by the use of broad-spectrum antibiotics to which *P. aeruginosa* is resistant, and invasive infection may follow in the compromised host. *P. aeruginosa* septicemia is associated with high mortality rates.

P. aeruginosa can be typed by a variety of methods including several molecular methods (143). Many studies have shown that several different types may be in circulation during an apparent outbreak, and while person-to-person spread does occur, endogenous infection is common (144–146). Carriage of clinically undetectable resistant *P. aeruginosa* may be common in normal persons, and this resistant population may emerge under antibiotic pressure in hospitals to cause environmental colonization and endogenous infection (145,146).

P. aeruginosa tolerates a wide range of temperatures and is often found in wet hospital environmental sites such as sinks, disinfectants, humidifier water of ventilators and incubators, water baths, and suction apparatus (65). It is also a common contaminant of medicinal jellies and ointments. *P. aeruginosa* can multiply in these environmental sites and then gain access to compromised patients, leading to colonization of oropharyngeal and respiratory mucosa, bladder, wounds, skin, and bowel. It should be noted, however, that environmental sites can just as well be contaminated by patients as the reverse, and although sinks often contain multiply resistant pseudomonads, they are not often the source of patient infection (27,142).

P. aeruginosa is inherently resistant to most penicillins and cephalosporins, tetracyclines, chloramphenicol, sulfonamides, and nalidixic acid. It is naturally susceptible to the aminoglycosides, antipseudomonal penicillins and cephalosporins, quinolones, and carbapenems. However, acquired antibiotic resistance in *P. aeruginosa* is common. The microorganism can exchange antibiotic resistance plasmids with other gram-negative bacilli while colonizing patients (147,148), but acquired resistance to aminoglycosides and other agents is probably more often the result of changes in membrane permeability (149,150). Resistance to fluoroquinolones (due to mutations in DNA gyrase, membrane permeability, or both) has emerged relatively rapidly in *P. aeruginosa* and now about a third of hospital isolates are resistant (151) (Table 91.1). This microorganism can develop resistance to ceftazidime by mutation to constitutive production of chromosomal class I β-lactamase (134,135), and this may occur during treatment (152). It may also, though less readily, develop resistance to carbapenems such as imipenem and meropenem, usually by changes in membrane permeability (47,153, 154). In the NNIS studies between 1994–1998 and 1999, resistance to quinolones and carbapenems in ICU isolates of *P. aeruginosa* increased by 49% and 35%, respectively (Table 91.2).

Bacteremia is often a terminal event in highly immunocompromised patients dying from underlying disease, and it is the major cause of death in burn patients in some centers, in whom *P. aeruginosa* bacteremia has a mortality rate of more than 70% (155). Neutropenic and burn patients should be treated with a synergistic combination of an antipseudomonal β-lactam, such as ceftazidime, with an aminoglycoside (156–158).

Stenotrophomonas maltophilia

Stenotrophomonas maltophilia (formerly *Xanthomonas* or *Pseudomonas maltophilia*) is a free-living, opportunistic, gram-negative nonfermenter, less frequently isolated than *P. aeruginosa* but similar in its epidemiology and clinical presentation (159–161). However, *S. maltophilia* is more antibiotic-resistant, often showing resistance to all aminoglycosides and to carbapenems, although it is characteristically susceptible to cotrimoxazole and tetracyclines. Its ability to develop multiple acquired resistance is partly related to outer membrane impermeability and the production of inducible broad-spectrum β-lactamases (162). Because of these inherent and acquired multiple resistances, *S. maltophilia* is being seen with increasing frequency as an opportunistic pathogen in immunocompromised patients in intensive care and other high-dependency units, especially in areas of heavy imipenem use (94). *S. maltophilia* infections have been treated successfully with combinations of cotrimoxazole, antipseudomonal penicillins and cephalosporins, and tetracyclines, but sensitivities need to be confirmed at the start of therapy and monitored during treatment.

Burkholderia cepacia

Burkholderia cepacia (formerly known as *Pseudomonas cepacia* or *Pseudomonas multivorans*) is a cause of endemic and epidemic hospital-acquired infection, usually associated with contamination of wet hospital environments, especially disinfectants (163–165) and intensive care equipment (35,166). This microorganism can colonize mucous membranes and, like other pseudomonads, occasionally produces invasive infection in immunocompromised patients, but *B. cepacia* appears to be even less pathogenic than *P. aeruginosa,* and the differentiation between colonization and infection is often difficult. *B. cepacia* is characteristically resistant to aminoglycosides and most β-lactam antibiotics, but it is normally susceptible to cotrimoxazole and chloramphenicol. However, additional acquired multiple resistance is becoming more common (167), and the choice of therapy for true *B. cepacia* infection should be guided by the results of sensitivity tests. Multiply resistant *B. cepacia* causing colonization and severe lung infections has been seen in cystic fibrosis patients, sometimes associated with a high mortality rate (168, 169). In these patients, cross-infection may sometimes occur in both the community and the hospital (166,170).

Ralstonia pickettii

This microorganism was previously known as *Pseudomonas pickettii* or *Pseudomonas thomasii,* but later transferred to the genus *Burkholderia* (171) and then *Ralstonia* (172). It is of low virulence and a relatively uncommon cause of human and hospital infection, but may be associated with outbreaks caused by contamination of supposedly sterile fluids for injection or infusion (173). Like other such opportunists, the microorganism may cause pseudobacteremias or multistrain outbreaks. It is of low virulence, usually causing mucosal colonizations and sometimes bacteremias and other more serious infections. Isolates are usually resistant to aminoglycosides, ampicillin, and colistin but susceptible to chloramphenicol and newer cephalosporins.

Achromobacter xylosoxidans

The taxonomic position of this microorganism is confused. DNA homology studies suggest that it and *Alcaligenes denitrificans* should be classified together as two subspecies of *Alcaligenes xylosoxidans* (174). *A. xylosoxidans* subspecies *xylosoxidans* (*Achromobacter xylosoxidans*) is very disinfectant-resistant and can survive in cetrimide (like *P. aeruginosa*) and in 1% chlorhexidine for 10 minutes or more (175). Not surprisingly, therefore, it has caused a number of hospital outbreaks associated with contaminated disinfectants and other wet sites (174,176). It is characteristically susceptible to cotrimoxazole, ceftazidime, and fluoroquinolones but resistant to aminoglycosides. It resembles *P. aeruginosa* in its epidemiology but appears to be rather less pathogenic. Although some reports suggest that this microorganism is being isolated with increasing frequency (176), in the 20-year study of more than 4,000 episodes of septicemia at St. Thomas's Hospital in London, there were only two episodes of *Achromobacter* septicemia and one of *Alcaligenes* (71).

Acinetobacter baumannii

Acinetobacter species are nonfermenting gram-negative coccobacilli found widely distributed as free-living saprophytes in soil and water. They also colonize the skin and mucous membranes in about 25% of normal people (177,178). The classification and nomenclature of this group have undergone frequent changes, and until recently only one species was recognized with various biochemical variants. The most frequently isolated *Acinetobacter,* the one most likely to acquire multiple antibiotic resistance, and the commonest cause of hospital outbreaks, is *Acinetobacter baumannii* (179), formerly known as *Acinetobacter calcoaceticus* var. *anitratus* and in the past allocated to other genera such as *Mima, Herellea, Achromobacter,* and *Moraxella.* Hospital outbreaks originate from contaminated environmental sources or follow hand transmission from the skin of colonized patients (180,181). These microorganisms can also survive for long periods on dry surfaces (182–184) and can probably be transmitted via dust and fomites (185–187). Most clinical isolates represent colonization rather than infection (181), but serious and sometimes fatal infections occur in compromised patients, including septicemia, endocarditis, meningitis, and pneumonia (178,188).

In the early 1970s, *Acinetobacter* species were usually susceptible to many common antimicrobials, including gentamicin and the cephalosporins, and they were relatively uncommon hospital pathogens (189). By the mid-1980s, however, hospital outbreaks with multiply resistant *Acinetobacter* strains were being frequently reported (178,190) and were dubbed "bacteria resistant to everything" (191). Many hospital strains are now resistant to the aminoglycosides and to older and newer cephalosporins, and some have developed resistance to the quinolones (192,193) and carbapenems (194). *A. baumannii* is usually susceptible *in vitro* to β-lactamase inhibitors such as clavulanic acid and, thus, to co-amoxiclav (amoxicillin plus cluvulanic acid), ampicillin plus sulbactam, and piperacillin plus tazobactam, but these agents may not be effective clinically. The mechanisms and genetics of resistance in this species are complex and difficult to investigate (195), but they involve several plasmid-borne β-lactamases and aminoglycoside-modifying enzymes as well as alterations in membrane permeability and penicillin-binding proteins (PBPs) (189,194–197). The ability of *A. baumannii* to acquire multiple resistances, as well as to survive on skin and in the environment, undoubtedly contributes to its success as a nosocomial pathogen.

Gram-Positive Bacteria

Staphylococcus aureus

Staphylococcus aureus is usually the second most common bacterial isolate in hospital laboratories after *E. coli* and is associated with wound infections and septicemia (71). Surface isolates often represent colonization, but invasive infection causes high morbidity and may be fatal. *S. aureus* is naturally susceptible to many classes of antimicrobials, including penicillins, cephalosporins, macrolides, sulfonamides, trimethoprim, tetracyclines, chloramphenicol, lincosamines, aminoglycosides, quinolones, and glycopeptides, but it has great ability to develop resistance to many of these drugs simultaneously. Antibiotic resistance facilitates the survival and spread of these microorganisms in the hospital environment, and multiresistant strains are often responsible for large and serious outbreaks of nosocomial infection. Since the 1950s, many different resistance problems have been encountered (66,67). Penicillin resistance due to the production of plasmid-mediated penicillinase appeared in *S. aureus* soon after penicillin was introduced (198) and increased to 85% by the late 1970s (199). During the 1950s, multiresistant strains of *S. aureus* began to appear, and large epidemics of hospital infection with microorganisms resistant to penicillin, tetracycline, erythromycin, chloramphenicol, and other drugs were seen throughout the world. Many of these outbreaks were caused by virulent microorganisms of phage type 80/81, a group that became known as "the hospital staphylococcus" (200–203). The hospital staphylococcus was greatly feared, because infections were often untreatable and outbreaks were associated with high mortality rates.

Gentamicin resistance was uncommon in the 1960s, but some hospitals experienced outbreaks with gentamicin-resistant *S. aureus* in the 1970s (204), and during this time gentamicin resistance was used as a marker of potentially epidemic strains. In general, however, the incidence of hospital infection with multiply resistant staphylococci gradually declined during the 1960s and 1970s (42,199,205–207). The exact reasons for this are unclear, but the decline was associated with the introduction in the 1960s of the penicillinase-stable semisynthetic penicillins, methicillin, nafcillin, oxacillin, and cloxacillin (which are active against penicillinase-producing staphylococci), an apparent loss of virulence in the phage type 80/81 strains, and improvements in hospital infection control (66,67).

Strains of MRSA were noted soon after methicillin was introduced into clinical practice (208), but they were generally rare until the 1980s despite widespread use of methicillin, cloxacillin, and related drugs (42). In the late 1970s, however, MRSA emerged as a major pathogen of hospital infection in most countries and regions of the world (209). In both the U.S. and Europe, around 30% to 50% of hospital isolates of *S. aureus* are now methicillin resistant (87,151) (Table 91.1), although in the Netherlands and Scandinavia rates are less than 1% (87).

In a given population of MRSA, not all daughter cells may express methicillin resistance. This is called "heterogeneous resistance," and commonly, under routine culture conditions, less than 1% of cells may be phenotypically resistant (210,211). To improve detection during *in-vitro* susceptibility testing, special conditions are required to increase the proportion of cells expressing methicillin resistance. These include reducing the incubation temperature to 30° or 35°C, prolonging the incubation time to 48 hours, and making the culture medium more hypertonic—for example, by increasing the NaCl content to 5% (212, 213). If these special test conditions are not used, laboratories may fail to identify some methicillin-resistant strains.

Methicillin resistance is mediated primarily by the production of an abnormal PBP called PBP-2a or PBP-2′ (214–216). β-Lactam antibiotics bind to normal bacterial PBPs and inhibit their activity, preventing proper formation of cell wall peptidoglycan and leading to cell death by osmotic lysis. PBP-2a binds poorly with most β-lactams and can fulfill the functions of the so-called essential PBPs 1, 2, and 3 (217). Microorganisms producing PBP-2a are thus resistant to most available β-lactams, including methicillin and the isoxazolyl penicillins. Although they may appear susceptible to some β-lactams *in vitro,* the agents so far tested are clinically ineffective and should not be used for therapy.

The production of PBP-2a is encoded by the *mecA* gene located on the chromosome. This gene appears to have been derived from coagulase-negative staphylococci, hospital strains of which are now frequently methicillin-resistant (218). Recent genetic studies suggest that MRSA has repeatedly emerged from methicillin-sensitive *S. aureus* (MSSA) at different times in different parts of the world (219,220).

MRSA strains are resistant to methicillin, oxacillin, and other penicillinase-stable β-lactams including the carbapenems, and to several other classes of antibiotic. Following the rapid emergence of resistance to quinolones (221–224), many strains of MRSA remain susceptible only to the glycopeptides vancomycin and teicoplanin, and vancomycin is the drug of choice for serious infection (225,226). There are a number of new drugs under development for the treatment of multiresistant gram-positive bacteria, including new glycopeptides, quinolones, ketolides, oxazolidinones, and the streptogramin combination quinupristin/dalfopristin, but the role of these agents in the treatment of MRSA remains to be elucidated (217,226).

Because of the present importance of vancomycin and teicoplanin in the treatment of severe MRSA sepsis, the emergence of glycopeptide resistance in MRSA is greatly feared. Unfortunately, several types of glycopeptide resistance have emerged in MRSA in recent years.

The glycopeptides are normally slowly bactericidal for *S. aureus.* However, some recent isolates of MRSA exhibit glycopeptide tolerance, that is, they are inhibited by normal concentrations of these agents but are not killed (227,228). Tolerance has been associated with treatment failures, but its exact clinical significance is unclear. Glycopeptide tolerance is not routinely tested, and tolerant strains usually go undetected.

There have been some reports of *S. aureus* strains with reduced vancomycin susceptibility from Japan, North America, and Europe (229–231). These strains have non–plasmid-mediated low-level or "intermediate" resistance to vancomycin, with vancomycin minimum inhibitory concentration (MIC) of 8 μg/mL, and have been associated with treatment failures. They have been designated "vancomycin-intermediate *S. aureus*" (VISA). In Japan, some strains showing "heterogeneous" vancomycin resistance have affected many hospitals (232). In a given population of these strains, the majority have vancomycin MICs of 2 to 4 μg/mL, but there is a subpopulation with MICs of 5 to 9 μg/mL that may emerge under glycopeptide pressure. The mechanism of vancomycin resistance in these microorganisms has not been fully elucidated but may result from increased amounts of normal D-Ala–D-Ala residues in the cell wall that absorb therapeutic concentrations of vancomycin (233). These VISA strains appear to be rare and their true clinical significance is uncertain. As with glycopeptide tolerance, GISA strains are not routinely identified in the laboratory but may be identified retrospectively after treatment failure (234).

High-level, inducible, transferable resistance to both vancomycin and teicoplanin is now seen quite commonly in enterococci, and is encoded by a series of genes, including *vanA* (see below). This *vanA* resistance is usually plasmid-borne and was transferred to *S. aureus* in the laboratory in 1992 (235). Ten years later, two clinical isolates of MRSA that contained the *vanA* gene and had vancomycin MICs of >128μg/mL and teicoplanin MICs of 32 μg/mL, were reported from the U.S. (236, 237). Such strains are still exceptionally rare, but since both MRSA and vancomycin-resistant enterococci (VRE) are widespread in hospitals throughout the world, there is fear that fully glycopeptide-resistant MRSA will become common nosocomial pathogens in the near future. It is essential to avoid any unnecessary use of glycopeptides that might encourage the emergence of such strains, to maintain vigilant surveillance for their appearance, and to strictly isolate any cases that do occur to prevent further spread.

There has been debate over the clinical significance of MRSA, some holding that these microorganisms are merely opportunistic commensals of low pathogenicity that colonize highly compromised patients but contribute little to morbidity or mortality (238). Nevertheless, MRSA strains appear similar to methicillin-sensitive strains in their abilities to produce invasive infection in humans and animals (225,239) and to cause deep infections such as septicemia, osteomyelitis, severe pneumonia, and brain abscesses. Mortality rates in MRSA septicemia are high, partly due to the poor prognosis of the underlying diseases seen in these patients but also to the failure of standard antimicrobial therapy against these microorganisms. Most authors with experience in MRSA outbreaks would agree with Waldvogel (240) that "data clearly define MRSA as a major pathogen, fully equipped to produce infections and death," and conclude with Casewell (241) that "the clinical importance of MRSA is now indisputable."

MRSA strains are primarily hospital pathogens and are usually seen in tertiary referral centers. However, MRSA also readily colonize elderly patients in nursing homes (242–244). These institutions may act as reservoirs of MRSA, continually reseeding acute care hospitals with resistant staphylococci carried by patient transfers. Some MRSA strains have particular abilities to spread in hospitals (and sometimes into the community) and have been called "epidemic methicillin-resistant *S. aureus*" (EMRSA) strains to distinguish them from other MRSA strains (245,246).

Within hospitals, the sources of cross-infection with MRSA are usually infected or asymptomatic patients who may be colonized in the nose, pharynx, rectum, wounds, and chronic skin lesions. Nasal carriage by staff members is usually low, on the order of 1% to 8%, but staff members may transfer MRSA between patients by hand contact, either directly from patient to patient or via fomites (247,248). Although MRSA may be spread by airborne transmission, this appears to be less common than with methicillin-sensitive strains. The risk of colonization and infection with MRSA increases with length of hospitalization, severity of underlying disease, number of operations or manipulations, and previous exposure to antibiotics, especially cephalosporins and aminoglycosides (249,250). Although some types of MRSA appear sporadically and rarely cause outbreaks, epidemic strains spread rapidly in hospitals and may become endemic.

Once established within a hospital, MRSA may be very difficult to eradicate (251). Nevertheless, most authorities believe that vigorous efforts should be made to control outbreaks of MRSA, especially if infection is not yet endemic. A U.K. working party of the British Society for Antimicrobial Chemotherapy, the Hospital Infection Society, and the Infection Control Nurses Association has published detailed guidelines for the control of epidemic and endemic MRSA (252). Briefly, infected patients should be isolated; others on the ward should be screened for carriage, and colonized patients should be isolated in cohorts or discharged home; infected patients should be treated systemically, if necessary, with glycopeptides; nasal carriage should be cleared by topical agents, and skin carriage by disinfectant baths; if the outbreak is not brought quickly under control, staff members should be screened and carriers removed from critical areas until they have been cleared. Cohorting of new cases as they appear and strict attention to hand washing are of the utmost importance. The control of moderately sized or large outbreaks may require the closure and cleaning of affected wards; control may be facilitated by having a dedicated infection isolation ward (253).

Despite such control policies, many hospitals are now affected by endemic MRSA. Eradication is difficult, because colonized patients are often readmitted after discharge and in tertiary referral centers colonized patients are constantly being admitted from other institutions. Under these circumstances many authorities believe that attempts to control all MRSA colonizations is not cost-effective, and instead efforts should be directed toward control in high-risk wards such as orthopedics, cardiothoracic surgery, and intensive care (252).

Topical mupirocin is widely used for the clearance of nasal carriers of MRSA during outbreaks (247,254,255). Susceptible strains have MICs of less than 1 μg/mL, and the ointment contains 20,000 μg/mL. Resistance to mupirocin is uncommon, but rates tend to be higher in patients given prolonged treatment such as those in dermatology clinics and during outbreaks of mupirocin-resistant strains. Mupirocin acts by inhibiting bacterial isoleucyl–transfer RNA (tRNA) synthetase, and resistance appears to be mediated by the production of modified enzymes. Isolates showing low-level resistance have a single chromosomally encoded modified synthetase, whereas those with high-level resistance also have a second enzyme encoded on a plasmid (256–258). Staphylococci can be trained to low levels of mupirocin resistance (MICs <64 μgm/L *in vitro,* and similar low-level resistance may emerge during therapy. The clinical significance of such resistance is uncertain, since topical mupirocin concentrations are very much higher than these MICs, and carriage of low-level resistant strains can be eradicated with normal mupirocin therapy (254). More important are isolates showing high-level resistance (MICs >1,024 μg/mL), which cannot be cleared by mupirocin therapy (259). This type of resistance may be carried on a conjugative plasmid or transposon and can transfer to other microorganisms (260). Since mupirocin is so useful in the management of *S. aureus* outbreaks, the use of this agent should be carefully controlled to preserve its effectiveness.

MRSA strains are usually brought into hospitals by asymptomatic carriers, either patients or staff members. An important control measure is to screen patients admitted from other hospitals and keep them in isolation until they are shown not to be carriers. Similarly, new staff members who have recently worked at other hospitals (including agency staff members) should not be allowed to work until they have been shown to be free of MRSA. It is also good practice to inform other hospitals if infected or colonized patients are to be transferred to them.

Coagulase-Negative Staphylococci

There are many species of coagulase-negative staphylococci, of which the commonest isolated from clinical material is *S.*

epidermidis. At one time, coagulase-negative staphylococci were regarded as insignificant pathogens of humans, but they are now recognized as increasingly important causes of infection in hospitalized and compromised patients. Many of these microorganisms are multiply antibiotic-resistant (78,261–263) and can produce an extracellular "slime" that allows them to stick to plastic prostheses and survive on foreign surfaces within a protective biofilm (72–74,264). As a result, infections with coagulase-negative staphylococci are being seen with increasing frequency in compromised patients. These include bacteremia (associated with intravascular catheters and vascular grafts), endocarditis (prosthetic heart valves), meningitis (ventricular shunts), peritonitis (peritoneal dialysis catheters), and infection of joint prostheses. Coagulase-negative staphylococci are now common isolates from blood cultures (71), usually associated with vascular lines, especially indwelling and long-term ones such as Hickman lines (72,264,265).

About half the strains isolated in hospitals show multiple antibiotic resistance, including resistance to methicillin (and other β-lactams) and gentamicin. Methicillin-resistant strains tend to be more multiply resistant than methicillin-sensitive ones. Healthy individuals are normally colonized by relatively sensitive microorganisms, primarily *S. epidermidis*. After admission to the hospital, and especially after exposure to multiple courses of antibiotics or surgical prophylaxis, patients become colonized with multiply resistant strains and with other more resistant coagulase-negative species such as *Staphylococcus hemolyticus* (266–268). Resistance in coagulase-negative staphylococci appears to be increasing, probably under pressure of antibiotic use (269,270). Sensitive staphylococci may receive plasmid-borne resistance factors from other microorganisms during contact on the skin surface, and there is evidence that coagulase-negative staphylococci may be a reservoir of resistance genes that can be transferred to *S. aureus* (271,272).

Because of extensive multiple resistance in coagulase-negative staphylococci, the glycopeptides vancomycin and teicoplanin are often used for therapy and prophylaxis in high-risk patients. Low-level resistance to glycopeptides has appeared in hospital isolates of coagulase-negative staphylococci, and such resistance can be produced by exposure to increasing drug concentrations *in vitro*. Teicoplanin resistance is easier to produce than vancomycin resistance, and MICs are higher (273). Similar low-level teicoplanin-resistant, vancomycin-sensitive strains are being increasingly isolated from clinical specimens (274–276). There is some evidence that *S. hemolyticus* is more likely to exhibit teicoplanin resistance than are other coagulase-negative species, but not all studies have shown this. Glycopeptide resistance is probably related to the increasing use of these drugs, and the emergence of resistant strains following intraperitoneal vancomycin treatment of chronic ambulatory peritoneal dialysis (CAPD) peritonitis has been reported (277).

Epidemiologic investigations were previously hampered by the lack of good typing systems, but new molecular methods have revealed clusters of hospital infection with indistinguishable strains of coagulase-negative staphylococci (278–281). In most instances, however, the sources and routes of transmission of the outbreak strains are unclear.

In general, therefore, infection with coagulase-negative staphylococci should be regarded as endogenous unless clustering of unusually resistant isolates is noted. Colonization and infection with resistant strains are more likely with prolonged hospitalization and multiple courses of antibiotic therapy, and these should be avoided when possible. Eradication of infection usually requires the removal of the colonized catheter or prosthesis.

Multiply Resistant Coryneform Bacteria

Johnson and Kaye (282) were the first to describe clinical isolates of multiply antibiotic-resistant coryneforms that became known as the JK group of corynebacteria and were later distinguished by the species name *Corynebacterium jeikeium* (283).

These microorganisms are inherently resistant to many common antibiotics, hospital isolates often being sensitive only to vancomycin (284–286). They are found on the skin of healthy individuals, more often in men and postmenopausal women, in whom the fatty acid composition of epidermal fats may favor the survival of these microorganisms. Hospitalized patients tend to become colonized with multiply resistant strains, especially after multiple courses of antibiotic treatment, and may remain carriers for weeks or months. Staff members in high-risk units such as oncology departments may also become colonized with multiply resistant coryneforms (287). These microorganisms are classic opportunistic pathogens, having low virulence for healthy individuals, but causing local skin sepsis and bacteremia in the compromised, especially those with hematologic and other malignancies. They may also cause bacteremia and endocarditis in association with vascular catheterization and prosthetic implants such as heart valves (288,289). Thus, in many respects, *C. jeikeium* behaves clinically like multiply resistant coagulase-negative staphylococci, producing primarily endogenous infection in highly compromised patients after prolonged hospitalization, often in association with vascular and prosthetic foreign bodies. The prevention of such resistant infections is also similar: the likelihood of colonization can be reduced by avoiding unnecessary antibiotic use, and the theoretic possibility of spread to others can be limited by isolating colonized patients and emphasizing hand washing by staff members.

Enterococci

Enterococci are found in the stools of most normal people and sometimes in other sites such as the mouth and vagina. *Enterococcus faecalis* and *Enterococcus faecium* predominate, with *E. faecalis* usually being the most common. Other enterococcal species are infrequent human commensals. The enterococci typically cause endogenous infections, most commonly of the urinary tract, but also of the abdomen and pelvis, where they are usually mixed with other bowel flora. They are relatively poor pathogens but may go on to cause invasive disease in compromised patients, causing cholangitis, septicemia, endocarditis, and meningitis (290). Multiresistant strains of enterococci cause hospital outbreaks in which they colonize the bowels of asymptomatic patients and are transferred between patients on staff members' hands (290,291).

The enterococci are typically susceptible to ampicillin/amoxicillin but intrinsically relatively resistant to benzylpenicillin and other β-lactams such as cloxacillin, the cephalosporins, and the carbapenems. They are also usually resistant to trimethoprim and the sulfonamides, the quinolones, low levels of aminoglycosides, and low levels of clindamycin. Furthermore, these microorganisms have a remarkable ability to acquire new resistances to ampicillin/amoxicillin and other drugs that might be used against gram-positive bacteria, including chloramphenicol, erythromycin, tetracycline, high levels of aminoglycosides and clindamycin, and now the glycopeptides vancomycin and teicoplanin. *E. faecium* is inherently more resistant to penicillin and ampicillin than *E. faecalis,* and hospital isolates have tended to show increasing high-level resistance (292). This high-level ampicillin resistance is probably due to changes in affinity of the enterococcal PBPs and contributes to the growing importance of *E. faecium* as a nosocomial pathogen.

Transferable β-lactamase–mediated ampicillin resistance has been reported in *E. faecalis,* and although such strains have caused several large hospital outbreaks (293,294), they are usually rare in clinical material.

Because the enterococci are intrinsically resistant to the most commonly used antimicrobials, they have become increasingly important as causes of infection and superinfection in hospitalized patients (75,295). Nosocomial enterococcal infections are increasing in prevalence and now cause 10% to 12% of all hospital-acquired infection, 10% to 20% of hospital-acquired urinary tract infections, and 5% to 10% of hospital-acquired bacteremias (76,296). Most hospital infections are endogenous, arising from the patient's own bowel, but outbreaks of cross-infection via staff hands or by environmental contamination does occur (297–301).

Because of their great ability to acquire multiple resistances, the enterococci are one of the few bacterial groups that can become resistant to all available antibiotics. Many of these resistances are borne on transferable plasmids, and it has been demonstrated *in vitro* that the enterococci have the potential to transfer them to streptococci and staphylococci as well as to other enterococci. For these reasons, the enterococci have fulfilled the prediction that they were set to become the most important and problematic nosocomial pathogens of the 1990s (302).

Glycopeptide-Resistant Enterococci

The glycopeptides inhibit synthesis of gram-positive cell walls by binding to the amide bond of the D-alanyl–D-alanine terminal sequences of the muramyl pentapeptide of the elongating peptidoglycan polymer. The large glycopeptide molecules then impede the action of both the polymerase that extends the peptidoglycan backbone and the transpeptidase that cross-links the growing chain to the existing cell wall (303,304).

Most clinically important gram-positive bacteria are naturally susceptible to the glycopeptides vancomycin and teicoplanin. Vancomycin resistance can be divided into low-level (MICs of 8–32 μg/mL) and high-level (MICs ≥64 μg/mL). Acquired glycopeptide resistance is rare but is most frequently seen in enterococci, which exhibit at least four resistance phenotypes (303,305): (a) *vanA,* high-level transferable resistance to both vancomycin and teicoplanin, associated with the production of a 38- to 40-kd membrane protein; (b) *vanB,* inducible low-level resistance to vancomycin alone that, in some strains, is associated with a 39.5-kd membrane protein; (c) *vanC,* constitutive low-level vancomycin resistance seen in some strains of *Enterococcus gallinarum*; and (d) *vanD,* described in only a few strains of *E. faecium,* with constitutive resistance to vancomycin (MICs ~64 μg/mL) and to low levels of teicoplanin (MICs ~4 μg/mL). *Enterococcus casseliflavus/Enterococcus flavescens* appear to have intrinsic low-level resistance unrelated to that of the other phenotypes. As more glycopeptide-resistant strains are investigated, an increasingly wider range of resistant phenotypes are being described, some resulting from alterations or deletions of the genes encoding the more common types.

Low-level resistance usually involves only one of the glycopeptides and is encoded on the chromosome. The *vanA* phenotype of high-level resistance to both vancomycin and teicoplanin is usually encoded on a transferable plasmid and is a potentially more serious clinical problem. *vanA* strains have vancomycin MICs of 64 to more than 1,024 μg/mL and teicoplanin MICs usually one or two times lower than this. This phenotype has been seen so far only in clinical isolates of enterococci, most frequently in *E. faecium,* sometimes in *E. faecalis,* and rarely in *Enterococcus avium.* The *vanA* gene encodes an abnormal D-Ala–D-Ala ligase, which results in the replacement of the normal D-Ala–D-Ala termini of peptidoglycan precursors by D-Ala–D-lactate, which cannot bind glycopeptides (305–309). The successful production of the *vanA* glycopeptide resistance phenotype is dependent on the cooperative activity of the products of seven genes, which in *E. faecium* BM4147 are contained in a transposon *Tn*1546 (307) that is usually encoded on a plasmid but sometimes transfers to the chromosome. The mechanisms and genetics of the other vancomycin resistance phenotypes have not been so well elucidated, but they all seem to result from the production of altered ligases. The *vanB* phenotype is encoded by a similar gene cluster encoded on a transposon *Tn*1547 and containing the *vanB* gene (310–312). The gene product *vanB* encodes a ligase that has a 76% amino-acid identity with *vanA* and is presumably responsible for the formation of D-Ala–D-Lac (313). Enterococci expressing *vanB* are resistant to vancomycin but remain susceptible to teicoplanin, presumably because teicoplanin does not induce resistance. *vanC* in *E. gallinarum* encodes a ligase that substitutes D-Ala–D-Ser for the normal D-Ala–D-Ala in peptidoglycan precursors. The *vanD* gene encodes a D-Ala–D-Lac ligase related to *vanA* and *vanB* (314, 315).

The *vanA* gene is variably transferable by conjugation or transformation *in vitro* to other gram-positive bacteria, including *S. aureus* (235), but it has not, until recently, been passed to other genera naturally. However, as described above, there were reports from the U.S. in 2002 of two unrelated clinical isolates of MRSA that had acquired the *vanA* gene, presumably from enterococci, and expressed high-level vancomycin and teicoplanin resistance (236). Continuing surveillance will reveal whether such strains will increase in prevalence in the future.

Vancomycin has been used for several decades, but acquired resistance was rare until a multiple strain outbreak of vancomycin and teicoplanin resistant enterococci appeared in London in 1986 (316). Since then, such strains have been seen throughout the world. They are common in the U.S., where the NNIS system survey found a 20-fold increase in nosocomial VRE isolates during the period 1989–1993 (317), and a 47% increase in ICU isolates between 1994–1998 and 1999 (13). In U.S. ICUs, about 12% of hospital isolates of enterococci are VRE. They are much less common in Europe, where only about 1% of blood isolates of *E. faecalis* (range in different countries 0–7%) and 5% of *E. faecium* (range 0–21%) are resistant (87). Twelve of the 20 European countries surveyed by EARSS reported no VRE from the blood.

The reservoir of enterococci is the colonized bowel of patients, and most infections are endogenous. Thus the increasing isolation of enterococci is usually caused by the multiple endogenous strains rather than outbreaks of cross-infection. Nevertheless, epidemic infection does occur, and microorganisms probably spread from patient to patient on staff hands (297–300). During outbreaks of both vancomycin-sensitive enterococci (VSE) and VRE, there is extensive colonization of patient and staff bowel and asymptomatic carriage may persist for months (301,318,319). Colonization of other mucous membranes such as throat, stomach, and vagina, and skin colonization of moist sites such as groins may occur. Microorganisms may then be transferred from these sites by hand contact. Evidence for this is provided by the isolation of outbreak strains of VRE and VSE from environmental surfaces likely to have had hand contact such as telephones, stethoscopes, instrument dials, and doorknobs. Boyce et al. (301) found that during an outbreak of enterococci carrying transferable *VanB* resistance, there was extensive contamination of the environment, which was significantly more widespread around colonized patients who also had diarrhea.

After experimental inoculation VSE and VRE survive on fingers for about 30 minutes. Washing with soap and water fails to remove these microorganisms. Aqueous chlorhexidine and povidone iodine are also unreliable but alcohol and alcoholic chlorhexidine are effective (320,321).

Large hospital outbreaks with VRE have a number of similarities. Patients are usually on renal, pediatric, oncologic, intensive care, or other special units in which glycopeptides are used. Although cross-infection does occur, multiple enterococcal strains are often involved, usually of more than one species, and outbreaks often appear to be caused by multiple microorganisms that have acquired resistance via transposons. Asymptomatic stool carriage is common, often lasting weeks or months, and may contribute to the spread of resistant strains into the community. Although most isolates represent colonization or minor infection, septicemia and other serious invasive infection does occur and may be associated with fatalities.

Outbreaks should be dealt with by isolation and hand washing; antibiotic pressure should be reduced by restricting the use of glycopeptides, and methods should be sought to eliminate stool carriage of resistant microorganisms.

Although the origin of the vancomycin-resistance transposons is obscure, the emergence of this resistance has occurred during a time when the glycopeptides have been increasingly used for the treatment of multiresistant staphylococci, enterococci, and *Clostridium difficile*–associated diarrhea (322). Furthermore, outbreaks of nosocomial VRE are most common in renal, liver, hematology, and intensive care units where glycopeptide therapy is common.

A further source of glycopeptide "pressure" is the use of the antibiotic avoparcin in animal husbandry. Avoparcin is a glycopeptide related to vancomycin that is not used in human therapy but that is added in small amounts to animal feeds in Europe. Several studies suggest that in farms where avoparcin additives are used, animal and human bowels become colonized with *vanA*-type VRE, and frozen chickens in supermarkets may be a source of VRE for people unexposed to hospitals or glycopeptides (323,324). After admission to hospital, treatment with glycopeptides may select these microorganisms from the bowel with resulting nosocomial infection (325). As a result of these studies, several European countries have now banned avoparcin feed supplements, but this issue remains controversial. Avoparcin is not used in the U.S., which has the greatest incidence of VRE and where transmission appears to be mainly healthcare-associated. The reasons for the differences in epidemiology of VRE between Europe and the U.S. has not been fully elucidated (326,327).

Multiply Resistant Pneumococci

Streptococcus pneumoniae is the most common cause of bacterial pneumonia, the second most common cause of meningitis, the third most common cause of septicemia, and an important pathogen of otitis media (71,328); all of these are predominantly community-acquired infections. Until recently, the pneumococcus was fully sensitive to benzylpenicillin and not often considered an important hospital pathogen. However, the pneumococcus does cause hospital cross-infection (329), and hospital outbreaks with multiply resistant strains (which are more readily recognized) are being reported with increasing frequency. Transmission is presumably by droplet spread, and ideally, infected patients should be nursed in side rooms (329).

S. pneumoniae frequently acquires resistance to tetracycline and sometimes to sulfonamides, erythromycin, lincomycin, or chloramphenicol. Pneumococci are normally relatively resistant to aminoglycosides (MICs of streptomycin 8 μg/mL), but some strains show high-level resistance (>2,000 μg/mL) (287). Penicillin resistance was first reported in 1967 from Papua New Guinea, and since then has been seen with increasing frequency in many countries (328,330). Multiple resistance is an increasing problem, the most commonly seen patterns being resistance to penicillin and tetracycline and resistance to penicillin, tetracycline, and chloramphenicol.

Sensitive strains of pneumococci have penicillin MICs of 0.006 to 0.008 μg/mL. The first penicillin-resistant isolates showed low-level resistance with MICs of 0.1 to 1.0 μg/mL, but in 1977 pneumococci were isolated in South Africa showing high-level resistance with penicillin MICs of more than 1 μg/mL (331). Penicillin resistance results from the stepwise acquisition of multiple genetic changes that produce various alterations in pneumococcal PBPs (332). The variant sequences inserted into the PBP genes appear to have been derived by transformation from oral streptococcal species (333). Although many penicillin-resistant isolates of pneumococci are sensitive to newer β-lactams such as cefotaxime, some strains are resistant to these drugs by producing simultaneous changes in more than one penicillin-binding protein (334,335). Penicillin resistance in pneumococci may not be detected by routine sensitivity-testing methods, and for disk testing, a 1-mg oxacillin disk is recommended (336,337).

The geographic variation in the distribution of resistant strains of pneumococci is considerable, even between different cities in the same country, but accurate data are lacking. In the EARSS (87) study of resistance rates in European blood isolates, the rates of reduced penicillin susceptibility in pneumococci varied from <3% (usually in Northern European countries) to >30% (usually in Mediterranean countries). In the NNIS system surveillance report for 2002 (Table 91.1), penicillin resistance rates in nosocomial isolates were around 20% for both ICU and non-ICU patients. In some places there have been dramatic increases in penicillin resistance rates; in Cadiz, Spain, for example, high-level penicillin resistance was 29% in 1991 and 75% in 1995; in Hong Kong, China, penicillin-resistance was seen in 6.6% of sputum isolates in the first quarter of 1993 and in 56% of isolates in the second quarter of 1995; and in Kentucky, 53% of childhood community isolates were penicillin-resistant and 33% high-level resistant (338–340). Penicillin-resistant strains of pneumococci are also usually multiply resistant to other antibiotics.

Since the early 1980s, many reports have appeared of hospital outbreaks of penicillin-resistant pneumococci (328,341–345). These outbreaks often involve children or the elderly in daycare or chronic-care centers. In these age groups, nasal carriage is common, and during outbreaks other patients, staff members, and family members may become rapidly colonized by resistant pneumococci after casual contact with affected patients. Carriage may persist for several months, and the microorganisms may then disseminate further within the community.

The prevention and control of hospital outbreaks depend on early detection, isolation, and treatment of infected cases. Infected patients should be isolated, and strict attention should be paid to hand washing. Visitors should be carefully supervised. During an outbreak, patients and staff members should be screened for nasopharyngeal carriage, and carriers should be cohorted or removed, as in the control of MRSA. Attempts should be made to eliminate nasal carriage with topical agents such as mupirocin and erythromycin, depending on the microorganism's sensitivity.

Respiratory infections with strains of pneumococci showing low-level penicillin resistance can be treated with high doses of penicillin. Meningitis and infections with high-level resistant strains have been successfully treated with vancomycin or third-generation cephalosporins such as cefotaxime or ceftriaxone (346,347). However, resistance to third-generation cephalosporins has increased dramatically in some areas (348), and there have been failures with these regimes in meningitis, and the combination of vancomycin with cephalosporins, meropenem, or rifampin has been recommended (349). Treatment with other antistaphylococcal agents such as erythromycin, chloramphenicol, lincomycin, or rifampin should be guided by the results of sensitivity testing.

CONTROL OF ANTIBIOTIC-RESISTANT NOSOCOMIAL INFECTION

Control of Antibiotic Use

The correct use of antibiotics, as for all therapeutic drugs, includes the choice of agents that are necessary, effective, and safe. However, antibiotic therapy is unique, because it is directed against bacteria rather than patients, because it may be used to prevent as well as to cure disease, and because every treatment disturbs the human and environmental microflora of the hospital. In particular, correct use must take account of the potential effects on the development of antibiotic resistance. McGowan (18), in his extensive review of antibiotic use and antibiotic resistance, concluded, "Consensus rarely exists on topics in infectious disease. Yet, authors of virtually all of the papers reviewed here [68 references] agree on the need for careful, discriminating use of antibiotics as being the keystone of our attempts to control resistant bacteria in the hospital."

Nevertheless, many studies have shown that antibiotic use in hospitals is far from ideal (350,351). Reports from U.S. hospitals have shown that 25% to 40% of hospital patients receive systemic antibiotics, with the proportions tending to rise in later surveys (351–359). Many patients receive antibiotics unnecessarily, and on surgical units 38% to 48% of treated patients have no evidence of infection (353). Similar patterns of use have been noted in British hospitals, in which about 20% to 30% of patients receive antibiotics and about 40% of courses are for prophylaxis (360–363). In U.S. studies, 30% to 70% of all antibiotic courses were judged inappropriate (353). Other studies have shown that intravenous and prophylactic therapy is often unnecessarily prolonged and that the timing of prophylaxis is often inappropriate (312,357,358,364).

Some of this antibiotic misuse results from inadequate knowledge and poor understanding of antimicrobial therapy on the part of physicians. This can be attributed both to failures of education in medical schools and hospitals and the influence of specific product-related information from the pharmaceutical industry. Physicians probably get most of their information on antibiotics from pharmaceutical companies, and this needs to be balanced by impartial guidance from independent microbiologists and infectious diseases physicians (354). The results of educational programs aimed at improving use have varied, but they can be successful, especially when they are combined with audit of antibiotic use and feedback of results (365).

Numerous strategies have been proposed to improve antibiotic use in hospitals (351,353,354,366–368). A multidisciplinary group of experts in the U.S. was formed to develop strategies to prevent and control the emergence of antibiotic resistant microorganisms in hospitals (369). They proposed five strategic goals to optimize antimicrobial use, to optimize antimicrobial prophylaxis for surgery, to optimize choice and duration of empirical therapy, to improve prescribing by education, to monitor and feedback information on antimicrobial resistance rates, and to produce protocols for antibiotic usage.

Most authorities recommend the publication of a formulary that limits the agents available for prescription from the hospital pharmacy, and this may be supplemented by specific written antibiotic guidelines or a hospital antibiotic policy. Separate policies may be needed for specialized units such as intensive care or hematology/oncology. Since antibiotic policies imply some loss of individual clinical freedom for the benefit of the hospital as a whole, they should be overseen by a hospital committee consisting of senior physicians, surgeons, microbiologists, and pharmacists, and with the power to implement its decisions. The committee needs to meet regularly to revise and update the hospital policy, which will change with changing circumstances. To facilitate such revisions, the committee should receive regular audit reports of antibiotic use (and expenditure) in different clinical services as well as trends in antibiotic resistance in nosocomial pathogens.

Most hospital prescribing is done by junior staff members who have limited experience in antibiotic therapy. Antibiotic policies usually restrict the number of agents available from a given antibiotic class; this reduces confusion, allows staff members to gain expertise in a smaller number of drugs, helps preserve the effectiveness of newer agents, and reduces pharmacy costs. Older, cheaper, and well-established "first-line" antibiotics are unrestricted and can be prescribed by all staff members for simple infections. Prescriptions for the more expensive and powerful "second-line" or "reserve" drugs may require the countersignature of senior physicians, clinical justification to the pharmacy, or, as is often the case in North America, consultation with the infectious diseases service.

Another effective way to promote sensible antibiotic prescribing is by "intelligent" laboratory reporting facilitated by pathology computer systems. First, the laboratory should test a limited number of appropriate antibiotics for each significant isolate. Second, only a few of the agents tested should be reported, if the microorganism is reasonably sensitive, beginning with the recommended first-line agents. Third, if the microorganism is unusually resistant, or if the isolate is likely to be clinically insignificant, a "please consult" message should be given on the report form in place of the microorganism sensitivities; this will reduce the temptation to treat isolates rather than infections and encourage consultation on the use of second- and third-line agents.

Even when an antibiotic prescription is justified, therapy may be unnecessarily prolonged. One way to reduce the length of treatment is to implement "stop" policies in which the pharmacy automatically cancels an antibiotic prescription after 3 to 5 days unless it is specifically renewed by the ward physician. A large proportion of antibiotic use and misuse is for prophylaxis, and it is especially important to have clear policies in this area. The hospital antibiotic committee should review the scientific literature in each area of prophylaxis and issue guidelines for the choice of agent and the timing of administration. For most surgical prophylaxis, the antibiotic should be given just before surgery and continue for no more than 24 hours. Limitation of prophylaxis in this way will greatly reduce the pressure on antibiotic resistance as well as produce considerable cost savings.

There is evidence in the literature that formal policies of rotation—or complete withdrawal—of certain antibiotics were useful in the past for dealing with the emergence of multiresistant microorganisms (370–372). Such policies usually were applied to problems of resistance in gram-negative bacteria at a time when relatively few effective agents were available. Nowadays, several antibiotic groups are active against gram-negative microorganisms, and such policies are not often required. Nevertheless, in some areas where gentamicin resistance in Enterobacteriaceae and pseudomonads has been a problem, but where microorganisms have remained susceptible to amikacin, hospitals have adopted a policy of exclusive use of amikacin (373–375). In these centers, this policy has resulted in a decrease in gentamicin resistance without a concomitant increase in amikacin resistance. However, most hospitals now find multiply resistant gram-positive bacteria to be the major problem in hospital infection. There may be a need in the future to rotate or restrict agents active against gram-positive bacteria in order to preserve the effectiveness of reserve drugs such as vancomycin.

Hospital antibiotic policies emphasize restriction and conservation, especially of newer and more expensive agents. Pharmaceutical representatives inevitably have rather different goals. Open communication between physicians and the pharmaceutical industry is mutually beneficial and should be encouraged, but this should be monitored to ensure that commercial activity does not conflict with the established hospital antibiotic policy (354).

Experience with antibiotic policies has shown that attempts to enforce restriction on antibiotic use will only ever have limited success. Rather, it is education that is the keystone of an effective antibiotic policy (356,361). "Knowing when not to use an antibiotic is as important as knowing which antibiotic to choose" (366).

Control of Hospital Infection

After the reduction of unnecessary antibiotic use, the control of resistant bacteria in hospitals depends on the implementation of rational programs of infection control. As hospital pathogens become increasingly antibiotic-resistant, prevention of infection and spread assumes ever-greater importance. Infection control programs are the same for both sensitive and resistant bacteria and are dealt with in detail elsewhere in this book. However, several areas are of particular importance for the control of resistant microorganisms and are emphasized here.

The U.S. consensus group that drew up five strategic goals for optimizing antimicrobial use referred to previously also proposed five strategic goals to detect, report, and prevent transmission of antibiotic resistant microorganisms in hospitals (369): to develop systems to recognize and report trends in resistance within hospitals; to develop systems to rapidly detect, report, and act on the presence of resistant microorganisms in individual patients; to improve compliance with basic infection control procedures and policies; to incorporate the detection, prevention, and control of antimicrobial resistance into institutional strategic goals; and to develop plans for identifying, transferring, discharging, and readmitting patients colonized with resistant microorganisms.

Patients who have infection or asymptomatic colonization with antibiotic-resistant bacteria should be carefully assessed and isolated if necessary, and staff should pay strict attention to hand washing. Urinary catheterization is associated with considerable risk of cross-infection with resistant microorganisms, and staff members should follow hospital policies for urinary catheter care. Similarly, policies for the insertion, management, and removal of vascular catheters should be followed to reduce infection with resistant skin bacteria.

As described previously, gram-negative opportunistic pathogens are often inherently antibiotic- and disinfectant-resistant and may survive and proliferate in nutritionally poor environments. Thus, they contaminate diluted disinfectants and medications and wet environmental sites such as ventilator, humidifiers, water systems, sinks, and drains. Programs should be instituted to ensure clean and safe disinfectants (376); reliable methods to decontaminate hospital equipment and environmental sites should be established; and single-use or individual medications, creams, jellies, and ointments should be employed.

The value of surveillance or screening cultures is debated. Most authorities believe that routine environmental cultures are unnecessary and that environmental screening should be done only during searches for the source of an outbreak, and then only under the supervision of the infection control staff. It should be remembered that infected or colonized patients are often the sources of environmental contamination and that random sampling may reveal resistant environmental microorganisms that have no clinical significance. Screening of patients, and sometimes of staff members, is more useful. During an outbreak, many patients and staff members may become asymptomatic carriers of resistant microorganisms—for example, with MRSA or multiply resistant *Klebsiella.* Control of such epidemics requires that colonized patients and staff members be isolated (or removed from work) until cleared of carriage. Under these circumstances, screens should be repeated until all carriers have been eliminated and the outbreak has been controlled. Surveillance screening in the absence of an outbreak is more contentious (377). It is well recognized that patients and staff members from other hospitals known or suspected of being affected by epidemic-resistant pathogens with high epidemic potential such as MRSA should be screened for carriage before being allowed in general ward areas. When patients are admitted from other hospitals to high-risk areas such as oncology or intensive care units, they should also be screened for stool carriage of multiply resistant, gram-negative bacteria. Some specialized wards such as neonatal or bone marrow transplantation units, especially those that have recurrent problems with multiply resistant pathogens, might wish to screen patients (nasopharynx, moist skin sites, rectum, and vagina) at weekly intervals. This should be done only after discussion with the infection control team, and the specific pathogens being sought should be carefully defined (377).

SELECTIVE DECONTAMINATION OF THE DIGESTIVE TRACT

In intensive care patients, the most common site of infection is the lower respiratory tract, common pathogens are multiresistant aerobic gram-negative bacilli, and the most common source is the patient's own oropharynx colonized by microorganisms from the hospital environment. Some colonization may be due to endogenous multiresistant microorganisms brought in by the patient from the community and then encouraged to proliferate by hospital antibiotic pressure (61,107,144,378). This type of infection carries a high mortality rate in compromised patients, and attempts have been made to reduce its incidence by selective decontamination of the digestive tract (SDD). In this procedure, intravenous and topical antibiotics are used in high-risk patients (especially ventilated patients on ICUs) to prevent colonization of the oropharynx and gut by potentially pathogenic bacteria and yeasts. SDD regimes are designed to kill aerobic gram-negative bacteria and (often) fungi while preserving the normal anaerobic flora.

Most SDD regimes are successful in reducing oropharyngeal colonization with aerobic gram-negative bacteria and encouraging their replacement with gram-positive aerobes (379,380). Because of this, gram-negative infections may be replaced by gram-positive ones, including infection with multiply resistant strains (381–383), and some authorities now recommend the addition of vancomycin to standard regimes (382). Some studies and meta-analyses of SDD have shown a reduction in the rates of respiratory tract infection and mortality (384) but some double-blind trials have indicated no obvious benefit (385). Unfortunately, many different SDD regimes are used, and many studies of their effectiveness have been poorly designed. The value of the new vancomycin regimes needs to be properly assessed by controlled trials, and the danger that the widespread use of SDD antibiotics might encourage, rather than prevent, the emergence of resistant bacteria in ICUs needs further study.

The case for routine SDD to prevent multiresistant gram-negative infections in high-risk patients has not yet been proven. SDD may turn out to be more useful for controlling established outbreaks of resistant bacteria (386,387).

CONCLUSION

Antimicrobial resistance, often multiple, has spared few nosocomial pathogens, and despite overreporting, is increasing inexorably. Some have suggested that the emergence of essentially untreatable nosocomial pathogens, such as multiresistant gram-negative bacilli and VRE, signifies a crisis for antimicrobial therapy and heralds the end of the antibiotic era (1,47,388). One lesson that should have been learned is that increasing antimicrobial use is associated with increasing antimicrobial resistance. The management and control of resistant infections in hospitals will depend more on the control of hospital infection and of unnecessary antimicrobial therapy than on the availability of yet more powerful antibiotics.

REFERENCES

1. Cohen ML. Epidemiology of drug resistance: implications for a post-antimicrobial era. *Science* 1992;257:1050–1055.
2. Maré IJ. Incidence of R factors among gram negative bacteria in drug-free human and animal communities. *Nature* 1968;220:1046–1047.
3. Gardner P, Smith DH, Beer H, et al. Recovery of resistance (R) factors from a drug-free community. *Lancet* 1969;2:774–776.
4. Datta N. Drug resistance and R factors in the bowel bacteria of London patients before and after hospital admission. *Br Med J* 1969;2: 407–411.
5. Linton KB, Richmond MH, Bevan R, et al. Antibiotic resistance and

R factors in coliform bacilli isolated from hospital and domestic sewage. *J Med Microbiol* 1974;7:91–103.
6. French GL, Ling JML. Influence of a new hospital on antibiotic resistance in sewage bacteria in Hong Kong. In: Ishigami J, ed. *Recent advances in chemotherapy (Proceedings of the 14th International Congress in Chemotherapy, Kyoto).* Tokyo: University of Tokyo Press, 1985: 397–398.
7. National Committee for Clinical Laboratory Standards. *Analysis and presentation of cumulative antimicrobial susceptibility test data—proposed guideline M39-P.* Wayne, PA: NCCLS, 2000;16SS:19–24.
8. Shannon KP, French GL. Validation of the NCCLS proposal to use results only from the first isolate of a species per patient in the calculation of susceptibility frequencies. *J Antimicrob Chemother* 2002;50(6): 965–969.
9. Shannon KP, French GL. Antibiotic resistance: effect of different criteria for classifying isolates as duplicates on apparent resistance frequencies. *J Antimicrob Chemother* 2002;49(1):201–204.
10. Fridkin SK, Edwards JR, Tenover FC, et al. Intensive Care Antimicrobial Resistance Epidemiology (ICARE) Project. National Nosocomial Infections Surveillance (NNIS) System Hospitals. Antimicrobial resistance prevalence rates in hospital antibiograms reflect prevalence rates among pathogens associated with hospital-acquired infections. *Clin Infect Dis* 2001;33(3):324–330.
11. Archibald L, Phillips L, Monnet D, et al. Antimicrobial resistance in isolates from inpatients and outpatients in the United States: increasing importance of the intensive care unit. *Clin Infect Dis* 1997;24(2): 211–215.
12. Vincent JL, Bihari DJ, Suter PM, et al. The prevalence of nosocomial infection in intensive care units in Europe. Results of the European Prevalence of Infection in Intensive Care (EPIC) Study. EPIC International Advisory Committee. *JAMA* 1995;274(8):639–644.
13. National Nosocomial Infections Surveillance. System Report, Data Summary from January 1990–May 1999, Issued June 1999. *Am J Infect Control* 1999;27:520–532.
14. van Belkum A, Struelens M, de Visser A, et al. Role of genomic typing in taxonomy, evolutionary genetics, and microbial epidemiology. *Clin Microbiol Rev* 2001;14(3):547–560.
15. van Belkum A. High-throughput epidemiologic typing in clinical microbiology. *Clin Microbiol Infect* 2003;9(2):86–100.
16. Tenover FC, Lancaster MV, Hill BC, et al. Characterization of staphylococci with reduced susceptibility to vancomycin and other glycopeptides. *Antimicrob Agents Chemother* 1998;36:1020–1027.
17. Stefani S, Agodi A. Molecular epidemiology of antibiotic resistance. *Int J Antimicrob Agents* 2000;13(3):143–153.
18. McGowan JE. Antimicrobial resistance in hospital organisms and its relation to antibiotic use. *Rev Infect Dis* 1983;5:1033–1048.
19. Phillips I, Eykyn S, Laker M. Outbreak of hospital infection caused by contaminated autoclaved fluids. *Lancet* 1972;1:1258–1260.
20. Black HJ, Holt EJ, Kitson K, et al. Contaminated hospital water supplies. *Br Med J* 1979;1:1564–1565.
21. Newsom SWB. Hospital infection from contaminated ice. *Lancet* 1968;2:620–622.
22. Abrutyn E, Goodhart GL, Roos K, et al. *Acinetobacter calcoaceticus* outbreak associated with peritoneal dialysis. *Am J Epidemiol* 1978; 107:328–335.
23. Casewell MW, Slater NGP, Cooper JE. Operating theatre waterbaths as a cause of Pseudomonas septicaemia. *J Hosp Infect* 1981; 2: 237–240.
24. Muyldermans et al. 1998.
25. Ayliffe GAJ, Babb JR, Collins BJ, et al. *Pseudomonas aeruginosa* in hospital sinks. *Lancet* 1974;2:578–581.
26. Perryman FA, Flournoy DJ. Prevalence of gentamicin- and amikacin-resistant bacteria in sink drains. *J Clin Microbiol* 1980;12:79–83.
27. Levin MH, Olson B, Nathan C, et al. Pseudomonas in the sinks in an intensive care unit: relation to patients. *J Clin Pathol* 1984;37: 424–427.
28. Murray AE, Bartzokas CA, Shepherd AJ, et al. Blood transfusion-associated *Pseudomonas fluorescens* septicaemia: is this an increasing problem? *J Hosp Infect* 1987;9:243–248.
29. Stiles GM, Singh L, Imazaki G, et al. Thermodilution cardiac output studies as a cause of prosthetic valve bacterial endocarditis. *J Thorac Cardiovasc Surg* 1984;88:1035–1037.
30. Alvarado CJ, Stolz SM, Maki DG. Nosocomial infections from contaminated endoscopes: a flawed automated endoscope washer. An investigation using molecular epidemiology. *Am J Med* 1991;91: 272S–280S.
31. Schelenz S, French G. An outbreak of multidrug-resistant Pseudomonas aeruginosa infection associated with contamination of bronchoscopes and an endoscope washer-disinfector. *J Hosp Infect* 2000;46: 23–30.
32. Maki DG, Martin WT. Nationwide epidemic of septicaemia caused by contaminated infusion products. IV. Growth of microbial pathogens in fluids for intravenous infusion. *J Infect Dis* 1975;131: 267–272.
33. Maki DG, Rhame FS, Mackel DC, et al. Nationwide epidemic of septicaemia caused by contaminated intravenous products. I. Epidemiologic and clinical features. *Am J Med* 1976;60:471–485.
34. Gaston MA. *Enterobacter*: an emerging nosocomial pathogen. *J Hosp Infect* 1988;11:197–208.
35. Phillips I, Eykyn S, Curtis MA, et al. *Pseudomonas cepacia* (*multovorans*) septicaemia in an intensive care unit. *Lancet* 1971;1:375–377.
36. Mermel LA, Maki DG. Epidemic bloodstream infections from hemodynamic pressure monitoring: signs of the times. *Infect Control Hosp Epidemiol* 1989;10:47–53.
37. Hoffman PN. The significance of bacterial contamination of fibreoptic endoscopes. *J Hosp Infect* 1981;2:392–394.
38. Donowitz LG, Marsik FJ, Fisher KA, et al. Contaminated breast milk: a source of *Klebsiella* bacteremia in a newborn intensive care unit. *Rev Infect Dis* 1981;3:716–720.
39. Gransden WR, Webster M, French GL, et al. An outbreak of *Serratia marscescens* transmitted by contaminated breast pumps in a special care baby unit. *J Hosp Infect* 1986;7:149–154.
40. Casewell MW, Cooper JE, Webster M. Enteral feeds contaminated with *Enterobacter* cloacae as a cause of septicaemia. *Br Med J* 1981; 282:973.
41. Simmons NA. Hazards of naso-enteric feeds. *J Hosp Infect* 1981;2: 276–278.
42. Cookson B, Phillips I. Methicillin-resistant staphylococci. *J Appl Bacteriol* 1990;(Symposium suppl):55S–70S.
43. Leelaporn A, Paulsen IT, Tennent JM, et al. Multidrug resistance to antiseptics and disinfectants in coagulase-negative staphylococci. *J Med Microbiol* 1994;40:214–220.
44. McGowan JE. Environmental factors in nosocomial infection—a selective focus. *Rev Infect Dis* 1981;3:760–769.
45. Maki DG, Alvarado CJ, Hassemer CA, et al. Relation of the inanimate hospital environment to endemic nosocomial infection. *N Engl J Med* 1982;307:1562–1566.
46. Jacoby GA, Archer GL. New mechanisms of bacterial resistance to antimicrobial agents. *N Engl J Med* 1991;324:601–612.
47. Neu HC. The crisis in antibiotic resistance. *Science* 1992;257: 1064–1072.
48. Rice LB. Association of different mobile elements to generate novel integrative elements. *Cell Mol Life Sci* 2002;59:2023–2032.
49. Leverstein-van Hall MA, Blok MHE, Donders TAR, et al. Multidrug resistance among Enterobacteriaceae is strongly associated with the presence of integrons and is independent of species and isolate origin. *J Infect Dis* 2003;187:251–259.
50. Leverstein-van Hall MA, Paauw A, Box ATA, et al. Presence of integron-associated resistance in the community is widespread and contributes to multidrug resistance in the hospital. *J Clin Microbiol* 2002; 40(8):3038–3040.
51. Canton R, Coque TM, Baquero F. Multiresistant Gram-negative bacilli: from epidemics to endemics. *Curr Opinion Infect Dis* 2003;164; 315–325.
52. O'Brien TF, Ross DG, Guzman MA, et al. Dissemination of an antibiotic resistance plasmid in hospital patient flora. *Antimicrob Agents Chemother* 1980;17:537–542.
53. Markowitz SM, Veazly JM, Macrina FL, et al. Sequential outbreaks of infection due to *Klebsiella pneumoniae* in a neonatal intensive care

unit: implication of a conjugative R plasmid. *J Infect Dis* 1980;142: 106–112.
54. Knight S, Casewell M. The dissemination of resistance plasmids among gentamicin-resistant enterobacteria from hospital patients. *Br Med J* 1981;283:755–756.
55. Thomas FEJ, Jackson RT, Melly A, et al. Sequential hospital-wide outbreaks of resistant *Serratia* and *Klebsiella* infections. *Arch Intern Med* 1977;137:581–584.
56. Tompkins et al. 1980.
57. Casewell MW, Talsania HG, Knight S. Gentamicin-resistant *Klebsiella aerogenes* as a clinically significant source of transferable antibiotic resistance. *J Antimicrob Chemother* 1981;8:153–160.
58. Mayer KH, Hopkins JD, Gilleece ES, et al. Molecular evolution, species distribution, and clinical consequences of an endemic aminoglycoside resistance plasmid. *Antimicrob Agents Chemother* 1986;29: 628–633.
59. Gould JC. *Pseudomonas pyocyanea*. In: Williams REO, Shooter RA, eds. *Infection in hospitals, epidemiology and control.* Oxford: Blackwell Scientific, 1963:119–130.
60. Ayliffe GAJ. Use of antibiotics and resistance. In: Geddes AM, Williams JD, eds. *Current antibiotic therapy.* Edinburgh: Churchill Livingstone, 1976:53–60.
61. Weinstein RA. Endemic emergence of cephalosporin-resistant *Enterobacter*: relation to prior therapy. *Infect Control Hosp Epidemiol* 1986; 7(suppl):120–123.
62. Kernodle DS, Barg NL, Kaiser AB. Low-level colonization of hospitalized patients with methicillin-resistant coagulase-negative staphylococci and emergence of the organisms during surgical antimicrobial prophylaxis. *Antimicrob Agents Chemother* 1988;32:202–208.
63. Finland M, Jones WF, Barnes MW. Occurrence of serious bacterial infections since introduction of antibacterial agents. *JAMA* 1959;170: 2188–2197.
64. Phillips et al. 1974.
65. Morrison AJ, Wenzel RP. Epidemiology of infections due to *Pseudomonas aeruginosa. Rev Infect Dis* 1984;6(suppl 3):S627–S642.
66. Shanson DC. Antibiotic resistance in *Staphylococcus aureus*. In: Cafferkey MT, ed. *Methicillin-resistant Staphylococcus aureus.* New York: Marcel Dekker, 1992:11–20.
67. Shanson DC. Antibiotic resistance in *Staphylococcus aureus. J Hosp Infect* 1981;2:11–36.
68. McGowan JE. Gram-positive bacteria: spread and antimicrobial resistance in university and community hospitals in the USA. *J Antimicrob Chemother* 1988;21(suppl C):49–55.
69. Haley RW, Hightower AW, Khabbaz RF, et al. The emergence of methicillin-resistant *Staphylococcus aureus* infections in United States hospitals. *Ann Intern Med* 1982;97:297–308.
70. Keane CT, Cafferkey MT. Re-emergence of methicillin-resistant *Staphylococcus aureus* causing severe infection. *J Infect* 1984;9:6–16.
71. Eykyn S, Gransden WR, Phillips I. The causative organisms of septicaemia and their epidemiology. *J Antimicrob Chemother* 1990; 25(suppl C):41–58.
72. Christensen GD, Bisno AL, Parisi JT, et al. Nosocomial septicaemia due to multiply antibiotic-resistant *Staphylococcus epidermidis. Ann Intern Med* 1982;96:1–10.
73. Peters G, Locci R, Pulverer G. Adherence and growth of coagulase-negative staphylococci on surfaces of intravenous catheters. *J Infect Dis* 1982;146:479–482.
74. Peters G. New considerations in the pathogenesis of coagulase-negative staphylococcal foreign body infections. *J Antimicrob Chemother* 1988;21(suppl C):139–148.
75. Terpenning MS, Zervos MJ, Schaberg DR, et al. Enterococcal infections: an increasing problem in hospitalized patients. *Infect Control Hosp Epidemiol* 1988;9:457–461.
76. NNIS 1996.
77. NNIS 1997.
78. Phillips I, King A, Gransden WR, et al. The antibiotic sensitivity of bacteria isolated from the blood of patients in St Thomas's Hospital, 1969–1988. *J Antimicrob Chemother* 1990;25(suppl C):59–80.
79. Wiedemann B, Kliebe C, Kresken M. The epidemiology of β-lactamases. *J Antimicrob Chemother* 1989;24(suppl B):1–22.
80. Wu PJ, Shannon K, Phillips I. β-Lactamases and susceptibility to b-lactam antibiotics in *Escherichia coli. J Antimicrob Chemother* 1992; 30:868–871.
81. Stapleton P, Wu P-J, King A, et al. Incidence and mechanisms of resistance to the combination of amoxicillin and clavulanic acid in *Escherichia coli. Antimicrob Agents Chemother* 1995;39:2478–2483.
82. Datta N, Kontomichalou P. Penicillinase synthesis controlled by infectious R factors in *Enterobacteriaceae. Nature* 1965;208:239–241.
83. Shannon K, Williams H, King A, et al. Hyperproduction of TEM-1 beta-lactamase in clinical isolates of *Escherichia coli* serotype O15. *FEMS Microbiol Lett* 1990;67:319–324.
84. Wu PJ, Shannon K, Phillips, I. Effect of hyperproduction of TEM-1 β-lactamase on in vitro susceptibility of *Escherichia coli* to β-lactam antibiotics. *Antimicrob Agents Chemother* 1994;38:494–498.
85. Philippon A, Labia R, Jacoby G. Extended-spectrum β-lactamases. *Antimicrob Agents Chemother* 1989;33:1131–1136.
86. Schmitz FJ, Verhoef L, Fluit A. Geographical distribution of quinolone resistance among *Staphylococcus aureus, Escherichia coli* and *Klebsiella* spp. Isolates from 20 European University Hospitals. *J Antimicrob Chemother* 1999;43:431–434.
87. European Antimicrobial Resistance Surveillance System. Annual Report, 2001.
88. Fridkin SK, Hill HA, Volkova NV, et al., and the Intensive Care Antimicrobial Resistance Epidemiology (ICARE) Project Hospitals. Temporal changes in prevalence of antimicrobial resistance in 23 U.S. hospitals. *Emerg Infect Dis* 2002;8:697–701.
89. Hart CA, Gibson MF, Buckles AM. Variation in skin and environmental survival of hospital gentamicin-resistant *Enterobacteria*. *J Hyg* 1981;87:277–285.
90. Tullus K, Hörlin K, Svenson SB, et al. Epidemic outbreaks of acute pyelonephritis caused by nosocomial spread of P fimbriated *Escherichia coli* in children. *J Infect Dis* 1984;150:728–736.
91. Olesen B, Kolmos HJ, Orskov F, et al. Epidemic multiresistant *Escherichia coli* O78:H10 in Denmark. Abstract 963. 6th European Congress of Clinical Microbiology and Infectious Diseases, Seville, March 28–31, 1993.
92. Mayer KH. Review of epidemic aminoglycoside resistance worldwide. *Am J Med* 1986;80:56–64.
93. Mayer KH. The epidemiology of antibiotic resistance in hospitals. *J Antimicrob Chemother* 1986;18(suppl C):223–233.
94. Sanders CC, Sanders WC. Beta-Lactam resistance in gram-negative bacteria: global trends and clinical impact. *Clin Infect Dis* 1992;15: 824–839.
95. Sanders CC, Sanders WC. Microbial resistance to newer generation β-lactam antibiotics: clinical and laboratory implications. *J Infect Dis* 1985;151:399–406.
96. Leung M, Shannon K, French G. Rarity of transferable β-lactamase production by *Klebsiella* species. J Antimicrob Chemother 1997.
97. Cooke EM, Brayson JC, Aedmonson AS, et al. An investigation into the incidence and source of *Klebsiella* infections in hospital patients. *J Hyg* 1979;82:473–480.
98. Cooke EM, Pool R, Brayson JC, et al. Further studies on the sources of *Klebsiella* aerogenes in hospital patients. *J Hyg* 1979;83:391–395.
99. Seldon R, Lees, Wang WLL, et al. Nosocomial *Klebsiella* infections: intestinal colonization as a reservoir. *Ann Intern Med* 1971;74: 657–664.
100. Casewell MW, Dalton MT, Webster M, et al. Gentamicin-resistant *Klebsiella aerogenes* in a urological ward. *Lancet* 1977;2:444–446.
101. Casewell MW, Phillips I. Hands as route of transmission for *Klebsiella* species. *Br Med J* 1977;2:1315–1317.
102. Noreiga ER, Leibowitz RE, Richmond AS, et al. Nosocomial infection caused by gentamicin-resistant streptomycin-sensitive Klebsiella. *J Infect Dis* 1975;131(suppl):S45–S50.
103. Rennie RP, Duncan IBR. Emergence of gentamicin-resistant *Klebsiella* in a general hospital. *Antimicrob Agents Chemother* 1977;11: 179–184.
104. Forbes I, Gray A, Hurse A, et al. The emergence of gentamicin-resistant *Klebsiellae* in a large general hospital. *Med J Aust* 1977;1: 14–16.
105. Curie K, Speller DCE, Simpson RA, et al. A hospital epidemic caused

by a gentamicin-resistant *Klebsiella aerogenes*. *J Hyg* 1978;80: 115–123.

106. Gerding DN, Buxton AE, Hughes RA, et al. Nosocomial multiply resistant *Klebsiella pneumoniae*: epidemiology of an outbreak of apparent index case origin. *Antimicrob Agents Chemother* 1979;15:608–615.
107. Weinstein RA, Nathan C, Gruensfelder R, et al. Endemic aminoglycoside resistance in Gram-negative bacilli: epidemiology and mechanisms. *J Infect Dis* 1974;141:338–345.
108. Shah P, Stille W. *E. coli* and *K. pneumoniae* strains more susceptible to cefoxitin than to third-generation cephalosporins. *J Antimicrob Chemother* 1983;11:597–598.
109. Knothe H, Shah P, Krcmeryery V, et al. Transferrable resistance to cefotaxime, cefoxitin, cefamandole and cefuroxime in clinical isolates of *Klebsiella pneumoniae* and *Serratia marcescens*. *Infection* 1983;11: 315–317.
110. Sirot D, Sirot J, Labia R, et al. Transferrable resistance to third-generation cephalosporins in clinical isolates of *Klebsiella pneumoniae*: identification of CTX-1, a novel β-lactamase. *J Antimicrob Chemother* 1987;20:323–334.
111. Shannon K, Stapleton P, Xiaoqin X, et al. Extended-spectrum β-lactamase-producing *Klebsiella pneumoniae* strains causing nosocomial outbreaks of infection in the United Kingdom. *J Clin Microbiol* 1998; 36:3105–3110.
112. Fernandez-Rodriguez A, Canton R, Perez-Diaz JC, et al. Aminoglycoside-modifying enzymes in clinical isolates harboring extended-spectrum β-lactamases. *Antimicrob Agents Chemother* 1992;36: 2563–2538.
113. French GL, Shannon KP, Simmons N. Hospital outbreak of *Klebsiella pneumoniae* resistant to broad-spectrum cephalosporins and β-lactam-β-lactamase inhibitor combinations by hyperproduction of SHV-5 β-lactamase. *J Clin Microbiol* 1996;34:358–363.
114. Xiaoqin Xiang, Shannon K, French G. Mechanism and stability of hyperproduction of the extended-spectrum beta-lactamase SHV-5 in *Klebsiella pneumoniae. Antimicrob Agents Chemother* 1997.
115. Sader HS, Pfaller MA, Jones RN. Prevalence of important pathogens and the antimicrobial activity of parenteral drugs at numerous medical centers in the United States. II study of the intra- and interlaboratory dissemination of extended-spectrum β-lactamase-producing *Enterobacteriaceae. Diag Microbiol Infect Dis* 1994;20:203–208.
116. Brun-Buisson C, Legrand P, Phillipon A, et al. Transferrable enzymatic resistance to third-generation cephalosporins during nosocomial outbreak of multiresistant *Klebsiella pneumoniae. Lancet* 1987;2: 302–306.
117. Arlet G, Sanson-le Pors MJ, Rouveau M, et al. Outbreak of nosocomial infections due to *Klebsiella pneumoniae* producing SHV-4 beta-lactamase. *Eur J Clin Microbiol Infect Dis* 1990;9:797–803.
118. De Champs C, Rouby D, Guelon D, et al. A case-control study of an outbreak of infections caused by *Klebsiella pneumoniae* strains producing CTX-1 (TEM-3) beta-lactamase. *J Hosp Infect* 1991;18: 5–13.
119. Johnson AP, Weinbren MJ, Ayling-Smith B, et al. Outbreak of infection in two UK hospitals caused by a strain of *Klebsiella pneumoniae* resistant to cefotaxime and ceftazidime. *J Hosp Infect* 1992;20: 97–103.
120. Naumovski L, Quinn JP, Miyashiro D, et al. Outbreak of ceftazidime resistance due to a novel extended-spectrum beta-lactamase in isolates from cancer patients. *Antimicrob Agents Chemother* 1992;36: 1991–1996.
121. Bauernfeind A, Rosenthal E, Eberlein E, et al. Spread of *Klebsiella pneumoniae* producing SHV-5 beta-lactamase among hospitalized patients. *Infection* 1993;21:18–22.
122. Meyer KS, Urban C, Eagan JA, et al. Nosocomial outbreak of *Klebsiella* infection resistant to late generation cephalosporins. *Ann Intern Med* 1993;119:353–358.
123. Marchese A, Arlet G, Schito GC, et al. Detection of SHV-5 extended-spectrum beta-lactamase in *Klebsiella pneumoniae* strains isolated in Italy. *Eur J Clin Microbiol Infect Dis* 1996;15:245–248.
124. Hobson RP, MacKenzie FM, Gould IM. An outbreak of multiply-resistant *Klebsiella pneumoniae* in the Grampian region of Scotland. *J Hosp Infect* 1996;33:249–262.
125. Shannon K, Fung K, Anthony R, et al. A hospital outbreak of extended-spectrum β-lactamase-producing *Klebsiella pneumoniae* investigated by RAPD typing and analysis of the genetics and mechanisms of resistance. *J Hosp Infect* 1998;39:291–300.
126. Macrae MB, Shannon KP, Rayner DM, et al. A simultaneous outbreak on a neonatal unit of two strains of multiply antibiotic resistant *Klebsiella pneumoniae* controllable only by ward closure. *J Hosp Infect* 2001;49:183–192.
127. Legakis NJ, Tzouvelekis LS, Hatzoudis G, et al. *Klebsiella pneumoniae* infections in Greek hospitals. Dissemination of plasmids encoding an SHV-5 type β-lactamase. *J Hosp Infect* 1995;31:177–187.
128. Yuan M, Aucken H, Hall LM, et al. Epidemiological typing of klebsiellae with extended-spectrum beta-lactamases from European intensive care units. *J Antimicrob Chemother* 1998;41:527–539.
129. Jain K, Radsak K, Mannheim W. Differentiation of the Oxytocum group from *Klebsiella* by deoxyribonucleic acid–deoxyribonucleic acid hybridisation. *Int J Syst Bacteriol* 1974;24:402.
130. Morgan ME, Hart CA, Cooke RW. *Klebsiella* infection in a neonatal intensive care unit: role of bacteriological surveillance. *J Hosp Infect* 1984;5:377–385.
131. Alverez S, Stinnett JA, Shell CG, et al. *Klebsiella oxytoca* isolates in a general hospital. *Infect Control* 1985;6:310–313.
132. Payne DJ, Marriott MS, Amyes SG. Mutants of the TEM-1 beta-lactamase conferring resistance to ceftazidime. *J Antimicrob Chemother* 1989;24:103–110.
133. Chow JW, Fine MJ, Shlaes DM, et al. *Enterobacter* bacteremia: clinical features and emergence of antibiotic resistance during therapy. *Ann Intern Med* 1991;115:585–590.
134. Livermore DM. Clinical significance of β-lactamase induction and stable derepression in gram-negative rods. *Eur J Clin Microbiol* 1987; 6:439–445.
135. Lodge JM, Piddock LJV. The control of class I β-lactamase expression in *Enterobacteriaceae* and *Pseudomonas aeruginosa. J Antimicrob Chemother* 1991;28:167–172.
136. Phillips I, Shannon K. The emergence of resistance and the therapy of septicaemia. *Chemiotherapia* 1985;4:90–94.
137. Editorial. The importance of *Serratia marscescens. Lancet* 1977;1: 636–637.
138. Bouza E, Garcia de la Torre M, Erice A, et al. *Serratia* bacteremia. *Diagn Microbiol Infect Dis* 1987;7:237–247.
139. Watanakunakorn C. *Serratia* bacteremia: a review of 44 episodes. Scand *J Infect Dis* 1989;21:477–483.
140. Saito H, Elting L, Bodey GP, et al. *Serratia* bacteremia: review of 118 cases. *Rev Infect Dis* 1989;11:912–920.
141. Kusek et al. 1981.
142. Griffith SJ, Nathan C, Selander RK, et al. The epidemiology of *Pseudomonas aeruginosa* in oncology patients in a general hospital. *J Infect Dis* 1989;160:1030–1036.
143. Poh CL, Yeo CC. Recent advances in typing of *Pseudomonas aeruginosa. J Hosp Infect* 1993;24:175–181.
144. Noone MR, Pitt TL, Bedder M, et al. *Pseudomonas aeruginosa* colonization in an intensive therapy unit: role of cross infection and host factors. *Br Med J* 1983;286:341–344.
145. Olson B, Weinstein RA, Nathan C, et al. Epidemiology of *Pseudomonas aeruginosa*: why infection control efforts have failed. *J Infect Dis* 1984;150:808–816.
146. Olson B, Weinstein RA, Nathan C, et al. Occult aminoglycoside resistance in *Pseudomonas aeruginosa*: epidemiology and implications for therapy and control. *J Infect Dis* 1985;152:769–774.
147. Roe E, Jones RJ, Lowbury EJL. Transfer of antibiotic resistance between *Pseudomonas aeruginosa, Escherichia coli,* and other Gram-negative bacilli in burns. *Lancet* 1971;1:149–152.
148. Maliwan N, Grieble HG, Bird TJ. Hospital *Pseudomonas aeruginosa*: surveillance of resistance of gentamicin and transfer of amino-glycoside R factor. *Antimicrob Agents Chemother* 1975;8:415–420.
149. Price et al. 1981.
150. Sabath LD. Biochemical and physiologic basis for susceptibility and resistance of *Pseudomonas aeruginosa* to antimicrobial agents. *Rev Infect Dis* 1984;6(suppl 3):S643–S656.
151. National Nosocomial Infections Surveillance. System Report, data

summary from January 1992 to June 2002, issued August 2002. *Am J Infect Control* 2002;30:458–475.

152. King A, Shannon K, Eykyn S, et al. Reduced sensitivity to β-lactam antibiotics arising during ceftazidime treatment of *Pseudomonas aeruginosa* infections. *J Antimicrob Chemother* 1983;12:363–370.
153. Quinn JP, Studemeister AE, DiVincenzo CA, et al. Resistance to imipenem in *Pseudomonas aeruginosa*: clinical experience and biochemical mechanisms. *Rev Infect Dis* 1988;10:892–898.
154. Gaynes RP, Culver DH. Resistance to imipenem among selected gram-negative bacilli in the United States. *Infect Control Epidemiol* 1992;13:10–14.
155. McManus AT, Mason AD, McManus WF, et al. Twenty-five year review of *Pseudomonas aeruginosa* bacteremia in a burn center. *Eur J Clin Microbiol* 1985;4:219–223.
156. Love LJ, Schimpff SC, Schiffer CA, et al. Improved prognosis for granulocytopenic patients with gram-negative bacteremia. *Am J Med* 1980;68:643–648.
157. DeJongh CA, Joshi JH, Newman KA, et al. Antibiotic synergism and response in gram-negative bacteremia in granulocytopenic cancer patients. *Am J Med* 1986;80(suppl 5C):96–100.
158. Hilf M, Yu VL, Sharp JA, et al. Antibiotic therapy for *Pseudomonas aeruginosa* bacteremia: outcome correlations in a prospective study of 200 patients. *Am J Med* 1989;87:540–546.
159. Morrison AJ, Hoffmann KK, Wenzel RP. Associated mortality and clinical characteristics of nosocomial Pseudomonas maltophilia in a university hospital. *J Clin Microbiol* 1986;24:52–55.
160. Muder RR, Yu VL, Dunner JS, et al. Infections caused by *Pseudomonas maltophilia.* Expanding clinical spectrum. *Arch Intern Med* 1987;147: 1672–1674.
161. Schoch PE, Cunha BA. *Pseudomonas maltophilia. Infect Control* 1987; 8:169–172.
162. Mett H, Rosta S, Schacher B, et al. Outer membrane permeability and β-lactamase content in *Pseudomonas maltophilia* clinical isolates and laboratory mutants. *Rev Infect Dis* 1988;10:765–769.
163. Martone WJ, Tablan OC, Jarvis WR. The epidemiology of nosocomial epidemic *Pseudomonas cepacia* infections. *Eur J Epidemiol* 1987; 3:222–232.
164. Goldmann DA, KLinger JD. *Pseudomonas cepacia*: biology, mechanisms of virulence, epidemiology. *J Pediatr* 1986;108:806–812.
165. Panllilio AL, Beck-Sague CM, Siegel JD, et al. Infections and pseudoinfections due to povidone-iodine solution contaminated with *Pseudomonas cepacia. Clin Infect Dis* 1992;14:1078–1083.
166. Burge DR, Nakielna EM, Noble MA. Case-control and vector studies of nosocomial acquisition of *Pseudomonas cepacia* in adult patients with cystic fibrosis. *Infect Control Hosp Epidemiol* 1993;14:127–130.
167. Aronoff SC. Outer membrane permeability in *Pseudomonas cepacia*: diminished porin content in a β-lactam–resistant mutant and in resistant cystic fibrosis isolates. *Antimicrob Agents Chemother* 1988;32: 1636–1639.
168. Tablan OC, Martone WJ, Jarvis WR. The epidemiology of *Pseudomonas cepacia* in patients with cystic fibrosis. *Eur J Epidemiol* 1987;3: 336–342.
169. Taylor RF, Gaya H, Hodson ME. *Pseudomonas cepacia*: pulmonary infection in patients with cystic fibrosis. *Respir Med* 1993;87: 187–192.
170. Govan JR, Brown PH, Maddison J, et al. Evidence of transmission of *Pseudomonas cepacia* by social contact in cystic fibrosis. *Lancet* 1993; 342:15–19.
171. Yabuuchi E, Kosako Y, Oyaizu H, et al. Proposal of *Burkholderia* gen nov. and transfer of seven species of the genus *Pseudomonas* homology group II to the new genus, with the type species *Burkholderia cepacia* (Pelleroni and Holmes 1981) comb. Nov. *Microbiol Immunol* 1992; 36:1251–1275.
172. Yabuuchi E, Kosako Y, Yano I, et al. Transfer of two *Burkholderia* and an *Alcaligenes* species to *Ralstonia* gen. Nov. *Microbiol Immunol* 1995;39:897–904.
173. Baird RM, Elhag KM, Shaw EJ. *Pseudomonas thomasii* in a hospital distilled-water supply. *J Med Microbiol* 1976;9:493–495.
174. Holmes B. Other non-fermentative gram-negative rods. In: Parker MT, Collier LH, eds. *Topley and Wilson's principles of bacteriology, virology and immunity,* 8th ed. London: Edward Arnold, 1990: 289–302.
175. Shigeta S, Yasunaga Y, Honzumi K, et al. Cerebral ventriculitis associated with *Achromobacter xylosoxidans. J Clin Pathol* 1978;31:156–161.
176. Schoch PE, Cunha BA. Topics in clinical microbiology: nosocomial *Achromobacter xylosoxidans* infections. *Infect Control Hosp Epidemiol* 1988;9:984–987.
177. Taplin D, Rebell G, Zaias N. The human skin as a source of Mima-Herellea infections. *JAMA* 1963;186:952–955.
178. Bergogne-Berezin E, Joly-Guillon ML, Vieu JF. Epidemiology of nosocomial infections due to *Acinetobacter calcoaceticus. J Hosp Infect* 1987;10:105–113.
179. Bouvet PJM, Grimont PAD. Taxonomy of the genus *Acinetobacter* with the recognition of *Acinetobacter baumannii* sp. nov., *Acinetobacter haemolyticus* sp. nov., *Acinetobacter johnsonii* sp. nov. and *Acinetobacter junii* sp. nov. and emended descriptions of *Acinetobacter calcoaceticus* and *Acinetobacter lwofi. Int J Syst Bacteriol* 1986;36:228–240.
180. Buxton AE, Anderson RL, Werdegar D, et al. Nosocomial respiratory tract infection and colonization with *Acinetobacter calcoaceticus.* Epidemiologic characteristics. *Am J Med* 1978;65:507–513.
181. French GL, Casewell MW, Roncoroni AJ, et al. A hospital outbreak of antibiotic-resistant *Acinetobacter anitratus*: epidemiology and control. *J Hosp Infect* 1980;1:125–131.
182. Getchell-White SI, Donowitz LG, Groschel DH. The inanimate environment of an intensive care unit as a potential source of nosocomial bacteria: evidence for long survival of *Acinetobacter calcoaceticus. Infect Control Hosp Epidemiol* 1989;10:402–407.
183. Wendt C, Dietze B, Dietz E, et al. Survival of Acinetobacter baumannii on dry surfaces. *J Clin Microbiol* 1997;35:1394–1397.
184. Jawad A, Seifert H, Snelling AM, et al. Survival of Acinetobacter baumannii on dry surfaces: comparison of outbreak and sporadic isolates. *J Clin Microbiol* 1998;36:1938–1941.
185. Allen KD. Green HT. Hospital outbreak of multi-resistant Acinetobacter anitratus: an airborne mode of spread? *J Hosp Infect* 1987;9: 110–119.
186. Catalano M, Quelle LS, Jeric PE, et al. Survival of Acinetobacter baumannii on bed rails during an outbreak and during sporadic cases. *J Hosp Infect* 1999;42:27–35.
187. Weernink A, Severin WP, Tjernberg I, et al. Pillows, an unexpected source of Acinetobacter. *J Hosp Infect* 1995;29:189–199.
188. Ramphal R, Kluge RM. *Acinetobacter calcoaceticus* variety *anitratus*: an increasing nosocomial problem. *Am J Med Sci* 1979;277:57–66.
189. Bergogne-Berezin E, Joly-Guillon ML. An underestimated nosocomial pathogen, *Acinetobacter calcoaceticus. J Antimicrob Chemother* 1985;16:535–538.
190. Rosenthal SL. *Acinetobacter*: new name in the microbial game. *Ann Intern Med* 1978; 88:123–124.
191. Soussy JC, Denoyer MC, Duval J, et al. Les bactèries rèsistantes à tout existent-elles? *Med Mal Infect* 1974;4:341–348.
192. Seifert H, Baginski R, Schulze A, et al. Antimicrobial susceptibility of *Acinetobacter* species. *Antimicrob Agents Chemother* 1993;37: 750–753.
193. Shalit I, Dan M, Gutman R, et al. Cross resistance to ciprofloxacin and other antimicrobial agents among clinical isolates of *Acinetobacter calcoaceticus* biovar *anitratus. Antimicrob Agents Chemother* 1990;34: 494–495.
194. Gehrlein M, Leying H, Cullmann W, et al. Imipenem resistance in *Acinetobacter baumannii* is due to altered penicillin-binding proteins. *Chemotherapy* 1991;37:405–412.
195. Vivian A, Hinchliffe E, Fewson CA. *Acinetobacter calcoaceticus*: some approaches to a problem. *J Hosp Infect* 1981;2:199–203.
196. Murray BE, Moellering RC. Evidence of plasmid-mediated production of aminoglycoside-modifying enzymes not previously described in *Acinetobacter. Antimicrob Agents Chemother* 1980;17:30–36.
197. Villa J, Marcos A, Marco F, et al. In vitro antimicrobial production of beta-lactamases, aminoglycoside-modifying enzymes, and chloramphenicol acetyltransferase by and susceptibility of clinical isolates of *Acinetobacter baumannii. Antimicrob Agents Chemother* 1993;37: 138–141.

198. North EA, Christie R. Acquired resistance of staphylococci to the action of penicillin. *Med J Aust* 1946;1:176–179.
199. Gransden WR, Atkinson D, Stead KC, et al. Antibiotic resistance of *Staphylococcus aureus* 1969–1981. *Proc 13th Intl Congr Chemother* 1983;8:74/36–39.
200. Rountree PM, Freeman BM. Infections caused by a particular phage type of *Staphylococcus aureus. Med J Aust* 1955;2:157–161.
201. Byynoe ET, Elder RH, Camptois RD. Phage typing and antibiotic resistance of staphylococci isolated in a general hospital. *Can J Microiol* 1956;2:246–358.
202. Williams REO. Epidemic staphylococci. *Lancet* 1958;1:190–195.
203. Parker MT, Jevons MP. Hospital strains of staphylococci. In: Williams REO, Shooter RA, eds. *Infection in hospitals, epidemiology and control.* Oxford: Blackwell Scientific, 1963:3–56.
204. Speller DCE, Raghanath D, Stephens M, et al. Epidemic infection by gentamicin resistant *Staphylococcus aureus* in three hospitals. *Lancet* 1976;1:464–466.
205. Bulger R, Sherris JC. Decreased incidence of antibiotic resistance among *Staphylococcus aureus*: a study in a university hospital over a nine year period. *Ann Intern Med* 1968;69:1099–1108.
206. Jepsen OB. The demise of the "old" methicillin-resistant *Staphylococcus aureus. J Hosp Infect* 1986;7(suppl A):13–17.
207. Ayliffe GAJ, Lilly HA, Lowbury EJL. Decline of the hospital staphylococcus? Incidence of multiresistant *Staph. aureus* in three Birmingham hospitals. *Lancet* 1979;2:538–541.
208. Jevons MP. Celbenin-resistant staphylococci. *Br Med J* 1961;1:124.
209. Brumfitt W, Hamilton-Miller J. Methicillin-resistant *Staphylococcus aureus. N Engl J Med* 1989;320:1188–1196.
210. Matthews PR, Stuart PR. Resistance heterogeneity in methicillin-resistant *Staphylococcus aureus. FEMS Microbiol Lett* 1984;22:161–166.
211. Hartman BJ, Tomasz A. Expression of methicillin resistance in heterogeneous strains of *Staphylococcus aureus. Antimicrob Agents Chemother* 1986;29:85–92.
212. French GL, Ling JL, Hui Y-W, et al. Determination of methicillin resistance in *Staphylococcus aureus* by agar dilution and disc diffusion methods. *J Antimicrob Chemother* 1987;20:599–608.
213. Oppenheim BA. Laboratory methods for the detection of methicillin-resistant *Staphylococcus aureus.* In: Cafferkey MT, ed. *Methicillin-Resistant Staphylococcus aureus.* New York: Marcel Dekker, 1992:57–75.
214. Brown DFJ, Reynolds PE. Intrinsic resistance to beta-lactam antibiotics in *Staphylococcus aureus. FEBS Lett* 1980;122:275–278.
215. Georgopapadakou NH, Smith SA, Bonner DP. Penicillin-binding proteins in a *Staphylococcus aureus* strain resistant to specific beta-lactam antibiotics. *Antimicrob Agents Chemother* 1982;22:172–175.
216. Hartman BJ, Tomasz A. Low-affinity penicillin-binding protein associated with beta-lactam resistance in *Staphylococcus aureus. J Bacteriol* 1984;158:513–516.
217. Chambers HF. Methicillin resistance in staphylococci: molecular and biochemical basis and clinical implications. *Clin Microbiol Rev* 1997; 10:781–791.
218. Ubukata K, Nonoguchi R, Song MD, et al. Homology of *mecA* gene in methicillin-resistant *Staphylococcus haemolyticus* and *Staphylococcus simulans* to that of *Staphylococcus aureus. Antimicrob Agents Chemother* 1990;34:170–172.
219. Hiramatsu K, Cui L, Kuroda M, et al. The emergence and evolution of methicillin-resistant Staphylococcus aureus. *Trends Microbiol* 2001; 9:486–493.
220. Enright MC, Robinson DA, Randle G, et al. The evolutionary history of methicillin-resistant Staphylococcus aureus (MRSA). *Proc Natl Acad Sci USA* 2002;99:7687–7692.
221. Isaacs RD, Kunke PJ, Cohen RL, et al. Ciprofloxacin resistance in epidemic methicillin-resistant *Staphylococcus aureus. Lancet* 1988;2: 843.
222. Schaefler S. Methicillin-resistant strains of *Staphylococcus aureus* resistant to quinolones. *J Clin Microbiol* 1989;27:335–336.
223. Anonymous. Epidemic methicillin-resistant *Staphylococcus aureus. Comm Dis Rep Weekly* 1995;5:165.
224. Sader HS, Pignatari AC, Hollis RJ, et al. Oxacillin- and quinolone-resistant *Staphylococcus aureus* in São Paulo, Brazil: a multicenter molecular epidemiology study. *Infect Control Hosp Epidemiol* 1993;14: 260–264.
225. French GL, Cheng AFB, Ling JML, et al. Hong Kong strains of methicillin-resistant and methicillin-sensitive *Staphylococcus aureus* have similar virulence. *J Hosp Infect* 1990;15:117–125.
226. Michel M, Gutmann L. Methicillin-resistant *Staphylococcus aureus* and vancomycin-resistant enterococci: therapeutic realities and possibilities. *Lancet* 1997;349:1901–1906.
227. May J, Shannon K, King A, et al. Glycopeptide tolerance in *Staphylococcus aureus. J Antimicrob Chemother* 1998;42:189–197.
228. Perry JD, Jones AL, Gould FK. Glycopeptide tolerance in bacteria causing endocarditis. *J Antimicrob Chemother* 1999;44:121–124.
229. Hiramatsu K, Aritaka N, Hanaki H, et al. Dissemination in Japanese hospitals of strains of *Staphylococcus aureus* heterogeneously resistant to vancomycin. *Lancet* 1997;350:1670–1673.
230. CDC (Centers for Disease Prevention and Control). *Staphylococcus aureus* with reduced susceptibility to vancomycin—United States, 1997. *MMWR* 1997;46:765–766.
231. Ploy MC, Grelaud C, Martin C, et al. First clinical isolate of vancomycin-intermediate *Staphylococcus aureus* in a French hospital. *Lancet* 1998;351:1212–1212.
232. Hiramatsu K, Hanaki H, Ino T, et al. Methicillin-resistant *Staphylococcus aureus* clinical strain with reduced vancomycin susceptibility. *J Antimicrob Chemother* 1997;40:135–136.
233. Tenover FC, Arbeit RD, Goering RV. How to select and interpret molecular strain typing methods for epidemiological studies of bacterial infections: a review for healthcare epidemiologists. Molecular Typing Working Group of the Society for Healthcare Epidemiology of America. *Infect Control Hosp Epidemiol* 1997;18(6):426–439.
234. Burnie J, Matthews R, Jiman-Fatami A, et al. Analysis of 42 cases of septicemia caused by an epidemic strain of methicillin-resistant Staphylococcus aureus: evidence of resistance to vancomycin. *Clin Infect Dis* 2000;31:684–689.
235. Noble WC, Virani Z, Cree RGA. Co-transfer of vancomycin and other resistance genes from *Enterococcus faecalis* NCTC 12201 to *Staphylococcus aureus. FEMS Microbiol Lett* 1992;93:195–198.
236. CDC (Centers for Disease Prevention and Control). Vancomycin-resistant *Staphylococcus aureus* —Pennsylvania, 2002. *MMWR* 2002(Oct 11);902.
237. Anonymous. From the Centers for Disease Control and Prevention. Vancomycin resistant Staphylococcus aureus—Pennsylvania, 2002. *JAMA* 2002;288(17):2116.
238. Lacey RW. Multi-resistant *Staphylococcus aureus*—a suitable case for inactivity? *J Hosp Infect* 1987;9:103–105.
239. Humphreys H. Comparison of infections caused by methicillin-sensitive and methicillin-resistant *Staphylococcus aureus.* In: Cafferkey MT, ed. *Methicillin-resistant Staphylococcus aureus.* New York: Marcel Dekker, 1992:77–90.
240. Waldvogel FA. Treatment of infections due to methicillin-resistant *Staphylococcus aureus. J Hosp Infect* 1986;7(suppl A):37–46.
241. Casewell MW. Epidemiology and control of the "modern" methicillin-resistant *Staphylococcus aureus. J Hosp Infect* 1986;7(suppl A): 1–11.
242. Storch GA, Radcliff JL, Meyer PL, et al. Methicillin-resistant *Staphylococcus aureus* in a nursing home. *Infect Control* 1987;8:24–29.
243. Kauffman CA, Bradley SF, Terpenning MS. Methicillin-resistant *Staphylococcus aureus* in long-term care facilities. *Infect Control Hosp Epidemiol* 1990;11:600–603.
244. Thomas JC, Bridge J, Waterman S, et al. Transmission and control of methicillin-resistant *Staphylococcus aureus* in a skilled nursing facility. *Infect Control Hosp Epidemiol* 1989;10:106–110.
245. Cooke EM, Marples RR. Outbreaks of staphylococcal infection. *PHLS Microbiol Dig* 1985;2:62–64.
246. Cookson B, Phillips I. Epidemic methicillin-resistant *Staphylococcus aureus. J Antimicrob Chemother* 1988;21(suppl C):57–65.
247. Cookson B, Peters B, Webster M, et al. Staff carriage of epidemic methicillin-resistant *Staphylococcus aureus. J Clin Microbiol* 1989;27: 1471–1476.
248. Crossley KB, Thurn JR. Control measures for MRSA—can the cost

be reduced? In: Cafferkey MT, ed. *Methicillin-resistant Staphylococcus aureus*. New York: Marcel Dekker, 1992:187–196.

249. Thompson et al. 1982.
250. Klimek et al. 1976.
251. Boyce JM. Methicillin-resistant *Staphylococcus aureus*: detection, epidemiology and control measures. *Infect Dis Clin North Am* 1989;3: 901–913.
252. Combined Working Party. Revised guidelines for the control of methicillin-resistant *Staphylococcus aureus* infection in hospitals. *J Hosp Infect* 1998;39:253–290.
253. Duckworth GJ, Lothian JLE, Williams JD. Methicillin-resistant *Staphylococcus aureus*: report of an outbreak in a London teaching hospital. *J Hosp Infect* 1988;11:1–5.
254. Hudson IRB. The efficacy of intranasal mupirocin in the prevention of staphylococcal infections: a review of recent experience. *J Hosp Infect* 1994;27:81–98.
255. Hill RLR, Duckworth GJ, Casewell MW. Elimination of nasal carriage of methicillin-resistant *Staphylococcus aureus* with mupirocin during a hospital outbreak. *J Antimicrob Chemother* 1988;22: 377–384.
256. Farmer TH, Gilbart J, Elson SW. Biochemical basis of mupirocin resistance in strains of *Staphylococcus aureus*. *J Antimicrob Chemother* 1992;30:587–596.
257. Gilbart J, Perry CR, Slocombe B. High level mupirocin resistance in *Staphylococcus aureus*: evidence for two distinct isoleucyl-tRNA synthetases. *Antimicrob Agents Chemother* 1993;37:32–38.
258. Cookson B. Mupirocin resistance in staphylococci. *J Antimicrob Chemother* 1990;25:497–503.
259. Rahman M, Noble WC, Cookson B. Mupirocin-resistant *Staphylococcus aureus*. *Lancet* 1987;2:387.
260. Rahman M, Noble WC, Cookson B. Transmissible mupirocin resistance in *Staphylococcus aureus*. *Epidemiol Infect* 9;102:261–270.
261. Deighton MA, Franklin JC, Spicer WJ, et al. Species identification, antibiotic sensitivity and slime production of coagulase-negative staphylococci isolated from clinical specimens. *Epidemiol Infect* 1988; 101:99–113.
262. Hansen-Nord M, Gahrn-Hansen B, Siboni K. Studies of clinical isolates of coagulase-negative staphylococci resistant to methicillin. *APMIS* 1988;96:133–140.
263. Refsahl K, Andersen BM. Clinically significant coagulase-negative staphylococci: identification and resistance patterns. *J Hosp Infect* 1992;22:19–31.
264. Elliott TSJ. Intravascular-device infections. *J Med Microbiol* 1988;27: 161–167.
265. Ponce de Leon S, Wenzel RP. Hospital-acquired bloodstream infections with *Staphylococcus epidermidis*. Review of 100 cases. *Am J Med* 1984;77:639–644.
266. Crossley KB, Ross J. Colonization of hospitalized patients by *Staphylococcus aureus, Staphylococcus epidermidis* and enterococci. *J Hosp Infect* 1985;6:179–186.
267. Riben PD, Horsman GB, Rayner E, et al. Emergence of tobramycin-resistant *S. epidermidis* possessing aminoglycoside modifying enzymes and bacteremic superinfection during empiric therapy of febrile neutropenic episodes. *Clin Invest Med (Med Clin Exp)* 1985;8:272–285.
268. Thurn JR, Crossley KB, Gerdts A, et al. Dynamics of coagulase-negative staphylococcal colonization in patients and employees in a surgical intensive care unit. *J Hosp Infect* 1992;20:247–255.
269. George RC, Ball LC, Norbury PB. Susceptibility to ciprofloxacin of nosocomial gram-negative bacteria and staphylococci isolated in the UK. *J Antimicrob Chemother* 1990;26(suppl F):145–156.
270. Lyytikainen O, Vaara M, Jarviluoma E, et al. Increased resistance among *Staphylococcus epidermidis* isolates in a large teaching hospital over a 12-year period. *Eur J Clin Microbiol Infect Dis* 1996;15: 133–138.
271. Archer GL. Molecular epidemiology of multiresistant *Staphylococcus epidermidis*. *J Antimicrob Chemother* 1988;21(suppl C):133–138.
272. Jaffe HW, Sweeney HM, Nathan C, et al. Identity and interspecific transfer of gentamicin-resistance plasmids in *Staphylococcus aureus* and *Staphylococcus epidermidis*. *J Infect Dis* 1980;141:738–747.
273. Watanakunakorn C. In-vitro induction of resistance in coagulase-negative staphylococci to vancomycin and teicoplanin. *J Antimicrob Chemother* 1988;22:321–324.
274. Schwalbe RS, Stapleton JT, Gilligan, PH. Emergence of vancomycin resistance in coagulase-negative staphylococci. *N Engl J Med* 1987; 316:927–931.
275. Greenwood D. Microbiological aspects of teicoplanin. *J Antimicrob Chemother* 1988;21(suppl A):1–13.
276. Wilson APR, O'Hare MD, Felmingham D, et al. Teicoplanin-resistant coagulase-negative Staphylococcus. *Lancet* 1986;2:973.
277. Sanyal D, Williams AJ, Johnson AP, et al. The emergence of vancomycin resistance in renal dialysis. *J Hosp Infect* 1993;24:167–173.
278. Houang ET, Marples RR, Weir I, et al. Problems in the investigation of an apparent outbreak of coagulase-negative staphylococcal septicaemia following cardiac surgery. *J Hosp Infect* 1986;8:224–232.
279. Boyce JM, Potter-Bynoe G, Opal SM, et al. A common-source outbreak of *Staphylococcus epidermidis* infections among patients undergoing cardiac surgery. *J Infect Dis* 1990;161:493–499.
280. Carlos CC, Ringertz S, Rylander M, et al. Nosocomial *Staphylococcus epidermidis* septicaemia among very low birth weight neonates in an intensive care unit. *J Hosp Infect* 1991;19:201–217.
281. Menzies R, MacCulloch D, Comere B. Investigation of nosocomial valve endocarditis due to antibiotic-resistant *Staphylococcus epidermidis*. *J Hosp Infect* 1991;19:107–114.
282. Johnson WD, Kaye D. Serious infections caused by diphtheroids. *Ann NY Acad Sci* 1970;174:568–576.
283. Jackman PJH, Pitcher DG, et al. Classification of corynebacteria associated with endocarditis (group JK) as *Corynebacterium jeikeium* SP-NOV. *Syst Appl Microbiol* 1987;9:83–90.
284. Hande KR, Witebsky FG, Brown MS, et al. Sepsis with a new species of *Corynebacterium*. *Ann Intern Med* 1976;85:423–426.
285. Stamm WE, Tompkins LS, Wagner KF, et al. Infection due to *Corynebacterium* species in marrow transplant patients. *J Intern Med* 1979; 91:167–173.
286. Gill VJ, Manning C, Lamson M, et al. Antibiotic-resistant group JK bacteria in hospitals. *J Clin Microbiol* 1981;13:472–477.
287. Horn WA, Larson EL, McGineley KJ, et al. Microbial flora on the hands of health care personnel: differences in composition and antibacterial resistance. *Infect Control Hosp Epidemiol* 1988;9:189–193.
288. Davis A, Binder MJ, Burroughs JT, et al. Diphtheroid endocarditis after cardiopulmonary bypass surgery for the repair of cardiac valvular defects. *Antimicrob Agents Chemother* 1963;3:643–655.
289. Van Scoy RE, Cohen SN, Geraci JE, et al. Coryneform bacterial endocarditis. Difficulties in diagnosis and treatment, presentation of three cases, and review of the literature. *Mayo Clin Proc* 1977;52: 216–219.
290. Murray BE. The life and times of the enterococcus. *Clin Microbiol Rev* 1990;3:46–65.
291. Gray JW, Pedler SJ. Antibiotic-resistant enterococci. *J Hosp Infect* 1992;21:1–14.
292. Bush LM, Calmon J, Cherney CL, et al. High-level penicillin resistance among isolates of enterococci: implications for treatment of enterococcal infections. *Ann Intern Med* 1989;110:515–520.
293. Murray BE. β-Lactamase–producing enterococci. *Antimicrob Agents Chemother* 1992;37:2355–2359.
294. Wells VD, Wong ES, Murray BE, et al. Infections due to beta-lactamase-producing high-level gentamicin-resistant *Enterococcus faecalis*. *Ann Intern Med* 1992;116:285–289.
295. Zervos MJ, Bacon AE, Patterson JE, et al. Enterococcal superinfection in patients treated with ciprofloxacin. *J Antimicrob Chemother* 1988; 21:113–115.
296. Anonymous. 1986.
297. Coudron PE, Mayhall CG, Facklam RR, et al. *Streptococcus faecium* outbreak in a neonatal intensive care unit. *J Clin Microbiol* 1984;20: 1044–1048.
298. Zervos MJ, Kauffman CA, Therasse PM, et al. Nosocomial infection by gentamicin-resistant *Streptococcus faecalis*—an epidemiologic study. *Ann Intern Med* 1987;106:687–691.
299. Zervos MJ, Terpenning MS, Schaberg DR, et al. High-level aminoglycoside-resistant enterococci—colonization of nursing home and acute care hospital patients. *Arch Intern Med* 1987;147:1591–1594.

300. Rhinehart E, Smith NE, Wennersten C, et al. Rapid dissemination of β-lactamase-producing, aminoglycoside-resistant *Enterococcus faecalis* among patients and staff in an infant-toddler surgical ward. *N Engl J Med* 1990;323:1814–1818.
301. Boyce JM, Opal SM, Chow JW, et al. Outbreak of multidrug-resistant Enterococcus faecium with transferable vanB class vancomycin resistance. *J Clin Microbiol* 1994;32:1148–1153.
302. Spera RV, Farber BF. Multiply-resistant *Enterococcus faecium*. The nosocomial pathogen of the 1990s. *JAMA* 1992;268:2563–2564.
303. Reynolds PE. Glycopeptide resistance in Gram-positive bacteria. *J Med Microbiol* 1992;36:14–17.
304. Reynolds PE. Structure, biochemistry and mechanism of action of glycopeptide antibiotics. *Eur J Clin Microbiol Infect Dis* 1989;8: 943–950.
305. Arthur M, Courvalin P. Genetics and mechanisms of glycopeptide resistance in enterococci. *Antimicrob Agents Chemother* 1993;37: 1563–1571.
306. Arthur M, Molinas C, Bugg TDH, et al. Evidence for in vivo incorporation of D-lactate into peptidoglycan precursors of vancomycin-resistant enterococci. *Antimicrob Agents Chemother* 1992;36:867–869.
307. Arthur M, Molinas C, Depardieu, et al. Characterization of *Tn*1546, a *Tn*3-related transposon conferring glycopeptide resistance by synthesis of depsipeptide peptidoglycan precursors in *Enterococcus faecium* BM4147. *J Bacteriol* 1993;175:117–127.
308. Messer J, Reynolds PE. Modified peptidoglycan precursors produced by glycopeptide-resistant enterococci. *FEMS Microbiol Lett* 1992;94: 195–200.
309. Allen NE, Hobbs JN, Richardson JM, et al. Biosynthesis of modified peptidoglycan precursors by vancomycin resistant *Enterococcus faecium. FEMS Microbiol Lett* 1992;98:109–16.
310. Evers S, Courvalin P. Regulation of VanB-type vancomycin resistance gene expression by the VanS(B)-VanR(B) two-component regulatory system in *Enterococcus* faecalis V583. *J Bacteriol* 1996;178: 1302–1309.
311. Evers S, Reynolds PE, Courvalin P. Sequence of the *vanB* and *ddl* genes encoding D-alanine:D-lactate and D-alanine:D-alanine ligases in vancomycin-resistant *Enterococcus faecalis* V583. *Gene* 1994;140: 97–102.
312. Quinitiliani R, Evers S, Courvalin P. The *vanB* gene confers various levels of self-transferable resistance to vancomycin in enterococci. *J Infect Dis* 1993;167:1220–1223.
313. Billot-Klein D, Shlaes D, Bryant D, et al. Peptidoglycan structure of *Enterococcus faecium* expressing vancomycin resistance of the VanB type. *Biochem J* 1996;313:711–715.
314. Leclerq R, Dutka-Malen S, Duval J, et al. Vancomycin resistance gene *vanC* is specific to *Enterococcus gallinarum. Antimicrob Agents Chemother* 1992;36:2005–2008.
315. Perichon B, Reynolds P, Courvalin P. VanD-type glycopeptide-resistant *Enterococcus faecium* BM4339. *Antimicrob Agents Chemother* 1997;41:2016–2018.
316. Uttley AHC, George RC, Naidoo J, et al. High-level vancomycin-resistant enterococci causing hospital infections. *Epidemiol Infect* 1989;103:173–181.
317. Anonymous. Nosocomial enterococci resistant to vancomycin—United States, 1989–1993. *MMWR* 1993;42:597–599.
318. Livornese LL, Dias S, Samuel C, et al. Hospital-acquired infection with vancomycin-resistant *Enterococcus faecium* transmitted by electronic thermometers. *Ann Intern Med* 1992;117:112–116.
319. Rubin LG, Tucci V, Cerenado E, et al. Vancomycin-resistant *Enterococcus* faecium in hospitalized children. *Infect Control Hosp Epidemiol* 1992;13:700–705.
320. Wade JC, Schimpff SC, Newman KA, et al. *Staphylococcus epidermidis*: an increasing cause of infection in patients with granulocytopenia. *Ann Intern Med* 1982;97:503–508.
321. Kjolen H, Andersen BM. Handwashing and disinfection of heavily contaminated hands—effective or ineffective? *J Hosp Infect* 1992;21: 61–71.
322. Kirst HA, Thompson DG, Nicas TI. Historical yearly usage of Vancomycin. *Antimicrob Agents Chemother* 1998;42:1303–1304.
323. Bates J. Epidemiology of vancomycin-resistant enterococci in the community and the relevance of farm animals to human infection. *J Hosp Infect* 1997;37:89–101.
324. Witte W. Selective pressure by antibiotic use in livestock. *Int J Antimicrob Agents*
325. Endtz HP, van den Braak N, van Belkum A, et al. Fecal carriage of vancomycin-resistant enteroccocci in hospitalized patients and those living in the community in the
326. Martone WJ. Spread of vancomycin-resistant enterococci: why did it happened in the United States. *Infect Control Hosp Epidemiol* 1998; 19:539–545.
327. Mayhall CG. The epidemiology and control of VRE: still struggling to come of age. *Infect Control Hosp Epidemiol* 1999;20:650–652.
328. Allen KD. Penicillin-resistant pneumococci. *J Hosp Infect* 1991;17: 31–13.
329. Davies AJ, Hawkey PM, Simpson RA, et al. Pneumococcal cross-infection in hospital. *Br Med J* 1984;288:1195.
330. Jacobs MR, Koornhoof MJ, Robins-Braine PM, et al. Emergence of multiply resistant pneumococci. *N Engl J Med* 1978;299:735–740.
331. Appelbaum PC, Bhamjee A, Scragg JN, et al. *Streptococcus pneumoniae* resistant to penicillin and chloramphenicol. *Lancet* 1977;2:995–997.
332. Markiewicz Z, Tomasz A. Variation in penicillin-binding protein patterns of penicillin-resistant clinical isolates of pneumococci. *J Clin Microbiol* 1989;27:405–410.
333. Dowson CG, Coffey TJ, Kell C, et al. Evolution of penicillin resistance in *Streptococcus pneumoniae*; the role of *Streptococcus mitis* in the formation of a low affinity PBP2B in *S. pneumoniae. Mol Microbiol* 1993;9:635–643.
334. Muñoz R, Dowson CG, Daniels M, et al. Genetics of resistance to third-generation cephalosporins in clinical isolates of *Streptococcus pneumoniae. Mol Microbiol* 1992;6:2461–2465.
335. Koornhof HJ, Klugman KP. Evolution of extended spectrum cephalosporin resistance in the pneumococcus. *J Antimicrob Chemother* 1997; 39:837–838.
336. Dixon JMS, Lipinski AE, Graham MEP. Detection and prevalence of pneumococci with increased resistance to penicillin. *Can Med Assoc J* 1977;117:1159–1161.
337. Swenson JM, Hill BC, Thornsberry C. Screening pneumococci for penicillin resistance. *J Clin Microbiol* 1986;24:749–752.
338. Lyon DJ, Scheel O, Fung KS, et al. Rapid emergence of penicillin-resistant pneumococci in Hong Kong. *Scand J Infect Dis* 1996;28: 375–376.
339. Garcia-Martos P, Galan F, Marin P, et al. Increase in high-level resistance to penicillin of clinical isolates of *Streptococcus pneumoniae* in Cadiz, Spain. *Chemotherapy* 1997;43:179–181.
340. Duchin JS, Breiman RF, Diamond A, et al. High prevalence of multidrug-resistant *Streptococcus pneumoniae* in a rural Kentucky community. *Pediatr Infect Dis J* 1995;14:745–750.
341. Gould FK, Magee JG, Ingham HR. A hospital outbreak of antibiotic-resistant *Streptococcus pneumoniae. J Infect* 1987;15:77–79.
342. Moore EP, Williams EW. Hospital transmission of multiply antibiotic-resistant *Streptococcus pneumoniae. J Hosp Infect* 1988;16: 199–200.
343. Willett LD, Dillon HC, Gray BM. Penicillin-intermediate pneumococci in a children's hospital. *Am J Dis Child* 1985;139:1054–1057.
344. Millar MR, Brown NM, Tobin GW, et al. Outbreak of infection with penicillin-resistant *Streptococcus pneumoniae* in a hospital for the elderly. *J Hosp Infect* 1994;27:99–104.
345. Radetsky MS, Istre GR, Johansen TL, et al. Multiply antibiotic-resistant pneumococcus causing meningitis: its epidemiology within a day-care centre. *Lancet* 1981;2:771–773.
346. Rubinstein E, Rubinovitch B. Treatment of severe infections caused by penicillin-resistant pneumococci. Role of third generation cephalosporins. *Infection* 1994;22(suppl 3):S161–S166.
347. Grimwood K, Collingnon PJ, Currie BJ, et al. Antibiotic management of pneumococcal infections in an era of increased resistance. *J Paediatr Child Health* 1997;33:287–295.
348. Friedland IR, Klugman KP. Antibiotic-resistant pneumococcal disease in South African children. *Am J Dis Child* 1992;146:920–923.
349. Bradley JS, Scheld WM. The challenge of penicillin-resistant *Strepto-*

coccus pneumoniae meningitis: current antibiotic therapy in the 1990s. *Clin Infect Dis* 1997;24(suppl 2):S213–S221.

350. Simmons HE, Stolley PD. Trends and consequences of antibiotic use in the United States. *JAMA* 1974;227:1023–1028.
351. Cooke DM, Salter AJ, Phillips I. Antimicrobial misuse, antibiotic policies and information resources. *J Antimicrob Chemother* 1980;6: 435–443.
352. Scheckler WE, Bennett JV. Antibiotic use in seven community hospitals. *JAMA* 1970;213:264–267.
353. Kunin CM, Tupasi T, Craig WA. Use of antibiotics. A brief exposition of the problem and some tentative solutions. *Ann Intern Med* 1973;79:555–560.
354. Kunin CM. Evaluation of antibiotic use: a comprehensive look at alternative approaches. *Rev Infect Dis* 1981;3:745–753.
355. McGowan JE, Finland M. Infection and antibiotic use at Boston City Hospital: changes in prevalence during the decade. *J Infect Dis* 1974; 129:421–428.
356. Buckwold FJ, Ronald AR. Antimicrobial misuse: effects and suggestions for control. *J Antimicrob Chemother* 1979;5:129–136.
357. Shapiro M, Townsend TR, Rosner B, et al. Use of antimicrobial drugs in general hospitals. II: Analysis of patterns of use. *J Infect Dis* 1979; 139:698–706.
358. Shapiro M, Townsend TR, Rosner B, et al. Use of antimicrobial drugs in general hospitals: patterns of prophylaxis. *N Engl J Med* 1979;301: 351–355.
359. Stevens GP, Jacobson JA, Burke JP. Changing patterns of hospital infections and antibiotic use. Prevalence surveys in a community hospital. *Arch Intern Med* 1981;141:587–592.
360. Lawson DH, MacDonald S. Antibacterial therapy in general medical wards. *Postgrad Med J* 1977;53:206–309.
361. Moss EM, McNicol MW, McSwiggan DA, et al. Survey of antibiotic prescribing in a district general hospital. *Lancet* 1981;2: 349–352,407–409,461–462.
362. Geddes AM. The impact on clinical practice of antibiotic-resistant micro-organisms. In: Stuart-Harris CH, Harris DM, eds. *The control of antibiotic-resistant bacteria.* London: Academic Press, 1982:1–16.
363. Cooke DM, Salter AJ, Phillips I. The impact of antibiotic policy on prescribing in a London teaching hospital. A one-day prevalence survey as an indicator of antibiotic use. *J Antimicrob Chemother* 1983; 11:447–453.
364. Clausen DC, Evans RS, Pretotnik SL, et al. The timing of prophylactic antibiotics and the risk of surgical wound infection. *N Engl J Med* 1992;326:281–286.
365. Hirschman SZ, Meyers BR, Bradbury K, et al. Use of antimicrobial agents in a university teaching hospital. Evolution of a comprehensive control program. *Arch Intern Med* 1988;148:2001–2007.
366. Phillips I. Antibiotic policies. In: Reeves D, Geddes A, eds. *Recent advances in infection.* Edinburgh: Churchill Livingstone, 1979: 151–123.
367. Phillips I, Cooke D. The control of antibiotic prescribing in a London teaching hospital. In: Stuart-Harris CH, Harris DM, eds. *The control of antibiotic-resistant bacteria.* London: Academic Press, 1982: 201–209.
368. Bryan CS. Strategies to improve antibiotic use. *Infect Dis Clin North Am* 1989;3:723–734.
369. Goldman DA, Weinstein RA, Wenzel RP, et al. Strategies to prevent and control the emergence and spread of antimicrobial-resistant microorganism in hospitals: a challenge to hospital leadership. *JAMA* 1996;275:234–240.
370. Ridley M, Barrie D, Lynn R, et al. Antibiotic-resistant *Staphylococcus aureus* and hospital antibiotic policies. *Lancet* 1970;1:230–233.
371. Price DJE, Sleigh JD. Control of infection due to *Klebsiella aerogenes* in a neurosurgical unit by withdrawal of all antibiotics. *Lancet* 1970; 2:1213–1215.
372. Lowbury EJL, Babb JR, Roe E. Clearance from a hospital of gram-negative bacilli that transfer carbenicillin-resistance to *Pseudomonas aeruginosa. Lancet* 1972;2:941–945.
373. Ruiz-Palacios GM, Ponce de Leon S, Sifuentes J, et al. Control of emergence of multi-resistant gram-negative bacilli by exclusive use of amikacin. *Am J Med* 1986;80(6b):71–75.
374. Gerding DN, Larson TA. Resistance surveillance programs and the incidence of gram-negative bacillary resistance to amikacin from 1967 to 1985. *Am J Med* 1986;80(6b):22–28.
375. Young EJ, Sewell CM, Koza MA, et al. Antibiotic resistance patterns during aminoglycoside restriction. *Am J Med Sci* 1985;290:223–227.
376. Coates D, Hutchinson DN. How to produce a hospital disinfection policy. *J Hosp Infect* 1994;26:57–68.
377. Jolley AE. The value of surveillance cultures on neonatal intensive care units. *J Hosp Infect* 1993;25:153–159.
378. Flynn DM, Weinstein RA, Nathan C, et al. Patients' endogenous flora as the source of "nosocomial" *Enterobacter* in cardiac surgery. *J Infect Dis* 1987;156:363–368.
379. First European Consensus Conference in Intensive Care Medicine. Selective decontamination in intensive care unit patients. *Intensive Care Med* 1992;18:182–188.
380. Occhipinti DJ, Itokazu G, Danzinger LH. Selective decontamination of the digestive tract as an infection-control measure in intensive care unit patients. *Pharmacotherapy* 1992;12(suppl):50S–63S.
381. Daschner F. Emergence of resistance during selective decontamination of the digestive tract. *Eur J Clin Microbiol Infect Dis* 1992;11: 1–3.
382. van Saene HKF, Unertl KE, Alcock SR, et al. Emergence of antibiotic resistance during selective digestive decontamination? *J Hosp Infect* 1992;24:158–161.
383. Webb CH. Antibiotic resistance associated with selective decontamination of the digestive tract. *J Hosp Infect* 1992;22:1–5.
384. D'Amico R, Pifferi S, Leonetti C, et al. Effectiveness of antibiotic prophylaxis in critically ill adult patients: systematic review of randomised controlled trials. *Br Med J* 1998;316:1275–1285.
385. Hammond JMJ, Potgeiter PD, Saunders GL, et al. Double-blind study of selective decontamination of the digestive tract in intensive care. *Lancet* 1992;340:5–9.
386. Brun-Buisson C, Legrand P, Rauss A, et al. Intestinal decontamination for control of nosocomial multiresistant Gram-negative bacilli. Study of an outbreak in an intensive care unit. *Ann Intern Med* 1989; 110:837–881.
387. Weinstein RA. Selective intestinal decontamination—an infection control measure whose time has come? *Ann Intern Med* 1989;110: 853–855.
388. Kunin CM. Resistance to antimicrobial drugs—a worldwide calamity. *Ann Intern Med* 1993;118:557–566.

xxx. Anonymous. Vancomycin resistant enterococci in hospitals in the United Kingdom. *Comm Dis Rep CDR Weekly* 1995;50:281.
xxx. Casewell M, Phillips I. Food as a source of *Klebsiella* species for colonization and infection of intensive care patients. *J Clin Pathol* 1978;31:845–849.
xxx. De Champs C, Sirot D, Chanal C, et al. Concomitant dissemination of three extended-spectrum beta-lactamases among different Enterobacteriaceae isolated in a French hospital. *J Antimicrob Chemother* 1991;27:441–457.
xxx. Hamory BH, Parisis JT, Hutton JP. *Staphylococcus epidermidis*: a significant nosocomial pathogen. *Am J Infect Control* 1987;15:59–74.
xxx. Mazurek G. Modern typing methods for the investigation of nosocomial infections. *Curr Opin Infect Dis* 1993;6:538–543.
xxx. Netherlands. *J Clin Microbiol* 1997;35:3026–3031.
xxx. Price EH. *Staphylococcus epidermidis* infections of cerebrospinal fluid shunts. *J Hosp Infect* 1984;5:7–17.
xxx. Quintiliani R, Cooper BW, Briceland LL, et al. Economic impact of streamlining antibiotic administration. *Am J Med* 1987;82(suppl 4A):391–394.
xxx. Reynolds PE, Fuller C. Methicillin-resistant strains of *Staphylococcus aureus*: presence of identical additional penicillin-binding protein in all strains examined. *FEMS Microbiol Lett* 1986;33:251–254.
xxx. United States. *Infect Control Hosp Epidemiol* 1998;19:539–545.
xxx. Willems RJL, Top J, van den Braak N, et al. Molecular diversity and evolutionary .

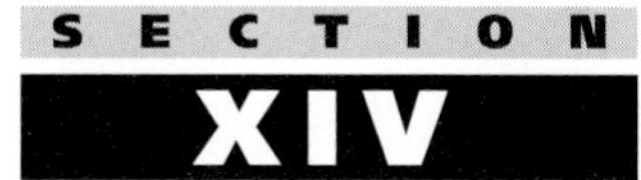

SECTION XIV

THE LITERATURE IN HOSPITAL EPIDEMIOLOGY AND INFECTION CONTROL

92

SEARCHING THE LITERATURE IN HOSPITAL EPIDEMIOLOGY AND INFECTION CONTROL

CYNTHIA J. WALKER
K. ANN MCKIBBON
FIONA SMAILL
R. BRIAN HAYNES

Since the second edition of this book was published in 1999, access to healthcare literature has continued to become easier, faster, and more widespread. The Internet features prominently as a primary repository for healthcare information. Indeed, many of the traditional forms of literature such as journal articles and books are available in their entirety on the Internet. More quality-filtered and patient-ready resources are available to help streamline the search for information. Finally, a new form of technology has invaded the information scene: the handheld or personal digital assistant (PDA).

In this updated chapter, we explore the improvements in information access to evidence-based resources with relevance to infection control. We review these new resources and improvements in old ones as they relate to three areas in which a healthcare professional would require high-quality information: (a) solving clinical problems, (b) keeping up-to-date, and (c) setting clinical policy.

USING THE LITERATURE TO SOLVE CLINICAL PROBLEMS

Quick and efficient access to high-quality reliable information is never so important as when faced with a pressing clinical problem. This is especially true in the rapidly changing field of infection control in which practices and policies are subject to frequent changes and amendments. To make informed clinical decisions, recent reports are needed of systematic reviews or major preplanned human investigations relevant to the clinical setting. One could rely on one's colleague down the hall—if one has a colleague and he or she is more up to date and has time when one needs them . . . or one can search the literature to find the current best evidence by carefully defining the clinical question, choosing the most appropriate information source, and designing a search strategy (1).

Until recently, textbooks were often sources for basic information that did not change quickly (2). Anatomy plus physiology and other such basic science subjects lend themselves well to the publication pace of textbooks. With the publication potential of the Internet, however, clinical practice textbooks have entered an "evidence-based era." Many textbooks are now available on the Internet and integrate evidence-based information with specific clinical problems. In addition, they are updated more or less regularly. *Up-To-Date (www.uptodate.com)* is an evidence-based electronic textbook [Web-based and compact disc read-only memory (CD-ROM)] for general internal medicine and a growing number of other specialties. *WebMD Scientific American Medicine www.samed.com)* is also available on the Internet and CD-ROM.

Clinical Evidence, from the BMJ Publishing Group, is a dynamic electronic synthesis of evidence from randomized trials, published in print, on CD-ROM, and on the Internet in unabridged, concise, and PDA formats. Organized by clinical area, the focus of each section is a selection of clinical questions and answers most often related to therapies. New and updated topics are posted online each month. The questions in *Clinical Evidence* concern the benefits and harms of preventative and therapeutic interventions, with emphasis on outcomes that matter to patients.

The Physicians' Information and Education Resource (PIER) is a new Web-based service from the American College of Physicians-American Society of Internal Medicine (ACP-ASIM) *(pier-.acponline.org).* Volunteer physician editorial consultants review the literature and prepare PIER modules for specific topics. The consultants are given recent citations to relevant articles obtained through filtered electronic searches. The modules are updated quarterly and made available on the Internet. Coverage includes diseases, screening and prevention, complementary and alternative medicine, ethical and legal issues, and procedures. The design of *Clinical Evidence* and PIER also make them useful for keeping up with the medical literature and for providing basic knowledge on healthcare topics.

The Cochrane Library contains the collected work of the Cochrane Collaboration, an international organization that prepares, maintains, and disseminates systematic reviews of controlled trials of healthcare interventions (note that topics such as diagnosis and prognosis are not covered). Within the Cochrane Library, the Cochrane Database of Systematic Reviews (CDSR) contains reviews that have high standards for finding, rating, summarizing, and reporting the evidence from trials (1). The Cochrane Library is searchable, contains almost exclusively controlled trials and systematic reviews, and is much smaller than MEDLINE, so that methodologic filtering is not needed and a simple, even one-word, search strategy will likely retrieve high-quality evidence with a clinical bottom line. Furthermore, the Cochrane Library is cumulative, and the reviews are regularly updated or tagged as no longer current, if not updated within a specified period. The Cochrane Library also contains summaries of non-Cochrane systematic reviews, citations on how to do systematic reviews, and a huge database of citations of clinical trials, many of them not available on MEDLINE. The Cochrane Library is available on CD-ROM and the Internet as a stand-alone resource and in other services, such as Ovid's "Evidence-Based Medicine Reviews." If one choose not to subscribe to it, one's health sciences or hospital library likely does. Abstracts of Cochrane reviews and the abstracts of other systematic reviews (but not the rest of the library) are also available for free on the Internet at the U.K. Cochrane site *(http://www.cochrane.org)* and other Web sites.

MEDLINE is the most likely general source to turn to when one's specific information sources fail or when one is faced with a nonroutine clinical problem. It should not be consulted first if one knows of a specific source that is current, of high quality, and tailored to the problem being dealt with, as we describe later. MEDLINE is the largest readily available database of biomedical journal citations and is now available in full or subset form for free on many Web sites, one of them produced by the U.S. National Library of Medicine (NLM). It is also more up-to-date than ever, with leading journals providing electronic copy for close to date-of-publication posting.

PubMed *(www.ncbi.nlm.nih.gov/entrez/)* is the MEDLINE search interface produced by the NLM in conjunction with the U.S. National Center for Biotechnology Information. PubMed provides on-line access to literature citations and links to full-text journals at Web sites of participating publishers. (User registration, a subscription fee, or some other type of fee may be required to access the full text of articles for some journals.) PubMed also contains PREMEDLINE citations: basic citation information and abstracts are entered or downloaded daily before the full records that contain MeSH terms, publication types, and other indexing data are prepared and added to MEDLINE. Furthermore, it has a clinical query feature *(http://www.ncbi.nlm.nih.gov/entrez/query/static/clinical.html)* that allows a search strategy to be fine tuned using methodologic terms so that retrieval will be more clinically applicable. For example, if one's question has to do with the cause, course, diagnosis, prevention, or treatment of a clinical problem, one could go directly to the clinical query screen and indicate the study category in which one is interested and whether one would like a "sensitive" (maximal retrieval of relevant articles, with a high rate of false-positive articles) or "specific" (lower retrieval of relevant articles with fewer false positives) approach. After content words on the clinical problem of interest are entered, one proceeds with the search and complex pretested search strategies are automatically invoked, optimizing the yield of clinically relevant studies (3). In the near future, updated clinical queries will be available. These queries will be expanded from therapy, diagnosis, prognosis, and etiology to include clinical prediction guides, economics, qualitative studies, and systematic reviews (4).

PubMed also has a "related articles" feature that allows the searcher to view citations related to an individual citation retrieved in a search without having to do another search. Thus, if one finds a study that is right on target, one can click on the [Related Articles] link and retrieve more articles on the same topic sorted in order of relevance.

Although powerful and free, MEDLINE is not the only large biomedical database. EMBASE/Excerpta Medica and the Cumulative Index to Nursing and Allied Health Literature (CINAHL) are also available and are useful to the infection control professional in search of information. Both EMBASE and CINAHL (as well as MEDLINE) are available on the Internet through Ovid *(www.ovid.com)*. Ovid provides a front-end search engine that has user fees, but many health sciences and hospital libraries provide it because it offers access to several different databases using the same user-friendly search interface and integration of database searching with a strong collection of full-text clinical journals. In addition to databases of citations to articles, Ovid provides access to books, a diagnosis program, and Evidence-Based Medicine Reviews, a multifile database that allows simultaneous searching of evidence-based medicine databases including *ACP Journal Club* and databases within the Cochrane Library.

Case Scenario: Solving a Problem of Treatment

An aggressive, bottom-line obsessed administrator in your hospital is looking for ways to save money. She requests that you consider reverting from antimicrobial-coated catheters in the intensive care unit to less expensive, uncoated catheters. She demands that you show that the coated catheters are worth their higher cost. You seek to do so as quickly as possible.

Because you are pushed for time and you know that you want high-quality, patient-centered information, you start with *ACP Journal Club (acpjc.org)*. Your initial search is effective using two words—"catheter" and "infection." You retrieve 30 hits, most of them directly relevant. Two very relevant studies (5,6) show that the coated catheters are effective. The systematic review by Mermel (5) showed that they are more effective than noncoated catheters and Veenstra et al. (6) provided data that showed that the coated ones are cost effective.

Although the *acpjc.org* search was successful, it is worth taking a quick look in the Cochrane Library, another high-quality information source. You call up the Cochrane Library online, and in the "searchphrase" window you type "impregnated catheter." There is one review in the CDSR, but it is not very relevant, because it pertains to umbilical artery catheters in newborns in the neonatal intensive care unit (7). In the Cochrane Central Register of Controlled Trials (CENTRAL), there are citations with abstracts to five randomized trials, all from 1997 to 1999. Running the search again with "coated catheter" you find no systematic reviews but 11 more randomized trials in the CENTRAL database. CENTRAL contains specialized registers of citations submitted by Cochrane groups and other organizations from many journals and other sources that are not included in MEDLINE. Potential records from CENTRAL are assessed with quality control procedures to ensure that only reports of definite randomized controlled trials or controlled clinical trials are included.

Just to make sure that you did not miss any important studies on coated catheters, you go on the Internet and pull up the clinical query option for PubMed. You pick the therapy category, select the "sensitivity" search option, and then type "impregnated central venous catheters" in the search window. You retrieve 23 citations, several of which look relevant including the already seen systematic review by Mermel (5) and the cost-effectiveness study by Veenstra et al. (6).

Another method for effective clinical-based searching is to search only for articles that are clinical trials. For an article to be indexed with the publication type "clinical trial," it must be a "preplanned, usually controlled clinical study of the efficacy, safety, or optimum dosage schedule of one or more therapeutic, diagnostic, or prophylactic drugs, devices, or techniques in humans selected according to predetermined criteria of eligibility and observed for predefined evidence of favorable and unfavorable effects" (8). The citations you retrieve using the clinical query feature in PubMed or the publication type "clinical trial" are more likely to be ready for clinical application and to help you make an informed patient-care decision than if you had not included any methodologic filtering in your search strategy.

The previous scenario illustrates a search for quality-filtered prevention literature. Reports of applied clinical research have two features in common: they are designed in advance to follow a study protocol and they are comparative. Criteria exist for studies from each of the four categories of therapy and prevention, diagnosis, etiology and causation, and prognosis and natural history, as well as economic evaluations, decision analysis, quality of life, clinical utilization, reviews, guidelines, clinical prediction, and qualitative studies (9).

Searching on the Internet is another route to take to help solve patient problems. However, only a small proportion of the content has been peer reviewed or provides enough information so that you can do your own evaluation on the material found. One of the most effective, and certainly the most used, search engines is Google *(http://www.google.com/)*. No single search engine searches more than 30% to 40% of the current Web content, so a variety of search approaches may be warranted for comprehensive Internet searching. Google's search function lets you type in words or concepts of interest and then retrieves Web sites that contain these terms ranked in the order of how many other sites have linked to the original site—sort of a quality indicator. Typing in the very specific phrase "intravascular catheter infections prevention" provided access to 3,030 Web pages in 0.14 seconds. The first two link to the U.S. Centers for Disease Control and Prevention (CDC) "2002 Guidelines for the Prevention of Intravascular Catheter-Related Infections" (10). This 36-page guideline includes an analysis of previous studies and cites both the Mermel and Veenstra et al. studies along with many original studies. O'Grady et al. (10) stated that although the coated catheters are more expensive, they reduce infections and costs. All the evidence found to date seems to support the added initial expense of the coated catheters.

Another approach to searching the Internet is to use one of the new question-answering systems (e.g., AskJeeves at *www.ask.com* or AnswerBus at *http://www.coli.uni-sb.de/~zheng/answerbus/*). Asking Jeeves "How do I prevent intravascular infections?" produced links to both U.S. and Canadian guidelines. The AnswerBus did not provide links to any site.

KEEPING UP WITH THE MEDICAL LITERATURE

Health professionals typically rate journal reading as their preferred means of keeping current, but more than 15 years ago, Covell et al. (11) demonstrated that this was highly overrated as a method for keeping up-to-date. Journal reading is still recommended for keeping up-to-date but with a "critical appraisal" approach, so that a reader quickly and systematically detects the original studies and reviews that are more likely to be useful to his or her practice (12). The medical literature has continued to grow at an increasing rate since the mid-1980s, so the challenge of keeping up-to-date might be considered greater than ever. However, substantial improvements have occurred in information processing as well to compensate somewhat for the increased amount of publication.

We consider the journal literature first. Publishing in peer-reviewed print journals is still the most common form of spreading the word about advances in medicine, although this may change with the advent of on-line journals. *ACP Journal Club,* a bimonthly publication of the ACP, contains 25 structured abstracts and accompanying commentaries of original studies and systematic reviews of interest to general internal medicine, including infectious diseases. The articles, both original studies and systematic reviews, are selected from approximately 115 journals according to explicit rules of sound methodology and pertain to the treatment or prevention, diagnosis, prognosis, or etiology of disease (13). Also included are sound studies of clinical prediction, economics, differential diagnosis, and quality improvement. Following our clinical example, studies and reviews of catheter infections and their prevention have appeared several times a year in *ACP Journal Club* and include the Mermel and Veenstra et al. articles (5,6).

Evidence-Based Nursing is a quarterly journal published by the BMJ Publishing Group that aims to bring high quality studies and reviews to the attention of nurses attempting to keep pace with important advances in their profession. It follows a production procedure similar to that of *ACP Journal Club. Evidence-Based Medicine,* also published by the BMJ Publishing Group and aimed at primary care physicians, abstracts studies in family medicine, pediatrics, surgery, psychiatry and psychology, and obstetrics and gynecology, in addition to internal medicine. The abstracts for these journals are prepared by research staff with methodologic expertise and report enough information about the methods of the studies that readers can judge for themselves the strength of the research and the applicability of the findings to their own patients.

Furthermore, in many instances, additional numerical results not provided in the original article are obtained or calculated and included in the abstract, such as relative risk reductions, confidence intervals, and numbers needed to treat to prevent a bad outcome or achieve a good outcome. The abstracts and commentaries have several steps in the production process to ensure their accuracy (13). *ACP Journal Club, Evidence-Based Nursing,*, and *Evidence-Based Medicine* are also available on the Web sites of their respective publishers (*http://www.acpjc.org/, http://ebn.bmjjournals.com/*, and *http://ebm.bmjjournals.com/*). *ACP Journal Club* is also available on Ovid in the "Evidence-Based Medicine Reviews."

MEDLINE can also be used to keep up to date, because it is updated frequently: weekly for most on-line or Internet versions and daily in the PubMed system. Searchers can thus run frequent broad-based searches to obtain the most recent citations on a topic they want to follow. "Catheter infection" might be a useful search to run weekly if one wanted to keep current with all the research on the topic. For example, on January 13, 2003 we ran this search and found another relevant guideline that had been entered into the MEDLINE system on January 9, 2003 (14).

Most healthcare organizations have a "Web presence" and many have current awareness features that one can tap into to keep up to date. The Web site for the Society for Healthcare Epidemiology of America, Inc. (SHEA) *(www.shea-online.org)* is a good starting point for Web searching because it provides a page of links to other infection control sites including government (state, national, and international), other organizations, and related information resources. Furthermore, many of the various organizations have e-mail discussion lists (listservs) that one can join to receive and participate in correspondence on topics of interest. One should note that these discussion lists are anecdotal in nature and are simply exchanges of opinions among health professionals. It is up to the reader to judge the validity of individual comments.

The CDC Web site *(www.cdc.gov)* provides a wide array of documents including the CDC prevention guidelines, the *Morbidity and Mortality Weekly Reports,* and links to many other health resources, both within the United States, including the state departments of health services, and worldwide. The CDC Web site allows searches using boolean logic in an advanced search mode (and's and or's), so that a searcher can combine words to expand or pinpoint retrieval.

For keeping up to date, one can subscribe to a CDC mailing list and receive only the tables of contents or the entire documents for such items as the *Journal of Emerging Infectious Diseases,* human immunodeficiency virus (HIV)/acquired immunodeficiency syndrome publications, and *Morbidity and Mortality Weekly Report.* The Division of Healthcare Quality Promotion provides information on the prevention and control of nosocomial infections *(http://www.cdc.gov/ncidod/hip).* It has guidelines, recommendations, and answers to frequently asked questions on topics such as outbreaks, occupational exposure to HIV, needlestick injuries, and child care. Of note is their "2002 Guideline for Prevention of Intravascular Catheter-Related Infections" *(http://www.cdc.gov/ncidod/hip/IV/IV.HTM)* already identified in our Internet search. The CDC Web site also indicates which documents have recently been added and which are expected soon. It ranks its top challenge as reducing catheter-associated adverse events by 50% among patients in healthcare settings.

The Web site for the Hospital Infection Society *(http://www.his.org.uk)* in the United Kingdom includes the abstracts of articles in the *Journal of Hospital Infection,* lists future scientific meetings, and has an e-mail discussion list. The Web site for the Faculty of Medicine at Université Catholique de Louvain in Brussels *(http://www.md.ucl.ac.be/entites/esp/hosp/infcon.htm)* has a database of many hundreds of selected articles with abstracts in the area of infection control that is updated quarterly. It also links to journals on infection control and hospital epidemiology for scanning tables of contents to identify potentially relevant citations.

The Association for Professionals in Infection Control and Epidemiology (APIC) has a Web site *(http://www.apic.org)* that updates professionals about courses and educational activities, upcoming conferences, and publications (such as the APIC Text of Infection Control) that can be ordered from the Internet. Professional resources provided on the APIC Web site include a discussion forum in which infection control professionals can discuss issues with each other; find or list job postings; and access a resource list, a searchable abstract database, and an open e-mail list server.

The Program for Monitoring Emerging Diseases (ProMED) *(www.fas.org/promed)* is a free electronic conferencing system formed by the Federation of American Scientists to create a global system of early detection and response to disease outbreaks. It also has a search engine for archived e-mail correspondence.

Individual clinicians can keep in touch with a variety of health organizations through Web sites as an increasing number of organizations post their latest information on the Internet. By subscribing to some of the many list servers and discussion lists of the aforementioned organizations, one can participate in real time discussions on topics of interest, and current information such as the latest journal contents or knowledge of outbreaks comes automatically. Unfortunately, for most of these services, one will need to do an assessment of the validity and relevance of the information. The relevance check is pretty easy, but checking the sources for scientific merit requires skill and time.

Several of the aforementioned resources are now available in a format for the latest in computer gadgetry: the handheld or PDA. PDAs have been embraced by many in the medical community, because they can store surprisingly large amounts of information and can be used in any location by virtue of their small size and portability (15,16). Many sources of information exist for clinicians interested in PDAs and one such site is Evidence-Based Medicine Tools for the PDA *(http://www.ils.unc.edu/~caham/ebmtools/ebmtools.html).* Categories of applications and services include drug information (especially ePocrates *http://www.epocrates.com/*), news and abstracting services, healthcare literature summaries and full text, guidelines and summaries, textbook information, diagnostic aids, statistical and numerical calculators, and clinical prediction guides. A listing of available resources in this chapter would not be very helpful because of the rapid rate of change, so we urge those who are interested in acquiring a PDA to consult peers and use the Internet to learn about and acquire clinical resources for downloading.

SETTING CLINICAL POLICY

Clinical practice guidelines have metamorphosed from their first appearance on the healthcare stage, as small local health plans or care maps developed to reduce variability in care, into a healthcare industry. Practice guidelines have become ubiquitous and are promoted for a number of reasons, including improving the quality of healthcare, optimizing patient outcomes, discouraging the use of ineffective or harmful interventions, improving the consistency of care, identifying gaps in evidence, helping to balance costs and outcomes, or simply cutting costs. Clinical practice guidelines for screening, diagnosis, prevention, and treatment are produced by diverse organizations, from government departments (such as the U.S. Agency for Healthcare Research and Quality or the CDC), healthcare associations and specialty societies (such as the American College of Physicians, the Society for Healthcare Epidemiology of America, and the Infectious Disease Society of America), and local hospitals. The definition from the Institute of Medicine in 1990 (17) still applies, however, at all levels: "Practice guidelines are systematically developed statements to assist practitioner and patient decisions about appropriate healthcare for specific clinical circumstances." Three useful Internet sites that list guidelines are the National Guideline Clearinghouse *(http://www.guideline.gov/index.asp)*, Agency for Healthcare Research and Quality *(http://www.ahcpr.gov/clinic/cpgsix.htm)*, and the Canadian Medical Association *(http://www.cma.ca/cma/common/displayPopup.do?tab=422&skin=125&pMenuId=4)*. The first site, the U.S. National Guideline Clearinghouse, is a valuable site for access to almost any local, regional, national, or international guideline. It not only lists guidelines and provides access to the full text of many but also has the capability of comparing two guidelines in a tabular format.

Infection control is particularly suited to the use of clinical practice guidelines. If based on sound current evidence, guidelines can greatly reduce the amount of work of infection control specialists in searching the literature. Guidelines published in the journal literature are searchable in MEDLINE by using the publication type field "guideline" for administrative procedural guidelines and "practice guideline" for specific healthcare guidelines. The Internet is also an excellent source in which to locate guidelines, particularly because the entire document is usually posted on the Web site, whereas in MEDLINE only the citation and possibly the abstract to the document is available. The Future Health Care Web site *(http://www.futurehealthcare.com/pages/guidetobestpractices.htm)* is particularly useful for helping to define "best practices" for quality assurance activities (18).

We have already identified a recent and relevant clinical practice guideline on our intravascular coated catheters (10) so we will identify any more, although several less recent ones exist.

CONCLUSIONS

To conclude our clinical scenario, you give your administrator the data you find. She is duly impressed with your evidence that the more expensive coated catheters are actually saving the hospital money and reducing infections. She thanks you and as you return to your office and mentally review your information trek. You wonder if this is just the first of many such evidence assessments you will be asked to perform.

Persons involved with hospital epidemiology and infection control have many diverse information needs that include medical and other health-related clinical materials, basic science information, management and educational resources, and policy documents from regional and national agencies. Today, clinicians are working in a rapidly changing environment with new discoveries, scarce resources, and new challenges presented by the changing model of healthcare delivery, multiresistant microorganisms, emerging pathogens, and outbreak detection. To succeed, one must develop rapid and efficient ways of acquiring new relevant information. By investing time in experimenting with the different resources available, one will be able to develop an individual strategy for dealing with new clinical problems, keeping up-to-date, and effectively implementing new policies. Clinicians are indeed fortunate that as the need for information increases, the means for acquiring it continue to evolve and improve.

REFERENCES

1. Sackett DL, Straus SE, Richardson WS, et al. *Evidence-based medicine: how to practice & teach EBM,* 2nd ed. Edinburgh: Churchill Livingstone, 2000.
2. Richardson WS, Wilson MC. Textbook descriptions of disease—where's the beef? [editorial]. *ACP J Club* 2002 Jul–Aug;137: A11–A15.
3. Haynes RB, Wilczynski N, McKibbon KA, et al. Developing optimal search strategies for detecting clinically sound studies in MEDLINE. *J Am Med Inform Assoc* 1994;1:447–458.
4. Wilczynski NL, Haynes RB. Robustness of empirical search strategies for clinical content in MEDLINE. *Proc AMIA Symp* 2002;904–908.
5. Mermel LA. Prevention of intravascular catheter-related infections. *Ann Intern Med* 2000;132:391–402.
6. Veenstra DL, Saint S, Sullivan SD. Cost-effectiveness of antiseptic-impregnated central venous catheters for the prevention of catheter-related bloodstream infection. *JAMA* 1999;282:554–560.
7. Barrington KJ. Umbilical artery catheters in the newborn: effects of catheter materials. Cochrane Review [updated 18 Nov 1998]. In: *The Cochrane library.* Oxford: Update Software.
8. National Library of Medicine. Medical Subject Headings, Annotated Alphabetic List. 1998. Distributed by the National Technical Information Service, U.S. Department of Commerce. PB98-964801.
9. Guyatt G, Rennie D, eds. The Evidence-Based Medicine Working Group. *Users' guides to the medical literature: a manual for evidence-based clinical practice.* Chicago, 2002.
10. O'Grady NP, Alexander M, Dellinger EP, et al. Guidelines for the prevention of intravascular catheter-related infections, 2002. *MMWR Morb Mortal Wkly Rep* 2002;51:RR-10 available at *http://www.cdc.gov/ncidod/hip/IV/IV.HTM* (accessed).
11. Covell D, Uman G, Manning P. Information needs of office practice: are they being met? *Ann Intern Med* 1985;103:596–599.
12. Sackett DL, Haynes RB, Guyatt GH, et al. *Clinical epidemiology: a basic science for clinical medicine,* 2nd ed. Boston: Little, Brown and Company, 1991.
13. Sackett DL, Haynes RB. 13 steps, 100 people, and 1,000,000 thanks [editorial]. *ACP J Club* 1997 Jul–Aug;127:A14.
14. O'Grady NP, Alexander M, Dellinger EP, et al. Guidelines for the prevention of intravascular catheter-related infections. *Infect Control Hosp Epidemiol* 2002;23:759–769.
15. Richardson WS, Durdette SD. Practice corner: taking evidence in hand [editorial]. *ACP J Club* 2003 Jan–Feb;138:A12.
16. Rao G. Introduction of handheld computing to a family practice residency program. *J Am Board Fam Med* 2002;15:118–122.
17. Field MJ, Lohr KN. *Clinical practice guidelines.* Washington, DC: National Academy Press, 1990.
18. Kibbe DC, Smith PP, LaVallee R, et al. A guide to finding and evaluating best practices health care information on the Internet: the truth is out there? *Jt Comm J Qual Improv* 1997;23:678–689.

93

A METHODOLOGICALLY FOCUSED REVIEW OF THE LITERATURE IN HOSPITAL EPIDEMIOLOGY AND INFECTION CONTROL

MATTHEW SAMORE
STEPHAN HARBARTH

The use of appropriate epidemiologic methods in experimental design and data analysis is recognized as an important aspect of generating sound scientific evidence. This chapter discusses methodologies relevant to epidemiologic, outcome, and intervention studies, as they are applied to problems of healthcare-associated infections. We stress common pitfalls and focus particularly on limitations of the published literature in hospital epidemiology.

Although many of the basic ideas of hospital epidemiology can be traced back to Semmelweis (1), the formal application of epidemiologic methods in infection control received a substantial boost during the 1970s and 1980s, with the publication of a number of methodologically oriented articles that brought innovation to the field (2–7). These influential, seminal articles covered topics such as the relationship between prevalence and incidence, matched cohort study design, confounding, and effect modification. Based on the assumption that nosocomial infections have causal and preventive factors that can be identified through systematic investigation, these articles demonstrated convincingly that epidemiologic methods add important knowledge to reduce the rates of hospital-acquired infections. Thus, the conceptual framework was laid for many interventional and observational studies in the field.

This chapter elaborates on this seminal body of work and brings to the readers' attention newer methodologies and principles. Recent advances in the conceptual underpinnings of epidemiology and selection of statistical models that facilitate causal inference may not have garnered widespread attention by infection control professionals and hospital epidemiologists. Using selected articles as examples, the quality of methods in the infection control literature is discussed and opportunities for improvement are highlighted. By necessity, our review of articles and choice of topics is selective. The criticisms and suggestions, which complement the information presented in Chapters 1 to 4, are intended to be constructive. Some of our arguments may even challenge conventional wisdom, and in the process stimulate a fresh perspective on the literature in infection control and hospital epidemiology.

The chapter is organized into five sections, based on specific recommendations for improving the quality of observational research in infection control and translating that research into action:

1. Use terminology clearly and precisely.
2. Search for and destroy confounding (as much as possible).
3. Recognize selection bias in all of its guises.
4. Account for timing of exposures and time at risk.
5. Develop guidelines according to explicit rules.

RECOMMENDATION 1: USE TERMINOLOGY CLEARLY AND PRECISELY

Fundamental to scientific reasoning is the correct use of terminology. Several expressions used in hospital epidemiology are misnomers, well embedded in everyday use. Table 93.1 summarizes several commonly misused terms and suggests more accurate terms.

Confusion in Classification of Study Design and Use of Terms *Case* and *Control*

Misnomers regarding terminology appear to be particularly common in conjunction with studies that examine outcomes of infections and other adverse events. If patients with a nosocomial infection are being compared to patients without nosocomial infection with respect to an outcome such as length of stay, mortality, or medical costs, a *cohort study* is being conducted, assuming that patients are selected on the basis of the presence or absence of infection. The infection constitutes the exposure. Similarly, studies in which outcomes of patients with a resistant microorganism are compared to outcomes of patients with the susceptible form of the microorganism are following a cohort design. If exposed and nonexposed subjects are matched on other criteria, such as age and severity of illness, the study is a *matched cohort study.* The distinction between matched cohort and

TABLE 93.1. TERMINOLOGY: COMMONLY USED PROBLEMATIC AND AMBIGUOUS TERMS

Commonly Used Name	More Appropriate Term	Explanation
Prevalence rate	Prevalence or prevalence proportion	Prevalence is the proportion of a specified population with a condition or disease at a defined point in time. A rate is the magnitude of change of one entity divided by another entity. Rates have different units in the numerator and denominator. *Prevalence rate* is an example of a term in which the word *rate* is used inappropriately to mean proportion.
Matched case-control study	Matched cohort study	Retrospective studies assessing the impact of nosocomial infections are comparing outcomes (deaths, costs) as the principal study measurement. Since the exposure is known (presence or absence of an infection) and the outcome unknown, it's a cohort study by definition.
Mortality rate	Case-fatality proportion or fraction	*Mortality rate* is often used as a synonym for the incidence proportion of deaths in a study cohort due to the disease of interest. Similar to the term *prevalence rate*, it would be more accurate to use the terms *case-fatality proportion* or *case-fatality fraction*.
Attributable fraction	Excess fraction	If the term *attributable fraction* is taken to mean the fraction of disease (or deaths) in which exposure was a contributory cause of disease, strong biologic assumptions are required. To avoid this problem, the term *excess fraction* is preferred.

matched case-control studies is not just a semantic one. In a matched case-control study, it is necessary to perform a matched analysis if the matching factors are associated with exposure, even if they are not associated with the outcome, whereas in a matched cohort study this requirement does not exist (8).

Abundant examples exist in which the terms *case* and *control* are used in the context of a matched cohort study, leading to confusion about the study design (9,10). For instance, a recent study (10) about the "attributable mortality rate" of bacteremia due to methicillin-resistant *Staphylococcus aureus* (MRSA) claimed to perform a "retrospective cohort analysis and two independent case-control analyses." As outlined above, this terminology is incorrect, since in all three analyses outcomes were compared and thus the term *matched cohort studies* would have been more appropriate.

Multiple Meanings of the Term *Attributable*

Perhaps nowhere is terminology in hospital epidemiology more confusing than in the use of the word *attributable* (11–13). This word is included in a myriad of epidemiologic terms with meanings that vary widely. The dictionary definition of *attributable* is "ascribed to" and, in epidemiology, it is frequently taken to be synonymous with "caused by." However, there are two types of causation that often are not distinguished. During a defined follow-up period, an exposure may either shorten the interval to occurrence of disease or cause a disease case to occur that otherwise would not have occurred (14). The former is an accelerated disease case, whereas the latter is an excess case. If exposure prevents disease, this may be restated to indicate that exposure either lengthens the interval to occurrence of disease or averts a case from happening that otherwise would have occurred.

The rationale for constructing formulas to measure the *attributable fraction* is that not all disease in exposed patients is necessarily due to exposure: some exposed individuals would have developed disease, even at the same time, if they had not been exposed. It is also evident that the ratio of exposed patients belonging to these two causal types, accelerated or excess cases, depends on the duration of the follow-up. It can be shown that, compared to the enumeration of excess cases, deriving an estimate of the number of accelerated cases relies on additional, more tenuous assumptions about the form of the causal relationship between exposure and disease. Hence, rather than attempting to estimate the fraction of exposed cases that are caused by exposure, it is generally preferred to restrict attention to excess cases. The occurrence of excess cases can be estimated by simply comparing the incidence proportion in exposed individuals to the incidence proportion in nonexposed individuals, assuming that confounding is absent. Due to these considerations, Greenland and Robins (15,16) recommend use of the term *excess fraction* in place of *attributable fraction* when the objective is to quantify the fraction of exposed cases that are excess cases caused by exposure (15,16). They reserve the term *etiologic fraction* to indicate the proportion of exposed cases caused by exposure, including both types of causation. The *population excess fraction* is an estimate of the fraction of all cases in the population that are excess cases due to exposure. The set of terms that cover these concepts are referred to as the family of *attributable fractions* (15,17).

RECOMMENDATION 2: SEARCH FOR AND DESTROY CONFOUNDING

This section discusses the central challenge in epidemiology, namely, how to reduce confounding. Informative examples from the published literature that have relevance to key aspects of the problem of confounding have been selected for pedagogic purposes. Prior to evaluating the quality of the methods used in these investigations, we provide an in-depth explanation of why confounding is important and how it arises. There are four research questions covered by the articles, reworded here to be as explicit as possible:

1. Does prolonged postoperative antimicrobial use increase the risk of nosocomial bloodstream infection compared to short postoperative antimicrobial prophylaxis?

2. How much does inadequate antimicrobial treatment of bloodstream infection in critically ill patients heighten the risk of death compared to adequate antimicrobial treatment?
3. Among patients with bloodstream infections due to *Staphylococcus aureus*, does methicillin-resistance increase the risk of mortality compared to methicillin-susceptible infection?
4. Does perioperative antimicrobial prophylaxis decrease the risk of wound infection after clean surgery compared to no prophylaxis?

Background

The surgeon who explains that the reason her patients have a higher infection rate is that she operates on sicker patients demonstrates an informal grasp of the concept of confounding. However, when it is necessary to conduct and analyze an epidemiologic investigation, this intuitive understanding of confounding reveals its limitations. We begin by offering two core principles that may run somewhat counter to conventional wisdom:

1. It is not possible to use *statistical criteria alone* to recognize confounding, or determine whether it has been removed.
2. Confounding is identifiable only in the context of a *causal model* (18–20).

Confounding is present when there is discordance between the *true causal effect* of an exposure on disease or other outcome in a target population and the *measured association* between exposure and disease (21). Thus, an exploration of confounding starts with an exposition on causation. What is meant by *true causal effect*?

Causation is best understood in terms of the question, What would have happened if the exposure had not occurred? Stated another way, the causal effect of exposure in exposed individuals is represented by the difference between their actual disease status and what would have happened if everything else had been the same up until the time of exposure, but that they had then not been exposed or exposed to a different degree (21). Under this formulation, causation is defined on the basis of a comparison between outcomes under mutually exclusive conditions, exposed and unexposed or, alternatively, varied levels of exposure. However, in any single patient, only one of these conditions is observed. In the absence of time machines to replay experience under dissimilar exposure conditions, a straightforward way to directly measure causal effects is not available. When exposure is randomly allocated, it is possible to derive an estimate of the unconfounded, average causal effect of exposure, with a random error correlated with sample size. In the absence of random allocation of exposure, causal inference relies on untestable beliefs regarding causal relationships and unmeasured confounders (22).

It is useful to depict assumptions about causal relationships in a graphical format to identify potential sources of confounding. The causal effects of exposure on disease may be visualized as arrows aiming from exposure to disease (Fig. 93.1). These arrows represent the postulated causal mechanisms or pathways by which exposure affects the outcome or disease. Causal pathways that link exposure (E) and disease (D) may be direct or indirect. An indirect pathway is characterized by the presence of an "intermediate variable" (I) that mediates a causal effect, whereas a direct effect lacks an intermediate variable (23). The causal null hypothesis is the assumption that there are no indirect or direct causal pathways pointing from exposure to disease. Graphical representations of causal relationships are called *directed acyclic graphs* (DAGs) (18,24–26).

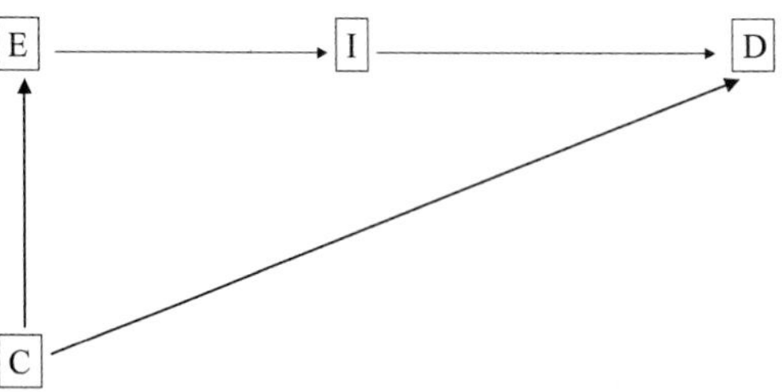

Figure 93.1. Graphical representation of causal relationships illustrated by *directed acyclic graphs* (DAGs). An exposure (E) has both direct and indirect effects on disease (D). The indirect effects are mediated by an intermediate variable (I). A confounding factor (C) is a cause of both the exposure (E) and the disease (D).

Confounding arises when direct or indirect causes of exposure are also direct or indirect causes of disease status. When exposure is a type of treatment and confounding is due to factors that influence treatment selection, the term *confounding by indication* is sometimes used (27). Causes of exposure can be visualized as arrows pointing toward exposure. If these inputs into exposure also have outputs connecting to disease through paths that do not include exposure, noncausal pathways from exposure to disease exist. The labeling of a pathway as noncausal is done from the perspective of exposure and disease. If research questions pertain to multiple exposures, the postulated connections between each factor of interest and disease may, in turn, be divided into causal or noncausal pathways. Noncausal pathways create an association between exposure and disease, one that is not a consequence of exposure, hence the need to block the noncausal pathways if the goal is to estimate the true causal effects of exposure. Factors located within these noncausal pathways are usually associated both with exposure and disease, although in any given study these associations may themselves be obscured by confounding, and therefore not manifested (21,28).

Successful randomization eliminates confounding by breaking the causal inputs into exposure or treatment. It makes the exposure or treatment actually received independent of what would have happened had exposure been absent or altered. This principle, which is surprisingly difficult to grasp, is another way to define the absence of confounding. The goal of epidemiology is to attempt to accomplish this feat with respect to measured confounders, using appropriate design and analytic strategies (28).

Perhaps what poses the most difficulty to individuals conducting epidemiologic research and readers of the literature is the myriad of statistical techniques available to analyze data. These statistical methods are not reviewed in detail here. Detailed recommendations for conducting methodologically sound multivariable analyses of observational studies have been summarized elsewhere (29–31). Rather, our goal is to emphasize the distinction between the statistical evaluation of association and the identification of confounding. Contrary to widespread belief, the *p*-value is not a useful test of confounding. Even the comparison of crude and adjusted measures of association is an inadequate approach by itself to detect confounding. Depending on the causal model, the adjusted measure of association may be more or less confounded than the crude measure. The judgment of whether an adjusted association is less confounded than a crude association relies on assumptions about the causal relationships between exposure, outcome, and the adjustment variables (25).

Example 1: Prolonged Antimicrobial Prophylaxis

The first step toward reducing confounding in observational research on causal effects is to recognize its potential existence and to obtain measurements on potential confounders or to account for potential confounding during the design phase of the study. Sometimes these initial steps are omitted, as the following example illustrates.

Many investigators have examined the effect of antimicrobials on subsequent occurrence of infection. Under certain conditions, systemic antibiotic use may decrease the risk of nosocomial infection. For instance, this has been demonstrated in clinical trials of nosocomial pneumonia in ventilated patients (32–34). An opposite effect of antimicrobial prophylaxis was suggested in a study that found that duration of antimicrobial prophylaxis after major surgery was associated with a significantly increased risk of nosocomial bloodstream infection (BSI) (35). The authors of this study observed six cases of BSI among 180 patients receiving short antibiotic prophylaxis, compared with 16 cases of BSI in 94 patients with extended antibiotic prophylaxis [crude odds ratio (OR), 5.9]. These results were presented without any consideration of the possibility of confounding.

In an observational study we conducted of the relationship between duration of antimicrobial prophylaxis and infections (36), we also found a strong association between prolonged antibiotic prophylaxis and subsequent nosocomial BSI in the crude analysis. A total of 2,641 patients undergoing cardiac surgery were included in the study, divided into those in whom antimicrobial prophylaxis was short (<48 hours) and those in whom antibiotic prophylaxis was prolonged (>48 hours) (36). The unadjusted analysis revealed an odds ratio of 3.3, based on the occurrence of 27 cases of nosocomial BSI (1.8%) after 1,478 procedures using short antibiotic prophylaxis compared with 65 cases of nosocomial BSI (5.7%) after 1,139 operations with prolonged antibiotic prophylaxis. The problem with this crude analysis was that length of follow-up and intensive care unit (ICU) stay affected the likelihood of receiving prolonged antimicrobial prophylaxis.

Using survival analysis methods removed confounding related to differences in length of follow-up; the apparent association appeared smaller [hazard ratio (HR), 1.7] based on Cox proportional hazards regression. Seventy-seven percent of cases of nosocomial BSI occurred in patients who stayed more than 4 days in the ICU. Similarly, extended antibiotic prophylaxis was correlated with longer ICU stay. After stratifying for length of ICU stay, prolonged antibiotic prophylaxis was not associated with a significantly increased risk of BSI (HR, 1.4). In an additional analysis, we showed that prolonged antibiotic prophylaxis did not decrease the incidence of surgical site infection; however, it increased the risk of isolation of resistant gram-negative bacteria and vancomycin-resistant enterococci (37). In summary, these results demonstrate confounding of the crude association between prolonged antibiotic prophylaxis and nosocomial BSI by differences in follow-up and length of ICU stay (36).

Example 2: Inadequate Antimicrobial Therapy

More often, investigators do attempt to address confounding, but use analytic methods that are suboptimal. A common error is to identify confounders primarily on the basis of the statistical significance of the association between the outcome and potential confounders. This tactic is inappropriate when the purpose of the regression model is to estimate the magnitude of the causal effect of an exposure on an outcome.

As an example, consider studies that have examined the impact of inadequate antimicrobial treatment of infection on patient outcomes (38–43). This is a research question that is not amenable to direct testing in a randomized trial, since it would be unethical to willingly expose patients to inappropriate treatment. To answer the question, therefore, we have to rely on observational studies. On the face of it, it is highly likely that inadequate antimicrobial therapy does have some negative effect on outcome in critically ill patients. The key objective of an observational study, then, is to remove as much of the confounding as possible so as to obtain an unbiased estimate of the magnitude of effect of inadequate therapy. In one such widely cited study of patients in the ICU with BSI, therapy was defined as inadequate if the antimicrobials being given to the patient were ineffective against the causative pathogen at the time that identification and susceptibility results were reported by the clinical microbiologic laboratory (44). The crude relative risk for mortality after inadequate therapy compared to adequate therapy equaled 2.2, corresponding to a crude odds ratio of 4.1 (44). The "adjusted" effect estimate of inadequate antimicrobial treatment of BSI on hospital mortality had an odds ratio of 6.9, after including use of vasopressors, age, organ dysfunctions, and severity of illness, along with inadequate therapy, in a multivariable logistic regression model.

A major limitation with this analysis was that the factors included in the logistic regression model were only those found to be significantly associated with mortality. A stepwise variable selection approach was used, with a *p*-value of .05 as the limit for the acceptance or removal of new terms. The problem is that this method does not remove confounding by factors not selected into the model. Many characteristics were identified that distinguished patients with inappropriate and appropriate antimicrobial use, such as time in the hospital prior to BSI, prior use of antimicrobials, and serum albumin. Presumably, these were factors that directly or indirectly influenced the probability that treatment was inadequate or were proxies for such factors. Some of these factors were also associated with the outcome, but not always to a statistically significant degree. Not including these factors in the model likely contributed to an exaggerated estimate of effect (44).

All observational research is limited by the possibility of residual confounding due to unmeasured variables, but given a postulated causal model and a set of measured variables, some analytic strategies are less prone to confounding than others (25,45). The key point is that confounders do not have to be statistically significantly associated with the outcome to be confounders. As stated in the background section, the results of statistical hypothesis testing are tangential to the recognition of confounding. To some extent, the notion that confounders should be significantly associated with the outcome reflects the belief that the only "true" associations are ones that are statistically significant. Instead of focusing on statistical significance, the analysis should be directed toward a careful consideration of the potential sources of confounding and deriving the least biased estimate of the true causal effect.

A frequently overlooked problem with conventional regression models is that they impose assumptions regarding the form of the relationship between the additional model factors and the outcome, and between these additional factors and the exposure, which, if incorrect, may increase confounding (31). The association parameter derived from the regression model provides an estimate of the unconfounded causal effect of exposure only when all of the assumptions of the multivariable model are correct. In addition, automated variable selection methods completely ignore the relationship between the putative confounders and the exposure. If the factors selected into the model are affected by exposure, their inclusion may also be deleterious with respect to confounding. This problem is discussed in more detail below.

Traditional stratification methods have an advantage over regression models because they involve fewer assumptions, but they lead to sparse numbers within strata when multiple confounders are present (46). Newer analytic strategies have been developed that overcome some of these types of problems and allow improved causal inference. These more robust methods start with specification of the exposure of interest and build on an explicit structural model of causal relationships (45,47). Another recent advance in epidemiology is the use of simulation to increase the flexibility of sensitivity analyses of confounding and other types of bias (48,49).

One analytic method that has gained widespread application is the use of propensity scores, particularly for point exposures that are dichotomous or categorical (50). The propensity score is the probability of exposure or treatment based on factors that influence treatment, and thus lies between 0 and 1 (51,52). A multivariable logistic regression model is typically used to estimate this probability and, most commonly, the propensity score is used as either a matching or stratification variable to remove confounding by indication due to measured factors (53). The propensity score method relies on assumptions about the form of the relationship between the confounder and exposure but is less susceptible than traditional models to bias by misspecification of the relationship between the confounders and the outcome (54).

Example 3: Excess Mortality Due to MRSA Bloodstream Infection

Including a variable for adjustment sometimes increases confounding rather than reduces it. This happens when the adjuster is a consequence of the exposure of the interest, and either lies on one of the causal paths between exposure and the outcome or also is an effect of the outcome (26).

A number of investigators have compared outcomes in patients with resistant and susceptible infection (10,55,56). In such studies, it is especially crucial to precisely specify the causal hypothesis of interest. Often, it pertains to the virulence of the microorganism: Do infections due to the resistant form of the microorganism have worse, similar, or better outcomes than infections due to the susceptible form of the microorganism? One such study measured mortality following BSI, comparing infections due to MRSA and to methicillin-susceptible *S. aureus* (57). One of the control variables included in the logistic regression model was the presence of shock, presumably measured at the time of detection of BSI. The problem is that one path by which methicillin-resistance may raise the mortality rate is by increasing the risk of shock. Controlling for shock produces bias in the estimate of effect of methicillin-resistance toward the null by blocking one of the causal pathways linking the exposure and outcome. More suitable adjusters would be measures of severity of illness, such as APACHE score, taken prior to onset of symptoms and signs of infection.

On the other hand, if the study goals were to address the question whether inadequate therapy of methicillin resistance caused an increase in mortality compared to adequate therapy of methicillin-resistant or methicillin-susceptible infection, shock at the time of detection of infection, prior to initiation of therapy, would be an appropriate adjuster. In this situation, shock is no longer causally downstream of the exposure of interest.

Example 4: Antimicrobial Prophylaxis in Clean Surgery

The final example is of a publication in which confounding was addressed in an appropriate fashion (58). The purpose of the study was to evaluate the effect of antimicrobial prophylaxis on surgical site infection after clean surgery. Control variables included in the analysis were factors that possibly influenced both the decision to prescribe antibiotic prophylaxis and the outcome of interest (surgical site infection in clean surgery). The observational study, of patients undergoing herniorrhaphy or selected breast surgery procedures, was done in conjunction with a randomized clinical trial of perioperative prophylaxis (59). Patients were included in the observational cohort if they did not participate in the clinical trial. Thirty-four percent of patients (1,077/3,202) received prophylaxis at the discretion of the surgeon; 86 surgical site infections (2.7%) were identified. The unadjusted odds ratio for infection comparing prophylaxis recipients with nonrecipients was 0.85 (26/1,077 vs. 60/2,125). The odds ratio after adjustment for duration of surgery and type of procedure was substantially lower, at 0.59, indicating a 41% reduction in the odds of surgical site infection following prophylaxis. Additional adjustment for age, body mass index, the presence of drains, diabetes, and exposure to corticosteroids did not change the magnitude of this effect meaningfully. The conclusion of the investigators was that the clinical criteria individual surgeons were using to decide which patients should receive prophylaxis were successfully targeting patients within the clean surgery group who were at higher risk for infection. Thus, this study confirmed results from the randomized study (59), and showed that after correct adjustment for confounders, prophylactic antibiotics were beneficial in the nonrandomized patients.

RECOMMENDATION 3: RECOGNIZE SELECTION BIAS IN ALL OF ITS GUISES

Selection bias occurs when the selection of study subjects induces a noncausal association between exposure and disease. Thus, the end result is similar to confounding: it leads to distortion of the measured association between exposure and disease away from the true causal effect (60,61).

For a variety of reasons, selection bias tends to be more common in case-control studies than cohort studies, although this need not be the case if the case-control study is rigorously conducted (60,61). In the case-control study, subjects are chosen for inclusion according to case status (e.g., presence or absence of a resistant microorganism). The key principle is that controls should be an unbiased sample of the source population with respect to exposure (60,61). Just as in a cohort study, it is necessary to delineate the source population or study base—individuals who would be classified as cases if they developed the disease, or alternatively, the person-time experience during which there is eligibility to become a case. The failure to select subjects independently of exposure status distorts the causal relationship between exposure and disease. If subject selection is influenced by a factor that is associated with exposure, the consequence is selection bias. The result is that distribution of exposure in controls will differ in a systematic way from that of the entire study base. The sampled exposed and unexposed individuals will no longer be comparable with respect to disease incidence; a noncausal exposure-disease association is induced.

Antimicrobial Use and Risk of Infection with Resistant Microorganisms

Case-control studies on antibiotic-resistant microorganisms typically aim to determine risk factors (e.g., specific antimicrobial agents) causally related to colonization or infection with resistant pathogens (62–68). The choice of appropriate controls is central to the validity of results in those studies (69,70).

We will look at studies of antimicrobial risk factors for infection with vancomycin-resistant enterococci (VRE), which have been plagued by suboptimal selection of controls (69). If the exposure of interest in a case-control study of VRE acquisition is vancomycin use, then controls should be selected that are representative of vancomycin exposure in the entire cohort of hospitalized patients. Controls should not be intentionally limited to certain wards where vancomycin use is low since this would falsely overestimate the odds ratio obtained for vancomycin. Often, for convenience reasons, patients with vancomycin-susceptible enterococci (VSE) are selected as the control group. The reason the choice of patients with susceptible microorganisms as the control group leads to a biased estimate of relative risk is that a distorted estimate of exposure frequency in the source population is obtained. The selection bias introduced by using control patients with susceptible microorganisms is likely to have the strongest impact on estimating the effect of exposure to antibiotics that are active against susceptible (but not resistant) microorganisms, which is often the exposure of greatest interest. The reason for this particular bias is that treatment with active antibiotics likely inhibits the growth of susceptible microorganisms, therefore making this exposure less frequent among patients who are culture positive for susceptible microorganisms than among patients in the source population.

Thus, vancomycin therapy may be identified as an individual risk factor not because it is a risk factor for development of VRE but because fewer patients in the VSE comparison group received vancomycin. Vancomycin may be causal only with respect to its killing effect on VSE, not to its effect to enhance risk of VRE acquisition (71). The selection bias associated with this type of control group selection was demonstrated in a meta-analysis that aimed to assess whether vancomycin therapy was a risk factor for development of VRE (72). Studies that used a control group of patients with VSE identified vancomycin therapy as a risk factor (pooled OR, 10.7), whereas studies that used a second control group (no patients with VRE and not limited to patients with VSE, therefore similar to the base population of hospital admissions) revealed a far weaker association (OR 2.7). This weaker association was then eliminated when the analysis was limited to studies that also controlled for time at risk prior to the outcome (72).

Another situation in which selection bias may be a problem results from the use of clinical cultures to identify patients with a resistant microorganism. If the exposure influences performance of the test used to identify the resistant microorganism or is itself influenced by a factor that affects culturing, the consequence is selection bias. This is similar to the well-described selection bias that occurred when investigators attempted to study the effect of estrogen replacement therapy on uterine cancer (18). The disease and the exposure both affected vaginal bleeding, a symptom that influenced the likelihood of detection of uterine cancer. In the example of studies of resistant microorganisms, when the exposure of interest is antimicrobial use, factors that may influence both future culturing practices and prescribing of antimicrobials are the initial symptoms and signs of infection. Adjusting for the clinical manifestations of infection and other indications for antimicrobial use can remove this selection bias.

RECOMMENDATION 4: ACCOUNT FOR TIMING OF EXPOSURE AND TIME AT RISK

Time at Risk

There are two common ways that time is misunderstood or mishandled in epidemiologic studies within the field of infection control. One pertains to the concept of *time at risk* and the other to time-varying exposures. The key role of time in the occurrence and detection of disease is worth emphasizing. First, time at risk serves as the stage on which other causes act. For instance, the longer the patient is hospitalized, the greater the opportunity for the patient to experience the use of invasive medical devices that are causes of nosocomial infection and the higher the cumulative probability of occurrence of a nosocomial infection. Second, even for those causes that are experienced at a single point of time, for instance, ingestion of food contaminated by *Listeria* (73), time is important because of the induction period. If the follow-up time is shorter than the maximum interval from exposure to onset of symptoms (incubation period), the case may not be detected. Third, time at risk itself may act as an intermediate variable, mediating the effects of other causes of disease. One of the indirect pathways by which high illness severity leads to higher infection risk is by increasing the length of hospital stay. Fourth, exposures may not be constant during the period of risk; accounting for time-varying exposures poses additional problems discussed in more detail below.

Consider what actually constitutes the time at risk for nosocomial infections, using the situation in which only the initial infection is studied. An individual's time at risk for a nosocomial BSI begins when he or she is admitted to the hospital and ends at the time of occurrence of the first BSI or at discharge. More precisely, information about the presumed incubation period may be used to modify the start and stop times of this interval. The first 48 hours after hospitalization is "immortal time" in the sense that, by the usual case definition, events with onset during that interval are excluded. Conversely, infections detected up to a certain number of days after discharge may be included as cases, and so the follow-up time may extend for a brief period postdischarge (74). Notwithstanding these subtleties, the time at risk is approximately the hospital length of stay for individuals who do not experience a BSI and the interval from admission to occurrence of the infection for those that do.

When the time at risk varies substantially from individual to individual, the incidence rate, denominated by person-time experience, is the appropriate measure of disease frequency. This concept is widely understood in infection control and forms the basis for measures of disease frequency such as number of catheter-related infections per 1,000 catheter days (75,76). However, the implication of variation in time at risk for the choice of the target measure of effect is less often recognized. Generally, if there is a need for adjustment on time-at-risk, the target parameter of an epidemiologic analysis should be person-time based, usually the incidence rate ratio or hazard ratio (HR) (77,78). Analyses of data from case-control or cohort studies using logistic regression often neglect this issue (79–81). Sometimes in such analyses, the time at risk is treated as a conventional risk factor (82,83). Although this approach may be less biased than not accounting for time at risk at all, it neglects the distinction between time at risk and other types of confounders (84). A related limitation is to use hospital length of stay for all patients, regardless of case status, as the adjustment variable (85). A comparable type of inaccuracy is to calculate incidence densities using total person-time instead of person-time at risk (86).

Time-Varying Exposures and Matched Cohort Studies

The analytic techniques that account for variation in time at risk are particularly valuable when exposures change over time (87). An exposure is considered time varying when its value changes in a meaningful way during follow-up. In outcome studies of nosocomial infections or other adverse events, in which the aim is to estimate the causal effect of infection on endpoints such as mortality or costs, the infection is a time-varying exposure. Infected patients are deemed exposed after onset of the infection. Prior to infection, patients are unexposed, as are patients who never experience infection. The interval from start of follow-up to onset of infection differs from patient to patient.

The most commonly used method to estimate excess morbidity and mortality caused by nosocomial infection or other adverse event is to perform a matched cohort study, in which patients with the adverse event are matched to one or more reference patients who did not experience the adverse event (88–91). Infected and uninfected patients are usually matched for age, the underlying disease, as well as additional variables that may have contributed to excess morbidity and extra length of hospital stay (Fig. 93.2).

This study design has several limitations because of the time-varying nature of the exposure. One source of bias occurs when infected and uninfected patients are compared with regard to *total* hospital costs or *total* hospital length of stay (88,91,92). For infected patients, only those costs incurred after the occurrence of the nosocomial infection are possibly secondary to infection. Prior to occurrence of infection, patients are unexposed. The association between preinfection outcome and infection is entirely noncausal from the perspective of measuring the excess burden of infection. Therefore, combining preinfection outcomes with postinfection outcomes dramatically amplifies confounding.

Modifying the analysis such that average postinfection length of stay in infected patients is compared with average total length of stay in noninfected patients does not completely remove confounding by time (93). Bias persists even in matched cohort studies in which noninfected patients are selected to have a hospital length of stay at least as long as the interval to infection

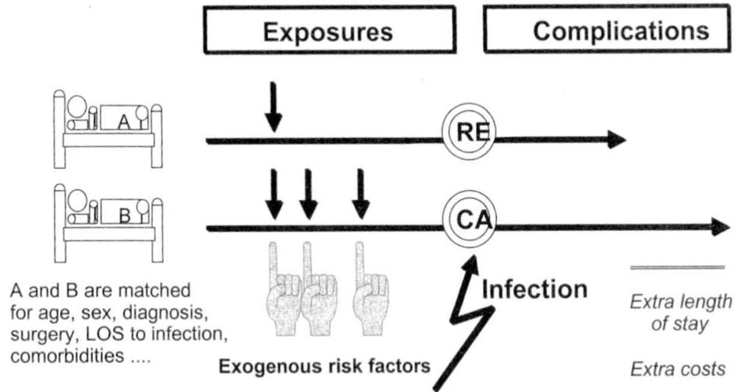

Figure 93.2. A schematic design of a matched cohort study. *Arrows* indicate exposure to risk factors for infection after admission. Patient A is considered as uninfected reference patient ("RE") for "case" patient B ("CA") who developed nosocomial infection indicated by the *broken arrow*.

in the corresponding infected patient, irrespective of differences in severity of illness. The reason for this bias is that conditioning on presence or absence of infection induces an association between the time to infection and time to discharge.

Several recent studies have demonstrated the effect of this bias. Outcome analyses that did not account for the time prior to the occurrence of the infection or adverse event yielded different results than studies that did account for the time prior to the infection. As shown in Table 93.2, there is an important difference in excess length of stay between conventional matching approaches and methods that adequately model the timing of events (94). Schulgen et al. (95) tested different methods and showed that the use of unmatched or matched comparisons between noninfected and infected patients led to an overestimation of the excess length of stay due to surgical site infections or nosocomial pneumonia, compared to analyses based on a structural formulation of transitions between different states (Table 93.2). Similarly, Asensio and Torres (96) found that regression models yielded lower estimates of the excess length of stay and cost due to nosocomial infection than a matched-pair comparison.

Another approach to estimating cost and length of stay effects of adverse events is to apply survival models, in which the adverse event is incorporated as a time-dependent variable (97). This strategy can be applied to costs as well as length of stay (97).

Even when the time-varying nature of the exposure is accounted for, it is still necessary to adequately adjust for traditional confounders, those factors that both increase risk of infection and affect the outcome of interest (98). For instance, Soufir et al. (13) investigated the excess risk of death due to catheter-related bloodstream infection (CR-BSI) in a cohort of critically ill patients. The crude case-fatality ratio was 50% and 21% in patients with and without CR-BSI. The statistical method of adjustment was based on Cox proportional hazards regression, with inclusion of matching variables and prognostic factors for mortality. CR-BSI remained associated with mortality following adjustment for prognostic factors at ICU admission (HR, 2.0; $p = .03$). However, after controlling for severity scores calculated 1 week before CR-BSI, the increased mortality was no longer significant in the Cox model (HR, 1.4; $p = .27$).

In summary, nosocomial infections unquestionably have substantial effects on morbidity and mortality. However, the matched cohort study design produces bias in the estimation of the effects of nosocomial infection on length of stay and costs. Cost effects or excess length of stay are likely to be overestimated if the interval to onset of nosocomial infection is not properly accounted for in the study design or analysis (95,99). Finally, appropriate statistical methods are important in analysis of excess costs associated with nosocomial infections, because informed decisions and policy developments may depend on them (98). Additionally, exaggeration of excess costs may lead to unintentional errors in the economic analysis of intervention programs.

RECOMMENDATION 5: DEVELOP GUIDELINES ACCORDING TO EXPLICIT RULES

Translating research in infection control into practice guidelines involves as the first step a rigorous review of evidence. Although expert opinion is a critical component of the development of recommendations and guidelines, it is important, whenever possible, to use results of the highest quality studies possible as the basis for infection control policy (100). This is crucial, because many practices in infection control have not been validated by controlled clinical trials. For instance, due to the lack of randomized studies, misconceptions about the value of alcohol-based hand disinfection widely persisted during the 20th century in most English-speaking countries (101). Alcohol-based hand gels have now been introduced in the United States and other English-speaking countries, although no controlled clinical trial has been published to determine whether alcohol-based hand gels are as effective as alcohol-based hand rinses. Only *in vitro* experiments have been conducted, and these have generated substantial controversies (102,103). There are numerous other examples about scientific uncertainty in infection control. Unfortunately, there are many important questions in infection control for which we may never obtain data from randomized trials because of limitations in funding, lack of feasibility, and ethical dilemmas (104).

TABLE 93.2. ESTIMATED DURATION OF EXTRA STAY IN DAYS PER INFECTED PATIENT AND 95% CONFIDENCE INTERVAL (CI) FOR TWO STUDIES ON THE EFFECT OF SURGICAL SITE INFECTION (STUDY I) AND ON NOSOCOMIAL PNEUMONIA (STUDY II)

	Surgical Site Infection (Study I)		Nosocomial Pneumonia (Study II)	
Approach	Estimated Extra Hospital Stay	95% CI	Estimated Extra Stay in ICU	95% CI
Two-group comparison	20.7	18.4–23.0	14.4	10.7–18.2
Confounder matching	16.9[a]	12.9–20.9	12.3	9.7–14.9
Confounder and time matching	11.4[b]	7.1–15.7	8.2	5.9–10.5
Method 1	9.8	5.7–13.8	3.4	0.8–6.0
Method 2	11.5	8.9–14.0	4.0	1.5–6.1

[a] Matching for age, sex, diagnosis, and degree of contamination of wound.
[b] Matching for age, sex, diagnosis, degree of contamination of wound, and time to infection.
Study I used a Markov transition state model and study II used a structural nested failure time model. Both studies account for the time from admission to nosocomial infection in the estimation of the effect of nosocomial infection on subsequent length of stay.
Adapted from Schulgen G, Kropec A, Kappstein I, et el. Estimation of extra hospital stay attributable to nosocomial infections: heterogeneity and timing of events. *J Clin Epidemiol* 2000;53(4):409–417.

Methodologic Quality of Guidelines in Infection Control

Guidelines are widely used and cited, because they attempt to summarize and critically appraise currently available evidence and give recommendations for daily practice (105). By contrast, individual trials are often conflicting or nondefinitive, because of their small sample size or other methodologic limitations. Many guidelines rely on reviews that were either previously published or created by guideline developers. Systematic reviews can aid in guideline development, because they involve selecting, critically appraising, and summarizing the results of primary research. The more rigorous the review method used and the higher the quality of the primary research that is synthesized, the more evidence-based the practice guideline is likely to be (106). Conversely, the quality of a review is compromised if a comprehensive search is not made to ensure that all potentially relevant articles are considered for inclusion, if the selection of studies is not reproducible or is open to bias, if the methodologic quality of the primary studies is not evaluated, or if possible reasons for the variability in results are not explored (107). Table 93.3 summarizes the most commonly used levels of evidence of preventive or therapeutic interventions, and the grading scale for recommendations made in practice guidelines.

Many guidelines in the infection control literature are not following the highest possible methodologic standards for development of guidelines, as suggested by the Cochran review group (108). For instance, the new guideline on preventing catheter-related infections published in 2002 named about eight different groups involved in the task force, but did not outline how the data were assembled or judged (109). The recently published hand hygiene guideline (110), an otherwise exemplary appraisal of the evidence, also did not include a detailed description of the systematic review process. Finally, the new Society for Hospital Epidemiology of America (SHEA) guideline for preventing nosocomial transmission of multiresistant *Staphylococcus* and *Enterococcus* may have upgraded the level of evidence generated by studies arguing in favor of screening cultures (111). Thus, these guidelines leave uncertain the study selection criteria, data extraction process, and quality of the included studies. To improve the quality of evidence, investigators assembling consensus guidelines should add more systematic information about the search methods, data sources, study selection criteria, and details about study designs, interventions, settings, and the quality of studies included in their recommendations. These recommendations have been followed in several practice guidelines published recently (112,113).

TABLE 93.3. LEVELS OF EVIDENCE AND GRADES OF RECOMMENDATIONS FOR PREVENTIVE OR THERAPEUTICAL INTERVENTIONS

Quality of evidence	
I	Evidence obtained from at least one properly randomized clinical trial with high power
II-1	Evidence obtained from clinical trials with low power or without randomization
II-2	Evidence obtained from well-designed cohort or case control studies
II-3	Evidence obtained from studies using historical cohort comparisons
III	Descriptive case series without controls or opinions of respected authorities
Strength of recommendation	
A	Good evidence to support a recommendation
B	Fair evidence to support a recommendation
C	Insufficient evidence to recommend for or against a recommendation
D	Fair evidence to withhold a recommendation
E	Good evidence to withhold a recommendation

Adapted from the rating scale used by the U.S. Preventive Services Task Force.

CONCLUSION

We have critically assessed selected articles from the hospital epidemiology and infection control literature to highlight methodologic limitations and areas in need of improvement. We hope that this review will act as a stimulus to further research, based on sound methodologic tools, and that the resulting body of work will advance new hypotheses for the prevention of nosocomial infections. Assuming that healthcare-associated infections have causal and preventive factors that can be identified through systematic investigation of different populations, epidemiology has the potential to contribute substantially to the understanding of the effectiveness of infection control measures and act as a driver of practice change. As in any scientific endeavor, the fundamental challenge in hospital epidemiology is to ask the important questions and then select the right methods to answer them. The availability of systematic epidemiologic methods for use in infection control provides an opportunity for more complete prevention of nosocomial infections in the next millennium.

ACKNOWLEDGMENTS

We thank Michael Rubin and Marc Lipsitch for helpful comments and Didier Pittet for providing Figure 93.2.

REFERENCES

1. Harbarth S. Epidemiologic methods for the prevention of nosocomial infections. *Int J Hyg Environ Health* 2000;203(2):153–157.
2. Haley RW, Schaberg DR, Von Allmen SD, et al. Estimating the extra charges and prolongation of hospitalization due to nosocomial infections: a comparison of methods. *J Infect Dis* 1980;141:248–257.
3. Haley RW, Quade D, Freeman HE, et al. Study on the efficacy of nosocomial infection control (SENIC Project). Summary of study design. *Am J Epidemiol* 1980;111(5):472–485.
4. Freeman J, McGowan JE Jr. Methodologic issues in hospital epidemiology. II. Time and accuracy in estimation. *Rev Infect Dis* 1981; 3(4):668–677.
5. Freeman J, McGowan JE Jr. Methodologic issues in hospital epidemiology. I. Rates, case-finding, and interpretation. *Rev Infect Dis* 1981;3(4):658–667.
6. Freeman J, McGowan JE Jr. Differential risk of nosocomial infection. *Am J Med* 1981;70(4):915–918.
7. Townsend TR, Wenzel RP. Nosocomial bloodstream infections in a newborn intensive care unit—a matched-case control study of morbidity, mortality and risk. *Am J Epidemiol* 1981;114:73–80.
8. Rothman KJ, Greenland S. Matching. In: Rothman KJ, Greenland

S, eds. *Modern epidemiology,* vol 2. Philadelphia: Lippincott-Raven, 1998:147–162.
9. Classen DC, Pestotnik SL, Evans RS, et al. Adverse drug events in hospitalized patients. Excess length of stay, extra costs, and attributable mortality. *JAMA* 1997;277(4):301–306.
10. Blot SI, Vandewoude KH, Hoste EA, et al. Outcome and attributable mortality in critically Ill patients with bacteremia involving methicillin-susceptible and methicillin-resistant Staphylococcus aureus. *Arch Intern Med* 2002;162(19):2229–2235.
11. Landry SL, Kaiser DL, Wenzel RP. Hospital stay and mortality attributed to nosocomial enterococcal bacteremia: a controlled study. *Am J Infect Control* 1989;17:323–329.
12. Fagon JY, Novara A, Stephan F, et al. Mortality attributable to nosocomial infections in the ICU. *Infect Control Hosp Epidemiol* 1994; 15:428–434.
13. Soufir L, Timsit JF, Mahe C, et al. Attributable morbidity and mortality of catheter-related septicemia in critically ill patients: a matched, risk-adjusted, cohort study. *Infect Control Hosp Epidemiol* 1999;20(6): 396–401.
14. Greenland S. Relation of probability of causation to relative risk and doubling dose: a methodologic error that has become a social problem. *Am J Public Health* 1999;89(8):1166–1169.
15. Greenland S, Robins J. Conceptual problems in the definition and interpretation of attributable fractions. *Am J Epidemiol* 1988;128: 1185–1197.
16. Robins JM, Greenland S. Estimability and estimation of excess and etiologic fractions. *Stat Med* 1989;8(7):845–859.
17. Rothman KJ, Greenland S. Measures of Effect and Association. In: Rothman KJ, Greenland S, eds. *Modern epidemiology,* vol 2. Philadelphia: Lippincott-Raven, 1998:47–64.
18. Robins JM. Data, design, and background knowledge in etiologic inference. *Epidemiology* 2001;12(3):313–320.
19. Robins JM, Greenland S. The role of model selection in causal inference from nonexperimental data. *Am J Epidemiol* 1986;123(3): 392–402.
20. Robins J. A graphical approach to the identification and estimation of causal parameters in mortality studies with sustained exposure periods. *J Chronic Dis* 1987;40(suppl 2):139S–161S.
21. Greenland S, Brumback B. An overview of relations among causal modelling methods. *Int J Epidemiol* 2002;31(5):1030–1037.
22. Maldonado G, Greenland S. Estimating causal effects. *Int J Epidemiol* 2002;31(2):422–429.
23. Robins JM, Greenland S. Identifiability and exchangeability for direct and indirect effects. *Epidemiology* 1992;3(2):143–155.
24. Greenland S, Pearl J, Robins JM. Causal diagrams for epidemiologic research. *Epidemiology* 1999;10(1):37–48.
25. Hernan MA, Hernandez-Diaz S, Werler MM, et al. Causal knowledge as a prerequisite for confounding evaluation: an application to birth defects epidemiology. *Am J Epidemiol* 2002;155(2):176–184.
26. Cole SR, Hernan MA. Fallibility in estimating direct effects. *Int J Epidemiol* 2002;31(1):163–165.
27. Carmeli Y, Castro J, Eliopoulos GM, et al. Clinical isolation and resistance patterns of and superinfection with 10 nosocomial pathogens after treatment with ceftriaxone versus ampicillin-sulbactam. *Antimicrob Agents Chemother* 2001;45(1):275–279.
28. Greenland S, Morgenstern H. Confounding in health research. *Annu Rev Public Health* 2001;22:189–212.
29. Concato J, Feinstein AR, Holford TR. The risk of determining risk with multivariable models. *Ann Intern Med* 1993;118(3):201–210.
30. Katz MH. Multivariable analysis: a primer for readers of medical research. *Ann Intern Med* 2003;138:644–650.
31. Greenland S. Modeling and variable selection in epidemiologic analysis. *Am J Public Health* 1989;79(3):340–349.
32. Sirvent J, Torres A, El-Ebiary M, et al. Protective effect of intravenously administered cefuroxime against nosocomial pneumonia in patients with structural coma. *Am J Respir Crit Care Med* 1997;155: 1729–1734.
33. Cook D, Walter S, Cook R, et al. Incidence of and risk factors for ventilator-associated pneumonia in critically ill patients. *Ann Intern Med* 1998;129:433–440.
34. Krueger WA, Lenhart FP, Neeser G, et al. Influence of combined intravenous and topical antibiotic prophylaxis on the incidence of infections, organ dysfunctions, and mortality in critically ill surgical patients: a prospective, stratified, randomized, double-blind, placebo-controlled clinical trial. *Am J Respir Crit Care Med* 2002;166(8): 1029–1037.
35. Namias N, Harvill S, Ball S, et al. Cost and morbidity associated with antibiotic prophylaxis in the ICU. *J Am Coll Surg* 1999;188(3): 225–230.
36. Harbarth S, Samore MH, Lichtenberg D, et al. Is prolonged antibiotic prophylaxis after major surgery associated with an increased risk of nosocomial bloodstream infection? *J Am Coll Surg* 2000;190(4): 503–504.
37. Harbarth S, Samore MH, Lichtenberg D, et al. Prolonged antibiotic prophylaxis after cardiovascular surgery and its effect on surgical site infections and antimicrobial resistance. *Circulation* 2000;101(25): 2916–2921.
38. Leibovici L, Shraga I, Drucker M, et al. The benefit of appropriate empirical antibiotic treatment in patients with bloodstream infection. *J Intern Med* 1998;244(5):379–386.
39. Kollef MH, Sherman G, Ward S, et al. Inadequate antimicrobial treatment of infections: a risk factor for hospital mortality among critically ill patients. *Chest* 1999;115(2):462–474.
40. Hanon FX, Monnet DL, Sorensen TL, et al. Survival of patients with bacteraemia in relation to initial empirical antimicrobial treatment. *Scand J Infect Dis* 2002;34(7):520–528.
41. Harbarth S, Garbino J, Pugin J, et al. Inappropriate initial antimicrobial therapy and its effect on survival in a clinical trial of immunomodulating therapy for severe sepsis. *Am J Med* 2003;115:529.
42. Zaragoza R, Artero A, Camarena J, et al. The influence of inadequate empirical antimicrobial treatment on patients with bloodstream infections in an intensive care unit. *Clin Microbiol Infect* 2003;9:412–418.
43. Dupont H, Montravers P, Gauzit R, et al. Outcome of postoperative pneumonia in the EOLE study. *Intensive Care Med* 2003;29(2): 179–188.
44. Ibrahim EH, Sherman G, Ward S, et al. The influence of inadequate antimicrobial treatment of bloodstream infections on patient outcomes in the ICU setting. *Chest* 2000;118(1):146–155.
45. Robins JM, Hernan MA, Brumback B. Marginal structural models and causal inference in epidemiology. *Epidemiology* 2000;11(5): 550–560.
46. Freeman J, Goldmann DA, McGowan JE. Methodologic issues in hospital epidemiology. IV. Risk ratios, confounding, effect modification, and the analysis of multiple variables. *Rev Infect Dis* 1988;10(6): 1118–1141.
47. Hernan MA, Brumback B, Robins JM. Marginal structural models to estimate the causal effect of zidovudine on the survival of HIV-positive men. *Epidemiology* 2000;11(5):561–570.
48. Phillips CV. Quantifying and reporting uncertainty from systematic errors. *Epidemiology* 2003;14(4):459–466.
49. Lash TL, Fink AK. Semi-automated sensitivity analysis to assess systematic errors in observational data. *Epidemiology* 2003;14(4): 451–458.
50. Cepeda MS, Boston R, Farrar JT, et al. Comparison of logistic regression versus propensity score when the number of events is low and there are multiple confounders. *Am J Epidemiol* 2003;158(3): 280–287.
51. Rubin D. Estimating causal effects from large data sets using propensity scores. *Ann Intern Med* 1997;127:757–763.
52. Braitman L, Rosenbaum P. Rare outcomes, common treatments: analytic strategies using propensity scores. *Ann Intern Med* 2002;137: 693–695.
53. Carmeli Y, Eliopoulos G, Mozaffari E, et al. Health and economic outcomes of vancomycin-resistant enterococci. *Arch Intern Med* 2002; 162(19):2223–2228.
54. D'Agostino RB Jr. Propensity score methods for bias reduction in the comparison of a treatment to a non-randomized control group. *Stat Med* 1998;17(19):2265–2281.
55. Harbarth S, Rutschmann O, Sudre P, et al. Impact of methicillin

resistance on the outcome of patients with bacteremia caused by Staphylococcus aureus. *Arch Intern Med* 1998;158(2):182–189.
56. Cosgrove SE, Sakoulas G, Perencevich EN, et al. Comparison of mortality associated with methicillin-resistant and methicillin-susceptible Staphylococcus aureus bacteremia: a meta-analysis. *Clin Infect Dis* 2003;36(1):53–59.
57. Soriano A, Martinez JA, Mensa J, et al. Pathogenic significance of methicillin resistance for patients with Staphylococcus aureus bacteremia. *Clin Infect Dis* 2000;30(2):368–373.
58. Platt R, Zucker JR, Zaleznik DF, et al. Prophylaxis against wound infection following herniorrhaphy or breast surgery. *J Infect Dis* 1992; 166(3):556–560.
59. Platt R, Zaleznik DF, Hopkins CC, et al. Perioperative antibiotic prophylaxis for herniorrhaphy and breast surgery. *N Engl J Med* 1990; 322(3):153–160.
60. Wacholder S, McLaughlin JK, Silverman DT, et al. Selection of controls in case-control studies. I. Principles. 1992;135(9):1019–1028.
61. Wacholder S, Silverman DT, McLaughlin JK, et al. Selection of controls in case-control studies. II. Types of controls. 1992;135(9): 1029–1041.
62. Lipsitch M. Measuring and interpreting associations between antibiotic use and penicillin resistance in Streptococcus pneumoniae. *Clin Infect Dis* 2001;32(7):1044–1054.
63. Troillet N, Carmeli Y, Venkataraman L, et al. Epidemiological analysis of imipenem-resistant Serratia marcescens in hospitalized patients. 1999;42(1):37–43.
64. Morris JG Jr, Shay DK, Hebden JN, et al. Enterococci resistant to multiple antimicrobial agents, including vancomycin. Establishment of endemicity in a university medical center. *Ann Intern Med* 1995; 123(4):250–259.
65. Bonten MJ, Slaughter S, Ambergen AW, et al. The role of "colonization pressure" in the spread of vancomycin-resistant enterococci: an important infection control variable. *Arch Intern Med* 1998;158(10): 1127–1132.
66. Wenzel RP, ed. *Prevention and control of nosocomial infections,* 4th ed: Philadelphia: Lippincott Williams & Wilkins, 2003.
67. Carmeli Y, Eliopoulos GM, Samore MH. Antecedent treatment with different antibiotic agents as a risk factor for vancomycin-resistant Enterococcus. *Emerg Infect Dis* 2002;8(8):802–807.
68. Cetinkaya Y, Falk PS, Mayhall CG. Effect of gastrointestinal bleeding and oral medications on acquisition of vancomycin-resistant Enterococcus faecium in hospitalized patients. *Clin Infect Dis* 2002;35(8): 935–942.
69. Harris AD, Karchmer TB, Carmeli Y, et al. Methodological principles of case-control studies that analyzed risk factors for antibiotic resistance: a systematic review. *Clin Infect Dis* 2001;32(7):1055–1061.
70. Harris AD, Samore MH, Lipsitch M, et al. Control-group selection importance in studies of antimicrobial resistance: examples applied to Pseudomonas aeruginosa, Enterococci, and Escherichia coli. *Clin Infect Dis* 2002;34(12):1558–1563.
71. Ostrowsky BE, Venkataraman L, D'Agata EM, et al. Vancomycin-resistant enterococci in intensive care units: high frequency of stool carriage during a non-outbreak period. *Arch Intern Med* 1999; 159(13):1467–1472.
72. Carmeli Y, Samore MH, Huskins C. The association between antecedent vancomycin treatment and hospital-acquired vancomycin-resistant enterococci: a meta-analysis. *Arch Intern Med* 1999;159(20): 2461–2468.
73. Elsner HA, Tenschert W, Fischer L, et al. Nosocomial infections by Listeria monocytogenes: analysis of a cluster of septicemias in immunocompromised patients. *Infection* 1997;25(3):135–139.
74. Hugonnet S, Eggimann P, Sax H, et al. Intensive care unit-acquired infections: is postdischarge surveillance useful? *Crit Care Med* 2002; 30(12):2636–2638.
75. Eggimann P, Harbarth S, Constantin MN, et al. Impact of a prevention strategy targeted at vascular-access care on incidence of infections acquired in intensive care. *Lancet* 2000;355(9218):1864–1868.
76. Zuschneid I, Schwab F, Geffers C, et al. Reducing central venous catheter-associated primary bloodstream infections in intensive care units is possible: data from the German nosocomial infection surveillance system. *Infect Control Hosp Epidemiol* 2003;24(7):501–505.
77. Harbarth S, Liassine N, Dharan S, et al. Risk factors for persistent carriage of methicillin-resistant Staphylococcus aureus. *Clin Infect Dis* 2000;31(6):1380–1385.
78. Harbarth S, Harris AD, Carmeli Y, et al. Parallel analysis of individual and aggregated data on antibiotic exposure and resistance in gram-negative bacilli. *Clin Infect Dis* 2001;33(9):1462–1468.
79. Papazian L, Bregeon F, Thirion X, et al. Effect of ventilator-associated pneumonia on mortality and morbidity. *Am J Respir Crit Care Med* 1996;154(1):91–97.
80. Barbut F, Corthier G, Charpak Y, et al. Prevalence and pathogenicity of Clostridium difficile in hospitalized patients. A French multicenter study. *Arch Intern Med* 1996;156(13):1449–1454.
81. Cunnion KM, Weber DJ, Broadhead WE, et al. Risk factors for nosocomial pneumonia: comparing adult critical-care populations. *Am J Respir Crit Care Med* 1996;153(1):158–162.
82. Leu HS, Kaiser DL, Mori M, et al. Hospital-acquired pneumonia. Attributable mortality and morbidity. *Am J Epidemiol* 1989;129: 1258–1267.
83. Singh-Naz N, Sprague BM, Patel KM, et al. Risk factors for nosocomial infection in critically ill children: a prospective cohort study. *Crit Care Med* 1996;24(5):875–878.
84. de Irala-Estevez J, Martinez-Concha D, Diaz-Molina C, et al. Comparison of different methodological approaches to identify risk factors of nosocomial infection in intensive care units. *Intensive Care Med* 2001;27(8):1254–1262.
85. Gleason TG, Crabtree TD, Pelletier SJ, et al. Prediction of poorer prognosis by infection with antibiotic-resistant gram-positive cocci than by infection with antibiotic-sensitive strains. *Arch Surg* 1999; 134(10):1033–1040.
86. Eggimann P, Hugonnet S, Sax H, et al. Ventilator-associated pneumonia: caveats for benchmarking. *Intensive Care Med* 2003;29(11): 2086.
87. Fisher LD, Lin DY. Time-dependent covariates in the Cox proportional-hazards regression model. *Annu Rev Public Health* 1999;20: 145–157.
88. Wey SB, Motomi M, Pfaller MA, et al. Hospital-acquired candidemia. The attributable mortality and excess length of stay. *Arch Intern Med* 1988;148:2642–2645.
89. Martin MA, Pfaller MA, Wenzel RP. Coagulase-negative staphylococcal bacteremia. Mortality and hospital stay. *Ann Intern Med* 1989; 110:9–16.
90. Coello R, Glenister H, Fereres J, et al. The cost of infection in surgical patients: a case-control study. *J Hosp Infect* 1993;25(4):239–250.
91. Pittet D, Tarara D, Wenzel RP. Nosocomial bloodstream infection in critically ill patients: excess length of stay, extra costs, and attributable mortality. *JAMA* 1994;271:1598–1601.
92. Kirkland KB, Briggs JP, Trivette SL, et al. The impact of surgical-site infections in the 1990s: attributable mortality, excess length of hospitalization, and extra costs. *Infect Control Hosp Epidemiol* 1999; 20(11):725–730.
93. Samore M. How to improve outcome studies. In: ASM, ed. ICAAC. Chicago: ASM, 2003: abstract 1786, session 177.
94. Hosmer D, Lomeshow S. *Applied survival analysis: regression modeling of time to event data.* New York: John Wiley, 1999.
95. Schulgen G, Kropec A, Kappstein I, et al. Estimation of extra hospital stay attributable to nosocomial infections: heterogeneity and timing of events. *J Clin Epidemiol* 2000;53(4):409–417.
96. Asensio A, Torres J. Quantifying excess length of postoperative stay attributable to infections: a comparison of methods. *J Clin Epidemiol* 1999;52(12):1249–1256.
97. Harbarth S, Burke JP, Lloyd JF, et al. Clinical and economic outcomes of conventional amphotericin B-associated nephrotoxicity. *Clin Infect Dis* 2002;35(12):E120–127.
98. Rello J. Impact of nosocomial infections on outcome: myths and evidence. *Infect Control Hosp Epidemiol* 1999;20(6):392–394.
99. Frank U, Daschner FD, Schulgen G, et al. Incidence and epidemiology of nosocomial infections in patients infected with human immunodeficiency virus. *Clin Infect Dis* 1997;25(2):318–320.
100. Gastmeier P, Daschner F, Ruden H. Guidelines for infection preven-

tion and control in Germany: evidence- or expert-based? *J Hosp Infect* 1999;43(suppl):S301–305.

101. Harbarth S. Handwashing—the Semmelweis lesson misunderstood? *Clin Infect Dis* 2000;30(6):990–991.
102. Kramer A, Rudolph P, Kampf G, et al. Limited efficacy of alcohol-based hand gels. *Lancet* 2002;359(9316):1489–1490.
103. Boyce JM, Larson EL, Weinstein RA. Alcohol-based hand gels and hand hygiene in hospitals. *Lancet* 2002;360(9344):1509–1510; author reply 1511.
104. Harbarth S, Pittet D. Control of nosocomial methicillin-resistant Staphylococcus aureus: where shall we send our hospital director next time? *Infect Control Hosp Epidemiol* 2003;24(5):314–316.
105. Natsch S, van der Meer JW. The role of clinical guidelines, policies and stewardship. *J Hosp Infect* 2003;53(3):172–176.
106. Cook DJ, Greengold NL, Ellrodt AG, et al. The relation between systematic reviews and practice guidelines. *Ann Intern Med* 1997; 127(3):210–216.
107. Nathwani D. From evidence-based guideline methodology to quality of care standards. *J Antimicrob Chemother* 2003;51(5):1103–1107.
108. Jadad AR, Cook DJ, Jones A, et al. Methodology and reports of systematic reviews and meta-analyses: a comparison of Cochrane reviews with articles published in paper-based journals. *JAMA* 1998; 280(3):278–280.
109. O'Grady NP, Alexander M, Dellinger EP, et al. Guidelines for the prevention of intravascular catheter-related infections. Centers for Disease Control and Prevention. *MMWR Recomm Rep* 2002;51(RR-10):1–29.
110. Boyce JM, Pittet D. Guideline for hand hygiene in health-care settings: recommendations of the Healthcare Infection Control Practices Advisory Committee and the HICPAC/SHEA/APIC/IDSA Hand Hygiene Task Force. *Infect Control Hosp Epidemiol* 2002;23(12 suppl):S3–40.
111. Muto CA, Jernigan JA, Ostrowsky BE, et al. Guideline for preventing nosocomial transmission of multidrug-resistant strains of *Staphylococcus aureus*and *Enterococcus. Infect Control Hosp Epidemiol* 2003;24: 362–386.
112. Pratt RJ, Pellowe C, Loveday HP, et al. The epic project: developing national evidence-based guidelines for preventing healthcare associated infections. Phase I: guidelines for preventing hospital-acquired infections. Department of Health (England). *J Hosp Infect* 2001; 47(suppl):S3–82.
113. Cooper BS, Stone SP, Kibbler CC, et al. Systematic review of isolation policies in the hospital management of MRSA: a review of the literature with epidemiological and economic modelling. *Health Technol Assess* 2003;7(39):1–194.

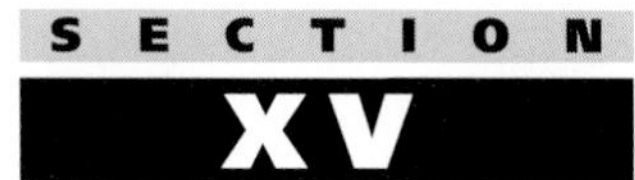

ORGANIZATION AND IMPLEMENTATION OF INFECTION CONTROL PROGRAMS

94

SURVEILLANCE OF NOSOCOMIAL INFECTIONS

TERESA C. HORAN
ROBERT P. GAYNES

Surveillance of nosocomial infections provides data useful for identifying infected patients, determining the site of infection, and identifying the factors that contribute to nosocomial infections. When infection problems are recognized, surveillance data allow the hospital to institute appropriate intervention measures and evaluate their efficacy. In addition, one can follow the trends of infections that are increasing in incidence, such as bloodstream infections (1). The landmark Study on the Efficacy of Nosocomial Infection Control (SENIC Project) demonstrated that to be effective, nosocomial infection control programs must include the following components: organized surveillance and control activities, an adequate number of trained infection control staff, and a system for reporting surgical site infection (SSI) rates to surgeons (2). Thus, the SENIC Project provided the scientific basis for the assertion that surveillance is an essential element of an infection control program.

Surveillance data can also be used to assess the quality of care in the hospital. Surveillance sometimes leads down new paths that indirectly aid in the understanding of the causes of nosocomial infections. If the data collected are to be most useful for decision making, the hospital should focus on its most important and predominant problems and use surveillance methodology that adheres to sound epidemiologic principles.

DEFINITION OF SURVEILLANCE

Surveillance is defined as "the ongoing, systematic collection, analysis, and interpretation of health data essential to the planning, implementation, and evaluation of public health practice, closely integrated with the timely dissemination of these data to those who need to know"(3). A nosocomial infection surveillance system may be sentinel event based, population based, or both. A sentinel infection is one that clearly indicates a failure in the hospital's efforts to prevent infections and, in theory, requires individual investigation (4,5). Denominator data are usually not collected in sentinel event-based surveillance. Sentinel event-based surveillance identifies only the most serious problems and should not be the only surveillance system in the hospital. Population-based surveillance, that is, surveillance of patients with similar risks, requires both a numerator (the infection) and denominator (number of patients or days of exposure to the risk). The essential elements of surveillance are shown in Table 94.1.

NATIONAL NOSOCOMIAL INFECTIONS SURVEILLANCE SYSTEM

Throughout this chapter, we use the Centers for Disease Control and Prevention's (CDC) National Nosocomial Infections Surveillance (NNIS) system to illustrate practical elements of surveillance. The NNIS system began in 1970 when selected U.S. hospitals began routinely reporting their nosocomial infection surveillance data to the CDC for aggregation into a national database. It is currently the only source of national data on the epidemiology of nosocomial infections in the United States. Hospitals participating in the NNIS system provide general medical-surgical inpatient services to adults or children requiring acute care. The identities of the more than 270 hospitals currently participating in the NNIS system are confidential.

All NNIS data are collected using four standardized protocols called surveillance components: adult and pediatric intensive care unit (ICU), high-risk nursery (HRN), surgical patient (6), and antimicrobial use and resistance (AUR). From October 1986 to December 1998, the hospital-wide component was used (all information reported for all patients; rates are calculated by ward using hospital discharges or patient-days as a denominator); however, because there was no way to risk-adjust the rates from this component it was discontinued. The components may be

TABLE 94.1. ESSENTIAL ELEMENTS OF SURVEILLANCE

- Assess the population
- Select the outcome (event) or process to survey
- Choose the surveillance method(s) keeping in mind the need for risk-adjustment of data
- Monitor for the event or process
- Apply surveillance definitions during monitoring
- Calculate rates and analyze surveillance data
- Report and use surveillance information

Adapted from Lee TB, Baker OG, Lee JT, et al. Recommended practices for surveillance. *Am J Infect Control* 1998;26:277–288, with permission.

used singly or simultaneously, but, once selected, they must be used for a minimum of one calendar month. All infections are categorized into major and specific infection sites, using standard CDC definitions that include laboratory and clinical criteria (7) (Appendix A).

Adult and Pediatric Intensive Care Unit Surveillance Component

Infection control professionals (ICPs) collect data on all sites of nosocomial infection in patients located in ICUs and ICU-specific denominator data. Site-specific infection rates can be calculated by using the number of patients at risk; total patient-days; and days of indwelling urinary catheterization, central vascular cannulation, or ventilator support as denominators.

High-Risk Nursery Surveillance Component

ICPs collect data on all sites of nosocomial infection in patients located in HRN and HRN-specific denominator data. Site-specific infection rates can be calculated by using as denominators the number of patients at risk, total patient-days, days of umbilical catheter and/or central line use, and days of ventilator assistance for each of four birth-weight categories (≤1,000, 1,001 to 1,500, 1,501 to 2,500, and >2,500 g).

Surgical Patient Surveillance Component

ICPs select from the NNIS operative procedure list (8) those procedures that they wish to follow and monitor the patients undergoing those procedures for all infections or SSIs only. A record on every patient undergoing the selected procedure is generated that includes information on risk factors for SSIs such as wound class (9), duration of operation, and American Society of Anesthesiology (ASA) score (10). Using a composite index for predicting the risk of SSI after surgery, ICPs can calculate rates by number of risk factors present (11).

Before 1986, only hospital-wide surveillance was performed by NNIS hospitals. However, as resources for this activity became more limited, interest in the more efficient targeted surveillance methods increased. One area targeted was the ICU. Donowitz et al. (12) showed that disproportionately more nosocomial infections of all types are found in ICU patients than patients in noncritical care areas. They also found that 33% to 45% of all nosocomial bloodstream infections occurred in patients in the ICU, although these patients occupied only 8% of the beds (11). By using the ICU component, hospitals are able to monitor patients whose care requires the use of devices that are associated with high infection risks. Similarly, the HRN surveillance component was developed because studies have shown that neonates in the HRN are among the most susceptible to nosocomial infections (13,14). Finally, the surgical patient component is based on the findings of the SENIC Project that patients who undergo surgical operations are three times more likely to develop a nosocomial infection than are nonsurgical patients (15) and that surveillance is effective in reducing the SSI rate, particularly when infection rates are fed back to surgeons (2, 16).

Antimicrobial Use and Resistance Component

Hospitals choosing the AUR component aggregate AUR data from at least three areas: one ICU or specialty care area (e.g., bone marrow transplant unit), all non-ICU inpatient areas combined, and all outpatient areas combined. Although collection of infection data is not required for this component, it is strongly recommended that the ICU component be used for the same ICU(s) and months as is being reported for the AUR component. The AUR component allows interhospital comparison of select antimicrobial use and antimicrobial resistance rates, which can be used in conjunction with the device-associated rates generated from the ICU component.

The lessons learned from more than 30 years of NNIS surveillance have proved useful in advising hospitals on effective methods for conducting surveillance of nosocomial infections. These methods are also potentially useful for assessing other adverse events associated with hospital care (17).

DEFINITIONS OF NOSOCOMIAL INFECTIONS

The ability of data collectors to define infections as nosocomial and identify their sites consistently is of paramount importance. Use of uniform definitions is critical if data from one hospital are to be compared with those of another hospital or with an aggregated database (e.g., the NNIS system) (7,18,19). The NNIS system defines a nosocomial infection as a localized or systemic condition that results from adverse reaction to the presence of an infectious agent(s) or its toxin(s) and that was not present or incubating at the time of admission to the hospital (7) (NNIS Manual, Section XIII, May 1994, unpublished data). For most bacterial nosocomial infections, this means that the infection usually becomes evident 48 hours (i.e., the typical incubation period) or more after admission. However, because the incubation period varies with the type of pathogen and to some extent with the patient's underlying condition, each infection must be assessed individually for evidence that links it to the hospitalization.

There are several other important principles on which nosocomial infection definitions are based (7). First, the information used to determine the presence and classification of an infection should be a combination of clinical findings and results of laboratory and other tests. Clinical evidence is derived from direct observation of the infection site or review of other pertinent sources of data, such as the patient's chart (detailed in a later section of this chapter). Laboratory evidence includes results of cultures, antigen or antibody detection tests, polymerase chain reaction (PCR), or microscopic visualization. Supportive data are derived from other diagnostic studies, such as x-ray, ultrasound, computed tomography, magnetic resonance imaging, radiolabeled scan, endoscopic procedure, biopsy, or needle aspiration. For infections whose clinical manifestations in neonates and infants are different from those in older persons, specific criteria apply.

Second, a physician's or surgeon's diagnosis of infection derived from direct observation during a surgical operation, endoscopic examination, or other diagnostic studies or from clinical judgment is an acceptable criterion for an infection, unless there is compelling evidence to the contrary (e.g., information written in the wrong patient's record, presumptive diagnosis that was not substantiated by subsequent studies). For certain sites of infection, however, a physician's clinical diagnosis in the absence of supportive data either must be accompanied by initiation of appropriate antimicrobial therapy to satisfy the criterion (e.g., bloodstream infection) or is not an acceptable criterion (e.g., pneumonia).

There are two special situations in which an infection is considered nosocomial: infection that is acquired in the hospital but does not become evident until after hospital discharge and infection in a neonate that results from passage through the birth canal. There are two special situations in which an infection is not considered nosocomial: infection that is associated with a complication or extension of infection already present on admission, unless a change in pathogen or symptoms strongly suggests the acquisition of a new infection, and, in an infant, an infection that is known or proved to have been acquired transplacentally (e.g., toxoplasmosis, rubella, cytomegalovirus, or syphilis) and becomes evident at or before 48 hours after birth.

There are two conditions that are not infections: colonization, which is the presence of microorganisms (on skin, mucous membranes, in open wounds, or in excretions or secretions) that are not causing adverse clinical signs or symptoms, and inflammation, which is a condition that results from tissue response to injury or stimulation by noninfectious agents, such as chemicals.

Appendix A-1 contains the criteria that comprise the definitions of nosocomial infections (NNIS Manual, Section XIII, May 1994, unpublished data). It lists the 13 major site categories and the 48 specific sites or types of infection for which criteria have been developed, beginning with the most frequently occurring sites of infection in hospitalized patients—urinary tract, surgical site, pneumonia, and primary bloodstream—followed by other sites of infection listed alphabetically by major site category (e.g., bone and joint, central nervous system). New criteria for defining pneumonia were adopted and have been used by NNIS hospitals since January 2002 (Appendix A-2).

Two additional points are important to understand with regard to definitions of nosocomial infections (20). First, the preventability or inevitability of an infection is not a consideration when determining whether it is nosocomial. For example, preventing the development of nosocomial *Clostridium difficile* gastroenteritis after extensive antibiotic treatment may not be possible. As another example, some would argue that neonatal infections acquired during vaginal delivery are inevitable and, therefore, should not be counted as nosocomial. However, as noted previously, these neonatal infections (e.g., group B streptococcal bacteremias with early onset) are considered nosocomial, they can be identified as maternally acquired, and the analysis of their incidence can be disseminated to obstetricians for intervention strategies. Second, surveillance definitions are not intended to define clinical disease for the purpose of making therapeutic decisions. Some true infections, therefore, are missed, whereas other conditions may erroneously be counted as infections.

PURPOSES OF SURVEILLANCE

A healthcare facility should have clear goals for doing surveillance. These goals must be reviewed and updated frequently to meet new infection risks in changing patient populations, such as the introduction of new high-risk medical interventions and changing pathogens and their resistance to antibiotics. The collection and analysis of surveillance data must be performed in conjunction with a prevention strategy. It is vital to identify and state objectives of surveillance before designing a system and starting surveillance.

Reducing Infection Rates within a Healthcare Facility

The most important purpose or goal of surveillance is to reduce the risks of acquiring nosocomial infections. To attain this goal, specific objectives for surveillance must be defined based on how the data are to be used and on the availability of financial and personnel resources for surveillance (21,22). Objectives for surveillance can be either outcome or process oriented. Outcome objectives are those activities aimed at reducing infection risks and costs, such as comparative rate analysis and feedback to patient care personnel. Process objectives, on the other hand, are activities necessary to achieving outcome objectives. Examples of process objectives are defining and identifying infections, analyzing and interpreting data, observing and evaluating patient care practices, monitoring equipment and the environment, and providing education. Much of the time spent performing surveillance is devoted to the process objectives. However, these activities are of limited value without clearly stated outcome objectives. Although there are other legitimate purposes for surveillance of nosocomial infections, the ultimate goal is to achieve the outcome objectives: decreases in infection rates, morbidity, mortality, and cost.

Establishing Endemic Baseline Rates

A basic use of surveillance data is the quantification of baseline rates of endemic nosocomial infections. This measurement provides hospitals with objective knowledge of the ongoing infection risks in hospitalized patients. Most nosocomial infections, perhaps 90% to 95%, are endemic, that is, not part of recognized outbreaks (23). Thus, surveillance activities should be viewed as a method of lowering the endemic rate. Although 91% of hospitals reported using surveillance data to establish endemic baseline rates, the mere act of collecting data does not usually influence infection risks appreciably unless it is linked with a prevention strategy (24). Otherwise, surveillance is no more than "bean counting," an expensive exercise without focus that today's hospitals can ill afford and that ICPs will ultimately find dissatisfying.

Identifying Outbreaks

Once endemic rates are established, one may be able to recognize deviations from the baseline that sometimes represent outbreaks of infection. The ability to compare baseline data with such deviations may help to confirm that an outbreak exists. This benefit must be balanced with the relatively time-consuming task of the ongoing collection of surveillance data, because only a small proportion of nosocomial infections, perhaps 5% to 10%, occurs in outbreaks (23). Moreover, outbreaks of nosocomial infections are often brought to the attention of infection control personnel by astute clinicians or laboratory personnel much more quickly than by the analysis of surveillance data. This lack of timeliness often limits the use of routine surveillance in identifying outbreaks in a hospital.

Convincing Medical Personnel

One of the most difficult tasks of an infection control program is convincing hospital personnel to adopt recommended preventive practices. Familiarity with the scientific literature on hospital epidemiology and infection control is only effective in influencing behavior if the hospital personnel believe the information is relevant to the specific situation in question. Often, studies in the literature do not address the many varied situations encountered in a particular hospital. Information on one's own hospital, used to influence personnel, is one of the most effective means of addressing a problem and applying the recommended techniques to prevent infection. If surveillance data are analyzed appropriately and routinely presented in a skillful manner, medical personnel usually come to rely strongly on them for guidance. The feedback of such information is often quite effective in persuading personnel to adopt recommended preventive practices (2).

Evaluating Control Measures

After a problem has been identified through surveillance data and control measures have been instituted, continued surveillance is needed to ensure that the problem has come under control. By continual monitoring, some control measures that seemed rational can be shown to be ineffective. For example, the use of daily meatal care to prevent nosocomial urinary tract infections seemed appropriate but did not control infection (25). Even after the initial success of control measures, breakdowns in applying them can occur, requiring a constant vigil, including the continued collection of surveillance data.

Satisfying Regulators

Satisfying the requirements of regulators such as the Joint Commission on Accreditation of Healthcare Organizations (JCAHO) is a very commonly reported use of surveillance data but one of the least justifiable if used only for that purpose. The collection of surveillance data merely to satisfy a surveyor who visits a hospital once every 3 years (or occasionally more often) is an extraordinary waste of resources. The JCAHO also viewed this process-oriented task of collecting data as unproductive when it altered its standards in 1990. Since 1992, hospitals have been required to use surveillance in a directed manner to bring about change in the risk of infection to patients (26). The JCAHO introduced the ORYX initiative in 1997 (see *http://www.jcaho.org/accredited+organizations/hospitals/oryx/index.htm*). This initiative attempts to integrate outcomes and other performance measurement data into the accreditation process. On July 1, 2002, accredited hospitals began to collect data on four initial, standardized- or core-performance measures for hospitals in the following areas: acute myocardial infarction, heart failure, community-acquired pneumonia, and pregnancy and related conditions. More core measures will be identified in the future. Based on the healthcare services it provides, hospitals are required to select core measure sets. Hospitals that do not provide services in these core measurement areas must select measures from performance measurement system(s) that have contracted with JCAHO for inclusion in the accreditation process. These performance measurement systems are quite varied; some include infection rates but most do not. A hospital will be expected to demonstrate, for each measure, the ability to collect data reliably, conduct credible analyses of the data, and initiate appropriate system and process improvements. Although this JCAHO requirement demands expert input on surveillance of healthcare-associated events, it is not yet clear how this initiative will affect infection control and surveillance or even the accreditation process.

Defending Malpractice Claims

Previously, one concern about the collection of surveillance data was that it would create a record that could be used against the hospital in a malpractice claim related to a nosocomial infection. Most legal experts now take the position that the presence of a strong surveillance component in an infection control program demonstrates that a hospital is attempting to detect problems rather than conceal them. This has proved to be an important defense against unwarranted claims. In addition, the records of infection control committees are considered privileged in most states and are not discoverable in civil court proceedings. Therefore, surveillance is often helpful in defending against malpractice claims; it is rarely, if ever, a hindrance. (See also Chapter 104.)

Comparing Infection Rates between Hospitals

Setting the priorities of an infection control program is a difficult and ever-changing task. One of the main purposes of comparing an infection rate of a hospital with those of other hospitals is to determine where the limited resources of the infection control program should be directed. The focus may be on all patients who are at risk for an infection at a particular site (e.g., the urinary tract) or on a smaller group or cohort of patients (e.g., those in an ICU). A "high" infection rate compared with other hospitals may give the infection control program the signal to investigate a potential problem. It does not define an infection control problem. Comparisons should be used only as an initial guide for setting priorities for further investigation. Two major difficulties, appropriate risk adjustment of infection rates and accurate data collection, result in many uncertainties when aggregating data from multiple hospitals. To adequately adjust infection rates, patients' intrinsic and extrinsic risks of infection must be examined (27,28) (refer to the section on Comparing Rates Among Patient Groups). Some progress in achieving suitable risk adjustment for infection rates has been made but requires the accumulation of more specific data (27,28). It must be emphasized that a single number expressing a hospital's overall nosocomial infection rate is not a valid measure of the efficacy of the infection control program (27,29,30). Therefore, a hospital's overall nosocomial infection rate, as currently derived, should not be used for interhospital comparison.

Data inaccuracy is another difficulty for hospitals and the organizations or institutions aggregating hospitals data. Assessing accuracy may entail reporting data back to the hospital in an effort to detect errors in data transmission. Aggregating organizations should examine a hospital's data for accuracy, for example, by screening for unusual patterns.

The independent determination of data accuracy, so-called validation, is an essential activity of any group that is aggregating data from multiple collectors. At issue is assessing the accuracy of case-finding of nosocomial infections by determining three factors: sensitivity, predictive value positive (PVP), and specificity. Ascertaining the sensitivity, PVP, and specificity of nosocomial infection case-finding by an independent trained observer will add to the credibility of the surveillance system, determine ways to adjust rates for hospitals that vary, and offer ways to improve surveillance.

Sensitivity is the percentage of all true infections that are reported. PVP is the percentage of infections reported deemed to be true infections. Specificity is expressed as the reported number of patients without nosocomial infections divided by the actual number of patients without nosocomial infections (31). Low sensitivity (i.e., missed infections) in a surveillance system is usually more common than low specificity (i.e., the patients reported to have infections who did not actually have infections).

Although the sensitivity, PVP, and specificity of all hospitals reporting are important to the credibility of the multihospital surveillance system, determining the variation in sensitivity and specificity of hospitals in a multihospital system may be even more important. Surveillance rarely achieves 100% accuracy. However, if one hospital is finding only 30% of all patients with nosocomial infections whereas a second hospital finds 90%, variations in infection rates between these hospitals may be entirely due to differences in case-finding sensitivity. Unfortunately, determining sensitivity and specificity is difficult and resource intensive. The NNIS Evaluation Study has suggested that data on nosocomial infections are generally accurately reported. Sensitivity (underreporting of infections), which ranged from 59% to 85% for the four major sites of nosocomial infection—bloodstream, pneumonia, urinary tract, and surgical site—was a more serious problem than other measures of accuracy. PVP ranged from 72% to 92% for these sites, and specificity ranged from 97.7% to 98.7% (32).

Hospitals considering participation in a multihospital system that aggregates data on nosocomial infections should inquire about that system's approach to data accuracy and risk adjustment before participation.

Some success in the surveillance of hospital-acquired infections has been achieved. The CDC reported substantial reductions in hospital-acquired infection rates from ICUs in hospitals that participate in the NNIS system. The report showed the value of NNIS as a model to prevent hospital-acquired infections. There were a number of elements critical for the rate reduction. These included (a) voluntary participation and confidentiality for NNIS hospitals; (b) standard definitions and protocols; (c) targeted, high-risk populations (e.g., intensive care and surgical patients); (d) site-specific, risk-adjusted infection rates comparable across institutions; (e) adequate numbers of trained ICPs; (f) data dissemination to healthcare providers; and (g) links between monitored rates and prevention efforts (33).

SURVEILLANCE METHODS

Case-finding Issues

Three questions related to case-finding must be answered before a specific method of surveillance is chosen (34). First, should infections be sought by passive or active means? In passive surveillance, persons who do not have a primary surveillance role, that is, persons other than ICPs, are relied on for identification and reporting of infections. For example, forms might be completed by physicians or nurses when a nosocomial infection is detected. Because these people's skills and knowledge are centered on patient care rather than surveillance, it is not surprising that problems associated with passive surveillance are misclassification, underreporting, and lack of timeliness of the data. Active surveillance is the process of vigorously looking for nosocomial infections using trained personnel, nearly always ICPs. ICPs seek out nosocomial infections by using various data sources to accumulate information and decide whether or not a nosocomial infection has occurred. Such personnel are likely to keep abreast of changes in surveillance definitions and reach beyond the nursing ward for clues to infection.

Second, should infection detection be patient- or laboratory-based? Patient-based surveillance includes counting nosocomial infections, assessing risk factors, and monitoring patient care procedures and practices for adherence to infection control principles. It requires ward rounds and discussions with caregivers. In laboratory-based surveillance, detection is based solely on the findings of laboratory studies of clinical specimens. Therefore, infections that are not cultured, that is, those based on physical signs and symptoms such as clinical sepsis would be missed; positive cultures without clinical confirmation may erroneously be called infections (e.g., the positives may represent colonization rather than infection).

Third, should infections be detected prospectively or retrospectively? Prospective surveillance refers to monitoring patients while they are still hospitalized and, for SSIs, includes the post-discharge period. Retrospective surveillance uses chart review after patient discharge as the sole means of identifying infections. The major advantages of prospective surveillance are that it can readily identify clusters of infection, provide increased visibility of ICPs on the wards, and facilitate timely analysis and feedback of data. One disadvantage is greater resource expense than retrospective surveillance.

TABLE 94.2. SUMMARY OF THE NNIS SURVEILLANCE COMPONENT PROTOCOLS

Surveillance Component	Population at Risk	Infection Sites	Denominator Data	Rates/Ratios
Required Data				
Intensive care unit	All patients on selected ICU(s). Follow patients for 48 hours after discharge from ICU	All infection sites with date of onset in the same month	For each ICU, number of • Patients • Patient-days • Urinary catheter-days • Central line-days • Ventilator-days • Patients present on first day of month and first day of next month	For each type of ICU • Overall ICU rate per 100 patients and 1,000 patient-days • Urinary catheter-associated UTI rate per 1,000 urinary catheter-days • Central line-associated BSI rate per 1,000 central line-days • Ventilator-associated pneumonia rate per 1,000 ventilator-days Device utilization ratios • Overall • Central line • Ventilator • Urinary catheter

High-risk nursery	All infants in level III or II/III nursery
	Follow patients for 48 hours after discharge from HRN
		All infection sites with date of onset in same month	Data collected for each of 4 birth-weight categories
			• $\leq$1,000 g
			• 1,001–1,500 g
			• 15,01–2,500 g
			• $>$2,500 g
			Number of
			• Patients
			• Patient-days
			• Central (umbilical) line-days
			• Ventilator-days
			• Infants present on first day of month and first day of next month
				Overall HRN rate per 100 patients at risk and 1,000 patient-days
				For each birth-weight category
				• Overall rate per 100 patients at risk and per 1,000 patient-days
				• Central (umbilical) line-associated BSI rate per 1,000 central line-days
				• Ventilator-associated pneumonia rate per 1,000 ventilator-days
				Device utilization ratios
				• Overall
				• For each birth-weight category
				  • Central (umbilical) line
				  • Ventilator

Surgical patient	All patients undergoing selected NNIS operative procedures Patients followed for infection until their discharge	All infection sites or surgical site infections only in patients who had their operation during the same month	Risk-specific data on every patient monitored • Operation date • NNIS operative procedure category • Patient ID number • Age • Sex • Duration of operation • Wound class • General anesthesia • ASA score • Emergency • Trauma • Multiple procedures • Endoscopic approach • Discharge date	SSI rates by • Procedure and risk index • Wound class Standardized infection ratios by procedure Rates by procedure and site
Optional Data				
Hospital-wide	All patients	All infection sites with date of onset in same month	Number of • Admissions or discharges from each hospital ward • Patient-days from each hospital ward	Rates per 1,000 patient-days or 100 admissions or discharges • Overall • Site-specific • Ward-specific • Site-specific by ward
Surgical patient	Same as for required data	Same as for required data	Name or code of surgeon	SSI rates by surgeon, procedure, and risk index
			Hospital-defined optional data	Standardized infection ratios by surgeon and procedure Rates by surgeon and site

ASA, American Society of Anesthesiology; BSI, bloodstream infection; HRN, high-risk nursery; ICU, intensive care unit; NNIS, National Nosocomial Infection, Surveillance; UTI, urinary tract infection.

TABLE 94.3. METHODS FOR SURVEILLANCE OF NOSOCOMIAL INFECTIONS: ADVANTAGES AND DISADVANTAGES

Method	Advantages	Disadvantages
Hospital-wide		
Ongoing	Provides data on all infections in all patients; identifies clusters	Expensive and labor intensive; interhospital comparison of rates not possible
Prevalence	Inexpensive and requires little effort; may also be done on a rotating basis	Overestimates patients' risk of acquiring infection; estimates not precise enough to detect important differences among patient populations
Targeted		
Site-directed	Flexible; can be mixed with other methods	May not have defined prevention objectives; denominator data may be inadequate; may miss clusters
Unit-directed	Focuses on patients at greater risk; may require fewer personnel	Continuous surveillance required to establish baseline rates; may miss clusters
Objective/priority-directed	Uses resources more effectively by focusing on user-defined prevention objectives	No baseline rates; may miss clusters
Limited periodic	Provides baseline data; less time-consuming than ongoing hospital-wide	May miss clusters
Postdischarge	Substantially increases SSI case finding	Problems with timeliness and accuracy of data and with patients lost to follow-up

SSI, surgical site infection.
Adapted from Perl TM. Surveillance, reporting, and the use of computers. In: Wenzel, RP, ed. *Prevention and control of nosocomial infections,* 2nd ed. Baltimore: Williams & Wilkins, 1993:152, with permission.

Participation in the NNIS system requires active, patient-based, prospective surveillance. The methods of surveillance used by NNIS participants have been described (6) and are updated in Table 94.2. The forms used are included in Appendix B. NNIS surveillance methods are a mix of several different strategies described in this section. Finally, all methods described in this section (Table 94.2) are designed to detect new or incident cases of nosocomial infection and generally will yield incidence rates or incidence density (refer to the section on Data Analysis).

Incidence Versus Prevalence in Hospital-Wide Surveillance

There are two types of hospital-wide surveillance: incidence and prevalence. Incidence surveillance is continual monitoring of all patients for new nosocomial infections of all kinds on all wards. It has also been termed "ongoing," "total," "housewide," or "comprehensive" surveillance (35,36). Hospital-wide surveillance has the advantage of providing a global view of what is happening in the hospital so that potential clusters of infection or antibiotic resistance can be detected anywhere. It does, however, require considerable time and personnel resources and may not be driven by clear objectives for prevention. Furthermore, denominators that adjust for case mix are not available for calculating risk-adjusted infection rates (27).

TABLE 94.4. ESSENTIAL DATA ON NOSOCOMIAL INFECTIONS

Demographic
Name
Age
Sex
Hospital identification number
Service
Ward/intensive care unit
Admission date
Infection
Onset date
Site of infection
Laboratory
Pathogen(s)
Antibiogram

Prevalence surveillance is surveillance for all active (existing and new) nosocomial infections in the hospital on a single day (point prevalence) or over several days (period prevalence); each bed is visited only once. It is usually performed by a team that has been trained to use surveillance definitions and uses chart review, discussion with caregivers, or direct assessment of patients to identify infections.

The advantage of prevalence surveillance is that it is a rapid inexpensive way to estimate the magnitude of nosocomial infection problems in a hospital (37). Data from a prevalence survey may be helpful when trying to establish the scope and magnitude of nosocomial infections in a hospital, stratified by hospital ward or service. There are two major disadvantages of prevalence surveillance. First, in small hospitals, the number of patients surveyed is insufficient to detect important differences among patient populations, for example, a difference between pneumonia rates on medical and surgical services. Second, patients' risk of infection is overestimated with the prevalence rate, which is calculated as the number of active infections on the day of the visit divided by the number of beds visited. This is due to the influence of the duration of infections (38), as is explained in the section on defining and calculating rates.

Prevalence surveillance data have been used in several ways with varying success. One study demonstrated that secular trends in the epidemiology of nosocomial infections in an institution may be estimated from repeatedly conducting prevalence surveys (39). However, the interpretation of the results was complicated by the small number of patients studied and variations in the types of prevalence rates calculated. Therefore, secular trends are best derived from ongoing prospective (incidence) surveillance methods.

Another use of prevalence surveys is to determine the approximate sensitivity of a hospital's ongoing prospective surveillance, that is, how well true infections are being detected (40). The assumption is made that the prevalence surveyors will detect and correctly identify 100% of infections. An estimate is derived of the percentage of true infections detected by routine surveillance; this has been termed the *efficiency-of-reporting score* or *efficiency factor* (40,41). The efficiency factor, which was found in one national study to be 65%, can then be used to adjust incidence rate estimates for the magnitude of underascertainment and, thus, yield a more accurate rate (41). This method and all incidence surveillance methods assume perfect specificity (1.0), that is, that patients without infection are identified as truly not having infection. In one study, it was shown that ICPs had more difficulty determining when an infection was not present than when one was (18), suggesting the need to adjust infection rates by this factor and by efficiency.

Before ongoing prospective surveillance attained widespread use in this country, some investigators used data from prevalence surveillance performed at regular intervals or from a single study to estimate the incidence of nosocomial infections (42–44). This use has not been widely applied, partly because of the statistical conversion necessary.

Some have used prevalence surveillance to estimate antimicrobial use and adherence to isolation practices and to monitor practices related to high-risk devices such as intravascular catheters (39,45). One group of investigators used sequential prevalence surveys to estimate the effectiveness of their infection control program on reducing the risks of nosocomial infection (37). Prevalence surveillance data have also been used to heighten the awareness of nosocomial infection problems in institutions without other surveillance methods in place and have been influential in helping establish ongoing prospective (incidence) surveillance.

Finally, using prevalence surveillance to establish a single overall rate for the purposes of interhospital comparison is not recommended for the same reasons that overall rates generated from incidence surveillance are inappropriate (27).

Targeted Surveillance

Surveillance strategies that demanded more efficiency of ICPs began to emerge in the late 1970s. These strategies focused or targeted efforts on certain areas in the hospitals (e.g., ICUs), patient groups (e.g., surgical patients), or infection sites (e.g., bloodstream infections). These targeted efforts have become increasingly common in this decade not only because of their positive impact on resource management but because they have the potential for yielding more meaningful results than hospital-wide surveillance. A disadvantage of these limited strategies is that clusters of infection in areas not under surveillance may be missed.

Site-directed targeted surveillance focuses on detecting one or more specific sites of infection (e.g., bloodstream infections) occurring among all hospitalized patients. This method may easily be combined with other strategies. Two potential disadvantages, however, are that clearly defined prevention objectives may not have been established and that adequate denominator data may not be readily available across the entire hospital (such as number of device-specific days).

Unit-directed surveillance targets specific units or wards with the highest risks of nosocomial infection (e.g., ICU and bone marrow transplant units) (40). The ICU and HRN components are examples of unit-directed surveillance in the NNIS system. Usually, patients are monitored for the presence of all types of infection, although some hospitals may choose to focus only on a particular infection (e.g., ventilator-associated pneumonia). Because a geographically smaller area is covered during unit-directed surveillance, theoretically less time is needed for this type of surveillance. However, because patients in these units are among the most ill in the hospital, they also have extensive records. Therefore, time spent per patient's record reviewed with this method actually may be greater than for other surveillance strategies.

Objective/Priority-Directed Surveillance

This method, also called surveillance by objective, was promulgated by Haley in the mid-1980s (21,22). Infections are prioritized for prevention efforts—the more serious the infection, the more effort expended. In determining which infections to rank highest, Haley suggested considering more than just the relative frequency of occurrence. Factors to assess include morbidity and mortality, extra costs associated with the infection, and preventability (46–48). Accordingly, SSIs and pneumonias would be allocated the most surveillance resources (one half and one third, respectively), with much less for bloodstream and urinary tract infections. The surgical patient component of the NNIS system allows hospitals the opportunity to follow patients undergoing selected operations for nosocomial infections in a priority-directed manner. Objectives for surveillance should be evaluated annually and adjusted as necessary. The obvious advantage of this method is that specific measurable objectives are set and attainment is carefully evaluated. Therefore, ICP time and effort are directed in a very productive manner. A potential disadvantage is undetected outbreaks, although Haley recommended that the ICP train other hospital staff to be alert for and report unusual clustering (49).

Limited Periodic Surveillance

This method is a combination of hospital-wide and site-specific targeted surveillance. Chelgren and LaForce (50) used total surveillance for 1 month per quarter and targeted bloodstream infection surveillance during the other 8 months. Although the potential for missing clusters is less than for targeted methods, it still exists during two thirds of the year.

Postdischarge Surveillance

There is currently no standard method for following patients for evidence of infection once they have left the hospital. The impetus for tracking patients during the postdischarge period stems from the decrease in patients lengths of stay after surgery that has been largely due to the adoption of the prospective payment system and implementation of diagnosis-related groups (51–53). Because of the shorter postoperative stay, it is estimated that as many as 50% of SSIs may be missed if a formal postdischarge surveillance system is not in place (54). The techniques for case-finding used include one or more of the following: patient contact by telephone or mail; physician contact by telephone or mail; observation in clinic by surgeon, nurse, or ICP; and detection on readmission (55–68). Significant methodologic problems with postdischarge surveillance include reliance on physicians to return information on patients to the ICP in a timely manner, patients' inability to accurately diagnose infection (69), and determination of how to handle patients lost to follow-up. More recently, efforts focusing on antimicrobial use in surgical patients after discharge have improved case finding in this setting and demonstrated the poor sensitivity of other methods of postdischarge surveillance such as mailed questionnaires to surgeons or patients (70). However, refinements in this approach are needed, especially because many institutions are unable to examine antimicrobial use in their outpatient populations in a systematic way. Until a standard method for postdischarge surveillance is developed and validated, the Surgical Wound Infection Task Force recommended in 1992 that hospitals use a method that accommodates their resources and data needs (19). Some progress has been made since that recommendation. Monitoring outpatient antibiotic use (70) or automated medical records (71) has proven more efficient than some more traditional approaches of postdischarge surveillance but may not be widely applicable (72).

DATA COLLECTION

Numerator

What Data to Collect

Three categories of data comprise the usual information collected on a patient with a nosocomial infection: demographic, infection, and laboratory data. Table 94.4 shows the most essential data. Information describing important risk factors for infection should also be collected but only if it will be analyzed and used by the hospital. For example, timing, dosage, and route of administration of preoperative antibiotics may be collected if such data will be used to help understand and guide the practice of surgical prophylaxis. Risk factors specific for certain types of infection are also useful, such as an indwelling urinary catheter for urinary tract infection, central intravascular or peripheral lines for primary bloodstream infection, or a ventilator for pneumonia. Where feasible, corresponding denominator data should also be collected so that risk-adjusted infection rates can be calculated (e.g., ventilator-associated pneumonia rates per 1,000 ventilator-days in a specific type of ICU). In the NNIS system, information on adverse outcomes of nosocomial infection are also collected, such as development of a secondary bloodstream infection and whether the patient died. If the patient died, the ICP must make a determination of the relationship of infection to death, which is helpful in understanding one outcome of nosocomial infections.

For infected surgical patients, it may be useful to collect risk factors associated with the operation. In the NNIS system, the following are reported for infections noted in patients being monitored under the surgical patient surveillance component: operative procedure category; date, duration, and wound class of the operation; ASA score; whether general anesthesia was given, an endoscopic approach was used, or multiple procedures were done through the same incision on the same trip to the operating room; and whether the procedure was an emergency or was done as a result of traumatic injury to the patient. In addition, the date of discharge is reported so that length of postoperative stay can be determined. When these data are also collected on all surgical patients being monitored (denominators), specific rates can be calculated (Table 94.2).

Whenever possible, the data should be entered and analyzed with the aid of a computer and securely stored. Included in Appendix B is the NNIS Infection Worksheet, the infection data collection form used by hospitals in the NNIS system. Appendix C lists the definitions of some key terms used in the NNIS system.

Who Should Collect the Data

The ICP should be responsible for identifying nosocomial infections because of her or his knowledge of the criteria for defining infections and skill at finding them. Others who interact with patients or review charts on a regular basis may be able to provide the ICP with assistance, but they should not make the decision as to presence or absence of infection.

Sources of Data

Many sources of data are used to perform surveillance, depending on the type of patients served by the hospital (35,73). The ICP should have ready access to every area of the hospital and the full cooperation of hospital staff to perform surveillance or conduct an outbreak investigation (20). The first step should be initial case finding. This usually begins with the admission department, microbiology laboratory records, patient wards, or other areas to determine which patients' charts should be reviewed.

Computerized Patient Records

Information technology is rapidly evolving. Computerized patient records are available in a number of hospitals in the United States. This technology will eventually have a significant impact on surveillance. Using computerized data, ICPs will be able to identify a signal that suggests that an adverse event might be present, which can then be investigated. Although this approach also typically involves going to the chart to verify the event, it is much less costly than review of unscreened charts. Such a process may already be used at hospitals for microbiology data, but the computerized medical record will allow monitoring of clinical events such as fevers, radiologic findings such as new pulmonary infiltrates, or antimicrobial use. Because only a small proportion of charts need to be reviewed, the review can be highly focused saving up to 65% of an ICP's time (74–76).

The second step is case confirmation. The most important internal source for confirmation is the patient's chart, which contains results of laboratory, radiology, and pathology studies; nursing and physician's notes and consults; the admission diagnosis; history and physical examination findings; records of diagnostic and surgical interventions; a temperature chart; and information on administration of antibiotics. Patient care staff, including nurses, physicians, and respiratory therapists, are excellent adjunctive data sources. Several departments can also provide information that may be helpful in identifying clusters or trends: laboratory, admissions, pharmacy, radiology, and pathology. External sources of data such as health departments or the CDC may be helpful in alerting the ICP to newly emerging infections and strategies for prevention and control.

How to Collect the Data

Regardless of the active prospective surveillance method used (see next section), collecting data on infected patients is essentially the same. The usual way to collect the data is to review laboratory data and then the patient's record (77,78). When access to computerized data sources exists, the ICP can perform many case-finding activities at her or his desk. However, there is no substitute for frequent visits to the laboratory and patient care areas.

Usually, case-finding begins with the ICP screening admission lists for patients admitted with infection (either community-acquired or nosocomial from a previous visit) and those whose diagnoses put them at risk of acquiring nosocomial infection (e.g., diabetes or severe immunosuppressive disorders). Next, a visit to the laboratory to review culture reports can help better define the list of patients whose records require review. On the ward, a quick screening of nursing care reports, temperature charts, antibiotic administration sheets, and Kardexes, plus conversations with nurses and physicians, can expand or narrow the list further. Regular visits to both the microbiology laboratory and patient wards give the ICP the chance to frequently interact with these staff members to pick up clues on infected patients and to provide on-the-spot infection control education. Finally, records are reviewed for evidence of infection, and infection data collection forms are completed. Physicians progress notes and nurses notes are particularly helpful and should be reviewed first.

Denominator

What Data to Collect

The denominators of infection rates are a tabulation of the cohorts of patients at risk of acquiring nosocomial infections. For comparative purposes, the traditional denominators of patients admitted to or discharged from the hospital, ward, or service have largely been replaced by those that better account for the differences in the risks of the monitored patients, such as number of days of device exposure. Examples of denominators currently used in NNIS hospitals using the ICU surveillance component are total number of patients and patient-days in the unit and total number of ventilator-days, central-line days, and urinary catheter-days. Table 94.2 lists required and optional denominator data for each of the NNIS surveillance components.

Data Sources and Collection Techniques

The ICP should enlist the help of others to collect denominator data. Operating room staff keep detailed logs of each procedure performed and should be encouraged to send daily reports to the ICP. Alternatively, if the operating room records are computerized, these data can be downloaded directly into the infection control department's computer. Similarly, a ward clerk in the ICU or HRN can easily be trained to perform daily counts of the number of patients admitted and the number of commonly used devices associated with nosocomial infections (e.g., urinary catheters). The midnight census can be used as the source of the number of patients in the ICU, and a copy should be obtained daily by the ICP.

DATA ANALYSIS

Defining and Calculating Rates

A rate is an expression of probability of occurrence of an event. It usually takes the form $(x/y)k$, where x, the numerator, is the number of times an event has occurred during a specified time period; y, the denominator, equals the population from which those experiencing the event were derived during the same time period; and k is the base or a round number (e.g., 100, 1,000, or 10,000) that can help express the rate as a whole integer. The time period must be specified and be identical for the numerator and denominator for the rate to be meaningful.

Three kinds of rates are used in nosocomial infection surveillance or, in reality, any surveillance: incidence, prevalence, and incidence density. Incidence is the number of new cases of disease that occur in a defined population during a specified period of time. For nosocomial infection incidence, it is simply the number of new nosocomial infections in a given time period divided by the number of patients at risk during that time period.

Prevalence is the total number of active (existing and new) cases of the disease in a defined population either during a specified period of time (period prevalence) or at a specified point in time (point prevalence). The point prevalence nosocomial infection rate is calculated simply by dividing the number of active nosocomial infections in patients surveyed by the number of patients surveyed.

Rhame described the relationship between incidence and prevalence rates as follows: $I = P[LA/(LN - INTN)]$, where I is the incidence rate, P is the prevalence rate, LA is the mean length of hospital stay for all patients, LN is the mean length of hospital stay for patients with one or more nosocomial infections, and $INTN$ is the mean interval from admission to the first nosocomial infection in those patients with one or more nosocomial infections (38,79). In the hospital setting, prevalence rates almost always overestimate the infection risk, because the length of stay of uninfected patients is usually shorter than for those with infection. This can be seen more readily by rearranging the equation as $P = I(LN - INTN)/LA$, such that prevalence equals incidence times infection duration.

Incidence density is the instantaneous rate at which disease is occurring, relative to the size of the disease-free population. Incidence density is measured in units of the number of cases of disease per person per unit of time. An example of an incidence density that is commonly used in healthcare settings is the number of nosocomial infections per 1,000 patient-days. Incidence density is useful essentially in two situations. First, it is useful when the infection rate is a linear function of the length of time a patient is exposed to a risk factor (i.e., the longer the patient is exposed, the greater the chance of acquiring infection). For example, rate 1, number of urinary catheter-associated urinary tract infections divided by the number of indwelling urinary catheter-days, is more useful than rate 2, number of urinary catheter-associated urinary tract infections divided by the number of patients with urinary catheters, because rate 1 controls for the length of time a patient is exposed to the risk factor—the indwelling urinary catheter—which is linearly related to the infection risk.

One other rate that is often used is the attack rate, which is a special type of incidence rate. It is usually expressed as a percentage, where $k = 100$, and is used almost exclusively for describing outbreaks of infection where particular populations are exposed for short periods of time.

Importance of Computer Assistance

Surveillance is a time-consuming process requiring nearly half of an ICP's time (80). The principal reason for considering computer support for surveillance is efficiency in analysis. The data volume and detail and analytic complexity make the use of a computer essential to all but the smallest hospital. In addition, a surveillance system should have the flexibility to deal not only with current difficulties but other areas that may become problems in the future.

Advice for selecting a computer-based system has been given elsewhere (81). Briefly, an ICP or hospital epidemiologist cannot function properly in their position without the help of a computer. Computer networks in hospitals now allow data on patient census, test results, and other information to be transferred electronically. Specialized software for infection control is available from a variety of vendors but is often expensive. It is possible to collect and analyze surveillance data using applications that are supplied on most computers, but the process can be simplified by infection control software. Most importantly, the decision on specific software should follow a careful examination of a program's needs. Any decisions on computer hardware should follow the decision on software. (See also Section III.)

Comparing Rates among Patient Groups

The denominator of a rate must reflect the population at risk. To compare a rate among patient groups within a hospital, over time, or across hospitals, ICPs must adjust the rate for the variations in the major risk factor(s) that leads to the infection. The importance of risk adjustment was demonstrated when the former Health Care Financing Administration failed to adjust for the major risk factor predicting mortality, severity of illness. This failure made these rates uninterpretable to most hospital administrators (82,83).

A patient's predisposition for becoming infected is strongly influenced by certain risk factors such as personal characteristics and exposures. These risk factors are roughly divided into two categories, intrinsic and extrinsic factors (20,27). Intrinsic risk factors are those that are inherent in the patient, such as underlying disease conditions and advanced age (20). Knowledge of the intrinsic risk factors is useful, because separate risk-specific rates can be calculated that permit the comparison of rates among patients with similar risks in different hospitals or different time periods. There has been considerable discussion but limited progress on the difficult task of developing a practical risk index that can be used to adjust the overall nosocomial infection rate (84). The Acute Physiologic and Chronic Health Evaluation (APACHE II) and diagnosis-related groups are two well-known indices for severity of illness and are used to predict the risk of death among ICU patients and resource utilization, respectively. They are less useful when applied to nosocomial infections, because the factors associated with increased mortality and resource utilization apparently are not the same as those that increase the risk of infection. Patients with very high APACHE II scores probably do not survive long enough to acquire a nosocomial infection. A recent review suggests that no current severity of illness scoring system consistently risk adjusts for nosocomial infections (85). Basic studies are needed to describe simple objective measures of severity of illness and/or underlying diseases that correlate with site-specific nosocomial infections. These efforts should also control for extrinsic risk factors for nosocomial infections, such as device exposure.

Extrinsic risk factors may be patient care staff based (practices of an individual caregiver) or institution based (practices in an entire hospital). Although many extrinsic factors contribute to nosocomial infections, the factors that have been most frequently implicated and studied are certain high-risk medical interventions such as surgical operations or the use of invasive devices (23,86–90). There are numerous reasons why the nosocomial infection rate in patients exposed to certain devices is many times greater than among those not exposed to the devices (27). Patients who require invasive devices may have more severe underlying disease conditions that increase their susceptibility to infections. These devices also provide a pathway for microorganisms from the environment to enter the body; facilitate the transfer of pathogens from one part of the patient's body to another; and act as inanimate foci where pathogens can proliferate, protected from the patient's immune defenses.

The risk of SSI is related to a number of factors. Among the most important are the operative procedure performed, the degree of microbiologic contamination of the operative field, duration of operation, and the intrinsic risk of the patient (11, 89). Because infection control practices cannot ordinarily alter or eliminate these risks, SSI rates must be adjusted for these risks before the rates can be used for comparative purposes. Two SSI risk indices—basic and modified—that effectively adjusts SSI rates for most operations have been developed by the NNIS system (11,91).

Figure 94.1 more fully illustrates the effect of risk adjustment when comparing infection rates of various patient groups in hospital ICUs. The rate for Hospital Unit A, which uses the number of patients in the denominator, was nearly five times higher than the median for similar ICUs. However, Hospital Unit A had the highest central line use, that is, more than 80% of patient-days were also central line-days. Using central line-days as the denominator of the rate helps to take into account this high use of central lines; thus, Hospital Unit A's device-

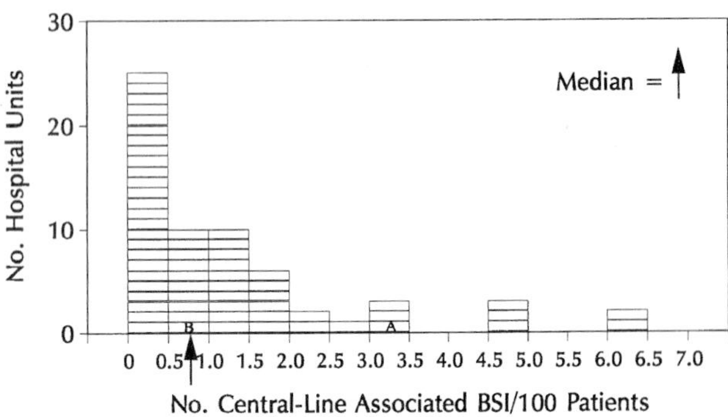

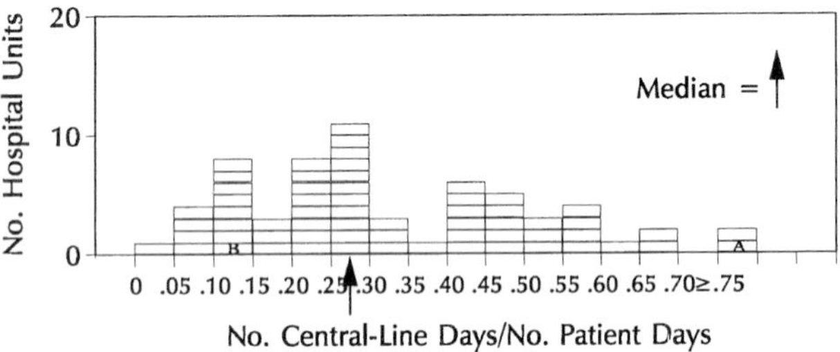

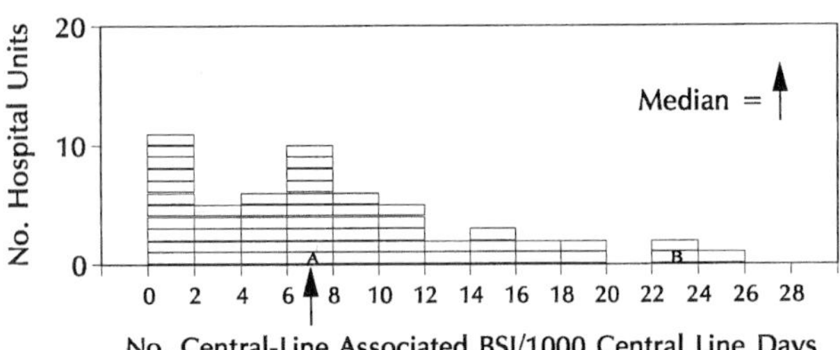

Figure 94.1. Comparison of the distributions of bloodstream infection (BSI) rates (based on patients and on central line-days) and central line use in combined coronary and medical intensive care units (ICUs). **A** and **B** indicate the specific location of individual hospital unit rates. ICU Component, NNIS System, October 1986 to December 1990. (Adapted from Jarvis WR, Edwards JR, Culver DH, et al. Nosocomial infection rates in adult and pediatric intensive care units in the United States. National Nosocomial Infections Surveillance System. *Am J Med* 1991;91(Suppl 3B):185S5–191S5, with permission.)

associated device-day bloodstream infection rate was slightly lower than the median. Although using Hospital Unit A's device-associated, device-day bloodstream infection rate eliminated its high outlier status, the unit's high central line use may need to be reviewed for appropriateness. On the other hand, for Hospital Unit B, the central line-associated bloodstream infection patient rate was near the median and the central line use was low. When Hospital Unit B's rate was calculated using central line-days in the denominator, it was quite high, possibly suggesting the need to review central line insertion and maintenance practices.

Comparing Rates Over Time

The same issues that require risk adjustment when comparing rates among patient groups are evident when comparing rates over time. The epidemiology of nosocomial infections has been affected by the introduction of the prospective payment system that changed the economics of healthcare delivery in the United States (92–94). Patients admitted to hospitals are different from what they were only a few years ago. More surgical operations are performed in outpatient settings, and patients are more seriously ill at the time of admission or require sophisticated and sometimes high-risk procedures that can be performed only on inpatients. Paradoxically, they are usually discharged from the hospital earlier than in previous years (95), and their care is usually continued at home or in skilled nursing or rehabilitation facilities. With increasing average severity of illness among hospitalized patients, the infection rate is also expected to increase. The task of the infection control program to monitor the infection rate is complicated by the difficulty of detecting infections in patients after discharge from the hospital. Postdischarge surveillance for certain infection sites may be necessary for a quality surveillance system and is being urged by some experts (53). Because these factors can be correlated with nosocomial infection rates, controlling for these changes over time is just as important as it is when one compares two populations of patients who have different severities of illness.

Comparing Infection Rates

Hospitals use surveillance data to assess their infection control program by comparing their infection rates with similar patient populations within the hospital (two separate ICUs) or with external benchmark rates or by comparing changes in rates over time in their own hospital. However, such comparisons can only be made if the rates control for variations in the distribution of the major risk factors associated with the infections. This process of developing comparable rates requires that the rates are site specific, that uniform definitions and surveillance protocols are used to collect the data, that there is consistent and accurate case-finding, and that the risks are similar or controlled for by risk-adjustment methods (such as stratification or standardization) (96). The NNIS system uses a population-based surveillance system that provides risk-adjusted rates that can be used for interhospital comparisons (27,97).

Testing for significance among infection rates is the subject of Chapter 3. However, the interpretation of those statistical tests should be carefully considered. Many hospitals assume that any difference in the rates represents success or failure in the patient care staff or institutional practices to prevent nosocomial infections. Although this may be true, there are other factors that could account for the differences in the rates. First, surveillance definitions or techniques may not be uniform among the hospitals or they may be used inconsistently over time, causing variations to occur in sensitivity and specificity of infection case-finding. Second, inaccurate or insufficient information about clinical and laboratory evidence of infections in the patient's medical record may seriously affect the validity and utility of the infection rate.

Third, the rates may not be adjusted for patients' intrinsic risks for infection. These risks are usually outside of the control of the hospital and vary from hospital to hospital but are important factors in determining whether patients will develop infections. For example, a hospital with a large proportion of immunocompromised patients would be expected to have a population at higher intrinsic risk for infection than a hospital without such a population of patients. The unsuccessful attempts to compare unadjusted mortality rates (82,83) are reminders to those comparing infection rates that they must also take care to risk adjust nosocomial infection rates. Finally, the size of the population at risk (e.g., number of patients, admissions and discharges, patient-days, or operations) may not be large enough to calculate rates that adequately estimate the true rates for the hospital.

Although it may not be possible to fully correct for these factors, hospitals should be aware of how these factors affect the infection rate and take them into consideration when interpreting the data.

Identifying Outbreaks

An epidemic is defined as an unusual statistically significant increase in the incidence of a particular disease. This definition does not automatically send a signal to those who analyze surveillance data as to when to initiate an investigation. However, there are important implications for analyzing surveillance data when considering this definition. The opportunity to determine an infection rate's change over time to detect an "unusual statistically significant increase" implies that the information is already being collected. This is often not the case. An astute clinician or laboratory worker may report the apparent increase in the incidence of an infection, but proving the existence of an outbreak may require additional baseline data. However, if the data are already available, considerable time can be saved.

One popular approach has been the "setting of a threshold rate" for initiating an investigation. This cannot be done without considerable experience with data. Using an arbitrary number or a rate for establishing a threshold for initiating an investigation is usually an inefficient use of resources, because it is sometimes set so low that excessive investigation occurs. Worse, an extremely high threshold may exclude initiating a needed investigation. The use of aggregate data from a source such as the NNIS system may help determine whether an investigation is needed. However, a high rate does not define a problem for the reasons noted previously.

Assessing Appropriateness of Medical Care

Device utilization (DU) can be defined as the number of device-days divided by the number of patient-days. For the adult and pediatric ICU component of the NNIS system, device-days consist of the total number of ventilator-days, central line-days, and urinary catheter-days. The DU of an ICU is one measure of the unit's invasive practices that constitute an extrinsic risk factor for nosocomial infection. As such, DU may also serve as a marker for severity of illness of patients in the unit, that is, patients intrinsic susceptibility to infection. The unit's DU is independent of the device-associated device-day infection rate. An ICP's attention should not focus solely on infection rates in hospitals. Those responsible for delivery of quality medical care must ask whether patients' exposures to interventions (e.g., devices or operative procedures) that increase risks of nosocomial infection have been minimized wherever possible. For ICUs and HRNs, the extent of DU of an ICU or HRN may have to be examined. For surgical patients undergoing specific procedures, the distribution of patients among the risk categories may provide valuable information (27). For example, it may help in determining whether appropriate classification has occurred. Examining the appropriateness of an intervention may also aid in determining whether patient exposure was minimized. However, once the decision is made to use a device (i.e., place the patient at higher risk for a nosocomial infection), the infection rate is independent of the DU.

DATA DISSEMINATION

Surveillance is not complete until the data are disseminated to those who will use it to prevent and control infections. Because of its sensitive nature, information containing identifiers of patients or patient care staff should be carefully handled. In some states such data are confidential. Data should not be used for punitive purposes but rather to augment quality improvement efforts.

It is customary for the ICP to provide, on a regular basis, a narrative summary and tabular and graphic reports of surveillance data to the hospital's infection control committee. The ICP should only include infection rates for which there are sufficient denominator data to calculate meaningful estimates of risk. Therefore, in many small hospitals or when small numbers of patients are at risk in larger institutions (e.g., for certain low-volume operations), monthly rate tabulation will not be practical. Rates may have to be calculated quarterly, semiannually, or annually, depending on the size of the denominator. In addition, a thorough analysis of numerator data (i.e., the nosocomial infections) can be performed to gain insight into their epidemiology, including information on pathogens and risk factors.

APPLICATION OF SURVEILLANCE METHODS TO NONINFECTIOUS OUTCOMES OF HOSPITALIZATION

Nearly all of the considerations in monitoring hospital-acquired infections can be applied to noninfectious outcomes of hospitalization. The characteristics of a successful monitoring and reporting system include the system being nonpunitive, confidential, independent, timely, systems-oriented, and responsive and having expert analysis (98). Indeed, one expert has cited the NNIS system as a model for reporting such events (98). ICPs experienced in monitoring hospital-acquired infections can lend considerable expertise to colleagues monitoring other adverse events and attempting to improve the quality of care throughout the institution. Because the collection of reliable data is an essential element of this evaluation process, nosocomial infection surveillance can make an important contribution to continuous quality improvement in the hospital. Examination of complication rates (a more general approach than merely examining infection rates) and the "appropriateness" of medical interventions are of major interest to quality assurance personnel (99,100). NNIS data suggest that interhospital comparison of indicators of quality of medical care will be more useful if these indicators examine the use of practices that increase patients' extrinsic risk and rates of adverse outcomes that attempt to control for exposure to the major risk factor(s) among patients with similar intrinsic risk-adjusted rates of adverse outcomes. Failure to do so will certainly make interhospital comparisons meaningless or even misleading (27).

APPENDIX A-1. CDC DEFINITIONS OF NOSOCOMIAL INFECTIONS [EXCLUDING PNEUMONIA (SEE APPENDIX A-2)]

Listing of Major and Specific Site Codes and Descriptions

UTI **Urinary Tract Infection**
- SUTI Symptomatic urinary tract infection
- ASB Asymptomatic bacteriuria
- OUTI Other infections of the urinary tract

SSI **Surgical Site Infection**
- SKIN Superficial incisional site, except after CBGB[1]
- SKNC After CBGB, report SKNC for superficial incisional infection at chest incision site
- SKNL After CBGB, report SKNL for superficial incisional infection at leg (donor) site
- ST Deep incisional surgical site infection, except after CBGB
- STC After CBGB, report STC for deep incisional surgical site infection at chest incision site
- STL After CBGB, report STL for deep incisional surgical site infection at leg (donor) site
- Organ/Space Surgical Site Infection
  Indicate specific site:
  BONE, BRST, CARD, DISC, EAR, EMET, ENDO, EYE, GIT, IAB, IC, JNT, LUNG, MED, MEN, ORAL, OREP, OUTI, SA, SINU, UR, VASC, VCUP.

PNEU **Pneumonia (See Appendix A:2)**
- PNU 1
- PNU 2
- PNU 3

BSI **Bloodstream Infection**
- LCBI Laboratory-confirmed bloodstream infection
- CSEP Clinical sepsis

BJ **Bone and Joint Infection**
- BONE Osteomyelitis
- JNT Joint or bursa
- DISC Disc space

CNS **Central Nervous System Infection**
- IC Intracranial infection
- MEN Meningitis or ventriculitis
- SA Spinal abscess without meningitis

CVS **Cardiovascular System Infection**
- VASC Arterial or venous infection
- ENDO Endocarditis
- CARD Myocarditis or pericarditis
- MED Mediastinitis

EENT **Eye, Ear, Nose, Throat, or Mouth Infection**
- CONJ Conjunctivitis
- EYE Eye Other than conjunctivitis
- EAR Ear Mastoid
- ORAL Oral Cavity (mouth, tongue, or gums)
- SINU Sinusitis
- UR Upper respiratory tract, pharyngitis, laryngitis, epiglottitis

GI **Gastrointestinal System Infection**
- GE Gastroenteritis
- GIT Gastrointestinal (GI) tract
- HEP Hepatitis
- IAB Intraabdominal, not specified elsewhere
- NEC Necrotizing enterocolitis

LRI **Lower Respiratory Tract Infection, Other Than Pneumonia**
- BRON Bronchitis, tracheobronchitis, tracheitis, without evidence of pneumonia
- LUNG Other infections of the lower respiratory tract

REPR **Reproductive Tract Infection**
- EMET Endometritis
- EPIS Episiotomy
- VCUF Vaginal cuff
- OREP Other infections of the male or female reproductive tract

SST **Skin and Soft Tissue Infection**
- SKIN Skin
- ST Soft tissue
- DECU Decubitus ulcer
- BURN Burn
- BRST Breast abscess or mastitis
- UMB Omphalitis
- PUST Infant pustulosis
- CIRC Newborn circumcision

SYS **Systemic Infection**
- DI Disseminated infection

Definitions of Infection Sites

INFECTION SITE: Symptomatic urinary tract infection
CODE: UTI-SUTI
DEFINITION: A symptomatic urinary tract infection must meet at least one of the following criteria:

Criterion 1: Patient has at least *one* of the following signs or symptoms with no other recognized cause: fever (>38°C), urgency, frequency, dysuria, or suprapubic tenderness
and
patient has a positive urine culture, that is, $\geq 10^5$ microorganisms per cm^3 of urine with no more than two species of microorganisms.

Criterion 2: Patient has at least *two* of the following signs or

[1] CBGB, coronary artery bypass graft with both chest and donor site incisions.

symptoms with no other recognized cause: fever (>38°C), urgency, frequency, dysuria, or suprapubic tenderness
and
at least *one* of the following:
a. Positive dipstick for leukocyte esterase and/or nitrate
b. Pyuria (urine specimen with ≥10 WBC/mm^3 or ≥3 WBC/high power field of unspun urine)
c. Organisms seen on Gram stain of unspun urine
d. At least *two* urine cultures with repeated isolation of the same uropathogen (gram-negative bacteria or *S. saprophyticus*) with ≥10^2 colonies/mL in nonvoided specimens
e. ≤10^5 colonies/mL of a single uropathogen (gram-negative bacteria or *S. saprophyticus*) in a patient being treated with an effective antimicrobial agent for a urinary tract infection
f. Physician diagnosis of a urinary tract infection
g. Physician institutes appropriate therapy for a urinary tract infection

Criterion 3: Patient ≤1 year of age has at least *one* of the following signs or symptoms with no other recognized cause: fever (>38°C), hypothermia (<37°C), apnea, bradycardia, dysuria, lethargy, or vomiting
and
patient has a positive urine culture, that is, ≥10^5 microorganisms per cm^3 of urine with no more than two species of microorganisms.

Criterion 4: Patient ≤1 year of age has at least *one* of the following signs or symptoms with no other recognized cause: fever (>38°C), hypothermia (<37°C), apnea, bradycardia, dysuria, lethargy, or vomiting
and
at least *one* of the following:
a. Positive dipstick for leukocyte esterase and/or nitrate
b. Pyuria (urine specimen with ≥10 WBC/mm^3 or ≥3 WBC/high power field of unspun urine)
c. Organisms seen on Gram stain of unspun urine
d. At least *two* urine cultures with repeated isolation of the same uropathogen (gram-negative bacteria or *S. saprophyticus*) with ≥10^2 colonies/mL in nonvoided specimens
e. ≤10^5 colonies/mL of a single uropathogen (gram-negative bacteria or *S. saprophyticus*) in a patient being treated with an effective antimicrobial agent for a urinary tract infection
f. Physician diagnosis of a urinary tract infection
g. Physician institutes appropriate therapy for a urinary tract infection

COMMENTS:

- A positive culture of a urinary catheter tip is *not* an acceptable laboratory test to diagnose a urinary tract infection.
- Urine cultures must be obtained using appropriate technique, such as clean catch collection or catheterization.
- In infants, a urine culture should be obtained by bladder catheterization or suprapubic aspiration; a positive urine culture from a bag specimen is unreliable and should be confirmed by a specimen aseptically obtained by catheterization or suprapubic aspiration.

INFECTION SITE: Asymptomatic bacteriuria
CODE: UTI-ASB
DEFINITION: An asymptomatic bacteriuria must meet at least one of the following criteria:

Criterion 1: Patient has had an indwelling urinary catheter within 7 days before the culture
and
patient has a positive urine culture, that is, ≥10^5 microorganisms per cm^3 of urine with no more than two species of microorganisms
and
patient has *no* fever (>38°C), urgency, frequency, dysuria, or suprapubic tenderness.

Criterion 2: Patient has *not* had an indwelling urinary catheter within 7 days before the first positive culture
and
patient has had at least *two* positive urine cultures, that is, ≥10^5 microorganisms per cm^3 of urine with repeated isolation of the same microorganism and no more than two species of microorganisms
and
patient has *no* fever (>38°C), urgency, frequency, dysuria, or suprapubic tenderness.

COMMENTS:

- A positive culture of a urinary catheter tip is *not* an acceptable laboratory test to diagnose bacteriuria.
- Urine cultures must be obtained using appropriate technique, such as clean catch collection or catheterization.

INFECTION SITE: Other infections of the urinary tract (kidney, ureter, bladder, urethra, or tissues surrounding the retroperitoneal or perinephric spaces)
CODE: SUTI-OUTI
DEFINITION: Other infections of the urinary tract must meet at least one of the following criteria:

Criterion 1 Patient has organisms isolated from culture of fluid (other than urine) or tissue from affected site.

Criterion 2: Patient has an abscess or other evidence of infection seen on direct examination, during a surgical operation, or during a histopathologic examination.

Criterion 3: Patient has at least *two* of the following signs or symptoms with no other recognized cause: fever (>38°C), localized pain, or localized tenderness at the involved site
and
at least *one* of the following:
a. Purulent drainage from affected site

b. Organisms cultured from blood that are compatible with suspected site of infection
c. Radiographic evidence of infection, for example, abnormal ultrasound, computed tomography (CT), magnetic resonance imaging (MRI), or radiolabel scan (gallium, technetium)
d. Physician diagnosis of infection of the kidney, ureter, bladder, urethra, or tissues surrounding the retroperitoneal or perinephric space
e. Physician institutes appropriate therapy for an infection of the kidney, ureter, bladder, urethra, or tissues surrounding the retroperitoneal or perinephric space

Criterion 4: Patient ≤1 year of age has at least one of the following signs or symptoms with no other recognized cause: fever (>38°C), hypothermia (<37°C), apnea, bradycardia, lethargy, or vomiting
and
at least *one* of the following:
a. Purulent drainage from affected site
b. Organisms cultured from blood that are compatible with suspected site of infection
c. Radiographic evidence of infection, for example, abnormal ultrasound, CT, MRI, or radiolabel scan (gallium, technetium)
d. Physician diagnosis of infection of the kidney, ureter, bladder, urethra, or tissues surrounding the retroperitoneal or perinephric space
e. Physician institutes appropriate therapy for an infection of the kidney, ureter, bladder, urethra, or tissues surrounding the retroperitoneal or perinephric space

REPORTING INSTRUCTION:

- Report infections following circumcision in newborns as SST-CIRC.

INFECTION SITE: Surgical site infection (superficial incisional)
CODE: SSI-(SKIN) except following the NNIS operative procedure, CBGB. For CBGB[a] only, if infection is at chest site, use SKNC (skin-chest) or if at leg (donor) site, use SKNL (skin-leg)
DEFINITION: A superficial SSI must meet the following criteria:
Infection occurs within 30 days after the operative procedure
and
involves only skin and subcutaneous tissue of the incision
and
patient has at least *one* of the following:
a. Purulent drainage from the superficial incision
b. Organisms isolated from an aseptically obtained culture of fluid or tissue from the superficial incision
c. At least one of the following signs or symptoms of infection: pain or tenderness, localized swelling, redness, or heat, *and* superficial incision is deliberately opened by surgeon, *unless* incision is culture-negative
d. Diagnosis of superficial incisional SSI by the surgeon or attending physician

REPORTING INSTRUCTIONS:

- Do *not* report a stitch abscess (minimal inflammation and discharge confined to the points of suture penetration) as an infection.
- Do not report a localized stab wound infection as SSI, instead report as skin or soft tissue infection, depending on its depth.
- Report infection of the circumcision site in newborns as SST-CIRC. Circumcision is not an NNIS operative procedure.
- Report infection of the episiotomy site as REPR-EPIS. Episiotomy is not an NNIS operative procedure.
- Report infected burn wound as SST-BURN.
- If the incisional site infection involves or extends into the fascial and muscle layers, report as a deep incisional SSI.
- Classify infection that involves *both* superficial and deep incision sites as deep incisional SSI.
- Report culture specimen from superficial incisions as ID (incisional drainage).

INFECTION SITE: Surgical site infection (deep incisional)
CODE: SSI-[ST (soft tissue)] except following the NNIS operative procedure, CBGB. For CBGB only, if infection is at chest site, use STC (soft tissue-chest) or if at leg (donor) site, use STL (soft tissue-leg)
DEFINITION: A deep incisional SSI must meet the following criteria:
Infection occurs within 30 days after the operative procedure if no implant[b] is left in place or within 1 year if implant is in place and the infection appears to be related to the operative procedure
and
involves deep soft tissues (e.g., fascial and muscle layers) of the incision
and
patient has at least *one* of the following:
a. Purulent drainage from the deep incision but not from the organ/space component of the surgical site
b. A deep incision spontaneously dehisces or is deliberately opened by a surgeon when the patient has at least one of the following signs or symptoms: fever (>38°C) or localized pain or tenderness, *unless* incision is culture-negative
c. An abscess or other evidence of infection involving the deep incision is found on direct

[a] CBGB, coronary artery bypass graft with both chest and donor site incisions.

[b] A nonhuman-derived implantable foreign body (e.g., prosthetic heart valve, nonhuman vascular graft, mechanical heart, or hip prosthesis) that is permanently placed in a patient during surgery.

examination, during reoperation, or by histopathologic or radiologic examination

d. Diagnosis of a deep incisional SSI by a surgeon or attending physician

REPORTING INSTRUCTIONS:

- Classify infection that involves *both* superficial and deep incision sites as deep incisional SSI.
- Report culture specimen from deep incisions as ID.

INFECTION SITE: Surgical site infection (organ/space)
CODE: SSI-(Specific site of organ/space)
DEFINITION: An organ/space SSI involves any part of the body, excluding the skin incision, fascia, or muscle layers, that is opened or manipulated during the operative procedure. Specific sites are assigned to organ/space SSI to further identify the location of the infection. Listed later are the specific sites that must be used to differentiate organ/space SSI. An example is appendectomy with subsequent subdiaphragmatic abscess, which would be reported as an organ/space SSI at the intraabdominal specific site (SSI-IAB).
An organ/space SSI must meet the following criteria:
Infection occurs within 30 days after the operative procedure if no implant[b] is left in place or within 1 year if implant is in place and the infection appears to be related to the operative procedure
and
infection involves any part of the body, excluding the skin incision, fascia, or muscle layers, that is opened or manipulated during the operative procedure
and
patient has at least *one* of the following:

a. Purulent drainage from a drain that is placed through a stab wound into the organ/space
b. Organisms isolated from an aseptically obtained culture of fluid or tissue in the organ/space
c. An abscess or other evidence of infection involving the organ/space that is found on direct examination, during reoperation, or by histopathologic or radiologic examination
d. Diagnosis of an organ/space SSI by a surgeon or attending physician

REPORTING INSTRUCTIONS:

- Occasionally, an organ/space infection drains through the incision. Such infection generally does not involve reoperation and is considered a complication of the incision. Therefore, it is classified as a deep incisional SSI.
- Report culture specimen from organ/space as DD (deep drainage).

The following are specific sites of an organ/space SSI:

Code	Site
BONE	Osteomyelitis
BRST	Breast abscess or mastitis
CARD	Myocarditis or pericarditis
DISC	Disc space
EAR	Ear, mastoid
EMET	Endometritis
ENDO	Endocarditis
EYE	Eye, other than conjunctivitis
GIT	GI tract
IAB	Intraabdominal, not specified elsewhere
IC	Intracranial, brain abscess or dura
JNT	Joint or bursa
LUNG	Other infections of the lower respiratory tract
MED	Mediastinitis
MEN	Meningitis or ventriculitis
ORAL	Oral cavity (mouth, tongue, or gums)
OREP	Other male or female
OUTI	Other infections of the urinary tract
SA	Spinal abscess without meningitis
SINU	Sinusitis
UR	Upper respiratory tract
VASC	Arterial or venous infection
VCUF	Vaginal cuff

INFECTION SITE: Pneumonia (See Appendix A-2)
INFECTION SITE: Laboratory-confirmed bloodstream infection
CODE: BSI-LCBI
DEFINITION: Laboratory-confirmed bloodstream infection must meet at least one of the following criteria:

Criterion 1: Patient has a recognized pathogen cultured from one or more blood cultures
and
organism cultured from blood is *not* related to an infection at another site.

Criterion 2: Patient has at least *one* of the following signs or symptoms: fever (>38°C), chills, or hypotension
and
at least *one* of the following:

a. Common skin contaminant (e.g., diphtheroids, *Bacillus* sp., *Propionibacterium* sp., coagulase-negative staphylococci, or micrococci) is cultured from two or more blood cultures drawn on separate occasions
b. Common skin contaminant (e.g., diphtheroids, *Bacillus* sp., *Propionibacterium* sp., coagulase-negative staphylococci, or micrococci) is cultured from at least one blood culture from a patient with an intravascular line, and the physician institutes appropriate antimicrobial therapy
c. Positive antigen test on blood (e.g., *Haemophilus influenzae, Streptococcus pneumoniae, Neisseria meningitidis,* or group B *Streptococcus*)

and
signs and symptoms and positive laboratory results are *not* related to an infection at another site.

Criterion 3: Patient ≤1 year of age has at least *one* of the following signs or symptoms: fever (>38°C), hypothermia (<37°C), apnea, or bradycardia
and
at least *one* of the following:

a. Common skin contaminant (e.g., diphtheroids, *Bacillus* sp., *Propionibacterium* sp., coagulase-negative staphylococci, or micrococci) is cultured from *two* or more blood cultures drawn on separate occasions

b. Common skin contaminant (e.g., diphtheroids, *Bacillus* sp., *Propionibacterium* sp., coagulase-negative staphylococci, or micrococci) is cultured from at least one blood culture from a patient with an intravascular line, and physician institutes appropriate antimicrobial therapy

c. Positive antigen test on blood (e.g., *H. influenzae, S. pneumoniae, N. meningitidis,* or group B *Streptococcus*)

and

signs and symptoms and positive laboratory results are *not* related to an infection at another site.

REPORTING INSTRUCTIONS:

- Report purulent phlebitis confirmed with a positive semi-quantitative culture of a catheter tip, but with either negative or no blood culture, as CVS-VASC.
- Report organisms cultured from blood as BSI-LCBI when no other site of infection is evident.
- Pseudobacteremias are not nosocomial infections.

INFECTION SITE: Clinical sepsis
CODE: BSI-CSEP
DEFINITION: Clinical sepsis must meet at least one of the following criteria:

Criterion 1: Patient has at least *one* of the following clinical signs or symptoms with no other recognized cause: fever (>38°C), hypotension (systolic pressure ≤ 90 mm Hg), or oliguria (<20 cm^3/hr)

and

blood culture *not* done or *no* organisms or antigen detected in blood

and

no apparent infection at another site

and

physician institutes treatment for sepsis.

Criterion 2: Patient ≤1 year of age has at least *one* of the following clinical signs or symptoms with no other recognized cause: fever (>38°C), hypothermia (<37°C), apnea, or bradycardia

and

blood culture *not* done or *no* organisms or antigen detected in blood

and

no apparent infection at another site

and

physician institutes treatment for sepsis.

REPORTING INSTRUCTION:

- Report culture-positive infections of the bloodstream as BSI-LCBI.

INFECTION SITE: Osteomyelitis
CODE: BJ-BONE
DEFINITION: Osteomyelitis must meet at least one of the following criteria:

Criterion 1: Patient has organisms cultured from bone.

Criterion 2: Patient has evidence of osteomyelitis on direct examination of the bone during a surgical operation or histopathologic examination.

Criterion 3: Patient has at least *two* of the following signs or symptoms with no other recognized cause: fever (>38°C), localized swelling, tenderness, heat, or drainage at suspected site of bone infection

and

at least *one* of the following:

a. Organisms cultured from blood
b. Positive blood antigen test (e.g., *H. influenzae, S. pneumoniae*)
c. Radiographic evidence of infection, for example, abnormal findings on x-ray, CT, MRI, radiolabeled scan (gallium, technetium, etc.)

INFECTION SITE: Joint or bursa
CODE: BJ-JNT
DEFINITION: Joint or bursa infections must meet at least one of the following criteria:

Criterion 1: Patient has organisms cultured from joint fluid or synovial biopsy.

Criterion 2: Patient has evidence of joint or bursa infection seen during a surgical operation or histopathologic examination.

Criterion 3: Patient has at least *two* of the following signs or symptoms with no other recognized cause: joint pain, swelling, tenderness, heat, evidence of effusion or limitation of motion

and

at least *one* of the following:

a. Organisms *and* white blood cells seen on Gram stain of joint fluid
b. Positive antigen test on blood, urine, or joint fluid
c. Cellular profile and chemistries of joint fluid compatible with infection and *not* explained by an underlying rheumatologic disorder
d. Radiographic evidence of infection, for example, abnormal findings on x-ray, CT, MRI, radiolabel scan (gallium, technetium, etc.)

INFECTION SITE: Disc space
CODE: BJ-DISC
DEFINITION: Vertebral disc space infection must meet at least one of the following criteria:

Criterion 1: Patient has organisms cultured from vertebral disc space tissue obtained during a surgical operation or needle aspiration.

Criterion 2: Patient has evidence of vertebral disc space infection seen during a surgical operation or histopathologic examination.

Criterion 3: Patient has fever (>38°C) with no other recog-

nized cause or pain at the involved vertebral disc space
and
radiographic evidence of infection, e.g., abnormal findings on x-ray, CT, MRI, radiolabel scan with gallium or technetium.
Criterion 4: Patient has fever (>38°C) with no other recognized cause and pain at the involved vertebral disc space
and
positive antigen test on blood or urine (e.g., *H. influenzae, S. pneumoniae, N. meningitidis,* or group B *Streptococcus*)

INFECTION SITE: Intracranial infection (brain abscess, subdural or epidural infection, encephalitis)
CODE: CNS-IC
DEFINITION: Intracranial infection must meet at least one of the following criteria:

Criterion 1: Patient has organisms cultured from brain tissue or dura.

Criterion 2: Patient has an abscess or evidence of intracranial infection seen during a surgical operation or histopathologic examination.

Criterion 3: Patient has at least *two* of the following signs or symptoms with no other recognized cause: headache, dizziness, fever (>38°C), localizing neurologic signs, changing level of consciousness, or confusion
and
if diagnosis is made antemortem, physician institutes appropriate antimicrobial therapy
and
at least *one* of the following:
a. Organisms seen on microscopic examination of brain or abscess tissue obtained by needle aspiration or by biopsy during a surgical operation or autopsy
b. Positive antigen test on blood or urine
c. Radiographic evidence of infection, for example, abnormal findings on ultrasound, CT, MRI, radionuclide brain scan, or arteriogram
d. Diagnostic single antibody titer (IgM) or fourfold increase in paired sera (IgG) for pathogen

Criterion 4: Patient ≤1 year of age has at least *two* of the following signs or symptoms with no other recognized cause: fever (>38°C), hypothermia (<37°C), apnea, bradycardia, localizing neurologic signs, or changing level of consciousness
and
if diagnosis is made antemortem, physician institutes appropriate antimicrobial therapy
and
at least *one* of the following:
a. Organisms seen on microscopic examination of brain or abscess tissue obtained by needle aspiration or by biopsy during a surgical operation or autopsy
b. Positive antigen test on blood or urine
c. Radiographic evidence of infection, for example, abnormal findings on ultrasound CT, MRI, radionuclide brain scan, or arteriogram
d. Diagnostic single antibody titer (IgM) or fourfold increase in paired sera (IgG) for pathogen

REPORTING INSTRUCTION:

- If meningitis and a brain abscess are present together, report the infection as IC.

INFECTION SITE: Meningitis or ventriculitis
CODE: CNS-MEN
DEFINITION: Meningitis or ventriculitis must meet at least one of the following criteria:

Criterion 1: Patient has organisms cultured from cerebrospinal fluid (CSF).

Criterion 2: Patient has at least *one* of the following signs of symptoms with no other recognized cause: fever (>38°C), headache, stiff neck, meningeal signs, cranial nerve signs, or irritability
and
if diagnosis is made antemortem, physician institutes appropriate antimicrobial therapy
and
at least *one* of the following:
a. Increased white cells, elevated protein and/or decreased glucose in CSF
b. Organisms seen on Gram stain of CSF
c. Organisms cultured from blood
d. Positive antigen test of CSF, blood, or urine
e. Diagnostic single antibody titer (IgM) or fourfold increase in paired sera (IgG) for pathogen

Criterion 3: Patient ≤1 year of age has at least *one* of the following signs or symptoms with no other recognized cause: fever (>38°C), hypothermia (<37°C), apnea, bradycardia, stiff neck, meningeal signs, cranial nerve signs, or irritability
and
if diagnosis is made antemortem, physician institutes appropriate antimicrobial therapy
and
at least *one* of the following:
a. Positive CSF examination with increased white cells, elevated protein, and/or decreased glucose
b. Positive Gram stain of CSF
c. Organisms cultured from blood
d. Positive antigen test of CSF, blood, or urine
e. Diagnostic single antibody titer (IgM) or fourfold increase in paired sera (IgG) for pathogen

REPORTING INSTRUCTIONS:

- Report meningitis in the newborn as nosocomial *unless* there is compelling evidence indicating the meningitis was acquired transplacentally.
- Report CSF shunt infection as SSI-MEN if it occurs ≤1 year of placement; if later, report as CNS-MEN.
- Report meningoencephalitis as MEN.
- Report spinal abscess with meningitis as MEN.

INFECTION SITE: Spinal abscess without meningitis
CODE: CNS-SA
DEFINITION: An abscess of the spinal epidural or subdural space, without involvement of the CSF or adjacent bone structures, must meet at least one of the following criteria:

Criterion 1: Patient has organisms cultured from abscess in the spinal epidural or subdural space.

Criterion 2: Patient has an abscess in the spinal epidural or subdural space seen during a surgical operation or at autopsy of evidence of an abscess seen during a histopathologic examination.

Criterion 3: Patient has at least *one* of the following signs or symptoms with no other recognized cause: fever (>38°C), back pain, focal tenderness, radiculitis, paraparesis, or paraplegia
and
if diagnosis is made antemortem, physician institutes appropriate antimicrobial therapy
and
at least *one* of the following:
a. Organisms cultured from blood
b. Radiographic evidence of a spinal abscess, for example, abnormal findings on myelography, ultrasound, CT, MRI, or other scans (gallium, technetium, etc.)

REPORTING INSTRUCTION:

- Report spinal abscess *with* meningitis as MEN.

INFECTION SITE: Arterial or venous infection
CODE: CVS-VASC
DEFINITION: Arterial or venous infection must meet at least one of the following criteria:

Criterion 1: Patient has organisms cultured from arteries or veins removed during a surgical operation
and
blood culture *not* done or *no* organisms cultured from blood.

Criterion 2: Patient has evidence of arterial or venous infection seen during a surgical operation or histopathologic examination.

Criterion 3: Patient has at least *one* of the following signs or symptoms with no other recognized cause: fever (>38°C), pain, erythema, or heat at involved vascular size
and
more than 15 colonies cultured from intravascular cannula tip using semiquantitative culture method
and
blood culture *not* done or *no* organisms cultured from blood.

Criterion 4: Patient has purulent drainage at involved vascular site
and
blood culture *not* done or *no* organisms cultured from blood.

Criterion 5: Patient ≤1 year of age has at least *one* of the following signs or symptoms with no other recognized cause: fever (>38°C), hypothermia (<37°C), apnea, bradycardia, lethargy, or pain, erythema, or heat at involved vascular site
and
more than 15 colonies cultured from intravascular cannula tip using semiquantitative culture method
and
blood culture *not* done or *no* organisms cultured from blood.

REPORTING INSTRUCTIONS:

- Report infections of an arteriovenous graft, shunt, or fistula or intravascular cannulation site without organisms cultured from blood as CVS-VASC.
- Report intravascular infections with organisms cultured from the blood as BSI-LCBI.

INFECTION SITE: Endocarditis involving either a natural or prosthetic heart valve
CODE: CVS-ENDO
DEFINITION: Endocarditis of a natural or prosthetic heart valve must meet at least one of the following criteria:

Criterion 1: Patient has organisms cultured from valve or vegetation.

Criterion 2: Patient has *two* or more of the following signs or symptoms with no other recognized cause: fever (>38°C), new or changing murmur, embolic phenomena, skin manifestations (i.e., petechiae, splinter hemorrhages, painful subcutaneous nodules), congestive heart failure, or cardiac conduction abnormality
and
if diagnosis is made antemortem, physician institutes appropriate antimicrobial therapy
and
at least *one* of the following:
a. Organisms cultured from *two* or more blood cultures
b. Organisms seen on Gram stain of valve when culture is negative or *not* done
c. Valvular vegetation seen during a surgical operation or autopsy
d. Positive antigen test on blood or urine (e.g., *H. influenzae, S. pneumoniae, N. meningitidis,* or group B *Streptococcus*)
e. Evidence of new vegetation seen on echocardiogram

Criterion 3: Patient ≤1 year of age has *two* or more of the following signs or symptoms with no other recognized cause fever (>38°C), hypothermia (<37°C), apnea, bradycardia, new or changing murmur, embolic phenomena skin manifestations (i.e., petechiae, splinter hemorrhages, painful subcutaneous nodules), congestive heart failure, or cardiac conduction abnormality
and
if diagnosis is made antemortem, physician institutes appropriate antimicrobial therapy

and
at least *one* of the following:
a. Organisms cultured from *two* or more blood cultures
b. Organisms seen on Gram stain of valve when culture is negative or *not* done
c. Valvular vegetation seen during a surgical operation or autopsy
d. Positive antigen test on blood or urine (e.g., *H. influenzae, S. pneumoniae, N. meningitidis,* or group B *Streptococcus*)
e. Evidence of new vegetation seen on echocardiogram

INFECTION SITE: Myocarditis or pericarditis
CODE: CVS-CARD
DEFINITION: Myocarditis or pericarditis must meet at least one of the following criteria:

Criterion 1: Patient has organisms cultured from pericardial tissue or fluid obtained by needle aspiration or during a surgical operation.

Criterion 2: Patient has at least *two* of the following signs or symptoms with no other recognized cause: fever (>38°C), chest pain, paradoxical pulse, or increased heart size
and
at least *one* of the following:
a. Abnormal electrocardiogram (ECG) consistent with myocarditis or pericarditis
b. Positive antigen test on blood (e.g., *H. influenzae, S. pneumoniae*)
c. Evidence of myocarditis or pericarditis on histologic examination of heart tissue
d. Fourfold rise in type-specific antibody with or without isolation of virus from pharynx or feces
e. Pericardial effusion identified by echocardiogram, CT, MRI, or angiography

Criterion 3: Patient ≤1 year of age has at least *two* of the following signs of symptoms with no other recognized cause: fever (>38°C), hypothermia (<37°C), apnea, bradycardia, paradoxical pulse, or increased heart size
and
at least *one* of the following:
a. Abnormal ECG consistent with myocarditis or pericarditis
b. Positive antigen test on blood (e.g., *H. influenzae, S. pneumoniae*)
c. Histologic examination of heart tissue shows evidence of myocarditis or pericarditis
d. Fourfold rise in type-specific antibody with or without isolation of virus from pharynx or feces
e. Pericardial effusion identified by echocardiogram, CT, MRI, or angiography

COMMENT:

- Most cases of postcardiac surgery or postmyocardial infarction pericarditis are not infectious.

INFECTION SITE: Mediastinitis
CODE: CVS-MED
DEFINITION: Mediastinitis must meet at least one of the following criteria:

Criterion 1: Patient has organisms cultured from mediastinal tissue or fluid obtained during a surgical operation or needle aspiration.

Criterion 2: Patient has evidence of mediastinitis seen during a surgical operation of histopathologic examination.

Criterion 3: Patient has at least *one* of the following signs or symptoms with no other recognized cause: fever (>38°C), chest pain, or sternal instability
and
at least *one* of the following:
a. Purulent discharge from mediastinal area
b. Organisms cultured from blood or discharge from mediastinal area
c. Mediastinal widening on x-ray

Criterion 4: Patient ≤1 year of age has at least *one* of the following signs or symptoms with no other recognized cause: fever (>38°C), hypothermia (<37°C), apnea, bradycardia, or sternal instability
and
at least one of the following:
a. Purulent discharge from mediastinal area
b. Organisms cultured from blood or discharge from mediastinal area
c. Mediastinal widening on x-ray

REPORTING INSTRUCTION:

- Report mediastinitis following cardiac surgery that is accompanied by osteomyelitis as SSI-MED rather than SSI-BONE.

INFECTION SITE: Conjunctivitis
CODE: EENT-CONJ
DEFINITION: Conjunctivitis must meet at least one of the following criteria:

Criterion 1: Patient has pathogens cultured from purulent exudate obtained from the conjunctiva or contiguous tissues, such as eyelid, cornea, meibomian glands, or lacrimal glands.
Criterion 2: Patient has pain or redness of conjunctiva or around eye
and
at least *one* of the following:
a. WBCs and organisms seen on Gram stain of exudate
b. Purulent exudate
c. Positive antigen test [e.g., enzyme-linked immunosorbent assay (ELISA) or immunofluorescence (IF) for *Chlamydia trachomatis,* herpes simplex virus, adenovirus) on exudate or conjunctival scraping
d. Multinucleated giant cells seen on microscopic examination of conjunctival exudate or scrapings
e. Positive viral culture
f. Diagnostic single antibody titer (IgM) or fourfold increase in paired sera (IgG) for pathogen

REPORTING INSTRUCTIONS:

- Report other infections of the eye as EYE.
- Do *not* report chemical conjunctivitis caused by silver nitrate ($AgNO_3$) as a nosocomial infection.
- Do *not* report conjunctivitis that occurs as a part of a more widely disseminated viral illness (e.g., measles, chickenpox, or a URI).

INFECTION SITE: Eye, other than conjunctivitis
CODE: EENT-EYE
DEFINITION: An infection of the eye, other than conjunctivitis, must meet at least one of the following criteria:
Criterion 1: Patient has organisms cultured from anterior or posterior chamber of vitreous fluid.
Criterion 2: Patient has at least *two* of the following signs or symptoms with no other recognized cause: eye pain, visual disturbance, or hypopyon
and
at least *one* of the following:
a. Physician's diagnosis of an eye infection
b. Positive antigen test on blood (e.g., *H. influenzae, S. pneumoniae*)
c. Organisms cultured from blood

INFECTION SITE: Ear, mastoid
CODE: EENT-EAR
DEFINITION: Ear and mastoid infections must meet the following applicable criteria:
Otitis externa must meet at least one of the following criteria:
Criterion 1: Patient has pathogens cultured from purulent drainage from ear canal.
Criterion 2: Patient has at least *one* of the following signs or symptoms with no other recognized cause: fever (>38°C), pain, redness, or drainage from ear canal
and
organisms seen on Gram stain of purulent drainage.
Otitis media must meet at least one of the following criteria:
Criterion 1: Patient has organisms cultured from fluid from middle ear obtained by tympanocentesis or at surgical operation.
Criterion 2: Patient has at least *two* of the following signs or symptoms with no other recognized cause: fever (>38°C) pain in the eardrum, inflammation, retraction or decreased mobility of eardrum, or fluid behind eardrum.
Otitis interna must meet at least one of the following criteria:
Criterion 1: Patient has organisms cultured from fluid from inner ear obtained at surgical operation.
Criterion 2: Patient has a physician's diagnosis of inner ear infection.
Mastoiditis must meet at least one of the following criteria:
Criterion 1: Patient has organisms cultured from purulent drainage from mastoid.
Criterion 2: Patient has at least *two* of the following signs or symptoms with no other recognized cause: fever (>38°C), pain, tenderness, erythema, headache, or facial paralysis
and
at least *one* of the following:
a. Organisms seen on Gram stain of purulent material from mastoid
b. Positive antigen test on blood

INFECTION SITE: Oral cavity (mouth, tongue, or gums)
CODE: EENT-ORAL
DEFINITION: Oral cavity infections must meet at least one of the following criteria:
Criterion 1: Patient has organisms cultured from purulent material from tissues of oral cavity.
Criterion 2: Patient has an abscess or other evidence of oral cavity infection seen on direct examination, during a surgical operation, or during a histopathologic examination.

Criterion 3: Patient has at least *one* of the following signs or symptoms with no other recognized cause: abscess, ulceration, or raised white patches on inflamed mucosa, or plaques on oral mucosa
and
at least *one* of the following:
a. Organisms seen on Gram stain
b. Positive potassium hydroxide (KOH) stain
c. Multinucleated giant cells seen on microscopic examination of mucosal scrapings
d. Positive antigen test on oral secretions
e. Diagnostic single antibody titer (IgM) or fourfold increase in paired sera (IgG) for pathogen
f. Physician diagnosis of infection and treatment with topical or oral antifungal therapy

REPORTING INSTRUCTION:

- Report nosocomial primary herpes simplex infections of the oral cavity as ORAL; recurrent herpes infections are *not* nosocomial.

INFECTION SITE: Sinusitis
CODE: EENT-SINU
DEFINITION: Sinusitis must meet at least one of the following criteria:
Criterion 1: Patient has organisms cultured from purulent material obtained from sinus cavity.
Criterion 2: Patient has at least *one* of the following signs or symptoms with no other recognized cause: fever (>38°C), pain or tenderness over the involved sinus, headache, purulent exudate, or nasal obstruction
and
at least *one* of the following:
a. Positive transillumination
b. Positive radiographic examination

INFECTION SITE: Upper respiratory tract, pharyngitis, laryngitis, epiglottitis
CODE: EENT-UR
DEFINITION: Upper respiratory tract infections must meet at least one the following criteria:
Criterion 1: Patient has at least *two* of the following signs or

symptoms with no other recognized cause: fever (>38°C), erythema of pharynx, sore throat, cough, hoarseness, of purulent exudate in throat
and
at least *one* of the following:
a. Organisms cultured from the specific site
b. Organisms cultured from blood
c. Positive antigen test on blood or respiratory secretions
d. Diagnostic single antibody titer (IgM) or fourfold increase in paired sera (IgG) for pathogen
e. Physician's diagnosis of an upper respiratory infection

Criterion 2: Patient has an abscess seen on direct examination, during a surgical operation, or during a histopathologic examination.

Criterion 3: Patient ≤1 year of age has at least *two* of the following signs or symptoms with no other recognized cause: fever (>38°C), hypothermia (<37°C), apnea, bradycardia, nasal discharge, or purulent exudate in throat
and
at least *one* of the following:
a. Organisms cultured from the specific site
b. Organisms cultured from blood
c. Positive antigen test on blood or respiratory secretions
d. Diagnostic single antibody titer (IgM) or fourfold increase in paired sera (IgG) for pathogen
e. Physician's diagnosis of an upper respiratory infection

INFECTION SITE: Gastroenteritis
CODE: GI-GE
DEFINITION: Gastroenteritis must meet at least one of the following criteria:

Criterion 1: Patient has an acute onset of diarrhea (liquid stools for more than 12 hours) with or without vomiting or fever (>38°C) and no likely noninfectious cause (e.g., diagnostic tests, therapeutic regimen, acute exacerbation of a chronic condition, or psychologic stress).

Criterion 2: Patient has at least *two* of the following signs or symptoms with no other recognized cause: nausea, vomiting, abdominal pain, or headache
and
at least *one* of the following:
a. An enteric pathogen is cultured from stool or rectal swab
b. An enteric pathogen is detected by routine or electron microscopy
c. An enteric pathogen is detected by antigen or antibody assay on blood or feces
d. Evidence of an enteric pathogen is detected by cytopathic changes in tissue culture (toxin assay)
e. Diagnostic single antibody titer (IgM) or fourfold increase in paired sera (IgG) for pathogen

INFECTION SITE: GI tract (esophagus, stomach, small and large bowel, and rectum) excluding gastroenteritis and appendicitis
CODE: GI-GIT
DEFINITION: Gastrointestinal tract infections, excluding gastroenteritis and appendicitis, must meet at least one of the following criteria:

Criterion 1: Patient has an abscess or other evidence of infection seen during a surgical operation or histopathologic examination.

Criterion 2: Patient has at least *two* of the following signs or symptoms with no other recognized cause and compatible with infection of the organ or tissue involved: fever (>38°C), nausea, vomiting, abdominal pain, or tenderness
and
at least *one* of the following:
a. Organisms cultured from drainage or tissue obtained during a surgical operation or endoscopy or from a surgically placed drain
b. Organisms seen on Gram or KOH stain or multinucleated giant cells seen on microscopic examination of drainage or tissue obtained during a surgical operation or endoscopy or from a surgically placed drain
c. Organisms cultured from blood
d. Evidence of pathologic findings on radiologic examination
e. Evidence of pathologic findings on endoscopic examination (e.g., *Candida* esophagitis or proctitis)

INFECTION SITE: Hepatitis
CODE: GI-HEP
DEFINITION: Hepatitis must meet the following criterion:
Patient has at least *two* of the following signs or symptoms with no other recognized cause: fever (>38°C), anorexia, nausea, vomiting, abdominal pain, jaundice, or history of transfusion within the previous 3 months
and
at least *one* of the following:
a. Positive antigen or antibody test for hepatitis A, hepatitis B, hepatitis C, or delta hepatitis
b. Abnormal liver function tests (e.g., elevated alanine/aspartate aminotransferases, bilirubin)
c. Cytomegalovirus detected in urine or oropharyngeal secretions

REPORTING INSTRUCTIONS:

- Do *not* report hepatitis or jaundice of noninfectious origin (alpha-1 antitrypsin deficiency, etc.).
- Do *not* report hepatitis or jaundice that results from exposure to hepatotoxins (alcoholic or acetaminophen-induced hepatitis, etc.).
- Do *not* report hepatitis or jaundice that results from biliary obstruction (cholecystitis).

INFECTION SITE: Intraabdominal, including gallbladder, bile ducts, liver (excluding viral hepatitis), spleen, pancreas, perito-

neum, subphrenic or subdiaphragmatic space, or other intraabdominal tissue or area *not* specified elsewhere
CODE: GI-IAB
DEFINITION: Intraabdominal infections must meet at least one of the following criteria:
Criterion 1: Patient has organisms cultured from purulent material from intraabdominal space obtained during a surgical operation or needle aspiration.
Criterion 2: Patient has abscess or other evidence of intraabdominal infection seen during a surgical operation or histopathologic examination.
Criterion 3: Patient has at least *two* of the following signs or symptoms with no other recognized cause: fever (>38°C), nausea, vomiting, abdominal pain, or jaundice
and
at least *one* of the following:
a. Organisms cultured from drainage from surgically placed drain (e.g., closed suction drainage system, open drain, T-tube drain)
b. Organisms seen on Gram stain of drainage or tissue obtained during surgical operation or needle aspiration
c. Organisms cultured from blood and radiographic evidence of infection, for example, abnormal findings on ultrasound, CT, MRI, or radiolabel scans (gallium, technetium, etc.) or on abdominal x-ray

REPORTING INSTRUCTION:

- Do *not* report pancreatitis (an inflammatory syndrome characterized by abdominal pain, nausea, and vomiting associated with high serum levels of pancreatic enzymes) unless it is determined to be infectious in origin.

INFECTION SITE: Necrotizing enterocolitis
CODE: GI-NEC
DEFINITION: Necrotizing enterocolitis in infants must meet the following criteria:
Infant has at least *two* of the following signs or symptoms with no other recognized cause: vomiting, abdominal distention, or prefeeding residuals
and
persistent microscopic or gross blood in stools
and
at least *one* of the following abdominal radiographic abnormalities:
a. Pneumoperitoneum
b. Pneumatosis intestinalis
c. Unchanging "rigid" loops of small bowel

INFECTION SITE: Bronchitis, tracheobronchitis, bronchiolitis, tracheitis, without evidence of pneumonia
CODE: LRI-BRON
DEFINITION: Tracheobronchial infections must meet at least one of the following criteria:
Criterion 1: Patient has *no* clinical or radiographic evidence of pneumonia
and
patient has at least *two* of the following signs or symptoms with no other recognized cause: fever (>38°C), cough, new or increased sputum production, rhonchi, wheezing
and
at least *one* of the following:
a. Positive culture obtained by deep tracheal aspirate or bronchoscopy
b. Positive antigen test on respiratory secretions
Criterion 2: Patient ≤1 year of age has *no* clinical or radiographic evidence of pneumonia
and
patient has at least *two* of the following signs or symptoms with no other recognized cause: fever (>38°C), cough, new or increased sputum production, rhonchi, wheezing, respiratory distress, apnea, or bradycardia
and
at least *one* of the following:
a. Organisms cultured from material obtained by deep tracheal aspirate or bronchoscopy
b. Positive antigen test on respiratory secretions
c. Diagnostic single antibody titer (IgM) or fourfold increase in paired sera (IgG) for pathogen

REPORTING INSTRUCTION:

- Do *not* report chronic bronchitis in a patient with chronic lung disease as an infection unless there is evidence of an acute secondary infection, manifested by change in organism.

INFECTION SITE: Other infections of the lower respiratory tract
CODE: LRI-LUNG
DEFINITION: Other infections of the lower respiratory tract must meet at least one of the following criteria:
Criterion 1: Patient has organisms seen on smear or cultured from lung tissue or fluid, including pleural fluid.
Criterion 2: Patient has a lung abscess or empyema seen during a surgical operation or histopathologic examination.
Criterion 3: Patient has an abscess cavity seen on radiographic examination of lung.

REPORTING INSTRUCTIONS:

- Report concurrent lower respiratory tract infection and pneumonia with the same organism(s) as PNEU.
- Report lung abscess or empyema without pneumonia as LUNG.

INFECTION SITE: Endometritis
CODE: REPR-EMET
DEFINITION: Endometritis must meet at least one of the following criteria:
Criterion 1: Patient has organisms cultured from fluid or tissue from endometrium obtained during surgical operation, by needle aspiration, or by brush biopsy.
Criterion 2: Patient has at least *two* of the following signs or symptoms with no other recognized cause: fever

(>38°C), abdominal pain, uterine tenderness, or purulent drainage from uterus.

REPORTING INSTRUCTION:

- Report postpartum endometritis as a nosocomial infection *unless* the amniotic fluid is infected at the time of admission or the patient was admitted 48 hours after rupture of the membrane.

INFECTION SITE: Episiotomy
CODE: REPR-EPIS
DEFINITION: Episiotomy infections must meet at least one of the following criteria:
Criterion 1: Postvaginal delivery patient has purulent drainage from the episiotomy.
Criterion 2: Postvaginal delivery patient has an episiotomy abscess.

REPORTING INSTRUCTION:

- Episiotomy is not a NNIS operative procedure; do not report as an SSI.

INFECTION SITE: Vaginal cuff
CODE: REPR-VCUF
DEFINITION: Vaginal cuff infections must meet at least one of the following criteria:
Criterion 1: Posthysterectomy patient has purulent drainage from the vaginal cuff.
Criterion 2: Posthysterectomy patient has an abscess at the vaginal cuff.
Criterion 3: Posthysterectomy patient has pathogens cultured from fluid or tissue obtained from the vaginal cuff.

REPORTING INSTRUCTION:

- Most vaginal cuff infections are SSI-VCUF.
- Report only late onset (>30 days after hysterectomy) VCUF as REPR-VCUF.

INFECTION SITE: Other infections of the male or female reproductive tract (epididymis, testes, prostate, vagina, ovaries, uterus, or other deep pelvic tissues, excluding endometritis or vaginal cuff infections)
CODE: REPR-OREP
DEFINITION: Other infections of the male or female reproductive tract must meet at least one of the following criteria:
Criterion 1: Patient has organisms cultured from tissue or fluid from affected site.
Criterion 2: Patient has an abscess or other evidence of infection of affected site seen during a surgical operation or histopathologic examination.
Criterion 3: Patient has *two* of the following signs or symptoms with no other recognized cause: fever (>38°C), nausea, vomiting, pain, tenderness, or dysuria
and
at least *one* of the following:
a. Organisms cultured from blood
b. Diagnosis by physician

REPORTING INSTRUCTIONS:

- Report endometritis as EMET.
- Report vaginal cuff infections as VCUF.

INFECTION SITE: Skin
CODE: SST-SKIN
DEFINITION: Skin infections must meet at least one of the following criteria:
Criterion 1: Patient has purulent drainage, pustules, vesicles, or boils.
Criterion 2: Patient has at least *two* of the following signs or symptoms with no other recognized cause: pain or tenderness, localized swelling, redness, or heat
and
at least *one* of the following:
a. Organisms cultured from aspirate or drainage from affected site; if organisms are normal skin flora (e.g., coagulase negative staphylococci, micrococci, diphtheroids) they must be a pure culture
b. Organisms cultured from blood
c. Positive antigen test performed on infected tissue or blood (e.g., herpes simplex, varicella zoster, *H. influenzae, N. meningitidis*)
d. Multinucleated giant cells seen on microscopic examination of affected tissue
e. Diagnostic single antibody titer (IgM) or fourfold increase in paired sera (IgG) for pathogen

COMMENT:

- Nosocomial skin infections may be the result of exposure to a variety of procedures performed in the hospital. Superficial incisional infections after surgery are identified separately as SSI-SKIN unless the operative procedure is a CBGB. If the chest incision site after a CBGB becomes infected, the specific site is denoted SKNC; if the donor site becomes infected, the specific site is denoted SKNL. Other skin infections associated with important exposures are identified with their own sites and are listed in the section on reporting instructions.

REPORTING INSTRUCTIONS:

- Report omphalitis in infants as UMB.
- Report infections of the circumcision site in newborns as CIRC.
- Report pustules in infants as PUST.
- Report infected decubitus ulcers as DECU.
- Report infected burns as BURN.
- Report breast abscesses or mastitis as BRST.

INFECTION SITE: Soft tissue (necrotizing fascitis, infectious gangrene, necrotizing cellulitis, infectious myositis, lymphadenitis, or lymphangitis)
CODE: SST-ST
DEFINITION: Soft tissue infections must meet at least one of the following criteria:
Criterion 1: Patient has organisms cultured from tissue or drainage from affected site.
Criterion 2: Patient has purulent drainage at affected site.
Criterion 3: Patient has an abscess or other evidence of infec-

tion seen during a surgical operation or histopathologic examination.

Criterion 4: Patient has at least *two* of the following signs of symptoms at the affected site with no other recognized cause: localized pain or tenderness, redness, swelling, or heat
and
at least *one* of the following:
a. Organisms cultured from blood
b. Positive antigen test performed on blood or urine (e.g., *H. influenzae, S. pneumoniae, N. meningitidis,* group B *Streptococcus, Candida* sp.)
c. Diagnostic single antibody titer (IgM) or fourfold increase in paired sera (IgG) for pathogen

REPORTING INSTRUCTIONS:

- Report surgical site infections that involve both the skin and deep soft tissue (at or beneath the fascial or muscle layer) as SSI-ST (soft tissue) unless the operative procedure is a CBGB. For CBGB, if skin and deep soft tissue at the chest incision site become infected, the specific site is STC and if skin and deep soft tissue at the donor site become infected, the specific site is STL.
- Report infected decubitus ulcers as DECU.
- Report infection of deep pelvic tissues as OREP.

INFECTION SITE: Decubitus ulcer, including both superficial and deep infections
CODE: SST-DECU
DEFINITION: Decubitus ulcer infections must meet the following criterion:
Patient has at least *two* of the following signs or symptoms with no other recognized cause: redness, tenderness, or swelling of decubitus wound edges
and
at least *one* of the following:
a. Organisms cultured from properly collected fluid or tissue (see later)
b. Organisms cultured from blood

COMMENTS:

- Purulent drainage alone is not sufficient evidence of an infection.
- Organisms cultured from the surface of a decubitus ulcer are not sufficient evidence that the ulcer is infected. A properly collected specimen from a decubitus ulcer involves needle aspiration of fluid or biopsy of tissue from the ulcer margin.

INFECTION SITE: Burn
CODE: SST-BURN
DEFINITION: Burn infections must meet one of the following criteria:

Criterion 1: Patient has a change in burn wound appearance or character, such as rapid eschar separation; dark brown, black, or violaceous discoloration of the char; or edema at wound margin
and
histologic examination of burn biopsy shows invasion of organisms into adjacent viable tissue.

Criterion 2: Patient has a change in burn wound appearance or character, such as rapid eschar separation; dark brown, black, or violaceous discoloration of the eschar; or edema at wound margin
and
at least *one* of the following:
a. Organisms cultured from blood in the absence of other identifiable infection
b. Isolation of herpes simplex virus, histologic identification of inclusions by light or electron microscopy or visualization of viral particles by electron microscopy in biopsies or lesion scrapings

Criterion 3: Patient with a burn has at least *two* of the following signs or symptoms with no other recognized cause: fever (>38°C) or hypothermia (<36°C), hypotension, oliguria (<20 cm^3/hr), hyperglycemia at previously tolerated level of dietary carbohydrate, or mental confusion
and
at least *one* of the following:
a. Histologic examination of burn biopsy shows invasion of organisms into adjacent viable tissue
b. Organisms cultured from blood
c. Isolation of herpes simplex virus, histologic identification of inclusions by light or electron microscopy, or visualization of viral particles electron microscopy in biopsies or lesion scrapings

COMMENTS:

- Purulence alone at the burn wound site is *not* adequate for the diagnosis of burn infection; such purulence may reflect incomplete wound care.
- Fever alone in a burn patient is *not* adequate for the diagnosis of a burn infection because fever may be the result of tissue trauma or the patient may have an infection at another site.
- Surgeons in Regional Burn Centers who take care of burn patients exclusively, may require Criterion 1 for diagnosis burn infection.
- Hospitals with Regional Burn Centers may further divide burn infections into the following: burn wound site, burn graft site, burn donor site, burn donor site-cadaver; the NNIS system, however, will code all of these as BURN.

INFECTION SITE: Breast abscess or mastitis
CODE: SST-BRST
DEFINITION: A breast abscess or mastitis must meet at least one of the following criteria:

Criterion 1: Patient has a positive culture of affected breast tissue or fluid obtained by incision and drainage or needle aspiration.

Criterion 2: Patient has a breast abscess or other evidence of infection seen during a surgical operation or histopathologic examination.

Criterion 3: Patient has fever (>38°C) and local inflammation of the breast
and
physician's diagnosis of breast abscess.

COMMENT:

- Breast abscesses occur most frequently after childbirth. Those that occur within 7 days after childbirth should be considered nosocomial.

INFECTION SITE: Omphalitis
CODE: SST-UMB
DEFINITION: Omphalitis in a newborn (≤30 days old) must meet at least one of the following criteria:
Criterion 1: Patient has erythema and/or serous drainage from umbilicus
and
at least *one* of the following:
a. Organisms cultured from drainage or needle aspirate
b. Organisms cultured from blood.
Criterion 2: Patient has both erythema and purulence at the umbilicus.

REPORTING INSTRUCTIONS:

- Report infection of the umbilical artery or vein related to umbilical catheterization as CVS-VASC if blood culture is negative or not done.
- Report as nosocomial if infection occurs in a newborn within 7 days of hospital discharge.

INFECTION SITE: Infant pustulosis
CODE: SST-PUST
DEFINITION: Pustulosis in an infant (≤12 months old) must meet at least one of the following criteria:
Criterion 1: Infant has *one* or more pustules
and
physician diagnosis of skin infection.
Criterion 2: Infant has *one* or more pustules
and
physician institutes appropriate antimicrobial therapy.

REPORTING INSTRUCTIONS:

- Do *not* report erythema toxicum and noninfectious causes of pustulosis.
- Report as nosocomial if pustulosis occurs in an infant within 7 days of hospital discharge.

INFECTION SITE: Newborn circumcision
CODE: SST-CIRC
DEFINITION: Circumcision infection in a newborn (≤30 days old) must meet at least one of the following criteria:
Criterion 1: Newborn has purulent drainage from circumcision site.
Criterion 2: Newborn has at least *one* of the following signs or symptoms with no other recognized cause at circumcision site: erythema, swelling, or tenderness
and
pathogen cultured from circumcision site.
Criterion 3: Newborn has at least *one* of the following signs or symptoms with no other recognized cause at circumcision site: erythema, swelling, or tenderness
and
skin contaminant (coagulase-negative staphylococci, diphtheroids, *Bacillus* sp., or micrococci) is cultured from circumcision site
and
physician diagnosis of infection or physician institutes appropriate therapy.

REPORTING INSTRUCTION:

- Newborn circumcision is not an NNIS operative procedure; do not report as an SSI.

INFECTION SITE: Disseminated infection
CODE: SYS-DI
DEFINITION: Disseminated infection is infection involving multiple organs or systems, without an apparent single site of infection, usually of viral origin, and with signs or symptoms with no other recognized cause and compatible with infectious involvement of multiple organs or systems.

REPORTING INSTRUCTIONS:

- This code should be used primarily for viral infections involving multiple organ systems (e.g., measles, mumps, rubella, varicella, erythema infectiosum). These infections often can be identified by clinical criteria alone. Do *not* use this code for nosocomial infections with multiple metastatic sites, such as with bacterial endocarditis; only the primary site of these infections should be reported.
- Do not report fever of unknown origin (FUO) as DI-SYS.
- Report neonatal "sepsis" as BSI-CSEP.
- Report viral exanthems or rash illness as DI-SYS.

APPENDIX A-2. CRITERIA FOR DEFINING NOSOCOMIAL PNEUMONIA

General Comments Applicable to All Pneumonia Specific Site Criteria

1. Physician's diagnosis of pneumonia alone is *not* an acceptable criterion for nosocomial pneumonia.
2. Although specific criteria are included for infants and children, pediatric patients may meet any of the other pneumonia specific site criteria.
3. Ventilator-associated pneumonia (i.e., pneumonia in persons who had a device to assist or control respiration continuously through a tracheostomy or by endotracheal intubation within the 48-hour period before the onset of infection) should be so designated when reporting pneumonia data.
4. When assessing a patient for presence of pneumonia, it is important to distinguish between changes in clinical status resulting from other conditions such as myocardial infarction, pulmonary embolism, respiratory distress syndrome, atelectasis, malignancy, chronic obstructive pulmonary disease, hyaline membrane disease, bronchopulmonary dysplasia, and so forth. Also, care must be taken when assessing intubated patients to distinguish between tracheal colonization, upper

respiratory tract infections (e.g., tracheobronchitis), and early onset pneumonia. Finally, it should be recognized that it may be difficult to determine nosocomial pneumonia in the elderly, infants, and immunocompromised patients because such conditions may mask typical signs or symptoms associated with pneumonia. Alternate specific criteria for the elderly, infants and immunocompromised patients have been included in this definition of nosocomial pneumonia.

5. Nosocomial pneumonia can be characterized by its onset: early or late. Early onset pneumonia occurs during the first 4 days of hospitalization and is often caused by *Moraxella catarrhalis, H. influenzae,* and *S. pneumoniae.* Causative agents of late onset pneumonia are frequently gram-negative bacilli or *Staphylococcus aureus,* including methicillin-resistant *S. aureus.* Viruses (e.g., influenza A and B or respiratory syncytial virus) can cause early and late onset nosocomial pneumonia, whereas yeasts, fungi, legionellae, and *Pneumocystis carinii* are usually pathogens of late onset pneumonia.
6. Pneumonia resulting from gross aspiration (e.g., in the setting of intubation in the emergency room or operating room) is considered nosocomial if it meets any specific criteria and was not clearly present or incubating at the time of admission to the hospital.
7. Multiple episodes of nosocomial pneumonia may occur in critically ill patients with lengthy hospital stays. When determining whether to report multiple episodes of nosocomial pneumonia in a single patient, look for evidence of resolution of the initial infection. The addition of or change in pathogen alone is *not* indicative of a new episode of pneumonia. The combination of new signs and symptoms and radiographic evidence or other diagnostic testing is required.
8. Positive Gram stain for bacteria and positive KOH mount for elastin fibers and/or fungal hyphae from appropriately collected sputum specimens are important clues that point toward the etiology of the infection. However, sputum samples are frequently contaminated with airway colonizers and, therefore, must be interpreted cautiously. In particular, *Candida* is commonly seen on stain but infrequently causes nosocomial pneumonia.

Abbreviations

BAL—bronchoalveolar lavage
EIA—enzyme immunoassay
FAMA—fluorescent-antibody staining of membrane antigen
IFA—immunofluorescent antibody
LRT—lower respiratory tract
PCR—polymerase chain reaction
PMN—polymorphonuclear leukocyte
RIA—radioimmunoassay

Reporting Instructions

- There is a hierarchy of specific site categories within the major site pneumonia. Even if a patient meets criteria for more than one specific site, report only one:
  - If a patient meets criteria for both PNU1 and PNU2, report PNU2.
  - If a patient meets criteria for both PNU2 and PNU3, report PNU3.
  - If a patient meets criteria for both PNU1 and PNU3, report PNU3.
- Report concurrent lower respiratory tract infection (e.g., abscess or empyema) and pneumonia with the same organism(s) as pneumonia.
- Report lung abscess or empyema *without* pneumonia as LUNG.
- Report acute bronchitis, tracheitis, tracheobronchitis, or bronchiolitis *without* pneumonia as BRON.

APPENDIX A-2. PNEUMONIA ALGORITHMS

Major Site: Pneumonia (PNEU)
Site-Specific Algorithms for Clinically Defined Pneumonia (PNU1)

Radiology	Signs/symptoms/laboratory	Code
Two or more serial chest radiographs with at least *one* of the following[1,2]: • New or progressive • *and* persistent infiltrate • Consolidation • Cavitation • Pneumatoceles, in infants ≤1 year old NOTE: In patients without underlying pulmonary or cardiac disease (e.g., respiratory distress syndrome, bronchopulmonary dysplasia, pulmonary edema, or chronic obstructive pulmonary disease), *one definitive* chest radiograph is acceptable[1].	FOR ANY PATIENT, at least *one* of the following: • Fever (>38°C or >100.4°F) with no other recognized cause • Leukopenia (<4,000 WBC/mm³) *or* leukocytosis (≥12,000 WBC/mm³) • For adults ≥70 years old, altered mental status with no other recognized cause *and* At least *two* of the following: • New onset of purulent sputum[3], or change in character of sputum[4], or increased respiratory secretions, or increased suctioning requirements • New onset or worsening cough, or dyspnea, or tachypnea[5] • Rales[6] or bronchial breath sounds • Worsening gas exchange (e.g., O_2 desaturations [e.g., $PaO_2/FiO_2 \leq 240$][7], increased oxygen requirements, or increased ventilation demand) ALTERNATE CRITERIA FOR INFANT ≤1 YEAR OLD: Worsening gas exchange (e.g., O_2 desaturations, increased oxygen requirements, or increased ventilator demand) *and* at least *three* of the following: • Temperature instability with no other recognized cause • Leukopenia (<4,000 WBC/mm³) *or* leukocytosis (≥15,000 WBC/mm³) and left shift (≥10% band forms) • New onset of purulent sputum[3], or change in character of sputum[4], or increased respiratory secretions, or increased suctioning requirements • Apnea, tachypnea[5], nasal flaring with retraction of chest wall, or grunting • Wheezing, rales[6], or rhonchi • Cough • Bradycardia (<100 beats/min) or tachycardia (>170 beats/min) ALTERNATE CRITERIA FOR CHILD >1 OR ≤12 YEARS OLD, at least *three* of the following: • Fever (>38.4°C or >101.1°F) or hypothermia (<37°C or <97.7°F) with no other recognized cause • Leukopenia (<4,000 WBC/mm³) *or* leukocytosis (≥15,000 WBC/mm³) • New onset of purulent sputum[3], or change in character of sputum[4], or increased respiratory secretions, or increased suctioning requirements • New onset or worsening cough or dyspnea, apnea, or tachypnea[5] • Rales[6] or bronchial breath sounds • Worsening gas exchange (e.g., O_2 desaturations [e.g., pulse oximetry <94%], increased oxygen requirements, or increased ventilation demand)	PNU1

Major Site: Pneumonia (PNEU)
Specific Site Algorithms for Pneumonia with Common Bacterial or Filamentous Fungal Pathogens and Specific Laboratory Findings (PNU2)

Radiology	Signs/symptoms	Laboratory	Code
Two or more serial chest radiographs with at least *one* of the following[1,2]: • New or progressive *and* persistent infiltrate • Consolidation • Cavitation NOTE: In patients without underlying pulmonary or cardiac disease (e.g., respiratory distress syndrome, bronchopulmonary dysplasia, pulmonary edema, or chronic obstructive pulmonary disease), *one definitive* chest radiograph is acceptable[1].	At least *one* of the following: • Fever (>38°C or >100.4°F) with no other recognized cause • Leukopenia (<4,000 WBC/mm³) *or* leukocytosis (≥12,000 WBC/mm³) • For adults ≥70 years old, altered mental status with no other recognized cause *and* At least *one* of the following: • New onset of purulent sputum[3], or change in character of sputum[4], or increased respiratory secretions, or increased suctioning requirements • New onset or worsening cough, or dyspnea, or tachypnea[5] • Rales[6] or bronchial breath sounds • Worsening gas exchange (e.g., O_2 desaturations [e.g., $PaO_2/FiO_2 \leq 240$][7], increased oxygen requirements, or increased ventilation demand)	At least *one* of the following: • Positive growth in blood culture[8] not related to another source of infection • Positive growth in culture of pleural fluid • Positive quantitative culture[9] from minimally contaminated LRT specimen (e.g., BAL or protected specimen brushing) • ≥5% BAL-obtained cells contain intracellular bacteria on direct microscopic exam (e.g., Gram stain) • Histopathologic exam shows at least *one* of the following evidences of pneumonia: Abscess formation or foci of consolidation with intense PMN accumulation in bronchioles and alveoli Positive quantitative culture[9] of lung parenchyma Evidence of lung parenchyma invasion by fungal hyphae or pseudohyphae	PNU2

Major Site: Pneumonia (PNEU)
Specific Site Algorithms for Pneumonia with Viral, *Legionella, Chlamydia, Mycoplasma*, and Other Uncommon Pathogens and Specific Laboratory Findings (PNU2)

Radiology	Signs/symptoms	Laboratory	Code
Two or more serial chest radiographs with at least *one* of the following[1,2]: • New or progressive *and* persistent infiltrate • Consolidation • Cavitation NOTE: In patients without underlying pulmonary or cardiac disease (e.g., respiratory distress syndrome, bronchopulmonary dysplasia, pulmonary edema, or chronic obstructive pulmonary disease), *one definitive* chest radiograph is acceptable[1].	At least *one* of the following: • Fever (>38°C or >100.4°F) with no other recognized cause • Leukopenia (<4,000 WBC/mm^3) *or* leukocytosis (≥12,000 WBC/mm^3) • For adults ≥70 years old, altered mental status with no other recognized cause *and* At least *one* of the following: • New onset of purulent sputum[3], or change in character of sputum[4], or increased respiratory secretions, or increased suctioning requirements • New onset or worsening cough, dyspnea, or tachypnea[5] • Rales[6] or bronchial breath sounds • Worsening gas exchange (e.g., O_2 desaturations [e.g., $PaO_2/FiO_2 \leq 240$][7], increased oxygen requirements, or increased ventilation demand)	At least *one* of the following[10–12]: • Positive culture of virus or *Chlamydia* from respiratory secretions • Positive detection of viral antigen or antibody from respiratory secretions (e.g., EIA, FAMA, shell vial assay, PCR) • Fourfold rise in paired sera (IgG) for pathogen (e.g., influenza viruses, *Chlamydia*) • Positive PCR for *Chlamydia* or *Mycoplasma* • Positive micro-IF test for *Chlamydia* • Positive culture or visualization by micro-IF of *Legionella* spp. from respiratory secretions or tissue • Detection of *Legionella pneumophila* serogroup 1 antigens in urine by RIA or EIA • Fourfold rise in *L. pneumophila* serogroup **1** antibody titer to ≥1 : 128 in paired acute and convalescent sera by indirect IFA	PNU2

Major Site: Pneumonia (PNEU)
Specific Site Algorithm for Pneumonia in Immunocompromised Patients (PNU3)

Radiology	Signs/symptoms	Laboratory	Code
Two or more serial chest radiographs with at least *one* of the following[1,2]: • New or progressive *and* persistent infiltrate • Consolidation • Cavitation NOTE: In patients without underlying pulmonary or cardiac disease (e.g., respiratory distress syndrome, bronchopulmonary dysplasia, pulmonary edema, or chronic obstructive pulmonary disease), *one definitive* chest radiograph is acceptable[1].	Patient who is immunocompromised[13] has at least *one* of the following: • Fever (>38°C or >100.4°F) with no other recognized cause • For adults ≥70 years old, altered mental status with no other recognized cause • New onset of purulent sputum[3], or change in character of sputum[4], or increased respiratory secretions, or increased suctioning requirements • New onset or worsening cough, or dyspnea, or tachypnea[5] • Rales[6] or bronchial breath sounds • Worsening gas exchange (e.g., O_2 desaturations [e.g., $PaO_2/FiO_2 \leq 240$][7], increased oxygen requirements, or increased ventilation demand) • Hemoptysis • Pleuritic chest pain	At least *one* of the following: • Matching positive blood and sputum cultures with *Candida* spp.[14,15] • Evidence of fungi or *Pneumocytis carinii* from minimally contaminated LRT specimen (e.g., BAL or protected specimen brushing) from *one* of the following: – Direct microscopic exam – Positive culture of fungi Any of the following from: LABORATORY CRITERIA DEFINED UNDER PNU2	PNU3

1. Occasionally, in nonventilated patients, the diagnosis of nosocomial pneumonia may be quite clear on the basis of symptoms, signs, and a single definitive chest radiograph. However, in patients with pulmonary or cardiac disease (e.g., interstitial lung disease or congestive heart failure), the diagnosis of pneumonia may be particularly difficult. Other noninfectious conditions (e.g., pulmonary edema from decompensated congestive heart failure) may simulate the presentation of pneumonia. In these more difficult cases, serial chest radiographs must be examined to help separate infectious from noninfectious pulmonary processes. To help confirm difficult cases, it may be useful to review radiographs on the day of diagnosis, 3 days prior to the diagnosis, and on days 2 and 7 after the diagnosis. Pneumonia may have rapid onset and progression but does not resolve quickly. Radiographic changes of pneumonia persist for several weeks. As a result, rapid radiograph resolution suggests that the patient does *not* have pneumonia but rather a noninfectious process such as atelectasis or congestive heart failure.
2. Note that there are many ways of describing the radiographic appearance of pneumonia. Examples include, but are not limited to, air-space disease, focal opacification, and patchy areas of increased density. Although perhaps not specifically delineated as pneumonia by the radiologist, in the appropriate clinical setting these alternative descriptive wordings should be seriously considered as potentially positive findings.
3. Purulent sputum is defined as secretions from the lungs, bronchi, or trachea that contain ≥25 neutrophils and ≤10 squamous epithelial cells per low power field (×100). If your laboratory reports these data qualitatively (e.g., many WBCs or few squames), be sure their descriptors match this definition of purulent sputum. This laboratory confirmation is required because written clinical descriptions of purulence are highly variable.
4. A single notation of either purulent sputum or change in character of the sputum is not meaningful; repeated notations over a 24-hour period would be more indicative of the onset of an infectious process. Change in character of sputum refers to the color, consistency, odor, and quantity.

Footnotes Continued.

5. In adults, tachypnea is defined as respiration rate >25 breaths per minute. Tachypnea is defined as >75 breaths per minute in premature infants born at <37 weeks' gestation and until the 40th week; >60 breaths per minute in patients <2 months old; >50 breaths per minute in patients 2–12 months old; and >30 breaths per minute in children >1 year old.
6. Rales may be described as crackles.
7. This measure of arterial oxygenation is defined as the ratio of the arterial tension (PaO_2) to the inspiratory fraction of oxygen (FiO_2).
8. Care must be taken to determine the etiology of pneumonia in a patient with positive blood cultures and radiographic evidence of pneumonia, especially if the patient has invasive devices in place such as intravascular lines or an indwelling urinary catheter. In general, in an immunocompetent patient, blood cultures positive for coagulase negative staphylococci, common skin contaminants, and yeasts will not be the etiologic agent of the pneumonia.
9. Refer to Table A-2.1 for threshold values of bacteria from cultured specimens. An endotracheal aspirate is not a minimally contaminated specimen. Therefore, an endotracheal aspirate does not meet the laboratory criteria.
10. Once laboratory-confirmed cases of pneumonia due to respiratory syncytial virus (RSV), adenovirus, or influenza virus have been identified in a hospital, clinician's presumptive diagnosis of these pathogens in subsequent cases with similar clinical signs and symptoms is an acceptable criterion for presence of nosocomial infection.
11. Scant or watery sputum is commonly seen in adults with pneumonia due to viruses and *Mycoplasma* although sometimes the sputum may be mucopurulent. In infants, pneumonia due to RSV or influenza yields copious sputum. Patients, except premature infants, with viral or mycoplasmal pneumonia may exhibit few signs or symptoms, even when significant infiltrates are present on radiographic exam.
12. Few bacteria may be seen on stains of respiratory secretions from patients with pneumonia due to *Legionella* spp, *Mycoplasma*, or viruses.
13. Immunocompromised patients include those with neutropenia (absolute neutrophil count <500/mm^3), leukemia, lymphoma, HIV with CD4 count <200, or splenectomy; those who are in their transplant hospital stay; and those who are on cytotoxic chemotherapy, high dose steroids, or other immunosuppressives daily for >2 weeks [e.g., >40mg of prednisone or its equivalent (>160mg hydrocortisone, >32mg methylprednisolone, >6mg dexamethasone, >200mg cortisone)].
14. Blood and sputum specimens must be collected within 48 hours of each other.
15. Semiquantitative or nonquantitative cultures of sputum obtained by deep cough, induction, aspiration, or lavage are acceptable. If quantitative culture results are available, refer to algorithms that include such specific laboratory findings.

TABLE A-2.1. THRESHOLD VALUES FOR CULTURED SPECIMENS USED IN THE DIAGNOSIS OF PNEUMONIA

Specimen Collection/Technique	Values	Comment
Lung parenchyma	$\geq 10^4$ CFU/g tissue	1
Bronchoscopically (B) obtained specimens		
Bronchoalveolar lavage (B-BAL)	$\geq 10^4$ CFU/mL	
Protected BAL (B-PBAL)	$\geq 10^4$ CFU/mL	
Protected specimen brushing (B-PSB)	$\geq 10^3$ CFU/mL	
Nonbronchoscopically (NB) obtained (blind) specimens		
NB-BAL	$\geq 10^4$ CFU/mL	
NB-PSB	$\geq 10^3$ CFU/mL	

1, open-lung biopsy specimens and immediate postmortem specimens obtained by transthoracic or transbronchial biopsy; CFU, colony-forming units; g, gram; mL, milliliter.

OMB No. 0920-0012
Exp. Date 09-30-2003

NATIONAL NOSOCOMIAL INFECTIONS SURVEILLANCE SYSTEM
INFECTION WORKSHEET

NNID #: ______________ **Infection ID #:** ____-__________ **Type:** N ________
Patient ID #: ______________ **Patient name:** ______________ **Sex:** M F
Admission date: ____-____-____ (mm dd yy) **Age:** ________ (years/months/days)

Service: BUR GU OPH TRA GYN ORT CS MED PED ENT NS PLS GS ONC

HRN - Maternally acquired: Y N
Birthweight in grams: (A1) ≤ 1000 (A2) 1001-1500 (B) 1501-2500 (C) >2500
OB – Vaginal Delivery: Y N
WBN – Maternally acquired: Y N

Ward: ____________ **ICU:** Y N **Type of ICU:** B C CT M MS N NS P R S T O: ________
Opt1: ____________________________

Surgical Risk Factors

Operation: Y N
Procedure: AMP APPY BILI CARD CBGB CBGC CHOL COLO CRAN CSEC FUSN FX GAST HER HN HPRO HYST KPRO LAM MAST NEPH OBL OCVS OENT OES OEYE OGIT OGU OMS ONS OOB OPRO ORES OSKN PRST SB SKGR SPLE THOR TP VHYS VS VSHN XLAP

Date of operation: ____-____-____ (mm dd yy) **Duration of operation:** ______hrs. ______min.
Wound class: C CC CO D U **Surgeon:** ______________
General anesthesia: Y N **ASA classification:** 1 2 3 4 5
Emergency: Y N **Trauma:** Y N **Implant:** Y N
Endoscopic approach: Y N **Multiple procedures:** Y N
Opt2: ____________________________

Infections and Their Related Risk Factors

Infection date: ____-____ (mm dd)

UTI: ASB SUTI OUTI
Indwelling urinary catheter: Y N
Other bladder instrumentation: Y N

PNEU: PNU1 PNU2 PNU3
CXR: Def Ventilator: Y N

SSI: Indicate specific site: ______________
Detected during: A P R

BSI: LCBI CSEP
Central line(s): Y N TPN: Y N
Peripheral line(s): Y N Umbilical catheter: Y N

Infections other than UTI, SSI, PNEU, BSI: Major site: __________ Specific site: __________
Invasive device/procedure: Y N

Outcomes

Secondary bloodstream infection: Y N **Died:** Y N **Relationship to death:** CA CO NR U
Opt3: ____________________________

Assurance of Confidentiality: The information obtained in this surveillance system that would permit identification of any individual or institution is collected with a guarantee that it will be held in strict confidence, will be used only for the purposes stated, and will not otherwise be disclosed or released without the consent of the individual, or the institution in accordance with Sections 304, 306 and 308(d) of the Public Health Service Act (42 USC 242b, 242k, and m(d)).

Public reporting burden of this collection of information is estimated to average 32 minutes per response, including the time for reviewing instructions, searching existing data sources, gathering and maintaining the data needed, and completing and reviewing the collection of information. An agency may not conduct or sponsor, and a person is not required to respond to a collection of information unless it displays a currently valid OMB control number. Send comments regarding this burden estimate or any other aspect of this collection of information, including suggestions for reducing this burden to CDC/ATSDR Reports Clearance Officer; 1600 Clifton Road NE, MS D-24, Atlanta, Georgia 30333; ATTN: PRA (0920-0012).

CDC 57.58D (Front) REV. 9-00 IDEAS Version 6.06

Figure 94–B.1. National Nosocomial Infections Surveillance System infection worksheet (front).

OMB No. 0920-0012
Exp. Date 09-30-2003

Laboratory Data

NNID#: ________ **Infection ID#:** ____-____________

Laboratory diagnosis: C A V N

Culture specimen: B BX CSF DD ID NSD R S ST U VC OTH ________________

Opt4: ____

Antibiogram

Antibiotic agent	Pathogen code: Pathogen1	Pathogen2	Pathogen3	Pathogen4
Pathogen code:	______	______	______	______
Amikacin	______	______	______	
Amoxicillin/Clavulanic Acid	______	______	______	
Ampicillin	______	______	______	
Ampicillin/Sulbactam	______	______	______	
Aztreonam	______	______	______	
Carbenicillin or Ticarcillin	______	______	______	
Cefaclor	______	______	______	
Cefamandole	______	______	______	
Cefazolin	______	______	______	
Cefepime	______	______	______	
Cefixime	______	______	______	
Cefmetazole	______	______	______	
Cefonicid	______	______	______	
Cefoperazone	______	______	______	
Cefotaxime	______	______	______	
Cefotetan	______	______	______	
Cefoxitin	______	______	______	
Ceftazidime	______	______	______	
Ceftizoxime	______	______	______	
Ceftriaxone	______	______	______	
Cefuroxime	______	______	______	
Cephalothin	______	______	______	
Chloramphenicol	______	______	______	
Ciprofloxacin	______	______	______	
Clindamycin	______	______	______	
Erythromycin	______	______	______	
Gentamycin	______	______	______	
Imipenem	______	______	______	
Kanamycin	______	______	______	
Meropenem	______	______	______	
Methicillin	______	______	______	
Metronidazole	______	______	______	
Nafcillin	______	______	______	
Nalidixic Acid	______	______	______	
Netilmicin	______	______	______	
Nitrofurantoin	______	______	______	
Norfloxacin	______	______	______	
Ofloxacin	______	______	______	
Oxacillin	______	______	______	
Penicillin	______	______	______	
Piperacillin	______	______	______	
Piperacillin/Tazobactam	______	______	______	
Rifampin	______	______	______	
Sulfisoxazole	______	______	______	
Teicoplanin	______	______	______	
Tetracycline	______	______	______	
Ticarcillin/Clavulanic Acid	______	______	______	
Tobramycin	______	______	______	
Trimethoprim	______	______	______	
Trimethoprim/Sulfamethoxazole	______	______	______	
Vancomycin	______	______	______	

Additional Optional Fields

a1____	a3________	a5____________
b1____	b3________	b5____________
c1____	c3________	
d1____	d3________	
e1____	e3________	

CDC 57.58D (Back) REV. 9-00 IDEAS Version 6.06

Figure 94–B.2. National Nosocomial Infections Surveillance System infection worksheet (back).

OMB No. 0920-0012
Exp. 09/30/2003

NATIONAL NOSOCOMIAL INFECTIONS SURVEILLANCE SYSTEM
ADULT AND PEDIATRIC INTENSIVE CARE UNIT (ICU) MONTHLY REPORT FORM

NNID #________ **Month and Year**__________________ **Hospital's code for this ICU**______________

Circle type of ICU: Burn Coronary care CardioThoracic Medical Medical/Surgical Neurosurgical
Pediatric Respiratory Surgical Trauma Other (specify)__________________________

	First Day of Month	First Day of Next Month
Number of patients in ICU	________	________

			Number of patients with:		
Date	# New arrivals	# Patients	Indwelling urinary catheter	Central line(s)	Ventilator
1					
2					
3					
4					
5					
6					
7					
8					
9					
10					
11					
12					
13					
14					
15					
16					
17					
18					
19					
20					
21					
22					
23					
24					
25					
26					
27					
28					
29					
30					
31					
TOTAL					

Assurance of Confidentiality: The information obtained in this surveillance system that would permit identification of any individual or institution is collected with a guarantee that it will be held in strict confidence, will be used only for the purposes stated, and will not otherwise be disclosed or released without the consent of the individual, or the institution in accordance with Sections 304, 306 and 308(d) of the Public Health Service Act (42 USC 242b, 242k, and m(d)).

Public reporting burden of this collection of information is estimated to average 6 hours per response, including the time for reviewing instructions, searching existing data sources, gathering and maintaining the data needed, and completing and reviewing the collection of information. An agency may not conduct or sponsor, and a person is not required to respond to a collection of information unless it displays a currently valid OMB control number. Send comments regarding this burden estimate or any other aspect of this collection of information, including suggestions for reducing this burden to CDC/ATSDR Reports Clearance Officer; 1600 Clifton Road NE, MS D-24, Atlanta, Georgia 30333; ATTN: PRA (0920-0012).

CDC 57.58B REV. 9-00 IDEAS Version 6.06

Figure 94–B.3. National Nosocomial Infections Surveillance System adult and pediatric intensive care unit (ICU) monthly report form.

OMB No. 0920-0012
Exp. Date 09-30-2003

NATIONAL NOSOCOMIAL INFECTIONS SURVEILLANCE SYSTEM
HIGH RISK NURSERY (HRN) SURVEILLANCE
MONTHLY REPORT FORM

NNID #_______________ **Month and Year_______________**

Birthweight (BW) in grams	On the first day of the month — Number of patients	On the first day of the next month — Number of patients
≤1000	________	________
1001-1500	________	________
1501-2500	________	________
>2500	________	________

DO NOT LEAVE BLANKS; RECORD A ZERO WHERE APPROPRIATE

USE THE REVERSE SIDE TO COMPLETE THE DAILY TOTALS.

REPORT TO CDC THE ABOVE DATA AND THE SUM OF EACH COLUMN ON THE REVERSE SIDE.

Assurance of Confidentiality: The information obtained in this surveillance system that would permit identification of any individual or institution is collected with a guarantee that it will be held in strict confidence, will be used only for the purposes stated, and will not otherwise be disclosed or released without the consent of the individual, or the institution in accordance with Sections 304, 306 and 308(d) of the Public Health Service Act (42 USC 242b, 242k, and m(d)).

Public reporting burden of this collection of information is estimated to average 4 hours per response, including the time for reviewing instructions, searching existing data sources, gathering and maintaining the data needed, and completing and reviewing the collection of information. An agency may not conduct or sponsor, and a person is not required to respond to a collection of information unless it displays a currently valid OMB control number. Send comments regarding this burden estimate or any other aspect of this collection of information, including suggestions for reducing this burden to CDC/ATSDR Reports Clearance Officer; 1600 Clifton Road NE, MS D-24, Atlanta, Georgia 30333; ATTN: PRA (0920-0012).

CDC 57.58H (Front) REV. 9-00 IDEAS Version 6.06

Figure 94–B.4. National Nosocomial Infections Surveillance System high-risk nursery (HRN) surveillance monthly report form (front).

Date	BW ≤1000 grams				BW 1001-1500 grams				BW 1501-2500 grams				BW >2500 grams			
	# new arrivals	# of pts	# of pts with: U/C	V	# new arrivals	# of pts	# of pts with: U/C	V	# new arrivals	# of pts	# of pts with: U/C	V	# new arrivals	# of pts	# of pts with: U/C	V
1																
2																
3																
4																
5																
6																
7																
8																
9																
10																
11																
12																
13																
14																
15																
16																
17																
18																
19																
20																
21																
22																
23																
24																
25																
26																
27																
28																
29																
30																
31																
Total																

U/C = # patients with umbilical catheter(s) or central line(s)

V = # patients on mechanical ventilation

DO NOT LEAVE BLANKS; RECORD A ZERO WHERE APPROPRIATE

CDC 57.58H (Back) REV. 9-00

IDEAS Version 6.06

Figure 94–B.5. National Nosocomial Infections Surveillance System high-risk nursery (HRN) surveillance monthly report form (back).

OMB No. 0920-0012
Exp. Date 09-30-2003

NATIONAL NOSOCOMIAL INFECTIONS SURVEILLANCE SYSTEM

SURGICAL PATIENT SURVEILLANCE

OPERATIVE PROCEDURE DAILY REPORT FORM

NNID #________________ Page_______ of _______

Operation Date (mm/dd/yy)	NNIS Code*	Patient ID#	Disch Date	Age˙	Sex	Duration Hrs:Min	Wound Class	Gen Anes	ASA Class	Em	Tr	Endo-Scope	Mult Proc	Optional Fields: Surgeon code (≤20 char) and Four ≤5 char fields
__/__/__	______	____________	__/__/__	___ M Y	M F	___:___	C CC CO D	Y N	1 2 3 4 5	Y N	Y N	Y N	Y N	____________ ____ ____ ____ ____
__/__/__	______	____________	__/__/__	___ M Y	M F	___:___	C CC CO D	Y N	1 2 3 4 5	Y N	Y N	Y N	Y N	____________ ____ ____ ____ ____
__/__/__	______	____________	__/__/__	___ M Y	M F	___:___	C CC CO D	Y N	1 2 3 4 5	Y N	Y N	Y N	Y N	____________ ____ ____ ____ ____
__/__/__	______	____________	__/__/__	___ M Y	M F	___:___	C CC CO D	Y N	1 2 3 4 5	Y N	Y N	Y N	Y N	____________ ____ ____ ____ ____
__/__/__	______	____________	__/__/__	___ M Y	M F	___:___	C CC CO D	Y N	1 2 3 4 5	Y N	Y N	Y N	Y N	____________ ____ ____ ____ ____
__/__/__	______	____________	__/__/__	___ M Y	M F	___:___	C CC CO D	Y N	1 2 3 4 5	Y N	Y N	Y N	Y N	____________ ____ ____ ____ ____
__/__/__	______	____________	__/__/__	___ M Y	M F	___:___	C CC CO D	Y N	1 2 3 4 5	Y N	Y N	Y N	Y N	____________ ____ ____ ____ ____
__/__/__	______	____________	__/__/__	___ M Y	M F	___:___	C CC CO D	Y N	1 2 3 4 5	Y N	Y N	Y N	Y N	____________ ____ ____ ____ ____
__/__/__	______	____________	__/__/__	___ M Y	M F	___:___	C CC CO D	Y N	1 2 3 4 5	Y N	Y N	Y N	Y N	____________ ____ ____ ____ ____
__/__/__	______	____________	__/__/__	___ M Y	M F	___:___	C CC CO D	Y N	1 2 3 4 5	Y N	Y N	Y N	Y N	____________ ____ ____ ____ ____

*NNIS operative procedure code

˙If age <1 year, enter age in months and circle M. If age is <1 month, enter 0 and circle M.
If age ≥1 year, enter age in years and circle Y.

Em = emergency
Tr = trauma

Assurance of Confidentiality: The information obtained in this surveillance system that would permit identification of any individual or institution is collected with a guarantee that it will be held in strict confidence, will be used only for the purposes stated, and will not otherwise be disclosed or released without the consent of the individual, or the institution in accordance with Sections 304, 306 and 308(d) of the Public Health Service Act (42 USC 242b, 242k, and m(d)).

Public reporting burden of this collection of information is estimated to average 40 hours per response, including the time for reviewing instructions, searching existing data sources, gathering and maintaining the data needed, and completing and reviewing the collection of information. An agency may not conduct or sponsor, and a person is not required to respond to a collection of information unless it displays a currently valid OMB control number. Send comments regarding this burden estimate or any other aspect of this collection of information, including suggestions for reducing this burden to CDC/ATSDR Reports Clearance Officer; 1600 Clifton Road NE, MS D-24, Atlanta, Georgia 30333; ATTN: PRA (0920-0012).

CDC 57.58G (Front) REV. 9-00 IDEAS Version 6.06

Figure 94–B.6. National Nosocomial Infections Surveillance System surgical patient surveillance operative procedure daily report form (front).

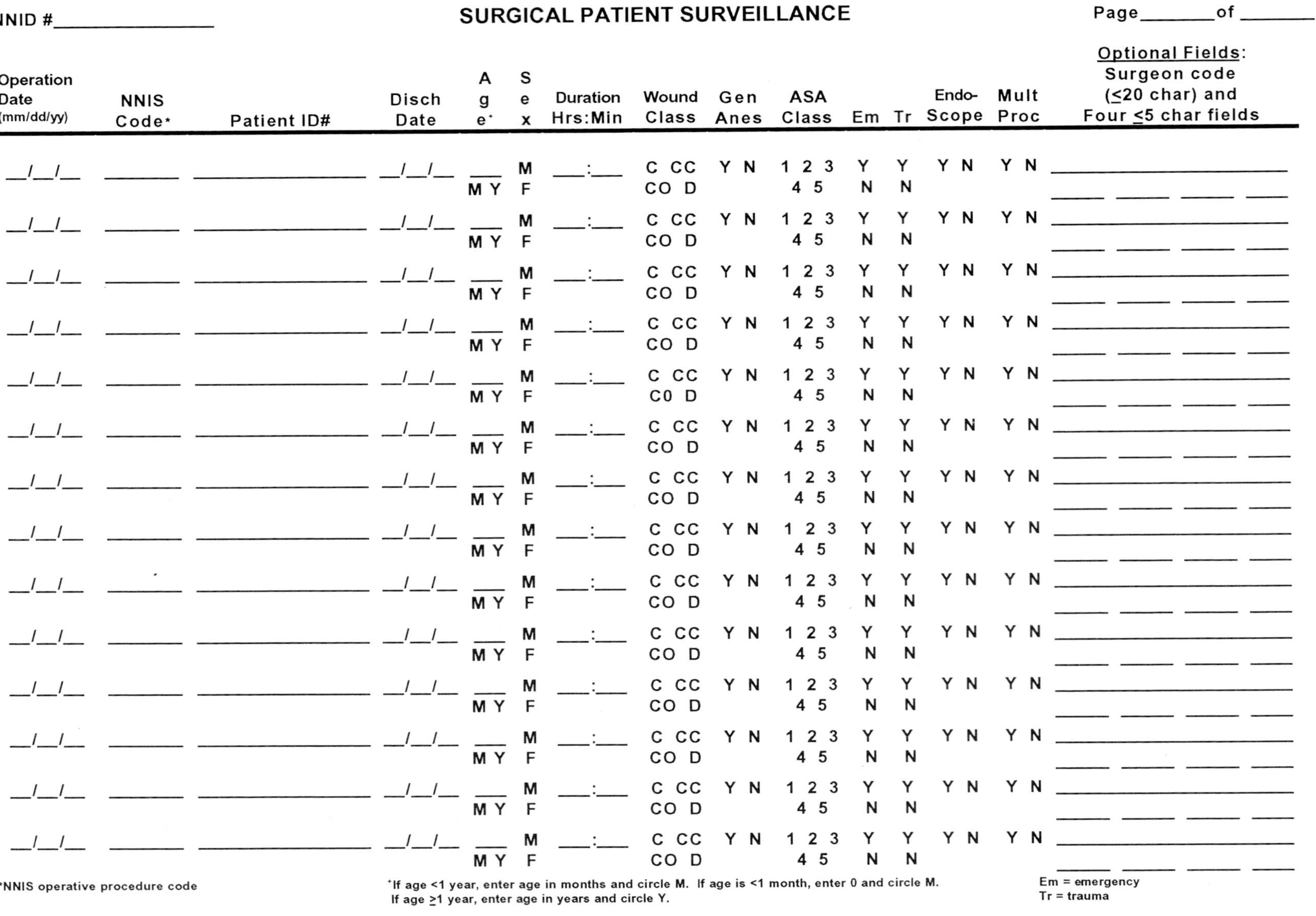

NNID # ______

SURGICAL PATIENT SURVEILLANCE

Page ______ of ______

Operation Date (mm/dd/yy)	NNIS Code*	Patient ID#	Disch Date	Age'	Sex	Duration Hrs:Min	Wound Class	Gen Anes	ASA Class	Em	Tr	Endo-Scope	Mult Proc	Optional Fields: Surgeon code (≤20 char) and Four ≤5 char fields
__/__/__			__/__/__	___ M Y	M F	__:__	C CC CO D	Y N	1 2 3 4 5	Y N	Y N	Y N	Y N	
__/__/__			__/__/__	___ M Y	M F	__:__	C CC CO D	Y N	1 2 3 4 5	Y N	Y N	Y N	Y N	
__/__/__			__/__/__	___ M Y	M F	__:__	C CC CO D	Y N	1 2 3 4 5	Y N	Y N	Y N	Y N	
__/__/__			__/__/__	___ M Y	M F	__:__	C CC CO D	Y N	1 2 3 4 5	Y N	Y N	Y N	Y N	
__/__/__			__/__/__	___ M Y	M F	__:__	C CC C0 D	Y N	1 2 3 4 5	Y N	Y N	Y N	Y N	
__/__/__			__/__/__	___ M Y	M F	__:__	C CC CO D	Y N	1 2 3 4 5	Y N	Y N	Y N	Y N	
__/__/__			__/__/__	___ M Y	M F	__:__	C CC CO D	Y N	1 2 3 4 5	Y N	Y N	Y N	Y N	
__/__/__			__/__/__	___ M Y	M F	__:__	C CC CO D	Y N	1 2 3 4 5	Y N	Y N	Y N	Y N	
__/__/__			__/__/__	___ M Y	M F	__:__	C CC CO D	Y N	1 2 3 4 5	Y N	Y N	Y N	Y N	
__/__/__			__/__/__	___ M Y	M F	__:__	C CC CO D	Y N	1 2 3 4 5	Y N	Y N	Y N	Y N	
__/__/__			__/__/__	___ M Y	M F	__:__	C CC CO D	Y N	1 2 3 4 5	Y N	Y N	Y N	Y N	
__/__/__			__/__/__	___ M Y	M F	__:__	C CC CO D	Y N	1 2 3 4 5	Y N	Y N	Y N	Y N	
__/__/__			__/__/__	___ M Y	M F	__:__	C CC CO D	Y N	1 2 3 4 5	Y N	Y N	Y N	Y N	
__/__/__			__/__/__	___ M Y	M F	__:__	C CC CO D	Y N	1 2 3 4 5	Y N	Y N	Y N	Y N	

*NNIS operative procedure code

'If age <1 year, enter age in months and circle M. If age is <1 month, enter 0 and circle M.
If age ≥1 year, enter age in years and circle Y.

Em = emergency
Tr = trauma

CDC 57.58G (Back) REV. 9-00

Figure 94–B.7. National Nosocomial Infections Surveillance System surgical patient surveillance operative procedure daily report form (back).

OMB No. 0920-0012
Exp. Date 09-30-2003

NATIONAL NOSOCOMIAL INFECTIONS SURVEILLANCE SYSTEM
ANTIMICROBIAL USE AND RESISTANCE (AUR) SURVEILLANCE COMPONENT
MONTHLY REPORT FORM

YEAR:_____	MONTH:_____	PATIENT GROUP: _____ (ICU, INP, OUT)	UNIT NAME: ______________ (for ICU or AUR specialty unit only)	PATIENT DAYS:_______

MICROBIOLOGY LAB DATA

Do not report duplicate isolates (i.e., the same bacteria in the same patient with the same antibiotic susceptibility pattern or surveillance cultures)

Total No. of CULTURES _______ (only clinical cultures processed for this month)	S*	I	R	Total Tested	Total Isolated
Staphylococcus aureus					
vancomycin					
methicillin or nafcillin or oxacillin					
Coagulase-negative staphylococci					
vancomycin					
methicillin or nafcillin or oxacillin					
***Enterococcus* spp.**					
vancomycin					
Streptococcus pneumoniae					
penicillin					
cefotaxime or ceftriaxone					
Escherichia coli					
ceftazidime or cefotaxime or ceftriaxone					
ciprofloxacin or ofloxacin or levofloxacin					
Klebsiella pneumoniae					
ceftazidime or cefotaxime or ceftriaxone					
***Enterobacter* spp.**					
ceftazidime or cefotaxime or ceftriaxone					
imipenem or meropenem					
Pseudomonas aeruginosa					
piperacillin					
ceftazidime					
imipenem					
meropenem					
ciprofloxacin					
ofloxacin					
levofloxacin					

CDC 57.68 (front) REV. 9-00

IDEAS Version 6.06

Figure 94–B.8. National Nosocomial Infections Surveillance System antimicrobial use and resistance (AUR) surveillance component monthly report form, microbiology lab data (front).

OMB No. 0920-0012
Exp. Date 09-30-2003

YEAR:_____	MONTH:_____	PATIENT GROUP: _____ (ICU, INP, OUT)	UNIT NAME: ______________ (for ICU or AUR specialty unit only)	PATIENT DAYS:_______

PHARMACY DATA

Parenteral Antibiotics

Antibiotic	Quantity Used	Antibiotic	Quantity Used
ampicillin	g	cefmetazole	g
ampicillin*/sulbactam	g	cefotaxime	g
nafcillin	g	ceftazidime	g
oxacillin	g	ceftizoxime	g
penicillin G	mill. I.U.	ceftriaxone	g
procaine pen. G	mill. I.U.	cefepime	g
pen. G benzathine	mill. I.U.	aztreonam	g
piperacillin	g	imipenem	g
piperacillin*/tazobacta	g	meropenem	g
ticarcillin	g	vancomycin	g
ticarcillin*/clav. acid	g	quinupristin/dalfopristin	g
cefazolin	g	ciprofloxacin	g
cephalothin	g	ofloxacin	g
cefotetan	g	trovafloxacin	g
cefoxitin	g	levofloxacin	g
cefuroxime	g	**trimethoprim***sulfamethoxazole	g

Oral Antibiotics

Antibiotic	Quantity Used	Antibiotic	Quantity Used
amoxicillin	g	cefixime	g
amoxicillin*/clav. acid	g	vancomycin	g
ampicillin	g	ciprofloxacin	g
dicloxacillin	g	norfloxacin	g
penicillin V	g	ofloxacin	g
cefadroxil	g	lomefloxacin	g
cephalexin	g	sparfloxacin	g
cefprozil	g	levofloxacin	g
cefaclor	g	tovafloxacin	g
cefuroxime axetil	g	**trimethoprim***sulfamethoxazole	g

*For combination drugs, record grams for the drug marked with the asterisk.

Figure 94–B.9. National Nosocomial Infections Surveillance System antimicrobial use and resistance (AUR) surveillance component monthly report form, microbiology lab data (back).

APPENDIX C. DEFINITIONS OF KEY TERMS USED IN THE NNIS SYSTEM

NNIS patient admission — A patient whose dates of hospital admission and discharge are different calendar days
and
who does *not* belong to any of the following patient groups:

- Psychiatry; physical medicine and rehabilitation; nursing home; or subacute, skilled nursing, or domiciliary care
- Outpatient (same-day, 1-day, or ambulatory) surgical or outpatient nonsurgical care

Service — A designation given to a group of patients who have similar disease conditions or who are receiving care by physicians with similar medical or surgical specialties. Examples include medicine, pediatrics, neurosurgery, and cardiac surgery.

NNIS operative procedure — A procedure performed on a patient who is a NNIS patient admission
and
takes place during an operation, which is a single trip to the operating room (OR), or delivery room if the procedure is a cesarean section, where a surgeon makes at least one incision through the skin or mucous membrane (including endoscopic or laparoscopic approaches), and closes the incision before the patient leaves the OR
and
is included in one of the operative procedure categories (8).

Duration of operation — Interval in hours and minutes between the skin incision and skin closure.

Multiple procedures — More than one NNIS operative procedure performed through the same incision during the same trip to the OR.

NNIS intensive care unit (ICU) — A nursing care area that provides intensive observation and diagnostic and therapeutic procedures for adults and/or children who are critically ill. An ICU *excludes* bone marrow transplant units and nursing areas that provide step-down, intermediate care, or telemetry only. The type of ICU is determined by the service of the majority of patients cared for by the unit. That is, if 80% of the patients are on a certain service (e.g., general surgery), then the ICU is designated as that type of unit (e.g., surgical ICU). (See ICU form in Appendix B for types of NNIS ICUs.)

NNIS ICU patient — A patient who is a NNIS patient admission
and
is admitted to a NNIS ICU.

ICU-associated infection — An infection in a NNIS ICU patient that was not present or incubating at the time of the patients' admission to the ICU but became apparent during the ICU stay or within 48 hours after transfer from the ICU.

Ventilator — A device to assist or control respiration continuously through a tracheostomy or by endotracheal intubation. Lung expansion devices such as intermittent positive pressure breathing (IPPB), nasal positive end-expiratory pressure (PEEP), and continuous nasal positive airway pressure (CPAP, hypoCPAP) are *not* considered ventilators unless delivered via tracheostomy or nasotracheal intubation (e.g., ET-CPAP).

Central line (central vascular cannula/vascular infusion device) — A vascular infusion device that terminates at or close to the heart or in one of the great vessels. An umbilical artery or vein catheter is considered a central line. Pacemaker wires and other noninfusion devices inserted into central blood vessels or the heart are *not* considered central lines.

Great vessel — The following are considered great vessels for the purpose of reporting central-line infections and counting central line-days in the NNIS system: aorta, vena cava, brachiocephalic veins, internal jugular veins, and subclavian veins. Note that neither the location of the insertion site nor the type of device may be used to determine if a line qualifies as a central line (e.g., a femorally inserted line is only considered to be a central line if the tip of the catheter lies in one of the vessels described previously). The device must terminate in one of these vessels or in or near the heart to qualify it as a central line.

Indwelling urinary catheter — A drainage tube that is inserted into the urinary bladder through the urethra, is

	left in place, and is connected to a closed collection system; also called a Foley catheter. Does not include straight in-and-out catheters.
Device-associated infection	An infection in a patient with a device, that is, ventilator or central line, that was used within the 48-hour period before its onset. If the time interval is longer than 48 hours, there must be compelling evidence that the infection was associated with use of the device. For catheter-associated urinary tract infection (UTI), the indwelling urinary catheter must have been in place within the 7-day period before positive laboratory results or signs and symptoms meeting the criteria for UTI were evident.
Secondary bloodstream infection	A culture-confirmed bloodstream infection (BSI) associated with nosocomial infection at another site. Secondary BSI must yield culture of same organism and exhibit same antibiogram as the primary nosocomial infection site. For example, if blood culture is positive in a patient with nosocomial UTI and organisms and antibiograms of both blood and urine specimens are identical, infection is reported as UTI with secondary BSI. Secondary BSI is not reported separately.

REFERENCES

1. Banerjee SN, Emori TG, Culver DH, et al. Secular trends in nosocomial primary bloodstream infections in the United States, 1980–1989. *Am J Med* 1991;91(Suppl 3B):86S–89S.
2. Haley RW, Culver DH, White JW, et al. The efficacy of infection surveillance and control programs in preventing nosocomial infections in U.S. hospitals. *Am J Epidemiol* 1985;212:182–205.
3. Centers for Disease Control and Prevention. *CDC surveillance update.* Atlanta: Centers for Disease Control and Prevention, 1988.
4. Scheckler WE. Continuous quality improvement in a hospital system: implications for hospital epidemiology. *Infect Control Hosp Epidemiol* 1992;13:288–292.
5. Seligman PJ, Frazier TM. Surveillance: the sentinel health event approach. In: Halperin W, Baker EL, eds. *Public health surveillance.* New York: Van Nostrand Reinhold, 1992:16–25.
6. Emori TG, Culver DH, Horan TC, et al. National nosocomial infections surveillance system (NNIS): description of surveillance methods. *Am J Infect Control* 1991;19:19–35.
7. Garner JS, Jarvis WR, Emori TG, et al. CDC definitions for nosocomial infections, 1988. *Am J Infect Control* 1988;16:28–40.
8. Horan TC, Emori TG. Definitions of key terms used in the NNIS system. *Am J Infect Control* 1997;25:112–116.
9. Garner JS. CDC guideline for prevention of surgical wound infections, 1985. *Infect Control* 1986;7:193–200.
10. Owens WD, Felts JA, Spitznagel EL Jr. ASA physical status classification: a study of consistency of ratings. *Anesthesiology* 1978;49: 239–243.
11. Culver DH, Horan TC, Gaynes RP, et al. Surgical wound infection rates by wound class, operative procedure, and patient risk index. *Am J Med* 1991;91(Suppl 3B):152S–157S.
12. Donowitz LG, Wenzel RP, Hoyt JW. High risk of hospital-acquired infection in the ICU patient. *Crit Care Med* 1982;10:355–357.
13. Hemming VG, Overall JC Jr, Britt MR. Nosocomial infections in a newborn intensive-care unit. *N Engl J Med* 1976;294:1310–1316.
14. Goldmann DA, Durbin WA, Freeman J. Nosocomial infections in a neonatal intensive care unit. *J Infect Dis* 1981;144:449–459.
15. Haley RW, Hooton TM, Culver DH. Nosocomial infections in U.S. hospitals, 1975–1976. *Am J Med* 1981;70:947–959.
16. Cruse PJE. Wound infection surveillance. *Rev Infect Dis* 1981;3: 734–737.
17. Burke JP. Infection control—a problem for patient safety. *N Engl J Med* 2003;348:651–656.
18. Larson E, Horan T, Cooper B, et al. Study of the definitions of nosocomial infections (SDNI). *Am J Infect Control* 1991;19:259–267.
19. Sherertz RJ, Garibaldi RA, Marosok RD, et al. Consensus paper on the surveillance of surgical wound infections. *Am J Infect Control* 1992;20:263–270.
20. Emori TG, Gaynes RP. An overview of nosocomial infections, including the role for the microbiology laboratory. *Clin Microbiol Rev* 1993; 6:428–442.
21. Haley RW. Surveillance by objective: a new priority-directed approach to the control of nosocomial infections. *Am J Infect Control* 1985;13:78–89.
22. Haley RW. *Managing hospital infection control for cost-effectiveness.* Chicago: American Hospital Publishing, 1986.
23. Stamm WE, Weinstein RA, Dixon RE. Comparison of endemic and epidemic nosocomial infections. *Am J Med* 1981;70:393–397.
24. Emori TG, Haley RW, Garner JS. Techniques and uses of nosocomial infection surveillance in U.S. hospitals, 1976–1977. *Am J Med* 1981; 70:933–940.
25. Stamm WE. Catheter-associated urinary tract infections: epidemiology, pathogenesis, and prevention. *Am J Med* 1991;91(Suppl 3B): 65S–71S.
26. Joint Commission on Accreditation of Healthcare Organizations. *Accreditation manual for hospitals, 1992.* Oakbrook Terrace, IL: Joint Commission on Accreditation of Healthcare Organizations, 1991.
27. National Nosocomial Infections Surveillance System. Nosocomial infection rates for interhospital comparison: limitations and possible solutions. *Infect Control Hosp Epidemiol* 1991;12:609–621.
28. Joint Commission on Accreditation of Healthcare Organizations. *A brief overview of the Joint Commission's agenda for change.* Chicago: Joint Commission on Accreditation of Healthcare Organizations, 1987.
29. Britt MR, Schleupner VJ, Matsumiya S. Severity of underlying disease as a predictor of nosocomial infection: utility in the control of nosocomial infection. *JAMA* 1978;239:1047–1051.
30. Fuchs PC. Will the real infection rate please stand up? *Infect Control* 1987;8:235–236.
31. Kleinbaum DG, Kupper LL, Morgenstern H. *Epidemiologic research: principles and quantitative methods.* Belmont, CA: Wadsworth, 1982: 221–222.
32. Emori TG, Edwards JR, Culver DH, et al. Accuracy of reporting nosocomial infections in intensive care unit patients to the National Nosocomial Infections Surveillance (NNIS) system: a pilot study. *Infect Control Hosp Epidemiol* 1998;19:308–316.
33. Centers for Disease Control and Prevention. Monitoring hospital-acquired infections to promote patient safety—United States, 1990–1999. *MMWR Morb Mortal Wkly Rep* 2000;49:149–153.
34. Abrutyn E, Talbot GH. Surveillance strategies: a primer. *Infect Control* 1987;8:459–464.
35. Freeman J, McGowan JE Jr. Methodologic issues in hospital epidemiology. I. Rates, case-finding, and interpretation. *Rev Infect Dis* 1981;3:658–667.
36. Wenzel RP, Osterman CA, Hunting KJ, et al. Hospital acquired infections. I. Surveillance in a university hospital. *Am J Epidemiol* 1976;103:251–260.
37. French GL, Cheng AF, Wong SL, et al. Repeated prevalence surveys

for monitoring effectiveness of hospital infection control. *Lancet* 1989; 2:1021–1023.

38. Rhame FS, Sudderth WD. Incidence and prevalence as used in the analysis of the occurrence of nosocomial infections. *Am J Epidemiol* 1981;113:1–11.
39. McGowan JE Jr, Finland M. Infection and usage of antibiotics at Boston City Hospital: changes in prevalence during the decade 1964–1973. *J Infect Dis* 1974;129:421–428.
40. Haley RW, Aber RC, Bennett JV. Surveillance of nosocomial infections. In: Bennett JV, Brachman PS, eds. *Hospital infections,* 2nd ed. Boston: Little, Brown and Company, 1986:51–71.
41. Bennett JV, Scheckler WE, Maki DG, et al. Current national patterns: United States of America. In: Brachman PS, Eickhoff TC, eds. *Proceedings of the international conference on nosocomial infections.* Chicago: American Hospital Association, 1971:42–49.
42. Wenzel RP, Osterman CA, Hunting KJ, et al. Hospital-acquired infections. I. Surveillance in a university hospital. *Am J Epidemiol* 1976; 103:251–255.
43. Wenzel RP, Thompson RL, Landry SM, et al. Hospital-acquired infections in intensive care unit patients: an overview with emphasis on epidemics. *Infect Control* 1983;4:371–375.
44. Freeman J, McGowan JE Jr. Day-specific incidence of nosocomial infection estimated from a prevalence survey. *Am J Epidemiol* 1981; 114:888–892.
45. Scheckler WE, Garner JS, Kaiser AB, et al. Prevalence of infections and antibiotic usage in eight community hospitals. In: Brachman PS, Eickhoff TC, eds. *Proceedings of the international conference on nosocomial infections.* Chicago: American Hospital Association, 1971: 299–305.
46. Haley RW, Schaberg DR, Crossley KB, et al. Extra charges and prolongation of stay attributable to nosocomial infections: a prospective interhospital comparison. *Am J Med* 1981;70:51–58.
47. Haley RW, White JW, Culver DH, et al. The financial incentive for hospitals to prevent nosocomial infections under the prospective payment system. *JAMA* 1987;257:1611–1614.
48. Centers for Disease Control and Prevention. Public health focus: surveillance, prevention, and control of nosocomial infections. *MMWR Mortal Morb Wkly Rep* 1992;41:783–787.
49. Haley RW, Gaynes RP, Aber RC, et al. Surveillance of nosocomial infections. In: Bennett JV, Brachman PS, eds. *Hospital infections,* 3rd ed. Boston: Little, Brown and Company, 1992:103.
50. Chelgren G, LaForce FM. Limited periodic surveillance proves practical and effective. *Hospitals* 1978;52:151–154.
51. Rubenstein E, Green M, Modan M, et al. The effects of nosocomial infections on the length and costs of hospital stay. *J Antimicrob Chemother* 1982;9:93–100.
52. Kerstein M, Flower M, Harkavy LM, et al. Surveillance for postoperative wound infections: practical aspects. *Am Surg* 1978;44:210–215.
53. Holtz TH, Wenzel RP. Postdischarge surveillance for nosocomial wound infection: a brief review and commentary. *Am J Infect Control* 1992;20:206–213.
54. Weigelt JA, Dryer D, Haley RW. The necessity and efficiency of wound surveillance after discharge. *Arch Surg* 1992;127:77–82.
55. Olson MM, O Connor M, Schwartz ML. Surgical wound infections: a 5-year prospective study of 20,193 wounds at the Minneapolis VA Medical Center. *Ann Surg* 1984;199:253–259.
56. Zoutman D, Pearce P, McKenzie M, et al. Surgical wound infections occurring in day surgery patients. *Am J Infect Control* 1990;18: 277–282.
57. Salem RJ, Johnson J, Devitt P. Short term metronidazole therapy contrasted with povidone-iodine spray in the prevention of wound infection after appendectomy. *Br J Surg* 1979;66:430–431.
58. Bates T, Touguet VLR, Tutton MK, et al. Prophylactic metronidazole in appendectomy: a controlled trial. *Br J Surg* 1980;67:547–550.
59. Burns SJ, Dippe SE. Postoperative wound infections detected during hospitalization and after discharge in a community hospital. *Am J Infect Control* 1982;10:60–65.
60. Brown RM, Bradley S, Opitz E, et al. Surgical wound infections documented after hospital discharge. *Am J Infect Control* 1987;15: 54–58.
61. Rosendorf LL, Octavio J, Estes JP. Effect of methods of postdischarge wound infection surveillance on reported infection rates. *Am J Infect Control* 1983;11:226–229.
62. Polk FB, Shapiro M, Goldstein P, et al. Randomized clinical trial of perioperative cefazolin in preventing infection after hysterectomy. *Lancet* 1980;1:437–441.
63. Cruse PJE, Foord R. A five-year prospective study of 23,649 wounds. *Arch Surg* 1973;107:206–210.
64. Condon RE, Schulte WJ, Malangoni MA, et al. Effectiveness of a surgical wound surveillance program. *Arch Surg* 1983;118:303–307.
65. Reimer K, Gleed C, Nicolle LE. The impact of postdischarge infection on surgical wound infection rates. *Infect Control* 1987;8:237–240.
66. Manian FA, Meyer L. Comprehensive surveillance of surgical wound infections in outpatient and inpatient surgery. *Infect Control Hosp Epidemiol* 1990;11:515–520.
67. Holbrook KF, Nottebart VF, Hameed SR, et al. Automated postdischarge surveillance for postpartum and neonatal nosocomial infections. *Am J Med* 1991;91(Suppl 3B):125S–130S.
68. Hulton LJ, Olmstead RN, Treston-Aurand J, et al. Effect of postdischarge surveillance on rates of infectious complications after cesarean section. *Am J Infect Control* 1992;20:198–201.
69. Seaman M, Lammers R. Inability of patients to self-diagnose wound infections. *J Emerg Med* 1991;9:215–219.
70. Sands K, Vineyard G, Platt R. Surgical site infections occurring after hospital discharge. *J Infect Dis* 1996;173:963–970.
71. Sands K, Vineyard G, Livingston J, et al. Efficient identification of postdischarge surgical site infections using automated medical records. *J Infect Dis* 1999;179;434–441.
72. Platt R. Progress in surgical site infection surveillance. *Infect Control Hosp Epidemiol* 2002;22:361–363.
73. Centers for Disease Control and Prevention. *Outline for surveillance and control of nosocomial infections.* Atlanta: Centers for Disease Control and Prevention, 1972.
74. Evans RS, Larsen RA, Burke JP, et al. Computer surveillance of hospital-acquired infections and antibiotic use. *JAMA* 1986;256: 1007–1011.
75. Kahn MG, Steib SA, Fraser VJ, et al. An expert system for culture-based infection control surveillance. *Proc Annu Symp Comput Appl Med Care* 1993;171–175.
76. Bates DW, Evans RS, Murff H, et al. Detecting adverse events using information technology. *J Am Med Inform Assoc* 2003;10(2): 115–128.
77. Gross PA, Beaugard A, VanAntwerpen C. Surveillance for nosocomial infections: can the sources of data be reduced? *Infect Control* 1980; 1:233–236.
78. Glenister H, Taylor L, Bartlett C, et al. An assessment of selective surveillance methods for detecting hospital-acquired infection. *Am J Med* 1991;91(Suppl 3B):121S–124S.
79. Rhame FS. Surveillance objectives: descriptive epidemiology. *Infect Control* 1987;8:454–458.
80. Bjerke NB, Fabrey LJ, Johnson CB, et al. Job analysis 1992: infection control practitioner. *Am J Infect Control* 1993;21:51–57.
81. Gaynes RP, Friedman C, Thiele G, et al. A methodology for selecting a computer-based surveillance system for nosocomial infections. *Am J Infect Control* 1989;12:48–60.
82. Green J, Wintfeld N, Sharkey P, et al. The importance of severity of illness in assessing hospital mortality. *JAMA* 1990;263:241–246.
83. Jencks SF, Daley J, Draper D, et al. Interpreting hospital mortality data: the role for clinical risk adjustment. *JAMA* 1988;260: 3611–3616.
84. Gross PA. Striving for benchmark infection rates: progress in control for patient mix. *Am J Med* 1991;91(Suppl 3B):16S–20S.
85. Keita-Perse O, Gaynes RP. Severity of illness scoring systems to adjust nosocomial infection rates: a review and commentary. *Am J Infect Control* 1996;24:429–434.
86. Kunin CM, McCormick RD. Prevention of catheter-induced urinary-tract infections by sterile closed drainage. *N Engl J Med* 1966;274: 1155–1161.
87. Maki DG, Goldmann DA, Rhame FS. Infection control in intravenous therapy. *Ann Intern Med* 1973;79:867–887.

88. Maki DG. Nosocomial bacteremia: an epidemiologic overview. *Am J Med* 1981;70:719–732.
89. Nichols RL. Surgical wound infection. *Am J Med* 1991;91(Suppl 3B): 54S– 64S.
90. Wenzel RP, Osterman CA, Donowitz LG, et al. Identification of procedure-related nosocomial infections in high-risk patients. *Rev Infect Dis* 1981;3:701–706.
91. Gaynes RP, Culver DH, Horan TC, et al. Surgical site infection (SSI) rates in the United States, 1992-1998: the National Nosocomial Infections Surveillance System basic risk index. *Clin Infect Dis* 2001; 33(Suppl 2):S69–77.
92. Kahn KL, Keeler EB, Sherwood MJ, et al. Comparing outcomes of care before and after implementation of the DRG-based prospective payment system. *JAMA* 1990;264:1984–1988.
93. Keeler EB, Kahn KL, Draper D, et al. Changes in sickness at admission following the introduction of the prospective payment system. *JAMA* 1990;264:1962–1968.
94. Kosecoff J, Kahn KL, Rogers WH, et al. Prospective payment system and impairment at discharge. *JAMA* 1990;264:1980–1988.
95. Graves EJ. National hospital discharge survey: annual summary 1990. National Center for Health Statistics. *Vital Health Stat* 1992;13(112): 1–62.
96. Gaynes R. Surveillance of nosocomial infections: a fundamental ingredient for quality. *Infect Control Hosp Epidemiol* 1997;18:475–478.
97. Gaynes, RP, Solomon S. Improving hospital-acquired infection rates: the CDC experience. *J Qual Improve* 1996;22:457-67.
98. Leape LL. Reporting of adverse events. *N Engl J Med* 2002;347: 1633–1638.
99. Donabedian A. The quality of medical care. *Science* 1978;200: 856–863.
100. Roper WL, Winkenwerder W, Hackbarth GM, et al. Effectiveness in health care: an initiative to evaluate and improve medical practice. *N Engl J Med* 1988;319:1197–1202.

95

ISOLATION OF PATIENTS WITH COMMUNICABLE DISEASES

JAN EVANS PATTERSON

Despite advances in the control of infectious diseases in the last century, there is more interest than ever in the use of isolation precautions to control emerging diseases such as multidrug resistant bacteria, multidrug resistant tuberculosis, severe acute respiratory syndrome (SARS), and others. These precautions are particularly important in the institutional setting, due to the proximity and potential common exposures of patients who have communicable diseases with other patients. The terminology for isolation precautions has changed and developed in recent years. Although the universal implementation of standard precautions has simplified isolation policies to some degree, the terms used for isolation precautions have varied among institutions, and some confusion has ensued (1,2). In addition, some of the situations outlined above may call for additional measures not in "universal precautions" as originally defined. The most recent revision of the Centers for Disease Control and Prevention's (CDC) guidelines for isolation has approached isolation as transmission based and has clarified some confusing issues (3). Still, the infection control professional is frequently called regarding the appropriate use of isolation precautions.

HISTORICAL PERSPECTIVE

The concept of isolating persons with communicable diseases was in practice even in ancient times according to biblical accounts of leper colonies, even though we now know that leprosy is not highly communicable and that the leprosy of biblical times may have been other skin diseases (4). In modern times, hospital construction before 1850 featured crowded open wards (5). As a consequence, cross-infection was common, and mortality rates were high in urban hospitals (6). Florence Nightingale's observations from the Crimean War (7) led her to advocate small pavilion-type wards joined by open-air corridors. Nightingale emphasized the importance of asepsis and a clean environment. Her teachings were called "fever nursing" and varied from popular concepts of disease at the time, because fever nursing implicated transmission by contact with body substances rather than the environment (8).

The germ theory of infection was accepted in U.S. hospitals in the late 1800s, after the influence of Lister and Pasteur, and conditions began to improve as overcrowding decreased and antisepsis increased (6). Communicable disease hospitals were using individual and group isolation as early as 1889 (9). By the turn of the century, general hospitals were beginning to isolate patients with communicable diseases in an individual room with the use of separate utensils and disinfectants (8,10). Grancher in Paris promoted the theory of communicability by contact rather than airborne spread for most diseases and allowed patients with communicable diseases to be housed in general wards but with separation by wire screens (8). This separated the patient from other patients and served as a reminder for staff members to gown and wash their hands. Thus, began the trend in the United States from the isolation hospital to care of communicable diseases in a general hospital setting.

In the early 20th century, Charles V. Chapin of Providence City Hospital used individual isolation cubicles for patients with communicable diseases and documented that fumigation had no effect on secondary cases (11). His work was very important in emphasizing the roles of persons rather than things as spreaders of disease and helped to end the miasmatic theory of transmission (12). Richardson, the physician superintendent of Providence City Hospital, used the barrier method and the cubicle method for isolation of patients, allowing some patients with communicable diseases to be housed in the same room as other patients (8). A card outlining the barrier technique needed was placed on the patient's bed.

The emergence of *Staphylococcus aureus* as a hospital pathogen in the 1950s and 1960s prompted the development of infection control programs in U.S. hospitals. In 1968, the first edition of the American Hospital Association's manual (12) presented a simple barrier precautions scheme for patients with communicable diseases, listing the need for gloves, gowns, masks, and visitor screening.

EARLY RECOMMENDATIONS FROM CENTERS FOR DISEASE CONTROL AND PREVENTION

While conducting nosocomial outbreak investigations in the 1960s, the CDC recognized that standardized policies for isolating hospitalized patients with communicable diseases were lacking (13). A group of experts convened in 1967 to develop the first CDC isolation recommendations, published in 1970 (14).

The isolation techniques described were based on seven categories of isolation: strict isolation, respiratory isolation, enteric precautions, wound and skin precautions, discharge precautions, blood precautions, and protective isolation. Even in this initial manual, the philosophy behind the more recently developed universal precautions was expressed. Many procedures discussed in the manual are applicable when ministering to the needs of any hospitalized patient, not just those with infectious diseases. Personnel could be lulled into a false sense of security when applying these principles to infected patients and practice poor techniques when handling uninfected patients (14). Updated editions of this manual were published in 1975 and 1978. By 1976, a survey showed that 93% of hospitals in the U.S. were using the category-specific approach to isolation (15).

Substantial changes were made in the 1983 CDC recommendations (16). First, the title of the isolation recommendations included the word *guideline*, and these isolation guidelines became part of the CDC series *Guidelines for the Prevention and Control of Nosocomial Infections.* Another notable change was the elimination of three categories of isolation (drainage precautions, blood precautions, and protective isolation) and expansion/modification to include four new categories of isolation: contact isolation, tuberculosis [acid-fast bacillus (AFB)] isolation, drainage/secretion precautions, and blood/body fluid precautions. In addition, this guideline introduced disease-specific isolation as an alternative to category-specific isolation. Disease-specific isolation was offered as an alternative for hospitals wanting a more economic system that directed precautions at preventing transmission of a specific disease while avoiding unnecessary isolation precautions for some diseases. The guidelines stated that hospitals could choose the category-specific or the disease-specific system or design their own systems.

The CDC first published five categories of isolation in 1970 (14). The most recent category-specific guidelines for isolation were published by the CDC in 1983 (16) and included seven categories of isolation: strict isolation, respiratory isolation, enteric precautions, contact isolation, tuberculosis (AFB) isolation, drainage/secretion precautions, and blood and body fluid precautions. These isolation categories grouped diseases that require the same isolation precautions. After the more recently revised transmission-based guidelines from CDC, these categories are now of historical interest, but the terms are still commonly used and confused by some healthcare workers. Infection control professionals may be called on to clarify and compare these previous categories with the newer guidelines.

Strict Isolation

Strict isolation was used to prevent transmission of diseases spread by both air and contact. Specifications for strict isolation include a private room with the door closed. Masks, gowns, and gloves were indicated for all persons entering the room. This category has now been replaced with the use of standard precautions (for all patients) or contact precautions combined with airborne precautions in the new guidelines.

Contact Isolation

Contact isolation was a category designed to prevent the transmission of epidemiologically important microorganisms causing infection or colonization or highly transmissible microorganisms that do not warrant strict isolation. Conditions in this category are spread by direct or close contact. This category has been replaced by contact precautions in the new transmission-based guidelines.

Respiratory Isolation

Respiratory isolation was used to prevent droplet nuclei transmission, that is, transmission of diseases over long distances through the air. In the newer guidelines, this category has been replaced by droplet precautions.

Tuberculosis Isolation (Acid-Fast Bacillus Isolation)

Tuberculosis isolation was referred to as AFB isolation on the standard instruction card to protect patient confidentiality (16). Airborne precautions have replaced this category in the new guideline. However, there are still many issues pertinent to tuberculosis that warrant special consideration regarding isolation, and these are discussed below (see Duration of Isolation, in section Tuberculosis Precautions: Special Considerations).

Enteric Precautions

Enteric precautions were used to prevent infections transmitted by feces. Examples would be hepatitis A or bacterial diarrhea. Enteric precautions are now included in standard precautions or, in the case of diapered or incontinent patients, contact precautions.

Drainage/Secretion Precautions

Drainage/secretion precautions were used to prevent transmission of infection by direct or indirect contact with drainage from an infected body site or from purulent material. This isolation category was newly created for the 1983 guidelines and used for many infections isolated under wound and skin precautions or discharge and secretion precautions in the previous guideline. Minor skin, wound, or burn infections that can be adequately covered by a dressing previously included in this category are now covered by standard precautions. Major infections not covered or not adequately covered by a dressing are now covered under standard precautions, or contact precautions, depending on the clinical setting.

Blood and Body Fluid Precautions

Blood and body fluid precautions were designed to prevent the transmission of blood-borne pathogens. This category is now only for historical reference, because universal precautions superseded it. Precautions used for blood and body fluids are now recommended in the standard precautions, which should be used for the care of all patients.

Comments

The advantage of category-specific isolation was that the grouping of diseases with similar routes of transmission was relatively easy to teach to personnel. It consisted of seven categories (six, if blood and body fluid precautions was excluded) that could be adopted and the diseases grouped accordingly. A disadvantage of the system was that it was diagnosis or disease recognition driven, and depended on the caregiver to identify the presence or suspected presence of a disease. In addition, drainage/secretion precautions could be confused with contact isolation and vice versa. Universal precautions recommended barriers to prevent contact with blood and certain body fluids; body substance isolation (BSI) recommends barrier protection for contact with all body fluids or open skin lesions. Because standard precautions recommend both, many categories in category-specific isolation are superfluous. Strict isolation, respiratory isolation, and AFB isolation are exceptions but are categorized differently in the new guidelines.

DISEASE-SPECIFIC ISOLATION

Disease-specific isolation was one of two isolation systems recommended by the CDC in 1983 (16). In this system, communicable diseases were considered individually as to mode of transmission and infective material, and accordingly, precautions are specified for each disease. The purported advantage of this system is that because precautions are specific for each disease, there are no unnecessary barriers used, and this lowers the cost of isolation. It may also enhance compliance by physicians who more readily understand the need for specific precautions for each disease. The disadvantage of this system is that because diseases are not grouped by category, it is more difficult to train staff who are not familiar with specific diseases. Each disease is referenced in a table in the 1983 guidelines, where specific precautions are listed and infective material is identified. Another disadvantage is that, like category-specific isolation, this system is diagnosis driven, and isolation precautions are often important early in the patient's hospital stay before a diagnosis is made or even suspected.

IMPACT OF THE ACQUIRED IMMUNODEFICIENCY SYNDROME EPIDEMIC

The recognition of the acquired immunodeficiency syndrome (AIDS) epidemic in the mid-1980s affected isolation policies in healthcare institutions unlike any other event in modern medicine. Before 1987, most hospitals placed patients in isolation, based on diagnosis or suspected diagnosis, according to the category-specific or disease-specific precautions as outlined by the aforementioned CDC guideline (16). As it became apparent that transmission of human immunodeficiency virus (HIV) could occur from patient to healthcare worker, new guidelines were established to minimize exposure to blood-borne pathogens from all patients, not just patients with a diagnosis or suspected diagnosis of HIV infection (17). In contrast to the 1983 CDC guideline, the 1987 CDC document (17) recommended blood and body fluid precautions for all patients, regardless of known HIV status. The belief that such precautions were unnecessary in patients not known to have blood-borne pathogens was gone. Specifically, barrier precautions were recommended to prevent contact with blood, certain body fluids, and body fluids containing blood. The application of blood and body fluid precautions to all patients was referred to as "universal blood and body fluid precautions" or "Universal Precautions." In 1988, the CDC published an updated Universal Precautions for the prevention of transmission of HIV, hepatitis B virus, and other blood-borne pathogens to supplement the 1987 publication (18). This document made it clear that transmission of other blood-borne pathogens, such as hepatitis B, should be prevented as well as that of HIV. In a new precedent for the healthcare industry, the Occupational Safety and Health Administration (OSHA) became involved in regulating and enforcing these guidelines (19). Now healthcare institutions were mandated to apply and enforce what was, in effect, blood and body fluid precautions as a minimum standard for protection of the healthcare worker.

Infection control programs recognized the potential benefit of this universal concept as a means of preventing cross-transmitted pathogens (blood-borne and non–blood-borne) among patients and healthcare workers. It became clear very quickly that an additional isolation system was needed to reduce the risk of transmitting non–blood-borne pathogens, because the CDC-defined Universal Precautions were primarily for preventing transmission of blood-borne pathogens. In the CDC 1988 update (18), category-specific or disease-specific isolation precautions are recommended to fill this need as described in the 1983 CDC guidelines. Infection control professionals at Harborview Medical Center in Seattle, Washington, recognized the problem early. They implemented a BSI system at Harborview in 1984 to control cross-transmission of non–blood-borne pathogens. This system designated all body fluids and tissue as potentially infectious (20). In 1987 and 1990, Lynch et al. (21,22) described their system and its advantages in preventing the transmission of both blood-borne and non–blood-borne pathogens. This system provided an alternative to the category-specific or disease-specific systems. Some confusion ensued, because the term *universal precautions* was sometimes used to apply to barrier precautions for all body fluids, not just blood and certain body fluids as originally defined (1,2). Characteristics and comparisons of the four major systems (category-specific, disease-specific, universal precautions, and BSI) are summarized in Tables 95.1 and 95.2. Although the more recent 1996 CDC guideline for isolation precautions in hospitals includes concepts of both Universal Precautions and BSI, these isolation systems are described briefly below because of their impact on the current practices. Universal Precautions are also described in Chapter 79.

UNIVERSAL PRECAUTIONS

In 1985 and 1986, the CDC published recommendations to prevent the transmission of HIV in the workplace (23,24). In 1987, a more comprehensive document (17) was published in response to increasing concern from healthcare workers about occupational exposure to HIV. These guidelines recommended the application of blood and body fluid precautions to all patients and designated this policy "Universal Precautions" or "universal blood and body fluid precautions."

TABLE 95.1. CHARACTERISTICS OF ISOLATION SYSTEMS

System (Reference)	Description	Advantages	Disadvantages
Category-specific (CDC, 1983) (16)	Six categories; each with a different set of precautions	Relatively simple Diseases are grouped	Diseases in same category may have different modes of transmission; distinction between use of contact isolation and drainage/secretion precautions may be confusing
Disease-specific (CDC, 1983) (16)	Individual precautions for each disease based on mode of transmission and infective material	Minimizes "overisolation" for some diseases May encourage compliance Potentially more costly for supplies	Dependent on diagnosis or clinical suspicion Difficult to teach
Universal Precautions (CDC update, 1988) (18)	Barrier precautions for blood and certain body fluids of all patients and all visibly bloody body fluids	Now standard for all patients (OSHA regulations) Protects worker and patient against blood-borne pathogen transmission	Sometimes difficult to determine at bedside if specimen is "visibly bloody" Terminology has been confusing Does not protect against non–blood-borne pathogens Must use category-specific or disease-specific precautions in combination for some situations
Body substance isolation (Lynch and Jackson, 1987) (20,21)	Barrier precautions used for blood, all body fluids, and substances of all patients	Easy to teach Universally applicable Isolates substances, not people Protects worker and patient against non–blood-borne and blood-borne pathogens	Potentially more costly for supplies May have less compliance if some see as "overisolation" Initial emphasis on gloves vs. hand washing Need to use respiratory isolation category in addition for some diseases
Transmission-based precautions (CDC, 1996) (3)	Two tiers of precautions: Standard Precautions for all patients Transmission-based precautions: airborne, droplet, contact	Combines major features of Universal Precautions and body substance isolation Standard Precautions apply to all patients Simplifies categories of isolation into three sets of precautions based on transmission	Terminology new to staff Special measures may be needed for some multidrug-resistant microorganisms

OSHA, Occupational Safety and Health Administration.

Universal Precautions as presented by the CDC in 1987 (17) include the following concepts:

1. Healthcare workers should use appropriate barrier precautions to avoid skin and mucous membrane exposure when contact with blood or body fluids from any patient is anticipated. Gloves are to be worn for contact with blood and body fluids, mucous membranes, or nonintact skin; when handling surfaces or items soiled with blood or body fluids; or for venipuncture or other procedures involving vascular access. Gloves should be changed after each patient contact. Masks and protective eyewear or face shields should be worn when procedures are likely to generate aerosols or droplets of blood or other body fluids. Gowns should be worn for procedures that are likely to soil clothing.
2. Hands or skin contaminated with blood or body fluids should be washed immediately. Hands should be washed after removing gloves.
3. Precautions should be taken to prevent sharps or needlestick injuries. Needles should not be recapped, removed from disposable syringes, or manipulated by hand. After use, needles, disposable syringes, scalpels, and other disposable sharp instruments should immediately be placed in a designated puncture-resistant container.
4. Mouthpieces and resuscitation devices should be readily available for use in areas where resuscitation procedures may be anticipated.
5. Healthcare workers with exudative skin lesions should not be involved in direct patient care or handle patient care equipment until the condition has resolved.

Precautions for Invasive Procedures

These were also outlined in the 1987 document and included routine surgical and obstetric procedures and outpatient physician and dentist office procedures. An invasive procedure was defined as surgical entry into tissues, cavities, or organs or repair of major traumatic injuries in an operating or delivery room, emergency department, or outpatient setting, including both physician and dentist offices; cardiac catheterization and angiographic procedures; vaginal or cesarean delivery or other invasive obstetric procedure during which bleeding may occur; or the

TABLE 95.2. COMPARING FOUR SYSTEMS FOR INFECTION PRECAUTIONS

Type of Infection	Category-Specific (CDC, 1983) (16)	Universal Precautions (CDC Update, 1988) (18)	Body Substance Isolation 1984–1987 (20,21)	Transmission-Based, (CDC 1996) (3)
Diagnosed blood-borne pathogen infection	Blood/body fluid precautions now standard with Universal Precautions	Gloves and other protective barriers for contact with blood or certain body fluids Trash and linen bagged to prevent leakage	Gloves for contact with blood or body substances Gown if soiling likely Private room if poor hygiene Mask/eye protection if splashing Trash/linen bagged to prevent leakage	Standard Precautions: gloves for contact with blood, all body fluids (except sweat) whether or not they are bloody Gown if soiling likely Mask/eye protection if splashing Trash/linen bagged to prevent leakage
Undiagnosed blood-borne pathogen infection	Same as above	Same as above	Same as above	Same as above
Diagnosed enteric infection (e.g., salmonellosis)	Enteric precautions	Enteric precautions; universal precautions do not apply to feces unless visibly bloody	Same as above	Same as above Contact Precautions if patient is diapered or incontinent
Undiagnosed enteric infection	No special precautions	Universal precautions do not apply except as above	Same as above	Same as above Contact Precautions if patient is diapered or incontinent
Known MRSA infection	Contact isolation	Universal precautions do not apply except as above	Same as above	Contact Precautions (determined by institution)
Unrecognized MRSA infection or colonization	No special precautions	Universal precautions do not apply except as above	Same as above	Standard Precautions
Infection spread by airborne route				
Disseminated varicella	Strict isolation	Strict isolation	Immune personnel—same as above	Airborne and Contact Precautions; restrict entry of susceptibles
Tuberculosis	Airborne precautions	AFB isolation	AFB isolation	Airborne Precautions
Meningococcal meningitis	Respiratory isolation	Respiratory isolation		Droplet Precautions

CDC, Centers for Disease Control and Prevention; MRSA, methicillin-resistant *Staphylococcus aureus*; AFB, acid-fast bacillus.
Modified from Jackson MM, Lynch P. An attempt to make an issue less murky: a comparison of four systems for infection precautions. *Infect Control Hosp Epidemial* 1991;12:448–450, with permission.

manipulation, cutting, or removal of any oral or perioral tissues, including tooth structure, during which bleeding occurs or the potential for bleeding exists. Healthcare workers participating in such procedures should routinely use barrier precautions as needed to prevent skin and mucous membrane exposure to blood and body fluids from all patients. This includes not only gloves and surgical masks for invasive procedures but also protective eyewear or face shields for procedures that are anticipated to generate droplets or splashing of blood or body fluids. Effective barrier gowns should be worn when splashing is anticipated. Healthcare workers in obstetrics should use appropriate barrier precautions during deliveries. If a glove is torn or a sharps injury occurs, the glove should be replaced with a new glove. The needle or sharp instrument involved should also be removed from the sterile field.

Precautions for Dentistry

Blood, saliva, and gingival fluid from all dental patients should be considered potentially infective in both institutional and noninstitutional settings. Dental workers should wear gloves for contact with oral mucous membranes and, in addition, surgical masks and protective eyewear or face shields for procedures in which splashing of blood or body fluids is likely. Handpieces should be sterilized after each patient use. Handpieces that cannot be sterilized should at least be flushed, cleaned with a chemical germicide, and rinsed after each patient use. Contaminated dental materials (impressions, bite registration) should be cleaned and disinfected before being handled in the dental laboratory and before being placed in another patient's mouth. Infection control precautions for dentistry are more specifically outlined and updated in later recommendations (25) (see also Chapter 54).

Precautions for Autopsies or Mortician Services

Persons participating in postmortem procedures should wear appropriate barrier protective equipment. Equipment and surfaces contaminated during such procedures should be cleaned with an appropriate chemical germicide (see Chapter 85).

Precautions for Dialysis

Blood and body fluid precautions are to be used when dialyzing all hemodialysis patients, not just those identified as hepatitis B surface antigen positive or HIV positive. HIV-infected patients do not need to be isolated from other patients during hemodialysis. The dialyzer may be discarded after use. Institutions that reuse dialyzers may designate a specific single-use dialyzer to a specific patient for reuse after appropriate cleaning and disinfection on the same patient only. HIV-infected patients may be included in the reuse programs; individual dialyzers must never be used on more than one patient (see Chapter 64).

Precautions for Laboratories

Blood and other body fluid specimens from all patients are considered infective. Specimens should be placed in a well-constructed container with a secure lid to avoid leakage. Contamination of the outside of the container or the laboratory form should be avoided. Personnel who process specimens should wear gloves. Other barrier protection should be used as needed if splashing or aerosolization is anticipated. Biologic safety cabinets should be used for procedures that are likely to generate droplets or aerosols. After specimen processing, gloves should be changed and hands washed. Mechanical devices should be used for pipetting; mouth pipetting should never be done. Laboratory work surfaces and laboratory equipment should be decontaminated with an appropriate chemical germicide after blood or body fluid spills and when work is completed. Before leaving the laboratory, personnel should remove protective clothing and wash their hands (see Chapter 82).

ENVIRONMENTAL CONSIDERATIONS FOR HUMAN IMMUNODEFICIENCY VIRUS TRANSMISSION

Disinfection and Sterilization

Environmental transmission of HIV has not been documented; however, environmental considerations are reviewed, and the same precautions are recommended for all patients. Standard disinfection and sterilization procedures for equipment are recommended for inpatient and outpatient settings, as previously described in the CDC guidelines for environmental control (26). Semicritical items, or items that contact mucous membranes such as endoscopes and bronchoscopes, should be sterilized or undergo high-level disinfection after each patient use. Chemical germicides registered with the U.S. Environmental Protection Agency (EPA) as sterilants may be used for high-level disinfection or sterilization depending on contact time (see Chapter 85). Under such guidelines, instruments used on HIV-positive patients do not require separate processing because high-level disinfection or sterilization should take place after use on any patient.

Housekeeping

Cleaning of environmental surfaces should be done after contamination by any patient; special cleaning is not required for patients with blood-borne pathogen infections. Horizontal surfaces should be cleaned when spills or soilage occurs and when patients are discharged. EPA-registered disinfectant-detergents should be used. Spills of blood or body fluids should be cleaned up immediately. Personnel should wear gloves. Broken glass and any other sharp objects should first be removed using tongs or forceps and placed in a sharps container. Then, visible fluid should be wiped up, the absorbent materials discarded as infectious waste, and the area decontaminated with a chemical germicide that is tuberculocidal and EPA approved as a hospital disinfectant. For large spills, the contaminated area should be treated first with the chemical germicide and then cleaned and fresh germicide used for decontamination.

Laundry

Soiled linen should be handled in the same way for all patients with a minimum of agitation; linen should be bagged at the location where it was used. Linen with blood or body fluid soilage should be transported in leak-proof bags. Linen should be laundered with detergent in hot water (71°C, 160°F) for 25 minutes. If a lower temperature is used, suitable chemicals for low-temperature washing must be used.

Infective Waste

Special precautions are recommended for handling certain hospital wastes that may be infective such as microbiology laboratory waste, pathology waste, and blood specimens or blood products. There has been disagreement on whether to classify communicable disease isolation waste as infectious waste. The CDC does not consider such waste as infectious, but before the Medical Waste Tracking Act of 1988, the EPA classified such waste as infectious waste. In the Medical Waste Tracking Act, however, the EPA modified its position and included only certain highly communicable disease waste from patients with infections due to biosafety level 4 etiologic agents (e.g., viral hemorrhagic fevers, such as Marburg, Lassa, and Ebola) as regulated medical waste (27). Bulk blood, body fluids, or excretions may be disposed of through the sanitary sewer system (see Chapter 100).

Implementation

These recommendations also stated that employers should ensure that workers receive initial orientation and continuing education and training on the transmission and prevention of blood-borne infections and routine application of universal precautions in the care of all patients. Personal protective equipment should be provided by the employer, and monitoring of compliance to the recommended protective measures should be followed.

Other Isolation Categories

With regard to other isolation categories as outlined in the 1983 guideline, the implementation of universal precautions superseded the need for a separate category of blood and body fluid precautions. Other isolation precautions, however, were recommended as needed for conditions such as infectious diarrhea (enteric precautions) or tuberculosis (AFB precautions).

UPDATE: UNIVERSAL PRECAUTIONS, 1988

After the recommendations for Universal Precautions were published in 1987, hospitals scurried to write their own institutional policies and implement training for their personnel in the prevention of blood-borne diseases in the workplace. In 1988, the CDC published an update to Universal Precautions that indicated these precautions were also for the prevention of other blood-borne pathogens such as hepatitis B and specified that only specific body fluids implicated in the transmission of blood-borne pathogens needed to be included under Universal Precautions. Many hospitals already had policies in place and employees trained by this time, which contributed to confusion in the use of the term *Universal Precautions.* A variety of different systems carried this term in individual institutions (28). The 1988 update also included further clarification on the use of protective barriers, the use of gloves for phlebotomy, the selection of gloves, and waste management.

Body Fluids to Which Universal Precautions Apply

In terms of occupational exposures, blood is the most important source of hepatitis B, HIV, and other blood-borne pathogens. Infection control efforts aimed at preventing occupationally acquired blood-borne infections must emphasize prevention of exposures to blood and promotion of hepatitis B virus immunization. Universal Precautions apply to semen, vaginal secretions, cerebrospinal fluid, synovial fluid, pleural fluid, peritoneal fluid, pericardial fluid, amniotic fluid, and any body fluid containing visible blood.

Body Fluids to Which Universal Precautions Do Not Apply

According to the 1988 update, Universal Precautions do not apply to feces, nasal secretions, sputum, sweat, tears, urine, and vomitus unless they contain visible blood. The risk of blood-borne pathogen transmission from these fluids is very low or nonexistent. The 1983 CDC guidelines (category-specific or disease-specific isolation) are cited for the prevention of non–blood-borne pathogen transmission. Universal Precautions do not routinely apply to saliva; however, special precautions are reiterated for dentistry because contamination of saliva with blood is predictable with dental procedures.

Use of Protective Barriers

The types of barriers needed for different procedures and clinical situations vary, so the healthcare worker must use judgment. Barrier precautions do not prevent sharps injuries; thus, caution in handling needles and sharps instruments, as previously outlined, is also necessary. Protective barriers should be used when exposure to blood or the above-named body fluids is anticipated. Hands or other surfaces contaminated with blood or the specified body fluids should be washed immediately.

Glove Use for Phlebotomy

Although gloves may reduce the amount of blood contaminating hands during venipuncture, they do not prevent needlestick injuries. The likelihood of exposure during phlebotomy depends on the skill of the personnel, the cumulative risk of the worker, whether the procedure is in a routine or emergency setting, and the prevalence of blood-borne pathogens in the patient population. Even though blood from all patients is considered infectious, the prevalence of HIV or hepatitis B virus in volunteer blood donor centers is known to be low. Some centers, therefore, have not routinely recommended gloves for phlebotomy in these settings. Gloves should always be available for workers who choose to use them, however. Gloves should always be used for phlebotomy when the healthcare worker has scratches, cuts, or other breaks in the skin; when hand contamination with blood is anticipated, such as when phlebotomy is done on an uncooperative patient; for finger or heel sticks on infants or children; and when personnel are receiving phlebotomy training.

Glove Selection

The Center for Devices and Radiological Health, Food and Drug Administration (FDA), is responsible for the regulation of the medical glove industry. Medical gloves include sterile surgical or nonsterile examination gloves made of vinyl or latex. The gloves selected should be task appropriate, and the following are general guidelines. Sterile gloves should be used for contact with sterile body areas. Nonsterile examination gloves may be used for contact with nonsterile body areas or other procedures that do not require aseptic technique. Gloves should be changed between patient contacts. Gloves should not be washed or disinfected between patients. Exposing the gloves to surfactants used for washing may cause increased penetration of liquids through unseen holes in the glove (wicking). Disinfectants may damage the gloves. General-purpose utility gloves (rubber household gloves) should be used for housekeeping activities and instrument cleaning in which contact with blood or specified body fluids is anticipated. These gloves can be reused after decontamination but should be discarded if torn or visibly damaged. Since the publication of this 1988 update, there have been many studies published evaluating glove integrity (see below, Are Gloves an Effective Barrier?).

Waste Management

Guidelines on waste management remained unchanged from the 1987 recommendations, but state and local regulations in many areas now supersede these recommendations, and this was acknowledged.

Comment

Universal Precautions have the advantage of protecting the healthcare worker against unidentified blood-borne pathogen risk. Also, this system is simpler than the traditional systems because the blood and body fluid isolation category applies to all patients. However, the 1988 update, which was intended to clarify which body fluids are infectious, only served to confuse the issue, because it is often difficult at the bedside to discern whether a body fluid contains blood. Furthermore, it is sometimes difficult to know the origin of a body fluid at the bedside, and even more so when the specimen is removed from the bedside. BSI addresses some of these issues. Even so, the issue of cost and compliance in using Universal Precautions may also present a problem (see below, Impact of Universal Precautions and Body Substance Isolation).

ARE GLOVES AN EFFECTIVE BARRIER?

At the time of the publication of the 1988 CDC update, there were no published data on the preference of latex versus vinyl gloves. Since that time, there have been numerous studies addressing the integrity of gloves in general and latex versus vinyl gloves in particular. The standards for testing the integrity of latex gloves were established by the American Society for Testing and Materials (ASTM) of the FDA, and compliance with them is voluntary. In 1977, the standard allowed no more than 15 defects per 1,000 (1.5%) as determined by the watertight method of testing (29) for sterile unused latex surgical gloves and 25 per 1,000 (2.5%) for latex examination gloves (29). In 1989, the FDA method for testing gloves improved and the standards changed to an allowable defect rate of 2.5% for surgeon's gloves and 4.0% for examination gloves (30). There are no standards for vinyl gloves. Concern regarding occupational exposure to HIV raised the issue of glove integrity in the clinical setting. In addition, some cases of herpetic whitlow in intensive care unit (ICU) nurses who used gloves focused more attention on this issue (31). Scanning of gloves by electron microscopy has documented inapparent pits from 30 to 50 μm in size, suggesting the possibility that viruses could penetrate this barrier (32).

In addition, several studies have documented leakage rates higher than the ASTM standard of 1.5% to 2.5%. DeGroot-Kosolcharoen and Jones (33) showed that whereas several brands of sterile latex surgical gloves were impermeable to water and blood, some brands showed leakage rates of up to 8%. Nonsterile latex and vinyl gloves showed leakage rates of 0% to 52%. Nonsterile packaging or packaging in suction kits increased leakage rates. Korniewicz et al. (34) studied gloves stressed by conditions mimicking those encountered in patient care and found that 63% of vinyl gloves leaked a stock solution of bacteriophage compared with 7% of latex gloves. Korniewicz et al. (35) also documented the penetration of 20% of latex gloves and 34% of vinyl gloves by *Serratia marcescens.* These studies indicate that gloves reduce the risk of gross soilage from blood or body fluids but that they are not 100% effective.

Doebbeling et al. (36) showed that washing gloved hands was not effective for decontamination, and, in fact, 5% to 50% of hands were contaminated after gloves were removed. Washing gloves has also been shown to decrease their integrity (37). Thus, gloves should not be washed and reused between patients. These studies affirm that although gloves can be used as a barrier to reduce gross contamination from blood and body fluids, antisepsis after glove removal remains very important because occult breaks in gloves can and do occur.

The surgical literature has long been concerned with perforations in gloves during surgical procedures. In 1899, Bovie (38) stated that careful hand washing was needed, because gloves could be punctured accidentally during an operation. More recent studies have quantitated the number and location of inapparent perforations that may occur in gloves during surgical or dental procedures. Albin et al. (39) showed a 33% leak rate of latex gloves randomly studied after surgical procedures. These authors also documented a leak rate of up to 5.5% in unused gloves. Gloves studied sequentially showed a leak rate of 58.5% at the end of surgical procedures and 32% at the end of dental procedures. Double gloving decreased the leak rate to 25%. In the sequential surgical study, 52% of the leaks occurred in the first 75 minutes; in the sequential dental study, 75% of the leaks occurred in the first 30 minutes. Gloves used in cardiovascular, orthopedic, abdominal, and oral surgical procedures had leak rates of more than 50%. The frequency of occult glove perforation has been noted to be as high as 10% after interventional radiologic procedures (40). In the Albin et al. study evaluating surgical and dental procedures, leak rates for gloves were evaluated for various members of the surgical team and were found to be highest for the surgeon (52%), followed next by the first assistant (29%), and then the scrub nurse (25%) (39). Most perforations (60%) occurred in the thumb or index finger of the glove. Other studies have also documented that the largest number of perforations occur in the thumb, index finger, and middle finger (41,42).

BODY SUBSTANCE ISOLATION

Jackson and Lynch (20) responded early on to the concern that unrecognized or undiagnosed cases resulted in unsafe exposures for healthcare workers. As early as 1984, these authors pointed out that many infectious agents are transmitted from patients who have only mild symptoms or no symptoms, and recommended barrier precautions for anticipated contact with blood or any body fluids from all patients, and reemphasized the important role of hand washing. Recognizing the limitations of the diagnosis-driven, category-specific, and disease-specific isolation systems, they systematically outlined an alternative system called "body substance isolation" (21). This approach was similar to the CDC Universal Precautions in that it presumed that all patients were potentially infectious, but it differed in that barrier precautions are used to prevent contact with all body fluids and tissue, not just certain body fluids and blood-tinged body fluids, as recommended in the 1988 CDC update. The term *body substance* rather than *body fluid* is used to emphasize that barrier precautions should be used to prevent contact with solids such as tissue and feces and body fluids. BSI contains six major components (21):

1. Gloves should be used for anticipated contact with blood, mucous membranes, nonintact skin, secretions, and moist body substances of all patients. The 1987 article stated that hand washing is not necessary unless hands are visibly soiled from breaks in gloves. Gloves should be changed between patients.
2. After other types of patient contact without gloves, hand washing, which is effective in removing transient flora from the hands, should be done (10 seconds of soap and friction followed by rinse with running water).
3. Other barriers such as gowns, plastic aprons, masks, or goggles should be worn as needed when soiling of clothing and/or skin or mucous membranes is anticipated.
4. Soiled reusable items, linen, and trash should be contained such that no leakage occurs. Double bagging is not needed unless the outside of the bag is soiled.
5. Needles and sharps should be placed in rigid puncture-resistant containers. Needles should not be recapped.
6. Private rooms are indicated for patients with diseases transmissible by the airborne route and for patients who may soil the environment with body substances.

Operational Issues

A single universal reminder sign—"Body substance isolation is for all patient care"—is placed in every patient room or at every bedside. This sign defines body substances and uses graphics and words to indicate when gloves, gowns, masks, or eye protection should be used. A stop sign alert is used on the door of patients with airborne diseases. This sign indicates that persons should check with the floor nurse before entering the room. The floor nurse will determine if the person is immune and need not wear a mask (e.g., measles, chickenpox) or instruct the person to wear a mask (e.g., tuberculosis). Nonsterile gloves must be accessible near the bedside, and other barriers must be available on the nursing unit. As with Universal Precautions, some judgment by healthcare workers is required in determining when exposures may be anticipated.

Comment

Body substance isolation is like Universal Precautions in that it protects workers and patients against transmission of bloodborne pathogens. BSI is easier to teach to staff and to apply at the bedside than Universal Precautions as clarified in 1988, because barrier precautions apply to all body fluids not just certain body fluids. BSI has the advantage of protecting against non–bloodborne pathogens as well. Use of gloves has been shown to control cross-transmission of multidrug-resistant enteric gram-negative rods (43). Appropriate use of BSI has indeed been documented to reduce colonization and infection with sentinel microorganisms such as *Pseudomonas aeruginosa, S. marcescens,* and aminoglycoside-resistant gram-negative bacilli (22). In addition, BSI also has the advantage of lessening the psychological trauma of isolation by emphasizing the isolation of body substances rather than the isolation of people (44). That is, because barrier precautions are used for all patients, additional restrictive isolation practices are not needed for most diseases, except those communicable by the respiratory route.

The system as it was published in 1987 suggested that hand washing was unnecessary when gloves were used for barrier precautions (21). This prompted criticism of the system by those stating that the wearing of gloves for contact with blood or body fluids did not eliminate the need for hand washing (13,45). Studies have documented that hands can be contaminated with microorganisms even though gloves are worn (36,46). When the system was described in later publications, gloving was not emphasized as a substitute for hand washing. In fact, hand washing is recommended when hands are soiled and between patient contacts (22). Many institutions that have adopted that BSI require hand washing after glove removal (28).

IMPACT OF UNIVERSAL PRECAUTIONS AND BODY SUBSTANCE ISOLATION

Universal Precautions are now a minimum standard in U.S. hospitals as a result of OSHA regulations. Many hospitals also have BSI or some modification of BSI in place because of increasing emphasis on the potential infectiousness of body fluids from all patients, and the increasing rate of multidrug-resistant pathogens. To review the advantages of these systems over category-specific or disease-specific isolation, the latter systems may be inconsistently or incorrectly applied, whereas precautions that are used for all patients not only are easier to implement but also protect cross-transmission from patients who may lack signs or symptoms of a disease. Furthermore, there is less psychological trauma for individual patients identified as having a microorganism transmissible by blood or body fluids, because all patients are treated in a standard manner. Because of healthcare worker concern about HIV in particular, this system at least theoretically eliminates the need for routine screening of all patients and personnel for HIV at periodic intervals, a process that would prove extremely costly (47).

Some disadvantages of the Universal concept have been proposed. Because gloves were used more extensively for barrier precautions in BSI and in Universal Precautions, some healthcare workers have sometimes neglected to change gloves between patients (43,45), and such practices have been associated with cross-transmission of microorganisms (48,49). Education and reinforcement of appropriate use of gloves and changing gloves between patients can be successful in reducing such practices (22,48).

The CDC has stated that each institution may design its own system of isolation (16). Indeed, as hospitals have tailored universal precautions or BSI to their own institutional needs, each system has incorporated elements of the other and the terms have been used interchangeably, even though there are real and philosophical differences between the two systems (2). Consequently, confusion has ensued regarding the term *Universal Precautions* in particular (1). The primary purpose of Universal Precautions is to reduce healthcare worker exposure to bloodborne pathogens, whereas the primary intent of BSI is to reduce cross-transmission of microorganisms between patients by transient carriage on the hands of personnel. An additional benefit is the protection of the healthcare worker from the patient's microorganisms (2). Those institutions adopting CDC-defined Universal Precautions may use category-specific or disease-specific isolation precautions (18), whereas category-specific and disease-specific systems are not necessary under BSI. Some institutions have instituted policies using both terminologies, because the universal term has been so widely accepted (28). In an attempt to lessen confusion over the terms and systems, Jackson and Lynch (2) published a table comparing the four most widely used systems of isolation precautions, and the table has been modified for additional comparisons (Table 95.2).

The effectiveness of Universal Precautions has been evaluated using the frequency of personnel nonparenteral exposures to blood and body fluids (including sputum, urine, feces) as a monitor. Fahey et al. (50) and Wong et al. (51) documented a significant decrease in nonparenteral exposures to blood and body substances after the implementation of Universal Precautions. Saghafi et al. (52) also documented a reduction in exposure of unprotected skin to blood, but the rate of needlestick exposures remained unchanged. So it appears that although Universal Precautions or BSI may significantly reduce nonparenteral exposures to blood or body fluids, other measures such as engineering controls are needed to reduce parenteral exposures such as needlesticks.

As Universal Precautions or BSI systems were implemented throughout the country, glove use increased substantially and cost became a concern. Doebbeling and Wenzel (53) evaluated the costs of using Universal Precautions, and McPherson et al. (54) evaluated the cost of BSI. Universal Precautions increased the total annual costs for isolation materials at a large university teaching hospital by $350,900, an increase, adjusted for inflation, from $13.70 to $22.89 (67%) per admission. Although BSI theoretically could be more costly, it caused an unadjusted increase in cost of 147% for isolation materials compared with an unadjusted increase of cost of 167% for Universal Precautions (53,54). There was an approximately 80% increase in the use of gloves for BSI compared with a 64% increase in glove use for universal precautions. Doebbeling et al. estimated that universal precautions cost approximately $269 million annually nationwide (in 1989 dollars) in hospitals alone and approximately $67 million in the outpatient setting, accounting for $336 million total per year nationwide (53).

Although these systems are expensive, the alternatives must be considered. The alternative of testing all patients admitted to U.S. hospitals each year is estimated to be $2.6 billion, or approximately eight times the cost of Universal Precautions (55). Thus, Universal Precautions are less expensive than universal testing. In addition, a decrease in nosocomial infection rates has been documented after implementation of Universal Precautions and BSI (2,53), providing further evidence for the cost benefit of these systems in the U.S.

NEW CENTERS FOR DISEASE CONTROL AND PREVENTION GUIDELINES

The CDC's isolation guidelines were revised by the CDC's Healthcare Infection Control Practices Advisory Committee and were published in draft guideline format for public comment in 1994 (56) and in final form in 1996 (3) (Table 95.3). The guideline contains three important changes from previous recommendations. First, "Standard Precautions" combines the major features of universal precautions and BSI. These precautions apply to all patients regardless of diagnosis or known infection status. Standard Precautions are applicable to blood, all body fluids, secretions, and excretions, whether or not they contain visible blood. This first tier of precautions is used to decrease the risk of transmission from recognized or unrecognized infection. Second, the previous categories of isolation (strict isolation, contact isolation, respiratory isolation, enteric precautions, drainage/secretion precautions) and the previous disease-specific precautions are superseded by the three types of transmission-based precautions. These precautions are based on routes of transmission for patients known or suspected to be infected or colonized with highly transmissible or epidemiologically significant pathogens. Third, the new guideline lists specific syndromes in adult and pediatric patients that are suspicious for infection and indicate which precautions to use on an empiric basis pending diagnosis. As with previous guidelines, the CDC recognized that no guideline adequately addresses each hospital's needs. Individual hospitals and healthcare systems are encouraged to review the recommendations and modify them according to their own needs and resources.

General Principles

Antisepsis

Hand washing is the still the single most important method for preventing nosocomial transmission of infection. It is regrettable that compliance with hand washing may be only about 40%, even in critical care units (57,58). Such information must encourage, rather than discourage, infection control professionals to continue to reinforce this basic control measure. Easy access to hand washing sinks or antiseptics may increase compliance and should be available, especially in high-risk areas (59). Hands should be washed even when gloves are used, because small tears in the glove may be present and contamination can occur when the glove is removed (3). In addition, failing to change gloves between patients has been implicated in cross-transmission of hospital pathogens (48). Several studies have shown reduced rates of nosocomial infections, including resistant pathogens with improved hand hygiene (60). However, noncompliance with this simple measure has been documented

TABLE 95.3. TYPES OF ISOLATION PRECAUTIONS

Standard Precautions
- Use for the care of all patients

Airborne Precautions
- In addition to standard precautions, use airborne precautions for patients known or suspected to have serious illnesses transmitted by airborne droplet nuclei; examples of such illnesses:
  - Measles
  - Varicella (including disseminated zoster); also use contact precautions for patient with primary or disseminated zoster
  - Tuberculosis; see specific guidelines (74)

Droplet Precautions
- In addition to standard precautions, use droplet precautions for patients known or suspected to have serious illnesses transmitted by large-particle droplets; examples of such illnesses:
  - Invasive Haemophilus influenzae type b disease, including meningitis, pneumonia, epiglottitis, and sepsis
  - Invasive Neisseria meningitidis disease, including meningitis, pneumonia, and sepsis
  - Invasive multidrug-resistant Streptococcus pneumoniae disease, including meningitis, pneumonia, sinusitis, and otitis media
  - Other serious bacterial respiratory infections spread by droplet transmission, including
  - Diphtheria (pharyngeal)
  - Mycoplasma pneumonia
  - Pertussis
  - Pneumonic plague
  - Streptococcal pharyngitis, pneumonia, or scarlet fever in infants and young children
  - Serious viral infections spread by droplet transmission:
    - Adenovirus
    - Influenza
    - Mumps
    - Parvovirus B19
    - Rubella

Contact Precautions
- In addition to standard precautions, use contact precautions for patients known or suspected to have serious illnesses easily transmitted by direct patient contact or by contact with items in the patient's environment. Examples of such illnesses:
- Gastrointestinal, respiratory, skin, or wound infections or colonization with multidrug-resistant bacteria judged by the infection control program, based on current state, regional, or national recommendations, to be of special clinical and epidemiologic significance
- Enteric infections with a low infectious dose or prolonged environmental survival:
  - *Clostridium difficile*
  - For diapered or incontinent patients: enterohemorrhagic *Escherichia coli* O 157:H7, *Shigella,* hepatitis A, or rotavirus
  - Respiratory syncytial virus, parainfluenza virus, or enteroviral infections in infants and young children
  - Skin infections that are highly contagious or that may occur on dry skin:
  - Diphtheria (cutaneous)
  - Herpes simplex virus (neonatal or mucocutaneous)
  - Impetigo
  - Major (noncontained) abscesses, cellulitis, or decubiti
  - Pediculosis
  - Scabies
  - Staphylococcal furunculosis in infants and young children
  - Staphylococcal scalded skin syndrome
  - Zoster (disseminated or in the immunocompromised host)
  - Viral/hemorrhagic conjunctivitis
  - Viral hemorrhagic fevers (Lassa fever or Marburg virus)

From Garner JS, the Hospital Infection Control Practices Advisory Committee. Guideline for isolation precautions in hospitals. *Infect Control Hosp Epidemiol* 1996;17:53–80, with permission.

repeatedly (61,62). Risk factors for noncompliance with hand hygiene include being a physician and a high demand for handwashing, i.e. high workload. Although the lack of physician compliance remains inexplicable, high workload is a serious problem, particularly in an ICU, where there may be as many as 40 opportunities for hand hygiene in a 1-hour period (63,64). Handwashing at the sink is effective but is time-consuming compared to antiseptic hand rub, and frequent handwashing can also result in skin reactions (65). These factors have led to the studies that have documented the efficacy of antiseptic hand rubs as a method for hand hygiene. Pittet et al. (65) documented an improvement in hand hygiene compliance from 48% to 66% with use of the hand rub, and documented a consistent decrease in nosocomial infection rates hospital-wide, including decreased rates of methicillin-resistant *S. aureus* (MRSA) (65). For such reasons, the antiseptic hand rub is becoming increasingly accepted, particularly in high-risk units such as the ICU. Recent CDC guidelines on antisepsis have also recommended this method (66). If hands are visibly soiled, handwashing at the sink should still be used.

Patient Placement and Transport

A private room is recommended for patients with some infections that are highly transmissible or when patient hygiene is poor. The private room serves as a physical barrier and helps to reinforce antisepsis before exiting the room. Private rooms used for isolation should also contain bath and toilet facilities. If a private room is not available, patients infected or colonized with the same microorganisms may share a room. Grouping or cohorting with other infected or colonized patients is useful in an outbreak situation or when private rooms are scarce. There may be circumstances when a patient with a transmissible infection must share a room with a noninfected patient. An appropriate roommate should be selected who is not likely to become infected or in whom consequences of infection would likely not be severe. In these cases, an infection control professional should evaluate the situation to assist in selecting roommates carefully. Personnel caring for these patients should be aware of modes of transmission and take appropriate precautions to prevent spread of the microorganism.

Construction features and ventilation of isolation rooms are outlined in other publications (67–69). A private room with special ventilation (as outlined below) is necessary for those with diseases transmitted by the airborne route. An anteroom between the room and the hallway may be advantageous (although not required) for housing patients in Airborne Precautions by decreasing the possibility of the spread of airborne agents from the room into the hall (see also Chapter 89).

In the acute care setting, limiting the movement of the patient in isolation precautions limits the potential for spread of the transmissible epidemiologically significant pathogen. Thus, it is recommended that these patients leave their room only for medically necessary purposes. When transport is required, the appropriate barriers (dressings, masks, etc.) should be in place, and the personnel in the receiving department should be aware of the patient's isolation precautions and measures to reduce transmission. When possible, the patient should be educated about ways they can assist in minimizing spread of the microorganism. In the extended care or rehabilitation setting, residents or patients must leave their rooms for rehabilitation and socialization. There have been modified Contact Precautions recommended in this setting that will be discussed below.

Face Barrier Protection

Besides gloves (discussed above) and gowns, barrier protection is also required to protect the face and mucous membranes when splashing of blood or body fluids is anticipated. Various kinds of mask protection, goggles, and face shields may be used as barriers to protect the eyes, nose, and mouth from exposures. This protection is required by the OSHA blood-borne pathogen final rule (3,19). A surgical mask can provide protection against large-particle droplets that are transmitted by close contact and travel short distances, as in those diseases covered by Droplet Precautions (see below). A major issue in the past few years has been the controversy over appropriate respiratory protection for *Mycobacterium tuberculosis*. Respiratory protection for tuberculosis is discussed below under Airborne Precautions.

Gowns

Gowns that are impermeable to liquids should be worn when splashing is anticipated. Leg coverings or shoe covers should be used when splashing is expected to be extensive. The wearing of gowns and protective apparel under such circumstances is mandated by the OSHA blood-borne pathogens final rule (3, 19). Gowns are used with gloves for Contact Precautions, and have been shown to decrease institutional spread of multidrug-resistant microorganisms (70,71).

Equipment

Whether special handling of equipment or articles is needed depends on the likelihood that the article is contaminated and the ability of the particular microorganism to survive in the environment (72). Articles that are visibly contaminated or likely to be contaminated should be bagged. One bag is sufficient if it is sturdy and does not allow leakage and the outside of the bag is not contaminated when the article is placed in the bag (73). Equipment may be disposable or reusable. Disposable equipment has the advantage of reducing the possibility of equipment becoming a vehicle for transmission of the agent, but use of disposable equipment may increase costs. Equipment that is reused between patients should be appropriately cleaned and disinfected (see Chapter 85). Waste should be handled according to the institutional policy on waste disposal (see Chapter 100). Generally, double bagging is not indicated for waste or articles from isolation rooms.

Linen, Laundry, and Eating Utensils

Soiled linen should be handled with a minimum of agitation and placed in a laundry bag in the patient's room or at the location where it was used. It should be transported in bags that prevent leakage. Disposable dishes and eating utensils are not required for patients on isolation. Reusable dishes may be used for patients in isolation, because the combination of dishwasher detergents and water temperature adequately decontaminates dishes (3,72).

Housekeeping

Routine daily cleaning procedures should be used in rooms with patients on most isolation precautions. Exceptions are those patients with microorganisms known to be hardy in the environment (*Clostridium difficile*, vancomycin-resistant enterococci). Special measures for these microorganisms include cleaning of the immediate patient environment (bed rails, bedside tables, commodes, doorknobs, horizontal surfaces) daily with an EPA-approved germicide. Terminal cleaning should include items that have been in direct contact with the patient or the patient's infective material. Housekeeping personnel use the same barrier precautions that would be indicated if the patient were still in the room. Horizontal surfaces and floors should be cleaned with a disinfectant-detergent solution. With the possible exception of the tuberculosis (AFB) isolation room, airing of a room or delay in admitting the next patient after an isolated patient's discharge is not needed (16,72,74).

Standard Precautions

Standard Precautions are the first tier of precautions in the new guideline and combine the major features of Universal Precautions (designed to prevent blood-borne pathogen transmission) and BSI (designed to prevent pathogen transmission from moist body surfaces). These precautions are used for all patients and apply to blood and to all body fluids, including secretions and excretions (except sweat), whether or not they contain visible blood.

For Standard Precautions, hands should be washed using a plain (nonantimicrobial) soap, or an instant antiseptic. Use gloves when contacting blood, body fluids, and contaminated items. Remove gloves before touching noncontaminated items or before going to another patient and wash hands immediately. Use mask and eye protection or a face shield to protect the eyes, nose, and mouth during activities that may generate splashing of blood or body fluids. Wear a gown to protect skin and prevent soiling of clothing during such activities as well. Reusable equipment should be cleaned and reprocessed before being used on another patient. Ensure adequate cleaning of environmental surfaces. Handle soiled equipment and laundry in a manner to avoid exposures and transfer of microorganisms to other patients and the environment.

Care should be taken to avoid sharps injuries. Never recap used needles, or use a technique that involves directing the point of the needle toward any part of the body. Place used sharps in a puncture-resistant container. Use mouthpieces or resuscitation bags instead of mouth-to-mouth resuscitation in areas where the need for cardiopulmonary resuscitation is predictable.

A patient who contaminates the environment or who cannot assist in using appropriate hygiene should be placed in a private room. If a private room is not available, seek consultation from an infection control professional regarding placement.

Transmission-Based Precautions

The second tier of precautions is for patients with documented or suspected transmissible or epidemiologically significant pathogens that require more than standard precautions to prevent cross-transmission. Hospital-acquired pathogens may be transmitted by five major routes: contact, droplet, airborne, vector-borne, and common vehicle. The isolation guidelines are not generally relevant to vector-borne and common vehicle routes. Transmission-based precautions are of three types: Airborne Precautions, Droplet Precautions, and Contact Precautions. Types may be combined for diseases with multiple routes of transmission, and each type is used in addition to Standard Precautions. Another feature of the new guidelines is a list of specific syndromes in adult and pediatric patients that should be considered possibly infectious along with a listing of the type of transmission-based precautions that should be used empirically pending diagnosis (Table 95.4).

Airborne Precautions

Airborne diseases are spread by small airborne droplets (<5 mm) suspended in the air or by dust particles containing the microorganism. These pathogens are easily dispersed widely by air currents and may be inhaled by a susceptible host in the same room or in an area with shared air circulation. For this reason, special air handling and ventilation are required. Diseases in this category include tuberculosis, varicella (chicken pox or disseminated varicella), and rubeola (measles). Ventilation requirements are similar to those published previously for AFB isolation. The patient should be in a private room with monitored negative airflow, a minimum of 6 to 12 air changes per hour, and direct exhaust to the outside or high-efficiency particulate air (HEPA) filtration if the exhaust is recirculated. The door should be kept closed, and the patient should leave the room for essential purposes only. If the patient must be transported, he or she should wear a surgical mask. Respiratory protection should be worn when entering the room of a patient with known or suspected pulmonary tuberculosis. Persons susceptible to measles or varicella (chickenpox or disseminated varicella) should avoid entering the room of patients with these infections. If susceptible persons must enter the room, they should wear respiratory protection (75).

Additional considerations for preventing transmission of tuberculosis are discussed in detail below.

Droplet Precautions

This category of transmission-based precautions is intended to reduce droplet transmission of infectious pathogens. Droplet

TABLE 95.4. CLINICAL SYNDROMES OR CONDITIONS WARRANTING ADDITIONAL EMPIRIC PRECAUTIONS

Clinical Syndrome or Condition	Potential Pathogens	Empiric Precautions
Diarrhea		
Acute diarrhea with a likely infectious cause in an incontinent or diapered patient	Enteric pathogens	Contact
Diarrhea in an adult with a history of broad-spectrum or long-term antibiotics	*Clostridium difficile*	Contact
Meningitis		
Rash or exanthems, generalized, etiology unknown	*Neisseria meningitides*	Droplet
Petechial/ecchymotic with fever	*Neisseria meningitidis*	Airborne and contact
Vesicular	Varicella	
Maculopapular with coryza and fever	Rubeola (measles)	Airborne
Respiratory infections		
Cough/fever/upper lobe pulmonary infiltrate in an HIV-negative patient or a patient at low risk for HIV infection	*Mycobacterium tuberculosis*	Airborne
Cough/fever/pulmonary infiltrate in any lung location in an HIV-infected patient or at high risk for HIV infection	*Mycobacterium tuberculosis*	Airborne
Paroxysmal or severe persistent cough during periods of pertussis activity	*Bordetella pertussis*	Droplet
Respiratory infections, particularly bronchiolitis and croup, in infants and young children	Respiratory syncytial or parainfluenza virus	Contact
Risk of multidrug-resistant microorganisms		
History of infection or colonization with multidrug-resistant organisms	Resistant bacteria	Contact
Skin, wound, or urinary tract infection in a patient with a recent hospital or nursing home stay in a facility where multidrug-resistant organisms are prevalent	Resistant bacteria	Contact
Skin or wound infection		
Abscess or draining wound that cannot be covered	*Staphylococcus aureus*, group A streptococcus	Contact

HIV, human immunodeficiency virus.

transmission occurs when large-particle droplets (>5 mm in diameter) from an infectious person make contact with the mucous membranes of the nose, mouth, or conjunctivae of a susceptible person. Droplets may be generated in the course of talking, coughing, or sneezing and during procedures involving the airway, such as intubation or bronchoscopy. Transmission via large droplets differs from airborne transmission in that the former requires close contact (within 3 feet) between the source and the recipient person and because large droplets do not remain suspended in the air and usually travel only short distances. Examples of diseases for which droplet precautions are recommended are meningococcal meningitis, multidrug-resistant pneumococcal meningitis or pneumonia, pertussis, streptococcal pharyngitis or pneumonia, influenza, and parvovirus B19 (for patients with aplastic crisis or chronic infection). The patient should be placed in a private room. If a private room is not available, patients with infection due to the same microorganism may be cared for in the same room (cohorted). If both private rooms and cohorting are unavailable, there must be spatial separation of at least 3 feet between the infected patient and other patients and visitors. A mask should be worn when one is within 3 feet of the patient. Logistically, it may be most practical to wear a mask upon entering the room. The patient should leave the room only when necessary and should wear a surgical mask when doing so.

Contact Precautions

These precautions are used for patients with known or suspected multidrug-resistant or epidemiologically significant pathogen infection or colonization. These are for such pathogens transmitted by direct patient contact (i.e., hand or skin-to-skin contact) that occurs during routine patient care or indirect contact (touching) with environmental surfaces. The patient should be placed in a private room when possible. If this is not possible, cohorting with other infected or colonized patients is acceptable. If neither a private room nor cohorting is possible, the epidemiology of the microorganism must be considered and infection control professionals consulted before placement. Gloves should be used as a barrier, as with Standard Precautions, for contact with blood and body substances. Also, under contact precautions, gloves should be changed after contacting infective material with high concentrations of microorganisms (e.g., feces and wound drainage). Gloves should be removed before one leaves the patient's room, and hands should immediately be cleansed with an antiseptic agent. A clean nonsterile gown should be worn if substantial contact with the patient is anticipated, the patient is incontinent of stool, or the patient has wound drainage that is not well contained by a dressing. The gown should be removed before one leaves the patient's environment. In the acute care setting, movement of the patient from the room should be for essential purposes only, and precautions should be maintained by the receiving department. When feasible, the use of noncritical equipment should be dedicated to a single patient or a cohort of patients. If equipment must be shared, it should be disinfected before use by another patient.

Examples of diseases for which Contact Precautions are recommended include infection or colonization with multidrug-resistant bacteria, *C. difficile* colitis, respiratory syncytial virus (RSV) infection in children, and skin infections due to scabies, impetigo, and varicella zoster. Some diseases that are communicable by contact and by the respiratory route require contact precautions in combination with droplet or airborne precautions. Examples include viral hemorrhagic fevers such as Lassa fever or Marburg virus (contact and droplet precautions), disseminated varicella (Contact and Airborne Precautions), and smallpox (Contact and Airborne Precautions).

Vancomycin-Resistant Enterococci

Vancomycin-resistant enterococci have emerged and are quite prevalent in some areas of the U.S. and much less common in others. Patients colonized or infected with these microorganisms may be handled under contact precautions. Guidelines from the CDC for preventing transmission of vancomycin-resistant enterococci have also been published (76) and emphasize the principles of Contact Precautions. Environmental cleaning is also quite important for control of this microorganism due to its hardiness on environmental surfaces. For this reason, a daily cleaning of the patient's immediate environment (bed rails, bedside table, commode, doorknobs, horizontal surfaces) with an EPA-approved germicide is indicated.

A multifactorial approach in controlling this microorganism is recommended, such as antibiotic utilization efforts including appropriate vancomycin use by both the oral and the parenteral routes (76). In some institutions, restriction of broad-spectrum cephalosporins has been helpful for control of vancomycin-resistant enterococci as well as other multidrug-resistant pathogens such as extended-spectrum β-lactamase–producing *Klebsiella pneumoniae* (77).

Vancomycin-Intermediate and Vancomycin-Resistant *Staphylococcus Aureus*

Vancomycin-intermediate (or glycopeptide-intermediate) *S. aureus* (VISA) [minimum inhibitory concentration (MIC) 8 μg/mL) was initially reported from Japan in 1996 and was subsequently reported from the U.S. Although these isolates showed reduced susceptibility to vancomycin rather than complete resistance, VISA was a concern because most reported patients required alternative therapy other than vancomycin. The CDC published interim guidelines for the prevention and control of staphylococcal infection associated with reduced susceptibility to vancomycin in 1997 (78). These guidelines reiterate conservative use of vancomycin as a preventive measure. In addition, laboratory methods for susceptibility testing of these strains have been revised for more accurate detection. For preventing the spread of these microorganisms, the laboratory should immediately notify infection control personnel and the patient's attending physician. Infection control personnel, in conjunction with the state health department and the CDC, should initiate an epidemiologic investigation. Contact Precautions should be strictly enforced in the care of the patient. The number of personnel caring for the patient should be minimized, and specific healthcare workers should be assigned to the care of the colonized/infected patient or patients. Infection control personnel should inform healthcare workers regarding the epidemiologic significance of VISA and assist in monitoring compliance with contact precautions and other control measures. In coordination with public health officials as above, baseline surveillance cultures of the anterior nares and hands of those exposed to the patient, including healthcare workers and roommates, may be indicated to determine whether transmission has already occurred. Transfer of the patient within the facility or between facilities should be avoided. If transfer is necessary, the receiving unit or institution should be fully informed. Additional recommendations have been published by Wenzel and Edmond (79) that include excluding healthcare workers at risk for staphylococcal colonization from caring for patients with VISA and the use of mupirocin for eradication of nasal *S. aureus* colonization (see also Chapter 28).

Surprisingly, as of June 2002, there have been only eight patients in the U.S. with VISA clinical infections, so it has not emerged widely as initially anticipated. However, a more serious problem emerged in 2002, with the report of two isolates that were fully resistant (MIC >32 μg/mL) to vancomycin (80). The concern with these isolates not only is the complete resistance to vancomycin, but also genetic analysis suggests conjugative transfer of the *vanA* resistance gene from *Enterococcus* species to *S. aureus.* Thus, this may become a more significant problem than VISA. The CDC recommends the same guidelines for control of vancomycin-resistant *S. aureus* VRSA as for VISA, emphasizing strict Contact Precautions.

TUBERCULOSIS PRECAUTIONS: SPECIAL CONSIDERATIONS

There has been a substantial increase in tuberculosis cases since the mid-1980s, primarily in association with the HIV epidemic. In 1990 and 1991, several nosocomial outbreaks of multidrug-resistant tuberculosis (MDR-TB) were documented (81, 82). In each outbreak, a delay or lapse in AFB isolation was a major factor in transmission. This recent resurgence of tuberculosis, emergence of strains of *M. tuberculosis* resistant to isoniazid and rifampin, and documentation of nosocomial outbreaks of *M. tuberculosis* prompted the expansion and revision of CDC AFB isolation guidelines in 1990 (83). In 1993, expanded updated guidelines were published in draft form in the Federal Register (84), and more extensive guidelines were published in 1994 (74). Due to enhanced containment and directly observed therapy, the national trend is now a decrease in tuberculosis cases, but some areas are still experiencing sustained increased rates compared to the 1980s.

Major changes in AFB isolation include requirements for a high-efficiency filtration mask and duration of isolation based on clinical improvement and an emphasis on ventilation controls. Although special ventilation requirements were mentioned in the 1983 CDC guidelines for tuberculosis and certain diseases under strict isolation, the 1990 and subsequent guidelines emphasize these as particularly important control measures. Hospitals with older ventilation systems, which include many public hospitals with patients at risk for tuberculosis, have looked at ways to retrofit isolation rooms to meet the ventilation criteria outlined. In addition, the 1990 guidelines recommended special ventilation in bronchoscopy and areas where cough-inducing procedures, such as aerosolized pentamidine treatments, are performed. Infection control programs have also experienced OSHA involvement in this area, because healthcare workers were involved in nosocomial outbreaks.

Respiratory Protection

Respiratory protection for tuberculosis has been an area of major controversy in recent years. The 1983 guidelines for AFB isolation stated that a (surgical) mask should be worn if the patient is coughing and does not reliably cover his or her mouth (16). One report suggests that poorly fitting standard surgical masks are not protective (85); but data on the efficacy of well-fitted masks (high-efficiency filtration or otherwise) in the clinical setting are lacking. The standard surgical masks used before the 1990 guidelines are adequate for barrier precautions but are not designed to seal tightly on the face and filter small particles. Disposable particulate respirators were originally designed for industrial use and filter particles 1 to 5 μm in size. They provide a better fit and filtration capability.

The 1990 guidelines stated that persons entering the room should wear a mask and specify that it should be a disposable, valveless, particulate respirator (83). The 1993 draft guidelines called for a HEPA filtration mask (84). The guidelines stated that the HEPA respirator mask is currently the only National Institute for Occupational Safety and Health (NIOSH)-certified mask meeting all suggested performance criteria regarding fit and filtration. NIOSH-certified dust-mist or dust, fume, and mist respirators had not been evaluated for these criteria. There was much controversy, discussion, and public comment regarding the need for these much more costly and uncomfortable masks in the clinical setting, particularly because the role of respiratory protection devices in preventing transmission of tuberculosis is not known. After a public comment period, guidelines were published in 1994 (74) with respirator criteria unchanged; however, in 1995, NIOSH subsequently revised the respirator certification to allow a broader range of respirator alternatives (73). NIOSH indicated that the N95 (N category at 95% efficiency) meets CDC performance criteria for a tuberculosis respirator, and this respiratory protection is now widely used.

Duration of Isolation

Before 1990, the duration of isolation for tuberculosis patients was 2 to 3 weeks after beginning antituberculous therapy (16,86,87). However, even the 1983 guidelines state that isolation should be continued until there is a clinical response and a decrease in the number of microorganisms on smear (16). This qualification is further emphasized in recent guidelines because of failures of empiric therapy in MDR-TB cases in nosocomial outbreaks in the late 1980s (83). The guidelines now state that AFB isolation precautions may be discontinued and the patient placed in a private room when cough is decreased substantially, the number of microorganisms on smear is decreased, and there is overall clinical improvement. For a patient with suspected or confirmed MDR-TB, AFB isolation should continue until there is clinical improvement and the smear is negative for AFB. The guidelines also state that it is not advisable to place a tuberculosis patient in a room with other patients until the AFB smear is negative on three consecutive days.

Barrier Protection

Gowns are needed only if soiling of clothing is anticipated. Gloves are not indicated except, as dictated under universal precautions, for contact with blood or certain body fluids. As with other types of isolation, hands should be washed after touching the patient or potentially contaminated articles and before contact with another patient.

Decontamination

It is rare for inanimate articles to be involved in tuberculosis transmission. Procedures for cleaning, disinfecting, or sterilizing an item should be determined by its intended use. As for items used on any patient, critical items should be sterilized, semicritical items should undergo high-level disinfection or sterilization, and noncritical items should be cleaned (see Chapter 85). Recent guidelines from the Association for Professionals in Infection Control and Epidemiology have recommended a 20-minute disinfection time for semicritical instruments such as bronchoscopes to ensure tuberculocidal activity. Exceptional terminal cleaning to disinfect environmental surfaces is rarely needed. Routine cleaning with a hospital-grade EPA-approved germicide/disinfectant is recommended (26). Routine daily cleaning procedures should be used to clean patient rooms on AFB precautions.

Ventilation

The American Society of Heating, Refrigerating, and Air Conditioning Engineers (ASHRAE) and the Federal Health Resources and Services Administration have published standard recommendations for indoor air quality in healthcare facilities (67–69). Special ventilation requirements for a patient on AFB precautions include negative pressure in relation to the hallway or anteroom; a minimum of six to 12 air changes per hour, including two outside air exchanges per hour; and direct exhaust to the outside or HEPA filtration if the air is recirculated (69, 74). The negative pressure room maintains airflow into the room from the hallway to minimize potential spread of tuberculosis bacilli into surrounding areas. The door must be kept closed to maintain negative pressure, and the direction of airflow should be monitored while the room is used for AFB isolation. A separate anteroom is not required but, if used, may serve as an airlock to minimize spread of droplet nuclei into the hallway. The anteroom should also have directional airflow. Direct exhaust to the outside must be away from intake vents, people, and animals in accordance with federal, state, and local regulations for environmental discharges.

The 1994 guidelines also address ventilation in patient waiting areas. Emergency room waiting areas should have at least ten air changes per hour, as recommended by ASHRAE. The guidelines also suggest that air from clinics with patients at high risk for tuberculosis not be recirculated except through a HEPA filter. Because this may be very difficult to achieve in many clinic areas, early identification of patients with suspected tuberculosis followed by placement of the patient in a designated isolation room in the clinic or emergency room will assist prevention (see also Chapter 89).

Patient Management

Patient management issues arise for all types of isolation but may be particularly difficult for patients on AFB precautions. Patient and family education is particularly important when AFB isolation is implemented so that the patient understands the rationale for isolation and the psychological aspects and stigma of isolation can be minimized. The patient should be educated about coughing into a tissue and wearing a mask when it is necessary to leave the room. In general, the patient should not leave the room except for medically necessary procedures.

SPECIAL CONSIDERATIONS IN PEDIATRIC PATIENTS

Because pediatric hospitalizations are often due to communicable diseases, isolation guidelines are particularly relevant for this group of patients. Previous guidelines have stated that infants and very young children with pulmonary tuberculosis do not require isolation precautions because cough is rare and AFB in bronchial secretions is minimal. Exceptions could include pediatric patients with cavitary disease and patients with positive AFB smears. Concerns have also been raised recently about HIV-infected pediatric patients with tuberculosis. The 1993 guidelines state that pediatric patients with suspected or confirmed tuberculosis should be evaluated in the same manner as adults for potential infectiousness (84). (See Chapter 37 for additional information on control of tuberculosis in healthcare facilities.)

The psychosocial effects of isolation of hospitalized children have not been extensively studied, but a Swedish study suggests that isolation does not have a negative effect on a child as long as that child can observe the staff (88). As in adult patients, Standard Precautions are used, and thus the category of blood and body fluid precautions is no longer necessary. Transmission-based precautions are currently recommended in addition, but disease-specific or category-specific isolation may be used, depending on the institution's choice. The recent Report of the Committee on Infectious Diseases (the Red Book) recommends transmission-based precautions, according to current CDC recommendations (89). Some institutions may choose BSI instead of transmission-based precautions. In the category-specific system, several pediatric diseases, which are grouped under Contact isolation, include acute respiratory infections in infants and young children due to croup, bronchitis, adenovirus, influenza, and parainfluenza viruses.

Under the new transmission-based guidelines, Droplet Precautions and Airborne Precautions are used more frequently on the pediatric ward because of the more common occurrence of airborne illnesses such as varicella, pertussis, measles, and erythema infectiosum. In the category-specific system, varicella is included under strict isolation. *Haemophilus influenzae* pneumonia requires respiratory isolation in children but not in adults (16).

Isolation Precautions for Newborns and Infants

The 1983 CDC guidelines outline modifications for the newborn or infant requiring isolation (16). Such modifications are needed because generally only a small number of private rooms are available for this group of patients and because it is frequently necessary to cohort newborns and infants when outbreaks occur. Private rooms for isolation of newborns and infants are seldom indicated (or available), provided the following conditions are met: an adequate number of nursing and medical personnel are on duty and have sufficient time for appropriate hand washing, sufficient space is available for a 4- to 6-foot aisle or area between newborn stations, an adequate number of sinks for hand washing are available in each nursery room or area, and continuing instruction is given to personnel about the mode of transmission of infections. When these criteria are not met, a separate room with hand washing facilities may be indicated (16).

Forced-air incubators do not substitute for private rooms, because they filter incoming air but not air being discharged into the nursery. In addition, the surfaces of incubators can become contaminated with nosocomial microorganisms and can colonize the hands and forearms of personnel caring for infants through portholes. Thus, forced-air incubators provide some protective isolation for the infants but do not prevent cross-transmission.

Cohorts of well newborns are also useful in minimizing cross-transmission of infection in a large nursery setting:

- A cohort usually consists of all well newborns from the same 24- or 48-hour birth period; these newborns are admitted to and kept in a single nursery room and ideally are taken care of by a single group of personnel who do not take care of any other cohort during the same shift. After the newborns in a cohort have been discharged, the room is thoroughly cleaned and prepared to accept the next cohort.
- Cohorting is not practical as a routine for small nurseries or in neonatal ICUs or graded in care nurseries. It is useful in these nurseries, however, as a control measure during outbreaks or for managing a group of infants or newborns colonized or infected with a multidrug-resistant or epidemiologically significant pathogen. Under these circumstances, having a separate room for each cohort is ideal but not mandatory for many kinds of infections if cohorts can be kept separate within a single large room and if personnel are assigned to take care of only those in the cohort.
- During outbreaks, newborns or infants with overt infection or colonization and personnel who are carriers, if indicated, should be identified rapidly and placed in cohorts; if rapid identification is not possible, exposed newborns or infants should be placed in a cohort separate from those with disease and separate from unexposed infants and newborns and new admissions. The success of cohorting depends largely on the willingness and ability of nursing and ancillary personnel to adhere strictly to the cohort system and to meticulously follow patient care practices (16).

Specific recommendations regarding the design of newborn nurseries are available (90,91) and specify the amount of floor space that should be allowed per bassinet for adequate separation of infants. Barrier precautions should be followed according to standard precautions for all patients and according to BSI in institutions that have this policy. The routine use of an overgown in the nursery has not been shown to decrease nosocomial infection rates or intravascular catheter colonization rates or to change hand-washing practices (92). Policies regarding gown use in nurseries vary between institutions, and nurseries should establish their own guidelines based on what is most appropriate for their personnel and problems. Gowns may be useful in decreasing the spread of microorganisms transmitted by droplets (see below, Respiratory Syncytial Virus) and should be used in those situations. A barrier such as a blanket or gown should be used when the infant comes into contact with staff, such as during a feeding (92). Personnel do not need to wear masks, caps, and hair nets routinely.

Equipment shared by infants in a unit should be disinfected between uses with alcohol or a bleach solution. Nebulizers should be sterilized by autoclaving or gas sterilization at every shift. Soiled linens are handled as in other areas and removed from the nursery at every shift (92).

Respiratory Syncytial Virus

Another special consideration in pediatric patients is RSV, a major lower respiratory tract pathogen causing community-acquired or nosocomial infection in infants and children. Large community epidemics occur characteristically from mid-winter to early spring. Bronchiolitis due to RSV is included in contact isolation under the category-specific system, which recommends a gown when soiling of clothes is likely. The updated CDC transmission-based guidelines recommend droplet and contact precautions for pediatric and adult RSV disease (56). Several studies have suggested that special precautions are beneficial in preventing cross-transmission of this microorganism. Viruses such as RSV and rhinovirus can be transmitted by close person-to-person contact by large droplet spread, which occurs during coughing and sneezing (93,94). In addition, respiratory secretions are also spread by hand-to-hand contact or by contaminated fomites (93,95). Persistent shedding of RSV is common after infection, and RSV persists for a long period of time on environmental surfaces as well (94). Thus, it is easy to see why RSV is transmitted easily in both the community and hospital settings and has been documented to cause symptomatic infections in 40% to 60% of infant contacts and 50% of hospital staff (96). Control measures are particularly important in newborn nurseries that house premature infants and infants with pulmonary disease. In these high-risk hosts, mortality from RSV may be 35% to 50% (97).

Disposable eye-nose goggles decreased nosocomial RSV transmission in patients and staff during a 3-week period in one study (95). When goggles were used, 5% of staff and 6% of infants acquired RSV disease, compared with 34% of staff and 43% of infants when goggles were not used. Another study observed a 5% rate of disease in staff members using goggles versus 61% in those not using goggles (98). Long-term efficacy, compliance, and cost-effectiveness of these goggles have not been evaluated.

The use of gowns and masks has not been effective in reducing cross-transmission (99,100). The use of gowns and gloves has been effective as evaluated in a long-term interventional study in which compliance was also followed (101). The infection rate before intervention, when compliance with gown and glove isolation precautions was only 40%, was three times the rate of infection after intervention when compliance had increased to 80%. Glove and gown precautions have also been effective in other studies (102).

Parvovirus

Human parvovirus B19 is the etiologic agent of erythema infectiosum (fifth disease), a common childhood exanthem resulting in a slapped cheek appearance. It occurs in the community sporadically and in outbreaks. In addition to causing asymptomatic or mildly symptomatic disease in healthy adults, human parvovirus B19 may cause chronic anemia in immunodeficient patients and aplastic crisis in patients who have hematologic conditions with accelerated red blood cell turnover such as sickle cell anemia, hereditary spherocytosis, β-thalassemia, pyruvate kinase deficiency, and autoimmune hemolytic anemia (103). This agent is transmitted by contact with respiratory secretions. Persons with erythema infectiosum, the most common form of infection due to this agent, do not require Droplet Precautions when admitted to the hospital, because they are unlikely to transmit infection after the onset of the characteristic rash (87,89). However, patients acutely infected with parvovirus B19 during aplastic crises can transmit the virus to patients and staff in the healthcare setting through contact with respiratory secretions, although this is uncommon (102,103). Patients with chronic parvovirus B19 infection are probably less likely to transmit the virus in the nosocomial setting, perhaps because of lower levels of viremia (104–106).

The following recommendations are suggested for the control of nosocomial transmission of parvovirus B19. Patients who have hereditary or acquired chronic hemolytic anemias presenting with aplastic crisis and immunosuppressed persons with aplastic crisis should be evaluated for parvovirus B19 infection (107, 108). Persons with suspected or proven acute or chronic infection (other than erythema infectiosum) should be on Droplet Precautions (3,103,106,107) (see also Chapter 51).

Burkholderia cepacia in Cystic Fibrosis Patients

Burkholderia cepacia is a multidrug-resistant gram-negative bacillus that chronically colonizes and may infect the respiratory tract of some cystic fibrosis patients. Colonization or infection with *B. cepacia* in cystic fibrosis patients is significant, because colonization is difficult to eradicate and infection often results in rapid decline in pulmonary function and earlier death (109). Several studies have suggested that person-to-person transmission is important (110–112) both inside and outside the hospital. In the hospital, *B. cepacia*–positive cystic fibrosis patients should not be housed in the same room as *B. cepacia*–negative cystic fibrosis patients. Contact Precautions or BSI should be used in the care of *B. cepacia*–positive cystic fibrosis patients.

PROTECTIVE ISOLATION

Although the technique for protective isolation was outlined in previous editions of the CDC Isolation Techniques for Use in Hospitals, the 1983 CDC guidelines eliminated this isolation category. Protective isolation requiring the use of gown, gloves, and mask for all persons entering the room of a patient immunocompromised by hematologic malignancy, chemotherapy-induced granulocytopenia, or solid organ transplant has not been shown to reduce infection risk (16,113,114). Nauseef and Maki (113) studied acute nonlymphocytic leukemia patients with chemotherapy-induced granulocytopenia and found that protective isolation did not decrease rates of infection, time of onset to first infection, or days with fever. In fact, there was a higher rate of bacteremia in isolated patients, perhaps because of neglected intravenous catheter care in this group. Walsh et al. (114) studied the value of protective isolation in cardiac transplant patients. There was no difference in isolated versus nonisolated patients in infection rate, infection-related deaths, types of infection, or overall outcome.

The lack of demonstrable beneficial effect from protective isolation may result from the fact that infections in these patients are often due to their own endogenous flora; to transmission of microorganisms by unwashed hands of personnel; to the use of nonsterile items in routine protective isolation such as patient-care equipment, food, or water; and to the presence of nonsterile air (16). CDC guidelines state that in general, compromised patients should be taken care of by using precautions that are not different from routine good patient care techniques, but for these patients, routine techniques must be emphasized and enforced. Healthcare workers involved in the care of these patients should be meticulous about hand washing before and after each patient contact. Such immunocompromised patients should be in a private room, when possible, and should be housed separately from infected patients or those likely to have an infection (16).

The total protected environment (TPE) has shown efficacy, however, in preventing infections in patients with prolonged granulocytopenia (115). TPE includes a private room; HEPA filtration; disinfection or sterilization of all objects coming in contact with the patient; the use of sterile gowns, masks, gloves, caps, and boots by hospital personnel and visitors entering the room; the use of sterile water and semisterile or low microbial count food; and decontamination of the gastrointestinal tract (115). This approach is expensive and may have poor patient acceptance (115–119). Although TPE has been shown to lower the incidence of infection, the rate of survival may not differ in patients in TPE as compared with a standard hospital room (119). This is largely due to improved management of infections and makes TPE a cost-benefit issue. Invasive aspergillosis is an infection that is often refractory to therapy and has a high mortality in these patients (120). For this reason, the use of HEPA filtration and a private room is recommended for patients with prolonged granulocytopenia, such as bone marrow transplant patients (121) (see also Chapter 60).

SPECIAL CONSIDERATIONS FOR PATIENTS IN EXTENDED CARE OR REHABILITATION

As the number of elderly patients in extended care grows and as rehabilitation programs continue to proliferate, there are an increasing number of patients with multidrug-resistant microorganisms in these settings. These patients have often been in the acute care setting for extended periods of time or for frequent readmissions and have had multiple opportunities to acquire microorganisms such as MRSA, vancomycin-resistant *E. faecium* (VRE), and multidrug-resistant *K. pneumoniae.* Rehabilitation and socialization in these settings are critical to maintaining or increasing functional status, and keeping patients restricted to their room in the Contact Precautions as outlined for acute care may not be practical. Studies have documented that MRSA colonization is common in the nursing home, but infections are not frequent. This may also be the case with VRE as the data are accumulating (122). The Long-Term-Care Committee of the Society for Healthcare Epidemiology of American has published guidelines recommending minor modifications of Contact Precautions in the long-term care setting (122). This approach recommends education of personnel in these units regarding basic infection control measures and VRE. Surveillance cultures may be used in an outbreak of infection but are not cost-effective in the non-outbreak setting. When a resident is transferred to another unit or facility, the receiving party should be aware of VRE colonization.

A private room is recommended when possible or if necessary. If this is not feasible, the patient who is colonized with VRE and is continent without diarrhea or an open wound that is infected or colonized with VRE may be placed with another patient. The roommate should be selected with care and should not be severely immunocompromised, have open wounds, and preferably should not be receiving antibiotics or have an indwelling urinary catheter or drainage device. Gloves should be used for contact with the patients and their environment. Because soap may not adequately remove VRE from hands, chlorhexidine or an alcohol-containing antiseptic should be used after caring for VRE infected or colonized patients. Gowns are recommended if contact is anticipated with the patient, the patient's secretions, or the environment. VRE-infected or colonized residents may leave their room, provided that they can understand and are compliant with basic personal hygiene, continent of stool (or diapered to contain stool), and wear clean clothing. Resident education is particularly important, as much as is feasible, regarding good hygiene and hand washing. Patient care equipment should be dedicated when possible and the use of individual thermometers is recommended. In the rehabilitation unit, where equipment may be central, the patient may be scheduled at the end of the day and equipment disinfected after use. As with recommendations for VRE in acute care, daily environmental cleaning with a germicide is recommended. Vancomycin and cephalosporin use should be prudent.

Such modified Contact Precautions may be used as a model for other problematic multidrug-resistant microorganisms in the extended care setting. A similar protocol has been used in a unit with VRE and multidrug-resistant *K. pneumoniae.* Stool surveillance prevalence studies from 1 year compared with the next showed no significant increase in these microorganisms using these principles of modified precautions (123).

CATEGORY A BIOTERRORISM AGENTS AND ISOLATION

Since potential bioterrorist diseases are not routinely seen, the hospital epidemiologist and infection control department must be aware of whether and what type of isolation precautions are needed, particularly for the category A agents, deemed the most likely bioterrorist agents.

Anthrax

Person-to-person transmission of anthrax is not a concern (124). The natural life cycle is that hoofed animals inhale or ingest infective spore forms of *Bacillus anthracis* from soil or dust. The spore forms then germinate to become vegetative forms as they multiply, causing massive infection and toxin release associated with edema, hemorrhagic necrosis, and death. The carcass then decomposes, vegetative spores are exposed to oxygen, and the spore forms are regenerated. Humans can be an incidental host by skin contact with the spore forms; 95% of natural anthrax cases are cutaneous. Humans can also become an incidental host by inhalation of spores, occurring primarily by wool-sorting in endemic areas. Since the vegetative forms cause the disease in the body, anthrax is not transmissible person to person. The intentional anthrax attacks in October 2001 caused cutaneous cases from mail handling and inhalation cases from aerosolization of spores from mail-sorting equipment. There was no person-to-person transmission from these cases (123). Standard Precautions is the only isolation category recommended for anthrax (see also Chapter 111).

Smallpox

Transmission of smallpox (variola) has generally occurred only in close contacts, but nosocomial spread has been reported. Droplet spread is the major mode of transmission, but airborne transmission through fine particle aerosol can occur, particularly in severely ill patients (125). The skin lesions of smallpox are also contagious, and, unlike varicella, are contagious until the scabs separate. Contact Precautions and Airborne Precautions should be instituted immediately when there is high suspicion for smallpox, and public health officials should be notified. Masks of N95 quality of higher, disposable gloves, gowns, and shoe covers should be used for all contact with patients. Personnel should remove and dispose of protective garb before contact with others. Reusable bedding and clothing should be autoclaved or laundered in hot water with bleach to inactivate the virus. If smallpox is confirmed, these isolation precautions should continue until the scabs are separated. Clinical specimens should not be sent through the pneumatic tube system, and should be carefully packaged for referral to a public health laboratory (see also Chapter 112).

Botulism

Botulism is a toxin-mediated disease due to botulinum toxin produced by *Clostridium botulinum,* and thus is not transmitted person to person. Botulinum toxin can be detected in stool and serum and if accidentally ingested or inhaled could cause disease. Standard precautions should be used in the handling of blood and body fluids (126,127) (see also Chapter 111).

Plague

Natural cases of plague, due to infection by *Yersinia pestis,* are usually bubonic, associated with the characteristic buboes as a result of transmission from the bites of infected fleas. Primary plague pneumonia is uncommon in natural disease, but would be the expected form of intentional, or bioterrorist, plague. Person-to-person spread of pneumonic plague may occur by respiratory droplets. Therefore, Droplet Precautions are recommended for cases of pneumonic plague for until at least 48 hours of appropriate antibiotic therapy is administered and the patient shows clinical improvement (128). Patients with natural cases of bubonic plague without secondary pneumonic plague require only Standard Precautions (see also Chapter 111).

Viral Hemorrhagic Fevers

This diverse group of viruses, including Ebola, Marburg, and Lassa, are spread in a variety of ways, but may be transmitted by the respiratory route or as a blood-borne pathogen. Droplet and Contact Precautions should be used (56) for these patients. Equipment should not be shared between patients, and materials contaminated with body fluids should be disinfected with a bleach solution or phenolics. Special laboratory handling is required, including a biosafety cabinet and barrier precautions. Laboratory personnel should be notified when this disease is suspected (see also Chapter 111).

Tularemia

The most common form of natural disease due to *Francisella tularensis* is ulceroglandular disease with associated lymphadenopathy; natural tularemic pneumonia is less common. Bioterrorist disease would be expected to be tularemic pneumonia, however, due to intentional aerosolization. Person-to-person transmission does not occur, so only Standard Precautions are required. However, this disease is transmitted quite easily in the laboratory, and should be handled under a biosafety cabinet; therefore the laboratory should be notified if tularemia is suspected (129) (see also Chapter 111).

CONCLUSION

Isolation guidelines have changed tremendously in recent years, largely because of the AIDS epidemic and the small but recognized risk of nosocomial transmission. The positive aspect of this change is that guidelines designed to protect against blood-borne pathogen transmission are now standard for all patients. Precautions to prevent non–blood-borne pathogen transmission, including multidrug-resistant pathogens are now more widely used and are standard in many institutions. The revision of CDC isolation guidelines has addressed some of the confusion in terminology that occurred with implementation of Universal Precautions. Two tiers of precautions are used: Standard Precautions for the care of all patients, and a second tier of transmission-based precautions (Airborne Precautions, Droplet Precautions, and Contact Precautions) for patients with known or suspected diseases spread by these routes.

REFERENCES

1. Birnbaum D, Schulzer M, Mathias RG, et al. Adoption of guidelines for universal precautions and body substance isolation in Canadian acute-care hospitals. *Infect Control Hosp Epidemiol* 1990;11:465–472.
2. Jackson MM, Lynch P. An attempt to make an issue less murky: a comparison of four systems for infection precautions. *Infect Control Hosp Epidemiol* 1991;12:448–450.
3. Garner JS, the Hospital Infection Control Practices Advisory Committee. Guideline for isolation precautions in hospitals. *Infect Control Hosp Epidemiol* 1996;17:53–80.
4. Smith DT. Mycobacteriaceae. In: Joklik WK, Willet HP, eds. *Zinsser's microbiology,* 16th ed. New York: Appleton-Century-Crofts, 1976: 502–509.
5. Wylie WG. *Hospitals: their history, organization and construction.* New York: D. Appleton, 1877.
6. Bordley J, Harvey AM. *Two centuries of American medicine, 1776–1976.* Philadelphia: WB Saunders, 1976.
7. Richardson DL. Aseptic fever nursing. *Am J Nurs* 1915;15: 1082–1093.
8. Morrison ST, Arnold CR, eds. *Communicable diseases by Landon and Sider,* 9th ed. Philadelphia: FA Davis, 1969.
9. Aronson SP. *Communicable disease nursing.* Garden City, NY: Medical Examination Publishing, 1978.
10. Chapin CV. *The sources and modes of infection,* 2nd ed. New York: John Wiley, 1912.
11. Anderson GW, Arnstein MG. *Ancient concepts of transmission. Communicable disease control,* 3rd ed. New York: Macmillan, 1953.12. *Infection control in the hospital.* Chicago: American Hospital Association, 1968.
13. Garner JS, Hughes JM. Options for isolation precautions. *Ann Intern Med* 1987;107:248–250.
14. Centers for Disease Control. *Isolation techniques for use in hospitals.* DHEW publication no. (PHS) 70-2054. Washington, DC: U.S. Government Printing Office, 1970.
15. Haley RW, Shactman RH. The emergence of infection surveillance and control programs in U.S. hospitals: an assessment, 1976. *Am J Epidemiol* 1980;111:574–591.
16. Garner JS, Simmons BP. Guideline for isolation precautions in hospitals. *Infect Control* 1983;4:245–325.
17. Centers for Disease Control. Recommendations for prevention of HIV transmission in health-care settings. *MMWR* 1987;36(suppl 2S): 1S–18S.
18. Centers for Disease Control. Update: universal precautions for prevention of transmission of human immunodeficiency virus, hepatitis B virus, and other bloodborne pathogens in health-care settings. *MMWR* 1988;37:377–382,387–388.

19. Department of Labor, Occupational Safety and Health Administration. Occupational exposure to bloodborne pathogens; final rule. *Fed Reg* 1991;56:64175–64182.
20. Jackson MM, Lynch P. Infection control too much or too little? *Am J Nurs* 1984;84:208–210.
21. Lynch P, Jackson MM, Cummings MJ, et al. Rethinking the role of isolation practices in the prevention of nosocomial infections. *Ann Intern Med* 1987;107:243–246.
22. Lynch P, Cummings MJ, Roberts PL, et al. Implementing and evaluating a system of generic infection precautions: body substance isolation. *Am J Infect Control* 1990;18:1–12.
23. Centers for Disease Control. Recommendations for preventing transmission of infection with human T-lymphotropic virus type III/lymphadenopathy-associated virus in the workplace. *MMWR* 1985;34:1–8.
24. Centers for Disease Control. Recommendations for preventing transmission of infection with human T-lymphotropic virus type III/lymphadenopathy-associated virus during invasive procedures. *MMWR* 1986;35:221–223.
25. Centers for Disease Control. Recommended infection control practices for dentistry. *MMWR* 1993;42:1–12.
26. Garner JS, Favero MS. *Guideline for hand washing and hospital environmental control.* HHS publication no. 99-1117. Atlanta, GA: U.S. Department of Health and Human Services, Public Health Service, CDC, 1985.
27. Rutala WA, Mayhall CG. Position paper: medical waste. *Infect Control Hosp Epidemiol* 1992;13:38–48.
28. Pugliese G, Lynch P, Jackson MM, eds. *Universal precautions.* Chicago: American Hospital Publishing, 1991.
29. American Society for Testing and Materials. Standard specification for rubber and latex examination gloves. In: *Annual book of ASTM standards,* vol 37. Philadelphia: American Society for Testing and Materials, 1977:1–10.
30. Department of Health and Human Services, Food and Drug Administration. Medical devices: patient examination and surgeons gloves; adulteration. *Fed Reg* 1989(Nov 21);54. Proposed rules, 48218.
31. Kotilainen RH, Brinker J, Avato J, et al. Latex and vinyl examination gloves: quality control procedures and implications for healthcare workers. *Arch Intern Med* 1989;149:2749–2753.
32. Arnold S, Whitman J. Latex gloves not enough to exclude viruses. *Nature* 1988;335:19.
33. DeGroot-Kosolcharoen J, Jones JM. Permeability of latex and vinyl gloves to water and blood. *Am J Infect Control* 1989;17:196–201.
34. Korniewicz D, Laughon BE, Cyr WH, et al. Leakage of virus through used vinyl and latex examination gloves. *J Clin Microbiol* 1990;28:787–788.
35. Korniewicz D, Laughon B, Butz A, et al. Integrity of vinyl and latex procedure gloves. *Nurs Res* 1989;38:144–146.
36. Doebbeling BN, Pfaller MA, Houston AK, et al. Removal of nosocomial pathogens from the contaminated glove. *Ann Intern Med* 1988;109:394–398.
37. Martin MV, Dunn HM, Field EA, et al. A physical and microbiological evaluation of the re-use of non-sterile gloves. *Br Dent J* 1988;165;321–324.
38. Bovie JW. The use of gloves in abdominal surgery. *Am J Obstet* 1899;40:491.
39. Albin MS, Bunegin L, Duke ES, et al. Anatomy of a defective barrier: sequential glove leak detection in a surgical and dental environment. *Crit Care Med* 1992;20:170–184.
40. Hansen ME, McIntire DD, Miller GL III. Occult glove perforations: frequency during interventional radiologic procedures. *AJR* 1992;159:131–135.
41. Burke JT, Wilson NHF. The incident of undiagnosed punctures in non-sterile gloves. *Br Dent J* 1990;168:67–72.
42. Otis LL, Cottone JA. Prevalence of perforations in disposable latex gloves during routine dental treatment. *J Am Dent Assoc* 1989;118:321–324.
43. Weinstein RA, Kabins SA. Strategies for prevention and control of multiple drug-resistant nosocomial infection. *Am J Med* 1981;70:449–454.
44. Jackson MM, Lynch P. An alternative to isolating patients. *Geriatr Nurs* 1987;8:308–311.
45. Weinstein RA, Kabins SA. Isolation practices in hospitals. *Ann Intern Med* 1987;107:781–782.
46. Olson B, Weinstein RA, Nathan C, et al. Occult aminoglycoside resistance in *Pseudomonas aeruginosa*: epidemiology and implications for therapy and control. *J Infect Dis* 1985;152:769–774.
47. Gerberding JL. Expected costs of implementing a mandatory HIV and hepatitis B virus testing and restriction program for healthcare workers performing invasive procedures. *Infect Control Hosp Epidemiol* 1991;12:443–447.
48. Patterson JE, Vecchio J, Pantelick EL, et al. Association of contaminated gloves with transmission of *Acinetobacter calcoaceticus* var. *anitratus* in an intensive care unit. *Am J Med* 1991;91:479–483.
49. Maki DG, McCormick RD, Zilz MA, et al. An MRSA outbreak in a SICU during universal precautions: new epidemiology for nosocomial MRSA; downside for universal precautions (abstract 41). Third Decennial International Conference on Nosocomial Infections, July 31–August 3, 1990, Atlanta, GA.
50. Fahey BJ, Koziol DE, Banks SM, et al. Frequency of nonparenteral occupational exposures to blood and body fluids before and after universal precautions training. *Am J Med* 1991;90:145–153.
51. Wong ES, Stotka JL, Chinchilli VM, et al. Are universal precautions effective in reducing the number of occupational exposures among health care workers? *JAMA* 1991;265:1123–1128.
52. Saghafi L, Raselli P, Francillon C, et al. Exposure to blood during various procedures: results of two surveys before and after the implementation of universal precautions. *Am J Infect Control* 1992;20:53–57.
53. Doebbeling BN, Wenzel RP. The direct costs of universal precautions in a teaching hospital. *JAMA* 1990;264:2083–2087.
54. McPherson DC, Jackson MM, Rogers JC. Evaluating the cost of the body substance isolation system. *J Healthc Mater Manage* 1988;6:20–28.
55. Gordin FM, Gilgert C, Hawley HP, et al. Prevalence of human immunodeficiency virus and hepatitis B virus in unselected hospital admissions: implications for mandatory testing and universal precautions. *J Infect Dis* 1990;161:14–17.
56. Garner JS, and HICPAC, Centers for Disease Control and Prevention. Guideline for isolation precautions in hospitals. *Infect Control Hosp Epidemiol* 1996;17:53–80 and *Am J Infect Control* 1996;24:24–52. *http://www.cdc.gov/ncidod/hip/ISOLAT/isolate.htm.*
57. Albert RK, Condie F. Handwashing patterns in medical intensive-care units. *N Engl J Med* 1981;304:1465–1466.
58. Doebbeling BN, Stanley GL, Sheetz CT, et al. Comparative efficacy of alternative hand-washing agents in reducing nosocomial infections in intensive care units. *N Engl J Med* 1992;327:88–93.
59. Bishoff WE, Reynolds TM, Sessler CN, et al. Handwashing compliance by health care workers: the impact of an education and awareness program (abstract 22). In: Abstracts of the Society for Healthcare Epidemiology, Orlando, 1998.
60. Larson EL. APIC guideline for handwashing and hand antisepsis in healthcare settings. *Am J Infect Control* 1995;23:251–269.
61. Albert RK, Condie F. Handwashing patterns in medical intensive care units. *N Engl J Med* 1981;304:1465–1466.
62. Pittet D, Mourouga P, Perneger TV. Complicance with handwashing in a teaching hospital infection control program. *Ann Intern Med* 1999;130;126–130.
63. Vandenbroucke-Grauls CM. Clean hands closer to the bedside. *Lancet* 2000;356:1290–1291.
64. Voss A, Widmer AF. No time for handwashing!? Handwashing versus alcoholic rub: can we afford 100% compliance? *Infect Control Hosp Epidemiol* 1997;18:205–208.
65. Pittet D, Hugonnet S, Harbarth S, et al. Effectiveness of a hospital-wide programme to improve compliance with hand hygiene. Infection Control Programme. *Lancet* 2000;356:1307–1312.
66. Boyce JM, Pittet D, HICPAC and the HICPAC/SHEA/APIC/IDSA Hand Hygiene Task Force. *MMWR* 2002;51(RR-16):1–44. *http://www.cdc.gov/mmwr/preview/mmwrhtml/rr5116a1.htm.*
67. Health Resources and Services Administration. *Guidelines for construc-*

tion and equipment of hospital and medical facilities. PHS publication no. (HRSA) 84-14500. Rockville, MD: U.S. Department of Health and Human Services, Public Health Service, 1984.

68. American Institute of Architects, Committee on Architecture for Health. General hospital. In: *Guidelines for construction and equipment of hospital and medical facilities.* Washington, DC: American Institute of Architects Press, 1993.
69. American Society of Heating, Refrigerating, and Air Conditioning Engineers. Health facilities. In: *1991 Application handbook.* Atlanta, GA: American Society of Heating, Refrigerating, and Air Conditioning Engineers, 1991.
70. Srinivasan A, Song X, Ross T, et al. A prospective study to determine whether cover gowns in addition to gloves decrease nosocomial transmission of vancomycin-resistant enterococci in an intensive care unit. *Infect Control Hosp Epidemiol* 2002;23:424–435.
71. Byers KE, Anglim AM, Anneski CJ, et al. A hospital epidemic of vancomycin-resistant *Enterococcus*: risk factors and control. *Infect Control Hosp Epidemiol* 2001;22:140–147.
72. Garner JS, Hierholzer WJ. Controversies in isolation policies and practices. In: Wenzel RP, ed. *Prevention and control of nosocomial infections,* 2nd ed. Baltimore: Williams & Wilkins, 1993:70–81.
73. Maki DG, Alvarado C, Hassemer C. Double-bagging of items from isolation rooms is unnecessary as an infection control measure: a comparative study of surface contamination with single- and double-bagging. *Infect Control* 1986;7:535–537.
74. Centers for Disease Control and Prevention. Guidelines for preventing the transmission of tuberculosis in health-care facilities, 1994. *MMWR* 1994;43:1–132 and *Fed Reg* 1994;59:54242–54303.
75. Department of Health and Human Services, Department of Labor. Respiratory protective devices: final rules and notice. *Fed Reg* 1995; 60:30336–30402.
76. Hospital Infection Control Practices Advisory Committee. Recommendations for preventing the spread of vancomycin resistance. *Infect Control Hosp Epidemiol* 1995;16:105–113.
77. Quale J, Landman D, Saurina G, et al. Manipulation of a hospital antimicrobial formulary to control an outbreak of vancomycin-resistant enterococci. *Clin Infect Dis* 1996;23;1020–1025.
78. Centers for Disease Control and Prevention. Interim guidelines for prevention and control of staphylococcal infections associated with reduced susceptibility to vancomycin. *MMWR* 1997;46: 626–628,635.
79. Wenzel RP, Edmond MB. Vancomycin-resistant *Staphylococcus aureus*: infection control considerations. *Clin Infect Dis* 1998;27: 245–251.
80. Centers for Disease Control and Prevention. *Staphylococcus aureus* resistant to vancomycin—United States, 2002. *MMWR* 2002;51(26): 565–567.
81. Centers for Disease Control. Nosocomial transmission of multidrug-resistant tuberculosis among HIV-infected persons Florida and New York, 1988–1991. *MMWR* 1991;40:585–591.
82. Fischl MA, Uttamchandani RB, Daikos GL, et al. An outbreak of tuberculosis caused by multiple-drug-resistant tubercle bacilli among patients with HIV infection. *Ann Intern Med* 1992;117:177–183.
83. Centers for Disease Control. Guidelines for preventing the transmission of tuberculosis in health-care settings, with special focus on HIV-related issues. *MMWR* 1990;30:1–29.
84. Department of Health and Human Services. Centers of Disease Control and Prevention (CDC). Draft guidelines for preventing the transmission of tuberculosis in health-care facilities. Second edition: notice of comment rule. *Fed Reg* 1993;58:52810–52854.
85. Pippen DJ, Verderame RA, Weber KK. Efficacy of face masks in preventing inhalation of airborne contaminants. *Oral Maxillofac Surg* 1987;45:319–323.
86. Des Prez RM, Heim CR. *Mycobacterium tuberculosis.* In: Mandel GL, Douglas RG, Bennett JE, eds. *Principles and practice of infectious diseases.* New York: Churchill Livingston, 1990:1877–1906.
87. Benenson AS, ed. *Control of communicable diseases in man,* 15th ed. Washington, DC: American Public Health Association, 1990.
88. Putsep E. Pediatric patients. In: Putsep E, ed. *Modern hospital.* London: Lloyd-Luke, 1981:86–88.
89. American Academy of Pediatrics. Infection control for hospitalized children. In: Pickering LK, ed. *2000 Red Book: Report of the Committee on Infectious Diseases,* 25th ed. Elk Grove Village, IL: American Academy of Pediatrics; 2000:127–137.
90. *Planning and design for perinatal and pediatric facilities.* Columbus, OH: Ross Laboratories, 1977.
91. Frigoletto FD, Little GA. *American Academy of Pediatrics and American College of Obstetricians and Gynecologists guidelines for perinatal care,* 2nd ed. Evanston, IL: American Academy of Pediatrics, 1988.
92. Donowitz LG. Failure of the overgown to prevent nosocomial infection in a pediatric intensive care unit. *Pediatrics* 1986;77:35.
93. Brawley RL. Infection control practices for preventing respiratory syncytial virus infections. *Infect Control Hosp Epidemiol* 1988;9:103–104.
94. Hall CB, Douglas RG Jr. Modes of transmission of respiratory syncytial virus. *J Pediatr* 1981;99:100.
95. Gala CL, Hall CB, Schnable KC, et al. The use of eye-nose goggles to control nosocomial respiratory syncytial virus infection. *JAMA* 1986;256:2706–2708.
96. Hall CB. The nosocomial spread of respiratory syncytial viral infection. *Annu Rev Med* 1983;34:311–319.
97. Anderson LJ, Parker RA, Strikas RL. Association between respiratory syncytial virus outbreaks and lower respiratory tract deaths of infants and young children. *J Infect Dis* 1990;161:640–646.
98. Agah R, Cherry JD, Garakian AJ, et al. Respiratory syncytial virus (RSV) infection rate in personnel caring for children with RSV infections. *Am J Dis Child* 1987;141:695–697.
99. Hall CB, Douglas RG Jr. Nosocomial respiratory syncytial virus infections: should gowns and masks be used? *Am J Dis Child* 1981;135: 512–515.
100. Murphy D, Tood JK, Chao RK, et al. The use of gowns and masks to control respiratory illness in pediatric hospital personnel. *J Pediatr* 1981;99:746–750.
101. Leclair JM, Freeman J, Sullivan BF, et al. Prevention of nosocomial respiratory syncytial virus infections through compliance with glove and gown isolation precautions. *N Engl J Med* 1987;317:329–334.
102. Tucker JA, Meservey M, Grossi L, et al. Prevention of nosocomial infections by isolation procedures [letter]. *N Engl J Med* 1988;318: 326–327.
103. Koziol DE, Kurtzman G, Ayub J, et al. Nosocomial human parvovirus B19 infection: lack of transmission from a chronically infected patient to hospital staff. *Infect Control Hosp Epidemiol* 1992;13:343–348.
104. Evans JPM, Rossiter MA, Kumaran TO, et al. Human parvovirus aplasia: case due to cross infection in a ward. *Br Med J* 1984;288: 681.
105. Bell LM, Naides SJ, Stoffman P, et al. Human parvovirus B19 infection among hospital staff members after contact with infected patients. *N Engl J Med* 1989;321:485–491.
106. Naides SJ. Infection control measures for human parvovirus B19 in the hospital setting. *Infect Control Hosp Epidemiol* 1989;10:326–329.
107. Graeve JL, de Alarcon PA, Naides SJ. Parvovirus B19 infection in patients receiving cancer chemotherapy: the expanding spectrum of disease. *Am J Pediatr Hematol Oncol* 1989;11:441–444.
108. Centers for Disease Control. Risks associated with human parvovirus B19 Infection. *MMWR* 1989;38:81–97.
109. Tablan OC, Martone WJ, Doershuk CF, et al. Colonization of the respiratory tract with *Pseudomonas cepacia* in cystic fibrosis: risk factors and outcomes. *Chest* 1987;91:527–532.
110. Tablan OC, Chorba TL, Schidlow DV, et al. *Pseudomonas cepacia* colonization in patients with cystic fibrosis: risk factors and clinical outcome. *J Pediatr* 1985;107:382–387.
111. LiPuma JJ, Dasen TD, Nielson DW, et al. Person-to-person transmission of *Pseudomonas cepacia* between patients with cystic fibrosis. *Lancet* 1990;336:1094–1096.
112. Centers for Disease Control. Cooperative agreements for human immunodeficiency virus (HIV); prevention projects program announcement and availability of funds for fiscal year 1993. *Fed Reg* 1992;57: 40675–40683.
113. Nauseef WM, Maki DG. A study of the value of simple protective isolation in patients with granulocytopenia. *N Engl J Med* 1981;304: 448–453.

114. Walsh TR, Guttendorf J, Dummer S, et al. The value of protective isolation procedures in cardiac allograft recipients. *Ann Thorac Surg* 1989;47:539–545.
115. Pizzo PA, Schimpff SC. Strategies for the prevention of infection in the myelosuppressed or immunosuppressed cancer patient. *Cancer Treat Rep* 1983;67:223–234.
116. Pizzo PA. The value of protective isolation in preventing nosocomial infections in high risk patients. *Am J Med* 1981;70:631–637.
117. Pizzo PA. Do results justify the expense of protected environments? In: Wiernik PH, ed. *Controversies of oncology.* New York: John Wiley, 1982:271.
118. Engelhard D, Marks MI, Good RA. Infections in bone marrow transplant recipients. *J Pediatr* 1986;108:335–345.
119. Pizzo PA. Considerations for the prevention of infectious complications in patients with cancer. *Rev Infect Dis* 1989;11(suppl 7): 1551–1563.
120. Denning DW, Stevens DA. The treatment of invasive aspergillosis: surgery and antifungal therapy of 2,121 published cases. *Rev Infect Dis* 1990;12:1147–1201.
121. Rhame FS. Nosocomial aspergillosis: how much protection for which patients? *Infect Control Hosp Epidemiol* 1989;10:296–298.
122. Crossley K, the Long-Term-Care Committee of the Society for Healthcare Epidemiology of America. Vancomycin-resistant enterococci in long-term care facilities. *Infect Control Hosp Epidemiol* 1998; 19:521–525.
123. Grota P, Shoe S, Patterson J. Management of multiple drug resistant organisms in a VA nursing home. *Am J Infect Control* 1998;188(abst).
124. Inglesby TV, Henderson DA, Bartlett JG, et al. Anthrax as a biological weapon. *JAMA* 1999;281:1735–1745.
125. Inglesby TV, O'Toole T, Henderson DA, et al. Anthrax as a biological weapon, 2002. Updated recommendations for management. *JAMA* 2002;288:2236–2252.
126. Centers for Disease Control and Prevention. Smallpox Response Plan and Guidelines, version 3.0, 2002. *http://www.healthpolicyinstitute.org/projects/disaster response/guidance document.pdf.*
127. Arnon SS, Schecter R, Inglesby TV, et al. Botulinum toxin as a biological weapon. *JAMA* 285:1059–1070.
128. Inglesby TV, Dennis DT, Henderson DA, et al. Plague as a biological weapon. *JAMA* 2000;283:2281–2290.
129. Dennis DT, Inglesby TV, Henderson DA, et al. tularemia as a biological weapon. *JAMA* 2001;285:2763–2773.

96

HAND WASHING AND HAND DISINFECTION

MANFRED L. ROTTER

Although the importance of hands for the transmission of infectious diseases was not demonstrable before the 19th century when medicine began to adopt scientific ways of thinking, an idea of their role must have existed long before the Hungarian obstetrician Ignaz Philipp Semmelweis made his epidemiologic observations on the horrible spread of puerperal fever, which caused maternal mortality rates of up to 18% in some months at a Vienna, Austria, lying-in hospital during the years 1841–1847. At least from examples of the historical tradition, it may be concluded that hand washing is an old cultural heritage of human civilization. The idea has been handed down to us that this procedure not only served for the removal of dirt but also to deliver people symbolically from physical and moral evils, such as illness and sin. It is characteristic of the efficacy of modern scientific methodology that hands were identified as transmitters of disease even at a time when microorganisms were not yet recognized as a cause of infection. Semmelweis applied epidemiologic rather than microbiologic methods to test his hypothesis that preventing hands from introducing a fatal something into the maternal birth canal during vaginal examination would also end the hyperendemic situation of puerperal fever at his hospital. His attention was especially drawn to the markedly lower maternal mortality at the second obstetric department of the same hospital where, in contrast to his working place, usually midwives conducted deliveries (Fig. 96.1) (1). He identified the distinguishing moment in the incidence of puerperal fever by the fact that midwives had no contact with the autopsy room where, he postulated, hands were contaminated with the fatal etiologic agent.

Although the role of hands in the transmission of puerperal fever had been recognized in 1795 by Alexander Gordon and in 1843 by Oliver Wendell Holmes (2), Semmelweis was the first to take appropriate action by introducing hand disinfection into clinical practice in May 1847. A little later and probably without knowledge of Semmelweis's findings, the Scottish surgeon Joseph Lister tested and proved Louis Pasteur's hypothesis that microorganisms not only cause fermentation and putrefaction but may also initiate suppuration in living tissues. By inactivating and keeping the causative microorganisms away from the surgical site, he prevented postoperative infection. Among other vehicles and sources, he also recognized the importance of the hands of the surgical team and consequently tried to eliminate their microbial flora before surgery.

MICROBIAL FLORA OF HANDS

Although it is not always feasible to do so (3,4), three groups of microorganisms may be distinguished on the skin: (a) microorganisms that reside on the skin, which the American surgeon Price (5) termed "resident" flora; (b) those that happen to be there as contaminants, which Price termed "transient" flora; and (c) pathogens that cause infections on the hands, such as panaritium digiti or paronychia, which can be called "infectious" flora.

Resident Flora

Except for the anaerobic propionibacteria that are located mainly at the ducts of sebaceous glands, most of these microorganisms reside on the uppermost part of the stratum corneum (6, 7) on corneocytes and embedded in a mass of lipids and cell

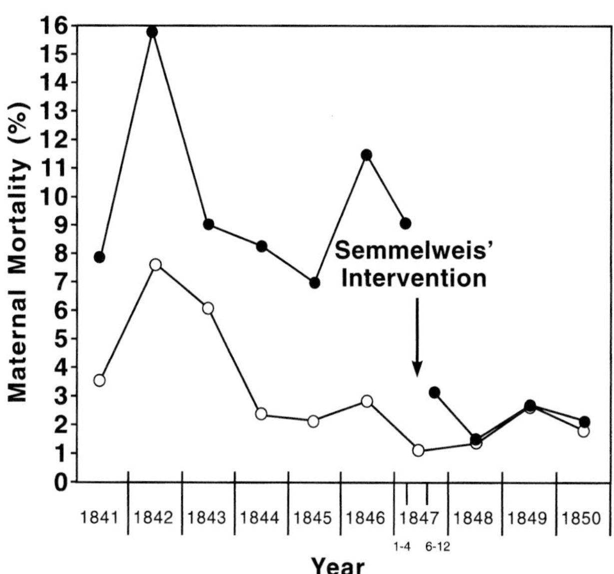

Figure 96.1. Maternal mortality at the First and Second Imperial-Royal Obstetric Department of the General Hospital in Vienna, Austria, 1841–1850. ●, First department; ○, second department. (From Rotter ML. Semmelweis' sesquicentennial: a little noted anniversary of hand washing. *Curr Opin Infect Dis* 1998;11:457–460, with permission.)

detritus of the pars disjuncta (8,9). They multiply in the upper regions of the hair follicle (10). The deeper regions of the skin are not colonized, as are the ducts of eccrine and apocrine glands (11). The composition of skin flora has been described in several reviews (12–19). It varies qualitatively and quantitatively with body site, gender, age, health condition, hospitalization, and season (6,11,20–22). Except for areas with large numbers of sebaceous glands where propionibacteria prevail, the main portion of the skin flora is made up of Micrococcaceae such as staphylococcal species (*Staphylococcus epidermidis, S. hominis, S. capitis,* etc.) and micrococci. Also, *S. aureus* may temporarily colonize the skin, especially the perineal region, the nose, hands, face, and neck. This occurs more often with children than with adults (3), but healthcare personnel are especially prone to this colonization; the prevalence of colonization with *S. aureus* in healthcare personnel was reported by Larson et al. (23) to reach 18%. In the intensive care unit (ICU) of a German teaching hospital, Hofmann et al. (24) found *S. aureus* on 18.4% of nurses' hands and on 36% of doctors' hands. These data more likely reflect, however, a state of repeated contamination rather than true long-term carriage. Lipophilic and nonlipophilic corynebacteria are common inhabitants of the skin, the former usually in hairy regions, the latter more in bald regions (6). The antibiotic-resistant *Corynebacterium jeikeium* may cause therapeutically difficult nosocomial infections in high-risk patients. Although the most common site of isolation is the perineum (22), it may occur also on the hands. *Propionibacterium acnes* and *P. granulosum,* the latter of which is less often isolated, multiply at sebaceous body sites (11,25). They can, however, also be found in small numbers on the hands, although most likely as transients (9).

Gram-negative bacteria such as *Acinetobacter* and *Enterobacter* species may be isolated mainly from moist skin areas (25–28) but also regularly from the hands, where they may be regarded as residents (29). Larson (30) found that 80% of persons outside the hospital and 21% of hospital personnel persistently carried *Acinetobacter* species and members of the *Klebsiella-Enterobacter* group. Males were significantly more likely to be carriers than females, and persons who washed their hands less than eight times per day were more likely to persistently carry the same gram-negative species than those who washed more than eight times. Well known is the report by Casewell and Phillips (31) of a hospital outbreak with *Klebsiella* colonizing the hands of hospital personnel. Attendants with close patient contact, as in ICUs, were especially likely to carry gram-negative bacteria on their hands (32).

On the hands, the population density of resident skin bacteria ranges somewhere between 10^2 and 10^3 colony-forming units (CFU)/cm^2 (1) and remains remarkably stable for each individual over long periods of time (5,20,33,34). Only diseases of the skin and agents interfering with the biozenosis such as antibiotics or disinfectants may cause long-term alterations (6,14,25,35). The greatest short-term fluctuations (1 to 2 hours) are seen after intense contact with water (36).

The normal microbial skin flora fulfills the important function of colonization resistance, thereby preventing colonization with other and potentially more pathogenic microorganisms. The influencing factors are the presence of free fatty acids liberated from skin lipids by bacterial metabolism, the presence of bacteriocins and other antibiotic-like bacterial secretions, and the low water content of the stratum corneum (3,17,37). The pH value and osmotic conditions are less important (20). Unless introduced into body tissue by trauma or in the presence of foreign bodies such as catheters or implants, the pathogenic potential of the resident flora is usually regarded as low (38,39). Resident flora are difficult to remove by mechanical means. Washing hands with soap and water reduces the release of skin bacteria every 5 minutes by only 50% (5,40–42).

Transient Flora

Members of this group are characterized by their inability to multiply on the skin. They occur as skin contaminants. Among them, microorganisms with a high pathogenic potential may also be found. Usually transient flora does not survive for very long. Besides the above-mentioned factor of colonization resistance, the inhospitable physicochemical environment may be another reason for the failure of transient flora to survive. Medical personnel, however, should never rely on this. In contrast to natural microbial skin flora, transient flora is easily removed by mechanical means such as hand washing. If hands are washed for 1 minute with soap and water, the bacterial release is reduced by two to three orders of magnitude (43–49). Even rubbing hands with water alone is effective (47).

Infectious Flora

This group includes the etiologic agents of actual infections such as abscesses, panaritium, paronychia, and infected eczema on the hands. They are of proven pathogenicity. *S. aureus* and β-hemolytic streptococci are the species most often encountered.

STRATEGIES OF HAND HYGIENE

Strategies for the prevention of hand-associated microbial transfer must take into consideration the fact that it is much easier to reduce the release of transient flora from the hands than that of resident flora, and that, more than ever, infectious lesions must be healed before the hands may be regarded as safe. Therefore, the choice of preventive measures depends on which group of microbial flora is to be attacked. The precautions proposed in Table 96.1 are discussed below.

If microbial contamination is to be expected, the strategy is to *keep* hands clean, because this is much easier to do than to *make* them clean. If used intelligently, both the no-touch technique (use instruments rather than fingers) and protective gloves are suitable remedies against microbial transfer. This implies, of course, that instruments and gloves are changed after every patient. Although it was reported that transient bacteria were washed from gloves more easily than from hands (44) and that used gloves can be successfully cleaned of adhering microorganisms (50,51) and even of hepatitis B virus (HBV) antigen (50) by washing or disinfecting gloved hands for 30 to 120 seconds, this could not be confirmed by Doebbeling et al. (52) under

TABLE 96.1. STRATEGIES FOR THE PREVENTION OF MICROBIAL TRANSFER BY HANDS

Objective Situation	Strategy
To reduce the release of transient flora	Keep hands clean (noncontamination)
Hands are still clean	No-touch technique Gloves (protective)
Hands are contaminated	Render hands clean (elimination of transients)
After contacts without known or suspected "dangerous" contamination (Fulkerson scale 5–7)	Hand wash or Hygienic hand wash or Hygienic hand rub
After known or suspected contacts with patient secretions, excretions, blood, and infected sites (Fulkerson scale 8–15)	Hygienic hand rub
After working in a microbiology laboratory	Hygienic hand rub
To reduce or prevent the release of transient and resident flora	Prevent microbial release
Before surgical activity	Surgical hand disinfection and gloves (surgical)
Before patient care in protective isolation	Hygienic hand wash and gloves (sterile)
Colonization of hands with pathogens	Treat the diseased skin Chemotherapy (?) Antiseptic washings (?)
To avoid transmission of pathogens from infected lesions on the hands	Refrain from activities involving infectious hazard (e.g., surgery, handling foodstuffs and pharmaceuticals)

conditions more appropriate to clinical practice with various treatments of only 10 seconds. The authors recultured the microorganisms used for artificial contamination not only from 4% to 100% of the gloves in counts between 0 and 4.7 log, but also from the hands after removal of gloves. They concluded that it may not be prudent to wash and reuse gloves between patients and that hand washing or disinfection should be strongly encouraged after removal of protective gloves (52).

If hands are known to be or are suspected of being contaminated, the undesired transient microbial flora must be eliminated to render the hands safe for the next patient contact. This may be achieved by washing or disinfecting the hands. If, in contrast to an ordinary hand wash, a postcontamination treatment of hands involves the application of an antimicrobial preparation (detergent or rub), it is termed "hygienic" (hygienic hand wash, hygienic hand rub) in Europe, to indicate that these measures aim only at the contaminating transient flora without consideration of the number and fate of the resident skin flora.

Recently, an excellent guideline was published in the United States that delineates indications and details for hand washing (53). Below, some additional perspectives are considered. The decision to use one of the above measures in a particular situation depends on the probability that hands may have become contaminated by pathogens during a potential or known exposure. The higher this risk, the more important it is to use a postcontamination treatment that is effective and safe. In this context, "effective" means efficiently reducing the release of transients, and "safe" means that the treatment itself should not disseminate pathogens to be eliminated onto other sites. It has indeed been demonstrated that vigorous hand washing can disperse pathogenic microorganisms such as *Salmonella typhi* into the environment and onto the person who is washing (54,55). Because hygienic hand rubs will kill most transients still on the hands, rub-on techniques can avoid microbial dispersal and therefore should be used after all contagious contacts in the microbiology laboratory and in patient care such as those ranked as "very dirty" on the Fulkerson scale (56,57) (Table 96.2) when they involve infected sites (ranks 13 to 15). Often, however, hygienic rubs are used not because of a specific indication but for purely practical reasons, such as availability and the simplicity of their application (36). All other dirty contacts (ranks 8 to 12) may be followed by hand washing with unmedicated soap, but it should be realized that the complete procedure including the journey to and from the wash place makes a very uneconomic use of time because it takes three times as long as a hygienic hand rub with an alcoholic solution delivered from a dispenser next to the patient's bed (58). This may also be one of the reasons for poor compliance of healthcare workers with hand washing. Hygienic hand washes with an antiseptic detergent are designed to rapidly wash off most of the transient flora by their mechanical detergent effect and to exert an additional sustained antimicrobial activity on the remaining hand flora. Usually, the multiplication of the resident flora will be retarded too, so that hygienic hand washes may be useful in areas where microbiologically clean hands are desired during extended periods such as in

TABLE 96.2. FULKERSON SCALE RANKING CONTACTS OF NURSING PERSONNEL FROM CLEAN TO DIRTY

Rank[a]	Contact with
1	Sterile or autoclaved materials
2	Thoroughly cleaned or washed materials
3	Materials not necessarily cleaned but free from patient contact (e.g., papers)
4	Objects contacted by patients either infrequently or not expected to be contaminated (e.g., patient furniture)
5	Objects intimately associated with patients, but not known to be contaminated (e.g., patient gowns, linens, dishes, bedside rails)
6	Patient, but minimal and limited (e.g., shaking hands, taking pulse)
7	Objects in contact with patient secretions
8	Patient secretions or mouth, nose, genitoanal area, etc.
9	Materials contaminated by patient urine
10	Patient urine
11	Materials contaminated with feces
12	Feces
13	Materials contaminated with secretions or excretions from infected sites
14	Secretions or excretions from infected sites
15	Infected patient sites (e.g., wounds, tracheotomy)

[a] "Clean" activities, 1–7; "dirty" activities, 8–15.
From Fox MK, Langner SB, Wells RW. How good are handwashing practices? *Am J Nurs* 1974;74:1676–1678, and Larson E, Lusk E. Evaluating handwashing technique. *J Adv Nurs* 1985;10:547–552, with permission.

protective isolation, in the food and pharmaceutical industries, and in surgery.

In these indications, not only is the role of the hands that of microbial vector, they may act also as an important source of undesired microorganisms multiplying in and being shed from the skin. The strategy to prevent these microflora from reaching sensitive areas such as wounds, foodstuffs, or pharmaceuticals is to reduce the microbial release from the hands. This is best attained by the use of (sterile) gloves. Surgical hand disinfection can greatly reduce the release of transient and resident skin flora and is usually used as an adjunct to surgical gloves in case they become punctured or torn. Scrubbing hands with unmedicated soap alone removes transient flora efficiently but has only a negligible effect on the release of resident skin bacteria (see below). For preoperative preparation of the surgeon's hands, prolonged scrubbing with unmedicated soap is therefore worth neither the effort nor the strain on the skin. Helpful recommendations for surgical hand scrubs have been provided by the Association of Operating Room Nurses (AORN) (59).

Antiseptic hand washing may also be used therapeutically to clear carriers of pathogenic resident flora (60). Hands with infected purulent lesions are very dangerous sources of microbial flora with proven pathogenicity. Therefore, the only effective strategy is to prohibit any activity involving infectious risks such as engaging in surgery and other types of patient care or handling foodstuffs and pharmaceuticals.

METHODS OF ELIMINATING MICROORGANISMS FROM THE HANDS

Mechanical and chemical methods for the reduction of microbial release from the hands are summarized in the following subsections.

Hand Washing

Whereas in German-speaking countries this term is exclusively reserved for the use of unmedicated soap and water (with or without a brush), in other parts of the world it also implies the application of antiseptic soaps (disinfectants-detergents). In this chapter, the term is applied *sensu strictu* to washing hands with unmedicated detergent and water.

The objective of hand washing is to remove dirt (consisting of extraneous substances, sweat, skin lipids, epithelial debris, etc.) and loosely adhering microbial skin flora, which will include most of the transient but only a small part of the resident flora. In fields of application where the microbiologic aspect dominates, the aim, of course, is to reduce microbial release from hands to an extent that may be considered safe for the intended purpose. In the medical field, this purpose is usually to prevent hand-borne infection.

The efficacy of a hand wash depends on the time taken and the technique. Unfortunately, this period is usually rather (too?) short in normal hospital work. The average duration was reported by several authors to be between 8 and 20 seconds (23, 61). This period of time, however, does not include the additional time needed to approach and return from the wash place. Therefore, the complete process takes much longer. In fact, it has been measured to take 40 to 80 seconds (58). Table 96.3 indicates how effectively the release of transient bacteria from artificially contaminated hands can be reduced by hand washing. The greatest reduction is achieved within the first 30 seconds; it ranges between 0.6 and 1.1 log after 15 seconds and 1.8 and 2.8 log at the end of 30 seconds. Extending the washing time to 1 minute results in reductions of 2.7 to 3.0 log. A further prolongation of the procedure is not worth the effort, because after 2 minutes the reduction increases negligibly to only 3.3 log and after 4 minutes to only 3.7 log.

Although in most instances these reductions are probably sufficient to prevent infection-generating transmission of pathogens (46,48,62–65), this is not always the case. Semmelweis, for instance, observed that normal hand washing did not always prevent the spread of fatal infection. Eleven parturient women died of puerperal fever after having been examined immediately after contact with a patient suffering from a foully discharging medullary carcinoma (66) by attendants who in between had washed their hands only with soap and water. After this experience, Semmelweis extended his order to disinfect hands in a solution of chlorinated lime, from before entering the delivery or patient room, to use of the solution before each vaginal examination (66–69). It is important to understand that some procedures of hand disinfection are significantly more efficient in reducing bacterial release from hands than hand washing.

Although highly sophisticated wash places with fully automated functions have been shown to be counterproductive rather than motivating healthcare personnel to adhere to hand washing rules (70), certain requirements for wash places must be fulfilled for minimal compliance. Wash basins should be conveniently located; no overflow or plug is necessary because hands should be washed only under running water. A mixer tap helps to provide water of comfortable temperature that, under the best conditions, is controlled thermostatically. Operation of the water flow without using the hands (elbow, knee, foot, automatic) may be desirable in certain critical areas. Suitable dispensers for soap, disinfectant (rub is better than detergent), hand lotion, and one-way towels are accepted requirements. There must also be a container for used towels. If liquid soap is used, dispensers must either be easily removable and heat resistant for thermal reprocessing or they should be disposable containers. Liquid soap dispensed from refillable containers should be bacte-

TABLE 96.3. REDUCTION OF THE RELEASE OF TEST BACTERIA FROM ARTIFICIALLY CONTAMINATED HANDS BY WASHING WITH SOAP AND WATER

Duration	Mean Log_{10} Reduction	Reference
15 s	0.6–1.1	62
30 s	1.8	45, 63
	2.3–2.5	48
	2.5–2.8	43, 44
1 min	2.7	49
	3.0	47, 64
2 min	3.3	47
4 min	3.7	47

riostatic to prevent microbial growth; topping off these containers should be strictly prohibited.

An appropriate hand washing technique includes adjusting the water flow and the temperature (both activities can be accelerated by suitable technical devices), wetting hands, taking soap, rubbing hands to produce a lather without splashing, and performing wash movements that include rubbing palm to palm, right palm over left dorsum and vice versa, palm to palm with fingers interlaced, backs of fingers to opposing palm with fingers interlocked, rotational rubbing of right thumb clasped in left palm and vice versa, rotational rubbing with clasped fingers of right hand in palm of left hand and with changed roles. This technique was proposed by Ayliffe et al. (71) as a standard technique when testing antiseptic hand washes. It could, however, represent a routine hand wash technique for every day. Finally, hands are rinsed with fingertips up, and the water is cautiously shaken off. This procedure should take not less than 30 seconds, a goal difficult to attain. The subungual spaces harbor by far the main part of the bacterial hand flora (72). The importance of this observation for the transmission of nosocomial infections by medical personnel is unknown, however. After washing, the hands are dried with a disposable towel (paper or textile). Unless the water is turned off by an automatic device, the water should be turned off using the disposable towel rather than by the freshly washed hands (73). The towel is discarded in the appropriate container and hand lotion is applied to the hands. This latter step is extremely important to prevent chapping. Electric hand dryers are useless in hospitals, because hand drying takes too long with them, and because they lack the friction of towels to remove remaining soap from the skin.

No matter how well and detailed hand washing techniques may be described, Larson and Kretzer (74) are probably right in suggesting that of much greater concern is how to motivate personnel to wash their hands in the first place, because hand washing practices still remain suboptimal.

Hygienic Hand Rub

The objective of the hygienic hand rub is to reduce the release of transient pathogens with maximum efficacy and speed, so that hands can be rendered safe after known or suspected contamination. This should be done in a way that avoids microbial dispersal into the environment. A sustained effect is not required. The fate of the resident skin flora is disregarded in this procedure.

The technique of hygienic hand rubs includes rubbing small portions (3 to 5 mL) of a fast-acting antiseptic preparation onto both hands. This can be a very convenient way of treating hands after known or suspected contamination, because dispensers for hand rubs can easily be made available wherever necessary; for instance, they may be placed in the vicinity of every patient bed in high-risk areas. All areas of the hands must be covered by the disinfectant, but this is often not done (61).

The antimicrobial spectrum necessary for hygienic hand rubs depends on the intended use. Commonly, the antimicrobial spectrum required includes bacterial and fungal pathogens. There is no need for sporicidal activity in hand disinfectants. An activity against mycobacteria is required only at certain places such as in tuberculosis hospitals, wards for acquired immunodeficiency syndrome patients, and pathology and microbiology laboratories. The antituberculous effect must be proven and stated on the label. The same is true for virucidal activity. A general claim for virucidal activity is justified only if the antiviral spectrum also includes enteroviruses such as polio or hepatitis A virus after a reasonable exposure time.

Possible agents for hand rubs are highly concentrated alcohols, used alone or mixed with other antiseptics; aqueous solutions containing halogens such as chlorine or iodine; chlorhexidine; quaternary ammonium compounds; phenolics; triclosan; aldehydes; metallo-organic compounds; and oxidizing agents such as peracetic acid. Except for the alcohols and the aqueous solutions of chlorine, povidone-iodine, and chlorhexidine, the other agents are used as adjuncts to alcohols (quaternary ammonium and ampholytic compounds, phenolics), are contained in antiseptic detergents (phenol derivatives, triclosan), or are not used at all because of poor efficacy, allergenicity, irritant or toxic potential or ecologic considerations (aldehydes, metallo-organic and oxidizing agents). There is no doubt that alcohols are much more comfortable to rub onto the skin than aqueous solutions because of specific features such as excellent spreading and quick evaporation.

Table 96.4 summarizes results on general antibacterial efficacy, which was assessed in tests simulating practical conditions on artificially contaminated hands of volunteers (75–88). As demonstrated, the alcohols *n*-propanol, isopropanol, and ethanol, and the halogens sodium tosylchloramide and povidone-iodine appear superior to aqueous solutions of chlorhexidine diacetate, chlorocresol, and hydrogen peroxide. Within the results of the alcohols, there is a clear positive association between the extent of bacterial reduction and the concentration used. If the mean log reductions obtained with the three alcohols are compared with each other at equal concentrations, *n*-propanol is the most and ethanol the least effective alcohol. The efficacy of aqueous solutions of sodium tosylchloramide and povidone-iodine compares well with that of isopropanol at a concentration of 60% v/v.

Tuberculocidal activity has been demonstrated for the alcohols mentioned (89–94), although with prolonged exposure (90). Several recommendations suggest disinfection times of 1 to 5 minutes with 70% ethanol, 60% to 70% isopropanol, or 50% to 70% *n*-propanol (88,95). The halogen-based preparations are also regarded as active (54,95).

The virucidal activity of alcohols is generally good with enveloped viruses (96,97) with the exception of rabies, which is reported to be ethanol resistant (98); it is effective against human immunodeficiency virus (HIV) (75). Naked viruses, such as enteroviruses, are inactivated by high concentrations of alcohols (99); the most effective of which is reported to be ethanol (97, 100). *In vivo* tests have shown that the effectiveness of alcohols against some difficult viruses such as entero- and rotavirus is significantly better than that of hand washing with unmedicated soap (100–104). Absolute ethanol reduced, for instance, the viral release from the hands by 3.2 log, 80% ethanol (v/v) by 2.2 log, and absolute *n*-propanol by 2.4 log (101). In contrast, individual hand washing for 10 to 55 seconds caused a reduction of only 1 log.

TABLE 96.4. HYGIENIC HAND RUB: EFFICACY OF VARIOUS AGENTS IN REDUCING THE RELEASE OF TEST BACTERIA FROM ARTIFICIALLY CONTAMINATED HANDS

			Mean Log Reduction Exposure Time (min)			
Agent	**Concentration[a](%)**	**Test Bacterium**	**0.5**	**1.0**	**2.0**	**Reference**
n-Propanol	100	*E. coli*		5.8		76
	60			5.5		77
	50			5.0		77, 78
			3.7	4.7	4.9	77
	40			4.3		77
Isopropanol	70	*E. coli*		4.9		77
				4.8		80
			3.5			71
	60			4.4		78
				4.3		80, 81
				4.2		82
				4.0		83
		S. marcescens		4.1		84
	50	*E. coli*	3.4	3.9	4.4	77
Ethanol	80	*E. coli*		4.5		77
	70			4.3	5.1	85
				4.3	4.9	47
				4.0		78
			3.6	3.8	4.5	77
			3.4	4.1		48
		S. aureus	3.7			48
			2.6			86
		S. saprophyticus	3.5			48
	60	*E. coli*		3.8		77
Tosylchloramide (aq. sol.)	2.0[b]	*E. coli*		4.2		75
Povidone-iodine (aq. sol.)	1.0[b]	*E. coli*		4.0–4.3		79
Chlorhexidine diacetate (aq. sol.)	0.5[b]	*E. coli*		3.1		44
Chloro-cresol (aq. sol.)	1.0[b]	*E. coli*		3.6		9, 87
Hydrogen peroxide	7.5	*E. coli*		3.6		88

[a] If not stated otherwise, v/v.
[b] w/v.
From Rotter ML, Kramer A. Hygienische Händeantiseptik. In: Kramer A, Gröschel D, Heeg P, et al., eds. *Klinische Antiseptik*. Berlin, Heidelberg, New York: Springer-Verlag, 1993:67–82, with permission (75).

Schürmann and Eggers (99) concluded that the commercial high-alcohol content preparation tested by them was effective against enteroviruses only under favorable environmental conditions (high temperature, large disinfectant-to-virus volume ratio, low protein load). The reduction in the release of human rotavirus strains from the hands by 70% ethanol (v/v) or 70% isopropanol (v/v) was approximately 100 times that of the reduction attainable by tap water or liquid soap (102). A reduction of >3 log by a 60% ethanol preparation was demonstrated *in vivo* with the nonenveloped rota-, adeno-, and rhinoviruses (103).

For years, the HBV was thought to be extremely resistant to the action of chemical disinfectants. Dried or liquid human plasma containing high-titer HBV, however, did not cause hepatitis if the sera were treated before inoculation into susceptible chimpanzees with 70% isopropanol for 10 minutes, 80% ethanol for 2 minutes, 0.1% glutaraldehyde for 5 minutes, povidone-iodine with 0.8% available iodine for 10 minutes, or hypochlorite solution with 500 mg/L free chlorine for 10 minutes, whereas the control animals receiving untreated plasma developed the disease (105,106). In another test system, the so-called morphology alteration and disintegration test, the HBV appeared significantly altered and disintegrated after exposure to 82% ethanol (107). In combination with agents such as hexachlorophene, quaternary ammonium compounds, octenidine, biphenylol, or hydrogen peroxide, ethanol was reported active against HBV at a concentration as low as 70% (106–110).

Hepatitis C virus (HCV) is likely to be inactivated by concentrations of 60% to 70% ethanol (111).

As is evident from the above, alcoholic rubs are very well suited for hygienic hand disinfection, because their antimicrobial performance is excellent and fast, thus saving time; no wash basin is necessary for their use and they can be positioned next to every patient bed; and their application does not cause microbial contamination of nurses' uniforms. However, one must bear in mind that the antimicrobial efficacy of alcohols is very sensitive to dilution with water and is therefore vulnerable to inactivation, especially with the small volumes (3 to 6 mL) distributed over both hands for hygienic hand rubs. If, for instance, 60% (v/v) isopropanol were rubbed onto wet hands in two portions of 3 mL, each for 30 seconds, the mean log bacterial reduction achieved would be 3.7, as opposed to 4.3 with dry hands (112, 113). Although it is not as comfortable to apply, an aqueous solution of povidone-iodine may be used as an alternative hand rub, if necessary, for any reason.

Recently, there is a trend toward gel formulations, mainly in North America. Comparative tests between liquid and gel formulations of alcoholic hand rubs revealed, however, that the bactericidal efficacy of gels is significantly lower than that of the rinses. Kramer et al. (114) compared the efficacy of ten commercial gels and four rinses using the method of the European standard EN 1500. No single gel met the requirements within 30 seconds of application, whereas all rinses did. This correlates with the experience of the Vienna group that tested five other gels with the same results. From a recent report by Kampf et al. (115), it appears, however, that gels with a very high alcohol content can meet the requirement of EN 1500. A new gel containing 85% (by weight) ethanol proved to be bactericidal in suspension (when tested according to prEN 12054) and on volunteers' hands (EN 1500); furthermore, in suspension tests the gel was shown to be fungicidal (EN 1275), tuberculocidal (test according to the German Society of Hygiene and Microbiology with *Mycobacterium terrae* as a surrogate mycobacterium for *M. tuberculosis*), and virucidal, defined as a 4 log reduction, within different exposure times with orthopox and herpes simplex 1 and 2 viruses (15 seconds), rotavirus and HIV (30 seconds), and adeno- (2 minutes), polio- (3 minutes) and papova-virus (15 minutes). Despite the high alcohol concentration, the user acceptability was described as excellent. Together with the ease of performing a hygienic hand disinfection, this offers a chance to improve the compliance of medical personnel with hand hygiene.

Hygienic Hand Wash

The objective of the hygienic hand wash is to reduce the release of transient flora by a washing procedure of significantly stronger efficacy than that of an ordinary hand wash with unmedicated soap. Even if the effect on the resident flora is usually disregarded in most indications, a residual effect may be desirable in some areas, such as in protective isolation, during hospital outbreaks (60,71), and for handling foodstuffs. The technique is similar to that of the normal hand wash, but is performed according to the instructions of the manufacturer. As with the hygienic hand rub, the antimicrobial spectrum required depends on the area of intended use. But, in general, an antituberculous or antiviral activity is not necessarily expected from these antiseptics.

Agents most often used today are detergent preparations containing iodophors, chlorhexidine gluconate, triclosan, biphenylol, and chloroxylenol. Hexachlorophene should not be used anymore because of transdermal absorption (116,117), neurotoxic activity (116,118,119), and its poor activity against gram-negative bacteria (44,47,120). Amphotensides and quaternary ammonium compounds are more suited to being used as adjuncts to alcohols than to being used on their own, because they are easily neutralized by anionic detergents and—at least for the quaternary ammonium compounds—by protein.

Table 96.5 summarizes results on general antibacterial efficacy as assessed by the test method of the European standard EN 1499 (83,121). It can be seen that of five antiseptic detergents tested, only povidone-iodine liquid soap would have met the pass criterion. Chlorhexidine gluconate detergent was better

TABLE 96.5. HYGIENIC HAND WASH: EFFICACY OF VARIOUS ANTISEPTIC DETERGENTS IN REDUCING THE RELEASE OF TEST BACTERIA FROM ARTIFICIALLY CONTAMINATED HANDS

Detergent	Concentration (%)	Mean Log Reduction
Povidone-iodine	0.75[a]	3.5[b]
Chlorhexidine gluconate	4.0[a]	3.1
Triclosan	0.1[c]	2.8
2-Biphenylol	2.0[c]	2.6
Octenidine	0.5[c]	2.5
Soft soap	20.0[a]	2.7

Duration of treatment: 1 min.
[a] w/v.
[b] Significantly better than soft soap.
[c] w/w.
From Rotter ML, Koller W. A European test for the evaluation of the efficacy of procedures of the antiseptic handwash. *Hyg Med* 1991;16:4–12, with permission.

than soft soap, although not quite significantly, in this test (83). It is important to note that the hygienic hand rub with 60% isopropanol, tested as a control in the same experiment, caused a significantly stronger bacterial reduction (4.0 log) than any of the hand washes (83). These results compare well with those of Ayliffe et al. (71), who found that alcoholic preparations, particularly *n*-propanol and isopropanol, were the most effective, followed by chlorhexidine and povidone-iodine detergent preparations, all of which were significantly more effective than nonmedicated soap. However, triclosan-containing soaps were no more effective than nonmedicated soap. In these experiments, the chlorhexidine detergent was found to be significantly more effective than the povidone-iodine preparation.

These results demonstrate clearly that compared with other methods of postcontamination hand treatment, alcoholic hand rubs are, at present, the most effective measure to quickly reduce the release of transient flora from the hands. Consequently, it may be inferred that alcohol-treated hands are less likely to transfer bacteria than washed hands. Indeed, this has been shown by Ehrenkranz and Alfonso (122), who demonstrated that after contact with heavily colonized patient groins, hand washing failed to prevent the transfer of aerobic gram-negative bacilli by healthcare workers' hands to urinary catheters in 11 of 12 experiments; after hand treatment with 70% (v/v) isopropanol, bacteria were transferred in only two of 12 experiments. Furthermore, soap failed to stop subsequent colonization in each of the 12 experiments, whereas alcohol failed in only five. The authors concluded that soap was generally ineffective in preventing hand transfer of gram-negative bacilli to catheters after contact with a heavy contamination source, whereas alcohol was generally effective.

In another clinical trial it was shown that measures of hand hygiene prior to the insertion of peripheral venous catheters significantly influenced the relative risk of infectious complications, in that local reddening, swelling, pain, purulence, or fever of unknown origin occurred only in 51% or 61% when gloves were worn or hands were rubbed with an alcoholic rinse, respectively, as compared to no measure of hand hygiene or washing hands with plain soap (123).

Unfortunately, definitions for requirements of the effectiveness of procedures for both hand rub and hand wash can hardly be based on sound epidemiologic data. Besides Semmelweis's experience that soap and water was not sufficient for some situations (66,68), only a few, more or less well-controlled field trials relate the use of certain hand washing procedures to the infection rate (124–128). Even if one or another detail in these studies may be criticized, they all indicate that the use of disinfectants results in reduced infection rates as compared with the use of unmedicated soap or with no hand washing. If this is translated into terms of disinfectant testing, which is easier to do (71,113), one might be tempted to speculate that disinfectant-detergents, exerting an antimicrobial effect similar to that of chlorhexidine detergent or better, may have the potential to reduce the rate of hospital infections more efficiently than ordinary soap. Indeed, the European Committee for Standardization has decided that as a pass criterion for hygienic hand washes, the bacterial reduction assessed in a test simulating practical conditions shall be significantly greater than that obtained with unmedicated soap. This shall be tested in parallel with the same volunteers, on the same day and in a crossover design as a reference (121).

For hygienic hand rubs, few clinical correlates to results from disinfectant testing exist. In one controlled study trying to relate the use of alcoholic rubs to infection rates (127), isopropanol was used in a way that cannot be regarded as a real hygienic hand rub, namely with average volumes of 0.9 mL, which is much too small to cover both hands and to remain there long enough to exert bactericidal effects, and after visible contamination, as an adjunct to a preceding hand wash, therefore acting, if at all, on wet or moist hands. The study demonstrates, however, that the hygienic hand wash with chlorhexidine detergent, which was also tested, is clinically more effective than an individual hand wash with soap (followed by rubbing a bit of alcohol into the hands) and that despite a preceding intensive education program, it seems very difficult to persuade and motivate medical personnel to obey the simplest rules for the most efficient procedure in the prevention of hospital-acquired infections. Because hand rubs have a high antimicrobial potential, they can also be used in situations where direct contact with dangerous pathogens has occurred, such as after spillage in a microbiology laboratory or after touching infectious lesions. A high-level requirement, therefore, is justified. With this perspective, a requirement was formulated by the Austrian and German Microbiological Societies and finally by the European Committee for Standardization, choosing among the best-acting rubs available. From these, 60% isopropanol (v/v) was taken, arbitrarily, as an agent to be used in two portions of 3 mL each, during a total disinfection period of 60 seconds, for a reference hand rub. The reduction of transient flora assessed with a hand rub shall not be significantly smaller than that with the reference rub tested in parallel with the same volunteers, on the same day, and in a crossover fashion (128–130).

However, as Larson (73) stressed a decade ago, even the most effective procedure for removal of transient microbial flora from the hands is futile, if it is not carried out by healthcare personnel. Thus, compliance with the rules of hand hygiene is equally important for preventing the transmission of pathogens via hands and consequently the emergence of nosocomial infections. By changing behavioral patterns of the staff and by creating an organizational climate, in which hand hygiene was a definite goal, Larson et al. (131) succeeded, as a positive example, to reduce the incidence of infections due to methicillin-resistant *S. aureus* (MRSA) and vancomycin-resistant enterococci (VRE) by considerably improving compliance to hand hygiene in two critical-care units of the intervention hospital as compared with the situation in comparable units of a control hospital.

In a similar attempt to promote hand hygiene by implementing a program with emphasis on alcohol-based hand rubs, Pittet et al. (132) improved the compliance of the staff from 48% to 66% within 3 years. As a consequence, the overall ratio of nosocomial infections decreased from 16.9% to 9.9%. Also the transmission frequency of MRSA decreased from 2.16 to 0.93 episodes per 10,000 patient days.

To understand motives and attitudes and to identify reasons for poor compliance, studies have been carried out since the early 1980s. They were recently summarized by Pittet and Boyce (133). An analysis of their own data by Pittet et al. (134) revealed that although varying greatly, the average compliance was found to range below 50%. Doctors were less compliant than nurses and the following risk factors for poor compliance were found: being a doctor [odds ration (OR) 2.8 vs. nurse] or a nursing assistant (OR 1.3 vs. nurse), working during the week (OR 1.7 vs. weekend), activities with high-risk of cross-contamination (OR 1.8 vs. low risk), working in ICU (OR 2.0 vs. internal medicine units), and high intensity of patient care (OR up to 2.1 vs. low intensity).

Surgical Hand Disinfection

The objective of surgical hand disinfection is to reduce the release of skin bacteria from the hands of the surgical team for the duration of an operation in case the surgical glove is punctured or torn. The intention is thus to bring down the bioburden of glove juice as low as possible to keep the infectious inoculum in the surgical site below the threshold for induction of infection. This varies, however, and is unknown in the individual case, because it depends not only on the kind and virulence of bacteria entering the surgical site but also on the effectiveness of the host's defense mechanisms. These mechanisms, however, can be impaired by circumstances determined by the type of surgery (such as implantation of foreign bodies), by the need to operate on some patients with immunodeficiency, and by a failure to remove all necrotic tissue.

Although at least one outbreak of surgical site infections was reported when an antiseptic scrub was replaced by a nonantimicrobial soap (135), in contrast to hygienic hand disinfection, rub or wash, surgical hand disinfection has never been proved to be necessary or clinically effective, in a controlled study. Nevertheless, it is justified, because it is an integral part of the concept of aseptic surgery, the value of which can be regarded as having been proved by Lister's findings. Indeed, indirect evidence for the necessity of a precaution in addition to the surgical glove can be drawn from results compiled by Cruse and Foord (136), who reported for clean surgical sites an infection rate of 1.7% if gloves remained intact but of 5.7% for operations where holes were noted in gloves. To keep the bacterial load low on the skin beneath the glove therefore is an important goal. Because latex gloves are vulnerable, they cannot be relied on. Hoborn (137) reported in a study on glove perforations that 38% of all gloves used by the surgical team in orthopedic surgery were perforated. The following details are of interest: left-hand gloves were more often perforated (47%) than right-hand gloves (29%). The surgeons' gloves were most often damaged (53%), followed by those of the operating nurse (41%) and the assistant (19%). The index finger of the left hand was the most endangered site (29%), followed by the palm (24%). The left index finger was involved in 43% of all specifically surgeon-associated perforations. In soft tissue surgery, glove punctures were found at a significantly lower frequency. The overall ratio was 16%; left-hand gloves were involved in 22% and right-hand ones in 11%. The sequence of persons was the same as above: surgeon, 28%; operating nurse, 16%; assistant, 4%. These data confirm those reported earlier by Furuhashi and Miyamae (138). A later study by Palmer and Rickett (139) arrived at similar conclusions.

The bacterial leakage through pinholes in gloves has been found experimentally to range between 10^3 and 10^4 CFU (137, 138). In contrast, when the hands were disinfected before donning gloves, the bacterial counts from the leaking gloves did not exceed 100 CFU (138). In fact, clinical indications show a causal link between hand preparation of the surgical team and the incidence of surgical site infections (135).

Although the aim of surgical hand disinfection is to render hands microbiologically clean with as little microbial release as possible, the antimicrobial spectrum need not include tuberculocidal, fungicidal, or virucidal activity, because pathogens belonging to these groups of microorganisms do not usually cause surgical site infections. However, agents for surgical hand disinfection must be active against the resident flora and bacteria associated with surgical site infection.

With regard to antimicrobial effects, an immediate effect must be distinguished from sustained, cumulative, and persistent effects (140), the occurrence of which depends on the frequency of contacts with the antiseptic, as follows:

- After a single contact, the *sustained effect* is defined as short-term antimicrobial activity, further reducing or maintaining the bacterial count under the glove.
- After multiple contacts, the *cumulative effect* is a microbial reduction that increases with every application of the antiseptic.
- With regular contact, the *persistent effect* is the progressive reduction of skin flora.

Because the surgeon's hands should be safe at the time of the first operation after the weekend or after a vacation, neither cumulative nor persistent effects are really advantageous. Furthermore, in the interest of colonization resistance, it would not be desirable to completely eliminate the resident skin flora by multiple or regular use of a highly active antiseptic. Admittedly, to attain this would be very difficult. In contrast, a sustained effect may be desirable to keep the bacterial numbers low under the glove during an operation, especially if preparations with only moderate immediate effect are used for surgical disinfection. Because most operations are completed within 3 hours and because during long-lasting operations gloves will be changed, 3 hours may be a reasonable time span to check on this feature in disinfectant testing. To test every hour up to 6 hours as proposed in a guideline of the U.S. Food and Drug Administration (141) may not be necessary.

Because the technique of surgical hand disinfection is of considerable influence on the release of skin flora, it is described here in detail. Useful guidelines for the surgical hand scrub have also been published by AORN (59). On entering the operating suite, hands should first be treated as if contaminated and transients removed with a social hand wash or, preferably, with an alcoholic hand rub. Then, the subungual spaces should be cleaned with soft wooden sticks because most bacterial flora resides under the nails (72). Long-lasting wash procedures with unmedicated soap and scrubbing are counterproductive, because they cause skin damage without significantly reducing the release of resident skin bacteria (5,41,42,79). In fact, a preceding treatment with soap may even hamper the effect of an alcohol treatment (142–144). For this reason, clean hands should not be washed before applying an alcohol rub. A (soft) brush should be used only to brush the nails and subungual spaces but not the skin because skin damage may result. Sterile disposable sponges may also be used. Fingertips should always point upward, with elbows down, to avoid recontamination of clean fingers and hands by water running down from contaminated proximal areas. If hands were (pre)washed, drying them is of great importance if an alcohol rub is to be used subsequently, to avoid its dilution. In this case, the towels, paper or textile, need not be sterile but only clean.

There are two principal techniques of surgical hand disinfection, both of which have advantages and drawbacks. If performed with a suitable antiseptic, the *surgical hand rub* is very efficient in reducing the skin flora and hands need not be dried afterward. It lacks, however, the cleaning function provided by a surgical hand wash. This, in turn, requires hand drying and is less efficient.

Surgical hand rubs are performed by pouring small volumes of a suitable antiseptic, usually an alcohol preparation, into the cupped dry hands, rubbing it onto the entire surface of hands and forearms, keeping them wet for the scheduled time by adding further portions as necessary, and carrying out wash movements. Usually, 15 to 25 mL is needed for a 5-minute period. All other techniques, such as bathing hands in a bowl with an antiseptic solution, either are wasteful and create an increased risk of skin damage and fire hazard or their antimicrobial effect is poor, as with alcohol wipes and sprays. In contrast, brushing an alcoholic preparation into the subungual spaces increases the effect considerably (143). Alcohol-wet hands should not be gloved but air-dried before donning gloves to avoid skin damage. During and between operations, surgical rubs can easily be performed after removal of gloves.

Surgical hand washes are performed with antiseptic detergents according to the instructions of the manufacturer. Drying hands with sterile towels or drapes is usually necessary before donning surgical gloves.

A combined two-phase technique that includes a surgical hand wash followed by a surgical hand rub may also be used. If the antimicrobial agents are properly chosen, hands may be cleaned with an antiseptic detergent without reducing the antimicrobial efficacy of the subsequent hand rub, as is the case when an alcohol rub immediately follows a hand wash with unmedicated soap (144,145). A hand rub should never be followed by a hand wash, because this has been shown to considerably lessen the effect of the rub (146).

The duration of any preoperative treatment of the surgical team's hands should be kept as short as possible but as long as necessary to attain the goal of a low bacterial load in the glove. From the literature and from results of our own experiments (147), it can be shown that the antimicrobial effectiveness of both surgical hand rub and hand wash is significantly associated with the duration of the procedure (Tables 96.6 and 96.7). Times of 3 to 5 minutes are common today for preoperative hand treatment.

There is only a limited list of possible agents that can be used for the surgical hand rub. An indication of their antimicrobial efficacy is shown in Table 96.6, in which results obtained by comparable test methods are compiled from the literature. A clear association of the bacterial reduction with the nature and the concentration of the antiseptic and with the application time can be seen (41,42,46,79,80,82,138,145,147–155). Similar data have been produced also by more recent studies (156,157). As with the hygienic hand rub, *n*-propanol is the most active of the agents listed, followed by isopropanol, ethanol, povidone-iodine solution, and peracetic acid. An aqueous solution of chlorhexidine gluconate alone exerts only a mediocre immediate effect but is the only agent listed with a definite sustained activity. In combination with alcohol (ethanol 61% w/w, in this case), however, the results are considerably more favorable (156,157), although in one study (157) the magnitude of an immediate reduction of 2.5 log within approximately 2.0 to 2.5 minutes raises the suspicion of incomplete neutralization of chlorhexidine

TABLE 96.6. SURGICAL HAND RUB: EFFICACY OF VARIOUS RUBS IN REDUCING THE RELEASE OF RESIDENT SKIN FLORA FROM CLEAN HANDS

Rub	Concentration[a] (%)	Time (min)	Mean Log Reduction		Reference
			Immediate	Sustained (3 hr)	
n-Propanol	60	5	2.9[b]	1.6[b]	79
		5	2.7[b]	NA	41
		5	2.5[b]	1.8[b]	145
		5	2.3[b]	1.6[b]	147
		3	2.9[c]	NA	149
		3	2.0[b]	1.0[b]	147
		1	1.1[b]	0.5[b]	147
Isopropanol	90	3	2.4[c]	1.4[c]	148
	80	3	2.3[c]	1.2[c]	148
	70	5	2.4[b]	2.1[b]	150
		5	2.1[b]	1.0[b]	147
		3	2.0[c]	0.7[c]	148
		3	1.7[c]	NA	149
		3	1.5[b]	0.8[b]	147
		2	1.2	0.8	151
		1	0.7[b]	0.2	147
		1	0.8	NA	152
	60	5	1.7	1.0	80,150
Isopropanol + chlorhexidine gluc. (w/v)	70 + 0.5	5	2.5[b]	2.7[b]	150
		2	1.0	1.5	151
Ethanol	95	2	2.1	NA	153
	85	3	2.4[c]	NA	149
	80	2	1.5	NA	154
	70	2	1.0	0.6	151
	61 (w/w)	approx. 2–2.5	1.1	1.4	157
Ethanol + chlorhexidine gluc. (w/v)	95 + 0.5	2	1.7	NA	46
	77 + 0.5	5	2.0	1.5[d]	42
	70 + 0.5	2	0.7	1.4	151
		1.0	0,9	NA	156
	61 (w/w)	approx. 2–2.5	2.5	2.9	157
Chlorhexidine gluc. (aq. sol., w/v)	0.5	2	0.4	1.2	151
Povidone-iodine (aq. sol., w/v)	1.0	5	1.9[b]	0.8[b]	82
Peracetic acid (w/v)	0.5	5	1.9	NA	155

NA, not available.
[a] v/v unless otherwise stated.
[b] Tested according to Deutsche Gesellschaft für Hygiene, und Mikrobiologie (DGHM)-German Society of Hygiene and Microbiology method (129).
[c] Tested according to European Standard prEN 12791.
[d] After 4 hours.
From Rotter M. Chirurgische Händedesinfektion. In, Kramer A, Gröschel D, Heeg P, et al., eds. *Klinische Antiseptik*. Berlin, Springer-Verlag, 1993:67–82, with permission (158).

TABLE 96.7. SURGICAL HAND WASH: EFFICACY OF VARIOUS (ANTISEPTIC) DETERGENTS IN REDUCING THE RELEASE OF RESIDENT SKIN FLORA FROM CLEAN HANDS

			Mean Log Reduction		
Detergent	Concentration[a] (%)	Time (min)	Immediate	Sustained (3 hr)	References
Unmedicated		5	0.4[b]	−0.1[b]	79
		5	0.4[b]	NA	41
		5	0.4	0.0[c]	42
Povidone-iodine	0.8	5	1.1	0.3[c]	42
		5	1.0	NA	41
		5	1.0[b]	0.2[b]	82
		5	0.9[b]	0.2[b]	80
		2	0.5	NA	159
Chlorhexidine gluconate	4.0	6	1.2	NA	138
		5	0.9[b]	0.9[b]	79
		5	0.9	0.6	42
		3	1.2[d]	1.4	160
		3	0.9[d]	NA	149
		3	0.8[b]	1.0[b]	79
		3	0.8[b]	0.8[b]	80
		3	0.8	NA	156
		3	1.6	1.8	157
		2	0.9	1.6	161
		5	1.6	2.0	162
Hexachlorophene	3.0	4	0.3	1.0	140
Benzethonium chloride	10.0	6	1.3	NA	138
		3	0.9	NA	138
Zephirol	0.1	2	0.4	NA	154
		2	0.3	NA	159
Cetrimide	1.0	2	0.4	NA	159
Chloro-cresol	0.3	2	0.4	NA	159
Triclosan	1.0	5	0.6	0.5[c]	42
	2.0	5	0.8	1.1	162

NA, not available.
[a] w/v.
[b] Tested according to DGHM method (129).
[c] After 4 hours.
[d] Tested according to European Standard prEN 12791.
From Rotter M. Chirurgische Händedesinfektion. In, Kramer A, Gröschel D, Heeg P, et al., eds. *Klinische Antiseptik*. Berlin, Springer-Verlag, 1993:67–82, with permission (158).

gluconate (Table 96.6). The immediate effect of an aqueous povidone-iodine solution compares well with that of 60% isopropanol (v/v). Peracetic acid must be disregarded for toxicologic reasons.

As with products for the hygienic hand disinfection, the incorporation of antimicrobial agents into gels is a new trend. And indeed, one gel containing 85% (w/w) ethanol was found to pass the strict requirement of prEN 12791, the European norm for testing products for surgical hand disinfection (Kampf et al., 2003, submitted).

The efficacy of frequently used antiseptic detergents is shown in Table 96.7 and compared with that of unmedicated soap (41, 42,79,80,82,138,140,149,154,159–162). Here again, the association between bacterial reduction and duration of hand wash can be seen, although it is not as strong as that seen with the rubs. Unmedicated soap, used for 5 minutes, has only a poor immediate and no sustained effect, whereas povidone-iodine liquid soap causes a significantly stronger immediate reduction but also without noticeable sustained action. A chlorhexidine gluconate (4%) detergent was found, to be as active as the former immediately after disinfection, but, in addition, demonstrated prolonged activity.

In one of the more recent studies mentioned above (157), an initial (first day) preoperative scrub resulted in an unusually high immediate bacterial reduction of 1.6 log and a first-day 3-hour value of 1.8 log raising the suspicion of an incomplete neutralization (Table 96.7).

For toxicologic reasons hexachlorophene should no longer be used for surgical hand wash. In contrast to the immediate effect, which is the same as that of unmedicated soap, it possesses strong sustained activity. Quaternary ammonium compounds such as benzethonium chloride, benzalkonium chloride, and cetrimide all have similar activity. They are not used alone anymore but, like chlorhexidine gluconate, are frequently added as supplements to alcohol rubs for synergistic and sustained effects that are, for instance, clearly demonstrable for chlorhexidine-alcohol preparations (Table 96.6). Triclosan has some sustained activity, but even with five scrubs, each of 3 minutes, the bacterial reductions reported are rather disappointing.

From the above results, it is evident that the antimicrobial effectiveness of all antiseptic detergents currently available on the European market is significantly inferior to that of alcohol rubs or povidone-iodine aqueous solution. This is also depicted in Figure 96.2, which contains results that, except for hexachlorophene, were obtained by the same test method (163; updated 1993). From there, it can be seen that highly concentrated short-chain aliphatic alcohols, such as iso- and *n*-propanol, are up to 100 times more effective in reducing the release of skin bacteria. With this strong immediate effect, the question arises whether a sustained action, which is not demonstrable for alcohols, is needed and desired, as after extensive reduction it takes the resident skin flora several hours to become completely restored (Fig. 96.2).

The consecutive use of a detergent and isopropanol, both containing chlorhexidine, results in a significant increase in effectiveness compared with unmedicated soap and alcohol (138, 145) (Table 96.8).

To develop a standard for the efficacy of surgical hand disinfection is difficult, because epidemiologic information on the effect of various procedures on the ratio of surgical site infections is not available. Therefore, it has been decided arbitrarily by the expert authorities in some European countries (129,164) to choose a reference procedure for efficacy that ensures maximum reduction of skin flora at tolerable levels of skin strain and time expenditure. Efficacy, thus, is defined not by a numerically fixed measure of microbial reduction but by the mean reduction achieved by a reference disinfection procedure that is tested in parallel with the surgical disinfection to be evaluated with the same volunteers in two experiments that are carried out in a crossover design. Each volunteer acts as his or her own control. The requirement is then that the mean bacterial reduction assessed with the procedure under evaluation shall not be significantly smaller than that of the reference. This procedure involves rubbing and keeping hands wet with 60% (v/v) *n*-propanol (for details, see ref. 165). For the new tentative European standard prEN 12791 on surgical hand disinfection (166), a disinfection period of 3 minutes was chosen. With a well-trained team, the mean reduction in bacterial release will reach a magnitude of up to 2.9 log (Table 96.6). It is, however, unknown whether *in vivo* laboratory test results correlate with the ratio of surgical site infections. The results of one study comparing the clinical effect of a 75% alcoholic rub with that of surgical scrubs with either povidone-iodine or chlorhexidine (4%) gluconate detergents throw some doubts on this assumption: Although the bacterial reduction of skin flora achievable with the alcoholic rub was significantly superior to that assessed with the two scrubs, the clinical outcome of clean and clean-contaminated operations was virtually the same (167). But more data will have to be generated before a final conclusion will be possible.

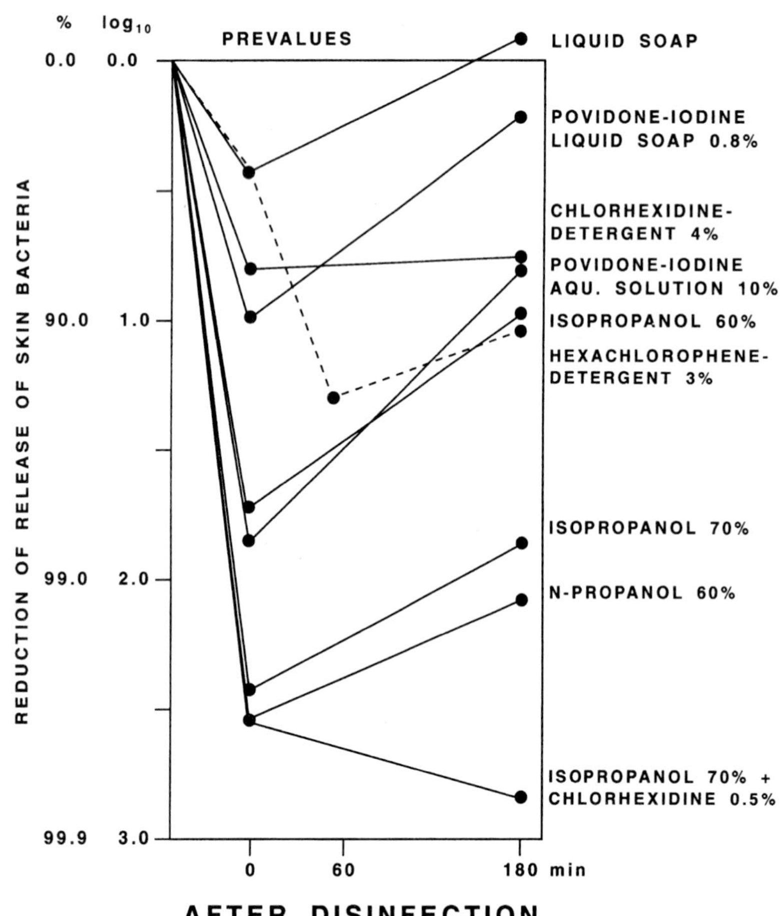

Figure 96.2. Killing curves showing the efficacy of various antiseptics for surgical hand disinfection (163; updated 1993) as assessed by the test model of the Austrian (164) and German (129) Societies for Hygiene and Microbiology and (for hexachlorophene, 4 minutes) according to the results of Michaud et al. (140).

TABLE 96.8. SURGICAL HAND DISINFECTION: EFFICACY OF CONSECUTIVE USE OF CHLORHEXIDINE (4%)-DETERGENT AND CHLORHEXIDINE (0.5%)-ISOPROPANOL (60%) AS COMPARED WITH UNMEDICATED SOAP AND ALCOHOL

		Mean Log Reduction	
Washing (3 min)	Rubbing in (4 min)	Immediate	Sustained (3 hr)
Unmedicated soap	Isopropanol	1.7	1.1
CHG-detergent	Isopropanol + CHG	2.5[a]	1.7[a]

CHG, chlorhexidine gluconate.
[a] $p < .1$.
From Rotter ML, Koller W. Surgical hand disinfection: effect of sequential use of two chlorhexidine preparations. *J Hosp Infect* 1990;16:161–166, with permission.

ACCEPTABILITY OF HAND WASHING AND HAND DISINFECTION PROCEDURES

To ensure compliance with hand washing rules, detergents and antiseptic preparations must be acceptable to the user (168). Healthcare personnel often complain of dry skin, skin irritation, or even frank symptoms of acute irritative dermatitis, which increase the risk of colonization with potential pathogens from the hospital environment (22,169). Suitable preparations, therefore, should have minimal toxicity of any kind, including allergenic and irritant properties. Only a few chemicals meet this requirement to an acceptable degree.

Frequent application of alcohol preparations may cause skin drying and, in some persons, irritative dermatitis (170). Defatting is sometimes suspected as one of the possible reasons (42), but this seems more likely to occur with detergents that indeed remove skin lipids, whereas evaporating alcohols leave dissolved fats behind. On the whole, skin dryness from frequent alcohol application is usually mild and may be easily prevented by the addition of suitable emollients to alcoholic hand antiseptics. Even after extensive usage of alcohol rubs, a blinded dermatologic expert had difficulty identifying any differences in the condition of the skin (170). Contrary to the general opinion in countries where alcohols are not much used for hand disinfection, they have been found quite acceptable to healthcare personnel with less drying than, for instance, chlorhexidine detergents (156,157,167,171–175). Short-chain aliphatic alcohols are usually nonallergenic.

In contrast, it seems that most antimicrobials contained in detergents possess a certain allergenic potential. But the reports on the acceptability of the various agents are contradictory (22, 71). This may signify that variables other than the antiseptic agents themselves may be involved in reported adverse reactions.

For chlorhexidine gluconate the allergenic potential seems proven (176). Reports on adverse reactions after application of chlorhexidine-containing preparations, however, do not always permit conclusions to be drawn as to whether they were the consequence of true allergies or other reactions (177). Otherwise, chlorhexidine preparations received more or less positive ratings in comparative studies (22,42).

Povidone-iodine– and triclosan-containing products were judged differently, depending on the individual preparation (22, 71,178). Therefore, a general comparative judgment does not seem possible. In one report, the acceptability of triclosan detergents was comparable with that of soap and of a chlorhexidine detergent and better than that of ethanol and povidone-iodine liquid soap; the latter was considered especially harsh (42). In another report, a triclosan preparation, among 14 products, was noticed to be especially harsh, whereas two other triclosan detergents did not cause noticeable skin damage (71). Chloroxylenol is a proven allergen. The incidence of allergic reactions is reported by the North American Contact Dermatitis group to be 1% (22).

A list of potentially allergenic agents used as hand antiseptics was published by Lautier et al. (179) in 1978. The list contains relevant agents and indices for primary inflammation and surface irritancy according to dermatologic criteria.

AGENTS USED FOR DISINFECTION OF HANDS

This section summarizes the agents most often used for hand disinfection. Hexachlorophene is not included, because it is no longer an accepted ingredient of hand and skin antiseptics.

Alcohols

Only short-chain aliphatic alcohols that are completely miscible with water are used as the main carrier of antimicrobial activity in hand rubs. These are ethanol and iso- and *n*-propanol. Although it is also a member of this group, methanol is seldom used. Low concentrations of higher alcohols such as butanol and aromatic alcohols such as benzylalcohol are sometimes contained in alcoholic preparations as synergistic supplements.

The antimicrobial effects of alcohols are based on protein denaturation. Alcohols have excellent and the most rapid bactericidal and fungicidal activity of all agents used in hand disinfection. They also possess good mycobactericidal activity. Enveloped viruses including HIV are readily inactivated, rabies virus being the only exception. Inactivation of naked viruses such as picornavirus takes longer and requires higher concentrations (from 80% v/v upward), as does HBV. Dry bacterial spores may survive in various alcohols for long periods of time (180). Alcohols evaporate quickly from the skin and do not have a sustained activity. Because of their extraordinarily high bactericidal activity, including good activity against the resident skin flora, this is, in fact, seldom needed. It takes the resident flora several hours to regrow after a 3- to 5-minute exposure to high concentrations of iso- or *n*-propanol (Fig. 96.2). As shown in Tables 96.4 and 96.5, the bactericidal activity decreases in the order *n*-propanol > isopropanol > ethanol. From the available data (181), it appears that identical bactericidal activity can be expected on the skin at the following concentrations (v/v): 42% *n*-propanol = 60% isopropanol = 77% ethanol. Methanol is infrequently used because of its toxicity and because of its relatively poor activity (182).

The addition of some chemicals may increase the immediate effect of alcohols significantly or provide a substantive effect. With a supplement of 1% (v/v) hydrogen peroxide, the activity of ethanol was, for instance, increased by 0.26 log (183). The alcohol may even become sporicidal (184). A combination with 1% to 2% iodine is classic. It must be removed from the skin after drying, however, because of possible skin irritation (141). We could not find a noticeable effect of low concentrations of iodophor used as a supplement in alcohols (79). Additions of chlorhexidine, quaternary ammonium compounds, ampholytic and phenolic compounds, triclosan, and octenidine serve mainly to furnish the alcohol with sustained activity (75). Organic matter diminishes the antimicrobial activity of alcohols only slightly (88). With blood, a bacterial reduction of 3.6 log resulting from a short-time rub (30 seconds) was diminished by 0.1 to 0.4 log, and one of 3.8 to 4.4 log after a longer rub (60 seconds) was diminished by 0.2 to 0.7 log (183).

The above alcohols are flammable. Because in most countries, strict fire regulations exist, which require special storage conditions for liquids with a flash point less than 21°C ("easily flammable"), it may be wise to shift the flash point of alcoholic preparations above this critical temperature. Products such as these are categorized as "flammable," can be stored in larger volumes and at less stringent conditions, and meet the requirement at the following (or lower) concentrations (v/v), which have been assessed according to EN 22719: ethanol ≤68%, isopropanol ≤70%, and *n*-propanol ≤82%. Mixtures of ethanol or isopropanol with the latter alcohol increase both the flash point and the antimicrobial efficacy.

In the applications discussed above, alcohols are nontoxic; they also lack any allergenic potential. Skin drying and irritant skin reactions may be avoided by adding suitable emollients such as glycerol, volatile silicone oils, refattening agents, and probably most importantly, rehydrating agents.

Iodophors

The use of elemental iodine as (alcoholic) tincture of iodine or as an aqueous solution of potassium iodine (Lugol solution) has been replaced by preparations containing complexed iodine, usually with polyvinylpyrrolidone, polyether glycols, or polyoxyethanol derivatives, for better acceptability. The main mechanism of microbicidal activity is based on the oxidizing potential of iodine. It is important to note that the strongest antimicrobial effect occurs with dilute rather than concentrated iodophor solutions (185,186), which have harbored live bacteria (187). As can be noted in Tables 96.4, 96.5, and 96.6, an aqueous solution of povidone-iodine, the most commonly used iodophor, is approximately as effective in reducing skin flora as 60% isopropanol, but preparations in liquid soap are much less active.

The antimicrobial spectrum of iodine preparations is wide, even including bacterial spores (188). But this latter activity is too slow to be useful in hand disinfection (44,189). There are, however, important holes in the spectrum, especially with enteroviruses (190). The sustained effect is small and only short lived (80,191). Organic matter reduces antimicrobial activity slightly (186), but blood may abolish the antimicrobial effect altogether (183,192). One gram of hemoglobin can inactivate 58 mg of iodine (193). Unless special precautions are taken, the antimicrobial efficacy of povidone preparations wanes during storage (186).

Because iodine is absorbed through the intact skin of neonates and across mucous membranes, the use of iodine-containing preparations may be associated with undesired side effects such as hypothyroidism and allergic reactions. But this is seldom a problem with iodophors in the field of application discussed here. In contrast, skin irritation and damage occur rather often and may thus adversely influence compliance with hand disinfection (42,194). But acceptability may vary with the type of preparation and brand.

Chlorhexidine

Chemically, chlorhexidine is a cationic bisbiguanide compound. Its most commonly used water-soluble form is the digluconate salt, but the acetate has also been used (195,196). There are also aqueous and alcohol solutions and detergent preparations. The hydrochloride is used in a powder preparation. There is incompatibility with some non-ionogenic chemicals such as Tween 80 and with some anions such as soap, phosphates, and nitrates. Some protein-containing solutions such as pus, blood, serum, or milk interfere slightly with the antimicrobial effect, which is best at pH 8 (195,197). Chlorhexidine exerts its antimicrobial activity by increasing the permeability of the microbial cell, causing cell disruption and precipitation of the cellular contents. The antimicrobial spectrum is broad. There are, however, gaps that should be known. The activity against gram-positive is better than the activity against gram-negative bacteria and against fungi; activity against mycobacteria is poor. Chlorhexidine has no sporicidal activity. It is effective against lipophilic viruses (197) but hardly active against nonenveloped viruses such as entero-, rota-, and adenoviruses (53).

The immediate antibacterial activity is definitely slower than that of alcohols (80), but the residual effect of chlorhexidine, because of its strong affinity for surfaces, is probably the best of any antiseptic available (197,198). This feature has been successfully used in surgical hand disinfection to extend the antimicrobial activity of alcohols under the glove (Table 96.6 and Fig. 96.2) and to build up an antimicrobial layer by consecutive use of detergent and alcohol, both containing chlorhexidine (145). In a clinical study, the rate of central catheter–associated infections was significantly reduced by preparation and regular care of the site at the catheter entrance with chlorhexidine as compared with alcohol or povidone-iodine treatment (199). When chlorhexidine was used for routine hygienic hand washes in ICUs as opposed to hand washing with unmedicated soap, a reduction of hospital infections was observed (124–127,200).

Except for ototoxicity when instilled into the middle ear

(201), chlorhexidine is regarded as a safe antiseptic, even when used regularly on the skin of newborn infants (202,203). There is no indication of absorption by the skin (203,204). Skin irritation is usually regarded as low (188), although not always (177).

Triclosan

This trichlorinated dioxydiphenylether (Irgasan DP-300) is poorly soluble in water but dissolves well in alcohols and various detergents, such as anionic soaps. It is incompatible with lecithin and some non-ionogenic detergents such as Tween 80 (205). It probably acts on the cytoplasmic membrane of the microbial cell. Except for *Pseudomonas aeruginosa,* the antibacterial spectrum is broad, mainly bacteriostatic, with minimal inhibitory concentrations between 0.1 and 10 mg/L but minimal bactericidal concentrations of 25 to 500 mg/L at 10 minutes of exposure (205). Acceptable mycobactericidal activity has been reported (194). Fungistatic (10 mg/L) and fungicidal (25 mg/L per 10 minutes) activities toward *Candida* species are good (206) but poor against molds such as *Aspergillus* species (minimal inhibitory concentration 100 mg/L). Triclosan is contained in detergents (0.4% to 2%) and in alcohols (0.2% to 0.5%) used for hygienic and surgical hand or preoperative skin disinfection and in soaps and deodorants. Compared with alcohols and even iodophors and chlorhexidine, its immediate effect is slow but more rapid than that of hexachlorophene. Although not as strong as that of chlorhexidine gluconate (207), there is a definite sustained effect (Table 96.7) that is minimally affected by organic matter or blood (208). There is no indication in the literature that triclosan has a toxic, allergenic, mutagenic, or carcinogenic potential. Acceptability of use on the hands was rated differently.

Phenol Derivatives

Only a short synopsis is given here, inasmuch as phenol derivatives are less used today than in past decades because of ecologic concerns.

2-Phenylphenol (2-Biphenylol, 2-Hydroxybiphenyl)

This agent is similar to chlorocresol and is incompatible with non-ionogenic detergents, quaternary ammonium compounds, and proteins. It has a broad antimicrobial spectrum, including mycobacteria, fungi, and viruses such as adenovirus, herpes, and influenza but not enteroviruses; in combination with propanols and detergents, 2-phenylphenol is active against HBV. Fields of application include hygienic hand wash (2%), skin antisepsis (0.2%), and preservation of cosmetics. Rotter and Koller (83) did not observe activity significantly different from that of unmedicated soap when used for 1-minute hand washes. A sustained antimicrobial effect has been reported (205). It is well tolerated and nontoxic.

Chlorocresol (4-Chloro-3-Methylphenol)

This agent is poorly soluble (0.4%) in water but dissolves well in alcohols. It is incompatible with non-ionogenic detergents and quaternary ammonium compounds. Chlorocresol is usually used in combination with other phenol derivatives in alcohols or soap for hygienic hand disinfection. It is a weak allergen, has low toxicity, and is well tolerated (205).

Chloroxylenol (Para-Chloro-Meta-Xylenol)

This agent is similar to chlorocresol but has slightly better antimicrobial activity because of enzyme inactivation and cell wall alteration. It has a broad antimicrobial spectrum, including mycobacteria and some viruses (e.g., vaccinia). The immediate effect is less than that noted for chlorhexidine and iodophors (209,210). It has a substantive effect. Organic matter has little impact on its effectiveness. It is used for hygienic hand washes in concentrations of 0.5% to 1%. The highest allowable concentration as a preservative in cosmetics in European countries of the Common Market is 0.5%, but in toilet and deodorant soaps it may be used at a concentration of 2% (193). It is less toxic than chlorocresol and has been documented to be a mild allergen.

Quaternary Ammonium Compounds

Common properties of this group of agents, which include benzalkonium chloride, benzethonium chloride, cetrimide, and cetylpyridinium chloride (205), are as follows: They are mainly bacteriostatic and fungistatic and microbiocidal only in high concentrations, especially against gram-negative bacteria (*P. aeruginosa*); they have no activity against mycobacteria but are active against some viruses, especially in combination with alcohols (lipophilic viruses, rabies); and they are incompatible with anionic detergents and have reduced effectiveness in the presence of organic matter and ion-rich water. These compounds are seldom used alone today for skin and hand disinfection but rather are used in combination with other antiseptics such as alcohols to confer on them a sustained effect. Quaternary ammonium compounds have low allergenic and toxicity potentials, but these are usually three to ten times higher than the substituted phenol derivatives discussed above (205).

REFERENCES

1. Rotter ML. Semmelweis' sesquicentennial: a little noted anniversary of hand washing. *Curr Opin Infect Dis* 1998;11:457–460.
2. Stewart DB, Williams JG. Bleeding and purging: a cure for puerperal fever? *J Hosp Infect* 1996;34:691–709.
3. Woodroffe RCS, Shaw DA. Natural control and ecology of microbial populations on skin and hair. In: Skinner FA, Carr JG, eds. *The normal microbial flora of man.* London, New York: Academic Press, 1974:3–34.
4. Ayliffe GAJ. The effect of antibacterial agents on the flora of the skin. *J Hosp Infect* 1980;1:11–124.
5. Price PB. The bacteriology of normal skin: a new quantitative test applied to a study of the bacterial flora and the disinfectant action of mechanical cleansing. *J Infect Dis* 1938;63:301–318.
6. Marples RP, Williamson P. Effect of systemic dimethyltetracycline on human cutaneous microflora. *Appl Microbiol* 1969;18:228–234.
7. Beetz HM. Zur Tiefenverteilung der Hautbakterien im Stratum corneum. *Arch Dermatol Forsch* 1972;244:76–80.
8. Gibbs BM, Stuttard LW. Evaluation of skin germicides. *J Appl Bacteriol* 1967;30:66–77.

9. Evans CA, Stevens RL. Differential quantitation of surface and subsurface bacteria of normal skin by the combined use of the cotton swab and the scrub methods. *J Clin Microbiol* 1976;3:576–581.
10. Montes LF, Wilbourne WH. Location of bacterial skin flora. *Br J Dermatol* 1969;81:23–26.
11. Kligman AM. The bacteriology of normal skin. In: Maibach HI, Hildick-Smith G, eds. *Skin bacteria and their role in infection.* New York: McGraw-Hill, 1965:13–31.
12. Evans CA, Smith WM, Johnston EA, et al. Bacterial flora of the normal human skin. *J Invest Dermatol* 1950;15:305–324.
13. Rosebury T. *Microorganisms indigenous to man.* New York: McGraw-Hill, 1962.
14. Marples MJ. *The ecology of the human skin.* Springfield, IL: Charles C Thomas, 1965.
15. Maibach HI, Hildick-Smith G. *Skin bacteria and their role in infection.* New York, Sydney, Toronto, London: McGraw-Hill, 1965.
16. Lowbury EJL. Gram negative bacilli on the skin. *Br J Dermatol* 1969; 81:55–61.
17. Marples RP. The effect of hydration on the bacterial flora of the skin. In: Maibach HI, Hildick-Smith G, eds. *Skin bacteria and their role in infection.* New York: McGraw-Hill, 1965:33–41.
18. Noble WC, Somerville DA. *Microbiology of human skin.* London: WB Saunders, 1974.
19. McBride ME, Ducan WC, Knox JM. The environment and the microbial ecology of human skin. *Appl Environ Microbiol* 1977;33: 603–608.
20. Blank IH. Survival of bacteria on the skin. In: Maibach HI, Hildick-Smith G, eds. *Skin bacteria and their role in infection.* New York: McGraw-Hill, 1965:43–47.
21. Davies J, Babb JR, Ayliffe GAJ, et al. The effect on the skin flora of bathing with antiseptic solutions. *J Antimicrob Chemother* 1977;3: 473–481.
22. Larson E, Leyden JJ, McGinley KJ, et al. Physiologic and microbiologic changes in skin related to frequent handwashing. *Infect Control* 1986;7:59–63.
23. Larson E, McGinley KJ, Grove GL, et al. Physiologic, microbiologic, and seasonal effects of handwashing on the skin of healthcare personnel. *Am J Infect Control* 1986;14:51–59.
24. Hofmann E, Mlangeni D, Grundmann HJ, et al. Das Problem der infektiösen Enteritiden als Aufgabe für Klinikhygieniker und Betriebsarzt. In: Hofmann F, ed. *Infektiologie.* Landsberg, Germany: Ecomed Verlags GesmbH, 1991:20–25.
25. Marples MJ. The normal microbial flora of the skin. In: Skinner FA, Carr JG, eds. *The normal microbial flora of man.* London: Academic Press, 1974:7–12.
26. Reber H. Versagen der Händedesinfektion bei Besiedlung von *Cloaca cloaca. Pathol Microbiol* 1960;23:587–593.
27. Noble WC, Savin JA. Gram-negative infections of the skin. *Br J Dermatol* 1971;85:286–289.
28. Al-Khoja MS, Darrell JH. The skin as source of *Acinetobacter* and *Moraxella* species occurring in blood cultures. *J Clin Pathol* 1979;32: 497–499.
29. Hoffmann PN, Cooke EM, McCarville MR, et al. Microorganisms isolated from skin under wedding rings worn by hospital staff. *Br Med J* 1985;290:206–207.
30. Larson E. Persistent carriage of gram-negative bacteria on hands. *Am J Infect Control* 1981;9:112–119.
31. Casewell M, Phillips I. Hands as route of transmission of *Klebsiella* species. *Br Med J* 1977;2:1315–1317.
32. Polk HC, Lopez JF. Bacterial ecology of hands of intensive care unit nurses cleansed with povidone-iodine. In: Polk H, Ehrenkranz NJ, eds. *Medical and surgical antisepsis with betadine microbicides.* New York: Purdue Frederick, 1972:41–45.
33. Borneff J. Die Testung chirurgischer Händedesinfektionsmittel nach der Handschuhmethode. *Arch Hyg* 1966;150:281–293.
34. Evans CA. Persistent individual differences in the bacterial flora of the skin of the forehead: numbers of propionibacteria. *J Invest Dermatol* 1975;64:42–46.
35. Marples RR, Kligman AM. Methods for evaluating topical antibacterial agents on human skin. *Antimicrob Agents Chemother* 1974;5: 323–329.
36. Meers PD, Yeo GA. Shedding of bacteria and skin squames after handwashing. *J Hyg* 1978;81:99–105.
37. Marsh DD, Selwyn S. Studies on antagonism between human skin bacteria. *J Med Microbiol* 1977;10:161–169.
38. Selwyn S, Ellis H. Skin bacteria and skin disinfection reconsidered. *Br Med J* 1972;1:136–140.
39. Skinner PR, Taylor AJ, Coakham H. Propionibacteria as a cause of shunt and postneurosurgical infection. *J Clin Pathol* 1978;31: 1085–1090.
40. Rotter M, Koller W, Wewalka G. Eignung von Chlorhexidinglukonat- und PVC-Jodhaltigen Präparationen zur Händedesinfektion. *Hyg Med* 1981;6:425–430.
41. Heeg P, Oswald W, Schwenzer N. Wirksamkeitsvergleich von Desinfektionsverfahren zur chirurgischen Händedesinfektion unter experimentellen und klinischen Bedingungen. *Hyg Med* 1986;11:107–11.
42. Larson EL, Butz AM, Gullette DL, et al. Alcohol for surgical scrubbing. *Infect Control Hosp Epidemiol* 1990;11:139–143.
43. Lowbury EJL, Lilly HA. Disinfection of the hands of surgeons and nurses. *Br Med J* 1960;1:1445–1450.
44. Lowbury EJL, Lilly HA, Bull JP. Disinfection of hands: removal of transient organisms. *Br Med J* 1964;2:230–233.
45. Marples RR, Towers AG. A laboratory model for the investigation of contact transfer of microorganisms. *J Hyg Camb* 1979;82:237–248.
46. Ayliffe GAJ, Babb JR, Bridges K, et al. Comparison of two methods for assessing the removal of total organisms from the skin. *J Hyg Camb* 1975;75:259–274.
47. Mittermayer H, Rotter M. Vergleich der Wirkung von Wasser, einigen Detergentien und Äthylalkohol auf die transiente Flora der Hände. *Zentralbl Bakteriol Hyg I Abt Orig B* 1975;160:163–172.
48. Ayliffe GAJ, Babb JR, Quoraishi AH. A test for hygienic hand disinfection. *J Clin Pathol* 1978;31:923–928.
49. Rotter ML, Koller W. A European test for the evaluation of the efficacy of procedures for the antiseptic handwash. *Hyg Med* 1991; 16:4–12.
50. Mitchell R, Cumming CG, Mac Lennan ED, et al. The use of operating gloves in dental practice. *Br Dent J* 1983;154:372–374.
51. Gobetti JP, Cerminaro M, Shipman CJR. Hand asepsis. The efficacy of different soaps in the removal of bacteria from sterile, gloved hands. *J Am Dent Assoc* 1986;113:291–292.
52. Doebbeling BN, Pfaller MA, Houston AK, et al. Removal of nosocomial pathogens from the contaminated glove. *Ann Intern Med* 1988; 109:394–398.
53. Boyce JM, Pittet D. Guideline for Hand hygiene in Health-care settings. Recommendations of the healthcare infection control practices advisory committee and the HICPAC/SHEA/APIC/IDSA hand hygiene task force. Centers for Disease Control and Prevention. *MMWR* 2002;51(RR-16):1–45.
54. Börnstein P. Versuche über die Möglichkeit, infizierte Hände durch einfache Verfahren zu desinfizieren. *Z Hyg* 1915;79:145–169.
55. Günther A, Schwab R, Eberhard T. Zur Kontamination der Umgebung beim Waschen infizierter Hände. In: Horn H, Weuffen W, eds. *Vorträge des VII. Kongresses über Sterilisation, Desinfektion und Antiseptik—Kurzfassungen.* Berlin: Gesellschaft für die gesamte Hygiene der DDR, 1980:24–25.
56. Fox MK, Langner SB, Wells RW. How good are handwashing practices? *Am J Nurs* 1974;74:1676–1678.
57. Larson E, Lusk E. Evaluating handwashing technique. *J Adv Nurs* 1985;10:547–552.
58. Voss A, Widmer AF. No time for handwashing? Handwashing versus alcoholic rub: can we afford 100% compliance? *Infect Control Hosp Epidemiol* 1997;18:205–208.
59. AORN. *Recommended practices for surgical hand scrubs. Standards recommended practices and guidelines.* Denver: AORN, 1997:197–202.
60. Lowbury EJL, Ayliffe GAJ, Geddes AM, et al. *Control of hospital infection.* London: Chapman and Hall, 1975.
61. Taylor LS. An evaluation of handwashing techniques. *Nurs Times* 1978;74:54–55, 108–111.
62. Ojajärvi J. Effectiveness of hand washing and disinfection methods

in removing transient bacteria after patient nursing. *J Hyg Camb* 1980;85:193–203.
63. Lilly HA, Lowbury EJL. Transient skin flora—their removal by cleansing or disinfection in relation to their mode of deposition. *J Clin Pathol* 1978;31:919–922.
64. Rotter ML, Koller W. Test models for hygienic handrub and hygienic handwash: the effects of two different contamination and sampling techniques. *J Hosp Infect* 1992;20:163–171.
65. Gruendemann BJ, Larson E. Antisepsis in current practice. In: Rutala WA, ed. *Disinfection, sterilization and antisepsis in health care.* Washington, DC: Association of Professionals in Infection Control and Epidemiology, and Champlain, NY: Polyscience Publications, 1998:183–195.
66. Hebra F. Höchst wichtige Erfahrungen über die Ätiologie des in Gebäranstalten epidemischen Puerperalfiebers. *Z Ges Ärzte Wien* 1848;5:64–65.
67. Sinclair WJ. *Semmelweis. His life and doctrines.* Manchester, England: Manchester University Press, 1909.
68. Newsom SWB. Pioneers in infection control: Ignaz Philipp Semmelweis. *J Hosp Infect* 1993;23:175–187.
69. Rotter MI. 150 years of hand disinfection—Semmelweis' heritage. *Hyg Med* 1997;22:332–339.
70. Larson E, McGeer A, Quraishi ZA, et al. Effect of an automated sink on handwashing practices and attitudes in high-risk units. *Infect Control Hosp Epidemiol* 1991;12:422–428.
71. Ayliffe GAJ, Babb JR, Davies JG, et al. Hand disinfection: a comparison of various agents in laboratory studies and ward studies. *J Hosp Infect* 1988;11:226–243.
72. McGinley KJ, Larson E, Leyden JJ. Composition and density of microflora in the subungual space of the hand. *J Clin Microbiol* 1988;26:950–953.
73. Larson E. Skin cleansing. In: Wenzel R, ed. *Prevention and control of nosocomial infections,* 2nd ed. Baltimore: Williams & Wilkins, 1993:450–459.
74. Larson E, Kretzer EK. Compliance with handwashing and barrier precautions. *J Hosp Infect* 1995;30(suppl):88–106.
75. Rotter ML, Kramer A. Hygienische Händeantiseptik. In: Kramer A, Gröschel D, Heeg P, et al., eds. *Klinische Antiseptik.* Berlin, Heidelberg, New York: Springer-Verlag, 1993:67–82.
76. Wewalka G, Rotter M, Koller W, et al. Wirkungsvergleich von 14 Verfahren zur Hygienischen Händedesinfektion. *Zentralbl Bakteriol Hyg I Abt Orig B* 1977;165:242–249.
77. Rotter M, Koller W, Kundi M. Weitere Untersuchungen zur Wertbestimmung von Verfahren zur Hygienischen Händedesinfektion: Ermittlung eines Vergleichsstandards. *Mitt Österr San Verw* 1977;78:170–172.
78. Rotter M, Koller W, Wewalka G, et al. Evaluation of procedures for hygienic hand disinfection: controlled parallel experiments on the Vienna test model. *J Hyg Camb* 1986;96:27–37.
79. Rotter M, Koller W, Wewalka G. Eignung von Chlorhexidinglukonat- und PVP-Jodhaltigen Präparationen zur Händedesinfektion. *Hyg Med* 1981;6:425–430.
80. Rotter ML, Koller W, Wewalka G. Povidone-iodine and chlorhexidine gluconate-containing detergents for disinfection of hands. *J Hosp Infect* 1980;1:149–158.
81. Rotter ML, Koller W. Test models for hygienic handrub and hygienic handwash: the effects of two different contamination and sampling techniques. *J Hosp Infect* 1992;20:163–171.
82. Rotter M, Koller W, Wewalka G. Über die Wirksamkeit von PVP-Jod-haltigen Präparationen bei der Händedesinfektion. *Hyg Med* 1980;5:553–553.
83. Rotter ML, Koller W. A European test for the evaluation of the efficacy of procedures of the antiseptic handwash. *Hyg Med* 1991;16:4–12.
84. Rotter M, Wewalka G, Koller W. Einfluss einiger Variablen auf die Ergebnisse von Prüfungen Hygienischer Händedesinfektionsverfahren. *Hyg Med* 1982;7:157–166.
85. Koller W, Rotter M, Mittermayer H, et al. Zur Kinetik der Keimabgabe von der künstlich kontaminierten Hand. *Zentralbl Bakteriol Hyg I Abt Orig B* 1976;163:509–523.
86. Lilly HA, Lowbury EJL. Transient skin flora-their removal by cleansing or disinfection in relation to their mode of deposition. *J Clin Pathol* 1978;31:919–922.
87. Grün L, Schopner R. Erwartung und Leistung bei der Hygienischen Händedesinfektion. *Z Hyg* 1957;143:521–532.
88. Rotter M. Händedesinfektion. In: Horn H, Privora J, Weuffen W, eds. *Handbuch der Desinfektion und Sterilisation.* Band IV. Berlin: VEB Verlag Volk und Gesundheit, 1984:62–143.
89. Frobisher M Jr, Sommermeyer L. A study of alcohols on tubercle bacilli and other bacteria in sputum. *Am Rev Tubercul* 1953;68:419–424.
90. Hailer E, Heicken M. Die Abtötung von Tuberkelbazillen in dünner Auswurfschicht (Händedesinfektion). *Beitr Klin Tuberk* 1939;93:1–10.
91. Hailer E. Die Einwirkung keimtötender Stoffe auf Tuberkelbazillen des Typus humanus und bovinus. *Z Hyg Infektionskr* 1929;110:22–36.
92. Smith CR. Alcohol as a disinfectant against the tubercle bacillus. *Public Health Rep* 1947;62:1285–1295.
93. Hare R, Raik E, Gash S. Efficiency of antiseptics when acting on dried organism. *Br Med J* 1993;1:496–500.
94. Shaffer CH Jr, Ortenzio LF, Stuart LS. Activity of phenol, ethyl alcohol, and isopropyl alcohol in the AOAC official, first action tuberculocidal test. *J Assoc Off Anal Chem* 1967;50:765–769.
95. Bundesgesundheitsamt. Liste der vom Bundesgesundheitsamt geprüften und anerkannten Desinfektionsmittel und -verfahren. (List of disinfectants and disinfection procedures tested and recognized by the Federal Office of Health [BGA], Germany). *Bundesgesundheitsblatt* 1990;11:504–516.
96. Groupé V, Engle CG, Gaffney PE, et al. Virucidal activity of representative antiinfective agents against influenza A and vaccinia viruses. *Appl Microbiol* 1955;3:333–336.
97. Klein M, Deforest A. Antiviral action of germicides. *Soap Chem Specialities* 1963;34:70–72,95–97.
98. Jaeger O, Barth R, Tusch W. Zur Wirksamkeit von Desinfektionsmitteln gegenüber dem Tollwutvirus. *Zentralbl Bakteriol Hyg I Abt Orig B* 1978;167:183–192.
99. Schürmann W, Eggers H. Antiviral activity of an alcoholic hand disinfectant, comparison of the in vitro test with in vivo experiments on hands, and on individual fingers. *Antiviral Res* 1983;3:25–41.
100. Steinmann J, Nehrkorn R, Meyer A, et al. Two in-vivo protocols for testing virucidal efficacy of handwashing and hand disinfection. *Zentralbl Hyg Umweltmed* 1995;196:425–436.
101. Steinmann J, Nehrkorn R, Lösche E, et al. Viruswirksamkeit der hygienischen Händedesinfektion. *Hyg Med* 1990;15:7–14.
102. Ansari SA, Sattar SA, Springthorpe VS, et al. In vivo protocol for testing efficacy of hand-washing agents against viruses and bacteria: experiments with rotavirus and Escherichia coli. *Appl Environ Microbiol* 1989;55:3113–3118.
103. Sattar SA, Abebe M, Bueti AJ, et al. Activity of an alcohol-based hand gel against human adeno-, rhino-, and rotaviruses using the fingerpad method. *Infect Control Hosp Epidemiol* 2000;21:516–519.
104. Schürmann W, Eggers HJ. An experimental study on the epidemiology of enteroviruses: water and soap washing of poliovirus 1–contaminated hands, its effectiveness and kinetics. *Med Microbiol Immunol* 1985;174:221–336.
105. Bond WW, Favero MS, Petersen NJ, et al. Inactivation of hepatitis B virus by intermediate-to-high-level disinfectant chemicals. *J Clin Microbiol* 1983;18:535–538.
106. Kobayashi H, Tsuzuki M, Koshimizu K, et al. Susceptibility of hepatitis B virus to disinfectants or heat. *J Clin Microbiol* 1984;20:214–216.
107. Kuwert EK, Thraenhart O, Dermitzel R, et al. *Zur Hepatitis-B-Virus-Wirksamkeit und Hepatoviruzidie von Desinfektionsverfahren auf der Grundlage des MADT,* 3rd ed. Wiesbaden: mhp-Verlag, 1983.
108. Kuwert EK, Scheiermann N, Thraenhart O. *Transmission der Hepatitis-Viren Hepatitis A, B sowie NonA/NonB.* Wiesbaden: mhp-Verlag, 1982.
109. Howard CR, Dixon J, Young P, et al. Chemical inactivation of hepatitis B virus: the effect of disinfectants on virus-associated DNA poly-

merase activity, morphology and infectivity. *J Virol Methods* 1983;7: 135–148.

110. Kramer A, Schuster G, Hauthal HG. Emulgator E39-ein oberflächenaktiver Kombinationspartner für antimikrobielle Zubereitungen. In: Kramer A, Weuffen W, Krasilnikow AP, et al., eds. *Handbuch der Antiseptik,* vol 2, part 3. Stuttgart: G Fischer, 1987:423–446.
111. Sattar SA, Tetro J, Springthorpe VS, et al. Preventing the spread of Hepatitis B and C viruses: where are germicides relevant? *Am J Infect Control* 2001;29:187–197.
112. Rotter M, Wewalka G, Koller W. Einfluss einiger Variablen auf die Ergebnisse von Prüfungen Hygienischer Händedesinfektionsverfahren. *Hyg Med* 1982;7:157–166.
113. Rotter M. Hygienic hand disinfection. *Infect Control* 1983;5:18–22.
114. Kramer A, Rudolph P, Kampf G, et al. Limited efficacy of alcohol-based hand gels. *Lancet* 2002;359:1489–1490.
115. Kampf G, Rudolf M, Labadie J-C, et al. Spectrum of antimicrobial activity and user acceptability of the hand disinfectant agent Sterillium gel. *J Hosp Infect* 2002;S2:141–147.
116. Curley A, Hawk RE, Kimbrough RD, et al. Dermal absorption of hexachlorophane in infants. *Lancet* 1971;2:296–297.
117. U.S. General Services Administration. O-T-C topical antimicrobial products and drug and cosmetic products. *Fed Reg* 1974;33:102–141.
118. Kimbrough RD, Gaines TB. Hexachlorophene effects on the rat brain. *Arch Environ Health* 1971;23:114–118.
119. Innes JRM. Status spongiosus and hexachlorophene toxicity in children, experimental monkeys, rats and other species. *Bull Soc Pharmacol Environ Pathol* 1973;2:8–9.
120. Sprunt K, Redman W, Leidy G. Antibacterial effectiveness of routine hand washing. *Pediatrics* 1973;52:264–271.
121. European Committee for Standardization (CEN). *Hygienic handwash. EN 1499: chemical disinfectants and antiseptics.* Brussels: European Committee for Standardization, 1998.
122. Ehrenkranz NJ, Alfonso BL. Failure of handwashing to prevent hand transfer of patient bacteria to urethral catheters. *Infect Control Hosp Epidemiol* 1991;12:654–662.
123. Hirschmann H, Fux L, Podusel J, et al. The influence of hand hygiene prior to insertion of peripheral venous catheters on the frequency of complications. *J Hosp Infect* 2001;49:199–203.
124. Black RE, Dykes AC, Anderson KE, et al. Handwashing to prevent diarrhea in day-care centers. *Am J Epidemiol* 1981;113:445–451.
125. Maki D, Hecht J. Antiseptic containing handwashing agents reduce nosocomial infections: a prospective study. In: Abstracts of the 22nd Interscience Conference on Antimicrobial Agents and Chemotherapy, Miami Beach, FL, October 4–6, 1982. Washington, DC: American Society of Microbiology, 1982:188.
126. Massanari RM, Hierholzer WJ Jr. A crossover comparison of antiseptic soaps on nosocomial infection rates in intensive care units. *Am J Infect Control* 1984;12:247–248(abst).
127. Doebbeling BN, Stanley GL, Sheetz CT, et al. Comparative efficacy of alternative handwashing agents in reducing nosocomial infections in intensive care units. *N Engl J Med* 1992;327:88–93.
128. Österreichische Gesellschaft für Hygiene, Mikrobiologie und Präventivmedizin. Richtlinie der Österreichischen Gesellschaft für Hygiene, Mikrobiologie und Präventivmedizin (ÖGHMP) vom November 4, 1980 zur Prüfung der Desinfektionswirkung von Verfahren für die Hygienische Händedesinfektion. *Österr Krankenhausz* 1981;22: 23–31 and *Hyg Med* 1981;6:4–9.
129. Deutsche Gesellschaft für Hygiene und Mikrobiologie. Richtlinien für die Prüfung und Bewertung chemischer Desinfektionsverfahren. *Zentralbl Bakteriol Hyg I Abt Orig B* 1981;172:528–556.
130. European Committee for Standardization. *Hygienic handrub. EN 1500: chemical disinfectants and antiseptics.* Brussels: European Committee for Standardization, 1998.
131. Larson EL, Early E, Cloonan P, et al. An organizational climate intervention associated with increased handwashing and decreased nosocomial infections. *Behav Med* 2000;26:14–22.
132. Pittet D, Hugonnet S, Harbarth S, et al. Effectiveness of a hospital-wide programme to improve compliance with hand hygiene. *Lancet* 2000;356:1307–1312.
133. Pittet D, Boyce JM. Hand hygiene and patient care: pursuing the Semmelweis legacy. *Lancet Infect Dis* 2001;1:9–20.
134. Pittet D, Mourouga P, Pernegger TV, and the members of the Infection Control Programme. Compliance with handwashing in a teaching hospital. *Ann Intern Med* 1999;130:126–130.
135. Grinbaum RS, deMendonca JS, Cado DM. An outbreak of handscrubbing-related surgical site infections in vascular surgery procedures. *Infect Control Hosp Epidemiol* 1995;16:198–202.
136. Cruse PJE, Foord R. A five-year prospective study of 23,649 surgical wounds. *Arch Surg* 1973;107:206–210.
137. Hoborn J. Transmission of aerobic skin organisms via contact. In: Hoborn J, ed. *Humans as dispersers of microorganisms—dispersion pattern and prevention [thesis].* Göteborg, Sweden: University of Göteborg, 1981:65–85.
138. Furuhashi M, Miyamae T. Effect of preoperative hand scrubbing and influence of pinholes appearing in surgical rubber gloves during operation. *Bull Tokyo Med Dent Univ* 1979;26:73–80.
139. Palmer JD, Rickett JWS. The mechanisms and risks of surgical glove perforation. *J Hosp Infect* 1992;22:279–286.
140. Michaud RN, McGrath MB, Goss WA. Application of a gloved-hand model for multiparameter measurements of skin-degerming activity. *J Clin Microbiol* 1976;3:406–413.
141. U.S. General Services Administration. O-T-C drugs generally recognized as safe, effective and not misbranded: tentative final order. *Fed Reg* 1978;43:1210–1249.
142. Blech MF, Hartemann P, Paquin JL. Activity of non-antiseptic soaps and ethanol for hand disinfection. *Zentralbl Bakteriol Hyg [B]* 1985; 181:496–512.
143. Heeg P, Ulmer R, Schwenzer N. Verbessern Händewaschen und Verwendung der Handbürste das Ergebnis der Chirurgischen Händedesinfektion? *Hyg Med* 1988;13:270–272.
144. Rotter ML, Koller W. Sequential use of chlorhexidine detergent and alcohol for surgical hand disinfection. Second International Conference of the Hospital Infection Society, London, September 1990, Poster no. 0073.
145. Rotter ML, Koller W. Surgical hand disinfection: effect of sequential use of two chlorhexidine preparations. *J Hosp Infect* 1990;16: 161–166.
146. Lilly HA, Lowbury EJL, Wilkins MD. Limits to progressive reduction of resident skin bacteria by disinfection. *J Clin Pathol* 1979;32: 382–385.
147. Rotter ML, Koller W. Surgical hand disinfection: the influence of time on the effectiveness. 24th Congress of the Austrian Soc. Hygiene, Microbiol., Prevent. Med., Salzburg, May 22–24, 1994.
148. Rotter ML, Simpson RA, Koller W. Surgical hand disinfection with alcohols at various concentrations—parallel experiments using the new proposed European standards (CEN) method. *Infect Control Hosp Epidemiol* 1998;19:778–781.
149. Rotter ML, Stoklasek B, Koller W, et al. Surgical hand disinfection: intra laboratory reproducibility of the test model according to prEN 12791. 26th Congress of the Austrian Soc. Hygiene, Microbiology, Prevent. Med., Millstatt (A), May 26–28, 1998.
150. Wewalka G, Rotter M, Koller W. Wirksamkeit verschiedener Mittel zur chirurgischen Händedesinfektion und präoperativen Hautdesinfektion. In: Porpaczy R, ed. *10 Jahre Ludwig-Boltzmann-Institut zur Erforschung von Infektionen und Geschwülsten des Harntraktes.* Wien: Egermann, 1980:9–15.
151. Lowbury EJL, Lilly HA, Ayliffe GAJ. Preoperative disinfection of surgeons hands: use of alcoholic solutions and effects of gloves on skin flora. *Br Med J* 1974;1:369–372.
152. Aly R, Maybach HI. Comparative study on the antimicrobial effect of 0.5% chlorhexidine gluconate and 70% isopropyl alcohol on the normal flora of hands. *Appl Environ Microbiol* 1979;37:610–613.
153. Lilly HA, Lowbury EJL, Wilkins D. Detergents compared with each other and with antiseptics as skin, degerming agents. *J Hyg Camb* 1979;82:89–93.
154. Altemeier WA. Surgical antisepsis. In: Block SS, ed. *Disinfection, sterilization and preservation,* 2nd ed. Philadelphia: Lea & Febiger, 1977: 641–653.
155. Hasek P, Kupfer M, Schreiber M. Neue Methoden der chirurgischen

Händedesinfektion—Kombination von Wofasteril und Fesia-cito. In: Winkler H, Kramer A, Wigert H, eds. *Beiträge zur Krankenhaushygiene und zur experimentellen und praktischen Keimtötung.* Leipzig: Barth, 1980:176–177.

156. Larson EL, Aiello A, Heilmann J, et al. Comparison of different regimens for surgical hand preparation. *AORN J* 2001;73:412–432.
157. Mulberry G, Snyder AT, Heilman J, et al. Evaluation of a waterless scrubbles chlorhexidine gluconate/ethanol surgical scrub for antimicrobial efficacy. *Am J Infect Control* 2001;29:377–382.
158. Rotter M. Chirurgische Händedesinfektion. In: Kramer A, Gröschel D, Heeg P, et al., eds. *Klinische antiseptik.* Berlin: Springer-Verlag, 1993:67–82.
159. Lilly HA, Lowbury EJL. Disinfection of the skin: an assessment of some new preparations. *Br Med J* 1971;3:674–676.
160. Holloway PM, Platt JH, Reybrouck G, et al. A multicenter evaluation of two chlorhexidine-containing formulations for surgical hand disinfection. *J Hosp Infect* 1990;16:151–159.
161. Lowbury EJL, Lilly HA, Bull JP. Disinfection of hands: removal of resident bacteria. *Br Med J* 1963;1:1252–1256.
162. Bendig JWA. Surgical hand disinfection: comparison of 4% chlorhexidine detergent solution and 2% triclosan detergent solution. *J Hosp Infect* 1990;15:143–148.
163. Rotter ML. Povidone-iodine and chlorhexidine gluconate containing detergents for disinfection of hands [letter]. *J Hosp Infect* 1981;2: 273–276.
164. Österreichische Gesellschaft für Hygiene, Mikrobiologie und Präventivmedizin. Richtlinie der Österreichischen Gesellschaft für Hygiene, Mikrobiologie und Präventivmedizin (ÖGHMP) vom November 4, 1980 zur Prüfung der Desinfektionswirkung von Verfahren für die Chirurgische Händedesinfektion. *Hyg Med* 1981;6:10–16.
165. Rotter ML. Are models useful for testing hand antiseptics? *J Hosp Infect* 1988;11(suppl A):236–243.
166. European Committee for Standardization (CEN). *Surgical hand disinfection. prEN 12791: chemical disinfectants and antiseptics.* Brussels: European Committee for Standardization, 1997.
167. Parienti JJ, Thibon P, Heller R, et al. Hand-rubbing with an aqueous alcoholic solution vs traditional surgical hand-scrubbing and 30-day surgical site infection rates. *JAMA* 2002;288:722–727.
168. Larson E, Killien M. Factors influencing hand washing behaviour of patient care personnel. *Am J Infect Control* 1982;10:93–99.
169. Larson E. Handwashing and skin: physiologic and bacteriologic aspects. *Infect Control* 1985;6:14–23.
170. Rotter ML, Koller W, Neumann R. The influence of cosmetic additives on the acceptability of alcohol based hand disinfectants. *J Hosp Infect* 1991;18(suppl B):57–63.
171. Boyce JM, Kellihers S, Vallande N. Skin irritation and dryness associated with two hand-hygiene regimens: soap-and-water handwashing versus hand antisepsis with an alcoholic gel. *Infect Control Hosp Epidemiol* 2000;21:442–448.
172. Grove GL, Zerweck CR, Heilmann JM, et al. Methods for evaluation changes in skin condition due to the effects of antimicrobial hand cleansers: Two studies comparing a new waterless chlorhexidine gluconate/ethanol-emollient antiseptic preparation with a conventional water-applied product. *Am J Infect Control* 2001;29:377–382.
173. Pittet D, Boyce JM. Handhygiene and patient care: pursuing the Semmelweis legacy. *Lancet Infect Dis* 2001;1:9–20.
174. Kampf G, Muscatiello M, Häntschel D, et al. Dermal tolerance and effect on skin hydration of a new ethanol-based hand gel. *J Hosp Infect* 2002;52:297–301.
175. Kramer A, Bernig T, Kampf G. Clinical double blind trial on the dermal tolerance and user acceptability of six alcohol-based hand disinfectants for hygienic hand disinfection. *J Hosp Infect* 2002;51: 114–120.
176. Osmundsen PE. Contact dermatitis to chlorhexidine. *Contact Dermatitis* 1982;8:81–83.
177. Ojajärvi J, Mäkelä P, Rantasalo I. Failure of hand disinfection with frequent washing: a need for prolonged field studies. *J Hyg Camb* 1977;79:107–119.
178. Webster J. Handwashing in a neonatal intensive care nursery: product acceptability and effectiveness of chlorhexidine gluconate 5% and triclosan 1%. *J Hosp Infect* 1992;21:137–141.
179. Lautier F, Razafitsalma D, Lavillaureix J. Hautentzündungstest zur Untersuchung der Toxizität antiseptischer Lösungen. *Zentralbl Bakteriol Hyg [B]* 1978;167:193–205.
180. Coulthard CE, Sykes G. Germicidal effect of alcohol with special reference on bacterial spores. *Pharm J* 1936;137:79–81.
181. Rotter M, Koller W, Kundi M. Eignung dreier Alkohole für eine Standarddesinfektionsmethode in der Wertbestimmung von Verfahren für die Hygienische Händedesinfektion. *Zentralbl Bakteriol Hyg [B]* 1977;164:428–438.
182. Tanner FW, Wilson FL. Germicidal action of aliphatic alcohols. *Proc Soc Exp Biol Med* 1943;52:138–140.
183. Renner P, Unger G, Peters J. Efficacy of hygienic hand disinfectants in the presence of blood. *Hyg Med* 1993;18:153–158.
184. Weuffen W, Hemanek R, Berling H. Beitrag zur Eliminierung von Sporen aus Ethanol. In: Kramer W, Wigert H, Kemter B, eds. *Mikrobielle Umwelt und antimikrobielle Maßnahmen,* vol 8. Leipzig: Barth, 1984:246–250.
185. Berkelman RL, Holland BW, Anderson RL. Increased bactericidal activity of dilute preparations of povidone-iodine solutions. *J Clin Microbiol* 1982;15:635–639.
186. Gottardi W. Iodine and iodine compounds. In: Block SS, ed. *Disinfection, sterilization, and preservation,* 3rd ed. Philadelphia: Lea & Febiger, 1983:183–196.
187. Centers For Disease Control. Contaminated povidone-iodine solution—northeastern United States. *MMWR* 1980;29:553–555.
188. Reybrouck G. Handwashing and hand disinfection. *J Hosp Infect* 1986;8:919–922.
189. Gershenfeld L. Povidone-Iodine as a sporicide. *Am J Pharm* 1962; 134:78–81.
190. Mahnel H. Desinfektion von Viren. *Zentralbl Veterinarmed* 1983;30: 81–96.
191. Koller W, Rotter M, Gottardi W, et al. Langzeitwirkung eines PVP-Jodpräparates bei der Händedesinfektion. *Hyg Med* 1991;16: 111–114.
192. Ghogawala Z, Futardo D. In vitro and in vivo bactericidal activities of 10%, 2.5% and 1% povidone iodine. *Am J Hosp Pharm* 1990;47: 1562–1566.
193. Lacey RW. Antibacterial activity of povidone-iodine towards non-sporing bacteria. *J Appl Bacteriol* 1979;46:443–449.
194. Steere AC, Mallison F. Handwashing practices for the prevention of nosocomial infections. *Ann Intern Med* 1975;83:683–690.
195. Davies GE, Francis J, Martin AR, et al. 1:6-Di-4-Chlorophenyl-diguanidohexan (Hibitane). Laboratory investigation of a new antibacterial agent of high potency. *Br J Pharmacol* 1954;9:192–196.
196. Rose FL, Swain G. Bisdiguanidines having anti-bacterial activity. *J Chem Soc* 1956;4422–4425.
197. Gardner JF, Gray KB. Chlorhexidine. In: Block SS, ed. *Disinfection, sterilization, and preservation,* 3rd ed. Philadelphia: Lea & Febiger, 1983:251–270.
198. Smylie HG, Logie JRC, Smith G. From pHisoHex to Hibiscrub. *Br Med J* 1973;4:586–589.
199. Maki DG, Ringer M, Alvarado CJ. Prospective randomised trial of povidone-iodine, alcohol and chlorhexidine for prevention of infection associated with central venous or arterial catheters. *Lancet* 1991; 338:339–343.
200. Maki D, Zilz MA, Alvarado CJ. Evaluation of antibacterial efficacy of four agents for handwashing. Proceedings of the 11th International Congress on Chemotherapy. *Curr Chemother Infect Dis* 1979;11: 1089.
201. Morizono T, Johnston BM, Hadjar E. The ototoxicity of antiseptics. *J Otolargyngol Soc Aust* 1973;3:550–559.
202. Bygdeman S, Hambraeus A, Henningsson A, et al. Influence of ethanol with and without chlorhexidine on the bacterial colonization of the umbilicus of newborn infants. *Infect Control* 1984;5:275–278.
203. Alder VG, Burman D, Simpson RA, et al. Comparison of hexachlorophene and chlorhexidine powders in prevention of neonatal infection. *Arch Dis Child* 1980;55:277–280.
204. Gongwer LE, Hubben K, Lenkiewicz RS, et al. The effects of daily

bathing of neonatal rhesus monkeys with an antimicrobial skin cleanser containing chlorhexidine gluconate. *Toxicol Appl Pharmacol* 1980;52:255–261.

205. Kramer A, Wallhäusser KH. Wirkungsspektrum und Anwendungseigenschaften angewandter Antiseptika. In: Kramer A, Gröschel D, Heeg P, et al., eds. *Klinische Antiseptik.* Berlin, Heidelberg, New York, London: Springer-Verlag, 1993:23–65.
206. Räuchle A. Triclosan. In: Kramer A, Gröschel D, Heeg P, et al., eds. *Handbuch der Antiseptik, vol 2. Antiseptika, part 3. Antibakterielle, antifungielle und antivirale Antiseptik—ausgewählte Wirkstoffe.* Leipzig: VEB Verlag Volk und Gesundheit, 1987:527–546.
207. Faoagali J, Fong J, George N, et al. Comparison of the immediate residual, and cumulative antibacterial effects of Novaderm, Novascrub, Betadine surgical srub, Hibiclens and liquid soap. *Am J Infect Control* 1995;23:337–343.
208. Marzulli FN, Bruch M. Antimicrobial soaps: benefits versus risks. In: Maibach H, Aly R, eds. *Skin microbiology: relevance to clinical infection.* New York: Springer-Verlag, 1981:125–134.
209. Davies J, Babb JR, Ayliffe GAJ, et al. Disinfection of the skin of the abdomen. *Br J Surg* 1978;65:855–858.
210. Sheena AZ, Stiles ME. Efficacy of germicidal handwashing agents in hygienic hand disinfection. *J Food Protect* 1982;45:713–720.

97

EVALUATING AND SELECTING PRODUCTS THAT HAVE INFECTION CONTROL IMPLICATIONS

ROBYN R. M. GERSHON
KRISTINE A. QURESHI
MARTHA J. GRIMES
JUDITH MCKENZIE

Healthcare technology has become increasingly sophisticated, with a rapid increase in the past three decades in both the number and variety of medical devices and other products designed for the healthcare industry. During this same period of time, medical devices have become smaller and more complex. With the ever-increasing use of advanced medical devices and products, patients' healthcare has improved. However, a potential side effect of these advances is the increased risk of nosocomial infections and healthcare worker exposure to potential pathogens. Approximately 45% of all nosocomial infections in the United States are related to the use of medical devices (1), and there are an estimated 150,000 cases of nosocomial bacteremia in the U.S. annually (2,3). Every day, new products continue to flood the healthcare market. It has been estimated that, for example, large medical centers may have in excess of 140,000 types of products in inventory from more than 8,000 different vendors (4). Adding to the complexity created by the multitude of choices is the current dual emphasis on cost containment and quality in healthcare. The total cost of a product includes not only the direct cost but also the indirect costs, such as the storage, maintenance, and cost of any related adverse outcomes (e.g., nosocomial infection and exposure follow-up). Another major hidden cost is the training and maintenance of competency of the personnel who use the product.

Healthcare cost containment has placed additional constraints on limited hospital budgets, and to reduce costs, facilities often switch to less expensive products. Unfortunately, indirect costs are rarely calculated in the analysis of cost-effectiveness. Thus, for the protection of both patients and healthcare workers, and for improving quality of care, infection control input to product evaluation is essential.

Since 1976, the Joint Commission on Accreditation of Healthcare Organizations (JCAHO) has recommended that infection control personnel be consulted on the purchase of all equipment and supplies used for sterilization, disinfection, and decontamination (5). Today, most hospitals standardize the purchase of products by using designated committees such as product standardization or value analysis committees. The infection control professional (ICP), who is generally a member of these committees, is responsible for the evaluation of any product having infection control implications (for both patients and healthcare workers) before a decision to purchase is made. Reduction of the risk of nosocomial infections among patients and personnel are not the only benefits realized when the ICP works with departments or product selection committees; significant cost savings related to reduced potential for nosocomial infections and healthcare worker exposure can often be achieved as well.

This chapter discusses the "tools" and information necessary for ICPs and others with infection control responsibilities to be effective internal consultants, and outlines a method for evaluating and selecting products that have infection control implications.

ROLE OF INFECTION CONTROL

There are several ways in which ICPs can take part in product consultation. One way is for ICPs to become involved in the formal acquisition process for medical-surgical products. Most hospitals have some form of a product evaluation and standardization committee, but if this is not available, then ICPs should use the JCAHO standards to work with the staff who select new products. The person with whom the ICP works might be a materials manager or purchasing agent who regulates the purchase of equipment and supplies. It may also be a person outside of the hospital who is making corporate decisions for multiple participating facilities within the healthcare system.

Another avenue could be to incorporate the requirement for ICP consultation or approval of products with infection control implications into the hospital's infection control policies. For example, the housekeeping department could have a policy requiring ICP approval of cleaning and disinfecting agents, and central sterile supply could have a policy on approval of all products for reprocessing, e.g., sterilization and disinfection. In any case, the ICP is often the uniquely qualified individual to assess the risks and costs associated with infection control-related items. The risk of a medical device is a function of (a) past response, (b) device failure, and (c) user failure (6). The ICP needs to consider each of these areas when evaluating a medical device. To assess these risks, however, items with infection control–related risks need to be identified to begin with, and the ICP needs the necessary tools and information as described below.

Tools

By "tools" we mean (a) an understanding of the risk factors associated with infection for the product under consideration (e.g., routes of transmission, risk identification, etc.); (b) rates of infection for the old device versus the new (proposed) device or rates of infection for no device versus the new device as when new technology is introduced; and (c) cost-effectiveness analysis. To apply a cost-effectiveness analysis to the problem, the ICP must have a wide variety of information available (see Cost and Standardization, below).

PRODUCTS RELATED TO INFECTION CONTROL

Since 1994 all of the JCAHO standards have recommended that persons qualified in infection surveillance, prevention, and control provide consultation regarding the purchase of all equipment and supplies used for sterilization, disinfection, and decontamination purposes and that they be consulted on any major changes in cleaning products or techniques (5). Included among these products are any cleaners or disinfectants used by the housekeeping department and hand washing products. Hand washing is the most important practice for preventing nosocomial infections. Thus, providing a mild soap that has undergone a hospital evaluation by the staff using it is a priority. The hand washing agent used by the facility should be approved by the infection control department (which seeks the approval of the infection control committee). Antiseptics used for hand sanitation and skin disinfection should also be approved by the infection control department. Sterilization and high-level disinfection systems, and process indicators related to their assurance (e.g., biologic indicators), should also be approved by the ICP.

Other items that relate to infection control should also be reviewed, including those touching mucous membranes or penetrating the skin, such as suction catheters; indwelling Foley catheters; urine drainage systems; intravenous catheters; intravenous administration sets; respiratory therapy equipment; wound drainage systems, etc. Personal protective devices such as masks, gowns, and gloves, and other equipment, including protective intravenous devices, should be evaluated as well.

METHODS FOR EVALUATING AND SELECTING PRODUCTS

Sources of Information

Product information regarding new devices on the market can be obtained from a variety of sources. The most informative resource is often the manufacturers' representatives. To streamline the process and continue representative access to staff and managers, some hospitals route these representatives through the purchasing department. Within the last few years, most facilities have established vendor policies, and it would be wise to be familiar with them. If an ICP is interested in a product, information can first be obtained from the company, and then a decision can be made whether to acquire further information from a representative. Another source of information about the latest products is journal advertisements or Web sites. Some national educational conferences or meetings, such as those sponsored by the Association for Professionals in Infection Control and Epidemiology, Inc. *(http://www.apic.org/)* and the Society for Healthcare Epidemiology of America *(http://www.shea-online.org/),* offer excellent opportunities for actually viewing new products. Another form of journal advertisement is the complimentary product magazines sponsored by manufacturers.

Information on product evaluations is frequently published in the materials management or nursing management journals. Readers can benefit from the Emergency Care Research Institute's (ECRI) product comparisons, some of which are reprinted in the *Journal of Health Care Material Management.* The ECRI is an independent nonprofit agency that is committed to improving the safety, efficacy, and cost-effectiveness of healthcare technology. Biomedical departments often subscribe to one of the ECRI's many publications, including *Product Comparison Systems.* Information derived from product testing is published in the ECRI journal *Health Devices* and in derivative newsletters for medical and surgical specialists. Reviewing the literature can be very time consuming and possibly expensive; therefore, many ICPs network with others in their field to be more efficient.

Many different disciplines of the hospital staff can request new products. Nurses usually are frequently involved in identifying potentially useful new products. Nurses attending conventions and trade shows, such as the American Association of Critical Care Nurses and the Association of Operating Room Nurses meetings, often view exhibits about new products (7,8). Therefore, another good source of product information can be hospital staff.

It is essential that the hospital have a clearly defined process for the evaluation of new products. Staff should not be allowed to try out samples of new products without the formal approval of the Product Evaluation and Standardization Committee.

Evaluation Criteria

Membership on the Product Evaluation and Standardization Committee by infection control staff is to ensure that products and equipment supports good technique with minimal risk to the patient as well as the healthcare providers. Although there are few articles on the evaluation of products, the ECRI provides some of this information in its *Product Comparison Systems* (see Sources of Information, above). The ECRI does not permit manufacturers or distributors of medical devices to exploit its product evaluations that are published in *Health Devices* to support marketing and sales. Seven criteria have been identified as being the most important in terms of evaluating new products: quality, efficacy, safety, cost, standardization, serviceability, and availability (9).

Quality

How can we determine the quality of a product? According to one study on product evaluation, *quality* refers to the extent to which the product performs its defined function (10). To determine the quality of a product, one has to return to the sources of data on the product and examine each of them for quality, keeping in mind the following question: Will this product provide better patient care without contributing to nosocomial infections? A manufacturer is understandably biased about the quality of its products, so it is the responsibility of the potential customer to objectively evaluate the company's product literature. Will the manufacturer's claims be substantiated in a clinical setting? Are instructions for use of the product clear and simple to understand? To assess another hospital's experience with a product, it is especially important to obtain detailed data on not only the product but also the evaluation criteria that were used, because it may differ significantly from your hospital's approach.

Efficacy

Efficacy of a product refers to how effectively the product meets its specified function. To measure this, some products are evaluated by independent laboratory testing (e.g., face masks undergo testing for filtering efficiency). Hospitals generally are not really equipped to do product testing. Manufacturers, therefore, should provide the data on their products for review, preferably with data from articles published in peer-reviewed journals (see Chapter 92). Another measure of efficacy is through the U.S. Food and Drug Administration (FDA), which regulates not only products used as drugs but also chemical sterilants and antiseptics in hand products (11). The U.S. Environmental Protection Agency (EPA) also registers hospital-level disinfectants (see Environmental Protection Agency Registration of Chemicals for Disinfection and Food and Drug Administration Approval of Antiseptics, below). Because both the FDA and EPA have regulatory powers, their efficacy data are usually reliable. Finally, efficacy data are also provided by ECRI (see Quality, above).

Whenever feasible, new products should be evaluated by the hospital, for example, a clinical research protocol might be used to evaluate efficacy. Evaluation of new (premarket) products requires research protocols. Any research involving the evaluation of a device must have the approval of an institutional review board before the device may be used in a study (12). For example, a hospital might be interested in using a medical device that has not been field-tested. Before the product can be used on patients, a research protocol would have to be prepared and approved by the institutional review board. The study design, protocol, and product testing is often a cooperative effort between the hospital and the manufacturer (13).

The Medical Device Amendments to the Federal Food, Drug, and Cosmetic Act (passed in 1976) gave the FDA authority to regulate new and existing medical devices (14–16). The amendments provided for three regulatory classes. Class I devices (e.g., tongue depressors and band-aids) require only good manufacturing practices. Class II devices (e.g., x-ray machines and some lasers) require establishing standards for design and performance. Class III devices (e.g., implantable devices and lithotriptors) must undergo scientific evaluation known as premarket approval. If a medical device investigation is conducted in accordance with the applicable requirements of the regulation, an investigational device exemption may be granted. The device is then exempt from certain requirements of the amendments to which it would normally be subject, such as premarket approval, performance standards, and premarket notification.

Safety

The safety of a product is an extremely important criterion in product selection, and consideration must be given to the patient as well as the healthcare worker. The challenge is how to determine a product's safety. First, product instructions should be simple and easy to understand, so that the user can apply them without difficulty. Second, a review of the manufacturer's safety data should be conducted. Third, a survey of current users of the product (e.g., other hospitals) should be conducted to identify any potential safety hazard.

The Safe Medical Devices Act of 1990, which became effective on November 28, 1991, gave the FDA the authority to assess new technologic characteristics, required manufacturers to conduct postmarketing surveillance, and mandated the reporting of device-related injuries and deaths (17). Safety is a concern not only during the initial use of a new product but also throughout the life of a product.

Companies must notify users about product recalls. In addition to recalls, there are two other ways to learn about product failures: the publication from the FDA called *The Medical Bulletin,* which carries this information, and alerts that are available from the ECRI. Each facility should have an identified person responsible for receiving and logging information on recalls, as well as maintaining a log of those persons who have been notified and the products removed from use. The ICP is an invaluable resource for this person when establishing/providing alternate products or alternate techniques.

Cost and Standardization

Today, more than ever, cost is an integral factor in determining product acquisition. Although cost-analysis information is rarely found in the literature, companies often supply a cost analysis for their product. When the prices of two items are compared, the fact that the price of one is lower than the price of the other does not necessarily mean that the item costs less. Price and cost analyses are not exactly the same. Price analysis looks at what the hospital pays for the equipment and supplies. A cost analysis also takes into account hidden expenses such as time and the other factors needed to support the new product, such as storage space and staff training. Institutions that try to reduce costs by introducing new products from the lowest bidder should be reminded that the cost of staff training can often offset savings based on price alone.

The Centers for Disease Control and Prevention (CDC) addresses cost-effectiveness by referring to a framework for assessing the effectiveness of diseases and injury prevention (18). The CDC offers a formula for cost-effectiveness (Fig. 97.1). This formula can help the ICP conduct a cost analysis. For example, if the annual cost of a new butterfly needle is $140,000 and the old device costs $100,000, the following indirect cost data can be used to justify its cost. As an estimate, if there are 20 needlesticks that require treatment per year at a cost of $3,000 per needlestick treatment (this does not include other costs such as lost work time, etc.), the total cost of the needlestick treatments is on average $60,000 per year. If the old device is used, the net cost equals the cost of the device plus the side effect, which in this case adds $60,000. For the new device, which will prevent needlesticks, the net cost is the device minus $60,000. Even though the direct cost of the new device costs more, an overall savings of $80,000 may be realized:

$$\text{Net cost}^{\text{old device}}\ \$100{,}000 + 60{,}000 = \$160{,}000$$
$$\text{Net cost}^{\text{new device}}\ \$140{,}000 - 60{,}000 = \$80{,}000$$

Many tactics can be used to reduce cost. For instance, a group of hospitals can buy medical devices and supplies in large volume. Alternatively, some hospitals have found that leasing equipment results in a cost savings (19). Overall, standardization of products usually results in significant cost saving for the institution. For example, at one hospital, using only one type of contrast media saved over $100,000, and using standards in orthopedic surgery sets in the operating room saved over $500,000. A reusable piece of equipment may appear to cost less than a disposable one until the cost of reprocessing is included (see Reusable Versus Disposable Products, below). Aber and O'Brien (20) recommend avoiding the compulsion to buy the "cadillac" (top of the line) product if the "chevrolet" product will get the job done without sacrificing the quality of care.

Cost analysis for infection control products is unique in that a higher cost for a better product can be justified when cost-effectiveness is taken into account, namely, the cost effectiveness of preventing nosocomial infections or occupational exposures. Needle devices that decrease the risk of a needlestick injury often cost more than devices that offer no protection. However, the expense (not to mention the pain and suffering) of treating needlestick injuries more than justifies the added cost. Today, the use of these engineering controls are mandated, in part by the need to comply with the regulations of the Occupational Safety and Health Administration (OSHA) to prevent exposure of healthcare workers to blood-borne pathogens (21).

$$\text{Cost effectiveness} = \frac{\text{Net Cost}}{\text{Adverse Outcomes Adverted}}$$

where

$$\text{Net Cost} = \text{Cost}_{\text{Program}} + \text{Cost}_{\text{Side effects}} - \text{Cost}_{\text{Disease}} \text{-} \text{Cost}_{\text{Indirect}}$$

Figure 97.1. Formula for calculating cost-effectiveness. (From Daschner F. The hospital and pollution: role of hospital epidemiologist in protecting the environment. In: Wenzel RP, ed. *Prevention and control of nosocomial infections,* 2nd ed. Baltimore: Williams & Wilkins, 1993:993–1000, with permission.)

Serviceability and Availability

Finally, in evaluating a new product, one must determine how serviceable and available it is. Serviceability refers to the ease of use and maintenance, user acceptability, and durability of a product when compared with similar products (4). Not only must a product be serviceable, it must also be available in sufficient quantity for the hospital's need. Products that are continuously back-ordered are unacceptable.

FEDERAL, STATE, AND LOCAL STANDARDS

The ICP should check with local and state governments to see if they have standards for products. For example, there may be regulations on the thickness or color of a plastic trash bag for hazardous waste or for what type of needle container may be used. Before the advent of safe work practices, referred to as universal precautions, now known as standard precautions, the federal government had no regulations on types of products required for healthcare; the CDC had only infection control recommendations. Today, OSHA requires that all hospitals provide certain infection control products to minimize the risk of exposure to pathogens. There are also standards on what type of respirator to wear for respiratory protection against tuberculosis and other airborne pathogens or chemicals (22).

Environmental Protection Agency Registration of Chemicals for Disinfection

The EPA registers chemical germicides based on efficacy and on other data obtained from the manufacturer. Because of concerns in the public health community and issues raised in a 1990 General Accounting Office report on the EPA's antimicrobial program, the EPA initiated a testing program to confirm efficacy claims of registered products on the market. Hotlines and clearinghouses are now available for technical information, reports, documents, and questions through the EPA Library and Information Center as well as through the EPA Web site (23).

Food and Drug Administration Approval of Antiseptics

Food and Drug Administration approval is required for skin antiseptics and other skin products. The Antimicrobial Panel Report to the FDA, published in the *Federal Register,* September 13, 1974, proposed seven categories of skin antiseptics:

1. Skin antiseptic
2. Patient preoperative skin preparation
3. Surgical hand scrub
4. Healthcare personnel hand wash
5. Skin wound cleanser
6. Skin wound protectant
7. Antimicrobial soap (used in the home)

The use of alcohol-based gel antiseptics for hand hygiene is becoming increasingly popular and should be thoroughly evaluated by the ICP prior to introduction into regular practice (24,

25,26). (See Chapter 96 for more information on the use of skin antiseptics in the decontamination of healthcare workers' hands).

REUSABLE VERSUS DISPOSABLE PRODUCTS

The 1980s and 1990s were the age of the disposable product. In many cases, it is easier and more cost-effective to discard a product rather than to reprocess it. However, one must consider the environmental impact and the cost for disposing of these products (27).

Whether to reprocess an item marked as single use only is an individual hospital's decision. Facilities that do so must strictly follow the guidelines established by the FDA (28). The decision to reprocess and reuse devices sold for single use only should be made only after a careful assessment of the risks and benefits (see Chapter 87). Even when the labor and cost of reprocessing are considered, using such items is often less expensive (29–32).

SELECTION OF NEW PRODUCTS BY A COMMITTEE

Most hospitals appoint a multidisciplinary committee, often called either the Product Evaluation and Standardization Committee or the Value Analysis Committee, to address product acquisition and review. There is usually a separate committee to evaluate new drugs.

Because nurses are direct users of many medical device products, they should always be included on the committee (33). These committees function to ensure four main objectives: (a) that required products are available; (b) that safe, reliable products are selected; (c) that the number of brands of the same item is limited; and (d) that unnecessary costs are reduced. If a committee meets the first three objectives, costs will usually be reduced. Providing the staff with the best, most efficient products to accomplish the task increases efficiency. Use of safe, reliable products serves to decrease iatrogenic complications, including nosocomial infections. Standardization of products and equipment reduces costs in several ways, including (a) decreasing the number of stock items; (b) increasing opportunities to purchase in large quantities and achieve bulk cost savings; and (c) decreasing the number of items for which staff may need training, which will lessen the likelihood of user errors.

For example, standardization of the type of electrocardiogram machines (ECG) throughout a hospital results in (a) the need for only one type of machine use training program; (b) bulk purchase of ECG paper and electrodes; (c) units readily sharing supplies during times of shortage; and (d) correct machine use by staff, especially those who are floated from other units. The result is lower costs to the facility and better quality ECG readings, which benefits patient care.

When a product review committee is established, policies and procedures for its operation should be written (34,35). There must be a concise delineation of its purpose and its objectives, which must be understood by all committee members. The committee's permanent members should meet at least monthly, and other staff members should be included as needed. One of the tasks of the committee should be to develop an approved product list. Souhrada (36) conducted a survey of product committees and found that, on average, 42.3% of such committees review about 20 to 49 products per year and 56.1% have ten or fewer members.

The Role of Purchasing

The purchasing department plays a key role in product acquisition. For standardization to be most effective, the purchasing department must have the authority to reject new product orders that have not received Product Evaluation and Standardization Committee approval. Purchasing should also be the liaison between the facility and the manufacturer. Purchasing representatives should know the details of the facility's procedures for obtaining bids and should be involved in identifying the cost of the item as well as assisting the committee with performing the cost analysis.

Before a new product can be obtained, precise specifications for the item must be determined. An important aspect of this process is review of any published scientific data on the product. The next step would be to determine whether other products could perform the same function. New equipment should be evaluated by the biomedical engineering department to test performance and electrical safety. The manufacturer should be required to provide a list of comparable facilities using their product or equipment. These facilities should be called to determine their level of satisfaction with the item. For larger facilities, it is also important to know whether the manufacturer can supply a sufficient quantity of the item to meet the needs of the facility.

INTRODUCTION OF NEW PRODUCTS

New products can be categorized as either (a) a completely new product never used in the facility, or (b) a change from one brand of product to another (e.g., buying a syringe from a different manufacturer). A completely new product should always undergo a thorough evaluation (Fig. 97.2). Although the new product may seem appropriate for use, the end users must be involved in its evaluation. Products used in multiple hospital areas should be evaluated in each area. For example, to introduce a new intravenous catheter, evaluations should be performed by a sample of users in different areas of the hospital and on all types of patients. Often, products for adults cannot be used on pediatric patients. For products to be evaluated, there should be a written evaluation form. When changing products, you will rarely get 100% approval; remember Pritchett's (37) "20-50-30" rule: only 20% of the population is change friendly, 30% are resistant to change, and 50% are neutral. Some hospitals require the written approval of the medical and nursing directors for affected units before a change can be made in a clinical product.

After a product has had a positive evaluation, a decision should be made by the committee for its approval. Once it is approved, the next step is to introduce the new product. No

GLOVE EVALUATION

PLEASE EVALUATE GLOVES FOR AN ENTIRE WORKDAY

Number of pairs evaluated=______

Please check one:

1. The glove was acceptable: ☐
2. The glove was not acceptable: ☐
   (please indicate a reason(s) below)

poor fit
ease of putting on/taking off
tactile sensation is lost
irritating to hands
poor integrity/tore easily
cuff fits too loosely
cuff too short
patient care compromised
patient acceptance poor
storage unacceptable

COMMENTS: ______

optional information

Name: ______

Unit: ______

Title: ______

Figure 97.2. Sample form for evaluation of a new product.

matter how simple a new product may seem, it must be introduced into the hospital with some form of staff education. Depending on hospital policy, the manufacturer may be required to provide around-the-clock in-service training for all users. The ICP should conduct surveillance to rapidly identify nosocomial infections that may be related to the use of a new medical device (38). The process of evaluation does not end once a new product is obtained. A product must always be available and safe, and perform its intended function.

CONCLUSION

As healthcare institutions' budgets continue to be contained, the drive to use less expensive products will continue. The ICP must be the hospital's conscience, mediating between the hospital's need to be competitive and the patients' need for quality care. Product safety for the patient and the healthcare worker must always be of prime concern. The ICP has an important role in guiding purchasing decisions wisely.

ACKNOWLEDGMENTS

Special thanks are extended to Kevin Butchez at the FDA and Cynthia Szymanski and Barbara Mandula at the EPA for providing up-to-date information.

REFERENCES

1. Stamm WE. Infections due to medical devices. Part 2. *Ann Intern Med* 1978;89:764–769.
2. Nettleman MD. Institutional epidemiologists' role in evaluating medical devices. *Clin Perform Qual Healthcare* 1999;7(2)104–106.
3. Darouiche RO, Raad II, Heard SO, et al. A comparison of two antimicrobial-impregnated central venous catheters. Catheter Study Group. *N Engl J Med* 1999;340:1–8.
4. Larson E, Maciorowski L. Rational product evaluation. *J Nurs Admin* 1986;16:31–36.
5. Joint Commission on Accreditation of Hospitals. Infection control. In: *Accreditation manual for hospitals.* Chicago: JCAH, 2004.
6. Callahan TJ, Marlowe D. Risk assessment and management as related to evaluation of medical devices: a view from the FDA. *J Long-Term Effects Med Implants* 1993;3(4):269–276.
7. Dix K. ICPs, nurse managers play critical role in product selection. *Infection control today.* Available at: *http://www.infectioncontroltoday.-com/articles/2bltopics.html.*
8. Carroll P. Nursing input into the purchase decision reveals costs not included in the price tag. *Hosp Mater Manage Q* 1992;12:63–68.
9. Berkowitz DA, Diamond JF, Montagnolo AJ. Maximizing purchase decision factors other than price. *Hosp Mater Manage Q* 1992;13: 27–41.
10. Larson EL, Peters DA. Integrating cost analyses in quality assurance. *J Nurs Qual Assur* 1986;1(1):1–7.
11. Haggar B. How do regulatory agencies ensure the release of a safe medical device? *Clin Perform Qual Healthcare* 1999;7(2):100–103.
12. Caley LM, Scharf L. Protecting patient safety in new product evaluation. *Nurs Manage* 1992;23:49–56.
13. Kennedy RS. Clinical investigations with medical devices. *JAMA* 1981; 245:2052–2055.
14. Pilot LR. FDA enforcement policies: a 20-year perspective. *Med Device Diagn Ind* 1996. Available at: *http://www.devicelink.com/mmddi/archive/96/05/016.html.*
15. Friedman M. Testimony on FDA's Medical Device Program.April 30, 1997. Available at: *http://www.hhs.gov/asl/testify/t970430a.html.*
16. Lally R. Achieving systematic compliance with the medical device directive. *Med Device Technol* 1996;7:28–33.
17. Schremp PS. Safe medical devices act: reporting requirements and risk management concerns. Available at: *http://www.allnight.com/prtfolio/omic/riskmanagement/deskref/medicaloffice/general/2.*
18. Centers for Disease Control. Public health service: a framework for assessing the effectiveness of disease and injury prevention. *MMWR* 1992;41:1–10.
19. Gapenski LC, Langland-Orban B. Leasing capital assets and durable goods: opinions and practices in Florida hospitals. *Health Care Manage Rev* 1991;16:73–81.
20. Aber RC, O'Brien WE. Organizing and managing product evaluation. In: Wenzel RP, ed. *Prevention and control of nosocomial infections.* Baltimore: Williams & Wilkins, 1987:243–249.
21. U.S. Department of Labor. Occupational Safety and Health Administration. 29 CFR Part 1910.1030. Occupational exposure to bloodborne pathogens: final rule. *Fed Reg* 1991;56:64004–64182.
22. Code of Federal Register: Personal Practitioner Standard. 29 CFR 1910.134.
23. Environmental Protection Agency. Available at: *http://www.epa.gov.*
24. The Antimicrobial Panel Report to the FDA. *Fed Reg* 39 FR 33103 and 33114.
25. Boyce JM, Larson EL, Weinstein RA. Alcohol-based hand gels and hand hygiene in hospitals. *Lancet* 2002;360(9344):1509–1510.
26. Bruch MK. Methods of testing antiseptics: antimicrobials used topically in humans and procedures for hand scrubs. In: Block S, ed. *Disinfection, sterilization, and preservation,* 4th ed. Malvern, PA: Lea & Febiger, 1991:1028–1029.
27. Daschner F. The hospital and pollution: role of hospital epidemiologist in protecting the environment. In: Wenzel RP, ed. *Prevention and control of nosocomial infections,* 2nd ed. Baltimore: Williams & Wilkins, 1993:993–1000.

28. U.S. Food and Drug Administration. Reuse of single devices. Available at: *http://www.fda.gov/cdrh/Reuse/reuse-documents.html.*
29. Martin L. Basin sets: recycling is best. *Hosp Mater Manage Q* 1991; 13:61–65.
30. Souhrada L. Reusables may slow rising tide of laparoscopic surgery costs. *Mater Manage* 1993;2:22.
31. Gordon L. Switching back to reusable underpads. *Hosp Mater Manage Q* 1992;14:15–17.
32. Becker GE. Are sterilization containers cost-effective? *J Health Mater Manage* 1992;42:44–46.
33. Silva L. Who makes up the standardization committee? *Hosp Mater Manage Q* 1983;5:18–22.
34. Freed DH. Why product standardization fails. *J Health Mater Manage* 1993;2:30–35.
35. Housley CD. *Strategies in hospital material management. Product standardization.* Gaithersburg, MD: Aspen, 1985:213–232.
36. Souhrada L. Product committees try to be productive—and to prove it. *Mater Manage* 1994:12:26–30.
37. Pritchett P. *Resistance moving beyond the barriers to change.* Dallas, TX: Pritchett Pub. Co: 1996:3–4.
38. Pittet D. Compliance with hand disinfection and its impact on hospital-acquired infections. *J Hosp Infect* 2001;48:S40–S46.

SUGGESTED READING

Valenti WM, Herwaldt LA. Product evaluation. *Infect Control Hosp Epidemiol 1997;18:722–727.*

HELPFUL WEB SITES

Single use/reprocessing: Canadian reference: *http://www.braytonlaw.com/news/mednews/060702 bronchoscope.htm*

Single use: *http://www.hc-sc.gc.ca/pphb-dgspsp/publicat/ccdr-rmtc/01vol27/dr2723ea.html*

Form for product evaluation, click on two links: *http://www.noharm.org/greenPurchasing/pecs*

98

EDUCATION OF HEALTHCARE WORKERS IN THE PREVENTION OF HEALTHCARE-ASSOCIATED INFECTIONS

KAREN K. HOFFMANN
EVA P. CLONTZ

In the healthcare setting, ongoing education is required for several reasons. First, all healthcare providers need to participate in ongoing education to remain abreast of the scientific innovations in the field of infection control. Figure 98.1 illustrates the growth of the scientific literature that provides the database for infection control. Second, technologic innovation demands learning new skills. Examples include the increasing use of computers in managing and analyzing nosocomial infection surveillance data and the increasing use of molecular epidemiology to evaluate healthcare-associated outbreaks. Third, regulatory bodies [e.g., Occupational Safety and Health Administration (OSHA), the Joint Commission on Accreditation of Healthcare Organizations (JCAHO)] now require that workers receive ongoing training in a variety of areas depending on their job duties. Such training includes instruction on isolation techniques, aseptic practices, prevention of blood and body fluid exposure, and proper handling of hazardous chemicals.

The results of the national certification examination job analysis survey, administered to infection control professionals (ICPs) between 1982 and 2002 by the Certification Board of Infection Control and Epidemiology (CBIC), has consistently identified the task of education as one of the major areas of responsibility for infection control professionals (Table 98.1).

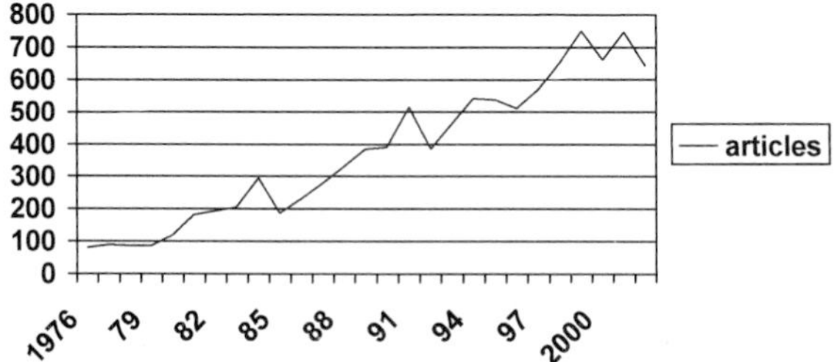

Figure 98.1. Journal articles published in a 25-year period from 1978 through 2002, indexed on Medline as "infection control."

This chapter discusses education of staff for the prevention of healthcare-associated infections, and reviews educational requirements mandated by government and licensing agencies and research findings regarding education about specific areas in infection control. The chapter also includes a brief introduction to human factors engineering, learning theory, and the educational program planning process.

INFECTION CONTROL EDUCATION FOR HEALTHCARE WORKERS

Regulatory Educational Standards

The JCAHO expects that new employees will receive orientation that covers the organization's infection control program and the individual's role in the prevention of infection. Another suggested activity is that continuing education be part

TABLE 98.1. ASSOCIATION FOR PROFESSIONALS IN INFECTION CONTROL AND EPIDEMIOLOGY (APIC) MAJOR EDUCATIONAL TASKS CITED BY INFECTION CONTROL PROFESSIONALS

Assess educational needs of healthcare workers
Develop goals, objectives, and plans
Use principles of adult learning
Assess physical environment, size of audience, resources
Review prepared educational tools and audiovisual
Prepare, present, or coordinate educational workshop
Instruct staff; evaluate
Participate in orientation program
Disseminate information and literature on infection control
Assess needs of patients/families
Instruct patients/families
Serve as a public educator to the community

From Goldrick BA, Dingle DA, Gilmore GK, et al. Practice analysis for infection control and epidemiology in the new millennium. *Am J Infect Control* 2002 : 30 : 437–448.

of a problem-oriented or outbreak response. When infection rates are not reduced by the feedback of surveillance rates alone, JCAHO suggests using innovative educational approaches beyond the routine or standard in-services. Another expectation is for at least yearly education and training of all personnel to maintain or improve knowledge and skills based on findings from infection control activities such as healthcare-associated infection rates or outbreak investigations (2).

The OSHA Occupational Exposure to Bloodborne Pathogens: Final Rule requires appropriate training for any employees who are reasonably anticipated to come into contact with blood or other potentially infectious materials in the performance of their job duties. The standard mandates training initially upon an employee's assignment and annually thereafter (Tables 98.2 and 98.3). The OSHA Compliance Directive CPL 2.106 Enforcement Procedures and Scheduling for Occupational Exposure to Tuberculosis (TB) requires worker training and information to ensure appropriate recognition and isolation of tuberculosis-infected patients (Tables 98.3 and 98.4). Specific training elements must be included for each of these standards. Training records for blood-borne pathogens must be maintained for 3 years and must include dates, contents of the training program or a summary, the trainer's name and qualification, and names and job titles of all persons attending the sessions (3).

TABLE 98.2. OCCUPATIONAL EXPOSURE TO BLOODBORNE PATHOGENS: FINAL RULE REQUIRED TRAINING

The training program shall contain at a minimum the following elements (summary):

A. Accessible copy of the regulatory text of this standard and an explanation of its contents
B. Explanation of the epidemiology and symptoms of blood-borne diseases
C. Explanation of the modes of transmission of blood-borne pathogens
D. Explanation of the employer's exposure control plan and the means by which the employee can obtain a copy of the written plan
E. Explanation of the appropriate methods for recognizing tasks and other activities that may involve exposure to blood and other potentially infectious materials
F. Explanation of the use and limitations of methods that will prevent or reduce exposure
G. Information on the types, proper use, location, removal, handling, decontamination, and disposal of personal protective equipment
H. Explanation of the basis for selection of personal protective equipment
I. Information on the hepatitis B vaccine
J. Information on the appropriate actions to take and persons to contact in an emergency involving blood or other potentially infectious materials
K. Explanation of the procedure to follow if an exposure incident occurs
L. Information on the postexposure evaluation and follow-up
M. Explanation of the signs and labels and/or color coding required
N. An opportunity for interactive questions and answers with the person conducting the training session

See complete list in 29 CFR Part 1910.1030, Occupational Exposure to Bloodborne Pathogens: Final Rule, December 6, 1992.

TABLE 98.3. PREVENTING THE TRANSMISSION OF *MYCOBACTERIUM TUBERCULOSIS*—REQUIRED TRAINING

The program may include the following elements (summary):

- Basic concepts of *M. tuberculosis* transmission, pathogenesis, and diagnosis
- Potential for occupational exposure to persons who have infectious TB in the healthcare facility
- Principles and practices of infection control that reduce the risk for transmission of *M. tuberculosis*
- Purpose of PPD skin testing, the significance of a positive PPD test result, and the importance of participating in the skin-test program
- Principles of preventive therapy for latent TB infection
- Healthcare worker's responsibility to seek prompt medical evaluation if a PPD test conversion occurs or if symptoms develop that could be caused by TB
- Principles of drug therapy for active TB
- Importance of notifying the facility if the HCW is diagnosed with active TB so that contact investigation procedures can be initiated
- Responsibilities of the facility to maintain the confidentiality of the HCW while ensuring that the HCW who has TB receives appropriate therapy and is noninfectious before returning to duty
- Higher risks associated with TB infection in persons who have HIV infection or other causes of severely impaired cell-mediated immunity
- Potential development of cutaneous anergy as immune function (as measured by $CD4^+$ T-lymphocyte counts) declines
- Information regarding the efficacy and safety of BCG vaccination and the principles of PPD screening among BCG recipients
- Facility's policy on voluntary work reassignment options for immunocompromised healthcare workers

See complete list in Guidelines for Preventing the Transmission of *Mycobacterium Tuberculosis* in Health-Care Facilities, 1994.
BCG, Bacille Calmette–Guérin; HCW, healthcare worker; PPD, purified protein derivative.

Educational Offerings Designed for Infection Control

Formal education specifically designed for the training of healthcare professionals in infection control began with a course offered by the Centers for Disease Control and Prevention (CDC) in 1968 (5). This course plus additional training courses were offered by the CDC for many years but were discontinued in 1988 (6). In 1989, the Association for Professionals in Infection Control and Epidemiology (APIC) assumed responsibility for offering training courses for infection control, and education remains the organization's top priority (7). In addition to APIC, sponsors of infection control conferences and workshops include APIC chapters in states and regions and specialized training programs, such as at the University of North Carolina at Chapel Hill. The Study on the Efficacy of Nosocomial Infection Control Project (SENIC) findings emphasized the need for physician training in infection control. In response, the Society for Healthcare Epidemiology of America (SHEA) and the CDC provide a training course in hospital epidemiology for physicians (8).

A survey by the National APIC Education Committee investigated the use of outdated infection control practices or rituals. Outdated practices were more likely to be used by persons who were not certified by the CBIC and who worked in long-term-care facilities or in smaller hospitals rather than larger hospitals.

TABLE 98.4. GENERAL CHARACTERISTICS OF INSTRUCTIONAL METHODS

Methods	Domain	Learner Role	Teacher Role	Advantages	Limitations
Lecture	Cognitive	Passive	Presents information	Cost-effective Targets large groups	Not individualized
Group discussion	Affective Cognitive	Active, if learner participates	Guides and focuses discussion	Stimulates sharing ideas and emotions	Shy or dominant member
One-to-one instruction	Cognitive Affective Psychomotor	Active	Presents information and facilitates individualized learning	Tailored to individual's needs and goals	High levels of diversity Labor-intensive Isolates learner
Demonstration	Cognitive	Passive	Models skill or behavior	Preview of "exact" skill/behavior	Small groups needed to facilitate visualization
Return demonstration	Psychomotor	Active	Individualizes feedback to refine performance	Immediate individual guidance	Labor-intensive to view individual performance
Gaming	Cognitive Affective	Active, if learner participates	Oversees pacing Referees Debriefs	Captures learner enthusiasm	Environment too competitive for some learners
Simulation	Cognitive Psychomotor	Active	Designs environment Facilitates process Debriefs	Practice "reality" in safe setting	Labor-intensive Equipment costs
Role-playing	Affective	Active	Designs format Debriefs	Develops understanding of others	Exaggeration or underdevelopment of role
Role-modeling	Affective Cognitive	Passive	Models skill or behavior	Helps with socialization to role	Requires rapport
Self-instruction	Cognitive Psychomotor	Active	Designs package Gives individual feedback	Self-packed Cost-effective Consistent	Procrastination Requires literacy
Computer-assisted instruction	Cognitive	Active	Purchases or designs program Provides individual feedback	Immediate and continuous feedback Private Individualized	Costly to design or purchase Must have hardware
Distance learning	Cognitive	Passive	Presents information Answers questions	Targets learners who are at varying distances from expert	Lack of personal contact Accessibility

From Bastable SB. *Nurse as educator: principles of teaching and learning for nursing practice*. Sudbury, MA: Jones and Bartlett, 2003, with permission (*WWW.jbpub.com.*).

However, certified respondents were no more likely than noncertified to be interested in changing any rituals (9).

The CBIC administers the process for Certification in Infection Control (CIC). APIC founded CBIC in 1981, and the first exam was administered in 1983. CBIC is a voluntary, autonomous, multidisciplinary board that provides direction for professionals in infection control and applied epidemiology. The principal purpose of CBIC is to provide public protection by providing and measuring a standard of knowledge desirable for practicing professionals, to encourage professional growth and individual study, and to recognize individuals who fulfill the requirements for certification. Eligibility requirements include at least 2 years' experience of defined infection control practice and a current license or registration as a medical technologist, physician, or registered nurse, or a minimum of a baccalaureate degree. To use the designation CIC, the professional must meet the eligibility requirements and pass an examination. To maintain certification, professionals must recertify every 5 years (10).

APIC provides numerous educational resources, most importantly the curriculum manual, *APIC Text of Infection Control and Epidemiology*, and *Certification Study Guide.*

The Area Health Education Centers (AHEC) concept was enacted into law by Congress in 1971 to develop regional educational interventions. This program, which has expanded from the original 11 university health science centers that received the initial AHEC funding to centers in over 40 states, has been a means for providing continuing education in infection control across the United States, including medically underserved areas (11).

Infection control education begins in college programs for healthcare workers; however, this subject is inadequately presented before clinical experience. Instruction in microbiology (the basis for understanding transmission of infectious diseases) is not required in many schools of nursing, and when infection control material is presented, it is frequently presented by someone lacking the expertise of an infection control professional (12).

Although manufacturers are not routinely classified as sources of educational programs for healthcare professionals, they provide information in marketing their products. Such information must always be critically examined as to whether it is reliable and supported by scientific evidence. Manufacturers also provide training for use of their equipment, provide grants to support lectures, and produce products designed specifically for educational purposes, such as videotapes and slides. These materials should be carefully evaluated for completeness of information and evidence of objectivity.

Targeted Infection Control Education

Blood and Body Fluid Precautions

Misinformation and confusion about the transmission of blood-borne pathogens have given impetus to infection control education. Studies of human immunodeficiency virus (HIV)/ hepatitis B virus (HBV) blood-borne pathogens have emphasized the difficulty of changing behaviors and have shown that knowledge does not necessarily translate into changed behaviors. Several studies have recognized that the desired outcome has not been reached through in-service educational programs that provide the standard information on risk behavior and ways to reduce that risk (13–15). A 5-year study found a decrease in the number of needlesticks through a combination of more convenient placement of needle disposal containers, communication, and education, but this study did not single out effectiveness of education (16). A variety of interventions tested on personnel in an emergency department improved compliance with universal precautions, including making gloves and eyewear more accessible, signage reminders, and hands-on training (17,18).

Hand Washing/Compliance

A lack of compliance with the CDC hand washing standards has plagued infection control efforts using traditional strategies for education. In a longitudinal study of hospital workers, it was found that, despite a comprehensive educational and promotional campaign, hand washing frequencies returned to precampaign levels in 6 months. The authors concluded that a lack of motivation (failure to change attitudes), rather than a lack of education, was the most important cause of poor compliance (19). Similarly, Larson and Killien (20) found that current methods of focusing on the benefits of hand washing with a public relations approach (i.e., signs, lectures, or posters describing the importance of hand washing) missed the significant reasons given for infrequent hand washing, such as being too busy. Two sequential studies of intensive care unit (ICU) personnel found that education alone did not have a sustained effect, but that maintaining education and providing feedback on hand washing performance were critical to having a continuing effect on motivation (21,22).

More recently a hospital-wide education program demonstrated that adherence to hand hygiene recommendations improved significantly (48% to 66%). The program involved using posters and other visual displays that promoted the use of bedside hand rubs. The posters featured messages submitted by healthcare workers that were then graphically illustrated in cartoons. The creativity of this program may be one reason for its success, giving recognition and ownership to local healthcare workers (23).

An evaluation of a patient-empowering model for increasing healthcare worker hand washing compliance on a 24-bed inpatient unit effectively increased compliance 56% and was sustained over 3 months. Compliance was measured through soap usage per resident day. The intervention was that patients asked their healthcare workers if they had washed hands before providing care. Interestingly, patients reported asking nurses 65% of the time to only 35% for doctors (24).

Noncompliance with the basic tenets of healthcare is evident in other areas of infection control practice, including aseptic technique, isolation, and universal precautions techniques. Ching and Seto (25) found that patient care practices for urinary catheter care were significantly improved when a nurse from the ward was chosen to act as an infection control liaison, promoting control measures and providing teaching, as compared to nurses receiving only in-service lectures. Two studies report successful outcomes in reducing either ventilator-associated pneumonia or central line venous catheter infections. Both used a multidisciplinary task force to develop self-study modules, lectures, pre- and posttesting, and posted fact sheets as posters through the ICU. The studies, using a multiintervention approach, showed significant reductions of 50% (26) to 66% (27) in hospital infection rates. These reports suggest a variety of educational methods may be needed to achieve and maintain adherence (23).

Human Factors Engineering

Well-trained and educated healthcare workers continue not to comply with infection control mandates. Alvarado has stated that the educational methods themselves are at fault. "Search for the individual bad actor keeps us from looking at the design of the overall system"(28). The traditional way of "simply telling them" assumes that the healthcare workers have the information, that learning has taken place, and that they will change to the desired behavior. It may be time to consider multifaceted approaches that will achieve good and sustained results, for example, human factors engineering (HFE), which has its origins in the Industrial Revolution (29). It looks at the causes and effects of human error and was originally applied to the design of increasingly complex airplane cockpits (30). HFE has been applied to numerous diverse systems such as software and computer control. In healthcare HFE has been applied to the problem that 70% to 80% of adverse anesthetic events in the operating room involve human error (30). Evaluating the differences between visual and manual activities using the HFE model removed the problems and reduced the errors (31).

The goal of HFE is a systematic approach to designing safer processes and products rather than relying on education alone. It relies on communication; training; fatigue and scheduling; environment and equipment; rules, policies, and procedures; barriers (safeguards); and tasks and technology tools (32). The human factors model is to write down the characteristic of each aspect of performance expectations and then consider the effect of each characteristic on the individual whose behavior needs changing and alter the model so that the desired outcome is reached (33). Ultimately, it has been demonstrated to reduce the need for training and seeks to achieve optimum performance.

The continuing problem in infection control is that healthcare workers do not consistently comply with critical practices such as proper hand washing, administering preoperative antibiotics at the appropriate time, precleaning and disinfecting endoscopes correctly, following isolation precautions, using aseptic practices, and wearing appropriate personal protective equipment. HFE focuses on the user interface. Bagian et al. (32)

state, "It is essential to design and implement a system that takes into account the concerns of the frontline personnel and is aimed at being a tool for learning, not accountability." The objective of HFE is to design devices or procedures that users accept willingly and operate safely in realistic conditions (30). An example is the improved compliance of healthcare workers with hand hygiene policies with use of waterless hand agents as an alternative to soap and water under certain conditions.

Alvarado (33) suggests comprehensive blame-free programs to analyze near misses as well as crashes. Lapses in infection control reflect system flaws rather than human incompetence.

Education for Specific Groups of Healthcare Workers

Effective programs must be customized to meet the needs of the group for which they are given. Studying a specific group of healthcare providers or targeting a learner population can assist the educator in developing programs that meet the unique interests of the group based on professional experience, intellectual maturity, and group readiness (34). Factors to consider regarding the participants include the general educational background, reasons for attending, current level of knowledge on topic, and level in the decision-making structure of the institution (35).

Seto (36) found that the differing responses to "social power" by nurses and housekeepers have implications for their training. Social power is defined as "the potential ability of an influencing agent to affect the cognition attitudes or behavior of another person (the target) in infection control." Studies found that nurses respond best to informational and expert power. This finding suggests that effective education for nurses should include relevant references and convincing information (e.g., surveillance rates) given by a perceived "expert" in the field. Housekeepers were responsive to legitimate power (the target's acceptance of a role relationship that obligates the target to comply with the agent's request) and coercive power (ability of the influencing agent to mediate punishment for the target), but less responsive to informational power. It therefore would be prudent for this group to have acknowledgment of the supervisor's endorsement of the educational content (36).

Hospital personnel with academic preparation in healthcare begin their employment with varying educational backgrounds in infection control. In addition to providing on-the-job training, the challenge is for infection control professionals to advocate changes in basic education in the curricula of schools of nursing and medicine so that healthcare personnel enter their professions with basic knowledge in infection control (37). Dembry and Hierholzer (38) consider changes in the role of the hospital epidemiologist over the years, and recommend that infectious diseases programs in medical schools should include training in infection control.

Reports have demonstrated significant benefits by focusing on physician-in-training for specific educational interventions (39,40). An observation that few physicians were using a full-size drape during central venous line insertion led to a nonrandomized pre- and postobservational trial in six ICUs and a step-down unit. A 1-day didactic course on infection control practices and procedures for third-year medical students and first-year residents resulted in a significant increase ($p < .001$) of full-size drape use, and a significant reduction in catheter-related infections (40). Another report using stations for training house staff on safety issues (needlesticks, back injuries, TB exposures) resulted in reduction or elimination of each adverse outcome (39).

LEARNING THEORY AND BEHAVIORAL SCIENCES

Knowledge of learning theory and relevant fields in the behavioral sciences should guide the educator in planning educational activities for infection control. Learning theories have some elements in common, including the idea that learning produces a relatively permanent behavior change and is an internal process that varies from person to person. Both biologic factors (e.g., heredity, sensory structures) and the intelligence that results from experience, education, and cultural background influence learning (41).

Seto (36) has investigated social psychology, a field of study in behavioral sciences that is relevant for infection control education. The reasoned action model assumes that people's behavioral intent is a good predictor of actual behavior. A study testing this theory on the infection control policy to stop recapping of needles divided nurses into three groups of three wards each, using an initial survey to categorize those who would comply with practice as "agreeables" and those who would not as "nonagreeables." The authors then utilized three methods to introduce the policy: (a) by announcement only, (b) by announcement and passive (posters and pamphlets), and (c) passive plus active (e.g., in-service lectures). Behavioral change was assessed by another survey. The results suggested that the agreeables had significant improvement in compliance (85%) using the announcement and passive method compared to the nonagreeables (21% compliance). The nonagreeables reached 83% compliance when passive plus active methods were used. Before the introduction of a new policy or procedure, a survey can be used to assess the proportion of staff already with behavioral intent to comply. If these are the majority, then an in-service program is not needed and the passive method would be sufficient (36).

Research in another social psychology theory, consumer behavior, has found that there are individuals called opinion leaders who can exert significant influence over others within their social/work groups). These opinion leaders can also influence how effectively new information is accepted by the group. Before and after direct observation of practice was made on two groups of ward nurses using new urinary catheter care guidelines as the infection control monitor. After both groups received the standard in-service education, opinion leaders provided tutorial demonstration to one group. There was a significant difference ($p < .01$) in compliance by the group receiving the opinion leaders' additional training (36,42). ICPs should consider whether ward staff opinion leaders may promote or assist education.

PLANNING EDUCATIONAL PROGRAMS

The ICP and other healthcare professionals are engaged in education in informal settings such as responding to questions on the telephone or in the hallway; however, scheduled programs that meet institutional requirements or specific needs necessitate planning that is based on teaching-learning principles. Planning an educational program, activities, or displays includes the following steps: (a) assess learner needs; (b) define goals or purpose; (c) formulate objectives; (d) develop a plan—determine the setting, organize the content, choose the format, choose teaching materials, and establish a climate conducive to learning; (e) prepare an evaluation; and (f) implement, evaluate, and revise the program (43).

Needs Assessment

Planning for educational programs begins with determining what knowledge is needed (e.g., what the discrepancy is between the present and required levels of competency). This needs assessment may be based on the needs of the individual learner (e.g., a hospital employee who fears catching a communicable disease) or on the needs of the institution (e.g., passing the JCAHO survey or implementing decisions of the infection control committee).

Methods of determining the educational needs include interviews (both structured and informal, such as asking nurses and doctors what is perceived to be harming their patients), surveillance, environmental rounds, questionnaires, tests, observations, group meetings for problem analysis (e.g., discussion of isolation techniques), and medical/hospital records and reports (e.g., healthcare-associated infection rates). Seto et al. (44) used a written survey and found that the educational needs for nurses were not the same as those for the entire hospital, and identified the specific needs of nurses in various units. Long-term-care facility ICPs responded to Leinback and English's (45) statewide needs assessment indicating that training is needed, especially if it is comprehensive, accessible, and focused on long-term care. Weinstein et al.'s (46) study made use of observation in a hands-on exercise for needs assessment in basic infection control practice. Observation was also used in Fernsebner's (47) study for educational needs assessment through the use of mock surgery for operating room staff to identify breaks in aseptic technique. Another way to identify needs is to review new infection control guidelines to focus on only the practices that require change and to evaluate barriers for staff compliance (48).

Goals and Objectives

Needs assessment determines the goal or purpose of the learning activity and leads to formulation of objectives that assist the educator and the learner in planning, conducting, and evaluating the learning process. Goals tend to be descriptive global statements, whereas instructional objectives describe a performance the learners will be able to exhibit in order to be competent. An objective is the specific observable, measurable behavioral outcome of instruction. Mager (49) identifies three characteristics of an instructional objective: performance, conditions, and criterion. For performance, the objective describes what a learner is expected to be able to do using specific action words. Any conditions or constraints are described in the objective. Finally, the criterion states how well the learner must perform or what the criterion level is for mastery (49).

Objectives may be classified into categories using classification systems such as one developed by Benjamin Bloom identifying three domains (affective, cognitive, and psychomotor). The affective domain includes interests, values, and attitudes. The cognitive domain includes knowledge, intellectual skills, and problem-solving abilities. The psychomotor domain includes manipulations and motor skills. The value of such a classification system for the educator is that it assists in communicating objectives clearly to the learner and in understanding the level of difficulty of the objectives (50).

A learning objective clarifies what will be learned, gives guidance to choosing appropriate formats and teaching methods, and specifies what is to be assessed in the evaluation of the learner (49).

Instructional Formats

The objectives guide the educator in choosing the most appropriate instructional format or combination of formats, including large groups, small groups and seminars, individualized instruction, or experiential learning, to facilitate student learning.

Another consideration in choosing the format is the preferred teaching style of the instructor/facilitator and the preferred learning style of the participant. Teachers have a preference for teaching styles, such as formal lecture, small group discussion, or a mentor role working individually with learners, but they frequently adapt to a less preferred style, because the objectives and educational needs influence the format. Kolb's classification system of learning styles combines two of four learning processes [concrete experience (feeling), active experimentation (doing), abstract conceptualization (thinking), reflective observation (watching)] for each of the four learning styles in his system. Goldrick et al.'s (51) study of nurses in three specialized groups (critical care, operating room, and infection control) found that 64% of the respondents preferred the abstract, reflective self-directed, discovery approach. Rakoczy and Money's (52) study of nursing students' preferred learning style produced similar results; students preferred abstract/reflective learning. Another study examining the cognitive style preferences of staff registered nurses found the majority expressed agreement with making decisions by rule or policy, preferred focusing on learning one task at a time and rated high a commitment to a group of principles or set of values (53).

Large Groups

The lecture-discussion method has been widely used and accepted by the educational community and is useful for groups larger than 15 people. It is an efficient way to transmit material to a large group in a short time and provides a specialist as a role model. However, this method is inconsistent with some principles of adult learning, and its disadvantages include the following: the student's role is passive; feedback is slow; individual differences cannot be accommodated; and attitude changes and reasoning skills are not developed (54).

The qualities of a good lecturer/instructor include more than knowing the subject well. The speaker must organize the presentation logically with an introduction, body, and summary, and then communicate that information effectively. Personal characteristics of the speaker such as a sense of humor, spontaneity, and even dramatic ability help to maintain the attention of the learners. Butler (55) found that the students perceive the traditional didactic lecture as the least effective learning method. However, varying the lecture format with handouts or experiential tasks that involve active participation by students greatly enhances student learning. Cooper et al.'s (56) study of infection control training needs of medical students found that the 30-minute lecture/discussion was not effective in teaching about infection control guidelines in relationship to perceived risks of acquiring human immunodeficiency virus (HIV). A comparison of traditional classroom lecture with computer-managed instruction and keypad questions in a nursing course found no statistically significant difference in achievement between the two groups (57).

Small Groups and Seminars

The small group instruction format is useful for groups of 15 or fewer participants. The small group is called a "seminar" when led by an instructor. When the group is student-centered, eight should be the maximum number of participants, and the instructor should serve as a resource person. Small groups and seminars are effective for attitude change, developing collaboration and problem-solving skills, applying concepts, and promoting peer interaction. The disadvantages of this method are that the groups require a great deal of time for careful management and planning by a competent facilitator, and evaluating individual progress is difficult (54).

ICPs can maximize time and individualize educational offerings for specialized departmental needs by using departmental liaisons who learn from the ICPs and take messages and programs back to their departments. To save travel and meeting time for distant locations, the Internet or teleconferences can be utilized (58).

Individualized Instruction

Individualized instruction designed to meet the exact needs of the individual student is ideal in that it accommodates individual differences, provides immediate feedback, and allows the learner to be an active participant. However, this method is difficult to use with large groups of people and with students who are not motivated, and is less effective for learning that involves changes in attitude. Developing materials for individualized instruction can be extremely time-consuming. Individualized instruction is applied through the use of such methods as independent study, correspondence study, manuals or syllabuses, videotapes, programmed instruction, and computer-assisted instruction (54). Lieb et al. (59) developed self-paced learning stations for tuberculosis respirator training that was effective and time-efficient.

Programmed instruction consists of a series of frames that are carefully sequenced so that learners will proceed at their own pace toward the desired behavior. This method is useful for teaching facts and skills but is less appropriate for teaching concepts and relationships (60). Studies by Goldrick (61) concluded that the programmed instruction unit (PIU) is an effective alternative to classroom lectures for teaching basic infection control principles and resulted in cost savings. Application to infection control was tested on a randomized population of senior nursing students. A comparison was made of those receiving a PIU in the basic principles of infection control with those given tests only or those given tests and another PIU that did not cover infection control material. The study reported significantly improved scores for those given a PIU in infection control and an additional finding that 68% of students preferred this type of learning to a lecture (61). In addition, a study of nurses and a study of third-year baccalaureate nursing students indicated that those who took a PIU covering the basic principles of infection control scored higher on posttests than those who attended a lecture, regardless of their pretest scores, educational level, and experience (62,63).

Experiential Learning

Experiential learning includes internships, student-initiated projects, and student participation in scholarship or research. This method is time-consuming for the educator and requires a supervisor for each student, but it offers effective individualized and specialized learning. Instructional methods are summarized in Table 98.4 (64).

Teaching Aids

Materials and Media

Media and teaching materials can assist in achieving the objectives of an educational program but should be used only if they serve an educational purpose. Comprehension and retention can be dramatically increased with visual aids, because as much as 83% of the data people gather may be from sight (65). Available media include print (e.g., handout, manual, textbook), chalkboards or flip charts, computer-assisted instruction, overhead transparencies, slides, audiotapes, videotapes, films, television, games and simulations, and manipulative materials.

When selecting teaching materials, the educator determines if the quality and potential effectiveness will enhance learning. The selection of materials must also be based on availability of equipment and money and compatibility with the educational setting (e.g., format, staff, space, time). Guidelines for evaluating media include the following: (a) Is the information appropriate for the level of the learners? (b) Is the information accurate and current? (c) Is there consistency between the learning objectives and the material? (d) Is the material organized and presented in a logical sequence? (e) Is the visual and verbal information simple? and (f) Is the technical quality good?

Slides provide colored visual stimuli, are appropriate for large groups, and are easily transported. The following principles should be applied when designing or using slides: (a) clarity—address one point and present limited information so that it is clearly visible; (c) focus—select data that fit the objectives and synthesize the data; (c) appropriateness—present information that is appropriate to the level of understanding of the audience; do not present highly detailed and complex information to a general audience and do not oversimplify for an advanced-level audience; (d) accuracy—the slides should present correct information, using correct spelling; (e) purpose—select only slides that match the focus of the presentation; eliminate information that is not directly relevant (66).

Technologic Resources

Technology is a powerful tool that enables the educator to provide a dynamic learning environment. The creative educator can facilitate learning using technologic resources such as computers and telecommunications. Computers provide software for learners to explore and gain information using nonlinear, nonsequential searching techniques to link facts and ideas in a way best suited to that person's needs. Technologic advances such as virtual reality systems (a computer-based platform using a helmet-like apparatus to project a video image that gives the illusion of reality) have potential for useful application in education in healthcare.

Computer-assisted instruction and interactive video are useful aids for educating healthcare workers. In computer-assisted instruction, the learner interacts with a computer program that presents information in small steps. This method provides immediate feedback and allows learners to advance at their own pace. Interactive video (controlling a video by the computer) allows the learner to respond and interact. One study showed that computer-assisted instruction resulted in marked improvement in universal precautions–related behaviors in nurses (67). Cohen and Dacanay (68) conducted a meta-analysis on computer-based instruction (CBI). The majority of the studies favored CBI over traditional methods of instruction, although few studies reported on retention, attitudes, and time to learn. The authors found large positive effects for interactive video applications of CBI that simulates clinical settings, requires involvement, and gives immediate feedback. Jamison and Brannigan (69) suggest that people with medical knowledge, as well as computer specialists, are needed for the process of implementing interactive video in medical education to make it most effective.

Establishing an Environment Conducive to Learning

Principles of adult learning applied to educational programs result in an environment that is conducive to learning. In addition to a comfortable physical environment, the interpersonal and organizational climate influence learning (33). Some guidelines that facilitate a positive learning setting include the following: (a) adults are generally participating voluntarily in educational activities and do not respond well to coercive practices; (b) effective education is based on the mutual respect of instructors and learners; (c) collaboration, not competition, contributes to effective adult education; (d) active involvement followed by reflection is essential; and (e) adult learning is most effective when it is self-directed (34).

Evaluation

Evaluation is essential in the educational process in that its purposes are to improve the learner's performance, the instructor/facilitator's performance, and the educational program itself. Evaluation is accomplished in informal ways as well as through the use of formal evaluation instruments to collect data. No single evaluation method is suitable for all purposes, but available methods include anecdotal records, self-evaluations, checklists, rating scales, tests, questionnaires, and interviews.

The first step in the evaluation is to determine the purpose of the evaluation. Questions to consider to guide the establishment of an evaluation process include: (a) Who is to be evaluated (e.g., learner, instructor, or program)? (b) When is the evaluation to occur? (c) What is to be examined (e.g., learners, instructors, instructional formats, or materials and teaching aids)?

When learners are to be evaluated, they need to know what is expected of them. The objectives for an educational program state what is to be accomplished and are the guide for constructing an instrument to measure the extent of learning. A pretest may be administered to assess the learner's level of competence at the beginning of an educational program, and then a posttest indicates the progress made. When instructors are to be evaluated, constructive feedback results in improvement in teaching. Evaluation of an educational program may be formative or summative, depending on the purpose. Formative evaluation occurs during the program and provides for modification of the program while it is being conducted. Summative evaluation occurs after the program is completed and focuses on accountability, indicating whether a program should be continued, modified, or discontinued (72).

> "I believe that education is the principal component of infection control. Without education, every other activity of our specialty is just so much meaningless busy work."—Sandra J. Pfaff (37), Third Annual Carole de Mille Lecture

REFERENCES

1. Goldrick BA, Dingle DA, Gilmore GK, et al. Practice analysis for infection control and epidemiology in the new millennium. *Am J Infect Control* 2002;30:437–438.
2. Joint Commission on Accreditation of Healthcare Organizations. *Comprehensive accreditation manual for hospitals.* Washington, DC: Joint Commission on Accreditation of Healthcare Organizations, 2003.
3. Occupational Safety and Health Administration. Occupational exposure to bloodborne pathogens; final rule. *Fed Reg* 1991;56: 64003–64182.
4. OSHA. CPL 2.106—Enforcement procedures and scheduling for occupational exposure to tuberculosis. February 9, 1966.
5. Haley RW. The development of infection surveillance and control programs. In: Bennett JV, Brachman PS, eds. *Hospital infections,* 3rd ed. Boston: Little, Brown, 1992:63–77.
6. Abbott D. Association news: president's message. *Am J Infect Control* 1989;17:25A–28A.
7. Laxton CE. Infection control: an idea whose time has come. *Am J Infect Control* 1997;25:34–37.

8. Centers for Disease Control. Public health focus: surveillance, prevention, and control of nosocomial infections. *MMWR* 1992;41:783–787.
9. Pirwitz S, Manian F. Prevalence of use of infection control rituals and outdated practices: education committee survey results. *Am J Infect Control* 1997;25:28–33.
10. Docken L. ICP certification: looking back, looking forward. *Hospital Infection Control* March 1998.
11. Nichols AW. The evolution of the AHEC program: from Carnegie Commission Report to a national resource. *Natl AHEC Bull* 1990;8: 3–5,23.
12. Goetz A, Yu CM, Muder RR. Microbiology, infection control, immunizations, and infectious disease exposure: education and practices in United States nursing schools. *Am J Infect Control* 1992;20:115–121.
13. Linnemann CC, Cannon C, DeRonde M, et al. Effect of educational programs, rigid sharps containers, and universal precautions on reported needlestick injuries in healthcare workers. *Infect Control Hosp Epidemiol* 1991;12:214–219.
14. Krasinski K, LaCouture R, Holzman RS. Effect of changing needle disposal systems on needle puncture injuries. *Infect Control* 1987;8: 59–62.
15. Whitby M, Stead P, Najman JM. Needlestick injury: impact of a recapping device and an associated education program. *Infect Control Hosp Epidemiol* 1991;12:220–225.
16. Haiduven DJ, DeMaio TM, Stevens DA. A five-year study of needlestick injuries: significant reduction associated with communication, education, and convenient placement of sharps containers. *Infect Control Hosp Epidemiol* 1992;13:265–271.
17. Kim L, Freeman B, Jaffe D, et al. Educational intervention improves compliance with universal precautions in the operating room for two years after training. Presented at the 10th annual meeting of the Society for Healthcare Epidemiology of America, Atlanta, March 5–9, 2000.
18. Kim LE, Evanoff BA, Parks RL, et al. Compliance with Universal Precautions among emergency department personnel: Implications for prevention programs. *Am J Infect Control* 1999;27:453–455.
19. Williams E, Buckles A. A lack of motivation. *Nurs Times* 1988;84: 60,63–64.
20. Larson E, Killien M. Factors influencing handwashing behavior of patient care personnel. *Am J Infect Control* 1982;10:93–99.
21. Conly JM, Hill S, Ross J, et al. Handwashing practices in an intensive care unit: the effects of an educational program and its relationship to infection rates. *Am J Infect Control* 1989;17:330–339.
22. Dubbert PM, Dolce J, Richter W, et al. Increasing ICU staff handwashing: effects of education and group feedback. *Infect Control Hosp Epidemiol* 1990;11:191–193.
23. Pittet D, Hugonnet S, Harbarth S, et al. Effectiveness of a hospital-wide programme to improve compliance with hand hygiene. *Lancet* 2000;356:1307–1312.
24. McGuckin M, Taylor A, Martin V, et al. Evaluation of a patient empowering model for increasing hand-washing compliance on an inpatient rehabilitation unit (abstract 244). Presented at the annual meeting of the Society for Healthcare Epidemiology of America. Washington, DC, April 2003.
25. Ching TY, Seto WH. Evaluating the efficacy of the infection control liaison nurse in the hospital. *J Adv Nurs* 1990;15:1128–1131.
26. Coopersmith CM, Rebmann TI, Zack JE, et al. Effect of an education program on decreasing catheter-related bloodstream infections in the surgical intensive care unit. *Crit Care Med* 2002;30:59–64.
27. Zack JE, Garrison T, Trovillion E, et al. Effect of an education program aimed at reducing the occurrence of ventilator-associated pneumonia. *Crit Care Med* 2002;30:2407–2412.
28. Scheckler WE, Brimhall D, Buck AS, et al. Requirements for infrastructure and essential activities of infection control and epidemiology in hospitals: a consensus panel report. *Am J Infect Control* 1998;26:47–60.
29. The University of Texas Human Factors Research Project. Research into Medical Human Factors and Human Error in Medicine. *http://homepage.psy.utexas.edu/homepage/group/HelmreichLAB/Medicine/medicine.html.*
30. Welch DL. Human error and human factors engineering in healthcare. *Biomed Instrum Technol* 1997;31:627–31.
31. Calkins JM. Why new delivery systems? *Contemp Anesth Pract* 1984; 8:3–8.
32. Bagian JP, Lee C, Gosbee J, et al. Developing and deploying a patient safety program in a large healthcare delivery system: you can't fix what you don't know about. *Joint Commission J Qual Improvement* 2001; 27:522–532.
33. Alvarado CJ. Infection control errors: don't fix blame, fix the system. In: *Touch, infection control newsletter.* Cincinnati: Sci-Health Communications, 1999.
34. Hinson PL. Education and training. In: *APIC test of infection control and epidemiology.* Washington, DC: Association for Professionals in Infection Control and Epidemiology, 2000:8/1–8/21.
35. Jackson MM, Lynch P. Education of the adult learner: a practical approach for the infection control practitioner. *Am J Infect Control* 1986;14:257–271.
36. Seto, WH. Staff compliance with infection control practices: application of behavioural sciences. *J Hosp Infect* 1995;30(suppl):107–115.
37. Pfaff SJ. Education—past, present, and future. *Infect Control* 1982; 10:133–137.
38. Dembry LM, Hierholzer WJ Jr. Educational needs and opportunities for the hospital epidemiologist. *Infect Control Hosp Epidemiol* 1996; 17:188–192.
39. DeBaum B, McGuire T, McLemore C, et al. Impact of an interactive health and safety fair: personalizing house staff orientation (abstract). Association for Professionals in Infection Control, Seattle WA, June 2001.
40. Sherertz RJ, Ely WE, Westbrook DM, et al. Education of physicians in-training can decrease the risk of vascular catheter infection. *Ann Intern Med* 2000;132:641–648.
41. Kidd JR. *How adults learn.* New York: Association Press, 1973.
42. Seto WH, Ching TY, Yuen KY, et al. The enhancement of infection control in-service education by ward opinion leaders. *Am J Infect Control* 1991;19:86–91.
43. Knowles M. *The modern practice of adult education.* Chicago: Association Press, Follett Publishing, 1980.
44. Seto WH, Ong SG, Ching TY, et al. Educational needs in patient care practices in Hong Kong. *Am J Infect Control* 1988;16:19–25.
45. Leinbach RM, English AJ. Training needs of infection control professionals in long-term care facilities in Virginia. *Am J Infect Control* 1995; 23:73–77.
46. Weinstein SA, Kotilainen HR, Gantz NM. Nursing assessment program in infection control procedures. *Am J Infect Control* 1987;15: 238–244.
47. Fernsebner B. Infection control education: identifying breaks in aseptic techniques. *AORN J* 1986;43:898–899.
48. Seto WH. Training the work force—models for effective education in infection control. *J Hosp Infect* 1995;30(suppl):241–247.
49. Mager RF. *Preparing instructional objectives,* 2nd ed. Belmont, CA: Pitman Learning, 1975.
50. Bloom BS. *Taxonomy of educational objectives. Handbook I: cognitive domain.* New York: David McKay, 1956.
51. Goldrick B, Gruendemann B, Larson E. Learning styles and teaching/learning strategy preferences: implications for educating nurses in critical care, the operating room, and infection control. *Heart Lung* 1993; 22:176–182.
52. Rakoczy M, Money S. Learning styles of nursing students: a 3-year cohort longitudinal study. *J Prof Nurs* 1995;11:170–174.
53. Nortridge JA, Bell ML. Recognizing RNs' cognitive style preferences. *Nurs Manage* 1996;27:40–44.
54. Stritter FT. Managing the educational process. In: Ridky J, Sheldon G, eds. *Managing in academics: a health center model.* St. Louis: Quality Medical Publishing, 1993.
55. Butler JA. Use of teaching methods within the lecture format. *Med Teach* 1992;14:11–25.
56. Cooper GS, Vincent DS, Harvey J, et al. A study of infection control training needs of medical students. *Am J Infect Control* 1990;18: 126–127.
57. Halloran L. A comparison of two methods of teaching: computer managed instruction and keypad questions versus traditional classroom lecture. *Comput Nurs* 1995;13:285–288.

58. Shimkus J. Spreading the word: grass-roots infection education. *Health Facilities Management* December 1997;33–34.
59. Lieb VA, Kozinn WP, Baxter P. Self-paced learning stations for tuberculosis respirator training: report of a pilot program. *Am J Infect Control* 1996;24:299–303.
60. Cross KP. *Accent on learning.* San Francisco: Jossey-Bass, 1976.
61. Goldrick BA. Effectiveness of an infection control programmed unit of instruction in nursing education. *Am J Infect Control* 1987;15:16–19.
62. Goldrick BA. Programmed instruction revisited: a solution to infection control inservice education. *J Contin Educ Nurs* 1989;20:222–227.
63. Goldrick B, Appling-Stevens S, Larson E. Infection control programmed instruction: an alternative to classroom instruction in baccalaureate nursing education. *J Nurs Educ* 1990;29:20–25.
64. Bastable SB. *Nurse as educator: principles of teaching and learning for nursing practice.* Sudbury, MA: Jones and Bartlett, 2003.
65. Smith TC. *Making successful presentations: a self-teaching guide.* New York: John Wiley, 1984.
66. Beery MP. Visuals for written and oral presentations. In: McGaghie WC, Frey JJ, eds. *Handbook for the academic physician.* New York: Springer, 1986:312–333.
67. Wright BJ, Turner JG, Daffin P. Effectiveness of computer-assisted instruction in increasing the rate of universal precautions-related behavior. *Am J Infect Control* 1997;25:426–429.
68. Cohen PA, Dacanay LS. A meta-analysis of computer-based instruction in nursing education. *Comput Nurs* 1994;12:89–97.
69. Jamison JP, Brannigan P. Interactive video in medical education: a program on jugular venous pressure and the cardiac cycle. *Med Educ* 1991;25:160–164.
70. Axnick KJ. Education. In: Axnick KJ, Yarbrough M, eds. *Infection control: an integrated approach.* St. Louis: CV Mosby, 1984:216–252.
71. McGaghie WC, Stritter FT. Principles of clinical education. *Alcohol Health Res World* 1989;13:28–31.
72. McGaghie WC. Evaluation of learners. In: McGaghie WC, Frey JJ, eds. *Handbook for the academic physician.* New York: Springer, 1986:125–146.

99

INFECTION CONTROL AND THE EMPLOYEE HEALTH SERVICE

PAMELA S. FALK

Hospitals, although traditionally a refuge for the sick and injured, not only are very dangerous environments for healthcare workers, but also can be dangerous for patients. Hospital-based employee health programs are charged with diagnosing, treating, and preventing infectious diseases in healthcare workers. Because of this, a hospital-based employee health service plays an important role in the infection control program and is a key element in protecting patients from nosocomial infections.

Clear lines of communication need to be established between the employee health service and the infection control department. Infection control and employee health staff should meet on a routine basis and should communicate (telephone, notes, fax, e-mail) as needed for integration of activities. Protocols for triage, evaluation, prophylaxis, and follow-up after exposures should be developed and the roles and responsibilities of employee health and infection control should be carefully defined.

CONTROL AND PREVENTION OF SPECIFIC INFECTIOUS DISEASES IN THE HEALTHCARE SETTING

Varicella-Zoster Virus

The varicella-zoster virus (VZV) causes two diseases, varicella (chickenpox) and herpes zoster (shingles). Chickenpox is a common childhood disease. For the approximately 1% to 10% of adults who are susceptible to VZV (1–7), exposure poses a significant risk of infection.

Assessment of Healthcare Worker Immune Status

A common goal of all infection control programs is to protect patients from healthcare workers who may be incubating infectious diseases after exposure in the community or in the hospital. All employees should, on their post-offer employee screening, be asked about a history of chickenpox. A healthcare worker with a positive history of chickenpox can be considered immune (5–19). If the healthcare worker denies having had the disease or has an uncertain history for chickenpox, a serologic test, if deemed cost-effective by the institution, may be done to determine his or her immune status (see Chapter 81).

Institutions should develop guidelines for managing healthcare personnel eligible for the varicella vaccine (20). If the healthcare worker is not immune (either by history or serologic test), the varicella vaccine should be offered (16–20). Serologic testing for postvaccination antibodies is not required (16–19). Personnel who develop a rash after receiving the varicella vaccine may need to refrain from patient contact until the rash clears (15). Recent vaccinees with or without a rash should avoid contact with patients who are at greater risk from varicella infections, including immunocompromised patients, newborns, and pregnant women (15).

Nonimmune healthcare workers for whom the vaccine is contraindicated should be educated about the risk they pose to patients should they be exposed to VZV. They should not be assigned to the care of any patient with chickenpox or herpes zoster. They should be asked at the time of their annual health evaluation whether they had chickenpox in the past year and, if not, can they now receive the varicella vaccine. This should be documented in their employee health record.

Exposures to Varicella-Zoster Virus

After a case of chickenpox has been confirmed in a patient or healthcare worker, infection control professionals should compile a list of personnel and patients exposed to the index case. The names of exposed employees are provided to the employee health service so that the immune status of those exposed can be determined. Exposed healthcare workers who are not immune should be furloughed. The period of contagiousness of infected persons is estimated to begin 1 to 2 days before the onset of the rash and to end when all lesions are crusted (18). Thus, furlough should begin 10 days after the first day of exposure and extend through day 21 after the last day of exposure (6,7,14,15,18,20).

It is very important that nonimmune employees report chickenpox exposures whether they occur in the community or in the hospital. Employers should furlough healthcare workers with pay for exposures that occur within the institution. Without this policy, employees are reluctant to report their exposures. Although employees are strongly encouraged to report community exposures, few institutions furlough employees with pay after exposures in the community.

Although the risk of infection with VZV is less after exposure to a patient with herpes zoster than after exposure to a patient with chickenpox, the clinical manifestations of chickenpox are the same after acquisition of infection by either type of exposure (12). Nonimmune healthcare workers who have direct physical contact with draining vesicles of patients with herpes zoster should also be considered exposed and furloughed from work (12). Nonimmune healthcare workers should refrain from working with patients with herpes zoster (12).

Often, the source of exposure to VZV is a healthcare worker. One of the most important functions for the employee health service during the investigation of a VZV exposure episode is to confirm VZV infection in the index case. Once VZV infection has been confirmed, the employee must be furloughed until all lesions are crusted (12). Although the furlough may be instituted by either the infection control department or the employee health service, the employee must return to the employee health service to be cleared before returning to work.

Prophylaxis using varicella-zoster immune globulin should be considered for nonimmune exposed healthcare workers who are at high risk for complications of varicella-zoster infection (pregnant and immunosuppressed employees) (21) (see Chapters 42 and 80).

Tuberculosis

The American Thoracic Society issued a statement in 1967 recommending that all hospitals have a "consistent program of tuberculin testing . . . of all employees who may be subject to exposure" (22). By 1983, the Centers for Disease Control and Prevention (CDC) recognized that all healthcare workers were not at equal risk for acquiring tuberculosis (TB) and recommended skin testing based on individual classification of risk for a facility and the location and prevalence of untreated TB in the community, in the institution, and among personnel (23,24).

Because of these recommendations, many hospitals in the late 1980s discontinued or restricted their purified protein derivative (PPD) skin testing program. However, since 1988, there has been a dramatic increase in TB in the United States that is largely related to the human immunodeficiency virus (HIV) epidemic (24–26). Hospitals have had to reassess their TB surveillance plans and develop mandatory skin testing policies for healthcare workers. These programs should include baseline TB skin tests upon employment, periodic retesting for at-risk employees, postexposure evaluation, preventive therapy as indicated, and employee education (24) (see Chapter 37).

Healthcare workers with a positive TB skin test on initial testing or with a skin test conversion after exposure should be evaluated for active TB by the employee health service. Persons with symptoms suggestive of TB should be evaluated regardless of skin test results. If TB is diagnosed, appropriate therapy should be instituted. Healthcare workers with a reactive skin test but without disease should be educated about the signs and symptoms of disease and instructed to report immediately to the employee health service for evaluation should they develop any of these signs and symptoms.

Healthcare workers who have active pulmonary or laryngeal TB pose a risk to patients and staff. Therefore, the CDC recommends that they be excluded from work until adequate treatment has been instituted, cough has resolved, and sputum has been found free of acid-fast bacilli on three consecutive smears taken on different days (15,24). Healthcare workers with TB at sites other than the lungs or larynx do not need to be excluded from work if concurrent pulmonary TB has been ruled out. Personnel with pulmonary TB who discontinue treatment before the recommended course of therapy has been completed should not be allowed to work until treatment is resumed, adequate response to therapy is documented, and they have three consecutive negative sputum smears taken on different days. Healthcare workers without evidence of active pulmonary tuberculosis who are receiving preventive treatment for latent TB infection should be allowed to continue usual work activities.

Healthcare workers who cannot take or do not accept or complete a full course of preventive therapy should have their work situations evaluated to determine whether reassignment is indicated (24). Work restrictions may not be necessary for otherwise healthy persons who do not accept or do not complete preventive therapy. These persons should be counseled about the risk of reactivation of infection and development of disease and should be instructed to seek evaluation promptly if symptoms develop that may be due to TB.

Annual and postexposure tuberculin skin test results should be monitored routinely. Results of skin tests should be placed in the healthcare worker's medical records and recorded in an aggregate form for analysis of skin test conversion patterns in various areas of the hospital. The aggregate data set should include information about each skin test conversion such as job classification, work location, date of first PPD, and date of positive PPD. Analysis of the aggregate data set is done by the infection control department to determine whether personnel in any area or service in the hospital have an increased incidence of skin test conversions. An increased incidence of skin test conversions in a given area or service may indicate that the infection control procedures to prevent transmission of TB in that area or service need to be improved.

Influenza

Since 1984, the recommendations of the Advisory Committee on Immunization Practices (ACIP) for immunization against influenza have included healthcare workers as a group, because they may transmit influenza to patients (27). The 2002 ACIP recommendations for the prevention and control of influenza state that the following groups should be vaccinated (28): (a) physicians, nurses, and other personnel in both hospital and outpatient-care settings, including medical emergency response workers (e.g., paramedics and emergency medical technicians); (b) employees of nursing homes and chronic-care facilities who have contact with patients or residents; (c) employees of assisted living and other residences for persons in groups at high risk from influenza; (d) persons who provide home care to persons in groups at high risk; and (e) household members (including children) of persons in groups at high risk.

All healthcare institutions should develop a policy to enhance the delivery of influenza vaccine to healthcare workers for the following reasons (28): (a) nosocomial outbreaks occur during the influenza season, and a well-immunized work force is less likely to transmit influenza to the patients under their care; (b) immunizations should minimize absenteeism during influenza outbreaks; and (c) influenza can be a serious disease and should not be confused with a cold or "intestinal flu." Immunization provides the best personal protection for each employee.

The vaccine should be offered beginning in October of each year. The employee health service and the infection control department need to collaborate in the education of healthcare workers about the importance of immunization against influenza. Measures should be taken to provide all healthcare workers, regardless of shift or work location, convenient access to influenza vaccinations at the work site, free of charge, as part of the employee health program (20). The risk of introducing influenza into high-risk groups, such as those with compromised cardiopulmonary or immune systems or infants in the neonatal intensive care unit, should be reduced by targeted vaccination programs of these medical personnel.

In addition to a vaccination program, monitoring the community for influenza activity and monitoring healthcare workers for influenza may help prevent nosocomial transmission of influenza. When healthcare workers have signs and symptoms of influenza, they should be evaluated by the employee health service, and if possible, viral cultures and serologic tests for antibodies to influenza should be obtained.

To reduce the spread of virus to persons at high risk during community or institutional outbreaks, chemoprophylaxis during peak influenza activity can be considered for unvaccinated persons who have frequent contact with persons at high risk. Persons with frequent contact include employees of hospitals, clinics, and chronic-care facilities, household members, visiting nurses and volunteer workers. If an outbreak is caused by a variant strain of influenza that might not be controlled by the vaccine, chemoprophylaxis should be considered for all such persons, regardless of their vaccination status (28) (see Chapter 41). In addition, the employee health service would be responsible for education of healthcare workers about the side effects of the prophylactic drugs, and for evaluation of healthcare workers for possible side effects of these medications. Healthcare workers with active disease should be relieved from duty, because it is estimated that viral shedding in the nasal secretions usually continues up to 7 days after the onset of illness (13,15). Healthcare workers should be cleared by the employee health service before returning to work.

Blood-Borne Diseases

All healthcare institutions should have a plan to follow-up all occupational exposures to blood-borne pathogens (29). Healthcare workers must be educated about the importance of promptly reporting exposures. Ideally, each institution should have a triage system available by telephone 24 hours a day. Such a triage service could be provided by the infection control department, by the employee health service, or jointly by both services. This system provides immediate triage, initial evaluation, and early prophylaxis if needed. It also permits early counseling for anxious healthcare workers after exposure. If the exposed healthcare worker is seen in urgent care or the emergency department at night or on weekends or holidays, he or she should be instructed to report to the employee health service on the next business day.

The interval within which postexposure prophylaxis for HIV should be started for optimal efficacy is unknown. An occupational exposure should be regarded as an urgent medical concern and postexposure prophylaxis started as soon as possible after the exposure (i.e., within a few hours rather than days) (30). In the author's hospital, the policy is to start prophylaxis within 2 hours of exposure.

Prompt reporting of all exposures is necessary for the timely administration of postexposure prophylaxis. Source patients should be evaluated for a history of high-risk behavior and should have serologic tests performed for viral hepatitis and HIV as soon as possible after the exposure. Infection control personnel should conduct the risk assessment. Once the risk assessment has been completed, the information should be shared with the employee health service so that postexposure prophylaxis can be administered as soon as possible after exposure (15) (see also Chapters 78 and 79).

Measles, Mumps, and Rubella

Healthcare workers are considered at higher risk of acquiring measles (rubeola), mumps, or rubella than the general population because of their chance exposure to either ambulatory or hospitalized patients being treated for these diseases (31). An effective immunization program for healthcare workers can markedly reduce this risk. In addition to protection for healthcare workers, such immunization programs can be expected to have institutional benefits, such as prevention of transmission of infectious diseases to patients and visitors, reduction of workers' sick days, and improved efficiency in the management of outbreaks and exposures.

When developing a measles, mumps, and rubella (MMR) vaccination program, the most accessible population for vaccination is the healthcare workers who are being seen for their post-offer evaluations. All healthcare workers who do not have documentation of physician-diagnosed measles, laboratory evidence of measles immunity, or contraindications to the MMR vaccine and who have not already received two doses should be vaccinated with MMR before starting work. All healthcare workers should be assessed during their annual physical/visit to the employee health service. If a healthcare worker had a contraindication to MMR vaccine during the last employee health service visit, that healthcare worker should be reassessed and the vaccine given if possible. If patients or personnel are exposed to measles, mumps or rubella, the following should be considered (31):

1. If the index case is an employee, the infection should be confirmed by the employee health service. Serum should be obtained for acute and convalescent antibody titers to help establish the diagnosis. However, results of serologic tests are usually not immediately available, and the response to most exposure incidents must be based on a clinical diagnosis. It must be remembered that measles, mumps, and rubella are no longer common childhood diseases, and each can easily be misdiagnosed by relying on clinical signs alone. Consultation

with a physician experienced in the diagnosis of measles, mumps, or rubella, such as a dermatologist, pediatrician, or infectious diseases specialist, should be considered if the diagnosis is unclear.
2. The activities of the index case, such as contact with coworkers on his/her unit and social contact with other healthcare workers in areas in which the employee has worked (e.g., nursing units, various departments, clinics), should be documented. A list of exposed healthcare workers should be sent to the employee health service.
3. Exposed healthcare workers with documentation of immunity by vaccination or positive serologic tests should be considered immune and not at risk for clinical disease.
4. Those without documented immunity should be vaccinated as soon as possible, if there are no contraindications, and furloughed as necessary. Exposure to measles requires a furlough from 5 days after the date of first exposure to 21 days from the date of last exposure (15–20,32,33). Those exposed to rubella should be furloughed from the seventh day after the first exposure to the 21st day after the last exposure (15, 20,34), and those exposed to mumps should be furloughed from the 12th day after the first exposure to the 26th day after the last exposure (12,13,15).
5. Exposure to measles or rubella is not a contraindication to vaccination. An emergency MMR vaccination program may be implemented if there is evidence that many employees are susceptible to the disease in question. Such an emergency program may be needed to prevent an outbreak of infections among employees.
6. During an outbreak of measles, all healthcare workers with direct patient contact who were born after 1957 should receive one dose of measles vaccine unless they can provide proof of immunity or document previous receipt of two doses of the measles vaccine (33) (see also Chapter 51).

Pertussis

Multiple outbreaks of pertussis in healthcare facilities have been reported in the literature. These outbreaks have resulted from failure to recognize and isolate infected infants and children, failure to treat the disease in staff members, and failure to quickly institute certain measures. Nosocomial acquisition of pertussis by healthcare workers has occurred during several outbreaks (34).

Recommendations and protocols for management of pertussis in healthcare facilities include postexposure prophylaxis for all asymptomatic exposed employees. Symptomatic employees should be treated and furloughed for the first 5 days of their therapy (35).

Therapy of infected patients and chemoprophylaxis of exposed healthcare workers has been successful in terminating outbreaks in healthcare institutions. Erythromycin has been the antibiotic of choice for both treatment and prophylaxis. Clarithromycin and azithromycin may be effective alternatives for prophylaxis; however, the latter antimicrobial agents have been studied only as treatment regimens (35) (see Chapters 80 and 81).

Meningococcal Exposure

Healthcare workers may be exposed to the meningococcus. Source patients with *Neisseria meningitidis* in their blood, spinal fluid, or respiratory secretions can be considered to be colonized with the microorganism in their oropharynx. Transmission is probably by way of large droplets. Exposure in a healthcare setting should be defined as an individual who has had close contact with the source patient with meningococcal disease. Close contact is defined as exposure to the patient's respiratory secretions (i.e., mouth-to-mouth resuscitation endotracheal intubation, or endotracheal tube management) but not as routine patient care activities (e.g., making beds, taking blood pressures) (36).

In the microbiology laboratory, care should be taken whenever droplet formation or aerosolization is possible (subculturing and serogrouping). It is recommended that all work manipulations be done in a biologic safety cabinet. Some states are now requiring those who perform testing on this microorganism receive the quadrivalent meningococcal polysaccharide vaccination for *N. meningitidis* types A, C, Y, and W-135 (37,38). Therefore, personnel in the microbiology laboratory must be considered for prophylaxis during the investigation of an exposure to *N. meningitidis.*

Infection control personnel should investigate every possible exposure, interview healthcare workers regarding possible exposure, and refer healthcare workers with exposures to the employee health service for prophylaxis (see Chapter 47).

Herpes Simplex Virus

Personnel with active herpes simplex virus infections pose certain problems for infection control. Healthcare workers with draining oral lesions need to be educated about the importance of good hand washing, use of barrier protection for the infected site (e.g., mask), and avoiding care of high-risk patients (e.g., immunocompromised patients, newborns). Healthcare workers with herpetic whitlow may transmit the virus even when wearing gloves (39). These healthcare workers should be excluded from patient care until the lesions are healed (2,15,38). There is no evidence that healthcare workers with genital herpes need work restrictions.

All healthcare workers should be educated about the need to seek evaluation at the employee health service for diagnosis, treatment, and potential reassignment or furlough for herpetic lesions. It is the responsibility of the infection control department to educate healthcare workers about their risk of acquiring and transmitting the herpes simplex virus and the importance of hand washing after contact with herpetic lesions in patients (see Chapter 43).

Ectoparasites

The most difficult part of dealing with healthcare workers who have been exposed, or presumably exposed, to an ectoparasite is contending with their hysteria. The employee health service and infection control department should work together and follow a consistent protocol for prophylaxis. In general, prophylaxis is not recommended for exposure to lice (sans bed mates).

Healthcare workers who have had prolonged skin-to-skin contact with patients with scabies may benefit from prophylactic treatment (i.e., permethrin 5%, lindane 1%, or crotamiton) (15). All healthcare workers must be made aware of the signs and symptoms of infestation, regardless of source of exposure, and must be instructed to report to the employee health service for treatment if such manifestations appear (see Chapter 46).

SYNDROMES THAT MAY BE DUE TO INFECTIOUS DISEASES

Diarrhea

An employee health policy should be developed that requires all employees with diarrhea to report to the employee health service for evaluation and clearance before reporting for work. Any employee with acute diarrhea should be relieved from work until it is determined whether there is an infectious etiology. The elements of good hand washing, especially after using the restroom, must be stressed.

Diarrhea in a food handler may be cause for concern. Because of the fecal-oral route of transmission for many bacterial and viral pathogens, the food handler may be the source of a hospital outbreak. It is very important that all food handlers report to the employee health service when they have diarrhea. They should comply with the hand washing policy after using the restroom and before handling food. They should also understand the proper use of gloves.

Skin Eruptions of Undetermined Cause

Many viral diseases such as chickenpox, measles, rubella, and Rocky Mountain spotted fever present with the sudden onset of a rash. Healthcare workers with a new-onset skin eruption should be instructed to report to the employee health service for diagnosis and clearance before reporting for work. Hospital-based outbreaks may be caused by a healthcare worker who does not report an eruption to the employee health service and continues to work, exposing patients and other healthcare workers.

The employee health service should play a pivotal role in the triage of all healthcare workers with a rash. Healthcare workers should be seen in the employee health service in a timely manner and evaluated by an experienced practitioner. Employees who have a communicable disease should be furloughed from work. All employees who have a rash that may be a manifestation of a communicable disease should be reported to the infection control department so that postexposure control measures may be instituted. Employees with skin eruptions may be sources of exposure for diseases associated with significant morbidity and mortality in hospitalized patients.

DERMATITIS

Frequent hand washing is stressed extensively in infection control educational programs. One consequence of this is development of dermatitis of the hands. It is probably more risky to provide patient care with weeping dermatitis than it is to forgo hand washing all together. Furthermore, transient microbial flora on the hands acquired by contact with patients and environmental surfaces cannot be removed by hand washing when healthcare workers have dermatitis of their hands.

Dermatitis can be caused by a variety of factors, but in healthcare workers it is most commonly caused by excessive hand washing, harsh hand soaps, and use of gloves. Healthcare workers who scrub for operative procedures often react to the harshness of the scrub brushes. In addition, the unavailability of moisturizing lotion can lead to dry and cracked skin, especially during the cooler winter season.

Infection control professionals should encourage not only good hand washing but also good hand maintenance. When employees develop hand dermatitis, they should be instructed to report to the employee health service. Protecting the hands of healthcare workers from dermatitis is important for the health of the healthcare worker and for patients. The employee health service can help prevent nosocomial infections by consulting with infection control regarding reported cases of hand dermatitis and offering healthcare workers education and alternatives regarding daily hand maintenance.

Latex Allergy

Latex is liquid sap from the commercial rubber tree. Latex contains naturally occurring impurities (e.g., plant proteins and peptides), which are believed to be responsible for allergic reactions. Latex is processed to form natural rubber latex and dry natural rubber. Dry natural rubber and natural rubber latex might contain the same plant impurities as latex but in lesser amounts. Natural rubber latex is used to produce medical gloves, catheters, and other products. Dry natural rubber is used in syringe plungers, vial stoppers, and injection ports on intravascular tubing. Synthetic rubber and synthetic latex also are used in medical gloves, syringe plungers, and vial stoppers. Synthetic rubber and synthetic latex do not contain natural rubber or natural latex, and therefore do not contain the impurities linked to allergic reactions (40).

Reactions Associated with Latex Exposure

1. *Contact irritant dermatitis:* This is the most common type of reaction. It is not an allergic reaction that involves the immune system. Symptoms often present as skin irritations (e.g., dry, itchy, cracked, and reddened). Latex allergens may be absorbed through the openings in the skin and could progress to a true allergy (41).
2. *Type IV delayed hypersensitivity (allergic contact dermatitis):* This is the second most common type of reaction reported due to latex exposure. This type of allergic reaction is mediated by T cells and is typically characterized by swelling, burning, itching, and rashes on hands when using gloves containing natural rubber latex (NRL). The reaction can occur in as little as 6 hours and up to 48 hours after an exposure to the offensive allergens. Allergic contact dermatitis associated with poison ivy exposure is an example of a type IV reaction. Generally, allergic contact dermatitis may spread

beyond the area that has been exposed to the offensive allergen. Conversely, irritant contact dermatitis generally does not extend beyond the area of contact. Type IV reactions can progress to type I reactions with repeated exposure (41).

3. *Type I immediate hypersensitivity:* This is the least common type of reaction but is the most serious and potentially life threatening. It is an immune response to a foreign substance (latex protein) and produces such symptoms as edema of the exposed site(s), nausea, vomiting, sneezing, nasal congestion, or systemic reactions. Reactions typically begin within minutes, but may take several hours to manifest. The airways can close down, which may result in respiratory arrest. If not handled properly by medical personnel during such a reaction, anaphylactic type reactions can be fatal. Fatal reactions have been reported from exposure to NRL even when patients have no history of latex allergy (41).

Recognized Routes of Latex Exposure

1. *Cutaneous* exposure can occur while wearing latex gloves or touching other latex products.
2. *Percutaneous* exposure can occur if the latex protein gets under the skin as with dry, irritated, and cracked skin.
3. *Mucosal* exposure occurs when touching a latex balloon to one's lips and mouth while blowing it up or having a dental procedure with a rubber dental dam.
4. *Parenteral* exposure occurs when medications are injected through a latex IV port or with a syringe with a dry rubber latex (DRL)-tipped plunger. In this way, allergens are injected into the body or bloodstream.
5. *Aerosol* exposure may occur when an individual enters a room in which someone has donned powered latex gloves (causing proteins to be airborne) and protein particles are inhaled into the lungs.

At-Risk Healthcare Workers

Healthcare workers may be at increased risk of developing a latex allergy if they work in a clinical environment where latex products are frequently used. Healthcare workers with a history of multiple allergies, especially foods such as bananas, chestnuts, kiwi, avocados, or other tropical fruits, also are at risk. Asthma, allergic rhinitis, and hand dermatitis in a latex glove wearer also raises the risk of developing latex allergy.

The American Academy of Allergy and Immunology (AAAI) determined that because there is no known cure for this allergy, it would be beneficial to implement regulations early to prevent the allergy from becoming widespread. On September 30, 1997, the Food and Drug Administration (FDA) ruled that "All medical devices containing latex [MUST] be labeled as such and [MUST] carry a caution that latex can cause allergic reactions" (42).

The National Institute of Occupational Safety and Health issued comprehensive recommendations regarding latex in 1997. The recommendation was aimed at the employer and the employee. The healthcare facility was encouraged to use nonlatex gloves when latex was not absolutely necessary. It also encouraged education about latex allergies and periodic screening of high-risk employees. It was recommended that the employees take the initiative to rid the work environment of latex containing dust (42).

In studies of healthcare workers, self-reported hypersensitivity is fairly common and closely associated with the use of medical gloves. There are no diagnostic tests or standardized criteria to diagnosis latex allergy. It is recommended that each institution assess the use of latex products and try to minimize it. Also, education is recommended for all healthcare workers about their personal risk and the risk they pose to their patients.

SPECIAL EMPLOYEE POPULATIONS

Day-Care Centers Associated with Hospitals

As competition among healthcare institutions grows, more institutions are offering on-site day-care centers for the children of healthcare workers. Employees in day-care centers may be exposed to a greater variety of infections compared with their counterparts in the main healthcare facility (see Chapter 53). Infection control departments and employee health services are frequently charged with providing services for associated day-care facilities.

Diseases Commonly Encountered in Day Care

Enteric Diseases

Fecal-oral transmission of pathogens such as *Salmonella, Shigella, Escherichia coli, Campylobacter,* hepatitis A, rotavirus, and a variety of parasites are common in day-care centers. It is imperative that the infection control department educate the staff frequently on proper hygienic practices such as hand washing, diapering, and infant feeding. Employees in this area must understand the importance of reporting to the employee health service for any gastrointestinal signs and symptoms and/or diarrhea to avoid spread of disease in this highly susceptible population.

Respiratory Infections

Children with respiratory infections may shed viruses before the onset of symptoms, making control of infections due to respiratory syncytial virus, parainfluenza virus, adenovirus, and other respiratory viruses difficult. Although infection control professionals need to educate the employees on hand washing, the employee health service can also help prevent the spread of diseases by diagnosing communicable diseases in employees and furloughing them during the infectious stage of their illness. Because the day-care center employees are asked to report to the employee health service for symptoms of any respiratory infection, the employee health service should document each case and share data on respiratory infections with infection control. In the event a higher than expected rate of disease is discovered in the day-care center, infection control professionals can investigate and implement control measures.

Skin and Cutaneous Infections

As in the hospitalized population, lice and scabies pose a unique problem to employees in the day-care center. Employees or day-care center attendees may also contract and expose others to herpes simplex virus or bacterial pathogens such as group A β-hemolytic streptococci. It is important that both the infection control department and the employee health service are notified in the event of a case of cutaneous infection. The infection control department should investigate the exposure, and the employee health service should evaluate employees, provide treatment, and determine whether employees can continue to work or should be furloughed.

Day-Care Center Employee Health Policies

Policies for the prevention of infections in the day-care setting and adherence to these policies are important for effective infection control in day-care centers. The policies must be in compliance with the appropriate regulatory agency guidelines. The policies relating to employee health should require (a) documented evidence of immunity to tetanus, measles, mumps, rubella, diphtheria, and poliomyelitis in caregivers either by immunization or serologic evidence of prior infection; (b) TB screening within 1 month of starting work and then annually, and appropriate follow-up protocols for PPD skin test converters; (c) annual updating for immunizations; and (d) guidelines for work restrictions if an employee has a communicable disease (i.e., furloughed from direct child care or excluded from work until the disease is no longer contagious).

Prehospital Healthcare Workers

Today, firefighters, emergency medical technicians, police officers, and others often are exposed to infectious diseases during patient care and transport to the hospital. The receiving hospital is often called on to triage and treat these prehospital healthcare workers or at least to ensure that their exposures are managed appropriately.

For the most part, prehospital healthcare workers transport patients with undiagnosed diseases. Therefore, when a patient has a disease transmitted by the airborne route, such as TB or chickenpox, or by large droplets, such as meningococcal disease, prehospital healthcare workers may be inadvertently exposed. It is important that infection control professionals include prehospital healthcare workers in investigations of exposures. Prehospital healthcare workers may be evaluated, prophylaxed, and followed up by the hospital employee health service just as the hospital's healthcare workers are evaluated, prophylaxed, and followed up after exposures to communicable diseases. If a separate healthcare provider has been established for the prehospital healthcare workers, the infection control department should communicate directly with that provider.

Prehospital healthcare workers are most at risk for exposures to blood and body fluids via needlesticks and splashes to mucous membranes. A system of reporting such exposures must be developed and included either in the hospital employee health program or by the outside healthcare provider. Education of the prehospital healthcare workers about reporting all exposures is important to the success of such programs. All prehospital healthcare workers need to know the mechanism for reporting exposures and fully understand the importance of postexposure evaluation, prophylaxis, and follow-up (see Chapter 83).

Emergency Department: An After-Hours Employee Health Service

Traditionally, employee health services operate during the day Monday through Friday. However, employees who sustain an exposure after hours, on weekends, or on holidays usually report to the emergency department. Thus, the emergency department is often an extension of the employee health service, and communication between the emergency department and the employee health service and interaction with the infection control department is important to provide continuity of care for exposed employees.

Protocols for meningococcal exposure prophylaxis, hepatitis B vaccination and hepatitis B immune globulin administration, prophylaxis for exposure to HIV, and diagnosis of diseases such as chickenpox and measles are extremely helpful to emergency room doctors and nurses who are triaging an employee. Consistency in delivering care is the goal. Although the initial diagnosis or prophylaxis may occur in the emergency department, employees receive their follow-up care at the employee health service and their records are permanently filed in that location.

Although protocols outline the various interventions that are needed postexposure, it is important that emergency department physicians document the following: (a) complete description of the exposure; (b) completed employee occurrence report; (c) type of prophylaxis administered (e.g., hepatitis B vaccine, hepatitis B immune globulin) and schedule of additional doses if required; (d) clear communication to employee regarding furlough status (after communication with the infection control department); and (e) referral to the employee health service, as soon as possible, to arrange follow-up care for any exposed or ill employee.

REFERENCES

1. Alter SJ, Hammond JA, McVey CJ, et al. Susceptibility to varicella-zoster virus among adults at high risk for exposure. *Infect Control* 1986;7:448–451.
2. Lievens W, Taylor-Wiedeman J, Brunell PA. Immunity of young adults to childhood diseases. *Pediatr Res* 1984;18:185A(abst).
3. Morens DM, Bregman DJ, West CM, et al. An outbreak of varicella zoster virus infection among cancer patients 1980. *Ann Intern Med* 1980;93:414–419.
4. Murray DL, Cleveland RP, Keefe C. Varicella-zoster dilemma: common sense in medical education. *Am J Public Health* 1986;76:1362–1363.
5. Steele RW, Coleman MA, Fiser M, et al. Varicella zoster in hospital personnel: skin test reactivity to monitor susceptibility. *Pediatrics* 1982;70:604–608.
6. McKinney WP, Horowitz MM, Battiola RJ. Susceptibility of hospital-based healthcare personnel to varicella-zoster virus infections. *Am J Infect Control* 1989;17:26–30.
7. Hoffman KK, Weber DJ, Rutala WA. Infection control strategies relevant to employee health. *AAOHN J* 1991;39:167–181.
8. Myers MG, Rasley DA, Hierholzer WJ. Hospital infection control for varicella zoster virus infection. *Pediatrics* 1982;70:199–202.
9. Shehab ZM, Burnell PA. Susceptibility of hospital personnel to varicella virus. *J Infect Dis* 1984;150:786.

10. Weber DJ, Rutala WA, Parham C. Impact and cost of varicella prevention in a university hospital 1988. *Am J Public Health* 1988;78:19–23.
11. Krasinki K, Holzman RS, LaCuture R, et al. Hospital experience with varicella-zoster virus. *Infect Control* 1986;7:312–316.
12. Williams WW. CDC guidelines for infection control in hospital personnel. *Infect Control* 1983;4:326–347.
13. Peter G, ed. *2000 Red book: report of the Committee on Infectious Diseases*, 25th ed. Elk Grove Village, IL: American Academy of Pediatrics, 2000.
14. Centers for Disease Control. Varicella-zoster immunoglobulin for the prevention of chickenpox. *Ann Intern Med* 1984;100:859–865.
15. Bolyard E, Tablao, Williams W, et al. Guideline for infection control in healthcare personnel, 1998. *Infect Control Hosp Epidemiol* 1998;26: 289–327.
16. Lyznicki J, Berman R, Genel M. Report on the Council on Scientific Affairs of the American Medical Association, immunization of healthcare workers with varicella vaccine. *Infect Control Hosp Epidemiol* 1998;19:348–353.
17. Weber D, Rutala W, Hamilton H. Prevention and control of varicella-zoster infections in healthcare facilities. *Infect Control Hosp Epidemiol* 1996;17:694–705.
18. Centers for Disease Control and Prevention. Prevention of varicella: recommendations of the Advisory Committee on Immunization Practices (ACIP). *MMWR* 1996;45:1–36.
19. U.S. Preventive Services Task Force. Adult immunization. In: *Guide to clinical preventive services,* 2nd ed. Baltimore: Williams & Wilkins, 1996:791–814.
20. Centers for Disease Control and Prevention. Immunization of healthcare workers: recommendations of the Advisory Committee on Immunization Practices (APIC) and the Hospital Infection Control Practices Advisory Committee (HICPAC). *MMWR* 1997;46(RR-18);25.
21. Gardner P, Eickhoff T, Poland G, et al. Adult immunizations. *Ann Intern Med* 1996;124:35–40.
22. American Thoracic Society. Infectiousness of tuberculosis: a statement of the Ad Hoc Committee on Treatment of Tuberculosis Patients in Hospitals. *Am Rev Respir Dis* 1967;96:836–837.
23. Centers for Disease Control. *Guidelines for prevention of TB transmission in hospitals.* Atlanta: U.S. Public Health Service, 1982;82:8371.
24. Centers for Disease Control and Prevention. Guidelines now for preventing the transmission of Mycobacterium tuberculosis in healthcare facilities, 1994. *MMWR* 1994;43(RR-13):2–55.
25. Centers for Disease Control. Tuberculosis mortality in the United States: final data, 1990. *MMWR* 1991;40:23–27.
26. Centers for Disease Control. Tuberculosis and human immunodeficiency virus infection: recommendation of the Advisory Committee for the Elimination of Tuberculosis (ACET). *MMWR* 1989;38: 236–238,243–250.
27. Centers for Disease Control. Recommendations of the Immunization Practices Advisory Committee (APIC), prevention and control of influenza. *MMWR* 1984;33:253–266.
28. Centers for Disease Control and Prevention. Prevention and control of influenza: recommendations of the Advisory Committee on Immunization Practices. *MMWR* 2002;51(RR-3):1–36.
29. Occupational Safety and Health Administration. Final rule on occupational exposure to bloodborne pathogens. *Fed Reg* 1991;56: 64004–64182.
30. Centers for Disease Control and Prevention. Public Health Service guidelines for the management of health-care worker exposures to HIV and recommendations for postexposure prophylaxis. *MMWR* 1998;47: 18.
31. Centers for Disease Control and Prevention. Measles, mumps, and rubella—vaccine use and strategies for elimination of measles, rubella, and congenital rubella syndrome and control of mumps: recommendations of the Advisory Committee on Immunization Practices (ACIP). *MMWR* 1998;47(RR-8):1–58.
32. Davis DM, Orenstein WA, Frank JA Jr, et al. Transmission of measles in a medical setting. *JAMA* 1986;255:1295–1298.
33. Centers for Disease Control. Measles prevention: recommendations of the Immunization Practices Advisory Committee (ACIP). *MMWR* 1989;38:5–9.
34. Centers for Disease Control. Rubella prevention: recommendations of the Immunization Practices Advisory Committee (ACIP). *MMWR* 1990;39:1–18.
35. Weber DJ, Rutala WA. Pertussis: a continuing hazard for healthcare facilities. *Infect Control Hosp Epidemiol* 2001;22:736–740.
36. Centers for Disease Control and Prevention. Control and prevention of meningococcal disease and control and prevention of serogroup C meningococcal disease: evaluation and management of suspected outbreaks: recommendations of the Advisory Committee on Immunization Practices (ACIP). *MMWR* 1997;46(RR-5):6–7..
37. Risk of exposure to meningococcal disease in the laboratory. *TDH* 2002;62(7):1–3.
38. Centers for Disease Control and Prevention. Laboratory-acquired meningococcal disease—United States, 2000. *MMWR* 2002;51(7): 380–383.
39. Simmon BP, Gelfand MS. Herpes simplex virus. *Infect Control* 1986; 7:380–383.
40. Atkinson WL, Pickering LK, Schwartz B, et al. Centers for Disease Control. General recommendations on immunization. Recommendations of the Advisory Committee on Immunization Practices (ACIP) and the American Academy of Family Physicians (AAFP). *MMWR* 2002:51(RR-02):1–36.
41. Thurlow KL. Latex allergies: management and clinical responsibilities. *Home Healthcare Nurse* 2001;19(6):369.
42. Zaglaniczny K. Latex allergy: are you at risk? *AANA* 2001;69(5).

100

MEDICAL WASTE MANAGEMENT

JUDITH G. GORDON
PETER A. REINHARDT
GERALD A. DENYS

Until fairly recently, medical waste management was generally not considered an issue, and it had no special relevance for infection control, occupational safety, the public health, or the environment. Only wastes from microbiology laboratories had traditionally received special handling. In the 1980s and 1990s, concerns about exposure to the human immunodeficiency virus (HIV) and hepatitis B virus (HBV) led to questions about potential risks inherent in medical wastes. Laws and regulations to control medical wastes were promulgated at the federal and state levels. In response, institutional waste management programs were expanded, and specialized commercial services for disposal of medical waste became available. The cost of medical waste management increased substantially. We hope that refined regulations will better reflect our knowledge of the risks actually present in medical waste.

This chapter generally uses the term *medical waste*—a term that is more appropriate than *infectious waste*, because there is no safe and simple method to test waste for infectiousness. Furthermore, this category also includes waste that presents a physical hazard (e.g., sharps) and waste that has the potential to cause a nuisance or lead to aesthetic degradation of the environment if disposed of carelessly. It is common practice to define medical waste by source and type rather than by detrimental characteristics. Nevertheless, the term *infectious waste* sometimes is cited in this chapter because federal agencies use the term.

This chapter provides guidance for infection control in healthcare institutions with respect to the management of medical waste, medical waste being the discarded materials that serve no further purpose and are considered to be wastes, designated for disposal. For information on the management, disinfection, reuse of reusable items and supplies, and reuse of disposable items, see Chapters 74, 85, and 87.

The term *waste management* is used rather than *waste disposal* because our discussion is much broader than just the disposal process. For waste management to be efficient, the waste should be managed at every step: from acquisition of materials that eventually become waste, to waste generation, discard, collection, containment, handling, accumulation, storage, transport, treatment, and finally disposal. "Disposal" refers to the final disposition of waste or waste treatment products, such as placement in a solid waste landfill. (In this sense, "solid waste" refers to ordinary trash, garbage, refuse, etc.)

The rationale for special management of medical waste is based on three considerations. First, it has long been standard practice among healthcare institutions to take additional precautions with certain wastes that appear to be more hazardous than the rest of the waste stream. For example, it has been standard practice to contain, and often treat, waste from the microbiology laboratory and waste soaked with blood or other potentially infectious materials, such as operating room waste. Second, some federal, state, and local laws regulate the management of medical waste with the goals of minimizing risks to workers who handle waste and of minimizing any possible adverse environmental effects as well as aesthetic degradation of the environment. These laws reflect the concern of the general public, to which healthcare institutions are extremely sensitive. The third consideration in managing medical waste is the lack of epidemiologic evidence that medical waste poses a risk to public health, which argues against extreme control measures.

When choosing medical waste management practices, therefore, healthcare practitioners must weigh what they judge to be prudent practice, the need to meet legal requirements, and the scientific basis for their chosen waste management practices. This chapter seeks that balance; it is meant to aid the practitioner in making sound legal medical waste management decisions.

DEFINING AND CHARACTERIZING MEDICAL WASTE

Waste from healthcare institutions consists of all the wastes generated during the care, diagnosis, and treatment of patients and during medical and pharmaceutical research. Such waste is varied, consisting of infectious, chemical [some of which is hazardous according to the Resource Conservation and Recovery Act (RCRA) regulations], radioactive, and multihazardous wastes (i.e., wastes that are infectious and chemically hazardous and/or radioactive). Medical facilities also generate wastewater, food wastes, and general trash. This discussion is limited to medical wastes because the focus of this chapter is on the infection control aspects of medical waste. (For comprehensive coverage of all wastes from healthcare institutions, see refs. 1, 2, and 3.)

Infectious waste acquired new importance with passage of

RCRA in 1976 when Congress used the term *infectious characteristics* in the definition of "hazardous waste" (4). This legislation evoked concern in the medical community about the effect hazardous waste regulations might have on the practices and costs of infectious waste management. (For a discussion of relevant regulations, see Regulatory Considerations, below.)

The development of infectious waste regulations at the federal and state levels was accompanied by a proliferation of the terms used to describe this type of waste, with no uniform terminology being adopted or achieving universal usage. These terms included *infectious, infective, red bag, medical, biomedical, biologic, contaminated,* and *biohazardous.* The particular types of waste that were classified as infectious also varied with the agency and the jurisdiction.

Types of Infectious Waste

Even federal agencies have not defined infectious waste uniformly. It is important to realize that these differences are attributable to the unique mission of each federal agency. Also, the infection control aspects were not always, and sometimes were rarely, a factor in an agency's approach to infectious waste management.

Thus, the Centers for Disease Control and Prevention (CDC), in guidelines for prevention of the transmission of HIV, HBV, and hepatitis C virus, listed types of infective waste generated by patients with these diseases (5–8). The U.S. Occupational Safety and Health Administration (OSHA) addressed infectious waste as an aspect of occupational exposure to blood-borne pathogens (9). The U.S. Environmental Protection Agency (EPA) was concerned with protection of the environment from waste mismanagement and related environmental degradation (10–12). Table 100.1 compares the types of waste listed as infectious by these agencies. Medical waste regulated under the OSHA blood-borne pathogens standard is called "regulated waste" (13). The EPA medical waste tracking regulations referred to "regulated medical waste" (14), whereas the EPA hospital/medical/infectious waste incinerator regulations refer to "medical/infectious" waste and to "hospital" waste (15). The U.S. Department of Transportation (DOT) recently issued regulations for transport of "regulated medical waste" (16).

Select Agents

Select agents are biologic agents that have significant potential for misuse, either inadvertently or as the result of a terrorist or criminal act. Select agents may be used or found in research, diagnosis, verification, and proficiency testing. The U.S. Department of Health and Human Services (DHHS) and the U.S. Department of Agriculture have identified these agents and specified notification and destruction procedures (17). Cultures and stocks as well as wastes that contain select agents are subject to these regulations.

Infectious Waste from Isolation Rooms

For several centuries, hospitals have used isolation precautions for patients with either suspected or known infectious diseases. The CDC and others have published various guidelines on isolation precautions for hospitals (6,18,19), the most recent being that published in 1996 by the CDC Hospital Infection Control Practices Advisory Committee (HICPAC) (19). However, none of the new isolation precautions guidelines altered the basic disposal recommendations for medical waste generated in any patient care area.

TABLE 100.1. TYPES OF INFECTIOUS WASTE LISTED BY FEDERAL AGENCIES

Waste Type	CDC[a]	OSHA[b]	EPA[c]	EPA[d,e]
Microbiologic laboratory waste	Yes	Yes[f]	Yes	Yes
Pathology waste	Yes	Yes[f]	Yes	Yes
Human blood specimens and blood products	Yes	Yes	Yes	Yes
Sharps (i.e., needles, blades, etc.), contaminated	Yes	Yes[g]	Yes	Yes
Sharps, uncontaminated	No	No	No	Yes
Isolation waste	No	No	Yes	Yes
Cultures and stocks and associated biologics	No	Maybe[h]	Yes	Yes
Contaminated animal carcasses, body parts, and bedding	No	Maybe[h]	Yes	Yes
Contaminated wastes from surgery and autopsy	No	Maybe[i]	Optional	Maybe[j]
Contaminated laboratory wastes	No	Maybe[i]	Optional	Maybe[j]
Dialysis unit wastes	No	Yes	Optional	Maybe[j]
Contaminated equipment	No	Maybe[i]	Optional	No

[a] Centers for Disease Control and Prevention's "infective wastes" (5–8).
[b] U.S. Occupational Safety and Health Administration's bloodborne pathogen rule refers to "blood and other potentially infectious materials" (13).
[c] U.S. Environmental Protection Agency's guidance manual classifies infectious waste categories as recommended or optional (10).
[d] U.S. Environmental Protection Agency's medical waste tracking regulations lists classes of "regulated medical waste" (14).
[e] U.S. Environmental Protection Agency's hospital/medical/infectious waste incinerator regulations define "medical/infectious waste" (15) to correspond to the definition of "regulated medical waste" in the medical waste tracking regulations (14).
[f] If the waste contains blood or other potentially infectious materials.
[g] If contaminated with blood or other potentially infectious materials.
[h] If from a research laboratory or production facility that produces or uses human immunodeficiency virus (HIV) or hepatitis B virus (HBV).
[i] If the waste can release liquid, semiliquid, or dried blood or other potentially infectious material during handling.
[j] Items that are saturated and/or dripping with human blood and items that were saturated and/or dripping with human blood that are now caked with dried human blood; may be included in another category of regulated medical waste or medical/infectious waste.

Under isolation precautions, as in any healthcare setting, disposable syringes with attached needles, scalpel blades, and other sharp items capable of causing injury must be placed into designated puncture-resistant containers located as close as is practical to the item's point of use. Bulk blood or other body fluids may be carefully poured down a drain or other plumbing connected to a sanitary sewer. According to the HICPAC guidelines, disposable items or articles soiled with infective material may be placed with the patient's general waste in a bag or in a container that prevents leaking and that is not easily torn or penetrated in transport (19).

The EPA has taken a more rigid stand than the CDC on classifying waste from patients in isolation precautions. Isolation wastes were classified as "regulated medical waste" under the EPA medical waste tracking regulations (14) and as "medical/infectious waste" under the EPA's hospital/medical/infectious waste incinerator regulations (15). This category refers specifically to waste from patients with contagious highly communicable diseases such as those caused by certain etiologic agents (e.g., Lassa, Marburg, and Ebola viruses). Reports of Lassa fever in the United States suggest that the spread of Lassa fever virus can be prevented by the use of accepted barrier techniques such as standard precautions or body substance isolation, which includes waste management (20,21).

These findings and the CDC guidelines negate the rationale for the EPA requirements. However, some states adopted EPA's medical waste tracking regulations, and in these states, compliance with the regulations is mandatory even if a scientific basis is lacking.

Medical Waste in the Home Care Setting

Because patients are now being discharged from the acute care setting to the home care setting at a much earlier time in their recovery, patients, family members, and/or home healthcare providers must deliver patient care in the home. Also, many procedures that were previously performed on an inpatient basis or during a clinic visit are now administered in the patient's home. Instructions for home healthcare are given by the healthcare facility or by the home healthcare agency; these instructions should include procedures for disposal of all medical wastes that are generated in the home. Wastes from the home (households) are generally not regulated, but appropriate waste management practices should be encouraged because of the protection they provide to waste handlers (22,23).

Handling and disposing of medical waste generated in the home becomes the responsibility, theoretically if not physically, of all involved—the healthcare facility, the home healthcare agency, and/or the patient and the patient's caregivers. The handling and disposal of such waste may be subject to state requirements. Most states allow medical waste generated in the home to be disposed of in the regular household garbage. However, some states do regulate the handling and disposal of medical waste generated in the home by the personnel of home healthcare agencies (24).

Every year Americans use more than one billion sharp objects in their homes to administer healthcare. These "sharps" include lancets, needles, and syringes. If not disposed of in puncture-resistant containers, sharps pose a risk of injury to trash handlers and others. Although not proven to be an infectious risk in household garbage, contaminated materials such as bandages, dressings, disposable sheets, and soiled medical gloves certainly could have a deleterious effect on the environment aesthetically.

Needles, syringes, lancets, and other sharps should be placed in hard plastic or metal containers. Many home healthcare facilities provide sharps containers and offer medical waste disposal for their clients as part of the treatment contract. Commercial medical sharps containers can be purchased for use in the home. Alternatively, many containers found in the household are also suitable for use for the disposal of medical sharps (22,23). For example, large, empty, hard plastic laundry detergent bottles with screw-on lids make excellent sharps disposal containers for the home. Because most communities with waste recycling programs recycle this type of plastic container, a container used for sharps disposal must be kept out of the recycling waste stream. Furthermore, it must be marked "Not Recyclable" or "Do Not Recycle."

Soiled bandages, disposable sheets, medical gloves, or other nonsharp disposable medical items should be placed in plastic bags that are securely fastened and disposed of in the garbage with other household waste. Color-coded or labeled bags are not necessary, and it is not necessary to identify this waste. Rather, the objective is to contain the waste and to protect others from contact with the waste. This barrier precaution is easily accomplished with commercially available, securely fastened, plastic garbage bags.

Blood, feces, urine, or other body fluids can be disposed of in the sewer system (toilet) without containment or additional treatment.

In 1993, the EPA published tips on disposal for home healthcare for both the healthcare professional (22) and the patient (23). The two brochures provide information on how to properly dispose of medical sharps and other medical waste generated during home healthcare. The brochures are available from EPA's National Center for Environmental Publications and Information (1-800-490-9198), through e-mail at *RCRA-Docket@epamail.epa.gov,* or on the Internet at *http://www.epa.gov.*

Safe disposal of medical wastes begins at the point of generation (25). As patient care moves from hospitals and clinics to the patient's home, the same precautions used for sharps disposal in the traditional patient care setting should be used. The home healthcare agency must be aware of state and local laws and regulations pertaining to medical waste generated during home healthcare, and they should develop a medical waste disposal program. Their personnel should be encouraged to educate patients and clients on how to safely dispose of sharps in their homes. (See Chapter 107 for more information on infection control in the home healthcare setting.)

Multihazardous Waste

Multihazardous waste includes waste that is infectious and that contains radionuclides and/or hazardous chemicals. An example is waste contaminated with blood or body fluids and with a chemotherapy drug. Multihazardous waste is best managed and treated separately from other infectious waste.

It should be noted that mercury thermometers are not infectious waste, and they should not be classified and managed as such. All unwanted or broken mercury thermometers should be managed and disposed of as hazardous chemical waste. They should never be placed in sharps containers.

Microbiology of Medical Waste

Practically it is impossible to ascertain the microbial load of medical waste because of the difficulties in obtaining representative samples and in providing all the required conditions for culture of all the microorganisms that may be present. In addition, such activity is not recommended because of biosafety considerations.

Based on the literature to date, no conclusions can be drawn. Management decisions, therefore, should be based on the potential risk that is posed by medical waste.

HEALTH IMPLICATIONS OF MEDICAL WASTE

Even though hospitals are subject to elaborate regulation of medical waste, very little disease transmission from medical waste has been documented.

Risk to Healthcare Workers from Medical Waste

The potential for infection from contact with nonsharp medical waste is virtually nonexistent (26,27). The only medical waste that has been associated with infectious diseases transmission is contaminated sharps. Obviously, this potential for transmission exists when infectious sharps are mishandled and are not properly discarded or contained (28). The OSHA blood-borne pathogens standard specifies requirements for the handling, discard, and containment of contaminated sharps (9) (see Containing Medical Waste, below).

Risk to Handlers of Medical Waste

Waste handlers incur risks of exposure from medical waste that are similar to those of healthcare workers. Improperly contained, contaminated sharps pose the greatest infectious risk associated with hospital waste. There is also a theoretical health risk to medical waste handlers from pathogens that may be aerosolized during the compacting, grinding, or shredding process that is associated with certain medical waste management/treatment practices (29).

Another potential health risk for medical waste handlers is physical injury due to handling heavy and cumbersome waste containers. Physical and health hazards are also associated with the high operating temperatures of incinerators and steam sterilizers and with toxic gases vented into the atmosphere after waste treatment (29).

Risk to the Public from Medical Waste

Medical waste poses virtually no infectious hazard to the public or the environment (26,30). Public impacts of medical waste disposal are confined to aesthetic degradation of the environment from careless disposal (e.g., improper containment and medical litter) and the environmental impact of improperly operated incinerators or other medical waste treatment equipment.

MEDICAL WASTE MANAGEMENT: SEGREGATION, CONTAINMENT, HANDLING, STORAGE, AND TRANSPORT

Figure 100.1 depicts the options available for medical waste management, starting with purchasing decisions and then following the waste pathway from point of waste generation to treatment to ultimate disposal (1–3,31,32). Storage is not included in the figure, because waste can be stored at any point along the management pathway.

Medical waste should be managed according to its type and characteristics. Therefore, it is prudent to keep different waste types separate. Waste containers are usually handled manually, so protection of waste handlers is key to reducing risks of exposure. Protection is best accomplished through proper containment of the waste and prompt waste treatment.

Source Separation and Waste Segregation

Source separation of waste means separating, at the point of generation and discard, wastes with distinct characteristics into separate waste streams (such as infectious waste, radioactive waste, etc.). Separation is usually accomplished by using different and distinct waste collection containers for each type of waste. For example, medical waste and normal trash should be kept separate. Sharps must be placed into special puncture-resistant containers, and, to further facilitate source separation, these containers should be easily accessible to personnel and must be located as close as feasible to the immediate area where sharps are used (33). In addition, it is prudent to separate recyclable items, such as aluminum cans and newspapers.

Such separation is best done when materials are discarded as waste (at the point of waste generation), because the person who discards the waste is generally most knowledgeable about its nature. Brief instructions at the point of discard (e.g., posted above the waste container) facilitate compliance with source separation, as does placing containers for the different waste types as close as possible to the point of waste generation, even though this may require the use of several collection containers at a particular point of waste generation. Source separation eliminates the need for subsequent sorting of wastes (which could be hazardous) as well as the extra effort and expense that such sorting entails.

Waste segregation means keeping waste streams separate from the point of generation through collection and handling, accumulation, storage, transport, and treatment. Source separation and waste segregation permit efficient waste management through the application of methods that are specific to each waste stream. Therefore, waste handlers should keep the different waste streams segregated in order to enhance efficiency.

For source separation and waste segregation to be successful, there must be an explicit label on each waste receptacle and a

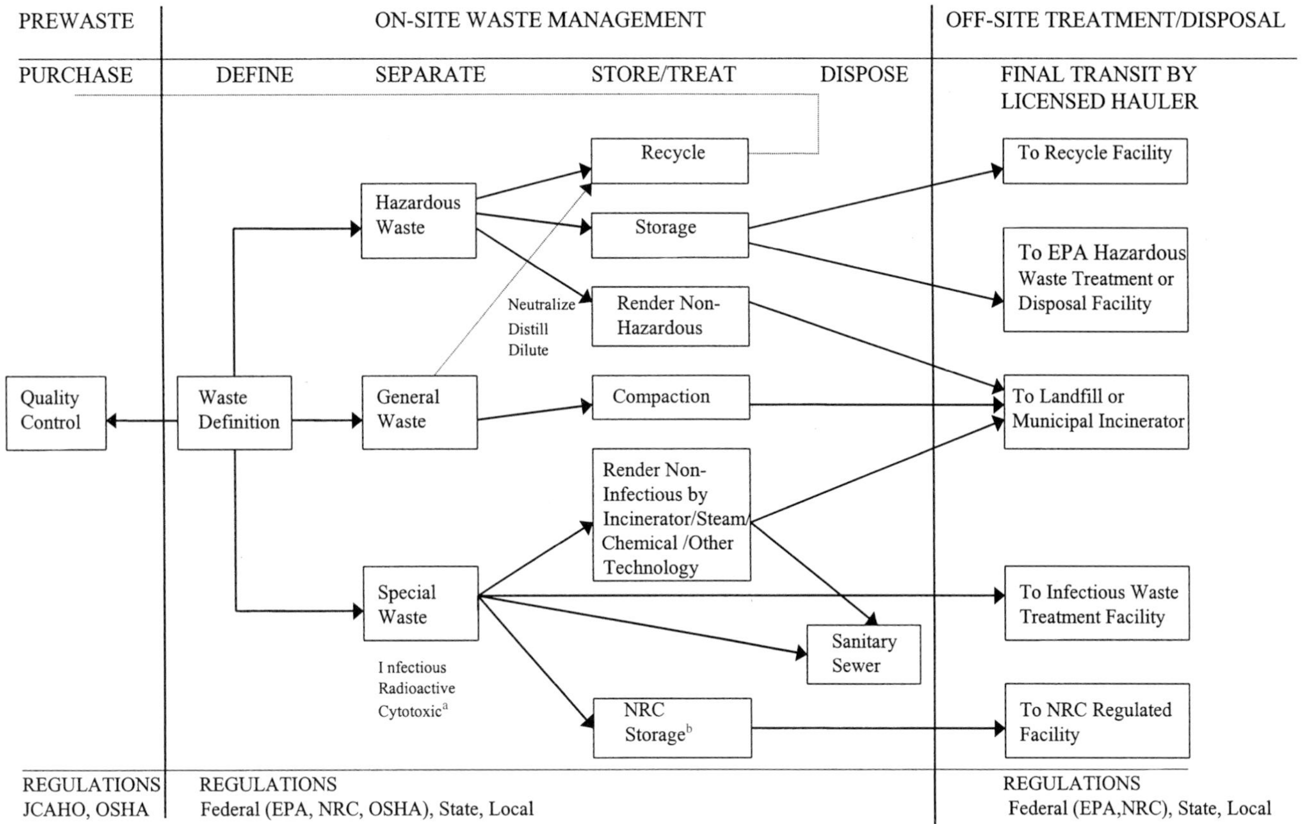

Figure 100.1. Medical waste management planning and implementation process. [a], Some cytotoxic waste must be managed as hazardous waste. [b], After decay in storage (DIS), waste can be disposed of as nonregulated waste. (Adapted from Denys GA. Infectious waste management. In: Lederberg J, ed. *Encyclopedia of microbiology,* vol 2, 2nd ed. Orlando, FL: Academic Press, 2000:782–796.)

clear understanding by waste generators and handlers as to what each label means. Labels should both identify and warn. A waste container should be identified by content (as medical waste) and also by waste type (e.g., by a sharps label). The biohazard symbol, the marking "biohazard," and red containers (i.e., color coding) are commonly used and are now required by OSHA regulations (9,34).

Containing Medical Waste

Proper containment of medical waste is critical to minimize the risk of occupational exposure to infectious agents present in the waste. The people who discard the medical waste are responsible for maintaining the integrity of the containers by not ripping or overfilling them.

Containment of sharps presents a special challenge. OSHA regulations require that contaminated sharps be discarded into containers that can be closed and that are puncture resistant and leak-proof on the sides and bottom (33). It is important to select sharps containers that are designed to minimize the risk of injury when sharps are placed into the container and to minimize the possibility of removal or spilling of the contained sharps.

At most institutions, red plastic bags are used to contain most types of nonsharp infectious medical waste. OSHA requires that waste collection containers for regulated waste can be closed and that they are constructed so as to contain all contents and prevent leakage of fluids during handling, storage, and transport (34).

Considerations When Handling Medical Waste

The primary factor to be considered when establishing procedures for the handling of medical waste is the risk of worker exposure. Minimization of worker exposure can be achieved by ensuring containment of the waste and maintenance of the integrity of the waste container. Before removal from the point of generation, waste containers should be closed and sealed to prevent spillage and the risk of exposure during handling and movement of containers.

Collection containers must be removed or replaced frequently enough to prevent overfilling. Waste handlers must also maintain container integrity during handling and segregation by closing containers before pickup to prevent spillage or protrusion of contents during handling, storage, and transport. Torn, damaged, or leaking containers should be overpacked (i.e., placed within a second container).

If waste containers are distinctly labeled, unopened containers of the same waste type may be grouped to reduce the handling effort. Bags of waste should never be opened nor waste transferred between containers because of the risk of exposure.

Efficient waste management also requires that waste handlers help maintain the quality of the waste management program by reporting any discrepancies with policies and procedures.

Waste Accumulation and Storage

Waste accumulation and storage can occur between the point of waste generation and the site of waste treatment or disposal. Accumulation refers to the temporary holding of small quantities of waste near the point of generation. An accumulation area can serve multiple waste generation points so that a sufficient quantity of waste can be accumulated before removal in order to promote efficient waste handling.

Storage of waste is characterized by longer holding periods and larger waste quantities. Storage areas are usually located near where waste is treated, loaded for transport (i.e., a loading dock), or disposed of. Any off-site holding of waste is also considered storage. Any designated area, room, or separate facility may be used for storage of medical waste.

Because of the larger waste volumes and longer holding times, special design and operation precautions are prudent for a medical waste storage facility. Containment is the key design feature of a medical waste storage area. This may require special ventilation features, such as use of high-efficiency particulate air (HEPA) filters. To contain spills, storage areas should not have floor drains and should be recessed or diked to hold liquids. Floors and walls should be impervious to liquids and easy to clean. Access should be limited to authorized personnel. Storage areas should be disinfected regularly. Refrigeration may be appropriate (or required) for prolonged storage of putrescible and other wastes. Storage areas should be posted with explicit signs.

Transportation of Medical Waste

When medical waste is not treated on site, untreated waste must be transported from the generating facility to another site for treatment and/or disposal. DOT regulates the commercial transport of medical waste (see Federal Regulations/U.S. Department of Transportation, below, and ref. 35). In addition, some states regulate the transport of untreated medical waste, and their regulations include specifications for containers and labels, types of vehicles, driver training and appropriate licensure, and emergency plans.

TREATMENT OPTIONS FOR MEDICAL WASTE

Medical waste generators have various treatment and disposal choices despite recent consolidations within the medical waste treatment industry (1–3,36). There are many options, because medical waste varies in its characteristics and degree of risk and because treatment methods vary in their capabilities, cost, availability to generators, and impacts on the environment. Table 100.2 provides an overview of medical waste treatment technologies that are in use or under development. Not all of these technologies are available for on-site treatment of medical waste, and some are now used only at off-site commercial facilities. Some are no longer commercially available in the U.S.

Traditional treatment methods are incineration and steam sterilization (autoclaving). New alternative technologies include chemical, thermal (low and high temperature), and ionizing radiation processes. Since the EPA's new emission standards in 1997 for reducing pollution from medical incinerators, many healthcare facilities have discontinued using existing units. As a result, other on-site alternative treatment technologies or off-site commercial waste treatment and disposal services are being used.

Alternative treatment systems combine treatment with other processes that are designed to address potential problems. Most of the new treatment systems incorporate mechanical grinding or shredding, either before or after treatment, to improve the effectiveness of treatment and/or to alter the appearance of the treated waste. Other systems provide compaction or encapsulation of the treated waste (2,3,36).

Disposal Without Treatment

In some states and localities, medical waste can be disposed of in a sanitary landfill without pretreatment. According to the U.S. Public Health Service, Agency for Toxic Substances and Disease Registry, untreated medical waste can be disposed of in sanitary landfills, provided established procedures to prevent worker contact with this waste during handling and disposal operations are strictly followed (26). Disposal without treatment is not recommended for human tissue, sharps, and cultures from clinical laboratories. Liquid waste should not be landfilled.

Sanitary Sewer Disposal

Most medical facilities dispose of their wastewater through a sanitary sewer system to a publicly owned treatment works (POTW). Sewage systems and treatment works are designed to treat biologic wastes. As a result, disposal to a sanitary sewer system is an option for bulk blood, body fluids, and other aqueous liquids unless such disposal is prohibited in your jurisdiction (37). Some institutions also grind pathologic waste for disposal to the sanitary sewer system.

Sewer disposal of infectious liquids poses risks of occupational exposure from splashing and aerosols that occur during the emptying of waste containers. Use of personal protective equipment (e.g., full face shields) and engineering controls (e.g., splash guards) can minimize such risks, but employees must be informed of the potential for exposure and the precautions that must be taken to avoid exposure. Sewer disposal of blood and body fluids should be done in a sink used only for that purpose.

Use of a sanitary sewer system is subject to the rules of the local POTW. These rules may limit discharges of certain wastes. Contact your local POTW to determine which wastewater discharges are permitted. Wastewater systems that lead to septic and storm water systems are not appropriate for disposing of medical waste because of the possibility of exposure to untreated waste. During periods of heavy rain, for example, combined sanitary sewer/storm water systems might overflow and release untreated wastewater.

TABLE 100.2. COMPARISON OF ON-SITE MEDICAL WASTE TREATMENT TECHNOLOGIES[a]

	Traditional Methods		Alternative Treatment Methods		
Factor	Incineration	Steam/Autoclave	Steam/Mechanical	Steam/Compaction	Steam/Heat/Alkali
Type of waste[b]	RMW/P/C	RMW	RMW/P	RMW	RMW/P/C
Equipment operation	Complex	Easy	Easy/automated	Easy/automated	Easy/automated
Operator requirement	Trained and certified	Trained	Trained	Trained	Trained
Load standardization	Needed[c]	Needed[c]	Needed[c]	Needed[c]	Needed
Capacity[d]	1,200 lb/hr	200 lb/hr	200–1,370 lb/hr	25–2,000 lb/hr	10–10,000 lb/hr
Effect of waste treatment	Burned	Unchanged	Shredded/ground	Compacted	Digested
Volume reduction	85–95%	30%	85–90%	60–80%	98%
Potential side benefits	Energy recovery	None	Yes[e]	Yes[e]	Yes[e]
Disposal of residue					
Liquids	Treated[f]	Sanitary sewer[g]	Sanitary sewer[g]	Sanitary sewer[g]	Sanitary sewer[g]
Solids	Hazardous ash[h]	Sanitary landfill[i]	Sanitary landfill	Sanitary landfill	Sanitary landfill

	Alternative Treatment Methods				
Factor	Chlorine Dioxide/ Mechanical	Peracetic Acid/ Mechanical	Electrothermal/ Mechanical	Microwave/ Mechanical	Pyrolysis/ Oxidation
Type of waste[b]	RMW/P	RMW	RMW	RMW	RMW/P/C
Equipment operation	Easy	Easy	Complex	Easy	Easy/automated
Operator requirement	Trained	Trained	Trained	Trained	Trained
Load standardization	Needed[c]	Needed[c]	Needed[c]	Needed[c]	Needed
Capacity[d]	600 lb/hr	20 lb/hr	n/a	550–900 lb/hr	100–2,500 lb/hr
Effect of waste treatment	Shredded	Pulverized	Shredded	Shredded	Vaporized
Volume reduction	85–95%	Up to 85%	Up to 85%	Up to 85%	99%
Potential side benefit	Yes[e]	Yes[e,j]	Yes[e]	Yes[e]	Energy recovery[e]
Disposal of residue					
Liquids	Sanitary sewer[g,k]	Sanitary sewer[g]	None[l]	None[l]	Sanitary sewer[g]
Solids	Sanitary landfill	Sanitary landfill	Sanitary landfill	Sanitary landfill	Sanitary landfill

[a] Information provided by manufacturers.
[b] Infectious waste types: RMW, regulated medical waste; P, pathologic waste; C, chemotherapeutic waste. Waste segregation may be needed to eliminate pathologic, chemotherapeutic, and/or nontreatable waste from the waste stream.
[c] To eliminate bulk fluids such as dialysis fluid or to ensure that sufficient solid waste is present in the load together with the bulk fluid.
[d] Includes a range of models.
[e] No harmful by-products; lower volume to commercial waste streams.
[f] If there is scrubber water present, it must be treated at publicly owned treatment works (POTW) or on site.
[g] Low volume or intermittent drain to sanitary sewer.
[h] Resource Conservation and Recovery Act (RCRA)-permitted landfill.
[i] Potential problem with recognizable red-bag waste.
[j] Point of generation treatment.
[k] Potential formation of carcinogenic compounds in chlorine-based systems.
[l] Moisture retained in solids or held within the unit.

Incineration

Incineration is very effective in treating most medical wastes. Modern incinerators ensure the destruction of infectious agents and can recover useful energy from the combustion of high-BTU paper and plastics, which are common components of medical waste (38). Incinerated medical waste becomes indistinguishable ash, and so incineration is ideal for the disposal of human tissue.

Not all wastes from healthcare institutions can be safely treated by incineration. Toxic metals can concentrate in the ash; so, for example, mercury thermometers should not be disposed of with medical or infectious waste that will be incinerated. Some units cannot handle large amounts of glass or liquids, such as bulk blood or other body fluids. Chlorinated plastics cause hydrochloric acid emissions.

Incineration is the most appropriate way to treat most types of chemotherapy drug waste, including empty drug containers and spill residues and drug-contaminated infectious wastes such as delivery sets, syringes, and gloves. Most other infectious waste treatment methods are not appropriate for chemotherapy waste. All unemptied source containers of chemotherapy drugs should be disposed of with hazardous chemical waste—not with other chemotherapy waste (39,40).

Incineration impacts the environment through its ash, air emissions, and effluents to the sewer (41). Federal regulation of hospital/medical/infectious waste incinerators severely limits emissions and/or requires expensive pollution control measures (12) (see discussion below under Federal Regulations/U.S. Environmental Protection Agency). State regulations may be more stringent. Because of the federal regulations, a number of institutions no longer use on-site incineration and instead are contracting with commercial vendors for the treatment and disposal of their medical waste.

Medical waste incineration is controversial (besides being regulated), and siting and permitting can be difficult. Complexity and the expense of compliance usually make large units with high throughput most cost-efficient. However, new incineration technology does offer the prospect of smaller, less polluting units that may be appropriate for on-site incineration of medical waste.

Steam Sterilization

Microbiology laboratories have long used the autoclave to sterilize contaminated waste, and the quality assurance protocol is well developed (42). A variety of chemical and biologic indicators are available commercially for routine testing of the effectiveness of treatment. Steam sterilizers range in size from small bench-top models to large commercial units. Some commercial treatment facilities use large high-temperature high-pressure retorts for steam sterilization of large quantities of medical waste.

Many types of medical waste can be difficult to treat effectively by steam sterilization on a smaller scale. Steam sterilization requires that infectious agents be in direct contact with saturated steam for sufficient time and temperature (2,43,44). Steam sterilization is suitable for waste that is easily penetrated by steam, but plastic bags and other containers can interfere with steam penetration. Because bags of medical waste are filled with a great variety of discarded items, it is difficult to standardize loads and to ensure consistent conditions for sterilization. Types of waste that should not be autoclaved include antineoplastic agents, toxic chemicals, radioisotopes, and volatile chemicals. Another disadvantage of steam sterilization is that the treated waste is recognizable and can be offensive aesthetically, which requires an additional step (e.g., shredding or compaction) in the treatment system.

Chemical Treatment and Disinfection

Chemical decontamination and disinfection is a proven technique suitable for treatment of certain medical wastes (2,45,46). Chemical disinfection requires that the infectious agent be in contact with disinfectant of sufficient concentration for a sufficient period of time. Wastes suitable for chemical treatment are those with only surface contamination and those that can be easily penetrated by the disinfectant. Moisture and organic matter in the waste can diminish the effectiveness of certain disinfectants.

Chemical disinfection has many applications in treating medical waste. On a small scale, disposable items can be soaked overnight in a fresh 10% bleach solution. Some treatment systems use high-level disinfectant solutions in combination with grinding or shredding of the waste to provide sufficient contact between infectious agents in the waste and the disinfectant (sodium hypochlorite, chlorine dioxide, or peracetic acid). Grinding also renders the waste unrecognizable. Reduction cremation by alkaline hydrolysis is an alternative to incineration for the treatment and disposal of infectious animal and pathologic waste (47).

Small chemical treatment units are suitable for a laboratory or a medical office. Large units can treat most types of medical waste from an institution.

Thermal Treatment

Alternative thermal processes are available that operate at low or high temperatures. Low temperature systems (300°F/149°C) incorporate specialized equipment for compacting, grinding, or shredding the waste. Examples of these technologies include high-vacuum autoclave with rotating drum and shredder; high-vacuum autoclave with compactor or shredder; continuous feed, chemically enhanced autoclave with shredder; microwave heat-generating unit with shredder; and microwave (electrothermal deactivation) heat-generating unit with shredder. The order of operation in these systems is usually as follows: introduction of the waste into a treatment unit or chamber, physical destruction of the waste either pre- or post-heating, and discharge of the final unrecognizable end product into a dumpster for shipment to a landfill for disposal. Commercial systems and prototypes differ in size and capabilities.

High-temperature technologies operate at 2,000–20,000°F (1,093–11,093° C). They use pyrolysis and oxidation, plasma, and plasma pyrolysis for treatment and disposal of the medical waste.

Irradiation

Ionizing radiation from an electron beam source has been adapted for off-site treatment of medical waste. Penetration of the electrons is limited, however, so only a thin layer of material can be treated. Irradiation systems must incorporate posttreatment shredding to render the waste unrecognizable and to reduce the waste volume.

Criteria for Selecting Treatment and Disposal Methodologies

The following criteria should be considered when selecting treatment and disposal methods for medical waste. These are listed in approximate order of importance:

- *Suitability of method for waste type.* For example, the sanitary sewer is suitable for the disposal of liquid infectious waste, because the sanitary sewer is designed for the disposal of liquids and the degradation of biologic waste. Incineration is most suitable for pathologic wastes, because it eliminates aesthetic concerns. Some state laws specify which treatment methods must be used for certain waste types.
- *Risk.* It is prudent to minimize handling risks associated with sharps and with waste that contains a highly infectious agent. Steam sterilization can minimize risks, because it is often used close to the point of generation (so there is less handling and storage) and because quality control procedures are well established to ensure effectiveness of treatment.
- *Effectiveness.* Treatment effectiveness varies with the characteristics of the waste and the need to prepare the waste for its ultimate route of disposal. Sterilization of medical waste is rarely necessary. Disinfection usually reduces microbiologic loads sufficiently for safe disposal in the normal trash; some states have set criteria for microbial inactivation (kill efficacy) of specific microorganisms. Destruction of sharps reduces the risk of injury during handling and disposal. For putrescible

waste to be disposed of in the normal trash, treatment must first prevent it from becoming a nuisance. Regardless of the treatment method, final disposal of treated waste must not cause aesthetic degradation of the environment.

- *Consistent quality.* A waste treatment process should reliably deliver a satisfactory level of effectiveness. Reliable treatment quality requires measurable operational parameters and effectiveness (e.g., temperature and burndown for incineration) and standardization of procedures. Any new technology should include standards and methodology to maintain treatment quality.
- *Cost.* Cost is always an important factor, but it is usually evaluated after the treatment methods under consideration have met the minimum standards for other criteria that are important to the waste generator. Costs include all capital and operating costs of the treatment unit and startup costs. Be sure that cost and labor estimates are accurate by evaluating data from similar installations.

Other selection criteria for treatment methods include record of success at other installations, appearance of the treated waste, occupational risks, environmental impacts, and reductions in waste volume and weight. State and local laws, regulatory burden (e.g., permitting costs), and community opinion (e.g., opposition to incinerators) often influence the relative importance of these criteria.

On-Site Versus Off-Site Treatment of Medical Waste

On-site treatment is favored by generators who produce small volumes of medical waste and by those who want more control over the treatment and disposal of their wastes and their associated liabilities. On-site treatment is also the choice of institutions that are distant from a commercial service area so that commercial disposal is unavailable or prohibitively expensive. Of course, on-site waste treatment has the burden and costs of operation, maintenance, and final disposal of the treated waste. Except for the largest institutions, on-site incineration may not take full advantage of the economies of scale.

Off-site medical waste treatment is more likely in states and urban locations where medical waste is subject to greater regulatory scrutiny and community concern. Off-site treatment and disposal entails the use of either a commercial or a cooperatively owned facility. In some regions, economies of scale and competition can keep the cost of commercial disposal in check.

Medical institutions retain liability for certain aspects of off-site management of their waste, even when the waste is in the control of another entity. Therefore, it is prudent to choose waste hauling, treatment, and disposal firms carefully.

DISPOSAL OF TREATED MEDICAL WASTE

After treatment, medical waste is usually disposed of as ordinary solid waste with the normal trash, garbage, and refuse. Depending on the institution's solid waste disposal firm, treated waste is ultimately disposed of in a solid waste landfill or used as refuse-derived fuel in a solid waste incinerator. As mentioned above, some treatment and disposal methods involve discharging wastes to a sanitary sewer system.

Increasingly, normal trash is sorted to recover recyclable materials, so there may be special handling considerations when treated medical waste is disposed of in the normal trash. Your disposal facility should be contacted to determine its requirements and concerns for handling treated waste.

Incinerator ash may be subject to special disposal requirements. Some states regulate incinerator ash as chemically hazardous waste if the ash has a high content of toxic metals. A few states have designated a small number of specially designed landfills for disposal of ash.

WASTE MINIMIZATION METHODS

Waste minimization is an important aspect of medical waste management. This importance derives from a variety of considerations, including regulatory requirements to reduce and to minimize the quantities of wastes generated, cost savings that can be realized when smaller quantities of waste must be managed and disposed of as medical waste, cost savings that can be realized when some wastes are reused or recycled, increased environmental awareness by the institution and its employees, and institutional concerns about community relations.

Waste minimization in hospitals is best implemented through a waste management program that emphasizes source reduction and recycling of wastes (48). There are many opportunities in the hospital for minimization of all types of waste (e.g., also see ref. 48 for a discussion of waste minimization in the medical laboratory). This section pertains mainly to the minimization of infectious waste.

Source reduction means reducing the quantities of waste generated. One approach is through strict definition of waste types accompanied by source separation of the different waste streams (1–3,10,48). Such a policy reduces the quantities of special wastes generated, because it specifies exactly which wastes comprise each category of waste (e.g., infectious, chemical, radioactive, normal trash, uncontaminated recyclable material, etc.); this ensures that all special wastes are placed in the designated containers, whereas other wastes are excluded. This policy also enhances regulatory compliance by ensuring that all special wastes are properly managed while reducing the costs of regulatory compliance by excluding from these streams those wastes that do not require special handling. Medical waste, normal trash, and recyclables should be kept segregated during handling and storage.

Source reduction is also achieved by product substitution, that is, the substitution of products that generate less waste. One example in the hospital setting is the use of devices such as needleless intravenous systems that reduce sharps generation and protect healthcare workers from exposure to blood-borne pathogens (49). Another example is the substitution of reusable items for the single-use items that gained wide acceptance, because they eliminated the need for on-site reprocessing. This latter approach to waste reduction requires careful evaluation of such factors as reprocessing requirements, quality control, biosafety of agents used in reprocessing, infection risk, practicality, availability of personnel for reprocessing activities, and comparative costs of disposable and reusable items (see Chapter 87). The actual total cost of reuse is difficult to ascertain, because it includes the costs of reprocessing, disposal, labor, and storage space. There is no consensus yet about the relative costs of single-use and reusable items.

Product substitution is also important in minimizing the quantities of chemical and radioactive wastes generated in various laboratory analyses. Examples include the use of new technology such as miniaturization, which reduces sample size and the quantities of waste generated (including infectious waste from excess sample material), new methods in which nonhazardous reagents have replaced hazardous ones, and new methods that are nonradiometric (48).

Recycling reduces the quantities of wastes generated by reusing certain materials, with or without prior reprocessing, rather than discarding them. The concept of recycling has increased interest in the possibility of reprocessing and reusing items that were intended to be used only once before disposal. This approach requires reprocessing of the used contaminated materials, which necessitates consideration of the factors mentioned above relative to the substitution of reusable for single-use items. This type of recycling also requires decisions regarding the type of item (i.e., reusable or single use) that is most suitable for reprocessing (see Chapter 87).

Other wastes that lend themselves to recycling are solvents, packaging materials, paper, and aluminum cans. Many solvents can be redistilled for reuse (50). An alternative approach for some solvents is incineration with heat recovery. Some manufacturers are now packaging their products in usable containers. Other packaging materials (e.g., corrugated cardboard and some plastics) are recyclable. Aluminum cans and many paper products (e.g., newspaper and office bond paper) can also be recycled.

Proper management is essential for implementation of a waste minimization program. The good management program includes an employee awareness program, employee training, purchasing strategies, and inventory control. It is important to let vendors know that you prefer products that produce less waste as well as those that can be cost-effectively reused or recycled.

REGULATORY CONSIDERATIONS

There are regulations for the management of medical wastes at the federal and state levels (and in some areas, at the local level as well). Compliance with all regulatory requirements is mandatory, and penalties can be imposed for noncompliance. Some federal and state agencies have also issued guidelines for medical waste management; these guidelines are recommendations and therefore are voluntary rather than mandatory. Certain guidelines must be followed in order to achieve accreditation from the state or from professional organizations such as the Joint Commission on Accreditation of Healthcare Organizations (51) and the American College of Pathologists (3).

Federal Regulations

At the federal level, three agencies of government have at various times issued regulations that pertain to medical waste: EPA (11,12), OSHA (9), and DOT (35). In addition, the CDC has issued guidelines (not regulations) that include sections pertaining to medical waste management (5–8,19,20,37,52). The EPA has also issued guidelines for infectious waste management (10).

U.S. Environmental Protection Agency

The jurisdiction of the EPA is environmental issues. The EPA has authority under RCRA to regulate infectious waste as a hazardous waste (4) but has chosen not to do so. Instead of regulations, EPA issued guidelines for infectious waste management in 1982 and 1986 (10,53).

The Medical Waste Tracking Act directed EPA to institute a 2-year demonstration program during which medical waste was to be tracked and the data collected and analyzed in order to ascertain the real extent of the medical waste problem (54). This demonstration program was in effect from June 1989 to June 1991 in five jurisdictions: Connecticut, New Jersey, New York, Rhode Island, and Puerto Rico (11). The EPA and the Agency for Toxic Substances and Disease Registry have published certain mandated reports to Congress (26,29,55).

The Clean Air Act Amendments of 1990 directed EPA to regulate waste incinerators (56). The EPA applied its definition of "regulated medical waste" from the medical waste tracking regulations (14) to "medical/infectious waste" (15) (Table 100.1) and promulgated regulations for new and existing incinerators that burn this waste (12). All hospital/medical/infectious waste incinerators are now subject to emission limits and to requirements for operator training, testing and monitoring of emissions, record keeping, and reporting. New incinerators are subject to siting requirements and even lower emission limits. The regulations also require preparation of a waste management plan. Human remains intended for interment or cremation are not regulated as hospital/medical/infectious waste under these rules. "Pathological waste" and "chemotherapeutic waste" are defined, and some may also meet the EPA's definition of hospital/medical/infectious waste. Separate standards will be promulgated for crematories and for the incineration of pathologic and chemotherapeutic waste. Rural incinerators and co-fired combustors are subject to less stringent regulatory requirements.

U.S. Occupational Safety and Health Administration

Under its jurisdiction of occupational safety and health (57), OSHA addressed the issue of occupational exposure to blood-borne pathogens (9). The blood-borne pathogen rules include many regulatory requirements that pertain specifically to medical waste (9,58), such as the handling of sharps (33) and container specifications (34). Relevant sections of the OSHA regulations are listed in Table 100.3.

U.S. Department of Transportation

DOT rules for bulk shipments of regulated medical waste became effective in 2003 (35). [See also DOT's Hazardous Materials Table (59) for additional relevant information.] The

TABLE 100.3. SECTIONS OF THE OSHA BLOODBORNE PATHOGEN RULE RELEVANT TO HANDLING OF MEDICAL WASTE

Section of 29 CFR 1910.1030	Subject
(d)(2)	Methods of compliance
	Engineering and work practice controls
(d)(2)(vii)	Contaminated needles and other sharps
(d)(2)(viii)	Sharps containers
(d)(4)(ii)	Housekeeping
	Cleaning and decontamination
(d)(4)(ii)(D)	Broken glassware
(d)(4)(iii)	Regulated waste
(d)(4)(iii)(A)	Contaminated sharps
(d)(4)(iii)(B)	Other regulated waste
(d)(4)(iii)(C)	Disposal of regulated waste
(e)	HIV and HBV research laboratories and production facilities
(e)(2)(ii)(B)	Contaminated materials
(e)(2)(ii)(H)	Decontamination of all waste
(e)(2)(ii)(J)	Use, discard, and decontamination of hypodermic needles and syringes
(e)(3)(ii) laboratories	Autoclave for decontamination in research
(g)	Communication of hazards to employees
(g)(1)(i)(A)	Labels on containers of regulated waste
(g)(1)(i)(B-E)	Requirements for labels
(g)(1)(i)(I)	Decontaminated regulated waste

OSHA, Occupational Safety and Health Administration; HIV, human immunodeficiency virus; HBV, hepatitis B virus.

DOT regulations include specifications for the containers used to transport regulated medical waste as well as requirements for marking and bulk packaging (60). Containers must be rigid, leak resistant, impervious to moisture, of sufficient strength to prevent tearing or bursting under normal conditions of use and handling, puncture resistant for sharps, and break resistant. When fluids are present in quantities greater than 20 cm^3, the containers must be tightly lidded or stoppered. Also, containers must be sealed to prevent leakage during transport.

U.S. Department of Health and Human Services

Select agents used in proficiency testing must be destroyed within 90 days of receipt. Select agents identified through diagnosis or verification must be reported and destroyed on-site within 7 days, unless managed otherwise according to law. When a registered activity is discontinued, written notice must be provided to DHHS prior to destruction of a select agent (17).

State Regulations

State regulations that control the management of medical waste are quite diverse (61). There is no commonality in the terms used in the definitions and specifications of which wastes are regulated. Some states have regulatory requirements for handling, treatment, transport, and disposal of medical waste, and these differ. For example, some states specify requirements for red bags (bag thickness or passing of the dart test) (62), containers, and transport vehicles, and for approval of treatment technologies. Landfill disposal of untreated waste is allowed in some jurisdictions but banned in others. Furthermore, all states that were included in the federal medical waste tracking demonstration program have adopted state regulations that continue the tracking, even though it is no longer required on the federal level.

It is therefore essential to ascertain which regulations are in effect in your particular jurisdiction so that you can establish waste management policies and procedures that are in compliance with all relevant state regulations.

Local Regulations

Many local jurisdictions have ordinances that can affect medical waste management; examples are ordinances that pertain to POTWs and landfills. The local POTW usually determines which types of wastewater may be discharged into the sewer system, and it may permit or may ban the discharge of liquid medical waste. Landfill operations are also subject to local regulation, and the requirements vary greatly. Many jurisdictions ban the landfilling of untreated medical waste, whereas it is allowed in others. Most jurisdictions classify treated medical waste as ordinary trash, but some localities specify requirements for the landfilling of all medical waste including that which has been treated.

Local regulations must be given the same consideration as those at the state and federal levels when waste management decisions are made.

ECONOMIC CONSIDERATIONS

Cost is often the decisive factor in decisions pertaining to medical waste management. The costs of various alternatives should always be evaluated, but these are often difficult to ascertain or quantify.

For example, source separation at the point of generation makes it possible to manage and dispose of waste most efficiently. However, labor shortages or time constraints (e.g., in the operating room or the emergency room) can make it infeasible to separate the discarded waste. Similarly, solvent recycling has proven to be cost-effective in many institutions, but some hospitals cannot afford the costs of space, specialized recycling equipment, and labor. Reusable items may be more expensive than single-use items because of the total cost of reprocessing. The costs of the various treatment and disposal options are complex and can be difficult to determine, especially when off-site alternatives are also considered.

Nevertheless, because of the importance of cost, it is essential to carefully evaluate the total cost of each option in the management scheme (63). Only then can a cost-effective medical waste management program be developed.

CONCLUSION

Hospital epidemiologists and infection control professionals agree that there is little risk of disease transmission from prudently managed medical waste. It is very important that they lend their expertise in hospital and community policymaking to ensure the acceptance of appropriate and cost-effective waste management procedures. As hospitals return to the use of non-disposable medical equipment to facilitate recycling, reuse, and medical waste reduction, the infection control team will play a large role in establishing safe and effective methods. Furthermore, it is important that hospital epidemiologists and infection control personnel express their professional opinions whenever any new regulations are being developed, whether at the federal, state, or local level.

Medical wastes are most easily managed through a comprehensive waste management system that incorporates management plans for the different types of medical waste that are generated (1–3,31). A comprehensive system includes all aspects of waste management: definition of waste types; source separation and segregation of waste streams; containment, handling, storage, transport, treatment, and disposal of wastes; procedures to ensure quality control; training; and waste minimization. Such a system provides the benefits of risk minimization, regulatory compliance, cost containment, liability reduction, and promotion of good community relations.

REFERENCES

1. Reinhardt PA, Gordon JG. *Infectious and medical waste management.* Chelsea: Lewis, 1991.
2. Gordon JG, Denys GA. Infectious wastes: efficient and effective management. In: Block SS, ed. *Disinfection, sterilization, and preservation,* 5th ed. Philadelphia: Lippincott Williams & Wilkins, 2001: 1139–1157.
3. National Committee for Clinical Laboratory Standards (NCCLS). 2nd ed. #GP5-A2. Wayne, PA: NCCLS, 2002.
4. The Resource Conservation and Recovery Act, PL 94-580, October 21, 1976.
5. U.S. Department of Health and Human Services, Centers for Disease Control. Recommendations for prevention of HIV transmission in health-care settings. *MMWR* 1987;36(suppl 2S):1s–18s.
6. U.S. Department of Health and Human Services, Centers for Disease Control. Update: universal precautions for prevention of transmission of human immunodeficiency virus, hepatitis B virus, and other bloodborne pathogens in health-care settings. *MMWR* 1988;37: 377–388.
7. U.S. Department of Health and Human Services, Centers for Disease Control. Guidelines for prevention and transmission of human immunodeficiency virus and hepatitis B virus to health care and public-safety workers. *MMWR* 1989;38(suppl 5–6):1–37.
8. U.S. Department of Health and Human Services, Centers for Disease Control and Prevention. Recommendations for prevention and control of hepatitis C virus (HCV) infection and HCV-related chronic disease. *MMWR* 1998;47(RR-19):1–39.
9. U.S. Department of Labor, Occupational Safety and Health Administration. Occupational exposure to bloodborne pathogens; final rule. *Fed Reg* 1991;56(235):64003–64182 (codified as Title 29, Code of Federal Regulations, Section 1910.1030, Bloodborne Pathogens).
10. U.S. Environmental Protection Agency. *EPA guide for infectious waste management,* EPA/530-SW-86-014. Washington: EPA, May 1986.
11. U.S. Environmental Protection Agency. Standards for the tracking and management of medical waste; interim final rule and request for comments. *Fed Reg* 1989;54(56):12325–12395 (codified as Title 40, Code of Federal Regulations, Part 259, Standards for the Tracking and Management of Medical Waste).
12. U.S. Environmental Protection Agency. Standards for performance for new stationary sources and emission guidelines for existing sources. Hospital/medical/infectious waste incinerators; final rule. *Fed Reg* 1997;62(178):48347–48391 (codified as Title 40, Code of Federal Regulations, Part 60, Standards of performance for new stationary sources, subpart Ce, emission guidelines and compliance times for hospital/medical/infectious waste incinerators, and subpart Ec, standards of performance for hospital/medical/infectious waste incinerators for which construction commenced after June 20, 1997).
13. U.S. Department of Labor, Occupational Safety and Health Administration. Title 29, Code of Federal Regulations, Section 1910.1030(b), Definitions, Regulated Waste. 1991.
14. U.S. Environmental Protection Agency. Title 40, Code of Federal Regulations, Section 259.30, Definition of Regulated Medical Waste. 1989.
15. U.S. Environmental Protection Agency. Title 40, Code of Federal Regulations, Section 60.51c, Definitions, Medical/Infectious Waste. 1997.
16. U.S. Department of Transportation. Title 49, Code of Federal Regulations, Section 173.134(a)(5), Regulated Medical Waste. 2003.
17. U.S. Department of Health and Human Services, Centers for Disease Control and Prevention, Office of Inspector General HHS. Title 42, Code of Federal Regulations, Part 73, Possession, Use, and Transfer of Select Agents and Toxins. 2003.
18. Lynch P, Cummings MJ, Roberts PL, et al. Implementing and evaluating a system of generic infection precautions: body substance isolation. *Am J Infect Control* 1990;18:1–12.
19. Garner JS. The Hospital Infection Control Practices Advisory Committee: guidelines for isolation precautions in hospitals. *Infect Control Hosp Epidemiol* 1996;17:53–80.
20. U.S. Department of Health and Human Services, Centers for Disease Control. Management of patients with suspected viral hemorrhagic fever. *MMWR* 1988;37(suppl S3):1–16.
21. Holmes GP, McCormick JB, Trock SC, et al. Lassa fever in the United States: investigation of a case and new guidelines for management. *N Engl J Med* 1990;323:1120–1123.
22. U.S. Environmental Protection Agency. Disposal tips for home health care (a professional brochure). EPA/530-F-93-027A. Washington, DC: EPA, November 1993.
23. U.S. Environmental Protection Agency. Disposal tips for home health care (a patient flyer), EPA/530-F-93-027B. Washington, DC: EPA, November 1993.
24. Thomas CS. Management of infectious waste in the home care setting. *J Intravenous Nurs* 1997;20:188–192.
25. Keene JH. Regulated medical waste. In: Abrutyn E, Goldman DA, Scheckler WE, eds. *Saunders infection control reference service.* Philadelphia: WB Saunders, 1998:729.
26. U.S. Department of Health and Human Services, Agency for Toxic Substances and Disease Registry. *The public health implications of medical waste: a report to Congress.* PB91-100271. Atlanta: ATSDR, September 1990.
27. Lichtveld MY, Rodenbeck SE, Lybarger JA. The findings of the Agency for Toxic Substances and Disease Registry Medical Waste Tracking Act report. *Environ Health Perspect* 1992;98:243–250.
28. National Committee for Clinical Laboratory Standards (NCCLS). *Protection of laboratory workers from instrument biohazards and infectious disease transmitted by blood, body fluids, and tissue: approved guideline.* #M29-A. Villanova, PA: NCCLS, 1997.
29. U.S. Environmental Protection Agency. *Medical waste management in the United States: second interim report to Congress.* EPA/530-SW-90-O87A. Washington, DC: EPA, 1990.
30. Rutala WA, Mayhall CG. The Society for Hospital Epidemiology of America. Position paper: Medical waste. *Infect Control Hosp Epidemiol* 1992;13:38–48.
31. Denys GA. Infectious waste management. In: Lederberg J, ed. *Encyclopedia of microbiology,* vol 2, 2nd ed. Orlando, FL: Academic Press, 2000:782–796.
32. Gordon JG. Safety in waste management: a comprehensive plan for infectious waste management. In: *Clinical microbiology procedures handbook,* suppl 1, section 14.6. Washington, DC: American Society for Microbiology, 1994:14.6.1–14.6.6.
33. U.S. Department of Labor, Occupational Safety and Health Administration. Title 29, Code of Federal Regulations, Section

1910.1030(d)(4)(iii)(A), Contaminated Sharps Discarding and Containment. 1991.

34. U.S. Department of Labor, Occupational Safety and Health Administration. Title 29, Code of Federal Regulations, Section 1910.1030(d)(4)(iii)(B), Other Regulated Waste Containment. 1991.
35. U.S. Department of Transportation. Title 49, Code of Federal Regulations, Section 173.197, Regulated Medical Waste. 2003.
36. Marsik FJ, Denys GA. Sterilization, decontamination and disinfection procedures for the microbiology laboratory. In: Murray TR, Baron EJ, Pfaller MA, et al., eds. *Manual of clinical microbiology,* 6th ed. Washington, DC: American Society for Microbiology, 1995:86–98.
37. Garner JS, Favero MS. *Guideline for handwashing and hospital environmental control.* PB85-923404. Atlanta: U.S. Department of Health and Human Services, 1985:15–16,99–117.
38. Cross FL, Hesketh HE, Rykowski PK. *Infectious waste management.* Lancaster, PA: Technomic, 1990.
39. Vaccari PL, Tonat K, DeChristoforo R, et al. Disposal of antineoplastic wastes at the National Institutes of Health. *Am J Hosp Pharm* 1984; 41:87–93.
40. U.S. Department of Labor, Occupational Safety and Health Administration, OSHA Office of Science and Technology Assessment. Controlling occupational exposure to hazardous drugs. Instruction TED 1.15, section V, chapter 3. 1995.
41. U.S. Congress, Office of Technology Assessment. *Issues in medical waste management.* Background paper. OTA-BP-O-49. Washington, DC: U.S. Government Printing Office, October 1988.
42. Cooney TE. *Techniques for steam sterilizing laboratory waste. Waste processing technical report.* Erie, PA: AMSCO, 1988.
43. Rutala WA, Stiegel MM, Sarubbi FA Jr. Decontamination of laboratory microbiological waste by steam sterilization. *Appl Environ Microbiol* 1982;43:1311–1416.
44. Lauer JL, Battles DR, Vesley D. Decontaminating infectious waste by autoclaving. *Appl Environ Microbiol* 1982;44:690–694.
45. Favero MS, Bond WW. Sterilization, disinfection, and antisepsis in the hospital. In: *Manual of clinical microbiology.* Washington, DC: American Society for Microbiology, 1991:183–300.
46. Rutala WA, Weber DJ. Uses of inorganic hypochlorite (bleach) in health-care facilities. *Clin Microbiol Rev* 1997;(4)597–610.
47. Kaye GI, Weber PB, Evans A, et al. Efficacy of alkaline hydrolysis as an alternative method for treatment and disposal of infectious animal waste. *Contemp Topics* 1998;37(3):43–46.
48. Gordon JG, Denys GA. Minimization of waste generation in medical laboratories. In: Reinhardt PA, Leonard KL, Ashbrook PC, eds. *Pollution prevention and waste minimization in laboratories.* Boca Raton, FL: CRC/Lewis, 1996:163–193.
49. Rutowski J, Peterson SL. A needleless intravenous system: an effective risk management strategy. *Infect Control Hosp Epidemiol* 1993;14: 226–227.
50. Gibbs LM. Recovery of waste organic solvents in a health care institution. *Am Clin Products Rev* 1983;Nov/Dec.
51. Joint Commission on Accreditation of Healthcare Organizations (JCAHO). *Hospital accreditation standards: standards, intents.* Chicago: JCAHO.
52. U.S. Department of Health and Human Services, Public Health Service, Centers for Disease Control and Prevention, and National Institutes of Health. *Biosafety in microbiological and biomedical laboratories,* 4th ed. HHS publication (CDC)93-8395. Washington, DC: U.S. Government Printing Office, 1999.
53. U.S. Environmental Protection Agency. *Draft manual for infectious waste management.* SW-957. Washington, DC: EPA, September 1982.
54. Medical Waste Tracking Act of 1988. PL 100-582. November 1, 1988.
55. U.S. Environmental Protection Agency. *Medical waste management in the United States. First interim report to Congress.* EPA/530-SW-90-051A and EPA/530-SW-90-051B. Washington, DC: EPA, May 1990.
56. Clean Air Act Amendments of 1990. PL101-549. November 15, 1990.57 Occupational Safety and Health Act. PL 91-596. December 29, 1970.
58. U.S. Department of Labor, Occupational Safety and Health Administration. See the Compliance Assistance section of *www.osha.gov* for OSHA's most recent compliance directives.
59. U.S. Department of Transportation. Title 49, Code of Federal Regulations, Section 172.101, Hazardous Materials Table. 2003.
60. U.S. Department of Transportation. Title 49, Code of Federal Regulations, Part 178, Packaging. 2003.
61. State and Territorial Association on Alternative Treatment Technologies. Technical assistance manual: state regulatory oversight of medical waste treatment technologies. December 1998.
62. American Society for Testing and Materials (ASTM). ASTM Standard D1709-01. Standard test methods for impact resistance of plastic film by the free-falling dart method. West Conshohocken, PA: ASTM, 2001.
63. Garcia R. Effective cost-reduction strategies in the management of regulated medical waste. *Am J Infect Control* 1999;27(2):165–175.

101

EPIDEMIOLOGY AND PREVENTION OF NOSOCOMIAL INFECTIONS ASSOCIATED WITH ANIMALS IN THE HOSPITAL

DAVID J. WEBER
WILLIAM A. RUTALA

Americans keep a wide variety of animals as household pets. Common pets include cats, dogs, birds, and fish; however, increasingly more exotic animals are being kept as pets, including other felines, ferrets, monkeys and other primates, rabbits, reptiles, rodents, and wolves. In addition, a variety of farm animals may be kept as pets, such as cattle, chickens, horses, pigs, and sheep. In 2001, 36.1% of households owned a dog, 31.6% owned a cat, and 4.6% owned a pet bird (1). The total number of animals owned was 61.6 million dogs, 70.8 million cats, and 10.1 million birds. An estimated 20 million American homes have aquariums (2). Retail trade in pet food alone totaled $8.7 billion in 1996 (3).

Hospitalized patients may come into contact with animals for two main reasons: the use of animals for pet—facilitated therapy and the use of service animals, such as guide dogs for the blind and primates for persons with impaired motion. This chapter focuses on the benefits and potential risks of animal use in the hospital, especially pet therapy. This review covers only the most common animals kept as pets and the major zoonotic diseases. Readers interested in a comprehensive review of zoonotic diseases or in rare and exotic zoonotic diseases are referred to several comprehensive monographs (4–13) and review articles (14–16). Several excellent reviews of infections associated with pets have appeared in the general medical literature (17–29). The frequency of type of allergic reactions to pets has also been reviewed (23,24). The clinical diseases associated with specific zoonotic agents and their therapy are well covered in several infectious diseases textbooks (30,31). Finally, the infectious hazards associated with the use of animals in medical research have also been reviewed (32).

Many potential bioterrorist agents are zoonotic pathogens including *Bacillus anthracis* (anthrax), *Coxiella burnetii* (Q fever), *Francisella tularensis* (tularemia), and *Yersinia pestis* (plague) (33–40). Bioterrorist agents are discussed in Section XVII Bioterrorism. In the future, zoonotic pathogens may be introduced into humans via the use of xenotransplantation (41–46). Xenotransplantation is discussed in Chapter 73.

POTENTIAL HAZARDS OF ANIMALS IN THE HOSPITAL

More than 200 infectious diseases of animals can be transmitted to humans. Strictly speaking, zoonoses refer only to those diseases that are transmitted from vertebrate animals to humans. In most cases, humans are accidentally infected and are dead-end hosts. Other pathogens also share maintenance of their life cycle with both animals and humans. In addition, the ectoparasites of some domestic animals carry pathogenic microorganisms, which may spread to humans through close association with infested animals.

Humans may come into contact with animals through many activities, including pet ownership; leisure pursuits such as camping, hunting, and hiking; travel to remote regions; and via occupations such as animal husbandry, medical research, veterinary medicine, animal control, and handling of agricultural products or animal hides (47). This chapter reviews only the diseases most likely to be transmitted by domesticated animals that serve as pets or service animals, because these animals are most likely to be encountered in the hospital (Table 101.1). These common pets include birds; cats; dogs; rodents such as mice, rats, gerbils, and hamsters; and fish, turtles, snakes, and rabbits. Nonhuman primates, that may be used to aid disabled persons, are also discussed.

Potential Pathogens

Animals commonly used as pets can serve as the reservoir or source for a significant number of diseases that potentially could be transmitted to humans in the healthcare setting (Table 101.2). These animals are also involved in the life cycles of an even wider variety of diseases in which nosocomial transmission is either rare or impossible (e.g., echinococcosis, leishmaniasis, schistosomiasis, and trypanosomiasis). New zoonotic pathogens continue to be recognized either because the microbial agent is newly isolated or because its potential to cause human disease is newly recognized (48–52). For example, newly recognized

TABLE 101.1. DISEASES POTENTIALLY TRANSMITTED BY PETS IN THE HEALTHCARE SETTING

Infectious Disease	Cats	Dogs	Fish	Fowl/birds	Primates	Rabbits	Reptiles[a]	Rodents[b]
Cat scratch disease	+++	+						
Ehrlichiosis		+						
Erysipeloid			+	+				+
Leptospirosis		+		+		+		+
Listeriosis		+		+		+	+	
Murine typhus								+
Mycobacteriosis *(Mycobacterium marinum)*			+++					
Pasteurellosis	+++	++		+		+++		+
Plague	+							+
Psittacosis				+++				
Q fever	++							
Rat bite fever								+++
Rocky Mountain spotted fever		++						
Salmonellosis	+	+		+++	+	+++	+++	+++
Tuberculosis	+	+			+	+		
Tularemia	++	+				++		+
Vibriosis			+					
Yersiniosis		+		+	+	++	++	++
Parasites								
Cryptosporidiosis	+	+		+				
Dipylidiasis	+	+						
Dirofilariasis		+						
Echinococcosis		+						
Fleas	+	+						
Giardia lamblia	+	+		+				
Mites (scabies)	+	+						
Toxocariasis	++	+						
Toxoplasmosis	+++							
Mycotic								
Dermatophytosis	+	++			+++		+++	

[a] Reptiles include lizards, snakes, and turtles.
[b] Rodents include hamsters, mice, and rats.
+, rare zoonoses; ++, occasional zoonoses; +++, most common zoonoses.
Adapted from refs. 5, 17, 19–21.

zoonotic pathogens (reservoir) include Hendra virus (horses) (53), Nipah virus (pigs) (54), and the coronavirus (civet) that causes the severe acute respiratory syndrome (55). (See also Chapter 113.)

Nosocomial Hazards of Animals in the Hospital

Zoonotic diseases can be transmitted to humans through animal trauma (bites, scratches, and stings); direct contact; arthropod vectors; aerosols; and contamination of food, water, or milk (5,47,56,57) (Table 101.3). Physicians should be aware of the major clinical syndromes associated with zoonotic diseases and their potential to cause nosocomial infection (58) (Table 101.2).

Hospitalized patients often have altered host defenses that may increase their susceptibility to a zoonotic infection and/or increase the severity of clinical disease (Table 101.4).

In addition to direct transmission from animal to human, hospital epidemiologists and infection control professionals should be aware that some zoonotic diseases may be transmitted from human to human, whereas others may represent a hazard in the microbiology laboratory (Table 101.4) (see Chapter 82).

Unfortunately, few scientific studies have addressed the potential risks of animal-to-human transmission in the healthcare setting. Furthermore, because animals have, in general, been excluded from hospitals, experience gained by means of case reports and outbreak investigations is minimal. Scott et al. (59) described an epidemic of methicillin-resistant *Staphylococcus aureus* (MRSA) on a rehabilitation geriatric ward. The paws and fur of a cat that roamed the ward were heavily colonized by MRSA, and the cat was considered to be a possible vector for the transmission of MRSA. Lyons et al. (60) described an outbreak of *Salmonella heidelberg* in a hospital nursery that was traced to infected calves on a dairy farm where the mother of the index patient lived. An outbreak of *Rhodococcus* (Gordona) *bronchialis* sternal surgical site infections after coronary artery bypass surgery was linked to a nurse whose hands, scalp, and vagina were colonized with the epidemic pathogen (61). Although cultures of neck-scruff skin of two of her three dogs were also positive, whether the animals were the source for colonizing the nurse or whether both the animals and nurse were colonized from an environmental reservoir could not be determined. An evaluation of a large outbreak of *Malassezia pachydermatis* in an intensive care nursery discovered that the isolates from all 15 case patients, 9 additional colonized infants, 1 healthcare worker, and 3 pet dogs owned by healthcare workers had identical patterns of restriction fragment length polymorphisms (RFLPs) (62). The authors believed it likely that *M. pachydermatis* was introduced into the intensive care nursery from the

TABLE 101.2. MEDICALLY IMPORTANT ZOONOTIC DISEASES

Pathogen	Disease	Medical illness(es)
Viral		
Coronavirus	SARS	Pneumonia (mortality 10–15%)
Herpesvirus simiae (B virus)	B virus infection	Erythema, vescicles, ulcers, and local pain at site of inoculation. Rapidly progressive ascending neuropathy and encephalitis
Lymphocytic choriomeningitis (LCM)	LCM meningitis	Influenza-like illness; occasional meningitis
Orbivirus	Colorado tick fever	Biphasic disease: sudden onset of fever, prostration, headache, photophobia, muscle and joint pains; followed by 2- to 3-day remission; then second episode of fever, rash (10%)
Orthopoxvirus	Monkeypox	Variola-like skin eruption with lymphyadenopathy (mortality ~10%)
Rhabdovirus	Rabies	Encephalitis (mortality ~100%)
Rotavirus	Rotavirus	Enteritis
Bacterial		
Aeromonas species	Aeromonas	Gangrenous wound infection; gastroenteritis; pneumonia
Bacillus anthracis	Woolsorter's disease	Localized skin lesions; mediastinal or intestinal infection (rare) leading to sepsis
Borrelia burgdorferi	Lyme arthritis	Three stages: (1) localized characterized by skin rash (erythema chronicum migrans); (2) disseminated characterized by musculoskeletal symptoms, neurologic or cardiac abnormalities, arthritis; (3) persistent infection with chronic skin, nervous system, or joint involvement
Borrelia species	Relapsing fever	Systemic disease marked by periods of fever alternating with afebrile episodes; erythema, petechia, jaundice may occur
Brucella species	Brucellosis	Systemic disease with acute or insidious onset, characterized by fever, headache, weakness, sweating, chills, arthralgia, weight loss
Campylobacter jejuni	Campylobacteriosis	Gastroenteritis
Capnocytophaga canimorsus	Septicemia	Sepsis with multiorgan failure, cutaneous gangrene
Rochalimaea henselae	Cat scratch disease	Lymphadenitis; Parinaud's syndrome; meningo-encephalitis; bacillary angiomatosis in HIV-infected patients
Chlamydia psittaci	Psittacosis	"Atypical" pneumonia
Ehrlichia species	Ehrlichiosis	Multisystem disease; may have rash
Erysipelothrix insidiosa	Erysipeloid	Skin infection (localized pain, erythema, edema surrounding wound); arthritis; sepsis (rare)
Francisella tularensis	Tularemia	Indolent ulcer and adenopathy (ulceroglandular); pneumonia; systemic symptoms (typhoidal); pharyngitis, abdominal pain, diarrhea, vomiting (gastrointestinal); conjunctivitis and adenopathy (oculoglandular)
Leptospira interrogans	Leptospirosis	Variable disease; biphasic illness—sudden onset with fever, headache, severe myalgias, conjunctival suffusion; rash, meningitis, hepatorenal failure, CNS involvement
Listeria monocytogenes	Listeriosis	Variable disease; meningitis; abortion
Mycobacterium marinum	Skin granulomas	Local ulcerative disease
Mycobacterium tuberculosis	Tuberculosis	Pneumonia; disseminated infection; meningitis
Pasteurella multocida	Pasteurellosis	Cellulitis, septic arthritis, osteomyelitis; pneumonia; meningitis; endocarditis; sepsis; intraabdominal infection
Pseudomonas pseudomallei	Melioidosis	Fever, pneumonia, gastroenteritis; chronic cases may have necrotic and granulomatous soft tissue or bone lesions
Coxiella burnetii	Q fever	Variation in severity and duration; onset may be sudden with chills, headache, weakness, and malaise; pneumonitis and endocarditis may occur
Rickettsia rickettsii	Rocky Mt. spotted fever	Systemic illness with fever, headache, rash, meningitis, multiorgan failure
Salmonella enteriditis	Salmonellosis	Gastroenteritis; sepsis (occasionally); osteomyelitis
Staphylococcus aureus	Staphylococcal infection	Skin and soft tissue infections; osteomyelitis; endocarditis; toxic shock syndrome; gastroenteritis (toxin mediated)
Streptococcus pyogenes	Streptococcal infection	Pharyngitis, cellulitis; streptococcal toxic shock syndrome
Streptobacillus moniliformis	Haverhill or rat bite fever	Systemic illness characterized by sudden onset fever and chills, headache and muscle pain, followed by rash, polyarthritis, and rarely endocarditis
Vibrio parahemolyticus	Vibriosis	Acute gastroenteritis
Yersinia enterocolitica	Yersiniosis	Acute ileitis; peritonitis may occur; rarely septicemia, reactive arthritis
Yersinia pestis	Plague	Systemic disease with multiple manifestations: lymphadenitis (bubonic); pneumonia (pneumonic); sepsis
Fungal		
Dermatophytes	Ringworm	Skin disease (ringworm)
Parasitic		
Babesia microti	Babesiosis	Sepsis with fever, shaking chills, headache, gastrointestinal symptoms, arthralgias; hemolytic anemia
Cryptosporidia species	Cryptosporidiosis	Gastroenteritis (self-limited in normal host, may become chronic in immunocompromised host)
Ehrlichia risticii	Ehrlichiosis	Systemic illness similar to Rocky Mt. spotted fever without rash
Giardia lamblia	Giardiasis	Chronic diarrhea
Toxoplasma gondii	Toxoplasmosis	Usually asymptomatic; lymphadenopathy; chorioretinitis; encephalitis (immunocompromised host)

CNS, central nervous system; HIV, human immunodeficiency virus.
Adapted from refs. 5–7, 9, 10, 30, 31.

TABLE 101.3. TRANSMISSION OF IMPORTANT ZOONOTIC DISEASES

Disease	Aerosol	Ingestion	Contact	Animal trauma	Arthropod-vector
Viral					
B virus infection		Saliva		Primate bite	
LCM meningitis	Infected aerosols	Food, water			
Colorado tick fever					Tick
Rabies	Probably bat caves, laboratory		Secretions, corneal tranplant	Wild animals, dog, cat	
Bacterial					
Aeromonas species	Fresh water drowning	Food, water	Water	Fish, reptile	
Anthrax	Spores in hides, spores in raw wool	Spores in contaminated meat	Spores in hides or environment	Contact with lesions on animals	
Brucellosis	Inhalation while handling animals or products	Goat cheese and milk	Animal and food products		
Campylobacteriosis		Meat, poultry, milk, water	Puppies with diarrhea		
Capnocytophaga canimorsus sepsis				Dog bite	
Cat scratch disease				Cat scratch	
Erysipeloid			Fish slime, shellfish	Lobster or crab pinch	
Leptospirosis	Secretions, wild and domestic animals	Water, milk	Contaminated water		
Listeriosis		Vegetables, water, cheese			
Lyme arthritis					Tick
Melioidosis			Rodents		
Monkeypox	From infected animals		Primates, rodents		
Mycobacteriosis *(Mycobacterium marinum)*			Water, fish tanks		
Pasteurellosis	Respiratory secretions		Cat, dog secretions	Feline bites and scratches, dog bites	
Plague	Inhalation—infected material		Infected animals	Cat scratch	Rodent flea
Psittacosis	Dried excreta from birds				
Q fever	Endospores from animal-contaminated soil, cat afterbirth		Infected animals		
Rat bite fever		Water, milk contaminated by infected urine		Lab and wild rodents	
Rocky Mountain spotted fever	Laboratory accident		Engorged tick		Tick
Relapsing fever					Tick
Salmonellosis		Food esp. poultry, eggs, shellfish, water	Fecal material reptile/amphibians		Cockroaches, bed bugs
Tuberculosis	Respiratory secretions	Milk *(Mycobacterium bovis)*			
Tularemia	Droplet particles, dead birds, animals	Food including meat	Dressing squirrels, muskrats, etc.	Cat bite (rare)	Tick
Vibriosis		Shellfish			
Yersiniosis		Milk, water	Farm animals		
Fungal					
Dermatophytes			Dogs, cats		
Parasitic					
Babesiosis					Tick
Cryptopsoridiosis		Cysts in water, ice			
Ehrlichiosis					Tick
Giardiasis		Cysts in water			
Toxoplasmosis		Oocysts from cat feces, tissue cysts from uncooked meat			

Adapted from ref. 5, 45, 56, 57.

TABLE 101.4. ZOONOTIC DISEASES WITH SPECIAL NOSOCOMIAL CONCERN

			Compromised Hosts with Increased Susceptibility	
Disease	Human-to-human transmission	Important lab hazard	At-risk population[a]	Disease
Viral				
LCM meningitis	Not described	Yes	Not described	
Colorado tick fever	Not described	No	Not described	
Rabies	Anecdotal reports; corneal transplants	Yes	Not described	
Bacterial				
Aeromonas infection	Yes (contact, fecal-oral)	No	Not described	
Anthrax	Yes (contact)	Yes	Not described	
Brucellosis	Not described	Yes	Not described	
Campylobacteriosis	Yes (fecal-oral)	No	Not described	
C. canimorsus sepsis	Not described	No	Asplenia	Sepsis
Cat scratch disease	Not described	No	HIV infection	Bacillary angiomatosis, Bacillary peliosis
Erysipeloid	Not described	No	Not described	
Leptospirosis	Not described	Yes	Not described	
Listeriosis	Not described	No	Organ transplant, chemotherapy	Sepsis, meningitis Sepsis, meningitis
Lyme disease	Not described	No	Not described	
Melioidosis	Yes (contact)	No	Not described	
Mycobacterium marinum granuloma	Not described	No	Not described	
Monkeypox	Yes	Yes	Not described	
Pasteurellosis	Not described	No	Lung disease	Pneumonia
			Prosthetic joint	Septic arthritis
Plague	Yes (aerosol)	Yes	Not described	
Psittacosis	Yes (aerosol)	Yes	Not described	Chronic infection
Q fever	Yes (aerosol during birth)	Yes	Cancer	
Rat bite fever	Not described	No	Not described	
Relapsing fever	Not described	Yes	Not described	
Rocky Mountain spotted fever	Not described	Yes	G6PD deficiency	Death from infection
Salmonellosis	Yes (contact, fecal-oral)	Yes	Achlorhydria	Sepsis
			HIV infection	Prolonged infection, sepsis
			Hemoglobinopathy	Osteomyelitis
Tuberculosis	Yes (aerosol)	Yes	Organ transplant	Pneumonia, disseminated disease
			Chemotherapy	Pneumonia, disseminated disease
			HIV infection	Pneumonia, disseminated disease
Tularemia	Not described	Yes	Not described	
Vibriosis	Yes (fecal-oral)	No	Cirrhosis (*Vibrio vulnificus*)	Sepsis
Yersiniosis	Yes (fecal-oral)	No	Not described	
Fungal				
Dermatophytes	Yes (contact)	Yes	Not described	
Parasitic				
Babesiosis	Yes (transfusion)	No	Asplenia	Sepsis (death)
Cryptosporidiosis	Yes (fecal-oral)	No	HIV infection	Chronic gastroenteritis
Ehrlichiosis	Not described	No	Not described	
Giardiasis	Yes (fecal-oral)	No	Not described	
Toxoplasmosis	Yes (transfusion)	Yes	Organ transplant	Pneumonia
			HIV infection	Encephalitis

G6PD, glucose 6-phosphate dehydrogenase; HIV, human immunodeficiency virus.
[a] Lack of a described risk should not be taken to imply that immunocompromised patients are not in fact at higher risk for disease acquisition or progression.

healthcare worker's hands after being colonized from pet dogs at home and then persisted in the nursery through patient-to-patient transmission. Patient infections were not benign and included eight bloodstream infections, two urinary tract infections, one case of meningitis, and four asymptomatic colonizations. Three nosocomial outbreaks of *Microsporum canis* (ringworm) with person-to-person transmission have been described in newborn nurseries (63,64) or neonatal intensive care units (65). In the latter case, the source of infection was a nurse likely infected from her pet cat.

Outbreaks of Q fever have been described in a secondary school in which infected goats were maintained for teaching purposes (66), in a psychiatric institution in which patients and staff worked with goats on a farm (67), and in a university department in which sheep placentas were used for fetal respiratory studies (68). There are two reports of postmortem examinations leading to transmission of *C. burnetii* to pathologists, mortuary technicians, doctors, and a medical student (69,70). Person-to-person transmission of Q fever within a family that affected five members has been reported (71). Nosocomial transmission has also been reported. There have been several reports of hospital staff who acquired Q fever via exposure to infected patients (69,72,73). In the latter case, Q fever developed in an obstetrician 7 days after he cared for a women undergoing a spontaneous abortion at 24 weeks. *C. burnetii* was identified in the fetal spleen and kidney, and the placenta, but not the lung. Probable patient-to-patient transmission has also been described (74).

ANIMAL USE IN THE HOSPITAL

Service Animals as Aids for Disabled Persons

The Americans with Disabilities Act (ADA) of 1990 is a federal civil rights law that protects persons with disabilities from discrimination in areas of employment, public services, public accommodations, services operated by private entities, and telecommunications (75). Title III of the ADA mandates that persons with disabilities accompanied by service animals generally must be allowed access with their service animals into places of public accommodation, including restaurants, public transportation, and healthcare facilities. The responsibilities of healthcare institutions under the Act have been extensively reviewed in a guidance document by the Association for Professionals in Infection Control and Epidemiology (75). *Disability,* as defined in the ADA is any physical or mental impairment that substantially limits one or more major life activities such as breathing, hearing, or caring for oneself. *Service animal* is a legal term defined in the ADA. A service animal is any animal individually trained to do work or perform tasks for the benefit of a person with a disability. A service animal is not considered a "pet," because it is specially trained to help a person overcome the limitations caused by his or her disability (75).

Dogs are most often trained for service work (75). In the United States, an estimated 5,000 working dogs guide the visually impaired, more than 2,500 working dogs assist the hearing impaired, and more than 2,500 working dogs aid the physically challenged (76). Service animals provide several valuable services, including enhanced mobility, dignity, decreased anxiety, improved confidence, and independence (77). Not surprisingly, visually challenged persons have a close relationship with their dogs. The importance of guide dogs is well recognized, and they are often exempt from public health regulations governing dogs in general. Animals may also be used to aid the hearing disabled and physically disabled patient; however, these uses are less well described than guide dogs.

Healthcare facilities as places of public accommodation are required to permit the use of service animals by a person with a disability as defined by the ADA, unless doing so would create a fundamental alteration or a direct threat to the safety of others or the facility (75). It is not permissible to require that a service animal wear special equipment or tag nor is it permissible to require "certification" or proof of an animal's training or a person's disability.

To ensure compliance with the ADA, healthcare facilities should have a written policy regarding the use of service animals by employees, patients, and visitors. This policy should ensure that service dogs and their owners have general access to the institution. The service animal policy should include the following topics (75,78). First, the locations in the hospital from which the service animal is prohibited. Such areas would include those that pose a risk to patients, especially areas that require the use of sterile or clean precautions such as operating rooms, pharmacy, and kitchens. Also the service animal should be prohibited from areas that pose a risk to the animal such as pathology and radiology. Second, facilities should not permit handlers with service animals to act as self-appointed animal-assisted therapy (AAT) ("pet therapy") providers. Third, employees, visitors, and patients should be educated to understand that service animals should not be allowed to come in contact with any patient's nonintact skin (e.g., surgical wounds, drainage tube, etc.). Fourth, there should be a mechanism to screen persons other than the handler (e.g., roommate) who may come into contact with the service animal for allergies or fears regarding the service animal. Fifth, the policy should define conditions on which the service animal may be removed, restricted, or denied access to an area. Such conditions might include aggressive behavior (i.e., biting), inability to contain excretions, or apparent illness. Evaluation of a potentially ill animal should be made by a veterinarian. Sixth, care and feeding of the service animal should be the responsibility of owner or handler or their designee rather than healthcare personnel. The facility may elect to provide temporary care such as during a short operative procedure but would need to have available trained personnel. Legal services should be consulted regarding any formal consent needed when the handler transfers responsibility for service animal stewardship to a facility representative. Finally, a mechanism should be in place for determining the appropriate use of a service animal on a case-by-case basis.

Differences Between Service Animals and Therapy Animals

Therapy animals and their handlers are trained to provide specific human populations with appropriate contact with animals (79). They are usually personal pets of the handlers and accompany their handlers to the sites they visit, but they may also reside at a facility. Animals must meet specific criteria for health, grooming, and behavior. Therapy animals are usually not service animals. Federal law, which protects the rights of qualified persons with disabilities, has no provision for people to be accompanied by therapy animals in places of public accommodation that have "no pets" policies. *Animal-assisted therapy (AAT)* is a goal-directed intervention in which an animal is incorporated as an integral part of the clinical healthcare treatment process. *Animal-assisted activities (AAAs)* provide opportunities for motivational, educational, and/or recreational benefits to enhance a person's quality of life. Both AAT and AAA are delivered by a trained person.

Animal-Assisted Therapy

AAT is designed to promote improvement in the physical, psychosocial, and/or cognitive function of people who are being medically treated (80). Other terms used in the literature for AAT are "pet therapy" or "pet-facilitated therapy." In a review of pet-facilitated therapy as an aid to psychotherapy, Draper et al. (81) noted that a literature review conducted in 1987 revealed more than 1,000 articles on the human-animal bond. As of 1983, however, only six studies of the therapeutic value of pets in which controls were used had been reported. They concluded that the benefits of pet therapy rely heavily on anecdotal reports and the widespread attachment of persons with animals. More recently, Allen (82) performed a critical appraisal of the literature from 1986 through 1997 and concluded that most reports describing the effects of human-canine interactions fell into the lowest category of scientific studies (i.e., descriptive studies and expert opinion). Newer research has provided evidence that companion animals provide health benefits in the home setting. However, there continues to be a paucity of well-designed clinical trials evaluating the benefits of AAT in the hospital.

The benefits of AAT have been reviewed (83–89). AAT has been most commonly reported to be beneficial among the chronically mentally ill (85,90,91), geriatric patients (92–94), patients with hypertension or coronary artery disease (95), and human immunodeficiency virus (HIV)-infected persons (96).

Several recent articles have reviewed the potential risks associated with AAT in healthcare facilities (97–101). Risks fall into three general areas; animal bites or scratches, allergies, and transmission of a zoonotic infection. The potential risks of bites or acquisition of a zoonotic disease are reviewed later. However, to date there have been no reports of illness or disease among hospitalized patients associated with a well-designed program that provides AAT.

DISEASES TRANSMITTED BY ANIMAL BITES

Animal bites are a major public health problem (102). National estimates based on a 1994 national telephone survey of randomly selected households revealed 4.7 million dog bites, of which approximately 799,700 necessitated medical attention (103). These numbers corresponded to an annual incidence rate of 18 per 1,000 and bites requiring medical attention 3 per 1,000 (adults 2 per 1,000 vs. children 6.4 per 1,000). Although most bite wounds are trivial and most victims do not seek medical attention (104), bite wounds have been reported to account for approximately 1% of all emergency room visits in the United States (105–108). More precise population-based estimates are available from a 1992 to 1994 National Center for Health Statistics survey, which reported that 334,000 dog-related injuries were seen in United States emergency departments for a rate of 129 per 100,000 persons (106). More recent data from the National Electronic Surveillance System-All Injury Program for the year 2001 revealed that an estimated 368,245 persons were treated in U.S. emergency departments for dog bite-related injuries (rate: 129.3 per 10,000 population) (109). These injuries constituted 0.4% of all emergency department visits during the study period. Although most bites produce only minor injury, at least 10% require suturing (110), and 1% to 5% required hospitalization (106,110–114). An estimated 5,991 hospitalizations resulted from dog bites in 1994 (114). Attacks by dogs resulted in at least 25 deaths between 1995 and 1996 (115) and 27 deaths between 1997 and 1998 (116). In summary, dog bites result annually in an estimated 17 deaths, nearly 6,000 hospitalizations, and more than 330,000 emergency department visits, with the total costs of treating these injuries of $235,600,000 to $253,700,000 (114). Because of its medical importance, the epidemiology, clinical management, and prevention of bite wounds has been extensively reviewed (104,107, 112,117–128).

Epidemiology

Only the epidemiology of bites relevant to risks associated with the use of animals in the hospital is reviewed here. Dog bites account for 70% to 93% of animal bites, and cat bites account for 3% to 15% (107,112,129–131). Dog bites more commonly involve the lower extremities, followed by the hands, arms, face, and trunk (104,107,112,119,132). A survey of dog bite wounds treated in the emergency department in 2001 revealed that 45% of injuries occurred to the arm and hand but that injuries to the extremity increased with age and accounted for 86.2% of injuries treated in persons 15 years of age (109). Cat bites more commonly involve the hands, followed by the arms, lower extremities, face, and trunk (107,119,133). The peak incidence of bites occurs in persons 5 to 9 years of age (104, 106,109–111,132). Compared with older children and adults, young children have a higher risk of being bitten and of suffering fatal injuries from bites (113,115,134–136); bites are more likely to involve the face, head, or neck (106,109, 134); bites are more likely to occur at home and to be caused by the child's pet (106,113,135); and the attacking dog is less likely to have a previous history of biting (113).

About two thirds of bites occur when interacting with a dog (e.g., petting, feeding, playing) or when on the dog owner's property (132,137). Only about 25% of victims, however, report direct interaction with the dog, such as feeding, playing, or petting (132). Only a small proportion of bites occur when the dog has been teased or abused. Large dogs are more commonly involved in attacks than small dogs. Shepherds and mixed breeds are most commonly named as the biting animal (107,137,138).

During 1995 to 1996 and 1997 to 1998, Rottweilers were the most commonly reported breed involved in fatal attacks (115, 116).

Etiologic Agents of Infection

The infection rate from penetrating dog bites has generally been reported in the range of 5% to 15% (107,108,118,122, 139). Cat bites are more likely to become infected than dog bites (107,140). Factors that increase the risk of infection after a dog or cat bite include (a) full-thickness puncture; (b) hand or lower extremity wounds; (c) wounds requiring surgical debridement; (d) wounds involving joints, tendons, ligaments, or fractures; and (e) wounds in patients who are high-risk hosts (122).

A large number of aerobes and anaerobes have been isolated from the gingival flora of cats and dogs (141,142). Pathogenic microorganisms derived from the normal oral flora of cats and dogs can be isolated from approximately 90% of clinically infected wounds (118,143). Most infections that develop after a cat or dog bite are polymicrobial (143–145). Goldstein, Talan, and associates (144–148) have studied the microbial agents associated with animal bite infections. The most common aerobic microorganisms isolated from infected dog bites were *Pasteurella* species 50%, *Streptococcus* species 46%, *Staphylococcus* species 46%, and *Neisseria* species 16% (145). The most common aerobic microorganisms isolated from infected cat bites were *Pasteurella* species 75%, *Streptococcus* species 46%, *Moraxella* species 35%, *Staphylococcus* species 35%, and *Cornyebacterium* species 28% (145). Anaerobic microorganisms are commonly isolated from both cat bite and dog bite wounds. In addition to these microorganisms, others included: *Enterococcus* species, *Eikenella corrodens,* EF-4a and 4b, *Micrococcus* species, *Acinetobacter actinomycetemcomitans,* and *Haemophilus aphrophilus.* Rarely, gram-negative bacilli, such as *Proteus mirabilis, Enterobacter cloacae,* and *Pseudomonas fluorescens,* have been isolated from infected wounds. Of particular importance is *Capnocytophaga canimorsus,* which has been associated with severe sepsis and a high case fatality rate. Unusual infections following dog bites have included blastomycosis (149), leptospirosis (150), brucellosis (151), and salmonellosis (152). Unusual infections transmitted by cat bites or scratches have included tularemia (153–165) and plague (166–168).

The anaerobic bacteria isolated from dog bite wounds may include species of *Actinomyces, Bacteroides, Fusobacterium, Peptostreptococcus, Eubacterium, Veillonella,* and *Leptotrichia.* The constituents of the oral flora of animals may occasionally be β-lactamase producers (118).

A large number of pathogens may occur in infections that complicate the bites of animals other than dogs and cats (117); however, a few generalizations may be made. All felines, including lions, cougars, panthers, and tigers, may transmit *Pasteurella multocida. P. multocida* may also be transmitted by other animals, including pigs, rabbits, rats, opossums, and wolves. The agents of rat bite fever, *Streptobacillus moniliformis* and *Spirillum minor,* may be transmitted by several small rodents, such as the rat, mouse, and gerbil (170). Bites inflicted in the water or by aquatic animals or reptiles (alligators, snakes, piranhas) may become infected with *Aeromonas hydrophila, Vibrio* species or *Edwardsiella tarda.* Although most cases of tularemia follow the handling of rabbits, infection may be transmitted by the bites from other animals, such as the cat, coyote, pig, and squirrel. Ferrets have become a popular pet in recent years. Ferret attacks are common and may lead to severe injury and even death, especially among young infants (171,172). Ferrets have been the source of viral influenza (173) and *Mycobacterium bovis* chronic wound infection (174). Potential zoonotic diseases include leptospirosis, listeriosis, salmonellosis, campylobacteriosis, tuberculosis, rabies, cryptosporidiosis, dermatophytosis, scabies, and various helminth infections (visceral larva migrans, cutaneous larva migrans, dipylidiasis, and dirofilariasis) (175).

More than 80 strains of aerobic bacteria have been isolated from the mouths of rhesus monkeys (176,177). Nonhuman primate bites can result in infection with herpes B virus, *Eikenella corrodens, Corynebacterium* species, α-hemolytic streptococci, and occasionally Enterobacteriaceae (178). Nonhuman primates may become infected with bunyaviruses (Marituba fever, Caraparu fever, Oropouche virus), poxviruses (tanapox, monkeypox), rhabdoviruses (Marburg disease), togaviruses (Kyasanur forest virus, yellow fever, Zika fever), hepatitis A, hepatitis B, *Campylobacter, Salmonella, Shigella, Mycobacterium tuberculosis, Yersinia* species, *Giardia, Cryptosporidia,* filaria *(Brugei malayi),* flukes *(Paragonimus westermani),* and flatworms *(S. japonicum).* Transmission to humans for some pathogens (e.g., *B. malayi*) may require the presence of specific arthropod vectors. Other agents may be transmitted by the respiratory route (e.g., *M. tuberculosis*) or fecal-oral route (e.g., hepatitis A). Of these pathogens, laboratory personnel have acquired Marburg virus, Ebola virus, monkeypox, hepatitis A, *Shigella,* tuberculosis, and herpes B virus infection. To date, more than 25 cases of herpes B virus infection in humans have been reported (179–182), with a case fatality rate of greater than 50%. A guideline designed to prevent herpes B virus infection in monkey handlers has been published (183).

PATHOGENS OF SPECIAL IMPORTANCE

Pasteurella species

Epidemiology and Microbiology

Pasteurella spp. are small, nonmotile, nonspore-forming, gram-negative coccobacilli. On Gram-stained smear, the microorganisms generally appear as a single bacillus but may occur in pairs or chains. They frequently show bipolar staining. The microorganisms are aerobic, facultatively anaerobic, and grow well at 37°C on blood, chocolate, and Mueller-Hinton agar but not on MacConkey's agar. Growth is facilitated by enriched media and increased CO_2. More than 17 species of *Pasteurella* are known, *P. multocida* subspecies *multocida, P. multocida* subspecies*septica, Pasteurella canis, Pasteurella stomatis,* and *Pasteurella dogmatis* are the most common pathogens in humans (184). One author noted that *P. multocida* subspecies *septica* was more likely to be isolated from wounds and *P. multocida* subspecies *multocida* from the respiratory tract (184). However, a larger study reported that for both cat- and dog-associated bite wounds, *P. multocida* subspecies *multocida* was more commonly isolated than *P. multocida* subspecies *septica* (145).

P. multocida has been isolated from the digestive system or respiratory tract of domestic cats and dogs, rats, mice, rabbits, cattle, sheep, swine, horses, and monkeys. Carriage rates of *P. multocida* in the oral or nasal secretions of various apparently well animals are high: 70% to 90% in cats, 50% to 66% in dogs, 51% in pigs, and 14% in Norway rats.

Most human infections result from direct inoculation by bites or scratches. Infections following animal exposure in the absence of bites or scratches probably stem from contact with animal secretions. *Pasteurella multocida* infections are frequently associated with impaired host defenses and include the following localized infections (host defense defects): septic arthritis (prosthetic joints or joints damaged by degenerative or rheumatoid arthritis), meningitis (children younger than 1 year of age or elderly persons), spontaneous bacterial peritonitis (cirrhosis), sepsis (alcoholism, diabetes mellitus), lower respiratory tract infections (chronic obstructive pulmonary disease, bronchiectasis), urinary tract (underlying structural and/or functional alterations), and endocarditis (prosthetic valve). Human-to-human spread of infection has not been documented, and contaminated food or water has not been implicated as a source of infection.

Clinical Features of Disease and Diagnosis

Infections with *P. multocida* may be divided into three categories (185). First, soft tissue infections may follow animal bites or scratches (186–189). Rapidly spreading cellulitis is the most common presentation. Joint or bone penetration may lead to septic arthritis or osteomyelitis (190). Prosthetic joints may be seeded by more distal injury with infection (191,192). Second, *P. multocida* may cause respiratory tract colonization or infections such as acute pneumonia, chronic pneumonitis, or empyemas (186,188,193–195). Most infected patients have underlying pulmonary diseases, including bronchitis, chronic obstructive pulmonary disease, or bronchiectasis. A history of animal contact is common, but actual bites or scratches are rare. Finally, *P. multocida* may cause serious systemic diseases such as endocarditis (196,197), meningitis (198–200), intraabdominal infection (188,201,202), urinary tract infection (203), and sepsis (204,205).

Definitive diagnosis requires isolation of the microorganism. However, *P. multocida* should be considered a potential pathogen in any skin or soft tissue infection after an animal bite, especially that of a cat or a dog.

Capnocytophaga Canimorsus

Epidemiology and Microbiology

Capnocytophaga canimorsus [dysgonic fermentor-2 (DF-2)' is a fastidious, gram-negative, opportunistic pathogen that can cause serious multiorgan disease in humans. More than 100 cases have been described in recent reviews (206–214).

C. canimorsus is a thin nonspore-forming rod 1 to 3 μ long. The microorganism exhibits gliding motility and is oxidase- and catalase-positive but negative for nitrate reduction, urease, and indole. It is a fastidious, slow-growing microorganism that, depending on the culture method used, may take from 3 to 11 days to form mature colonies.

C. canimorsus has a worldwide distribution. Studies suggest that it is part of the normal gingival flora of cats and dogs. Although infected patients have ranged from infants to persons older than 75 years, 60% of infections have been reported in adults older than 50 years.

Approximately 80% of patients reported in the literature have a predisposing condition, most commonly splenectomy. Other predisposing conditions have included Hodgkin's disease, trauma, idiopathic thrombocytopenic purpura, alcohol abuse, steroid therapy, and chronic lung disease. Forty percent of the cases of sepsis, however, have occurred in persons with no predisposing condition. Sepsis is the most common clinical infection. *C. canimorsus* infections range from mild to fulminant, with shock, respiratory distress, and disseminated intravascular coagulation. Meningitis may occur (215,216). Dermatologic lesions (maculopapular rash, purpura) or gangrene are common. The overall mortality is approximately 30%.

Infection is strongly associated with dog bites. More than 50% of patients have reported dog bites before clinical infection. Infections have also followed cat bites or scratches (213,217, 218), scratches from dogs, and contact with wild animals. An additional 20% of patients have reported exposure to dogs without a history of an actual bite or scratch.

Clinical Features of Disease and Diagnosis

The clinical syndrome in humans is characterized by disseminated intravascular coagulation, cellular necrosis in certain organs such as kidneys and adrenal glands, cutaneous gangrene, thrombocytopenia, hypotension, hemorrhagic diathesis with purpuric skin lesions and petechiae, and renal failure with oliguria and anuria. The case fatality rate is approximately 25%. Death has not been confined to immunocompromised patients.

Infection with *C. canimorsus* should be considered in patients who have a compatible clinical syndrome with a history of a dog bite or animal exposure. Definitive diagnosis requires isolation of the microorganism from blood or other body fluids or tissues. Empiric therapy should be instituted based on the clinical presentation. In patients who show high-grade bacteremia, the microorganism has been demonstrated in peripheral blood smears (219,220). Therefore, all patients suspected of having *C. canimorsus* sepsis, especially splenectomized patients, should have a Gram stain of their buffy coat.

Cat Scratch Disease

Epidemiology and Microbiology

Bartonella and *Afipia* are closely related genera. *Afipia* species differ from *Bartonella* in that they are urease and oxidase positive. Eight species of *Bartonella* have been demonstrated to be pathogenic for humans. Clinical syndromes caused by these bacteria (etiologic agents) include the following: Oroya fever and verruga peruana *(Bartonella bacilliformis),* bacteremia and endocarditis *(Bartonella quintana, Bartonella henselae),* bacillary angiomatosis and peliosis *(B. quintana, B. henselae),* HIV-associated neurologic syndromes *(B. quintana),* and cat scratch disease (CSD) (*B. henselae, Bartonella clarridgeiae,* and *Afipia felis*) (221–228). *B. henselae* is considered the primary agent of CSD.

The syndrome of regional lymphadenopathy after a cat scratch was first described in 1932 by Lee Foshay in the United States and Robert Debre in France. Debre and Lamy provided the definitive description of CSD in 1950. A clinical diagnosis of CSD was considered established by the presence of three of four criteria including (a) a history of animal (in 99% of cases a cat or dog) contact with an abrasion, scratch, or ocular lesion; (b) a positive cat scratch skin test; (c) negative results of laboratory studies for other causes of lymphadenopathy; and (d) characteristic histopathology of the lymph node.

Infection with *Bartonella* species results in disease syndromes of variable severity, ranging from lymphadenopathy only (CSD) to systemic disease. As noted by Anderson and Neuman (226), the severity and presentation of disease are related to immune status. In general (excluding *B. bacilliformis*), immunocompetent patients who are otherwise healthy tend to present with classic CSD when infected with *B. henselae*. Patients who are immunocompromised by having acquired immunodeficiency syndrome (AIDS), chronic alcoholism, immunosuppression, or other serious health problems tend to have systemic disease; however, there have been rare reports of systemic disease, including bacillary angiomatosis, in immunocompetent persons (229).

Clinical Features of Disease and Diagnosis

CSD most commonly occurs among children and adolescents. Typically, it begins 4 to 6 days after animal contact (most commonly a scratch by a cat, especially a kitten) with the formation of a 2- to 3-mm macule at the site of inoculation, which progresses to a papule or pustule. Inoculation papules are described in 50% to 76% of reports (230). Approximately 3 weeks after inoculation, regional adenopathy develops (range 5 to 50 days). About 80% of involved nodes are located in the head, neck, or upper extremities. The node is tender in 80% of patients and suppurates in 15% of patients. Fever and malaise each accompany the illness in about 30% of patients. Resolution occurs spontaneously in 2 to 6 months. Less common clinical findings include rash, hepatosplenomegaly, lytic bone lesions, granulomatous conjunctivitis, pneumonitis, endocarditis, and central nervous system involvement (231). *B. henselae* has been shown to be the third most common cause of fever of unknown origin in children, accounting for approximately 55% of cases.

Manifestations of *Bartonella* infection in the immunocompromised patient include cutaneous bacillary angiomatosis (BA), extracutaneous lesions, bacillary peliosis hepatitis, and fever with bacteremia (232–234). BA is the most common clinical manifestation of *Bartonella* infection in the immunocompromised person. Clinical findings associated with BA include elevated, friable, firm, bright red papules (~67% of cases); subcutaneous nodules (~50%); and cellulitis plaques (~5% to 10%). Extracutaneous manifestations may be present and include visceral lesions in the respiratory or gastrointestinal mucosa, heart, liver, spleen, bone marrow, muscles or lymph nodes.

CSD is diagnosed by its distinctive clinical picture and the characteristic histology of lymph node biopsies. Bacillary angiomatosis similarly is diagnosed by its clinical syndrome and characteristic histology of skin or liver biopsies. Polymerase chain reaction and indirect immunofluorescence assays for antibodies to *B. henselae* are predominantly used for clinical studies and are not routinely available.

Prevention of Animal Bites in the Hospital

Hospital personnel and owners of seeing eye dogs should be notified to discourage petting of the guide dogs. Petting and playing with dogs distracts them from their primary responsibility and might lead to injury.

Animals used for pet therapy should be carefully screened and all encounters should be carefully supervised. Patients who might benefit from pet therapy should be carefully screened as well. Toddlers, patients with psychiatric difficulties, and active children are probably at higher risk for bites and should either be excluded from pet therapy or carefully supervised. Guidelines for the prevention of animal bites have been published (235, 236). Immunocompromised patients, including functionally asplenic patients and HIV-infected patients, also should not interact directly with animals. All patients bitten or scratched in the hospital should be appropriately evaluated.

DISEASES TRANSMITTED BY DIRECT CONTACT

Ectoparasites

Animals may be infested with ectoparasites, which harbor microorganisms potentially pathogenic for humans, either transiently or chronically. Animals that are allowed outdoors, such as cats and dogs, are at special risk for becoming infested. Once infested, close contact with humans may allow transmission of infection. Of most concern are tick-borne diseases, which in the United States include babesiosis, Colorado tick fever, ehrlichiosis, Lyme disease, relapsing fever, Rocky Mountain spotted fever, and tularemia (237–241). In general, the reservoir for these diseases are small animals, such as rodents or rabbits. Only in the case of ehrlichiosis is the dog believed to be a possible reservoir. In other cases, the dog acts as a passive carrier of the infected tick. Pets may become ill with leptospirosis, Rocky Mountain spotted fever, and tularemia.

As with humans, pets should be inspected twice daily for ticks. Removal is best accomplished by grasping the head of the tick with a forceps and gently pulling until it is removed (242). Care should be taken to avoid crushing attached ticks, spraying blood from engorged ticks, and excoriating the area. After removal, the area should be cleansed with soap and water or a disinfectant.

Cats and dogs could also be agents for transmitting plague to humans via its rodent flea vector. Plague causes a self-limited disease in dogs, but cats are susceptible to severe and often fatal infection. Animal fleas are best eradicated by flea dips. Pets should not be allowed to forage in areas where *Y. pestis* is prevalent.

Scabies is caused by a subspecies of the mite *Sarcoptes scabiei* (243). The subspecies that infects cats and dogs can occasionally be transmitted to humans. These mites can cause intensely pruritic, papular, excoriated lesions but do not cause burrows, because the animal subspecies cannot complete their life cycle in humans. Hence, disease is a manifestation of hypersensitivity in the human host. Diagnosis is by clinical presentation, because skin scrapings are negative.

Fleas from infested animals, as well as those in the environment, will feed on humans (243). They also carry the intermediate stage of the tapeworm, *Dipylidium caninum* (human infestation occurs via ingestion of infected fleas).

Pathogenic Bacteria

Animals may harbor pathogenic *Staphylococcus* species (244) or *Streptococcus* species (245) on their fur or in their pharynx. MRSA has been isolated from the skin of cats (246). Occasionally, humans may become infected as a result of animal contact. For example, a household cat or dog has occasionally served as the reservoir for household infections with the group A *Streptococcus* (247).

Dermatomycoses

Zoophilic dermatophytes occasionally cause disease in humans. *M. canis* (less commonly *Microsporum gypseum* and *Trichophyton mentagrophytes*) produces most superficial fungus infections of dogs and cats and may cause tinea capitis or ringworm in humans (17,247); however, cats, the major reservoir for *M. canis,* often have inconspicuous or subclinical infections. These infections may not be suspected until lesions appear on human contacts. Ten percent to 30% of cases of human dermatophytoses in urban settings are estimated to be of animal origin.

The spectrum of disease is variable and can include circular alopecia, scaling and crusting lesions, or ulcers and nodules. Ringworm is characterized by an annular, expanding, erythematous area with central scaling, crusting or healing, and surrounding follicular papules. An exudative secondary bacterial infection may occur. Wood's light examination of hairs demonstrates *Microsporum* infection by showing blue-green fluorescence. Zoophilic fungal infections may also be demonstrated by scraping the lesions followed by examination with 20% potassium hydroxide. Exact identification of pathogens requires culture on fungal media.

Aquariums and Water-Related Diseases

A large number of bacterial infections may be acquired by trauma sustained in water or by injuries caused by water-dwelling animals (248). The most important of these pathogens are *A. hydrophila, E. tarda, Erysipelothrix rhusiopathiae, Mycobacterium marinum, Vibrio cholerae* non-O1, *Vibrio parahaemolyticus,* and *Vibrio vulnificus.* Aquarium-acquired *Plesiomonas shigelloides* infection has been reported in a 14-month-old girl (249). Cercarial dermatitis occurred in a 33-year-old man who stocked his aquarium with local snails (250).

M. marinum causes granulomatous, papular cutaneous lesions in humans. Deep tissue infections may also occur and include tenosynovitis, septic arthritis, and osteomyelitis. Many cases result from injuries sustained while cleaning fish tanks (251–258).

Erysipeloid is a skin infection of pig handlers, abattoir workers, and fish workers worldwide. Infection usually results when the microorganism contaminates cuts and abrasions. Infection is characterized by erythema with pain and edema of skin spreading peripherally. Septic arthritis may develop.

Severe cellulitis, including gangrenous soft tissue infection, may result from infection with *A. hydrophila* or *V. vulnificus. Aeromonas* infection has also followed the use of medicinal leeches (see following section).

A large number of marine animals may injure humans via bites or stings or when humans ingest them (259–264).

Because aquariums may harbor the aforementioned pathogens, aquariums, if present in a medical facility, should be cleaned only by trained medical personnel. In addition, because water may serve as a reservoir for multiple antibiotic-resistant gram-negative bacilli, aquariums should not be maintained in areas frequented by immunocompromised or intensive care patients.

Francisella tularensis

Epidemiology and Microbiology

F. tularensis is capable of infecting more than 100 species of wild and domestic animals and more than 100 species of invertebrates (265). Natural infection has also been found in ticks, mosquitoes, horseflies, fleas, and lice that parasitize lagomorphs (rabbits) and rodents. Natural foci of infection are found in the Northern Hemisphere. Both sporadic (266) and epidemic cases occur (267).

Tularemia may be acquired via multiple routes including (a) direct contact with infected animals, including bites, scratches, and contact with nonintact skin or mucous membranes; (b) arthropod bite (most commonly an infected tick); (c) inhalation of contaminated animal products in the laboratory; and (d) ingestion of contaminated food or water (268–275). Crushing of infected ticks living on dogs may also lead to infection (276).

Clinical Features of Disease and Diagnosis

The incubation period is 3 to 5 days (range 1 to 21 days). Multiple clinical forms have been described; they are determined principally by the agent's route of entry (272–276). Tularemia usually starts abruptly, with onset of fever, chills, headache, anorexia, malaise, and fatigue. Other symptoms include myalgia, cough, vomiting, pharyngitis, abdominal pain, and diarrhea. Fever typically lasts several days, remits for a brief period, and then recurs (277,278). Presentations of tularemia include the following:

1. Ulceroglandular (21% to 78% of cases)—The most common presentation of tularemia is the ulceroglandular form, which accounts for about 85% of cases in the Western Hemisphere. A local lesion is seen at the site of entry (an arthropod bite or an injury inflicted by a contaminated sharp), which progresses to a necrotic ulceration accompanied by swelling of the nearby lymph node. The node frequently suppurates, ulcerates, and becomes sclerotic.
2. Oculoglandular (0% to 5% of cases)—This form develops when infective material comes into contact with the conjunc-

tiva. The primary lesion consists of an ulcerated papule on the lower eyelid that is associated with regional adenopathy (279).

3. Glandular (3% to 20% of cases)—Occasionally, lymphadenopathy may occur in the absence of an ulcerative local lesion. The course is similar to ulceroglandular fever.
4. Pulmonary (7% to 20% of cases)—Pneumonia may result from inhalation of an infected aerosol from handling dead animals or examining pets that are ill with respiratory infections and when laboratory workers attempt to isolate the pathogen on agar plates (280–283). During septicemia, the microorganisms can lodge in pulmonary tissues and give rise to secondary tularemic pneumonia. Symptoms include cough and high fever, occasional pleurisy, and rarely dyspnea. The chest radiograph may demonstrate disproportionately extensive disease compared with the physical examination.
5. Typhoidal (5% to 30% of cases)—The typhoidal form, which is uncommon, results from ingestion of contaminated food (usually rabbit meat) or water. Symptoms include fever, prostration, and gastroenteritis. Ulcerative lesions are found in the mucosa of the gastrointestinal tract.
6. Miscellaneous—Uncommon forms of tularemia include oropharyngeal (0% to 12% of cases), caused by ingestion of contaminated food or water, and meningitis (rare) (284). Infection of a central nervous system shunt has been reported (285).

Tularemia may be a serious disease. The case fatality rate in untreated patients for the pneumonic and typhoidal forms is between 40% and 60%.

The diagnosis is often suspected on the basis of an appropriate exposure history or with an eschar at the site of an arthropod bite; it may be confirmed by serologic testing.

RESPIRATORY INFECTIONS TRANSMITTED FROM ANIMALS

The diagnosis of a lower respiratory tract infection is relatively simple in most cases. The major symptoms are fever, productive or nonproductive cough, chest pain that may be pleuritic, and shortness of breath. Headache and myalgias are common. Physical examination and chest radiography can confirm the diagnosis. Despite the relative ease of diagnosis, defining the etiologic agent of pneumonia remains difficult. Etiologic agents are commonly grouped into "typical" and "atypical" agents. Typical agents include *Streptococcus pneumoniae, Streptococcus* species, *S. aureus,* and *Haemophilus influenzae.* Atypical agents most commonly include respiratory viruses, mycoplasma, *Chlamydia pneumoniae,* and *Legionella pneumophila;* however, a variety of zoonotic pneumonias that are community-acquired must be considered in the differential diagnosis of "atypical pneumonia" (286,287).

Etiologic Agents and Epidemiology

Several zoonotic agents transmitted from pets may produce significant respiratory symptoms. Diseases transmitted by the aerosol route include anthrax, brucellosis, plague, psittacosis, Q fever, and tularemia. Other zoonotic agents that may involve the lungs include CSD, dirofilariasis, echinococcosis, ehrlichiosis, leptospirosis, melioidosis, pasteurellosis, Rocky Mountain spotted fever, toxocariasis, and toxoplasmosis. Of these, the pathogens most likely to be transmitted during pet therapy would be *Chlamydia psittaci* from infected birds, *C. burnetii* by infected cats, and *P. multocida* by close animal contact.

Pets, especially dogs, can develop fungal pneumonia following exposure to an environmental source with *Blastomyces dermatitidis, Coccidioides immitis, Histoplasma capsulatum,* and *Cryptococcus neoformans.* Common-source outbreaks involving humans and dogs of both histoplasmosis and blastomycosis have been described. In general, animal-to-human transmission does not occur; however, animal-to-human transmission of blastomycosis has been reported after dog bites.

The etiologic agents of mammalian tuberculosis *(M. tuberculosis, Mycobacterium bovis* and *Mycobacterium africanum(* can infect animals, and, rarely, animal-to-human transmission has been described. The main reservoir of *M. bovis* infection in mammals are cattle, but badgers, foxes, nonhuman primates, bison, and opossums have been found to be infected (288–290). Transmission to humans is usually via milk from infected cattle. Pasteurization and destruction of infected cattle has eliminated human *M. bovis* infection in the United States, but *M. bovis* infection remains a major public health problem worldwide. The main reservoir for *M. tuberculosis* is the human, but other animals including monkeys, large apes, and dogs can become infected.

Mycobacteriuam avium complex are of most consequence for birds but are also pathogenic for swine, cattle, sheep, dogs, cats, and humans. Other mycobacterial species, such as *Mycobacterium fortuitum, Mycobacterium chelonae, Mycobacterium kansasii,* and *M. marinum* have only infrequently been isolated from exotic and cold-blooded animals.

Prevention

Of the zoonotic agents that may cause pneumonia, only plague (291), *M. bovis* (292), Q fever, and possibly psittacosis (293) may be transmitted between humans. Patients with respiratory infections with these agents, therefore, should be placed on airborne precautions. Birds, especially psittacine birds, should be excluded from the hospital. Patients with respiratory infections consistent with tuberculosis should be maintained on airborne precautions and be prohibited from interacting with animals.

Q Fever

Epidemiology and Microbiology

Q fever is the only rickettsial microorganism spread primarily by the aerosol route rather than by an arthropod intermediate (294–308). In the United States, a variety of domestic farm animals may be infected, including goats, sheep, and cattle. Microorganisms are shed with placental tissues, feces, urine, and uterine discharges. Domestic animals may become infected from contact with contaminated tissues during parturition (309). Parturient cats have been the source of multiple outbreaks (310–312). A parturient dog has also been reported as the source of an outbreak (313).

Clinical Features of Disease and Diagnosis

Most patients with Q fever are asymptomatic, and disease is usually self-limited. The spectrum of Q fever includes isolated fever, flulike illness, atypical pneumonia, hepatitis, fever and rash, pericarditis, myocarditis, meningoencephalitis, and infection during pregnancy (314). Pneumonia is highly variable, occurring in up to 90% of cases (315,316). Acute disease typically manifests as a pneumonitis with malaise, anorexia, muscular pain, and usually an intense preorbital headache and fever; defervescence usually occurs within 1 or 2 weeks. Extrapulmonary complications include granulomatous hepatitis, pericarditis, myocarditis, uveitis, meningitis, and subacute bacterial endocarditis. Of these, endocarditis is the most common complication (317). Infection of vascular grafts has been reported (318). Chronic infection in patients with cancer has been described (319). As in animals, infection in pregnant women may result in maternal illness, prematurity, or abortion (320,321). Epidemiologic clues and serologic testing are the keys for proper diagnosis (322).

Prevention

Immunization with inactivated vaccine prepared from *C. burnetii* (Phase I)-infected yolk sac is available in Australia and Eastern European countries. It has proven useful in protecting laboratory workers and should also be considered for use by abattoir workers and others in hazardous occupations.

Chlamydia Psittaci

Epidemiology and Microbiology

C. psittaci is pathogenic for most avian species and is capable of widespread dissemination to humans who have pet birds, who visit pet shops, or who care for birds (323–327). During the 1980s, approximately 70% of the psittacosis cases with a known source of infection resulted from human exposure to caged pet birds (328). Other persons at risk include employees in poultry slaughtering and processing plants, veterinarians, laboratory workers, farmers, and zoo workers. Spread to humans occurs by inhalation of microorganisms persisting in dried feces, contact with bird feather dust, and exposure to birds flapping their wings for exercise. Outbreak investigations suggest that human-to-human transmission occurs in addition to animal-to-human transmission (329). Nosocomial outbreaks have been reported (293,330), but the accurate identification of the causative agent as *C. psittaci* has been questioned, because serologic tests may cross-react with *C. pneumoniae* (331). Infection with feline *C. psittaci* has been reported in a man with a cat (332).

Clinical Features of Disease and Diagnosis

C. psittaci causes infections in humans ranging from a severe systemic illness to an asymptomatic infection (333–338). Symptomatic psittacosis is characterized by high fever, chills, headache, myalgias, dry cough, and, sometimes, respiratory compromise. Extrapulmonary manifestations are common and include cardiac, neurologic, hematologic, hepatic, and renal changes. Case fatality rates as high as 40% have been reported, but with treatment mortality is usually less than 1%.

Similar to Q fever, the diagnosis is suggested by an epidemiologic exposure and compatible disease course and is confirmed by serology.

Yersinia pestis

Epidemiology and Microbiology

Most cases of plague result from humans coming into contact with sylvatic sources of disease and being bitten by an infected flea. Pneumonic plague may occur following hematogenous spread of bacteria during bacteremia in patients with bubonic or septicemic plague, or by inhalation of bacteria after coming into contact with a person or animal (most commonly a cat) with plague pneumonia. Acquisition of pneumonic plague via droplet transmission from an infected cat has been reported (339–343). Pneumonic plague in humans is believed to be highly contagious via droplet transmission. However, the last case of secondary pneumonic plague in the United States was reported in 1925 (344).

Clinical Features of Disease and Diagnosis

Inhalation plague pneumonia begins with a painless cough and shortness of breath (345–348). Pathologically, plague pneumonia is a bronchiolitis and alveolitis causing lobar consolidation and evolves into lobar consolidation with areas of hemorrhage. Patients with hematogenous plague pneumonia present with fever, lymphadenopathy, cough, hemoptysis, and chest pain. Diagnosis is via isolation of the causative pathogen from sputum.

GASTROINTESTINAL INFECTIONS ACQUIRED FROM ANIMAL RESERVOIRS

Many gastrointestinal pathogens of humans have animal reservoirs. These pathogens may then be acquired by humans via ingestion of contaminated surface waters; raw milk; and uncooked or undercooked foods, such as shellfish, fish, poultry, and meat. Enteric bacterial pathogens acquired from pets include *A. hydrophila, P. shigelloides, Campylobacter jejuni, E. tarda, Salmonella, Yersinia enterocolitica,* and *Yersinia pseudotuberculosis* (349). Parasites include *Cryptospordium, D. caninum, Giardia, Isospora belli,* and *Strongyloides* species (349).

Of the zoonotic infections, *Salmonella* is the greatest public health concern. Nontyphoidal *Salmonella* have been isolated from many domestic animals, including cats, dogs, birds, reptiles, hamsters, and monkeys. In the recent past, turtles were recognized as an important source of human salmonellosis (350). Pet turtles cause an estimated 14% of all cases of *Salmonella* infections in the United States for a total of 2,000,000 cases per year. Reptiles continue to be a source of human salmonellosis (351,352). Multiple outbreaks of *Salmonella* have been reported in hospitals involving person-to-person transmission, common-source outbreaks (e.g., food), and use of contaminated instruments (e.g., gastrointestinal endoscopes) (353).

Bacterial gastroenteritis linked to pets has been demonstrated for *A. hydrophila, P. shigelloides, Y. enterocolitica* (354), and *C. jejuni* (355–357). All of these pathogens have been isolated from many animals, including dogs, cats, reptiles, hamsters, and monkeys. In humans, all of these pathogens may cause gastroenteritis characterized by fever, chills, nausea, vomiting, and diarrhea.

Cryptosporidia is now recognized as an important gastrointestinal pathogen. In normal hosts, it generally causes an episode of self-limited diarrhea. However, in patients immunocompromised by HIV infection, it may cause chronic diarrhea with severe fluid losses and malnutrition. Multiple outbreaks among veterinarians have been described. Hospital (358–361) and veterinary school outbreaks (362) have also been described. Cats and dogs can likely transmit infective oocysts to humans.

Although most dogs and cats harbor *D. caninum,* human infections are uncommon (288). Infections are acquired by ingestion of an infected flea, which acts as an intermediate host. Infection may be asymptomatic or associated with abdominal pain, diarrhea, irritability, and anal pruritus. Passage of proglottids that resemble grains of rice in the stool may lead to presentation to a physician (363).

Toxocara canis and *Toxocara cati* are helminth parasites that affect dogs and cats, respectively. Animals may be infected *in utero* and transplacentally or may become infected by ingestion of infested feces. Once passed in animal feces, the ova take several weeks to mature but can remain viable for months. Humans are infected by ingestion of the ova. This situation usually occurs in children younger than 6 years who play in areas where cats and dogs defecate. Contamination of sandboxes used by daycare centers has been demonstrated. In humans, most infections are asymptomatic but may present as cough and wheezing from pulmonary migration, or with abdominal pain, hepatomegaly, and peripheral eosinophilia.

The reservoir for *Giardia* are wild animals. The role of pets in the transmission of giardiasis to humans has not been well defined; however, there have been isolated reports of giardiasis related to dog or cat exposure.

Fang et al. (349) have summarized several rules to help prevent the acquisition of enteric infections from pets. These rules include (a) wash hands after handling an animal, (b) keep cages and pens clean to avoid attracting fleas, (c) do not use waste material from pets as fertilizer, (d) cover children's sandboxes when not in use, (e) consult a veterinarian regarding illness in a pet, (f) deworm dogs and cats regularly and do not allow them to defecate on playgrounds, (g) remove animal feces on a lawn frequently, (h) dispose of cat litter daily, (i) treat affected pets and their areas with powders and sprays on alternate weeks for effective flea control, and (j) do not keep turtles as pets.

GUIDELINES FOR PREVENTION OF TRANSMISSION OF ZOONOTIC DISEASES

Service Animals

Service animals such as guide dogs provide an important health service for the disabled. Prohibiting service animals access to a public facility violates the ADA. Recommendations for the use of guide dogs in hospitals have been published (Table 101.5).

Pet-Facilitated Therapy

An extensive literature supports the use of pet-facilitated therapy. Benefits cited by advocates include improved self-esteem, increased knowledge and practice of caring from pets, increased socialization by sharing animal experiences, increased empathy, production of feelings of being liked unconditionally, enhanced nurturing behaviors, increased feelings of control, increased independence, and increased ability to follow directions. Unfortunately, these reported benefits are almost entirely based on anecdotal reports rather than on controlled clinical trials. Additional research is required to determine scientifically which patients would benefit from pet-facilitated therapy and the best form of animal-human interaction.

Animals within the hospital pose a potential risk; however, with the use of a carefully developed and implemented policy,

TABLE 101.5. RECOMMENDATIONS FOR THE USE OF SERVICE ANIMALS IN HOSPITALS

1. Healthcare facilities should have a policy regarding the use of service animals by emplopyees, visitors, and patients.
2. Service animals should not be allowed into the hospital if they are unhealthy; feverish; or suffering from gastroenteritis, fleas, or skin lesions. Such animals should be evaluated by a veterinarian.
3. Healthy, well-groomed dogs that are guiding their owners may enter all areas of a hospital that are generally accessible to the public, such as lobbies and cafeterias, and may proceed to nursing stations on unrestricted wards. There the owner should inquire about the possibility of visiting a patient. Depending on the condition of the patient, a healthcare provider will give the owner permission to proceed with the dog.
4. Service animals should defecate outside of the hospital. Use standard precautions (gloves) and EPA approved surface disinfectants to clean any soiled areas.
5. Petting and playing with the guide dog by hospital personnel or patients should be prohibited.
6. After settling their animal, disabled people should wash their hands before coming into direct contact with patients.
7. Service animals should not be allowed to come into direct contact with nonintact skin (e.g., wounds).
8. Consideration should be given to restricting visits by persons using service aninmals in the following circumstances (decide on a case-by-case basis):
   a. The patient is in isolation for respiratory, enteric, or other infectious diseases or is on protective isolation.[a]
   b. The patient, although not on protective isolation, is immunocompromised or has an immunocompromised roommate.
   c. The patient is in an intensive care unit, burn unit, or other restricted-access unit of the hospital.
   d. The patient or a roommate has an allergy to dogs or a severe phobia.
   e. The patient or roommate is psychotic, hallucinating, or confused, or has an altered perception of reality and is not amenable to rational explanations.

EPA, Environmental Protection Agency.
[a] Patient is in a laminar air-flow room or similar protected environment designed to protect patients with high levels of immunosuppression, such as bone marrow transplant patients.

TABLE 101.6. MODEL PET VISITATION/THERAPY PROTOCOL

I. Purpose

To allow hospitalized children the opportunity to interact with animals in an effort to reduce the stress incurred by hospitalization and to provide hospitalized children with the opportunity to enhance their task and social skills.

II. Procedure

Potential pet volunteers and their dogs will be screened by the local animal protection shelter (APS) and volunteer veterinarians using appropriate health and behavioral screening tools. Records of the microorganisms recovered in cultures will be maintained by the APS and forwarded to infection control for review.

Volunteers will attend the hospital's volunteer orientation and will also meet with members of the hospital's recreation therapy team.

Trained volunteers and their dogs will be allowed to visit the hospitalized children in a designated central area on a monthly basis. The dogs must pass a behavioral and medical screen before participating in this program.

The behavioral screen, which will occur twice a year, includes assessment of the dogs' response to a new environment; the approach of, physical contact with, and interaction with a stranger; response to an unexpected loud noise; response to painful stimulation; and reaction to an unexpected event.

The medical screening includes proof of up-to-date immunizations (distemper, parainfluenza, hepatitis, parvovirus, and rabies), having fecal and nasal cultures every 4 months, receiving routine medication for the prevention of heartworm, and following a flea prevention routine.

Animals positive for any of the following microorganisms will be excluded until one negative culture (negative stool examination for *Giardia*) has been obtained after treatment for the specific microorganism: *Giardia*, group A streptococcus, *Shigella*, *Salmonella*, and *Campylobacter*.

The dog must also be bathed with a flea shampoo and receive an antiflea dip on the day before or the day of the hospital visit. The dog must also wear a designated shirt to identify it as a canine volunteer and to reduce the spread of dog hair. The dog must be on a leash and under the direct supervision of the owner at all times.

On the day of the hospital visit, the pet volunteer and dog will be met by a recreation therapist at the front door of the hospital. The pair will be escorted to the elevators and then to the final hospital location. The escort and pet visitation pair must be the only occupants of the elevator. Pets on antibiotic therapy for an infection, with skin or ear infections, wearing a bandage, or experiencing any gastrointestinal upset will be excluded from visiting.

As part of the hospital admission packet, the parent(s) of children admitted to the hospital will be asked to sign a consent form allowing their child to participate in the pet visitation program. In addition, the attending physician must write an order in the medical record (chart) for the child to participate in the pet visitation program. Hospitalized children with the following ailments will be excluded from participating in the pet visitation program: (1) children with open sores on exposed areas of skin, (2) children exhibiting aggressive behavior, (3) neutropenic children (WBC $<$1,000), (4) HIV-infected children; and (5) children with immunoglobulin deficiencies.

The animals will not be permitted to play with the children's toys.

HIV, human immunodeficiency virus; WBC, white blood cell.

animals can probably be used with minimal risk (Table 101.6). Infection control guidelines for AAAs and AAT are also available from the Delta Society (79,364,365). Similar to the perceived benefits of pet therapy, the risks have been incompletely assessed. In a recent study, however, 2,361 visits to 1,158 patients by dogs under "strict guidelines" did not result in any incidents of zoonotic infections or evidence that the dogs acted as fomites in the transmission of microorganisms from patient to patient (366). Additional studies are warranted, especially before immunocompromised patients are allowed contact with animals. The Delta Society provides a directory listing of AAT and AAA programs in hospitals (Web site: *www.deltasociety.org*).

More detailed guidelines regarding the evaluation of patients suitable for AAT, medical clearance procedures for animals considered for pet therapy, and protocols for the management of pet therapy in healthcare facilities have been published (79,97, 101,364).

OTHER USES OF ANIMALS IN HOSPITALS

Medicinal Leeches

Leeches have been used in medicine for centuries. The word *leech* is likely derived from the Old English *laece* meaning physician (367). Leeches continue to be used in modern medicine in the management of acute problems related to vascular congestion in patients with reimplantation of digits and ears and in reconstruction using cutaneous or muscle flaps (368–372). Leeches are useful in reducing vascular congestion, because they are capable of ingesting up to ten times their body weight in blood. The process of absorbing blood is aided by the production of hirudin, which inhibits the thrombin-catalyzed conversion of fibrinogen to fibrin, hyaluronidase, proteinase inhibitors, and a vasodilator.

The most common leech used is *Hirudo medicinalis.* Wound infections are an important hazard with the use of medicinal leeches. The most common pathogen is *A. hydrophila* (373–375), but infection with *Vibrio fluvialis* has also been reported (376). The incidence of wound infections has been reported to be 7% (273) and 20% (377). Multiple potential pathogens have been isolated from *H. medicinalis,* including *A. hydrophila, Staphylococcus* species, *Alcaligenes* species, *Pseudomonas putida,* and *Fusobacterium varium* (378). *A. hydrophila* obtained from the gut of *H. medicinalis* has been found to be susceptible to third-generation cephalosporins and tetracycline (379). Systemic antibiotics administered to patients have been found to penetrate into leeches and to significantly reduce the rate of *A. hydrophila* isolation compared with controls (i.e., 12% versus 100%) (380). For this reason, suppression of leech enteric bacteria by antibiotic administration has been recommended as possibly an effective strategy to prevent invasive infection with

A. hydrophila. Additional clinical trials have been recommended, however, to assess the efficacy of prophylactic antibiotic administration (380).

Medicinal leeches should not be reused between patients because of the risk of cross-infection. Syphilis, puerperal fever, and erysipelas have occurred from reuse of medicinal leeches (367). Furthermore, laboratory studies have indicated that many parasites, such as *Toxoplasma gondii* and *Trypanosoma brucei,* not only survive but also multiply inside the gut of the leech (381). Once used, medicinal leeches are a biohazard and should be discarded in a manner consistent with Occupational Safety and Health Administration (OSHA) guidelines.

CONCLUSIONS

The use of service animals provides a valuable function for the disabled. Adherence to the ADA with regard to service animals can be safely managed in the hospital setting. The benefits of a well-managed AAT program remain inadequately demonstrated by scientific studies. However, the risks have proved largely theoretical. Pets have been associated with nosocomial infections and should be prohibited from hospitals. All healthcare facilities should have policies regarding service animals and the visitation by personal pets.

REFERENCES

1. American Veterinary Medical Association. *U.S. pet ownership and demographics sourcebook.* Schaumburg, IL: American Veterinary Medical Association, 2002.
2. Gratzeck JB. Tropical fish: keeping a giant industry healthy. In: *Animal health, 1984 yearbook of agriculture.* 347–357.
3. Anonymous. Dog and cat food represent an $8.7 billion opportunity. *Food People* 1998 March:14.
4. Hubbert WT, McCulloch WF, Schnurrenberger PR. *Diseases transmitted from animals to man,* 6th ed. Springfield, IL: Charles C. Thomas, 1975.
5. Acha PN, Szyfres B. *Zoonoses and communicable diseases common to man and animals,* 2nd ed. Scientific publication no. 503. Washington DC: Pan American Health Organization, 1987.
6. Zoonosis update. *J Am Vet Med Assoc* 1990.
7. Bell JC, Palmer SR, Payne JM. *The zoonoses: infections transmitted from animals to man.* Baltimore: Edward Arnold, 1988.
8. Weinberg AN, Weber DJ. Animal-associated human infections. *Infect Dis Clin North Am* 1991;5:1–181.
9. Beran GW, Steele JH. *Handbook of zoonoses,* 2nd ed. *Section A: bacterial, rickettsial, chlamydial, and mycotic.* Boca Raton, FL: CRC Press, 1994.
10. Beran GW, Steele JH. *Handbook of zoonoses,* 2nd ed. *Section B: viral.* Boca Raton, FL: CRC Press, 1994.
11. Palmer SR, Soulsby L, Simpson DIH. *Zoonoses: biology, clinical practice, and public health control.* Oxford, UK:Oxford Press, 1998.
12. Langley RL. Animal handlers. *Occupational Medicine* 1999;14(2): 1–478.
13. Krauss H, Weber A, Appel M, et al. *Zoonoses,* 3rd ed. Washington DC: American Society for Microbiology Press, 2003.
14. Sanford JP. Humans and animals: increasing contacts, increasing infections. *Hosp Pract* 1990;25:123–130, 133–134, 137–140.
15. Hart CA, Trees AJ, Duerden BI. Zoonoses: introduction. *J Med Microbiol* 1997;46:4–6, 28–33.
16. Sellman J, Bender J. Zoonotic infections in travelers to the tropics. *Primary Care Clin Office Pract* 2002;29:907–929.
17. Elliot DL, Tolle SW, Goldberg L, et al. Pet-associated illness. *N Engl J Med* 1985;313:985–995.
18. Chretien JH, Garagusi VF. Infections associated with pets. *Am Fam Physician* 1990;41:831–845.
19. Marx MB. Parasites, pets, and people. *Primary Care* 1991;18: 153–165.
20. Goldstein EJ. Household pets and human infections. *Infect Dis Clin North Am* 1991;5:117–130.
21. Chomel BB. Zoonoses of house pets other than dogs, cats and birds. *Pediatr Infect Dis J* 1992;11:479–487.
22. Harris JM. Zoonotic diseases of birds. *Vet Clin North Am* 1991;21: 1289–1298.
23. Riordan A, Tarlow M. Pets and diseases. *Br J Hosp Med* 1996;56: 321–324.
24. Plaut M, Zimmerman EM, Goldstein RA. Health hazards to humans associated with domestic pets. *Annu Rev Public Health* 1996;17: 221–245.
25. Tan JS. Human zoonotic infections transmitted by dogs and cats. *Arch Intern Med* 1997;157:1933–1943.
26. Steele RW. Sizing up the risks of pet-transmitted diseases. *Contemp Pediatr* 1997;14:43–44, 49, 54–56, 59, 60, 65, 68.
27. Glaser C, Lewis P, Wong S. Pet-, animal-, and vector-borne infections. *Pediatr Rev* 2000;21:219–232.
28. Morrison G. Zoonotic infections from pets. Understanding the risks and treatment. *Postgrad Med* 2001;110:24–26, 29–30, 35–36.
29. Kravetz JD, Federman DG. Cat-associated zoonoses. *Arch Intern Med* 2002;162:1945–1952.
30. Mandell GL, Douglas RG, Bennett JE. *Principles and practice of infectious diseases,* 6th ed. New York: Churchill Livingstone *(in press).*
31. Gorbach SL, Bartlett JG, Blacklow NR. *Infectious diseases,* 2nd ed. Philadelphia: WB Saunders, 1998.
32. Fox JG, Lipman NS. Infections transmitted by large and small laboratory animals. *Infect Dis Clin North Am* 1991;5:131–163.
33. Franz DR, Jahrling PB, Friedlander AM, et al. Clinical recognition and management of patients exposed to biological warfare agents. *JAMA* 1997;278:399–411.
34. Atlas RM. The medical threat of biological weapons. *Crit Rev Microbiol* 1998;24:157–168.
35. Centers for Disease Control and Prevention. Biological and chemical terrorism: strategic plan for preparedness and response. *MMWR Morb Mortal Wkly Rep* 2000;49(RR-4).
36. Franz DR, Jahrling PB, McClain DJ, et al. Clinical recognition and management of patients exposed to biological warfare agents. *Clin Lab Med* 2001;21:435–473.
37. Bronze MS, Huycke MM, Machado LJ, et al. Viral agents as biological weapons and agents of bioterrorism. *Am J Med Sci* 2002;323: 316–325.
38. Greenfield RA, Drevets DA, Machado LJ, et al. Bacterial pathogens as biological weapons and agents of bioterrorism. *Am J Med Sci* 2002; 323:299–315.
39. Darling RG, Catlett CL, Huebner KD, et al. Threats in bioterrorism. I: CDC category A agents. *Emerg Med Clin North Am* 2002;20: 273–309.
40. Moran GJ. Threats in bioterrorism. I: CDC category B and C agents. *Emerg Med Clin North Am* 2002;20:311–330.
41. Fishman JA. Infection and xenotransplantation. Developing strategies to minimize the risk. *Ann N Y Acad Sci* 1998;862:52–66.
42. Fishman JA. Infections in xenotransplantation.*BMJ* 2000;321: 717–718.
43. Onions DE, Witt CJ. Xenotransplantation: an overview of microbiological risks and potential for risk management. *Revue Scientifique Technique* 2000;19:289–301.
44. Fishman JA. Infection in xenotransplantation. *J Cardiac Surg* 2001; 16:363–373.
45. Boneva RS, Folks TM, Chapman LE. Infectious diseases issues in xenotransplantation. *Clin Microbiol Rev* 2001;14:1–14.
46. Chapman LE. Xenotransplantation: public health risks—patient vs. society in an emerging field. *Curr Top Microbiol Immunol* 2003;278: 23–45.
47. Weinberg A. Ecology and epidemiology of zoonotic pathogens. *Infect Dis Clin North Am* 1991;5:1–6.

48. Walker DH, Barbour AG, Oliver JH, et al. Emerging bacterial zoonotic and vector-borne diseases. *JAMA* 1996;275:463–469.
49. Murphy FA. Emerging zoonoses. *Emerg Infect Dis* 1998;4:429–435.
50. Mahy BW, Brown CC. Emerging zoonoses: crossing the species barrier. *Revue Scientifique Technique* 2000;19:33–40.
51. Weiss RA. Cross-species infections. *Curr Top Microbiol Immunol* 2003;278:47–71.
52. Smolinski MS, Hamburg MA, Lenderbeg J. *Microbial threats to health.* Institute of Medicine, 2003.
53. Westbury HA. Hendra virus disease in horses. *Revue Scientifique Technique* 2000;19:151–159.
54. Wong KT, Shieh WJ, Zaki SR, et al. Nipah virus infection, an emerging paramyxoviral zoonosis. *Springer Semin Immunopathol* 2002;24: 215–228.
55. Guan Y, Zheng BJ, He YQ, et al. Isolation and characterization of viruses related to SARS coronavirus from animals in southern China. *Science* 2003;302:276–278.
56. Yu V, Meissner C. Zoonoses. In: Schaechter M, Medoff G, Schlessinger D, eds. *Mechanisms of microbial diseases.* Baltimore: Williams & Wilkins, 1989:749–764.
57. Ryan KJ. Some bacteria causing zoonotic diseases. In: Sherris JC, ed. *Medical microbiology,* 2nd ed. New York: Elsevier, 1990:489–498.
58. Marcus LC, Marcus E. Nosocomial zoonoses. *N Engl J Med* 1998; 338:757–759.
59. Scott GM, Thomson R, Malone-Lee J, et al. Cross-infection between animals and man: possible feline transmission of *Staphylococcus aureus* infection in humans? *J Hosp Infect* 1988;12:29–34.
60. Lyons RW, Samples CL, DeSilva HN, et al. An epidemic of resistant *Salmonella* in a nursery: animal-to-human spread. *JAMA* 1980;243: 546–547.
61. Richet HM, Craven PC, Brown JM, et al. A cluster of *Rhodococcus (Gordona) bronchialis* sternal-wound infections after coronary-artery bypass surgery. *N Engl J Med* 1991;324:104–109.
62. Chang HJ, Miller HL, Watkins N, et al. An epidemic of *Malassezia pachydermatis* in an intensive care nursery associated with colonization of health care workers' pet dogs. *N Engl J Med* 1998;338:706–711.
63. Mossovitch M, Mossovitch B, Alkan M. Nosocomial dermatophytosis caused by *Microsporum canis* in a newborn department. *Infect Control* 1986;7:593–595.
64. Snider R, Lander S, Levy ML. The ringworm riddle: an outbreak of *Microsporum canis* in the nursery. *Pediatr Infect Dis J* 1993;12: 145–148.
65. Drusin LM, Ross BG, Rhodes KH, et al. Nosocomial ringworm in a neonatal intensive care unit: a nurse and her cat. *Infect Control Hosp Epidemiol* 2000;21:605–607.
66. Jorm LR, Lightfoot NF, Morgan KL. An epidemiological study of an outbreak of Q fever in a secondary school. *Epidemiol Infect* 1990; 104:467–477.
67. Fishbein DB, Raoult D. A cluster of *Coxiella burnetii* infections associated with exposure to vaccinated goats and their unpasteurized dairy products. *Am J Trop Med Hyg* 1992;47:35–40.
68. Hamadeh GN, Turner BW, Trible W, et al. Laboratory outbreak of Q fever. *J Fam Pract* 1992;35:683–685.
69. Hartman JB. Q fever in Great Britain. Clinical account of eight cases. *Lancet* 1949;ii:1028–1030.
70. Gerth H, Leidig U, Reimenschneider T. Q-fiever epidemie in einem Institut fur Humanpathologie. *Dtch Med Wochenschr* 1982;107: 1391–1395.
71. Mann JS, Douglas JG, Inglis JM, et al. Q fever: person-to-person transmission within a family. *Thorax* 1986;41:974–975.
72. Deutch DL, Peterson ET. Q fever: transmission from one human to others. *JAMA* 1950;143:348–350.
73. Raoult DL, Stein A. Q fever during pregnancy-a risk fro women, fetuses, and obstetrician [Letter]. *N Engl J Med* 1994;330:371.
74. Osorio S, Sarria C, Gonzalez-Ruano P, et al. Nosocomial transmission of Q fever. *J Hosp Infect* 2003;54:162–168.
75. Duncan SL. APIC state-of-the art report: the implications of service animals in health care settings. *Am J Infect Control* 2000;29:170–180.
76. Sandler JL. Care and treatment of service dogs and their owners. *JAVMA* 1996;208:1979–1981.
77. Hardy GJ. The seeing-eye dog: an infection risk in hospital. *CMAJ* 1981;124:698–700.
78. Houghtalen RP, Doody J. After the ADA: service dogs on inpatient psychiatric units. *Bull Am Acad Psychiatr Law* 1995;23:211–217.
79. Delta Society. *Animal-assisted therapy: therapeutic interventions.* Renton, WA: Delta Society, 1997.
80. Carpenter S. Therapeutic roles of animals. *JAVMA* 1997;211:154.
81. Draper RJ, Gerber GJ, Layng EM. Defining the role of pet animals in psychotherapy. *Psychiatr J Univ Ottawa* 1990;15:169–172.
82. Allen DT. Effects of dogs on human health. *JAVMA* 1997;210: 1136–1139.
83. Edney ATB. Companion animals and human health: an overview. *J R Soc Med* 1995;88:704–708.
84. Beck AM, Meyers NM. Health enhancement and companion animal ownership. *Ann Rev Pub Health* 1996;17:247–257.
85. Willis DA. Animal therapy. *Rehabil Nurs* 1997;22:78–81.
86. Jorgenson J. Therapeutic use of companion animals in health care. *Image* 1997;29:249–254.
87. Gammonley J, Howie AR, Kirwin S, et al. *Animal-assisted therapy: therapeutic interventions.* Renton, WA: Delta Society, 1997.
88. Brodie SJ, Biley FC. An exploration of the potential benefits of pet-facilitated therapy. *J Clin Nurs* 1999;8:329–337.
89. Hooker SD, Freeman LH, Stewart P. Pet therapy research: a historical review. *Holist Nurs Pract* 2003;17:17–23.
90. Hundley J. Pet project: the use of pet-facilitated therapy among the chronically mentally ill. *J Psychosoc Nurs* 1991;29:23–26.
91. Edney ATB. Companion animals and human health. *Vet Record* 1992; 130:285–287.
92. Anonymous. Patients' best friend? *Nurs Times* 1991;87:34–35.
93. Glickman LT. Implications of the human/animal bond for human health and veterinary practice. *JAVMA* 1992;201:848–851.
94. Laun. Benefits of pet therapy in dementia. *Home Healthcare Nurse* 2003;21:49–52.
95. Patronek GJ, Glickman LT. Pet ownership protects against the risks and consequences of coronary heart disease. *Med Hypotheses* 1993; 40:245–249.
96. Carmack BJ. The role of companion animals for persons with AIDS/ HIV. *Holist Nurs Pract* 1991;5:24–31.
97. Khan MA, Farrag N. Animal-assisted activity and infection control implications in a healthcare setting. *J Hosp Infect* 2000;46:4–11.
98. Owen OG. Paws for thought. *Nurs Times* 2001;97:28–29.
99. Guay DR. Pet-assisted therapy in the nursing home setting: potential for zoonosis. *Am J Infect Control* 2001;29:178–186.
100. Donowitz LG. Pet therapy. *Pediatr Infect Dis J* 2002;21:64–66.
101. Brodie SJ, Biley FC, Shewring M. An exploration of the potential risks associated with using pet therapy in healthcare settings. *J Clin Nurs* 2002;11:444–4356.
102. Overall KL, Love M. Dog bites to humans—demography, epidemiology, injury, and risk. *JAVMA* 2001;218:1923—1934.
103. Sacks JJ, Kresnow M, Houston B. Dog bites: how big a problem? *Injury Prev* 1996;2:52–54.
104. Lauer EA, White WC, Lauer BA. Dog bites. *Am J Dis Child* 1982; 136:202–204.
105. Kizer KW. Epidemiologic and clinical aspects of animal bite injuries. *J Am Coll Emerg Phys* 1979;8:134–141.
106. Weiss HB, Friedman DI, Coben JH. Incidence of dog bite injuries treated in emergency departments. *JAMA* 1998;279:51–53.
107. Douglas LG. Bite wounds. *Am Fam Physician* 1975;11:93–99.
108. Aghababian RV, Conte JE. Mammalian bite wounds. *Ann Emerg Med* 1980;9:79–83.
109. Centers for Disease Control and Prevention. Nonfatal dog bite-related injuries treated in hospital emergency departments—United States, 2001. *MMWR Morb Mortal Wkly Rep* 2003;52:605–608, 610.
110. Berzon DR, DeHoff JB. Medical costs and other aspects of dog bites in Baltimore. *Public Health Rep* 1974;89:377–381.
111. Graham WP, Calabretta AM, Miller SH. Dog bites. *Am Fam Physician* 1977;15:132–137.
112. Maetz HM. Animal bites, a public health problem in Jefferson County, Alabama. *Public Health Rep* 1979;94:528–534.

113. Chun Y-T, Berkelhamer JE, Herold TE. Dog bites in children less than 4 years old. *Pediatrics* 1982;69:119–120.
114. Quinlan KP, Sacks JJ. Hospitalizations for dog bite injuries. *JAMA* 1999;281:232–233.
115. Centers for Disease Control and Prevention. Dog bite—related fatalities—United States, 1995–96. *MMWR Morb Mortal Wkly Rep* 1997; 46:463–467.
116. Sacks JJ, Sinclair L, Gilchrist J, et al. Breeds of dogs involved in fatal human attacks in the United States between 1979 and 1998. *JAVMA* 2000;217:836–840.
117. Weber DJ, Hansen AR. Infections resulting from animal bites. *Infect Dis Clin North Am* 1991;5:663–680.
118. Goldstein EJC. Bite wounds and infection. *Clin Infect Dis* 1992;14: 633–640.
119. Beck AM. The epidemiology and prevention of animal bites. *Semin Vet Med Surg* 1991;6:186–191.
120. Goldstein EJC. Infectious complications and therapy of bite wounds. *J Am Podiatr Med Assoc* 1989;79:486–491.
121. Anderson CR. Animal bites: guidelines to current management. *Postgrad Med* 1992;92:134–149.
122. Dire DJ. Emergency management of dog and cat bite wounds. *Emerg Med Clin North Am* 1992;4:719–736.
123. Hagan M, Goldstein E, Sanford JP. Bites from pet animals. *Hosp Pract* 1993;28:79–86, 90.
124. Griego RD, Rosen T, Orengo IF, et al. Dog, cat, and human bites: a review. *J Am Acad Dermatol* 1995;33:1019–1029.
125. Dinman S, Jarosz DA. Managing serious dog bite injuries in children. *Pediatr Nurs* 1996;22:413–417.
126. Kelleher AT, Gordon SM. Management of bite wounds and infection in primary care. *Cleve Clin J Med* 1997;64:137–141.
127. Goldstein EJC. Current concepts on animal bites: bacteriology and therapy. *Curr Clin Top Infect Dis* 1999;19:99–111.
128. Presutti RJ. Prevention and treatment of dog bites. *Am Fam Physician* 2001;63:1567–1572.
129. Berzon DR. The animal bite epidemic in Baltimore, Maryland: review and update. *Am J Public Health* 1978;68:593–595.
130. Berzon DR, Farber RE, Gordon J, et al. Animal bites in a large city—a report on Baltimore, Maryland. *Am J Public Health* 1972;62: 422–426.
131. Moore RM, Zehmer RB, Moulthrop JI, et al. Surveillance of animal-bite cases in the United States, 1971–1972. *Arch Environ Health* 1977;32:267–270.
132. Spence G. A review of animal bites in Delaware—1989 to 1990. *Del Med J* 1990;62:1425–1433.
133. Wright JC. Reported cat bites in Dallas: characteristics of the cats, the victims, and the attack events. *Public Health Rep* 1990;105:420–424.
134. Karlson TA. The incidence of facial injuries from dog bites. *JAMA* 1984;251:3265–3267.
135. Bernardo LM, Gardner MJ, O'Connor J, et al. Dog bites in children treated in a pediatric emergency department. *JSPN* 2000;5:87–95.
136. Bernardo LM, Gardner MJ, Rosenfield RL, et al. A comparison of dog bite injuries in younger and older children treated in a pediatric emergency department. *Pediatr Emerg Care* 2002;18:247–249.
137. Shewell PC, Nancarrow JD. Dogs that bite. *BMJ* 1991;303: 1512–1513.
138. Levene S. Dog bites to children [Letter]. *BMJ* 1991;303:466.
139. Callaham ML. Treatment of common dog bites: infection risk factors. *J Am Coll Emerg Phys* 1978;7:83–87.
140. Dire DJ. Cat bite wounds: risk factors for infection. *Ann Emerg Med* 1991;20:973–979.
141. Rayan GM, Downard D, Cahill S, et al. A comparison of human and animal mouth flora. *J Okla State Med Assoc* 1991;84:510–515.
142. Bailie WE, Stowe EC, Schmitt AM. Aerobic bacterial flora of oral and nasal fluids of canines with reference to bacteria associated with bites. *J Clin Microbiol* 1978;7:223–231.
143. Ordog GJ. The bacteriology of dog bite wounds on initial presentation. *Ann Emerg Med* 1986;15:1324–1329.
144. Goldstein EJC, Reinhardt JF, Murray PM, et al. Outpatient therapy of bite wounds. *Int J Dermatol* 1987;26:123–127.
145. Talan DA, Citron DM, Abrahamian FM, et al. Bacteriologic analysis of infected dog and cat bites. *N Engl J Med* 1999;340:85–92.
146. Talan DA, Staatz D, Staatz A, et al. *Staphylococcus intermedius* in canine gingiva and canine-inflicted human wound infections: laboratory characterization of a newly recognized zoonotic pathogen. *J Clin Microbiol* 1989;27:78–81.
147. Goldstein EJC, Citron DM, Finegold SM. Dog bite wounds and infection: a prospective clinical study. *Ann Emerg Med* 1980;9: 508–512.
148. Goldstein EJC, Citron DM, Wield B, et al. Bacteriology of human and animal bite wounds. *J Clin Microbiol* 1978;8:667–672.
149. Scott MJ. Cutaneous blastomycosis: report of a case following dog bite. *Northwest Med* 1955;54:255–257.
150. Parry WH, Seymour MW. An unusual case of leptospirosis. *Practitioner* 1973;210:791–793.
151. Robertson MG. *Brucella* infection transmitted by dog bite. *JAMA* 1973;225:750–751.
152. Bimbaum M, Miller K, Sratigos GT. *Salmonella typhi* facial infection. *Oral Surg Oral Med Oral Pathol* 1980;49:219–220.
153. Collins MM. The transmission of tularemia by the domestic cat. New Orleans *Med Surg J* 1933;86:105–106.
154. Rudesill CL. Tularemia from bite of a nursing kitten. *JAMA* 1937; 108:2118.
155. Jungherr E. Latent feline tularemia apparently responsible for a human infection. *J Bacteriol* 1942;43:643.
156. Miller LD, Mongomergy EL. Human tularemia transmitted by bite of cat. *JAVMA* 1957;130:314.
157. Shaffer JH. Tularemia: a report of four cases with unusual contacts. *Ann Intern Med* 1943;18:72–80.
158. Cooper WR, Ewell NM. Cat scratch induced tularemia. *Virginia Med Monthly* 100:640–642.
159. Quenzer RW, Mostow SR, Emerson JK. Cat-bite tularemia. *JAMA* 1977;238:1845.
160. Gallivan MVE, Davis WA, Garagusi VF, et al. Fatal cat-transmitted tularemia: demonstration of the organism in tissue. *South Med J* 1980; 73:240–242.
161. Evans ME, McGee ZA, Hunter PT, et al. Tularemia and the tomcat. *JAMA* 1981;246:1343.
162. Rohrback BW. Tularemia. *JAVMA* 1988;193:428–432.
163. Liles WC, Burger RJ. Tularemia from domestic cats. *West J Med* 1993;158:619–622.
164. Capellan J, Fong IW. Tularemia from a cat bite: case report and review of feline-associated tularemia. *Clin Infect Dis* 1993;16: 472–475.
165. Arav-Boger R. Cat-bite tularemia in a seventeen-year-old girl treated with ciprofloxacin. *Pediatr Infect Dis J* 2000;19:583–584.
166. Centers for Disease Control and Prevention. Human plague associated with domestic cats—California, Colorado. *MMWR Morb Mortal Wkly Rep* 1981;30:265–266.
167. Weniger BG, Warren AJ, Forseth V, et al. Human bubonic plague transmitted by a domestic cat scratch. *JAMA* 1984;251:927–928.
168. Eidson M, Tierney LA, Rollag OJ, et al. Feline plague in New Mexico: risk factors and transmission to humans. *Am J Public Health* 1988; 78:1333–1335.
169. Centers for Disease Control and Prevention. Human plague—United States, 1993–1994 *MMWR Morb Mortal Wkly Rep* 1994;43: 242–246.
170. Ordog GJ. Rat bites: fifty cases. *Ann Emerg Med* 1985;14:126–130.
171. Kizer KW, Constantine DG. Pet ferrets—a hazard to public health and wildlife. *West J Med* 1989;150:466.
172. Applegate JA, Walhout MF. Childhood risks from the ferret. *J Emerg Med* 1998;16:425–427.
173. Smith W, Stuart-Harris CH. Influenza infection of man from the ferret. *Lancet* 1936;231:121–123.
174. Jones JW, Pether JVS, Rainey HA, et al. Recurrent *Mycobacterium bovis* infection following a ferret bite. *J Infect* 1993;26:225–226.
175. Marini RP, Adkins JA, Fox JG. Proven or potential zoonotic diseases of ferrets. *JAVMA* 1989;195:990–994.
176. Rayan GM, Flournoy DJ, Cahill SL. Aerobic mouth flora of the rhesus monkey. *J Hand Surg* 1987;12A:299–301.

177. Janda DH, Ringler DH, Hilliard J, et al. Nonhuman primate bites. *J Orthoped Res* 1990;8:146–150.
178. Goldstein EJC, Pryor EP, Citron DM. Simian bites and bacterial infection. *Clin Infect Dis* 1995;20:1551–1552.
179. Holmes GP, Hilliar JK, Klontz KC, et al. B virus Herpesvirus simiae infection in humans: epidemiologic investigation of a cluster. *Ann Intern Med* 1990;112:833–839.
180. Weigler BJ. Biology of B virus in macaque and human hosts: a review. *Clin Infect Dis* 1992;14:555–567.
181. Davenport DS, Johnson DR, Holmes GP, et al. Diagnosis and management of human B virus (Herpesvirus simiae) infections in Michigan. *Clin Infect Dis* 1994;19:33–41.
182. Ostrowski SR, Leslie MJ, Parrott T, et al. B-virus from pet macaque monkeys: an emerging threat in the United States? *Emerg Infect Dis* 1998;4:117–121.
183. Cohen JI, Davenport DS, Stewart JA, et al. Recommendations for prevention and therapy for exposure to B virus (cercophithcine herpesvirus 1). *Clin Infect Dis* 2002;35:1191–1203.
184. Chen HI, Hulten K, Clarridge JE. Taxonomic subgroups of *Pasteruella multocida* correlate with clinical presentation. *J Clin Microbiol* 2002;40:3438–3441.
185. Weber DJ, Wolfson JS, Swartz MN, et al. *Pasteurella multocida* infections: report of 34 cases and review of the literature. *Medicine* 1984; 63:133–154.
186. Hubbert WT, Rosen MN. I. *Pasteurella multocida* infection due to animal bite. *Am J Public Health* 1970;60:1103–1108.
187. Holloway WJ, Scott EG, Adams YB. *Pasteurella multocida* infection in man. *Am J Clin Pathol* 1969;51:705–708.
188. Furie RA, Cohen RP, Hartman BJ, et al. *Pasteurella multocida* infection: report in urban setting and review of spectrum of human disease. *N Y State J Med* 1980;80:1597–1602.
189. Francis DP, Holmes MA, Brandon G. *Pasteurella multocida:* infections after domestic animal bites and scratches. *JAMA* 1975;233: 42–45.
190. Ewing R, Fainstein V, Musher DM, et al. Articular and skeletal infections caused by *Pasteurella multocida. South Med J* 1980;73: 1349–1352.
191. Maradona JA, Asensi V, Carton JA, et al. Prosthetic joint infection by *Pasteurella multocida. Eur J Clin Microbiol Infect Dis* 1997;16: 623–625.
192. Guion TL, Sculco TP. *Pasteurella multocida* infection in total knee arthroplasty. *J Arthroplasty* 1992;7:157–160.
193. Hubbert WT, Rosen MN. II. *Pasteurella multocida* infection in man unrelated to animal bite. *Am J Public Health* 1970;60:1109–1117.
194. Nelson SC, Hammer GS. *Pasteurella multocida* empyema: case report and review of the literature. *Am J Med Sci* 1981;281:43–49.
195. Klein NC, Cunha BA. *Pasteurella multocida* pneumonia. *Semin Respir Infect* 1997;12:54–56.
196. Hombal SM, Dincsoy HP. *Pasteurella multocida* endocarditis. *Am J Clin Pathol* 1992;98:565–568.
197. Nettles RE, Sexton DJ. *Pasteurella multocida* prosthetic valve endocarditis: case report and review. *Clin Infect Dis* 1997;25:920–921.
198. Kumar A, Devlin HR, Vellend H. *Pasteurella multocida* meningitis in an adult: case report and review. *Rev Infect Dis* 1990;12:440–448.
199. Controni G, Jones RS. *Pasteurella* meningitis: a review of the literature. *Am J Med Technol* 1967;33:379–386.
200. Green BT, Ramsey KM, Nolan PE. *Pasteurella multocida*meningitis: case report and review of the last 11 y. *Scand J Infect Dis* 2002;34: 213–217.
201. Elsey RM, Carson RW, Dubose TD. *Pasteurella multocida* peritonitis in an HIV-positive patient on continuous cycling peritoneal dialysis. *Am J Nephrol* 1991;11:61–63.
202. Koch CA, Mabee CL, Robyn JA, et al. Exposure to domestic cats: risk factors for *Pasteurella multocida* peritonitis in liver cirrhosis? *Am J Gastroenterol* 1996;91:1447–1449.
203. Lie W, Chemaly RF, Tuohy MJ, et al. *Pasteurella multocida* urinary tract infection with molecular evidence of zoonotic transmission. *Clin Infect Dis* 2003;36:e58–60.
204. Gowda RV, Stout R. *Pasteurella multocida* infection in a post-chemotherapy neutropenic host following cat exposure. *Clin Oncol* 2002; 14:497–498.
205. Laupland KB, Rimmer KP, Gregson DB, et al. Spontaneous empyema and overwhelming septic shock due to *Pasteurella multocida. Scand J Infect Dis* 2003;35:132–133.
206. Kuliberg B-J, Westendorp RGJ, van't Wout JW, et al. Purpura fulminans and symmetrical peripheral gangrene caused by *Capnocytophaga canimorsus* (formerly DF-2) septicemia—a complication of dog bite. *Medicine* 1991;70:287–292.
207. Hicklin H, Verghese A, Alvarez S. Dysgonic fermenter 2 septicemia. *Rev Infect Dis* 1987;9:884–890.
208. Job L, Horman JT, Grigor JK, et al. Dysgonic fermenter–2: a clinico-epidemiologic review. *J Emerg Med* 1989;7:185–192.
209. Krol-van Straaten MJ, Landheer JE, et al. *Capnocytophaga canimorsus* (formerly DF-2) infections: review of the literature. *Neth J Med* 1990; 36:304–309.
210. Zumla A, Lipscomb G, Corbett M, et al. Dysgonic fermenter-type 2: an emerging zoonosis: report of two cases and review. *Q J Med* 1988;68:741–752.
211. Bilgrami S, Bergstrom SK, Peterson DE, et al. *Capnocytophaga* bacteremia in a patient with Hodgkin's disease following bone marrow transplantation: case report and review. *Clin Infect Dis* 1992;14: 1045–1049.
212. Pers C, Gahrn-Hansen B, Frederiksen W. *Capnocytophaga canimorsus* septicemia in Denmark, 1982–1995: review of 39 cases. *Clin Infect Dis* 1996;23:71–75.
213. Lion C, Escande F, Burdin JC. *Capnocytophaga canimorsus* infections in human: review of the literature and cases report. *Eur J Epidemiol* 1996;12:521–533.
214. Hovenga S, Tulleken JE, Moller LV, et al. Dog-bite induced sepsis: a report of four cases. *Intensive Care Med* 1997;23:1179–1180.
215. Rosenman JR, Reynolds JK, Kleiman MB. *Capnocytophaga canimorsus* meningitis in a newborn: an avoidable infection.*Pediatr Infect Dis J* 2003;22:204–205.
216. Le Moal G, Grollier G, Robert R, et al. Meningitis due to *Capnocytophaga canimorsus* after receipt of a dog bite: case report and review of the literature. *Clin Infect Dis* 2003;36:e42–46.
217. Mahrer S, Raik E. *Capnocytophaga canimorsus* septicemia associated with cat scratch. *Pathology* 1992;24:194–196.
218. Valtonen M, Lauhio A, Carlson P, et al. *Capnocytophaga canimorsus* septicemia: fifth report of a cat-associated infection and five other cases. *Eur J Clin Microbiol Infect Dis* 1995;14:520–523.
219. Sawmiller CJ, Dudrick SJ, Hamzi M. Postsplenectomy *Capnocytophaga canimorsus* sepsis presenting as acute abdomen. *Arch Surg* 1998; 133:1362–1365.
220. Mossad SB, Lichtin AE, Hall G, et al. Diagnosis: *Capnocytophaga canimorsus* septicemia. *Clin Infect Dis* 1997;24:123, 267.
221. Adal KA, Cockerell CJ, Petri WA. Cat scratch disease, bacillary angiomatosis, and other infections due to *Rochalimaea. N Engl J Med* 1994;330:1509–1515.
222. Midani S, Ayoub EM, Anderson B. Cat-scratch disease. *Adv Pediatr* 1996;43:397–422.
223. Maurin M, Raoult D. *Bartonella (Rochalimaea) quintana* infections. *Clin Microbiol Rev* 1996;9:273–292.
224. Koehler JE. *Bartonella* infections. *Adv Pediatr Infect Dis* 1996;11: 1–27.
225. Williams A, Sheldon CD, Riordan T. Cat scratch disease. *BMJ* 2002; 324:1199–1200.
226. Anderson BE, Neuman MA. *Bartonella* spp. as emerging human pathogens. *Clin Microbiol Rev* 1997;10:203–219.
227. Spach DH, Koehler JE. *Bartonella*-associated infections. *Infect Dis Clin North Am* 1998;12:137–155.
228. Koehler JE. *Bartonella:* an emerging human pathogen. In: Scheld WM, Armstrong D, Hughes JM, eds. *Emerging infections.* Washington, DC: American Society for Microbiology Press, 1998.
229. Tappero JW, Koehler JE, Berger TG, et al. Bacillary angiomatosis and bacillary splenitis in immunocompetent adults. *Ann Intern Med* 1993;118:363–365.
230. Schwartzman WA. Infections due to *Rochalimaea*: the expanding clinical spectrum. *Clin Infect Dis* 1992;15:893–902.

231. Margileth AM, Wear DJ, English CK. Systemic cat scratch disease: report of 23 patients with prolonged or recurrent severe bacterial infection. *J Infect Dis* 1987;155:390–402.
232. Schwartzman WA, Marchevsky A, Meyer RD. Epithelioid angiomatosis or cat scratch disease with splenic and hepatic abnormalities in AIDS: case report and review of literature. *Scand J Infect Dis* 1990; 22:121–133.
233. LeBoit PE. Bacillary angiomatosis: a systemic opportunistic infection with prominent cutaneous manifestations. *Semin Dermatol* 1991;10: 194–198.
234. Kemper CA, Lombard CM, Deresinski SC, et al. Visceral bacillary epithelioid angiomatosis: possible manifestations of disseminated cat scratch disease in the immunocompromised host: a report of two cases. *Am J Med* 1990;89:216–222.
235. Mofenson HC, Greensher J, Teitelbaum H. How to avoid animal bites. *Med Times* 1972;100:92–98.
236. Anonymous. Dog bites. *Missouri Med* 1991;88:217–218.
237. Hoskins JD. Tick-borne zoonoses: Lyme disease, ehrlichiosis and Rocky Mountain spotted fever. *Semin Vet Med Surg* 1991;6:236–243.
238. Grist N. Ticks are topical. *J Infect* 1992;24:117–121.
239. Telford SR, Pollack RJ, Spielman A. Emerging vector-borne infections. *Infect Dis Clin North Am* 1991;5:7–17.
240. Spach DH, Liles WC, Campbell GL, et al. Tick-borne diseases in the United States. *N Engl J Med* 1993;329:936–947.
241. Parola P, Raoult D. Tick and tickborne bacterial diseases in human: an emerging infectious threat. *Clin Infect Dis* 2001;32:897–928.
242. Needham GR. Evaluation of five popular methods for tick removal. *Pediatrics* 1985;75:997–998.
243. Thomsett L. Zoonotic skin diseases. *Practitioner* 1990;234:52–55.
244. Devriese LA. Staphylococci in healthy and diseased animals. *J Appl Bacteriol Symp Suppl* 1990;19:71S–80S.
245. Falck G. Group A streptococci in household pets' eyes—a source of infections in humans? *Scand J Infect Dis* 1997;29:469–471.
246. Lilenbaum W, Nunes EL, Azeredo MA. Prevalence and antimicrobial susceptibility of staphylococci isolated from the skin surface of clinically normal cats. *Lett Appl Microbiol* 1998;27:224–228.
247. Radentz WH. Fungal skin infections associated with animal contact. *Am Fam Physician* 1991;43:1253–1256.
248. Czachor JS. Unusual aspects of bacterial water-borne illnesses. *Am Fam Physician* 1992;46:797–804.
249. Centers for Disease Control and Prevention. Aquarium-associated *Plesiomonas shigelloides* infection—Missouri. *MMWR Morb Mortal Wkly Rep* 1989;38:617–619.
250. Bastert J, Sing A, Wollenberg A, et al. Aquarium dermatitis: cercarial dermatitis in an aquarist. *Dermatology* 1998;197:84–86.
251. Vincenzi C, Bardazzi F, Tosti A, et al. Fish tank granuloma: report of a case. *Cutis* 1992;49:275–276.
252. Gray SF, Smith RS, Reynolds NJ, et al. Fish tank granuloma. *BMJ* 1990;300:1069–1070.
253. Ries KM, White GL, Murdock RT. Atypical mycobacterial infection caused by *Mycobacterium marinum. N Engl J Med* 1990;322:633.
254. Huminer D, Pitlik SD, Block C, Kaufman L, et al. Aquarium-borne *Mycobacterium marinum* skin infection. *Arch Dermatol* 1986;122: 698–703.
255. Ljungberg B, Christensson B, Grubb R. Failure of doxycycline treatment in aquarium-associated *Mycobacterium marinum* infections. *Scand J Infect Dis* 1987;19:539–543.
256. Lambertus MW, Mathisen GE. *Mycobacterium marinum* infection in a patient with cryptosporidiosis and the acquired immunodeficiency syndrome. *Cutis* 1988;42:38–40.
257. Alinovi A, Vecchini F, Bassissi P. Sporothricoid mycobacterial infection. *Acta DermatoVenereologica* 1993;73:146–147.
258. Brady RC, Sheth A, Mayer T, et al. Facial sporotrichoid infection with *Mycobacterium marinum. J Pediatr* 1997;130:324–326.
259. Auerbach PS. Marine envenomations. *N Engl J Med* 1991;325: 486–493.
260. Brown CK, Shepherd SM. Marine trauma, envenomations, and intoxications. *Emerg Med Clin North Am* 1992;10:385–408.
261. McGoldrick J, Marx JA. Marine envenomations; Part I: vertebrates. *J Emerg Med* 1991;9:497–502.
262. McGoldrick J, Marx JA. Marine envenomations; Part II: invertebrates. *J Emerg Med* 1992;10:71–77.
263. Eastaugh J, Shepherd S. Infectious and toxic syndromes from fish and shellfish consumption. *Arch Intern Med* 1989;149:1735–1740.
264. Hawdon GM, Winkel KD. Venomous marine creatures. *Aust Fam Physician* 1997;26:1369–1374.
265. Evans ME, Gregory DW, Schaffner W, et al. Tularemia: a 30-year experience with 88 cases. *Medicine* 1985;64:251–269.
266. Langley R, Campbell R. Tularemia in North Carolina, 1965–1990. *N C Med J* 1995;56:314–317.
267. Teutsch SM, Martone WJ, Brink EW, et al. Pneumonic tularemia on Martha's Vineyard. *N Engl J Med* 1979;301:826–828.
268. Craven RB, Barnes AM. Plague and tularemia. *Infect Dis Clin North Am* 1991;5:165–175.
269. Jacobs RF. Tularemia. *Adv Pediatr Infect Dis* 1997;12:55–69.
270. Jacobs RF, Narain JP. Tularemia in children. *Pediatr Infect Dis J* 1983;2:487–491.
271. Ohara Y, Sato T, Homma M. Arthropod-borne tularemia in Japan: clinical analysis of 1,374 cases observed between 1924 and 1996. *J Med Entomol* 1998;35:471–473.
272. Dennis DT, Inglesby TV, Henderson DA, et al. Tularemia as a biological weapon. *JAMA* 2001;285:2763–2773.
273. Ellis J, Oyston PCF, Green M, et al. Tularemia. *Clin Microbiol Rev* 2002;15:631–646.
274. Feldman KA. Tularemia. *JAVMA* 2003;222:725–730.
275. Tamvik A, Berglund L. Tularemia. *Eur Respir J* 2003;21:361–373.
276. Ohara Y, Sato T, Fujita H, et al. Clinical manifestations of tularemia in Japan—analysis of 1,355 cases observed between 1924 and 1987. *Infection* 1991;19:14–17.
277. Uhari M, Syrjala H, Salminen A. Tularemia in children caused by *Francisella tularensis* biovar *palaearctica. Pediatr Infect Dis J* 1990;9: 80–83.
278. Cross JT. Tularemia in the United States. *Infect Med* 1997;14: 881–882, 885–886, 889–890.
279. Steinemann TL, Sheikholeslami MR, Brown HH, et al. Oculoglandular tularemia. *Arch Ophthalmol* 1999;117:132–133.
280. Halsted CC, Kulasinghe HP. Tularemia pneumonia in urban children. *Pediatrics* 1978;61:660–662.
281. Roy TM, Fleming D, Anderson WH. Tularemic pneumonia mimicking Legionnaires disease with false-positive direct fluorescent antibody stains for Legionella. *South Med J* 1989;82:1429–1431.
282. Miller RP, Bates JH. Pleuropulmonary tularemia. *Am Rev Respir Dis* 1969;99:31–41.
283. Gill V, Cunha BA. Tularemia pneumonia. *Semin Resp Infect* 1997; 12:61–67.
284. Tarnvik A, Sandstrom G, Sjostedt A. Infrequent manifestations of tularaemia in Sweden. *Scand J Infect Dis* 1997;29:443–446.
285. Pittman T, Williams D, Friedman AD. A shunt infection caused by *Francisella tularensis. Pediatr Neurosurg* 1996;24:50–51.
286. Weinberg AN. Respiratory infections transmitted from animals. *Infect Dis Clin North Am* 1991;5:649–661.
287. Winer-Muram HT, Rubin SA. Pet-associated lung diseases. *J Thorac Imaging* 1991;6:14–30.
288. O'Reilly LM, Daborn CJ. The epidemiology of *Mycobacterium bovis* infections in animals and man: a review. *Tubercle Lung Dis* 1995; 76(Suppl 1):1–46.
289. Moda G, Daborn CJ, Grange JM, et al. The zoonotic importance of *Mycobacterium bovis. Tubercle Lung Dis* 1996;77:103–108.
290. Cosivi O, Grange JM, Daborn CJ, et al. Zoonotic tuberculosis due to *Mycobacterium bovis* in developing countries. *Emerg Infect Dis* 1998; 4:59–70.
291. Meyer KF. Pneumonic plague. *Bact Rev* 1961;25:249–261.
292. Bouvet E, Casalino E, Mendoza-Sassi G, et al. A nosocomial outbreak of multi drug-resistant *Mycobacterium bovis* among HIV-infected patients. *AIDS* 1993;7:1453–1460.
293. Hughes C, Maharg P, Rosario P, et al. Possible nosocomial transmission of psittacosis. *Infect Control Hosp Epidemiol* 1997;18:165–168.
294. Raoult D. Host factors in the severity of Q fever. *Ann N Y Acad Sci* 1990;590:33–38.

295. Baca OG. Pathogenesis of rickettsial infections: emphasis on Q fever. *Eur J Epidemiol* 1991;7:222–228.
296. Sawyer LA, Fishbein DB, McDade JE. Q fever: current concepts. *Rev Infect Dis* 1987;9:935–946.
297. Spelman DW. Q Fever: a study of 111 consecutive cases. *Med J Aust* 1982;1:547–553.
298. Aitken ID, Bogel K, Cracea E, et al. Q fever in Europe: current aspects of aetiology, epidemiology, human infection, diagnosis and therapy. *Infection* 1987;15:323–327.
299. Raoult D, Marrie T. Q fever. *Clin Infect Dis* 1995;20:489–496.
300. Garner MG, Longbottom HM, Cannon RM, et al. A review of Q fever in Australia 1991–1994. *Aust N Z J Public Health* 1997;21:722–730.
301. McQuiston JH, Childs JE. Q fever in humans and animals in the United States. *Vector Borne Zoonotic Dis* 2002;2:179–191.
302. Kovacova E, Kazar J. Q fever—still a query and underestimated infectious disease. *Acta Virologica* 2002;46:193–210.
303. Marrie TJ, Raoult D. Update on Q fever, including Q fever endocarditis. *Curr Clin Top Infect Dis* 2002;22:97–124.
304. Cutler SJ, Paiba GA, Howells J, et al. Q fever—forgotten disease? *Lancet Infect Dis* 2002;2:717–718.
305. McQuiston JH, Childs JE. Q fever. *JAVMA* 2002;221:796–799.
306. Sampere M, Font B, Font J, et al. Q fever in adults: review of 66 clinical cases. *Eur J Clin Microbiol Infect Dis* 2003;22:108–110.
307. Marrie TJ. *Coxiella burnetii* pneumonia. *Eur Resp J* 2003;21:713–719.
308. Alcarcon A, Villanueva JL, Viciana P, et al. Q fever: epidemiology, clinical features and prognosis. *J Infect* 2003;47:110–116.
309. Welsh HH, Lennette EH, Abinanti FR, et al. Air-borne transmission of Q fever: the role of parturition in the generation of infective aerosols. *Ann N Y Acad Sci* 1957;70:528–540.
310. Pinsky RL, Fishbein DB, Greene CR, et al. An outbreak of cat-associated Q fever in the United States. *J Infect Dis* 1991;164:202–204.
311. Embil J, Williams JC, Marrie TJ. The immune response in a cat-related outbreak of Q fever as measured by the indirect immunofluorescence test and the enzyme-linked immunosorbent assay. *Can J Microbiol* 1990;36:292–296.
312. Marrie TJ, Durant H, Williams JC, et al. Exposure to parturient cats: a risk factor for acquisition of Q fever in maritime Canada. *J Infect Dis* 1998;158:101–108.
313. Buhariwalla F, Cann B, Marrie TJ. A dog-related outbreak of Q fever. *Clin Infect Dis* 1996;23:753–755.
314. Dupont HT, Raoult D, Brouqui P, et al. Epidemiologic features and clinical presentation of acute Q fever in hospitalized patients: 323 French cases. *Am J Med* 1992;93:427–434.
315. Antony SJ, Schaffner W. Q fever pneumonia. *Semin Resp Infect* 1997;12:2–6.
316. Caron F, Meurice JC, Ingrand P, et al. Acute Q fever pneumonia: a review of 80 hospitalized patients. *Chest* 1998;114:808–813.
317. Siegman-Igra Y, Kaufman O, Keysary A, et al. Q fever endocarditis in Israel and a worldwide review. *Scand J Infect Dis* 1997;29:41–49.
318. Fournier P-E, Casalta J-P, Piquet P, et al. *Coxiella burnetii* infection of aneurysms or vascular grafts: report of seven cases and review. *Clin Infect Dis* 1998;26:116–121.
319. Raoult D, Brouqui P, Marchou B, et al. Acute and chronic Q fever in patients with cancer. *Clin Infect Dis* 1992;14:127–130.
320. Ludlam H, Wreghitt TG, Thornton S, et al. Q fever in pregnancy. *J Infect* 1997;34:75–78.
321. Stein A, Raoult D. Q fever during pregnancy: a public health problem in southern France. *Clin Infect Dis* 1998;27:592–596.
322. Fournier P-E, Marrie T, Raoult D. Diagnosis of Q fever. *J Clin Microbiol* 1998;36:1823–1834.
323. Centers for Disease Control and Prevention. Human psittacosis linked to a bird distributor in Mississippi—Massachusetts and Tennessee, 1992. *MMWR Morb Mortal Wkly Rep* 1992;41:794–797.
324. Weston VC, Mansell P, Allison SP. Family outbreak of psittacosis. *Lancet* 1990;335:1226–1227.
325. Morrison WM, Hutchison RB, Thomason J, et al. An outbreak of psittacosis. *J Infect* 1991;22:71–75.
326. Schlossberg D, Delgado J, Moore M, et al. An epidemic of avian and human psittacosis. *Arch Intern Med* 1993;153:2594–2596.
327. Eidson M. Psittacosis/avian chlamydiosis. *JAVMA* 2002;221:1710–1712.
328. Centers for Disease Control and Prevention. Compendium of measures to control *Chlamydia psittaci* infection among humans (psittacosis) and pet birds (avian chlamydiosis). *MMWR Morb Mortal Wkly Rep* 1998;47(RR-10):1–14.
329. Ito I, Ishida T, Mishima M, et al. Familial cases of psittacosis: possible person-to-person transmission. *Intern Med* 2002;41:580–583.
330. Broholm KA, Bottiger M, Jernelius H, et al. Ornithosis as a nosocomial infection. *Scand J Infect Dis* 1977;9:263–267.
331. Schaffner W. Birds of a feather—do they flock together? *Infect Control Hosp Epidemiol* 1997;18:162–164.
332. Cotton MM, Partidge MR. Infection with feline *Chlamydia psittaci*. *Thorax* 1998;53:75–76.
333. Grayston JT, Thom DH. The chlamydial pneumonias. *Curr Clin Top Infect Dis* 1991;11:1–18.
334. Crosse BA. Psittacosis: a clinical review. *J Infect Dis* 1990;21:251–259.
335. Hirschmann JV. Psittacosis. *Med Grand Rounds* 1982;1:57–66.
336. Vergweij PE, Meis JFGM, Eijk R, et al. Severe human psittacosis requiring artificial ventilation: case report and review. *Clin Infect Dis* 1995;20:440–442.
337. Gregory DW, Schaffner W. Psittacosis. *Semin Resp Infect* 1997;12:7–11.
338. Kirchner JT. Psittacosis: is contact with birds causing your patient's pneumonia? *Postgrad Med* 1997;102:181–182, 187–188, 193–194.
339. Werner SB, Weidmer CE, Nelson BC, et al. Primary plague pneumonia contracted from a domestic cat at South Lake Tahoe, California. *JAMA* 1984;251:929–931.
340. Centers for Disease Control and Prevention. Plague—Arizona, Colorado, New Mexico. *MMWR Morb Mortal Wkly Rep* 1977;26:215–216.
341. Centers for Disease Control and Prevention. Human plague—United States, 1993–1994. *MMWR Morb Mortal Wkly Rep* 1994;43:242–246.
342. Centers for Disease Control and Prevention. Prevention of plague: recommendations of the Advisory Committee on Immunization Practices (ACIP). *MMWR Morb Mortal Wkly Rep* 1996;45(RR-14):1–15.
343. Centers for Disease Control and Prevention. Fatal human plague—Arizona and Colorado, 1996. *MMWR Morb Mortal Wkly Rep* 1997;46:617–620.
344. Cleri DJ, Vernaleo JR, Lombardi LJ, et al. Plague pneumonia: disease caused by *Yersinia pestis*. *Semin Resp Infect* 1997;12:12–23.
345. Inglesby TV, Dennis DT, Henderson DA, et al. Plague as a biological weapon. *JAMA* 2000;283:2281–2290.
346. Putzker M, Sauer H, Sobe D. Plague and other human infections by *Yersinia* species. *Clin Lab* 2001;47:453–466.
347. Rollins SE, Rollins SM, Ryan ET. *Yersinia pestis* and the plague. *Am J Clin Pathol* 2003;119(Suppl):S78–85.
348. Orloski KA, Lathrop SL. Plague: a veterinary perspective. *JAVMA* 2003;222:444–448.
349. Fang G, Araujo V, Guerrant RL. Enteric infections associated with exposure to animals or animal products. *Infect Dis Clin North Am* 1991;5:681–701.
350. Altman R, Gorman JC, Bernhardt LL, et al. Turtle-associated salmonellosis. *Am J Epidemiol* 1972;95:518–520.
351. Woodward DL, Khakhria R, Johnson WM. Human salmonellosis associated with exotic pets. *J Clin Microbiol* 1997;35:2786–2790.
352. Austin CC, Wilkins MJ. Reptile-associated salmonellosis. *JAVMA* 1998;212:866–867.
353. Weber DJ, Rutala WA, Li E. Public health for medical staff. In: Yamada T, ed. *Textbook of gastroenterology*, vol. 1. Philadelphia: JB Lippincott, 1991:1042–1064.
354. Wilson HD, McCormick JB, Feeley JC. *Yersinia enterocolitica* infection in a 4-month-old infant associated with infection in household dogs. *J Pediatr* 1975;89:767–769.
355. Saeed AM, Harris NV, DiGiacomo RF. The role of exposure to ani-

mals in the etiology of *Campylobacter jejuni/coli* enteritis. *Am J Epidemiol* 1993;137:108–114.

356. Blaser MJ, Weiss SH, Barrett TJ. *Campylobacter* enteritis associated with a healthy cat. *JAMA* 1982;247:816.
357. Fox JG, Moore R, Ackerman JI. Canine and feline campylobacteriosis: epizootiology and clinical and public health features. *JAVMA* 1983; 183:1420–1424.
358. Ravn P, Lundren JD, Kjaeldgaard P, et al. Nosocomial outbreak of cryptosporidiosis in AIDS patients. *BMJ* 1991;302:277–280.
359. Martino P, Gentile G, Caprioli A, et al. Hospital-acquired cryptosporidiosis in a borne marrow transplantation unit. *J Infect Dis* 1988;158: 647–648.
360. Baxby D, Hart CA, Taylor C. Human cryptosporidiosis: a possible case of hospital cross infection. *BMJ* 1983;287:1760.
361. Dryjanski J, Gold JW, Ritchie MT, et al. Cryptosporidiosis: case report in a health team worker. *Am J Med* 1986;80:751.
362. Reif JS, Wimmer L, Smith JA, et al. Human cryptosporidiosis associated with an epizootic in calves. *Am J Public Health* 1989;79: 1528–1530.
363. Hamrick HJ, Drake R, Jones HM, et al. Two cases of dipylidiasis (dog tapeworm infection) in children: update on an old problem. *Pediatrics* 1983;72:114–117.
364. *Animals in institutions* (AAT110). Renton, WA: Delta Society, xxxx.
365. *Standards of practice for animal-assisted activities and therapy.* Renton, WA: Delta Society, 1996.
366. Wallace S, Pfau H, Bideshi D, et al. Safety of dog visits for patients in an acute hospital setting. In: Program and abstracts of the 32nd Interscience Conference on Antimicrobial Agents and Chemotherapy, Anaheim, CA, October 11–14, 1992(abst).
367. Adams SL. The medicinal leech. *Ann Intern Med* 1988;109:399–405.
368. Wade JW, Brabham RF, Allen RJ. Medicinal leeches: once again at the forefront of medicine. *South Med J* 1990;83:1168–1173.
369. Valauri FA. The use of medicinal leeches in microsurgery. *Blood Coag Fibrinolysis* 1991;2:185–187.
370. Lineaweaver WC, O'Hara M, Stridde B, et al. Clinical leech use in a microsurgical unit: the San Francisco experience. *Blood Coag Fibrinolysis* 1991;2:189–192.
371. Dabb RW, Malone JM, Leverett LC. The use of medicinal leeches in the salvage of flaps with venous congestion. *Ann Plast Surg* 1992; 29:250–256.
372. Wells MD, Manktelow RT, Boyd JB, et al. The medical leech: an old treatment revisited. *Microsurgery* 1993;14:183–186.
373. Lineaweaver WC. *Aeromonas hydrophila* infections following clinical use of medicinal leeches: a review of published cases. *Blood Coag Fibrinolysis* 1991;2:201–203.
374. Lineaweaver WC, Hill MK, Buncke GM, et al. *Aeromonas hydrophila* infections following use of medicinal leeches in reimplantation and flap surgery. *Ann Plast Surg* 1992;29:238–244.
375. Sartor C, Limouzin-Perotti F, Legre R, et al. Nosocomial infection with *Aeromonas hydrophila* from leeches. *Clin Infect Dis* 2002;35: e1–5.
376. Varghese MR, Farr RW, Wax MK, et al. *Vibrio fluvialis* wound infection associated with the medicinal leech therapy. *Clin Infect Dis* 1996; 22:709–710.
377. Mercer NSG, Beere DM, Bornemisza AJ, et al. Medical leeches as sources of wound infection. *BMJ* 1987;294:937.
378. Kraemer BA, Korber KE, Aquino TI, et al. Use of leeches in plastic and reconstructive surgery: a review. *J Reconstructive Microsurg* 1988; 4:381–386.
379. Hermansdorfer J, Lineaweaver W, Follansbee S, et al. Antibiotic sensitivities of *Aeromonas hydrophila* cultured from medicinal leeches. *Br J Plastic Surg* 1988;41:649–651.
380. Lineaweaver WC, Furnas H, Follansbee S, et al. Postprandial *Aeromonas hydrophila* cultures and antibiotic levels of enteric aspirates from medicinal leeches applied to patients receiving antibiotics. *Ann Plastic Surg* 1992;29:245–249.
381. Nehili M, Ilk C, Mehlhorn H, Ruhnau K, et al. Experiments on the possible role of leeches as vectors of animal and human pathogens: a light and electron microscopy study. *Parasitol Res* 1994;80:277–290.

102

ROLE OF THE MICROBIOLOGY LABORATORY IN HOSPITAL EPIDEMIOLOGY AND INFECTION CONTROL

CHARLES W. STRATTON IV
JOHN N. GREENE

In the late nineteenth century, early microbiologists such as Pasteur and Koch demonstrated that infections were due to specific microorganisms and that these microbes could be isolated by appropriate cultures. Another early microbiologist, Lister, recognized the principle that certain chemicals antagonized microbes. Lister then applied this principle to infection control by using phenol to sterilize surgical instruments and dressings to reduce the morbidity and mortality associated at that time with surgery (1). Thus began the association of microbiology with antibiosis and infection control.

The relationship of microbiology with infection control was formally recognized in the early 1970s by the Centers for Disease Control and Prevention (CDC), which developed standard definitions for nosocomial infections and methods for infection surveillance (2). Infection control committees incorporated these CDC recommendations into practice at that time. The result was a shift from unproductive environmental sampling (3) to more directed surveillance and intervention when established baseline endemic rates of infection were exceeded. However, unless these baseline endemic rates of infection were exceeded, the surveillance process was, for the most part, passive.

As humans enter the twenty-first century, infection control strategies continue to evolve. First, microbiologic surveillance has shifted away from general categories of medical service, infection site, and hospital-wide infection rates and is focusing instead on problem categories (4,5). These focused categories include high-risk areas such as intensive care units (ICUs) (6), preventable high-risk infections such as intravascular device-related infections (7), the surveillance and control of microbial resistance (8–12), and emerging pathogens (8,13). Second, infection control strategies today are more proactive, which simply means that active intervention for prevention of infections and control of resistance has an equal priority to simply monitoring for changes in these parameters (6,7,14,15). Third, it is now recognized that a key component in this proactive strategy is the need for ongoing and constant education of hospital and infection control personnel as well as education of infectious diseases fellows (16). Such educational efforts are becoming important functions of an infection control committee with the assistance of the microbiology laboratory. Fourth, implementation of efficient infection control requires the construction of a computerized information network that ideally includes the hospital, the community, and the nation (17–19). Such a network that includes guidelines, microbiologic surveillance data, and full-text references available on the Internet ultimately will become the cornerstone of infection control.

The interaction of the microbiology laboratory with hospital epidemiology and infection control continues to evolve as an integral part of a nationwide concerted effort to develop and improve infection control practices and programs. This process began with the National Nosocomial Infections Surveillance (NNIS) system developed by the CDC. This system provides risk-specific infection rates for use by hospitals and national healthcare planners to set priorities for their infection control programs and to evaluate the effectiveness of their effort (20). The Division of Healthcare Quality Promotion (DHQP) at the CDC through NNIS continues to provide relevant surveillance information on nosocomial infections (21). In addition, the DHQP is expanding to provide relevant information for other healthcare facilities such as dialysis centers (19). The Study on the Efficacy of Nosocomial Infection Control (SENIC) conducted by the CDC in the 1970s found hospitals had lower rates of nosocomial infections if levels of surveillance activities were increased (22). Thus, many infection control programs received additional support to increase the number of infection control professionals (ICPs).

Meanwhile, the focus and procedures of microbiology laboratories were changing because of multiple factors that included increasing resistance, emerging pathogens, and new technology (8,13,23). For example, the need for clinical microbiology laboratories to detect emerging antimicrobial resistance (24) has resulted in new approaches and technology for this purpose (25). All of these factors have resulted in important changes in the role of the microbiology laboratory in hospital epidemiology and infection control.

The microbiology laboratory has always been recognized as

an essential element in the control of nosocomial infection (3) and has long served as an early warning system for nosocomial infections by identifying clusters of microbes with unique phenotypic characteristics and communicating this information to ICPs (26,27). In the past, such hospital epidemiology and infection control activities did not place a great demand on the microbiology laboratory.

Today, however, the work done by the microbiology laboratory is increasingly complex and demanding. Much of this has direct implications on hospital epidemiology and infection control. Microbiology laboratories now must be able to detect, identify, and characterize an expanded array of microbes, including newly emerging pathogens (8). Some of these pathogens, such as fungal microorganisms, may be important causes of nosocomial infections but difficult to detect (28,29). Fortunately, traditional methods using cultures for isolation, identification, and susceptibility testing of pathogens have been supplemented by highly sensitive, rapid, and specific molecular biologic techniques in which unique DNA or RNA sequences can be directly detected (8,10,13,25,30–35). These and other molecular techniques have enabled microbiology laboratories to "fingerprint" microbes, thereby facilitating studies of nosocomial transmission (36). Finally, the microbiology laboratory's role in monitoring and controlling resistance has become critical because of the increasing frequency with which resistant pathogens are causing nosocomial infections (8,10–12,37). This role today may include not only the accurate detection of resistance per se but also the determination of the molecular epidemiology of the resistant isolates. The amount of work by the microbiology laboratory to support hospital epidemiology and infection control has greatly increased.

The role of the microbiology laboratory in hospital epidemiology and infection control continues to expanded. For example, ICPs today often augment their surveillance efforts by the use of computer-generated focused microbiologic surveillance reports from the microbiology laboratory. Problems thus detected may require molecular methods as a part of their evaluation. If the problems involve resistance, additional susceptibility testing and molecular methods may be required. Finally, the microbiology laboratory has become recognized as an important resource for the microbiologic training and education of hospital and infection control personnel. Indeed, the interactions of infection control committees with the microbiology laboratory are now so complex and important that most committees require that a representative of the microbiology laboratory serve as an active member to ensure the appropriate advice, education, coordination, and technical support. This chapter examines these various facets of the changing and increasingly critical role of the microbiology laboratory in hospital epidemiology and infection control.

SURVEILLANCE

The key to an effective infection control program continues to be effective surveillance, which the SENIC has defined as an ICP using basic epidemiologic techniques to perform surveillance on clinical ward rounds, to analyze rates of infection, and to incorporate the data generated in decision making (20). Such surveillance for nosocomial infections involves identifying patients who are colonized or infected, assessing the risk of transmission of infection between patients, proving transmission of a given strain from one patient to another, and, more generally, detecting hospital outbreaks (38). However, to recognize the existence of an outbreak, baseline endemic rates of infection must be determined for each type of infection within a given institution.

Defining endemic rates (the number of infections divided by the number of patient-days or patients at risk) for services, sites of infection, microorganisms, and procedures can be accomplished in each hospital by an active surveillance system coordinated by the ICP and the microbiology laboratory. Clusters and epidemics can be investigated when endemic threshold rates are exceeded, when unusual or new microorganisms are isolated, and when new sites of infection are identified. Collection of surveillance data, usually by the ICP, consists of reviewing microbiology reports generated by the laboratory. If trends of increasing or unusual infection rates are discovered, then chart review and discussion with personnel involved in patient care should follow to determine the significance of these isolates. The importance of active surveillance is seen with the recent outbreak of severe acute respiratory syndrome (SARS) (39). SARS is an example of emerging and reemerging infectious diseases that must be monitored with ongoing surveillance strategies and new diagnostic methods (40,41). (See also Chapter 113.)

With increasing resistance and the fact that many nosocomial infections are caused by resistant microbes, surveillance and control of resistance has become critical (8,10–12,18,24,25). Susceptibility patterns can be monitored for emergence of resistant microorganisms; when resistant microorganisms are identified, appropriate isolation precautions should be instituted. Moreover, control of antimicrobial use has become important for controlling resistance (8,11,12). For this reason, the antibiotic subcommittee of the pharmacy and therapeutics committee should be included as a part of the infection control program for preventing resistance. One practical way to do this is for a representative of the microbiology laboratory to be a voting member of both the infection control committee and the antibiotic subcommittee. In addition, one or more members of the antibiotic subcommittee should be a member(s) of the infection control committee.

Today, almost all microbiology laboratories have a computerized reporting system. Computer-generated microbiology reports are usually sorted by site of isolation, type of microorganism, and location of the patient, but they can be programmed to focus on any particular problem. Reports are generated daily and cumulatively. These reports are used to detect trends of increasing infection rates or increasing resistance and are reviewed daily by the ICP. In addition, the ICP often participates in daily clinical microbiology rounds in which new positive cultures at each bench station are reviewed.

The microbiology laboratory receives appropriate hospital demographic information on any culture request and often is able to use this information to recognize clusters of similar isolates. In addition, the availability of laboratory computer systems allows specific types of patients (e.g., transplant patients) or specific locations (e.g., ICUs) to be easily grouped and reviewed. When such focused microbiologic surveillance is desired, the microbiology laboratory should have the capability to provide such reports. In the past, a computerized reporting system did not necessarily mean that focused surveillance reports could be easily obtained. Often, some degree of computer programming was needed; therefore, this programming capability should be readily available. Once obtained, these focused surveillance reports for specific units should be incorporated as a routine surveillance method with these reports also provided to the medical director of the specific unit(s) (5,8).

Once the microbiology reports have been reviewed and prioritized, charts of the patients with the microorganisms of interest should be analyzed to evaluate the significance of the isolates as potential causes of nosocomial colonization and infection. Susceptibility trends should be analyzed. By defining baseline endemic rates for various infections and resistance problems through effective surveillance, unusual disease and resistance activity will trigger disease control and prevention efforts (8, 10–12,24,25). In summary, an active surveillance system assists the clinician in making an accurate diagnosis and prescribing therapy by providing the knowledge of disease occurrence and antibiotic resistance patterns.

IDENTIFICATION OF OUTBREAKS

An investigation of a potential outbreak of nosocomial infections must first determine if these infections are related in any way (20,38). Most often, this determination involves recognition of the microbial pathogen causing the outbreak and differentiation from those microorganisms of the same genus or species that, although isolated from some patients, are not involved in the outbreak (20,38,42). However, an outbreak may involve resistance rather than an increased incidence of infections. For example, an outbreak might actually consist of only one strain of vancomycin-resistant *Staphylococcus aureus* because of the implications of such an isolate (43). If the outbreak can be linked to infection by a single strain (also called a clone), exposure to a common source or reservoir or transmission from patient to patient would be inferred.

Traditionally, the epidemic strain has been defined with phenotypic methods, which include genus, species, biotype, serotype, phage type, bacteriocin production, and antimicrobial susceptibility patterns (44). Phenotypic methods reflect genetic traits and may be quite specific. When a given phenotype is rarely found in a microbial strain, that phenotype alone may provide convincing evidence of transmission between patients (e.g., *Escherichia coli* 0157:H7) (44). However, microorganisms with commonly expressed phenotypic characteristics may require additional subtyping (32,34–36). Sometimes, isolates share phenotypic markers but are actually genotypically different; this implies the presence of two separate strains and infection from two different sources (32). The limitations of phenotypic techniques are presented in Table 102.1.

When microbial pathogens are nontypeable by phenotypic methods or have only a few types, the poor discriminatory power precludes the use of these typing methods. This has led to the use of genotypic methods for typing. This approach has been extremely successful and is now termed *molecular epidemiology* (23,27,32,34,35,45). These molecular epidemiologic methods most often involve genotyping of microbial plasmid or chromosomal DNA and go far beyond the current limitations of phenotyping and provide more accurate data during outbreak investigation (32). Moreover, outbreaks of viruses (46) and free-living microorganisms can now be adequately studied with current molecular epidemiologic methods.

TABLE 102.1. LIMITATIONS OF PHENOTYPIC METHODS

Influenced by environmental selective pressure
Unstable antigenic traits may be altered by random mutation
Resistance patterns are strongly influenced by the selective pressure of antibiotic use
Bacteria predictably alter the expression of the characteristic being assessed
Necessary reagents may not be commercially available, which limits the number of tests available for phenotypic testing
Phenotypic traits may not have sufficient discriminatory power to distinguish each strain of a species

Data from refs. 23, 27, 32, 34, 35, 45.

However, combining methods of microorganism identification provides stronger evidence for the presumed relationship between isolates. Such was the case with an outbreak of neonatal meningitis caused by *Enterobacter sakazakii* (47). Biotypes, plasmid DNA profiles, and antibiograms of isolates from patients and the environment were identical, establishing the means of transmission from a powdered milk preparation. On the other hand, multiple typing systems may show dissimilarity among strains, casting uncertainty on the relatedness of isolates. This was illustrated when widespread colonization of personnel with methicillin-resistant coagulase-negative staphylococci (MRCNS) at a Veterans Affairs hospital was investigated (48). Antimicrobial susceptibility profiles, biotyping, phage typing, plasmid profiles, restriction fragment length polymorphism (RFLP), and plasmid hybridization with a DNA probe showed dissimilarity among strains. Because of the absence of strain similarity that has been found using the various methods, the role of human reservoirs of MRCNS as a source for infections in hospitalized patients remains obscure (48).

Identification of a microorganism by any means requires thorough knowledge of the unique attributes of the microorganism to distinguish it from the large background of nonepidemic, nonpathogenic strains (45). Specific strain identification can be critical in identifying outbreaks of infection (45). This can be seen with the speciation of coagulase-negative staphylococci. *Staphylococcus schleiferi* is a new species of coagulase-negative staphylococci that is pathogenic in humans, causes abscesses, and has been described in an outbreak of wound infections (49). Isolation and speciation of this pathogen from a cluster of surgical site infections would have far greater impact than the isolation and report of coagulase-negative staphylococci from the same cluster, as the latter would be interpreted as likely representing various coagulase-negative species and thus skin contaminants. As the ability to characterize strains improves, the number of differences detected between strains will likely increase (45).

An important feature of an epidemiologic evaluation is the determination of clonality of the suspected pathogen regardless of the mode of transmission. A clone is a set of isolates that have been recovered independently from different sources, in different locations, and possibly at different times but that show so many identical phenotypic and genetic traits that the most likely explanation for this identity is a common origin (45,50). Clonality among isolates in an outbreak must be established before it can be concluded that the outbreak originated from a common source (45). Successful clone identification requires knowledge of the genetic stability of the microorganism, the selective pressure of the environment, and the discriminatory power of the given procedure used to characterize the isolate (45). The judgment of nonclonality eliminates an isolate from consideration as one involved in a particular chain of transmission (45). A judgment of probable clonality strengthens the case for either a common-source outbreak or an outbreak resulting from person-to-person transmission in proportion to the rareness of that clone in the environment (45). Following a given clone throughout its travels by surveillance methods has documented the worldwide spread of multiresistant strains of penicillin-resistant *Streptococcus pneumoniae* (PRSP) (51) and methicillin-resistant *S. aureus* (MRSA) (52).

Host responses to invading microorganisms may also be used to identify and track infections that are difficult to investigate using current phenotypic and genotypic methods. For instance, serology may be used to determine infection rates during outbreaks, particularly when cultures have not been obtained or are obtained after initiating treatment or when routine cultures may not detect infection (e.g., pneumonia). This was seen with group A *Streptococcus* (GAS) infections in a nursing home (53). Nine (56%) of the 16 cases of GAS disease or infection in residents were confirmed by serologic testing (anti-DNase B titers) alone (53). The identification of a single serotype (M-1, T-1) from the four available isolates and epidemiologic correlation suggested that a single strain of GAS was introduced into the nursing home by the index patient, with subsequent person-to-person transmission. Similarly, pulsed-field gel electrophoresis (PFGE) has been used to document a community outbreak of invasive GAS infection in Minnesota (54). Field inversion gel electrophoresis is another electrophoretic typing method similar to PFGE that has been developed for GAS (55). These electrophoretic methods are able to identify differences between and within M types of GAS. Another molecular method for distinguishing GAS is fluorescent amplified fragment length polymorphism (AFLP) analysis (56). Finally, the *emm* gene for the M protein has proven useful for typing GAS (57).

When investigating a possible outbreak, the hospital epidemiologist or ICP, who formulates a hypothesis based on clinical and epidemiologic evidence, must collaborate with a microbiology laboratory to provide microbiologic data to either support or refute the hypothesis (23,26,27,36). Isolates from multiple patients are examined to determine whether the infections are related. Establishing similarities or differences among epidemic isolates is not always sufficient to determine the source or the mode of dissemination (58). Data derived from epidemiologic studies are also needed. Cultures and molecular typing without an epidemiologic study often lead to uninterpretable results. However, when molecular typing is combined with an epidemiologic study, the two methods are complementary in confirming transmission of a single or multiple strains (59).

EPIDEMIOLOGIC TYPING

Currently, there are a vast number of epidemiologic typing systems available (23,60–62). These include molecular methods that are clearly useful for the epidemiologic analysis of infectious disease outbreaks (32,62,63). However, to gain acceptance and be routinely applied in clinical situations, molecular epidemiologic methods must be easy to perform, rapid, reproducible, and cost-effective and provide additional information not obtained from traditional typing techniques (58,59). Also, it is important with high-resolution typing systems to distinguish between comparative epidemiologic typing systems that are used in outbreak investigations and library epidemiologic typing systems that are used in surveillance systems (61). Most of the currently available molecular typing systems are comparative methods that are reproducible in single assay, have high discrimination ($D>0.95$), and are used to compare isolates from a suspected outbreak and distinguish them from sporadic isolates. Such comparative methods include RFLP, PFGE, and arbitrarily primed and randomly amplified polymorphic polymerase chain reaction (PCR) analysis. Library typing systems, in contrast, are reproducible over time and between laboratories, have discrimination power balanced against evolutionary stability, and are used for long-term surveillance. Library methods include serotyping, insertion sequence fingerprinting, ribotyping, PFGE, AFLP, infrequent-restriction-site amplification PCR, interrepetitive element PCR typing (rep-PCR), and PCR-RFLP of polymorphic loci. Finally, a typing method cannot be considered valid unless it is capable of discriminating among randomly chosen isolates (58–63).

The basic premise inherent in any typing system is that epidemiologically related isolates are derived from the clonal expression of a single precursor and share characteristics that differ from epidemiologically unrelated isolates (32). The utility of a particular characteristic for typing is related to its stability within a strain and its diversity within the species (64). The most clinically relevant isolates or those with characteristics that provide for increased virulence or resistance are often the most difficult to differentiate (64). The strength of typing depends on the discriminatory power of the method used (64). When strains are nontypeable or have only a few serotypes, such poor discriminatory power precludes the use of certain typing methods. Ideally, a typing method will recognize each unrelated isolate as unique. In practice, the technique is considered useful if the most common type it detects occurs in less than 5% of the population (64). There is currently no gold standard or definitive typing system or even an authoritatively validated collection of isolates against which a new method can be evaluated (64). Nevertheless, bacterial typing systems are applied clinically to address one fundamental question: Are two isolates the same or different (64)?

One of the earliest phenotypic methods used in hospitals for outbreak investigations was biotyping. Biotyping refers to establishing the pattern of activity of cellular enzymes. Most microbiology laboratories identify bacteria with an automated biotype system (65). The ability of biotyping to differentiate among unrelated strains (discriminatory power) is poor. However, Maki et al. (66) successfully used biotyping to implicate contaminated intravenous fluid preparations as the means of transmitting *Enterobacter agglomerans* to patients. However, if the same strain differs in one or more biochemical reactions because of mutations in gene expression or a random mutation, then the strains may be mistakenly reported as unrelated (64). Also, specific testing reagents are often difficult and expensive to develop and characterize or are not available in most microbiology laboratories (64). Because of these limitations, new methods to characterize epidemic strains were developed. The different but complementary epidemiologic typing techniques are reviewed in the chronologic order of their development.

ANTIMICROBIAL SUSCEPTIBILITY TESTING

Antimicrobial susceptibility testing (AST) is an inexpensive, easy to use, and readily available means that often is used to characterize microorganisms. The ICP frequently reviews daily and cumulative antimicrobial susceptibility reports (antibiograms) for emerging patterns of resistance. A new or unusual trend of antibiotic resistance from isolates from different patients may raise the suspicion of an outbreak. For example, the rate of ampicillin resistance in *Haemophilus influenzae* isolates from adults was higher than expected in a Georgia community when all isolates were analyzed over a given time, alerting local physicians to the possibility of treatment failure (67).

AST has been used successfully in the investigation of several outbreaks. Review of antimicrobial susceptibility patterns implicated vancomycin-resistant *Enterococcus faecium* as the cause of an outbreak in a cardiothoracic surgery ICU (68). AST is frequently all that is required in the investigation of an outbreak of MRSA in a hospital where the microorganism is not endemic. However, this has become the exception rather than the rule. In an era of multidrug resistant pathogens, AST has become less sensitive. The shortcomings of AST for epidemic typing are well known. The use of AST is limited in epidemiologic studies because of phenotypic variations and because changes in antibiotic resistance occur frequently under the extraordinary selective pressure caused by the extensive use of antimicrobials in hospitals today.

Resistance can rapidly evolve within a strain or be readily acquired from other strains. An example of this phenomenon is resistance to vancomycin in enterococci that is inducible and may not be readily identified by automated susceptibility testing or agar disk diffusion (69–71). For this reason, approved methods are now described by the National Committee on Clinical Laboratory Standards (NCCLS) and include disk diffusion and both agar and broth minimal inhibitory concentration (MIC) testing methods. The E-test (AB Biodisk) has also been used to reliably perform susceptibility testing on enterococci. Finally, the Food and Drug Administration (FDA) has approved a modification of the Vitek method for testing enterococci that shows improved detection of significant resistance to vancomycin and high-level resistance to aminoglycosides.

Many susceptibility tests do not detect β-lactamase–mediated resistance in strains of *Enterobacter* species and other Enterobacteriaceae; this may give rise to a false sense of security when a reportedly sensitive strain is resistant (72–74). Limitations of disk diffusion testing were demonstrated when Meyer et al. (75) studied a nosocomial outbreak of ceftazidime-resistant *Klebsiella pneumoniae.* Isolates that appeared sensitive by routine disk diffusion testing were shown to be inhibited but not killed when broth macrodilution MIC and minimum bacteriocidal concentration (MBC) tests were performed. This problem with disk diffusion susceptibility testing has been addressed in a number of ways. Standard disk diffusion or broth dilution testing of cefpodoxime appears to be a useful way to screen for extended spectrum β-lactamases (74). Alternatively, a 5-μg ceftazidime disk has recently been proposed. Finally, a clavulanate double-disk potentiation procedure has been successfully used to detect extended-spectrum β-lactamases (74).

BACTERIOPHAGE AND BACTERIOCIN TYPING

Bacteriophages are viruses capable of infecting and lysing bacterial cells. When used in epidemiologic investigations, their susceptibility or resistance to lysis characterizes isolates by each member of a panel of bacteriophages (75). For *S. aureus* and *Salmonella* species, phage typing was the mainstay of strain discrimination in the past (75). The problem with this method is that it is very demanding, subject to biologic variability, and available only at reference laboratories because of the need to maintain stocks of phages and control strains (75). DNA-based techniques have thus replaced bacteriophage typing as the authoritative system.

Bacteriocin typing depends on the susceptibility of the test microorganism to toxins produced by other bacteria. This method has limitations similar to those of phage typing and is rarely used today.

PLASMID PROFILE ANALYSIS

The first genotypic method applied to epidemiologic study involved the analysis of plasmids. Plasmid profile analysis (PPA) or plasmid fingerprinting involves the extraction of plasmid DNA followed by the separation of plasmid molecules by agarose gel electrophoresis (76). Initially, the isolation of plasmid DNA required liters of bacterial broth cultures and relied on sophisticated ultracentrifugational techniques (77). Currently, PPA is simple to perform, requires a minimum of equipment and expense, and is well suited for the study of outbreaks of infection (23). This technique has been used successfully for the isolation of plasmid DNA from most Enterobacteriaceae, *Streptococcus* species, *Staphylococcus* species, *Legionella, Vibrio* species, *Plesiomonas, Pseudomonas* species, and *Campylobacter* species (23,77).

Plasmid fingerprinting by agarose gel electrophoresis is a useful means of identifying epidemic strains in outbreaks of nosocomial infections and following endemic antibiotic resistance patterns and the spread of specific resistance genes (76). PPA has been used to identify epidemic strains of gram-negative bacilli

(GNB). In one study, PPA for all epidemic isolates of GNB were the same, whereas co-isolates (controls) showed different DNA patterns, although the antibiograms failed to show a difference (78). Plasmid profiles were found to be better than antibiograms in identifying epidemic strains of *Salmonella typhimurium* and slightly better than phage typing (77). An epidemic of *Pseudomonas aeruginosa* causing wound and peritoneal infections in hemodialysis patients was traced with PPA to an iodophor solution (79). Two outbreaks of infection resulting from *Enterobacter cloacae* that occurred 6 years apart in the same burn unit were attributed to two different strains by plasmid fingerprinting (80). An outbreak of infections caused by an aminoglycoside-resistant strain of *Acinetobacter calcoaceticus* in an intensive care setting was investigated with plasmid fingerprinting (81). All isolates from patients and the environment were identical, thus suggesting a means of transmission (81).

Because plasmids can spread from one bacterial species or strain to another by conjugation, it is occasionally the plasmid rather than the bacterial strain that is epidemic (82). An epidemic plasmid may be found in several different bacterial species or serotypes (82). These epidemic plasmids can enter a hospital in one or a few strains and subsequently spread by conjugation to other strains present in the flora of hospitalized patients (82). Whenever possible, it is extremely important for one to compare epidemic strains with nonepidemic control strains (23,77). However, the presence of one or more plasmids may be unique to a particular strain of a pathogen and, therefore, be used to incriminate that microorganism in an epidemic, especially if the plasmid is stable through time and environmental stress (23,77).

PPA has significant limitations inherent in the fact that plasmids are mobile, extrachromosomal elements rather than the chromosomal genotype that defines the host microorganism. Moreover, plasmids can exist in different molecular forms such as supercoiled (closed circle), nicked (open circle), and linear; each form migrates differently during gel electrophoresis. Both the reproducibility and discriminatory power of plasmid analysis can be greatly improved by digesting the plasmids with restriction endonuclease enzymes. The resulting restriction fragments are then analyzed by electrophoresis. Restriction enzyme analysis (see later) (83) of plasmids is now the method of choice when plasmid analysis is desired. Tables 102.2 and 102.3 show the advantages and limitations of PPA, respectively. Usually, PPA is most effective in studies that are restricted in time and place (e.g., an acute outbreak at one institution) (84).

TABLE 102.2. ADVANTAGES OF PLASMID PROFILE ANALYSIS

Applicable to many bacterial strains
Entire analysis can be completed in 1 day
Twenty-four or more cultures can be processed at one time
Gene expression (i.e., production of surface antigen or specific protein) is not necessary
Cultures too "rough" to serotype are easily analyzed
Microtechniques conserve reagents and space
Rapid, inexpensive, and reproducible

Data from refs. 23, 78.

TABLE 102.3. LIMITATIONS OF PLASMID PROFILE ANALYSIS

The epidemic strain may contain no plasmid DNA or a plasmid that is difficult to isolate
Strains unrelated to the outbreak may contain the epidemic profile
The presence of a plasmid does not provide evidence that it codes for a specific factor (i.e., toxin, antigen, or resistance)
Many plasmids (especially R-plasmids) are readily lost or acquired
Plasmids are subject to rearrangements
As extrachromosomal elements, plasmids do not reflect the stable genotype of the microorganism

Data from refs. 23, 45, 63, 78.

RESTRICTION ENDONUCLEASE ANALYSIS

Restriction endonuclease analysis (REA) relies on enzymes that recognize unique plasmid or chromosomal DNA sequences and cleaves the double-stranded DNA at specific sites within the target (23,85). The separation of these fragments by size in agarose gel produces a restriction endonuclease profile (REP) (86). Unlike PPA, small differences in bacterial strains with identical profiles can be detected with REA, as can acquisition of a new plasmid. If two plasmids are of the same size and yield identical fragment patterns on REA, especially if two or more restriction enzymes are used, they may be assumed to be identical or nearly so (82). Thus, two plasmids may be the same size but produce different patterns of fragments, identifying two different strains. Such was the case when large plasmids of similar size were found in both strains of *K. pneumoniae* causing infection in an intensive care nursery a year apart, suggesting they were similar strains (86). However, REA showed that the two plasmids were from two different strains causing two separate outbreaks (86).

REA of plasmid DNA was used to implicate rectal probes of electronic thermometers in the transmission of vancomycin-resistant *E. faecium* between patients during an outbreak (87). In another study using REA, spread of MRSA in a hospital was traced to a healthcare worker (HCW) with chronic sinusitis (88). The plasmid DNA of isolates from affected patients and a respiratory therapist yielded the same pattern on restriction endonuclease digestion. Epidemiologic methods led to the control of the outbreak without extensive culturing of specimens from patients, personnel, or environmental surfaces or requiring other expensive and labor-intensive resources.

The role of asymptomatic fecal excretors treated with antibiotics in the epidemiology of nosocomial *Clostridium difficile* diarrhea was clarified with REA typing of the strains cultured from stool specimens. Johnson et al. (89) found that asymptomatic fecal excretion of *C. difficile* was transient in most patients. Treatment with metronidazole was not effective. Although treatment with vancomycin was temporarily effective, it was associated with a significantly higher rate of *C. difficile* carriage 2 months after treatment. In five instances, the recurrent *C. difficile* excretion represented acquisition of new strains (reinfection) based on REA typing of the isolates, and three patients began excreting the same REA strain after initial eradication with vancomycin. In another study, the epidemiology and relatedness of

C. difficile isolates in two geographically separated hospitals in a large city were studied using REA (90). A high degree of similarity among isolates from these different hospitals suggested the possibility of an extended outbreak with subsequent genetic drift at the two different institutions. Comparisons of REA typing with other methods such as immunoblot, bacteriophage and bacteriocin, ribotyping, protein profile analysis, arbitrarily primed polymerase chain reaction (AP-PCR), and toxinotyping for *C. difficile* have noted that REA (along with AP-PCR and toxinotyping) is among the most discriminating of the techniques in establishing strain differences (91–93). The REA for *C. difficile* strains is among the most reliable typing methods for current use by clinical laboratories.

Molecular epidemiology can also be used to study resistance patterns resulting from selective pressure from antibiotics. REA of chromosomal DNA has been used to demonstrate that resistance to ciprofloxacin in strains of *Serratia marcescens* and *Proteus mirabilis* (94) and to imipenem in strains of *Enterobacter aerogenes* (95) arose from endemic susceptible strains.

REA can be combined with other methods to strengthen the association between isolates during outbreak investigations. PPA and REA were used to trace an outbreak of multiresistant *Salmonella newport* infections to animals fed subtherapeutic doses of antibiotics (96). Another example involved the use of plasmid profiles and restriction endonuclease digestion to show that a MRSA outbreak was caused by a single strain introduced by an employee 15 months before an outbreak on a vascular surgery service (76). Strains from patients and employees were found to be identical with this technique.

In addition to plasmid DNA, reproducible REA patterns of chromosomal DNA can be detected. REA is especially useful for examining viruses, protozoans, and bacterial strains that lack plasmids (97). REA recognizes specific sites on the chromosome, and the pattern is unique for each isolate (97). Different strains of the same bacterial species can be shown to have different REA profiles. Despite phenotypic dissimilarity, REA of chromosomal DNA of group B *Neisseria meningitidis* identified isolates from the throat that were genetically similar to an epidemic strain (98). However, if, genotypically, all strains appear similar, including the random endemic isolates (controls), then additional restriction digestions with at least two other enzymes that are able to discriminate outbreak strains from endemic strains are likely to be useful in typing isolates (58). The outbreak strains can be considered to belong to the same clone if a second enzyme shows identity among the outbreak strains (58).

RFLP produced by restriction endonucleases has proved useful for strain identification of mycobacteria, for detecting cross-contamination, and for tracing epidemics (99,100). For example, RFLP was used effectively to study an outbreak of tuberculosis with accelerated progression among human immunodeficiency virus (HIV)-infected patients (101). An outbreak of 60 cases of tuberculosis in the Netherlands associated with one physician's office was successfully investigated using RFLP (102). Ongoing uses of RFLP include determining whether the emergence of a multidrug-resistant tuberculosis isolate is clonal or whether reinfection occurs with different RFLP types and analyzing strains on a geographic basis (103). The results of such studies are changing the traditional concepts of tuberculosis transmission. For example, tuberculosis in elderly persons has been generally thought to be the result of reactivation. However, two recent studies have found that a high proportion (30% or more) of tuberculosis cases in elderly people appear to be due to recent infection rather than reactivation (104,105). This has important implications for control of tuberculosis.

The limitation of having enough DNA to analyze (which requires 6 or more weeks of growth of the isolate) can now be overcome by combining RFLP with PCR (which requires short periods of growth by amplifying small quantities of DNA) (103). However, the expense and the labor-intensive and time-consuming requirements of RFLP limits its use to research facilities.

Invasive aspergillosis is a well-known infection with a high mortality that affects immunosuppressed patients. Nosocomial outbreaks have been associated with contaminated ventilation systems and construction within or near hospitals that have immunosuppressed patients (106). Although airborne transmission has been suggested by epidemiologic studies, an accurate typing system, until recently, has not existed to confirm this hypothesis. Biotyping methods are unreliable in differentiating strains because of variable phenotypic expression under different environmental conditions. RFLP of total DNA, digested by particular restriction enzymes, is able to discriminate strains of *Aspergillus fumigatus* to some degree (107). Girardin et al. (108) used Southern blot hybridization of moderately repeated DNA sequences to fingerprint strains of *A. fumigatus* isolated from patients with invasive aspergillosis and from their hospital environment. They demonstrated that some strains persist in the hospital environment for at least 6 months and found suggestive evidence of nosocomial spread of *A. fumigatus* in two patients (108). Thus, the nosocomial origin of infection can be demonstrated if environmental strains identical to the strains from patients are isolated in a prospective survey a few days before the patient's aspergillosis is diagnosed (108). More recent studies done by other molecular methods (109,110) have confirmed this link.

The major advantage of REA is that it allows for differentiation of one strain from another without relying on the expression of a given phenotype (83). The major limitation of REA has been that the number of chromosomal bands produced (approximately 103) is so large and overlapping that the specific bands are difficult to identify; thus, it does not lend itself to a comparison of various isolates (83,84). This limitation of REA has largely been overcome by using PFGE instead of agarose gel electrophoresis (see later discussion).

PULSED FIELD GEL ELECTROPHORESIS

PFGE of chromosomal DNA is a variation of agarose gel electrophoresis that allows analysis of bacterial DNA fragments over and above conventional REA (62). Although it is more expensive and demanding than conventional REA, a highly reproducible restriction profile is provided with PFGE that shows distinct, well-resolved fragments representing the entire bacterial chromosome in a single gel. PFGE banding patterns can readily discriminate among endemic and epidemic strains, especially for *E. coli* and *Mycobacterium avium-intracellulare* but not for MRSA and *H. influenzae* serotype b. RFLP patterns of *Mycobac-*

terium species can be easily interpreted with PFGE, unlike the pattern obtained with routine electrophoresis (99).

Back et al. (111) investigated a recurrent epidemic of erythromycin-resistant *S. aureus* infection in a well-baby nursery. Initial traditional epidemiologic techniques suggested that these were two separate outbreaks. However, REA of plasmid DNA along with genomic DNA typing by PFGE of the isolates demonstrated that the two epidemics resulted from the same strain. A nursing assistant was assumed to be responsible for the first epidemic, because she carried a *S. aureus* strain with the same antibiogram. However, she was infected with an unrelated strain, as assessed by REA with PFGE. Instead, a physician who attended on the unit during both epidemics had the same epidemic strain and was the most likely source of the outbreaks. The authors concluded that traditional epidemic investigations might engender misleading conclusions that can be avoided with molecular epidemiologic techniques. The cost for epidemiologic typing of this outbreak was $1,000 for REA and $1,500 for REA with PFGE.

REA of genomic DNA with PFGE provides DNA fingerprinting of various microorganisms, especially *S. aureus,* which is highly discriminatory and stable enough to reliably characterize many strains (112,113). Such molecular typing has been used recently to identify and characterize the rapid emergence of a new strain of MRSA in Ontario, Canada (114,115). This strain is known as the Ontario epidemic (OE) strain and creates several important problems as follows. Clinical microbiology laboratories in the province of Ontario have noted a striking increase in the rate of isolation of MRSA, from 4.3 isolates per 10,000 admissions in 1994 to 52 per 10,000 admissions in 1997. Molecular typing has shown that this increase is almost exclusively due to the dissemination of a single newly recognized clone of MRSA—the OE strain.

The OE strain is characterized by a colonial morphology that resembles that of coagulase-negative staphylococci in that colonies are chalk-white and γ-hemolytic. Like coagulase-negative staphylococci and unlike *S. aureus,* the OE strain is pyrrolidonyl arylamidase (PYR) positive. DNAase production has been found to be weak or absent in half of the OE strains tested. The tube coagulase test has been found to be relatively sensitive and specific (approximately 90% for each) but often takes 18 hours to become positive. Most rapid slide agglutination tests that were used to identify *S. aureus* have been found to be unreliable when challenged with isolates of the OE clone. Only one commercially available slide agglutination test (Staphaurex Plus, Murex Diagnostics, Norcross, GA) has been found to be 100% sensitive and specific; this kit detects clumping factor, protein A, and capsular polysaccharides (116).

Not only is the OE strain difficult to detect in the microbiology laboratory but also this clone has other attributes that contribute to its rapid spread. The OE strain has a tendency to initially colonize patients at sites other than the anterior nares. Nasal screening alone may fail to identify many colonized individuals. Unexpectedly high rates of isolation of the OE strain from the urinary tract have been noted. Colonization of the rectum and wounds has been seen as well. Initiation of a screening program for this OE strain at Vanderbilt University Hospital in Nashville, Tennessee, resulted in identification of one OE strain within the first 2 weeks.

With the prevalence of community-acquired MRSA steadily increasing, differentiation from nosocomial cases is needed. Clonal expansion of community-acquired MRSA was identified in a Native American community using PFGE analysis (117). This technique identified 31 or 32 isolates of MRSA from the community that were highly related, yet distinguishable from 32 hospital-acquired MRSA strains.

In another study, endemic MRSA in a Veterans Administration medical center was evaluated using PFGE analysis (118). A large amount of strain variation was detected and 40% of patients observed over time were colonized or infected with more than one strain of MRSA. This form of molecular typing was very useful in evaluating the epidemiology of MRSA in this setting.

PFGE has also been useful in studying the spread of GAS in an outbreak setting. Nosocomial transmission of GAS occurred from a single source patient to 24 HCWs in a hospital (119). PFGE analysis revealed that all of the isolates were identified to that of the source patient. The 24 HCWs developed symptoms of pharyngitis less than 4 days after exposure to the source patient. Rapid identification, early treatment, and adherence to infection control practices were able to control the outbreak.

Outbreaks from gram-negative bacilli have been successfully evaluated with PFGE. Multidrug resistant *K. pneumoniae* caused an outbreak in a university hospital in Lisbon, Portugal (120). PFGE identified an endemic strain that presented in different wards in the hospital. In another study, a nosocomial outbreak of *K. pneumoniae* producing extended-spectrum β-lactamase was shown by PFGE to be of the same clone (121).

PFGE of chromosomal DNA was found to be a reliable method for epidemiologic typing of *Serratia odorifera* (122). In this investigation, neither biotype nor antibiogram was useful in differentiating strains. Although no source for the microorganisms or mode of transmission was identified, the isolates from the two patients in a cardiothoracic surgery unit were identical by PFGE of chromosomal DNA, suggesting possible nosocomial transmission.

PFGE of genomic DNA combined with clinical epidemiologic analysis was successfully used to investigate an outbreak of *Mycobacterium abscessus* pseudoinfection (123). Fifteen patients had positive cultures for *M. abscessus* without evidence of infection following endoscopy. Environmental and case-patient isolates had identical large restriction fragment patterns of genomic DNA separated by PFGE. An automated endoscope washer was implicated as the source of the pseudoepidemic. A similar outbreak of pseudoinfection by *M. abscessus* was detected by molecular typing (RA-PCR in this instance) in which the use of in-house prepared distilled water was the source of a pseudo-outbreak (124).

Phenotypic differences among strains of the same *Candida* species may not reflect true strain differences because *Candida* is able to switch phenotypes. Because different phenotypes can coexist at the same site of infection, genotyping techniques were developed (125). REA with PFGE has shown that isolates of the same *Candida* strain share the same DNA profile, whereas epidemiologically unrelated isolates have patterns that are distinctly different (125). RFLP has also been used to delineate specific strains of *Candida* species for epidemiologic studies (125). By the use of DNA content as an epidemiologic marker of strain identity, studies have shown that transmission of *Candida albicans* probably occurs through indirect contact between patients by way of the hands of HCWs (125). Vazquez et al. (126) found that REA patterns of chromosomal DNA from *C. albicans* isolates cultured from patients who were geographically and temporally associated were identical. This study also suggested that nosocomial acquisition of *C. albicans* occurs by way of indirect contact between patients. More recently, Vazquez et al. (127) have found similar molecular epidemiologic evidence that indirect contact between patients is an important factor in nosocomial colonization by *Candida glabrata*. Finally, *Candida inconspicua* has been identified by similar molecular typing techniques as a nosocomial pathogen in patients with hematologic malignancies and appears to emanate from a common source within the hospital environment (128).

Combining several isolate-typing methods may allow for surveying a large population consisting of many different microorganisms. Chetchotisakd et al. (129) used PPA (for *E. coli, K. pneumoniae,* and *E. cloacae*), REA of plasmid DNA (for *S. aureus*), and/or PFGE of chromosomal DNA (for *S. aureus*, enterococci, *P. aeruginosa,* and other bacteria) to demonstrate that endemic bacterial cross-transmission in ICUs is relatively infrequent. DNA typing of these isolates found cross-transmitted bacteria not to be common causes of endemic ICU-related nosocomial infections.

DNA HYBRIDIZATION

Genetic probing or DNA hybridization involves denaturing double-stranded DNA into single-stranded DNA. The single strands from the isolate can be joined to the complementary single-stranded DNA probe that is labeled with a marker, such as P_{32}. The hybrids formed are then measured. The primary requirement for a successful probe is that the sequence be both unique and conserved in the group of microbes to be identified (64). For diagnostic tests, useful probes are prepared by cloning specific DNA sequences from the microorganism to be probed (78). The stringent requirement for complementarity as a precondition for strand reassociation is the basis for the great specificity of the DNA hybridization probe test (78).

DNA probes can be used with the method of Southern hybridization for epidemiologic studies and have been used successfully to investigate the epidemiology of infections caused by *Vibrio cholera, Yersinia enterocolitica,* enteroadherent *E. coli,* enteroinvasive *E. coli, Salmonella* species, *P. aeruginosa,* and *Legionella pneumophila* (64,77). The genes that encode *E. coli* enterotoxins have been cloned from toxigenic strains and used as probes to detect the presence of the target gene in a clinical isolate (78). These probes are important in differentiating pathogenic *E. coli* from nonpathogenic *E. coli* found in the stool of ill and healthy patients (77).

Because small amounts of homologous DNA can be detected, DNA hybridization is useful when isolation of a pathogen is impossible, insensitive, or too time-consuming (78). See Table 102.4 for additional advantages of using the DNA hybridization technique.

Besides toxin production genes, antibiotic resistance genes have been analyzed with DNA probes. DNA hybridization determined the extent of homology between two plasmids that suggested transfer of antibiotic resistance among different species (82). Through the use of DNA probes, *E. coli* plasmid DNA was shown to have a high degree of relatedness with plasmid DNA from tobramycin-resistant strains of *E. cloacae* and *K. pneumoniae* that had been isolated from burn patients (130). This pattern suggested that interbacterial transfer of the plasmid between different species had probably occurred on the burn ward. Interbacterial transfer of a plasmid mediating gentamicin resistance was first described in 1981. In this report, separate outbreaks involving *P. aeruginosa* and *S. marcescens* followed by *K. pneumoniae* and *S. marcescens* were related by the presence of plasmids that contained a common transposable sequence. This suggested transfer of a transposon (translocatable DNA sequence) between plasmids as the mechanism for transmission of gentamicin resistance (131). Recent work suggests that dissemination of resistant genes carried on transposable elements may be important in vancomycin-resistant enterococci (132).

DNA probes have also been used to characterize other microorganisms than bacteria such as mycobacteria, viruses, and fungi. DNA hybridization has identified fingerprint patterns to help define the epidemiology of infections caused by *C. albicans* (133). The DNA probe can be used for mycobacterial cultures but is not sufficiently sensitive to detect microorganisms directly from clinical specimens (134). Identification of individual *Mycobacterium tuberculosis* (MTB) strains is now possible through DNA fingerprinting (134). Because most MTB strains share common drug susceptibility patterns and bacteriophage types, it has been difficult to document transmission of specific strains from person to person (134). However, DNA fingerprints of individual MTB strains remain relatively stable over time and permit delineation of patterns of tuberculosis transmission (134). Not only are DNA probes available for MTB but also for *M. avium-intracellulare, Mycobacterium kansasii,* and *Mycobacterium gordonae*; these probes used with the Bactec system can provide identification within 2 to 4 weeks (135). Despite the many uses of DNA hybridization, a few drawbacks exist. DNA hybridization is costly, slow to perform, and cumbersome.

TABLE 102.4. ADVANTAGES OF DNA HYBRIDIZATION

Does not require the pathogen to be propagated or be viable
Able to safely handle difficult to grow and highly pathogenic (hazardous) microorganisms
Reduces the number of bands for analysis with restriction endonuclease and highlights specific
DNA restriction sites
Can distinguish individual strains of bacteria
Can detect pathogens (CMV, rotavirus, papilloma virus, chlamydia, and mycoplasma) in clinical specimens that are abundant but difficult to cultivate
Can track transposon movement

CMV, cytomegalovirus.
Data from refs. 23. 45. 83. 84.

TABLE 102.5. DISADVANTAGES OF DNA HYBRIDIZATION

Costly, slow to perform, and cumbersome
Often less sensitive than culture when done on an individual basis
Radioisotopes may be required for use

Data from refs. 23, 45, 83, 84.

It is often less sensitive than culture when done on an individual basis, and radioisotopes may be required for its use (Table 102.5) (63,77,82).

RIBOTYPING

Ribosomal RNA (rRNA) represents highly conserved nucleotide sequences that are found in most microorganisms. Probes have been produced based on rRNA that are unique to species, genus, and groups like all gram-negative bacilli and the intracellular pathogen *Legionella* (77). Fingerprinting of rRNA has been valuable for typing strains of *Salmonella typhi, Campylobacter* species, *Pasteurella multocida,* and various *Staphylococcus* species (58,77). REA of rRNA can be used to distinguish isolates of *Staphylococcus* species and strains of *H. influenzae, Providencia stuartii,* and *Candida* species (136). Ribosomal RNA gene restriction patterns were used to show that *H. influenzae* isolates cultured from the trachea and blood of an infant and from the mother's cervix were identical, indicating that the mode of transmission was from mother to child (136).

Ribotyping was found to be a more reliable technique than biochemical typing when evaluating *S. marcescens* strains. Identical ribotypes of *S. marcescens* were found colonizing 12 children in five different hospital wards over a 20-day period (137). Combining epidemiologic findings with the ribotype patterns suggested cross-contamination between the patients on four of the wards.

Epidemiologic studies of *E. cloacae* have relied primarily on the study of phenotypic traits such as biochemical profiles; antibiotic resistance; and serologic, bacteriocin, and phage typing (138). Because of insufficient discrimination, poor reproducibility, or low typeability, these methods are unsatisfactory for analyzing *E. cloacae.* Using RFLP of total DNA and ribotyping, Lambert-Zechovsky et al. (138) were able to document endogenous bacteremia and meningitis resulting from *E. cloacae* that originated from colonization of the gastrointestinal tract in an infant. Each of the five isolates from the infant had identical ribotypes, whereas the comparison strains exhibited different unique ribotype patterns. This case study supports the use of RFLP analysis of total DNA and ribotyping to study the epidemiology of nosocomial infections resulting from *E. cloacae* strains.

Ribotyping and PFGE can be used to characterize multidrug-resistant gram-negative bacilli. The prevalence of carbapenem-resistant *Acinetobacter baumannii* and *P. aeruginosa* in Brooklyn, New York was determined by ribotyping and PFGE on 419 and 823 isolates, respectively (139). Ribotyping revealed a single clone accounted for 62% of the samples and was isolated from patients at all 15 hospitals in the area. Ribotyping revealed that 3 clones accounted for nearly half of the isolates and were shared by most hospitals.

In another study, ribotyping and PFGE was used to characterize a foodborne outbreak. Acute gastroenteritis developed in 21 nursing home patients with two deaths after consumption of minced beef heart contaminated with *Clostridium perfringens* (140). PFGE was not able to characterize a majority of the *C. perfringens* isolates. However, ribotyping successfully distinguished four different groups of *C. perfringens.* The same ribopattern was detected in a food sample, autopsy samples from the two deceased patients, and stool samples from six further patients who had fallen ill with diarrhea.

Besides outbreak investigations, rRNA has been very useful in phylogenetic analysis. The gene sequence in ribosomal DNA was pivotal in the discovery of the causative agents of bacillary angiomatosis, human ehrlichiosis, Whipple's disease, and Tyzzer's disease (141).

POLYMERASE CHAIN REACTION

PCR is the repetitive cycling of three simple reactions in a semiautomated, self-contained system capable of amplifying a single strand of DNA or RNA with 50 to more than 2,000 base pairs more than a million-fold in only a few hours (142). More than 22 different microorganisms that grow slowly or not at all on routine culture media can now be detected using PCR (141). With this tool, the hospital epidemiologist can rapidly diagnose an otherwise difficult to detect pathogen and, thus, initiate specific infection control measures promptly (143).

By virtue of its speed and high degree of sensitivity and specificity, rapid and reliable detection of microbes present in small numbers is now possible. For diagnosis, PCR goes beyond the detection of microorganism-specific immunoglobulin M (IgM) or antibodies in serum, demonstration of seroconversion to a microorganism on testing acute and convalescent sera, or detection of microorganisms in clinical specimens using cultures or antigen assays (144). Pathogens that are difficult to culture, are in the latent stage, or require an antibody response to be detected can potentially be detected with PCR (145). PCR is useful when other tests provide ambiguous results or are subject to technical failures. See Table 102.6 for the benefits of PCR use in epidemiologic investigations. Like other detection systems, PCR has some limitations and pitfalls. The nucleic acid sequence of the pathogens to be detected must be known to develop the appropriate primer. If the sequence is known, and the microorganism is detected, the significance of a positive test result still depends on the clinical situation. For example, cytomegalovirus (CMV) viremia detected by PCR or by culture could indicate asymptomatic shedding versus active infection, making clinical correlation an essential part of the investigation.

PCR has been used in several outbreak investigations and sheds new light on the pathogenesis and spread of difficult-to-detect microorganisms. Enterotoxigenic *E. coli,* a very difficult microorganism to separate from nontoxigenic strains, was successfully detected and identified with the PCR technique (146).

PCR along with other techniques can evaluate infection control surveillance systems. PPA combined with PFGE and PCR

TABLE 102.6. BENEFITS OF POLYMERASE CHAIN REACTION (PCR) IN AN EPIDEMIOLOGIC INVESTIGATION

Direct typing for specific microorganisms
Detection of genes that code for toxins, virulence factors, and antimicrobial resistance
Rapid diagnosis
Detection of microorganisms in low numbers
Detection of microorganisms that are slow-growing or do not grow at all *in vitro*
Does not require an antibody response to the infecting agent
Does not require active replication; latent stage is able to be detected
Able to study the reservoirs and modes of transmission of difficult-to-track pathogens
Detection of microorganisms in body fluids (CSF, ocular fluid, fetal blood)

CSF, cerebrospinal fluid.
Data from refs. 23, 142–145.

was used to study the utility of surveillance for multidrug resistant Enterobacteriaceae in the absence of an outbreak in new organ transplant patients (147). The authors conclude that this form of surveillance is costly and provides little or no benefit for infection control or predicting clinical infections in this population. However, surveillance of colonization may play a greater role in the event that a clonal outbreak is identified.

PCR can also verify the accuracy of other techniques such as PFGE used in outbreak investigations. An outbreak of vancomycin-resistant *E. faecium* was identified in a teaching hospital in Medillin, Columbia using PFGE. PCR identified all 23 isolates as identical, thus complimenting the use of PFGE. (148).

The reservoirs and modes of transmission of nosocomial *Legionella* infection have been further elucidated using newer molecular techniques such as PCR methodology (149–151). An indoor hot tub at a resort condominium complex was implicated as the source of an outbreak of Pontiac fever by using PCR (152). Although cultures of water for *Legionella* were negative, direct fluorescent antibody and PCR were positive, thus incriminating nonviable and nonculturable *L. pneumophila.*

PCR was used to study two outbreaks of infection with a hypervirulent strain of hepatitis B virus (HBV) that was associated with a high mortality (153,154). Mutations in the HBV genome were detected from the index patients and their contacts but absent from unrelated infectious patients, thus implicating the virulent strain as the cause of the outbreaks. The most notable outbreak investigation using PCR involved HIV transmission from a dentist to five of his patients in a healthcare setting (155).

With the recent surge in the incidence of tuberculosis, rapid and accurate diagnosis is becoming increasingly important. As few as one or two microorganisms in a given *Mycobacterium* species can be detected with the PCR method (99). This method can diagnose pulmonary tuberculosis (TB) when acid-fast bacilli (AFB) smears and cultures are negative (99). Eisenach et al. (156) reported a sensitivity of 100% and a specificity of 99% when using PCR techniques to analyze sputum from patients with and without TB. Kirschner et al. (157) over a longer 18-month period noted a sensitivity of only 84.5% and a specificity of 99.5%.

In addition to REA with PFGE and RFLP, PCR has also been used to type *Candida* species. van Belkum et al. (158) successfully typed *C. albicans* strains with PCR amplification of variable DNA domains. They suggest that all colonies of *C. albicans* isolated from clinical specimens can be typed by PCR both prospectively and longitudinally. With this technique, suspected outbreaks resulting from *Candida* species can be investigated more thoroughly to clarify the role of exogenous transmission versus endogenous colonization leading to infection.

A novel variant of conventional PCR, AP-PCR, or random amplified polymorphic DNA (RAPD), has been used successfully in several outbreak investigations. With this new technique, arbitrarily selected primer DNA is annealed to the template DNA under low stringency conditions for the initial cycles of DNA replication (159). This step requires no prior knowledge of the sequences to be amplified. The products of the initial cycles of low-stringency polymerization are amplified under high-stringency conditions, as in conventional PCR, and separated by gel electrophoresis (159). The pattern generated is highly reproducible and specific for a given strain; furthermore, it can be used to distinguish different strains within a single species (160).

Current typing schemes for meningococci include serogrouping of capsular polysaccharides or outer membrane proteins, multilocus enzyme electrophoresis of metabolic enzymes, and genomic restriction endonuclease digestion with or without PFGE (161). An outbreak of meningococcal meningitis at a college campus was successfully investigated using AP-PCR (161). All three disease isolates and 7 of 11 carrier isolates were identical, as found by using four different primers, and were easily distinguishable from unrelated isolates. AP-PCR further demonstrated the clonal nature of meningococcal disease outbreaks in which most disease isolates are of the same clone (161).

Nosocomial transmission of multidrug-resistant gram-negative bacilli in intensive care settings has been elucidated with RA-PCR. A burn unit experienced an outbreak of multidrug-resistant *P. aeruginosa.* RA-PCR identified two predominant genotypes that were responsible for recurrent outbreaks (162). One of the strains was endemic to the burn ward and developed multidrug resistance at the end of the study period. In another study, two outbreaks of multidrug-resistant *K. pneumoniae* in an ICU were analyzed by RA-PCR (163). The first outbreak was caused by two different types of *K. Pneumoniae.* RA-PCR identified yet a different strain that caused the second outbreak. The authors conclude that RA-PCR is easy to perform, highly reproducible, and had a high discriminatory power.

Typing of *C. difficile* to differentiate highly pathogenic from nonpathogenic strains has been accomplished with a number of techniques including bacteriophage, bacteriocin, toxinotyping, and REA of DNA (91–93). Complex and difficult to interpret DNA patterns are sometimes produced with REA of DNA. Silva et al. (164) successfully used AP-PCR to genotype *C. difficile* isolates from various sources. Two strains isolated from patients on the same floor but different wards had the same DNA banding patterns, suggesting a common source of cross-infection through hospital contact. Others have found AP-PCR to be useful for genotyping *C. difficile* (92).

The epidemiology of *Staphylococcus* species can be characterized using RA-PCR. Neonates are susceptible to infections caused by methicillin-resistant coagulase-negative *Staphylococcus.* Dissemination of one particular clone was identified using the RA-PCR technique among a group of neonates on a hospital ward (165). In addition, persistence of the isolate and reinfection was effectively identified with this methodology. In another study, PFGE and PCR were used to characterize colonization of children and their guardians with *S. aureus* (166). When both members of the child-guardian pair were colonized with *S. aureus,* transmission within the family was implicated, because 67% of the colonizing isolates were the same strain.

An outbreak of MRSA in a burn unit was investigated with AP-PCR and restriction endonuclease analysis of plasmid (REAP) DNA (160). Complementary evidence of a clonal relationship among isolates from patients and staff in the burn unit was established with these techniques. MRSA isolates from other hospital wards were clearly distinguishable from the epidemic isolates. The authors concluded that the combination of AP-PCR and REAP may be a useful means of tracking the nosocomial spread of microbial strains and their mobile genetic elements (160). Conventional epidemiologic methods may be inadequate in some outbreak investigations, as this study suggests.

The ability of the hospital epidemiologist or ICP to identify patterns of MRSA spread is dependent on distinguishing the epidemic strain from unrelated MRSA strains (167). During the investigation of the MRSA outbreak in the burn unit mentioned previously, antimicrobial susceptibility patterns suggested a general grouping of MRSA strains, but definitive typing was not possible with this method. However, REAP analysis (plasmid fingerprinting) yielded useful information for strain typing but resulted in some ambiguities that were resolved by AP-PCR (160).

Mycobacterium and *Candida* transmission has been documented with AP-PCR. An outbreak of *M. abscessus* from benzalkonium chloride antiseptic solution was investigated with RA-PCR and PFGE (168). Joint and periarticular soft tissue infections developed after steroid injection from the same physician. Clinical and antiseptic solution strains of *M. abscessus* were indistinguishable by RA-PCR.

After the occurrence of two chronologically related cases of *Candida tropicalis* fungemia in a neonatal ICU, a prospective study of fungal colonization and infection was initiated (169). RFLP and RA-PCR identified fungemia more commonly in colonized than in noncolonized neonates, and no environmental source was found. The authors conclude that these molecular diagnostic tests can improve our understanding of the epidemiology of *Candida* infections, including the mode of transmission. It is likely that techniques for epidemiologic typing for application during outbreak investigations will continue to advance in the age of the evolving PCR technique.

SELECTIVE CULTURE MEDIA AND SPECIAL MICROBIOLOGIC TECHNIQUES

Selective Culture Media

Selective culture media, which inhibit microorganisms in the clinical sample that might obscure or inhibit the growth of the desired strain, may be used during outbreak investigations. For example, the ideal medium for stool specimens would inhibit the competing microorganisms from the normal flora and select out the pathogenic strain desired for analysis. *E. coli* 0157:H7, the cause of severe bloody diarrhea and hemolytic uremic syndrome, was first linked to human illness in 1982. Modified MacConkey medium containing sorbitol allows for culture of stool specimens to diagnose *E. coli* 0157:H7 infection (170).

The laboratory diagnosis of antibiotic-associated colitis caused by *C. difficile* usually requires the detection of cytotoxin or enterotoxin in stool. However, investigations of *C. difficile*-induced outbreaks of colitis require the isolation of strains for comparison. Selective medium was developed for isolating *C. difficile* in the late 1970s, with cefoxitin-cycloserine fructose agar (CCFA) deemed most satisfactory (171). Various modifications of the original formulation of CCFA now exist for selective culturing of *C. difficile* for use in epidemiologic studies (172).

When investigating MRSA outbreaks, the ideal medium allows the growth of MRSA or clearly differentiates between MRSA and multiresistant coagulase-negative staphylococci (173). Currently, the best discriminating medium to select for MRSA is mannitol salt agar (7.5% sodium chloride) or Mueller-Hinton medium supplemented with 4% sodium chloride, each containing methicillin, oxacillin, or both (174).

A selective medium consisting of Mueller-Hinton agar with vancomycin (20 μg/mL), polymyxin (100 μg/mL), and streptomycin (100 μg/mL) was successfully used to culture for vancomycin-resistant *E. faecium* from rectal and environmental swabs during an outbreak investigation (87).

Special Microbiologic Techniques

Susceptibility testing for penicillin-resistant pneumococci has rapidly evolved. Previously, this was done in most microbiology laboratories using the NCCLS method with Mueller-Hinton agar containing added sheep blood and a 1-μg oxacillin disk to screen for penicillin resistance (175). Today, disk diffusion and/or E-test methods are preferred (176). In the future, PCR may become the standard (177).

Traditionally, specimens for isolation of mycobacteria have been inoculated on Lowenstein-Jensen American Thoracic Society medium or Middlebrook 7H10 or 7H11 medium. Incubation for 4 to 6 weeks is required to detect growth with these methods. A more recent approach is to inoculate a thinly poured plate of Middlebrook 7H11 medium and examine with a conventional microscope (99). This allows for slow-growing mycobacteria to be detected in as few as 3 days and identified in 7 to 10 days (99). A biphasic broth culture system, the Roche Septi-Chek AFB system (Roche, Rockwell, MD), is comparable to the Bactec system (99). Another newer method now available is the mycobacteria growth indicator tube (MGIT) [Baltimore Biological Laboratory (BBL)]. The MGIT system consists of a modified Middlebrook 7H9 broth and a sensor embedded in silicone on the bottom of a tube. The appearance of orange-colored fluorescence in the sensor when excited indicates the growth of mycobacteria (178).

Antimicrobial susceptibilities for mycobacteria are generally determined by comparing the amount of growth in the media containing known drug concentrations with growth in the control media (99). Traditionally, antimicrobial susceptibility results obtained by using Middlebrook 7H10 or 7H11 agar with the antituberculosis agents added at specific concentrations takes about 4 weeks of incubation. Currently, the Bactec radiometric system for mycobacterial susceptibility testing can provide results in a week or less (99). The MGIT offers equal speed for mycobacterial susceptibility testing (179).

CONCLUSIONS

The microbiology laboratory has become an integral part of a hospital epidemiology and infection control program. The constantly changing spectrum of nosocomial pathogens and their susceptibilities and the availability of newer technologies require constant communication, cooperation, and collaboration between microbiology personnel and ICPs. In the twenty-first century, this relationship is more critical than at any time in the past.

The key to effective hospital epidemiology and infection control efforts in the twenty-first century will be the proper application of diverse phenotypic and genotypic methods for detection, identification, susceptibility testing, and typing of nosocomial pathogens. Phenotypic methods, although readily available, are frequently misleading and, therefore, have limited value in epidemiologic studies today. Genotyping has overcome almost all of the limitations of phenotyping and now provides very effective tools for the hospital epidemiologist and ICP to use in epidemiologic investigations. Important genotypic methods are briefly summarized.

One of the first genotypic methods, PPA, is well suited for the analysis of outbreaks that occur over a relatively short period. This technique is convenient for use in diagnostic laboratories and requires a minimum of equipment and expense. Because many bacterial species harbor plasmids infrequently and because plasmids can be gained or lost, PPA may not be satisfactory for long-term follow-up studies.

REA of plasmid or chromosomal DNA has been very useful for typing many microorganisms in epidemiologic studies. RFLP profiles produced by REA can detect different strains of the same species because of variation in their DNA sequences. The advantages of total DNA RFLP include universal applicability, high sensitivity, and ease of performance. Because some REA patterns were too large and indistinct when obtained with agarose gel electrophoresis, PFGE was developed to provide clearer patterns with better discriminatory power. PFGE appears to give the best results for investigating staphylococci, enterococci, and *P. aeruginosa.*

DNA hybridization with Southern blotting is another molecular method that uses a labeled DNA probe to reduce the number of visible fragments to a manageable number and, thus, produces a clearer fingerprint of the microorganism.

Ribotyping has taken advantage of highly conserved sequences that are found in most microorganisms to delineate the epidemiology of a number of outbreaks. Ribotyping with rDNA is the method of choice when evaluating Enterobacteriaceae, *Burkholderia cepacia,* and *Stenotrophomonas maltophilia*; this method takes about 5 days.

Finally, the most sensitive of all molecular typing methods, PCR, has allowed the identification of new entities and discrimination of nearly identical appearing strains. AP-PCR is the most rapid method (1–2 days) and is also the least expensive method that soon may be applicable to all bacteria.

The rapid development and use of genotypic typing techniques has significantly expanded the understanding of the epidemiology of many nosocomial pathogens. The challenge for the microbiology laboratory in the twenty-first century is to make these techniques readily available (in-house or from a reference laboratory) and affordable. With such tools, the hospital epidemiologist and the ICP should be able to achieve more effective investigations of outbreaks and, thus, will be able to develop better prevention strategies.

REFERENCES

1. Ashhurst AP. The centenary of Lister (1827–1927). A tale of sepsis and antisepsis. *Ann Med Hist* 1927;9:205–211.
2. Centers for Disease Control and Prevention. Infection surveillance and control programs in U.S. hospitals: an assessment, 1976. *MMWR Morb Mortal Wkly Rep* 1976;27:139–145.
3. Mallison GF. Monitoring of sterility and environmental sampling in programs for the control of nosocomial infections. In: Cundy KR, Ball W, eds. *Infection control in health care facilities: microbiological surveillance.* Baltimore: University Park Press, 1977:23–31.
4. Stratton CW, Ratner H, Johnston PE, et al. Focused microbiologic surveillance by specific hospital unit as a sensitive means of defining antimicrobial resistance problems. *Diagn Microbiol Infect Dis* 1992; 15(Suppl):S11–S18.
5. Stratton CW, Ratner H, Johnston PE, et al. Focused microbiologic surveillance by specific hospital unit: practical application and clinical utility. *Clin Ther* 1993;15(Suppl A):S12–S20.
6. Eggimann P, Pittet D. Infection control in the ICU. *Chest* 2001;120: 2059–2093.
7. O'Grady NP, Alexander M, Dellinger EP, et al. Guidelines for the prevention of intravascular catheter-related infections. *Infect Control Hosp Epidemiol* 2001;23:759–769.
8. Pfaller MA, Herwaldt LA. The clinical microbiology laboratory and infection control: emerging pathogens, antimicrobial resistance, and new technology. *Clin Infect Dis* 1997;25:858–870.
9. McDonald LC, Jarvis WR. Linking antimicrobial use to nosocomial infections: the role of a combined laboratory-epidemiology approach. *Ann Intern Med* 1998;129:245–247.
10. Bergeron MG, Ouellette M. Preventing antibiotic resistance through rapid genotypic identification of bacteria and their antibiotic resistance genes in the clinical microbiology laboratory. *J Clin Microbiol* 1998;36:2169–2172.
11. Tenover FC. Development and spread of bacterial resistance to antimicrobial agents: an overview. *Clin Infect Dis* 2001;33(Suppl 3): S108–S115.
12. Finch R. Antibiotic resistance—from pathogen to disease surveillance. *Clin Microbiol Infect* 2002;8:317–320.
13. Relman DA. New technologies, human-microbe interactions, and the search for previously unrecognized pathogens. *J Infect Dis* 2002; 186(Suppl 2):S254–S258.
14. Bonten MJ, Weinstein RA. Infection control in intensive care units and prevention of ventilator-associated pneumonia. *Semin Respir Infect* 2000;15:327–335.
15. Friedman ND, Kaye KS, Stout JE, et al. Health care—associated bloodstream infections in adults: a reason to change the accepted definition of community-acquired infections. *Ann Intern Med* 2002; 137:791–797.

16. Joiner KA, Dismukes WE, Britigan BE, et al. Adequacy of fellowship training: results of a survey of recently graduated fellows. *Clin Infect Dis* 2001;32:255–262.
17. Reagan DR. Microcomputers in hospital epidemiology. *Infect Control Hosp Epidemiol* 1997;18:440–448.
18. Stratton CW. Get a handle on resistance before it gets a handle on you: the PROTEKT US Surveillance Study. *South Med J* 2001;94: 891–892.
19. Tokars JI, Miller ER, Stein G. New national surveillance system for hemodialysis-associated infections: initial results. *Am J Infect Control* 2002;30:288–295.
20. Emori TG, Culver DH, Horan TC, et al. National nosocomial infections surveillance system (NNIS): description of surveillance methods. *Am J Infect Control* 1991;19:19–35.
21. Richards MJ, Edwards JR, Culver DH, et al. Nosocomial infections in medical intensive care units in the United States. National Nosocomial Infections Surveillance System. *Crit Care Med* 1999;27: 887–892.
22. Haley RW, Culver DH, White JW, et al. The efficacy of infection surveillance and control programs in preventing nosocomial infections in university hospitals. *Am J Epidemiol* 1985;121:182–205.
23. Soll DR, Lockhart SR, Pujol C. Laboratory procedures for the epidemiological analysis of microorganisms. In: Murray PR, Baron EJ, Jorgensen JH, et al., eds. *Manual of clinical microbiology,* 8th ed. Washington DC: American Society for Microbiology, 2003: 139–161.
24. Steward CD, Wallace D, Hubert SK, et al. Ability of laboratories to detect emerging antimicrobial resistance in nosocomial pathogens: a survey of project ICARE laboratories. *Diagn Microbiol Infect Dis* 2000; 38:59–67.
25. Peterson LR, Noskin GA. New technology for detecting multidrug-resistant pathogens in the clinical microbiology laboratory. *Emerg Infect Dis* 2001;7:306–311.
26. McGowan JE Jr, Metchock BG. Basic microbiologic support for hospital epidemiology. *Infect Control Hosp Epidemiol* 1996;17:298–303.
27. Diekema DJ, Pfaller MA. Infection control epidemiology and clinical microbiology. In: Murray PR, Baron EJ, Jorgensen JH, et al., eds. *Manual of clinical microbiology,* 8th ed. Washington DC: American Society for Microbiology, 2003:129–138.
28. Pfaller MA. Epidemiology and control of fungal infections. *Clin Infect Dis* 1994;19(Suppl 1):S8–S12.
29. Petignat C, Blanc DS, Francioli P. Occult nosocomial infections. *Infect Control Hosp Epidemiol* 1998;19:593–596.
30. Jungkind D. Molecular testing for infectious disease. *Science* 2001; 284:1553–1555.
31. Wolk D, Mitchell S, Patel R. Principles of molecular microbiology testing methods. *Infect Dis Clin North Am* 2001;15:1157–1204.
32. Versalovic J, Lupski JF. Molecular detection and genotyping of pathogens: more accurate and rapid answers. *Trends Microbiol* 2002; 10(Suppl):S15–S21.
33. Nissen MD, Sloots TP. Rapid diagnosis in pediatric infectious diseases: the past, the present and the future. *Pediatr Infect Dis* 2002; 21:605–612.
34. Gilbert GL. Molecular diagnostics in infectious diseases and public health microbiology: cottage industry to postgenomics. *Trends Molec Microbiol* 2002;8:280–287.
35. Nolte FS, Caliendo AM. Molecular detection and identification of microorganisms. In: Murray PR, Baron EJ, Jorgensen JH, et al., eds. *Manual of clinical microbiology,* 8th ed. Washington DC: American Society for Microbiology, 2003:234–256.
36. Weber S, Pfaller MA, Herwaldt LA. Role of molecular epidemiology in infection control. *Infect Dis Clin North Am* 1997;11:257–278.
37. Schentag JJ, Hyatt JM, Carr JR, et al. Genesis of methicillin-resistant *Staphylococcus aureus* (MRSA), how treatment of MRSA infections has selected for vancomycin-resistant *Enterococcus faecium,* and the importance of antibiotic management and infection control. *Clin Infect Dis* 1998;26:1204–1214.
38. Thacker SB, Choi K, Brachman PS. The surveillance of infectious diseases. *JAMA* 1983:249:1181–1185.
39. Centers for Disease Control and Prevention. Update: outbreak of severe acute respiratory syndrome—worldwide, 2003. *MMWR Morb Mortal Wkly Rep* 2003;52:241–246.
40. Feldmann H, Czub M, Jones S, et al. Emerging and re-emerging infectious diseases. *Med Microbiol Immunol* 2002;191:63–74.
41. Snell NJC. Examining unmet needs in infectious disease. *Drug Discov Today* 2003;8:22–30.
42. Wachsmuth K. Molecular epidemiology of bacterial infections: examples of methodology and of investigations of outbreaks. *Rev Infect Dis* 1986;8:682–692.
43. Smith TL, Pearson ML, Wilcox KR, et al. Emergence of vancomycin resistance in *Staphylococcus aureus. N Engl J Med* 1999;340:493–501.
44. Pfaller MA. Typing methods for epidemiologic investigation. In: Balows A, Hausler WJ Jr, Herrman K, et al., eds. *Manual of clinical microbiology,* 5th ed. Washington DC: American Society for Microbiology, 1991:171–182.
45. Eisenstein BI. New molecular techniques for microbial epidemiology and the diagnosis of infectious diseases. *J Infect Dis* 1990;161: 595–602.
46. Zambon M, Bull T, Sadler CJ, et al. Molecular epidemiology of two consecutive outbreaks of parainfluenza 3 in a bone marrow transplant unit. *J Clin Microbiol* 1998;36:2289–2293.
47. Biering G, Karlsson S, Clark NC, et al. Three cases of neonatal meningitis caused by *Enterobacter sakazakii* in powdered milk. *J Clin Microbiol* 1989;27:2054–2056.
48. John JF, Grieshop TJ, Atkins LM, et al Widespread colonization of personnel at a Veterans Affairs medical center by methicillin-resistant, coagulase-negative *Staphylococcus. Clin Infect Dis* 1993;17:380–388.
49. Kluytmans J, Berg H, Steegh P, et al. Outbreak of *Staphylococcus schleiferi* wound infections: strain characterization by randomly amplified polymorphic DNA analysis, PCR ribotyping, conventional ribotyping, and pulsed-field gel electrophoresis. *J Clin Microbiol* 1998; 36:2214–2219.
50. Versalovic J, Koeuth T, Lupski JR. Distribution of repetitive DNA sequences in eubacteria and application of fingerprinting of bacterial genomes. *Nucleic Acids Res* 1991;19:6823–6831.
51. McGee L, Klugman KP, Friedland D, et al. Spread of the Spanish multi-resistant serotype 23F clone of *Streptococcus pneumoniae* to Seoul, Korea. *Microb Drug Resist* 1997;3:253–257.
52. Aires de Sousa M, Santos Sanches I, Ferro ML, et al. Intercontinental spread of a multidrug-resistant methicillin-resistant *Staphylococcus aureus* clone. *J Clin Microbiol* 1998;36:2590–2596.
53. Auerbach SB, Schwartz B, Williams D, et al. Outbreak of invasive group A streptococcal infections in a nursing home. *Arch Intern Med* 1992;152:1017–1022.
54. Cockerill FR III, Thompson RL, Musser JM, et al. Molecular, serological, and clinical features of 16 consecutive cases of invasive streptococcal disease. *Clin Infect Dis* 1998;26:1448–1458.
55. Martin JM, Ward ER, Green M. Field inversion gel as a typing system for group A streptococcus. *J Infect Dis* 1998;177:504–507.
56. Desai M, Tanna A, Wall R, et al. Fluorescent amplified-fragment length polymorphism analysis of an outbreak of group A streptococcal invasive disease. *J Clin Microbiol* 1998;36:3133–3137.
57. Facklam R, Beall B, Efstrtious A, et al. *emm* typing and validation of provisional M types for group A streptococci. *Emerg Infect Dis* 1999;5:247–253.
58. Barg NL. An introduction to molecular hospital epidemiology. *Infect Control Hosp Epidemiol* 1993;14:395–396.
59. Jarvis WR. Usefulness of molecular epidemiology for outbreak investigations. *Infect Control Hosp Epidemiol* 1994;15:500–503.
60. Maslow J, Mulligan ME. Epidemiologic typing systems. *Infect Control Hosp Epidemiol* 1996;17:595–604.
61. Tenover FC, Arbeit RD, Coering RV, et al. How to select and interpret molecular typing methods for epidemiological studies of bacterial infections: a review for healthcare epidemiologists. *Infect Control Hosp Epidemiol* 1997;18:426–429.
62. Wu F, Della-Latta P. Molecular typing strategies. *Semin Perinatol* 2002;26:357–366.
63. Lupski JR. Molecular epidemiology and its clinical application. *JAMA* 1993;270:1363–1364.
64. Engleberg NC, Eisenstein BI. The impact of new cloning techniques

on the diagnosis and treatment of infectious diseases. *N Engl J Med* 1984;311:892–901.

65. Woods GL. Automation in clinical microbiology. *Am J Clin Pathol* 1992;98(Suppl 1):S22–S30.
66. Maki DG, Rhame FS, Mackel DC, et al. Nationwide epidemic of septicemia caused by contaminated intravenous products. I. Epidemiologic and clinical features. *Am J Med* 1976;60:471–485.
67. Farley MM, Stephens DS, Brachman PS, et al. Invasive *Haemophilus influenzae* disease in adults: a perspective, population-based surveillance. *Ann Intern Med* 1992;116:806–812.
68. Karanfil LV, Murphy M, Josephson A, et al. A cluster of vancomycin-resistant *Enterococcus faecium* in an intensive care unit. *Infect Control Hosp Epidemiol* 1992;13:195–200.
69. Kohner PC, Patel R, Uhl JR, et al. Comparison of agar dilution, broth microdilution, E-test, disk diffusion, and automated Vitek methods for testing susceptibilities of *Enterococcus* sp. to vancomycin. *J Clin Microbiol* 1997;35:3258–3263.
70. Hawley HB, Elder BL. Multiple-drug resistant enterococci: laboratory identification, prevention, and treatment. *Antimcrob Infect Dis Newslett* 1997;16:65–68.
71. Tenover FC. Laboratory methods for surveillance of vancomycin-resistant enterococci. *Clin Microbiol Newslett* 1998;20:1–5.
72. Sanders CC, Iaconis JP, Bodey GP, et al. Resistance to ticarcillin-potassium clavulanate among clinical isolates of the family *Enterobacteriaceae*: role of PSE-1 beta-lactamase and high levels of TEM-1 and SHV-1 and problems with false susceptibility in disk diffusion tests. *Antimicrob Agents Chemother* 1988;32:1365–1369.
73. Sanders CC. New beta-lactams: new problems for the internist. *Ann Intern Med* 1991;115:650–651.
74. Patterson JE, Rech M, Jorgensen JH. Extended-spectrum beta-lactamases: dilemmas in detection and therapy. *Antimicrob Infect Dis Newslett* 1997;16:57–61.
75. Meyer KS, Urban C, Eagen JA, et al. Nosocomial outbreak of *Klebsiella* infection resistant to late-generation cephalosporins. *Ann Intern Med* 1993;119:353–358.
76. Shlaes DM, Currie-McCumber CA. Plasmid analysis in molecular epidemiology: a summary and future directions. *Rev Infect Dis* 1986; 8:738–746.
77. Wachsmuth K. Molecular epidemiology of bacterial infections: examples of methodology and of investigations of outbreaks. *Rev Infect Dis* 1986;8:682–692.
78. Eisenstein BI, Engleberg NC. Applied molecular genetics: new tools for microbiologists and clinicians. *J Infect Dis* 1986;153:416–430.
79. Parrott PL, Terry PM, Whitworth EN, et al. *Pseudomonas aeruginosa* peritonitis associated with contaminated poloxamer-iodine solution. *Lancet* 1982;2(8300):683–685.
80. Markowitz SM, Smith SM, Williams DS. Retrospective analysis of plasmid patterns in a study of a burn unit outbreak of infection due to *Enterobacter cloacae. J Infect Dis* 1983;148:18–23.
81. Girgis I, Isenberg JS, Ozuner G, et al. An outbreak of aminoglycoside-resistant *Acinetobacter calcoaceticus* in an intensive care setting. *Infect Med* 1992;28:33–35.
82. Farrar WE. Molecular analysis of plasmids in epidemiologic investigation. *J Infect Dis* 1983; 148:1–6.
83. Stull TL, LiPuma JJ, Edlind TD. A broad-spectrum probe for molecular epidemiology of bacteria: ribosomal RNA. *J Infect Dis* 1988;157: 280–286.
84. Maslow JN, Mulligan ME, Arbeit RD. Molecular epidemiology: application of contemporary techniques to the typing of microorganisms. *Clin Infect Dis* 1993;17:153–164.
85. Sader HS, Hollis RJ, Pfaller MA. The use of molecular techniques in the epidemiology and control of infectious diseases. *Clin Lab Med* 1995;2:407-431.
86. John JF, McKee KT, Twitty JA, et al. Molecular epidemiology of sequential nursery epidemics caused by multi-resistant *Klebsiella pneumoniae. J Pediatr* 1983;102:825–830.
87. Livornese LL, Dias S, Samel C, et al. Hospital-acquired infection with vancomycin-resistant *Enterococcus faecium* transmitted by electronic thermometers. *Ann Intern Med* 1992;117:112–116.
88. Boyce JM, Opal SM, Potter-Boynoe G, et al. Spread of methicillin-resistant *Staphylococcus aureus* in a hospital after exposure to a health care worker with chronic sinusitis. *Clin Infect Dis* 1993;17:496–504.
89. Johnson S, Homann SR, Bettin KM, et al. Treatment of asymptomatic *Clostridium difficile* carriers (fecal excretors) with vancomycin or metronidazole. *Ann Intern Med* 1992;117:297–302.
90. Mekonen E, Gerding DN, Sambol SP, et al. Predominance of a single restriction endonuclease analysis group with intrahospital subgroup diversity among *Clostridium difficile* isolates at two Chicago hospitals. *Infect Control Hosp Epidemiol* 2002;23:648–652.
91. Peterson LR, Kelly PJ. The role of the clinical microbiology laboratory in the management of *Clostridium difficile*–associated diarrhea. *Infect Dis Clin North Am* 1993;7:277–293.
92. Rafferty ME, Baltch AL, Smith RP, et al. Comparison of restriction enzyme analysis, arbitrarily primed PCR, and protein profile analysis typing for epidemiologic investigation of an ongoing *Clostridium difficile* outbreak. *J Clin Microbiol* 1998;36:2957–2963.
93. Rupnik M, Avesani V, Janc M, et al. A novel toxinotyping scheme and correlation of toxinotypes with serogroups of *Clostridium difficile* isolates. *J Clin Microbiol* 1998;36:2240–2247.
94. Yee YC, Muder RR, Hsieh MH, et al. Molecular epidemiology of endemic ciprofloxacin-susceptible and -resistant *Enterobacteriaceae. Infect Control Hosp Epidemiol* 1992;13:706–710.
95. De Gheldre Y, Maes N, Rost F, et al. Molecular epidemiology of an outbreak of multidrug-resistant *Enterobacter aerogenes* infections and in vivo emergence of imipenem resistance. *J Clin Microbiol* 1997;35: 152–160.
96. Holmberg SD, Osterholm MT, Senger KA, et al. Drug-resistant *Salmonella* from animals fed antimicrobials. *N Engl J Med* 1984;311: 617–622.
97. Tompkins LS. The use of molecular methods in infectious diseases. *N Engl J Med* 1992;327:1290–1297.
98. Kristiansen B, Sorensen B, Bjorvatn B, et al. An outbreak of group B meningococcal disease: tracing of the causative strains of *Neisseria meningitidis* by DNA fingerprinting. *J Clin Microbiol* 1986;23: 764–767.
99. Stratton CW. Tuberculosis, infection control, and the microbiology laboratory. *Infect Control Hosp Epidemiol* 1993;14:481–487.
100. Behr MA, Small PM. Molecular fingerprinting of *Mycobacterium tuberculosis*: how it can help the clinician? *Clin Infect Dis* 1997;25: 806–810.
101. Daley CL, Small PM, Schecter GF, et al. An outbreak of tuberculosis with accelerated progression among persons infected with the human immunodeficiency virus. Analysis using restriction-fragment-length-polymorphisms. *N Engl J Med* 1992;326:231–235.
102. Van Soolingen D, Hermans PWM, de Haas PEW, et al. Occurrence and stability of insertion sequences in *Mycobacterium tuberculosis* complex strains: evaluation of an insertion sequence-dependent DNA polymorphism as a tool in the epidemiology of tuberculosis. *J Clin Microbiol* 1991; 29:2578–2586.
103. Snider DE, La Montagne JR. The neglected global tuberculosis problem: a report of the 1992 World Congress on tuberculosis. *J Infect Dis* 1994;169:1189–1196.
104. Bauer J, Yang Z, Poulsen S, et al. Results from 5 years of nationwide DNA fingerprinting of *Mycobacterium tuberculosis* complex isolates in a country with a low incidence of *M. tuberculosis* infection. *J Clin Microbiol* 1998;36:305–308.
105. Gurierrez MC, Vincent V, Aubert D, et al. Molecular fingerprinting of *Mycobacterium tuberculosis* and risk factors for tuberculosis transmission in Paris, France, and surrounding areas. *J Clin Microbiol* 1998; 36:486–492.
106. Walsh TJ, Dixon DM. Nosocomial aspergillosis: environmental microbiology, hospital epidemiology, diagnosis and treatment. *Eur J Epidemiol* 1989;5:131–142.
107. Denning DW, Clemons KV, Hanson LH, et al. Restriction endonuclease analysis of total cellular DNA of *Aspergillus fumigatus* isolates of geographically and epidemiologically diverse origin. *J Infect Dis* 1990;162:1151–1158.
108. Girardin H, Sarfati J, Traore F, et al. Molecular epidemiology of nosocomial invasive aspergillosis. *J Clin Microbiol* 1994;32:684–690.
109. Chazalet V, Debeaupuis J-P, Sarfati J, et al. Molecular typing of envi-

ronmental and patient isolates of *Aspergillus fumigatus* from various hospital settings. *J Clin Microbiol* 1998;36:1494–1500.

110. Radford SA, Johnson EM, Leeming JP, et al. Molecular epidemiological study of *Aspergillus fumigatus* in a bone marrow transplantation unit by PCR amplification of ribosomal intergenic spacer sequences. *J Clin Microbiol* 1998;36:1294–1299.
111. Back NA, Linnemann CC, Pfaller MA, et al. Recurrent epidemics caused by a single strain of erythromycin-resistant *Staphylococcus aureus*: the importance of molecular epidemiology. *JAMA* 1993;270: 1329–1333.
112. Hartstein AI, Morthland VH, Eng S, et al. Restriction enzyme analysis of plasmid DNA and bacteriophage typing of paired *Staphylococcus aureus* blood culture isolates. *J Clin Microbiol* 1989;27:1874–1879.
113. Pfaller MA, Wakefield DS, Hollis R, et al. The clinical microbiology laboratory as an aid in infection control: the application of molecular techniques in epidemiologic studies of methicillin-resistant *Staphylococcus aureus. Diagn Microbiol Infect Dis* 1991;14:209–217.
114. Green K, Fleming CA, McGeer A, et al. Dramatic emergence of methicillin-resistant *Staphylococcus aureus* (MRSA) in Ontario, Canada. Abstract E-127. In: *Proceedings of the 37th ICCAC, Toronto, Ontario, Canada.* Washington DC: American Society for Microbiology, 1997:136.
115. McGeer A, Low DE, Conly J, et al. The rapid emergence of a new strain of MRSA in Ontario: laboratory and infection control implications. *Lab Proficiency Testing Program Newslett* 1996;190.
116. Papasian CJ, Garrison B. Evaluation of a rapid slide agglutination test for identification of *Staphylococcus aureus. Diagn Microbiol Infect Dis* 1999;33:201–203.
117. Fey PD, Said-Salim B, Rupp ME, et al. Comparative molecular analysis of community or hospital acquired methicillin-resistant *Staphylococcus aureus. Antimicrobiol Agents Chemother* 2003;47:196–203.
118. Herwaldt LA, Pottinger JM, Coffman S, et al. Molecular epidemiology of methicillin-resistant *Staphylococcus aureus* in a Veterans Administration medical center. *Infect Control Hosp Epidemiol* 2002;23: 502–505.
119. Kakis A, Gibbs L, Eguia J, et al. An outbreak of group A streptococcal infection among health care workers. *Clin Infect Dis* 2002;35: 1353–1359.
120. Durarte A, Boavida F, Grosso F, et al. Outbreak of GES-1 B-lactamase-producing multidrug-resistant *Klebsiella pneumoniae* in a university hospital in Lisbon, Portugal. *Antimicrobial Agent Chemother* 2003; 47:1481–1482.
121. Gruteke P, Goessens W, van Gils J, et al. Patterns of resistance associated with integrons, the extended-spectrum B-lactamase SHV-5 gene, and a multidrug efflux pump of *Klebsiella pneumoniae* causing a nosocomial outbreak. *J Clin Microbiol* 2003;41:1161–1166.
122. Sader HS, Perl TM, Hollis RJ, et al. Nosocomial transmission of *Serratia odorifera* biogroup 2: case report demonstration by macrorestriction analysis of chromosomal DNA using pulsed-field gel electrophoresis. *Infect Control Hosp Epidemiol* 1994;15:390–393.
123. Maloney S, Welbel S, Daves B, et al. *Mycobacterium abscessus* pseudoinfection traced to an automated endoscope washer: utility of epidemiologic and laboratory investigation. *J Infect Dis* 1994;169: 1166–1169.
124. Lai KK, Brown BA, Westerling JA, et al. Long-term laboratory contamination by *Mycobacterium abscessus* resulting in two pseudo-outbreaks: recognition with use of random amplified polymorphic DNA (RAPD) polymerase chain reaction. *Clin Infect Dis* 1998;27:169–175.
125. Dembry LM, Vazquez JA, Zervos MJ. DNA analysis in the study of the epidemiology of nosocomial candidiasis. *Infect Control Hosp Epidemiol* 1994;15:48–53.
126. Vazquez JA, Sanchez V, Dmuchowski C, et al. Nosocomial acquisition of *Candida albicans*: an epidemiologic study. *J Infect Dis* 1993; 168:195–201.
127. Vazquez JA, Dembry LM, Sanchez V, et al. Nosocomial *Candida glabrata* colonization: an epidemiologic study. *J Clin Microbiol* 1998; 36:421–426.
128. D'Antonio D, Violante B, Mazzoni A, et al. A nosocomial cluster of *Candida inconspicua* infections in patients with hematological malignancies. *J Clin Microbiol* 1998;36:792–795.
129. Chetchotisakd P, Phelps CL, Hartstein AI. Assessment of bacterial cross-transmission as a cause of infections in patients in intensive care units. *Clin Infect Dis* 1994;18:929–937.
130. Elwell LP, Inamine JM, Minshew BH. Common plasmid specifying tobramycin-resistance found in two enteric bacteria isolated from burn patients. *Antimicrob Agents Chemother* 1978;13:312–317.
131. Rubens CE, Farrar WE, McGee ZA, et al. Evolution of a plasmid mediating resistance to multiple antimicrobial agents during a prolonged epidemic of nosocomial infections. *J Infect Dis* 1981;143: 170–181.
132. van den Braak N, van Belkum A, van Keulen M, et al. Molecular characterization of vancomycin-resistant enterococci from hospitalized patients and poultry products in the Netherlands. *J Clin Microbiol* 1998;36:1927–1932.
133. Fox BC, Mobley HLT, Wade JC. The use of a DNA probe for epidemiologic studies of candidiasis in immunocompromised hosts. *J Infect Dis* 1989;159:488–494.
134. Barnes PF, Barrows SA. Tuberculosis in the 1990s. *Ann Intern Med* 1993;119:400–410.
135. Peterson EM, Lu R, Floyd C, et al. Direct identification of *Mycobacterium tuberculosis, Mycobacterium avium,* and *Mycobacterium intracellulare* from amplified cultures in Bactec media using DNA probes. *J Clin Microbiol* 1989;27:1543–1547.
136. Thomson-Carter FM, Carter PE, Pennington TH. Differentiation of staphylococcal species and strains by ribosomal RNA gene restriction patterns. *J Gen Microbiol* 1989;135:2093–2097.
137. Bingen EH, Mariani-Kurkdjian P, Lambert-Zechovsky NY, et al. Ribotyping provides efficient differentiation of nosocomial *Serratia marcescens* isolates in a pediatric hospital. *J Clin Microbiol* 1992;30: 2088–2091.
138. Lambert-Zechovsky N, Bingen E, Denamur E, et al. Molecular analysis provides evidence for the endogenous origin of bacteremia and meningitis due to *Enterobacter cloacae* in an infant. *Clin Infect Dis* 1992;15:30–32.
139. Landman D, Quale JM, Mayorga D, et al. Citywide clonal outbreak of multiresistant *Acinetobacter baumannii* and *Pseudomonas aeruginosa* in Brooklyn, N.Y. *Arch Intern Med* 2002;162:1515–1520.
140. Schalch B, Bader L, Schau HP, et al. Molecular typing of *Clostridium perfringens* from a food-borne disease outbreak in a nursing home: ribotyping versus pulsed-field gel electrophoresis. *J Clin Microbiol* 2003;41:892–895.
141. Wilson KH. Detection of culture-resistant bacterial pathogens by amplification and sequencing of ribosomal DNA. *Clin Infect Dis* 1994; 18:958–962.
142. Eisenstein BI. The polymerase chain reaction: a new method of using molecular genetics for medical diagnosis. *N Engl J Med* 1990;322: 178–183.
143. Templeton NS. The polymerase chain reaction: history, methods and applications. *Diag Molec Pathol* 1992;1:58–72.
144. Jungkind D. Automation of laboratory testing for infectious diseases using polymerase chain reaction: our past, our present, our future. *J Clin Virol* 2001;20:1–6.
145. Peter JB. The polymerase chain reaction: amplifying our options. *Rev Infect Dis* 1991;13:166–171.
146. Olive DM. Detection of enterotoxigenic *Escherichia coli* after polymerase chain reaction amplification with a thermostable DNA polymerase. *J Clin Microbiol* 1989;27:261–265.
147. Gardam MA, Burrows LL, Kus JV, et al. Is surveillance for multidrug-resistant Enterobacteriaceae an effective infection control strategy in the absence of an outbreak? *J Infect Dis* 2002;186:1754–1760.
148. Panesso D, Ospina S, Robledo J, et al. First characterization of a cluster of vanA-type glycopeptide-resistant *Enterococcus faecium,* Colombia. *Emerg Infect Dis* 2002;8:961–966.
149. Starnbach MN, Falkow S, Tompkins LS. Species-specific detection of *Legionella pneumophila* in water by DNA amplification and hybridization. *J Clin Microbiol* 1989;27:1257–1261.
150. Riffard S, Presti FL, Vandenesch F, et al. Comparative analysis of infrequent-restriction-site PCR and pulsed-field gel electrophoresis for epidemiological typing of *Legionella pneumophila* serogroup 1 strains. *J Clin Microbiol* 1998;36:161–167.

151. Fiore AE, Muorti JP, Levine OS, et al. Epidemic Legionnaires' disease two decades later: old sources, new diagnostic methods. *Clin Infect Dis* 1998;26:426–433.
152. Miller LA, Beebe JL, Butler JC, et al. Use of polymerase chain reaction in an epidemiologic investigation of Pontiac fever. *J Infect Dis* 1993; 168:769–772.
153. Omata M, Ehata T, Yokosuka O, et al. Mutations in the precore region of hepatitis B virus DNA in patients with fulminant and severe hepatitis. *N Engl J Med* 1991; 324:1699–1704.
154. Liang TJ, Hasegawa K, Rimon N, et al. A hepatitis B virus mutant associated with an epidemic of fulminant hepatitis. *N Engl J Med* 1991;324:1705–1709.
155. Centers for Disease Control and Prevention. Prevention update: transmission of HIV infection during an invasive dental procedure—Florida. *MMWR Morb Mortal Wkly* 1991;40:21–27, 33.
156. Eisenach KD, Sifford MD, Cave MD, et al. Detection of *Mycobacterium tuberculosis* complex strains by polymerase chain reaction. *J Clin Microbiol* 1990;28:1204–1213.
157. Kirschner P, Rosenau J, Springer B, et al. Diagnosis of mycobacterial infections by nucleic acid amplification: 18-month prospective study. *J Clin Microbiol* 1996;34:304–312.
158. van Belkum A, Melchers W, de Pauw BE, et al. Genotypic characterization of sequential *Candida albicans* isolates from fluconazole-treated neutropenic patients. *J Infect Dis* 1994;169:1062–1070.
159. Welsh J, McClelland M. Fingerprinting genomes using PCR with arbitrary primers. *Nucleic Acids Res* 1990;18:7213–7218.
160. Fang FC, McClelland M, Guiney DG, et al. Value of molecular epidemiologic analysis in a nosocomial methicillin-resistant *Staphylococcus aureus* outbreak. *JAMA* 1993;270:1323–1328.
161. Woods JP, Kersulyte D, Tolan RW, et al. Use of arbitrarily primed polymerase chain reaction analysis to type disease and carrier strains of *Neisseria meningitidis* isolated during a university outbreak. *J Infect Dis* 1994;169:1384–1389.
162. Pirnay JP, De Vos D, Cochez C, et al. Molecular epidemiology of *Pseudomonas aeruginosa* colonization in a burn unit: persistence of a multidrug-resistant clone and a silver sulfadiazine-resistant clone. *J Clin Microbiol* 2003;41:1192–1202.
163. van der Zee A, Steer N, Thijssen E, et al. Use of multienzyme multiplex PCR amplified fragment length polymorphism typing in analysis of outbreaks of multiresistant *Klebsiella pneumoniae* in an intensive care unit. *J Clin Microbiol* 2003;41:798–802.
164. Silva J, Yajarayma JT, Gumerlock PH. Genotyping of *Clostridium difficile* isolates. *J Infect Dis* 1994;169:661–664.
165. Bogado I, Limansky A, Sutich E, et al. Molecular characterization of methicillin-resistant coagulase-negative staphylococci from a neonatal intensive care unit. *Infect Control Hosp Epidemiol* 2002;23:447–451.
166. Shopsin B, Mathema B, Alcabes P, et al. Prevalence of agr specificity groups among *Staphylococcus aureus* strains colonizing children and their guardians. *J Clin Microbiol* 2003;41:456–459.
167. Roberts RB, de Lancastre, Eisner W, et al. Molecular epidemiology of methicillin-resistant *Staphylococcus aureus* in 12 New York hospitals. *J Infect Dis* 1998;178:164–171.
168. Tiwari TS, Ray B, Jost KC Jr, et al. Forty years of disinfectant failure: outbreak of postinjection *Mycobacterium abscessus* infection caused by contamination of benzalkonium chloride. *Clin Infect Dis* 2003;36: 954–962.
169. Roilides E, Farmaki E, Evdoridou J, et al. *Candida tropicalis* in a neonatal intensive care unit; epidemiologic and molecular analysis of an outbreak of infection with an uncommon neonatal pathogen. *J Clin Microbiol* 2003;41:735–741.
170. Centers for Disease Control and Prevention. Preliminary report: foodborne outbreak of *Escherichia coli* 0157:H7 infections from hamburgers—western United States, 1993. *MMWR Morb Mortal Wkly Rep* 1993;42:85–86.
171. George WL, Sutter VL, Citron D, et al. Selective and differential medium for isolation of *Clostridium difficile. J Clin Microbiol* 1979; 9:214–219.
172. Brazier JS. Role of the laboratory in investigation of *Clostridium difficile* diarrhea. *Clin Infect Dis* 1993;16:S228–S233.
173. Brumfitt W, Hamilton-Miller J. Methicillin-resistant *Staphylococcus aureus. N Engl J Med* 1989;320:1188–1196.
174. Kampf G, Lecke C, Cimbal A-K, et al. Evaluation of mannitol salt agar for detection of oxacillin resistance in *Staphylococcus aureus* by disk diffusion and agar screening. *J Clin Microbiol* 1998;36: 2254–2257.
175. Caputo GM, Appelbaum PC, Liu HH. Infections due to penicillin-resistant pneumococci: clinical, epidemiologic, and microbiologic features. *Arch Intern Med* 1993;153:1301–1310.
176. Jones RN, Wilson WR. Epidemiology, laboratory detection, and therapy of penicillin resistant streptococcal infections. *Diagn Microbiol Infect Dis* 1998;31:453–459.
177. de Plessis M, Smith AM, Klugman KP. Rapid detection of penicillin-resistant *Streptococcus pneumoniae* in cerebrospinal fluid by a seminested-PCR strategy. *J Clin Microbiol* 1998;36:453–457.
178. Chew WK, Lasaitis RM, Schio FA, et al. Clinical evaluation of the mycobacteria growth indicator tube (MGIT) compared with radiometric (Bactec) and solid media for isolation of *Mycobacterium* species. *J Med Microbiol* 1998;47:821–827.
179. Bergmann JS, Woods GL. Reliability of mycobacterial growth indicator tube for testing susceptibility of *Mycobacterium tuberculosis* to ethambutol and streptomycin. *J Clin Microbiol* 1997;35:3325–3327.

103

DETERMINING THE COST-EFFECTIVENESS OF HEALTHCARE EPIDEMIOLOGY AND INFECTION CONTROL PROGRAMS

LINDA M. MUNDY
VICTORIA J. FRASER

Nosocomial infections contribute significant costs above and beyond what is expected from patients' underlying disease states (1–3). Over the past 2 decades, there has been growing recognition of the economic impact of nosocomial infections across the continuum of care, which compounds the substantial costs of healthcare in general (4,5). In estimates of hospital reimbursements, hospitals receive additional payments that account for less than 5% of the actual costs of care to treat nosocomial infections (6,7).

Despite the ongoing development and expansion of technologic advances in healthcare systems, efforts to control and maintain healthcare costs focus mostly on optimizing resource utilization, reducing waste, and identifying duplication of services. Continued reductions in healthcare budgets have particularly impacted healthcare epidemiology and infection control programs, which do not generate revenue and are challenged to prove their worth. Although the methods used to determine the costs of nosocomial infections have been analyzed in detail (8,9), justifying healthcare epidemiology and infection control services through cost-effectiveness analysis (CEA) is less frequently performed. CEA is an analytic tool in which costs and effects of an intervention or program and at least one alternative approach are calculated and presented in a ratio of incremental cost to incremental effect, with the effect being a measurable health outcome. The core purpose of a CEA is to provide a relative value to different healthcare interventions and to relate the value of the impact of these interventions to the value of specific health outcomes.

In 1993, the United States Public Health Service convened the Panel on Cost-Effectiveness in Health and Medicine. The panel members gave two broad recommendations for conducting studies to improve quality and encourage comparability (9). The first recommendation emphasized that in healthcare studies, the focus should be on CEA rather than cost-benefit analysis, because in the latter type of study the effect is monetary rather than health outcomes. The second recommendation emphasized that decision making for resource allocations should be society based using reference case analysis. The societal perspective attempts to incorporate all costs and health effects regardless of who incurs the costs and who obtains the effects. These recommendations are applicable to healthcare epidemiology and infection control programs and are expanded on in this chapter.

Given that the mission of healthcare epidemiology and infection control programs is to provide a safe healthcare environment for patients, families, and employees, diverse and dynamic skills and infrastructures are required to succeed in this mission. In the early 1970s, the Study on the Efficacy of Nosocomial Infection Control (SENIC) project confirmed that hospital-based infection control programs with strategies for surveillance, feedback to surgeons on surgical site infection rates, and competent infection control staff were able to reduce nosocomial infection rates by 32% (10). In more recent years, healthcare epidemiology programs are challenged to exceed the SENIC perspective and to prevent, control, and monitor nosocomial health outcomes across the continuum of healthcare. Economic evaluations in technical and administrative reports help to measure the success of these goals.

This chapter, intended for hospital epidemiologists, infection control professionals (ICPs), and administrative staff, describes how to incorporate economic evaluations into the design, implementation, and evaluation of healthcare epidemiology and infection control programs. In healthcare, five types of economic evaluations are commonly used. A cost-minimization analysis includes the incremental costs of alternatives that achieve the same outcome. A cost-consequence analysis considers the incremental costs and effects that achieve the same outcome, without an attempt to aggregate the costs and effects. The two major economic evaluations, the cost-benefit and cost-effectiveness analyses, are described in greater detail in the chapter. Lastly, the cost-utility analysis is a special type of CEA, in which quality of life is also considered as part of the outcome.

COST-BENEFIT ANALYSIS

Nosocomial infections are complications of hospitalization that by definition were not present or incubating on admission.

In addition to morbidity and mortality, nosocomial infections significantly increase use of societal resources. In the 1970s and 1980s, methods for estimating costs and benefits of nosocomial infections were identified:

1. Estimations of cost. Estimations of cost for nosocomial infections require that the incremental costs associated with diagnosing and treating the infection be distinguished from the costs attributable to diagnosis and management of the primary medical problem. Incremental costs of nosocomial infections include costs allocated for laboratory, pharmacy, procedures, and additional hospital days. Haley et al. (11) reported in 1981 that approximately half of the additional costs of treating nosocomial infections were accounted for by extra days of hospital stay. Several methods for estimating costs by estimating incremental excess length of stay resulting from nosocomial infections have been identified: implicit physician assessment, unmatched group comparison, matched group comparison, and an appropriateness evaluation protocol (AEP) method (8,12).
   a. Implicit physician assessment. In this method, a chart review by a designated person is conducted via an outlined protocol. This method is limited by subjectivity and, in comparison with other methods, consistently underestimates the true incremental costs of nosocomial infections (13).
   b. Unmatched group comparison. In this method the total number of hospital days attributable to nosocomial infections is determined by comparing patients with and without nosocomial infections. This method is limited, because there is no adjustment for severity of illness, and hence this method consistently overestimates additional incremental costs of nosocomial infections.
   c. Matched control comparison. In this method, the total number of extra hospital days resulting from the nosocomial infection is determined by matching patients with nosocomial infections with uninfected patients who have comparable age, severity of illness, and underlying disease (14,15). This method is likely to give the most accurate assessment of the additional incremental costs of nosocomial infections.
   d. AEP-based method. This method distinguishes original causes of hospitalization from those related to a nosocomial infection (8,16). Each day of hospital care is linked to one or both of these categories. Objective categorization protocols are designed for this method. This method is labor intensive.
2. Estimations of benefits. Benefits of infection control strategies include subjective and objective determinations of the decrease in the occurrence or effects of infections resulting from infection control interventions. Such benefits may include a decrease in the number of hospital days or a decrease in nosocomial infection rates (17).
3. Cost-benefit analysis. A cost-benefit analysis is an analytic tool for estimating the net societal benefit of a program or intervention. This is measured as the incremental benefit of the program minus the incremental cost, with all benefits and costs measured in dollars (9). The goal in using a cost-benefit analysis is twofold: to eliminate procedures when the cost outweighs the benefit and to facilitate or encourage implementation of the procedure when the benefit outweighs the cost (18). The two major limitations of this method are determining the level at which the benefit is significant enough to implement the intervention and its lack of a societal perspective (19,20).

COST-EFFECTIVE ANALYSIS

In contrast to cost-benefit analysis, which compares the monetary cost of a program with the monetary benefit, CEA does not require that costs and benefits be reduced to a common denominator. As a methodology, CEA evaluates outcomes and costs of interventions designed to improve health. Such analyses aid decision-making processes that pertain to resource allocations but are limited by not necessarily being able to incorporate all variables relevant to such decisions.

Comparison of CEAs in various medical and public heath disciplines is notable for wide variation in cost-effectiveness ratios. To put CEAs for infection control into perspective with studies of cancer screening and coronary artery disease, some traditionally accepted healthcare interventions save money, whereas others cost more than $1 million per year of life gained. Cost-effectiveness ratios for annual mammography screening of women aged 55 to 65 ranges from $32,000 to $120,000, based on the Breast Cancer Detection Demonstration Project and Health Insurance Plan Study, respectively (21,22). In applying quality weights to the years of additional life anticipated from colorectal cancer screening, a cost-effectiveness ratio of $18,000 per quality-adjusted life year (QALY) has been estimated (21, 23). Somewhat intuitively, as the frequency of cervical cancer screening increases, the cost-effectiveness ratio becomes less favorable. Screening women aged 20 to 75 years every 4 years compared with no screening yielded a cost-effectiveness ratio of $260,000 per life-year saved, whereas screening annually has an incremental cost-effectiveness ratio of greater than $1 million per life-year saved (21,24). Two examples of CEAs from the cardiovascular literature demonstrate wide variations in cost-effectiveness ratios. In one comparison of percutaneous transluminal coronary angioplasty and coronary artery bypass graft (CABG), CABG was more expensive yet more effective, at an incremental cost-effectiveness ratio of $26,000 per life-year saved (25). Another investigation identified the cost-effectiveness ratios of CABG as ranging from $17,500 to $45,000 for patients aged 45 to 74 with prior myocardial infarction and exercise-induced ischemia (26).

1. Cost-effectiveness ratio. Cost-effectiveness analyses use the cost-effectiveness ratio. This is a mathematical ratio in which the numerator includes all changes in resource utilization relative to at least one stated alternative, and the denominator includes all the health effects of an intervention relative to the stated alternative(s). Ultimately, the CEA provides ratios that show the cost (in monetary terms) of achieving one unit of health outcome (27).
   a. Numerator. Variables for the numerator should include

the costs of healthcare services, patient time expended for the intervention, paid and unpaid caregiving services, costs associated with lost productivity or illness (e.g., travel, child care, missed employment), costs linked to the nonhealth impact of the intervention (e.g., the environment), and time spent seeking an intervention.
   b. Denominator. Variables for the denominator include those that are effects of the health intervention, such as subsequent morbidity and length of life.
2. Costs.
   a. Direct costs. Direct costs are the value of all resources, goods, and services consumed in the provision of an intervention or in dealing with the consequences of the intervention. Such costs may be medical or nonmedical.
   b. Indirect costs. In CEA, indirect costs pertain to productivity gains or losses related to illness or death.
   c. Marginal costs. Marginal costs are the extra amount of resource consumption incurred for providing a service as compared with the costs of not providing the same service.
   d. Incremental costs. Incremental costs are the costs of one alternative (comparator) minus the cost of another alternative. The incremental cost-effectiveness ratio is the difference in costs between two alternatives compared with the difference in effectiveness between the same two alternatives.
3. Discounting. Discounting is the process of converting future dollars and future health outcomes to a present value.
4. Reference case analysis. When a CEA will contribute to decisions that pertain to broad or societal allocation of resources, a reference case analysis is recommended (9). A reference case analysis includes a baseline computation of the cost-effectiveness ratio along with a meaningful set of sensitivity analyses that allows for comparison of the results with other published studies. This reference case analysis should include validated measurement of health-related quality of life that can incorporate the effects of morbidity on productivity and leisure. In addition, the health intervention of interest should be compared with existing practice rather than an unattainable alternative.

COMPONENTS OF HEALTH OUTCOME ANALYSES

The outcomes evaluation process begins with the identification of one or more desired outcomes. The measures of health outcomes most commonly employed are the number of lives, life-years, QALYs, and disability-adjusted life years (DALYs). If an intervention varies in intensity or periodicity, incremental cost-effectiveness ratios are calculated that express the additional cost per each additional unit of outcome obtained.

1. Outputs versus outcomes. Outputs are the number of service units that a program delivers. Outcomes are the results of the specific intervention. In setting up a health outcomes analysis, it is imperative that long-term outcomes be distinguished from intermediate and short-term outcomes to better characterize the study design.
2. Structured and process measures. Structured measures assess organizational or programmatic features that are perceived to influence performance. Process measures assess the ways in which the intervention occurs.
3. QALYs. Quality of life is a rather broad construct that attempts to comprise all valued aspects of an individual's existence (e.g., aspects of health, economics, environment, politics, culture, and spiritual values). In health outcomes measurement, QALYs are assigned to each time period of evaluation with a weight, ranging between 0 and 1, that corresponds to the health-related measure during that period (9). In analysis, a weight of 1 corresponds to optimal health, whereas a weight of 0 corresponds to a health state judged equivalent to death (9). Such weights are further described in the Beaver Dam Health Outcomes Study and in the Functional Capacity Index (28,29). The major assumption that must be addressed with this measure is that a QALY may not be of equal value to all who gain from it, and the gain may not be equal during all components of the lifespan.
4. Utility and patient preference. In health-related quality of life measurement, utility refers to the preference for a particular health outcome. Patient preference for a particular health outcome can be quantified with standardized metrics and expressed as utility functions or preferences for a particular outcome and incorporated into CEAs. Common patient preference measures include standard gamble and time trade-off.
   a. Standard gamble. Standard gamble is a determination of patient preference, or utility, for a particular outcome. A comparison is made between the probability of a particular health state (e.g., assured perfect health) versus an alternative health state (e.g., chronic infection, bed-bound, or death). In measurement of the gamble, the probability p is varied until the preference for the assured health state is equal to the preference for the alternative $(1 - p)$.
   b. Time trade-off. In this patient preference metric, a patient is asked to trade off years of life in a state of less than perfect health for a shorter lifespan in a state of perfect health (9). Although occasionally patients will not trade any years of life for less than perfect health, this time trade-off measurement is calculated as the ratio of the number of years in perfect health equivalent to the often longer span in less than perfect health.
5. Cost perspectives. The cost-effectiveness construct and the ultimate results obtained from it depend on the perspective taken from the population affected by the intervention. Such perspectives include the patient, payer, provider, and society.
   a. Patient. Costs to the patient include copayments, lost time from work, and lost value or even years of life if there is a health status change.
   b. Payer perspective. Payers are accountable for contracted rates for services that often depend more on the contract than on the actual services delivered.
   c. Provider perspective. For providers, profit must be considered. Short-term decisions are measured as the difference between receipts and the variable cost of providing the service, whereas long-term decisions are measures that include fixed and variable costs.

   d. Societal perspective. The 1993 U.S. Public Health Service expert panel on cost-effectiveness recommended that, if the nature of the problem is broad, the perspective of the CEA should be equally broad and reflect the societal perspective (9). In such an analysis, everyone affected by the intervention and all significant health outcomes and costs that flow from the intervention must be included in the analysis. Society is interested in a balance that ensures that resources are allocated in such a way that each unit is put to its most productive use. This rarely happens, so on a more practical basis, society prefers options that produce more output for a given amount of resources. Although health outcomes are often represented by years of life gained in CEA using the societal perspective, the measure of outcomes should be defined more broadly. In application of the reference case analysis, economic evaluation may vary between countries and the societal perspective must be that of the country in which the intervention is performed.

POTENTIAL COMPONENTS OF A COST-EFFECTIVENESS ANALYSIS FOR HEALTHCARE EPIDEMIOLOGY AND INFECTION CONTROL PROGRAMS

In preparation for a CEA of a project in healthcare epidemiology or infection control, several specific issues should be considered, which are detailed in the following:

1. Type of institution. As the site of an episode of healthcare becomes a continuum from the acute to alternative care settings, measurement of risks and resource allocations become more complicated for healthcare epidemiology and infection control programs.
   a. Acute care institution. Resource allocations for a hospital epidemiology program are often determined by hospital size (licensed bed number). In 1995, the estimated cost of an ideal infection control program in a 250-bed hospital was $200,000 (30). This estimate included supplies, overhead, and the salaries of a part-time physician, nurse, secretary, and data programmer. Based on this program budget, cost-effectiveness estimates for mortality and cost-benefit estimates of morbidity were determined. Using these estimates of preventable deaths, the years of life saved and the costs of treating infections can be calculated to estimate the marginal cost per infection and the break-even point for a healthcare epidemiology program (30).
   b. Long-term care facility. An algorithm, or formula, for the minimal resource allocation for an infection control program in long-term care has not been established. The intensity and degree of infection control surveillance, infrastructure, and regulations in long-term care are not necessarily parallel to those identified for acute care. In addition, these strategies vary depending on the type of setting, patient's acuity of illness, state regulations, and other factors. As an example, the recommendations from the Society for Healthcare Epidemiology of America for the prevention and control of multidrug-resistant pathogens in long-term care facilities allow for a wide range of strategies to be potentially implemented (31).
   c. Home care and other alternative settings. Home health agencies accounted for the fastest growing personal healthcare expenditures during the 1980s (32). Mid-1990 estimates from the Health Care Financing Administration suggest that expenditures for the provision of home healthcare will increase from almost $2 billion in 1988 to $25 billion in 1999 (33). The role of infection control in home care is often collapsed into the general responsibilities and resources available to nurses within the individual home care organization. Few studies have yet evaluated the additional but sometimes unrecognized costs of home healthcare on nosocomial infections (34).
2. Endemic versus epidemic infection control strategies. As the majority of healthcare epidemiology efforts are dedicated to the control of endemic infections, rather than epidemic infections, resource allocations should parallel this distribution of activity. Cost-effectiveness analyses in infection control need to distinguish between these two very different control strategies and eventually identify estimates of burden incurred from the societal perspective. The CDC recommends four key components for infection control programs targeted to control the spread of multidrug-resistant pathogens: surveillance, applied research, prevention and control strategies, and development or expansion of infrastructure (35). Cost-effective analysis of such infection control programs should take these components into consideration.
   a. Surveillance. The degree of pathogen surveillance within a healthcare setting can range from none to epidemic-intense specimen procurement, reporting, and evaluation. The surveillance plan may vary, contingent on the identified pathogen, intervention, and goals of the program. For healthcare systems dedicated to the prevention and control of the spread of multidrug-resistant microorganisms, the options for surveillance span from a threshold alert on clinical isolates, to use of a suppressed or routine passive surveillance system (i.e., screen for vancomycin-resistant enterococci in stools submitted for another clinical indication), to elaborate programs with formalized active surveillance.
   b. Applied research. To adequately assess the impact of infection control programs, resource allocation is needed for molecular testing of microbiology specimens, data programming and analysis from information systems, and CEAs.
   c. Prevention and control strategies. The strategies employed in healthcare epidemiology and infection control programs are myriad. Such strategies may be categorized as environmental (disinfectants, enhanced cleaning, changes in the physical plant), educational, behavioral (observations of compliance to contact precautions, monitoring of traffic control in operating rooms, surgeon-specific feedback of surgical site infection rates), and pharmacologic (cyclic rotation of antimicrobial agents, formulary restrictions, vaccine administration).
   d. Development or expansion of existing infrastructure. A

secure and well-functioning infrastructure is crucial for an effective healthcare epidemiology or infection control program. ICPs in large and small programs need access to administrative leadership, database management support, and performance monitoring systems. As a program or hospital department, infection control programs are accountable for patients, healthcare workers, and the public health components of their immediate environment. During times of accreditation, healthcare epidemiologists and ICPs are often expected to report on performance and update policies and procedures for the Joint Commission on Accreditation of Healthcare Organizations, Health Care Financing Administration, and other federal and state regulatory agencies.

3. Interventions. Infection control interventions may focus on either prevention or treatment. The types of interventions that are best as candidates for widespread implementation are those that are readily modifiable and feasible. Primary prevention interventions involve strategies to reduce risk factors or prevent exposure. Interventions in secondary prevention reduce the effects of the risk or exposure. Treatment interventions treat the insult resulting from the risk or exposure.

PUBLISHED STUDIES OF HEALTHCARE EPIDEMIOLOGY AND INFECTION CONTROL: COST-ESTIMATES, COST-BENEFIT, AND COST-EFFECTIVENESS ANALYSIS

Few studies in healthcare epidemiology and infection control have focused on in-depth cost analysis. Use of a reference case analysis has been limited to evaluations of immunization programs. A summary of economic evaluation studies in the field of healthcare epidemiology and infection control categorized as cost-estimates, cost-benefit analyses, and CEAs is given in the following:

1. Cost estimates. Although high, the attributable costs of nosocomial infections are not well determined. In general, nosocomial infections have a mean attributable cost of $13,973; targeted intervention costs approximately $1,138. (36–39). Published studies with economic evidence of the attributable costs of specific nosocomial infections are summarized in the following.
   a. Bloodstream infections. The excess duration of hospitalization secondary to bloodstream infections is 7 to 21 days, estimated attributable mortality is 16% to 35%, and the average costs are $3,061 to $40,000 (2,6,15,40–42). The costs attributed to bloodstream infections vary widely with the host comorbidities, severity of illness, and the specific pathogen.
   b. Surgical site infections. Surgical site infection rates vary by surgical procedure and patient risk (43,44). The excess duration of hospitalization secondary to surgical site infections range from 7 to 8 days and increase costs by an average of $690 to $2,734 (37,45). Costs attributed to incisional and organ/space sternal surgical site infections after cardiothoracic surgery are estimated to be much higher, whereas other surgeries vary in costs and benefits (46–48).
   c. Urinary tract infections. Nosocomial urinary tract infections prolong hospitalization by at least 1 day at an average cost ranging from $589 to $700 (40,42,49,50). A relatively large study identified a 32% reduction in urinary tract infections with the use of silver alloy coated catheters. A cost model of catheter use suggested an overall savings in a hospital setting (50).
   d. Ventilator-associated pneumonia. Nosocomial pneumonia is often associated with mechanical ventilation. These infections prolong hospitalization by an average of 6 days and increase costs by an average of $4,947 (6,40).
   e. Dressing changes of central venous catheters. In a recent comparative study of central venous catheter dressing changes by ward nurses (case) versus an infusion team (control group), catheter-related bacteremia rates were 1.7% among cases and 1.4% among controls (51). There were also no differences in catheter site infection rates, and the investigators estimated a cost savings in excess of $90,000 per year by delegation of this dressing change to the ward nurses.
   f. Antimicrobial drug use. The relationship between antimicrobial control programs and antimicrobial resistance patterns is complex. A few institutions have shown an increase in susceptibility to antimicrobial agents following intensive control or monitoring of antimicrobial drug use (52–54). Cost estimates have not been well established for these efforts.
2. Cost-benefit analyses.
   a. Surgical-site infections. In one study, patients with cancer and confirmed postsurgical infection had a mean increase in costs of $12,542 per patient. Interestingly, the workup of postoperative fever had a mean increase in costs of $145 per patient and was six times more common than postsurgical infections. Hence, the overall management of suspected infection cost the hospital more than the management of confirmed infection (55).
   b. Endemic control of *Staphylococcus aureus* infections.
      i. In a study from 1982 to 1985, cost calculations attributable to *S. aureus* nosocomial infections were calculated for laboratory, antibiotic use, and per diem costs using the AEP (56). In the evaluation of 58 patients, laboratory costs accounted for 2%, antibiotics for 21%, and per diem costs for 77% of the total infection-related costs. Although only 45% of the patients were hospitalized for additional days specifically because of *S. aureus* infections, those with prolonged stay had an average of 18 extra hospital days.
      ii. Nasal carriage of *S. aureus* is considered a significant risk factor for the development of *S. aureus* infections. An intervention study on a cardiothoracic surgical unit evaluated the effect of perioperative mupirocin nasal ointment on the incident rate of surgical site infections (48). Mupirocin had a 62% effect on reducing surgical site infections with an estimated cost-effectiveness ratio of $16,633 per infection prevented.

TABLE 103.1. COMPARISON OF THREE STUDIES OF COST-EFFECTIVENESS ANALYSIS FOR HEPATITIS B PREVENTION

Age Group	Cost-effectiveness ratio	Study
Perinatal (0–12 months)	$3,300 per QALY	Margolis et al. (60)
Infants (1–5 years)	$25,000 per QALY	
Youth (≥6 years)	$33,000 per QALY	
Newborns	$52,000 per QALY	Bloom et al. (61)
Adolescents	$137,000 per QALY	
Adults	$385,000 per QALY	
Infants	$35,000–40,000 per life-year	Krahn and Detsky (62)

QALY, quality-adjusted life year.

3. Cost-effectiveness analyses. Although a cost-benefit analysis is of interest when health effects are valued in terms of willingness to pay, the CEA allows decision making for health protection at identified costs. Nonetheless, assessment of CEA, as with any new tool, requires recognition of assets and limitations. One recent review of published studies using CEA reported that the majority of these studies support strategies requiring additional expenditures, thus implicating potential bias in the focus of CEAs (57). Although the 1993 Panel on Cost-Effectiveness in Health and Medicine has helped to standardize an approach to CEAs, greater uniformity in analytic practices is still needed if CEAs are to become a more influential tool in debates of resources utilization in the decades to come. For hospital epidemiology and infection control programs, recognizing the impact of our efforts on the expanding episodes of care and emerging multidrug-resistant pathogens may allow for sophisticated CEAs in the years to come. Some of the best CEAs in infection control have been performed as a component of primary prevention studies with vaccines and subsequent immunization programs.
   a. Varicella immunization. From the societal perspective, a CEA of routine varicella immunization of U.S. children confirmed that the program would save more than $5 for every dollar invested in vaccination (58). From the health payer's perspective, the program would cost $2 per case of varicella prevented or $2,500 per life-year saved and be a relatively cost-effective intervention compared with other preventive health programs.
   b. Pneumococcal immunization. In a CEA of pneumococcal vaccination compared with no vaccination from the societal perspective, investigators used base case estimates and a sensitivity analysis (best and worst cases) (59). Patients 65 years and older in three U.S. geographic areas were enrolled to determine whether or not vaccination reduced medical expenses and the risk of pneumococcal bacteremia. Pneumococcal vaccinations saved $8.27 and gained 1.21 QALY for each person vaccinated. Excluding future medical costs of survivors, the cost per QALY gained was $3,597 for those aged 65 to 74 years, $6,464 for those aged 75 to 84, and $100,742 for those 85 years of age or older.
   c. Hepatitis B immunization. Three studies have used CEA in hepatitis B prevention strategies (60–62). Given varying methods and results, the findings from the CEAs have also varied. Using quality of life weights, Graham et al. (63) summarized these studies (Table 103.1).

REPORTING COST-BENEFIT AND COST-EFFECTIVENESS STUDIES AND RESULTS

The contribution of a cost-benefit analysis or a CEA through clinical and policy decision-making is linked to the clarity, organization, and ability of the report to facilitate a comparison of the relative value of the intervention. The information must be readily understandable by all users of the report and may be presented in the format of either a journal or technical report (9). The different types of cost reports are summarized in the following:

1. Journal report. The journal report is one well known to academicians and to those involved in hospital epidemiology and infection control. The outline usually includes an introduction, addresses methods (which includes the framework of the analysis outcomes, values, costs, and sensitivity analysis) and results, and concludes with a discussion. The intervention used in the CEA must be detailed enough for application of the intervention by others, and a reasonable determination must be made of the incremental cost-effectiveness ratio obtained. The perspective of the analyses is a key feature of the report as it will define the costs and effects relevant to the analyses.
2. Technical report. The technical report may well complement the journal report. The technical report contains additional information with a detailed description of the analyses.

MAKING THE BUSINESS CASE FOR HEALTHCARE EPIDEMIOLOGY

The use of cost-benefit analyses and CEA can help healthcare epidemiologists and ICPs understand the economic impact of nosocomial infections and the benefits of decreasing the risk of infections. To maintain or obtain additional programmatic resources to reduce infection rates it is often necessary to present a business model to the healthcare administration. This plan may require regular meetings with the senior executives and the development of reports of infection rates that focus on the financial impact converted to dollars, excess length of stay, and mortality (64,65). Demonstrating the attributable costs and excess lengths of stay resulting from hospital-acquired infections, using either reports from the literature or one's own data, is likely to make a greater impact on the administration than reports outlining only the infection rates.

In most institutions the resources spent on infection control is usually a fraction of what is lost to nosocomial infections. Of historic note, Haley calculated that prevention of just 6% of nosocomial infections would offset the cost of an inexpensive $60,000 infection control program for a 250-bed hospital (6, 10–12). Prevention of 30% to 50% of nosocomial infections would save, at minimum, $70,000 to $340,000 in 1995 dollars at a 250-bed hospital.(6,10–12,30) Helping administrators understand the financial impact and scope of the institution's nosocomial infections is essential. Ample data exist in the literature demonstrating the cost benefit of infection control departments that have been successful at lowering infection rates. These data must be used at infection control committee meetings, in reports to the administration, in departmental budget planning, and in making the business case for ongoing and future programmatic resources.

REFERENCES

1. Pittett D, Taraara D, Wenzel RP. Nosocomial bloodstream infection in critically ill patients. Excess length of stay, extra costs, and attributable mortality. *JAMA* 1994;271:1598–1601.
2. Wakefield DS. Understanding the costs of nosocomial infections. In: Wenzel RP, ed. *Prevention and control of nosocomial infections,* 2nd ed. Baltimore, MD: Williams & Wilkins, 1993:21–41.
3. Shadel B, Mundy L, Puzniak L, et al. Comparison of active versus passive surveillance for vancomycin-resistant enterococci: rates, costs, and implications. Fortieth annual meeting of the Infectious Diseases Society of America, Chicago, IL, October 24–27, 2002, abstract no. 404.
4. Wenzel RP, Rohrer JE. The iron triangle of health care reform. *Clin Perform Qual Health Care* 1994;2:7–9.
5. Wenzel RP. Instituting health care reform and preserving quality: role of the hospital epidemiologist. *Clin Infect Dis* 1993;17:831–834.
6. Haley RW, White JW, Culver D, et al. The financial incentive for hospitals to prevent nosocomial infections under the prospective payment system. *JAMA* 1987;257:1611–1614.
7. Massanari RM, Wilkerson K, Streed SA, et al. Reliability of reporting of nosocomial infections in the discharge abstracts and implications for receipt of revenues under prospective reimbursement. *Am J Public Health* 1987;77:561–564.
8. Wakefield DS, Pfaller MA, Hammons GT, et al. Use of the appropriateness evaluation protocol for estimating the incremental costs associated with nosocomial infections. *Med Care* 1987;25:481–488.
9. Gold MR, Siegel JE, Russell LB, et al. *Cost effectiveness in health and medicine.* New York: Oxford University Press, 1996.
10. Haley RW, Culver DH, White JW, et al. The efficacy of infection surveillance and control programs in preventing nosocomial infections in U.S. hospitals. *Am J Epidemiol* 1985;121:182–205.
11. Haley RW, Schaberg DR, Crossley KB, et al. Extra changes and prolongation of stay attributable to nosocomial infections: a prospective interhospital comparison. *Am J Med* 1981:70:51.
12. Haley RW, Schaberg DR, von Allmen SD, et al. Estimating the extra changes and prolongation of hospitalization due to nosocomial infections: a comparison of methods. *J Infect Dis* 1980;141:248–257.
13. McGowan JE. Cost and benefit a critical issue for hospital infection control. *Am J Infect Control* 1982;10:100.
14. Scheckler WE. Hospital costs of nosocomial infections: a prospective three-month study in a community hospital. *Infect Control* 1980;1: 150.
15. Townsend TR, Wenzel RP. Nosocomial blood stream infections in a newborn intensive care unit: a case-matched control study of morbidity, morality, and risk. *Am J Epidemiol* 1981;114:73.
16. Gertman PM, Restuccia JD. The appropriateness evaluation protocol: a technique for assessing unnecessary days of hospital care. *Med Care* 1981;19:855.
17. Freeman J, Rosner BA, McGowan JE. Adverse effects of nosocomial infection. *J Infect Dis* 1979;140:732–740.
18. McGowan JE Jr. Cost and benefit in control of nosocomial infection: methods for analysis. *Rev Infect Dis* 1981;3:790–797.
19. Boden LI. Cost-benefit analysis caveat emptor. *Am J Public Health* 1979;69:1210–1211.
20. Gross PA, Neu HC, Aswapokee P, et al. Deaths from nosocomial infections: experience in a university hospital and a community hospital. *Am J Med* 1980;68:219–223.
21. Graham JD, Corso PS, Morris JM, et al. Evaluating the cost-effectiveness of clinical and public health measures. *Annu Rev Public Health* 1998;19:125–152.
22. Eddy DM. Screening for breast cancer. *Ann Intern Med* 1989;111: 389–399.
23. Eddy DM. Screening for colorectal cancer. *Ann Intern Med* 1990;113: 373–384.
24. Eddy DM. Screening for cervical cancer. *Ann Intern Med* 1990;113: 214–226.
25. Hlatky MA, Rogers WJ, Johnstone I, et al. Medical care costs and quality of life after randomization to coronary angioplasty or coronary bypass surgery. *N Engl J Med* 1997;336:92–99.
26. Kuntz KM, Tsevat J, Goldman L, et al. Cost-effectiveness of routine coronary angiography after acute myocardial infarction. *Circulation* 1996;94:957–965.
27. Weinstein MC, Stason WB. Foundations of cost-effectiveness analysis for health and medical practices. *N Engl J Med* 1977;296:716–721.
28. Fryback DG, Dasbach EJ, Klein R, et al. The Beaver Dam health outcomes study: initial catalog of health-state quality factors. *Med Decis Making* 1993;13:89–102.
29. MacKenzie EJ, Damiano AM, Miller TR, et al. The development of the functional capacity index. *J Trauma* 1996;41:799–807.
30. Wenzel RP. The economics of nosocomial infections. *J Hosp Infect* 1995;31:79–87.
31. Nicolle LE, Bentley D, Garibaldi R, et al. SHEA Long-Term-Care Committee. Antimicrobial use in long-term-care facilities. *Infect Control Hosp Epidemiol* 1996;17:119–128.
32. Levit K, Lazenby H, Cowan C, et al. National health expenditures, 1990. *Health Care Financing Rev* 1991;13:29–54.
33. Vladeck BC. From the Health Care Financing Administration: Medicare home health initiative. *JAMA* 1994;271:1566.
34. Prescott PA, Soeken KL, Griggs M. Identification and referral of hospitalized patients in need of home care. *Res Nurs Health* 1995;18:85–95.
35. Hospital Infection Control Practices Advisory Committee. Recommendations for preventing the spread of vancomycin resistance. *Infect Control Hosp Epidemiol* 1995;16:105–113.
36. Berg DE, Hershow RC, Ramirez CA, et al. Control of nosocomial infections in an intensive care unit in Guatemala City. *Clin Infect Dis* 1995;21:588–593.
37. Coello R, Glenister H, Fereres J, et al. The cost of infection in surgical patients: a case-control study. *J Hosp Infect* 1993;25:239–250.
38. Hacek DM, Suriano T, Noskin GA, et al. Medical and economic benefit of a comprehensive infection control program that includes routine determination of microbial clonality. *Am J Clin Pathol* 1999; 111:647–654.
39. Price J, Ekleberry A, Grover A, et al. Evaluation of clinical practice guidelines on outcome of infection in patients in the surgical intensive care unit. *Crit Care Med* 1999;27:2118–2124.
40. Haley RW, Culver DH, White JW, et al. The nationwide nosocomial infection rate. A new need for vital statistics. *Am J Epidemiol* 1985; 121:159–167.
41. Fagon JY, Novara A, Stephan F, et al. Mortality attributable to nosoco-

mial infections in the ICU. *Infect Control Hosp Epidemiol* 1994;15: 428–434.
42. Fagon JY, Chastre J, Vuagnat A, et al. Nosocomial pneumonia and mortality among patients in intensive care units. *JAMA* 1996;275: 866–869.
43. Haley RW, Culver DH, Morgan WM, et al. Identifying patients at high risk of surgical wound infection: a simple multivariate index of patient susceptibility and wound contamination. *Am J Epidemiol* 1985; 121:206–215.
44. Culver DH, Horan TC, Gaynes RP, et al. Surgical wound infection rates by wound class, operative procedure, and patient risk index. *Am J Med* 1991;91:152S–157S.
45. Haley RW, White JW, Culver DH, et al. The financial incentive for hospitals to prevent nosocomial infections under the prospective payment system: an empirical determination from a nationally representative sample. *JAMA* 1987;257:1611–1614.
46. Franchi M, Salvatore S, Zanaboni F, et al. Infectious morbidity in gynecologic oncologic surgery. A clinical and economic evaluation. *Clin Exp Obstet Gynecol* 1993;20:23–26.
47. Persson U, Persson M, Malchau H. The economics of preventing revisions in total hip replacement. *Acta Orthopaed Scand* 1999;70: 163–169.
48. VandenBergh MF, Kluytmans JA, van Hout BA, et al. Cost-effectiveness of perioperative mupirocin nasal ointment in cardiothoracic surgery. *Infect Control Hosp Epidemiol* 1996;17:786–792.
49. Duffy LM, Cleary J, Ahern S, et al. Clean intermittent catheterization: safe, cost-effective bladder management for male residents of VA nursing homes. *J Am Geriatr Soc* 1995;43:865–670.
50. Tambyah PA, Knasinski V, Maki DG. The direct costs of nosocomial catheter-associated urinary tract infection in the era of managed care. *Infect Control Hosp Epidemiol* 2002;23:27–31.
51. Abi-Said D, Raad I, Umphrey J, et al. Infusion therapy team and dressing changes of central venous catheters. *Infect Control Hosp Epidemiol* 1999;20:101–105.
52. Stratton CW, Ratner H, Johnston PE, et al. Focused microbiologic surveillance by specific hospital unit as a sensitive means of defining antimicrobial resistance problems. *Diagn Microbiol Infect Dis* 1992;15: 11S–18S.
53. Stratton CW IV, Ratner H, Johnston PE, et al. Focused microbiologic surveillance by specific hospital unit: practical application and clinical utility. *Clin Ther* 1993;15(Suppl A):12–20.
54. Ballow CH, Schentag JJ. Trends in antibiotic utilization and bacterial resistance. Report of the National Nosocomial Resistance Surveillance Group. *Diagn Microbiol Infect Dis* 1992;15:37S–42S.
55. Shulkin DJ, Kinosian B, Glick H, et al. The economic impact of infections: an analysis of hospital costs and charges in surgical patients with cancer. *Arch Surg* 1993;128:449–452.
56. Wakefield DS, Helms CM, Massanari RM, et al. Cost of nosocomial infection: relative contributions of laboratory, antibiotic, and per diem costs in serious *Staphylococcus aureus* infections. *Am J Infect Control* 1988;1615:192.
57. Azimi NA, Welch HG. The effectiveness of cost-effectiveness analysis in containing costs. *J Gen Intern Med* 1998;13:664–669.
58. Lieu TA, Cochi SL, Black SB, et al. Cost-effectiveness of a routine varicella vaccination program for US children. *JAMA* 1994;271: 375–381.
59. Sisk JE, Moskowitz AJ, Whang W, et al. Cost effectiveness of vaccination against pneumococcal bacteremia among elderly people. *JAMA* 1997;278:1333–1339.
60. Margolis HS, Coleman PJ, Brown RE, et al. Prevention of hepatitis B virus transmission by immunization. *JAMA* 1995;274:1201–1208.
61. Bloom BS, Hillman AL, Fendrisk AM, et al. A reappraisal of hepatitis B virus vaccination strategies using cost-effectiveness analysis. *Ann Intern Med* 1993;118:298–306.
62. Krahn M, Detsky AS. Should Canada and the United States universally vaccinate infants against hepatitis B? A cost-effectiveness analysis. *Med Decis Making* 1993;13:4–20.
63. Graham JD, Corso PS, Morris JM, et al. Evaluating the cost-effectiveness of clinical and public health measures. *Annu Rev Public Health* 1998;19:125–152.
64. Murphy DM, From expert data collectors to interventionists: changing the focus for infection control professionals. *Am J Infect Control* 2002; 30:120–132.
65. Fraser VJ, Olsen, MA, The business of healthcare epidemiology: creating a vision for service excellence. *Am J Infect Control* 2002;30:77–85.

104

LEGAL ISSUES IN HOSPITAL EPIDEMIOLOGY AND INFECTION CONTROL

MARY ANNE BOBINSKI

Public awareness of the importance of epidemiology and hospital infection control increased in 2003 because of concerns about bioterrorism and emerging diseases such as severe acute respiratory syndrome (SARS) (1,2). Infection control is a major issue even leaving aside these new threats because millions of people acquire nosocomial infections each year in hospitals and some of these infections will be caused by drug-resistant infectious agents (3,4). Public health authorities, hospitals, physicians, and others use a number of strategies to reduce or eliminate the threat of infection. Efforts to reduce the risk of infection are medically appropriate; however, they also have serious legal implications. A hospital's infection control practices often are as focused on limiting legal liability as they are attentive to the need to preserve life and health.[1]

In many cases, of course, the two goals of preventing injury and limiting liability overlap. Thus, standard epidemiologic and infection control policies both protect health and serve to reduce or eliminate legal liability. The legal landscape is complicated. Legal obligations can be created at different levels of government (federal, state, and local) and promulgated in different ways (statutes, regulations, and court decisions). Some legal rules explicitly address infection control policies, other rules (e.g., those governing medical confidentiality and discrimination against persons with disabilities) have an indirect but important impact on infection control regimens. Persons who work with hospital epidemiology or infection control policies, therefore, must have an understanding of both the legal and medical implications of their work.

The hospital setting creates risks for three different groups of persons: hospital patients, hospital workers, and persons who come into contact with either patients or workers. Hospital patients are most clearly at risk: surgical incisions can become infected, for example, or patients may suffer from nosocomial infections transmitted by other patients or healthcare workers (5). Hospital workers, too, face risks in the healthcare environment. Workers may come into contact with patients suffering from a wide range of communicable diseases, of which SARS, tuberculosis (TB), viral hepatitis, and infection with the human immunodeficiency virus (HIV) are currently among the most common examples (2,5). The risk of infection is also present for others, such as family members or other hospital visitors (6).

The legal system responds to the risk of infection or injury in two major ways. First, state licensure standards, federal provider eligibility standards, and federal worker safety regulations each impose specific duties on hospitals and hospital employees to reduce the risk of infection. Second, the legal system allows persons injured by hospital-related infections to sue for damages. Courts throughout the country have been willing to hold hospitals liable for lapses in infection control procedures. These liability decisions, often called common law rules, indirectly define standards or duties for hospitals. A court decision that holds a hospital liable for its failure to provide a piece of equipment, for example, implicitly suggests that other hospitals wishing to avoid liability should acquire the same equipment.

Statutory, regulatory, and common law duties are often interrelated: A jury might find, for example, that a hospital was negligent in its administration of an infection control plan, because the hospital failed to meet standards established in a state licensure statute. The legal rules can also appear to be in conflict, such as when a hospital has to implement its duty to prevent transmission of illness while meeting its legal obligations to protect the confidentiality of patients and the employment rights of its workers. Understanding the sources, scope, and limits of these legal rules is an important task.

THE HOSPITAL'S DUTY TO PROTECT PATIENTS AND VISITORS

Hospitals must comply with several types of legal rules designed to protect patients. These rules can be found in federal or state statutes and regulations, in the standards of private accrediting organizations, and in the judgments of juries holding hospitals liable in tort cases. This complex regulatory structure can create an intricate and sometimes contradictory web of duties.

[1] This chapter provides general information about some of the legal issues raised by epidemiology and infection control policies. A licensed attorney should always be consulted for specific legal advice.

Hospital Regulation

There are several different types of hospital regulation. All hospitals in the United States are subject to state licensure requirements (7). Hospitals seeking reimbursement from the Medicare and Medicaid programs must also meet standards established under federal and state law (7,8). Important standards also are established by public health authorities, such as the Centers for Disease Control and Prevention (CDC) and the CDC's Healthcare Infection Control Practices Advisory Committee (HICPAC) (5,9) and by private accrediting groups, such as the Joint Commission on the Accreditation of Healthcare Organizations (JCAHO) (10).

Hospital licensure statutes are designed to protect patients. These statutes generally require that hospitals reduce the risks of infection to patients, staff, or others by maintaining appropriate equipment, employing persons with specialized training, and implementing mechanisms to reduce the risk of infection. The Florida statute provides, for example, that hospital regulators must adopt "reasonable and fair minimum standards for ensuring that" hospitals implement "[i]nfection control, housekeeping, sanitary conditions, and medical record procedures that will adequately protect patient care and safety" (11).

The guidelines of public health entities such as the CDC and HICPAC are important even though they may not be incorporated into a specific statute or regulation, because they might be used, explicitly or implicitly, by licensing authorities or others (5). The JCAHO's hospital accreditation requirements are incorporated into many state licensure statutes (12) and the federal Medicare and Medicaid regulations (13). The end result is that hospitals are subject to specific performance-based standards designed to ensure that they monitor and reduce the risk of infection. The CDC's National Nosocomial Infections Surveillance (NNIS) system also creates the opportunity for benchmarking the results of hospital infections control policies (14).

These general infection control standards are supplemented by more specific requirements for some diseases. The special rules governing HIV and hepatitis B virus (HBV) are particularly important. Several states have enacted statutes designed to protect hospital patients from HIV or HBV infection. Under federal law, states generally must implement the CDC's recommendations to reduce the risk of HIV or HBV transmission from healthcare workers to patients (15). The CDC's 1991 recommendations require healthcare workers who perform "exposure-prone procedures" to know their HIV and HBV status and to refrain from engaging in those procedures without the consent of an expert review panel (16). Depending on state law, hospitals may have a role in implementing these recommendations by defining which procedures are exposure prone or through establishing expert review panels that can advise HIV- or HBV-infected practitioners (16,17). It has been difficult for hospitals to implement these regulations in the absence of consensus about either the degree of actual risk posed by HIV-infected healthcare workers or the identification of exposure-prone procedures (15, 18).

A hospital's compliance with government regulations, public health guidelines, and private accreditation requirements can be very important in three respects. First, hospitals that fail to meet these requirements risk suspension of licensure, the imposition of civil fines, and the attendant bad publicity. Second, hospitals without effective infection control policies might lose eligibility for Medicare reimbursement, an important source of revenue. Third, a hospital's failure to comply with these public or private regulatory schemes increases the risk of tort liability. Injured patients will be able to claim that a hospital's violation of a particular statutory or regulatory requirement is evidence that the hospital was negligent in providing for the welfare of its patients.

Hospital Tort Liability

Hospitals and healthcare professionals are increasingly concerned about tort liability. The charitable or governmental immunity that long protected hospitals from lawsuits has crumbled over the past 30 years (19,20). The tort system requires a defendant to compensate a plaintiff when the plaintiff can show that the defendant's negligence caused the plaintiff's injury (21). *Negligence* is a legal term meaning that a defendant failed to exercise the degree of care owed to the plaintiff (21). Generally, individuals or institutions have the duty to exercise reasonable care (21). In the healthcare context, hospitals are often required to observe the standard of care that would be exercised by other hospitals under similar circumstances (21). Statutes, regulations, or accreditation requirements can be used to define a hospital's required standard of care (22).

There are several different types of hospital liability (23). Hospitals are generally held liable for the negligent acts of hospital employees under the doctrine of respondeat superior (21). Hospitals also are directly liable for institutional negligence, such as for failing to have equipment necessary to prevent nosocomial infections or for failing to establish policies or procedures designed to reduce the risk of infection. Matters are complicated somewhat by the fact that hospital patients are often treated by private physicians who are not hospital employees. A hospital generally will not be held liable for the negligence of a private physician so long as it is clear to patients that the physician is not a hospital employee (21). However, the hospital can be held liable if its employees knew or should have known of the risk of infection and failed to take appropriate action, even if the patient is also under the care of a private physician.[2]

There are four elements to a patient's tort claim against a healthcare professional or hospital. The plaintiff must show that the defendant owed her or him a duty to provide a particular standard of care, that the defendant failed to meet the required standard of care (negligence), that the breach of the standard of care caused the plaintiff's injury, and that the plaintiff's injury is of a type that deserves compensation (21). The plaintiff must prove these four elements by a preponderance of the evidence.

The first element has two parts: The hospital must have a duty to the plaintiff to provide a particular standard of care. In general, a hospital has a duty to protect persons who are forseea-

---

[2] Individual healthcare professionals can be held personally liable for their negligent acts' however, the focus of this chapter is on institutional liability for errors in hospital epidemiology and infection control.

bly at risk for harm from the hospital's conduct. This is a relatively easy element for plaintiffs to prove. Patients are under the care and control of the hospital, and it is foreseeable that the hospital's failure to take care in the provision of its services could cause its patients harm. A hospital's duty to protect its patients from infection also arises from the statutes, regulations, and standards discussed previously. Hospitals clearly have a duty to protect patients from the risk of infection (22–24). Hospitals have an additional duty to protect nonpatients who are the foreseeable victims of hospital negligence. A hospital may be held liable, for example, for injuries sustained by the family members or visitors of infected patients (23,25,26). Most courts hold that physicians owe a duty to the fetus of a pregnant patient although there is sometimes disagreement about the basis of the duty, that is, whether fetuses of pregnant patients should be treated as patients themselves or as foreseeably affected third parties (27).

The first element also requires plaintiffs to establish the hospital's required standard of care. For hospitals, the standard of care is measured by what other hospitals would do under like or similar circumstances. Sometimes the standard of care can be determined by examining the relevant statutes or regulations. In Ford v. Saint Francis Hospital, Inc. (28), for example, a patient who contracted staphylococcal infection of his aortic valve while hospitalized for heart surgery alleged that the defendant hospital was negligent per se, because it was violating federal regulations governing infection control. The hospital was able to defend the action by showing that it had passed a state agency's surprise inspection shortly before the surgery took place.

Plaintiffs and defendants might also rely on the guidelines issued by public health authorities, such as the CDC and the HICPAC, to establish the standard of care. Both sides may also present testimony about the customary practices of other hospitals as a method of establishing the required standard of care (22). The testimony of medical experts generally is used to establish the standard of care against which the hospital's conduct will be measured (23,29). Newly recognized threats, such as SARS or the threat of bioterrorism, may complicate the situation because healthcare institutions and physicians must rapidly identify and implement a newly emerging standard of care.

The second element of the plaintiff's cause of action requires proof that the defendant breached the standard of care. This is often a difficult task for the plaintiff who may not be able to present evidence showing that a particular hospital employee failed to use the sterile technique required by the standard of care. Courts sometimes use the legal doctrine of *res ipsa loquitur* ("the thing speaks for itself") to assist plaintiffs who cannot identify the specific act of negligence committed by the defendant (21). Under *res ipsa loquitur,* the jury might be permitted to presume the existence of a breach of the standard of care under some circumstances, such as where the patient's infection is rare and difficult to acquire in the absence of negligence (21). Courts have rejected the application of *res ipsa loquitur* and have required plaintiffs to prove a breach of the standard of care in cases alleging injury from some common types of infections. When patients have sued for damages based on hospital-acquired staphylococcal infection, for example, many courts have held that the infection in and of itself does not prove negligent conduct, because staphylococcal infections can occur in the absence of negligence (24,30–32).

The first two elements of a negligence claim, therefore, require the plaintiff to prove that the defendant hospital breached a duty it owed to the plaintiff to provide a particular standard of care. There have been a number of cases analyzing a hospital's duty to protect its patients or visitors from infection; several examples can be used to illustrate how the first two legal elements apply in the typical hospital setting.

The first example involves the scope of a hospital's duty to exercise care in selecting and assigning staff. In Taaje v. St. Olaf Hospital (33) the court held a hospital liable for an infant's death from TB based on a nursing supervisor's failure to "exercise due care to see that her nurses were free from communicable disease." Despite this decision, hospitals do not have an absolute continuing duty to screen all employees for all communicable diseases. The hospital's duty to screen—the standard of care governing screening—is established by medical knowledge and community practice at the time the patient received care. In one 1962 case, for example, the court refused to find a hospital liable for the transmission of *Staphylococcus aureus,* in part, because the standard of care did not require employee screening during the relevant time period (30).

The debate about hospital duties to screen and select employees currently is focused on the risks presented by HIV- or HBV-infected healthcare workers. As noted previously, hospitals are required to follow the CDC's 1991 HIV- and HBV-infected healthcare worker guidelines (15,16). These guidelines impose the duty on healthcare workers to know their own HIV and HBV status rather than requiring hospitals to screen healthcare workers (16). Could a hospital avoid liability altogether by implementing even stricter restrictions on the continued practice of HIV- or HBV-infected healthcare workers? The answer is no. Healthcare workers infected with contagious diseases are considered persons with disabilities who are protected by federal and state laws prohibiting discrimination based on disability. Hospitals may only discriminate against an infected healthcare worker when the worker presents a significant risk to the health or safety of others, such as that identified in the CDC guidelines (34). Workers who present minute or insignificant risks are protected from discrimination (15,35).

The second example of litigation about the standard of care involves hospital decisions regarding the acquisition and maintenance of equipment and facilities. In Bush v. Board of Managers of Binghamton City Hospital (36), the plaintiff claimed that his wife had died from diphtheria acquired in the course of her hospital stay. The court held that the hospital defendant could not be held liable for the woman's death, in part because the evidence indicated that its facilities were "suitable, adequate, and safe for the purposes in the manner used; that the means of sterilization and disinfecting employed were safe and adequate; and that the rooms were surgically clean" (36).

The third type of standard of care litigation involves disputes over the adequacy of hospital policies designed to identify and respond to the presence of infection. In Helman v. Sacred Heart Hospital (37), the plaintiff claimed that he had acquired a staphylococcal infection from his hospital roommate. The plaintiff presented evidence on the required standard of care, including the existence of "hospital . . . rules . . . requiring isolation of all patients known to be infected with staphylococci and requiring all medical personnel to report open sores, boils and pimples, which emitted purulent drainage, among both patients and hospital personnel" (37). The plaintiff also presented evidence that hospital employees had breached this standard of care by failing to "observe the sterile techniques prescribed by the hospital in cases where infection is suspected; they [also] did not wash their hands or leave the room between administering to the patients, even after the plaintiff's roommate experienced a boil with purulent drainage" (37). The plaintiff, thus, presented evidence defining the required standard of care and demonstrated that the defendant had violated this standard of conduct.

In other cases, however, defendants have avoided liability by showing that hospital personnel followed standard practice in caring for a patient (38). In Roark v. St. Paul Fire & Marine Ins. Co. (24), the plaintiff claimed that he had acquired a staphylococcal infection because of the negligence of the Glenwood Hospital. The defendant was able to avoid liability because

> Evidence introduced at trial show[ed] plaintiff was given a shower with antiseptic soap, and that the surgical site was scrubbed with antiseptics prior to surgery. The standard procedures employed by the hospital to establish the sterility of the supplies, instruments, and environment were also detailed. The evidence show[ed] that the procedures employed me[t] or exceed[ed] national standards (24).

Similar results have been achieved in transfusion-related HIV transmission cases; most jurisdictions have shielded hospitals from liability so long as the hospital blood banking organization followed the standard of care in effect at the time the transfusion took place (39,40).

The degree of care required may vary with the type of patient. A hospital has a heightened duty to protect patients who it knows are particularly vulnerable to infection. In Kapuschinsky v. United States (41), for example, the hospital was held to a greater duty to exercise care, because premature infants were particularly susceptible to infection. Hospitals generally have a heightened duty to protect immunocompromised patients.

The discussion of tort liability thus far has focused on the first two elements of the plaintiff's claim: establishing that the hospital has breached a required standard of care. The third element of a plaintiff's case is causation. The plaintiff must show that the defendant's negligence was the actual and legal cause of the plaintiff's injury (21). The causation requirement is another source of protection for hospital defendants and another source of problems for plaintiffs. Common infections, such as those resulting from staphylococci, present particular difficulties of proof for plaintiffs, because there are multiple possible sources of infection (42). Medical tests designed to determine the source of infection are extremely important. In the early 1990s, researchers relied on a genetic analysis of HIV in determining that dentist David Acer was the source of HIV infection for five of his patients (43). Other techniques, such as contact tracing, historically have been used to identify possible sources of other nosocomial infections (44).

Causation can also be difficult to prove because of the lack of evidence linking the hospital's conduct to the plaintiff's injury (45). In Contreras v. St. Luke's Hospital (46), for example, Solomon Contreras brought suit against St. Luke's Hospital and his surgeon after he sustained a surgical site infection caused by enterococci. The court held that the evidence was insufficient to impose liability, because "there is no evidence that th[e] delay [in removing a bedpan] or understaffing had any connection with the infection. Similarly, there is nothing to indicate that the failure of the nurses to trim the plaintiff's ingrown toenail had anything to do with the infection" (46). Mere negligence and injury are not sufficient; the plaintiff must be able to show that the defendant's wrongful acts actually caused the injury.

The fourth and final element of the plaintiff's tort claim is the requirement of a legally recognized injury. Often the plaintiff will seek compensation for the extra expenses associated with a lengthened hospital stay or for the additional pain and suffering accompanying the negligently inflicted infection. Occasionally, the patient dies from the infection, and the patient's estate and beneficiaries will bring survival and wrongful death claims. In Jistarri v. Nappi (47), for example, the decedent's estate sued the defendant doctors and hospital, claiming that a series of negligent acts during the decedent's treatment for a broken wrist had allowed staphylococci to enter the decedent's bloodstream, after which it weakened her heart and eventually caused her death.

Courts currently are struggling with whether to permit plaintiffs to recover damages for their fear of acquiring a disease when transmission does not actually occur. The cases largely arise in the context of HIV: Patients who might have been exposed to HIV in the healthcare environment argue that they should be compensated for experiencing fear about the risk of HIV transmission. Courts are divided on whether the fear of disease transmission is a legally compensable injury.

A small number of courts have adopted a liberal standard under which plaintiffs are permitted to recover for their fear of transmission so long as it is "reasonable." In Faya v. Almaraz (48), for example, the plaintiffs learned from news reports that their oncologic surgeon had HIV infection. They became afraid that the surgeon might have infected them with HIV during surgery. Both plaintiffs underwent HIV-antibody testing; both tested negative. They then sought compensation for their emotional distress from the physician's estate and from the hospital in which the physician had practiced. The Maryland Court of Appeals upheld the plaintiffs' complaint, noting that "we cannot say that [the plaintiffs'] alleged fear of acquired AIDS was initially unreasonable as a matter of law, even though the averments of the complaints did not identify any actual channel of transmission of the AIDS virus" (48). The court did restrict the plaintiffs to receiving compensation "for the period constituting their reasonable window of anxiety—the period between which they learned of Almaraz's illness and received their HIV-negative results" (48).

The New Jersey Supreme Court added a refinement to this approach. In Williamson v. Waldman (49) the court held that plaintiffs could recover for fear of HIV transmission even without proof of actual exposure to HIV so long as current medically accurate information about HIV would lead a reasonable person to experience substantial emotional distress about the risk of HIV transmission in a similar situation.

These cases represent the minority view. Most courts have placed serious restrictions on acquired immunodeficiency syndrome (AIDS) phobia claims. There are three major types of requirements: plaintiffs must show "actual exposure" to HIV-infected body fluids (50,51), they must show that the alleged exposure followed a medically recognized channel of transmission (52), and/or they must show a high probability that HIV transmission could have occurred (53).

The Minnesota Supreme Court's decision in K.A.C. v. Benson (50) illustrates the "actual exposure" principle. In this case, a plaintiff argued that she had suffered severe emotional injuries after learning that Dr. Benson had performed gynecologic procedures on her while he was infected with HIV. The plaintiff repeatedly tested negative for HIV antibodies. The court rejected the plaintiff's claims for damages associated with her fear of acquiring HIV, in part because she could not prove that actual exposure to HIV had occurred during the medical procedures (50). Similarly, the Tennessee Supreme Court rejected a claim brought by a patient in an alcohol and drug treatment center who was not informed that his roommate had HIV infection. The plaintiff argued that he had used the room's toilet while suffering from an open sore and that he had shared his roommate's disposable razor. The court held that this did not constitute evidence of an actual exposure (52).

Courts may also require the plaintiff to show a medically accepted "channel" for transmission of the virus. The Supreme Court of New Mexico recently applied this restriction in a suit brought by a woman whose hands with unhealed cuts were exposed to medical samples containing blood (52). In this case, the court permitted the plaintiff's claims to go forward, because she alleged a medically appropriate channel of potential transmission.

Finally, some courts require plaintiffs seeking compensation for the fear of a disease to prove that transmission of the disease is highly probable. In Kerins v. Hartley (53), a patient of an HIV-infected surgeon sued for damages based on her fear that she had acquired HIV during surgery. The court rejected the claim, holding that the plaintiff was required to show that it was "more likely than not" that she would become HIV positive as a result of the surgery. This standard is clearly very difficult for plaintiffs to meet in HIV-exposure cases, because the risk of transmission is usually very small.

Most jurisdictions thus have severely restricted AIDS phobia claims. Hospitals and healthcare professionals should recognize, however, that the law remains in flux and that plaintiffs claiming AIDS phobia may be able to recover significant damage awards in some jurisdictions (55).

As noted previously, a hospital's tort liability for patient or visitor injuries rests on the plaintiff's ability to prove that a hospital had a duty to observe a particular standard of care, that the hospital breached that standard, and that the breach caused the plaintiff's injuries. The hospital might have some defenses to the plaintiff's claims. For example, the hospital's liability might be reduced if the patient's own negligent conduct contributed to the injury (21). A patient may have failed to follow postoperative instructions, for example. However, it often will be difficult for hospitals to prove that a patient's own negligence contributed to her or his injury.

Healthcare workers and hospital administrators concerned with liability issues should understand these general tort rules. The best method for reducing the risk of liability is to reduce the risk of injury to patients and visitors. Hospitals should review their policies to ensure they meet national standards of hospital epidemiology and infection control as reflected in statutes, regulations, public health standards, national accreditation standards, and the practices of other hospitals. The special risks of infection for immunosuppressed persons should be considered. The development of appropriate policies is not sufficient, however. Hospitals must ensure that the policies are followed in practice and that appropriate records are maintained. A hospital's ability to prove that it met the standard of care and to present an appropriate defense ultimately will depend on whether appropriate documentation can be produced at trial.

THE DUTY TO PROTECT HEALTHCARE WORKERS

Hospitals also have a duty to protect their workers from harm. This duty is created under federal and state law. Breach of the duty can lead to licensure suspension, civil penalties, and civil liability. The regulations designed to protect healthcare workers can be divided into roughly two types: those imposed to prevent injury and those designed to provide compensation to healthcare workers who are injured in the course of their employment.

Regulations Designed to Protect Healthcare Workers

The federal government regulates the safety of workplaces under the Occupational Safety and Health Act, which is enforced by the Occupational Safety and Health Administration (OSHA) (see Chapter 79). All private hospitals are subject to OSHA regulation, and all federal hospitals are subject to equivalent standards (56). State and local government hospitals are exempt from OSHA regulations, although many states have laws or regulations imposing safety and health standards similar to those imposed by OSHA (57,58).

Under OSHA, an employer must provide a workplace that is "free from recognized hazards that are causing or are likely to cause death or serious physical harm to his employees" (59). In addition, employers must comply with all OSHA standards and regulations (60). Therefore, hospitals must comply with specific standards issued to protect healthcare workers. Employees are also required to comply with OSHA regulations, but the statute does not impose penalties or other sanctions on noncompliant employees, only on noncompliant employers (61).

OSHA has issued an extremely important regulation designed to reduce the risk of transmission of blood-borne pathogens in healthcare settings (62). Hospitals must comply with the blood-borne pathogen standard along with other standards governing the use of personal protective equipment (63), the use of biohazard warning signs (64), the proper implementation of sanitation and waste disposal (65), and housekeeping (66). OSHA recently withdrew a proposed rule designed to limit occupational exposure to TB (67) The blood-borne pathogen standard explicitly requires that hospitals implement a variety of programs designed to reduce the risk of infection for employees. This standard can be divided into three major parts.

First, the regulation requires hospitals to analyze all employment positions to determine which employees have "reasonably anticipated" exposures to blood or other potentially infectious materials and to design an exposure control plan that specifies how employee exposures are to be eliminated or minimized (68). Employees must be provided with adequate training to implement and update the exposure control plan (69).

Second, the blood-borne pathogen standard directly requires the implementation of specified mechanisms to reduce the risk of infection for workers. Hospitals must implement universal precautions (70). They must provide free and ready access to hand washing facilities and personal protective equipment such as gowns, masks, and gloves (71). The standard specifies certain work practices that are forbidden, such as the recapping of used needles or the improper disposal of potentially infectious materials (72). Employers must provide free and voluntary HBV vaccination to certain employees (see Chapter 78). All employees are to be offered voluntary and confidential postexposure incident evaluation and follow-up care (70,71). After an exposure incident, the blood of the potential source of infection may be tested only if the source consents or if consent is not required under state law (71).

Third, hospitals are required to observe certain monitoring and recordkeeping requirements (71,72). Employers must keep records for each employee with an exposure incident for the duration of employment plus 30 years. The records are to be confidential and released to others only with the employee's consent (72). The OSHA rules are consistent with the CDC's recommendations governing the management of occupational exposures to HBV, hepatitis C virus (HCV), and HIV (73).

OSHA can impose hefty penalties for violations (74). Nonserious and serious violations can draw up to $7,000 in civil fines per incident; willful violations have a minimum penalty of $5,000 and can reach $70,000. A willful disregard of an OSHA standard that results in a death can be prosecuted criminally with convictions resulting in imprisonment or fines. Hospitals seeking to limit OSHA liability should establish programs to comply with all OSHA requirements and, as importantly, should monitor employee compliance.

Injured Healthcare Workers and the Tort and Workers Compensation Systems

Injured healthcare workers can bring claims under either workers' compensation or tort law. Most persons injured in the course of their employment are forced to seek compensation under the workers' compensation scheme established in each state or, for some types of employment, under the compensation system established under federal law (75). The workers' compensation laws generally provide relatively quick access to preset levels of reimbursement for medical expenses and lost wages. Persons who are not covered by the workers' compensation scheme can pursue ordinary tort claims. The tort system generally provides higher levels of compensation to injured persons, but it is more difficult for injured workers to successfully pursue their claims because of the larger number of defenses available to defendants (76).

Generally, workers' compensation laws create a "no-fault" system in which injured workers do not have to prove their employers were negligent to receive compensation and in which an employee's own negligence is not likely to bar recovery (76). The workers' compensation rules also cover occupational diseases (77). Employees usually have the most difficulty proving that the disease is "occupational." Coverage under the workers' compensation system is contingent on proving that the disease was acquired during the course of employment because of the particular risks created by that employment.

In many jurisdictions, it is not enough for an employee to show that she or he was exposed to an illness on the job; she or he must show that the employment creates some special risk of acquiring this illness. In Paider v. Park East Movers (78), for example, a truck driver sought workers' compensation benefits after acquiring TB from a co-worker. The driver argued that he was exposed to TB, because his employment required that he be confined in the cab of the truck with his co-worker. The New York Court of Appeals rejected this contention, holding that the claimant's disease resulted not from the ordinary and generally recognized hazards incident to a particular employment but rather from the general risks common to every individual regardless of the employment in which he is engaged. The claimant's illness, therefore, was not an occupational disease (78). Fortunately for injured healthcare workers, certain types of illness, such as TB or hepatitis, are often covered under the workers' compensation laws as ordinary and generally recognized hazards of employment in hospitals (78,79).

However, even where a particular illness is recognized as an occupational hazard, healthcare workers often must present proof that they actually acquired their illness on the job (80). There is some disagreement about the nature of proof required. Sometimes courts have upheld workers' compensation awards based on evidence that the disease was an occupational hazard and that it was unlikely to be acquired in the employee's nonwork environment (77,81). Other courts seem to require additional evidence of workplace exposure, such as evidence that the healthcare worker came into contact with a particular patient suffering from the disease or condition (80,82).

The tort system provides compensation to injured healthcare workers who are not covered by state or federal workers' compensation schemes. Nonemployee physicians, for example, might be able to bring their claims under tort law rules (83). These healthcare workers must prove the four basic elements of a tort claim discussed previously (21). The worker must prove that the hospital had a duty to observe a particular standard of care, that the hospital breached its duty, that the breach caused harm, and that the harm was of a type recognized as deserving compensation (21). Hospitals can defend these claims by arguing that one or more of these four elements are absent; they can also reduce their liability by arguing that the injury was caused by the healthcare worker's own negligence.

It is clear that hospitals have a duty to protect their employees from foreseeable injuries, such as occupationally acquired infectious diseases (21). The scope of this duty can be defined in the same way as the scope of the hospital's duty to its patients. The applicable standard of care can be derived from licensure codes, occupational safety and health regulations, accreditation standards, and the general practices of other hospitals (21,22).

The employee must prove that the defendant hospital breached the standard of care. In John Doe v. Kaiser (84), for example, a surgeon sued the hospital in which he practiced, claiming that it "did not enforce Universal Precautions or provide its medical staff with materials or training on those precautions." In Prego v. City of New York (85), an unpaid extern working at Kings County Hospital brought suit against the hospital, contending that it had breached its duty by providing "inadequate disposal facilities for contaminated needles."

The employee must prove that the defendant's breach of the standard of care actually caused the employee's injury. This may present problems for healthcare workers who cannot identify specific sources of infection. Thus, the surgeon in the John Doe v. Kaiser case contended that the hospital's conduct caused his HIV infection. The hospital argued in response that there was no proof connecting the surgeon's HIV infection to his work at the hospital; it noted that "[d]uring the seven months that the surgeon worked at Kaiser before testing HIV positive, he did not report being exposed to body fluids or encountering lapses in Kaiser's Universal Precautions policies" (84). In contrast, Veronica Prego had documented evidence of two different exposures to blood from HIV-infected patients (85). Healthcare workers should be attentive to the need to document potential exposures.

Healthcare workers must also meet the legal injury requirement. A healthcare worker who acquires TB, hepatitis, or HIV infection easily meets this requirement. This leaves claims by workers based on the fear of transmission alone. Court rulings here follow the general trends noted above. Some jurisdictions have adopted a liberal approach that permits disease phobia claims based on reasonable fears. Most jurisdictions have imposed some additional requirements, such as proof of actual exposure (48–55).

Hospital defendants in tort suits brought by healthcare workers who are not covered by the workers' compensation system may reduce their liability by arguing that the employee was contributorily negligent (21). The hospital must show that the employee's negligent conduct contributed to her or his injury. This claim is likely to be asserted whenever the healthcare worker has failed to observe a workplace policy. Healthcare workers who acquire hepatitis or HIV infection after failing to use universal precautions or attempting to recap a needle would be particularly vulnerable to this type of hospital defense. However, courts might excuse an employee's deviation from required practices, particularly where the employee is injured while responding to an emergency situation (86).

Hospitals seeking to reduce liability to healthcare workers, either under the workers' compensation or tort systems, should implement hospital epidemiology and infection control programs that meet all federal, state, and community standards. This should reduce the number of claims made under the workers' compensation system, because it will reduce the total number of injuries. Appropriate implementation will additionally limit tort liability, because the hospital will be able to demonstrate compliance with the required standard of care. Hospitals should devote resources to updating policies, as necessary, and to documenting the implementation of all policies.

CONFLICTS BETWEEN THE DUTY TO MAINTAIN CONFIDENTIALITY AND THE DUTY TO PREVENT INJURY

This discussion of the legal rules governing hospital epidemiology and infection control has revealed a complex regulatory framework that places many demands on healthcare institutions. These legal obligations can come into apparent conflict. The most difficult problems are raised by the hospital's ability, or even its legal duty, to prevent injury by warning third parties of the risk of infection. Conflicts between confidentiality and risk reduction can arise in the relationship between the hospital and its patients or in the relationship between the hospital and its employees.

Historically, the duty to preserve the confidentiality of medical information was derived from constitutional law (for public entities) (87), common law (88), or statute (89). These traditional confidentiality rules were applied to hospitals and to individual healthcare providers such as physicians. Many states also enacted specific statutes protecting the confidentiality of certain types of information, such as HIV status (90). Although still important, these traditional approaches have been eclipsed by the federal government's new HIPAA privacy rule (91). The HIPAA privacy rule restricts "covered entities" (including hospitals) from using or disclosing "protected health information" except as permitted by the regulation (92). The federal rules create a "floor" for protection—weaker state confidentiality protections will be preempted, but stronger state confidentiality rules can still be enforced.

Despite its wide and deep legal underpinnings, the duty to maintain confidentiality is not absolute. What happens when this right to confidentiality is pitted against the hospital's duty to protect others from the risk of infection? There are two different paradigmatic examples of this conflict: In the first the hospital is concerned with a patient's infectious condition; in the second the hospital must respond to the medical condition of an employee.

In the first case, the hospital may wish to disclose the patient's contagious condition to employees or other third parties whom it knows might be put at risk of infection. Both federal and state rules permit the disclosure of otherwise confidential medical information to third parties where the goal is to prevent the transmission of disease. Under the HIPAA privacy rule, for example, a covered entity may disclose individual healthcare information "to carry out treatment . . . or payment operations" without securing patient consent (93). Texas law provides an example of a common state law approach to the protection of healthcare providers. The statute permits physicians to disclose otherwise confidential medical information to "another physician or other personnel acting under the direction of the physician who participate in the diagnosis, evaluation, or treatment of the patient" (94). A hospital is also authorized to provide information to third parties. Under HIPAA, "[a] covered entity may disclose protected health information for the public health . . . to . . . a person who may have been exposed to a communicable disease or may otherwise be at risk of contracting or spreading a disease or condition, if the covered entity . . . is authorized by law to notify such person . . .." (95). Many states have similar rules derived from statutes or court decisions (87–89).

There is a distinction between permitting and requiring disclosures. The fact that a hospital or healthcare provider is permitted to disclose healthcare information to protect third parties does not mean that it will be held liable for failing to make the disclosure. Courts have expressed concern about whether healthcare providers should owe a duty of care for nonpatients (96). Even if there is a duty, it is not clear that the standard of care would require providers to breach confidentiality by disclosing information to a third party. The healthcare provider's duty might be discharged by counseling the patient about how to avoid transmitting the condition to others (97).

Despite these caveats, healthcare workers infected by patients occasionally bring suit against hospitals for failing to disclose a patient's contagious condition (98). Healthcare facilities tempted to permit disclosures of patient status to healthcare workers should monitor the process to restrict unwarranted disclosures of information (99) and to ensure that healthcare workers do not unlawfully discriminate against a patient based on that patient's disabling illnesses (100,101).

Similar arguments apply to claims brought by nonpatients and nonemployees against healthcare providers for an allegedly negligent failure to disclose confidential information about a patient's contagious condition. In Lemon v. Stewart (102), for example, an HIV-infected patient's extended family sued a hospital for failing to disclose the patient's HIV status. The court rejected the claim, noting that there was no duty to disclose, despite the fact that the plaintiffs alleged that they had been exposed to the patient's urine, feces, saliva, blood, and serum. Although there is no general rule resolving the conflict between the patient's right to confidentiality and the hospital's duty to protect others, the most straightforward solution is to secure the patient's consent to any proposed disclosure.

The second paradigmatic situation involves conflicts between the hospital's duty to protect patients and its obligations to protect the confidentiality of its employees and to refrain from discriminating against employees who have disabling illnesses. HIPAA excludes records held by the hospital in its role as an employer from the scope of "protected health information" (92). Employees nonetheless have a right to confidentiality and a right to nondiscriminatory treatment that is protected by a variety of laws, including the OSHA blood-borne pathogen rule (62) and the Americans with Disabilities Act (103).

Despite these protections, two courts have held that the need to protect patients can outweigh the healthcare worker's rights. In one case, the court upheld a trial court order authorizing the release of certain information about an HIV-positive surgeon to his colleagues and patients (104). The court found that the hospital had demonstrated a compelling need for the disclosure because of the need to warn patients of the risk of HIV exposure (104). Similarly, in Estate of Behringer v. The Medical Center at Princeton (99), the court upheld a hospital policy that required an HIV-infected surgeon to disclose his status to his patients before performing surgery. These cases may represent judicial and medical overreaction to the risks of HIV transmission by healthcare workers (18), but they nonetheless indicate a trend toward diminished confidentiality protections for healthcare workers (see Chapter 79).

LEGAL ASPECTS OF EMERGING DISEASES AND THE RISK OF BIOTERRORISM

The recent emergence of new health threats, such as SARS and West Nile virus have created additional stresses for epidemiology and infection control. These diseases have spread across national borders and created diagnostic and treatment challenges (2). At the same time, the public and private healthcare systems are focusing on the need to prepare for possible bioterrorism events, such as the release of smallpox or some other highly contagious and destructive agent (1). These events have created three different sorts of legal issues.

First, it may be difficult for healthcare providers and patients to determine *ex ante* the standard of care for identifying and treating these newly dispersed diseases. The standard of care is developing quite rapidly and may or may not be captured well by periodic updates in on-line journals, traditional medical journals, and the reports and guidelines issued by advisory groups and public health authorities. As one example, providers did not initially realize that the West Nile virus could be transmitted by blood transfusion. Was the initial failure to screen donors for symptoms of West Nile virus negligent? The answer will depend on the testimony of medical experts before a judge and jury in some future litigation (105).

The second set of issues involves a reexamination of the relationship between public health law and public health policy. SARS and fears about bioterrorism have combined to make private and public health entities more conscious of the need to understand when and how individual liberties can be constrained to protect the public health. Would a renewed SARS epidemic or the threat of smallpox justify the imposition of mandatory medical examinations, vaccinations, treatment, or isolation and quarantine? Would private healthcare entities be required to seek a court order in these cases or would public health authorities intervene? Can public health authorities require healthcare providers to collect and to report on a wide range of health data to facilitate efforts to identify a public health threat? How will public and private entities interact in a public health emergency? Many public and private organizations are working on responses to these important questions (1,2,106,107). A detailed review of the state of the law is beyond the scope of this chapter. In general terms, public health authorities are likely to be given whatever power is needed to address a serious health crisis, including the power to impose serious restrictions on individual liberty.

The third area of legal concern relates to the need to build an infrastructure of public and private healthcare facilities, which will be prepared to provide services in public health emergencies. The difficulties can be demonstrated with the small but significant example of recent efforts to use smallpox vaccinations to create a nationwide team of healthcare workers who would be able to provide immediate support in the event of an outbreak (108). Despite a massive public relations campaign and concerted effort at the federal, state, and local levels, very few healthcare workers had undergone vaccination as of October 2003 (109). Legal concerns about compensation for vaccine-related injuries appeared to be at least one factor in the slow implementation of the project, although criticism of the risk-to-benefit calculations underlying the program undoubtedly played a larger role (110).

CONCLUSIONS

No one can be sure what threats to public health will emerge in the coming years. The legal rules governing hospital epidemiology and infection control policies are complicated and sometimes conflicting. Hospitals have a duty to protect patients and third parties from the risk of infection. A hospital's failure to meet this obligation can result in sanctions under licensing statutes and in civil liability. Hospitals also have a duty to protect their employees from the risks of infection. Breaches of this duty can also result in administrative sanctions and in civil liability. Hospitals seeking to meet their obligation to prevent transmission of disease also must be conscious of the need to safeguard confidentiality and to prevent discrimination against persons with disabling illnesses. Hospitals must also focus attention on documenting compliance with all relevant legal standards. Finally, the emergence of new public health threats has created new areas of legal concern for professionals engaged in epidemiology and infection control.

REFERENCES

1. Centers for Disease Control and Prevention. Emergency preparedness and response. Available at *http://www.bt.cdc.gov/* (accessed October 23, 2003).
2. Centers for Disease Control and Prevention. Draft, public health guidance for community-level preparedness and response to severe acute respiratory syndrome (SARS) (October 23, 2003). Available at *http://www.cdc.gov/ncidod/sars/sarsprepplan.htm* (accessed October 25, 2003).
3. Centers for Disease Control and Prevention. Monitoring hospital-acquired infections to promote patient safety—United States, 1990–1999. *MMWR Mortal Morb Wkly Rep* 2000;49:149–153.
4. Fidler DP. Legal issues associated with antimicrobial drug resistance. *Emerg Infect Dis* [serial online]. April–June 1998;4. Available at *http://www.cdc.gov/ncidod/eid/vol4no2/fidler.htm* (accessed October 23, 2003).
5. Bolyard EA, Tablan OC, Williams WW et al. Guidelines for infection control in health care personnel, 1998. *Am J Infect Control* 1998;26: 289–354.
6. Shepard v. Redford Community Hospital, 151 Mich. App. 242, 390 N.W.2d 239 (1986).
7. Grad FP. *The public health law manual,* 2nd ed., Washington DC: American Public Health Association, 1990:111–112.
8. 42 C.F.R. §482.1 (2003) (conditions for hospital Medicare and Medicaid participation).
9. Centers for Disease Control and Prevention. Healthcare Infection Control Practices Advisory Committee, Centers for Disease Control and the Hospital Infection Control Practices Advisory Committee. Available at *http://www.cdc.gov/ncidod/hip/HICPAC/Hicpac.htm* (accessed October 26, 2003).
10. The Joint Commission on Accreditation of Healthcare Organizations. *2004 Comprehensive accreditation manual for hospitals: the official handbook.* Chicago: The Joint Commission on Accreditation of Healthcare Organizations, 2004.
11. Fla. Stat. Ann. §395.1055(1)(b) (West 2003).
12. Alaska Stat. §18.20.080(2002) (Joint Commission accreditation can replace state's annual inspection in some circumstances).
13. 42 C.F.R. §488.5 (2003) (institutions with JCAHO or AOA accreditation deemed to meet Medicare criteria with several exceptions).
14. Centers for Disease Control and Prevention. About NNIS. Available at *http://www.gov/ncidod/hip/NNIS/@nnis.htm* (accessed October 28, 2003).
15. Bobinski MA. Risk and rationality: the Centers for Disease Control and the regulation of HIV-infected health care workers. *St Louis Univ Law J* 1992;36:213–307.
16. Centers for Disease Control and Prevention. Recommendations for preventing transmission of human immunodeficiency virus and hepatitis B virus to patients during exposure-prone invasive procedures. *MMWR Mortal Morb Wkly Rep* 1991;40:1–9.
17. Tex. Health & Safety Code §85.201-.206 (West 2003).
18. Gostin, LO. A proposed national policy on health care workers living with HIV/AIDS and other blood-borne pathogens. *JAMA* 2000;284: 1965–1970.
19. Bing v. Thunig, 2 N.Y.2d 656, 163 N.Y.S.2d 3, 143 N.E.2d 3 (1957).
20. Showalter JS. *The law of healthcare administration,* 4th ed. Health Administration Press, 2003.
21. Hall MA, Bobinski MA, Orentlicher D. *Health care law and ethics,* 6th ed. Aspen Publishers, 2003.
22. Darling v. Charleston Community Memorial Hospital, 33 Ill.2d 326, 211 N.E.2d 253, cert. denied 383 U.S. 946 (1966).
23. Kraut J. Annotation: hospital's liability for exposing patient to extraneous infection or contagion. 96 A.L.R.2d 1205-12 (1964 and supplements).
24. Roark v. St. Paul Fire & Marine Ins. Co., 415 So.2d 295, 297, 299 (La. App. 1982).
25. Bateman T. Annotation: liability of doctor or other health practitioner to third party contracting contagious disease from doctor's patient, 3 A.L.R. 5th 370–393 (1993 and supplements).
26. Bolieu v. Sisters of Providence in Washington, 953 P.2d 1233 (Alaska 1998) (facility owed duty to spouses of nursing assistants to prevent spread of staph infections).
27. Nold v. Binyon, 31 P.3d 274 (Kansas 2001) (physician caring for pregnant woman who intends to carry her pregnancy to term also has duty to fetus; physician had duty to communicate information about woman's contagious disease which could be transmitted during delivery).
28. Ford v. Saint Francis Hospital, Inc., 490 S.E.2d 415 (Ga. Ct. App. 1997).
29. Ardoin v. Mills, 780 So2d 1265 (La. App. 3 Cir. 2001) (example of Daubert challenge to medical expert testimony).
30. Thompson v. Methodist Hospital, 367 S.W.2d 134, 135 (Tenn. 1962).
31. Mahan v. Bethesda Hospital, Inc., 84 Ohio App.3d 520, 617 N.E.2d 714 (1992).
32. Neary v. Charleston Area Medical Center, Inc., 460 S.E.2d 464 (W.Va. 1995).
33. Taaje v. St. Olaf Hospital, 271 N.W. 109, 115 (Minn. 1937).
34. Waddell v. Valley Forge Dental Associates, 276 F.3d 1275 (11th Cir. 2001) (HIV-infected dental hygienist poses direct threat to patients; ADA does not prohibit employer from precluding contact with patients), cert. denied 535 U.S. 1096 (2002).
35. Americans with Disabilities Act of 1990, 42 U.S.C.A. §12101 et seq. (West 2003).
36. Bush v. Board of Managers of Binghamton City Hospital, 297 N.Y.S. 991, 993, 996 (1937).
37. Helman v. Sacred Heart Hospital, 381 P.2d 605, 606, 608 (Wash. 1963).
38. Harris v. State Through Huey P. Long Memorial Hospital, 378 So.2d 383, 388–389 (La. 1979).

39. Kozup v. Georgetown University, 663 F.Supp. 1048 (D.D.C. 1987), aff'd in part, vacated in part, 851 F.2d 437 (D.C. Cir. 1988).
40. Zitter JM. Annotation: liability of hospital, physician, or other individual medical practitioner for injury or death resulting from blood transfusion. 20 A.L.R.4th 136 (1983 and supplements).
41. Kapuschinsky v. United States, 248 F. Supp. 732, 739 (D.S.C. 1966).
42. Robinson v. Intermountain Health Care, 740 P.2d 262 (Utah App. 1987).
43. Centers for Disease Control and Prevention. Update: transmission of HIV infection during invasive dental procedures. *MMWR Mortal Morb Wkly Rep* 1991;40:377–381.
44. Spearing NM, Horvarth RL, McCormack JG. Pertussis: adults as a source in health care settings. *MJA* 2002;177:568–569.
45. Harvey v. Washington, 95 S.W.2d 93 (Missouri 2003) (example of "but for" causation in infection case).
46. Contreras v. St. Luke's Hospital, 78 Cal. App. 3d 919, 929, 144 Cal. Rptr. 647, 654 (1st Dist. Ct. App. Div. 1 1978).
47. Jistarri v. Nappi, 549 A.2d 210, 212 (Pa. Super. 1988).
48. Faya v. Almaaraz, 620 A.2d 327 (Md. 1993).
49. Williamson v. Waldman, 696 A.2d 14 (N.J. 1997).
50. K.A.C. v. Benson, 527 N.W.2d 553 (Minn. 1995) (The Minnesota Supreme Court also noted that the defendant physician had followed the guidelines for continued practice established by the Minnesota Board of Medical Examiners).
51. Majca v. Beekil, 701 N.E.2d 1084 (Ill. 1998) (Illinois requires actual exposure but does not require plaintiff to demonstrate likelihood of developing HIV if actual exposure has occurred).
52. Bain v. Wells, 936 S.W.2d 618 (Tenn. 1997).
53. Madrid v. Lincoln County Medical Center, 923 P.2d 1154 (N.M. 1996).
54. Kerins v. Hartley, 33 Cal. Rptr.2d 172, 179 (Cal. App. 2 Dist. 1994) (" [I]n the absence of physical injury or illness, damages for fear of AIDS may be recovered only if the plaintiff is exposed to HIV . . . and the plaintiff's fear stems from a knowledge, corroborated by reliable medical or scientific opinion, that it is more likely than not he or she will become HIV seropositive and develop AIDS due to the exposure").
55. Fisher, ES. AIDSphobia: A National Survey of Emotional Distress Claims for the Fear of Contracting AIDS. *Torts and Insurance LJ* 1997;33:169–226.
56. 29 U.S.C.A. §668 (West 2003).
57. 29 U.S.C.A. §652(5) (West 2003).
58. 29 U.S.C.A. §667 (West 2003) (OSHA and approval of state plans).
59. 29 U.S.C.A. §654(a)(1) (West 2003).
60. 29 U.S.C.A. §654(a)(2) (West 2003).
61. 29 U.S.C.A. §654(b) (West 2003).
62. 29 C.F.R. §1910.1030 (2003).
63. 29 C.F.R. §1910.132 (2003).
64. 29 C.F.R. §1910.145(e)(2003).
65. 29 C.F.R. §1910.141 (2003).
66. 29 C.F.R. §1910.22(a) (2003).
67. OSHA, 1827. Occupational Exposure to Tuberculosis, 68 Fed. Reg. 30588-89 (May 27, 2003) (withdrawing proposed TB exposure rule).
68. 29 C.F.R. §1910.1030(b),(c) (2003).
69. 29 C.F.R. §1910.1030(g) (2003).
70. 29 C.F.R. §1910.1030(d) (2003).
71. 29 C.F.R. §1910.1030(f) (2003).
72. 29 C.F.R. §1910.1030(h) (2003).
73. Centers for Disease Control and Prevention. Updated U.S. Public Health Service Guidelines for the management of occupational exposures to HBV, HCV, and HIV and recommendations for postexposure prophylaxis. *MMWR Morb Mortal Wkly Rep* 2001;50(RR11): 1–42.
74. Occupational Safety and Health Act, Civil and Criminal Penalties, 15 U.S.C.A. §666 (West 2003).
75. Federal Employers Liability Act (FELA), 45 U.S.C.A. §§ 51–60 (2003).
76. Haas TF. On reintegrating workers' compensation and employers liability. Ga L Rev 1987;21:843–899.
77. Flor v. Holguin, 9 P.3d 382 (Hawaii 2000) (dental hygienist permitted to pursue workers' compensation claim against former employers for Hepatitis C transmission despite inability to prove precise date of infection).
78. Paider v. Park East Movers, 19 N.Y.2d 373, 280 N.Y.S.2d 140, 144 (1967).
79. Booker v. Duke Medical Center, 297 N.C. 458, 256 S.E.2d 189–205 (1979) (hepatitis covered as occupational illness under North Carolina statute).
80. Drouillard v. City of Vinton Police Dep't, 815 So.2d 398 (La. App. 3 Cir. 2002) (former police officer failed to establish reasonable probability of occupational transmission of hepatitis C).
81. Browning-Ferris Industries of Pennsylvania v. Workmens Compensation Appeal Board (Jones), 617 A.2d 846 (Pa. Commw. 1992) (refuse collector's hepatitis infection entitled to statutory presumption that infection acquired during course of health care-related employment).
82. Sperling v. Industrial Commission, 129 Ill.2d 416, 544 N.E.2d 290–294 (Ill. 1989) (court refuses to reverse an arbitrator's decision holding that an operating room nurse had failed to show that her hepatitis infection was contracted in her employment).
83. Doe v. Yale University, 748 A.2d 834 (Conn. 2000) (medical resident attempts to bring negligence action for HIV acquired during residency).
84. Surgeon sues hospital for failure to protect him from HIV infection. *AIDS Policy Law* 1992;7:6–7.
85. Prego v. City of New York, 147 A.D.2d 165, 541 N.Y.S.2d 995 (2d Dept. 1989).
86. Doe v. State, 588 N.Y.S.2d 698 (Ct. Cl. 1992), modified on other grounds and remanded, 595 N.Y.S. 2d 592 (1993).
87. Whalen v. Roe, 429 U.S. 589 (1977).
88. Horne v. Patton, 291 Ala. 701, 287 So.2d 824 (1973).
89. Texas Occupations Code §159.002-.003 (West 2003).
90. Bobinski MA. Autonomy and privacy: protecting patients from their physicians. *Univ Pitt Law Rev* 1994;55:330–339.
91. Office of Civil Rights, U.S. Dep't of Health and Human Services, Standards for Privacy of Individually Identifiable Health Information, 45 C.F.R. §160.500-.534 (West 2003).
92. 45 C.F.R. §§160.103, 164.502 (West 2003).
93. 45 C.F.R. §164.506 (West 2003).
94. Texas Occupations Code §159.004 (West 2003).
95. 45 C.F.R. §164.512(b)(1)(iv) (West 2003).
96. McNulty v. City of New York, 792 N.E.2d 162 (N.Y. 2003) (defendants owed no duty to friend of patient treated for meningitis to advise her to seek treatment).
97. Troxel v. A.I. Dupont Institute, 675 A.2d 314 (Pa. Super. 1996) (physicians' duty to third parties was to inform patient about contagious nature of disease and how to avoid its spread).
98. Juneau v. Humana, Inc., 657 So.2d 457 (La. App. 3 Cir. 1995) (nurse sues hospital and fellow employee for failing to disclose HIV status of patient; nurse allegedly acquired HIV infection from patient).
99. Estate of Behringer v. The Medical Center at Princeton, 592 A.2d 1251 (N.J. Super. Ct. 1991).
100. Americans with Disabilities Act, 42 U.S.C.A §§12181–12182 (West 2003) (rules prohibiting discrimination against persons with disabilities in places of public accommodation).
101. Bragdon v. Abbott, 524 U.S. 624 (1998).
102. Lemon v. Stewart, 682 A.2d 1177 (Md. App. 1996).
103. 42 U.S.C.A. §12112(d) (West 2003).
104. In re Milton S. Hershey Medical Center, 634 A.2d 159 (Pa. 1993).
105. CDC report: CDC investigates possible West Nile virus transmission through organ transplant. Available at *http://www.injuryboard.com/view.cfm/Article=1652* (accessed October 29, 2003) (Web site sponsored by law firms).
106. The Center for Law and the Public's Health is a joint project of Georgetown and Johns Hopkins Universities and a CDC Collaborating Center. The Center's Web site includes materials about the Model State Emergency Health Powers Act and other resources related to public health law and bioterrorism. Center for Law and the Public's Health, available at *http://www.publichealthlaw.net/* (accessed October 29, 2003).
107. National Advisory Committee on SARS and Public Health. Learning

from SARS: renewal of public health in Canada, October 2003. Available at *http://www.hc-sc.gc.ca/english/protection/warnings/sars/learning.html* (accessed October 29, 2003).

108. Centers for Disease Control and Prevention. Protecting Americans: smallpox vaccination program. Dec. 13, 2002. Available at *http://www.bt.cdc.gov/agent/smallpox/vaccination/vaccination-program-statement.asp* (accessed October 29, 2003).
109. Institute of Medicine. Smallpox vaccination program implementation. Available at *http://www.iom.edu/project.asp?id=4781* (accessed October 29, 2003) (includes periodic reports and recommendations on the program).
110. Richards EP, Rathbun KC. Smallpox vaccine injury and law guide, 19 May 2003. Available at *http://biotech.law.lsu.edu/blaw/bt/smallpox/svlaw.htm* (accessed October 29, 2003).

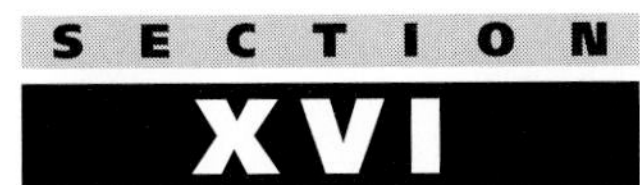

HOSPITAL EPIDEMIOLOGY AND INFECTION CONTROL IN SPECIAL SETTINGS FOR HEALTHCARE DELIVERY

105

HOSPITAL EPIDEMIOLOGY AND INFECTION CONTROL IN SMALL HOSPITALS

WILLIAM E. SCHECKLER

For purposes of this chapter, attention is focused on acute care, short-term, general hospitals with 99 beds or less, the "small" hospital. Because of their size and usual rural small-town location, very little has been published about any aspect of infection control and hospital epidemiology in such settings. Recommendations for infection control have been based entirely on data from large institutions. The same is true for the recent profusion of Occupational Safety and Health Administration (OSHA) standards. More information on the reality of nosocomial infections in small hospitals would be very useful. However, since this chapter was written for the second edition, very little new, useful information about nosocomial infection data was discovered in a February 2003 literature search. Based on my own experience in the broad field of hospital epidemiology and actual work done in small hospitals, I outline recommendations for infection control and epidemiologic approaches to problems in these institutions. These recommendations may still be viewed in light of Joint Commission on the Accreditation of Healthcare Organizations (JCAHO) reviews of small hospital infection control programs (1) and of a 1998 Consensus Panel report (2).

PROFILE OF THE SMALL HOSPITAL

The 2003 edition of *Hospital Statistics* from the American Hospital Association (3) provides interesting data about the status of small hospitals in 2001 compared with the 1996 information provided in the second edition of this chapter. The 2001 data are the most recent available and are summarized in Table 105.1. Despite the continued discussions of the demise of small hospitals, change has been minimal. There are only 29 less hospitals of 99 beds or less, a decline of only 1%. Total admissions are up 12% and total births up 0.5%. Combined inpatient and outpatient surgeries are up 25%. Considering the national trends in mergers and closings of urban hospitals, the small hospital changes suggest stability and growth since 1996.

Small hospitals continue to be important economic engines in their communities. Seventy percent of these hospitals are rural in location. The total economic impact of these 2,267 small hospitals is considerable. They employ about 384,000 full-time and 171,000 part-time employees. Their total net revenue in 2001 was more than $38.6 billion. Although they may account for only about 14% of the acute care beds provided in the United States, they are important economic and medical anchors in the communities that they serve (4).

AVAILABLE LITERATURE ABOUT NOSOCOMIAL INFECTIONS AND INFECTION CONTROL IN SMALL HOSPITALS

Very little has been published about infection control issues in small hospitals. The Study on the Efficacy of Nosocomial Infection Control (5), undertaken by the Centers for Disease Control and Prevention (CDC) over 2 decades ago, excluded hospitals of less than 50 beds and had only a very small sample of hospitals of 50 to 100 beds. The other major ongoing CDC project evaluating nosocomial infections is the National Nosocomial Infection Surveillance (NNIS) system. The system has excluded hospitals of less than 100 beds on statistical grounds (6). Britt et al. (7) published data from 18 prevalence surveys of small hospitals in the intermountain West. They conducted prevalence studies and looked at laboratory and infection control practices in these small institutions in the early 1970s. Few had infection

TABLE 105.1. 2001 PROFILE OF 6- TO 99-BED GENERAL HOSPITALS UNITED STATES

Total number of hospitals	2,267
Location[a]	
Urban	677 (30)
Rural	1,590 (70)
Hospital ownership[a]	
State and local government	787 (39)
Not for profit	1,157 (48)
Investor owned	323 (13)
Total number of beds	117,851
Total admissions	3,592,780
Total inpatient days	21,187,165
Total inpatient surgeries	817,628
Total outpatient surgeries	2,354,170
Total births	359,678

[a] Values are total number with percents in parentheses.

TABLE 105.2. INCIDENCE PER 100 DISCHARGES OF NOSOCOMIAL INFECTIONS IN 15 RURAL WISCONSIN HOSPITALS[a]

Service	Number of nosocomial infections	Number of discharges	Incidence of nosocomial infections	1984 NNIS hospitals (*n* = 60) incidence of nosocomial infections per 100 discharges
Medicine	64	6,759	0.95	3.57
Surgery	116	2,878	4.03	4.48
Gynecology	19	385	4.94	2.67
Obstetrics	17	1,411	1.20	1.46
Newborn	4	1,241	0.32	1.38
Pediatrics	0	746	0	1.28
Total	220	13,420	1.64	3.24

NNIS, National Nosocomial Infection Surveillance system.
[a] Data based on comprehensive prospective surveillance for 6 consecutive months in each of the 15 hospitals between May 1, 1984 and April 30, 1985.

control programs. In some institutions, even basic services such as Gram stains for microbiologic review were not available on site. The level of infection control could best be characterized as primitive. However, because these data are now more than 20 years old, they are unlikely to be valid today. Our studies of nosocomial infection in 15 rural hospitals in southwestern Wisconsin have constituted the principal information available in this area. Despite the fact that these data are now aging and do not represent targeted surveillance, they are reviewed here, because little more recent published data from small hospitals are available (8,9).

The Wisconsin data set was collected in several stages from the members of the Rural Wisconsin Hospital Cooperative. An initial survey was made of the hospital, and basic information about its range of activities, laboratories, infection control policies and data, personnel, and other relevant areas was collected in a structured questionnaire. These data were validated on a visit by the two investigators who conducted a comprehensive chart review prevalence survey of all patients in the hospital the day of the survey. An infection control professional (ICP) was identified in each institution and trained in the use of NNIS definitions of nosocomial infections and surveillance techniques. Then each ICP completed 6 months of comprehensive hospital-wide nosocomial infection surveillance using NNIS methodology and forms. These data were analyzed by the author with NNIS computer software.

Tables 105.2 and 105.3 are reproduced from the 1986 Wisconsin report (9). Because of the small numbers available for 6 months of hospital-wide surveillance in 15 different institutions, the data were combined for purposes of analysis. Both tables also compare NNIS data from the same time period from larger hospitals. The results demonstrate that the overall incidence of nosocomial infections was 1.6% in the small hospitals compared with 3.2% in the NNIS group. The two groups were most similar for surgical and gynecology patients and for surgical site infections. There were many fewer nosocomial infections in medical patients and none at all in pediatric patients in the small hospitals—a striking difference from the NNIS data.

Other data from the Wisconsin hospitals were also of considerable interest. Contrary to an earlier Virginia study (10), which suggested that higher procedure-specific surgical site infection rates were correlated with operations being done in smaller numbers in smaller hospitals, the Wisconsin data suggested very low rates for several types of procedures. The author replicated the same Wisconsin findings a year later from the same institutions. These findings do not support the widely held belief that quality

TABLE 105.3. NUMBER AND INCIDENCE OF NOSOCOMIAL INFECTIONS BY SERVICE AND MAJOR SITE: 6 MONTHS OF PROSPECTIVE SURVEILLANCE IN 15 RURAL WISCONSIN HOSPITAL

Service	UTI	Surgical site	Pneumonia	Primary bacteremia	Gastrointestinal	Vaginitis	Upper respiratory	Bronchitis	Empyema	Vein	Other cutaneous	Total	% Total
Surgery	45	38	15	1	2	1	1	2	2	5	4	116	52.7
Gynecology	9	10										19	8.7
Medicine	29		19	2	2	1	2			5	4	64	29.1
Obstetrics	4	13										17	7.7
Newborn			1								3	4	1.8
Pediatrics												0	0
Total	87	61	35	3	4	2	3	2	2	10	11	220	100.0
% of total	39.6	27.7	16.0	1.3	1.8	.9	1.3	.9	.9	4.6	5.0	100.0	
Incidence per 100 discharges	0.65	0.46	0.26	0.02	0.03	0.01	0.02	0.01	0.01	0.07	0.08	1.64	
1984 NNIS incidence per 100 discharges	1.25	0.54	0.58[a]	0.25	0.03	0.07[b]	0.04	[a]	[a]	0.09	0.19	3.24	

[a] All lower respiratory.
[b] All gynecologic.
NNIS, National Nosocomial Infection Surveillance system; UTI, urinary tract infection.

care can only be delivered if large quantities of care are provided. Age was associated with an increased incidence of nosocomial infection, however. The incidence of nosocomial infections was 2.7% for Medicare admissions and 0.9% for patients younger than 65 years (9).

NEW INFORMATION FROM RURAL WISCONSIN HOSPITALS

To update information for the second edition, a two-page survey was sent to 18 hospital ICPs in June 1998. Nine ICPs responded. They were asked to provide basic data about their hospitals, their job duties, infection control activities, and key areas of infection control the past year. They were also asked to comment on the utility of reference services available to them, including the first edition of this chapter, which was sent with the survey.

Results of the survey are summarized in Table 105.4. As noted in 1992 and in 1996, the ICPs continue to have multiple roles. A combination of infection control and employee health duties was present in eight of nine respondents. The other respondent spent her entire time in infection control activities in the hospital, a nursing home, 2-day care units, home care, and in two community-based residential facilities. Other ICP duties included staff and postanesthesia care unit (PACU), nursing utilization review, and drug utilization and pharmacy studies; one was also director of ancillary services.

Several of the ICPs commented on the need to have some type of useful comparison data for any of the surveillance data they collect, whether hospital-wide or targeted. None of them are using nosocomial infection data for the outcome measures (ORYX Initiative) of the JCAHO. All of the ICPs focused on surgical site infections, including day care surgeries, and all had some type of postdischarge surveillance in place.

The ICPs were also asked to list "three of your infection control activities from 1997 or 1998 that you consider most important." The answers showed many parallels. Most common were policy and procedure reviews, including meeting CDC and

TABLE 105.4. RESULTS FROM 1998 SURVEY OF NINE RURAL WISCONSIN HOSPITAL INFECTION CONTROL PROFESSIONALS (ICPs)

General data	Range	Average
Number of active beds	23–100	49
Number of swing beds	0–20	10 in 5 hospitals
Average daily census	4–38	19
ICP job information		
% of full time as ICP	25–65%	46%
% of full time in employee health	0–50%	20%
Surveillance type—these categories overlap		
Hospital-wide	8 of 9	
Targeted	8 of 9	
Postdischarge surveillance		
Active	6 of 9	
Passive	8 of 9	

the OSHA standards. New employee orientation and continuing education of staff in infection control and hand washing was frequently noted. Several commented on new innovations such as postdischarge surveillance using a new clinic computer system; establishing a communication link with public health to improve communication with hospital, public health, nursing homes, and other care facilities and agencies; establishing influenza vaccination programs for employees; and implementing an antibiotic prophylaxis protocol.

All reporting ICPs were enthusiastic about their access, as members of the Association for Professionals in Infection Control and Epidemiology (APIC), to their local and state chapter programs and those supplied by the University of Wisconsin. Compared with the 1984 study period noted earlier, great strides have been made among these rural hospitals. It would not be wise to assume what is true in rural Wisconsin is true elsewhere in the country, but the framework of what works and what must be done are clear from these data.

NEW DATA FROM THE WESTERN UNITED STATES

A collaborative group consisting of the Centers for Medicare and Medicaid Services; the Medicare quality improvement organizations for Idaho, Nevada, Utah, and Washington; the CDC; and the Division of Clinical Epidemiology from the University of Utah School of Medicine funded and completed a quality improvement survey of smaller hospitals in the four-state area in July 2000. Inclusion criteria for the survey required at least two of these three criteria be met: less than 150-patient daily census, rural location, and less than 20% of the state Medicare admissions. The final survey included four sections: (a) basic demographics, (b) microbiology laboratory testing, (c) pharmacy management of antimicrobial use, and (d) the infection surveillance and control program.

Results from the survey have been presented at several recent national meetings of the Society for Healthcare Epidemiology of America, APIC, and the Infectious Diseases Society of America as abstracts (11). Seventy-six of the 100 eligible hospitals in the four states responded to the survey. The median bed size was 26 (range 4 to 206).

Several of the results are of value when thinking about the recommendations at the end of this chapter. The good news is that 97% of the hospitals had at least one ICP. Most of these ICPs conducted surveillance of nosocomial infections using NNIS and CDC definitions. They also participated in data analysis, policy development, staff education, and infection control activities very similar to the 1990s Wisconsin data for ICPs. However, there was less use of referral of microbiology laboratory specimens to a reference laboratory when resistance was thought to be present than in the Wisconsin experience. Only about half of the 76 hospitals had computer information systems that could link pharmacy use data, microbiology lab results, and infection control information together. Also unlike the Wisconsin systems, not all hospitals had easy access to the Internet. However, compared with the Britt data from the 1970s in the same geographic area, striking improvements have occurred. The new data from these four states do validate the recommendations made at the end of this chapter. It will be useful to see what this group publishes in the future from their important project (11).

COMMENTS

Other than the abstracts cited previously, I was unable to find any other data of note on nosocomial infections in small hospitals published since the Wisconsin studies in 1986 (8,9). It would be quite inappropriate to suggest that all small hospitals are the same. Even other rural, midwestern, acute care, nonprofit hospitals may be different from the Wisconsin group. The Wisconsin group is not homogeneous either. There are no available data on small federal, state, or local government hospitals or on for-profit institutions. Therefore, a huge gap exists between what is known about these institutions and what regulators have assumed about them. JCAHO rules, CDC and Healthcare Infection Control Practices Advisory Committee (HICPAC) guidelines, and OSHA requirements make no distinctions and no special acknowledgment of the issues of smaller institutions. It is regrettable that very little new data have been developed between 1993 and 2003.

It is worth considering some plausible explanations for the substantially lower rates of nosocomial infections in small hospitals, even though a substantial body of rigorously collected data are not available. In rural Wisconsin, the distances to larger referral centers are relatively small, much less so than in the Britt et al. study. The roads are in good condition. Complex procedures are done, and critically ill patients are treated in the accessible regional centers. Emergency helicopter transportation is now available to transport critically ill patients of any age to a tertiary center if required. Thus, most invasive procedures associated with substantial risk of nosocomial infections are not performed in small hospitals. Endotracheal intubations, multiple vascular access lines, and complex immune-suppressing therapy are all the province of the larger centers, although some of these procedures may be initiated in the smaller hospital before referral transport.

There also has been a revolution in access to diagnostic technology and medical information in the past 20 years. Most family physicians in our study hospitals are residency trained and board certified. They all have access to a medical interlibrary system connected by telephone and computer to the database search services now available even to physicians on their home computers. In the microbiology laboratory, standardization and automation of culture methods and biochemical and sensitivity testing are now easily implemented, even in small laboratories. More complex tests are done promptly in nearby regional centers. Computed tomography and magnetic resonance imaging can be obtained from mobile units on semitrailer trucks. The networks described in the Wisconsin study were greatly facilitated by the existence of the Rural Wisconsin Hospital Cooperative.

A number of issues that may be problems elsewhere are also dealt with easily in Wisconsin. ICPs have access to regular continuing education at 2½-day seminars at the University of Wisconsin and numerous APIC chapter meetings. Iowa also has a strong program at its University Medical Center for training ICPs. Because of a substantial number of group practice and managed care networks, physicians in Wisconsin also have access to infectious diseases and epidemiologic consultation as needed. Such networks will doubtless become more common in the future.

A thoughtful chapter on the applicability of JCAHO standards was recently published as a book chapter (1). The survey standards are applied to all acute care hospitals in a consistent fashion while evaluating infection control activities. In 1993, when the JCAHO had 47 individual infection control standards, 10% of hospitals of 1 to 99 beds had minimal or noncompliance with the 47 standards. In hospitals of 100 to 299 beds this figure dropped to 6%, and in larger hospitals it was only 2%. Similarly, partial compliance was found in 41% of the small hospitals, 36% of the medium-sized, and 32% of the large hospital groups. Clearly, in 1993, the JCAHO survey suggested that small hospitals could substantially improve their infection control programs. The Wisconsin experience suggests that is quite possible.

A major issue of some importance facing smaller hospitals is deciding what type of surveillance makes the most sense. No matter the type of surveillance, even more critical is the value and validity of rate calculations. Current science in hospital epidemiology, well documented by the NNIS studies, suggests that surveillance should be focused on specific risks in populations carefully defined. Thus, hospital-wide surveillance of all nosocomial infections, measured as an incidence of infections per 100 discharges or per 1,000 patient-days, is no longer recommended as useful. If this is true for the larger hospitals with higher rates of nosocomial infections, then on statistical grounds alone it is even more true for the smaller hospital. The same is true of crude surgical site infection rates, even if stratified in the "clean" and "clean contaminated" wound classification categories. The recent Wisconsin data suggest that vigorous postdischarge surveillance can uncover more nosocomial infections, but the rates will still be low. Of more potential value may be assessing the frequency or incidence of invasive procedures known to be associated with nosocomial infections. Therefore, surveillance of indwelling Foley catheter use, central line use, and endotracheal intubations could be tracked and evaluated for their appropriateness rather than just finding the patient who had these procedures and then developed an infection. Other types of infection control practices might also be surveyed, such as tuberculosis skin test studies and hepatitis B immunization of hospital medical staff and hospital employees. Antibiotic use might be evaluated for patients with bacteremia or pneumonia—both nosocomial and community acquired—to check for appropriateness, using medical staff-approved guidelines. All these ideas are plausible but need further evaluation in small hospitals.

RECOMMENDATIONS

Based on the available data and the preceding comments, there are some conclusions available from the Wisconsin experience that might prove useful. These are developed as a set of specific recommendations for epidemiology and infection control in small hospitals:

1. All small hospitals should have an ICP with training in infection control. Membership in the local APIC chapter is strongly advised. Ten to 20 hours per week should be dedicated to infection control duties.
2. An infection control team or committee should be constituted and consist of
   a. A medical staff physician with an interest in epidemiology and infectious diseases
   b. The ICP
   c. A representative of the microbiology laboratory
   d. A representative of hospital administration, preferably nursing administration
   e. Someone with pharmacy expertise.

   This is the minimum; this group should meet at least every other month. They can be part of a larger quality improvement (QI) effort but must maintain their own identity.
3. The infection control team should
   a. Collect and analyze appropriate nosocomial infection surveillance data for their institution with a view toward improving patient care
   b. Develop, recommend, and monitor infection control policy
   c. Identify means of educating the employees and staff of the hospital about infection control
   d. Report their activities to the medical staff and hospital administration on a regular basis, at least quarterly.
4. The infection control team should develop expertise in epidemiologic principles and serve in a facilitator capacity for other quality improvement activities in the institution.
5. Appropriate nosocomial infection surveillance should focus on the profile of the institution. Known risk groups include the Medicare population; all those receiving surgical procedures; and all receiving invasive devices, such as central venous catheters and indwelling urinary catheters. Monitoring the frequency of use of invasive procedures may be more productive than just focusing on nosocomial infections associated with those procedures. Attention to intensive care unit patients may also be appropriate.
6. Calculation of nosocomial infection rates from hospital-wide surveillance, by site, or by service should be done with great caution or not at all. Such rates should never be used as a basis for comparison with other institutions, unless the data are accurate, are adjusted for patient risk groups, and are part of a study to define the problem of nosocomial infections in smaller institutions. No credible benchmark rates for nosocomial infections currently exist for small hospitals. The Wisconsin data described in this chapter are merely an example of the meager available literature in the area.
7. Networks of small hospitals and ICP groups working together through the Rural Wisconsin Hospital Cooperative or an APIC chapter constitute important mechanisms of sharing data and concerns. In addition, the infection control team should establish links with the infection control and hospital epidemiologic expertise in their area. Conferences and periodic visits to colleagues are a good way to keep in touch with changes in the field.
8. The recommendations of the Consensus Panel on the infrastructure and essential activities of a hospital epidemiology and infection control program should be carefully reviewed and implemented (2). These recommendations were specifically developed to include hospitals of all sizes and would meet current JCAHO requirements if implemented in any hospital.

THE FUTURE

Guidelines and regulatory bodies need comprehensive data about infection control and hospital epidemiology in small hospitals. The Wisconsin studies still need to be replicated in other locations to test for general applicability. The new data from Idaho, the Utah group, is promising. The HICPAC of the CDC, the JCAHO, OSHA, and other groups should be cognizant of the realities of small hospitals and should be careful about "one size fits all" requirements. Continued access to care in small hospitals with quality programs in infection control should be part of healthcare reform. Small-town and rural institutions should be retained as important geographic links to medical care.

REFERENCES

1. Schyve PM, Patterson CH. Special considerations in small hospitals: the Joint Commission Standards. In: Abrutyn E, Goldmann DA, Scheckler WE, eds. *Saunders infection control reference service.* Philadelphia: WB Saunders, 1998:59–70.
2. Scheckler WE, Brimhall D, Buck AS, et al., of the Society for Healthcare Epidemiology of America Consensus Panel. Requirements for infrastructure and essential activities of infection control and epidemiology in hospitals: a consensus panel report. *Infect Control Hosp Epidemiol* 1998;19:114–124.
3. *Hospital statistics.* Chicago: Health Forum, AHA, 2003:10–16.
4. McDermott RE, Cornia GC, Parsons RJ. The economic impact of hospitals in rural communities. *J Rural Health Spring* 1991;7:117–133.
5. Haley RW, Culver DH, White JW, et al. The efficacy of infection surveillance and control programs in preventing nosocomial infections in US hospitals. *Am J Epidemiol* 1985;121:182–205.
6. Gaynes RP, Culver DH, Emori TG, et al. The National Nosocomial Infections Surveillance systems: plans for the 1990's and beyond. *Am J Med* 1991;91(Suppl 3B):116s–120s.
7. Britt MR, Burke JP, Nordquist AG, et al. Infection control in small hospitals prevalence surveys in 18 institutions. *JAMA* 1976;236: 1700–1703.
8. Scheckler WE, Peterson PJ. Nosocomial infection prevalence, risk and control in small community and rural hospitals. *Infect Control* 1986; 7(Suppl):144–148.
9. Scheckler WE, Peterson PJ. Nosocomial infections in 15 rural Wisconsin hospitals results and conclusions from 6 months of comprehensive surveillance. *Infect Control* 1986;7:397–402.
10. Farber BF, Kaiser DL, Wenzel RP. Relation between surgical volume and incidence of postoperative wound infection. *N Engl J Med* 1981; 305:200–204.
11. Personal Communication, Kurt Stevenson, MD, MPH, Qualis Health, Boise ID—from 2001 and 2002 meeting abstracts SHEA, APIC, and IDSA.

106

EPIDEMIOLOGY AND PREVENTION OF INFECTIONS IN RESIDENTS OF LONG-TERM CARE FACILITIES

LARRY J. STRAUSBAUGH
CAROL L. JOSEPH

Older adults in the United States have many options for residential long-term care, ranging from semi-independent apartments to foster care in single-family homes to more traditional institutional settings such as nursing homes (NHs). The latter are inpatient facilities for persons who require nursing care and related medical or psychosocial services. This chapter focuses primarily on infections that occur in this setting, because they account for the majority of long-term care facilities (LTCFs) in the United States. Moreover, most medical literature on infections in LTCFs derives from studies originating in NHs. When possible, this chapter includes observations and data from other types of LTCFs, but the description of infections in these other settings is meager. Finally, this chapter largely concentrates on the LTCF experience in the United States.

DEMOGRAPHICS

In 1999, the U.S. NHs numbered 18,000 (1). On any given day during that year, these facilities cared for approximately 1.6 million individuals, of whom 90% were elderly. During the course of that year, 2.5 million Americans were discharged from NHs. These numbers are expected to grow as the population ages. In the United States, the percentage of the population aged ≥65 years is projected to increase from 12.4% in 2000 to 19.6% in 2030 (2). Concomitantly, it is estimated that 5.3 million Americans will reside in NHs in 2030 (3).

RELATIONSHIP OF LONG-TERM CARE FACILITIES TO OTHER COMPONENTS OF THE MEDICAL SYSTEM

The relationship between hospitals and LTCFs is complex and dynamic. Since the 1980s, the Medicare Prospective Payment System has resulted in shifting of sicker and more dependent residents to NHs (4). Long-term care is often viewed as a less costly alternative to hospitalization, with the result that increasingly sicker and more dependent persons receive care in NHs. Such patients also have greater risks for infection (5). Infections have been implicated in up to 54% of acute medical problems in the NH and in 63% of deaths (6,7).

Most NH residents are now admitted from acute care hospitals, and nearly half are discharged to a hospital within the first 6 months of their NH stay (1,8). Infections are most often the cause of NH to hospital transfers, accounting for 17% to 49% of cases; conversely, continued treatment of hospital-acquired infections is a frequent reason for NH admission (9–11). There is also a significant interface between NHs and other LTCFs and the community. Approximately 30% of NH discharges (excluding deaths) are to a private or semiprivate residence, whereas 15% are to another NH or healthcare facility (12).

ETIOLOGY OF INFECTION

Spectrum of Pathogens

In many ways, LTCFs occupy an intermediate position between the hospital and the community. Not surprisingly, the etiologies and types of infections in these facilities reflect a mixture ranging from classic community-acquired infections (e.g., pneumococcal pneumonia) to those that are usually hospital acquired [e.g., catheter-associated urinary tract infections (UTIs) caused by *Pseudomonas aeruginosa*]. Crowding; socialization; medical care; and common sources of air, food, and water within a community populated by persons with assorted risk factors also influence this mixture of infections. Thus, in addition to the expected sporadic infections seen in all human populations, clusters of pneumococcal pneumonia or catheter-associated UTIs caused by multidrug-resistant strains of *Streptococcus pneumoniae* and *P. aeruginosa,* respectively, may be observed, as well as outbreaks of tuberculosis or staphylococcal food poisoning.

The spectrum of etiologies and types of infections also varies considerably from one LTCF to another. This is obvious when the experience of a skilled nursing facility is compared with that of a psychiatric hospital or when one contemplates the likely experience in small foster care homes. However, it is also true within a given category, such as NHs. The occurrence of outbreaks can magnify these differences (13).

TABLE 106.1. COMMONLY REPORTED ENDEMIC PATHOGENS IN NURSING HOMES

Bacteria
- Staphylococci: *Staphylococcus aureus, Staphylococcus epidermidis,* and other coagulase-negative species
- Streptococci: *Streptococcus pneumoniae, Streptococcus agalactiae*
- Enterococci: *Enterococcus faecalis, Enterococcus faecium*
- Gram-negative microorganisms: Enterobacteriaceae (*Escherichia coli, Klebsiella pneumoniae, Proteus mirabilis,* etc.), *Pseudomonas aeruginosa, Acinetobacter* species *Stenotrophomonas maltophila, Moraxella catarrhalis,* and *Haemophilus influenzae*
- Anaerobes: *Bacteroides fragilis, Clostridium* species including *Clostridium difficile,* and others

Yeasts
- *Candida albicans, Torulopsis glabrata*

Viruses
- Herpes simplex virus, varicella-zoster virus

Endemic Pathogens

The range of endemic pathogens reported from surveillance studies performed in NHs includes a number of common bacteria, fungi, and viruses (Table 106.1) (14–35). Pathogens recovered in Veterans Affairs (VA) facilities parallel those isolated in community NHs.

Epidemic Pathogens

The list of bacterial, viral, and parasitic agents causing outbreaks in LTCFs continues to grow (Table 106.2) (13, 36–101). Agents causing respiratory and gastrointestinal outbreaks predominate, but antimicrobial-resistant bacteria and bacteria causing skin and soft tissue infections (SSTIs) cause outbreaks with some frequency (13). Most outbreak reports arise from NHs, but some have issued from psychiatric facilities, homes for the mentally retarded, and pediatric units. Many pathogens listed also cause disease in nonoutbreak settings, especially the antimicrobial-resistant bacteria.

TABLE 106.2. ETIOLOGY OF OUTBREAKS IN NURSING HOMES AND OTHER LONG-TERM CARE FACILITIES

Bacteria
- Staphylococci: methicillin-resistant and enterotoxigenic *Staphylococcus aureus* (37–42)
- Streptococci: *Streptococcus pyogenes* (43), *Streptococcus pneumoniae* including drug-resistant strains (44,45)
- Enterococci: vancomycin-resistant enterococci (46–49,54) and high-level gentamicin-resistant enterococci (40)
- Gram-negative: *Escherichia coli* O157:H7 (50), *Salmonella* (42,51,56–59,66,82), *Shigella* (42,51,56,57,60,82,85), *Bordetella pertussis* (62), *Haemophilus influenzae* (52), *Campylobacter jejuni* (42,59,82), *Aeromonas hydrophila* (64), *Legionella* species (63,92), *Chlamydia pneumoniae* (53), *C. psittaci* (57) and antimicrobial-resistant gram-negative bacilli (40,61,65)
- Anaerobes: *Clostridium perfringens* (42,68), *Clostridium difficile* (67)
- Miscellaneous: *Mycobacterium tuberculosis* (70–72), *Bacillus cereus* (42)

Viruses
- Influenza virus A and B (55,74,76–78,95–98), parainfluenza virus (55,73,93), respiratory syncytial virus (36), adenovirus (87,94), rhinovirus (79), coronavirus (36,13), coxsackievirus (80), cytomegalovirus (81), rotavirus (55,83,90), caliciviridae (75,82,88,89), astroviruses (13) and hepatitis virus A and B (68,84,99)

Parasites
- *Giardia lamblia* (13,57), *Entamoeba histolytica* (13,57), *Cryptosporidium* (13), *Sarcoptes scabiei* var. hominis (86,101)

Antimicrobial-resistant Pathogens

NHs play an important role in the problem of antimicrobial resistance. The most common and worrisome resistant pathogens in LTCFs are methicillin-resistant *Staphylococcus aureus* (MRSA), vancomycin-resistant enterococci (VRE), and Enterobacteriaceae producing extended-spectrum beta-lactamases (ESBLs) (26,37–41,46–49,54,61,65,102–112). Less common concerns include aminoglycoside-resistant gram-negative bacilli (40,105), high level aminoglycoside-resistant enterococci (40, 111), multidrug-resistant pneumococci (44,45,104), and fluoroquinolone-resistant gram-negative bacilli (66,104,109).

The frequency of antimicrobial-resistant pathogens in LTCFs varies by location and interfaces with acute care facilities. For example, Scheckler and Peterson (17) found antimicrobial resistance to be rare in their survey of eight small rural NHs in Wisconsin. Likewise, Mylotte et al. (112) found antimicrobial-resistant pathogens uncommonly (in <20% of admissions) in residents of community NHs admitted to an inpatient geriatric service in Buffalo. In contrast, a number of large urban facilities have reported high frequencies of resistant pathogens. For example, Trick et al. (102) found at least one antimicrobial-resistant bacterial isolate in 43% of 117 LTCF residents screened in one urban facility in Illinois. Of the 50 culture-positive residents, 24% harbored MRSA, 18% ESBL-producing *Klebsiella pneumoniae,* 15% ESBL-producing *Escherichia coli,* and 3.5% VRE. Studies in similar types of facilities frequently receiving colonized or infected patients from acute care units or tertiary care medical centers have yielded comparable results (26,40,110,111).

In the LTCF, high frequencies of antibiotic use and high prevalences of infections that are not easily eradicated (e.g., bacteriuria in catheterized individuals) facilitate proliferation and persistence of resistant strains, which usually become endemic within the facility (26,40,104,113,114). Risk factors for colonization or infection with antimicrobial-resistant strains include serious underlying disease, poor functional status, cutaneous wounds such as pressure sores, presence of invasive devices, and prior antimicrobial therapy (26,37,38,40,46,61,65,102,105, 110,111). NH residents can remain colonized for months to years and reintroduce resistant microbes into hospitals when management of acute illnesses necessitates their transfer (26,40, 107,108).

TYPES OF INFECTION

The types of infection observed in LTCFs are diverse (Table 106.3). They represent a mixture of common community-acquired and hospital-acquired infections, with additional contributions from outbreaks arising from the introduction of new pathogens into relatively closed societies. In general, the most

TABLE 106.3. TYPES OF INFECTION COMMONLY ENCOUNTERED IN LONG-TERM CARE FACILITIES

- **I. Skin and soft tissue infections**
  - A. Endemic
    - 1. Infected pressure ulcers
    - 2. Cellulitis and cutaneous abscesses
    - 3. Conjunctivitis
    - 4. Herpetic infections
    - 5. Candidiasis
  - B. Endemic or epidemic
    - 1. Cellulitis
    - 2. Scabies
    - 3. Conjunctivitis
- **II. Respiratory tract infections**
  - A. Endemic
    - 1. Sinusitis
    - 2. Otitis media or externa
    - 3. Bronchitis
    - 4. Pneumonia
  - B. Endemic or epidemic
    - 1. Pharyngitis
    - 2. Common cold
    - 3. Influenza
    - 4. Tuberculosis
- **III. Urinary tract infections (endemic)**
  - A. Bacteriuria
  - B. Symptomatic urinary tract infection
    - 1. Lower (cystitis)
    - 2. Upper (pyelonephritis)
- **IV. Bacteremia (predominantly endemic)**
  - A. Primary
  - B. Secondary
- **V. Gastrointestinal tract infections (endemic or epidemic)**
  - A. Acute gastroenteritis
  - B. *Clostridium difficile* colitis
  - C. Viral hepatitis

common types of infection in NHs are UTIs; lower respiratory tract infections (LRTIs), especially pneumonia; and SSTIs, principally cellulitis and infected pressure sores (10,14–27,35). These are usually endemic infections, though clusters are not unknown. Their relative frequency varies considerably from one facility to another, but they invariably predominate.

Patient characteristics, such as underlying disease, mobility, and presence of urinary catheters and other invasive devices, influence the relative frequencies of these types of infection in any given institution. The frequency of pneumonia, for example, is influenced by outbreaks of viral respiratory diseases that predispose to bacterial invasion of the lung (30,93). Outbreaks of other infections (e.g., gastroenteritis) add diversity to the overall picture of infection within a facility and may occasionally skew an institution's rates to obscure the importance of UTIs, LRTIs, and SSTIs.

Other types of infections occur in NH residents—meningitis, brain abscess, endocarditis, osteomyelitis, septic arthritis, cholecystitis, diverticulitis, prostatitis, and vaginitis—but they are relatively uncommon. With few exceptions, none of these other infections is even mentioned in the major NH surveillance studies (10,14–27,35). They may account for a few of the undelineated "other infections" reported in some studies, but they constitute only a small percentage of the total. Because of their low frequency and the paucity of epidemiologic data, these infections are not considered further. Opportunistic infections associated with the acquired immunodeficiency syndrome (AIDS) are also not considered. In those facilities that admit patients with AIDS, the unique infections of this patient group (e.g., toxoplasmosis or pneumocystosis) may enter the case mix. However, in one surveillance study of human immunodeficiency virus (HIV)-infected patients in long-term care, the three most common infections were *Clostridium difficile*-associated diarrhea, primary bacteremias, and UTIs (115). These data may reflect the efficacy of prophylaxis for opportunistic infections.

PATHOGENESIS OF INFECTION

The pathogenesis of specific infections is discussed in previous chapters, but some special considerations arise in the LTCF setting.

Effect of Aging on Adaptive Immunity

Aging produces a number of changes in immune response (referred to as immune senescence or immune dysregulation) that result in increased vulnerability to infection (116,117). Cell-mediated immunity is primarily affected, but humoral immunity declines as well. For the most part, changes in T-lymphocyte function and decreased production of the cytokine interleukin-2 are thought to underlie the major clinical consequences of immune senescence. Recent studies, however, suggest that age-related immune defects are more widespread than previously thought. (118). Because of these changes, cell-mediated immunity and antibody production in response to new antigens are decreased in elderly persons. The result is increased vulnerability to viral, fungal, and mycobacterial diseases such as tuberculosis (119). Diminished antibody production may also result in inadequate response to immunizations with pneumococcal polysaccharide, tetanus toxoid, hepatitis B, and influenza vaccines (118). Some investigators have reported increased mortality among NH residents with impairment in cell-mediated immunity (120).

Effect of Aging on Nonadaptive Immunity

Many of the age-related changes that occur in all organ systems predispose the elderly to infection (Table 106.4).

Additional Predisposing Factors

Malnutrition

Protein calorie malnutrition is estimated to affect 52% to 85% of NH residents (121). Malnutrition is associated with impaired immune function manifested by a decrease in cell-mediated immunity. The consequences of malnutrition such as delayed wound healing, decreased level of consciousness, and decline in functional status also increase the risk of infection. Concomitant vitamin and mineral deficiency, particularly zinc, may also play a role in depressed host resistance (122).

TABLE 106.4. CHANGES IN NONADAPTIVE IMMUNITY WITH AGING

Aging Changes	Consequences
Skin	
Epidermal thinning	Increased susceptibility to trauma, pressure ulcers
Flattening of dermoepidermal junction	
Decreased elasticity	
Decreased subcutaneous tissue	
Decreased vascularity	Delayed wound healing
Respiratory	
Decline in cough reflex	Aspiration
Diminished immunoglobin A secretion	Increased susceptibility to pathogens
Loss of elastic tissue	Decreased lung expansion
Decreased mucociliary transport	Decreased clearance of secretions
Increased gram-negative colonization of oropharynx	Increased risk of gram-negative lower respiratory infection
Urinary	
Hormonal changes (female)	Perineal colonization, vaginitis
Prostate enlargement	Urinary stasis, bacterial colonization
Decreased prostatic secretions	Decreased antibacterial activity
Decreased uromucoid secretions	
Increased bacterial adherence to uroepithelial cells	Increased bacterial colonization of bladder
Decreased renal ability to excrete acid or urea, or to maintain high osmolality	
Gastrointestinal	
Decreased gastric acidity	Increased susceptibility to salmonellae and other enteric pathogens
Decreased intestinal motility	

Medical Illness

The most commonly reported diagnoses among NH residents in 1999 were circulatory system disease, such as hypertension, and cardiac disease (26%); mental disorders including Alzheimer's disease (26%); and diseases of the respiratory system (11%) (1). Diabetes mellitus affects 20% to 30% of NH residents and has been implicated in immune dysfunction and a host of target organ impairments (123). These underlying chronic illnesses predispose the NH resident to LRTIs, SSTIs, and UTIs.

Functional Impairment

Functional impairments such as immobility, incontinence, and dysphagia have been reported to increase the risk for infections (124). In 1999, 95% of NH residents needed assistance with at least one self-care activity, and 75% were dependent in three to five such activities (1). Many NH residents suffer from arthritis, strokes, or other forms of paralysis; 62% use a wheelchair; almost half are incontinent of urine (1). This combination or decreased mobility and incontinence places them at high risk for URIs, SSTIs and UTIs.

Medications

NH residents take an average of six to eight different medications (125). Frequently prescribed drugs include sedatives, neuroleptics, and narcotic analgesics, which may depress the level of consciousness and increase the risk for LRTIs. Tricyclic antidepressants, some antihypertensives, and antianginal medications can precipitate urinary retention and subsequent UTIs. Other commonly used medications in the long-term care setting include H_2 blockers, which may predispose to infection by decreasing gastric acidity; corticosteroids, which reduce immune function; and antibiotics, which encourage colonization with resistant microorganisms.

Invasive Devices

Invasive medical devices such as urinary catheters, feeding tubes, tracheostomies, and intravenous catheters further breech the already compromised host defenses of the chronically ill NH resident. Although some devices (e.g., intravenous catheters) are encountered less frequently in the LTCF than in the hospital, others, such as urinary drainage systems, are used in 5% to 10% of NH residents (126).

CLINICAL MANIFESTATIONS

Atypical Presentations

The classic presenting signs and symptoms of infection are often blunted, altered, or absent in elderly NH residents. As a result of cognitive impairment or reluctance to complain, NH residents may not draw attention to infectious problems (127, 128). Furthermore, comorbid conditions can mask the symptoms of infection or make them difficult to interpret. For example, incontinence may mask irritative symptoms of a UTI, or chronic osteomyelitis may be confused with degenerative joint disease. Alternatively, decline in functional status may be the chief herald of serious infection. Thus, UTIs may present with confusion rather than dysuria; pneumonia with a fall not a cough (129). Compared with younger patients, older persons with bacteremia are less likely to develop chills, diaphoresis, altered mental state, physical complaints, or lymphopenia (130). The signs of infection are often subtle and appreciated only by staff members who know the resident well.

Altered Inflammatory Response

Temperature elevations may be blunted or absent in as many as one third of elderly persons, despite serious bacterial infection (128–132). Potential explanations for altered fever responses in the elderly include deficits in immune response and lymphokine production, depressed cellular and hypothalamic response to endogenous pyrogens (e.g., interleukin-1 and tumor necrosis factor), and diminished ability to regulate body heat (11,127,133). A subset of elderly NH residents may have lower basal body temperatures. Hence, even a normal temperature elevation with infection results in low-grade fevers of 37.3°C to 37.8°C, which may be mistakenly dismissed (131). Castle et al. (134) found that an oral temperature of 37.8°C had a sensitivity of 70% among NH patients with clinical infections, whereas setting the threshold for significant fever at 38.3°C reduced sensitivity to only 40%. In addition, measuring oral or axillary temperatures may miss up to three fourths of fevers in elderly persons (135). Likewise, frequently used clinical signs of infection, such as leukocytosis and a "left shift," may also be absent in the elderly (129,132). Up to 40% of elderly NH residents have a white blood cell count of less than 10,000 per μL in the presence of bacteremia (136,137). Not surprisingly, guidelines from the Infectious Diseases Society of America emphasize the need for a strong index of suspicion in the clinical evaluation of elderly NH residents (138).

Fever of Unexplained Significance

In surveillance studies that include febrile episodes in their statistics, fever without localizing findings accounts for 2% to 48% of all events (10,18,139). Some unexplained febrile episodes may be due to noninfectious etiologies, but most are attributed to undiagnosed infections (10,139). For example, Orr et al. (139) attributed only 1% of fevers to noninfectious sources in their study of two Canadian NHs. They attributed all of the other febrile episodes to infections, although nearly half had no identifiable source.

DIAGNOSIS OF INFECTION

In general, the diagnosis of infection in LTCF residents conforms to the principles and criteria used for nosocomial infections. It should be noted, however, that LTCFs often lack ready access to laboratory and radiologic services, and physicians may not be present to diagnose infections as they occur. Accordingly, investigators performing surveillance studies in such facilities have often modified the Centers for Disease Control and Prevention's (CDC's) definitions for nosocomial infections to make them more applicable to the NH environment. McGeer et al. (140) offered a comprehensive set of definitions for surveillance in LTCFs that account for the unique circumstances of these institutions (Table 106.5). Although appealing and widely used, these criteria have yet to be validated in prospective studies.

TABLE 106.5. DEFINITIONS OF INFECTION FOR SURVEILLANCE IN LTCFS

I. Skin and soft tissue infections
- A. Cellulitis/soft tissue/wound infection–pus at a wound, skin, or soft tissue site or four of the following: (a) fever (>38.0°C) or worsening mental/functional status and/or at the affected site, the presence of new or increasing (b) heat, (c) redness, (d) swelling, (e) tenderness or pain, (f) serous drainage
- B. Fungal skin infection—both a maculopapular rash and either physician diagnosis or laboratory confirmation
- C. Herpes simplex and herpes zoster infection—both vesicular rash and either physician diagnosis or laboratory confirmation
- D. Scabies—both a maculopapular and/or itching rash and either physician diagnosis or laboratory confirmation
- E. Conjunctivitis—pus appearing from one or both eyes for at least 24 hr or new or increased conjunctival redness, with or without itching or pain, for at least 24 hr

II. Respiratory tract infections
- A. Common cold syndromes/pharyngitis—two of the following new signs or symptoms: runny nose or sneezing; stuffy nose (congestion); sore throat, hoarseness, or difficulty swallowing; dry cough, swollen or tender glands in the neck
- B. Influenza-like illness–fever (>38.0°C) and three of the following during influenza season: chills, new headache or eye pain, myalgias, malaise or loss of appetite, sore throat, or new or increased dry cough
- C. Bronchitis or tracheobronchitis—a negative chest radiograph (or no chest radiograph was taken) and three of the following: new or increased cough; new or increased sputum production; fever (>38.0°C); pleuritic chest pain; new or increased findings on exam (rales, rhonchi, wheezes, bronchial breathing); and new or increased shortness of breath, respiratory rate >25 per minute, worsening mental status, or worsening functional status
- D. Pneumonia—two of the signs listed under bronchitis or tracheobronchitis and a chest radiograph demonstrating pneumonia, probable pneumonia, or an infiltrate
- E. Ear infection—either a physician's diagnosis or drainage from one or both ears (ear pain or redness also required if drainage is not purulent)
- F. Sinusitis—physician diagnosis
- G. Mouth and perioral infection—physician or dentist diagnosis

III. Urinary tract infection
- A. The resident who does not have an indwelling urinary catheter must have three of the following: fever (>38.0°C) or chills; new or increased burning pain on urination, frequency, or urgency; new flank or suprapubic pain or tenderness; change in character of urine; worsening of mental or functional status (may be new or increased incontinence)
- B. The resident who has an indwelling catheter must have two of the following: fever (>38.0°C) or chills, new flank or suprapubic pain or tenderness, change in character of urine, worsening of mental or functional status

IV. Primary bloodstream infection—either two or more blood cultures positive for the same microorganism or a single positive culture with a microorganism not thought to be a contaminant and one of the following: fever (>38.0°C), new hypothermia (<34.5°C), a drop in systolic blood pressure >30 mm Hg from baseline, worsening mental or functional status

V. Gastroenteritis—one of the following: two or more loose or watery stools above what is normal within a 24-hr period, two or more episodes of vomiting in a 24-hr period, or a stool culture positive for *Salmonella, Shigella, Escherichia coli* O157:H7, or *Campylobacter* or a toxin assay positive for *Clostridium difficile* toxin and one symptom or sign of gastrointestinal infection (nausea, vomiting, abdominal pain or tenderness, or diarrhea)

VI. Unexplained febrile episode—fever (>38.0°C) on two or more occasions at least 12 hr apart in any 3-day period with no known infectious or noninfectious cause.

LTCF, long-term care facility.
Adapted from McGeer A, Campbell B, Emori T, et al. Definitions of infection for surveillance in long-term care facilities. *Am J Infect Control* 1991;19:1–7, with permission.

EPIDEMIOLOGY

General Considerations

Available Studies and Their Variation

Although outbreaks in LTCFs have been recognized for a long time, more comprehensive studies of infections in these settings have only appeared since 1980. Most of these studies have focused on NHs, and, taken together, they offer a fairly complete picture of infection in that environment. Nevertheless, the data vary considerably. Some of this variation reflects differences in the types of institutions under study: large versus small, urban versus rural, hospital-affiliated versus independent, and VA versus community. Some of the variation reflects differences in the patient populations under study, for example, differences in gender, severity of underlying disease, and prevalence of risk factors such as invasive devices. The role of outbreaks in this variation has been noted previously. Other factors influencing the observed variation include differences in surveillance definitions (e.g., counting or not counting asymptomatic bacteriuria as an infection) and differences in surveillance methodology (e.g., surveillance based largely on chart review, which is notoriously unreliable, vs. surveillance based on regular visits by a nurse practitioner).

Almost no surveillance data are available for LTCFs other than NHs, but it seems likely that they have lower rates. A survey of 103 private psychiatric hospitals supports this conception (141). The hospitals reported an average length of stay of 66 days. Twenty-eight of 103 responding hospitals reported annual facility-acquired infection rates calculated on the basis of patient discharges. The mean for reported rates was 0.05, and the median was 0.04 infections per patient discharged. These data indicate that infectious morbidity is much lower in psychiatric hospitals than in NHs.

Reports from surveillance studies can be confusing and difficult to compare, because infection rates have been expressed in a number of terms that are not readily interchanged: percentage of residents at risk found to be infected in a given period (point and period prevalences), percentage of infected patients in relation to numbers of patients admitted or discharged, infections per 100 resident-months, infections per 100 resident-years, and infections per 1,000 resident care days. In the last decade, infections per 1,000 resident (or patient) care days has become the most common reported measure of incidence. Schicker et al. (19) emphasized the utility of this calculation, which yields rates that vary less than census-based figures and accommodates data from individuals with prolonged lengths of stay. The Society for Healthcare Epidemiology of America (SHEA)/Association for Professionals in Infection Control and Epidemiology (APIC) position paper for LTCFs suggest using infections per 1,000 resident-days to calculate and express incidence data (142).

Incidence of Infection in Nursing Homes

The overall incidence of infection in various types of Canadian and U.S. facilities has ranged from 1.8 to 9.4 infections per 1,000 resident care days (Table 106.6). Considering the different types of facilities and resident populations involved and the different surveillance methodologies used, it seems remarkable that most rates fall within the tenfold range of one to ten infections per 1,000 resident care days. The 7.2 rate reported by Jackson et al. (18) is probably the most defensible single number for non-VA NHs. This rate does not include cases of asymptomatic bacteriuria; it reflects the use of definitions carefully tailored to the NH setting and intensive surveillance by a nurse practitioner, who visited all residents two to four times per month. Other studies probably underestimated the true fre-

TABLE 106.6. INCIDENCES OF INFECTIONS IN LONG-TERM CARE FACILITIES

Ref.	Date of Study (duration in months)	Types of LTCFs and location	% Men	Incidence of Infection[a]			
				Overall	UTIs	LRTIs	SSTIs
16	1983–84 (12)	Large, urban NHs in MD					
		(a) NH-A	28	3.6	1.2[b]	1.1[c]	0.2
		(b) NH-B	18	3.8	1.3[b]	1.2[c]	0.5
17	1984–85 (6)	Eight rural NHs in WI, 7 adjacent to hospital	24	3.6	1.6	0.6	0.5
18	1984–87 (36)	Large, free-standing proprietary NH in CA	25	7.1	1.3	2.6	1.2
19	1985–86 (12)	VA NH in WI—hospital-based	>95	5.4	1.9	1.6	0.6
20	1985–86 (9)	VA NH in WA	99	2.6	1.0	0.8	0.4
21	1987 (12)	VA NH in FL	96	4.6	1.9	1.0	0.9
15	1987–89 (24)	Geriatric LTCF in Ontario					
		(a) chronic care unit	30	1.8	0.3	0.3	0.3
		(b) skilled care unit	40	9.4	1.5	1.3	2.1
27	1989 (3–4)	7 skilled nursing facilities in CA	26	6.1	2.8	1.6	0.9
143	1996–98 (6–24)	6 skilled nursing facilities in ID	NS	4.2	1.5	1.3	1.0

LRTI, lower respiratory tract infection; LTCF, long-term care facility; NH, nursing home; NS, not stated; SSTI, skin and soft tissue infection; UTI, urinary tract infection; VA, Veterans Affairs.
[a] Number of infections per 1,000 resident care days.
[b] Includes asymptomatic bacteriuria with symptomatic UTIs.
[c] Rate includes URTIs and LRTIs.

quency of infection. For example, the 2.6 incidence rate reported by Jacobson and Strausbaugh (20) did not include patients with upper respiratory tract infections (URTIs) or bronchitis. Other studies using the CDC definitions for nosocomial infection may have underestimated their rates, because laboratory and radiologic data were insufficient for diagnosis.

Several other observations are also of interest. First, the 2.6 to 5.4 per 1,000 resident care days range for incidence rates in VA facilities with a predominantly male population was not dissimilar from the 1.8 to 9.4 per 1,000 resident care days range in non-VA homes, wherein women predominate. Second, the mean incidence rate in eight rural Wisconsin NHs including several facilities with fewer than 100 beds (3.6 infections per 1, 000 resident days) was similar to the mean rate for six mostly rural NHs in Idaho (4.22 infections per 1,000 resident days) (17,143). In turn, these rates were generally comparable to those observed in two large urban NHs in Maryland (3.6 and 3.8 infections per 1,000 resident days and seven NHs in Orange County, California (range 4.1 to 6.6 infections per 1,000 resident days) (16,27). Finally, incidence rates for infection are higher in LTCFs that offer a higher level of skilled nursing care and presumably care for more debilitated patients. For example, Darnowski et al. (15) observed a 1.8 incidence rate in one unit and a 9.4 incidence rate in another unit that delivered a more aggressive level of care. Similar observations were made in one VA study with different types of units (14).

An estimated 1.6 million Americans currently reside in NHs, which translates to 584,000,000 resident care days each year. This figure for resident care days combined with the incidence rates in Table 106.6 project an annual incidence of NH-acquired infections ranging from 1.1 to 5.5 million infections. This range narrows to a more probable 1.8 to 4.1 million infections per year when only incidence rates from the more recent and better designed studies are considered—three to seven infections per 1,000 resident care days (144). These projections for NH-acquired infections rival or exceed the 2.1 million hospital-acquired infections that are estimated to occur in the United States each year (145). Similar projections also indicate that NH-acquired infections account for 153,000 to 306,000 hospital admissions (transfers from NHs) and 23,100 to 70,000 deaths each year (144).

Prevalence of Infection in Nursing Homes

During the last 2 decades, a number of 1-day prevalence studies have been conducted in LTCFs (Table 106.7). Most have focused on NHs or other specific units for the elderly. Some have examined more than one facility or different types of units at once. Some have summarized the results of multiple 1-day prevalence surveys (14,23). The prevalence of infection on the day of study in all surveys ranged from 2.4% to 18.4%. This broad range reflected methodologic differences, especially differing criteria for infection. For example, two studies (14, 146), including the one with the highest rate, counted asymptomatic bacteriuria as an infection, whereas other studies did not. Steinmiller et al. (24), who used the CDC's definitions for nosocomial infections, thought they underestimated the true prevalence of infection in their LTCF. Of interest, the only two studies (17,22) that used identical definitions observed similar prevalences of infection on the day of study—16.2% and 13.9%, even though one was conducted in urban Utah and the other was conducted in rural Wisconsin. Overall, these data from prevalence studies indicate that, on any given day

TABLE 106.7. ONE-DAY PREVALENCE STUDIES IN LONG-TERM CARE FACILITIES

				Prevalence of infection[a]			
Ref.	Date of Study	Types of LTCFs and Location	% Men	Overall	UTIs	LRTIs	SSTIs
22	1980–1981	7 skilled care NHs in urban UT	36	16.2	2.6	2.1	6.0
14	1983	VA Medical Center in TN					
		(a) two ICWs	>95	10.6[b]	1.6[c]	5.8	1.7
		(b) one NH ward	>95	2.4[b]	1.2[c]	0.3	0.9
17	1984	8 rural NHs in WI & adjacent to hospital	24	13.9	3.5	2.5	5.5
23	Pub. 1985	9 LTC units of county hospital in NJ	26	12.2[b]	4.7	2.3	5.6
24	Pub. 1991	4 VA combined ICW and NH units in PA	>95	9.8	2.8	2.5	2.8
146	1996	One-day survey of geriatric wards in 77 hospitals in northern France	30				
		(a) Geriatric rehabilitation wards (*n* = 50)		18.4	7.3	9.9	5.9
		(b) Geriatric LTC wards (*n* = 198)		9.4	3.2	4.7	2.6

[a] Prevalence = number of residents with infection/number of residents in LTCF × 100%.
[b] Includes asymptomatic bacteriuria with symptomatic UTIs.
[c] Summary data for multiple 1-day prevalence surveys. ICW, intermediate care ward; LRTI, lower respiratory tract infection; LTCF, long-term care facility; NH, nursing home; SSTI, skin and soft tissue infection; UTI, urinary tract infection; VA, Veterans Affairs.
NH, nursing home; SSTI, skin and soft tissue infection; UTI, urinary tract infection; VA, Veterans Affairs.

in the United States, 5% to 15% of NH residents are infected—80,000 to 240,000 residents.

The results of the prevalence studies parallel the results of the incidence studies in several respects. First, rates in VA facilities, which range from 2.4% to 10.6%, overlap those in non-VA facilities, which range from 9.4% to 18.4%. As noted earlier, rates in urban and rural facilities appear comparable. Finally, higher prevalence rates prevail in units delivering higher levels of care, presumably because patients are sicker and more susceptible to infection (14,146).

Skin and Soft Tissue Infections

Most SSTIs encountered in LTCFs are endemic, although some, such as scabies or infections caused by *Streptococcus pyogenes,* can occur in outbreaks. Infected ulcers, cellulitis, cutaneous abscesses, and conjunctivitis occur most frequently, but the range of potential infections includes such diverse conditions as herpes zoster and surgical site infections.

For the purposes of surveillance, most studies have relied on CDC definitions of SSTIs, sometimes with minor modifications to accommodate the long-term care setting. SSTIs are frequently reported in the aggregate without listing statistics for each infection separately. The overall incidence of NH-acquired cutaneous infections is reported to be 0.2 to 2.1 per 1,000 resident care days (14,16–18,21). The chronicity of some skin infections results in their overrepresentation in prevalence surveys. Thus, point prevalence studies have identified SSTIs in 1% to 6% of NH residents (Table 106.7), and in several studies they have accounted for 33% to 39% of all NH-acquired infections (17,22, 23). In incidence studies, however, SSTIs make up a more modest percentage of infections (14,15,10,17,20,21).

Definitions

Infected Pressure Ulcers

Skin ulcers in LTCFs may be caused by diabetes mellitus, vascular insufficiency, vasculitis, malignancy, or pressure. Most institutional surveillance studies have concentrated on infected pressure ulcers, using the CDC criterion—purulent exudate—as the indication of infection. Reported frequencies of infected ulcers vary markedly by surveillance methodology. In point prevalence studies, they range from 24% to 33% of LTCF infections, whereas, in incidence studies, they represent less than 5% of reported infections (10,17,20,22). Pressure ulcers often start in the hospital before NH transfer, so some pressure ulcer infections may be hospital-acquired rather than LTCF-acquired (147). The few studies that have assessed LTCF-acquired pressure ulcer infections specifically report incidences of 0.2 to 1.4 per 1,000 resident care days (17,148). Bacterial species isolated from pressure ulcers vary depending on host characteristics, environmental setting, culture methods, and condition of the wound. Wound cultures usually yield polymicrobial growth with a mixture of gram-positive and gram-negative aerobic and anaerobic flora (149,150). Frequent isolates include *Proteus mirabilis,* Group D streptococci, *E. coli, Staphylococcus* species, *Pseudomonas* species, *Peptostreptococcus* species, *Peptococcus* species, *Bacteroides fragilis,* and *Clostridium perfringens* (150,151). Rarely, tetanus may arise from pressure ulcers in NH residents (152). Complications of infected pressure ulcers in LTCFs are similar to those in other settings and include local infection, cellulitis, osteomyelitis, and bacteremia (see Chapter 56).

Cellulitis and Cutaneous Abscesses

Cellulitis and cutaneous abscesses accounted for less than 10% of NH infections in the few studies that reported separate statistics for these conditions (10,18,20). Skin microorganisms are the usual etiology of cellulitis (i.e., *S. pyogenes* or *S. aureus*). However, in NHs, where a large proportion of the residents are diabetic, elderly, or immunocompromised, other gram-positive bacteria, gram-negative bacilli (especially *E. coli, Proteus* species, *Klebsiella* species, *Enterobacter* species, *Serratia marcescens,* and *Bacteroides* species), or fungi may cause cellulitis (149). Cellulitis has been prominent in several *S. pyogenes* outbreaks in NHs (13, 32,43) (see Chapter 31). Streptococcal toxic shock syndrome has been observed in some of these outbreaks with associated renal failure and adult respiratory distress syndrome. Case fatality rates have approached 60%.

Conjunctivitis

In some studies, conjunctivitis has the highest incidence and prevalence among SSTI in LTCFs (18). Incidence rates range from 0.075 to 3.5 per 1,000 resident care days, and prevalence rates range from 3.9% to 13% (10,16,18,20,21,100,153). Conjunctivitis may be acute or chronic, sporadic or epidemic. *S. pneumoniae* and *S. aureus* cause acute bacterial conjunctivitis most commonly, but many other bacteria, viruses, and fungi have also been implicated (87,100,152). Both *S. pyogenes* and MRSA have caused outbreaks of conjunctivitis in NH (13,154).

Herpetic Infections

Herpes simplex virus (HSV) causes a variety of mucocutaneous lesions: facial-oral infection ("cold sores"), gingivostomatitis, genital infection, and herpetic whitlow. Their incidence in LTCFs has received little attention. However, in one 3-year surveillance study, HSV infections accounted for less than 1% of all new infections in a community NH (18).

Varicella-zoster virus (VZV) infections would be expected to occur in LTCFs at a rate comparable to that among community-dwelling elderly, particularly considering the age and general frailty of NH inhabitants. Because nosocomial transmission of VZV manifesting as chickenpox (not shingles) has been well documented, outbreaks would also be expected (155). Nevertheless, only one NH surveillance study mentions VZV infections. During the 3 years of observation, nine new episodes of shingles occurred (18). These infections accounted for less than 1% of infections during the study period. In the elderly and immunosuppressed, VZV infections often run a more protracted course, with deeper lesions that scar. Dissemination also occurs more commonly. Other complications include postherpetic neuralgia, which may be more severe in the aged; encephalitis; motor neuropathies; and pneumonitis (32,33,56).

Candidiasis

Candida causes a vast array of clinical diseases (see Chapter 39). Those commonly seen in LTCFs include lesions such as "thrush" (acute pseudomembranous candidiasis) and "denture stomatitis" (chronic atrophic candidiasis), intertriginous infections, vulvovaginitis, balanitis, and nail infections (34,56,156). In a 3-year surveillance study, candidal infections accounted for 4% of all NH-acquired infections, with an incidence of 0.28 per 1,000 resident care days (18). However, the prevalence of unrecognized oral candidal infections in LTCFs is probably much higher. An oral examination of 137 residents in an LTCF in Glasgow, Scotland, revealed that 47% had oral candidal infections (156,157). A similar study conducted in Denmark among residents of eight NHs and five LTCFs uncovered denture stomatitis in approximately one third of participants. *Candida albicans, Candida parapsilosis, Candida tropicalis, Candida pseudotropicalis,* and *Torulopsis glabrata* have all been cultured from residents of LTCFs with chronic atrophic candidiasis (156,157).

Scabies

Scabies outbreaks have been frequently documented in LTCFs (86,158,159) (see Chapter 46). Seventeen percent of Michigan's 725 NHs reported scabies in the facility during a 1-year period (86). The mite *Sarcoptes scabiei* causes the infections. A clinical variant, Norwegian scabies, which typically occurs in persons with immunodeficiency, also occurs more frequently in residents of NHs and homes for the mentally retarded (159, 160). Extensive lesions with crusting that mimics dermatitis or psoriasis and nail involvement with nail dystrophy or nail loss characterize this variant. In the elderly and physically debilitated, scabies lesions may be seen in atypical locations and distributions, further hampering diagnosis (160).

Reservoirs and Sources

Infected Pressure Ulcers

Pathogens infecting pressure ulcers are frequently endogenous, arising from microorganisms colonizing the skin or from fecal contamination and possibly from the urinary tract of incontinent bacteriuric NH residents. They may derive from the patient's normal flora or from that of other infected or colonized residents or staff members. Occasionally, environmental surfaces or equipment (e.g., bathtubs and bedpans) serve as reservoirs. Contaminated whirlpool baths, for example, have been implicated in the development of *P. aeruginosa* infections (161). Infected pressure ulcers may harbor MRSA and multiply resistant gram-negative bacilli too, thus facilitating intrafacility and interfacility spread of these resistant microorganisms.

Cellulitis and Cutaneous Abscesses

The reservoirs and sources for microorganisms associated with cellulitis and cutaneous abscesses are similar to those described for infected pressure ulcers. In addition, staff members, visitors, or new residents with streptococcal skin or URTIs or colonization may introduce *S. pyogenes* into LTCFs (13) (see Chapter 31).

Conjunctivitis

Microorganisms implicated in conjunctival infections may derive from sites of extraocular infection or colonization in the resident or others. A variety of eye preparations, drops, and ointments may serve as additional sources for infection (see Chapter 26). Epidemic keratoconjunctivitis has spread to NH residents from contaminated optic solutions at eye clinics during outpatient appointments and outbreaks of epidemic keratoconjunctivitis caused by adenovirus 37 have been reported (100). Environmental surfaces in NHs may harbor infectious virus for up to a week (100).

Herpetic Infections

Persons with active herpetic infections—residents, staff, or visitors—are the main source of HSV infection in LTCFs. Persons with shingles may be a source for chickenpox (VZV) infection until the lesions are crusted over. Because shingles take longer to heal in the elderly and immunocompromised (up to 2 to 4 weeks), NH residents with VZV infections may pose a greater risk to other immunocompromised residents or to susceptible staff members.

Candidiasis

Reservoirs for *Candida* infection in the LTCF are many and varied. *Candida* is ubiquitous; it can readily be cultured from the skin and mucous membranes of NH residents and staff members or from environmental surfaces and personal items such as dentures. Colonization rates for *C. albicans,* determined monthly, averaged 35% among residents of a VA LTCF over the course of a 2-year prospective study (162).

Scabies

Scabies may enter LTCFs via infected residents, staff members, or visitors. NH residents with Norwegian scabies may harbor thousands of mites. Scabies mites are known to survive 34 hours under normal room conditions and have been recovered live from bed linens of NH residents (158). Other fomites include rehabilitative walking belts, skin creams, ointments, and mineral oil (13).

Transmission

Infected Pressure Ulcers

Some of the microorganisms causing infected pressure ulcers are transmitted via direct contact with other residents, staff members, and possibly environmental surfaces.

Cellulitis and Cutaneous Abscesses

Transmission of streptococcal infections may occur either by direct person-to-person contact or by respiratory droplet spread from residents or staff members with streptococcal skin infections or URTIs, respectively (43). Outbreak investigations have not implicated fomites in transmission.

Conjunctivitis

Conjunctivitis usually spreads via direct contact with the hands of residents or staff members, but contaminated eye preparations may transfer bacteria from extraocular to intraocular sites or from one patient to another (153). Outbreak investigations suggest that epidemic keratoconjunctivitis may be spread by fomites (100).

Herpetic Infections

Herpes simplex infections are transmitted through direct contact with active lesions. Herpetic whitlow in a healthcare worker may pose a particular problem because of the potential for spread of infection (see Chapter 43). VZV may be transmitted from person to person by direct contact with open lesions or via the droplet and airborne routes (155). Direct contact with open zoster lesions may lead to chickenpox in susceptible individuals. Persons with disseminated zoster or immunocompromised persons with dermatomal zoster may also transmit chickenpox by the droplet or airborne routes (155). Transmission of shingles itself has not been demonstrated (see Chapter 42).

Candidiasis

Clusters of candidal UTIs in NHs suggest that person-to-person transmission may occur.

Scabies

Transmission of scabies infections occurs most often by direct person-to-person contact, but transmission may also occur by contact with mite-contaminated objects (e.g., bed linens). Index cases of Norwegian scabies have resulted in infection of 50% of patients in the same NH ward and 78% of roommates (159).

Risk Factors

Residents of LTCFs with their fragile skin, tenuous nutritional status, and mobility deficits are particularly vulnerable to SSTIs (Table 106.4). Few studies have addressed other risk factors.

Infected Pressure Ulcers

Risk factors for developing pressure ulcers are well delineated, but the reason why some ulcers become infected is not (31,150, 163). Incontinence is generally regarded as a risk factor for skin infections. However, a case control study conducted among 4,259 residents in 53 Maryland NHs did not confirm this hypothesis. Residents with multiple or deep ulcers, however, were more likely to have skin ulcer infections (10).

Cellulitis and Cutaneous Abscesses

Cutaneous trauma and underlying skin lesions such as pressure sores, vascular insufficiency, chronic edema, and stasis dermatitis predispose NH residents to cellulitis and cutaneous abscesses. Advanced age appears to confer susceptibility to *S. pyogenes* infections, which have a higher incidence in the elderly (43). Outbreak investigations have identified proximity to infected residents and lapses in infection control procedures as additional risk factors for streptococcal infection in NHs (43).

Conjunctivitis

The risk of developing conjunctivitis increases in NH residents with physical impairments or prior ocular problems, such as ectropion, entropion, or glaucoma (153). In one NH outbreak, residents with MRSA conjunctivitis frequently exhibited colonization at extraocular sites (154).

Herpetic Infections

Herpetic infections in elderly LTCF residents most often represent reactivation of prior herpes virus infections. Although risk factors for reactivation of VZV infection in LTCFs have not been addressed specifically, they are likely similar to those described in other settings (e.g., advanced age, immunosuppression, radiotherapy, malignancy, corticosteroids) (see Chapters 42 and 43).

Candidiasis

Candida infections are generally opportunistic and have been associated with diabetes, obesity, antibiotic use, and immunosuppression. Oral candidiasis in LTCF residents is highly associated with dentures, poor oral hygiene, cigarette smoking, and possibly by using medications that cause xerostomia (156,157).

Scabies

The enforced proximity of institutional living and need for direct personal care places LTCF residents and staff members at high risk for infection during scabies outbreaks. Infestation of nursing staff members working with crusted scabies patients ranges from 40% to 70% (56).

Respiratory Tract Infections

Description

Upper Respiratory Tract Infections

The common cold syndrome and, to a lesser extent, pharyngitis, sinusitis, and otitis occur with measurable frequency in LTCFs, as they do in other population groups. Their occurrence may be endemic or epidemic. Incidence studies in four LTCFs, principally NHs, have reported rates for generic (i.e., otherwise not delineated) URTIs ranging from 0.3 to 1.6 infections per 1,000 days of resident care (15,17–19). This variation undoubtedly reflects the different surveillance definitions and techniques used in these studies and the occurrence of outbreaks during the study period. The results from prevalence studies also have varied considerably. Garibaldi et al. (22) noted a 1-day prevalence rate for URTIs of 1.5% in seven Salt Lake City, Utah, NHs. Scheckler and Peterson (17) observed a 0.5% 1-day prevalence rate in eight rural Wisconsin NHs. Several prevalence studies reported no URTIs on the day of survey. In both incidence and prevalence studies that have specifically noted URTIs, these infections have generally accounted for 3% to 10% of the total infections. Rates of infection, especially for infections caused by viruses, typically increase during winter months.

The etiology of URTIs in LTCFs has been most clearly defined in outbreaks. Outbreaks are not uncommon and they occur year-round with no seasonal pattern (36). They usually involve both residents and staff members and may have attack rates in the 20% to 30% range. Outbreaks caused by rhinoviruses, respiratory syncytial virus, and parainfluenza virus types 1 and 3 have been reported in NHs, and outbreaks caused by adenoviruses and enteroviruses have been reported in pediatric LTCFs (13,55,79,80,94). An outbreak of adenovirus 35 among adult residents and staff of a chronic care psychiatric facility has been reported (164). Pertussis outbreaks have been reported in NHs and facilities for the developmentally disabled (62,165). Pharyngitis and other URTIs have also occurred during outbreaks caused by *S. pyogenes* in NHs (43). Most of these outbreak pathogens also account for some of the endemic disease. Other studies on URTIs in LTCFs have also identified a role for *Mycoplasma pneumoniae, Chlamydia pneumoniae,* influenza virus, rhinoviruses, respiratory syncytial virus, parainfluenza virus, and coronaviruses in the endemic setting (139,166).

Influenza

Influenza is occasionally recognized as a cause of endemic disease in LTCFs. In their year-long study of URTIs in a VA NH, Arroyo et al. (166) isolated influenza B virus from 2 of their 59 cases. They also found serologic evidence for influenza B infection in six additional cases and for influenza A in two cases. More frequently, influenza is recognized in epidemic form, and the medical literature is dominated by outbreak reports (see Chapter 41). Influenza outbreaks in LTCFs usually occur in the late fall or winter as they do in the community at large. H1N1 and H3N2 strains of influenza A and various strains of influenza B have caused outbreaks with attack rates ranging from 15% to 70%, depending to some extent on vaccination status of residents and staff members (13,36,56,57,74,76–78,95–98,139, 167,168). During the decade 1988 to 1998, 16 outbreaks involving more than 1,000 residents and at least 20 facilities were reported (74). Attack rates in these outbreaks ranged from 20% to 30% but exceeded 40% in two.

In their older review of nine influenza A outbreaks in NHs housing 2,419 residents, Cesario and Yousefi (167) calculated an overall attack rate of 29%—704 residents developed an influenza-like illness. These authors noted that 91 patients (13%) developed pneumonia and that 67 died (9%). In their review of two influenza B outbreaks in NHs, these authors found that 143 of 449 exposed residents developed an influenza-like illness, 5 (3%) developed pneumonia, and 1 died.

Lower Respiratory Tract Infections

With few exceptions, most surveillance studies in LTCFs have used the term LRTI in accordance with the CDC's definition for nosocomial infection without delineating specific entities (i.e., bronchitis, pneumonia, lung abscess, or other pulmonary infection). A few studies have reported only pneumonias. The 3-year study reported by Jackson et al. (18) clearly delineated bronchitis and pneumonia cases. In that study, 60% of the 286 LRTIs were due to pneumonia and 40% were due to bronchitis. In the point prevalence study reported by Steinmiller et al. (24), 18% of the 40 infections were due to pneumonia and 8% of the infections were due to bronchitis, tracheobronchitis, or tracheitis. Despite uncertainties about these percentages in other studies, it is nevertheless clear that LRTIs are quite common in NHs. They are consistently among the top three causes of infectious morbidity in this setting. LRTIs usually occur most frequently in the late fall and winter, probably reflecting the role of viral respiratory infections in their pathogenesis.

In reported studies, the incidence of LRTIs has ranged from 0.3 to 2.6 infections per 1,000 resident care days (Table 106.6). The median value in these studies is 1.1 case per 1,000 resident care days, which accords with the median value reported by Muder (169) in his review of these and other series and rates observed in recent studies (18,27,143,170). In 1-day prevalence studies, the percentage of LRTIs has ranged from 0.3% to 9.9% (Table 106.7). In incidence studies, LRTIs have accounted for 13% to 53% of all infections. In prevalence studies, they have accounted for 6% to 48% of all infections.

As judged by studies in the literature, which have almost exclusively relied on culture results from expectorated sputum specimens, the etiology of LRTIs in LTCFs falls in between the patterns usually observed in the community and the hospital. In NHs, pneumonia caused by *S. aureus* and aerobic gram-negative bacilli, especially *K. pneumoniae,* are more common than in the community at large (169,171–176). At the same time, pneumonias caused by *S. pneumoniae* and *Haemophilus influenzae* are also common, being observed more frequently in this setting than in the hospital (44,45). Other pathogens commonly recognized in NHs include other members of the family Enterobacteriaceae, *Moraxella catarrhalis,* various streptococci, and *P. aeruginosa.* Other causes of pneumonia, recognized primarily in outbreaks, include *C. pneumoniae, Legionella* species, and multidrug-resistant *S. pneumoniae* (45,53,63,92). Respiratory viral infections, especially influenza A, can involve the lower respiratory tract directly, but their role as the sole cause of pneumonia and bronchitis in LTCF residents has not been clearly elucidated.

Pneumonia is an important cause of morbidity and mortality in residents of NHs. Although blood cultures may not be obtained regularly on patients with pneumonia in this setting, bacteremia is frequently mentioned in published reports. For example, 5 (23%) of 22 patients with pneumonia were bacteremic in one VA study (20). Moreover, in three studies of NH-acquired bacteremias, LRTIs were the second and third leading causes, accounting for 10% to 11% of cases (5,177,178). Pneumonias are frequently associated with clinical deterioration necessitating transfer to hospital. Nine percent to 51% of patients acquiring pneumonia in NHs require transfer to acute care facilities, and NH transfers account for 10% to 18% of community-acquired pneumonia cases (169,170,179).

Pneumonias are frequently fatal in this population. In the three NH surveillance studies that commented on mortality resulting from pneumonia, case fatality rates ranged from 6% to 23% (17,18,20). More recently, a study from Nova Scotia found that the 32% in-hospital mortality rate for patients with NH-acquired pneumonia differed significantly from the 14% rate for other patients admitted with community-acquired pneumonia (173). Pneumonia is also a marker for future recurrences and subsequent mortality. In a prospective study of outcomes in a VA LTCF, the 14-day, 12-month, and 24-month mortality figures for 108 residents with pneumonia were 19%, 59%, and 75%, respectively (180). Of the 87 residents who survived the first episode of pneumonia, 43% had additional episodes during the subsequent 6 months.

Tuberculosis

The incidence of tuberculosis is increased in residents and staff members of NHs (see Chapter 37). In a CDC-sponsored survey of 15,379 routinely reported cases of tuberculosis from 29 states, 8% of the 4,919 cases that occurred among elderly persons involved residents of NHs, yielding an incidence rate of 39.2 per 100,000 person-years (72,181). In contrast, the incidence of tuberculosis among elderly persons living in the community was 21.5 cases per 100,000 person-years, and the incidence among all other age groups averaged 9.3 cases per 100,000 person-years. The rate of tuberculosis among NH employees was three times the expected rate in employed adults of similar age, race, and sex. Reports by Stead and colleagues (182) have delineated even higher rates of tuberculosis among NH residents in Arkansas. Based on cases reported to the Arkansas Department of Health during the period 1981 to 1983, the incidence in elderly NH residents was 234 cases per 100,000, a rate four times higher than that for persons older than 65 years residing at home.

Outbreaks of tuberculosis in NHs have received most attention in the medical literature. A recent report from Arkansas exemplifies the problem (71). It describes an outbreak that started in one NH and subsequently spread to another NH, a local hospital, and the community before it was recognized. Investigators ultimately traced the outbreak to a 91-year-old NH resident who remained undiagnosed for more than 8 months. During this period she infected 52 NH employees, 23 NH residents, and one visitor. The authors of this report speculate that such occurrences are not uncommon although they may be infrequently recognized. Periodic reports from the CDC support this contention (181).

Endemic cases have not received as much attention. Cases of active tuberculosis were rarely noted in the major NH surveillance studies, but the surveillance techniques may not have been optimal. The studies by Stead and colleagues in Arkansas NHs suggest that many NHs encounter tuberculosis in an endemic form (182). They observed the transmission of tuberculosis in 32% of 227 NHs in Arkansas during an 8-year period. Age-specific case rates in male NH residents were fairly comparable during this period, ranging from 943 per 100,000 in the 80- to 89-year age group to 1,181 per 100,000 in the older than 90-year age group. Rates in female NH residents were lower and more related to age, ranging from 183 per 100,000 in the 50- to 59-year age group to 695 per 100,000 in the older than 90-year age group. The case rate was lowest in NHs with zero to one case during the period of observation (173 per 100,000) and highest in NHs with ten or more cases (1,998 per 100, 000). Each case of active disease was associated with skin test conversions in five to seven other fellow residents or staff members.

Reservoirs and Sources

Upper Respiratory Tract Infections

Staff members and visitors usually introduce upper respiratory tract pathogens circulating in the community into LTCFs (56,57). As these pathogens spread to other staff members and residents, they, in turn, become the source of infection for others. Environmental surfaces contaminated with viruses or bacteria sometimes transiently serve as a reservoir.

Influenza

Staff members, visitors, and, possibly, newly admitted residents who have been infected elsewhere bring influenza into LTCFs (74,96,98). For a few days, these individuals are the source. As residents and staff members become infected, they become the sources for additional cases. Influenza virus may also persist for several hours in dried mucus, permitting mucus-contaminated objects to briefly serve as an additional source of infection.

Lower Respiratory Tract Infections

Bacterial infections of the lower respiratory tract in LTCFs generally arise from the residents endogenous flora, the bacteria colonizing the upper airway. Although not well studied, colonization in NH residents is thought to be a dynamic process, with residents acquiring new flora predominantly as a result of contact with other residents and staff members. The role played by other patients and staff members is usually only appreciated in outbreaks. Environmental objects freshly contaminated with respiratory secretions sometimes serve as transient reservoirs. Aspiration is the predominant mechanism for delivering bacteria to the lower airways (169,172,174–176).

Tuberculosis

As in other situations, the main reservoirs for tuberculosis in LTCFs are patients with active disease, especially those with cavitary lung disease who have not been previously identified, isolated, or treated (70–72,181,182). To a lesser extent, tuberculin-positive patients who have never been treated with isoniazid (INH) serve as potential reservoirs, because they may develop active disease as their immunity wanes. Data from the Arkansas NH studies indicate that only 10% to 20% of new residents are tuberculin positive, and two-step or "booster" tuberculin testing procedures are required to identify all of these previously infected individuals (183). Rates are generally higher in men than in women and higher in nonwhites than in whites.

Transmission

Upper Respiratory Tract Infections

For the most part, upper respiratory tract pathogens spread from person to person via direct contact, either by touching or by direct projection of droplet spray (e.g., from a sneeze or cough) onto a susceptible mucous membrane. Small-particle aerosols may also play a role in some situations.

Influenza

Influenza is predominantly spread by indirect contact with large droplets produced by infectious persons. Whether airborne spread or direct contact with mucus-soiled objects plays a role in LTCFs is unclear, but the former route may be important where crowding and poor ventilation coexist, and the latter may be important in pediatric facilities.

Lower Respiratory Tract Infection

The spread of *S. aureus* and aerobic gram-negative bacilli in NHs is thought to parallel the spread that occurs in the hospital and is easily envisioned in residents who require endotracheal suctioning or other direct handling of the airway. Clusters of pneumonia caused by *S. pneumoniae* have been observed in NHs, and at least one report has suggested a role for person-to-person spread (45). Whether this involves indirect contact via droplet spray or direct contact by touching or contact with articles freshly soiled with respiratory secretions remains uncertain.

Tuberculosis

Residents with active pulmonary or laryngeal tuberculosis transmit this infection to susceptible persons via airborne droplet nuclei, which arise during the course of coughing, laughing, singing, or other forceful expiratory efforts.

Risk Factors

Upper Respiratory Tract Infections

Risk factors for URTIs in LTCFs have not been delineated, but they presumably do not differ from those operative in other settings. The common cold and pharyngitis probably predispose residents to the subsequent development of sinusitis and, to a lesser extent, otitis media.

Influenza

The nonvaccinated state and low preinfection antibody titers are generally regarded as risk factors, although the former is controversial (74,77,96,98,184). In a meta-analysis predominantly using studies conducted in NH residents, the risk for respiratory illness in vaccinated patients was 44% that of control subjects (confidence interval, 32% to 61%; $p < .00001$) (185). However, NH outbreaks involving large numbers of vaccinated patients are well documented (77). Failure of vaccination to induce hemagglutination-inhibition antibody titers of 1:40 or greater may account for the low efficacy of vaccination in some outbreaks (185). Residence in LTCFs with low rates of vaccination among healthcare workers also appears to be a risk factor for influenza (186,187). Although publications from the CDC have suggested that vaccination rates among NH residents in excess of 80% may protect facilities from outbreaks, several reports indicate that protection is not insured (13,97).

Lower Respiratory Tract Infections

Several studies have examined risk factors using univariate techniques. Observed statistical associations may be artifactual because of the large number of comparisons performed. Nevertheless, many observed associations conform to common expectations. Risk factors identified include chronic obstructive pulmonary disease, inability to eat independently, presence of a nasogastric or gastrostomy feeding tube, bladder and bowel incontinence, tracheostomy and need for tracheal suctioning, low Karnofsky score, unstable medical condition, decubitus ulcers, intravenous lines, absence of pneumococcal vaccine, smoking, and use of neuroleptic agents (20,22,23).

Studies using multivariable techniques have identified the following risk factors for pneumonia: poor functional status, presence of nasogastric tubes, difficulties swallowing, witnessed aspiration, occurrence of unusual events defined as confusion, agitation, falls, or wandering, receipt of tranquilizers, chronic lung disease, tracheostomy, increasing age, lack of influenza vaccine, and male sex (169,170,174–176,188). Several of these factors point to the primacy of aspiration in the pathogenesis of NH-acquired pneumonia.

A prospective study of pulmonary aspiration in an LTCF offered confirmatory data (172). During the 8-month study period, 98 aspirations occurred in 69 residents—1.6 aspirations per 1,000 resident days. Fifty-six percent of the aspiration events progressed to roentgenographically proven cases of pneumonia. Multivariable analysis identified tube feeding, presence of a hyperextended neck or contractures, malnutrition, and the use of benzodiazepines and anticholinergics as risk factors for aspiration.

Tuberculosis

Asymptomatic, tuberculin-positive residents of LTCFs, especially the elderly in NHs, are at risk for active disease as their general state of health and immunity decline. Active disease may appear at any time after admission to LTCFs and eventually occurs in 2% to 3% of these residents (181).

Residents who are tuberculin negative at the time of admission to an LTCF are clearly most susceptible to subsequent infection with the tubercle bacillus, and those who are infected are at increased risk for active disease if they are not treated with preventive therapy (70,72). The risk for these tuberculin-negative individuals increases demonstrably when cases of active disease are present in the facility. In the studies conducted in Arkansas NHs, the annual purified protein derivative skin test conversion rate was 5% in NHs with active cases of tuberculosis and 3.5% in NHs without recognized cases. The risk of active tuberculosis in these converters was 8% for women and 12% for men; most cases of active disease occurred within 1 or 2 years of skin test conversion. Active disease was more likely to occur in residents with large zones of reaction to their tuberculin tests—reactions more than 12 mm larger than the reaction from their last negative test (72,182,183).

Preventive therapy with INH reduces the risk of active disease in purified protein derivative-positive individuals residing in NHs. This effect is most apparent in newly infected persons. In one of their Arkansas NH studies, Stead et al. (189) reported that only 1 of 605 documented converters (0.16%) who received preventive therapy developed active disease in contrast to 45 of 757 recent converters (5.9%) who did not receive preventive therapy. Therefore, the lack of preventive therapy in tuberculin-positive residents, especially those with recent infection, is a risk factor for developing active disease.

Urinary Tract Infections

Ascertaining the actual frequency of UTIs in LTCFs is complicated by problems of definition: many studies report asymptomatic and symptomatic bacteriuria together as UTIs, bacteriuria can be either continuous or intermittent, data for catheterized and noncatheterized residents are often lumped together, and the clinical diagnosis of upper tract infection is difficult and likely to be unreliable, particularly in the NH setting.

Description

Asymptomatic Bacteriuria

Surveillance studies in LTCFs have generally used the CDC definition of asymptomatic bacteriuria (i.e., >100,000 microorganisms/mL of urine without manifestations of infection). Bacteriuria is very common in residents of LTCFs, with prevalences of 15% to 50% in noncatheterized elderly NH residents and an incidence of 1.1 episodes per 1,000 resident care days (190–193). In NHs, the prevalence of asymptomatic bacteriuria is 15% to 35% in men and 25% to 50% in women (194). Five percent to 10% of U.S. NH residents have indwelling urethral catheters (195). Among residents with indwelling catheters, bacteriuria is universal (196). Likewise, NH residents using external or intermittent catheterization are at very high risk for bacteriuria. Up to 87% of male NH residents who use external catheters continuously have at least one episode of bacteriuria (197). In a study of elderly hospital and NH patients undergoing intermittent urethral catheterization, 88.6% developed bacteriuria (198).

Gram-negative bacilli are the predominate isolates from noncatheterized NH residents with asymptomatic bacteriuria, but gram-positive microorganisms (e.g., *Enterococcus faecalis*) also are isolated frequently. Multiple species are isolated about one third of the time (190). Among NH residents with indwelling catheters, bacteriuria is often polymicrobial and characterized by frequently changing microorganisms although certain species, for example, *E. coli* and *Providencia stuartii* may persist for long periods (192,196,199).

Asymptomatic bacteriuria does not correlate with nonspecific symptoms such as fatigue, malaise, anorexia, or sleep difficulties nor has it been convincingly linked to renal failure, hypertension, or increased mortality (190). In uncatheterized NH residents with fever, bacteriuria has a positive predictive value of only 9% for clinical UTI (200). Treatment of asymptomatic bacteriuria with antimicrobial agents does not decrease the frequency of symptomatic UTI, improve survival, or decrease chronic incontinence (191). Thus, surveillance with routine urine cultures is not necessary.

Symptomatic Urinary Tract Infection

Surveillance studies have generally used the CDC definition of UTI, requiring the presence of symptoms (e.g., fever, dysuria, costovertebral angle, or suprapubic tenderness) and more than 10,000 microorganisms/mL of urine or more than ten white blood cells per high-power field in an uncentrifuged urine specimen. In point prevalence studies, symptomatic UTIs have made up 12% to 25% of NH infections, affecting 2.6% to 3.5% of NH residents (10,14,17,22). Rates in incidence studies have varied more widely, with symptomatic UTIs accounting for 16% to 42% of infections (15,18,20,21). Variations in methodology, setting, and patient risk factors affect the rates reported in these studies. Reported incidences of symptomatic UTIs in LTCFs vary between 0.3 and 2.8 per 1,000 resident care days (Table 106.6).

The use of urinary drainage devices, especially indwelling catheters, has been associated with an increase in symptomatic UTIs. A 1-year study of male VA NH residents with urethral and suprapubic catheters yielded an incidence of seven symptomatic UTIs per 1,000 resident care days at risk (201). Warren et al. (202) reported 11 febrile episodes of possible urinary tract origin per 1,000 resident care days among institutionalized women with indwelling catheters. Among male NH patients who used external catheters continuously, Ouslander et al. (197) reported 2.7 episodes of symptomatic UTI per 1,000 resident care days. In a study of elderly hospital and NH patients undergoing intermittent urethral catheterization, 11% had symptomatic urinary infections (197).

Predominant urinary pathogens vary in different facilities. In general, *E. coli* remains a frequent isolate, but in some facilities, especially VA LTCFs with a preponderance of male residents, *Proteus* and *Providencia* species are found more often (21). *Klebsiella* species, *P. aeruginosa,* and *Enterococcus* species are more common in the LTCF resident than in noninstitutionalized persons (191). In a study of Nebraska NHs, the most frequent isolates from LTCF residents with indwelling catheters were *Enterococcus* species and *P. aeruginosa* (28). Multiresistant bacteria and unusual microorganisms, such as fungi, are also observed (29,34,40,162).

In contrast to asymptomatic bacteriuria, symptomatic UTIs can have serious consequences among residents of the LTCF. Symptomatic UTIs are the leading source of bacteremia in LTCF residents and an important cause of gram-negative sepsis and death among the elderly (5,11,177,202).

Upper and lower UTIs cannot be reliably distinguished by clinical criteria, and surveillance studies have not reported separate statistics for upper tract infections. However, two studies have attempted to localize urinary infections in NH residents. Their findings suggest that upper tract involvement may not be uncommon (203,204).

Reservoirs and Sources

Most UTIs arise from endogenous bowel and perineal flora. Extrinsic sources are also important, particularly in the catheterized resident, and include microorganisms on the hands of NH personnel, urinary drainage devices, contaminated antiseptic solutions, and nonsterile irrigation fluids. Colonized residents and equipment such as urinals, urometers, and bedpans have served as a source for outbreaks of UTIs with multiresistant microorganisms (57,190).

Transmission

UTIs have often occurred in clusters in LTCFs, and transmission from one resident to another by staff members has been described repeatedly (205). Multiresistant gram-negative microorganisms may be carried from one facility to another via persons with UTIs. In one outbreak, condom catheters proved to be a reservoir for multiresistant microorganisms that were transmitted when nursing staff members emptied the drainage bags into urinals and redistributed the urinals among the residents sharing a room (206).

Risk Factors

General predisposing factors for UTIs commonly encountered among residents of LTCFs include conditions that interfere with bladder emptying (e.g., neurogenic bladder or prostatic hypertrophy), kidney and bladder stones, diabetes, and prior antibiotic use (207).

Asymptomatic Bacteriuria

Case-control and cohort studies in NH residents have shown an association between asymptomatic bacteriuria and urinary and fecal incontinence, dementia, and decline in functional status (208).

Symptomatic Urinary Tract Infections

In a retrospective review of data collected from the 20,479 LTCFs participating in the 1985 National NH study, the presence of an indwelling catheter was the strongest predictor of symptomatic UTI (relative risk = 6.6) (209). In Denmark, national efforts have successfully reduced indwelling catheter use with a resulting decrease in the number of catheter-associated UTIs by one half (210).

Bacteremias

Description

The definition of LTCF-acquired bacteremia varies from study to study. Some authors accept a single positive blood culture as an indication of bacteremia, whereas others require at least two positive cultures and/or symptoms and signs consistent with bloodstream infection. There are also reasons to expect that bacteremias are underestimated in the LTCF. First, resources for obtaining blood cultures are often limited. Second, the criterion for obtaining blood cultures is usually fever, and up to 13% of elderly persons may have afebrile bacteremia (211). Despite these caveats and methodologic variations, the reported incidence and prevalence of bacteremias in LTCFs are remarkably consistent.

In surveillance studies, bacteremias account for about 2% to 7% of infectious episodes (10,14,18,21). The reported incidence of bacteremias among NH residents ranges from 0.2 to 0.36 episodes per 1,000 resident care days and has been shown to parallel the overall infection rate (5,14,177,212,213).

Primary Bacteremia

Primary bacteremias related to intravascular devices are reported infrequently in LTCFs, reflecting the lower use of invasive devices in this setting. In a series of 163 episodes of bacteremia that occurred over a 5-year period in a 432-bed VA LTCF, only four primary bacteremias were identified (5). Similarly, Setia et al. (177) reported only one primary bacteremia in a series of 100 consecutive LTCF patients with bloodstream infections during a 24-month period. Data are insufficient to describe the etiology of LTCF-acquired primary bacteremias; however, the spectrum of pathogens is probably similar to that encountered in the hospital.

Secondary Bacteremia

The most frequent source for bloodstream infections among NH residents is the urinary tract, which is the portal of entry for about 56% of bacteremias (5,177,178,212). Other frequent sources include the respiratory tract (7% to 11%) and SSTIs (7% to 14%). No source is identifiable for 7% to 22% of NH bacteremias.

Fifty-nine percent to 67% of microorganisms isolated from bacteremic NH residents are gram-negative, reflecting their predominantly urinary tract origin. *E. coli, Providencia* species, *Klebsiella* species, and *Proteus* species are the most frequent isolates. Gram-positive microorganisms make up 24% to 35% of isolates, with *S. aureus* and *Enterococcus* species accounting for the greatest number. A significant number of bloodstream infections are polymicrobial (9% to 22%) (5,177,178,212). *S. pyogenes* bacteremia has been reported in conjunction with NH outbreaks (43). Fungemia, an increasingly frequent nosocomial infection in the United States, has also been reported in the NH (5,34). In pediatric chronic care facilities, *H. influenzae* type b has been associated with outbreaks of bacteremia (214). Bacteremia is associated with a disproportionately high mortality rate relative to its prevalence in the LTCF. In the NH, the overall mortality rate has been reported to be 21% to 35% (5,177,178,212). However, the case fatality rate for subsets of residents can be even higher. In one series, a respiratory source for bacteremia was associated with a 50% mortality rate (5). Polymicrobial bacteremia may also carry a worse prognosis (178,212).

Reservoirs and Sources

Primary Bacteremia

Endogenous flora of the resident and possibly bacteria acquired from other residents or staff members are the major source of pathogens for primary bacteremias.

Secondary Bacteremia

Sources for secondary bacteremia are those identified for UTIs, LRTIs, and SSTIs.

Transmission

Primary Bacteremia

Direct contact with other residents and staff members or with contaminated equipment may supply the microbes that subsequently infect an intravascular device.

Secondary Bacteremia

Transmission follows that noted for UTIs, LRTIs, and SSTIs.

Risk Factors

Primary Bacteremia

Risk factors for primary bacteremia in LTCFs have not been described but presumably are similar to those in the hospital setting.

Secondary Bacteremia

Urinary catheterization and urinary incontinence are significantly associated with bacteremia in NH residents (177,212, 213). Pressure ulcers have been associated with polymicrobial bacteremia. Risk factors for bacteremia identified in multivariable analysis include advanced Alzheimer's disease, chronic UTI, hypoalbuminemia, hypocholesterolemia, anemia, and elevated blood glucose (212,213).

Gastrointestinal Tract Infections

Description

Acute Gastroenteritis

Outbreaks of gastrointestinal tract infections receive most of the attention in LTCFs, but acute gastroenteritis is, nevertheless, a common endemic problem in NHs and probably in other types of LTCFs. In NH surveillance studies, gastroenteritis defined in terms of the CDC criteria for nosocomial infections or various combinations of diarrhea, nausea, vomiting, and abdominal pain has occurred with frequencies ranging up to 2.5 infections per 1,000 resident care days (14,16–21). In most studies in which it was specifically mentioned, the gastroenteritis rate was greater than 0.1 but less than 1.0 episodes per 1,000 resident care days. In these incidence studies, gastroenteritis accounted for 1% to 17% of all infections observed. The higher rates were observed in NHs that experienced outbreaks during the study period. Gastroenteritis has also been noted in 1-day prevalence studies. Garibaldi et al. (22) reported a 1.3% prevalence rate of diarrhea in seven Salt Lake City, Utah, NHs; Scheckler and Peterson (17) reported a 0.5% prevalence rate in eight rural Wisconsin NHs. Gastroenteritis accounted for 7% and 4% of all infections in these two studies, respectively.

The etiology of acute gastroenteritis in NH surveillance studies has not usually been specified, reflecting both the difficulties in diagnosing enteric diseases and the limited laboratory backup in many facilities. In contrast, the etiologic agents are more frequently identified in outbreaks. Reported causes of gastroenteritis outbreaks in NHs include *Salmonella* species, *Shigella* species, *S. aureus, C. perfringens, E. coli* O157:H7, *Aeromonas hydrophila, Campylobacter jejuni, Bacillus cereus,* caliciviruses (Norwalk and Norwalk-like agents), astroviruses, rotaviruses, and *Giardia lamblia* (13,42,50,55–57,59,64,82,215). How frequently these pathogens cause endemic disease remains to be established.

Outbreaks of gastroenteritis often involve foodborne pathogens. A report by Levine et al. (42) from the CDC denoted 115 outbreaks of foodborne disease affecting NHs in 26 states during the period 1975 through 1987. Altogether, 4,944 persons became ill during these outbreaks, and 51 persons died. An etiologic agent was established in about half of the outbreaks. *Salmonella* species accounted for 52% of the outbreaks and 81% of the deaths. Eggs were frequently implicated in the spread of salmonellosis. *S. aureus* was the next most commonly identified cause, accounting for 23% of outbreaks.

Less is known about gastroenteritis in other types of LTCFs, but the available information indicates that they are not spared (56,216). *Salmonella* species have caused outbreaks in psychiatric hospitals and institutions for the retarded. An outbreak caused by *G. lamblia* has been reported in a residential facility for the mentally retarded. Institutional outbreaks of amebiasis have also been recognized (see also Chapter 24).

***Clostridium Difficile*–Associated Diarrhea**

Although *C. difficile* has rarely been mentioned in surveillance studies performed in NHs, several reports published in the last decade suggest that *C. difficile*-associated diarrhea occurs in both endemic and epidemic form in LTCFs (see Chapter 36). In 1986, Bender et al. (217) reported on 7 months of surveillance in a chronic care hospital ward of an LTCF in Baltimore. Their study was prompted by the occurrence of six cases of *C. difficile*-associated diarrhea within a 2-week period. At the beginning of their study, 28% of the 40 patients were toxin positive and 33% were culture positive. At each subsequent sampling time, 14% to 30% of patients were toxin positive. Twenty-two percent of 40 patients tested on admission were toxin positive, and 19% of 31 patients who were negative on admission subsequently became toxin positive. Fifteen percent of environmental cultures were positive for *C. difficile.* Approximately one third of the toxin-positive patients had diarrhea. Control efforts, including treatment of toxin-positive patients, failed to alter the high prevalence rates.

In a follow-up study conducted in a 233-bed LTCF, the same group of investigators evaluated *C. difficile* infection in residents receiving antimicrobial therapy over a 6-month period (218). Of the 36 residents studied after their first course of therapy, 12 (33%) proved to have *C. difficile* infection. Seven residents had positive toxin assays, and 11 had positive stool cultures. Only one of the infected patients had diarrhea.

Other authors have reported outbreaks, clusters, and endemic cases of *C. difficile* in LTCFs (67). In their surveillance study in a 120-bed VA NH, Jacobson and Strausbaugh (20) observed four symptomatic patients with positive toxin assays who were housed in adjacent rooms on one wing of their facility over a 7-month period. Three facility-wide surveys conducted during 1 year in a large Canadian NH and chronic care hospital revealed prevalences ranging from 2.1% to 8.1% and 7.1% to 14.7%, respectively (219). Only 17% of these cases had diarrhea at the time that *C. difficile* was detected. Finally, after finding electronic rectal thermometers contaminated with *C. difficile,* Brooks et al. (220) studied the frequency of *C. difficile*-associated diarrhea in a 538-bed chronic care skilled nursing facility before and after the replacement of electronic thermometers with single-use disposable thermometers. There were 40 cases of *C. difficile*-associated diarrhea in the 6 months before the intervention and only 11 in the subsequent 6 months. When electronic thermometers were in use, *C. difficile*-associated diarrhea occurred with a frequency of 0.41 cases per 1,000 resident care days. After the disposable thermometers were introduced, the frequency dropped to 0.27 cases per 1,000 resident care days, a highly significant reduction.

These reports suggest that *C. difficile*-associated diarrhea is common in LTCFs, especially NHs. However, puzzling questions remain. Why is the frequency of *C. difficile* colonization so high in residents of LTCFs? Why is the frequency of diarrheal disease in patients with toxin-positive stool specimens so low in some studies? These questions await answers in the results of future studies.

Viral Hepatitis

Outbreaks of viral hepatitis have occasionally occurred in LTCFs, primarily in facilities for mentally retarded children (57, 84) but also in NHs (69,99) (see Chapter 45). Both hepatitis A and hepatitis B have been recognized in these settings. Attack rates of 60% to 70% are common for hepatitis A in institutions for mentally retarded children. One small outbreak of hepatitis

B has been described in a Scandinavian home for the elderly (57). A seroprevalence study of 199 residents in three St. Louis NHs found prevalences of 80%, 24%, and 4% for antibodies to hepatitis A, hepatitis B, and hepatitis C, respectively (221). The prevalence of chronic hepatitis C infection as established by positive recombinant immunoblot and polymerase chain reaction assays was 2.5% in one intermediary care facility for the developmentally challenged (222). Hepatitis has received no comment in the NH surveillance studies. Taken as a whole, these observations suggest that viral hepatitis is not a common problem in NHs, but the potential is present. Contamination of food or drink by a foodhandler infected with hepatitis A can have major repercussions in LTCFs.

Reservoirs and Sources

Acute Gastroenteritis

Infected patients or staff members and contaminated food or drink are the major sources of pathogens in LTCFs, as they are in the hospital (see Chapter 24).

***Clostridium Difficile*–Associated Diarrhea**

As in the hospital, colonized or infected individuals and probably, to some extent, spores in the environment constitute the reservoir of *C. difficile* in LTCFs (see Chapter 36).

Viral Hepatitis

Infected residents or staff members constitute the main reservoir for hepatitis viruses in LTCFs, as they do in hospitals (see Chapter 45).

Transmission

Acute Gastroenteritis

In LTCFs, as in other settings, microorganisms causing acute gastroenteritis may be transmitted person to person by the fecal-oral route or by ingestion of contaminated food or drink (see Chapter 24). Fomites may play a role in some situations.

***Clostridium Difficile*–Associated Diarrhea**

Residents in LTCFs probably acquire *C. difficile* as a result of person-to-person spread via the fecal-oral route or from contaminated objects in the environment (see Chapter 36). As noted previously, electronic rectal thermometers were implicated in disease transmission in one LTCF study (220).

Viral Hepatitis

Hepatitis A virus is generally transmitted person to person by the fecal-oral route. Contaminated food or drink often plays a role in outbreaks. Hepatitis B virus is generally transmitted person to person as a result of direct contact between infected blood or serum-derived body fluids with mucosal surfaces or nonintact skin of susceptible individuals (see Chapter 45). Contamination of diabetic care supplies resulted in one outbreak of hepatitis B in a skilled nursing facility (99). Hepatitis C virus generally requires contact with infected blood for transmission.

Risk Factors

Acute Gastroenteritis

No specific risk factors for gastroenteritis have been identified in prospective studies conducted in LTCFs, but they are probably similar to those identified in hospital patients (see Chapter 24). It seems highly likely that decreased gastric acidity because of age, disease, or medications; decreased gastrointestinal tract motility resulting from narcotic use; disturbances of normal gastrointestinal flora because of antimicrobial therapy; and fecal incontinence are major predisposing factors.

***Clostridium Difficile*–Associated Diarrhea**

Thomas et al. (218) examined risk factors for *C. difficile* infection in LTCF residents receiving antimicrobial therapy. Stool incontinence and residence on a chronic care ward that had been the site of a previous outbreak were the only significant differences between the infected and uninfected groups. Infected patients, however, tended to be older, to have diagnosed dementia, to have lower mean Mini-Mental State Examination scores, to have pressure sores, and to have lower body mass indices. Along similar lines, Simor et al. (219) found that previous antibiotic treatment within 8 weeks, presence of a feeding tube, urinary and fecal incontinence, and presence of more than three underlying diseases were statistically independent variables associated with *C. difficile* infection in their NH and chronic care hospital residents.

Viral Hepatitis

Specific risk factors for viral hepatitis have not been delineated for residents of LTCFs, but presumably they do not differ from those established for hospitalized patients (see Chapter 45). Absence of serum antibody against hepatitis A and B viruses is clearly important, establishing a rationale for vaccination in high-risk residents (e.g., children in institutions for the mentally retarded).

PREVENTION AND CONTROL

Immunizations and Prophylactic Therapy

Effective immunization and prophylaxis are available for a variety of diseases (Table 106.8). However, primary disease prevention is generally underused in LTCFs.

Influenza

Studies regarding the effectiveness of influenza vaccine in NHs have yielded conflicting results. Influenza vaccination has been shown to produce protective antibody titers in as few as 17% and as many as 69% of NH residents in different studies (11,223). However, controlled trials have demonstrated substantial benefit in the form of reducing hospitalization and complications such as pneumonia and death (74,78,184,223–226). NHs should vaccinate all residents in October and November and continue vaccinations into March for newly admitted residents as long as vaccine is available (227). Immunization of more than 80% of NH residents provides a degree of "herd immunity"

TABLE 106.8. VACCINATION AND PROPHYLAXIS RECOMMENDATIONS FOR LONG-TERM CARE FACILITIES

Vaccine/Prophylaxis (ref)	Recommendation
Influenza vaccine (227) Inactivated split virus; 0.5 mL IM annually	Optimal time for nursing home vaccination is October–November. Immunization of unvaccinated residents should continue as long as vaccine is available Contraindication—anaphylactic hypersensitivity to eggs
Influenza antiviral medications (227,233)	1. When influenza vaccination is contraindicated: administer throughout influenza season or during peak community influenza activity 2. Adjunct to immunization: administer to NH residents who are vaccinated after a community outbreak of influenza has begun until immunity has developed (approximately 2 weeks) 3. Institutional outbreaks: administer to all residents regardless of immunization status for at least 2 weeks, continuing for 1 week after the end of the outbreak and as an adjunct to immunization if influenza is noted in the community before vaccination
Influenza A	Amantadine 100 mg/day or less (reduce dosage for creatinine clearance less than 50 mL/min) Rimantadine 100 mg/day
Influenza A and B	Zanamivir (approved for treatment only, not prophylaxis) 10 mg twice daily via inhalation Oseltamivir 75 mg/day (reduce dosage for creatinine clearance less than 30 mL/min)
Pneumococcal polysaccharide vaccine (238) 23 valent One dose IM	Consider immunization for any LTCF resident All residents 65 and older and anyone with a chronic condition that increases the risk of pneumococcal disease (i.e., chronic lung disease, heart disease, diabetes, renal failure, alcoholism) Revaccination—persons 65 or older first vaccinated before age 65 should be given a one-time revaccination 5 years after initial vaccination
Tetanus-diphtheria toxoid (Adult Td) (239) unimmunized—two doses IM 1—2 months apart; third dose 6–12 months later Everyone—booster every 10 years	Unimmunized/history unknown administer full series All other residents, booster every 10 years Clean wounds—Td if >10 years since last vaccination Dirty wounds, puncture, frostbite—Td if fully immunized and >5 years since last booster dose; If unimmunized, inadequate primary series (<3 doses) or history unknown, tetanus immune globulin + primary immunization series Contraindications—neurologic reaction or hypersensitivity to previous dose
Latent tuberculosis (241) Isoniazid 300 mg (with pyridoxine) Daily	TB skin test >10mm induration, no fibrotic lesions *or* TB skin test >5mm induration + fibrotic lesions on chest x-ray no evidence of active disease, no prior treatment for TB: isoniazid for 9 months

IM, intramuscular; LTCF, long-term care facility; NH, nursing home.

and, thus, protects against institutional outbreaks. This strategy has been associated with a decreased risk for influenza outbreaks in some studies, but even institutions with high vaccination rates have experienced epidemics (13,77,78,226). Immunizing NH employees may be the most effective preventive measure. Studies in the United Kingdom demonstrated that facilities with substantial vaccination rates among healthcare workers (61%) experienced significant reductions in patient mortality and influenza-like illness independent of patient immunization status (186, 187).

In addition to vaccination, antiviral drugs should be used for persons in whom influenza vaccine is contraindicated, for prophylaxis during institutional outbreaks regardless of immunization status, and as an adjunct to immunization if influenza is noted in the community before vaccination (227). In the United States there are four antiviral agents licensed for use, amantadine, rimantadine, zanamivir, and oseltamivir. Prophylaxis with amantadine and rimantadine have demonstrated 70% to 90% effectiveness in preventing illness from influenza A infection (226–229). Drawbacks to amantadine use include its side effects, inactivity against influenza B, and rapid appearance of amantadine-resistance in influenza A isolates (76). NH residents appear to tolerate rimantadine better (223,228). In contrast to amantadine and rimantadine, zanamivir and oseltamivir have activity against both influenza A and B viruses (227). Although only oseltamivir has an indication for prophylaxis, one study reported zanamivir use in quelling an outbreak of amantadine-resistant influenza. It was well tolerated and temporally associated with termination of the outbreak (229). Clinical studies have demonstrated oseltamivir's safety and effectiveness in frail older adults in LTCFs too. In a double-blind, randomized, controlled trial involving 572 elderly senior care home residents, the oseltamivir treated group suffered fewer cases of influenza and fewer influenza-related complications (230).

The decision to institute antiviral prophylaxis in LTCFs requires weighing the potential risk of an institutional outbreak against likely side effects of the prophylactic agents and their costs (231). Delays in instituting prophylaxis may be disastrous for frail, older adults. Drinka et al. (232) studied the consequences of delaying prophylaxis in NHs over the course of six influenza seasons. From their observations, these authors concluded that NHs need to start antivirals as soon as the first NH case is confirmed by a rapid, on-site test when culture-confirmed influenza is present in the community. All NH residents regardless of vaccination status should receive antiviral therapy for at least 2 weeks or until 1 week after the last case appears (227, 233).

Pneumococcal Infections

The morbidity and mortality associated with pneumococcal disease remain high despite appropriate antibiotic therapy. Fatality rates in bacteremic pneumococcal disease range from 25% to 40% in persons older than 50 and in those with chronic illnesses (45,234). The currently available 23-valent vaccine contains the capsular polysaccharides of serotypes that account for approximately 90% of bacteremic infections. Although the vaccine is effective in young healthy persons, its efficacy in the elderly and infirm is controversial. A protective effect (53% to 64%) has been reported among immunocompetent elderly persons with underlying chronic diseases (235). However, a randomized, controlled trial among elderly patients in Sweden failed to demonstrate that vaccination prevented pneumococcal pneumonia (236). Because any protective effect is short-lived in the elderly and immunocompromised, a one-time revaccination is recommended for persons 65 years and older 5 years after initial vaccination if they were younger than 65 when first vaccinated (237,238) (Table 106.8).

Tetanus and Diphtheria

Although tetanus is now a rare disease in the United States, with an incidence of less than 100 cases per year, over half of the cases occur in persons aged 60 and older. The elderly also have the highest mortality, with a case fatality rate of 60% (152). Older persons are particularly likely to lack immunity, because routine immunization only started in the 1940s.

Tetanus has been reported in association with chronic wounds such as skin ulcers, surgical site infections, abscesses, and gangrene, placing NH residents at increased risk. Studies have shown that NH residents achieve protective levels of antitoxin in response to immunization (152). Tetanus immunization should be part of routine care in NHs.

Antibody studies indicate that at least 50% of adults in the United States are susceptible to diphtheria, and the percentage is higher in the elderly. Diphtheria immunization should be combined with tetanus toxoid for NH residents and given on the same schedule (223,239).

Hepatitis B

Thirty percent to 80% of residents in institutions for the mentally retarded have serologic evidence of hepatitis B infection, likely because of frequent exposure to open skin lesions, saliva, and other contaminated body fluids (223). Screening for hepatitis B on admission is recommended as is vaccination of susceptible individuals.

Hepatitis A

Immunoglobulins for prevention of hepatitis A may be considered for institutional outbreaks wherein fecal-oral transmission is likely (223). Hepatitis A vaccine may also be useful in outbreaks and in residents of institutions for the developmentally challenged (240).

Tuberculosis

Tuberculosis infection in elderly NH residents generally results from reactivation of latent infection (70). Resistant tuberculosis is rare in the LTCF, and INH remains the drug of choice in this setting. INH prophylaxis can effectively prevent clinical tuberculosis (241). Among Arkansas NH residents treated with INH, 98.4% of recent skin test converters were protected from clinical tuberculosis (242). However, the usefulness of INH among the elderly is limited by the side effect of hepatitis, which increases in frequency with age and is potentially life threatening. In the NH, treatment with INH causes hepatic toxicity in 4% to 5% of residents and other side effects in 6% (242). Nevertheless, available data support giving INH to NH residents with newly reactive tuberculin skin tests regardless of age. Data also suggest that INH preventive therapy may aid in the management of NH residents with positive tuberculin skin tests and fibrotic lesions on their chest radiographs (243). Less is known about the impact of treating NH residents with positive skin tests and other clinical risk factors such as diabetes, steroid administration, and malnutrition. Contraindications to INH include previous INH-associated hepatic injury, other acute liver disease, or other severe adverse reaction to INH (see also Chapter 37).

Infection Control Program

Infection control in LTCFs has drawn increased attention over the last 20 years (244,245). Although surveys performed in several states during the late 1980s pointed to a number of deficiencies (26,246), more recent surveys have found considerable improvement. For example, a 1995 survey of 136 New England skilled nursing LTCFs found that 98% had personnel responsible for infection control (247). Ninety percent of these persons were registered nurses, and more than 50% had received formal training in infection control. These individuals spent a median of 8 hours per week on activities related to infection control. Moreover, survey results identified improvement in virtually all categories since 1988.

Regulatory considerations continue to drive efforts to improve infection control in LTCFs. In the United States, the Health Care Financing Administration, the Occupational Safety and Health Administration (OSHA), the Joint Commission on Accreditation of Healthcare Organizations, and various state and local health departments have issued standards and regulations that address infection control practices in LTCFs (248). The Minister of National Health and Welfare has circulated guidelines for Canadian facilities (249). Working together, SHEA and APIC have published detailed guidelines for infection control in LTCFs (142,250).

Other aspects of LTCF infection control programs have also received attention in recent years. The Nebraska Infection Control Network has developed a 2-day basic skills training program for LTCF infection control professionals (251). Evaluation of the first 17 courses conducted between 1986 and 1990 at three different sites indicated that course attendance had favorably influenced infection control activities in the professional's facility (252). Results of a more recent survey suggested a sustained effect by course graduates on their institutions' infection control program (253). Other publications have outlined the specific contributions that hospital-based infection control professionals, physicians, hospital epidemiologists, nurses' aides, and microbiology laboratories can make to infection control programs in LTCFs (254–258).

The essential elements of an infection control program for LTCFs have been organized and conceptualized in a number of different but overlapping frameworks (142,247,250,259–261). The following description of key components in LTCF infection control programs is taken, for the most part, from the SHEA/APIC position paper (142). The authors of this paper envision the program being implemented by well-trained infection control professionals who report to and function under the auspices of a multidisciplinary oversight committee that meets on a regular basis. Specific program elements are outlined briefly here. This position paper, like the more recent and generic infrastructure paper (250), gives specific recommendations for each element and rates each one in accordance with the strength and quality of evidence supporting their use.

Surveillance

Data about LTCF-acquired infections are essential to plan control activities and educational programs and to prevent epidemics. Good surveillance requires well-defined criteria for infection (Table 106.5) and sensitive case finding methods. Walking rounds in the LTCF one or more times per week is recommended for case finding in conjunction with review of reports from nurses, charts, laboratory reports, medication records, and cardexes. Data need to be compiled and analyzed on a regular, usually monthly, basis. Data regarding infectious morbidity are optimally presented in terms of incidence rates (e.g., the number of infections per 1,000 resident care days). Distribution of this information to appropriate committees and personnel and storage of the records are also important.

Outbreak Control

Routine surveillance facilitates the recognition of outbreaks. Once an outbreak is suspected, the infection control professional may need to gather additional data to confirm the existence of an outbreak, develop a case definition, analyze the pattern of disease occurrence, formulate hypotheses regarding transmission, design control measures, evaluate control measures, consult with an experienced epidemiologist, or prepare reports for local authorities and supervisors.

Isolation and Precautions

LTCFs need defined policies for identifying and containing the risks of disease transmission posed by infected residents, staff members, and visitors. Some facilities use one of the major systems developed for use in the hospital, whereas other facilities develop their own. The availability of private rooms for patients requiring contact precautions or respiratory isolation rooms to prevent transmission of airborne pathogens is an important consideration in developing local policies. Meeting OSHA standards for blood-borne pathogens is also an essential requirement of any facility's policies. Specific guidelines for dealing with antimicrobial-resistant pathogens in LTCFs have been published in two SHEA position papers (40,262).

Policies and Procedures

As in the hospital, the development and regular updating of infection control procedures to cover such topics as hand hygiene, laundry, dietetic services, physical therapy, disinfectant and antiseptic use, medical devices, pets (see Chapter 101), visitors, and disposal of infectious wastes form an integral part of the infection control program. Pet-assisted therapy warrants specific policies in LTCFs that use this approach (263).

Education

As in the hospital, staff education is a pivotal component of infection control programs in LTCFs. Information regarding patterns of infectious morbidity, disease transmission, isolation and precautions, recognition of infection, and hand washing can help the staff function more safely. An orientation to infection control is essential for new employees, and periodic in-service programs serve as a review for other employees.

Resident Health Program

Comprehensive resident health programs ensure administration of appropriate vaccines; secure admission, annual and post-exposure tuberculin skin tests; and address risk reduction in residents prone to aspiration, obstructive uropathy, pressure sores, and other medical conditions that may be complicated by infection.

Employee Health Program

Employee health programs ensure that all employees are free of communicable diseases at the time of employment. They also ensure that tuberculin skin tests are administered annually and as indicated after exposure, that appropriate vaccines are offered, and that exposures to certain infections (e.g., tuberculosis or HIV infection) are managed properly. (See Chapters 78, 79 and 99.)

Antibiotic Review

Resistant pathogens, high levels of use, and inappropriate use are well-recognized problems associated with antimicrobial agents in NHs (40,264). For that reason, regular review of antimicrobial use and patterns of resistance is recommended. Presentation of this information to the medical staff can guide practice patterns and decrease the prevalence of resistant pathogens.

Product Review and Evaluation

Selection of disinfectants, antiseptics, medical devices, and other products commonly used in LTCFs may be difficult for the uninitiated, warranting the input of a knowledgeable infection control professional or an infectious diseases consultant (see Chapters 85 and 97).

Disease Reporting

LTCFs, like other healthcare organizations, are obligated to notify public health authorities in a timely manner about the occurrence of reportable infections within the facility.

Quality Management

Infection control is an important aspect of any quality management program within LTCFs. As in the hospital, the infection control professional in LTCFs, by virtue of training, experience, and focus, can uniquely contribute to the facility's quality management program.

REFERENCES

1. Jones A. The National Nursing Home Survey: 1999 summary. National Center for Health Statistics. *Vital Health Stat* 2002;13(152).
2. Centers for Disease Control and Prevention. Trends in aging—United States and worldwide. *MMWR Morb Mortal Wkly Rep* 2003;52:101–106.
3. National Center for Health Statistics. *Highlights of trends in the health of older Americans: United States, 1994.* Washington DC: US Department of Health and Human Services, 1995.
4. Hing E. Effects of the prospective payment system on nursing homes. Vital and health statistics, series 13: data from the National Health Survey. Hyattsville, MD: US Department of Health and Human Services, 1989.
5. Muder RR, Brennen C, Wagener MM, et al. Bacteremia in a long-term-care facility: a five-year prospective study of 163 consecutive episodes. *Clin Infect Dis* 1992;14:647–654.
6. Mott P, Barker W. Treatment decisions for infections occurring in nursing home residents. *J Am Geriatr Soc* 1988;36:820–824.
7. Kerr H, Byrd J. Nursing home patients transferred by ambulance to a VA emergency department. *J Am Geriatr Soc* 1991;39:132–136.
8. Frijters DH, Mor V, Dupaquier JN, et al. Transitions across various continuing care settings. *Age Ageing* 1997;26(Suppl 2):73–76.
9. Rubenstein L, Ouslander J, Wieland D. Dynamics and clinical implications of the nursing home-hospital interface. *Clin Geriatr Med* 1988; 4:471–491.
10. Magaziner J, Tenney J, DeForge B, et al. Prevalence and characteristics of nursing home-acquired infections in the aged. *J Am Geriatr Soc* 1991;39:1071–1078.
11. Woodson C, Sachs G. Prevention, diagnosis, and management of infection in the nursing home. *Clin Geriatr Med* 1988;4:507–525.
12. Sekscenski E. Discharges from nursing homes: 1985 National Nursing Home Survey. Vital and health statistics, series 13: data from the National Health Survey. 1990;103:1–87.
13. Strausbaugh LJ, Sukumar SR, Joseph CL. Outbreaks in nursing homes: unappreciated hazard for the frail elderly. *Clin Infect Dis* 2003; 36:870–876.
14. Alvarez S, Shell C, Woolley T, et al. Nosocomial infections in long-term facilities. *J Gerontol* 1988;43:M9–M17.
15. Darnowski S, Gordon M, Simor A. Two years of infection surveillance in a geriatric long-term care facility. *Am J Infect Control* 1991;19: 185–190.
16. Vlahov D, Tenney J, Cervino K, et al. Routine surveillance for infections in nursing homes: experience at two facilities. *Am J Infect Control* 1987;15:47–53.
17. Scheckler W, Peterson P. Infections and infection control among residents of eight rural Wisconsin nursing homes. *Arch Intern Med* 1986;146:1981–1984.
18. Jackson M, Fierer J, Barrett-Connor E, et al. Intensive surveillance for infections in a three-year study of nursing home patients. *Am J Epidemiol* 1992;135:685–696.
19. Schicker J, Franson T, Duthie E Jr, et al. Comparison of methods for calculation and depiction of incidence infection rates in long-term care facilities. *J Clin Epidemiol* 1988;41:757–761.
20. Jacobson C, Strausbaugh L. Incidence and impact of infection in a nursing home care unit. *Am J Infect Control* 1990;18:151–159.
21. Hoffman N, Jenkins R, Putney K. Nosocomial infection rates during a one-year period in a nursing home care unit of a Veterans Administration hospital. *Am J Infect Control* 1990;18:55–63.
22. Garibaldi R, Brodine S, Matsumiya R. Infections among patients in nursing homes: policies, prevalence, and problems. *N Engl J Med* 1981;305:731–735.
23. Setia U, Serventi I, Lorenz P. Nosocomial infections among patients in a long-term care facility: spectrum, prevalence, and risk factors. *Am J Infect Control* 1985;13:57–62.
24. Steinmiller A, Robb S, Muder R. Prevalence of nosocomial infection in long-term-care Veterans Administration medical centers. *Am J Infect Control* 1991;19:143–146.
25. Beck-Sague C, Villarino E, Giuliano D, et al. Infectious diseases and death among nursing home residents: results of surveillance in 13 nursing homes. *Infect Control Hosp Epidemiol* 1994;15:494–496.
26. Nicolle LE, Strausbaugh LJ, Garibaldi RA. Infections and antibiotic resistance in nursing homes. *Clin Microbiol Rev* 1996;9:1–17.
27. Lee Y-L, Thrupp LD, Friis RH, et al. Nosocomial infection and antibiotic utilization in geriatric patients: a pilot prospective surveillance program in skilled nursing facilities. *Gerontology* 1992;38:223–232.
28. Smith PW, Seip CW, Schaefer SC, et al. Microbiologic survey of long-term care facilities. *Am J Infect Control* 2000;28:8–13.
29. Nicolle LE. Urinary tract infections. In: Yoshikawa TT, Ouslander JG, eds. *Infection management for geriatrics in long-term care facilities.* New York: Marcel Dekker, 2002:173–195.
30. Mylotte JM. Pneumonitis and bronchitis. In: Yoshikawa TT, Ouslander JG, eds. *Infection management for geriatrics in long-term care facilities.* New York: Marcel Dekker, 2002:223–243.
31. Livesley N, Chow AW. Infected pressure ulcers. In: Yoshikawa TT, Ouslander JG, eds. *Infection management for geriatrics in long-term care facilities.* New York: Marcel Dekker, 2002:257–281.
32. Schmader K, Twersky J. Herpes zoster, cellulitis, and scabies. In: Yoshikawa TT, Ouslander JG, eds. *Infection management for geriatrics in long-term care facilities.* New York: Marcel Dekker, 2002:28300-303.
33. Schmader K. Herpes zoster in the elderly: issues related to geriatrics. *Clin Infect Dis* 1999;28:736–739.
34. Kauffman CA, Hedderwick SA. Candida and other fungi. In: Yoshikawa TT, Ouslander JG, eds. *Infection management for geriatrics in long-term care facilities.* New York: Marcel Dekker, 2002:449–472.
35. Smith MA, Duke WM. A retrospective review of nosocomial infections in an acute rehabilitative and chronic population at a large skilled nursing facility. *J Am Geriatr Soc* 1994;42:45–49.
36. Loeb M, McGeer A, McArthur M, et al. Surveillance for outbreaks of respiratory tract infections in nursing homes. *CMAJ*2000;162: 1133–1137.
37. Strausbaugh LJ. Methicillin-resistant *Staphylococcus aureus.* In: Yoshikawa TT, Ouslander JG, eds. *Infection management for geriatrics in long-term care facilities.* New York: Marcel Dekker, 2002:383–409.
38. Bradley SF. Methicillin-resistant *Staphylococcus aureus*: long-term care concerns. *Am J Med* 1999;106(5A):2S–10S.
39. Kotilainen P, Routamaa M, Peltonen R, et al. Eradication of methicillin-resistant *Staphylococcus aureus* from a health center ward and associated nursing home. *Arch Intern Med* 2001;161:859–863.
40. Strausbaugh LJ, Crossley KB, Nurse BA, et al. Antimicrobial resistance in long-term care facilities. *Infect Control Hosp Epidemiol* 1996; 17:129–140.
41. Stover B, Duff A, Adams G, et al. Emergence and control of methicillin-resistant *Staphylococcus aureus* in a children's hospital and pediatric long-term care facility. *Am J Infect Control* 1992;20:248–255.
42. Levine W, Smart J, Archer D, et al. Foodborne disease outbreaks in nursing homes, 1975 through 1987. *JAMA* 1991;266:2105–2109.
43. Schwartz B, Ussery X. Group A streptococcal outbreaks in nursing homes. *Infect Control Hosp Epidemiol* 1992;13:742–747.
44. Gleich S, Morad Y, Echague R, et al. *Streptococcus pneumoniae* serotype 4 outbreak in a home for the aged: report and review of recent outbreaks. *Infect Control Hosp Epidemiol* 2000;21:711–717.
45. Nuorti JP, Butler JC, Crutcher JM, et al. An outbreak of multidrug-resistant pneumococcal pneumonia and bacteremia among unvaccinated nursing home residents. *N Engl J Med* 1998;338:1861–1868.
46. Mody L, McNeil SA, Bradley SF. Vancomycin (Glycopeptide)-resistant enterococci. In: Yoshikawa TT, Ouslander JG, eds. *Infection management for geriatrics in long-term care facilities.* New York: Marcel Dekker, 2002:411–428.

47. Bonilla HF, Zervos MA, Lyons MJ, et al. Colonization with vancomycin-resistant *Enterococcus faecium*: comparison of a long-term care unit with an acute-care hospital. *Infect Control Hosp Epidemiol* 1997;18: 333–339.
48. Silverblatt FJ, Tibert C, Mikolich D, et al. Preventing the spread of vancomycin-resistant enterococci in a long-term care facility. *J Am Geriatr Soc* 2000;48:1211–1215.
49. Ostrowsky BE, Trick WE, Sohn AH, et al. Control of vancomycin-resistant enterococcus in health care facilities in a region. *N Engl J Med* 2001;344:1427–1433.
50. Carter A, Borczyk A, Carlson J, et al. A severe outbreak of *Escherichia coli* O157:H7-associated hemorrhagic colitis in a nursing home. *N Engl J Med* 1987;317:1496–1500.
51. Aktar AJ. Infectious diarrheas. In: Yoshikawa TT, Ouslander JG, eds. *Infection management for geriatrics in long-term fare facilities.* New York: Marcel Dekker, 2002:305–312.
52. Smith PF, Stricof RL, Shayegani M, et al. Cluster of *Haemophilus influenzae* Type b infections in adults. *JAMA*1988;260:1446–1449.
53. Troy CJ, Peeling RW, Ellis AG, et al. *Chlamydia pneumoniae* as a new source of infectious outbreaks in nursing homes. *JAMA* 1997; 27:1214–1218.
54. Armstrong-Evans M, Litt M, McArthur MA, et al. Control of transmission of vancomycin-resistant *Enterococcus faecium* in a long-term–care facility. *Infect Control Hosp Epidemiol* 1999;20:312–317.
55. Jackson M, Fierer J. Infections and infection risk in residents of long-term care facilities: a review of the literature, 1970–1984. *Am J Infect Control* 1985;13:63–77.
56. Verghese A, Berk S, eds. *Infections in nursing homes and long-term care facilities.* Basel: Karger, 1990.
57. Smith PW, ed. *Infection control in long-term care facilities,* 2nd ed. Albany, NY: Delmar Publishers Inc., 1994.
58. Standaert S, Hutchesen R, Schaffner W. Nosocomial transmission of salmonella gastroenteritis to laundry workers in a nursing home. *Infect Control Hosp Epidemiol* 1994;15:22–26.
59. Layton MC, Calliste SG, Gomez TM, et al. A Mixed foodborne outbreak with *Salmonella heidelberg* and *Campylobacter jejuni* in a nursing home. *Infect Control Hosp Epidemiol* 1997;18:115–121.
60. McCall B, Stafford R, Cherian S, et al. An outbreak of multi-resistant *Shigella sonnei* in a long-stay geriatric nursing centre. *Comm Dis Intel* 2000;24:272–275.
61. Dhawan VK. Gram-negative bacteria. In: Yoshikawa TT, Ouslander JG, eds. *Infection management for geriatrics in long-term care facilities.* New York: Marcel Dekker, 2002:429–448.
62. Addiss D, Davis J, Meade B, et al. A pertussis outbreak in a Wisconsin nursing home. *J Infect Dis* 1991;164:704–710.
63. Stout JE, Brennen C, Muder RR. Legionnaires' disease in a newly constructed long-term care facility. *J Am Geriatr Soc* 2000;48: 1589–1592.
64. Bloom H, Bottone E. *Aeromonas hydrophila* diarrhea in a long-term care setting. *J Am Geriatr Soc* 1990;38:804–806.
65. Wiener J, Quinn JP, Bradford PA, et al. Multiple antibiotic-resistant *Klebsiella* and *Escherichia coli* in nursing homes. *JAMA* 1999;287: 517–523.
66. Olsen SJ, DeBess EE, McGivern TE, et al. A nosocomial outbreak of fluoroquinolone-resistant salmonella infection. *N Engl J Med* 2001; 344:1572–1579.
67. Simor A, Bradley, SF, Strausbaugh LJ, et al. SHEA position paper: *Clostridium difficile* in long-term-care facilities for the elderly. *Infect Control Hosp Epidemiol* 2002;23:696–703.
68. Tallis G, Ng S, Ferreira C. A Nursing home outbreak of *Clostridium perfringens* associated with pureed food. *Aust N Z J Public Health* 1999;23:421–423.
69. Harrington DW, Barrett PV. Hepatitis. In: Yoshikawa TT, Ouslander JG, eds. *Infection management for geriatrics in long-term care facilities.* New York: Marcel Dekker, 2002:305–312.
70. Rajagopalan S, Yoshikawa TT. Tuberculosis in long-term-care facilities. *Infect Control Hosp Epidemiol* 2000;21:611–615.
71. Ijaz K, Dillaha JA, Yang Z, et al. Unrecognized tuberculosis in a nursing home causing death with spread of tuberculosis to the community. *J Am Geriatr Soc* 2002;50:1213–1218.
72. Bentley D. Tuberculosis in long-term care facilities. *Infect Control Hosp Epidemiol* 1990;11:42–46.
73. Faulks JT, Drinka PJ, Shult P. A serious outbreak of parainfluenza type 3 on a nursing unit. *J Am Geriat Soc* 2000;48:1216–1218.
74. Bradley SF, Long-Term-Care Committee for the Society of Healthcare Epidemiology of America. Prevention of influenza in long-term-care facilities. *Infect Control Hosp Epidemiol* 1999;20:629–637.
75. Green KY, Belliot GT, Taylor JL et al. A predominant role for Norwalk-like viruses as agents of epidemic gastroenteritis in Maryland nursing homes for the elderly. *J Infect Dis* 2002;185:133–146.
76. Mast EE, Harmon MW, Gravenstein S, et al. Emergence and possible transmission of amantadine-resistant viruses during nursing home outbreaks of influenza A (H3N2). *Am J Epidemiol* 1991;134: 988–997.
77. Morens DM, Rash VM. Lessons from a nursing home outbreak of influenza A. *Infect Control Hosp Epidemiol* 1995;16:275–280.
78. Libow LS, Neufeld RR, Olson E, et al. Sequential outbreak of influenza A and B in a nursing home: efficacy of vaccine and amantadine. *J Am Geriatr Soc* 1996;44:1153–1157.
79. Wald TG, Shult P, Krause P, et al. A rhinovirus outbreak among residents of a long-term care facility. *Ann Intern Med* 1995;123: 588–593.
80. Johnson I, Hammond GW, Verma MR. Nosocomial coxsackie B4 virus infections in two chronic-care pediatric neurological wards. *J Infect Dis* 1985;151:1153–1156.
81. Demmler GJ, Yow MD, Spector SA, et al. Nosocomial cytomegalovirus infections within two hospitals caring for infants and children. *J Infect Dis* 1987;156:9–16.
82. Bennett RG. Diarrhea among residents of long-term care facilities. *Infect Control Hosp Epidemiol*1993;14:397–404.
83. Lambert M, Patton T, Chudzio T, et al. An outbreak of rotaviral gastroenteritis in a nursing home for senior citizens. *Can J Public Health* 1991;82:351–353.
84. Tassopoulos NC, Roumeliotou-Karayannis A, Sakka M, et al. An epidemic of hepatitis A in an institution for young children. *Am J Epidemiol* 1987;125:302–307.
85. Mahoney FJ, Farley TA, Burbank DF, et al. Evaluation of an intervention program for the control of an outbreak of shigellosis among institutionalized persons. *J Infect Dis* 1993;168:1177–1180.
86. Degelau J. Scabies in long-term care facilities. *Infect Control Hosp Epidemiol* 1992;13:421–425.
87. Piednoir E, Bureau-Chalot F, Gotzamanis A, et al. Direct costs associated with a nosocomial outbreak of adenoviral conjunctivitis infection in a long-term care institution. *Am J Infect Control* 2002;30:407–410.
88. Marx A, Shay DK, Noel JS, et al. An outbreak of acute gastroenteritis in a geriatric long-term-care facility: combined application of epidemiological and molecular diagnostic methods. *Infect Control Hosp Epidemiol* 1999;20:306–311.
89. Fankhauser RL, Monroe SS, Noel JS, et al. Epidemiologic and molecular trends of "Norwalk-like viruses" associated with outbreaks of gastroenteritis in the United States. *J Infect Dis* 2002;186:1–7.
90. Griffin DD, Fletcher M, Levy ME, et al. Outbreaks of adult gastroenteritis traced to a single genotype of rotavirus. *J Infect Dis* 2002;185: 1502–1505.
91. Centers for Disease Control and Prevention. Norovirus activity—United States, 2002. *MMWR Morb Mortal Wkly Rep* 2003;52: 41–45.
92. Loeb M, Simor AE, Mandell L, et al. Two nursing home outbreaks of respiratory infection with *Legionella sainthelensi. J Am Geriatr Soc* 1999;47:547–552.
93. Fiore AE, Iverson C, Messmer T, et al. Outbreak of pneumonia in a long-term care facility: antecedent human parainfluenza virus 1 infection may predispose to bacterial pneumonia. *J Am Geriatr Soc* 1998; 46:1112–1117.
94. Gerber SI, Erdman DD, Pur SL, et al. Outbreak of adenovirus genome type 7d2 infection in a pediatric chronic-care facility and tertiary-care hospital. *Clin Infect Dis* 2001;32:694–700.
95. Fine AD, Bridges CB, De Guzman AM, et al. Influenza A among patients with human immunodeficiency virus: an outbreak of infec-

tion at a residential facility in New York City. *Clin Infect Dis* 2001; 32:1784–1791.
96. Arden NH. Control of influenza in the long-term-care facility: a review of established approaches and newer options. *Infect Control Hosp Epidemiol* 2000;21:59–64.
97. Drinka PJ, Gravenstein S, Krause P, et al. Outbreaks of influenza A and B in a highly immunized nursing home population. *J Fam Pract* 1997;45:509–514.
98. Simor AE. Influenza outbreaks in long-term-care facilities: how can we do better? *Infect Control Hosp Epidemiol* 2002;23:564–567.
99. Khan AJ, Cotter SM, Schulz B, et al. Nosocomial transmission of hepatitis B virus infection among residents with diabetes in a skilled nursing facility. *Infect Control Hosp Epidemiol* 2002;23:313–318.
100. Buffington J, Chapman LE, Stobierski MG, et al. Epidemic keratoconjunctivitis in a chronic care facility: risk factors and measures for control. *J Am Geriatr Soc* 1993;41:1177–1181.
101. Andersen BM, Haugen H, Rasch M, et al. Outbreak of scabies in Norwegian nursing homes and home care patients: control and prevention. *J Hosp Infect* 2000;45:160–164.
102. Trick WE, Weinstein RA, DeMarais PL, et al. Colonization of skilled-care facility residents with antimicrobial-resistant pathogens. *J Am Geriatr Soc* 2001;49:270–276.
103. Drinka P, Faulks JT, Gauerke C, et al. Adverse events associated with methicillin-resistant *Staphylococcus aureus* in a nursing home. *Arch Intern Med* 2001;161:2371–2377.
104. Bonomo RA. Multiple antibiotic-resistant bacteria in long-term-care facilities: an emerging problem in the practice of infectious diseases. *Clin Infect Dis* 2000;31:1414–1422.
105. Bradley SF. Issues in the management of resistant bacteria in long-term-care facilities. *Infect Control Hosp Epidemiol* 1999;20:362–366.
106. Brennen C, Wagener MM, Muder RR. Vancomycin-resistant *Enterococcus faecium* in a long-term care facility. *J Am Geriatr Soc* 1998;46: 157–160.
107. Elizaga ML, Weinstein RA, Hayden MK. Patients in long-term care facilities: a reservoir for vancomycin-resistant enterococci. *Clin Infect Dis* 2002;34:441–446.
108. Baden LR, Thiemke W, Skolnik A, et al. Prolonged colonization with vancomycin-resistant *Enterococcus faecium* in long-term care patients and the significance of "clearance". *Clin Infect Dis* 2001;33: 1654–1660.
109. Lee Y-L, Cesario T, McCauley V, et al. Low-level colonization and infection with ciprofloxacin-resistant gram-negative bacilli in a skilled nursing facility. *Am J Infect Control* 1998;26:552–557.
110. Muder RR, Brennen C, Drenning SD, et al. Multiply antibiotic-resistant gram-negative bacilli in a long-term care facility: a case-control study of patient risk factors and prior antibiotic use. *Infect Control Hosp Epidemiol* 1997;18:809–813.
111. Terpenning MS, Bradley SF, Wan JY, et al. Colonization and infection with antibiotic-resistant bacteria in a long-term care facility. *J Am Geriatr Soc* 1994;42:1062–1069.
112. Mylotte JM, Goodnough S, Tayara A. Antibiotic-resistant organisms among long-term care facility residents on admission to an inpatient geriatrics unit: retrospective and prospective surveillance. *Am J Infect Control* 2001;29:139–144.
113. Mylotte JM. Antimicrobial prescribing in long-term care facilities: prospective evaluation of potential antimicrobial use and cost indicators. *Am J Infect Control* 1999;27:10–19.
114. Loeb M. Antibiotic use in long-term-care facilities: many unanswered questions. *Infect Control Hosp Epidemiol* 2000;21:680–683.
115. DeMarais PL, Gertzen J, Weinstein RA. Nosocomial infections in human immunodeficiency virus-infected patients in a long-term care setting. *Clin Infect Dis* 1997;25:1230–1232.
116. Yoshikawa TT. Perspective: aging and infectious diseases: past, present, and future. *J Infect Dis* 1997;176:1053–1057.
117. Yung RL. Changes in immune function with age. *Rheum Dis Clin North Am* 2000;26:455–473.
118. Castle SC. Clinical relevance of age-related immune dysfunction. *Clin Infect Dis* 2000;31:578–585.
119. Ben-Yehuda A, Weksler M. Host resistance and the immune system. *Clin Geriatr Med* 1992;8:701–712.
120. Cohn J, Hohle C, Buckley E. The relationship between cutaneous cellular immune responsiveness and mortality in a nursing home population. *J Am Geriatr Soc* 1983;31:808–809.
121. Henderson C. Nutrition and malnutrition in the elderly nursing home patient. *Clin Geriatr Med* 1988;4:527–547.
122. Thompson J, Robbins J, Cooper J. Nutrition and immune function in the geriatric population. *Clin Geriatr Med* 1987;3:309–318.
123. Ouslander J. Medical care in the nursing home. *JAMA* 1989;262: 2582–2590.
124. Olive K, Berk S. Infections in the nursing home. *Clin Geriatr Med* 1992;8:821–834.
125. Beers M, Avorn J, Soumerai S, et al. Psychoactive medication in an intermediate care facility. *JAMA* 1988;260:3016–3020.
126. Nicolle LE. The Chronic indwelling catheter and urinary infection in long-term-care facility residents. *Infect Control Hosp Epidemiol* 2001;22:316–321.
127. Norman D, Toledo S. Infections in elderly persons: an altered clinical presentation. *Clin Geriatr Med* 1992;8:713–719.
128. Yoshikawa TT, Norman DC. Approach to fever and infection in the nursing home. *J Am Geriatr Soc* 1996;44:74–82.
129. Harper C, Newton P. Clinical aspects of pneumonia in the elderly veteran. *J Am Geriatr Soc* 1989;37:867–872.
130. Chassagne P, Perol M-B, Doucet J, et al. Is presentation of bacteremia in the elderly the same as in younger patients? *Am J Med* 1996;100: 65–70.
131. Castle S, Norman D, Yeh M, et al. Fever response in elderly nursing home residents: are the older truly colder? *J Am Geriatr Soc* 1991; 39:853–857.
132. Wasserman M, Levinstein M, Keller E, et al. Utility of fever, white blood cells, and differential count in predicting bacterial infections in the elderly. *J Am Geriatr Soc* 1989;37:537–543.
133. Norman DC. Fever in the elderly. *Clin Infect Dis* 2000;31:148–151.
134. Castle SC, Yeh M, Toledo S, et al. Lowering the temperature criterion improves detection of infection in nursing home residents. *Aging Immunol Infect Dis* 1993;4:67–76.
135. Downton J, Andrews E, Puxty J. Silent pyrexia in the elderly. *Age Ageing* 1987;16:41–44.
136. Meyers B, Sherman E, Mendelson M, et al. Bloodstream infections in the elderly. *Am J Med* 1989;86:379–384.
137. Bender B. Sepsis. *Clin Geriatr Med* 1992;8:913–923.
138. Bentley DW, Bradley S, High K, et al. Practice guideline for evaluation of fever and infection in long-term care facilities. *Clin Infect Dis* 2000;31:640–653.
139. Orr PH, Peeling RW, Fast M, et al. Serological study of responses to selected pathogens causing respiratory tract infection in the institutionalized elderly. *Clin Infect Dis* 1996;23:1240–1245.
140. McGeer A, Campbell B, Emori T, et al. Definitions of infection for surveillance in long-term care facilities. *Am J Infect Control* 1991;19: 1–7.
141. Loving P, Porter S, Stuifbergen A, et al. Surveillance of nosocomial infection in private psychiatric hospitals: an exploratory study. *Am J Infect Control* 1992;20:149–155.
142. Smith P, Rusnak P. SHEA/APIC position paper—infection prevention and control in the long-term-care facility. *Infect Control Hosp Epidemiol* 1997;18:831–849.
143. Stevenson KB. Regional data set of infection rates for long-term care facilities: description of a valuable benchmarking tool. *Am J Infect Control* 1999;27:20–26.
144. Strausbaugh LJ, Joseph CL. The burden of infection in long-term care. *Infect Control Hosp Epidemiol* 2000;21:674–679.
145. Jarvis WR. Selected aspects of the socioeconomic impact of nosocomial infections: morbidity, mortality, cost, and prevention. *Infect Control Hosp Epidemiol* 1996;17:552–557.
146. Golliot F, Astagneau P, Cassou B, et al. Nosocomial infections in geriatric long-term-care and rehabilitation facilities: exploration in the development of a risk index for epidemiological surveillance. *Infect Control Hosp Epidemiol* 2001;22:746–753.
147. Shepard M, Parker D, DeClerque N. The under-reporting of pressure sores in patients transferred between hospital and nursing home. *J Am Geriatr Soc* 1987;35:159–160.

148. Nicolle LE, Orr P, Dickworth H, et al. Prospective study of decubitus ulcers in two long term care facilities. *Can J Infect Control* 1994;9: 35–38.
149. Lertzman BH, Gaspari AA. Drug treatment of skin and soft tissue infections in elderly long-term care residents. *Drugs Aging* 1996;9: 109–121.
150. Livesley NJ, Chow AW. Infected pressure ulcers in elderly individuals. *Clin Infect Dis* 2002;35:1390–1396.
151. Allman R. Pressure ulcers among the elderly. *N Engl J Med* 1989; 320:850–853.
152. Richardson JP. Tetanus and tetanus immunization in long-term care facilities. *Infect Control Hosp Epidemiol* 1993;14:591–594.
153. Boustcha E, Nicolle LE. Conjunctivitis in a long-term care facility. *Infect Control Hosp Epidemiol* 1995;16:210–216.
154. Brennen C, Muder R. Conjunctivitis associated with methicillin-resistant *Staphylococcus aureus* in a long-term-care facility. *Am J Med* 1990;88(Suppl 5):14N–17N.
155. Weber DJ, Rutala WA, Hamilton H. Prevention and control of varicella-zoster infections in healthcare facilities. *Infect Control Hosp Epidemiol* 1996;17:694–705.
156. Kreher JM, Graser GN, Handelman SL, et al. Oral yeasts, mucosal health, and drug use in an elderly denture-wearing population. *Spec Care Dentist* 1991;11:222–226.
157. Abu-Elteen KH, Abu-Alteen RM. The prevalence of *Candida albicans* populations in the mouths of complete denture wearers. *New Microbiol* 1998;21:41–48.
158. Arlian L, Estes S, Vyszenski-Moher DL. Prevalence of *Sarcoptes scabiei* in the homes and nursing homes of scabietic patients. *J Am Acad Dermatol* 1988;19:806–811.
159. Jimenez-Lucho VE, Fallon F, Caputo C, et al. Role of prolonged surveillance in the eradication of nosocomial scabies in an extended care Veterans Affairs medical center. *Am J Infect Control* 1995;23: 44–49.
160. Wilson M-MG, Philpott CD, Breer WA. Atypical presentation of scabies among nursing home residents. *J Gerontol* 2001;56A: M424–M427.
161. Hollyoak V, Allison D, Summers J. Pseudomonas aeruginosa wound infection associated with a nursing home's whirlpool bath. *Commun Dis Rep CDR Rev* 1995;5:R100–R102.
162. Hedderwick SA, Wan JY, Bradley SF, et al. Risk factors for colonization with yeast species in a Veterans Affairs long-term care facility. *J Am Geriatr Soc* 1998;46:849–853.
163. Goode P, Allman R. The prevention and management of pressure ulcers. *Med Clin North Am* 1989;73:1511–1524.
164. Sanchez MP, Erdman DD, Torok TJ, et al. Outbreak of adenovirus 35 pneumonia among adult residents and staff of a chronic care psychiatric facility. *J Infect Dis* 1997;176:760–763.
165. Steketee RW, Wassilak GF, Adkins WN Jr, et al. Evidence for a high attack rate and efficacy of erythromycin prophylaxis in a pertussis outbreak in a facility for the developmentally disabled. *J Infect Dis* 1988;157:434–440.
166. Arroyo J, Jordan W, Milligan L. Upper respiratory tract infection and serum antibody responses in nursing home patients. *Am J Infect Control* 1988;16:152–158.
167. Cesario T, Yousefi S. Viral infections. *Clin Geriatr Med* 1992;8: 735–743.
168. Drinka PJ, Krause P, Schilling M, et al. Report of an outbreak: nursing home architecture and influenza-A attack rates. *J Am Geriatr Soc* 1996; 44:910–913.
169. Muder RR. Pneumonia in residents of long-term care facilities: epidemiology, etiology, management, and prevention. *Am J Med* 1998; 105:319–330.
170. Loeb M, McGeer A, McArthur M, et al. Risk factors for pneumonia and other lower respiratory tract infections in elderly residents of long-term care facilities. *Arch Intern Med* 1999;159:2058–2064.
171. McDonald A, Dietsche L, Litsche M, et al. A retrospective study of nosocomial pneumonia at a long-term care facility. *Am J Infect Control* 1992;20:234–238.
172. Pick N, McDonald A, Bennett N, et al. Pulmonary aspiration in a long-term care setting: clinical and laboratory observations and an analysis of risk factors. *J Am Geriatr Soc* 1996;44:763–768.
173. Marrie TJ, Blanchard W. A comparison of nursing home-acquired pneumonia patients with patients with community-acquired pneumonia and nursing home patients without pneumonia. *J Am Geriatr Soc* 1997;45:50–55.
174. Medina-Walpole AM, Katz PR. Nursing home-acquired pneumonia. *J Am Geriatr Soc* 1999;47:1005–1015.
175. Mylotte JM. Nursing home-acquired pneumonia. *Clin Infect Dis* 2002;35:1205–1211.
176. Marrie TJ. Pneumonia in the long-term-care facility. *Infect Control Hosp Epidemiol* 2002;23:159–164.
177. Setia U, Serventi I, Lorenz P. Bacteremia in a long-term care facility. *Arch Intern Med* 1984;144:1633–1635.
178. Mylotte JM, Tayara A, Goodnough S. Epidemiology of bloodstream infection in nursing home residents: evaluation in a large cohort from multiple homes. *Clin Infect Dis* 2002;35:1481–1490.
179. Irvine P, Van Buren N, Crossley K. Causes for hospitalization of nursing home residents: the role of infection. *J Am Geriatr Soc* 1984; 32:103–107.
180. Muder RR, Brennen C, Swenson DL, et al. Pneumonia in a long-term care facility—a prospective study of outcome. *Arch Intern Med* 1996;156:2365–2370.
181. Hutton MD, Cauthen GM, Bloch AB. Results of 29-state survey of tuberculosis in nursing homes and correctional facilities. *Public Health Rep* 1993;108:305–314.
182. Dutt AK, Stead WW. Tuberculosis. *Clin Geriatr Med* 1992;8: 761–775.
183. Stead W, To T. The significance of the tuberculin skin test in elderly persons. *Ann Intern Med* 1987;107:837–842.
184. Gross PA, Hermogenes AW, Sacks, HS, et al. The efficacy of influenza vaccine in elderly persons a meta-analysis and review of the literature. *Ann Intern Med* 1995;123:518–527.
185. Gross P, Quinnan G, Rodstein M, et al. Association of influenza immunization with reduction in mortality in an elderly population. *Arch Intern Med* 1988;148:562–565.
186. Potter J, Stott DJ, Roberts MA, et al. Influenza vaccination of healthcare workers in long-term-care hospitals reduces the mortality of elderly patients. *J Infect Dis* 1997;175:1–6.
187. Carman WF, Elder AG, Wallace LS, et al. Effects of influenza vaccination of health-care workers on mortality of elderly people in long-term care: a randomised controlled trial. *Lancet*2000;355:93–97.
188. Vergis EN, Brennen C, Wagener M, et al. Pneumonia in long-term care: a prospective case-control study of risk factors and impact on survival. *Arch Intern Med* 2001;161:2378–2381.
189. Stead W, Logfren J, Warren E, et al. Tuberculosis as an endemic and nosocomial infection among the elderly in nursing homes. *N Engl J Med* 1985;312:1483-1487.
190. Nicolle L, Bjornson J, Harding G, et al. Bacteriuria in elderly institutionalized men. *N Engl J Med* 1983;309:1420–1425.
191. Nicolle L. Urinary tract infections in long-term care facilities. *Infect Control Hosp Epidemiol*1993;14:220–225.
192. Nicolle LE. Urinary tract infections in long-term-care facilities. *Infect Control Hosp Epidemiol* 2001;22;167–175.
193. Nicolle LE. Urinary tract infection in long-term-care facility residents. *Clin Infect Dis* 2000:31:757–761.
194. Nicolle LE. Asymptomatic bacteriuria in the elderly. *Infect Dis Clin North Am* 1997;11:647–662.
195. Moseley CB. The impact of federal regulations on urethral catheterization in Virginia nursing homes. *Am J Med Qual* 1996;11:222–226.
196. Breitenbucher R. Bacterial changes in the urine samples of patients with long-term indwelling catheters. *Arch Intern Med* 1984;144: 1585–1588.
197. Ouslander J, Greengold B, Chen S. External catheter use and urinary tract infections among incontinent male nursing home patients. *J Am Geriatr Soc* 1987;35:1063–1070.
198. Terpenning M, Allada R, Kauffman C. Intermittent urethral catheterization in the elderly. *J Am Geriatr Soc* 1989;37:411–416.
199. Warren JW. Catheter-associated bacteriuria in long-term care facilities. *Infect Control Hosp Epidemiol* 1994;15:557–562.

200. Orr PH, Nicolle LE, Duckworth H, et al. Febrile urinary infection in the institutionalized elderly. *Am J Med* 1996;100:71–77.
201. Ouslander J, Greengold B, Chen S. Complications of chronic indwelling urinary catheters among male nursing home patients: a prospective study. *J Urol* 1987;138:1191–1195.
202. Warren J, Damron D, Tenney J, et al. Fever, bacteremia, and death as complications of bacteriuria in women with long-term urethral catheters. *J Infect Dis* 1987;155:1151–1158.
203. Warren J, Muncie H Jr, Hall-Craggs M. Acute pyelonephritis associated with bacteriuria during long-term catheterization: a prospective clinicopathological study. *J Infect Dis* 1988;158:1341–1346.
204. Nicolle L, Muir P, Harding G, et al. Localization of urinary tract infection in elderly institutionalized women with asymptomatic bacteriuria. *J Infect Dis* 1988;157:65–70.
205. Fryklund B, Haeggman S, Burman LG. Transmission of urinary bacterial strains between patients with indwelling catheter-nursing in the same room and in separate rooms compared. *J Hosp Infect* 1997;36: 147–153.
206. Fierer J, Ekstrom M. An Outbreak of *Providencia stuartii* urinary tract infections: patients with condom catheters are a reservoir of the bacteria. *JAMA* 1981;245:1553–1555.
207. Lloyd S, Zervos M, Rula M, et al. Risk factors for enterococcal urinary tract infection and colonization in a rehabilitation facility. *Am J Infect Control* 1998;265:35–39.
208. Nicolle L, Henderson E, Bjornson J, et al. The association of bacteriuria with resident characteristics and survival in elderly institutionalized men. *Ann Intern Med* 1987;106:682–686.
209. Beck-Sague C, Banerjee S, Jarvis WR. Infectious diseases and mortality among US NH residents. *Am J Public Health* 1993;83:1739–1742.
210. Zimakoff J, Stickler DJ, Pontoppidan B, et al. Bladder management and urinary tract infection in Danish hospitals, nursing homes, and home care: a national prevalence study. *Infect Control Hosp Epidemiol*1996;17:215–221.
211. Gleckman R, Hibert D. Afebrile bacteremia: a phenomenon in geriatric patients. *JAMA* 1982;248:1478–1481.
212. Rudman D, Hontanosas A, Cohen C, et al. Clinical correlates of bacteremia in a Veterans Administration extended care facility. *J Am Geriatr Soc* 1988;36:726–732.
213. Richardson JP, Hricz L. Risk factors for the development of bacteremia in nursing home patients. *Arch Fam Med* 1995;4:785–789.
214. Bachrach S. An outbreak of *Haemophilus influenzae* type b bacteremia in an intermediate care hospital for children. *J Hosp Infect* 1988;11: 121–126.
215. Rodriquez EM, Parrott C, Rolka H, et al. An outbreak of viral gastroenteritis in a nursing home: importance of excluding ill employees. *Infect Control Hosp Epidemiol* 1996;17:587–592.
216. Ahmad F, Bray G, Prescott RWG, et al. Use of ciprofloxacin to control a *Salmonella* outbreak in a long-stay psychiatric hospital. *J Hosp Infect* 1991;17:171–178.
217. Bender BS, Laughon BE, Gaydos C, et al. Is *Clostridium difficile* endemic in chronic-care facilities? *Lancet*1986;2:11–13.
218. Thomas D, Bennett R, Laughon B, et al. Postantibiotic colonization with *Clostridium difficile* in nursing home patients. *J Am Geriatr Soc* 1990;38:415–420.
219. Simor AE, Yake SL, Tsimidis K. Infection due to *Clostridium difficile* among elderly residents of a long-term-facility. *Clin Infect Dis* 1993; 17:672–678.
220. Brooks S, Veal R, Kramer M, et al. Reduction in the incidence of *Clostridium difficile* associated diarrhea in an acute care hospital and a skilled nursing facility following replacement of electronic thermometers with single use disposables. *Infect Control Hosp Epidemiol* 1992; 13:98–103.
221. Chien NT, Dundoo G, Mohamad H, et al. Seroprevalence of viral hepatitis in an older nursing home population. *J Am Geriatr Soc* 1999; 47:1110–1113.
222. Nowicki MJ, Ahmad N, Schmidt RE, et al. Prevalence of hepatitis C virus in a chronic care facility. *Pediatr Infect Dis J* 1994;13:151–152.
223. American College of Physicians. *Guide for adult immunization,* 3rd ed. Philadelphia: American College of Physicians, 1994.
224. Monto AS, Hornbuckle K, Ohmit, SE. Influenza vaccine effectiveness among elderly nursing home residents: a cohort study. *Am J Epidemiol* 2001;154:155–160.
225. Deguchi Y, Nishimura K. Efficacy of influenza vaccine in elderly persons in welfare nursing homes: reduction in risks of mortality and morbidity during an influenza A (H3N2) epidemic. *J Gerontol* 2001; 59:M 391–394.
226. Arden N, Monto AS, Ohmit SE. Vaccine use and the risk of institutional outbreaks in a sample of nursing homes during a type A (H3N2) influenza epidemic. *Am J Public Health* 1995;85:399–401.
227. Centers for Disease Control and Prevention. Prevention and control of influenza: recommendations of the advisory committee on immunization practices (ACIP). *MMWR Morb Mortal Wkly Rep* 2002; 51(RR03):1–31.
228. Douglas R. Prophylaxis and treatment of influenza. *N Engl J Med* 1990;322:443–450.
229. Lee C, Loeb M, Phillips A, et al. Zanamivir use during transmission of amantadine-resistant influenza A in a nursing home. *Infect Control Hosp Epidemiol* 2000;21:700–704.
230. Peters PH, Gravenstein S, Norwood P, et al. Long-term use of oseltamivir for the prophylaxis of influenza in a vaccinated frail older population. *J Am Geriatr Soc* 2001;49:1025–1031.
231. Gomolin IH, Leib HB, Arden NH, et al. Control of influenza outbreaks in the nursing home: guidelines for diagnosis and management. *J Am Geriatr Soc* 1996;44:74–82.
232. Drinka PJ, Krause P, Nest L, et al. Delays in the application of outbreak control prophylaxis for influenza A in a nursing home. *Infect Control Hosp Epidemiol* 2002;23:600–603.
233. Drinka PJ, Gravenstein S, Schilling M, et al. Duration of antiviral prophylaxis during nursing home outbreaks of influenza A: a comparison of 2 protocols. *Arch Intern Med* 1998;158:2155–2159.
234. Bentley D. Vaccinations. *Clin Geriatr Med* 1992;8:745–760.
235. Shapiro E, Berg A, Austrian R, et al. The protective effect of polyvalent pneumococcal polysaccharide vaccine. *N Engl J Med* 1991;325: 1453–1460.
236. Ortquist A, Hedlund J, Burman L-A, et al. Randomised trial of 23-valent pneumococcal capsular polysaccharide vaccine in prevention of pneumonia in middle-aged and elderly people. *Lancet* 1998;351: 399–403.
237. Centers for Disease Control and Prevention. Outbreak of pneumococcal pneumonia among unvaccinated residents of a nursing home—New Jersey, April 2001. *MMWR Morb Mortal Wkly Rep* 2001;50:707–710.
238. Centers for Disease Control and Prevention. Prevention of pneumococcal disease: recommendations of the advisory committee on Immunization Practices (ACIP). *MMWR Morb Mortal Wkly Rep* 1997; 46(RR-8):1–24.
239. Centers for Disease Control and Prevention. Diphtheria, tetanus, and pertussis: recommendations of the Advisory Committee on Immunization Practices (ACIP). *MMWR Morb Mortal Wkly Rep* 1991; 40(RR10):1–28.
240. Centers for Disease Control and Prevention. Prevention of hepatitis A through active or passive immunization: recommendations of the Advisory Committee on Immunization Practices (ACIP). *MMWR Morb Mortal Wkly Rep*1996;45:1–30.
241. Centers for Disease Control and Prevention. Targeted tuberculin testing and treatment of latent tuberculosis. *MMWR Morb Mortal Wkly Rep* 2000;49(RR06):1–54.
242. Stead W, To T, Harrison R, et al. Benefit-risk considerations in preventive treatment for tuberculosis in elderly persons. *Ann Intern Med* 1987;107:843–845.
243. Cooper J. Decision analysis for tuberculosis preventive treatment in nursing homes. *J Am Geriatr Soc* 1986;34:814–817.
244. Nicolle LE. Infection control in long-term care facilities. *Clin Infect Dis* 2000;31:752–756.
245. Stone SP, Kibbler CC, Bowman C, et al. Controlling infection in British nursing homes: it is time for a national strategy. *BMJ* 2001; 322:506.
246. Goldrick BA. Infection control programs in long-term-care facilities: structure and process. *Infect Control Hosp Epidemiol* 1999;20: 764–769.

247. Goldrick BA. Infection control programs in skilled nursing long-term care facilities: an assessment, 1995. *Am J Infect Control* 1999;27:4–9.
248. Smith PW. Nursing home infection control: a status report. *Infect Control Hosp Epidemiol* 1998;19:366–369.
249. Campbell B. Surveillance and control of infections in long-term care: the Canadian experience. *Am J Med* 1991;91(Suppl 3B):286S–288S.
250. Friedman C. Barnette M, Buck AS, et al. Requirements for infrastructure and essential activities of infection control and epidemiology in out-of-hospital settings: a consensus panel report. *Infect Control Hosp Epidemiol* 1999;20:695–705.
251. Smith P, Daly P, Rusnak P, et al. Design and dissemination of a multiregional long-term care infection control training program. *Am J Infect Control* 1992;20:275–277.
252. Daly P, Smith P, Rusnak P, et al. Impact on knowledge and practice of a multiregional long-term care facility infection control training program. *Am J Infect Control* 1992;20:225–233.
253. Smith PW, Helger V, Sonksen D. Survey of infection control training program graduates: long-term care facility and small hospital practitioners. *Am J Infect Control* 2002;30:311–313.
254. Satterfield N. Infection control in long-term care facilities: the hospital-based practitioner's role. *Infect Control Hosp Epidemiol* 1993;14: 40–47.
255. Bentley DW, Cheney L. Infection control in the nursing home: the physician's role. *Geriatrics* 1990;45:59–66.
256. Mylotte J. The hospital epidemiologist in long-term care: practical considerations. *Infect Control Hosp Epidemiol* 1991;12:439–442.
257. Jackson MM, Schafer K. Identifying clues to infections in nursing home residents: the role of the nurses aide. *J Gerontol Nurs* 1993;19: 33–42.
258. Simor AE. The role of the laboratory in infection prevention and control programs in long-term-care facilities for the elderly. *Infect Control Hosp Epidemiol* 2001;22:459–463.
259. Ahlbrecht H, Shearen C, Degelau J, et al. Team approach to infection prevention and control in the nursing home setting. *Am J Infect Control* 1999;27:64–70.
260. Makris AT, Morgan L, Gaber DJ, et al. Effect of a comprehensive infection control program on the incidence of infections in long-term care facilities. *Am J Infect Control* 2000;28:3–7.
261. Rubino JR. Infection control practices in institutional settings. *Am J Infect Control* 2001;29:241–243.
262. Crossley K, The long-term-care committee of the Society for Healthcare Epidemiology of America. Vancomycin-resistant enterococci in long-term-care facilities. *Infect Control Hosp Epidemiol* 1998; 19:521–525.
263. Guay DRP. Pet-assisted therapy in the nursing home setting: potential for zoonosis. *Am J Infect Control* 2001;29:178–186.
264. Nicolle LE, Bentley DW, Garibaldi R, et al. Antimicrobial use in long-term-care facilities. *Infect Control Hosp Epidemiol* 2000;21:537–545.

107

EPIDEMIOLOGY AND PREVENTION OF INFECTIONS IN HOME HEALTHCARE

PHILIP W. SMITH
JANE S. ROCCAFORTE

BACKGROUND

The Home Healthcare Field

Home healthcare is the most rapidly growing segment of the healthcare delivery system; about as many persons in the United States receive healthcare in the home as in acute care settings (1). More than 20,000 agencies deliver home care to 7.6 million individuals, generating about $40 billion in expenditures (1). Medicare is the largest payer of home health services (2). The most commonly used services are skilled nursing care, personal care, and physical therapy.

Home healthcare specialists provide many services traditionally given in the hospital or in a long-term care facility (LTCF). The number and types of patients who receive professional care in the home setting are increasing; major categories of home care services include infusion therapy, respiratory therapy, dialysis, diabetic monitoring, wound care, other skilled nursing care, physical therapy, nutritional therapy, occupational therapy, social services, and hospice care. Also included in these general categories are patients requiring special nursing support by virtue of medical needs (e.g., enteral nutrition) or disease complexity (e.g., acquired immunodeficiency syndrome). In total, about 670,000 persons are employed in the home healthcare industry, mostly home care aides and registered nurses (2). Other professionals including respiratory therapists, physical therapists, social service workers, speech therapists, pharmacists and durable medical equipment suppliers are also involved in providing home healthcare.

Infections and Risk Factors in Home Healthcare Patients

Many patients cared for at home have underlying conditions such as organ transplants that compromise the immune system. They may have multiple invasive devices such as intravenous (IV) catheters, urinary tract catheters, and tracheostomies. A survey of home healthcare patients revealed that these predominantly elderly individuals had an average of 3.6 comorbid conditions; 12% had invasive devices (3). The leading comorbid conditions were hypertension, congestive heart failure, diabetes, pressure ulcers, chronic obstructive pulmonary disease, and cerebrovascular disease. Many infections acquired in the home are related to devices or breaks in local defenses (Table 107.1). The leading invasive devices noted were urethral or suprapubic catheters (12%), nasogastric tubes (10.8%), IV catheters (6.3%), and tracheostomies (2.3%). In another survey (4), it was found that 34% of home care patients had invasive devices on the day of the survey (21% had a urinary catheter, 17% a central venous catheter, 7% a gastrostomy tube, and 1% a mechanical ventilator). Although comparative data are not available, the home healthcare patient is presumably less immunosuppressed than the typical hospital or LTCF patient but more at risk for infection than other community-dwelling individuals.

Home healthcare patients may have a variety of infectious diseases that have implications for infection control in the home. One prevalence survey (3) found that 20.6% of home healthcare patients had an infection on the day surveyed. One fourth of these infections occurred during the home healthcare period, including urinary tract, respiratory tract, and wound infections. Another more recent prevalence survey found an overall infection rate of 16% in the home with 8% of these infections homecare acquired, 16% hospital-acquired, 41% community-acquired, and 35% unknown (4). The most common infections were urinary tract (27%), respiratory tract (24%), skin and soft tissue (24%), surgical wound (12%), and bloodstream (2%) infections. The incidence, risk factors, types of infections, and preventability of infections in the home healthcare setting still remain largely to be defined.

TABLE 107.1. INFECTIONS OF IMPORTANCE IN HOME HEALTH

Infection	Associated Condition or Device
Bacteremia	Intravenous access device
Urinary tract infection	Bladder catheters
Pneumonia	Nasogastric tube, tracheostomy
Peritonitis	Peritoneal dialysis catheter
Wound infection	Recent surgery

HOME INFUSION THERAPY

The home infusion industry has grown rapidly, greatly advanced by the development and widespread availability of devices to secure long-term venous access. Antibiotic therapy, parenteral nutrition, hydration therapy, chemotherapy, and pain medications account for most IV home medications.

Infections in Home Infusion Therapy

Most infections in home infusion therapy are related to vascular access devices. In a study of 300 home IV patients, Graham et al. (5) found a rate of bacteremia of 4.6 cases per 10,000 catheter days or 6.0 per 10,000 home care days, with all bacteremias related to vascular access devices. Others have noted rates of 7 to 21 bacteremias per 10,000 catheter days (6–9). Noninfectious complications of venous access in the home environment include thrombophlebitis, bleeding, and air embolism (5).

Infections related to indwelling vascular access devices can present as sepsis or fever without localizing signs or symptoms. Alternately, one may see signs of exit-site infection (erythema, tenderness, or purulent discharge at the catheter exit site) or a tunnel infection (erythema, tenderness, and induration along the subcutaneous tract). Catheter-related sepsis and tunnel infections often require catheter removal (7). The most common microorganisms associated with these infections are coagulase-negative staphylococci, *Staphylococcus aureus,* aerobic gram-negative bacilli (such as *Klebsiella pneumoniae* and *Pseudomonas aeruginosa*), and *Candida* species. In one report, gram-negative microorganisms were responsible for a greater proportion of central line-related bacteremias in pediatric oncology patients receiving home care than in those in the hospital (8). The mean time between catheter insertion and bacteremia was 133 days.

Risk factors for bloodstream infections in patients receiving home infusion therapy include bone marrow transplantation, parenteral nutrition, use of multilumen catheters, and reception of an infusion at a hospital clinic or physician's office (10). Needleless devices have been associated with bloodstream infections in the home setting, especially when changed only weekly (11).

Home Parenteral Nutrition

One special area of home infusion therapy is home parenteral nutrition (HPN). Most infections in HPN are related to the indwelling vascular catheter. In one study, catheter-related bacteremia in HPN patients occurred at a rate of 2.1 infections per 1,000 HPN days (12). The leading microorganisms were coagulase-negative staphylococci, *K. pneumoniae, Escherichia coli, S. aureus,* and *Candida* species.

Infusate-related bacteremia from contaminated parenteral nutrition fluids is relatively uncommon but remains a concern. A variety of microorganisms have been shown to proliferate in parenteral nutrition solutions, particularly gram-negative bacteria and *Candida* species. Other pathways of infection may occur; nine HPN patients had bacteremia resulting from contamination of preslit injection caps in a needleless IV system (13).

Preventive Aspects

Infection control recommendations for home infusion therapy pertain mainly to the prevention of vascular access-associated infections. Guidelines for preventing IV-related infections in the hospital have been published (14). The guidelines address frequency of catheter and administration set change, aseptic technique during catheter insertion, and length of hang time for lipid-containing solutions. The guidelines also provide definitions of catheter-related infections for surveillance purposes. The home care agency is responsible for ensuring sterility of solutions prepared for IV infusion.

Both the patient and the home healthcare provider need to be familiar with the signs and symptoms of infection, the side effects of infusion therapy, and the maintenance and care of vascular access devices. Lack of education is a risk factor for line-related bacteremia in the home (11). See Chapter 18 for more information on the use of IV devices inserted for long-term vascular access.

HOME RESPIRATORY CARE

Technologic advances have had a great impact on home healthcare patients with chronic respiratory conditions. Home care of patients with tracheostomies has become an accepted practice; this raises questions regarding aseptic technique when performing tracheostomy care and tracheal suctioning. Sophisticated respiratory care equipment is used in the home and requires meticulous maintenance to prevent bacterial contamination and respiratory tract infection by inhalation. Finally, chronic ventilatory support may be provided with in-home ventilators, requiring adaptation of standard acute care hospital respiratory care techniques to the home care setting. Home respiratory care patients are at particular risk for respiratory tract infections because of underlying pulmonary diseases and devices such as tracheostomies that bypass upper airway defenses.

Infection Control Aspects of Airway Management

There are no controlled studies of the risk of infection or of infection control methods for these patients in the home environment. Recommendations are based on extrapolations from current hospital practices (see Chapter 22). Areas of concern are listed in Table 107.2.

TABLE 107.2. INFECTION CONTROL CONCERNS IN HOME RESPIRATORY CARE

Tracheostomy care
Changing of inner cannula
Tracheostomy site care
Suctioning technique
Reuse of suction catheters
Disinfection of respiratory care equipment
Ventilator circuits
Ventilator apparatus
Humidifiers
Nebulization equipment
Oxygen delivery systems

A tracheostomy is required for all individuals using positive pressure ventilators in the home. The goal of tracheostomy site care is to maintain a clean site. The tracheostomy should be cleaned with a lintless piece of gauze or a cotton-tipped applicator dipped in 3% hydrogen peroxide. Both the tracheostomy dressing and the tracheostomy tie should be changed when they are soiled. Clean gloves should be worn during care of the tracheostomy site (15).

Likewise, tracheal suctioning is a clean rather than a sterile technique. Home cleaning and disinfection of suction catheters includes cleaning with soapy water, rinsing, boiling, and flushing with hydrogen peroxide. These measures are effective at decreasing bacterial growth, allowing for reuse of tracheal suction catheters in home healthcare (15). Tracheostomy cannulas may also be cleaned with soap and water, soaked in hydrogen peroxide or alcohol, and boiled for 15 minutes.

Home Ventilator and Equipment Care

For patients receiving assisted ventilation in the home, cleaning of the ventilatory circuits is important. Several circuits should be provided, and the circuits (including tubing, manifold, and humidifier) not in use should be cleaned and dried before being stored. Adequate precleaning of equipment is an important part of the disinfection process.

Room humidifiers that produce a fine spray of water droplets are frequently used in the home and are often contaminated with bacteria. Although high-level disinfection is recommended (16), these humidifiers are difficult to clean and pose significant risk to immunocompromised patients. Drying between uses decreases bacterial contamination. Humidifiers that work by simple evaporation are safer than those that produce a fine mist spray.

Preventive Aspects

Guidelines for prevention of nosocomial pneumonia (17) have some relevance for home care, including immunization recommendations (pneumococcal vaccine, influenza vaccine), suctioning, ventilator care, aspiration prevention after enteral feeding, and humidifier care. The American Association of Respiratory Care has a Web site that lists clinical practice guidelines for home suctioning, home ventilation, postural drainage, and ventilator circuit changes (16).

HOME DIALYSIS CARE

Technologic advances have resulted in the ability of many patients with chronic renal failure to receive dialysis at home. Both peritoneal dialysis and hemodialysis may be administered in the home setting. Most infections in dialysis patients are related to access devices.

Infections in Home Dialysis

One of the most serious problems associated with peritoneal dialysis is infection involving either the catheter exit site through the skin or the peritoneal cavity itself. The former infection, analogous to indwelling central IV access device infections, may involve either the exit site or the tunnel. The latter generally presents as peritonitis. The incidence of infectious complications related to continuous ambulatory peritoneal dialysis (CAPD) is about 1.1 to 1.3 episodes per patient-year (18). Recurrent peritonitis is a leading cause of CAPD failure.

Most bacteria causing CAPD-related peritonitis are gram-positive bacteria (specifically, coagulase-negative staphylococci and *S. aureus*), reflecting the important role of skin flora in catheter-related peritonitis (18). Polymicrobial infections and gram-negative bacteria suggest a bowel perforation by the catheter. Nasal carriage of *S. aureus* may be a risk factor for catheter exit-site infections by this microorganism.

Home hemodialysis may be complicated by pyrogenic reactions, but the most important infection is vascular access-related infection.

Preventive Aspects

A key to minimizing CAPD peritonitis is care of the exit site and surrounding skin. Initial care after catheter placement has been described and consists of cleaning the exit site and surrounding skin with an antiseptic agent, drying the skin, covering the exit site with a sterile gauze dressing, and securing with surgical tape. After the exit site has healed, routine care includes daily examination of the exit site and tunnel for signs of infection and cleaning of the exit site. Cleaning with soap and water may be adequate. The catheter should be protected from mechanical stress (19).

The potential exists for contamination of the peritoneal dialysis system when the system is opened to connect or disconnect bags of fluid. Devices have been developed to reduce the risk of contamination; ultraviolet light applied to the connections may decrease the risk of peritonitis. Infections in peritoneal dialysis are discussed in greater depth in Chapter 65.

A guideline for preventing infection transmission in chronic hemodialysis patients discusses some aspects relevant to home care, such as cleaning and disinfection of equipment (20). Hemodialysis and related complications are discussed in Chapter 64.

INFECTION CONTROL ASPECTS OF OTHER TYPES OF HOME HEALTHCARE

Urinary Catheterization in the Home

The home healthcare patient may use continuous or intermittent urinary catheterization. Intermittent catheterization is usually limited to individuals with neurogenic bladders who are able to actively participate in their own care. Clean rather than sterile catheter technique is appropriate (21). It is recommended that indwelling catheters be placed with aseptic technique using sterile equipment and be properly secured.

A study of indwelling urinary catheters in the home setting demonstrated that most patients had infected urine after 4 weeks of catheterization (22). This is similar to what would be expected in a hospital or LTCF setting. Bacteremia was demonstrated after 20 of 197 changes of urethral catheters and after 1 of 19 changes of suprapubic catheters. Other investigators found an infection rate of 4.5 symptomatic urinary tract infections (UTIs) per 1,000 catheter days (9). A survey of home care patients with urinary catheters during a 6-month period found the mean duration of catheterization to be about 300 days (23). One fourth had a UTI at the start of catheterization, and 43% of the remainder acquired infection during the study period. Frequent catheter change was an infection risk.

Guidelines for prevention of UTI associated with indwelling catheters can be found in the literature (24) and in Chapter 20. They emphasize aseptic catheter insertion, maintenance of unobstructed flow, use of a closed drainage system, and minimization of drainage tube disconnections. Leg bags should be emptied, cleaned, disinfected with an agent such as a 1:10 dilution of bleach, and dried between uses (21). One method for disinfecting reusable urinary catheters for intermittent catheterization is to boil the catheter in water for 15 minutes or microwave after cleaning the catheter with soap and water.

Home Wound Care

A Michigan prevalence survey found that 36.3% of a large sample of home care patients had wounds present—most commonly surgical wounds, pressure ulcers, and vascular leg ulcers. Of patients with wounds, 41% had multiple wounds (25). In another survey, 9% of home care patients had a stage II or deeper pressure ulcer, and one third had more than one ulcer (26).

Generally, fresh surgical wounds are not encountered in the home setting; thus, clean technique is adequate for most wound care. Proper wound care involves the use of gloves or the "no touch" technique for clean wounds, the use of gloves for infected or draining wounds, and proper disposal of soiled dressings. The patient, the family, and the home healthcare provider need to be alert for signs and symptoms of wound infection, such as fever, pain, swelling, induration, erythema, and warmth. Guidelines for pressure ulcer prevention are available (27).

Enteral Feedings in the Home

Enteral feeding via nasogastric or another enteral tube is often undertaken in the home setting. The risk of infection is primarily related to the potential for aspiration resulting from the presence of the nasogastric tube. The possibility of bacterial contamination of enteral feeding solutions must also be considered (28).

In general, clean technique is appropriate for preparing and administering enteral feedings. To minimize contamination of the enteral feeding solution, raw meats, uncooked eggs, and unpasteurized milk should be avoided when making feedings (21). It is recommended that this solution be changed every 24 hours if a premixed commercial solution is used and every 8 hours if a commercial feeding solution requiring mixing and reconstitution is used. After each feeding session, the tube should be flushed with 25 to 100 mL of lukewarm water. The feeding bag and tubing must be washed, rinsed, and thoroughly dried periodically. To minimize the risk of aspiration pneumonia, tube placement should be confirmed and the patient should be kept in the erect or semierect position during the feeding and for 1 hour afterward (17).

THE HOME HEALTH INFECTION CONTROL PROGRAM

There is a trend toward formalizing infection control efforts in home health (29). The functions of an infection control program in this setting are listed in Table 107.3. The basic elements of infection control for out-of-hospital settings are (a) managing data, (b) developing control efforts, (c) preventing of infections, and (d) training (30).

An administrative structure should identify a designated infection control professional (ICP) who is responsible for the program, and the program may have a formal infection control committee (31). Ideally, the ICP is available to conduct infection control activities from within the agency. An infectious diseases physician with experience in infection control should be available on a consultative basis.

Communication with other healthcare organizations is important, especially because many home care patients have recently been in acute care hospitals or LTCFs. Exchange of microbiologic and clinical information is helpful for medical decision making by healthcare providers and for infection control planning. Communication includes disease reporting to health departments and nosocomial infection reporting to the patients' institutions of recent residence. This is one aspect of regulatory compliance. Surveillance data facilitate detection of epidemics and adverse events and are key to quality improvement efforts.

Employee protection begins with a basic employee health program, addressing such issues as tuberculosis skin testing, postexposure protocols, and immunizations. Policies and procedures for infection control measures are designed to minimize infection transmission; they deal with asepsis, disinfection, and hygiene, including hand washing and waste disposal. Barrier protection methods are also part of employee protection and may vary depending on the patient's infectious condition (e.g., colonization with antibiotic-resistant bacteria) and level of compliance. The ICP plays an important role in prevention of cross-infection in the home by education of patients and families.

Most agencies have policies and procedures for standard pre-

TABLE 107.3. FACETS OF A HOME HEALTHCARE INFECTION CONTROL PROGRAM

1. Administrative structure
2. Communication
3. Disease reporting
4. Regulatory compliance
5. Surveillance system
6. Quality improvement
7. Employee health
8. Policies and procedure
9. Asepsis, disinfection, and hygiene
10. Waste disposal
11. Barrier protection
12. Education of patients and families

cautions, hand washing, handling sharps and needles, and cleaning or disinfecting equipment (32). A Missouri survey found that 90% of 95 home care agencies had written infection control policies, and 95% had a system for reporting exposures, injuries, or infections in their personnel (33). Seventy percent of the agencies conducted infection surveillance (most used standard definitions, used standard data collection forms, and calculated infection rates). Two thirds had a routine process for checking the antimicrobial sensitivities of pathogens, but only about half had a designated ICP.

Surveillance

The first step in developing an infection control program is to create a surveillance system for infections acquired in home healthcare and for employee exposures. Surveillance for home care-associated infections is a difficult task. Unlike the hospital or LTCF patient, the home care patient has contact with healthcare providers for a very small amount of time (a few minutes per visit, with contact perhaps not occurring daily). It is, therefore, not always clear which infections occur as a result of normal daily life (community-acquired) and which are related to care received in the home (home care-associated).

Both numerator and denominator data may be problematic (34), the former requiring sharing of data by hospitals and laboratories and collection of information by home care nurses in the field. Device-related denominator data is not readily obtained if devices are inserted or removed at various facilities without notification of the home care nurses. Surveillance has been advanced by publication of draft definitions of infections for the home care setting (35), although the definitions have not been validated. Of necessity, these definitions rely more heavily on clinical signs and symptoms and tests that can be performed at the bedside like urine dipstick testing (29). Denominator data permitting calculation of rates per 1,000 device days (eg, urinary catheter, central venous catheter) are preferable (36) but not always readily obtained.

Surveillance data should be collected and reviewed by the ICP. Data can be used to provide valuable information to healthcare providers about the patient's condition, such as detection of febrile episodes in home care patients with hematologic malignancies. Surveillance in the home is also useful for detection of home care-associated outbreaks such as bloodstream infections (37). This is the ideal setting for focused surveillance, collecting data on a few select infections such as IV-related infections, wound infections, or UTIs.

Asepsis, Disinfection, and Hygiene

Perhaps the most important infection control measure in the home setting is hand washing. A recent guideline recommends a 15-second soap and water scrub or using an alcohol-based rub until dry (38). Waterless agents may be preferable, and running water is not always available. Adherence to hand hygiene should be monitored.

Reusable objects that touch mucous membranes, such as suction catheters and glass thermometers, should be limited to use on one patient and may be disinfected between uses on the same patient. A discussion of disinfectants is available (39); bleach, 70% alcohol, and 3% hydrogen peroxide are good disinfectants for the home setting. Clorox and Lysol are the household disinfectants with activity against virtually all agents tested, including polioviruses (40).

The home care provider should educate patients and families in the basics of hygiene and asepsis to minimize the risk of infection transmission. This risk was demonstrated by acquisition of hepatitis C by a hemophiliac child from his mother during infusion of clotting factor concentrate in the home (41). One survey of hemophiliac patients found inadequate infection control practices in the home (42); frequent needlestick injuries were noted (often during recapping) and gloves were often not used for cleaning up blood spills or during blood product infusions.

The home nursing bag is an important piece of equipment for the home health professional (Fig. 107.1); the bag should be considered a clean piece of equipment. Contaminated items that cannot be cleaned or discarded in the home should be placed in an impervious container in the nursing bag, and hands should be washed before handling equipment inside the bag (21). The bag should contain a spill kit to deal with large volume blood or body fluid spills.

Isolation Issues

Isolation techniques used in the home should follow the general principles of standard precautions (43). Basic protective measures are indicated for use with all patients. This includes wearing gloves for contact with blood and body fluids, wearing masks for contact with a patient who is coughing frequently or unable to control secretions, and using a cover gown or apron if soiling with blood or body fluids is likely. Goggles should be available to protect the eyes from splattering of blood or body fluids. Blood spills should be cleaned up, after donning gloves, with a 1:10 to 1:100 solution of fresh bleach, and good handwashing technique should be followed.

Transmission-based precautions are additional barriers needed for patients with certain contagious diseases. For example, masks are also necessary for contact with a patient who has a contagious disease such as tuberculosis, influenza, mumps, measles, chickenpox, or pertussis. The importance of barrier precautions is enhanced by the high prevalence of carriers of antimicrobial-resistant bacteria; vancomycin-intermediate *S. aureus* colonization was discovered in a home healthcare patient who had received long-term antibiotics (44). Items such as gloves, goggles, gowns and masks should be in the home nursing bag (Fig. 107.1). See Chapter 95 for more information on isolation precautions for patients with communicable diseases.

Waste Disposal

State regulations for medical waste vary considerably and may require the healthcare provider to remove medical waste generated in the home (45). Liquid wastes, such as urine, can be flushed down the toilet, with care being taken to avoid splashing during disposal. Used needles and other sharp objects should be placed in a puncture-resistant container such as a portable sharps

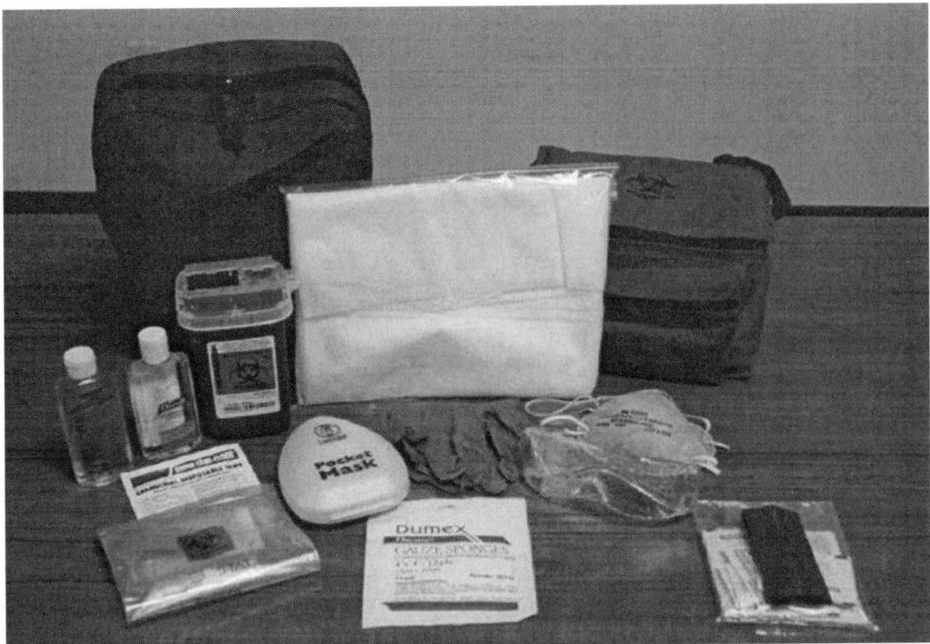

Figure 107.1. Home nursing bag. Contents relevant to infection control: hand-washing agents, antiseptic wipes, biohazard bags, sharps disposal container, resuscitation mask, gown, gloves, gauze sponges, goggles, N95 mask, and biohazard transport bag. (Courtesy Bridget Young and Eleanor Bistline, Visiting Nurse Association of the Midlands, Omaha, NE.)

container. Other contaminated materials can be placed in a plastic bag that is sealed and discarded in the routine trash disposal system. An Environmental Protection Agency (EPA) Web site provides information on waste disposal in the home care environment (46). Medical waste is covered in Chapter 100.

Employee Health Program

Employee health information for hospital employees is available in the medical literature and in many cases is applicable to the home healthcare professional (47,48). The employee should have updated immunizations, including tetanus, diphtheria, measles, mumps, rubella, influenza, and hepatitis B (47). The varicella immune status should be known. Baseline and periodic tuberculosis skin testing should be performed. Other issues to be addressed include a protocol for postexposure prophylaxis for exposures to blood or body fluids containing human immunodeficiency virus (HIV) and hepatitis B or C (49) and recommendations for work restrictions for ill employees. (See Chapters 78, 79, 80, and 99.)

Employee education in infection control is an important part of employee protection. A study of blood contacts among home healthcare workers found that most blood exposures could have been prevented by simple glove use (50). Employees need to be educated in standard precautions, barrier precautions for specific contagious diseases, and reporting of exposures.

Quality Improvement

Quality improvement principles can be applied to home healthcare as well as to the hospital and LTCF. The Joint Commission on Accreditation of Healthcare Organizations (JCAHO) has proposed standards for patient safety in home care (51) as part of its ORYX initiative. This is an error-reduction program in which data collected are incorporated into performance improvement initiatives. Elements to be studied include infection control, surveillance, and disease reporting. Measurable outcome indicators should be selected, such as immunization levels, compliance with infection control practices, employee exposures, medication errors, or home care-associated infection incidence.

The Center for Medicare and Medicaid Services in collaboration with the Centers for Health Policy Research has developed the Outcome and Assessment Information Set (OASIS) to measure patient outcomes and improve quality in home care. The OASIS reports are available on line (52), and examine variables such as inpatient facility admissions (and reason for admission), sanitation standards in the patient's home, and patient medical status (e.g., pressure ulcers). There are problems with both ORYX and OASIS data sets regarding standardization of definitions and completeness of data (53). (See Chapters 9 to 13 in Section II.)

Disease Reporting and Regulatory Compliance

Proper reporting is an important issue to be considered by the home health professional. Home care-associated infections may be initially detected by the visiting home health practitioner and should be reported to the patient's physician for consideration of therapy and to the appropriate hospital or LTCF (if they are nosocomial). Contagious diseases (e.g., hepatitis, tuberculosis, impetigo, pertussis, and scabies) are especially important to report, and certain diseases are reportable to the health department. A proper home healthcare medical record should be kept.

The ICP needs to be aware of regulatory compliance issues including Medicare, the JCAHO (54), the Occupational Safety and Health Administration (OSHA), and state and local regulations that affect home care.

REFERENCES

1. Jarvis WR. Infection control and changing health-care delivery systems. *Emerg Infect Dis* 2001;7:170–173.
2. National Association for Home Care. *Basic statistics about home care.* Available at *www.nahc.org.*
3. White MC. Infections and infection risks in home care settings. *Infect Control Hosp Epidemiol* 1992;13:525–529.
4. Manangan LM, Schantz M, Pearson ML, et al. Prevalence of infections among patients in home care. *Infect Control Hosp Epidemiol* 2000;21:114(abst).
5. Graham DR, Keldermans MM, Klemm LW, et al. Infectious complications among patients receiving home intravenous therapy with peripheral, central, or peripherally placed central venous catheters. *Am J Med* 1991;91(Suppl):95–100.
6. White MC, Ragland KE. Surveillance of intravenous catheter-related infections among home care clients. *Am J Infect Control* 1993;21:231–235.
7. Gilbert DN, Dworkin RJ, Raber SR, et al. Outpatient parenteral antimicrobial drug therapy. *N Engl J Med* 1997;337:829–839.
8. Shah SS, Manning ML, Leahy E, et al. Central venous catheter-associated bloodstream infections in pediatric oncology home care. *Infect Control Hosp Epidemiol* 2002;23:99–101.
9. Rosenheimer L, Embry FC, Sanford J, et al. Infection surveillance in home care: device related incidence rates. *Am J Infect Control* 1998;26:359–363.
10. Tokars JI, Cookson ST, McArthur MA, et al. Prospective evaluation of risk factors for bloodstream infection in patients receiving home infusion therapy. *Ann Intern Med* 1999;131:340–347.
11. Do AN, Ray BJ, Banerjee SN, et al. Bloodstream infection associated with needleless device use and the importance of infection-control practices in the home health care setting. *J Infect Dis* 1999;179:442–448.
12. Colomb V, Fabeiro M, Dabbas M, et al. Central venous catheter-related infections in children on long-term home parenteral nutrition: incidence and risk factors. *Clin Nutr* 2000;19:355–359.
13. Danzig LE, Short LJ, Collins K, et al. Bloodstream infections associated with a needleless intravenous infection system in patients receiving home infusion therapy. *JAMA* 1995;173:1862–1864.
14. Hospital Infection Control Practices Advisory Committee. Guidelines for the prevention of intravascular catheter-related infections. *MMWR Morb Mortal Wkly Rep* 2002;51:1–32.
15. Luebbert PP. Home care In: *APIC text of infection control and epidemiology.* Washington, DC: APIC, Inc. 2000;44:1–11.
16. American Association of Respiratory Care. AARC clinical practice guidelines. Available at *www.aarc.org.*
17. Hospital Infection Control Practices Advisory Committee. Guideline for prevention of nosocomial pneumonia. *Am J Infect Control* 1994;22:247–292.
18. Keane WF, Bailie GR, Boeschoten E, et al. Peritoneal dialysis-related peritonitis treatment recommendations: 2000 update. International Society for Peritoneal Dialysis. Available at *www.ispd.org/guidelines.*
19. Prowant BF, Twardowski ZJ. Recommendations for exit site care. *Perit Dial Int* 1996;16(Suppl):S94–S99.
20. Centers for Disease Control and Prevention. Recommendations for preventing transmission of infections among chronic hemodialysis patients. *MMWR Morb Mortal Wkly Rep* 2001;50:1–43.
21. Simmons B, Trusler M, Roccaforte J, et al. Infection control for home health. *Infect Control Hosp Epidemiol* 1990;11:362–370.
22. Jewes LA, Gillespie WA, Leadbetter A, et al. Bacteriuria and bacteraemia in patients with long-term indwelling catheters a domiciliary study. *J Med Microbiol* 1988;26:61–65.
23. White MC, Ragland KE. Urinary catheter-related infections among home care patients. *J Wound Ost Cont Soc* 1995;22:286–290.
24. Kunin CM. *Detection, prevention and management of urinary tract infections,* 5th ed. Philadelphia: Lea & Febiger, 1997.
25. Pieper B, Templin TN, Dobal M, et al. Wound prevalence, types, and treatments in home care. *Adv Wound Care* 1999;12:117–126.
26. Ferrell BA, Josephson K, Norvid P, et al. Pressure ulcers among patients admitted to home care. *JAGS* 2000;48:1042–1047.
27. Panel for the Prediction and Prevention of Pressure Ulcers in Adults. Pressure ulcers in adults: prediction and prevention. Clinical practice guideline, Number 3. Rockville, MD: Agency for Health Care Policy and Research, Public Health Service, U.S. Department of Health and Human Services, 1992; AHCPR publications no. 92-0047.
28. Oie S, Kamiya A, Hironaga K, et al. Microbial contamination of enteral feeding solution and its prevention. *Am J Infect Control* 1993;21:34–38.
29. Rhinehart E. Infection control in home care. *Emerg Infect Dis* 2001;7:208–211.
30. Friedman C, Barnette M, Buck AS, et al. Requirements for infrastructure and essential activities of infection control and epidemiology in out-of-hospital-settings: a consensus panel report. *Infect Control Hosp Epidemiol* 1999;20:695–705.
31. Rhinehart E. Friedman MM. *Infection control in home care.* Gaithersburg, MD: Aspen Publishers, 1999.
32. White MC, Smith W. Infection control in home care agencies. *Am J Infect Control* 1993;21:146–150.
33. Manangan LP, Schantz M, Pearson M, et al. Assessment of infection control resources in the home care setting. *Infect Control Hosp Epidemiol* 2000;21:114(abst).
34. Manangan LP, Pearson ML, Tokars JI, et al. Feasibility of national surveillance of health-care-associated infections in home-care settings. *Emerg Infect Dis* 2002;8:233–236.
35. APIC Home Care Membership Section. Draft definitions for surveillance of infections in home health care. *Am J Infect Control* 2000;28:449–453.
36. Rosenheimer L, Embry FC, Sanford J, et al. Infection surveillance in home care: device related incidence rates. *Am J Infect Control* 1998;26:359–363.
37. Jarvis WR. The evolving world of healthcare-associated bloodstream infection surveillance and prevention: is your system as good as you think? *Infect Control Hosp Epidemiol* 2002;23:236–238.
38. Hospital Infection Control Practices Advisory Committee. Guideline for hand hygiene in health care settings. *MMWR Morb Mortal Wkly Rep* 2002;51:1–44.
39. Rutala WA. APIC guideline for selection and use of disinfectants. *Am J Infect Control* 1996;24:313–342.
40. Rutala WA, Barbee SL, Aguiar NC, et al. Antimicrobial activity of home disinfectants and natural products against potential human pathogens. *Infect Control Hosp Epidemiol* 2000;21:33–38.
41. Centers for Disease Control and Prevention. Transmission of hepatitis C virus infection associated with home infusion therapy for hemophilia. *MMWR Morb Mortal Wkly Rep* 1997;46:597–599.
42. Lobato MN, Oxtoby MJ, Augustyniak L, et al. Infection control practices in the home: a survey of households of HIV-infected persons with hemophilia. *Infect Control Hosp Epidemiol* 1996;17:721–725.
43. Hospital Infection Control Practices Advisory Committee. Guideline for isolation precautions in hospitals. *Infect Control Hosp Epidemiol* 1996;17:53–80.
44. Hageman JC, Pegues DA, Jepson C, et al. Vancomycin-intermediate *Staphylococcus aureus* in a home health-care patient. *Emerg Infect Dis* 2001;7:1023–1025.
45. Thomas CS. Management of infectious waste in the home care setting. *J Intraven Nurs* 1997;20:188–192.
46. Disposal tips for home health care. U.S. EPA Web site. Available at *www.epa.gov/epaoswer/other/medical/dispose2.*
47. Hospital Infection Control Practices Advisory Committee. Guideline for infection control in health care personnel, 1998. *Infect Control Hosp Epidemiol* 1998;19:407–463.

48. Herwaldt LA, Pottinger JM, Carter CD, et al. Exposure workups. *Infect Control Hosp Epidemiol* 1997;18:850–871.
49. Centers for Disease Control and Prevention. Updated US Public Health Service guidelines for the management of occupational exposures to HBV, HCV, HIV and recommendations for postexposure prophylaxis. *MMWR Morb Mortal Wkly Rep* 2001;50:1–52.
50. Beltrami MD, McArthur MA, McGeer A, et al. The nature and frequency of blood contacts among home healthcare workers. *Infect Control Hosp Epidemiol* 2000;21:765–770.
51. Joint Commission on Accreditation of Healthcare Organizations Web site. *www.jcaho.org.*
52. Health Care Financing Administration, OASIS Web site. *www.hcfa.gov/medicaid/oasis/osishmp.htm.*
53. Zimay DL. Standardizing the definition and measurement of catheter-related infections in home care: a proposed outcome measurement system. *J Med Syst* 1999;23:189–199.
54. *JCAHO 2004–2005 comprehensive accreditation manual for home care.* Oakbrook Terrace, IL: JCAMO.

108

INFECTION CONTROL IN COUNTRIES WITH LIMITED RESOURCES

W. CHARLES HUSKINS
EDWARD J. O'ROURKE
EMILY RHINEHART
DONALD A. GOLDMANN

Substantial progress has been made in the past decade in improving infection control in hospitals in countries with limited resources.[1] National infection control initiatives have made considerable progress in Latin America, Asia, Eastern Europe, and the newly independent states of the former Soviet Union and are gaining momentum in Africa. These initiatives have been driven in part by clinicians who recognize the need to reduce the unnecessary morbidity and mortality and the substantial waste of scarce healthcare resources caused by preventable nosocomial infections. In addition, many governmental and nongovernmental organizations engaged in improving healthcare in these countries have recognized that they must also improve the basic infection control infrastructure to achieve their specific missions (1, 2). The Centers for Disease Control and Prevention (CDC) has played an important role in solving outbreaks of nosocomial infections and is conducting other epidemiologic projects related to the prevention of nosocomial infections in many countries (3). Finally, the World Health Organization (WHO) has devoted significant attention to the problem by publishing introductory guides and manuals and by including basic infection control principles and practices in key international collaborations to address injection safety, antimicrobial resistance, and nosocomial spread of *Mycobacterium tuberculosis,* hemorrhagic fever viruses, and severe acute respiratory syndrome-associated coronavirus (4–10).

These initiatives have been successful in increasing public and professional awareness of the need for organized infection control programs, establishing training courses and reference centers for infection control professionals, and promulgating guidelines. Model surveillance and control programs have been developed and demonstrate that reductions in nosocomial infection rates can be achieved (11–15).

However, well-organized, effective infection control programs are often confined to select hospitals, typically academic institutions and well-funded government and private hospitals, whereas many hospitals farther removed from urban centers and/or with fewer resources have programs that may exist in name only or have no program at all. Strategies that will facilitate implementation of basic, cost-effective prevention and control measures in hospitals of all types, especially those with the fewest resources, are desperately needed.

This need is acute. The risk of nosocomial infection after basic healthcare interventions such as intravenous therapy, childbirth, and simple surgical procedures is unacceptably high. Moreover, sophisticated medical care, such as intensive care, open heart and solid organ transplant surgery, intensive chemotherapy, and even hematopoietic stem cell transplantation, is being offered in more hospitals; however, many hospitals do not have the infection control infrastructure necessary to minimize the substantial nosocomial infection risk associated with this care. Widespread use and misuse of antimicrobial agents has resulted in the emergence of highly resistant gram-positive and gram-negative bacteria, and ineffective infection control practices have facilitated intrahospital and interhospital dissemination of these microorganisms. Nosocomial spread of communicable infections such as gastrointestinal infections, respiratory infections, and measles remain a major problem, particularly among pediatric patients. Nosocomial transmission of *M. tuberculosis* is a significant threat to hospitalized patients and healthcare workers alike, especially when multidrug resistant strains are involved. Finally, the worldwide explosion of human immunodeficiency virus (HIV) infection has dramatically illustrated the risk of transmission of blood-borne infections to patients and hospital personnel.

Hospitals in many countries face many challenges in responding to these problems, including financial challenges. Hospitals consume most healthcare funds in most countries; however, most of the services they provide are substantially less cost-effective than those provided by community and preventive healthcare programs. Hospitals are being forced to decrease costs and become more efficient; however, hospital administrators may lack the experience and skills to effectively manage the hospital during these changes. Against this backdrop, broad-

[1] In this chapter, "countries with limited resources" are defined as countries with low- and middle-income economies in Africa, Asia, Latin America, the Middle East, and countries that comprise territories included in the formerly socialist economies of Europe.

based national and regional economic downturns inevitably have an independent negative impact on hospital resources.

The urgent need to improve the cost-effectiveness of hospital care is undeniable. However, it should be remembered that hospitals provide acute care unavailable in other settings; therefore, they represent a critical component of overall healthcare delivery. Indeed, improving access of patients who require hospital care to appropriate institutions is a major goal of many basic health programs, for instance Safe Motherhood programs. Simply reducing the funds available to hospitals is likely to exacerbate existing problems that indirectly contribute to the occurrence of nosocomial infections, such as understaffing and inadequate supplies.

Instead, there must be a broad-based effort to assist hospitals in improving the effectiveness, efficiency, and quality of care. The development of organized, effective infection control programs in all hospitals is fundamental to this effort. Indeed, the authors have argued that nosocomial infection control is an ideal model for nascent efforts to improve the quality of hospital care because of its proven efficacy in reducing the occurrence of infections that compromise patient outcomes and increase costs (16).

The primary goal of this chapter is to provide a framework for practical nosocomial infection prevention and control efforts in countries with limited resources. To lay the foundation for this discussion, key studies regarding the epidemiology of nosocomial infections in countries with limited resources are reviewed, and our experience performing infection control surveys in a variety of hospitals around the world is discussed. Organizational strategies, program priorities, and practical infection control interventions are discussed, recognizing that the ultimate design and implementation of prevention and control measures must always take into account existing local conditions and resources. Areas in which additional research is critically needed are highlighted.

EPIDEMIOLOGY OF NOSOCOMIAL INFECTIONS IN COUNTRIES WITH LIMITED RESOURCES

International, National, and Hospital Surveys of Nosocomial Infections

A prevalence study in 47 hospitals in 14 countries in 1983 to 1985 sponsored by the WHO is the only worldwide survey of nosocomial infections (17). The survey was performed by local teams of physicians and nurses on all hospital wards (excluding "long-stay wards") using a standard protocol that included definitions of infections. Because of practical limitations, the study organizers recognized from the outset that the sample of hospitals surveyed would not necessarily be representative nor was it possible to determine interobserver reliability or to independently verify the accuracy of data from individual hospitals. Nonetheless, the results of this study emphasize the worldwide importance of nosocomial infections. The mean prevalence of nosocomial infection in hospitals surveyed was 8.7% (range 3% to 21%). An additional report from this survey reports the prevalence of infection in different regions of the world, although figures from individual countries are not provided (18). Hospitals in Eastern Mediterranean and Southeast Asian countries reported a higher prevalence of nosocomial infection than hospitals in European and Western Pacific countries, although it is not stated whether this is a statistically significant difference (18).

Surveys of nosocomial infections conducted in national samples of hospitals from Latin America, Asia, and Eastern Europe, many of which date from the late 1980s to the mid-1990s, have been summarized in a previous edition of this chapter (19). More recently, a 1-day prevalence survey in 254 adult intensive care units (ICUs) in Mexico demonstrated that 23% of patients in these units developed a nosocomial infection (20). These surveys provide estimates of the magnitude of the nosocomial infection problem, but further interpretation of the data is difficult because of methodologic issues, and comparisons of rates among countries are likely to be misleading. Even when surveillance methods have been standardized, data are usually collected by personnel from the participating hospitals and are not subjected to rigorous assessments of reliability and validity. Variation in the quality of clinical documentation and the availability of microbiologic support may affect the sensitivity and specificity of surveillance. Finally, data from many hospitals are combined, obscuring potentially critical differences among hospitals and their patients. Patient populations in these hospitals may differ widely in terms of their demographics, underlying diseases, severity of illness, duration of hospitalization, and exposure to invasive procedures and devices, all of which may affect the risk of infection.

Despite these limitations, national surveys have served an important purpose. They have dramatized the impact of nosocomial infections to health policymakers and medical professionals, stimulated the initiation of infection control programs in individual hospitals, and contributed to the training of health professionals in surveillance methodology. Moreover, prospective nationwide surveillance programs can facilitate monitoring of trends in infection rates, the emergence of new pathogens, changes in antimicrobial resistance, and the identification of outbreaks.

Surveys conducted in individual hospitals are less subject to some of the methodologic difficulties outlined previously, although assessments of the reliability and accuracy of data collection are described in only a few studies (12,14,21–34). These studies report data primarily from large urban and/or university hospitals; few data are available from rural and district hospitals (hospitals of first referral) (31,33,35).

Nosocomial Infections at Specific Sites and in Specific Patient Populations

Surgical site infections (SSIs), urinary tract infections, lower respiratory infections, and bloodstream infections are the most common nosocomial infections (12,14,21–32,36,37). Skin and soft tissue infections and gastrointestinal infections are also common (12,21,23–25,29,32). The importance of nosocomial diarrhea, including diarrhea caused by *Clostridium difficile,* has been emphasized by a number of studies (38–42).

Ward-specific nosocomial infection rates are consistently highest in ICUs, because these units, by definition, care for the most severely ill patients and because the care of these individuals often requires use of invasive devices and procedures (14,23–32, 36,37,43). A handful of studies have reported specifically on device-associated infections (12,13,34,44–47). Using the CDC's National Nosocomial Infection Surveillance (NNIS) system surveillance methods to survey device-associated infection rates in six ICUs in four hospitals in Brazil, Starling found that rates of central line-associated bloodstream infections were comparable to NNIS system benchmarks, but rates of ventilator-associated pneumonia and catheter-associated urinary tract infection were substantially higher in some units. In a study involving patients undergoing major surgical procedures in a teaching hospital in Thailand, Narong et al. (34) reported rates that were higher than the NNIS system for catheter-associated urinary tract infections but comparable rates of central line-associated bloodstream infections and ventilator-associated pneumonia. A study conducted in three ICUs in Argentina found high rates for all types of device-associated infections (47). A study in Guatemala reported high rates of ventilator-associated pneumonia in an ICU (13). Avila-Figueroa et al. (46) have reported data regarding device-associated infections in pediatric patients in a network of hospitals in Mexico and also demonstrated high rates of ventilator-associated pneumonia.

SSIs have been examined in more detail (12,34,48–55). Numerous investigators have used NNIS system methods and reported risk-adjusted, procedure-specific infection rates (12,34, 51–53,55). Compared with NNIS system benchmarks, most of these studies have reported higher rates of infection, although not necessarily for all procedures examined. Several investigators reported that the duration of surgery in their surveys were substantially different from that in the NNIS system (51–53). The impact of this finding on standardized methods for international SSI surveillance is not clear.

Nosocomial acquisition of common communicable infections is particularly problematic for pediatric patients. Although somewhat dated, a report from the general pediatric wards of a hospital in South Africa is still illustrative (56). In that study, 14.3% of hospitalized patients developed a nosocomial infection. Communicable respiratory infections, including croup, bronchitis, bronchiolitis, and upper respiratory tract infections, accounted for more than 20% of the infections. Gastroenteritis and systemic viral infections (measles, varicella, and mumps) represented 13% and 7% of infections, respectively. Other studies have emphasized the threat of nosocomial measles, particularly in sub-Saharan Africa (57–60). Sizable outbreaks of hospital-acquired salmonellosis and cholera on pediatric wards have also been described (61–68), and nosocomial rotavirus and respiratory syncytial virus infection are endemic problems throughout the world (69–74).

A number of studies have shown that nosocomial transmission of communicable infections can also be the direct cause of some community outbreaks. Patients who acquired *Vibrio cholerae,* measles virus, Ebola virus, and severe acute respiratory syndrome-associated coronavirus in the hospital, but were in the incubation phase of their disease at the time of discharge, have been implicated in causing outbreaks of these infections in the community (59,61,75–78). Using molecular epidemiology techniques, a study in São Paulo, Brazil demonstrated that "endemic" salmonellosis in the community was in fact a series of small outbreaks of infection caused by antibiotic-resistant *Salmonella typhimurium* spread from the hospital to the community by recently discharged patients (79). Transmission of a multidrug-resistant strain of *Streptococcus pneumoniae* among hospitalized children in Slovakia was responsible for the subsequent spread of this strain into the community (80). Dissemination of hospital-acquired strains of multidrug-resistant *M. tuberculosis* is also a serious threat (81).

Nosocomial infections associated with childbirth are a major cause of morbidity among women, although a limited number of studies have examined this problem (12,15,82–84). Postpartum endometritis, SSI after cesarean section, and episiotomy infections are the most common infections.

The importance of nosocomial infections in newborn infants, particularly premature infants who are often cared for in crowded ICUs, is emphasized by a large number of studies. There are numerous reports of bloodstream infection, meningitis, and pneumonia, usually linked to the use intravascular catheters and mechanical ventilation and in association with substantial mortality (85–99). Many outbreaks of nosocomial gastroenteritis, bacteremia, and meningitis caused by *Salmonella* species have been reported (67,100–105), and nosocomial listeriosis has also been described (106,107). Infections in healthy full-term newborns are also a problem. A longitudinal study of neonatal diarrhea in a large urban maternity hospital in Burma found that the rate of diarrhea in infants born by cesarean section was five times that of infants born vaginally (108). This difference was attributed to the fact that infants born vaginally were cared for by their mothers (rooming-in), whereas infants born by cesarean section were cared for by nurses in the nursery. Skin and soft tissue infections resulting from *Staphylococcus aureus* also appear to be relatively common (personal observation).

Studies of nosocomial infections in other patient populations have been reported in a previous edition of this chapter (19), including oncology patients, patients with burns, patients undergoing hemodialysis, and cardiac surgery patients.

Etiologic Agents

In studies discussed in the previous section, bacteria caused most nosocomial infections associated with the use of invasive devices or procedures. *S. aureus* and coagulase-negative staphylococci are the most common gram-positive bacteria. Infections caused by enterococci are reported infrequently, although this may represent reporting bias or incomplete microbiologic evaluation. Infections caused by group A streptococci are rare. The most commonly reported gram-negative bacteria include *Pseudomonas aeruginosa, Escherichia coli, Klebsiella* species, *Enterobacter* species, *Proteus* species, and a variety of nonfermenting gram-negative bacteria. *Salmonella* species are common causes of gastrointestinal and systemic infection, particularly among newborn infants (40,42,65–67,100–103,105). *Shigella* species and other enteric bacteria are less common causes of gastrointestinal infection (40,109).

The worldwide crisis of antibiotic resistance among bacteria is an on-going, extremely serious problem (110–113). International surveys of antibiotic resistance among hospital isolates are available (114–116), and there are data from hospitals in countries with limited resources in these and other reports (117–123). The SENTRY Antimicrobial Surveillance Program has been particularly active in Latin America (124–128). The International Network for the Study and Prevention of Emerging Antimicrobial Resistance (INSPEAR) was formed by the collaborative effort of the CDC and microbiologists and epidemiologists in the United States and Western Europe, but it has subsequently expanded to involve more than 160 facilities in 40 countries (116). WHONET, a computer program to facilitate the analysis of trends in antimicrobial resistance developed in collaboration with the WHO, is being applied in an increasing number of hospitals around the world (129).

Existing data paint a bleak picture. Infections with methicillin-resistant *S. aureus* are well documented in many countries (130). Multiply resistant isolates of coagulase-negative staphylococci are also commonplace (95,99,119). In contrast to the situation in the United States, vancomycin-resistant enterococci appear to not be a significant problem, although there have been few systematic surveys (127,131). Nosocomial infections caused by penicillin-resistant *S. pneumoniae* are a long-standing problem in South Africa and are becoming more frequent in other regions (56,132–134). Gram-negative bacteria (e.g., *Klebsiella* species, *P. aeruginosa, Enterobacter* species, *Serratia marcescens,* and *E. coli*) that produce extended-spectrum beta-lactamases and also manifest resistance to aminoglycosides are widespread (135, 136), and resistance to fluoroquinolones among these bacteria is also increasing (137). In Latin America, multidrug-resistant gram-negative rods are a very significant problem (121, 124–128,138).

Given the prevalence of active tuberculosis, the presence of highly susceptible HIV-infected patients on hospital wards, and inadequate infection control practices, one can assume that nosocomial transmission of *M. tuberculosis* is commonplace. A few reports document this threat (8,81,139). Ritacco et al. (81) described a large, extended outbreak of nosocomial multidrug-resistant tuberculosis (MDR-TB) among HIV-infected patients in an infectious diseases hospital in Buenos Aires. Other studies have illustrated the potential for occupational *M. tuberculosis* infection among healthcare workers (8,140–142).

The burden of nosocomial infection caused by respiratory and gastrointestinal viruses is large, although the limited availability of diagnostic tests to identify these viruses hampers detection in many settings. Respiratory syncytial virus and a variety of gastrointestinal viruses, most notably rotavirus, are the primary causes of these infections (69–73,143,144). Viral infections diagnosed by clinical criteria, such as measles, varicella, mumps, and rubella, are a serious problem on pediatric wards, especially in areas where immunization rates are suboptimal (56,60).

Nosocomial transmission of blood-borne viruses is a major but often underappreciated problem (145–148). Blood transfusions and contaminated needles and syringes have been documented as a cause of HIV infection in Africa, in the former Soviet republic of Kalmykia, and in Romania (149–151). Nosocomial transmission of HIV and hepatitis C virus has been demonstrated among hemodialysis patients (152–155).

Some arbovirus infections are an uncommon but serious threat to patients and hospital personnel. Nosocomial transmission has been documented for Lassa virus, Ebola virus, Crimean-Congo virus, Marburg virus, Andes virus, and West Nile virus (75–77,156–162).

Evidenced by several reports, nosocomial fungal infections are common. *Candida* species are reported commonly among intensive care and immunocompromised patients (163–169). *Aspergillus* species as a cause of infected burns and pneumonia in leukemia patients has been reported (163,164).

Nosocomial infections caused by protozoa, helminths, and arthropods have been extensively reviewed in a series of publications (170–172). Giardiasis, amebiasis, and cryptosporidiosis are highly transmissible intestinal protozoa infections with the potential for nosocomial spread; amebiasis and cryptosporidiosis have been specifically reported in hospitalized patients (38,173, 174). Despite the high prevalence of infection with intestinal helminths in many countries, these organisms are unlikely causes of nosocomial infection, because most require an intermediate, nonhuman host or extrinsic maturation of excreted eggs or larvae (170). *Enterobius vermicularis, Strongyloides stercoralis, Hymenolepis nana,* and *Taenia solium* may be transmitted from person to person, but only *E. vermicularis* has been demonstrated in the hospital setting (170).

Infections caused by protozoa from blood transfusions, percutaneous exposures, and organ transplantation include *Plasmodium* species, *Trypanosoma cruzi, Trypanosoma brucei, Toxoplasma,* and *Leishmania* (171,175,176). Helminthic infections causing a chronic microfilaremia could conceivably be transmitted by blood transfusion, but clinical infections have not been documented (171,177).

Scabies and myiasis are well-documented nosocomial ectoparasitic infections (22,172). A hospital in El Salvador reported myiasis in 0.2% of discharged patients (22).

Host Risk Factors for Nosocomial Infection

There are few data describing specific host risk factors for nosocomial infections in countries with limited resources. Studies to identify risk factors require a comparison of infected patients and noninfected patients by performing an appropriate case-referent study with multivariable analysis to control for potentially confounding variables. Although some studies from countries with limited resources have described risk factors for specific infections, typically these reports do not control for age, underlying diseases, surgical procedures, or duration of period at risk in their analyses.

The distribution of underlying illnesses is different. Infectious diseases and traumatic injuries are more common and chronic, noninfectious diseases are less common in hospitalized patients in countries with limited resources compared with the United States and Western Europe. The impact of these differences on the risk of nosocomial infections has not been studied.

Likewise, the impact of severity of illness on the risk of nosocomial infection in countries with limited resources has been assessed only by broad measures, such as the likelihood of imminent death (178). Patients are hospitalized for long periods in some hospitals; the reasons for this are not clear but may be related to greater use of inpatient stays for diagnostic evaluations, longer convalescent periods after acute illness or surgery, the lack of alternatives for community- or home-based care, and/

or social considerations. Consequently, in some situations the average severity of illness may be lower among these patients compared with those in industrialized nations, reducing the risk of nosocomial infection.

Studies of nosocomial infections in malnourished children reveal a high cumulative incidence of infection (range 17% to 49%) (56,179–181), although the independent contribution of malnutrition per se to nosocomial infection has not been adequately examined. The reason for the apparent susceptibility of malnourished children to nosocomial infection is undetermined, although one can speculate that diminished immune function, compromised integrity of skin or mucosal barriers, and factors related to inpatient care (e.g., use of parenteral and enteral nutrition solutions) may all play a role. Whether vitamin A deficiency is a risk factor for nosocomial infection has not been explored.

Anemia was noted to be a risk factor for nosocomial infection in one study (182). Anemia had not been established as a risk factor for nosocomial infection in previous studies, and it is difficult to postulate why anemia alone would predispose patients to nosocomial infection. Anemia is an extremely common finding in children and in women of childbearing age in countries with limited resources and may be a marker for other host factors, such as malnutrition, that may increase the risk of nosocomial infection. Severe anemia increases the use of blood transfusions and has been associated with an increased incidence of transfusion-related HIV infection in Africa (149,183).

Factors Related to Hospital Facilities, Equipment, Supplies, Procedures, and Patient Care Practices that Increase the Risk of Nosocomial Infection

Information regarding hospital facilities, equipment, supplies, procedures, and patient care practices that have an impact on the risk of nosocomial infections in countries with limited resources is largely qualitative (184,185), including that summarized here. To better understand the existing status of hospital infection control in these countries, we have performed comprehensive infection control surveys in a variety of philanthropic and publicly funded hospitals in Central and South America, Asia, and Eastern Europe. We have noted a great deal of variability. Hospitals with exceptional infection control programs certainly exist. However, in hospitals with very limited resources and hospitals in which infection control programs have not been developed or have not had substantial influence, we have identified a number of factors related to hospital facilities, equipment, supplies, procedures, and patient care practices that are likely to increase the risk of nosocomial infection substantially. In the following discussion, we do not imply that these problems are present in every hospital or that they invariably represent a significant risk for nosocomial infection; nonetheless, they are encountered with substantial frequency and should be evaluated as a part of any comprehensive infection control assessment.

Hand Hygiene

Alcohol-based, waterless hand-washing agents are not available or are underused. In some older facilities or facilities where maintenance has been inadequate, sinks are not always functional (e.g., no running water or no drain). More commonly, there is simply an inadequate number of sinks (one sink for a large, multiple-bed ward). Sinks are also often inconveniently placed, making compliance with hand washing difficult for persons providing direct patient care.

The water supply may be contaminated with large numbers of gram-negative bacteria (186). Water filters are used in some hospitals, but the filters themselves may become heavily contaminated unless they are maintained scrupulously. Chlorination of the water supply is an effective, low-cost solution (187), but it may be inconsistently maintained or at insufficient concentration. One study found an association of an outbreak of gram-negative bacteremia in a neonatal ICU with contamination of the hospital water supply during a period when the hospital's water chlorination system was not functional (91), and another study correlated an increased risk of parenteral infusate contamination in wards with inadequate water chlorine levels (188).

Supplies of plain or antiseptic soap and paper towels are often inadequate. Some hospitals use single-use, small cloth hand towels that are laundered between uses. However, large, multiple-use cloth towels are more commonly used. These towels become damp during extended use and can harbor gram-negative rods (186). Some hospitals have installed hot-air hand dryers, but these appear to be used irregularly, presumably because of their noise and the duration of time required for drying wet hands.

Given the lack of facilities and supplies for hand hygiene, it is understandable that compliance with hand hygiene is poor, even among motivated personnel. In addition, even if sufficient facilities and supplies are available, it is likely that some personnel do not fully appreciate the importance of hand hygiene in reducing the spread of nosocomial pathogens.

Standard and Isolation Precautions

The large, open, overcrowded wards in many hospitals facilitate direct contact transmission and droplet and airborne spread of microorganisms. Although most hospitals have access to published guidelines for isolation precautions, these precautions are not often used effectively, because the guidelines are not available to physicians and nurses caring for patients, the responsibility for assessing the need for precautions is not clearly assigned, infection control personnel do not supervise and enforce precautions, supplies of barriers (e.g., gloves, masks, eye protection, gowns) are insufficient, and the physical plant does not support isolation requirements. In addition, even the most capable microbiology laboratories tend to be underused and may lack the resources or expertise to reliably identify specific communicable pathogens and/or antibiotic-resistant bacteria. Many hospitals also do not have policies for the identification and exclusion of hospital personnel or visitors with transmissible infections.

Few hospitals have rooms specifically designed for the isolation of patients with infections spread by the airborne route, because this requires special ventilation systems that can maintain negative air pressure relative to the hallway. Some hospitals use wall-mounted fans to exhaust room air outdoors. In tropical climates, rooms are often open to the outside air and may have excellent ventilation, but there is no control of the direction of air currents relative to the rest of the hospital.

Lacking specifically designed isolation rooms, most hospitals designate a single-bed room or a suite of rooms as isolation rooms. Patients with communicable infections are often cohorted in these rooms together, regardless of the specific infection and route of transmission. Many pediatric wards have large multibed rooms designated for care of patients with any gastrointestinal infection or any respiratory infection. When combined with the use of appropriate barriers and hand washing, such cohorting is an effective practice during seasonal outbreaks of a specific disease in the community, for instance, during outbreaks of viral gastrointestinal infection. However, more often than not, children with different infections are cohorted together, and when use of barriers and hand washing are inconsistent, this practice facilitates transmission of these infections to other susceptible children in the same room.

Barriers for use in isolation precautions systems, specifically gloves, masks, eye protection, and gowns, are often of poor quality, in short supply, or used incorrectly. Gloves are often reprocessed for reuse, increasing the likelihood that they have small, inconspicuous breaks or tears that result in increased hand contamination. Personnel using gloves often fail to remove them promptly after use, facilitating the spread of microorganisms. Cloth masks and gowns become moist easily, diminishing their effectiveness as barriers. Respirator masks and goggles or masks with face shields are very infrequently available.

Except in severely impoverished facilities, most healthcare workers are aware of the need to use barrier precautions to prevent exposure to blood. However, the use of barriers during contact with body fluids, mucous membranes, and nonintact skin, as prescribed by the CDC's Standard Precautions, has not been adopted widely or practiced routinely. In some facilities, the equivalent of "blood and body fluid precautions" is still practiced and barrier precautions are used only for patients who are identified as being infected with HIV or hepatitis B virus. Unfortunately, hepatitis B virus infection is so prevalent in some regions that many personnel tend to minimize the risk of hepatitis B virus infection to patients and themselves. Barriers for protection of mucous membranes from splashes of blood or other body fluids (e.g., face shields or masks and goggles) are not available or used routinely.

Although effective use of barriers at "the point of care" is frequently lacking, it is not unusual to encounter units, especially neonatal ICUs, requiring the use of gowns and booties or changes in footwear merely for entry to the unit.

Invasive Devices and Procedures

The use of invasive devices, such as indwelling urinary catheters, intravascular catheters, and mechanical ventilators, may be life-saving, but inappropriate use increases the risk of life-threatening nosocomial infections. This is a particular problem in tertiary care centers that use invasive medical technologies extensively. This was dramatically demonstrated by our experience in a pediatric ICU in Southeast Asia, where nosocomial infections related to the overuse of invasive devices contributed significantly to mortality (186). Others have demonstrated similar findings. A retrospective study in six pediatric ICUs in Mexico and Ecuador documented that children with low severity of illness scores (Pediatric Risk of Mortality score ≤ 10) underwent central venous catheterization and endotracheal intubation with mechanical ventilation more commonly than in a comparison pediatric ICU in the United States (189). The mortality rate among children with low severity of illness scores in the ICUs in Mexico and Ecuador was four times higher than predicted by their score.

Overuse may occur in two forms: (a) use of invasive devices when noninvasive alternatives would serve equally well, as in the use of indwelling urinary catheters instead of external bag urine collectors in pediatric patients, and (b) use of invasive devices for unnecessarily long periods, as in the failure to aggressively wean and extubate mechanically ventilated patients. Insufficient access to supporting equipment, such as pulse oximeters and blood gas analyzers to facilitate more aggressive weaning and earlier extubation of patients, is an issue in many hospitals. Overuse of invasive devices is undoubtedly also due to a lack of appreciation of the risk associated with these devices.

Intravascular Catheters, Intravenous Fluids, and Medications

Intravascular catheters are the most commonly used invasive devices. Many hospitals use metal intravenous catheters ("butterflies" or scalp vein needles) for short-term infusions. These catheters are associated with a low risk of phlebitis and local and systemic catheter-related infection, in part because they infiltrate easily and need to be changed frequently (190). Polyurethane or Teflon peripheral intravenous catheters, which have a longer dwell time, are available in many hospitals, but their expense may prohibit use in some settings.

Percutaneous central venous catheters (CVCs) are a much more significant problem. These catheters are commonly used in ICUs for infusions of fluids, medications, and parenteral nutrition and, more rarely, for hemodynamic monitoring. CVCs in use range from sophisticated silicon and polyurethane catheters to "home-made" silastic catheters manufactured locally from rolls of silastic tubing and hubs taken from peripheral catheters to stiff, polyvinyl chloride (PVC) nasogastric tubes. PVC catheters are likely to carry a much higher risk of thrombosis, suppurative thrombophlebitis, and bloodstream infection. In addition, because home-made silastic and PVC catheters cannot be inserted percutaneously, they must be inserted by cut-down (venous dissection), which also increases the risk of infection. Indeed, a study from Mexico found that insertion of CVCs by venous dissection independently increased the risk of bloodstream infection nearly threefold (191). In most instances, insertion sites are covered with gauze and tape; however, in some hospitals the insertion site is left exposed. Protocols for assessment of insertion sites, site change, or criteria for removal may be present but are often inconsistently applied. CVCs that are associated with a low risk of bloodstream infection such as tunneled (e.g., Hickman, Broviac) or totally implanted CVCs are rarely used.

In our experience, hemodynamic monitoring with pressure transducers is performed only in select tertiary care hospitals;

consequently, arterial and pulmonary artery (Swan-Ganz) catheters are not commonly used. When pulmonary artery catheters or cardiac catheters are used, they are often reused after ethylene oxide sterilization. Central venous pressure is sometimes monitored with a hydrostatic fluid column, which represents a site for contaminating microorganisms to multiply and potentially gain access to the bloodstream. Umbilical venous catheters are used frequently in premature or ill full-term infants, sometimes for long duration. Umbilical artery catheters are used much less frequently, usually in tertiary care centers with neonatal ICUs where blood gas analysis is readily available and used heavily.

Many hospitals use intravenous fluids manufactured by large multinational companies with high-quality manufacturing processes. However, many others rely on local manufacturers or even produce their own intravenous fluids on-site. An outbreak of sepsis and death in a newborn nursery in Brazil attributed to endotoxin contamination of locally manufactured intravenous fluids illustrates the consequences of breakdowns in proper manufacturing technique (192). Although the risk of bloodstream infection or pyrogenic reactions attributable to intrinsic contamination of intravenous fluids is likely to be low, detection of such a problem would be difficult. Written records of lot numbers are often inconsistently maintained, microbiology laboratories in many hospitals are unable to perform adequate cultures of intravenous fluids, and assays of endotoxin levels are expensive and not easily available. We have not encountered intravenous fluid containers with screw tops, which were linked to widespread contamination of intravenous fluids in the United States and, more recently, in Greece (193,194). The quality of plastics used in intravenous fluid containers, and their potential to develop small holes that might permit contamination, is a potential problem. We have observed fungus balls in plastic intravenous fluid containers in storage. In hospitals manufacturing their own intravenous fluids and storing them in reused glass containers, cracks in the glass and improper sealing theoretically could predispose to contamination.

Extrinsic contamination of intravenous fluids and medications is a more likely problem. Cross-sectional surveys of intravenous infusate contamination in Mexico have demonstrated contamination rates of 0% to 19% in individual hospitals (188, 195,196). Gram-negative rods, primarily of the tribe *Klebsielleae,* represent the majority of the isolates.

Potential sources of extrinsic contamination are multiple. Some hospitals use plastic intravenous fluid containers with access ports that must be cut open with scissors or another sharp instrument before the infusion set can be connected. Single-use sterile instruments for this purpose are not typically used. Instead, one instrument may be used multiple times and stored between uses in paper wrapping, a sterile container, or containers of disinfectant solution. Some hospitals use intravenous infusion systems from a variety of manufacturers that have incompatible connections, facilitating leakage and potential contamination (186).

In some hospitals, admixture of intravenous fluids and preparation of intravenous medications is performed in a room dedicated for this purpose or in the pharmacy; however, the availability of a laminar air flow hood is a rarity. More commonly, these tasks are performed on individual wards, and may occur in the midst of busy units in close proximity to potential sources of contamination, such as sinks and storage/cleaning areas for contaminated items. Many types of multidose vials are in use with variable methods for storage between uses. Glass ampules may be left standing open, with needles in the top, or covered with gauze and tape or tape alone. Refrigeration for multidose vials or prepared solutions is not always available. Protocols for disposal of opened vials, intravenous fluid containers, and infusion sets at routine intervals exist in some institutions, although it is difficult to assess compliance. Intravenous infusion sets are changed at a variety of time intervals ranging from 24 to 72 hours. Although the 72-hour interval is comparable to that recommended in United States hospitals (197), cost-effectiveness studies performed in countries with limited resources are needed to determine the optimal interval in this setting given the higher risk of extrinsic contamination of the infusate.

The use of parenteral nutrition deserves additional comment. A prospective study in Brazil found that receipt of parenteral nutrition was an independent risk factor for nosocomial infections in pediatric ICU patients (37). Small numbers of microorganisms can multiply in these solutions, particularly in lipid emulsions (198,199). Although these solutions are widely used, preparation rarely occurs under conditions designed to minimize the likelihood of contamination, such as in a dedicated clean room under a laminar air flow hood. In addition, because lipid emulsions are particularly costly, an individual bottle may be divided into infusions for multiple patients, increasing the likelihood of contamination during manipulation. Infusions may continue until containers are empty, regardless of the duration of infusion. This is unlikely to exceed 24 hours in adults, but individual containers and infusion sets may be in use for extended periods in premature infants.

Mechanical Ventilation and Respiratory Equipment

Nosocomial pneumonia poses a significant risk in severely ill, mechanically ventilated ICU patients, even under the best of circumstances. There is evidence that rates of ventilator-associated pneumonia are higher in countries with limited resources (12,13,46,200), although the lack of specificity in the definition of pneumonia makes it difficult to be confident of this assertion (200).

A number of factors are likely to exacerbate the problem of cross-colonization of the respiratory tract of intubated patients. In some units, suctioning is performed by designated personnel moving from bed to bed through the unit. Unless hand washing and proper suctioning technique are followed scrupulously, microorganisms can easily be spread by this practice. Other practices facilitate transmission of gram-negative bacteria because of their ability to survive and grow on wet surfaces and in solutions. Individual suction catheters are sometimes used for multiple suctioning episodes during a single nursing shift and are stored at each bedside in open containers of saline or other solutions (13). Saline used for instillation into the trachea is dispensed from large multidose containers, which may become contaminated unless handled with scrupulous care.

Respiratory equipment represents another potential reservoir for the propagation and transmission of gram-negative bacteria.

Large-volume nebulizers and mechanical nebulizers, which are associated with a high risk of infection because they generate aerosols that can carry contaminating bacteria to the distal airways (201,202), are uncommon. However, small nebulizers and multidose containers of aerosolized medications can also become contaminated (203,204), and potential risks associated with their use are often underappreciated. Although "bubble-through" and cascade humidifiers used with mechanical ventilators do not generate aerosols, in many hospitals these humidifiers do not have the capacity to heat the reservoir water, increasing the potential for contaminating gram-negative bacteria to flourish in these reservoirs. Filtered, distilled, or tap water, rather than sterile water, is occasionally used to fill these humidifiers, and reservoirs may be topped off instead of being cleaned and disinfected before refilling. Because ventilator tubing with heating coils to warm inspiratory gas are generally not available, large volumes of condensate can accumulate in the ventilator tubing, and personnel are often unaware of the risk of allowing this potentially contaminated fluid to reflux into the trachea. The number of reusable ventilator tubing circuits is often limited, so routine changes occur at intervals longer than every 72 hours and sometimes do not occur at all. There is no evidence that this practice has a significant impact on the risk of pneumonia, but specific investigations in this setting are needed to address this question.

Adequate high-level disinfection of respiratory and anesthesia equipment is not uniformly practiced.

Urinary Catheters and Urine Drainage Systems

Several risk factors for urinary tract infection among patients with indwelling urinary catheters are encountered commonly in countries with limited resources. Catheters and urine drainage systems used in many hospitals do not have ports for obtaining urine specimens. Consequently, the catheter is often disconnected from the drainage system to obtain a urine sample or to irrigate the catheter. The use of open urine drainage systems is also very common. Urine drainage systems are often emptied using a common collection container, facilitating cross-colonization among patients. In some settings, the urinary drainage system and/or the urinary catheter are changed at routine intervals, which disrupts the integrity of the catheter–drainage system junction and is unnecessarily costly.

Surgery and Wound Care

A number of factors increase the risk for SSI. Preoperative stays may be long, especially for patients in referral hospitals who do not live in the city where the hospital is located. Shaving of the skin the evening before surgery is routinely performed, despite the increased risk of SSI associated with this practice (205–207). Perioperative antibiotic prophylaxis is commonly used, but prophylaxis is often underused and administration may occur long after the optimal time (15). Agents used for the surgical scrub and skin antisepsis before surgery are generally adequate, although appropriate application of these agents can only be determined by detailed observational studies. Surgical linens (e.g., gowns and drapes) are typically used and resterilized many times, potentially decreasing their effectiveness as barriers to penetration of bacteria. Finally, many hospitals have room air conditioners in the operating rooms and others have only window ventilation. Although there are no data that indicate that this increases the risk of SSI, the number of air exchanges in these rooms is likely to be very low.

Colonization of open surgical sites and nonsurgical wounds may be facilitated by practices on the wards. Supplies used for surgical site and wound care are often organized on dressing carts that are wheeled from bed to bed, increasing the potential for indirect contact transmission of bacteria. Some hospitals use individually wrapped sterile instruments; however, in hospitals where these items are in short supply, instruments are submerged in disinfectant solutions (usually chlorhexidine-containing solutions) between uses. This process is unlikely to provide reliable disinfection for these instruments. Benzalkonium chloride, furazolidone, and mercurial and nitrofurantoin solutions, which are easily contaminated and are less effective than alcohol or povidone-iodine preparations, are used as skin antiseptics in some hospitals (85). Antiseptics stored in large containers and used for long periods of time increase the risk of contamination, especially when empty containers are refilled without first being thoroughly cleaned and dried.

Sterilization and Disinfection

Many items used in patient care are reused in hospitals with limited resources. Some items are specifically designed for reuse, such as glass syringes, metal-hub needles, and red rubber nasogastric tubes. However, many other items intended and manufactured for single use (so-called disposable items) are also reused, including plastic-hub needles, plastic syringes, indwelling urinary catheters, urine collection systems, nasogastric tubes, wound drains, endotracheal tubes, suction catheters, and latex gloves. Most of these items undergo steam or ethylene oxide sterilization before reuse, although it is difficult to assess compliance with proper reprocessing methods. There are a number of examples of outbreaks of blood-borne infections occurring as the result of reuse of needles and syringes without proper reprocessing (151,152,176). The impact of reprocessing on the integrity, safety, and function of single-use items is unknown. (See also Chapter 87.)

Organizational problems regarding reprocessing are often encountered. The responsibility for supervising reprocessing may be assigned to a nurse who may lack the requisite technical training. Reference materials and advice from more experienced personnel at referral hospitals may be available, but tradition is often the strongest determinant of the procedures in use, particularly in smaller hospitals. Reprocessing of patient care items is often performed in a variety of places in the hospital, including patient care units, ICUs, and clinics, despite the existence of better equipped and supervised central supply departments.

Even in central supply departments, quality control may be lacking. Because of the volume of materials that require daily reprocessing, autoclaves can be overloaded or may not be loaded properly (for gravity displacement autoclaves). Sterilization parameters such as time, temperature, and pressure are not always monitored. In some cases, this is because the temperature and pressure gauges are not functional. More commonly, gauges are working, but they are not routinely monitored or, in the case of newer autoclaves with functional chart recorders, chart paper is unavailable or not changed. Chemical indicator tape is appropriately used to identify items that have undergone sterilization, but in some cases is mistakenly regarded as an indication of sterilization efficacy. Biologic indicators to verify the adequacy of sterilization are used variably. Preventive maintenance of equipment is often not performed routinely.

Sterilization of critical items that cannot withstand high temperatures for steam or dry heat sterilization is a very difficult problem for many hospitals. Some hospitals have ethylene oxide sterilizers; others send materials to facilities that can perform this service, substantially prolonging turnaround time. Many small hospitals are forced to use other methods. Chemical sterilization using glutaraldehyde solutions is an acceptable alternative, although difficulties with adequate rinsing, storage, and potential occupational exposure complicate its use. In addition, in some instances equipment may not be adequately cleaned, exposure of all equipment surfaces to solution for recommended times is not ensured, and the solution may not be changed at recommended intervals. Other disinfection and sterilization methods for which efficacy has not been established are commonly used, such as the use of formaldehyde tablets or liquid for sterilization of delicate or heat-sensitive equipment. New technologies for low-temperature sterilization, such liquid peracetic acid and plasma sterilization, are generally not available because of the expensive equipment that is required.

Reprocessing of endoscopes is particularly problematic. Favero and Pugliese (208) emphasized the substantial gap between published guidelines for adequate reprocessing of endoscopes and actual practices around the world. A report from Brazil found that only 1 of 39 hospitals surveyed in São Paulo used adequate disinfection methods for gastrointestinal endoscopes, although this report did not find an association between a prior history of endoscopy and *Helicobacter pylori* infection (209).

Standardized, effective reprocessing protocols are particularly difficult to implement for expensive equipment purchased by individual physicians. Physicians may reprocess this equipment themselves in their offices with little guidance or quality control, or they may dictate the reprocessing methods to be used in the hospital, which may be inadequate.

Procedures for reprocessing anesthesia and respiratory equipment are often insufficient. Masks and anesthesia circuits used during surgery may only be cleaned, rather than disinfected, between cases. When more intensive reprocessing methods are used, there is often confusion regarding the minimum requirements of the process. In some hospitals, ethylene oxide sterilization is used. Although ethylene oxide sterilization is certainly adequate, high-level disinfection is sufficient and is likely to be accomplished at lower cost and with a faster turnaround time. In hospitals using chemical disinfection, exposure time to glutaraldehyde is often excessively long, frequently up to 24 hours, instead of the much shorter periods recommended in standard references (210). Rinsing is sometimes performed with filtered water, distilled, or tap water, instead of sterile water, as is generally recommended (210). Although it is not clear that rinsing with sterile water is absolutely necessary, nonsterile water supplies in hospitals in countries with limited resources may contain unacceptably high concentrations of enteric and/or nonenteric gram-negative rods, making them unsuitable for this purpose.

Many of the deficiencies and problem areas described previously were illustrated in a survey of sterilization and disinfection practices in 22 hospitals in Mexico performed by Zaidi et al. (85). They found that exposure times for steam and dry heat sterilization were often too short, low-level disinfectants were used for reprocessing critical and semicritical items, and biologic indicators were infrequently used to monitor the efficacy of steam, dry heat, and ethylene oxide sterilization.

Food and Water

Investigations of foodborne outbreaks in United States hospitals have identified several common food-handling errors: use of potentially contaminated foodstuffs, inadequate cooking, improper holding temperatures, contaminated equipment, and poor personal hygiene (211). These deficiencies are likely to be found in some hospitals in countries with limited resources as well.

Contamination of infant formula and enteral feedings is an area of particular concern. Most hospitals have special areas and designated equipment for preparation of special solutions, although, in some instances, infant formula may be prepared in nurseries. Terminal sterilization is commonly performed as a means of eliminating bacterial contamination from infant formula. Although adequate to kill contaminating microorganisms, this practice may degrade the nutritional value of the formula. As with regular foods, improper holding temperatures, contamination of equipment used to prepare these items, and poor hygienic practices of workers are also likely to be significant problems unless the process is closely supervised.

Because most hospitals use municipal water supplies, the suitability of this water for human consumption is an important consideration. Although outbreaks of nosocomial infection in hospitals conclusively tied to consumption of contaminated municipal water have not been reported, it is prudent to provide patients with water that has been treated secondarily (e.g., boiling or filtration) to ensure its potability.

Inanimate Environment

Newly established infection control programs are usually excessively concerned with microorganisms in the environment, as was the case in United States hospitals when infection control programs were being established. However, in specific circumstances, environmental microorganisms may pose a substantial risk.

Even if the municipal water supply does not contain any coliform bacteria, it is likely to contain nonenteric gram-negative bacteria. Hospitals often filter municipal water or distill water in an effort to provide water with a lower total microbial concentration for specific purposes (e.g., rinsing of semicritical items after high-level chemical disinfection). However, there is often no routine maintenance of filtering equipment, which may allow overgrowth of bacteria in the filter. There is significant risk associated with using water that is heavily contaminated by nonenteric gram-negative bacteria (e.g., *P. aeruginosa*) for hand washing in ICUs or for rinsing semicritical items after high-level chemical disinfection.

Given its propensity to colonize aging water distribution systems, nosocomial infection resulting from *Legionella pneumophila* is a potential problem, although there are no reports of pneumonia attributable to this pathogen specifically from countries with limited resources, probably because the methodology for identifying this microorganism is beyond the capabilities of most microbiology laboratories and systematic serologic studies have not been performed.

Although hemodialysis is widely used in countries with limited resources, some dialysis units do not quantitatively monitor the microbial content of the water or dialysate used in this process, as is recommended to prevent gram-negative bacteremia or endotoxin reactions (212). Water tubs used for hydrotherapy or burn wound debridement may represent a significant source of cross-colonization of patients unless disinfection procedures are performed carefully.

Airborne fungi are a significant cause of pneumonia in immunocompromised patients. Although these microorganisms are ubiquitous and exposure is likely to occur at least as commonly in the community as in the hospital, nosocomial transmission is a particular concern in tertiary care hospitals using intensive chemotherapeutic regimens and even bone marrow transplantation. These hospitals are unlikely to have the sophisticated air handling equipment [high-efficiency particulate air (HEPA) filtration] recommended to filter fungal spores (212). Environmental contamination with fungi is increased by chronic dampness, inadequate facility maintenance, and renovation or construction activity within the hospital or in the surrounding areas.

Although environment does not play a significant role in the spread of most bacterial pathogens, heavy environmental contamination has been noted in outbreaks of infection resulting from *C. difficile,* methicillin-resistant *S. aureus,* and antibiotic-resistant *Enterococcus* species. Respiratory syncytial virus and hepatitis B virus can survive for long periods on environmental surfaces. This emphasizes the need for good housekeeping with attention to specific products used for cleaning and disinfection of noncritical items and surfaces.

Mortality, Prolongation of Stay, and Costs of Nosocomial Infections

Information regarding mortality, prolongation of stay, and costs associated with nosocomial infections in countries with limited resources are important to emphasize the public health importance of improving nosocomial infection prevention. However, studies using matching or multivariable analysis to control for confounding variables have not been performed. Nonetheless, some crude estimates are available.

Ponce de Leon has extrapolated surveillance data from several hospitals to venture some startling estimates of the magnitude of the national burden of nosocomial infections in Mexico and in the world (184,213). Based on the occurrence of an estimated 450,000 nosocomial infections in the country each year and an attributable mortality of 5%, an estimated 32 deaths per 100,000 inhabitants are attributable to nosocomial infections. This estimate would rank nosocomial infections as the third most common cause of death in Mexico, behind only intestinal infections and pneumonia. Based on an average prolongation of stay of 10 days and an average bed-day cost of $100, the estimated yearly cost of nosocomial infections in Mexico approaches $450 million (213). On a global basis, he estimates that 1.5 million deaths and an expenditure of $1.5 billion per year are attributable to nosocomial infection (184).

A retrospective study from Thailand of 300 deaths occurring on the medical wards of a university hospital over a year and a half found that nosocomial infections were associated with 36% of deaths (214). Septicemia and pneumonia accounted for 60% of the infections in these patients. Infections were regarded as causing death in 43% and contributing to death in 32% of infected patients, although rigorous definitions were not used and many of the patients were judged to have underlying diseases that were likely to be "rapidly fatal" or "ultimately fatal."

An additional case-control study from a large teaching hospital in Turkey found that length of hospital stay was approximately 10 days longer for patients with nosocomial infections and that the average cost per infection was nearly $1,500 (215). The attributable mortality of nosocomial infection was 16% in this study.

PREVENTION AND CONTROL OF NOSOCOMIAL INFECTIONS IN COUNTRIES WITH LIMITED RESOURCES

The following sections discuss the development, organization, and activity of infection control programs and specific infection control interventions that are pertinent for areas of the world where resources are scarce and hospital infection control programs are a relatively new phenomenon. These sections recapitulate many issues discussed in more detail elsewhere in this text and readers should refer to other relevant chapters. Areas of particular relevance for hospitals in countries with limited resources are emphasized. A number of other publications and on-line training courses provide useful recommendations for infection control programs in countries with limited resources (1, 2,4,5,184,216–220).

Political, Economic, and Social Forces

The ultimate responsibility for infection control rests within individual hospitals, but external political, economic, and social forces may have a significant impact on the development of these programs.

Government regulations requiring hospitals to establish infection control programs have been promulgated in many countries, and training courses for personnel responsible for managing these programs have been developed (11,221). However, independent verification of compliance with regulations, for instance, as a component of a hospital accreditation process, is an important component of such an approach and is often not performed as systematically as necessary. Uncontrolled prospective observations suggest that this approach can have a positive impact on the development of hospital infection control programs (221). In contrast, some countries (e.g., Russia) have had outdated regulations for hospital hygiene that paradoxically prevented the adoption of new infection control policies and practices.

Initiatives to improve infection control have a powerful appeal to ministries of health because of their potential to reduce the costs of hospital-based healthcare. In addition to the cost estimates of Ponce de Leon noted previously (184,213), Nettleman (222) has estimated that the potential cost savings from reduced rates of nosocomial infection in South American hospitals could range from $300 million to more than $1 billion per year. The estimate for cost savings for Brazil alone ranged from $175 million to $840 million. These estimates are based on a cumulative incidence of infection of 8%, bed occupancy of 90%, additional hospital costs of $382 to $1,833 per infection (based on estimates from studies in Costa Rica and the United States), and a 32% reduction in rates of infection. These figures do not take into account the costs associated with establishing and maintaining infection control programs, and some of the underlying assumptions are likely to be overestimates; nonetheless, they provide an indication of the potential magnitude of savings.

Incentives for individual hospitals to reduce costs may also be important in stimulating development of infection control programs. Such incentives are present in capitated reimbursement systems that are being implemented in many countries. A diagnosis-related group (DRG)-based system has been in place in Brazil for more than a decade and, in combination with economic difficulties in the early 1990s, provided powerful incentives for cost-saving (221,223). In such settings, savings are likely to accrue from cost-effective use of antibiotics, antiseptics, and disinfectants and from prevention of nosocomial infections. Accordingly, Starling et al. (12) in Brazil report that their combined infection control and antibiotic control program saved their hospital $1.8 million over nearly 4 years. Another hospital program in Brazil has reported substantial cost savings by reducing rates of infection, reducing unnecessary use of antibiotics, and discontinuing wasteful practices such as environmental culturing and the use of expensive disinfectants for general cleaning (224). The methodology used to calculate these figures is not described in detail in either report.

The degree of authority that hospital administrators have over their budgets is also important. Although budgetary authority is becoming increasingly decentralized, many public hospitals still operate under fixed budgets determined at the local, regional, or federal level. Consequently, if cost savings are realized in one area, individual hospital administrators may not have the authority to shift funds to other areas. Supplies and equipment may be purchased centrally, and individual hospital administrators may be unable to authorize purchases of alternative devices that lower the risk of nosocomial infection (e.g., closed urine drainage systems).

Cultural factors may also have considerable impact on the vigor with which infection control efforts are pursued. Class, ethnic, racial, and religious differences between patients and caregivers may affect practices. The perception of the patient as a consumer of medical care, instead of a passive recipient of care, is a relatively recent but growing phenomenon in most countries. It can be expected that the general public and lay press will put increasing pressure on hospitals to provide assurance that patients are protected from avoidable complications of medical care, including nosocomial infections. Likewise, medical malpractice suits are also likely to become more common and will put additional pressure on hospitals to improve their risk management, quality management, and infection control programs.

Infection Control Programs and Committees

In the 1970s, the Study of the Efficacy of Nosocomial Infection Control (SENIC) demonstrated the efficacy of U.S. hospital infection control programs in reducing nosocomial infection rates (225). More recently, Danchaivijitr and colleagues offer evidence of the efficacy of hospital infection control programs in Thailand (11). Prevalence surveys of nosocomial infections were performed in a random sample of hospitals with more than 200 beds in Thailand during 1988 and 1992 using a protocol developed by the WHO for a previous international survey (17). In 1988, infection control committees (ICCs) and infection control nurses (ICNs) were present, and surveillance of nosocomial infections was performed in a small minority of the 23 hospitals surveyed. By 1992, these criteria were present in all of the 33 hospitals surveyed. The overall prevalence of nosocomial infection decreased from 11.7% in 1988 to 7.3% in 1992, a 38% reduction. Reduced infection rates were noted in all types of hospitals, across a wide spectrum of hospital services, and for all sites of nosocomial infection. This study does not prove that the infection control programs were responsible for the observed decrease in infection rates nor does it describe the characteristics of programs associated with the largest decreases. Nonetheless, it does provide persuasive, if indirect, evidence of the efficacy of these programs.

Hospital infection control programs are highly cost-effective. Wenzel (226) documented that these programs rank favorably with other key public health interventions in terms of their cost per quality-adjusted life year saved. Starling et al. (12) report that their combined nosocomial infection and antibiotic control program saved more than $1.8 million in antibiotic costs alone in a large Brazilian hospital over a 4-year period, a figure eight times higher than the cost of the entire program during this period.

Although these studies demonstrate the value of hospital infection control programs, only one study—the SENIC—has examined the structure and activities of these programs in relation to their efficacy (225). The SENIC identified the following features as characterizing highly effective programs: organized surveillance and control activities; a trained, effectual infection control physician; one ICN per 250 beds; and a system for reporting infection rates to practicing surgeons.

However, there is difficulty in directly applying this model in many resource-limited settings. First, it is often difficult to find trained individuals to serve as a hospital epidemiologist or an ICN. Second, the nursing profession may not have sufficient stature in some countries for ICNs to exercise the responsibilities and authority traditionally assigned to this position. Third, although ICCs are regarded as essential components of infection control programs by some, it is not clear that ICCs are always appropriate or effective in other settings, especially in hospitals where organizational structure is not rigidly defined and there are few, if any, other hospital committees. In some hospitals, for example, policy is determined by a few key physicians or administrators. On the other hand, established infection control models may be appropriate for large tertiary care hospitals with greater human resources and a more complex organizational structure.

In 1998, a consensus panel provided updated recommendations regarding the infrastructure and essential activities of hospital infection control and epidemiology programs (227). Specific recommendations are offered in the following areas: management of critical data and information (e.g., surveillance and clinical performance indicators); development, implementation, and monitoring of policies and procedures relevant to infection control and prevention; compliance with existing regulations, guidelines, and accreditation requirements; collaboration with the employee health program to ensure the health and safety of healthcare workers; direct interventions to prevent transmission of infectious diseases; education and training of healthcare workers; and resources available to the programs. The recommendations are a useful guide for program development and may serve as a foundation for hospital accreditation standards in many countries. However, employee health programs do not exit in many hospitals and recommendations related to program resources are likely to be out of reach.

Medical professionals with specific training in infection control are scarce in many countries with limited resources. Therefore, it is presumptuous to propose specific credentials for infection control personnel. However, a few simple guidelines may be helpful. At least one physician and one nurse should be a part of the infection control team to facilitate close ties between the program and the clinical services. It is preferable that these individuals have considerable patient care experience. Of course, it is helpful if the physician has training in epidemiology, infectious diseases, and/or microbiology. Recognizing the wide variation in educational preparation of nurses, it is preferable for the ICN to have a university nursing degree that will enable him or her to work as both a supervisor and educator for other nurses. Excellent interpersonal skills are essential to ensure productive working relationships with other hospital personnel.

The director of the infection control program is very likely to be a physician and is often an individual with considerable seniority. Certainly, programs can benefit from the legitimacy and authority provided by a senior physician. However, often this responsibility, thrust on a senior physician whose other duties prevent him or her from committing the required effort to the program, particularly in its early stages; this may result in a program that lacks direction and is unable to solve day-to-day problems. If a senior physician is required to lend status to the program, consideration should be given to assigning this individual an advisory role in setting programmatic goals and priorities, while a more junior physician assumes the primary responsibility for day-to-day efforts.

Most infection control programs in countries with limited resources are understaffed, as judged by the SENIC criteria and by even casual observation of the activities of program staff. In addition, many infection control personnel are not compensated directly for their infection control work and have this responsibility added to their other duties. Although this is understandable, it has a direct negative impact on the effectiveness of the program. Undercompensated and overworked personnel tend to leave the program, compounding the understaffing problem and taking with them any experience or training they have received. The staffing ratio of ICNs to hospital beds (one ICN to 250 acute care beds) established by the SENIC study is a useful rule of thumb (225) because this study was performed in hospitals with newly established infection control programs, a situation analogous to that in many hospitals in countries with limited resources. However, circumstances in individual hospitals may justify a higher or lower staffing ratio.

Aside from a physician and a nurse, the infection control program may benefit from the skills and experience of other professionals and disciplines. Persons with training in microbiology are particularly helpful. In some countries, community health officials are associated with hospitals. Although these individuals may have little experience in hospital infection control, they often have useful training in infectious diseases, epidemiology, and general disease control strategies. Computer specialists may provide assistance with surveillance data collection, entry, and analysis. Administrative and/or secretarial support is critical in providing infection control personnel more time to complete their work.

If an ICC is a part of the infection control program, appropriate membership is crucial. In addition to the personnel performing the day-to-day infection control work, representatives from the following departments should be included: hospital administration, medical staff (including a surgeon and an obstetrician, if appropriate), nursing (including a representative from the nursing administration and an operating room nurse), microbiology, central supply, and pharmacy. Representatives from other departments or wards, especially ICUs, and/or ad hoc members should be included as necessary. Assigning department chiefs to the ICC lends authority to the committee but is problematic if they do not have sufficient time to devote to the committee. Staff members with a genuine interest in infection control and detailed knowledge of clinical care and other work processes in their departments are preferable. Committee meetings should be held regularly, at least bimonthly, with minutes of the meetings recorded and distributed.

A direct reporting line by the infection control program to hospital administration is critical. Because the program is responsible for infection control in all areas of the hospital, it should report to the person or management committee that is responsible for the overall operation of the hospital. Some programs report to a department head, usually the nursing director. Although it is not clear that this is an ineffective approach, it may limit the scope and authority of the program, which should be hospital-wide.

Given the daunting task of implementing and/or improving infection control in hospitals with limited resources, it is crucial for new programs to establish a track record of problem solving. Hospital personnel often do not understand the role of the infection control program and may regard its work as unnecessary and intrusive. Unfortunately, this perception is strengthened when infection control personnel are seen primarily as regulators or policemen. By sharing data, educating patient care staff, and involving them in the identification of problems and the design of potential solutions, the program can foster its image as a problem-solver and an important ally in patient care.

Surveillance

The surveillance methodology used by the NNIS system (228–231) is being applied increasingly in other countries, particularly in South America (12,49,50,52,53,232). In Hungary, the Hospitals in Europe Link for Infection Control through Surveillance (HELICS) protocol (a protocol consistent with NNIS methods) was used to perform prospective surveillance of SSI in a cross section of 20 public hospitals (51). The latter study emphasized that nosocomial infection surveillance is an excellent model for outcome measurement in hospitals with little or no experience in quality improvement methods. However, the validity of surveillance data collected by networks of hospitals and the adequacy of risk adjustment indices, such as the NNIS SSI risk index, must be evaluated in more detail before nosocomial infection rates can be used widely as benchmarks for quality improvement efforts in countries with limited resources.

Unfortunately, these active surveillance systems are also labor intensive. Although some hospitals have sufficient personnel for this activity, many do not. In our experience, infection control personnel frequently spend more than half of their time collecting surveillance data on the wards. Although this activity promotes interaction with the clinical staff, it severely limits time for other critical activities. Clerical and computer support for analysis of the data and generation of reports is often unavailable, adding to the burden.

A simple solution is to ensure that data collection focuses only on information critical to the analysis and reporting of infection rates. Often times a large volume of detailed clinical information is collected but never analyzed, wasting precious time and effort. Additional time can be saved by eliminating the surveillance of community-acquired infections—a common practice, but one of limited value unless confined to specific diseases with important public health implications.

Time dedicated to surveillance can be used most efficiently by focusing on wards with high-risk patient populations (e.g., ICUs), patients with specific risk factors (e.g., CVCs), or types of infections with the highest mortality risk or cost (e.g., bacteremia or ventilator-associated pneumonia). Lima et al. (27) in Brazil reported an evaluation of a program designed to identify patients at higher risk for nosocomial infections. Incoming residents were given training in the epidemiology and identification of nosocomial infections and were required to record the occurrence of risk factors for nosocomial infection (a set of specified procedures and treatments and defined signs and symptoms of infection) on forms maintained on each ward. The ICN reviewed these forms to identify patients with risk factors and subsequently followed these patients prospectively, using bedside surveillance. A record review of a 5% sample of all hospitalized patients performed on three occasions by infectious diseases specialists was used as the gold standard against which this surveillance system was evaluated (although it should be noted that concurrent bedside surveillance would have been a more accurate gold standard). The sensitivity of the system was 74% [95% confidence interval (CI), 54% to 93%], the specificity was 99.7% (95% CI, 99% to 100%), the positive predictive value of a single risk factor was 93% (95% CI, 81% to 100%), and the negative predictive value was 99% (95% CI, 97% to 100%). A review of the forms revealed that 36% were incomplete and that 30% of the patients who had incomplete records (11% of patients overall) had unrecorded risk factors. Use of clinical microbiology laboratory reports alone to identify infected patients would have identified only 20% of the patients with nosocomial infections, all of whom had either a urinary tract or bloodstream infection. Although imperfect, this system reduced the number of patients followed by the ICN by approximately 50%.

Ponce de Leon and Macias (184) have recommended focusing on nosocomial bacteremia, because it is common, is associated with substantial morbidity and mortality, and is frequently associated with defects in infection control procedures that facilitate extrinsic contamination of intravenous fluids.

Other approaches can be used when human resources are very limited. Surveillance may be conducted on specific wards on a regularly scheduled, rotating basis. Surveillance may also be performed to collect data that will be used to answer a specific question or measure the impact of an infection control intervention.

Repeat prevalence surveys using the same methodology are another alternative, but these surveys tend to overestimate the frequency of infections with a long duration, and rates are not as precise as incidence rates because of random fluctuation in the number of infections present at the time of the survey. Prevalence rates can be converted to incidence data if the duration of infection is known (233). A study examining the correlation of concurrently collected incidence and prevalence data in a Mexican hospital found that the observed incidence rate of 4.5 infections per 100 discharges correlated well with the expected incidence of 4 infections per 100 discharges calculated from prevalence data and the date of onset of the infection (234). It is important to further note that this approach assumes a steady state in the population under study and may not be very sensitive for detecting outbreaks.

Prevalence surveys are useful for other purposes, such as evaluating the sensitivity and specificity of case finding by prospective surveillance efforts. They may also be used to evaluate characteristics of the hospital's patient population, the use of invasive devices and other risk factors for nosocomial infection, compliance with isolation precautions, and patterns of antibiotic use. Prospective surveillance can also evaluate these factors, but the volume of data collection may become overwhelming without yielding any more useful information.

Passive reporting systems have poor sensitivity and are not recommended. Laboratory-based surveillance also have poor sensitivity in hospitals where the microbiologic laboratory support is limited or underused, a common situation in many regions. If the infection control program is so understaffed that one of these approaches must be used, it is helpful to at least have some estimate of the degree of underreporting as determined by a prevalence survey as described previously.

Infection control personnel should review microbiology results on a regular basis as a routine part of their activity. Simply by reviewing microbiology logbooks during our surveys, we have identified several outbreaks of nosocomial bloodstream infection that infection control programs had not fully appreciated through their bedside surveillance efforts. Emergence of new pathogens and trends in antibiotic resistance may be appreciated more quickly if results of all cultures of hospitalized patients are reviewed rather than relying solely on bedside surveillance of clinical infections. Early detection of colonized patients can facilitate efforts to limit the spread of such microorganisms. The use of selective media to screen patients for antibiotic-resistant bacteria is particularly useful but can be accomplished only if there is good collaboration between the infection control personnel and the microbiology laboratory.

A collaborative relationship between the infection control program and the microbiology laboratory has other advantages. Infection control personnel in countries with limited resources may have little background in microbiology and can benefit from the expertise that microbiologists bring to the overall infection control effort. In turn, infection control personnel can serve as an important bridge between the microbiology laboratory and the clinical services. For example, they can help improve specimen collection and labeling on the wards, develop systems for more useful and timely reporting of culture results to clinicians, and compile annual summaries of antimicrobial susceptibility results for common nosocomial and community pathogens as an aid for physicians prescribing empiric antimicrobial therapy.

For hospitals initiating infection control programs, establishing baseline rates of nosocomial infections is especially important because these data will be used to demonstrate the burden of nosocomial infections to medical professionals and hospital administrators, to determine whether future clusters of infection represent significant outbreaks, and to guide implementation of specific interventions and determine their effect. The methodology used to determine baseline rates of infection should be based on the level of sophistication of the hospital and infection control personnel resources. If possible, tertiary care hospitals should invest the time and effort to perform prospective, ongoing surveillance to determine incidence rates, particularly in high-risk wards and ICUs. Baseline data should be collected over a sufficient period of time such that monthly and seasonal variation in infection rates can be determined; in most instances, this requires at least 1 year of baseline data collection. In hospitals with lower risk patients, prospective ongoing surveillance is useful, but repeat prevalence surveys performed at various times of the year may suffice.

Most importantly, the infection control program must develop a surveillance plan that addresses the needs of the institution. The goals and methods of surveillance must be reviewed at least yearly. Consideration should be given to the usefulness of the data in detecting patterns of infection, including potential outbreaks; the spectrum of nosocomial pathogens, including infection and colonization by antibiotic-resistant bacteria; and its impact in the design and evaluation of future infection control interventions. In some countries, national initiatives to improve infection control have mandated specific surveillance strategies. Although there are benefits to this approach, particularly in the early stages of infection control program development, some flexibility is needed lest surveillance becomes an exercise in fulfilling requirements instead of a process of data collection and analysis that addresses specific institutional needs and improves patient care.

Prompt, careful investigation of potential outbreaks is also critical. As demonstrated by a summary of 14 years of experience with nosocomial infection outbreaks of in a tertiary center in Mexico (235), these infections often occur in highly vulnerable patients and are associated with high mortality rates. Common-source outbreaks resulting from contamination of equipment, solutions, and medications remain a major threat in hospitals with limited resources. Personnel in these hospitals often do not fully appreciate the ability of gram-negative rods to proliferate in virtually anything wet. Recognition of the importance of such contaminated reservoirs led to enormous reductions in the risk of gram-negative bacterial infection in United States hospitals in the 1960s and 1970s, particularly in nurseries and ICUs. It is reasonable to hypothesize that attention to this important source of infection would have a dramatic impact in countries with limited resources as well.

Additional research and discussion regarding appropriate surveillance methodologies for use in countries with limited resources is desperately needed. Such methods must use human resources efficiently and use definitions of infections that are useful in settings with limited laboratory support.

Policies and Procedures

A major priority for newly established infection control programs is the development and implementation of infection control policies and procedures. A complete review of all of the policies and procedures that should be addressed by the infection control program is beyond the scope of this chapter, but a few of the most important issues are mentioned briefly in this section, accompanied by recommendations for practical interventions in hospitals with limited resources in the next section.

Infection control policies and procedures should focus on preventing (a) transmission of infectious agents from infected or colonized patients, healthcare workers, and visitors or from the environment of care to susceptible hosts and (b) infections usually caused by patients' endogenous flora that gain access to sterile body sites through the use of invasive devices or procedures. Accordingly, core policies and procedures for preventing transmission of potentially infectious agents should address hand hygiene, standard precautions and isolation precautions, occupational health issues for healthcare workers, visitor policies, injection practices, reprocessing reused materials, and environmental cleaning and sanitation. Policies and procedures for preventing infections associated with invasive devices and procedures should focus, at a minimum, on safe use of intravascular catheters, mechanical ventilation and other respiratory equipment, urinary catheters, and surgical procedures.

Infection control personnel should work with physicians and supervisory nurses to establish written protocols for these key policies and procedures. In addition to providing a reference for future training, this process will help to identify areas for improvement in practices and promote standardization of practices.

Practical Interventions to Reduce the Risk of Nosocomial Infections

In this section, we recommend a number of practical interventions directed at potential problem areas identified previously (in the section about factors related to hospital facilities, equipment, supplies, procedures, and care practices that increase the risk of nosocomial infection). These interventions are based on evidence-based guidelines from the CDC's Healthcare Infection Control Practices Advisory Committee (HICPAC) and other professional societies (197,210,212,236–241), CDC and WHO publications (4,8–10), published investigations, and our practical experience. In some cases, these recommendations represent significant adaptations of existing guidelines when necessitated by limited resources. They have not been reviewed or endorsed by any official body. Some of the recommendations are interventions with well-established efficacy, others have the potential to reduce the risk of nosocomial infection, although efficacy has not been clearly established, and others represent what may best be termed "good practice." The rationale for these recommendations and applicable references are noted.

It is naive to assert that the implementation of these interventions is a simple task, and additional expenditures may be required in some cases. Nonetheless, many of these basic interventions are within the means of many hospitals and are likely to be cost-effective, although this determination can only be assessed completely at the local level.

Finally, implementation is much more likely to be successful if it is undertaken in the context of a coordinated multidisciplinary effort to improve care and if specific process and outcome measures are used to monitor the effect of the intervention and feedback this information to those who need to know (15,16).

Hand Hygiene

Use of alcohol-based, waterless hand antiseptics have become the preferred method for hand hygiene when hands are not visibly soiled (240). Compared with hand washing with soap and water, these antiseptics have greater efficacy in reducing bacterial counts on the hands, are more convenient for healthcare workers to use, and reduce skin dryness and irritation (240). Use of these agents is an excellent way to facilitate compliance with hand hygiene, especially in hospitals with an inadequate number of accessible sinks in patient care areas (Table 108.1). A number of commercial solutions are available for this purpose. Cheaper alternatives, such as an alcohol and emollient solution (for 1 L of solution, mix 980 mL of 70% isopropyl alcohol with 20 mL of glycerin; adjust the amount of glycerin added from 10 to 30 mL according to the preferences of healthcare workers), can be formulated locally. Waterless hand antiseptics should be dispensed in small, pour-top or squeeze bottles. Open basins used for hand "dipping" should not be used. Portable containers are particularly well suited for use by caregivers moving from patient to patient on large crowded wards. They can also be used for hand hygiene before performing invasive procedures or contact with patients at high risk for nosocomial infections

For hand washing, a source of clean, running water, either from a tap or a bucket or cistern, and plain soap must be available to remove organic material. An adequate method for drying hands is also essential. Paper towels are the most convenient method for hand drying. If hospitals are unable to afford paper towels, single-use cloth hand towels that are laundered between uses are an acceptable alternative. Towels left beside sinks for use by multiple personnel are strongly discouraged. Some hospitals use hot air dryers for hand drying, but personnel may avoid their use because of their noise during operation and the relatively long period of time necessary to adequately dry hands. This equipment also requires a larger initial capital expense, consumes energy, and is subject to mechanical breakdown.

For a surgical scrub, an antiseptic with persistent activity should be used. Use of either a waterless agent containing alcohol and chlorhexidine or a scrub using water and soap containing chlorhexidine or povidone-iodine are suitable agents (240).

TABLE 108.1. HAND HYGIENE: POTENTIAL PROBLEM AREAS IN HOSPITALS WITH LIMITED RESOURCES, PRACTICAL INTERVENTIONS, AND RATIONALE

Potential Problem Area	Practical Intervention	Rationale
No sinks or sinks without running water	Provide source of clean, running water	Soap and running water are needed to remove visible blood, other body fluids, or proteinaceous material from hands
	Provide an alcohol-based, waterless hand antiseptic (see text for recipe)	Use of a waterless, alcohol-based hand antiseptic is the preferred method for hand hygiene when visible soiling is not present (240)
Sinks not conveniently located in patient care areas	Same as above	Same as above
Soap not available	Provide plain soap	Soap and running water are needed to remove visible blood, other body fluids, or proteinaceous material from hands
Multiple-use towel or no hand drying method available	Provide paper towels or single-use cloth hand towels	Multiple-use cloth towels may become contaminated (186)
Poor adherence	Ensure availability of basic supplies	Compliance will be poor until basic supplies are available
	Provide education, promotion, role modeling by physician and nursing leaders, and feedback on adherence	Multidimensional interventions can improve compliance (240)

sion of nosocomial pathogens, proper hand washing technique and use of waterless hand antiseptics, and motivational activities to improve compliance with hand washing guidelines should be emphasized. Several studies have demonstrated that the behavior of role models can significantly influence hand hygiene practices by others (240).

Standard Precautions and Transmission-Based Isolation Precautions

In the "Guideline for Isolation Precautions in Hospitals" published in 1996, the CDC/HICPAC emphasized use of standard precautions to prevent transmission of blood-borne pathogens, multidrug resistant bacteria, and other pathogens from patients who are not recognized to be infected or colonized with these agents (242). Standard Precautions are technically appropriate for use in all settings, a point reinforced by the WHO in its infection control manual and the CDC in its manual for control of viral hemorrhagic fevers in Africa (5,9). However, full use of Standard Precautions requires ready access to gloves, gowns, face and eye protection, and footwear that is well beyond the capacity of many hospitals in low-resource settings. A study from Thailand published in 1997 reported the average overall cost for protective equipment was \$5.37 per inpatient stay and \$0.15 per outpatient visit (243).

Consequently, hospitals may need to devise alternative strategies (Table 108.2). They should focus on hand hygiene using a alcohol-based, waterless hand antiseptic and use available supplies of barriers preferentially in high-risk areas (e.g., operating and delivery rooms, emergency department). Plastic bags can be used as barriers in dire circumstances (Table 108.2). In very high risk situations (e.g., treating a patient with suspected viral hemorrhagic fever) where gloves are in very limited supply, healthcare workers can dip their gloved hands into a solution of diluted (1:100) household bleach for 1 minute between contacts (if soiled, gloved hands should be washed with soap and water first) (9).

A practical isolation precaution system is an essential compo-

TABLE 108.2. STANDARD AND TRANSMISSION-BASED ISOLATION PRECAUTIONS: POTENTIAL PROBLEM AREAS IN HOSPITALS WITH LIMITED RESOURCES, PRACTICAL INTERVENTIONS, AND RATIONALE

Potential Problem Area	Practical Intervention	Rationale
No system for SP or IP	Develop and apply system for SP and IP	Concepts of SP and IP are applicable in all settings, although they may need local adaptation due to insufficient supplies (see below) (5,9,242)
SP and IP underutilized or overused	Educate HCWs	Many HCWs lack knowledge of the modes of transmission of infectious agents
Unable to specifically identify infections because microbiology testing limited or not available	Base IP on identification of clinical syndromes	Clinical syndromes can be used to determine appropriate IP in most situations (242)
Incomplete or slow initiation of IP	Assign responsibility for initiating IP Include screening questions with decision regarding need for IP as a part of the admission procedure Monitor completeness and time to initiation of IP	Optimize the system for initiating IP (242)
Insufficient supplies (e.g., gloves, gowns, masks, goggles) not addressed by conservation and reuse	Emphasize hand hygiene, including use of alcohol-based, waterless hand antiseptic	Alcohol is active against gram-positive and gram-negative vegetative bacteria, including multidrug-resistant bacteria, various fungi, many enveloped viruses and some nonenveloped viruses (240)
	Prioritize available supplies for use in high-risk areas (e.g., operating and delivery rooms, emergency department)	Locations where invasive procedures are performed or where ill patients who potentially have transmissible infections present for care are the highest risk areas
	Use plastic bags on hands or feet	Bags are a physical barrier (9)
	Dip gloved hands with diluted household bleach (1 : 100) for 1 minute between contacts (if soiled, wash gloved hands with soap and water first)	Hypochlorite solution inactivates blood-borne viruses and many gram-positive and gram-negative vegetative bacteria (9)
No negative pressure rooms	Cohort patients with the same airborne disease (e.g., measles, multidrug resistant tuberculosis)	Cohorting is an adjunctive strategy if substantial numbers of patients with the same infection are encountered (242)
	Avoid cough inducing procedures	Decrease generation of droplet nuclei (8)
	Ensure adequate natural ventilation	Fresh air reduces the concentration of droplet nuclei (8)
	Close doors and use out-facing window or wall fans	Direct airflow out of the building (8)
	UVGI may be appropriate in some situations when natural ventilation is impossible	UVGI can kill *Mycobacterium tuberculosis* (8)

HCW, healthcare worker; IP, isolation precautions; SP, Standard Precautions; UVGI, ultraviolet germicidal irradiation.

nent of any infection control program (Table 108.2). As previously noted, transmission-based isolation precautions outlined in the CDC/HICPAC guideline are technically appropriate for use anywhere (242). Recommendations for isolation precautions based on clinical syndromes included in this guideline are useful in settings where diagnostic microbiologic support is lacking (242). However, as noted for standard precautions, the practical application of the CDC/HICPAC system may be constrained by limited supplies of barriers. In addition, recommendations for use of negative pressure rooms and respirator masks to prevent the spread of tuberculosis are impractical in many settings and local adaptations are needed.

Infection control programs should focus on making clinical staff aware of the indications for precautions and on monitoring compliance. The responsibility for assessing the need for isolation precautions must be clearly assigned, preferably to the admitting physician and the nurse performing the initial nursing assessment. Admitting departments also should be aware of the isolation precautions policy to ensure placement of patients in appropriate wards and rooms. Simple algorithms may be developed and posted in clearly visible places to facilitate this process. Once the need for isolation precautions has been identified, the appropriate precautions must be determined. Written guidelines must be accessible for easy reference, infection control personnel must be available to provide consultation, and the necessary supplies must be at hand.

The problem of tuberculosis deserves additional comment, although readers should consult the WHO guideline for a comprehensive discussion of this topic (8). Preventing the spread of *M. tuberculosis* in healthcare settings requires at three-tier approach including administrative and environmental controls and the use of personal protective equipment (8). Administrative controls, which include prompt recognition of potentially infectious patients, separation or isolation of infectious patients, and initiation of effective antituberculous therapy, are within the capacity of many low-resource facilities. Experience in Peru has emphasized that even multidrug-resistant tuberculosis can be treated effectively in low-resource settings (244). Environmental controls that emphasize natural ventilation and simple methods to direct air flow are also achievable in many settings (Table 108.2). These interventions may be applicable to preventing the spread of other airborne infections, such as measles. Ultraviolet germicidal irradiation is an adjunctive environmental control for *M. tuberculosis* when natural ventilation is not possible (8). Personal protective equipment, including personal respirators, are likely to be too expensive for widespread use but may be used in very high risk settings (i.e., tuberculosis clinic or ward.).

Occupational Health Issues for Healthcare Workers

Given the multitude of other important tasks, infection control programs cannot usually assume primary responsibility for administering an occupational health program. Nonetheless, infection control personnel can assist in developing practical guidelines for (a) exclusion criteria for hospital personnel with communicable diseases, (b) prophylaxis and counseling for hospital personnel with occupational exposure to communicable diseases (including blood-borne pathogens), and (c) interventions to prevent exposure to blood-borne pathogens. Published guidelines are generally applicable for hospitals with limited resources (238), but specific recommendations are likely to require adaptation based on knowledge of the local epidemiology of the particular infectious diseases and practical considerations.

A systematic evaluation of practices that contribute to needlesticks and other percutaneous exposures should be undertaken, particularly in the operating theater, the ICUs, the emergency room, delivery rooms, and the clinical laboratories. Discussions with hospital personnel may identify changes in practices that will reduce the likelihood of exposure.

Provision of hepatitis B vaccine free of charge to all at-risk, susceptible hospital employees is beyond the means of many hospitals in countries with limited resources. However, an approach targeted toward high-risk, hepatitis B surface antigen (HbsAg)-negative personnel may be feasible in some settings. Postexposure chemoprophylaxis for HIV is expensive but is available in some countries and hospitals. On the other hand, postexposure counseling can be provided, and hospitals may be able to provide follow-up serologic testing for HIV and HBsAg.

Injection Practices

The WHO has developed the Safe Injections Global Network (SIGN) Alliance, an extensive program to ensure safe and appropriate injection practices (6). Key elements of the program at a local level are behavior change strategies to decrease injection overuse; ensuring that adequate equipment and supplies, including autodisposable syringes for immunization and appropriate syringes and needles (sterilizable, disposable, or auto-disposable) for curative care, are available in sufficient supply; and ensuring that sharps waste is handled in an efficient, safe, environmentally friendly manner (6). A "toolbox" of practical policy management and technical tools and additional resources is available on the WHO Web site (245).

Intravascular Catheters, Intravenous Fluids, and Medications

Intravascular catheters, particularly percutaneously inserted CVCs, should be used only when central venous access is absolutely necessary and should be removed as soon as possible (Table 108.3). CVCs should be inserted using an effective antiseptic at the site of insertion and maximal sterile barrier precautions, and the insertion site should be appropriately dressed (e.g., covered with gauze) (197). Protocols for routine assessment of the insertion site and criteria for removal of the catheter should be established and followed. Although high-quality CVCs made of pliable, biocompatible materials (e.g., silicon, polyurethane) are expensive, the relatively small numbers of these catheters in use in most hospitals make the extra expense justifiable, especially when compared with the cost of treatment for thrombophlebitis and/or catheter-related bloodstream infection. CVCs should be inserted percutaneously whenever possible; cut-downs should be avoided.

Several measures can be implemented to reduce the risk of contamination of intravenous fluids (Table 108.3). Equipment should be selected to ensure that connections between the intra-

TABLE 108.3. INTRAVASCULAR CATHETERS, INTRAVENOUS FLUIDS, AND MEDICATIONS: POTENTIAL PROBLEM AREAS IN HOSPITALS WITH LIMITED RESOURCES, PRACTICAL INTERVENTIONS, AND RATIONALE

Potential Problem Area	Practical Intervention	Rationale
Intravascular catheters used when less invasive alternatives exist or for unnecessarily long periods of time	Use less invasive alternatives whenever possible and remove catheter as soon as possible	Reduces exposure risk
Inadequate technique for insertion and care of intravascular catheters	Use maximal sterile barrier precautions, an effective antiseptic, and aseptic technique during insertion	Demonstrated to be effective in reducing catheter colonization and bloodstream infection (255,256)
CVCs made of inferior materials (e.g., polyvinyl chloride) and inserted by cut-down (venous dissection)	Use catheters made of high-quality material; insert catheters percutaneously whenever possible	Reduces incidence of thrombosis, catheter-related phlebitis, local infection of the insertion site, and catheter-related BSI (197)
Incompatible connections of IV fluid containers and/or infusion sets	Obtain supplies with compatible connections	Reduces risk of extrinsic contamination
IV fluids and medications prepared by multiple different personnel on wards in close proximity to sources of contamination	Utilize premixed IV fluids whenever possible	Same as above (197)
	Prepare IV fluids and medications in designated area (preferably in laminar air flow hood) away from potential sources of contamination	Same as above (197)
	Allow only specially trained individuals to prepare fluids, especially parenteral nutrition solutions	Same as above (197)
Access ports of IV fluid containers opened with multiple-use, nonsterile instrument	Open access ports aseptically using sterile single-use instrument	Same as above (197)
Multidose vials exposed to environmental contamination between uses	Minimize use of multidose vials	Same as above (197)
	Mark with date and time of opening Use aseptic technique during handling Use sterile device when accessing vial Prevent exposure to environmental contamination Store according to manufacturer's guidelines	
Parenteral and/or lipid emulsion containers and infusion sets changed irregularly or only when empty	Use parenteral nutrition and lipid emulsion solutions promptly	Parenteral nutrition and lipid emulsions, in particular, facilitate growth of contaminating microorganisms (197–199)
	Complete the infusion of lipid-containing solutions within 24 hours When lipid emulsions are given alone, complete the infusion within 12 hours	

BSI, primary bloodstream infection; CVC, central venous catheter; IV, intravenous.

venous fluid container and all components of the infusion set are compatible and can be maintained. Qualified personnel should perform preparation of intravenous fluids and medications in a quiet, clean area. Insertion of the infusion set into the access port of the intravenous fluid container must be performed using aseptic technique. This requires that a single-use sterile instrument be used to open the access port, if this is necessary. The use of multidose medication vials should be minimized. If multidose vials are used, they should be labeled with an expiration time, protected from potential sources of environmental contamination, and stored according to manufacturer's guidelines. Admixtures of parenteral nutrition or lipid emulsions should be used promptly after preparation and discarded within 24 hours, regardless of whether they are empty.

Mechanical Ventilation and Respiratory Equipment

Mechanical ventilation should only be used when absolutely necessary and should be discontinued as soon as possible (Table 108.4). Nonemergent use of mechanical ventilation requires that equipment for monitoring oxygenation and ventilation is available to ensure that weaning of ventilatory support and extubation occur in a timely fashion. Measurements of respiratory mechanics may also help to identify patients that can be extubated safely.

Procedures used for suctioning of mechanically ventilated patients should minimize the potential for cross-colonization of the respiratory tract (Table 108.4) (237). Suction catheters should be used once and either discarded or reprocessed. If this

TABLE 108.4. MECHANICAL VENTILATION AND RESPIRATORY EQUIPMENT: POTENTIAL PROBLEM AREAS IN HOSPITALS WITH LIMITED RESOURCES, PRACTICAL INTERVENTIONS, AND RATIONALE

Potential Problem Area	Practical Intervention	Rationale
MV used when less invasive alternatives exist or for unnecessarily long periods of time	Use less invasive alternatives whenever possible and extubate as soon as possible	Reduces exposure risk
	Provide monitoring equipment (oxygen saturation monitors, blood gas analyzers)	Better monitoring may allow more aggressive weaning and earlier extubation
Inadequate technique for suctioning	Provide appropriate supplies and emphasize aseptic technique	Reduces risk of cross-colonization (237)
Suction catheters used for multiple suctioning episodes and stored at the bedside between uses in bottles of saline or other solutions	Dispose or reprocess suction catheters after use or rinse and store in dry, covered container and dispose or reprocess after every nursing shift	Reduces risk of cross-colonization if suction catheters must be reused (13)
	Eliminate bedside reservoirs of saline or other solutions	Eliminate potential reservoirs of gram-negative bacteria (13)
Sterile saline for suctioning drawn from large reservoirs	Use single-dose containers of saline or dispense saline from large reservoir into small, single-use containers and discard reservoir daily	Minimize potential reservoirs of gram-negative bacteria if use of single-dose containers of saline is not possible (13)
Large amounts of condensate collect in ventilator tubing and may drain into the trachea	Prevent drainage of condensate into the trachea; dispose of condensate appropriately	Condensate may contain high concentrations of bacteria (237)
No protocols for use of nebulizers	Use only small-volume nebulizers; do not use large-volume nebulizers	Nebulizers can generate bacteria-containing aerosols; large-volume nebulizers have been associated with outbreaks of pneumonia (201,202)
	Use sterile saline for small volume nebulizers	Minimize the potential for contamination of small-volume nebulizer and nebulized medications (237)
	Rinse and store nebulizers dry	
	Store nebulized medications according to manufacturer's guidelines	
	Discard or reprocess small-volume nebulizers at least every 24 hours	
No protocols for care during enteral feeding	Elevate the head of the bed during enteral feeding and avoid large boluses	Minimize the potential for reflux of gastric contents into the oropharynx
Inadequate reprocessing of respiratory and anesthesia equipment	Clean equipment thoroughly and then EtO or HLD	Prevent transmission of contaminating microorganisms to other patients (237)

EtO, ethylene oxide sterilization; HLD, high-level disinfection; MV, mechanical ventilation.

is not possible, catheters should be rinsed with sterile water; stored in a dry, covered container; and discarded or reprocessed at the end of every nursing shift. Bedside containers of saline or other solutions may serve as potential reservoirs of gram-negative bacteria and should be avoided. Sterile saline for suctioning and sterile water used for rinsing catheters should be dispensed in small containers, which are discarded or reprocessed between uses. Large containers of saline used for suctioning may also serve as reservoirs and should be eliminated whenever possible or discarded at regular intervals. Hospital personnel should be educated to prevent reflux of ventilator tubing condensate into the trachea and to dispose of collected condensate appropriately.

Nebulizers can generate bacteria-containing aerosols that can reach distal airways (201). Large-volume nebulizers have clearly been associated with gram-negative pneumonia and should not be used (202) (Table 108.4), but the use of small-volume medication nebulizers is unavoidable. To minimize the potential for contamination of small-volume nebulizers, only sterile water and medications should be used, medications should be stored according to manufacturer's guidelines, and nebulizers should be discarded or reprocessed every 24 hours (237).

Contaminated ventilator humidifier reservoirs and humidifiers for wall oxygen or oxygen tanks are an unlikely cause of pneumonia because they do not generate aerosols. However, it is reasonable to take simple steps to avoid the possibility for build-up of large concentrations of bacteria in these reservoirs. Sterile water should be used to fill the reservoir, and reservoirs should be cleaned and disinfected before refilling. Humidifier reservoirs should be cleaned and disinfected between uses.

In-use ventilator circuits become contaminated by microbial flora colonizing the upper respiratory tract in a matter of hours. Therefore, it is unclear whether there is any benefit to changing ventilator circuits at a specific interval. If circuits are changed, it does not appear necessary to change them more frequently than once per week (237). This is an extremely important issue for hospitals with limited resources because of the limited number of available ventilator circuits and the expense and effort required for reprocessing these items. For these reasons, this issue trations of bacteria into the oropharynx and potentially into the trachea appears to increase the risk of pneumonia in mechanically ventilated patients, appropriate measures to decrease this risk have not been universally accepted. Raising the head of the bed and avoiding large boluses of enteral feedings are simple measures that may be helpful (Table 108.4). Other measures including the use of duodenal versus gastric feeding tubes and specific regimens for gastric ulcer prophylaxis have not been demonstrated to be effective. A meta-analysis demonstrated that antibiotic prophylaxis (including systemic and topical antibiotics administered via the digestive tract) reduces ventilator-associated pneumonia and mortality rates (246); however, this strategy for infection prevention remains controversial and is expensive, and its effect on antimicrobial resistance has not be determined.

All respiratory and anesthesia equipment should be subjected to ethylene oxide sterilization or high-level disinfection before reuse (Table 108.4) (237). Individual hospitals must determine which of these methods is most efficient and economical. Although high-level disinfection is likely to be cheaper and provides faster turnaround time, it is also potentially more labor intensive and error-prone, requiring more direct supervision. Because both methods have a potential for exposing workers to toxic fumes, the capability of facilities to provide a safe working environment for either of the processes may also determine which method is preferred. Research regarding the application of new low temperature sterilization technologies in limited resource settings is needed.

Urinary Catheters and Urine Drainage Systems

Indwelling urinary catheters should be used only when absolutely necessary to monitor urine output in critically ill patients and to relieve functional or anatomic obstruction to urine outflow (Table 108.5) (236). They should never be used for incontinence alone. In patients requiring chronic catheterization, intermittent straight catheterization may be preferable. Only closed urinary drainage systems should be used, because open drainage systems increase the risk of urinary tract infection (236,247). Indwelling urinary catheters with aspiration and irrigation ports should be used to eliminate the need for disruption of the catheter-collection system junction. If catheters with aspiration and irrigation ports are not available, urine specimens should be obtained by aspirating urine from the catheter using a needle and syringe. A small supply of triple-lumen irrigation catheters should be available for use in patients undergoing urologic surgeries for whom frequent irrigation is needed. Clean, individual patient containers should be used to drain the urine from drainage systems to prevent cross-colonization (236). Urine collection systems should be suspended off the floor and kept below the level of the bladder to prevent reflux of urine (236).

Surgery and Wound Care

A number of interventions can reduce the risk of SSI (Table 108.6). Preoperative stays should be minimized. Routine shaving of patients the night before surgery should not be performed (205–207,239). If hair removal is absolutely necessary, it should be done as close to the time of surgery as possible (239). Hair clippers should be used instead of razors; clipper heads should be disinfected between uses. If shaving is absolutely required, disposable razors should be used to eliminate the potential for transmission of blood-borne pathogens (239). Appropriate perioperative antibiotic prophylaxis should be given within 2 hours preceding the start of surgery, and additional doses should be administered as necessary to ensure that adequate tissue levels of antibiotic are maintained throughout the surgery (239,248, 249). The duration of prophylaxis should not exceed 24 hours (239).

The use of dressing carts with containers of disinfectants in which instruments are submerged between uses should be eliminated, given the potential for contamination of these disinfectants. Sterile instruments should be provided in individually wrapped sterile packages. Ineffective antiseptics or antiseptics that may easily become contaminated, such as benzalkonium

TABLE 108.5. INDWELLING URINARY CATHETERS AND URINE DRAINAGE SYSTEMS: POTENTIAL PROBLEM AREAS IN HOSPITALS WITH LIMITED RESOURCES, PRACTICAL INTERVENTIONS, AND RATIONALE

Potential Problem Area	Practical Intervention	Rationale
UCs used when less invasive alternatives exist or for unnecessarily long periods of time	Use less invasive alternatives whenever possible; remove UC as soon as possible	Reduces exposure risk
Inadequate technique for insertion of UC	Provide appropriate supplies and emphasize aseptic technique during insertion and care	Reduce risk of UTI by minimizing potential for contamination of catheter (236)
Open UDS used	Use only closed UDS	Reduces the incidence of UTI (247)
UC/UDS with aspiration/irrigation ports not available; frequent disruption of UC/UDS junction to obtain urine specimen or for irrigation	Use UC/UDS with aspiration/irrigation ports or obtain urine specimen by using a sterile needle and syringe to aspirate from UC/UDS Minimize irrigation	Reduces risk of UTI by maintaining integrity of UC/UDS junction (236)
Common urine measuring container used to drain UDS from multiple patients	Use a separate container for each patient	Reduces risk of cross-colonization (236)

UC, indwelling urinary catheter; UDS, urine drainage system; UTI, urinary tract infection.

TABLE 108.6. PREOPERATIVE AND POSTOPERATIVE CARE OF SURGICAL PATIENTS: POTENTIAL PROBLEM AREAS IN HOSPITALS WITH LIMITED RESOURCES, PRACTICAL INTERVENTIONS, AND RATIONALE

Potential Problem Area	Practical Intervention	Rationale
Long preoperative stay	Minimize preoperative stay	Reduces incidence of SSI (206,239)
Patients shaved the night before surgery	Do not remove hair or remove hair with clipper or disposable razor immediately before surgery	Same as above (205–207,239)
Choice, timing, and number of doses of perioperative antibiotic prophylaxis may not be optimal	Administer appropriate perioperative antibiotic prophylaxis within 2 hours before the start of surgery; repeat doses to maintain tissue levels during surgery	Appropriate choice and timing of antibiotic dosing is critical to achieving and maintaining effective tissue levels throughout surgery (239,248,249)
	Limit prophylaxis to <24 hours	Continuing prophylaxis for >24 hours postop is unnecessary and wasteful (239)
Dressing carts with instruments submerged in disinfectants	Use individually wrapped sterile instruments	Reduce potential for cross-colonization
Ineffective antiseptics used (benzalkonium chloride, furazolidone, and nitrofurantoin solutions)	Use only effective antiseptics	Antiseptic with a broad spectrum of activity more likely to be effective
Large containers of antiseptics are used and may be refilled without cleaning	Use small containers of antiseptics	Minimizes the risk of contamination
	Clean and completely dry containers before reuse	

SSI, surgical site infection.

tants. Sterile instruments should be provided in individually wrapped sterile packages. Ineffective antiseptics or antiseptics that may easily become contaminated, such as benzalkonium chloride, should be not be used. Antiseptics should be supplied in small containers, which should be cleaned and dried thoroughly before refilling.

Sterilization and Disinfection

The infection control program should review reprocessing procedures because so many patient care items are reused in hospitals in countries with limited resources. This requires close collaboration with the supervisor of the central supply department and supervisors and staff in other areas in the hospital where reprocessing occurs. The review should examine the following components of the reprocessing process: (a) cleaning methods; (b) sterilization methods for critical items; (c) sterilization or high-level disinfection methods for semicritical items; (d) intermediate or low-level disinfection for noncritical items; (e) packaging, storage, and shelf life of reprocessed items; and (f) quality control. Standard references (210,241,250) and manufacturer's recommendations should be used as guides for determining adequate reprocessing methods.

It is critically important that decisions regarding reprocessing methods be based on adequate information (Table 108.7) (210, 241,250). This is particularly important because new sophisticated devices that cannot withstand standard reprocessing methods, such as fiberoptic endoscopes, are being used more frequently. A number of sources may be used to determine adequate reprocessing methods: standard texts and references; government, professional, and industry guidelines; and individual manufacturers' recommendations (210,241,250).

Items designed for single-use (disposables) present a more difficult problem, because guidelines for reprocessing these items are not available and manufacturers are unlikely to provide recommendations. Although this practice cannot be endorsed, some general guidelines are necessary because reuse of single-use items is so widespread. First, the need for reuse should be incorporated into purchasing decisions; in other words, items specifically designed for reuse should be purchased preferentially over disposable items. Second, items that cannot be cleaned or reprocessed adequately should be discarded. Third, reprocessing methods must be adequate for the intended use of the item (i.e., critical items must be sterilized). Fourth, because many single-use items are not designed for reprocessing, the integrity and function of these items must be routinely evaluated. Although simple tests are often used (e.g., filling latex gloves with air or water to look for leaks), they may not be sufficiently sensitive. Finally, reusing items for purposes other than those for which they were designed (i.e., reusing glass medication vials as specimen containers) may be very reasonable in some situations but may pose hazards in other situations (i.e., use of intravenous infusion tubing as a part of an improvised open urine drainage system). (See also Chapter 87.)

Supervision of reprocessing activities is critical. The volume of materials requiring steam sterilization may exceed the capacity of available autoclaves. Proper loading and placement of items (for gravity autoclaves) in the autoclave must be ensured. Quality control in reprocessing is a multistep process. Parameters of the reprocessing method, such as monitoring time, temperature, and pressure of autoclave cycles, should be routinely monitored. This obviously requires working gauges and chart recorders (if available). Chemical indicators are useful to identify items that have been sterilized by steam, dry heat,

TABLE 108.7. STERILIZATION AND DISINFECTION: POTENTIAL GENERAL PROBLEM AREAS IN HOSPITALS WITH LIMITED RESOURCES, PRACTICAL INTERVENTIONS AND RATIONALE

Potential Problem Area	Practical Intervention	Rationale
Standard references and/or guidelines are not used to determine adequate reprocessing methods	Use standard references, published guidelines, and manufacturer's recommendations	Only methods with established efficacy should be used
Nonstandard methods used to sterilize heat or moisture sensitive critical and semicritical items	Follow guidelines in standard references, published guidelines, and/or manufacturer's recommendations	Same as above
Single-use ("disposable") items are reprocessed and reused	Discard items that cannot be cleaned completely or reprocessed adequately	Inadequate data to determine whether reprocessing and reuse of disposable items is safe, but is frequently done out of practical necessity
	Reprocessing methods must be adequate for the type of device and its use (i.e., critical items must be sterilized)	
	Assess the integrity and function of reprocessed items	
Overloading of autoclave	Maintain appropriate size loads in autoclave	General principles of sterilization
	Package and place items appropriately in gravity autoclave	
Inadequate quality control	Monitor and record sterilization parameters (time, temperature, pressure)	General principles of sterilization
	Use chemical indicators to show that item was autoclaved	
	Use biologic indicators to verify adequacy of sterilization	
No preventive maintenance	Follow manufacturer's guidelines for preventive maintenance	Preventive maintenance is likely to improve performance of equipment
Reprocessed items stored near potential sources of contamination	Package and store away from potential sources of contamination	Prevent contamination before reuse

or ethylene oxide, but biologic indicators are needed to verify that sterilization was effective. Biologic indicators for steam sterilization should be used at least on a weekly basis and in every load in which implantable materials are included; biologic indicators should be used for every load sterilized using ethylene oxide. Many hospitals may not be able to perform testing with this frequency; however, a routine schedule for testing should be used. Finally, preventive maintenance is necessary to ensure proper functioning of all equipment.

Reprocessed items should be stored in areas that prevent or minimize the potential for contamination. Most hospitals wrap steam-sterilized items only in muslin, but resterilize these items at predetermined intervals if they have not been used. Because inventories of equipment are low in many hospitals, long-term storage is unlikely. Hospitals with larger inventories and adequate storage facilities may move to event-related reprocessing. (See also Chapter 74.)

Alternative approaches for solving problems associated with reprocessing reused instruments and equipment in low-resource settings are desperately needed. Barone et al. (251) described their adaptation and testing of a portable steam sterilizer for instruments and supplies used for intrauterine device insertion in a community-based family planning program in Bangladesh (251). The sterilizer is a commercially available device originally designed to sterilize needles and syringes for use in the WHO's Expanded Programme on Immunization. Other uses of this type of device could be devised and tested. Recently developed methods of low-temperature sterilization (e.g., liquid peracetic acid and plasma sterilization) are attractive options (250), but the equipment necessary to use these processes is likely to be too expensive for most hospitals.

The infection control program should also determine which disinfectants and antiseptics are available in the hospital, their specific uses, and the procedures used to prepare and dispense these agents. If possible, these agents should be prepared in a centralized area and dispensed through an exchange program (e.g., empty containers exchanged for full containers). Containers should be thoroughly cleaned and dried before refilling.

In very resource poor areas, simple household bleach (5.0% chlorine concentration) can be used as an effective disinfectant. A 1:100 solution (0.05% final concentration) can be used to disinfect surfaces, medical equipment, plastic bedding, and reusable protective barriers (9).

Environmental Cleaning and Sanitation

General cleaning agents and procedures should be also reviewed. In hospitals that have received donations of medical supplies, expensive disinfectants may occasionally be used to clean floors and walls. Procedures should be standardized and wasteful or unnecessary practices, such as fogging or closure of operating rooms after "infected" surgeries, should be eliminated.

Education of Hospital Personnel

An education program for hospital personnel is necessary to increase awareness of nosocomial infections, improve knowledge of basic infection control principles, and provide instruction for implementation of specific interventions such as those discussed previously. Training should be incorporated into institutional orientation programs for new personnel and for ongoing educational activities.

Infection control personnel frequently do not have sufficient time to provide training for all of the personnel in the hospital, so they need to take advantage of opportunities where they exist. Informal infection control education can be performed during routine surveillance on the wards and can be a valuable adjunct to more structured programs. In addition, infection control personnel should concentrate on educating supervisory nurses, many of whom have nursing degrees and readily appreciate the need for improvement in infection control practices. In many hospitals, these nurses perform most of the sophisticated patient care and invasive procedures, supervise other nurses performing routine patient care, and provide on-the-job training for nursing personnel. Nurses and physicians working in ICUs represent another target group. In hospitals with residency training programs, house staff should have formal infection control training and on-the-job exposure to infection control personnel, because many of these physicians subsequently will practice in hospitals with no infection control program.

Educational activities should focus on a core of important infection control topics, including hand hygiene practices, use of invasive devices (including limiting the duration of use of these devices and use of noninvasive alternatives), aseptic technique, procedures for preparation and use of intravenous fluids and medications, care of ventilated patients, care of patients with indwelling urinary catheters, wound care and use of antiseptic solutions, standard precautions and other isolation precautions, effective use of microbiology laboratory services, and appropriate use of antimicrobials.

Antimicrobial Use Monitoring and Control

Monitoring the prescription of antimicrobial agents, particularly expensive and/or broad-spectrum agents, is critical because of the impact these agents have on hospital microbial ecology and hospital costs. Antimicrobial control policies are frequently instituted primarily for cost control, but, from an infection control point of view, controlling the use of broad-spectrum antibiotics is critical to limiting the emergence of antibiotic resistance.

Decisions regarding which antibiotics should be subjected to restrictions will be guided by the hospital's patient population, regional and local antibiotic resistance patterns, and the cost and availability of specific agents. From the standpoint of preventing the emergence of antibiotic resistance, strong consideration should be given to controlling prescription of second- and third-generation cephalosporins, carbapenems, monobactams, vancomycin, amikacin, quinolones, and linezolid. Restricted access to the newer systemic antifungals and intravenous antiviral agents may be needed from a cost standpoint.

A variety of methods can be used to manage the prescription of antimicrobial agents, but there are few comparative data to guide the selection of the most effective approach (252,253). A management policy administered by one or more knowledgeable physicians is likely to be effective not only in restricting access to specific antibiotics but also in providing other physicians with expert guidance in alternative antibiotic selection. However, the expertise required for this task may not be readily available, except in reference hospitals or academic centers. Infection control physicians may be unwilling to undertake this challenge in the early phases of implementing an infection control program, especially if they detect resistance among the clinical staff.

Other approaches may be useful and are less labor intensive (252,253). Special order forms can be designed to direct physicians to specific preferred agents, dosages and dosing intervals, and duration of therapy. These forms are most likely to be useful for perioperative antibiotic prophylaxis and empiric therapy for common infectious processes. Forms that allow prescription of specified antibiotics for a limited number of doses or "automatic stop orders" may discourage extended use without specific justification. Forms that require a statement regarding the reason for treatment and supporting culture information may provide additional constraints on inappropriate use but require review by a physician expert and tend to be ignored unless rigorously enforced. Education programs conducted by outside experts may improve the prescribing habits of practicing physicians, but their effect generally wanes quickly unless continuously reinforced.

Several other inexpensive approaches may also be useful in hospitals with limited resources. First, a review of the formulary can eliminate duplication among classes of antibiotics and identify cheaper alternatives. Second, antibiotic susceptibility testing can be restricted to a limited number of antibiotics. Finally, restricting the marketing activities of pharmaceutical representatives in the hospital may be helpful, especially in training centers.

Intervention programs that include multiple interventions are likely to be the most successful (254). We have found that perioperative antimicrobial prophylaxis is a good initial target for efforts to improve antimicrobial use in resource-limited settings (15). Arguments in favor of this strategy include the following: (a) evidence-based guidelines for perioperative prophylaxis are well-accepted and widely available, (b) appropriate and inappropriate use can be defined and measured, (c) problems in systems for ordering and administering prophylaxis can be identified easily and solutions are relatively straightforward, and (d) improvements may be correlated with lower infection rates and/or lower costs. A successful program to improve perioperative prophylaxis may also help to facilitate acceptance of additional efforts to improve use of antimicrobial agents by physicians.

CONCLUSIONS

Substantial progress has been made in improving infection prevention measures in hospitals in countries with limited resources. Many dedicated physicians and nurses around the world have recognized this need and have been working toward this goal, often with little if any support. Projects that stress the cultivation of local and national expertise, development of basic standards, and additional study of cost-effective prevention and control measures are likely to have a substantial long-term effect. Research regarding methods to facilitate implementation of effective improvements in a broad range of hospitals not just in referral and academic hospitals is desperately needed. By focusing on infection control, countries with limited resources can develop a blueprint for broader strategies to improve the quality of hospital care in the future.

ACKNOWLEDGMENTS

Supported in part by the Thrasher Research Fund, People-to-People Foundation (Project Hope), the International Society for Infectious Diseases, and the United States Agency for International Development. We thank Carol O'Boyle, R.N., Ph.D., and Barbara Soule, R.N., M.P.A., C.I.C., for their assistance in performing surveys of hospital infection control. We thank the many physicians, nurses, and other hospital personnel who have participated in these surveys.

REFERENCES

1. Tietjen L, Bossemeyer D, McIntosh N. *Infection prevention: guidelines for healthcare facilities with limited resources.* Baltimore: JHPIEGO Corporation, 2003.
2. EngenderHealth. Infection prevention: online course. 2003.
3. Manangan LP, Archibald LK, Pearson ML, et al. Selected global health care activities of the Hospital Infections Program, Centers for Disease Control and Prevention. *Am J Infect Control* 1999;27: 270–274.
4. Ducel G, Fabry J, Nicolle L. *Prevention of hospital-acquired infections: a practical guide.* Geneva: World Health Organization, 2002.
5. World Health Organization Regional Office for Africa, Commonwealth Regional Health Community Secretariat, East CaSACoN. *Manual of infection prevention and control: policies and guidelines.* Harare, 2003.
6. World Health Organization. The SIGN Alliance. 2003.
7. Nicolle L. *Infection control programmes to contain antimicrobial resistance,.* Geneva: World Health Organization, 2001.
8. World Health Organization. *Guidelines for the prevention of tuberculosis in health care facilities in resource limited settings,* 1999.
9. Centers for Disease Control and Prevention, World Health Organization. *Infection control for viral haemorrhagic fevers in the African health care setting.* Atlanta, GA: Centers for Disease Control and Prevention, 1998:1–198.
10. World Health Organization. *Hospital infection control guidance for severe acute respiratory syndrome,* 2003.
11. Danchaivijitr S, Tangtrakool T, Waitayapiches S, et al. Efficacy of hospital infection control in Thailand 1988–1992. *J Hosp Infect* 1996; 32:147–153.
12. Starling CE, Couto BR, Pinheiro SM. Applying the Centers for Disease Control and Prevention and National Nosocomial Surveillance system methods in Brazilian hospitals. *Am J Infect Control* 1997;25: 303–311.
13. Berg DE, Hershow RC, Ramirez CA, et al. Control of nosocomial infections in an intensive care unit in Guatemala City. *Clin Infect Dis* 1995;21:588–593.
14. Ponce de Leon S, Rangel-Frausto MS, Elias-Lopez JI, et al. Nosocomial infections: secular trends of a control program in Mexico. *Salud Publica Mex* 1999;41:S5–11.
15. Weinberg M, Fuentes JM, Ruiz AI, et al. Reducing infections among women undergoing cesarean section in Colombia by means of continuous quality improvement methods. *Arch Intern Med* 2001;161: 2357–2365.
16. Huskins WC, Soule BM, O'Boyle C, et al. Hospital infection prevention and control: a model for improving the quality of hospital care in low and middle income countries. *Infect Control Hosp Epidemiol* 1998;19:125–135.
17. Mayon-White RT, Ducel G, Kereseselidze T, et al. An international survey of the prevalence of hospital acquired infection. *J Hosp Infect* 1988;11:43–48.
18. Tikomirov E. WHO programme for the control of hospital infections. *Chemioterapia* 1987;6:148–151.
19. Huskins WC, O'Rourke EJ, Rhinehart E, et al. Infection control in countries with limited resources. In: Mayhall CG, ed. *Hospital epidemiology and infection control.* Philadelphia: Lippincott Williams & Wilkins, 1999:1489–1513.
20. Ponce de Leon-Rosales SP, Molinar-Ramos F, Dominguez-Cherit G, et al. Prevalence of infections in intensive care units in Mexico: a multicenter study. *Crit Care Med* 2000;28:1316–1321.
21. Daniel SO. An epidemiological study of nosocomial infections at the Lagos University Teaching Hospital. *Public Health* 1977;91:13–18.
22. Cáceres JAM, Sotello Y. Infection control in El Salvador: the Hospital Rosales experience. *Infect Control* 1987;8:495–500.
23. Srisupan V, Pichiansathien W, Senaratana W, et al. Nosocomial infections in Maharaj Nakhon Chiang Mai Hospital. *J Med Assoc Thai* 1989;72:7–11.
24. Sithikesorn J, Bunma P, Lumpikanon P, et al. Nosocomial infections in Srinagarind Hospital. *J Med Assoc Thai* 1989;72:12–14.
25. Wagner MB, Petrillo V, Gay V, et al. A prevalence survey of nosocomial infection in a Brazilian hospital. *J Hosp Infect* 1990;15:379–381.
26. Abussaud MJI. Prevalence of nosocomial infections in a Saudi Arabian teaching hospital. *J Hosp Infect* 1990;17:235–238.
27. Lima NL, Pereira CRB, Souza IC, et al. Selective surveillance for nosocomial infections in a Brazilian hospital. *Infect Control Hosp Epidemiol* 1993;14:197–202.
28. Kraisriwatana J, Reongroj M, Tachapiroj K. Prevalence of nosocomial infections in Udornthanee Hospital 1990. *J Med Assoc Thai* 1995; 78:S50–S52.
29. Pitaksiripan S, Butpongsapan S, Tepsuporn M, et al. Nosocomial infections in Lampang Hospital. *J Med Assoc Thai* 1995;78:S53–S56.
30. Valinteliene R, Jurkuvenas V, Jepsen OB. Prevalence of hospital-acquired infection in a Lithuanian hospital. *J Hosp Infect* 1996;34: 321–329.
31. Orrett FA, Brooks PJ, Richardson EG. Nosocomial infections in a rural regional hospital in a developing country: infection rates by site, service, cost, and infection control practices. *Infect Control Hosp Epidemiol* 1998;19:136–140.
32. Durmaz B, Durmaz R, Otlu B, Sonmez E. Nosocomial infections in a new medical center, Turkey. *Infect Control Hosp Epidemiol* 2000; 21:534–536.
33. de Lourdes Garcia-Garcia M, Jimenez-Corona A, Jimenez-Corona ME, et al. Nosocomial infections in a community hospital in Mexico. *Infect Control Hosp Epidemiol* 2001;22:386–388.
34. Narong MN, Thongpiyapoom S, Thaikul N, et al. Surgical site infections in patients undergoing major operations in a university hospital: using standardized infection ratio as a benchmarking tool. *Am J Infect Control* 2003;31:274–279.
35. Lederer W. Infection control in a small rural hospital in Uganda. *J Hosp Infect* 1997;35:91–95.
36. Kumarasinghe G, Goh H, Tan KN. Hospital acquired infections in a Singapore Hospital: 1985–1992. *Malays J Pathol* 1995;17:17–21.
37. Gilio AE, Stape A, Pereira CR, et al. Risk factors for nosocomial infections in a critically ill pediatric population: a 25-month prospective cohort study. *Infect Control Hosp Epidemiol* 2000;21:340–342.
38. Zaidi M, Ponce de Leon S, Ortiz RM, et al. Hospital-acquired diarrhea in adults a prospective case control study in Mexico. *Infect Control Hosp Epidemiol* 1991;12:349–355.
39. Martirosian G, Polanski JA, Szubert A, et al. *Clostridium difficile* in a department of surgery. *Mater Med Pol* 1993;25:145–147.
40. Dutta P, Mitra U, Rasaily R, et al. Prospective study of nosocomial enteric infections in a pediatric hospital, Calcutta. *Indian Pediatr* 1993;30:187–194.
41. Soyletir G, Eskiturk A, Kilic G, et al. *Clostridium difficile* acquisition

rate and its role in nosocomial diarrhoea at a university hospital in Turkey. *Eur J Epidemiol* 1996;12:391–394.

42. Das AS, Mazumder DN, Pal D, et al. A study of nosocomial diarrhea in Calcutta. *Indian J Gastroenterol* 1996;15:12–13.
43. Merchant M, Karnard R, Kanbur AA. Incidence of nosocomial pneumonia in a medical intensive care unit and general medical ward patients in a public hospital in Bombay, India. *J Hosp Infect*1998;38: 143–148.
44. Jamulitrat S, Meknavin U, Thongpiyapoom S. Factors affecting mortality outcome and risk of developing nosocomial bloodstream infection. *Infect Control Hosp Epidemiol* 1994;15:163–170.
45. Thanamee N, Sujaritjan N, Techasena W. Pneumonia in mechanically ventilated patients in Nan Hospital intensive care unit. *J Med Assoc Thai* 1995;78:S102–S104.
46. Avila-Figueroa C, Garcia Gaytan E, Becerril R, et al. Surveillance of the utilization of invasive devices and device-related infections in pediatric hospitals in Mexico. Thirty-sixth annual meeting of the Infectious Diseases Society of America, Denver, CO, 1998.
47. Rosenthal VD, Guzman S, Orellano PW. Nosocomial infections in medical-surgical intensive care units in Argentina: attributable mortality and length of stay. *Am J Infect Control* 2003;31:291–295.
48. Abussaud MJ. Incidence of wound infection in three different departments and the antibiotic sensitivity pattern of the isolates in a Saudi Arabian hospital. *Acta Microbiol Immunol Hung* 1996;43:301–305.
49. Santos KR, Fonseca LS, Bravo Neto GP, et al. Surgical site infection: rates, etiology and resistance patterns to antimicrobials among strains isolated at Rio de Janeiro University Hospital. *Infection* 1997;25: 217–220.
50. Wagner MB, da Silva NB, Vinciprova AR, et al. Hospital-acquired infections among surgical patients in a Brazilian hospital. *J Hosp Infect* 1997;35:277–285.
51. Gulacsi L, Kiss ZT, Goldmann DA, et al. Risk-adjusted infection rates in surgery: a model for outcome measurement in hospitals developing new quality improvement programmes. *J Hosp Infect* 2000;44: 43–52.
52. Campos ML, Cipriano ZM, Freitas PF. Suitability of the NNIS index for estimating surgical-site infection risk at a small university hospital in Brazil. *Infect Control Hosp Epidemiol* 2001;22:268–272.
53. Soleto L, Pirard M, Boelaert M, et al. Incidence of surgical-site infections and the validity of the National Nosocomial Infections Surveillance System risk index in a general surgical ward in Santa Cruz, Bolivia. *Infect Control Hosp Epidemiol* 2003;24:26–30.
54. Porras-Hernandez JD, Vilar-Compte D, Cashat-Cruz M, et al. A prospective study of surgical site infections in a pediatric hospital in Mexico City. *Am J Infect Control* 2003;31:302–308.
55. Pishori T, Siddiqui AR, Ahmed M. Surgical wound infection surveillance in general surgery procedures at a teaching hospital in Pakistan. *Am J Infect Control* 2003;31:296–301.
56. Cotton MF, Berkowitz FE, Berkowitz Z, et al. Nosocomial infection in black South African children. *Pediatr Infect Dis J* 1989;8:676–683.
57. Aaby P, Bukh J, Lisse IM, et al. Introduction of measles into a highly immunized West African community the role of health care institutions. *J Epidemiol Community Health* 1985;39:113–116.
58. Glyn-Jones R. Measles vaccine: gamma globulin in the prevention of cross infection with measles in a acute paediatric ward. *Cent Afr J Med* 1972;18:4–9.
59. Reynolds LGB, Klein M. The hospital as a vector of measles in the community. *S Afr Med J* 1987;71:637–638.
60. Marshall TM, Hlatswayo D, Schoub B. Nosocomial outbreaks—a potential threat to the elimination of measles? *J Infect Dis* 2003;187: S97–101.
61. Mhalu FS, Mtango FD, Msengi AE. Hospital outbreaks of cholera transmitted through close person-to-person contact. *Lancet* 1984; 2(8394):82–84.
62. Cliff, JL, Zinkin P, Martelli A. A hospital outbreak of cholera in Maputo, Mozambique. *Trans R Soc Trop Med Hyg* 1986;80:473–476.
63. Ryder RW, Mizanur Rahman ASM, Alim ARMA, et al. An outbreak of nosocomial cholera in a rural Bangladesh hospital. *J Hosp Infect* 1986;8:275–282.
64. Swaddiwudhipong W, Kunasol P. An outbreak of nosocomial cholera in a 755-bed hospital. *Trans R Soc Trop Med Hyg* 1989;83:279–281.
65. Shi J. A survey of nosocomial infection by *Salmonella typhimurium. Chung Hua Liu Hsing Ping Hsueh Tsa Chih* 1990;11:284–287.
66. Saha MR, Sircar BK, Dutta P, et al. Occurrence of multi-resistant *Salmonella typhimurium* infection in a pediatric hospital at Calcutta. *Indian Pediatr* 1992;29:307–311.
67. Asensi MD, Solari CA, Hofer E. A *Salmonella agona* outbreak in a pediatric hospital in the city of Rio de Janeiro, Brazil. *Mem Inst Oswaldo Cruz* 1994;89:1–4.
68. Hernandez JE, Mejia CR, Cazali IL, et al. Nosocomial infection due to *Vibrio cholerae* in two referral hospitals in Guatemala. *Infect Control Hosp Epidemiol* 1996;17:371–372.
69. Avendaño LF, Larrañaga C, Palomino MA, et al. Community- and hospital-acquired respiratory syncytial virus infection in Chile. *Pediatr Infect Dis J* 1991;10:564–568.
70. Abiodun PO, Omoigberale A. Prevalence of nosocomial rotavirus infection in hospitalized children in Benin City, Nigeria. *Ann Trop Paediatr* 1994;14:85–88.
71. Gusmao RH, Mascarenhas JD, Gabbay YB, et al. Rotaviruses as a cause of nosocomial, infantile diarrhoea in northern Brazil: pilot study. *Mem Inst Oswaldo Cruz* 1995;90:743–749.
72. Desikan P, Daniel JD, Kamalarathnam CN, et al. Molecular epidemiology of nosocomial rotavirus infection. *J Diarrhoeal Dis Res* 1996; 14:12–15.
73. Kilgore PE, Unicomb LE, Gentsch JR, et al. Neonatal rotavirus infection in Bangladesh: strain characterization and risk factors for nosocomial infection. *Pediatr Infect Dis J* 1996;15:672–677.
74. Kamalaratnam CN, Kang G, Kirubakaran C, et al. A prospective study of nosocomial enteric pathogen acquisition in hospitalized children in South India. *J Trop Pediatr* 2001;47:46–49.
75. Baron RC, McCormick JB, Zubeir OA. Ebola virus disease in southern Sudan: hospital dissemination and intrafamilial spread. *Bull World Health Organ* 1983;61:997–1003.
76. Ndambi R, Akamituna P, Bonnet MJ, et al. Epidemiologic and clinical aspects of the Ebola virus epidemic in Mosango, Democratic Republic of the Congo, 1995. *J Infect Dis* 1999;179:S8–10.
77. Muyembe-Tamfum JJ, Kipasa M, Kiyungu C, et al. Ebola outbreak in Kikwit, Democratic Republic of the Congo: discovery and control measures. *J Infect Dis* 1999;179:S259–262.
78. Centers for Disease Control and Prevention. Severe acute respiratory syndrome—Singapore, 2003. *MMWR Morb Mortal Wkly Rep* 2003; 52:405–411.
79. Riley LW, Ceballos BSO, Trabulsi LR, et al. The significance of hospitals as reservoirs for endemic multiresistant *Salmonella typhimurium* causing infection in urban Brazilian children. *J Infect Dis* 1984; 150:236–241.
80. Reichler MR, Rakovsky J, Slacikova M, et al. Spread of multidrug-resistant *Streptococcus pneumoniae* among hospitalized children in Slovakia. *J Infect Dis* 1996;173:374–379.
81. Ritacco V, Di Lonardo M, Reniero A, et al. Nosocomial spread of human immunodeficiency virus-related multidrug-resistant tuberculosis in Buenos Aires. *J Infect Dis* 1997;176:637–642.
82. Gedebou M, Habte-Gabr E, Kronvall G, et al. Hospital-acquired infections among obstetric and gynaecological patients at Tikur Anbessa Hospital, Addis Ababa. *J Hosp Infect* 1988;11:50–59.
83. Figueroa-Damian R, Ortiz-Ibarra FJ, Arredondo-Garcia JL. Nosocomial infections of gynecologic-obstetrical origin at a perinatal care hospital. *Salud Publica Mex* 1994;36:10–16.
84. Balkhy HH, Memish ZA, Almuneef MA. Effect of intensive surveillance on cesarean-section wound infection rate in a Saudi Arabian hospital. *Am J Infect Control* 2003;31:288–290.
85. Zaidi M, Sifuentes J, Bobadilla M, et al. Epidemic of *Serratia marcescens* bacteremia and meningitis in a neonatal unit in Mexico City. *Infect Control Hosp Epidemiol* 1989;10:14–20.
86. Centron Garcia D, Ruiz T, Botto L, et al. An outbreak of multiply resistant *Pseudomonas aeruginosa*in a neonatal unit: plasmid pattern analysis. *J Hosp Infect* 1989;14:99–105.
87. Coovadia YM, Johnson AP, Bhana RH, et al. Multiresistant *Klebsiella pneumoniae* in a neonatal nursery the importance of maintenance of

infection control policies and procedures in the prevention of outbreaks. *J Hosp Infect* 1992;22:197–205.

88. Raman TS, Jayaprakash DG, Singh D, et al. *Citrobacter*septicemia in neonates. *Indian Pediatr* 1993;30:516–520.
89. Adeyemo AA, Akindele JA, Omokhodion SI. *Klebsiella*septicaemia, osteomyelitis and septic arthritis in neonates in Ibadan, Nigeria. *Ann Trop Paediatr* 1993;13:285–289.
90. Aihara M, Sakai M, Iwasaki M, et al. Prevention and control of nosocomial infection caused by methicillin-resistant *Staphylococcus aureus* in a premature infant ward—preventive effect of a povidone-iodine wipe of neonatal skin. *Postgrad Med J* 1993;69:S117–S121.
91. Pegues DA, Arathoon EG, Samayoa B, et al. Epidemic gram-negative bacteremia in a neonatal intensive care unit in Guatemala. *Am J Infect Control* 1994;22:163–171.
92. Boo NY, Chor CY. Six year trend of neonatal septicaemia in a large Malaysian maternity hospital. *J Paediatr Child Health* 1994;30: 23–27.
93. Tan KW, Tay L, Lim SH. An outbreak of methicillin-resistant *Staphylococcus aureus* in a neonatal intensive care unit in Singapore: a 20-month study of clinical characteristics and control. *Singapore Med J* 1994;35:277–282.
94. Koutouby A, Habibullah J. Neonatal sepsis in Dubai, United Arab Emirates. *J Trop Pediatr* 1995;41:177–180.
95. Camargo LF, Strabelli TM, Ribeiro FG, et al. Epidemiologic investigation of an outbreak of coagulase-negative *Staphylococcus*primary bacteremia in a newborn intensive care unit. *Infect Control Hosp Epidemiol* 1995;16:595–596.
96. Flidel-Rimon O, Leibovitz E, Juster-Reicher A, et al. An outbreak of antibiotic multiresistant *Klebsiella*at the neonatal intensive care unit, Kaplan Hospital, Rehovot, Israel, November 1991 to April 1992. *Am J Perinatol* 1996;13:99–102.
97. Bhutta ZA. *Enterobacter*sepsis in the newborn—a growing problem in Karachi. *J Hosp Infect* 1996;34:211–216.
98. Pengsaa K, Lumbiganon P, Taksaphan S, et al. Risk factors for neonatal *Klebsiella*septicemia in Srinagarind Hospital. *Southeast Asian J Trop Med Public Health* 1996;27:102—106.
99. Mehta G, Kumari S. Multi-resistant *Staphylococcus haemolyticus* in a neonatal unit in New Delhi. *Ann Trop Paediatr* 1997;17:15–20.
100. Joseph AT, Rammurty DV, Srivastava L, et al. *Salmonella senftenberg* outbreak in a neonatal unit. *Indian Pediatr* 1990;27:157–160.
101. Ayyagari A, Chander J, Narang A, et al. Outbreak of *Salmonella worthington* meningitis and septicaemia in a hospital at Chandigarh (north India). *Indian J Med Res* 1990;91:15–17.
102. Gupta P, Ramachandran VG, Sharma PP, et al. *Salmonella senftenberg*-septicemia: a nursery outbreak. *Indian Pediatr* 1993;30:514–516.
103. Wu SX, Tang Y. Molecular epidemiologic study of an outbreak of *Salmonella typhimurium*infection at a newborn nursery. *Chin Med J* 1993;106:423–427.
104. Pawa AK, Ramji S, Prakash K, et al. Neonatal nosocomial infection: profile and risk factors. *Indian Pediatr* 1997;34:297–302.
105. Gupta P, Talwar V, Revathi G, et al. Nosocomial *Salmonella bareilly* septicemia: a nursery outbreak. *Indian Pediatr* 1997;34:144–146.
106. Sethi SK, Ghafoor MA, Vandepitte J. Outbreak of neonatal listeriosis in a regional hospital in Kuwait. *Eur J Pediatr* 1989;148:368–370.
107. Schuchat A, Lizano C, Broome CV, et al. Outbreak of neonatal listeriosis associated with mineral oil. *Pediatr Infect Dis J* 1991;10:183–189.
108. Aye DT, Bact D, Sack DA, et al. Neonatal diarrhea at a maternity hospital in Rangoon. *Am J Public Health* 1991;81:480–481.
109. Pillay DG, Karas JA, Pillay A, et al. Nosocomial transmission of *Shigella dysenteriae* type 1. *J Hosp Infect* 1997;37:199–205.
110. Kunin CM. Resistance to antimicrobial drugs—a worldwide calamity. *Ann Intern Med* 1993;118.
111. O'Brien TF. The global epidemic nature of antimicrobial resistance and the need to monitor and manage it locally. *Clin Infect Dis* 1997; 24:S2–S8.
112. Goldmann DA, Huskins WC. Control of nosocomial antimicrobial-resistant bacteria: a strategic priority for hospitals worldwide. *Clin Infect Dis* 1997;24:S139–S145.
113. Hart CA, Kariuki S. Antimicrobial resistance in developing countries. *BMJ* 1998;317:647–650.
114. Pfaller MA, Jones RN, Doern GV, et al. Bacterial pathogens isolated from patients with bloodstream infection: frequencies of occurrence and antimicrobial susceptibility patterns from the SENTRY antimicrobial surveillance program (United States and Canada, 1997). *Antimicrob Agents Chemother* 1998;42:1762–1770.
115. Jones ME, Jones RN, Sader H, et al., Sentry Antimicrobial Surveillance Program. Current susceptibilities of staphylococci to glycopeptides determined as part of an international resistance surveillance programme. *J Antimicrob Chemother* 1998;42:119–121.
116. Richet HM, Mohammed J, McDonald LC, et al. Building communication networks: international network for the study and prevention of emerging antimicrobial resistance. *Emerg Infect Dis* 2001;7: 319–322.
117. Turnidge J. Epidemiology of quinolone resistance: Eastern hemisphere. *Drugs* 1995;49(Suppl 2):43–47.
118. Wallace MR, Johnson AP, Daniel M, et al. Sequential emergence of multi-resistant *Klebsiella pneumoniae* in Bahrain. *J Hosp Infect* 1995; 31:247–252.
119. Mehta A, Rodrigues C, Kumar R, et al. A pilot programme of MRSA surveillance in India. *J Postgrad Med* 1996;42:1–3.
120. Vahaboglu H, Ozturk R, Aygun G, et al. Widespread detection of PER-1-type extended-spectrum beta-lactamases among nosocomial *Acinetobacter* and *Pseudomonas aeruginosa* isolates in Turkey: a nationwide multicenter study. *Antimicrob Agents Chemother* 1997;41: 2265–2269.
121. Bello H, Gonzalez G, Dominguez M, et al. Activity of selected beta-lactams, ciprofloxacin, and amikacin against different *Acinetobacter baumannii* biotypes from Chilean hospitals. *Diagn Microbiol Infect Dis* 1997;28:183–186.
122. Durmaz B, Durmaz R, Sahin K. Methicillin-resistance among Turkish isolates of *Staphylococcus aureus* strains from nosocomial and community infections and their resistance patterns using various antimicrobial agents. *J Hosp Infect* 1997;37:325–329.
123. Hariharan S, Nanduri SB, Moseley HSL, et al. Spectrum of microbes and antimicrobial resistance in a surgical intensive care unit, Barbados. *Am J Infect Control* 2003;31:280–287.
124. Gales AC, Jones RN, Forward KR, et al. Emerging importance of multidrug-resistant *Acinetobacter* species and *Stenotrophomonas maltophilia* as pathogens in seriously ill patients: geographic patterns, epidemiological features, and trends in the SENTRY Antimicrobial Surveillance Program (1997-1999). *Clin Infect Dis* 2001;32: S104–113.
125. Gales AC, Sader HS, Jones RN. Urinary tract infection trends in Latin American hospitals: report from the SENTRY antimicrobial surveillance program (1997–2000). *Diagn Microbiol Infect Dis* 2002; 44:289–299.
126. Sader HS, Jones RN, Silva JB. Skin and soft tissue infections in Latin American medical centers: four-year assessment of the pathogen frequency and antimicrobial susceptibility patterns. *Diagn Microbiol Infect Dis* 2002;44:281–288.
127. Sader HS, Jones RN, Andrade-Baiocchi S, Biedenbach DJ. Four-year evaluation of frequency of occurrence and antimicrobial susceptibility patterns of bacteria from bloodstream infections in Latin American medical centers. *Diagn Microbiol Infect Dis* 2002;44:273–280.
128. Andrade SS, Jones RN, Gales AC, et al. Increasing prevalence of antimicrobial resistance among Pseudomonas aeruginosa isolates in Latin American medical centres: 5 year report of the SENTRY Antimicrobial Surveillance Program (1997–2001). *J Antimicrob Chemother* 2003;52:140–141.
129. Stelling JM, O'Brien TF. Surveillance of antimicrobial resistance: the WHONET program. *Clin Infect Dis* 1997;24:S157–S168.
130. Ayliffe GA. The progressive intercontinental spread of methicillin-resistant *Staphylococcus aureus. Clin Infect Dis* 1997;24:S74–79.
131. Dalla Costa LM, Souza DC, Martins LT, et al. Vancomycin-resistant *Enterococcus faecium*: first case in Brazil. *Braz J Infect Dis* 1998;2: 160–163.
132. Jacobs MR, Koornhof HJ, Robins-Browne RM, et al. Emergence of multiply resistant pneumococci. *N Engl J Med* 1978;299:735–740.
133. Friedland IR, Klugman KP. Antibiotic-resistant pneumococcal disease in South African children. *Am J Dis Child* 1992;146:920–923.

134. Tomasz A. Antibiotic resistance in *Streptococcus pneumoniae. Clin Infect Dis* 1997;24:S85–88.
135. Medeiros AA. Evolution and dissemination of beta-lactamases accelerated by generations of beta-lactam antibiotics. *Clin Infect Dis* 1997; 24:S19–S45.
136. Miller GH, Sabatelli FJ, Hare RS, et al. The most frequent aminoglycoside resistance mechanisms—changes with time and geographic area: a reflection of aminoglycoside usage patterns? *Clin Infect Dis* 1997;24:S46–S62.
137. Acar JF, Goldstein FW. Trends in bacterial resistance to fluoroquinolones. *Clin Infect Dis* 1997;24:S67–S73.
138. Sader HS, Mendes CF, Pignatari AC, et al. Use of macrorestriction analysis to demonstrate interhospital spread of multiresistant *Acinetobacter baumannii* in Sao Paulo, Brazil. *Clin Infect Dis* 1996;23: 631–634.
139. Sacks LV, Pendle S, Orlovic D, et al. A comparison of outbreak- and nonoutbreak-related multidrug-resistant tuberculosis among human immunodeficiency virus-infected patients in a South African hospital. *Clin Infect Dis* 1999;29:96–101.
140. Harries AD, Kamenya A, Namarika D, et al. Delays in diagnosis and treatment of smear-positive tuberculosis and the incidence of tuberculosis in hospital nurses in Blantyre, Malawi. *Trans R Soc Trop Med Hyg* 1997;91:15–17.
141. Wilkinson D, Crump J, Pillay M, et al. Nosocomial transmission of tuberculosis in Africa documented by restriction fragment length polymorphism. *Trans R Soc Trop Med Hyg* 1997;91:318.
142. Tan LH, Kamarulzaman A, Liam CK, et al. Tuberculin skin testing among healthcare workers in the University of Malaya Medical Centre, Kuala Lumpur, Malaysia. *Infect Control Hosp Epidemiol* 2002; 23:584–590.
143. Dutta P, Bhattacharya EK, Saha MR, et al. Nosocomial rotavirus diarrhea in two medical wards of a pediatric hospital in Calcutta. *Indian Pediatr* 1992;29:701–706.
144. Unicomb LE, Banu NN, Azim T, et al. Astrovirus infection in association with acute, persistent and nosocomial diarrhea in Bangladesh. *Pediatr Infect Dis J* 1998;17:611–614.
145. Hu DJ, Kane MA, Heymann DL. Transmission of HIV, hepatitis B virus and other bloodborne pathogens in health care settings: a review of risk factors and guidelines for prevention. *Bull World Health Organ* 1991;69:623–630.
146. Aylward B, Kane M, McNair-Scott R, et al. Model-based estimates of the risk of human immunodeficiency virus and hepatitis B virus transmission through unsafe injections. *Int J Epidemiol* 1995;24: 446–452.
147. Sagoe-Moses C, Pearson RD, Perry J, et al. Risks to health care workers in developing countries. *N Engl J Med* 2001;345:538–541.
148. Gisselquist D, Rothenberg R, Potterat J, et al. Non-sexual transmission of HIV has been overlooked in developing countries. *BMJ* 2002; 324:235.
149. Greenberg AE, Phuc ND, Mann JM, et al. The association between malaria blood transfusions and HIV seropositivity in a pediatric population in Kinshasa, Zaire. *JAMA* 1988;259:545—49.
150. Beldescu N, Apetrei R, Calumfirescu A. Nosocomial transmission of HIV in Romania, Sixth International Conference on AIDS, San Francisco, June 20–21, 1990.
151. Pokrovsky V, Eramova EU. Nosocomial outbreak of HIV infection in Elista, USSR, Fifth International Conference on AIDS, Montréal, June 4–9, 1989.
152. Velandia M, Fridkin SK, Cardenas V, et al. Transmission of HIV in dialysis centre. *Lancet*1995;345:1417–1422.
153. Pujol FH, Ponce JG, Lema MG, et al. High incidence of hepatitis C virus infection in hemodialysis patients in units with high prevalence. *J Clin Microbiol* 1996;34:1633–1636.
154. Seme K, Poljak M, Zuzec-Resek S, et al. Molecular evidence for nosocomial spread of two different hepatitis C virus strains in one hemodialysis unit. *Nephron* 1997;77:273–278.
155. Abdelnour GE, Matar GM, Sharara HM, et al. Detection of anti-hepatitis C-virus antibodies and hepatitis C-virus RNA in Lebanese hemodialysis patients. *Eur J Epidemiol* 1997;13:863–867.
156. White HA. Lassa fever: a study of 23 hospital cases. *Trans R Soc Trop Med Hyg* 1972;66:390–398.
157. Monath TP, Mertens PE, Patton R, et al. A hospital epidemic of Lassa fever in Zorzor, Liberia, March–April 1972. *Am J Epidemiol* 1973;22:773–779.
158. Burney MI, Ghafoor A, Saleen M, et al. Nosocomial outbreak of viral hemorrhagic fever caused by Crimean-Congo hemorrhagic fever virus in Pakistan, January 1976. *Am J Trop Med Hyg*1980;29:941–947.
159. Smith DH, Isaacson M, Johnson KM. Marburg-virus disease in Kenya. *Lancet* 1982;1(8276):816–820.
160. Fisher-Hoch SP, Tomori O, Nasidi A, et al. Review of cases of nosocomial Lassa fever in Nigeria: the high price of poor medical practice. *BMJ* 1995;311:857–859.
161. Padula PJ, Edelstein A, Miguel SD, et al. Hantavirus pulmonary syndrome outbreak in Argentina: molecular evidence for person-to-person transmission of Andes virus. *Virology* 1998;241:323–330.
162. Iwamoto M, Jernigan DB, Guasch A, et al. Transmission of West Nile virus from an organ donor to four transplant recipients. *N Engl J Med* 2003;348:2196–2203.
163. Awidi A. Infection in adults with cancer in a developing country: a three year prospective study. *Eur J Cancer* 1991;27:423–426.
164. Chakrabarti A, Nayak N, Sampath Dumar P, et al. Surveillance of nosocomial fungal infections in a burn care unit. *Infection* 1992;20: 132–135.
165. Al Soub H, Estinoso W. Hospital-acquired candidaemia: experience from a developing country. *J Hosp Infect* 1997;35:141–147.
166. Chiu NC, Chung YF, Huang FY. Pediatric nosocomial fungal infections. *Southeast Asian J Trop Med Public Health* 1997;28:191–195.
167. Narang A, Agrawal PB, Chakrabarti A, et al. Epidemiology of systemic candidiasis in a tertiary care neonatal unit. *J Trop Pediatr* 1998;44: 104–108.
168. Pacheco-Rios A, Avila-Figueroa C, Nobigrot-Kleinman D, et al. Mortality associated with systemic candidiasis in children. *Arch Med Res* 1997;28:229–232.
169. Weinberger M, Sacks T, Sulkes J, et al. Increasing fungal isolation from clinical specimens: experience in a university hospital over a decade. *J Hosp Infect* 1997;35:185–195.
170. Lettau LA. Nosocomial transmission and infection control aspects of parasitic and ectoparasitic diseases: I. introduction/enteric parasites. *Infect Control Hosp Epidemiol* 1991;12:59–65.
171. Lettau LA. Nosocomial transmission and infection control aspects of parasitic and ectoparasitic diseases: II. blood and tissue parasites. *Infect Control Hosp Epidemiol* 1991;12:111–121.
172. Lettau LA. Nosocomial transmission and infection control aspects of parasitic and ectoparasitic diseases: III. ectoparasites/summary and conclusions. *Infect Control Hosp Epidemiol* 1991;12:179–185.
173. Navarrete S, Avila C, Stetler H, et al. Nosocomial outbreak of *Cryptosporidium* diarrhea in a pediatric hospital and its relationship to AIDS. Program and abstracts of the 29th Interscience Conference on Antimicrobial Agents and Chemotherapy, Houston, TX, 1989. American Society for Microbiology.
174. Roncoroni AJ, Gomez MA, Mera J, et al. *Cryptosporidium*infection in renal transplant patients. *J Infect Dis* 1989;160:559.
175. Bruce-Chwatt LJ. Transfusion malaria. *Bull World Health Organ* 1974;50:337–346.
176. Abulrahi HA, Bohlega EA, Fontaine RE, et al. *Plasmodium falciparum*malaria transmitted in hospital through heparin locks. *Lancet* 1997; 349:23–25.
177. Akinoboye DO, Ogunrinade AF. Malaria and loaisis among blood donors at Ibadan, Nigeria. *Trans R Soc Trop Med Hyg* 1987;81: 398–399.
178. Al-Orainey IO, Al-Nasser MN, Saeed ES, et al. Nosocomial bacteraemia in a teaching hospital in Saudi Arabia. *J Hosp Infect* 1989;14: 201–207.
179. Berkowitz FE. Infections in children with severe protein-energy malnutrition. *Ann Trop Paediatr* 1983;3:79–83.
180. Berkowitz FE. Bacteremia in hospitalized black South African children. *Am J Dis Child* 1984;138:551–556.
181. Isaack H, Mbise RL, Hirji KF. Nosocomial bacterial infections among

children with severe protein energy malnutrition. *East Afr Med J* 1992; 69:433–436.

182. Habte-Gabr E, Gedebou M, Kronvall G. Hospital-acquired infections among surgical patients in Tikur Anbessa Hospital, Addis Ababa, Ethiopia. *Am J Infect Control* 1988;16:7–13.
183. Allen S, Van de Perre P, Serufilira A, et al. Human immunodeficiency virus and malaria in a representative sample of childbearing women in Kigali. *J Infect Dis* 1991;164:67–71.
184. Ponce-de-León-Rosales S, Macias AE. Global perspectives of infection control. In: Wenzel RP, ed. *Prevention and control of nosocomial infections.* Philadelphia: Lippincott Williams & Wilkins, 2003:14–32.
185. Starling C. Infection control in developing countries. Curr Opin Infect Dis. 2001;14:461-466.
186. Rhinehart E, Goldmann DA, O'Rourke EJ. Adaptation of the Centers for Disease Control Guidelines for the prevention of nosocomial infection in a pediatric intensive care unit in Jakarta, Indonesia. *Am J Med* 1991;91:213S–220S.
187. Rutala WA, Weber DJ. Uses of inorganic hypochlorite (bleach) in health-care facilities. *Clin Microbiol Rev* 1997;10:597–610.
188. Macias AE, Munoz JM, Bruckner DA, et al. Parenteral infusions bacterial contamination in a multi-institutional survey in Mexico: considerations for nosocomial mortality. *Am J Infect Control* 1999; 27:285–290.
189. Earle M, Jr., Martinez Natera O, Zaslavsky A, et al. Outcome of pediatric intensive care at six centers in Mexico and Ecuador. *Crit Care Med* 1997;25:1462–1467.
190. Tully JL, Friedland GH, Baldini LM, et al. Complications of intravenous therapy with steel needles and Teflon catheters a comparative study. *Am J Med* 1981;70:702–706.
191. Perez-Delgadillo MA, Cashat-Cruz M, Avila-Figueroa C. Central IV-catheter related infections in a pediatric hospital in Mexico. Thirty-fifth annual meeting of the Infectious Diseases Society of America, San Francisco, CA, 1997.
192. Centers for Disease Control and Prevention. Clinical sepsis and death in a newborn nursery associated with contaminated parenteral medications—Brazil, 1996. *MMWR Morb Mortal Wkly Rep* 1998;47: 610–612.
193. Maki DG, Rhame FS, Mackel DC, et al. Nationwide epidemic of septicemia caused by contaminated intravenous products: I. epidemiologic and clinical features. *Am J Med* 1976;60:471–485.
194. Matsaniotis NS, Syriopoulou VP, Theodoridou MC, et al. *Enterobacter*sepsis in infants and children due to contaminated fluids. *Infect Control* 1984;5:471–477.
195. Macias-Hernandez AE, Hernandez-Ramos I, Munoz-Barrett JM, et al. Pediatric primary gram-negative nosocomial bacteremia: a possible relationship with infusate contamination. *Infect Control Hosp Epidemiol* 1996;17:276–280.
196. Hernandez-Ramos I, Gaitan-Meza J, Garcia-Gaitan E, et al. Extrinsic contamination of intravenous infusates administered to hospitalized children in Mexico. *Pediatr Infect Dis J* 2000;19:888–890.
197. O'Grady NP, Alexander M, Dellinger EP, et al. Guideline for the prevention of intravascular catheter-related infections. *MMWR* 2002; 51(RR-10)1–29.
198. Goldmann DA, Martin WT, Worthington JW. Growth of bacteria and fungi in total parenteral nutrition solutions. *Am J Surg* 1973; 126:314–318.
199. Gilbert M, Gallagher SC, Eads M, et al. Microbial growth patterns in a total parenteral nutrition formulations containing lipid emulsion. *J Parenter Enter Nutr* 1986;10:494–497.
200. Hasan R, Babar SI. Nosocomial and ventilator-associated pneumonias: developing country perspective. *Curr Opin Pulm Med* 2002;8: 188–194.
201. Pierce AK, Sanford JP. Bacterial contamination of aerosols. *Arch Intern Med* 1973;131:156–159.
202. Smith PW, Massanari RM. Room humidifiers as the source of *Acinetobacter*infections. *JAMA* 1977;237:795–797.
203. Sanders CV Jr, Luby JP, Johanson WG Jr, et al. *Serratia marcescens* infections from inhalation therapy medication: nosocomial outbreak. *Ann Intern Med* 1970;73:15–21.
204. Mertz JJ, Scharer L, McClement JH. A hospital outbreak of *Klebsiella* pneumonia from inhalation therapy with contaminated aerosol solutions. *Am Rev Respir Dis* 1967;95:454–460.
205. Seropian R, Reynolds BM. Wound infection after preoperative debilatory versus razor preparation. *Am J Surg* 1971;121:251–254.
206. Cruse PJ, Foord R. The epidemiology of wound infection: a 10-year prospective study of 62,939 wounds. *Surg Clin North Am* 1980;60: 27–40.
207. Alexander JW, Fisher JE, Boyajian M, et al. The influence of hair removal methods on wound infections. *Arch Surg* 1983;118:347–352.
208. Favero MS, Pugliese G. Infections transmitted by endoscopy: an international problem. *Am J Infect Control* 1996;24:343–345.
209. Silveira Rohr MR, Castro R, Morais M, et al. Risk of *Helicobacter pylori* transmission by upper gastrointestinal endoscopy. *Am J Infect Control* 1998;26:12–15.
210. Rutala WA, 1994 and 1996 APIC Guidelines Committee, Association for Professionals in Infection Control and Epidemiology Inc. APIC guideline for selection and use of disinfectants. *Am J Infect Control* 1996;24:313–342.
211. Villarino ME, Vugia DJ, Bean NH, et al. Foodborne disease prevention in health care facilities. In: Bennett JV, Brachman PS, eds. *Hospital infections.* Boston: Little, Brown and Company, 1992:345–358.
212. Centers for Disease Control and Prevention. Guidelines for environmental infection control in health-care facilities: recommendations of CDC and the Healthcare Infection Control Practices Advisory Committee. *MMWR Morb Mortal Wkly Rep* 2003;52 (RR-16):1–44.
213. Ponce de Leon S. The needs of developing countries and the resources required. *J Hosp Infect* 1991;18:376–381.
214. Awaspokee N, Chongsuvivatwong V, Wanasaeng S, et al. Fatal nosocomial infection in medical wards of a university hospital. *J Med Assoc Thai* 1988;71(Suppl 3):22–27.
215. Yalcin AN, Hayran M, Unal S. Economic analysis of nosocomial infections in a Turkish university hospital. *J Chemother* 1997;9: 411–414.
216. Mehtar S. *Hospital infection control: setting a cost-effective programme.* New York: Oxford University Press, 1992.
217. Tietjen L, Cronin W, McIntosh N. *Infection prevention for family planning service programs: a problem-solving reference manual.* Durant, OK: Essential Medical Information Systems, 1992.
218. Ponce-de-León RS, Baridó ME, Rangel-Frausto MS. *Manual de prevención y control de infecciones nosocomiales.* Washington DC: Organización Panaméricana de la Salud, 1996.
219. Lynch P, Jackson M, Preston GA, et al. *Infection prevention with limited resources: a handbook for infection committees.* Chicago: ETNA Communications, 1997.
220. Wenzel R, Edmond M, Pittet D, et al. *A guide to infection control in the hospital.* Hamilton: BC Decker, 1998.
221. Pannuti CS, Grinbaum RS. An overview of nosocomial infection control in Brazil. *Infect Control Hosp Epidemiol* 1995;16:170–174.
222. Nettleman MD. The global impact of infection control. In: Wenzel RP, ed. *Prevention and control of nosocomial infections.* Baltimore: Williams & Wilkins, 1993:13–20.
223. Wey SB. Infection control in a country with annual inflation of 3,600%. *Infect Control Hosp Epidemiol* 1995;16:175–178.
224. Cavalcante MDA, Braga OB, Teofilo CH, et al. Cost improvements through establishment of prudent infection control practices in a Brazilian general hospital: 1986–1989. *Infect Control Hosp Epidemiol* 1991;12:649–653.
225. Haley RW, Culver DH, White JW, et al. The efficacy of infection surveillance and control programs in preventing nosocomial infections in US hospitals. *Am J Epidemiol* 1985;121:182–205.
226. Wenzel RP. The Lowbury Lecture. The economics of nosocomial infections. *J Hosp Infect* 1995;31:79–87.
227. Scheckler WE, Brimhall D, Buck AS, et al. Requirements for infrastructure and essential activities of infection control and epidemiology in hospitals: a consensus panel report. *Infect Control Hosp Epidemiol* 1998;19:114–124.
228. Garner JG, Jarvis WR, Emori TG, et al. CDC definitions for nosocomial infections, 1988. *J Infect Control* 1988;16:128–140.
229. Horan TC, Gaynes RP, Martone WJ, et al. CDC definitions of nosocomial surgical site infections, 1992: a modification of CDC defini-

tions of surgical wound infections. *Am J Infect Control* 1992;20: 271–274.

230. Emori TG, Culver DH, Horan TC, et al. National nosocomial infections surveillance system (NNIS): description of surveillance methods. *Am J Infect Control* 1991;19:19–35.
231. Horan TC, Emori TG. Definitions of key terms used in the NNIS System. *Am J Infect Control* 1997;25:112–116.
232. Velasco E, Thuler LC, Martins CA, et al. Nosocomial infections in an oncology intensive care unit. *Am J Infect Control* 1997;25:458–462.
233. Freeman J, Hutchison GB. Prevalence incidence and duration. *Am J Epidemiol* 1980;112:707–723.
234. García-García ML, Gómez-Morales E, Sánchez-García G. Validación de un programa de vigilancia de infecciones nosocomiales. *Salud Publica Mex* 1989;31:481–492.
235. Ostrosky-Zeichner L, Baez-Martinez R, Rangel-Frausto MS, et al. Epidemiology of nosocomial outbreaks: 14-year experience at a tertiary-care center. *Infect Control Hosp Epidemiol* 2000;21:527–529.
236. Wong E. *Guideline for prevention of catheter-associated urinary tract infections.* Atlanta: Centers for Disease Control and Prevention, 1981.
237. Tablan OC, Anderson LJ, Arden NH, et al. Guideline for prevention of nosocomial pneumonia. *Infect Control Hosp Epidemiol* 1994;15: 587–627.
238. Bolyard EA, Tablan OC, Williams WW, et al. Guideline for infection control in healthcare personnel, 1998. *Infect Control Hosp Epidemiol* 1998;19:407–463.
239. Mangram AJ, Horan TC, Pearson ML, et al., Hospital Infection Control Practices Advisory Committee. Guideline for prevention of surgical site infection, 1999. *Am J Infect Control* 1999;27:97–132.
240. Centers for Disease Control and Prevention. Guideline for hand hygiene in healthcare settings: recommendations of the Healthcare Infection Control Practices Advisory Committee and the HICPAC/SHEA/APIC/IDSA Hand Hygiene Task Force. *MMWR Morb Mortal Wkly Rep* 2002;51(RR-16):1–48.
241. Nelson DB, Jarvis WR, Rutala WA, et al. Position statement: multisociety guideline for reprocessing flexible gastrointestinal endoscopes. *Am J Infect Control* 2003;31:309–315.
242. Garner JS, Hospital Infection Control Practices Advisory Committee. Guideline for isolation precautions in hospitals. *Infect Control Hosp Epidemiol* 1996;17:53–80.
243. Danchaivijitr S, Tangtrakool T, Chokloikaew S, T et al. Universal precautions: costs for protective equipment. *Am J Infect Control* 1997; 25:44–50.
244. Mitnick C, Bayona J, Palacios E, et al. Community-based therapy for multidrug-resistant tuberculosis in Lima, Peru. *N Engl J Med* 2003; 348:119–128.
245. World Health Organization. *Injection safety toolbox,* 2003.
246. Liberati A, D'Amico R, Pifferi S, et al. Antibiotic prophylaxis for respiratory tract infections in adult patients in intensive care units (Cochrane Review). In: *The Cochrane library,* vol. Issue 3. Oxford: Update Software, 1998.
247. Sanford JP. Hospital-acquired urinary tract infections. *Ann Intern Med* 1964;60:903–914.
248. Anonymous. Antimicrobial prophylaxis in surgery. *Med Lett Drugs Ther* 2001;43:92–97.
249. Classen DC, Evans RS, Pestotnik SL, et al. The timing of prophylactic administration of antibiotics and the risk of surgical-wound infection. *N Engl J Med* 1992;326:281–286.
250. Rutala WA. Disinfection and sterilization of patient-care items. *Infect Control Hosp Epidemiol* 1996;17:377–384.
251. Barone MA, Faisel AJ, Andrews L, et al. Adaptation and validation of a portable steam sterilizer for processing intrauterine device insertion instruments and supplies in low-resource settings. *Am J Infect Control* 1997;25:350–356.
252. Shlaes DM, Gerding DN, John JF Jr., et al. Society for Healthcare Epidemiology of America and Infectious Diseases Society of America Joint Committee on the Prevention of Antimicrobial Resistance: guidelines for the prevention of antimicrobial resistance in hospitals. *Clin Infect Dis* 1997;25:584–599.
253. McGowan JE Jr, Tenover FC. Control of antimicrobial resistance in the health care system. *Infect Dis Clin North Am* 1997;11:297–311.
254. Bantar C, Sartori B, Vesco E, et al. A hospitalwide intervention program to optimize the quality of antibiotic use: impact on prescribing practice, antibiotic consumption, cost savings, and bacterial resistance. *Clin Infect Dis* 2003;37:180–186.
255. Maki DG, Ringer M, Alvarado CJ. Prospective randomised trial of povidone-iodine, alcohol, and chlorhexidine for prevention of infection associated with central venous and arterial catheters. *Lancet* 1991; 338:339–343.
256. Raad I, Hohn DC, Gilbreath BJ, et al. Prevention of central venous catheter-related infections by using maximal sterile barrier precautions during insertion. *Infect Control Hosp Epidemiol* 1994;15:231–238.

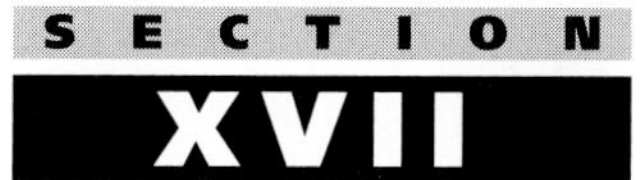

BIOTERRORISM

109

BIOLOGIC TERRORISM: AN OVERVIEW

MARGARET A. HAMBURG
C. J. PETERS

Once considered a remote concern, the possibility that biologic agents might be intentionally used to cause widespread panic, disruption, disease, and death is now widely recognized. Neither technical barriers nor moral repugnance can protect us from their use. Future attacks could occur again at any time, from many potential sources and using many possible biologic agents. Whether an unsophisticated delivery system with a limited number of infections, as we experienced in the United States in 2001 with the letters laced with anthrax, or a more technologically advanced and carefully orchestrated attack with mass casualties, the prospects are frightening. Further, we must recognize that this evolving threat presents the medical, public health, and scientific community with a set of difficult and pressing challenges.

By its very nature, the biologic weapons threat—with its close links to naturally occurring infectious agents and disease—requires a different paradigm than that for conventional terrorism, military strikes, or attacks caused by other weapons of mass destruction. A biologic event could well unfold as a disease epidemic, spread out in time and place before authorities even realize that an attack has occurred. What is more, opportunities for access to dangerous pathogens can be relatively routine, significant damage can be done even without large quantities of material or an elaborate delivery mechanism, and new possibilities for exploitation are embedded in the very science and technology advances that hold great promise for health.

There is an urgent need for systematic study and action concerning what is needed to control the development, proliferation, and use of biologic weapons, as well as the crucial elements of response should an attack occur. Clearly, this requires both new thinking about how to define and implement meaningful solutions, and the full engagement of the biomedical community (1).

This chapter offers an overview of the threat of bioterrorism, and discusses some of the critical issues that need to be addressed as the United States prepares to deal with this disturbing and potentially catastrophic threat. Subsequent chapters in this section discuss the specific elements of preparedness and response at the national, state, and local level, such as the identification and management of many biologic agents of particular concern.

WHAT IS BIOTERRORISM?

Terrorism can be most simply defined as "warfare deliberately waged against civilians with the purpose of destroying their will to support either leaders or policies" (2); however, the term as commonly used includes the implicit connotations that some weaker group attempts to gain international support or tumble the government targeted in order to achieve their goals, and that it often employs an element of fear in the targeted noncombatant population (3). The use of these tactics is probably as old as organized governments and has been traced back as far as the third century B.C. tactics of Hannibal or the spectacular murders by the eleventh century assassin cult. In any case, this approach has continued to the present day and is evolving according to available technology. Today's terrorists use the Internet and cellular phones, and incorporate the most modern destructive weapons.

Bioterrorism refers to terrorism carried out using biologic weapons. The international definition of biologic weapons includes replicating microorganisms such as bacteria and viruses as well as toxins derived from microorganisms. This definition includes a wide variety of attacks using any of a huge selection of microorganisms. Many of these events would be of lesser impact and might be of little more consequence than a crime or assassination executed with firearms (4,5). However, the element of terror is an important part of the impact. For example, the consequences of cyanide poisoning of analgesics or of imported grapes (3) had far reaching consequences in the public mind and economy. Only 21 anthrax cases with five deaths in 2001 resulted in a great deal of fear in the involved areas, paralyzed mail communications, and handicapped government functioning. Even hoaxes can be highly disruptive and expensive.

There is a much more serious side to the threat of bioterrorism, and it is best understood through the history of biologic warfare. Attempts at biologic attacks date back far in history. For example, in the 1300s, the bodies of plague-infected victims were catapulted over the city walls during the Tatar siege of Kaffa. In the 1700s, during the French and Indian War, native American adversaries were given "gifts" of smallpox-contaminated blankets by the British that decimated their numbers (6).

The development of a more modern approach to biologic

weapons dates to the early decades of the 20th century. During the 1930s and 1940s, the Japanese conducted extensive experiments and large-scale field trials—primarily involving contaminated food and water supplies—on unwitting civilians and prisoners of war in occupied Manchuria. In fact, during World War II, every major combatant had a biologic weapons program, although Japan is the only country that is generally agreed to have used biologic weapons during the course of the conflict (6,7).

The United States began its bioweapons program in 1943, partially in response to the research programs established by the Japanese and the Germans as well. But in 1969, President Nixon renounced the use of biologic weapons and ordered that our offensive program be ceased and all stockpiles destroyed (8,9). This decision paved the way for negotiation of the Biologic and Toxin Weapons Convention (BWC) treaty, which prohibits possessing, stockpiling, or transferring bioweapons. The treaty was concluded in 1972, and subsequently ratified by more than 140 countries. The signing of the BWC represented a very important commitment to abandon pursuit of biologic agents as weapons, but it did not—and still does not—contain explicit monitoring, inspection, or enforcement requirements (10).

As the 20th century closed, several events gave bioweapons greater prominence on the national security agenda. The first strong indication came from the accident at a Soviet bioweapons factory in Sverdlovsk; a human error led to the accidental release of weaponized anthrax with resulting cases in humans and cattle in the city. The source of the epidemic was suspected in the military and intelligence community but was denied by the Soviets and some American academics. Later investigations and Soviet admissions confirmed that it was, indeed, an epidemic of inhalation anthrax, practically pathognomonic of a biologic weapon in the pattern observed (9,11). As the Soviet Union broke up in the 1980s there were startling revelations about the magnitude and scope of the bioweapons program in the former Soviet Union, which began in full force the same year it signed on to the BWC. At the height of its program, more than 50 institutes were involved, employing tens of thousands of workers, including an estimated 7,000 scientists deemed security risks on the basis of their knowledge and expertise (12), and making ton quantities of weaponized anthrax, smallpox, and other microorganisms, as well as developing resistant strains and new pathogen variants, and experimenting with innovative strategies to cause disease, including recombinant microorganisms such as *Escherichia coli*–expressing neuromodulators (9,13).

Concerns were further heightened by the disclosure of an ambitious bioweapons program mounted by Iraq (14,15), and by the findings that Aum Shinrikyo, the Japanese group that released nerve gas in the Tokyo subway, had also experimented with botulism and anthrax, and had sent teams to Zaire in an effort to obtain Ebola virus for use as a weapon (16,17). Episodes in the U.S. involving extremist groups or individuals who were able to obtain dangerous pathogens such as ricin, anthrax, and *Yersinia pestis* for dubious purposes added to the growing perception of risk (18). The final breach of the barrier to use of biologic agents for terrorism or weapons came with the anthrax attacks in October 2001.

WHAT IS THE REAL THREAT OF BIOTERRORISM?

Any discussion of bioterrorism must begin with a consideration of the scenario: Who is executing the attack, why are they doing it, and what are their resources? This delineation allows us to focus on the scope, sophistication, and possible modalities of the attack or defense. A lone person with little microbiologic expertise poses a lower risk with microbes than with an automatic weapon. But a state-sponsored program is the other end of the threat spectrum and could result in many thousands of deaths. It is possible that the terrorist's desired outcome is merely that the turnout for voting is diminished, as occurred with a sect in Oregon that contaminated salad bars with *Salmonella* (19), or it may be more lethal such as Aum Shinrikyo's goals (16,17).

Certainly, attacks on a limited scale have occurred and will occur again (17,20). Terrorists or nation states have noted the remarkable success of the 2001 anthrax attacks, and will attempt to repeat them. In fact, anthrax is the most likely agent to be used in the future, because the microorganism is readily available in nature worldwide, the spores are stable in storage and in aerosol without special preparation, and *Bacillus anthracis* is easily grown and purified. It is particularly worrisome that the Federal Bureau of Investigation still has not caught the perpetrator of the 2001 anthrax weapon or determined how it was prepared (21).

However, most attention has been focused on attacks that carry the threat of very large numbers of casualties. It is easiest to analyze these attacks according to how the agent would be disseminated (Table 109.1). Direct injection has been used (22) as an assassination tool with ricin, but is impractical in any large-scale attack. Water is often mentioned and could be a risk on a small scale, but dilution and residual chlorine make it impractical on a large scale. Arthropods or rodents could be used with some agents such as tularemia or yellow fever, and indeed plague-infected fleas were used by the Japanese in World War II (7). However, the biology of such attacks can be difficult to predict or manage, as anyone who followed the arguments about the persistence of West Nile virus after its introduction into North America can attest. Food sources have been increasingly recognized as sources of multistate outbreaks and must be regarded as a vulnerable link, but we are also responding to them more effectively so that surveillance could give early warning and food lots could be recalled unless the dissemination occurred in a setting in which many consume the product synchronously. Clearly, protection of the food supply at the source is an increas-

TABLE 109.1. METHODS OF DISSEMINATION OF A BIOTERRORIST AGENT AND SOME OF THEIR DRAWBACKS

Injection-limited numbers
Water-purification plants, residual chlorine, and dilution
Arthropods, rodents-tricky biology
Food-access, synchronization, wide coverage
Interhuman spread-will the agent really do it?
Aerosol-relatively few agents useful, technical difficulties in preparing for stable, efficient delivery

ingly important consideration (23). The most efficient approach to infecting a large number of target humans would be to use an agent that would spread from person to person after the initial infections; only smallpox can actually do this. Influenza strains have been suggested, but they lack "directionality" toward an enemy and the immediacy required in most scenarios. That does not detract from the fact that influenza A is the greatest natural threat we face and that new strains could be responsible for millions of deaths worldwide (18). Other infections such as plague and viral hemorrhagic fevers have a limited possibility for spread and will not cause secondary infections beyond possibly limited numbers of close personal contacts and a few in the medical setting.

This leaves aerosol dissemination on the list (Table 109.1); however, there are only a few agents that can be grown to high titer, are infectious by the aerosol route, and cause severe and fatal disease. The small particle aerosols are subject to ultraviolet inactivation in most cases, can be carried away by wind currents, and require special preparation and skill in dissemination. They have some advantages: they can be disseminated at night under inversion conditions and with attention to meteorologic variables and be carried silently down wind to expose large numbers of people and/or animals. In fact, this approach was exactly that chosen by both the U.S. and the Soviet Union for their biologic warfare programs, and the testing suggested that it would be highly effective (24). The U.S. program was tested in each step, ranging from indoor and outdoor tests of aerosols, actual determination of the minimal infectious dose in humans for selected agents, and extensive animal testing. The testing showed that aerosols of simulated microorganisms (microorganisms that resemble the one to be used as a weapon but of minimal virulence) or powders with similar aerosol properties could be disseminated over large areas and would have the potential to produce tens or hundreds of thousands of casualties (25). Thus, each step of the use of such weapons was in place and there is no doubt that they would have been effective (8,9,22).

There is considerable argument over exactly which microorganisms belong in this "rogues' gallery" of aerosol infectious agents with lethal outcome. The Centers for Disease Control and Prevention (CDC) has proposed a grouping of categories A, B, and C, with category A being those of most concern (Table 109.2) (26). They were selected because of their catastrophic public health consequences with the expectation that, properly delivered, they would induce mass casualties that would overwhelm medical systems and carry with them a high mortality; no one would quarrel that these agents belong in the highest priority category. Smallpox has the additional threat that it would be contagious and spread among the unvaccinated populace. Botulism may have less potential as a mass casualty agent, but it certainly has a need for public health preparedness to manage the expected respiratory paralysis. This list has been the template for an enhanced defensive public health agenda. There are many arguments about what other microorganisms may be sufficiently dangerous to warrant consideration. Table 109.3 lists some of these, but there are differing opinions among the various authorities.

If aerosol delivery of biologic agents is so effective, why was it not used in warfare and why did the U.S. renounce its use? There are multiple considerations, but it is worthwhile to note that the Soviet program began in earnest around that time. The U.S. remained confident of the utility of nuclear weapons, and the Soviets were concerned about U.S. superiority and therefore were seeking other weapons of mass destruction. Another powerful reason comes out of the analysis of why lethal chemical agents were not used by the major powers after World War I; support by the military establishment requires that it understands the capabilities of a weapon and has a systematic doctrine for its use (27). This was not the case within the U.S. military establishment, which began to take biologic warfare defense seriously only after the Desert Storm operation in Kuwait and Iraq in 1991 put them in the arena with an adversary that may have had effective biologic weapons and was believed to be capable of using them if the situation demanded. The ability of biologic weapons to strengthen the capability of an otherwise poorly armed Third World country's military with attainable financial and expertise requirements fits into the doctrine of "asymmetric warfare." Biologic weapons are much cheaper and more easily produced than the equivalent nuclear capability, so they can provide weapons of mass destruction for countries that do not follow the nuclear route.

This discussion begs the question of how much expertise is needed for terrorists to mount such an attack should they not

TABLE 109.2. CATEGORY A BIOTERRORIST AGENTS DEFINED BY THE CDC

Variola major (Smallpox)
Bacillus anthracis (Anthrax)
Yersinia pestis (Plague)
Francisella tularensis (Tularemia)
Botulinum toxin (Botulism)
Viral hemorrhagic fevers
  Filoviruses (Ebola and Marburg)
  Arenaviruses (South American hemorrhagic fevers, Lassa fever)

Rotz, et al[26]. All are capable of efficient aerosol delivery. Only smallpox is also highly transmissible person-to-person

TABLE 109.3. OTHER MICROORGANISMS OF CONCERN IN BIOTERRORISM DEFENSE

VIRUSES
Other viral hemorrhagic fevers
  Rift Valley fever
  Tick-borne flaviviruses
Monkeypox virus
Alphaviruses Venezuelan equine encephalitis (VEE) virus
Nipah virus
(SARS) coronavirus
BACTERIA
Typhus and other critical rickettsiae
Glanders
OTHER
Crop agents
Veterinary pathogens
Bioengineered microorganisms

The agents above are often mentioned in lists of formerly weaponized microorganisms or microorganisms suspected of having that potential.

acquire weapons from a sympathetic country. Obtaining many of the most dangerous agents from nature is not difficult for a determined person with the microbiologic knowledge needed to produce a significant weapon. Their propagation in simple media or animals is straightforward for an experienced microbiologist, and the equipment and supplies needed are readily available. However, a limiting step is converting this slurry of potentially lethal microorganisms into a form that is stable and readily disseminated in aerosols. One example of a terrorist group's attempt is the failed effort of Aum Shinrikyo to prepare lethal anthrax and botulinum toxin weapons. Adequate financing, equipment, and a locale were available, but the principal players had such a lack of microbiologic expertise that a vaccine strain of *B. anthracis* was selected for their "weapon" (16,17). We cannot depend on the ineptitude of terrorists for our protection.

Before the terrorist attacks on September 11, 2001, several important commissions examined the vulnerability of the U.S. to terrorism and found the likelihood of a serious attack to be very high. The Bremer (28), Rudman and Hart (29), and Gilmore (30) commissions warned of catastrophic terrorist events including bioterrorist attacks, and indeed they were essentially correct in their assessments. Later reports from the Gilmore Commission (20) conclude that the post-9/11 status is still precarious. There are indications that Al Qaeda has interests in anthrax as a weapon (31). Thus, the continuing escalation of terrorists dedicated to extreme lethal events and expert assessments suggest that the risks of biologic attacks continue to be very real.

PREVENTION OF BIOTERRORISM

The fundamental approach would be to eliminate the seeds of terrorism, but this remedy does not seem to be forthcoming in the foreseeable future (32). The next step would be to design international arms control regimens that would stop the proliferation of biologic weapons in state programs. Unlike nuclear and chemical threats, biologic weapons do not emit radioactivity or have unique precursors or equipment for manufacture. The prospect of complete control by such a regimen is small, although it is an important and useful counter-proliferation modality to have treaties such as the BWC in place and to be seeking improved ways to pursue enforcement and surveillance activities (10).

Another approach has been to deny access of unauthorized persons to the microorganisms that might be used to produce weapons of mass destruction, and this has been pursued through establishing a list of select agents and stringently limiting access to these microorganisms. This clearly will have utility in preventing the use of hard-to-obtain agents such as smallpox, Ebola, or Marburg viruses. It is ineffectual and expensive when applied to agents such as anthrax, plague, and tularemia, which are widely available from nature worldwide. In fact, it is counterproductive, as it fosters unrealistic public attitudes about the danger, and the small research quantities of these agents limit the research and discourage scientists from working with them.

One might also attempt to protect the public by limiting effective processing of biothreat agents for aerosol dissemination, but much of the knowledge and equipment could be available through the pharmaceutical, cosmetic, agricultural, paint, and other manufacturing industries. Probably the most potentially dangerous people are those who worked in the Soviet biowarfare program because they have specific knowledge about processing, stabilization, and other manipulations for preparing infectious agents for aerosolization.

The strongest approach in the short term is to utilize the intelligence community in the U.S. and abroad to detect the next attack. Although this approach is likely to be successful in many instances, we cannot depend on it to intercept every bioterrorist attack before its execution, and thus a medical defense will be needed as well.

In the long run, we must recognize that those same advances in science and technology that hold enormous promise for improving health and combating bioterrorism also present many opportunities for misapplication or inadvertent harm. We need to ensure that the tools of modern genomic biology are not used to create new and more dangerous microorganisms. This is a complex challenge, for no one would want to impede the progress of legitimate and important science. However, we also have a responsibility to face up to the very real concern of the potential misuse of the biotechnologic tools increasingly available to those who want to do harm.

With leadership from the scientific community, we must begin to examine the context and conduct of modern science, and what opportunities may exist to constructively reduce this emerging threat. A recent report from the National Research Council of the National Academies emphasizes that "biologic scientists have an affirmative moral duty to avoid contributing to the advancement of biowarfare or bioterrorism." The report goes on to state that "scientists can and should take reasonable steps to minimize this possibility," indicating that it is the "the responsibility of the research community, including scientific societies and organizations, to define what these reasonable steps entail and to provide scientists with the education, skills, and support they need to honor these steps" (32). On a policy level, such prevention efforts will require a global approach, including the development and implementation of international standards, norms, or guidelines for biosecurity and the practice of biomedical research.

MEDICAL DEFENSE AGAINST BIOLOGIC THREATS

Because of the diversity of threats, one must settle on defined scenarios for response planning. Uses of biologic agents to cause disease in small numbers of people are probably best dealt with by alert medical and public health communities that will recognize the possibility that such outbreaks are due to human intervention and respond accordingly (4,5). At the current stage of national planning, most effort has gone into preparations for mass casualty situations. The scenario usually envisaged is not a "lights and sirens" kind of attack. Most likely there would be no announcement—no envelope saying, "This is anthrax, take penicillin." Without a fortuitous discovery early on, there would be no discrete signal that an attack had occurred; no site you can cordon off while you take care of the casualties, search for clues, and eventually clean up and repair the damage. Instead, this type of event would probably unfold as a disease epidemic, spread out in time and place before authorities even recognize that an attack has occurred. We would know we had been attacked only when people began appearing in doctors' offices or emergency rooms with unusual symptoms or inexplicable disease. The "first responders" to a bioterrorism event would not be hazardous materials (Hazmat) teams but rather public health officials and healthcare workers. "Ground zero" would be hospitals, labs, and healthcare facilities. Unfortunately, in many scenarios, diagnosis of the problem may be delayed, because medical providers and laboratories are not equipped to recognize and deal with the diseases of greatest concern. What is more, effective medical interventions may be limited, and where they exist, the window of opportunity for successful intervention would be narrow.

The response to such events must involve above all a strong public health system, an element in the national infrastructure that has been severely neglected and in need of repair for bioterrorism response, protection from emerging infectious diseases, and even dealing with established quotidian disease threats (18). Strengthening surveillance systems will be among the most important elements of the early warning systems. Many innovative ideas such as syndromic surveillance through a variety of electronic means are in urgent need of evaluation for sensitivity and specificity (33) (see Chapter 110). Some of these approaches may prove more useful for reassurance about nonevents or assessing ongoing attacks than for early detection. It is absolutely clear that effective surveillance requires a large investment in basic epidemiologic investigation of case clusters, but it is by no means clear that the trained manpower and resources for this effort exist. In addition, improved communication—including computer connectivity—is essential to quickly collect, analyze, and share information among public health and other officials at local, state, and federal levels, as well as other essential partners.

One of the important elements of the response is an enhanced laboratory capability in the public health and clinical arenas. The importance of high-volume testing was abundantly clear during the 2001 anthrax episodes, and the CDC's strengthening of the Laboratory Response Network was an important component of bringing existing resources on-line to respond. In the hospital laboratory there are two important considerations. First, the most dangerous bacterial bioterrorism agents are not necessarily optimally cultivated in the systems used and may even be discarded from considerations by some of the automated processing. Second, the distribution of infectious diseases is generally log-normal and characterized by the median and the dispersion (34). One consequence of this is that the number of cases is skewed toward the earlier times, and so early recognition is important to yield an increased therapeutic and prophylactic window of time. The only way we will be likely to achieve this is if point-of-care diagnostics are available for many of the threat agents, particularly plague.

It is worth noting that the front line for recognition of a bioterrorist attack will likely be the clinician. This was true in the 2001 anthrax attack, in which a Florida clinician used the classic tools of infectious diseases diagnosis to recognize a case of inhalation anthrax with secondary meningitis (35); it is true in most emerging infectious disease outbreaks; and it will likely hold for the next bioterrorist attack. The implications for clinician education and awareness are obvious.

Once an outbreak is recognized, treatment and postexposure prophylaxis will be paramount. In the late 1990s, a National Pharmaceutical Stockpile was established to address this concern (36). The response capability of a stockpile of vital medical supplies, including selected drugs, vaccines, antidotes, and medical equipment was demonstrated in several recent tragedies, including the World Trade Center attack and the 2001 anthrax attacks. Responsibility to maintain and oversee use of this stockpile, now called the National Strategic Stockpile (NSS), has been transferred from the CDC to the new Department of Homeland Security. The NSS is cached in selected locations across the country to be delivered within 12 hours to any place in the nation that requires assistance. The nature and quantities of materials maintained in the stockpile needs to be reviewed and extended.

OTHER CONSIDERATIONS

There are many issues undergoing rapid development that are beyond the scope of this chapter. Some are discussed in the following chapters in this section. Here is a list of some of these issues:

1. Acute-care hospitals have an insufficient surge capacity. With the improved efficiency in bed utilization in today's hospitals we have lost the ability to respond to the room and staff demands that would be expected from any significant bioterrorist attack. This is evident in the frequent diversion of ambulances and closure of emergency rooms in response to even a moderate increase in influenza A cases. The experience with severe acute respiratory syndrome (SARS) in several foreign cities in 2003 has demonstrated how easily healthcare systems elsewhere can be overwhelmed, and how the breakdown of care and services can contribute to ongoing and international spread of disease.
2. Some progress has been made in improving the legal underpinnings of quarantine and other emergency decisions that might be important in dealing with a bioterrorist situation, but this remains geographically spotty and generally untested.
3. Uses of drugs and diagnostics that are unlicensed or perhaps licensed for other indications is a major concern. The Food and Drug Administration (FDA) and others are working positively in this area (37), but we are far from resolving the issues that surround diseases that are not commonly seen in the U.S., and in some cases anywhere in the world.
4. Communications are always cited as a problem, but the scope of needed improvements in the biodefense field is immense. Obvious basic concerns about sharing information among public health and medical personnel during evolving situations are complicated by the need to extend this to civil authorities, law enforcement, the public, and the media. Some of the issues are not merely solved by computers or

phone lists; there are deep cultural divides among these compartments and issues of control. To deal with such an emergency, there will be no substitute for having an informed cadre of reporters who understand the issues and have some rapport with the public health authorities; this will facilitate dealing with the anxious, the incubating, and the sick with minimal public panic.

5. Although public education might be subsumed under the rubric of "communication," this aspect is so important that we mention it separately. An appreciation of the basic facts of infectious diseases and bioterrorism will be essential in obtaining an effective response to an attack and in engendering support for the counterterrorist agenda. We must begin now.
6. Infectious agents can be directed against crops or domestic animals. Even without the loss of one human life, it is resoundingly clear that terrorists could achieve their goals of producing mass panic, economic damage, and the undermining of public confidence in government by an attack on animals or crops. If the agent is Rift Valley fever, for example, which is both an agricultural pathogen and a human pathogen, the complications will be multiplied (38).
7. The research agenda is enormous. It ranges from the psychological effects of bioterrorism to operations research to the most basic molecular biology. Most of the biothreat microorganisms are emerging infectious diseases and/or regional threats outside the U.S. However, through global neglect of these agents, we have a poor understanding of their basic biology and treatment. We have not begun to think through some of the trade-offs in our attempts to medically protect the civilian population from bioterrorism. As one example, traditional infectious diseases control as well as protection of the military against biologic warfare regards vaccines as the gold standard. However, in today's world with multiple threat agents and no certainty of the use of any one of them, vaccines present an inherent risk that may not be acceptable. It may be preferable to rely on drugs in many situations; even though they have their own side effects and treatment may not be as effective as vaccine prevention, at least they would be used in the presence of a known risk (39). Certainly, vaccines will be important for a communicable disease such as smallpox, to protect at-risk laboratory workers and selected populations or circumstances (40).
8. The aerosol mode of delivery presents us with a discipline that is both familiar and yet strangely forgotten. At one time, aerosols were studied as important mechanisms of spread of tuberculosis, measles, and other diseases; in the last two decades much of this knowledge has eroded from the medical curriculum. We need to resurrect this information and add new research findings. The importance in defense against catastrophic bioterrorism is undeniable. Observations on the use of *Bacillus thuringiensis* to kill arthropods have provided a chilling example of large area coverage by this relative of *B. anthracis* (41,42). Older observations based on liquid and powder aerosol biologic warfare agents have given us a good perspective on the dissemination of airborne infection (22, 24). However, the properties of the fine, hydrophobic powders that were the most dangerous weapons developed are not well understood by the medical community (5), and the knowledge of their properties to form secondary aerosols is an area of some ignorance to all (43).

CONCLUSION

The U.S. is just beginning a long march toward effective biodefense measures. We should not suppose that this threat will disappear or that it is not significant because of the failure to find biologic weapons in Iraq. The process will be expensive but will yield dividends through strengthening our national security, our posture toward emerging infectious diseases, and the public health system that protects us every day (18). We still need a national dialogue and deeper thinking to resolve the elements of this complex problem (20,44).

FURTHER READING

The best single source for the principles of dissemination, history of biologic warfare, and several of the diseases is the *Textbook of Military Medicine* edited by Sidell, Takafuji, and Franz (45). Because many of the diseases are emerging or tropical diseases, the literature in that area often has a more expansive treatment than texts oriented toward North American considerations (46). The series of articles from the Johns Hopkins Center for Civilian Biodefense are excellent treatments of category A agents and are available through its Web site (*http://www.upmc-biosecurity.org/*). Some excellent Web-based aids are available at *www.cidrap.umn.edu*. Good popular books about biowarfare and bioterrorism cover the older history (8) and more recent events (9). An excellent book for the intelligent layman who needs background is *Living Terrors: What America Needs to Know to Survive the Coming Bioterrorist Catastrophe* (47). It would be of interest to many to read at least one of the pre-9/11 commission reports predicting catastrophic terrorism and bioterrorism (28–30), as well as some of the more recent thinking on where we need to be going in biodefense (44).

REFERENCES

1. Hamburg MA. Bioterrorism: a challenge to public health and medicine. In: Knobler SL, Mahmoud AAF, Pray LA, eds. *Biological threats and terrorism.* Washington, DC: National Academy Press, 2000:38–44.
2. Carr C. *The lessons of terror. A history of warfare against civilians.* New York: Random House, 2003.
3. Simon JD. *The terrorist trap. America's experience with terrorism.* Bloomington and Indianapolis, IN: Indiana University Press, 1994.
4. Kolavic SA, Kirmura A, Simons SL, et al. An outbreak of Shigella dysenteriae type 2 among laboratory workers due to intentional food contamination. In: Lederberg J, ed. *Biological weapons: limiting the threat.* Cambridge, MA: MIT Press, 1999:185–192.
5. Torok TJ, Tauxe RV, Wise RP, et al. A large community outbreak of salmonellosis caused by intentional contamination of restaurant salad bars. In: Lederberg J, ed. *Biological weapons: limiting the threat.* Cambridge, MA: MIT Press, 1999:167–184.
6. Christopher GW, Cieslak TJ, Pavlin JA, et al. Biological warfare. A historical perspective. In: Knobler SL, Mahmoud AAF, Pray LA, eds.

Biological threats and terrorism. Washington, DC: National Academy Press, 1997:412–417.

7. Harris S. *Factories of death. Japanese biological warfare, 1932–45, and the American cover-up.* London: Routledge, 1995.
8. Harris R, Paxman J. *A higher form of killing.* New York: Hill and Wang, 1982.
9. Miller J, Engelberg S, Broad W. *Germs: biological weapons and America's secret war.* New York: Simon & Shuster, 2001.
10. Kadlec RP, Zelicoff AP, Vrtis AM. Biological weapons control: prospects and implications for the future. In: Lederberg J, ed. *Biological weapons: limiting the threat.* Cambridge, MA: MIT Press, 1999: 95–111.
11. Meselson M, Guillemin J, Hugh-Jones M, et al. The Sverdlovsk Anthrax outbreak of 1979. *Science* 1994;266:1202–1208.
12. Smithson AE. *Toxic archipelago: preventing proliferation from the former Soviet chemical and biological weapons complexes.* Washington, DC: Henry L. Stimson Center, 1999.
13. Alibek K, Handelman S. *Biohazard.* New York: Random House, 1999.
14. Ekeus R. U.N. biological inspections in Iraq. In: Drell SD, ed. *The new terror: facing the threat of biological and chemical weapons.* Stanford, CA: Hoover Institution Press, 1999:237–254.
15. Davis CJ. Nuclear blindness: an overview of the biological weapons programs of the Former Soviet Union and Irag. *Emerg Infect Dis* 1999; 5:509–512.
16. Olson KB. Aum Shinrikyo: once and future threat. *Emerg Infect Dis* 1999;5:513–516.
17. Smithson AE, Levy LA. *Ataxia: the chemical and biological terrorism threat and the US Response.* Washington, DC: Henry L. Stimson Center, 2000:35.
18. Institute of Medicine of the National Academies. *Microbial threats to health.* Washington, DC: National Academies Press, 2003.
19. Torok TJ, Tauxe RV, Wise RP, et al. A large community outbreak of salmonellosis caused by intentional contamination of restaurant salad bars. In: Knobler SL, Mahmoud AAF, Pray LA, eds. *Biological threats and terrorism.* Washington, DC: National Academy Press, 1997: 389–395.
20. Gilmore JS. *Fourth annual report of the advisory panel. Implementing the national strategy.* 2002.
21. Matsumoto G. Anthrax powder: state of the art? *Science* 2003;302: 1492–1497.
22. *Medical aspects of chemical and biological warfare.* Washington, DC: Office of the Surgeon General, 1997.
23. Khan AS, Swerdlow DL, Juranek DD. Precautions against biological and chemical terrorism directed at food and water supplies. In: Knobler SL, Mahmoud AAF, Pray LA, eds. *Biological threats and terrorism.* Washington, DC: National Academy Press, 2001:3–14.
24. Peters CJ, Spertzel R, Patrick W. Aerosol technology and biological weapons. In: Knobler SL, Mahmoud AAF, Pray LA, eds. *Biological threats.* Washington, DC: National Academy Press, 2002:66–77.
25. McDermott J. *The killing winds. The menace of biological warfare.* New York: Arbor House, 1987.
26. Rotz LD, Khan AS, Lillibridge SC, et al. Public health assessment of potential biological terrorism agents. *Emerg Infect Dis* 2003;8: 225–230.
27. Brown FJ. *Chemical warfare. A study in restraints.* Princeton, NJ: Princeton University Press, 1968.
28. Bremer LP. Countering the changing threat of international terrorism. Report of the National Commission on Terrorism. Washington, DC: National Commission on Terrorism, 2000.
29. Rudman WB, Hart G. *The U.S. Commission on National Security for the 21st Century.* 1999.
30. Gilmore JS. *First annual report of the Advisory Panel to Assess Domestic Response Capabilities for Terrorism Involving Weapons of Mass Destruction.* 1999.
31. Anthrax linked to Al Qaeda. *Washington Post* 2003 Oct 11:A13.
32. Committee on Research Standards and Practices to Prevent the Destructive Application of Biotechnology of the National Research Council of the National Academies. *Biotechnology research in an age of terrorism: confronting the dual use dilemma.* Washington, DC: National Academies Press, 2003.
33. Buehler JW, Berkelman RL, Harley DM, et al. Syndromic surveillance and bioterrorism-related epidemics. *Emerg Infect Dis* 2003;9: 1197–1204.
34. Sartwell PE. The distribution of incubation periods of infectious diseases. *Am J Hyg* 1950;51:310–318.
35. Bush LM, Abrams BH, Beall A, et al. Index case of fatal inhalational anthrax due to bioterrorism in the United States. *N Engl J Med* 2001; 345:1607–1610.
36. Office of Management and Budget. *Annual report to Congress on combating terrorism.* Washington, DC: Government Printing Office, 2001.
37. Goodman JL. Meeting the regulatory and product development challenges for vaccines and other biologics to address terrorism. In: Knobler SL, Mahmoud AAF, Pray LA, eds. *Biological threats and terrorism.* Washington, DC: National Academy Press, 2002:105–110.
38. Peters CJ. Are hemorrhagic fever viruses practical agents for biological terrorism? In: Scheld WM, Craig WA, Hughes JM, eds. *Emerging infections.* Washington, DC: ASM Press, 2000:203–211.
39. Peters CJ. The role of antivirals in responding to biological threats. In: Knobler SL, Mahmoud AAF, Pray LA, eds. *Biological threats and terrorism.* Washington, DC: National Academy Press, 2002:119–130.
40. Russell PK. Vaccines for threatening agents: ensuring the availability of countermeasures for bioterrorism. In: Knobler SL, Mahmoud AAF, Pray LA, eds. *Biological threats and terrorism.* Washington, DC: National Academy Press, 2002:87–90.
41. Levin DB, Valadares de Amorim G. Potential for aerosol dissemination of biological weapons: lessons form biological control of insects. *Biosecurity and Bioterrorism* 2003;1:37–42.
42. Hartley DM, Peters CJ. Aerosols from insect control measures show dangers of bioterrorism. *Biosecurity and Bioterrorism: Biodefense Strategy, Practice, and Science* 2003;1:221–222.
43. Weis CP, Intrepido AJ, Miller AK, et al. Secondary aerosolization of viable bacillus anthracis spores in a contaminated US senate office. *JAMA* 2002;288:2853–285.
44. Danzig R. *Catastrophic bioterrorism—what is to be done?* Washington, DC: Center for Technology and National Security Policy at the National Defense University, 2003.
45. Sidell, Takafuji, and Franz. *Textbook of military medicine.*
46. Guerrant RL, Walker DH, Weller PF. *Essentials of tropical infectious diseases.* Philadelphia: Churchill Livingstone, 2001.
47. Osterholm MT, Schwartz J. *Living terrors: what America needs to know to survive the coming bioterrorist satastrophe.* New York: Delacorte Press, 2000.

110

THE STATE AND LOCAL RESPONSE TO BIOTERRORISM

MARCELLE LAYTON
ELSIE LEE
DON WEISS
DEBRA BERG
SARA BEATRICE
JOEL ACKELSBERG

Since the tragic events of the Fall of 2001, bioterrorism preparedness planning efforts have accelerated at local and state public health agencies, similar to the efforts taking place in the medical care sector and at the federal level. The local and state public health response to a large-scale, covert bioterrorist event requires rapid recognition that an unusual disease manifestation or a clustering and/or increase in infectious disease illnesses is occurring, followed by prompt epidemiologic and laboratory investigations to determine the etiologic agent and whether this finding represents a true outbreak, and, if so, whether the source may have been intentional (e.g., terrorist act) versus a natural cause. If a potential bioterrorist event is suspected, public health authorities will need to mobilize rapidly to identify the time and site of the initial attack and conduct ongoing surveillance and epidemiologic investigations to monitor the extent of the outbreak. At the same time, health authorities will need to address public and provider concerns and provide frequent updates as the outbreak evolves and new information becomes available. There will be a need to determine whether antibiotic or vaccine prophylaxis is indicated and, if so, to coordinate with emergency management agencies and the healthcare community to provide medications to potentially exposed persons, which depending on the circumstances of the event may involve the entire population of the jurisdiction. The enhanced capacities and infrastructure required for a rapid and successful response to a large, covert bioterrorist event (Table 110.1) also ensure that public health agencies are able to respond to natural infectious diseases threats, such as pandemic influenza or the severe acute respiratory syndrome (SARS).

An effective public health response to bioterrorism also requires that local and state public health departments are closely coordinated with the appropriate governmental agencies at the local and state (e.g., emergency management, police, emergency medical services), regional (neighboring state and county authorities, especially public health counterparts), and federal (e.g., Health and Human Services, Department of Homeland Security, Department of Defense, and Department of Justice) levels. Lastly, and most importantly, the successful detection and response to a bioterrorism event relies heavily on linkages that should already be in place between local and state public health officials and the local healthcare provider, hospital, and laboratory communities within their jurisdictions.

STATE AND LOCAL HEALTH DEPARTMENTS IN THE UNITED STATES

Public health authority in the United States resides mostly at the state and local levels, with the powers of our federal public health agencies being limited and specific to certain key areas (e.g., international and interstate quarantine or regulation of drugs and vaccines). At the state level, the public health role focuses on ensuring that statutory authority is in place for both routine and emergency health activities, monitoring statewide disease surveillance in coordination with local health units, developing policy and guidelines for disease control activities, providing reference laboratory services, and supporting local public health agencies through financial or technical assistance. In contrast, local public health activities focus more directly on the collection of disease surveillance data; case and contact management activities to control disease spread (e.g., provision of immune globulin for hepatitis A contacts or directly observed therapy for tuberculosis); and in some localities, direct provision of healthcare (1). However, great heterogeneity exists with respect to personnel capacity, services offered, and organizational structure among state and local health departments in the United States. In some states, public health is decentralized, with most activities and services occurring at the local level and with state officials providing more of an oversight and advisory role. In other states, there are no local health units and all public health activities are conducted by the state. An even greater diversity of capacity and services exists among local health departments;

TABLE 110.1. BIOTERRORISM PREPAREDNESS CHECKLIST FOR LOCAL AND STATE PUBLIC HEALTH AGENCIES

1. Coordination and communication.
   a. Development and maintenance of an up-to-date contact list, with built-in redundancy, for all key personnel at responding local, state, and federal agencies (e.g., emergency management, police, fire, regional public health partners, FBI, and CDC)
   b. Regular interagency meetings with emergency management, law enforcement, and hazardous material responders to ensure that public health planning efforts are integrated with other agencies' plans
   c. Prepreparation of response protocols for various potential bioterrorist scenarios (e.g., threat incidents involving suspicious environmental samples vs. covert large-scale attack)
   d. Regular tabletop exercises and drills (include representatives from medical and laboratory communities)
2. Surveillance
   a. All potential bioterrorist agents should be included on the notifiable disease list; in addition, a clause to ensure that any unusual disease clusters or manifestations are reportable should be included in the local and/or state health code
   b. Ongoing outreach efforts to maintain or increase physician awareness regarding the clinical presentations of the likely bioterrorist agents, *and the* requirement that all notifiable diseases and any unusual disease manifestations be reported to the local health department
   c. Periodic bulletins on disease reporting and bioterrorism, with an emphasis on 24-hour telephone contact information for reporting suspect cases of urgent concern
   d. Training clinical microbiologists on the preliminary diagnosis of bacterial bioterrorist agents
   e. 24-hour/7-day response capability with appropriately trained medical staff to triage calls from providers regarding potential cases of public health concern
   f. Consider establishing syndrome-based or unexplained illness/death surveillance with protocols in place outlining response mechanisms if unusual disease activity is identified
3. Epidemiologic capacity
   a. Contingency plans for calling-up health department staff to assist in a large-scale epidemiologic investigation
   b. Preprepared template questionnaire forms, study protocols, and database
   c. Preestablished guidelines for conducting epidemiologic investigations, in coordination with the criminal investigations of the local police and FBI
   d. Planning to integrate environmental health assessments into the surveillance and epidemiologic response
4. Laboratory capacity
   a. Education of clinical microbiologists at local hospitals regarding criteria for reporting suspicious laboratory findings and protocols for proper collection, packaging, and transport of specimens for reference laboratory testing that meet federal chain of custody requirements
   b. Public health laboratories should be registered as at least a Level B (ideally a Level C) laboratory in the CDC's Laboratory Response Network and function as reference laboratories for confirmation of bioterrorist agents, using both conventional microbiologic and molecular methodologies
5. Guidance regarding clinical management of illness due to bioterrorist agents
   a. Pre-prepared protocols for the medical management of the likely bioterrorist agents
   b. Communication infrastructure to ensure rapid distribution of these protocols to providers and hospitals, if needed (e.g., broadcast facsimile and electronic mail, Web site, and Health Alert Network secure Internet sites)
   c. Preplanning for establishing a medical hotline to assist clinicians in the management of patients and contacts and to triage reports on suspect cases
6. Mass medical and mortuary care
   a. Contingency plans for enhancing capacity for acute medical care and mass mortuary needs (including plans for how federal DMAT and DMORT teams will be used)
   b. Contingency plans for rapidly establishing and maintaining community-based clinics for mass prophylaxis using vaccines and/or antibiotics (including plans for providing prophylaxis to difficult-to-reach populations, such as the homebound and homeless)
   c. Determination of need and feasibility of establishing a local antibiotic stockpile to ensure adequate supplies while awaiting federal reserves (antibiotic stockpiles need to include alternative regimens for pediatric, pregnant, and immunocompromised patients, when indicated)
   d. Prepreparation of multilingual patient information sheets and vaccine consent forms
   e. Contingency plans for establishing and enforcing quarantine of potentially infectious contacts (e.g., contacts of smallpox cases)
   f. Guidelines for local medical care institutions for preparing a surge capacity response plan to a citywide infectious disease disaster, including how individual institution plans need to be integrated into regional response planning
   g. Contingency plans for mass mortuary care including tracking, storage, and disposal of potentially infectious corpses
7. Communication and mental health issues
   a. In coordination with other responding agencies, predesignation of primary spokesperson and/or agency
   b. Preprepared fact sheets on the potential bioterrorist agents for the general public
   c. Adequate capacity to rapidly establish telephone hotlines for the general public and medical providers
   d. In partnership with mental health agencies, develop plans for providing surge capacity for crisis counseling for potential victims, their families, first responders, the medical and public health community, and the general public
   e. Broadcast facsimile and electronic mail capacity and secure Internet connections (Health Alert Network) to facilitate urgent communications and notifications of the medical community
8. General infrastructure issues
   a. Establishment of a public health incident management system with training of all staff regarding their expected emergency response roles and responsibilities
   b. Sufficient capacity for communication (cellular phones, two-way radios), transportation, information technology, and personal protective equipment

CDC, Centers for Disease Control and Prevention; DMAT, Disaster Medical Assistance Team; DMORT, Disaster Mortuary Relief Team; FBI, Federal Bureau of Investigation.

in some large urban areas, the local health agencies are larger than many state health departments and function independently, whereas in more rural counties, resources may be quite limited with minimal professionally trained staff, thus requiring a greater reliance on state-level support.

ROUTINE LINKAGES BETWEEN PUBLIC HEALTH AND THE HEALTHCARE SECTOR

One of the core missions of public health agencies is the control of communicable diseases. This legal mandate has prompted public health officials to work closely with local healthcare providers and hospital and laboratory communities. Traditionally, disease surveillance activities depend on prompt reporting by healthcare providers and laboratorians concerning suspect or confirmed cases of notifiable diseases to local and state health departments. Case investigations by public health officials often require frequent communication with the reporting clinician or hospital infection control personnel to obtain more detailed clinical and epidemiologic data or to help facilitate obtaining appropriate clinical specimens for testing at public health reference laboratories (e.g., rabies or botulism). For certain contagious diseases (e.g., hepatitis A or invasive meningococcal disease), public health officials may request assistance in providing prophylaxis to contacts at high risk for secondary transmission. The successful implementation of public health prevention campaigns also relies on close partnerships between health departments and the medical community. Recent examples of this successful partnership include the response to the epidemic of multidrug-resistant tuberculosis in the early 1990s (2); perinatal hepatitis B prevention programs; and HIV counseling, testing, and partner notification programs.

From a surveillance and control perspective, one of the most important linkages at the local level is between public health officials, infection control professionals (ICPs), and hospital epidemiologists. ICPs and hospital epidemiologists serve as the primary points of contact in hospitals for surveillance and disease control activities during both community and nosocomial outbreaks and, as such, serve a critical role in any hospital's ability to respond to a bioterrorist event.

BIOTERRORISM PREPAREDNESS REQUIRES ENHANCED LINKAGES

Bioterrorism preparedness requires building on the existing linkages between the public health and hospital and medical care sectors that are already in place to confront routine public health problems, such as influenza, tuberculosis, and new or emerging infectious diseases (e.g., SARS). Key aspects of plans that need to be in place for the public health response to bioterrorism parallel what needs to be in place for naturally occurring infectious diseases outbreaks and include detection, epidemiologic investigation, active surveillance, laboratory testing, communication, and prophylaxis. The areas in which relationships with the hospital and medical communities are key include the initial detection of the event, provision of care to the victims, isolation of potentially contagious patients, provision of prophylaxis to those potentially exposed, and providing timely and effective education to the public regarding the medical aspects of the event. All clinicians and laboratorians should be familiar with the legal requirements under their local and state health codes, including which diseases are listed as notifiable in their state and mechanisms for disease reporting.

As with any emergency, it is essential that the local medical and public health communities are familiar with each other ahead of time. Medical providers and key hospital staff (e.g., infection control and microbiology staff) should be aware of both their local and state health departments' 24-hour, 7-day a week emergency contact numbers and Web site information and should be registered and familiar with any existing public health electronic communication systems (e.g., Health Alert Network, broadcast facsimile, and electronic mail health alert systems) that provide urgent notification of the healthcare community during acute events.

DETECTION OF A BIOTERRORISM EVENT: TRADITIONAL AND NONTRADITIONAL SURVEILLANCE SYSTEMS

Concern has been raised regarding the possible delays in recognizing an outbreak resulting from bioterrorism and the subsequent impact that this could have on morbidity and mortality if treatment or preventive measures were delayed. The diseases caused by many of the potential bioterrorist agents may not be accurately diagnosed until late in their course because the initial presentations may be nonspecific (e.g., influenza-like prodrome of anthrax), most physicians in the United States have little or no clinical experience with these agents (e.g., anthrax or smallpox), and the laboratory diagnosis for some agents may require days or even weeks for a positive or presumptive identification (e.g., tularemia). Therefore, alternative or early warning surveillance systems for recognizing unusual disease manifestations or clusters may be needed to improve the ability to detect a biologic terrorist event as rapidly as possible. Prompt recognition is necessary to expedite mobilization of an effective public health response, including rapid testing at a public health or other reference laboratory to identify the etiologic agent (along with susceptibility results for bacterial agents); enhanced or active surveillance for additional cases; epidemiologic investigations to determine the cause (natural vs. intentional source), the time and site of a suspected release, and event reconstruction to identify those still at-risk; and initiation of treatment and prophylaxis measures.

State and local public health officials need to be alert to potential scenarios that may represent the initial evidence of a bioterrorist event. A *possible* bioterrorist event, from the health department's perspective, could include any of the following:

1. A single, definitively diagnosed or strongly suspected case of an illness resulting from a recognized bioterrorist agent occurring in a patient without a plausible explanation for his or her illness (e.g., a case of plague in the absence of a recent travel history to a recognized endemic area).

2. A cluster of patients presenting with a similar clinical syndrome with either unusual characteristics (unusual age distribution) or unusually high morbidity or mortality, without an obvious etiology or explanation.
3. An *unexplained* increase in the incidence of a common syndrome above seasonally expected levels (e.g., a marked increase in influenza-like illness during the summer with both rapid and conventional virology tests being negative for influenza or other common respiratory viruses).

In the event that a potential bioterrorist event is suspected, an investigation should be initiated immediately to confirm the suspected diagnosis, ensure that there are no other explanations for the illness(es), and determine the likely source of infection. Because these case definitions are nonspecific for bioterrorism and would also apply to natural outbreaks of known or new infectious diseases, it is essential that bioterrorism be considered as part of all routine case and/or outbreak investigations, until a natural cause is established. Prior outbreaks of *Salmonella* in a community (3) and *Shigella* among employees of a hospital laboratory (4) were eventually found to be due to intentional contamination of food items when the initial epidemiologic and laboratory investigation revealed concerning features that would not have been expected if the infections had occurred naturally.

There are several surveillance methodologies for detecting a bioterrorist event that focus on ensuring the prompt recognition of (a) a suspected or confirmed case or cluster resulting from a recognized bioterrorist agent; (b) community-wide or localized increases in influenza-like illness activity or other nonspecific syndromes, or increases in potential markers of early prodromal illness (e.g., over-the-counter drug sales); (c) an increase in unexplained, severe infectious illnesses or deaths; or (d) detection of select bacteria or viruses in air samples obtained through routine environmental biomonitoring programs.

Traditional Public Health Surveillance

Traditional public health surveillance for bioterrorism relies on enhancing the medical and laboratory communities' awareness of bioterrorism to improve reporting of (a) suspect cases of illness potentially caused by a bioterrorist agent or (b) unusual disease manifestations or clusters. Most local and state health codes require that physicians, hospitals, and laboratories report a defined list of notifiable infectious diseases. With recent concerns regarding the threat of bioterrorism, most state public health agencies have added all Centers for Disease Control and Prevention (CDC) Category A and most Category B agents that were not already included on their reportable disease lists (5). In addition, recognizing the need to detect newly emergent diseases that are not yet listed on the health code, most states also require reporting of any unusual disease clusters or manifestations.

Early recognition of a bioterrorist event depends in large part on astute clinicians and laboratorians recognizing one of the index cases based on a suspicious clinical, radiologic, or laboratory presentation (e.g., a febrile illness associated with a widened mediastinum on chest radiograph in an otherwise healthy adult has a limited differential diagnosis besides anthrax). Isolated cases presenting at separate hospitals will not be recognized as a potential outbreak, unless each case is reported promptly to the local health department, where the perspective exists to detect population-based aberrations in disease trends. Previous examples of astute clinicians recognizing and reporting unusual disease clusters or manifestations that led to the detection of a more widespread outbreak include an outbreak of Legionnaires' disease associated with the whirlpool on a cruise ship (6), an outbreak of *Cyclospora* associated with contaminated raspberries imported from Guatemala (7), and the initial outbreak of West Nile virus in New York City in 1999 (8) Similarly, the initial detection of the intentional anthrax outbreak in 2001 was due to a public health responsive physician who recognized a suspect case of inhalational and meningeal anthrax in Florida after noting large gram-positive rods in the cerebrospinal fluid of his patient and promptly reported his concerns to local and state public health authorities (9).

To educate clinicians and laboratorians regarding their essential role in recognizing and reporting a suspected case of bioterrorism or other unusual infectious diseases occurrences, public health officials need to promote the importance of disease reporting through ongoing educational efforts. For bioterrorism concerns, targeted outreach efforts should focus on specialists in key areas, such as infectious diseases, infection control, microbiology, emergency medicine, dermatology, and neurology. Educational outreach should emphasize the clinical presentations and diagnostic clues for specific bioterrorist agents (e.g., anthrax, plague, smallpox) and unusual illness patterns suggestive of a potential bioterrorist event. One of the lessons learned during the 2001 anthrax attack was the need to maintain awareness of all potential clinical manifestations of the bioterrorist agents, such as cutaneous disease, and not simply focus on illness resulting from inhalational routes of exposure. Educational materials should emphasize prompt reporting of any unusual disease clusters or manifestations to the local or state health department as paramount to the early recognition of natural and intentional outbreaks. Educational outreach is also needed for key members of the local first responder community (HAZMAT, police, emergency medical services).

The following mechanisms may be used to help increase awareness of bioterrorism in the medical and laboratory communities:

1. Oral presentations targeting specialists in internal medicine, emergency medicine, pediatrics, dermatology, neurology, family practice, infectious diseases, pathology, laboratory medicine, intensive care, pulmonary, radiology, and primary care physicians; physicians-in-training and medical students; medical examiners; veterinarians and microbiologists.
2. Public health bulletins, newsletters, posters, or pocket cards on bioterrorism, which provide an overview of the clinical aspects of the potential bioterrorist agents (e.g., clinical presentation, laboratory diagnosis, treatment, and prophylaxis) and emphasize the importance of promptly reporting any unusual disease clusters or manifestations to the local and state health departments. These educational materials must be repeated and updated periodically to maintain ongoing awareness of the threat of bioterrorism.

3. Posting educational materials on the health department's Web site with links to other useful sites (10), including the CDC *(www.cdc.gov),* the Infectious Disease Society of American *(www.idsociety.org),* and the American Society of Microbiology *(www.asm.org).*
4. Development of teaching slides and videos that can be distributed to academic and community-based physicians for presentations on bioterrorism (train-the-trainer modules). Because many health departments may not have sufficient staff with the expertise or time to meet every request for a talk on bioterrorism, efforts should be made to provide teaching materials (e.g., slide presentations with speaker notes) to interested colleagues in infectious diseases, infection control. or other specialties to do presentations to medical staff at their own institutions or organizations.

Improving the overall relationship between the health department and the medical community is an important element in ensuring that providers report promptly. Therefore, efforts to improve provider relations and ease the burden of physician reporting should be prioritized [e.g., having a single telephone number (e.g., by implementing 1-800 provider hotlines, such as 1-800-MD-REPORT) for physician reporting to ensure easy access to health department staff and a dedicated office, with clinically trained professionals, for handling telephone inquiries from the medical and laboratory community]. The medical and laboratory communities are more likely to report if the process is streamlined and there is a positive perception of the public health responsiveness to disease and/or outbreak reporting. Routine dissemination of surveillance data and prompt feedback are essential for fostering an ongoing, collaborative relationship between public health and the medical and laboratory communities. These efforts have the additional benefit of improving all aspects of local public health surveillance.

Recent experiences with the West Nile virus (11) and monkeypox (12) outbreaks have highlighted the need for public health officials to establish and maintain similar active linkages with the animal health community. Because many potential bioterrorist agents cause zoonotic disease (e.g., anthrax and plague), the first indication of an aerosolized release may be illness or death in animals or rodents. Historically, with the exception of rabies-related issues, local and state infectious diseases epidemiologists have not had strong relationships with clinical veterinarians and wildlife specialists in their community. However, with the continued emergence of new zoonotic disease threats, and the concerns about bioterrorism, this has needed to change. Many states and local health departments have recently added or expanded current disease reporting requirements for animal health specialists to notify public health officials of any suspect or confirmed illness in an animal that may be due to a potential bioterrorist agent. Similar to the list of notifiable diseases in humans, these regulations often require reporting of any unusual disease clusters or manifestations in animals as well.

Nontraditional Surveillance Systems (Syndromic Surveillance)

The recent bioterrorist attacks associated with the intentional release of *Bacillus anthracis* spores have increased interest in the potential value of enhanced public health surveillance systems for early detection of epidemics caused by biologic terrorism. In the event of a covert large-scale biologic attack with the potential to cause hundreds to thousands of casualties, rapid detection, and characterization of the outbreak would be of the utmost importance. Rapid mobilization of surveillance and epidemiologic resources to determine the place and time of the attack would facilitate targeting preventive measures to those at-risk, speed the epidemiologic and criminal investigation, and reduce public panic. For diseases such as inhalational anthrax, with short incubation periods, the window of opportunity to mobilize a response to mitigate morbidity and mortality is quite small, being a matter of days. Therefore, surveillance systems that provide early and enhanced recognition of a covert bioterrorist event are advantageous.

The traditional public health surveillance system, based on passive reporting of a limited number of defined, notifiable diseases, may not be sufficient for early detection of a bioterrorist event. Certain potential bioterrorist agents (e.g., tularemia) have nonspecific clinical presentations and/or laboratory diagnosis may be difficult. Thus, alternative systems that allow prompt recognition of unusual disease manifestations, illness clusters, increases above seasonal levels of common syndromes (e.g., influenza-like illnesses), or deaths resulting from infectious causes prior to suspicion or confirmation of the causative agent(s) are potentially useful components of bioterrorism surveillance.

Although increasing provider education on bioterrorism and improved communication among public health officials, clinicians, and laboratorians is an essential component of enhanced traditional surveillance, surveillance for nonspecific clinical syndromes using data available in existing electronic health databases is also now considered a potentially valuable adjunct system for the timely detection of large-scale bioterrorist events. Although many of the most concerning infections (e.g., anthrax, plague, smallpox, and viral hemorrhagic fever) have distinct clinical characteristics and diagnostic criteria once the disease is full blown, the first signs of illness for many of these agents is a nonspecific prodrome with respiratory and constitutional symptoms similar to influenza-like illness. Because most medical providers and laboratories in the United States have little experience with these pathogens, the diagnoses may be delayed. Therefore, the first indication that a large-scale attack has taken place might be an increase in nonspecific symptoms at the community level. Surveillance for these increases in nonspecific syndromes (e.g., respiratory or gastrointestinal) constitutes the cornerstone of syndromic surveillance. (13).

The ideal features of a syndromic surveillance system for early detection of a covert bioterrorist attack include the ability to detect changes in disease trends that are based on health event information available continuously or at least in 12- to 24-hour increments. Health event information is most timely when it is electronic, gathered routinely for other purposes, and not limited by diagnostic or recording delays. Syndromic surveillance systems based on clinical data have proven most popular, but other sources such as over-the-counter drug sales may also have utility.

Electronic data that may provide a reflection of communitywide illness is increasingly available, including for example, emergency department visit logs (14), ambulances dispatches

(15), ambulatory care encounters (16), volume of specimen submissions to commercial clinical laboratories, and sales of prescription and over-the-counter pharmaceuticals. Because of the challenges in requiring additional efforts by physicians or other providers, the most reliable electronic data sources probably are those that already exist and that do not rely on additional collection or reporting of data by medical providers. In many systems, these data include geographic information (e.g., home or work zip code or location of store), theoretically enabling the detection of localized disease outbreaks.

Important features to consider when evaluating potential syndromic surveillance systems include presence of computerized data that already is categorized into clinical syndromes, can be made available to health authorities on at least a daily basis (including weekends and holidays), and is geographically representative of the population. Ideally, the operation of these systems for public health surveillance purposes should include at least daily electronic transfer of data that has been de-linked of personal identifiers and that uses statistical algorithms to rapidly detect increases in disease syndromes compared with expected seasonal trends (17). Some systems have the additional sensitivity to detect spatial aberrancies or unexpected geographic clusters (18) Hospitals and medical care systems may be able to share such data sources with their local or state health departments, including information on emergency department or primary care clinic visits or hospital admissions; if the data does not contain confidential information on patients (e.g., data, limited to age, date of visit, chief complaint, or provider diagnosis), then potential restrictions in the Health Information Privacy and Accountability Act would not apply (19).

When an aberration in a particular syndrome is identified, either a jurisdiction-wide increase or a geographic-specific signal, public health officials need to assess the situation to determine if the finding truly represents worrisome illness in the community and, if so, conduct an investigation. Similar to traditional outbreak investigations, syndromic signal investigations attempt to determine if the aberration represents a common illness with or without a common exposure. To assist in determining if the aberration is a real event versus a statistical anomaly, it is generally assumed that a continued rise in the incidence of the syndrome is evidence of a real event. Interim data from the involved facilities (e.g., a 12-hour chief complaint log), although often difficult to obtain, can be useful in this evaluation. Inspection of the aberrant data will reveal any unexpected coding mistakes and the presence of commonalities in demographic variables. Although anecdotal, calls to emergency department staff, as directed by geographic clustering, can be reassuring. When signals contain concerning features, as determined by the particular syndrome and parameters such as size of the cluster or magnitude of the increase, age clustering, seasonality, and syndrome overlap, staff can be dispatched to review medical records, conduct interviews, or telephone follow-up on discharged patients. Prospective surveillance is implemented with augmented diagnostic testing for newly presenting patients, as indicated by the syndrome of concern (e.g., rapid antigen tests for influenza, chest radiographs, or blood cultures).

One of the challenges to syndromic surveillance has been establishing the definitive microbiologic cause when an increase in an infectious disease syndrome is identified. Limitations in obtaining clinical specimens, particularly in outpatient settings, and in being able to perform full diagnostic testing, especially for viruses, renders interpretation of signals and evaluation of syndromic systems difficult. Because the primary objective of syndromic surveillance is early outbreak detection, there is a need to link the use of rapid diagnostics (especially for viral agents, such as influenza, and ideally the bioterrorist agents as well) to investigations of syndromic surveillance signals.

Although the initial objectives for many of the current syndromic systems was early detection of a large, aerosolized covert bioterrorist attack, these systems also offer the ability to monitor for both natural infectious diseases outbreaks and trends in noninfectious events of public health importance. In New York City, syndromic surveillance has been in place since 2000 and currently includes multiple data sources, including ambulance dispatches, emergency department visits, pharmaceutical sales from a large retail chain, and employee absenteeism. Because an aberration in one system may represent an artifact (e.g., an increase in antidiarrheals being caused by a promotional sale at the pharmacy chain), when multiple systems are in place, an increase in more than one system is considered more concerning and may prompt a more intensive investigation. These New York City systems have provided the earliest warning of influenza-like activity at the start of each season, allowing earlier notification of the medical community of the need to prioritize completion of vaccination campaigns (Fig. 110.1, Panel A). In addition, New York City's syndromic surveillance systems provided early warning of the 2002 norovirus outbreak and detected a city-wide increase in diarrheal illness in the days following the August 2003 blackout (See Fig. 110.1, Panel B).

Health officials in New York City also have found syndromic surveillance useful for providing reassurance that medium to large outbreaks are not being missed during times of heightened concern. During the international outbreak of severe acute respiratory syndrome (SARS) the absence of a persistent city-wide increase or geographic clustering of respiratory or febrile syndromes in any of the current systems in place in New York City provided some assurance that unrecognized SARS transmission was not occurring in the city. Similarly, when cases of inhalational anthrax (20) and bubonic plague (21) were confirmed in New York City, the lack of signals from these systems suggested that these were isolated, not city-wide, events. Lastly, syndromic surveillance data in New York City has been used to monitor trends in noninfectious diseases or conditions of public health concern. Recent uses include estimating the burden of domestic violence by neighborhood using emergency department visit data, monitoring sales of nicotine prevention products in the retail pharmacy system after implementation of an increase in the local cigarette sales tax, and looking for increases in asthma-like symptoms presenting to emergency departments in areas where pesticides have been applied to control mosquito activity as part of the West Nile viral prevention program.

Over the past few years, there has been great interest in establishing syndromic surveillance in both the private and public sectors, but these systems remain untested with respect to their ability to detect a bioterrorist event. Although early indications support the potential usefulness of these systems, more formal

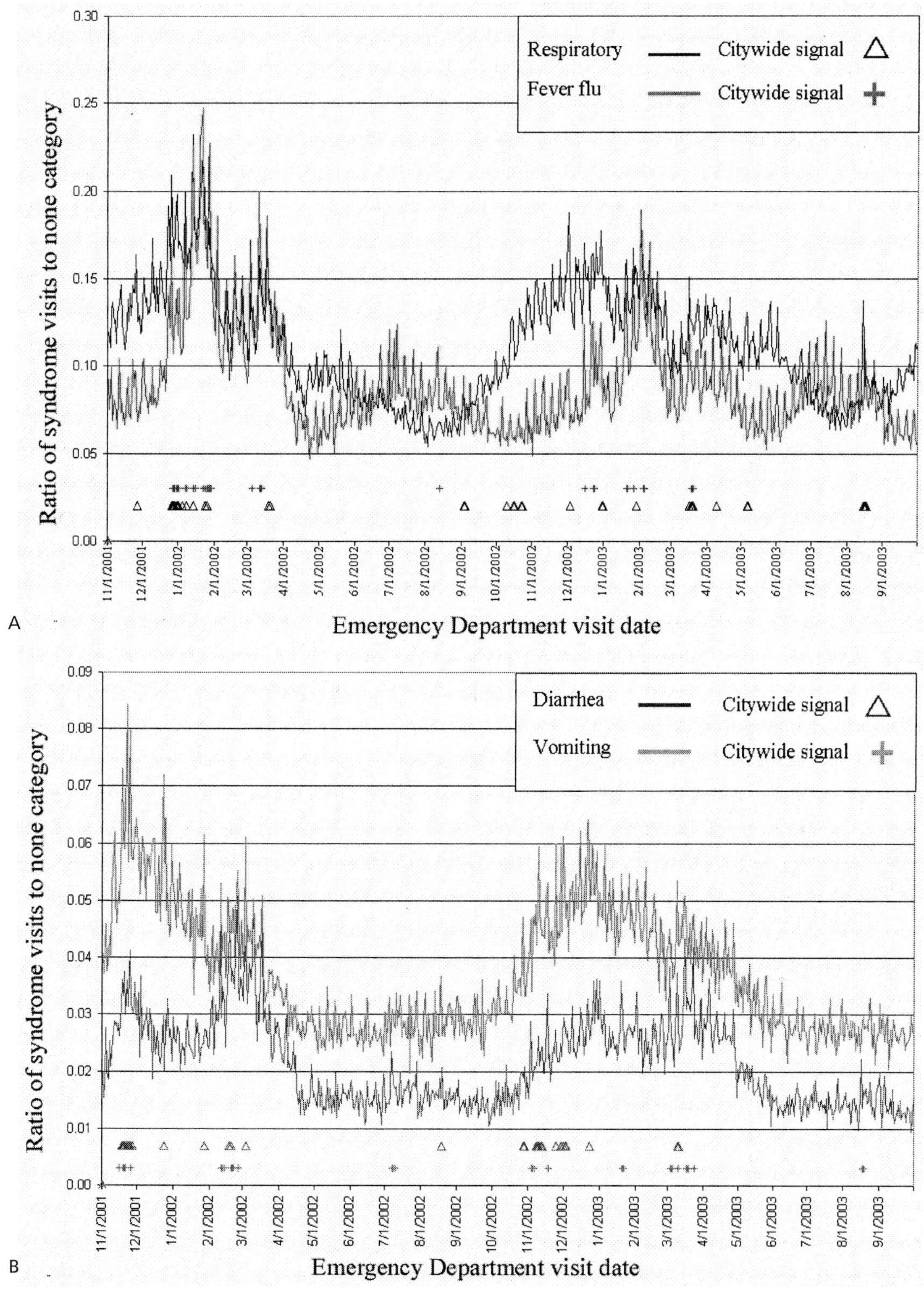

Figure 110.1. **A:** Ratio of respiratory and fever flu emergency department visits, November 2001 to September 2003. **B:** Ratio of vomiting and diarrhea emergency department visits, November 2001 to September 2003. Signals denote days where log likelihood ratio exceeds that of the preceding 14-day baseline.

evaluation is needed to ensure that the significant investment of funding and staff resources in these systems is warranted. Most importantly, these systems complement but can not replace traditional disease surveillance based on disease reporting from astute medical providers. Most of the major outbreaks of public health importance in recent years have been detected after a concerned physician rapidly notified the local or state public health authorities. (20,21)

Integrated syndromic surveillance systems may represent reasonable investments for large metropolitan public health departments but may not be practical or advisable in smaller jurisdictions. New systems are being developed (e.g., BioSense) that may have the capacity to identify local and regional illness trends from large national data sets, allowing smaller local and state agencies to make use of syndromic surveillance technology. As this interest in nontraditional public health surveillance continues, it is important to keep in mind its limitations. Syndromic surveillance, generating signals before or at the moment when persons seek medical care, is a public health early warning system suggesting that a serious public health concern may be evolving. As such, it requires a response, no less than a smoke alarm calls for a rapid assessment and the possible intervention by firefighters. It would be unwise to invest in syndromic surveillance at the expense of core, traditional surveillance and epidemiology infrastructure—the public health epidemiologists or nurses who would investigate natural or intentional disease outbreaks. Similarly, it would make little sense for public health departments or hospitals to focus on syndromic surveillance before concerted efforts had been expended to enhance traditional public health surveillance.

UNEXPLAINED DEATHS AND ILLNESSES POTENTIALLY RESULTING FROM INFECTIOUS CAUSES

Other surveillance systems that may potentially be useful for bioterrorism detection involve surveillance for unexplained deaths or severe illnesses that may be due to unrecognized infectious causes. Sources of data include intensive care unit admissions, medical examiner referrals, and vital records, as long as death certificates are available within 24 hours of filing. These systems also have potential usefulness for detecting new or reemerging infectious diseases, such as hantavirus pulmonary syndrome or SARS.

Existing systems focus on potentially infectious deaths or illnesses among otherwise healthy adults, between the ages of 18 to 65, because unexplained infectious deaths are less common in this age group.(22) Surveillance for unexplained infectious illness requires establishing collaborations with the critical care community and ICPs; providing clear criteria for reporting suspect cases; and ideally including a strong laboratory component that encourages submission of appropriate clinical samples, including tissue biopsies, for comprehensive testing at reference laboratories. Similar collaborations should be in place with the local medical examiner for unexplained infectious death surveillance, with protocols in place to obtain tissue samples from multiple organs for microbiologic and immunohistochemical testing.

Simpler systems for monitoring for potentially infectious deaths involve the use of death certificate data, which are already being collected at the state and some local health department levels. These systems require clear criteria regarding which causes of death should be included as potentially infectious (e.g., sepsis without a specific etiology). However, the timeliness of detecting an outbreak is currently limited with this method of surveillance by the typical 2- to 3-day delay between the time of death and filing of the death certificate, the lack of electronic death certificate data in most jurisdictions, and the fact that these systems are unable to detect clusters at the time of illness onset because the data are restricted to fatal cases only. The usefulness of these systems are also limited because of the concerns regarding the reliability and accuracy of cause of death data and the inability to obtain additional diagnostic testing unless clinical specimens are still available or autopsies were performed.

Although these systems in and of themselves may not be useful for the initial detection of a bioterrorist event, they have potential usefulness as adjunct systems. In the event that a suspicious case or cluster is detected, it is valuable to have these systems already in place to quickly assess whether there have been any recent fatalities with similar presentations that may be part of the larger outbreak. Finally, these systems allow public health officials to forge relationships with partners in the intensive care and medical examiner communities that may not have been in place beforehand, which are invaluable to have established ahead of time in the event of a large, infectious disease outbreak of public health concern, whether intentional or natural.

ENVIRONMENTAL MONITORING FOR COVERT BIOLOGIC RELEASES

First-generation environmental biosurveillance systems have recently been deployed in some urban centers to routinely test for certain select biologic agents. This technology currently relies on air sample collection onto filter media and transport to local or state public health laboratories for polymerase chain reaction analyses. Second-generation systems are in development that will be more automated, decreasing the potential impact that biosurveillance systems would have on public health laboratory resources.

Although biodetectors have been deployed successfully in combat environments, their use in civilian settings is new. Technical limitations include cost, impacts on public health laboratory resources, and the potential for disruptive false-positive results. As these barriers are overcome, it will be important to deploy these systems with forethought and care. Not all jurisdictions live under the same level of ongoing threat, and not all locations within a city are likely targets for attack. Threat assessments by local, state, and federal law enforcement agencies can guide a rational strategy for the deployment of environmental biomonitors. Essential to the use of these new systems will be effective and coordinated multidisciplinary planning among local agencies (including public health, law enforcement, and emergency management) for the potential response strategies that would be implemented depending on which potential bioterrorist agent is detected and the number and distribution of sites that test positive. These response plans need to include the surveillance, environmental, laboratory, and forensic assessments that would be initiated to determine if a positive environmental finding has implications for human health, as well as whether environmental results alone will prompt communication to the public and media and clinical interventions, such as antibiotic or vaccine prophylaxis.

COORDINATION AND LAW ENFORCEMENT

A suspect or confirmed bioterrorist outbreak is a criminal event and requires the involvement of law enforcement including the Federal Bureau of Investigation (FBI) and local and state police. The primary agency charged with leading the forensic investigation is the FBI, with support from local and state law enforcement. Because these disciplines have not historically worked closely with the public health community, relationships must be established, especially at the local level. One of the lessons learned during the anthrax attack of 2001 was the value of public health and law enforcement officials knowing each other ahead of time as opposed to first meeting at the time of a crisis. (23)

At both the local and federal levels, public health and law enforcement officials should establish consensus protocols regarding how they will communicate and coordinate during any investigations of a suspect bioterrorist attack. These protocols should address the mutual importance of early notification to the other discipline when there is concern or suspicion of a potential event. If law enforcement officials become aware that terrorists known or suspected to have access to biologic weapons are present locally, the health department should be notified to be alert to any suspicious disease occurrence, including lowering the threshold for investigating any aberrations in existing syndromic surveillance systems or reports of an unusual disease case or cluster. In certain circumstances, the health department might notify hospitals, so that active surveillance could be enhanced. Likewise, if public health officials detect sporadic disease or a small disease cluster potentially caused by a bioterrorist agent, this information may need to be shared confidentially with law enforcement to evaluate whether the victims or close contacts are associated with any known terrorist group. The threshold for providing law enforcement with confidential patient information must be high and consistent with local, state, and federal statutes and regulations, and criteria for a potential bioterrorist disease and cluster must be well defined. Open communication links with clearly designated points of contact should be established between these respective disciplines at both local and federal agencies so that intelligence or disease-specific information can be shared confidentially and securely.

Once a suspected covert bioterrorist event is detected, public health and law enforcement staff must conduct joint epidemiologic and forensic investigations of potential victims and their close contacts to determine the exact site, time, and circumstances of the initial release. This may require joint interviews of patients and families in hospitals, sharing of data, and active participation in each other's meetings to discuss findings of both epidemiologic and criminal and intelligence information. Any laboratory specimens obtained as part of the investigation, including both clinical and environmental samples, must be considered potential evidence and must be collected with full attention to chain of custody documentation requirements.

INITIAL INVESTIGATION AND NOTIFICATION OF ALL KEY PARTNERS IN THE EVENT OF A SUSPECT OR CONFIRMED BIOTERRORIST EVENT

In the event that public health officials are notified or become aware of a potential bioterrorist event, protocols should be in place that outline the initial response for determining if an emergency situation is occurring. Separate protocols may be needed to address the response to at least four potential scenarios: (a) an unusual disease cluster or manifestation reported by a physician or laboratorian (e.g., patient with suspected anthrax in the absence of obvious risk exposures), (b) statistical aberrations detected by syndromic or unexplained infectious illness surveillance systems (e.g., increases in influenza-like illnesses reported to 911 or unexplained infectious deaths), (c) a suspicious environmental sample identified in the field (e.g., mail containing a suspicious powder and a written threat that this material contains a bioterrorist agent, such as anthrax or plague), or (d) a positive laboratory result from an environmental biomonitoring system.

In the event of the first two scenarios, an initial rapid clinical, epidemiologic, and laboratory assessment of the situation should be performed to determine if an outbreak is occurring and whether the findings suggest a potential bioterrorist event. This initial assessment also may require rapid laboratory testing of clinical samples from the index case-patients to determine the potential causative agent(s). If the findings from this initial evaluation suggest the possibility that a bioterrorist event has occurred, the response protocol should include a list outlining who must be notified within the local health department, at other local agencies (e.g., the mayor's office, police, fire, and emergency management), at the state and federal levels (e.g., the CDC and FBI), and within the local medical and laboratory communities. Notification of federal authorities will likely include a request for support, such as epidemiologic and laboratory assistance from the CDC, calling up the Disaster Medical Assistance Teams (DMATs) and Disaster Mortuary Relief Teams (DMORTs), and mobilization of medical, pharmaceutical, and/or vaccine supplies from federal stockpiles (Strategic National Stockpile).

Response protocols should address the following issues: arranging for rapid diagnostic testing to confirm the etiologic agent; providing disease-specific information to the healthcare community on medical management of case-patients and potentially exposed persons; implementation of active surveillance and epidemiologic investigations; initiating mass medical care and prophylaxis, when indicated; setting up communication hotline capacity for the media and general public; and addressing mental health concerns. Emergency call-up lists should be in place to ensure sufficient public health surge capacity to assist in all aspects of the disaster response.

Unlike a disease outbreak detected by traditional or syndromic surveillance, the response to a suspicious environmental sample is more like a hazardous material event with the involvement of first responders from the fire, police, and emergency management agencies at the scene. The protocol for evaluating suspicious environmental samples should address: (a) coordination with other responding local agencies (e.g., emergency management, police, and fire hazmat); (b) protocols for collecting, packaging, and transporting samples for rapid testing at predesignated reference laboratories; (c) appropriate protective gear for first responders; and (d) guidelines for determining if and when there is a need for decontamination and prophylaxis of potentially exposed persons. Although there are rapid field test kits commercially available for biologic agents, the lack of sensitivity and specificity of these immunoassays is concerning, and currently the CDC and FBI advise against using these kits in the field because of the risk of both a false-positive and false-negative result. Because reference laboratory testing at state or local public health laboratories is available within a matter of hours in most jurisdictions, it is currently advised to withhold any preventive measures, such as antibiotics or vaccinations, pending test results, unless there are extenuating circumstances that suggest that a bioterrorist attack is likely (e.g., intelligence information or suspicious disseminating device found at the scene). Similarly, full-body decontamination in the field is rarely required after potential exposure to a suspected biologic agent. Persons who came into contact with the suspected material typically should be instructed to wash any exposed skin with soap and water. Grossly contaminated clothing can be removed, bagged, and laundered on returning home, and potentially exposed persons also can shower and shampoo at that time. Personnel at the scene should obtain 24-hour emergency contact information for all victims so that they can be contacted rapidly in the event that the test results are positive for a potential bioterrorist agent. It also is unlikely that these individuals would need to be evaluated at hospitals following potential exposure to a suspected environmental substance unless symptomatic. If they do present to hospitals, antimicrobial prophylaxis would rarely be indicated and should not be started without first consulting the local health department and/or awaiting results of laboratory testing. Educational sessions and mental health counseling may also be required on-site and should be included in the interagency response plan to suspicious environmental samples.

PUBLIC HEALTH REFERENCE LABORATORY TESTING OF SUSPICIOUS CLINICAL AND/OR ENVIRONMENTAL SAMPLES

A close and active partnership between the public health laboratory and local clinical laboratories is essential to any infectious disease emergency response. Clinical laboratories must be aware of how to reach local or state health departments on a 24-hour basis in the event that a test result of potential public health importance is identified. Protocols on the proper procedures for packaging and transport of clinical specimens must be in place between the hospital laboratories and local and state health departments and between the health departments and CDC.

Current capacity at local clinical microbiology laboratories for diagnosing the microorganisms that could potentially be used as bioterrorist agents should be assessed. Some hospital microbiology laboratories may have (or could develop) the capacity for *preliminary* identification of the bacterial bioterrorist agents.

The CDC and the Association of Public Health Laboratories (APHL) have developed a tiered-response national laboratory system, the Laboratory Response Network (LRN), for handling the testing and confirmation of potential bioterrorist agents. Level A laboratories include many hospital and commercial laboratories and require the use of established protocols for the initial testing of suspicious specimens and the ability to "rule out" a bioterrorist agent. Appropriate training materials and slides are available via the LRN to educate hospital laboratory staff regarding the staining properties, growth characteristics on routine media, and preliminary biochemical test results for the bacterial agents and the need to report immediately to the local health department and to arrange for confirmatory testing if a potential bioterrorist agent is suspected. Suspicious samples must be referred to Level B or C laboratories that involve federal, state, and some local health departments. Level B and C laboratories have protocols and reagents for "ruling in" select agents. Level D laboratories, include the CDC and Department of Defense laboratories, which have biosafety Level 4 capabilities and can provide final confirmatory testing, especially for the initial victims of a suspected bioterrorist event.

Symposiums on the laboratory diagnosis and biosafety precautions for biologic weapons of mass destruction (WMDs) and chain of custody requirements are being offered by state and local health departments, with the target audience being clinical microbiologists at local hospitals. All training materials and programs emphasize the critical potential role of the clinical microbiology laboratory in early recognition of a bioterrorist event and that prompt reporting to the local or state health department is essential to the success of the public health response in the event of an attack.

Protocols for ensuring rapid collection and packaging of specimens from clinical laboratories and safe transport to public health reference laboratories that meet forensic chain of custody requirements must be in place and well understood by clinical laboratory staff at hospital-based and commercial laboratories.

If a potential bioterrorist event is suspected or recognized, the medical and public health response will require rapid confirmation of the etiologic agent so that disease-specific recommendations regarding medical management can be provided to clinicians and laboratorians. Because neither hospital nor commercial microbiology laboratories have the technical capability (LRN reagents and protocols are not available to Level A laboratories) to confirm bioterrorist agents (e.g., anthrax, smallpox, tularemia), suspicious bacterial cultures or other clinical specimens require rapid and safe transport to a public health reference laboratory for confirmatory testing. Antibiotic susceptibility data for the bacterial bioterrorist agents is also essential so that the appropriate recommendations regarding antimicrobial therapy and prophylaxis can be provided to medical providers who are caring for victims and/or exposed persons.

In the event of a large-scale outbreak, local clinical laboratory facilities must implement plans for managing surge capacity needs. Execution of these plans must occur rapidly to manage the likely marked increase in requests for clinical and confirmatory testing that will occur once an outbreak is recognized (e.g., the large number of requests for testing "suspicious powders" that occurred immediately after the finding of the first anthrax threat letter at a major television news outlet in New York City was reported to the national media). To avoid overwhelming reference laboratory capacity with unnecessary test requests once a bioterrorist attack is identified, clear criteria for who (or what) should be tested, the recommended specimens to be obtained, and proper handling and shipping procedures should be shared with the medical and laboratory community via a public health alert system.

ACTIVE SURVEILLANCE AND EPIDEMIOLOGIC INVESTIGATIONS AFTER THE INITIAL DETECTION OF A CONFIRMED BIOTERRORIST EVENT

Once a bioterrorist event is recognized and then confirmed by laboratory testing, public health officials will be primarily responsible for (a) tracking the number of cases to define the scope of the incident and (b) performing epidemiologic investigations to determine the common source(s) and site(s) of exposure. After detection of an unannounced bioterrorist event, it will be essential to determine where and when the attack occurred and who else may have been exposed (either at the event or because of down-wind distribution of the aerosol if an outdoor release occurred) and thus would require antimicrobial prophylaxis. The epidemiologic investigation will need to be coordinated with local and federal law enforcement officials, with joint interviews and sharing of the data collected. Because a large bioterrorist event in an urban setting will likely result in cases throughout the metropolitan area, and potentially in distant states and countries, there will be a need for interstate and international coordination of the epidemiologic investigation. If the attack was covert, outlier cases occurring among residents of neighboring or other jurisdictions may provide valuable information to help identify the site and time of release.

Active surveillance must be initiated rapidly once a bioterrorist event is recognized. Prereadied materials are invaluable to ensure the ability to expedite an investigation including (a) surveillance instruments (e.g., ready-to-go generic questionnaires for case ascertainment and risk exposure histories that can be rapidly modified to the specific circumstances under investigation); (b) a sampling strategy to use when conducting a rapid, large-scale epidemiologic investigation; (c) a centralized database system with linkages to the laboratory to facilitate tracking the outbreak and data analysis; and (d) a communication system and protocols for mobilizing and deploying active surveillance teams to area hospitals.

Generic surveillance instruments should include variables on patient demographics, clinical illness, home residence(s), work location(s), exposure to ill contacts, usual commuter route (e.g., subway or bus routes), and a detailed diary that includes the times at all known locations and the way that the patient transited to any of these places during the incubation period of the suspected agent (including stores, restaurants, theaters, museums, tourist attractions, sports events, parks, places of worship, school attendance, and any other special events he or she attended during this time period). Both paper and electronic copies of these surveillance materials should be readily available.

Data management is one of the highest priorities and challenges during an acute, high-profile epidemiologic investigation of a potentially large outbreak. Effective outbreak data management requires the linking of clinical and epidemiologic data with laboratory information, including whether appropriate specimens have been obtained, their test results, and the patient's case status (i.e., suspect or laboratory-confirmed). Appropriate public health decisions depend on having up-to-date, accurate information about the evolving outbreak, and political leaders, the news media, and the public need accurate information describing the impact of the event. This requires having flexible, tested databases that can be modified to the specific event. These systems should be exercised during routine outbreak investigations to facilitate efficient use during emergencies.

GUIDANCE FOR HOSPITAL AND MEDICAL PROVIDERS

Most medical and laboratory professionals in the United States have had minimal clinical experience with the most worrisome bioterrorist agents (e.g., anthrax, smallpox, and plague). In the event of a bioterrorist event, public health authorities must provide timely information on the medical management of these diseases and how to coordinate with local, state, and federal public health partners.

Disease-specific protocols should be prepared ahead of time for the biologic agents of greatest concern (e.g., anthrax, smallpox, tularemia, Q fever, botulism, and plague). These protocols should address clinical presentations, diagnosis, therapy, patient isolation and waste disposal, biosafety issues for handling clinical specimens, and preventive therapy. These draft protocols can then be modified to the specific circumstances of the event and rapidly distributed. Additional information that should be included in guidelines for hospitals and medical providers include clear criteria for reporting suspect cases (including clinical and epidemiologic features that meet the public health case definition), instructions for submitting laboratory samples for testing at the public health reference laboratory, details regarding mass prophylaxis plans being coordinated by the local or state authorities, and mechanisms to obtain current patient information materials being prepared by the health department. These protocols must be updated as new information becomes available. Electronic and paper copies of these disease specific protocols should be readily accessible in several sites for rapid distribution in the event of an emergency. These protocols would be distributed once a bioterrorist event has been confirmed using existing emergency communication systems that should already be in place and that link public health and local hospital and medical communities. Communication methods might include public health alert systems (e.g., broadcast facsimile and electronic mail systems configured to transmit public health alerts to key partners in hospitals and outpatient settings), the health department's public Web site, and emergency transportation of written documents (including posters and bulletins) to local hospitals. Frequent public health alerts to provide updates on the evolving outbreak and any changes in public health recommendations should be provided as often as needed.

Health departments also must be able to rapidly mobilize medical hotlines using clinically trained staff (e.g., physicians and nurses), who would be available to triage calls regarding suspect cases and answer questions regarding the medical management of cases, their close contacts, and potentially exposed persons who are not yet symptomatic. The staffing, training, and telephone equipment needs for this unit should be predefined. Ideally, preexisting provider hotlines that are already in place for routine public health issues should be used. However, given the potential for a marked increase in calls to this hotline during times of emergency, planning should address the need for enhancing staff and telephone line capacity and the hotline staff's training needs when an event is rapidly unfolding and information and guidance may change frequently.

PLANNING FOR MASS MEDICAL AND MORTUARY CARE AND MASS PROPHYLAXIS

Local and state public health authorities should play an active role in planning for how mass medical care will be addressed and coordinated from a jurisdiction-wide perspective, in coordination with area hospitals, emergency medical services, and emergency management agencies. Essential to planning efforts is up-to-date information on existing bed capacity, including isolation capacity, and key equipment inventories, such as ventilators, for all acute care facilities within the jurisdiction. Local public health officials should work with area medical care facilities to test response plans using tabletop and/or field exercises to assess institutional response to a bioterrorist disaster, with a focus on addressing those areas where close coordination between hospital and public health authorities are key to an effective response.

In the event of a successful release of an aerosolized bioterrorist agent, there is a potential for mass casualties on a scale that could easily overwhelm local hospital capacity. Therefore, contingency plans for how mass casualties will be handled, with special attention to isolation and infection control issues if an agent with potential person-to-person transmission is involved, must be developed. Individual hospitals or hospital networks must develop institutional-specific plans for how they will respond to a large infectious disease outbreak (e.g., activating the hospital's incident management system, triaging massive numbers of visits to and admissions from the emergency department, canceling all nonemergent admissions, transferring nonacute patients, calling in additional staff, rapid reopening of wards that have been closed because decreasing census, and establishing emergency isolation units).

Difficult issues that must be addressed ahead of time include whether and how specific hospitals will be designated to care for victims of a bioterrorist event, how limited resources will be distributed if insufficient supplies are available (e.g., ventilators), establishment of alternate sites for triage of patients with less severe symptoms, and emergency credentialing procedures to allow nonaffiliated staff to work in local hospitals. Mass care planning should be coordinated with local relief agencies, such as the American Red Cross, and public health authorities in neighboring states and counties. Preestablished memoranda of understanding for sharing resources are useful to have in place before emergencies, as has been done among fire departments and other traditional first responders. Finally, because there will likely be a need to call in federal support (e.g., DMATs), determination of how and where these teams will be deployed must be planned ahead of time.

Mass mortuary issues (including, tracking, storage, and disposal of victims) must be addressed by the local and state medical examiners, in coordination with local public health officials, emergency management, and hospital associations. Guidance for the handling and disposal of potentially infectious remains should be developed. For most potential bioterrorist agents, routine infection control practices should be sufficient to protect pathologists, medical examiner staff, and persons involved in preparing the body for burial or cremation. However, in the event of a smallpox attack, these professionals should be prioritized for receiving smallpox vaccine if not already vaccinated. In addition, reducing the potential for disease transmission should be a priority. Certain procedures (e.g., embalming) should be ended temporarily and recommendations for use of sealed caskets or cremation should be considered by local authorities. Because a bioterrorist event is a criminal act, an efficient mechanism must be established urgently to ensure that all deaths resulting from the outbreak are reported to the appropriate local authorities, such as the medical examiner or coroner's office.

In addition to medical care for ill patients, there may be a need to provide mass prophylaxis to potentially exposed persons and/or close contacts for certain bioterrorist agents (e.g., anthrax and smallpox). Planning for the rapid provision of antibiotics or vaccines to large populations requires the involvement of public health and emergency management officials, with input from the local medical community. Efforts should focus on (a) predetermination of which antibiotics and vaccines may be needed (including recommendations for special populations, such as children and pregnant women) and (b) how these medications will be mobilized and distributed rapidly in the event of a bioterrorist event. Although there is currently a federal stockpile of medications and supplies, the Strategic National Stockpile, local and state officials ought to consider whether a smaller stockpile should also be maintained locally to ensure supplies are available in the first hours or days after an attack is detected, given cost issues and limited shelf life of many pharmaceutical agents. Specifically, contingency plans for setting up community-based, mass prophylaxis clinics that address staffing resources and equipment and space requirements and procedures that outline patient flow must be developed ahead of time. (24) Many jurisdictions are creating a reserve corp of medical volunteers to help support these clinics and providing training on expected roles and responsibilities in the event that such clinics are required.

Multilingual medical information sheets and vaccine informed consent forms should be prepared, and multiple mechanisms for rapid mass reproduction identified. Risk communication strategies should be developed to ensure that persons at-risk understand the need for compliance with prevention messages and, as importantly, that those not at-risk understand the need to avoid overwhelming hospitals and clinics if they do not have an exposure or symptoms of concern. Mass prophylaxis plans need to consider the specific challenges in distributing antibiotics and vaccine to difficult-to-reach populations, such as the homeless and homebound.

INTERAGENCY AND INTERSECTOR COORDINATION AND COMMUNICATION

The response to a large biologic disaster, whether a bioterrorist event or natural outbreak such as pandemic influenza or SARS, requires successful coordination and communication between public health agencies; other relevant local, state (e.g., emergency management, police, fire/Hazmat), and federal (e.g., CDC, FBI) agencies; and the healthcare sector (both in-patient and out-patient). A centralized emergency operating center is essential to facilitate coordination and communication. In the event of an emergency, predesignated representatives from all involved agencies and any local or state hospital associations should be assigned to this center to ensure effective coordination of the overall response.

The public health sector's communication, transportation, and other equipment or infrastructure needs for disaster response should be assessed ahead of time. Essential resources include reliable and redundant communication capacity (e.g., cellular telephones, laptop computers with modem, two-way and 800-megahertz radios or satellite telephones); broadcast facsimile and electronic mail capability; secure Internet sites (e.g., Health Alert Network) to rapidly notify and inform the healthcare sector regarding events of public health concern; and computer systems that are networked between the local and state health department, the local emergency management command center, and appropriate state and federal agencies. Back-up generators should be available as well as alternative locations to meet if the primary emergency operations center is damaged because of the disaster.

Ongoing training for public health staff should not just include the clinical, laboratory, and epidemiologic features of the bioterrorist agents but also focus on the agency's emergency response command system, with an emphasis on staff's expected roles and responsibilities during the health department's response to a bioterrorism event. One of the more effective training tools are tabletop and field exercises, with involvement of representatives from all key local, state, and federal agencies and representatives from the local medical and laboratory communities. These exercises provide the opportunity to test assumptions in existing plans and work out issues related to decision-making authority and respective roles and responsibilities among the various disciplines that would be involved in responding to a bioterrorist attack. A successful exercise highlights gaps in preparedness that should be addressed through follow-up meetings and revision of written plans, if indicated, and reevaluated with repeat exercises.

LEGAL ISSUES RELATED TO THE PUBLIC HEALTH RESPONSE TO BIOTERRORISM OR OTHER INFECTIOUS DISEASE EMERGENCIES

Many state and local public health laws have not undergone major revisions since the middle of the last century. Although current regulations are adequate for routine public health concerns, the response to a bioterrorist event may require emergency powers beyond existing legislative or executive authority. In 2002, the CDC in collaboration with Georgetown University School of Law developed a model state public health law for jurisdictions to use to assess their current regulations and implement modifications to those areas that were not yet adequately addressed. (25) In addition to ensuring sufficient authority to collect disease surveillance data, conduct contact tracing, and provide preventive measures to those at risk, public health laws must provide health officials with the authority to implement isolation and quarantine measures if needed to control a severe and virulent contagious communicable disease outbreak. Isolation and quarantine regulations should include the components needed to establish and enforce a large-scale quarantine including who has this authority, what criteria need to be met, the legal mechanism for rapid implementation in the event of an emergency, and who will be responsible for enforcement and should provide for due process measures to protect those affected. In addition to the legal aspects of isolation and quarantine measures, public health officials need to ensure that plans address the operational aspects of implementing and enforcing these regulations. Specific issues include developing criteria for the use of home quarantine versus removal of contacts to separate facilities, identification of potential facilities that might be used to isolate contagious patients or quarantine close contacts, determination of how detained persons will be fed and cared for, and mechanisms to compensate detainees for lost wages.

ENVIRONMENTAL ISSUES

Public health agencies also need to have plans and staff expertise to assess the environmental impact of an attack and determine if remediation efforts are needed to decontaminate the affected site(s). Environmental health specialists should work closely with their counterparts in infectious diseases epidemiology to plan for how epidemiologic and environmental investigations will be coordinated, especially if the attack was covert and these investigations are needed to identify the initial site of release.

The anthrax attacks of 2001 revealed the lack of knowledge regarding the environmental impact of weaponized bioterrorist agents in indoor settings. At that time, no public health agency at the local, state, or federal levels had sufficient expertise or experience regarding methods for collecting and testing environmental samples of weapons-grade anthrax in workplace-type settings, interpreting these findings to assess ongoing risk, or optimal methods for decontamination and remediation of affected environments. Fortunately, this experience did lead to the development of federal guidelines for assessing environmental contamination resulting from weaponized anthrax. Now, similar efforts need to address the other potential bioterrorist agents, especially regarding whether there are any ongoing environmental risks when agents that do not have a spore form are released.

MENTAL HEALTH PREPAREDNESS AND RESPONSE

Both the World Trade Center attack and the outbreak of intentional anthrax resulting from contamination of the mail highlighted the dramatic psychologic effects that a terrorist event can have on the public, even in areas far removed from the actual events. One of the primary targets of terrorism is the public's mental health, with the potential impact lasting beyond the immediate event and affecting persons far from the area affected. The media often plays an unwitting role in facilitating this with constant replays and graphic images shown frequently on television and in newspapers in the immediate aftermath of an event.

In New York City, soon after the World Trade Center attacks, a telephone survey revealed that between 7.5% and 40% of Manhattan residents had symptoms consistent with posttraumatic stress disorder; the prevalence was higher among those closer to the site or among those who had witnessed the attacks (26). As impressive, a similar survey conducted nationwide within a week of the attack revealed that 44% of adults and 35% of children had one or more stress symptoms (27). The tremendous subsequent number of "powder incidents" illustrated that one does not need sophisticated weapon delivery systems to cause public panic. In many of the affected jurisdictions, it was not the outbreak response at the affected worksite locations that overwhelmed local public health and emergency response authorities but the hundreds to thousands of calls regarding concerns about potential "powder threats." This illustrated the impact that the worried well can have on the public health and medical care systems, and many jurisdictions did not anticipate nor were they prepared for the response needed to manage these calls.

Unfortunately, mental health preparedness is an area that many local and state public health agencies have minimal staff expertise or experience addressing. It is essential that a community's bioterrorism response plan address the community's mental health response to terrorism both before and after an event. Preplanning efforts for mental health preparedness should include development of a risk communication strategy with training of all potential public health spokespersons and the establishment of surge capacity for mental health services after an event occurs (28). Ideally, the public and media should be educated ahead of time about the risk of bioterrorism and relevant details of their local government response plans, so that they know what steps can be taken to improve personal, family, and community preparedness and what to do in the event of an attack.

Planning for the potential demands for mental health counseling should not be limited just to the actual victims of the attack but also should address the needs of the victims' families and friends; those responding to the event, including traditional first responders and the medical provider community; and the general public. Strategies could include plans for rapidly establishing crisis hotlines and referral sites and for mobilizing additional assistance through creation of a mental health reserve corp. Involvement of community-based organizations, religious leaders, and local government officials in both preplanning and response efforts is essential. Given the potential for the worried well to overwhelm medical care services, as was seen in the immediate days after the anthrax attack was first recognized, a proactive, clear, and effective risk communication strategy should be prioritized to ensure that the public understands what is known about the event; who is at risk; which symptoms suggest the need for medical evaluation; the importance of not seeking medical care if one does not have these symptoms, to avoid overwhelming local hospitals and clinics; and who needs antibiotic prophylaxis and where and when to go to obtain it, if indicated.

COMMUNICATION WITH THE GENERAL PUBLIC

As with any major disaster, one of the most important components of the governmental response is a proactive, effective, communication strategy. An essential component of a communication strategy is having preexisting and effective communication links with the media (including local and national print, radio, and television outlets). The multidisciplinary involvement in the response to a bioterrorist event will require coordination of media outreach through a joint information center that includes local, state, and federal officials. Public affairs staff at hospitals should coordinate any public messages with their counterparts at the local and state health departments.

Ideally, there should be one primary predesignated spokesperson to provide consistent messages throughout the disaster response. This spokesperson should be clearly in charge (e.g., the top elected official); an effective, clear, and concise communicator; and available for frequent press briefings. Although the primary spokesperson does not have to be a medical or public health official, it is essential that persons with such expertise be present to answer or clarify health-related questions or issues. One of the most difficult risk communication challenges following a bioterrorist event is communicating uncertainty, given that it may take days or weeks before the full circumstances of the event is known. It is important for spokespersons to be ready to admit what they do not know, yet also be able to reassure the public by providing detailed information regarding what is being done to answer all key questions. Frequent updates should be provided to the news media and public when new information becomes available.

The communication response to the 2001 anthrax attack taught us that public confidence can be lost quickly and that spokespersons need to be credible and believable. Trying to reassure the public that the index case of inhalational anthrax may have been due to natural causes had a decidedly negative public impact. Once the public and news media's trust has been lost due to minimizing the situation or misinformation, it is difficult to regain.

Although the most efficient mechanism for communicating

to the general public is through the news media, public health officials also need to be prepared to provide additional information through other mechanisms to be able to address the numerous questions and concerns that the news media stories will generate among the public. Fact sheets on the likely bioterrorist agents should be prepared ahead of time for the general public, posted on the agency's public Web site and then tailored to the specific events. During the emergency, these informational sheets should be widely distributed to multiple venues. In most parts of the country, translations into one or more languages will be needed.

In addition to written materials, contingency plans for establishing a hotline for the general public should be a key component of the public health response planning efforts. Hotlines will likely need surge capacity for the immediate hours and days after an acute event, with respect to both staff and telephone infrastructure. Staff used for hotline support need to be trained for handling acute calls from a concerned public, and mechanisms need to be in place to provide ongoing training and updates, because information about the outbreak and public health recommendations will likely evolve rapidly over the course of the event.

SUMMARY

After the terrorist events of 2001, there was nationwide recognition of the importance of improving and maintaining the public health infrastructure at local, state, and federal levels as a primary defense against bioterrorism. On January 31, 2001, the Department of Health and Human Services announced the availability of $1.1 billion in federal funding that would be made available to all states and four large urban areas (Chicago, District of Columbia, Los Angeles, and New York City) in federal fiscal year 2003. This level of funding was continued for at least a second year in 2004. This has provided an unprecedented opportunity to address critical gaps in current bioterrorism public health preparedness plans.

Jurisdictions have used these funds to address the following key areas: emergency planning and response for biologic or chemical terrorism events, as well as for natural disease outbreaks; enhancing surveillance and epidemiologic capacity; expanding reference laboratory services, especially for confirmation of the CDC Category A and B agents; developing or enhancing environmental health expertise; planning for large-scale antibiotic and vaccine distribution clinics; developing or expanding secure electronic communication links with key partners at the local level; establishing or enhancing local and state legal authorities for implementing and enforcing isolation and quarantine; ensuring that communication mechanisms and strategies are in place to provide up-to-date information to the medical community and general public; providing risk communication and media training for key public health staff; training of medical providers on the clinical aspects of the potential bioterrorist agents; and mental health preparedness planning.

Integration of bioterrorism-related surveillance, laboratory, environmental, and communication efforts into routine public health activities will improve the core public health functions, which in a crisis need to function well. This will have the dual benefit of improving local and state public health responses to natural disease disasters, as well, such as would be required to respond to pandemic influenza or SARS. Although significant advances have been made in the past 2 years, there are concerns about how long-lasting these will be, if federal support is withdrawn or decreased over time. Enhancing our public health infrastructure is a long-term investment, one that will have long-lasting impact in protecting the public's health from natural and intentional disease threats

REFERENCES

1. Pickett G, Hanlon JJ, eds. *Public health: administration and practice,* 9th ed. St. Louis: Times Mirror/Mosby College Publishing, 1990:97–120.
2. Frieden TR, Fujiwara PI, Washko RM, et al. Tuberculosis in New York City—turning the tide. *N Engl J Med* 1995;333:229–233.
3. Torok TJ, Tauxe RV, Wise RP, et al. A large community outbreak of salmonellosis caused by intentional contamination of restaurant salad bars *JAMA* 1997;278:389–395.
4. Kolavic SA, Kimura A, Simons SL, et al. An outbreak of *Shigella dysenteriae* type 2 among laboratory workers due to intentional food contamination *JAMA* 1997;278:396–398.
5. Rotz LD, Khan AS, Lillibridge SR, et al. Public health assessment of potential biological terrorism agents. *Emerg Infect Dis* 2002;8: 225–230.
6. Jernigan DB, Hofmann J, Cetron MS, et al. Outbreak of Legionnaires' disease among cruise ship passengers exposed to a contaminated whirlpool spa. *Lancet* 1996:347:494–499.
7. Herwaldt BL, Ackers M-L, and the Cyclospora Working Group. An outbreak in 1996 of cyclosporiasis associated with imported raspberries. *N Engl J Med* 1997;336:1548–1556.
8. Nash D, Mostashari F, Fine A, et al. The outbreak of West Nile virus infection in the New York City area in 1999. *N Engl J Med* 2001; 344:1807–1814.
9. Bush LM, Abrams BH, Johnson CC. Index case of fatal inhalational anthrax due to bioterrorism in the United States. *N Engl J Med* 2001; 345:1607–1610.
10. Ferguson NE, Steele L, Crawford CY, et al. Bioterrorism Web site resources for infectious disease clinicians and epidemiologists. *Clin Infect Dis* 2003;36:1458–1473.
11. United States General Accounting Office. West Nile virus outbreak: lessons for public health preparedness. September 2000. GAO/HEHS-00-180.
12. Centers for Disease Control and Prevention. Multistate outbreak of monkeypox—Illinois, Indiana, and Wisconsin, 2003. *MMWR Morb Mortal Wkly Rep* 2003;52:54:537–540.
13. Mostashari F, Hartman J. Syndromic surveillance—a local perspective. *J Urban Health* 2003;80:i1–i7.
14. Babcock Irvin C, Patrelia Nouhan P, et al. Syndromic analysis of computerized emergency department patients' chief complaints: an opportunity for bioterrorism and influenza surveillance. *Ann Emerg Med* 2003;41:447–452.
15. Mostashari F, Fine A, Das D, et al. Use of ambulance dispatch data as an early warning system for community wide influenza like illness, New York City. *J Urban Health* 2003:80:i43–i49.
16. Lazarus R, Kleinman K, Dashevsky I, et al. Use of automated ambulatory care encounters for detection of acute illness clusters, including potential bioterrorist events. *Emerg Infect Dis* 2002;8:753–760.
17. Hutwagner L, Thompson W, Seeman CG, et al. The bioterrorism and response early aberration reporting system (EARS). *J Urban Health* 2003;80:i89–i96.
18. Burkam HS. Biosurveillance applying scan statistics with multiple, disparate data sources. *J Urban Health* 2003;80:i57–i65.
19. Lopez W. New York City and state legal authorities related to syndromic surveillance. *J Urban Health* 2003;80:i23–i24.

20. Holtz T, Ackelsberg J, Kool JL, et al. Isolated case of bioterrorism-related inhalational anthrax. New York City, 2001. *Emerg Infect Dis* 2003;9:689–696.
21. Centers for Disease Control and Prevention. Imported plague—New York City, 2002. *MMWR Morb Mortal Wkly Rep* 2003;52:725–728.
22. Hajjeh RA, Relman D, Cieslak P, et al. Surveillance for unexplained deaths and critical illnesses due to possibly infectious causes, United States, 1995–1998. *Emerg Infect Dis* 2002;8:145–153.
23. Butler JC, Cohen ML, Friedman CR, et al. Collaboration between public health and law enforcement: new paradigms and partnerships for bioterrorism planning and response. *Emerg Infect Dis* 2002;8: 1152–1156.
24. Blank S, Moskin LC, Zucker JR. An ounce of prevention is a ton of work: mass antibiotic prophylaxis for anthrax, New York City, 2001. *Emerg Infect Dis* 2003;9:615–622.
25. Gostin LO, Sapsin JD, Teret SP, et al. The Model State Emergency Health Powers Act: planning for and response to bioterrorism and naturally occurring infectious diseases. *JAMA* 2002;288:622–628.
26. Galea S, Ahern J, Resnick H, et al. Psychological sequelae of the September 11 terrorist attacks in New York City. *N Engl J Med* 2002; 346:982–987.
27. Galea S, Ahern J, Resnick H, et al. Psychological sequelae of the September 11 terrorist attacks in New York City. *N Engl J Med* 2002; 346:982–987.
28. Glass TA, Schoch-Spana M. Bioterrorism and the people: how to vaccinate a city against panic. *Clin Infect Dis* 2002;34:xx–xx.

111

THE AGENTS OF BIOTERRORISM

MICHAEL OSTERHOLM
ELIZABETH LINNER MCCLURE
C.J. PETERS

THE HISTORY OF BIOTERRORISM

The weaponization of biologic agents is as old as recorded history (1). Serpents, tossed onto enemy ships, were used in ancient times as weapons of warfare. The Tartar army, in 1346, used the bodies of plague victims as weapons of war, catapulting them into the city of Caffa. In 1763, the British army intentionally infected Delaware Indians by providing them with blankets used by smallpox victims. Various human and animal pathogens were used on a limited scale as biologic weapons in both World War I and World War II.

Both twentieth century World Wars stimulated research and development of biologic weapons. Although many countries, including the United States, Canada, the United Kingdom, and the Soviet Union continued the development of biologic agents as weapons following World War II, most of these programs were abandoned in the late 1960s and early 1970s. In 1972, the Biologic Weapons Convention Treaty (BWCT) was ratified by more than 140 nations. This treaty prohibited the possession, stockpile, or use of biologic weapons, although no provisions for monitoring, inspection, or enforcement were made within that treaty.

In the mid-1990s, it became evident that the Soviet Union had secretly continued an aggressive program to weaponize biologic agents (2). Major aspects of that program included the production of large amounts of smallpox virus and research surrounding a means to weaponize it. Other biologic weapons were developed by the Soviets and included *Bacillus anthracis* spores and botulinum toxin (3).

The dissolution of the Soviet Union increased the vulnerability of the world to bioterrorism. Soviet scientists left the Soviet Union and have been actively recruited by rogue nations such as Iraq, Iran, Syria, and North Korea. Stockpiles of biologic agents from the Soviet program are also missing or inadequately contained (4).

After the Gulf War, there was concern that Iraq may be developing an extensive biologic weapons program predominately involving anthrax and botulism. There is also concern that both Iraq and North Korea may have obtained smallpox virus.

Today, there is little doubt that biologic weapons of mass destruction lie within the grasp of many nations and groups. The recent terrorist attack on the United States in 2001 with aerosolized anthrax is just one example of the reality of biologic agents as weapons. Several commissions have recently reviewed the threat of bioterrorism on the United States (United States Commission on National Security/21st Century, 2001; National Commission on Terrorism, 2000; Gilmore Commission, 2000). In November 2001, the Institute of Medicine convened a workshop on bioterrorism—"Biologic Threats and Terrorism: Assessing the Science and Response Capabilities." All of these expert panels have uniformly concluded that the United States is highly vulnerable to another bioterrorist attack potentially much more massive in scale than the anthrax attacks of 2001.

BIOLOGIC AGENTS AS WEAPONS

What are the agents that would be used as biologic weapons or instruments of terrorism? One way to analyze the problem is to narrow the problem according to the scenarios that are most damaging. The modes of dissemination of a biologic agent are numerous, but the optimal way to infect large numbers of persons with a lethal agent is to use infectious aerosols. This conclusion allows one to narrow the spread of agents of concern to those that can be grown in large quantities and that are infectious in aerosols, a relatively small subset of the total number of microorganisms that a terrorist might use. Contamination of the food supply is another possible route of infection that is of great concern but probably not as potentially severe as an aerosol attack. Other means of infection could be imagined, but none seem to be so effective in producing mass casualties by direct infection. Smallpox is particularly concerning, however, because in addition to its direct aerosol transmission it can be spread person-to-person in ever-widening circles and, thus, could be a highly effective terror weapon even if the initial number of persons infected were relatively small. The Centers for Disease Control and Prevention (CDC) published a list of biologic agents in 2000 selected for their needs for public health preparedness and their likely health and social impact (5). The list is divided into categories A, B, and C. Category A agents are characterized as being easily disseminated or transmitted person to person. They are capable of causing high mortality leading to public panic and government destabilization. They also require rapid

TABLE 111.1. CRITICAL BIOLOGIC AGENTS FOR USE IN BIOTERRORISM

Category A agents: Bacillus anthracis (anthrax), *Clostridium botulinum* toxin (botulism), *Yersinia pestis* (plague), *Francisella tularensis* (tularemia), Variola major virus (smallpox), Ebola, Marburg, Lassa, and South American hemorrhagic fever viruses (viral hemorrhagic fevers)

Category B agents: Coxiella burnetii (Q fever), *Brucella* species (brucellosis), *Burkholderia mallei* (glanders), Alphaviruses (Venezuelan encephalomyelitis and eastern and western equine encephalomyelitis), Ricin toxin from *Ricinus communis* (castor beans), Epsilon toxin of *Clostridium perfringens, Staphylococcus* enterotoxin B. Foodborne or waterborne agents also are included under Category B. These pathogens include but are not limited to: *Salmonella* species, *Shigella* species, *Escherichia coli* O157:H7, *Vibrio cholerae, Cryptosporidium parvum*

Category C agents: Nipah virus, Hantaviruses, Tickborne hemorrhagic fever viruses, Tickborne encephalitis viruses, Yellow fever virus, Multidrug-resistant *Mycobacterium tuberculosis*

Source: CDC. Biological and chemical terrorism (see References).

public health response and preparedness. Category B agents are moderately easy to disseminate. They cause lower morbidity and mortality and require important public health diagnostic capability and disease surveillance. Category C agents include emerging biologic agents that could be weaponized in the future because of their availability, ease of production and dissemination, and high morbidity and mortality (Table 111.1). This chapter focuses on CDC Category A agents including *B. anthracis, Clostridium botulinum* toxin, *Yersinia pestis, Francisella tularensis,* Variola major virus (smallpox), and the viral hemorrhagic fever (VHF) viruses. Major clinical, microbiologic, and epidemiologic factors are addressed particularly within the context of the suitability of each agent as a potential biologic weapon. This list is by no means comprehensive. There are many other known biologic agents suitable for weaponization that could become the source of a bioterrorist attack in the future. The Soviet Union alone is known to have weaponized at least 30 biologic agents, some of which focus on vaccine or drug resistance (4).

ROUTES OF DISSEMINATION

Many different bioterrorist attack scenarios are possible. As noted previously, two important modes of transmission include aerosol and foodborne attacks. Aerosols are an efficient mode of transport to a wide geographic area. The inhalation of small particles (1 to 5 μ) causes deposition deep in lung tissue, and some agents are capable of very efficiently setting up a systemic infection from that site. There are basically two mechanisms for developing these aerosols. One involves the generation of the particles from liquids energized by passage of air over a nozzle, and the other is the production of fine powders that are treated to be electrically neutral and readily propelled into the air by small energy input and to continue to be carried by the air currents. Potentially available means for wide-scale dissemination of aerosolized particles could include the use crop-dusting planes, small aerosolizing generators in closed spaces such as shopping mall or subways, the dissemination of particles through the ventilation systems of large buildings, and the contamination of items in the environment by fine powders as was the case with the recent anthrax attacks on the United States in 2001.

Foodborne bioterrorism, which could encompass a variety of biologic agents, is also a real threat. These agents are relatively easy to obtain, and some agents can cause mortality at very low doses. They are also readily available in the environment and may be the easiest bioterrorism agents to disseminate. Contamination of water sources is much less likely to be effective because the dilutional effect would be too great and most agents are vulnerable to chlorine, a standard additive to potable water.

ANTHRAX

Agent

B. anthracis is a large gram-positive bacillus. It forms long chains *in vitro* but exists in single cells or short chains *in vivo.* It is a nonmotile, catalase-positive aerobe or facultative anaerobe. Colonies are fast growing and exhibit a ground-glass appearance. *B. anthracis* also exists as a spore. These spores germinate, forming vegetative cells in nutrient-rich environments. Anthrax bacilli are vulnerable and readily inactivated outside mammalian hosts and will sporulate when nutrients in their environment are exhausted. These spores are highly stable, existing in the environment for years. Spores have been shown to survive in the environment for more than 40 years (6).

Laboratory diagnostic procedures beyond culture are not well standardized. Blood cultures are usually positive in serious cases, but automated systems may reject the early-growing bacillus as a contaminant. Late in infection, direct smears of peripheral blood or cerebrospinal fluid (CSF) usually show the microorganism directly. Autopsy findings are pathognomonic, and tissue Gram stains are positive. Polymerase chain reaction (PCR) of tissues and direct tests for toxin in the blood are promising experimental approaches to microbiologic diagnosis. Convalescent patients usually develop antibodies to anthrax toxins such as protective antigen (PA).

Modes of Transmission

Anthrax is primarily a disease of livestock or other herbivores. Infection is acquired through consumption of soil or feed containing *B. anthracis* spores. Illness in humans most often occurs following exposure to infected animals. Exposure to infected animals occurs from contact with contaminated tissue; the consumption of undercooked, contaminated meat; or the vigorous handling of tainted wool, hides, or other animal byproducts during processing. Person-to-person transmission has occurred rarely with cutaneous anthrax but not with gastrointestinal (GI) or inhalational disease (7,8). Cutaneous disease from laboratory inoculation with *B. anthracis* has also been recognized (9).

Clinical Syndromes

Naturally occurring anthrax infection in humans can present as cutaneous anthrax, inhalational anthrax, or GI anthrax. The cutaneous manifestation is the most common presentation. Inhalational anthrax is the disease associated with aerosol dissemination in a bioterrorist attack, although cutaneous disease might result from environmental contamination.

Inhalational Anthrax

Inhaled *B. anthracis* spores are deposited deep in the lung. Endospores are then phagocytosed by macrophages and transported to regional lymph nodes. Within the lymph nodes, spores germinate into vegetative cells, multiply, and enter the bloodstream. Bacteremia leads to septic shock and toxemia. Hemorrhagic mediastinitis and massive pleural effusions frequently occur. Secondary meningitis or involvement of other lymph nodes can be seen. The chest x-ray is a critical part of the diagnostic workup because of the typical widened mediastinum from regional lymph involvement (10). It has become apparent that use of thoracic computed tomography (CT) scans is a more sensitive way to detect and quantify the pathognomic node involvement and the effusions.

Illness may be biphasic, with an initial prodrome of fever and malaise. If left untreated, a second phase follows characterized by a sudden increase in fever and rapid onset respiratory distress and cardiovascular collapse. Case-fatality rates decrease with prompt and aggressive antibiotic therapy.

The ID50 for inhalational anthrax has been estimated at 8,000 to 50,000 spores (11), although the minimum infective does may be considerably less. Extrapolation of dose-response curves from cynomolgus monkeys predict that the LD10 in humans may be as low as 50 to 98 spores, and the LD1 may be only a single spore (12). Host factors may affect susceptibility as well.

Cutaneous Anthrax

Cutaneous anthrax is largely a localized infection caused by the introduction of endospores into a break in the skin. Germination at the site of entry causes localized infection, which appears as a papule with localized edema. Ulceration occurs after 1 to 2 days followed by the formation of a black eschar over the ulcerated lesion. These lesions heal without scarring in 80% to 90% of patients. Rarely, a more generalized lymphadenitis can occur; patients with multiple bullae deteriorate secondary to severe edema and shock. The overall case-fatality rate is extremely low with proper antibiotic therapy. Before the era of antibiotics, the case-fatality rate approached 20%. The infective dose for cutaneous anthrax is not known (13).

Gastrointestinal Anthrax

GI anthrax is rare, and its etiology is poorly understood. Unlike the other forms of anthrax in which the endospore is the infecting agent, GI anthrax is thought to be secondary to the ingestion of vegetative cells from undercooked meat taken from ruminants dying of anthrax (13). Patients infected with anthrax via the GI tract may exhibit symptoms ranging from oropharyngeal involvement to widespread edema, ascites, hemorrhage, and shock. The overall case-fatality rate is between 25% and 60%. The impact of early antibiotic therapy is not known.

Epidemiology

B. anthracis can be found in the soil of many areas around the world, particularly those that experience episodic periods of heavy rainfall followed by drought. It is a disease of animals primarily and is endemic in most areas of the Middle East, equatorial Africa, Mexico, Central and South America, and some Asian countries (14). Globally, several thousand cases of anthrax are reported each year (15). These are mostly cutaneous; inhalational and GI anthrax occur at much lower rates.

In the United States, naturally occurring anthrax is relatively rare in humans. Approximately ten cases of human disease were reported in the United States each year since the late 1960s, a number that has declined from more than 100 cases per year in the early 1900s. Since 1990, only two cases of naturally occurring anthrax were reported—one in 1990 and one in 2000. Both were cases of cutaneous anthrax (16). Livestock and wild ruminant disease is common, particularly in the western states.

Anthrax as a Biologic Weapon

B. anthracis is an ideal biologic agent for weaponization. It is stable in spore form, making it easy to store, transport, and aerosolize (13). It is readily available in nature and has a long history of development as a weapon of mass destruction since the early 1940s. The impact of a massive aerosolized anthrax release attack is not known, but several agencies have conducted hypothetical scenarios that predict extremely large casualties. The Office of Technology Assessment (OTA) in 1993, for example, concluded that deaths of more than 3 million could occur following a 100-kg aerosol release dissemination of *B. anthracis.*

Although aerosol release of anthrax spores is the most likely mechanism for its use as a biologic weapon, deliberate contamination of food is also a possibility. During World War II, the Japanese reportedly impregnated chocolate with anthrax to kill Chinese children. The apartheid government of South Africa also experimented with anthrax in chocolate (17).

Weaponized anthrax has been the cause of disease outbreaks twice in history. In 1979, an accidental release of weaponized anthrax from a laboratory weapons factory in the Soviet Union caused 75 cases of inhalational anthrax and 2 cases of cutaneous anthrax. The overall case-fatality rate was 86% (18). The release dose amount of anthrax was estimated by investigators to be as low as a few milligrams.

The United States, in 2001, experienced an outbreak of anthrax involving the intentional contamination of mail with anthrax spores. Four letters containing up to 2 g of powder, with more than 500 billion spores per gram, were mailed from Trenton, New Jersey, over a 3-week period. Twenty-two cases of anthrax (11 inhalational and 11 cutaneous) were reported. All cases involved the Ames strain of *B. anthracis* and shared identical molecular subtyping. The case-fatality rate for inhalational anthrax was 45% (19,20).

Following recognition of anthrax in postal workers, the U.S. Postal Service initiated a pilot program called the Biohazard

Detection System in July 2003 that involves placing anthrax detection systems at selected mail-processing centers around the country.

Therapeutic Countermeasures for Weaponized Anthrax Release

Vaccine

Currently, Bioport Corporation manufactures a cell-free anthrax vaccine called AVA (Biothrax) (21). Seroconversion following three doses of the vaccine is reported (in one study) to be 95% (22); however, the correlation between antibody titer and protection against infection has not been defined. The duration of vaccine efficacy is also unknown but thought to be approximately 1 to 2 years.

Biothrax is not available to the general public. Persons who should receive a preexposure vaccination series include the following: members of the military (or other select populations with a risk of exposure to weaponized anthrax), laboratory workers engaged in production of *B. anthracis* cultures, veterinarians or other high-risk persons handling potentially contaminated meat or animal products, and workers who may be making repeated entries into a *B. anthracis* contaminated site after a bioterrorist attack (23,24). Anthrax vaccine is not currently recommended for postexposure use; thus, it must be given under an investigational new drug (IND) application with the Food and Drug Administration (FDA).

Recent Advisory Committee on Immunization Practices (ACIP) guidelines recommend the use of anthrax vaccine in combination with antibiotics following an inhalational exposure to *B. anthracis*. Exposed persons should receive a three-dose regimen of Biothrax and a 30-day course of antibiotic therapy (25).

Antibiotics

The FDA has approved doxycycline, ciprofloxacin, and penicillin G procaine for use in postexposure prophylaxis against aerosolized anthrax. Prophylactic antibiotic therapy is recommended for persons exposed to an air space contaminated with a suspicious material that may contain anthrax spores or those exposed to an airspace with known anthrax release. This includes unvaccinated laboratory workers exposed to suspected aerosolized *B. anthracis* in culture. Antibiotic prophylaxis is not recommended for autopsy personnel, for medical personnel caring for anthrax victims, or for the prevention of cutaneous anthrax (25).

In the event of a massive aerosolized release of anthrax spores, rapid delivery of prophylactic antibiotics would be crucial in preventing large casualties (26). States can request antibiotic and medical supplies from the Strategic National Stockpile through the CDC. State and local health departments should activate their bioterrorism preparedness plans to distribute antibiotics rapidly.

Implications for Healthcare Workers

Standard Precautions are considered adequate for patients with inhalational, GI, and oropharyngeal anthrax because person-to-person transmission for these forms of the disease has not been reported (13). Although people with inhalational anthrax may have residual contamination of hair and clothing from their exposure event on presentation to a medical facility, this does not appear to be a transmission concern to healthcare workers. Standard Precautions are also recommended by most sources for cutaneous anthrax; however, because person-to-person transmission has occurred rarely for this type of anthrax, Contact Precautions have also been recommended (7,27).

Complete information regarding the use of personal protective equipment for first responders and other healthcare workers can be found in documents from the CDC and the Occupational Safety and Health Administration (OSHA) (25,28):

- CDC: protecting investigators performing environmental sampling for *B. anthracis*: personal protective equipment
- OSHA: anthrax in the workplace
- OSHA: fact sheet and references on worker health and safety for anthrax exposure

BOTULINUM TOXIN

Agent

Botulinum Toxin

Botulinum toxins are the most lethal human toxins known. They are colorless, odorless, and tasteless at concentrations that are lethal. The toxins are produced by vegetative cells following the germination of *C. botulinum* spores and released by cell lysis. In the case of wound botulism or infant botulism the microorganisms may be present in the wound or the bowel, but in foodborne disease or bioterrorist events the toxin is released from the microorganism before the intoxication. Several distinct antigenic toxin types are produced by *C. botulinum* and other *Clostridium* species. Types A, B, E, and F cause natural disease in humans; toxin type F accounts for less than 1% of naturally occurring disease. Other antigenic subtypes, including toxin types C, D, and G can cause disease in other mammals and birds. Botulinum toxin is inactivated by heating it to 85°C for 5 minutes (29). It is important to note that in the event of an intentional dissemination of botulinum toxin, the causative (vegetative) microorganisms may not be present.

Diagnostic procedures usually rely on the toxicity for mice confirmed by neutralization of the toxin by antiserum. Toxin can be detected in food, gastric contents, or serum. Antibodies do not usually develop in convalescence because of the very small lethal dose.

Clostridium botulinum

C. botulinum is a gram-positive spore-forming bacillus. It is "sluggishly" motile, anaerobic, and found in soil and aquatic sediments. There are several strains of *C. botulinum*; subtyping is based on metabolic characteristics of the microorganism. Groups I and II are responsible for the toxin production that is lethal to humans.

C. botulinum spores are resilient, resisting destruction with prolonged boiling at high temperatures and desiccation. They have been shown to survive in a dry state for more than 30 years. The spores are susceptible to chlorine in dilute concentrations (as in chlorinated water). They undergo germination most readily by exposure to heat ("heat shocking") of 80°C for 10 to 20 minutes (30).

Botulism Pathophysiology and Clinical Presentation

Botulinum toxin can enter the body via ingestion or inhalation. Exposure can also occur through local production in the GI tract or necrotic tissue at the site of a wound. Botulinum toxin is activated by proteolytic cleavage; the activated structure contains a heavy and light polypeptide chain. The toxin is carried through the bloodstream to the neuromuscular junction where the heavy chain binds to presynaptic receptors causing permanent inhibition of acetylcholine release. After several months, muscle function is regained based largely on the production of new synapses at the neuromuscular junction.

Clinically, patients present with neuromuscular weakness, ranging from mild cranial nerve dysfunction to complete flaccid paralysis. The severity of disease corresponds to the toxin dose and the toxin subtype; type A creates a more severe clinical presentation than types B or E. The major differential diagnoses include Guillain-Barré syndrome, Eaton-Lambert syndrome, and polyneuropathies such as the recently recognized West Nile syndrome. Botulism is characteristically distinguished by initiation of involvement with the cranial nerves and descending in the neuraxis as it progresses.

Loss of respiratory and pharyngeal muscle function can require a prolonged period of mechanical ventilation. Death often results from complications of prolonged ventilatory support. Before mechanical ventilation, death rates approached 50% (31). Case-fatality rates are now lower because of the advent of adequate supportive care including advanced respiratory support capabilities. The current overall case-fatality rate is 5% to 10% for foodborne disease and somewhat higher for wound botulism (31,32).

Modes of Transmission and Epidemiology

Foodborne Botulism

Botulinum toxin can be produced in food items that are contaminated with *C. botulinum* spores. Conditions, including an anaerobic environment, acidic pH, minimum temperature of 10°C, and availability of a water source, must exist to facilitate germination of spores and production of botulinum toxin (33). Food containing the neurotoxin that is not sufficiently reheated to at least 85°C for 5 minutes becomes a potent toxin delivery source for humans (29).

A single case of foodborne botulism is considered an outbreak and declared a public health emergency. All cases of botulism must be reported to the CDC immediately. In the United States, an average of nine outbreaks per year was seen in the late 1990s, with approximately two to three cases per outbreak (33). Improperly home-canned vegetables are the most common source of foodborne botulism; however, over the past 20 years, a variety of commercially produced, preservative-free foods have caused outbreaks. Garlic in oil, baked potatoes in foil, jarred peanuts, and commercially processed cheese sauce have been associated with outbreaks (34–38).

Botulinum toxin is rapidly inactivated by the chlorine that is a standard additive to potable water. For this reason, cases of botulism have not been associated with contaminated water (39, 40).

Wound Botulism

C. botulinum infection is usually associated with traumatic injuries of the extremities, especially those which involve contact with soil or another natural *C. botulinum* source. Although seen more rarely, cases of botulism following a postoperative infection, the use of intravenous (IV) or intranasal illicit drugs, or dental abscess have also been reported. Wound botulism is a rare event; only 78 cases were reported to the CDC for the period of 1986 to 1996 (33).

Inhalational Botulism

Inhalational botulism is caused by inhalation of aerosolized preformed botulinum toxin into the lungs and, subsequently, the circulation. It is a very rare exposure event, occurring only once in a veterinary laboratory setting in Germany in 1962 (39). Inhalational disease has also been produced experimentally in primates. Results of this study showed disease onset occurring 12 to 80 hours after exposure (41).

Botulinum Toxin as a Biologic Weapon

Botulinum toxin has been manufactured as a potential biologic weapon since World War II. The United States produced the toxin during that time period but abandoned production after signing the BWTC in 1972 renouncing use, stockpiling, or production of biologic weapons. The Soviet Union, however, continued production into the early 1990s. At the time of the Gulf War, Iraq had produced over 19,000 L of botulinum toxin, some of which was weaponized (42). On three occasions between 1990 and 1995, the Japanese cult Aum Shinrikyo attempted to use aerosolized botulinum toxin in Japanese cities but was not successful.

Botulinum toxin could be disseminated via the deliberate contamination of food or beverages or as an aerosol. Experts believe that the foodborne route represents the most likely bioterrorist scenario. Deliberate contamination of a large source of commercially available and distributed food or beverage product, particularly one in which adequate heating would be unlikely, could cause massive extensive casualties across the country. The widespread nature of the attack would also create significant panic, economic loss, and social disruption.

The dispersal of aerosolized toxin is also possible and could result in extremely large numbers of casualties, in this instance concentrated in a single urban setting. One gram of aerosolized botulinum toxin could theoretically kill 1.5 million people (43);

however it is likely that, for practical considerations, the effects of a botulinum toxin attack would be relatively limited compared with one of the infectious agents.

Contamination of a water source is unlikely because of dilution as well as the vulnerability of the toxin to chlorine, a standard additive to potable water.

Therapeutic Countermeasures for Weaponized Botulinum Toxin

Botulinum Antitoxin

Botulinum antitoxin is of equine origin and has traditionally been developed for use against subtypes A, B, and E. The use of this trivalent antitoxin has recently been suspended by the FDA. Currently available antitoxin formulations include equine antitoxin against types A and B and a second formulation against type E. The antitoxin does not reverse the blockade of acetylcholine at the neuromuscular junction but prevents binding of any circulating neurotoxin. The CDC maintains an active surveillance program for cases of botulism and is responsible through state health departments for the distribution of antitoxin in suspected cases (39,41).

In the event of a bioterrorist attack with botulinum toxin, it is possible that other subtypes will be weaponized. The U.S. Army has developed an equine Fabantitoxin effective against all botulinum toxin types, but its efficacy in humans is not clear. In addition, as for the licensed product, it carries with it the potential for serious allergic reaction.

The dose of antitoxin required to reduce the effects of the neurotoxin varies with the inoculating dose. In the event of a mass release of weaponized botulinum toxin, the scarcity of antitoxin would be highly likely (39).

Botulinum Toxoid Vaccine

Vaccination with botulinum toxoid is currently recommended for laboratory personnel who work with *C. botulinum* and military personnel at risk for exposure to weaponized botulinum toxin (44). The vaccine is not considered a viable countermeasure against a bioterrorist attack. It is not effective against all subtypes, it is painful to receive and requires a yearly booster, and it also disallows the recipient from receiving botulinum antitoxin therapy for life.

Emergency Response to a Mass Exposure

A single case of botulism is considered a public health emergency (45). In the event of a suspected botulism outbreak, public health officials will assist with appropriate laboratory testing to confirm diagnosis, authorize use of antitoxin, and conduct aggressive surveillance investigations to identify the source of an outbreak to determine if there is evidence to suggest a bioterrorism-related event.

In the event of a mass exposure, such as a widespread aerosol release of botulinum toxin, the rapid administration of antitoxin to ill persons would be indicated. Although antitoxin does not reverse existing paralysis, it binds remaining circulating toxin, mitigating progression of the disease. Rapid mobilization of mechanical ventilators and other ancillary supportive care tools would be critical to successful management of any mass-exposure botulism outbreak.

Implications for Healthcare Workers

In the hospital setting, Standard Precautions are adequate for patents with botulism because person-to-person transmission does not occur. In the laboratory setting, *C. botulinum* toxin detection should only be performed by trained individuals at level C or higher LRN laboratories (46). The FDA also released biosafety recommendations for laboratories that test for *C. botulinum.* A partial list includes the following: placement of biohazard signage, the use appropriate laboratory safety apparel including coats and safety glasses, restriction of solo work shifts, immediate autoclaving of all toxic material, and ready access to information on the location of an antitoxin source. (47).

PLAGUE

Agent

Y. pestis is the causative agent of plague. It is a pleomorphic gram-negative bacillus, existing as single cells or short chains in direct smears. It is a nonmotile, nonsporulating facultative anaerobe that is slow-growing in culture. At 48 to 72 hours of incubation on solid media, colonies have a raised, "fried egg" appearance. Data banks for many commercial laboratory identification systems do not include *Y. pestis* (48).

Y. pestis is thought to have evolved from *Yersinia pseudotuberculosis* 1,500 to 20,000 years ago (49). Recent data suggest the continued evolution of the bacillus through the emergence of several new genotypes (50).

Modes of Transmission

Humans are an incidental hosts for *Y. pestis* and are not part of its natural life cycle. Many different animal species (mostly wild rodents) are natural reservoirs for the bacillus (51). Like humans, other nonrodent mammalian species serve as incidental hosts for *Y. pestis.* These animals, however, can serve as sources of human exposure. Disease occurrence in humans is dependent on the frequency of infection in local rodent populations. Human outbreaks are usually preceded by epizootics with increased deaths in susceptible animal hosts (52,53).

The vector for *Y. pestis* is the flea. More than 1,500 species of flea exist; approximately 30 are known to be vectors for *Y. pestis* (53).

Humans can become infected with *Y. pestis* via the bite of an infected flea, a bite or scratch from an infected incidental host mammal such as a cat, or the direct contact with infected animal carcasses or products. Inhalation of respiratory droplets from infected animals or humans can also cause infection (54).

Pathogenesis and Clinical Syndromes

The classic forms of plague are bubonic plague, pneumonic plague, and septicemic plague. Rarely, plague can be manifested as meningitis, pharyngitis, or pestis minor, a milder form of bubonic plague.

Bubonic Plague

Bubonic plague is transmitted to humans via the bite of an infected flea, a bite or scratch from an infected animal, or direct contact with infected animal carcasses. Between 25,000 and 100,000 *Y. pestis* microorganisms are inoculated into the skin after a bite from an infected flea (55). The microorganisms migrate through the cutaneous lymphatics to regional lymph nodes. Once in the lymph nodes they are phagocytized by polymorphonuclear leukocytes (PMNs) and mononuclear phagocytes. Microorganisms phagocytized by PMNs are largely destroyed, whereas those phagocytized by mononuclear cells proliferate intracellularly and are released when cell lysis occurs (53). Initially, affected nodes contain a thick exudate composed of plague bacilli, PMNs, and lymphocytes. This pattern gives way to hemorrhagic necrosis, which creates the clinical picture of swollen, painful buboes that are characteristic of bubonic plague. Microorganisms also enter the bloodstream causing hemorrhagic lesions in other lymph nodes and organs throughout the body. Eventually septicemia, disseminated intravascular coagulation (DIC), and shock ensues. Without prompt antibiotic therapy, death usually results from overwhelming septicemia.

Pneumonic Plague

Y. pestis can enter the lungs directly through direct inhalation (primary pneumonic plague) or via hematogenous spread of bubonic plague (secondary pneumonic plague). Primary pneumonic plague is acquired by inhalation of approximately 100 to 500 microorganisms (13). Clinically, patients present with fulminant lobar or multilobular pneumonia. Marked edema and congestion of the lungs are also common. Death from overwhelming sepsis, DIC, and multiorgan failure occurs rapidly without prompt antibiotic therapy. Untreated, mortality approaches 100% (53).

Septicemic Plague

Primary septicemic plague is defined as systemic toxicity caused by *Y. pestis* infection without apparent lymph node involvement. Secondary septicemic plague occurs commonly as part of bubonic or pneumonic plague. Septicemia is the syndrome that leads to multiorgan failure, DIC, and death. In the late stages of the disease, high-density bacteremia often occurs, with ready identification of microorganisms on peripheral blood smears (52).

Epidemiology

Historical Perspective

Three plague pandemics have occurred during recorded history causing an estimated 200 million deaths (56). The first recorded pandemic began in Egypt in 542 AD and spread throughout Europe, Central and Southern Asia, and Africa, killing more than 100 million people. The second pandemic, widely known as the Black Death began in Italy in 1347 and spread rapidly across Europe killing one third of the population. The most recent pandemic began in China in 1894 and spread throughout the world over a 10-year period, presumably facilitated by ship travel. This pandemic was responsible for an estimated 12 million deaths, most occurring in India.

Naturally Occurring Plague in the United States

Plague was first introduced to the United States in 1900 as part of the third pandemic and created an epidemic in the early 1900s in San Francisco (57).

It was sporadically epidemic largely in urban settings secondary to infected rat populations (58). After 1926, plague became endemic in wild animal populations in the western United States. Cases have also been associated with infected domestic cats (54).

Today plague remains endemic in the United States. It is usually seasonal, with a higher case incidence during summer months (57,58). From 1947 through 1996, 390 cases of plague were reported to the CDC with an overall case fatality rate of 15.4% (59). Bubonic plague accounted for 83.9% of those reported cases. An average of 8.9 cases per year were reported to the CDC from 1990 to 1999 (60,61). Many of these cases developed secondary pneumonia, but no transmission to contacts has been seen. The disjunct between the pneumonic transmission, which occurred during the Manchurian epidemics early in the century, and the uncommon documentation of pneumonic spread in other settings may reflect the crowding and lack of basic hygiene during earlier epidemics.

Plague as a Biologic Weapon

Y. pestis is a potentially suitable agent for use as a biologic weapon, because it can be aerosolized and/or transmitted person to person. The pneumonic form of plague is highly fatal, and its communicability could generate widespread fear and panic. Plague was used as a biologic weapon in the Middle Ages when armies catapulted the bodies of plague victims into cities to spread the disease (1). In World War II Japan used plague against the Chinese by dropping plague-infested fleas over populated areas causing outbreaks of the disease (1,62). *Y. pestis* has also been weaponized by the United States and the former Soviet Union, the latter having also engineered *Y. pestis* for increased virulence and microbial resistance (63,64).

In 1970, the World Health Organization (WHO) modeled a biologic warfare attack with *Y. pestis.* This report estimated that the aerosol dissemination of 50 kg of dried powder containing 6×10^{15} *Y. pestis* microorganisms over a city of 5 million people would generate 150,000 cases and 36,000 deaths. They speculated that subsequent person-to-person transmission would create another 500,000 cases and 100,000 deaths, but the actual pneumonic spread is not clearly established in modern times (65).

The primary clinical presentation of persons infected by aerosolized *Y. pestis* would be pneumonic plague although septicemic disease might occur. Previously healthy patients would present with severe and rapidly progressive multilobular pneumonia. Hemoptysis, GI symptoms, evidence of DIC, and a fulminant clinical course would be highly suspicious for pneumonic plague. Notably, characteristic buboes, associated with bubonic plague would be absent, and patients would not necessarily present with risk factors for plague exposure. This disease requires intensive medical and nursing support with rapid isolation and antibiotic therapy followed by hospitalization for several weeks of convalescence.

Therapeutic Countermeasures for Aerosol Dissemination of Plague

A rapid, coordinated public health response is essential to minimize casualties during a bioterrorist attack of weaponized plague. The Working Group on Civilian Biodefense developed consensus-based recommendations for the treatment of pneumonic plague for two scenarios: In a setting with limited potential casualties, and an adequate medical care delivery system, parenteral antibiotics (streptomycin or gentamicin) should be administered to all patients whenever possible. In a mass casualty setting, in which the medical care resources are outstripped, oral antibiotics (doxycycline or ciprofloxacin) should be administered for a period of 10 days. Antibiotics must be administered early in the course of the infection (perhaps within 24 to 48 hours of onset) or death occurs in 3 to 6 days. In addition, close contacts of untreated patients should also receive prophylactic oral antibiotics for a period of 7 days (63).

Plague Vaccine

A licensed, killed whole-cell vaccine was available in the United States until 1999 (66). It was used by the military and showed some efficacy against bubonic plague but not pneumonic plague. It is no longer manufactured, and its lack of efficacy against pneumonic plague would limit its usefulness in the event of a bioterrorist attack. A live, attenuated vaccine was developed in the early 1900s and has been used in some parts of the world. The vaccine strain is not avirulent, however, and is associated with significant safety concerns.

Research is ongoing to develop new plague vaccines. Two approaches include the development of a live, attenuated mutant *Y. pestis* vaccine strain and the use of antigenic subunit vaccine (67,68). This recombinant vaccine has shown the best protection against both bubonic and pneumonic plague. It is currently unavailable, but research is ongoing.

Decontamination

In general, environmental decontamination following an aerosol event has not been recommended, because experts have estimated that an aerosol of *Y. pestis* microorganisms would be infectious for only about 1 hour (63). A recent study demonstrated that *Y. pestis* can survive on selected environmental surfaces for at least several days, although the potential for reaerosolization of these microorganisms was not addressed (69).

Implications for Healthcare Workers

Healthcare workers need to be protected from transmission of *Y. pestis.* Droplet Precautions with eye protection in addition to Standard Precautions are indicated for patients with pneumonic plague (70). Patients should be considered infectious for 48 to 72 hours after appropriate antibiotic therapy has been initiated with evidence of clinical improvement (9,64). The detailed mechanisms of transmission of pneumonic plague are unknown. The Manchurian and Indian epidemics early in the twentieth century were associated with crowding and a lack of hygiene and are thought to reflect droplet spread, a conclusion supported by the protection provided to medical staff by surgical masks. There has been no interhuman transmission of plague in the United States since 1924 despite numerous bubonic and a smaller number of pneumonic cases. The possibility of aerosol transmission of pneumonic plague, particularly in the unexplored setting of a bioterrorist attack, is unknown but believed to be unlikely (70). Nevertheless, medical staff, like other contacts, who are in close contact with plague patients should receive antibiotic prophylaxis.

SMALLPOX

Agent

Variola viruses are orthopoxviruses from the family Poxviridae. They are DNA viruses, brick shaped, and large in size (200 nm diameter). The average genome is 200 kbp, and several strains have been completely sequenced. Efforts are ongoing to determine genetic diversity of existing variola viruses (71). Variola viruses have been classified as variola major or variola minor based on the severity of their clinical manifestations.

Many viruses in the Poxviridae family do not include humans as a natural host. Some, however, in addition to variola virus, can cause natural human infection. These include members of the Orthopoxvirus species, including monkeypox, vaccinia, and cowpox viruses. Other poxviruses that cause human infection include yatapoxviruses, parapoxviruses, and Molluscipoxvirus (the causative agent of molluscum contagiosum).

Laboratory diagnosis is most readily made from skin lesions by electron microscopy, which can correctly identify viruses as orthopoxviruses, and by PCR and sequencing, which can arrive at a species identification. Cultivation of virus and other approaches are also useful.

Epidemiology and Modes of Transmission

Smallpox virus no longer exists in nature. Several important epidemiologic properties of the virus helped facilitate its eradication in the 1970s. Of primary significance is the fact that humans represent the only natural reservoir for the virus. In addition, the infectivity of naturally occurring smallpox is not generally as high as that for other common exanthems such as measles, usually requiring close contact for transmission. Maximal infectivity also occurs during the height of clinical illness, a time during which infected persons are bedridden and severely ill, limiting contact with uninfected populations. After recovery, infectivity wanes with the resolution of pustules; smallpox cannot exist in a chronic carrier state (72). Currently, declared variola major virus exists in only two WHO-approved facilities: the CDC in Atlanta and the Russian State Centre for Research on Virology and Biotechnology in Novosibirsk (73).

Smallpox is transmitted person to person via large droplet nuclei or aerosols generated from oropharyngeal secretions of smallpox victims (72). Airborne transmission is unusual but was documented in two hospital outbreaks in Germany in the 1960s (74). Transmission of the virus via fomites has also occurred. This was an intentional transmission mode during the French-Indian wars of the mid-1700s (75).

Smallpox is a moderately contagious disease. The infectious dose is presumed to be low (10 to 100 microorganisms) (13). Unlike some other viruses, persons with the disease are not considered infectious in the prodromal stage of the disease (76). The highest risk for transmission occurs 1 week after the onset of rash when oral lesions ulcerate and release large amounts of virus into the saliva. Patients should be considered infectious at the time of fever onset, however, because some virus may be present in oral secretions shortly before the onset of the rash. Virus is present in skin lesions and scabs, so communicability lasts until the pustules have scabbed over and fallen off.

In the pre-eradication era, the average number of cases infected by a primary case was approximately 3.5 to 6 (77). The secondary attack rate among close contacts varied from 37% to more than 70% (78–80). Transmission outside the family and the hospital (patients and medical staff) was uncommon. Random spread to less intimate contacts was not a feature of the European epidemiology in the era in which vaccination was waning and occasional introductions occurred.

Clinical Features

Variola major virus can cause several distinct clinical disease manifestations. In the pre-eradication period, distinguishing between these types was based on rash pattern, clinical illness, epidemiology, and laboratory findings. Major types are reviewed briefly. Monkeypox, a related orthopoxvirus, has some similarities in presentation and is also reviewed.

Ordinary Smallpox

Ordinary smallpox accounted for more than 90% of variola major infections in the pre-eradication period. After a 10- to 13-day incubation period, a prodrome of fever, chills, and prostration ensues. This lasts 2 to 4 days and is often followed by the appearance of a few skin lesions on the face called "herald spots." Painful, hard lesions progress synchronously on the face and distal extremities including the palms and soles. Fewer lesions are found on the trunk. These are initially maculopapular then vesicular and finally pustular, leaving pitting scars after recovery.

Patients may undergo massive fluid shifts, hemodynamic instability, and skin desquamation, resembling a massive burn clinically. The overall case-fatality rate is 15% to 45% in unvaccinated persons (72).

Flat-type (Malignant) Smallpox

Flat-type smallpox is a highly fatal disease, affecting children primarily. It accounted for less than 10% of variola major presentations in the pre-eradication period. Malignant smallpox has a similar incubation period and clinical prodrome to ordinary smallpox. In this disease, however, lesions develop slowly and have a confluent, flat, velvety pattern. The nonpustular appearance of the rash can obscure the diagnosis. This type of smallpox is almost uniformly fatal.

Hemorrhagic Smallpox

Hemorrhagic smallpox was very rare in the pre-eradication period, accounting for less than 5% of overall cases. Pregnant women experienced the greatest mortality among patients with this type of smallpox. The clinical picture of hemorrhagic smallpox is that of DIC, shock, and organ failure. The case-fatality rate for hemorrhagic smallpox exceeds 96%, and death can occur before the development of the rash (81). Because of the atypical presentation and the very high virus levels in blood and throat wash, this clinical form is particularly dangerous epidemiologically.

Monkeypox

Monkeypox virus is an orthopoxvirus that causes an infection similar to smallpox but generally milder. It occurs sporadically in Western and Central Africa.

Clinically, patients experience a similar prodrome (fever, chills, headache, backache) to smallpox (82). After 1 to 3 days, a smallpox-like rash appears, which lasts 2 to 4 weeks. Lymphadenopathy is a more prominent feature in monkeypox than smallpox (82–84).

The case-fatality rate for monkeypox is lower, reflecting a milder clinical course. In two reported outbreaks the case-fatality rate varied form 3% to 11%. All deaths in these two outbreaks involved children younger than age 10 with no prior smallpox vaccination (82).

Monkeypox virus can be spread from animal reservoirs (squirrels, rabbits, rodents, prairie dogs) or person to person. The secondary attack rate for household contacts is low; rates ranging from 7% to 15% have been reported among unvaccinated close contacts (83,85,86).

In June, 2003, an outbreak of monkeypox occurred in the United States. The outbreak was traced back to infected prairie dogs which had contracted the virus by close contact during shipping with imported Gambian rats from Africa. Seventy-one cases were reported; 26% were hospitalized, but no deaths occurred. Thirty exposed persons received smallpox vaccine to prevent monkeypox; one of these was later confirmed with the disease (87).

Smallpox as a Bioweapon

Smallpox has been considered the most devastating of all global infectious diseases, and its intentional reintroduction would be a "crime of unprecedented proportions" (4). This fact alone makes it an attractive agent of terror.

Smallpox has several features that enhance its potential as a biologic weapon: it is contagious, and, at this point in time, most of the population has no immunity to the disease; it can be aerosolized; the virus carries a high rate of morbidity and mortality and would undoubtedly cause wide-spread panic and social disruption (88,89). Ongoing global vigilance is necessary to detect any recurrence of smallpox through accidental or intentional release (84).

Therapeutic Countermeasures for Weaponized Smallpox

Treatment

Supportive care including fluid management, pain alleviation, and surveillance for bacterial superinfection is the only available treatment for patients with smallpox. In the pre-eradication period there was no available antiviral therapy against smallpox. Today, there have been more than 200 antiviral compounds tested for therapeutic benefit against variola virus and other orthopoxviruses (72). Among those tested, cidofovir, adefovir, dipivoxil, and ribavirin have shown significant *in vitro* activity (13). Animal model testing is the next stage toward the development of a clinically effective antiviral therapy. At least one study has suggested that cidofovir might be useful in postexposure prophylaxis or perhaps treatment.

Vaccination

The vaccinia vaccine has been available since the 1970s in a lyophilized preparation called Dryvax (Wyeth Laboratories). It is an infectious vaccinia virus containing the antibiotics polymyxin B, streptomycin, tetracycline, and neomycin. Existing Dryvax vaccine produced in the 1970s has retained potency in its lyophilized state; currently there are approximately 15.4 million doses available (72). Although studies have shown that the vaccine can be diluted 1:5 and 1:10 with relatively high vaccination responses among study subjects (90–92), the CDC has no plans to dilute the vaccine at this time, because the margin of excess virus (especially in the 1:10 dilution) could lead to a large number of vaccine failures in the field if any mishandling of the vaccination procedure occurs.

CDC is the only vaccine distributor for civilians. In addition to the Dryvax vaccine, an additional 85 million doses of a smallpox vaccine using the Dryvax strain but stored frozen have been produced and donated by Aventis to the federal government. Studies are ongoing to determine efficacy of this vaccine in a 1:5 dilution. Diluted stores of this vaccine in addition to the Dryvax vaccine will bring the United States stockpile to more than 400 million doses.

A new cell culture-derived vaccinia vaccine is being produced by Acambis (ACAM100) and Acambis-Baxter (ACAM200) under contract with the federal government. Two hundred nine million doses of smallpox vaccine produced in cell culture are undergoing development; however, clinical trials for efficacy are also ongoing.

It must be borne in mind that there are, as yet, no accurate animal models that could quantitatively predict human protection, although these products are sufficiently close to the original vaccine so that one can expect good protection. More attenuated vaccines are under development for protection of persons with contraindications to vaccination such as the immunosuppressed, but one cannot be certain of their efficacy.

Use of Vaccine for Postexposure Prophylaxis

Immunity to variola virus generally develops within 8 to 11 days after vaccination. Because the incubation period for smallpox averages 12 days, vaccination soon after exposure (up to 4 days) may confer some immunity and reduce overall mortality. This may be particularly true for persons who received smallpox vaccination in the pre-eradication period because of the anamnestic immune response that occurs with revaccination (93). The true efficacy and timing of postexposure vaccination prophylaxis remains unclear.

Use of Vaccine During a Smallpox Emergency

A "ring vaccination" strategy has been used successfully during the smallpox eradication campaign and is the approach incorporated by the current CDC Smallpox Plan (94). This strategy involves rapid identification and isolation of smallpox cases, identification and vaccination of contacts with monitoring for symptoms, and vaccination of household members of contacts (where no contraindications exist). In addition to ring vaccinations, rapid voluntary vaccination of a large population may be necessary to aid containment control strategies. Large-scale voluntary vaccination would only be initiated in certain situations under the recommendation from the Secretary of Health and Human Services. Vaccination of the general population before the threat of a smallpox attack is better defined; it would be associated with an unacceptable number of serious and fatal adverse effects.

Vaccination only provides solid immunity if given within the previous 3 to 5 years. However, there is amelioration of severity and protection from mortality for many years, depending on the number of vaccinations. Because infection with rash and spread of virus may occur and because some patients with distant vaccination will be expected to die, history of vaccination should not dissuade revaccination when indicated for protection.

Targeted quarantine of selected high-risk exposures would be expected to have a place in control of smallpox under certain circumstances. Wide-scale quarantine of communities would likely not be effective and is not recommended (95).

Implications for Healthcare Workers

Patients with suspected smallpox should be cared for using strict isolation procedures including placement in negative pressure rooms with external air exhaust or high-efficiency particulate air (HEPA) filters where available. In the event of a massive outbreak, smallpox patients should be cohorted and isolated. All healthcare workers caring for patients with suspected smallpox should be vaccinated immediately (96).

Current Recommendations for Vaccination of Healthcare Workers

In October 2002, the ACIP and the Healthcare Infection Control Practices Advisory Committee (HICPAC) at the CDC made the following recommendations for smallpox vaccination of healthcare workers in the pre-event setting:

- Smallpox vaccination is recommended for persons designated by the appropriate bioterrorism and public health authorities to conduct investigation and follow-up of initial smallpox cases (i.e., smallpox response teams). These teams might include medical team leaders, public health advisors, medical epidemiologists, disease investigators, diagnostic laboratory scientists, nurses, personnel who would administer smallpox vaccines, and security and law enforcement personnel.
- Each acute care hospital should identify a group of healthcare workers (i.e., smallpox healthcare teams) who should be vaccinated and trained to provide direct medical care for the first few smallpox patients requiring hospital admission and to evaluate and manage patients who present to the emergency department with suspected smallpox. These teams should have a wide range of expertise and should include emergency department physicians and nurses, intensive care unit staff, general medical unit staff, primary care house staff, medical subspecialists (including infectious diseases specialists, medical consultants with smallpox experience, dermatologists, ophthalmologists, pathologists, surgeons, and anesthesiologists), infection control professionals, respiratory therapists, radiology technicians, security personnel, and housekeeping staff. Ideally, each hospital should have enough vaccinated personnel from each occupational category to ensure continuity of care (95).

Contraindications for the vaccination of healthcare workers included history of eczema or atopic dermatitis, persons with other exfoliative skin diseases or burns, immunocompromised patients, and patients with known cardiac risk factors (97).

TULAREMIA

Agent

F. tularensis is the causative agent of tularemia. It is a small gram-negative rod, often mistaken visually on Gram stain for *Haemophilus* species. It is a nonsporulating, nonmotile aerobe. There are several subspecies of *F. tularensis* that are differentiated by biochemical tests and antimicrobial resistance. These microorganisms flourish in moist environments (water, mud, animal carcasses) and can survive for extended periods of time in these settings (98–100). There are several biovars, but the *F. tularensis* biovar tularensis or Type A is the most virulent.

Laboratory diagnosis is possible by cultivation from blood or other relevant clinical samples, although growth may be slow and conventional media may not be optimum. Investigational techniques include PCR and antigen detection.

Epidemiology and Modes of Transmission

The primary vectors for *F. tularensis* are ticks, mosquitoes, and biting flies (101,102). The principal reservoirs include a variety of small animal species including rabbits, rats and mice, lemmings, squirrels, and aquatic rodents (101–103). Humans and other mammals and some species of birds, fish, and amphibians serve as incidental hosts. An outbreak of tularemia in commercially distributed prairie dogs was reported in the United States in 2002 but did not result in human cases (104).

F. tularensis can be transmitted to humans by several routes: the bite of an infected arthropod vector (105), ingestion of contaminated food or water (106,107), the handling of infected animal tissue (108), the inhalation of aerosolized bacteria during the mowing of hay or grass (109,110), or during processing of bacteria in the laboratory (111). The average incubation period is 3 to 5 days; *F. tularensis* is highly infectious but not contagious person to person.

Most cases in the United States in recent years have been associated with bites from infected arthropods, although animal exposure continues to be a common source of infection in the southeastern United States (112). States with the highest number of reported cases include Arkansas, Kansas, Missouri, Montana, Oklahoma, and South Dakota (113). Most cases occur in rural or semirural settings and show seasonality, presenting between May and August. Sporadic cases may rarely occur in urban settings with no identifiable source but would justify additional scrutiny.

Although the number of cases reported each year is declining, tularemia can occur in outbreaks, the most recent of which occurred in Martha's Vineyard in 2000. Fifteen cases of primarily pneumonic tularemia occurred, presumably secondary to aerosolized exposure to *F. tularensis* via lawn mower clippings. There was one fatality in that series (110). Worldwide, tularemia is seen most often in Scandinavian countries and Russia (101). It is endemic in latitudes that include North America, Europe, states of the Russian Federation, China, and Japan (101). Outbreaks have been reported intermittently in Europe as well.

Clinical Syndromes

Infection with *F. tularensis* can cause several clinical syndromes ranging from a mild, localized infection to a life-threatening systemic illness. Poor outcomes occur in patients with significant comorbidity or in those in whom diagnosis and antibiotic therapy has been delayed (101).

Glandular, ulceroglandular, and pneumonic tularemia are the most common naturally occurring manifestations of tularemia. Other rare presentations of *F. tularensis* include oculoglandular and oropharyngeal tularemia (101). Typhoidal tularemia is a term used historically to describe pneumonic tularemia. Experts in this field now recommend the term "typhoidal tularemia" to denote systemic infections with *F. tularensis* that lack a clear anatomic focus.

Glandular and Ulceroglandular Tularemia

Ulceroglandular tularemia is the most common manifestation of *F. tularensis* infection accounting for more than half of all clinical presentations of *F. tularensis* infection. Glandular tularemia represents 25% of cases. In both illness, manifestations microorganisms enter the body through inapparent breaks in the skin or via the bite of an infected arthropod. The infectious dose for humans following percutaneous or inhalational inoculation is 10 to 50 microorganisms (11). Patients with these forms of tularemia usually present with a painful, localized cutaneous infection and tender, regional lymphadenopathy. Fever, chills, axillary adenopathy, and myalgias are also common. Complications of this type of infection include secondary pneumonia, hematogenous spread to other organs, and rarely sepsis. Glandular tularemia is distinguished by lymph node involvement but lack of an ulceration at the site of inoculation (99). The case-fatality rate is generally low (<2%), but some subtypes are more virulent than others.

Pneumonic Tularemia

Pneumonia caused by *F. tularensis* can result from inhalation of infectious aerosols or via hematogenous spread. Primary pneumonic tularemia often presents as an atypical pneumonia unresponsive to conventional therapy. Symptoms include fever, nonproductive cough, myalgias, and occasionally nausea and vomiting. The disease course is extremely variable. Complications include the adult respiratory distress syndrome (ARDS), lung abscesses, sepsis, or involvement of other organs through hematogenous spread. Recovery is prolonged, and relapses can occur even with antibiotic therapy. The case-fatality rate with prompt antibiotic treatment has been reported at less than 3%.

Secondary pneumonia occurs frequently in patients with typhoidal tularemia. Case-fatality rates of this pneumonia presentation have approached 50% in the preantibiotic era but are significantly reduced with appropriate antibiotic treatment.

Tularemia as a Biologic Weapon

There is information and evidence to support the use of *F. tularensis* as a biologic weapon (112). During World War II, the Japanese conducted research on *F. tularensis* as a biologic weapon. *F. tularensis* was also investigated for weaponization by the United States in the 1950s and 1960s, although these stockpiles were destroyed in 1973 as part of the BWTC act. The former Soviet Union also weaponized *F. tularensis,* including the development of antibiotic-resistant strains. In 1969, A WHO modeling scenario estimated that a 50-kg release with dissemination of *F. tularensis* over a city of 5 million people would cause 250,000 illnesses and 19,000 deaths (114).

A bioterrorist attack with aerosolized *F. tularensis* would be expected to cause primarily pneumonic tularemia; however, some cases of typhoidal (nonspecific) and glandular tularemia may occur as well. Tularemia is highly infectious and it should be assumed that weaponized *F. tularensis* would be selected for high virulence and engineered for antimicrobial resistance and high virulence.

An outbreak of tularemia from a bioterrorist attack would be differentiated from a natural occurring outbreak in that persons infected would have no known exposure to the bacteria, and cases would likely present in an urban rather than rural setting (112).

Therapeutic Countermeasures for Weaponized Tularemia Exposure

Postexposure Prophylaxis

The prompt initiation of a prophylactic antibiotic treatment regimen is critical for reducing morbidity and mortality and for providing a community-wide sense of calm and control. One challenge study involving volunteer subjects using tetracycline demonstrated that antibiotic postexposure prophylaxis can prevent disease if administered within 24 hours of exposure (115).

Current recommendations by the Working Group on Civilian Biodefense include the use of oral antibiotics (doxycycline or ciprofloxacin) for persons in the exposed population and for cases resulting from suspected *F. tularensis* release for a period of 14 days. In a situation of a known terrorist attack with documented clinical cases, all persons should be watched for signs of fever; any person who develops fever or flu-like symptoms should be placed on parenteral antibiotics if available or oral antibiotics in mass casualty settings (112).

Antibiotic Treatment

Antibiotic therapy for patients with documented tularemia is similar to prophylactic treatment regimens. The Working Group on Civilian Biodefense has made the following recommendations for treatment during a bioterrorist attack: If parenteral therapy is available, patients should be given streptomycin or gentamicin intramuscular (IM) for 10 days. In a situation of mass casualties in which the medical delivery system in unable to meet patient care demands, oral antibiotics should be administered for a period of 14 days. It is important to watch for posttreatment relapse and consider the possibility that a weaponized form of *F. tularensis* may be engineered for antimicrobial resistance (112).

Tularemia Vaccine

There is no vaccine currently available for tularemia. A live-attenuated vaccine has been shown effective against experimental aerosol challenge and has been used extensively in the former Soviet Union. This vaccine was available for laboratory workers until recently and is currently under further consideration by the United States Department of Agriculture and the FDA.

Postexposure vaccination against tularemia is not a feasible strategy; the short incubation period of the disease (3 to 5 days) negates the benefit of vaccine-based immunity, which requires 14 days to develop after injection.

Implications for Healthcare Workers

Healthcare workers exposed to aerosolized *F. tularensis* should undergo postexposure prophylaxis as described previously. In caring for patients with diagnosed tularemia, the use of Standard Precautions (70) are adequate because the agent, although highly infectious, is not contagious person to person.

F. tularensis does pose a significant potential threat in the laboratory setting because tularemia can be easily aerosolized and requires an extremely small dose for infectivity. In addition, the agent may be present in virtually any human specimen (116). A recent report described the exposure of 12 laboratory workers after a delay in identification of *F. tularensis* (117). This led to a recommendation by the authors that any bacterial microorganisms with properties suggestive of *F. tularensis* on initial evaluation be evaluated under a biologic safety cabinet until the microorganism is further identified.

VIRAL HEMORRHAGIC FEVER

Agents

Hemorrhagic fever (HF) viruses are a collection of taxonomically distinct viruses that cause the HF syndrome. Because the clinical presentation of these viruses is similar they are all considered HF viruses.

They share commonalities in composition; they are all single-stranded RNA viruses and possess a characteristic lipid envelope. The four taxonomic families represented in this clinical group include Filoviridae, Flaviviridae, Arenaviridae, and Bunyaviridae. Some key characteristics of specific HF viruses within these families are shown in Table 111.2 (118–125).

Laboratory diagnosis is specialized and can be achieved by detection of viral RNA through reverse transcriptase polymerase chain reaction (RT-PCR) or viral antigen by enzyme-linked immunosorbent assay (ELISA). Viral isolation is also useful in a longer time frame. After the disappearance of virus-related markers as the patient enters convalescence, IgM appears. Hantaviruses are an exception in that patients present with IgM antibodies in serum.

Clinical Syndromes and Epidemiology

Although each virus family has unique clinical and epidemiologic characteristics, the overall clinical picture for the group of HF viruses is similar (1267). The infectious dose for HF viruses appears to be extremely low (1 to 10 microorganisms) (11). Regardless of the route of infection, they induce a systemic illness with fever, capillary dysfunction, prostration, and in their most severe manifestations shock and central nervous system dysfunction. Many patients experience hemorrhagic manifestations that occur as a result of thrombocytopenia or severe platelet dysfunction along with endothelial dysfunction (126). A hemorrhagic or purpuric rash, epistaxis, menometrorrhagia, hematemesis, hemoptysis, blood in stools, and nondependent petechiae are common bleeding manifestations.

The Working Group on Civilian Biodefense has compiled a list of HF viruses that pose the most serious threat as biologic agents of terror. Notable clinical features of these specific viruses are reviewed briefly (127).

Ebola Hemorrhagic Fever

Ebola belongs to the Filoviridae family of viruses. It is an important emerging infectious disease, with increasingly frequent outbreaks documented in central Africa since its discovery in 1976 (128). Much about the transmission, reservoirs, and

TABLE 111.2. CHARACTERISTICS OF HEMORRHAGIC FEVER VIRUSES

Family	Agents	Characteristics
Filoviridae	Ebola virus Marburg Virus	– Filamentous virions (from the Latin "filo" for "thread" – Genome contains single stranded nonsegmented RNA – Size: 19 kbp, 80 nm in diameter, variable length – Transmembrane spike glycoprotein produces antigenically distinct viral species
Arenaviridae	Old World arenaviruses: – Lassa virus New World arenaviruses: – Junin virus (Argentine hemorrhagic fever) – Machupo virus (Bolivian hemorrhagic fever) – Guanarito virus (Venezuelan hemorrhagic fever) – Sabia virus (Brazilian hemorrhagic fever) – Whitewater Arroyo virus	– Spherical or pleomorphic virions with "sandy", granular ultrastructural appearance – Genome contains single stranded RNA with 2 segments – Size: 11 kbp, generally 110–130 nm in diameter – Distinct club shaped or spike glycoprotein projections on viral envelope – Lassa fever viruses exhibit 4 distinct genetic lineages (3 in Nigeria, and 1 in Guinea, Liberia, and Sierra Leone) – New World arenaviruses differ by neutralization tests and rodent reservoirs
Bunyaviridae	Phlebovirus (Rift Valley fever virus) Nairo virus (Crimean Congo hemorrhagic fever) Hanta virus (Hantaan virus; Sin nombre virus)	– Spherical or slightly pleomorphic virions – Genome contains single-stranded RNA with 3 segments – Size: 11–19kbp, 80–120 nm in diameter
Flaviviridae	Yellow Fever virus Kyanasur Forest disease virus Omsk hemorrhagic fever virus Dengue virus (primary infection only rarely causes hemorrhagic fever)	– Family name from Latin "flavus" for "yellow" – Icosahedral virions – Single-stranded nonsegmented RNA Size: 10–12 kbp, 40–50 nm in diameter Virions covered with surface projections comprised of M (membrane) and E (envelope) glycoproteins

(References 118–125).

pathogenesis of this disease remain unclear; however, its high case-fatality rate (50% to 90%) and its potential for weaponization have made it an increasing focus of public health interest in recent years.

Clinically, Ebola HF presents with fever, maculopapular rash (especially on the trunk), myalgias, chest pain, jaundice, and severe prostration. After several days, bleeding ensues, followed by DIC, shock, and end-organ failure. Death occurs usually within 10 days of symptom onset (128,129).

Modes of transmission in nature include person to person, contact with blood or body fluids (including semen), or direct contact with nonhuman primates and possibly via aerosolization (130–132).

Marburg Hemorrhagic Fever

Marburg virus is a member of the Filoviridae family and shares many similarities to Ebola virus. It was discovered in 1967 following an outbreak in laboratory workers in Marburg, Germany (as well as in Yugoslavia) (133). It has been responsible for several outbreaks in central Africa, the largest in the Democratic Republic of the Congo in 1998 (134).

It has a similar but less lethal clinical picture than Ebola virus; case-fatality rates are generally less than 25%. Like Ebola, its pathogenesis, modes of transmission, and reservoirs have not been completely elucidated.

Lassa fever

Lassa fever virus is a member of the Arenaviridae family of viruses. It is a disease that has become endemic in West Africa over the past 30 years. It was discovered in 1969 in northern Nigeria and has been responsible for 100,000 to 300,000 yearly infections since that time (135). Occasionally, it is imported into the United States or other Western countries (136).

Clinically, Lassa fever is characterized by a prodrome of fever and general malaise, followed by severe exudative pharyngitis; occasionally maculopapular rash and prostration; and, in about ⅓ of cases, bleeding manifestations. The case-fatality rate is about 15%. Ribavirin therapy is helpful in management of severe cases.

New World Arenavirus Hemorrhagic Fevers

Several different viruses from the Arenaviridae family are responsible for the New World HFs. Most cases occur in South America, although one strain, Whitewater Arroyo virus, has been identified as a cause of disease in California (137). The virus is transmitted from asymptomatic, infected rodents that serve as a reservoir for the virus. The disease is common in the endemic regions of Bolivia and Argentina; however, some viruses have been responsible for only a very small number of cases.

New World HF viruses that cause disease in humans include Junin virus (Argentine HF), Machupo virus (Bolivian HF), Guanarito virus (Venezuelan HF), Sabia virus (Brazilian HF), and Whitewater Arroyo virus.

Clinically, they are similar; most cases are notable for fever, sore throat, myalgias, conjunctivitis, petechiae and other bleeding manifestations, neurologic involvement, and occasionally shock. Recovery occurs over 2 to 3 weeks; the overall case-fatality rate is 15% to 30% (138).

Rift Valley Fever

Mosquitoes serve as the vector for Rift Valley fever virus, a Bunyavirus (Family Bunyaviridae, genus Phlebovirus), which is endemic in sub-Saharan and North Africa. The disease virus was first discovered in sheep in 1930 in Kenya (139). Livestock and humans are most often affected. Epizootics in animals characteristically involve high rates of prenatal sheep or cattle mortality and spontaneous, high rates of abortions. Outbreaks are episodic and most often follow heavy rainfall that results in flooding of previously dry areas, allowing for extensive hatching of the primary mosquito vector (140).

Human illness is usually relatively mild, although most infections are subclinically evident. In less than 1% of cases, VHF with marked hepatitis and bleeding manifestations can occur. Encephalitis is also an infrequent manifestation of the disease. Retinitis occurs in perhaps 10% of cases, is associated with secondary blindness, and may be associated with permanent visual impairment. The overall case-fatality rate is less than 1% but is as high as 50% in cases of HF.

Yellow Fever

Yellow fever virus is a member of the Flaviviridae family of viruses. It has been described as early as the 1600s and continues to be endemic in sub-Saharan Africa and tropical South America (141). A variety of mosquito species serve as vectors for yellow fever virus. The WHO estimates 200,000 cases per year and 30,000 deaths worldwide, although many of these are unreported.

Many cases of yellow fever are mild or even subclinical. Cases of severe disease are characterized by fulminant hepatitis, bleeding, renal failure, shock, and death. The overall case-fatality rate is from 5% to about 20% but increases to 50% or more for patients with severe disease.

Kyasanur Forest Disease and Omsk Hemorrhagic Fever

Kyasanur Forest disease is a rare, tick-borne infection found only in one region of India. Outbreaks occur periodically and parallel epizootics are found in the local monkey population. Omsk HF is also a rare form of VHF, limited to regions of Central Asia and Siberia. It is associated with episodic outbreaks that have been documented since the 1940s and 1950s (142).

The clinical picture is similar to other HF viruses; many cases are mild, but severe disease can be associated with meningoencephalitis and VHF. The overall case-fatality rate for Kyasanur Forest disease is 3% to 10% and for Omsk HF is 0.5% to 10%.

Hemorrhagic Fever Viruses as Biologic Weapons

VHF viruses have been the subject of considerable research and development as biologic weapons; the United States, before

1972, conducted research on a variety of agents, and the Soviet Union weaponized Marburg virus and conducted research on Ebola, Lassa, and Rift Valley fever viruses and others. There is concern that North Korea may have weaponized yellow fever virus (143).

These viruses have characteristics that make them attractive as biologic agents of terror: They are infectious by aerosols at low doses and can be aerosolized, they can cause high fatality rates with a dramatic clinical syndrome that could contribute to subsequent wide-spread panic and social destabilization, and many are readily available and have been extensively researched by several countries. In addition, treatment options are limited or nonexistent.

The CDC, in 2000, listed Ebola, Marburg, and Lassa viruses and New World arenaviruses as Category A agents; those most likely to cause mass casualties if deliberately disseminated. In 2002, the Working Group on Civilian Biodefense added Rift Valley Fever virus, yellow fever virus, Kyasanur Forest disease virus, and Omsk HF virus to the list compiled by the CDC (127).

Therapeutic Countermeasures for Weaponized Viral Hemorrhagic Fever

Treatment

The mainstay of treatment for VHF is supportive, intensive care as indicated by the complications of the disease. Management of bleeding diatheses is controversial but generally involves the administration of blood and clotting factor components as indicated by the laboratory findings. Heparin or tissue factor antagonists may be useful therapeutic choices in cases of DIC (144). Steroids have not been shown to be effective but should be considered with evidence of adrenal involvement (145,146).

Ribavirin has some *in vitro* activity against members of the Arenaviridae and Bunyaviridae (127,147–150). *In vivo,* the major established therapeutic use of the drug is in the Arenavirus HFs. Human data are available for Lassa fever, but for the Bolivian, Argentine, and Brazilian viruses there are only animal data with anecdotal clinical reports (151–154). There are a number of experimental approaches that are impractical or insufficiently developed, including passive antibody therapy or interferon prophylaxis. Antiviral agents have not been shown to be effective against diseases caused by filoviruses or flaviviruses (127).

Postexposure Prophylaxis

There is no effective postexposure prophylaxis for asymptomatic persons exposed to weaponized HF virus. The Working Group on Civilian Biodefense instead recommends that exposed populations be placed under surveillance for signs of fever or other symptoms suggestive of VHF. In the event of a documented fever higher than 101°F, persons should be given intravenous ribavirin unless the agent is a confirmed filovirus or flavivirus (155). This is an off-label use, and intravenous ribavirin is mainly accessible for compassionate use. Surveillance should continue for 21 days following exposure (127).

Vaccine

The only effective licensed vaccine against VHF is yellow fever vaccine. It is a live-virus vaccine and has been associated with many adverse events including fever, jaundice, and multiple organ system failure on rare occasions. The vaccine is in limited supply and is only recommended for travelers to areas endemic for yellow fever and laboratory personnel with an ongoing exposure risk to yellow fever (156).

In the event of a bioterrorist attack, yellow fever vaccine would not be effective as a prophylactic treatment following exposure, because the disease incubation period is significantly shorter than the time required for developing immunity following vaccination (127,157).

Vaccines against Argentine HF and Rift Valley fever are known to be efficacious but are available only as investigational drugs (158). Efforts to develop additional vaccines against various HF viruses are ongoing (159–161).

Implications for Healthcare Workers

Transmission within healthcare settings has been documented for several VHFs, including Ebola, Marburg, Lassa, Machupo, and Crimean-Congo viruses (7). Nosocomial transmission has usually occurred by contact with infected body fluids or blood (162,163). Needlesticks or the reuse of needles has also been associated with viral transmission (159,164). Although these viruses form stable infectious aerosols, person-to-person airborne transmission is distinctly uncommon, the potential for airborne transmission in a healthcare setting cannot be ruled out (127,165). There is one documented case of airborne transmission of Machupo virus to a nursing student observing a bed linen change. The student had no physical contact with the patient or any associated fomites (166). Contact with cadavers has also been a documented source of infection during outbreaks with Ebola HF (167).

Healthcare workers must exercise appropriate isolation procedures for patients with suspected or confirmed VHF including a combination of Airborne and Contact Precautions (7). The Working Group on Civilian Biodefense recommends the following precautions for healthcare settings (127):

- All healthcare workers must have appropriate personal protective equipment, including N95 masks or personal air-purifying respirators (PAPR).
- Patients must be placed in a negative pressure room, with restriction of nonessential staff and visitors.
- All healthcare workers who have had high-risk close contact with patients suspected of having VHF should be placed under medical surveillance for 21 days following exposure (127).
- If multiple patients suspected of having VHF are admitted to a healthcare facility, they should be cohorted to minimize exposure to healthcare workers and other patients.

All cases of suspected VHF should be reported immediately to state or local public health officials, according to disease reporting requirements.

REFERENCES

1. Osterholm MT, Schwartz J. *Living terrors: what America needs to know to survive the coming bioterrorist catastrophe.* New York: Delacorte Press, 2000.
2. Miller J, Engelberg S, Broad W. *Germs: biological weapons and America's secret war.* New York: Simon & Schuster, 2001.
3. Meselson M, Guillemin J, Hugh-Jones M, et al. The Sverdlovsk anthrax outbreak of 1979. *Science* 1994;266:1202–1208.
4. Henderson DA. The looming threat of bioterrorism. *Science* 1999; 283:1279–1282.
5. Centers for Disease Control and Prevention. Biological and chemical terrorism: strategic plan for preparedness and response: recommendations of the CDC strategic planning workgroup. *MMWR Morb Mortal Wkly Rep* 2000:49(RR04):1–14.
6. Manchee RJ, Broster MG, Stagg AJ, et al. Out of Gruinard Island. *Salisbury Med Bull* 1990;68(Special Suppl):17–18.
7. Weber DJ, Rutala WA. Risks and prevention of nosocomial transmission of rare zoonotic diseases. *Clin Infect Dis* 2001;32:446–456.
8. Weber DJ, Rutala WA. Recognition and management of anthrax [Letter]. *N Engl J Med* 2002;346:943–946.
9. Centers for Disease Control and Prevention. Investigation of bioterrorism-related anthrax and interim guidelines for clinical evaluation of persons with possible anthrax. *MMWR Morb Mortal Wkly Rep* 2001;50;941–948.
10. Abramova FA, Grinberg LM, Yampolskaya OV. Pathology of inhalational anthrax in 42 cases from the Sverdlovsk outbreak of 1979. *Proc Natl Acad Sci* 1993;90:2291–2294.
11. Franz DR, Jahrling PB, Friedlander AM, et al. Clinical recognition and management of patients exposed to biological warfare agents. *JAMA* 1997;278:399–411.
12. Peters CJ, Hartley DM. Anthrax inhalation and lethal human infection. *Lancet* xxxx;359:710–711.
13. Inglesby TV, O''Toole, T, Henderson DA, et al. for the Working Group on Civilian Biodefense. Anthrax as a biological weapon, 2002: updated recommendations for management. *JAMA* 2002;287: 2236–2252.
14. WHOCC. World anthrax data site [Home page].
15. Brachman PS. Anthrax. In: Warren KS, Mahmoud AF, eds. *Tropical and geographic medicine.* New York: McGraw-Hill, 1984:826–830.
16. Centers for Disease Control and Prevention. Human anthrax associated with an epizootic among livestock—North Dakota, 2000. *MMWR Morb Mortal Wkly Rep* 2001;50:677–680.
17. Sirisanthana T, Brown AE. Anthrax of the gastrointestinal tract. *Emerg Infect Dis* 2002;8(7).
18. Brookmeyer R, Blades N, Hugh-Jones M, et al. The statistical analysis of truncated data: application to the Sverdlovsk anthrax outbreak. *Biostatistics* 2001;2:233–247.
19. Jernigan DB, Raghunathan PL, Bell BP, et al. investigation of bioterrorism-related anthrax, United States, 2001; epidemiologic findings. *Emerg Infect Dis* 2002;8:1019–1028.
20. Brookmeyer R, Blades N. Prevention of inhalational anthrax in the US outbreak. *Science* 2002;295:1861.
21. BioPort Corporation. Anthrax vaccine adsorbed (Biothrax) [Package Insert].
22. Turnbull PCB, Broster MG, Carman JA, et al. Development of antibodies to protective antigen and lethal factor components of anthrax toxin in humans and guinea pigs and their relevance to protective immunity. *Infect Immun* 1986;52:356–363.
23. Centers for Disease Control and Prevention. Use of anthrax vaccine in response to terrorism: supplemental recommendations of the Advisory Committee on Immunization Practices. *MMWR Morb Mortal Wkly Rep* 2002;51:1024–1026.
24. Centers for Disease Control and Prevention. Investigation of anthrax associated with intentional exposure and interim public health guidelines, October 2001. *MMWR Morb Mortal Wkly Rep* 2001;50: 889–93.
25. Centers for Disease Control and Prevention. Interim guidelines for investigation of and response to *Bacillus anthracis* exposures. *MMWR Morb Mortal Wkly Rep* 2001;50:987–990.
26. Wein LM, Craft DL, Kaplan EH. Emergency response to an anthrax attack. *Proc Natl Acad Sci* 2003;100:4346–4351.
27. Swartz MN. Current concepts: recognition and management of anthrax—an update. *N Engl J Med* 2001;345:1621–1626.
28. Occupational Safety and Health Administration. Fact sheet and references on worker health and safety for anthrax exposure [Web page].
29. Siegel LS. Human immune response to botulinum pentavalent (ABCDE) toxoid determined by a neutralization test and by an enzyme-linked immunosorbent assay. *J Clin Microbiol* 1988;26; 2341–2346.
30. Smith LDS. The occurrence of *Clostridium botulinum* and *Clostridium tetani* in the soil of the United States. *Health Lab Sci* 1978;15(12): 74–80.
31. Shapiro RL, Hatheway C, Becher J, et al. Botulism surveillance and emergency response: a public health strategy for a global challenge. *JAMA* 1997;278:433–435.
32. Werner SB, Passaro K, McGee J, et al. Wound botulism in California, 1951–1998: recent epidemic in heroin injectors. *Clin Infect Dis* 2000; 31:1018–1024.
33. Centers for Disease Control and Prevention. *Botulism in the United States, 1899–1996. Handbook for epidemiologists, clinicians, and laboratory workers.* Atlanta, GA: Centers for Disease Control and Prevention, 1998.
34. Angulo FJ, Getz J, Taylor JP, et al. A large outbreak of botulism: the hazardous baked potato. *J Infect Dis* 1998;178:172–177.
35. Chou JH, Hwant PH, Malison MD. An outbreak of type A foodborne botulism in Taiwan due to commercially preserved peanuts. *Int J Epidemiol* 1988;17:899–902.
36. St Louis ME, Peck SHS, Bowering D, et al. Botulism from chopped garlic: delayed recognition of a major outbreak. *Ann Intern Med* 1988; 108:363–368.
37. Townes JM, Cieslak PR, Hatheway CL, et al. An outbreak of type A botulism associated with a commercial cheese sauce. *Ann Intern Med* 1996;125:558–563.
38. MacDonald KL, Spengler RF, Hatheway CL, et al. Type A botulism from sauteed onions: clinical and epidemiologic observations. *JAMA* 1985;253:1275–1278.
39. Arnon SS, Schechter R, Inglesby TV, et al. Botulinum toxin as a biological weapon: medical and public health management. *JAMA* 2001;285:1059—1081.
40. Siegel 1993.
41. Franz DR, Pitt LM, Clayton MA, et al. Efficacy of prophylactic and therapeutic administration of antitoxin for inhalation botulism. In: DasGupta BR, ed. *Botulism and tetanus neurotoxins: neurotransmission and biomedical aspects.* New York: Plenum Press, 1993:473–476.42.
43. Shapiro RL, Hatheway C, Swerdlow DL. Botulism in the United States: a clinical and epidemiologic review. *Ann Intern Med* 1998; 129:221–228.
44. Centers for Disease Control and Prevention. *Biosafety in microbiological and biomedical laboratories (BMBL),* 4th ed. Atlanta, GA: Centers for Disease Control and Prevention, 1999.
45. MacDonald KL, Cohen ML, Blake PA. The changing epidemiology of botulism in the United States. *Am J Epidemiol* 1986;124:794–799.
46. Gilchrist MJR. The progress, priorities and concerns of public health laboratories. Presented at the Forum on Infections, Biological Threats and Terrorism, Institute of Medicine, November 28, 2001.
47. Solomon HM, Lilly T Jr. *Clostridium botulinum.* In: Jackson GH, Merker RI, Bandler R, project coordinators. *Bacteriological analytical manual online.* Washington DC: FDA CFSAN, 2001.
48. Centers for Disease Control and Prevention. Level A laboratory procedures for identification of *Yersinia pestis.*
49. Achtman M, Zurth K, Morelli G, et al. *Yersinia pestis,* the cause of plague, is a recently emerged clone of *Yersinia pseudotuberculosis* (erratum in *Proc Natl Acad Sci* 2000;97:8192). *Proc Natl Acad Sci* 1999;96:14043–14048.
50. Guiyoule A, Rasoamanana B, Buchrieser C, et al. Recent emergence of new variants of *Yersinia pestis* in Madagascar. *J Clin Microbiol* 1997; 35:2826–2833.
51. Dennis D, Meier F. Plague. In: Horsburgh CR, Nelson AM, eds.

Pathology of emerging infections. Washington DC: ASM Press, 1997: 21–47.
52. Butler T. Plague. In: Strickland GT, ed. *Tropical medicine.* Philadelphia: WB Saunders, 1991:408–416.
53. Perry RD, Fetherston JD. *Yersina pestis*—etiologic agent of plague. Clin Microbiol Rev 1997;10(1):35–66.
54. Gage KL, Dennis DT, Orloski KA, et al. Cases of cat-associated human plague in the Western US, 1977–1998. *Clin Infect Dis* 2000; 30:893–900.
55. Reed WP, Palmer DL, Williams RC Jr, et al. Bubonic plague in the southwestern United States: a review of recent experience. *Medicine (Balt)* 1970;49:465–486.
56. World Health Organization. Plague. In: *WHO report on global surveillance of epidemic-prone infectious diseases, 2000.*
57. Caten JL, Kartman L. Human plague in the United States, 1900–1966. *JAMA* 1968;205:333–336.
58. Kaufmann AF, Boyce JM, Martone W. Trends in human plague in the United States. *J Infect Dis*1980;141:522–524.
59. Centers for Disease Control and Prevention. Fatal human plague—Arizona and Colorado, 1996. *MMWR Morb Mortal Wkly Rep* 1997;46:617–620.
60. Centers for Disease Control and Prevention. Summary of notifiable diseases—United States, 2000. *MMWR Morb Mortal Wkly Rep* 2002; 49(53):1–120.
61. Centers for Disease Control and Prevention. Human plague—United States, 1993–1994. *MMWR Morb Mortal Wkly Rep* 1994;43: 242–246.
62. McGovern TW, Friedlander AM. Plague. In: Zajtchuk R, Bellamy RF, eds. *Textbook of military medicine: medical aspects of chemical and biological warfare.* Washington DC: Office of the Surgeon General, Borden Institute, Walter Reed Army Medical Center, 1997.
63. Inglesby TV, Dennis DT, Henderson DA, et al. for the Working Group on Civilian Biodefense. Plague as a biological weapon: medical and public health management. *JAMA* 2000;283:2281–290.
64. Inglesby TV, Grossman R, O"Toole T. A plague on your city: observations from TOPOFF. *Biodefense Q* 2000;(2).
65. World Health Organization. *Health aspects of chemical and biological weapons.* Geneva, Switzerland: World Health Organization, 1970: 98–109.
66. Advisory Committee on Immunization Practices /Centers for Disease Control and Prevention. Prevention of plague: recommendations of the Advisory Committee on Immunization Practices (ACIP). *MMWR Morb Mortal Wkly Rep* 1996;45(RR14):1–15.
67. Anderson GW Jr, Heath DG, Bolt CR, et al. Short- and long-term efficacy of single-dose subunit vaccines against *Yersinia pestis* in mice. *Am J Trop Med Hyg* 1998;58:793–799.
68. Titball RW, Williamson ED. Vaccination against bubonic and pneumonic plague. *Vaccine* 2001;19:4175–4184.
69. Rose LJ, Donlan R, Banerjee SN, et al. Survival of *Yersinia pestis* on environmental surfaces. *Appl Environ Microbiol* 2003;69:2166–2171.
70. Centers for Disease Control and Prevention/Hospital Infection Control Practices Advisory Committee. Recommendations for isolation precautions in hospitals. *Am J Infect Control* 1996;24:24–52.
71. LeDuc JW, Jahrling PB. Strengthening national preparedness for smallpox; an update. *Emerg Infect Dis* 2001;7:155–157.
72. Fenner F, Henderson DA, Arita I, et al. *Smallpox and its eradication.* Geneva, Switzerland: World Health Organization, 1988
73. World Health Organization. Smallpox eradication: destruction of variola virus stocks. Executive Board Documentation, Dec 20, 2001.
74. Wehrle PF, Posch J, Richter KH, et al. An airborne outbreak of smallpox in a German hospital and its significance with respect to other recent outbreaks in Europe. *Bull WHO* 1970;43:669–679.
75. Stearn EW, Stearn AE. *The effect of smallpox on the destiny of the Amerindian.* Boston: Bruce Humphries, 1945.
76. Henderson DA, Inglesby TV, Bartlett JG, et al. Smallpox as a biological weapon: medical and public health management. *JAMA* 1999; 281:2127–2139.
77. Gani R, Leach S. Transmission potential of smallpox in contemporary populations. *Nature* 2001;414:748–751.
78. Rao AR, Jacob ES, Kamalakshi S, et al. Epidemiological studies in smallpox: a study of intrafamilial transmission in a series of 254 infected families. *Indian J Med Res* 1968;56:1826–1854.
79. Arnt N, Morris L. Smallpox outbreaks in two Brazilian villages: epidemiologic characteristics. *Am J Epidemiol* 1972;95:363–370.
80. Heiner GG, Fatima N, McCrumb FR. A study of intrafamilial transmission of smallpox. *Am J Epidemiol* 1971;94:316–326.
81. Henderson DA. Smallpox: clinical and epidemiologic features. *Emerg Infect Dis* 1999;5:537–539.
82. Jezek Z, Szczeniowski M, Paluku KM, et al. Human monkeypox: clinical features of 282 patients. *J Infect Dis* 1987;156:293–298.
83. Arita I, Jezek Z, Khodakevich L, et al. Human monkeypox: a newly emerged orthopoxvirus zoonosis in the tropical rain forests of Africa. *Am J Trop Med Hyg* 1985;34:781–789.
84. Breman JG, Arita I, Fenner F. Preventing the return of smallpox. *N Engl J Med* 2003;348:463–466.
85. Jezek Z, Grab B, Szczeniowski MV, et al. Human monkeypox: secondary attack rates. *Bull WHO* 1988;66:465–470.
86. Jezek Z, Marennikova SS, Mutumbo M, et al. Human monkeypox: a study of 2,510 contacts of 214 patients. *J Infect Dis* 1986;154: 551–555.
87. Centers for Disease Control and Prevention. Preliminary report: multistate outbreak of monkeypox in persons exposed to pet prairie dogs. Jun 9, 2003.
88. Henderson DA. Bioterrorism as a public health threat. *Emerg Infect Dis* 1998;4:488–492.
89. O"Toole T, Mair M, Inglesby TV. Shining light on "Dark Winter." *Clin Infect Dis* 2002;34:972–983.
90. Frey SE, Couch RB, Tacket CO, et al. Clinical responses to undiluted and diluted smallpox vaccine. *N Engl J Med* 2002;346:1265–1274.
91. Frey SE, Newman FK, Cruz J, et al. Dose-related effects of smallpox vaccine. *N Engl J Med* 2002;346:1275–1280.
92. Frey SE, Newman FK, Yan L, et al. Response to smallpox vaccine in persons immunized in the distant past. *JAMA* 2003;289:3295–3299.
93. Henderson DA, Fenner F. Recent events and observations pertaining to smallpox virus destruction in 2002. *Clin Infect Dis* 2001;33: 1057–1059.
94. Centers for Disease Control and Prevention. Smallpox response plan and guidelines, Nov 26, 2002. Version 3.0.
95. Barbera J, Macintyre A, Gostin L, et al. Large-scale quarantine following biological terrorism in the United States: scientific examination, logistic and legal limits, and possible consequences. *JAMA* 2001;286: 2711–2717.
96. Centers for Disease Control and Prevention. Recommendations for using smallpox vaccine in a pre-event smallpox vaccination program. Supplemental recommendations of ACIP and HICPAC. *MMWR Morb Mortal Wkly Rep* xxxx;52(RR07):1–16.
97. Centers for Disease Control and Prevention. Supplemental recommendations on adverse events following smallpox vaccine in the pre-event vaccination program: recommendations of the Advisory Committee on Immunization Practices. *MMWR Morb Mortal Wkly Rep* 2003;52(13):282–284.
98. Centers for Disease Control and Prevention. Level A laboratory procedures for identification of *Francisella tularensis.* Laboratory Response Network. Rev Dec 13, 2001.
99. Cross JT, Penn RL. *Francisella tularensis.* In: Mandell GL, Bennett JE, Dolin R, eds. *Principles and practice of infectious diseases,* 5th ed. New York: Churchill Livingstone, 2000:2393–2402.
100. Sneath PH, Mair NS, Sharpe ME et al, eds. *Bergey's manual of systematic bacteriology,* vol 2. Baltimore: Williams & Wilkins, 1986.
101. Dennis DT. Tularemia. In: Wallace RB, ed. *Public health and preventive medicine,* 14th ed. Stamford, CT: Appleton & Lange; 1998: 354–357.
102. Hopla CE. The ecology of tularemia. *Adv Vet Sci Comp Med* 1974; 18:25–53.
103. Gelman AG. The ecology of tularemia. In: May JM, ed. *Studies in disease ecology.* New York: Hafner Publishing Co, 1961:89–108.
104. Centers for Disease Control and Prevention. Outbreak of tularemia among commercially distributed prairie dogs, 2002. *MMWR Morb Mortal Wkly Rep* 2002;51(31):688, 699.

105. Klock LE, Olsen PF, Fukushima T. Tularemia epidemic associated with the deerfly. *JAMA* 1973;226:149–152.
106. Mignani E, Palmieri E, Fontana M, et al. Italian epidemic of waterborne tularaemia. *Lancet*1988;2:1423.
107. Reintjes R, Dedusha I, Gjini A, et al. Tularemia outbreak investigation in Kosovo: case control and environmental studies. *Emerg Infect Dis* 2002;8:69–73.
108. Young LS, Bicknell DS, Archer BG, et al. Tularemia epidemic: Vermont 1968. Forty-seven cases linked to contact with muskrats. *N Engl J Med* 1969;280:1253–1260.
109. Dahlstrand S, Ringertz O, Zetterberg B. Airborne tularemia in Sweden. *Scand J Infect Dis* 1971;3:7–16.
110. Feldman KA, Enscore RE, Lathrop SL, et al. An outbreak of primary pneumonic tularemia on Martha's Vineyard. *N Engl J Med* 2001; 345:1601–1606.
111. Overholt EL, Tibertt WD, Kadull PJ, et al. An analysis of forty-two cases of laboratory-acquired tularemia. *Am J Med* 1961;30:785–806.
112. Dennis DT, Inglesby TV, Henderson DA, et al. Tularemia as a biological weapon: medical and public health management. *JAMA* 2001; 285:2763–2773.
113. Centers for Disease Control and Prevention. Summary of notifiable diseases—United States, 2000. *MMWR Morb Mortal Wkly Rep* 2002; 49(53):1–120.
114. World Health Organization. *Health aspects of chemical and biological weapons.* Geneva, Switzerland: World Health Organization, 1970:98.
115. Sawyer WD, Dangerfield HG, Hogge AL, et al. Antibiotic prophylaxis and therapy of airborne tularemia. *Bacteriol Rev* 1966;30:542–548.
116. Pike RM. Laboratory-associated infections: summary and analysis of 3921 cases. *Health Lab Sci* 1976;13(2):105–114.
117. Shapiro DS, Schwartz DR. Exposure of laboratory workers to *Francisella tularensis* despite a bioterrorism procedure. *J Clin Microbiol* 2002; 40:2278–2281.
118. Peters CJ. Marburg and Ebola virus hemorrhagic fevers. In: Mandell GL, Bennett JE, Dolin R, eds. *Principles and practice of infectious diseases,* 5th ed. New York: Churchill Livingstone, 2000:1821–1822.
119. Feldman H, Volchkov VE, Volchcova VA, et al. The glycoproteins of Marburg and Ebola virus and their potential roles in pathogenesis. *Arch Virol* 1999;159(Suppl):159–169.
120. Jahrling PB, Geisbert TW, Geisbert JB, et al. Evaluation of immune globulin and recombinant interferon-alpha2b for treatment of experimental Ebola virus infections. *J Infect Dis* 1999;179(Suppl 1): S224–S234.
121. Sanchez A, Trappier SG, Mahy BW, et al. The virion glycoproteins of Ebola viruses are encoded in two reading frames and are expressed through transcriptional editing. *Proc Natl Acad Sci U S A* 1996;93: 3602–3607.
122. Sanchez A, Yang ZY, Xu L, et al. Biochemical analysis of the secreted and virion glycoproteins of Ebola virus. *J Virol* 1998;72:6442–6447.
123. Sanchez A, Ksiazek TG, Rollin PE, et al. Detection and molecular characterization of Ebola viruses causing disease in human and nonhuman primates. *J Infect Dis* 1999;179(Suppl 1):S164–S169.
124. Tsai TF. Arboviruses. In: Murray PR, Baron EJ, Pfaller MA, et al., eds. *Manual of clinical microbiology,* 7th ed. Washington DC: American Society for Microbiology Press, 1999:1107–1124.
125. Tsai TF. Flaviviruses (yellow fever, Dengue, Dengue hemorrhagic fever, Japanese encephalitis, St. Louis encephalitis, tick-borne encephalitis). In: Mandell GL, Bennett JE, Dolin R, eds. *Principles and practice of infectious diseases,* 5th ed. New York: Churchill Livingstone, 2000:1855–1873.
126. Peters CJ, Zaki SR. Role of the endothelium in viral hemorrhagic fevers. *Crit Care Med* 2002;30(5 Suppl):S268–S273.
127. Borio L, Inglesby T, Peters CJ, et al. Hemorrhagic fever viruses as biological weapons: medical and public health management. *JAMA* 2002;287:2391–2405.
128. Peters CJ, LeDuc JW. An introduction to Ebola: the virus and the disease. *J Infect Dis* 1999;179(Suppl 1):ix–xvi .
129. Gubler DJ, Zaki SR. Dengue and other viral hemorrhagic fevers. In: Nelson AM, Horsburgh CR, eds. *Pathology of emerging infections 2.* Washington DC: American Society of Microbiology Press, 1998: 43–71.
130. Johnson E, Jaax N, White J, et al. Lethal experimental infections of rhesus monkeys by aerosolized Ebola virus. *Int J Exp Pathol* 1995; 76:227–236.
131. Kenyon RH, McKee KT Jr, Sack PM, et al. Aerosol infection of rhesus macaques with Junin virus. *Intervirology* 1992;33(1):23–31.
132. Stephenson EH, Larson EW, Dominik JW. Effect of environmental factors on aerosol-induced Lassa virus infection. *J Med Virol* 1984; 14:295–303.
133. Martini GA, Sieger R, eds. *Marburg virus disease.* Berlin: Springer-Verlag, 1971.
134. World Health Organization. Outbreak News Index: Hemorrhagic fever.
135. McCormick JB, Webb PA, Krebs JW, et al. A prospective study of the epidemiology and ecology of Lassa fever. *J Infect Dis* 1987;155: 437–444.
136. Isaacson M. Viral hemorrhagic fever hazards for travelers in Africa. *Clin Infect Dis* 2001;33:1707–1712.
137. Centers for Disease Control and Prevention. Fatal illness associated with a New World arenavirus—California, 1999-2000. *MMWR Morb Mortal Wkly Rep* 2000;49(31):709–711.
138. Centers for Disease Control and Prevention. Bolivian hemorrhagic fever—El Beni Department, Bolivia, 1994. *MMWR Morb Mortal Wkly Rep* 1994;43(50):943–946.
139. Daubney R, Hudson JR, Garnham PC. Enzootic hepatitis or Rift Valley fever: an undescribed virus disease of sheep, cattle, and man from East Africa. *J Pathol Bacteriol* 1931;34:545–579.
140. LeDuc JW. Epidemiology of hemorrhagic fever viruses. *Rev Infect Dis* 1989;11(Suppl 4):S730–735.
141. World Health Organization. Fact sheets: yellow fever. Dec 2000.
142. World Health Organization. Viral hemorrhagic fevers: report of a WHO expert committee, 1984.
143. Monterey Institute of International Studies: Center for Nonproliferation Studies. Chemical and biological weapons possession and programs past and present. November 2000.
144. Jahrling P. Viral hemorrhagic fevers. In: Zajtchuk R, Bellamy RF, eds. *Textbook of military medicine: medical aspects of chemical and biological warfare.*Washington DC: Office of the Surgeon General, Borden Institute, Walter Reed Army Medical Center, 1997.
145. Abraham E, Evans T. Corticosteroids and septic shock [Editorial]. *JAMA* 2002;288:886—887.
146. Annane D, Sebille V, Charpentier C, et al. Effect of treatment with low doses of hydrocortisone and fludrocortisone on mortality in patients with septic shock. *JAMA* 2002:288:862–871.
147. Enria DA, Maiztegui JI. Antiviral treatment of Argentine hemorrhagic fever. *Antivirol Res*1994;23:23–31.
148. Huggins JW. Prospects for treatment of viral hemorrhagic fevers with ribavirin, a broad-spectrum antiviral drug. *Rev Infect Dis* 1989; 11(Suppl 4):S750–S761.
149. Kilgore PE, Ksiazek TB, Rollin PE, et al. Treatment of Bolivian hemorrhagic fever with intravenous ribavirin. *Clin Infect Dis* 1997;24: 718–722.
150. McCormick JB, King IJ, Webb PA, et al. A case-control study of the clinical diagnosis and course of Lassa fever. *J Infect Dis* 1987;155: 445–455.
151. Enria D, Maiztegui JI. Antiviral treatment of Argentine hemorrhagic fever. *Antivirol Res* 1994;23:23–31.
152. McCormick JB, King IJ, Webb PA, et al. Lassa fever. Effective therapy with ribavirin. *N Engl J Med* 1986:314:20–26.
153. Barry M, Russi M, Armstrong L, et al. Treatment of a laboratory-acquired Sabia virus infection. *N Engl J Med* 1995;333:294–296.
154. Kilgore PE, Ksiazek TG, Rollin PE, et al. Treatment of Bolivian hemorrhagic fever with intravenous ribavirin. *J Infect Dis* 1997;24: 718–722.
155. Enria D, Peters CJ. Other viruses and emerging viruses of concern. In: Boucher CAB, Galasso GA, eds. *Practical guidelines in antiviral therapy.* Amsterdam: Elsevier, 2002:279–301.
156. Centers for Disease Control and Prevention. Yellow fever vaccine recommendations of the Advisory Committee on Immunization Practices (ACIP), 2002. *MMWR Morb Mortal Wkly Rep* 2002;51(RR17): 1–10.

157. Monath TP. Yellow fever: an update. *Lancet Infect Dis* 2001;1:11–20.
158. Maiztegui JI, McKee KT, Barrera Oro JG, et al. Protective efficacy for a live attenuated vaccine against Argentine Hemorrhagic Fever. *J Infect Dis* 1998;177:277–283.
159. Fisher-Hoch SP, Hutwagner L, Brown B, et al. Effective vaccine for Lassa fever. *J Virol* 2000;74:6777–6783.
160. Geisbert TW, Pushko P, Anderson K, et al. Evaluation in nonhuman primates of vaccines against Ebola virus. *Emerg Infect Dis* 2002;8: 503–507.
161. Sullivan NJ, Geisbert TW, Geisbert JB, et al. Accelerated vaccination for Ebola virus haemorrhagic fever in non-human primates. *Nature* 424:681–684.
162. Dowell SF, Mukundu R, Ksiazek TG, et al. Transmission of Ebola hemorrhagic fever: a study of risk factors in family members, Kikwit, Democratic Republic of the Congo, 1995. *J Infect Dis* 1999; 179(Suppl 1):S87–S91.
163. Monath TP. Lassa fever: review of epidemiology and epizootiology. *Bull World Health Organ* 1975;52:577–592.
164. Guimard Y, Bwaka MA, Colebunders R, et al. Organization of patient care during the Ebola hemorrhagic fever epidemic in Kikwit, Democratic Republic of the Congo, 1995. *J Infect Dis* 1999;179(Suppl 1): S268–S273.
165. Peters CJ, Jahrling PB, Khan AS. Management of patients infected with high-hazard viruses: scientific basis for infection control. *Arch Virol* 1996;(Suppl 11):1–28.
166. Peters CJ, Kuehne RW, Mercado RR, et al. Hemorrhagic fever in Cochabamba, Bolivia, 1971. *Am J Epidemiol* 1974;99:425–433.
167. Roels TH, Bloom AS, Buffington J, et al. Ebola hemorrhagic fever, Kikwit, Democratic Republic of the Congo: risk factors for patients without a reported exposure. *J Infect Dis* 1999;179(Suppl 1): S92–S97.

112

PREPAREDNESS FOR A BIOTERRORIST ATTACK WITH SMALLPOX

MICHAEL ALBERT
DANIEL R. LUCEY
JOEL G. BREMAN

Smallpox is a highly infectious disease caused by the variola virus. Although evidence of the existence of smallpox dates back to antiquity, the disease ceased to be a natural threat following its eradication in 1977 (1). Inoculation (initially with cowpox and later with vaccinia virus) as a means of preventing smallpox, had been widely utilized since the British physician, Edward Jenner (2), reported successful results in his famous *Inquiry* in 1798. In the 1960s the World Health Organization (WHO) began the Intensified Smallpox Eradication Programme, an international campaign that was based on immunization, surveillance, and containment of disease. Eradication of smallpox was possible because of certain features related to its control: the lack of an animal reservoir for variola; the production of a characteristic rash that was readily identifiable; the efficacy of a stable vaccine; and the 10- to 14-day incubation period, which resulted in a relatively slow development of epidemics (3). From 1967 to 1973, the number of countries or territories in which smallpox was endemic shrank from 33 to six (4). The last endemic case occurred in Somalia in October 1977, and two additional cases resulted from a laboratory accident in Birmingham, England, in 1978. In December 1979, a special commission of the WHO concluded that smallpox eradication had been achieved throughout the world (4).

Although there have been no cases of smallpox in 25 years, there is concern today about the potential use of variola virus as an agent of bioterrorism or biologic warfare. The number of laboratories retaining variola virus decreased from 76 in 1980 to two in 1984—one each in the United States and the Soviet Union (5). The virus is currently known to exist only at the Centers for Disease Control and Prevention (CDC) in Atlanta, and the State Research Center of Virology and Biotechnology (Vektor Institute) in Novosibirsk, Russia. However, a former deputy director of the Soviet Union's civilian bioweapons program alleged that in the 1980s the Soviet government initiated a program to produce the virus in large quantities and to weaponize it in bombs and intercontinental ballistic missiles (6). This has heightened speculation over the possibility that variola virus may exist outside its known locations and could fall into the hands of rogue states or terrorists. The use of variola in bioterrorism is particularly feared because of its transmissibility from person to person, high case-fatality rate, and the fact that the vast majority of the world's population is now susceptible to smallpox.

In the fall of 2001, envelopes containing *Bacillus anthracis* spores were sent through the U.S. mail, resulting in 22 related cases of anthrax, with five fatalities (7). These attacks, which occurred in the months following terrorist attacks in New York City and Washington, D.C., illustrated the dangers posed by bioterrorism. In response, there has been an intensive effort to prepare for public health emergencies resulting from the use of biologic agents. The threat of the deliberate release of variola is lessened by preparedness including awareness of the disease by clinicians, vaccination of selected healthcare workers and other first responders, the availability of a large stock of vaccine, and emergency guidelines for the control and prevention of smallpox in the event of an epidemic. This chapter reviews the clinical manifestations, diagnosis, epidemiology, control, and prevention of smallpox, and describes how a hospital might manage suspected and confirmed smallpox patients.

ETIOLOGY AND EPIDEMIOLOGY OF SMALLPOX

Variola virus belongs to the Poxviridae family and the genus *Orthopoxvirus* (3). This genus also includes related animal viruses such as the species vaccinia virus, cowpox virus, monkeypox virus, ectromelia virus, camelpox virus, taterapox virus, raccoonpox virus, and Uasin Gishu disease virus. Several benign skin diseases in humans are caused by poxviruses. The most common of these is molluscum contagiosum, frequently encountered in children and young adults, with widespread lesions sometimes occurring in immunosuppressed individuals (8). Other localized conditions resulting from poxviruses occur in individuals exposed to infected animals and include cowpox, milker's nodules, and orf. In central and western Africa, monkeypox is endemic and there are occasional outbreaks of this potentially serious zoonotic disease, which resembles smallpox clinically but differs biologically and epidemiologically (9). A recent outbreak of monkeypox in the U.S. resulted from contact with infected pet prairie dogs that had been housed or transported with imported African rodents (10,10a).

Poxvirus virions are large (approximately 300 × 250 × 200 nm) and rectangular, appearing brick-shaped by electron microscopy (11). The genome of all orthopoxviruses consist of single, linear, double-stranded DNA, ranging in size from approximately 165-kilobase (kb) pairs to 210-kb pairs, with a low guanine and cytosine content (3). The complete genomic sequences for numerous isolates of variola virus have recently been determined (12). Viral replication occurs in the cell cytoplasm, and eosinophilic cytoplasmic inclusion bodies are apparent histologically in infected cells (13). Vaccinia virus, used for smallpox vaccination, shares more than 96% of its nucleotide identity with variola, and essential virion proteins share more than 98% of their amino acid identity (14).

Human-to-human transmission of smallpox usually occurs by virus-laden respiratory droplets, with initial infection of the upper respiratory tract and draining lymph nodes (11). The virus then seeds the reticuloendothelial system, where it multiplies during a clinically latent period of 4 to 14 days before a secondary viremia leads to the onset of cutaneous manifestations. Variola elicits both a cellular and humoral immune response. Cell-mediated immunity is believed to be most important in clearing infection, whereas neutralizing antibodies prevent reinfection (15). Neutralizing antibodies and hemagglutinin-inhibiting antibodies usually appear during the first week of illness and may be detectable for years (3,11).

Smallpox cases are generally considered infectious from the onset of the enanthem until all scabs have separated; however, patient infectivity decreases after the second week of the eruption as oropharyngeal lesions heal (3). Reported secondary attack rates of variola major during the global eradication program ranged from 37% to 88% for unvaccinated household contacts and 1% to 26% for vaccinated household contacts (3). Smallpox is less commonly transmitted from contact with skin lesions or fomites. Smallpox inoculated into the skin usually results in a milder course than when acquired by the respiratory route; indeed, prior to Jenner's introduction of vaccination, intentional variola inoculation in the skin (variolation) was practiced in various cultures (1).

Indirect aerosol transmission of smallpox has occasionally been reported. A well-documented episode occurred in Meschede, Germany, in 1970 (16). Following the hospitalization of a patient with smallpox, 17 of 19 additional cases were determined to be infected by airborne spread of virus over a considerable distance within a single hospital building. Features that were important in viral dissemination in this outbreak were the index patient's extensive rash, severe bronchitis, cough, and the very low relative humidity and strong air currents that existed within the hospital (16).

CLINICAL DISEASE

A 7- to 17-day incubation period (mean 10 to 14 days) precedes the development of signs and symptoms in individuals infected with variola. This is followed by a 1- to 4-day prodromal period. The most common prodromal symptoms in a large patient population studied in Bombay were fever (100%), headache (90%), backache (90%), chills (60%), and vomiting (50%) (17). Pharyngitis, diarrhea, delirium, abdominal colic, and convulsions each occurred in 15% or less of patients. The eruptive period starts with an enanthem appearing in the mouth and oropharynx with small erythematous macules evolving over several days into papules and then vesicles. The skin eruption follows the enanthem by 1 to 2 days, beginning on the face and spreading over the body in a centrifugal distribution, with greater involvement of the face and distal extremities (Figs. 112.1 and 112.2) than the trunk and proximal extremities. The smallpox rash is characterized by lesions that evolve together (monomorphic) over approximately 18 days (Figs. 112.3 to 112.6) as erythematous macules, papules, vesicles, pustules, and crusts. By about day 5 of the rash (Fig. 112.4), vesicles have evolved into pustules, which are deep-seated and may display a characteristic central umbilication. In more severe cases, lesions on the face and extremities may become confluent. The eruption resolves during the third week, with lesions of the palms and soles persisting longest (Fig. 112.2). Recovery from smallpox results in elimination of the virus from the body, and there is no risk of recurrence.

Viral bronchitis or pneumonitis is not uncommon in severe cases of smallpox. Arthritis more commonly occurs in children, primarily resulting from viral infection of the metaphyses of growing bones (3). Other potential complications include keratitis, corneal ulceration, encephalitis, and orchitis. Secondary bacterial infection may also occur, including pneumonia, osteomyelitis, joint infections, septicemia, skin abscesses, and impetiginized skin lesions (15). The most common sequela of smallpox is pitted scars, which have a predilection for the face and occur in more than half of severe cases (11). The cause of death from smallpox is not well understood, but may result from the cytopathic effects of the virus in the lungs, kidneys, and other organs (18). The mortality rate for unvaccinated individuals is approximately 20% to 30% for variola major. Patients with smallpox who have a prior history of vaccination have increased survival and tend to have milder disease (17,19–21). Infants and the elderly have a higher case fatality rate, and pregnant women and persons with immunodeficiency are also at risk for severe disease and death (3,20).

The WHO classified smallpox (variola major) into five clinical types (3): ordinary, modified, hemorrhagic, flat, and variola sine eruptione. Ordinary smallpox constituted almost 90% of cases in unvaccinated individuals. The modified type generally occurred in previously vaccinated individuals and was characterized by an accelerated clinical course with fewer and smaller lesions, and a low mortality. Hemorrhagic smallpox, more prevalent in pregnant women, was associated with hemorrhages into the skin and mucous membranes either early or late in the disease. In the flat type, the skin often had a cobblestone-like appearance, with lesions coalescing, remaining flat, and not progressing to pustules. This rare type occurred primarily in children and was thought to reflect a deficient cellular immune response to variola (15). The hemorrhagic and flat variants were usually fatal. Variola sine eruptione occurred in vaccinated individuals who developed constitutional symptoms but not a rash. Variola minor was a mild variety of smallpox that accounted for >95% of cases in the U.S. during the 20th century and was prominent in parts of South America and eastern and southern Africa (3). Patients with variola minor frequently had smaller lesions that evolved more rapidly, and they did not usually become seriously ill; their mortality rate was less than 1%.

DIAGNOSIS

The differential diagnosis for smallpox includes varicella (chickenpox); a drug hypersensitivity reaction; disseminated herpes zoster; disseminated herpes simplex; contact dermatitis; impetigo; erythema multiforme minor or major; hand, foot, and mouth disease; scabies; arthropod bites; molluscum contagiosum; and human monkeypox (11,22). Prior to its eradication, smallpox was most commonly confused with varicella. Distinguishing clinical features of varicella include a mild or absent febrile prodrome; lesions that are superficial, appear in crops, rapidly evolve, and are present in different stages of development (polymorphic); a concentration of lesions on the trunk; and infrequent involvement of the palms and soles (22). Primary cases of human monkeypox, which may resemble smallpox clinically, are presumed to be infected from an animal source; the virus has a low attack rate and transmission rate for humans (9).

Handling and transport of laboratory specimens of a suspected case of smallpox must be coordinated with local, state, and federal health agencies in accordance with CDC guidelines (23). Laboratory confirmation of smallpox has traditionally relied on isolation of the virus on the chorioallantoic membrane of the chick embryo. Today, polymerase chain reaction (PCR) methods may be employed for rapidly identifying variola virus. PCR strategies may detect both conserved genes of orthopoxviruses as well as variola-specific genes (14). Electron microscopy analysis can be used to identify orthopoxvirus, although the findings are not species specific. Other methods for confirming orthopoxvirus infection include immunohistochemistry and serologic detection of viral antigen (14).

EMERGENCY REPORTING AND RESPONSE

A suspected case of smallpox is a public health emergency that should be reported immediately to state and federal officials. Following prompt isolation of the patient, interviews are conducted to identify close contacts (11). If a case of smallpox is confirmed, surveillance of the health status of contacts is undertaken immediately to identify any additional cases. Those who have been in close contact with the patient since the onset of symptoms and the household members of such persons are vaccinated following exposure in an effort to prevent or modify disease (see below). Symptomatic contacts should be counseled and reported as suspected cases (24). Individuals in the community should be directed to specific facilities for evaluation if they develop a fever and rash (see CDC Plan in 2003: Type C, Type X, and Type R Facilities, below). In addition, hospitals in the area should review recent cases of patients who had symptoms compatible with smallpox. Persons with whom the patient had contact in the 3 weeks prior to onset of signs and symptoms are traced to determine the source of infection.

Because smallpox is no longer naturally occurring, the likely scenarios for its reappearance would include accidental laboratory-associated cases or deliberate release as an act of bioterrorism (24). The surveillance-containment strategy used successfully in the smallpox eradication program in the 1960s and 1970s would be utilized (3). In the event of bioterrorism, large-scale voluntary vaccination may be recommended in the areas affected. Recent guidelines for a model vaccination clinic addressed logistical considerations for postevent large-scale vaccination and provided an example with an output goal of administering vaccine to 1 million individuals over a 10-day period (25).

VACCINATION

The smallpox vaccine available in the U.S. is Dryvax, a lyophilized calf lymph containing the New York City Board of Health (NYCBH) strain of live vaccinia virus. In addition, the CDC recently contracted for the manufacture of a cell culture-grown vaccinia vaccine, available as investigational new drug (IND) product (12,26). Prospective studies are currently being performed to evaluate the reactogenicity of newer vaccine (27). Attenuated vaccines, including the modified vaccinia Ankara vaccine and Japanese strain LC16m8 vaccine, might result in fewer adverse effects, and are also under investigation (26).

Successful primary vaccination induces protective immunity against smallpox in more than 95% of patients (11). Vaccination results in both humoral and cellular immune responses with the induction of neutralizing antibodies, which may be long-lived, as well as vaccinia virus-specific $CD8^+$ cytotoxic T lymphocytes and interferon-γ (IFN-γ)–producing T-cell responses (3,28). Protective immunity generally begins to wane after a period of 5 years following primary vaccination, although the duration of immunity may be longer following successful revaccination (29). Vaccination can also prevent smallpox if given within 3 to 4 days of exposure, and likely offers some protection if performed 4 to 7 days after exposure (29,30,30a).

The standard site of vaccination is the outer aspect of the upper right arm. Vaccination is performed by dipping the tip of a sterile bifurcated needle (Fig. 112.7) into reconstituted vaccine and rapidly making perpendicular strokes (three for primary vaccination and 15 for revaccination) to the skin overlying a 5-mm-diameter area (31). The appearance of a trace of blood indicates that the strokes have been sufficiently vigorous. If successful, an erythematous papule normally develops at the vaccination site within 3 to 4 days, frequently with associated pruritus (32). The papule evolves into a vesicle (day 5 to 6) and then a pustule (day 8 to 9), which crusts over. The scab falls off by about 21 days after vaccination, usually leaving a scar (Fig. 112.8). Response to vaccination should be evaluated (Figs. 112.8 and 112.9) on postvaccination day 6 to 8 (27). Accelerated or modified reactions may occur in persons who have been previously vaccinated.

It is important that a gauze bandage be used to cover the vaccination site until the scab has separated to avoid secondary transmission of vaccinia virus to unvaccinated contacts. Vaccinees who work in a healthcare setting should cover the vaccination site with gauze as well as semipermeable dressing and a shirt (33). Vaccinia-contaminated bandages should be sealed in a plastic bag prior to throwing them away, and careful attention should be paid to hand washing after touching anything that might have become contaminated with virus (33). There have been numerous reports in the medical literature of nosocomial and family outbreaks of vaccinia, although the rate and route of vaccinia transmission remain unknown (34).

The Advisory Committee on Immunization Practices (ACIP) and CDC have listed numerous contraindications to smallpox vaccination (34a). Vaccination is contraindicated when either potential vaccinees or their household contacts have immunodeficiency or immunosuppression from any cause; a history of atopic dermatitis or Darier's disease; acute or chronic dermatologic conditions causing a loss of skin integrity; or pregnancy (35). In addition, vaccination is contraindicated in patients who have an allergy to components of the smallpox vaccine (Dryvax contains polymyxin B sulfate, streptomycin sulfate, chlortetracycline hydrochloride, neomycin sulfate, and phenol), have moderate or severe acute illness, are less than 12 months of age, or are breast-feeding mothers (35). Except when a vaccination program is undertaken to counter a smallpox outbreak, smallpox vaccination is not recommended in persons less than 18 years old or above 65 years old, or those who have inflammatory eye diseases requiring corticosteroid eyedrops (36). Recent reports of myopericarditis and ischemic cardiac events following smallpox vaccination (see below) have added heart disease to the list of contraindications (37). Vaccination should also be avoided in patients with three or more of the following cardiac risk factors: hypertension, hypercholesterolemia, diabetes, cigarette smoking, or a first-degree relative with onset of heart disease under age 50 (37). However, there are no absolute contraindications to vaccination in patients who have confirmed exposure to variola.

Routine smallpox vaccination was discontinued in the U.S. in 1972 and elsewhere by the 1980s upon recommendation of the WHO at the time that smallpox eradication was confirmed. Because of concern about the possible use of variola as a bioterrorism agent, a smallpox vaccination program was reinstituted by President George W. Bush in 2002 (38). Under this plan, voluntary vaccination is being offered to healthcare and other emergency workers who would be the first to respond in the event of an outbreak (Table 112.1). By June 2003, over 37,000 civilian healthcare and public health workers had received smallpox vaccination (39). In addition, vaccination was administered to over 450,000 selected military personnel who were or might be deployed in high-risk areas (40). As initially outlined, approximately 440,000 healthcare responders would be voluntarily vaccinated in phase 1 of the program, followed by up to an additional 10 million medical and emergency workers in phase 2 (26). Because the threat of the deliberate release of variola is considered very low, mass vaccination of the general public is not recommended at present. However, phase 3 of the program would eventually make vaccine available to "those adult members of the general public without medical contraindications who insist on being vaccinated" (38). It is possible the original goals of the smallpox vaccination program will need to be revised due to a lack of volunteers, resistance from labor unions, and concerns over reported cardiac adverse events following smallpox vaccination (see below) (41,42).

TABLE 112.1. RECOMMENDED MEMBERS OF SMALLPOX RESPONSE TEAMS (PER ACIP AND HICPAC)

1. Emergency Department Staff, including physicians and nurses caring for children and adults
2. Intensive care unit staff, including physicians and nurses, and in hospitals that care for infants and children, pediatricians and pediatric intensive care specialists.
3. General medical unit staff, including nurses, internists, pediatricians, hospitalists (physicians whose practice emphasizes providing care for hospitalized patients), and family physicians in institutions where these persons are the essential providers of inpatient medical care.
4. Primary-care house staff (i.e., medical, pediatric, and family physicians)
5. Medical subspecialists, including Infectious Diseases specialists
6. Infection control professionals
7. Respiratory therapists
8. Radiology technicians
9. Security personnel
10. Housekeeping staff (e.g., those staff involved in maintaining the health-care environment and decreasing the risk for fomite transmission).

Adapted from CDC. Recommendation for using smallpox vaccine in a pre-event vaccination program. MMWR. 2003;52(RR-07):1–16
ACIP, Advisory Committee on Immunization Practices; HICPAC, Healthcare Infection Control Practices Advisory Committee

ADVERSE REACTIONS TO SMALLPOX VACCINATION

Local reactions are common in primary vaccination and may include edema, inflammation, and pain at the vaccination site; the appearance of satellite lesions; and swelling and tenderness of regional lymph nodes (43). Common systemic reactions include fever, malaise, and myalgia. A recent study of 680 adults undergoing primary vaccination found that 36.4% were sufficiently ill to miss work, school, or recreational activities, or to have trouble sleeping (44). Among studied military personnel, 0.5–3.0% of vaccine recipients required short-term sick leave (40).

Other potential complications include inadvertent inoculation of the virus at another body site. Inoculation of vaccinia in the cornea (Fig. 112.10) may result in vaccinia keratitis, which can lead to corneal scarring and vision loss. Hypersensitivity reactions, including erythema multiforme (Fig. 112.11), may occur following vaccination. Generalized vaccinia (Fig. 112.12) is believed to result from hematogenous spread of vaccinia, although it is self-limited in the immunocompetent host (27). Patients with either active or inactive atopic dermatitis are at risk for developing eczema vaccinatum (Fig. 112.13), an often severe complication resulting from the spread of vaccinia. Vaccinia necrosum (or progressive vaccinia) (Figs. 112.14 and 112.15) is a rare but life-threatening complication in immunocompromised persons, in which necrosis occurs at the vaccination site, and often other areas of the body (45,46). Postvaccinial

TABLE 112.2. ADVERSE EVENTS FROM VACCINATION

RATES OF COMPLICATIONS FROM PRIMARY VACCINIA VACCINATION AND INDICATIONS FOR VACCINIA IMMUNOGLOBIN (VIG)

Complication	No. of events/1 million[a]	VIG Treatment[b]
Accidental infection	529	May be indicated in ocular inoculation without vaccinial keratitis
Generalized vaccinia	242	May be indicated in patients who are severely ill or have serious underlying illness
Erythema multiforme	165	Not indicated
Eczema vaccinatum	39	Indicated in severe cases
Postvaccinial encephalitis	12	Not indicated
Progressive vaccinia	2	May be effective, depending on immune defect
Other	266	Not indicated

[a] Data from: Lane JM, Ruben FL, Neff JM, Millar JD. Complications of smallpox vaccination, 1968: results of ten statewide surveys. J Infect Dis 1970;122:303–9.
[b] Recommendations from: Vaccinia (Smallpox) Vaccine Recommendations of the Advisory Committee on Immunization Practices (ACIP), 2001.

encephalitis is another severe complication, which has an approximately 15% to 25% mortality rate and results in permanent neurologic sequelae in about 25% of survivors (43). Although rare, fetal vaccinia may result from smallpox vaccination given during pregnancy or shortly before conception and frequently leads to fetal or neonatal death (27).

An analysis of reported complications in a ten-state survey for 1968 estimated a complication rate of 1,250 per million persons receiving primary vaccination and 110 per million for persons receiving revaccination (Table 112.2) (47). Among primary vaccinees, accidental inoculation of vaccinia at other body sites was the most frequently reported complication (42%), with the eyelid being the most commonly affected site. Generalized vaccinia accounted for 19% of complications. Other complications included erythema multiforme (13%), eczema vaccinatum (3%), postvaccinial encephalitis (1%), and vaccinia necrosum (<1%). An additional 21% of complications consisted of other adverse effects, such as bacterial superinfection or pain at the vaccination site. One probable case of fetal vaccinia was also reported.

In the U.S., during the years 1959–66 and 1968, there were 82 reported fatalities from complications of smallpox vaccination; one study determined 68 of these to be truly vaccinia-related, with an estimated fatality rate of 1 per 1,000,000 primary vaccinations (48). Of these, 36 deaths were associated with postvaccinial encephalitis, 19 with vaccinia necrosum, 12 with eczema vaccinatum, and one with Stevens-Johnson syndrome. All 12 deaths from eczema vaccinatum occurred in children who were not vaccinated themselves but acquired vaccinia from contact with recently vaccinated persons.

More recent data on vaccination following the recently implemented smallpox vaccination program suggests myopericarditis may occur as an adverse effect of vaccination at a higher rate than had previously been recognized. Following 450,293 vaccinations of selected military personnel from December 2002 through May 2003, 37 suspected, probable, or confirmed cases of acute myopericarditis occurred (40). All cases were in male primary vaccinees aged 21 to 33 years, and all occurred from 7 to 19 days after vaccination. In a report that described the initial 18 cases of myopericarditis in this patient population, the authors concluded that a causal relationship between vaccination and myopericarditis was supported by close temporal clustering, wide geographic and temporal distribution, and occurrence in only primary vaccinees (49). Additional cardiac events reported in military personnel included four cases of myocardial infarction, two cases of angina, one case of coronary artery spasm, and one case of atrial fibrillation (40). Among over 37,000 civilian healthcare and public health workers vaccinated from January 2003 through June 2003, 21 suspected or probable cases of myopericarditis were reported (39). Other cardiac events included five cases of myocardial infarction, three cases of angina, and two cases of cardiomyopathy. At present, smallpox vaccination and reported ischemic events or cardiomyopathy are not known to be causally associated (39,40).

A recent retrospective analysis of cardiac deaths after the 1947 mass smallpox vaccination campaign of 6.4 million persons in New York City did not reveal any increased number of cardiac deaths, including those caused by myo/pericarditis, when compared to the same time frames in 1946 and 1948 (50). However, surveillance was probably not as comprehensive then as performed recently. In an effort to prevent myopericarditis and pericarditis after smallpox vaccination the CDC has added detailed specific screening questions to avoid vaccination of persons who might be at increased risk for cardiac adverse events (Table 112.3). Moreover, myocarditis and pericarditis have been included in the federal smallpox vaccine injury table in terms of liability provisions (Table 112.4) (53) within a defined time period after vaccination.

Vaccinia immune globulin (VIG), derived from the serum of individuals vaccinated with vaccinia, is available from the CDC as an IND for treating certain severe complications (Table 112.2). It may be indicated in eczema vaccinatum, progressive vaccinia, severe generalized vaccinia, and autoinoculation of the eye or eyelid without vaccinial keratitis (15). VIG is not effective for postvaccinial encephalitis and is contraindicated in cases of vaccinial keratitis, because it may worsen corneal scarring. The antiviral drug cidofovir (see below) is also being evaluated under an IND protocol as a secondary treatment for vaccinia-related complications that are unresponsive to VIG (27).

PATIENT MANAGEMENT

There is no proven effective treatment for smallpox, and management is largely supportive. Patients are placed in a negative-

TABLE 112.3. CDC UPDATED (NOV 15, 2003) SMALLPOX GUIDELINES FOR "SMALLPOX PRE-VACCINATION INFORMATION PACKET: CONTENTS AND INSTRUCTIONS". "SMALLPOX VACCINATION PATIENT MEDICAL HISTORY AND CONSENT FORM". HEART PROBLEMS

1. Have you ever been diagnosed by a doctor as having a heart condition with or without symptoms such as a previous myocardial infarction (heart attack), angina (chest pain caused by a lack of blood flow to the heart), congestive heart failure, or cardiomyopathy?
2. Have you ever had a stroke or transient ischemic attack (a "mini-stroke" that produces stroke-like symptoms but no lasting damage)?
3. Do you have chest pain or shortness of breath when you exert yourself (such as when you walk up stairs)?
4. Do you have any other heart condition for which you are under the care of a doctor?
5. Do you have three or more of the following risk factors?
   a. You have been told by a doctor that you have high blood pressure.
   b. You have been told by a doctor that you have high blood cholesterol.
   c. You have been told by a doctor that you have diabetes or high blood sugar.
   d. You have a first-degree relative (for example, mother, father, brother, or sister) who had a heart condition before the age of 50).
   e. You smoke cigarettes now.

pressure room (if available) under strict respiratory and contact isolation (15). Fluid and electrolyte balance should be maintained, particularly in patients with poor oral intake, fever, or widespread skin breakdown. Symptomatic care may be necessary for nausea, vomiting, or diarrhea. Systemic antibiotics are administered to treat complications from secondary bacterial infection, with therapy guided by culture confirmation of the causative microorganism. Severe respiratory complications may require intubation and mechanical ventilation. Topical idoxuridine, or newer ophthalmic antiviral agents such as trifluridine, may be considered to treat corneal lesions, although they are of unproven efficacy for smallpox. Patients with hemorrhagic smallpox should be evaluated for disseminated intravascular coagulation.

TABLE 112.4. SMALLPOX (VACCINIA) VACCINE INJURY TABLE

Injury or condition in Vaccine Recipient, or in a Contact of the Recipient.

1. Significant Local Skin Reaction
2. Stevens-Johnson Syndrome
3. Inadvertent Inoculation
4. Generalized Vaccinia
5. Eczema Vaccinatum
6. Progressive Vaccinia
7. Postvaccinial Encephalopathy, Encephalitis or Encephalomyelitis
8. Fetal Vaccinia
9. Secondary Infection
10. Anaphylaxis or Anaphylactic Shock
11. Vaccinial Myocarditis, Pericarditis, or Myopericarditis
12. Death resulting from an injury referred to above in which the injury arose within the time interval referred to (in this Federal Register document).

[a] Adapted from Federal Register 2003;68:51492–51499.

Potential antiviral drugs for smallpox are currently under investigation. The nucleotide analog cidofovir inhibits viral DNA polymerase by competitive inhibition and is approved by the Food and Drug Administration for the treatment of cytomegalovirus retinitis in patients with acquired immune deficiency syndrome (54). Cidofovir has broad-spectrum activity against DNA viruses including *in vitro* activity against variola (12). In addition, animal studies indicated that cidofovir protected immunocompetent mice from fatal infection with vaccinia or cowpox, if administered 24 hours after infection (55,56). Cidofovir is administered intravenously and is associated with renal and ocular toxicity. Coadministration with probenecid and hydration before and after cidofovir therapy may lessen renal toxicity. More than 20 additional antiviral drugs have been identified as having *in vitro* activity against orthopoxviruses, and will be further tested in animal models (12). Another treatment under investigation in animal studies is immunotherapy with neutralizing monoclonal antibodies; (57).

HOSPITAL PREPAREDNESS FOR A SMALLPOX OUTBREAK

This section discusses hospital care of the patient with smallpox and the "smallpox hospital" from three perspectives. First, an historical perspective is summarized. Second, the current plan and guidelines from the CDC that address medical facilities for use in a smallpox outbreak are reviewed. Third, specific aspects of planning at one of our own (Washington, D.C.) city hospitals and regional communities are presented, and potential measures to be taken in the event of a bioterrorism-linked return of smallpox to the human population are discussed.

An Historical Synopsis

A thorough historical review of the smallpox hospital is found in Dixon's (58) 30-page chapter on the subject in his 1962 book on smallpox. He reviews the history of smallpox hospitals as conventional hospital structures, floating hospital ships, or temporary emergency structures such as large airplane hangars. He discusses the use of ships as isolation hospitals for smallpox patients, particularly in England. In 1885, all smallpox patients in London were sent directly from their homes to the river wharves where boats termed "river ambulances" were used to transport them to the larger ships being used exclusively as smallpox isolation and treatment wards.

Dixon emphasizes the importance of having security at these facilities strictly enforced to minimize the number of persons entering the smallpox hospital, being certain they are vaccinated, keeping a written record of everyone who enters the facility, and as much as possible not allowing any visitors in the smallpox hospital. Dixon also highlights the critical role of the control-of-infection committee, with a designated representative who interacts bilaterally each day with the department or ministry of health to provide information on the patients in the hospital and their contacts in the community, as well as to convey and implement the directives of the department of health for the hospital.

In Fenner et al.'s (3) 1988 classic text on smallpox and its eradication, smallpox hospitals, with some exceptions as far back as 10th century Japan, are noted to have been unusual in most parts of the world prior to the 20th century. In fact, most smallpox patients were generally not admitted to a hospital. By contrast, during a 1901–1903 smallpox epidemic in Boston, all patients, except those too sick to be moved, were required to be admitted to one of two special detention hospitals, one of which was located on Gallops Island in Boston Harbor (59). As recently as the 1970s, Germany and England still had hospitals for patients returning with smallpox from endemic areas of the world (3).

Recent Guidelines for Medical and Public Health Responses

Working Group on Civilian Biodefense

In 1999 Henderson et al. (60) published consensus guidelines on medical and public health management of smallpox if the virus were used as a bioweapon. The size of an outbreak would impact the types of facilities in which smallpox patients would be managed. For example, if only a small number of patients (defined locally but generally <10) had smallpox, then they could be admitted to existing hospitals that had negative-pressure airborne infectious isolation rooms with high-efficiency particulate air (HEPA) filtration. In "larger outbreaks, home isolation and care should be the objective for most patients." In recognition of the reality that home care will not be a feasible option for some patients, this Working Group on Civilian Biodefense also recommended that "authorities should consider the possibility of designating a specific hospital or hospitals for smallpox care." Patients placed into such a smallpox isolation hospital and everyone who worked in the facility should be immediately vaccinated (60).

CDC Plan in 2003: Type C, Type X, and Type R Facilities

The CDC smallpox response plan draft guide C discusses infection control measures for healthcare and community settings (61). It distinguishes among three types of medical facilities that will be needed for use in a smallpox outbreak: type C (contagious), type X (uncertain diagnosis), and type R (residential) (Table 112.5). In apparent distinction from the 1999 consensus guidelines by Henderson et al.'s (60) Working Group on Civilian Biodefense, the type R residential facility, which the CDC states "may be the person's own home," is not the recommended objective for the care of most patients with smallpox. In fact, the CDC states, "It is expected that once a large outbreak of smallpox is confirmed, all confirmed or suspected smallpox patients will be isolated in a type C facility that has been designated for the isolation of such patients."

The CDC specifies three groups of persons, all of whom are asymptomatic contacts rather than symptomatic smallpox patients, for management in type R residential facilities: (a) afebrile vaccinated contacts; (b) afebrile vaccinated persons who were exposed to one or more smallpox patients 10 to 18 days before the onset of the rash (i.e., possible common exposure); and (c) contacts of smallpox patients who for whatever reason refuse vaccination. If asymptomatic contacts cannot be housed in their own homes, for individual or societal reasons, then alternative type R facilities such as motels or hotels or similarly equipped facilities must be used (61).

In a type R residential facility the noninfectious, asymptomatic contacts must measure their temperatures twice each day for 18 days after their last exposure or until 14 days after successful vaccination, whichever comes first. If two successive fevers ≥38°C (≥100.4°F) are recorded while under this fever surveillance period, then this person must notify the health department with which he or she should already be in daily communication by phone, or if feasible daily site visits by health staff. In addition, febrile persons in residential facilities must remain in their home while awaiting transfer to a type X or type C facility for medical evaluation to determine the cause of the fever. Afebrile individuals in their homes can maintain their routine activities outside the facility, given that infectiousness begins with onset of a rash that follows several days of fever; these persons will remain within 20 miles of their city of residence. If cohort isolation of noninfectious individuals in an alternative type R facility is needed, however, outside an individual's home, then the contacts should remain in the facility during the fever surveillance period. All persons entering the alternative type R facility must be vaccinated against smallpox.

A type X facility is primarily for isolation and observation of persons with uncertain diagnosis who have been vaccinated, do not have a rash, and are febrile contacts of smallpox patients.

TABLE 112.5. THREE TYPES OF FACILITIES FOR USE IN A SMALLPOX EMERGENCY: TYPE R, TYPE X, AND TYPE C

1. Type R facility (R = "Residential"):
   a. Use: For persons who were exposed to smallpox, but are without fever or any symptoms ("asymptomatic contacts"), and therefore are not infectious to other people. Includes afebrile vaccinated persons and contacts who refuse vaccination.
   b. Location: May be the residence (e.g., home) of these asymptomatic persons.
2. Type X facility (X= "Uncertain diagnosis"):
   a. Use: For isolation of persons who were exposed to smallpox, and recently vaccinated against smallpox, who now have a fever but no rash.
   b. Location: Any medical facility that meets the same isolation requirements of a type C facility except that only basic medical care such as monitoring of vital signs is required, because patients are all stable at time of admission.
3. Type C facility: (C = "Contagious"):
   a. Use: For isolation of persons who have suspected, probable, or confirmed smallpox and thus are infectious to other people.
   b. Location: A dedicated medical facility equipped to provide complex medical care and strict infection control precautions to prevent transmission of smallpox.

Adapted from CDC. Smallpox Response Plan. Draft Guide C., Part I. Infection control measures for healthcare and community settings, April 2, 2003.

Such patients will have had a fever of ≥38°C (100.4°F) on two successive measurements. If their numbers are small, then another option is to transfer them to a type C hospital with known smallpox patients, given that they have recently been vaccinated. If there are many such patients, however, then the CDC recommends use of additional type X facilities to observe these patients for development of a rash consistent with smallpox, or manifestations of a different disease and the exclusion of smallpox. If a rash does not develop in the vaccinated febrile patient in a type X facility, and the fever is attributable to a non-smallpox diagnosis, then the patient can return home to complete the required period of fever surveillance as described above (61).

If a rash appears, however, then the patient should be transferred to a type C facility for further management to decrease the risk of transmitting variola to other persons in the type X facility. Patients in a type X facility need only have their vital signs monitored, but the same isolation requirements are needed as for a type C facility (see below). To minimize the risk of variola transmission, isolation of persons as soon as fever begins is recommended. This policy optimizes the chance that the patient will be isolated by the time the infectious stage, coincident with onset of the smallpox rash, occurs following the 2 to 3 days of the febrile prodrome.

The type C facility is designed to "house cases of smallpox and thus minimize the exposure of susceptible individuals to contagious individuals." Importantly, the CDC recommends that all persons entering a type C facility as patients or workers, including patients already considered to be smallpox cases, must be vaccinated with vaccinia. The rationale for vaccinating all patients upon entrance to the type C facility is that diagnostic errors can result in susceptible patients without smallpox being admitted and exposed to smallpox in the facility. Since chickenpox (varicella) can be confused clinically with smallpox, testing for varicella is advised, if feasible, using a direct fluorescent assay in persons without either a history of chickenpox or varicella vaccination. Of note, if a patient with varicella is admitted to a smallpox medical facility, then an outbreak of varicella can occur in the facility.

Table 112.6 summarizes the requirements for a type C facility (61). A hospital in the traditional sense is not necessary, per se. Candidate alternative buildings include adequately equipped motels, college dormitories, ships, or a separate building of a hospital. All patients, healthcare workers, persons handling laundry and waste, and any visitors allowed to enter the facility must be vaccinated beforehand. Until a successful vaccine "take" has been demonstrated 6 to 8 days after vaccination, all personnel working in the facility must measure their temperature twice each day and report to a designated supervisor any fever or illness. Standard, contact, and airborne precautions, to include fit-tested N-95 respirators, must be used. Once a successful vaccine take has been documented, then "the care provider is no longer required to wear an N-95 mask. Standard Precautions and Contact Precautions should be maintained." Specific chemical decontamination recommendations for variola virus have been provided by the CDC based on studies using vaccinia virus (Table 112.7). Additional infection control measures and decontamination measures include the following (62): All laundry and linens should be placed in biohazard bags and laundered in the facility. If nonvaccinated personnel must process the laundry, then it should be autoclaved first, after being taken out of the biohazard bags. Food should be prepared within the facility or brought in in disposable containers. Preferably, a laboratory diagnosis should be made for probable and suspected cases of smallpox to optimize patient management. For example, if an illness other than smallpox is diagnosed, then as soon as a successful vaccine "take" is documented, the patient can be discharged from a type C facility. If smallpox is confirmed, then a prognosis can be estimated, and survivors can be discharged after 3 to 4 weeks or when all scabs have separated. Given the gravity of the clinical and public health decision to discharge a patient from a type C or type X facility, final approval to do so should be made only by the state epidemiologist or health officer, or someone officially

TABLE 112.6. CDC REQUIREMENTS FOR A TYPE C CONTAGIOUS SMALLPOX FACILITY

1. A building with nonshared air, heating, and ventilation systems with 100% of exhaust air to the outside through a HEPA filter, ***OR*** is a minimum of 100 yards away from any other occupied area.
2. Water, electricity, heating, cooling, and closed-window ventilation for daily activities and medical care.
3. A dependable communication system within and outside the facility
4. Controllable access e.g., a secure fence around the building or monitored entrances to prevent unvaccinated persons from coming into the facility.
5. Ability to provide medical care within the facility including:
   a. IV fluids, antibiotics, other supportive care
   b. Skin care
   c. Oxygen monitoring (pulse oximetry), and an oxygen supply (in-line or portable)
   d. Vital signs monitoring
   e. Cardiac and respiratory resuscitation
   f. Ventilatory support and suctioning equipment
   g. Routine laboratory assays such as complete blood count, and chemistries.
   h. Portable chest x-rays
   i. Staffing resources

Adapted from CDC. Smallpox Response Plan. Draft Guide C., Part I. Infection control measures for healthcare and community settings, April 2, 2003.

TABLE 112.7. CHEMICAL INACTIVATION OF VACCINIA VIRUS ON SURFACES AFTER 10 MINUTES AT ROOM TEMPERATURE

Chemical Disinfectant	Minimum concentration required for Inactivation
Ethyl alcohol	40%
Isopropyl alcohol	30%
Benzalkonium chloride	100 parts per million (ppm)
Sodium hypochlorite	200 ppm
Ortho-phenyphenol	0.12%
Iodophor	75 ppm

Adapted from CDC. Smallpox Response Plan. Guide F—environmental control of smallpox virus. March 20, 2003.
ppm, parts per million

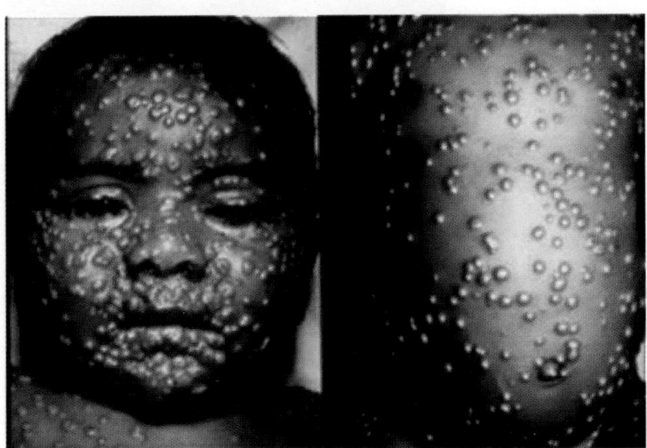

Figure 112.1 Smallpox pustules: density on the face exceeds that on the abdomen [World Health Organization (WHO)].

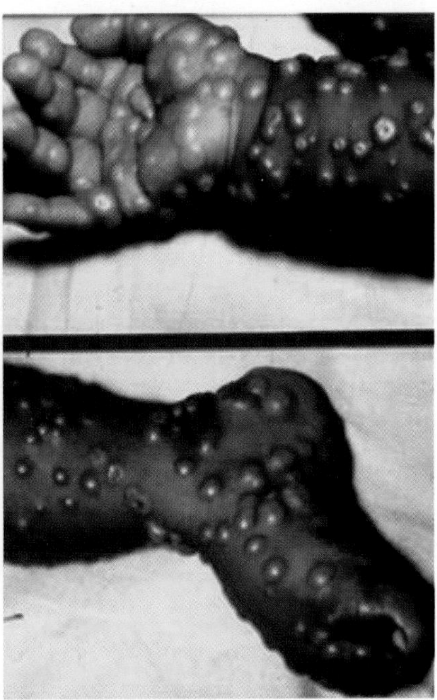

Figure 112.2 Smallpox: lesions on the palms and soles (WHO).

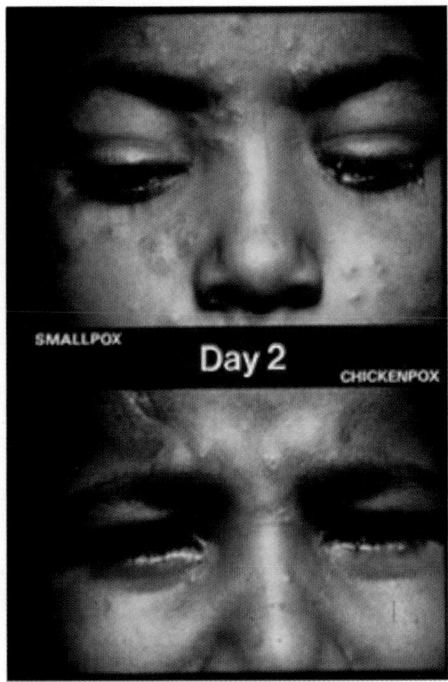

Figure 112.3 Day 2. Smallpox vs. chickenpox: smallpox (top) vs. chickenpox (bottom).

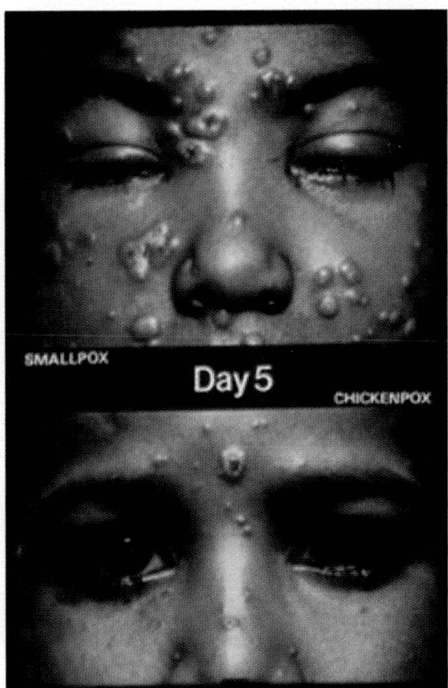

Figure 112.4 Day 5 of rash: smallpox (top) vs. chickenpox (bottom) (WHO).

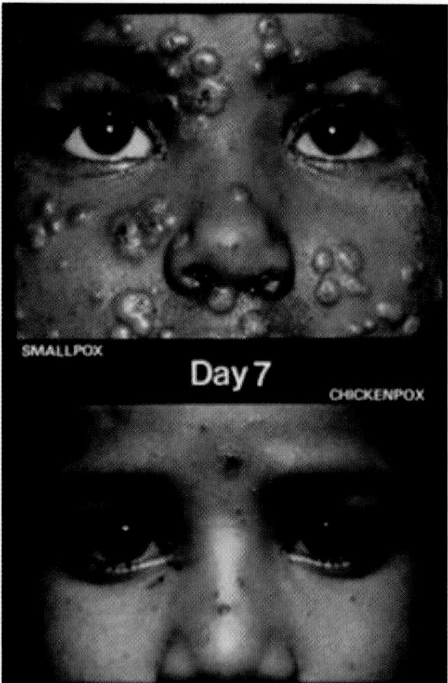

Figure 112.5 Day 7 of rash: smallpox (top) vs. chickenpox (bottom) (WHO).

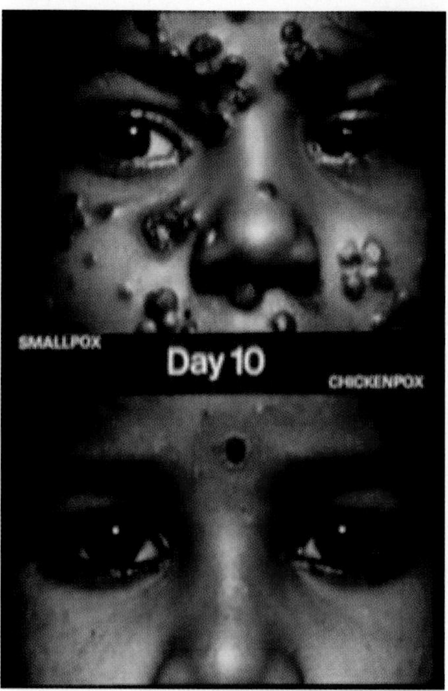

Figure 112.6 Day 10 of rash: smallpox (top) vs. chickenpox (bottom) (WHO).

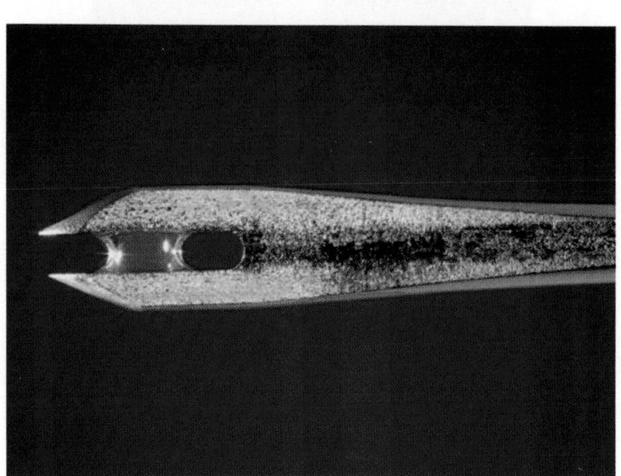

Figure 112.7 Bifurcated needle [(Centers for Disease Control and Prevention (CDC)].

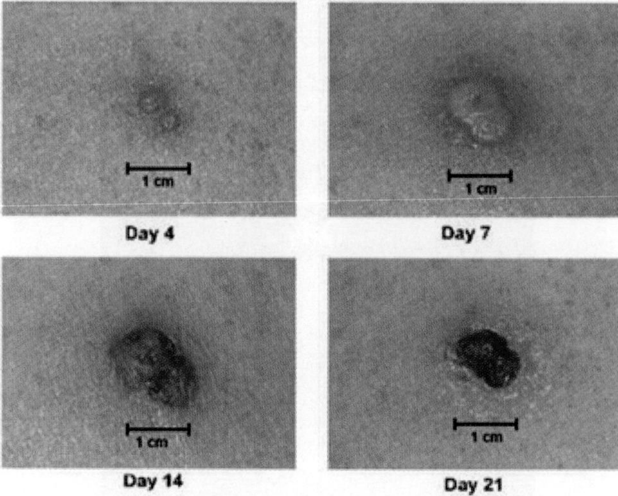

Figure 112.8 Normal vaccinia site reaction days 4, 7 (successful take), 14, and 21 (CDC).

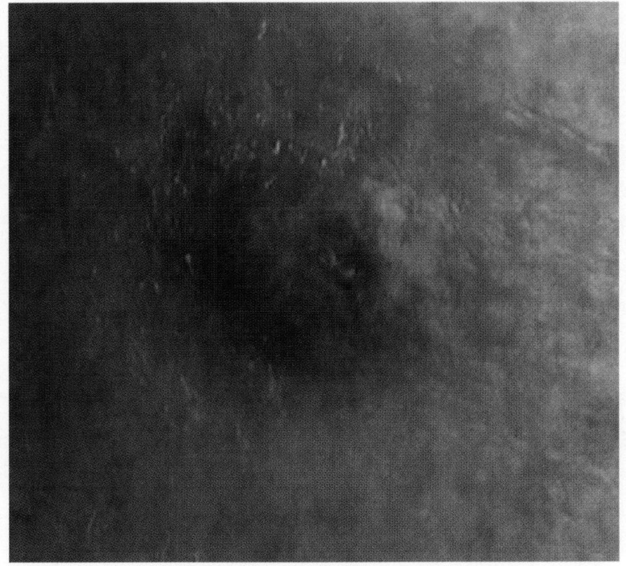

Figure 112.9 Day 6 vaccination site in a revaccinee (DRL): March 9 2003.

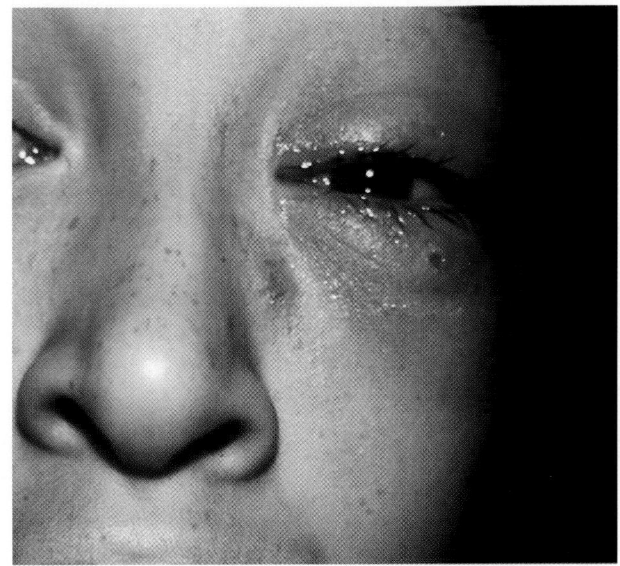

Figure 112.10 Vaccinia infection of the cornea (CDC).

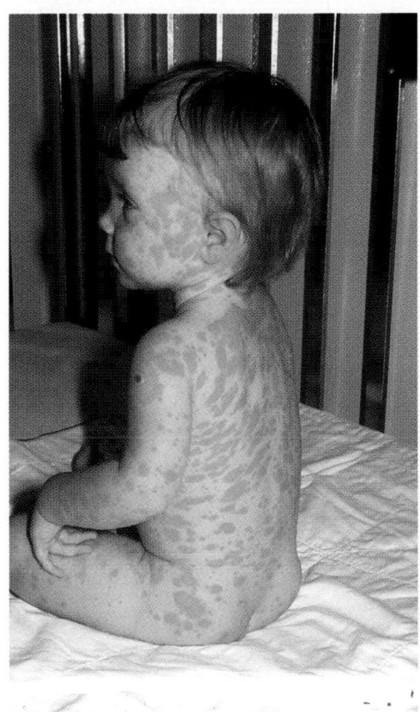

Figure 112.11 Erythema multiforme (CDC).

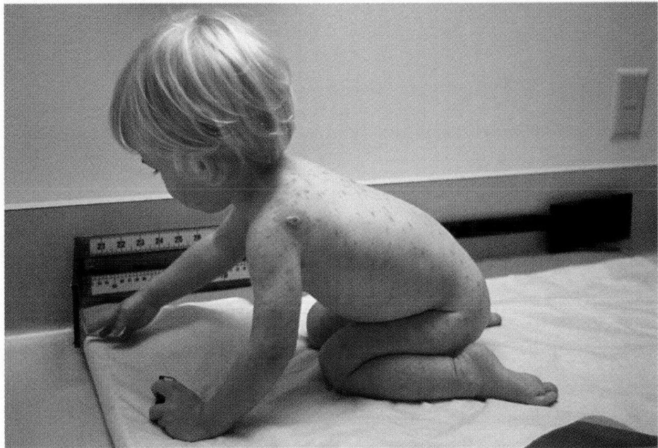

Figure 112.12 Generalized vaccinia in an apparently normal child. Recovered without sequelae (CDC).

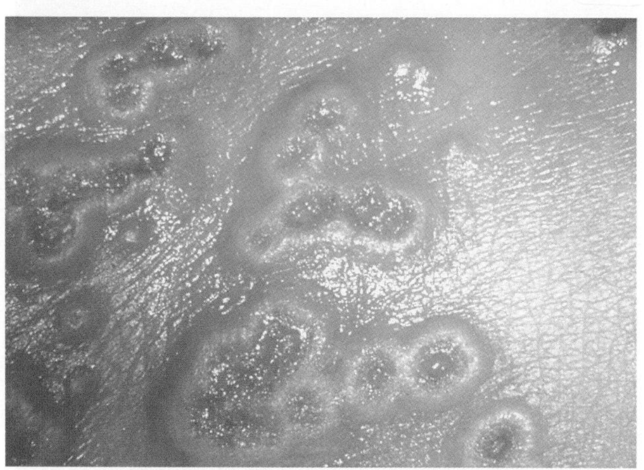

Figure 112.13 Eczema vaccinatum (CDC).

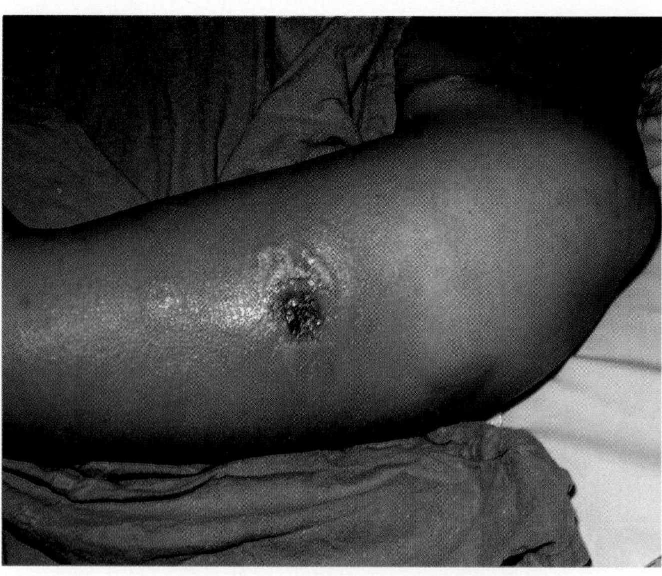

Figure 112.14 Progressive vaccinia (CDC).

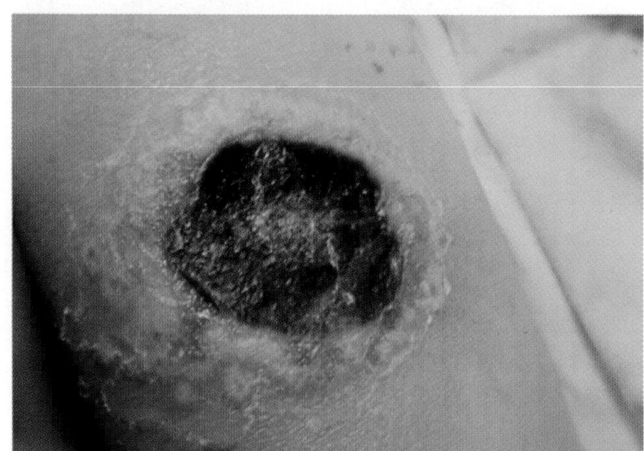

Figure 112.15 Progressive vaccinia (CDC).

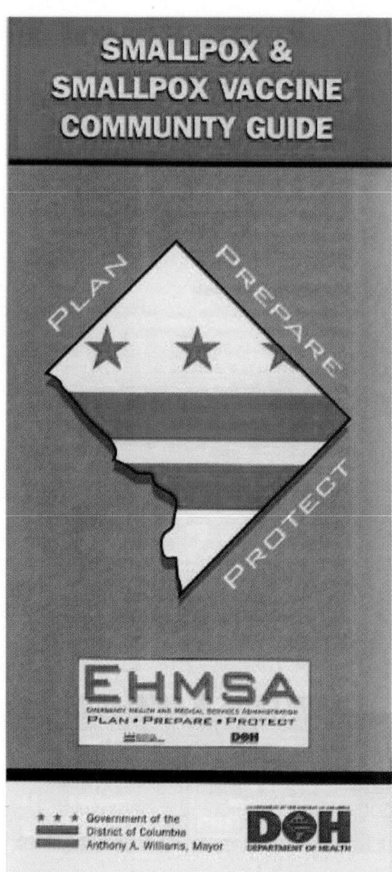

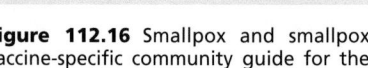

Figure 112.16 Smallpox and smallpox vaccine-specific community guide for the District of Columbia (D.C.).

TABLE 112.8. INFECTION CONTROL MEASURES FOR EVALUATING POTENTIAL SMALLPOX PATIENTS IN A CONVENTIONAL HOSPITAL ALREADY TREATING PATIENTS WITHOUT SMALLPOX

1. Minimize any close contact between the patient with suspected smallpox and other patients and health care workers who are not (yet) wearing appropriate personal protective equipment (PPE).
2. Place a surgical mask and a linen sheet on the patient with suspected smallpox in order to decrease the risk of transmission by droplets to other patients or health care workers.
3. Have a planned route for transport of the patient from the site of entry to the hospital, e.g., Emergency Room or outpatient clinic, to an airborne infection isolation (AII) room with negative pressure. Activate the plan, including use of a nonpublic, designated elevator(s) if needed.
4. Follow Airborne, Contact, and Standard Precautions including use of a fit-tested N-95 respirator, gowns, gloves, and protective eyewear.
5. The linen sheet used to transport the patient and all PPE should be placed in biohazard bags for disposal before leaving the patient's room.
6. All persons entering the patient's room should have been vaccinated recently against smallpox.
7. Maintain detailed written records, preferably computerized, of everyone who enters the patient's room or may possibly be exposed to the patient in any other location.
8. Severely restrict the number of persons entering the room to only essential personnel and do not allow the patient to travel within the hospital unless absolutely necessary. For example, if transfer to an intensive care unit is required, then as on initial admission to the hospital, clear the route of transport of any non-essential persons, cover the patient with a linen sheet, and place a surgical mask.
9. Consult with the jurisdictional Department of Health for guidance on whether to vaccinate and monitor for fever all or only designated hospital workers.

Adapted from CDC. Smallpox Response Plan. Draft Guide C., Part I. Infection control measures for healthcare and community settings, April 2, 2003.

designated (61). Prior to establishment of a type C facility, the initial patients with suspected smallpox will be admitted to a non-smallpox hospital. Table 112.8 summarizes CDC infection control precautions that should be implemented immediately in this situation (61).

How does a hospital in 2004 implement a smallpox response plan? As an example, our Washington, D.C., city hospital's plan has evolved over several years and been modified as further information and guidelines have become available from the CDC and through regional multidisciplinary planning efforts. By 1999, our hospital had a written bioterrorism preparedness plan that included smallpox. Very limited national supplies of smallpox vaccine were recognized as one of the many potential problems in the event of a smallpox attack. By noon on September 11, 2001, just 3 hours after the terrorist attacks, a rapid education program about the major bioterrorism agents, including smallpox, had begun in the Department of Medicine, including house staff and fellow trainees, and the Division of Nursing. This educational effort was begun by Infectious Diseases and Infection Control Services, and before the end of September 2001 involved many other disciplines and most of the hospital, including the administration and media relations office. Photographic and written information regarding the clinical recognition and diagnosis of smallpox, the access issues related to smallpox vaccine and bifurcated needles to administer the vaccine, and infection control issues to prevent transmission of variola were discussed. By September 21, thousands of N-95 respirators had been stockpiled (as well as thousands of doses of doxycycline for management of potential non-smallpox bioterrorism threats). A reiterative, multidimensional educational program about bioterrorism including smallpox was initiated throughout the hospital. These training efforts included lectures; written handouts; posters [in the hospital wards, library, and intensive care units (ICUs)]; PDA-compatible tabular information on diagnosis, prophylaxis, and treatment; and Internet sources of practical information and updates. Coordinated planning with pediatric services was done to facilitate care of both adults and children.

Information on the potential off-label use of the antiviral drug cidofovir for therapy of variola or vaccinia was obtained. By December 2001, a protocol was submitted to the hospital institutional review board (IRB) for use of cidofovir for smallpox, or severe vaccinia reactions not resolved with VIG. This protocol was written by the infectious diseases staff and included involvement of a nephrologist to guarantee precautions to prevent and mitigate the potential renal toxicities of cidofovir.

By December 2001, a detailed written protocol for the management of patients with suspected or confirmed smallpox was completed by the infection control and infectious diseases services in coordination with the multidisciplinary bioterrorism preparedness task force working closely with the Department of Emergency Medicine. This protocol contained detailed information about the following issues: (a) strict airborne respiratory precautions procedures, with personal protective equipment (PPE) to include N-95 respirator and eye protection, HEPA filters, and transport of admitted patients covered with a sheet and a mask; (b) notification lists of specific personnel and pager numbers with responsibility for contacting the local Department of Health (in Washington, D.C.) as per routine by the infection control service of the hospital; (c) prioritization of personnel to care for smallpox patients, with preference given to persons vaccinated at least once in the past, and without medical conditions that would be contraindications to vaccination in the absence of exposure to smallpox; (d) transport and handling of laboratory specimens, including never using the pneumatic tube system and always calling the laboratory technologist in charge (a technologist would be available 24 hours a day, 7 days a week) before sending any patient specimens to the laboratory to minimize both risk and anxiety within the clinical laboratory environment; all laboratory diagnostics for variola would be done only outside the hospital, at a Laboratory Response Network laboratory or the CDC initially under Biosafety Level 4 precautions; (e) tracking of all patients and their contacts in the hospital using a standardized form, and evaluation of all exposed healthcare workers; and (f) specific guidelines for patients identified prior to arrival at the hospital (e.g., in an ambulance), or patients identified in the emergency department (where two negative-pressure rooms existed), or patients identified only after being admitted to a hospital ward or ICU. Standardized forms were included that were required to be posted outside the patient's room for strict airborne precautions, and sign in/sign out of all personnel entering the room.

In early January 2002 a series of 17 monthly bioterrorism continuing medical education public forums for regional hospitals, clinics, and public health officials was begun. The initial and multiple subsequent monthly meetings included presentations and discussions on smallpox and smallpox vaccination. At a later date, a 270-person regional tabletop exercise on smallpox and smallpox vaccination was organized involving multiple disciplines including clinicians, public health departments, fire/EMS, and security organizations. By June 2002, the monthly biodefense meetings included demonstrations and hands-on opportunities to use the bifurcated needle required for smallpox vaccination on an artificial skin-covered deltoid teaching device (or a piece of fruit, or a mannequin arm covered with DuoDerm-like material). These hands-on training sessions were combined with a standardized Powerpoint slide presentation and expanded to healthcare settings across the region, including private clinics, hospitals, and the local physician medical society. The training slides were posted on a biodefense Web site we initiated (*www.bepast.org*), along with other information and references to smallpox. Soon the Washington, D.C., Department of Health began to cosponsor these training exercises and to issue laminated smallpox immunization technician certification cards for over 300 persons completing these hands-on educational sessions. The Department of Health initiated a written record of contact information for recipients of these training certificates, anticipating that in the event of a smallpox emergency these persons could volunteer to assist the Department of Health with vaccination efforts. Some members of the nascent regional medical reserve corps also were trained in these smallpox vaccine administration and education sessions.

In addition, the director and senior nurses in this hospital were trained in these same hands-on sessions, and copies of the training slides provided for "train-the-trainer" exercises with other nurses. Importantly, members of a large regional Visiting Nurse Association (VNA) also were trained in how to use the bifurcated needle in the event they were needed for large-scale hospital or community-based smallpox vaccinations. The VNA could be particularly valuable in this regard in that it is already well known in the community for giving the annual influenza vaccinations.

By June 2002, an illustrated teaching guide for the diagnosis and management of the six CDC category A bioterrorism agents, including smallpox, was created. This poster was disseminated throughout the hospital, and several thousand were provided to regional and national hospitals, clinics, public health facilities, fire/EMS stations, and posted on the Web site (*www.bepast.org*). By December 2002, a smallpox and smallpox vaccine–specific illustrated guide was coauthored with the Washington, D.C., Department of Health for persons in the medical and nonmedical community (Fig. 112.16). This training guide was subse-

TABLE 112.9. A PROPOSED HOSPITAL RESPONSE PLAN GIVEN ONE PATIENT WITH SMALLPOX IN THE WORLD

1. Communicate with local jurisdictional Department of Health and request guidance.
2. Contact Hospital Administration, Infection Control Service, and Facility Engineers (ventilation) as part of the activation of the multidisciplinary hospital response plan for smallpox and smallpox vaccination (assuming consistent with Department of Health).
3. Begin to distribute Personal Protective Equipment (PPE) for smallpox including N-95 respirators, and begin to offer smallpox vaccination to hospital workers based on specific prioritization guidance from the Department of Health.
4. Activate the hospital plan to "*Look Within*" the hospital for possible patients with unrecognized smallpox, including the febrile prodrome without rash.
5. Establish security for the hospital entrances, as well as outpatient clinics and the Emergency Department, and activate surveillance to "Look Without" for patients entering the hospital with possible smallpox.
6. Follow the CDC algorithm for diagnosing patients with possible smallpox and distinguishing them from chickenpox and other diseases in the differential diagnosis.
7. Evaluate all patients with rash. Focus initially on the face and palms of the hands. Specifically search for the typical smallpox rash, but also evaluate all patients with a rash consistent with hemorrhagic or flat smallpox.
8. Ask for epidemiologic clues such as any travel or other epidemiologic link to the possible (global) outbreak location. Determine if the patient with a suspicious rash is either pregnant or immunocompromised since atypical smallpox rashes are more likely to appear in such patients.
9. Any patients with possible smallpox must be immediately isolated from other patients in a negative pressure room airborne isolation (AII) room, reported to the Infection Control Service, and by them to the Department of Health.
10. A (computerized) list of suspected smallpox patients and all their potential contacts must be continually updated and coordinated with the Department of Health.
11. Contact the Hospital Blood Bank about possible blood donations prior to donors being vaccinated against smallpox, and about possible "look-back" at any recent donors later if any are identified as suspected smallpox patients.
12. Communicate with Department of Health about:
    a. any changes in recommendations in terms of vaccine contraindications or paperwork requirements, particularly if large numbers of vaccinations within days becomes necessary.
    b. dilution of vaccine 1 : 5 for either naive or revaccinees,
    c. voluntary rapid testing for HIV or pregnancy,
    d. IND use of any non-FDA licensed smallpox vaccine
13. Communicate daily with Hospital Media Relations Office and Hospital Administration.
14. If any patients identified in the hospital, outpatient clinic, or Emergency Department, then anticipate possible need for urgent vaccination of large numbers of health care workers, and possibly other patients if they were in contact with suspected cases.
15. f large numbers of potential vaccinees are anticipated, then keep vaccination site(s) in hospital open 24 hours a day and, if needed, immediately train more vaccinators and personnel to expedite the vaccination process safely and efficiently.
16. Anticipate that health care workers will request that their family members, and household contacts, be offered smallpox vaccine.
17. Anticipate the need for follow-up of vaccinees for local or systemic reactions.
18. Work with Department of Health to activate plan for transfer of patients with suspected, probable, or confirmed smallpox to the designated medical facility dedicated exclusively to the care of patients with smallpox (if such a facility exists in that region's jurisdiction).

quently distributed widely in the District of Columbia by the Department of Health. The guide was posted on the department's Web site, *www.bt.dc.gov*, and on *www.bepast.org*. This document has been translated into five languages, including Spanish and Chinese.

In early March 2003 a small number of persons (four) volunteered to be the first vaccinated against smallpox by the Washington, D.C., Department of Health. After documenting a successful take, two of the authors then vaccinated 40 healthcare workers on March 20th, gaining valuable experience in the prevaccination screening process and in the actual, rather than simulated, use of the bifurcated needle. Also in March 2003 a proposed hospital response plan was written, subsequently updated (Table 112.9), and distributed regionally for specific actions a hospital should take in the event of even a single patient with smallpox being diagnosed anywhere in the world, in concert with the jurisdictional Department of Health.

CONCLUSION

Local and national preparedness for smallpox has improved markedly since September 2001. The civilian smallpox vaccination program, however, has markedly slowed in the last half of 2003. This fact highlights the need to be able to respond rapidly to a smallpox outbreak in terms of hospital readiness for vaccinating more healthcare workers on short notice and operation of medical facilities (type C and type X) and residential-home (type R) facilities for patients as recommended by the CDC. Traditional surveillance and containment measures, sometimes referred to as "ring vaccination," will likely be used initially to control the outbreak. Whether additional, more extensive population "targeted" or "mass" vaccinations will be necessary may well depend on the nature of the smallpox outbreak, e.g., if an aerosol release in multiple cities occurs. A detailed analysis of the multiple models published to date on how best to prepare and respond to a smallpox outbreak has recently been reviewed (63). Finally, it should be emphasized that to prepare for a potential bioterrorism agent such as smallpox is also to prepare simultaneously for an emerging disease such as severe acute respiratory syndrome (SARS) (see Chapter 113), or pandemic influenza, or another new respiratory infectious disease in terms of similarities in disease transmission, personal protective equipment, and public health response.

REFERENCES

1. Hopkins DR. *Princes and peasants: smallpox in history.* Chicago: University of Chicago Press, 1983.
2. Jenner E. *An inquiry into the causes and effects of variolae vaccinae, a disease discovered in some of the western counties of England, particularly Gloucestershire, and known by the name of cow pox.* London: S. Low, 1798.
3. Fenner F, Henderson DA, Arita I, et al. Smallpox and its eradication. In: *History of international public health,* no. 6. Geneva: World Health Organization, 1988.
4. Breman JG, Arita I. The confirmation and maintenance of smallpox eradication. *N Engl J Med* 1980;303:1263–1273.
5. Breman JG, Henderson DA. Poxvirus dilemmas—monkeypox, smallpox, and biologic terrorism. *N Engl J Med* 1998;339:556–559.
6. Alibek K. *Biohazard.* New York: Delta, 2000.
7. Jernigan DB, Raghunathan PL, Bell BP, et al., and the National Anthrax Epidemiologic Team. Investigation of bioterrorism-related anthrax, United States, 2001: epidemiologic findings. *Emerg Infect Dis* 2002;8:1019–1028.
8. Sterling JC, Kurtz JB. Viral infections. In: Champion RH, Burton JL, Burns DA, et al., eds. *Rook/Wilkinson/Ebling textbook of dermatology,* 6th ed. Oxford: Blackwell Science, 1998:995–1095.
9. Breman JG. Monkeypox: an emerging infection for humans? In: Scheld WM, Craig WA, Hughes JM, eds. *Emerging infections,* vol 4. Washington, DC: ASM Press, 2000:45–67.
10. Update: multistate outbreak of monkeypox—Illinois, Indiana, Kansas, Missouri, Ohio, and Wisconsin, 2003. *MMWR* 2003;52:642–646.

10a. Reed KD, Mels JW, Graham MB, et al. The initial detection of human monkeypox in the western hemiphere. *N Engl J Med* 2004 (in press).

11. Breman JG, Henderson DA. Diagnosis and management of smallpox. *N Engl J Med* 2002;346:1300–1308.
12. LeDuc JW, Damon I, Meegan JM, et al. Smallpox research activities: U.S. interagency collaboration, 2001. *Emerg Infect Dis* 2002;8: 743–745.
13. Lever WF, Schaumburg-Lever G. *Histopathology of the skin,* 7th ed. Philadelphia: JB Lippincott, 1990.
14. Damon I, Li Y, Kline R, et al. Variola virus and smallpox: past, present, or future tense? Available at Centers for Disease Control and Prevention Web site: *http://ftp.cdc.gov/pub/infectious diseases/iceid/2002/pdf/regnery.pdf.*
15. Centers for Disease Control and Prevention. Smallpox response plan and guidelines. Annex 1: overview of smallpox, clinical presentations, and medical care of smallpox patients. Available at: *http://www.bt.cdc.gov/agent/smallpox/response-plan/index.asp.*
16. Wehrle PF, Posch J, Richter KH, et al. An airborne outbreak of smallpox in a German hospital and its significance with respect to other recent outbreaks in Europe. *Bull WHO* 1970;43:669–679.
17. Rao AR. *Smallpox.* Bombay, India: Kothari Book Depot, 1972.
18. Martin DB. The cause of death in smallpox: an examination of the pathology record. *Milit Med* 2002;167:546–551.
19. Mack TM. Smallpox in Europe, 1950–1971. *J Infect Dis* 1972;125: 161–169.
20. Albert MR, Ostheimer KG, Liewehr DJ, et al. Smallpox manifestations and survival during the Boston epidemic of 1901 to 1903. *Ann Intern Med* 2002;137:993–1000.
21. Baxby D. Studies in smallpox and vaccination. *Rev Med Virol* 2002; 12:201–209.
22. Centers for Disease Control and Prevention. Evaluating patients for smallpox. Available at: *http://www.bt.cdc.gov/agent/smallpox/diagnosis/pdf/spox-poster-full.pdf.*
23. Centers for Disease Control and Prevention. Smallpox response plan and guidelines. Guide D: specimen collection and transport guidelines. Available at: *http://www.bt.cdc.gov/agent/smallpox/response-plan/index.asp.*
24. Centers for Disease Control and Prevention. Smallpox response plan and guidelines. Draft guide A: smallpox surveillance and case reporting; contact identification, tracing, vaccination, and surveillance; and epidemiologic investigation. Available at: *http://www.bt.cdc.gov/agent/smallpox/response-plan/index.asp.*
25. Centers for Disease Control and Prevention. Smallpox response plan and guidelines. Annex 3: smallpox vaccination clinic guide. Available at: *http://www.bt.cdc.gov/agent/smallpox/response-plan/index.asp.*
26. Bartlett J, Borio L, Radonovich L, et al. Smallpox vaccination in 2003: key information for clinicians. *Clin Infect Dis* 2003;36:883–902.
27. Cono J, Casey CG, Bell DM, Centers for Disease Control and Prevention. Smallpox vaccination and adverse reactions: guidance for clinicians. *MMWR Recomm Rep* 2003;52:1–28.
28. Ennis FA, Cruz J, Demkowicz WE, et al. Primary induction of human CD8+ cytotoxic T lymphocytes and interferon-γ-producing T cells after smallpox vaccination. *J Infect Dis* 2002;185:1657–1659.
29. Centers for Disease Control and Prevention. Smallpox fact sheet: vac-

cination overview. Available at: *http://www.bt.cdc.gov/agent/smallpox/vaccination/facts.asp.*
30. Sommer A. The 1972 smallpox outbreak in Khulna Municipality, Bangladesh. II. Effectiveness of surveillance and containment in urban epidemic control. *Am J Epidemiol* 1974;99:303–313.
30a. Massoudi MS, Barker L, Schwartz B. Effectiveness of postexposure Vaccination for the prevention of smallpox: results of a delphi analysis. *J Infect Dis* 2003;188:973–976.
31. Centers for Disease Control and Prevention. Smallpox fact sheet: smallpox vaccination method. Available at: *http://www.bt.cdc.gov/agent/smallpox/vaccination/vaccination-method.asp.*
32. Centers for Disease Control and Prevention. Smallpox vaccination and adverse events training module. Available at: *http://www.bt.cdc.gov/training/smallpoxvaccine/reactions/normal.html.*
33. Centers for Disease Control and Prevention. Smallpox vaccine information statement supplement B: vaccination site appearance and care. Available at: *http://www.bt.cdc.gov/agent/smallpox/vaccination/site-care-vis.asp.*
34. Sepkowitz KA. How contagious is vaccinia? *N Engl J Med* 2003;248: 439–446.
34a. Wharton M, Strikas RA, Harpaz R, et al. Recommendations for using smallpox vaccine in a pre-event vaccination program. *MMWR* 2003; 52(RR07):1–16.
35. Centers for Disease Control and Prevention. Smallpox fact sheet: smallpox (vaccinia) vaccine contraindications. Available at: *http://www.bt.cdc.gov/agent/smallpox/vaccination/contraindications-clinic.asp.*
36. Centers for Disease Control and Prevention. Smallpox fact sheet: people who should not get the smallpox vaccine. Available at: *http://www.bt.cdc.gov/agent/smallpox/vaccination/contraindications-public.asp.*
37. Centers for Disease Control and Prevention. Interim smallpox fact sheet: smallpox vaccine and heart problems. Available at: *http://www.bt.cdc.gov/agent/smallpox/vaccination/heartproblems.asp.*
38. Centers for Disease Control and Prevention. Protecting Americans: smallpox vaccination program. Available at: *http://www.bt.cdc.gov/agent/smallpox/vaccination/vaccination-program-statement.asp.*
39. Update: cardiac and other adverse events following civilian smallpox vaccination—United States, 2003. *MMWR* 2003;52:639–642.
40. Grabenstein JD, Winkenwerder W. US military smallpox vaccination program experience. *JAMA* 2003;289:3278–3282.
41. Enserink M. Smallpox vaccination campaign in the doldrums. *Science* 2003;300:880–881.
42. Couzin J. Panel urges caution over heart problems. *Science* 2003;300: 2013–2014.
43. Centers for Disease Control and Prevention. Smallpox fact sheet: adverse reactions following smallpox vaccination. Available at: *http://www.bt.cdc.gov/agent/smallpox/vaccination/reactions-vacc-clinic.asp.*
44. Frey SE, Couch RB, Tacket CO, et al. Clinical responses to undiluted and diluted smallpox vaccine. *N Engl J Med* 2002;346:1265–1274.
45. Bray M, Wright ME. Progress vaccinia. *Clin Infect Dis* 2003;36: 766–774.
46. Dropulic LK, Rubin RH, Bartlett JG. Smallpox vaccination and the patient with an organ transplant. *Clin Infect Dis* 2003;36:786–788.
47. Lane JM, Ruben FL, Neff JM, et al. Complications of smallpox vaccination, 1968: results of ten statewide surveys. *J Infect Dis* 1970;122: 303–309.
48. Lane JM, Ruben FL, Abrutyn E, et al. Deaths attributable to smallpox vaccination, 1959 to 1966, and 1968. *JAMA* 1970;212:441–444.
49. Halsell JS, Riddle JR, Atwood JE, et al. Myopericarditis following smallpox vaccination among vaccinia-naive US military personnel. *JAMA* 2003;289:3283–3289.
50. CDC. Cardiac deaths after a mass smallpox vaccination campaign—New York City, 1947. *MMWR* 2003;52(39):933–936.
51. Reference deleted in proofs.
52. Reference deleted in proofs.
53. Health Resources and Services Administration. Department of Health and Human Services. Smallpox vaccine injury compensation program: Smallpox (Vaccinia) vaccine injury table. *Fed Reg* 2003;68(166): 51492–51499.
54. Havens PL. Smallpox treatment 2002: topics for speculation. (2002). From Centers for Disease Control and Prevention Web site: *http://ftp.cdc.gov/pub/infectious diseases/iceid/2002/pdf/havens.pdf.*
55. Smee DF, Bailey KW, Sidwell RW. Treatment of lethal vaccinia virus respiratory infections in mice with cidofovir. *Antiviral Chem Chemother* 2001;12:71–76.
56. Bray M, Martinez M, Smee DF, et al. Cidofovir protects mice against lethal aerosol or intranasal cowpox virus challenge. *J Infect Dis* 2000; 181:10–19.
57. Ramírez JC, Tapia E, Esteban M. Administration to mice of a monoclonal antibody that neutralizes the intracellular mature virus form of vaccinia virus limits virus replication efficiently under prophylactic and therapeutic conditions. *J Gen Virol* 2002;83:1059–1067.
58. Dixon CW. The smallpox hospital. In: *Smallpox.* Boston: Little, Brown, 1962:361–390.
59. Albert MR, Ostheimer KG, Breman JG. The last smallpox epidemic in Boston and the vaccination controversy, 1901–1903. *N Eng J Med* 2001;344:375–379.
60. Henderson DA, Inglesby TV, Bartlett JG et al. Smallpox as a biological weapon. Medical and public health management. *JAMA* 1999;281: 2127–2137.
61. CDC. Smallpox response plan. Draft guide C, part 1. Infection control measures for healthcare and community settings, April 2, 2003.
62. CDC. Smallpox response plan. Guide F—environmental control of smallpox virus, March 20, 2003.
63. Ferguson NM, Keeling MJ, Edmunds WJ, et al. Planning for smallpox outbreaks. *Nature* 2003;425:681–685.

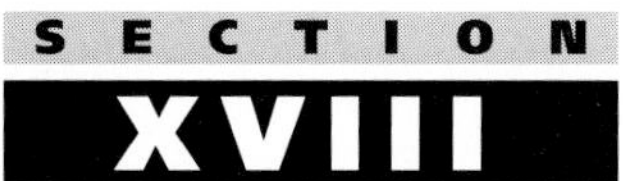

EMERGING INFECTIOUS DISEASES AND HEALTHCARE EPIDEMIOLOGY

113

SEVERE ACUTE RESPIRATORY SYNDROME

JAY C. BUTLER
JOHN A. JERNIGAN

BACKGROUND

In February 2003, the World Health Organization (WHO) received the first reports of an outbreak of atypical pneumonia in Guangdong Province of southern China. Some 305 cases were known to have occurred since November 2002. In late February, an ill physician who had treated patients in Guangdong Province traveled to Hong Kong where the infection was transmitted to at least 10 other guests at the hotel where he stayed (1,2). These guests subsequently transmitted infection as they continued their travels or returned home, resulting in direct spread of the illness from Hong Kong to Vietnam, Singapore, and Canada. A particularly disturbing characteristic of the illness was the apparent ease of transmission in healthcare facilities. On March 12, 2003, the WHO issued a global health alert about the disease that soon became known as severe acute respiratory syndrome (SARS). Before the end of March 2003, scientists working in a collaborative network of 11 laboratories found evidence of infection with a previously unknown coronavirus in patients with SARS (3–8). The remarkable speed in identifying the clusters of illness outside of China, identifying an infectious agent, and instituting control measures is gratifying. Nonetheless, by early July 2003, when the WHO declared that there was no more known person-to-person transmission of SARS in the world and that the initial epidemic was over, over 8,000 cases, resulting in nearly 800 deaths had been reported from 30 countries.

Much has been learned from the initial outbreak of SARS in 2003. This chapter reviews what has been learned during that period about the transmission, pathogenesis, clinical manifestations, diagnosis, epidemiology, and control and prevention of SARS. However, as with any newly recognized clinical entity, the body of knowledge for SARS is evolving, and recommendations for prevention and control may change as additional data become available. In addition to the information presented in this chapter, the reader may wish to consult the Internet sites listed at the end of the chapter.

TRANSMISSION AND PATHOGENESIS

The causative role of the SARS-associated coronavirus (SARS-CoV) has been confirmed by replication of SARS-like illness and reisolation of SAR-CoV in experimentally infected macaques (9,10). Two coronaviruses previously recognized as causing illness in humans, OC43 and 229E, are common causes of mild upper respiratory tract infections (11–16). Serious lower respiratory tract disease caused by OC43 and 229E is observed mainly in persons with underlying cardiopulmonary diseases or immunocompromising conditions (17,18). Transmission of OC43 and 229E is primarily by respiratory droplet.

The mode of transmission of SARS-CoV has not been confirmed, but in most instances transmission appears to have occurred when symptomatic infected persons spread infection via large respiratory droplets or by direct contact with a person ill with SARS (19–21). Airborne transmission is plausible and at this time cannot be excluded in certain circumstances. In one report, nine healthcare workers were infected by participating in the care of a SARS patient immediately before, during, or after administration of noninvasive positive pressure ventilation, followed by endotracheal intubation and high-frequency oscillatory ventilation (22). SARS developed in these healthcare workers despite use of personal protective equipment (PPE) that would have been expected to prevent droplet or contact transmission. In a cohort study of intensive care unit (ICU) nurses caring for SARS patients in Toronto, acquisition of SARS was associated with providing assistance during endotracheal intubation, suctioning of the airway before intubation, and manipulation of the patient's oxygen mask (23). Use of an N-95 respirator appeared to afford greater protection when compared to simple surgical masks, suggesting that airborne transmission of SARS-CoV may have occurred in that setting. A study of 40 infected healthcare workers in Hong Kong suggested that surgical masks did not provide adequate protection (21). However, the linear growth of the 2003 epidemic over time suggests that close contact is required for transmission in most circumstances. If SARS were transmitted primarily by the airborne route, exponential growth in the number of cases would be expected (24). Another epidemiologic study of healthcare workers found that wearing either a surgical mask or an N-95 respirator reduced the risk of infection, and the investigators interpreted these data as suggesting that transmission is most often by respiratory droplet (25). Direct contact may also play a role in transmission. In a study of 69 ICU staff exposed to a patient with SARS, six of seven

SARS cases occurred among those who entered the patient's room, and all six performed procedures that involved direct contact with the patient's mucous membranes or respiratory secretions (26). Use of gloves appeared to be highly protective in that study. SARS-CoV is relatively stable on inanimate surfaces (27), suggesting that indirect contact transmission via infectious fomites could also occur.

Other modes of transmission appear unlikely at this time. Spread via an animal vector has been proposed to explain clustering of cases in a housing complex in Hong Kong, but remains unproven (28). Of five infants born to women infected with SARS-CoV, no evidence of perinatal transmission was found (29). SARS-CoV RNA has been detected in blood specimens from patients with SARS (4); however, viremia has not been documented in asymptomatic persons, and transmission through transfusion of blood products has not been reported.

The site of initial infection with SARS-CoV is unknown, and the pathogenesis of SARS is incompletely understood at present. In lung tissue collected at autopsy from patients dying from SARS, SARS-CoV was detected by reverse-transcriptase polymerase chain reaction (RT-PCR), and particles with coronavirus morphology were found by electron microscopy (30). Pathologic findings in the lungs included pneumocyte proliferation and desquamation, hyaline membrane formation, mixed inflammatory infiltrate, and intraalveolar edema early (<10 days) in the course of illness. Diffuse alveolar damage is seen in cases of longer duration. Giant cells that stained for CD68, a macrophage marker, were also observed. Examination of biopsy and postmortem lung tissue specimens from six SARS patients led Nicholls et al. (30) to conclude that proinflammatory cytokines released by stimulated alveolar macrophages have a prominent role in the pathogenesis of SARS. The role of immunopathogenic mechanisms in SARS is the subject of ongoing investigations. Lymphopenia is common among patients with SARS. In a cohort of 38 SARS patients, CD4 T-lymphocyte counts were reduced in all, but reductions in circulating levels of CD8 T lymphocytes, B lymphocytes, and natural killer cells were also common (31). CD4 and CD8 lymphocyte counts fall early in the course of illness, and low CD4 and CD8 levels have been associated with more severe illness (32).

Death from SARS usually occurs late in the course of illness (>1 week after onset) and has been attributed to adult respiratory distress syndrome (ARDS), multiorgan failure, thromboembolic complications, secondary infections, and septic shock (33,34). Co-infection with human metapneumovirus has been reported among patients with laboratory confirmed SARS (35); however, the role of co-infection or superinfection in amplifying the pathogenicity of SARS-CoV is unknown at this time.

CLINICAL MANIFESTATIONS

Investigation of SARS cases occurring after a single known contact indicate that illness usually begins 2 to 10 days after exposure. The most common initial symptom is fever, often accompanied by headache, myalgias, malaise, chills, and rigor (2, 4,19,35–39). In some patients, headache, myalgia, and malaise precede the onset of fever by up to 1 day, and fever may resolve by the time respiratory symptoms, such as cough and dyspnea, appear. Respiratory symptoms typically do not begin until 2 to 7 days following illness onset, although they are among the initial symptoms in up to 30% of patients. The most common respiratory complaints are nonproductive cough and dyspnea; however, productive cough is reported in up to 25% of patients. Upper respiratory complaints, such as rhinorrhea or sore throat, are less common and are reported in <25% of patients (2,19,35–37, 40). The prevalence of gastrointestinal symptoms at presentation has varied by report, but nausea, vomiting, and/or diarrhea have generally been reported in up to 25% of patients (2,4,19,35–38, 41). In one series, 73% of patients developed diarrhea at some point in the course of illness (39). Fever and diarrhea have been the dominant presenting symptoms in some patients (42). Asymptomatic infection with SARS-CoV appears to be uncommon (43,44).

Elderly patients and those with underlying chronic illnesses such as renal failure may not present with typical symptoms of SARS (42,45,46). SARS was relatively uncommon among children during 2003, and compared with adults, illness appeared to be generally milder among children with SARS (47, 48). For patients in these groups who have strong epidemiologic risk factors for SARS, a strong index of suspicion is appropriate, even in the absence of typical clinical features.

Physical findings in patients with SARS include tachypnea and tachycardia, which have been reported in 40% to 75% of patients upon admission to the hospital (2,4,35,36), but may be less common among patients who present earlier in the course of illness (38). As many as 15% to 44% of patients have a normal body temperature at the time of presentation (35,36). Rales or rhonchi have been detected by auscultation in the majority of patients in some series, and less commonly in others (2,36,38, 49). Some have observed a paucity of auscultatory findings despite marked infiltration on chest radiography (38,49).

Hypoxemia is a common finding in patients with respiratory symptoms of SARS (2,35). Hematologic abnormalities are among the most consistent laboratory findings reported; most patients have total white blood counts that are normal or slightly low, and 70% to 95% of patients have lymphopenia (2,32, 35–37,39). Platelet counts are mildly depressed in 30% to 50% of patients. Prolongation of the activated partial thromboplastin time can be observed in 40% to 60% of patients, but disseminated intravascular coagulation is uncommon (32,37). Other common abnormal laboratory findings include elevated lactate dehydrogenase levels in 70% to 90%, elevated alanine aminotransferase or aspartate aminotransferase levels in 20% to 30%, and elevated creatine phosphokinase in 30% to 40% (37–39, 50).

Although the full understanding of the spectrum of radiographic manifestations of SARS requires additional information, the available data suggest that almost all reported patients with laboratory evidence of SARS-CoV infection have radiographic evidence of pneumonia at some point during the course of illness (35,38,51). However, chest radiographs may be normal at the time of presentation in up to 30% of patients with a clinical diagnosis of SARS (36,39,52–54). In reports from China during 2003, radiographic changes consistent with pneumonia were detected in 67% to 80% by day 3 of illness, 97% to 100% by day

7 of illness, and in 100% by day 10 of illness (53,54). Among 144 patients with illness meeting the surveillance case definition of SARS in Toronto, 10% did not have pulmonary infiltrates documented (36). The lesions typically begin as an isolated focal lesion found predominately in a peripheral location, often in the lower lobes. In 75% of patients the lesions progress over several days to involve additional lobes or both lungs (52,54).

Computed tomography (CT) of the chest appears to be more sensitive than conventional chest radiography for detecting pneumonia. SARS patients who have normal chest radiographic findings early in their clinical course often have evidence of pneumonia by CT (37,55). Common thin-section CT findings are ground-glass opacification with a lower lobe and peripheral distribution (55).

As with other causes of bacterial and viral pneumonia, clinical findings in patients with SARS cannot always predict the etiologic agent. Further study is required to determine whether a constellation of clinical findings alone can be used to discriminate accurately between SARS and other respiratory illnesses (especially viral respiratory illnesses). Many of the clinical and laboratory features of SARS are similar to other forms of viral pneumonia (49,56). Several clinical features, however, may be helpful in facilitating recognition of patients with SARS (Table 113.1) (57).

Severity of illness and risk of death from SARS increases with advanced age and in the presence of certain underlying medical conditions. Severity of illness was independently associated with advanced age and chronic hepatitis B virus infection treated with lamivudine among SARS patients in Hong Kong (32,37,39). In multivariable analysis of 144 patients in Canada, the risk of death or admission to intensive care was associated with age ≥60 years and the presence of diabetes mellitus and other comorbid conditions (36,58). Mortality for SARS patients aged 60 years and older in 2003 was 43% to 54%, compared with 3% to 13% for persons aged <60 years (19,59).

TABLE 113.1. COMMON CLINICAL FEATURES OF SEVERE ACUTE RESPIRATORY SYNDROME (SARS)

- Presenting symptoms
  - Nonrespiratory prodrome lasting 2 to 7 days characterized by one or more of the following:
    - Fever
    - Rigors
    - Headache
    - Malaise
    - Myalgia
    - Diarrhea
  - Respiratory phase beginning 2 to 7 days after onset characterized by:
    - Nonproductive cough
    - Dyspnea
    - Absence of upper respiratory symptoms
- Laboratory findings
  - Normal or low total white blood cell count
  - Lymphopenia
  - Mildly depressed platelet count
  - Elevated lactate dehydrogenase levels
  - Elevated creatine phospokinase levels
  - Elevated transaminase levels
  - Prolonged activated partial thromboplastin time
- Radiographic findings
  - Abnormal chest x-ray in almost all patients by the second week of illness

DIAGNOSIS

The diagnosis of SARS is based on either detection of the virus in clinical specimens or the finding of antibodies directed against SARS-CoV in serum. Isolation of the virus in Vero E6 cells and morphologic characterization of the virus by electron microscopy provided the initial evidence for the role of a previously unrecognized coronavirus in SARS. However, viral culture is not recommended for routine diagnosis because of low sensitivity and because isolation of SARS-CoV requires biosafety level (BSL)-3 facilities and work practices. In general, manipulation of untreated clinical specimens from patients with SARS may be performed in BSL-2 laboratories using BSL-3 work practices. Any procedure with the potential to generate fine particulate aerosols (e.g., vortexing or sonication of specimens in an open tube) should be performed in a biologic safety cabinet, and consideration should be given to use of respiratory protection using a properly fitted National Institute for Occupational Safety and Health (NIOSH)-approved respirator (N-95 or higher). Work surfaces and equipment should be decontaminated using agents that are effective against lipid-enveloped viruses.

RT-PCR has provided a powerful tool for the diagnosis of SARS. A highly sensitive real-time RT-PCR assay that can detect as few as one to ten copies is available. The assay targets three sites in the nucleocapsid and polymerase genes, and amplification of at least two targets is required for a test to be considered positive. All positive tests should be confirmed by testing of a second specimen and by testing in a reference laboratory. Shedding of virus in respiratory secretions is greatest early in the second week of illness (39,60); therefore, specimens collected in the first few days after onset may be falsely negative because of low numbers of virions.

Antibodies to SARS-CoV may be detected by enzyme immunosorbent assay (EIA) as early as the end of the first week of illness. However, delayed seroconversions have been reported (39,61); therefore, serologic assays for SARS should not be considered negative until a specimen collected at least 28 days after onset has been tested. The EIA for SARS-CoV appears to be highly specific. No cross-reactions have been documented with coronavirus OC43 or 229E. No antibodies to SARS-CoV were detected among blood donors from the U.S. during 2003 (3). The duration of the antibody response to SARS-CoV has not yet been determined.

Body fluids that should be submitted for testing from patients with suspected SARS include respiratory tract secretions, serum, whole blood, and stool. Lower respiratory tract specimens (e.g., sputum, bronchial alveolar lavage fluid) appear to have higher yield than upper respiratory tract specimens (e.g., nasal or pharyngeal aspirates or swabs). Collection of multiple specimens during the course of illness may be required to confirm the diagnosis, particularly if presentation is early after illness onset. SARS-CoV may be detected in whole blood by RT-PCR in the first few days after illness onset. SARS-CoV may be detected in respiratory secretions and stool during convalescence and for 3 or more weeks after illness onset.

Based on experience with SARS during 2003, three epidemiologic clues should increase clinical suspicion for SARS: (a) travel to an areas where SARS has been known to be transmitted or exposure to a person with SARS, (b) clustering of cases with clinical manifestations suggestive of SARS, or (c) exposure to a healthcare facility. If all three of these epidemiologic clues are missing, the likelihood of SARS is very low, and the risk of a false-positive test for SARS-CoV is increased. When no SARS transmission is known to be occurring anywhere in the world, testing for SARS-CoV should be restricted to persons with a suggestive clinical presentation and at least one of these three epidemiologic clues. Unusual circumstances, such as a clinically compatible illness in a person working with SARS-CoV in a research laboratory, may also justify testing for SARS.

Laboratory evaluation and management of patients with suspected SARS should include consideration of other common respiratory pathogens, particularly if the clinical or epidemiologic picture is not highly suggestive of SARS. Respiratory pathogens that were commonly identified among patients with illness meeting the case definition of SARS in the U.S. during March to July 2003 included *Mycoplasma pneumoniae,* picornaviruses, influenza viruses, human metapneumovirus, adenovirus, and human parainfluenza viruses (62). *Streptococcus pneumoniae* and infection with other pyogenic bacteria were also diagnosed among patients with suspected SARS. In addition to the clinical and epidemiologic picture, the predictive value of the tests utilized must be considered before assuming an alternative diagnosis and discontinuing infection control precautions for patients with possible SARS. For example, serologic test results from a single specimen suggesting infection with another microorganism or isolation of bacteria from sputum without Gram stain indicating the same microorganism in a specimen of good quality have occurred in cases of laboratory-confirmed SARS cases, and results of these tests can be quite misleading.

New diagnostic tests will likely become available in the near future. A particular challenge is development of tests that can provide a definitive diagnosis early in the course of illness. An immunohistochemical stain for SARS-CoV has been developed and has been used for documenting SARS-CoV antigen in infected Vero cells from culture; however, at the time of this writing, immunohistochemical staining of tissue from persons with SARS have not provided clinically useful information. Newer serologic assays, including a SARS-CoV specific immunoglobulin M (IgM) assay are under evaluation and may provide valuable tools for earlier diagnosis and epidemiologic investigations (63).

EPIDEMIOLOGY

The epidemiology of SARS has been quite variable in different regions of the world. In Singapore, Vietnam, and Canada, transmission occurred primarily among household members and in healthcare facilities, and almost all cases can be linked to close contact with a person who is ill with SARS. In Hong Kong and China, transmission was much more widespread and a large number of cases occurred among persons with no known history of exposure to other SARS patients. China accounted for over half of all SARS cases reported in the world during 2003, with cases reported from 24 of China's 31 provinces (64). Over 2,500 cases occurred in Beijing alone during March to July 2003, representing an attack rate of 19 cases/100,000 population (65).

The epidemiology of SARS in China has provided clues for ongoing investigation into the origin of SARS-CoV. In Guangdong Province during November 2002 to February 2003, some of the earliest SARS cases occurred among persons who handle, kill, or sell food animals or those who prepare and serve food (64,66). A coronavirus with 99% homology with human SARS-CoV isolates has been recovered from Himalayan palm civets (also known as civet cats, *Paguma larvata*) and a raccoon-dog (*Nyctereutes procyonoides*) sold live for food in markets in Guangzhou, Guangdong Province (67). Of 508 animal traders in three Guangzhou animal markets tested in 2003, 6% to 20% had antibody to SARS-CoV, and the animal traders were significantly more likely to have antibodies compared with control groups of healthcare workers, public health staff, and healthy adults (68). Although investigations in other areas suggest that asymptomatic infection with SARS-CoV is rare (43), none of the seropositive animal traders in Guangzhou reported illness suggestive of SARS. Taken together, these observations support the hypothesis that SARS-CoV was first transmitted from wild animals used for food to humans, with subsequent person-to-person transmission. Most coronaviruses cause disease in only one host species (69); however, the possible role of ongoing zoonotic transmission cannot be excluded at present.

A small minority of persons with SARS appear to be very efficient in transmitting SAR-CoV to susceptible persons under certain circumstances, leading to so-called super-spreading events. Super-spreading events have occurred in a number of settings including the hotel in Hong Kong where transmission occurred in February 2003, an apartment complex in Hong Kong, and hospitals in Hong Kong, Taiwan, Vietnam, Singapore, and Canada (1,19,35,46,59,70,71). Factors contributing to super-spreading events are poorly defined. It is not known whether transmission by a mode other than respiratory droplets, such as airborne spread, contributes to super-spreading events.

Mathematical modeling of data from Hong Kong and Singapore suggest that without control measures, each SARS case will lead to 2.2 to 3.7 secondary cases in a susceptible population (72,73). Although these numbers suggest a lower level of infectivity and a greater likelihood of success with control measures than would be expected for influenza or measles, they also indicate that in the absence of infection control precautions, SARS has the potential to spread very widely. Additionally, the models are based on limited data and may not adequately address the role of super-spreading events in global transmission. In fact, one of the models excludes super-spreading events from the estimation altogether (72).

Transmission of SARS-CoV from infected persons without symptoms of SARS was not documented in 2003. Thus, the period of communicability is thought to begin after onset of symptoms. Quantitative RT-PCR testing of nasopharyngeal aspirates indicates that the greatest level of viral shedding and, presumably, communicability occurs early in the second week of illness (39,60). Virus has been detected by RT-PCR in clinical specimens more than 3 weeks after onset, but transmission from SARS patients late in convalescence has not been reported.

Healthcare workers were particularly affected by SARS during 2003, and transmission to healthcare workers was common prior to institution of infection control precautions in hospitals evaluating patients with SARS. Factors that possibly facilitated spread of SARS in hospitals and from hospitals into communities have included transfer of SARS patients to other healthcare facilities (42), admission of large numbers of infectious patients during a short period (70), use of personal attendants (persons hired by families to provide care for inpatients) who are not supplied with and trained in the use of appropriate PPE (42), delay in hospitalization and institution of isolation until late in the course of illness (72), delay in instituting isolation because SARS is not considered in the differential diagnosis (59), uncontrolled access for visitors to isolation wards (20), lack of strict policy for direct admission of suspected SARS patients to isolation (20), atypical clinical presentations causing a delay in diagnosis and isolation (45,71), heavy exposure to infectious aerosols during intubation, bronchoscopy, or airway manipulation (26,59,71), unrecognized SARS in healthcare personnel (42,46,74), and inadequate training in use of PPE (71).

CONTROL AND PREVENTION

General

In the absence of a vaccine, effective drugs, or natural immunity to SARS-CoV, the only currently available strategies to limit the spread of SARS are based on traditional public health tools used to prevent the transmission of any infectious disease. These measures include global and community surveillance, detection and isolation of cases, identification and monitoring of contacts, adherence to infection control precautions, and, in some instances, measures to restrict the movement of asymptomatic but potentially infected persons (e.g., quarantine). Once patients suspected of having SARS are identified, they should be rapidly isolated to separate them from healthy persons and to restrict their movement to prevent transmission to others. Isolation may take place within a healthcare facility, home, or other facility in the community, depending on the patient's medical needs.

A critical component of community prevention strategies is establishing a system to rapidly and efficiently identify, evaluate, and monitor contacts of patients with SARS. In limited outbreaks, asymptomatic contacts need not be restricted in their activities. In more extensive outbreak settings, quarantine of exposed persons may be considered as a means of further reducing exposures that might occur during the interval between onset of symptoms and institution of appropriate precautions. In some situations, depending on the extent of the outbreak and the availability of resources, implementation of more extensive community-based control measures that decrease social interaction and make inadvertent SARS exposures less likely may be considered, such as cancellation of public events and closure of schools.

Timely dissemination of information on extent and manner of SARS transmission to the public health and healthcare communities and to the public is critical for development of appropriate control policies at the local, regional, and national levels. Other measures that may be important in control of SARS outside of healthcare settings include issuance of travel alerts/advisories, screening of ill travelers at airports, and other border control measures to prevent international spread.

Healthcare Settings

Healthcare facilities have played a central role in the epidemiology of SARS. Once SARS-CoV is introduced into a community, infected patients may present to healthcare facilities. If not recognized and isolated early, these patients likely will transmit SARS-CoV to healthcare workers and other patients. Persons who work in healthcare settings were among the earliest and most severely affected populations in almost every major outbreak during 2003 (37,42,59). For example, in Toronto and Singapore, 43% and 41%, respectively, of the SARS cases occurred in healthcare workers (75). When cases among patients and visitors are considered, greater than 50% of all SARS cases reported in some regions were likely acquired in healthcare settings (36,46). Prevention of transmission of SARS-CoV within healthcare settings will play a crucial role in preventing and controlling future SARS outbreaks.

At the time of this writing, there remain unanswered questions regarding the epidemiology and transmission of SARS-CoV. Current infection control recommendations are based on the experience to date, and may change as new data become available.

Preventing Droplet and Contact Transmission

The predominant mode of transmission of SARS-CoV in the healthcare setting appears to be through large respiratory droplets or direct contact (25,59). Droplet transmission involves contact of the conjunctivae or the mucous membranes of the nose or mouth of a susceptible person with large-particle droplets (larger than 5 μm in size) containing microorganisms generated from a person who is infected with SARS-CoV. Droplets are generated primarily during coughing, sneezing, or talking and during the performance of certain procedures such as suctioning and bronchoscopy. Transmission via large-particle droplets requires close contact between source and recipient persons, because droplets do not remain suspended in the air and generally travel only short distances through the air.

Standard Precautions, including hand hygiene, and precautions that adequately protect against transmission by both the droplet and contact routes should be employed when caring for patients with SARS. Protection against droplet transmission requires that healthcare personnel wear a mask when working within 1 m of the patient. Generally, a surgical mask is used for Droplet Precautions, but in the case of SARS, where protection against airborne transmission is also recommended (see below), devices that provide respiratory protection (e.g., N-95 respirators) should serve the same purpose. Contact Precautions are designed to reduce the risk of transmitting infectious agents by direct or indirect contact with an infectious person and involve placing the patient in a private room, if possible, and the use of gloves and gowns when entering the patient's room. In addition, dedicated use of noncritical patient-care equipment to a single patient should be considered to avoid sharing between patients. If use of common equipment or items is unavoidable, then they should be adequately cleaned and disinfected before use for another patient.

Eye protection has been recommended for use by healthcare personnel caring for SARS patients (76). The additional protective impact of this recommendation is not yet known, but there is theoretical rationale to support it. Epidemiologic study of other viral illnesses, such as rhinovirus infection, suggest that autoinoculation of the conjunctival mucosa via contaminated hands is an efficient means of viral transmission (77). Given the high attack rate of SARS among exposed healthcare workers and the potentially severe morbidity and mortality associated with the infection, use of eye protection may be prudent pending further epidemiologic study.

Cleaning and disinfection of environmental surfaces may be important components of preventing transmission of SARS in healthcare facilities. Those surfaces that are touched frequently may become contaminated. Preliminary data suggest that SARS-CoV loses infectivity after exposure to commonly used disinfectants (27). Therefore, frequently touched surfaces should be cleaned and disinfected with an approved hospital disinfectant effective against enveloped viruses daily and when visible soiling/contamination occurs.

Preventing Possible Airborne Transmission

Although the primary mode of transmission in the healthcare setting appears to be via large respiratory droplets or contact (25,59), airborne transmission cannot be ruled out as an occasional mode of transmission. Airborne transmission occurs by dissemination of infectious airborne nuclei of evaporated droplets, generally <5 μm in diameter, that may remain suspended in the air for periods of time longer than that of larger respiratory droplets. Microorganisms carried in this manner can be dispersed by air currents or ventilation systems and may be inhaled by or deposited on a susceptible host some distance from the source patient. Occasional reports suggest that transmission of SARS-CoV by the airborne route may have occurred, particularly in the setting of aerosol-generating medical procedures involving the respiratory tract such as endotracheal intubation (22, 23,26,59,71).

Based on these and similar events in which transmission by the airborne route cannot be ruled out, Airborne Precautions should be employed when possible in the care of patients with SARS until the epidemiology of transmission is better understood. Airborne Precautions include placing the patient in an airborne infection isolation room that has negative pressure relative to the surrounding area, and use of respiratory protection (N-95 particulate respirator or other respirators with equivalent or higher levels of respiratory protection) when entering the patient's room. Adherence to Airborne Precautions should also protect against spread by the droplet route.

Because aerosol-generating procedures may pose a greater risk of SARS transmission (22,23,26,59,71), additional precautions should be considered for those performing and attending procedures such as administration of aerosolized or nebulized medications, diagnostic sputum induction, bronchoscopy, airway suctioning, endotracheal intubation, positive pressure ventilation via face mask [e.g., bi-level positive airway pressure (BiPAP), continuous positive airway pressure (CPAP)], and high-frequency oscillatory ventilation. Healthcare facilities should review their strategies to protect healthcare personnel during aerosol-generating procedures, including the use of PPE and safe work practices such as limiting performance of aerosol-generating procedures on SARS patients to those procedures that are considered medically essential; using clinically appropriate sedation during intubation and bronchoscopy to minimize resistance and coughing during the procedure; limiting the healthcare personnel present in the room during an aerosol-generating procedure to those essential for patient care and support; performing aerosol-generating procedures in an airborne infection isolation room, or if an airborne infection isolation room is not available, performing the procedure in a private room, away from other patients; and using bacterial/viral filters on exhalation valves of mechanical ventilators to prevent contaminated aerosols from entering the environment.

Disposable particulate respirators (e.g., N-95, N-99, or N-100) are sufficient for routine respiratory protection for Airborne Precautions and are the minimum level of respiratory protection for healthcare personnel who are performing aerosol-generating procedures. To ensure adequate protection, healthcare personnel must be fit-tested to the respirator model that they will wear, and also know how to check their face-piece seal. A fit-check to ensure an appropriate seal between the mask and face should be performed each time the respirator is donned, prior to entering the patient room. If disposable respirators cannot be fit-tested to the healthcare provider, a higher level of respiratory protection should be used.

Healthcare facilities in some SARS affected areas have used higher levels of respiratory protection, such as powered air purifying respirators or full face-piece elastomeric negative pressure (i.e., nonpowered) respirators with N-, R-, or P-100 filters, for persons present during aerosol-generating procedures on SARS patients (71). It is unknown whether these higher levels of respiratory protection further reduce transmission. Factors that should be considered in choosing respirators in this setting include availability, impact on mobility and communication, comfort, and the potential for reusable respirators to serve as fomites for transmission.

The optimal combination of PPE other than respiratory protective devices for preventing transmission of SARS during aerosol-generating procedures has not been determined. It is possible that the increased risk of transmission during such procedures is due not to airborne transmission, but rather to extensive contamination of the environment by respiratory secretions. Under such conditions it is possible that autoinoculation of mucosal surfaces occurs via hands that become contaminated after contacting contaminated PPE during removal or after contact with exposed areas of skin or hair that were contaminated during the procedure. For this reason, some have recommended additional PPE to protect all exposed areas of skin or hair. It may also be important to provide training on a proper PPE removal procedure that guards against self-inoculation from contaminated items such as gloves, masks, or gowns.

Discontinuing Precautions

Patients suspected of having SARS should remain under appropriate isolation precautions for the duration of the period of communicability, or until convincing evidence against SARS is documented. During 2003, the isolation of patients until 10 days after resolution of fever provided that respiratory symptoms were improving seemed an effective method to prevent additional transmission, and no cases of transmission during convalescence were documented (76,78).

The Centers for Disease Control and Prevention (CDC) currently recommends hospitalization for SARS patients based on medical need, not on the need for infection control (76). Patients can be isolated at home or other non-healthcare facilities if sufficient infection control measures can be established to keep household members and the community at minimal risk of exposure. Minimum requirements for home isolation might include the availability of a primary caregiver to assist the patient with basic needs, a separate bedroom that will be occupied only by the SARS patient during the isolation period, access to a bathroom designated for use only by the SARS patient, and adequate PPE for patient and contacts (e.g., gloves, surgical masks) with instructions for proper use. If possible, a SARS patient should wear a surgical mask during close contact with uninfected persons to prevent the spread of infectious droplets. When a SARS patient is unable to wear a surgical mask, household members should wear surgical masks when in close contact with the patient.

Preparedness Planning

Surveillance and Triage

Although unanswered questions remain regarding the epidemiology of SARS, it appears that the standard infection control measures discussed above can dramatically reduce transmission of SARS-CoV (25,59,79,80). The most difficult challenge in preventing transmission, however, is not preventing transmission from known or suspected SARS patients, but rather early recognition of patients with SARS from among the large population of patients with fever and respiratory illness. In every region in which major outbreaks were reported in 2003, a substantial proportion of cases resulted from delays in clinical recognition and isolation of SARS among patients, visitors, and healthcare workers (37,42,46,59,79). Studies of the transmission dynamics in Hong Kong, Singapore, and Canada all suggest that early case detection will be a critical component in controlling future outbreaks of SARS (72,73,80,81).

Therefore, healthcare facilities should develop strategies to identify patients at risk for SARS as soon as possible after presenting for care. A graded approach to early recognition based on the level of SARS activity in the world, the surrounding community, and within the facility will be needed (57). At the time of this writing there are no widely available rapid diagnostic tests that can be used at the point of care to rule out SARS among patients presenting with febrile respiratory illnesses. Because the early clinical features can be similar to other viral infections, rapid recognition of patients with SARS from among the much larger population of patients with more common respiratory illnesses presents clinicians and infection control professionals with a dilemma. Screening methods that are not sufficiently sensitive may result in uncontrolled transmission of SARS, whereas nonspecific screening methods could lead to unnecessary isolation of large numbers of persons. This in turn could rapidly overburden the already limited resources of both the healthcare and public health systems. A balanced approach to early recognition of SARS requires that clinicians not only look for suggestive clinical features, but also routinely include questions in the medical history that may provide epidemiologic clues suggesting exposure to other persons with SARS-CoV infection.

The clinical and epidemiologic clues that should trigger suspicion may vary depending on the level of documented SARS activity in the surrounding community and the world. In the absence of any documented SARS cases worldwide, the overall likelihood that a given patient being evaluated for fever or respiratory illness has SARS-CoV infection will be exceedingly low unless there are both typical clinical findings and some accompanying epidemiologic evidence that raises the index of suspicion for SARS-CoV infection. Therefore, one approach would be to consider the diagnosis only among patients with both unexplained pneumonia and one of the following: an epidemiologic link to a cluster of cases of unexplained pneumonia, a history of contact with ill persons during recent travel to a previously SARS-affected area (or close contact with an ill traveler with such a history), or some unusual exposure history, such as working in a laboratory where SARS-CoV is propagated. Patients who have such risk factors may still have a low likelihood of having SARS. Rather than placing all such patients in Airborne Precautions, Droplet Precautions should be applied during further clinical and epidemiologic investigation. Healthcare facilities should consider initiating a policy of universal respiratory hygiene/cough etiquette, in which surgical masks or tissues are provided to all patients presenting with respiratory symptoms, and such patients are separated from other patients as soon as possible, either by placing them directly into an examination room or by providing a separate area of the waiting room. The use of Droplet Precautions (i.e., surgical masks when working within 1 m of the patient) by healthcare personnel during evaluation of any patient with respiratory illness should also be considered (82).

Once SARS activity has been documented anywhere in the world, the positive predictive value of clinical symptoms, although still low (38), is more acceptable if used in combination with an epidemiologic link to settings in which SARS has been documented. Therefore, after SARS transmission has been documented in the world, all patients with fever or respiratory symptoms should be screened for a history of close contact to persons with SARS, travel to areas or epidemiologic settings in which SARS transmission is suspected, or contact with ill persons with such a travel or exposure history. Patients with a clinical syndrome compatible with SARS and one of these risk factors should be placed on Airborne and Contact Precautions pending further workup (57).

Preparedness planning should include strategies to ensure that clinicians and intake and triage staff are familiar with the appropriate procedures for screening, triage, and placement of patients with possible SARS within the outpatient facility and that they know where and how to report a potential SARS case. In addition, plans should include a mechanism for providing regular updates to clinicians and staff on the status of SARS activity locally, nationally, and internationally (82).

If the number of patients presenting with SARS is limited, such as in the setting of no or limited local transmission of SARS, evaluation and triage should be feasible within the existing patient intake infrastructures. In the event that community outbreaks of SARS become extensive, healthcare facilities and communities may need to plan for a separate designated space for a SARS evaluation center, which may be a temporary structure or part of an existing facility. The purpose is to separate potential SARS patients from other patients seeking healthcare. Planning for these specialized evaluation centers should include determining appropriate traffic routes and modes of transport for patients who must be taken from the evaluation center to the healthcare facility for further evaluation or inpatient care (82). Extensive transmission in the community may also necessitate limiting visitors and establishing a mechanism for actively screening all persons entering the facility for symptoms and signs of a febrile or respiratory illness.

Patient Placement, Isolation, and Cohorting

Appropriate patient placement is a significant component of effective SARS control. Each healthcare facility should develop a strategy and procedures to (a) quickly separate potential SARS patients from other patients, and (b) implement appropriate isolation procedures. In outpatient facilities that have limited or no airborne infection isolation rooms, transmission may be substantially decreased by simple procedures such as placing a surgical mask on potential SARS patients and moving them to a private examination room as soon as feasible while awaiting availability of airborne isolation rooms. In some inpatient settings, a lack of sufficient airborne isolation rooms and the need to concentrate infection control efforts and resources may lead to a strategy of cohorting patients in individual rooms on the same floor, rather than placing them in airborne isolation rooms throughout the hospital. This strategy physically isolates SARS patients from non-SARS patients and also makes it possible to dedicate resources and appropriately trained staff to their care. Part of SARS preparedness planning should include identification of an area of the hospital that could serve this purpose and determining whether non-airborne isolation rooms or areas designated for SARS care might be modified to achieve appropriate airflow (82). Healthcare facilities should develop a patient transport plan to safely move SARS patients within the facility and identify routes to segregate SARS patients from main traffic paths as much as possible (82).

Exposure Reporting and Evaluation Among Healthcare Personnel

Unrecognized SARS-CoV infection among healthcare workers may have contributed substantially to nosocomial transmission during 2003 (42,46,74). Therefore, a critical component of preventing transmission in the healthcare setting is assuring that mechanisms are in place to rapidly report unprotected exposures of healthcare providers to patients with SARS and to evaluate and manage exposed workers. Various approaches to management of exposed healthcare workers have been used. In some outbreak settings, healthcare workers were excluded from duty following unprotected exposures, whereas in other settings exposed healthcare personnel were allowed to continue work while being actively monitored (e.g., daily interview and temperature measurement) for symptoms and signs that might suggest early manifestations of SARS. The optimal approach is currently unknown. The CDC currently recommends excluding from duty only those healthcare workers with unprotected high-risk exposures, such as being in the same room as a SARS patient during an aerosol generating procedure when infection control precautions were absent or breached. Healthcare workers with lower risk exposures need not be excluded from duty, but should be under active surveillance for development of fever or respiratory symptoms (82).

Staffing, Resources, and Communication

A SARS outbreak has the potential to challenge a healthcare facility's ability to meet staffing and resource needs. During an outbreak of any size, existing staffing shortages may be amplified by illness among staff members or their families, fear and concern about SARS, and quarantine of exposed staff members. Staffing shortages are also likely to escalate as an outbreak progresses. During the preparedness period, it is important to plan for how to meet the range of staffing needs that might be required to manage a SARS outbreak. Potential strategies include relocating healthcare workers to different settings or modifying the type of services they usually provide. Non-healthcare workers or retired healthcare workers may be utilized to provide supplementary services. Volunteers will also be a potential human resource during an emergency response. Use of alternative staffing will require training in the details of SARS infection control and exposure management (82).

Both consumable (e.g., PPE) and durable (e.g., ventilators) supplies will be needed to care for SARS patients. Experience during 2003 indicates that a SARS outbreak may not only strain a facility's stock of these resources but also affect the ability to order replacement supplies. As part of preparedness planning, healthcare facilities should determine the current availability of and anticipated need for supplies and equipment that would be used in a SARS outbreak (82).

When SARS is present in the community surrounding a healthcare facility, preventing unrecognized SARS patients from entering the facility is essential. Appropriate surveillance and screening measures might include establishing criteria and protocols for limiting hospital admissions, transfers, and discharges, in accordance with local/state recommendations and regulations. Healthcare facilities should also establish criteria and protocols for limiting hospital visitors, and in the case of extensive community outbreaks, screening all persons entering the facility for signs and symptoms of a febrile or respiratory illness (82).

Because early recognition of SARS depends on identifying the epidemiologic linkage to SARS-affected persons or places, clinicians must remain updated with current information regarding the locations of SARS activity in order to obtain the appropriate history from patients with fever or respiratory illness. Mechanisms for rapid communication among healthcare facilities, clinicians, and public health agencies must be in place so that frequent updates can be obtained as outbreaks evolve both locally and globally. Rapid communication is also important in helping public health agencies more rapidly identify emerging areas of activity, such as clusters of illness or spread of infection into new geographic areas. Similarly, communication between healthcare facilities within the community is essential. Rapid communication of the epidemiologic details of SARS activity in a particular affected location or facility greatly informs assessment of risk of exposure for patients presenting to other healthcare facilities.

UNANSWERED QUESTIONS AND LESSONS LEARNED

A number of questions remain about optimal methods for prevention and control of SARS in healthcare settings. Defining the relative importance of masks, gowns, eye shields, and hand hygiene is critical for controlling the spread of SARS, particularly in developing countries where resources and availability of PPE may be limited. Better understanding of the mode of transmission and factors contributing to super-spreading events also will allow more efficient use of PPE. The role of environmental contamination and spread of SARS-CoV by fomites, and determining optimal methods of environmental disinfection are the subject of ongoing research. Refined screening criteria are needed to identify infectious patients and institute isolation as early as possible in the period of communicability (38,57). More data are needed to determine the exact period of communicability so that isolation is not extended longer than is needed and to determine the role of quarantine for healthy persons who are well but have had a high-risk exposure. Preexposure and postexposure prophylaxis require development of vaccines and antiviral agents active against SARS-CoV.

The control of SARS in 2003 is testimony to the power of basic public health and infection control tools—surveillance, isolation and quarantine, use of appropriate PPE, and basic epidemiologic investigation. However, the future of SARS is unknown. Ongoing low-level transmission among persons with few or no symptoms, spread of SARS-CoV from infected mammals, or accidental or intentional release of SARS-CoV from a laboratory could lead to a return of epidemic SARS. Of the many lessons learned from SARS during 2003, perhaps the most important is the critical role of the infection control professional to prevent spread of infection among patients, visitors, and staff within healthcare facilities. In addition to preventing infection, effective infection control practices play a critical role in minimizing the psychological impact of epidemic disease on healthcare facility staff and in ensuring continuing hospital operations (40,83). Our ability to learn from the experience of SARS in 2003 will have a profound effect on prevention and control of the next microbial threat in healthcare settings, whether that be a resurgence of SARS, emergence of another new infectious disease, the intentional release of smallpox or plague, transmission of multidrug-resistant nosocomial pathogens, or pandemic spread of a new influenza virus.

ADDITIONAL INFORMATION

CDC SARS Website: *http://www.cdc.gov/ncidod/sars/*

HealthCanada SARS Website: *http://www.hc-sc.gc.ca/pphb-dgspsp/sars-sras/index.html*

WHO SARS Website: *http://www.who.int/csr/sars/en/*

ACKNOWLEDGMENTS

The authors would like to thank Rita Helfand, Donald Low, Arjun Srinivasan, and other members of the Centers for Disease Control and Prevention SARS Preparedness Task Force for their contributions to CDC's "Public Health Guidance for Community-Level Preparedness and Response to Severe Acute Respiratory Syndrome" (82), which formed the basis of many of the prevention and control concepts described in this chapter.

REFERENCES

1. Centers for Disease Control and Prevention. Update: outbreak of severe acute respiratory syndrome—worldwide, 2003. *MMWR* 2003;52:241–246,248.
2. Tsang KW, Ho PL, Ooi GC, et al. A cluster of cases of severe acute respiratory syndrome in Hong Kong. *N Engl J Med* 2003;348:1977–1985.
3. Ksiazek TG, Erdman D, Goldsmith CS, et al. A novel coronavirus associated with severe acute respiratory syndrome. *N Engl J Med* 2003;348:1953–1966.
4. Drosten C, Gunther S, Preiser W, et al. Identification of a novel coronavirus in patients with severe acute respiratory syndrome. *N Engl J Med* 2003;348:1967–1976.
5. Peiris JS, Lai ST, Poon LL, et al. Coronavirus as a possible cause of severe acute respiratory syndrome. *Lancet* 2003;361:1319–1325.
6. World Health Organization Multicentre Collaborative Network for Severe Acute Respiratory Syndrome (SARS) Diagnosis. A multicentre collaboration to investigate the cause of severe acute respiratory syndrome. *Lancet* 2003;361:1730–1733.
7. Rota PA, Oberste MS, Monroe SS, et al. Characterization of a novel coronavirus associated with severe acute respiratory syndrome. *Science* 2003;300:1394–1399.
8. Marra MA, Jones SJ, Astell CR, et al. The genome sequence of the SARS-associated coronavirus. *Science* 2003;300:1399–1404.
9. Fouchier RA, Kuiken T, Schutten M, et al. Koch's postulates fulfilled for SARS virus. *Nature* 2003;423:240.
10. Kuiken T, Fouchier RA, Schutten M, et al. Newly discovered coronavirus as the primary cause of severe acute respiratory syndrome. *Lancet* 2003;362:263–270.
11. Kapikian AZ, James HD Jr, Kelly SJ, et al. Isolation from man of "avian infectious bronchitis virus-like" viruses (coronaviruses) similar to 229E virus, with some epidemiological observations. *J Infect Dis* 1969;119:282–290.
12. McIntosh K, Becker WB, Chanock RM. Growth in suckling-mouse brain of "IBV-like" viruses from patients with upper respiratory tract disease. *Proc Natl Acad Sci USA* 1967;58:2268–2273.
13. Hendley JO, Fishburne HB, Gwaltney JM Jr. Coronavirus infections in working adults. Eight-year study with 229 E and OC 43. *Am Rev Respir Dis* 1972;105:805–811.
14. McIntosh K, Kapikian AZ, Turner HC, et al. Seroepidemiologic studies of coronavirus infection in adults and children. *Am J Epidemiol* 1970;91:585–592.
15. Monto AS, Lim SK. The Tecumseh study of respiratory illness. VI. Frequency of and relationship between outbreaks of coronavirus infection. *J Infect Dis* 1974;129:271–2716.
16. Vabret A, Mourez T, Gouarin S, et al. An outbreak of coronavirus

OC43 respiratory infection in Normandy, France. *Clin Infect Dis* 2003;36:985–989.

17. El-Sahly HM, Atmar RL, Glezen WP, et al. Spectrum of clinical illness in hospitalized patients with "common cold" virus infections. *Clin Infect Dis* 2000;31:96–100.
18. Pene F, Merlat A, Vabret A, et al. Coronavirus 229E-related pneumonia in immunocompromised patients. *Clin Infect Dis* 2003;37:929–932.
19. Donnelly CA, Ghani AC, Leung GM, et al. Epidemiological determinants of spread of causal agent of severe acute respiratory syndrome in Hong Kong. *Lancet* 2003;361:1761–1766.
20. Chan-Yeung M, Seto WH, Sung JJ. Severe acute respiratory syndrome: patients were epidemiologically linked. *Br Med J* 2003;326:1393.
21. Ho AS, Sung JJY, Chan-Yeung M. An outbreak of severe acute respiratory syndrome among hospital workers in a community hospital in Hong Kong. *Ann Intern Med* 2003;139:564–567.
22. Centers for Disease Control and Prevention. Cluster of severe acute respiratory syndrome cases among protected health-care workers—Toronto, Canada, April 2003. *MMWR* 2003;52:433–436.
23. Loeb M, Henry B, Ofner M, et al. Risk factors for severe acute respiratory syndrome among critical care nurses, 43rd Interscience Conference on antimicrobial agents and chemotherapy, American Society of Microbiology, Chicago, 2003.
24. Vogel G. SARS outbreak. Modelers struggle to grasp epidemic's potential scope. *Science* 2003;300:558–559.
25. Seto WH, Tsang D, Yung RW, et al. Effectiveness of precautions against droplets and contact in prevention of nosocomial transmission of severe acute respiratory syndrome (SARS). *Lancet* 2003;361:1519–1520.
26. Scales DC, Green K, Chan AK, et al. Illness in intensive care staff after brief exposure to severe acute respiratory syndrome. *Emerg Infect Dis* 2003;9:1205–1210.
27. World Health Organization. First data on stability and resistance of SARS coronavirus compiled by members of WHO laboratory network. 2003. Available at: *http://www.who.int/csr/sars/survival_2003_05_04/en/index.html.*
28. Ng SK. Possible role of an animal vector in the SARS outbreak at Amoy Gardens. *Lancet* 2003;362:570–572.
29. Shek CC, Ng PC, Fung GP, et al. Infants born to mothers with severe acute respiratory syndrome. *Pediatrics* 2003;112:e254–256.
30. Nicholls JM, Poon LL, Lee KC, et al. Lung pathology of fatal severe acute respiratory syndrome. *Lancet* 2003;361:1773–1778.
31. Cui W, Fan Y, Wu W, et al. Expression of lymphocytes and lymphocyte subsets in patients with severe acute respiratory syndrome. *Clin Infect Dis* 2003;37:857–859.
32. Wong RS, Wu A, To KF, et al. Haematological manifestations in patients with severe acute respiratory syndrome: retrospective analysis. *Br Med J* 2003;326:1358–1362.
33. Lew TW, Kwek TK, Tai D, et al. Acute respiratory distress syndrome in critically ill patients with severe acute respiratory syndrome. *JAMA* 2003;290:374–380.
34. Wang H, Ding Y, Li X, et al. Fatal aspergillosis in a patient with SARS who was treated with corticosteroids. *N Engl J Med* 2003;349:507–508.
35. Poutanen SM, Low DE, Henry B, et al. Identification of severe acute respiratory syndrome in Canada. *N Engl J Med* 2003;348:1995–2005.
36. Booth CM, Matukas LM, Tomlinson GA, et al. Clinical features and short-term outcomes of 144 patients with SARS in the greater Toronto area. *JAMA* 2003;289:2801–2809.
37. Lee N, Hui D, Wu A, et al. A major outbreak of severe acute respiratory syndrome in Hong Kong. *N Engl J Med* 2003;348:1986–1994.
38. Rainer TH, Cameron PA, Smith D, et al. Evaluation of WHO criteria for identifying patients with severe acute respiratory syndrome out of hospital: prospective observational study. *Br Med J* 2003;326:1354–1358.
39. Peiris JS, Chu CM, Cheng VC, et al. Clinical progression and viral load in a community outbreak of coronavirus-associated SARS pneumonia: a prospective study. *Lancet* 2003;361:1767–1772.
40. Avendano M, Derkach P, Swan S. Clinical course and management of SARS in health care workers in Toronto: a case series. *Can Med Assoc J* 2003;168:1649–1660.
41. Zhao Z, Zhang F, Xu M, et al. Description and clinical treatment of an early outbreak of severe acute respiratory syndrome (SARS) in Guangzhou, PR China. *J Med Microbiol* 2003;52:715–720.
42. Centers for Disease Control and Prevention. Severe acute respiratory syndrome—Taiwan, 2003. *MMWR* 2003;52:461–466.
43. Chan PKS, Ip M, Ng KC, et al. Severe acute respiratory syndrome-associated coronovirus infection. *Emerg Infect Dis* 2003;9:1453–1454.
44. Gold WL, Mederski B, Rose D, et al. Prevalence of asymptomatic infection by severe acute respiratory syndrome coronavirus in exposed healthcare workers. Abstract K-1315c. 43rd Interscience Conference on Antimicrobial Agents and Chemotherapy (ICAAC), Chicago, 2003.
45. Fisher DA, Lim TK, Lim YT, et al. Atypical presentations of SARS. *Lancet* 2003;361:1740.
46. Centers for Disease Control and Prevention. Severe acute respiratory syndrome—Singapore, 2003. *MMWR* 2003;52:405–411.
47. Hon KL, Leung CW, Cheng WT, et al. Clinical presentations and outcome of severe acute respiratory syndrome in children. *Lancet* 2003;361:1701–1703.
48. Bitnun A, Allen U, Heurter H, et al. Children hospitalized with severe acute respiratory syndrome-related illness in Toronto. *Pediatrics* 2003;112:e261–268.
49. Hsu LY, Lee CC, Green JA, et al. Severe acute respiratory syndrome (SARS) in Singapore: clinical features of index patient and initial contacts. *Emerg Infect Dis* 2003;9:713–717.
50. Antonio GE, Wong KT, Hui DS, et al. Thin-section CT in patients with severe acute respiratory syndrome following hospital discharge: preliminary experience. *Radiology* 2003;228:810–815.
51. Wang T, Jang T, Huong C, et al. Establishing a clinical decision rule of severe acute respiratory syndrome at emergency department. *Ann Emerg Med* 2004;43:17–22.
52. Wong KT, Antonio GE, Hui DS, et al. Severe acute respiratory syndrome: radiographic appearances and pattern of progression in 138 patients. *Radiology* 2003;228:401–406.
53. Wang H, Li Y, Sun T. Study of roentgenigraphy in 102 patients with severe acute respiratory syndrome, Proceedings of International Science Symposium on SARS, Beijing, China, July 2003.
54. Xue X, Gao Z, Xu Y, et al. Clinical analysis of 45 patients with severe acute respiratory syndrome. *Chin Med J* 2003;116:819–822.
55. Wong KT, Antonio GE, Hui DS, et al. Thin-section CT of severe acute respiratory syndrome: evaluation of 73 patients exposed to or with the disease. *Radiology* 2003;228:395–400.
56. Klinger JR, Sanchez MP, Curtin LA, et al. Multiple cases of life-threatening adenovirus pneumonia in a mental health care center. *Am J Respir Crit Care Med* 1998;157:645–649.
57. Jernigan JA, Low DE, Helfand RF. Combining clinical and epidemiologic features for early recognition of SARS. *Emerg Infect Dis* 2004;10:327–333.
58. Fowler RA, Lapinsky SE, Hallett D, et al. Critically ill patients with severe acute respiratory syndrome. *JAMA* 2003;290:367–373.
59. Varia M, Wilson S, Sarwal S, et al. Investigation of a nosocomial outbreak of severe acute respiratory syndrome (SARS) in Toronto, Canada. *Can Med Assoc J* 2003;169:285–292.
60. Tsang OT, Chau T, Choi K, et al. Coronavirus-positive nasopharyngeal aspirate as predictor for severe acute respiratory syndrome mortality. *Emerg Infect Dis* 2003;9:1381–1387.
61. Hsueh PR, Hsiao CH, Yeh SH, et al. Microbiologic characteristics, serologic responses, and clinical manifestations in severe acute respiratory syndrome, Taiwan. *Emerg Infect Dis* 2003;9:1163–1167.
62. Schrag S, Brooks J, Van Beneden C, et al. SARS surveillance during emergency public health response United States, March–July, 2003. *Emerg Infect Dis* 2004;10:185.
63. Li G, Chen X, Xu A. Profile of specific antibodies to the SARS-associated coronavirus. *N Engl J Med* 2003;349:508–509.
64. Breiman R, Evans M, Pereiser W, et al. Role of China in the quest to define and control severe acute respiratory syndrome. *Emerg Infect Dis* 2003;9:1037–1041.
65. Centers for Disease Control and Prevention. Efficiency of quarantine during an epidemic of severe acute respiratory syndrome—Beijing, China, 2003. *MMWR* 2003;52:1037–1040.
66. Zhong N, Zheng B, Li Y, et al. Epidemiology and cause of severe acute

respiratory syndrome (SARS) in Guangdong, People's Republic of China, in February 2003. *Lancet* 2003;362:1353–1358.

67. Guan Y, Zheng B, He Y, et al. Isolation and characterization of viruses related to the SARS Coronavirus from animals in Southern China. *Science* 2003;302:276–278.
68. Centers for Disease Control and Prevention. Prevalence of IgG Antibody to SARS-associated coronavirus in animal traders—Guangdong Province, China, 2003. *MMWR* 2003;52:986–987.
69. Holmes KV. SARS-associated coronavirus. *N Engl J Med* 2003;348: 1948–1951.
70. Chan-Yeung M, Yu WC. Outbreak of severe acute respiratory syndrome in Hong Kong Special Administrative Region: case report. *Br Med J* 2003;326:850–852.
71. Singh KS, Hsu LY, Villacian JS, et al. Severe acute respiratory syndrome: lessons from Singapore. *Emerg Infect Dis* 2003;9: 1294–1298.
72. Riley S, Fraser C, Donnelly CA, et al. Transmission dynamics of the etiological agent of SARS in Hong Kong: impact of public health interventions. *Science* 2003;300:1961–1966.
73. Lipsitch M, Cohen T, Cooper B, et al. Transmission dynamics and control of severe acute respiratory syndrome. *Science* 2003;300: 1966–1970.
74. Centers for Disease Control and Prevention. Update: severe acute respiratory syndrome—Toronto, Canada, 2003. *MMWR* 2003;52: 547–550.
75. World Health Organization. Cumulative number of reported probable cases of severe acute respiratory syndrome (SARS). August 15, 2003. Available at: *http://www.who.int/csr/sars/country/2003_08)15/en/.*
76. Centers for Disease Control and Prevention. SARS infection control and exposure management. September 23, 2003. Available at: *http://www.cdc.gov/ncidod/sars/ic.htm.*
77. Gwaltney JM Jr, Moskalski PB, Hendley JO. Hand-to-hand transmission of rhinovirus colds. *Ann Intern Med* 1978;88:463–467.
78. Centers for Disease Control and Prevention. Update: severe acute respiratory syndrome—United States, June 11, 2003. *MMWR* 2003;52: 550.
79. Tomlinson B, Cockram C. SARS: experience at Prince of Wales Hospital, Hong Kong. *Lancet* 2003;361:1486–1487.
80. Chowell G, Fenimore PW, Castillo-Garsow MA, et al. SARS outbreaks in Ontario, Hong Kong and Singapore: the role of diagnosis and isolation as a control mechanism. *J Theor Biol* 2003;224:1–8.
81. Dye C, Gay N. Epidemiology. Modeling the SARS epidemic. *Science* 2003;300:1884–1885.
82. Centers for Disease Control and Prevention. Draft public health guidance for community level preparedness and response to severe acute respiratory syndrome, 2003. November 3, 2003. Available at: *http://www.cdc.gov/ncidod/sars/sarsprepplan.htm.*
83. Maunder R, Hunter J, Vincent L, et al. The immediate psychological and occupational impact of the 2003 SARS outbreak in a teaching hospital. *Can Med Assoc J* 2003;168:1245–1251.

INDEX

Note: Page numbers followed by f indicate figures; those followed by t indicate tables.

C

D

F

G

H

I

M

O

S

U